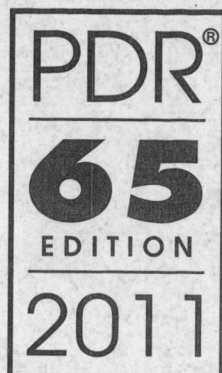

PDR® 65 EDITION 2011

PHYSICIANS' DESK REFERENCE®

CEO: Edward Fotsch, MD
President: David Tanzer
Chief Medical Officer: Christine Côté, MD
Chief Technology Officer: Nick Krym
Chief Financial Officer: Dawn Carfora

Vice President, Product Management & Operations: Valerie Berger
Vice President, Emerging Products: Debra Del Guidice
Vice President, Corporate Development, Copy Sales & General Counsel: Andrew Gelman
Vice President, Sales: John Loucks
Vice President, Marketing: Julie Baker
Vice President, Business Development: Tom Dieker

Director of Sales: Eileen Bruno
Business Manager: Karen Fass
Senior Account Executives: Marjorie A. Jaxel, Philip Molinaro
Account Executives: Nick W. Clark, Carlos Cornejo, Caryn Trick
Associate Account Executives: Carol Levine, Janet Wallendal
Sales Coordinator: Dawn McPartland

Senior Director, Operations & Client Services: Stephanie Struble
Senior Director, Editorial & Publishing: Bette Kennedy
Director, Clinical Services: Sylvia Nashed, PharmD
Director, Marketing: Kim Marich

Senior Manager, Client Services: Lisa Caporuscio
Manager, Clinical Services: Nermin Kerolous, PharmD
Senior Drug Information Specialist, Database Management: Christine Sunwoo, PharmD
Senior Drug Information Specialist, Product Development: Anila Patel, PharmD
Drug Information Specialists: Peter Leighton, PharmD; Kristine Mecca, PharmD; See-Won Seo, PharmD
Manager, Editorial Services: Lori Murray
Associate Editor: Jennifer Reed
Manager, Art Department: Livio Udina
Electronic Publication Designer: Carrie Spinelli Faeth

Director, PDR Production: Jeffrey D. Schaefer
Associate Director, Manufacturing & Distribution: Thomas Westburgh
Production Manager, PDR: Steven Maher
Operations Database Manager: Noel Deloughery
Senior Index Editor: Allison O'Hare
Index Editor: Julie L. Cross
Senior Production Coordinator: Yasmin Hernández
Production Coordinators: Eric Udina, Christopher Whalen
Format Editor: Dan Cappello
Fulfillment Management Specialist: Gary Lew
Manager, Customer Service: Todd Taccetta

ISBN: 978-1-56363-780-3

FOREWORD TO THE 65th EDITION

PDR Network, LLC

As the nation's leading distributor of drug labeling information, product safety alerts, and REMS programs, PDR Network is committed to ensuring that prescribers have access to the right information at the point of prescribing. PDR Network includes *Physicians' Desk Reference®* ("*PDR®* "), the most highly trusted and commonly used drug information reference available in the U.S.; PDR.net®, the online home of PDR; *mobile*PDR®; and the Health Care Notification Network ("HCNN"), the only specialty-specific service that provides electronic delivery of FDA-approved Drug Alerts to physicians and other healthcare professionals.

By improving communication of important medication information and FDA-approved Drug Alerts, PDR Network's unique services enhance patient safety and may help to reduce medical liability. For more information or to sign up for electronic PDR® Drug Alerts, visit **PDR.net**.

About *PDR*

PDR is published by PDR Network, LLC (the "Publisher") in cooperation with participating manufacturers, and contains U.S. Food and Drug Administration ("FDA")-approved product labeling. In accordance with current FDA policies, *PDR* also includes prescribing information provided by manufacturers for products marketed without FDA approval, as well as information on some dietary supplements and other products.

New features for this edition include color-coded indices (designated with white, pink, or blue pages at the front of the book), and a Generic/Brand Cross Reference Table in Section 2, which can help you quickly locate the brand names associated with specific active ingredients as well as the associated product indications. In addition, manufacturer-supplied information on dietary supplements is now listed separately in Section 6.

Each full-length product entry in *PDR* provides you with an exact, formatted copy of the product's FDA-approved or other manufacturer-supplied labeling. Under the Federal Food, Drug and Cosmetic (FD&C) Act, a drug approved for marketing may be labeled, promoted, and advertised by the manufacturer for only those uses for which the drug's safety and effectiveness have been established. The Code of Federal Regulations [Title 21 Section 201.100(d)(1)] pertaining to labeling for prescription products requires that for *PDR* content "indications, effects, dosages, routes, methods, and frequency and duration of administration, and any relevant warnings, hazards, contraindications, side effects, and precautions" must be "*same in language and emphasis*" as the approved labeling for the products. The FDA regards the words *same in language and emphasis* as requiring VERBATIM use of the approved labeling providing such information. Furthermore, information that is emphasized in the FDA-approved labeling by the use of type set in a box, or in capitals, boldface, or italics, must be given the same emphasis in *PDR*.

The FDA has also recognized that the FD&C Act does not, however, limit the manner in which a physician may use an approved drug. Once a product has been approved for marketing, a physician may choose to prescribe it for uses or in treatment regimens or patient populations that are not included in approved labeling. The FDA also observes that accepted medical practice includes drug use that is not reflected in approved drug labeling. In addition, the dietary supplements listed in Section 6 are marketed under the Dietary Supplement Health and Education Act of 1994 (DSHEA). Products marketed under the DSHEA do not receive formal evaluation or approval from the FDA. The following disclaimer applies to all product information listed in Section 6, as mandated by the federal government: *These statements have not been evaluated by the Food and Drug Administration. This product is not intended to diagnose, treat, cure, or prevent any disease.*

The function of the Publisher is the compilation, organization, and distribution of this information. All product information appearing in *PDR* is made possible through the courtesy of the manufacturers whose products appear in it. The information concerning each product has been provided by such manufacturers and in each instance fully approved by such manufacturers prior to publication by the Publisher. In organizing and presenting the material in *PDR*, the Publisher does not warrant or guarantee any of the products described, or perform any independent analysis in connection with any of the product information contained herein. The Publisher does not assume, and expressly disclaims, any obligation to obtain and include any information other than that provided to it by the manufacturers. It should be understood that by making this material available, the Publisher is not advocating the use of any product described herein, nor is the Publisher responsible for misuse of a product due to typographical error. Additional information on any product may be obtained from the manufacturer.

PDR Updates

This print edition of *PDR* contains the latest information available when the book went to press. As new drugs are released and new research data, clinical findings, and safety information emerge throughout the year, it is the responsibility of the manufacturer to provide that information to the medical community and revise that information accordingly in the *PDR* database. These revisions are published six times annually in the *PDR Update Insert Cards*, more regularly on PDR.net and *mobile*PDR, and emailed monthly to prescribers via PDR Network's *eDrug Update*. To be certain that you have the most current data, always consult the *PDR Update Insert Cards*, PDR.net, *mobile*PDR, and the *eDrug Update* before prescribing or administering any product described in the following pages.

Electronic *PDR* Resources

PDR.net®, a web portal designed specifically for healthcare professionals, provides trusted, professional drug information, including full FDA-approved labeling as well as concise point-of-care drug information. PDR.net provides prescribers with online access to the authoritative drug information they need to support their treatment decisions, and free Continuing Medical Education (CME) credits are available to qualified prescribers who read product labeling and FDA-approved Drug Alerts on **PDR.net**.

*mobile*PDR® provides the only source for FDA-approved full product labeling and concise point-of-care drug information from the *PDR* database directly on a mobile device. Information on over 2,400 drugs, full-color product images, and weekly updates provide up-to-date drug information. *mobile*PDR is free for U.S.-based MDs, DOs, NPs, and PAs in full-time patient practice and can be downloaded at **PDR.net**. *mobile*PDR is available for all major mobile platforms.

PDR® Drug Alerts

FDA-approved Drug Alerts are delivered electronically to physicians and other prescribers who register to receive them at **PDR.net**, through participating medical societies, or by returning the verification form distributed with complimentary copies of *PDR*. Free to all licensed U.S. physicians and their staffs, these alerts are delivered via the Health Care Notification Network (HCNN), a service of PDR Network. By ensuring that this service is used exclusively for the rapid delivery of PDR Drug Alerts—not advertising or marketing—PDR Network fulfills FDA guidance for electronic delivery of alerts, improves patient safety, and may help to reduce liability.

RxEvent Adverse Drug Event Reporting System

To date, adverse drug and device event reporting has been challenging. Now, through a new service, you can more easily and effectively report adverse drug and device events and help contribute significantly to increased drug and device safety. For more information, visit **RxEvent.org**.

Electronic Health Records (EHR) Safety Event Reporting System

Physicians and other healthcare providers are increasingly relying on EHR systems for the practice of medicine. As EHR systems are adopted, it is important to track and understand issues of safety and accuracy as they develop, such as software issues and insufficient or incorrect information. Reporting issues will allow for improvement in EHRs and patient safety and may also result in liability reduction, since medical professional insurance carriers support this initiative and encourage reporting. For more information, visit **EHRevent.org**.

Other Products from *PDR*

PDR® Pharmacopoeia Pocket Dosing Guide provides quick dosage confirmation in a convenient and portable print format. Only slightly larger than an index card and just half an inch thick, it fits easily into any pocket and provides you with FDA-approved dosing recommendations for more than 1,500 drugs. Unlike other condensed drug references, the information in the **PDR Pharmacopoeia Pocket Dosing Guide** is drawn exclusively from the FDA-approved drug labeling as published in *PDR* or supplied by the manufacturer.

PDR® on CD-ROM is another source of *PDR* prescribing information. This Windows®-compatible disc provides users with a complete database of *PDR* prescribing information, electronically searchable for instant retrieval. This product includes *PDR*'s sophisticated search software and an extensive file of chemical structures, illustrations, and full-color product photographs. For anyone who wants to double-check a proposed prescription, there is also the **PDR® Drug Interactions and Side Effects System**, a software capable of automatically screening a 20-drug regimen for conflicts, then proposing alternatives for any problematic medication. This unique decision-making tool comes free with **PDR on CD-ROM**.

PDR® for Nutritional Supplements, Second Edition helps provide counsel for patients who use over-the-counter supplements, and offers scientific consensus on hundreds of popular products, including amino acids, fatty acids, probiotics, phytoestrogens, phytosterols, over-the-counter hormones, and much more. Focused on the scientific evidence for each supplement's claims, this unique reference offers you a detailed, informed, and objective overview of a burgeoning area in the field of self-treatment.

PDR® for Herbal Medicines, Fourth Edition includes science-based assessments of more than 700 botanicals, and is designed to help counsel patients who favor herbal remedies. Indexed by scientific and common names (as well as Western, Asian, and homeopathic indications), this volume also includes a Side Effects Index, a Drug/Herb Interactions Guide, an Herb Identification Guide with nearly 400 color photos, and a Safety Guide that lists herbs to be avoided during pregnancy and those to be used only under professional supervision. Although botanical products are not officially regulated or monitored in the United States, *PDR for Herbal Medicines* provides you with authoritative information, including the findings of the German Regulatory Authority's expert committee on herbal medicines, Commission E.

For more information on these or any other members of the growing family of *PDR* products, please call toll-free 800-232-7379; fax 201-722-2680; or visit *PDRbookstore.com*. A special professional discount is available for subsequent copies of *PDR* and all other titles at *PDRbookstore.com/discount*. When ordering, simply enter code: G9005PD10.

Any portion of *PDR* that is reproduced, duplicated, copied, downloaded, sold, resold, or otherwise exploited for any commercial purpose without the express written consent of *PDR* is prohibited. Any use of trademarks, logos, or other proprietary information (including images, text, page layout, and form) of *PDR* and/or its affiliates without the express written consent of *PDR* is also prohibited. For more information about licensing *PDR* content, please contact Andrew Gelman at 201-358-7540 or andrew.gelman@pdr.net.

CONTENTS

SECTION 1

MANUFACTURERS' INDEX

Listed in this index are all manufacturers participating in PHYSICIANS' DESK REFERENCE®. It is through their courtesy that PDR® is brought to the medical profession.

Each company's entry includes the address, phone, and fax number of its headquarters and regional offices, as well as contacts for inquiries, orders, and medical emergency information. Products with entries in the Product Information section are listed with their page numbers. Other products available from the manufacturer are listed following the described products.

If an entry in the index lists multiple page numbers, the first ones shown refer to photographs of the product, the last one to its prescribing information.

■ **Bold page numbers** indicate full prescribing information.

■ *Italic page numbers* signify partial information.

■ The ◆ symbol marks drugs shown in the Product Identification Guide.

4LIFE RESEARCH USA, LLC   **3544**
9850 South 300 West
Sandy, Utah 84070

Direct Inquiries to:
(801) 562-3600
Fax: (801) 562-3611
productsupport@4life.com
www.4life.com

Products Described:
4Life Transfer Factor Tri-Factor
  Formula 3544

Other Products Available:
4Life Transfer Factor Belle Vie
4Life Transfer Factor Cardio
4Life Transfer Factor Chewable
  Tri-Factor Formula
4Life Transfer Factor GluCoach
4Life Transfer Factor Immune Spray
4Life Transfer Factor KBU
4Life Transfer Factor Kids
4Life Transfer Factor MalePro
4Life Transfer Factor Plus Tri-Factor
  Formula
4Life Transfer Factor ReCall
4Life Transfer Factor RioVida Tri-Factor
  Formula

ABBOTT LABORATORIES   **303, 402**
Pharmaceutical Products Division
North Chicago, IL 60064, U.S.A.

Pharmaceutical Products Division—
Direct Inquiries to:
  Customer Service:
  (800) 255-5162
  Patient Access Program:
  (800) 441-4987
For Medical Information Contact:
  Generally:
  (800) 633-9110
  or www.abbottmedinfo.com
  Adverse experiences or side effects
  (for all Abbott drug products):
  (800) 633-9110
  or rxabbott.com
Sales and Ordering:
  (800) 255-5162

Products Described:
Abbo-Code Index *402*
◆Advicor Tablets **303, 402**
◆Biaxin Filmtab Tablets **303, 412**
◆Biaxin Granules **303, 412**
◆Biaxin XL Filmtab Tablets..... **303, 412**
Calcijex Injection **422**
◆Cardizem LA Extended
  Release Tablets............... **303, 423**
◆Depakene Capsules *303, 402*
◆Depakote Delayed Release
  Tablets...................... *303, 402*
◆Depakote ER Extended
  Release Tablets............... **303, 425**
◆Depakote Sprinkle Capsules.... *303, 402*
◆E.E.S. 400 Filmtab Tablets..... **303, 437**
E.E.S. Granules **437**
EryPed 200 & EryPed 400 Oral
  Suspension..................... **434**

◆Gengraf Capsules **303, 439**
◆Humira Injection Syringe and
  Pen......................... **303, 448**
◆Kaletra Oral Solution.......... **303, 458**
◆Kaletra Tablets............... **303, 458**
◆Lupron Depot 3.75 mg......... **303, 473**
◆Lupron Depot 7.5 mg.......... **303, 477**
◆Lupron Depot— 3 Month
  11.25 mg.................... **303, 479**
◆Lupron Depot— 3 Month
  22.5 mg.................... **303, 483**
◆Lupron Depot— 4 Month
  30 mg **303, 485**
◆Lupron Depot-PED 7.5 mg,
  11.25 mg and 15 mg **303, 488**
◆Mavik Tablets................. **303, 489**
◆Meridia Capsules.............. **303, 492**
◆Niaspan Extended-Release
  Tablets..................... **303, 498**
Nimbex Injection................. **504**
◆Norvir Oral Solution **304, 521**
◆Norvir Soft Gelatin Capsules ... **304, 510**
◆Norvir Tablets................ **304, 521**
◆Simcor Tablets............... **304, 537**
◆Synthroid Tablets.............. **304, 542**
◆Tarka Tablets................. **304, 547**
◆Teveten Tablets............... **304, 552**
◆Teveten HCT Tablets........... **304, 554**
◆Tricor Tablets................ **304, 558**
◆Trilipix Delayed Release
  Capsules **304, 562**
Ultane Volatile Liquid for
  Inhalation **568**
◆Vicodin Tablets **304, 573**
◆Vicodin ES Tablets............ **304, 575**
◆Vicodin HP Tablets............ **304, 576**
◆Vicoprofen Tablets **304, 578**
◆Zemplar Capsules............. **304, 581**
Zemplar Injection **585**

The following products, described in
this edition of the PDR, have been
discontinued as of PDR press time:
Azmacort Inhalation Aerosol **408**
E.E.S. 200 Liquid **437**
E.E.S. 400 Liquid **437**
EryPed Drops...................... **434**
◆Omnicef Capsules.............. **304, 532**
◆Omnicef for Oral Suspension .. **304, 532**

Other Products Available:
Depakene Oral Solution
Ery Tab Tablets
Erythrocin Stearate Filmtab
Erythromycin Base Filmtab
Erythromycin Delayed Release Capsules
Gengraf Oral Solution
K-Tab Tablets
PCE Tablets

ADOLOR CORPORATION   **304, 588**
700 Pennsylvania Drive
Exton, PA 19341

Direct Inquiries to:
(866) 4ADOLOR (866-423-6567)

Products Described:
◆Entereg Capsules.............. **304, 588**

ALCON LABORATORIES, INC.   **591**
Alcon Laboratories, Inc.
And its affiliates
Corporate Headquarters
6201 South Freeway
Fort Worth, TX 76134

Direct Inquiries to:
(800) 757-9195
Outside the U.S. call (817) 568-6725
medinfo@alconlabs.com

Products Described:
Ciprodex Otic Suspension **591**
Pataday Ophthalmic Solution....... **592**
Patanase Nasal Spray.............. **593**
Systane Balance Lubricant Eye
  Drops..................... **596**
Systane Ultra Lubricant Eye Drops.. **597**
Travatan Z Ophthalmic Solution.... **597**
Vigamox Ophthalmic Solution...... **598**

Other Products Available:
Alcaine Ophthalmic Solution
Alomide Ophthalmic Solution
Atropine Sulfate Ophthalmic Solution,
  1%
Azopt Ophthalmic Suspension
Betadine 5% Sterile Ophthalmic Prep
  Solution
Betoptic S Ophthalmic Suspension
BSS and BSS Plus Irrigation Solution
  Administration Set
BSS Plus Sterile Irrigation Solution
  (250 mL, 500 mL)
BSS Sterile Irrigation Solution (15 mL,
  30 mL, 250 mL, 500 mL)
Cellugel Ophthalmic Viscosurgical
  Device
Ciloxan Ophthalmic Ointment
Ciloxan Ophthalmic Solution
Cipro HC Otic Suspension
Cyclogyl Ophthalmic Solution
Cyclomydril Ophthalmic Solution
DisCoVisc Ophthlamic Viscosurgical
  Device
DuoVisc Viscoelastic System (.35 mL,
  .40 mL, .5 mL, .55 mL)
Durezol Ophthalmic Emulsion
Emadine Ophthalmic Solution
Enuclene Cleaning/Lubricating Solution
  for Artificial Eyes
Eye-Stream Eye Irrigating Solution
Flarex Ophthalmic Suspension
Fluorescite Injection
Iopidine Ophthalmic Solution
Isopto Atropine Ophthalmic Solution
Isopto Carbachol Ophthalmic Solution
Isopto Carpine Ophthalmic Solution
Isopto Homatropine Ophthalmic Solution
Isopto Hyoscine Ophthalmic Solution
Isopto Tears Ophthalmic Solution
Maxidex Ophthalmic Suspension
Maxitrol Ophthalmic Ointment
Maxitrol Ophthalmic Suspension
Miostat Intraocular Miotic Solution
Mydfrin Ophthalmic Solution
Mydriacyl Ophthalmic Solution
Naphcon Solution
Natacyn Ophthalmic Suspension
Nevanac Ophthalmic Suspension
Omnipred Ophthalmic Suspension
Patanol Ophthalmic Solution
Pilocarpine Hydrochloride Ophthalmic
  Solution

Pilopine HS Gel
ProVisc Ophthalmic Viscosurgical
  Device (.44 mL, .55 mL, .85 mL)
Schirmer Tear Test Strips
Tetracaine Hydrochloride 0.5%
TobraDex Ophthalmic Ointment
TobraDex Ophthalmic Suspension
TobraDex ST Ophthalmic Suspension
Tobrex Ophthalmic Ointment
Tobrex Ophthalmic Solution
Travatan Ophthalmic Solution
Triesence Suspension
Vexol Ophthalmic Suspension
Viscoat Ophthalmic Viscosurgical Device
  (.5 mL, .75 mL)

ALLERGAN, INC.   **304, 599**
2525 Dupont Drive
P.O. Box 19534
Irvine, CA 92623-9534

Direct Inquiries to:
For Medical Information, Contact:
  Outside CA: (800) 433-8871
  CA: (714) 246-4500
Sales and Ordering:
  Outside CA: (800) 377-7790
  CA: (714) 246-4500

Products Described:
◆Aczone Gel 5% **304, 599**
◆Alphagan P Ophthalmic
  Solution.................... **304, 602**
BOTOX for Injection................ **603**
◆Combigan Ophthalmic
  Solution.................... **305, 610**
◆Lumigan Ophthalmic Solution.. **305, 613**
◆Restasis Ophthalmic Emulsion.. **305, 614**
Sanctura XR Capsules............. **615**

Other Products Available:
Betagan Ophthalmic Solution
Bleph-10 Ophthalmic Solution
FML Forte Ophthalmic Suspension
FML Ophthalmic Ointment
FML Ophthalmic Suspension
Ocufen Ophthalmic Solution
Poly-Pred Ophthalmic Suspension
Pred Forte Ophthalmic Suspension
Pred-G Ophthalmic Ointment
Pred-G Ophthalmic Suspension
Pred Mild Ophthalmic Suspension
Refresh Celluvisc Lubricant Eye Drops
Refresh Liquigel Lubricant Eye Drops
Refresh Plus Lubricant Eye Drops
Refresh P.M. Lubricant Eye Ointment
Refresh Tears Lubricant Eye Drops

ALTO   **305, 3545**
PHARMACEUTICALS,
INC.
P.O. Box 271150
Tampa, FL 33688-1150
3172 Lake Ellen Drive
Tampa, FL 33618

Direct Inquiries to:
John J. Cullaro
Customer Service
altopharm@aol.com
Tel: (800) 330-2891
Fax: (813) 968-0527

Products Described:
◆Zinc-220 Capsules............ **305, 3545**

AMGEN INC. 305, 619
Amgen Inc.
One Amgen Center Drive
Thousand Oaks, CA 91320-1799

For Product Inquiries and Adverse Event Reporting Contact:
Amgen Medical Information
(800) 772-6436
FAX: (866) 292-6436
www.amgen.com
Sales and Ordering:
Amgen Trade Operations
(800) 282-6436
FAX: (866) 292-6436

Products Described:
◆Aranesp for Injection 305, 619
◆Enbrel Solution for
   Subcutaneous Injection 305, 630
◆Epogen for Injection 305, 646
◆Neulasta 305, 657
◆Neupogen for Injection 305, 660
◆Nplate for Subcutaneous
   Injection 306, 669
◆Prolia Injection 306, 673
◆Sensipar Tablets 306, 678
◆Vectibix Injection for
   Intravenous Use 306, 681

AMYLIN 306, 684
PHARMACEUTICALS, INC.
9360 Towne Centre Drive
San Diego, CA 92121

Direct Inquiries to:
Ph: (858) 552-2200
FAX: (858) 552-2212

Products Described:
◆Byetta Injection 306, 684
◆Symlin Injection 690
◆SymlinPen 306, 690

ANGELINI LABOPHARM 321, 3446
LLC
202 Carnegie Center, Suite 107
Princeton, NJ 08540

Direct Inquiries to:
(877) 345-6177

Products Described:
◆Oleptro Extended-Release
   Tablets 321, 3446

ASTRAZENECA LP 306, 321, 695
Wilmington, DE 19850-5437

**For Product Full Prescribing
Information, Business Information,
Medical Information, Adverse Drug
Experiences, and Customer Service:**
Information Center 1-800-236-9933

For Product Ordering:
Trade Customer Service 1-800-842-9920

**For Product Full Prescribing
Information:**
Internet: www.astrazeneca-us.com

Products Described:
◆Atacand Tablets 321, 3451
◆Atacand HCT 16-12.5
   Tablets 321, 3455
◆Atacand HCT 32-12.5
   Tablets 321, 3455
◆Nexium Delayed-Release
   Capsules 306, 695
◆Nexium for Delayed-Release
   Oral Suspension 306, 695
◆Nexium I.V. 306, 702
◆Pulmicort Flexhaler 306, 705
◆Symbicort 80/4.5 Inhalation
   Aerosol 306, 712
◆Symbicort 160/4.5 Inhalation
   Aerosol 306, 712
◆Toprol-XL Tablets 306, 724

Other Products Available:
Prilosec

ASTRAZENECA 306, 728
PHARMACEUTICALS LP
1800 Concord Pike
Wilmington, DE 19850-5437 USA
General Number: (302) 886-3000

**For Medical Information Contact:
For Product Full Prescribing
Information, Business Information,
Medical Information, Adverse Drug
Experiences, and Customer Service:**
Generally:
Information Center
(302) 886-8000
(800) 236-9933

◆ **Shown in Product Identification Guide**

**After Hours and Weekend Emergencies:
For Product Ordering:**
Trade Customer Service
(302) 886-3000

Adverse Drug Experiences:
(800) 842-9920

**For Product Full Prescribing
Information:**
Sales Contact and Ordering:
(800) 842-9920
www.astrazeneca-us.com

Products Described:
◆Crestor Tablets 306, 728
◆Seroquel Tablets 306, 735
◆Seroquel XR
   Extended-Release Tablets 306, 748
◆Vimovo Delayed-Release
   Tablets 306, 760
Zomig Nasal Spray 768
Zomig Tablets 773
Zomig-ZMT Tablets 773

Other Products Available:
Tenoretic
Tenormin I.V. Injection
Tenormin Tablets
Zestoretic Tablets
Zestril Tablets

AXCAN PHARMA U.S., INC. 306, 778
22 Inverness Center Parkway
Birmingham, AL 35242

Direct Inquiries to:
Customer Service
FAX: (205) 991-8426

Products Described:
◆Canasa Rectal Suppositories 306, 778
Carafate Suspension 780
◆Photofrin for Injection 306, 781
Pylera Capsules 788

Other Products Available:
ADEKs Multivitamin Supplement
ADEKs Pediatric Drops
Bentyl Capsules
Bentyl Injection
Bentyl Syrup
Bentyl Tablets
Carafate Tablets
FLUTTER
SCANDICAL
SCANDISHAKE
SCANDISHAKE — Lactose Free
SCANDISHAKE — Sweetened with
   Aspartame
Urso 250 Tablets
Urso Forte Tablets

AXCAN SCANDIPHARM INC.
(See AXCAN PHARMA U.S.,
INC.)

BAUSCH & LOMB 792
INCORPORATED
One Bausch & Lomb Place
Rochester, NY 14604
7 Giralda Farms
Madison, NJ 07940

Direct Inquiries to:
(800) 323-0000
Consumer Affairs
(800) 553-5340

Products Described:
Besivance Ophthalmic
   Suspension 792

BAXTER HEALTHCARE 793
CORPORATION
BioScience
One Baxter Way
Westlake Village, CA 91362

For Medical Information Contact:
Baxter Healthcare Corporation
Baxter Bioscience Medical Information
(866) 424-6724

Products Described:
Advate 793
Aralast NP Solvent Detergent ... 800
Buminate 25% Solution 803
Feiba NF 804
Flexbumin 25% Solution 807
Gammagard Liquid 808
Gammagard S/D 812
Hemofil M 816
Recombinate 817

BAXTER HEALTHCARE 821
**CORPORATION ANESTHESIA
& CRITICAL CARE**
95 Spring Street
New Providence, NJ 07974

Direct Inquiries to:
Professional Services Department
(800) ANA-DRUG
(800) 262-3784

For Medical Emergencies Contact:
(800) ANA-DRUG
(800) 262-3784

Sales and Ordering:
To place an order, call or fax:
(800) 667-0959
FAX: (877) 702-3580

Products Described:
Suprane Volatile Liquid for
   Inhalation 821

BAYER HEALTHCARE 307, 825
PHARMACEUTICALS INC.
6 West Belt
Wayne, NJ 07470

Direct Inquiries to:
(888) 84-BAYER
(888) 842-2937
www.bayerhealthcare.com

For Medical Information contact:
Vice President, Medical Communications
(888) 84-Bayer (888) 842-2937

Products Described:
◆Angeliq Tablets 307, 825
◆Climara Transdermal System ... 307, 830
◆Climara Pro Transdermal
   System 307, 835
Menostar Transdermal System ... 842
◆Mirena Intrauterine System ... 307, 848
◆Natazia Tablets 307, 854
◆Yasmin 28 Tablets 307, 859
◆Yaz Tablets 307, 868

BEACH 307, 878
PHARMACEUTICALS
Division of Beach Products, Inc.
5220 S. Manhattan Avenue
Tampa, FL 33611

Direct Inquiries to:
Richard Stephen Jenkins
(813) 839-6565
FAX: (813) 837-2511

Manufacturing and Distribution:
1700 Perimeter Road
Greenville, SC 29605
(800) 845-8210

Products Described:
◆Beelith Tablets 307, 3545
◆K-Phos Original (Sodium
   Free) Tablets 307, 879
K-Phos M.F. Tablets 878
◆K-Phos Neutral Tablets 307, 878
K-Phos No. 2 Tablets 878
◆Uroqid-Acid No. 2 Tablets 307, 879

BERTEK
PHARMACEUTICALS INC.
(See MYLAN
PHARMACEUTICALS INC.)

BOEHRINGER INGELHEIM 307, 880
A subsidiary of Boehringer Ingelheim
   Corporation
900 Ridgebury Road
P.O. Box 368
Ridgefield, CT 06877-0368

Direct Inquiries to:
(800) 243-0127
TTY (800) 246-6196
**For medical information or to report
an adverse drug experience contact:**
(800) 542-6257 (option 4)
TTY (800) 459-9906
us.boehringer-ingelheim.com

Products Described:
◆Aggrenox Capsules 307, 880
◆Spiriva HandiHaler 307, 885

BRISTOL-MYERS SQUIBB 321, 3458
COMPANY
P.O. Box 4500
Princeton, NJ 08543-4500

For Medical Information Contact:
Generally:
Bristol-Myers Squibb Medical
   Information Department
P.O. Box 4500
Princeton, NJ 08543-4500
(800) 321-1335 between 8:00 AM -
   8:00 PM EST

**To report SUSPECTED ADVERSE
REACTIONS, Contact Bristol-Myers
Squibb Company at**
(800) 721-5072
Sales and Ordering:
Orders may be placed by:
Calling your purchase orders in toll-free
   between 8:30 AM - 5:00 PM EST:
(800) 631-5244
Mailing your purchase orders to:
Bristol-Myers Squibb U.S.
   Pharmaceuticals
Attn: Customer Service
P.O. Box 4500
Princeton, NJ 08543-4500
Faxing your puchase orders in:
(800) 277-0988

Products Described:
◆Abilify Injection 321, 3458
◆Abilify Oral Solution 321, 3458
◆Abilify Discmelt Orally
   Disintegrating Tablets 321, 3458
◆Abilify Tablets 321, 3458
◆Atripla Tablets 321, 3471
   Baraclude Oral Solution 3484
◆Baraclude Tablets 321, 3484
◆Erbitux 321, 3490
◆Onglyza Tablets 321, 3495
◆Orencia Powder for
   Intravenous Infusion 321, 3501
◆Plavix Tablets 322, 3506
◆Reyataz Capsules 322, 3511
◆Sprycel Tablets 322, 3527
◆Sustiva Capsules 322, 3532
◆Sustiva Tablets 322, 3532

BRISTOL-MYERS SQUIBB 891
**COMPANY & GILEAD
SCIENCES, LLC**
333 Lakeside Drive
Foster City, CA 94404

For Medical Information Contact:
1-888-547-4267
Medicalinformation@BMS-Gilead.com
To Report Adverse Events, Contact:
1-800-445-3235 press option 3
For Business Operations Contact:
1-800-445-3235 press option 8

Products Described:
Atripla Tablets 891

J. R. CARLSON 307, 3545
LABORATORIES, INC.
15 College Drive
Arlington Heights, IL 60004-1985

Direct Inquiries to:
Customer Service
(888) 234-5656
FAX: (847) 255-1605
www.carlsonlabs.com
For Medical Information Contact:
In Emergies:
Customer Service
(888) 234-5656
FAX: (847) 255-1605

Products Described:
◆Ddrops Dietary Supplement ... 307, 3545
Med Omega Fish Oil 2800 3545
Norwegian Cod Liver Oil 3545
Super Omega-3 Gems Softgels ... 3546

CELLTECH
**PHARMACEUTICALS,
INC.**
(See UCB, INC.)

CENTOCOR ORTHO 307, 904
BIOTECH INC.
800 Ridgeview Drive
Horsham, PA 19044
USA
www.centocororthobiotech.com

Direct General Inquiries to:
Ph: (610) 651-6000
FAX: (610) 651-6100

For Medical Emergencies Contact:
Ph: (800) 457-6399

**For Medical Information/Adverse
Experience Reporting Contact:**
Medical Information
Ph: (800) 457-6399

Products Described:
◆Remicade for IV Injection 307, 904
◆Simponi Injection 307, 916
◆Stelara Injection 307, 926

Other Products Available:
ReoPro Vials
Sporanox Oral Solution

◆ **Shown in Product Identification Guide**   *Italic Page Number* **Indicates Brief Listing**

GLENWOOD   310, 1660

111 Cedar Lane
Englewood, NJ 07631

Direct Inquiries to:
Professional Services Department
(201) 569-0050
(800) 542-0772
For Medical Information Contact:
In Emergencies:
Professional Services Department
(201) 569-0050
(800) 542-0772

Products Described:
◆Potaba Capsules............ 310, 1660
◆Potaba Tablets 310, 1660

Other Products Available:
Yodoxin Tablets

GORDON LABORATORIES 310, 1660

6801 Ludlow Street
Upper Darby, PA 19082

Direct Inquiries to:
Customer Service
(610) 734-2011
Fax: (610) 734-2049
Website: http://www.gordonlabs.net
E-mail: gordonlabs@att.net

◆ Shown in Product Identification Guide

For medical emergencies contact:
David Dercher
(610) 734-2011
Fax: (610) 734-2049

Products Described:
◆Formadon Solution............ 310, 1660
◆Gordochom Solution.......... 310, 1660

Other Products Available:
Abscents Deodorizing Powder
Aloe Grande Creme
Aloe Grande Lotion
Bromi-Lotion
Bromi-Talc Powder
Bromi-Talc Plus Powder
Calicylic Creme
Emollia Creme
Emollia Lotion
Forma-Ray Solution
Gordobalm Massage Lotion
Gordofilm Wart Remover
Gordomatic Crystals
Gordon's Boro-Packs
Gordon's No. Five Spray Foot Powder
Gordon's Urea 40% Ointment
Gordon's Vite A Creme
Gordon's Vite A Lotion
Gordon's Vite E Creme
Gordo-Pool Whirlpool Drops
Gormel Creme
Gormel Ten Lotion
Lugol's Strong Iodine Solution
Monsel's Ferric Subsulfate Solution
Mycomist Shoe & Boot Spray
Potassium Hydroxide Solution 5%
Silver Nitrate Solution 10%, 25%, 50%
Sodium Hydroxide Solution 10%
Sorbidon Hydrate Creme
Stik It Ampules
Tri-Chlor Solution
Vita-Ray Creme

GRACEWAY   1661
PHARMACEUTICALS, LLC

340 Martin Luther King Jr. Blvd.,
  Suite 500
Bristol, TN 37620

Direct Inquiries to:
(800) 328-0255
www.gracewaypharma.com

Products Described:
Zyclara Cream, 3.75%............. 1661

GRIFOLS BIOLOGICALS INC.   1664

5555 Valley Boulevard
Los Angeles, CA 90032

Direct Inquiries to:
CONTACTS:
All services incl.
24-Hour Ordering
(888) GRIFOLS or (888) 474-3657
Direct Inquiries:
(323) 225-2221
Fax: (323) 441-7698
Website: www.grifolsusa.com

Products Described:
Albutein 5% Solution.............. 1664
Albutein 25% Solution............ 1665
Alphanate......................... 1666
AlphaNine SD..................... 1671
Flebogamma 5% DIF 1674
Flebogamma 10% DIF 1678
Profilnine SD..................... 1683

HEEL INC.   1684

10421 Research Road SE
Albuquerque, NM 87123

Direct Inquiries to:
Medical Department
(800) 621-7644
Fax: (800) 217-6934
www.heelusa.com
info@heelusa.com

Products Described:
Traumeel Ear Drops................ 1684
Traumeel Gel...................... 1684
Traumeel Injection Solution....... 1684
Traumeel Ointment................. 1684
Traumeel Oral Drops............... 1684
Traumeel Oral Liquid in Vials...... 1684
Traumeel Tablets.................. 1684
Zeel Injection Solution............ 1685

Other Products Available:
Engystol Tablets
Gripp-Heel Tablets
Lymphomyosot Tablets
Sinusin Nasal Spray
Vertigoheel Tablets (Rx)
Zeel Ointment
Zeel Tablets

HEMISPHERX   310, 1686
BIOPHARMA, INC.

One Penn Center
1617 JFK Boulevard
Philadelphia, PA 19103-1806

Direct Inquiries to:
(732) 249-3250 (Alferon N Injection)
or
(215) 988-0080

Products Described:
◆Alferon N Injection 310, 1686

HIGH CHEMICAL   310, 1688
COMPANY

3901-A Nebraska Street
Levittown, PA 19056
www.sarapin.com

Direct Inquiries to:
(800) 447-8792
(215) 788-3113
sarapin@gmail.com

Products Described:
◆Sarapin Vials 310, 1688

IMMUNOTEC INC.   3547

300 Joseph Carrier
Vaudreuil-Dorion, QC
Canada J7V 5V5

For Direct Inquiries Contact:
(450) 424-9992 Ext 4453

Products Described:
Immunocal Powder Sachets........ 3547

INSPIRE PHARMACEUTICALS,   1689
INC.

4222 Emperor Boulevard, #200
Durham, NC 27703

Direct Inquiries to:
Telephone: 919-941-9777
Fax: 919-941-9797
E-mail: info@inspirepharm.com
For AzaSite:
Patient/Physician Questions:
  1-888-881-4696

Products Described:
AzaSite Ophthalmic Drops......... 1689

INTENDIS, INC.   310, 1690

36 Columbia Road
P.O. Box 1941
Morristown, NJ 07962-1941

Direct Inquiries to:
1-(866) 463-3634

**For Medical Information and to report
  adverse drug events:**
1-(866) 463-3634

Products Described:
◆Desonate Gel 310, 1690
◆Finacea Gel 310, 1692
◆NeoBenz Micro SD.......... 310, 1693
◆NeoBenz Micro Wash........ 310, 1693

INTERMUNE, INC.   1694

3280 Bayshore Boulevard
Brisbane, CA 94005

For Direct Inquiries Contact:
Medical Information:
(888) 486-6411
Corporate Offices:
(415) 466-2200
Corporate Fax:
(415) 466-2300

Products Described:
Actimmune....................... 1694

JACOBUS PHARMACEUTICAL   1696
CO., INC.

37 Cleveland Lane
P.O. Box 5290
Princeton, NJ 08540

Direct All Inquiries to:
(609) 921-7447
FAX: (609) 799-1176

Products Described:
Dapsone Tablets USP.............. 1696
Paser Granules.................... 1697

JAZZ PHARMACEUTICALS,   1698
INC.

3180 Porter Drive
Palo Alto, CA 94304

Direct Inquiries to:
(650) 496-3777
FAX: (650) 496-3781
customercare@jazzpharma.com
For medical information:
jazzpharma@medcomsol.com
For media information:
mediainfo@jazzpharma.com

Products Described:
Xyrem Oral Solution.............. 1698

JOHNSON & JOHNSON •   1703
**MERCK CONSUMER
PHARMACEUTICALS CO.**

Camp Hill Road
Fort Washington, PA 19034

Direct Inquiries to:
Consumer Relationship Center
Fort Washington, PA 19034
1-800-755-4008

Products Described:
Original Strength Pepcid AC
  Tablets........................ 1703
Maximum Strength Pepcid AC
  Tablets........................ 1703
Pepcid Complete Chewable
  Tablets........................ 1704

KING   310, 1704
**PHARMACEUTICALS,
INC.**

501 Fifth Street
Bristol, TN 37620

Direct Inquiries to:
Customer Service:
Tel: (888) 358-6436
Fax: (866) 990-0545
**To Report an Adverse
  Drug Experience:**
Tel: (800) 546-4905
Fax: (423) 990-8351
www.kingpharm.com

Products Described:
Altace Capsules................... 1704
◆Avinza Capsules.............. 310, 1708
Bicillin L-A Injection 1712
Cytomel Tablets.................. 1714
◆Embeda Extended Release
  Capsules.................... 310, 1716
◆Flector Patch................. 310, 1723
◆Levoxyl Tablets.............. 310, 1727
◆Skelaxin Tablets............. 310, 1732

Other Products Available:
Neosporin Ophthalmic Solution Sterile
Viroptic Ophthalmic Solution, 1% Sterile

KOWA   310, 1733
**PHARMACEUTICALS
AMERICA, INC.**

530 Industrial Park Boulevard
Montgomery, AL 36117

Direct Inquiries:
(344) 288-1288
Fax: (344) 288-2788
info@kowapharma.com

Products Described:
◆Livalo Tablets................ 310, 1733

KYOWA WELLNESS CO.,   310, 3548
LTD. S-S-I CO., LTD.

Ishikura Bldg. 3F3
5-2 Oodenma-Cho, Nihonbashi,
Chuo-Ku, Tokyo 103-001, Japan

Direct Inquiries to:
Consumer Relations
Tel: +81-3-3660-1235
Fax: +81-3-3660-1236
URL: http://www.s-s-i.jp

Products Described:
◆Sen-Sei-Ro Liquid Gold....... 310, 3548
◆Sen-Sei-Ro Liquid Royal...... 310, 3548
◆Sen-Sei-Ro Powder Gold...... 310, 3548

LEGACY FOR LIFE, LLC   310, 3548

P.O. Box 14510
Oklahoma City, OK 73113

Direct Inquiries to:
(800) 557-8477
info@legacyforlife.net
www.LegacyforLife.net
www.HyperimmuneEgg.org

Italic Page Number **Indicates Brief Listing**

Products Described:
◆i26 Dietary Supplement
  Powder 310, 3548
i26 Capsules 3548
i26 Chewables 3548
i26 Complete Support Dietary
  Supplement 3548
i26 Fit Dietary Supplement 3548

ELI LILLY AND COMPANY
310, 1737

For Medical Information Contact:
Customer Services
Lilly Corporate Center
Indianapolis, IN 46285
(800) 545-5979
(800) LILLY-RX

Direct Inquiries to:
Lilly Corporate Center
Indianapolis, IN 46285
(317) 276-2000
www.lilly.com

Products Described:
Alimta for Injection 1737
Byetta for Injection (See
  AMYLIN
  PHARMACEUTICALS, INC.) ... 1747
Capastat Sulfate for Injection 1747
◆Cialis Tablets 310, 1749
◆Cymbalta Delayed-Release
  Capsules 310, 1759
Effient Tablets 1768
◆Evista Tablets 310, 1774
◆Forteo for Injection 310, 1781
Gemzar for Injection 1787
Glucagon for Injection Vials and
  Emergency Kit 1795
◆Humalog-Pen and KwikPen .. 311, 1797
◆Humalog Mix50/50-Pen and
  KwikPen 311, 1801
◆Humalog Mix75/25-Pen and
  KwikPen 311, 1804
Humulin 70/30 Vial 1807
Humulin N Vial 1809
Humulin R 1812
Humulin R (U-500) 1813
◆Prozac Pulvules 311, 1816
◆Prozac Weekly Capsules 311, 1816
Seromycin Capsules 1827
◆Strattera Capsules 311, 1828
◆Symbyax Capsules 311, 1835
◆Zyprexa Tablets 311, 1850
◆Zyprexa IntraMuscular 311, 1850
◆Zyprexa ZYDIS Orally
  Disintegrating Tablets 311, 1850
◆Zyprexa Relprevv 311, 1865

Other Products Available:
Adcirca Tablets
Humatrope Vials and Cartridges
Quinidine Gluconate Injection, USP
ReoPro Vials
Xigris Powder for Intravenous Infusion

LUNDBECK INC.
311, 1876

Four Parkway North
Deerfield, IL 60015

Direct Inquiries to:
(847) 282-1000
Fax: (847) 282-1001
info@lundbeck.com

Products Described:
NeoProfen Injection 1876
◆Panhematin for Injection 311, 1878
◆Sabril for Oral Solution 311, 1879
◆Sabril Tablets 311, 1886
◆Xenazine Tablets 311, 1893

LUPIN PHARMACEUTICALS, INC.
1898

Harbor Place Tower
111 South Calvert Street, 21st Floor
Baltimore, MD 21202

Direct Inquiries to:
Phone (410) 576-2000

Products Described:
Suprax for Oral Suspension 1898
Suprax Tablets 1898

McNEIL CONSUMER HEALTHCARE
1901

Division of McNeil-PPC, Inc.
Fort Washington, PA 19034

Direct Inquiries to:
Consumer Relationship Center
Fort Washington, PA 19034
(800) 962-5357

Products Described:
Benadryl Allergy Ultratab Tablets .. 1901
Children's Benadryl Allergy
  Liquid 1901

Imodium A-D Liquid, Caplets,
  and EZ Chews 1901
Imodium Multi-Symptom Relief
  Caplets and Chewable Tablets...... 1902
Motrin IB Tablets and Caplets...... 1902
Children's Motrin Dosing Chart.... 1902
Children's Motrin Oral
  Suspension 1903
Infants' Motrin Concentrated
  Drops 1903
Junior Strength Motrin Caplets
  and Chewable Tablets 1903
Motrin PM Caplets 1904
Precise Cream 1904
Precise Patches 1904
St. Joseph 81 mg Aspirin
  Chewable and Enteric Coated
  Tablets......................... 1905
Children's Sudafed Non-Drowsy
  Nasal Decongestant Liquid...... 1907
Sudafed Congestion Tablets........ 1907
Sudafed PE Congestion Tablets..... 1907
Children's Sudafed PE Nasal
  Decongestant Liquid 1907
Regular Strength Tylenol Tablets ... 1910
Tylenol Arthritis Pain Extended
  Release Gelcaps/Caplets......... 1910
Tylenol 8 Hour Extended Release
  Caplets 1910
Extra Strength Tylenol Rapid
  Release Gels.................... 1910
Extra Strength Tylenol Caplets
  and EZ Tabs.................... 1910
Extra Strength Tylenol Adult
  Rapid Blast Liquid 1910
Extra Strength Tylenol PM
  Caplets 1910
Children's Tylenol Dosing Chart ... 1910
Children's Tylenol Meltaways...... 1908
Children's Tylenol Suspension
  Liquid.......................... 1908
Concentrated Tylenol Infants'
  Drops........................... 1908
Jr. Tylenol Meltaways............. 1908
Zyrtec Allergy Tablets and Liquid
  Gels............................ 1912
Children's Zyrtec Allergy Syrup.... 1912
Zyrtec Itchy Eye Drops........... 1912
Zyrtec-D Allergy & Congestion
  Extended-Release Tablets........ 1913

MEDICIS PHARMACEUTICAL CORPORATION
1913

7720 N. Dobson Road
Scottsdale, AZ 85256

**For updates to the product information
listed, please visit:**
www.Medicis.com
For Medical Information Contact:
Phone: (602) 808-8800
FAX: (602) 808-0822

Products Described:
Dysport for Injection 1913
Solodyn Extended Release
  Tablets......................... 1919
Vanos Cream 0.1%................. 1923

Other Products Available:
Ammonul (sodium phenylacetate and
  sodium benzoate) Injection 10%/10%
Buphenyl (sodium phenylbutyrate)
  Tablets and Powder
Ziana (clindamycin phosphate 1.2% and
  tretinoin 0.025%) Gel

MEDIMMUNE, LLC
311, 1924

One MedImmune Way
Gaithersburg, MD 20878

**For all inquiries, including emergencies
(24 hours), medical information,
adverse drug experiences, product
sales and ordering, and customer
service, please contact:**
(877) 633-4411
www.medimmune.com

Products Described:
◆FluMist Vaccine.............. 311, 1924
◆Synagis Intramuscular
  Solution 311, 1929

MERCK
311, 1931

One Merck Drive
P.O. Box 100
Whitehouse Station, NJ 08889

**For updates to the product information
listed below, please check the Merck
Web site, http://www.merck.com, or
call 1-866-342-5683.**

**Direct Inquiries, including 24-hour
emergency information to healthcare
professionals, to:**
The Merck National Service Center
(800) NSC-MERCK
(800) 672-6372

Merck U.S. operating companies
include:
Merck, Sharp & Dohme Corp.
Schering Corporation

Products Described:
Aminohippurate Sodium "PAH"
  Injection 1931
Antivenin (Black Widow Spider
  Antivenin) 1932
◆Asmanex Twisthaler......... 311, 1932
◆Avelox I.V. 311, 1939
◆Avelox Tablets 311, 1939
Cancidas for Injection 1947
◆Cipro I.V. 312, 1965
◆Cipro Oral Suspension 312, 1956
◆Cipro Tablets 312, 1956
◆Cipro XR Tablets 312, 1974
◆Clarinex Syrup 312, 1981
◆Clarinex Tablets 312, 1981
◆Clarinex Reditabs Tablets ... 312, 1981
◆Clarinex-D 12 Hour
  Extended Release Tablets... 312, 1984
Clarinex-D 24 Hour
  Extended-Release Tablets...... 1988
◆Clinoril Tablets 312, 1993
Comvax 1997
◆Cozaar Tablets 312, 2001
◆Crixivan Capsules 312, 2007
◆Diprolene Lotion 0.05%..... 312, 2017
◆Diprolene Ointment 0.05%... 312, 2019
◆Diprolene AF Cream 0.05%... 312, 2016
◆Dulera Inhalation Aerosol 312, 2020
◆Elocon Cream 0.1%......... 312, 2029
◆Elocon Lotion 0.1%......... 312, 2030
◆Elocon Ointment 0.1%...... 312, 2032
◆Emend Capsules 312, 2033
Emend for Injection............. 2042
◆Follistim AQ Cartridge...... 312, 2049
◆Foradil Aerolizer 312, 2058
Fosamax Oral Solution 2065
◆Fosamax Tablets 312, 2065
◆Fosamax Plus D Tablets..... 313, 2074
Gardasil Injection 2081
◆Hyzaar 50-12.5 Tablets..... 313, 2091
◆Hyzaar 100-12.5 Tablets.... 313, 2091
◆Hyzaar 100-25 Tablets...... 313, 2091
◆Implanon Implant 313, 2097
◆Integrilin Injection 313, 2104
◆Intron A for Injection 313, 2108
Invanz for Injection............. 2127
◆Isentress Tablets 313, 2134
◆Janumet Tablets 313, 2142
◆Januvia Tablets 313, 2151
◆Levitra Tablets 313, 2158
◆Lotrisone Cream 313, 2164
◆Lotrisone Lotion 313, 2164
◆Maxalt Tablets 313, 2170
◆Maxalt-MLT Orally
  Disintegrating Tablets 313, 2170
◆Mevacor Tablets 313, 2175
M-M-R II 2166
◆Nasonex Nasal Spray 313, 2180
◆Nitro-Dur Transdermal
  Infusion System............ 313, 2186
◆Noroxin Tablets 313, 2188
◆Noxafil Oral Suspension 313, 2193
◆NuvaRing 313, 2202
PedvaxHIB Liquid............. 2209
◆PegIntron Powder for
  Injection 313, 2212
◆Pepcid Tablets 313, 2228
Pneumovax 23 2231
Primaxin I.M................... 2233
Primaxin I.V................... 2236
◆Prinivil Tablets 313, 2241
◆Prinzide Tablets 313, 2246
◆Propecia Tablets 313, 2250
ProQuad 2254
◆Proscar Tablets 313, 2263
◆Proventil HFA Inhalation
  Aerosol 313, 2268
◆Rebetol Capsules 313, 2271
◆Rebetol Oral Solution 313, 2271
Recombivax HB 2278
◆Remeron Tablets 314, 2282
◆RemeronSolTab Tablets ... 314, 2286
RotaTeq 2291
◆Saphris Tablets 314, 2296
Singulair Chewable Tablets...... 2302
Singulair Oral Granules 2302
◆Singulair Tablets 314, 2302
◆Stromectol Tablets 314, 2309
◆Temodar Capsules 314, 2311
Temodar Injection.............. 2311
◆Tice BCG................. 314, 2319
Trusopt Sterile Ophthalmic
  Solution 2322
Vaqta 2324
Varivax 2331
◆Vytorin 10/10 Tablets...... 314, 2335
◆Vytorin 10/20 Tablets...... 314, 2335
◆Vytorin 10/40 Tablets...... 314, 2335
◆Vytorin 10/80 Tablets...... 314, 2335
◆Zemuron Injection 314, 2344
◆Zetia Tablets 314, 2350
◆Zocor Tablets 314, 2357
◆Zolinza Capsules 314, 2363
Zostavax Injection 2367

MERCK SCHERING PLOUGH PHARMACEUTICALS INC.
(See MERCK)

MERICON INDUSTRIES, INC.
314, 3549

8819 N. Pioneer Road
Peoria, IL 61615

Direct Inquiries to:
William R. Connelly
(309) 693 2150
FAX: (309) 693-2158
E-mail: mericon@sbcglobal.net
www.mericon-industries.com
Sales & Ordering:
(800) 242-6464

Products Described:
◆Florical Capsules............ 314, 3549
Florical Tablets 3549
Meribin Capsules 3549

MERZ PHARMACEUTICALS
2371

Division of Merz, Inc.
4215 Tudor Lane (27410)
P.O. Box 18806
Greensboro, NC 27419

Direct Inquiries to:
Medical/Regulatory Affairs
(336) 856-2003
Fax: (336) 217-2439
For Medical Information Contact:
(336) 856-2003
Fax: (336) 217-2439

Products Described:
Naftin Cream 2371
Naftin Gel 2371

Other Products Available:
Appearex Tablets
Mederma Cream Plus SPF 30
Mederma for Kids Topical Gel
Mederma Topical Gel
Nu-Iron 150 Capsules

MILLENNIUM PHARMACEUTICALS, INC.
314, 2372

40 Landsdowne Street
Cambridge, MA 02139

Direct Inquiries to:
Medical Information:
Call 1-866-VELCADE

Products Described:
◆Velcade for Injection.......... 314, 2372

MISSION PHARMACAL COMPANY
2380

10999 IH 10 West, Suite 1000
San Antonio, TX 78230-1355

Direct All Inquiries to:
P.O. Box 786099
San Antonio, TX 78278-6099
Toll Free: (800) 292-7364
Customer Service (M-W 7A-5:30P C.T.,
  Th 7:30A-5P C.T.)
(210) 696-8400
FAX: (210) 696-6010

Products Described:
CitraNatal Assure Capsules........ 2380
CitraNatal Assure Tablets.......... 2380
CitraNatal B-Calm Tablets 2380
CitraNatal 90 DHA Capsules....... 2380
CitraNatal 90 DHA Tablets........ 2380
CitraNatal Harmony Gel Caps...... 2381
Ferralet 90 Tablets 2381
Tindamax Tablets 2381
Urocit-K Tablets 2385

Other Products Available:
Calcet Tablets
Calcet Creamy Bites Chewable Pieces
Calcet Plus Tablets
CitraNatal DHA Capsules
CitraNatal DHA Tablets
CitraNatal Rx Tablets
Compete Tablets
Dr. Smith's Diaper Ointment
Dr. Smith's Rash-N-All Ointment
Fosfree Tablets
Iromin-G Tablets
Lithostat Tablets
Mission Prenatal H.P. Tablets
Mission Prenatal Tablets
Mission Prenatal F.A. Tablets
NataChew Prenatal Tablets
NataFort Prenatal Tablets
Oncovite Tablets
Thera-Gesic Creme
Thera-Gesic Plus Creme
Thiola Tablets

MANUFACTURERS' INDEX

MONARCH PHARMACEUTICALS

(See KING PHARMACEUTICALS, INC.)

MYLAN PHARMACEUTICALS INC.   2387

781 Chestnut Ridge Road
P.O. Box 4310
Morgantown, WV 26504-4310

Direct Inquiries to:
(304) 599-2595

For Medical Information Contact:
Clinical Research Department
(877) 446-3679
(877) 4INFO-RX

Sales and Ordering:
Sales Department
(800) RX-MYLAN

Other Products Available:
Biobrane Temporary Wound Dressing
Flexzan Wound Dressing
Hydrocol Hydrocolloid Wound Dressing
Proderm
Sorbsan Wound Dressing

NOVARTIS CONSUMER HEALTH, INC.   314, 2447

200 Kimball Drive
Parsippany, NJ 07054-0622

Direct Inquiries to:
Novartis Consumer Relationship Center
(800) 452-0051
Fax: (973) 503-8400
or write to 200 Kimball Drive
Parsippany, NJ 07054-0622

NOVARTIS PHARMACEUTICALS CORPORATION   314, 2450

One Health Plaza
East Hanover, NJ 07936
(for branded products)

For Information Contact (branded products):
Customer Response Department
(888) NOW-NOVA (888-669-6682)
www.novartis.com

Other Products Available:
Lopressor Injection
Lopressor Tablets
Lopressor HCT Tablets
Lotensin Tablets
Lotensin HCT Tablets
Methergine Injection
Methergine Tablets
Parlodel Injection
Parlodel Tablets
Tegretol XR Tablets
Trileptal Oral Suspension
Trileptal Tablets

◆ **Shown in Product Identification Guide**   *Italic Page Number* **Indicates Brief Listing**

NOVO NORDISK INC.   316, 2640
100 College Road West
Princeton, NJ 08540

Direct Inquiries to:
Novo Nordisk Inc.
(800) 727-6500
8:30 AM - 6:00 PM EST M-F

In Emergencies after hours & weekends:
(609) 987-5800

Products Described:
Levemir Injection.................. 2640
NovoLog Injection................. 2646
NovoLog Mix 70/30............... 2655
NovoSeven RT Lyophilized
  Powder...................... 2662
◆Victoza Injection............. 316, 2668

ORTHO-McNEIL-JANSSEN   316, 2678
**PHARMACEUTICALS,
INC.**
1000 Route 202
P.O. Box 300
Raritan, NJ 08869-0602
and
1125 Trenton-Harbourton Road
P.O. Box 200
Titusville, NJ 08560-0200

For Medical Information Contact:
Generally:
(800) 682-6532
In Emergencies:
(908) 218-7325
For Customer Service (Sales and
Ordering):
(800) 631-5273

Products Described:
Axert Tablets...................... 2678
◆Concerta Extended-Release
  Tablets.................316, 2678
Doribax Injection.................. 2678
◆Duragesic Transdermal
  System 316, 2684
Elmiron Capsules.................. 2678
Haldol Injection................... 2678
Haldol Decanoate IM Injection..... 2678
◆Invega Extended-Release
  Tablets.................316, 2691
◆Invega Sustenna
  Extended-Release
  Injectable Suspension.......316, 2698
◆Levaquin Injection........316, 2707
◆Levaquin Oral Solution 316, 2707
◆Levaquin Tablets..........316, 2707
◆Levaquin in 5% Dextrose
  Injection...............316, 2707
Modicon Tablets................... 2678
Natrecor for Injection............. 2678
◆Nucynta Tablets...........317, 2720
Ortho Diaphragm Kits............. 2678
◆Ortho Evra Transdermal
  System 316, 2725
Ortho Micronor.................... 2678
Ortho Tri-Cyclen Lo Tablets....... 2678
Ortho Tri-Cyclen Tablets.......... 2678
Ortho-Cept Tablets................ 2678
Ortho-Cyclen Tablets.............. 2678
Ortho-Novum Tablets.............. 2678
Ortho-Novum 1/50 Tablets......... 2678
◆Pancreaze Delayed-Release
  Capsules...............317, 2737
Parafon Forte DSC................. 2678
Razadyne Oral Solution............ 2678
Razadyne Tablets.................. 2678
Razadyne ER Extended-Release
  Capsules...................... 2678
Risperdal M-Tab................... 2678
Risperdal Oral Solution............ 2678
Risperdal Tablets.................. 2678
◆Risperdal Consta
  Long-Acting Injection......317, 2741
Terazol 3 Vaginal Cream........... 2678
Terazol 3 Vaginal Suppositories ... 2678
Terazol 7 Vaginal Cream........... 2678
Tolectin 200/400/600.............. 2678
Topamax Sprinkle Capsules........ 2678
Topamax Tablets.................. 2678
◆Tylenol with Codeine Tablets..317, 2750
Tylox Capsules.................... 2678
Ultracet Tablets................... 2678
Ultram Tablets.................... 2678
Ultram ER Extended-Release
  Tablets....................... 2678

OTSUKA AMERICA   2751
PHARMACEUTICAL, INC.
2440 Research Boulevard
Rockville, MD 20850

Direct Medical Inquiries to:
Medical Affairs
Otsuka America Pharmaceutical, Inc.
(800) 441-6763
Fax: (301) 721-7044

To Request Routine or Emergency
Medical Information, or to Report an
Adverse Experience:
(800) 438-9927

Products Described:
Samsca Tablets.................... 2751

PAR PHARMACEUTICAL,   317, 2756
INC.
One Ram Ridge Road
Spring Valley, NY 10977

Direct Inquiries to:
Customer Representative
(800) 828-9393

Products Described:
Megace ES Oral Suspension........ 2756
◆Nascobal Nasal Spray......... 317, 2759
◆Oravig Buccal Tablets......... 317, 2761
◆Zuplenz Oral Soluble Film.... 317, 2765

PARKE-DAVIS   2770
A Division of Warner-Lambert
  Company LLC
A Pfizer Company
235 East 42nd Street
New York, NY 10017-5755
For updates to the product information
  listed below, please check the
  Pfizer Web site,
  http://www.pfizerpro.com, or call
  (800) 438-1985.

For Medical Information, Contact:
(800) 438-1985
24 hours a day, 7 days a week
Distribution:
1855 Shelby Oaks Drive North
Memphis, TN 38134
(901) 387-5200
Customer Service
(800) 533-4535

Products Described:
Lipitor Tablets.................... 2770

Other Products Available:
Accupril Tablets
Accuretic Tablets
Celontin Capsules
Dilantin Capsules
Dilantin Infatabs
Dilantin-125 Oral Suspension
Lopid Tablets
Nardil Tablets
Neurontin Capsules
Neurontin Oral Solution
Neurontin Tablets
Nitrostat Tablets
Zarontin Capsules

PBM   317, 2777
**PHARMACEUTICALS,
INC.**
204 North Main Street
Gordonsville, VA 22942

Direct Inquiries to:
Customer Service
(866) 366-6282
FAX: (866) 435-1487

Products Described:
◆Animi-3 Capsules............. 317, 2777
◆Donnatal Extentabs 317, 2777

**PFIZER CONSUMER
HEALTHCARE, PFIZER
INC.**
(See McNEIL CONSUMER
HEALTHCARE)

PFIZER INC.   2778
235 East 42nd Street
New York, NY 10017-5755
For updates to the product information
  listed below, please check the
  Pfizer Web site
  http://www.pfizerpro.com or call
  (800) 438-1985.

For Medical Information, Contact:
(800) 438-1985
24 hours a day, 7 days a week
Distribution:
1855 Shelby Oaks Drive North
Memphis, TN 38134
(901) 387-5200
Customer Service:
(800) 533-4535
Pfizer Companies Include:
Agouron Pharmaceuticals
Parke-Davis (see PAKE-DAVIS)
Pharmacia & Upjohn (see PHARMACIA
  & UPJOHN)

G.D. Searle & Co. (see G.D. SEARLE &
  CO.)
Wyeth Pharmaceuticals (see WYETH
  PHARMACEUTICALS)

Products Described:
Caduet Tablets.................... 2778
Chantix Tablets................... 2788
Geodon Capsules 2793
Geodon for Injection.............. 2793
Lyrica Capsules 2802
Lyrica Oral Solution.............. 2802
Sutent Capsules.................. 2812
Toviaz Extended-Release Tablets ... 2819
Viagra Tablets 2823

Other Products Available:
Antivert, Antivert/25, & Antivert/50
  Tablets
Cardura Tablets
Cardura XL Tablets
Diflucan Injection
Diflucan Oral Suspension
Diflucan Tablets
Eraxis for Injection
Feldene Capsules
Glucotrol Tablets
Glucotrol XL Extended Release Tablets
Inspra Tablets
Minipress Capsules
Norvasc Tablets
Pfizerpen for Injection
Procardia Capsules
Procardia XL Extended Release Tablets
Relpax Tablets
Rescriptor Tablets
Revatio Tablets
Tikosyn Capsules
Unasyn
VFEND I.V.
VFEND Oral Suspension
VFEND Tablets
Vibramycin Calcium Oral Suspension
  Syrup
Vibramycin Hyclate Capsules
Vibramycin Monohydrate for Oral
  Suspension
Vibra-Tabs Film Coated Tablets
Viracept Oral Powder
Viracept Tablets
Vistaril Capsules
Zithromax for Oral Suspension, 1g
Zithromax for Oral Suspension, 300 mg,
  600 mg, 900 mg, 1200 mg
Zithromax IV
Zithromax Tablets, 250 mg, 500 mg
Zithromax Tablets, 600 mg
Zithromax Tri-Pak
Zithromax Z-Pak
Zmax for Oral Suspension
Zoloft Oral Concentrate
Zoloft Tablets

PHARMACEUTICAL   2829
ASSOCIATES, INC.
A Subsidiary of Beach Products, Inc.
201 Delaware Street
Greenville, SC 29605

Direct Inquiries to:
Clete Harmon, Sr. Vice President
(800) 845-8210
(864) 277-7282
FAX: (864) 236-0116
www.paipharma.com

Products Described:
Acetaminophen Oral Solution
  USP...................... 2829
Acetaminophen Oral Suspension
  USP...................... 2829
Acetaminophen and Codeine
  Phosphate Oral Solution USP.... 2829
Aluminum Hydroxide Gel USP..... 2829
Aluminum Hydroxide Gel
  Concentrate................... 2829
Amantadine Hydrochloride Oral
  Solution USP................. 2829
Calcium Carbonate Oral
  Suspension................... 2829
Cetirizine Hydrochloride Syrup..... 2829
Chloral Hydrate Oral Solution
  USP...................... 2829
Cimetidine Hydrochloride Oral
  Solution 2829
Diphenhydramine Hydrochloride
  Oral Solution USP............. 2829
Docusate Sodium Liquid 2829
Docusate Sodium Syrup USP....... 2829
Ethosuximide Syrup............... 2829
Ferrous Sulfate Oral Solution
  USP...................... 2829
Fluoxetine Oral Solution USP..... 2829
Fluphenazine Hydrochloride
  Elixir USP................... 2829
Fluphenazine Hydrochloride Oral
  Solution USP (Concentrate) 2829
Guaifenesin Oral Solution USP..... 2829
Guaifenesin and Codeine
  Phosphate Oral Solution........ 2829

Guaifenesin Syrup and
  Dextromethorphan.............. 2829
Guaifenesin Syrup and
  Dextromethorphan (Maximum
  Strength)..................... 2829
Haloperidol Oral Solution USP
  (Concentrate) 2829
Hydrocodone Bitartrate and
  Acetaminophen Oral Solution
  7.5 mg/500 mg/15 mL 2829
Hydrocodone Bitartrate and
  Acetaminophen Oral Solution
  10 mg/325 mg/15 mL 2829
Hydrocodone Bitartrate and
  Homatropine Methylbromide
  Syrup....................... 2829
Ibuprofen Oral Suspension USP.... 2829
Lactulose Solution USP............ 2829
Levetiracetam Oral Solution 2829
MAG-AL Liquid.................. 2829
MAG-AL Plus.................... 2829
MAG-AL Plus XS................. 2829
MAG-AL Ultimate Strength....... 2829
Megestrol Acetate Oral
  Suspension................... 2829
Metoclopramide Oral Solution
  USP...................... 2829
Milk of Magnesia (8%
  Suspension).................. 2829
Milk of Magnesia Concentrate
  (24% Suspension)............. 2829
Mineral Oil 2829
Nortriptyline Hydrochloride Oral
  Solution USP................. 2829
Nystatin Oral Suspension USP..... 2829
Oxybutynin Chloride Syrup USP... 2829
Phenobarbital Oral Solution USP... 2829
Pink Bismuth 2829
Potassium Chloride Oral Solution
  USP 10%................... 2829
Potassium Chloride Oral Solution
  USP 20%................... 2829
Potassium Citrate and Citric Acid
  Oral Solution USP............. 2829
Prednisolone Sodium Phosphate
  Oral Solution 15 mg/mL......... 2829
Promethazine Hydrochloride and
  Codeine Phosphate Syrup........ 2829
Pseudoephedrine Hydrochloride
  Oral Solution USP............. 2829
Ranitidine Syrup (Oral Solution
  USP)...................... 2829
Senna Syrup..................... 2829
Sodium Citrate and Citric Acid
  Oral Solution USP............. 2829
Sorbitol Solution USP............. 2829
Sore Throat Spray................. 2829
Sucralfate Suspension............. 2829
Sulfamethoxazole and
  Trimethoprim Oral Suspension
  USP...................... 2829
Theophylline Oral Solution........ 2829
Tricitrates Oral Solution............ 2829
Tricitrates SF Oral Solution........ 2829
Trihexyphenidyl Hydrochloride
  Elixir USP................... 2829
Valproic Acid Oral Solution USP... 2829

PHARMACIA & UPJOHN   2830
A Division of Pfizer
235 East 42nd Street
New York, NY 10017-5755
For updates to the product information
  listed below, please check the
  Pfizer Web site,
  http://www.pfizerpro.com, or call
  (800) 438-1985.

For Medical Information, Contact:
(800) 438-1985
24 hours a day, 7 days a week
Distribution:
1855 Shelby Oaks Drive North
Memphis, TN 38134
(901) 387-5200
Customer Service:
(800) 533-4535

Products Described:
Aromasin Tablets 2830
Detrol LA Capsules 2838
Detrol Tablets.................... 2835
Genotropin Lyophilized Powder.... 2842
Zyvox for Oral Suspension........ 2848
Zyvox Injection.................. 2848
Zyvox Tablets.................... 2848

Other Products Available:
Aldactazide Tablets
Aldactone Tablets
Atgam Sterile Solution
Azulfidine Tablets
Azulfidine EN-Tabs Tablets
Calan Tablets
Calan SR Caplets
Camptosar Injection
Caverject Impulse Injection
Caverject Sterile Powder
Cleocin HCl Capsules
Cleocin Pediatric for Oral Solution, USP
Cleocin Phosphate Sterile Solution
Cleocin T Topical Gel
Cleocin T Topical Lotion
Cleocin T Topical Solution

◆ **Shown in Product Identification Guide**

Italic Page Number **Indicates Brief Listing**

SECTION 2

BRAND AND GENERIC NAME INDEX

This index includes all entries in the Product Information section. Products are listed alphabetically by both brand and generic name. Generic names are underlined; brand names are not. Under each generic name, you will find a list of the brands that contain it. This enables you to find a product by either of its names. For example, the brand Aciphex appears once in the A's, and again under its generic name, rabeprazole sodium.

Each time a brand name appears, it is followed by the manufacturer's name and the page number to consult

for further information. If multiple page numbers appear, the first ones refer to photos of the product, the last one to its prescribing information. Under a generic heading, all fully described brands are listed first, followed by those with only partial information.

- **Bold page numbers** indicate full prescribing information.
- *Italic page numbers* signify partial information.
- The ◆ symbol marks drugs shown in the Product Identification Guide.

A

ABACAVIR SULFATE
Epzicom Tablets *(ViiV)*................. 3296
Trizivir Tablets *(ViiV)*................ 3340
Ziagen Oral Solution *(ViiV)*............ 3346
Ziagen Tablets *(ViiV)*................. 3346

ABATACEPT
Orencia Powder for Intravenous Infusion *(Bristol-Myers Squibb)*.................. 321, 3501

ABBO-CODE INDEX *(Abbott)*........ *402*

ABELCET INJECTION
(Sigma-Tau)....................... 3111

◆ABILIFY INJECTION
(Bristol-Myers Squibb)......... 321, 3458

◆ABILIFY ORAL SOLUTION
(Bristol-Myers Squibb)......... 321, 3458

◆ABILIFY DISCMELT ORALLY DISINTEGRATING TABLETS *(Bristol-Myers Squibb)*................ 321, 3458

◆ABILIFY TABLETS
(Bristol-Myers Squibb)........ 321, 3458

ABOBOTULINUMTOXINA
Dysport for Injection *(Medicis)*.......... 1913

ACEBUTOLOL HYDROCHLORIDE
Acebutolol Hydrochloride Capsules *(Mylan)*...................... *2387*

◆ACETADOTE INJECTION
(Cumberland).................. 308, 986

ACETAMINOPHEN
Percocet Tablets *(Endo)*............ 309, 1096
Regular Strength Tylenol Tablets *(McNeil Consumer)*................. 1910
Tylenol Arthritis Pain Extended Release Gelcaps/Caplets *(McNeil Consumer)*...................... 1910
Tylenol 8 Hour Extended Release Caplets *(McNeil Consumer)*.......... 1910
Extra Strength Tylenol Rapid Release Gels *(McNeil Consumer)*............. 1910
Extra Strength Tylenol Caplets and EZ Tabs *(McNeil Consumer)*.......... 1910
Extra Strength Tylenol Adult Rapid Blast Liquid *(McNeil Consumer)*....... 1910
Extra Strength Tylenol PM Caplets *(McNeil Consumer)*................. 1910
Tylenol with Codeine Tablets *(Ortho-McNeil-Janssen)*......... 317, 2750
Children's Tylenol Meltaways *(McNeil Consumer)*................. 1908
Children's Tylenol Suspension Liquid *(McNeil Consumer)*................. 1908
Concentrated Tylenol Infants' Drops *(McNeil Consumer)*................. 1908
Jr. Tylenol Meltaways *(McNeil Consumer)*...................... 1908
Vicodin Tablets *(Abbott)*........... 304, 573

Vicodin ES Tablets *(Abbott)*......... 304, 575
Vicodin HP Tablets *(Abbott)*......... 304, 576
Zydone Tablets *(Endo)*............ 309, 1113
Acetaminophen Oral Solution USP *(Pharmaceutical Associates)*.......... *2829*
Acetaminophen Oral Suspension USP *(Pharmaceutical Associates)*.......... *2829*
Acetaminophen and Codeine Phosphate Oral Solution USP *(Pharmaceutical Associates)*.......... *2829*
Hydrocodone Bitartrate and Acetaminophen Oral Solution 10 mg/325 mg/15 mL *(Pharmaceutical Associates)*.......... *2829*
Hydrocodone Bitartrate and Acetaminophen Oral Solution 7.5 mg/500 mg/15 mL *(Pharmaceutical Associates)*.......... *2829*
Oxycodone and Acetaminophen Tablets *(Mylan)*................... *2387*
Propoxyphene Hydrochloride and Acetaminophen Tablets *(Mylan)*....... *2387*
Propoxyphene Napsylate and Acetaminophen Tablets *(Mylan)*....... *2387*
Tramadol Hydrochloride and Acetaminophen Tablets *(Mylan)*....... *2387*

ACETYLCYSTEINE
Acetadote Injection *(Cumberland)*................ 308, 986

ACETYL-L-CARNITINE HYDROCHLORIDE
Sanitin/Cericar/Carmentin/Demencerin Capsules *(CPH)*.................... 3546

ACETYLSALICYLIC ACID
(see under: ASPIRIN)

ACHILLEA MILLEFOLIUM
Traumeel Injection Solution *(Heel)*........ 1684

◆ACIPHEX TABLETS *(Eisai)*.... 308, 993

ACITRETIN
Soriatane Capsules *(Stiefel)*........ 319, 3138

ACONITUM NAPELLUS
Traumeel Injection Solution *(Heel)*....... 1684

◆ACTEMRA INJECTION
(Genentech)................. 309, 1142

◆ACTICIN CREAM *(Mylan)* *2387*

ACTIMMUNE *(InterMune)* 1694

ACTIVE CALCIUM TABLETS
(Usana)....................... 3554

ACTONEL TABLETS *(Warner Chilcott)*..................... 3352

ACTOPLUS MET TABLETS
(Takeda)....................... 3159

◆ACTOPLUS MET XR EXTENDED-RELEASE TABLETS *(Takeda)*........... 320, 3159

◆ACTOS TABLETS *(Takeda)*.... 319, 3168

ACYCLOVIR
Zovirax Capsules *(GlaxoSmithKline)*...... 1650
Zovirax Suspension *(GlaxoSmithKline)*................. 1650
Zovirax Tablets *(GlaxoSmithKline)*..... 1650
Acyclovir Capsules and Tablets *(Mylan)*...................... *2387*

◆ACZONE GEL 5% *(Allergan)*.... 304, 599

ADALIMUMAB
Humira Injection Syringe and Pen *(Abbott)*.................. 303, 448

ADEFOVIR DIPIVOXIL
Hepsera Tablets *(Gilead)*.......... 309, 1158

◆ADIPEX-P CAPSULES *(Teva Biologics and Specialty)*........... 3205

◆ADIPEX-P TABLETS *(Teva Biologics and Specialty)*........... 3205

ADVAIR DISKUS 100/50
(GlaxoSmithKline)................ 1189

ADVAIR DISKUS 250/50
(GlaxoSmithKline)................ 1189

ADVAIR DISKUS 500/50
(GlaxoSmithKline)................ 1189

ADVAIR HFA 45/21 INHALATION AEROSOL
(GlaxoSmithKline)................ 1202

ADVAIR HFA 115/21 INHALATION AEROSOL
(GlaxoSmithKline)................ 1202

ADVAIR HFA 230/21 INHALATION AEROSOL
(GlaxoSmithKline)................ 1202

ADVATE *(Baxter Healthcare)* 793

◆ADVICOR TABLETS *(Abbott)* ... 303, 402

◆AEROCHAMBER PLUS FLOW-VU AND AEROCHAMBER PLUS FLOW-VU WITH MASK *(Forest)*.................. 309, 1124

AESCULUS
Topricin Pain Relief and Healing Cream *(Topical Biomedics)*................. 320, 3248
Topricin Foot Therapy Cream *(Topical Biomedics)*............. 320, 3248
Topricin Junior *(Topical Biomedics)*................. 320, 3248

◆AFINITOR TABLETS
(Novartis)................. 314, 2450

AGARICUS BLAZEI MURILL MUSHROOM
Sen-Sei-Ro Liquid Gold *(Kyowa)*.................... 310, 3548
Sen-Sei-Ro Liquid Royal *(Kyowa)*.................... 310, 3548
Sen-Sei-Ro Powder Gold *(Kyowa)*.................... 310, 3548

◆AGGRENOX CAPSULES *(Boehringer Ingelheim)*....... 307, 880

ALA (ALPHA-LINOLENIC ACID)
Norwegian Cod Liver Oil *(Carlson)*....... 3545

ALBENDAZOLE
Albenza Tablets *(GlaxoSmithKline)*...... 1212

ALBENZA TABLETS
(GlaxoSmithKline)................ 1212

ALBUMIN (HUMAN)
Albutein 5% Solution *(Grifols)*.......... 1664
Albutein 25% Solution *(Grifols)*......... 1665
Buminate 25% Solution *(Baxter Healthcare)*..................... 803
Flexbumin 25% Solution *(Baxter Healthcare)*..................... 807

ALBUTEIN 5% SOLUTION
(Grifols)....................... 1664

ALBUTEIN 25% SOLUTION
(Grifols)....................... 1665

ALBUTEROL
Albuterol Tablets *(Mylan)*.............. *2387*

ALBUTEROL SULFATE
ProAir HFA Inhalation Aerosol *(Teva Respiratory)*............... 320, 3219
Proventil HFA Inhalation Aerosol *(Merck)*............. 313, 2268
Ventolin HFA Inhalation Aerosol *(GlaxoSmithKline)*................ 1599
Albuterol Sulfate Extended-release Tablets *(Mylan)*................. *2387*
Albuterol Sulfate Inhalation Solution *(Mylan)*...................... *2387*
Ipratropium Bromide and Albuterol Sulfate Inhalation Solution *(Mylan)*...... *2387*

ALENDRONATE SODIUM
Fosamax Oral Solution *(Merck)*.......... 2065
Fosamax Tablets *(Merck)*.......... 312, 2065
Fosamax Plus D Tablets *(Merck)*.................. 313, 2074
Alendronate Sodium Tablets *(Mylan)*...... *2387*

◆ALFERON N INJECTION
(Hemispherx).................. 310, 1686

ALFUZOSIN
Uroxatral Extended-Release Tablets *(sanofi-aventis)*.................. 3064

ALIMTA FOR INJECTION
(Lilly)....................... 1737

ALISKIREN
Tekamlo Tablets *(Novartis)*............. 2598
Tekturna Tablets *(Novartis)*........ 316, 2604
Tekturna HCT Tablets *(Novartis)*.................. 316, 2608
Valturna Tablets *(Novartis)*........ 316, 2617

ALITRETINOIN
Panretin Gel 0.1% *(Eisai)*.............. 1038

ALKERAN FOR INJECTION
(GlaxoSmithKline)................ 1213

ALKERAN TABLETS
(GlaxoSmithKline)................ 1215

◆ALLEGRA ODT ORALLY DISINTEGRATING TABLETS *(sanofi-aventis)*..... 318, 2915

◆ALLEGRA ORAL SOLUTION *(sanofi-aventis)* ... 318, 2915

◆ALLEGRA TABLETS
(sanofi-aventis)............. 318, 2915

◆ALLEGRA-D 12 HOUR EXTENDED-RELEASE TABLETS *(sanofi-aventis)*..... 318, 2919

◆ **Shown in Product Identification Guide**   <u>Underline</u> Denotes Generic Name   *Italic Page Number* **Indicates Brief Listing**

BRAND AND GENERIC NAME INDEX

BRAND AND GENERIC NAME INDEX

◆ **Shown in Product Identification Guide**   <u>Underline Denotes Generic Name</u>   *Italic Page Number* **Indicates Brief Listing**

DEHYDROEPIANDROSTERONE
Tofipan/Tofipan-Z/Fibrinase-PMS/
Andromon Capsules (CPH) 3547

DELATESTRYL INJECTION
(Endo) 1079

DELAVIRDINE MESYLATE
Rescriptor Tablets (ViiV) 3313

DENAVIR CREAM (Novartis
Consumer) 2447

DENILEUKIN DIFTITOX
Ontak Vials (Eisai) 308, 1036

DENOSUMAB
Prolia Injection (Amgen) 306, 673

◆**DEPAKENE CAPSULES**
(Abbott) 303, 402

◆**DEPAKOTE DELAYED
RELEASE TABLETS**
(Abbott) 303, 402

◆**DEPAKOTE ER EXTENDED
RELEASE TABLETS**
(Abbott) 303, 425

◆**DEPAKOTE SPRINKLE
CAPSULES** (Abbott) 303, 402

DEPRENYL
(see under: **SELEGILINE
HYDROCHLORIDE**)

DESFLURANE
Suprane Volatile Liquid for Inhalation
(Baxter Anesthesia) 821

DESLORATADINE
Clarinex Syrup (Merck) 312, 1981
Clarinex Tablets (Merck) 312, 1981
Clarinex Reditabs Tablets
(Merck) 312, 1981
Clarinex-D 12 Hour Extended
Release Tablets (Merck) 312, 1984
Clarinex-D 24 Hour Extended-Release
Tablets (Merck) 1988

◆**DESONATE GEL** (Intendis) 310, 1690

DESONIDE
Desonate Gel (Intendis) 310, 1690
Verdeso Foam (Stiefel) 3148

DESVENLAFAXINE
Pristiq Extended-Release
Tablets (Wyeth) 321, 3409

DETROL LA CAPSULES
(Pharmacia & Upjohn) 2838

DETROL TABLETS
(Pharmacia & Upjohn) 2835

DEXAMETHASONE
Ciprodex Otic Suspension (Alcon) 591

**DEXEDRINE SPANSULE
SUSTAINED-RELEASE
CAPSULES** (GlaxoSmithKline) 1342

◆**DEXILANT DELAYED
RELEASE CAPSULES**
(Takeda) 320, 3178

DEXLANSOPRAZOLE
Dexilant Delayed Release
Capsules (Takeda) 320, 3178

**DEXMETHYLPHENIDATE
HYDROCHLORIDE**
Focalin XR Capsules (Novartis) 315, 2530

DEXTROAMPHETAMINE SULFATE
Dexedrine Spansule
Sustained-Release Capsules
(GlaxoSmithKline) 1342

**DEXTROMETHORPHAN
HYDROBROMIDE**
Guaifenesin Syrup and
Dextromethorphan (Pharmaceutical
Associates) 2829

DHA (DOCOSAHEXAENOIC ACID)
(see under: **DOCOSAHEXAENOIC ACID
(DHA)**)

DIAZEPAM
Diazepam Tablets (Mylan) 2387

DIAZOXIDE
Proglycem Capsules (Teva Biologics
and Specialty) 3206
Proglycem Suspension (Teva
Biologics and Specialty) 3206

DIBASIC SODIUM PHOSPHATE
Fleet Enema (Fleet) 1119
Fleet Enema Extra (Fleet) 1119
Fleet Enema for Children (Fleet) 1119
Fleet Pedia-Lax Enema (Fleet) 1119
Fleet Prep Kit 3 (Fleet) 1122
OsmoPrep Tablets (Salix) 318, 2908

◆**DIBENZYLINE CAPSULES**
(WellSpring) 321, 3366

DICLOFENAC EPOLAMINE
Flector Patch (King) 310, 1723

DICLOFENAC POTASSIUM
Diclofenac Potassium Tablets (Mylan) 2387

DICLOFENAC SODIUM
Diclofenac Sodium Delayed-release
Tablets (Mylan) 2387
Diclofenac Sodium Extended-release
Tablets (Mylan) 2387

DICYCLOMINE HYDROCHLORIDE
Dicyclomine Hydrochloride Capsules
and Tablets (Mylan) 2387

DIDANOSINE
Didanosine Delayed-release Capsules
(Mylan) 2387

DIDRONEL TABLETS (Warner
Chilcott) 3364

DIENOGEST
Natazia Tablets (Bayer
HealthCare Pharmaceuticals) 307, 854

DIETARY SUPPLEMENT
Immunizen Capsules (Unicity) 3553
Mega Antioxidant Tablets (Usana) 3554

DIGESTIVE ENZYMES
(see under: **PANCRELIPASE**)

DIGOXIN
Lanoxin Injection (GlaxoSmithKline) 1460
Lanoxin Injection Pediatric
(GlaxoSmithKline) 1464
Lanoxin Tablets (GlaxoSmithKline) 1468

◆**DILAUDID INJECTION**
(Purdue Pharma) 317, 2876

◆**DILAUDID ORAL LIQUID**
(Purdue Pharma) 317, 2873

◆**DILAUDID TABLETS**
(Purdue Pharma) 317, 2873

◆**DILAUDID-HP INJECTION**
(Purdue Pharma) 317, 2876

◆**DILAUDID-HP
LYOPHILIZED POWDER
250 MG** (Purdue Pharma) 317, 2876

DILTIAZEM HYDROCHLORIDE
Cardizem LA Extended Release
Tablets (Abbott) 303, 423
Diltiazem Hydrochloride
Extended-release Capsules
(once-a-day) (Mylan) 2387
Diltiazem Hydrochloride
Extended-release Capsules
(twice-a-day) (Mylan) 2387
Diltiazem Hydrochloride Tablets
(Mylan) 2387

DINOPROSTONE
Cervidil Vaginal Insert (Forest) 309, 1128

**DIOCTYL SODIUM
SULFOSUCCINATE**
(see under: **DOCUSATE SODIUM**)

◆**DIOVAN TABLETS**
(Novartis) 314, 2465

◆**DIOVAN HCT TABLETS**
(Novartis) 315, 2470

DIPHENHYDRAMINE CITRATE
Motrin PM Caplets (McNeil
Consumer) 1904

**DIPHENHYDRAMINE
HYDROCHLORIDE**
Benadryl Allergy Ultratab Tablets
(McNeil Consumer) 1901
Children's Benadryl Allergy Liquid
(McNeil Consumer) 1901
Extra Strength Tylenol PM Caplets
(McNeil Consumer) 1910
Diphenhydramine Hydrochloride Oral
Solution USP (Pharmaceutical
Associates) 2829

**DIPHENOXYLATE
HYDROCHLORIDE**
Diphenoxylate Hydrochloride and
Atropine Sulfate Tablets (Mylan) 2387

DIPHENYLHYDANTOIN
(see under: **PHENYTOIN SODIUM**)

**DIPHTHERIA & TETANUS
TOXOIDS AND ACELLULAR
PERTUSSIS VACCINE ADSORBED**
Boostrix Vaccine (GlaxoSmithKline) 1312
Infanrix Injection Vaccine
(GlaxoSmithKline) 1420

**DIPHTHERIA & TETANUS
TOXOIDS AND ACELLULAR
PERTUSSIS VACCINE ADSORBED,
HEPATITIS B (RECOMBINANT)
AND INACTIVATED POLIOVIRUS
VACCINE COMBINED**
Pediarix Injection Vaccine
(GlaxoSmithKline) 1512

**DIPHTHERIA AND TETANUS
TOXOIDS AND ACELLULAR
PERTUSSIS ADSORBED AND
INACTIVATED POLIOVIRUS
VACCINE**
Kinrix Injection Vaccine
(GlaxoSmithKline) 1433

◆**DIPROLENE LOTION
0.05% (Merck)** 312, 2017

◆**DIPROLENE OINTMENT
0.05% (Merck)** 312, 2019

◆**DIPROLENE AF CREAM
0.05% (Merck)** 312, 2016

DIPYRIDAMOLE
Aggrenox Capsules (Boehringer
Ingelheim) 307, 880

DIVALPROEX SODIUM
Depakote ER Extended Release
Tablets (Abbott) 303, 425
Depakote Delayed Release
Tablets (Abbott) 303, 402
Depakote Sprinkle Capsules
(Abbott) 303, 402
Divalproex Sodium Delayed-release
Tablets (Mylan) 2387
Divalproex Sodium Extended-release
Tablets (Mylan) 2387

◆**DIVIGEL 0.1%**
(Upsher-Smith) 321, 3276

DL-ALPHA TOCOPHERYL ACETATE
CitraNatal Harmony Gel Caps
(Mission) 2381

DOCETAXEL
Taxotere Injection Concentrate
(sanofi-aventis) 3050

DOCOSAHEXAENOIC ACID (DHA)
Animi-3 Capsules (PBM) 317, 2777
CitraNatal Assure Capsules (Mission) 2380
CitraNatal 90 DHA Capsules
(Mission) 2380
CitraNatal Harmony Gel Caps
(Mission) 2381
Med Omega Fish Oil 2800 (Carlson) 3545
Norwegian Cod Liver Oil (Carlson) 3545
OmegaLife-3 Supplementation
(Unicity) 3553
Prenate Essentials Softgels (Shionogi) 3092
PreNexa Premier Capsules
(Upsher-Smith) 321, 3285
Sanitin/Cericar/Carmentin/Demencerin
Capsules (CPH) 3546
Super Omega-3 Gems Softgels
(Carlson) 3546
Xantasil/Neoastor/Vasculax/Choroxan
Capsules (CPH) 3547

DOCUSATE SODIUM
CitraNatal Assure Tablets (Mission) 2380
CitraNatal 90 DHA Tablets (Mission) 2380
CitraNatal Harmony Gel Caps
(Mission) 2381
Ferralet 90 Tablets (Mission) 2381
Fleet Pedia-Lax Liquid Stool Softener
(Fleet) 1121
PreNexa Premier Capsules
(Upsher-Smith) 321, 3285
Docusate Sodium Liquid
(Pharmaceutical Associates) 2829
Docusate Sodium Syrup USP
(Pharmaceutical Associates) 2829

DOLASETRON MESYLATE
Anzemet Injection
(sanofi-aventis) 318, 2934
Anzemet Tablets
(sanofi-aventis) 318, 2937

DONEPEZIL HYDROCHLORIDE
Aricept Tablets (Eisai) 308, 1004
Aricept ODT Tablets (Eisai) 308, 1004

◆**DONNATAL EXTENTABS**
(PBM) 317, 2777

DORIBAX INJECTION
(Ortho-McNeil-Janssen) 2678

**DORYX DELAYED-RELEASE
TABLETS** (Warner Chilcott) 3352

DORZOLAMIDE HYDROCHLORIDE
Trusopt Sterile Ophthalmic Solution
(Merck) 2322

DOXAZOSIN MESYLATE
Doxazosin Tablets (Mylan) 2387

DOXEPIN HYDROCHLORIDE
Doxepin Hydrochloride Capsules
(Mylan) 2387

◆**DOXIL INJECTION** (Centocor
Ortho Biotech) 307, 929

**DOXORUBICIN HYDROCHLORIDE
LIPOSOME**
Doxil Injection (Centocor Ortho
Biotech) 307, 929

DOXYCYCLINE
Doxycycline Tablets (Mylan) 2387

DOXYCYCLINE HYCLATE
Doryx Delayed-Release Tablets
(Warner Chilcott) 3352

DRONEDARONE
Multaq Tablets (sanofi-aventis) 319, 3030

DROSPIRENONE
Angeliq Tablets (Bayer
HealthCare Pharmaceuticals) 307, 825
Yasmin 28 Tablets (Bayer
HealthCare Pharmaceuticals) 307, 859
Yaz Tablets (Bayer HealthCare
Pharmaceuticals) 307, 868

DUAC TOPICAL GEL (Stiefel) 3131

◆**DUETACT TABLETS**
(Takeda) 320, 3182

◆**DULERA INHALATION
AEROSOL** (Merck) 312, 2020

DULOXETINE HYDROCHLORIDE
Cymbalta Delayed-Release
Capsules (Lilly) 310, 1759

◆**DURAGESIC
TRANSDERMAL SYSTEM**
(Ortho-McNeil-Janssen) 316, 2684

DUTASTERIDE
Avodart Soft Gelatin Capsules
(GlaxoSmithKline) 1293
Jalyn Capsules (GlaxoSmithKline) 1427

DYAZIDE CAPSULES
(GlaxoSmithKline) 1344

**DYNACIRC CR
CONTROLLED RELEASE
TABLETS** (GlaxoSmithKline) 1347

◆**DYRENIUM CAPSULES**
(WellSpring) 321, 3367

DYSPORT FOR INJECTION
(Medicis) 1913

E

ECHINACEA
Topricin Pain Relief and
Healing Cream (Topical
Biomedics) 320, 3248
Topricin Foot Therapy Cream
(Topical Biomedics) 320, 3248
Topricin Junior (Topical
Biomedics) 320, 3248

ECHINACEA ANGUSTIFOLIA
Traumeel Injection Solution (Heel) 1684

ECHINACEA PURPUREA
Traumeel Injection Solution (Heel) 1684

E.E.S. 200 LIQUID (Abbott) 437

E.E.S. 400 LIQUID (Abbott) 437

◆**E.E.S. 400 FILMTAB
TABLETS** (Abbott) 303, 437

E.E.S. GRANULES (Abbott) 437

EFAVIRENZ
Atripla Tablets (Bristol-Myers
Squibb) 321, 3471
Atripla Tablets (Bristol-Myers Squibb
& Gilead Sciences) 891
Sustiva Capsules (Bristol-Myers
Squibb) 322, 3532
Sustiva Tablets (Bristol-Myers
Squibb) 322, 3532

EFFIENT TABLETS (Lilly) 1768

EGG PRODUCT, HYPERIMMUNE
i26 Dietary Supplement Powder
(Legacy for Life) 310, 3548
i26 Capsules (Legacy for Life) 3548
i26 Chewables (Legacy for Life) 3548
i26 Complete Support Dietary
Supplement (Legacy for Life) 3548
i26 Fit Dietary Supplement (Legacy
for Life) 3548

BRAND AND GENERIC NAME INDEX

BRAND AND GENERIC NAME INDEX

BRAND AND GENERIC NAME INDEX

◆ **Shown in Product Identification Guide**   <u>Underline</u> Denotes Generic Name   *Italic Page Number* **Indicates Brief Listing**

BRAND AND GENERIC NAME INDEX

BRAND AND GENERIC NAME INDEX

BRAND AND GENERIC NAME INDEX

BRAND AND GENERIC NAME INDEX

BRAND AND GENERIC NAME INDEX

BRAND AND GENERIC NAME INDEX

GENERIC/BRAND CROSS-REFERENCE TABLE

This table includes a list of over 200 of the top prescribed products used in the retail setting. For ease of use, products are listed alphabetically by generic name with reference to the corresponding brand name(s) available on the market. Additionally, the table contains indications for each product; if indications differ either by the way the drug is supplied (i.e., injection, cream, etc.) or by specific brand, this is noted.

Products with full prescribing information listed in *PDR* are in **boldface** in the Brand column. Please go to **PDR.net** to see prescribing information on a particular product.

GENERIC	BRAND(S)	INDICATION(S)
Acetaminophen/Butalbital/Caffeine	Esgic, Esgic-Plus, Fioricet	migraine/tension headache
Acetaminophen/Codeine Phosphate	**Tylenol with Codeine**	pain
Acetaminophen/Hydrocodone Bitartrate	Anexsia, Lorcet, Lortab, Maxidone, Norco, **Vicodin, Vicodin ES, Vicodin HP, Zydone**	pain
Acetaminophen/Oxycodone HCl	Endocet, **Percocet**, Roxicet, Tylox	pain
Acetaminophen/Propoxyphene Napsylate	Darvocet A500, Darvocet-N	pain
Acetaminophen/Tramadol HCl	Ultracet	pain
Acyclovir	Zovirax Cream, Zovirax Ointment, **Zovirax Oral**	Cream/Ointment: herpes; infections, viral/topical. Oral: chickenpox; herpes; infections, viral/systemic; shingles.
Acyclovir Sodium	Zovirax Injection	Injection: herpes; infections, viral/systemic; shingles
Albuterol Sulfate Nebulizer Solution	AccuNeb	asthma, bronchospasm
Alendronate Sodium	**Fosamax**	osteoporosis, Paget's disease
Allopurinol	Zyloprim	chemotherapy adjunct, gout, hyperuricemia, hyperuricosuria, renal calculi
Allopurinol Sodium	Aloprim	chemotherapy adjunct, hyperuricemia, hyperuricosuria
Alprazolam	Niravam, Xanax, Xanax XR	Niravam, Xanax: anxiety, panic disorder. Xanax XR: panic disorder.
Amiodarone HCl	Cordarone, Nexterone IV, Pacerone	arrhythmia
Amitriptyline HCl	Amitriptyline HCl (generic)	depression
Amlodipine Besylate	Norvasc	angina; angina—reduce risk; coronary artery disease; hypertension; revascularization—reduce risk
Amlodipine Besylate/Benazepril HCl	Lotrel	hypertension
Amoxicillin	**Amoxil**, DisperMox, **Moxatag**	Amoxil, DisperMox: gonorrhea; *H. pylori* eradication; infections (bacterial/skin, bacterial/respiratory tract, otic, urinary tract); otitis media; ulcer, GI. Moxatag: pharyngitis, tonsillitis.
Amoxicillin/Potassium Clavulanate	**Augmentin, Augmentin ES-600, Augmentin XR**	Augmentin: infections (bacterial/respiratory tract, bacterial/skin, otic, urinary tract); otitis media; sinusitis. Augmentin ES-600: infections, otic; otitis media. Augmentin XR: infections, bacterial/respiratory tract; pneumonia, bacterial; sinusitis.
Aspirin, enteric-coated	Bayer Aspirin, Bayer Aspirin Extra Strength, Ecotrin, Halfprin, St. Joseph 81mg Aspirin	Bayer Aspirin/Ecotrin: angina; ankylosing spondylitis; osteoarthritis; rheumatoid arthritis; lupus erythematosus; myocardial infarction postmanagement; stroke. Bayer Aspirin Extra Strength: arthritis, fever, pain. Halfprin: myocardial infarction; myocardial infarction postmanagement; stroke. St. Joseph 81 mg Aspirin: angina; ankylosing spondylitis; osteoarthritis; rheumatoid arthritis; lupus erythematosus; pain; stroke.
Atenolol	Tenormin	angina; hypertension; myocardial infarction postmanagement
Atenolol/Chlorthalidone	Tenoretic	hypertension
Atropine Sulfate/Diphenoxylate HCl	Lomotil, Lonox	diarrhea
Azathioprine	Azasan, Imuran	rheumatoid arthritis, organ transplant rejection
Azithromycin	**Azasite**, Zmax, Zithromax	Azasite: conjunctivitis; infections; bacterial/ophthalmic. Zmax: infections, bacterial/respiratory tract; pneumonia, bacterial; sinusitis. Zithromax: cervicitis; COPD; infections (bacterial/respiratory tract, bacterial/skin, gynecological, otic, urinary tract); mycobacterium avium complex; otitis media; pharyngitis; pneumonia, bacterial; sinusitis; tonsillitis; urethritis.

Please go to **PDR.net** to view prescribing information for these and other products.

GENERIC	BRAND(S)	INDICATION(S)
Baclofen	Lioresal Intrathecal	Baclofen: multiple sclerosis, muscle spasm. Lioresal Intrathecal: musculoskeletal conditions.
Benazepril HCl	Lotensin	hypertension
Benazepril HCl/Hydrochlorothiazide	Lotensin HCT	hypertension
Benzonatate	Tessalon	cough
Benztropine Mesylate	Cogentin	extrapyramidal disorder, Parkinson's disease
Betamethasone Dipropionate	**Diprolene, Diprolene AF**	dermatitis; inflammation, topical; pruritus, topical
Betamethasone Dipropionate/Clotrimazole	**Lotrisone**	athlete's foot; infections, fungal/topical
Bisoprolol Fumarate/Hydrochlorothiazide	Ziac	hypertension
Bumetanide Non-Injection	Bumex	congestive heart failure, edema
Buproprion Hydrobromide ER	**Aplenzin**	major depressive disorder
Bupropion HCl	**Wellbutrin**	depression
Bupropion HCl ER	Wellbutrin XL	depression
Bupropion HCl SR	**Wellbutrin SR, Zyban**	Wellbutrin SR: depression. Zyban: smoking cessation.
Buspirone HCl	BuSpar	anxiety
Calcitriol	**Calcijex,** Rocaltrol, Vectical	Calcijex: hypocalcemia. Rocaltrol: hyperparathyroidism, hypocalcemia, hypoparathyroidism. Vectical: psoriasis.
Carbamazepine	**Carbatrol,** Epitol, Equetro, Tegretol, Tegretol-XR	Carbatrol, Epitol, Tegretol, Tegretol-XR: pain, seizures, trigeminal neuralgia. Equetro: bipolar disorder.
Carbidopa/Levodopa	Atamet, Parcopa, Sinemet, Sinemet CR	Parkinson's disease
Carisoprodol	Soma	muscle spasm, musculoskeletal conditions, pain
Carvedilol	**Coreg**	congestive heart failure; hypertension; myocardial infarction postmanagement
Carvedilol Phosphate	**Coreg CR**	congestive heart failure; hypertension; myocardial infarction postmanagement
Cefdinir	**Omnicef**	bronchitis; infections (bacterial/respiratory tract, bacterial/skin, otic); otitis media; pharyngitis; pneumonia, bacterial; sinusitis; tonsillitis
Cefprozil	Cefzil	bronchitis; infections (bacterial/respiratory tract, bacterial/skin, otic); otitis media; pharyngitis; sinusitis; tonsillitis
Cefuroxime Axetil	**Ceftin**	bronchitis; gonorrhea; impetigo; infections (bacterial/skin, bacterial/respiratory tract, otic, urinary tract); Lyme disease; otitis media; pharyngitis; sinusitis; tonsillitis
Cephalexin	Cephalexin (generic), Keflex	infections (bacterial/bone, bacterial/respiratory tract, bacterial/skin, otic, urinary tract); otitis media; prostatitis
Chlorhexidine Gluconate	Peridex, PerioGard	gingivitis
Chlorpheniramine Maleate/ Dextromethorphan Hydrobromide/ Phenylephrine HCl	C-Phen DM, Rondec DM Oral Drops, Rondec DM Syrup	allergy; congestion, nasal; cough
Cilostazol	Pletal	intermittent claudication
Ciprofloxacin HCl	Cetraxal, Ciloxin, **Cipro Oral, Cipro XR,** Proquin XR	Cetraxal: infections, otic; otitis externa. Ciloxin: conjunctivitis; corneal ulcer; infections, bacterial/ophthalmic. Cipro Oral: anthrax; bronchitis; diarrhea; gonorrhea; infections (bacterial/bone, bacterial/respiratory tract, bacterial/skin, bacterial/systemic, gynecological, intra-abdominal, urinary tract); prostatitis; sinusitis; typhoid fever. Cipro XR: infections, urinary tract. Proquin XR: infections, urinary tract.
Citalopram Hydrobromide	Celexa	depression
Clarithromycin	**Biaxin, Biaxin XL**	Biaxin: AIDS adjunct; bronchitis; *H. pylori* eradication; infections (bacterial/respiratory tract, bacterial/skin, otic); mycobacterium avium complex; otitis media; pharyngitis; pneumonia, bacterial; sinusitis; tonsillitis; ulcer, gastrointestinal. Biaxin XL: bronchitis; infections, bacterial/respiratory tract; pneumonia, bacterial; sinusitis.
Clindamycin HCl Systemic	Cleocin	infections (bacterial/respiratory tract, bacterial/skin, bacterial/systemic, gynecological, intra-abdominal); septicemia

Please go to **PDR.net** to view prescribing information for these and other products.

GENERIC	BRAND(S)	INDICATION(S)
Clindamycin Phosphate Systemic	Cleocin	infections (bacterial/respiratory tract, bacterial/skin, bacterial/systemic, gynecological, intra-abdominal); septicemia
Clindamycin Phosphate Topical	Clindamycin Phosphate (generic), Cleocin Vaginal, Cleocin Vaginal Ovules, Cleocin T, Clindagel, Clindamax, Clindamax Vaginal, Clindesse, **Evoclin**	Cleocin Vaginal, Cleocin Vaginal Ovules, Clindamax Vaginal, Clindesse: vaginosis, bacterial. Clindamycin Phosphate, Cleocin T, Clindagel, Clindamax, Evoclin: acne.
Clobetasol Propionate	Clobetasol Propionate (generic), Clobevate, Clobex, Cormax, Olux, **Olux-E**, Temovate, Temovate Scalp, Temovate-E	Clobetasol Propionate, Clobevate, Cormax, Olux-E: dermatitis; inflammation, topical; pruritus, topical Clobex, Olux, Temovate, Temovate Scalp, Temovate-E: dermatitis; inflammation, topical; pruritus, topical; psoriasis.
Clonazepam	Clonazepam ODT, Klonopin	panic disorder, seizures
Clonidine HCl	Catapres, Catapres-TTS, Clonidine ER, Duraclon Injection, Jenloga	Catapres, Catapres-TTS, Jenloga: hypertension. Duraclon Injection: cancer pain; pain, neuropathic.
Codeine Phosphate/Guaifenesin	Cheratussin AC, Halotussin AC	cough, expectorant
Codeine Phosphate/Promethazine HCl	Promethazine with Codeine	allergy; congestion, nasal; cough
Colchicine	Colcrys	gout
Cyanocobalamin	**Nascobal**	AIDS adjunct, anemia, vitamin/mineral supplements
Cyclobenzaprine HCl	**Amrix**, Flexeril	muscle spasm, musculoskeletal conditions, pain
Dexamethasone Oral	Dexamethasone (generic)	allergy, arthritis, dermatitis, diagnostic aid, edema, meningitis, tuberculosis
Dexamethasone/Tobramycin Ophthalmic	TobraDex	infections, bacterial/ophthalmic; inflammation, ophthalmic
Dextromethorphan Hydrobromide/ Promethazine HCl	Promethazine DM	allergy; congestion, nasal; cough
Diazepam	Diazepam Injection, Diastat, Valium	Diazepam Injection: alcohol withdrawal management, anxiety, muscle spasm, seizures, surgical adjunct/aid. Diastat: seizures. Valium: alcohol withdrawal management, anxiety, muscle spasm, seizures.
Diclofenac Sodium SR	Voltaren-XR	ankylosing spondylitis; osteoarthritis; rheumatoid arthritis
Dicyclomine HCl	Bentyl	irritable bowel syndrome
Digoxin	**Lanoxin**	arrhythmia, heart failure
Diltiazem HCl	Cardizem, Diltiazem Injection	Cardizem: angina. Diltiazem Injection: arrhythmia.
Diltiazem HCl CD	Cardizem CD	angina, hypertension
Diltiazem HCl SR	**Cardizem LA**, Cardizem SR, Dilacor XR, Diltia XT, Taztia XT, Tiazac	Cardizem LA, Dilacor XR, Diltia XT, Taztia XT, Tiazac: angina, hypertension. Cardizem SR: hypertension.
Diphenhydramine HCl Tablets	Benadryl Allergy, Simply Sleep Caplets	Benadryl Allergy: allergy. Simply Sleep Caplets: insomnia.
Divalproex Sodium	Depakote, **Depakote ER**	bipolar disorder, mania, migraine/tension headache, seizures
Dorzolamide HCl/Timolol Maleate	**Cosopt**	glaucoma/IOP
Doxazosin Mesylate	Cardura, Cardura XL	Cardura: benign prostatic hypertrophy, hypertension. Cardura XL: benign prostatic hypertrophy.
Doxepin HCl	Doxepin HCl (generic), Silenor, Zonalon	Doxepin HCl (generic): anxiety, depression. Silenor: insomnia. Zonalon: dermatitis; inflammation, topical; pruritus, topical.
Doxycycline	Oracea	rosacea
Doxycycline Calcium	Vibramycin	acne; actinomycosis; anthrax; bartonellosis; brucellosis; chancroid; chlorea; conjunctivitis; gonorrhea; infections (bacterial/ophthalmic, bacterial/respiratory tract, bacterial/skin, gynecological, intra-abdominal, urinary tract); listeriosis; malaria; plague; psittacosis; Rocky Mountain spotted fever; syphilis; trachoma; tularemia; typhus; urethritis; yaws
Doxycycline Hyclate	Doryx, Doxycycline IV, Periostat, Vibramycin, Vibra-Tabs	Doryx: acne; anthrax; conjunctivitis; infections (bacterial/endocervical, bacterial/ophthalmic, bacterial/rectal, bacterial/respiratory tract, bacterial/skin, bacterial/systemic, gynecological, intra-abdominal, urinary tract); malaria; syphilis; urethritis; yaws. Doxycycline IV: anthrax; gonorrhea; infections (bacterial/ophthalmic, bacterial/respiratory tract, bacterial/systemic, gynecological, intra-abdominal, urinary tract); syphilis. Periostat: periodontitis. Vibramycin, Vibra-Tabs: acne; actinomycosis; anthrax; bartonellosis; brucellosis; chancroid; chlorea; conjunctivitis; gonorrhea; infections (bacterial/ophthalmic, bacterial/respiratory tract, bacterial/skin, gynecological, intra-abdominal, urinary tract); listeriosis; malaria; plague; psittacosis; Rocky Mountain spotted fever; syphilis; trachoma; tularemia; typhus; urethritis; yaws.

Please go to **PDR.net** to view prescribing information for these and other products.

GENERIC	BRAND(S)	INDICATION(S)
Doxycycline Monohydrate	Adoxa, Monodox, Vibramycin	Adoxa: acne; actinomycosis; bartonellosis; brucellosis; chancroid; cholera; conjunctivitis; gonorrhea; infections (bacterial/skin, bacterial/respiratory tract, urinary tract); listeriosis; plague; psittacosis; Rocky Mountain spotted fever; syphilis; trachoma; tularemia; typhus; urethritis; yaws. Monodox: acne; anthrax; gonorrhea; infections (bacterial/ophthalmic, bacterial/respiratory tract, bacterial/skin, gynecological, intra-abdominal, urinary tract); syphilis. Vibramycin: acne; actinomycosis; anthrax; bartonellosis; brucellosis; chancroid; chlorea; conjunctivitis; gonorrhea; infections (bacterial/ophthalmic, bacterial/respiratory tract, bacterial/skin, gynecological, intra-abdominal, urinary tract); listeriosis; malaria; plague; psittacosis; Rocky Mountain spotted fever; syphilis; trachoma; tularemia; typhus; urethritis; yaws.
Enalapril Maleate	Vasotec	heart failure, hypertension
Erythromycin Ophthalmic	Erythromycin Ophthalmic (generic)	infections, bacterial/ophthalmic
Estradiol Oral	Estrace, Estradiol Tablets	cancer, breast; cancer, prostate; hypoestrogenism; menopause; osteoporosis; atrophic vaginitis
Estradiol Acetate Oral	Femtrace	menopause
Ethinyl Estradiol/Ferrous Fumarate/Norethindrone Acetate	Gildess Fe 1/20, Junel Fe 1/20, Loestrin Fe 1/20, Microgestin Fe 1/20	contraception
Ethinyl Estradiol/Norgestimate	Ortho Tri-Cyclen, Tri-Previfem, Tri-Sprintec, Trinessa	acne, contraception
Etodolac	Etodolac (generic), Etodolac ER	Etodolac (generic): osteoarthritis; rheumatoid arthritis; pain. Etodolac ER: osteoarthritis; rheumatoid arthritis.
Famotidine	**Pepcid**, Pepcid AC, Pepcid Complete, Pepcid Oral Suspension	Pepcid, Pepcid Oral Suspension: erosive esophagitis; GERD; hypersecretory conditions; ulcer, GI; Zollinger-Ellison syndrome. Pepcid AC, Pepcid Complete: GERD, heartburn.
Felodipine ER	Plendil	hypertension
Fenofibrate	Antara, Fenoglide, Lipofen, Lofibra, **Tricor**, Triglide	hypercholesterolemia, hyperlipidemia, hypertriglyceridemia
Fentanyl Transdermal	**Duragesic**	pain
Ferrous Sulfate	Feosol (Ferrous Sulfate-Iron Carbonyl)	anemia, iron deficiency
Fexofenadine HCl	**Allegra**	allergy, rhinitis, urticaria
Finasteride	**Propecia, Proscar**	Propecia: alopecia. Proscar: benign prostatic hypertrophy.
Fluconazole	Diflucan	bone marrow transplant; candidemia; candidiasis (esophageal, oropharyngeal, vaginal); infections (fungal/systemic, fungal/vaginal, gynecological, urinary tract); meningitis; peritonitis; pneumonia, fungal
Fluocinonide	Fluocinonide, Fluocinonide-E, **Vanos**	dermatitis; inflammation, topical; pruritus, topical; psoriasis
Fluocinonide Acetonide	Capex, Derma-Smoothe/FS, Fluocinolone Acetonide, Retisert	Capex: dermatitis, seborrheic. Derma-Smoothe/FS: dermatitis, atopic; psoriasis. Fluocinolone Acetonide: dermatitis; inflammation, topical; pruritus, topical; psoriasis.
Fluoxetine HCl	**Prozac, Prozac Weekly**, Sarafem	Prozac: bipolar disorder (in combination with olanzapine), bulimia, major depressive disorder, obsessive-compulsive disorder, panic disorder. Prozac Weekly: major depressive disorder. Sarafem: premenstrual dysphoric disorder.
Fluticasone Furoate Nasal	**Veramyst**	allergy, rhinitis
Fluticasone Propionate Nasal	**Flonase**	allergy, rhinitis
Folic Acid	Folic Acid (generic)	anemia; anemia, megaloblastic
Fosinopril Sodium	Monopril	congestive heart failure, hypertension
Furosemide Oral	Lasix	congestive heart failure, edema, hypertension
Gabapentin	Neurontin	pain, neuropathic; seizures
Gemfibrozil	Lopid	coronary artery disease, hypercholesterolemia, hyperlipidemia, hypertriglyceridemia
Glimepiride	Amaryl	diabetes
Glipizide	Glucotrol	diabetes
Glipizide ER	Glucotrol XL	diabetes
Glyburide	DiaBeta, Glynase PresTab, Micronase	diabetes
Glyburide/Metformin HCl	Glucovance	diabetes
Haloperidol	Haloperidol (generic)	behavioral problems, psychosis, schizophrenia, Tourette's disorder
Haloperidol Decanoate	Haldol Decanoate, Haldol Injection	psychosis, schizophrenia

Please go to **PDR.net** to view prescribing information for these and other products.

GENERIC	BRAND(S)	INDICATION(S)
Haloperidol Lactate	Haldol, Haloperidol Lactate (generic)	psychosis, schizophrenia
Hydralazine HCl	Hydralazine HCl (generic)	hypertension
Hydrochlorothiazide	Microzide	hypertension
Hydrochlorothiazide/Lisinopril	**Prinzide**, Zestoretic	hypertension
Hydrochlorothiazide/Triamterene	**Dyazide**, Maxzide, Maxzide-25	edema, hypertension
Hydrocodone Bitartrate/Ibuprofen	Reprexain, **Vicoprofen**	pain
Hydrocortisone/Neomycin Sulfate/Polymyxin B Sulfate	Neomycin/Polymyxin B/Hydrocortisone Otic, Pediotic	infections, otic; otitis externa
Hydrocortisone Topical Rx	Anusol-HC Cream, Colocort, Hytone 1%, Hytone 2.5%, Proctocream HC, Proctosol HC, Proctozone-HC	Anusol-HC Cream, Proctocream HC, Proctosol HC, Proctozone-HC: dermatitis; inflammation, topical; pruritus, topical; psoriasis. Hytone 1%: bites; dermatitis, seborrheic; eczema; inflammation, topical; pruritus, topical; psoriasis. Hytone 2.5%: dermatitis; inflammation, topical; pruritus, topical. Colocort: colitis, ulcerative; proctitis.
Hydrocortisone Acetate Topical Rx	Alacort, Anucort HC, Anusol-HC Suppository, Cortifoam, Hemorrhoidal HC, Proctocort Suppository, Tucks Hydrocortisone Anti-Itch Ointment	Alacort: dermatitis; inflammation, topical; pruritus, topical. Anucort HC, Anusol-HC Suppository, Hemorrhoidal HC, Proctocort Suppository: colitis, ulcerative; hemorrhoids; inflammation, topical; proctitis; pruritus, topical. Cortifoam: proctitis.
Hydrocortisone Butyrate Topical Rx	Locoid	dermatitis; dermatitis, seborrheic; inflammation, topical; pruritus, topical; psoriasis
Hydrocortisone Probutate Topical Rx	Pandel	dermatitis; inflammation, topical; pruritus, topical; psoriasis
Hydrocortisone Valerate Topical Rx	Westcort	dermatitis; inflammation, topical; pruritus, topical; psoriasis
Hydromorphone HCl	**Dilaudid**, **Dilaudid-HP**, Exalgo, Palladone	pain
Hydroxychloroquine Sulfate	Plaquenil	rheumatoid arthritis; lupus erythematosus; malaria
Hydroxyzine HCl	Hydroxyzine HCl (generic)	allergy; anxiety; pruritus, topical; sedation, preoperative
Hydroxyzine Pamoate	Hydroxyzine Pamoate (generic), Vistaril	allergy; anxiety; pruritus, topical; sedation; sedation, preoperative
Ibuprofen	Advil Migraine, **Caldolor**, Motrin, Motrin (Children's, Infant's, Junior's), Motrin IB, Motrin Migraine, **Neoprofen**, Nuprin	Advil Migraine, Motrin Migraine: migraine/tension headache. Caldolor: fever, pain. Motrin (Children's, Infant's, Junior's): fever, influenza, pain. Motrin, Motrin IB: osteoarthritis; rheumatoid arthritis; dysmenorrhea; fever; pain. Neoprofen: ductus arteriosus. Nuprin: arthritis, fever, pain.
Ibuprofen Liquid	Motrin, Motrin (Children's, Infant's, Junior's)	Motrin: osteoarthritis; rheumatoid arthritis; dysmenorrhea; fever; pain. Motrin (Children's, Infant's, Junior's): fever, influenza, pain.
Indomethacin	Indomethacin (generic), Indocin	ankylosing spondylitis, arthritis, bursitis, gout, pain, tendinitis
Indomethacin Sodium Trihydrate	Indocin I.V.	ductus arteriosis
Isosorbide Mononitrate	Imdur, Ismo, Monoket	angina
Ketoconazole Topical	**Extina**, Ketoconazole Topical, Nizoral A-D, Nizoral Shampoo, **Xolegel**	Extina, Xolegel: dermatitis, seborrheic. Ketoconazole Topical: athlete's foot; dandruff; dermatitis, seborrheic; infections, fungal/topical. Nizoral A-D: dandruff; dermatitis, seborrheic. Nizoral Shampoo: dandruff; dermatitis, seborrheic; infections, fungal/topical.
Labetalol HCl	Labetalol HCl (generic), Trandate	hypertension
Lactulose	Constulose, Enulose, Generlac, **Kristalose**, Lactulose (generic)	constipation
Lamotrigine	**Lamictal**, **Lamictal CD**, **Lamictal ODT**, **Lamictal XR**	Lamictal, Lamictal CD, Lamictal ODT: bipolar disorder, seizures. Lamictal XR: seizures.
Levetiracetam	Keppra, **Keppra XR**	seizures
Levothyroxine Sodium	Levothroid, **Levoxyl**, **Synthroid**, Unithroid	Levothroid: cancer, thyroid; diagnostic aid; goiter; hypothyroidism; surgical adjunct/aid; thyrotoxicosis; TSH suppression. Levoxyl, Synthroid, Unithroid: cancer, thyroid; goiter; hypothyroidism; surgical adjunct/aid; TSH suppression.
Lisinopril	**Prinivil**, Zestril	heart failure; hypertension; myocardial infarction postmanagement
Lithium Carbonate	Lithium Carbonate (generic), Lithobid	bipolar disorder, mania
Lorazepam	Ativan, Ativan Injection	Ativan: anxiety, depression. Ativan Injection: anesthesia, adjunct; seizures.

Please go to **PDR.net** to view prescribing information for these and other products.

GENERIC	BRAND(S)	INDICATION(S)
Lovastatin	Altoprev, **Mevacor**	Altoprev: angina—reduce risk; coronary artery disease; hypercholesterolemia; hyperlipidemia; hypertriglyceridemia; myocardial infarction—reduce risk; revascularization—reduce risk. Mevacor: angina—reduce risk; coronary artery disease; hypercholesterolemia; hyperlipidemia; myocardial infarction—reduce risk; revascularization—reduce risk.
Meclizine HCl	Antivert, Dramamine Less Drowsy Tablets	Antivert: motion sickness, nausea, vertigo, vomiting. Dramamine Less Drowsy Tablets: motion sickness, nausea, vomiting.
Medroxyprogesterone Acetate Injection	Depo-Provera, Depo-Provera Contraceptive, Depo-SubQ Provera 104	Depo-Provera: cancer, endometrial; cancer, renal. Depo-Provera Contraceptive: contraception. Depo-SubQ Provera 104: contraception, endometriosis.
Medroxyprogesterone Acetate Tablet	Provera	amenorrhea; endometrial hyperplasia; uterine bleeding, abnormal
Meloxicam	Mobic	osteoarthritis; rheumatoid arthritis
Metformin HCl	Glucophage, Riomet	diabetes
Metformin HCl ER	Fortamet, Glumetza, Glucophage XR	diabetes
Methadone HCl Non-Injectable	Dolophine, Methadone (generic), Methadose	detoxification, methadone maintenance, pain
Methocarbamol	Robaxin, Robaxin Injection, Robaxin-750	musculoskeletal conditions, pain
Methotrexate	Methotrexate (generic), Rheumatrex	arthritis; cancer (bone, breast, head and neck, lung); leukemia; lymphoma; psoriasis
Methylphenidate	Daytrana	ADHD
Methylphenidate HCl	**Concerta**, **Metadate CD**, Metadate ER, Methylin, Methylin ER, Ritalin, Ritalin LA, Ritalin SR	Concerta, Metadate CD, Ritalin LA: ADHD. Metadate ER, Methylin, Methylin ER, Ritalin, Ritalin SR: ADHD, narcolepsy.
Methylprednisolone Tablets	Medrol, Medrol Dosepak	allergy; arthritis; arthritis, gouty; osteoarthritis; rheumatoid arthritis; bursitis; colitis, ulcerative; dermatitis; edema; meningitis; trichinosis; tuberculosis
Metoclopramide	Metoclopramide (generic), **Metozolv ODT**, Reglan, Reglan Injection	chemotherapy adjunct, diagnostic aid, gastroparesis, GERD, nausea, vomiting
Metolazone	Zaroxolyn	congestive heart failure, edema, hypertension
Metoprolol Succinate	**Toprol-XL**	angina, heart failure, hypertension
Metoprolol Tartrate	Lopressor	angina, hypertension, myocardial infarction
Metronidazole Tablets	Flagyl, Flagyl ER	Flagyl: cervicitis; endocarditis; infections (bacterial/bone, bacterial/endocervical, bacterial/respiratory tract, bacterial/skin, bacterial/systemic, gynecological, intra-abdominal, urinary tract); meningitis; peritonitis; pneumonia, bacterial; septicemia; vaginosis, bacterial. Flagyl ER: bacterial vaginosis.
Minocycline HCl	Arestin, Dynacin, Minocin, **Solodyn**	Arestin: periodontitis. Dynacin: acne; anthrax; bartonellosis; brucellosis; chancroid; cholera; conjunctivitis; gonorrhea; infections (bacterial/endocervical, bacterial/rectal, bacterial/respiratory tract, bacterial/skin, gynecological, urinary tract); listeriosis; meningitis; plague; psittacosis; Rocky Mountain spotted fever; syphilis; trachoma; tularemia; typhus; urethritis; yaws. Minocin: acne; anthrax; bartonellosis; brucellosis; chancroid; cholera; conjunctivitis; gonorrhea; infections (bacterial/respiratory tract, bacterial/skin, bacterial/endocervical, gynecological, bacterial/rectal, urinary tract); listeriosis; meningitis; plague; psittacosis; Rocky Mountain spotted fever; syphilis; trachoma; tularemia; typhus; urethritis; yaws. Solodyn: acne.
Mirtazapine	**Remeron, RemeronSolTab**	depression, major depressive disorder
Mometasone Furoate Topical	**Elocon**	dermatitis; inflammation, topical; pruritus, topical
Morphine Sulfate ER	**Avinza**, Kadian, MS Contin, Oramorph SR	pain
Mupirocin	**Bactroban**	impetigo; infections, bacterial/skin
Mupirocin Calcium	**Bactroban Nasal**	infections, bacterial/skin
Nabumetone	Nabumetone (generic)	osteoarthritis; rheumatoid arthritis
Nadolol	**Corgard, Nadolol (generic)**	angina, hypertension
Naproxen	Naprosyn, EC-Naprosyn	Naprosyn: ankylosing spondylitis; osteoarthritis; rheumatoid arthritis; bursitis; dysmenorrhea; gout; pain; tendinitis. EC-Naprosyn: ankylosing spondylitis; osteoarthritis; rheumatoid arthritis.
Naproxen Sodium	Aleve, Anaprox, Anaprox DS, Naprelan	Aleve: arthritis, fever, pain. Anaprox, Anaprox DS, Naprelan: ankylosing spondylitis; osteoarthritis; rheumatoid arthritis; bursitis; dysmenorrhea; gout; pain; tendinitis.
Nifedipine XL	Procardia XL	angina, hypertension

GENERIC/BRAND CROSS-REFERENCE TABLE

Please go to **PDR.net** to view prescribing information for these and other products.

GENERIC	BRAND(S)	INDICATION(S)
Nifedipine	Adalat, Nifedipine (generic), Procardia	angina
Nifedipine ER	Adalat CC, Afeditab CR	hypertension
Nitrofurantoin Macrocrystals	Macrodantin	infections, urinary tract
Nitrofurantoin Monohydrate	Macrobid	infections, urinary tract
Nitroglycerin	Minitran, Nitrek, Nitro-Bid, **Nitro-Dur**, Nitrolingual Spray, NitroMist, Nitroquick, Nitrostat	angina
Nortriptyline HCl	Pamelor	depression
Nystatin Systemic	Nystatin Oral	candidiasis, oropharyngeal
Nystatin Topical	Nystatin Topical, Nystop	infections, fungal/topical
Nystatin/Triamcinolone Acetonide	Nystatin/Triamcinolone Acetonide (generic)	infections, fungal/topical
Omeprazole Magnesium	Prilosec, Prilosec OTC	Prilosec: erosive esophagitis; GERD; *H. pylori* eradication; hypersecretory conditions; ulcer, gastrointestinal; Zollinger-Ellison syndrome. Prilosec OTC: heartburn.
Ondansetron	**Zuplenz**	chemotherapy adjunct, nausea, radiotherapy adjunct, vomiting
Ondansetron HCl	**Zofran**	chemotherapy adjunct, nausea, radiotherapy adjunct, vomiting
Ondansetron HCl ODT	**Zofran ODT**	chemotherapy adjunct, nausea, vomiting
Oxcarbazepine	Trileptal	seizures
Oxybutynin Chloride	Ditropan, Gelnique	bladder, overactive; urinary incontinence
Oxybutynin Chloride ER	Ditropan XL	bladder, overactive; urinary incontinence
Pantoprazole Sodium	Protonix, Protonix IV	erosive esophagitis, GERD, heartburn, hypersecretory conditions, Zollinger-Ellison syndrome
Paroxetine HCl	**Paxil, Paxil CR**	Paxil: anxiety, major depressive disorder, obsessive-compulsive disorder; panic disorder; posttraumatic stress disorder. Paxil CR: anxiety, major depressive disorder, panic disorder, premenstrual dysphoric disorder.
Paroxetine Mesylate	Pexeva	anxiety, depression, major depressive disorder, obsessive-compulsive disorder, panic disorder
Penicillin V Potassium	Penicillin VK (generic), Veetids	infections (bacterial/respiratory tract, bacterial/skin, bacterial/systemic)
Phenobarbital	Phenobarbital (generic)	anxiety, insomnia, seizures
Phentermine HCl	**Adipex-P**, Phentermine HCl (generic)	obesity
Phenytoin Sodium ER	Dilantin, Dilantin Kapseals, **Phenytek**	seizures
Piroxicam	Feldene	osteoarthritis; rheumatoid arthritis
Polyethylene Glycol	MiraLax	constipation
Polymyxin B Sulfate/Trimethoprim Sulfate	Polytrim	conjunctivitis; infections, bacterial/ophthalmic
Potassium Chloride	K-Lor, K-Lyte/CL, K-Lyte/CL 50	K-Lor: digitalis toxicity, hypokalemia. K-Lyte/CL, K-Lyte/CL 50: digitalis toxicity, hypochloremia, hypokalemia.
Potassium Chloride ER	**Klor-Con, Klor-Con M**, Klotrix, K-Dur, K-Tab, Micro-K	digitalis toxicity, hypokalemia
Pravastatin Sodium	Pravachol	coronary artery disease; hypercholesterolemia; hyperlipidemia; hypertriglyceridemia; myocardial infarction—reduce risk; revascularization—reduce risk; stroke—reduce risk; TIA—reduce risk
Prednisolone Sodium Phosphate Oral	Orapred, **Orapred ODT**, Pediapred	Orapred, Orapred ODT: AIDS adjunct, allergy, arthritis, asthma, bursitis, dermatitis, edema, meningitis, multiple sclerosis, tuberculosis. Pediapred: AIDS adjunct; allergy; anemia; arthritis; asthma; bursitis; colitis, ulcerative; dermatitis; edema; leukemia; meningitis; multiple sclerosis; tuberculosis.
Prednisolone Acetate Ophthalmic	Pred Forte, Pred Mild	Pred Mild: inflammation, ophthalmic. Pred Forte: conjunctivitis; inflammation, ophthalmic.
Prednisone Oral	Prednisone	allergy, arthritis, dermatitis, edema, meningitis, tuberculosis
Prochlorperazine Maleate	Prochlorperazine (generic)	anxiety, nausea, psychosis, schizophrenia, vomiting
Promethazine HCl Tablets	Phenergan, Promethazine HCl (generic)	allergy; anaphylaxis; conjunctivitis; motion sickness; nausea; pain; rhinitis; sedation; sedation, preoperative; urticaria; vomiting
Propranolol HCl	Inderal, Inderal XL, **Innopran XL**	Inderal: angina; arrhythmia; hypertension; hypertrophic subaortic stenosis; migraine/tension headache; myocardial infarction postmanagement; pheochromocytoma; tremor. Inderal XL: angina, hypertension, hypertrophic subaortic stenosis, migraine/tension headache. Innopran XL: hypertension.
Quinapril HCl	Accupril	heart failure, hypertension

Please go to **PDR.net** to view prescribing information for these and other products.

GENERIC/BRAND CROSS-REFERENCE TABLE

GENERIC	BRAND(S)	INDICATION(S)
Ramipril	**Altace**	congestive heart failure; hypertension; myocardial infarction postmanagement; myocardial infarction—reduce risk; stroke—reduce risk
Ranitidine HCl	**Zantac**, Zantac OTC, Zantac 75, **Zantac 150**	Zantac: erosive esophagitis; GERD; hypersecretory conditions; ulcer, GI; Zollinger-Ellison syndrome. Zantac OTC, Zantac 75, Zantac 150: heartburn.
Risperidone	Risperdal, **Risperdal Consta**, Risperdal M-Tab	Risperdal, Risperdal M-Tab: autistic disorder, irritability; bipolar disorder; mania; psychosis; schizophrenia. Risperdal Consta: bipolar disorder, psychosis, schizophrenia.
Ropinirole HCl	**Requip, Requip XL**	Requip: Parkinson's disease, restless legs syndrome (RLS). Requip XL: Parkinson's disease.
Sertraline HCl	Zoloft	anxiety, depression, obsessive-compulsive disorder, major depressive disorder, panic disorder, posttraumatic stress disorder, premenstrual dysphoric disorder
Simvastatin	**Zocor**	coronary artery disease; hypercholesterolemia; hyperlipidemia; hypertriglyceridemia; myocardial infarction—reduce risk; revascularization—reduce risk; stroke—reduce risk
Sodium Fluoride	Luride, PreviDent, PreviDent 5000 Plus	dental caries, fluoride supplement
Sotalol HCl	Betapace, Betapace AF	arrhythmia
Spironolactone	Aldactone	congestive heart failure, edema, hyperaldosteronism, hypertension, hypokalemia
Sucralfate	**Carafate**	ulcer, GI
Sumatriptan Succinate Oral	**Imitrex**	migraine/tension headache
Tamoxifen Citrate	Soltamox, Tamoxifen Citrate (generic)	cancer, breast
Temazepam	Restoril	insomnia
Terazosin HCl	Terazosin HCl (generic)	benign prostatic hypertrophy, hypertension
Terbinafine HCl	Lamisil, Lamisil AT	Lamisil: infections, fungal/topical; onychomycosis. Lamisil AT: athlete's foot; infections, fungal/topical.
Terconazole	Terazol 3, Terazol 7, Zazole	candidiasis, vaginal; infections (fungal/vaginal, gynecological)
Tetracycline HCl	Sumycin	acne; anthrax; brucellosis; chancroid; cholera; gonorrhea; infections (bacterial/endocervical, bacterial/ophthalmic, bacterial/rectal, bacterial/respiratory tract, bacterial/skin, gynecological, intra-abdominal, urinary tract); listeriosis; plague; psittacosis; syphilis; trachoma; urethritis
Theophylline SR	Theo-24, Uniphyl	asthma, bronchitis, emphysema
Timolol Maleate Ophthalmic	Istalol, Timolol GFS, Timoptic, Timoptic in Ocudose, Timoptic-XE	glaucoma/IOP
Tizanidine HCl	Zanaflex	muscle spasm
Topiramate	Topamax, Topamax Sprinkle Capsules	migraine/tension headache, seizures
Torsemide	Demadex	congestive heart failure, edema, hypertension
Tramadol HCl	Rybix ODT, **Ryzolt**, Ultram, Ultram ER	pain
Trazodone HCl	**Oleptro**	major depressive disorder
Tretinoin	Atralin, Avita, Renova, Retin-A, Retin-A Micro	Atralin, Avita, Retin-A, Retin-A Micro: acne. Renova: hyperpigmentation; wrinkles, facial.
Triamcinolone Acetonide Topical	Kenalog	Kenalog: dermatitis; inflammation, topical; pruritus, topical; psoriasis
Triazolam	Halcion	insomnia
Sulfamethoxazole/Trimethoprim	Bactrim, Bactrim DS, Septra, Septra DS, Sulfatrim Pediatric	Bactrim, Bactrim DS, Septra, Septra DS, Sulfatrim Pediatric: AIDS adjunct; bronchitis; diarrhea; infections (bacterial/respiratory tract, intra-abdominal, otic, urinary tract); otitis media; *pneumocystis carinii* pneumonia.
Venlafaxine HCl	Effexor, Effexor ER	Effexor: depression, major depressive disorder. Effexor ER: anxiety, depression, major depressive disorder, panic disorder.
Verapamil HCl SR	Calan SR, Covera-HS, Isoptin SR, Verelan, Verelan PM	Calan SR, Isoptin SR, Verelan, Verelan PM: hypertension. Covera-HS: angina, hypertension.
Warfarin Sodium	Coumadin, Jantoven	myocardial infarction postmanagement; myocardial infarction—reduce risk; pulmonary embolism; stroke—reduce risk; thrombosis prevention
Zolpidem Tartrate	**Ambien, Ambien CR**, Edluar, Zolpimist	insomnia

GENERIC/BRAND CROSS-REFERENCE TABLE

Please go to **PDR.net** to view prescribing information for these and other products.

SECTION 3

PRODUCT CATEGORY INDEX

This index lists products by prescribing category, allowing you to quickly and easily identify all agents with a given therapeutic use or mechanism of action. Categories are based on the latest medical terminology and are comprehensively cross-referenced. Included are all fully described products in the Product Information section of PDR®.

If an entry in the index lists multiple page numbers, the first ones shown refer to photographs of the product, the last one to its prescribing information.

A

ACE INHIBITORS
(see under:
CARDIOVASCULAR AGENTS
ANGIOTENSIN CONVERTING ENZYME
(ACE) INHIBITORS
ANGIOTENSIN CONVERTING ENZYME
(ACE) INHIBITORS WITH CALCIUM
CHANNEL BLOCKERS
ANGIOTENSIN CONVERTING ENZYME
(ACE) INHIBITORS WITH DIURETICS)

ACETYLCHOLINE AGONISTS
Chantix Tablets (Pfizer) 2788

ACNE PREPARATIONS
(see under:
**SKIN & MUCOUS MEMBRANE
AGENTS**
ACNE PREPARATIONS)

**ACQUIRED IMMUNE
DEFICIENCY SYNDROME
THERAPY**
(see under:
**AIDS/HIV ADJUNCT AGENTS
ANTI-INFECTIVE AGENTS,
SYSTEMIC**
AIDS ADJUNCT ANTI-INFECTIVES
AIDS CHEMOTHERAPEUTIC AGENTS)

ACROMEGALY AGENTS
Sandostatin Injection (Novartis) 315, 2576
Sandostatin LAR Depot (Novartis) .. 316, 2578

AIDS THERAPY
(see under:
**AIDS/HIV ADJUNCT AGENTS
ANTI-INFECTIVE AGENTS,
SYSTEMIC**
AIDS ADJUNCT ANTI-INFECTIVES
AIDS CHEMOTHERAPEUTIC AGENTS)

AIDS/HIV ADJUNCT AGENTS
(see also under:
**ANTI-INFECTIVE AGENTS,
SYSTEMIC**
AIDS ADJUNCT ANTI-INFECTIVES)
Epogen for Injection (Amgen) 305, 646
Intron A for Injection (Merck) 313, 2108
Megace ES Oral Suspension (Par) 2756
Orapred ODT Orally Disintegrating Tablets
(Shionogi) 3088
Procrit for Injection (Centocor Ortho
Biotech) 307, 943
Serostim for Injection (EMD Serono) 1075

ALPHA ADRENERGIC AGONISTS
(see under:
OPHTHALMIC PREPARATIONS
SYMPATHOMIMETICS & COMBINATIONS)

ALTERNATIVE MEDICINE
(see under:
HOMEOPATHIC REMEDIES)

**ALZHEIMER'S DISEASE
MANAGEMENT**
Aricept Tablets (Eisai) 308, 1004
Aricept ODT Tablets (Eisai) 308, 1004
Exelon Capsules (Novartis) 315, 2484
Exelon Oral Solution (Novartis) 2484
Exelon Patch (Novartis) 315, 2489
Namenda Oral Solution (Forest) 309, 1137
Namenda Tablets (Forest) 309, 1137

AMEBICIDES
(see under:
**ANTI-INFECTIVE AGENTS,
SYSTEMIC**
AMEBICIDES)

AMINO ACIDS
(see under:
DIETARY SUPPLEMENTS
AMINO ACIDS & COMBINATIONS)

AMPHETAMINES
(see under:
**CENTRAL NERVOUS SYSTEM
STIMULANTS**
AMPHETAMINES)

**AMYOTROPHIC LATERAL
SCLEROSIS THERAPEUTIC
AGENTS**
Rilutek Tablets (sanofi-aventis) 319, 3047

ANALEPTIC AGENTS
(see under:
**CENTRAL NERVOUS SYSTEM
STIMULANTS)**

ANALGESICS
(see also under:
**GOUT PREPARATIONS
MIGRAINE PREPARATIONS
MUSCLE RELAXANTS**
SKELETAL MUSCLE RELAXANTS &
COMBINATIONS
**SKIN & MUCOUS MEMBRANE
AGENTS**
ANALGESICS & COMBINATIONS
ANESTHETICS & COMBINATIONS)
**ACETAMINOPHEN &
COMBINATIONS**
(see also under:
**ANTIHISTAMINES &
COMBINATIONS**
RESPIRATORY AGENTS
DECONGESTANTS & COMBINATIONS)
Percocet Tablets (Endo) 309, 1096
Regular Strength Tylenol Tablets (McNeil
Consumer) 1910
Tylenol Arthritis Pain Extended Release
Gelcaps/Caplets (McNeil Consumer) .. 1910
Tylenol 8 Hour Extended Release Caplets
(McNeil Consumer) 1910
Extra Strength Tylenol Rapid Release Gels
(McNeil Consumer) 1910
Extra Strength Tylenol Caplets and EZ
Tabs (McNeil Consumer) 1910
Extra Strength Tylenol Adult Rapid Blast
Liquid (McNeil Consumer) 1910
Extra Strength Tylenol PM Caplets
(McNeil Consumer) 1910
Tylenol with Codeine Tablets
(Ortho-McNeil-Janssen) 317, 2750
Children's Tylenol Meltaways (McNeil
Consumer) 1908
Children's Tylenol Suspension Liquid
(McNeil Consumer) 1908
Concentrated Tylenol Infants' Drops
(McNeil Consumer) 1908
Jr. Tylenol Meltaways (McNeil Consumer). 1908
CENTRALLY ACTING ANALGESICS
Cymbalta Delayed-Release Capsules
(Lilly) 310, 1759
Lyrica Capsules (Pfizer) 2802
Lyrica Oral Solution (Pfizer) 2802
Nucynta Tablets
(Ortho-McNeil-Janssen) 317, 2720
Ryzolt Extended-Release Tablets
(Purdue Pharma) 317, 2886
**MISCELLANEOUS ANALGESIC
AGENTS**
Carbatrol Capsules (Shire US) 319, 3095
Hyalgan Solution (sanofi-aventis) ... 319, 2994
Sarapin Vials (High Chemical) 310, 1688

NARCOTICS
**NARCOTIC
AGONIST-ANTAGONIST &
COMBINATIONS**
Embeda Extended Release
Capsules (King) 310, 1716
NARCOTICS & COMBINATIONS
Avinza Capsules (King) 310, 1708
Butrans Transdermal System
(Purdue Pharma) 317, 2864
Dilaudid Injection (Purdue
Pharma) 317, 2876
Dilaudid Oral Liquid (Purdue
Pharma) 317, 2873
Dilaudid Tablets
(Purdue Pharma) 317, 2873
Dilaudid-HP Injection (Purdue
Pharma) 317, 2876
Dilaudid-HP Lyophilized Powder
250 mg (Purdue Pharma) ... 317, 2876
Duragesic Transdermal System
(Ortho-McNeil-Janssen) 316, 2684
Fentanyl Transdermal System Patches
(Mylan) 2403
Fentora Tablets (Cephalon) 308, 957
Opana Tablets (Endo) 308, 1085
Opana ER Tablets (Endo) 309, 1090
OxyContin Tablets (Purdue
Pharma) 317, 2879
Percocet Tablets (Endo) 309, 1096
Percodan Tablets (Endo) 309, 1099
Tylenol with Codeine Tablets
(Ortho-McNeil-Janssen) 317, 2750
Vicodin Tablets (Abbott) 304, 573
Vicodin ES Tablets (Abbott) 304, 575
Vicodin HP Tablets (Abbott) 304, 576
Vicoprofen Tablets (Abbott) 304, 578
Zydone Tablets (Endo) 309, 1113

**NONSTEROIDAL
ANTI-INFLAMMATORY DRUGS
(NSAIDS) & COMBINATIONS**
Caldolor Injection (Cumberland) 308, 989
Celebrex Capsules (Searle) 3072
Clinoril Tablets (Merck) 312, 1993
Flector Patch (King) 310, 1723
Motrin IB Tablets and Caplets (McNeil
Consumer) 1902
Children's Motrin Oral Suspension
(McNeil Consumer) 1903
Infants' Motrin Concentrated Drops
(McNeil Consumer) 1903
Junior Strength Motrin Caplets and
Chewable Tablets (McNeil Consumer) . 1903
Motrin PM Caplets (McNeil Consumer) ... 1904
Treximet Tablets (GlaxoSmithKline) 1578
Vimovo Delayed-Release Tablets
(AstraZeneca Pharmaceuticals) .. 306, 760

SALICYLATES
ASPIRIN & COMBINATIONS
Percodan Tablets (Endo) 309, 1099
St. Joseph 81 mg Aspirin Chewable and
Enteric Coated Tablets (McNeil
Consumer) 1905

ANEMIA PREPARATIONS
(see under:
BLOOD MODIFIERS
HEMATINICS)

ANESTHETICS
(see also under:
**SKIN & MUCOUS MEMBRANE
AGENTS**
ANESTHETICS & COMBINATIONS)

GENERAL ANESTHETICS
Suprane Volatile Liquid for Inhalation
(Baxter Anesthesia) 821
Ultane Volatile Liquid for Inhalation
(Abbott) 568
LOCAL ANESTHETICS
Lidoderm Patch (Endo) 308, 1084
MISCELLANEOUS ANESTHETICS
Lusedra Injection (Eisai) 308, 1030

**ANGIOTENSIN CONVERTING
ENZYME INHIBITORS**
(see under:
CARDIOVASCULAR AGENTS
ANGIOTENSIN CONVERTING ENZYME
(ACE) INHIBITORS
ANGIOTENSIN CONVERTING ENZYME
(ACE) INHIBITORS WITH CALCIUM
CHANNEL BLOCKERS
ANGIOTENSIN CONVERTING ENZYME
(ACE) INHIBITORS WITH DIURETICS)

**ANGIOTENSIN II RECEPTOR
ANTAGONISTS**
(see under:
CARDIOVASCULAR AGENTS
ANGIOTENSIN II RECEPTOR
ANTAGONISTS
ANGIOTENSIN II RECEPTOR
ANTAGONISTS WITH DIURETICS)

ANORETICS
(see under:
OBESITY MANAGEMENT)

ANOREXIANTS
(see under:
OBESITY MANAGEMENT)

ANTACIDS
(see under:
GASTROINTESTINAL AGENTS
ANTACIDS)

ANTHELMINTICS
(see under:
**ANTI-INFECTIVE AGENTS,
SYSTEMIC**
ANTHELMINTICS)

ANTIARTHRITICS
(see under:
ANALGESICS
NONSTEROIDAL ANTI-INFLAMMATORY
DRUGS (NSAIDS) & COMBINATIONS
SALICYLATES
**ANTIRHEUMATIC AGENTS
GOUT PREPARATIONS
HORMONES**
GLUCOCORTICOIDS
**SKIN & MUCOUS MEMBRANE
AGENTS**
ANALGESICS & COMBINATIONS)

ANTIBIOTICS
(see under:
**ANTI-INFECTIVE AGENTS,
SYSTEMIC**
ANTIBIOTICS
ANTINEOPLASTICS
ANTIBIOTICS
NASAL PREPARATIONS
ANTIBIOTICS & COMBINATIONS
OPHTHALMIC PREPARATIONS
ANTI-INFECTIVES
ANTIBIOTICS & COMBINATIONS
OTIC PREPARATIONS
ANTIBIOTIC & STEROID COMBINATIONS
**SKIN & MUCOUS MEMBRANE
AGENTS**
ANTI-INFECTIVES
ANTIBIOTICS & COMBINATIONS)

W

WART PREPARATIONS
(see under:
  **SKIN & MUCOUS MEMBRANE
  AGENTS**
    WART PREPARATIONS)

**WEIGHT CONTROL
PREPARATIONS**
(see under:
  OBESITY MANAGEMENT)

Key to Controlled Substances Categories

Products listed with the symbols shown below are subject to the Controlled Substances Act of 1970. These drugs are categorized according to their potential for abuse. The greater the potential, the more severe the limitations on their prescription.

CATEGORY   INTERPRETATION

Ⓒ II   **HIGH POTENTIAL FOR ABUSE.** Use may lead to severe physical or psychological dependence.

Ⓒ III   **SOME POTENTIAL FOR ABUSE.** Use may lead to low-to-moderate physical dependence or high psychological dependence.

Ⓒ IV   **LOW POTENTIAL FOR ABUSE.** Use may lead to limited physical or psychological dependence.

Ⓒ V   **SUBJECT TO STATE AND LOCAL REGULATION.** Abuse potential is low.

Key to FDA Use-in-Pregnancy Ratings

The U.S. Food and Drug Administration's use-in-pregnancy rating system weighs the degree to which available information has ruled out risk to the fetus against the drug's potential benefit to the patient. The ratings, and their interpretation, are as follows:

CATEGORY   INTERPRETATION

A   **CONTROLLED STUDIES SHOW NO RISK.** Adequate, well-controlled studies in pregnant women have failed to demonstrate a risk to the fetus in any trimester of pregnancy.

B   **NO EVIDENCE OF RISK IN HUMANS.** Adequate, well-controlled studies in pregnant women have not shown increased risk of fetal abnormalities despite adverse findings in animals, or, in the absence of adequate human studies, animal studies show no fetal risk. The chance of fetal harm is remote, but remains a possibility.

C   **RISK CANNOT BE RULED OUT.** Adequate, well-controlled human studies are lacking, and animal studies have shown a risk to the fetus or are lacking as well. There is a chance of fetal harm if the drug is administered during pregnancy, but the potential benefits may outweigh the potential risk.

D   **POSITIVE EVIDENCE OF RISK.** Studies in humans, or investigational or post-marketing data, have demonstrated fetal risk. Nevertheless, potential benefits from the use of the drug may outweigh the potential risk. For example, the drug may be acceptable if needed in a life-threatening situation or serious disease for which safer drugs cannot be used or are ineffective.

X   **CONTRAINDICATED IN PREGNANCY.** Studies in animals or humans, or investigational or post-marketing reports, have demonstrated positive evidence of fetal abnormalities or risk which clearly outweighs any possible benefit to the patient.

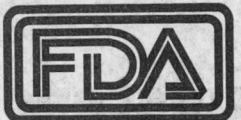

U.S. FOOD AND DRUG ADMINISTRATION

Medical Product Reporting Programs

MedWatch (24-hour service)... **800-332-1088**
Reporting of problems with drugs, devices, biologics (except vaccines), medical foods, and dietary supplements.

Vaccine Adverse Event Reporting System (24-hour service).................................. **800-822-7967**
Reporting of vaccine-related problems.

Mandatory Medical Device Reporting... **800-332-1088**
Reporting required from user facilities regarding device-related deaths and serious injuries.

Veterinary Adverse Drug Reaction Program... **888-332-8387**
Reporting of adverse drug events in animals.

Information for Health Professionals

Center for Drug Evaluation and Research Drug Information Hotline....................... **888-463-6332**
Information on human drugs including hormones.

Center for Biologics Office of Communications... **800-835-4709**
Information on biological products including vaccines and blood.

Center for Devices and Radiological Health... **800-638-2041**
Automated request for information on medical devices and radiation-emitting products.

Division of Drug Marketing, Advertising, and Communication (DDMAC)............... **301-796-1200**
Inquiries from health professionals regarding product promotion.

Emergency Operations... **866-300-4374**
Emergencies involving FDA-regulated products, tampering reports, and emergency Investigational New Drug requests.

Office of Orphan Products Development.. **800-300-7469**
Information on products for rare diseases.

General Information

General Consumer Inquiries.. **888-463-6332**
Consumer information on regulated products/issues.

Freedom of Information.. **301-827-6567**
Requests for publicly available FDA documents.

Office of Public Affairs.. **301-827-6250**
Interviews/press inquiries on FDA activities.

Center for Food Safety and Applied Nutrition.. **888-723-3366**
Information on food safety, seafood, dietary supplements, women's nutrition, and cosmetics.

Consumer Information Service, Center for Devices and Radiological Health......... **800-638-2041**
Information on medical devices, mammography facilities, and radiation-emitting products.

POISON CONTROL CENTERS

The American Association of Poison Control Centers (AAPCC) uses a single, nationwide **emergency** number to automatically link callers with their regional poison center. This toll-free number, **800-222-1222**, also works for **teletype lines (TTY)** for the hearing-impaired and **telecommunication devices (TTD)** for individuals who are deaf. However, a few local poison centers and the ASPCA/Animal Poison Control Center are not part of this nationwide system and continue to use separate numbers.

Most of the centers listed below are accredited by the AAPCC. **Certified centers are marked by an asterisk after the name.**

Each has to meet certain criteria. It must, for example, serve a large geographic area; it must be open 24 hours a day and provide direct-dial or toll-free access; it must be supervised by a medical director; and it must have registered pharmacists or nurses available to answer questions from the public.

Within each state, centers are listed alphabetically by city. Some state poison centers also list their original emergency numbers (including TTY/TDD) that only work within that state. For these listings, callers may use either the state number or the nationwide 800 number.

ALABAMA

BIRMINGHAM

Regional Poison Control Center (*)
Children's Health System

1600 7th Ave. South
Birmingham, AL 35233
Business: 205-939-9100
Emergency: 800-222-1222
www.chsys.org

TUSCALOOSA

Alabama Poison Center (*)

2503 Phoenix Dr.
Tuscaloosa, AL 35405
Business: 800-462-0800
Emergency: 800-222-1222
              800-462-0800 (AL)
www.alapoisoncenter.org

ALASKA

JUNEAU

Alaska Poison Control System
Section of Injury Prevention
and EMS

410 Willoughby Ave., Room 103
Box 110616
Juneau, AK 99811-0616
Business: 907-465-3027
Emergency: 800-222-1222
www.chems.alaska.gov

(PORTLAND, OR)

Oregon Poison Center (*)
Oregon Health and Science
University

3181 SW Sam Jackson Park Rd.
CB550
Portland, OR 97239
Business: 503-494-8600
Emergency: 800-222-1222
www.oregonpoison.com

ARIZONA

PHOENIX

Banner Poison Control Center (*)
Banner Good Samaritan
Medical Center

1111 E. McDowell Rd.
Phoenix, AZ 85006
Business: 602-839-2000
Emergency: 800-222-1222
www.bannerpoisoncontrol.com

TUCSON

Arizona Poison and Drug
Information Center (*)
Arizona Health Sciences Center

1295 N. Martin Ave.
PO Box 210202
Tucson, AZ 85721
Business: 520-626-7899
Emergency: 800-222-1222
www.pharmacy.arizona.edu/
outreach/poison

ARKANSAS

LITTLE ROCK

Arkansas Poison and Drug
Information Center (*)
College of Pharmacy - UAMS

4301 West Markham St.
Mail Slot 522-2
Little Rock, AR 72205-7122
Business: 501-686-5540
Emergency: 800-222-1222
              800-376-4766 (AR)
TDD/TTY: 800-641-3805

ASPCA/
ANIMAL POISON
CONTROL CENTER

1717 South Philo Rd.
Suite 36
Urbana, IL 61802
Business: 217-337-5030
Emergency: 888-426-4435
              800-548-2423
www.aspca.org/apcc

CALIFORNIA

FRESNO/MADERA

California Poison Control
System-Fresno/Madera Div. (*)
Children's Hospital Central
California

9300 Valley Children's Place, MB 15
Madera, CA 93636-8762
Business: 559-353-3000
Emergency: 800-222-1222
              800-876-4766 (CA)
TDD/TTY: 800-972-3323
www.calpoison.org

SACRAMENTO

California Poison Control
System-Sacramento Div. (*)
UC Davis Medical Center

2315 Stockton Blvd.
Sacramento, CA 95817
Business: 916-227-1400
Emergency: 800-222-1222
              800-876-4766 (CA)
TDD/TTY: 800-972-3323
www.calpoison.org

SAN DIEGO

California Poison Control
System-San Diego Div. (*)
UC San Diego Medical Center

200 West Arbor Dr.
San Diego, CA 92103-8925
Business: 858-715-6300
Emergency: 800-222-1222
              800-876-4766 (CA)
TDD/TTY: 800-972-3323
www.calpoison.org

SAN FRANCISCO

California Poison Control
System-San Francisco Div. (*)
University of California
San Francisco

Box 1369
San Francisco, CA 94143-1369
Business: 415-502-6000
Emergency: 800-222-1222
              800-876-4766 (CA)
TDD/TTY: 800-972-3323
www.calpoison.org

COLORADO

DENVER

Rocky Mountain Poison
and Drug Center (*)

777 Bannock St., Mail Code 0180
Denver, CO 80204-4507
Business: 303-389-1100
Emergency: 800-222-1222
TDD/TTY: 303-739-1127 (CO)
www.RMPDC.org

CONNECTICUT

FARMINGTON

**Connecticut Poison Control
Center (*)
University of Connecticut
Health Center**

263 Farmington Ave.
Farmington, CT 06030-5365
Business: 860-679-4540
Emergency: 800-222-1222
TDD/TTY: 866-218-5372
http://poisoncontrol.uchc.edu

DELAWARE

(PHILADELPHIA, PA)

**The Poison Control Center (*)
Children's Hospital of Philadelphia**

34th St. & Civic Center Blvd.
Philadelphia, PA 19104-4399
Business: 215-590-1000
Emergency: 800-222-1222
TDD/TTY: 215-590-8789
www.poisoncontrol.chop.edu

DISTRICT OF COLUMBIA

WASHINGTON, DC

National Capital Poison Center (*)

3201 New Mexico Ave., NW
Suite 310
Washington, DC 20016
Business: 202-362-3867
Emergency: 800-222-1222
www.poison.org

FLORIDA

JACKSONVILLE

**Florida Poison Information
Center-Jacksonville (*)**

655 West 8th St.
Box C23
Jacksonville, FL 32209
Business: 904-244-4465
Emergency: 800-222-1222
http://fpicjax.org

MIAMI

**Florida Poison Information
Center (*)
University of Miami,
Dept. of Pediatrics**

P.O. Box 016960 (R-131)
Miami, FL 33101
Business: 305-585-5250
Emergency: 800-222-1222
www.med.miami.edu/poisoncontrol

TAMPA

**Florida Poison Information
Center (*)
Tampa General Hospital**

P.O. Box 1289
Tampa, FL 33601-1289
Business: 813-844-7044
Emergency: 800-222-1222
www.poisoncentertampa.org

GEORGIA

ATLANTA

**Georgia Poison Center (*)
Hughes Spalding Children's
Hospital, Grady Health System**

80 Jesse Hill Jr. Dr., SE
P.O. Box 26066
Atlanta, GA 30303-3050
Business: 404-616-9237
Emergency: 800-222-1222
404-616-9000 (Atlanta)
TDD: 404-616-9287
www.georgiapoisoncenter.org

HAWAII

(DENVER, CO)

**Rocky Mountain Poison
and Drug Center (*)**

777 Bannock St., Mail Code 0180
Denver, CO 80204
Business: 303-389-1100
Emergency: 800-222-1222
TDD/TTY: 303-739-1127 (CO)
www.RMPDC.org

IDAHO

(DENVER, CO)

**Rocky Mountain Poison
and Drug Center (*)**

777 Bannock St., Mail Code 0180
Denver, CO 80204
Business: 303-389-1392
Emergency: 800-222-1222
TDD/TTY: 303-739-1127 (CO)
www.RMPDC.org

ILLINOIS

CHICAGO

Illinois Poison Center (*)

222 South Riverside Plaza
Suite 1900
Chicago, IL 60606
Business: 312-906-6136
Emergency: 800-222-1222
TDD/TTY: 312-906-6185
www.mchc.org/ipc

INDIANA

INDIANAPOLIS

**Indiana Poison Control Center (*)
Methodist Hospital,
Emergency Medicine
& Trauma Center**

I-65 at 21st St.
P.O. Box 1367
Indianapolis, IN 46206-1367
Business: 317-962-2335
Emergency: 800-222-1222
800-382-9097
317-962-2323
(Indianapolis)
www.clarian.org/poisoncontrol

IOWA

SIOUX CITY

**Iowa Statewide Poison
Control Center (*)
Iowa Health System and the
University of Iowa Hospitals
and Clinics**

401 Douglas St., Suite 402
Sioux City, IA 51101
Business: 712-279-3710
Emergency: 800-222-1222
712-277-2222 (IA)
www.iowapoison.org

KANSAS

KANSAS CITY

**University of Kansas
Poison Control Hospital Center**

3901 Rainbow Blvd.
Delp - Room 4043
Kansas City, KS 66160-7231
Business: 913-588-6638
Emergency: 800-222-1222
800-332-6633 (KS)
www.kumed.com/poison

KENTUCKY

LOUISVILLE

**Kentucky Regional Poison
Center (*)
Medical Towers South**

234 E Gray St, Suite 847
Louisville, KY 40202
Business: 502-629-7246
Emergency: 800-222-1222
www.krpc.com

LOUISIANA

SHREVEPORT

**Louisiana Poison Center (*)
LSUHSC - Shreveport
Dept. of Emergency Medicine
Section of Clinical Toxology**

1455 Wilkinson St
Shreveport, LA 71130
Business: 318-813-3314
Emergency: 800-222-1222

MAINE

PORTLAND

**Northern New England Poison
Center (*)**

22 Bramhall St.
Portland, ME 04102-3175
Business: 207-662-0111
Emergency: 800-222-1222
800-442-6035
877-339-3107
207-871-2879 (ME)
TDD/TTY: 207-662-4900 (ME)
www.nnepc.org

MARYLAND

BALTIMORE

Maryland Poison Center (*)
University of Maryland at
Baltimore School of Pharmacy

220 Arch St.
Office Level 01
Baltimore, MD 21201
Business: 410-706-7604
Emergency: 800-222-1222
TDD: 410-528-7530
www.mdpoison.com

(WASHINGTON, DC)

National Capital Poison Center (*)

3201 New Mexico Ave., NW
Suite 310
Washington, DC 20016
Business: 202-362-3867
Emergency: 800-222-1222
www.poison.org

MASSACHUSETTS

BOSTON

Regional Center for Poison
Control and Prevention (*)
(Serving Massachusetts
and Rhode Island)

300 Longwood Ave.
Boston, MA 02115
Business: 617-355-6609
Emergency: 800-222-1222
TDD/TTY: 888-244-5313
www.maripoisoncenter.com

MICHIGAN

DETROIT

Regional Poison Control Center (*)
Children's Hospital of Michigan

3901 Beaubien
Detroit, MI 48201
Business: 313-745-5437
Emergency: 800-222-1222
TDD/TTY: 800-356-3232
www.mitoxic.org/pcc

MINNESOTA

MINNEAPOLIS

Hennepin Regional Poison
Control Systems (*)
Hennepin County Medical Center

701 Park Ave.
Mail Code RL
Minneapolis, MN 55415
Business: 612-873-3144
Emergency: 800-222-1222
www.mnpoison.org

MISSISSIPPI

JACKSON

Mississippi Regional Poison
Control Center
University of Mississippi
Medical Center

2500 North State St.
Jackson, MS 39216
Business: 601-984-1680
Emergency: 800-222-1222
http://poisoncontrol.umc.edu

MISSOURI

ST. LOUIS

Missouri Regional Poison
Center (*)
SM Cardinal Glennon Children's
Medical Center

1465 S. Grand Blvd.
St. Louis, MO 63104-1095
Business: 314-577-5600
Emergency: 800-222-1222
www.cardinalglennon.com

MONTANA

(DENVER, CO)

Rocky Mountain Poison
and Drug Center (*)

777 Bannock St., Mail Code 0180
Denver, CO 80204
Business: 303-389-1100
Emergency: 800-222-1222
TDD/TTY: 303-739-1127 (CO)
www.RMPDC.org

NEBRASKA

OMAHA

Nebraska Regional Poison
Center (*)

8401 W. Dodge Rd., Suite 115
Omaha, NE 68114
Business: 402-390-5555
Emergency: 800-222-1222
www.nebraskapoison.com

NEVADA

(DENVER, CO)

Rocky Mountain Poison
and Drug Center (*)

777 Bannock St., Mail Code 0180
Denver, CO 80204 -4028
Business: 303-389-1100
Emergency: 800-222-1222
TDD/TTY: 303-739-1127 (CO)
www.RMPDC.org

NEW HAMPSHIRE

(PORTLAND, ME)

Northern New England Poison
Center
Maine Medical Center

22 Bramhall St.
Portland, ME 04102-3175
Business: 207-662-0111
                   877-339-3107
TTY: 207-662-4900
Emergency: 800-222-1222
www.nnepc.org

NEW JERSEY

NEWARK

New Jersey Poison Information
and Education System (*)
UMDNJ

140 Bergen St.
Suite G1600
PO Box 1709
Newark, NJ 07101-1709
Business: 973-972-9280
Emergency: 800-222-1222
TDD/TTY: 973-926-8008
www.njpies.org

NEW MEXICO

ALBUQUERQUE

New Mexico Poison
and Drug Information Center (*)

MSC09/5080
1 University of New Mexico
Albuquerque, NM 87131-0001
Business: 505-272-4261
Emergency: 800-222-1222
http://hsc.unm.edu/pharmacy/poison

NEW YORK

MINEOLA

Long Island Regional Poison
and Drug Information Center (*)
Winthrop University Hospital

259 First St.
Mineola, NY 11501
Business: 516-663-2650
Emergency: 800-222-1222
www.lirpdic.org

NEW YORK CITY

New York City Poison
Control Center (*)
NYC Bureau of Public Health

455 First Ave., Room 123, Box 81
New York, NY 10016-9102
Business: 212-447-8152
Emergency: 800-222-1222
(English)   212-340-4494
                   212-POISONS
                   (212-764-7667)
Emergency: 212-venenos
(Spanish)   (212-836-3667)
TDD: 212-689-9014
www.nyc.gov/html/doh/html/poison/
poison.shtml

ROCHESTER

The Ruth A. Lawrence
Regional Poison and Drug
Information Center (*)
University of Rochester
Medical Center

601 Elmwood Ave.
Box 321
Rochester, NY 14642
Business: 585-273-4155
Emergency: 800-222-1222
TTY: 585-273-3854
www.fingerlakespoison.org

SYRACUSE

Upstate New York Poison Center (*)
SUNY Upstate Medical University

750 East Adams St.
Syracuse, NY 13210
Business: 315-464-7078
Emergency: 800-222-1222
TTY: 315-464-5424
www.upstatepoison.org

NORTH CAROLINA

CHARLOTTE

Carolinas Poison Center (*)

PO Box 32861
Charlotte, NC 28232-2861
Business: 704-512-3795
Emergency: 800-222-1222
www.ncpoisoncenter.org

NORTH DAKOTA

(MINNEAPOLIS, MN)

Minnesota Poison Control Center (*)
Hennepin County Medical Center

701 Park Ave., Mail Code RL
Minneapolis, MN 55415
Business: 612-873-3144
Emergency: 800-222-1222
www.mnpoison.org

OHIO

CINCINNATI

Cincinnati Drug and Poison Information Center (*)

3333 Burnet Ave., MLC 9004
Cincinnati, OH 45229-3039
Business: 513-636-4200
               513-636-5111
Emergency: 800-222-1222
TTY: 513-636-4900
www.cincinnatichildrens.org/dpic

CLEVELAND

Northern Ohio Poison Center
Rainbow Babies and Children's Hospital

11100 Euclid Ave.
B261 MP 6007
Cleveland, OH 44106-6010
Business: 216-844-8447
Emergency: 800-222-1222
www.uhhospitals.org/rainbowchildren/
tabid/195/Default.aspx

COLUMBUS

Central Ohio Poison Center (*)

700 Children's Dr.
Columbus, OH 43205
Business: 614-355-0463
Emergency: 800-222-1222
TTY: 866-688-0088
www.bepoisonsmart.com

OKLAHOMA

OKLAHOMA CITY

Oklahoma Poison Control Center (*)
OU Health Sciences Center

940 NE 13th St.
Room 3N3510
Oklahoma City, OK 73104
Business: 405-271-5062
Emergency: 800-222-1222
www.oklahomapoison.org

OREGON

PORTLAND

Oregon Poison Center (*)
Oregon Health and Science University

3181 S.W. Sam Jackson Park Rd.
CB550
Portland, OR 97239
Business: 503-494-8600
Emergency: 800-222-1222
www.ohsu.edu/poison

PENNSYLVANIA

PHILADELPHIA

The Poison Control Center (*)
Children's Hospital of Philadelphia

34th Street & Civic Center Blvd.
Philadelphia, PA 19104
Business: 215-590-1000
Emergency: 800-222-1222
               215-386-2100 (PA)
TDD/TTY: 215-590-8789
www.poisoncontrol.chop.edu

PITTSBURGH

Pittsburgh Poison Center (*)
University of Pittsburgh

200 Lothrop Street
Pittsburgh, PA 15213
Business: 412-390-3300
Emergency: 800-222-1222
               412-681-6669
www.upmc.com/services/
poisoncenter

RHODE ISLAND

(BOSTON, MA)

Regional Center for Poison Control and Prevention (*)
(Serving Massachusetts and Rhode Island)
Children's Hospital of Boston

300 Longwood Ave.
Boston, MA 02115
Business: 617-355-6609
Emergency: 800-222-1222
TDD/TTY: 888-244-5313
www.maripoisoncenter.com

SOUTH CAROLINA

COLUMBIA

Palmetto Poison Center (*)
South Carolina College of Pharmacy
University of South Carolina

USC Columbia, SC 29208
Business: 803-777-7909
Emergency: 800-222-1222
http://poison.sc.edu

SOUTH DAKOTA

(MINNEAPOLIS, MN)

Minnesota Poison Control Center (*)
Hennepin County Medical Center

701 Park Ave., Mail Code RL
Minneapolis, MN 55415
Business: 612-873-3141
Emergency: 800-222-1222
www.mnpoison.org

TENNESSEE

NASHVILLE

Tennessee Poison Center (*)

1161 21st Ave. South
501 Oxford House
Nashville, TN 37232-4632
Business: 615-936-0760
Emergency: 800-222-1222
www.tnpoisoncenter.org

TEXAS

AMARILLO

Texas Panhandle Poison Center (*)

1501 S. Coulter Dr.
Amarillo, TX 79106 -1770
Business: 806-354-1630
Emergency: 800-222-1222
www.poisoncontrol.org

DALLAS

North Texas Poison Center (*)
Texas Poison Center Network
Parkland Health & Hospital Systems

5201 Harry Hines Blvd.
Dallas, TX 75235
Business: 214-589-0911
Emergency: 800-222-1222
www.poisoncontrol.org

EL PASO

West Texas Regional Poison Center (*)
At University Medical Center of El Paso

4815 Alameda Ave.
El Paso, TX 79905
Business: 915-534-3800
Emergency: 800-222-1222
www.poisoncontrol.org

GALVESTON

Southeast Texas Poison Center (*)
The University of Texas Medical Branch

301 University Blvd.
3.112 Trauma Center
Galveston, TX 77555-1175
Business: 409-772-3332
Emergency: 800-222-1222
www.utmb.edu/setpc

SAN ANTONIO

South Texas Poison Center (*)
The University of Texas Health
Science Center–San Antonio
Dept. of Surgery

7703 Floyd Curl Dr., MSC 7849
San Antonio, TX 78229-3900
Business: 210-567-5762
Emergency: 800-222-1222
TTY: 1-800-222-1222
www.texaspoison.com

TEMPLE

Central Texas Poison Center (*)
Scott & White Memorial Hospital

2401 South 31st St.
Temple, TX 76508
Business: 254-724-7405
Emergency: 800-222-1222
http://www.sw.org/web/
patientsAndVisitors/iwcontent/
public/poison/en_us/html/poison.jsp

UTAH

SALT LAKE CITY

Utah Poison Control Center (*)
University of Utah

585 Komas Dr. Suite #200
Salt Lake City, UT 84108-1234
Business: 801-587-0600
Emergency: 800-222-1222
http://uuhsc.utah.edu/poison

VERMONT

(PORTLAND, ME)

Northern New England
Poison Center (*)
Maine Medical Center

22 Bramhall St.
Portland, ME 04102-3175
Business: 207-662-0111
               877-339-3107
Emergency: 800-222-1222
TTY   207-662-4900
www.nnepc.org

VIRGINIA

CHARLOTTESVILLE

Blue Ridge Poison Center (*)
Jefferson Park Place

1222 Jefferson Park Ave.
Charlottesville, VA 22908-0774
Business: 434-924-0347
Emergency: 800-222-1222
www.healthsystem.virginia.edu/brpc

RICHMOND

Virginia Poison Center (*)
Virginia Commonwealth University
Medical Center

600 E. Broad St.
Suite 640
P.O. Box 980522
Richmond, VA 23298-0522
Business: 804-828-4780
Emergency: 800-222-1222
www.poison.vcu.edu

WASHINGTON

SEATTLE

Washington Poison Center (*)

155 NE 100th St.
Seattle, WA 98125-8007
Business: 206-517-2359
Emergency: 800-222-1222
TDD/TTY: 1-800-222-1222
www.wapc.org

WEST VIRGINIA

CHARLESTON

West Virginia Poison Center (*)
Robert C. Byrd
Health Sciences Center
Charleston Division

3110 MacCorkle Ave. SE
Charleston, WV 25304
Business: 304-347-1212
Emergency: 800-222-1222
www.wvpoisoncenter.org

WISCONSIN

MILWAUKEE

Wisconsin Poison Center

Mail Station 660
P.O. Box 1997
Milwaukee, WI 53201-1997
Business: 414-266-6973
Emergency: 800-222-1222
www.wisconsinpoison.org

WYOMING

(OMAHA, NE)

Nebraska Regional Poison
Center (*)

8401 W. Dodge St., Suite 115
Omaha, NE 68114
Business: 402-390-5555
Emergency: 800-222-1222
www.nebraskapoison.com

COMMON LABORATORY TEST VALUES

Listed below are generally accepted normal values for a selection of common laboratory assays conducted on serum, plasma, and blood. Remember that norms may vary from laboratory to laboratory in accordance with the methodology and quality control measures employed by the facility.

When in doubt, check with the laboratory that performed the analysis.

"SI range" refers to Système International d'Unités, a uniform system of reporting numerical values that permits interchangeability of information among nations and disciplines.

Test	US Range	SI Range
Acid phosphatase	≤2.5 ng/mL	≤2.5 µg/L
Prostatic Total	≤5.8 U/L	<97 nkat/L
Alanine aminotransferase [ALT] (SGPT)	≤48 U/L	≤0.8 µkat/L
Albumin, serum	3.5-5.5 g/dL	35-55 g/L
Alkaline phosphatase	20-125 U/L	0.33-2.08 µkat/L
Ammonia [NH_3^+]	10-80 µg/dL	6-47 µmol/L
Amylase, serum	60-180 U/L	0.8-3.2 µkat/L
Antinuclear antibodies (ANA)	Negative at 1:40 dilution	
Aspartate aminotransferase (AST) (SGOT)	≤42 U/L	<0.7 µkat/L
Bilirubin		
Total	0.3-1.0 mg/dL	5.1-17 µmol/L
Direct	0.1-0.3 mg/dL	1.7-5.1 µmol/L
Indirect	0.2-0.7 mg/dL	3.4-12 µmol/L
Blood urea nitrogen/creatinine ratio	10:1-20:1	Average 15:1
Calcium, plasma	9-10.5 mg/dL	2.2-2.6 mmol/L
Calcium, ionized	4.5-5.6 mg/dL	1.1-1.4 mmol/L
Chloride, serum	95-108 mEq/L	95-108 mmol/L
Cholesterol (total plasma)		
Desirable level	<200 mg/dL	<5.20 mmol/L
Moderate risk	200-240 mg/dL	5.2-6.3 mmol/L
High risk	>240 mg/dL	>6.3 mmol/L
Copper	70-140 µg/dL	11-22 µmol/L
Cortisol, serum		
0800 hours	5-25 µg/dL	140-690 nmol/L
1600 hours	3-12 µg/dL	80-330 nmol/L
Creatinine kinase (CK)		
Isoenzymes	CK-MM: 97-100% of total	CK-MM: 0.97-1.00 of total
	CK-MB: <3% of total	CK-MB: <0.03 of total
	CK-BB: 0% of total	CK-BB: 0 of total
Total	Male: ≤235 U/L	Male: ≤3.92 µkat/L
	Female: ≤190 U/L	Female: ≤3.17 µkat/L
Creatinine, serum	<1.5 mg/dL	<133 µmol/L
Creatinine clearance	75125 mL/min	1.2-4-2.08 mL/sec
Digoxin		
Therapeutic	0.8-2.0 ng/mL	1.0-2.6 nmol/L
Toxic	>2.5 ng/mL	>3.2 nmol/L

Test	US Range	SI Range
Erythrocyte count (RBC)	4.1-54.90 × 10⁶/mm³	4.15-4.90 × 10¹²/L
Erythrocyte sedimentation rate (ESR)		
Male	0-20 mm/hr	0-20 mm/hr
Female	0-30 mm/hr	0-30 mm/hr
Ferritin		
Male	15-400 ng/mL	15-400 µg/L
Female	10-200 ng/mL	10-200 µg/L
Folic acid	3-16 ng/mL	7-36 nmol/L
Follicle-stimulating hormone (FSH)		
Female	1.4-9.6 mIU/mL	1.4-9.6 IU/L
Ovulation	2.3-21 mIU/mL	2.3-21 IU/L
Postmenopausal	34-96 mIU/mL	34-96 IU/L
Male	0.9-15 mIU/mL	0.9-15 IU/L
Gamma-glutamyl transferase (GGT)		
Male	≤65 U/L	≤1.08 µkat/L
Female	≤45 U/L	≤0.75 µkat/L
Gases, arterial blood		
pO_2	80-100 mmHg	11-13 kPa
pCO_2	35-45 mmHg	4.7-6 kPa
Glucose, plasma		
Fasting	75-115 mg/dL	4.2-6.4 mmol/L
Postprandial (2 h)	<140 mg/dL	<7.8 mmol/L
Immunoglobulins (Ig)		
IgG	800-1500 mg/dL	8.0-15.0 g/L
IgA	90-325 mg/dL	0.9-3.2 g/L
IgM	45-150 mg/dL	0.45-1.5 g/L
IgD	0-8 mg/dL	0-0.08 g/L
IgE	<0.025 mg/dL	<0.00025 g/L
Iron, serum	50-150 µg/dL	9-27 µmol/L
Iron binding capacity	250-370 µg/dL	45-66 µmol/L
Iron saturation	20-45%	
Lactic acid (plasma, venous)	9-16 mg/dL	1.0-1.8 mmol/L
Lactic dehydrogenase (LDH)	100-190 U/L	1.7-3.2 µkat/L
Lead	<20 µg/dL	1.0 µmol/L
Leukocyte count (WBC)	4.3-10.8 × 10³	4.3-10.8 × 10⁹/L
Lipase	0-160 U/L	0-2.66 µkat/L
Lipoproteins (desirable levels)		
Low density (LDL)	<130 mg/dL	<3.36 mmol/L
High density (HDL)	>60 mg/dL	>1.55 mmol/L
Lithium ion (therapeutic)	0.6-1.2 mEq/L	0.6-1.2 mmol/L
Luteinizing hormone		
Female	0.8-26 mIU/mL	0.8-26 IU/L
Ovulation	25-57 mIU/mL	25-57 IU/L
Postmenopausal	40-104 mIU/mL	40-104 IU/L
Male	1.3-13 mIU/mL	1.3-13 IU/L

Test	US Range	SI Range
Osmolality, plasma	285-295 mOsm/kg	285-295 mmol/kg
Phenytoin		
Therapeutic	10-20 mg/L	40-80 µmol/L
Toxic	>30 mg/L	>120 µmol/L
Phosphorus, serum	2.5-4.5 mg/dL	0.8-1.45 mmol/L
Potassium, serum	3.5-5 mEq/L	3.5-5 mmol/L
Prolactin	2-15 ng/mL	2-15 µg/L
Prostate-specific antigen (PSA)	≤4 ng/mL	≤4 µg/L
Protein		
Total	5.5-8.0 g/dL	55-80 g/L
Albumin	3.5-5.5 g/dL	35-55 g/L
Globulin	2.0-3.5 g/dL	20-35 g/L
Reticulocyte count	0.5-2.3% of RBCs	0.005-0.023 of RBCs
Rheumatoid factor	<40 IU/mL	<40 kIU/L
Sodium, serum	136-145 mEq/L	136-145 mmol/L
Theophylline (therapeutic)	10-20 mg/L	55-110 µmol/L
Thyroxine-binding globulin (TBG)	16-34 mg/L	16-34 mg/L
Thyroid-stimulating hormone (TSH)	0.4-5 µU/mL	0.4-5 mU/L
Thyroxine (T_4)		
Free	0.8-1.8 ng/dL	10-23 pmol/L
Total	4.5-12.5 µg/dL	58-161 nmol/L
Transferrin	230-390 µg/dL	2.3-3.9 mg/L
Triglycerides	<160 µg/dL	<1.8 mmol/L
Triiodothyronine (T_3)	70-190 ng/dL	1.1-2.9 nmol/L
T_3 uptake	25-35%	0.25-0.35 (proportion of 1.0)
Urea nitrogen, blood (BUN)	7-30 mg/dL	2.5-10.7 mmol/L
Uric acid		
Male	4.0-8.5 mg/dL	238-506 µmol/L
Female	2.5-7.5 mg/dL	149-446 µmol/L
Vitamin B_{12}	200-600 pg/mL	148-443 pmol/L

SOURCES:

Beers MH, Porter RS, Jones TV, et al. *Merck Manual of Diagnosis and Therapy*, ed 18. Whitehouse Station, NJ: Merck Research Laboratories; 2006.

Cahill M. *Illustrated Guide to Diagnostic Tests*, ed 2. Springhouse, PA: Springhouse Corporation; 1998.

Fauci AS, Braunwald E, Kasper DL, et al. *Harrison's Principles of Internal Medicine*, ed 17. New York, NY: McGraw Hill; 2008.

Goldman L, Ausiello D. *Cecil Medicine*, ed 23. Philadelphia, PA: Saunders Elsevier; 2008.

Sacher RA, McPherson RA, Campos JM. *Wildmann's Clinical Interpretation of Laboratory Tests*. Philadelphia, PA: FA Davis Company; 2000.

SECTION 5

PRODUCT INFORMATION

This edition of *PDR®* contains the latest information available when the book went to press. Listings are arranged alphabetically by manufacturer; late submissions appear alphabetically by manufacturer at the end of this section. As new drugs are released, and new research data, clinical findings, and safety information emerge throughout the year, it is the responsibility of the manufacturer to provide that information to the medical community and revise that information in the *PDR* database accordingly. These revisions are published six times annually in the *PDR Update Insert Cards*, more regularly on PDR.net and *mobilePDR®*, and emailed monthly via the *eDrug Update*. To be certain that you have the most current data, always consult PDR.net, *mobilePDR*, *eDrug Update*, or the *PDR Update Insert Cards* before prescribing or administering any product described in the following pages.

Abbott Laboratories
Pharmaceutical Products Division
NORTH CHICAGO, IL 60064, U.S.A.

Pharmaceutical Products Division—
Direct Inquiries to:
Customer Service:
(800) 255-5162
Patient Access Program:
(800) 441-4987
For Medical Information Contact:
(800) 633-9110 or www.abbottmedinfo.com
Adverse experiences or side effects
(for all Abbott drug products):
(800) 633-9110 or rxabbott.com
Sales and Ordering:
(800) 255-5162

ABBO–CODE™ INDEX

The Abbo-Code identification system provides positive identification of a drug and dosage strength. The following Abbott products are imprinted or debossed with an Abbo-Code designation:

PRODUCT	ABBO-CODE
Advicor® Tablet (niacin extended-release/lovastatin tablets)	
1000 mg/20 mg	a 1002
1000 mg/40 mg	a 1004
750 mg/20 mg	a 752
500 mg/20 mg	a 502
Biaxin® Filmtab® Tablets (clarithromycin tablets, USP)	
250 mg	KT
500 mg	KL
Biaxin® XL Filmtab® Tablets (clarithromycin extended-release tablets)	
500 mg	KJ
Depakene® Capsules (valproic acid capsules, USP)	
250 mg	DEPAKENE
Depakote® ER Tablets (divalproex sodium EXTENDED-RELEASE tablets)	
500 mg	HC
250 mg	HF
Depakote® Sprinkle Capsules (divalproex sodium coated particles in capsules)	
125 mg	↑THIS END UP DEPAKOTE SPRINKLE 125 mg
Depakote® Tablets (divalproex sodium delayed-release tablets)	
125 mg	NT
250 mg	NR
500 mg	NS
Ery-Tab® Enteric-Coated Tablets (erythromycin delayed-release tablets, USP)	
250 mg	EC
333 mg	EH
500 mg	ED
Erythrocin® Stearate Filmtab® Tablets (erythromycin stearate tablets, USP)	
250 mg erythromycin activity	ES
500 mg erythromycin activity	ET
Erythromycin Base Filmtab® Tablets (erythromycin tablets, USP)	
250 mg	EB
500 mg	EA
Erythromycin Delayed-release Capsules, USP	
250 mg	ER
Erythromycin Ethylsuccinate Tablets, USP	
400 mg erythromycin activity	74 ZE
Gengraf® Capsules (cyclosporine capsules, USP [MODIFIED])	
25 mg	OR 25 mg
100 mg	OT 100 mg
Kaletra® **(lopinavir/ritonavir)**	
133.3 mg lopinavir/33.3 mg ritonavir	PK
Kaletra® Tablet (lopinavir/ritonavir)	
200 mg lopinavir/50 mg ritonavir	KA
K ·Tab® Filmtab® Tablets (potassium chloride extended-release tablets, USP)	
10 mEq (750 mg)	K-TAB
Mavik® Tablets (trandolapril)	
1 mg	FT
2 mg	FX
4 mg	FZ

Meridia® Capsules Ⓒⓥ **(sibutramine hydrochloride monohydrate)**	
5 mg	MERIDIA 5
10 mg	MERIDIA 10
15 mg	MERIDIA 15
Niaspan® (niacin extended-release tablets) [film-coated]	
500 mg	Niaspan 500
750 mg	Niaspan 750
1000 mg	Niaspan 1000
Norvir® **(ritonavir capsules) Soft Gelatin**	
100 mg	DS 100
PCE® Dispertab® Tablets (erythromycin particles in tablets)	
333 mg	PCE
500 mg	EK
Simcor® Tablet (niacin extended-release/simvastatin tablets)	
500 mg/20 mg	a 500-20
500 mg/40 mg	a 500-40
750 mg/20 mg	a 750-20
1000 mg/20 mg	a 1000-20
1000 mg/40 mg	a 1000-40
Synthroid® Tablets **(levothyroxine sodium tablets, USP)**	
25 mcg (0.025 mg)	SYNTHROID 25
50 mcg (0.05 mg)	SYNTHROID 50
75 mcg (0.075 mg)	SYNTHROID 75
88 mcg (0.088 mg)	SYNTHROID 88
100 mcg (0.1 mg)	SYNTHROID 100
112 mcg (0.112 mg)	SYNTHROID 112
125 mcg (0.125 mg)	SYNTHROID 125
137 mcg (0.137 mg)	SYNTHROID 137
150 mcg (0.15 mg)	SYNTHROID 150
175 mcg (0.175 mg)	SYNTHROID 175
200 mcg (0.2 mg)	SYNTHROID 200
300 mcg (0.3 mg)	SYNTHROID 300
Tarka® Tablets **(trandolapril/verapamil hydrochloride ER)**	
2 mg/180 mg	182Δ
1 mg/240 mg	241Δ
2 mg/240 mg	242Δ
4 mg/240 mg	244Δ
Tricor® (fenofibrate tablets)	
48 mg	FI
54 mg	TA
145 mg	FO
160 mg	TC
Trilipix™ Capsules (fenofibric acid delayed release capsules)	
45 mg	a 45
135 mg	a 135
Vicodin® Tablet Ⓒⓘⓘ	VICODIN
(hydrocodone bitartrate and acetaminophen tablets, USP)	
hydrocodone bitartrate	5 mg
acetaminophen	500 mg
Vicodin ES® Tablet Ⓒⓘⓘ	VICODIN ES
(hydrocodone bitartrate and acetaminophen tablets, USP)	
hydrocodone bitartrate	7.5 mg
acetaminophen	750 mg
Vicodin HP® Tablet Ⓒⓘⓘ	VICODIN HP
(hydrocodone bitartrate and acetaminophen tablets, USP)	
hydrocodone bitartrate	10 mg
acetaminophen	660 mg
Vicoprofen® Tablet Ⓒⓘⓘ	VP
(hydrocodone bitartrate and ibuprofen tablets)	
hydrocodone bitartrate	7.5 mg
ibuprofen	200 mg
Zemplar® Capsules (paricalcitol)	
1 mcg	ZA
2 mcg	ZF
4 mcg	ZK

ADVICOR®
[ăd-vĭ-kŏr]
(niacin extended-release/lovastatin tablets)

℞

DESCRIPTION
ADVICOR® (niacin extended-release and lovastatin) is intended to facilitate the daily administration of its individual components, Niaspan® and lovastatin, when used together for the intended patient population (see **INDICATIONS AND USAGE** and **DOSAGE AND ADMINISTRATION**). ADVICOR contains niacin extended-release and lovastatin in combination. Lovastatin, an inhibitor of 3-hydroxy-3-methylglutaryl-coenzyme A (HMG-CoA) reductase, and niacin are both lipid-altering agents.
Niacin is nicotinic acid, or 3-pyridinecarboxylic acid. Niacin is a white, nonhygroscopic crystalline powder that is very soluble in water, boiling ethanol and propylene glycol. It is insoluble in ethyl ether. The empirical formula of niacin is

$C_6H_5NO_2$ and its molecular weight is 123.11. Niacin has the following structural formula:

Lovastatin is [1S-[1(alpha)(R*), 3(alpha), 7(beta), 8(beta)(2S*, 4S*), 8a(beta)]]-1,2,3, 7,8,8a-hexahydro-3,7-dimethyl-8-[2-(tetrahydro-4-hydroxy-6-oxo-2H-pyran-2-yl) ethyl]-1-naphthalenyl 2-methylbutanoate. Lovastatin is a white, nonhygroscopic crystalline powder that is insoluble in water and sparingly soluble in ethanol, methanol, and acetonitrile. The empirical formula of lovastatin is $C_{24}H_{36}O_5$ and its molecular weight is 404.55. Lovastatin has the following structural formula:

ADVICOR tablets contain the labeled amount of niacin and lovastatin and have the following inactive ingredients: hypromellose, povidone, stearic acid, polyethylene glycol, titanium dioxide, polysorbate 80.
The individual tablet strengths (expressed in terms of mg niacin/mg lovastatin) contain the following coloring agents:
ADVICOR 500 mg/20 mg—Iron Oxide Yellow, Iron Oxide Red.
ADVICOR 750 mg/20 mg—FD&C Yellow #6/Sunset Yellow FCF Aluminum Lake.
ADVICOR 1000 mg/20 mg—Iron Oxide Red, Iron Oxide Yellow, Iron Oxide Black.
ADVICOR 1000 mg/40 mg—Iron Oxide Red.

CLINICAL PHARMACOLOGY
A variety of clinical studies have demonstrated that elevated levels of total cholesterol (TC), low-density lipoprotein cholesterol (LDL-C), and apolipoprotein B-100 (Apo B) promote human atherosclerosis. Similarly, decreased levels of high-density lipoprotein cholesterol (HDL-C) are associated with the development of atherosclerosis. Epidemiological investigations have established that cardiovascular morbidity and mortality vary directly with the level of TC and LDL-C, and inversely with the level of HDL-C.
Cholesterol-enriched triglyceride-rich lipoproteins, including very low-density lipoproteins (VLDL), intermediate-density lipoproteins (IDL), and their remnants, can also promote atherosclerosis. Elevated plasma triglycerides (TG) are frequently found in a triad with low HDL-C levels and small LDL particles, as well as in association with non-lipid metabolic risk factors for coronary heart disease (CHD). As such, total plasma TG have not consistently been shown to be an independent risk factor for CHD.
As an adjunct to diet, the efficacy of niacin and lovastatin in improving lipid profiles (either individually, or in combination with each other, or niacin in combination with other statins) for the treatment of dyslipidemia has been well documented. The effect of combined therapy with niacin and lovastatin on cardiovascular morbidity and mortality has not been determined.

Effects on lipids
ADVICOR
ADVICOR reduces LDL-C, TC, and TG, and increases HDL-C due to the individual actions of niacin and lovastatin. The magnitude of individual lipid and lipoprotein responses may be influenced by the severity and type of underlying lipid abnormality.
Niacin
Niacin functions in the body after conversion to nicotinamide adenine dinucleotide (NAD) in the NAD coenzyme system. Niacin (but not nicotinamide) in gram doses reduces LDL-C, Apo B, Lp(a), TG, and TC, and increases HDL-C. The increase in HDL-C is associated with an increase in apolipoprotein A-I (Apo A-I) and a shift in the distribution of HDL subfractions. These include an increase in the HDL_2:HDL_3 ratio, and an elevation in lipoprotein A-I (Lp A-I, an HDL-C particle containing only Apo A-I). In addition, preliminary reports suggest that niacin causes favorable LDL particle size transformations, although the clinical relevance of this effect is not yet clear.
Lovastatin
Lovastatin has been shown to reduce both normal and elevated LDL-C concentrations. Apo B also falls substantially during treatment with lovastatin. Since each LDL-C particle contains one molecule of Apo B, and since little Apo B is found in other lipoproteins, this strongly suggests that

lovastatin does not merely cause cholesterol to be lost from LDL-C, but also reduces the concentration of circulating LDL particles. In addition, lovastatin can produce increases of variable magnitude in HDL-C, and modestly reduces VLDL-C and plasma TG. The effects of lovastatin on Lp(a), fibrinogen, and certain other independent biochemical risk markers for coronary heart disease are not well characterized.

Mechanism of Action

Niacin

The mechanism by which niacin alters lipid profiles is not completely understood and may involve several actions, including partial inhibition of release of free fatty acids from adipose tissue, and increased lipoprotein lipase activity (which may increase the rate of chylomicron triglyceride removal from plasma). Niacin decreases the rate of hepatic synthesis of VLDL-C and LDL-C, and does not appear to affect fecal excretion of fats, sterols, or bile acids.

Lovastatin

Lovastatin is a specific inhibitor of 3-hydroxy-3-methylglutaryl-coenzyme A (HMG-CoA) reductase, the enzyme that catalyzes the conversion of HMG-CoA to mevalonate. The conversion of HMG-CoA to mevalonate is an early step in the biosynthetic pathway for cholesterol. Lovastatin is a prodrug and has little, if any, activity until hydrolyzed to its active beta-hydroxyacid form, lovastatin acid. The mechanism of the LDL-lowering effect of lovastatin may involve both reduction of VLDL-C concentration and induction of the LDL receptor, leading to reduced production and/or increased catabolism of LDL-C.

Pharmacokinetics

Absorption and Bioavailability

ADVICOR

In single-dose studies of ADVICOR, rate and extent of niacin and lovastatin absorption were bioequivalent under fed conditions to that from NIASPAN® (niacin extended-release tablets) and Mevacor® (lovastatin) tablets, respectively. After administration of two ADVICOR 1000 mg/20 mg tablets, peak niacin concentrations averaged about 18 mcg/mL and occurred about 5 hours after dosing; about 72% of the niacin dose was absorbed according to the urinary excretion data. Peak lovastatin concentrations averaged about 11 ng/mL and occurred about 2 hours after dosing.

The extent of niacin absorption from ADVICOR was increased by administration with food. The administration of two ADVICOR 1000 mg/20 mg tablets under low-fat or high-fat conditions resulted in a 22 to 30% increase in niacin bioavailability relative to dosing under fasting conditions. Lovastatin bioavailability is affected by food. Lovastatin C_{max} was increased 48% and 21% after a high- and a low-fat meal, respectively, but the lovastatin AUC was decreased 26% and 24% after a high- and a low-fat meal, respectively, compared to those under fasting conditions.

A relative bioavailability study results indicated that ADVICOR tablet strengths (i.e., two tablets of 500 mg/20 mg and one tablet of 1000 mg/40 mg) are not interchangeable.

Niacin

Due to extensive and saturable first-pass metabolism, niacin concentrations in the general circulation are dose dependent and highly variable. Peak steady-state niacin concentrations were 0.6, 4.9, and 15.5 mcg/mL after doses of 1000, 1500, and 2000 mg NIASPAN once daily (given as two 500 mg, two 750 mg, and two 1000 mg tablets, respectively).

Lovastatin

Lovastatin appears to be incompletely absorbed after oral administration. Because of extensive hepatic extraction, the amount of lovastatin reaching the systemic circulation as active inhibitors after oral administration is low (<5%) and shows considerable interindividual variation. Peak concentrations of active and total inhibitors occur within 2 to 4 hours after Mevacor® administration.

Lovastatin absorption appears to be increased by at least 30% by grapefruit juice; however, the effect is dependent on the amount of grapefruit juice consumed and the interval between grapefruit juice and lovastatin ingestion.

With a once-a-day dosing regimen, plasma concentrations of total inhibitors over a dosing interval achieved a steady-state between the second and third days of therapy and were about 1.5 times those following a single dose of Mevacor®.

Although the mechanism is not fully understood, cyclosporine has been shown to increase the AUC of HMG-CoA reductase inhibitors. The increase in AUC for lovastatin and lovastatin acid is presumably due, in part, to inhibition of CYP3A4.

Distribution

Niacin

Niacin is less than 20% bound to human serum proteins and distributes into milk. Studies using radiolabeled niacin in mice show that niacin and its metabolites concentrate in the liver, kidney, and adipose tissue.

Table 2. LDL-C mean percent change from baseline

Week	ADVICOR			NIASPAN			Lovastatin		
	n*	Dose (mg/mg)	LDL	n*	Dose (mg)	LDL	n*	Dose (mg)	LDL
Baseline	57	-	190.9 mg/dL	61	-	189.7 mg/dL	61	-	185.6 mg/dL
12	47	1000/20	-30%	46	1000	-3%	56	20	-29%
16	45	1000/40	-36%	44	1000	-6%	56	40	-31%
20	42	1500/40	-37%	43	1500	-12%	54	40	-34%
28	42	2000/40	-42%	41	2000	-14%	53	40	-32%

*n = number of patients remaining in the trial at each timepoint

Lovastatin

Both lovastatin and its beta-hydroxyacid metabolite are highly bound (>95%) to human plasma proteins. Distribution of lovastatin or its metabolites into human milk is unknown; however, lovastatin distributes into milk in rats. In animal studies, lovastatin concentrated in the liver, and crossed the blood-brain and placental barriers.

Metabolism

Niacin

Niacin undergoes rapid and extensive first-pass metabolism that is dose-rate specific and, at the doses used to treat dyslipidemia, saturable. In humans, one pathway is through a simple conjugation step with glycine to form nicotinuric acid (NUA). NUA is then excreted, although there may be a small amount of reversible metabolism back to niacin. The other pathway results in the formation of NAD. It is unclear whether nicotinamide is formed as a precursor to, or following the synthesis of, NAD. Nicotinamide is further metabolized to at least N-methylnicotinamide (MNA) and nicotinamide-N-oxide (NNO). MNA is further metabolized to two other compounds, N-methyl-2-pyridone-5-carboxamide (2PY) and N-methyl-4-pyridone-5-carboxamide (4PY). The formation of 2PY appears to predominate over 4PY in humans.

Lovastatin

Lovastatin undergoes extensive first-pass extraction and metabolism by cytochrome P450 3A4 in the liver, its primary site of action. The major active metabolites present in human plasma are the beta-hydroxyacid of lovastatin (lovastatin acid), its 6′-hydroxy derivative, and two additional metabolites.

Elimination

ADVICOR

Niacin is primarily excreted in urine mainly as metabolites. After a single dose of ADVICOR, at least 60% of the niacin dose was recovered in urine as unchanged niacin and its metabolites. The plasma half-life for lovastatin was about 4.5 hours in single-dose studies.

Niacin

The plasma half-life for niacin is about 20 to 48 minutes after oral administration and dependent on dose administered. Following multiple oral doses of NIASPAN, up to 12% of the dose was recovered in urine as unchanged niacin depending on dose administered. The ratio of metabolites recovered in the urine was also dependent on the dose administered.

Lovastatin

Lovastatin is excreted in urine and bile, based on studies of Mevacor®. Following an oral dose of radiolabeled lovastatin in man, 10% of the dose was excreted in urine and 83% in feces. The latter represents absorbed drug equivalents excreted in bile, as well as any unabsorbed drug.

Special Populations

Hepatic

No pharmacokinetic studies have been conducted in patients with hepatic insufficiency for either niacin or lovastatin (see **WARNINGS, Liver Dysfunction**).

Renal

No information is available on the pharmacokinetics of niacin in patients with renal insufficiency.

In a study of patients with severe renal insufficiency (creatinine clearance 10 to 30 mL/min), the plasma concentrations of total inhibitors after a single dose of lovastatin were approximately two-fold higher than those in healthy volunteers.

ADVICOR should be used with caution in patients with renal disease.

Gender

Plasma concentrations of niacin and metabolites after single- or multiple-dose administration of niacin are generally higher in women than in men, with the magnitude of the difference varying with dose and metabolite. Recovery of niacin and metabolites in urine, however, is generally similar for men and women, indicating similar absorption for both genders. The gender differences observed in plasma niacin and metabolite levels may be due to gender-specific differences in metabolic rate or volume of distribution. Data from clinical trials suggest that women have a greater hypolipidemic response than men at equivalent doses of NIASPAN and ADVICOR.

In a multiple-dose study, plasma concentrations of active and total HMG-CoA reductase inhibitors were 20 to 50% higher in women than in men. In two single-dose studies with ADVICOR, lovastatin concentrations were about 30% higher in women than men, and total HMG-CoA reductase inhibitor concentrations were about 20 to 25% greater in women.

In a multi-center, randomized, double-blind, active-comparator study in patients with Type IIa and IIb hyperlipidemia, ADVICOR was compared to single-agent treatment (NIASPAN and lovastatin). The treatment effects of ADVICOR compared to lovastatin and NIASPAN differed for males and females with a significantly larger treatment effect seen for females. The mean percent change from baseline at endpoint for LDL-C, TG, and HDL-C by gender are as follows (Table 1):

Table 1. Mean percent change from baseline at endpoint for LDL-C, HDL-C and TG by gender

	ADVICOR 2000 mg/40 mg		NIASPAN 2000 mg		Lovastatin 40 mg	
	Women (n=22)	Men (n=30)	Women (n=28)	Men (n=28)	Women (n=21)	Men (n=38)
LDL-C	-47%	-34%	-12%	-9%	-31%	-31%
HDL-C	+33%	+24%	+22%	+15%	+3%	+7%
TG	-48%	-35%	-25%	-15%	-15%	-23%

Clinical Studies

In a multi-center, randomized, double-blind, parallel, 28-week, active-comparator study in patients with Type IIa and IIb hyperlipidemia, ADVICOR was compared to each of its components (NIASPAN and lovastatin). Using a forced dose-escalation study design, patients received each dose for at least 4 weeks. Patients randomized to treatment with ADVICOR initially received 500 mg/20 mg. The dose was increased at 4-week intervals to a maximum of 1000 mg/20 mg in one-half of the patients and 2000 mg/40 mg in the other half. The NIASPAN monotherapy group underwent a similar titration from 500 mg to 2000 mg. The patients randomized to lovastatin monotherapy received 20 mg for 12 weeks titrated to 40 mg for up to 16 weeks. Up to a third of the patients randomized to ADVICOR or NIASPAN discontinued prior to Week 28. In this study, ADVICOR decreased LDL-C, TG and Lp(a), and increased HDL-C in a dose-dependent fashion (Tables 2, 3, 4 and 5 below). Results from this study for LDL-C mean percent change from baseline (the primary efficacy variable) showed that:

1. LDL-lowering with ADVICOR was significantly greater than that achieved with lovastatin 40 mg only after 28 weeks of titration to a dose of 2000 mg/40 mg (p<.0001)
2. ADVICOR at doses of 1000 mg/20 mg or higher achieved greater LDL-lowering than NIASPAN (p<.0001) The LDL-C results are summarized in Table 2.

[See table 2 above]

ADVICOR achieved significantly greater HDL-raising compared to lovastatin and NIASPAN monotherapy at all doses (Table 3).

[See table 3 at top of next page]

In addition, ADVICOR achieved significantly greater TG-lowering at doses of 1000 mg/20 mg or greater compared to lovastatin and NIASPAN monotherapy (Table 4).

[See table 4 at top of next page]

The Lp(a) lowering effects of ADVICOR and NIASPAN were similar, and both were superior to lovastatin (Table 5). The

Information on the Abbott Pharmaceutical Products listed on these pages is from the prescribing information in use as of June 1, 2010. For more information, please visit rxabbott.com or call 1-800-633-9110.

independent effect of lowering Lp(a) with NIASPAN or ADVICOR on the risk of coronary and cardiovascular morbidity and mortality has not been determined.
[See table 5 at right]

ADVICOR Long-Term Study

A total of 814 patients were enrolled in a long-term (52-week), open-label, single-arm study of ADVICOR. Patients were force dose-titrated to 2000 mg/40 mg over 16 weeks. After titration, patients were maintained on the maximum tolerated dose of ADVICOR for a total of 52 weeks. Five hundred-fifty (550) patients (68%) completed the study, and fifty-six percent (56%) of all patients were able to maintain a dose of 2000 mg/40 mg for the 52 weeks of treatment. The lipid-altering effects of ADVICOR peaked after 4 weeks on the maximum tolerated dose, and were maintained for the duration of treatment. These effects were comparable to what was observed in the double-blind study of ADVICOR (Tables 2-4).

INDICATIONS AND USAGE

Therapy with lipid-altering agents should be only one component of multiple risk-factor intervention in individuals at significantly increased risk for atherosclerotic vascular disease due to hypercholesterolemia. Drug therapy is indicated as an adjunct to diet when the response to a diet restricted in saturated fat and cholesterol and other nonpharmacologic measures alone has been inadequate (see also Table 7 and the NCEP treatment guidelines[1]).

ADVICOR

ADVICOR (niacin extended-release and lovastatin) is indicated for use when treatment with both NIASPAN and lovastatin is appropriate. As described in the labeling for Niaspan and lovastatin below, the components of ADVICOR are both indicated for the treatment of hypercholesterolemia. Patients receiving treatment with ADVICOR should be on a standard cholesterol-lowering diet and should continue on this diet during treatment.

NIASPAN (niacin extended-release)

Hypercholesterolemia

NIASPAN is indicated as an adjunct to diet for reduction of elevated TC, LDL-C, Apo B and TG levels, and to increase HDL-C in patients with primary hypercholesterolemia (heterozygous familial and nonfamilial) and mixed dyslipidemia (Frederickson Types IIa and IIb; Table 6), when the response to an appropriate diet has been inadequate.

Secondary Prevention of Cardiovascular Events

In patients with a history of myocardial infarction and hypercholesterolemia, niacin is indicated to reduce the risk of recurrent nonfatal myocardial infarction.

Hypertriglyceridemia

Niacin is also indicated as adjunctive therapy for treatment of adult patients with very high serum triglyceride levels (Types IV and V hyperlipidemia; Table 6) who present a risk of pancreatitis and who do not respond adequately to a determined dietary effort to control them. Such patients typically have serum TG levels over 2000 mg/dL and have elevations of VLDL-C as well as fasting chylomicrons (Type V hyperlipidemia; Table 6). Patients who consistently have total serum or plasma TG below 1000 mg/dL are unlikely to develop pancreatitis. Therapy with niacin may be considered for those patients with TG elevations between 1000 and 2000 mg/dL who have a history of pancreatitis or of recurrent abdominal pain typical of pancreatitis. Some Type IV patients with TG under 1000 mg/dL may, through dietary or alcohol indiscretion, convert to a Type V pattern with massive TG elevations accompanying fasting chylomicronemia, but the influence of niacin therapy on risk of pancreatitis in such situations has not been adequately studied. Drug therapy is not indicated for patients with Type I hyperlipoproteinemia, who have elevations of chylomicrons and plasma TG, but who have normal levels of VLDL-C. Inspection of plasma refrigerated for 14 hours is helpful in distinguishing Types I, IV, and V hyperlipoproteinemia.[2]

Lovastatin

Hypercholesterolemia

Lovastatin is indicated as an adjunct to diet for the reduction of elevated TC and LDL-C levels in patients with primary hypercholesterolemia (Frederickson Types IIa and IIb; Table 6), when the response to diet restricted in saturated fat and cholesterol and to other nonpharmacological measures alone has been inadequate.

Primary Prevention of Cardiovascular Events

In individuals without symptomatic cardiovascular disease, average to moderately elevated TC and LDL-C, and below average HDL-C, lovastatin is indicated to reduce the risk of:
- Myocardial infarction
- Unstable angina
- Coronary revascularization procedures

Secondary Prevention of Cardiovascular Events

Lovastatin is also indicated to slow the progression of coronary atherosclerosis in patients with coronary heart disease as part of a treatment strategy to lower TC and LDL-C to target levels.

Table 3. HDL-C mean percent change from baseline

Week	ADVICOR			NIASPAN			Lovastatin		
	n*	Dose (mg/mg)	HDL	n*	Dose (mg)	HDL	n*	Dose (mg)	HDL
Baseline	57	-	45 mg/dL	61	-	47 mg/dL	61	-	43 mg/dL
12	47	1000/20	+20%	46	1000	+14%	56	20	+3%
16	45	1000/40	+20%	44	1000	+15%	56	40	+5%
20	42	1500/40	+27%	43	1500	+22%	54	40	+6%
28	42	2000/40	+30%	41	2000	+24%	53	40	+6%

*n = number of patients remaining in the trial at each timepoint

Table 4. TG median percent change from baseline

Week	ADVICOR			NIASPAN			Lovastatin		
	n*	Dose (mg/mg)	TG	n*	Dose (mg)	TG	n*	Dose (mg)	TG
Baseline	57	-	174 mg/dL	61	-	186 mg/dL	61	-	171 mg/dL
12	47	1000/20	-32%	46	1000	-22%	56	20	-20%
16	45	1000/40	-39%	44	1000	-23%	56	40	-17%
20	42	1500/40	-44%	43	1500	-31%	54	40	-21%
28	42	2000/40	-44%	41	2000	-31%	53	40	-20%

*n = number of patients remaining in the trial at each timepoint

Table 5. Lp(a) median percent change from baseline

Week	ADVICOR			NIASPAN			Lovastatin		
	n*	Dose (mg/mg)	Lp(a)	n*	Dose (mg)	Lp(a)	n*	Dose (mg)	Lp(a)
Baseline	57	-	34 mg/dL	61	-	41 mg/dL	60	-	42 mg/dL
12	47	1000/20	-9%	46	1000	-8%	55	20	+8%
16	45	1000/40	-9%	44	1000	-12%	55	40	+8%
20	42	1500/40	-17%	43	1500	-22%	53	40	+6%
28	42	2000/40	-22%	41	2000	-32%	52	40	0%

*n = number of patients remaining in the trial at each timepoint

The National Cholesterol Education Program (NCEP) Treatment Guidelines are summarized below:

Table 6. Classification of Hyperlipoproteinemias

Type	Lipoproteins Elevated	Lipid Elevations Major	Minor
I (rare)	Chylomicrons	TG	↑→TC
IIa	LDL	TC	-
IIb	LDL, VLDL	TC	TG
III (rare)	IDL	TC/TG	-
IV	VLDL	TG	↑→TC
V (rare)	Chylomicrons, VLDL	TG	↑→TC

TC = total cholesterol; TG = triglycerides; LDL = low-density lipoprotein; VLDL = very low-density lipoprotein; IDL = intermediate-density lipoprotein ↑→ = increased or no change

General Recommendations

Prior to initiating therapy with a lipid-lowering agent, secondary causes for hypercholesterolemia (e.g., poorly controlled diabetes mellitus, hypothyroidism, nephrotic syndrome, dysproteinemias, obstructive liver disease, other drug therapy, alcoholism) should be excluded, and a lipid profile performed to measure TC, HDL-C, and TG. For patients with TG < 400 mg/dL, LDL-C can be estimated using the following equation:

$$LDL-C = TC - [(0.20 \times TG) + HDL-C]$$

For TG levels > 400 mg/dL, this equation is less accurate and LDL-C concentrations should be determined by ultracentrifugation. Lipid determinations should be performed at intervals of no less than 4 weeks and dosage adjusted according to the patient's response to therapy. The NCEP Treatment Guidelines are summarized in Table 7.
[See table 7 at bottom of next page]
After the LDL-C goal has been achieved, if the TG is still ≥200 mg/dL, non-HDL-C (TC minus HDL-C) becomes a secondary target of therapy. Non-HDL-C goals are set 30 mg/dL higher than LDL-C goals for each risk category.

CONTRAINDICATIONS

ADVICOR is contraindicated in patients with a known hypersensitivity to niacin, lovastatin or any component of this medication, active liver disease or unexplained persistent elevations in serum transaminases (see WARNINGS), active peptic ulcer disease, or arterial bleeding.

Pregnancy and lactation—Atherosclerosis is a chronic process and the discontinuation of lipid-lowering drugs during pregnancy should have little impact on the outcome of long-term therapy of primary hypercholesterolemia. Moreover, cholesterol and other products of the cholesterol biosynthesis pathway are essential components for fetal development, including synthesis of steroids and cell membranes. Because of the ability of inhibitors of HMG-CoA reductase, such as lovastatin, to decrease the synthesis of cholesterol and possibly other products of the cholesterol biosynthesis pathway, ADVICOR is contraindicated in women who are pregnant and in lactating mothers. ADVICOR may cause fetal harm when administered to pregnant women. ADVICOR should be administered to women of childbearing age only when such patients are highly unlikely to conceive. If the patient becomes pregnant while taking this drug, ADVICOR should be discontinued immediately and the patient should be apprised of the potential hazard to the fetus (see PRECAUTIONS, Pregnancy).

WARNINGS

ADVICOR should not be substituted for equivalent doses of immediate-release (crystalline) niacin. For patients switching from immediate-release niacin to NIASPAN, therapy with NIASPAN should be initiated with low doses (i.e., 500 mg once daily at bedtime) and the NIASPAN dose should then be titrated to the desired therapeutic response (see DOSAGE AND ADMINISTRATION).

Liver Dysfunction

Cases of severe hepatic toxicity, including fulminant hepatic necrosis, have occurred in patients who have substituted sustained-release (modified-release, timed-release) niacin products for immediate-release (crystalline) niacin at equivalent doses.

ADVICOR should be used with caution in patients who consume substantial quantities of alcohol and/or have a past history of liver disease. Active liver disease or unexplained transaminase elevations are contraindications to the use of ADVICOR.

Niacin preparations and lovastatin preparations have been associated with abnormal liver tests. In studies using NIASPAN alone, 0.8% of patients were discontinued for transaminase elevations. In studies using lovastatin alone, 0.2% of patients were discontinued for transaminase elevations.[4] In three safety and efficacy studies involving titration to final daily ADVICOR doses ranging from 500 mg/10 mg to 2500 mg/40 mg, ten of 1028 patients (1.0%) experienced reversible elevations in AST/ALT to more than 3 times the upper limit of normal (ULN). Three of ten elevations occurred at doses outside the recommended dosing limit of 2000 mg/40 mg; no patient receiving 1000 mg/20 mg had 3-fold elevations in AST/ALT.

In clinical studies with ADVICOR, elevations in transaminases did not appear to be related to treatment duration; elevations in AST and ALT levels did appear to be dose related. Transaminase elevations were reversible upon discontinuation of ADVICOR.

Liver function tests should be performed on all patients during therapy with ADVICOR. Serum transaminase levels, including AST and ALT (SGOT and SGPT), should be monitored before treatment begins, every 6 to 12 weeks for the first 6 months, and periodically thereafter (e.g., at approximately 6-month intervals). Special attention should be paid to patients who develop elevated serum transaminase levels, and in these patients, measurements should be repeated promptly and, if confirmed, then performed more frequently. If the transaminase levels show evidence of progression, particularly if they rise to 3 times ULN and are persistent, or if they are associated with symptoms of nausea, fever, and/or malaise, the drug should be discontinued.

Skeletal Muscle

Lovastatin

Lovastatin and other inhibitors of HMG-CoA reductase occasionally cause myopathy, which is manifested as muscle pain or weakness associated with grossly elevated creatine kinase (> 10 times ULN). **Rhabdomyolysis, with or without acute renal failure secondary to myoglobinuria, has been reported rarely and can occur at any time.** In a large, long-term, clinical safety and efficacy study (the EXCEL study)[5,6] with lovastatin, myopathy occurred in up to 0.2% of patients treated with lovastatin 20 to 80 mg for up to 2 years. When drug treatment was interrupted or discontinued in these patients, muscle symptoms and creatine kinase (CK) increases promptly resolved. The risk of myopathy is increased by concomitant therapy with certain drugs, some of which were excluded by the EXCEL study design.

Potent inhibitors of CYP3A4: The risk of myopathy appears to be increased by high levels of HMG-CoA reductase inhibitory activity in plasma. Lovastatin is metabolized by the cytochrome P450 isoform 3A4. Certain drugs which share this metabolic pathway can raise the plasma levels of lovastatin and may increase the risk of myopathy. These include cyclosporine, itraconazole, ketoconazole and other antifungal azoles, the macrolide antibiotics erythromycin and clarithromycin, and the ketolide antibiotic telithromycin, HIV protease inhibitors, the antidepressant nefazodone, or large quantities of grapefruit juice (>1 quart daily).

ADVICOR

Myopathy and/or rhabdomyolysis have been reported when lovastatin is used in combination with lipid-altering doses (≥ 1g/day) of niacin. Physicians contemplating the use of ADVICOR, a combination of lovastatin and niacin, should weigh the potential benefits and risks, and should carefully monitor patients for any signs and symptoms of muscle pain, tenderness, or weakness, particularly during the initial month of treatment or during any period of upward dosage titration of either drug. Periodic CK determinations may be considered in such situations, but there is no assurance that such monitoring will prevent myopathy.

In clinical studies, no cases of rhabdomyolysis and one suspected case of myopathy have been reported in 1079 patients who were treated with ADVICOR at doses up to 2000 mg/40 mg for periods up to 2 years.

Patients starting therapy with ADVICOR should be advised of the risk of myopathy, and told to report promptly unexplained muscle pain, tenderness, or weakness. A CK level above 10 times ULN in a patient with unexplained muscle symptoms indicates myopathy. ADVICOR therapy should be discontinued if myopathy is diagnosed or suspected.

In patients with complicated medical histories predisposing to rhabdomyolysis, such as preexisting renal insufficiency, dose escalation requires caution. Also, as there are no known adverse consequences of brief interruption of therapy, treatment with ADVICOR should be stopped for a few days before elective major surgery and when any major acute medical or surgical condition supervenes.

Use of ADVICOR with other Drugs

Gemfibrozil, particularly with higher doses of lovastatin: The incidence and severity of myopathy may be increased by concomitant administration of ADVICOR with drugs that can cause myopathy when given alone, such as gemfibrozil and other fibrates. The dose of lovastatin should not exceed 20 mg daily in patients receiving concomitant medication with gemfibrozil.

The use of ADVICOR in combination with fibrates should be avoided unless the benefit of further alterations in lipid levels is likely to outweigh the increased risk of this drug combination.

Cyclosporine or danazol, with higher doses of lovastatin: In patients taking concomitant cyclosporine, danazol or fibrates, the dose of ADVICOR should generally not exceed 1000 mg/20 mg (see DOSAGE AND ADMINISTRATION), as the risk of myopathy may increase at higher doses. Interruption of ADVICOR therapy during a course of treatment with a systemic antifungal azole or a macrolide antibiotic, or a ketolide antibiotic should be considered.

PRECAUTIONS

General

Before instituting therapy with a lipid-altering medication, an attempt should be made to control dyslipidemia with appropriate diet, exercise, and weight reduction in obese patients, and to treat other underlying medical problems (see **INDICATIONS AND USAGE**).

Patients with a past history of jaundice, hepatobiliary disease, or peptic ulcer should be observed closely during ADVICOR therapy. Frequent monitoring of liver function tests and blood glucose should be performed to ascertain that the drug is producing no adverse effects on these organ systems.

Diabetic patients may experience a dose-related rise in fasting blood sugar (FBS). In three clinical studies, which included 1028 patients exposed to ADVICOR (6 to 22% of whom had diabetes type II at baseline), increases in FBS above normal occurred in 46 to 65% of patients at any time during study treatment with ADVICOR. Fourteen patients (1.4%) were discontinued from study treatment: 3 patients for worsening diabetes, 10 patients for hyperglycemia and 1 patient for a new diagnosis of diabetes. In the studies in which lovastatin and NIASPAN were used as active controls, 24 to 41% of patients receiving lovastatin and 43 to 58% of patients receiving NIASPAN also had increases in FBS above normal. One patient (1.1%) receiving lovastatin was discontinued for hyperglycemia. Diabetic or potentially

diabetic patients should be observed closely during treatment with ADVICOR, and adjustment of diet and/or hypoglycemic therapy may be necessary.

In one long-term study of 106 patients treated with ADVICOR, elevations in prothrombin time (PT) >3 times ULN occurred in 2 patients (2%) during study drug treatment. In a long-term study of 814 patients treated with ADVICOR, 7 patients were noted to have platelet counts <100,000 during study drug treatment. Four of these patients were discontinued, and one patient with a platelet count <100,000 had prolonged bleeding after a tooth extraction. Prior studies have shown that NIASPAN can be associated with dose-related reductions in platelet count (mean of −11% with 2000 mg) and increases of PT (mean of approximately +4%). Accordingly, patients undergoing surgery should be carefully evaluated. In controlled studies, ADVICOR has been associated with small but statistically significant dose-related reductions in phosphorus levels (mean of ~10% with 2000 mg/40 mg). Phosphorus levels should be monitored periodically in patients at risk for hypophosphatemia. In clinical studies with ADVICOR, hypophosphatemia was more common in males than in females. The clinical relevance of hypophosphatemia in this population is not known.

Niacin

Caution should also be used when ADVICOR is used in patients with unstable angina or in the acute phase of MI, particularly when such patients are also receiving vasoactive drugs such as nitrates, calcium channel blockers, or adrenergic blocking agents.

Elevated uric acid levels have occurred with niacin therapy; therefore, in patients predisposed to gout, niacin therapy should be used with caution. Niacin is rapidly metabolized by the liver, and excreted through the kidneys. ADVICOR is contraindicated in patients with significant or unexplained hepatic dysfunction (see **CONTRAINDICATIONS** and **WARNINGS**) and should be used with caution in patients with renal dysfunction.

Lovastatin

Lovastatin may elevate creatine phosphokinase and transaminase levels (see **WARNINGS** and **ADVERSE REACTIONS**). This should be considered in the differential diagnosis of chest pain in a patient on therapy with lovastatin. *Endocrine function*—HMG-CoA reductase inhibitors interfere with cholesterol synthesis and as such might theoretically blunt adrenal and/or gonadal steroid production. Results of clinical studies with drugs in this class have been inconsistent with regard to drug effects on basal and reserve steroid levels. However, clinical studies have shown that lovastatin does not reduce basal plasma cortisol concentration or impair adrenal reserve, and does not reduce basal plasma testosterone concentration. Another HMG-CoA reductase inhibitor has been shown to reduce the plasma testosterone response to human chorionic gonadotropin (HCG). In the same study, the mean testosterone response to HCG was slightly but not significantly reduced after treatment with lovastatin 40 mg daily for 16 weeks in 21 men. The effects of HMG-CoA reductase inhibitors on male fertility have not been studied in adequate numbers of male patients. The effects, if any, on the pituitary-gonadal axis in premenopausal women are unknown. Patients treated with lovastatin who develop clinical evidence of endocrine dysfunction should be evaluated appropriately. Caution should also be exercised if an HMG-CoA reductase inhibitor or other agent used to lower cholesterol levels is administered to patients also receiving other drugs (e.g., ketoconazole, spironolactone, cimetidine) that may decrease the levels or activity of endogenous steroid hormones.

CNS toxicity—Lovastatin produced optic nerve degeneration (Wallerian degeneration of retinogeniculate fibers) in clinically normal dogs in a dose-dependent fashion starting at 60 mg/kg/day, a dose that produced mean plasma drug levels about 30 times higher than the mean drug level in humans taking the highest recommended dose (as measured by total enzyme inhibitory activity). Vestibulocochlear Wallerian-like degeneration and retinal ganglion cell chromatolysis were also seen in dogs treated for 14 weeks at 180 mg/kg/day, a dose which resulted in a mean plasma drug level (C_{max}) similar to that seen with the 60 mg/kg/day dose.

CNS vascular lesions, characterized by perivascular hemorrhage and edema, mononuclear cell infiltration of perivascular spaces, perivascular fibrin deposits and necrosis of small vessels, were seen in dogs treated with lovastatin at a dose of 180 mg/kg/day, a dose which produced plasma drug levels (C_{max}) which were about 30 times higher than the mean values in humans taking 80 mg/day.

Table 7. NCEP Treatment Guidelines: LDL-C Goals and Cutpoints for Therapeutic Lifestyle Changes and Drug Therapy in Different Risk Categories

Risk Category	LDL Goal (mg/dL)	LDL Level at Which to Initiate Therapeutic Lifestyle Changes (mg/dL)	LDL Level at Which to Consider Drug Therapy (mg/dL)
CHD[†] or CHD risk equivalents (10-year risk >20%)	< 100	≥ 100	≥ 130 (100-129:drug optional)[††]
2+ Risk factors (10-year risk ≤20%)	< 130	≥ 130	10-year risk 10%-20%: ≥ 130 / 10-year risk <10%: ≥ 160
0-1 Risk factors[†††]	< 160	≥ 160	≥ 190 (160-189: LDL-lowering drug optional)

† CHD, coronary heart disease

†† Some authorities recommend use of LDL-lowering drugs in this category if an LDL-C level of <100 mg/dL cannot be achieved by therapeutic lifestyle changes. Others prefer use of drugs that primarily modify triglycerides and HDL-C, e.g., nicotinic acid or fibrate. Clinical judgement also may call for deferring drug therapy in this subcategory.

††† Almost all people with 0-1 risk factor have 10-year risk <10%; thus, 10-year risk assessment in people with 0-1 risk factor is not necessary.

Information on the Abbott Pharmaceutical Products listed on these pages is from the prescribing information in use as of June 1, 2010. For more information, please visit rxabbott.com or call 1-800-633-9110.

Similar optic nerve and CNS vascular lesions have been observed with other drugs of this class.

Cataracts were seen in dogs treated with lovastatin for 11 and 28 weeks at 180 mg/kg/day and 1 year at 60 mg/kg/day.

Information for Patients

Patients should be advised of the following:

- to report promptly unexplained muscle pain, tenderness, or weakness (see **WARNINGS, Skeletal Muscle**);
- to take ADVICOR at bedtime, with a low-fat snack. Administration on an empty stomach is not recommended;
- to carefully follow the prescribed dosing regimen (see **DOSAGE AND ADMINISTRATION**);
- that flushing is a common side effect of niacin therapy that usually subsides after several weeks of consistent niacin use. Flushing may last for several hours after dosing, may vary in severity, and will, by taking ADVICOR at bedtime, most likely occur during sleep. If awakened by flushing, especially if taking antihypertensives, rise slowly to minimize the potential for dizziness and/or syncope;
- that taking aspirin (up to approximately 30 minutes before taking ADVICOR) may minimize flushing;
- to avoid ingestion of alcohol, hot beverages and spicy foods around the time of ADVICOR administration, to minimize flushing;
- should not be administered with grapefruit juice;
- that if ADVICOR therapy is discontinued for an extended length of time, their physician should be contacted prior to re-starting therapy; re-titration is recommended (see **DOSAGE AND ADMINISTRATION**);
- to notify their physician if they are taking vitamins or other nutritional supplements containing niacin or related compounds such as nicotinamide (see **Drug Interactions**);
- to notify their physician if symptoms of dizziness occur;
- if diabetic, to notify their physician of changes in blood glucose;
- that ADVICOR tablets should not be broken, crushed, or chewed, but should be swallowed whole.

Drug Interactions

Niacin

Antihypertensive Therapy—Niacin may potentiate the effects of ganglionic blocking agents and vasoactive drugs resulting in postural hypotension.

Aspirin: Concomitant aspirin may decrease the metabolic clearance of niacin. The clinical relevance of this finding is unclear.

Bile Acid Sequestrants—An *in vitro* study was carried out investigating the niacin-binding capacity of colestipol and cholestyramine. About 98% of available niacin was bound to colestipol, with 10 to 30% binding to cholestyramine. These results suggest that 4 to 6 hours, or as great an interval as possible, should elapse between the ingestion of bile acid-binding resins and the administration of ADVICOR.

Other—Concomitant alcohol or hot drinks may increase the side effects of flushing and pruritus and should be avoided around the time of ADVICOR ingestion. Vitamins or other nutritional supplements containing large doses of niacin or related compounds such as nicotinamide may potentiate the adverse effects of ADVICOR.

Lovastatin

Serious skeletal muscle disorders, e.g., rhabdomyolysis, have been reported during concomitant therapy of lovastatin or other HMG-CoA reductase inhibitors with cyclosporine, danazol, itraconazole, ketoconazole, gemfibrozil, niacin, erythromycin, clarithromycin, telithromycin, nefazodone or HIV protease inhibitors. (See **WARNINGS, Skeletal Muscle**).

Coumarin Anticoagulants—In a small clinical study in which lovastatin was administered to warfarin-treated patients, no effect on PT was detected. However, another HMG-CoA reductase inhibitor has been found to produce a less than two seconds increase in PT in healthy volunteers receiving low doses of warfarin. Also, bleeding and/or increased PT have been reported in a few patients taking coumarin anticoagulants concomitantly with lovastatin. It is recommended that in patients taking anticoagulants, PT be determined before starting ADVICOR and frequently enough during early therapy to insure that no significant alteration of PT occurs. Once a stable PT has been documented, PT can be monitored at the intervals usually recommended for patients on coumarin anticoagulants. If the dose of ADVICOR is changed, the same procedure should be repeated.

Antipyrine—Lovastatin had no effect on the pharmacokinetics of antipyrine or its metabolites. However, since lovastatin is metabolized by the cytochrome P450 isoform 3A4 enzyme system, this does not preclude an interaction with other drugs metabolized by the same isoform.

Propranolol—In normal volunteers, there was no clinically significant pharmacokinetic or pharmacodynamic interaction with concomitant administration of single doses of lovastatin and propranolol.

Digoxin—In patients with hypercholesterolemia, concomitant administration of lovastatin and digoxin resulted in no effect on digoxin plasma concentrations.

Oral Hypoglycemic Agents—In pharmacokinetic studies of lovastatin in hypercholesterolemic, non-insulin dependent diabetic patients, there was no drug interaction with glipizide or with chlorpropamide.

Drug/Laboratory Test Interactions

Niacin may produce false elevations in some fluorometric determinations of plasma or urinary catecholamines. Niacin may also give false-positive reactions with cupric sulfate solution (Benedict's reagent) in urine glucose tests.

Carcinogenesis, Mutagenesis, Impairment of Fertility

No studies have been conducted with ADVICOR regarding carcinogenesis, mutagenesis, or impairment of fertility.

Niacin

Niacin, administered to mice for a lifetime as a 1% solution in drinking water, was not carcinogenic. The mice in this study received approximately 6 to 8 times a human dose of 3000 mg/day as determined on a mg/m[2] basis. Niacin was negative for mutagenicity in the Ames test. No studies on impairment of fertility have been performed.

Lovastatin

In a 21-month carcinogenic study in mice, there was a statistically significant increase in the incidence of hepatocellular carcinomas and adenomas in both males and females at 500 mg/kg/day. This dose produced a total plasma drug exposure 3 to 4 times that of humans given the highest recommended dose of lovastatin (drug exposure was measured as total HMG-CoA reductase inhibitory activity in extracted plasma). Tumor increases were not seen at 20 and 100 mg/kg/day, doses that produced drug exposures of 0.3 to 2 times that of humans at the 80 mg/day dose. A statistically significant increase in pulmonary adenomas was seen in female mice at approximately 4 times the human drug exposure. (Although mice were given 300 times the human dose on a mg/kg body weight basis, plasma levels of total inhibitory activity were only 4 times higher in mice than in humans given 80 mg of lovastatin.)

There was an increase in incidence of papilloma in the non-glandular mucosa of the stomach of mice beginning at exposures of 1 to 2 times that of humans. The glandular mucosa was not affected. The human stomach contains only glandular mucosa.

In a 24-month carcinogenicity study in rats, there was a positive dose-response relationship for hepatocellular carcinogenicity in males at drug exposures between 2 to 7 times that of human exposure at 80 mg/day (doses in rats were 5, 30, and 180 mg/kg/day).

An increased incidence of thyroid neoplasms in rats appears to be a response that has been seen with other HMG-CoA reductase inhibitors.

A drug in this class chemically similar to lovastatin was administered to mice for 72 weeks at 25, 100, and 400 mg/kg body weight, which resulted in mean serum drug levels approximately 3, 15, and 33 times higher than the mean human serum drug concentration (as total inhibitory activity) after a 40 mg oral dose. Liver carcinomas were significantly increased in high-dose females and mid- and high-dose males, with a maximum incidence of 90% in males. The incidence of adenomas of the liver was significantly increased in mid- and high-dose females. Drug treatment also significantly increased the incidence of lung adenomas in mid- and high-dose males and females. Adenomas of the Harderian gland (a gland of the eye of rodents) were significantly higher in high-dose mice than in controls.

No evidence of mutagenicity was observed in a microbial mutagen test using mutant strains of *Salmonella typhimurium* with or without rat or mouse liver metabolic activation. In addition, no evidence of damage to genetic material was noted in an *in vitro* alkaline elution assay using rat or mouse hepatocytes, a V-79 mammalian cell forward mutation study, an *in vitro* chromosome aberration study in CHO cells, or an *in vivo* chromosomal aberration assay in mouse bone marrow.

Drug-related testicular atrophy, decreased spermatogenesis, spermatocytic degeneration and giant cell formation were seen in dogs starting at 20 mg/kg/day. Similar findings were seen with another drug in this class. No drug-related effects on fertility were found in studies with lovastatin in rats. However, in studies with a similar drug in this class, there was decreased fertility in male rats treated for 34 weeks at 25 mg/kg body weight, although this effect was not observed in a subsequent fertility study when this same dose was administered for 11 weeks (the entire cycle of spermatogenesis, including epididymal maturation). In rats treated with this same reductase inhibitor at 180 mg/kg/day, seminiferous tubule degeneration (necrosis and loss of spermatogenic epithelium) was observed. No microscopic changes were observed in the testes from rats of either study. The clinical significance of these findings is unclear.

Pregnancy

Pregnancy Category X— See **CONTRAINDICATIONS**.

ADVICOR should be administered to women of childbearing potential only when such patients are highly unlikely to conceive and have been informed of the potential hazard. Safety in pregnant women has not been established and there is no apparent benefit to therapy with ADVICOR during pregnancy (see **CONTRAINDICATIONS**). Treatment should be immediately discontinued as soon as pregnancy is recognized.

Niacin

Animal reproduction studies have not been conducted with niacin or with ADVICOR. It is also not known whether niacin at doses typically used for lipid disorders can cause fetal harm when administered to pregnant women or whether it can affect reproductive capacity. If a woman receiving niacin or ADVICOR for primary hypercholesterolemia (Types IIa or IIb) becomes pregnant, the drug should be discontinued.

Lovastatin

Rare reports of congenital anomalies have been received following intrauterine exposure to HMG-CoA reductase inhibitors. In a review[7] of approximately 100 prospectively followed pregnancies in women exposed to lovastatin or another structurally related HMG-CoA reductase inhibitor, the incidences of congenital anomalies, spontaneous abortions and fetal deaths/stillbirths did not exceed what would be expected in the general population. The number of cases is adequate only to exclude a 3- to 4-fold increase in congenital anomalies over the background incidence. In 89% of the prospectively followed pregnancies, drug treatment was initiated prior to pregnancy and was discontinued at some point in the first trimester when pregnancy was identified. Lovastatin has been shown to produce skeletal malformations at plasma levels 40 times the human exposure (for mouse fetus) and 80 times the human exposure (for rat fetus) based on mg/m[2] surface area (doses were 800 mg/kg/day). No drug-induced changes were seen in either species at multiples of 8 times (rat) or 4 times (mouse) based on surface area. No evidence of malformations was noted in rabbits at exposures up to 3 times the human exposure (dose of 15 mg/kg/day, highest tolerated dose).

Labor and Delivery

No studies have been conducted on the effect of ADVICOR, niacin or lovastatin on the mother or the fetus during labor or delivery, on the duration of labor or delivery, or on the growth, development, and functional maturation of the child.

Nursing Mothers

No studies have been conducted with ADVICOR in nursing mothers.

Because of the potential for serious adverse reactions in nursing infants from lipid-altering doses of niacin and lovastatin (see **CONTRAINDICATIONS**), ADVICOR should not be taken while a woman is breastfeeding. Niacin has been reported to be excreted in human milk. It is not known whether lovastatin is excreted in human milk. A small amount of another drug in this class is excreted in human breast milk.

Pediatric Use

No studies in patients under 18 years-of-age have been conducted with ADVICOR. Because pediatric patients are not likely to benefit from cholesterol lowering for at least a decade and because experience with this drug or its active ingredients is limited, treatment of pediatric patients with ADVICOR is not recommended at this time.

Geriatric Use

Of the 214 patients who received ADVICOR in double-blind clinical studies, 37.4% were 65 years-of-age and older, and of the 814 patients who received ADVICOR in open-label clinical studies, 36.2% were 65 years-of-age and older. Responses in LDL-C, HDL-C, and TG were similar in geriatric patients. No overall differences in the percentage of patients with adverse events were observed between older and younger patients. No overall differences were observed in selected chemistry values between the two groups except for amylase which was higher in older patients.

ADVERSE REACTIONS

Overview

In controlled clinical studies, 40/214 (19%) of patients randomized to ADVICOR discontinued therapy prior to study completion. Of the 214 patients enrolled 18 (8%) discontinued due to flushing. In the same controlled studies, 9/94 (10%) of patients randomized to lovastatin and 19/92 (21%) of patients randomized to NIASPAN also discontinued treatment prior to study completion secondary to adverse events. Flushing episodes (i.e., warmth, redness, itching and/or tingling) were the most common treatment-emergent adverse events, and occurred in 53% to 83% of patients treated with ADVICOR. Spontaneous reports with NIASPAN and clinical studies with ADVICOR suggest that flushing may also be accompanied by symptoms of dizziness or syncope, tachycardia, palpitations, shortness of breath, sweating, burning sensation/skin burning sensation, chills, and/or edema.

Adverse Reactions Information

Because clinical studies are conducted under widely varying conditions, adverse reaction rates observed in clinical studies of a drug cannot be directly compared to rates in the clinical studies of another drug and may not reflect the rates observed in clinical practice. The adverse reaction information from clinical studies does, however provide a basis for identifying the adverse events that appear to be related to drug use and for approximating rates.

The data described in this section reflect the exposure to ADVICOR in two double-blind, controlled clinical studies of 400 patients. The population was 28 to 86 years-of-age, 54% male, 85% Caucasian, 9% Black, and 7% Other, and had mixed dyslipidemia (Frederickson Types IIa and IIb).

In addition to flushing, other adverse events occurring in 5% or greater of patients treated with ADVICOR are shown in Table 8 below.

[See table 8 at right]

The following adverse events have also been reported with niacin, lovastatin, and/or other HMG-CoA reductase inhibitors, but not necessarily with ADVICOR, either during clinical studies or in routine patient management.

Body as a Whole:	chest pain; abdominal pain; edema; chills; malaise
Cardiovascular:	atrial fibrillation; tachycardia; palpitations, and other cardiac arrhythmias; postural hypotension, orthostasis; hypotension; syncope
Eye:	toxic amblyopia; cystoid macular edema; ophthalmoplegia; eye irritation, blurred vision
Gastrointestinal:	activation of peptic ulcers and peptic ulceration; dyspepsia; vomiting; anorexia; constipation; flatulence, pancreatitis; hepatitis; fatty change in liver; jaundice; and rarely, cirrhosis, fulminant hepatic necrosis, and hepatoma, eructation
Metabolic:	gout, decreased glucose tolerance
Musculoskeletal:	muscle cramps; myopathy; rhabdomyolysis; arthralgia, myalgia
Nervous:	dizziness; insomnia; dry mouth; paresthesia; anxiety; tremor; vertigo; memory loss; peripheral neuropathy; psychic disturbances; dysfunction of certain cranial nerves, nervousness, burning sensation/skin burning sensation
Skin:	hyper-pigmentation; acanthosis nigricans; urticaria; alopecia; dry skin; sweating; and a variety of skin changes (e.g., nodules, discoloration, dryness of mucous membranes, changes to hair/nails), vesiculobullous rash, maculopapular rash
Respiratory:	dyspnea; rhinitis
Urogenital:	gynecomastia; loss of libido; erectile dysfunction
Hypersensitivity reactions:	An apparent hypersensitivity syndrome has been reported rarely, which has included one or more of the following features: anaphylaxis, angioedema, tongue edema, larynx edema, face edema, peripheral edema, laryngismus, lupus erythematous-like syndrome, polymyalgia rheumatica, vasculitis, purpura, thrombocytopenia, leukopenia, hemolytic anemia, positive ANA, ESR increase, eosinophilia, arthritis, arthralgia, urticaria, asthenia, photosensitivity, fever, chills, flushing, malaise, dyspnea, toxic epidermal necrolysis, erythema multiforme, including Stevens-Johnson syndrome
Other:	migraine

Clinical Laboratory Abnormalities

Chemistry

Elevations in serum transaminases (see **WARNINGS - Liver Dysfunction**), CPK and fasting glucose, and reductions in phosphorus. Niacin extended-release tablets have been associated with slight elevations in LDH, uric acid, total bilirubin, amylase and creatine kinase. Lovastatin and/or

Table 8. Treatment-Emergent Adverse Events in ≥ 5% of Patients
(Events Irrespective of Causality; Data from Controlled, Double-Blind Studies)

Adverse Event	ADVICOR	NIASPAN	Lovastatin
Total Number of Patients	214	92	94
Cardiovascular	**163 (76%)**	**66 (72%)**	**24 (26%)**
Flushing	152 (71%)	60 (65%)	17 (18%)
Body as a Whole	**104 (49%)**	**50 (54%)**	**42 (45%)**
Asthenia	10 (5%)	6 (7%)	5 (5%)
Flu Syndrome	12 (6%)	7 (8%)	4 (4%)
Headache	20 (9%)	12 (13%)	5 (5%)
Infection	43 (20%)	14 (15%)	19 (20%)
Pain	18 (8%)	3 (3%)	9 (10%)
Pain, Abdominal	9 (4%)	1 (1%)	6 (6%)
Pain, Back	10 (5%)	5 (5%)	5 (5%)
Digestive System	**51 (24%)**	**26 (28%)**	**16 (17%)**
Diarrhea	13 (6%)	8 (9%)	2 (2%)
Dyspepsia	6 (3%)	5 (5%)	4 (4%)
Nausea	14 (7%)	11 (12%)	2 (2%)
Vomiting	7 (3%)	5 (5%)	0
Metabolic and Nutrit. System	**37 (17%)**	**18 (20%)**	**13 (14%)**
Hyperglycemia	8 (4%)	6 (7%)	6 (6%)
Musculoskeletal System	**19 (9%)**	**9 (10%)**	**17 (18%)**
Myalgia	6 (3%)	5 (5%)	8 (9%)
Skin and Appendages	**38 (18%)**	**19 (21%)**	**11 (12%)**
Pruritus	14 (7%)	7 (8%)	3 (3%)
Rash	11 (5%)	11 (12%)	3 (3%)

Note: Percentages are calculated from the total number of patients in each column.

HMG-CoA reductase inhibitors have been associated with elevations in alkaline phosphatase, γ-glutamyl transpeptidase and bilirubin, and thyroid function abnormalities.

Hematology

Niacin extended-release tablets have been associated with slight reductions in platelet counts and prolongation in PT (see **WARNINGS**).

DRUG ABUSE AND DEPENDENCE

Neither niacin nor lovastatin is a narcotic drug. ADVICOR has no known addiction potential in humans.

OVERDOSAGE

Information on acute overdose with ADVICOR in humans is limited. Until further experience is obtained, no specific treatment of overdose with ADVICOR can be recommended. The patient should be carefully observed and given supportive treatment.

Niacin

The s.c. LD50 of niacin is 5 g/kg in rats.

The signs and symptoms of an acute overdose of niacin can be anticipated to be those of excessive pharmacologic effect: severe flushing, nausea/vomiting, diarrhea, dyspepsia, dizziness, syncope, hypotension, possibly cardiac arrhythmias and clinical laboratory abnormalities. Insufficient information is available on the potential for the dialyzability of niacin.

Lovastatin

After oral administration of lovastatin to mice the median lethal dose observed was >15 g/m^2.

Five healthy human volunteers have received up to 200 mg of lovastatin as a single dose without clinically significant adverse experiences. A few cases of accidental overdose have been reported; no patients had any specific symptoms, and all patients recovered without sequelae. The maximum dose taken was 5 to 6 g. The dialyzability of lovastatin and its metabolites in man is not known at present.

DOSAGE AND ADMINISTRATION

The patient should be placed on a standard cholesterol-lowering diet before receiving ADVICOR or its individual active components and should continue on this diet during treatment with lipid-altering therapy (see NCEP Treatment Guidelines for details on dietary therapy).

ADVICOR

ADVICOR should be taken at bedtime, with a low-fat snack. ADVICOR tablets should be taken whole and should not be broken, crushed, or chewed before swallowing. Patients not currently on NIASPAN must start ADVICOR at the lowest initial ADVICOR dose, a single 500 mg/20 mg tablet once daily at bedtime. The dose of ADVICOR should not be increased by more than 500 mg daily (based on the NIASPAN component) every 4 weeks. The dose of ADVICOR should be individualized based on targeted goals for cholesterol and triglycerides, and on patient response. Doses of ADVICOR greater than 2000 mg/40 mg daily are not recommended. If ADVICOR therapy is discontinued for an extended period (>7 days), reinstitution of therapy should begin with the lowest dose of ADVICOR.

Flushing of the skin (see **ADVERSE REACTIONS**) may be reduced in frequency or severity by pretreatment with aspirin up to the recommended dose of 325 mg (taken up to approximately 30 minutes prior to ADVICOR dose). Flushing,

pruritus, and gastrointestinal distress are also greatly reduced by slowly increasing the dose of niacin and avoiding administration on an empty stomach.

Equivalent doses of ADVICOR may be substituted for equivalent doses of NIASPAN but should not be substituted for other modified-release (sustained-release or time-release) niacin preparations or immediate-release (crystalline) niacin preparations (see WARNINGS). Patients previously receiving niacin products other than NIASPAN should be started on NIASPAN with the recommended NIASPAN titration schedule, and the dose should subsequently be individualized based on patient response. A relative bioavailability study results indicated that ADVICOR tablet strengths (i.e. two tablets of 500 mg/20 mg and one tablet of 1000 mg/40 mg) are not interchangeable.

NIASPAN

NIASPAN should be taken at bedtime, after a low-fat snack, and doses should be individualized according to patient response. Therapy with NIASPAN must be initiated at 500 mg qhs in order to reduce the incidence and severity of side effects which may occur during early therapy. NIASPAN must be titrated and the dose should not be increased by more than 500 mg every 4 weeks up to a maximum dose of 2000 mg a day. The recommended dose escalation is shown in Table 9 below. Patients already receiving a stable dose of NIASPAN may be switched directly to a niacin-equivalent dose of ADVICOR.

[See table 9 at top of next page]

Maintenance Dose:

The daily dosage of NIASPAN should not be increased by more than 500 mg in any 4-week period. The recommended maintenance dose is 1000 mg (two 500 mg tablets) to 2000 mg (two 1000 mg tablets or four 500 mg tablets) once daily at bedtime. Doses greater than 2000 mg daily are not recommended. Women may respond at lower NIASPAN doses than men.

Flushing of the skin (see **ADVERSE REACTIONS**) may be reduced in frequency or severity by pretreatment with aspirin up to the recommended dose of 325 mg (taken 30 minutes prior to NIASPAN dose). Tolerance to this flushing develops rapidly over the course of several weeks. Flushing, pruritus, and gastrointestinal distress are also greatly reduced by slowly increasing the dose of niacin and avoiding administration on an empty stomach. Concomitant alcoholic, hot drinks or spicy foods may increase the side effects of flushing and pruritus and should be avoided around the time of ADVICOR ingestion.

Equivalent doses of NIASPAN should **not** be substituted for sustained-release (modified-release, timed-release) niacin preparations or immediate-release (crystalline) niacin (see **WARNINGS**). Patients previously receiving other niacin products should be started with the recommended NIASPAN titration schedule (see Table 9), and the dose should subsequently be individualized based on patient re-

---

Information on the Abbott Pharmaceutical Products listed on these pages is from the prescribing information in use as of June 1, 2010. For more information, please visit rxabbott.com or call 1-800-633-9110.

Table 9. Recommended Dosing

	Week(s)	Daily dose	NIASPAN Dosage
INITIAL TITRATION SCHEDULE	1 to 4	500 mg	1 NIASPAN 500 mg tablet at bedtime
	5 to 8	1000 mg	2 NIASPAN 500 mg tablets at bedtime
	*	1500 mg	2 NIASPAN 750 mg tablets or 3 NIASPAN 500 mg tablets at bedtime
	*	2000 mg	2 NIASPAN 1000 mg tablets or 4 NIASPAN 500 mg tablets at bedtime

*After Week 8, titrate to patient response and tolerance. If response to 1000 mg daily is inadequate, increase dose to 1500 mg daily; may subsequently increase dose to 2000 mg daily. Daily dose should not be increased more than 500 mg in a 4-week period, and doses above 2000 mg daily are not recommended. Women may respond at lower doses than men.

sponse. Single-dose bioavailability studies have demonstrated that NIASPAN tablet strengths are not interchangeable.

If NIASPAN therapy is discontinued for an extended period, reinstitution of therapy should include a titration phase (see Table 9).

NIASPAN tablets should be taken whole and should not be broken, crushed or chewed before swallowing.

Concomitant Therapy

Concomitant Therapy with Lovastatin

Patients already receiving a stable dose of lovastatin who require further TG-lowering or HDL-raising (e.g., to achieve NCEP non-HDL-C goals), may receive concomitant dosage titration with NIASPAN per NIASPAN recommended initial titration schedule (see Table 9, **DOSAGE AND ADMINISTRATION** section). For patients already receiving a stable dose of NIASPAN who require further LDL-lowering (e.g., to achieve NCEP LDL-C goals; Table 7), the usual recommended starting dose of lovastatin is 20 mg once a day. Dose adjustments should be made at intervals of 4 weeks or more. Combination therapy with NIASPAN and lovastatin should not exceed doses of 2000 mg and 40 mg daily, respectively.

Dosage in Patients with Renal or Hepatic Insufficiency

Use of NIASPAN in patients with renal or hepatic insufficiency has not been studied. NIASPAN is contraindicated in patients with significant or unexplained hepatic dysfunction (see **WARNINGS, PRECAUTIONS**). NIASPAN should be used with caution in patients with renal insufficiency (see **CLINICAL PHARMACOLOGY**).

Lovastatin

The usual recommended starting dose is 20 mg once a day given with the evening meal. The recommended dosing range is 10-80 mg/day in single or two divided doses; the maximum recommended dose is 80 mg/day. Doses should be individualized according to the recommended goal of therapy (see NCEP Guidelines and **CLINICAL PHARMACOLOGY**). Patients requiring reductions in LDL cholesterol of 20% or more to achieve their goal (see **INDICATIONS AND USAGE**) should be started on 20 mg/day of lovastatin. A starting dose of 10 mg may be considered for patients requiring smaller reductions. Adjustments should be made at intervals of 4 weeks or more.

Cholesterol levels should be monitored periodically and consideration should be given to reducing the dosage of lovastatin if cholesterol levels fall significantly below the targeted range.

Dosage in Patients taking Cyclosporine or Danazol

In patients taking cyclosporine or danazol concomitantly with lovastatin (see **WARNINGS, Myopathy/Rhabdomyolysis**), therapy should begin with 10 mg of lovastatin and should not exceed 20 mg/day.

Dosage in Patients taking Amiodarone or Verapamil

In patients taking amiodarone or verapamil concomitantly with lovastatin, the dose should not exceed 40 mg/day (see **WARNINGS, Myopathy/Rhabdomyolysis** and **PRECAUTIONS, Drug Interactions, Other drug interactions**).

Dosage in Patients with Renal Insufficiency

In patients with severe renal insufficiency (creatinine clearance <30 mL/min), dosage increases above 20 mg/day should be carefully considered and, if deemed necessary, implemented cautiously (see **CLINICAL PHARMACOLOGY** and **WARNINGS, Myopathy/Rhabdomyolysis**).

HOW SUPPLIED

ADVICOR is an unscored capsule-shaped tablet containing either 500, 750, or 1000 mg of extended-release niacin, and 20 mg of immediate-release lovastatin (ADVICOR 500 mg/20 mg, 750 mg/20 mg, 1000 mg/20 mg), or 1000 mg

of extended-release niacin and 40 mg of immediate-release lovastatin (ADVICOR 1000 mg/40 mg). Tablets are color-coated and printed with the Abbott "ᗡ" logo and a code number specific to the tablet strength on the same side. ADVICOR 500 mg/20 mg tablets are light yellow, code "502". ADVICOR 750 mg/20 mg tablets are light orange, code "752". ADVICOR 1000 mg/20 mg tablets are dark pink/light purple, code "1002". ADVICOR 1000 mg/40 mg tablets are reddish brown, code "1004." Tablets are supplied in bottles of 90 tablets as shown below.

500 mg/20 mg tablets: bottles of 90-NDC# 0074-3005-90
750 mg/20 mg tablets: bottles of 90-NDC# 0074-3072-90
1000 mg/20 mg tablets: bottles of 90-NDC# 0074-3007-90
1000 mg/40 mg tablets: bottles of 90-NDC# 0074-3010-90
Store at room temperature (20° to 25°C or 68° to 77°F).

NIASPAN is a registered trademark of Abbott Laboratories, and Mevacor is a registered trademark of Merck & Co., Inc.

REFERENCES

1. Executive Summary of the Third Report of the National Cholesterol Education Program (NCEP) Expert Panel on Detection, Evaluation, and Treatment of High Blood Cholesterol in Adults (Adult Treatment Panel III). *JAMA* 2001; 285:2486-2497.
2. Nikkila EA. In: *The Metabolic Basis of Inherited Disease*, 5th ed., Chap 30, 622-642, 1983.
3. Grundy SM, et al. *Circulation* 2004; 110:227-239.
4. Downs JR, et al. *JAMA* 1998; 279:1615-1622.
5. Bradford RH, et al. *Arch Intern Med* 1991;151:43-49.
6. Bradford RH, et al. *Am J Cardiol* 1994; 74:667-673.
7. Manson JM, et al. *Reprod Toxicol* 1996; 10(6): 439-446.

Manufactured by Abbott Pharmaceuticals PR Ltd., Barceloneta, PR 00617
for Abbott Laboratories, North Chicago, IL 60064, U.S.A.
© 2010 Abbott Laboratories
U.S. Patent Nos. 6,080,428; 6,129,930; 6,406,715 B1; 6,676,967; 6,746,691; 6,818,229; 7,011,848; and other patents pending.
Ref. 03-A331-Revised February, 2010
Shown in Product Identification Guide, page 303

AZMACORT®   ℞
[ăz-mă-kŏrt]
(triamcinolone acetonide)
Inhalation Aerosol
Rx only
For Oral Inhalation Only
Shake Well Before Using

DESCRIPTION

Triamcinolone acetonide, USP, the active ingredient in **Azmacort®** Inhalation Aerosol, is a corticosteroid with a molecular weight of 434.5 and with the chemical designation 9-Fluoro-11β,16α,17,21-tetrahydroxypregna-1,4-diene-3,20-dione cyclic 16,17-acetal with acetone. ($C_{24}H_{31}FO_6$).

Azmacort Inhalation Aerosol is a metered-dose aerosol unit containing a microcrystalline suspension of triamcinolone acetonide in the propellant dichlorodifluoromethane and dehydrated alcohol USP 1% w/w. Each canister contains 60 mg

triamcinolone acetonide. The canister must be primed prior to the first use. After an initial priming of 2 actuations, each actuation delivers 200 mcg triamcinolone acetonide from the valve and 75 mcg from the spacer-mouthpiece under defined *in vitro* test conditions. The canister will remain primed for 3 days. If the canister is not used for more than 3 days, then it should be reprimed with 2 actuations. There are at least 240 actuations in one **Azmacort** Inhalation Aerosol canister. **After 240 actuations, the amount delivered per actuation may not be consistent and the unit should be discarded.**

CLINICAL PHARMACOLOGY

Triamcinolone acetonide is a more potent derivative of triamcinolone. Although triamcinolone itself is approximately one to two times as potent as prednisone in animal models of inflammation, triamcinolone acetonide is approximately 8 times more potent than prednisone.

The precise mechanism of the action of glucocorticoids in asthma is unknown. However, the inhaled route makes it possible to provide effective local anti-inflammatory activity with reduced systemic corticosteroid effects. Though highly effective for asthma, glucocorticoids do not affect asthma symptoms immediately. While improvement in asthma may occur as soon as one week after initiation of **Azmacort** Inhalation Aerosol therapy, maximum improvement may not be achieved for 2 weeks or longer.

Based upon intravenous dosing of triamcinolone acetonide phosphate ester, the half-life of triamcinolone acetonide was reported to be 88 minutes. The volume of distribution (Vd) reported was 99.5 L (SD ± 27.5) and clearance was 45.2 L/hour (SD ± 9.1) for triamcinolone acetonide. The plasma half-life of glucocorticoids does not correlate well with the biologic half-life.

The pharmacokinetics of radiolabeled triamcinolone acetonide [14C] were evaluated following a single oral dose of 800 mcg to healthy male volunteers. Radiolabeled triamcinolone acetonide was found to undergo relatively rapid absorption following oral administration with maximum plasma triamcinolone acetonide and [14C]-derived radioactivity occurring between 1.5 and 2 hours. Plasma protein binding of triamcinolone acetonide appears to be relatively low and consistent over a wide plasma triamcinolone acetonide concentration range as a function of time. The overall mean percent fraction bound was approximately 68%.

The metabolism and excretion of triamcinolone acetonide were both rapid and extensive with no parent compound being detected in the plasma after 24 hours post-dose and a low ratio (10.6%) of parent compound $AUC_{0-\infty}$ to total [14C] radioactivity $AUC_{0-\infty}$. Greater than 90% of the oral [14C]-radioactive dose was recovered within 5 days after administration in 5 out of the 6 subjects in the study. Of the recovered [14C]-radioactivity, approximately 40% and 60% were found in the urine and feces, respectively.

Three metabolites of triamcinolone acetonide have been identified. They are 6β-hydroxytriamcinolone acetonide, 21-carboxytriamcinolone acetonide and 21-carboxy-6β-hydroxytriamcinolone acetonide. All three metabolites are expected to be substantially less active than the parent compound due to (a) the dependence of anti-inflammatory activity on the presence of a 21-hydroxyl group, (b) the decreased activity observed upon 6-hydroxylation, and (c) the markedly increased water solubility favoring rapid elimination. There appeared to be some quantitative differences in the metabolites among species. No differences were detected in metabolic pattern as a function of route of administration.

CLINICAL TRIALS

Double-blind, placebo-controlled efficacy and safety studies have been conducted in asthma patients with a range of asthma severities, from those patients with mild disease to those with severe disease requiring oral steroid therapy. The efficacy and safety of **Azmacort** Inhalation Aerosol given twice daily was demonstrated in two placebo-controlled clinical trials. In two separate studies, 222 asthmatic patients were randomized to receive either **Azmacort** Inhalation Aerosol 300 mcg twice daily or matching placebo for a treatment period of 6 weeks. Patients were adult asthmatics who were using inhaled beta₂-agonists on more than an occasional basis (at least three times weekly), either without or with inhaled corticosteroids, for control of their asthma symptoms. For the combined studies, 48% (52/109) patients randomized to placebo and 41% (46/113) patients randomized to **Azmacort** Inhalation Aerosol treatment were previously treated with inhaled corticosteroids.

Results of weekly lung function tests (FEV_1) from one of these trials is presented graphically below. Results of the second study are presented in tabular form as the changes in asthma measures from baseline to the end of the treatment period.

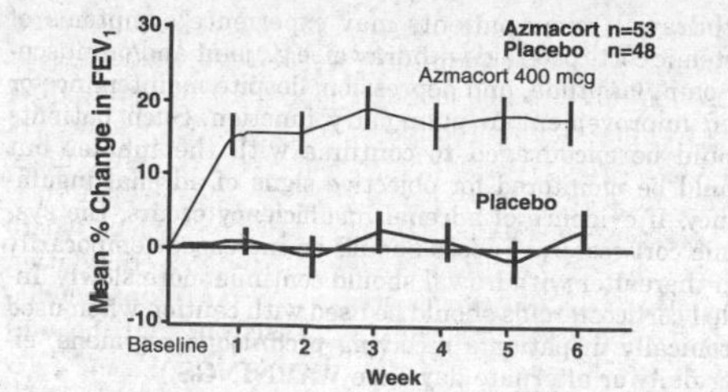

Mean Changes in Asthma Measures from Baseline to Endpoint[a] All-Treated Patients Results from a Placebo-Controlled, 6 Week Study

Asthma Measure	Placebo (N=61)	Azmacort 300 mcg bid (N=60)
Percent Change in FEV_1(%)	2.8%	17.5%
Increase in Morning Peak Flow Rate (L/min)	6.7	45.9
Decrease in Albuterol Use (puffs/day)	0.6	3.4
Decrease in Daily Asthma Symptom Score (units/day)[b]	0.5	2.3

[a] Endpoint results are obtained from the last evaluable data, regardless of whether the patient completed 6 weeks of treatment

[b] Scale (0-6) with 0 = no symptom: Maximum Score (AM + PM) = 12

In both studies, treatment with **Azmacort** Inhalation Aerosol (300 mcg twice daily) resulted in significant improvements in all clinical asthma measures (lung functions, asthma symptoms, use of as-needed $beta_2$-agonist medications) when compared to placebo.

INDICATIONS

Azmacort Inhalation Aerosol is indicated in the maintenance treatment of asthma as prophylactic therapy.
Azmacort Inhalation Aerosol is also indicated for asthma patients who require systemic corticosteroid administration, where adding **Azmacort** may reduce or eliminate the need for the systemic corticosteroids.
Azmacort Inhalation Aerosol is NOT indicated for the relief of acute bronchospasm.

CONTRAINDICATIONS

Azmacort Inhalation Aerosol is contraindicated in the primary treatment of status asthmaticus or other acute episodes of asthma where intensive measures are required.
Hypersensitivity to triamcinolone acetonide or any of the other ingredients in this preparation contraindicates its use.

WARNINGS

Particular care is needed in patients who are transferred from systemically active corticosteroids to **Azmacort** Inhalation Aerosol because deaths due to adrenal insufficiency have occurred in asthmatic patients during and after transfer from systemic corticosteroids to aerosolized steroids in recommended doses. After withdrawal from systemic corticosteroids, a number of months is usually required for recovery of hypothalamic-pituitary-adrenal (HPA) function. For some patients who have received large doses of oral steroids for long periods of time before therapy with **Azmacort** Inhalation Aerosol is initiated, recovery may be delayed for one year or longer. During this period of HPA suppression, patients may exhibit signs and symptoms of adrenal insufficiency when exposed to trauma, surgery, or infections, particularly gastroenteritis or other conditions with acute electrolyte loss. Although **Azmacort** Inhalation Aerosol may provide control of asthmatic symptoms during these episodes, in recommended doses it supplies only normal physiological amounts of corticosteroid systemically and does NOT provide the increased systemic steroid which is necessary for coping with these emergencies.
During periods of stress or a severe asthmatic attack, patients who have been recently withdrawn from systemic corticosteroids should be instructed to resume systemic steroids (in large doses) immediately and to contact their physician for further instruction. These patients should also be instructed to carry a warning card indicating that they may need supplementary systemic steroids during periods of stress or a severe asthma attack.
Localized infections with *Candida albicans* have occurred infrequently in the mouth and pharynx. These areas should be examined by the treating physician at each patient visit. The percentage of positive mouth and throat cultures for *Candida albicans* did not change during a year of continuous therapy. The incidence of clinically apparent infection is low (2.5%). These infections may disappear spontaneously or may require treatment with appropriate antifungal therapy or discontinuance of treatment with **Azmacort** Inhalation Aerosol.
Children who are on immunosuppressant drugs are more susceptible to infections than healthy children. Chickenpox and measles, for example, can have a more serious or even fatal course in children on immunosuppressant doses of corticosteroids. In such children, or in adults who have not had these diseases, particular care should be taken to avoid exposure. If exposed, therapy with varicella zoster immune globulin (VZIG) or pooled intravenous immunoglobulin (IVIG), as appropriate, may be indicated. If chickenpox develops, treatment with antiviral agents may be considered.
Azmacort Inhalation Aerosol is not to be regarded as a bronchodilator and is not indicated for rapid relief of bronchospasm.
As with other inhaled asthma medications, bronchospasm may occur with an immediate increase in wheezing following dosing. If bronchospasm occurs following use of **Azmacort** Inhalation Aerosol, it should be treated immediately with a fast-acting inhaled bronchodilator. Treatment with **Azmacort** Inhalation Aerosol should be discontinued and alternative treatment should be instituted.
Patients should be instructed to contact their physician immediately when episodes of asthma which are not responsive to bronchodilators occur during the course of treatment with **Azmacort** Inhalation Aerosol. During such episodes, patients may require therapy with systemic corticosteroids.
The use of **Azmacort** Inhalation Aerosol with systemic prednisone, dosed either daily or on alternate days, could increase the likelihood of HPA suppression compared to a therapeutic dose of either one alone. Therefore, **Azmacort** Inhalation Aerosol should be used with caution in patients already receiving prednisone treatment for any disease.
Transfer of patients from systemic steroid therapy to **Azmacort** Inhalation Aerosol may unmask allergic conditions previously suppressed by the systemic steroid therapy, e.g., rhinitis, conjunctivitis, and eczema.

PRECAUTIONS

Orally inhaled corticosteroids may cause a reduction in growth velocity when administered to pediatric patients (see **PRECAUTIONS, Pediatric Use**). Because of the possibility of systemic absorption of inhaled corticosteroids, patients treated with these drugs should be observed carefully for any evidence of systemic corticosteroid effects including suppression of growth in children. Particular care should be taken in observing patients postoperatively or during periods of stress for evidence of a decrease in adrenal function.
During withdrawal from oral steroids, some patients may experience symptoms of systemically active steroid withdrawal, e.g., joint and/or muscular pain, lassitude, and depression, despite maintenance or even improvement of respiratory function. (See **DOSAGE AND ADMINISTRATION**.) Although steroid withdrawal effects are usually transient and not severe, severe and even fatal exacerbation of asthma can occur if the previous daily oral corticosteroid requirement had significantly exceeded 10 mg/day of prednisone or equivalent.
In responsive patients, inhaled corticosteroids will often permit control of asthmatic symptoms with less suppression of HPA function than therapeutically equivalent oral doses of prednisone. Since triamcinolone acetonide is absorbed into the circulation and can be systemically active, the beneficial effects of **Azmacort** Inhalation Aerosol in minimizing or preventing HPA dysfunction may be expected only when recommended dosages are not exceeded.
Suppression of HPA function has been reported in volunteers who received 4000 mcg daily of triamcinolone acetonide by oral inhalation. In addition, suppression of HPA function has been reported in some patients who have received recommended doses for as little as 6 to 12 weeks. Since the response of HPA function to inhaled corticosteroids is highly individualized, the physician should consider this information when treating patients.
When used at excessive doses or at recommended doses in a small number of susceptible individuals, systemic corticosteroid effects such as hypercorticoidism and adrenal suppression may appear. If such changes occur, **Azmacort®** Inhalation Aerosol should be discontinued slowly, consistent with accepted procedures for reducing systemic steroid therapy and for management of asthma symptoms.
Azmacort Inhalation Aerosol should be used with caution, if at all, in patients with active or quiescent tuberculosis infection of the respiratory tract; untreated systemic fungal, bacterial, parasitic, or viral infections; or ocular herpes simplex.
The long-term local and systemic effects of **Azmacort** Inhalation Aerosol in human subjects are still not fully known. While there has been no clinical evidence of adverse experiences, the effects resulting from chronic use of **Azmacort** Inhalation Aerosol on developmental or immunologic processes in the mouth, pharynx, trachea, and lung are unknown.

Information for Patients: Patients being treated with **Azmacort** Inhalation Aerosol should receive the following information and instructions. This information is intended to aid them in the safe and effective use of this medication. It is not a complete disclosure of all possible adverse or intended effects.
Patients should use **Azmacort** Inhalation Aerosol at regular intervals as directed. Results of clinical trials indicate that significant improvement in asthma may occur by 1 week, but maximum benefit may not be achieved for 2 weeks or more. The patient should not increase the prescribed dosage but should contact the physician if symptoms do not improve or if the condition worsens.
In clinical studies and post-marketing experience with **Azmacort** Inhalation Aerosol, local infections of the oropharynx with *Candida albicans* have occurred. When such an infection develops, it should be treated with appropriate local or systemic (i.e., oral antifungal) therapy while remaining on treatment with **Azmacort** Inhalation Aerosol. However, at times therapy with **Azmacort** Inhalation Aerosol may need to be interrupted.
Patients should be instructed to track their use of **Azmacort** Inhalation Aerosol and to dispose of the canister after 240 actuations since reliable dose delivery cannot be assured after 240 doses.
Patients who are on immunosuppressant doses of corticosteroids should be warned to avoid exposure to chickenpox or measles and, if exposed, to obtain medical advice.

Carcinogenesis, Mutagenesis, Impairment of Fertility: No evidence of treatment-related carcinogenicity was demonstrated after two years of once daily gavage of triamcinolone acetonide at doses of 0.05, 0.2, and 1.0 mcg/kg (approximately 0.02, 0.07, and 0.4% of the maximum recommended human daily inhalation dose on a mcg/m^2 basis) in the rat and 0.1, 0.6, and 3.0 mcg/kg (approximately 0.02, 0.1, and 0.6% of the maximum recommended human daily inhalation dose on a mcg/m^2 basis) in a mouse.
Mutagenesis studies with triamcinolone acetonide have not been carried out.
No evidence of impaired fertility was manifested when oral doses of up to 15.0 mcg/kg (8% of the maximum recommended human daily inhalation dose on a mcg/m^2 basis) were administered to female and male rats. However, triamcinolone acetonide at oral doses of 8 mcg/kg (approximately 4% of the maximum recommended human daily inhalation dose on a mcg/m^2 basis) caused dystocia and prolonged delivery and at oral doses of 5.0 mcg/kg (approximately 2.5% of the maximum recommended human daily inhalation dose on a mcg/m^2 basis) and above caused increases in fetal resorptions and stillbirths and decreases in pup body weight and survival. At a lower dose of 1.0 mcg/kg (approximately 0.5% of the maximum recommended human daily inhalation dose on a mcg/m^2 basis) it did not induce the above mentioned effects.

Pregnancy: Pregnancy Category C. Triamcinolone acetonide has been shown to be teratogenic at inhalational doses of 20, 40, and 80 mcg/kg in rats (approximately 0.1, 0.2, and 0.4 times the maximum recommended human daily inhalation dose on a mcg/m^2 basis, respectively), in rabbits at the same doses (approximately 0.2, 0.4, and 0.8 times the maximum recommended human daily inhalation dose on a mcg/m^2 basis, respectively) and in monkeys, at an inhalational dose of 500 mcg/kg (approximately 5 times the maximum recommended human daily inhalation dose on a mcg/m^2 basis). Dose related teratogenic effects in rats and rabbits included cleft palate and/or internal hydrocephaly and axial skeletal defects whereas the teratogenic effects observed in the monkey were CNS and/or cranial malformations. There are no adequate and well controlled studies in pregnant women. Triamcinolone acetonide should be used during pregnancy only if the potential benefit justifies the potential risk to the fetus.
Experience with oral glucocorticoids since their introduction in pharmacologic as opposed to physiologic doses suggests that rodents are more prone to teratogenic effects from glucocorticoids than humans. In addition, because there is a natural increase in glucocorticoid production during pregnancy, most women will require a lower exogenous steroid dose and many will not need glucocorticoid treatment during pregnancy.

Nonteratogenic Effects: Hypoadrenalism may occur in infants born of mothers receiving corticosteroids during pregnancy. Such infants should be carefully observed.

Information on the Abbott Pharmaceutical Products listed on these pages is from the prescribing information in use as of June 1, 2010. For more information, please visit rxabbott.com or call 1-800-633-9110.

Nursing Mothers: It is not known whether triamcinolone acetonide is excreted in human milk. Because other corticosteroids are excreted in human milk, caution should be exercised when **Azmacort** Inhalation Aerosol is administered to nursing women.

Pediatric Use: Safety and effectiveness have not been established in pediatric patients below the age of 6.

Controlled clinical studies have shown that orally inhaled corticosteroids may cause a reduction in growth velocity in pediatric patients. In these studies, the mean reduction in growth velocity was approximately one centimeter (cm) per year (range 0.3 to 1.8 cm per year; 0.12 to 0.71 inches) and appears to depend upon dose and duration of exposure. [The specific growth effects of **Azmacort** have also been studied in a controlled clinical trial (see data below)]. This effect was observed in the absence of laboratory evidence of hypothalamic-pituitary-adrenal (HPA) axis suppression, suggesting that growth velocity is a more sensitive indicator of systemic corticosteroid exposure in pediatric patients than some commonly used tests of HPA axis function.

To assess if **Azmacort** has an effect on growth, a one-year, randomized, open-label study of pre-pubescent boys and girls ages 6-11 with moderate to severe asthma was conducted. Children with moderate asthma were randomized to a nonsteroidal treatment or to **Azmacort**, children with severe asthma to **Azmacort** plus prednisone or just prednisone alone. A sex and age matched group of healthy non-asthmatic children was also included. The average daily dose of **Azmacort** was 400 mcg (range 75 to 1600 mcg/day, dose adjustments were permitted). Non-asthmatic children (mean 8.2 years) grew 5.93 cm/year (n=96). In the moderate asthma groups, the **Azmacort** children (mean 8.2 years) grew 5.34 cm/year (n=101) and the nonsteroidal children (mean 8.5 years) grew 6.13 cm/year (n=95). In the severe groups, the **Azmacort** plus prednisone children (mean 8.2 years) grew 5.46 cm/year (n=33) and the prednisone only children (mean 8.0 years) grew 5.59 cm/year (n=31). Due to low enrollment in the severe patient groups, there was insufficient power to interpret the statistical analyses on these groups.

The long-term effects of this reduction in growth velocity associated with orally inhaled corticosteroids, including the impact on final adult height, are unknown. The potential for "catch up" growth following discontinuation of treatment with orally inhaled corticosteroids has not been adequately studied. The growth of children and adolescents receiving orally inhaled corticosteroids, including **Azmacort**, should be monitored routinely (e.g. via stadiometry). The potential growth effects of prolonged treatment should be weighed against the clinical benefits obtained and the risk associated with alternative therapies. To minimize the systemic effects of orally inhaled corticosteroids, including **Azmacort**, each patient should be titrated to the lowest dose that effectively controls his/her symptoms.

Geriatric Use: Clinical studies of **Azmacort** Inhalation Aerosol did not include sufficient numbers of subjects aged 65 and over to determine whether they respond differently from younger subjects. Other reported clinical experience has not identified differences in responses between the elderly and younger patients. In general, dose selection for an elderly patient should be cautious, usually starting at the low end of the dosing range, reflecting the greater frequency of decreased hepatic, renal, or cardiac function, and of concomitant disease or other drug therapy.

ADVERSE REACTIONS

The table below describes the incidence of common adverse experiences based upon three placebo-controlled, multicenter US clinical trials of 507 patients (297 female and 210 male adults (age range 18-64)). These trials included asthma patients who had previously received inhaled beta₂-agonists alone, as well as those who previously required inhaled corticosteroid therapy for the control of their asthma. The patients were treated with **Azmacort** Inhalation Aerosol (including doses ranging from 150 to 600 mcg twice daily for 6 weeks) or placebo.

Adverse Events Occurring at an Incidence of Greater Than 3% and Greater Than Placebo

Adverse Event	Azmacort Dose 150 mcg bid (n=57)	Azmacort Dose 300 mcg bid (n=170)	Azmacort Dose 600 mcg bid (n=57)	Placebo (n=167)
Sinusitis	5 (9%)	7 (4%)	1 (2%)	6 (4%)
Pharyngitis	4 (7%)	42 (25%)	10 (18%)	19 (11%)
Headache	4 (7%)	35 (21%)	7 (12%)	24 (14%)
Flu Syndrome	2 (4%)	8 (5%)	1 (2%)	5 (3%)
Back Pain	2 (4%)	3 (2%)	2 (4%)	3 (2%)

Adverse events that occurred at an incidence of 1-3% in the overall **Azmacort** Inhalation Aerosol treatment group and greater than placebo included:

Body as a whole: facial edema, pain, abdominal pain, photosensitivity

Digestive system: diarrhea, oral monilia, toothache, vomiting

Metabolic and Nutrition: weight gain

Musculoskeletal system: bursitis, myalgia, tenosynovitis

Nervous system: dry mouth

Organs of special sense: rash

Respiratory system: chest congestion, voice alteration

Urogenital system: cystitis, urinary tract infection, vaginal monilia

In older controlled clinical trials of steroid dependent asthmatics, urticaria was reported rarely. Anaphylaxis was not reported in these controlled trials. Typical steroid withdrawal effects including muscle aches, joint aches, and fatigue were noted in clinical trials when patients were transferred from oral steroid therapy to **Azmacort** Inhalation Aerosol. Easy bruisability was also noted in these trials. Hoarseness, dry throat, irritated throat, dry mouth, facial edema, increased wheezing, and cough have been reported. These adverse effects have generally been mild and transient. Cases of oral candidiasis occurring with clinical use have been reported. (See **WARNINGS**.) Cases of growth suppression have been reported for orally inhaled corticosteroids (see **PRECAUTIONS, Pediatric Use** section).

Post Marketing: In addition to adverse events reported from clinical trials, the following events have been identified during post approval use of **Azmacort** Inhalation Aerosol where these events were reported voluntarily from a population of unknown size, and the frequency of occurrence cannot be determined precisely. These include rare reports of anaphylaxis, cataracts, glaucoma and very rare reports of bone mineral density loss and osteoporosis, especially with prolonged use, which may lead to an increased risk of fractures.

OVERDOSAGE

There are no data available on the effects of acute or chronic overdose. However, acute overdosing with **Azmacort** Inhalation Aerosol is unlikely in view of the total amount of active ingredient present and the route of administration. The maximum total daily dose (1200 mcg) has been well tolerated when administered as a single dose of 16 consecutive inhalations to adult asthmatics in a controlled clinical trial. Chronic overdosage may result in signs/symptoms of hypercorticoidism. (See **PRECAUTIONS**.) The risk of candidiasis could also be increased.

DOSAGE AND ADMINISTRATION

Adults: The usual recommended dosage is two inhalations (150 mcg) given three to four times a day or four inhalations (300 mcg) given twice daily. The maximal daily intake should not exceed 16 inhalations (1200 mcg) in adults. Higher initial doses (12 to 16 inhalations per day) may be considered in patients with more severe asthma.

Children 6 to 12 Years of Age: The usual recommended dosage is one or two inhalations (75 to 150 mcg) given three to four times a day or two to four inhalations (150 to 300 mcg) given twice daily. The maximal daily intake should not exceed 12 inhalations (900 mcg) in children 6 to 12 years of age. Insufficient clinical data exist with respect to the safety and efficacy of the administration of **Azmacort** Inhalation Aerosol to children below the age of 6. The long-term effects of inhaled steroids, including **Azmacort** Inhalation Aerosol, on growth are still not fully known. Rinsing the mouth after inhalation is advised.

Different considerations must be given to the following groups of patients in order to obtain the full therapeutic benefit of **Azmacort** Inhalation Aerosol:

Note: In all patients, it is desirable to titrate to the lowest effective dose once asthma stability has been achieved.

Patients Not Receiving Systemic Corticosteroids: Patients who require maintenance therapy of their asthma may benefit from treatment with **Azmacort** Inhalation Aerosol at the doses recommended above. In patients who respond to **Azmacort** Inhalation Aerosol, improvement in pulmonary function is usually apparent within one to two weeks after the initiation of therapy.

Patients Maintained on Systemic Corticosteroids: Clinical studies have shown that **Azmacort** Inhalation Aerosol may be effective in the management of asthmatics dependent or maintained on systemic corticosteroids and may permit replacement or significant reduction in the dosage of systemic corticosteroids.

The patient's asthma should be reasonably stable before treatment with **Azmacort** Inhalation Aerosol is started. Initially, **Azmacort** Inhalation Aerosol should be used concurrently with the patient's usual maintenance dose of systemic corticosteroid. After approximately one week, gradual withdrawal of the systemic corticosteroid is started by reducing the daily or alternate daily dose. Reductions may be made after an interval of one or two weeks, depending on the response of the patient. A slow rate of withdrawal is strongly recommended. Generally, these decrements should not exceed 2.5 mg of prednisone or its equivalent. During

withdrawal, some patients may experience symptoms of systemic corticosteroid withdrawal, e.g., joint and/or muscular pain, lassitude, and depression, despite maintenance or even improvement in pulmonary function. Such patients should be encouraged to continue with the inhaler but should be monitored for objective signs of adrenal insufficiency. If evidence of adrenal insufficiency occurs, the systemic corticosteroid doses should be increased temporarily and thereafter withdrawal should continue more slowly. Inhaled corticosteroids should be used with caution when used chronically in patients receiving prednisone regimens, either daily or alternate day. (See **WARNINGS**.)

During periods of stress or a severe asthma attack, transfer patients may require supplementary treatment with systemic corticosteroids.

Directions for Use: An illustrated leaflet of patient instructions for proper use accompanies each package of **Azmacort** Inhalation Aerosol.

HOW SUPPLIED

Azmacort Inhalation Aerosol contains 60 mg triamcinolone acetonide in a 20 gram package which delivers at least 240 actuations. It is supplied with a white plastic actuator, a white plastic spacer-mouthpiece and patient's leaflet of instructions: box of one. NDC 0074–3014–60. Each actuation delivers 200 mcg triamcinolone acetonide from the valve and 75 mcg from the spacer-mouthpiece under defined *in vitro* test conditions.

Avoid spraying in eyes.

For best results, the canister should be at room temperature before use.

Shake well before using.

CONTENTS UNDER PRESSURE. Do not puncture. Do not use or store near heat or open flame. Exposure to temperatures above 120°F may cause bursting. Never throw canister into fire or incinerator. Keep out of reach of children unless otherwise prescribed. Store at Controlled Room Temperature 20 to 25°C (68 to 77°F) [see USP].

Note: The indented statement below is required by the Federal government's Clean Air Act for all products containing or manufactured with chlorofluorocarbons (CFCs):

WARNING: Contains CFC-12, a substance which harms public health and the environment by destroying ozone in the upper atmosphere.

A notice similar to the above WARNING has been placed in the "Information For The Patient" portion of this package insert under the Environmental Protection Agency's (EPA's) regulations. The patient's warning states that the patient should consult his or her physician if there are questions about alternatives.

©2007 Abbott Laboratories
Ref: 03-A020-R1
Rev. September, 2007
Manufactured for:
Abbott Laboratories
North Chicago, IL 60064 U.S.A.

INFORMATION FOR THE PATIENT

Your Guide to the
Azmacort®
(triamcinolone acetonide)
Inhalation Aerosol
Special Delivery System
Ref: 03-A020-R1
Rev. September, 2007
Rx Only

Your doctor has prescribed **Azmacort®** (triamcinolone acetonide) Inhalation Aerosol to help control your asthma. Your **Azmacort** Inhalation Aerosol is one of the most efficient and easy-to-use devices available to help you take your prescribed medication. Used properly, it will effectively and reliably relieve your asthma symptoms.

To receive the maximum benefit, **it is very important that you carefully read and follow all the instructions contained in this booklet** for the daily use and care of your **Azmacort** Inhalation Aerosol.

IMPORTANT NOTE: If you've used other metered-dose inhalers before, you may expect the **Azmacort** Inhalation Aerosol to deliver a noticeable "blast" of medication into your mouth.

Your AZMACORT Inhalation Aerosol, however, is designed to provide a gentle mist, not a "blast," when used.

This gentle action makes it possible for your medication to be more effectively delivered into the passageways to your lungs, with very little left to linger in your mouth. In fact, you may not even feel the medication entering your mouth, but rest assured, that is how the **Azmacort** Inhalation Aerosol works.

IMPORTANT: Please read all instructions in this guide carefully before using your **Azmacort** Inhalation Aerosol.

BEFORE STARTING TO TAKE THIS MEDICINE, TELL YOUR DOCTOR:
• If you are pregnant or intending to become pregnant.
• If you are breast-feeding a baby.

- If you are allergic to **Azmacort** Inhalation Aerosol or any other orally inhaled glucocorticoid.
- If you are taking other medications. In some circumstances, this medication may not be suitable and your doctor may wish to give you a different medicine.

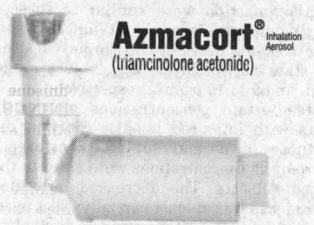

Azmacort® Inhalation Aerosol
(triamcinolone acetonide)

PREPARE YOUR AZMACORT INHALATION AEROSOL INHALER FOR USE

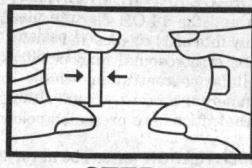

STEP 1

1. Line up the arrows on the inhaler.

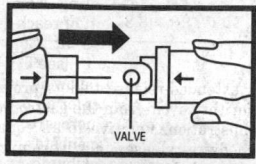

VALVE

STEP 2

2. Gently pull the inhaler to its fully extended position. You will see the valve (small hole) where the medication will come out.

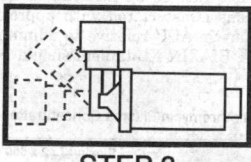

STEP 3

3. Adjust the inhaler into an "L" shape. It is hinged to swing in one direction only.

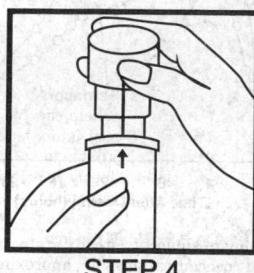

STEP 4

4. The ridge on the top part of the inhaler should fit into the notch on the bottom part.

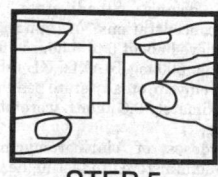

STEP 5

5. Remove the mouthpiece cap. To prepare your **Azmacort** Inhalation Aerosol for use, the inhaler must be primed prior to the first use. To prime, hold the inhaler upright, with the mouthpiece facing away from you. Shake the inhaler gently, then press the canister firmly and quickly. Repeat this procedure again so a total of 2 puffs are released. Your **Azmacort** Inhalation Aerosol is now ready for use. Repriming is only necessary when your inhaler has not been used for more than 3 days. To reprime, shake the inhaler and release one puff. Repeat this procedure again so a total of two puffs are released.

USING YOUR AZMACORT INHALATION AEROSOL INHALER

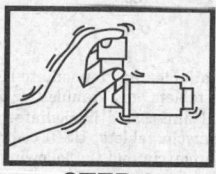

STEP 6

6. The metal **Azmacort** canister has already been inserted into the inhaler. Once you have opened the inhaler, shake it well before each use. **IMPORTANT: You must shake the inhaler each and every time before inhaling the medication.** If your doctor has instructed you to take more than one breath of medication at a time, **you must shake the inhaler EACH TIME before each inhalation of medication, NOT JUST ONCE.**

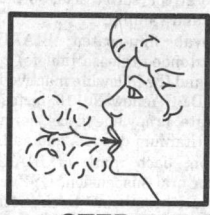

STEP 7

7. Breathe out to empty your lungs completely before using the inhaler! This is important to make sure that you can breathe the medication deeply into your lungs.

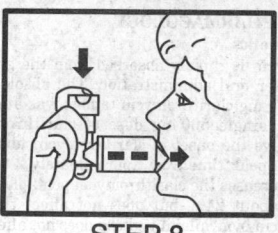

STEP 8

8. Place mouthpiece into your mouth, and close your lips tightly around it. Press down firmly and steadily on the metal canister while breathing in slowly and deeply **THROUGH YOUR MOUTH ONLY.** (If necessary, pinch your nose closed.) Be sure to release your finger pressure from the top of the canister after the medication is released. Remember, the **Azmacort** Inhalation Aerosol delivers a **gentle mist** of medication, so don't be surprised if you hardly feel it.

Do not remove the inhaler from your mouth after breathing in the medication. Hold your breath for 10 seconds with the inhaler STILL in your mouth, THEN remove the inhaler and breathe out very slowly.

Unlike the other inhalers you may have used, you will not feel the medication impact the back of your mouth. This is because of the unique design of the **Azmacort** Inhalation Aerosol delivery system.

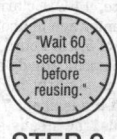

"Wait 60 seconds before reusing."

STEP 9

9. If your doctor has told you to take more than one breath of medication at a time: **WAIT AT LEAST 60 SECONDS** between each one, then start again at Step 6.
[See figure at top of next column.]

10. After the prescribed number of inhalations, thoroughly rinse out your mouth with water. **NOTE:** If your mouth becomes sore or develops a rash, be sure to mention this to your physician, but do not stop using your inhaler unless instructed to do so.

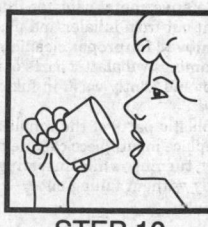

STEP 10

DOSAGE: USE ONLY AS DIRECTED BY YOUR PHYSICIAN
WARNING: Azmacort® (triamcinolone acetonide) Inhalation Aerosol contains medication that is intended for treatment of your asthma. It does *not* contain medication intended to provide rapid relief of your breathing difficulties during an asthma attack.

It is very important that you use **Azmacort** Inhalation Aerosol regularly at the intervals recommended by your doctor, and not as an emergency measure. Your physician will decide whether other medication is needed, should you require immediate relief.

CAUTION: CONTENTS OF CANISTER UNDER PRESSURE. Do not puncture. Do not store near heat or open flame. Exposure to temperatures above 120°F may cause bursting. Never throw canisters into a fire or incinerator. Please keep out of the reach of children.

Note: The indented statement below is required by the Federal government's Clean Air Act for all products containing or manufactured with chlorofluorocarbons (CFCs):

This product contains CFC-12, a substance which harms the environment by destroying ozone in the upper atmosphere.

Your physician has determined that this product is likely to help your personal health. **USE THIS PRODUCT AS DIRECTED, UNLESS INSTRUCTED TO DO OTHERWISE BY YOUR PHYSICIAN.** If you have any questions about alternatives, consult with your physician.

IMPORTANT TIPS FOR USING YOUR AZMACORT INHALATION AEROSOL INHALER

- Always use only as directed by your physician. Do not use it more often than instructed; do not skip doses.
- Follow all instructions in this booklet very closely and carefully for best results, especially those for use and cleaning.
- Remember, repriming is only necessary when the inhaler has not been used for more than 3 days. To reprime, shake the inhaler gently and release one puff. Repeat this procedure again so that a total of two puffs have been released. Do not reprime between more frequent usage.
- **Please Note:**
You will receive a new **Azmacort** Inhalation Aerosol unit each time you refill your prescription. This is done to assure optimal working order of the unique **Azmacort** Inhalation Aerosol spacer device/delivery system. In addition, a new **Azmacort** Inhalation Aerosol unit will guard against a build-up of the drug on the barrel portion of the device, maximizing the cleanliness of your unit. The cost of **Azmacort** Inhalation Aerosol is MINIMALLY affected by including a new inhaler with each prescription.

STORING YOUR AZMACORT INHALATION AEROSOL INHALER

- Keep your inhaler **out of the reach of children**, unless otherwise prescribed.
- Store your **Azmacort** Inhalation Aerosol, including the metal canister, at room temperature.
- Protect from freezing temperatures and direct sunlight.
- For best results, the canister should be at room temperature before use.
- **DO NOT** use after the date shown as "EXP" on the label or box.
- **Azmacort** Inhalation Aerosol canisters are for use with **Azmacort** Inhalation Aerosol actuators and spacer-mouthpieces only. The actuator and spacer-mouthpiece should not be used with other aerosol medications.
- **REMEMBER: This medicine has been prescribed for you by your doctor. DO NOT give this medicine to anyone else.**

DAILY CARE OF YOUR AZMACORT INHALATION AEROSOL INHALER

Your **Azmacort** Inhalation Aerosol **MUST** be cleaned in lukewarm water only once each day to avoid build-up of medication particles in the inhaler that can block the puff of medication and interfere with proper operation. The use of soap, detergents, or disinfectants is unnecessary.

Information on the Abbott Pharmaceutical Products listed on these pages is from the prescribing information in use as of June 1, 2010. For more information, please visit rxabbott.com or call 1-800-633-9110.

1. **IMPORTANT: Remove metal canister from inhaler.** Pull canister straight out from inhaler and place aside. **Canister must be removed for proper cleaning of inhaler.**
2. Pull apart remaining two plastic parts of inhaler, remove mouthpiece cap, and gently wash in lukewarm water. **Dry thoroughly.**
3. Snap the two plastic parts of the inhaler back together; push closed. Replace mouthpiece cap. Reinsert metal canister by gently turning while inserting. The canister should fit snugly without falling out.

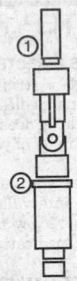

HOW TO CHECK CONTENTS OF YOUR CANISTER

Shaking the canister will **NOT** give you a good estimate of how much **Azmacort®** (triamcinolone acetonide) Inhalation Aerosol is left.

We have included a convenient check-off chart to assist you in keeping track of medication puffs used. This will help assure that you receive the 240 "Full Puffs" of medication present.

Azmacort® Inhalation Aerosol 240 Puff Check-Off

- Retain with medication or affix to convenient location.
- Starting with puff #1, check off one circle for each puff used.
- **DISCARD MEDICATION AFTER 240 PUFFS.**

FURTHER INFORMATION

- This leaflet does not contain the complete information about your medication.
- *If you have any further questions, or are not sure about something, you should ask your doctor or pharmacist.*
- You may want to read this leaflet again. Please **DO NOT THROW IT AWAY** until you have finished this canister.

©2007 Abbott Laboratories
Manufactured for:
Abbott Laboratories
North Chicago, IL 60064 U.S.A.
Ref: 03-A020-R1
Rev. September, 2007
Please check the Abbott website, www.rxabbott.com, or call (800) 633-9110 for full prescribing information.

BIAXIN® FILMTAB®   R̥

[bī´ax ən]
(clarithromycin tablets, USP)

BIAXIN® XL FILMTAB®

(clarithromycin extended-release tablets)

BIAXIN® GRANULES

(clarithromycin for oral suspension, USP)

To reduce the development of drug-resistant bacteria and maintain the effectiveness of BIAXIN and other antibacterial drugs, BIAXIN should be used only to treat or prevent infections that are proven or strongly suspected to be caused by bacteria.

DESCRIPTION

Clarithromycin is a semi-synthetic macrolide antibiotic. Chemically, it is 6-0-methylerythromycin. The molecular formula is $C_{38}H_{69}NO_{13}$, and the molecular weight is 747.96. The structural formula is:

[See chemical structure at top of next column]

Clarithromycin is a white to off-white crystalline powder. It is soluble in acetone, slightly soluble in methanol, ethanol, and acetonitrile, and practically insoluble in water.

BIAXIN is available as immediate-release tablets, extended-release tablets, and granules for oral suspension. Each yellow oval film-coated immediate-release BIAXIN tablet (clarithromycin tablets, USP) contains 250 mg or 500 mg of clarithromycin and the following inactive ingredients:

250 mg tablets: hypromellose, hydroxypropyl cellulose, croscarmellose sodium, D&C Yellow No. 10, FD&C Blue No. 1, magnesium stearate, microcrystalline cellulose, povidone, pregelatinized starch, propylene glycol, silicon dioxide, sorbic acid, sorbitan monooleate, stearic acid, talc, titanium dioxide, and vanillin.

500 mg tablets: hypromellose, hydroxypropyl cellulose, colloidal silicon dioxide, croscarmellose sodium, D&C Yellow No. 10, magnesium stearate, microcrystalline cellulose, povidone, propylene glycol, sorbic acid, sorbitan monooleate, titanium dioxide, and vanillin.

Each yellow oval film-coated BIAXIN XL tablet (clarithromycin extended-release tablets) contains 500 mg of clarithromycin and the following inactive ingredients: cellulosic polymers, D&C Yellow No. 10, lactose monohydrate, magnesium stearate, propylene glycol, sorbic acid, sorbitan monooleate, talc, titanium dioxide, and vanillin.

After constitution, each 5 mL of BIAXIN suspension (clarithromycin for oral suspension, USP) contains 125 mg or 250 mg of clarithromycin. Each bottle of BIAXIN granules contains 1250 mg (50 mL size), 2500 mg (50 and 100 mL sizes) or 5000 mg (100 mL size) of clarithromycin and the following inactive ingredients: carbomer, castor oil, citric acid, hypromellose phthalate, maltodextrin, potassium sorbate, povidone, silicon dioxide, sucrose, xanthan gum, titanium dioxide and fruit punch flavor.

CLINICAL PHARMACOLOGY

Pharmacokinetics

Clarithromycin is rapidly absorbed from the gastrointestinal tract after oral administration. The absolute bioavailability of 250 mg clarithromycin tablets was approximately 50%. For a single 500 mg dose of clarithromycin, food slightly delays the onset of clarithromycin absorption, increasing the peak time from approximately 2 to 2.5 hours. Food also increases the clarithromycin peak plasma concentration by about 24%, but does not affect the extent of clarithromycin bioavailability. Food does not affect the onset of formation of the antimicrobially active metabolite, 14-OH clarithromycin or its peak plasma concentration but does slightly decrease the extent of metabolite formation, indicated by an 11% decrease in area under the plasma concentration-time curve (AUC). Therefore, BIAXIN tablets may be given without regard to food.

In nonfasting healthy human subjects (males and females), peak plasma concentrations were attained within 2 to 3 hours after oral dosing. Steady-state peak plasma clarithromycin concentrations were attained within 3 days and were approximately 1 to 2 µg/mL with a 250 mg dose administered every 12 hours and 3 to 4 µg/mL with a 500 mg dose administered every 8 to 12 hours. The elimination half-life of clarithromycin was about 3 to 4 hours with 250 mg administered every 12 hours but increased to 5 to 7 hours with 500 mg administered every 8 to 12 hours. The nonlinearity of clarithromycin pharmacokinetics is slight at the recommended doses of 250 mg and 500 mg administered every 8 to 12 hours. With a 250 mg every 12 hours dosing, the principal metabolite, 14-OH clarithromycin, attains a peak steady-state concentration of about 0.6 µg/mL and has an elimination half-life of 5 to 6 hours. With a 500 mg every 8 to 12 hours dosing, the peak steady-state concentration of 14-OH clarithromycin is slightly higher (up to 1 µg/mL), and its elimination half-life is about 7 to 9 hours. With any of these dosing regimens, the steady-state concentration of this metabolite is generally attained within 3 to 4 days.

After a 250 mg tablet every 12 hours, approximately 20% of the dose is excreted in the urine as clarithromycin, while after a 500 mg tablet every 12 hours, the urinary excretion of clarithromycin is somewhat greater, approximately 30%. In comparison, after an oral dose of 250 mg (125 mg/5 mL) suspension every 12 hours, approximately 40% is excreted in urine as clarithromycin. The renal clearance of clarithromycin is, however, relatively independent of the dose size and approximates the normal glomerular filtration rate. The major metabolite found in urine is 14-OH

clarithromycin, which accounts for an additional 10% to 15% of the dose with either a 250 mg or a 500 mg tablet administered every 12 hours.

Steady-state concentrations of clarithromycin and 14-OH clarithromycin observed following administration of 500 mg doses of clarithromycin every 12 hours to adult patients with HIV infection were similar to those observed in healthy volunteers. In adult HIV-infected patients taking 500- or 1000-mg doses of clarithromycin every 12 hours, steady-state clarithromycin C_{max} values ranged from 2 to 4 µg/mL and 5 to 10 µg/mL, respectively.

The steady-state concentrations of clarithromycin in subjects with impaired hepatic function did not differ from those in normal subjects; however, the 14-OH clarithromycin concentrations were lower in the hepatically impaired subjects. The decreased formation of 14-OH clarithromycin was at least partially offset by an increase in renal clearance of clarithromycin in the subjects with impaired hepatic function when compared to healthy subjects. The pharmacokinetics of clarithromycin was also altered in subjects with impaired renal function. (See **PRECAUTIONS** and **DOSAGE AND ADMINISTRATION**.)

Clarithromycin and the 14-OH clarithromycin metabolite distribute readily into body tissues and fluids. There are no data available on cerebrospinal fluid penetration. Because of high intracellular concentrations, tissue concentrations are higher than serum concentrations. Examples of tissue and serum concentrations are presented below.

CONCENTRATION (after 250 mg q12h)

Tissue Type	Tissue (µg/g)	Serum (µg/mL)
Tonsil	1.6	0.8
Lung	8.8	1.7

Clarithromycin extended-release tablets provide extended absorption of clarithromycin from the gastrointestinal tract after oral administration. Relative to an equal total daily dose of immediate-release clarithromycin tablets, clarithromycin extended-release tablets provide lower and later steady-state peak plasma concentrations but equivalent 24-hour AUC's for both clarithromycin and its microbiologically-active metabolite, 14-OH clarithromycin. While the extent of formation of 14-OH clarithromycin following administration of BIAXIN XL tablets (2 × 500 mg once daily) is not affected by food, administration under fasting conditions is associated with approximately 30% lower clarithromycin AUC relative to administration with food. Therefore, BIAXIN XL tablets should be taken with food.

Steady-State Clarithromycin Plasma Concentration-Time Profiles

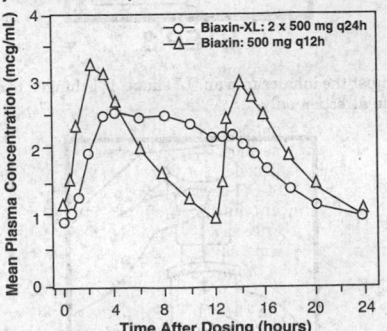

In healthy human subjects, steady-state peak plasma clarithromycin concentrations of approximately 2 to 3 µg/mL were achieved about 5 to 8 hours after oral administration of 2 × 500 mg BIAXIN XL tablets once daily; for 14-OH clarithromycin, steady-state peak plasma concentrations of approximately 0.8 µg/mL were attained about 6 to 9 hours after dosing. Steady-state peak plasma clarithromycin concentrations of approximately 1 to 2 µg/mL were achieved about 5 to 6 hours after oral administration of a single 500 mg BIAXIN XL tablet once daily; for 14-OH clarithromycin, steady-state peak plasma concentrations of approximately 0.6 µg/mL were attained about 6 hours after dosing.

When 250 mg doses of clarithromycin as BIAXIN suspension were administered to fasting healthy adult subjects, peak plasma concentrations were attained around 3 hours after dosing. Steady-state peak plasma concentrations were attained in 2 to 3 days and were approximately 2 µg/mL for clarithromycin and 0.7 µg/mL for 14-OH clarithromycin when 250-mg doses of the clarithromycin suspension were administered every 12 hours. Elimination half-life of clarithromycin (3 to 4 hours) and that of 14-OH clarithromycin (5 to 7 hours) were similar to those observed at steady state following administration of equivalent doses of BIAXIN tablets.

For adult patients, the bioavailability of 10 mL of the 125 mg/5 mL suspension or 10 mL of the 250 mg/5 mL suspension is similar to a 250 mg or 500 mg tablet, respectively.

In children requiring antibiotic therapy, administration of 7.5 mg/kg q12h doses of clarithromycin as the suspension generally resulted in steady-state peak plasma concentrations of 3 to 7 µg/mL for clarithromycin and 1 to 2 µg/mL for 14-OH clarithromycin.

In HIV-infected children taking 15 mg/kg every 12 hours, steady-state clarithromycin peak concentrations generally ranged from 6 to 15 µg/mL.

Clarithromycin penetrates into the middle ear fluid of children with secretory otitis media.

CONCENTRATION (after 7.5 mg/kg q12h for 5 doses)

Analyte	Middle Ear Fluid (µg/mL)	Serum (µg/mL)
Clarithromycin	2.5	1.7
14-OH Clarithromycin	1.3	0.8

In adults given 250 mg clarithromycin as suspension (n = 22), food appeared to decrease mean peak plasma clarithromycin concentrations from 1.2 ($\pm$ 0.4) µg/mL to 1.0 ($\pm$ 0.4) µg/mL and the extent of absorption from 7.2 ($\pm$ 2.5) hr•µg/mL to 6.5 ($\pm$ 3.7) hr•µg/mL.

When children (n = 10) were administered a single oral dose of 7.5 mg/kg suspension, food increased mean peak plasma clarithromycin concentrations from 3.6 ($\pm$ 1.5) µg/mL to 4.6 ($\pm$ 2.8) µg/mL and the extent of absorption from 10.0 ($\pm$ 5.5) hr•µg/mL to 14.2 ($\pm$ 9.4) hr•µg/mL.

Clarithromycin 500 mg every 8 hours was given in combination with omeprazole 40 mg daily to healthy adult males. The plasma levels of clarithromycin and 14-hydroxy-clarithromycin were increased by the concomitant administration of omeprazole. For clarithromycin, the mean C_{max} was 10% greater, the mean C_{min} was 27% greater, and the mean AUC_{0-8} was 15% greater when clarithromycin was administered with omeprazole than when clarithromycin was administered alone. Similar results were seen for 14-hydroxy-clarithromycin, the mean C_{max} was 45% greater, the mean C_{min} was 57% greater, and the mean AUC_{0-8} was 45% greater. Clarithromycin concentrations in the gastric tissue and mucus were also increased by concomitant administration of omeprazole.

[See first table above]

For information about other drugs indicated in combination with BIAXIN, refer to the **CLINICAL PHARMACOLOGY** section of their package inserts.

Microbiology

Clarithromycin exerts its antibacterial action by binding to the 50S ribosomal subunit of susceptible microorganisms resulting in inhibition of protein synthesis.

Clarithromycin is active *in vitro* against a variety of aerobic and anaerobic gram-positive and gram-negative microorganisms as well as most *Mycobacterium avium* complex (MAC) microorganisms.

Additionally, the 14-OH clarithromycin metabolite also has clinically significant antimicrobial activity. The 14-OH clarithromycin is twice as active against *Haemophilus influenzae* microorganisms as the parent compound. However, for *Mycobacterium avium* complex (MAC) isolates the 14-OH metabolite is 4 to 7 times less active than clarithromycin. The clinical significance of this activity against *Mycobacterium avium* complex is unknown.

Clarithromycin has been shown to be active against most strains of the following microorganisms both *in vitro* and in clinical infections as described in the **INDICATIONS AND USAGE** section:

Aerobic Gram-positive Microorganisms
Staphylococcus aureus
Streptococcus pneumoniae
Streptococcus pyogenes
Aerobic Gram-negative Microorganisms
Haemophilus influenzae
Haemophilus parainfluenzae
Moraxella catarrhalis
Other Microorganisms
Mycoplasma pneumoniae
Chlamydia pneumoniae (TWAR)
Mycobacteria
Mycobacterium avium complex (MAC) consisting of:
Mycobacterium avium
Mycobacterium intracellulare

Beta-lactamase production should have no effect on clarithromycin activity.

Clarithromycin Tissue Concentrations 2 hours after Dose (µg/mL)/(µg/g)

Treatment	N	antrum	fundus	N	mucus
Clarithromycin	5	10.48 ± 2.01	20.81 ± 7.64	4	4.15 ± 7.74
Clarithromycin + Omeprazole	5	19.96 ± 4.71	24.25 ± 6.37	4	39.29 ± 32.79

Clarithromycin Susceptibility Test Results and Clinical/Bacteriological Outcomes[a]

Clarithromycin Pretreatment Results	Clarithromycin Post-treatment Results				
	H. pylori negative - eradicated	H. pylori positive - not eradicated Post-treatment susceptibility results			
		S[b]	I[b]	R[b]	No MIC
Omeprazole 40 mg q.d./clarithromycin 500 mg t.i.d. for 14 days followed by omeprazole 20 mg q.d. for another 14 days (M93-067, M93-100)					
Susceptible[b]	108	72	1	26	9
Intermediate[b]	1			1	
Resistant[b]	4			4	
Ranitidine bismuth citrate 400 mg b.i.d./clarithromycin 500 mg t.i.d. for 14 days followed by ranitidine bismuth citrate 400 mg b.i.d. for another 14 days (H2BA3001)					
Susceptible[b]	124	98	4	14	8
Intermediate[b]	3	2			1
Resistant[b]	17	1		15	1
Ranitidine bismuth citrate 400 mg b.i.d./clarithromycin 500 mg b.i.d. for 14 days followed by ranitidine bismuth citrate 400 mg b.i.d. for another 14 days (H2BA3001)					
Susceptible[b]	125	106	1	12	5
Intermediate[b]	2	2			
Resistant[b]	20	1		19	
Omeprazole 20 mg b.i.d./clarithromycin 500 mg b.i.d./amoxicillin 1 g b.i.d. for 10 days (126, 127, M96-446)					
Susceptible[b]	171	153	7	3	8
Intermediate[b]					
Resistant[b]	14	4	1	6	3
Lansoprazole 30 mg b.i.d./clarithromycin 500 mg b.i.d./amoxicillin 1 g b.i.d. for 14 days (M95-399, M93-131, M95-392)					
Susceptible[b]	112	105			7
Intermediate[b]	3	3			
Resistant[b]	17	6		7	4
Lansoprazole 30 mg b.i.d./clarithromycin 500 mg b.i.d./amoxicillin 1 g b.i.d. for 10 days (M95-399)					
Susceptible[b]	42	40	1		1
Intermediate[b]					
Resistant[b]	4	1		3	

a Includes only patients with pretreatment clarithromycin susceptibility tests
b Susceptible (S) MIC < 0.25 µg/mL, Intermediate (I) MIC 0.5-1.0 µg/mL, Resistant (R) MIC > 2 µg/mL

NOTE: Most strains of methicillin-resistant and oxacillin-resistant staphylococci are resistant to clarithromycin.

Omeprazole/clarithromycin dual therapy; ranitidine bismuth citrate/clarithromycin dual therapy; omeprazole/clarithromycin/amoxicillin triple therapy; and lansoprazole/clarithromycin/amoxicillin triple therapy have been shown to be active against most strains of *Helicobacter pylori* in *vitro* and in clinical infections as described in the **INDICATIONS AND USAGE** section.

Helicobacter
Helicobacter pylori
Pretreatment Resistance

Clarithromycin pretreatment resistance rates were 3.5% (4/113) in the omeprazole/clarithromycin dual therapy studies (M93-067, M93-100) and 9.3% (41/439) in the omeprazole/clarithromycin/amoxicillin triple therapy studies (126, 127, M96-446). Clarithromycin pretreatment resistance was 12.6% (44/348) in the ranitidine bismuth citrate/clarithromycin b.i.d. versus t.i.d. clinical study (H2BA3001). Clarithromycin pretreatment resistance rates were 9.5% (91/960) by E-test and 11.3% (12/106) by agar dilution in the lansoprazole/clarithromycin/amoxicillin triple therapy clinical trials (M93-125, M93-130, M93-131, M95-392, and M95-399).

Amoxicillin pretreatment susceptible isolates (< 0.25 µg/mL) were found in 99.3% (436/439) of the patients in the omeprazole/clarithromycin/amoxicillin clinical studies (126, 127, M96-446). Amoxicillin pretreatment minimum inhibitory concentrations (MICs) > 0.25 µg/mL occurred in 0.7% (3/439) of the patients, all of whom were in the clarithromycin/amoxicillin study arm. Amoxicillin pretreatment susceptible isolates (< 0.25 µg/mL) occurred in 97.8% (936/957) and 98.0% (98/100) of the patients in the lansoprazole/clarithromycin/amoxicillin triple-therapy clinical trials by E-test and agar dilution, respectively. Twenty-one of the 957 patients (2.2%) by E-test and 2 of 100 patients (2.0%) by agar dilution had amoxicillin pretreatment MICs of > 0.25 µg/mL. Two patients had an unconfirmed pretreatment amoxicillin minimum inhibitory concentration (MIC) of > 256 µg/mL by E-test.

[See second table above]

Patients not eradicated of *H. pylori* following omeprazole/clarithromycin, ranitidine bismuth citrate/clarithromycin, omeprazole/clarithromycin/amoxicillin, or lansoprazole/clarithromycin/amoxicillin therapy would likely have clarithromycin resistant *H. pylori* isolates. Therefore, for patients who fail therapy, clarithromycin susceptibility testing should be done, if possible. Patients with clarithromycin resistant *H. pylori* should not be treated with any of the following: omeprazole/clarithromycin dual therapy; ranitidine bismuth citrate/clarithromycin dual therapy; omeprazole/clarithromycin/amoxicillin triple therapy; lansoprazole/clarithromycin/amoxicillin triple therapy; or other regimens which include clarithromycin as the sole antimicrobial agent.

Amoxicillin Susceptibility Test Results and Clinical/Bacteriological Outcomes

In the omeprazole/clarithromycin/amoxicillin triple-therapy clinical trials, 84.9% (157/185) of the patients who had pretreatment amoxicillin susceptible MICs (< 0.25 µg/mL) were eradicated of *H. pylori* and 15.1% (28/185) failed therapy. Of the 28 patients who failed triple therapy, 11 had no post-treatment susceptibility test results, and 17 had post-treatment *H. pylori* isolates with amoxicillin susceptible MICs. Eleven of the patients who failed triple therapy also had post-treatment *H. pylori* isolates with clarithromycin resistant MICs.

In the lansoprazole/clarithromycin/amoxicillin triple-therapy clinical trials, 82.6% (195/236) of the patients that had pretreatment amoxicillin susceptible MICs (< 0.25 µg/mL) were eradicated of *H. pylori*. Of those with pretreatment amoxicillin MICs of > 0.25 µg/mL, three of six had the *H. pylori* eradicated. A total of 12.8% (22/172) of the patients failed the 10- and 14-day triple-therapy regimens. Post-treatment susceptibility results were not obtained on 11 of the patients who failed therapy. Nine of the 11 patients with amoxicillin post-treatment MICs that failed the triple-therapy regimen also had clarithromycin resistant *H. pylori* isolates.

The following *in vitro* data are available, **but their clinical significance is unknown.** Clarithromycin exhibits *in vitro* activity against most strains of the following microorganisms; however, the safety and effectiveness of clarithromycin in treating clinical infections due to these

Information on the Abbott Pharmaceutical Products listed on these pages is from the prescribing information in use as of June 1, 2010. For more information, please visit rxabbott.com or call 1-800-633-9110.

microorganisms have not been established in adequate and well-controlled clinical trials.

Aerobic Gram-positive Microorganisms
Streptococcus agalactiae
Streptococci (Groups C, F, G)
Viridans group streptococci
Aerobic Gram-negative Microorganisms
Bordetella pertussis
Legionella pneumophila
Pasteurella multocida
Anaerobic Gram-positive Microorganisms
Clostridium perfringens
Peptococcus niger
Propionibacterium acnes
Anaerobic Gram-negative Microorganisms
Prevotella melaninogenica (formerly *Bacteriodes melaninogenicus*)

Susceptibility Testing Excluding Mycobacteria and Helicobacter

Dilution Techniques
Quantitative methods are used to determine antimicrobial minimum inhibitory concentrations (MICs). These MICs provide estimates of the susceptibility of bacteria to antimicrobial compounds. The MICs should be determined using a standardized procedure. Standardized procedures are based on a dilution method[1] (broth or agar) or equivalent with standardized inoculum concentrations and standardized concentrations of clarithromycin powder. The MIC values should be interpreted according to the following criteria:

For testing Staphylococcus spp.

MIC (µg/mL)	Interpretation
≤ 2.0	Susceptible (S)
4.0	Intermediate (I)
≥ 8.0	Resistant (R)

For testing Streptococcus spp. including Streptococcus pneumoniae[a]

MIC (µg/mL)	Interpretation
≤ 0.25	Susceptible (S)
0.5	Intermediate (I)
≥ 1.0	Resistant (R)

a These interpretive standards are applicable only to broth microdilution susceptibility tests using cation-adjusted Mueller-Hinton broth with 2-5% lysed horse blood.

For testing Haemophilus spp.[b]

MIC (µg/mL)	Interpretation
≤ 8.0	Susceptible (S)
16.0	Intermediate (I)
≥ 32.0	Resistant (R)

b These interpretive standards are applicable only to broth microdilution susceptibility tests with Haemophilus spp. using Haemophilus Testing Medium (HTM).[1]

Note: When testing *Streptococcus* spp., including *Streptococcus pneumoniae*, susceptibility and resistance to clarithromycin can be predicted using erythromycin.

A report of "Susceptible" indicates that the pathogen is likely to be inhibited if the antimicrobial compound in the blood reaches the concentrations usually achievable. A report of "Intermediate" indicates that the result should be considered equivocal, and, if the microorganism is not fully susceptible to alternative, clinically feasible drugs, the test should be repeated. This category implies possible clinical applicability in body sites where the drug is physiologically concentrated or in situations where high dosage of drug can be used. This category also provides a buffer zone which prevents small uncontrolled technical factors from causing major discrepancies in interpretation. A report of "Resistant" indicates that the pathogen is not likely to be inhibited if the antimicrobial compound in the blood reaches the concentrations usually achievable; other therapy should be selected.

Standardized susceptibility test procedures require the use of laboratory control microorganisms to control the technical aspects of the laboratory procedures. Standard clarithromycin powder should provide the following MIC values:

Microorganism		MIC (µg/mL)
S. aureus	ATCC 29213	0.12 to 0.5
S. pneumoniae[c]	ATCC 49619	0.03 to 0.12
Haemophilus influenzae[d]	ATCC 49247	4 to 16

c This quality control range is applicable only to *S. pneumoniae* ATCC 49619 tested by a microdilution procedure using cation-adjusted Mueller-Hinton broth with 2-5% lysed horse blood.
d This quality control range is applicable only to *H. influenzae* ATCC 49247 tested by a microdilution procedure using HTM[1].

Diffusion Techniques
Quantitative methods that require measurement of zone diameters also provide reproducible estimates of the susceptibility of bacteria to antimicrobial compounds. One such standardized procedure[2] requires the use of standardized inoculum concentrations. This procedure uses paper disks impregnated with 15-µg clarithromycin to test the susceptibility of microorganisms to clarithromycin.
Reports from the laboratory providing results of the standard single-disk susceptibility test with a 15-µg clarithromycin disk should be interpreted according to the following criteria:

For testing Staphylococcus spp.

Zone diameter (mm)	Interpretation
≥ 18	Susceptible (S)
14 to 17	Intermediate (I)
≤ 13	Resistant (R)

For testing Streptococcus spp. including Streptococcus pneumoniae[e]

Zone diameter (mm)	Interpretation
≥ 21	Susceptible (S)
17 to 20	Intermediate (I)
≤ 16	Resistant (R)

e These zone diameter standards only apply to tests performed using Mueller-Hinton agar supplemented with 5% sheep blood incubated in 5% CO_2.

For testing Haemophilus spp.[f]

Zone diameter (mm)	Interpretation
≥ 13	Susceptible (S)
11 to 12	Intermediate (I)
≤ 10	Resistant (R)

f These zone diameter standards are applicable only to tests with *Haemophilus* spp. using HTM[2].

Note: When testing *Streptococcus* spp., including *Streptococcus pneumoniae*, susceptibility and resistance to clarithromycin can be predicted using erythromycin.

Interpretation should be as stated above for results using dilution techniques. Interpretation involves correlation of the diameter obtained in the disk test with the MIC for clarithromycin.
As with standardized dilution techniques, diffusion methods require the use of laboratory control microorganisms that are used to control the technical aspects of the laboratory procedures. For the diffusion technique, the 15-µg clarithromycin disk should provide the following zone diameters in this laboratory test quality control strain:

Microorganism		Zone diameter (mm)
S. aureus	ATCC 25923	26 to 32
S. pneumoniae[g]	ATCC 49619	25 to 31
Haemophilus influenzae[h]	ATCC 49247	11 to 17

g This quality control range is applicable only to tests performed by disk diffusion using Mueller-Hinton agar supplemented with 5% defibrinated sheep blood.
h This quality control limit applies to tests conducted with *Haemophilus influenzae* ATCC 49247 using HTM[2].

In vitro Activity of Clarithromycin against Mycobacteria
Clarithromycin has demonstrated *in vitro* activity against *Mycobacterium avium* complex (MAC) microorganisms isolated from both AIDS and non-AIDS patients. While gene probe techniques may be used to distinguish *M. avium* species from *M. intracellulare*, many studies only reported results on *M. avium* complex (MAC) isolates.
Various *in vitro* methodologies employing broth or solid media at different pH's, with and without oleic acid-albumin-dextrose-catalase (OADC), have been used to determine clarithromycin MIC values for mycobacterial species. In general, MIC values decrease more than 16-fold as the pH of Middlebrook 7H12 broth media increases from 5.0 to 7.4. At pH 7.4, MIC values determined with Mueller-Hinton agar were 4- to 8-fold higher than those observed with Middlebrook 7H12 media. Utilization of oleic acid-albumin-dextrose-catalase (OADC) in these assays has been shown to further alter MIC values.
Clarithromycin activity against 80 MAC isolates from AIDS patients and 211 MAC isolates from non-AIDS patients was evaluated using a microdilution method with Middlebrook 7H9 broth. Results showed an MIC value of ≤ 4.0 µg/mL in 81% and 89% of the AIDS and non-AIDS MAC isolates, respectively. Twelve percent of the non-AIDS isolates had an MIC value ≤ 0.5 µg/mL. Clarithromycin was also shown to be active against phagocytized *M. avium* complex (MAC) in mouse and human macrophage cell cultures as well as in the beige mouse infection model.
Clarithromycin activity was evaluated against *Mycobacterium tuberculosis* microorganisms. In one study utilizing the agar dilution method with Middlebrook 7H10 media, 3 of 30 clinical isolates had an MIC of 2.5 µg/mL. Clarithromycin inhibited all isolates at > 10.0 µg/mL.
Susceptibility Testing for *Mycobacterium avium* Complex (MAC)
The disk diffusion and dilution techniques for susceptibility testing against gram-positive and gram-negative bacteria should not be used for determining clarithromycin MIC values against mycobacteria. *In vitro* susceptibility testing methods and diagnostic products currently available for determining minimum inhibitory concentration (MIC) values against *Mycobacterium avium* complex (MAC) organisms have not been standardized or validated. Clarithromycin MIC values will vary depending on the susceptibility testing method employed, composition and pH of the media, and the utilization of nutritional supplements. Breakpoints to determine whether clinical isolates of *M. avium* or *M. intracellulare* are susceptible or resistant to clarithromycin have not been established.
Susceptibility Test for *Helicobacter pylori*
The reference methodology for susceptibility testing of *H. pylori* is agar dilution MICs.[3] One to three microliters of an inoculum equivalent to a No. 2 McFarland standard (1×10^7-1×10^8 CFU/mL for *H. pylori*) are inoculated directly onto freshly prepared antimicrobial containing Mueller-Hinton agar plates with 5% aged defibrinated sheep blood (> 2-weeks old). The agar dilution plates are incubated at 35°C in a microaerobic environment produced by a gas generating system suitable for *Campylobacter* species. After 3 days of incubation, the MICs are recorded as the lowest concentration of antimicrobial agent required to inhibit growth of the organism. The clarithromycin and amoxicillin MIC values should be interpreted according to the following criteria:

Clarithromycin MIC (µg/mL)[i]	Interpretation
< 0.25	Susceptible (S)
0.5-1.0	Intermediate (I)
> 2.0	Resistant (R)

Amoxicillin MIC (µg/mL)[i,j]	Interpretation
< 0.25	Susceptible (S)

i These are tentative breakpoints for the agar dilution methodology, and they should not be used to interpret results obtained using alternative methods.
j There were not enough organisms with MICs > 0.25 µg/mL to determine a resistance breakpoint.

Standardized susceptibility test procedures require the use of laboratory control microorganisms to control the technical aspects of the laboratory procedures. Standard clarithromycin and amoxicillin powders should provide the following MIC values:
[See table at top of next page]

INDICATIONS AND USAGE

BIAXIN Filmtab (clarithromycin tablets, USP) and BIAXIN Granules (clarithromycin for oral suspension, USP) are indicated for the treatment of mild to moderate infections caused by susceptible strains of the designated microorganisms in the conditions as listed below:

Adults (BIAXIN Filmtab Tablets and Granules for Oral Suspension)

Pharyngitis/Tonsillitis due to *Streptococcus pyogenes* (The usual drug of choice in the treatment and prevention of streptococcal infections and the prophylaxis of rheumatic fever is penicillin administered by either the intramuscular or the oral route. Clarithromycin is generally effective in the eradication of *S. pyogenes* from the nasopharynx; however, data establishing the efficacy of clarithromycin in the subsequent prevention of rheumatic fever are not available at present).

Acute maxillary sinusitis due to *Haemophilus influenzae, Moraxella catarrhalis,* or *Streptococcus pneumoniae.*

Acute bacterial exacerbation of chronic bronchitis due to *Haemophilus influenzae, Haemophilus parainfluenzae, Moraxella catarrhalis,* or *Streptococcus pneumoniae.*

Community-Acquired Pneumonia due to *Haemophilus influenzae, Mycoplasma pneumoniae, Streptococcus pneumoniae,* or *Chlamydia pneumoniae* (TWAR).

Uncomplicated skin and skin structure infections due to *Staphylococcus aureus,* or *Streptococcus pyogenes* (Abscesses usually require surgical drainage).

Disseminated mycobacterial infections due to *Mycobacterium avium,* or *Mycobacterium intracellulare*

BIAXIN (clarithromycin) Filmtab tablets in combination with amoxicillin and PREVACID (lansoprazole) or PRILOSEC (omeprazole) Delayed-Release Capsules, as triple therapy, are indicated for the treatment of patients with *H. pylori* infection and duodenal ulcer disease (active or five-year history of duodenal ulcer) to eradicate *H. pylori.*

BIAXIN Filmtab tablets in combination with PRILOSEC (omeprazole) capsules or TRITEC (ranitidine bismuth citrate) tablets are also indicated for the treatment of patients with an active duodenal ulcer associated with *H. pylori* infection. However, regimens which contain clarithromycin as the single antimicrobial agent are more likely to be associated with the development of clarithromycin resistance among patients who fail therapy. Clarithromycin-containing regimens should not be used in patients with known or suspected clarithromycin resistant isolates because the efficacy of treatment is reduced in this setting.

In patients who fail therapy, susceptibility testing should be done if possible. If resistance to clarithromycin is demonstrated, a non-clarithromycin-containing therapy is recommended. (For information on development of resistance see **Microbiology** section.) The eradication of *H. pylori* has been demonstrated to reduce the risk of duodenal ulcer recurrence.

Children (BIAXIN Filmtab Tablets and Granules for Oral Suspension)

Pharyngitis/Tonsillitis due to *Streptococcus pyogenes.*

Community-Acquired Pneumonia due to *Mycoplasma pneumoniae, Streptococcus pneumoniae,* or *Chlamydia pneumoniae* (TWAR)

Acute maxillary sinusitis due to *Haemophilus influenzae, Moraxella catarrhalis,* or *Streptococcus pneumoniae*

Acute otitis media due to *Haemophilus influenzae, Moraxella catarrhalis,* or *Streptococcus pneumoniae*

NOTE: For information on otitis media, see **CLINICAL STUDIES - Otitis Media.**

Uncomplicated skin and skin structure infections due to *Staphylococcus aureus,* or *Streptococcus pyogenes* (Abscesses usually require surgical drainage.)

Disseminated mycobacterial infections due to *Mycobacterium avium,* or *Mycobacterium intracellulare*

Adults (BIAXIN XL Filmtab Tablets)

BIAXIN XL Filmtab (clarithromycin extended-release tablets) are indicated for the treatment of adults with mild to moderate infection caused by susceptible strains of the designated microorganisms in the conditions listed below:

Acute maxillary sinusitis due to *Haemophilus influenzae, Moraxella catarrhalis,* or *Streptococcus pneumoniae*

Acute bacterial exacerbation of chronic bronchitis due to *Haemophilus influenzae, Haemophilus parainfluenzae, Moraxella catarrhalis,* or *Streptococcus pneumoniae*

Community-Acquired Pneumonia due to *Haemophilus influenzae, Haemophilus parainfluenzae, Moraxella catarrhalis, Streptococcus pneumoniae, Chlamydia pneumoniae* (TWAR), or *Mycoplasma pneumoniae*

THE EFFICACY AND SAFETY OF BIAXIN XL IN TREATING OTHER INFECTIONS FOR WHICH OTHER FORMULATIONS OF BIAXIN ARE APPROVED HAVE NOT BEEN ESTABLISHED.

Prophylaxis

BIAXIN Filmtab tablets and BIAXIN Granules for oral suspension are indicated for the prevention of disseminated *Mycobacterium avium* complex (MAC) disease in patients with advanced HIV infection.

To reduce the development of drug-resistant bacteria and maintain the effectiveness of BIAXIN and other antibacterial drugs, BIAXIN should be used only to treat or prevent infections that are proven or strongly suspected to be caused by susceptible bacteria. When culture and susceptibility information are available, they should be considered in selecting or modifying antibacterial therapy. In the absence of such data, local epidemiology and susceptibility patterns may contribute to the empiric selection of therapy.

Microorganisms		Antimicrobial Agent	MIC (µg/mL)[k]
H. pylori	ATCC 43504	Clarithromycin	0.015-0.12 µg/mL
H. pylori	ATCC 43504	Amoxicillin	0.015-0.12 µg/mL

k These are quality control ranges for the agar dilution methodology and they should not be used to control test results obtained using alternative methods.

CONTRAINDICATIONS

Clarithromycin is contraindicated in patients with a known hypersensitivity to clarithromycin, erythromycin, or any of the macrolide antibiotics.

Concomitant administration of clarithromycin and any of the following drugs is contraindicated: cisapride, pimozide, astemizole, terfenadine, and ergotamine or dihydroergotamine (see **Drug Interactions**). There have been postmarketing reports of drug interactions when clarithromycin and/or erythromycin are coadministered with cisapride, pimozide, astemizole, or terfenadine resulting in cardiac arrhythmias (QT prolongation, ventricular tachycardia, ventricular fibrillation, and torsades de pointes) most likely due to inhibition of metabolism of these drugs by erythromycin and clarithromycin. Fatalities have been reported.

For information about contraindications of other drugs indicated in combination with BIAXIN, refer to the **CONTRAINDICATIONS** section of their package inserts.

WARNINGS

CLARITHROMYCIN SHOULD NOT BE USED IN PREGNANT WOMEN EXCEPT IN CLINICAL CIRCUMSTANCES WHERE NO ALTERNATIVE THERAPY IS APPROPRIATE. IF PREGNANCY OCCURS WHILE TAKING THIS DRUG, THE PATIENT SHOULD BE APPRISED OF THE POTENTIAL HAZARD TO THE FETUS. CLARITHROMYCIN HAS DEMONSTRATED ADVERSE EFFECTS OF PREGNANCY OUTCOME AND/OR EMBRYO-FETAL DEVELOPMENT IN MONKEYS, RATS, MICE, AND RABBITS AT DOSES THAT PRODUCED PLASMA LEVELS 2 TO 17 TIMES THE SERUM LEVELS ACHIEVED IN HUMANS TREATED AT THE MAXIMUM RECOMMENDED HUMAN DOSES. (See PRECAUTIONS - Pregnancy.)

Clostridium difficile associated diarrhea (CDAD) has been reported with use of nearly all antibacterial agents, including BIAXIN, and may range in severity from mild diarrhea to fatal colitis. Treatment with antibacterial agents alters the normal flora of the colon leading to overgrowth of *C. difficile.*

C. difficile produces toxins A and B which contribute to the development of CDAD. Hypertoxin producing strains of *C. difficile* cause increased morbidity and mortality, as these infections can be refractory to antimicrobial therapy and may require colectomy. CDAD must be considered in all patients who present with diarrhea following antibiotic use. Careful medical history is necessary since CDAD has been reported to occur over two months after the administration of antibacterial agents.

If CDAD is suspected or confirmed, ongoing antibiotic use not directed against *C. difficile* may need to be discontinued. Appropriate fluid and electrolyte management, protein supplementation, antibiotic treatment of *C. difficile,* and surgical evaluation should be instituted as clinically indicated.

There have been post-marketing reports of colchicine toxicity with concomitant use of clarithromycin and colchicine, especially in the elderly, some of which occurred in patients with renal insufficiency. Deaths have been reported in some such patients. (See **PRECAUTIONS**.)

For information about warnings of other drugs indicated in combination with BIAXIN, refer to the **WARNINGS** section of their package inserts.

PRECAUTIONS
General

Prescribing BIAXIN in the absence of a proven or strongly suspected bacterial infection or a prophylactic indication is unlikely to provide benefit to the patient and increases the risk of the development of drug-resistant bacteria.

Clarithromycin is principally excreted via the liver and kidney. Clarithromycin may be administered without dosage adjustment to patients with hepatic impairment and normal renal function. However, in the presence of severe renal impairment with or without coexisting hepatic impairment, decreased dosage or prolonged dosing intervals may be appropriate.

Clarithromycin in combination with ranitidine bismuth citrate therapy is not recommended in patients with creatinine clearance less than 25 mL/min. (See **DOSAGE AND ADMINISTRATION**.)

Clarithromycin in combination with ranitidine bismuth citrate should not be used in patients with a history of acute porphyria.

Exacerbation of symptoms of myasthenia gravis and new onset of symptoms of myasthenic syndrome has been reported in patients receiving clarithromycin therapy.

For information about precautions of other drugs indicated in combination with BIAXIN, refer to the **PRECAUTIONS** section of their package inserts.

Information to Patients

Patients should be counseled that antibacterial drugs including BIAXIN should only be used to treat bacterial infections. They do not treat viral infections (e.g., the common cold). When BIAXIN is prescribed to treat a bacterial infection, patients should be told that although it is common to feel better early in the course of therapy, the medication should be taken exactly as directed. Skipping doses or not completing the full course of therapy may (1) decrease the effectiveness of the immediate treatment and (2) increase the likelihood that bacteria will develop resistance and will not be treatable by BIAXIN or other antibacterial drugs in the future.

Diarrhea is a common problem caused by antibiotics which usually ends when the antibiotic is discontinued. Sometimes after starting treatment with antibiotics, patients can develop watery and bloody stools (with or without stomach cramps and fever) even as late as two or more months after having taken the last dose of the antibiotic. If this occurs, patients should contact their physician as soon as possible. BIAXIN may interact with some drugs; therefore patients should be advised to report to their doctor the use of any other medications.

BIAXIN tablets and oral suspension can be taken with or without food and can be taken with milk; however, BIAXIN XL tablets should be taken with food. Do **NOT** refrigerate the suspension.

Drug Interactions

Clarithromycin use in patients who are receiving theophylline may be associated with an increase of serum theophylline concentrations. Monitoring of serum theophylline concentrations should be considered for patients receiving high doses of theophylline or with baseline concentrations in the upper therapeutic range. In two studies in which theophylline was administered with clarithromycin (a theophylline sustained-release formulation was dosed at either 6.5 mg/kg or 12 mg/kg together with 250 or 500 mg q12h clarithromycin), the steady-state levels of C_{max}, C_{min}, and the area under the serum concentration time curve (AUC) of theophylline increased about 20%.

Hypotension, bradyarrhythmias, and lactic acidosis have been observed in patients receiving concurrent verapamil, belonging to the calcium channel blockers drug class.

Concomitant administration of single doses of clarithromycin and carbamazepine has been shown to result in increased plasma concentrations of carbamazepine. Blood level monitoring of carbamazepine may be considered.

When clarithromycin and terfenadine were coadministered, plasma concentrations of the active acid metabolite of terfenadine were threefold higher, on average, than the values observed when terfenadine was administered alone. The pharmacokinetics of clarithromycin and the 14-OH-clarithromycin were not significantly affected by coadministration of terfenadine once clarithromycin reached steady-state conditions. Concomitant administration of clarithromycin with terfenadine is contraindicated. (See **CONTRAINDICATIONS**.)

Clarithromycin 500 mg every 8 hours was given in combination with omeprazole 40 mg daily to healthy adult subjects. The steady-state plasma concentrations of omeprazole were increased (C_{max}, AUC_{0-24}, and $t_{1/2}$ increases of 30%, 89%, and 34%, respectively), by the concomitant administration of clarithromycin. The mean 24-hour gastric pH value was 5.2 when omeprazole was administered alone and 5.7 when coadministered with clarithromycin.

Coadministration of clarithromycin with ranitidine bismuth citrate resulted in increased plasma ranitidine concentrations (57%), increased plasma bismuth trough concentrations (48%), and increased 14-hydroxy-clarithromycin plasma concentrations (31%). These effects are clinically insignificant.

Simultaneous oral administration of BIAXIN tablets and zidovudine to HIV-infected adult patients may result in decreased steady-state zidovudine concentrations. Because

Information on the Abbott Pharmaceutical Products listed on these pages is from the prescribing information in use as of June 1, 2010. For more information, please visit rxabbott.com or call 1-800-633-9110.

clarithromycin appears to interfere with absorption of simultaneously administered oral zidovudine, this interaction can be largely avoided by staggering the doses of clarithromycin and zidovudine. This interaction does not appear to occur in pediatric HIV-infected patients taking clarithromycin suspension with zidovudine or dideoxyinosine. Similar interaction studies have not been conducted with clarithromycin extended release and zidovudine.

Simultaneous administration of BIAXIN tablets and didanosine to 12 HIV-infected adult patients resulted in no statistically significant change in didanosine pharmacokinetics.

Concomitant administration of fluconazole 200 mg daily and clarithromycin 500 mg twice daily to 21 healthy volunteers led to increases in the mean steady-state clarithromycin C_{min} and AUC of 33% and 18%, respectively. Steady-state concentrations of 14-OH clarithromycin were not significantly affected by concomitant administration of fluconazole. No clarithromycin dose adjustment is necessary.

Concomitant administration of clarithromycin and ritonavir (n = 22) resulted in a 77% increase in clarithromycin AUC and a 100% decrease in the AUC of 14-OH clarithromycin. Clarithromycin may be administered without dosage adjustment to patients with normal renal function taking ritonavir. However, for patients with renal impairment, the following dosage adjustments should be considered. For patients with CL_{CR} 30 to 60 mL/min, the dose of clarithromycin should be reduced by 50%. For patients with CL_{CR} < 30 mL/min, the dose of clarithromycin should be decreased by 75%.

Spontaneous reports in the post-marketing period suggest that concomitant administration of clarithromycin and oral anticoagulants may potentiate the effects of the oral anticoagulants. Prothrombin times should be carefully monitored while patients are receiving clarithromycin and oral anticoagulants simultaneously.

Digoxin is thought to be a substrate for the efflux transporter, P-glycoprotein (Pgp). Clarithromycin is known to inhibit Pgp. When clarithromycin and digoxin are administered together, inhibition of Pgp by clarithromycin may lead to increased exposure to digoxin. Elevated digoxin serum concentrations in patients receiving clarithromycin and digoxin concomitantly have also been reported in post-marketing surveillance. Some patients have shown clinical signs consistent with digoxin toxicity, including potentially fatal arrhythmias. Serum digoxin concentrations should be carefully monitored while patients are receiving digoxin and clarithromycin simultaneously.

Colchicine is a substrate for both CYP3A and the efflux transporter, P-glycoprotein (Pgp). Clarithromycin and other macrolides are known to inhibit CYP3A and Pgp. When clarithromycin and colchicine are administered together, inhibition of Pgp and/or CYP3A by clarithromycin may lead to increased exposure to colchicine. Patients should be monitored for clinical symptoms of colchicine toxicity. (See **WARNINGS**.)

Co-administration of clarithromycin, known to inhibit CYP3A, and a drug primarily metabolized by CYP3A may be associated with elevations in drug concentrations that could increase or prolong both therapeutic and adverse effects of the concomitant drug.

Clarithromycin should be used with caution in patients receiving treatment with other drugs known to be CYP3A enzyme substrates, especially if the CYP3A substrate has a narrow safety margin (e.g., carbamazepine) and/or the substrate is extensively metabolized by this enzyme. Dosage adjustments may be considered, and when possible, serum concentrations of drugs primarily metabolized by CYP3A should be monitored closely in patients concurrently receiving clarithromycin.

The following are examples of some clinically significant CYP3A based drug interactions. Interactions with other drugs metabolized by the CYP3A isoform are also possible.

Carbamazepine and Terfenadine

Increased serum concentrations of carbamazepine and the active acid metabolite of terfenadine were observed in clinical trials with clarithromycin.

Efavirenz, Nevirapine, Rifampicin, Rifabutin, and Rifapentine

Strong inducers of the cytochrome P450 metabolism system such as efavirenz, nevirapine, rifampicin, rifabutin, and rifapentine may accelerate the metabolism of clarithromycin and thus lower the plasma levels of clarithromycin, while increasing those of 14-OH-clarithromycin, a metabolite that is also microbiologically active. Since the microbiological activities of clarithromycin and 14-OH-clarithromycin are different for different bacteria, the intended therapeutic effect could be impaired during concomitant administration of clarithromycin and enzyme inducers.

Sildenafil, Tadalafil, and Vardenafil

Each of these phosphodiesterase inhibitors is metabolized, at least in part, by CYP3A, and CYP3A may be inhibited by concomitantly administered clarithromycin. Co-administration of clarithromycin with sildenafil, tadalafil, or vardenafil would likely result in increased phosphodiesterase inhibitor exposure. Reduction of sildenafil, tadalafil and vardenafil dosages should be considered when these drugs are co-administered with clarithromycin.

Tolterodine

The primary route of metabolism for tolterodine is via the 2D6 isoform of cytochrome P450 (CYP2D6). However, in a subset of the population devoid of CYP2D6, the identified pathway of metabolism is via CYP3A. In this population subset, inhibition of CYP3A results in significantly higher serum concentrations of tolterodine. A reduction in tolterodine dosage may be necessary in the presence of CYP3A inhibitors, such as clarithromycin in the CYP2D6 poor metabolizer population.

Triazolobenzodiazepines (e.g., alprazolam, midazolam, triazolam)

When midazolam was co-administered with clarithromycin tablets (500 mg twice daily), midazolam AUC was increased 2.7-fold after intravenous administration of midazolam and 7-fold after oral administration. Concomitant administration of oral midazolam and clarithromycin should be avoided. If intravenous midazolam is co-administered with clarithromycin, the patient must be closely monitored to allow dose adjustment.

The same precautions should also apply to other benzodiazepines that are metabolized by CYP3A, including triazolam and alprazolam. For benzodiazepines which are not dependent on CYP3A for their elimination (temazepam, nitrazepam, lorazepam), a clinically important interaction with clarithromycin is unlikely. There have been post-marketing reports of drug interactions and central nervous system (CNS) effects (e.g., somnolence and confusion) with the concomitant use of clarithromycin and triazolam. Monitoring the patient for increased CNS pharmacological effects is suggested.

Atazanavir

Both clarithromycin and atazanavir are substrates and inhibitors of CYP3A, and there is evidence of a bi-directional drug interaction. Co-administration of clarithromycin (500 mg twice daily) with atazanavir (400 mg once daily) resulted in a 2-fold increase in exposure to clarithromycin and a 70% decrease in exposure to 14-OH-clarithromycin, with a 28% increase in the AUC of atazanavir.

Because of the large therapeutic window for clarithromycin, no dosage reduction should be necessary in patients with normal renal function. For patients with moderate renal function (creatinine clearance 30 to 60 mL/min), the dose of clarithromycin should be decreased by 50%. For patients with creatinine clearance <30 mL/min, the dose of clarithromycin should be decreased by 75% using an appropriate clarithromycin formulation. Doses of clarithromycin greater than 1000 mg per day should not be co-administered with protease inhibitors.

Itraconazole

Both clarithromycin and itraconazole are substrates and inhibitors of CYP3A, leading to a bi-directional drug interaction. Clarithromycin may increase the plasma levels of itraconazole, while itraconazole may increase the plasma levels of clarithromycin. Patients taking itraconazole and clarithromycin concomitantly should be monitored closely for signs or symptoms of increased or prolonged pharmacologic effects.

Saquinavir

Both clarithromycin and saquinavir are substrates and inhibitors of CYP3A, and there is evidence of a bi-directional drug interaction. Concomitant administration of clarithromycin (500 mg bid) and saquinavir (soft gelatin capsules, 1200 mg tid) to 12 healthy volunteers resulted in steady-state AUC and C_{max} values of saquinavir which were 177% and 187% higher than those seen with saquinavir alone. Clarithromycin AUC and C_{max} values were approximately 40% higher than those seen with clarithromycin alone. No dose adjustment is required when the two drugs are co-administered for a limited time at the doses/formulations studied. Observations from drug interaction studies using the soft gelatin capsule formulation may not be representative of the effects seen using the saquinavir hard gelatin capsule. Observations from drug interactions studies performed with saquinavir alone may not be representative of the effects seen with saquinavir/ritonavir therapy. When saquinavir is co-administered with ritonavir, consideration should be given to the potential effects of ritonavir on clarithromycin (see **PRECAUTIONS — Drug Interactions**).

The following CYP3A based drug interactions have been observed with erythromycin products and/or with clarithromycin in post-marketing experience:

Antiarrhythmics

There have been post-marketing reports of torsades de pointes occurring with concurrent use of clarithromycin and quinidine or disopyramide. Electrocardiograms should be monitored for QTc prolongation during coadministration of clarithromycin with these drugs. Serum concentrations of these medications should also be monitored.

Ergotamine/Dihydroergotamine

Post-marketing reports indicate that coadministration of clarithromycin with ergotamine or dihydroergotamine has been associated with acute ergot toxicity characterized by vasospasm and ischemia of the extremities and other tissues including the central nervous system. Concomitant administration of clarithromycin with ergotamine or dihydroergotamine is contraindicated (see **CONTRAINDICATIONS**).

Triazolobenziodidiazepines (Such as Triazolam and Alprazolam) and Related Benzodiazepines (Such as Midazolam)

Erythromycin has been reported to decrease the clearance of triazolam and midazolam, and thus, may increase the pharmacologic effect of these benzodiazepines. There have been post-marketing reports of drug interactions and CNS effects (e.g., somnolence and confusion) with the concomitant use of clarithromycin and triazolam.

HMG-CoA Reductase Inhibitors

As with other macrolides, clarithromycin has been reported to increase concentrations of HMG-CoA reductase inhibitors (e.g., lovastatin and simvastatin). Rare reports of rhabdomyolysis have been reported in patients taking these drugs concomitantly.

Sildenafil (Viagra)

Erythromycin has been reported to increase the systemic exposure (AUC) of sildenafil. A similar interaction may occur with clarithromycin; reduction of sildenafil dosage should be considered. (See Viagra package insert.)

There have been spontaneous or published reports of CYP3A based interactions of erythromycin and/or clarithromycin with cyclosporine, carbamazepine, tacrolimus, alfentanil, disopyramide, rifabutin, quinidine, methylprednisolone, cilostazol, bromocriptine and vinblastine.

Concomitant administration of clarithromycin with cisapride, pimozide, astemizole, or terfenadine is contraindicated (see **CONTRAINDICATIONS**.)

In addition, there have been reports of interactions of erythromycin or clarithromycin with drugs not thought to be metabolized by CYP3A, including hexobarbital, phenytoin, and valproate.

Carcinogenesis, Mutagenesis, Impairment of Fertility

The following *in vitro* mutagenicity tests have been conducted with clarithromycin:

Salmonella/Mammalian Microsomes Test
Bacterial Induced Mutation Frequency Test
In Vitro Chromosome Aberration Test
Rat Hepatocyte DNA Synthesis Assay
Mouse Lymphoma Assay
Mouse Dominant Lethal Study
Mouse Micronucleus Test

All tests had negative results except the *In Vitro* Chromosome Aberration Test which was weakly positive in one test and negative in another.

In addition, a Bacterial Reverse-Mutation Test (Ames Test) has been performed on clarithromycin metabolites with negative results.

Fertility and reproduction studies have shown that daily doses of up to 160 mg/kg/day (1.3 times the recommended maximum human dose based on mg/m^2) to male and female rats caused no adverse effects on the estrous cycle, fertility, parturition, or number and viability of offspring. Plasma levels in rats after 150 mg/kg/day were 2 times the human serum levels.

In the 150 mg/kg/day monkey studies, plasma levels were 3 times the human serum levels. When given orally at 150 mg/kg/day (2.4 times the recommended maximum human dose based on mg/m^2), clarithromycin was shown to produce embryonic loss in monkeys. This effect has been attributed to marked maternal toxicity of the drug at this high dose.

In rabbits, *in utero* fetal loss occurred at an intravenous dose of 33 mg/m^2, which is 17 times less than the maximum proposed human oral daily dose of 618 mg/m^2.

Long-term studies in animals have not been performed to evaluate the carcinogenic potential of clarithromycin.

Pregnancy

Teratogenic Effects

Pregnancy Category C

Four teratogenicity studies in rats (three with oral doses and one with intravenous doses up to 160 mg/kg/day administered during the period of major organogenesis) and two in rabbits at oral doses up to 125 mg/kg/day (approximately 2 times the recommended maximum human dose based on mg/m^2) or intravenous doses of 30 mg/kg/day administered during gestation days 6 to 18 failed to demonstrate any teratogenicity from clarithromycin. Two additional oral studies in a different rat strain at similar doses and similar conditions demonstrated a low incidence of cardiovascular anomalies at doses of 150 mg/kg/day administered during gestation days 6 to 15. Plasma levels after 150 mg/kg/day were 2 times the human serum levels. Four studies in mice revealed a variable incidence of cleft palate following oral doses of 1000 mg/kg/day (2 and 4 times the recommended maximum human dose based on mg/m^2, respectively) during gestation days 6 to 15. Cleft palate was also seen at 500 mg/kg/day. The 1000 mg/kg/day exposure resulted in plasma levels 17 times the human serum levels. In monkeys, an oral dose of 70 mg/kg/day (an approximate equidose of the recommended maximum human dose based on mg/m^2) produced fetal growth retardation at plasma levels that were 2 times the human serum levels.

There are no adequate and well-controlled studies in pregnant women. Clarithromycin should be used during pregnancy only if the potential benefit justifies the potential risk to the fetus. (See **WARNINGS**.)

Nursing Mothers

It is not known whether clarithromycin is excreted in human milk. Because many drugs are excreted in human milk, caution should be exercised when clarithromycin is administered to a nursing woman. It is known that clarithromycin is excreted in the milk of lactating animals and that other drugs of this class are excreted in human milk. Preweaned rats, exposed indirectly via consumption of milk from dams treated with 150 mg/kg/day for 3 weeks, were not adversely affected, despite data indicating higher drug levels in milk than in plasma.

Pediatric Use

Safety and effectiveness of clarithromycin in pediatric patients under 6 months of age have not been established. The safety of clarithromycin has not been studied in MAC patients under the age of 20 months. Neonatal and juvenile animals tolerated clarithromycin in a manner similar to adult animals. Young animals were slightly more intolerant to acute overdosage and to subtle reductions in erythrocytes, platelets and leukocytes but were less sensitive to toxicity in the liver, kidney, thymus, and genitalia.

Geriatric Use

In a steady-state study in which healthy elderly subjects (age 65 to 81 years old) were given 500 mg every 12 hours, the maximum serum concentrations and area under the curves of clarithromycin and 14-OH clarithromycin were increased compared to those achieved in healthy young adults. These changes in pharmacokinetics parallel known age-related decreases in renal function. In clinical trials, elderly patients did not have an increased incidence of adverse events when compared to younger patients. Dosage adjustment should be considered in elderly patients with severe renal impairment. (See **WARNINGS** and **PRECAUTIONS**.)

ADVERSE REACTIONS

The majority of side effects observed in clinical trials were of a mild and transient nature. Fewer than 3% of adult patients without mycobacterial infections and fewer than 2% of pediatric patients without mycobacterial infections discontinued therapy because of drug-related side effects. Fewer than 2% of adult patients taking BIAXIN XL tablets discontinued therapy because of drug-related side effects.

The most frequently reported events in adults taking BIAXIN tablets (clarithromycin tablets, USP) were diarrhea (3%), nausea (3%), abnormal taste (3%), dyspepsia (2%), abdominal pain/discomfort (2%), and headache (2%). In pediatric patients, the most frequently reported events were diarrhea (6%), vomiting (6%), abdominal pain (3%), rash (3%), and headache (2%). Most of these events were described as mild or moderate in severity. Of the reported adverse events, only 1% was described as severe.

The most frequently reported events in adults taking BIAXIN XL (Clarithromycin extended-release tablets) were diarrhea (6%), abnormal taste (7%), and nausea (3%). Most of these events were described as mild or moderate in severity. Of the reported adverse events, less than 1% were described as severe.

In the acute exacerbation of chronic bronchitis and acute maxillary sinusitis studies overall gastrointestinal adverse events were reported by a similar proportion of patients taking either BIAXIN tablets or BIAXIN XL tablets; however, patients taking BIAXIN XL tablets reported significantly less severe gastrointestinal symptoms compared to patients taking BIAXIN tablets. In addition, patients taking BIAXIN XL tablets had significantly fewer premature discontinuations for drug-related gastrointestinal or abnormal taste adverse events compared to BIAXIN tablets.

In community-acquired pneumonia studies conducted in adults comparing clarithromycin to erythromycin base or erythromycin stearate, there were fewer adverse events involving the digestive system in clarithromycin-treated patients compared to erythromycin-treated patients (13% vs 32%; p < 0.01). Twenty percent of erythromycin-treated patients discontinued therapy due to adverse events compared to 4% of clarithromycin-treated patients.

In two U.S. studies of acute otitis media comparing clarithromycin to amoxicillin/potassium clavulanate in pediatric patients, there were fewer adverse events involving the digestive system in clarithromycin-treated patients compared to amoxicillin/potassium clavulanate-treated pa-

tients (21% vs. 40%, p < 0.001). One-third as many clarithromycin-treated patients reported diarrhea as did amoxicillin/potassium clavulanate-treated patients.

Post-Marketing Experience

Allergic reactions ranging from urticaria and mild skin eruptions to rare cases of anaphylaxis, Stevens-Johnson syndrome and toxic epidermal necrolysis have occurred. Other spontaneously reported adverse events include glossitis, stomatitis, oral moniliasis, anorexia, vomiting, pancreatitis, tongue discoloration, thrombocytopenia, leukopenia, neutropenia, and dizziness. There have been reports of tooth discoloration in patients treated with BIAXIN. Tooth discoloration is usually reversible with professional dental cleaning. There have been isolated reports of hearing loss, which is usually reversible, occurring chiefly in elderly women. Reports of alterations of the sense of smell including smell loss, usually in conjunction with taste perversion or taste loss, have also been reported.

Transient CNS events including anxiety, behavioral changes, confusional states, convulsions, depersonalization, disorientation, hallucinations, insomnia, depression, manic behavior, nightmares, psychosis, tinnitus, tremor, and vertigo have been reported during post-marketing surveillance. Events usually resolve with discontinuation of the drug.

Hepatic dysfunction, including increased liver enzymes, and hepatocellular and/or cholestatic hepatitis, with or without jaundice, has been infrequently reported with clarithromycin. This hepatic dysfunction may be severe and is usually reversible. In very rare instances, hepatic failure with fatal outcome has been reported and generally has been associated with serious underlying diseases and/or concomitant medications.

There have been rare reports of hypoglycemia, some of which have occurred in patients taking oral hypoglycemic agents or insulin.

There have been post-marketing reports of BIAXIN XL tablets in the stool, many of which have occurred in patients with anatomic (including ileostomy or colostomy) or functional gastrointestinal disorders with shortened GI transit times.

As with other macrolides, clarithromycin has been associated with QT prolongation and ventricular arrhythmias, including ventricular tachycardia and torsades de pointes.

There have been reports of interstitial nephritis coincident with clarithromycin use.

There have been post-marketing reports of colchicine toxicity with concomitant use of clarithromycin and colchicine, especially in the elderly, some of which occurred in patients with renal insufficiency. Deaths have been reported in some such patients. (See **WARNINGS** and **PRECAUTIONS**.)

Changes in Laboratory Values

Changes in laboratory values with possible clinical significance were as follows:

Hepatic

Elevated SGPT (ALT) < 1%; SGOT (AST) < 1%; GGT < 1%; alkaline phosphatase < 1%; LDH < 1%; total bilirubin < 1%

Hematologic

Decreased WBC < 1%; elevated prothrombin time 1%

Renal

Elevated BUN 4%; elevated serum creatinine < 1%

GGT, alkaline phosphatase, and prothrombin time data are from adult studies only.

OVERDOSAGE

Overdosage of clarithromycin can cause gastrointestinal symptoms such as abdominal pain, vomiting, nausea, and diarrhea.

Adverse reactions accompanying overdosage should be treated by the prompt elimination of unabsorbed drug and supportive measures. As with other macrolides, clarithromycin serum concentrations are not expected to be appreciably affected by hemodialysis or peritoneal dialysis.

DOSAGE AND ADMINISTRATION

BIAXIN® Filmtab® (clarithromycin tablets, USP) and BIAXIN® Granules (clarithromycin for oral suspension, USP) may be given with or without food. BIAXIN® XL Filmtab® (clarithromycin extended-release tablets) should be taken with food. BIAXIN XL tablets should be swallowed whole and not chewed, broken or crushed.

[See table above]

H. pylori Eradication to Reduce the Risk of Duodenal Ulcer Recurrence

Triple therapy: BIAXIN/lansoprazole/amoxicillin
The recommended adult dose is 500 mg BIAXIN, 30 mg lansoprazole, and 1 gram amoxicillin, all given twice daily (q12h) for 10 or 14 days. (See **INDICATIONS AND USAGE** and **CLINICAL STUDIES** sections.)

Triple therapy: BIAXIN/omeprazole/amoxicillin
The recommended adult dose is 500 mg BIAXIN, 20 mg omeprazole, and 1 gram amoxicillin, all given twice daily (q12h) for 10 days. (See **INDICATIONS AND USAGE** and **CLINICAL STUDIES** sections.) In patients with an ulcer present at the time of initiation of therapy, an additional 18 days of omeprazole 20 mg once daily is recommended for ulcer healing and symptom relief.

Dual therapy: BIAXIN/omeprazole
The recommended adult dose is 500 mg BIAXIN given three times daily (q8h) and 40 mg omeprazole given once daily (qAM) for 14 days. (See **INDICATIONS AND USAGE** and **CLINICAL STUDIES** sections.) An additional 14 days of omeprazole 20 mg once daily is recommended for ulcer healing and symptom relief.

Dual therapy: BIAXIN/ranitidine bismuth citrate
The recommended adult dose is 500 mg BIAXIN given twice daily (q12h) or three times daily (q8h) and 400 mg ranitidine bismuth citrate given twice daily (q12h) for 14 days. An additional 14 days of 400 mg twice daily is recommended for ulcer healing and symptom relief. BIAXIN and ranitidine bismuth citrate combination therapy is not recommended in patients with creatinine clearance less than 25 mL/min. (See **INDICATIONS AND USAGE** and **CLINICAL STUDIES** sections.)

Children
The usual recommended daily dosage is 15 mg/kg/day divided q12h for 10 days.

Information on the Abbott Pharmaceutical Products listed on these pages is from the prescribing information in use as of June 1, 2010. For more information, please visit rxabbott.com or call 1-800-633-9110.

ADULT DOSAGE GUIDELINES

Infection	BIAXIN Tablets Dosage (q12h)	BIAXIN Tablets Duration (days)	BIAXIN XL Tablets Dosage (q24h)	BIAXIN XL Tablets Duration (days)
Pharyngitis/Tonsillitis due to				
S. pyogenes	250 mg	10	-	-
Acute maxillary sinusitis due to	500 mg	14	2 × 500 mg	14
H. influenzae				
M. catarrhalis				
S. pneumoniae				
Acute exacerbation of chronic bronchitis due to				
H. influenzae	500 mg	7-14	2 × 500 mg	7
H. parainfluenzae	500 mg	7	2 × 500 mg	7
M. catarrhalis	250 mg	7-14	2 × 500 mg	7
S. pneumoniae	250 mg	7-14	2 × 500 mg	7
Community-Acquired Pneumonia due to				
H. influenzae	250 mg	7	2 × 500 mg	7
H. parainfluenzae	-	-	2 × 500 mg	7
M. catarrhalis	-	-	2 × 500 mg	7
S. pneumoniae	250 mg	7-14	2 × 500 mg	7
C. pneumoniae	250 mg	7-14	2 × 500 mg	7
M. pneumoniae	250 mg	7-14	2 × 500 mg	7
Uncomplicated skin and skin structure	250 mg	7-14	-	-
S. aureus				
S. pyogenes				

Total Volume After Constitution	Clarithromycin Concentration After Constitution	Clarithromycin Contents Per Bottle	NDC
50 mL	125 mg/5 mL	1250 mg	0074-3163-50
100 mL	125 mg/5 mL	2500 mg	0074-3163-13
50 mL	250 mg/5 mL	2500 mg	0074-3188-50
100 mL	250 mg/5 mL	5000 mg	0074-3188-13

	Mortality		Reduction in Mortality on Clarithromycin
	Placebo	Clarithromycin	
6 month	9.4%	6.5%	31%
12 month	29.7%	20.5%	31%
18 month	46.4%	37.5%	20%

PEDIATRIC DOSAGE GUIDELINES

Based on Body Weight
Dosing Calculated on 7.5 mg/kg q12h

Weight Kg	lbs	Dose (q12h)	125 mg/5 mL	250 mg/5 mL
9	20	62.5 mg	2.5 mL q12h	1.25 mL q12h
17	37	125 mg	5 mL q12h	2.5 mL q12h
25	55	187.5 mg	7.5 mL q12h	3.75 mL q12h
33	73	250 mg	10 mL q12h	5 mL q12h

Clarithromycin may be administered without dosage adjustment in the presence of hepatic impairment if there is normal renal function. However, in the presence of severe renal impairment (CR_{CL} < 30 mL/min), with or without coexisting hepatic impairment, the dose should be halved or the dosing interval doubled.

Mycobacterial Infections

Prophylaxis

The recommended dose of BIAXIN for the prevention of disseminated *Mycobacterium avium* disease is 500 mg b.i.d. In children, the recommended dose is 7.5 mg/kg b.i.d. up to 500 mg b.i.d. No studies of clarithromycin for MAC prophylaxis have been performed in pediatric populations and the doses recommended for prophylaxis are derived from MAC treatment studies in children. Dosing recommendations for children are in the table above.

Treatment

Clarithromycin is recommended as the primary agent for the treatment of disseminated infection due to *Mycobacterium avium* complex. Clarithromycin should be used in combination with other antimycobacterial drugs that have shown *in vitro* activity against MAC or clinical benefit in MAC treatment. (See **CLINICAL STUDIES**.) The recommended dose for mycobacterial infections in adults is 500 mg b.i.d. In children, the recommended dose is 7.5 mg/kg b.i.d. up to 500 mg b.i.d. Dosing recommendations for children are in the table above.

Clarithromycin therapy should continue for life if clinical and mycobacterial improvements are observed.

Constituting Instructions

The table below indicates the volume of water to be added when constituting:

Total Volume After Constitution	Clarithromycin Concentration After Constitution	Amount of Water to be Added*
50 mL	125 mg/5 mL	27 mL
100 mL	125 mg/5 mL	55 mL
50 mL	250 mg/5 mL	27 mL
100 mL	250 mg/5 mL	55 mL

* see instructions below.

Add half the volume of water to the bottle and shake vigorously. Add the remainder of water to the bottle and shake. Shake well before each use. Oversize bottle provides shake space. Keep tightly closed. Do not refrigerate. After mixing, store at 15° to 30°C (59° to 86°F) and use within 14 days.

HOW SUPPLIED

BIAXIN® Filmtab® (clarithromycin tablets, USP) are supplied as yellow oval film-coated tablets in the following packaging sizes:

250 mg tablets: (imprinted in blue with the Abbott ⊐ logo and Abbo-Code KT)
Bottles of 60 (NDC 0074-3368-60) and ABBO-PAC unit dose strip packages of 100 (NDC 0074-3368-11).
Store BIAXIN 250 mg tablets at controlled room temperature 15° to 30°C (59° to 86°F) in a well-closed container. Protect from light.
500 mg tablets: (debossed with the Abbott ⊐ logo on one side and Abbo-Code KL on the opposite side)
Bottles of 60 (NDC 0074-2586-60) and ABBO-PAC unit dose strip packages of 100 (NDC 0074-2586-11).
Store BIAXIN 500 mg tablets at controlled room temperature 20° to 25°C (68° to 77°F) in a well-closed container.
BIAXIN® XL Filmtab® (clarithromycin extended-release tablets) are supplied as yellow oval film-coated

500 mg tablets debossed (on one side) with the Abbott ⊐ logo and a two-letter Abbo-Code designation, KJ in the following packaging sizes:
500 mg tablets:
Bottles of 60 (NDC 0074-3165-60), ABBO-PAC unit dose strip packages of 100 (NDC 0074-3165-11), and BIAXIN® XL PAC carton of 4 blister packages 14 tablets each (NDC 0074-3165-41).
Store BIAXIN XL tablets at 20° to 25°C (68° to 77°F). Excursions permitted to 15° to 30°C (59° to 86°F). [See USP Controlled Room Temperature.]
BIAXIN® Granules (clarithromycin for oral suspension, USP) is supplied in the following strengths and sizes:
[See table above]
Store BIAXIN granules for oral suspension at controlled room temperature 15° to 30°C (59° to 86°F) in a well-closed container. Do not refrigerate BIAXIN suspension.

CLINICAL STUDIES

Mycobacterial Infections

Prophylaxis

A randomized, double-blind study (561) compared clarithromycin 500 mg b.i.d. to placebo in patients with CDC-defined AIDS and CD_4 counts < 100 cells/µL. This study accrued 682 patients from November 1992 to January 1994, with a median CD_4 cell count at study entry of 30 cells/µL. Median duration of clarithromycin was 10.6 months vs. 8.2 months for placebo. More patients in the placebo arm than the clarithromycin arm discontinued prematurely from the study (75.6% and 67.4%, respectively). However, if premature discontinuations due to MAC or death are excluded, approximately equal percentages of patients on each arm (54.8% on clarithromycin and 52.5% on placebo) discontinued study drug early for other reasons. The study was designed to evaluate the following endpoints:

1. MAC bacteremia, defined as at least one positive culture for *M. avium* complex bacteria from blood or another normally sterile site.
2. Survival.
3. Clinically significant disseminated MAC disease, defined as MAC bacteremia accompanied by signs or symptoms of serious MAC infection, including fever, night sweats, weight loss, anemia, or elevations in liver function tests.

MAC Bacteremia

In patients randomized to clarithromycin, the risk of MAC bacteremia was reduced by 69% compared to placebo. The difference between groups was statistically significant (p < 0.001). On an intent-to-treat basis, the one-year cumulative incidence of MAC bacteremia was 5.0% for patients randomized to clarithromycin and 19.4% for patients randomized to placebo. While only 19 of the 341 patients randomized to clarithromycin developed MAC, 11 of these cases were resistant to clarithromycin. The patients with resistant MAC bacteremia had a median baseline CD_4 count of 10 cells/mm³ (range 2 to 25 cells/mm³). Information regarding the clinical course and response to treatment of the patients with resistant MAC bacteremia is limited. The 8 patients who received clarithromycin and developed susceptible MAC bacteremia had a median baseline CD_4 count of 25 cells/mm³ (range 10 to 80 cells/mm³). Comparatively, 53 of the 341 placebo patients developed MAC; none of these isolates were resistant to clarithromycin. The median baseline CD_4 count was 15 cells/mm³ (range 2 to 130 cells/mm³) for placebo patients that developed MAC.

Survival

A statistically significant survival benefit was observed.

Survival All Randomized Patients

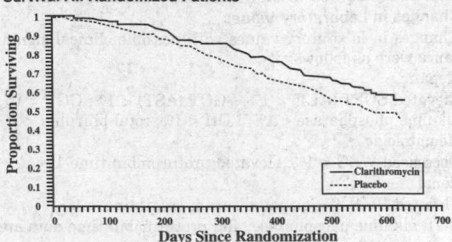

Since the analysis at 18 months includes patients no longer receiving prophylaxis the survival benefit of clarithromycin may be underestimated.

Clinically Significant Disseminated MAC Disease

In association with the decreased incidence of bacteremia, patients in the group randomized to clarithromycin showed reductions in the signs and symptoms of disseminated MAC disease, including fever, night sweats, weight loss, and anemia.

Safety

In AIDS patients treated with clarithromycin over long periods of time for prophylaxis against *M. avium*, it was often difficult to distinguish adverse events possibly associated with clarithromycin administration from underlying HIV disease or intercurrent illness. Median duration of treatment was 10.6 months for the clarithromycin group and 8.2 months for the placebo group.

Treatment-related* Adverse Event Incidence Rates (%) in Immunocompromised Adult Patients Receiving Prophylaxis Against *M. avium* Complex

Body System‡ Adverse Event	Clarithromycin (n = 339) %	Placebo (n = 339) %
Body as a Whole		
Abdominal pain	5.0%	3.5%
Headache	2.7%	0.9%
Digestive		
Diarrhea	7.7%	4.1%
Dyspepsia	3.8%	2.7%
Flatulence	2.4%	0.9%
Nausea	11.2%	7.1%
Vomiting	5.9%	3.2%
Skin & Appendages		
Rash	3.2%	3.5%
Special Senses		
Taste Perversion	8.0%	0.3%

* Includes those events possibly or probably related to study drug and excludes concurrent conditions.
‡ > 2% Adverse Event Incidence Rates for either treatment group.

Among these events, taste perversion was the only event that had significantly higher incidence in the clarithromycin-treated group compared to the placebo-treated group.

Discontinuation due to adverse events was required in 18% of patients receiving clarithromycin compared to 17% of patients receiving placebo in this trial. Primary reasons for discontinuation in clarithromycin treated patients include headache, nausea, vomiting, depression and taste perversion.

Changes in Laboratory Values of Potential Clinical Importance

In immunocompromised patients receiving prophylaxis against *M. avium*, evaluations of laboratory values were made by analyzing those values outside the seriously abnormal value (i.e., the extreme high or low limit) for the specified test.

[See table at top of next page]

Treatment

Three randomized studies (500, 577, and 521) compared different dosages of clarithromycin in patients with CDC-defined AIDS and CD_4 counts < 100 cells/µL. These studies accrued patients from May 1991 to March 1992. Study 500 was randomized, double-blind; Study 577 was open-label compassionate use. Both studies used 500 and 1000 mg b.i.d. doses; Study 500 also had a 2000 mg b.i.d. group. Study 521 was a pediatric study at 3.75, 7.5, and 15 mg/kg b.i.d. Study 500 enrolled 154 adult patients, Study 577 enrolled 469 adult patients, and Study 521 enrolled 25 patients between the ages of 1 to 20. The majority of patients had CD_4 cell counts < 50/µL at study entry. The studies were designed to evaluate the following end points:

1. Change in MAC bacteremia or blood cultures negative for *M. avium*.
2. Change in clinical signs and symptoms of MAC infection including one or more of the following: fever, night sweats, weight loss, diarrhea, splenomegaly, and hepatomegaly.

The results for the 500 study are described below. The 577 study results were similar to the results of the 500 study.

Percentage of Patients[a] Exceeding Extreme Laboratory Value in Patients Receiving Prophylaxis Against *M. avium* Complex

		Clarithromycin 500 mg b.i.d.	Placebo
Hemoglobin	< 8 g/dL	4/118 3%	5/103 5%
Platelet Count	< 50 × 10^9/L	11/249 4%	12/250 5%
WBC Count	< 1 × 10^9/L	2/103 4%	0/95 0%
SGOT	> 5 × ULN[b]	7/196 4%	5/208 2%
SGPT	> 5 × ULN[b]	6/217 3%	4/232 2%
Alk. Phos.	> 5 × ULN[b]	5/220 2%	5/218 2%

(a) Includes only patients with baseline values within the normal range or borderline high (hematology variables) and within the normal range or borderline low (chemistry variables).
(b) ULN = Upper Limit of Normal

	Resolution of Fever			Resolution of Night Sweats	
b.i.d. dose (mg)	% ever afebrile	% afebrile ≥ 6 weeks	b.i.d. dose (mg)	% ever resolving	% resolving ≥ 6 weeks
500	67%	23%	500	85%	42%
1000	67%	12%	1000	70%	33%
2000	62%	22%	2000	72%	36%

	Weight Gain > 3%			Hemoglobin Increase >1 gm	
b.i.d. dose (mg)	% ever gaining	% gaining ≥ 6 weeks	b.i.d. dose (mg)	% ever increasing	% increasing ≥ 6 weeks
500	33%	14%	500	58%	26%
1000	26%	17%	1000	37%	6%
2000	26%	12%	2000	62%	18%

Results with the 7.5 mg/kg b.i.d. dose in the pediatric study were comparable to those for the 500 mg b.i.d. regimen in the adult studies.

Study 069 compared the safety and efficacy of clarithromycin in combination with ethambutol versus clarithromycin in combination with ethambutol and clofazimine for the treatment of disseminated MAC (dMAC) infection.[4] This 24-week study enrolled 106 patients with AIDS and dMAC, with 55 patients randomized to receive clarithromycin and ethambutol, and 51 patients randomized to receive clarithromycin, ethambutol, and clofazimine. Baseline characteristics between study arms were similar with the exception of median CFU counts being at least 1 log higher in the clarithromycin, ethambutol, and clofazimine arm.

Compared to prior experience with clarithromycin monotherapy, the two-drug regimen of clarithromycin and ethambutol was well tolerated and extended the time to microbiologic relapse, largely through suppressing the emergence of clarithromycin resistant strains. However, the addition of clofazimine to the regimen added no additional microbiologic or clinical benefit. Tolerability of both multidrug regimens was comparable with the most common adverse events being gastrointestinal in nature. Patients receiving the clofazimine-containing regimen had reduced survival rates; however, their baseline mycobacterial colony counts were higher. The results of this trial support the addition of ethambutol to clarithromycin for the treatment of initial dMAC infections but do not support adding clofazimine as a third agent.

MAC Bacteremia

Decreases in MAC bacteremia or negative blood cultures were seen in the majority of patients in all dose groups. Mean reductions in colony forming units (CFU) are shown below. Included in the table are results from a separate study with a four drug regimen[5] (ciprofloxacin, ethambutol, rifampicin, and clofazimine). Since patient populations and study procedures may vary between these two studies, comparisons between the clarithromycin results and the combination therapy results should be interpreted cautiously.

Mean Reductions in Log CFU from Baseline (After 4 Weeks of Therapy)

500 mg b.i.d. (N = 35)	1000 mg b.i.d. (N = 32)	2000 mg b.i.d. (N = 26)	Four Drug Regimen (N = 24)
1.5	2.3	2.3	1.4

Although the 1000 mg and 2000 mg b.i.d. doses showed significantly better control of bacteremia during the first four weeks of therapy, no significant differences were seen beyond that point. The percent of patients whose blood was sterilized as shown by one or more negative cultures at any time during acute therapy was 61% (30/49) for the 500 mg

b.i.d. group and 59% (29/49) and 52% (25/48) for the 1000 and 2000 mg b.i.d. groups, respectively. The percent of patients who had 2 or more negative cultures during acute therapy that were sustained through Day 84 was 25% (12/49) in both the 500 and 1000 mg b.i.d. groups and 8% (4/48) for the 2000 mg b.i.d. group. By Day 84, 23% (11/49), 37% (18/49), and 56% (27/48) of patients had died or discontinued from the study, and 14% (7/49), 12% (6/49), and 13% (6/48) of patients had relapsed in the 500, 1000, and 2000 mg b.i.d. dose groups, respectively. All of the isolates had an MIC < 8 µg/mL at pre-treatment. Relapse was almost always accompanied by an increase in MIC. The median time to first negative culture was 54, 41, and 29 days for the 500, 1000, and 2000 mg b.i.d. groups, respectively. The time to first decrease of at least 1 log in CFU count was significantly shorter with the 1000 and 2000 mg b.i.d. doses (median equal to 16 and 15 days, respectively) in comparison to the 500 mg b.i.d. group (median equal to 29 days). The median time to first positive culture or study discontinuation following the first negative culture was 43, 59 and 43 days for the 500, 1000, and 2000 mg b.i.d. groups, respectively.

Clinically Significant Disseminated MAC Disease

Among patients experiencing night sweats prior to therapy, 84% showed resolution or improvement at some point during the 12 weeks of clarithromycin at 500 to 2000 mg b.i.d. doses. Similarly, 77% of patients reported resolution or improvement in fevers at some point. Response rates for clinical signs of MAC are given below:
[See second table above]
The median duration of response, defined as improvement or resolution of clinical signs and symptoms, was 2 to 6 weeks.

Since the study was not designed to determine the benefit of monotherapy beyond 12 weeks, the duration of response may be underestimated for the 25 to 33% of patients who continued to show clinical response after 12 weeks.

Survival

Median survival time from study entry (Study 500) was 249 days at the 500 mg b.i.d. dose compared to 215 days with the 1000 mg b.i.d. dose. However, during the first 12 weeks of therapy, there were 2 deaths in 53 patients in the 500 mg b.i.d. group versus 13 deaths in 51 patients in the 1000 mg b.i.d. group. The reason for this apparent mortality difference is not known. Survival in the two groups was similar beyond 12 weeks. The median survival times for these dosages were similar to recent historical controls with MAC when treated with combination therapies.[5]

Median survival time from study entry in Study 577 was 199 days for the 500 mg b.i.d. dose and 179 days for the 1000 mg b.i.d. dose. During the first four weeks of therapy, while patients were maintained on their originally assigned dose, there were 11 deaths in 255 patients taking 500 mg b.i.d. and 18 deaths in 214 patients taking 1000 mg b.i.d.

Safety

The adverse event profiles showed that both the 500 and 1000 mg b.i.d. doses were well tolerated. The 2000 mg b.i.d. dose was poorly tolerated and resulted in a higher proportion of premature discontinuations.

In AIDS patients and other immunocompromised patients treated with the higher doses of clarithromycin over long periods of time for mycobacterial infections, it was often difficult to distinguish adverse events possibly associated with clarithromycin administration from underlying signs of HIV disease or intercurrent illness.

The following analyses summarize experience during the first 12 weeks of therapy with clarithromycin. Data are reported separately for Study 500 (randomized, double-blind) and Study 577 (open-label, compassionate use) and also combined. Adverse events were reported less frequently in Study 577, which may be due in part to differences in monitoring between the two studies. In adult patients receiving clarithromycin 500 mg b.i.d., the most frequently reported adverse events, considered possibly or probably related to study drug, with an incidence of 5% or greater, are listed below. Most of these events were mild to moderate in severity, although 5% (Study 500: 8%; Study 577: 4%) of patients receiving 500 mg b.i.d. and 5% (Study 500: 4%; Study 577: 6%) of patients receiving 1000 mg b.i.d. reported severe adverse events. Excluding those patients who discontinued therapy or died due to complications of their underlying non-mycobacterial disease, approximately 8% (Study 500: 15%; Study 577: 7%) of the patients who received 500 mg b.i.d. and 12% (Study 500: 14%; Study 577: 12%) of the patients who received 1000 mg b.i.d. discontinued therapy due to drug-related events during the first 12 weeks of therapy. Overall, the 500 and 1000 mg b.i.d. doses had similar adverse event profiles.

Treatment-related* Adverse Event Incidence Rates (%) in Immunocompromised Adult Patients During the First 12 Weeks of Therapy with 500 mg b.i.d. Clarithromycin Dose

Adverse Event	Study 500 (n = 53)	Study 577 (n = 255)	Combined (n = 308)
Abdominal Pain	7.5	2.4	3.2
Diarrhea	9.4	1.6	2.9
Flatulence	7.5	0.0	1.3
Headache	7.5	0.4	1.6
Nausea	28.3	9.0	12.3
Rash	9.4	2.0	3.2
Taste Perversion	18.9	0.4	3.6
Vomiting	24.5	3.9	7.5

* Includes those events possibly or probably related to study drug and excludes concurrent conditions.

A limited number of pediatric AIDS patients have been treated with clarithromycin suspension for mycobacterial infections. The most frequently reported adverse events, excluding those due to the patient's concurrent condition, were consistent with those observed in adult patients.

Changes in Laboratory Values

In immunocompromised patients treated with clarithromycin for mycobacterial infections, evaluations of laboratory values were made by analyzing these values outside the seriously abnormal level (i.e., the extreme high or low limit) for the specified test.

Percentage of Patients[a] Exceeding Extreme Laboratory Value Limits During First 12 Weeks of Treatment 500 mg b.i.d. Dose[b]

		Study 500	Study 577	Combined
BUN	> 50 mg/dL	0%	< 1%	< 1%
Platelet Count	< 50 × 10^9/L	0%	< 1%	< 1%
SGOT	> 5 × ULN[c]	0%	3%	2%
SGPT	> 5 × ULN[c]	0%	2%	1%
WBC	< 1 × 10^9/L	0%	1%	1%

(a) Includes only patients with baseline values within the normal range or borderline high (hematology variables) and within the normal range or borderline low (chemistry variables)
(b) Includes all values within the first 12 weeks for patients who start on 500 mg b.i.d.
(c) ULN = Upper Limit of Normal

Otitis Media

In a controlled clinical study of acute otitis media performed in the United States, where significant rates

Information on the Abbott Pharmaceutical Products listed on these pages is from the prescribing information in use as of June 1, 2010. For more information, please visit rxabbott.com or call 1-800-633-9110.

of beta-lactamase producing organisms were found, clarithromycin was compared to an oral cephalosporin. In this study, very strict evaluability criteria were used to determine clinical response. For the 223 patients who were evaluated for clinical efficacy, the clinical success rate (i.e., cure plus improvement) at the post-therapy visit was 88% for clarithromycin and 91% for the cephalosporin.

In a smaller number of patients, microbiologic determinations were made at the pre-treatment visit. The following presumptive bacterial eradication/clinical cure outcomes (i.e., clinical success) were obtained:

U.S. Acute Otitis Media Study Clarithromycin vs. Oral Cephalosporin
EFFICACY RESULTS

PATHOGEN	OUTCOME
S. pneumoniae	clarithromycin success rate, 13/15 (87%), control 4/5
*H. influenzae**	clarithromycin success rate, 10/14 (71%), control 3/4
M. catarrhalis	clarithromycin success rate, 4/5, control 1/1
S. pyogenes	clarithromycin success rate, 3/3, control 0/1
Overall	clarithromycin success rate, 30/37 (81%), control 8/11 (73%)

* None of the *H. influenzae* isolated pre-treatment was resistant to clarithromycin; 6% were resistant to the control agent.

Safety
The incidence of adverse events in all patients treated, primarily diarrhea and vomiting, did not differ clinically or statistically for the two agents.

In two other controlled clinical trials of acute otitis media performed in the United States, where significant rates of beta-lactamase producing organisms were found, clarithromycin was compared to an oral antimicrobial agent that contained a specific beta-lactamase inhibitor. In these studies, very strict evaluability criteria were used to determine the clinical responses. In the 233 patients who were evaluated for clinical efficacy, the combined clinical success rate (i.e., cure and improvement) at the post-therapy visit was 91% for both clarithromycin and the control.

For the patients who had microbiologic determinations at the pre-treatment visit, the following presumptive bacterial eradication/clinical cure outcomes (i.e., clinical success) were obtained:

Two U.S. Acute Otitis Media Studies Clarithromycin vs. Antimicrobial/Beta-lactamase Inhibitor
EFFICACY RESULTS

PATHOGEN	OUTCOME
S. pneumoniae	clarithromycin success rate, 43/51 (84%), control 55/56 (98%)
*H. influenzae**	clarithromycin success rate, 36/45 (80%), control 31/33 (94%)
M. catarrhalis	clarithromycin success rate, 9/10 (90%), control 6/6
S. pyogenes	clarithromycin success rate, 3/3, control 5/5
Overall	clarithromycin success rate, 91/109 (83%), control 97/100 (97%)

* Of the *H. influenzae* isolated pre-treatment, 3% were resistant to clarithromycin and 10% were resistant to the control agent.

Safety
The incidence of adverse events in all patients treated, primarily diarrhea (15% vs. 38%) and diaper rash (3% vs. 11%) in young children, was clinically and statistically lower in the clarithromycin arm versus the control arm.

Duodenal Ulcer Associated with *H. pylori* Infection
Clarithromycin + Lansoprazole and Amoxicillin
H. pylori Eradication for Reducing the Risk of Duodenal Ulcer Recurrence
Two U.S. randomized, double-blind clinical studies in patients with *H. pylori* and duodenal ulcer disease (defined as an active ulcer or history of an active ulcer within one year) evaluated the efficacy of clarithromycin in combination with lansoprazole and amoxicillin capsules as triple 14-day therapy for eradication of *H. pylori*. Based on the results of these studies, the safety and efficacy of the following eradication regimen were established:
Triple therapy: BIAXIN (clarithromycin) 500 mg b.i.d. + lansoprazole 30 mg b.i.d. + amoxicillin 1 gm b.i.d.

Per-Protocol and Intent-to-Treat *H. pylori* Eradication Rates % of Patients Cured [95% Confidence Interval]

	Clarithromycin + omeprazole + amoxicillin		Clarithromycin + amoxicillin	
	Per-Protocol[†]	Intent-to-Treat[‡]	Per-Protocol[†]	Intent-to-Treat[‡]
Study 126	*77 [64, 86] (n = 64)	69 [57, 79] (n = 80)	43 [31, 56] (n = 67)	37 [27, 48] (n = 84)
Study 127	*78 [67, 88] (n = 65)	73 [61, 82] (n = 77)	41 [29, 54] (n = 68)	36 [26, 47] (n = 84)
Study M96-446	*90 [80, 96] (n = 69)	83 [74, 91] (n = 84)	33 [24, 44] (n = 93)	32 [23, 42] (n = 99)

† Patients were included in the analysis if they had confirmed duodenal ulcer disease (active ulcer studies 126 and 127; history of ulcer within 5 years, study M96-446) and *H. pylori* infection at baseline defined as at least two of three positive endoscopic tests from CLOtest®, histology, and/or culture. Patients were included in the analysis if they completed the study. Additionally, if patients dropped out of the study due to an adverse event related to the study drug, they were included in the analysis as failures of therapy. The impact of eradication on ulcer recurrence has not been assessed in patients with a past history of ulcer.
‡ Patients were included in the analysis if they had documented *H. pylori* infection at baseline and had confirmed duodenal ulcer disease. All dropouts were included as failures of therapy.
* p < 0.05 versus clarithromycin plus amoxicillin.

End-of-Treatment Ulcer Healing Rates Percent of Patients Healed (n/N)

Study	Clarithromycin + Omeprazole	Omeprazole	Clarithromycin
U.S. Studies			
Study 100	94% (58/62)[†]	88% (60/68)	71% (49/69)
Study 067	88% (56/64)[†]	85% (55/65)	64% (44/69)
Non-U.S. Studies			
Study 058	99% (84/85)	95% (82/86)	N/A
Study 812b[1]	100% (64/64)	99% (71/72)	N/A

† p < 0.05 for clarithromycin + omeprazole versus clarithromycin monotherapy.
1 In Study 812b patients received omeprazole 40 mg daily for days 15 to 28.

Treatment was for 14 days. *H. pylori* eradication was defined as two negative tests (culture and histology) at 4 to 6 weeks following the end of treatment.
The combination of BIAXIN plus lansoprazole and amoxicillin as triple therapy was effective in eradicating *H. pylori*. Eradication of *H. pylori* has been shown to reduce the risk of duodenal ulcer recurrence.
A randomized, double-blind clinical study performed in the U.S. in patients with *H. pylori* and duodenal ulcer disease (defined as an active ulcer or history of an ulcer within one year) compared the efficacy of clarithromycin in combination with lansoprazole and amoxicillin as triple therapy for 10 and 14 days. This study established that the 10-day triple therapy was equivalent to the 14-day triple therapy in eradicating *H. pylori*.

H. pylori Eradication Rates-Triple Therapy (BIAXIN/lansoprazole/amoxicillin) Percent of Patients Cured [95% Confidence Interval] (number of patients)

Study	Duration	Triple Therapy Evaluable Analysis*	Triple Therapy Intent-to-Treat Analysis#
M93-131	14 days	92[†] [80.0-97.7] (n = 48)	86[†] [73.3-93.5] (n = 55)
M95-392	14 days	86[‡] [75.7-93.6] (n = 66)	83[‡] [72.0-90.8] (n = 70)
M95-399[¶]	14 days	85 [77.0-91.0] (N = 113)	82 [73.9-88.1] (N = 126)
	10 days	84 [76.0-89.8] (N = 123)	81 [73.9-87.6] (N = 135)

* Based on evaluable patients with confirmed duodenal ulcer (active or within one year) and *H. pylori* infection at baseline defined as at least two of three positive endoscopic tests from CLOtest (Delta West LTD., Bentley, Australia), histology, and/or culture. Patients were included in the analysis if they completed the study. Additionally, if patients were dropped out of the study due to an adverse event related to the study drug, they were included in the analysis as evaluable failures of therapy.
# Patients were included in the analysis if they had documented *H. pylori* infection at baseline as defined above and had a confirmed duodenal ulcer (active or within one year). All dropouts were included as failures of therapy.
† (p < 0.05) versus BIAXIN/lansoprazole and lansoprazole/amoxicillin dual therapy.
‡ (p < 0.05) versus BIAXIN/amoxicillin dual therapy.

¶ The 95% confidence interval for the difference in eradication rates, 10-day minus 14-day, is (-10.5, 8.1) in the evaluable analysis and (-9.7, 9.1) in the intent-to-treat analysis.

Clarithromycin + Omeprazole and Amoxicillin Therapy
H. pylori Eradication for Reducing the Risk of Duodenal Ulcer Recurrence
Three U.S., randomized, double-blind clinical studies in patients with *H. pylori* infection and duodenal ulcer disease (n = 558) compared clarithromycin plus omeprazole and amoxicillin to clarithromycin plus amoxicillin. Two studies (Studies 126 and 127) were conducted in patients with an active duodenal ulcer, and the third study (Study 446) was conducted in patients with a duodenal ulcer in the past 5 years, but without an ulcer present at the time of enrollment. The dosage regimen in the studies was clarithromycin 500 mg b.i.d. plus omeprazole 20 mg b.i.d. plus amoxicillin 1 gram b.i.d. for 10 days. In Studies 126 and 127, patients who took the omeprazole regimen also received an additional 18 days of omeprazole 20 mg q.d. Endpoints studied were eradication of *H. pylori* and duodenal ulcer healing (studies 126 and 127 only). *H. pylori* status was determined by CLOtest®, histology, and culture in all three studies. For a given patient, *H. pylori* was considered eradicated if at least two of these tests were negative, and none was positive. The combination of clarithromycin plus omeprazole and amoxicillin was effective in eradicating *H. pylori*.
[See first table above]
Safety
In clinical trials using combination therapy with clarithromycin plus omeprazole and amoxicillin, no adverse reactions peculiar to the combination of these drugs have been observed. Adverse reactions that have occurred have been limited to those that have been previously reported with clarithromycin, omeprazole, or amoxicillin.
The most frequent adverse experiences observed in clinical trials using combination therapy with clarithromycin plus omeprazole and amoxicillin (n = 274) were diarrhea (14%), taste perversion (10%), and headache (7%).
For information about adverse reactions with omeprazole or amoxicillin, refer to the **ADVERSE REACTIONS** section of their package inserts.
Clarithromycin + Omeprazole Therapy
Four randomized, double-blind, multi-center studies (067, 100, 812b, and 058) evaluated clarithromycin 500 mg t.i.d. plus omeprazole 40 mg q.d. for 14 days, followed by omeprazole 20 mg q.d. (067, 100, and 058) or by omeprazole 40 mg q.d. (812b) for an additional 14 days in patients with active duodenal ulcer associated with *H. pylori*. Studies 067 and

100 were conducted in the U.S. and Canada and enrolled 242 and 256 patients, respectively. *H. pylori* infection and duodenal ulcer were confirmed in 219 patients in Study 067 and 228 patients in Study 100. These studies compared the combination regimen to omeprazole and clarithromycin monotherapies. Studies 812b and 058 were conducted in Europe and enrolled 154 and 215 patients, respectively. *H. pylori* infection and duodenal ulcer were confirmed in 148 patients in Study 812b and 208 patients in Study 058. These studies compared the combination regimen to omeprazole monotherapy. The results for the efficacy analyses for these studies are described below.

Duodenal Ulcer Healing
The combination of clarithromycin and omeprazole was as effective as omeprazole alone for healing duodenal ulcer. [See second table at top of previous page]

Eradication of H. pylori Associated with Duodenal Ulcer
The combination of clarithromycin and omeprazole was effective in eradicating *H. pylori*. [See first table above]

H. pylori eradication was defined as no positive test (culture or histology) at 4 weeks following the end of treatment, and two negative tests were required to be considered eradicated. In the per-protocol analysis, the following patients were excluded: dropouts, patients with major protocol violations, patients with missing *H. pylori* tests post-treatment, and patients that were not assessed for *H. pylori* eradication at 4 weeks after the end of treatment because they were found to have an unhealed ulcer at the end of treatment. Ulcer recurrence at 6-months following the end of treatment was assessed for patients in whom ulcers were healed post-treatment.
[See second table above]
Thus, in patients with duodenal ulcer associated with *H. pylori* infection, eradication of *H. pylori* reduced ulcer recurrence.

Safety
The adverse event profiles for the four studies showed that the combination of clarithromycin 500 mg t.i.d. and omeprazole 40 mg q.d. for 14 days, followed by omeprazole 20 mg q.d. (067, 100, and 058) or 40 mg q.d. (812b) for an additional 14 days was well tolerated. Of the 346 patients who received the combination, 12 (3.5%) patients discontinued study drug due to adverse events.
[See third table above]
Most of these events were mild to moderate in severity.

Changes in Laboratory Values
Changes in laboratory values with possible clinical significance in patients taking clarithromycin and omeprazole were as follows:
Hepatic—elevated direct bilirubin < 1%; GGT < 1%; SGOT (AST) < 1%; SGPT (ALT) < 1%.
Renal—elevated serum creatinine < 1%.
For information on omeprazole, refer to the **ADVERSE REACTIONS** section of the PRILOSEC package insert.

Clarithromycin + Ranitidine Bismuth Citrate Therapy
In a U.S. double-blind, randomized, multicenter, dose-comparison trial, ranitidine bismuth citrate 400 mg b.i.d. for 4 weeks plus clarithromycin 500 mg b.i.d. for the first 2 weeks was found to have an equivalent *H. pylori* eradication rate (based on culture and histology) when compared to ranitidine bismuth citrate 400 mg b.i.d. for 4 weeks plus clarithromycin 500 mg t.i.d. for the first 2 weeks. The intent-to-treat *H. pylori* eradication rates are shown below:
[See fourth table above]
H. pylori eradication was defined as no positive test at 4 weeks following the end of treatment. Patients must have had two tests performed, and these must have been negative to be considered eradicated of *H. pylori*. The following patients were excluded from the per-protocol analysis: patients not infected with *H. pylori* prestudy, dropouts, patients with major protocol violations, patients with missing *H. pylori* tests. Patients excluded from the intent-to-treat analysis included those not infected with *H. pylori* prestudy and those with missing *H. pylori* tests prestudy. Patients were assessed for *H. pylori* eradication (4 weeks following treatment) regardless of their healing status (at the end of treatment).
The relationship between *H. pylori* eradication and duodenal ulcer recurrence was assessed in a combined analysis of six U.S. randomized, double-blind, multicenter, placebo-controlled trials using ranitidine bismuth citrate with or without antibiotics. The results from approximately 650 U.S. patients showed that the risk of ulcer recurrence within 6 months of completing treatment was two times less likely in patients whose *H. pylori* infection was eradicated compared to patients in whom *H. pylori* infection was not eradicated.

Safety
In clinical trials using combination therapy with clarithromycin plus ranitidine bismuth citrate, no adverse reactions peculiar to the combination of these drugs (using clarithromycin twice daily or three times a day) were observed. Adverse reactions that have occurred have been lim-

H. pylori Eradication Rates (Per-Protocol Analysis) at 4 to 6 weeks Percent of Patients Cured (n/N)

Study	Clarithromycin + Omeprazole	Omeprazole	Clarithromycin
U.S. Studies			
Study 100	64% (39/61)†‡	0% (0/59)	39% (17/44)
Study 067	74% (39/53)†‡	0% (0/54)	31% (13/42)
Non-U.S. Studies			
Study 058	74% (64/86)‡	1% (1/90)	N/A
Study 812b	83% (50/60)‡	1% (1/74)	N/A

† Statistically significantly higher than clarithromycin monotherapy (p < 0.05).
‡ Statistically significantly higher than omeprazole monotherapy (p < 0.05).

Ulcer Recurrence at 6 months by H. pylori Status at 4-6 Weeks

	H. pylori Negative	H. pylori Positive
U.S. Studies		
Study 100		
Clarithromycin + Omeprazole	6% (2/34)	56% (9/16)
Omeprazole	- (0/0)	71% (35/49)
Clarithromycin	12% (2/17)	32% (7/22)
Study 067		
Clarithromycin + Omeprazole	38% (11/29)	50% (6/12)
Omeprazole	- (0/0)	67% (31/46)
Clarithromycin	18% (2/11)	52% (14/27)
Non-U.S.Studies		
Study 058		
Clarithromycin + Omeprazole	6% (3/53)	24% (4/17)
Omeprazole	0% (0/3)	55% (39/71)
Study 812b*		
Clarithromycin + Omeprazole	5% (2/42)	0% (0/7)
Omeprazole	0% (0/1)	54% (32/59)
***12-month recurrence rates:**		
Clarithromycin + Omeprazole	3% (1/40)	0% (0/6)
Omeprazole	0% (0/1)	67% (29/43)

Adverse Events with an Incidence of 3% or Greater

Adverse Event	Clarithromycin + Omeprazole (N = 346) % of Patients	Omeprazole (N = 355) % of Patients	Clarithromycin (N = 166) % of Patients *
Taste Perversion	15%	1%	16%
Nausea	5%	1%	3%
Headache	5%	6%	9%
Diarrhea	4%	3%	7%
Vomiting	4%	< 1%	1%
Abdominal Pain	3%	2%	1%
Infection	3%	4%	2%

* Studies 067 and 100, only.

H. pylori Eradication Rates in Study H2BA-3001

Analysis	RBC 400 mg + Clarithromycin 500 mg b.i.d.	RBC 400 mg + Clarithromycin 500 mg t.i.d.	95% CI Rate Difference
ITT	65% (122/188) [58%, 72%]	63% (122/195) [55%, 69%]	(-8%, 12%)
Per-Protocol	72% (117/162) [65%, 79%]	71% (120/170) [63%, 77%]	(-9%, 12%)

ited to those reported with clarithromycin or ranitidine bismuth citrate. (See **ADVERSE REACTIONS** section of the Tritec package insert.) The most frequent adverse experiences observed in clinical trials using combination therapy with clarithromycin (500 mg three times a day) with ranitidine bismuth citrate (n = 329) were taste disturbance (11%), diarrhea (5%), nausea and vomiting (3%). The most frequent adverse experiences observed in clinical trials using combination therapy with clarithromycin (500 mg twice daily) with ranitidine bismuth citrate (n = 196) were taste disturbance (8%), nausea and vomiting (5%), and diarrhea (4%).

ANIMAL PHARMACOLOGY AND TOXICOLOGY

Clarithromycin is rapidly and well-absorbed with dose-linear kinetics, low protein binding, and a high volume of distribution. Plasma half-life ranged from 1 to 6 hours and was species dependent. High tissue concentrations were achieved, but negligible accumulation was observed. Fecal clearance predominated. Hepatotoxicity occurred in all species tested (i.e., in rats and monkeys at doses 2 times greater than and in dogs at doses comparable to the maximum human daily dose, based on mg/m²). Renal tubular degeneration (calculated on a mg/m² basis) occurred in rats at

doses 2 times, in monkeys at doses 8 times, and in dogs at doses 12 times greater than the maximum human daily dose. Testicular atrophy (on a mg/m² basis) occurred in rats at doses 7 times, in dogs at doses 3 times, and in monkeys at doses 8 times greater than the maximum human daily dose. Corneal opacity (on a mg/m² basis) occurred in dogs at doses 12 times and in monkeys at doses 8 times greater than the maximum human daily dose. Lymphoid depletion (on a mg/m² basis) occurred in dogs at doses 3 times greater than and in monkeys at doses 2 times greater than the maximum human daily dose. These adverse events were absent during clinical trials.

REFERENCES

1. National Committee for Clinical Laboratory Standards, Methods for Dilution Antimicrobial Susceptibility Tests

Information on the Abbott Pharmaceutical Products listed on these pages is from the prescribing information in use as of June 1, 2010. For more information, please visit rxabbott.com or call 1-800-633-9110.

for Bacteria that Grow Aerobically - Fourth Edition. Approved Standard NCCLS Document M7-A4, Vol. 17, No. 2, NCCLS, Wayne, PA, January, 1997.
2. National Committee for Clinical Laboratory Standards, Performance Standards for Antimicrobial Disk Susceptibility Tests - Sixth Edition. Approved Standard NCCLS Document M2-A6, Vol. 17, No. 1, NCCLS, Wayne, PA, January, 1997.
3. National Committee for Clinical Laboratory Standards. Summary Minutes, Subcommittee on Antimicrobial Susceptibility Testing, Tampa, FL. January 11-13, 1998.
4. Chaisson RE, et al. Clarithromycin and Ethambutol with or without Clofazimine for the Treatment of Bacteremic *Mycobacterium avium* Complex Disease in Patients with HIV Infection. *AIDS.* 1997;11:311-317.
5. Kemper CA, et al. Treatment of *Mycobacterium avium* Complex Bacteremia in AIDS with a Four-Drug Oral Regimen. *Ann Intern Med.* 1992;116:466-472.

Filmtab – Film-sealed tablets, Abbott
Biaxin Filmtab 250 mg and 500 mg and Biaxin XL 500 mg
Mfd. by Abbott Pharmaceuticals PR Ltd., Barceloneta, PR 00617
Biaxin Granules for Oral Suspension, 125 mg/5 mL and 250 mg/5 mL
Mfd. by Abbott Laboratories, North Chicago, IL 60064
For Abbott Laboratories, North Chicago, IL 60064, U.S.A.
Ref. 03-A296-Revised August, 2009

Shown in Product Identification Guide, page 303

CALCIJEX® ℞
(calcitriol injection)
1 mcg/mL

DESCRIPTION

Calcijex (calcitriol injection) is synthetically manufactured calcitriol and is available as a sterile, isotonic, clear, colorless to yellow, aqueous solution for intravenous injection. Calcijex is available in 1 mL ampuls. Each 1 mL contains calcitriol, 1 mcg; Polysorbate 20, 4 mg; sodium ascorbate 2.5 mg added. May contain hydrochloric acid and/or sodium hydroxide for pH adjustment. pH is 6.5 (5.9 to 7.0). Contains no more than 1 mcg/mL of aluminum.
Calcitriol is a crystalline compound which occurs naturally in humans. It is soluble in organic solvents but relatively insoluble in water.
Calcitriol is chemically designated (5Z,7E)-9, 10-secocholesta-5,7,10(19)-triene-1α,3β,25-triol and has the following structural formula:

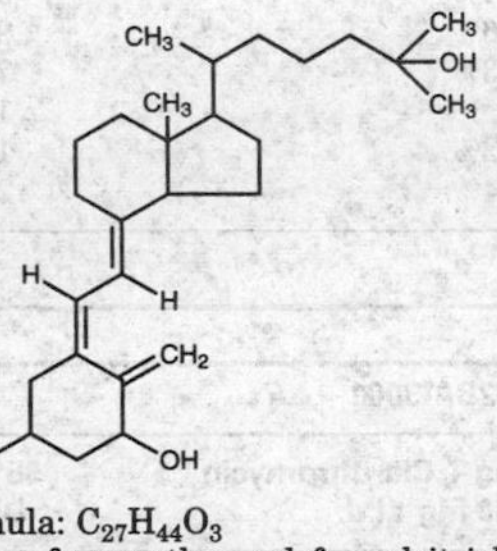

Molecular Formula: $C_{27}H_{44}O_3$
The other names frequently used for calcitriol are 1α,25-dihydroxycholecalciferol, 1α,25-dihydroxyvitamin D_3, 1,25-DHCC, 1,25$(OH)_2D_3$ and 1,25-diOHC.

CLINICAL PHARMACOLOGY

Calcitriol is the active form of vitamin D_3 (cholecalciferol). The natural or endogenous supply of vitamin D in man mainly depends on ultraviolet light for conversion of 7-dehydrocholesterol to vitamin D_3 in the skin. Vitamin D_3 must be metabolically activated in the liver and the kidney before it is fully active on its target tissues. The initial transformation is catalyzed by a vitamin D_3-25-hydroxylase enzyme present in the liver, and the product of this reaction is 25-$(OH)D_3$ (calcifediol). The latter undergoes hydroxylation in the mitochondria of kidney tissue, and this reaction is activated by the renal 25-hydroxyvitamin D_3-1-α-hydroxylase to produce 1,25-$(OH)_2D_3$ (calcitriol), the active form of vitamin D_3.
The known sites of action of calcitriol are intestine, bone, kidney and parathyroid gland. Calcitriol is the most active known form of vitamin D_3 in stimulating intestinal calcium transport. In acutely uremic rats, calcitriol has been shown to stimulate intestinal calcium absorption. In bone, calcitriol, in conjunction with parathyroid hormone, stimulates resorption of calcium; and in the kidney, calcitriol increases the tubular reabsorption of calcium. *In vitro* and *in vivo* studies have shown that calcitriol directly suppresses secretion and synthesis of PTH. A vitamin D-resistant state may exist in uremic patients because of the failure of the kidney to adequately convert precursors to the active compound, calcitriol.
Calcitriol when administered by bolus injection is rapidly available in the blood stream. Vitamin D metabolites are known to be transported in blood, bound to specific plasma proteins. The pharmacologic activity of an administered dose of calcitriol is about 3 to 5 days. Two metabolic pathways for calcitriol have been identified, conversion to 1,24,25-$(OH)_3D_3$ and to calcitroic acid.

INDICATIONS AND USAGE

Calcijex (calcitriol injection) is indicated in the management of hypocalcemia in patients undergoing chronic renal dialysis. It has been shown to significantly reduce elevated parathyroid hormone levels. Reduction of PTH has been shown to result in an improvement in renal osteodystrophy.

CONTRAINDICATIONS

Calcijex (calcitriol injection) should not be given to patients with hypercalcemia or evidence of vitamin D toxicity.

WARNINGS

Since calcitriol is the most potent metabolite of vitamin D available, vitamin D and its derivatives should be withheld during treatment.
A non-aluminum phosphate-binding compound should be used to control serum phosphorus levels in patients undergoing dialysis.
Overdosage of any form of vitamin D is dangerous (see also **OVERDOSAGE**). Progressive hypercalcemia due to overdosage of vitamin D and its metabolites may be so severe as to require emergency attention. Chronic hypercalcemia can lead to generalized vascular calcification, nephrocalcinosis and other soft-tissue calcification. The serum calcium times phosphate (Ca × P) product should not be allowed to exceed 70. Radiographic evaluation of suspect anatomical regions may be useful in the early detection of this condition.

PRECAUTIONS

General
Excessive dosage of Calcijex (calcitriol injection) induces hypercalcemia and in some instances hypercalciuria; therefore, early in treatment during dosage adjustment, serum calcium and phosphorus should be determined at least twice weekly. Should hypercalcemia develop, the drug should be discontinued immediately.
Calcijex should be given cautiously to patients on digitalis, because hypercalcemia in such patients may precipitate cardiac arrhythmias.

Information for the Patient
The patient and his or her parents should be informed about adherence to instructions about diet and calcium supplementation and avoidance of the use of unapproved nonprescription drugs, including magnesium-containing antacids. Patients should also be carefully informed about the symptoms of hypercalcemia (see **ADVERSE REACTIONS**).

Essential Laboratory Tests
Serum calcium, phosphorus, magnesium and alkaline phosphatase and 24-hour urinary calcium and phosphorus should be determined periodically. During the initial phase of the medication, serum calcium and phosphorus should be determined more frequently (twice weekly).
Adynamic bone disease may develop if PTH levels are suppressed to abnormal levels. If biopsy is not being done for other (diagnostic) reasons, PTH levels may be used to indicate the rate of bone turnover. If PTH levels fall below recommended target range (1.5 to 3 times the upper limit of normal), in patients treated with Calcijex, the Calcijex dose should be reduced or therapy discontinued. Discontinuation of Calcijex therapy may result in rebound effect, therefore, appropriate titration downward to a maintenance dose is recommended.

Drug Interactions
Magnesium-containing antacid and Calcijex should not be used concomitantly, because such use may lead to the development of hypermagnesemia.

Carcinogenesis, Mutagenesis, Impairment of Fertility
Long-term studies in animals have not been conducted to evaluate the carcinogenic potential of Calcijex (calcitriol injection). Calcitriol was not mutagenic *in vitro* in the Ames Test nor was oral calcitriol genotoxic *in vivo* in the Mouse Micronucleus Test. No significant effects on fertility and/or general reproductive performances were observed in a Segment I study in rats using oral calcitriol at doses of up to 0.3 mcg/kg.

Pregnancy
Teratogenic Effects
Pregnancy Category C
Calcitriol has been found to be teratogenic in rabbits when given orally at doses of 0.08 and 0.3 mcg/kg. All 15 fetuses in 3 litters at these doses showed external and skeletal abnormalities. However, none of the other 23 litters (156 fetuses) showed external and skeletal abnormalities compared with controls. Teratogenicity studies in rats at doses up to 0.45 mcg/kg orally showed no evidence of teratogenic potential. There are no adequate and well-controlled studies in pregnant women. Calcijex should be used during pregnancy only if the potential benefit justifies the potential risk to the fetus.
Nonteratogenic Effects
In the rabbit, oral dosages of 0.3 mcg/kg/day administered on days 7 to 18 of gestation resulted in 19% maternal mortality, a decrease in mean fetal body weight and a reduced number of newborns surviving to 24 hours. A study of the effects on orally administered calcitriol on peri-and postnatal development in rats resulted in hypercalcemia in the offspring of dams given calcitriol at doses of 0.08 or 0.3 mcg/kg/day, hypercalcemia and hypophosphatemia in dams given calcitriol at a dose of 0.08 or 0.3 mcg/kg/day and increased serum urea nitrogen in dams given calcitriol at a dose of 0.3 mcg/kg/day. In another study in rats, maternal weight gain was slightly reduced at an oral dose of 0.3 mcg/kg/day administered on days 7 to 15 of gestation.
The offspring of a woman administered oral calcitriol at 17 to 36 mcg/day during pregnancy manifested mild hypercalcemia in the first 2 days of life which returned to normal at day 3.

Nursing Mothers
It is not known whether this drug is excreted in human milk. Because many drugs are excreted in human milk and because of the potential for serious adverse reactions in nursing infants from calcitriol, a decision should be made whether to discontinue nursing or to discontinue the drug, taking into account the importance of the drug to the mother.

Pediatric Use
The safety and effectiveness of Calcijex were examined in a 12-week randomized, double-blind, placebo-controlled study of 35 pediatric patients, aged 13-18 years, with end-stage renal disease on hemodialysis. Sixty-six percent of the patients were male, 57% were African-American, and nearly all had received some form of vitamin D therapy prior to the study. The initial dose of Calcijex was 0.5 mcg, 1.0 mcg, or 1.5 mcg, 3 times per week, based on baseline iPTH level of less than 500 pg/mL, 500-1000 pg/mL, or greater than 1000 pg/mL, respectively. The dose of Calcijex was adjusted in 0.25 mcg increments based on the levels of serum iPTH, calcium, and Ca × P. The mean baseline levels of iPTH were 769 pg/mL for the 16 Calcijex-treated patients and 897 pg/mL for the 19 placebo-treated subjects. The mean weekly dose of Calcijex ranged from 1.0 mcg to 1.4 mcg. In the primary efficacy analysis, 7 of 16 (44%) subjects in the Calcijex group had 2 consecutive 30% decreases from baseline iPTH compared with 3 of 19 (16%) patients in the placebo group (95% CI for the difference between groups -6%, 62%). One Calcijex-treated patient experienced transient hypercalcemia (>11.0 mg/dL), while 6 of 16 (38%) Calcijex-treated patients vs. 2 of 19 (11%) placebo-treated patients experienced Ca × P >75.

Geriatric Use
Clinical studies of Calcijex did not include sufficient numbers of subjects aged 65 and over to determine whether they respond differently from younger subjects. Other reported clinical experience has not identified differences in responses between the elderly and younger patients. In general, dose selection for an elderly patient should be cautious, usually starting at the low end of the dosage range, reflecting the greater frequency of decreased hepatic, renal, or cardiac function, and of concomitant disease or other drug therapy.

ADVERSE REACTIONS

Adverse effects of Calcijex (calcitriol injection) are, in general, similar to those encountered with excessive vitamin D intake. The early and late signs and symptoms of vitamin D intoxication associated with hypercalcemia include:

Early
Weakness, headache, somnolence, nausea, vomiting, dry mouth, constipation, muscle pain, bone pain and metallic taste.

Late
Polyuria, polydipsia, anorexia, weight loss, nocturia, conjunctivitis (calcific), pancreatitis, photophobia, rhinorrhea, pruritus, hyperthermia, decreased libido, elevated BUN, albuminuria, hypercholesterolemia, elevated SGOT and SGPT, ectopic calcification, hypertension, cardiac arrhythmias and, rarely, overt psychosis.
Occasional mild pain on injection has been observed.

Post-Marketing Experience
Rare cases of hypersensitivity reactions have been reported, including anaphylaxis.

OVERDOSAGE

Administration of Calcijex (calcitriol injection) to patients in excess of their requirements can cause hypercalcemia, hypercalciuria and hyperphosphatemia. High intake of calcium and phosphate concomitant with Calcijex may lead to similar abnormalities.

Treatment of Hypercalcemia and Overdosage in Patients on Hemodialysis
General treatment of hypercalcemia (greater than 1 mg/dL above the upper limit of normal range) consists of immediate discontinuation of Calcijex therapy, institution of a low calcium diet and withdrawal of calcium supplements. Serum calcium levels should be determined daily until normocalcemia ensues. Hypercalcemia usually resolves in two to seven days. When serum calcium levels have returned to within normal limits, Calcijex therapy may be reinstituted at a dose 0.5 mcg less than prior therapy. Serum calcium levels should be obtained at least twice weekly after all dosage changes.
Persistent or markedly elevated serum calcium levels may be corrected by dialysis against a calcium-free dialysate.
Treatment of Accidental Overdosage of Calcitriol Injection
The treatment of acute accidental overdosage of Calcijex should consist of general supportive measures. Serial serum electrolyte determinations (especially calcium), rate of urinary calcium excretion and assessment of electrocardiographic abnormalities due to hypercalcemia should be obtained. Such monitoring is critical in patients receiving digitalis. Discontinuation of supplemental calcium and low calcium diet are also indicated in accidental overdosage. Due to the relatively short duration of the pharmacological action of calcitriol, further measures are probably unnecessary. Should, however, persistent and markedly elevated serum calcium levels occur, there are a variety of therapeutic alternatives which may be considered, depending on the patients' underlying condition. These include the use of drugs such as phosphates and corticosteroids as well as measures to induce an appropriate forced diuresis. The use of peritoneal dialysis against a calcium-free dialysate has also been reported.

DOSAGE AND ADMINISTRATION

The optimal dose of Calcijex (calcitriol injection) must be carefully determined for each patient.
The effectiveness of Calcijex therapy is predicated on the assumption that each patient is receiving an adequate and appropriate daily intake of calcium. The RDA for calcium in adults is 800 mg. To ensure that each patient receives an adequate daily intake of calcium, the physician should either prescribe a calcium supplement or instruct the patient in proper dietary measures.
The recommended initial dose of Calcijex, depending on the severity of the hypocalcemia and/or secondary hyperparathyroidism, is 1 mcg (0.02 mcg/kg) to 2 mcg administered three times weekly, approximately every other day. Doses as small as 0.5 mcg and as large as 4 mcg three times weekly have been used as an initial dose. If a satisfactory response is not observed, the dose may be increased by 0.5 to 1 mcg at two to four week intervals. During this titration period, serum calcium and phosphorus levels should be obtained at least twice weekly. If hypercalcemia or a serum calcium times phosphate product greater than 70 is noted, the drug should be immediately discontinued until these parameters are appropriate. Then, the Calcijex dose should be reinitiated at a lower dose. Doses may need to be reduced as the PTH levels decrease in response to the therapy. Thus, incremental dosing must be individualized and commensurate with PTH, serum calcium and phosphorus levels. The following is a suggested approach in dose titration:

PTH Levels	Calcijex Dose
the same or increasing	increase
decreasing by < 30%	increase
decreasing by > 30%, < 60%	maintain
decreasing by > 60%	decrease
one and one-half to three times the upper limit of normal	maintain

Parenteral drug products should be inspected visually for particulate matter and discoloration prior to administration, whenever solution and container permit.
Discard unused portion.

HOW SUPPLIED

Calcijex (calcitriol injection) is supplied as follows:

List	Container	Concentration	Fill
8110	Ampul	1 mcg/mL	1 mL

Protect from light.
Store at controlled room temperature 15° to 30°C (59° to 86°F).
Patent Pending.
Mfd. by:
Hospira, Inc.
Lake Forest, IL 60045 USA
For:
Abbott Laboratories
North Chicago, IL 60064 USA

EN-1498-Rev. July, 2007
Printed in USA
Please check the Abbott website, www.rxabbott.com, or call (800) 633-9110 for full prescribing information.

CARDIZEM® LA ℞

[*kär-dĭ-zĕm LA*]
(diltiazem hydrochloride)
Extended Release Tablets
℞ only
Once-a-Day Dosage
LB0024-07 Rev. 09/07
Nos. 3045, 3061, 3062, 3063, 3064, 3069

DESCRIPTION

Diltiazem hydrochloride is a calcium ion cellular influx inhibitor (slow channel blocker or calcium antagonist). Chemically, diltiazem hydrochloride is 1,5-benzothiazepin-4(5H)one,3-(acetyloxy)-5-[2-(dimethylamino)ethyl]-2, 3-dihydro-2-(4-methoxyphenyl)-, monohydrochloride, (+)-cis-. The structural formula is:

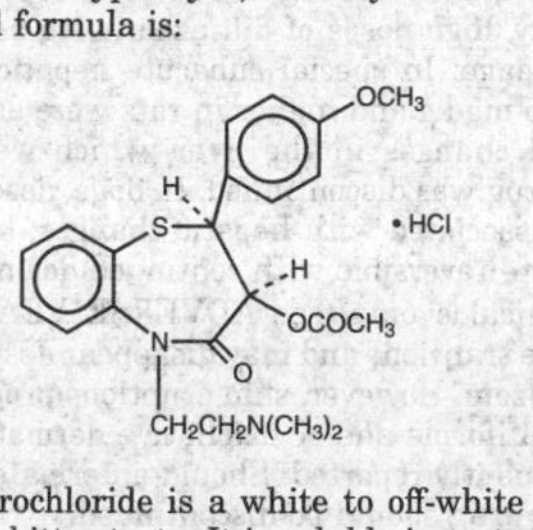

Diltiazem hydrochloride is a white to off-white crystalline powder with a bitter taste. It is soluble in water, methanol and chloroform. It has a molecular weight of 450.99. CARDIZEM® LA Tablets, for oral administration, are formulated as a once-a-day extended release tablet containing either 120 mg, 180 mg, 240 mg, 300 mg, 360 mg or 420 mg of diltiazem hydrochloride.
Also contains: Carnauba Wax NF, Colloidal Silicon Dioxide NF, Croscarmellose Sodium NF, Hydrogenated Vegetable Oil NF, Hypromellose USP, Magnesium Stearate NF, Microcrystalline Cellulose NF, Microcrystalline Wax NF, Pregelatinized Starch NF, Polyacrylate Dispersion 30%, Polyethylene Glycol NF, Polydextrose, Polysorbate NF, Povidone USP, Simethicone USP, Sodium Starch Glycolate NF, Sucrose Stearate, Talc USP, Titanium Dioxide USP.

CLINICAL PHARMACOLOGY

The therapeutic effects of diltiazem are believed to be related to its ability to inhibit the influx of calcium ions during membrane depolarization of cardiac and vascular smooth muscle.
Mechanisms of Action
Hypertension. Diltiazem produces its antihypertensive effect primarily by relaxation of vascular smooth muscle and the resultant decrease in peripheral vascular resistance. The magnitude of blood pressure reduction is related to the degree of hypertension; thus hypertensive individuals experience an antihypertensive effect, whereas there is only a modest fall in blood pressure in normotensives.
Angina. Diltiazem has been shown to produce increases in exercise tolerance, probably due to its ability to reduce myocardial oxygen demand. This is accomplished via reductions in heart rate and systemic blood pressure at submaximal and maximal work loads. Diltiazem has been shown to be a potent dilator of coronary arteries, both epicardial and subendocardial. Spontaneous and ergonovine-induced coronary artery spasms are inhibited by diltiazem.
In animal models, diltiazem interferes with the slow inward (depolarizing) current in excitable tissues. It causes excitation-contraction uncoupling in various myocardial tissues without changes in the configuration of the action potential. Diltiazem causes relaxation of coronary smooth muscle and dilation of both large and small coronary arteries at drug levels which cause little or no negative inotropic effect. The resultant increases in coronary blood flow (epicardial and subendocardial) occur in ischemic and nonischemic models and are accompanied by dose-dependent decreases in systemic blood pressure and decreases in peripheral resistance.
Pharmacokinetics and Metabolism
Diltiazem is well absorbed from the gastrointestinal tract and is subject to an extensive first-pass effect, giving an absolute bioavailability (compared to intravenous administration) of about 40%. Diltiazem undergoes extensive metabolism in which only 2% to 4% of the unchanged drug appears in the urine. Drugs which induce or inhibit hepatic microsomal enzymes may alter diltiazem disposition.
Total radioactivity measurement following short IV administration in healthy volunteers suggests the presence of other unidentified metabolites, which attain higher concentrations than those of diltiazem and are more slowly eliminated; half-life of total radioactivity is about 20 hours compared to 2 to 5 hours for diltiazem.
In vitro binding studies show diltiazem is 70% to 80% bound to plasma proteins. Competitive *in vitro* ligand binding studies have also shown diltiazem hydrochloride binding is not altered by therapeutic concentrations of digoxin, hydrochlorothiazide, phenylbutazone, propranolol, salicylic acid, or warfarin. The plasma elimination half-life following single or multiple drug administration is approximately 3.0 to 4.5 hours. Desacetyl diltiazem is also present in the plasma at levels of 10% to 20% of the parent drug and is 25% to 50% as potent as a coronary vasodilator as diltiazem. Minimum therapeutic plasma diltiazem concentrations appear to be in the range of 50 to 200 ng/mL. There is a departure from linearity when dose strengths are increased; the half-life is slightly increased with dose. A study that compared patients with normal hepatic function to patients with cirrhosis found an increase in half-life and a 69% increase in bioavailability in the hepatically impaired patients. A single study in patients with severely impaired renal function showed no difference in the pharmacokinetic profile of diltiazem compared to patients with normal renal function.
CARDIZEM LA Tablets. A single 360 mg dose of CARDIZEM LA results in detectable plasma levels within 3 to 4 hours and peak plasma levels between 11 and 18 hours; absorption occurs throughout the dosing interval. The apparent elimination half-life for CARDIZEM LA Tablets after single or multiple dosing is 6 to 9 hours. When CARDIZEM LA Tablets were coadministered with a high fat content breakfast, diltiazem peak and systemic exposures were not affected indicating that the tablet can be administered without regard to food. As the dose of CARDIZEM LA Tablets is increased from 120 to 240 mg, area-under-the-curve increases 2.5-fold.
Pharmacodynamics and Clinical Studies
Like other calcium channel antagonists, diltiazem decreases sinoatrial and atrioventricular conduction in isolated tissues and has a negative inotropic effect in isolated preparations. In the intact animal, prolongation of the AH interval can be seen at higher doses.
In man, diltiazem prevents spontaneous and ergonovine-provoked coronary artery spasm. It causes a decrease in peripheral vascular resistance and a modest fall in blood pressure in normotensive individuals and, in exercise tolerance studies in patients with ischemic heart disease, reduces the heart rate-blood pressure product for any given work load. Studies to date, primarily in patients with good ventricular function, have not revealed evidence of a negative inotropic effect; cardiac output, ejection fraction, and left ventricular end diastolic pressure have not been affected. Such data has no predictive value with respect to effects in patients with poor ventricular function, and increased heart failure has been reported in patients with preexisting impairment of ventricular function. There are as yet few data on the interaction of diltiazem and beta-blockers in patients with poor ventricular function. Resting heart rate is usually slightly reduced by diltiazem. Diltiazem decreases vascular resistance, increases cardiac output (by increasing stroke volume), and produces a slight decrease or no change in heart rate.
During dynamic exercise, increases in diastolic pressure are inhibited, while maximum achievable systolic pressure is usually reduced. Chronic therapy with diltiazem produces no change or an increase in plasma catecholamines. No increased activity of the renin-angiotensin-aldosterone axis has been observed. Diltiazem reduces the renal and peripheral effects of angiotensin II. Hypertensive animal models respond to diltiazem with reductions in blood pressure and increased urinary output and natriuresis without a change in urinary sodium/potassium ratio.
Intravenous diltiazem hydrochloride in doses of 20 mg prolongs AH conduction time and AV node functional and effective refractory periods by approximately 20%. In a study involving single oral doses of 300 mg of diltiazem hydrochloride in six normal volunteers, the average maximum PR prolongation was 14% with no instances of greater than first-degree AV block. Diltiazem associated prolongation of the AH interval is not more pronounced in patients with first-degree heart block. In patients with sick sinus syndrome, diltiazem significantly prolongs sinus cycle length (up to 50% in some cases).
Chronic oral administration of diltiazem hydrochloride to patients in doses of up to 540 mg/day has resulted in small increases in PR interval, and on occasion produces abnormal prolongation (see WARNINGS).

Information on the Abbott Pharmaceutical Products listed on these pages is from the prescribing information in use as of June 1, 2010. For more information, please visit rxabbott.com or call 1-800-633-9110.

Hypertension. In a randomized, double-blind, parallel-group, dose-response study involving 478 patients with essential hypertension, evening doses of CARDIZEM LA 120, 240, 360, and 540 mg were compared to placebo and to 360 mg administered in the morning. The mean reductions in diastolic blood pressure by ABPM at roughly 24 hours after the morning (4 AM-8 AM) or evening (6 PM-10 PM) administration (i.e., the time corresponding to expected trough serum concentrations) are shown in the table below:

Mean Change in Trough Diastolic Pressure by ABPM

Evening Dosing				Morning Dosing
120 mg	240 mg	360 mg	540 mg	360 mg
−2.0	−4.4	−4.4	−8.1	−6.4

A second randomized, double-blind, parallel-group, dose-response study (N=258) evaluated CARDIZEM LA following morning doses of placebo or 120, 180, 300, or 540 mg. Diastolic blood pressure measured by supine office cuff sphygmomanometer at trough (7 AM to 9 AM) decreased in an apparently linear manner over the dosage range studied. Group mean changes for placebo, 120 mg, 180 mg, 300 mg and 540 mg were −2.6, −1.9, −5.4, −6.1 and −8.6 mm Hg respectively.

Whether the time of administration impacts the clinical benefits of antihypertensive treatment is not known.

Postural hypotension is infrequently noted upon suddenly assuming an upright position. No reflex tachycardia is associated with the chronic antihypertensive effects.

Angina. The effects of Cardizem LA on angina were evaluated in a randomized, double-blind, parallel-group, dose-response trial of 311 patients with chronic stable angina. Evening doses of 180, 360 and 420 mg were compared to placebo and to 360 mg administered in the morning. All doses of Cardizem LA administered at night increased exercise tolerance when compared with placebo after 21 hours. The mean effect, placebo-subtracted, was 20 to 28 seconds for all three doses, and no dose-response was demonstrated. Cardizem LA, 360 mg, given in the morning, also improved exercise tolerance when measured 25 hours later. As expected, the effect was smaller than the effects measured only 21 hours following nighttime administration. Cardizem LA had a larger effect to increase exercise tolerance at peak serum concentrations than at trough.

INDICATIONS AND USAGE

CARDIZEM LA is indicated for the treatment of hypertension. It may be used alone or in combination with other antihypertensive medications.

CARDIZEM LA is indicated for the management of chronic stable angina.

CONTRAINDICATIONS

Diltiazem is contraindicated in (1) patients with sick sinus syndrome except in the presence of a functioning ventricular pacemaker, (2) patients with second- or third-degree AV block except in the presence of a functioning ventricular pacemaker, (3) patients with hypotension (less than 90 mm Hg systolic), (4) patients who have demonstrated hypersensitivity to the drug, and (5) patients with acute myocardial infarction and pulmonary congestion documented by x-ray on admission.

WARNINGS

1. **Cardiac Conduction.** Diltiazem prolongs AV node refractory periods without significantly prolonging sinus node recovery time, except in patients with sick sinus syndrome. This effect may rarely result in abnormally slow heart rates (particularly in patients with sick sinus syndrome) or second- or third-degree AV block (13 of 3290 patients or 0.40%). Concomitant use of diltiazem with beta-blockers or digitalis may result in additive effects on cardiac conduction. A patient with Prinzmetal's angina developed periods of asystole (2 to 5 seconds) after a single dose of 60 mg of diltiazem (see ADVERSE REACTIONS section).
2. **Congestive Heart Failure.** Although diltiazem has a negative inotropic effect in isolated animal tissue preparations, hemodynamic studies in humans with normal ventricular function have not shown a reduction in cardiac index nor consistent negative effects on contractility (dp/dt). An acute study of oral diltiazem in patients with impaired ventricular function (ejection fraction 24% ± 6%) showed improvement in indices of ventricular function without significant decrease in contractile function (dp/dt). Worsening of congestive heart failure has been reported in patients with preexisting impairment of ventricular function. Experience with the use of diltiazem in combination with beta-blockers in patients with impaired ventricular function is limited. Caution should be exercised when using this combination.
3. **Hypotension.** Decreases in blood pressure associated with diltiazem therapy may occasionally result in symptomatic hypotension.
4. **Acute Hepatic Injury.** Mild elevations of transaminases with and without concomitant elevation in alkaline phosphatase and bilirubin have been observed in clinical studies. Such elevations were usually transient and frequently resolved even with continued diltiazem treatment. In rare instances, significant elevations in enzymes such as alkaline phosphatase, LDH, SGOT, SGPT, and other phenomena consistent with acute hepatic injury have been noted. These reactions tended to occur early after therapy initiation (1 to 8 weeks) and have been reversible upon discontinuation of drug therapy. The relationship to diltiazem is uncertain in some cases, but probable in some (see PRECAUTIONS).

PRECAUTIONS

General

Diltiazem hydrochloride is extensively metabolized by the liver and excreted by the kidneys and in bile. As with any drug given over prolonged periods, laboratory parameters of renal and hepatic function should be monitored at regular intervals. The drug should be used with caution in patients with impaired renal or hepatic function.

In subacute and chronic dog and rat studies designed to produce toxicity, high doses of diltiazem were associated with hepatic damage. In special subacute hepatic studies, oral doses of 125 mg/kg and higher in rats were associated with histological changes in the liver, which were reversible when the drug was discontinued. In dogs, doses of 20 mg/kg were also associated with hepatic changes; however, these changes were reversible with continued dosing.

Dermatological events (see ADVERSE REACTIONS section) may be transient and may disappear despite continued use of diltiazem. However, skin eruptions progressing to erythema multiforme and/or exfoliative dermatitis have also been infrequently reported. Should a dermatologic reaction persist, the drug should be discontinued.

Drug Interactions. Due to the potential for additive effects, caution and careful titration are warranted in patients receiving diltiazem concomitantly with other agents known to affect cardiac contractility and/or conduction (see WARNINGS). Pharmacologic studies indicate that there may be additive effects in prolonging AV conduction when using beta-blockers or digitalis concomitantly with diltiazem (see WARNINGS).

As with all drugs, care should be exercised when treating patients with multiple medications. Diltiazem is both a substrate and an inhibitor of the cytochrome P-450 3A4 enzyme system. Other drugs that are specific substrates, inhibitors, or inducers of this enzyme system may have a significant impact on the efficacy and side effect profile of diltiazem. Patients taking other drugs that are substrates of CYP450, especially patients with renal and/or hepatic impairment, may require dosage adjustment when starting or stopping concomitantly administered diltiazem in order to maintain optimum therapeutic blood levels.

Buspirone. In nine healthy subjects, diltiazem significantly increased the mean buspirone AUC 5.5-fold and C_{max} 4.1-fold compared to placebo. The $T_{½}$ and T_{max} of buspirone were not significantly affected by diltiazem. Enhanced effects and increased toxicity of buspirone may be possible during concomitant administration with diltiazem. Subsequent dose adjustments may be necessary during coadministration, and should be based on clinical assessment.

Beta-Blockers. Controlled and uncontrolled domestic studies suggest that concomitant use of diltiazem and beta-blockers is usually well tolerated, but available data are not sufficient to predict the effects of concomitant treatment in patients with left ventricular dysfunction or cardiac conduction abnormalities.

Administration of diltiazem concomitantly with propranolol in five normal volunteers resulted in increased propranolol levels in all subjects and bioavailability of propranolol was increased approximately 50%. *In vitro*, propranolol appears to be displaced from its binding sites by diltiazem. If combination therapy is initiated or withdrawn in conjunction with propranolol, an adjustment in the propranolol dose may be warranted (see WARNINGS).

Cimetidine. A study in six healthy volunteers has shown a significant increase in peak diltiazem plasma levels (58%) and area-under-the-curve (53%) after a 1-week course of cimetidine at 1200 mg per day and a single dose of diltiazem 60 mg. Ranitidine produced smaller, nonsignificant increases. The effect may be mediated by cimetidine's known inhibition of hepatic cytochrome P-450, the enzyme system responsible for the first-pass metabolism of diltiazem. Patients currently receiving diltiazem therapy should be carefully monitored for a change in pharmacological effect when initiating and discontinuing therapy with cimetidine. An adjustment in the diltiazem dose may be warranted.

Digitalis. Administration of diltiazem with digoxin in 24 healthy male subjects increased plasma digoxin concentrations approximately 20%. Another investigator found no increase in digoxin levels in 12 patients with coronary artery disease. Since there have been conflicting results regarding the effect of digoxin levels, it is recommended that digoxin levels be monitored when initiating, adjusting, and discontinuing diltiazem therapy to avoid possible over- or under-digitalization (see WARNINGS).

Anesthetics. The depression of cardiac contractility, conductivity, and automaticity as well as the vascular dilation associated with anesthetics may be potentiated by calcium channel blockers. When used concomitantly, anesthetics and calcium blockers should be titrated carefully.

Benzodiazepines. Studies showed that diltiazem increased the AUC of midazolam and triazolam by 3- to 4-fold and the C_{max} by 2-fold, compared to placebo. The elimination half-life of midazolam and triazolam also increase (1.5- to 2.5-fold) during coadministration with diltiazem. These pharmacokinetic effects seen during diltiazem coadministration can result in increased clinical effects (e.g., prolonged sedation) of both midazolam and triazolam.

Cyclosporine. A pharmacokinetic interaction between diltiazem and cyclosporine has been observed during studies involving renal and cardiac transplant patients. In renal and cardiac transplant recipients, a reduction of cyclosporine dose ranging from 15% to 48% was necessary to maintain cyclosporine trough concentrations similar to those seen prior to the addition of diltiazem. If these agents are to be administered concurrently, cyclosporine concentrations should be monitored, especially when diltiazem therapy is initiated, adjusted, or discontinued.

The effect of cyclosporine on diltiazem plasma concentrations has not been evaluated.

Carbamazepine. Concomitant administration of diltiazem with carbamazepine has been reported to result in elevated serum levels of carbamazepine (40% to 72% increase), resulting in toxicity in some cases. Patients receiving these drugs concurrently should be monitored for a potential drug interaction.

Lovastatin. In a ten-subject study, coadministration of diltiazem (120 mg bid diltiazem SR) with lovastatin resulted in a 3- to 4-fold increase in mean lovastatin AUC and C_{max} versus lovastatin alone; no change in pravastatin AUC and C_{max} was observed during diltiazem coadministration. Diltiazem plasma levels were not significantly affected by lovastatin or pravastatin.

Quinidine. Diltiazem significantly increases the $AUC_{(0\to\infty)}$ of quinidine by 51%, $T_{½}$ by 36%, and decreases its CL_{oral} by 33%. Monitoring for quinidine adverse effects may be warranted and the dose adjusted accordingly.

Rifampin. Coadministration of rifampin with diltiazem lowered the diltiazem plasma concentrations to undetectable levels. Coadministration of diltiazem with rifampin or any known CYP 3A4 inducer should be avoided when possible, and alternative therapy considered.

Carcinogenesis, Mutagenesis, Impairment of Fertility. A 24-month study in rats at oral dosage levels of up to 100 mg/kg/day, and a 21-month study in mice at oral dosage levels of up to 30 mg/kg/day showed no evidence of carcinogenicity. There was also no mutagenic response *in vitro* or *in vivo* in mammalian cell assays or in vitro in bacteria. No evidence of impaired fertility was observed in a study performed in male and female rats at oral dosages of up to 100 mg/kg/day.

Pregnancy. Category C. Reproduction studies have been conducted in mice, rats, and rabbits. Administration of doses ranging from 4 to 6 times (depending on species) the upper limit of the optimum dosage range in clinical trials (480 mg q.d. or 8 mg/kg q.d. for a 60-kg patient) resulted in embryo and fetal lethality. These studies revealed, in one species or another, a propensity to cause fetal abnormalities of the skeleton, heart, retina, and tongue. Also observed were reductions in early individual pup weights, pup survival, as well as prolonged delivery times and an increased incidence of stillbirths.

There are no well-controlled studies in pregnant women; therefore, use diltiazem in pregnant women only if the potential benefit justifies the potential risk to the fetus.

Nursing Mothers. Diltiazem is excreted in human milk. One report suggests that concentrations in breast milk may approximate serum levels. If use of diltiazem is deemed essential, an alternative method of infant feeding should be instituted.

Pediatric Use. Safety and effectiveness in pediatric patients have not been established.

Geriatric Use. Clinical studies of diltiazem did not include sufficient numbers of subjects aged 65 and over to determine whether they respond differently from younger subjects. Other reported clinical experience has not identified differences in responses between the elderly and younger patients. In general, dose selection for an elderly patient should be cautious, usually starting at the low end of the dosing range, reflecting the greater frequency of decreased hepatic, renal, or cardiac function, and of concomitant disease or other drug therapy.

ADVERSE REACTIONS

Serious adverse reactions have been rare in studies carried out to date, but it should be recognized that patients with impaired ventricular function and cardiac conduction abnormalities have usually been excluded from these studies.

In the hypertension study, the following table presents adverse reactions more common on diltiazem than on placebo (but excluding events with no plausible relationship to treatment), as reported in placebo-controlled hypertension trials in patients receiving a diltiazem hydrochloride extended-release formulation (once-a-day dosing) up to 540 mg.

Adverse Reactions (MedDRA Term)	Placebo n = 120 # pts (%)	Diltiazem hydrochloride extended-release 120-360 mg n = 501 # pts (%)	540 mg n = 123 # pts (%)
Oedema lower limb	4 (3)	24 (5)	10 (8)
Sinus congestion	0 (0)	2 (1)	2 (2)
Rash NOS	0 (0)	3 (1)	2 (2)

In the angina study, the adverse event profile of CARDIZEM LA was consistent with what has been previously described for CARDIZEM LA and other formulations of diltiazem HCl. The most frequent adverse effects experienced by CARDIZEM LA-treated patients were edema lower-limb (6.8%), dizziness (6.4%), fatigue (4.8%), bradycardia (3.6%), first-degree atrioventricular block (3.2%), and cough (2%).

In clinical trials of other diltiazem formulations involving over 3200 patients, the most common events (i.e. greater than 1%) were edema (4.6%), headache (4.6%), dizziness (3.5%), asthenia (2.6%), first-degree AV block (2.4%), bradycardia (1.7%), flushing (1.4%), nausea (1.4%) and rash (1.2%).

In addition, the following events have been reported infrequently (less than 2%) in hypertension trials with other diltiazem products:

Cardiovascular: Angina, arrhythmia, AV block (second- or third-degree), bundle branch block, congestive heart failure, ECG abnormalities, hypotension, palpitations, syncope, tachycardia, ventricular extrasystoles.

Nervous System: Abnormal dreams, amnesia, depression, gait abnormality, hallucinations, insomnia, nervousness, paresthesia, personality change, somnolence, tinnitus, tremor.

Gastrointestinal: Anorexia, constipation, diarrhea, dry mouth, dysgeusia, mild elevations of SGOT, SGPT, LDH, and alkaline phosphatase (see hepatic warnings), nausea, thirst, vomiting, weight increase.

Dermatological: Petechiae, photosensitivity, pruritus.

Other: Albuminuria, allergic reaction, amblyopia, asthenia, CPK increase, crystalluria, dyspnea, ecchymosis, edema, epistaxis, eye irritation, headache, hyperglycemia, hyperuricemia, impotence, muscle cramps, nasal congestion, neck rigidity, nocturia, osteoarticular pain, pain, polyuria, rhinitis, sexual difficulties, gynecomastia.

The following postmarketing events have been reported infrequently in patients receiving diltiazem: allergic reactions, alopecia, angioedema (including facial or periorbital edema), asystole, erythema multiforme (including Stevens-Johnson syndrome, toxic epidermal necrolysis), exfoliative dermatitis, extrapyramidal symptoms, gingival hyperplasia, hemolytic anemia, increased bleeding time, leukopenia, purpura, retinopathy, and thrombocytopenia. In addition, events such as myocardial infarction have been observed which are not readily distinguishable from the natural history of the disease in these patients. A number of well-documented cases of generalized rash, some characterized as leukocytoclastic vasculitis, have been reported. However, a definitive cause and effect relationship between these events and diltiazem therapy is yet to be established.

OVERDOSAGE

The oral LD_{50}'s in mice and rats range from 415 to 740 mg/kg and from 560 to 810 mg/kg, respectively. The intravenous LD_{50}'s in these species were 60 and 38 mg/kg, respectively. The oral LD_{50} in dogs is considered to be in excess of 50 mg/kg, while lethality was seen in monkeys at 360 mg/kg.

The toxic dose in man is not known. Due to extensive metabolism, blood levels after a standard dose of diltiazem can vary over tenfold, limiting the usefulness of blood levels in overdose cases.

There have been 29 reports of diltiazem overdose in doses ranging from less than 1 g to 10.8 g. Sixteen of these reports involved multiple drug ingestions. Twenty-two reports indicated patients had recovered from diltiazem overdose ranging from less than 1 g to 10.8 g. There were seven reports with a fatal outcome; although the amount of diltiazem ingested was unknown, multiple drug ingestions were confirmed in six of the seven reports.

Events observed following diltiazem overdose included bradycardia, hypotension, heart block, and cardiac failure. Most reports of overdose described some supportive medical measure and/or drug treatment. Bradycardia frequently responded favorably to atropine as did heart block, although cardiac pacing was also frequently utilized to treat heart block. Fluids and vasopressors were used to maintain blood pressure, and in cases of cardiac failure, inotropic agents were administered. In addition, some patients received treatment with ventilatory support, gastric lavage, activated charcoal, and/or intravenous calcium. Evidence of the effectiveness of intravenous calcium administration to reverse the pharmacological effects of diltiazem overdose was conflicting.

In the event of overdose or exaggerated response, appropriate supportive measures should be employed in addition to gastrointestinal decontamination. Diltiazem does not appear to be removed by peritoneal or hemodialysis. Limited data suggest that plasmapheresis or charcoal hemoperfusion may hasten diltiazem elimination following overdose. Based on the known pharmacological effects of diltiazem and/or reported clinical experiences, the following measures may be considered:

Bradycardia: Administer atropine (0.60 to 1 mg). If there is no response to vagal blockage, administer isoproterenol cautiously.

High-Degree AV Block: Treat as for bradycardia above. Fixed high-degree AV block should be treated with cardiac pacing.

Cardiac Failure: Administer inotropic agents (isoproterenol, dopamine, or dobutamine) and diuretics.

Hypotension: Vasopressors (e.g., dopamine or norepinephrine).

Actual treatment and dosage should depend on the severity of the clinical situation and the judgment and experience of the treating physician.

DOSAGE AND ADMINISTRATION

CARDIZEM LA Tablets are an extended release formulation intended for once-a-day administration.

Patients controlled on diltiazem alone or in combination with other medications may be switched to CARDIZEM LA Tablets once-a-day at the nearest equivalent total daily dose. Higher doses of CARDIZEM LA Tablets once-a-day dosage may be needed in some patients. Patients should be closely monitored. Subsequent titration to higher or lower doses may be necessary and should be initiated as clinically warranted. There is limited general clinical experience with doses above 360 mg, but the safety and efficacy of doses as high as 540 mg have been studied in clinical trials. The incidence of side effects increases as the dose increases with first-degree AV block, dizziness, and sinus bradycardia bearing the strongest relationship to dose.

The tablet should be swallowed whole and not chewed or crushed.

Hypertension

Dosage needs to be adjusted by titration to individual patient needs. When used as monotherapy, reasonable starting doses are 180 to 240 mg once daily, although some patients may respond to lower doses. Maximum antihypertensive effect is usually observed by 14 days of chronic therapy; therefore, dosage adjustments should be scheduled accordingly. The dosage range studied in clinical trials was 120 to 540 mg once daily. The dosage may be titrated to a maximum of 540 mg daily.

CARDIZEM LA Tablets should be taken about the same time once each day either in the morning or at bedtime. The time of dosing should be considered when making dose adjustments based on trough effects.

Angina

Dosage for the treatment of angina should be individualized based on response. The initial dose of 180 mg once daily may be increased at intervals of 7-14 days if adequate response is not obtained. CARDIZEM LA doses above 360 mg appear to confer no additional benefit.

CARDIZEM LA can be given once daily, either in the evening or in the morning.

Concomitant Use with Other Cardiovascular Agents

1. **Sublingual NTG.** May be taken as required to abort acute anginal attacks during Diltiazem Hydrochloride Extended-release therapy.
2. **Prophylactic Nitrate Therapy.** Diltiazem Hydrochloride Extended Release Tablets may be safely coadministered with short-and long-acting nitrates.
3. **Beta-blockers.** (See WARNINGS and PRECAUTIONS.)
4. **Antihypertensives.** CARDIZEM LA has an additive antihypertensive effect when used with other antihypertensive agents. Therefore, the dosage of Diltiazem Hydrochloride Extended Release Tablets or the concomitant antihypertensives may need to be adjusted when adding one to the other.

HOW SUPPLIED

CARDIZEM LA is supplied as white, capsule-shaped tablets debossed with "B" on one side and the diltiazem content (mg) on the other.

Cardizem LA is available in the following packages

Strength	NDC # Bottles of 30	NDC # Bottles of 90
120 mg	NDC-0074-3045-30	NDC-0074-3045-90
180 mg	NDC-0074-3061-30	NDC-0074-3061-90
240 mg	NDC-0074-3062-30	NDC-0074-3062-90
300 mg	NDC-0074-3063-30	NDC-0074-3063-90
360 mg	NDC-0074-3064-30	NDC-0074-3064-90
420 mg	NDC-0074-3069-30	NDC-0074-3069-90

Storage conditions: Store at 25°C (77°F); excursions permitted to 15-30°C (59-86°F) [see USP Controlled Room Temperature].

Avoid excessive humidity and temperatures above 30°C (86°F).

Dispense in tight, light resistant container as defined in USP.

®Cardizem is a registered trademark of Biovail Laboratories International SRL.

Manufactured By:
Biovail Corporation
Mississauga, ON
L5N 8M5
Canada

Manufactured for:
Abbott Laboratories
North Chicago, IL 60064
USA

LB0024-07 Rev. 09/07

Shown in Product Identification Guide, page 303

DEPAKOTE® ER ℞

[dĕp' ă-kōte]

(divalproex sodium)

Tablet, Extended Release for Oral use

HIGHLIGHTS OF PRESCRIBING INFORMATION

These highlights do not include all the information needed to use Depakote ER safely and effectively. See full prescribing information for Depakote ER.

Depakote ER (divalproex sodium) Tablet, Extended Release for Oral use

Initial U.S. Approval: 2000

WARNING: LIFE THREATENING ADVERSE REACTIONS

See full prescribing information for complete boxed warning.

- **Hepatotoxicity, including fatalities, usually during first 6 months of treatment. Children under the age of two years are at considerably higher risk of fatal hepatotoxicity. Monitor patients closely, and perform liver function tests prior to therapy and at frequent intervals thereafter (5.1)**
- **Teratogenicity, including neural tube defects (5.2)**
- **Pancreatitis, including fatal hemorrhagic cases (5.3)**

RECENT MAJOR CHANGES

Warnings and Precautions (5.5) 4/2009
Warnings and Precautions (5.2) 11/2009

INDICATIONS AND USAGE

Depakote ER is indicated for:

- Acute treatment of manic or mixed episodes associated with bipolar disorder, with or without psychotic features (1.1)
- Monotherapy and adjunctive therapy of complex partial seizures and simple and complex absence seizures; adjunctive therapy in patients with multiple seizure types that include absence seizures (1.2)
- Prophylaxis of migraine headaches (1.3)

DOSAGE AND ADMINISTRATION

- Depakote ER is intended for once-a-day oral administration. Depakote ER should be swallowed whole and should not be crushed or chewed.
- Mania: - Initial dose is 25 mg/kg/day, increasing as rapidly as possible to achieve therapeutic response or desired plasma level (2.1). The maximum recommended dosage is 60 mg/kg/day. (2.1, 2.2)

Information on the Abbott Pharmaceutical Products listed on these pages is from the prescribing information in use as of June 1, 2010. For more information, please visit rxabbott.com or call 1-800-633-9110.

- Complex Partial Seizures: Start at 10 to 15 mg/kg/day, increasing at 1 week intervals by 5 to 10 mg/kg/day to achieve optimal clinical response; if response is not satisfactory, check valproate plasma level; see full prescribing information for conversion to monotherapy (2.2). The maximum recommended dosage is 60 mg/kg/day. (2.1, 2.2)
- Absence Seizures: Start at 15 mg/kg/day, increasing at 1 week intervals by 5 to 10 mg/kg/day until seizure control or limiting side effects (2.2). The maximum recommended dosage is 60 mg/kg/day. (2.1, 2.2)
- Migraine: The recommended starting dose is 500 mg/day for 1 week, thereafter increasing to 1000 mg/day (2.3)

——————DOSAGE FORMS AND STRENGTHS——————
Tablets: 250mg and 500mg (3)

——————————CONTRAINDICATIONS——————————
- Hepatic disease or significant hepatic dysfunction (4, 5.1)
- Known hypersensitivity to the drug (4, 5.10)
- Urea cycle disorders (4, 5.4)

—————————WARNINGS AND PRECAUTIONS—————————
- Hepatotoxicity; monitor liver function tests (5.1)
- Teratogenic effects; weigh Depakote ER benefits of use during pregnancy against risk to the fetus (5.2)
- Pancreatitis; Depakote ER should ordinarily be discontinued (5.3)
- Suicidal behavior or ideation; Antiepileptic drugs, including Depakote ER, increase the risk of suicidal thoughts or behavior (5.5)
- Thrombocytopenia; monitor platelet counts and coagulation tests (5.6)
- Hyperammonemia and hyperammonemic encephalopathy; measure ammonia level if unexplained lethargy and vomiting or changes in mental status, and also with concomitant topiramate use; consider discontinuation of valproate therapy (5.4, 5.7, 5.8)
- Hypothermia; Hypothermia has been reported during valproate therapy with or without associated hyperammonemia. This adverse reaction can also occur in patients using concomitant topiramate (5.9)
- Multi-organ hypersensitivity reaction; discontinue Depakote ER (5.10)
- Somnolence in the elderly can occur. Depakote ER dosage should be increased slowly and with regular monitoring for fluid and nutritional intake (5.12)

————————————ADVERSE REACTIONS————————————
- Most common adverse reactions (reported >5%) reported in adult studies are nausea, somnolence, dizziness, vomiting, asthenia, abdominal pain, dyspepsia, rash, diarrhea, increased appetite, tremor, weight gain, back pain, alopecia, headache, fever, anorexia, constipation, diplopia, amblyopia/blurred, ataxia, nystagmus, emotional lability, thinking abnormal, amnesia, flu syndrome, infection, bronchitis, rhinitis, ecchymosis, peripheral edema, insomnia, nervousness, depression, pharyngitis, dyspnea, tinnitus (6.1, 6.2, 6.3, 6.4).
- Most common, drug-related adverse reactions (reported >5% and twice the rate of placebo) reported in the controlled pediatric mania study are nausea, upper abdominal pain, somnolence, increased ammonia, gastritis and rash.

To report SUSPECTED ADVERSE REACTIONS, contact Abbott Laboratories at 1-800-633-9110 or FDA at 1-800-FDA-1088 or www.fda.gov/medwatch

—————————————DRUG INTERACTIONS—————————————
- Hepatic enzyme-inducing drugs (e.g., phenytoin, carbamazepine, primidone, phenobarbital, rifampin) can increase valproate clearance, while enzyme inhibitors (e.g., felbamate) can decrease valproate clearance. Therefore increased monitoring of valproate and concomitant drug concentrations and dose adjustment is indicated whenever enzyme-inducing or inhibiting drugs are introduced or withdrawn (7.1)
- Aspirin, carbapenem antibiotics: Monitoring of valproate concentrations are recommended (7.1)
- Co-administration of valproate can affect the pharmacokinetics of other drugs (e.g. diazepam, ethosuximide, lamotrigine, phenytoin) by inhibiting their metabolism or protein binding displacement (7.2)
- Dosage adjustment of amitryptyline/nortriptyline, warfarin, and zidovudine may be necessary if used concomitantly with Depakote ER (7.2)
- Topiramate: Hyperammonemia and encephalopathy (5.8, 7.3)

————————USE IN SPECIFIC POPULATIONS————————
- Pregnancy: Depakote ER can cause congenital malformations including neural tube defects (5.2, 8.1)
- Pediatric: Children under the age of two years are at considerably higher risk of fatal hepatotoxicity (5.1, 8.4)
- Geriatric: reduce starting dose; increase dosage more slowly; monitor fluid and nutritional intake, and somnolence (5.12, 8.5)

See 17 for PATIENT COUNSELING INFORMATION and FDA-approved patient labeling

Revised: 11/2009

FULL PRESCRIBING INFORMATION: CONTENTS*
BOXED WARNING
RECENT MAJOR CHANGES
* Sections or subsections omitted from the full prescribing information are not listed

FULL PRESCRIBING INFORMATION

BOXED WARNING
WARNING: LIFE THREATENING ADVERSE REACTIONS
Hepatotoxicity
Hepatic failure resulting in fatalities has occurred in patients receiving valproic acid and its derivatives. Children under the age of two years are at a considerably increased risk of developing fatal hepatotoxicity, especially those on multiple anticonvulsants, those with congenital metabolic disorders, those with severe seizure disorders accompanied by mental retardation, and those with organic brain disease. When Depakote ER is used in this patient group, it should be used with extreme caution and as a sole agent. The benefits of therapy should be weighed against the risks. The incidence of

fatal hepatotoxicity decreases considerably in progressively older patient groups.
These incidents usually have occurred during the first six months of treatment. Serious or fatal hepatotoxicity may be preceded by non-specific symptoms such as malaise, weakness, lethargy, facial edema, anorexia, and vomiting. In patients with epilepsy, a loss of seizure control may also occur. Patients should be monitored closely for appearance of these symptoms. Liver function tests should be performed prior to therapy and at frequent intervals thereafter, especially during the first six months [see Warnings and Precautions (5.1)].
Teratogenicity
Valproate can produce teratogenic effects such as neural tube defects (e.g., spina bifida). Accordingly, the use of Depakote ER in women of childbearing potential requires that the benefits of its use be weighed against the risk of injury to the fetus. This is especially important when the treatment of a spontaneously reversible condition not ordinarily associated with permanent injury or risk of death (e.g., migraine) is contemplated [see Warnings and Precautions (5.2)].
An information sheet describing the teratogenic potential of valproate is available for patients [see Patient Counseling Information (17.8)].
Pancreatitis
Cases of life-threatening pancreatitis have been reported in both children and adults receiving valproate. Some of the cases have been described as hemorrhagic with a rapid progression from initial symptoms to death. Cases have been reported shortly after initial use as well as after several years of use. Patients and guardians should be warned that abdominal pain, nausea, vomiting and/or anorexia can be symptoms of pancreatitis that require prompt medical evaluation. If pancreatitis is diagnosed, valproate should ordinarily be discontinued. Alternative treatment for the underlying medical condition should be initiated as clinically indicated [see Warnings and Precautions (5.3)].

1 INDICATIONS AND USAGE

1.1 Mania
Depakote ER is a valproate and is indicated for the treatment of acute manic or mixed episodes associated with bipolar disorder, with or without psychotic features. A manic episode is a distinct period of abnormally and persistently elevated, expansive, or irritable mood. Typical symptoms of mania include pressure of speech, motor hyperactivity, reduced need for sleep, flight of ideas, grandiosity, poor judgment, aggressiveness, and possible hostility. A mixed episode is characterized by the criteria for a manic episode in conjunction with those for a major depressive episode (depressed mood, loss of interest or pleasure in nearly all activities).
The efficacy of Depakote ER is based in part on studies of Depakote (divalproex sodium delayed release tablets) in this indication, and was confirmed in a 3-week trial with patients meeting DSM-IV TR criteria for bipolar I disorder, manic or mixed type, who were hospitalized for acute mania [see Clinical Studies (14.1)].
The effectiveness of valproate for long-term use in mania, i.e., more than 3 weeks, has not been demonstrated in controlled clinical trials. Therefore, healthcare providers who elect to use Depakote ER for extended periods should continually reevaluate the long-term risk-benefits of the drug for the individual patient.

1.2 Epilepsy
Depakote ER is indicated as monotherapy and adjunctive therapy in the treatment of adult patients and pediatric patients down to the age of 10 years with complex partial seizures that occur either in isolation or in association with other types of seizures. Depakote ER is also indicated for use as sole and adjunctive therapy in the treatment of simple and complex absence seizures in adults and children 10 years of age or older, and adjunctively in adults and children 10 years of age or older with multiple seizure types that include absence seizures.
Simple absence is defined as very brief clouding of the sensorium or loss of consciousness accompanied by certain generalized epileptic discharges without other detectable clinical signs. Complex absence is the term used when other signs are also present.

1.3 Migraine
Depakote ER is indicated for prophylaxis of migraine headaches. There is no evidence that Depakote ER is useful in the acute treatment of migraine headaches. Because it may be a hazard to the fetus, Depakote ER should be considered for women of childbearing potential only after this risk has been thoroughly discussed with the patient and weighed against the potential benefits of treatment [see Warnings and Precautions (5.2), Patient Counseling Information (17.3)].

2 DOSAGE AND ADMINISTRATION

Depakote ER is an extended-release product intended for once-a-day oral administration. Depakote ER tablets should be swallowed whole and should not be crushed or chewed.

2.1 Mania

Depakote ER tablets are administered orally. The recommended initial dose is 25 mg/kg/day given once daily. The dose should be increased as rapidly as possible to achieve the lowest therapeutic dose which produces the desired clinical effect or the desired range of plasma concentrations. In a placebo-controlled clinical trial of acute mania or mixed type, patients were dosed to a clinical response with a trough plasma concentration between 85 and 125 mcg/mL. The maximum recommended dosage is 60 mg/kg/day.

There is no body of evidence available from controlled trials to guide a clinician in the longer term management of a patient who improves during Depakote ER treatment of an acute manic episode. While it is generally agreed that pharmacological treatment beyond an acute response in mania is desirable, both for maintenance of the initial response and for prevention of new manic episodes, there are no data to support the benefits of Depakote ER in such longer-term treatment (i.e., beyond 3 weeks).

2.2 Epilepsy

Depakote ER (divalproex sodium) extended release tablets are administered orally, and must be swallowed whole. As Depakote ER dosage is titrated upward, concentrations of clonazepam, diazepam, ethosuximide, lamotrigine, tolbutamide, phenobarbital, carbamazepine, and/or phenytoin may be affected *[see Drug Interactions (7.2)]*.

Complex Partial Seizures

For adults and children 10 years of age or older.

Monotherapy (Initial Therapy)

Depakote ER has not been systematically studied as initial therapy. Patients should initiate therapy at 10 to 15 mg/kg/day. The dosage should be increased by 5 to 10 mg/kg/week to achieve optimal clinical response. Ordinarily, optimal clinical response is achieved at daily doses below 60 mg/kg/day. If satisfactory clinical response has not been achieved, plasma levels should be measured to determine whether or not they are in the usually accepted therapeutic range (50 to 100 mcg/mL). No recommendation regarding the safety of valproate for use at doses above 60 mg/kg/day can be made.

The probability of thrombocytopenia increases significantly at total trough valproate plasma concentrations above 110 mcg/mL in females and 135 mcg/mL in males. The benefit of improved seizure control with higher doses should be weighed against the possibility of a greater incidence of adverse reactions.

Conversion to Monotherapy

Patients should initiate therapy at 10 to 15 mg/kg/day. The dosage should be increased by 5 to 10 mg/kg/week to achieve optimal clinical response. Ordinarily, optimal clinical response is achieved at daily doses below 60 mg/kg/day. If satisfactory clinical response has not been achieved, plasma levels should be measured to determine whether or not they are in the usually accepted therapeutic range (50-100 mcg/mL). No recommendation regarding the safety of valproate for use at doses above 60 mg/kg/day can be made.

Concomitant antiepilepsy drug (AED) dosage can ordinarily be reduced by approximately 25% every 2 weeks. This reduction may be started at initiation of Depakote ER therapy, or delayed by 1 to 2 weeks if there is a concern that seizures are likely to occur with a reduction. The speed and duration of withdrawal of the concomitant AED can be highly variable, and patients should be monitored closely during this period for increased seizure frequency.

Adjunctive Therapy

Depakote ER may be added to the patient's regimen at a dosage of 10 to 15 mg/kg/day. The dosage may be increased by 5 to 10 mg/kg/week to achieve optimal clinical response. Ordinarily, optimal clinical response is achieved at daily doses below 60 mg/kg/day. If satisfactory clinical response has not been achieved, plasma levels should be measured to determine whether or not they are in the usually accepted therapeutic range (50 to 100 mcg/mL). No recommendation regarding the safety of valproate for use at doses above 60 mg/kg/day can be made.

In a study of adjunctive therapy for complex partial seizures in which patients were receiving either carbamazepine or phenytoin in addition to valproate, no adjustment of carbamazepine or phenytoin dosage was needed *[see Clinical Studies (14.3)]*. However, since valproate may interact with these or other concurrently administered AEDs as well as other drugs, periodic plasma concentration determinations of concomitant AEDs are recommended during the early course of therapy *[see Drug Interactions (7)]*.

Simple and Complex Absence Seizures

The recommended initial dose is 15 mg/kg/day, increasing at one week intervals by 5 to 10 mg/kg/day until seizures are controlled or side effects preclude further increases. The maximum recommended dosage is 60 mg/kg/day.

A good correlation has not been established between daily dose, serum concentrations, and therapeutic effect. However, therapeutic valproate serum concentration for most patients with absence seizures is considered to range from 50 to 100 mcg/mL. Some patients may be controlled with lower or higher serum concentrations *[see Clinical Pharmacology (12.3)]*.

As Depakote ER dosage is titrated upward, blood concentrations of phenobarbital and/or phenytoin may be affected *[see Drug Interactions (7.2)]*.

Antiepilepsy drugs should not be abruptly discontinued in patients in whom the drug is administered to prevent major seizures because of the strong possibility of precipitating status epilepticus with attendant hypoxia and threat to life.

2.3 Migraine

Depakote ER is indicated for prophylaxis of migraine headaches in adults.

The recommended starting dose is 500 mg once daily for 1 week, thereafter increasing to 1000 mg once daily. Although doses other than 1000 mg once daily of Depakote ER have not been evaluated in patients with migraine, the effective dose range of Depakote (divalproex sodium delayed-release tablets) in these patients is 500-1000 mg/day. As with other valproate products, doses of Depakote ER should be individualized and dose adjustment may be necessary. If a patient requires smaller dose adjustments than that available with Depakote ER, Depakote should be used instead.

2.4 Conversion from Depakote to Depakote ER

In adult patients and pediatric patients 10 years of age or older with epilepsy previously receiving Depakote, Depakote ER should be administered once-daily using a dose 8 to 20% higher than the total daily dose of Depakote (Table 1). For patients whose Depakote total daily dose cannot be directly converted to Depakote ER, consideration may be given at the clinician's discretion to increase the patient's Depakote total daily dose to the next higher dosage before converting to the appropriate total daily dose of Depakote ER.

Table 1. Dose Conversion

Depakote Total Daily Dose (mg)	Depakote ER (mg)
500*-625	750
750*-875	1000
1000*-1125	1250
1250-1375	1500
1500-1625	1750
1750	2000
1875-2000	2250
2125-2250	2500
2375	2750
2500-2750	3000
2875	3250
3000-3125	3500

* These total daily doses of Depakote cannot be directly converted to an 8 to 20% higher total daily dose of Depakote ER because the required dosing strengths of Depakote ER are not available. Consideration may be given at the clinician's discretion to increase the patient's Depakote total daily dose to the next higher dosage before converting to the appropriate total daily dose of Depakote ER.

There is insufficient data to allow a conversion factor recommendation for patients with DEPAKOTE doses above 3125 mg/day. Plasma valproate Cmin concentrations for DEPAKOTE ER on average are equivalent to DEPAKOTE, but may vary across patients after conversion. If satisfactory clinical response has not been achieved, plasma levels should be measured to determine whether or not they are in the usually accepted therapeutic range (50 to 100 mcg/mL) *[see Clinical Pharmacology (12.2)]*.

2.5 General Dosing Advice

Dosing in Elderly Patients

Due to a decrease in unbound clearance of valproate and possibly a greater sensitivity to somnolence in the elderly, the starting dose should be reduced in these patients. Starting doses in the elderly lower than 250mg can only be achieved by the use of Depakote. Dosage should be increased more slowly and with regular monitoring for fluid and nutritional intake, dehydration, somnolence, and other adverse reactions. Dose reductions or discontinuation of valproate should be considered in patients with decreased food or fluid intake and in patients with excessive somnolence. The ultimate therapeutic dose should be achieved on the basis of both tolerability and clinical response *[see Warnings and Precautions (5.12)]*.

Dose-Related Adverse Reactions

The frequency of adverse effects (particularly elevated liver enzymes and thrombocytopenia) may be dose-related. The probability of thrombocytopenia appears to increase significantly at total valproate concentrations of ≥ 110 mcg/mL (females) or ≥ 135 mcg/mL (males) *[see Warnings and Precautions (5.6)]*. The benefit of improved therapeutic effect with higher doses should be weighed against the possibility of a greater incidence of adverse reactions.

G.I. Irritation

Patients who experience G.I. irritation may benefit from administration of the drug with food or by slowly building up the dose from an initial low level.

Compliance

Patients should be informed to take Depakote ER every day as prescribed. If a dose is missed it should be taken as soon as possible, unless it is almost time for the next dose. If a dose is skipped, the patient should not double the next dose.

3 DOSAGE FORMS AND STRENGTHS

Depakote ER 250 mg is available as white ovaloid tablets with the corporate Abbott logo, and the Abbo-Code (HF). Each Depakote ER tablet contains divalproex sodium equivalent to 250 mg of valproic acid.

Depakote ER 500 mg is available as gray ovaloid tablets with the corporate Abbott logo, and the Abbo-Code (HC). Each Depakote ER tablet contains divalproex sodium equivalent to 500 mg of valproic acid.

4 CONTRAINDICATIONS

- Depakote ER should not be administered to patients with hepatic disease or significant hepatic dysfunction *[see Warnings and Precautions (5.1)]*.
- Depakote ER is contraindicated in patients with known hypersensitivity to the drug *[see Warnings and Precautions (5.10)]*.
- Depakote ER is contraindicated in patients with known urea cycle disorders *[see Warnings and Precautions (5.4)]*.

5 WARNINGS AND PRECAUTIONS

5.1 Hepatotoxicity

Hepatic failure resulting in fatalities has occurred in patients receiving valproic acid. These incidents usually have occurred during the first six months of treatment. Serious or fatal hepatotoxicity may be preceded by non-specific symptoms such as malaise, weakness, lethargy, facial edema, anorexia, and vomiting. In patients with epilepsy, a loss of seizure control may also occur. Patients should be monitored closely for appearance of these symptoms. Liver function tests should be performed prior to therapy and at frequent intervals thereafter, especially during the first six months. However, healthcare providers should not rely totally on serum biochemistry since these tests may not be abnormal in all instances, but should also consider the results of careful interim medical history and physical examination.

Caution should be observed when administering valproic acid products to patients with a prior history of hepatic disease. Patients on multiple anticonvulsants, children, those with congenital metabolic disorders, those with severe seizure disorders accompanied by mental retardation, and those with organic brain disease may be at particular risk. Experience has indicated that children under the age of two years are at a considerably increased risk of developing fatal hepatotoxicity, especially those with the aforementioned conditions. When Depakote ER is used in this patient group, it should be used with extreme caution and as a sole agent. The benefits of therapy should be weighed against the risks. Above this age group, experience in epilepsy has indicated that the incidence of fatal hepatotoxicity decreases considerably in progressively older patient groups.

The drug should be discontinued immediately in the presence of significant hepatic dysfunction, suspected or apparent. In some cases, hepatic dysfunction has progressed in spite of discontinuation of drug *[see Boxed Warning and Contraindications (4)]*.

5.2 Teratogenicity/Usage in Pregnancy

Use of Depakote ER during pregnancy can cause congenital malformations including neural tube defects. If this drug is used during pregnancy, or if the patient becomes pregnant while taking this drug, the patient should be apprised of the potential hazard to the fetus. Depakote ER should be considered for women of childbearing potential only after the risks have been thoroughly discussed with the patient and weighed against the potential benefits of treatment.

Data suggest that there is an increased incidence of congenital malformations associated with the use of valproate by women with seizure disorders during pregnancy when compared to the incidence in women with seizure disorders who do not use antiepileptic drugs during pregnancy, the incidence in women with seizure disorders who use other antiepileptic drugs, and the background incidence for the general population.

The data described below were gained almost exclusively from women who received valproate to treat epilepsy. There are multiple reports in the clinical literature that indicate

Information on the Abbott Pharmaceutical Products listed on these pages is from the prescribing information in use as of June 1, 2010. For more information, please visit rxabbott.com or call 1-800-633-9110.

Table 2. Risk by indication for antiepileptic drugs in the pooled analysis

Indication	Placebo Patients with Events Per 1000 Patients	Drug Patients with Events Per 1000 Patients	Relative Risk: Incidence of Events in Drug Patients/ Incidence in Placebo Patients	Risk Difference: Additional Drug Patients with Events Per 1000 Patients
Epilepsy	1.0	3.4	3.5	2.4
Psychiatric	5.7	8.5	1.5	2.9
Other	1.0	1.8	1.9	0.9
Total	2.4	4.3	1.8	1.9

the use of antiepileptic drugs during pregnancy results in an increased incidence of congenital malformations in offspring. Antiepileptic drugs, including valproate, should be administered to women of childbearing potential only if they are clearly shown to be essential in the management of their medical condition.

There have been reports of developmental delay, autism and/or autism spectrum disorder in the offspring of women exposed to valproate during pregnancy.

Antiepileptic drugs should not be discontinued abruptly in patients in whom the drug is administered to prevent major seizures because of the strong possibility of precipitating status epilepticus with attendant hypoxia and threat to life. In individual cases where the severity and frequency of the seizure disorder are such that the removal of medication does not pose a serious threat to the patient, discontinuation of the drug may be considered prior to and during pregnancy, although it cannot be said with any confidence that even minor seizures do not pose some hazard to the developing embryo or fetus *[see Boxed Warning and Use in Specific Populations (8.1)]*.

5.3 Pancreatitis

Cases of life-threatening pancreatitis have been reported in both children and adults receiving valproate. Some of the cases have been described as hemorrhagic with rapid progression from initial symptoms to death. Some cases have occurred shortly after initial use as well as after several years of use. The rate based upon the reported cases exceeds that expected in the general population and there have been cases in which pancreatitis recurred after rechallenge with valproate. In clinical trials, there were 2 cases of pancreatitis without alternative etiology in 2416 patients, representing 1044 patient-years experience. Patients and guardians should be warned that abdominal pain, nausea, vomiting, and/or anorexia can be symptoms of pancreatitis that require prompt medical evaluation. If pancreatitis is diagnosed, Depakote ER should ordinarily be discontinued. Alternative treatment for the underlying medical condition should be initiated as clinically indicated *[see Boxed Warning]*.

5.4 Urea Cycle Disorders

Depakote ER is contraindicated in patients with known urea cycle disorders (UCD). Hyperammonemic encephalopathy, sometimes fatal, has been reported following initiation of valproate therapy in patients with urea cycle disorders, a group of uncommon genetic abnormalities, particularly ornithine transcarbamylase deficiency. Prior to the initiation of Depakote ER therapy, evaluation for UCD should be considered in the following patients: 1) those with a history of unexplained encephalopathy or coma, encephalopathy associated with a protein load, pregnancy-related or postpartum encephalopathy, unexplained mental retardation, or history of elevated plasma ammonia or glutamine; 2) those with cyclical vomiting and lethargy, episodic extreme irritability, ataxia, low BUN, or protein avoidance; 3) those with a family history of UCD or a family history of unexplained infant deaths (particularly males); 4) those with other signs or symptoms of UCD. Patients who develop symptoms of unexplained hyperammonemic encephalopathy while receiving valproate therapy should receive prompt treatment (including discontinuation of valproate therapy) and be evaluated for underlying urea cycle disorders *[see Contraindications (4) and Warnings and Precautions (5.7)]*.

5.5 Suicidal Behavior and Ideation

Antiepileptic drugs (AEDs), including Depakote ER, increase the risk of suicidal thoughts or behavior in patients taking these drugs for any indication. Patients treated with any AED for any indication should be monitored for the emergence or worsening of depression, suicidal thoughts or behavior, and/or any unusual changes in mood or behavior. Pooled analyses of 199 placebo-controlled clinical trials (mono- and adjunctive therapy) of 11 different AEDs showed that patients randomized to one of the AEDs had approximately twice the risk (adjusted Relative Risk 1.8, 95% CI:1.2, 2.7) of suicidal thinking or behavior compared to patients randomized to placebo. In these trials, which had a median treatment duration of 12 weeks, the estimated incidence rate of suicidal behavior or ideation among 27,863 AED-treated patients was 0.43%, compared to 0.24% among 16,029 placebo-treated patients, representing an increase of approximately one case of suicidal thinking or behavior for every 530 patients treated. There were four suicides in

drug-treated patients in the trials and none in placebo-treated patients, but the number is too small to allow any conclusion about drug effect on suicide.

The increased risk of suicidal thoughts or behavior with AEDs was observed as early as one week after starting drug treatment with AEDs and persisted for the duration of treatment assessed. Because most trials included in the analysis did not extend beyond 24 weeks, the risk of suicidal thoughts or behavior beyond 24 weeks could not be assessed.

The risk of suicidal thoughts or behavior was generally consistent among drugs in the data analyzed. The finding of increased risk with AEDs of varying mechanisms of action and across a range of indications suggests that the risk applies to all AEDs used for any indication. The risk did not vary substantially by age (5-100 years) in the clinical trials analyzed.

Table 2 shows absolute and relative risk by indication for all evaluated AEDs.

[See table 2 above]

The relative risk for suicidal thoughts or behavior was higher in clinical trials for epilepsy than in clinical trials for psychiatric or other conditions, but the absolute risk differences were similar for the epilepsy and psychiatric indications.

Anyone considering prescribing Depakote ER or any other AED must balance the risk of suicidal thoughts or behavior with the risk of untreated illness. Epilepsy and many other illnesses for which AEDs are prescribed are themselves associated with morbidity and mortality and an increased risk of suicidal thoughts and behavior. Should suicidal thoughts and behavior emerge during treatment, the prescriber needs to consider whether the emergence of these symptoms in any given patient may be related to the illness being treated.

Patients, their caregivers, and families should be informed that AEDs increase the risk of suicidal thoughts and behavior and should be advised of the need to be alert for the emergence or worsening of the signs and symptoms of depression, any unusual changes in mood or behavior, or the emergence of suicidal thoughts, behavior, or thoughts about self-harm. Behaviors of concern should be reported immediately to healthcare providers.

5.6 Thrombocytopenia

The frequency of adverse effects (particularly elevated liver enzymes and thrombocytopenia) may be dose-related. In a clinical trial of valproate as monotherapy in patients with epilepsy, 34/126 patients (27%) receiving approximately 50 mg/kg/day on average, had at least one value of platelets $\leq 75 \times 10^9$/L. Approximately half of these patients had treatment discontinued, with return of platelet counts to normal. In the remaining patients, platelet counts normalized with continued treatment. In this study, the probability of thrombocytopenia appeared to increase significantly at total valproate concentrations of ≥ 110 mcg/mL (females) or ≥ 135 mcg/mL (males). The therapeutic benefit which may accompany the higher doses should therefore be weighed against the possibility of a greater incidence of adverse effects.

Because of reports of thrombocytopenia, inhibition of the secondary phase of platelet aggregation, and abnormal coagulation parameters, (e.g., low fibrinogen), platelet counts and coagulation tests are recommended before initiating therapy and at periodic intervals. It is recommended that patients receiving Depakote ER be monitored for platelet count and coagulation parameters prior to planned surgery. Evidence of hemorrhage, bruising, or a disorder of hemostasis/coagulation is an indication for reduction of the dosage or withdrawal of therapy.

5.7 Hyperammonemia

Hyperammonemia has been reported in association with valproate therapy and may be present despite normal liver function tests. In patients who develop unexplained lethargy and vomiting or changes in mental status, hyperammonemic encephalopathy should be considered and an ammonia level should be measured. Hyperammonemia should also be considered in patients who present with hypothermia *[see Warnings and Precautions (5.9)]*. If ammonia is increased, valproate therapy should be discontinued. Appropriate interventions for treatment of hyperammonemia should be initiated, and such patients should undergo investigation for underlying urea cycle disorders *[see Contraindications and Warnings and Precautions (4, 5.4, 5.8)]*.

During the placebo controlled pediatric mania trial, one (1) in twenty (20) adolescents (5%) treated with valproate developed increased plasma ammonia levels compared to no (0) patients treated with placebo.

Asymptomatic elevations of ammonia are more common and when present, require close monitoring of plasma ammonia levels. If the elevation persists, discontinuation of valproate therapy should be considered.

5.8 Hyperammonemia and Encephalopathy associated with Concomitant Topiramate Use

Concomitant administration of topiramate and valproic acid has been associated with hyperammonemia with or without encephalopathy in patients who have tolerated either drug alone. Clinical symptoms of hyperammonemic encephalopathy often include acute alterations in level of consciousness and/or cognitive function with lethargy or vomiting. Hypothermia can also be a manifestation of hyperammonemia *[see Warnings and Precautions (5.9)]*. In most cases, symptoms and signs abated with discontinuation of either drug. This adverse event is not due to a pharmacokinetic interaction. It is not known if topiramate monotherapy is associated with hyperammonemia. Patients with inborn errors of metabolism or reduced hepatic mitochondrial activity may be at an increased risk for hyperammonemia with or without encephalopathy. Although not studied, an interaction of topiramate and valproic acid may exacerbate existing defects or unmask deficiencies in susceptible persons. In patients who develop unexplained lethargy, vomiting, or changes in mental status, hyperammonemic encephalopathy should be considered and an ammonia level should be measured *[see Contraindications (4) and Warnings and Precautions (5.7)]*.

5.9 Hypothermia

Hypothermia, defined as an unintentional drop in body core temperature to < 35° C (95° F), has been reported in association with valproate therapy both in conjunction with and in the absence of hyperammonemia. This adverse reaction can also occur in patients using concomitant topiramate with valproate after starting topiramate treatment or after increasing the daily dose of topiramate *[see Drug Interactions (7.3)]*. Consideration should be given to stopping valproate in patients who develop hypothermia, which may be manifested by a variety of clinical abnormalities including lethargy, confusion, coma, and significant alterations in other major organ systems such as the cardiovascular and respiratory systems. Clinical management and assessment should include examination of blood ammonia levels.

5.10 Multi-Organ Hypersensitivity Reactions

Multi-organ hypersensitivity reactions have been rarely reported in close temporal association to the initiation of valproate therapy in adult and pediatric patients (median time to detection 21 days: range 1 to 40 days). Although there have been a limited number of reports, many of these cases resulted in hospitalization and at least one death has been reported. Signs and symptoms of this disorder were diverse; however, patients typically, although not exclusively, presented with fever and rash associated with other organ system involvement. Other associated manifestations may include lymphadenopathy, hepatitis, liver function test abnormalities, hematological abnormalities (e.g., eosinophilia, thrombocytopenia, neutropenia), pruritus, nephritis, oliguria, hepato-renal syndrome, arthralgia, and asthenia. Because the disorder is variable in its expression, other organ system symptoms and signs, not noted here, may occur. If this reaction is suspected, valproate should be discontinued and an alternative treatment started. Although the existence of cross sensitivity with other drugs that produce this syndrome is unclear, the experience amongst drugs associated with multi-organ hypersensitivity would indicate this to be a possibility.

5.11 Interaction with Carbapenem Antibiotics

Carbapenem antibiotics (ertapenem, imipenem, meropenem) may reduce serum valproic acid concentrations to subtherapeutic levels, resulting in loss of seizure control. Serum valproic acid concentrations should be monitored frequently after initiating carbapenem therapy. Alternative antibacterial or anticonvulsant therapy should be considered if serum valproic acid concentrations drop significantly or seizure control deteriorates *[see Drug Interactions (7.1)]*.

5.12 Somnolence in the Elderly

In a double-blind, multicenter trial of valproate in elderly patients with dementia (mean age = 83 years), doses were increased by 125 mg/day to a target dose of 20 mg/kg/day. A significantly higher proportion of valproate patients had somnolence compared to placebo, and although not statistically significant, there was a higher proportion of patients with dehydration. Discontinuations for somnolence were also significantly higher than with placebo. In some patients with somnolence (approximately one-half), there was associated reduced nutritional intake and weight loss. There was a trend for the patients who experienced these events to have a lower baseline albumin concentration, lower valproate clearance, and a higher BUN. In elderly patients, dosage should be increased more slowly and with regular monitoring for fluid and nutritional intake, dehydration, somnolence, and other adverse reactions. Dose reductions or discontinuation of valproate should be considered in patients with decreased food or fluid intake and in patients with excessive somnolence [see Dosage and Administration (2.4)].

5.13 Monitoring: Drug Plasma Concentration
Since valproic acid may interact with concurrently administered drugs which are capable of enzyme induction, periodic plasma concentration determinations of valproate and concomitant drugs are recommended during the early course of therapy [see Drug Interactions (7)].

5.14 Effect on Ketone and Thyroid Function Tests
Valproate is partially eliminated in the urine as a keto-metabolite which may lead to a false interpretation of the urine ketone test.
There have been reports of altered thyroid function tests associated with valproate. The clinical significance of these is unknown.

5.15 Effect on HIV and CMV Viruses Replication
There are in vitro studies that suggest valproate stimulates the replication of the HIV and CMV viruses under certain experimental conditions. The clinical consequence, if any, is not known. Additionally, the relevance of these in vitro findings is uncertain for patients receiving maximally suppressive antiretroviral therapy. Nevertheless, these data should be borne in mind when interpreting the results from regular monitoring of the viral load in HIV infected patients receiving valproate or when following CMV infected patients clinically.

6   ADVERSE REACTIONS
Because clinical studies are conducted under widely varying conditions, adverse reaction rates observed in the clinical studies of a drug cannot be directly compared to rates in the clinical studies of another drug and may not reflect the rates observed in practice.
Information on pediatric adverse reactions is presented in section 8.

6.1   Mania
The incidence of treatment-emergent events has been ascertained based on combined data from two three week placebo-controlled clinical trials of Depakote ER in the treatment of manic episodes associated with bipolar disorder.
Table 3 summarizes those adverse reactions reported for patients in these trials where the incidence rate in the Depakote ER-treated group was greater than 5% and greater than the placebo incidence.

Table 3. Adverse Reactions Reported by > 5% of Depakote-Treated Patients During Placebo-Controlled Trials of Acute Mania[1]

Adverse Event	Depakote ER (n=338)	Placebo (n=263)
Somnolence	26%	14%
Dyspepsia	23%	11%
Nausea	19%	13%
Vomiting	13%	5%
Diarrhea	12%	8%
Dizziness	12%	7%
Pain	11%	10%
Abdominal pain	10%	5%
Accidental injury	6%	5%
Asthenia	6%	5%
Pharyngitis	6%	5%

1. The following adverse reactions/event occurred at an equal or greater incidence for placebo than for Depakote ER: headache

The following additional adverse reactions were reported by greater than 1% but not more than 5% of the Depakote ER-treated patients in controlled clinical trials:
Body as a Whole: Back Pain, Flu Syndrome, Infection, Infection Fungal
Cardiovascular System: Hypertension
Digestive System: Constipation, Dry Mouth, Flatulence
Hemic and Lymphatic System: Ecchymosis
Metabolic and Nutritional Disorders: Peripheral Edema
Musculoskeletal System: Myalgia
Nervous System: Abnormal Gait, Hypertonia, Tremor
Respiratory System: Rhinitis

Skin and Appendages: Pruritus, Rash
Special Senses: Conjunctivitis
Urogenital System: Urinary Tract Infection, Vaginitis

6.2   Epilepsy
Based on a placebo-controlled trial of adjunctive therapy for treatment of complex partial seizures, Depakote was generally well tolerated with most adverse reactions rated as mild to moderate in severity. Intolerance was the primary reason for discontinuation in the Depakote-treated patients (6%), compared to 1% of placebo-treated patients.
Table 4 lists treatment-emergent adverse reactions which were reported by ≥ 5% of Depakote-treated patients and for which the incidence was greater than in the placebo group, in the placebo-controlled trial of adjunctive therapy for treatment of complex partial seizures. Since patients were also treated with other antiepilepsy drugs, it is not possible, in most cases, to determine whether the following adverse reactions can be ascribed to Depakote alone, or the combination of Depakote and other antiepilepsy drugs.

Table 4. Adverse Reactions Reported by ≥ 5% of Patients Treated with Valproate During Placebo-Controlled Trial of Adjunctive Therapy for Complex Partial Seizures

Body System/Event	Depakote (%) (N=77)	Placebo (%) (N=70)
Body as a Whole		
Headache	31	21
Asthenia	27	7
Fever	6	4
Gastrointestinal System		
Nausea	48	14
Vomiting	27	7
Abdominal pain	23	6
Diarrhea	13	6
Anorexia	12	0
Dyspepsia	8	4
Constipation	5	1
Nervous System		
Somnolence	27	11
Tremor	25	6
Dizziness	25	13
Diplopia	16	9
Amblyopia/Blurred Vision	12	9
Ataxia	8	1
Nystagmus	8	1
Emotional Lability	6	4
Thinking Abnormal	6	0
Amnesia	5	1
Respiratory System		
Flu Syndrome	12	9
Infection	12	6
Bronchitis	5	1
Rhinitis	5	4
Other		
Alopecia	6	1
Weight Loss	6	0

Table 5 lists treatment-emergent adverse reactions which were reported by ≥ 5% of patients in the high dose valproate group, and for which the incidence was greater than in the low dose group, in a controlled trial of Depakote monotherapy treatment of complex partial seizures. Since patients were being titrated off another antiepilepsy drug during the first portion of the trial, it is not possible, in many cases, to determine whether the following adverse reactions can be ascribed to Depakote alone, or the combination of valproate and other antiepilepsy drugs.

Table 5. Adverse Reactions Reported by ≥5% of Patients in the High Dose Group in the Controlled Trial of Valproate Monotherapy for Complex Partial Seizures[1]

Body System/Event	High Dose (%) (n=131)	Low Dose (%) (n=134)
Body as a Whole		
Asthenia	21	10
Digestive System		
Nausea	34	26
Diarrhea	23	19
Vomiting	23	15
Abdominal pain	12	9
Anorexia	11	4
Dyspepsia	11	10
Hemic/Lymphatic System		
Thrombocytopenia	24	1
Ecchymosis	5	4

Metabolic/Nutritional		
Weight Gain	9	4
Peripheral Edema	8	3
Nervous System		
Tremor	57	19
Somnolence	30	18
Dizziness	18	13
Insomnia	15	9
Nervousness	11	7
Amnesia	7	4
Nystagmus	7	1
Depression	5	4
Respiratory System		
Infection	20	13
Pharyngitis	8	2
Dyspnea	5	1
Skin and Appendages		
Alopecia	24	13
Special Senses		
Amblyopia/Blurred Vision	8	4
Tinnitus	7	1

1. Headache was the only adverse event that occurred in ≥5% of patients in the high dose group and at an equal or greater incidence in the low dose group.

The following additional adverse reactions were reported by greater than 1% but less than 5% of the 358 patients treated with valproate in the controlled trials of complex partial seizures:
Body as a Whole: Back pain, chest pain, malaise.
Cardiovascular System: Tachycardia, hypertension, palpitation.
Digestive System: Increased appetite, flatulence, hematemesis, eructation, pancreatitis, periodontal abscess.
Hemic and Lymphatic System: Petechia.
Metabolic and Nutritional Disorders: SGOT increased, SGPT increased.
Musculoskeletal System: Myalgia, twitching, arthralgia, leg cramps, myasthenia.
Nervous System: Anxiety, confusion, abnormal gait, paresthesia, hypertonia, incoordination, abnormal dreams, personality disorder.
Respiratory System: Sinusitis, cough increased, pneumonia, epistaxis.
Skin and Appendages: Rash, pruritus, dry skin.
Special Senses: Taste perversion, abnormal vision, deafness, otitis media.
Urogenital System: Urinary incontinence, vaginitis, dysmenorrhea, amenorrhea, urinary frequency.

6.3   Migraine
Based on two placebo-controlled clinical trials and their long term extension, valproate was generally well tolerated with most adverse reactions rated as mild to moderate in severity. Of the 202 patients exposed to valproate in the placebo-controlled trials, 17% discontinued for intolerance. This is compared to a rate of 5% for the 81 placebo patients. Including the long term extension study, the adverse reactions reported as the primary reason for discontinuation by ≥ 1% of 248 valproate-treated patients were alopecia (6%), nausea and/or vomiting (5%), weight gain (2%), tremor (2%), somnolence (1%), elevated SGOT and/or SGPT (1%), and depression (1%).
Table 6 includes those adverse reactions reported for patients in the placebo-controlled trial where the incidence rate in the Depakote ER-treated group was greater than 5% and was greater than that for placebo patients.

Table 6. Adverse Reactions Reported by >5% of Depakote ER-Treated Patients During the Migraine Placebo-controlled Trial with a Greater Incidence than Patients Taking Placebo[1]

Body System Event	Depakote ER (n=122)	Placebo (n=115)
Gastrointestinal System		
Nausea	15%	9%
Dyspepsia	7%	4%
Diarrhea	7%	3%
Vomiting	7%	2%
Abdominal Pain	7%	5%
Nervous System		
Somnolence	7%	2%

Information on the Abbott Pharmaceutical Products listed on these pages is from the prescribing information in use as of June 1, 2010. For more information, please visit rxabbott.com or call 1-800-633-9110.

Other		
Infection	15%	14%

1. The following adverse reactions occurred in greater than 5% of Depakote ER-treated patients and at a greater incidence for placebo than for Depakote ER: asthenia and flu syndrome.

The following additional adverse reactions were reported by greater than 1% but not more than 5% of Depakote ER-treated patients and with a greater incidence than placebo in the placebo-controlled clinical trial for migraine prophylaxis:
Body as a Whole: Accidental injury, viral infection.
Digestive System: Increased appetite, tooth disorder.
Metabolic and Nutritional Disorders: Edema, weight gain.
Nervous System: Abnormal gait, dizziness, hypertonia, insomnia, nervousness, tremor, vertigo.
Respiratory System: Pharyngitis, rhinitis.
Skin and Appendages: Rash.
Special Senses: Tinnitus.
Table 7 includes those adverse reactions reported for patients in the placebo-controlled trials where the incidence rate in the valproate-treated group was greater than 5% and was greater than that for placebo patients.

Table 7. Adverse Reactions Reported by > 5% of Valproate-Treated Patients During Migraine Placebo-Controlled Trials with a Greater Incidence than Patients Taking Placebo[1]

Body System Reaction	Depakote (n=202)	Placebo (n=81)
Gastrointestinal System		
Nausea	31%	10%
Dyspepsia	13%	9%
Diarrhea	12%	7%
Vomiting	11%	1%
Abdominal pain	9%	4%
Increased appetite	6%	4%
Nervous System		
Asthenia	20%	9%
Somnolence	17%	5%
Dizziness	12%	6%
Tremor	9%	0%
Other		
Weight gain	8%	2%
Back pain	8%	6%
Alopecia	7%	1%

1. The following adverse reactions occurred in greater than 5% of Depakote-treated patients and at a greater incidence for placebo than for Depakote: flu syndrome and pharyngitis.

The following additional adverse reactions were reported by greater than 1% but not more than 5% of the 202 valproate-treated patients in the controlled clinical trials:
Body as a Whole: Chest pain.
Cardiovascular System: Vasodilatation.
Digestive System: Constipation, dry mouth, flatulence, and stomatitis.
Hemic and Lymphatic System: Ecchymosis.
Metabolic and Nutritional Disorders: Peripheral edema.
Musculoskeletal System: Leg cramps.
Nervous System: Abnormal dreams, confusion, paresthesia, speech disorder, and thinking abnormalities.
Respiratory System: Dyspnea, and sinusitis.
Skin and Appendages: Pruritus.
Urogenital System: Metrorrhagia.

6.4 Other Patient Populations

Mania
The following adverse reactions not listed previously were reported by greater than 1% of Depakote-treated patients and with a greater incidence than placebo in placebo-controlled trials of manic episodes associated with bipolar disorder:
Body as a Whole: Chills, chills and fever, drug level increased, neck rigidity.
Cardiovascular System: Arrhythmia, hypotension, postural hypotension.
Digestive System: Dysphagia, fecal incontinence, gastroenteritis, glossitis, gum hemorrhage, mouth ulceration.
Hemic and Lymphatic System: Anemia, bleeding time increased, leucopenia.
Metabolic and Nutritional Disorders: Hypoproteinemia.
Musculoskeletal System: Arthrosis.
Nervous System: Agitation, catatonic reaction, dysarthria, hallucinations, hypokinesia, psychosis, reflexes increased, sleep disorder, tardive dyskinesia.
Respiratory System: Hiccup.
Skin and Appendages: Discoid lupus erythematosus, erythema nodosum, furunculosis, maculopapular rash, seborrhea, sweating, vesiculobullous rash.
Special Senses: Conjunctivitis, dry eyes, eye disorder, eye pain, photophobia, taste perversion.
Urogenital System: Cystitis, menstrual disorder.

Epilepsy
Adverse reactions that have been reported with all dosage forms of valproate from epilepsy trials, spontaneous reports, and other sources are listed below by body system.

Gastrointestinal
The most commonly reported side effects at the initiation of therapy are nausea, vomiting, and indigestion. These effects are usually transient and rarely require discontinuation of therapy. Diarrhea, abdominal cramps, and constipation have been reported. Both anorexia with some weight loss and increased appetite with weight gain have also been reported. In some patients, many of whom have functional or anatomic (including ileostomy or colostomy) gastrointestinal disorders with shortened GI transit times, there have been postmarketing reports of Depakote ER tablets in stool.

CNS Effects
Sedative effects have occurred in patients receiving valproate alone but occur most often in patients receiving combination therapy. Sedation usually abates upon reduction of other antiepileptic medication. Tremor (may be dose-related), hallucinations, ataxia, headache, nystagmus, diplopia, asterixis, "spots before eyes", dysarthria, dizziness, confusion, hypesthesia, vertigo, incoordination, and parkinsonism have been reported with the use of valproate. Rare cases of coma have occurred in patients receiving valproate alone or in conjunction with phenobarbital. In rare instances encephalopathy with or without fever has developed shortly after the introduction of valproate monotherapy without evidence of hepatic dysfunction or inappropriately high plasma valproate levels. Although recovery has been described following drug withdrawal, there have been fatalities in patients with hyperammonemic encephalopathy, particularly in patients with underlying urea cycle disorders *[see Warnings and Precautions (5.4)]*.
Several reports have noted reversible cerebral atrophy and dementia in association with valproate therapy.

Dermatologic
Transient hair loss, skin rash, photosensitivity, generalized pruritus, erythema multiforme, and Stevens-Johnson syndrome. Rare cases of toxic epidermal necrolysis have been reported including a fatal case in a 6 month old infant taking valproate and several other concomitant medications. An additional case of toxic epidermal necrosis resulting in death was reported in a 35 year old patient with AIDS taking several concomitant medications and with a history of multiple cutaneous drug reactions. Serious skin reactions have been reported with concomitant administration of lamotrigine and valproate *[see Drug Interactions (7)]*.

Psychiatric
Emotional upset, depression, psychosis, aggression, hyperactivity, hostility, and behavioral deterioration.

Musculoskeletal
Weakness.

Hematologic
Thrombocytopenia and inhibition of the secondary phase of platelet aggregation may be reflected in altered bleeding time, petechiae, bruising, hematoma formation, epistaxis, and frank hemorrhage *[see Warnings and Precautions (5.6) and Drug Interactions (7)]*. Relative lymphocytosis, macrocytosis, hypofibrinogenemia, leukopenia, eosinophilia, anemia including macrocytic with or without folate deficiency, bone marrow suppression, pancytopenia, aplastic anemia, agranulocytosis, and acute intermittent porphyria.

Hepatic
Minor elevations of transaminases (e.g., SGOT and SGPT) and LDH are frequent and appear to be dose-related. Occasionally, laboratory test results include increases in serum bilirubin and abnormal changes in other liver function tests. These results may reflect potentially serious hepatotoxicity *[see Warnings and Precautions (5.1)]*.

Endocrine
Irregular menses, secondary amenorrhea, breast enlargement, galactorrhea, and parotid gland swelling. Abnormal thyroid function tests *[see Warnings and Precautions (5.13)]*.
There have been rare spontaneous reports of polycystic ovary disease. A cause and effect relationship has not been established.

Pancreatic
Acute pancreatitis including fatalities *[see Warnings and Precautions (5.3)]*.

Metabolic
Hyperammonemia *[see Warnings and Precautions (5.7)]*, hyponatremia, and inappropriate ADH secretion.
There have been rare reports of Fanconi's syndrome occurring chiefly in children.
Decreased carnitine concentrations have been reported although the clinical relevance is undetermined.
Hyperglycinemia has occurred and was associated with a fatal outcome in a patient with preexistent nonketotic hyperglycinemia.

Genitourinary
Enuresis and urinary tract infection.

Special Senses
Hearing loss, either reversible or irreversible, has been reported; however, a cause and effect relationship has not been established. Ear pain has also been reported.

Other
Allergic reaction, anaphylaxis, edema of the extremities, lupus erythematosus, bone pain, cough increased, pneumonia, otitis media, bradycardia, cutaneous vasculitis, fever, and hypothermia.

7 DRUG INTERACTIONS

7.1 Effects of Co-Administered Drugs on Valproate Clearance

Drugs that affect the level of expression of hepatic enzymes, particularly those that elevate levels of glucuronosyltransferases, may increase the clearance of valproate. For example, phenytoin, carbamazepine, and phenobarbital (or primidone) can double the clearance of valproate. Thus, patients on monotherapy will generally have longer half-lives and higher concentrations than patients receiving polytherapy with antiepilepsy drugs.
In contrast, drugs that are inhibitors of cytochrome P450 isozymes, e.g., antidepressants, may be expected to have little effect on valproate clearance because cytochrome P450 microsomal mediated oxidation is a relatively minor secondary metabolic pathway compared to glucuronidation and beta-oxidation.
Because of these changes in valproate clearance, monitoring of valproate and concomitant drug concentrations should be increased whenever enzyme inducing drugs are introduced or withdrawn.
The following list provides information about the potential for an influence of several commonly prescribed medications on valproate pharmacokinetics. The list is not exhaustive nor could it be, since new interactions are continuously being reported.

Drugs for which a potentially important interaction has been observed

Aspirin
A study involving the co-administration of aspirin at antipyretic doses (11 to 16 mg/kg) with valproate to pediatric patients (n=6) revealed a decrease in protein binding and an inhibition of metabolism of valproate. Valproate free fraction was increased 4-fold in the presence of aspirin compared to valproate alone. The β-oxidation pathway consisting of 2-E-valproic acid, 3-OH-valproic acid, and 3-keto valproic acid was decreased from 25% of total metabolites excreted on valproate alone to 8.3% in the presence of aspirin. Whether or not the interaction observed in this study applies to adults is unknown, but caution should be observed if valproate and aspirin are to be co-administered.

Carbapenem antibiotics
A clinically significant reduction in serum valproic acid concentration has been reported in patients receiving carbapenem antibiotics (ertapenem, imipenem, meropenem) and may result in loss of seizure control. The mechanism of this interaction in not well understood. Serum valproic acid concentrations should be monitored frequently after initiating carbapenem therapy. Alternative antibacterial or anticonvulsant therapy should be considered if serum valproic acid concentrations drop significantly or seizure control deteriorates *[see Warnings and Precautions (5.11)]*.

Felbamate
A study involving the co-administration of 1200 mg/day of felbamate with valproate to patients with epilepsy (n=10) revealed an increase in mean valproate peak concentration by 35% (from 86 to 115 mcg/mL) compared to valproate alone. Increasing the felbamate dose to 2400 mg/day increased the mean valproate peak concentration to 133 mcg/mL (another 16% increase). A decrease in valproate dosage may be necessary when felbamate therapy is initiated.

Rifampin
A study involving the administration of a single dose of valproate (7 mg/kg) 36 hours after 5 nights of daily dosing with rifampin (600 mg) revealed a 40% increase in the oral clearance of valproate. Valproate dosage adjustment may be necessary when it is co-administered with rifampin.

Drugs for which either no interaction or a likely clinically unimportant interaction has been observed

Antacids
A study involving the co-administration of valproate 500 mg with commonly administered antacids (Maalox, Trisogel, and Titralac - 160 mEq doses) did not reveal any effect on the extent of absorption of valproate.

Chlorpromazine
A study involving the administration of 100 to 300 mg/day of chlorpromazine to schizophrenic patients already receiving valproate (200 mg BID) revealed a 15% increase in trough plasma levels of valproate.

Haloperidol
A study involving the administration of 6 to 10 mg/day of haloperidol to schizophrenic patients already receiving valproate (200 mg BID) revealed no significant changes in valproate trough plasma levels.
Cimetidine and Ranitidine
Cimetidine and ranitidine do not affect the clearance of valproate.

7.2 Effects of Valproate on Other Drugs
Valproate has been found to be a weak inhibitor of some P450 isozymes, epoxide hydrase, and glucuronosyltransferases.
The following list provides information about the potential for an influence of valproate co-administration on the pharmacokinetics or pharmacodynamics of several commonly prescribed medications. The list is not exhaustive, since new interactions are continuously being reported.
Drugs for which a potentially important valproate interaction has been observed
Amitriptyline/Nortriptyline
Administration of a single oral 50 mg dose of amitriptyline to 15 normal volunteers (10 males and 5 females) who received valproate (500 mg BID) resulted in a 21% decrease in plasma clearance of amitriptyline and a 34% decrease in the net clearance of nortriptyline. Rare postmarketing reports of concurrent use of valproate and amitriptyline resulting in an increased amitriptyline level have been received. Concurrent use of valproate and amitriptyline has rarely been associated with toxicity. Monitoring of amitriptyline levels should be considered for patients taking valproate concomitantly with amitriptyline. Consideration should be given to lowering the dose of amitriptyline/nortriptyline in the presence of valproate.
Carbamazepine/carbamazepine-10,11-Epoxide
Serum levels of carbamazepine (CBZ) decreased 17% while that of carbamazepine-10,11-epoxide (CBZ-E) increased by 45% upon co-administration of valproate and CBZ to epileptic patients.
Clonazepam
The concomitant use of valproic acid and clonazepam may induce absence status in patients with a history of absence type seizures.
Diazepam
Valproate displaces diazepam from its plasma albumin binding sites and inhibits its metabolism. Coadministration of valproate (1500 mg daily) increased the free fraction of diazepam (10 mg) by 90% in healthy volunteers (n=6). Plasma clearance and volume of distribution for free diazepam were reduced by 25% and 20%, respectively, in the presence of valproate. The elimination half-life of diazepam remained unchanged upon addition of valproate.
Ethosuximide
Valproate inhibits the metabolism of ethosuximide. Administration of a single ethosuximide dose of 500 mg with valproate (800 to 1600 mg/day) to healthy volunteers (n=6) was accompanied by a 25% increase in elimination half-life of ethosuximide and a 15% decrease in its total clearance as compared to ethosuximide alone. Patients receiving valproate and ethosuximide, especially along with other anticonvulsants, should be monitored for alterations in serum concentrations of both drugs.
Lamotrigine
In a steady-state study involving 10 healthy volunteers, the elimination half-life of lamotrigine increased from 26 to 70 hours with valproate co-administration (a 165% increase). The dose of lamotrigine should be reduced when coadministered with valproate. Serious skin reactions (such as Stevens - Johnson syndrome and toxic epidermal necrolysis) have been reported with concomitant lamotrigine and valproate administration. See lamotrigine package insert for details on lamotrigine dosing with concomitant valproate administration.
Phenobarbital
Valproate was found to inhibit the metabolism of phenobarbital. Co-administration of valproate (250 mg BID for 14 days) with phenobarbital to normal subjects (n=6) resulted in a 50% increase in half-life and a 30% decrease in plasma clearance of phenobarbital (60 mg single-dose). The fraction of phenobarbital dose excreted unchanged increased by 50% in presence of valproate.
There is evidence for severe CNS depression, with or without significant elevations of barbiturate or valproate serum concentrations. All patients receiving concomitant barbiturate therapy should be closely monitored for neurological toxicity. Serum barbiturate concentrations should be obtained, if possible, and the barbiturate dosage decreased, if appropriate.
Primidone, which is metabolized to a barbiturate, may be involved in a similar interaction with valproate.
Phenytoin
Valproate displaces phenytoin from its plasma albumin binding sites and inhibits its hepatic metabolism. Coadministration of valproate (400 mg TID) with phenytoin (250 mg) in normal volunteers (n=7) was associated with a 60% increase in the free fraction of phenytoin. Total plasma clearance and apparent volume of distribution of phenytoin increased 30% in the presence of valproate. Both the clearance and apparent volume of distribution of free phenytoin were reduced by 25%.
In patients with epilepsy, there have been reports of breakthrough seizures occurring with the combination of valproate and phenytoin. The dosage of phenytoin should be adjusted as required by the clinical situation.
Tolbutamide
From *in vitro* experiments, the unbound fraction of tolbutamide was increased from 20% to 50% when added to plasma samples taken from patients treated with valproate. The clinical relevance of this displacement is unknown.
Warfarin
In an *in vitro* study, valproate increased the unbound fraction of warfarin by up to 32.6%. The therapeutic relevance of this is unknown; however, coagulation tests should be monitored if valproic acid therapy is instituted in patients taking anticoagulants.
Zidovudine
In six patients who were seropositive for HIV, the clearance of zidovudine (100 mg q8h) was decreased by 38% after administration of valproate (250 or 500 mg q8h); the half-life of zidovudine was unaffected.
Drugs for which either no interaction or a likely clinically unimportant interaction has been observed
Acetaminophen
Valproate had no effect on any of the pharmacokinetic parameters of acetaminophen when it was concurrently administered to three epileptic patients.
Clozapine
In psychotic patients (n=11), no interaction was observed when valproate was co-administered with clozapine.
Lithium
Co-administration of valproate (500 mg BID) and lithium carbonate (300 mg TID) to normal male volunteers (n=16) had no effect on the steady-state kinetics of lithium.
Lorazepam
Concomitant administration of valproate (500 mg BID) and lorazepam (1 mg BID) in normal male volunteers (n=9) was accompanied by a 17% decrease in the plasma clearance of lorazepam.
Oral Contraceptive Steroids
Administration of a single-dose of ethinyloestradiol (50 mcg)/levonorgestrel (250 mcg) to 6 women on valproate (200 mg BID) therapy for 2 months did not reveal any pharmacokinetic interaction.

7.3 Topiramate
Concomitant administration of valproic acid and topiramate has been associated with hyperammonemia with and without encephalopathy *[see Contraindications and Warnings and Precautions (4, 5.7, 5.8)]*. **Concomitant administration of topiramate with valproic acid has also been associated with hypothermia in patients who have tolerated either drug alone. It may be prudent to examine blood ammonia levels in patients in whom the onset of hypothermia has been reported *[see Warnings and Precautions (5.7, 5.9)]*.**

8 USE IN SPECIFIC POPULATIONS

8.1 Pregnancy
Teratogenic Effects: Pregnancy Category D.
Use of Depakote ER during pregnancy can cause congenital malformations including neural tube defects. If this drug is used during pregnancy, or if the patient becomes pregnant while taking this drug, the patient should be apprised of the potential hazard to the fetus. Depakote ER should be considered for women of childbearing potential only after the risks have been thoroughly discussed with the patient and weighed against the potential benefits of treatment.
Human Data
Congenital Malformations
The North American Antiepileptic Drug Pregnancy Registry reported 16 cases of congenital malformations among the offspring of 149 women with epilepsy who were exposed to valproic acid monotherapy during the first trimester of pregnancy at doses of approximately 1,000 mg per day, for a prevalence rate of 10.7% (95% CI 6.3%-16.9%). Three of the 149 offspring (2%) had neural tube defects and 6 of the 149 (4%) had less severe malformations. Among epileptic women who were exposed to other antiepileptic drug monotherapies during pregnancy (1,048 patients) the malformation rate was 2.9% (95% CI 2.0% to 4.1%). There was a 4-fold increase in congenital malformations among infants with valproic acid-exposed mothers compared with those treated with other antiepileptic monotherapies as a group (Odds Ratio 4.0; 95% CI 2.1 to 7.4). This increased risk does not reflect a comparison versus any specific antiepileptic drug, but the risk versus the heterogeneous group of all other antiepileptic drug monotherapies combined. The increased teratogenic risk from valproic acid in women with epilepsy is expected to be reflected in an increased risk in other indications (e.g., migraine or bipolar disorder).
The strongest association of maternal valproate usage with congenital malformations is with neural tube defects (as discussed under the next subheading). However, other congenital anomalies (e.g. craniofacial defects, cardiovascular malformations and anomalies involving various body systems), compatible and incompatible with life, have been reported. Sufficient data to determine the incidence of these congenital anomalies are not available.
Neural Tube Defects
The incidence of neural tube defects in the fetus is increased in mothers receiving valproate during the first trimester of pregnancy. The Centers for Disease Control (CDC) has estimated the risk of valproic acid exposed women having children with spina bifida to be approximately 1 to 2%. The American College of Obstetricians and Gynecologists (ACOG) estimates the general population risk for congenital neural tube defects as 0.14% to 0.2%.
Tests to detect neural tube and other defects using currently accepted procedures should be considered a part of routine prenatal care in pregnant women receiving valproate.
Evidence suggests that pregnant women who receive folic acid supplementation may be at decreased risk for congenital neural tube defects in their offspring compared to pregnant women not receiving folic acid. Whether the risk of neural tube defects in the offspring of women receiving valproate specifically is reduced by folic acid supplementation is unknown. Dietary folic acid supplementation both prior to and during pregnancy should be routinely recommended to patients contemplating pregnancy.
Other Adverse Pregnancy Effects
Patients taking valproate may develop clotting abnormalities *[see Warnings and Precautions (5.6)]*. A patient who had low fibrinogen when taking multiple anticonvulsants including valproate gave birth to an infant with afibrinogenemia who subsequently died of hemorrhage. If valproate is used in pregnancy, the clotting parameters should be monitored carefully.
Patients taking valproate may develop hepatic failure *[see Warnings and Precautions (5.1)]*. Fatal hepatic failures, in a newborn and in an infant, have been reported following the maternal use of valproate during pregnancy.
There have been reports of developmental delay, autism and/or autism spectrum disorder in the offspring of women exposed to valproate during pregnancy.
Animal Data
Reproduction studies have demonstrated valproate-induced teratogenicity. Increased incidences of malformations, as well as intrauterine growth retardation and death, have been observed in mice, rats, rabbits, and monkeys following prenatal exposure to valproate. Malformations of the skeletal system are the most common structural abnormalities produced in experimental animals; however, neural tube closure defects were observed in mice exposed during organogenesis to maternal plasma valproate concentrations 2.3 times the upper limit of the human therapeutic range.
In pregnant rats, oral administration during organogenesis of a dose ≥0.5 times the maximum recommended daily human dose on a mg/m^2 basis (MRHD) produced malformations (e.g. skeletal, cardiac, and urogenital) and growth retardation in the offspring. These doses resulted in peak maternal plasma valproate levels of ≥ 3.4 times the upper limit of the human therapeutic range. Behavioral deficits have been reported in the offspring of rats given 0.5 times the MRHD on a mg/m^2 basis throughout most of pregnancy. Valproate produced skeletal and visceral malformations in the offspring of pregnant rabbits given an oral dose approximately 2 times the MRHD on a mg/m^2 basis during organogenesis. Skeletal malformations, growth retardation, and death were observed in rhesus monkeys following an oral dose equal to the MRHD on a mg/m^2 basis during organogenesis. This dose resulted in peak maternal plasma valproate levels 2.8 times the upper limit of the human therapeutic range.
Registry
To provide information regarding the effects of *in utero* exposure to Depakote ER, healthcare providers are advised to recommend that pregnant patients taking Depakote ER enroll in the North American Antiepileptic Drug (NAAED) Pregnancy Registry. This can be done by calling the toll free number 1-888-233-2334, and must be done by patients themselves. Information on the registry can also be found at the website http://www.aedpregnancyregistry.org/.

8.3 Nursing Mothers
Valproate is excreted in breast milk. Concentrations in breast milk have been reported to be 1-10% of serum concentrations. Because of the potential for adverse reactions in a nursing infant, a decision between the physician and

Information on the Abbott Pharmaceutical Products listed on these pages is from the prescribing information in use as of June 1, 2010. For more information, please visit rxabbott.com or call 1-800-633-9110.

the patient should be made on whether to discontinue nursing or consider an alternative drug treatment for the mother, as appropriate.

8.4 Pediatric Use

Depakote was studied in seven pediatric clinical trials. Two of the pediatric studies were placebo-controlled to evaluate the efficacy of Depakote ER for the indications of mania (150 patients aged 10 to 17 years, 76 of whom were on Depakote ER) and migraine (304 patients aged 12 to 17 years, 231 of whom were on Depakote ER).

Mania

A single 4-week outpatient, double-blind, placebo controlled study of 150 patients aged 10-17 years of age with pediatric bipolar disorder was conducted to evaluate the efficacy of Depakote ER in the treatment of pediatric bipolar disorder. Initial daily doses of 15mg/kg (max. 750mg/day) and flexible dosing was used to achieve a clinical response and/or a target serum valproate level of 80-125 mcg/ml with a maximum allowable dose set at 35mg/kg. Patients on stimulant medications at screening were allowed to continue and maintain current stimulant doses during the trial provided that doses were clinically stable. The trial efficacy endpoint was change from baseline on the YMRS scale at final visit. Results from the trial revealed that the mean maximum daily dose of 1457 mg (27.1 mg/kg) with a mean final serum valproate concentration of 80 mcg/ml was attained in this clinical trial.

Efficacy was not established in this study.

Migraine Prophylaxis

A single, double-blind, placebo-controlled, parallel-group, four equal armed (placebo, 250 mg, 500 mg and 1,000 mg) trial was performed to evaluate the efficacy of Depakote ER in adolescent patients with migraine (304 patients, ages 12-17 years old). The study consisted of a 4 week baseline period followed by a 12 week experimental period (including an initial 2 week titration phase). The primary endpoint was the reduction from baseline in the 4 week migraine headache rate. Placebo was compared to each dose.

Efficacy was not established in this migraine study.

Epilepsy

Depakote ER has not been proven to be safe and effective for epilepsy in children less than 10 years of age.

Pediatric Safety

Two six-month pediatric studies were conducted to evaluate the long-term safety of Depakote ER in the indication of mania (292 patients aged 10 to 17 years). Two twelve-month pediatric studies were conducted to evaluate the long-term safety of Depakote ER in the indication of migraine (353 patients aged 12 to 17 years). One twelve-month study was conducted to evaluate the safety of Depakote Sprinkles Capsules in the indication of partial seizures (169 patients aged 3 to 10 years).

Safety Studies-Mania

Safety Study-Controlled Mania Trial

The incidence of treatment-emergent events for the pediatric population was based on the data from the single placebo-controlled clinical trial of Depakote ER in the treatment of manic or mixed episodes associated with bipolar disorder.

Table 8 includes those adverse reactions reported for pediatric patients in the placebo-controlled mania trial where the incidence rate in the valproate-treated group was ≥5% and was at least twice the rate than that for placebo patients.

Table 8. Common, Drug-Related Adverse Reactions reported by >5% of Depakote-ER Treated Patients during Placebo Controlled Trials for Pediatric Acute Mania

Adverse Reaction-preferred term	Depakote ER (n=76)	Placebo (n=74)
Nausea	9%	1%
Upper abdominal Pain	8%	1%
Somnolence	7%	1%
Increased Ammonia	5%	0
Gastritis	5%	0
Rash	5%	1%

In addition, patients taking Depakote ER had a statistically significant 1.5 lbs mean increase in weight and 0.4 unit BMI mean increase from baseline values over placebo treated patients.

Safety Study-Open Label Mania Safety Data

In the two long-term (six month) safety studies in pediatric patients (n= 292) between the ages of 10 and 17 years old, no clinically meaningful differences in the adverse reaction profile were observed when compared to adults.

The safety and tolerability of Depakote ER in pediatric patients were shown to be comparable to those in adults *[see Adverse Reactions (6.1, 6.2, 6.3)]*.

Safety Studies-Epilepsy (open label)

Safety and tolerability in this study was found comparable to that observed in adult epilepsy studies.

Safety Studies-Migraine (controlled and open label)

Safety and tolerability in this study was found comparable to that observed in adult migraine studies.

Prior Safety Experience

Experience has indicated that pediatric patients under the age of two years are at a considerably increased risk of developing fatal hepatotoxicity, especially those with the aforementioned conditions *[see Boxed Warning, Warnings and Precautions (5.1)]*. When valproic acid is used in this patient group, it should be used with extreme caution and as a sole agent. The benefits of therapy should be weighed against the risks. Above the age of 2 years, experience in epilepsy has indicated that the incidence of fatal hepatotoxicity decreases considerably in progressively older patient groups.

The variability in free fraction limits the clinical usefulness of monitoring total serum valproic acid concentrations. Interpretation of valproic acid concentrations in children should include consideration of factors that affect hepatic metabolism and protein binding.

The safety and effectiveness of valproic acid for the treatment of acute mania has not been established in individuals below the age of 18 years.

The safety and effectiveness of valproic acid for the prophylaxis of migraines has not been studied in individuals below the age of 12 years.

Nonclinical Developmental Toxicology

The basic toxicology and pathologic manifestations of valproate sodium in neonatal (4-day old) and juvenile (14-day old) rats are similar to those seen in young adult rats. However, additional findings, including renal alterations in juvenile rats and renal alterations and retinal dysplasia in neonatal rats, have been reported. These findings occurred at a dose approximately equal to the maximum recommended daily human dose (MRHD). They were not seen at a dose 0.4 times the MRHD.

8.5 Geriatric Use

No patients above the age of 65 years were enrolled in double-blind prospective clinical trials of mania associated with bipolar illness. In a case review study of 583 patients, 72 patients (12%) were greater than 65 years of age. A higher percentage of patients above 65 years of age reported accidental injury, infection, pain, somnolence, and tremor. Discontinuation of valproate was occasionally associated with the latter two events. It is not clear whether these events indicate additional risk or whether they result from preexisting medical illness and concomitant medication use among these patients.

A study of elderly patients with dementia revealed drug related somnolence and discontinuation for somnolence *[see Warnings and Precautions (5.12)]*. The starting dose should be reduced in these patients, and dosage reductions or discontinuation should be considered in patients with excessive somnolence *[see Dosage and Administration (2.4)]*.

There is insufficient information available to discern the safety and effectiveness of valproic acid for the prophylaxis of migraines in patients over 65.

The capacity of elderly patients (age range: 68 to 89 years) to eliminate valproate has been shown to be reduced compared to younger adults (age range: 22 to 26 years) *[see Clinical Pharmacology (12.3)]*.

8.6 Effect of Disease

Liver Disease

[(See Boxed Warning, Contraindications (4), and Warnings and Precautions (5) and Clinical Pharmacology (12.3)]. Liver disease impairs the capacity to eliminate valproate.

10 OVERDOSAGE

Over dosage with valproate may result in somnolence, heart block, and deep coma. Fatalities have been reported; however patients have recovered from valproate levels as high as 2120 mcg/mL.

In overdose situations, the fraction of drug not bound to protein is high and hemodialysis or tandem hemodialysis plus hemoperfusion may result in significant removal of drug. The benefit of gastric lavage or emesis will vary with the time since ingestion. General supportive measures should be applied with particular attention to the maintenance of adequate urinary output.

Naloxone has been reported to reverse the CNS depressant effects of valproate over dosage. Because naloxone could theoretically also reverse the antiepileptic effects of valproate, it should be used with caution in patients with epilepsy.

11 DESCRIPTION

Divalproex sodium is a stable co-ordination compound comprised of sodium valproate and valproic acid in a 1:1 molar relationship and formed during the partial neutralization of valproic acid with 0.5 equivalent of sodium hydroxide. Chemically it is designated as sodium hydrogen bis(2-propylpentanoate). Divalproex sodium has the following structure:

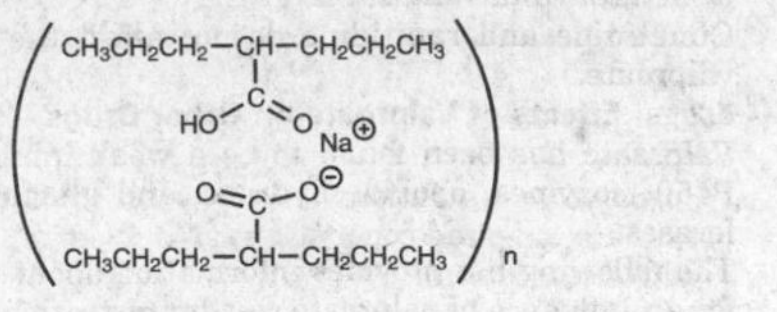

Divalproex sodium occurs as a white powder with a characteristic odor.

Depakote ER 250 and 500 mg tablets are for oral administration. Depakote ER tablets contain divalproex sodium in a once-a-day extended-release formulation equivalent to 250 and 500 mg of valproic acid.

Inactive Ingredients

Depakote ER 250 and 500 mg tablets: FD&C Blue No. 1, hypromellose, lactose, microcrystalline cellulose, polyethylene glycol, potassium sorbate, propylene glycol, silicon dioxide, titanium dioxide, and triacetin.

In addition, 500 mg tablets contain iron oxide and polydextrose.

12 CLINICAL PHARMACOLOGY

12.1 Mechanism of Action

Divalproex sodium dissociates to the valproate ion in the gastrointestinal tract. The mechanisms by which valproate exerts its therapeutic effects have not been established. It has been suggested that its activity in epilepsy is related to increased brain concentrations of gamma-aminobutyric acid (GABA).

12.2 Pharmacodynamics

The relationship between plasma concentration and clinical response is not well documented. One contributing factor is the nonlinear, concentration dependent protein binding of valproate which affects the clearance of the drug. Thus, monitoring of total serum valproate may not provide a reliable index of the bioactive valproate species as protein binding may be affected by age and disease state (e.g. hepatic or renal insufficiency, hyperlipidemia).

Epilepsy

The therapeutic range in epilepsy is commonly considered to be 50 to 100 mcg/mL of total valproate, although some patients may be controlled with lower or higher plasma concentrations.

Mania

In placebo-controlled clinical trials of acute mania, patients were dosed to clinical response with trough plasma concentrations between 85 and 125 mcg/mL *[see Dosage and Administration (2.1)]*.

12.3 Pharmacokinetics

Absorption/Bioavailability

The absolute bioavailability of Depakote ER tablets administered as a single dose after a meal was approximately 90% relative to intravenous infusion.

When given in equal total daily doses, the bioavailability of Depakote ER is less than that of Depakote (divalproex sodium delayed-release tablets). In five multiple-dose studies in healthy subjects (N=82) and in subjects with epilepsy (N=86), when administered under fasting and nonfasting conditions, Depakote ER given once daily produced an average bioavailability of 89% relative to an equal total daily dose of Depakote given BID, TID, or QID. The median time to maximum plasma valproate concentrations (C_{max}) after Depakote ER administration ranged from 4 to 17 hours. After multiple once-daily dosing of Depakote ER, the peak-to-trough fluctuation in plasma valproate concentrations was 10-20% lower than that of regular Depakote given BID, TID, or QID.

Conversion from Depakote to Depakote ER

When Depakote ER is given in doses 8 to 20% higher than the total daily dose of Depakote, the two formulations are bioequivalent. In two randomized, crossover studies, multiple daily doses of Depakote were compared to 8 to 20% higher once-daily doses of Depakote ER. In these two studies, Depakote ER and Depakote regimens were equivalent with respect to area under the curve (AUC; a measure of the extent of bioavailability). Additionally, valproate C_{max} was lower, and C_{min} was either higher or not different, for Depakote ER relative to Depakote regimens (see Table 9).

[See table 9 at top of next page]

Concomitant antiepilepsy drugs (topiramate, phenobarbital, carbamazepine, phenytoin, and lamotrigine were evaluated) that induce the cytochrome P450 isozyme system did not significantly alter valproate bioavailability when converting between Depakote and Depakote ER.

Distribution

Protein Binding

The plasma protein binding of valproate is concentration dependent and the free fraction increases from approximately 10% at 40 mcg/mL to 18.5% at 130 mcg/mL. Protein binding of valproate is reduced in the elderly, in patients with chronic hepatic diseases, in patients with renal impairment, and in the presence of other drugs (e.g., aspirin). Conversely, valproate may displace certain protein-bound drugs (e.g., phenytoin, carbamazepine, warfarin, and tolbutamide) [see Drug Interactions (7) for more detailed information on the pharmacokinetic interactions of valproate with other drugs].

CNS Distribution
Valproate concentrations in cerebrospinal fluid (CSF) approximate unbound concentrations in plasma (about 10% of total concentration).

Metabolism
Valproate is metabolized almost entirely by the liver. In adult patients on monotherapy, 30-50% of an administered dose appears in urine as a glucuronide conjugate. Mitochondrial β-oxidation is the other major metabolic pathway, typically accounting for over 40% of the dose. Usually, less than 15-20% of the dose is eliminated by other oxidative mechanisms. Less than 3% of an administered dose is excreted unchanged in urine.

The relationship between dose and total valproate concentration is nonlinear; concentration does not increase proportionally with the dose, but rather, increases to a lesser extent due to saturable plasma protein binding. The kinetics of unbound drug are linear.

Elimination
Mean plasma clearance and volume of distribution for total valproate are 0.56 L/hr/1.73 m² and 11 L/1.73 m², respectively. Mean plasma clearance and volume of distribution for free valproate are 4.6 L/hr/1.73 m² and 92 L/1.73 m². Mean terminal half-life for valproate monotherapy ranged from 9 to 16 hours following oral dosing regimens of 250 to 1000 mg.

The estimates cited apply primarily to patients who are not taking drugs that affect hepatic metabolizing enzyme systems. For example, patients taking enzyme-inducing antiepileptic drugs (carbamazepine, phenytoin, and phenobarbital) will clear valproate more rapidly. Because of these changes in valproate clearance, monitoring of antiepileptic concentrations should be intensified whenever concomitant antiepileptics are introduced or withdrawn.

Special Populations
Effect of Age
Pediatric
The valproate pharmacokinetic profile following administration of Depakote ER was characterized in a multiple-dose, non-fasting, open label, multi-center study in children and adolescents. Depakote ER once daily doses ranged from 250-1750 mg. Once daily administration of Depakote ER in pediatric patients (10-17 years) produced plasma VPA concentration-time profiles similar to those that have been observed in adults.
Elderly
The capacity of elderly patients (age range: 68 to 89 years) to eliminate valproate has been shown to be reduced compared to younger adults (age range: 22 to 26). Intrinsic clearance is reduced by 39%; the free fraction is increased by 44%. Accordingly, the initial dosage should be reduced in the elderly [see Dosage and Administration (2.4)].
Effect of Sex
There are no differences in the body surface area adjusted unbound clearance between males and females (4.8±0.17 and 4.7±0.07 L/hr per 1.73 m², respectively).
Effect of Race
The effects of race on the kinetics of valproate have not been studied.
Effect of Disease
Liver Disease
Liver disease impairs the capacity to eliminate valproate. In one study, the clearance of free valproate was decreased by 50% in 7 patients with cirrhosis and by 16% in 4 patients with acute hepatitis, compared with 6 healthy subjects. In that study, the half-life of valproate was increased from 12 to 18 hours. Liver disease is also associated with decreased albumin concentrations and larger unbound fractions (2 to 2.6 fold increase) of valproate. Accordingly, monitoring of total concentrations may be misleading since free concentrations may be substantially elevated in patients with hepatic disease whereas total concentrations may appear to be normal [see Boxed Warning, Contraindications (4), Warnings and Precautions (5.1)].
Renal Disease
A slight reduction (27%) in the unbound clearance of valproate has been reported in patients with renal failure (creatinine clearance < 10 mL/minute); however, hemodialysis typically reduces valproate concentrations by about 20%. Therefore, no dosage adjustment appears to be necessary in patients with renal failure. Protein binding in these patients is substantially reduced; thus, monitoring total concentrations may be misleading.

Table 9. Bioavailability of Depakote ER Tablets Relative to Depakote When Depakote ER Dose is 8 to 20% Higher

Study Population	Regimens Depakote ER vs. Depakote	Relative Bioavailability		
		AUC₂₄	C_max	C_min
Healthy Volunteers (N=35)	1000 & 1500 mg Depakote ER vs. 875 & 1250 mg Depakote	1.059	0.882	1.173
Patients with epilepsy on concomitant enzyme-inducing antiepilepsy drugs (N = 64)	1000 to 5000 mg Depakote ER vs. 875 to 4250 mg Depakote	1.008	0.899	1.022

13   NONCLINICAL TOXICOLOGY
13.1   Carcinogenesis, Mutagenesis, Impairment of Fertility
Carcinogenesis
Valproic acid was administered orally to Sprague Dawley rats and ICR (HA/ICR) mice at doses of 80 and 170 mg/kg/day (approximately 10 to 50% of the maximum human daily dose on a mg/m² basis) for two years. A variety of neoplasms were observed in both species. The primary findings were a statistically significant increase in the incidence of subcutaneous fibrosarcomas in high dose male rats receiving valproic acid and a statistically significant dose-related trend for benign pulmonary adenomas in male mice receiving valproic acid. The significance of these findings for humans is unknown.
Mutagenesis
Valproate was not mutagenic in an in vitro bacterial assay (Ames test), did not produce dominant lethal effects in mice, and did not increase chromosome aberration frequency in an in vivo cytogenetic study in rats. Increased frequencies of sister chromatid exchange (SCE) have been reported in a study of epileptic children taking valproate, but this association was not observed in another study conducted in adults. There is some evidence that increased SCE frequencies may be associated with epilepsy. The biological significance of an increase in SCE frequency is not known.
Fertility
Chronic toxicity studies in juvenile and adult rats and dogs demonstrated reduced spermatogenesis and testicular atrophy at oral doses of 400 mg/kg/day or greater in rats (approximately equivalent to or greater than the maximum human daily dose (MHD) on a mg/m² basis) and 150 mg/kg/day or greater in dogs (approximately 1.4 times the MHD or greater on a mg/m² basis). Fertility studies in rats have shown doses up to 350 mg/kg/day (approximately equal to the MHD on a mg/m² basis) for 60 days to have no effect on fertility. The effect of valproate on testicular development and on sperm production and fertility in humans is unknown.

14   CLINICAL STUDIES
14.1   Mania
The effectiveness of Depakote ER for the treatment of acute mania is based in part on studies establishing the effectiveness of Depakote (divalproex sodium delayed release tablets) for this indication. Depakote ER's effectiveness was confirmed in one randomized, double-blind, placebo-controlled, parallel group, 3-week, multicenter study. The study was designed to evaluate the safety and efficacy of Depakote ER in the treatment of bipolar I disorder, manic or mixed type, in adults. Adult male and female patients who had a current DSM-IV TR primary diagnosis of bipolar I disorder, manic or mixed type, and who were hospitalized for acute mania, were enrolled into this study. Depakote ER was initiated at a dose of 25 mg/kg/day given once daily, increased by 500 mg/day on Day 3, then adjusted to achieve plasma valproate concentrations in the range of 85-125 mcg/mL. Mean daily Depakote ER doses for observed cases were 2362 mg (range: 500-4000), 2874 mg (range: 1500-4500), 2993 mg (range: 1500-4500), 3181 mg (range: 1500-5000), and 3353 mg (range: 1500-5500) at Days 1, 5, 10, 15, and 21, respectively. Mean valproate concentrations were 96.5 mcg/mL, 102.1 mcg/mL, 98.5 mcg/mL, 89.5 mcg/mL at Days 5, 10, 15 and 21, respectively. Patients were assessed on the Mania Rating Scale (MRS; score ranges from 0-52).
Depakote ER was significantly more effective than placebo in reduction of the MRS total score.
14.2   Epilepsy
The efficacy of valproate in reducing the incidence of complex partial seizures (CPS) that occur in isolation or in association with other seizure types was established in two controlled trials.
In one, multiclinic, placebo controlled study employing an add-on design, (adjunctive therapy) 144 patients who continued to suffer eight or more CPS per 8 weeks during an 8 week period of monotherapy with doses of either carbamazepine or phenytoin sufficient to assure plasma concentrations within the "therapeutic range" were randomized to receive, in addition to their original antiepilepsy drug (AED),

either Depakote (divalproex sodium) or placebo. Randomized patients were to be followed for a total of 16 weeks. The following Table presents the findings.

Table 10. Adjunctive Therapy Study Median Incidence of CPS per 8 Weeks

Add-on Treatment	Number of Patients	Baseline Incidence	Experimental Incidence
Depakote	75	16.0	8.9*
Placebo	69	14.5	11.5

*Reduction from baseline statistically significantly greater for valproate than placebo at p ≤ 0.05 level.

Figure 1 presents the proportion of patients (X axis) whose percentage reduction from baseline in complex partial seizure rates was at least as great as that indicated on the Y axis in the adjunctive therapy study. A positive percent reduction indicates an improvement (i.e., a decrease in seizure frequency), while a negative percent reduction indicates worsening. Thus, in a display of this type, the curve for an effective treatment is shifted to the left of the curve for placebo. This Figure shows that the proportion of patients achieving any particular level of improvement was consistently higher for valproate than for placebo. For example, 45% of patients treated with valproate had a ≥ 50% reduction in complex partial seizure rate compared to 23% of patients treated with placebo.

Figure 1

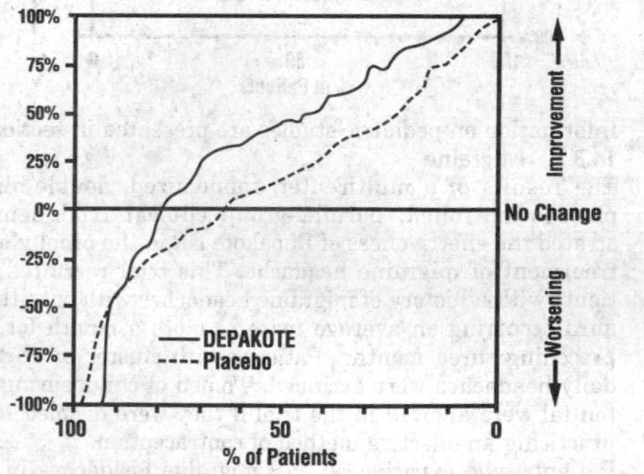

The second study assessed the capacity of valproate to reduce the incidence of CPS when administered as the sole AED. The study compared the incidence of CPS among patients randomized to either a high or low dose treatment arm. Patients qualified for entry into the randomized comparison phase of this study only if 1) they continued to experience 2 or more CPS per 4 weeks during an 8 to 12 week long period of monotherapy with adequate doses of an AED (i.e., phenytoin, carbamazepine, phenobarbital, or primidone) and 2) they made a successful transition over a two week interval to valproate. Patients entering the randomized phase were then brought to their assigned target dose, gradually tapered off their concomitant AED and followed for an interval as long as 22 weeks. Less than 50% of the patients randomized, however, completed the study. In patients converted to Depakote monotherapy, the mean total valproate concentrations during monotherapy were 71 and 123 mcg/mL in the low dose and high dose groups, respectively.
The following Table presents the findings for all patients randomized who had at least one post-randomization assessment.

Information on the Abbott Pharmaceutical Products listed on these pages is from the prescribing information in use as of June 1, 2010. For more information, please visit rxabbott.com or call 1-800-633-9110.

Table 11. Monotherapy Study Median Incidence of CPS per 8 Weeks

Treatment	Number of Patients	Baseline Incidence	Randomized Phase Incidence
High dose Valproate	131	13.2	10.7*
Low dose Valproate	134	14.2	13.8

*Reduction from baseline statistically significantly greater for high dose than low dose at p ≤ 0.05 level.

Figure 2 presents the proportion of patients (X axis) whose percentage reduction from baseline in complex partial seizure rates was at least as great as that indicated on the Y axis in the monotherapy study. A positive percent reduction indicates an improvement (i.e., a decrease in seizure frequency), while a negative percent reduction indicates worsening. Thus, in a display of this type, the curve for a more effective treatment is shifted to the left of the curve for a less effective treatment. This Figure shows that the proportion of patients achieving any particular level of reduction was consistently higher for high dose valproate than for low dose valproate. For example, when switching from carbamazepine, phenytoin, phenobarbital or primidone monotherapy to high dose valproate monotherapy, 63% of patients experienced no change or a reduction in complex partial seizure rates compared to 54% of patients receiving low dose valproate.

Figure 2

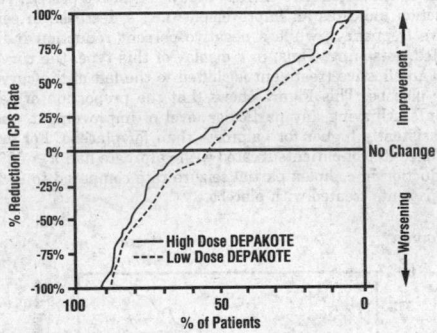

Information on pediatric studies are presented in section 8.

14.3 Migraine

The results of a multicenter, randomized, double-blind, placebo-controlled, parallel-group clinical trial demonstrated the effectiveness of Depakote ER in the prophylactic treatment of migraine headache. This trial recruited patients with a history of migraine headaches with or without aura occurring on average twice or more a month for the preceding three months. Patients with cluster or chronic daily headaches were excluded. Women of childbearing potential were allowed in the trial if they were deemed to be practicing an effective method of contraception.

Patients who experienced ≥ 2 migraine headaches in the 4-week baseline period were randomized in a 1:1 ratio to Depakote ER or placebo and treated for 12 weeks. Patients initiated treatment on 500 mg once daily for one week, and were then increased to 1000 mg once daily with an option to permanently decrease the dose back to 500 mg once daily during the second week of treatment if intolerance occurred. Ninety-eight of 114 Depakote ER-treated patients (86%) and 100 of 110 placebo-treated patients (91%) treated at least two weeks maintained the 1000 mg once daily dose for the duration of their treatment periods. Treatment outcome was assessed on the basis of reduction in 4-week migraine headache rate in the treatment period compared to the baseline period.

Patients (50 male, 187 female) ranging in age from 16 to 69 were treated with Depakote ER (N=122) or placebo (N=115). Four patients were below the age of 18 and 3 were above the age of 65. Two hundred and two patients (101 in each treatment group) completed the treatment period. The mean reduction in 4-week migraine headache rate was 1.2 from a baseline mean of 4.4 in the Depakote ER group, versus 0.6 from a baseline mean of 4.2 in the placebo group. The treatment difference was statistically significant (see Figure 3). [See figure 3 at top of next column]

16 HOW SUPPLIED/STORAGE AND HANDLING

Depakote ER 250 mg is available as white ovaloid tablets with the corporate Abbott ⊡ logo, and the Abbo-Code (HF). Each Depakote ER tablet contains divalproex sodium equivalent to 250 mg of valproic acid in the following package sizes:

Figure 3 Mean Reduction In 4-Week Migraine Headache Rates

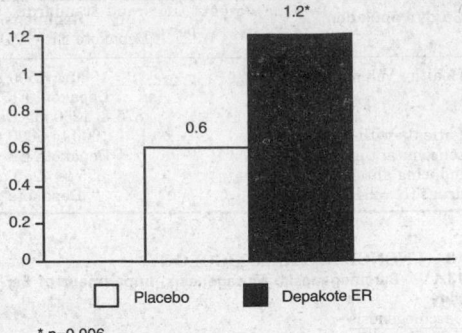

* p=0.006

Bottles of 60	(NDC 0074-3826-60).
Bottles of 100	(NDC 0074-3826-13).
Bottles of 500	(NDC 0074-3826-53).
ABBO-PAC unit dose packages of 100	(NDC 0074-3826-11).

Depakote ER 500 mg is available as gray ovaloid tablets with the corporate Abbott ⊡ logo, and the Abbo-Code (HC). Each Depakote ER tablet contains divalproex sodium equivalent to 500 mg of valproic acid in the following packaging sizes:

Bottles of 100	(NDC 0074-7126-13).
Bottles of 500	(NDC 0074-7126-53).
ABBO-PAC unit dose packages of 100	(NDC 0074-7126-11).

Recommended Storage

Store tablets at 25°C (77°F); excursions permitted to 15-30°C (59-86°F) [see USP Controlled Room Temperature].

17 PATIENT COUNSELING INFORMATION

See FDA-Approved Patient Labeling (17.8)

17.1 Hepatotoxicity

Patients and guardians should be warned that nausea, vomiting, abdominal pain, anorexia, diarrhea, asthenia, and/or jaundice can be symptoms of hepatotoxicity and, therefore, require further medical evaluation promptly [see Warnings and Precautions (5.1)].

17.2 Pancreatitis

Patients and guardians should be warned that abdominal pain, nausea, vomiting, and/or anorexia can be symptoms of pancreatitis and, therefore, require further medical evaluation promptly [see Warnings and Precautions (5.3)].

17.3 Teratogenicity/Usage in Pregnancy

Use of valproate during pregnancy increases the risk for neural tube defects and other malformations. Female patients of child-bearing age, who require therapy for epilepsy, bipolar disorder, or migraines, should be advised of the risks of valproate use during pregnancy and appropriate therapeutic options. This is particularly important when the treatment of a spontaneously reversible condition not ordinarily associated with permanent injury or risk of death (e.g. migraine) is considered. Patients should read the Patient Information Leaflet, which appears as the last section of the labeling [see Use in Specific Populations (8.1)].

Patients should be encouraged to enroll in the NAAED Pregnancy Registry if they become pregnant. This registry is collecting information about the safety of antiepileptic drugs during pregnancy. To enroll, patients can call the toll free number 1-888-233-2334 [see Use in Specific Populations (8.1)].

17.4 Suicidal Thinking and Behavior

Patients, their caregivers, and families should be counseled that AEDs, including Depakote ER, may increase the risk of suicidal thoughts and behavior and should be advised of the need to be alert for the emergence or worsening of symptoms of depression, any unusual changes in mood or behavior, or the emergence of suicidal thoughts, behavior, or thoughts about self-harm. Behaviors of concern should be reported immediately to the healthcare providers [see Warnings and Precautions (5.5)].

17.5 Hyperammonemia

Patients should be informed of the signs and symptoms associated with hyperammonemic encephalopathy and be told to inform the prescriber if any of these symptoms occur [see Warnings and Precautions (5.7, 5.8)].

17.6 CNS depression

Since valproate products may produce CNS depression, especially when combined with another CNS depressant (e.g., alcohol), patients should be advised not to engage in hazardous activities, such as driving an automobile or operating dangerous machinery, until it is known that they do not become drowsy from the drug.

17.7 Multi-organ Hypersensitivity Reaction

Patients should be instructed that a fever associated with other organ system involvement (rash, lymphadenopathy,

etc.) may be drug-related and should be reported to the physician immediately [see Warnings and Precautions (5.10)].

17.8 FDA–Approved Patient Labeling

Important Information for Women Who Could Become Pregnant About the Use of Depakote ER (divalproex sodium) extended release tablets.

Please read this leaflet carefully before you take any of this medication. This leaflet provides a summary of important information about taking this medication to women who could become pregnant. If you have any questions or concerns, or want more information about this medication, contact your doctor or pharmacist.

Information For Women Who Could Become Pregnant

You can only obtain this medication by prescription from your doctor. The decision to use this medicine should be made by you and your doctor based on your health needs and medical condition.

Before starting this medicine, you should know that using this medicine during pregnancy causes an increased chance of birth defects in your baby. These birth defects may include spina bifida and other defects where the spinal canal does not close normally. These defects usually occur in 1 to 2 out of every 1000 babies born in the United States. Studies show that for babies born to epileptic women who took valproate in the first 12 weeks of pregnancy, these defects occur in 1 to 2 out of every 100 babies.

Use of valproate during pregnancy also increases the chance of other birth defects such as of the heart, bones, and other parts of the body. Studies suggest that other medicines used to treat your condition may be less likely to cause these defects.

Information For Women Who Are Planning to Get Pregnant

Women using valproate who plan to get pregnant should discuss their treatment options with their doctor.

Information For Women Who Become Pregnant

If you become pregnant while taking valproate, you should contact your doctor immediately.

Other Important Information

• You should take your medicine exactly as prescribed by your doctor to get the most benefit from your medicine and reduce the risk of side effects.

• If you have taken more than the prescribed dose, contact your hospital emergency room or local poison center immediately.

• Your medicine was prescribed for your particular condition. Do not use it for another condition or give the drug to others.

Facts About Birth Defects

It is important to know that birth defects may occur even in children born to women who are not taking any medicines and do not have other risk factors.

This summary provides important information about the use of Depakote ER (divalproex sodium) extended release tablets to women who could become pregnant. If you would like more information, ask your doctor or pharmacist to let you read the professional labeling and then discuss it with them. If you have any questions or concerns about taking this medication, you should discuss them with your doctor.

Depakote ER 250 mg

Mfd. by Abbott Pharmaceuticals PR Ltd., Barceloneta, PR 00617

Depakote ER 500 mg

Mfd. by

Abbott Laboratories, North Chicago, IL 60064 U.S.A.

or

Abbott Pharmaceuticals PR Ltd., Barceloneta, PR 00617

Manufactured for

Abbott Laboratories

North Chicago, IL 60064 U.S.A.

Ref. 03-A308-R-13 Revised: November, 2009

Shown in Product Identification Guide, page 303

ERY-PED®   ℞

[erē′ ped]

(erythromycin ethylsuccinate, USP)

To reduce the development of drug-resistant bacteria and maintain the effectiveness of EryPed and other antibacterial drugs, EryPed should be used only to treat or prevent infections that are proven or strongly suspected to be caused by bacteria.

DESCRIPTION

Erythromycin is produced by a strain of *Saccharopolyspora erythraea* (formerly *Streptomyces erythraeus*) and belongs to the macrolide group of antibiotics. It is basic and readily forms salts with acids. The base, the stearate salt, and the esters are poorly soluble in water. Erythromycin ethylsuccinate is an ester of erythromycin suitable for oral administration. Erythromycin ethylsuccinate is known chemically as erythromycin 2′-(ethyl succinate). The molecular formula is $C_{43}H_{75}NO_{16}$ and the molecular weight is 862.06. The structural formula is:

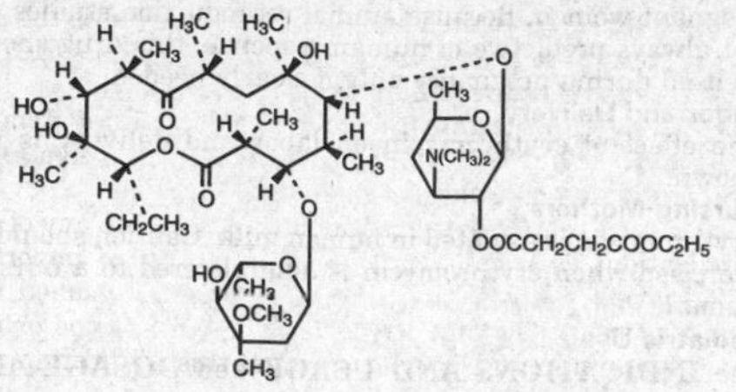

EryPed 200 and EryPed Drops (erythromycin ethylsuccinate for oral suspension) when reconstituted with water, forms a suspension containing erythromycin ethylsuccinate equivalent to 200 mg erythromycin per 5 mL (teaspoonful) or 100 mg per 2.5 mL (dropperful) with an appealing fruit flavor. EryPed 400 when reconstituted with water, forms a suspension containing erythromycin ethylsuccinate equivalent to 400 mg of erythromycin per 5 mL (teaspoonful) with an appealing banana flavor.

These products are intended primarily for pediatric use but can also be used in adults.

Inactive Ingredients

EryPed 200, EryPed 400 and EryPed Drops:

Caramel, polysorbate, sodium citrate, sucrose, xanthan gum and artificial flavors.

CLINICAL PHARMACOLOGY

Orally administered erythromycin ethylsuccinate suspension is readily and reliably absorbed under both fasting and nonfasting conditions.

Erythromycin diffuses readily into most body fluids. Only low concentrations are normally achieved in the spinal fluid, but passage of the drug across the blood-brain barrier increases in meningitis. In the presence of normal hepatic function, erythromycin is concentrated in the liver and excreted in the bile; the effect of hepatic dysfunction on excretion of erythromycin by the liver into the bile is not known. Less than 5 percent of the orally administered dose of erythromycin is excreted in active form in the urine.

Erythromycin crosses the placental barrier, but fetal plasma levels are low. The drug is excreted in human milk.

Microbiology

Erythromycin acts by inhibition of protein synthesis by binding 50 *S* ribosomal subunits of susceptible organisms. It does not affect nucleic acid synthesis. Antagonism has been demonstrated *in vitro* between erythromycin and clindamycin, lincomycin, and chloramphenicol.

Many strains of *Haemophilus influenzae* are resistant to erythromycin alone but are susceptible to erythromycin and sulfonamides used concomitantly.

Staphylococci resistant to erythromycin may emerge during a course of therapy.

Erythromycin has been shown to be active against most strains of the following microorganisms, both *in vitro* and in clinical infections as described in the **INDICATIONS AND USAGE** section.

Gram-positive organisms
Corynebacterium diphtheriae
Corynebacterium minutissimum
Listeria monocytogenes
Staphylococcus aureus (resistant organisms may emerge during treatment)
Streptococcus pneumoniae
Streptococcus pyogenes
Gram-negative organisms
Bordetella pertussis
Legionella pneumophila
Neisseria gonorrhoeae
Other microorganisms
Chlamydia trachomatis
Entamoeba histolytica
Mycoplasma pneumoniae
Treponema pallidum
Ureaplasma urealyticum

The following *in vitro* data are available, **but their clinical significance is unknown.**

Erythromycin exhibits *in vitro* minimal inhibitory concentrations (MIC's) of 0.5 µg/mL or less against most (≥ 90%) strains of the following microorganisms; however, the safety and effectiveness of erythromycin in treating clinical infections due to these microorganisms have not been established in adequate and well-controlled clinical trials.

Gram-positive organisms
Viridans group streptococci
Gram-negative organisms
Moraxella catarrhalis

Susceptibility Tests

Dilution Techniques

Quantitative methods are used to determine antimicrobial minimum inhibitory concentrations (MIC's). These MIC's provide estimates of the susceptibility of bacteria to antimicrobial compounds. The MIC's should be determined using a standardized procedure. Standardized procedures are based on a dilution method[1] (broth or agar) or equivalent with standardized inoculum concentrations and standardized concentrations of erythromycin powder. The MIC values should be interpreted according to the following criteria:

MIC (µg/mL)	Interpretation
≤ 0.5	Susceptible (S)
1-4	Intermediate (I)
≥ 8	Resistant (R)

A report of "Susceptible" indicates that the pathogen is likely to be inhibited if the antimicrobial compound in the blood reaches the concentrations usually achievable. A report of "Intermediate" indicates that the result should be considered equivocal, and, if the microorganism is not fully susceptible to alternative, clinically feasible drugs, the test should be repeated. This category implies possible clinical applicability in body sites where the drug is physiologically concentrated or in situations where high dosage of drug can be used. This category also provides a buffer zone which prevents small uncontrolled technical factors from causing major discrepancies in interpretation. A report of "Resistant" indicates that the pathogen is not likely to be inhibited if the antimicrobial compound in the blood reaches the concentrations usually achievable; other therapy should be selected.

Standardized susceptibility test procedures require the use of laboratory control microorganisms to control the technical aspects of the laboratory procedures. Standard erythromycin powder should provide the following MIC values:

Microorganism	MIC (µg/mL)
S. aureus ATCC 29213	0.12-0.5
E. faecalis ATCC 29212	1-4

Diffusion Techniques

Quantitative methods that require measurement of zone diameters also provide reproducible estimates of the susceptibility of bacteria to antimicrobial compounds. One such standardized procedure[2] requires the use of standardized inoculum concentrations. This procedure uses paper disks impregnated with 15-µg erythromycin to test the susceptibility of microorganisms to erythromycin.

Reports from the laboratory providing results of the standard single-disk susceptibility test with a 15-µg erythromycin disk should be interpreted according to the following criteria:

Zone Diameter (mm)	Interpretation
≥ 23	Susceptible (S)
14-22	Intermediate (I)
≤ 13	Resistant (R)

Interpretation should be as stated above for results using dilution techniques. Interpretation involves correlation of the diameter obtained in the disk test with the MIC for erythromycin.

As with standardized dilution techniques, diffusion methods require the use of laboratory control microorganisms that are used to control the technical aspects of the laboratory procedures. For the diffusion technique, the 15-µg erythromycin disk should provide the following zone diameters in these laboratory test quality control strains:

Microorganism	Zone Diameter (mm)
S. aureus ATCC 25923	22-30

INDICATIONS AND USAGE

To reduce the development of drug-resistant bacteria and maintain the effectiveness of Ery-Ped and other antibacterial drugs, Ery-Ped should be used only to treat or prevent infections that are proven or strongly suspected to be caused by susceptible bacteria. When culture and susceptibility information are available, they should be considered in selecting or modifying antibacterial therapy. In the absence of such data, local epidemiology and susceptibility patterns may contribute to the empiric selection of therapy.

Ery-Ped is indicated in the treatment of infections caused by susceptible strains of the designated organisms in the diseases listed below:

Upper respiratory tract infections of mild to moderate degree caused by *Streptococcus pyogenes*, *Streptococcus pneumoniae*, or *Haemophilus influenzae* (when used concomitantly with adequate doses of sulfonamides, since many strains of *H. influenzae* are not susceptible to the erythromycin concentrations ordinarily achieved). (See appropriate sulfonamide labeling for prescribing information.)

Lower-respiratory tract infections of mild to moderate severity caused by *Streptococcus pneumoniae* or *Streptococcus pyogenes*.

Listeriosis caused by *Listeria monocytogenes*.

Pertussis (whooping cough) caused by *Bordetella pertussis*. Erythromycin is effective in eliminating the organism from the nasopharynx of infected individuals rendering them noninfectious. Some clinical studies suggest that erythromycin may be helpful in the prophylaxis of pertussis in exposed susceptible individuals.

Respiratory tract infections due to *Mycoplasma pneumoniae*.

Skin and skin structure infections of mild to moderate severity caused by *Streptococcus pyogenes* or *Staphylococcus aureus* (resistant staphylococci may emerge during treatment).

Diphtheria: Infections due to *Corynebacterium diphtheriae*, as an adjunct to antitoxin, to prevent establishment of carriers and to eradicate the organism in carriers.

Erythrasma: In the treatment of infections due to *Corynebacterium minutissimum*.

Intestinal amebiasis caused by *Entamoeba histolytica* (oral erythromycins only). Extraenteric amebiasis requires treatment with other agents.

Acute Pelvic Inflammatory Disease Caused by *Neisseria gonorrhoeae*: As an alternative drug in treatment of acute pelvic inflammatory disease caused by *N. gonorrhoeae* in female patients with a history of sensitivity to penicillin. Patients should have a serologic test for syphilis before receiving erythromycin as treatment of gonorrhea and a follow-up serologic test for syphilis after 3 months.

Syphilis Caused by *Treponema pallidum*: Erythromycin is an alternate choice of treatment for primary syphilis in penicillin-allergic patients. In primary syphilis, spinal fluid examinations should be done before treatment and as part of follow-up after therapy.

Erythromycins are Indicated for the Treatment of the Following Infections Caused by *Chlamydia trachomatis*: Conjunctivitis of the newborn, pneumonia of infancy, and urogenital infections during pregnancy. When tetracyclines are contraindicated or not tolerated, erythromycin is indicated for the treatment of uncomplicated urethral, endocervical, or rectal infections in adults due to *Chlamydia trachomatis*.

When tetracyclines are contraindicated or not tolerated, erythromycin is indicated for the treatment of nongonococcal urethritis caused by *Ureaplasma urealyticum*.

Legionnaires' Disease caused by *Legionella pneumophila*. Although no controlled clinical efficacy studies have been conducted, *in vitro* and limited preliminary clinical data suggest that erythromycin may be effective in treating Legionnaires' Disease.

Prophylaxis

Prevention of Initial Attacks of Rheumatic Fever:

Penicillin is considered by the American Heart Association to be the drug of choice in the prevention of initial attacks of rheumatic fever (treatment of *Streptococcus pyogenes* infections of the upper respiratory tract, e.g., tonsillitis or pharyngitis). Erythromycin is indicated for the treatment of penicillin-allergic patients.[3] The therapeutic dose should be administered for 10 days.

Prevention of Recurrent Attacks of Rheumatic Fever:

Penicillin or sulfonamides are considered by the American Heart Association to be the drugs of choice in the prevention of recurrent attacks of rheumatic fever. In patients who are allergic to penicillin and sulfonamides, oral erythromycin is recommended by the American Heart Association in the long-term prophylaxis of streptococcal pharyngitis (for the prevention of recurrent attacks of rheumatic fever).[3]

CONTRAINDICATIONS

Erythromycin is contraindicated in patients with known hypersensitivity to this antibiotic.

Erythromycin is contraindicated in patients taking terfenadine, astemizole, pimozide, or cisapride. (See **PRECAUTIONS - Drug Interactions.**)

WARNINGS

There have been reports of hepatic dysfunction, including increased liver enzymes, and hepatocellular and/or cholestatic hepatitis, with or without jaundice, occurring in patients receiving oral erythromycin products.

There have been reports suggesting that erythromycin does not reach the fetus in adequate concentration to prevent

Information on the Abbott Pharmaceutical Products listed on these pages is from the prescribing information in use as of June 1, 2010. For more information, please visit rxabbott.com or call 1-800-633-9110.

congenital syphilis. Infants born to women treated during pregnancy with oral erythromycin for early syphilis should be treated with an appropriate penicillin regimen.

Clostridium difficile associated diarrhea (CDAD) has been reported with use of nearly all antibacterial agents, including Ery-Ped, and may range in severity from mild diarrhea to fatal colitis. Treatment with antibacterial agents alters the normal flora of the colon leading to overgrowth of *C. difficile*.

C. difficile produces toxins A and B which contribute to the development of CDAD. Hypertoxin producing strains of *C. difficile* cause increased morbidity and mortality, as these infections can be refractory to antimicrobial therapy and may require colectomy. CDAD must be considered in all patients who present with diarrhea following antibiotic use. Careful medical history is necessary since CDAD has been reported to occur over two months after the administration of antibacterial agents.

If CDAD is suspected or confirmed, ongoing antibiotic use not directed against *C. difficile* may need to be discontinued. Appropriate fluid and electrolyte management, protein supplementation, antibiotic treatment of *C. difficile*, and surgical evaluation should be instituted as clinically indicated.

Rhabdomyolysis with or without renal impairment has been reported in seriously ill patients receiving erythromycin concomitantly with lovastatin. Therefore, patients receiving concomitant lovastatin and erythromycin should be carefully monitored for creatine kinase (CK) and serum transaminase levels. (See package insert for lovastatin.)

PRECAUTIONS

General

Prescribing Ery-Ped in the absence of a proven or strongly suspected bacterial infection or a prophylactic indication is unlikely to provide benefit to the patient and increases the risk of the development of drug-resistant bacteria.

Since erythromycin is principally excreted by the liver, caution should be exercised when erythromycin is administered to patients with impaired hepatic function. (See CLINICAL PHARMACOLOGY and WARNINGS sections.)

Exacerbation of symptoms of myasthenia gravis and new onset of symptoms of myasthenic syndrome has been reported in patients receiving erythromycin therapy.

There have been reports of infantile hypertrophic pyloric stenosis (IHPS) occurring in infants following erythromycin therapy. In one cohort of 157 newborns who were given erythromycin for pertussis prophylaxis, seven neonates (5%) developed symptoms of non-bilious vomiting or irritability with feeding and were subsequently diagnosed as having IHPS requiring surgical pyloromyotomy. A possible dose-response effect was described with an absolute risk of IHPS of 5.1% for infants who took erythromycin for 8-14 days and 10% for infants who took erythromycin for 15-21 days.[4] Since erythromycin may be used in the treatment of conditions in infants which are associated with significant mortality or morbidity (such as pertussis or neonatal *Chlamydia trachomatis* infections), the benefit of erythromycin therapy needs to be weighed against the potential risk of developing IHPS. Parents should be informed to contact their physician if vomiting or irritability with feeding occurs.

Prolonged or repeated use of erythromycin may result in an overgrowth of nonsusceptible bacteria or fungi. If superinfection occurs, erythromycin should be discontinued and appropriate therapy instituted.

When indicated, incision and drainage or other surgical procedures should be performed in conjunction with antibiotic therapy.

Information for Patients

Patients should be counseled that antibacterial drugs including Ery-Ped should only be used to treat bacterial infections. They do not treat viral infections (e.g., the common cold). When Ery-Ped is prescribed to treat a bacterial infection, patients should be told that although it is common to feel better early in the course of therapy, the medication should be taken exactly as directed. Skipping doses or not completing the full course of therapy may (1) decrease the effectiveness of the immediate treatment and (2) increase the likelihood that bacteria will develop resistance and will not be treatable by Ery-Ped or other antibacterial drugs in the future.

Diarrhea is a common problem caused by antibiotics which usually ends when the antibiotic is discontinued. Sometimes after starting treatment with antibiotics, patients can develop watery and bloody stools (with or without stomach cramps and fever) even as late as two or more months after having taken the last dose of the antibiotic. If this occurs, patients should contact their physician as soon as possible.

Drug Interactions

Erythromycin use in patients who are receiving high doses of theophylline may be associated with an increase in serum theophylline levels and potential theophylline toxicity. In case of theophylline toxicity and/or elevated serum theoph-

ylline levels, the dose of theophylline should be reduced while the patient is receiving concomitant erythromycin therapy.

Hypotension, bradyarrhythmias, and lactic acidosis have been observed in patients receiving concurrent verapamil, belonging to the calcium channel blockers drug class.

Concomitant administration of erythromycin and digoxin has been reported to result in elevated digoxin serum levels.

There have been reports of increased anticoagulant effects when erythromycin and oral anticoagulants were used concomitantly. Increased anticoagulation effects due to interactions of erythromycin with various oral anticoagulants may be more pronounced in the elderly.

Erythromycin is a substrate and inhibitor of the 3A isoform subfamily of the cytochrome p450 enzyme system (CYP3A). Coadministration of erythromycin and a drug primarily metabolized by CYP3A may be associated with elevations in drug concentrations that could increase or prolong both the therapeutic and adverse effects of the concomitant drug. Dosage adjustments may be considered, and when possible, serum concentrations of drugs primarily metabolized by CYP3A should be monitored closely in patients concurrently receiving erythromycin.

The following are examples of some clinically significant CYP3A based drug interactions. Interactions with other drugs metabolized by the CYP3A isoform are also possible. The following CYP3A based drug interactions have been observed with erythromycin products in post-marketing experience:

Ergotamine/dihydroergotamine

Concurrent use of erythromycin and ergotamine or dihydroergotamine has been associated in some patients with acute ergot toxicity characterized by severe peripheral vasospasm and dysesthesia.

Triazolobenzodiazepines (such as triazolam and alprazolam) and Related Benzodiazepines

Erythromycin has been reported to decrease the clearance of triazolam and midazolam, and thus, may increase the pharmacologic effect of these benzodiazepines.

HMG-CoA Reductase Inhibitors

Erythromycin has been reported to increase concentrations of HMG-CoA reductase inhibitors (e.g., lovastatin and simvastatin). Rare reports of rhabdomyolysis have been reported in patients taking these drugs concomitantly.

Sildenafil (Viagra)

Erythromycin has been reported to increase the systemic exposure (AUC) of sildenafil. Reduction of sildenafil dosage should be considered. (See Viagra package insert.)

There have been spontaneous or published reports of CYP3A based interactions of erythromycin with cyclosporine, carbamazepine, tacrolimus, alfentanil, disopyramide, rifabutin, quinidine, methylprednisolone, cilostazol, vinblastine, and bromocriptine.

Concomitant administration of erythromycin with cisapride, pimozide, astemizole, or terfenadine is contraindicated. (See CONTRAINDICATIONS.)

In addition, there have been reports of interactions of erythromycin with drugs not thought to be metabolized by CYP3A, including hexobarbital, phenytoin, and valproate.

Erythromycin has been reported to significantly alter the metabolism of the nonsedating antihistamines terfenadine and astemizole when taken concomitantly. Rare cases of serious cardiovascular adverse events, including electrocardiographic QT/QT$_c$ interval prolongation, cardiac arrest, torsades de pointes, and other ventricular arrhythmias have been observed. (See CONTRAINDICATIONS.) In addition, deaths have been reported rarely with concomitant administration of terfenadine and erythromycin.

There have been post-marketing reports of drug interactions when erythromycin was co-administered with cisapride, resulting in QT prolongation, cardiac arrhythmias, ventricular tachycardia, ventricular fibrillation, and torsades de pointes most likely due to the inhibition of hepatic metabolism of cisapride by erythromycin. Fatalities have been reported. (See CONTRAINDICATIONS.)

Drug/Laboratory Test Interactions

Erythromycin interferes with the fluorometric determination of urinary catecholamines.

Carcinogenesis, Mutagenesis, Impairment of Fertility

Long-term (2-year) oral studies in rats with erythromycin ethylsuccinate and erythromycin base did not provide evidence of tumorigenicity. Mutagenicity studies have not been conducted. There was no apparent effect on male or female fertility in rats fed erythromycin (base) at levels up to 0.25% of diet.

Pregnancy

Teratogenic Effects

Pregnancy Category B

There is no evidence of teratogenicity or any other adverse effect on reproduction in female rats fed erythromycin base (up to 0.25% of diet) prior to and during mating, during gestation, and through weaning of two successive litters. There are, however, no adequate and well-controlled studies in

pregnant women. Because animal reproduction studies are not always predictive of human response, this drug should be used during pregnancy only if clearly needed.

Labor and Delivery

The effect of erythromycin on labor and delivery is unknown.

Nursing Mothers

Erythromycin is excreted in human milk. Caution should be exercised when erythromycin is administered to a nursing woman.

Pediatric Use

See INDICATIONS AND USAGE and DOSAGE AND ADMINISTRATION sections.

Geriatric Use

Elderly patients, particularly those with reduced renal or hepatic function, may be at increased risk for developing erythromycin-induced hearing loss. (See ADVERSE REACTIONS and DOSAGE AND ADMINISTRATION).

Elderly patients may be more susceptible to development of torsades de pointes arrhythmias then younger patients. (See ADVERSE REACTIONS).

Elderly patients may experience increased effects of oral anticoagulant therapy while undergoing treatment with erythromycin. (See PRECAUTIONS - Drug Interactions).

Ery-Ped 200 contains 117.5 mg (5.1 mEq) of sodium per individual dose.

Ery-Ped 400 contains 117.5 mg (5.1 mEq) of sodium per individual dose.

Based on the 200 mg/5 mL strength, at the usual recommended doses, adult patients would receive a total of 940 mg/day (40.8 mEq) of sodium. Based on the 400 mg/ 5 mL strength, at the usual recommended doses, adult patients would receive a total of 470 mg/day (20.4 mEq) of sodium. The geriatric population may respond with a blunted natriuresis to salt loading. This may be clinically important with regard to such diseases as congestive heart failure.

ERYPED® Drops contains 58.8 mg (2.6 mEq) of sodium per individual dose.

ADVERSE REACTIONS

The most frequent side effects of oral erythromycin preparations are gastrointestinal and are dose-related. They include nausea, vomiting, abdominal pain, diarrhea and anorexia. Symptoms of hepatitis, hepatic dysfunction and/or abnormal liver function test results may occur. (See WARNINGS section.)

Onset of pseudomembranous colitis symptoms may occur during or after antibacterial treatment. (See WARNINGS.)

Erythromycin has been associated with QT prolongation and ventricular arrhythmias, including ventricular tachycardia and torsades de pointes.

Allergic reactions ranging from urticaria to anaphylaxis have occurred. Skin reactions ranging from mild eruptions to erythema multiforme, Stevens-Johnson syndrome, and toxic epidermal necrolysis have been reported rarely.

There have been rare reports of pancreatitis and convulsions.

There have been isolated reports of reversible hearing loss occurring chiefly in patients with renal insufficiency and in patients receiving high doses of erythromycin.

OVERDOSAGE

In case of overdosage, erythromycin should be discontinued. Overdosage should be handled with the prompt elimination of unabsorbed drug and all other appropriate measures should be instituted.

Erythromycin is not removed by peritoneal dialysis or hemodialysis.

DOSAGE AND ADMINISTRATION

EryPed (erythromycin ethylsuccinate) oral suspensions may be administered without regard to meals.

Children

Age, weight, and severity of the infection are important factors in determining the proper dosage. In mild to moderate infections, the usual dosage of erythromycin ethylsuccinate for children is 30 to 50 mg/kg/day in equally divided doses every 6 hours. For more severe infections this dosage may be doubled. If twice-a-day dosage is desired, one-half of the total daily dose may be given every 12 hours. Doses may also be given three times daily by administering one-third of the total daily dose every 8 hours.

The following dosage schedule is suggested for mild to moderate infections:

Body Weight	Total Daily Dose
Under 10 lbs	30-50 mg/kg/day
	15-25 mg/lb/day
10 to 15 lbs	200 mg
16 to 25 lbs	400 mg
26 to 50 lbs	800 mg
51 to 100 lbs	1200 mg
over 100 lbs	1600 mg

Adults

400 mg erythromycin ethylsuccinate every 6 hours is the usual dose. Dosage may be increased up to 4 g per day according to the severity of the infection. If twice-a-day dosage is desired, one-half of the total daily dose may be given every 12 hours. Doses may also be given three times daily by administering one-third of the total daily dose every 8 hours.

For adult dosage calculation, use a ratio of 400 mg of erythromycin activity as the ethylsuccinate to 250 mg of erythromycin activity as the stearate, base or estolate.

In the treatment of streptococcal infections, a therapeutic dosage of erythromycin ethylsuccinate should be administered for at least 10 days. In continuous prophylaxis against recurrences of streptococcal infections in persons with a history of rheumatic heart disease, the usual dosage is 400 mg twice a day.

For treatment of urethritis due to _C. trachomatis_ or _U. urealyticum_

800 mg three times a day for 7 days.

For treatment of primary syphilis

Adults

48 to 64 g given in divided doses over a period of 10 to 15 days.

For intestinal amebiasis

Adults

400 mg four times daily for 10 to 14 days.

Children

30 to 50 mg/kg/day in divided doses for 10 to 14 days.

For use in pertussis

Although optimal dosage and duration have not been established, doses of erythromycin utilized in reported clinical studies were 40 to 50 mg/kg/day, given in divided doses for 5 to 14 days.

For treatment of Legionnaires' Disease

Although optimal doses have not been established, doses utilized in reported clinical data were 1.6 to 4 g daily in divided doses.

For the EryPed 200 unit dose, reconstitute with 2.9 mL of water. For the EryPed 400 unit dose, reconstitute with 2.7 mL of water.

HOW SUPPLIED

EryPed 200 (erythromycin ethylsuccinate for oral suspension, USP) is supplied in bottles of 100 mL (**NDC** 0074-6302-13), 200 mL (**NDC** 0074-6302-53), and 5 mL unit dose ABBO-PAC® packages of 100 bottles (**NDC** 0074-6302-05).

EryPed 400 (erythromycin ethylsuccinate for oral suspension, USP) is supplied in bottles of 60 mL (**NDC** 0074-6305-60), 100 mL (**NDC** 0074-6305-13), 200 mL (**NDC** 0074-6305-53), and 5 mL unit dose ABBO-PAC packages of 100 bottles (**NDC** 0074-6305-05).

EryPed Drops (erythromycin ethylsuccinate for oral suspension) is supplied in 50 mL bottles (**NDC** 0074-6303-50).

Recommended Storage

Store EryPed 200, EryPed 400, and EryPed Drops, prior to mixing, below 86°F (30°C). After reconstitution, EryPed 200, EryPed 400, and EryPed Drops must be stored at or below 77°F (25°C) and used within 35 days; refrigeration is not required.

REFERENCES

1. National Committee for Clinical Laboratory Standards, _Method for Dilution Antimicrobial Susceptibility Tests for Bacteria that Grow Aerobically_, Third Edition. Approved Standard NCCLS Document M7-A3, Vol. 13, No. 25. NCCLS, Villanova, PA, December 1993.
2. National Committee for Clinical Laboratory Standards, _Performance Standards for Antimicrobial Disk Susceptibility Tests_, Fifth Edition. Approved Standard NCCLS Document M2-A5, Vol. 13, No. 24. NCCLS, Villanova, PA, December 1993.
3. Committee on Rheumatic Fever, Endocarditis, and Kawasaki Disease of the Council on Cardiovascular Disease in the Young, the American Heart Association: Prevention of Rheumatic Fever. _Circulation._ 78(4):1082-1086, October 1988.
4. Honein, M.A., et.al.: Infantile hypertrophic pyloric stenosis after pertussis prophylaxis with erythromycin: a case review and cohort study. The Lancet 1999;354 (9196): 2101-5.

Abbott Laboratories

North Chicago, IL 60064, U.S.A.

Ref: 03-A168

Revised: November, 2008

Please check the Abbott website, www.rxabbott.com, or call (800) 633-9110 for full prescribing information for Ery-Tab® (erythromycin delayed-release tablets, USP), Erythrocin® Stearate (erythromycin stearate tablets, USP),

Erythromycin® Base Filmtab (erythromycin tablets, USP), and Erythromycin® Delayed-Release Capsules (erythromycin delayed-release capsules, USP).

E.E.S.® ℞

[ē-ē-s]

(erythromycin ethylsuccinate)

To reduce the development of drug-resistant bacteria and maintain the effectiveness of E.E.S. and other antibacterial drugs, E.E.S. should be used only to treat or prevent infections that are proven or strongly suspected to be caused by bacteria.

DESCRIPTION

Erythromycin is produced by a strain of _Saccharopolyspora erythraea_ (formerly _Streptomyces erythraeus_) and belongs to the macrolide group of antibiotics. It is basic and readily forms salts with acids. The base, the stearate salt, and the esters are poorly soluble in water. Erythromycin ethylsuccinate is an ester of erythromycin suitable for oral administration. Erythromycin ethylsuccinate is known chemically as erythromycin 2'-(ethylsuccinate). The molecular formula is $C_{43}H_{75}NO_{16}$ and the molecular weight is 862.06. The structural formula is:

E.E.S. Granules are intended for reconstitution with water. Each 5-mL teaspoonful of reconstituted cherry-flavored suspension contains erythromycin ethylsuccinate equivalent to 200 mg of erythromycin.

The pleasant tasting, fruit-flavored liquids are supplied ready for oral administration.

E.E.S. 200 Liquid: Each 5-mL teaspoonful of fruit-flavored suspension contains erythromycin ethylsuccinate equivalent to 200 mg of erythromycin.

E.E.S. 400 Liquid: Each 5-mL teaspoonful of orange-flavored suspension contains erythromycin ethylsuccinate equivalent to 400 mg of erythromycin.

Granules and ready-made suspensions are intended primarily for pediatric use but can also be used in adults.

E.E.S. 400® Filmtab® Tablets: Each tablet contains erythromycin ethylsuccinate equivalent to 400 mg of erythromycin.

The Filmtab® tablets are intended primarily for adults or older children.

Inactive Ingredients

E.E.S. 200 Liquid: FD&C Red No. 40, methylparaben, polysorbate 60, propylparaben, sodium citrate, sucrose, water, xanthan gum and natural and artificial flavors.

E.E.S. 400 Liquid: D&C Yellow No. 10, FD&C Yellow No. 6, methylparaben, polysorbate 60, propylparaben, sodium citrate, sucrose, water, xanthan gum and natural and artificial flavors.

E.E.S. Granules: Citric acid, FD&C Red No. 3, magnesium aluminum silicate, sodium carboxymethylcellulose, sodium citrate, sucrose and artificial flavor.

E.E.S. 400 Filmtab Tablets: Cellulosic polymers, confectioner's sugar (contains corn starch), corn starch, D&C Red No. 30, D&C Yellow No. 10, FD&C Red No. 40, magnesium stearate, polacrilin potassium, polyethylene glycol, propylene glycol, sodium citrate, sorbic acid, and titanium dioxide.

CLINICAL PHARMACOLOGY

Orally administered erythromycin ethylsuccinate suspensions and Filmtab tablets are readily and reliably absorbed. Comparable serum levels of erythromycin are achieved in the fasting and nonfasting states.

Erythromycin diffuses readily into most body fluids. Only low concentrations are normally achieved in the spinal fluid, but passage of the drug across the blood-brain barrier increases in meningitis. In the presence of normal hepatic function, erythromycin is concentrated in the liver and excreted in the bile; the effect of hepatic dysfunction on excretion of erythromycin by the liver into the bile is not known. Less than 5 percent of the orally administered dose of erythromycin is excreted in active form in the urine.

Erythromycin crosses the placental barrier, but fetal plasma levels are low. The drug is excreted in human milk.

Microbiology

Erythromycin acts by inhibition of protein synthesis by binding 50 S ribosomal subunits of susceptible organisms. It

does not affect nucleic acid synthesis. Antagonism has been demonstrated _in vitro_ between erythromycin and clindamycin, lincomycin, and chloramphenicol.

Many strains of _Haemophilus influenzae_ are resistant to erythromycin alone but are susceptible to erythromycin and sulfonamides used concomitantly.

Staphylococci resistant to erythromycin may emerge during a course of therapy.

Erythromycin has been shown to be active against most strains of the following microorganisms, both _in vitro_ and in clinical infections as described in the **INDICATIONS AND USAGE** section.

Gram-positive Organisms

Corynebacterium diphtheriae

Corynebacterium minutissimum

Listeria monocytogenes

Staphylococcus aureus (resistant organisms may emerge during treatment)

Streptococcus pneumoniae

Streptococcus pyogenes

Gram-negative Organisms

Bordetella pertussis

Legionella pneumophila

Neisseria gonorrhoeae

Other Microorganisms

Chlamydia trachomatis

Entamoeba histolytica

Mycoplasma pneumoniae

Treponema pallidum

Ureaplasma urealyticum

The following _in vitro_ data are available, **but their clinical significance is unknown**.

Erythromycin exhibits _in vitro_ minimal inhibitory concentrations (MIC's) of 0.5 μg/mL or less against most (≥ 90%) strains of the following microorganisms; however, the safety and effectiveness of erythromycin in treating clinical infections due to these microorganisms have not been established in adequate and well controlled clinical trials.

Gram-positive Organisms

Viridans group streptococci

Gram-negative Organisms

Moraxella catarrhalis

Susceptibility Tests

Dilution Techniques

Quantitative methods are used to determine antimicrobial minimum inhibitory concentrations (MIC's). These MIC's provide estimates of the susceptibility of bacteria to antimicrobial compounds. The MIC's should be determined using a standardized procedure. Standardized procedures are based on a dilution method[1] (broth or agar) or equivalent with standardized inoculum concentrations and standardized concentrations of erythromycin powder. The MIC values should be interpreted according to the following criteria:

MIC (μg/mL)	Interpretation
≤ 0.5	Susceptible (S)
1-4	Intermediate (I)
≥ 8	Resistant (R)

A report of "Susceptible" indicates that the pathogen is likely to be inhibited if the antimicrobial compound in the blood reaches the concentrations usually achievable. A report of "Intermediate" indicates that the result should be considered equivocal, and, if the microorganism is not fully susceptible to alternative, clinically feasible drugs, the test should be repeated. This category implies possible clinical applicability in body sites where the drug is physiologically concentrated or in situations where high dosage of drug can be used. This category also provides a buffer zone which prevents small uncontrolled technical factors from causing major discrepancies in interpretation. A report of "Resistant" indicates that the pathogen is not likely to be inhibited if the antimicrobial compound in the blood reaches the concentrations usually achievable; other therapy should be selected.

Standardized susceptibility test procedures require the use of laboratory control microorganisms to control the technical aspects of the laboratory procedures. Standard erythromycin powder should provide the following MIC values:

Information on the Abbott Pharmaceutical Products listed on these pages is from the prescribing Information in use as of June 1, 2010. For more information, please visit rxabbott.com or call 1-800-633-9110.

Microorganism	MIC (µg/mL)
S. aureus ATCC 25923	0.12-0.5
E. faecalis ATCC 29212	1-4

Diffusion Techniques

Quantitative methods that require measurement of zone diameters also provide reproducible estimates of the susceptibility of bacteria to antimicrobial compounds. One such standardized procedure[2] requires the use of standardized inoculum concentrations. This procedure uses paper disks impregnated with 15-µg erythromycin to test the susceptibility of microorganisms to erythromycin.

Reports from the laboratory providing results of the standard single-disk susceptibility test with a 15-µg erythromycin disk should be interpreted according to the following criteria:

Zone Diameter (mm)	Interpretation
≥ 23	Susceptible (S)
14-22	Intermediate (I)
≤ 13	Resistant (R)

Interpretation should be as stated above for results using dilution techniques. Interpretation involves correlation of the diameter obtained in the disk test with the MIC for erythromycin.

As with standardized dilution techniques, diffusion methods require the use of laboratory control microorganisms that are used to control the technical aspects of the laboratory procedures. For the diffusion technique, the 15-µg erythromycin disk should provide the following zone diameters in these laboratory test quality control strains:

Microorganism	Zone Diameter (mm)
S. aureus ATCC 25923	22-30

INDICATIONS AND USAGE

To reduce the development of drug-resistant bacteria and maintain the effectiveness of E.E.S. and other antibacterial drugs, E.E.S. should be used only to treat or prevent infections that are proven or strongly suspected to be caused by susceptible bacteria. When culture and susceptibility information are available, they should be considered in selecting or modifying antibacterial therapy. In the absence of such data, local epidemiology and susceptibility patterns may contribute to the empiric selection of therapy.

E.E.S. is indicated in the treatment of infections caused by susceptible strains of the designated organisms in the diseases listed below:

Upper respiratory tract infections of mild to moderate degree caused by *Streptococcus pyogenes, Streptococcus pneumoniae,* or *Haemophilus influenzae* (when used concomitantly with adequate doses of sulfonamides, since many strains of *H. influenzae* are not susceptible to the erythromycin concentrations ordinarily achieved). (See appropriate sulfonamide labeling for prescribing information.)

Lower-respiratory tract infections of mild to moderate severity caused by *Streptococcus pneumoniae* or *Streptococcus pyogenes.*

Listeriosis caused by *Listeria monocytogenes.*

Pertussis (whooping cough) caused by *Bordetella pertussis.* Erythromycin is effective in eliminating the organism from the nasopharynx of infected individuals rendering them noninfectious. Some clinical studies suggest that erythromycin may be helpful in the prophylaxis of pertussis in exposed susceptible individuals.

Respiratory tract infections due to *Mycoplasma pneumoniae.*

Skin and skin structure infections of mild to moderate severity caused by *Streptococcus pyogenes* or *Staphylococcus aureus* (resistant staphylococci may emerge during treatment).

Diphtheria: Infections due to *Corynebacterium diphtheriae,* as an adjunct to antitoxin, to prevent establishment of carriers and to eradicate the organism in carriers.

Erythrasma: In the treatment of infections due to *Corynebacterium minutissimum.*

Intestinal amebiasis caused by *Entamoeba histolytica* (oral erythromycins only). Extraenteric amebiasis requires treatment with other agents.

Acute pelvic inflammatory disease caused by *Neisseria gonorrhoeae:* As an alternative drug in treatment of acute pelvic inflammatory disease caused by *N. gonorrhoeae* in female patients with a history of sensitivity to penicillin.

Patients should have a serologic test for syphilis before receiving erythromycin as treatment of gonorrhea and a follow-up serologic test for syphilis after 3 months.

Syphilis caused by *Treponema pallidum:* Erythromycin is an alternate choice of treatment for primary syphilis in patients allergic to the penicillins. In treatment of primary syphilis, spinal fluid examinations should be done before treatment and as part of follow-up after therapy.

Erythromycins are indicated for the treatment of the following infections caused by *Chlamydia trachomatis:* conjunctivitis of the newborn, pneumonia of infancy, and urogenital infections during pregnancy. When tetracyclines are contraindicated or not tolerated, erythromycin is indicated for the treatment of uncomplicated urethral, endocervical, or rectal infections in adults due to *Chlamydia trachomatis.*

When tetracyclines are contraindicated or not tolerated, erythromycin is indicated for the treatment of nongonococcal urethritis caused by *Ureaplasma urealyticum.*

Legionnaires' Disease caused by *Legionella pneumophila.* Although no controlled clinical efficacy studies have been conducted, *in vitro* and limited preliminary clinical data suggest that erythromycin may be effective in treating Legionnaires' Disease.

Prophylaxis

Prevention of Initial Attacks of Rheumatic Fever

Penicillin is considered by the American Heart Association to be the drug of choice in the prevention of initial attacks of rheumatic fever (treatment of *Streptococcus pyogenes* infections of the upper respiratory tract, e.g., tonsillitis or pharyngitis). Erythromycin is indicated for the treatment of penicillin-allergic patients.[3] The therapeutic dose should be administered for 10 days.

Prevention of Recurrent Attacks of Rheumatic Fever

Penicillin or sulfonamides are considered by the American Heart Association to be the drugs of choice in the prevention of recurrent attacks of rheumatic fever. In patients who are allergic to penicillin and sulfonamides, oral erythromycin is recommended by the American Heart Association in the long-term prophylaxis of streptococcal pharyngitis (for the prevention of recurrent attacks of rheumatic fever).[3]

CONTRAINDICATIONS

Erythromycin is contraindicated in patients with known hypersensitivity to this antibiotic.

Erythromycin is contraindicated in patients taking terfenadine, astemizole, pimozide, or cisapride. (See **PRECAUTIONS - Drug Interactions.**)

WARNINGS

There have been reports of hepatic dysfunction, including increased liver enzymes, and hepatocellular and/or cholestatic hepatitis, with or without jaundice, occurring in patients receiving oral erythromycin products.

There have been reports suggesting that erythromycin does not reach the fetus in adequate concentration to prevent congenital syphilis. Infants born to women treated during pregnancy with oral erythromycin for early syphilis should be treated with an appropriate penicillin regimen.

Clostridium difficile associated diarrhea (CDAD) has been reported with use of nearly all antibacterial agents, including E.E.S., and may range in severity from mild diarrhea to fatal colitis. Treatment with antibacterial agents alters the normal flora of the colon leading to overgrowth of *C. difficile. C. difficile* produces toxins A and B which contribute to the development of CDAD. Hypertoxin producing strains of *C. difficile* cause increased morbidity and mortality, as these infections can be refractory to antimicrobial therapy and may require colectomy. CDAD must be considered in all patients who present with diarrhea following antibiotic use. Careful medical history is necessary since CDAD has been reported to occur over two months after the administration of antibacterial agents.

If CDAD is suspected or confirmed, ongoing antibiotic use not directed against *C. difficile* may need to be discontinued. Appropriate fluid and electrolyte management, protein supplementation, antibiotic treatment of *C. difficile,* and surgical evaluation should be instituted as clinically indicated.

Rhabdomyolysis with or without renal impairment has been reported in seriously ill patients receiving erythromycin concomitantly with lovastatin. Therefore, patients receiving concomitant lovastatin and erythromycin should be carefully monitored for creatine kinase (CK) and serum transaminase levels. (See package insert for lovastatin.)

PRECAUTIONS

General

Prescribing E.E.S. in the absence of a proven or strongly suspected bacterial infection or a prophylactic indication is unlikely to provide benefit to the patient and increases the risk of the development of drug-resistant bacteria.

Since erythromycin is principally excreted by the liver, caution should be exercised when erythromycin is administered to patients with impaired hepatic function. (See **CLINICAL PHARMACOLOGY** and **WARNINGS** sections.)

Exacerbation of symptoms of myasthenia gravis and new onset of symptoms of myasthenic syndrome have been reported in patients receiving erythromycin therapy.

There have been reports of infantile hypertrophic pyloric stenosis (IHPS) occurring in infants following erythromycin therapy. In one cohort of 157 newborns who were given erythromycin for pertussis prophylaxis, seven neonates (5%) developed symptoms of non-bilious vomiting or irritability with feeding and were subsequently diagnosed as having IHPS requiring surgical pyloromyotomy. A possible dose-response effect was described with an absolute risk of IHPS of 5.1% for infants who took erythromycin for 8-14 days and 10% for infants who took erythromycin for 15-21 days.[4] Since erythromycin may be used in the treatment of conditions in infants which are associated with significant mortality or morbidity (such as pertussis or neonatal *Chlamydia trachomatis* infections), the benefit of erythromycin therapy needs to be weighed against the potential risk of developing IHPS. Parents should be informed to contact their physician if vomiting or irritability with feeding occurs.

Prolonged or repeated use of erythromycin may result in an overgrowth of nonsusceptible bacteria or fungi. If superinfection occurs, erythromycin should be discontinued and appropriate therapy instituted.

When indicated, incision and drainage or other surgical procedures should be performed in conjunction with antibiotic therapy.

Information for Patients

Patients should be counseled that antibacterial drugs including E.E.S. should only be used to treat bacterial infections. They do not treat viral infections (e.g., the common cold). When E.E.S. is prescribed to treat a bacterial infection, patients should be told that although it is common to feel better early in the course of therapy, the medication should be taken exactly as directed. Skipping doses or not completing the full course of therapy may (1) decrease the effectiveness of the immediate treatment and (2) increase the likelihood that bacteria will develop resistance and will not be treatable by E.E.S. or other antibacterial drugs in the future.

Diarrhea is a common problem caused by antibiotics which usually ends when the antibiotic is discontinued. Sometimes after starting treatment with antibiotics, patients can develop watery and bloody stools (with or without stomach cramps and fever) even as late as two or more months after having taken the last dose of the antibiotic. If this occurs, patients should contact their physician as soon as possible.

Drug Interactions

Erythromycin use in patients who are receiving high doses of theophylline may be associated with an increase in serum theophylline levels and potential theophylline toxicity. In case of theophylline toxicity and/or elevated serum theophylline levels, the dose of theophylline should be reduced while the patient is receiving concomitant erythromycin therapy.

Hypotension, bradyarrhythmias, and lactic acidosis have been observed in patients receiving concurrent verapamil, belonging to the calcium channel blockers drug class.

Concomitant administration of erythromycin and digoxin has been reported to result in elevated digoxin serum levels.

There have been reports of increased anticoagulant effects when erythromycin and oral anticoagulants were used concomitantly. Increased anticoagulation effects due to interactions of erythromycin with various oral anticoagulants may be more pronounced in the elderly.

Erythromycin is a substrate and inhibitor of the 3A isoform subfamily of the cytochrome p450 enzyme system (CYP3A). Coadministration of erythromycin and a drug primarily metabolized by CYP3A may be associated with elevations in drug concentrations that could increase or prolong both the therapeutic and adverse effects of the concomitant drug. Dosage adjustments may be considered, and when possible, serum concentrations of drugs primarily metabolized by CYP3A should be monitored closely in patients concurrently receiving erythromycin.

The following are examples of some clinically significant CYP3A based drug interactions. Interactions with other drugs metabolized by the CYP3A isoform are also possible. The following CYP3A based drug interactions have been observed with erythromycin products in post-marketing experience:

Ergotamine/dihydroergotamine

Concurrent use of erythromycin and ergotamine or dihydroergotamine has been associated in some patients with acute ergot toxicity characterized by severe peripheral vasospasm and dysesthesia.

Triazolobenzodiazepines (such as triazolam and alprazolam) and related benzodiazepines

Erythromycin has been reported to decrease the clearance of triazolam and midazolam, and thus, may increase the pharmacologic effect of these benzodiazepines.

HMG-CoA Reductase Inhibitors
Erythromycin has been reported to increase concentrations of HMG-CoA reductase inhibitors (e.g., lovastatin and simvastatin). Rare reports of rhabdomyolysis have been reported in patients taking these drugs concomitantly.
Sildenafil (Viagra)
Erythromycin has been reported to increase the systemic exposure (AUC) of sildenafil. Reduction of sildenafil dosage should be considered. (See Viagra package insert.)
There have been spontaneous or published reports of CYP3A based interactions of erythromycin with cyclosporine, carbamazepine, tacrolimus, alfentanil, disopyramide, rifabutin, quinidine, methylprednisolone, cilostazol, vinblastine, and bromocriptine.
Concomitant administration of erythromycin with cisapride, pimozide, astemizole, or terfenadine is contraindicated. (See **CONTRAINDICATIONS**.)
In addition, there have been reports of interactions of erythromycin with drugs not thought to be metabolized by CYP3A, including hexobarbital, phenytoin, and valproate.
Erythromycin has been reported to significantly alter the metabolism of the nonsedating antihistamines terfenadine and astemizole when taken concomitantly. Rare cases of serious cardiovascular adverse events, including electrocardiographic QT/QT_c interval prolongation, cardiac arrest, torsades de pointes, and other ventricular arrhythmias have been observed. (See **CONTRAINDICATIONS**.) In addition, deaths have been reported rarely with concomitant administration of terfenadine and erythromycin.
There have been post-marketing reports of drug interactions when erythromycin is co-administered with cisapride, resulting in QT prolongation, cardiac arrhythmias, ventricular tachycardia, ventricular fibrillation, and torsades de pointes, most likely due to inhibition of hepatic metabolism of cisapride by erythromycin. Fatalities have been reported. (See **CONTRAINDICATIONS**.)

Drug/Laboratory Test Interactions
Erythromycin interferes with the fluorometric determination of urinary catecholamines.

Carcinogenesis, Mutagenesis, Impairment of Fertility
Long-term (2-year) oral studies in rats with erythromycin ethylsuccinate and erythromycin base did not provide evidence of tumorigenicity. Mutagenicity studies have not been conducted. There was no apparent effect on male or female fertility in rats fed erythromycin (base) at levels up to 0.25% of diet.

Pregnancy
Teratogenic Effects
Pregnancy Category B
There is no evidence of teratogenicity or any other adverse effect on reproduction in female rats fed erythromycin base (up to 0.25% of diet) prior to and during mating, during gestation, and through weaning of two successive litters. There are, however, no adequate and well controlled studies in pregnant women. Because animal reproduction studies are not always predictive of human response, this drug should be used during pregnancy only if clearly needed.

Labor and Delivery
The effect of erythromycin on labor and delivery is unknown.

Nursing Mothers
Erythromycin is excreted in human milk. Caution should be exercised when erythromycin is administered to a nursing woman.

Pediatric Use
See **INDICATIONS AND USAGE** and **DOSAGE AND ADMINISTRATION** sections.

Geriatric Use
Elderly patients, particularly those with reduced renal or hepatic function, may be at increased risk for developing erythromycin-induced hearing loss. (See **ADVERSE REACTIONS** and **DOSAGE AND ADMINISTRATION**).
Elderly patients may be more susceptible to the development of torsades de pointes arrhythmias than younger patients. (See **ADVERSE REACTIONS**).
Elderly patients may experience increased effects of oral anticoagulant therapy while undergoing treatment with erythromycin. (See **PRECAUTIONS - Drug Interactions**).
E.E.S.® Granules contains 25.9 mg (1.1 mEq) of sodium per individual dose.
E.E.S.® 200 Liquid and E.E.S.® 400 Liquid contain 23.7 mg/mL or 1.0 mEq/mL of sodium.
The geriatric population may respond with a blunted natriuresis to salt loading. This may be clinically important with regard to such diseases as congestive heart failure.
E.E.S. 400 Filmtab contains 47 mg (2 mEq) of sodium per tablet and 10.0 mg (0.3 mEq) of potassium per tablet.

ADVERSE REACTIONS

The most frequent side effects of oral erythromycin preparations are gastrointestinal and are dose-related. They include nausea, vomiting, abdominal pain, diarrhea and anorexia. Symptoms of hepatitis, hepatic dysfunction and/or abnormal liver function test results may occur. (See **WARNINGS**.)
Onset of pseudomembranous colitis symptoms may occur during or after antibiotic treatment. (See **WARNINGS**.)
Erythromycin has been associated with QT prolongation and ventricular arrhythmias, including ventricular tachycardia and torsades de pointes.
Allergic reactions ranging from urticaria to anaphylaxis have occurred. Skin reactions ranging from mild eruptions to erythema multiforme, Stevens-Johnson syndrome, and toxic epidermal necrolysis have been reported rarely.
There have been rare reports of pancreatitis and convulsions.
There have been isolated reports of reversible hearing loss occurring chiefly in patients with renal insufficiency and in patients receiving high doses of erythromycin.

OVERDOSAGE

In case of overdosage, erythromycin should be discontinued. Overdosage should be handled with the prompt elimination of unabsorbed drug and all other appropriate measures should be instituted.
Erythromycin is not removed by peritoneal dialysis or hemodialysis.

DOSAGE AND ADMINISTRATION

Erythromycin ethylsuccinate suspensions and Filmtab tablets may be administered without regard to meals.

Children
Age, weight, and severity of the infection are important factors in determining the proper dosage. In mild to moderate infections the usual dosage of erythromycin ethylsuccinate for children is 30 to 50 mg/kg/day in equally divided doses every 6 hours. For more severe infections this dosage may be doubled. If twice-a-day dosage is desired, one-half of the total daily dose may be given every 12 hours. Doses may also be given three times daily by administering one-third of the total daily dose every 8 hours.
The following dosage schedule is suggested for mild to moderate infections:

Body Weight	Total Daily Dose
Under 10 lbs	30-50 mg/kg/day 15-25 mg/kg/q 12 h
10 to 15 lbs	200 mg
16 to 25 lbs	400 mg
26 to 50 lbs	800 mg
51 to 100 lbs	1200 mg
over 100 lbs	1600 mg

Adults
400 mg erythromycin ethylsuccinate every 6 hours is the usual dose. Dosage may be increased up to 4 g per day according to the severity of the infection. If twice-a-day dosage is desired, one-half of the total daily dose may be given every 12 hours. Doses may also be given three times daily by administering one-third of the total daily dose every 8 hours.
For adult dosage calculation, use a ratio of 400 mg of erythromycin activity as the ethylsuccinate to 250 mg of erythromycin activity as the stearate, base or estolate.
In the treatment of streptococcal infections, a therapeutic dosage of erythromycin ethylsuccinate should be administered for at least 10 days. In continuous prophylaxis against recurrences of streptococcal infections in persons with a history of rheumatic heart disease, the usual dosage is 400 mg twice a day.

For Treatment of Urethritis Due to *C. trachomatis* or *U. urealyticum*
800 mg three times a day for 7 days.

For Treatment of Primary Syphilis
Adults: 48 to 64 g given in divided doses over a period of 10 to 15 days.

For Intestinal Amebiasis
Adults
400 mg four times daily for 10 to 14 days.
Children
30 to 50 mg/kg/day in divided doses for 10 to 14 days.

For Use in Pertussis
Although optimal dosage and duration have not been established, doses of erythromycin utilized in reported clinical studies were 40 to 50 mg/kg/day, given in divided doses for 5 to 14 days.

For Treatment of Legionnaires' Disease
Although optimal doses have not been established, doses utilized in reported clinical data were those recommended above (1.6 to 4 g daily in divided doses.)

HOW SUPPLIED

E.E.S. 200 LIQUID (erythromycin ethylsuccinate oral suspension, USP) is supplied in 1 pint bottles (**NDC** 0074-6306-16) and in 100-mL bottles (**NDC** 0074-6306-13).
E.E.S. 400® LIQUID (erythromycin ethylsuccinate oral suspension, USP) is supplied in 1 pint bottles (**NDC** 0074-6373-16) and in 100-mL bottles (**NDC** 0074-6373-13).
Both liquid products require refrigeration to preserve taste until dispensed. Refrigeration by patient is not required if used within 14 days.
E.E.S. GRANULES (erythromycin ethylsuccinate for oral suspension, USP) is supplied in 100-mL (**NDC** 0074-6369-02) and 200-mL (**NDC** 0074-6369-10) size bottles.
E.E.S. 400 Filmtab tablets (erythromycin ethylsuccinate tablets, USP) 400 mg, are supplied as pink tablets imprinted with the **Abbott logo**, and two letter Abbo-Code designation, EE, in bottles of 100 (**NDC** 0074-5729-13), 500 (**NDC** 0074-5729-53) and 1000 (**NDC** 0074-5729-19) and in ABBO-PAC unit dose strip packages of 100 (**NDC** 0074-5729-11).

Recommended storage
Store tablets below 86°F (30°C).
Store granules, prior to mixing, below 86°F (30°C). After mixing, refrigerate and use within 10 days.

REFERENCES

1. National Committee for Clinical Laboratory Standards, *Methods for Dilution Antimicrobial Susceptibility Tests for Bacteria that Grow Aerobically*, Third Edition. Approved Standard NCCLS Document M7-A3, Vol. 13, No. 25. NCCLS, Villanova, PA, December 1993.
2. National Committee for Clinical Laboratory Standards, *Performance Standards for Antimicrobial Disk Susceptibility Tests*, Fifth Edition. Approved Standard NCCLS Document M2-A5, Vol. 13, No. 24. NCCLS, Villanova, PA, December 1993.
3. Committee on Rheumatic Fever, Endocarditis, and Kawasaki Disease of the Council on Cardiovascular Disease in the Young, the American Heart Association: Prevention of Rheumatic Fever. *Circulation*. 78(4):1082-1086, October 1988.
4. Honein, M.A., et. al.: Infantile hypertrophic pyloric stenosis after pertussis prophylaxis with erythromycin: a case review and cohort study. The Lancet 1999;354 (9196): 2101-5.

Filmtab—Film-sealed tablets, Abbott.
Abbott Laboratories
North Chicago, IL 60064, U.S.A.
Ref. 03-A288-Revised June, 2009
Shown in Product Identification Guide, page 303

GENGRAF® CAPSULES ℞
[jen-graf]
(cyclosporine capsules USP [MODIFIED])

WARNING
Only physicians experienced in the management of systemic immunosuppressive therapy for the indicated disease should prescribe Gengraf (cyclosporine capsules, USP [**MODIFIED**]). At doses used in solid organ transplantation, only physicians experienced in immunosuppressive therapy and management of organ transplant recipients should prescribe Gengraf. Patients receiving the drug should be managed in facilities equipped and staffed with adequate laboratory and supportive medical resources. The physician responsible for maintenance therapy should have complete information requisite for the follow-up of the patient.
Gengraf, a systemic immunosuppressant, may increase the susceptibility to infection and the development of neoplasia. In kidney, liver, and heart transplant patients Gengraf may be administered with other immunosuppressive agents. Increased susceptibility to infection and the possible development of lymphoma and other neoplasms may result from the increase in the degree of immunosuppression in transplant patients.
Gengraf (cyclosporine capsules, USP [**MODIFIED**]) has increased bioavailability in comparison to Sandimmune®* (cyclosporine capsules, USP). Gengraf and Sandimmune* are not bioequivalent and cannot be used interchangeably without physician supervision. For a given trough concentration, cyclosporine exposure will be greater with Gengraf than with Sandimmune.* If a patient who is receiving exceptionally high doses of Sandimmune* is converted to Gengraf, particular cau-

Information on the Abbott Pharmaceutical Products listed on these pages is from the prescribing information in use as of June 1, 2010. For more information, please visit rxabbott.com or call 1-800-633-9110.

tion should be exercised. Cyclosporine blood concentrations should be monitored in transplant and rheumatoid arthritis patients taking Gengraf to avoid toxicity due to high concentrations. Dose adjustments should be made in transplant patients to minimize possible organ rejection due to low concentrations. Comparison of blood concentrations in the published literature with blood concentrations obtained using current assays must be done with detailed knowledge of the assay methods employed.

For Psoriasis Patients (see also BOXED WARNINGS above)

Psoriasis patients previously treated with PUVA and to a lesser extent, methotrexate or other immunosuppressive agents, UVB, coal tar, or radiation therapy, are at an increased risk of developing skin malignancies when taking Gengraf (cyclosporine capsules, USP [**MODIFIED**]).

Cyclosporine, the active ingredient in Gengraf, in recommended dosages, can cause systemic hypertension and nephrotoxicity. The risk increases with increasing dose and duration of cyclosporine therapy. Renal dysfunction, including structural kidney damage, is a potential consequence of cyclosporine, and therefore, renal function must be monitored during therapy.

DESCRIPTION

Gengraf (cyclosporine capsules, USP [**MODIFIED**]) is a modified oral formulation of cyclosporine that forms an aqueous dispersion in an aqueous environment.

Cyclosporine, the active principle in Gengraf, is a cyclic polypeptide immunosuppressant agent consisting of 11 amino acids. It is produced as a metabolite by the fungus species *Aphanocladium album*.

Chemically, cyclosporine is designated as [R-[R*,R*-(E)]]-cyclic-(L-alanyl-D-alanyl-N-methyl-L-leucyl-N-methyl-L-leucyl-N-methyl-L-valyl-3-hydroxy-N,4-dimethyl-L-2-amino-6-octenoyl-L-α-amino-butyryl-N-methylglycyl-N-methyl-L-leucyl-L-valyl-N-methyl-L-leucyl).

Gengraf Capsules (cyclosporine capsules, USP [**MODIFIED**]) are available in 25 mg and 100 mg strengths.

Each 25 mg capsule contains
cyclosporine, 25 mg, alcohol, USP, absolute, 12.8% v/v (10.1% wt/vol.).

Each 100 mg capsule contains
cyclosporine, 100 mg, alcohol, USP, absolute, 12.8% v/v (10.1% wt/vol.).

Inactive Ingredients
FD&C Blue No. 2, gelatin NF, polyethylene glycol NF, polyoxyl 35 castor oil NF, polysorbate 80 NF, propylene glycol USP, sorbitan monooleate NF, titanium dioxide.

The chemical structure for cyclosporine USP is:

$C_{62}H_{111}N_{11}O_{12}$ Mol. Wt. 1202.61

CLINICAL PHARMACOLOGY

Cyclosporine is a potent immunosuppressive agent that in animals prolongs survival of allogeneic transplants involving skin, kidney, liver, heart, pancreas, bone marrow, small intestine, and lung. Cyclosporine has been demonstrated to suppress some humoral immunity and to a greater extent, cell-mediated immune reactions such as allograft rejection, delayed hypersensitivity, experimental allergic encephalomyelitis, Freund's adjuvant arthritis, and graft vs. host disease in many animal species for a variety of organs.

The effectiveness of cyclosporine results from specific and reversible inhibition of immunocompetent lymphocytes in the G_0- and G_1-phase of the cell cycle. T-lymphocytes are preferentially inhibited. The T-helper cell is the main target, although the T-suppressor cell may also be suppressed. Cyclosporine also inhibits lymphokine production and release including interleukin-2.

No effects on phagocytic function (changes in enzyme secretions, chemotactic migration of granulocytes, macrophage migration, carbon clearance *in vivo*) have been detected in animals. Cyclosporine does not cause bone marrow suppression in animal models or man.

Pharmacokinetics
The immunosuppressive activity of cyclosporine is primarily due to parent drug. Following oral administration, absorption of cyclosporine is incomplete. The extent of absorption

Pharmacokinetic Parameters (mean ± SD)

Patient Population	Dose/day[1] (mg/d)	Dose/weight (mg/kg/d)	AUC[2] (ng·hr/mL)	C_{max} (ng/mL)	Trough[3] (ng/mL)	CL/F (mL/min)	CL/F (mL/min/kg)
De novo renal transplant[4] Week 4 (N = 37)	597 ± 174	7.95 ± 2.81	8772 ± 2089	1802 ± 428	361 ± 129	593 ± 204	7.8 ± 2.9
Stable renal transplant[4] (N = 55)	344 ± 122	4.10 ± 1.58	6035 ± 2194	1333 ± 469	251 ± 116	492 ± 140	5.9 ± 2.1
De novo liver transplant[5] Week 4 (N = 18)	458 ± 190	6.89 ± 3.68	7187 ± 2816	1555 ± 740	268 ± 101	577 ± 309	8.6 ± 5.7
De novo rheumatoid arthritis[6] (N = 23)	182 ± 55.6	2.37 ± 0.36	2641 ± 877	728 ± 263	96.4 ± 37.7	613 ± 196	8.3 ± 2.8
De novo psoriasis[6] Week 4 (N = 18)	189 ± 69.8	2.48 ± 0.65	2324 ± 1048	655 ± 186	74.9 ± 46.7	723 ± 186	10.2 ± 3.9

[1] Total daily dose was divided into two doses administered every 12 hours.
[2] AUC was measured over one dosing interval.
[3] Trough concentration was measured just prior to the morning cyclosporine (**MODIFIED**) dose, approximately 12 hours after the previous dose.
[4] Assay: TDx specific monoclonal fluorescence polarization immunoassay.
[5] Assay: Cyclo-trac specific monoclonal radioimmunoassay.
[6] Assay: INCSTAR specific monoclonal radioimmunoassay.

of cyclosporine is dependent on the individual patient, the patient population, and the formulation. Elimination of cyclosporine is primarily biliary with only 6% of the dose (parent drug and metabolites) excreted in urine. The disposition of cyclosporine from blood is generally biphasic, with a terminal half-life of approximately 8.4 hours (range 5 to 18 hours). Following intravenous administration, the blood clearance of cyclosporine (assay: HPLC) is approximately 5 to 7 mL/min/kg in adult recipients of renal or liver allografts. Blood cyclosporine clearance appears to be slightly slower in cardiac transplant patients.

The Gengraf Capsules (cyclosporine capsules, USP [**MODIFIED**]) and Gengraf Oral Solution (cyclosporine oral solution, USP [**MODIFIED**]) are bioequivalent.

The relationship between administered dose and exposure (area under the concentration versus time curve, AUC) is linear within the therapeutic dose range. The intersubject variability (total, % CV) of cyclosporine exposure (AUC) when cyclosporine (**MODIFIED**) or Sandimmune® is administered ranges from approximately 20% to 50% in renal transplant patients. This intersubject variability contributes to the need for individualization of the dosing regimen for optimal therapy (see **DOSAGE AND ADMINISTRATION**). Intrasubject variability of AUC in renal transplant recipients (% CV) was 9%-21% for cyclosporine (**MODIFIED**) and 19%-26% for Sandimmune®. In the same studies, intrasubject variability of trough concentrations (% CV) was 17%-30% for cyclosporine (**MODIFIED**) and 16%-38% for Sandimmune®.

Absorption
Cyclosporine (**MODIFIED**) has increased bioavailability compared to Sandimmune®. The absolute bioavailability of cyclosporine administered as Sandimmune® is dependent on the patient population, estimated to be less than 10% in liver transplant patients and as great as 89% in some renal transplant patients. The absolute bioavailability of cyclosporine administered as cyclosporine (**MODIFIED**) has not been determined in adults. In studies of renal transplant, rheumatoid arthritis and psoriasis patients, the mean cyclosporine AUC was approximately 20% to 50% greater and the peak blood cyclosporine concentration (C_{max}) was approximately 40% to 106% greater following administration of cyclosporine (**MODIFIED**) compared to following administration of Sandimmune®. The dose normalized AUC in *de novo* liver transplant patients administered cyclosporine (**MODIFIED**) 28 days after transplantation was 50% greater and C_{max} was 90% greater than in those patients administered Sandimmune®. AUC and C_{max} are also increased (cyclosporine [**MODIFIED**] relative to Sandimmune®) in heart transplant patients, but data are very limited. Although the AUC and C_{max} values are higher on cyclosporine (**MODIFIED**) relative to Sandimmune®, the pre-dose trough concentrations (dose-normalized) are similar for the two formulations.

Following oral administration of cyclosporine (**MODIFIED**), the time to peak blood cyclosporine concentrations (T_{max}) ranged from 1.5 to 2.0 hours. The administration of food with cyclosporine (**MODIFIED**) decreases the cyclosporine AUC and C_{max}. A high fat meal (669 kcal, 45 grams fat) consumed within one-half hour before cyclosporine (**MODIFIED**)

administration decreased the AUC by 13% and C_{max} by 33%. The effects of a low fat meal (667 kcal, 15 grams fat) were similar.

The effect of T-tube diversion of bile on the absorption of cyclosporine from cyclosporine (**MODIFIED**) was investigated in eleven *de novo* liver transplant patients. When the patients were administered cyclosporine (**MODIFIED**) with and without T-tube diversion of bile, very little difference in absorption was observed, as measured by the change in maximal cyclosporine blood concentrations from pre-dose values with the T-tube closed relative to when it was open: 6.9 ± 41% (range -55% to 68%).

[See table above]

Distribution
Cyclosporine is distributed largely outside the blood volume. The steady state volume of distribution during intravenous dosing has been reported as 3-5 L/kg in solid organ transplant recipients. In blood, the distribution is concentration dependent. Approximately 33%-47% is in plasma, 4%-9% in lymphocytes, 5%-12% in granulocytes, and 41%-58% in erythrocytes. At high concentrations, the binding capacity of leukocytes and erythrocytes becomes saturated. In plasma, approximately 90% is bound to proteins, primarily lipoproteins. Cyclosporine is excreted in human milk (see **PRECAUTIONS - Nursing Mothers**).

Metabolism
Cyclosporine is extensively metabolized by the cytochrome P-450 III-A enzyme system in the liver, and to a lesser degree in the gastrointestinal tract, and the kidney. The metabolism of cyclosporine can be altered by the coadministration of a variety of agents (see **PRECAUTIONS - Drug Interactions**). At least 25 metabolites have been identified from human bile, feces, blood, and urine. The biological activity of the metabolites and their contributions to toxicity are considerably less than those of the parent compound. The major metabolites (M1, M9, and M4N) result from oxidation at the 1-beta, 9-gamma, and 4-N-demethylated positions, respectively. At steady state following the oral administration of Sandimmune®, the mean AUCs for blood concentrations of M1, M9 and M4N are about 70%, 21%, and 7.5% of the AUC for blood cyclosporine concentrations, respectively. Based on blood concentration data from stable renal transplant patients (13 patients administered cyclosporine [**MODIFIED**] and Sandimmune® in a crossover study), and bile concentration data from *de novo* liver transplant patients (4 administered cyclosporine [**MODIFIED**], 3 administered Sandimmune®), the percentage of dose present as M1, M9, and M4N metabolites is similar when either cyclosporine (**MODIFIED**) or Sandimmune® is administered.

Excretion
Only 0.1% of a cyclosporine dose is excreted unchanged in the urine. Elimination is primarily biliary with only 6% of the dose (parent drug and metabolites) excreted in the urine. Neither dialysis nor renal failure alter cyclosporine clearance significantly.

Drug Interactions
(See **PRECAUTIONS - Drug Interactions**). When diclofenac or methotrexate was coadministered with cyclosporine in rheumatoid arthritis patients, the AUC of diclofenac and methotrexate, each was significantly in-

creased (see **PRECAUTIONS - Drug Interactions**). No clinically significant pharmacokinetic interactions occurred between cyclosporine and aspirin, ketoprofen, piroxicam, or indomethacin.

Special Population

Pediatric Population

Pharmacokinetic data from pediatric patients administered cyclosporine (**MODIFIED**) or Sandimmune® are very limited. In 15 renal transplant patients aged 3-16 years, cyclosporine whole blood clearance after IV administration of Sandimmune® was 10.6 ± 3.7 mL/min/kg (assay: Cyclo-trac specific RIA). In a study of 7 renal transplant patients aged 2-16, the cyclosporine clearance ranged from 9.8 to 15.5 mL/min/kg. In 9 liver transplant patients aged 0.6 to 5.6 years, clearance was 9.3 ± 5.4 mL/min/kg (assay: HPLC).

In the pediatric population, cyclosporine (**MODIFIED**) also demonstrates an increased bioavailability as compared to Sandimmune®. In 7 liver *de novo* transplant patients aged 1.4 to 10 years, the absolute bioavailability of cyclosporine (**MODIFIED**) was 43% (range 30% to 68%) and for Sandimmune® in the same individuals absolute bioavailability was 28% (range 17% to 42%).

[See table above]

Geriatric Population

Comparison of single dose data from both normal elderly volunteers (N = 18, mean age 69 years) and elderly rheumatoid arthritis patients (N = 16, mean age 68 years) to single dose data in young adult volunteers (N = 16, mean age 26 years) showed no significant difference in the pharmacokinetic parameters.

CLINICAL TRIALS

Rheumatoid Arthritis

The effectiveness of Sandimmune® and cyclosporine (**MODIFIED**) in the treatment of severe rheumatoid arthritis was evaluated in five clinical studies involving a total of 728 cyclosporine treated patients and 273 placebo treated patients.

A summary of the results is presented for the "responder" rates per treatment group, with a responder being defined as a patient having *completed* the trial with a 20% improvement in the tender and the swollen joint count and a 20% improvement in 2 of 4 of investigator global, patient global, disability, and erythrocyte sedimentation rates (ESR) for the Studies 651 and 652 and 3 of 5 of investigator global, patient global, disability, visual analog pain, and ESR for Studies 2008, 654, and 302.

Study 651 enrolled 264 patients with active rheumatoid arthritis with at least 20 involved joints, who had failed at least one major RA drug, using a 3:3:2 randomization to one of the following three groups: (1) cyclosporine dosed at 2.5 to 5 mg/kg/day, (2) methotrexate at 7.5 to 15 mg/week, or (3) placebo. Treatment duration was 24 weeks. The mean cyclosporine dose at the last visit was 3.1 mg/kg/day. See Graph below.

Study 652 enrolled 250 patients with active RA with > 6 active painful or tender joints who had failed at least one major RA drug. Patients were randomized using a 3:3:2 randomization to 1 of 3 treatment arms: (1) 1.5 to 5 mg/kg/day of cyclosporine, (2) 2.5 to 5 mg/kg/day of cyclosporine, and (3) placebo. Treatment duration was 16 weeks. The mean cyclosporine dose for group 2 at the last visit was 2.92 mg/kg/day. See Graph below.

Study 2008 enrolled 144 patients with active RA and > 6 active joints who had unsuccessful treatment courses of aspirin and gold or Penicillamine. Patients were randomized to one of two treatment groups: (1) cyclosporine 2.5 to 5 mg/kg/day with adjustments after the first month to achieve a target trough level and (2) placebo. Treatment duration was 24 weeks. The mean cyclosporine dose at the last visit was 3.63 mg/kg/day. See Graph below.

Study 654 enrolled 148 patients who remained with active joint counts of 6 or more despite treatment with maximally tolerated methotrexate doses for at least three months. Patients continued to take their current dose of methotrexate and were randomized to receive, in addition, one of the following medications: (1) cyclosporine 2.5 mg/kg/day with dose increases of 0.5 mg/kg/day at Weeks 2 and 4 if there was no evidence of toxicity and further increases of 0.5 mg/kg/day at Weeks 8 and 16 if a < 30% decrease in active joint count occurred without any significant toxicity; dose decreases could be made at any time for toxicity or (2) placebo. Treatment duration was 24 weeks. The mean cyclosporine dose at the last visit was 2.8 mg/kg/day (range: 1.3 to 4.1). See Graph below.

Study 302 enrolled 299 patients with severe active RA, 99% of whom were unresponsive or intolerant to at least one prior major RA drug. Patients were randomized to 1 of 2 treatment groups (1) cyclosporine (**MODIFIED**) and (2) Sandimmune® both of which were started at 2.5 mg/kg/day and increased after 4 weeks for inefficacy in increments of 0.5 mg/kg/day to a maximum of 5 mg/kg/day and decreased at any time for toxicity. Treatment duration was 24 weeks. The mean cyclosporine dose at the last visit was 2.91 mg/kg/day (range: 0.72 to 5.17) for cyclosporine (**MODIFIED**) and 3.27 mg/kg/day (range: 0.73 to 5.68) for Sandimmune®. See Graph below.

Pediatric Pharmacokinetic Parameters (mean ± SD)

Patient Population	Dose/day (mg/d)	Dose/weight (mg/kg/d)	AUC[1] (ng·hr/mL)	C_{max} (ng/mL)	CL/F (mL/min)	CL/F (mL/min/kg)
Stable liver transplant[2]						
Age 2-8, Dosed TID (N = 9)	101 ± 25	5.95 ± 1.32	2163 ± 801	629 ± 219	285 ± 94	16.6 ± 4.3
Age 8-15, Dosed BID (N = 8)	188 ± 55	4.96 ± 2.09	4272 ± 1462	975 ± 281	378 ± 80	10.2 ± 4.0
Stable liver transplant[3]						
Age 3, Dosed BID (N = 1)	120	8.33	5832	1050	171	11.9
Age 8-15, Dosed BID (N = 5)	158 ± 55	5.51 ± 1.91	4452 ± 2475	1013 ± 635	328 ± 121	11.0 ± 1.9
Stable renal transplant[3]						
Age 7-15, Dosed BID (N = 5)	328 ± 83	7.37 ± 4.11	6922 ± 1988	1827 ± 487	418 ± 143	8.7 ± 2.9

[1] AUC was measured over one dosing interval.
[2] Assay: Cyclo-trac specific monoclonal radioimmunoassay.
[3] Assay: TDx specific monoclonal fluorescence polarization immunoassay.

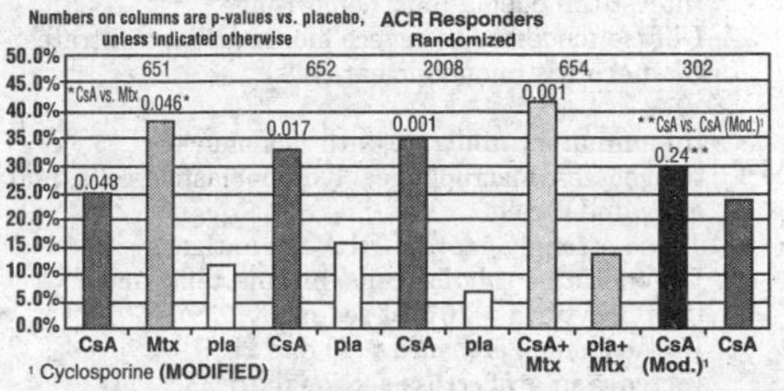

[1] Cyclosporine (**MODIFIED**)

INDICATIONS AND USAGE

Kidney, Liver and Heart Transplantation

Gengraf (cyclosporine capsules, USP [**MODIFIED**]) is indicated for the prophylaxis of organ rejection in kidney, liver, and heart allogeneic transplants. Cyclosporine (**MODIFIED**) has been used in combination with azathioprine and corticosteroids.

Rheumatoid Arthritis

Gengraf (cyclosporine capsules, USP [**MODIFIED**]) is indicated for the treatment of patients with severe active, rheumatoid arthritis where the disease has not adequately responded to methotrexate. Gengraf can be used in combination with methotrexate in rheumatoid arthritis patients who do not respond adequately to methotrexate alone.

Psoriasis

Gengraf (cyclosporine capsules, USP [**MODIFIED**]) is indicated for the treatment of *adult, nonimmunocompromised* patients with severe (i.e., extensive and/or disabling), recalcitrant, plaque psoriasis who have failed to respond to at least one systemic therapy (e.g., PUVA, retinoids, or methotrexate) or in patients for whom other systemic therapies are contraindicated, or cannot be tolerated.

While rebound rarely occurs, most patients will experience relapse with Gengraf as with other therapies upon cessation of treatment.

CONTRAINDICATIONS

General

Gengraf (cyclosporine capsules, USP [**MODIFIED**]) is contraindicated in patients with a hypersensitivity to cyclosporine or to any of the ingredients of the formulation.

Rheumatoid Arthritis

Rheumatoid arthritis patients with abnormal renal function, uncontrolled hypertension or malignancies should not receive Gengraf (cyclosporine capsules, USP [**MODIFIED**]).

Psoriasis

Psoriasis patients who are treated with Gengraf (cyclosporine capsules, USP [**MODIFIED**]) should not receive concomitant PUVA or UVB therapy, methotrexate or other immunosuppressive agents, coal tar or radiation therapy. Psoriasis patients with abnormal renal function, uncontrolled hypertension, or malignancies should not receive Gengraf.

WARNINGS

(See also **BOXED WARNINGS**).

All Patients

Cyclosporine, the active ingredient of Gengraf (cyclosporine capsules, USP [**MODIFIED**]), can cause nephrotoxicity and hepatotoxicity. The risk increases with increasing doses of cyclosporine. Renal dysfunction including structural kidney damage is a potential consequence of Gengraf and therefore renal function must be monitored during therapy. **Care should be taken in using cyclosporine with nephrotoxic drugs (see PRECAUTIONS).**

Patients receiving Gengraf require frequent monitoring of serum creatinine (see Special Monitoring under **DOSAGE AND ADMINISTRATION**). Elderly patients should be monitored with particular care, since decreases in renal function also occur with age. If patients are not properly monitored and doses are not properly adjusted, cyclosporine therapy can be associated with the occurrence of structural kidney damage and persistent renal dysfunction.

An increase in serum creatinine and BUN may occur during Gengraf therapy and reflect a reduction in the glomerular filtration rate. Impaired renal function at any time requires close monitoring, and frequent dosage adjustment may be indicated. The frequency and severity of serum creatinine elevations increase with dose and duration of cyclosporine therapy. These elevations are likely to become more pronounced without dose reduction or discontinuation.

Because Gengraf (cyclosporine capsules, USP [MODIFIED]) is not bioequivalent to Sandimmune (Cyclosporine Capsules), conversion from Gengraf to Sandimmune using a 1:1 ratio (mg/kg/day) may result in lower cyclosporine blood concentrations. Conversion from Gengraf to Sandimmune should be made with increased monitoring to avoid the potential of underdosing.

Kidney, Liver, and Heart Transplant

Cyclosporine, the active ingredient of Gengraf (cyclosporine capsules, USP [**MODIFIED**]), can cause nephrotoxicity and hepatotoxicity when used in high doses. It is not unusual for serum creatinine and BUN levels to be elevated during cyclosporine therapy. These elevations in renal transplant patients do not necessarily indicate rejection, and each patient must be fully evaluated before dosage adjustment is initiated.

Based on the historical Sandimmune® experience with oral solution, nephrotoxicity associated with cyclosporine had been noted in 25% of cases of renal transplantation, 38% of cases of cardiac transplantation, and 37% of cases of liver transplantation. Mild nephrotoxicity was generally noted 2-3 months after renal transplant and consisted of an arrest in the fall of the pre-operative elevations of BUN and creatinine at a range of 35-45 mg/dL and 2.0-2.5 mg/dL respectively. These elevations were often responsive to cyclosporine dosage reduction.

More overt nephrotoxicity was seen early after transplantation and was characterized by a rapidly rising BUN and creatinine. Since these events are similar to renal rejection episodes, care must be taken to differentiate between them. This form of nephrotoxicity is usually responsive to cyclosporine dosage reduction.

Although specific diagnostic criteria which reliably differentiate renal graft rejection from drug toxicity have not been found, a number of parameters have been significantly associated with one or the other. It should be noted however, that up to 20% of patients may have simultaneous nephrotoxicity and rejection.

[See table at top of next page]

A form of a cyclosporine-associated nephropathy is characterized by serial deterioration in renal function and morphologic changes in the kidneys. From 5% to 15% of transplant recipients who have received cyclosporine will fail to show a reduction in rising serum creatinine despite a decrease or discontinuation of cyclosporine therapy. Renal biopsies from these patients will demonstrate one or several of the following alterations: tubular vacuolization, tubular microcalcifications, peritubular capillary congestion, arteriolopathy, and a striped form of interstitial fibrosis with tubular atrophy. Though none of these morphologic changes is entirely specific, a diagnosis of cyclosporine-associated structural nephrotoxicity requires evidence of these findings.

When considering the development of cyclosporine-associated nephropathy, it is noteworthy that several authors have reported an association between the appearance of interstitial fibrosis and higher cumulative doses or persistently high circulating trough levels of cyclosporine. This is particularly true during the first 6 post-transplant months when the dosage tends to be highest and when, in

Information on the Abbott Pharmaceutical Products listed on these pages is from the prescribing information in use as of June 1, 2010. For more information, please visit rxabbott.com or call 1-800-633-9110.

Nephrotoxicity vs. Rejection

Parameter	Nephrotoxicity	Rejection
History	Donor > 50 years old or hypotensive Prolonged kidney preservation Prolonged anastomosis time Concomitant nephrotoxic drugs	Anti-donor immune response Retransplant patient
Clinical	Often > 6 weeks postop[b] Prolonged initial nonfunction (acute tubular necrosis)	Often < 4 weeks postop[b] Fever > 37.5°C Weight gain > 0.5 kg Graft swelling and tenderness Decrease in daily urine volume > 500 mL (or 50%)
Laboratory	CyA serum trough level > 200 ng/mL Gradual rise in Cr (< 0.15 mg/dL/day)[a] Cr plateau < 25% above baseline BUN/Cr ≥ 20	CyA serum trough level < 150 ng/mL Rapid rise in Cr (> 0.3 mg/dL/day)[a] Cr > 25% above baseline BUN/Cr < 20
Biopsy	Arteriolopathy (medial hypertrophy[a], hyalinosis, nodular deposits, intimal thickening, endothelial vacuolization, progressive scarring)	Endovasculitis[c] (proliferation[a], intimal arteritis[b], necrosis, sclerosis)
	Tubular atrophy, isometric vacuolization, isolated calcifications	Tubulitis with RBC[b] and WBC[b] casts, some irregular vacuolization
	Minimal edema	Interstitial edema[c] and hemorrhage[b]
	Mild focal infiltrates[c]	Diffuse moderate to severe mononuclear infiltrates[d]
	Diffuse interstitial fibrosis, often striped form	Glomerulitis (mononuclear cells)[c]
Aspiration Cytology	CyA deposits in tubular and endothelial cells Fine isometric vacuolization of tubular cells	Inflammatory infiltrate with mononuclear phagocytes, macrophages, lymphoblastoid cells, and activated T-cells These strongly express HLA-DR antigens
Urine Cytology	Tubular cells with vacuolization and granularization	Degenerative tubular cells, plasma cells, and lymphocyturia > 20% of sediment
Manometry	Intracapsular pressure < 40 mm Hg[b]	Intracapsular pressure > 40 mm Hg[b]
Ultrasonography	Unchanged graft cross sectional area	Increase in graft cross sectional area AP diameter ≥ Transverse diameter
Magnetic Resonance Imagery	Normal appearance	Loss of distinct corticomedullary junction, swelling image intensity of parachyma approaching that of psoas, loss of hilar fat
Radionuclide Scan	Normal or generally decreased perfusion Decrease in tubular function (^{131}I-hippuran) > decrease in perfusion (^{99m}Tc DTPA)	Patchy arterial flow Decrease in perfusion > decrease in tubular function Increased uptake of Indium 111 labeled platelets or Tc-99m in colloid
Therapy	Responds to decreased cyclosporine	Responds to increased steroids or antilymphocyte globulin

[a] $p < 0.05$,
[b] $p < 0.01$,
[c] $p < 0.001$,
[d] $p < 0.0001$

kidney recipients, the organ appears to be most vulnerable to the toxic effects of cyclosporine. Among other contributing factors to the development of interstitial fibrosis in these patients are prolonged perfusion time, warm ischemia time, as well as episodes of acute toxicity, and acute and chronic rejection. The reversibility of interstitial fibrosis and its correlation to renal function have not yet been determined. Reversibility of arteriolopathy has been reported after stopping cyclosporine or lowering the dosage.

Impaired renal function at any time requires close monitoring, and frequent dosage adjustment may be indicated.

In the event of severe and unremitting rejection, when rescue therapy with pulse steroids and monoclonal antibodies fail to reverse the rejection episode, it may be preferable to switch to alternative immunosuppressive therapy rather than increase the Gengraf dose to excessive levels.

Occasionally patients have developed a syndrome of thrombocytopenia and microangiopathic hemolytic anemia which may result in graft failure. The vasculopathy can occur in the absence of rejection and is accompanied by avid platelet consumption within the graft as demonstrated by Indium 111 labeled platelet studies. Neither the pathogenesis nor the management of this syndrome is clear. Though resolution has occurred after reduction or discontinuation of cyclosporine and 1) administration of streptokinase and heparin or 2) plasmapheresis, this appears to depend upon early detection with Indium 111 labeled platelet scans (see **ADVERSE REACTIONS**).

Significant hyperkalemia (sometimes associated with hyperchloremic metabolic acidosis) and hyperuricemia have been seen occasionally in individual patients.

Hepatotoxicity associated with cyclosporine use had been noted in 4% of cases of renal transplantation, 7% of cases of cardiac transplantation, and 4% of cases of liver transplantation. This was usually noted during the first month of therapy when high doses of cyclosporine were used and consisted of elevations of hepatic enzymes and bilirubin. The chemistry elevations usually decreased with a reduction in dosage.

As in patients receiving other immunosuppressants, those patients receiving cyclosporine are at increased risk for development of lymphomas and other malignancies, particularly those of the skin. Patients taking cyclosporine should be warned to avoid excess ultraviolet light exposure. The increased risk appears related to the intensity and duration of immunosuppression rather than to the use of specific agents. Because of the danger of oversuppression of the immune system resulting in increased risk of infection or malignancy, a treatment regimen containing multiple immunosuppressants should be used with caution. Some malignancies may be fatal. Transplant patients receiving cyclosporine are at increased risk for serious infection with fatal outcome.

Latent Viral Infections

Immunosuppressed patients are at increased risk for opportunistic infections, including activation of latent viral infections. These include BK virus-associated nephropathy which has been observed in patients receiving immunosuppressants, including Gengraf. This infection is associated with serious outcomes, including deteriorating renal function and renal graft loss. Patient monitoring may help detect patients at risk for BK virus-associated nephropathy. Reduction in immunosuppression should be considered for patients who develop evidence of BK virus-associated nephropathy.

There have been reports of convulsions in adult and pediatric patients receiving cyclosporine, particularly in combination with high dose methylprednisolone.

Encephalopathy has been described both in postmarketing reports and in the literature. Manifestations include impaired consciousness, convulsions, visual disturbances (including blindness), loss of motor function, movement disorders and psychiatric disturbances. In many cases, changes in the white matter have been detected using imaging techniques and pathologic specimens. Predisposing factors such as hypertension, hypomagnesemia, hypocholesterolemia, high-dose corticosteroids, high cyclosporine blood concentrations, and graft-versus-host disease have been noted in many but not all of the reported cases. The changes in most cases have been reversible upon discontinuation of cyclosporine, and in some cases improvement was noted after reduction of dose. It appears that patients receiving liver transplant are more susceptible to encephalopathy than those receiving kidney transplant. Another rare manifestation of cyclosporine-induced neurotoxicity, occurring in transplant patients more frequently than in other indications, is optic disc edema including papilloedema, with possible visual impairment, secondary to benign intracranial hypertension.

Care should be taken in using cyclosporine with nephrotoxic drugs (see **PRECAUTIONS**).

Rheumatoid Arthritis

Cyclosporine nephropathy was detected in renal biopsies of six out of 60 (10%) rheumatoid arthritis patients after the average treatment duration of 19 months. Only one patient, out of these 6 patients, was treated with a dose ≤ 4 mg/kg/day. Serum creatinine improved in all but one patient after discontinuation of cyclosporine. The "maximal creatinine increase" appears to be a factor in predicting cyclosporine nephropathy.

There is a potential, as with other immunosuppressive agents, for an increase in the occurrence of malignant lymphomas with cyclosporine. It is not clear whether the risk with cyclosporine is greater than that in rheumatoid arthritis patients or in rheumatoid arthritis patients on cytotoxic treatment for this indication. Five cases of lymphoma were detected: four in a survey of approximately 2,300 patients treated with cyclosporine for rheumatoid arthritis, and another case of lymphoma was reported in a clinical trial. Although other tumors (12 skin cancers, 24 solid tumors of diverse types, and 1 multiple myeloma) were also reported in this survey, epidemiologic analyses did not support a relationship to cyclosporine other than for malignant lymphomas.

Patients should be thoroughly evaluated before and during Gengraf (cyclosporine capsules, USP [**MODIFIED**]) treatment for the development of malignancies. Moreover, use of Gengraf therapy with other immunosuppressive agents may induce an excessive immunosuppression which is known to increase the risk of malignancy.

Psoriasis

(See also **BOXED WARNINGS** for Psoriasis)

Since cyclosporine is a potent immunosuppressive agent with a number of potentially serious side effects, the risks and benefits of using Gengraf (cyclosporine capsules, USP [**MODIFIED**]) should be considered before treatment of patients with psoriasis. Cyclosporine, the active ingredient in Gengraf, can cause nephrotoxicity and hypertension (see **PRECAUTIONS**) and the risk increases with increasing dose and duration of therapy. Patients who may be at increased risk such as those with abnormal renal function, uncontrolled hypertension or malignancies, should not receive Gengraf.

Renal dysfunction is a potential consequence of Gengraf, therefore renal function must be monitored during therapy.

Patients receiving Gengraf require frequent monitoring of serum creatinine (see Special Monitoring under **DOSAGE AND ADMINISTRATION**). Elderly patients should be monitored with particular care, since decreases in renal function also occur with age. If patients are not properly monitored and doses are not properly adjusted, cyclosporine therapy can cause structural kidney damage and persistent renal dysfunction.

An increase in serum creatinine and BUN may occur during Gengraf therapy and reflects a reduction in the glomerular filtration rate.

Kidney biopsies from 86 psoriasis patients treated for a mean duration of 23 months with 1.2 to 7.6 mg/kg/day of cyclosporine showed evidence of cyclosporine nephropathy in 18/86 (21%) of the patients. The pathology consisted of renal tubular atrophy and interstitial fibrosis. On repeat biopsy of 13 of these patients maintained on various dosages of cyclosporine for a mean of 2 additional years, the number with cyclosporine induced nephropathy rose to 26/86 (30%). The majority of patients (19/26) were on a dose of ≥ 5 mg/kg/day (the highest recommended dose is 4 mg/kg/day). The patients were also on cyclosporine for greater than 15 months (18/26) and/or had a clinically significant increase in serum creatinine for greater than 1 month (21/26). Creatinine levels returned to normal range in 7 of 11 patients in whom cyclosporine therapy was discontinued.

There is an increased risk for the development of skin and lymphoproliferative malignancies in cyclosporine-treated psoriasis patients. The relative risk of malignancies is comparable to that observed in psoriasis patients treated with other immunosuppressive agents.

Tumors were reported in 32 (2.2%) of 1439 psoriasis patients treated with cyclosporine worldwide from clinical trials. Additional tumors have been reported in 7 patients in cyclosporine postmarketing experience. Skin malignancies were reported in 16 (1.1%) of these patients; all but 2 of them had previously received PUVA therapy. Methotrexate was received by 7 patients. UVB and coal tar had been used by 2 and 3 patients, respectively. Seven patients had either a history of previous skin cancer or a potentially predisposing lesion was present prior to cyclosporine exposure. Of the

16 patients with skin cancer, 11 patients had 18 squamous cell carcinomas and 7 patients had 10 basal cell carcinomas. There were two lymphoproliferative malignancies; one case of non-Hodgkin's lymphoma which required chemotherapy, and one case of mycosis fungoides which regressed spontaneously upon discontinuation of cyclosporine. There were four cases of benign lymphocytic infiltration: 3 regressed spontaneously upon discontinuation of cyclosporine, while the fourth regressed despite continuation of the drug. The remainder of the malignancies, 13 cases (0.9%), involved various organs.

Patients should not be treated concurrently with cyclosporine and PUVA or UVB, other radiation therapy, or other immunosuppressive agents, because of the possibility of excessive immunosuppression and the subsequent risk of malignancies (see CONTRAINDICATIONS). Patients should also be warned to protect themselves appropriately when in the sun, and to avoid excessive sun exposure. Patients should be thoroughly evaluated before and during treatment for the presence of malignancies remembering that malignant lesions may be hidden by psoriatic plaques. Skin lesions not typical of psoriasis should be biopsied before starting treatment. Patients should be treated with Gengraf (cyclosporine capsules, USP [**MODIFIED**]) only after complete resolution of suspicious lesions, and only if there are no other treatment options (see **Special Monitoring for Psoriasis Patients**).

PRECAUTIONS

General

Hypertension

Cyclosporine is the active ingredient of Gengraf (cyclosporine capsules, USP [**MODIFIED**]). Hypertension is a common side effect of cyclosporine therapy which may persist (see **ADVERSE REACTIONS** and **DOSAGE AND ADMINISTRATION** for monitoring recommendations). Mild or moderate hypertension is encountered more frequently than severe hypertension and the incidence decreases over time. In recipients of kidney, liver, and heart allografts treated with cyclosporine, antihypertensive therapy may be required (see **Special Monitoring of Rheumatoid Arthritis and Psoriasis Patients**). However, since cyclosporine may cause hyperkalemia, potassium-sparing diuretics should not be used. While calcium antagonists can be effective agents in treating cyclosporine-associated hypertension, they can interfere with cyclosporine metabolism (see **PRECAUTIONS - Drug Interactions**).

Vaccination

During treatment with cyclosporine, vaccination may be less effective; and the use of live attenuated vaccines should be avoided.

Special Monitoring of Rheumatoid Arthritis Patients

Before initiating treatment, a careful physical examination, including blood pressure measurements (on at least two occasions) and two creatinine levels to estimate baseline should be performed. Blood pressure and serum creatinine should be evaluated every 2 weeks during the initial 3 months and then monthly if the patient is stable. It is advisable to monitor serum creatinine and blood pressure always after an increase of the dose of nonsteroidal anti-inflammatory drugs and after initiation of new nonsteroidal anti-inflammatory drug therapy during Gengraf (cyclosporine capsules, USP [**MODIFIED**]) treatment. If coadministered with methotrexate, CBC and liver function tests are recommended to be monitored monthly (see also **PRECAUTIONS - General, Hypertension**).

In patients who are receiving cyclosporine, the dose of Gengraf should be decreased by 25%-50% if hypertension occurs. If hypertension persists, the dose of Gengraf should be further reduced or blood pressure should be controlled with antihypertensive agents. In most cases, blood pressure has returned to baseline when cyclosporine was discontinued.

In placebo-controlled trials of rheumatoid arthritis patients, systolic hypertension (defined as an occurrence of two systolic blood pressure readings > 140 mmHg) and diastolic hypertension (defined as two diastolic blood pressure readings > 90 mmHg) occurred in 33% and 19% of patients treated with cyclosporine, respectively. The corresponding placebo rates were 22% and 8%.

Special Monitoring for Psoriasis Patients

Before initiating treatment, a careful dermatological and physical examination, including blood pressure measurements (on at least two occasions) should be performed. Since Gengraf (cyclosporine capsules, USP [**MODIFIED**]) is an immunosuppressive agent, patients should be evaluated for the presence of occult infection on their first physical examination and for the presence of tumors initially, and throughout treatment with Gengraf. Skin lesions not typical for psoriasis should be biopsied before starting Gengraf. Patients with malignant or premalignant changes of the skin should be treated with Gengraf only after appropriate treatment of such lesions and if no other treatment option exists.

Antibiotics	**Antineoplastics**	**Anti-inflammatory Drugs**	**Gastrointestinal Agents**
ciprofloxacin	melphalan	azapropazon	cimetidine
gentamicin		colchicine	ranitidine
tobramycin	**Antifungals**	diclofenac	
vancomycin	amphotericin B	naproxen	**Immunosuppressives**
trimethoprim with sulfamethoxazole	ketoconazole	sulindac	tacrolimus
			Other Drugs
			fibric acid derivatives (e.g., bezafibrate, fenofibrate)
			methotrexate

Calcium Channel Blockers	**Antifungals**	**Antibiotics**	**Glucocorticoids**	**Other Drugs**
diltiazem	fluconazole	azithromycin	methylprednisolone	allopurinol
nicardipine	itraconazole	clarithromycin		amiodarone
verapamil	ketoconazole	erythromycin		bromocriptine
	voriconazole	quinupristin/ dalfopristin		colchicine
				danazol
				imatinib
				metoclopramide
				nefazodone
				oral contraceptives

Baseline laboratories should include serum creatinine (on two occasions), BUN, CBC, serum magnesium, potassium, uric acid, and lipids.

The risk of cyclosporine nephropathy is reduced when the starting dose is low (2.5 mg/kg/day), the maximum dose does not exceed 4 mg/kg/day, serum creatinine is monitored regularly while cyclosporine is administered, and the dose of Gengraf is decreased when the rise in creatinine is greater than or equal to 25% above the patients pretreatment level. The increase in creatinine is generally reversible upon timely decrease of the dose of Gengraf or its discontinuation.

Serum creatinine and BUN should be evaluated every 2 weeks during the initial 3 months of therapy and then monthly if the patient is stable. If the serum creatinine is greater than or equal to 25% above the patient's pretreatment level, serum creatinine should be repeated within two weeks. If the change in serum creatinine remains greater than or equal to 25% above baseline, Gengraf should be reduced by 25%-50%. If at **any time** the serum creatinine increases by greater than or equal to 50% above pretreatment level, Gengraf should be reduced by 25%-50%. Gengraf should be discontinued if reversibility (within 25% of baseline) of serum creatinine is not achievable after two dosage modifications. It is advisable to monitor serum creatinine after an increase of the dose of nonsteroidal anti-inflammatory drug and after initiation of new nonsteroidal anti-inflammatory therapy during Gengraf treatment.

Blood pressure should be evaluated every 2 weeks during the initial 3 months of therapy and then monthly if the patient is stable, or more frequently when dosage adjustments are made. Patients without a history of previous hypertension before initiation of treatment with Gengraf, should have the drug reduced by 25%-50% if found to have sustained hypertension. If the patient continues to be hypertensive despite multiple reductions of Gengraf, then Gengraf should be discontinued. For patients with treated hypertension, before the initiation of Gengraf therapy, their medication should be adjusted to control hypertension while on Gengraf. Gengraf should be discontinued if a change in hypertension management is not effective or tolerable.

CBC, uric acid, potassium, lipids, and magnesium should also be monitored every 2 weeks for the first 3 months of therapy, and then monthly if the patient is stable or more frequently when dosage adjustments are made. Gengraf dosage should be reduced by 25%-50% for any abnormality of clinical concern.

In controlled trials of cyclosporine in psoriasis patients, cyclosporine blood concentrations did not correlate well with either improvement or with side effects such as renal dysfunction.

Information for Patients

Patients should be advised that any change of cyclosporine formulation should be made cautiously and only under physician supervision because it may result in the need for a change in dosage.

Patients should be informed of the necessity of repeated laboratory tests while they are receiving cyclosporine. Patients should be advised of the potential risks during pregnancy and informed of the increased risk of neoplasia. Patients should also be informed of the risk of hypertension and renal dysfunction.

Patients should be advised that during treatment with cyclosporine, vaccination may be less effective and the use of live attenuated vaccines should be avoided.

Patients should be advised to take Gengraf on a consistent schedule with regard to time of day and relation to meals. Grapefruit and grapefruit juice affect metabolism, increasing blood concentration of cyclosporine, thus should be avoided.

Laboratory Tests

In all patients treated with cyclosporine, renal and liver functions should be assessed repeatedly by measurement of serum creatinine, BUN, serum bilirubin, and liver enzymes. Serum lipids, magnesium, and potassium should also be monitored. Cyclosporine blood concentrations should be routinely monitored in transplant patients (see **DOSAGE AND ADMINISTRATION - Blood Concentration Monitoring in Transplant Patients**), and periodically monitored in rheumatoid arthritis patients.

Drug Interactions

All of the individual drugs cited below are well substantiated to interact with cyclosporine. In addition, concomitant non-steroidal anti-inflammatory drugs, particularly in the setting of dehydration, may potentiate renal dysfunction.

Drugs That May Potentiate Renal Dysfunction

[See first table above]

Drugs That Alter Cyclosporine Concentrations

Cyclosporine is extensively metabolized by CYP 3A isoenzymes, in particular CYP3A4, and is a substrate of the multidrug efflux transporter P-glycoprotein. Various agents are known to either increase or decrease plasma and whole blood of cyclosporine concentrations usually by inhibition or induction of CYP3A4 or P-glycoprotein transporter or both. Compounds that decrease cyclosporine absorption such as orlistat should be avoided. Monitoring of circulating cyclosporine concentrations and appropriate Gengraf (cyclosporine capsules, USP [**MODIFIED**]) dosage adjustment are essential when these drugs are used concomitantly (see **DOSAGE AND ADMINISTRATION - Blood Concentration Monitoring**).

Drugs That Increase Cyclosporine Concentrations

[See second table above]

The HIV protease inhibitors (e.g., indinavir, nelfinavir, ritonavir, and saquinavir) are known to inhibit cytochrome P-450 III-A and thus could potentially increase the concentrations of cyclosporine, however no formal studies of the interaction are available. Care should be exercised when these drugs are administered concomitantly.

Grapefruit and grapefruit juice affect metabolism, increasing blood concentrations of cyclosporine, thus should be avoided.

Drugs/Dietary Supplements That Decrease Cyclosporine Concentrations

Antibiotics	**Anticonvulsants**	**Other Drugs**
nafcillin	carbamazepine	bosentan
rifampin	oxcarbazepine	octreotide
	phenobarbital	orlistat
	phenytoin	sulfinpyrazone
		St. John's Wort
		terbinafine
		ticlopidine

There have been reports of a serious drug interaction between cyclosporine and the herbal dietary supplement, St.

Information on the Abbott Pharmaceutical Products listed on these pages is from the prescribing information in use as of June 1, 2010. For more information, please visit rxabbott.com or call 1-800-633-9110.

John's Wort. **This interaction has been reported to produce a marked reduction in the blood concentrations of cyclosporine, resulting in subtherapeutic levels, rejection of transplanted organs, and graft loss.**

Rifabutin is known to increase the metabolism of other drugs metabolized by the cytochrome P-450 system. The interaction between rifabutin and cyclosporine has not been studied. Care should be exercised when these two drugs are administered concomitantly.

Nonsteroidal Anti-inflammatory Drug (NSAID) Interactions
Clinical status and serum creatinine should be closely monitored when cyclosporine is used with nonsteroidal anti-inflammatory agents in rheumatoid arthritis patients (see **WARNINGS**).

Pharmacodynamic interactions have been reported to occur between cyclosporine and both naproxen and sulindac, in that concomitant use is associated with additive decreases in renal function, as determined by ^{99m}Tc-diethylenetriaminepentaacetic acid (DTPA) and (p-aminohippuric acid) PAH clearances. Although concomitant administration of diclofenac does not affect blood levels of cyclosporine, it has been associated with approximate doubling of diclofenac blood levels and occasional reports of reversible decreases in renal function. Consequently, the dose of diclofenac should be in the lower end of the therapeutic range.

Methotrexate Interaction
Preliminary data indicate that when methotrexate and cyclosporine were coadministered to rheumatoid arthritis patients (N = 20), methotrexate concentrations (AUCs) were increased approximately 30% and the concentrations (AUCs) of its metabolite,7-hydroxy methotrexate, were decreased by approximately 80%. The clinical significance of this interaction is not known. Cyclosporine concentrations do not appear to have been altered (N = 6).

Other Drug Interactions
Cyclosporine is an inhibitor of CYP3A4 and of the multidrug efflux transporter P-glycoprotein and may increase plasma concentrations of comedications that are substrates of CYP3A4 or P-glycoprotein or both.

Cyclosporine may reduce the clearance of digoxin, colchicine, prednisolone, and HMG-CoA reductase inhibitors (statins) and etoposide. Severe digitalis toxicity has been seen within days of starting cyclosporine in several patients taking digoxin. There are also reports on the potential of cyclosporine to enhance the toxic effects of colchicine such as myopathy and neuropathy, especially in patients with renal dysfunction. If digoxin or colchicine are used concurrently with cyclosporine, close clinical observation is required in order to enable early detection of toxic manifestations of digoxin or colchicine, followed by reduction of dosage or its withdrawal.

Literature and postmarketing cases of myotoxicity, including muscle pain and weakness, myositis, and rhabdomyolysis, have been reported with concomitant administration of cyclosporine with lovastatin, simvastatin, atorvastatin, pravastatin, and, rarely, fluvastatin. When concurrently administered with cyclosporine, the dosage of these statins should be reduced according to label recommendations. Statin therapy needs to be temporarily withheld or discontinued in patients with signs and symptoms of myopathy or those with risk factors predisposing to severe renal injury, including renal failure, secondary to rhabdomyolysis.

Cyclosporine may increase the plasma concentrations of repaglinide and thereby increase the risk of hypoglycemia. In 12 healthy male subjects who received two doses of 100 mg cyclosporine capsule orally 12 hours apart with a single dose of 0.25 mg repaglinide tablet (one half of a 0.5 mg tablet) orally 13 hours after the cyclosporine initial dose, the repaglinide mean C_{max} and AUC were increased 1.8 fold (range: 0.6-3.7 fold) and 2.4 fold (range 1.2-5.3 fold), respectively. Close monitoring of blood glucose level is advisable for a patient taking cyclosporine and repaglinide concomitantly.

Cyclosporine should not be used with potassium sparing diuretics because hyperkalemia can occur. Caution is also required when cyclosporine is coadministered with potassium sparing drugs (e.g. angiotensin converting enzyme inhibitors, angiotensin II receptor antagonists), potassium containing drugs as well as in patients on a potassium rich diet. Control of potassium levels in these situations is advisable.

Elevations in serum creatinine were observed in studies using sirolimus in combination with full-dose cyclosporine. This effect is often reversible with cyclosporine dose reduction. Simultaneous coadministration of cyclosporine significantly increases blood levels of sirolimus. To minimize increases in sirolimus blood concentrations, it is recommended that sirolimus be given 4 hours after cyclosporine administration.

During treatment with cyclosporine, vaccination may be less effective. The use of live vaccines should be avoided. Frequent gingival hyperplasia with nifedipine, and convulsions with high dose methylprednisolone have been reported.

Psoriasis patients receiving other immunosuppressive agents or radiation therapy (including PUVA and UVB) should not receive concurrent cyclosporine because of the possibility of excessive immunosuppression.

For additional information on Cyclosporine Drug Interactions please contact Abbott Laboratories Medical Information Department at 1-800-633-9110.

Carcinogenesis, Mutagenesis, Impairment of Fertility
Carcinogenicity studies were carried out in male and female rats and mice. In the 78-week mouse study, evidence of a statistically significant trend was found for lymphocytic lymphomas in females, and the incidence of hepatocellular carcinomas in mid-dose males significantly exceeded the control value. In the 24-month rat study, pancreatic islet cell adenomas significantly exceeded the control rate in the low dose level. Doses used in the mouse and rat studies were 0.01 to 0.16 times the clinical maintenance dose (6 mg/kg). The hepatocellular carcinomas and pancreatic islet cell adenomas were not dose related. Published reports indicate the co-treatment of hairless mice with UV irradiation and cyclosporine or other immunosuppressive agents shorten the time to skin tumor formation compared to UV irradiation alone.

Cyclosporine was not mutagenic in appropriate test systems. Cyclosporine has not been found to be mutagenic/genotoxic in the Ames Test, the V79-HGPRT Test, the micronucleus test in mice and Chinese hamsters, the chromosome-aberration tests in Chinese hamster bone-marrow, the mouse dominant lethal assay, and the DNA-repair test in sperm from treated mice. A recent study analyzing sister chromatid exchange (SCE) induction by cyclosporine using human lymphocytes in vitro gave indication of a positive effect (i.e., induction of SCE), at high concentrations in this system. In two published research studies, rabbits exposed to cyclosporine in utero (10 mg/kg/day subcutaneously) demonstrated reduced numbers of nephrons, renal hypertrophy, systemic hypertension and progressive renal insufficiency up to 35 weeks of age. Pregnant rats which received 12 mg/kg/day of cyclosporine intravenously (twice the recommended human intravenous dose) had fetuses with an increase incidence of ventricular septal defect. These findings have not been demonstrated in other species and their relevance for humans is unknown.

No impairment in fertility was demonstrated in studies in male and female rats.

Widely distributed papillomatosis of the skin was observed after chronic treatment of dogs with cyclosporine at 9 times the human initial psoriasis treatment dose of 2.5 mg/kg, where doses are expressed on a body surface area basis. This papillomatosis showed a spontaneous regression upon discontinuation of cyclosporine.

An increased incidence of malignancy is a recognized complication of immunosuppression in recipients of organ transplants and patients with rheumatoid arthritis and psoriasis. The most common forms of neoplasms are non-Hodgkin's lymphoma and carcinomas of the skin. The risk of malignancies in cyclosporine recipients is higher than in the normal, healthy population but similar to that in patients receiving other immunosuppressive therapies. Reduction or discontinuance of immunosuppression may cause the lesions to regress.

In psoriasis patients on cyclosporine, development of malignancies, especially those of the skin has been reported (see **WARNINGS**). Skin lesions not typical for psoriasis should be biopsied before starting cyclosporine treatment. Patients with malignant or premalignant changes of the skin should be treated with cyclosporine only after appropriate treatment of such lesions and if no other treatment option exists.

Pregnancy
Pregnancy Category C
Animal studies have shown reproductive toxicity in rats and rabbits. Cyclosporine gave no evidence of mutagenic or teratogenic effects in the standard test systems with oral application (rats up to 17 mg/kg and rabbits up to 30 mg/kg per day orally). Only at dose levels toxic to dams, were adverse effects seen in reproduction studies in rats. Cyclosporine has been shown to be embryo- and fetotoxic in rats and rabbits following oral administration at maternally toxic doses. Fetal toxicity was noted in rats at 0.8 and rabbits at 5.4 times the transplant doses in humans of 6 mg/kg, where dose corrections are based on body surface area. Cyclosporine was embryo- and fetotoxic as indicated by increased pre- and postnatal mortality and reduced fetal weight together with related skeletal retardation.

There are no adequate and well-controlled studies in pregnant women and, therefore, Gengraf (cyclosporine capsules, USP [**MODIFIED**]) should not be used during pregnancy unless the potential benefit to the mother justifies the potential risk to the fetus.

In pregnant transplant recipients who are being treated with immunosuppressants the risk of premature births is increased. The following data represent the reported outcomes of 116 pregnancies in women receiving cyclosporine during pregnancy, 90% of whom were transplant patients,

and most of whom received cyclosporine throughout the entire gestational period. The only consistent patterns of abnormality were premature birth (gestational period of 28 to 36 weeks) and low birth weight for gestational age. Sixteen fetal losses occurred. Most of the pregnancies (85 of 100) were complicated by disorders; including, pre-eclampsia, eclampsia, premature labor, abruptio placentae, oligohydramnios, Rh incompatibility and fetoplacental dysfunction. Pre-term delivery occurred in 47%. Seven malformations were reported in 5 viable infants and in 2 cases of fetal loss. Twenty-eight percent of the infants were small for gestational age. Neonatal complications occurred in 27%. Therefore, the risks and benefits of using Gengraf during pregnancy should be carefully weighed.

A limited number of observations in children exposed to cyclosporine in utero is available, up to an age of approximately 7 years. Renal function and blood pressure in these children were normal.

Because of the possible disruption of maternal-fetal interaction, the risk/benefit ratio of using Gengraf in psoriasis patients during pregnancy should carefully be weighed with serious consideration for discontinuation of Gengraf.

Nursing Mothers
Cyclosporine passes into breast milk. Mothers receiving treatment with Gengraf should not breast feed.

Pediatric Use
Although no adequate and well-controlled studies have been completed in children, transplant recipients as young as one year of age have received cyclosporine (**MODIFIED**) with no unusual adverse effects. The safety and efficacy of cyclosporine (**MODIFIED**) treatment in children with juvenile rheumatoid arthritis or psoriasis below the age of 18 have not been established.

Geriatric Use
In rheumatoid arthritis clinical trials with cyclosporine, 17.5% of patients were age 65 or older. These patients were more likely to develop systolic hypertension on therapy, and more likely to show serum creatinine rises ≥ 50% above the baseline after 3-4 months of therapy.

Clinical studies of cyclosporine oral solution (modified) in transplant and psoriasis patients did not include a sufficient number of subjects aged 65 and over to determine whether they respond differently from younger subjects. Other reported clinical experiences have not identified differences in response between the elderly and younger patients. In general, dose selection for an elderly patient should be cautious, usually starting at the low end of the dosing range, reflecting the greater frequency of decreased hepatic, renal, or cardiac function, and of concomitant disease or other drug therapy.

ADVERSE REACTIONS
Kidney, Liver, and Heart Transplantation
The principal adverse reactions of cyclosporine therapy are renal dysfunction, tremor, hirsutism, hypertension, and gum hyperplasia.

Hypertension, which is usually mild to moderate, may occur in approximately 50% of patients following renal transplantation and in most cardiac transplant patients.

Glomerular capillary thrombosis has been found in patients treated with cyclosporine and may progress to graft failure. The pathologic changes resembled those seen in the hemolytic-uremic syndrome and include thrombosis of the renal microvasculature, with platelet-fibrin thrombi occluding glomerular capillaries and afferent arterioles, microangiopathic hemolytic anemia, thrombocytopenia, and decreased renal function. Similar findings have been observed when other immunosuppressives have been employed post-transplantation.

Hypomagnesemia has been reported in some, but not all, patients exhibiting convulsions while on cyclosporine therapy. Although magnesium-depletion studies in normal subjects suggest that hypomagnesemia is associated with neurologic disorders, multiple factors, including hypertension, high dose methylprednisolone, hypocholesterolemia, and nephrotoxicity associated with high plasma concentrations of cyclosporine appear to be related to the neurological manifestations of cyclosporine toxicity.

In controlled studies, the nature, severity and incidence of the adverse events that were observed in 493 transplanted patients treated with cyclosporine (**MODIFIED**) were comparable with those observed in 208 transplanted patients who received Sandimmune® (cyclosporine capsules) in these same studies when the dosage of the two drugs was adjusted to achieve the same cyclosporine blood trough concentrations.

Based on the historical experience with Sandimmune®, the following reactions occurred in 3% or greater of 892 patients involved in clinical trials of kidney, heart, and liver transplants.
[See table at top of next page]

Among 705 kidney transplant patients treated with cyclosporine oral solution in clinical trials, the reason for treatment discontinuation was renal toxicity in 5.4%, infection in 0.9%, lack of efficacy in 1.4%, acute tubular necrosis in 1.0%, lymphoproliferative disorders in 0.3%, hypertension in 0.3%, and other reasons in 0.7% of the patients.

The following reactions occurred in 2% or less of Sandimmune®-treated patients: allergic reactions, anemia, anorexia, confusion, conjunctivitis, edema, fever, brittle fingernails, gastritis, hearing loss, hiccups, hyperglycemia, muscle pain, peptic ulcer, thrombocytopenia, tinnitus.

The following reactions occurred rarely: anxiety, chest pain, constipation, depression, hair breaking, hematuria, joint pain, lethargy, mouth sores, myocardial infarction, night sweats, pancreatitis, pruritus, swallowing difficulty, tingling, upper GI bleeding, visual disturbance, weakness, weight loss.

Patients receiving immunosuppressive therapies, including cyclosporine and cyclosporine-containing regimens, are at increased risk of infections (viral, bacterial, fungal, parasitic). Both generalized and localized infections can occur. Pre-existing infections may also be aggravated. Fatal outcomes have been reported (see **WARNINGS**).

[See table above]

Postmarketing Experience, Kidney, Liver and Heart Transplantation

BK virus associated nephropathy has been observed in patients receiving immunosuppressants, including Gengraf. This infection is associated with serious outcomes, including deteriorating renal function and renal graft loss (see **WARNINGS, Kidney, Liver and Heart Transplant**).

Rheumatoid Arthritis

The principal adverse reactions associated with the use of cyclosporine in rheumatoid arthritis are renal dysfunction (see **WARNINGS**), hypertension (see **PRECAUTIONS**), headache, gastrointestinal disturbances and hirsutism/hypertrichosis.

In rheumatoid arthritis patients treated in clinical trials within the recommended dose range, cyclosporine therapy was discontinued in 5.3% of the patients because of hypertension and in 7% of the patients because of increased creatinine. These changes are usually reversible with timely dose decrease or drug discontinuation. The frequency and severity of serum creatinine elevations increase with dose and duration of cyclosporine therapy. These elevations are likely to become more pronounced without dose reduction or discontinuation.

The following adverse events occurred in controlled clinical trials

[See table at top of next page]

In addition, the following adverse events have been reported in 1% to < 3% of the rheumatoid arthritis patients in the cyclosporine treatment group in controlled clinical trials.

Autonomic Nervous System
dry mouth, increased sweating;
Body as a Whole
allergy, asthenia, hot flushes, malaise, overdose, procedure NOS*, tumor NOS*, weight decrease, weight increase;
Cardiovascular
abnormal heart sounds, cardiac failure, myocardial infarction, peripheral ischemia;
Central and Peripheral Nervous System
hypoesthesia, neuropathy, vertigo;
Endocrine
goiter;
Gastrointestinal
constipation, dysphagia, enanthema, eructation, esophagitis, gastric ulcer, gastritis, gastroenteritis, gingival bleeding, glossitis, peptic ulcer, salivary gland enlargement, tongue disorder, tooth disorder;
Infection
abscess, bacterial infection, cellulitis, folliculitis, fungal infection, herpes simplex, herpes zoster, renal abscess, moniliasis, tonsillitis, viral infection;
Hematologic
anemia, epistaxis, leukopenia, lymphadenopathy;
Liver and Biliary System
bilirubinemia;
Metabolic and Nutritional
diabetes mellitus, hyperkalemia, hyperuricemia, hypoglycemia;
Musculoskeletal System
arthralgia, bone fracture, bursitis, joint dislocation, myalgia, stiffness, synovial cyst, tendon disorder;
Neoplasms
breast fibroadenosis, carcinoma;
Psychiatric
anxiety, confusion, decreased libido, emotional lability, impaired concentration, increased libido, nervousness, paroniria, somnolence;
Reproductive (Female)
breast pain, uterine hemorrhage;
Respiratory System
abnormal chest sounds, bronchospasm;
Skin and Appendages
abnormal pigmentation, angioedema, dermatitis, dry skin, eczema, nail disorder, pruritus, skin disorder, urticaria;

Special Senses
abnormal vision, cataract, conjunctivitis, deafness, eye pain, taste perversion, tinnitus, vestibular disorder;
Urinary System
abnormal urine, hematuria, increased BUN, micturition urgency, nocturia, polyuria, pyelonephritis, urinary incontinence.
* NOS = Not Otherwise Specified.

Psoriasis

The principal adverse reactions associated with the use of cyclosporine in patients with psoriasis are renal dysfunction, headache, hypertension, hypertriglyceridemia, hirsutism/hypertrichosis, paresthesia or hyperesthesia, influenza-like symptoms, nausea/vomiting, diarrhea, abdominal discomfort, lethargy, and musculoskeletal or joint pain.

In psoriasis patients treated in U.S. controlled clinical studies within the recommended dose range, cyclosporine therapy was discontinued in 1.0% of the patients because of hypertension and in 5.4% of the patients because of increased creatinine. In the majority of cases, these changes were reversible after dose reduction or discontinuation of cyclosporine.

There has been one reported death associated with the use of cyclosporine in psoriasis. A 27 year old male developed renal deterioration and was continued on cyclosporine. He had progressive renal failure leading to death.

Frequency and severity of serum creatinine increases with dose and duration of cyclosporine therapy. These elevations are likely to become more pronounced and may result in irreversible renal damage without dose reduction or discontinuation.

[See table at top of page 447]

The following events occurred in 1% to less than 3% of psoriasis patients treated with cyclosporine:

Body as a Whole
fever, flushes, hot flushes;
Cardiovascular
chest pain;
Central and Peripheral Nervous System
appetite increased, insomnia, dizziness, nervousness, vertigo;
Gastrointestinal
abdominal distention, constipation, gingival bleeding;
Liver and Biliary System
hyperbilirubinemia;
Neoplasms
skin malignancies [squamous cell (0.9%) and basal cell (0.4%) carcinomas];

Reticuloendothelial
platelet, bleeding, and clotting disorders, red blood cell disorder;
Respiratory
infection, viral and other infection;
Skin and Appendages
acne, folliculitis, keratosis, pruritus, rash, dry skin;
Urinary System
micturition frequency;
Vision
abnormal vision.

Mild hypomagnesemia and hyperkalemia may occur but are asymptomatic. Increases in uric acid may occur and attacks of gout have been rarely reported. A minor and dose related hyperbilirubinemia has been observed in the absence of hepatocellular damage. Cyclosporine therapy may be associated with a modest increase of serum triglycerides or cholesterol. Elevations of triglycerides (> 750 mg/dL) occur in about 15% of psoriasis patients; elevations of cholesterol (> 300 mg/dL) are observed in less than 3% of psoriasis patients. Generally these laboratory abnormalities are reversible upon dose reduction or discontinuation of cyclosporine.

OVERDOSAGE

There is a minimal experience with cyclosporine overdosage. Forced emesis and gastric lavage can be of value up to 2 hours after administration of Gengraf (cyclosporine capsules, USP [**MODIFIED**]). Transient hepatotoxicity and nephrotoxicity may occur which should resolve following drug withdrawal. Oral doses of cyclosporine up to 10 g (about 150 mg/kg) have been tolerated with relatively minor clinical consequences, such as vomiting, drowsiness, headache, tachycardia and, in a few patients, moderately severe, reversible impairment of renal function. However, serious symptoms of intoxication have been reported following accidental parenteral overdosage with cyclosporine in premature neonates. General supportive measures and symptomatic treatment should be followed in all cases of overdosage. Cyclosporine is not dialyzable to any great extent, nor is it cleared well by charcoal hemoperfusion. The oral dosage at which half of experimental animals are estimated to die is 31 times, 39 times and > 54 times the human

Body System	Adverse Reactions	Randomized Kidney Patients Sandimmune® (N = 227) %	Azathioprine (N = 228) %	Cyclosporine Patients (Sandimmune®) Kidney (N = 705) %	Heart (N = 112) %	Liver (N = 75) %
Genitourinary	Renal Dysfunction	32	6	25	38	37
Cardiovascular	Hypertension	26	18	13	53	27
	Cramps	4	<1	2	<1	0
Skin	Hirsutism	21	<1	21	28	45
	Acne	6	8	2	2	1
Central Nervous System	Tremor	12	0	21	31	55
	Convulsions	3	1	1	4	5
	Headache	2	<1	2	15	4
Gastrointestinal	Gum Hyperplasia	4	0	9	5	16
	Diarrhea	3	<1	3	4	8
	Nausea/Vomiting	2	<1	4	10	4
	Hepatotoxicity	<1	<1	4	7	4
	Abdominal Discomfort	<1	0	<1	7	0
Autonomic Nervous System	Paresthesia	3	0	1	2	1
	Flushing	<1	0	4	0	4
Hematopoietic	Leukopenia	2	19	<1	6	0
	Lymphoma	<1	0	1	6	1
Respiratory	Sinusitis	<1	0	4	3	7
Miscellaneous	Gynecomastia	<1	0	<1	4	3

Infectious Complications in Historical Randomized Studies in Renal Transplant Patients Using Sandimmune®

Complication	Cyclosporine Treatment (N = 227) % of Complications	Azathioprine with Steroids* (N = 228) % of Complications
Septicemia	5.3	4.8
Abscesses	4.4	5.3
Systemic Fungal Infection	2.2	3.9
Local Fungal Infection	7.5	9.6
Cytomegalovirus	4.8	12.3
Other Viral Infections	15.9	18.4
Urinary Tract Infections	21.1	20.2
Wound and Skin Infections	7.0	10.1
Pneumonia	6.2	9.2

*Some patients also received ALG.

Information on the Abbott Pharmaceutical Products listed on these pages is from the prescribing information in use as of June 1, 2010. For more information, please visit rxabbott.com or call 1-800-633-9110.

Cyclosporine (MODIFIED)/Sandimmune® Rheumatoid Arthritis Percentage of Patients with Adverse Events ≥ 3% in any Cyclosporine Treated Group

Body System	Preferred Term	Studies 651+652+2008 Sandimmune®† (N = 269)	Study 302 Sandimmune® (N = 155)	Study 654 Methotrexate & Sandimmune® (N = 74)	Study 654 Methotrexate & Placebo (N = 73)	Study 302 Cyclosporine (MODIFIED) (N = 143)	Studies 651+652+2008 Placebo (N = 201)
Autonomic Nervous System Disorders							
	Flushing	2%	2%	3%	0%	5%	2%
Body As A Whole - General Disorders							
	Accidental Trauma	0%	1%	10%	4%	4%	0%
	Edema NOS*	5%	14%	12%	4%	10%	<1%
	Fatigue	6%	3%	8%	12%	3%	7%
	Fever	2%	3%	0%	0%	2%	4%
	Influenza-like symptoms	<1%	6%	1%	0%	3%	2%
	Pain	6%	9%	10%	15%	13%	4%
	Rigors	1%	1%	4%	0%	3%	1%
Cardiovascular Disorders							
	Arrhythmia	2%	5%	5%	6%	2%	1%
	Chest Pain	4%	5%	1%	1%	6%	1%
	Hypertension	8%	26%	16%	12%	25%	2%
Central and Peripheral Nervous System Disorders							
	Dizziness	8%	6%	7%	3%	8%	3%
	Headache	17%	23%	22%	11%	25%	9%
	Migraine	2%	3%	0%	0%	3%	1%
	Paresthesia	8%	7%	8%	4%	11%	1%
	Tremor	8%	7%	7%	3%	13%	4%
Gastrointestinal System Disorders							
	Abdominal Pain	15%	15%	15%	7%	15%	10%
	Anorexia	3%	3%	1%	0%	3%	3%
	Diarrhea	12%	12%	18%	15%	13%	8%
	Dyspepsia	12%	12%	10%	8%	8%	4%
	Flatulence	5%	5%	5%	4%	4%	1%
	Gastrointestinal Disorder NOS*	0%	2%	1%	4%	4%	0%
	Gingivitis	4%	3%	0%	0%	0%	1%
	Gum Hyperplasia	2%	4%	1%	3%	4%	1%
	Nausea	23%	14%	24%	15%	18%	14%
	Rectal Hemorrhage	0%	3%	0%	0%	1%	1%
	Stomatitis	7%	5%	16%	12%	6%	8%
	Vomiting	9%	8%	14%	7%	6%	5%
Hearing and Vestibular Disorders							
	Ear Disorders NOS*	0%	5%	0%	0%	1%	0%
Metabolic and Nutritional Disorders							
	Hypomagnesemia	0%	4%	0%	0%	6%	0%
Musculoskeletal System Disorders							
	Arthropathy	0%	5%	0%	1%	4%	0%
	Leg Cramps/Involuntary Muscle Contractions	2%	11%	11%	3%	12%	1%
Psychiatric Disorders							
	Depression	3%	6%	3%	1%	1%	2%
	Insomnia	4%	1%	1%	0%	3%	2%
Renal							
	Creatinine elevations ≥ 30%	43%	39%	55%	19%	48%	13%
	Creatinine elevations ≥ 50%	24%	18%	26%	8%	18%	3%
Reproductive Disorders, Female							
	Leukorrhea	1%	0%	4%	0%	1%	0%
	Menstrual Disorder	3%	2%	1%	0%	1%	1%
Respiratory System Disorders							
	Bronchitis	1%	3%	1%	0%	1%	3%
	Coughing	5%	3%	5%	7%	4%	4%
	Dyspnea	5%	1%	3%	3%	1%	2%
	Infection NOS*	9%	5%	0%	7%	3%	10%
	Pharyngitis	3%	5%	5%	6%	4%	4%
	Pneumonia	1%	0%	4%	0%	1%	1%
	Rhinitis	0%	3%	11%	10%	1%	0%
	Sinusitis	4%	4%	8%	4%	3%	3%
	Upper Respiratory Tract	0%	14%	23%	15%	13%	0%
Skin and Appendages Disorders							
	Alopecia	3%	0%	1%	1%	4%	4%
	Bullous Eruption	1%	0%	4%	1%	1%	1%
	Hypertrichosis	19%	17%	12%	0%	15%	3%
	Rash	7%	12%	10%	7%	8%	10%
	Skin Ulceration	1%	1%	3%	4%	0%	2%
Urinary System Disorders							
	Dysuria	0%	0%	11%	3%	1%	2%
	Micturition Frequency	2%	4%	3%	1%	2%	2%
	NPN, Increased	0%	19%	12%	0%	18%	0%
	Urinary Tract Infection	0%	3%	5%	4%	3%	0%
Vascular (Extracardiac) Disorders							
	Purpura	3%	4%	1%	1%	2%	0%

† Includes patients in 2.5 mg/kg/day dose group only.
* NOS = Not Otherwise Specified.

maintenance dose for transplant patients (6 mg/kg; corrections based on body surface area) in mice, rats, and rabbits.
DOSAGE AND ADMINISTRATION
Gengraf (cyclosporine capsules, USP [MODIFIED]) has increased bioavailability in comparison to Sandimmune® (cyclosporine capsules). Gengraf and Sandimmune are not bioequivalent and cannot be used interchangeably without physician supervision.

The daily dose of Gengraf (cyclosporine capsules, USP [MODIFIED]) should always be given in two divided doses (BID). It is recommended that Gengraf be administered on a consistent schedule with regard to time of day and relation to meals. Grapefruit and grapefruit juice affect metabolism, increasing blood concentration of cyclosporine, thus should be avoided.

Newly Transplanted Patients

The initial oral dose of Gengraf (cyclosporine capsules, USP [MODIFIED]) can be given 4-12 hours prior to transplantation or be given postoperatively. The initial dose of Gengraf varies depending on the transplanted organ and the other immunosuppressive agents included in the immunosuppressive protocol. In newly transplanted patients, the initial oral dose of Gengraf is the same as the initial oral dose of Sandimmune®. Suggested initial doses are available from the results of a 1994 survey of the use of Sandimmune® in U.S. transplant centers. The mean ± SD initial doses were 9 ± 3 mg/kg/day for renal transplant patients (75 centers), 8 ± 4 mg/kg/day for liver transplant patients (30 centers), and 7 ± 3 mg/kg/day for heart transplant patients (24 centers). Total daily doses were divided into two equal daily doses. The Gengraf dose is subsequently adjusted to achieve a pre-defined cyclosporine blood concentration (see **DOSAGE AND ADMINISTRATION - Blood Concentration Monitoring in Transplant Patients**, below). If cyclosporine trough blood concentrations are used, the target range is the same for Gengraf as for Sandimmune®. Using the same trough concentration target range for Gengraf as for Sandimmune® results in greater cyclosporine exposure when Gengraf is administered (see **CLINICAL PHARMACOLOGY - Pharmacokinetics, Absorption**). Dosing should be titrated based on clinical assessments of rejection and tolerability. Lower Gengraf doses may be sufficient as maintenance therapy.

Adjunct therapy with adrenal corticosteroids is recommended initially. Different tapering dosage schedules of prednisone appear to achieve similar results. A representative dosage schedule based on the patient's weight started with 2 mg/kg/day for the first 4 days tapered to 1 mg/kg/day by 1 week, 0.6 mg/kg/day by 2 weeks, 0.3 mg/kg/day by 1 month, and 0.15 mg/kg/day by 2 months and thereafter as a maintenance dose. Steroid doses may be further tapered on an individualized basis depending on status of patient and function of graft. Adjustments in dosage of prednisone must be made according to the clinical situation.

Conversion from Sandimmune* (Cyclosporine) to Gengraf (Cyclosporine Capsules, USP [MODIFIED]) in Transplant Patients

In transplanted patients who are considered for conversion to Gengraf from Sandimmune* (cyclosporine), Gengraf should be started with the same daily dose as was previously used with Sandimmune* (cyclosporine) (1:1 dose conversion). The Gengraf dose should subsequently be adjusted to attain the pre-conversion cyclosporine blood trough concentration. Using the same trough concentration target range for Gengraf as for Sandimmune* (cyclosporine) results in greater cyclosporine exposure when Gengraf is administered (see **CLINICAL PHARMACOLOGY - Pharmacokinetics, Absorption**). Patients with suspected poor absorption of Sandimmune* (cyclosporine) require different dosing strategies (see **DOSAGE AND ADMINISTRATION - Transplant Patients with Poor Absorption of Sandimmune* (Cyclosporine)**, below). In some patients, the increase in blood trough concentration is more pronounced and may be of clinical significance.

Until the blood trough concentration attains the pre-conversion value, it is strongly recommended that the cyclosporine blood trough concentration be monitored every 4 to 7 days after conversion to Gengraf. In addition, clinical safety parameters such as serum creatinine and blood pressure should be monitored every two weeks during the first two months after conversion. If the blood trough concentrations are outside the desired range and/or if the clinical safety parameters worsen, the dosage of Gengraf must be adjusted accordingly.

Transplant Patients with Poor Absorption of Sandimmune* (Cyclosporine)

Patients with lower than expected cyclosporine blood trough concentrations in relation to the oral dose of Sandimmune* (cyclosporine) may have poor or inconsistent absorption of cyclosporine from Sandimmune* (cyclosporine). After conversion to Gengraf (cyclosporine capsules, USP [MODIFIED]), patients tend to have higher cyclosporine concentrations. **Due to the increase in bioavailability of cyclosporine following conversion to Gengraf, the cyclosporine blood trough concentration may exceed the target range. Particular caution should be exercised when converting patients to Gengraf at doses greater than 10 mg/kg/day.** The dose of Gengraf should be titrated individually based on cyclosporine trough concentrations, tolerability, and clinical response. In this population the cyclosporine blood trough concentration should be measured more frequently, at least twice a week (daily, if initial dose exceeds 10 mg/kg/day) until the concentration stabilizes within the desired range.

Rheumatoid Arthritis

The initial dose of Gengraf (cyclosporine capsules, USP [MODIFIED]) is 2.5 mg/kg/day, taken twice daily as a divided (BID) oral dose. Salicylates, nonsteroidal anti-inflammatory agents, and oral corticosteroids may be continued (see

Adverse Events Occurring in 3% or More of Psoriasis Patients in Controlled Clinical Trials

Body System* Preferred Term	Cyclosporine (MODIFIED) (N = 182)	Sandimmune® (N = 185)
Infection or Potential Infection	24.7%	24.3%
Influenza-like Symptoms	9.9%	8.1%
Upper Respiratory Tract Infections	7.7%	11.3%
Cardiovascular System	28.0%	25.4%
Hypertension**	27.5%	25.4%
Urinary System	24.2%	16.2%
Increased Creatinine	19.8%	15.7%
Central and Peripheral Nervous System	26.4%	20.5%
Headache	15.9%	14.0%
Paresthesia	7.1%	4.8%
Musculoskeletal System	13.2%	8.7%
Arthralgia	6.0%	1.1%
Body As a Whole – General	29.1%	22.2%
Pain	4.4%	3.2%
Metabolic and Nutritional	9.3%	9.7%
Reproductive, Female	8.5% (4 of 47 females)	11.5% (6 of 52 females)
Resistance Mechanism	18.7%	21.1%
Skin and Appendages	17.6%	15.1%
Hypertrichosis	6.6%	5.4%
Respiratory System	5.0%	6.5%
Bronchospasm, Coughing, Dyspnea, Rhinitis	5.0%	4.9%
Psychiatric	5.0%	3.8%
Gastrointestinal System	19.8%	28.7%
Abdominal Pain	2.7%	6.0%
Diarrhea	5.0%	5.9%
Dyspepsia	2.2%	3.2%
Gum Hyperplasia	3.8%	6.0%
Nausea	5.5%	5.9%
White cell and RES	4.4%	2.7%

* Total percentage of events within the system.
**Newly occurring hypertension = SBP ≥160 mm Hg and/or DBP ≥90 mm Hg.

WARNINGS and **PRECAUTIONS - Drug Interactions**). Onset of action generally occurs between 4 and 8 weeks. If insufficient clinical benefit is seen and tolerability is good (including serum creatinine less than 30% above baseline), the dose may be increased by 0.5 to 0.75 mg/kg/day after 8 weeks and again after 12 weeks to a maximum of 4 mg/kg/day. If no benefit is seen by 16 weeks of therapy, Gengraf therapy should be discontinued.

Dose decreases by 25%-50% should be made at any time to control adverse events, e.g., hypertension elevations in serum creatinine (30% above patient's pretreatment level) or clinically significant laboratory abnormalities (see **WARNINGS** and **PRECAUTIONS**).

If dose reduction is not effective in controlling abnormalities or if the adverse event or abnormality is severe, Gengraf should be discontinued. The same initial dose and dosage range should be used if Gengraf is combined with the recommended dose of methotrexate. Most patients can be treated with Gengraf doses of 3 mg/kg/day or below when combined with methotrexate doses of up to 15 mg/week (see **CLINICAL PHARMACOLOGY - Clinical Trials**).

There is limited long-term treatment data. Recurrence of rheumatoid arthritis disease activity is generally apparent within four weeks after stopping cyclosporine.

Psoriasis

The initial dose of Gengraf (cyclosporine capsules, USP [MODIFIED]) should be 2.5 mg/kg/day. Gengraf should be taken twice daily, as a divided (1.25 mg/kg BID) oral dose. Patients should be kept at that dose for at least 4 weeks, barring adverse events. If significant clinical improvement has not occurred in patients by that time, the patient's dosage should be increased at 2 week intervals. Based on patient response, dose increases of approximately 0.5 mg/kg/day should be made to a maximum of 4 mg/kg/day.

Dose decreases by 25%-50% should be made at any time to control adverse events, e.g., hypertension, elevations in serum creatinine (≥ 25% above the patient's pretreatment level), or clinically significant laboratory abnormalities.

If dose reduction is not effective in controlling abnormalities, or if the adverse event or abnormality is severe, Gengraf should be discontinued (see **PRECAUTIONS - Special Monitoring of Psoriasis Patients**).

Patients generally show some improvement in the clinical manifestations of psoriasis in 2 weeks. Satisfactory control and stabilization of the disease may take 12-16 weeks to achieve. Results of a dose-titration clinical trial with Gengraf indicate that an improvement of psoriasis by 75% or more (based on PASI) was achieved in 51% of the patients after 8 weeks and in 79% of the patients after 16 weeks. Treatment should be discontinued if satisfactory response cannot be achieved after 6 weeks at 4 mg/kg/day or the patient's maximum tolerated dose. Once a patient is adequately controlled and appears stable the dose of Gengraf should be lowered, and the patient treated with the lowest

dose that maintains an adequate response (this should not necessarily be total clearing of the patient). In clinical trials, cyclosporine doses at the lower end of the recommended dosage range were effective in maintaining a satisfactory response in 60% of the patients. Doses below 2.5 mg/kg/day may also be equally effective.

Upon stopping treatment with cyclosporine, relapse will occur in approximately six weeks (50% of the patients) to 16 weeks (75% of the patients). In the majority of patients rebound does not occur after cessation of treatment with cyclosporine. Thirteen cases of transformation of chronic plaque psoriasis to more severe forms of psoriasis have been reported. There were 9 cases of pustular and 4 cases of erythrodermic psoriasis. Long term experience with Gengraf in psoriasis patients is limited and continuous treatment for extended periods greater than one year is not recommended. Alternation with other forms of treatment should be considered in the long term management of patients with this life long disease.

Blood Concentration Monitoring in Transplant Patients

Transplant centers have found blood concentration monitoring of cyclosporine to be an essential component of patient management. Of importance to blood concentration analysis are the type of assay used, the transplanted organ, and other immunosuppressant agents being administered. While no fixed relationship has been established, blood concentration monitoring may assist in the clinical evaluation of rejection and toxicity, dose adjustments, and the assessment of compliance.

Various assays have been used to measure blood concentrations of cyclosporine. Older studies using a non-specific assay often cited concentrations that were roughly twice those of the specific assays. Therefore, comparison between concentrations in the published literature and an individual patient concentration using current assays must be made with detailed knowledge of the assay methods employed. Current assay results are also not interchangeable and their use should be guided by their approved labeling. A discussion of the different assay methods is contained in *Annals of Clinical Biochemistry* 1994;31:420-446. While several assays and assay matrices are available, there is a consensus that parent-compound-specific assays correlate best with clinical events. Of these, HPLC is the standard reference, but the monoclonal antibody RIAs and the monoclonal antibody FPIA offer sensitivity, reproducibility, and convenience. Most clinicians base their monitoring on trough cyclosporine concentrations. *Applied Pharmacokinetics, Principles of Therapeutic Drug Monitoring* (1992)

Information on the Abbott Pharmaceutical Products listed on these pages is from the prescribing information in use as of June 1, 2010. For more information, please visit rxabbott.com or call 1-800-633-9110.

contains a broad discussion of cyclosporine pharmacokinetics and drug monitoring techniques. Blood concentration monitoring is not a replacement for renal function monitoring or tissue biopsies.

HOW SUPPLIED

Gengraf Capsules (Cyclosporine Capsules, USP [MODIFIED])

25 mg
Oval, white imprinted in blue, the corporate Abbott ☐ logo, 25 mg, and the Abbo-Code OR. Packages of 30 unit-dose blisters. (NDC 0074-6463-32).

100 mg
Oval, white, with two blue stripes, imprinted in blue, the corporate Abbott ☐ logo, 100 mg, and Abbo-Code OT. Packages of 30 unit-dose blisters. (NDC 0074-6479-32).

Store and Dispense
In the original unit-dose container at controlled room temperature 68°-77°F (20°-25°C). (See USP Controlled Room Temperature).
*Sandimmune® is a registered trademark of Novartis Pharmaceuticals Corporation.
© Abbott
Abbott Laboratories, North Chicago, IL 60064, U.S.A.
Ref. 03-A325-R10 Revised January, 2010
Shown in Product Identification Guide, page 303

HUMIRA® ℞
[*hu-mare-ah*]
(adalimumab)
Injection, Solution for Subcutaneous use

HIGHLIGHTS OF PRESCRIBING INFORMATION
These highlights do not include all the information needed to use HUMIRA safely and effectively. See full prescribing information for HUMIRA.
HUMIRA (adalimumab) Injection, Solution for Subcutaneous use
Initial U.S. Approval: 2002

WARNINGS:
See full prescribing information for complete boxed warning.
SERIOUS INFECTIONS
• **Increased risk of serious infections leading to hospitalization or death, including tuberculosis (TB), bacterial sepsis, invasive fungal infections (such as histoplasmosis), and infections due to other opportunistic pathogens.**
• **HUMIRA should be discontinued if a patient develops a serious infection or sepsis during treatment.**
• **Perform test for latent TB; if positive, start treatment for TB prior to starting HUMIRA.**
• **Monitor all patients for active TB during treatment, even if initial latent TB test is negative. (5.1)**
MALIGNANCY
Lymphoma and other malignancies, some fatal, have been reported in children and adolescent patients treated with TNF blockers, of which HUMIRA is a member.

———RECENT MAJOR CHANGES———
Boxed Warning   11/2009
Warnings and Precautions, Serious Infections (5.1) 12/2008
Warnings and Precautions, Malignancies (5.2)   11/2009
———INDICATIONS AND USAGE———
HUMIRA is a tumor necrosis factor (TNF) blocker indicated for treatment of:
Rheumatoid Arthritis (RA) (1.1)
• Reducing signs and symptoms, inducing major clinical response, inhibiting the progression of structural damage, and improving physical function in adult patients with moderately to severely active disease.
Juvenile Idiopathic Arthritis (1.2)
• Reducing signs and symptoms of moderately to severely active polyarticular juvenile idiopathic arthritis in patients 4 years of age and older.
Psoriatic Arthritis (1.3)
• Reducing signs and symptoms of active arthritis, inhibiting the progression of structural damage, and improving physical function.
Ankylosing Spondylitis (1.4)
• Reducing signs and symptoms in patients with active disease.
Crohn's Disease (1.5)
• Reducing signs and symptoms and inducing and maintaining clinical remission in adult patients with moderately to severely active Crohn's disease who have had an inadequate response to conventional therapy. Reducing signs and symptoms and inducing clinical remission in these patients if they have also lost response to or are intolerant to infliximab.

Plaque Psoriasis (1.6)
• The treatment of adult patients with moderate to severe chronic plaque psoriasis who are candidates for systemic therapy or phototherapy, and when other systemic therapies are medically less appropriate.
———DOSAGE AND ADMINISTRATION———
HUMIRA is administered by subcutaneous injection.
Rheumatoid Arthritis, Psoriatic Arthritis, Ankylosing Spondylitis (2.1)
• 40 mg every other week. Some patients with RA not receiving methotrexate may benefit from increasing the frequency to 40 mg every week.
Juvenile Idiopathic Arthritis (2.2)
• 15 kg (33 lbs) to <30 kg (66 lbs): 20 mg every other week
• ≥30 kg (66 lbs): 40 mg every other week
Crohn's Disease (2.3)
• Initial dose (Day 1) is 160 mg (four 40 mg injections in one day or two 40 mg injections per day for two consecutive days), followed by 80 mg two weeks later (Day 15). Two weeks later (Day 29) begin a maintenance dose of 40 mg every other week.
Plaque Psoriasis (2.4)
• 80 mg initial dose, followed by 40 mg every other week starting one week after initial dose.
———DOSAGE FORMS AND STRENGTHS———
• 40 mg/0.8 mL in a single-use prefilled pen (HUMIRA Pen) (3)
• 40 mg/0.8 mL in a single-dose prefilled glass syringe (3)
• 20 mg/0.4 mL in a single-dose prefilled glass syringe (3)
———CONTRAINDICATIONS———
• None (4)
———WARNINGS AND PRECAUTIONS———
• Serious infections – do not start HUMIRA during an active infection. If an infection develops, monitor carefully, and stop HUMIRA if infection becomes serious (5.1)
• Malignancies – are seen more often than in controls, and lymphoma is seen more often than in the general population (5.2)
• Anaphylaxis or serious allergic reactions may occur (5.3)
• Hepatitis B virus reactivation – monitor HBV carriers during and several months after therapy. If reactivation occurs, stop HUMIRA and begin anti-viral therapy (5.4)
• Demyelinating disease, exacerbation or new onset, may occur (5.5)
• Cytopenias, pancytopenia – advise patients to seek immediate medical attention if symptoms develop, and consider stopping HUMIRA (5.6)
• Heart failure, worsening or new onset, may occur (5.8)
• Lupus-like syndrome – stop HUMIRA if syndrome develops (5.9)
———ADVERSE REACTIONS———
Most common adverse reactions (incidence >10%): infections (e.g. upper respiratory, sinusitis), injection site reactions, headache and rash (6.1)
To report SUSPECTED ADVERSE REACTIONS, contact Abbott Laboratories at 1-800-633-9110 or FDA at 1-800-FDA-1088 or www.fda.gov/medwatch
———DRUG INTERACTIONS———
• Anakinra – increased risk of serious infection (5.7, 7.1)
• Live vaccines – should not be given with HUMIRA (5.10, 7.2)
———USE IN SPECIFIC POPULATIONS———
• Pregnancy: Physicians are encouraged to enroll pregnant patients in the HUMIRA pregnancy registry by calling 1-877-311-8972 (8.1)
See 17 for PATIENT COUNSELING INFORMATION and Medication Guide

Revised: 11/2009

FULL PRESCRIBING INFORMATION: CONTENTS*
WARNINGS
RECENT MAJOR CHANGES
* Sections or subsections omitted from the full prescribing information are not listed

---

FULL PRESCRIBING INFORMATION

WARNINGS
SERIOUS INFECTIONS
Patients treated with HUMIRA are at increased risk for developing serious infections that may lead to hospitalization or death. Most patients who developed these infections were taking concomitant immunosuppressants such as methotrexate or corticosteroids.
HUMIRA should be discontinued if a patient develops a serious infection or sepsis.
Reported infections include:
• Active tuberculosis, including reactivation of latent tuberculosis. Patients with tuberculosis have frequently presented with disseminated or extrapulmonary disease. Patients should be tested for latent tuberculosis before HUMIRA use and during therapy. Treatment for latent infection should be initiated prior to HUMIRA use.
• Invasive fungal infections, including histoplasmosis, coccidioidomycosis, candidiasis, aspergillosis, blastomycosis, and pneumocystosis. Patients with histoplasmosis or other invasive fungal infections may present with disseminated, rather than localized, disease. Antigen and antibody testing for histoplasmosis may be negative in some patients with active infection. Empiric anti-fungal therapy should be considered in patients at risk for invasive fungal infections who develop severe systemic illness.
• Bacterial, viral and other infections due to opportunistic pathogens.
The risks and benefits of treatment with HUMIRA should be carefully considered prior to initiating therapy in patients with chronic or recurrent infection.
Patients should be closely monitored for the development of signs and symptoms of infection during and after treatment with HUMIRA, including the possible development of tuberculosis in patients who tested negative for latent tuberculosis infection prior to initiating therapy. *[See Warnings and Precautions (5.1) and Adverse Reactions (6.1)]*
MALIGNANCY
Lymphoma and other malignancies, some fatal, have been reported in children and adolescent patients treated with TNF blockers, of which HUMIRA is a member.

1   INDICATIONS AND USAGE

1.1   Rheumatoid Arthritis
HUMIRA is indicated for reducing signs and symptoms, inducing major clinical response, inhibiting the progression of structural damage, and improving physical function in adult patients with moderately to severely active rheumatoid arthritis. HUMIRA can be used alone or in combination with methotrexate or other disease-modifying antirheumatic drugs (DMARDs).

1.2 Juvenile Idiopathic Arthritis

HUMIRA is indicated for reducing signs and symptoms of moderately to severely active polyarticular juvenile idiopathic arthritis in patients 4 years of age and older. HUMIRA can be used alone or in combination with methotrexate.

1.3 Psoriatic Arthritis

HUMIRA is indicated for reducing signs and symptoms of active arthritis, inhibiting the progression of structural damage, and improving physical function in patients with psoriatic arthritis. HUMIRA can be used alone or in combination with DMARDs.

1.4 Ankylosing Spondylitis

HUMIRA is indicated for reducing signs and symptoms in patients with active ankylosing spondylitis.

1.5 Crohn's Disease

HUMIRA is indicated for reducing signs and symptoms and inducing and maintaining clinical remission in adult patients with moderately to severely active Crohn's disease who have had an inadequate response to conventional therapy. HUMIRA is indicated for reducing signs and symptoms and inducing clinical remission in these patients if they have also lost response to or are intolerant to infliximab.

1.6 Plaque Psoriasis

HUMIRA is indicated for the treatment of adult patients with moderate to severe chronic plaque psoriasis who are candidates for systemic therapy or phototherapy, and when other systemic therapies are medically less appropriate. HUMIRA should only be administered to patients who will be closely monitored and have regular follow-up visits with a physician [see Boxed WARNINGS and Warnings and Precautions (5)].

2 DOSAGE AND ADMINISTRATION

HUMIRA is administered by subcutaneous injection.

2.1 Rheumatoid Arthritis, Psoriatic Arthritis, and Ankylosing Spondylitis

The recommended dose of HUMIRA for adult patients with rheumatoid arthritis, psoriatic arthritis, or ankylosing spondylitis is 40 mg administered every other week. Methotrexate, glucocorticoids, salicylates, nonsteroidal anti-inflammatory drugs (NSAIDs), analgesics or other DMARDs may be continued during treatment with HUMIRA. In rheumatoid arthritis, some patients not taking concomitant methotrexate may derive additional benefit from increasing the dosing frequency of HUMIRA to 40 mg every week.

2.2 Juvenile Idiopathic Arthritis

The recommended dose of HUMIRA for patients 4 to 17 years of age with polyarticular juvenile idiopathic arthritis is based on weight as shown below. Methotrexate, glucocorticoids, salicylates, NSAIDs or analgesics may be continued during treatment with HUMIRA.

Pediatric Patients (4 to 17 years)	Dose
15 kg (33 lbs) to <30 kg (66 lbs)	20 mg every other week (20 mg Prefilled Syringe)
≥30 kg (66 lbs)	40 mg every other week (HUMIRA Pen or 40 mg Prefilled Syringe)

Limited data are available for HUMIRA treatment in pediatric patients with a weight below 15 kg.

2.3 Crohn's Disease

The recommended HUMIRA dose regimen for adult patients with Crohn's disease is 160 mg initially at Day 1 (given as four 40 mg injections in one day or as two 40 mg injections per day for two consecutive days), followed by 80 mg two weeks later (Day 15). Two weeks later (Day 29) begin a maintenance dose of 40 mg every other week. Aminosalicylates, corticosteroids, and/or immunomodulatory agents (e.g., 6-mercaptopurine and azathioprine) may be continued during treatment with HUMIRA. The use of HUMIRA in Crohn's disease beyond one year has not been evaluated in controlled clinical studies.

2.4 Plaque Psoriasis

The recommended dose of HUMIRA for adult patients with plaque psoriasis is an initial dose of 80 mg, followed by 40 mg given every other week starting one week after the initial dose. The use of HUMIRA in moderate to severe chronic plaque psoriasis beyond one year has not been evaluated in controlled clinical studies.

2.5 General Considerations for Administration

HUMIRA is intended for use under the guidance and supervision of a physician. A patient may self-inject HUMIRA if a physician determines that it is appropriate, and with medical follow-up as necessary, after proper training in subcutaneous injection technique.

The solution in the HUMIRA Pen or prefilled syringe should be carefully inspected visually for particulate matter and discoloration prior to subcutaneous administration. If particulates and discolorations are noted, the product should not be used. HUMIRA does not contain preservatives; therefore, unused portions of drug remaining from the syringe should be discarded. NOTE: The needle cover of the syringe contains dry rubber (latex), which should not be handled by persons sensitive to this substance.

Patients using the HUMIRA Pen or prefilled syringe should be instructed to inject the full amount in the syringe (0.8 mL), which provides 40 mg of HUMIRA, according to the directions provided in the Medication Guide [see Medication Guide (17)].

Patients (15 kg to <30 kg) using the pediatric pre-filled syringe, or their caregivers, should be instructed to inject the full amount in the syringe (0.4 mL), which provides 20 mg of HUMIRA, according to the directions provided in the Medication Guide.

Injection sites should be rotated and injections should never be given into areas where the skin is tender, bruised, red or hard.

3 DOSAGE FORMS AND STRENGTHS

• Pen

A single-use pen (HUMIRA Pen), containing a 1 mL prefilled glass syringe with a fixed 27 gauge ½ inch needle, providing 40 mg (0.8 mL) of HUMIRA.

• Prefilled Syringe

A single-dose, 1 mL prefilled glass syringe with a fixed 27 gauge ½ inch needle, providing 40 mg (0.8 mL) of HUMIRA.

A single-dose, 1 mL prefilled glass syringe with a fixed 27 gauge ½ inch needle, providing 20 mg (0.4 mL) of HUMIRA.

4 CONTRAINDICATIONS

None.

5 WARNINGS AND PRECAUTIONS

5.1 Serious Infections

(see also Boxed Warning)

Serious and sometimes fatal infections due to bacterial, mycobacterial, invasive fungal, viral, or other opportunistic pathogens have been reported in patients receiving TNF-blocking agents. Among opportunistic infections, tuberculosis, histoplasmosis, aspergillosis, candidiasis, coccidioidomycosis, listeriosis, and pneumocystosis were the most commonly reported. Patients have frequently presented with disseminated rather than localized disease, and are often taking concomitant immunosuppressants such as methotrexate or corticosteroids with HUMIRA.

Treatment with HUMIRA should not be initiated in patients with an active infection, including localized infections. The risks and benefits of treatment should be considered prior to initiating therapy in patients:

- with chronic or recurrent infection;
- who have been exposed to tuberculosis;
- who have resided or traveled in areas of endemic tuberculosis or endemic mycoses, such as histoplasmosis, coccidioidomycosis, or blastomycosis; or
- with underlying conditions that may predispose them to infection.

Cases of reactivation of tuberculosis or new tuberculosis infections have been observed in patients receiving HUMIRA, including patients who have previously received treatment for latent or active tuberculosis. Patients should be evaluated for tuberculosis risk factors and tested for latent infection prior to initiating HUMIRA and periodically during therapy.

Treatment of latent tuberculosis infection prior to therapy with TNF blocking agents has been shown to reduce the risk of tuberculosis reactivation during therapy. Induration of 5 mm or greater with tuberculin skin testing should be considered a positive test result when assessing if treatment for latent tuberculosis is needed prior to initiating HUMIRA, even for patients previously vaccinated with Bacille Calmette-Guerin (BCG).

Anti-tuberculosis therapy should also be considered prior to initiation of HUMIRA in patients with a past history of latent or active tuberculosis in whom an adequate course of treatment cannot be confirmed, and for patients with a negative test for latent tuberculosis but having risk factors for tuberculosis infection. Consultation with a physician with expertise in the treatment of tuberculosis is recommended to aid in the decision whether initiating anti-tuberculosis therapy is appropriate for an individual patient.

Tuberculosis should be strongly considered in patients who develop a new infection during HUMIRA treatment, especially in patients who have previously or recently traveled to countries with a high prevalence of tuberculosis, or who have had close contact with a person with active tuberculosis.

Patients should be closely monitored for the development of signs and symptoms of infection during and after treatment with HUMIRA, including the development of tuberculosis in patients who tested negative for latent tuberculosis infection prior to initiating therapy. Tests for latent tuberculosis infection may also be falsely negative while on therapy with HUMIRA.

HUMIRA should be discontinued if a patient develops a serious infection or sepsis. A patient who develops a new infection during treatment with HUMIRA should be closely monitored, undergo a prompt and complete diagnostic workup appropriate for an immunocompromised patient, and appropriate antimicrobial therapy should be initiated. For patients who reside or travel in regions where mycoses are endemic, invasive fungal infection should be suspected if they develop a serious systemic illness. Appropriate empiric antifungal therapy should be considered while a diagnostic workup is being performed. Antigen and antibody testing for histoplasmosis may be negative in some patients with active infection. When feasible, the decision to administer empiric antifungal therapy in these patients should be made in consultation with a physician with expertise in the diagnosis and treatment of invasive fungal infections and should take into account both the risk for severe fungal infection and the risks of antifungal therapy.

5.2 Malignancies

In the controlled portions of clinical trials of some TNF-blocking agents, including HUMIRA, more cases of malignancies have been observed among patients receiving those TNF blockers compared to control patients. During the controlled portions of HUMIRA trials in patients with rheumatoid arthritis, psoriatic arthritis, ankylosing spondylitis, Crohn's disease, and plaque psoriasis, malignancies, other than lymphoma and non-melanoma (basal cell and squamous cell) skin cancer, were observed at a rate (95% confidence interval) of 0.6 (0.3, 1.0)/100 patient-years among 3853 HUMIRA-treated patients versus a rate of 0.4 (0.2, 1.0)/100 patient-years among 2183 control patients (median duration of treatment of 5.5 months for HUMIRA-treated patients and 3.9 months for control-treated patients). The size of the control group and limited duration of the controlled portions of studies precludes the ability to draw firm conclusions. In the controlled and uncontrolled open-label portions of the clinical trials of HUMIRA, the more frequently observed malignancies, other than lymphoma and non-melanoma skin cancer, were breast, colon, prostate, lung, and melanoma. These malignancies in HUMIRA-treated and control-treated patients were similar in type and number to what would be expected in the general population.[1] During the controlled portions of HUMIRA rheumatoid arthritis, psoriatic arthritis, ankylosing spondylitis, Crohn's disease, and plaque psoriasis trials, the rate (95% confidence interval) of non-melanoma (basal cell and squamous cell) skin cancers was 0.9 (0.57, 1.35)/100 patient-years among HUMIRA-treated patients and 0.3 (0.08, 0.80)/100 patient-years among control patients. The potential role of TNF blocking therapy in the development of malignancies is not known.

Malignancies, some fatal, have been reported among children, adolescents, and young adults who received treatment with TNF-blocking agents (initiation of therapy ≤ 18 years of age), of which HUMIRA is a member. Approximately half the cases were lymphomas, including Hodgkin's and non-Hodgkin's lymphoma. The other cases represented a variety of different malignancies and included rare malignancies usually associated with immunosuppression and malignancies that are not usually observed in children and adolescents. The malignancies occurred after a median of 30 months of therapy (range 1 to 84 months). Most of the patients were receiving concomitant immunosuppressants. These cases were reported post-marketing and are derived from a variety of sources including registries and spontaneous postmarketing reports.

In the controlled portions of clinical trials of all the TNF-blocking agents, more cases of lymphoma have been observed among patients receiving TNF blockers compared to control patients. In controlled trials in patients with rheumatoid arthritis, psoriatic arthritis, ankylosing spondylitis, Crohn's disease, and plaque psoriasis, 2 lymphomas were observed among 3853 HUMIRA-treated patients versus 1 among 2183 control patients. In combining the controlled and uncontrolled open-label portions of these clinical trials with a median duration of approximately 2 years, including 6539 patients and over 16,000 patient-years of therapy, the observed rate of lymphomas is approximately 0.11/100 patient-years. This is approximately 3-fold higher than expected in the general population.[1] Rates in clinical trials for HUMIRA cannot be compared to rates of clinical trials of other TNF blockers and may not predict the rates observed in a broader patient population. Patients with rheumatoid arthritis, particularly those with highly active disease, are

Information on the Abbott Pharmaceutical Products listed on these pages is from the prescribing information in use as of June 1, 2010. For more information, please visit rxabbott.com or call 1-800-633-9110.

at a higher risk for the development of lymphoma. Cases of acute and chronic leukemia have been reported in association with postmarketing TNF-blocker use in rheumatoid arthritis and other indications. Even in the absence of TNF-blocker therapy, patients with rheumatoid arthritis may be at a higher risk (approximately 2-fold) than the general population for the development of leukemia.

5.3 Hypersensitivity Reactions

In postmarketing experience, anaphylaxis and angioneurotic edema have been reported rarely following HUMIRA administration. If an anaphylactic or other serious allergic reaction occurs, administration of HUMIRA should be discontinued immediately and appropriate therapy instituted. In clinical trials of HUMIRA in adults, allergic reactions overall (e.g., allergic rash, anaphylactoid reaction, fixed drug reaction, non-specified drug reaction, urticaria) have been observed in approximately 1% of patients.

5.4 Hepatitis B Virus Reactivation

Use of TNF blockers, including HUMIRA, may increase the risk of reactivation of hepatitis B virus (HBV) in patients who are chronic carriers of this virus. In some instances, HBV reactivation occurring in conjunction with TNF blocker therapy has been fatal. The majority of these reports have occurred in patients concomitantly receiving other medications that suppress the immune system, which may also contribute to HBV reactivation. Patients at risk for HBV infection should be evaluated for prior evidence of HBV infection before initiating TNF blocker therapy. Prescribers should exercise caution in prescribing TNF blockers for patients identified as carriers of HBV. Adequate data are not available on the safety or efficacy of treating patients who are carriers of HBV with anti-viral therapy in conjunction with TNF blocker therapy to prevent HBV reactivation. Patients who are carriers of HBV and require treatment with TNF blockers should be closely monitored for clinical and laboratory signs of active HBV infection throughout therapy and for several months following termination of therapy. In patients who develop HBV reactivation, HUMIRA should be stopped and effective anti-viral therapy with appropriate supportive treatment should be initiated. The safety of resuming TNF blocker therapy after HBV reactivation is controlled is not known. Therefore, prescribers should exercise caution when considering resumption of HUMIRA therapy in this situation and monitor patients closely.

5.5 Neurologic Reactions

Use of TNF blocking agents, including HUMIRA, has been associated with rare cases of new onset or exacerbation of clinical symptoms and/or radiographic evidence of demyelinating disease. Prescribers should exercise caution in considering the use of HUMIRA in patients with preexisting or recent-onset central nervous system demyelinating disorders.

5.6 Hematological Reactions

Rare reports of pancytopenia including aplastic anemia have been reported with TNF blocking agents. Adverse reactions of the hematologic system, including medically significant cytopenia (e.g., thrombocytopenia, leukopenia) have been infrequently reported with HUMIRA *[see Adverse Reactions (6)]*. The causal relationship of these reports to HUMIRA remains unclear. All patients should be advised to seek immediate medical attention if they develop signs and symptoms suggestive of blood dyscrasias or infection (e.g., persistent fever, bruising, bleeding, pallor) while on HUMIRA. Discontinuation of HUMIRA therapy should be considered in patients with confirmed significant hematologic abnormalities.

5.7 Use with Anakinra

Serious infections were seen in clinical studies with concurrent use of anakinra (an interleukin-1 antagonist) and another TNF-blocking agent, etanercept, with no added benefit compared to etanercept alone. Because of the nature of the adverse reactions seen with this combination therapy, similar toxicities may also result from combination of anakinra and other TNF blocking agents. Therefore, the combination of HUMIRA and anakinra is not recommended *[see Drug Interactions (7.1)]*.

5.8 Heart Failure

Cases of worsening congestive heart failure (CHF) and new onset CHF have been reported with TNF blockers. Cases of worsening CHF have also been observed with HUMIRA. HUMIRA has not been formally studied in patients with CHF; however, in clinical trials of another TNF blocker, a higher rate of serious CHF-related adverse reactions was observed. Physicians should exercise caution when using HUMIRA in patients who have heart failure and monitor them carefully.

5.9 Autoimmunity

Treatment with HUMIRA may result in the formation of autoantibodies and, rarely, in the development of a lupus-like syndrome. If a patient develops symptoms suggestive of a lupus-like syndrome following treatment with HUMIRA, treatment should be discontinued *[see Adverse Reactions (6.1)]*.

5.10 Immunizations

In a placebo-controlled clinical trial of patients with rheumatoid arthritis, no difference was detected in anti-pneumococcal antibody response between HUMIRA and placebo treatment groups when the pneumococcal polysaccharide vaccine and influenza vaccine were administered concurrently with HUMIRA. Similar proportions of patients developed protective levels of anti-influenza antibodies between HUMIRA and placebo treatment groups; however, titers in aggregate to influenza antigens were moderately lower in patients receiving HUMIRA. The clinical significance of this is unknown. Patients on HUMIRA may receive concurrent vaccinations, except for live vaccines. No data are available on the secondary transmission of infection by live vaccines in patients receiving HUMIRA.

It is recommended that juvenile idiopathic arthritis patients, if possible, be brought up to date with all immunizations in agreement with current immunization guidelines prior to initiating HUMIRA therapy. Patients on HUMIRA may receive concurrent vaccinations, except for live vaccines.

5.11 Immunosuppression

The possibility exists for TNF blocking agents, including HUMIRA, to affect host defenses against infections and malignancies since TNF mediates inflammation and modulates cellular immune responses. In a study of 64 patients with rheumatoid arthritis treated with HUMIRA, there was no evidence of depression of delayed-type hypersensitivity, depression of immunoglobulin levels, or change in enumeration of effector T- and B-cells and NK-cells, monocyte/macrophages, and neutrophils. The impact of treatment with HUMIRA on the development and course of malignancies, as well as active and/or chronic infections, is not fully understood *[see Warnings and Precautions (5.1, 5.2) and Adverse Reactions (6.1)]*. The safety and efficacy of HUMIRA in patients with immunosuppression have not been evaluated.

6 ADVERSE REACTIONS

6.1 Clinical Studies Experience

The most serious adverse reactions were *[see Warnings and Precautions (5)]*:

- Serious Infections
- Neurologic Reactions
- Malignancies

The most common adverse reaction with HUMIRA was injection site reactions. In placebo-controlled trials, 20% of patients treated with HUMIRA developed injection site reactions (erythema and/or itching, hemorrhage, pain or swelling), compared to 14% of patients receiving placebo. Most injection site reactions were described as mild and generally did not necessitate drug discontinuation.

The proportion of patients who discontinued treatment due to adverse reactions during the double-blind, placebo-controlled portion of Studies RA-I, RA-II, RA-III and RA-IV was 7% for patients taking HUMIRA and 4% for placebo-treated patients. The most common adverse reactions leading to discontinuation of HUMIRA were clinical flare reaction (0.7%), rash (0.3%) and pneumonia (0.3%).

Because clinical trials are conducted under widely varying and controlled conditions, adverse reaction rates observed in clinical trials of a drug cannot be directly compared to rates in the clinical trials of another drug and may not predict the rates observed in a broader patient population in clinical practice.

Infections

In placebo-controlled rheumatoid arthritis trials, the rate of infection was 1 per patient-year in the HUMIRA-treated patients and 0.9 per patient-year in the placebo-treated patients. The infections consisted primarily of upper respiratory tract infections, bronchitis and urinary tract infections. Most patients continued on HUMIRA after the infection resolved. The incidence of serious infections was 0.04 per patient-year in HUMIRA treated patients and 0.02 per patient-year in placebo-treated patients. Serious infections observed included pneumonia, septic arthritis, prosthetic and post-surgical infections, erysipelas, cellulitis, diverticulitis, and pyelonephritis *[see Warnings and Precautions (5.1)]*.

Tuberculosis and Opportunistic Infections

In completed and ongoing global clinical studies that include over 13,000 patients, the overall rate of tuberculosis is approximately 0.26 per 100 patient-years. In over 4500 patients in the US and Canada, the rate is approximately 0.07 per 100 patient-years. These studies include reports of miliary, lymphatic, peritoneal, as well as pulmonary. Most of the cases of tuberculosis occurred within the first eight months after initiation of therapy and may reflect recrudescence of latent disease. Cases of opportunistic infections have also been reported in these clinical trials at an overall rate of approximately 0.075/100 patient-years. Some cases of opportunistic infections and tuberculosis have been fatal *[see Warnings and Precautions (5.1)]*.

Malignancies

More cases of malignancy have been observed in HUMIRA-treated patients compared to control-treated patients in clinical trials *[see Warnings and Precautions (5.2)]*.

Autoantibodies

In the rheumatoid arthritis controlled trials, 12% of patients treated with HUMIRA and 7% of placebo-treated patients that had negative baseline ANA titers developed positive titers at week 24. Two patients out of 3046 treated with HUMIRA developed clinical signs suggestive of new-onset lupus-like syndrome. The patients improved following discontinuation of therapy. No patients developed lupus nephritis or central nervous system symptoms. The impact of long-term treatment with HUMIRA on the development of autoimmune diseases is unknown.

Immunogenicity

Patients in Studies RA-I, RA-II, and RA-III were tested at multiple time points for antibodies to adalimumab during the 6- to 12-month period. Approximately 5% (58 of 1062) of adult rheumatoid arthritis patients receiving HUMIRA developed low-titer antibodies to adalimumab at least once during treatment, which were neutralizing *in vitro*. Patients treated with concomitant methotrexate had a lower rate of antibody development than patients on HUMIRA monotherapy (1% versus 12%). No apparent correlation of antibody development to adverse reactions was observed. With monotherapy, patients receiving every other week dosing may develop antibodies more frequently than those receiving weekly dosing. In patients receiving the recommended dosage of 40 mg every other week as monotherapy, the ACR 20 response was lower among antibody-positive patients than among antibody-negative patients. The long-term immunogenicity of HUMIRA is unknown.

In patients with juvenile idiopathic arthritis, adalimumab antibodies were identified in 16% of HUMIRA-treated patients. In patients receiving concomitant methotrexate, the incidence was 6% compared to 26% with HUMIRA monotherapy.

In patients with ankylosing spondylitis, the rate of development of antibodies to adalimumab in HUMIRA-treated patients was comparable to patients with rheumatoid arthritis. In patients with psoriatic arthritis, the rate of antibody development in patients receiving HUMIRA monotherapy was comparable to patients with rheumatoid arthritis; however, in patients receiving concomitant methotrexate the rate was 7% compared to 1% in rheumatoid arthritis. In patients with Crohn's disease, the rate of antibody development was 2.6%. The immunogenicity rate was 8% for plaque psoriasis patients who were treated with HUMIRA monotherapy.

The data reflect the percentage of patients whose test results were considered positive for antibodies to adalimumab in an ELISA assay, and are highly dependent on the sensitivity and specificity of the assay. The observed incidence of antibody (including neutralizing antibody) positivity in an assay is highly dependent on several factors including assay sensitivity and specificity, assay methodology, sample handling, timing of sample collection, concomitant medications, and underlying disease. For these reasons, comparison of the incidence of antibodies to adalimumab with the incidence of antibodies to other products may be misleading.

Other Adverse Reactions

The data described below reflect exposure to HUMIRA in 2468 patients, including 2073 exposed for 6 months, 1497 exposed for greater than one year and 1380 in adequate and well-controlled studies (Studies RA-I, RA-II, RA-III, and RA-IV). HUMIRA was studied primarily in placebo-controlled trials and in long-term follow up studies for up to 36 months duration. The population had a mean age of 54 years, 77% were female, 91% were Caucasian and had moderately to severely active rheumatoid arthritis. Most patients received 40 mg HUMIRA every other week.

Table 1 summarizes reactions reported at a rate of at least 5% in patients treated with HUMIRA 40 mg every other week compared to placebo and with an incidence higher than placebo. Adverse reaction rates in patients treated with HUMIRA 40 mg weekly were similar to rates in patients treated with HUMIRA 40 mg every other week. In Study RA-III, the types and frequencies of adverse reactions in the second year open-label extension were similar to those observed in the one-year double-blind portion.

[See table 1 at top of next page]

Other Adverse Reactions

Other infrequent serious adverse reactions occurring at an incidence of less than 5% in rheumatoid arthritis patients treated with HUMIRA were:

Body As A Whole: Fever, infection, pain in extremity, pelvic pain, sepsis, surgery, thorax pain, tuberculosis reactivated

Cardiovascular System: Arrhythmia, atrial fibrillation, cardiovascular disorder, chest pain, congestive heart failure, coronary artery disorder, heart arrest, hypertensive encephalopathy, myocardial infarct, palpitation, pericardial effusion, pericarditis, syncope, tachycardia, vascular disorder

Collagen Disorder: Lupus erythematosus syndrome

Digestive System: Cholecystitis, cholelithiasis, esophagitis, gastroenteritis, gastrointestinal disorder, gastrointestinal hemorrhage, hepatic necrosis, vomiting

Endocrine System: Parathyroid disorder

Hemic And Lymphatic System: Agranulocytosis, granulocytopenia, leukopenia, lymphoma like reaction, pancytopenia, polycythemia *[see Warnings and Precautions (5.6)]*

Metabolic And Nutritional Disorders: Dehydration, healing abnormal, ketosis, paraproteinemia, peripheral edema

Musculo-Skeletal System: Arthritis, bone disorder, bone fracture (not spontaneous), bone necrosis, joint disorder, muscle cramps, myasthenia, pyogenic arthritis, synovitis, tendon disorder

Neoplasia: Adenoma, carcinomas such as breast, gastrointestinal, skin, urogenital, and others; lymphoma and melanoma

Nervous System: Confusion, multiple sclerosis, paresthesia, subdural hematoma, tremor

Respiratory System: Asthma, bronchospasm, dyspnea, lung disorder, lung function decreased, pleural effusion, pneumonia

Skin And Appendages: Cellulitis, erysipelas, herpes zoster

Special Senses: Cataract

Thrombosis: Thrombosis leg

Urogenital System: Cystitis, kidney calculus, menstrual disorder, pyelonephritis

Juvenile Idiopathic Arthritis Clinical Studies

In general, the adverse reactions in pediatric patients were similar in frequency and type to those seen in adult patients *[see Warnings and Precautions (5) and other sections under Adverse Reactions (6)]*. Important findings and differences from adults are discussed in the following paragraphs.

HUMIRA has been studied in 171 pediatric patients, 4 to 17 years of age, with polyarticular juvenile idiopathic arthritis. Severe adverse reactions reported in the study included neutropenia, streptococcal pharyngitis, increased aminotransferases, herpes zoster, myositis, metrorrhagia, appendicitis. Serious infections were observed in 4% of patients within approximately 2 years of initiation of treatment with HUMIRA and included cases of herpes simplex, pneumonia, urinary tract infection, pharyngitis, and herpes zoster.

A total of 45% of children experienced an infection while receiving HUMIRA with or without concomitant MTX in the first 16 weeks of treatment. The types of infections reported in juvenile idiopathic arthritis patients were generally similar to those commonly seen in outpatient JIA populations. Upon initiation of treatment, the most common adverse reactions occurring in the pediatric population treated with HUMIRA were injection site pain and injection site reaction (19% and 16%, respectively). A less commonly reported adverse event in children receiving HUMIRA was granuloma annulare which did not lead to discontinuation of HUMIRA treatment.

In the first 48 weeks of treatment, non-serious hypersensitivity reactions were seen in approximately 6% of children and included primarily localized allergic hypersensitivity reactions and allergic rash.

Isolated mild to moderate elevations of liver aminotransferases (ALT more common than AST) were observed in children with juvenile idiopathic arthritis exposed to HUMIRA alone; liver function tests (LFT) elevations were more frequent among those treated with the combination of HUMIRA and MTX. In general, these elevations did not lead to discontinuation of HUMIRA treatment.

In the juvenile idiopathic arthritis trial, 10% of patients treated with HUMIRA who had negative baseline anti-dsDNA antibodies developed positive titers after 48 weeks of treatment. No patient developed clinical signs of autoimmunity during the clinical trial.

Approximately 15% of children treated with HUMIRA developed mild-to-moderate elevations of creatine phosphokinase (CPK). Elevations exceeding 5 times the upper limit of normal were observed in several patients. CPK levels decreased or returned to normal in all patients. Most patients were able to continue HUMIRA without interruption.

Psoriatic Arthritis and Ankylosing Spondylitis Clinical Studies

HUMIRA has been studied in 395 patients with psoriatic arthritis in two placebo-controlled trials and in an open label study and in 393 patients with ankylosing spondylitis in two placebo-controlled studies. The safety profile for patients with psoriatic arthritis and ankylosing spondylitis treated with HUMIRA 40 mg every other week was similar to the safety profile seen in patients with rheumatoid arthritis, HUMIRA Studies RA-I through IV. In the clinical trials of patients with psoriatic arthritis and ankylosing spondylitis, elevations of aminotransferases were observed (ALT more common than AST) in a greater proportion of patients receiving HUMIRA than in controls, both when HUMIRA was given as monotherapy and when it was used in combination with other immunosuppressive agents. Most elevations of ALT and AST observed were in the range of 1.5 to 3 times the upper limit of normal. In general, patients who developed ALT and AST elevations were asymptomatic,

Table 1. Adverse Reactions Reported by ≥5% of Patients Treated with HUMIRA During Placebo-Controlled Period of Rheumatoid Arthritis Studies

Adverse Reaction (Preferred Term)	HUMIRA 40 mg subcutaneous Every Other Week (N=705) Percentage	Placebo (N=690) Percentage
Respiratory		
Upper respiratory infection	17	13
Sinusitis	11	9
Flu syndrome	7	6
Gastrointestinal		
Nausea	9	8
Abdominal pain	7	4
Laboratory Tests*		
Laboratory test abnormal	8	7
Hypercholesterolemia	6	4
Hyperlipidemia	7	5
Hematuria	5	4
Alkaline phosphatase increased	5	3
Other		
Injection site pain	12	12
Headache	12	8
Rash	12	6
Accidental injury	10	8
Injection site reaction**	8	1
Back pain	6	4
Urinary tract infection	8	5
Hypertension	5	3

* Laboratory test abnormalities were reported as adverse reactions in European trials

**Does not include erythema and/or itching, hemorrhage, pain or swelling

and the abnormalities decreased or resolved with either continuation or discontinuation of HUMIRA, or modification of concomitant medications.

Crohn's Disease Clinical Studies

HUMIRA has been studied in 1478 patients with Crohn's disease in four placebo-controlled and two open-label extension studies. The safety profile for patients with Crohn's disease treated with HUMIRA was similar to the safety profile seen in patients with rheumatoid arthritis.

Plaque Psoriasis Clinical Studies

HUMIRA has been studied in 1696 patients with plaque psoriasis in placebo-controlled and open-label extension studies. The safety profile for patients with plaque psoriasis treated with HUMIRA was similar to the safety profile seen in patients with rheumatoid arthritis with the following exceptions. In the placebo-controlled portions of the clinical trials in plaque psoriasis patients, HUMIRA-treated patients had a higher incidence of arthralgia when compared to controls (3% vs. 1%).

Elevations of aminotransferases were observed (ALT more common than AST) in a greater proportion of patients receiving HUMIRA than in controls. Most elevations of ALT and AST observed were in the range of 1.5 to 3 times the upper limit of normal. In general, patients who developed ALT and AST elevations were asymptomatic, and most of the abnormalities decreased or resolved with either continuation or discontinuation of HUMIRA.

6.2 Postmarketing Experience

Adverse reactions have been reported during post-approval use of HUMIRA. Because these reactions are reported voluntarily from a population of uncertain size, it is not always possible to reliably estimate their frequency or establish a causal relationship to HUMIRA exposure.

Hematologic reactions: Thrombocytopenia *[see Warnings and Precautions (5.6)]*

Hypersensitivity reactions: Anaphylaxis, angioneurotic edema *[see Warnings and Precautions (5.3)]*

Respiratory disorders: Interstitial lung disease, including pulmonary fibrosis

Skin reactions: Cutaneous vasculitis, erythema multiforme, new or worsening psoriasis (all sub-types including pustular and palmoplantar)

7 DRUG INTERACTIONS

7.1 Anakinra

Concurrent administration of anakinra (an interleukin-1 antagonist) and another TNF-blocking agent has been associated with an increased risk of serious infections, an increased risk of neutropenia and no additional benefit compared to these medicinal products alone. Therefore, the combination of anakinra with other TNF-blocking agents, including HUMIRA, may also result in similar toxicities *[see Warnings and Precautions (5.7)]*.

7.2 Live Vaccines

Live vaccines should not be given concurrently with HUMIRA *[see Warnings and Precautions (5.10)]*.

7.3 Methotrexate

HUMIRA has been studied in rheumatoid arthritis patients taking concomitant methotrexate. Although methotrexate reduced the apparent adalimumab clearance *[see Clinical Pharmacology (12.3)]*, the data do not suggest the need for dose adjustment of either HUMIRA or methotrexate.

8 USE IN SPECIFIC POPULATIONS

8.1 Pregnancy

Pregnancy Category B - An embryo-fetal perinatal developmental toxicity study has been performed in cynomolgus monkeys at dosages up to 100 mg/kg (266 times human AUC when given 40 mg subcutaneously with methotrexate every week or 373 times human AUC when given 40 mg subcutaneously without methotrexate) and has revealed no evidence of harm to the fetuses due to adalimumab. There are, however, no adequate and well-controlled studies in pregnant women. Because animal reproduction and developmental studies are not always predictive of human response, HUMIRA should be used during pregnancy only if clearly needed.

Pregnancy Registry: To monitor outcomes of pregnant women exposed to HUMIRA, a pregnancy registry has been established. Physicians are encouraged to register patients by calling 1-877-311-8972.

8.3 Nursing Mothers

It is not known whether adalimumab is excreted in human milk or absorbed systemically after ingestion. Because many drugs and immunoglobulins are excreted in human milk, and because of the potential for serious adverse reactions in nursing infants from HUMIRA, a decision should be made whether to discontinue nursing or to discontinue the drug, taking into account the importance of the drug to the mother.

8.4 Pediatric Use

Safety and efficacy of HUMIRA in pediatric patients for uses other than juvenile idiopathic arthritis have not been established.

Juvenile Idiopathic Arthritis

In the juvenile idiopathic arthritis study, HUMIRA was shown to reduce signs and symptoms of active polyarticular juvenile idiopathic arthritis in patients 4 to 17 years of age *[see Clinical Studies (14.2)]*. HUMIRA has not been studied in children less than 4 years of age, and there are limited data on HUMIRA treatment in children with weight <15 kg. Safety of HUMIRA in pediatric patients was generally similar to that observed in adults with certain exceptions *[see Adverse Reactions (6.1)]*.

8.5 Geriatric Use

A total of 519 rheumatoid arthritis patients 65 years of age and older, including 107 patients 75 years of age and older, received HUMIRA in clinical studies RA-I through IV. No overall difference in effectiveness was observed between these subjects and younger subjects. The frequency of serious infection and malignancy among HUMIRA treated sub-

---

Information on the Abbott Pharmaceutical Products listed on these pages is from the prescribing information in use as of June 1, 2010. For more information, please visit rxabbott.com or call 1-800-633-9110.

Table 2. ACR Responses in Studies RA-II and RA-III (Percent of Patients)

	Study RA-II Monotherapy (26 weeks)			Study RA-III Methotrexate Combination (24 and 52 weeks)	
Response	Placebo	HUMIRA 40 mg every other week	HUMIRA 40 mg weekly	Placebo/MTX	HUMIRA/MTX 40 mg every other week
	N=110	N=113	N=103	N=200	N=207
ACR20					
Month 6	19%	46%*	53%*	30%	63%*
Month 12	NA	NA	NA	24%	59%*
ACR50					
Month 6	8%	22%*	35%*	10%	39%*
Month 12	NA	NA	NA	10%	42%*
ACR70					
Month 6	2%	12%*	18%*	3%	21%*
Month 12	NA	NA	NA	5%	23%*

*p<0.01, HUMIRA *vs.* placebo

jects over 65 years of age was higher than for those under 65 years of age. Because there is a higher incidence of infections and malignancies in the elderly population in general, caution should be used when treating the elderly.

10 OVERDOSAGE

Doses up to 10 mg/kg have been administered to patients in clinical trials without evidence of dose-limiting toxicities. In case of overdosage, it is recommended that the patient be monitored for any signs or symptoms of adverse reactions or effects and appropriate symptomatic treatment instituted immediately.

11 DESCRIPTION

HUMIRA (adalimumab) is a recombinant human IgG1 monoclonal antibody specific for human tumor necrosis factor (TNF). HUMIRA was created using phage display technology resulting in an antibody with human derived heavy and light chain variable regions and human IgG1:k constant regions. Adalimumab is produced by recombinant DNA technology in a mammalian cell expression system and is purified by a process that includes specific viral inactivation and removal steps. It consists of 1330 amino acids and has a molecular weight of approximately 148 kilodaltons.

HUMIRA is supplied as a sterile, preservative-free solution of adalimumab for subcutaneous administration. The drug product is supplied as either a single-use, prefilled pen (HUMIRA Pen) or as a single-dose, 1 mL prefilled glass syringe. Enclosed within the pen is a single-use, 1 mL prefilled glass syringe. The solution of HUMIRA is clear and colorless, with a pH of about 5.2. Each prefilled syringe delivers 0.8 mL (40 mg) of drug product. Each 0.8 mL of HUMIRA contains 40 mg adalimumab, 4.93 mg sodium chloride, 0.69 mg monobasic sodium phosphate dihydrate, 1.22 mg dibasic sodium phosphate dihydrate, 0.24 mg sodium citrate, 1.04 mg citric acid monohydrate, 9.6 mg mannitol, 0.8 mg polysorbate 80, and Water for Injection, USP. Sodium hydroxide added as necessary to adjust pH. Each pediatric prefilled syringe delivers 0.4 mL (20 mg) of drug product. Each 0.4 mL of HUMIRA contains 20 mg adalimumab, 2.47 mg sodium chloride, 0.34 mg monobasic sodium phosphate dihydrate, 0.61 mg dibasic sodium phosphate dihydrate, 0.12 mg sodium citrate, 0.52 mg citric acid monohydrate, 4.8 mg mannitol, 0.4 mg polysorbate 80, and Water for Injection, USP. Sodium hydroxide added as necessary to adjust pH.

12 CLINICAL PHARMACOLOGY

12.1 Mechanism of Action

Adalimumab binds specifically to TNF-alpha and blocks its interaction with the p55 and p75 cell surface TNF receptors. Adalimumab also lyses surface TNF expressing cells *in vitro* in the presence of complement. Adalimumab does not bind or inactivate lymphotoxin (TNF-beta). TNF is a naturally occurring cytokine that is involved in normal inflammatory and immune responses. Elevated levels of TNF are found in the synovial fluid of rheumatoid arthritis, including juvenile idiopathic arthritis, psoriatic arthritis, and ankylosing spondylitis patients and play an important role in both the pathologic inflammation and the joint destruction that are hallmarks of these diseases. Increased levels of TNF are also found in psoriasis (Ps) plaques. In plaque psoriasis, treatment with HUMIRA may reduce the epidermal thickness and infiltration of inflammatory cells. The relationship between these pharmacodynamic activities and the mechanism(s) by which HUMIRA exerts its clinical effects is unknown.

Adalimumab also modulates biological responses that are induced or regulated by TNF, including changes in the levels of adhesion molecules responsible for leukocyte migration (ELAM-1, VCAM-1, and ICAM-1 with an IC_{50} of 1-2 × 10^{-10} M).

12.2 Pharmacodynamics

After treatment with HUMIRA, a decrease in levels of acute phase reactants of inflammation (C-reactive protein [CRP] and erythrocyte sedimentation rate [ESR]) and serum cytokines (IL-6) was observed compared to baseline in patients with rheumatoid arthritis. A decrease in CRP levels was also observed in patients with Crohn's disease. Serum levels of matrix metalloproteinases (MMP-1 and MMP-3) that produce tissue remodeling responsible for cartilage destruction were also decreased after HUMIRA administration.

12.3 Pharmacokinetics

The maximum serum concentration (C_{max}) and the time to reach the maximum concentration (T_{max}) were 4.7 ± 1.6 μg/mL and 131 ± 56 hours respectively, following a single 40 mg subcutaneous administration of HUMIRA to healthy adult subjects. The average absolute bioavailability of adalimumab estimated from three studies following a single 40 mg subcutaneous dose was 64%. The pharmacokinetics of adalimumab were linear over the dose range of 0.5 to 10.0 mg/kg following a single intravenous dose.

The single dose pharmacokinetics of adalimumab in rheumatoid arthritis (RA) patients were determined in several studies with intravenous doses ranging from 0.25 to 10 mg/kg. The distribution volume (V_{ss}) ranged from 4.7 to 6.0 L. The systemic clearance of adalimumab is approximately 12 mL/hr. The mean terminal half-life was approximately 2 weeks, ranging from 10 to 20 days across studies. Adalimumab concentrations in the synovial fluid from five rheumatoid arthritis patients ranged from 31 to 96% of those in serum.

In RA patients receiving 40 mg HUMIRA every other week, adalimumab mean steady-state trough concentrations of approximately 5 μg/mL and 8 to 9 μg/mL, were observed without and with methotrexate (MTX), respectively. MTX reduced adalimumab apparent clearance after single and multiple dosing by 29% and 44% respectively, in patients with RA. Mean serum adalimumab trough levels at steady state increased approximately proportionally with dose following 20, 40, and 80 mg every other week and every week subcutaneous dosing. In long-term studies with dosing more than two years, there was no evidence of changes in clearance over time.

Adalimumab mean steady-state trough concentrations were slightly higher in psoriatic arthritis patients treated with 40 mg HUMIRA every other week (6 to 10 μg/mL and 8.5 to 12 μg/mL, without and with MTX, respectively) compared to the concentrations in RA patients treated with the same dose.

The pharmacokinetics of adalimumab in patients with ankylosing spondylitis were similar to those in patients with RA.

In patients with Crohn's disease, the loading dose of 160 mg HUMIRA on Week 0 followed by 80 mg HUMIRA on Week 2 achieves mean serum adalimumab trough levels of approximately 12 μg/mL at Week 2 and Week 4. Mean steady-state trough levels of approximately 7 μg/mL were observed at Week 24 and Week 56 in Crohn's disease patients after receiving a maintenance dose of 40 mg HUMIRA every other week.

In patients with plaque psoriasis, the mean steady-state trough concentration was approximately 5 to 6 μg/mL during adalimumab 40 mg every other week monotherapy treatment.

Population pharmacokinetic analyses in patients with RA revealed that there was a trend toward higher apparent clearance of adalimumab in the presence of anti-adalimumab antibodies, and lower clearance with increasing age in patients aged 40 to >75 years.

Minor increases in apparent clearance were also predicted in RA patients receiving doses lower than the recommended dose and in RA patients with high rheumatoid factor or CRP concentrations. These increases are not likely to be clinically important.

No gender-related pharmacokinetic differences were observed after correction for a patient's body weight. Healthy volunteers and patients with rheumatoid arthritis displayed similar adalimumab pharmacokinetics.

No pharmacokinetic data are available in patients with hepatic or renal impairment.

In subjects with juvenile idiopathic arthritis (4 to 17 years of age), the mean steady-state trough serum adalimumab concentrations for subjects weighing <30 kg receiving 20 mg HUMIRA subcutaneously every other week as monotherapy or with concomitant methotrexate were 6.8 μg/mL and 10.9 μg/mL, respectively. The mean steady-state trough serum adalimumab concentrations for subjects weighing ≥30 kg receiving 40 mg HUMIRA subcutaneously every other week as monotherapy or with concomitant methotrexate were 6.6 μg/mL and 8.1 μg/mL, respectively.

13 NONCLINICAL TOXICOLOGY

13.1 Carcinogenesis, Mutagenesis, Impairment of Fertility

Long-term animal studies of HUMIRA have not been conducted to evaluate the carcinogenic potential or its effect on fertility. No clastogenic or mutagenic effects of HUMIRA were observed in the *in vivo* mouse micronucleus test or the *Salmonella-Escherichia coli* (Ames) assay, respectively.

14 CLINICAL STUDIES

14.1 Rheumatoid Arthritis

The efficacy and safety of HUMIRA were assessed in five randomized, double-blind studies in patients ≥18 years of age with active rheumatoid arthritis diagnosed according to American College of Rheumatology (ACR) criteria. Patients had at least 6 swollen and 9 tender joints. HUMIRA was administered subcutaneously in combination with methotrexate (MTX) (12.5 to 25 mg, Studies RA-I, RA-III and RA-V) or as monotherapy (Studies RA-II and RA-V) or with other disease-modifying anti-rheumatic drugs (DMARDs) (Study RA-IV).

Study RA-I evaluated 271 patients who had failed therapy with at least one but no more than four DMARDs and had inadequate response to MTX. Doses of 20, 40 or 80 mg of HUMIRA or placebo were given every other week for 24 weeks.

Study RA-II evaluated 544 patients who had failed therapy with at least one DMARD. Doses of placebo, 20 or 40 mg of HUMIRA were given as monotherapy every other week or weekly for 26 weeks.

Study RA-III evaluated 619 patients who had an inadequate response to MTX. Patients received placebo, 40 mg of HUMIRA every other week with placebo injections on alternate weeks, or 20 mg of HUMIRA weekly for up to 52 weeks. Study RA-III had an additional primary endpoint at 52 weeks of inhibition of disease progression (as detected by X-ray results). Upon completion of the first 52 weeks, 457 patients enrolled in an open-label extension phase in which 40 mg of HUMIRA was administered every other week for up to 5 years.

Study RA-IV assessed safety in 636 patients who were either DMARD-naive or were permitted to remain on their pre-existing rheumatologic therapy provided that therapy was stable for a minimum of 28 days. Patients were randomized to 40 mg of HUMIRA or placebo every other week for 24 weeks.

Study RA-V evaluated 799 patients with moderately to severely active rheumatoid arthritis of less than 3 years duration who were ≥18 years old and MTX naïve. Patients were randomized to receive either MTX (optimized to 20 mg/week by week 8), HUMIRA 40 mg every other week or HUMIRA/MTX combination therapy for 104 weeks. Patients were evaluated for signs and symptoms, and for radiographic progression of joint damage. The median disease duration among patients enrolled in the study was 5 months. The median MTX dose achieved was 20 mg.

Clinical Response

The percent of HUMIRA treated patients achieving ACR 20, 50 and 70 responses in Studies RA-II and III are shown in Table 2.

[See table 2 above]

The results of Study RA-I were similar to Study RA-III; patients receiving HUMIRA 40 mg every other week in Study RA-I also achieved ACR 20, 50 and 70 response rates of 65%, 52% and 24%, respectively, compared to placebo responses of 13%, 7% and 3% respectively, at 6 months (p<0.01).

The results of the components of the ACR response criteria for Studies RA-II and RA-III are shown in Table 3. ACR response rates and improvement in all components of ACR response were maintained to week 104. Over the 2 years in Study RA-III, 20% of HUMIRA patients receiving 40 mg every other week (EOW) achieved a major clinical response, defined as maintenance of an ACR 70 response over a 6-month period.

ACR responses were maintained in similar proportions of patients for up to 5 years with continuous HUMIRA treatment in the open-label portion of Study RA-III.
[See table 3 at right]

The time course of ACR 20 response for Study RA-III is shown in Figure 1.

In Study RA-III, 85% of patients with ACR 20 responses at week 24 maintained the response at 52 weeks. The time course of ACR 20 response for Study RA-I and Study RA-II were similar.

Figure 1: Study RA-III ACR 20 Responses over 52 Weeks

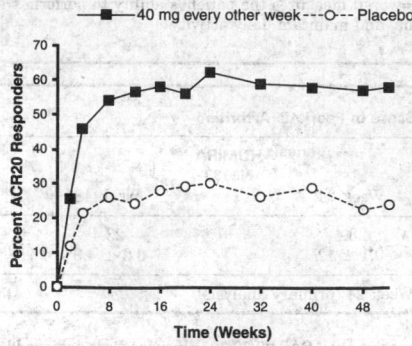

In Study RA-IV, 53% of patients treated with HUMIRA 40 mg every other week plus standard of care had an ACR 20 response at week 24 compared to 35% on placebo plus standard of care (p<0.001). No unique adverse reactions related to the combination of HUMIRA (adalimumab) and other DMARDs were observed.

In Study RA-V with MTX naïve patients with recent onset rheumatoid arthritis, the combination treatment with HUMIRA plus MTX led to greater percentages of patients achieving ACR responses than either MTX monotherapy or HUMIRA monotherapy at Week 52 and responses were sustained at Week 104 (see Table 4).

Table 4. ACR Response in Study RA-V (Percent of Patients)

Response	MTX[b] N=257	HUMIRA[c] N=274	HUMIRA/MTX N=268
ACR20			
Week 52	63%	54%	73%
Week 104	56%	49%	69%
ACR50			
Week 52	46%	41%	62%
Week 104	43%	37%	59%
ACR70			
Week 52	27%	26%	46%
Week 104	28%	28%	47%
Major Clinical Response[a]	28%	25%	49%

[a] Major clinical response is defined as achieving an ACR70 response for a continuous six month period
[b] p<0.05, HUMIRA/MTX vs. MTX for ACR 20
p<0.001, HUMIRA/MTX vs. MTX for ACR 50 and 70, and Major Clinical Response
[c] p<0.001, HUMIRA/MTX vs. HUMIRA

At Week 52, all individual components of the ACR response criteria for Study RA-V improved in the HUMIRA/MTX group and improvements were maintained to Week 104.
Radiographic Response
In Study RA-III, structural joint damage was assessed radiographically and expressed as change in Total Sharp Score (TSS) and its components, the erosion score and Joint Space Narrowing (JSN) score, at month 12 compared to baseline. At baseline, the median TSS was approximately 55 in the placebo and 40 mg every other week groups. The results are shown in Table 5. HUMIRA/MTX treated patients demonstrated less radiographic progression than patients receiving MTX alone at 52 weeks.
[See table 5 above]
In the open-label extension of Study RA-III, 77% of the original patients treated with any dose of HUMIRA were evaluated radiographically at 2 years. Patients maintained inhibition of structural damage, as measured by the TSS. Fifty-four percent had no progression of structural damage as defined by a change in the TSS of zero or less.

Table 3. Components of ACR Response in Studies RA-II and RA-III

	Study RA-II				Study RA-III			
	Placebo N=110		HUMIRA[a] N=113		Placebo/MTX N=200		HUMIRA[a]/MTX N=207	
Parameter (median)	Baseline	Wk 26	Baseline	Wk 26	Baseline	Wk 24	Baseline	Wk 24
Number of tender joints (0-68)	35	26	31	16*	26	15	24	8*
Number of swollen joints (0-66)	19	16	18	10*	17	11	18	5*
Physician global assessment[b]	7.0	6.1	6.6	3.7*	6.3	3.5	6.5	2.0*
Patient global assessment[b]	7.5	6.3	7.5	4.5*	5.4	3.9	5.2	2.0*
Pain[b]	7.3	6.1	7.3	4.1*	6.0	3.8	5.8	2.1*
Disability index (HAQ)[c]	2.0	1.9	1.9	1.5*	1.5	1.3	1.5	0.8*
CRP (mg/dL)	3.9	4.3	4.6	1.8*	1.0	0.9	1.0	0.4*

[a] 40 mg HUMIRA administered every other week
[b] Visual analogue scale; 0 = best, 10 = worst
[c] Disability Index of the Health Assessment Questionnaire; 0 = best, 3 = worst, measures the patient's ability to perform the following: dress/groom, arise, eat, walk, reach, grip, maintain hygiene, and maintain daily activity
*p<0.001, HUMIRA vs. placebo, based on mean change from baseline

Table 5. Radiographic Mean Changes Over 12 Months in Study RA-III

	Placebo/MTX	HUMIRA/MTX 40 mg every other week	Placebo/MTX-HUMIRA/MTX (95% Confidence Interval*)	P-value**
Total Sharp score	2.7	0.1	2.6 (1.4, 3.8)	<0.001
Erosion score	1.6	0.0	1.6 (0.9, 2.2)	<0.001
JSN score	1.0	0.1	0.9 (0.3, 1.4)	0.002

* 95% confidence intervals for the differences in change scores between MTX and HUMIRA.
** Based on rank analysis

Table 6. Radiographic Mean Change* in Study RA-V

		MTX[a] N=257	HUMIRA[a,b] N=274	HUMIRA/MTX N=268
52 Weeks	Total Sharp score	5.7 (4.2, 7.3)	3.0 (1.7, 4.3)	1.3 (0.5, 2.1)
	Erosion score	3.7 (2.7, 4.8)	1.7 (1.0, 2.4)	0.8 (0.4, 1.2)
	JSN score	2.0 (1.2, 2.8)	1.3 (0.5, 2.1)	0.5 (0.0, 1.0)
104 Weeks	Total Sharp score	10.4 (7.7, 13.2)	5.5 (3.6, 7.4)	1.9 (0.9, 2.9)
	Erosion score	6.4 (4.6, 8.2)	3.0 (2.0, 4.0)	1.0 (0.4, 1.6)
	JSN score	4.1 (2.7, 5.4)	2.6 (1.5, 3.7)	0.9 (0.3, 1.5)

* mean (95% confidence interval)
[a] p<0.001, HUMIRA/MTX vs. MTX at 52 and 104 weeks and for HUMIRA/MTX vs. HUMIRA at 104 weeks
[b] p<0.01, for HUMIRA/MTX vs. HUMIRA at 52 weeks

Fifty-five percent (55%) of patients originally treated with 40 mg HUMIRA every other week have been evaluated radiographically at 5 years. Patients had continued inhibition of structural damage with 50% showing no progression of structural damage defined by a change in the TSS of zero or less.
In Study RA-V, structural joint damage was assessed as in Study RA-III. Greater inhibition of radiographic progression, as assessed by changes in TSS, erosion score and JSN was observed in the HUMIRA/MTX combination group as compared to either the MTX or HUMIRA monotherapy group at Week 52 as well as at Week 104 (see Table 6).
[See table 6 above]
Physical Function Response
In studies RA-I through IV, HUMIRA showed significantly greater improvement than placebo in the disability index of Health Assessment Questionnaire (HAQ-DI) from baseline to the end of study, and significantly greater improvement than placebo in the health-outcomes as assessed by The Short Form Health Survey (SF 36). Improvement was seen in both the Physical Component Summary (PCS) and the Mental Component Summary (MCS).
In Study RA-III, the mean (95% CI) improvement in HAQ-DI from baseline at week 52 was 0.60 (0.55, 0.65) for the HUMIRA patients and 0.25 (0.17, 0.33) for placebo/MTX (p<0.001) patients. Sixty-three percent of HUMIRA-treated patients achieved a 0.5 or greater improvement in HAQ-DI at week 52 in the double-blind portion of the study. Eighty-two percent of these patients maintained that improvement through week 104 and a similar proportion of patients maintained this response through week 260 (5 years) of open-label treatment. Mean improvement in the SF-36 was maintained through the end of measurement at week 156 (3 years).
In Study RA-V, the HAQ-DI and the physical component of the SF-36 showed greater improvement (p<0.001) for the HUMIRA/MTX combination therapy group versus either the MTX monotherapy or the HUMIRA monotherapy group at Week 52, which was maintained through Week 104.

14.2   Juvenile Idiopathic Arthritis
The safety and efficacy of HUMIRA were assessed in a multicenter, randomized, withdrawal, double-blind, parallel-group study in 171 children (4 to 17 years of age) with polyarticular juvenile idiopathic arthritis (JIA). In the study, the patients were stratified into two groups: MTX-treated or non-MTX-treated. All subjects had to show signs of active moderate or severe disease despite previous treatment with NSAIDs, analgesics, corticosteroids, or DMARDS. Subjects who received prior treatment with any biologic DMARDS were excluded from the study.
The study included four phases: an open-label lead in phase (OL-LI; 16 weeks), a double-blind randomized withdrawal phase (DB; 32 weeks), an open-label extension phase (OLE-BSA; up to 136 weeks), and an open-label fixed dose phase (OLE-FD; 16 weeks). In the first three phases of the study, HUMIRA was administered based on body surface area at a dose of 24 mg/m² up to a maximum total body dose of 40 mg subcutaneously (SC) every other week. In the OLE-FD phase, the patients were treated with 20 mg of HUMIRA SC every other week if their weight was less than 30 kg and with 40 mg of HUMIRA SC every other week if their weight was 30 kg or greater. Patients remained on stable doses of NSAIDs and or prednisone (≤0.2 mg/kg/day or 10 mg/day maximum).
Patients demonstrating a Pediatric ACR 30 response at the end of OL-LI phase were randomized into the double blind (DB) phase of the study and received either HUMIRA or placebo every other week for 32 weeks or until disease flare. Disease flare was defined as a worsening of ≥30% from baseline in ≥3 of 6 Pediatric ACR core criteria, ≥2 active joints, and improvement of >30% in no more than 1 of the 6 criteria. After 32 weeks or at the time of disease flare during

Information on the Abbott Pharmaceutical Products listed on these pages is from the prescribing information in use as of June 1, 2010. For more information, please visit rxabbott.com or call 1-800-633-9110.

the DB phase, patients were treated in the open-label extension phase based on the BSA regimen (OLE-BSA), before converting to a fixed dose regimen based on body weight (OLE-FD phase).

Clinical Response

At the end of the 16-week OL-LI phase, 94% of the patients in the MTX stratum and 74% of the patients in the non-MTX stratum were Pediatric ACR 30 responders. In the DB phase significantly fewer patients who received HUMIRA experienced disease flare compared to placebo, both without MTX (43% vs. 71%) and with MTX (37% vs. 65%). More patients treated with HUMIRA continued to show pediatric ACR 30/50/70 responses at Week 48 compared to patients treated with placebo.

Pediatric ACR responses were maintained for up to two years in the OLE phase in patients who received HUMIRA throughout the study.

14.3   Psoriatic Arthritis

The safety and efficacy of HUMIRA was assessed in two randomized, double-blind, placebo controlled studies in 413 patients with psoriatic arthritis. Upon completion of both studies, 383 patients enrolled in an open-label extension study, in which 40 mg HUMIRA was administered every other week.

Study PsA-I enrolled 313 adult patients with moderately to severely active psoriatic arthritis (>3 swollen and >3 tender joints) who had an inadequate response to NSAID therapy in one of the following forms: (1) distal interphalangeal (DIP) involvement (N=23); (2) polyarticular arthritis (absence of rheumatoid nodules and presence of plaque psoriasis) (N=210); (3) arthritis mutilans (N=1); (4) asymmetric psoriatic arthritis (N=77); or (5) ankylosing spondylitis-like (N=2). Patients on MTX therapy (158 of 313 patients) at enrollment (stable dose of ≤30 mg/week for >1 month) could continue MTX at the same dose. Doses of HUMIRA 40 mg or placebo every other week were administered during the 24-week double-blind period of the study.

Compared to placebo, treatment with HUMIRA resulted in improvements in the measures of disease activity (see Tables 7 and 8). Among patients with psoriatic arthritis who received HUMIRA, the clinical responses were apparent in some patients at the time of the first visit (two weeks) and were maintained up to 88 weeks in the ongoing open-label study. Similar responses were seen in patients with each of the subtypes of psoriatic arthritis, although few patients were enrolled with the arthritis mutilans and ankylosing spondylitis-like subtypes. Responses were similar in patients who were or were not receiving concomitant MTX therapy at baseline.

Patients with psoriatic involvement of at least three percent body surface area (BSA) were evaluated for Psoriatic Area and Severity Index (PASI) responses. At 24 weeks, the proportions of patients achieving a 75% or 90% improvement in the PASI were 59% and 42% respectively, in the HUMIRA group (N=69), compared to 1% and 0% respectively, in the placebo group (N=69) (p<0.001). PASI responses were apparent in some patients at the time of the first visit (two weeks). Responses were similar in patients who were or were not receiving concomitant MTX therapy.

Table 7. ACR Response in Study PsA-I (Percent of Patients)

Response	Placebo N=162	HUMIRA* N=151
ACR20		
Week 12	14%	58%
Week 24	15%	57%
ACR50		
Week 12	4%	36%
Week 24	6%	39%
ACR70		
Week 12	1%	20%
Week 24	1%	23%

*p<0.001 for all comparisons between HUMIRA and placebo

[See table 8 above]

Similar results were seen in an additional, 12-week study in 100 patients with moderate to severe psoriatic arthritis who had suboptimal response to DMARD therapy as manifested by ≥3 tender joints and ≥3 swollen joints at enrollment.

Radiographic Response

Radiographic changes were assessed in the psoriatic arthritis studies. Radiographs of hands, wrists, and feet were obtained at baseline and Week 24 during the double-blind period when patients were on HUMIRA or placebo and at Week 48 when all patients were on open-label HUMIRA. A modified Total Sharp Score (mTSS), which included distal interphalangeal joints (i.e., not identical to the TSS used for rheumatoid arthritis), was used by readers blinded to treatment group to assess the radiographs.

Table 8. Components of Disease Activity in Study PsA-I

Parameter: median	Placebo N=162 Baseline	Placebo N=162 24 weeks	HUMIRA* N=151 Baseline	HUMIRA* N=151 24 weeks
Number of tender joints[a]	23.0	17.0	20.0	5.0
Number of swollen joints[b]	11.0	9.0	11.0	3.0
Physician global assessment[c]	53.0	49.0	55.0	16.0
Patient global assessment[c]	49.5	49.0	48.0	20.0
Pain[c]	49.0	49.0	54.0	20.0
Disability index (HAQ)[d]	1.0	0.9	1.0	0.4
CRP (mg/dL)[e]	0.8	0.7	0.8	0.2

*p<0.001 for HUMIRA vs. placebo comparisons based on median changes
[a] Scale 0-78
[b] Scale 0-76
[c] Visual analog scale; 0=best, 100=worst
[d] Disability Index of the Health Assessment Questionnaire; 0=best, 3=worst; measures the patient's ability to perform the following: dress/groom, arise, eat, walk, reach, grip, maintain hygiene, and maintain daily activity.
[e] Normal range: 0-0.287 mg/dL

Table 9. Change in Modified Total Sharp Score in Psoriatic Arthritis

	Placebo N=141 Week 24	HUMIRA N=133 Week 24	HUMIRA N=133 Week 48
Baseline mean	22.1	23.4	23.4
Mean Change ± SD	0.9 ± 3.1	-0.1 ± 1.7	-0.2 ± 4.9*

*<0.001 for the difference between HUMIRA, Week 48 and Placebo, Week 24 (primary analysis)

HUMIRA-treated patients demonstrated greater inhibition of radiographic progression compared to placebo-treated patients and this effect was maintained at 48 weeks (see Table 9).

[See table 9 above]

Physical Function Response

In Study PsA-I, physical function and disability were assessed using the HAQ Disability Index (HAQ-DI) and the SF-36 Health Survey. Patients treated with 40 mg of HUMIRA every other week showed greater improvement from baseline in the HAQ-DI score (mean decreases of 47% and 49% at Weeks 12 and 24 respectively) in comparison to placebo (mean decreases of 1% and 3% at Weeks 12 and 24 respectively). At Weeks 12 and 24, patients treated with HUMIRA showed greater improvement from baseline in the SF-36 Physical Component Summary score compared to patients treated with placebo, and no worsening in the SF-36 Mental Component Summary score. Improvement in physical function based on the HAQ-DI was maintained for up to 84 weeks through the open-label portion of the study.

14.4   Ankylosing Spondylitis

The safety and efficacy of HUMIRA 40 mg every other week was assessed in 315 adult patients in a randomized, 24-week double-blind, placebo-controlled study in patients with active ankylosing spondylitis (AS) who had an inadequate response to glucocorticoids, NSAIDs, analgesics, methotrexate or sulfasalazine. Active AS was defined as patients who fulfilled at least two of the following three criteria: (1) a Bath AS disease activity index (BASDAI) score ≥4 cm, (2) a visual analog score (VAS) for total back pain ≥ 40 mm, and (3) morning stiffness ≥ 1 hour. The blinded period was followed by an open-label period during which patients received HUMIRA 40 mg every other week subcutaneously for up to an additional 28 weeks.

Improvement in measures of disease activity was first observed at Week 2 and maintained through 24 weeks as shown in Figure 2 and Table 10.

Responses of patients with total spinal ankylosis (n=11) were similar to those without total ankylosis.

Figure 2: ASAS 20 Response By Visit, Study AS-I

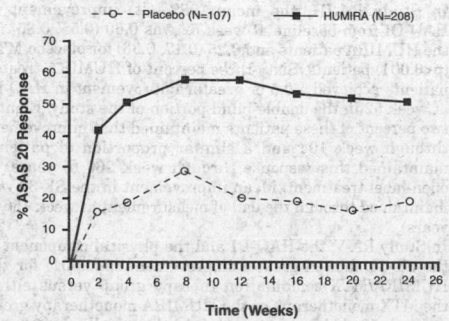

At 12 weeks, the ASAS 20/50/70 responses were achieved by 58%, 38%, and 23%, respectively, of patients receiving HUMIRA, compared to 21%, 10%, and 5% respectively, of patients receiving placebo (p <0.001). Similar responses were seen at Week 24 and sustained in patients receiving open-label HUMIRA for up to 52 weeks.

A greater proportion of patients treated with HUMIRA (22%) achieved a low level of disease activity at 24 weeks (defined as a value <20 [on a scale of 0 to 100 mm] in each of the four ASAS response parameters) compared to patients treated with placebo (6%).

[See table 10 at top of next page]

A second randomized, multicenter, double-blind, placebo-controlled study of 82 patients with ankylosing spondylitis showed similar results.

Patients treated with HUMIRA achieved improvement from baseline in the Ankylosing Spondylitis Quality of Life Questionnaire (ASQoL) score (-3.6 vs. -1.1) and in the Short Form Health Survey (SF-36) Physical Component Summary (PCS) score (7.4 vs. 1.9) compared to placebo-treated patients at Week 24.

14.5   Crohn's Disease

The safety and efficacy of multiple doses of HUMIRA were assessed in adult patients with moderately to severely active Crohn's disease (Crohn's Disease Activity Index (CDAI) ≥ 220 and ≤ 450) in randomized, double-blind, placebo-controlled studies. Concomitant stable doses of aminosalicylates, corticosteroids, and/or immunomodulatory agents were permitted, and 79% of patients continued to receive at least one of these medications.

Induction of clinical remission (defined as CDAI < 150) was evaluated in two studies. In Study CD-I, 299 TNF-blocker naïve patients were randomized to one of four treatment groups: the placebo group received placebo at Weeks 0 and 2, the 160/80 group received 160 mg HUMIRA at Week 0 and 80 mg at Week 2, the 80/40 group received 80 mg at Week 0 and 40 mg at Week 2, and the 40/20 group received 40 mg at Week 0 and 20 mg at Week 2. Clinical results were assessed at Week 4.

In the second induction study, Study CD-II, 325 patients who had lost response to, or were intolerant to, previous infliximab therapy were randomized to receive either 160 mg HUMIRA at Week 0 and 80 mg at Week 2, or placebo at Weeks 0 and 2. Clinical results were assessed at Week 4.

Maintenance of clinical remission was evaluated in Study CD-III. In this study, 854 patients with active disease received open-label HUMIRA, 80 mg at week 0 and 40 mg at Week 2. Patients were then randomized at Week 4 to 40 mg HUMIRA every other week, 40 mg HUMIRA every week, or placebo. The total study duration was 56 weeks. Patients in clinical response (decrease in CDAI ≥70) at Week 4 were stratified and analyzed separately from those not in clinical response at Week 4.

Induction of Clinical Remission

A greater percentage of the patients treated with 160/80 mg HUMIRA achieved induction of clinical remission versus

placebo at Week 4 regardless of whether the patients were TNF blocker naïve (CD-I), or had lost response to or were intolerant to infliximab (CD-II) (see Table 11).
[See table 11 at right]

Maintenance of Clinical Remission
In Study CD-III at Week 4, 58% (499/854) of patients were in clinical response and were assessed in the primary analysis. At Weeks 26 and 56, greater proportions of patients who were in clinical response at Week 4 achieved clinical remission in the HUMIRA 40 mg every other week maintenance group compared to patients in the placebo maintenance group (see Table 12). The group that received HUMIRA therapy every week did not demonstrate significantly higher remission rates compared to the group that received HUMIRA every other week.

Table 12. Maintenance of Clinical Remission in CD-III (Percent of Patients)

	Placebo N=170	40 mg HUMIRA every other week N=172
Week 26		
Clinical remission	17%	40%*
Clinical response	28%	54%*
Week 56		
Clinical remission	12%	36%*
Clinical response	18%	43%*

Clinical remission is CDAI score < 150; clinical response is decrease in CDAI of at least 70 points.

*p<0.001 for HUMIRA *vs.* placebo pairwise comparisons of proportions

Of those in response at Week 4 who attained remission during the study, patients in the HUMIRA every other week group maintained remission for a longer time than patients in the placebo maintenance group. Among patients who were not in response by Week 12, therapy continued beyond 12 weeks did not result in significantly more responses.

14.6   Plaque Psoriasis
The safety and efficacy of HUMIRA were assessed in randomized, double-blind, placebo-controlled studies in 1696 adult patients with moderate to severe chronic plaque psoriasis who were candidates for systemic therapy or phototherapy.
Study Ps-I evaluated 1212 patients with chronic plaque psoriasis with ≥10% body surface area (BSA) involvement, Physician's Global Assessment (PGA) of at least moderate disease severity, and Psoriasis Area and Severity Index (PASI) ≥12 within three treatment periods. In period A, patients received placebo or HUMIRA at an initial dose of 80 mg at Week 0 followed by a dose of 40 mg every other week starting at Week 1. After 16 weeks of therapy, patients who achieved at least a PASI 75 response at Week 16, defined as a PASI score improvement of at least 75% relative to baseline, entered period B and received open-label 40 mg HUMIRA every other week. After 17 weeks of open label therapy, patients who maintained at least a PASI 75 response at Week 33 and were originally randomized to active therapy in period A were re-randomized in period C to receive 40 mg HUMIRA every other week or placebo for an additional 19 weeks. Across all treatment groups the mean baseline PASI score was 19 and the baseline Physician's Global Assessment score ranged from "moderate" (53%) to "severe" (41%) to "very severe" (6%).
Study Ps-II evaluated 99 patients randomized to HUMIRA and 48 patients randomized to placebo with chronic plaque psoriasis with ≥10% BSA involvement and PASI ≥12. Patients received placebo, or an initial dose of 80 mg HUMIRA at Week 0 followed by 40 mg every other week starting at Week 1 for 16 weeks. Across all treatment groups the mean baseline PASI score was 21 and the baseline PGA score ranged from "moderate" (41%) to "severe" (51%) to "very severe" (8%).
Studies Ps-I and II evaluated the proportion of patients who achieved "clear" or "minimal" disease on the 6-point PGA scale and the proportion of patients who achieved a reduction in PASI score of at least 75% (PASI 75) from baseline at Week 16 (see Table 13 and 14).
Additionally, Study Ps-I evaluated the proportion of subjects who maintained a PGA of "clear" or "minimal" disease or a PASI 75 response after Week 33 and on or before Week 52.

Table 10. Components of Ankylosing Spondylitis Disease Activity

	Placebo N=107		HUMIRA N=208	
	Baseline mean	Week 24 mean	Baseline mean	Week 24 mean
ASAS 20 Response Criteria*				
Patient's Global Assessment of Disease Activity[a]*	65	60	63	38
Total back pain*	67	58	65	37
Inflammation[b]*	6.7	5.6	6.7	3.6
BASFI*	56	51	52	34
BASDAI[d] score*	6.3	5.5	6.3	3.7
BASMI[e] score*	4.2	4.1	3.8	3.3
Tragus to wall (cm)	15.9	15.8	15.8	15.4
Lumbar flexion (cm)	4.1	4.0	4.2	4.4
Cervical rotation (degrees)	42.2	42.1	48.4	51.6
Lumbar side flexion (cm)	8.9	9.0	9.7	11.7
Intermalleolar distance (cm)	92.9	94.0	93.5	100.8
CRP[f]*	2.2	2.0	1.8	0.6

[a] Percent of subjects with at least a 20% and 10-unit improvement measured on a Visual Analog Scale (VAS) with 0 = "none" and 100 = "severe"
[b] mean of questions 5 and 6 of BASDAI (defined in 'd')
[c] Bath Ankylosing Spondylitis Functional Index
[d] Bath Ankylosing Spondylitis Disease Activity Index
[e] Bath Ankylosing Spondylitis Metrology Index
[f] C-Reactive Protein (mg/dL)
* statistically significant for comparisons between HUMIRA and placebo at Week 24

Table 11. Induction of Clinical Remission in Studies CD-I and CD-II (Percent of Patients)

	CD-I		CD-II	
	Placebo N=74	HUMIRA 160/80 mg N=76	Placebo N=166	HUMIRA 160/80 mg N=159
Week 4				
Clinical remission	12%	36%*	7%	21%*
Clinical response	34%	58%**	34%	52%**

Clinical remission is CDAI score < 150; clinical response is decrease in CDAI of at least 70 points.
*p<0.001 for HUMIRA *vs.* placebo pairwise comparison of proportions
**p<0.01 for HUMIRA *vs.* placebo pairwise comparison of proportions

Table 13. Efficacy Results at 16 Weeks in Study Ps-I Number of Patients (%)

	HUMIRA 40 mg every other week N = 814	Placebo N = 398
PGA: Clear or minimal*	506 (62%)	17 (4%)
PASI 75	578 (71%)	26 (7%)

* Clear = no plaque elevation, no scale, plus or minus hyperpigmentation or diffuse pink or red coloration
Minimal = possible but difficult to ascertain whether there is slight elevation of plaque above normal skin, plus or minus surface dryness with some white coloration, plus or minus up to red coloration

Table 14. Efficacy Results at 16 Weeks in Study Ps-II Number of Patients (%)

	HUMIRA 40 mg every other week N = 99	Placebo N = 48
PGA: Clear or minimal*	70 (71%)	5 (10%)
PASI 75	77 (78%)	9 (19%)

* Clear = no plaque elevation, no scale, plus or minus hyperpigmentation or diffuse pink or red coloration
Minimal = possible but difficult to ascertain whether there is slight elevation of plaque above normal skin, plus or minus surface dryness with some white coloration, plus or minus up to red coloration

Additionally, in Study Ps-I, subjects on HUMIRA who maintained a PASI 75 were re-randomized to HUMIRA (N = 250) or placebo (N = 240) at Week 33. After 52 weeks of treatment with HUMIRA, more patients on HUMIRA maintained efficacy when compared to subjects who were re-randomized to placebo based on maintenance of PGA of "clear" or "minimal" disease (68% *vs.* 28%) or a PASI 75 (79% *vs.* 43%).

15   REFERENCES
1. National Cancer Institute. Surveillance, Epidemiology, and End Results Database (SEER) Program. SEER Incidence Crude Rates, 11 Registries, 1993-2001.

16   HOW SUPPLIED/STORAGE AND HANDLING
HUMIRA® (adalimumab) is supplied in prefilled syringes as a preservative-free, sterile solution for subcutaneous administration. The following packaging configurations are available.
• **HUMIRA Pen Carton**
HUMIRA is dispensed in a carton containing two alcohol preps and two dose trays. Each dose tray consists of a single-use pen, containing a 1 mL prefilled glass syringe with a fixed 27 gauge ½ inch needle, providing 40 mg (0.8 mL) of HUMIRA. The NDC number is 0074-4339-02.
• **HUMIRA Pen – Crohn's Disease Starter Package**
HUMIRA is dispensed in a carton containing 6 alcohol preps and 6 dose trays (Crohn's Disease Starter Package). Each dose tray consists of a single-use pen, containing a 1 mL prefilled glass syringe with a fixed 27 gauge ½ inch needle, providing 40 mg (0.8 mL) of HUMIRA. The NDC number is 0074-4339-06.
• **HUMIRA Pen – Psoriasis Starter Package**
HUMIRA is dispensed in a carton containing 4 alcohol preps and 4 dose trays (Psoriasis Starter Package). Each dose tray consists of a single-use pen, containing a 1 mL prefilled glass syringe with a fixed 27 gauge ½ inch needle, providing 40 mg (0.8 mL) of HUMIRA. The NDC number is 0074-4339-07.
• **Prefilled Syringe Carton – 40 mg**
HUMIRA is dispensed in a carton containing two alcohol preps and two dose trays. Each dose tray consists of a single-dose, 1 mL prefilled glass syringe with a fixed 27 gauge ½ inch needle, providing 40 mg (0.8 mL) of HUMIRA. The NDC number is 0074-3799-02.
• **Pediatric Prefilled Syringe Carton - 20 mg**
HUMIRA is supplied for pediatric use only in a carton containing two alcohol preps and two dose trays. Each dose tray consists of a single-dose, 1 mL pre-filled glass syringe with a fixed 27 gauge ½ inch needle, providing 20 mg (0.4 mL) of HUMIRA. The NDC number is 0074-9374-02.
• **Storage and Stability**
Do not use beyond the expiration date on the container. HUMIRA must be refrigerated at 2 to 8° C (36 to 46° F). DO

Information on the Abbott Pharmaceutical Products listed on these pages is from the prescribing information in use as of June 1, 2010. For more information, please visit rxabbott.com or call 1-800-633-9110.

NOT FREEZE. Protect the prefilled syringe from exposure to light. Store in original carton until time of administration.

17 PATIENT COUNSELING INFORMATION

See Medication Guide (17)

17.1 Patient Counseling

Patients should be advised of the potential benefits and risks of HUMIRA. Physicians should instruct their patients to read the Medication Guide before starting HUMIRA therapy and to reread each time the prescription is renewed.

• Immunosuppression

Inform patients that HUMIRA may lower the ability of their immune system to fight infections. Instruct the patient of the importance of contacting their doctor if they develop any symptoms of infection, including tuberculosis and reactivation of hepatitis B virus infections.

Patients should be counseled about the risk of lymphoma and other malignancies while receiving HUMIRA.

• Allergic Reactions

Patients should be advised to seek immediate medical attention if they experience any symptoms of severe allergic reactions. Advise latex-sensitive patients that the needle cap of the prefilled syringe contains latex.

• Other Medical Conditions

Advise patients to report any signs of new or worsening medical conditions such as heart disease, neurological disease, or autoimmune disorders. Advise patients to report any symptoms suggestive of a cytopenia such as bruising, bleeding, or persistent fever.

17.2 Instruction on Injection Technique

The first injection should be performed under the supervision of a qualified health care professional. If a patient or caregiver is to administer HUMIRA, he/she should be instructed in injection techniques and their ability to inject subcutaneously should be assessed to ensure the proper administration of HUMIRA [see Medication Guide (17)].

A puncture-resistant container for disposal of needles and syringes should be used. Patients or caregivers should be instructed in the technique as well as proper syringe and needle disposal, and be cautioned against reuse of these items.

MEDICATION GUIDE

HUMIRA® (HU-MARE-AH)

(adalimumab)

Read the Medication Guide that comes with HUMIRA before you start taking it and each time you get a refill. There may be new information. This Medication Guide does not take the place of talking with your doctor about your medical condition or treatment with HUMIRA.

What is the most important information I should know about HUMIRA?

HUMIRA is a medicine that affects your immune system. HUMIRA can lower the ability of the immune system to fight infections. **Serious infections have happened in patients taking HUMIRA. These infections include tuberculosis (TB) and infections caused by viruses, fungi or bacteria that have spread throughout the body. Some patients have died from these infections.**

• Your doctor should test you for TB before starting HUMIRA.

• Your doctor should monitor you closely for signs and symptoms of TB during treatment with HUMIRA.

Before starting HUMIRA, tell your doctor if you:

• think you have an infection. You should not start taking HUMIRA if you have any kind of infection.

• are being treated for an infection

• have signs of an infection, such as a fever, cough, or flu-like symptoms

• have any open cuts or sores on your body

• get a lot of infections or have infections that keep coming back

• have diabetes

• have TB, or have been in close contact with someone with TB

• were born in, lived in, or traveled to countries where there is more risk for getting TB. Ask your doctor if you are not sure.

• live or have lived in certain parts of the country (such as the Ohio and Mississippi River valleys) where there is an increased risk for getting certain kinds of fungal infections (histoplasmosis, coccidioidomycosis, or blastomycosis). If you do not know if you have lived in an area where histoplasmosis, coccidioidomycosis, or blastomycosis is common, ask your doctor.

• have or have had hepatitis B

• use the medicine Kineret (anakinra). You may have a higher chance for serious infections and a low white blood cell count when taking HUMIRA with Kineret.

• are scheduled to have major surgery

After starting HUMIRA, call your doctor right away if you have an infection, or any sign of an infection, including:

• a fever

• feel very tired

• a cough

• flu-like symptoms

• warm, red, or painful skin

• open cuts or sores on your body

HUMIRA can make you more likely to get infections or make any infection that you may have worse.

Certain types of Cancer.

• There have been cases of unusual cancers in children and teenage patients using TNF-blocking agents.

• For children and adults taking TNF-blocker medicines, including HUMIRA, the chances of getting lymphoma or other cancers may increase.

• Some patients receiving HUMIRA have developed types of cancer called non-melanoma skin cancer (basal cell cancer and squamous cell cancer of the skin), which are generally not life-threatening if treated. Tell your doctor if you have a bump or open sore that doesn't heal.

• Patients with RA, especially more serious RA, may have a higher chance for getting a kind of cancer called lymphoma.

See the section "What are the possible side effects of HUMIRA?" below for more information.

What is HUMIRA?

HUMIRA is a medicine called a Tumor Necrosis Factor (TNF) blocker. HUMIRA is used in adults or children (as indicated) to:

• Reduce the signs and symptoms of:

• **moderate to severe rheumatoid arthritis (RA)** in adults. HUMIRA can be used alone or with methotrexate or with certain other medicines. HUMIRA may prevent further damage to your bones and joints and may help your ability to perform daily activities.

• **moderate to severe polyarticular juvenile idiopathic arthritis (JIA)** in children 4 years of age and older. HUMIRA can be used alone or with methotrexate or with certain other medicines.

• **psoriatic arthritis (PsA).** HUMIRA can be used alone or with certain other medicines. HUMIRA may prevent further damage to your bones and joints and may help your ability to perform daily activities.

• **ankylosing spondylitis (AS)**

• **moderate to severe Crohn's disease (CD)** in adults who have not responded well to other treatments.

• **Treat moderate to severe chronic (lasting a long time) plaque psoriasis (Ps)** in adults who have the condition in many areas of their body and who may benefit from taking injections or pills (systemic therapy) or phototherapy (treatment using ultraviolet light alone or with pills).

People with these diseases have too much of a protein called tumor necrosis factor (TNF), in the affected areas of the body. HUMIRA can block the bad effects of TNF in those affected areas, but it can also lower the ability of the immune system to fight infections. See **"What is the most important information I should know about HUMIRA?"** and **"What are the possible side effects of HUMIRA?"**

What should I tell my doctor before taking HUMIRA?

Before starting HUMIRA, tell your doctor about all of your health conditions, including if you:

• have an infection. See "What is the most important information I should know about HUMIRA?"

• have any numbness or tingling or have a disease that affects your nervous system such as multiple sclerosis or Guillain-Barré syndrome.

• have heart failure or other heart conditions. If you have heart failure, it may get worse while you are taking HUMIRA.

• have recently received or are scheduled to receive a vaccine. Patients receiving HUMIRA should not receive live vaccines.

• are allergic to rubber or latex. The needle cover on the prefilled syringe contains dry natural rubber. Tell your doctor if you have any allergies to rubber or latex.

• are allergic to HUMIRA or to any of its ingredients. See the end of this Medication Guide for a list of ingredients in HUMIRA.

Tell your doctor if you are pregnant, planning to become pregnant, or breastfeeding. HUMIRA should only be used during a pregnancy if needed. Women who are breastfeeding should talk to their doctor about whether or not to use HUMIRA.

Pregnancy Registry: Abbott Laboratories has a registry for pregnant women who take HUMIRA. The purpose of this registry is to check the health of the pregnant mother and her child. Talk to your doctor if you are pregnant and contact the registry at 1-877-311-8972.

Tell your doctor about all the medicines you take, including prescription and non-prescription medicines, vitamins and herbal supplements. Especially, tell your doctor if you take Kineret (anakinra). You may have a higher chance for serious infections and a low white blood cell count when taking HUMIRA with Kineret. Also, tell your doctor if you are taking other medicines that suppress the immune system.

Know the medicines you take. Keep a list of your medicines with you to show your doctor and pharmacist each time you get a new medicine.

How should I take HUMIRA?

See the section, "How do I prepare and give an injection of HUMIRA?" at the end of this Medication Guide for complete instructions for use.

• HUMIRA is given by an injection under the skin. Your doctor will tell you how often to take an injection of HUMIRA. This is based on your condition to be treated. Do not inject HUMIRA more often than prescribed.

• Make sure you have been shown how to inject HUMIRA before you do it yourself. You can call your doctor or 1-800-4HUMIRA (448-6472) if you have any questions about giving yourself an injection. Someone you know can also help you with your injection.

• If you take more HUMIRA than you were told to take, call your doctor.

• Do not miss any doses of HUMIRA. If you forget to take HUMIRA, inject a dose as soon as you remember. Then, take your next dose at your regular scheduled time. This will put you back on schedule. To help you remember when to take HUMIRA, you can mark your calendar ahead of time with the stickers provided in the back of the Medication Guide.

What are the possible side effects of HUMIRA?

HUMIRA can cause serious side effects, including:

See "What is the most important information I should know about HUMIRA?"

• Serious infections.

Your doctor will examine you for TB and perform a test to see if you have TB. If your doctor feels that you are at risk for TB, you may be treated with medicine for TB before you begin treatment with HUMIRA and during treatment with HUMIRA. Even if your TB test is negative your doctor should carefully monitor you for TB infections while you are taking HUMIRA. Patients who had a negative TB skin test before receiving HUMIRA have developed active TB. Tell your doctor if you have any of the following symptoms while taking or after taking HUMIRA:

• cough that does not go away

• low grade fever

• weight loss

• loss of body fat and muscle (wasting)

• Allergic reactions. Signs of a serious allergic reaction include a skin rash, a swollen face, or trouble breathing.

• Hepatitis B virus reactivation in patients who carry the virus in their blood. In some cases patients have died as a result of hepatitis B virus being reactivated. Your doctor should monitor you carefully during treatment with HUMIRA if you carry the hepatitis B virus in your blood. Tell your doctor if you have any of the following symptoms:

• feel unwell

• poor appetite

• tiredness (fatigue)

• fever, skin rash, or joint pain

• Nervous system problems. Signs and symptoms of a nervous system problem include: numbness or tingling, problems with your vision, weakness in your arms or legs, and dizziness.

• Blood problems. Your body may not make enough of the blood cells that help fight infections or help to stop bleeding. Symptoms include a fever that does not go away, bruising or bleeding very easily, or looking very pale.

• New heart failure or worsening of heart failure you already have. Symptoms include shortness of breath or swelling of your ankles or feet or sudden weight gain.

• Immune reactions including a lupus-like syndrome. Symptoms include chest discomfort or pain that does not go away, shortness of breath, joint pain, or a rash on your cheeks or arms that gets worse in the sun. Symptoms may go away when you stop HUMIRA.

• Psoriasis. Some people using HUMIRA had new psoriasis or worsening of psoriasis they already had. Tell your doctor if you develop red scaly patches or raised bumps that are filled with pus. Your doctor may decide to stop your treatment with HUMIRA.

Call your doctor or get medical care right away if you develop any of the above symptoms. Your treatment with HUMIRA may be stopped.

Common side effects with HUMIRA include:

• **Injection site reactions** such as redness, rash, swelling, itching, or bruising. These symptoms usually will go away within a few days. If you have pain, redness or swelling around the injection site that doesn't go away within a few days or gets worse, call your doctor right away.

• **Upper respiratory infections** (including sinus infections)

• **Headaches**

• **Rash**

• **Nausea**

IMPORTANT NOTICE: Updated drug information is sent bi-monthly via the PDR® Update Insert. For *monthly* email updates, register at PDR.net.

These are not all the possible side effects with HUMIRA. Tell your doctor if you have any side effect that bothers you or that does not go away. Ask your doctor or pharmacist for more information.

How do I store HUMIRA?

- Store HUMIRA in a refrigerator at 36 to 46°F (2 to 8°C) in the original container until it is used. Protect from light. **Do not freeze HUMIRA.** Refrigerated HUMIRA remains okay to use until the expiration date printed on the pre-filled syringe or Pen. If you need to take HUMIRA with you, such as when traveling, store it in a cool carrier with an ice pack and protect it from light. If your HUMIRA has been frozen, do not use it, even after it has thawed. Do not use a Pen or prefilled syringe if the liquid is cloudy, dis-colored, or has flakes or particles in it. For additional information or questions, you can call 1-800-4HUMIRA (448-6472).
- Do not drop or crush HUMIRA. The prefilled syringe is glass.
- **Keep HUMIRA, injection supplies, and all other medicines out of the reach of children.**

General information about HUMIRA

Medicines are sometimes prescribed for purposes other than those listed in a Medication Guide. Do not use HUMIRA for a condition for which it was not prescribed. Do not give HUMIRA to other people, even if they have the same condition. It may harm them.

This Medication Guide summarizes the most important information about HUMIRA. If you would like more information, talk with your doctor. You can ask your doctor or pharmacist for information about HUMIRA that was written for healthcare professionals.

Call your doctor for medical advice about side effects. You may report side effects to FDA at 1-800-FDA-1088.

For more information go to www.HUMIRA.com or you can enroll in a patient support program by calling 1-800-4HUMIRA (448-6472).

What are the ingredients in HUMIRA?

Active ingredient: adalimumab

Inactive ingredients: sodium phosphate, sodium citrate, citric acid, mannitol, and polysorbate 80.

Patient Instructions for Use

What do I need to do to prepare and give an injection of HUMIRA?

HUMIRA comes as:

1. a single-use pen (HUMIRA PEN) containing a prefilled syringe
2. a single-dose prefilled syringe (HUMIRA)

Follow the directions below for your dose form.

IF YOU ARE USING THE HUMIRA PEN

1) Setting up for an injection

- Find a clean flat surface.
- Do not use if the seals on top and bottom of carton are broken or missing. Contact your pharmacist if the seals are broken.
- Take one dose tray containing a HUMIRA Pen from the refrigerator. Do not use a Pen that has been frozen or if it has been left in direct sunlight.

You will need the following items for each dose:
- 1 HUMIRA Pen
- 1 alcohol prep (swab)
- 1 cotton ball or gauze pad (not included in your HUMIRA box)

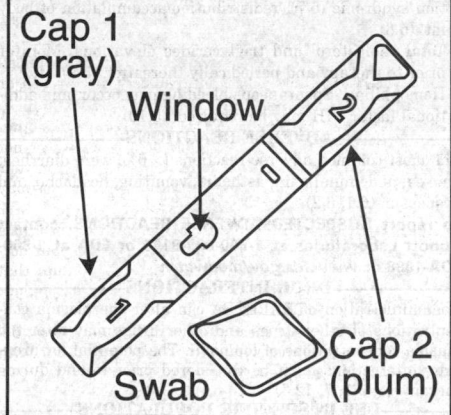

If you do not have all of the items you need to give yourself an injection, call your pharmacist. Use only the items provided in the box your HUMIRA comes in.
- Check and make sure the name HUMIRA appears on the dose tray and Pen label.
- Check the expiration date on the dose tray label and the Pen label to make sure the date has not passed. Do not use a Pen if the date has passed.

- Have a special sharps (puncture proof) container nearby for disposing of the used Pen.

For your protection, it is important that you follow these instructions.

2) Choosing and preparing an injection site
- Wash your hands well

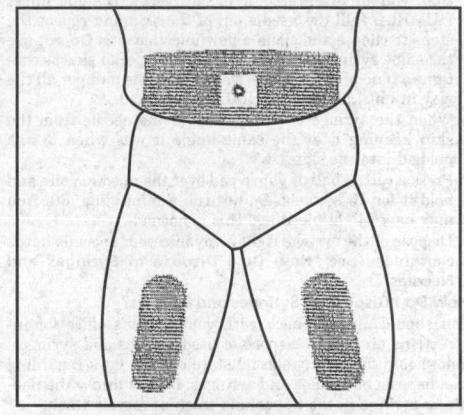

- Choose a site on the front of your thighs or your stomach area (abdomen). If you choose your abdomen, you should avoid the area 2 inches around your belly button (navel).
  - Choose a different site each time you give yourself an injection. Each new injection should be given at least one inch from a site you used before. **Never** inject into areas where the skin is tender, bruised, red or hard or where you have scars or stretch marks.
  - If you have psoriasis, you should try not to inject directly into any raised, thick, red or scaly skin patches or lesions.
  - You may find it helpful to keep notes on the location of your injection sites.
- Wipe the site where HUMIRA is to be injected with an alcohol prep (swab), using a circular motion. Do **not** touch this area again until you are ready to inject.

3) How to prepare your HUMIRA dose for injection with a HUMIRA Pen
- Hold the Pen with the gray cap pointing up. Check the solution through the windows on the side of the Pen to make sure the liquid is clear and colorless. Do not use a Pen if the liquid is cloudy or discolored or has flakes or particles in it. Do not use if frozen.

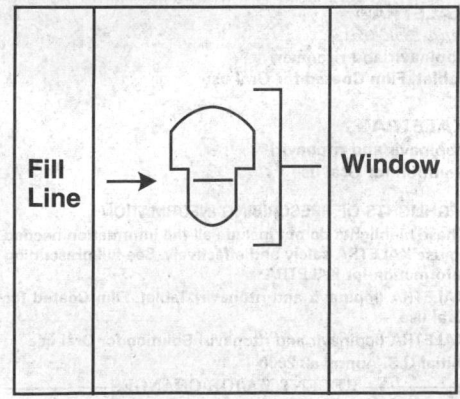

- Turn the Pen over and hold the Pen with the gray cap pointed down. Check to make sure that the amount of liquid in the Pen is the same or close to the fill line seen through the window. The fill line represents a full dose of the product. The top of the liquid may be curved. If the Pen does not have the full amount of liquid, **do not use that pen**. Call your pharmacist.

4) Injecting HUMIRA
- Hold the Pen with one hand. With your other hand, remove the gray cap (1) and discard cap. Pull the cap straight off. Do not twist the cap. Check that the small gray needle cover of the syringe has come off with the cap. After removal, the needle cover is held in the cap. Do not touch the needle. The white needle sleeve, which covers the needle, can now be seen. **Do not put the gray cap (1) back on** or you may damage the needle. Do not drop or crush the product as it contains a glass syringe that may break.
- Remove the plum colored safety cap (2) to expose the plum colored push button at the top. Pull the cap straight off. Do not twist the cap. The Pen is now ready to use. Please note that the Pen is activated after removing the plum

colored safety cap 2 and that pressing the button under the plum colored safety cap 2 will release the medicine from the syringe. Do not press the button until you are ready to inject HUMIRA. **Do not put the plum colored cap (2) back on the pen as this could cause medicine to come out of the syringe.**
- Hold the Pen so that the window can be seen.
- With your free hand, gently squeeze an area of the cleaned skin at the injection site. You will inject into this raised area of skin.
- Place the white end of the Pen straight (a 90° angle) and flat against the raised area of skin. Place the Pen so that it will not inject the needle into your fingers that are holding the raised skin.

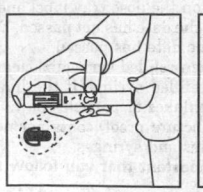 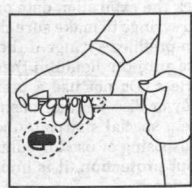

- With your first (index) finger, press the plum colored button to begin the injection. You may also use your thumb to press the plum colored button to begin the injection. Try not to cover the window. You will hear a 'click' when you press the button, which means the start of the injection. Keep pressing the button and continue to hold the Pen against the raised skin until all of the medicine is injected. This can take up to 10 seconds. It is important to keep holding the pen against the raised skin of your injection site for the whole time.
- You will know that the injection has finished when the yellow marker appears fully in the window view and stops moving.

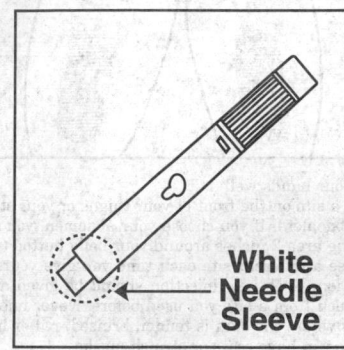

- When the injection is finished, pull the Pen from the skin. The white needle sleeve will move to cover the needle tip.
- Press a cotton ball or gauze pad over the injection site and hold it for 10 seconds. Do **not** rub the injection site. You may have slight bleeding. This is normal.
- Dispose of the Pen right away into your special sharps container.
- Do not try to touch the needle. The white needle sleeve is there to prevent you from touching the needle. (See "**How Do I Dispose of Syringes and Needles?**")

IF YOU ARE USING THE SINGLE-DOSE PREFILLED SYRINGE

1) Setting up for an injection
- Find a clean flat surface.
- Do not use if the seals on top and bottom of carton are broken or missing. Contact your pharmacist if the seals are broken.
- Take one dose tray containing a prefilled syringe of HUMIRA from the refrigerator. Do not use a prefilled syringe that has been frozen or if it has been left in direct sunlight.

You will need the following items for each dose:
- A dose tray containing a prefilled syringe of HUMIRA with a fixed needle
- 1 alcohol prep (swab)
- 1 cotton ball or gauze pad (not included in your HUMIRA box)

[See figure at top of next page]

If you do not have all of the items you need to give yourself an injection, call your pharmacist. Use only the items provided in the box your HUMIRA comes in.

Information on the Abbott Pharmaceutical Products listed on these pages is from the prescribing information in use as of June 1, 2010. For more information, please visit rxabbott.com or call 1-800-633-9110.

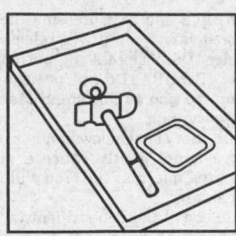

- Check and make sure the name HUMIRA appears on the dose tray and prefilled syringe label.
- Check the expiration date on the dose tray label and prefilled syringe to make sure the date has not passed. Do not use a prefilled syringe if the date has passed.
- Make sure the liquid in the prefilled syringe is clear and colorless. Do not use a prefilled syringe if the liquid is cloudy or discolored or has flakes or particles in it.
- Have a special sharps (puncture proof) container nearby for disposing of used needles and syringes.

For your protection, it is important that you follow these instructions.

2) Choosing and preparing an injection site

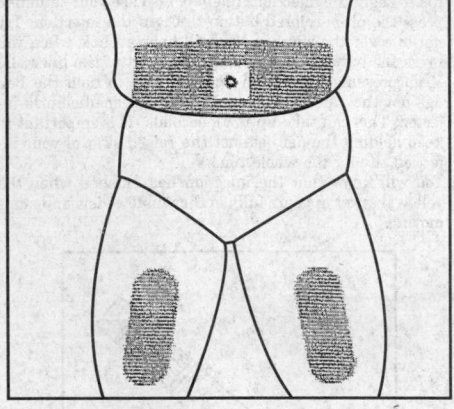

- Wash your hands well
- Choose a site on the front of your thighs or your stomach area (abdomen). If you choose your abdomen, you should avoid the area 2 inches around your belly button (navel).
  - Choose a different site each time you give yourself an injection. Each new injection should be given at least one inch from a site you used before. **Never** inject into areas where the skin is tender, bruised, red or hard or where you have scars or stretch marks.
  - If you have psoriasis, you should try not to inject directly into any raised, thick, red or scaly skin patches or lesions.
  - You may find it helpful to keep notes on the location of your injection sites.
- Wipe the site where HUMIRA is to be injected with an alcohol prep (swab), using a circular motion. Do **not** touch this area again until you are ready to inject.

3) How to prepare your HUMIRA dose for injection with a Prefilled Syringe

- Hold the syringe upright with the needle facing down. Check to make sure that the amount of liquid in the syringe is the same or close to the 0.8 mL line for the 40 mg prefilled syringe or the 0.4 mL line for the 20 mg pediatric prefilled syringe. The top of the liquid may be curved. If the syringe does not have the correct amount of liquid, **do not use that syringe**. Call your pharmacist.
- Remove the needle cover taking care not to touch the needle with your fingers or allow it to touch any surface.
- Turn the syringe so the needle is facing up and slowly push the plunger in to push the air in the syringe out through the needle. If a small drop of liquid comes out of the needle that is okay. Do not shake the syringe.

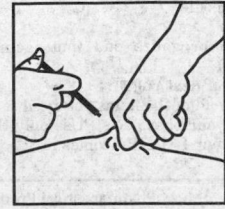

4) Injecting HUMIRA

- With your other hand, gently squeeze an area of the cleaned area of skin and hold it firmly. You will inject into

this raised area of skin. Hold the syringe like a pencil at about a 45° angle (see picture) to the skin.

- With a quick, short, "dart-like" motion, push the needle into the skin.
- After the needle is in, let go of the skin. Pull back slightly on the plunger. If blood appears in the syringe it means that you have entered a blood vessel. Do not inject HUMIRA. Pull the needle out of the skin and repeat the steps to choose and clean a new injection site. **Do not** use the same syringe. Dispose of it in your special sharps container. If no blood appears, slowly push the plunger all the way in until all of the HUMIRA is injected.
- When the syringe is empty, remove the needle from the skin keeping it at the same angle it was when it was pushed into the skin.
- Press a cotton ball or gauze pad over the injection site and hold it for 10 seconds. Do **not** rub the injection site. You may have slight bleeding. This is normal.
- Dispose of the syringe right away into your special sharps container. (See "How Do I Dispose of Syringes and Needles?")

How Do I Dispose of Syringes and Needles?

You should always check with your doctor's office for instructions on how to dispose of used needles and syringes. You should follow any special state or local laws regarding the disposal of needles and syringes. **Do not throw the needle or syringe in the household trash or recycle trash.**

- Place the used needles and syringes in a container made specially for disposing of used syringes and needles (called a "Sharps" container), or a hard plastic container with a screw-on cap or metal container with a plastic lid labeled "Used Syringes". Do not use glass or clear plastic containers.
- **Always keep the container out of the reach of children.**
- When the container is about two-thirds full, tape the cap or lid down so it does not come off and dispose of it as instructed by your doctor, nurse or pharmacist. **Do not throw the container in the household trash or recycle trash.**
- Used alcohol pads may be placed in the trash, unless otherwise instructed by your doctor, nurse or pharmacist. The dose tray and cover may be placed in your recycle trash.

U.S. Govt. Lic. No. 0043
Abbott Laboratories
North Chicago, IL 60064, U.S.A.
Ref. 03-A256-Revised November, 2009

Shown in Product Identification Guide, page 303

KALETRA®   ℞
[kuh-LEE-tra]
(lopinavir and ritonavir)
Tablet, Film Coated for Oral use

KALETRA®
(lopinavir and ritonavir)
Solution for Oral use

HIGHLIGHTS OF PRESCRIBING INFORMATION
These highlights do not include all the information needed to use KALETRA safely and effectively. See full prescribing information for KALETRA.

KALETRA (lopinavir and ritonavir) Tablet, Film Coated for Oral use
KALETRA (lopinavir and ritonavir) Solution for Oral use
Initial U.S. Approval: 2000

———————**RECENT MAJOR CHANGES**———————
Contraindications, Table 3 (4) 1/2010
Contraindications, Table 3 (4) 4/2010
Warnings and Precautions (5.3) 4/2010
Dosage and Administration, Adult Patients (2.1) 4/2010

———————**INDICATIONS AND USAGE**———————
KALETRA is an HIV-1 protease inhibitor indicated in combination with other antiretroviral agents for the treatment of HIV-1 infection. (1)

———————**DOSAGE AND ADMINISTRATION**———————
Do not use once daily administration of KALETRA in:
- HIV-1 infected patients with three or more of the following lopinavir resistance-associated substitutions: L10F/I/R/V, K20M/N/R, L24I, L33F, M36I, I47V, G48V, I54L/T/V, V82A/C/F/S/T, and I84V (2.1)
- Combination with efavirenz, nevirapine, amprenavir, nelfinavir, carbamazepine, phenobarbital, or phenytoin (2.1, 7.3)
- Pediatric patients (2.2)

Tablets: May be taken with or without food, swallowed whole and not chewed, broken, or crushed. (2)
Oral Solution: Must be taken with food. (2)

ADULT PATIENTS (2.1)
- 400/100 mg (two 200/50 mg tablets or 5 mL oral solution) twice daily or
- 800/200 mg (four 200/50 mg tablets or 10 mL oral solution) once daily in patients with less than three lopinavir resistance-associated substitutions.

PEDIATRIC PATIENTS (ages 14 days and older) (2.2)
- Twice daily dose is based on body weight or body surface area.

Concomitant Therapy in Adults and Pediatric Patients (2.1, 2.2)
- Dose adjustments of KALETRA may be needed when co-administering with efavirenz, nevirapine, amprenavir, or nelfinavir.

———————**DOSAGE FORMS AND STRENGTHS**———————
- Film-coated tablets: 200 mg lopinavir and 50 mg ritonavir (3)
- Film-coated tablets: 100 mg lopinavir and 25 mg ritonavir (3)
- Oral solution: 80 mg lopinavir and 20 mg ritonavir per milliliter (3)

———————**CONTRAINDICATIONS**———————
Hypersensitivity to KALETRA (e.g., Stevens-Johnson syndrome, erythema multiforme) or any of its ingredients, including ritonavir. (4)
Coadministration with:
- drugs highly dependent on CYP3A for clearance and for which elevated plasma levels may result in serious and/or life-threatening events. (4)
- potent CYP3A inducers where significantly reduced lopinavir plasma concentrations may be associated with the potential for loss of virologic response and possible resistance and cross resistance. (4)

———————**WARNINGS AND PRECAUTIONS**———————
The following have been observed in patients receiving KALETRA:
- Drug Interactions: Consider drug-drug interaction potential to reduce risk of serious or life-threatening adverse reactions. (5.1)
- Pancreatitis: Fatalities have occurred; suspend therapy as clinically appropriate. (5.2)
- Hepatotoxicity: Fatalities have occurred. Monitor liver function before and during therapy, especially in patients with underlying hepatic disease, including hepatitis B and hepatitis C, or marked transaminase elevations. (5.3, 8.6)
- PR interval prolongation may occur in some patients. Cases of second and third degree heart block have been reported. Use with caution in patients with pre-existing conduction system disease, ischemic heart disease, cardiomyopathy, underlying structural heart disease or when administering with other drugs that may prolong the PR interval. (5.1, 5.5, 12.3)
- QT interval prolongation and isolated cases of torsade de pointes have been reported although causality could not be established. Avoid use in patients with congenital long QT syndrome, those with hypokalemia, and with other drugs that prolong the QT interval. (5.1, 5.6, 12.3)
- Patients may develop new onset or exacerbations of diabetes mellitus, hyperglycemia (5.4), immune reconstitution syndrome (5.7), redistribution/accumulation of body fat. (5.8)
- Total cholesterol and triglycerides elevations. Monitor prior to therapy and periodically thereafter. (5.9)
- Hemophilia: Spontaneous bleeding may occur, and additional factor VIII may be required. (5.10)

———————**ADVERSE REACTIONS**———————
The most common adverse reactions (> 5%) were diarrhea, nausea, abdominal pain, asthenia, vomiting, headache, and dyspepsia. (6.1, 6.2)

To report SUSPECTED ADVERSE REACTIONS, contact Abbott Laboratories at 1-800-633-9110 or FDA at 1-800-FDA-1088 or www.fda.gov/medwatch

———————**DRUG INTERACTIONS**———————
Coadministration of KALETRA can alter the plasma concentrations of other drugs and other drugs may alter the plasma concentrations of lopinavir. The potential for drug-drug interactions must be considered prior to and during therapy. (4, 5.1, 7, 12.3)

———————**USE IN SPECIFIC POPULATIONS**———————
- Pregnancy: Physicians are encouraged to register patients in the Antiretroviral Pregnancy Registry by calling 1-800-258-4263. (8.1)
- Pediatric Use: The safety, efficacy, and pharmacokinetic profiles of KALETRA in pediatric patients below the age of 14 days have not been established. (8.4)

See 17 for PATIENT COUNSELING INFORMATION and Medication Guide

Revised: 04/2010

FULL PRESCRIBING INFORMATION: CONTENTS*

FULL PRESCRIBING INFORMATION

1   INDICATIONS AND USAGE

KALETRA is indicated in combination with other antiretroviral agents for the treatment of HIV-1 infection.

The following points should be considered when initiating therapy with KALETRA:

- The use of other active agents with KALETRA is associated with a greater likelihood of treatment response [see Clinical Pharmacology (12.4) and Clinical Studies (14)].
- Genotypic or phenotypic testing and/or treatment history should guide the use of KALETRA [see Clinical Pharmacology (12.4)]. The number of baseline lopinavir resistance-associated substitutions affects the virologic response to KALETRA [see Clinical Pharmacology (12.4)].
- Once daily administration of KALETRA is not recommended for any pediatric patients.

2   DOSAGE AND ADMINISTRATION

KALETRA tablets may be taken with or without food. The tablets should be swallowed whole and not chewed, broken, or crushed.

KALETRA oral solution must be taken with food.

2.1   Adult Patients

- KALETRA tablets 400/100 mg (given as two 200/50 mg tablets) twice daily.
- KALETRA oral solution 400/100 mg (5 mL) twice daily
- KALETRA tablets 800/200 mg (given as four 200/50 mg tablets) once daily in patients with less than three lopinavir resistance-associated substitutions.
- KALETRA oral solution 800/200 mg (10 mL) once daily in patients with less than three lopinavir resistance-associated substitutions.

Once daily administration of KALETRA is not recommended for adult patients with three or more of the following lopinavir resistance-associated substitutions: L10F/I/R/V, K20M/N/R, L24I, L33F, M36I, I47V, G48V, I54L/T/V, V82A/C/F/S/T, and I84V [see Clinical Pharmacology (12.4)]. KALETRA should not be administered once daily in combination with carbamazepine, phenobarbital, or phenytoin [see Drug Interactions (7.0)].

Concomitant Therapy: Efavirenz, Nevirapine, Amprenavir or Nelfinavir [see Clinical Pharmacology (12.3) and Drug Interactions (7.3)]

KALETRA tablets and oral solution should not be administered as a once daily regimen in combination with efavirenz, nevirapine, amprenavir, or nelfinavir.

- A dose increase is recommended for all patients who use KALETRA tablets. The recommended dose of KALETRA tablets is 500/125 mg (such as two 200/50 tablets and one 100/25 mg tablet) twice daily in combination with efavirenz, nevirapine, amprenavir or nelfinavir.
- A dose increase is recommended for all patients who use KALETRA oral solution. The recommended dose of KALETRA oral solution is 533/133 mg (6.5 mL) twice daily when used in combination with efavirenz, nevirapine, amprenavir or nelfinavir.

2.2   Pediatric Patients

KALETRA tablets and oral solution should not be administered once daily in pediatric patients < 18 years of age.

Healthcare professionals should pay special attention to accurate calculation of the dose of KALETRA, transcription of the medication order, dispensing information and dosing instructions to minimize the risk for medication errors, overdose, [see Overdosage (10)] and underdose.

Prescribers should calculate the appropriate dose of KALETRA for each individual child based on body weight (kg) or body surface area (BSA) and should not exceed the recommended adult dose.

Body surface area (BSA) can be calculated as follows:

$$\text{BSA (m}^2) = \sqrt{\frac{\text{Ht (Cm)} \times \text{Wt (kg)}}{3600}}$$

The KALETRA dose can be calculated based on weight or BSA:

Based on Weight:

Patient Weight (kg) × Prescribed lopinavir dose (mg/kg) = Administered lopinavir dose (mg)

Based on BSA:

Patient BSA (m²) × Prescribed lopinavir dose (mg/m²) = Administered lopinavir dose (mg)

If KALETRA oral solution is used, the volume (mL) of KALETRA solution can be determined as follows:

Volume of KALETRA solution (mL) = Administered lopinavir dose (mg) ÷ 80 (mg/mL)

The dose of the oral solution should be administered using a calibrated dosing syringe.

Before prescribing KALETRA 100/25 mg tablets, children should be assessed for the ability to swallow intact tablets. If a child is unable to reliably swallow a KALETRA tablet, the KALETRA oral solution formulation should be prescribed.

14 Days to 6 Months:

In pediatric patients 14 days to 6 months of age, the recommended dosage of lopinavir/ritonavir using KALETRA oral solution is 16/4 mg/kg or 300/75 mg/m² twice daily. Prescribers should calculate the appropriate dose based on body weight or body surface area.

Because no data exists for dosage when administered with efavirenz, nevirapine, amprenavir, or nelfinavir, it is recommended that KALETRA not be administered in combination with these drugs in patients < 6 months of age.

6 Months to 18 Years:

Without Concomitant Efavirenz, Nevirapine, Amprenavir or Nelfinavir

In children 6 months to 18 years of age, the recommended dosage of lopinavir/ritonavir using KALETRA oral solution without concomitant efavirenz, nevirapine, amprenavir, or nelfinavir is 230/57.5 mg/m² given twice daily, not to exceed the recommended adult dose. If weight-based dosing is preferred, the recommended dosage of lopinavir/ritonavir for patients < 15 kg is 12/3 mg/kg given twice daily and the dosage for patients ≥ 15 kg to 40 kg is 10/2.5 mg/kg given twice daily.

Table 1 provides the dosing recommendations for pediatric patients 6 months to 18 years of age based on body weight or body surface area for KALETRA tablets.

Table 1. Pediatric Dosing Recommendations for Patients 6 Months to 18 Years of Age Based on Body Weight or Body Surface Area for KALETRA Tablets Without Concomitant Efavirenz, Nevirapine, Amprenavir, or Nelfinavir

Body Weight (kg)	Body Surface Area (m²)*	Recommended number of 100/25 mg Tablets Twice Daily
15 to 25	≥0.6 to < 0.9	2
>25 to 35	≥0.9 to < 1.4	3
>35	≥1.4	4 (or two 200/50 mg tablets)

* KALETRA oral solution is available for children with a BSA less than 0.6 m² or those who are unable to reliably swallow a tablet.

Concomitant Therapy: Efavirenz, Nevirapine, Amprenavir, or Nelfinavir

A dose increase of KALETRA to 300/75 mg/m² is needed when co-administered with efavirenz, nevirapine, amprenavir, or nelfinavir in children (both treatment-naïve and treatment-experienced) 6 months to 18 years of age, not to exceed the recommended adult dose. If weight-based dosing is preferred, the recommended dosage for patients <15 kg is 13/3.25 mg/kg given twice daily and the dosage for patients >15 kg to 45 kg is 11/2.75 mg/kg given twice daily. Table 2 provides the dosing recommendations for pediatric patients 6 months to 18 years of age based on body weight or body surface area for KALETRA tablets when given in combination with efavirenz, nevirapine, amprenavir, or nelfinavir.

Table 2. Pediatric Dosing Recommendations for Patients 6 Months to 18 Years of Age Based on Body Weight or Body Surface Area for KALETRA Tablets With Concomitant Efavirenz†, Nevirapine, Amprenavir† or Nelfinavir†

Body Weight (kg)	Body Surface Area (m²)*	Recommended number of 100/25 mg Tablets Twice Daily
15 to 20	≥0.6 to < 0.8	2
>20 to 30	≥0.8 to < 1.2	3
>30 to 45	≥1.2 to <1.7	4 (or two 200/50 mg tablets)
>45	≥1.7	5 [see Dosage and Administration, Adult Patients (2.1)]

* KALETRA oral solution is available for children with a BSA less than 0.6 m² or those who are unable to reliably swallow a tablet.
† Please refer to the individual product labels for appropriate dosing in children.

3   DOSAGE FORMS AND STRENGTHS

- **KALETRA Tablets, 200 mg lopinavir/50 mg ritonavir**
Yellow, film-coated, ovaloid tablets debossed with the corporate logo ⊟ and the Abbo-Code KA providing 200 mg lopinavir/50 mg ritonavir.
- **KALETRA Tablets, 100 mg lopinavir/25 mg ritonavir**
Pale yellow, film-coated, ovaloid tablets debossed with the corporate logo ⊟ and the Abbo-Code KC providing 100 mg lopinavir/25 mg ritonavir.
- **KALETRA Oral Solution**
Light yellow to orange colored liquid containing 400 mg lopinavir/100 mg ritonavir per 5 mL (80 mg lopinavir/20 mg ritonavir per mL).

4   CONTRAINDICATIONS

- KALETRA is contraindicated in patients with previously demonstrated clinically significant hypersensitivity (e.g., Stevens-Johnson syndrome, erythema multiforme) to any of its ingredients, including ritonavir.
- Co-administration of KALETRA is contraindicated with drugs that are highly dependent on CYP3A for clearance and for which elevated plasma concentrations are associated with serious and/or life-threatening reactions.

Information on the Abbott Pharmaceutical Products listed on these pages is from the prescribing information in use as of June 1, 2010. For more information, please visit rxabbott.com or call 1-800-633-9110.

- Co-administration of KALETRA is contraindicated with potent CYP3A inducers where significantly reduced lopinavir plasma concentrations may be associated with the potential for loss of virologic response and possible resistance and cross-resistance. These drugs are listed in Table 3.
[See table 3 below]

5 WARNINGS AND PRECAUTIONS

5.1 Drug Interactions
See Tables 3 and 9 for listing of drugs that are contraindicated for use with KALETRA due to potentially life-threatening adverse events, significant drug interactions, or loss of virologic activity [see Contraindications (4) and Drug Interactions (7)].

5.2 Pancreatitis
Pancreatitis has been observed in patients receiving KALETRA therapy, including those who developed marked triglyceride elevations. In some cases, fatalities have been observed. Although a causal relationship to KALETRA has not been established, marked triglyceride elevations are a risk factor for development of pancreatitis [see Warnings and Precautions (5.9)]. Patients with advanced HIV-1 disease may be at increased risk of elevated triglycerides and pancreatitis, and patients with a history of pancreatitis may be at increased risk for recurrence during KALETRA therapy.

Pancreatitis should be considered if clinical symptoms (nausea, vomiting, abdominal pain) or abnormalities in laboratory values (such as increased serum lipase or amylase values) suggestive of pancreatitis occur. Patients who exhibit these signs or symptoms should be evaluated and KALETRA and/or other antiretroviral therapy should be suspended as clinically appropriate.

5.3 Hepatotoxicity
Patients with underlying hepatitis B or C or marked elevations in transaminase prior to treatment may be at increased risk for developing or worsening of transaminase elevations or hepatic decompensation with use of KALETRA. There have been postmarketing reports of hepatic dysfunction, including some fatalities. These have generally occurred in patients with advanced HIV-1 disease taking multiple concomitant medications in the setting of underlying chronic hepatitis or cirrhosis. A causal relationship with KALETRA therapy has not been established.

Elevated transaminases with or without elevated bilirubin levels have been reported in HIV-1 mono-infected and uninfected patients as early as 7 days after the initiation of KALETRA in conjunction with other antiretroviral agents. In some cases, the hepatic dysfunction was serious; however, a definitive causal relationship with KALETRA therapy has not been established.

Appropriate laboratory testing should be conducted prior to initiating therapy with KALETRA and patients should be monitored closely during treatment. Increased AST/ALT monitoring should be considered in the patients with underlying chronic hepatitis or cirrhosis, especially during the first several months of KALETRA treatment [see Use In Specific Populations (8.6)].

5.4 Diabetes Mellitus/Hyperglycemia
New onset diabetes mellitus, exacerbation of pre-existing diabetes mellitus, and hyperglycemia have been reported during post-marketing surveillance in HIV-1 infected patients receiving protease inhibitor therapy. Some patients required either initiation or dose adjustments of insulin or oral hypoglycemic agents for treatment of these events. In some cases, diabetic ketoacidosis has occurred. In those patients who discontinued protease inhibitor therapy, hyperglycemia persisted in some cases. Because these events have been reported voluntarily during clinical practice, estimates of frequency cannot be made and a causal relationship between protease inhibitor therapy and these events has not been established.

5.5 PR Interval Prolongation
Lopinavir/ritonavir prolongs the PR interval in some patients. Cases of second or third degree atrioventricular block have been reported. KALETRA should be used with caution in patients with underlying structural heart disease, pre-existing conduction system abnormalities, ischemic heart disease or cardiomyopathies, as these patients may be at increased risk for developing cardiac conduction abnormalities.

The impact on the PR interval of co-administration of KALETRA with other drugs that prolong the PR interval (including calcium channel blockers, beta-adrenergic blockers, digoxin and atazanavir) has not been evaluated. As a result, co-administration of KALETRA with these drugs should be undertaken with caution, particularly with those drugs metabolized by CYP3A. Clinical monitoring is recommended [see Clinical Pharmacology (12.3)].

5.6 QT Interval Prolongation
Postmarketing cases of QT interval prolongation and torsade de pointes have been reported although causality of KALETRA could not be established. Avoid use in patients with congenital long QT syndrome, those with hypokalemia, and with other drugs that prolong the QT interval [see Clinical Pharmacology (12.3)].

5.7 Immune Reconstitution Syndrome
Immune reconstitution syndrome has been reported in patients treated with combination antiretroviral therapy, including KALETRA. During the initial phase of combination antiretroviral treatment, patients whose immune system responds may develop an inflammatory response to indolent or residual opportunistic infections (such as Mycobacterium avium infection, cytomegalovirus, Pneumocystis jirovecii pneumonia [PCP], or tuberculosis) which may necessitate further evaluation and treatment.

5.8 Fat Redistribution
Redistribution/accumulation of body fat including central obesity, dorsocervical fat enlargement (buffalo hump), peripheral wasting, facial wasting, breast enlargement, and "cushingoid appearance" have been observed in patients receiving antiretroviral therapy. The mechanism and long-term consequences of these events are currently unknown. A causal relationship has not been established.

5.9 Lipid Elevations
Treatment with KALETRA has resulted in large increases in the concentration of total cholesterol and triglycerides [see Adverse Reactions (6.1)]. Triglyceride and cholesterol testing should be performed prior to initiating KALETRA therapy and at periodic intervals during therapy. Lipid disorders should be managed as clinically appropriate, taking into account any potential drug-drug interactions with KALETRA and HMG-CoA reductase inhibitors [see Contraindications (4) and Drug Interactions (7.3)].

5.10 Patients with Hemophilia
Increased bleeding, including spontaneous skin hematomas and hemarthrosis have been reported in patients with hemophilia type A and B treated with protease inhibitors. In some patients additional factor VIII was given. In more than half of the reported cases, treatment with protease inhibitors was continued or reintroduced. A causal relationship between protease inhibitor therapy and these events has not been established.

5.11 Resistance/Cross-resistance
Because the potential for HIV cross-resistance among protease inhibitors has not been fully explored in KALETRA-treated patients, it is unknown what effect therapy with KALETRA will have on the activity of subsequently administered protease inhibitors [see Clinical Pharmacology (12.4)].

6 ADVERSE REACTIONS
The following adverse reactions are discussed in greater detail in other sections of the labeling.
- PR Interval Prolongation, QT Interval Prolongation [see Warnings and Precautions (5.5, 5.6)]
- Drug Interactions [see Warnings and Precautions (5.1)]
- Pancreatitis [see Warnings and Precautions (5.2)]
- Hepatotoxicity [see Warnings and Precautions (5.3)]

Because clinical trials are conducted under widely varying conditions, adverse reactions rates observed in the clinical trials of a drug cannot be directly compared to rates in the clinical trials of another drug and may not reflect the rates observed in practice.

6.1 Adults - Clinical Trials Experience
The safety profile of KALETRA in adults is primarily based on 1964 HIV-1 infected patients in clinical trials.

The most common adverse reaction was diarrhea, which was generally of mild to moderate severity. In study 730, the incidence of diarrhea of any severity during 48 weeks of therapy was 60% in patients receiving KALETRA tablets once daily compared to 57% in patients receiving KALETRA tablets twice daily. More patients receiving KALETRA tablets once daily (14, 4.2%) had ongoing diarrhea at the time of discontinuation as compared to patients receiving KALETRA tablets twice daily (6, 1.8%). In study 730, discontinuations due to any adverse reaction were 4.8% in patients receiving KALETRA tablets once daily as compared to 3% in patients receiving KALETRA tablets twice daily. In study 802, the incidence of diarrhea of any severity during 48 weeks of therapy was 50% in patients receiving KALETRA tablets once daily compared to 39% in patients receiving KALETRA tablets twice daily. Moderate or severe drug-related diarrhea occurred in 14% of patients receiving KALETRA tablets once daily as compared to 11% in patients receiving KALETRA tablets twice daily. At the time of discontinuation, 19 (6.3%) patients receiving KALETRA tablets once daily had ongoing diarrhea, as compared to 11 (3.7%) patients receiving KALETRA tablets twice daily. Discontinuations due to any adverse reaction occurred in 4.3% of patients receiving KALETRA tablets once daily compared to 7.0% in patients receiving KALETRA tablets twice daily. In study 863, discontinuations of randomized therapy due to adverse reactions were 3.4% in KALETRA-treated and 3.7% in nelfinavir-treated patients.

Treatment-emergent clinical adverse reactions of moderate or severe intensity in ≥ 2% of patients treated with combination therapy for up to 48 weeks (Studies 863 and 730) and for up to 360 weeks (Study 720) are presented in Table 4 (treatment-naïve patients); and for up to 48 weeks (Studies 888 and 802), 84 weeks (Study 957) and 144 weeks (Study 765) in Table 5 (protease inhibitor-experienced patients).
[See table 4 at top of next page]
[See table 5 at top of page 462]

Less Common Adverse Reactions
Treatment-emergent adverse reactions occurring in less than 2% of adult patients receiving KALETRA in the clinical trials supporting approval and of at least moderate intensity are listed below by system organ class.

Blood and Lymphatic System Disorders
Anemia, leukopenia, lymphadenopathy, neutropenia, and splenomegaly.

Cardiac Disorders
Angina pectoris, atrial fibrillation, atrioventricular block, myocardial infarction, palpitations, and tricuspid valve incompetence.

Ear and Labyrinth Disorders
Hyperacusis, tinnitus, and vertigo.

Table 3. Drugs That Are Contraindicated With KALETRA

Drug Class	Drugs Within Class That Are Contraindicated With KALETRA	Clinical comments
Alpha 1-Adrenoreceptor antagonist	Alfuzosin	Potentially increased alfuzosin concentrations can result in hypotension.
Antimycobacterial	Rifampin	May lead to loss of virologic response and possible resistance to KALETRA or to the class of protease inhibitors or other co-administered antiretroviral agents [see Drug Interactions (7)].
Ergot Derivatives	Dihydroergotamine, ergonovine, ergotamine, methylergonovine	Potential for acute ergot toxicity characterized by peripheral vasospasm and ischemia of the extremities and other tissues.
GI motility agent	Cisapride	Potential for cardiac arrhythmias.
Herbal Products	St. John's Wort (hypericum perforatum)	May lead to loss of virologic response and possible resistance to KALETRA or to the class of protease inhibitors.
HMG-CoA Reductase Inhibitors	Lovastatin, simvastatin	Potential for myopathy including rhabdomyolysis.
PDE5 enzyme inhibitor	Sildenafil[a] (Revatio®) when used for the treatment of pulmonary arterial hypertension	A safe and effective dose has not been established when used with KALETRA. There is an increased potential for sildenafil-associated adverse events, including visual abnormalities, hypotension, prolonged erection, and syncope [see Drug Interactions (7)].
Neuroleptic	Pimozide	Potential for cardiac arrhythmias.
Sedative/Hypnotics	Triazolam; orally administered midazolam[b]	Prolonged or increased sedation or respiratory depression.

[a]see Drug Interactions (7) for coadministration of sildenafil in patients with erectile dysfunction.
[b]see Drug Interactions, Table 9 for parenterally administered midazolam.

Table 4. Percentage of Adult Patients with Selected Treatment-Emergent[1] Adverse Reactions of Moderate or Severe Intensity Reported in ≥ 2% of Adult Antiretroviral-Naïve Patients

	Study 863 (48 Weeks)		Study 720 (360 Weeks)	Study 730 (48 Weeks)	
	KALETRA 400/100 mg Twice Daily + d4T + 3TC (N = 326)	Nelfinavir 750 mg Three Times Daily + d4T + 3TC (N = 327)	KALETRA Twice Daily[2] + d4T + 3TC (N = 100)	KALETRA 800/200 mg Once Daily + TDF +FTC (N=333)	KALETRA 400/100 mg Twice Daily + TDF +FTC (N=331)
Endocrine Disorders					
Hypogonadism	0%	0%	2%	0%	0%
Gastrointestinal Disorders					
Diarrhea	16%	17%	28%	17%	15%
Nausea	7%	5%	16%	7%	5%
Vomiting	2%	2%	6%	3%	4%
Abdominal Pain	4%	3%	11%	1%	1%
Dyspepsia	2%	<1%	6%	0%	0%
Flatulence	2%	1%	4%	1%	1%
General Disorders and Administration Site Conditions					
Asthenia	4%	3%	9%	<1%	<1%
Infections and Infestations					
Bronchitis	0%	0%	2%	0%	<1%
Investigations					
Weight decreased	1%	<1%	2%	0%	<1%
Metabolism and Nutrition Disorders					
Anorexia	1%	<1%	2%	<1%	1%
Musculoskeletal and Connective Tissue Disorders					
Myalgia	1%	1%	2%	0%	0%
Nervous System Disorders					
Headache	2%	2%	6%	2%	2%
Paresthesia	1%	1%	2%	0%	0%
Psychiatric Disorders					
Insomnia	2%	1%	3%	1%	0%
Depression	1%	2%	0%	0%	0%
Libido decreased	<1%	<1%	2%	0%	<1%
Skin and Subcutaneous Tissue Disorders					
Rash	1%	2%	5%	<1%	1%
Vascular Disorders					
Vasodilation	0%	0%	3%	0%	0%

[1] Includes adverse reactions of possible or probable relationship to study drug.
[2] Includes adverse reaction data from dose group I (200/100 mg twice daily [N = 16] and 400/100 mg twice daily [N = 16]) and dose group II (400/100 mg twice daily [N = 35] and 400/200 mg twice daily [N = 33]). Within dosing groups, moderate to severe nausea of probable/possible relationship to KALETRA occurred at a higher rate in the 400/200 mg dose arm compared to the 400/100 mg dose arm in group II.
Definitions: d4T = Stavudine; 3TC = Lamivudine; TDF = Tenofovir Disoproxil Fumarate; FTC = Emtricitabine

Endocrine Disorders
Cushing's syndrome and hypothyroidism.
Eye Disorders
Eye disorder and visual disturbance.

Gastrointestinal Disorders
Abdominal discomfort, abdominal distension, abdomen pain lower, constipation, duodenitis, dry mouth, enteritis, enterocolitis, enterocolitis hemorrhagic, eructation, esophagitis,

fecal incontinence, gastric disorder, gastric ulcer, gastritis, gastroesophageal reflux disease, hemorrhoids, mouth ulceration, pancreatitis, periodontitis, rectal hemorrhage, stomach discomfort, and stomatitis.
General Disorders and Administration Site Conditions
Chest pain, cyst, drug interaction, edema, edema peripheral, face edema, fatigue, hypertrophy, and malaise.
Hepatobiliary Disorders
Cholangitis, cholecystitis, cytolytic hepatitis, hepatic steatosis, hepatitis, hepatomegaly, jaundice, and liver tenderness.
Immune System Disorders
Drug hypersensitivity, hypersitivity, and immune reconstitution syndrome.
Infections and Infestations
Bacterial infection, bronchopneumonia, cellulitis, folliculitis, furuncle, gastroenteritis, influenza, otitis media, perineal abscess, pharyngitis, rhinitis, sialoadenitis, sinusitis, and viral infection.
Investigations
Drug level increased, glucose tolerance decreased, and weight increased.
Metabolism and Nutrition Disorders
Decreased appetite, dehydration, diabetes mellitus, hypovitaminosis, increased appetite, lactic acidosis, lipomatosis, and obesity.
Musculoskeletal and Connective Tissue Disorders
Arthralgia, arthropathy, back pain, muscular weakness, osteoarthritis, osteonecrosis, and pain in extremity.
Neoplasms Benign, Malignant and Unspecified (incl Cysts and Polyps)
Benign neoplasm of skin, lipoma, and neoplasm.
Nervous System Disorders
Ageusia, amnesia, ataxia, balance disorder, cerebral infarction, convulsion, dizziness, dysgeusia, dyskinesia, encephalopathy, extrapyramidal disorder, facial palsy, hypertonia, migraine, neuropathy, neuropathy peripheral, somnolence, and tremor.
Psychiatric Disorders
Abnormal dreams, affect lability, agitation, anxiety, apathy, confusional state, disorientation, mood swings, nervousness, and thinking abnormal.
Renal and Urinary Disorders
Hematuria, nephritis, nephrolithiasis, renal disorder, urine abnormality, and urine odor abnormal.
Reproductive System and Breast Disorders
Breast enlargement, ejaculation disorder, erectile dysfunction, gynecomastia, and menorrhagia.
Respiratory, Thoracic and Mediastinal Disorders
Asthma, cough, dyspnea, and pulmonary edema.
Skin and Subcutaneous Tissue Disorders
Acne, alopecia, dermatitis acneiform, dermatitis allergic, dermatitis exfoliative, dry skin, eczema, hyperhidrosis, idiopathic capillaritis, nail disorder, pruritis, rash generalized, rash maculo-papular, seborrhea, skin discoloration, skin hypertrophy, skin striae, skin ulcer, and swelling face.
Vascular Disorders
Deep vein thrombosis, orthostatic hypotension, thrombophlebitis, varicose vein, and vasculitis.
Laboratory Abnormalities
The percentages of adult patients treated with combination therapy with Grade 3-4 laboratory abnormalities are presented in Table 6 (treatment-naïve patients) and Table 7 (treatment-experienced patients).
[See table 6 at top of page 463]
[See table 7 at top of page 464]
6.2 Pediatric Patients - Clinical Trials Experience
KALETRA oral solution dosed up to 300/75 mg/m² has been studied in 100 pediatric patients 6 months to 12 years of age. The adverse reaction profile seen during Study 940 was similar to that for adult patients.
Dysgeusia (22%), vomiting (21%), and diarrhea (12%) were the most common adverse reactions of any severity reported in pediatric patients treated with combination therapy for up to 48 weeks in Study 940. A total of 8 patients experienced adverse reactions of moderate to severe intensity. The adverse reactions meeting these criteria and reported for the 8 subjects include: hypersensitivity (characterized by fever, rash and jaundice), pyrexia, viral infection, constipation, hepatomegaly, pancreatitis, vomiting, alanine aminotransferase increased, dry skin, rash, and dysgeusia. Rash was the only event of those listed that occurred in 2 or more subjects (N = 3).
KALETRA oral solution dosed at 300/75 mg/m² has been studied in 31 pediatric patients 14 days to 6 months of age. The adverse reaction profile in Study 1030 was similar to that observed in older children and adults. No adverse reaction was reported in greater than 10% of subjects. Ad-

Information on the Abbott Pharmaceutical Products listed on these pages is from the prescribing information in use as of June 1, 2010. For more information, please visit rxabbott.com or call 1-800-633-9110.

verse drug reactions of moderate to severe intensity occurring in 2 or more subjects included decreased neutrophil count (N=3), anemia (N=2), high potassium (N=2), and low sodium (N=2).

KALETRA oral solution and soft gelatin capsules dosed at higher than recommended doses including 400/100 mg/m² (without concomitant NNRTI) and 480/120 mg/m² (with concomitant NNRTI) have been studied in 26 pediatric patients 7 to 18 years of age in Study 1038. Patients also had saquinavir mesylate added to their regimen at Week 4. Rash (12%), blood cholesterol abnormal (12%) and blood triglycerides abnormal (12%) were the only adverse reactions reported in greater than 10% of subjects. Adverse drug reactions of moderate to severe intensity occurring in 2 or more subjects included rash (N=3), blood triglycerides abnormal (N=3), and electrocardiogram QT prolonged (N=2). Both subjects with QT prolongation had additional predisposing conditions such as electrolyte abnormalities, concomitant medications, or pre-existing cardiac abnormalities.

Laboratory Abnormalities

The percentages of pediatric patients treated with combination therapy including KALETRA with Grade 3-4 laboratory abnormalities are presented in Table 8.

Table 8. Grade 3-4 Laboratory Abnormalities Reported in ≥ 2% Pediatric Patients in Study 940

Variable	Limit[1]	KALETRA Twice Daily + RTIs (N = 100)
Chemistry	**High**	
Sodium	> 149 mEq/L	3%
Total Bilirubin	≥ 3.0 × ULN	3%
SGOT/AST	> 180 U/L	8%
SGPT/ALT	> 215 U/L	7%
Total Cholesterol	> 300 mg/dL	3%
Amylase	> 2.5 × ULN	7%[2]
Chemistry	**Low**	
Sodium	< 130 mEq/L	3%
Hematology	**Low**	
Platelet Count	< 50 × 10⁹/L	4%
Neutrophils	< 0.40 × 10⁹/L	2%

[1] ULN = upper limit of the normal range.
[2] Subjects with Grade 3-4 amylase confirmed by elevations in pancreatic amylase.

6.3 Postmarketing Experience

The following adverse reactions have been reported during postmarketing use of KALETRA. Because these reactions are reported voluntarily from a population of unknown size, it is not possible to reliably estimate their frequency or establish a causal relationship to KALETRA exposure.

Body as a Whole

Redistribution/accumulation of body fat has been reported *[see Warnings and Precautions (5.8)].*

Cardiovascular

Bradyarrhythmias. First-degree AV block, second-degree AV block, third-degree AV block, QTc interval prolongation, torsades (torsade) de pointes *[see Warnings and Precautions (5.5, 5.6)].*

Skin and Appendages

Stevens-Johnson Syndrome and erythema multiforme.

7 DRUG INTERACTIONS

See also Contraindications (4), Clinical Pharmacology (12.3)

7.1 Potential for KALETRA to Affect Other Drugs

Lopinavir/ritonavir is an inhibitor of CYP3A and may increase plasma concentrations of agents that are primarily metabolized by CYP3A. Agents that are extensively metabolized by CYP3A and have high first pass metabolism appear to be the most susceptible to large increases in AUC (> 3-fold) when co-administered with KALETRA. Thus, co-administration of KALETRA with drugs highly dependent on CYP3A for clearance and for which elevated plasma concentrations are associated with serious and/or life-threatening events is contraindicated. Co-administration

Table 5. Percentage of Adult Patients with Selected Treatment-Emergent[1] Adverse Reactions of Moderate or Severe Intensity Reported in ≥ 2% of Adult Protease Inhibitor-Experienced Patients

	Study 888 (48 Weeks)		Study 957[2] and Study 765[3] (84-144 Weeks)	Study 802 (48 Weeks)	
	KALETRA 400/100 mg Twice Daily + NVP + NRTIs (N = 148)	Investigator-selected protease inhibitor(s) + NVP + NRTIs (N = 140)	KALETRA Twice Daily + NNRTI + NRTIs (N = 127)	KALETRA 800/200 mg Once Daily + NRTIs (N=300)	KALETRA 400/100 mg Twice Daily + NRTIs (N=299)
Gastrointestinal Disorders					
Diarrhea	7%	9%	23%	14%	11%
Nausea	7%	16%	5%	3%	7%
Vomiting	4%	12%	2%	2%	3%
Abdominal Pain	2%	2%	4%	2%	<1%
Abdominal Pain Upper	N/A	N/A	N/A	1%	2%
Dyspepsia	1%	1%	2%	1%	<1%
Flatulence	1%	2%	2%	1%	1%
Dysphasia	2%	1%	0%	0%	0%
General Disorders and Administration Site Conditions					
Asthenia	3%	6%	9%	<1%	<1%
Pyrexia	2%	1%	2%	0%	<1%
Chills	2%	0%	0%	0%	0%
Investigations					
Weight decreased	0%	1%	3%	<1%	<1%
Metabolism and Nutrition Disorders					
Anorexia	1%	3%	0%	0%	1%
Musculoskeletal and Connective Tissue Disorders					
Myalgia	1%	1%	2%	0%	0%
Nervous System Disorders					
Headache	2%	3%	2%	<1%	0%
Paresthesia	0%	1%	2%	0%	0%
Psychiatric Disorders					
Depression	1%	2%	3%	<1%	0%
Insomnia	0%	2%	2%	0%	<1%
Skin and Subcutaneous Tissue Disorders					
Rash	2%	1%	2%	0%	0%
Vascular Disorders					
Hypertension	0%	0%	2%	0%	0%

[1] Includes adverse reactions of possible or probable relationship to study drug.
[2] Includes adverse reaction data from patients receiving 400/100 mg twice daily (n = 29) or 533/133 mg twice daily (n = 28) for 84 weeks. Patients received KALETRA in combination with NRTIs and efavirenz.
[3] Includes adverse reaction data from patients receiving 400/100 mg twice daily (n = 36) or 400/200 mg twice daily (n = 34) for 144 weeks. Patients received KALETRA in combination with NRTIs and nevirapine.
Definitions: NVP = Nevirapine; NRTI = Nucleoside Reverse Transcriptase Inhibitors; NNRTI = Non-nucleoside Reverse Transcriptase Inhibitors

with other CYP3A substrates may require a dose adjustment or additional monitoring as shown in Table 9. Additionally, KALETRA induces glucuronidation.

7.2 Potential For Other Drugs To Affect Lopinavir

Lopinavir/ritonavir is a CYP3A substrate; therefore, drugs that induce CYP3A may decrease lopinavir plasma concentrations and reduce KALETRA's therapeutic effect. Although not observed in the KALETRA/ketoconazole drug interaction study, co-administration of KALETRA and other drugs that inhibit CYP3A may increase lopinavir plasma concentrations.

7.3 Established and Other Potentially Significant Drug Interactions

Table 9 provides a listing of established or potentially clinically significant drug interactions. Alteration in dose or regimen may be recommended based on drug interaction

studies or predicted interaction [see Clinical Pharmacology (12.3) for magnitude of interaction].
[See table 9 on pages 465 through 468]

7.4 Drugs with No Observed or Predicted Interactions with KALETRA

Drug interaction studies reveal no clinically significant interaction between KALETRA and desipramine (CYP2D6 probe), pravastatin, stavudine, lamivudine, omeprazole or ranitidine.

Based on known metabolic profiles, clinically significant drug interactions are not expected between KALETRA and fluvastatin, dapsone, trimethoprim/sulfamethoxazole, azithromycin, erythromycin, or fluconazole.

8 USE IN SPECIFIC POPULATIONS

8.1 Pregnancy

Pregnancy Category C.
No treatment-related malformations were observed when lopinavir in combination with ritonavir was administered to pregnant rats or rabbits. Embryonic and fetal developmental toxicities (early resorption, decreased fetal viability, decreased fetal body weight, increased incidence of skeletal variations and skeletal ossification delays) occurred in rats at a maternally toxic dosage. Based on AUC measurements, the drug exposures in rats at the toxic doses were approximately 0.7-fold for lopinavir and 1.8-fold for ritonavir for males and females that of the exposures in humans at the recommended therapeutic dose (400/100 mg twice daily). In a peri- and postnatal study in rats, a developmental toxicity (a decrease in survival in pups between birth and postnatal Day 21) occurred.
No embryonic and fetal developmental toxicities were observed in rabbits at a maternally toxic dosage. Based on AUC measurements, the drug exposures in rabbits at the toxic doses were approximately 0.6-fold for lopinavir and 1.0-fold for ritonavir that of the exposures in humans at the recommended therapeutic dose (400/100 mg twice daily). There are, however, no adequate and well-controlled studies in pregnant women. KALETRA should be used during pregnancy only if the potential benefit justifies the potential risk to the fetus.

Antiretroviral Pregnancy Registry: To monitor maternal-fetal outcomes of pregnant women exposed to KALETRA, an Antiretroviral Pregnancy Registry has been established. Physicians are encouraged to register patients by calling 1-800-258-4263.

8.3 Nursing Mothers

The Centers for Disease Control and Prevention recommend that HIV-1 infected mothers not breast-feed their infants to avoid risking postnatal transmission of HIV-1. Studies in rats have demonstrated that lopinavir is secreted in milk. It is not known whether lopinavir is secreted in human milk. Because of both the potential for HIV-1 transmission and the potential for serious adverse reactions in nursing infants, mothers should be instructed not to breast-feed if they are receiving KALETRA.

8.4 Pediatric Use

The safety, efficacy, and pharmacokinetic profiles of KALETRA in pediatric patients below the age of 14 days have not been established. KALETRA once daily has not been evaluated in pediatric patients.

An open-label, multi-center, dose-finding trial was performed to evaluate the pharmacokinetic profile, tolerability, safety and efficacy of KALETRA oral solution containing lopinavir 80 mg/mL and ritonavir 20 mg/mL at a dose of with 300/75 mg/m^2 twice daily plus two NRTIs in HIV-infected infants ≥14 days and < 6 months of age. Results revealed that infants younger than 6 months of age generally had lower lopinavir AUC$_{12}$ than older children (6 months to 12 years of age), however, despite the lower lopinavir drug exposure observed, antiviral activity was demonstrated as reflected in the proportion of subjects who achieved HIV-RNA <400 copies/mL at Week 24 [see Adverse Reactions (6.2), Clinical Pharmacology (12.3), Clinical Studies (14.4)].
Safety and efficacy in pediatric patients > 6 months of age was demonstrated in a clinical trial in 100 patients. The clinical trial was an open-label, multicenter trial evaluating the pharmacokinetic profile, tolerability, safety, and efficacy of KALETRA oral solution containing lopinavir 80 mg/mL and ritonavir 20 mg/mL in 100 antiretroviral naïve and experienced pediatric patients ages 6 months to 12 years. Dose selection for patients 6 months to 12 years of age was based on the following results. The 230/57.5 mg/m^2 oral solution twice daily regimen without nevirapine and the 300/75 mg/m^2 oral solution twice daily regimen with nevirapine provided lopinavir plasma concentrations similar to those obtained in adult patients receiving the 400/100 mg twice daily regimen (without nevirapine) [see Adverse Reactions (6.2), Clinical Pharmacology (12.3), Clinical Studies (14.4)].
A prospective multicenter, open-label trial evaluated the pharmacokinetic profile, tolerability, safety and efficacy of high-dose KALETRA with or without concurrent NNRTI therapy (Group 1: 400/100 mg/m^2 twice daily + ≥ 2 NRTIs;

Table 6. Grade 3-4 Laboratory Abnormalities Reported in ≥ 2% of Adult Antiretroviral-Naïve Patients

| Variable | Limit[1] | Study 863 (48 Weeks) | | Study 720 (360 Weeks) | Study 730 (48 Weeks) | |
		KALETRA 400/100 mg Twice Daily + d4T + 3TC (N = 326)	Nelfinavir 750 mg Three Times Daily + d4T + 3TC (N = 327)	KALETRA Twice Daily + d4T + 3TC (N = 100)	KALETRA Once Daily + TDF + FTC (N=333)	KALETRA Twice Daily + TDF + FTC (N=331)
Chemistry	**High**					
Glucose	> 250 mg/dL	2%	2%	4%	0%	<1%
Uric Acid	> 12 mg/dL	2%	2%	5%	<1%	1%
SGOT/AST[2]	> 180 U/L	2%	4%	10%	1%	2%
SGPT/ALT[2]	>215 U/L	4%	4%	11%	1%	1%
GGT	>300 U/L	N/A	N/A	10%	N/A	N/A
Total Cholesterol	>300 mg/dL	9%	5%	27%	4%	3%
Triglycerides	>750 mg/dL	9%	1%	29%	3%	6%
Amylase	>2 × ULN	3%	2%	4%	N/A	N/A
Lipase	>2 × ULN	N/A	N/A	N/A	3%	5%
Chemistry	**Low**					
Calculated Creatinine Clearance	<50 mL/min	N/A	N/A	N/A	2%	2%
Hematology	**Low**					
Neutrophils	<0.75 × 10^9/L	1%	3%	5%	2%	1%

[1] ULN = upper limit of the normal range; N/A = Not Applicable.
[2] Criterion for Study 730 was >5× ULN (AST/ALT).

Group 2: 480/120 mg/m^2 twice daily + ≥ 1 NRTI + 1 NNRTI) in children and adolescents ≥ 2 years to < 18 years of age who had failed prior therapy. Patients also had saquinavir mesylate added to their regimen. This strategy was intended to assess whether higher than approved doses of KALETRA could overcome protease inhibitor cross-resistance. High doses of KALETRA exhibited a safety profile similar to those observed in previous trials; changes in HIV-1 RNA were less than anticipated; three patients had HIV-1 RNA <400 copies/mL at Week 48. CD4+ cell count increases were noted in the eight patients who remained on treatment for 48 weeks [see Adverse Reactions (6.2), Clinical Pharmacology (12.3)].

8.5 Geriatric Use

Clinical studies of KALETRA did not include sufficient numbers of subjects aged 65 and over to determine whether they respond differently from younger subjects. In general, appropriate caution should be exercised in the administration and monitoring of KALETRA in elderly patients reflecting the greater frequency of decreased hepatic, renal, or cardiac function, and of concomitant disease or other drug therapy.

8.6 Hepatic Impairment

KALETRA is principally metabolized by the liver; therefore, caution should be exercised when administering this drug to patients with hepatic impairment, because lopinavir concentrations may be increased [see Warnings and Precautions (5.3) and Clinical Pharmacology (12.3)].

10 OVERDOSAGE

Overdoses with KALETRA oral solution have been reported. One of these reports described fatal cardiogenic shock in a 2.1 kg infant who received a single dose of 6.5 mL of KALETRA oral solution nine days prior. However, a causal relationship between the overdose and the outcome could not be established. Healthcare professionals should be aware that KALETRA oral solution is highly concentrated and therefore, should pay special attention to accurate calculation of the dose of KALETRA, transcription of the medication order, dispensing information and dosing instructions to minimize the risk for medication errors and overdose. This is especially important for infants and young children.
KALETRA oral solution contains 42.4% alcohol (v/v). Accidental ingestion of the product by a young child could result in significant alcohol-related toxicity and could approach the potential lethal dose of alcohol.
Human experience of acute overdosage with KALETRA is limited. Treatment of overdose with KALETRA should consist of general supportive measures including monitoring of vital signs and observation of the clinical status of the patient. There is no specific antidote for overdose with KALETRA. If indicated, elimination of unabsorbed drug should be achieved by emesis or gastric lavage. Administration of activated charcoal may also be used to aid in removal of unabsorbed drug. Since KALETRA is highly protein bound, dialysis is unlikely to be beneficial in significant removal of the drug.

11 DESCRIPTION

KALETRA® (lopinavir/ritonavir) is a co-formulation of lopinavir and ritonavir. Lopinavir is an inhibitor of the HIV-1 protease. As co-formulated in KALETRA, ritonavir inhibits the CYP3A-mediated metabolism of lopinavir, thereby providing increased plasma levels of lopinavir.
Lopinavir is chemically designated as [1S-[1R*,(R*), 3R*, 4R*]]-N-[4-[[(2,6-dimethylphenoxy)acetyl]amino]-3-hydroxy-5-phenyl-1-(phenylmethyl)pentyl]tetrahydro-alpha-(1-methylethyl)-2-oxo-1(2H)-pyrimidineacetamide. Its molecular formula is C$_{37}$H$_{48}$N$_4$O$_5$, and its molecular weight is 628.80. Lopinavir is a white to light tan powder. It is freely soluble in methanol and ethanol, soluble in isopropanol and practically insoluble in water. Lopinavir has the following structural formula:

Ritonavir is chemically designated as 10-hydroxy-2-methyl-5-(1-methylethyl)-1-[2-(1-methylethyl)-4-thiazolyl]-3,6-dioxo-8,11-bis(phenylmethyl)-2,4,7,12-tetraazatridecan-13-oic acid, 5-thiazolylmethyl ester, [5S-(5R*,8R*, 10R*,11R*)]. Its molecular formula is C$_{37}$H$_{48}$N$_6$O$_5$S$_2$, and its molecular weight is 720.95. Ritonavir is a white to light tan powder. It is freely soluble in methanol and ethanol, soluble in isopropanol and practically insoluble in water. Ritonavir has the following structural formula:

KALETRA film-coated tablets are available for oral administration in two strengths:

- Yellow tablets containing 200 mg of lopinavir and 50 mg of ritonavir
- Pale yellow tablets containing 100 mg of lopinavir and 25 mg of ritonavir.

The yellow, 200 mg lopinavir/50 mg ritonavir, tablets contain the following inactive ingredients: copovidone, sorbitan monolaurate, colloidal silicon dioxide, and sodium stearyl fumarate. The following are the ingredients in the film coating: hypromellose, titanium dioxide, polyethylene glycol 400, hydroxypropyl cellulose, talc, colloidal silicon dioxide, polyethylene glycol 3350, yellow ferric oxide E172, and polysorbate 80.

The pale yellow, 100 mg lopinavir/25 mg ritonavir, tablets contain the following inactive ingredients: copovidone, sorbitan monolaurate, colloidal silicon dioxide, and sodium stearyl fumarate. The following are the ingredients in the film coating: polyvinyl alcohol, titanium dioxide, talc, polyethylene glycol 3350, and yellow ferric oxide E172.

KALETRA oral solution is available for oral administration as 80 mg lopinavir and 20 mg ritonavir per milliliter with the following inactive ingredients: acesulfame potassium, alcohol, artificial cotton candy flavor, citric acid, glycerin, high fructose corn syrup, Magnasweet-110 flavor, menthol, natural & artificial vanilla flavor, peppermint oil, polyoxyl 40 hydrogenated castor oil, povidone, propylene glycol, saccharin sodium, sodium chloride, sodium citrate, and water. KALETRA oral solution contains 42.4% alcohol (v/v).

12   CLINICAL PHARMACOLOGY

12.1   Mechanism of Action

Lopinavir is an antiviral drug *[see Clinical Pharmacology (12.4)]*.

12.3   Pharmacokinetics

The pharmacokinetic properties of lopinavir co-administered with ritonavir have been evaluated in healthy adult volunteers and in HIV-1 infected patients; no substantial differences were observed between the two groups. Lopinavir is essentially completely metabolized by CYP3A. Ritonavir inhibits the metabolism of lopinavir, thereby increasing the plasma levels of lopinavir. Across studies, administration of KALETRA 400/100 mg twice daily yields mean steady-state lopinavir plasma concentrations 15- to 20-fold higher than those of ritonavir in HIV-1 infected patients. The plasma levels of ritonavir are less than 7% of those obtained after the ritonavir dose of 600 mg twice daily. The *in vitro* antiviral EC_{50} of lopinavir is approximately 10-fold lower than that of ritonavir. Therefore, the antiviral activity of KALETRA is due to lopinavir.

Figure 1 displays the mean steady-state plasma concentrations of lopinavir and ritonavir after KALETRA 400/100 mg twice daily with food for 3 weeks from a pharmacokinetic study in HIV-1 infected adult subjects (n = 19).

Figure 1. Mean Steady-State Plasma Concentrations with 95% Confidence Intervals (CI) for HIV-1 Infected Adult Subjects (N = 19)

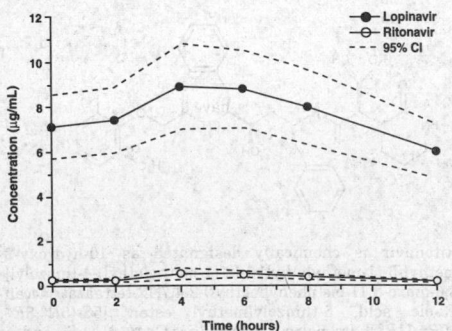

Absorption

In a pharmacokinetic study in HIV-1 positive subjects (n = 19), multiple dosing with 400/100 mg KALETRA twice daily with food for 3 weeks produced a mean ± SD lopinavir peak plasma concentration (C_{max}) of 9.8 ± 3.7 μg/mL, occurring approximately 4 hours after administration. The mean steady-state trough concentration prior to the morning dose was 7.1 ± 2.9 μg/mL and minimum concentration within a dosing interval was 5.5 ± 2.7 μg/mL. Lopinavir AUC over a 12 hour dosing interval averaged 92.6 ± 36.7 μg•h/mL. The

Table 7. Grade 3-4 Laboratory Abnormalities Reported in ≥ 2% of Adult Protease Inhibitor-Experienced Patients

Variable	Limit[1]	Study 888 (48 Weeks) KALETRA 400/100 mg Twice Daily + NVP + NRTIs (N = 148)	Study 888 (48 Weeks) Investigator-selected protease inhibitor(s) + NVP + NRTIs (N = 140)	Study 957[2] and Study 765[3] (84-144 Weeks) KALETRA Twice Daily + NNRTI + NRTIs (N = 127)	Study 802 (48 Weeks) KALETRA 800/200 mg Once Daily + NRTIs (N=300)	Study 802 (48 Weeks) KALETRA 400/100 mg Twice Daily + NRTIs (N=299)
Chemistry	**High**					
Glucose	>250 mg/dL	1%	2%	5%	2%	2%
Total Bilirubin	>3.48 mg/dL	1%	3%	1%	1%	1%
SGOT/AST[4]	>180 U/L	5%	11%	8%	3%	2%
SGPT/ALT[4]	>215 U/L	6%	13%	10%	2%	2%
GGT	>300 U/L	N/A	N/A	29%	N/A	N/A
Total Cholesterol	>300 mg/dL	20%	21%	39%	6%	7%
Triglycerides	>750 mg/dL	25%	21%	36%	5%	6%
Amylase	>2 × ULN	4%	8%	8%	4%	4%
Lipase	>2 × ULN	N/A	N/A	N/A	4%	1%
Creatine Phosphokinase	>4 × ULN	N/A	N/A	N/A	4%	5%
Chemistry	**Low**					
Calculated Creatine Clearance	<50 mL/min	N/A	N/A	N/A	3%	3%
Inorganic Phosphorus	<1.5 mg/dL	1%	0%	2%	1%	<1%
Hematology	**Low**					
Neutrophils	<0.75 ×10⁹/L	1%	2%	4%	3%	4%
Hemoglobin	<80 g/L	1%	1%	1%	1%	2%

[1] ULN = upper limit of the normal range; N/A = Not Applicable.
[2] Includes clinical laboratory data from patients receiving 400/100 mg twice daily (n = 29) or 533/133 mg twice daily (n = 28) for 84 weeks. Patients received KALETRA in combination with NRTIs and efavirenz.
[3] Includes clinical laboratory data from patients receiving 400/100 mg twice daily (n = 36) or 400/200 mg twice daily (n = 34) for 144 weeks. Patients received KALETRA in combination with NRTIs and nevirapine.
[4] Criterion for Study 802 was >5x ULN (AST/ALT).

absolute bioavailability of lopinavir co-formulated with ritonavir in humans has not been established. Under non-fasting conditions (500 kcal, 25% from fat), lopinavir concentrations were similar following administration of KALETRA co-formulated capsules and oral solution. When administered under fasting conditions, both the mean AUC and C_{max} of lopinavir were 22% lower for the KALETRA oral solution relative to the capsule formulation.

Plasma concentrations of lopinavir and ritonavir after administration of two 200/50 mg KALETRA tablets are similar to three 133.3/33.3 mg KALETRA capsules under fed conditions with less pharmacokinetic variability.

Effects of Food on Oral Absorption

KALETRA Tablets

No clinically significant changes in C_{max} and AUC were observed following administration of KALETRA tablets under fed conditions compared to fasted conditions. Relative to fasting, administration of KALETRA tablets with a moderate fat meal (500-682 Kcal, 23 to 25% calories from fat) increased lopinavir AUC and C_{max} by 26.9% and 17.6%, respectively. Relative to fasting, administration of KALETRA tablets with a high fat meal (872 Kcal, 56% from fat) increased lopinavir AUC by 18.9% but not C_{max}. Therefore, KALETRA tablets may be taken with or without food.

KALETRA Oral Solution

Relative to fasting, administration of KALETRA oral solution with a moderate fat meal (500-682 Kcal, 23 to 25% calories from fat) increased lopinavir AUC and C_{max} by 80 and 54%, respectively. Relative to fasting, administration of KALETRA oral solution with a high fat meal (872 Kcal, 56% from fat) increased lopinavir AUC and C_{max} by 130% and 56%, respectively. To enhance bioavailability and minimize pharmacokinetic variability KALETRA oral solution should be taken with food.

Distribution

At steady state, lopinavir is approximately 98-99% bound to plasma proteins. Lopinavir binds to both alpha-1-acid glycoprotein (AAG) and albumin; however, it has a higher af-

finity for AAG. At steady state, lopinavir protein binding remains constant over the range of observed concentrations after 400/100 mg KALETRA twice daily, and is similar between healthy volunteers and HIV-1 positive patients.

Metabolism

In vitro experiments with human hepatic microsomes indicate that lopinavir primarily undergoes oxidative metabolism. Lopinavir is extensively metabolized by the hepatic cytochrome P450 system, almost exclusively by the CYP3A isozyme. Ritonavir is a potent CYP3A inhibitor which inhibits the metabolism of lopinavir, and therefore increases plasma levels of lopinavir. A ¹⁴C-lopinavir study in humans showed that 89% of the plasma radioactivity after a single 400/100 mg KALETRA dose was due to parent drug. At least 13 lopinavir oxidative metabolites have been identified in man. Ritonavir has been shown to induce metabolic enzymes, resulting in the induction of its own metabolism. Pre-dose lopinavir concentrations decline with time during multiple dosing, stabilizing after approximately 10 to 16 days.

Elimination

Following a 400/100 mg ¹⁴C-lopinavir/ritonavir dose, approximately 10.4 ± 2.3% and 82.6 ± 2.5% of an administered dose of ¹⁴C-lopinavir can be accounted for in urine and feces, respectively, after 8 days. Unchanged lopinavir accounted for approximately 2.2 and 19.8% of the administered dose in urine and feces, respectively. After multiple dosing, less than 3% of the lopinavir dose is excreted unchanged in the urine. The apparent oral clearance (CL/F) of lopinavir is 5.98 ± 5.75 L/hr (mean ± SD, n = 19).

Once Daily Dosing

The pharmacokinetics of once daily KALETRA have been evaluated in HIV-1 infected subjects naïve to antiretroviral treatment. KALETRA 800/200 mg was administered in combination with emtricitabine 200 mg and tenofovir DF 300 mg as part of a once daily regimen. Multiple dosing of 800/200 mg KALETRA once daily for 4 weeks with food (n = 24) produced a mean ± SD lopinavir peak plasma con-

Table 9. Established and Other Potentially Significant Drug Interactions

Concomitant Drug Class: Drug Name	Effect on Concentration of Lopinavir or Concomitant Drug	Clinical Comment
HIV-1 Antiviral Agents		
Non-nucleoside Reverse Transcriptase Inhibitors: efavirenz*, nevirapine*	↓ lopinavir	KALETRA dose increase is recommended in all patients *[see Dosage and Administration (2.1) and Clinical Pharmacology (12.3)].* Increasing the dose of KALETRA tablets to 500/125 mg (given as two 200/50 mg tablets and one 100/25 mg tablet) twice daily co-administered with efavirenz resulted in similar lopinavir concentrations compared to KALETRA 400/100 mg (given as two 200/50 mg tablets) twice daily without efavirenz. Increasing the dose of KALETRA tablets to 600/150 mg (given as three 200/50 mg tablets) twice daily co-administered with efavirenz resulted in significantly higher lopinavir plasma concentrations compared to KALETRA tablets 400/100 mg twice daily without efavirenz. KALETRA should not be administered once daily in combination with efavirenz or nevirapine *[see Dosage and Administration (2.1) and Clinical Pharmacology (12.3)].*
Non-nucleoside Reverse Transcriptase Inhibitor: delavirdine	↑ lopinavir	Appropriate doses of the combination with respect to safety and efficacy have not been established.
Nucleoside Reverse Transcriptase Inhibitor: didanosine		KALETRA tablets can be administered simultaneously with didanosine without food. For KALETRA oral solution, it is recommended that didanosine be administered on an empty stomach; therefore, didanosine should be given one hour before or two hours after KALETRA oral solution (given with food).
Nucleoside Reverse Transcriptase Inhibitor: tenofovir	↑ tenofovir	KALETRA increases tenofovir concentrations. The mechanism of this interaction is unknown. Patients receiving KALETRA and tenofovir should be monitored for adverse reactions associated with tenofovir.
Nucleoside Reverse Transcriptase Inhibitor: abacavir zidovudine	↓ abacavir ↓ zidovudine	KALETRA induces glucuronidation; therefore, KALETRA has the potential to reduce zidovudine and abacavir plasma concentrations. The clinical significance of this potential interaction is unknown.
HIV-1 Protease Inhibitor: amprenavir*	↑ amprenavir ↓ lopinavir	KALETRA should not be administered once daily in combination with amprenavir *[see Dosage and Administration (2.1)].*
HIV-1 Protease Inhibitor: fosamprenavir/ritonavir	↓ amprenavir ↓ lopinavir	An increased rate of adverse reactions has been observed with co-administration of these medications. Appropriate doses of the combinations with respect to safety and efficacy have not been established.
HIV-1 Protease Inhibitor: indinavir*	↑ indinavir	Decrease indinavir dose to 600 mg twice daily, when co-administered with KALETRA 400/100 mg twice daily *[see Clinical Pharmacology (12.3)].* KALETRA once daily has not been studied in combination with indinavir.
HIV-1 Protease Inhibitor: nelfinavir*	↑ nelfinavir ↑ M8 metabolite of nelfinavir ↓ lopinavir	KALETRA should not be administered once daily in combination with nelfinavir *[see Dosage and Administration (2.1) and Clinical Pharmacology (12.3)].*
HIV-1 Protease Inhibitor: ritonavir*	↑ lopinavir	Appropriate doses of additional ritonavir in combination with KALETRA with respect to safety and efficacy have not been established.
HIV-1 Protease Inhibitor: saquinavir*	↑ saquinavir	The saquinavir dose is 1000 mg twice daily, when co-administered with KALETRA 400/100 mg twice daily. KALETRA once daily has not been studied in combination with saquinavir.
HIV-1 Protease Inhibitor: tipranavir	↓ lopinavir AUC and C_{min}	KALETRA should not be administered with tipranavir (500 mg twice daily) co-administered with ritonavir (200 mg twice daily).
HIV CCR5-antagonist: maraviroc	↑ maraviroc	Concurrent administration of maraviroc with KALETRA will increase plasma levels of maraviroc. When co-administered, patients should receive 150 mg twice daily of maraviroc. For further details see complete prescribing information for Selzentry® (maraviroc).

(Table continued on next page)

centration (C_{max}) of 11.8 ± 3.7 µg/mL, occurring approximately 6 hours after administration. The mean steady-state lopinavir trough concentration prior to the morning dose was 3.2 ± 2.1 µg/mL and minimum concentration within a dosing interval was 1.7 ± 1.6 µg/mL. Lopinavir AUC over a 24 hour dosing interval averaged 154.1 ± 61.4 µg•h/mL.

The pharmacokinetics of once daily KALETRA has also been evaluated in treatment experienced HIV-1 infected subjects. Lopinavir exposure (C_{max}, $AUC_{[0-24h]}$, C_{trough}) with once daily KALETRA administration in treatment experienced subjects is comparable to the once daily lopinavir exposure in treatment naïve subjects.

Effects on Electrocardiogram

QTcF interval was evaluated in a randomized, placebo and active (moxifloxacin 400 mg once daily) controlled crossover study in 39 healthy adults, with 10 measurements over 12 hours on Day 3. The maximum mean time-matched (95% upper confidence bound) differences in QTcF interval from placebo after baseline-correction were 5.3 (8.1) and 15.2 (18.0) mseconds (msec) for 400/100 mg twice daily and supratherapeutic 800/200 mg twice daily KALETRA, respectively. KALETRA 800/200 mg twice daily resulted in a Day 3 mean C_{max} approximately 2-fold higher than the mean C_{max} observed with the approved once daily and twice daily KALETRA doses at steady state.

PR interval prolongation was also noted in subjects receiving KALETRA in the same study on Day 3. The maximum mean (95% upper confidence bound) difference from placebo in the PR interval after baseline-correction were 24.9 (21.5, 28.3) and 31.9 (28.5, 35.3) msec for 400/100 mg twice daily and supratherapeutic 800/200 mg twice daily KALETRA, respectively *[see Warnings and Precautions (5.5, 5.6)].*

Special Populations

Gender, Race and Age

No gender related pharmacokinetic differences have been observed in adult patients. No clinically important pharmacokinetic differences due to race have been identified. Lopinavir pharmacokinetics have not been studied in elderly patients.

Pediatric Patients

The pharmacokinetics of KALETRA oral solution 300/75 mg/m² twice daily and 230/57.5 mg/m² twice daily have been studied in a total of 53 pediatric patients in Study 940, ranging in age from 6 months to 12 years *[see Clinical Studies (14.4)].* The 230/57.5 mg/m² twice daily regimen without nevirapine and the 300/75 mg/m² twice daily regimen with nevirapine provided lopinavir plasma concentrations similar to those obtained in adult patients receiving the 400/100 mg twice daily regimen (without nevirapine).

The mean steady-state lopinavir AUC, C_{max}, and C_{min} were 72.6 ± 31.1 µg•h/mL, 8.2 ± 2.9 and 3.4 ± 2.1 µg/mL, respectively after KALETRA oral solution 230/57.5 mg/m² twice daily without nevirapine (n = 12), and were 85.8 ± 36.9 µg• h/mL, 10.0 ± 3.3 and 3.6 ± 3.5 µg/mL, respectively, after 300/75 mg/m² twice daily with nevirapine (n = 12). The nevirapine regimen was 7 mg/kg twice daily (6 months to 8 years) or 4 mg/kg twice daily (> 8 years).

The pharmacokinetics of KALETRA oral solution at approximately 300/75 mg/m² twice daily have also been evaluated in infants at approximately 6 weeks of age (n = 9) and between 6 weeks and 6 months of age (n = 18) in Study 1030. The mean steady-state lopinavir AUC_{12}, C_{max}, and C_{12} were 43.4 ± 14.8 µg• h/mL, 5.2 ± 1.8 µg/mL and 1.9 ± 1.1 µg/mL, respectively, in infants at approximately 6 weeks of age, and 74.5 ± 37.9 µg• h/mL, 9.4 ± 4.9 and 3.1 ± 1.8 µg/mL, respectively, in infants between 6 weeks and 6 months of age after KALETRA oral solution was administered at approximately 300/75 mg/m² twice daily without concomitant NNRTI therapy.

The pharmacokinetics of KALETRA soft gelatin capsule and oral solution (Group 1: 400/100 mg/m² twice daily + 2 NRTIs; Group 2: 480/120 mg/m² twice daily + ≥ 1 NRTI + 1 NNRTI) have been evaluated in children and adolescents age ≥ 2 years to < 18 years of age who had failed prior therapy (n=26) in Study 1038. KALETRA doses of 400/100 and 480/120 mg/m² resulted in high lopinavir exposure, as almost all subjects had lopinavir AUC_{12} above 100 µg•h/mL. Both groups of subjects also achieved relatively high average minimum lopinavir concentrations.

KALETRA once daily has not been evaluated in pediatric patients.

Renal Impairment

Lopinavir pharmacokinetics have not been studied in patients with renal impairment; however, since the renal clearance of lopinavir is negligible, a decrease in total body clearance is not expected in patients with renal impairment.

Hepatic Impairment

Lopinavir is principally metabolized and eliminated by the liver. Multiple dosing of KALETRA 400/100 mg twice daily to HIV-1 and HCV co-infected patients with mild to moderate hepatic impairment (n = 12) resulted in a 30% increase in lopinavir AUC and 20% increase in C_{max} compared to HIV-1 infected subjects with normal hepatic function (n = 12). Additionally, the plasma protein binding of lopinavir was statistically significantly lower in both mild and moderate hepatic impairment compared to controls (99.09 vs. 99.31%, respectively). Caution should be exercised when administering KALETRA to subjects with he-

Information on the Abbott Pharmaceutical Products listed on these pages is from the prescribing information in use as of June 1, 2010. For more information, please visit rxabbott.com or call 1-800-633-9110.

patic impairment. KALETRA has not been studied in patients with severe hepatic impairment [see Warnings and Precautions (5.3) and Use In Specific Populations (8.6)].

Drug Interactions

KALETRA is an inhibitor of the P450 isoform CYP3A in vitro. Co-administration of KALETRA and drugs primarily metabolized by CYP3A may result in increased plasma concentrations of the other drug, which could increase or prolong its therapeutic and adverse effects [see Contraindications (4) and Drug Interactions (7)].

KALETRA does not inhibit CYP2D6, CYP2C9, CYP2C19, CYP2E1, CYP2B6 or CYP1A2 at clinically relevant concentrations.

KALETRA has been shown in vivo to induce its own metabolism and to increase the biotransformation of some drugs metabolized by cytochrome P450 enzymes and by glucuronidation.

KALETRA is metabolized by CYP3A. Drugs that induce CYP3A activity would be expected to increase the clearance of lopinavir, resulting in lowered plasma concentrations of lopinavir. Although not noted with concurrent ketoconazole, co-administration of KALETRA and other drugs that inhibit CYP3A may increase lopinavir plasma concentrations.

Drug interaction studies were performed with KALETRA and other drugs likely to be co-administered and some drugs commonly used as probes for pharmacokinetic interactions. The effects of co-administration of KALETRA on the AUC, C_{max} and C_{min} are summarized in Table 10 (effect of other drugs on lopinavir) and Table 11 (effect of KALETRA on other drugs). The effects of other drugs on ritonavir are not shown since they generally correlate with those observed with lopinavir (if lopinavir concentrations are decreased, ritonavir concentrations are decreased) unless otherwise indicated in the table footnotes. For information regarding clinical recommendations, see Table 9 in Drug Interactions (7).

[See table 10 on pages 469 and 470]
[See table 11 at top of page 471]

12.4 Microbiology

Mechanism of Action

Lopinavir, an inhibitor of the HIV-1 protease, prevents cleavage of the Gag-Pol polyprotein, resulting in the production of immature, non-infectious viral particles.

Antiviral Activity

The antiviral activity of lopinavir against laboratory HIV strains and clinical HIV-1 isolates was evaluated in acutely infected lymphoblastic cell lines and peripheral blood lymphocytes, respectively. In the absence of human serum, the mean 50% effective concentration (EC_{50}) values of lopinavir against five different HIV-1 subtype B laboratory strains ranged from 10-27 nM (0.006-0.017 μg/mL, 1 μg/mL = 1.6 μM) and ranged from 4-11 nM (0.003-0.007 μg/mL) against several HIV-1 subtype B clinical isolates (n = 6). In the presence of 50% human serum, the mean EC_{50} values of lopinavir against these five HIV-1 laboratory strains ranged from 65-289 nM (0.04-0.18 μg/mL), representing a 7- to 11-fold attenuation. Combination antiviral drug activity studies with lopinavir in cell cultures demonstrated additive to antagonistic activity with nelfinavir and additive to synergistic activity with amprenavir, atazanavir, indinavir, saquinavir and tipranavir. The EC_{50} values of lopinavir against three different HIV-2 strains ranged from 12-180 nM (0.008-113 μg/mL).

Resistance

HIV-1 isolates with reduced susceptibility to lopinavir have been selected in cell culture. The presence of ritonavir does not appear to influence the selection of lopinavir-resistant viruses in cell culture.

The selection of resistance to KALETRA in antiretroviral treatment naïve patients has not yet been characterized. In a study of 653 antiretroviral treatment naïve patients (Study 863), plasma viral isolates from each patient on treatment with plasma HIV-1 RNA > 400 copies/mL at Week 24, 32, 40 and/or 48 were analyzed. No evidence of resistance to KALETRA was observed in 37 evaluable KALETRA-treated patients (0%). Evidence of genotypic resistance to nelfinavir, defined as the presence of the D30N and/or L90M substitution in HIV-1 protease, was observed in 25/76 (33%) of evaluable nelfinavir-treated patients. The selection of resistance to KALETRA in antiretroviral treatment naïve pediatric patients (Study 940) appears to be consistent with that seen in adult patients (Study 863).

Resistance to KALETRA has been noted to emerge in patients treated with other protease inhibitors prior to KALETRA therapy. In studies of 227 antiretroviral treatment naïve and protease inhibitor experienced patients, isolates from 4 of 23 patients with quantifiable (> 400 copies/mL) viral RNA following treatment with KALETRA for 12 to 100 weeks displayed significantly reduced susceptibility to lopinavir compared to the corresponding baseline viral isolates. Three of these patients had previously received

treatment with a single protease inhibitor (indinavir, nelfinavir, or saquinavir) and one patient had received treatment with multiple protease inhibitors (indinavir, ritonavir, and saquinavir). All four of these patients had at least 4 substitutions associated with protease inhibitor resistance immediately prior to KALETRA therapy. Following viral rebound, isolates from these patients all contained additional substitutions, some of which are recognized to be associated with protease inhibitor resistance. However, there are insufficient data at this time to identify patterns of lopinavir resistance-associated substitutions in isolates from patients on KALETRA therapy. The assessment of these patterns is under study.

Cross-resistance - Preclinical Studies

Varying degrees of cross-resistance have been observed among HIV-1 protease inhibitors. Little information is available on the cross-resistance of viruses that developed decreased susceptibility to lopinavir during KALETRA therapy.

The antiviral activity in cell culture of lopinavir against clinical isolates from patients previously treated with a single protease inhibitor was determined. Isolates that displayed > 4-fold reduced susceptibility to nelfinavir (n = 13) and saquinavir (n = 4), displayed < 4-fold reduced susceptibility to lopinavir. Isolates with > 4-fold reduced susceptibility to indinavir (n = 16) and ritonavir (n = 3) displayed a mean of 5.7- and 8.3-fold reduced susceptibility to lopinavir, respectively. Isolates from patients previously treated with two or more protease inhibitors showed greater reductions in susceptibility to lopinavir, as described in the following paragraph.

Table 9 (cont.). Established and Other Potentially Significant Drug Interactions

Concomitant Drug Class: Drug Name	Effect on Concentration of Lopinavir or Concomitant Drug	Clinical Comment
Other Agents		
Antiarrhythmics: amiodarone, bepridil, lidocaine (systemic), and quinidine	↑ antiarrhythmics	Caution is warranted and therapeutic concentration monitoring (if available) is recommended for antiarrhythmics when co-administered with KALETRA.
Anticancer Agents: vincristine vinblastine	↑ anticancer agents	Concentrations of vincristine or vinblastine may be increased when co-administered with lopinavir/ritonavir (KALETRA) resulting in the potential for increased adverse events usually associated with these anticancer agents. Consideration should be given to temporarily withholding the ritonavir-containing antiretroviral regimen in patients who develop significant hematologic or gastrointestinal side effects when lopinavir/ritonavir (KALETRA) is administered concurrently with vincristine or vinblastine. If the antiretroviral regimen must be withheld for a prolonged period, consideration should be given to initiating a revised regimen that does not include a CYP3A or P-gp inhibitor.
Anticoagulant: warfarin		Concentrations of warfarin may be affected. It is recommended that INR (international normalized ratio) be monitored.
Anticonvulsants: carbamazepine, phenobarbital, phenytoin	↓ lopinavir ↓ phenytoin	KALETRA may be less effective due to decreased lopinavir plasma concentrations in patients taking these agents concomitantly and should be used with caution. KALETRA should not be administered once daily in combination with carbamazepine, phenobarbital, or phenytoin. In addition, co-administration of phenytoin and KALETRA may cause decreases in steady-state phenytoin concentrations. Phenytoin levels should be monitored when co-administering with KALETRA.
Antidepressant: bupropion	↓ bupropion ↓ active metabolite, hydroxybupropion	Concurrent administration of bupropion with KALETRA may decrease plasma levels of both bupropion and its active metabolite (hydroxybupropion). Patients receiving KALETRA and bupropion concurrently should be monitored for an adequate clinical response to bupropion.
Antidepressant: trazodone	↑ trazodone	Concomitant use of trazodone and KALETRA may increase concentrations of trazodone. Adverse reactions of nausea, dizziness, hypotension and syncope have been observed following co-administration of trazodone and ritonavir. If trazodone is used with a CYP3A4 inhibitor such as ritonavir, the combination should be used with caution and a lower dose of trazodone should be considered.
Anti-infective: clarithromycin	↑ clarithromycin	For patients with renal impairment, the following dosage adjustments should be considered: • For patients with CL_{CR} 30 to 60 mL/min the dose of clarithromycin should be reduced by 50%. • For patients with CL_{CR} < 30 mL/min the dose of clarithromycin should be decreased by 75%. No dose adjustment for patients with normal renal function is necessary.
Antifungals: ketoconazole*, itraconazole, voriconazole	↑ ketoconazole ↑ itraconazole ↓ voriconazole	High doses of ketoconazole (>200 mg/day) or itraconazole (> 200 mg/day) are not recommended. Co-administration of voriconazole with KALETRA has not been studied. However, a study has been shown that administration of voriconazole with ritonavir 100 mg every 12 hours decreased voriconazole steady-state AUC by an average of 39%; therefore, co-administration of KALETRA and voriconazole may result in decreased voriconazole concentrations and the potential for decreased voriconazole effectiveness and should be avoided, unless an assessment of the benefit/risk to the patient justifies the use of voriconazole. Otherwise, alternative antifungal therapies should be considered in these patients.

(Table continued on next page)

Table 9 (cont.). Established and Other Potentially Significant Drug Interactions

Concomitant Drug Class: Drug Name	Effect on Concentration of Lopinavir or Concomitant Drug	Clinical Comment
Other Agents (continued)		
Anti-gout: colchicine	↑ colchicine	Patients with renal or hepatic impairment should not be given colchicine with KALETRA. Treatment of gout flares-co-administration of colchicine in patients on KALETRA: 0.6 mg (1 tablet) × 1 dose, followed by 0.3 mg (half tablet) 1 hour later. Dose to be repeated no earlier than 3 days. Prophylaxis of gout flares-co-administration of colchicine in patients on KALETRA: If the original colchicine regimen was 0.6 mg twice a day, the regimen should be adjusted to 0.3 mg once a day. If the original colchicine regimen was 0.6 mg once a day, the regimen should be adjusted to 0.3 mg once every other day. Treatment of familial Mediterranean fever (FMF)-co-administration of colchicine in patients on KALETRA: Maximum daily dose of 0.6 mg (may be given as 0.3 mg twice a day).
Antimycobacterial: rifabutin*	↑ rifabutin and rifabutin metabolite	Dosage reduction of rifabutin by at least 75% of the usual dose of 300 mg/day is recommended (i.e., a maximum dose of 150 mg every other day or three times per week). Increased monitoring for adverse reactions is warranted in patients receiving the combination. Further dosage reduction of rifabutin may be necessary.
Antimycobacterial: rifampin	↓ lopinavir	May lead to loss of virologic response and possible resistance to KALETRA or to the class of protease inhibitors or other co-administered antiretroviral agents. A study evaluated combination of rifampin 600 mg once daily, with KALETRA 800/200 mg twice daily or KALETRA 400/100 mg + ritonavir 300 mg twice daily. Pharmacokinetic and safety results from this study do not allow for a dose recommendation. Nine subjects (28%) experienced a ≥ grade 2 increase in ALT/AST, of which seven (21%) prematurely discontinued study per protocol. Based on the study design, it is not possible to determine whether the frequency or magnitude of the ALT/AST elevations observed is higher than what would be seen with rifampin alone. [see Clinical Pharmacology (12.3) for magnitude of interaction].
Antiparasitic: atovaquone	↓ atovaquone	Clinical significance is unknown; however, increase in atovaquone doses may be needed.
Benzodiazepines: parenterally administered midazolam	↑ midazolam	Midazolam is extensively metabolized by CYP3A4. Increases in the concentration of midazolam are expected to be significantly higher with oral than parenteral administration. Therefore, KALETRA should not be given with orally administered midazolam [see Contraindications (4)]. If KALETRA is coadministered with parenteral midazolam, close clinical monitoring for respiratory depression and/or prolonged sedation should be exercised and dosage adjustment should be considered.
Calcium Channel Blockers, dihydropyridine: e.g., felodipine, nifedipine, nicardipine	↑ dihydropyridine calcium channel blockers	Caution is warranted and clinical monitoring of patients is recommended.
Contraceptive: ethinyl estradiol*	↓ ethinyl estradiol	Because contraceptive steroid concentrations may be altered when KALETRA is co-administered with oral contraceptives or with the contraceptive patch, alternative methods of nonhormonal contraception are recommended.
Corticosteroid: dexamethasone	↓ lopinavir	Use with caution. KALETRA may be less effective due to to decreased lopinavir plasma concentrations in patients taking these agents concomitantly.
disulfiram/metronidazole		KALETRA oral solution contains alcohol, which can produce disulfiram-like reactions when co-administered with disulfiram or other drugs that produce this reaction (e.g., metronidazole).

(Table continued on next page)

Clinical Studies - Antiviral Activity of KALETRA in Patients with Previous Protease Inhibitor Therapies

The clinical relevance of reduced susceptibility in cell culture to lopinavir has been examined by assessing the virologic response to KALETRA therapy in treatment-experienced patients, with respect to baseline viral genotype in three studies and baseline viral phenotype in one study.

Virologic response to KALETRA has been shown to be affected by the presence of three or more of the following amino acid substitutions in protease at baseline: L10F/I/R/V, K20M/N/R, L24I, L33F, M36I, I47V, G48V, I54L/T/V, V82A/C/F/S/T, and I84V. Table 12 shows the 48-week virologic response (HIV-1 RNA <400 copies/mL) according to the number of the above protease inhibitor resistance-associated substitutions at baseline in studies 888 and 765 [see Clinical Studies (14.2) and (14.3)] and study 957 (see below). Once daily administration of KALETRA for adult patients with three or more of the above substitutions is not recommended.

[See table 12 on page 472]

Virologic response to KALETRA therapy with respect to phenotypic susceptibility to lopinavir at baseline was examined in Study 957. In this study 56 NNRTI-naïve patients with HIV-1 RNA >1,000 copies/mL despite previous therapy with at least two protease inhibitors selected from indi-

navir, nelfinavir, ritonavir, and saquinavir were randomized to receive one of two doses of KALETRA in combination with efavirenz and nucleoside reverse transcriptase inhibitors (NRTIs). The EC_{50} values of lopinavir against the 56 baseline viral isolates ranged from 0.5- to 96-fold the wild-type EC_{50} value. Fifty-five percent (31/56) of these baseline isolates displayed >4-fold reduced susceptibility to lopinavir. These 31 isolates had a median reduction in lopinavir susceptibility of 18-fold. Response to therapy by baseline lopinavir susceptibility is shown in Table 13. [See table 13 on page 472]

13 NONCLINICAL TOXICOLOGY

13.1 Carcinogenesis, Mutagenesis, Impairment of Fertility

Lopinavir/ritonavir combination was evaluated for carcinogenic potential by oral gavage administration to mice and rats for up to 104 weeks. Results showed an increase in the incidence of benign hepatocellular adenomas and an increase in the combined incidence of hepatocellular adenomas plus carcinoma in both males and females in mice and males in rats at doses that produced approximately 1.6-2.2 times (mice) and 0.5 times (rats) the human exposure (based on AUC_{0-24hr} measurement) at the recommended dose of 400/100 mg KALETRA twice daily. Administration of lopinavir/ritonavir did not cause a statistically significant increase in the incidence of any other benign or malignant neoplasm in mice or rats.

Carcinogenicity studies in mice and rats have been carried out on ritonavir. In male mice, there was a dose dependent increase in the incidence of both adenomas and combined adenomas and carcinomas in the liver. Based on AUC measurements, the exposure at the high dose was approximately 4-fold for males that of the exposure in humans with the recommended therapeutic dose (400/100 mg KALETRA twice daily). There were no carcinogenic effects seen in females at the dosages tested. The exposure at the high dose was approximately 9-fold for the females that of the exposure in humans. There were no carcinogenic effects in rats. In this study, the exposure at the high dose was approximately 0.7-fold that of the exposure in humans with the 400/100 mg KALETRA twice daily regimen. Based on the exposures achieved in the animal studies, the significance of the observed effects is not known. However, neither lopinavir nor ritonavir was found to be mutagenic or clastogenic in a battery of in vitro and in vivo assays including the Ames bacterial reverse mutation assay using S. typhimurium and E. coli, the mouse lymphoma assay, the mouse micronucleus test and chromosomal aberration assays in human lymphocytes.

Lopinavir in combination with ritonavir at a 2:1 ratio produced no effects on fertility in male and female rats at levels of 10/5, 30/15 or 100/50 mg/kg/day. Based on AUC measurements, the exposures in rats at the high doses were approximately 0.7-fold for lopinavir and 1.8-fold for ritonavir of the exposures in humans at the recommended therapeutic dose (400/100 mg twice daily).

14 CLINICAL STUDIES

14.1 Patients Without Prior Antiretroviral Therapy

Study 863: KALETRA Capsules twice daily + stavudine + lamivudine compared to nelfinavir three times daily + stavudine + lamivudine

Study 863 was a randomized, double-blind, multicenter trial comparing treatment with KALETRA capsules (400/100 mg twice daily) plus stavudine and lamivudine versus nelfinavir (750 mg three times daily) plus stavudine and lamivudine in 653 antiretroviral treatment naïve patients. Patients had a mean age of 38 years (range: 19 to 84), 57% were Caucasian, and 80% were male. Mean baseline CD4+ cell count was 259 cells/mm^3 (range: 2 to 949 cells/mm^3) and mean baseline plasma HIV-1 RNA was 4.9 $\log_{10}$ copies/mL (range: 2.6 to 6.8 $\log_{10}$ copies/mL).

Treatment response and outcomes of randomized treatment are presented in Table 14.

Table 14. Outcomes of Randomized Treatment Through Week 48 (Study 863)

Outcome	KALETRA + d4T+ 3TC (N = 326)	Nelfinavir + d4T+ 3TC (N = 327)
Responder[1]	75%	62%
Virologic failure[2]	9%	25%
Rebound	7%	15%

Information on the Abbott Pharmaceutical Products listed on these pages is from the prescribing information in use as of June 1, 2010. For more information, please visit rxabbott.com or call 1-800-633-9110.

Never suppressed through Week 48	2%	9%
Death	2%	1%
Discontinued due to adverse events	4%	4%
Discontinued for other reasons[3]	10%	8%

[1] Patients achieved and maintained confirmed HIV-1 RNA < 400 copies/mL through Week 48.

[2] Includes confirmed viral rebound and failure to achieve confirmed < 400 copies/mL through Week 48.

[3] Includes lost to follow-up, patient's withdrawal, non-compliance, protocol violation and other reasons. Overall discontinuation through Week 48, including patients who discontinued subsequent to virologic failure, was 17% in the KALETRA arm and 24% in the nelfinavir arm.

Through 48 weeks of therapy, there was a statistically significantly higher proportion of patients in the KALETRA arm compared to the nelfinavir arm with HIV-1 RNA < 400 copies/mL (75% vs. 62%, respectively) and HIV-1 RNA < 50 copies/mL (67% vs. 52%, respectively). Treatment response by baseline HIV-1 RNA level subgroups is presented in Table 15.

[See table 15 on page 472]

Through 48 weeks of therapy, the mean increase from baseline in CD4+ cell count was 207 cells/mm³ for the KALETRA arm and 195 cells/mm³ for the nelfinavir arm.

Study 730: KALETRA Tablets once daily + tenofovir DF + emtricitabine compared to KALETRA Tablets twice daily + tenofovir DF + emtricitabine.

Study 730 was a randomized, open-label, multicenter trial comparing treatment with KALETRA 800/200 mg once daily plus tenofovir DF and emtricitabine versus KALETRA 400/100 mg twice daily plus tenofovir DF and emtricitabine in 664 antiretroviral treatment-naïve patients. Patients were randomized in a 1:1 ratio to receive either KALETRA 800/200 mg once daily (n = 333) or KALETRA 400/100 mg twice daily (n = 331). Further stratification within each group was 1:1 (tablet vs. capsule). Patients administered the capsule were switched to the tablet formulation at Week 8 and maintained on their randomized dosing schedule. Patients were administered emtricitabine 200 mg once daily and tenofovir DF 300 mg once daily. Mean age of patients enrolled was 39 years (range: 19 to 71); 75% were Caucasian, and 78% were male. Mean baseline CD4+ cell count was 216 cells/mm³ (range: 20 to 775 cells/mm³) and mean baseline plasma HIV-1 RNA was 5.0 $\log_{10}$ copies/mL (range: 1.7 to 7.0 $\log_{10}$ copies/mL).

Treatment response and outcomes of randomized treatment through Week 48 are presented in Table 16.

Table 16. Outcomes of Randomized Treatment Through Week 48 (Study 730)

Outcome	KALETRA Once Daily + TDF + FTC (n = 333)	KALETRA Twice Daily + TDF + FTC (n = 331)
Responder[1]	78%	77%
Virologic failure[2]	10%	8%
Rebound	5%	5%
Never suppressed through Week 48	5%	3%
Death	1%	<1%
Discontinued due to adverse events	4%	3%
Discontinued for other reasons[3]	8%	11%

[1] Patients achieved and maintained confirmed HIV-1 RNA < 50 copies/mL through Week 48.

[2] Includes confirmed viral rebound and failure to achieve confirmed < 50 copies/mL through Week 48.

[3] Includes lost to follow-up, patient's withdrawal, non-compliance, protocol violation and other reasons.

Through 48 weeks of therapy, 78% in the KALETRA once daily arm and 77% in the KALETRA twice daily arm achieved and maintained HIV-1 RNA < 50 copies/mL (95% confidence interval for the difference, -5.9% to 6.8%). Mean CD4+ cell count increases at Week 48 were 186 cells/mm³ for the KALETRA once daily arm and 198 cells/mm³ for the KALETRA twice daily arm.

14.2   Patients With Prior Antiretroviral Therapy

Study 888: KALETRA Capsules twice daily + nevirapine + NRTIs compared to investigator-selected protease inhibitor(s) + nevirapine + NRTIs

Study 888 was a randomized, open-label, multicenter trial comparing treatment with KALETRA capsules (400/100 mg twice daily) plus nevirapine and nucleoside reverse transcriptase inhibitors versus investigator-selected protease inhibitor(s) plus nevirapine and nucleoside reverse transcriptase inhibitors in 288 single protease inhibitor-experienced, non-nucleoside reverse transcriptase inhibitor (NNRTI)-naïve patients. Patients had a mean age of 40 years (range: 18 to 74), 68% were Caucasian, and 86% were male. Mean baseline CD4+ cell count was 322 cells/mm³ (range: 10 to 1059 cells/mm³) and mean baseline plasma HIV-1 RNA was 4.1 $\log_{10}$ copies/mL (range: 2.6 to 6.0 $\log_{10}$ copies/mL).

Table 9 (cont.). Established and Other Potentially Significant Drug Interactions

Concomitant Drug Class: Drug Name	Effect on Concentration of Lopinavir or Concomitant Drug	Clinical Comment
	Other Agents (continued)	
Endothelin receptor antagonists: bosentan	↑ bosentan	Co-administration of bosentan in patients on KALETRA: In patients who have been receiving KALETRA for at least 10 days, start bosentan at 62.5 mg once daily or every other day based upon individual tolerability. Co-administration of KALETRA in patients on bosentan: Discontinue use of bosentan at least 36 hours prior to initiation of KALETRA. After at least 10 days following the initiation of KALETRA, resume bosentan at 62.5 mg once daily or every other day based upon individual tolerability.
HMG-CoA Reductase Inhibitors: atorvastatin rosuvastatin	↑ atorvastatin ↑ rosuvastatin	Use lowest possible dose of atorvastatin or rosuvastatin with careful monitoring, or consider other HMG-CoA reductase inhibitors such as pravastatin or fluvastatin in combination with KALETRA.
Immunosuppressants: cyclosporine, tacrolimus, rapamycin	↑ immunosuppressants	Therapeutic concentration monitoring is recommended for immunosuppressant agents when co-administered with KALETRA.
Inhaled Steroid: fluticasone	↑ fluticasone	Concomitant use of fluticasone propionate and KALETRA may increase plasma concentrations of fluticasone propionate, resulting in significantly reduced serum cortisol concentrations. Systemic corticosteroid effects including Cushing's syndrome and adrenal suppression have been reported during post-marketing use in patients receiving ritonavir and inhaled or intranasally administered fluticasone propionate. Co-administration of fluticasone propionate and KALETRA is not recommended unless the potential benefit to the patient outweighs the risk of systemic corticosteroid side effect.
Long-acting beta-adrenoceptor agonist: salmeterol	↑ salmeterol	Concurrent administration of salmeterol and KALETRA is not recommended. The combination may result in increased risk of cardiovascular adverse events associated with salmeterol, including QT prolongation, palpitations and sinus tachycardia.
Narcotic Analgesic: methadone*	↓ methadone	Dosage of methadone may need to be increased when co-administered with KALETRA.
PDE5 inhibitors: sildenafil, tadalafil, vardenafil	↑ sildenafil ↑ tadalafil ↑ vardenafil	Particular caution should be used when prescribing sildenafil, tadalafil, or vardenafil in patients receiving KALETRA. Co-administration of KALETRA with these drugs is expected to substantially increase their concentrations and may result in an increase in PDE5 inhibitor associated adverse reactions including hypotension, syncope, visual changes and prolonged erection. Use of PDE5 inhibitors for pulmonary arterial hypertension (PAH): Sildenafil (Revatio®) is contraindicated when used for the treatment of pulmonary arterial hypertension (PAH) because a safe and effective dose has not been established when used with KALETRA [see Contraindications (4)]. The following dose adjustments are recommended for use of tadalafil (Adcirca™) with KALETRA: Co-administration of ADCIRCA in patients on KALETRA: In patients receiving KALETRA for at least one week, start ADCIRCA at 20 mg once daily. Increase to 40 mg once daily based upon individual tolerability. Co-administration of KALETRA in patients on ADCIRCA: Avoid use of ADCIRCA during the initiation of KALETRA. Stop ADCIRCA at least 24 hours prior to starting KALETRA. After at least one week following the initiation of KALETRA, resume ADCIRCA at 20 mg once daily. Increase to 40 mg once daily based upon individual tolerability. Use of PDE5 inhibitors for erectile dysfunction: It is recommended not to exceed the following doses: • Sildenafil: 25 mg every 48 hours • Tadalafil: 10 mg every 72 hours • Vardenafil: 2.5 mg every 72 hours Use with increased monitoring for adverse events.

*see Clinical Pharmacology (12.3) for Magnitude of Interaction.

Treatment response and outcomes of randomized treatment through Week 48 are presented in Table 17.
[See table 17 on page 472]

Through 48 weeks of therapy, there was a statistically significantly higher proportion of patients in the KALETRA arm compared to the investigator-selected protease inhibitor(s) arm with HIV-1 RNA < 400 copies/mL (57% vs. 33%, respectively).

Through 48 weeks of therapy, the mean increase from baseline in CD4+ cell count was 111 cells/mm³ for the KALETRA arm and 112 cells/mm³ for the investigator-selected protease inhibitor(s) arm.

Study 802: KALETRA Tablets 800/200 mg Once Daily Versus 400/100 mg Twice Daily when Coadministered with Nucleoside/Nucleotide Reverse Transcriptase Inhibitors in Antiretroviral-Experienced, HIV-1 Infected Subjects

M06-802 was a randomized open-label study comparing the safety, tolerability, and antiviral activity of once daily and twice daily dosing of KALETRA tablets in 599 subjects with detectable viral loads while receiving their current antiviral therapy. Of the enrolled subjects, 55% on both treatment arms had not been previously treated with a protease inhibitor and 81-88% had received prior NNRTIs as part of their anti-HIV treatment regimen. Patients were randomized in a 1:1 ratio to receive either KALETRA 800/200 mg once daily (n = 300) or KALETRA 400/100 mg twice daily (n = 299). Patients were administered at least two nucleoside/nucleotide reverse transcriptase inhibitors selected by the investigator. Mean age of patients enrolled was 41 years (range: 21 to 73); 51% were Caucasian, and 66% were male. Mean baseline CD4+ cell count was 254 cells/mm³ (range: 4 to 952 cells/mm³) and mean baseline plasma HIV-1 RNA was 4.3 log₁₀ copies/mL (range: 1.7 to 6.6 log₁₀ copies/mL). Treatment response and outcomes of randomized treatment through Week 48 are presented in Table 18.
[See table 18 at top of page 472]

Through 48 weeks of treatment, the mean change from baseline for CD4 + cell count was 135 cells/mm³ for the once daily group and 122 cells/mm³ for the twice daily group.

14.3 Other Studies Supporting Approval

Study 720: KALETRA twice daily + stavudine + lamivudine
Study 765: KALETRA twice daily + nevirapine + NRTIs

Study 720 (patients without prior antiretroviral therapy) and study 765 (patients with prior protease inhibitor therapy) were randomized, blinded, multi-center trials evaluating treatment with KALETRA at up to three dose levels (200/100 mg twice daily [720 only], 400/100 mg twice daily, and 400/200 mg twice daily). In Study 720, all patients switched to 400/100 mg twice daily between Weeks 48-72. Patients in study 720 had a mean age of 35 years, 70% were Caucasian, and 96% were male, while patients in study 765 had a mean age of 40 years, 73% were Caucasian, and 90% were male. Mean (range) baseline CD4+ cell counts for patients in study 720 and study 765 were 338 (3-918) and 372 (72-807) cells/mm³, respectively. Mean (range) baseline plasma HIV-1 RNA levels for patients in study 720 and study 765 were 4.9 (3.3 to 6.3) and 4.0 (2.9 to 5.8) log₁₀ copies/mL, respectively.

Through 360 weeks of treatment in study 720, the proportion of patients with HIV-1 RNA < 400 (< 50) copies/mL was 61% (59%) [n = 100]. Among patients completing 360 weeks of treatment with CD4+ cell count measurements [n=60], the mean (median) increase in CD4+ cell count was 501 (457) cells/mm³. Thirty-nine patients (39%) discontinued the study, including 13 (13%) discontinuations due to adverse reactions and 1 (1%) death.

Through 144 weeks of treatment in study 765, the proportion of patients with HIV-1 RNA < 400 (< 50) copies/mL was 54% (50%) [n = 70], and the corresponding mean increase in CD4+ cell count was 212 cells/mm³. Twenty-seven patients (39%) discontinued the study, including 5 (7%) discontinuations secondary to adverse reactions and 2 (3%) deaths.

14.4 Pediatric Studies

Study 1030 was an open-label, multicenter, dose-finding trial evaluating the pharmacokinetic profile, tolerability, safety and efficacy of KALETRA oral solution containing lopinavir 80 mg/mL and ritonavir 20 mg/mL at a dose of 300/75 mg/m² twice daily plus 2 NRTIs in HIV-1 infected infants ≥14 days and <6 months of age.

Ten infants, ≥14 days and <6 wks of age, were enrolled at a median (range) age of 5.7 (3.6-6.0) weeks and all completed 24 weeks. At entry, median (range) HIV-1 RNA was 6.0 (4.7-7.2) log₁₀ copies/mL. Seven of 10 infants had HIV-1 RNA <400 copies/mL at Week 24. At entry, median (range) CD4+ percentage was 41 (16-59) with a median decrease of 1% (95% CI: -10, 18) from baseline to week 24 in 6 infants with available data.

Twenty-one infants, between 6 weeks and 6 months of age, were enrolled at a median (range) age of 14.7 (6.9-25.7) weeks and 19 of 21 infants completed 24 weeks. At entry, median (range) HIV RNA level was 5.8 (3.7-6.9) log₁₀ copies/mL. Ten of 21 infants had HIV RNA <400 copies/mL at Week 24. At entry, the median (range) CD4+ percentage

was 32 (11-54) with a median increase of 4% (95% CI: -1, 9) from baseline to week 24 in 19 infants with available data.
See Clinical Pharmacology (12.3) for pharmacokinetic results.

Study 940 was an open-label, multicenter trial evaluating the pharmacokinetic profile, tolerability, safety and efficacy of KALETRA oral solution containing lopinavir 80 mg/mL and ritonavir 20 mg/mL in 100 antiretroviral naïve (44%) and experienced (56%) pediatric patients. All patients were non-nucleoside reverse transcriptase inhibitor naïve. Patients were randomized to either 230 mg lopinavir/57.5 mg ritonavir per m² or 300 mg lopinavir/75 mg ritonavir per m². Naïve patients also received lamivudine and stavudine. Experienced patients received nevirapine plus up to two nucleoside reverse transcriptase inhibitors.

Safety, efficacy and pharmacokinetic profiles of the two dose regimens were assessed after three weeks of therapy in each patient. After analysis of these data, all patients were continued on the 300 mg lopinavir/75 mg ritonavir per m² dose. Patients had a mean age of 5 years (range 6 months to 12 years) with 14% less than 2 years. Mean baseline CD4+ cell count was 838 cells/mm³ and mean baseline plasma HIV-1 RNA was 4.7 log₁₀ copies/mL.

Through 48 weeks of therapy, the proportion of patients who achieved and sustained an HIV-1 RNA < 400 copies/mL was 80% for antiretroviral naïve patients and 71% for antiretroviral experienced patients. The mean increase from baseline in CD4+ cell count was 404 cells/mm³ for antiretroviral naïve and 284 cells/mm³ for antiretroviral experienced patients treated through 48 weeks. At 48 weeks, two patients (2%) had prematurely discontinued the study. One antiretroviral naïve patient prematurely discontinued secondary to an adverse reaction, while one antiretroviral experienced patient prematurely discontinued secondary to an HIV-1 related event.

Dose selection in pediatric patients was based on the following:
• Among patients 14 days to 6 months of age receiving 300/75 mg/m² twice daily without nevirapine, plasma concentrations were lower than those observed in adults

---

Table 10. Drug Interactions: Pharmacokinetic Parameters for Lopinavir in the Presence of the Co-administered Drug for Recommended Alterations in Dose or Regimen

Co-administered Drug	Dose of Co-administered Drug (mg)	Dose of KALETRA (mg)	n	C_{max}	AUC	C_{min}
				Ratio (in combination with co-administered drug/alone) of Lopinavir Pharmacokinetic Parameters (90% CI); No Effect = 1.00		
Amprenavir	750 twice daily, 10 d	400/100 capsule twice daily, 21 d	12	0.72 (0.65, 0.79)	0.62 (0.56, 0.70)	0.43 (0.34, 0.56)
Efavirenz[1,10]	600 at bedtime, 9 d	400/100 capsule twice daily, 9 d	11, 7*	0.97 (0.78, 1.22)	0.81 (0.64, 1.03)	0.61 (0.38, 0.97)
	600 at bedtime, 9 d	500/125 tablet twice daily, 10 d	19	1.12 (1.02, 1.23)	1.06 (0.96, 1.17)	0.90 (0.78, 1.04)
	600 at bedtime, 9 d	600/150 tablet twice daily, 10 d	23	1.36 (1.28, 1.44)	1.36 (1.28, 1.44)	1.32 (1.21, 1.44)
Fosamprenavir[2]	700 twice daily plus ritonavir 100 twice daily, 14 d	400/100 capsule twice daily, 14 d	18	1.30 (0.85, 1.47)	1.37 (0.80, 1.55)	1.52 (0.72, 1.82)
Ketoconazole	200 single dose	400/100 capsule twice daily, 16 d	12	0.89 (0.80, 0.99)	0.87 (0.75, 1.00)	0.75 (0.55, 1.00)
Nelfinavir	1000 twice daily, 10 d	400/100 capsule twice daily, 21 d	13	0.79 (0.70, 0.89)	0.73 (0.63, 0.85)	0.62 (0.49, 0.78)
Nevirapine	200 twice daily, steady-state (> 1 yr)[3#]	400/100 capsule twice daily, steady-state	22, 19*	0.81 (0.62, 1.05)	0.73 (0.53, 0.98)	0.49 (0.28, 0.74)
	7 mg/kg or 4 mg/kg once daily, 2 wk; twice daily 1 wk[4]	(> 1 yr) 300/75 mg/m² oral solution twice daily, 3 wk	12, 15*	0.86 (0.64, 1.16)	0.78 (0.56, 1.09)	0.45 (0.25, 0.81)
Omeprazole	40 once daily, 5 d	400/100 tablet twice daily, 10 d	12	1.08 (0.99, 1.17)	1.07 (0.99, 1.15)	1.03 (0.90, 1.18)
	40 once daily, 5 d	800/200 tablet once daily, 10 d	12	0.94 (0.88, 1.00)	0.92 (0.86, 0.99)	0.71 (0.57, 0.89)
Pravastatin	20 once daily, 4 d	400/100 capsule twice daily, 14 d	12	0.98 (0.89, 1.08)	0.95 (0.85, 1.05)	0.88 (0.77, 1.02)
Rifabutin	150 once daily, 10 d	400/100 capsule twice daily, 20 d	14	1.08 (0.97, 1.19)	1.17 (1.04, 1.31)	1.20 (0.96, 1.65)
Ranitidine	150 single dose	400/100 tablet twice daily, 10 d	12	0.99 (0.95, 1.03)	0.97 (0.93, 1.01)	0.90 (0.85, 0.95)
	150 single dose	800/200 tablet once daily, 10 d	10	0.97 (0.95, 1.00)	0.95 (0.91, 0.99)	0.82 (0.74, 0.91)
Rifampin	600 once daily, 10 d	400/100 capsule twice daily, 20 d	22	0.45 (0.40, 0.51)	0.25 (0.21, 0.29)	0.01 (0.01, 0.02)
	600 once daily, 14 d	800/200 capsule twice daily, 9 d[5]	10	1.02 (0.85, 1.23)	0.84 (0.64, 1.10)	0.43 (0.19, 0.96)
	600 once daily, 14 d	400/400 capsule twice daily, 9 d[6]	9	0.93 (0.81, 1.07)	0.98 (0.81, 1.17)	1.03 (0.68, 1.56)

(Table continued on next page)

Information on the Abbott Pharmaceutical Products listed on these pages is from the prescribing information in use as of June 1, 2010. For more information, please visit rxabbott.com or call 1-800-633-9110.

or in older children. This dose resulted in HIV-1 RNA < 400 copies/mL in 55% of patients (70% in those initiating treatment at <6 weeks of age).

- Among patients 6 months to 12 years of age, the 230/57.5 mg/m² oral solution twice daily regimen without nevirapine and the 300/75 mg/m² oral solution twice daily regimen with nevirapine provided lopinavir plasma concentrations similar to those obtained in adult patients receiving the 400/100 mg twice daily regimen (without nevirapine). These doses resulted in treatment benefit (proportion of patients with HIV-1 RNA < 400 copies/mL) similar to that seen in the adult clinical trials.

- Among patients 12 to 18 years of age receiving 400/100 mg/m² or 480/120 mg/m² (with efavirenz) twice daily, plasma concentrations were 60-100% higher than among 6 to 12 year old patients receiving 230/57.5 mg/m². Mean apparent clearance was similar to that observed in adult patients receiving standard dose and in patients 6 to 12 years of age. Although changes in HIV-1 RNA in patients with prior treatment failure were less than anticipated, the pharmacokinetic data supports use of similar dosing as in patients 6 to 12 years of age, not to exceed the recommended adult dose.

- For all age groups, the body surface area dosing was converted to body weight dosing using the patient's prescribed lopinavir dose.

16 HOW SUPPLIED/STORAGE AND HANDLING

KALETRA® (lopinavir/ritonavir) Film-Coated tablets and Oral Solution are available in the following strengths and package sizes:

16.1 KALETRA Tablets, 200 mg lopinavir/50 mg ritonavir

Yellow film-coated ovaloid tablets debossed with the corporate logo ⊇ and the Abbo-Code KA:

Bottles of 120 tablets .... (NDC 0074-6799-22)
Recommended Storage

Store KALETRA film-coated tablets at 20°-25°C (68°-77°F); excursions permitted to 15°-30°C (59° to 86°F)[see USP controlled room temperature]. Dispense in original container or USP equivalent tight container (250 mL or less). For patient use: exposure of this product to high humidity outside the original container or USP equivalent tight container (250 mL or less) for longer than 2 weeks is not recommended.

16.2 KALETRA Tablets, 100 mg lopinavir/25 mg ritonavir

Pale yellow film-coated ovaloid tablets debossed with the corporate logo ⊇ and the Abbo-Code KC:

Bottles of 60 tablets .... (NDC 0074-0522-60)
Recommended Storage

Store KALETRA film-coated tablets at 20°-25°C (68°-77°F); excursions permitted to 15°-30°C (59° to 86°F) [see USP controlled room temperature]. Dispense in original container or USP equivalent tight container (100 mL or less). For patient use: exposure of this product to high humidity outside the original container or USP equivalent tight container (100 mL or less) for longer than 2 weeks is not recommended.

16.3 KALETRA Oral Solution

KALETRA (lopinavir/ritonavir) oral solution is a light yellow to orange colored liquid supplied in amber-colored multiple-dose bottles containing 400 mg lopinavir/100 mg ritonavir per 5 mL (80 mg lopinavir/20 mg ritonavir per mL) packaged with a marked dosing cup in the following size:

160 mL bottle .... (NDC 0074-3956-46)
Recommended Storage

Store KALETRA oral solution at 2°-8°C (36°-46°F) until dispensed. Avoid exposure to excessive heat. For patient use, refrigerated KALETRA oral solution remains stable until the expiration date printed on the label. If stored at room temperature up to 25°C (77°F), oral solution should be used within 2 months.

17 PATIENT COUNSELING INFORMATION

See Medication Guide
Information For Patients
Patients or parents of patients should be informed that:
General Information

□ They should pay special attention to accurate administration of their dose to minimize the risk of accidental overdose or underdose of KALETRA.

□ They should inform their healthcare provider if their children's weight changes in order to make sure that the child's KALETRA dose is the correct one.

□ They should take the prescribed dose of KALETRA as directed and to set up a daily routine in order to do so.

Table 10 *(cont.)*. Drug Interactions: Pharmacokinetic Parameters for Lopinavir in the Presence of the Co-administered Drug for Recommended Alterations in Dose or Regimen

Co-administered Drug	Dose of Co-administered Drug (mg)	Dose of KALETRA (mg)	Ratio (in combination with co-administered drug/alone) of Lopinavir Pharmacokinetic Parameters (90% CI); No Effect = 1.00			
			n	C_{max}	AUC	C_{min}
					Co-administration of KALETRA and rifampin is contraindicated. *[see Contraindications (4)]*	
Ritonavir[3]	100 twice daily, 3-4 wk[#]	400/100 capsule twice daily, 3-4 wk	8, 21*	1.28 (0.94, 1.76)	1.46 (1.04, 2.06)	2.16 (1.29, 3.62)
Tenofovir[7]	300 mg once daily, 14 d	400/100 capsule twice daily, 14 d	24	NC[†]	NC[†]	NC[†]
Tipranavir/ ritonavir[3]	500/200 mg twice daily (28 doses)[#]	400/100 capsule twice daily (27 doses)	21 69	0.53 (0.40, 0.69)[8]	0.45 (0.32, 0.63)[8]	0.30 (0.17, 0.51)[8] 0.48 (0.40, 0.58)[9]

All interaction studies conducted in healthy, HIV-1 negative subjects unless otherwise indicated.
[1] The pharmacokinetics of ritonavir are unaffected by concurrent efavirenz.
[2] Data extracted from the fosamprenavir package insert.
[3] Study conducted in HIV-1 positive adult subjects.
[4] Study conducted in HIV-1 positive pediatric subjects ranging in age from 6 months to 12 years.
[5] Titrated to 800/200 twice daily as 533/133 twice daily × 1 d, 667/167 twice daily × 1 d, then 800/200 twice daily × 7 d, compared to 400/100 twice daily × 10 days alone.
[6] Titrated to 400/100 twice daily to 400/200 twice daily × 1 d, 400/300 twice daily × 1 d, then 400/400 twice daily × 7 d, compared to 400/100 twice daily × 10 days alone.
[7] Data extracted from the tenofovir package insert.
[8] Intensive PK analysis.
[9] Drug levels obtained at 8-16 hrs post-dose.
[10] Reference for comparison is lopinavir/ritonavir 400/100 mg twice daily without efavirenz.
* Parallel group design; n for KALETRA + co-administered drug, n for KALETRA alone.
† NC = No change.
# For the nevirapine 200 mg twice daily study, ritonavir, and tipranavir/ritonavir studies, KALETRA was administered with or without food. For all other studies, KALETRA was administered with food.

□ KALETRA tablets may be taken with or without food. KALETRA oral solution should be taken with food to enhance absorption.

□ Sustained decreases in plasma HIV-1 RNA have been associated with a reduced risk of progression to AIDS and death. Patients should remain under the care of a physician while using KALETRA. Patients should be advised to take KALETRA and other concomitant antiretroviral therapy every day as prescribed. KALETRA must always be used in combination with other antiretroviral drugs. Patients should not alter the dose or discontinue therapy without consulting with their doctor. If a dose of KALETRA is missed patients should take the dose as soon as possible and then return to their normal schedule. However, if a dose is skipped the patient should not double the next dose.

□ KALETRA is not a cure for HIV-1 infection and that they may continue to develop opportunistic infections and other complications associated with HIV-1 disease. The long-term effects of KALETRA are unknown at this time. Patients should be told that there are currently no data demonstrating that therapy with KALETRA can reduce the risk of transmitting HIV-1 to others through sexual contact, sharing needles, or being exposed to their blood. For their health and the health of others, it is important that they always practice safer sex by using a latex or polyurethane condom or other barrier method to lower the chance of sexual contact with any body fluids such as semen, vaginal secretions, or blood. They should also be advised to never re-use or share needles.

Drug Interactions
□ KALETRA may interact with some drugs; therefore, patients should be advised to report to their doctor the use of any other prescription, non-prescription medication or herbal products, particularly St. John's Wort.

□ KALETRA tablets can be taken at the same time as didanosine without food. Patients taking didanosine should take didanosine one hour before or two hours after KALETRA oral solution.

□ If they are receiving sildenafil, tadalafil, or vardenafil, there may be an increased risk of associated adverse reactions including hypotension, visual changes, and sustained erection, and should promptly report any symptoms to their doctor.

□ If they are receiving estrogen-based hormonal contraceptives, additional or alternate contraceptive measures should be used during therapy with KALETRA.

□ If they are taking or before they begin using Serevent® (salmeterol) and KALETRA, they should talk to their doctor

about problems these two medications may cause when taken together. The doctor may choose not to keep someone on Serevent® (salmeterol).

□ If they are taking or before they begin taking Advair® (salmeterol in combination with fluticasone propionate) and KALETRA, they should talk to their doctor about problems these two medications may cause when taken together. The doctor may choose not to keep someone on Advair® (salmeterol in combination with fluticasone propionate).

Potential Adverse Effects
□ Skin rashes ranging in severity from mild to Stevens Johnson syndrome and Erythema multiforme have been reported in patients receiving KALETRA or its components lopinavir and/or ritonavir. Patients should be advised to contact their healthcare provider if they develop a rash while taking KALETRA. The healthcare provider will determine if treatment should be continued or an alternative antiretroviral regimen used.

□ Patients should be advised that appropriate liver function testing will be conducted prior to initiating and during therapy with KALETRA. Pre-existing liver disease including Hepatitis B or C can worsen with use of KALETRA. This can be seen as worsening of transaminase elevations or hepatic decompensation. Patients should be advised that their liver function tests will need to be monitored closely especially during the first several months of KALETRA treatment and that they should notify their healthcare provider if they develop the signs and symptoms of worsening liver disease including loss of appetite, abdominal pain, jaundice, and itchy skin.

□ New onset of diabetes or exacerbation of pre-existing diabetes mellitus, and hyperglycemia have been reported during KALETRA use. Patients should be advised to notify their healthcare provider if they develop the signs and symptoms of diabetes mellitus including frequent urination, excessive thirst, extreme hunger or unusual weight loss and/or an increased blood sugar while on KALETRA as they may require a change in their diabetes treatment or new treatment.

□ KALETRA might produce changes in the electrocardiogram (e.g., PR and/or QT prolongation). Patients should consult their physician if they experience symptoms such as dizziness, lightheadedness, abnormal heart rhythm or loss of consciousness.

□ They should seek medical assistance immediately if they develop a sustained penile erection lasting more than 4 hours while taking KALETRA and a PDE 5 Inhibitor such as Viagra, Cialis or Levitra.

Table 11. Drug Interactions: Pharmacokinetic Parameters for Co-administered Drug in the Presence of KALETRA for Recommended Alterations in Dose or Regimen

Co-administered Drug	Dose of Co-administered Drug (mg)	Dose of KALETRA (mg)	n	Ratio (in Combination with KALETRA/alone) of Co-administered Drug Pharmacokinetic Parameters (90% CI); No Effect = 1.00		
				C_{max}	AUC	C_{min}
Amprenavir[1]	750 twice daily, 10 d combo vs. 1200 twice daily, 14 d alone	400/100 capsule twice daily, 21 d	11	1.12 (0.91, 1.39)	1.72 (1.41, 2.09)	4.57 (3.51, 5.95)
Desipramine[2]	100 single dose	400/100 capsule twice daily, 10 d	15	0.91 (0.84, 0.97)	1.05 (0.96, 1.16)	N/A
Efavirenz	600 at bedtime, 9 d	400/100 capsule twice daily, 9 d	11, 12*	0.91 (0.72, 1.15)	0.84 (0.62, 1.15)	0.84 (0.58, 1.20)
Ethinyl Estradiol	35 µg once daily, 21 d (Ortho Novum®)	400/100 capsule twice daily, 14 d	12	0.59 (0.52, 0.66)	0.58 (0.54, 0.62)	0.42 (0.36, 0.49)
Fosamprenavir[3]	700 twice daily plus ritonavir 100 twice daily, 14 d	400/100 capsule twice daily, 14 d	18	0.42 (0.30, 0.58)	0.37 (0.28, 0.49)	0.35 (0.27, 0.46)
Indinavir[1]	600 twice daily, 10 d combo nonfasting vs. 800 three times daily, 5 d alone fasting	400/100 capsule twice daily, 15 d	13	0.71 (0.63, 0.81)	0.91 (0.75, 1.10)	3.47 (2.60, 4.64)
Ketoconazole	200 single dose	400/100 capsule twice daily, 16 d	12	1.13 (0.91, 1.40)	3.04 (2.44, 3.79)	N/A
Methadone	5 single dose	400/100 capsule twice daily, 10 d	11	0.55 (0.48, 0.64)	0.47 (0.42, 0.53)	N/A
Nelfinavir[1]	1000 twice daily, 10 d combo vs. 1250 twice daily 14 d alone	400/100 capsule twice daily, 21 d	13	0.93 (0.82, 1.05)	1.07 (0.95, 1.19)	1.86 (1.57, 2.22)
M8 metabolite				2.36 (1.91, 2.91)	3.46 (2.78, 4.31)	7.49 (5.85, 9.58)
Nevirapine	200 once daily, 14 d; twice daily, 6 d	400/100 capsule twice daily, 20 d	5, 6*	1.05 (0.72, 1.52)	1.08 (0.72, 1.64)	1.15 (0.71, 1.86)
Norethindrone	1 once daily, 21 d (Ortho Novum®)	400/100 capsule twice daily, 14 d	12	0.84 (0.75, 0.94)	0.83 (0.73, 0.94)	0.68 (0.54, 0.85)
Pravastatin	20 once daily, 4 d	400/100 capsule twice daily, 14 d	12	1.26 (0.87, 1.83)	1.33 (0.91, 1.94)	N/A
Rifabutin	150 once daily, 10 d; combo vs. 300 once daily, 10 d; alone	400/100 capsule twice daily, 10 d	12	2.12 (1.89, 2.38)	3.03 (2.79, 3.30)	4.90 (3.18, 5.76)
25-O-desacetyl rifabutin				23.6 (13.7, 25.3)	47.5 (29.3, 51.8)	94.9 (74.0, 122)
Rifabutin + 25-O-desacetyl rifabutin[4]				3.46 (3.07, 3.91)	5.73 (5.08, 6.46)	9.53 (7.56, 12.01)
Rosuvastatin[5]	20 mg once daily, 7 d	400/100 tablet twice daily, 7 d	15	4.66 (3.4, 6.4)	2.08 (1.66, 2.6)	1.04 (0.9, 1.2)
Tenofovir[6]	300 mg once daily, 14 d	400/100 capsule twice daily, 14 d	24	NC†	1.32 (1.26, 1.38)	1.51 (1.32, 1.66)

All interaction studies conducted in healthy, HIV-1 negative subjects unless otherwise indicated.
[1] Ratio of parameters for amprenavir, indinavir, and nelfinavir, are not normalized for dose.
[2] Desipramine is a probe substrate for assessing effects on CYP2D6-mediated metabolism.
[3] Data extracted from the fosamprenavir package insert.
[4] Effect on the dose-normalized sum of rifabutin parent and 25-O-desacetyl rifabutin active metabolite.
[5] Data extracted from the rosuvastatin package insert and results presented at the 2007 Conference on Retroviruses and Opportunistic Infection (Hoody, et al, abstract L-107, poster #564).
[6] Data extracted from the tenofovir package insert.
* Parallel group design; n for KALETRA + co-administered drug, n for co-administered drug alone.
N/A = Not available.
† NC = No change.

□ Redistribution or accumulation of body fat may occur in patients receiving antiretroviral therapy and that the cause and long term health effects of these conditions are not known at this time.
□ Patients should be informed that there may be a greater chance of developing diarrhea with the once daily regimen as compared with the twice daily regimen.

KALETRA Tablets, 200 mg lopinavir/50 mg ritonavir Manufactured by Abbott Pharmaceuticals PR Ltd., Barceloneta, PR 00617
for Abbott Laboratories, North Chicago, IL 60064, U.S.A.
KALETRA Tablets, 100 mg lopinavir/25 mg ritonavir and KALETRA Oral Solution
Abbott Laboratories, North Chicago, IL 60064, U.S.A.

MEDICATION GUIDE
KALETRA® (kuh-LEE-tra)
(lopinavir/ritonavir)
Tablets
KALETRA® (kuh-LEE-tra)
(lopinavir/ritonavir)
Oral Solution

Read the Medication Guide that comes with KALETRA before you start taking it and each time you get a refill. There may be new information. This information does not take the place of talking with your doctor about your medical condition or treatment. You and your doctor should talk about your treatment with KALETRA before you start taking it and at regular check-ups. You should stay under your doctor's care when taking KALETRA.

What is the most important information I should know about KALETRA?
KALETRA may cause serious side effects, including:
• **Interactions with other medicines. It is important to know the medicines that should not be taken with KALETRA.** Read the section "What should I tell my doctor before taking KALETRA?"
• **Changes in your heart rhythm and the electrical activity of your heart.** These changes may be seen on an EKG (electrocardiogram) and can lead to serious heart problems. Your risk for these problems may be higher if you:
  ○ already have a history of abnormal heart rhythm or other types of heart disease.
  ○ take other medicines that can affect your heart rhythm while you take KALETRA.

Tell your doctor right away if you have any of these symptoms while taking KALETRA:
• dizziness
• lightheadedness
• fainting
• sensation of abnormal heartbeats

See the section below "What are the possible side effects of KALETRA?" for more information about serious side effects.

What is KALETRA?
KALETRA is a prescription anti-HIV medicine that contains two medicines: lopinavir and ritonavir. KALETRA is called a protease inhibitor that is used with other anti-HIV-1 medicines to treat people with human immunodeficiency virus (HIV-1) infection. HIV-1 is the virus that causes AIDS (Acquired Immune Deficiency Syndrome).
It is not known if KALETRA is safe and effective in children under 14 days old.

Who should not take KALETRA?
• Do not take KALETRA if you are taking certain medicines. For more information about medicines you should not take with KALETRA, please see **"Can I take other medicines with KALETRA?"** and consult with your doctor about all other medicines you take.
• Do not take KALETRA if you have an allergy to KALETRA or any of its ingredients, including ritonavir and lopinavir.

What should I tell my doctor before taking KALETRA?
KALETRA may not be right for you. Tell your doctor about all your medical conditions, including if you:
• have any heart problems, including if you have a condition called Congenital Long QT Syndrome.
• have liver problems, including Hepatitis B or Hepatitis C.
• have diabetes.
• have hemophilia. People who take KALETRA may have increased bleeding.
• have low potassium in your blood.
• are pregnant or plan to become pregnant. It is not known if KALETRA will harm your unborn baby. Birth control pills or patches may not work as well while you take KALETRA. To prevent pregnancy while taking KALETRA, women who take birth control pills or use estrogen patch for birth control should either use a different type of birth control or an extra form of birth control. Talk to your doctor about how to prevent pregnancy while taking KALETRA.
• take KALETRA during pregnancy, talk with your doctor about how you can take part in an antiretroviral pregnancy registry. The purpose of the pregnancy registry is to follow the health of you and your baby.
• are breast-feeding. Do not breast-feed if you are taking KALETRA. You should not breast-feed if you have HIV-1. If you are a woman who has or will have a baby while taking KALETRA, talk with your doctor about the best way to feed your baby. If your baby does not already have HIV-1, there is a chance that HIV-1 can be passed to your baby through your breast milk.

Information on the Abbott Pharmaceutical Products listed on these pages is from the prescribing information in use as of June 1, 2010. For more information, please visit rxabbott.com or call 1-800-633-9110.

Tell your doctor about all the medicines you take, including prescription and non-prescription medicines, vitamins, and herbal supplements. Many medicines interact with KALETRA. Do not start taking a new medicine without telling your doctor or pharmacist. Your doctor can tell you if it is safe to take KALETRA with other medicines. Your doctor may need to change the dose of other medicines while you take KALETRA.

Medicines you should not take with KALETRA.
Serious problems or death can happen if you take these medicines with KALETRA:
- ergot containing medicines, including:
  - ergotamine tartrate (Cafergot®, Migergot, Ergomar, Ergostat, Medihaler Ergotamine, Wigraine, Wigrettes)
  - dihydroergotamine mesylate (D.H.E. 45®, Embolex, Migranal®)
  - ergonovine, ergonovine and methylergonovine (Ergotrate, Methergine), ergotamine and methylergonovine
  - Ergotrate Maleate, methylergonovine maleate (Methergine)
- triazolam (Halcion®), midazolam hydrochloride oral syrup
- pimozide (Orap®)
- the cholesterol lowering medicines lovastatin (Mevacor®) or simvastatin (Zocor®)
- sildenafil (Revatio®) only when used for the treatment of pulmonary arterial hypertension. (See "Medicines that may need changes" and "What are the possible side effects of Kaletra?" for information about the use of sildenafil for erectile problems.)
- alfuzosin (Uroxatral®)

Medicines that you should not take with KALETRA since they may make KALETRA not work as well:
- the herbal supplement St. John's Wort (hypericum perforatum)
- rifampin (Rimactane®, Rifadin®, Rifater®, or Rifamate®)

Medicines that may need changes:
- birth control pills that contain estrogen ("the pill") or the birth control (contraceptive) patches
- certain cholesterol lowering medicines, such as atorvastatin (Lipitor®) or rosuvastatin (Crestor®)
- certain other antiretroviral medicines, such as efavirenz (Atripla® and Sustiva®), nevirapine (Viramune®), amprenavir (Agenerase®), fosamprenavir calcium (Lexiva®) and nelfinavir (Viracept®)
- anti-seizure medicines, such as phenytoin (Dilantin®) carbamazepine, (Tegretol®), phenobarbital
- medicines for erectile problems, such as sildenafil (Viagra®, Revatio®), tadalafil (Cialis®), or vardenafil (Levitra®)
- medicines for tuberculosis (TB), such as rifabutin (Mycobutin®)
- inhaled steroid medicines, such as fluticasone propionate (Flonase®)
- inhaled medicines such as salmeterol (Serevent®) or salmeterol in combination with fluticasone propionate (Advair®). Your doctor may need to change to a different medicine.
- medicines for gout, such as colchicine (Colcrys®)
- medicines to treat pulmonary arterial hypertension (PAH), such as bosentan (Tracleer®) or tadalafil (Adcirca®)

If you are not sure if you are taking a medicine above, ask your doctor.

How should I take KALETRA?
- Take KALETRA every day exactly as prescribed by your doctor.
- It is very important to set up a dosing schedule and follow it every day.
- Do not change your treatment or stop treatment without first talking with your doctor.
- Swallow KALETRA tablets whole. Do not chew, break, or crush KALETRA tablets.
- KALETRA tablets can be taken with or without food.
- If you are taking both Videx® (didanosine) and KALETRA:
  - didanosine can be taken at the same time as KALETRA tablets, without food.
  - take didanosine either one hour before or two hours after taking KALETRA oral solution.
- Do not miss a dose of KALETRA. This could make the virus harder to treat. If you forget to take KALETRA, take the missed dose right away. If it is almost time for your next dose, do not take the missed dose. Instead, follow your regular dosing schedule by taking your next dose at its regular time. Do not take more than one dose of KALETRA at one time.
- If you take more than the prescribed dose of KALETRA, call your local poison control center or emergency room right away.
- Take KALETRA oral solution with food to help it work better.

- If KALETRA is being used for your child, tell your doctor if your child's weight changes.
- KALETRA should not be given one time each day in children. When giving KALETRA to your child, give KALETRA exactly as prescribed.
- KALETRA oral solution contains a large amount of alcohol.
  - If a young child drinks more than the recommended dose, it could make them sick from too much alcohol. Contact your local poison control center or emergency room right away.
  - Talk with your doctor if you take or plan to take metronidazole or disulfiram. You can have severe nausea and vomiting if you take these medicines with KALETRA.
- When your KALETRA supply starts to run low, get more from your doctor or pharmacy. It is important not to run out of KALETRA. The amount of HIV-1 virus in your blood may increase if the medicine is stopped for even a short time. The virus may become resistant to KALETRA and become harder to treat.
- KALETRA can be taken with acid reducing agents used for heartburn or reflux such as omeprazole (Prilosec®) and ranitidine (Zantac®) with no dose adjustment.
- KALETRA should not be administered once daily in combination with carbamazepine (Tegretol® and Epitol®), phenobarbital (Luminol®), or phenytoin (Dilantin®).
Avoid doing things that can spread HIV infection. KALETRA does not stop you from passing HIV infection to others. Do not share needles, other injection equipment or personal items that can have blood or body fluids on them, like toothbrushes and razor blades. Always practice safer sex by using a latex or polyurethane condom to lower the chance of sexual contact with semen, vaginal secretions, or blood.

Table 12. Virologic Response (HIV-1 RNA <400 copies/mL) at Week 48 by Baseline KALETRA Susceptibility and by Number of Protease Substitutions Associated with Reduced Response to KALETRA[1]

Number of protease inhibitor substitutions at baseline[1]	Study 888 (Single protease inhibitor-experienced[2], NNRTI-naïve) n=130	Study 765 (Single protease inhibitor-experienced[3], NNRTI-naïve) n=56	Study 957 (Multiple protease inhibitor-experienced[4], NNRTI-naïve) n=50
0-2	76/103 (74%)	34/45 (76%)	19/20 (95%)
3-5	13/26 (50%)	8/11 (73%)	18/26 (69%)
6 or more	0/1 (0%)	N/A	1/4 (25%)

[1] Substitutions considered in the analysis included L10F/I/R/V, K20M/N/R, L24I, L33F, M36I, I47V, G48V, I54L/T/V, V82A/C/F/S/T, and I84V.
[2] 43% indinavir, 42% nelfinavir, 10% ritonavir, 15% saquinavir.
[3] 41% indinavir, 38% nelfinavir, 4% ritonavir, 16% saquinavir.
[4] 86% indinavir, 54% nelfinavir, 80% ritonavir, 70% saquinavir.

Table 13. HIV-1 RNA Response at Week 48 by Baseline Lopinavir Susceptibility[1]

Lopinavir susceptibility[2] at baseline	HIV-1 RNA <400 copies/mL (%)	HIV-1 RNA <50 copies/mL (%)
< 10 fold	25/27 (93%)	22/27 (81%)
> 10 and < 40 fold	11/15 (73%)	9/15 (60%)
≥ 40 fold	2/8 (25%)	2/8 (25%)

[1] Lopinavir susceptibility was determined by recombinant phenotypic technology performed by Virologic.
[2] Fold change in susceptibility from wild type.

Table 15. Proportion of Responders Through Week 48 by Baseline Viral Load (Study 863)

Baseline Viral Load (HIV-1 RNA copies/mL)	KALETRA + d4T + 3TC			Nelfinavir + d4T + 3TC		
	<400 copies/mL[1]	<50 copies/mL[2]	n	<400 copies/mL[1]	<50 copies/mL[2]	n
< 30,000	74%	71%	82	79%	72%	87
≥ 30,000 to < 100,000	81%	73%	79	67%	54%	79
≥ 100,000 to < 250,000	75%	64%	83	60%	47%	72
≥ 250,000	72%	60%	82	44%	33%	89

[1] Patients achieved and maintained confirmed HIV-1 RNA < 400 copies/mL through Week 48.
[2] Patients achieved HIV-1 RNA < 50 copies/mL at Week 48.

Table 17. Outcomes of Randomized Treatment Through Week 48 (Study 888)

Outcome	KALETRA + nevirapine + NRTIs (n = 148)	Investigator-Selected Protease Inhibitor(s) + nevirapine + NRTIs (n = 140)
Responder[1]	57%	33%
Virologic failure[2]	24%	41%
Rebound	11%	19%
Never suppressed through Week 48	13%	23%
Death	1%	2%
Discontinued due to adverse events	5%	11%
Discontinued for other reasons[3]	14%	13%

[1] Patients achieved and maintained confirmed HIV-1 RNA < 400 copies/mL through Week 48.
[2] Includes confirmed viral rebound and failure to achieve confirmed < 400 copies/mL through Week 48.
[3] Includes lost to follow-up, patient's withdrawal, non-compliance, protocol violation and other reasons.

IMPORTANT NOTICE: Updated drug information is sent bi-monthly via the PDR® Update Insert. For *monthly* email updates, register at PDR.net.

Table 18. Outcomes of Randomized Treatment Through Week 48 (Study 802)

Outcome	KALETRA Once Daily + NRTIs (n = 300)	KALETRA Twice Daily + NRTIs (n = 299)
Virologic Success (HIV-1 RNA <50 copies/mL)	57%	54%
Virologic failure[1]	22%	24%
No virologic data in Week 48 window		
Discontinued study due to adverse event or death[2]	5%	7%
Discontinued study for other reasons[3]	13%	12%
Missing data during window but on study	3%	3%

[1] Includes patients who discontinued prior to Week 48 for lack or loss of efficacy and patients with HIV-1 RNA ≥ 50 copies/mL at Week 48.

[2] Includes patients who discontinued due to adverse events or death at any time from Day 1 through Week 48 if this resulted in no virologic data on treatment at Week 48.

[3] Includes withdrawal of consent, loss to follow-up, non-compliance, protocol violation and other reasons.

What are the possible side effects of KALETRA?
KALETRA can cause serious side effects.

• See "What is the most important information I should know about KALETRA?"

• **Liver problems.** Liver problems, including death, can happen in people who take KALETRA. Blood tests in people who take KALETRA may show possible liver problems. People with liver disease such as Hepatitis B and Hepatitis C who take KALETRA may have worsening liver disease. Tell your healthcare provider right away if you have any of these signs and symptoms of liver problems:
  ○ loss of appetite
  ○ yellow skin and whites of eyes (jaundice)
  ○ dark-colored urine
  ○ pale colored stools, itchy skin
  ○ stomach area (abdominal) pain.

• **Inflammation of the pancreas (pancreatitis).** Some people who take KALETRA get inflammation of the pancreas which may be serious and cause death. You have a higher chance of getting pancreatitis if you have had it before. Tell your doctor if you have nausea, vomiting, or abdominal pain while taking KALETRA. These may be signs of pancreatitis.

• **Increases in certain fat (triglycerides and cholesterol) levels in your blood.** Large increases of triglycerides and cholesterol can be seen in blood test results of some people who take KALETRA. The long-term chance of getting complications such as heart attacks or stroke due to increases in triglycerides and cholesterol caused by protease inhibitors is not known at this time.

• **Diabetes and high blood sugar (hyperglycemia).** Some people who take protease inhibitors including KALETRA get new or more serious diabetes, or high blood sugar. Tell your doctor if you notice an increase in thirst or urinate often while taking KALETRA.

• **Changes in body fat.** Changes in body fat in some people who take antiretroviral therapy. These changes may include increased amount of fat in the upper back and neck ("buffalo hump"), breast, and around the trunk. Loss of fat from the legs, arms and face may also happen. The cause and long-term health effects of these conditions are not known at this time.

• **Increased bleeding for hemophiliacs.** Some people with hemophilia have increased bleeding with protease inhibitors including KALETRA.

• **Increased risk of certain problems when you take medicines used for the treatment of erectile problems such as sildenafil (Viagra®), tadalafil (Cialis®), or vardenafil (Levitra®) with KALETRA:**
  ○ **low blood pressure.** If you get dizzy or faint, you need to lie down. Tell your doctor if you feel dizzy, or have fainting spells.
  ○ **vision changes.** Tell your doctor right away if you have vision changes.
  ○ **penis erection lasting more than 4 hours.** If you are a male and have an erection that lasts longer than 4 hours, get medical help right away to avoid permanent damage to your penis. Your doctor can explain these symptoms to you.

Common side effects of KALETRA include:
• diarrhea
• nausea
• stomach area (abdominal) pain
• feeling weak
• vomiting
• headache
• upset stomach

These are not all of the possible side effects of KALETRA. For more information, ask your doctor or pharmacist. Tell your doctor about any side effect that bothers you or that does not go away.

Call your doctor for medical advice about side effects. You may report side effects to FDA at 1-800-FDA-1088.

How should I store KALETRA?
KALETRA tablets:
• Store KALETRA tablets at room temperature, between 59°F to 86°F (15°C to 30°C).
• Do not keep KALETRA tablets out of the container it comes in for longer than 2 weeks, especially in areas where there is a lot of humidity. Keep the container closed tightly.

KALETRA oral solution:
• Store KALETRA oral solution in a refrigerator, between 36°F to 46°F (2°C to 8°C). KALETRA oral solution that is kept refrigerated may be used until the expiration date printed on the label.
• KALETRA oral solution that is stored at room temperature (less than 77°F or 25°C) should be used within 2 months.
• Keep KALETRA away from high heat.

Throw away any medicine that is out of date or that you no longer need.

Keep KALETRA and all medicines out of the reach of children.

General information about KALETRA
KALETRA does not cure HIV-1 or AIDS. The long-term effects of KALETRA are not known at this time. People taking KALETRA may still get opportunistic infections or other conditions that happen with HIV-1 infection. Some of these conditions are pneumonia, herpes virus infections, and *Mycobacterium avium* complex (MAC) infections.

Medicines are sometimes prescribed for purposes other than those listed in a Medication Guide. Do not use KALETRA for a condition for which it was not prescribed. Do not give KALETRA to other people, even if they have the same condition you have. It may harm them.

This Medication Guide summarizes the most important information about KALETRA. If you would like more information, talk with your doctor. You can ask your pharmacist or doctor for information about KALETRA that is written for health professionals. For more information about KALETRA call 1-800-633-9110 or go to www.KALETRA.com.

What are the ingredients in KALETRA?
Active ingredient: lopinavir and ritonavir
Inactive ingredients:

KALETRA 200 mg lopinavir and 50 mg ritonavir tablets: copovidone, sorbitan monolaurate, colloidal silicon dioxide, and sodium stearyl fumarate. The film coating contains: hypromellose, titanium dioxide, polyethylene glycol 400, hydroxypropyl cellulose, talc, colloidal silicon dioxide, polyethylene glycol 3350, yellow ferric oxide 172, and polysorbate 80.

KALETRA 100 mg lopinavir and 25 mg ritonavir tablets: copovidone, sorbitan monolaurate, colloidal silicon dioxide, and sodium stearyl fumarate. The film coating contains: polyvinyl alcohol, titanium dioxide, talc, polytheylene glycol 3350, and yellow ferric oxide E172.

KALETRA oral solution: acesulfame potassium, alcohol, artificial cotton candy flavor, citric acid, glycerin, high fructose corn syrup, Magnasweet-110 flavor, menthol, natural and artificial vanilla flavor, peppermint oil, polyoxyl 40 hydrogenated castor oil, povidone, propylene glycol, saccharin sodium, sodium chloride, sodium citrate, and water.

KALETRA oral solution contains 42.4% alcohol (v/v). "See How should I take KALETRA?".

KALETRA Tablets, 200 mg lopinavir/50 mg ritonavir
Manufactured by Abbott Pharmaceuticals PR Ltd., Barceloneta, PR 00617
for Abbott Laboratories, North Chicago, IL 60064, U.S.A.
KALETRA Tablets, 100 mg lopinavir/25 mg ritonavir and KALETRA Oral Solution

Abbott Laboratories, North Chicago, IL 60064, U.S.A.
2010, ALL RIGHTS RESERVED
* The brands listed are trademarks of their respective owners and are not trademarks of Abbott Laboratories. The makers of these brands are not affiliated with and do not endorse Abbott Laboratories or its products.
Ref 03-A363-R7 -Revised: April, 2010
This Medication Guide has been approved by the U.S. Food and Drug Administration.
Shown in Product Identification Guide, page 303

LUPRON DEPOT® 3.75 mg   ℞
[lew-prŏn]
(leuprolide acetate for depot suspension)
℞ only

This is combined labeling. Examples of different fonts appear below.
• General information
• Information on endometriosis
• Information on uterine fibroids

DESCRIPTION
Leuprolide acetate is a synthetic nonapeptide analog of naturally occurring gonadotropin-releasing hormone (GnRH or LH-RH). The analog possesses greater potency than the natural hormone. The chemical name is 5-oxo-L-prolyl-L-histidyl-L-tryptophyl-L-seryl-L-tyrosyl-D-leucyl-L-leucyl-L-arginyl-N-ethyl-L-prolinamide acetate (salt) with the following structural formula:
[See figure at top of next page]
LUPRON DEPOT is available in a prefilled dual-chamber syringe containing sterile lyophilized microspheres which, when mixed with diluent, become a suspension intended as a monthly intramuscular injection.
The front chamber of LUPRON DEPOT 3.75 mg prefilled dual-chamber syringe contains leuprolide acetate (3.75 mg), purified gelatin (0.65 mg), DL-lactic and glycolic acids copolymer (33.1 mg), and D-mannitol (6.6 mg). The second chamber of diluent contains carboxymethylcellulose sodium (5 mg), D-mannitol (50 mg), polysorbate 80 (1 mg), water for injection, USP, and glacial acetic acid, USP to control pH. During the manufacture of LUPRON DEPOT 3.75 mg, acetic acid is lost, leaving the peptide.

CLINICAL PHARMACOLOGY
Leuprolide acetate is a long-acting GnRH analog. A single monthly injection of LUPRON DEPOT 3.75 mg results in an initial stimulation followed by a prolonged suppression of pituitary gonadotropins. Repeated dosing at monthly intervals results in decreased secretion of gonadal steroids; consequently, tissues and functions that depend on gonadal steroids for their maintenance become quiescent. This effect is reversible on discontinuation of drug therapy.
Leuprolide acetate is not active when given orally. Intramuscular injection of the depot formulation provides plasma concentrations of leuprolide over a period of one month.
Pharmacokinetics
Absorption
A single dose of LUPRON DEPOT 3.75 mg was administered by intramuscular injection to healthy female volunteers. The absorption of leuprolide was characterized by an initial increase in plasma concentration, with peak concentration ranging from 4.6 to 10.2 ng/mL at four hours post-dosing. However, intact leuprolide and an inactive metabolite could not be distinguished by the assay used in the study. Following the initial rise, leuprolide concentrations started to plateau within two days after dosing and remained relatively stable for about four to five weeks with plasma concentrations of about 0.30 ng/mL.
Distribution
The mean steady-state volume of distribution of leuprolide following intravenous bolus administration to healthy male volunteers was 27 L. *In vitro* binding to human plasma proteins ranged from 43% to 49%.
Metabolism
In healthy male volunteers, a 1 mg bolus of leuprolide administered intravenously revealed that the mean systemic clearance was 7.6 L/h, with a terminal elimination half-life of approximately 3 hours based on a two compartment model.
In rats and dogs, administration of ^{14}C-labeled leuprolide was shown to be metabolized to smaller inactive peptides, a pentapeptide (Metabolite I), tripeptides (Metabolites II and III) and a dipeptide (Metabolite IV). These fragments may be further catabolized.
The major metabolite (M-I) plasma concentrations measured in 5 prostate cancer patients reached maximum con-

Information on the Abbott Pharmaceutical Products listed on these pages is from the prescribing information in use as of June 1, 2010. For more information, please visit rxabbott.com or call 1-800-633-9110.

centration 2 to 6 hours after dosing and were approximately 6% of the peak parent drug concentration. One week after dosing, mean plasma M-I concentrations were approximately 20% of mean leuprolide concentrations.

Excretion
Following administration of LUPRON DEPOT 3.75 mg to 3 patients, less than 5% of the dose was recovered as parent and M-I metabolite in the urine.

Special Populations
The pharmacokinetics of the drug in hepatically and renally impaired patients have not been determined.

Drug Interactions
No pharmacokinetic-based drug-drug interaction studies have been conducted with LUPRON DEPOT. However, because leuprolide acetate is a peptide that is primarily degraded by peptidase and not by cytochrome P-450 enzymes as noted in specific studies, and the drug is only about 46% bound to plasma proteins, drug interactions would not be expected to occur.

CLINICAL STUDIES
Endometriosis
In controlled clinical studies, LUPRON DEPOT 3.75 mg monthly for six months was shown to be comparable to danazol 800 mg/day in relieving the clinical sign/symptoms of endometriosis (pelvic pain, dysmenorrhea, dyspareunia, pelvic tenderness, and induration) and in reducing the size of endometrial implants as evidenced by laparoscopy. The clinical significance of a decrease in endometriotic lesions is not known at this time, and in addition laparoscopic staging of endometriosis does not necessarily correlate with the severity of symptoms.

LUPRON DEPOT 3.75 mg monthly induced amenorrhea in 74% and 98% of the patients after the first and second treatment months respectively. Most of the remaining patients reported episodes of only light bleeding or spotting. In the first, second and third post-treatment months, normal menstrual cycles resumed in 7%, 71% and 95% of patients, respectively, excluding those who became pregnant.

Figure 1 illustrates the percent of patients with symptoms at baseline, final treatment visit and sustained relief at 6 and 12 months following discontinuation of treatment for the various symptoms evaluated during two controlled clinical studies. This included all patients at end of treatment and those who elected to participate in the follow-up period. This might provide a slight bias in the results at follow-up as 75% of the original patients entered the follow-up study, and 36% were evaluated at 6 months and 26% at 12 months.

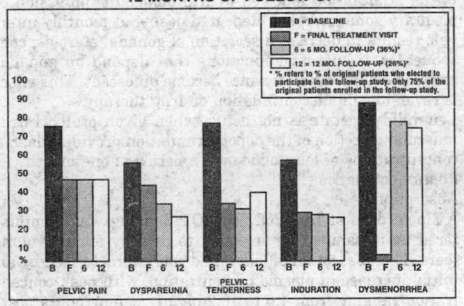

FIGURE 1–PERCENT OF PATIENTS WITH SIGN/SYMPTOMS AT BASELINE, FINAL TREATMENT VISIT, AND AFTER 6 AND 12 MONTHS OF FOLLOW-UP

Hormonal replacement therapy
Two clinical studies with a treatment duration of 12 months indicate that concurrent hormonal therapy (norethindrone acetate 5 mg daily) is effective in significantly reducing the loss of bone mineral density associated with LUPRON, without compromising the efficacy of LUPRON in relieving symptoms of endometriosis. (All patients in these studies received calcium supplementation with 1000 mg elemental calcium). One controlled, randomized and double-blind study included 51 women treated with LUPRON DEPOT alone and 55 women treated with LUPRON plus norethindrone acetate 5 mg daily. The second study was an open label study in which 136 women were treated with LUPRON plus norethindrone acetate 5 mg daily. This study confirmed the reduction in loss of bone mineral density that was observed in the controlled study. Suppression of menses was maintained throughout treatment in 84% and 73% of patients receiving LD/N in the controlled study and open label study, respectively. The median time for menses resumption after treatment with LD/N was 8 weeks. Figure 2 illustrates the mean pain scores for the LD/N group from the controlled study.

[See figure 2 at top of next column]

Uterine Leiomyomata (Fibroids)
In controlled clinical trials, administration of LUPRON DEPOT 3.75 mg for a period of three or six months was shown to decrease uterine and fibroid volume, thus allowing for relief of clinical symptoms (abdominal bloating, pelvic pain, and pressure). Excessive vaginal bleeding (menorrhagia and menometrorrhagia) decreased, resulting in improvement in hematologic parameters.

In three clinical trials, enrollment was not based on hematologic status. Mean uterine volume decreased by 41% and my-

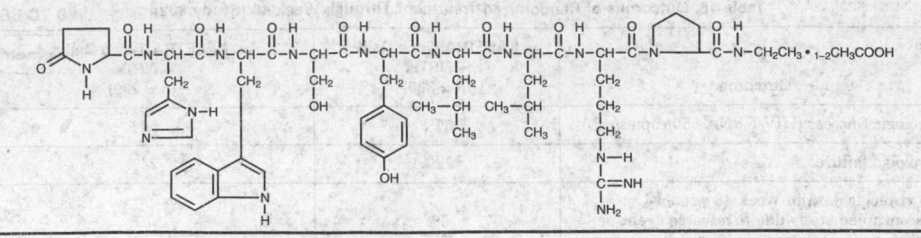

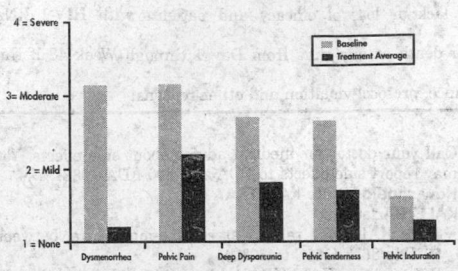

Figure 2
Treatment Period Mean Pain Scores for LD/N* Patients

* LD/N = LUPRON DEPOT 3.75 mg plus norethindrone acetate 5 mg daily

oma volume decreased by 37% at final visit as evidenced by ultrasound or MRI. These patients also experienced a decrease in symptoms including excessive vaginal bleeding and pelvic discomfort. Benefit occurred by three months of therapy, but additional gain was observed with an additional three months of LUPRON DEPOT 3.75 mg. Ninety-five percent of these patients became amenorrheic with 61%, 25%, and 4% experiencing amenorrhea during the first, second, and third treatment months respectively.

Post-treatment follow-up was carried out for a small percentage of LUPRON DEPOT 3.75 mg patients among the 77% who demonstrated a ≥ 25% decrease in uterine volume while on therapy. Menses usually returned within two months of cessation of therapy. Mean time to return to pretreatment uterine size was 8.3 months. Regrowth did not appear to be related to pretreatment uterine volume.

In another controlled clinical study, enrollment was based on hematocrit ≤ 30% and/or hemoglobin ≤ 10.2 g/dL. Administration of LUPRON DEPOT 3.75 mg, concomitantly with iron, produced an increase of ≥ 6% hematocrit and ≥ 2 g/dL hemoglobin in 77% of patients at three months of therapy. The mean change in hematocrit was 10.1% and the mean change in hemoglobin was 4.2 g/dL. Clinical response was judged to be a hematocrit of ≥ 36% and hemoglobin of ≥ 12 g/dL, thus allowing for autologous blood donation prior to surgery. At three months, 75% of patients met this criterion.

At three months, 80% of patients experienced relief from either menorrhagia or menometrorrhagia. As with the previous studies, episodes of spotting and menstrual-like bleeding were noted in some patients.

In this same study, a decrease of ≥ 25% was seen in uterine and myoma volumes in 60% and 54% of patients respectively. LUPRON DEPOT 3.75 mg was found to relieve symptoms of bloating, pelvic pain, and pressure.

There is no evidence that pregnancy rates are enhanced or adversely affected by the use of LUPRON DEPOT 3.75 mg.

INDICATIONS AND USAGE
Endometriosis
LUPRON DEPOT 3.75 mg is indicated for management of endometriosis, including pain relief and reduction of endometriotic lesions. LUPRON DEPOT monthly with norethindrone acetate 5 mg daily is also indicated for initial management of endometriosis and for management of recurrence of symptoms. (Refer also to norethindrone acetate prescribing information for WARNINGS, PRECAUTIONS, CONTRAINDICATIONS and ADVERSE REACTIONS associated with norethindrone acetate.) Duration of initial treatment or retreatment should be limited to 6 months.

Uterine Leiomyomata (Fibroids)
LUPRON DEPOT 3.75 mg concomitantly with iron therapy is indicated for the preoperative hematologic improvement of patients with anemia caused by uterine leiomyomata. The clinician may wish to consider a one-month trial period on iron alone inasmuch as some of the patients will respond to iron alone. (See Table 1.) LUPRON may be added if the response to iron alone is considered inadequate. Recommended duration of therapy with LUPRON DEPOT 3.75 mg is **up to** three months.

Experience with LUPRON DEPOT in females has been limited to women 18 years of age and older.

Table 1 PERCENT OF PATIENTS ACHIEVING HEMOGLOBIN ≥ 12 GM/DL

Treatment Group	Week 4	Week 8	Week 12
LUPRON DEPOT 3.75 mg with Iron	41*	71**	79*
Iron Alone	17	40	56

* P-Value < 0.01
** P-Value < 0.001

CONTRAINDICATIONS
1. Hypersensitivity to GnRH, GnRH agonist analogs or any of the excipients in LUPRON DEPOT.
2. Undiagnosed abnormal vaginal bleeding.
3. LUPRON DEPOT is contraindicated in women who are or may become pregnant while receiving the drug. LUPRON DEPOT may cause fetal harm when administered to a pregnant woman. Major fetal abnormalities were observed in rabbits but not in rats after administration of LUPRON DEPOT throughout gestation. There was increased fetal mortality and decreased fetal weights in rats and rabbits. (See **Pregnancy** section.) The effects on fetal mortality are expected consequences of the alterations in hormonal levels brought about by the drug. If this drug is used during pregnancy, or if the patient becomes pregnant while taking this drug, the patient should be apprised of the potential hazard to the fetus.
4. Use in women who are breast-feeding. (See **Nursing Mothers** section.)
5. Norethindrone acetate is contraindicated in women with the following conditions:
   - Thrombophlebitis, thromboembolic disorders, cerebral apoplexy, or a past history of these conditions
   - Markedly impaired liver function or liver disease
   - Known or suspected carcinoma of the breast

WARNINGS
Safe use of leuprolide acetate or norethindrone acetate in pregnancy has not been established clinically. Before starting treatment with LUPRON DEPOT, pregnancy must be excluded.

When used monthly at the recommended dose, LUPRON DEPOT usually inhibits ovulation and stops menstruation. Contraception is not insured, however, by taking LUPRON DEPOT. Therefore, patients should use non-hormonal methods of contraception. Patients should be advised to see their physician if they believe they may be pregnant. If a patient becomes pregnant during treatment, the drug must be discontinued and the patient must be apprised of the potential risk to the fetus.

During the early phase of therapy, sex steroids temporarily rise above baseline because of the physiologic effect of the drug. Therefore, an increase in clinical signs and symptoms may be observed during the initial days of therapy, but these will dissipate with continued treatment.

Symptoms consistent with an anaphylactoid or asthmatic process have been rarely reported post-marketing.

The following applies to co-treatment with LUPRON and norethindrone acetate:

Norethindrone acetate treatment should be discontinued if there is a sudden partial or complete loss of vision or if there is sudden onset of proptosis, diplopia, or migraine. If examination reveals papilledema or retinal vascular lesions, medication should be withdrawn.

Because of the occasional occurrence of thrombophlebitis and pulmonary embolism in patients taking progestogens, the physician should be alert to the earliest manifestations of the disease in women taking norethindrone acetate.

Assessment and management of risk factors for cardiovascular disease is recommended prior to initiation of add-back therapy with norethindrone acetate. Norethindrone acetate should be used with caution in women with risk factors, including lipid abnormalities or cigarette smoking.

PRECAUTIONS
Information for Patients
An information pamphlet for patients is included with the product. Patients should be aware of the following information:

1. Since menstruation usually stops with effective doses of LUPRON DEPOT, the patient should notify her physician if regular menstruation persists. Patients missing successive doses of LUPRON DEPOT may experience breakthrough bleeding.
2. Patients should not use LUPRON DEPOT if they are pregnant, breast feeding, have undiagnosed abnormal vaginal bleeding, or are allergic to any of the ingredients in LUPRON DEPOT.
3. Safe use of the drug in pregnancy has not been established clinically. Therefore, a non-hormonal method of contraception should be used during treatment. Patients should be advised that if they miss successive doses of LUPRON DEPOT, breakthrough bleeding or ovulation may occur with the potential for conception. If a patient becomes pregnant during treatment, she should discontinue treatment and consult her physician.
4. Adverse events occurring in clinical studies with LUPRON DEPOT that are associated with hypoestrogenism include: hot flashes, headaches, emotional lability, decreased libido, acne, myalgia, reduction in breast size, and vaginal dryness. Estrogen levels returned to normal after treatment was discontinued.
5. Patients should be counseled on the possibility of the development or worsening of depression and the occurrence of memory disorders.
6. The induced hypoestrogenic state **also** results in a loss in bone density over the course of treatment, some of which may not be reversible. For a period up to six months, this bone loss should not be clinically significant. Clinical studies show that concurrent hormonal therapy with norethindrone acetate 5 mg daily is effective in reducing loss of bone mineral density that occurs with LUPRON. (All patients received calcium supplementation with 1000 mg elemental calcium.) (See ***Changes in Bone Density*** section).
7. If the symptoms of endometriosis recur after a course of therapy, retreatment with a six-month course of LUPRON DEPOT and norethindrone acetate 5 mg daily may be considered. Retreatment beyond this one six month course cannot be recommended. It is recommended that bone density be assessed before retreatment begins to ensure that values are within normal limits. Retreatment with LUPRON DEPOT alone is not recommended.
8. In patients with major risk factors for decreased bone mineral content such as chronic alcohol and/or tobacco use, strong family history of osteoporosis, or chronic use of drugs that can reduce bone mass such as anticonvulsants or corticosteroids, LUPRON DEPOT therapy may pose an additional risk. In these patients, the risks and benefits must be weighed carefully before therapy with LUPRON DEPOT alone is instituted, and concomitant treatment with norethindrone acetate 5 mg daily should be considered. Retreatment with gonadotropin-releasing hormone analogs, including LUPRON is not advisable in patients with major risk factors for loss of bone mineral content.
9. Because norethindrone acetate may cause some degree of fluid retention, conditions which might be influenced by this factor, such as epilepsy, migraine, asthma, cardiac or renal dysfunctions require careful observation during norethindrone acetate add-back therapy.
10. Patients who have a history of depression should be carefully observed during treatment with norethindrone acetate and norethindrone acetate should be discontinued if severe depression occurs.

Laboratory Tests

See **ADVERSE REACTIONS** section.

Drug Interactions

See **CLINICAL PHARMACOLOGY, Pharmacokinetics.**

Drug/Laboratory Test Interactions

Administration of LUPRON DEPOT in therapeutic doses results in suppression of the pituitary-gonadal system. Normal function is usually restored within three months after treatment is discontinued. Therefore, diagnostic tests of pituitary gonadotropic and gonadal functions conducted during treatment and for up to three months after discontinuation of LUPRON DEPOT may be misleading.

Carcinogenesis, Mutagenesis, Impairment of Fertility

A two-year carcinogenicity study was conducted in rats and mice. In rats, a dose-related increase of benign pituitary hyperplasia and benign pituitary adenomas was noted at 24 months when the drug was administered subcutaneously at high daily doses (0.6 to 4 mg/kg). There was a significant but not dose-related increase of pancreatic islet-cell adenomas in females and of testicular interstitial cell adenomas in males (highest incidence in the low dose group). In mice, no leuprolide acetate-induced tumors or pituitary abnormalities were observed at a dose as high as 60 mg/kg for two years. Patients have been treated with leuprolide acetate for up to three years with doses as high as 10 mg/day and for two years with doses as high as 20 mg/day without demonstrable pituitary abnormalities.

Mutagenicity studies have been performed with leuprolide acetate using bacterial and mammalian systems. These studies provided no evidence of a mutagenic potential.

Clinical and pharmacologic studies in adults (>18 years) with leuprolide acetate and similar analogs have shown reversibility of fertility suppression when the drug is discontinued after continuous administration for periods of up to 24 weeks. Although no clinical studies have been completed in children to assess the full reversibility of fertility suppression, animal studies (prepubertal and adult rats and monkeys) with leuprolide acetate and other GnRH analogs have shown functional recovery.

Pregnancy

Teratogenic Effects

Pregnancy Category X (see **CONTRAINDICATIONS** section).

When administered on day 6 of pregnancy at test dosages of 0.00024, 0.0024, and 0.024 mg/kg (1/300 to 1/3 of the human dose) to rabbits, LUPRON DEPOT produced a dose-related increase in major fetal abnormalities. Similar studies in rats failed to demonstrate an increase in fetal malformations. There was increased fetal mortality and decreased fetal weights with the two higher doses of LUPRON DEPOT in rabbits and with the highest dose (0.024 mg/kg) in rats.

Nursing Mothers

It is not known whether LUPRON DEPOT is excreted in human milk. Because many drugs are excreted in human milk, and because the effects of LUPRON DEPOT on lactation and/or the breast-fed child have not been determined, LUPRON DEPOT should not be used by nursing mothers.

Pediatric Use

Experience with LUPRON DEPOT 3.75 mg for treatment of endometriosis has been limited to women 18 years of age and older. See LUPRON DEPOT-PED® (leuprolide acetate for depot suspension) labeling for the safety and effectiveness in children with central precocious puberty.

Geriatric Use

This product has not been studied in women over 65 years of age and is not indicated in this population.

ADVERSE REACTIONS

Clinical Trials

Estradiol levels may increase during the first weeks following the initial injection of LUPRON, but then decline to menopausal levels. This transient increase in estradiol can be associated with a temporary worsening of signs and symptoms (see **WARNINGS** section).

As would be expected with a drug that lowers serum estradiol levels, the most frequently reported adverse reactions were those related to hypoestrogenism.

Table 2 ADVERSE EVENTS REPORTED TO BE CAUSALLY RELATED TO DRUG IN ≥ 5% OF PATIENTS

	Endometriosis (2 Studies)						Uterine Fibroids (4 Studies)			
	LUPRON DEPOT 3.75 mg N=166		Danazol N=136		Placebo N=31		LUPRON DEPOT 3.75 mg N=166		Placebo N=163	
	N	(%)	N	(%)	N	(%)	N	(%)	N	(%)
Body as a Whole										
Asthenia	5	(3)	9	(7)	0	(0)	14	(8.4)	8	(4.9)
General pain	31	(19)	22	(16)	1	(3)	14	(8.4)	10	(6.1)
Headache*	53	(32)	30	(22)	2	(6)	43	(25.9)	29	(17.8)
Cardiovascular System										
Hot flashes/sweats*	139	(84)	77	(57)	9	(29)	121	(72.9)	29	(17.8)
Gastrointestinal System										
Nausea/vomiting	21	(13)	17	(13)	1	(3)	8	(4.8)	6	(3.7)
GI disturbances*	11	(7)	8	(6)	1	(3)	5	(3.0)	2	(1.2)
Metabolic and Nutritional Disorders										
Edema	12	(7)	17	(13)	1	(3)	9	(5.4)	2	(1.2)
Weight gain/loss	22	(13)	36	(26)	0	(0)	5	(3.0)	2	(1.2)
Endocrine System										
Acne	17	(10)	27	(20)	0	(0)	0	(0)	0	(0)
Hirsutism	2	(1)	9	(7)	1	(3)	1	(0.6)	0	(0)
Musculoskeletal System										
Joint disorder*	14	(8)	11	(8)	0	(0)	13	(7.8)	5	(3.1)
Myalgia*	1	(1)	7	(5)	0	(0)	1	(0.6)	0	(0)
Nervous System										
Decreased libido*	19	(11)	6	(4)	0	(0)	3	(1.8)	0	(0)
Depression/emotional lability*	36	(22)	27	(20)	1	(3)	18	(10.8)	7	(4.3)
Dizziness	19	(11)	4	(3)	0	(0)	3	(1.8)	6	(3.7)
Nervousness*	8	(5)	11	(8)	0	(0)	8	(4.8)	1	(0.6)
Neuromuscular disorders*	11	(7)	17	(13)	0	(0)	3	(1.8)	0	(0)
Paresthesias	12	(7)	11	(8)	0	(0)	2	(1.2)	1	(0.6)
Skin and Appendages										
Skin reactions	17	(10)	20	(15)	1	(3)	5	(3.0)	2	(1.2)
Urogenital System										
Breast changes/tenderness/pain*	10	(6)	12	(9)	0	(0)	3	(1.8)	7	(4.3)
Vaginitis*	46	(28)	23	(17)	0	(0)	19	(11.4)	3	(1.8)

The **monthly formulation of LUPRON DEPOT 3.75 mg** was utilized in controlled clinical trials that studied the drug in 166 endometriosis and 166 uterine fibroids patients. Adverse events reported in ≥5% of patients in either of these populations and thought to be potentially related to drug are noted in the following table.

[See table above]

In these same studies, symptoms reported in <5% of patients included: *Body as a Whole* - Body odor, Flu syndrome, Injection site reactions; *Cardiovascular System* - Palpitations, Syncope, Tachycardia; *Digestive System* - Appetite changes, Dry mouth, Thirst; *Endocrine System* - Androgen-like effects; *Hemic and Lymphatic System* - Ecchymosis, Lymphadenopathy; *Nervous System* – Anxiety*, Insomnia/Sleep disorders*, Delusions, Memory disorder, Personality disorder; *Respiratory System* - Rhinitis; *Skin and Appendages* - Alopecia, Hair disorder, Nail disorder; *Special Senses* - Conjunctivitis, Ophthalmologic disorders*, Taste perversion; *Urogenital System* - Dysuria*, Lactation, Menstrual disorders.

* = Possible effect of decreased estrogen.

In one controlled clinical trial utilizing the monthly formulation of LUPRON DEPOT, patients diagnosed with uterine fibroids received a higher dose (7.5 mg) of LUPRON DEPOT. Events seen with this dose that were thought to be potentially related to drug and were not seen at the lower dose included glossitis, hypesthesia, lactation, pyelonephritis, and urinary disorders. Generally, a higher incidence of hypoestrogenic effects was observed at the higher dose.

Table 3 lists the potentially drug-related adverse events observed in at least 5% of patients in any treatment group during the first 6 months of treatment in the add-back clinical studies.

In the controlled clinical trial, 50 of 51 (98%) patients in the LD group and 48 of 55 (87%) patients in the LD/N group reported experiencing hot flashes on one or more occasions during treatment. During Month 6 of treatment, 32 of 37 (86%) patients in the LD group and 22 of 38 (58%) patients in the LD/N group reported having experienced hot flashes. The mean number of days on which hot flashes were reported during this month of treatment was 19 and 7 in the LD and LD/N treatment groups, respectively. The mean maximum number of hot flashes in a day during this month of treatment was 5.8 and 1.9 in the LD and LD/N treatment groups, respectively.

Information on the Abbott Pharmaceutical Products listed on these pages is from the prescribing information in use as of June 1, 2010. For more information, please visit rxabbott.com or call 1-800-633-9110.

[See table 3 at right]

Changes in Bone Density

In controlled clinical studies, patients with endometriosis (six months of therapy) or uterine fibroids (three months of therapy) were treated with LUPRON DEPOT 3.75 mg. In endometriosis patients, vertebral bone density as measured by dual energy x-ray absorptiometry (DEXA) decreased by an average of 3.2% at six months compared with the pre-treatment value. Clinical studies demonstrate that concurrent hormonal therapy (norethindrone acetate 5 mg daily) and calcium supplementation is effective in significantly reducing the loss of bone mineral density that occurs with LUPRON treatment, without compromising the efficacy of LUPRON in relieving symptoms of endometriosis.

LUPRON DEPOT 3.75 mg plus norethindrone acetate 5 mg daily was evaluated in two clinical trials. The results from this regimen were similar in both studies. LUPRON DEPOT 3.75 mg was used as a control group in one study. The bone mineral density data of the lumbar spine from these two studies are presented in Table 4.

[See table 4 at right]

When LUPRON DEPOT 3.75 mg was administered for three months in uterine fibroid patients, vertebral trabecular bone mineral density as assessed by quantitative digital radiography (QDR) revealed a mean decrease of 2.7% compared with baseline. Six months after discontinuation of therapy, a trend toward recovery was observed. Use of LUPRON DEPOT for longer than three months (uterine fibroids) or six months (endometriosis) or in the presence of other known risk factors for decreased bone mineral content may cause additional bone loss **and is not recommended**.

Changes in Laboratory Values During Treatment

Plasma Enzymes

Endometriosis

During early clinical trials with LUPRON DEPOT 3.75 mg, regular laboratory monitoring revealed that AST levels were more than twice the upper limit of normal in only one patient. There was no clinical or other laboratory evidence of abnormal liver function.

In two other clinical trials, 6 of 191 patients receiving LUPRON DEPOT 3.75 mg plus norethindrone acetate 5 mg daily for up to 12 months developed an elevated (at least twice the upper limit of normal) SGPT or GGT. Five of the 6 increases were observed beyond 6 months of treatment. None were associated with elevated bilirubin concentration.

Uterine Leiomyomata (Fibroids)

In clinical trials with LUPRON DEPOT 3.75 mg, five (3%) patients had a post-treatment transaminase value that was at least twice the baseline value and above the upper limit of the normal range. None of the laboratory increases were associated with clinical symptoms.

Lipids

Endometriosis

In earlier clinical studies, 4% of the LUPRON DEPOT 3.75 mg patients and 1% of the danazol patients had total cholesterol values above the normal range at enrollment. These patients also had cholesterol values above the normal range at the end of treatment.

Of those patients whose pretreatment cholesterol values were in the normal range, 7% of the LUPRON DEPOT 3.75 mg patients and 9% of the danazol patients had post-treatment values above the normal range.

The mean (±SEM) pretreatment values for total cholesterol from all patients were 178.8 (2.9) mg/dL in the LUPRON DEPOT 3.75 mg groups and 175.3 (3.0) mg/dL in the danazol group. At the end of treatment, the mean values for total cholesterol from all patients were 193.2 mg/dL in the LUPRON DEPOT 3.75 mg group and 194.4 mg/dL in the danazol group. These increases from the pre-treatment values were statistically significant (p<0.03) in both groups. Triglycerides were increased above the upper limit of normal in 12% of the patients who received LUPRON DEPOT 3.75 mg and in 6% of the patients who received danazol.

At the end of treatment, HDL cholesterol fractions decreased below the lower limit of the normal range in 2% of the LUPRON DEPOT 3.75 mg patients compared with 54% of those receiving danazol. LDL cholesterol fractions increased above the upper limit of the normal range in 6% of the patients receiving LUPRON DEPOT 3.75 mg compared with 23% of those receiving danazol. There was no increase in the LDL/HDL ratio in patients receiving LUPRON DEPOT 3.75 mg but there was approximately a two-fold increase in the LDL/HDL ratio in patients receiving danazol.

In two other clinical trials, LUPRON DEPOT 3.75 mg plus norethindrone acetate 5 mg daily was evaluated for 12 months of treatment. LUPRON DEPOT 3.75 mg was used as a control group in one study. Percent changes from baseline for serum lipids and percentages of patients with serum lipid values outside of the normal range in the two studies are summarized in the tables below.

[See table 5 at top of next page]

Changes from baseline tended to be greater at Week 52. After treatment, mean serum lipid levels from patients with follow up data returned to pretreatment values.

[See table 6 at top of next page]

Low HDL-cholesterol (<40 mg/dL) and elevated LDL-cholesterol (>160 mg/dL) are recognized risk factors for cardiovascular disease. The long-term significance of the observed treatment-related changes in serum lipids in women with endometriosis is unknown. Therefore

Table 3 TREATMENT-RELATED ADVERSE EVENTS OCCURRING IN ≥ 5% OF PATIENTS

| | Controlled Study | | | | Open Label Study | |
| | LD - Only[1] N=51 | | LD/N[2] N=55 | | LD/N[2] N=136 | |
Adverse Events	N	(%)	N	(%)	N	(%)
Any Adverse Event	50	(98)	53	(96)	126	(93)
Body as a Whole						
Asthenia	9	(18)	10	(18)	15	(11)
Headache/Migraine	33	(65)	28	(51)	63	(46)
Injection Site Reaction	1	(2)	5	(9)	4	(3)
Pain	12	(24)	16	(29)	29	(21)
Cardiovascular System						
Hot flashes/sweats	50	(98)	48	(87)	78	(57)
Digestive System						
Altered Bowel Function	7	(14)	8	(15)	14	(10)
Changes in Appetite	2	(4)	0	(0)	8	(6)
GI Disturbance	2	(4)	4	(7)	6	(4)
Nausea/Vomiting	13	(25)	16	(29)	17	(13)
Metabolic and Nutritional Disorders						
Edema	0	(0)	5	(9)	9	(7)
Weight Changes	6	(12)	7	(13)	6	(4)
Nervous System						
Anxiety	3	(6)	0	(0)	11	(8)
Depression/Emotional Lability	16	(31)	15	(27)	46	(34)
Dizziness/Vertigo	8	(16)	6	(11)	10	(7)
Insomnia/Sleep Disorder	16	(31)	7	(13)	20	(15)
Libido Changes	5	(10)	2	(4)	10	(7)
Memory Disorder	3	(6)	1	(2)	6	(4)
Nervousness	4	(8)	2	(4)	15	(11)
Neuromuscular Disorder	1	(2)	5	(9)	4	(3)
Skin and Appendages						
Alopecia	0	(0)	5	(9)	4	(3)
Androgen-Like Effects	2	(4)	3	(5)	24	(18)
Skin/Mucous Membrane Reaction	2	(4)	5	(9)	15	(11)
Urogenital System						
Breast Changes/Pain/Tenderness	3	(6)	7	(13)	11	(8)
Menstrual Disorders	1	(2)	0	(0)	7	(5)
Vaginitis	10	(20)	8	(15)	11	(8)

[1] LD-Only = LUPRON DEPOT 3.75 mg
[2] LD/N = LUPRON DEPOT 3.75 mg plus norethindrone acetate 5 mg

Table 4 MEAN PERCENT CHANGE FROM BASELINE IN BONE MINERAL DENSITY OF LUMBAR SPINE

| | LUPRON DEPOT 3.75 mg | | LUPRON DEPOT 3.75 mg plus norethindrone acetate 5 mg daily | | | |
| | Controlled Study | | Controlled Study | | Open Label Study | |
	N	Change	N	Change	N	Change
Week 24[1]	41	-3.2%	42	-0.3%	115	-0.2%
Week 52[2]	29	-6.3%	32	-1.0%	84	-1.1%

[1] Includes on-treatment measurements that fell within 2-252 days after the first day of treatment.
[2] Includes on-treatment measurements >252 days after the first day of treatment.

assessment of cardiovascular risk factors should be considered prior to initiation of concurrent treatment with LUPRON and norethindrone acetate.

Uterine Leiomyomata (Fibroids)

In patients receiving LUPRON DEPOT 3.75 mg, mean changes in cholesterol (+11 mg/dL to +29 mg/dL), LDL cholesterol (+8 mg/dL to +22 mg/dL), HDL cholesterol (0 to +6 mg/dL), and the LDL/HDL ratio (-0.1 to +0.5) were observed across studies. In the one study in which triglycerides were determined, the mean increase from baseline was 32 mg/dL.

Other Changes

Endometriosis

The following changes were seen in approximately 5% to 8% of patients. In the earlier comparative studies, LUPRON DEPOT 3.75 mg was associated with elevations of LDH and phosphorus, and decreases in WBC counts. Danazol therapy was associated with increases in hematocrit, platelet count, and LDH. In the hormonal add-back studies LUPRON DEPOT in combination with norethindrone acetate was associated with elevations of GGT and SGPT.

Uterine Leiomyomata (Fibroids)

Hematology: (see CLINICAL STUDIES section) In LUPRON DEPOT 3.75 mg treated patients, although there were statistically significant mean decreases in platelet counts from baseline to final visit, the last mean platelet counts were within the normal range. Decreases in total WBC count and neutrophils were observed, but were not clinically significant.

Chemistry: Slight to moderate mean increases were noted for glucose, uric acid, BUN, creatinine, total protein, albumin, bilirubin, alkaline phosphatase, LDH, calcium, and phosphorus. None of these increases were clinically significant.

Postmarketing

During postmarketing surveillance, the following adverse events were reported. Like other drugs in this class, mood swings, including depression, have been reported. There have been rare reports of suicidal ideation and attempt. Many, but not all, of these patients had a history of depression or other psychiatric illness. Patients should be counseled on the possibility of development or worsening of depression during treatment with LUPRON.

Symptoms consistent with an anaphylactoid or asthmatic process have been rarely reported. Rash, urticaria, and photosensitivity reactions have also been reported.

Localized reactions including induration and abscess have been reported at the site of injection. Symptoms consistent with fibromyalgia (eg: joint and muscle pain, headaches, sleep disorder, gastrointestinal distress, and shortness of breath) have been reported individually and collectively. Other events reported are:

Cardiovascular System – Hypotension, Pulmonary embolism; *Hemic and Lymphatic System* - Decreased WBC; *Central/Peripheral Nervous System* - Convulsion, Peripheral neuropathy, Spinal fracture/paralysis; *Musculoskeletal System* - Tenosynovitis-like symptoms; *Urogenital System* - Prostate pain.

Pituitary apoplexy

During post-marketing surveillance, rare cases of pituitary apoplexy (a clinical syndrome secondary to infarction of the pituitary gland) have been reported after the administration of gonadotropin-releasing hormone agonists. In a majority of these cases, a pituitary adenoma was diagnosed,

Table 5 SERUM LIPIDS: MEAN PERCENT CHANGES FROM BASELINE VALUES AT TREATMENT WEEK 24

| | LUPRON | | LUPRON plus norethindrone acetate 5 mg daily | | | |
| | Controlled Study (n=39) | | Controlled Study (n=41) | | Open Label Study (n=117) | |
	Baseline Value*	Wk 24 % Change	Baseline Value*	Wk 24 % Change	Baseline Value*	Wk 24 % Change
Total Cholesterol	170.5	9.2%	179.3	0.2%	181.2	2.8%
HDL Cholesterol	52.4	7.4%	51.8	-18.8%	51.0	-14.6%
LDL Cholesterol	96.6	10.9%	101.5	14.1%	109.1	13.1%
LDL/HDL Ratio	2.0**	5.0%	2.1**	43.4%	2.3**	39.4%
Triglycerides	107.8	17.5%	130.2	9.5%	105.4	13.8%

* mg/dL
** ratio

Table 6 PERCENTAGE OF PATIENTS WITH SERUM LIPID VALUES OUTSIDE OF THE NORMAL RANGE

| | LUPRON | | LUPRON plus norethindrone acetate 5 mg daily | | | |
| | Controlled Study (n=39) | | Controlled Study (n=41) | | Open Label Study (n=117) | |
	Wk 0	Wk 24*	Wk 0	Wk 24*	Wk 0	Wk 24*
Total Cholesterol (>240 mg/dL)	15%	23%	15%	20%	6%	7%
HDL Cholesterol (<40 mg/dL)	15%	10%	15%	44%	15%	41%
LDL Cholesterol (>160 mg/dL)	0%	8%	5%	7%	9%	11%
LDL/HDL Ratio (>4.0)	0%	3%	2%	15%	7%	21%
Triglycerides (>200 mg/dL)	13%	13%	12%	10%	5%	9%

* Includes all patients regardless of baseline value.

with a majority of pituitary apoplexy cases occurring within 2 weeks of the first dose, and some within the first hour. In these cases, pituitary apoplexy has presented as sudden headache, vomiting, visual changes, ophthalmoplegia, altered mental status, and sometimes cardiovascular collapse. Immediate medical attention has been required.

See other LUPRON DEPOT and LUPRON Injection package inserts for other events reported in different patient populations.

OVERDOSAGE

In rats subcutaneous administration of 250 to 500 times the recommended human dose, expressed on a per body weight basis, resulted in dyspnea, decreased activity, and local irritation at the injection site. There is no evidence that there is a clinical counterpart of this phenomenon. In early clinical trials using daily subcutaneous leuprolide acetate in patients with prostate cancer, doses as high as 20 mg/day for up to two years caused no adverse effects differing from those observed with the 1 mg/day dose.

DOSAGE AND ADMINISTRATION

LUPRON DEPOT Must Be Administered Under The Supervision Of A Physician.
Endometriosis
The recommended duration of treatment with LUPRON DEPOT 3.75 mg alone or in combination with norethindrone acetate is six months. The choice of LUPRON DEPOT alone or LUPRON DEPOT plus norethindrone acetate therapy for initial management of the symptoms and signs of endometriosis should be made by the health care professional in consultation with the patient and should take into consideration the risks and benefits of the addition of norethindrone to LUPRON DEPOT alone.

If the symptoms of endometriosis recur after a course of therapy, retreatment with a six-month course of LUPRON DEPOT monthly and norethindrone acetate 5 mg daily may be considered. Retreatment beyond this one six-month course cannot be recommended. It is recommended that bone density be assessed before retreatment begins to ensure that values are within normal limits. LUPRON DEPOT alone is not recommended for retreatment. If norethindrone acetate is contraindicated for the individual patient, then retreatment is not recommended.

An assessment of cardiovascular risk and management of risk factors such as cigarette smoking is recommended before beginning treatment with LUPRON DEPOT and norethindrone acetate.
Uterine Leiomyomata (Fibroids)
*Recommended duration of therapy with LUPRON DEPOT 3.75 mg is **up to** 3 months.* The symptoms associated with uterine leiomyomata will recur following discontinuation of therapy. If additional treatment with LUPHON DEPOT 3.75 mg is contemplated, bone density should be assessed prior to initiation of therapy to ensure that values are within normal limits. The recommended dose of LUPRON DEPOT is 3.75 mg, incorporated in a depot formulation. The lyophilized microspheres are to be reconstituted and administered monthly

as a single intramuscular injection. *For optimal performance of the prefilled dual chamber syringe (PDS), read and follow the following instructions:*

1. The LUPRON DEPOT powder should be visually inspected and the syringe should NOT BE USED if clumping or caking is evident. A thin layer of powder on the wall of the syringe is considered normal. The diluent should appear clear.
2. To prepare for injection, screw the white plunger into the end stopper until the stopper begins to turn.
3. Hold the syringe UPRIGHT. Release the diluent by SLOWLY PUSHING (6 to 8 seconds) the plunger until the first stopper is at the blue line in the middle of the barrel.
4. Keep the syringe UPRIGHT. Gently mix the microspheres (powder) thoroughly to form a uniform suspension. The suspension will appear milky. If the powder adheres to the stopper or caking/clumping is present, tap the syringe with your finger to disperse. DO NOT USE if any of the powder has not gone into suspension.
5. Hold the syringe UPRIGHT. With the opposite hand pull the needle cap upward without twisting.
6. Keep the syringe UPRIGHT. Advance the plunger to expel the air from the syringe.
7. Inject the entire contents of the syringe intramuscularly at the time of reconstitution. The suspension settles very quickly following reconstitution; therefore, LUPRON DEPOT should be mixed and used immediately.
   NOTE: Aspirated blood would be visible just below the luer lock connection if a blood vessel is accidentally penetrated. If present, blood can be seen through the transparent LuproLoc™ safety device.
   AFTER INJECTION
8. Withdraw the needle. Immediately activate the LuproLoc™ safety device by pushing the arrow forward with the thumb or finger until the device is fully extended and a CLICK is heard or felt.

Since the product does not contain a preservative, the suspension should be discarded if not used immediately.

As with other drugs administered by injection, the injection site should be varied periodically.

HOW SUPPLIED

Each LUPRON DEPOT 3.75 mg kit (NDC 0074-3641-03) contains:
• one prefilled dual-chamber syringe
• one plunger
• two alcohol swabs
• instructions for how to mix and administer
• an information pamphlet for patients
• a complete prescribing information enclosure

Each syringe contains sterile lyophilized microspheres, which is leuprolide incorporated in a biodegradable copoly-

mer of lactic and glycolic acids. When mixed with diluent, LUPRON DEPOT 3.75 mg is administered as a single monthly IM injection.

Store at 25°C (77°F); excursions permitted to 15-30°C (59-86°F) [See USP Controlled Room Temperature]

U.S. Patent Nos. 4,652,441; 4,677,191; 4,728,721; 4,849,228; 4,917,893; 5,330,767; 5,476,663; 5,575,987; 5,631,020; 5,631,021; 5,716,640; 5,823,997; 5,980,488; and 6,036,976. Other patents pending.

Manufactured for
Abbott Laboratories
North Chicago, IL 60064
by Takeda Pharmaceutical Company Limited
Osaka, Japan 540-8645
™ - Trademark
® - Registered Trademark
(No. 3641)
03-A142 Revised: October, 2008
©2008, Abbott Laboratories

LUPRON DEPOT® 7.5 mg ℞
[lew-prŏn]
(leuprolide acetate for depot suspension)
Rx only

DESCRIPTION

Leuprolide acetate is a synthetic nonapeptide analog of naturally occurring gonadotropin-releasing hormone (GnRH or LH-RH). The analog possesses greater potency than the natural hormone. The chemical name is 5-oxo-L-prolyl-L-histidyl-L-tryptophyl-L-seryl-L-tyrosyl-D-leucyl-L-leucyl-L-arginyl-N-ethyl-L-prolinamide acetate (salt) with the following structural formula:
[See figure at top of next page]

LUPRON DEPOT is available in a prefilled dual-chamber syringe containing sterile lyophilized microspheres which, when mixed with diluent, becomes a suspension intended as a monthly intramuscular injection.

The front chamber of LUPRON DEPOT 7.5 mg prefilled dual-chamber syringe contains leuprolide acetate (7.5 mg), purified gelatin (1.3 mg), DL-lactic and glycolic acids copolymer (66.2 mg), and D-mannitol (13.2 mg). The second chamber of diluent contains carboxymethylcellulose sodium (5 mg), D-mannitol (50 mg), polysorbate 80 (1 mg), water for injection, USP, and glacial acetic acid, USP to control pH. During the manufacture of LUPRON DEPOT 7.5 mg, acetic acid is lost, leaving the peptide.

CLINICAL PHARMACOLOGY

Leuprolide acetate, an LH-RH agonist, acts as a potent inhibitor of gonadotropin secretion when given continuously and in therapeutic doses. Animal and human studies indicate that following an initial stimulation, chronic administration of leuprolide acetate results in suppression of ovarian and testicular steroidogenesis. This effect is reversible upon discontinuation of drug therapy. Administration of leuprolide acetate has resulted in inhibition of the growth of certain hormone dependent tumors (prostatic tumors in Noble and Dunning male rats and DMBA-induced mammary tumors in female rats) as well as atrophy of the reproductive organs.

In humans, administration of leuprolide acetate results in an initial increase in circulating levels of luteinizing hormone (LH) and follicle stimulating hormone (FSH), leading to a transient increase in levels of the gonadal steroids (testosterone and dihydrotestosterone in males, and estrone and estradiol in premenopausal females). However, continuous administration of leuprolide acetate results in decreased levels of LH and FSH. In males, testosterone is reduced to castrate levels. In premenopausal females, estrogens are reduced to postmenopausal levels. These decreases occur within two to four weeks after initiation of treatment. Castrate levels of testosterone in prostatic cancer patients have been demonstrated for up to 10 years. Leuprolide acetate is not active when given orally.
Pharmacokinetics
Absorption
Following a single injection of LUPRON DEPOT 7.5 mg to patients, mean plasma leuprolide concentration was almost 20 ng/mL at 4 hours and 0.36 ng/mL at 4 weeks. However, intact leuprolide and an inactive major metabolite could not be distinguished by the assay which was employed in the study. Nondetectable leuprolide plasma concentrations have been observed during chronic LUPRON DEPOT 7.5 mg administration, but testosterone levels appear to be maintained at castrate levels.

Information on the Abbott Pharmaceutical Products listed on these pages is from the prescribing information in use as of June 1, 2010. For more information, please visit rxabbott.com or call 1-800-633-9110.

Distribution
The mean steady-state volume of distribution of leuprolide following intravenous bolus administration to healthy male volunteers was 27 L. *In vitro* binding to human plasma proteins ranged from 43% to 49%.

Metabolism
In healthy male volunteers, a 1 mg bolus of leuprolide administered intravenously revealed that the mean systemic clearance was 7.6 L/h, with a terminal elimination half-life of approximately 3 hours based on a two compartment model.

In rats and dogs, administration of ^{14}C-labeled leuprolide was shown to be metabolized to smaller inactive peptides, a pentapeptide (Metabolite I), tripeptides (Metabolites II and III) and a dipeptide (Metabolite IV). These fragments may be further catabolized.

The major metabolite (M-I) plasma concentrations measured in 5 prostate cancer patients reached maximum concentration 2 to 6 hours after dosing and were approximately 6% of the peak parent drug concentration. One week after dosing, mean plasma M-I concentrations were approximately 20% of mean leuprolide concentrations.

Excretion
Following administration of LUPRON DEPOT 3.75 mg to 3 patients, less than 5% of the dose was recovered as parent and M-I metabolite in the urine.

Special Populations
The pharmacokinetics of the drug in hepatically and renally impaired patients have not been determined.

Drug Interactions
No pharmacokinetic-based drug-drug interaction studies have been conducted with LUPRON DEPOT. However, because leuprolide acetate is a peptide that is primarily degraded by peptidase and the drug is only about 46% bound to plasma proteins, drug interactions would not be expected to occur.

CLINICAL STUDIES

In an open-label, non-comparative, multicenter clinical study of LUPRON DEPOT 7.5 mg, 56 patients with stage D$_2$ prostatic adenocarcinoma and no prior systemic treatment were enrolled. The objectives were to determine if a 7.5 mg depot formulation of leuprolide injected once every 4 weeks would reduce and maintain serum testosterone to castrate range (≤50 ng/dL), to evaluate objective clinical response, and to assess the safety of the formulation. During the initial 24 weeks, serum testosterone was measured weekly, biweekly, or every four weeks and objective tumor response assessments were performed at Weeks 12 and 24. Once the patient completed the initial 24-week treatment phase, treatment continued at the investigator's discretion. Data from the initial 24-week treatment phase are summarized in this section.

In the majority of patients, serum testosterone increased by 50% or more above baseline during the first week of treatment. Serum testosterone suppressed to the castrate range within 30 days of the initial depot injection in 94% (51/54) of patients for whom testosterone suppression was achieved (2 patients withdrew prior to onset of suppression) and within 66 days in all 54 patients. Mean serum testosterone suppressed to castrate level by Week 3. The median dosing interval between injections was 28 days. One escape from suppression (2 consecutive testosterone values greater than 50 ng/dL after achieving castrate level) was noted at Week 18, associated with a substantial dosing delay. In this patient, serum testosterone returned to the castrate range at the next monthly measurement. Serum testosterone was minimally above the castrate range on a single occasion for 4 other patients. No clinical significance was attributed to these rises in testosterone.

**Lupron Depot 7.5 mg
Mean Serum Testosterone Concentrations**

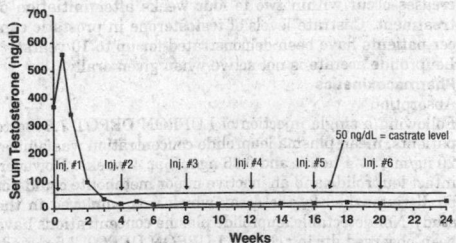

Secondary efficacy endpoints evaluated included objective tumor response, assessed by clinical evaluations of tumor burden (complete response, partial response, objectively stable, and progression), as well as changes in local disease status, assessed by digital rectal examination, and changes in prostatic acid phosphatase (PAP). These evaluations were performed at Weeks 12 and 24. The objective tumor response analysis showed a "no progression" (ie. complete or partial response, or stable disease) in 77% (40/52) of patients at Week 12, and in 84% (42/50) of patients at Week 24. Local disease improved or remained stable in all (42) patients evaluated at Week 12 and in 98% (41/42) of patients elevated at Week 24. PAP normalized or decreased at Week 12 and/or 24 in the majority of patients with elevated baseline PAP.

Periodic monitoring of serum testosterone and PSA levels is recommended, especially if the anticipated clinical or biochemical response to treatment has not been achieved. It should be noted that results of testosterone determinations are dependent on assay methodology. It is advisable to be aware of the type and precision of the assay methodology to make appropriate clinical and therapeutic decisions.

INDICATIONS AND USAGE

LUPRON DEPOT 7.5 mg is indicated in the palliative treatment of advanced prostatic cancer.

CONTRAINDICATIONS

1. Hypersensitivity to GnRH, GnRH agonist analogs or any of the excipients in LUPRON DEPOT. Reports of anaphylactic reactions to GnRH agonist analogs have been reported in the medical literature.[1,2]
2. All formulations of LUPRON DEPOT are contraindicated in women who are or may become pregnant while receiving the drug. LUPRON DEPOT may cause fetal harm when administered to a pregnant woman. Major fetal abnormalities were observed in rabbits but not in rats after administration of LUPRON DEPOT throughout gestation. There was increased fetal mortality and decreased fetal weights in rats and rabbits. The effects on fetal mortality are expected consequences of the alterations in hormonal levels brought about by this drug. Therefore, the possibility exists that spontaneous abortion may occur. If this drug is administered during pregnancy or if the patient becomes pregnant while taking any formulation of LUPRON DEPOT, the patient should be apprised of the potential hazard to the fetus.

WARNINGS

Initially, LUPRON DEPOT, like other LH-RH agonists, causes increases in serum levels of testosterone to approximately 50% above baseline during the first week of treatment. Transient worsening of symptoms, or the occurrence of additional signs and symptoms of prostate cancer, may occasionally develop during the first few weeks of LUPRON DEPOT treatment. A small number of patients may experience a temporary increase in bone pain, which can be managed symptomatically. As with other LH-RH agonists, isolated cases of ureteral obstruction and spinal cord compression have been observed, which may contribute to paralysis with or without fatal complications.

For patients at risk, initiation of therapy with daily LUPRON® (leuprolide acetate) Injection (see **DOSAGE AND ADMINISTRATION** section in the LUPRON Injection labeling) for the first two weeks to facilitate withdrawal of treatment may be considered. If spinal cord compression or renal impairment develops, standard treatment of these complications should be instituted.

PRECAUTIONS

Information for Patients
An information pamphlet for patients is included with the product.

General
Patients with metastatic vertebral lesions and/or with urinary tract obstruction should be closely observed during the first few weeks of therapy (see **WARNINGS** section).

Laboratory Tests
Response to LUPRON DEPOT 7.5 mg should be monitored by measuring serum levels of testosterone as well as prostate-specific antigen. In the majority of patients, testosterone levels increased above baseline during the first week, declining thereafter to baseline levels or below by the end of the second week. Castrate levels were reached within two to four weeks and once achieved were maintained for the duration of treatment in all 54 patients. Minimal and transient increases to above the castrate level occurred in eight patients (see **CLINICAL STUDIES** section).

Drug Interactions
(See **Pharmacokinetics**.)

Drug/Laboratory Test Interactions
Administration of LUPRON DEPOT in therapeutic doses results in suppression of the pituitary-gonadal system. Normal function is usually restored within three months after treatment is discontinued. Due to the suppression of pituitary-gonadal system by LUPRON DEPOT, diagnostic tests of pituitary gonadotropic and gonadal functions conducted during treatment and for up to three months after discontinuation of LUPRON DEPOT may be affected.

Carcinogenesis, Mutagenesis, Impairment of Fertility
Two-year carcinogenicity studies were conducted in rats and mice. In rats, a dose-related increase of benign pituitary hyperplasia and benign pituitary adenomas was noted at 24 months when the drug was administered subcutaneously at high daily doses (0.6 to 4 mg/kg). There was a significant but not dose-related increase of pancreatic islet-cell adenomas in females and of testicular interstitial cell adenomas in males (highest incidence in the low dose group). In mice, no leuprolide acetate-induced tumors or pituitary abnormalities were observed at a dose as high as 60 mg/kg for two years. Patients have been treated with leuprolide acetate for up to three years with doses as high as 10 mg/day and for two years with doses as high as 20 mg/day without demonstrable pituitary abnormalities.

Mutagenicity studies have been performed with leuprolide acetate using bacterial and mammalian systems. These studies provided no evidence of a mutagenic potential.

Clinical and pharmacologic studies in adults (≥ 18 years) with leuprolide acetate and similar analogs have shown reversibility of fertility suppression when the drug is discontinued after continuous administration for periods of up to 24 weeks.

Pregnancy Category X
See **CONTRAINDICATIONS** section.

Pediatric Use
See LUPRON DEPOT-PED® (leuprolide acetate for depot suspension) labeling for the safety and effectiveness of the monthly formulation in children with central precocious puberty.

Geriatric Use
In the clinical trials for LUPRON DEPOT, the majority (68%) of the subjects studied were at least 65 years of age. Therefore, the labeling reflects the pharmacokinetics, efficacy and safety of LUPRON DEPOT in this population.

ADVERSE REACTIONS

Clinical Trials
In the majority of patients, testosterone levels increased above baseline during the first week, declining thereafter to baseline levels or below by the end of the second week of treatment.

Potential exacerbations of signs and symptoms during the first few weeks of treatment is a concern in patients with vertebral metastases and/or urinary obstruction or hematuria which, if aggravated, may lead to neurological problems such as temporary weakness and/or paresthesia of the lower limbs or worsening of urinary symptoms (see **WARNINGS** section).

In a clinical trial of LUPRON DEPOT 7.5 mg, the following adverse reactions were reported in 5% or more of the patients during the initial 24-week treatment period regardless of causality.

LUPRON DEPOT 7.5 mg (N=56)		
	N	(%)
Body as a Whole		
General pain	13	(23.2)
Infection	3	(5.4)
Cardiovascular System		
Hot flashes/sweats*	32	(57.1)
Digestive System		
GI disorders	8	(14.3)
Metabolic and Nutritional Disorders		
Edema	8	(14.3)
Nervous System		
Libido decreased*	3	(5.4)

Respiratory System		
Respiratory disorder	6	(10.7)
Urogenital System		
Urinary disorder	7	(12.5)
Impotence*	3	(5.4)
Testicular atrophy*	3	(5.4)

*Due to the expected physiologic effect of decreased testosterone levels.

In this same study, the following adverse reactions were reported in less than 5% of the patients on LUPRON DEPOT 7.5 mg.
Body as a Whole - Asthenia, Cellulitis, Fever, Headache, Injection site reaction, Neoplasm; *Cardiovascular System* - Angina, Congestive heart failure; *Digestive System* - Anorexia, Dysphagia, Eructation, Peptic ulcer; *Hemic and Lymphatic System* - Ecchymosis; *Musculoskeletal System* - Myalgia; *Nervous System* - Agitation, Insomnia/sleep disorders, Neuromuscular disorders; *Respiratory System* - Emphysema, Hemoptysis, Lung edema, Sputum increased; *Skin and Appendages* - Hair disorder, Skin reaction; *Urogenital System* - Balanitis, Breast enlargement, Urinary tract infection.
Laboratory: Abnormalities of certain parameters were observed, but their relationship to drug treatment are difficult to assess in this population. The following were recorded in ≥5% of patients at final visit: Decreased albumin, decreased hemoglobin/hematocrit, decreased prostatic acid phosphatase, decreased total protein, decreased urine specific gravity, hyperglycemia, hyperuricemia, increased BUN, increased creatinine, increased liver function tests (AST, LDH), increased phosphorus, increased platelets, increased prostatic acid phosphatase, increased total cholesterol, increased urine specific gravity, leukopenia.
Postmarketing
During postmarketing surveillance, which includes other dosage forms and other patient populations, the following adverse events were reported.
Symptoms consistent with an anaphylactoid or asthmatic process have been rarely (incidence rate of about 0.002%) reported. Rash, urticaria, and photosensitivity reactions have also been reported.
Localized reactions including induration and abscess have been reported at the site of injection.
Symptoms consistent with fibromyalgia (eg, joint and muscle pain, headaches, sleep disorders, gastrointestinal distress, and shortness of breath) have been reported individually and collectively.
Cardiovascular System - Hypotension, Myocardial infarction, Pulmonary embolism; *Hemic and Lymphatic System* - Decreased WBC; *Central/Peripheral Nervous System* - Convulsion, Peripheral neuropathy, Spinal fracture/paralysis; *Endocrine System* – Diabetes; *Musculoskeletal System* - Tenosynovitis-like symptoms; *Urogenital System* - Prostate pain.
Changes in Bone Density: Decreased bone density has been reported in the medical literature in men who have had orchiectomy or who have been treated with an LH-RH agonist analog. In a clinical trial, 25 men with prostate cancer, 12 of whom had been treated previously with leuprolide acetate for at least six months, underwent bone density studies as a result of pain. The leuprolide-treated group had lower bone density scores than the nontreated control group. It can be anticipated that long periods of medical castration in men will have effects on bone density.
Pituitary apoplexy: During post-marketing surveillance, rare cases of pituitary apoplexy (a clinical syndrome secondary to infarction of the pituitary gland) have been reported after the administration of gonadotropin-releasing hormone agonists. In a majority of these cases, a pituitary adenoma was diagnosed, with a majority of pituitary apoplexy cases occurring within 2 weeks of the first dose, and some within the first hour. In these cases, pituitary apoplexy has presented as sudden headache, vomiting, visual changes, ophthalmoplegia, altered mental status, and sometimes cardiovascular collapse. Immediate medical attention has been required.
See other LUPRON DEPOT and LUPRON Injection package inserts for other events reported in women and pediatric populations.

OVERDOSAGE
In clinical trials using daily subcutaneous leuprolide acetate in patients with prostate cancer, doses as high as 20 mg/day for up to two years caused no adverse effects differing from those observed with the 1 mg/day dose.

DOSAGE AND ADMINISTRATION
LUPRON DEPOT Must Be Administered Under The Supervision Of A Physician.
The recommended dose of LUPRON DEPOT is 7.5 mg, incorporated in a depot formulation. The lyophilized microspheres are to be reconstituted and administered monthly

as a single intramuscular injection. *For optimal performance of the prefilled dual chamber syringe (PDS), read and follow the following instructions:*
1. The LUPRON DEPOT powder should be visually inspected and the syringe should NOT BE USED if clumping or caking is evident. A thin layer of powder on the wall of the syringe is considered normal. The diluent should appear clear.
2. To prepare for injection, screw the white plunger into the end stopper until the stopper begins to turn.
3. Hold the syringe UPRIGHT. Release the diluent by SLOWLY PUSHING (6 to 8 seconds) the plunger until the first stopper is at the blue line in the middle of the barrel.
4. Keep the syringe UPRIGHT. Gently mix the microspheres (powder) thoroughly to form a uniform suspension. The suspension will appear milky. If the powder adheres to the stopper or caking/clumping is present, tap the syringe with your finger to disperse. DO NOT USE if any of the powder has not gone into suspension.
5. Hold the syringe UPRIGHT. With the opposite hand pull the needle cap upward without twisting.
6. Keep the syringe UPRIGHT. Advance the plunger to expel the air from the syringe.
7. Inject the entire contents of the syringe intramuscularly at the time of reconstitution. The suspension settles very quickly following reconstitution; therefore, LUPRON DEPOT should be mixed and used immediately.
NOTE: Aspirated blood would be visible just below the luer lock connection if a blood vessel is accidentally penetrated. If present, blood can be seen through the transparent LuproLoc™ safety device.
AFTER INJECTION
8. Withdraw the needle. Immediately activate the LuproLoc™ safety device by pushing the arrow forward with the thumb or finger until the device is fully extended and a CLICK is heard or felt.
Since the product does not contain a preservative, the suspension should be discarded if not used immediately.
As with other drugs administered by injection, the injection site should be varied periodically.

HOW SUPPLIED
Each LUPRON DEPOT 7.5 mg kit (NDC 0074-3642-03) contains:
• one prefilled dual-chamber syringe
• one plunger
• two alcohol swabs
• instructions for how to mix and administer
• an information pamphlet for patients
• a complete prescribing information enclosure
The prefilled dual-chamber syringe contains sterile lyophilized microspheres of leuprolide acetate incorporated in a biodegradable lactic acid/glycolic acid copolymer. When mixed with 1 mL of accompanying diluent, LUPRON DEPOT 7.5 mg is administered as a single monthly intramuscular injection.
Store at 25°C (77°F); excursions permitted to 15–30°C (59–86°F) [See USP Controlled Room Temperature]

REFERENCES
1. Taylor, JD. Anaphylactic reaction to LHRH analogue, leuprorelin. *Med J Australia* 1994 Oct; 161(3): 455.
2. Letterie GS, *et al.* Recurrent anaphylaxis to a depot form of GnRH analogue. *Obstet Gynecol* 1991 Nov; 78: 943–946.
U.S. Patent Nos. 4,652,441; 4,677,191; 4,728,721; 4,849,228; 4,917,893; 5,330,767; 5,476,663; 5,575,987; 5,631,020; 5,631,021; 5,716,640; 5,823,997; 5,980,488; and 6,036,976. Other patents pending.
Manufactured for
Abbott Laboratories
North Chicago, IL 60064
By Takeda Pharmaceutical Company Limited
Osaka, JAPAN 540-8645
™—Trademark
®—Registered Trademark
(No. 3642)
Ref. 03-A143
Revised: October, 2008
©2008, Abbott Laboratories
Shown in Product Identification Guide, page 303

LUPRON DEPOT®–3 Month 11.25 mg ℞
[lew-prŏn]
(leuprolide acetate for depot suspension)
3-MONTH FORMULATION
Rx only

This is combined labeling. Examples of different fonts appear below
• General information
• Information on endometriosis
• Information on uterine fibroids

DESCRIPTION
Leuprolide acetate is a synthetic nonapeptide analog of naturally occurring gonadotropin-releasing hormone (GnRH or LH-RH). The analog possesses greater potency than the natural hormone. The chemical name is 5-oxo-L-prolyl-L-histidyl-L-tryptophyl-L-seryl-L-tyrosyl-D-leucyl-L-leucyl-L-arginyl-N-ethyl-L-prolinamide acetate (salt) with the following structural formula:
[See figure at top of next page]
LUPRON DEPOT–3 Month 11.25 mg is available in a prefilled dual-chamber syringe containing sterile lyophilized microspheres which, when mixed with diluent, become a suspension intended as an intramuscular injection to be given **ONCE EVERY THREE MONTHS**.
The front chamber of LUPRON DEPOT–3 Month 11.25 mg prefilled dual-chamber syringe contains leuprolide acetate (11.25 mg), polylactic acid (99.3 mg) and D-mannitol (19.45 mg). The second chamber of diluent contains carboxymethylcellulose sodium (7.5 mg), D-mannitol (75.0 mg), polysorbate 80 (1.5 mg), water for injection, USP, and glacial acetic acid, USP to control pH.
During the manufacture of LUPRON DEPOT–3 Month 11.25 mg, acetic acid is lost, leaving the peptide.

CLINICAL PHARMACOLOGY
Leuprolide acetate is a long-acting GnRH analog. A single injection of LUPRON DEPOT–3 Month 11.25 mg will result in an initial stimulation followed by a prolonged suppression of pituitary gonadotropins. Repeated dosing at quarterly (LUPRON DEPOT–3 Month 11.25 mg) intervals results in decreased secretion of gonadal steroids; consequently, tissues and functions that depend on gonadal steroids for their maintenance become quiescent. This effect is reversible on discontinuation of drug therapy.
Leuprolide acetate is not active when given orally.
Pharmacokinetics
Absorption
Following a single injection of the three month formulation of LUPRON DEPOT–3 Month 11.25 mg in female subjects, a mean plasma leuprolide concentration of 36.3 ng/mL was observed at 4 hours. Leuprolide appeared to be released at a constant rate following the onset of steady-state levels during the third week after dosing and mean levels then declined gradually to near the lower limit of detection by 12 weeks. The mean ($\pm$ standard deviation) leuprolide concentration from 3 to 12 weeks was 0.23 ± 0.09 ng/mL. However, intact leuprolide and an inactive major metabolite could not be distinguished by the assay which was employed in the study. The initial burst, followed by the rapid decline to a steady-state level, was similar to the release pattern seen with the monthly formulation.
Distribution
The mean steady-state volume of distribution of leuprolide following intravenous bolus administration to healthy male volunteers was 27 L. *In vitro* binding to human plasma proteins ranged from 43% to 49%.
Metabolism
In healthy male volunteers, a 1 mg bolus of leuprolide administered intravenously revealed that the mean systemic clearance was 7.6 L/h, with a terminal elimination half-life of approximately 3 hours based on a two compartment model.
In rats and dogs, administration of ^{14}C-labeled leuprolide was shown to be metabolized to smaller inactive peptides, a pentapeptide (Metabolite I), tripeptides (Metabolites II and III) and a dipeptide (Metabolite IV). These fragments may be further catabolized.
In a pharmacokinetic/pharmacodynamic study of endometriosis patients, intramuscular 11.25 mg LUPRON DEPOT (n=19) every 12 weeks or intramuscular 3.75 mg LUPRON DEPOT (n=15) every 4 weeks was administered for 24 weeks. There was no statistically significant difference in changes of serum estradiol concentration from baseline between the 2 treatment groups.
M-I plasma concentrations measured in 5 prostate cancer patients reached maximum concentration 2 to 6 hours after dosing and were approximately 6% of the peak parent drug concentration. One week after dosing, mean plasma M-I concentrations were approximately 20% of mean leuprolide concentrations.
Excretion
Following administration of LUPRON DEPOT 3.75 mg to 3 patients, less than 5% of the dose was recovered as parent and M-I metabolite in the urine.
Special Populations
The pharmacokinetics of the drug in hepatically and renally impaired patients have not been determined.

Information on the Abbott Pharmaceutical Products listed on these pages is from the prescribing information in use as of June 1, 2010. For more information, please visit rxabbott.com or call 1-800-633-9110.

Drug Interactions

No pharmacokinetic-based drug-drug interaction studies have been conducted with LUPRON DEPOT. However, because leuprolide acetate is a peptide that is primarily degraded by peptidase and not by cytochrome P-450 enzymes as noted in specific studies, and the drug is only about 46% bound to plasma proteins, drug interactions would not be expected to occur.

CLINICAL STUDIES

In a pharmacokinetic/pharmacodynamic study of healthy female subjects (N=20), the onset of estradiol suppression was observed for individual subjects between day 4 and week 4 after dosing. By the third week following the injection, the mean estradiol concentration (8 pg/mL) was in the menopausal range. Throughout the remainder of the dosing period, mean serum estradiol levels ranged from the menopausal to the early follicular range.

Serum estradiol was suppressed to ≤20 pg/mL in all subjects within four weeks and remained suppressed (≤40 pg/mL) in 80% of subjects until the end of the 12-week dosing interval, at which time two of these subjects had a value between 40 and 50 pg/mL. Four additional subjects had at least two consecutive elevations of estradiol (range 43-240 pg/mL) levels during the 12-week dosing interval, but there was no indication of luteal function for any of the subjects during this period.

LUPRON DEPOT–3 Month 11.25 mg induced amenorrhea in 85% (N=17) of subjects during the initial month and 100% during the second month following the injection. All subjects remained amenorrheic through the remainder of the 12-week dosing interval. Episodes of light bleeding and spotting were reported by a majority of subjects during the first month after the injection and in a few subjects at later time-points. Menses resumed on average 12 weeks (range 2.9 to 20.4 weeks) following the end of the 12-week dosing interval.

LUPRON DEPOT–3 Month 11.25 mg produced similar pharmacodynamic effects in terms of hormonal and menstrual suppression to those achieved with monthly injections of LUPRON DEPOT 3.75 mg during the controlled clinical trials for the management of endometriosis and the anemia caused by uterine fibroids.

Endometriosis

In a Phase IV pharmacokinetic/pharmacodynamic study of patients, LUPRON DEPOT–3 Month 11.25 mg (N=21) was shown to be comparable to monthly LUPRON DEPOT 3.75 mg (N=20) in relieving the clinical signs/symptoms of endometriosis (dysmenorrhea, nonmenstrual pelvic pain, pelvic tenderness and pelvic induration). In both treatment groups, suppression of menses was achieved in 100% of the patients who remained in the study for at least 60 days. Suppression is defined as no new menses for at least 60 consecutive days.

In controlled clinical studies, LUPRON DEPOT 3.75 mg monthly for six months was shown to be comparable to danazol 800 mg/day in relieving the clinical sign/symptoms of endometriosis (pelvic pain, dysmenorrhea, dyspareunia, pelvic tenderness, and induration) and in reducing the size of endometrial implants as evidenced by laparoscopy.

The clinical significance of a decrease in endometriotic lesions is not known at this time, and in addition laparoscopic staging of endometriosis does not necessarily correlate with the severity of symptoms.

LUPRON DEPOT 3.75 mg monthly induced amenorrhea in 74% and 98% of the patients after the first and second treatment months respectively. Most of the remaining patients reported episodes of only light bleeding or spotting. In the first, second and third post-treatment months, normal menstrual cycles resumed in 7%, 71% and 95% of patients, respectively, excluding those who became pregnant.

Figure 1 illustrates the percent of patients with symptoms at baseline, final treatment visit and sustained relief at 6 and 12 months following discontinuation of treatment for the various symptoms evaluated during the two controlled clinical studies. A total of 166 patients received LUPRON DEPOT 3.75 mg. Seventy-five percent (N=125) of these elected to participate in the follow-up period. Of these patients, 36% and 24% are included in the 6 month and 12 month follow-up analysis, respectively. All the patients who had a pain evaluation at baseline and at a minimum of one treatment visit, are included in the Baseline (B) and final treatment visit (F) analysis.

[See figure 1 at top of next column]

Hormonal add-back therapy

Two clinical studies with a treatment duration of 12 months indicate that concurrent hormonal therapy (norethindrone acetate 5 mg daily) is effective in significantly reducing the loss of bone mineral density associated with LUPRON, without compromising the efficacy of LUPRON in relieving symptoms of endometriosis. (All patients in these studies received calcium supplementation with 1000 mg elemental calcium). One controlled, randomized and double-blind study included 51 women treated with LUPRON DEPOT 3.75 mg alone and 55 women treated with LUPRON DEPOT 3.75 mg plus norethindrone acetate 5 mg (LD/N) daily. The second study was an open label study in which 136 women were treated with monthly LUPRON DEPOT 3.75 mg plus norethindrone acetate 5 mg daily. This study confirmed the reduction in loss of bone mineral density that was observed in the controlled study. Suppression of menses was maintained throughout

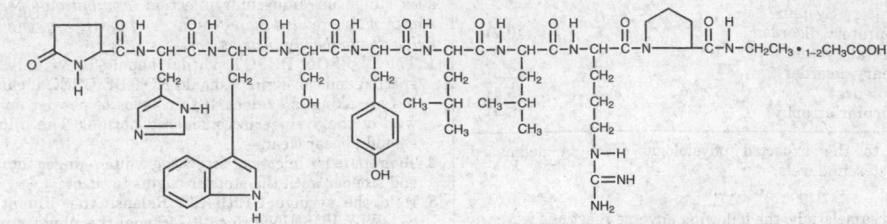

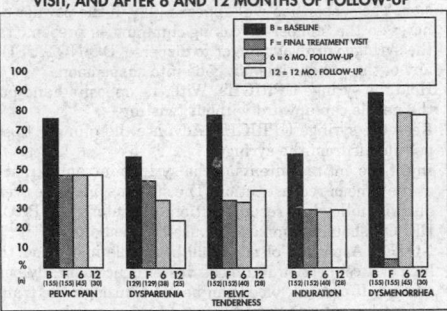

FIGURE 1 – PERCENT OF PATIENTS WITH SIGN/SYMPTOMS OF ENDOMETRIOSIS AT BASELINE, FINAL TREATMENT VISIT, AND AFTER 6 AND 12 MONTHS OF FOLLOW-UP

treatment in 84% and 73% of patients receiving LD/N, in the controlled study and open label study, respectively. The median time for menses resumption after treatment with LD/N was 8 weeks.

Figure 2 illustrates the mean pain scores for the LD/N group from the controlled study.

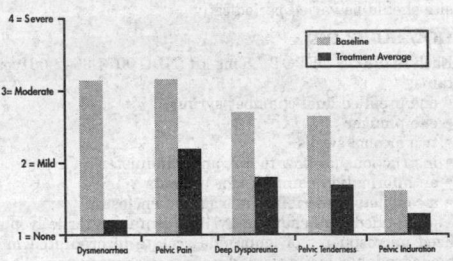

Figure 2
Treatment Period Mean Pain Scores for LD/N* Patients

* LD/N = LUPRON DEPOT 3.75 mg plus norethindrone acetate 5 mg daily

Uterine Leiomyomata (Fibroids)

LUPRON DEPOT 3.75 mg for a period of three to six months was studied in four controlled clinical trials.

In one of these clinical trials, enrollment was based on hematocrit ≤ 30% and/or hemoglobin ≤ 10.2 g/dL. Administration of LUPRON DEPOT 3.75 mg, concomitantly with iron, produced an increase of ≥ 6% hematocrit and ≥ 2 g/dL hemoglobin in 77% of patients at three months of therapy. The mean change in hematocrit was 10.1% and the mean change in hemoglobin was 4.2 g/dL. Clinical response was judged to be a hematocrit ≥ 36% and hemoglobin ≥ 12 g/dL, thus allowing for autologous blood donation prior to surgery. At two and three months respectively, 71% and 75% of patients met this criterion (Table 1). These data suggest however, that some patients may benefit from iron alone or 1 to 2 months of LUPRON DEPOT 3.75 mg.

Table 1 PERCENT OF PATIENTS ACHIEVING HEMATOCRIT ≥ 36% AND HEMOGLOBIN ≥ 12 GM/DL

Treatment Group	Week 4	Week 8	Week 12
LUPRON DEPOT 3.75 mg with Iron (N=104)	40*	71**	75*
Iron Alone (N=98)	17	39	49

* P-Value < 0.01
** P-Value < 0.001

Excessive vaginal bleeding (menorrhagia or menometrorrhagia) decreased in 80% of patients at three months. Episodes of spotting and menstrual-like bleeding were noted in 16% of patients at final visit.

In this same study, a decrease of ≥25% was seen in uterine and myoma volumes in 60% and 54% of patients respectively. The mean fibroid diameter was 6.3 cm at pretreatment and decreased to 5.6 cm at the end of treatment. LUPRON DEPOT 3.75 mg was found to relieve symptoms of bloating, pelvic pain, and pressure.

In three other controlled clinical trials, enrollment was not based on hematologic status. Mean uterine volume decreased by 41% and myoma volume decreased by 37% at final visit as evidenced by ultrasound or MRI. The mean fibroid diameter was 5.6 cm at pretreatment and decreased to 4.7 cm at the end of treatment. These patients also experienced a decrease in symptoms including excessive vaginal bleeding and pelvic discomfort. Ninety-five percent of these patients became amenorrheic with 61%, 25%, and 4% experiencing amenorrhea during the first, second, and third treatment months respectively.

In addition, posttreatment follow-up was carried out in one clinical trial for a small percentage of LUPRON DEPOT 3.75 mg patients (N=46) among the 77% who demonstrated a ≥ 25% decrease in uterine volume while on therapy. Menses usually returned within two months of cessation of therapy. Mean time to return to pretreatment uterine size was 8.3 months. Regrowth did not appear to be related to pretreatment uterine volume.

There is no evidence that pregnancy rates are enhanced or adversely affected by the use of LUPRON DEPOT.

INDICATIONS AND USAGE

Endometriosis

LUPRON DEPOT–3 Month 11.25 mg is indicated for management of endometriosis, including pain relief and reduction of endometriotic lesions. LUPRON DEPOT with norethindrone acetate 5 mg daily is also indicated for initial management of endometriosis and for management of recurrence of symptoms. (Refer also to norethindrone acetate prescribing information for WARNINGS, PRECAUTIONS, CONTRAINDICATIONS and ADVERSE REACTIONS associated with norethindrone acetate). Duration of initial treatment or retreatment should be limited to 6 months.

Uterine Leiomyomata (Fibroids)

LUPRON DEPOT–3 Month 11.25 mg concomitantly with iron therapy is indicated for the preoperative hematologic improvement of patients with anemia caused by uterine leiomyomata. The clinician may wish to consider a one-month trial period on iron alone inasmuch as some of the patients will respond to iron alone. (See Table 1, **CLINICAL STUDIES** section.) LUPRON may be added if the response to iron alone is considered inadequate. Recommended therapy is a single injection of LUPRON DEPOT–3 Month 11.25 mg. This dosage form is indicated only for women for whom three months of hormonal suppression is deemed necessary.

Experience with LUPRON DEPOT–3 Month 11.25 mg in females has been limited to women 18 years of age and older treated for no more than 6 months.

CONTRAINDICATIONS

1. Hypersensitivity to GnRH, GnRH agonist analogs or any of the excipients in LUPRON DEPOT.

2. Undiagnosed abnormal vaginal bleeding.

3. LUPRON DEPOT is contraindicated in women who are or may become pregnant while receiving the drug. LUPRON DEPOT may cause fetal harm when administered to a pregnant woman. Major fetal abnormalities were observed in rabbits but not in rats after administration of LUPRON DEPOT throughout gestation. There was increased fetal mortality and decreased fetal weights in rats and rabbits. (See **Pregnancy** section.) The effects on fetal mortality are expected consequences of the alterations in hormonal levels brought about by the drug. If this drug is used during pregnancy or if the patient becomes pregnant while taking this drug, the patient should be apprised of the potential hazard to the fetus.

4. Use in women who are breast-feeding. (See **Nursing Mothers** section.)

5. Norethindrone acetate is contraindicated in women with the following conditions:
   ○ Thrombophlebitis, thromboembolic disorders, cerebral apoplexy, or a past history of these conditions
   ○ Markedly impaired liver function or liver disease
   ○ Known or suspected carcinoma of the breast

WARNINGS

1. As the effects of LUPRON DEPOT–3 Month 11.25 mg are present throughout the course of therapy, the drug should only be used in patients who require hormonal suppression for at least three months.

2. Experience with LUPRON DEPOT–3 Month 11.25 mg in females has been limited to six months; therefore, exposure should be limited to six months of therapy.
3. Safe use of leuprolide acetate or norethindrone acetate in pregnancy has not been established clinically. Before starting treatment with LUPRON DEPOT pregnancy must be excluded.
4. When used at the recommended dose and dosing interval, LUPRON DEPOT usually inhibits ovulation and stops menstruation. Contraception is not insured, however, by taking LUPRON DEPOT. Therefore, patients should use nonhormonal methods of contraception. Patients should be advised to see their physician if they believe they may be pregnant. If a patient becomes pregnant during treatment, the drug must be discontinued and the patient must be apprised of the potential risk to the fetus. (See **CONTRAINDICATIONS** section.)
5. During the early phase of therapy, sex steroids temporarily rise above baseline because of the physiologic effect of the drug. Therefore, an increase in clinical signs and symptoms may be observed during the initial days of therapy, but these will dissipate with continued therapy.
6. Symptoms consistent with an anaphylactoid or asthmatic process have been rarely reported post-marketing.
7. The following applies to co-treatment with LUPRON and norethindrone acetate:

Norethindrone acetate treatment should be discontinued if there is a sudden partial or complete loss of vision or if there is sudden onset of proptosis, diplopia, or migraine. If examination reveals papilledema or retinal vascular lesions, medication should be withdrawn.

Because of the occasional occurrence of thrombophlebitis and pulmonary embolism in patients taking progestogens, the physician should be alert to the earliest manifestations of the disease in women taking norethindrone acetate.

Assessment and management of risk factors for cardiovascular disease is recommended prior to initiation of add-back therapy with norethindrone acetate. Norethindrone acetate should be used with caution in women with risk factors, including lipid abnormalities or cigarette smoking.

PRECAUTIONS

Information for Patients

An information pamphlet for patients is included with the product. Patients should be aware of the following information:

1. Since menstruation usually stops with effective doses of LUPRON DEPOT, the patient should notify her physician if regular menstruation persists. Patients missing successive doses of LUPRON DEPOT may experience breakthrough bleeding.
2. Patients should not use LUPRON DEPOT if they are pregnant, breast feeding, have undiagnosed abnormal vaginal bleeding, or are allergic to any of the ingredients in LUPRON DEPOT.
3. LUPRON DEPOT is contraindicated for use during pregnancy. Therefore, a non-hormonal method of contraception should be used during treatment. Patients should be advised that if they miss successive doses of LUPRON DEPOT, breakthrough bleeding or ovulation may occur with the potential for conception. If a patient becomes pregnant during treatment, she should discontinue treatment and consult her physician.
4. Adverse events occurring in clinical studies with LUPRON DEPOT that are associated with hypoestrogenism include: hot flashes, headaches, emotional lability, decreased libido, acne, myalgia, reduction in breast size, and vaginal dryness. Estrogen levels returned to normal after treatment was discontinued.
5. Patients should be counseled on the possibility of the development or worsening of depression and the occurrence of memory disorders.
6. The induced hypoestrogenic state **also** results in a loss in bone density over the course of treatment, some of which may not be reversible. For a period up to six months, this bone loss should not be clinically significant. Clinical studies show that concurrent hormonal therapy with norethindrone acetate 5 mg daily is effective in reducing loss of bone mineral density that occurs with LUPRON. (All patients received calcium supplementation with 1000 mg elemental calcium.) (See ***Changes in Bone Density*** section).
7. If the symptoms of endometriosis recur after a course of therapy, retreatment with a six-month course of LUPRON DEPOT and norethindrone acetate 5 mg daily may be considered. Retreatment beyond this one six-month course cannot be recommended. It is recommended that bone density be assessed before retreatment begins to ensure that values are within normal limits. Retreatment with LUPRON DEPOT alone is not recommended.
8. In patients with major risk factors for decreased bone mineral content such as chronic alcohol and/or tobacco use, strong family history of osteoporosis, or chronic use of drugs that can reduce bone mass such as anticonvulsants or corticosteroids, LUPRON DEPOT therapy may pose an additional risk. In these patients, the risks and benefits must be weighed carefully before therapy with LUPRON DEPOT alone is instituted, and concomitant treatment with norethindrone acetate 5 mg daily should be considered. Retreatment with gonadotropin-releasing hormone analogs, including LUPRON is not advisable in patients with major risk factors for loss of bone mineral content.
9. Because norethindrone acetate may cause some degree of fluid retention, conditions which might be influenced by this factor, such as epilepsy, migraine, asthma, cardiac or renal dysfunctions require careful observation during norethindrone acetate add-back therapy.
10. Patients who have a history of depression should be carefully observed during treatment with norethindrone acetate and norethindrone acetate should be discontinued if severe depression occurs.

Table 2 ADVERSE EVENTS REPORTED TO BE CAUSALLY RELATED TO DRUG IN ≥ 5% OF PATIENTS

	Endometriosis (2 Studies)						Uterine Fibroids (4 Studies)			
	LUPRON DEPOT 3.75 mg N=166		Danazol N=136		Placebo N=31		LUPRON DEPOT 3.75 mg N=166		Placebo N=163	
	N	(%)	N	(%)	N	(%)	N	(%)	N	(%)
Body as a Whole										
Asthenia	5	(3)	9	(7)	0	(0)	14	(8.4)	8	(4.9)
General pain	31	(19)	22	(16)	1	(3)	14	(8.4)	10	(6.1)
Headache*	53	(32)	30	(22)	2	(6)	43	(25.9)	29	(17.8)
Cardiovascular System										
Hot flashes/sweats*	139	(84)	77	(57)	9	(29)	121	(72.9)	29	(17.8)
Gastrointestinal System										
Nausea/vomiting	21	(13)	17	(13)	1	(3)	8	(4.8)	6	(3.7)
GI disturbances*	11	(7)	8	(6)	1	(3)	5	(3.0)	2	(1.2)
Metabolic and Nutritional Disorders										
Edema	12	(7)	17	(13)	1	(3)	9	(5.4)	2	(1.2)
Weight gain/loss	22	(13)	36	(26)	0	(0)	5	(3.0)	2	(1.2)
Endocrine System										
Acne	17	(10)	27	(20)	0	(0)	0	(0)	0	(0)
Hirsutism	2	(1)	9	(7)	1	(3)	1	(0.6)	0	(0)
Musculoskeletal System										
Joint disorder*	14	(8)	11	(8)	0	(0)	13	(7.8)	5	(3.1)
Myalgia*	1	(1)	7	(5)	0	(0)	1	(0.6)	0	(0)
Nervous System										
Decreased libido*	19	(11)	6	(4)	0	(0)	3	(1.8)	0	(0)
Depression/emotional lability*	36	(22)	27	(20)	1	(3)	18	(10.8)	7	(4.3)
Dizziness	19	(11)	4	(3)	0	(0)	3	(1.8)	6	(3.7)
Nervousness*	8	(5)	11	(8)	0	(0)	8	(4.8)	1	(0.6)
Neuromuscular disorders*	11	(7)	17	(13)	0	(0)	3	(1.8)	0	(0)
Paresthesias	12	(7)	11	(8)	0	(0)	2	(1.2)	1	(0.6)
Skin and Appendages										
Skin reactions	17	(10)	20	(15)	1	(3)	5	(3.0)	2	(1.2)
Urogenital System										
Breast changes/tenderness/pain*	10	(6)	12	(9)	0	(0)	3	(1.8)	7	(4.3)
Vaginitis*	46	(28)	23	(17)	0	(0)	19	(11.4)	3	(1.8)

Laboratory Tests

See **ADVERSE REACTIONS** section.

Drug Interactions

See **CLINICAL PHARMACOLOGY, Pharmacokinetics**.

Drug/Laboratory Test Interactions

Administration of LUPRON DEPOT in therapeutic doses results in suppression of the pituitary-gonadal system. Normal function is usually restored within three months after treatment is discontinued. Therefore, diagnostic tests of pituitary gonadotropic and gonadal functions conducted during treatment and for up to three months after discontinuation of LUPRON DEPOT may be misleading.

Carcinogenesis, Mutagenesis, Impairment of Fertility

A two-year carcinogenicity study was conducted in rats and mice. In rats, a dose-related increase of benign pituitary hyperplasia and benign pituitary adenomas was noted at 24 months when the drug was administered subcutaneously at high daily doses (0.6 to 4 mg/kg). There was a significant but not dose-related increase of pancreatic islet-cell adenomas in females and of testicular interstitial cell adenomas in males (highest incidence in the low dose group). In mice, no leuprolide acetate-induced tumors or pituitary abnormalities were observed at a dose as high as 60 mg/kg for two years. Patients have been treated with leuprolide acetate for up to three years with doses as high as 10 mg/day and for two years with doses as high as 20 mg/day without demonstrable pituitary abnormalities.

Mutagenicity studies have been performed with leuprolide acetate using bacterial and mammalian systems. These studies provided no evidence of a mutagenic potential.

Clinical and pharmacologic studies in adults (> 18 years) with leuprolide acetate and similar analogs have shown reversibility of fertility suppression when the drug is discontinued after continuous administration for periods of up to 24 weeks. Although no clinical studies have been completed in children to assess the full reversibility of fertility suppression, animal studies (prepubertal and adult rats and monkeys) with leuprolide acetate and other GnRH analogs have shown functional recovery.

Pregnancy

Teratogenic Effects

Pregnancy Category X (See **CONTRAINDICATIONS** section). When administered on day 6 of pregnancy at test dosages of 0.00024, 0.0024, and 0.024 mg/kg (1/300 to 1/3 of the human dose) to rabbits, LUPRON DEPOT produced a dose-related increase in major fetal abnormalities. Similar studies in rats failed to demonstrate an increase in fetal malformations. There was increased fetal mortality and decreased fetal weights with the two higher doses of LUPRON DEPOT in rabbits and with the highest dose (0.024 mg/kg) in rats.

Nursing Mothers

It is not known whether LUPRON DEPOT is excreted in human milk. Because many drugs are excreted in human milk, and because the effects of LUPRON DEPOT on lactation and/or the breast-fed child have not been determined, LUPRON DEPOT should not be used by nursing mothers.

Pediatric Use

Safety and effectiveness of LUPRON DEPOT–3 Month 11.25 mg have not been established in pediatric patients. Experience with LUPRON DEPOT for treatment of endometriosis has been limited to women 18 years of age and older. See LUPRON DEPOT-PED® (leuprolide acetate for depot suspension) labeling for the safety and effectiveness in children with central precocious puberty.

Geriatric Use

This product has not been studied in women over 65 years of age and is not indicated in this population.

ADVERSE REACTIONS

Clinical Trials

The **monthly formulation of LUPRON DEPOT 3.75 mg** was utilized in controlled clinical trials that studied the drug in 166 endometriosis and 166 uterine fibroids patients. Adverse events reported in ≥ 5% of patients in either of these populations and thought to be potentially related to drug are noted in the following table.

[See table 2 above]

In these same studies, symptoms reported in < 5% of patients included: *Body as a Whole* - Body odor, Flu syndrome,

Information on the Abbott Pharmaceutical Products listed on these pages is from the prescribing information in use as of June 1, 2010. For more information, please visit rxabbott.com or call 1-800-633-9110.

Table 3 TREATMENT-RELATED ADVERSE EVENTS OCCURRING IN ≥ 5% OF PATIENTS

	Controlled Study				Open Label Study	
	LD - Only[1] N=51		LD/N[2] N=55		LD/N[2] N=136	
Adverse Events	N	(%)	N	(%)	N	(%)
Any Adverse Event	50	(98)	53	(96)	126	(93)
Body as a Whole						
Asthenia	9	(18)	10	(18)	15	(11)
Headache/Migraine	33	(65)	28	(51)	63	(46)
Injection Site Reaction	1	(2)	5	(9)	4	(3)
Pain	12	(24)	16	(29)	29	(21)
Cardiovascular System						
Hot flashes/Sweats	50	(98)	48	(87)	78	(57)
Digestive System						
Altered Bowel Function	7	(14)	8	(15)	14	(10)
Changes in Appetite	2	(4)	0	(0)	8	(6)
GI Disturbance	2	(4)	4	(7)	6	(4)
Nausea/Vomiting	13	(25)	16	(29)	17	(13)
Metabolic and Nutritional Disorders						
Edema	0	(0)	5	(9)	9	(7)
Weight Changes	6	(12)	7	(13)	6	(4)
Nervous System						
Anxiety	3	(6)	0	(0)	11	(8)
Depression/Emotional Lability	16	(31)	15	(27)	46	(34)
Dizziness/Vertigo	8	(16)	6	(11)	10	(7)
Insomnia/Sleep Disorder	16	(31)	7	(13)	20	(15)
Libido Changes	5	(10)	2	(4)	10	(7)
Memory Disorder	3	(6)	1	(2)	6	(4)
Nervousness	4	(8)	2	(4)	15	(11)
Neuromuscular Disorder	1	(2)	5	(9)	4	(3)
Skin and Appendages						
Alopecia	0	(0)	5	(9)	4	(3)
Androgen-Like Effects	2	(4)	3	(5)	24	(18)
Skin/Mucous Membrane Reaction	2	(4)	5	(9)	15	(11)
Urogenital System						
Breast Changes/Pain/Tenderness	3	(6)	7	(13)	11	(8)
Menstrual Disorders	1	(2)	0	(0)	7	(5)
Vaginitis	10	(20)	8	(15)	11	(8)

[1] LD-Only = LUPRON DEPOT 3.75 mg
[2] LD/N = LUPRON DEPOT 3.75 mg plus norethindrone acetate 5 mg

Table 4 MEAN PERCENT CHANGE FROM BASELINE IN BONE MINERAL DENSITY OF LUMBAR SPINE

	LUPRON DEPOT 3.75 mg		LUPRON DEPOT 3.75 mg plus norethindrone acetate 5 mg daily			
	Controlled Study		Controlled Study		Open Label Study	
	N	Change	N	Change	N	Change
Week 24[1]	41	-3.2%	42	-0.3%	115	-0.2%
Week 52[2]	29	-6.3%	32	-1.0%	84	-1.1%

[1] Includes on-treatment measurements that fell within 2-252 days after the first day of treatment.
[2] Includes on-treatment measurements >252 days after the first day of treatment.

Injection site reactions; *Cardiovascular System* - Palpitations, Syncope, Tachycardia; *Digestive System* - Appetite changes, Dry mouth, Thirst; *Endocrine System* - Androgen-like effects; *Hemic and Lymphatic System* - Ecchymosis, Lymphadenopathy; *Nervous System* - Anxiety*, Insomnia/ Sleep disorders*, Delusions, Memory disorder, Personality disorder; *Respiratory System* - Rhinitis; *Skin and Appendages* - Alopecia, Hair disorder, Nail disorder; *Special Senses* - Conjunctivitis, Ophthalmologic disorders*, Taste perversion; *Urogenital System* - Dysuria*, Lactation, Menstrual disorders.

* = Possible effect of decreased estrogen.

In one controlled clinical trial utilizing the monthly formulation of LUPRON DEPOT, patients diagnosed with uterine fibroids received a higher dose (7.5 mg) of LUPRON DEPOT. Events seen with this dose that were thought to be potentially related to drug and were not seen at the lower dose included glossitis, hypesthesia, lactation, pyelonephritis, and urinary disorders. Generally, a higher incidence of hypoestrogenic effects was observed at the higher dose.

In a pharmacokinetic trial involving 20 healthy female subjects receiving LUPRON DEPOT–3 Month 11.25 mg, a few adverse events were reported with this formulation that were not reported previously. These included face edema, agitation, laryngitis, and ear pain.

In a Phase IV study involving endometriosis patients receiving LUPRON DEPOT 3.75 mg (N=20) or LUPRON DEPOT–3 Month 11.25 mg (N=21), similar adverse events were reported by the two groups of patients. In general the safety profiles of the two formulations were comparable in this study.

Table 3 lists the potentially drug-related adverse events observed in at least 5% of patients in any treatment group, during the first 6 months of treatment in the add-back clinical studies, in which patients were treated with monthly LUPRON DEPOT 3.75 mg with or without norethindrone acetate co-treatment.

[See table 3 above]

In the controlled clinical trial, 50 of 51 (98%) patients in the LD group (LUPRON DEPOT 3.75 mg) and 48 of 55 (87%) patients in the LD/N group (LUPRON DEPOT 3.75 mg plus norethindrone acetate 5 mg daily) reported experiencing hot flashes on one or more occasions during treatment. During Month 6 of treatment, 32 of 37 (86%) patients in the LD group and 22 of 38 (58%) patients in the LD/N group reported having experienced hot flashes. The mean number of days on which hot flashes were reported during this month of treatment was 19 and 7 in the LD and LD/N treatment groups, respectively. The mean maximum number of hot flashes per day during this month of treatment was 5.8 and 1.9 in the LD and LD/N treatment groups, respectively.

Changes in Bone Density

In controlled clinical studies, patients with endometriosis (six months of therapy) or uterine fibroids (three months of therapy) were treated with LUPRON DEPOT 3.75 mg. In endometriosis patients, vertebral bone density as measured by dual energy x-ray absorptiometry (DEXA) decreased by an average of 3.2% at six months compared with the pretreatment value. Clinical studies demonstrate that concurrent hormonal therapy (norethindrone acetate 5 mg daily) and calcium supplementation is effective in significantly reducing the loss of bone mineral density that occurs with LUPRON treatment, without compromising the efficacy of

LUPRON in relieving symptoms of endometriosis. LUPRON DEPOT 3.75 mg plus norethindrone acetate 5 mg daily was evaluated in two clinical trials. The results from this regimen were similar in both studies. LUPRON DEPOT 3.75 mg was used as a control group in one study. The bone mineral density data of the lumbar spine from these two studies are presented in Table 4.

[See table 4 at left]

In the Phase IV, six-month pharmacokinetic/pharmacodynamic study in endometriosis patients who were treated with LUPRON DEPOT 3.75 mg or LUPRON DEPOT–3 Month 11.25 mg, vertebral bone density measured by DEXA decreased compared with baseline by an average of 3.0% and 2.8% at six months for the two groups, respectively.

When LUPRON DEPOT 3.75 mg was administered for three months in uterine fibroid patients, vertebral trabecular bone mineral density as assessed by quantitative digital radiography (QDR) revealed a mean decrease of 2.7% compared with baseline. Six months after discontinuation of therapy, a trend toward recovery was observed. Use of LUPRON DEPOT for longer than three months (uterine fibroids) or six months (endometriosis) or in the presence of other known risk factors for decreased bone mineral content may cause additional bone loss **and is not recommended.**

Changes in Laboratory Values During Treatment

Liver Enzymes

Three percent of uterine fibroid patients treated with LUPRON DEPOT 3.75 mg, manifested posttreatment transaminase values that were at least twice the baseline value and above the upper limit of the normal range. None of the laboratory increases were associated with clinical symptoms.

In two other clinical trials, 6 of 191 patients receiving LUPRON DEPOT 3.75 mg plus norethindrone acetate 5 mg daily for up to 12 months developed an elevated (at least twice the upper limit of normal) SGPT or GGT. Five of the 6 increases were observed beyond 6 months of treatment. None were associated with an elevated bilirubin concentration.

Lipids

Triglycerides were increased above the upper limit of normal in 12% of the endometriosis patients who received LUPRON DEPOT 3.75 mg and in 32% of the subjects receiving LUPRON DEPOT–3 Month 11.25 mg.

Of those endometriosis and uterine fibroid patients whose pretreatment cholesterol values were in the normal range, mean change following therapy was +16 mg/dL to +17 mg/dL in endometriosis patients and +11 mg/dL to +29 mg/dL in uterine fibroid patients. In the endometriosis treated patients, increases from the pretreatment values were statistically significant (p<0.03). There was essentially no increase in the LDL/HDL ratio in patients from either population receiving LUPRON DEPOT 3.75 mg.

In two other clinical trials, LUPRON DEPOT 3.75 mg plus norethindrone acetate 5 mg daily were evaluated for 12 months of treatment. LUPRON DEPOT 3.75 mg was used as a control group in one study. Percent changes from baseline for serum lipids and percentages of patients with serum lipid values outside of the normal range in the two studies are summarized in the tables below.

[See table 5 at bottom of next page]

Changes from baseline tended to be greater at Week 52. After treatment, mean serum lipid levels from patients with follow up data returned to pretreatment values.

[See table 6 at bottom of next page]

Low HDL-cholesterol (<40 mg/dL) and elevated LDL-cholesterol (>160 mg/dL) are recognized risk factors for cardiovascular disease. The long-term significance of the observed treatment-related changes in serum lipids in women with endometriosis is unknown. Therefore assessment of cardiovascular risk factors should be considered prior to initiation of concurrent treatment with LUPRON and norethindrone acetate.

Chemistry

Slight to moderate mean increases were noted for glucose, uric acid, BUN, creatinine, total protein, albumin, bilirubin, alkaline phosphatase, LDH, calcium, and phosphorus. None of these increases were clinically significant. In the hormonal add-back studies LUPRON DEPOT in combination with norethindrone acetate was associated with elevations of GGT and SGPT in 6% to 7% of patients.

Postmarketing

During postmarketing surveillance with other dosage forms and in the same and/or different populations, the following adverse events were reported. Like other drugs in this class, mood swings, including depression, have been reported. There have been rare reports of suicidal ideation and attempt. Many, but not all, of these patients had a history of depression or other psychiatric illness. Patients should be counseled on the possibility of development or worsening of depression during treatment with LUPRON. Symptoms consistent with an anaphylactoid or asthmatic process have been rarely reported. Rash, urticaria, and photosensitivity reactions have also been reported.

Localized reactions including induration and abscess have been reported at the site of injection.

Symptoms consistent with fibromyalgia (eg: joint and muscle pain, headaches, sleep disorders, gastrointestinal distress, and shortness of breath) have been reported individually and collectively.

Other events reported are:

Cardiovascular System - Hypotension, Pulmonary embolism; *Hemic and Lymphatic System* - Decreased WBC; *Central/Peripheral Nervous System* - Convulsion, Peripheral neuropathy, Spinal fracture/paralysis; *Musculoskeletal System* - Tenosynovitis-like symptoms; *Urogenital System* - Prostate pain.

Pituitary apoplexy

During postmarketing surveillance, rare cases of pituitary apoplexy (a clinical syndrome secondary to infarction of the pituitary gland) have been reported after the administration of gonadotropin-releasing hormone agonists. In a majority of these cases, a pituitary adenoma was diagnosed, with a majority of pituitary apoplexy cases occurring within 2 weeks of the first dose, and some within the first hour. In these cases, pituitary apoplexy has presented as sudden headache, vomiting, visual changes, ophthalmoplegia, altered mental status, and sometimes cardiovascular collapse. Immediate medical attention has been required.

See other LUPRON DEPOT and LUPRON Injection package inserts for other events reported in the same and different patient populations.

OVERDOSAGE

In clinical trials using daily subcutaneous leuprolide acetate in patients with prostate cancer, doses as high as 20 mg/day for up to two years caused no adverse effects differing from those observed with the 1 mg/day dose.

DOSAGE AND ADMINISTRATION

LUPRON DEPOT Must Be Administered Under the Supervision of a Physician.

Endometriosis

The recommended duration of treatment with LUPRON DEPOT–3 Month 11.25 mg alone or in combination with norethindrone acetate is six months. The choice of LUPRON DEPOT alone or LUPRON DEPOT plus norethindrone acetate therapy for initial management of the symptoms and signs of endometriosis should be made by the health care professional in consultation with the patient and should take into consideration the risks and benefits of the addition of norethindrone to LUPRON DEPOT alone.

If the symptoms of endometriosis recur after a course of therapy, retreatment with a six-month course of LUPRON DEPOT and norethindrone acetate 5 mg daily may be considered. Retreatment beyond this one six-month course cannot be recommended. It is recommended that bone density be assessed before retreatment begins to ensure that values are within normal limits. LUPRON DEPOT alone is not recommended for retreatment. If norethindrone acetate is contraindicated for the individual patient, then retreatment is not recommended.

An assessment of cardiovascular risk and management of risk factors such as cigarette smoking is recommended before beginning treatment with LUPRON DEPOT and norethindrone acetate.

Uterine Leiomyomata (Fibroids)

The recommended dose of LUPRON DEPOT–3 Month 11.25 mg is one injection. The symptoms associated with uterine leiomyomata are to be reported following discontinuation of therapy. If additional treatment with LUPRON DEPOT–3 Month 11.25 mg is contemplated, bone density should be assessed prior to initiation of therapy to ensure that values are within normal limits.

Due to different release characteristics, a fractional dose of the 3-month depot formulation is not equivalent to the same dose of the monthly formulation and should not be given.

Incorporated in a depot formulation, the lyophilized microspheres are to be reconstituted and administered as a single intramuscular injection. *For optimal performance of the prefilled dual chamber syringe (PDS), read and follow the following instructions:*

1. The LUPRON DEPOT powder should be visually inspected and the syringe should NOT BE USED if clumping or caking is evident. A thin layer of powder on the wall of the syringe is considered normal. The diluent should appear clear.
2. To prepare for injection, screw the white plunger into the end stopper until the stopper begins to turn.
3. Hold the syringe UPRIGHT. Release the diluent by SLOWLY PUSHING (6 to 8 seconds) the plunger until the first stopper is at the blue line in the middle of the barrel.
4. Keep the syringe UPRIGHT. Gently mix the microspheres (powder) thoroughly to form a uniform suspension. The suspension will appear milky. If the powder adheres to the stopper or caking/clumping is present, tap the syringe with your finger to disperse. DO NOT USE if any of the powder has not gone into suspension.
5. Hold the syringe UPRIGHT. With the opposite hand pull the needle cap upward without twisting.
6. Keep the syringe UPRIGHT. Advance the plunger to expel the air from the syringe.
7. Inject the entire contents of the syringe intramuscularly at the time of reconstitution. The suspension settles very quickly following reconstitution; therefore, LUPRON DEPOT should be mixed and used immediately. NOTE: Aspirated blood would be visible just below the luer lock connection if a blood vessel is accidentally penetrated. If present, blood can be seen through the transparent LuproLoc™ safety device.

AFTER INJECTION

8. Withdraw the needle. Immediately activate the LuproLoc™ safety device by pushing the arrow forward with the thumb or finger until the device is fully extended and a CLICK is heard or felt.

Since the product does not contain a preservative, the suspension should be discarded if not used immediately.

As with other drugs administered by injection, the injection site should be varied periodically.

HOW SUPPLIED

Each LUPRON DEPOT – 3 Month 11.25 mg kit (NDC 0074-3663-03) contains:

• one prefilled dual-chamber syringe
• one plunger
• two alcohol swabs
• instructions for how to mix and administer
• an information pamphlet for patients
• a complete prescribing information enclosure

Each syringe contains sterile lyophilized microspheres which are leuprolide acetate incorporated in a biodegradable polymer of polylactic acid. When mixed with 1.5 mL of the diluent, LUPRON DEPOT–3 Month 11.25 mg is administered as a single IM injection EVERY THREE MONTHS.

Store at 25°C (77°F); excursions permitted to 15-30°C (59-86°F) [See USP Controlled Room Temperature]

U.S. Patent Nos. 4,728,721; 4,849,228; 5,330,767; 5,476,663; 5,480,656; 5,575,987; 5,631,020; 5,631,021; 5,643,607; 5,716,640; 5,814,342; 5,823,997; 5,980,488; and 6,036,976. Other patents pending.

Manufactured for
Abbott Laboratories, North Chicago, IL 60064
by Takeda Pharmaceutical Company Limited
Osaka, Japan 540-8645
™ - Trademark
® - Registered Trademark
(No. 3663)
03-A144-R16
Revised: October, 2008
©2008 Abbott Laboratories
Shown in Product Identification Guide, page 303

LUPRON DEPOT®–3 MONTH 22.5 MG ℞
[lū-prŏn]
(leuprolide acetate for depot suspension)
3–MONTH FORMULATION
Rx only

DESCRIPTION

Leuprolide acetate is a synthetic nonapeptide analog of naturally occurring gonadotropin-releasing hormone (GnRH or LH-RH). The analog possesses greater potency than the natural hormone. The chemical name is 5-oxo-L-prolyl-L-histidyl-L-tryptophyl-L-seryl-L-tyrosyl-D-leucyl-L-leucyl-L-arginyl-N-ethyl-L-prolinamide acetate (salt) with the following structural formula:

[See figure at top of next page]

LUPRON DEPOT–3 Month 22.5 mg is available in a prefilled dual-chamber syringe containing sterile lyophilized microspheres which, when mixed with diluent, become a suspension intended as an intramuscular injection to be given ONCE EVERY THREE MONTHS (84 days).

The front chamber of LUPRON DEPOT–3 Month 22.5 mg prefilled dual-chamber syringe contains leuprolide acetate (22.5 mg), polylactic acid (198.6 mg) and D-mannitol (38.9 mg). The second chamber of diluent contains carboxymethylcellulose sodium (7.5 mg), D-mannitol (75.0 mg), polysorbate 80 (1.5 mg), water for injection, USP, and glacial acetic acid, USP to control pH.

During the manufacture of LUPRON DEPOT–3 Month 22.5 mg, acetic acid is lost, leaving the peptide.

CLINICAL PHARMACOLOGY

Leuprolide acetate, an LH-RH agonist, acts as a potent inhibitor of gonadotropin secretion when given continuously and in therapeutic doses. Animal and human studies indicate that following an initial stimulation, chronic administration of leuprolide acetate results in suppression of ovarian and testicular steroidogenesis. This effect is reversible upon discontinuation of drug therapy. Administration of leuprolide acetate has resulted in inhibition of the growth of certain hormone dependent tumors (prostatic tumors in Noble and Dunning male rats and DMBA-induced mammary tumors in female rats) as well as atrophy of the reproductive organs.

In humans, administration of leuprolide acetate results in an initial increase in circulating levels of luteinizing hormone (LH) and follicle stimulating hormone (FSH), leading to a transient increase in levels of the gonadal steroids (testosterone and dihydrotestosterone in males, and estrone and estradiol in premenopausal females). However, continuous administration of leuprolide acetate results in decreased levels of LH and FSH. In males, testosterone is reduced to castrate levels. In premenopausal females, estrogens are reduced to postmenopausal levels. These decreases occur within two to four weeks after initiation of

Table 5 SERUM LIPIDS: MEAN PERCENT CHANGES FROM BASELINE VALUES AT TREATMENT WEEK 24

| | LUPRON DEPOT 3.75 mg | | LUPRON DEPOT 3.75 mg plus norethindrone acetate 5 mg daily | | | |
| | Controlled Study (n=39) | | Controlled Study (n=41) | | Open Label Study (n=117) | |
	Baseline Value*	Wk 24 % Change	Baseline Value*	Wk 24 % Change	Baseline Value*	Wk 24 % Change
Total Cholesterol	170.5	9.2%	179.3	0.2%	181.2	2.8%
HDL Cholesterol	52.4	7.4%	51.8	-18.8%	51.0	-14.6%
LDL Cholesterol	96.6	10.9%	101.5	14.1%	109.1	13.1%
LDL/HDL Ratio	2.0**	5.0%	2.1**	43.4%	2.3**	39.4%
Triglycerides	107.8	17.5%	130.2	9.5%	105.4	13.8%

* mg/dL
**ratio

Table 6 PERCENTAGE OF PATIENTS WITH SERUM LIPID VALUES OUTSIDE OF THE NORMAL RANGE

| | LUPRON DEPOT 3.75 mg | | LUPRON DEPOT 3.75 mg plus norethindrone acetate 5 mg daily | | | |
| | Controlled Study (n=39) | | Controlled Study (n=41) | | Open Label Study (n=117) | |
	Wk 0	Wk 24*	Wk 0	Wk 24*	Wk 0	Wk 24*
Total Cholesterol (>240 mg/dL)	15%	23%	15%	20%	6%	7%
HDL Cholesterol (<40 mg/dL)	15%	10%	15%	44%	15%	41%
LDL Cholesterol (>160 mg/dL)	0%	8%	5%	7%	9%	11%
LDL/HDL Ratio (>4.0)	0%	3%	2%	15%	7%	21%
Triglycerides (>200 mg/dL)	13%	13%	12%	10%	5%	9%

*Includes all patients regardless of baseline value.

Information on the Abbott Pharmaceutical Products listed on these pages is from the prescribing information in use as of June 1, 2010. For more information, please visit rxabbott.com or call 1-800-633-9110.

treatment, and castrate levels of testosterone in prostatic cancer patients have been demonstrated for more than five years.

Leuprolide acetate is not active when given orally.

Pharmacokinetics

Absorption

Following a single injection of the three month formulation of LUPRON DEPOT–3 Month 22.5 mg in patients, mean peak plasma leuprolide concentration of 48.9 ng/mL was observed at 4 hours and then declined to 0.67 ng/mL at 12 weeks. Leuprolide appeared to be released at a constant rate following the onset of steady-state levels during the third week after dosing, providing steady plasma concentrations through the 12-week dosing interval. However, intact leuprolide and an inactive major metabolite could not be distinguished by the assay which was employed in the study. Detectable levels of leuprolide were present at all measurement points in all patients. The initial burst, followed by the rapid decline to a steady-state level, was similar to the release pattern seen with the monthly formulation.

Distribution

The mean steady-state volume of distribution of leuprolide following intravenous bolus administration to healthy male volunteers was 27 L. *In vitro* binding to human plasma proteins ranged from 43% to 49%.

Metabolism

In healthy male volunteers, a 1 mg bolus of leuprolide administered intravenously revealed that the mean systemic clearance was 7.6 L/h, with a terminal elimination half-life of approximately 3 hours based on a two compartment model.

In rats and dogs, administration of ^{14}C-labeled leuprolide was shown to be metabolized to smaller inactive peptides, a pentapeptide (Metabolite I), tripeptides (Metabolites II and III) and a dipeptide (Metabolite IV). These fragments may be further catabolized.

The major metabolite (M-I) plasma concentrations measured in 5 prostate cancer patients reached maximum concentration 2 to 6 hours after dosing and were approximately 6% of the peak parent drug concentration. One week after dosing, mean plasma M-I concentrations were approximately 20% of mean leuprolide concentrations.

Excretion

Following administration of LUPRON DEPOT® 3.75 mg to 3 patients, less than 5% of the dose was recovered as parent and M-I metabolite in the urine.

Special Populations

The pharmacokinetics of the drug in hepatically and renally impaired patients have not been determined.

CLINICAL STUDIES

In clinical studies, serum testosterone was suppressed to castrate within 30 days in 87 of 92 (95%) patients and within an additional two weeks in three patients. Two patients did not suppress for 15 and 28 weeks, respectively. Suppression was maintained in all of these patients with the exception of transient minimal testosterone elevations in one of them, and in another an increase in serum testosterone to above the castrate range was recorded during the 12 hour observation period after a subsequent injection. This represents stimulation of gonadotropin secretion.

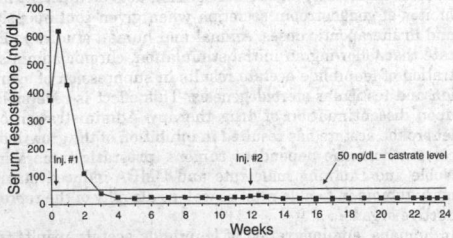

Lupron Depot – 3 Month 22.5 mg
Mean Serum Testosterone Concentrations

Note: Measurements were taken in a subset of patients from one study at Weeks 10.5, 11.5, 12.5, 22.5 and 23.5.

An 85% rate of "no progression" was achieved during the initial 24 weeks of treatment. A decrease from baseline in serum PSA of ≥90% was reported in 71% of the patients and a change to within the normal range (≤3.99 ng/mL) in 63% of the patients.

Periodic monitoring of serum testosterone and PSA levels is recommended, especially if the anticipated clinical or biochemical response to treatment has not been achieved. It should be noted that results of testosterone determinations are dependent on assay methodology. It is advisable to be aware of the type and precision of the assay methodology to make appropriate clinical and therapeutic decisions.

INDICATIONS AND USAGE

LUPRON DEPOT–3 Month 22.5 mg is indicated in the palliative treatment of advanced prostatic cancer. It offers an alternative treatment of prostatic cancer when orchiectomy or estrogen administration are either not indicated or unacceptable to the patient. In clinical trials, the safety and efficacy of LUPRON DEPOT–3 Month 22.5 mg were similar to that of the original daily subcutaneous injection and the monthly depot formulation.

CONTRAINDICATIONS

1. Hypersensitivity to GnRH, GnRH agonist analogs or any of the excipients in LUPRON DEPOT. Reports of anaphylactic reactions to GnRH agonist analogs have been reported in the medical literature.[1,2]
2. LUPRON DEPOT is contraindicated in women who are or may become pregnant while receiving the drug. When administered on day 6 of pregnancy at test dosages of 0.00024, 0.0024, and 0.024 mg/kg (1/600 to 1/6 of the human dose) to rabbits, the monthly formulation of LUPRON DEPOT produced a dose-related increase in major fetal abnormalities. Similar studies in rats failed to demonstrate an increase in fetal malformations. There was increased fetal mortality and decreased fetal weights with the two higher doses of the monthly formulation of LUPRON DEPOT in rabbits and with the highest dose in rats. The effects on fetal mortality are logical consequences of the alterations in hormonal levels brought about by this drug. Therefore, the possibility exists that spontaneous abortion may occur if the drug is administered during pregnancy.

WARNINGS

Isolated cases of worsening of signs and symptoms during the first weeks of treatment have been reported with LH-RH analogs. Worsening of symptoms may contribute to paralysis with or without fatal complications. For patients at risk, the physician may consider initiating therapy with daily LUPRON® (leuprolide acetate) Injection for the first two weeks to facilitate withdrawal of treatment if that is considered necessary.

PRECAUTIONS

Information for Patients

An information pamphlet for patients is included with the product.

General

Patients with metastatic vertebral lesions and/or with urinary tract obstruction should be closely observed during the first few weeks of therapy (see **WARNINGS** section).

Laboratory Tests

Response to LUPRON DEPOT–3 Month 22.5 mg should be monitored by measuring serum levels of testosterone, as well as prostate-specific antigen and prostatic acid phosphatase. In the majority of patients, testosterone levels increased above baseline during the first week, declining thereafter to baseline levels or below by the end of the second week. Castrate levels were reached within two to four weeks and once achieved were maintained for as long as the patients received their injections.

Drug Interactions

No pharmacokinetic-based drug-drug interaction studies have been conducted with LUPRON DEPOT. However, because leuprolide acetate is a peptide that is primarily degraded by peptidase and not by cytochrome P-450 enzymes as noted in specific studies, and the drug is only about 46% bound to plasma proteins, drug interactions would not be expected to occur.

Drug/Laboratory Test Interactions

Administration of LUPRON DEPOT 3.75 mg in women results in suppression of the pituitary-gonadal system. Normal function is usually restored within one to three months after treatment is discontinued. Therefore, diagnostic tests of pituitary gonadotropic and gonadal functions conducted during treatment and up to three months after discontinuation of LUPRON DEPOT 3.75 mg therapy may be misleading.

Carcinogenesis, Mutagenesis, Impairment of Fertility

Two-year carcinogenicity studies were conducted in rats and mice. In rats, a dose-related increase of benign pituitary hyperplasia and benign pituitary adenomas was noted at 24 months when the drug was administered subcutaneously at high daily doses (0.6 to 4 mg/kg). There was a significant but not dose-related increase of pancreatic islet-cell adenomas in females and of testicular interstitial cell adenomas in males (highest incidence in the low dose group).

In mice no pituitary abnormalities were observed at a dose as high as 60 mg/kg for two years. Patients have been treated with leuprolide acetate for up to three years with doses as high as 10 mg/day and for two years with doses as high as 20 mg/day without demonstrable pituitary abnormalities.

Mutagenicity studies have been performed with leuprolide acetate using bacterial and mammalian systems. These studies provided no evidence of a mutagenic potential.

Clinical and pharmacologic studies in adults (≥ 18 years) with leuprolide acetate and similar analogs have shown reversibility of fertility suppression when the drug is discontinued after continuous administration for periods of up to 24 weeks.

Pregnancy

Teratogenic Effects

Pregnancy Category X (see **CONTRAINDICATIONS** section).

Pediatric Use

See LUPRON DEPOT-PED® (leuprolide acetate for depot suspension) labeling for the safety and effectiveness of the monthly formulation in children with central precocious puberty.

Geriatric Use

In the clinical trials for LUPRON DEPOT – 3 Month 22.5 mg, the majority (80%) of the subjects studied were at least 65 years of age. Therefore, the labeling reflects the pharmacokinetics, efficacy and safety of LUPRON DEPOT in this population.

ADVERSE REACTIONS

Clinical Trials

In the majority of patients testosterone levels increased above baseline during the first week, declining thereafter to baseline levels or below by the end of the second week of treatment.

Potential exacerbations of signs and symptoms during the first few weeks of treatment is a concern in patients with vertebral metastases and/or urinary obstruction or hematuria which, if aggravated, may lead to neurological problems such as temporary weakness and/or paresthesia of the lower limbs or worsening of urinary symptoms (see **WARNINGS** section).

In two clinical trials of LUPRON DEPOT–3 Month 22.5 mg, the following adverse reactions were reported to have a possible or probable relationship to drug as ascribed by the treating physician in 5% or more of the patients receiving the drug. **Often, causality is difficult to assess in patients with metastatic prostate cancer.** Reactions considered not drug-related are excluded.

	LUPRON DEPOT–3 Month 22.5 mg N=94	(%)
Body As A Whole		
Asthenia	7	(7.4)
General Pain	25	(26.6)
Headache	6	(6.4)
Injection Site Reaction	13	(13.8)
Cardiovascular System		
Hot flashes/Sweats*	55	(58.5)
Digestive System		
GI Disorders	15	(16.0)
Musculoskeletal System		
Joint Disorders	11	(11.7)
Central/Peripheral Nervous System		
Dizziness/Vertigo	6	(6.4)
Insomnia/Sleep Disorders	8	(8.5)
Neuromuscular Disorders	9	(9.6)
Respiratory System		
Respiratory Disorders	6	(6.4)
Skin and Appendages		
Skin Reaction	8	(8.5)
Urogenital System		
Testicular Atrophy*	19	(20.2)
Urinary Disorders	14	(14.9)

In these same studies, the following adverse reactions were reported in less than 5% of the patients on LUPRON DEPOT–3 Month 22.5 mg.

Body As A Whole - Enlarged abdomen, Fever; *Cardiovascular System* - Arrhythmia, Bradycardia, Heart failure, Hypertension, Hypotension, Varicose vein; *Digestive System* - Anorexia, Duodenal ulcer, Increased appetite, Thirst/dry mouth; *Hemic and Lymphatic System* - Anemia, Lymphedema; *Metabolic and Nutritional Disorders* - Dehydration, Edema; *Central/Peripheral Nervous System* - Anxiety, Delusions, Depression, Hypesthesia, Libido decreased*, Nervousness, Paresthesia; *Respiratory System* - Epistaxis, Pharyngitis, Pleural effusion, Pneumonia; *Special Senses* - Abnormal vision, Amblyopia, Dry eyes, Tinnitus; *Urogenital System* - Gynecomastia, Impotence*, Penis disorders, Testis disorders.

* Physiologic effect of decreased testosterone.

Laboratory

Abnormalities of certain parameters were observed, but are difficult to assess in this population. The following were recorded in ≥5% of patients: Increased BUN, Hyperglycemia, Hyperlipidemia (total cholesterol, LDL-cholesterol, triglycerides), Hyperphosphatemia, Abnormal liver function tests, Increased PT, Increased PTT. Additional laboratory abnormalities reported were: Decreased platelets, Decreased potassium and Increased WBC.

Postmarketing

During postmarketing surveillance, which includes other dosage forms and other patient populations, the following adverse events were reported.

Symptoms consistent with an anaphylactoid or asthmatic process have been rarely (incidence rate of about 0.002%) reported. Rash, urticaria, and photosensitivity reactions have also been reported.

Localized reactions including induration and abscess have been reported at the site of injection.

Symptoms consistent with fibromyalgia (eg, joint and muscle pain, headaches, sleep disorders, gastrointestinal distress, and shortness of breath) have been reported individually and collectively.

Cardiovascular System – Hypotension, Myocardial infarction, Pulmonary embolism; *Hemic and Lymphatic System* - Decreased WBC; *Central/Peripheral Nervous System* - Convulsion, Peripheral neuropathy, Spinal fracture/paralysis; *Endocrine System* – Diabetes; *Musculoskeletal System* - Tenosynovitis-like symptoms; *Urogenital System* - Prostate pain.

Changes in Bone Density: Decreased bone density has been reported in the medical literature in men who have had orchiectomy or who have been treated with an LH-RH agonist analog. In a clinical trial, 25 men with prostate cancer, 12 of whom had been treated previously with leuprolide acetate for at least six months, underwent bone density studies as a result of pain. The leuprolide-treated group had lower bone density scores than the nontreated control group. It can be anticipated that long periods of medical castration in men will have effects on bone density.

Pituitary apoplexy: During post-marketing surveillance, rare cases of pituitary apoplexy (a clinical syndrome secondary to infarction of the pituitary gland) have been reported after the administration of gonadotropin-releasing hormone agonists. In a majority of these cases, a pituitary adenoma was diagnosed, with a majority of pituitary apoplexy cases occurring within 2 weeks of the first dose, and some within the first hour. In these cases, pituitary apoplexy has presented as sudden headache, vomiting, visual changes, ophthalmoplegia, altered mental status, and sometimes cardiovascular collapse. Immediate medical attention has been required.

See other LUPRON DEPOT and LUPRON Injection package inserts for other events reported in women and pediatric populations.

OVERDOSAGE

In rats subcutaneous administration of 250 to 500 times the recommended human dose, expressed on a per body weight basis, resulted in dyspnea, decreased activity, and local irritation at the injection site. There is no evidence at present that there is a clinical counterpart of this phenomenon. In early clinical trials with daily subcutaneous leuprolide acetate, doses as high as 20 mg/day for up to two years caused no adverse effects differing from those observed with the 1 mg/day dose.

DOSAGE AND ADMINISTRATION

LUPRON DEPOT Must Be Administered Under The Supervision Of A Physician.

The recommended dose of LUPRON DEPOT–3 Month 22.5 mg to be administered is one injection every three months **(84 days)**. Due to different release characteristics, a fractional dose of this 3-month depot formulation is not equivalent to the same dose of the monthly formulation and should not be given.

Incorporated in a depot formulation, the lyophilized microspheres are to be reconstituted and administered every three months as a single intramuscular injection. *For optimal performance of the prefilled dual chamber syringe (PDS), read and follow the following instructions:*

1. The LUPRON DEPOT powder should be visually inspected and the syringe should NOT BE USED if clumping or caking is evident. A thin layer of powder on the wall of the syringe is considered normal. The diluent should appear clear.
2. To prepare for injection, screw the white plunger into the end stopper until the stopper begins to turn.
3. Hold the syringe UPRIGHT. Release the diluent by SLOWLY PUSHING (6 to 8 seconds) the plunger until the first stopper is at the blue line in the middle of the barrel.
4. Keep the syringe UPRIGHT. Gently mix the microspheres (powder) thoroughly to form a uniform suspension. The suspension will appear milky. If the powder adheres to the stopper or caking/clumping is present, tap the syringe with your finger to disperse. DO NOT USE if any of the powder has not gone into suspension.
5. Hold the syringe UPRIGHT. With the opposite hand pull the needle cap upward without twisting.
6. Keep the syringe UPRIGHT. Advance the plunger to expel the air from the syringe.
7. Inject the entire contents of the syringe intramuscularly at the time of reconstitution. The suspension settles very quickly following reconstitution; therefore, LUPRON DEPOT should be mixed and used immediately.
   NOTE: Aspirated blood would be visible just below the luer lock connection if a blood vessel is accidentally penetrated. If present, blood can be seen through the transparent LuproLoc™ safety device.
   AFTER INJECTION
8. Withdraw the needle. Immediately activate the LuproLoc™ safety device by pushing the arrow forward with the thumb or finger until the device is fully extended and a CLICK is heard or felt.

Since the product does not contain a preservative, the suspension should be discarded if not used immediately.

As with other drugs administered by injection, the injection site should be varied periodically.

HOW SUPPLIED

Each LUPRON DEPOT–3 Month 22.5 mg kit (NDC 0074-3346-03) contains:

- one prefilled dual-chamber syringe
- one plunger
- two alcohol swabs
- instructions for how to mix and administer
- an information pamphlet for patients
- a complete prescribing information enclosure

The prefilled dual-chamber syringe contains sterile lyophilized microspheres of leuprolide acetate incorporated in a biodegradable lactic acid polymer. When mixed with 1.5 mL of accompanying diluent, LUPRON DEPOT–3 Month 22.5 mg is administered as a single intramuscular injection **EVERY THREE MONTHS (84 days)**.

Store at 25°C (77°F); excursions permitted to 15–30°C (59–86°F) [See USP Controlled Room Temperature]

REFERENCES

1. Taylor, JD. Anaphylactic reaction to LHRH analogue, leuprorelin. *Med J Australia* 1994 Oct; 161(3): 455.
2. Letterie GS, *et al.* Recurrent anaphylaxis to a depot form of GnRH analogue. *Obstet Gynecol* 1991 Nov; 78: 943–946.

U.S. Patent Nos. 4,728,721; 4,849,228; 5,330,767; 5,476,663; 5,480,656; 5,575,987; 5,631,020; 5,631,021; 5,643,607; 5,716,640; 5,814,342; 5,823,997; 5,980,488 and 6,036,976. Other patents pending.

Manufactured for:
Abbott Laboratories
North Chicago, IL 60064
by: Takeda Pharmaceutical Company Limited
Osaka, Japan 540-8645
™–Trademark
® – Registered trademark
(No. 3346)
03-A141-R15
Revised: October, 2008

Shown in Product Identification Guide, page 303

LUPRON DEPOT®–4 MONTH 30 mg ℞

[lew-prŏn]

(leuprolide acetate for depot suspension)
4-MONTH FORMULATION
Rx only

DESCRIPTION

Leuprolide acetate is a synthetic nonapeptide analog of naturally occurring gonadotropin-releasing hormone (GnRH or LH-RH). The analog possesses greater potency than the natural hormone. The chemical name is 5-oxo-L-prolyl-L-histidyl-L-tryptophyl-L-seryl-L-tyrosyl-D-leucyl-L-leucyl-L-arginyl-N-ethyl-L-prolinamide acetate (salt) with the following structural formula:

[See figure at top of next page]

LUPRON DEPOT-4 Month 30 mg is available in a prefilled dual-chamber syringe containing sterile lyophilized microspheres which, when mixed with diluent, become a suspension intended as an intramuscular injection to be given **ONCE EVERY FOUR MONTHS (16 weeks)**.

The front chamber of LUPRON DEPOT-4 Month 30 mg prefilled dual-chamber syringe contains leuprolide acetate (30 mg), polylactic acid (264.8 mg) and D-mannitol (51.9 mg). The second chamber of diluent contains carboxymethylcellulose sodium (7.5 mg), D-mannitol (75.0 mg), polysorbate 80 (1.5 mg), water for injection, USP, and glacial acetic acid, USP to control pH.

During the manufacture of LUPRON DEPOT-4 Month 30 mg, acetic acid is lost, leaving the peptide.

CLINICAL PHARMACOLOGY

Leuprolide acetate, an LH-RH agonist, acts as a potent inhibitor of gonadotropin secretion when given continuously and in therapeutic doses. Animal and human studies indicate that following an initial stimulation, chronic administration of leuprolide acetate results in suppression of ovarian and testicular steroidogenesis. This effect is reversible upon discontinuation of drug therapy. Administration of leuprolide acetate has resulted in inhibition of the growth of certain hormone dependent tumors (prostatic tumors in Noble and Dunning male rats and DMBA-induced mammary tumors in female rats) as well as atrophy of the reproductive organs.

In humans, administration of leuprolide acetate results in an initial increase in circulating levels of luteinizing hormone (LH) and follicle stimulating hormone (FSH), leading to a transient increase in levels of the gonadal steroids (testosterone and dihydrotestosterone in males, and estrone and estradiol in premenopausal females). However, continuous administration of leuprolide acetate results in decreased levels of LH and FSH. In males, testosterone is reduced to castrate levels. In premenopausal females, estrogens are reduced to postmenopausal levels. These decreases occur within two to four weeks after initiation of treatment. Castrate levels of testosterone in prostatic cancer patients have been demonstrated for more than five years.

Leuprolide acetate is not active when given orally.

Pharmacokinetics

Absorption

Following a single injection of LUPRON DEPOT-4 Month 30 mg in sixteen orchiectomized prostate cancer patients, mean plasma leuprolide concentration of 59.3 ng/mL was observed at 4 hours and the mean concentration then declined to 0.30 ng/mL at 16 weeks. The mean plasma concentration of leuprolide from weeks 3.5 to 16 was 0.44 ± 0.20 ng/mL (range: 0.20–1.06). Leuprolide appeared to be released at a constant rate following the onset of steady-state levels during the fourth week after dosing, providing steady plasma concentrations throughout the 16-week dosing interval. However, intact leuprolide and an inactive major metabolite could not be distinguished by the assay which was employed in the study. The initial burst, followed by the rapid decline to a steady-state level, was similar to the release pattern seen with the other depot formulations.

Distribution

The mean steady-state volume of distribution of leuprolide following intravenous bolus administration to healthy male volunteers was 27 L. *In vitro* binding to human plasma proteins ranged from 43% to 49%.

Metabolism

In healthy male volunteers, a 1 mg bolus of leuprolide administered intravenously revealed that the mean systemic clearance was 7.6 L/h, with a terminal elimination half-life of approximately 3 hours based on a two compartment model.

In rats and dogs, administration of ^{14}C-labeled leuprolide was shown to be metabolized to smaller inactive peptides, a pentapeptide (Metabolite I), tripeptides (Metabolites II and III) and a dipeptide (Metabolite IV). These fragments may be further catabolized.

The major metabolite (M-I) plasma concentrations measured in 5 prostate cancer patients reached maximum concentration 2 to 6 hours after dosing and were approximately 6% of the peak parent drug concentration. One week after dosing, mean plasma M-I concentrations were approximately 20% of mean leuprolide concentrations.

Information on the Abbott Pharmaceutical Products listed on these pages is from the prescribing information in use as of June 1, 2010. For more information, please visit rxabbott.com or call 1-800-633-9110.

Excretion
Following administration of LUPRON DEPOT® 3.75 mg to 3 patients, less than 5% of the dose was recovered as parent and M-I metabolite in the urine.
Special Populations
The pharmacokinetics of the drug in hepatically and renally impaired patients have not been determined.
Drug Interactions
No pharmacokinetic-based drug-drug interaction studies have been conducted with LUPRON DEPOT. However, because leuprolide acetate is a peptide that is primarily degraded by peptidase and the drug is only about 46% bound to plasma proteins, drug interactions would not be expected to occur.

CLINICAL STUDIES

In an open-label, noncomparative, multicenter clinical study of LUPRON DEPOT-4 Month 30 mg, 49 patients with stage D2 prostatic adenocarcinoma (with no prior treatment) were enrolled. The objectives were to determine whether a 30 mg depot formulation of leuprolide injected once every 16 weeks would reduce and maintain serum testosterone levels at castrate levels (≤ 50 ng/dL), and to assess the safety of the formulation. The study was divided into an initial 32-week treatment phase and a long-term treatment phase. Serum testosterone levels were determined biweekly or weekly during the first 32 weeks of treatment. Once the patient completed the initial 32-week treatment period, treatment continued at the investigator's discretion with serum testosterone levels being done every 4 months prior to the injection.

In the majority of patients, testosterone levels increased 50% or more above the baseline during the first week of treatment. Mean serum testosterone subsequently suppressed to castrate levels within 30 days of the first injection in 94% of patients and within 43 days in all 49 patients during the initial 32-week treatment period. The median dosing interval between injections was 112 days. One escape from suppression (two consecutive testosterone values greater than 50 ng/dL after castrate levels achieved) was noted at Week 16. In this patient, serum testosterone increased to above the castrate range following the second depot injection (Week 16) but returned to the castrate level by Week 18. No adverse events were associated with this rise in serum testosterone. A second patient had a rise in testosterone at Week 17, then returned to the castrate level by Week 18 and remained there through Week 32. In the long-term treatment phase two patients experienced testosterone elevations, both at Week 48. Testosterone for one patient returned to the castrate range at Week 52, and one patient discontinued the study at Week 48 due to disease progression.

Secondary efficacy endpoints evaluated in the study were the objective tumor response as assessed by clinical evaluations of tumor burden (complete response, partial response, objectively stable and progression) and evaluations of changes in prostatic involvement and prostate-specific antigen (PSA). These evaluations were performed at Weeks 16 and 32 of the treatment phase. The long-term treatment phase monitored PSA at each visit (every 16 weeks). The objective tumor response analysis showed "no progression" (i.e. complete or partial response, or stable disease) in 86% (37/43) of patients at Week 16, and in 77% (37/48) of patients at Week 32. Local disease improved or remained stable in all patients evaluated at Week 16 and/or 32. For patients with elevated baseline PSA, 50% (23/46) had a normal PSA (less than 4.0 ng/mL) at Week 16, and 51% (19/37) had a normal PSA at Week 32.

Periodic monitoring of serum testosterone and PSA levels is recommended, especially if the anticipated clinical or biochemical response to treatment has not been achieved. It should be noted that results of testosterone determinations are dependent on assay methodology. It is advisable to be aware of the type and precision of the assay methodology to make appropriate clinical and therapeutic decisions.

Using historical comparisons, the safety and efficacy of LUPRON DEPOT-4 Month 30 mg appear similar to the other LUPRON DEPOT formulations.

[See figure at top of next column]

INDICATIONS AND USAGE

LUPRON DEPOT-4 Month 30 mg is indicated in the palliative treatment of advanced prostatic cancer.

CONTRAINDICATIONS

1. Hypersensitivity to GnRH, GnRH agonist analogs or any of the excipients in LUPRON DEPOT. Reports of anaphylactic reactions to GnRH agonist analogs have been reported in the medical literature.[1,2]
2. This formulation is not indicated for use in women. (See LUPRON DEPOT 3.75 mg and LUPRON DEPOT®–3 Month 11.25 mg package inserts.)
3. All formulations of LUPRON DEPOT are contraindicated in women who are or may become pregnant while receiving the drug. LUPRON DEPOT may cause fetal harm

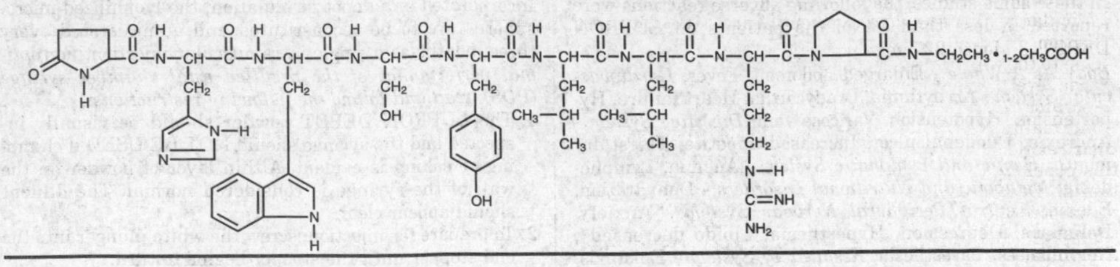

Lupron Depot – 4 Month 30 mg
Mean Serum Testosterone Concentrations

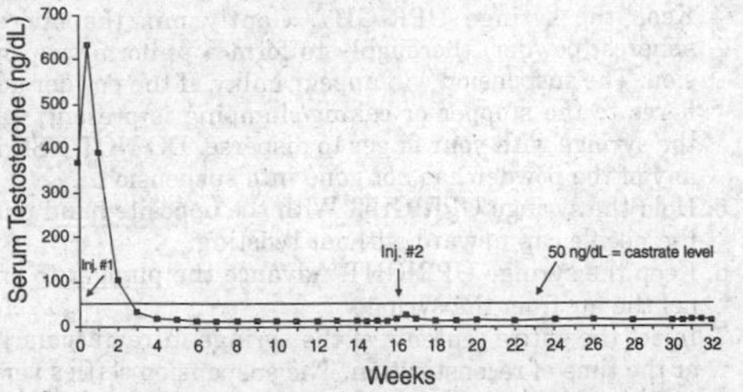

Note: Measurements were taken in a subset of patients at Weeks 14.5, 15.5, 16.5, 30.5, 31 and 31.5.

when administered to a pregnant woman. Major fetal abnormalities were observed in rabbits but not in rats after administration of LUPRON DEPOT throughout gestation. There was increased fetal mortality and decreased fetal weights in rats and rabbits. The effects on fetal mortality are expected consequences of the alterations in hormonal levels brought about by this drug. Therefore, the possibility exists that spontaneous abortion may occur. If this drug is used during pregnancy, or if the patient becomes pregnant while taking any formulation of LUPRON DEPOT, the patient should be apprised of the potential hazard to the fetus.

WARNINGS

Initially, LUPRON DEPOT, like other LH-RH agonists, causes increases in serum levels of testosterone to approximately 50% above baseline during the first week of treatment. Transient worsening of symptoms, or the occurrence of additional signs and symptoms of prostate cancer, may occasionally develop during the first few weeks of LUPRON DEPOT treatment. A small number of patients may experience a temporary increase in bone pain, which can be managed symptomatically. As with other LH-RH agonists, isolated cases of ureteral obstruction and spinal cord compression have been observed, which may contribute to paralysis with or without fatal complications.

For patients at risk, initiation of therapy with daily LUPRON® (leuprolide acetate) Injection (See **DOSAGE AND ADMINISTRATION** section in the LUPRON Injection labeling.) for the first two weeks to facilitate withdrawal of treatment may be considered. If spinal cord compression or renal impairment develops, standard treatment of these complications should be instituted.

PRECAUTIONS

Information for Patients
An information pamphlet for patients is included with the product.

General
Patients with metastatic vertebral lesions and/or with urinary tract obstruction should be closely observed during the first few weeks of therapy. (See **WARNINGS** section.)

Laboratory Tests
Response to LUPRON DEPOT-4 Month 30 mg should be monitored by measuring serum levels of testosterone, as well as prostate-specific antigen. In the majority of patients, testosterone levels increased above baseline during the first week, declining thereafter to baseline levels or below by the end of the second week. Castrate levels were reached within two to four weeks and once achieved were maintained in most (45/49) patients for as long as the patients received their injections. (See **CLINICAL STUDIES** and **ADVERSE REACTIONS**.)

Drug Interactions
See **CLINICAL PHARMACOLOGY, Pharmacokinetics.**

Drug/Laboratory Test Interactions
Administration of LUPRON DEPOT in therapeutic doses results in suppression of the pituitary-gonadal system. Normal function is usually restored within three months after treatment is discontinued. Due to the suppression of the pituitary-gonadal system by LUPRON DEPOT, diagnostic tests of pituitary gonadotropic and gonadal functions conducted during treatment and for up to three months after discontinuation of LUPRON DEPOT may be affected.

Carcinogenesis, Mutagenesis, Impairment of Fertility
Two-year carcinogenicity studies were conducted in rats and mice. In rats, a dose-related increase of benign pituitary hyperplasia and benign pituitary adenomas was noted at 24 months when the drug was administered subcutaneously at high daily doses (0.6 to 4 mg/kg). There was a significant but not dose-related increase of pancreatic islet-cell adenomas in females and of testicular interstitial cell adenomas in males (highest incidence in the low dose group). In mice no pituitary abnormalities were observed at a dose as high as 60 mg/kg for two years. Patients have been treated with leuprolide acetate for up to three years with doses as high as 10 mg/day and for two years with doses as high as 20 mg/day without demonstrable pituitary abnormalities.

Mutagenicity studies have been performed with leuprolide acetate using bacterial and mammalian systems. These studies provided no evidence of a mutagenic potential.

Clinical and pharmacologic studies in adults (≥ 18 years) with leuprolide acetate and similar analogs have shown reversibility of fertility suppression when the drug is discontinued after continuous administration for periods of up to 24 weeks.

Pregnancy
Teratogenic Effects
Pregnancy Category X (See **CONTRAINDICATIONS** section).

Pediatric Use
Safety and effectiveness of LUPRON DEPOT-4 Month 30 mg have not been established in pediatric patients. See LUPRON DEPOT-PED® (leuprolide acetate for depot suspension) labeling for the safety and effectiveness of the monthly formulation in children with central precocious puberty.

Geriatric Use
In the clinical trials for LUPRON DEPOT – 4 Month 30 mg, the majority (79%) of the subjects studied were at least 65 years of age. Therefore, the labeling reflects the pharmacokinetics, efficacy and safety of LUPRON DEPOT in this population.

ADVERSE REACTIONS

Clinical Trials
The 4-month formulation of LUPRON DEPOT 30 mg was utilized in clinical trials that studied the drug in 49 nonorchiectomized prostate cancer patients for 32 weeks or longer and in 24 orchiectomized prostate cancer patients for 20 weeks.

In the majority of nonorchiectomized patients, testosterone levels increased 50% or more above baseline during the first week of treatment with LUPRON DEPOT, declining thereafter to baseline levels or below by the end of the second week of treatment. Therefore, potential exacerbations of signs and symptoms during the first few weeks of treatment are of concern in patients with vertebral metastases and/or urinary obstruction or hematuria which, if aggravated, may lead to neurological problems such as temporary weakness and/or paresthesia of the lower limbs or worsening of urinary symptoms. (See **WARNINGS** section.)

In the above described clinical trials, the following adverse reactions were reported in ≥ 5% of the patients during the treatment period regardless of causality.

[See table at top of next page]

In these same studies, the following adverse reactions were reported in less than 5% of the patients on LUPRON DEPOT-4 Month 30 mg.

Body As a Whole - Abscess, Accidental injury, Allergic reaction, Cyst, Fever, Generalized edema, Hernia, Neck pain, Neoplasm; *Cardiovascular System* - Atrial fibrillation, Deep thrombophlebitis, Hypertension; *Digestive System* - Anorexia, Eructation, Gastrointestinal hemorrhage, Gingivitis, Gum hemorrhage, Hepatomegaly, Increased appetite, Intestinal obstruction, Periodontal abscess; *Hemic and Lymphatic System* - Lymphadenopathy; *Metabolic and Nutritional Disorders* - Healing abnormal, Hypoxia, Weight loss; *Musculoskeletal System* - Leg cramps, Pathological fracture, Ptosis; *Nervous System* - Abnormal thinking, Amnesia, Confusion, Convulsion, Dementia, Depression, Insomnia/sleep disorders, Libido decreased*, Neuropathy, Paralysis; *Respiratory System* - Asthma, Bronchitis, Hiccup, Lung disorder, Sinusitis, Voice alteration; *Skin and Appendages* - Herpes zoster, Melanosis; *Urogenital System* - Bladder carcinoma, Epididymitis, Impotence*, Prostate disorder, Testicular atrophy*, Urinary incontinence, Urinary tract infection.

* Due to the expected physiologic effects of decreased testosterone levels.

Laboratory

Abnormalities of certain parameters were observed, but their relationship to drug treatment is difficult to assess in this population. The following were recorded in ≥ 5% of patients: Decreased bicarbonate, Decreased hemoglobin/hematocrit/RBC, Hyperlipidemia (total cholesterol, LDL-cholesterol, triglycerides), Decreased HDL-cholesterol, Eosinophilia, Increased glucose, Increased liver function tests (ALT, AST, GGTP, LDH), Increased phosphorus. Additional laboratory abnormalities were reported: Increased BUN and PT, Leukopenia, Thrombocytopenia, Uricaciduria.

Postmarketing

During postmarketing surveillance, which includes other dosage forms and other patient populations, the following adverse events were reported.

Symptoms consistent with an anaphylactoid or asthmatic process have been rarely (incidence rate of about 0.002%) reported. Rash, urticaria, and photosensitivity reactions have also been reported.

Localized reactions including induration and abscess have been reported at the site of injection.

Symptoms consistent with fibromyalgia (eg, joint and muscle pain, headaches, sleep disorders, gastrointestinal distress, and shortness of breath) have been reported individually and collectively.

Cardiovascular System - Hypotension, Myocardial infarction, Pulmonary embolism; *Hemic and Lymphatic System* - Decreased WBC; *Central/Peripheral Nervous System* - Convulsion, Peripheral neuropathy, Spinal fracture/paralysis; *Endocrine System* – Diabetes; *Musculoskeletal System* - Tenosynovitis-like symptoms; *Urogenital System* - Prostate pain.

Changes in Bone Density: Decreased bone density has been reported in the medical literature in men who have had orchiectomy or who have been treated with an LH-RH agonist analog. In a clinical trial, 25 men with prostate cancer, 12 of whom had been treated previously with leuprolide acetate for at least six months, underwent bone density studies as a result of pain. The leuprolide-treated group had lower bone density scores than the nontreated control group. It can be anticipated that long periods of medical castration in men will have effects on bone density.

Pituitary apoplexy: During post-marketing surveillance, rare cases of pituitary apoplexy (a clinical syndrome secondary to infarction of the pituitary gland) have been reported after the administration of gonadotropin-releasing hormone agonists. In a majority of these cases, a pituitary adenoma was diagnosed, with a majority of pituitary apoplexy cases occurring within 2 weeks of the first dose, and some within the first hour. In these cases, pituitary apoplexy has presented as sudden headache, vomiting, visual changes, ophthalmoplegia, altered mental status, and sometimes cardiovascular collapse. Immediate medical attention has been required.

See other LUPRON DEPOT and LUPRON Injection package inserts for other events reported in women and pediatric populations.

OVERDOSAGE

In clinical trials using daily subcutaneous leuprolide acetate in patients with prostate cancer, doses as high as 20 mg/day for up to two years caused no adverse effects differing from those observed with the 1 mg/day dose.

DOSAGE AND ADMINISTRATION

LUPRON DEPOT Must Be Administered Under The Supervision Of A Physician.

The recommended dose of LUPRON DEPOT-4 Month 30 mg to be administered is one injection **EVERY FOUR MONTHS (16 weeks).** Due to different release characteristics, a fractional dose of this 4-month depot formulation is not equivalent to the same dose of the monthly formulation and should not be given.

Incorporated in a depot formulation, the lyophilized microspheres are to be reconstituted and administered **EVERY FOUR MONTHS (16 weeks)** as a single intramuscular injection. *For optimal performance of the prefilled dual chamber syringe (PDS), read and follow the following instructions:*

1. The LUPRON DEPOT powder should be visually inspected and the syringe should NOT BE USED if clumping or caking is evident. A thin layer of powder on the wall of the syringe is considered normal. The diluent should appear clear.
2. To prepare for injection, screw the white plunger into the end stopper until the stopper begins to turn.
3. Hold the syringe UPRIGHT. Release the diluent by SLOWLY PUSHING (6 to 8 seconds) the plunger until the first stopper is at the blue line in the middle of the barrel.
4. Keep the syringe UPRIGHT. Gently mix the microspheres (powder) thoroughly to form a uniform suspen-

sion. The suspension will appear milky. If the powder adheres to the stopper or caking/clumping is present, tap the syringe with your finger to disperse. DO NOT USE if any of the powder has not gone into suspension.
5. Hold the syringe UPRIGHT. With the opposite hand pull the needle cap upward without twisting.
6. Keep the syringe UPRIGHT. Advance the plunger to expel the air from the syringe.
7. Inject the entire contents of the syringe intramuscularly at the time of reconstitution. The suspension settles very quickly following reconstitution; therefore, LUPRON DEPOT should be mixed and used immediately.
NOTE: Aspirated blood would be visible just below the luer lock connection if a blood vessel is accidentally penetrated. If present, blood can be seen through the transparent LuproLoc™ safety device.
AFTER INJECTION
8. Withdraw the needle. Immediately activate the LuproLoc™ safety device by pushing the arrow forward with the thumb or finger until the device is fully extended and a CLICK is heard or felt.

Since the product does not contain a preservative, the suspension should be discarded if not used immediately.

As with other drugs administered by injection, the injection site should be varied periodically.

HOW SUPPLIED

Each LUPRON DEPOT–4 Month 30 mg kit (NDC 0074-3683-03) contains:
• one prefilled dual-chamber syringe
• one plunger
• two alcohol swabs
• instructions for how to mix and administer
• an information pamphlet for patients
• a complete prescribing information enclosure

The prefilled dual-chamber syringe contains sterile lyophilized microspheres of leuprolide acetate incorporated in a biodegradable lactic acid polymer. When mixed with 1.5 mL of accompanying diluent, LUPRON DEPOT–4 Month 30 mg is administered as a single intramuscular injection **EVERY FOUR MONTHS (16 weeks).**

Store at 25°C (77°F); excursions permitted to 15–30°C (59–86°F) [See USP Controlled Room Temperature]

REFERENCES

1. Taylor, JD. Anaphylactic reaction to LHRH analogue, leuprorelin. *Med J Australia* 1994 Oct; 161(3): 455.
2. Letterie GS, *et al.* Recurrent anaphylaxis to a depot form of GnRH analogue. *Obstet Gynecol* 1991 Nov; 78: 943–946.
U.S. Patent Nos. 4,728,721; 4,849,228; 5,330,767; 5,476,663; 5,480,656; 5,575,987; 5,631,020; 5,631,021; 5,643,607; 5,716,640; 5,814,342; 5,823,997; 5,980,488; and 6,036,976. Other patents pending.

Adverse Events Reported in ≥ 5% of Patients Regardless of Causality

LUPRON DEPOT-4 Month 30 mg

	Nonorchiectomized, N = 49 Study 013		Orchiectomized, N = 24 Study 012	
	N	(%)	N	(%)
Body As a Whole				
Asthenia	6	(12.2)	1	(4.2)
Flu Syndrome	6	(12.2)	0	(0.0)
General Pain	16	(32.7)	1	(4.2)
Headache	5	(10.2)	1	(4.2)
Injection Site Reaction	4	(8.2)	9	(37.5)
Cardiovascular System				
Hot flashes/Sweats*	23	(46.9)	2	(8.3)
Digestive System				
GI Disorders	5	(10.2)	3	(12.5)
Metabolic and Nutritional Disorders				
Dehydration	4	(8.2)	0	(0.0)
Edema	4	(8.2)	5	(20.8)
Musculoskeletal System				
Joint Disorder	8	(16.3)	1	(4.2)
Myalgia	4	(8.2)	0	(0.0)
Nervous System				
Dizziness/Vertigo	3	(6.1)	2	(8.3)
Neuromuscular Disorders	3	(6.1)	1	(4.2)
Paresthesia	4	(8.2)	1	(4.2)
Respiratory System				
Respiratory Disorder	4	(8.2)	1	(4.2)
Skin and Appendages				
Skin Reaction	6	(12.2)	0	(0.0)
Urogenital System				
Urinary Disorders	5	(10.2)	4	(16.7)

Manufactured for:
Abbott Laboratories
North Chicago, IL 60064
by: Takeda Pharmaceutical Company Limited
Osaka, Japan 540-8645
™– Trademark
® – Registered Trademark
(No. 3683)
Ref: 03-A145
Revised: October, 2008

Shown in Product Identification Guide, page 303

LUPRON DEPOT-PED® ℞

[lū-prŏn dē-pō ped]
(leuprolide acetate for depot suspension)
7.5 mg, 11.25 mg and 15 mg
Rx only

DESCRIPTION

Leuprolide acetate is a synthetic nonapeptide analog of naturally occurring gonadotropin-releasing hormone (GnRH or LH-RH). The analog possesses greater potency than the natural hormone. The chemical name is 5-oxo-L-prolyl-L-histidyl-L-tryptophyl-L-seryl-L-tyrosyl-D-leucyl-L-leucyl-L-arginyl-N-ethyl-L-prolinamide acetate (salt) with the following structural formula:

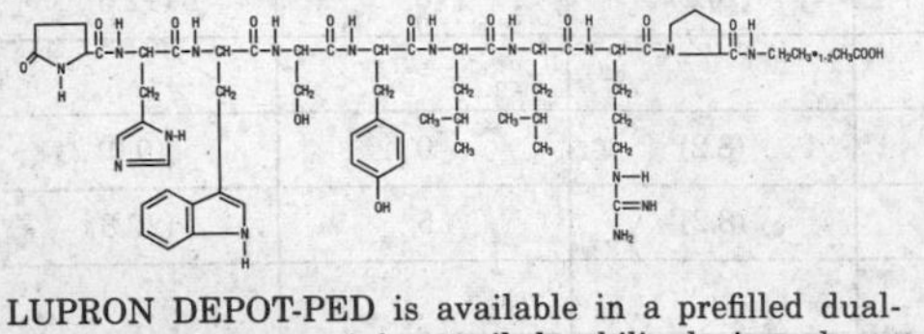

LUPRON DEPOT-PED is available in a prefilled dual-chamber syringe containing sterile lyophilized microspheres which, when mixed with diluent, become a suspension intended as a single intramuscular injection.

The front chamber of LUPRON DEPOT-PED 7.5 mg, 11.25 mg, and 15 mg prefilled dual-chamber syringe contains leuprolide acetate (7.5/11.25/15 mg), purified gelatin (1.3/1.95/2.6 mg), DL-lactic and glycolic acids copolymer (66.2/99.3/132.4 mg), and D-mannitol (13.2/19.8/26.4 mg). The second chamber of diluent contains carboxymethylcellulose sodium (5 mg), D-mannitol (50 mg), polysorbate 80 (1 mg), water for injection, USP, and glacial acetic acid, USP to control pH.

During the manufacture of LUPRON DEPOT-PED, acetic acid is lost, leaving the peptide.

CLINICAL PHARMACOLOGY

Leuprolide acetate, a GnRH agonist, acts as a potent inhibitor of gonadotropin secretion when given continuously and in therapeutic doses. Human studies indicate that following an initial stimulation of gonadotropins, chronic stimulation with leuprolide acetate results in suppression or "downregulation" of these hormones and consequent suppression of ovarian and testicular steroidogenesis. These effects are reversible on discontinuation of drug therapy.

Leuprolide acetate is not active when given orally.

Pharmacokinetics

Absorption

Following a single LUPRON DEPOT 7.5 mg injection to adult patients, mean peak leuprolide plasma concentration was almost 20 ng/mL at 4 hours and then declined to 0.36 ng/mL at 4 weeks. However, intact leuprolide and an inactive major metabolite could not be distinguished by the assay which was employed in the study. Nondetectable leuprolide plasma concentrations have been observed during chronic LUPRON DEPOT 7.5 mg administration, but testosterone levels appear to be maintained at castrate levels.

Distribution

The mean steady-state volume of distribution of leuprolide following intravenous bolus administration to healthy male volunteers was 27 L. *In vitro* binding to human plasma proteins ranged from 43% to 49%.

Metabolism

In healthy male volunteers, a 1 mg bolus of leuprolide administered intravenously revealed that the mean systemic clearance was 7.6 L/h, with a terminal elimination half-life of approximately 3 hours based on a two compartment model.

In rats and dogs, administration of ^{14}C-labeled leuprolide was shown to be metabolized to smaller inactive peptides, a pentapeptide (Metabolite I), tripeptides (Metabolites II and III) and a dipeptide (Metabolite IV). These fragments may be further catabolized.

The major metabolite (M-I) plasma concentrations measured in 5 prostate cancer patients reached maximum concentration 2 to 6 hours after dosing and were approximately 6% of the peak parent drug concentration. One week after dosing, mean plasma M-I concentrations were approximately 20% of mean leuprolide concentrations.

Excretion

Following administration of LUPRON DEPOT 3.75 mg to 3 patients, less than 5% of the dose was recovered as parent and M-I metabolite in the urine.

Special Populations

The pharmacokinetics of the drug in hepatically and renally impaired patients have not been determined.

CLINICAL STUDIES

In children with central precocious puberty (CPP), stimulated and basal gonadotropins are reduced to prepubertal levels. Testosterone and estradiol are reduced to prepubertal levels in males and females respectively. Reduction of gonadotropins will allow for normal physical and psychological growth and development. Natural maturation occurs when gonadotropins return to pubertal levels following discontinuation of leuprolide acetate.

The following physiologic effects have been noted with the chronic administration of leuprolide acetate in this patient population.

1. **Skeletal Growth.** A measurable increase in body length can be noted since the epiphyseal plates will not close prematurely.
2. **Organ Growth.** Reproductive organs will return to a prepubertal state.
3. **Menses.** Menses, if present, will cease.

In a study of 22 children with central precocious puberty, doses of LUPRON DEPOT were given every 4 weeks and plasma levels were determined according to weight categories as summarized below:

[See table below]

INDICATIONS AND USAGE

LUPRON DEPOT-PED is indicated in the treatment of children with central precocious puberty. Children should be selected using the following criteria:

1. Clinical diagnosis of CPP (idiopathic or neurogenic) with onset of secondary sexual characteristics earlier than 8 years in females and 9 years in males.
2. Clinical diagnosis should be confirmed prior to initiation of therapy:
   - Confirmation of diagnosis by a pubertal response to a GnRH stimulation test. The sensitivity and methodology of this assay must be understood.
   - Bone age advanced one year beyond the chronological age.
3. Baseline evaluation should also include:
   - Height and weight measurements.
   - Sex steroid levels.
   - Adrenal steroid level to exclude congenital adrenal hyperplasia.
   - Beta human chorionic gonadotropin level to rule out a chorionic gonadotropin-secreting tumor.
   - Pelvic/adrenal/testicular ultrasound to rule out a steroid secreting tumor.
   - Computerized tomography of the head to rule out intracranial tumor.

CONTRAINDICATIONS

1. Hypersensitivity to GnRH, GnRH agonist analogs or any of the excipients in LUPRON DEPOT. Reports of anaphylactic reactions to GnRH agonist analogs have been reported in the medical literature.[1,2]
2. LUPRON DEPOT-PED is contraindicated in women who are or may become pregnant while receiving the drug. When administered on day 6 of pregnancy at test dosages of 0.00024, 0.0024, and 0.024 mg/kg (1/1200 to 1/12 of the human pediatric dose) to rabbits, LUPRON DEPOT produced a dose-related increase in major fetal abnormalities. Similar studies in rats failed to demonstrate an increase in fetal malformations. There was increased fetal mortality and decreased fetal weights with the two higher doses of LUPRON DEPOT in rabbits and with the highest dose in rats. The effects on fetal mortality are logical consequences of the alterations in hormonal levels brought about by this drug. Therefore, the possibility exists that spontaneous abortion may occur if the drug is administered during pregnancy.

WARNINGS

During the early phase of therapy, gonadotropins and sex steroids rise above baseline because of the natural stimulatory effect of the drug. Therefore, an increase in clinical signs and symptoms may be observed. (See **CLINICAL PHARMACOLOGY** section.)

Noncompliance with drug regimen or inadequate dosing may result in inadequate control of the pubertal process. The consequences of poor control include the return of pubertal signs such as menses, breast development, and testicular growth. The long-term consequences of inadequate control of gonadal steroid secretion are unknown, but may include a further compromise of adult stature.

PRECAUTIONS

Laboratory Tests

Response to LUPRON DEPOT-PED should be monitored 1–2 months after the start of therapy with a GnRH stimulation test and sex steroid levels. Measurement of bone age for advancement should be done every 6–12 months.

Sex steroids may increase or rise above prepubertal levels if the dose is inadequate. (See **WARNINGS** section.) Once a therapeutic dose has been established, gonadotropin and sex steroid levels will decline to prepubertal levels.

Drug Interactions

No pharmacokinetic-based drug-drug interaction studies have been conducted. However, because leuprolide acetate is a peptide that is primarily degraded by peptidase and not by cytochrome P-450 enzymes as noted in specific studies, and the drug is only about 46% bound to plasma proteins, drug interactions would not be expected to occur.

Drug/Laboratory Test Interactions

Administration of LUPRON DEPOT 3.75 mg in women results in suppression of the pituitary-gonadal system. Normal function is usually restored within three months after treatment is discontinued. Therefore, diagnostic tests of pituitary gonadotropic and gonadal functions conducted during treatment and for up to three months after discontinuation of LUPRON DEPOT may be misleading.

Information for Parents

Prior to starting therapy with LUPRON DEPOT-PED, the parent or guardian must be aware of the importance of continuous therapy. Adherence to 4 week drug administration schedules must be accepted if therapy is to be successful.

- During the first 2 months of therapy, a female may experience menses or spotting. If bleeding continues beyond the second month, notify the physician.
- Any irritation at the injection site should be reported to the physician immediately.
- Report any unusual signs or symptoms to the physician.

Carcinogenesis, Mutagenesis, Impairment of Fertility

A two-year carcinogenicity study was conducted in rats and mice. In rats, a dose-related increase of benign pituitary hyperplasia and benign pituitary adenomas was noted at 24 months when the drug was administered subcutaneously at high daily doses (0.6 to 4 mg/kg). There was a significant but not dose-related increase of pancreatic islet-cell adenomas in females and of testicular interstitial cell adenomas in males (highest incidence in the low dose group). In mice, no leuprolide acetate-induced tumors or pituitary abnormalities were observed at a dose as high as 60 mg/kg for two years. Adult patients have been treated with leuprolide acetate for up to three years with doses as high as 10 mg/day and for two years with doses as high as 20 mg/day without demonstrable pituitary abnormalities.

Although no clinical studies have been completed in children to assess the full reversibility of fertility suppression, animal studies (prepubertal and adult rats and monkeys) with leuprolide acetate and other GnRH analogs have shown functional recovery. However, following a study with leuprolide acetate, immature male rats demonstrated tubular degeneration in the testes even after a recovery period. In spite of the failure to recover histologically, the treated males proved to be as fertile as the controls. Also, no histologic changes were observed in the female rats following the same protocol. In both sexes, the offspring of the treated animals appeared normal. The effect of the treatment of the parents on the reproductive performance of the F1 generation was not tested. The clinical significance of these findings is unknown.

Pregnancy

Teratogenic Effects

Pregnancy Category X

(See **CONTRAINDICATIONS** section.)

Nursing Mothers

It is not known whether leuprolide acetate is excreted in human milk. LUPRON should not be used by nursing mothers.

Patient Weight Range (kg)	Group Weight Average (kg)	Dose (mg)	Trough Plasma Leuprolide Level Mean ±SD (ng/mL)*
20.2 - 27.0	22.7	7.5	0.77±0.033
28.4 - 36.8	32.5	11.25	1.25±1.06
39.3 - 57.5	44.2	15.0	1.59±0.65

*Group average values determined at Week 4 immediately prior to leuprolide injection. Drug levels at 12 and 24 weeks were similar to respective 4 week levels.

IMPORTANT NOTICE: Updated drug information is sent bi-monthly via the PDR® Update Insert. For *monthly* email updates, register at PDR.net.

Geriatric Use

See also the labeling for LUPRON DEPOT 7.5 mg which is indicated for the palliative treatment of advanced prostate cancer. For LUPRON DEPOT-PED 11.25 mg and LUPRON DEPOT-PED 15 mg, no clinical information has been established for persons aged 65 and over.

ADVERSE REACTIONS

Clinical Trials

Potential exacerbation of signs and symptoms during the first few weeks of treatment (See **PRECAUTIONS** section) is a concern in patients with rapidly advancing central precocious puberty.

In two studies of children with central precocious puberty, in 2% or more of the patients receiving the drug, the following adverse reactions were reported to have a possible or probable relationship to drug as ascribed by the treating physician. Reactions which are not considered drug-related are excluded.

	Number of Patients N = 395	(%)
Body as a Whole		
General Pain	7	(2)
Integumentary System		
Acne/Seborrhea	7	(2)
Injection Site Reactions		
Including Abscess	21	(5)
Rash Including		
Erythema Multiforme	8	(2)
Urogenital System		
Vaginitis/Bleeding/		
Discharge	7	(2)

In those same studies, the following adverse reactions were reported in less than 2% of the patients.

Body as a Whole - Body Odor, Fever, Headache, Infection; *Cardiovascular System* - Syncope, Vasodilation; *Digestive System* - Dysphagia, Gingivitis, Nausea/Vomiting; *Endocrine System* - Accelerated Sexual Maturity; *Metabolic and Nutritional Disorders* - Peripheral Edema, Weight Gain; *Nervous System* - Emotional Lability, Nervousness, Personality Disorder, Somnolence; *Respiratory System* - Epistaxis; *Integumentary System* - Alopecia, Skin Striae; *Urogenital System* - Cervix Disorder, Gynecomastia/Breast Disorders, Urinary Incontinence.

Postmarketing

During postmarketing surveillance, which includes other dosage forms, the following adverse events were reported. Symptoms consistent with an anaphylactoid or asthmatic process have been rarely reported. Rash, urticaria, and photosensitivity reactions have also been reported.

Localized reactions including induration and abscess have been reported at the site of injection.

Cardiovascular System - Hypotension; *Hemic and Lymphatic System* - Decreased WBC; *Central/Peripheral Nervous System* - Peripheral neuropathy, Spinal fracture/paralysis; *Musculoskeletal System* - Tenosynovitis-like symptoms; *Urogenital System* - Prostate pain.

Pituitary apoplexy: During post-marketing surveillance, rare cases of pituitary apoplexy (a clinical syndrome secondary to infarction of the pituitary gland) have been reported after the administration of gonadotropin-releasing hormone agonists. In a majority of these cases, a pituitary adenoma was diagnosed, with a majority of pituitary apoplexy cases occurring within 2 weeks of the first dose, and some within the first hour. In these cases, pituitary apoplexy has presented as sudden headache, vomiting, visual changes, ophthalmoplegia, altered mental status, and sometimes cardiovascular collapse. Immediate medical attention has been required.

See other LUPRON DEPOT and LUPRON Injection package inserts for other events reported in different patient populations.

OVERDOSAGE

In rats, subcutaneous administration of 125 to 250 times the recommended human pediatric dose, expressed on a per body weight basis, resulted in dyspnea, decreased activity, and local irritation at the injection site. There is no evidence at present that there is a clinical counterpart of this phenomenon. In early clinical trials using leuprolide acetate in adult patients, doses as high as 20 mg/day for up to two years caused no adverse effects differing from those observed with the 1 mg/day dose.

DOSAGE AND ADMINISTRATION

LUPRON DEPOT-PED must be administered under the supervision of a physician.

The dose of LUPRON DEPOT-PED must be individualized for each child. The dose is based on a mg/kg ratio of drug to body weight. Younger children require higher doses on a mg/kg ratio.

For each dosage form, after 1–2 months of initiating therapy or changing doses, the child must be monitored with a GnRH stimulation test, sex steroids, and Tanner staging to confirm downregulation. Measurements of bone age for advancement should be monitored every 6–12 months. The dose should be titrated upward until no progression of the condition is noted either clinically and/or by laboratory parameters.

The first dose found to result in adequate downregulation can probably be maintained for the duration of therapy in most children. However, there are insufficient data to guide dosage adjustment as patients move into higher weight categories after beginning therapy at very young ages and low dosages. It is recommended that adequate downregulation be verified in such patients whose weight has increased significantly while on therapy.

Discontinuation of LUPRON DEPOT-PED should be considered before age 11 for females and age 12 for males.

The recommended starting dose is 0.3 mg/kg/4 weeks (minimum 7.5 mg) administered as a single intramuscular injection. The starting dose will be dictated by the child's weight.

≤ 25 kg	7.5 mg
>25-37.5 kg	11.25 mg
>37.5 kg	15 mg

If total downregulation is not achieved, the dose should be titrated upward in increments of 3.75 mg every 4 weeks. This dose will be considered the maintenance dose.

The lyophilized microspheres are to be reconstituted and administered as a single intramuscular injection. *For optimal performance of the prefilled dual chamber syringe (PDS), read and follow the following instructions:*

- The lyophilized microspheres are to be reconstituted and administered as a single intramuscular injection.
- Since LUPRON DEPOT-PED does not contain a preservative, the suspension should be discarded if not used immediately.

1. The LUPRON DEPOT powder should be visually inspected and the syringe should NOT BE USED if clumping or caking is evident. A thin layer of powder on the wall of the syringe is considered normal. The diluent should appear clear.
2. To prepare for injection, screw the white plunger into the end stopper until the stopper begins to turn.
3. Hold the syringe UPRIGHT. Release the diluent by SLOWLY PUSHING (6 to 8 seconds) the plunger until the first stopper is <u>at the blue line</u> in the middle of the barrel.
4. Keep the syringe UPRIGHT. Gently mix the microspheres (powder) thoroughly to form a uniform suspension. The suspension will appear milky. If the powder adheres to the stopper or caking/clumping is present, tap the syringe with your finger to disperse. DO NOT USE if any of the powder has not gone into suspension.
5. Hold the syringe UPRIGHT. With the opposite hand pull the needle cap upward without twisting.
6. Keep the syringe UPRIGHT. Advance the plunger to expel the air from the syringe.
   NOTE: Aspirated blood would be visible just below the luer lock connection if a blood vessel is accidentally penetrated. If present, blood can be seen through the transparent LuproLoc™ safety device. If blood is present remove the needle immediately. Do not inject the medication.
7. Inject the entire contents of the syringe intramuscularly at the time of reconstitution. The suspension settles very quickly following reconstitution; therefore, LUPRON DEPOT should be mixed and used immediately.
   AFTER INJECTION
8. Withdraw the needle. Immediately activate the LuproLoc™ safety device by pushing the arrow forward with the thumb or finger until the device is fully extended and a CLICK is heard or felt.

Since the product does not contain a preservative, the suspension should be discarded if not used immediately. As with other drugs administered by injection, the injection site should be varied periodically.

HOW SUPPLIED

LUPRON DEPOT-PED is packaged as follows:

Kit with prefilled dual-chamber syringe	7.5 mg	NDC 0074-2108-03
Kit with prefilled dual-chamber syringe	11.25 mg	NDC 0074-2282-03
Kit with prefilled dual-chamber syringe	15 mg	NDC 0074-2440-03

Each syringe contains sterile lyophilized microspheres of leuprolide acetate incorporated in a biodegradable lactic acid/glycolic acid copolymer. When mixed with 1 milliliter of accompanying diluent, LUPRON DEPOT-PED is administered as a single intramuscular injection.

Each kit contains:
- one prefilled dual-chamber syringe
- one plunger
- two alcohol swabs
- instructions for how to mix and administer
- an information pamphlet for patients
- a complete prescribing information enclosure

Store at 25°C (77°F); excursions permitted to 15–30°C (59–86°F) [See USP Controlled Room Temperature]

REFERENCES

1. Taylor, JD. Anaphylactic reaction to LHRH analogue, leuprorelin. *Med J Australia* 1994 Oct; 161(3): 455.
2. Letterie GS, *et al.* Recurrent anaphylaxis to a depot form of GnRH analogue. *Obstet Gynecol* 1991 Nov; 78: 943–946.

U.S. Patent Nos. 4,652,441; 4,677,191; 4,728,721; 4,849,228; 4,917,893; 5,330,767; 5,476,663; 5,823,997; 5,980,488; and 6,036,976. Other patents pending.

Manufactured for:
Abbott Laboratories
North Chicago, IL 60064
by: Takeda Pharmaceutical Company Limited
Osaka, Japan 540-8645
™ -Trademark
® -Registered Trademark
(Nos. 2108, 2282, 2440)
03-A140-R16
Revised: June, 2008
© 2008, Abbott Laboratories
Shown in Product Identification Guide, page 303

MAVIK®

[*MAH-vic*]

(trandolapril tablets)

℞

USE IN PREGNANCY

When used in pregnancy during the second and third trimesters, ACE inhibitors can cause injury and even death to the developing fetus. When pregnancy is detected, MAVIK® should be discontinued as soon as possible. See WARNINGS - Fetal/Neonatal Morbidity and Mortality.

DESCRIPTION

Trandolapril is the ethyl ester prodrug of a nonsulfhydryl angiotensin converting enzyme (ACE) inhibitor, trandolaprilat. Trandolapril is chemically described as (2S, 3aR, 7aS)-1-[(S)-N-[(S)-1-Carboxy-3-phenylpropyl]alanyl] hexahydro-2-indolinecarboxylic acid, 1-ethyl ester. Its empirical formula is $C_{24}H_{34}N_2O_5$ and its structural formula is

R = C₂ H₅, Trandolapril
= H, Trandolaprilat (diacid)

M.W. = 430.54

Melting Point = 125°C

Trandolapril is a white or almost white powder that is soluble (> 100 mg/mL) in chloroform, dichloromethane, and methanol. MAVIK tablets contain 1 mg, 2 mg, or 4 mg of trandolapril for oral administration. Each tablet also contains corn starch, croscarmellose sodium, hypromellose, iron oxide, lactose monohydrate, povidone, sodium stearyl fumarate.

CLINICAL PHARMACOLOGY

Mechanism of Action

Trandolapril is deesterified to the diacid metabolite, trandolaprilat, which is approximately eight times more active as an inhibitor of ACE activity. ACE is a peptidyl dipeptidase that catalyzes the conversion of angiotensin I to the vasoconstrictor, angiotensin II. Angiotensin II is a potent peripheral vasoconstrictor that also stimulates secretion of aldosterone by the adrenal cortex and provides negative

---

feedback for renin secretion. The effect of trandolapril in hypertension appears to result primarily from the inhibition of circulating and tissue ACE activity thereby reducing angiotensin II formation, decreasing vasoconstriction, decreasing aldosterone secretion, and increasing plasma renin. Decreased aldosterone secretion leads to diuresis, natriuresis, and a small increase of serum potassium. In controlled clinical trials, treatment with MAVIK alone resulted in mean increases in potassium of 0.1 mEq/L. (See **PRECAUTIONS.**)

ACE is identical to kininase II, an enzyme that degrades bradykinin, a potent peptide vasodilator; whether increased levels of bradykinin play a role in the therapeutic effect of trandolapril remains to be elucidated.

While the principal mechanism of antihypertensive effect is thought to be through the renin-angiotensin-aldosterone system, trandolapril exerts antihypertensive actions even in patients with low-renin hypertension. MAVIK was an effective antihypertensive in all races studied. Both black patients (usually a predominantly low-renin group) and non-black patients responded to 2 to 4 mg of MAVIK.

Pharmacokinetics and Metabolism

Pharmacokinetics

Trandolapril's ACE-inhibiting activity is primarily due to its diacid metabolite, trandolaprilat. Cleavage of the ester group of trandolapril, primarily in the liver, is responsible for conversion. Absolute bioavailability after oral administration of trandolapril is about 10% as trandolapril and 70% as trandolaprilat. After oral trandolapril under fasting conditions, peak trandolapril levels occur at about one hour and peak trandolaprilat levels occur between 4 and 10 hours. The elimination half-life of trandolapril is about 6 hours. At steady state, the effective half-life of trandolaprilat is 22.5 hours. Like all ACE inhibitors, trandolaprilat also has a prolonged terminal elimination phase, involving a small fraction of administered drug, probably representing binding to plasma and tissue ACE. During multiple dosing of trandolapril, there is no significant accumulation of trandolaprilat. Food slows absorption of trandolapril, but does not affect AUC or C_{max} of trandolaprilat or C_{max} of trandolapril.

Metabolism and Excretion

After oral administration of trandolapril, about 33% of parent drug and metabolites are recovered in urine, mostly as trandolaprilat, with about 66% in feces. The extent of the absorbed dose which is biliary excreted has not been determined. Plasma concentrations (C_{max} and AUC of trandolapril and C_{max} of trandolaprilat) are dose proportional over the 1-4 mg range, but the AUC of trandolaprilat is somewhat less than dose proportional. In addition to trandolaprilat, at least 7 other metabolites have been found, principally glucuronides or deesterification products.

Serum protein binding of trandolapril is about 80%, and is independent of concentration. Binding of trandolaprilat is concentration-dependent, varying from 65% at 1000 ng/mL to 94% at 0.1 ng/mL, indicating saturation of binding with increasing concentration.

The volume of distribution of trandolapril is about 18 liters. Total plasma clearances of trandolapril and trandolaprilat after approximately 2 mg IV doses are about 52 liters/hour and 7 liters/hour respectively. Renal clearance of trandolaprilat varies from 1-4 liters/hour, depending on dose.

Special Populations

Pediatric

Trandolapril pharmacokinetics have not been evaluated in patients < 18 years of age.

Geriatric and Gender

Trandolapril pharmacokinetics have been investigated in the elderly (> 65 years) and in both genders. The plasma concentration of trandolapril is increased in elderly hypertensive patients, but the plasma concentration of trandolaprilat and inhibition of ACE activity are similar in elderly and young hypertensive patients. The pharmacokinetics of trandolapril and trandolaprilat and inhibition of ACE activity are similar in male and female elderly hypertensive patients.

Race

Pharmacokinetic differences have not been evaluated in different races.

Renal Insufficiency

Compared to normal subjects, the plasma concentrations of trandolapril and trandolaprilat are approximately 2-fold greater and renal clearance is reduced by about 85% in patients with creatinine clearance below 30 ml/min and in patients on hemodialysis. Dosage adjustment is recommended in renally impaired patients. (See **DOSAGE AND ADMINISTRATION.**)

Hepatic Insufficiency

Following oral administration in patients with mild to moderate alcoholic cirrhosis, plasma concentrations of trandolapril and trandolaprilat were, respectively, 9-fold and 2-fold greater than in normal subjects, but inhibition of ACE activity was not affected. Lower doses should be considered in patients with hepatic insufficiency. (See **DOSAGE AND ADMINISTRATION.**)

Drug Interactions

Trandolapril did not affect the plasma concentration (predose and 2 hours post-dose) of oral digoxin (0.25 mg). Coadministration of trandolapril and cimetidine led to an increase of about 44% in C_{max} for trandolapril, but no difference in the pharmacokinetics of trandolaprilat or in ACE inhibition. Coadministration of trandolapril and furosemide led to an increase of about 25% in the renal clearance of trandolaprilat, but no effect was seen on the pharmacokinetics of furosemide or trandolaprilat or on ACE inhibition.

Pharmacodynamics and Clinical Effects

A single 2-mg dose of MAVIK produces 70 to 85% inhibition of plasma ACE activity at 4 hours with about 10% decline at 24 hours and about half the effect manifest at 8 days. Maximum ACE inhibition is achieved with a plasma trandolaprilat concentration of 2 ng/mL. ACE inhibition is a function of trandolaprilat concentration, not trandolapril concentration. The effect of trandolapril on exogenous angiotensin I was not measured.

Hypertension

Four placebo-controlled dose response studies were conducted using once-daily oral dosing of MAVIK in doses from 0.25 to 16 mg per day in 827 black and non-black patients with mild to moderate hypertension. The minimal effective once-daily dose was 1 mg in non-black patients and 2 mg in black patients. Further decreases in trough supine diastolic blood pressure were obtained in non-black patients with higher doses, and no further response was seen with doses above 4 mg (up to 16 mg). The antihypertensive effect diminished somewhat at the end of the dosing interval, but trough/peak ratios are well above 50% for all effective doses. There was a slightly greater effect on the diastolic pressure, but no difference on systolic pressure with b.i.d. dosing. During chronic therapy, the maximum reduction in blood pressure with any dose is achieved within one week. Following 6 weeks of monotherapy in placebo-controlled trials in patients with mild to moderate hypertension, once-daily doses of 2 to 4 mg lowered supine or standing systolic/diastolic blood pressure 24 hours after dosing by an average 7-10/4-5 mmHg below placebo responses in non-black patients. Once-daily doses of 2 to 4 mg lowered blood pressure 4-6/3-4 mmHg in black patients. Trough to peak ratios for effective doses ranged from 0.5 to 0.9. There were no differences in response between men and women, but responses were somewhat greater in patients under 60 than in patients over 60 years old. Abrupt withdrawal of MAVIK has not been associated with a rapid increase in blood pressure. Administration of MAVIK to patients with mild to moderate hypertension results in a reduction of supine, sitting and standing blood pressure to about the same extent without compensatory tachycardia.

Symptomatic hypotension is infrequent, although it can occur in patients who are salt- and/or volume-depleted. (See **WARNINGS.**) Use of MAVIK in combination with thiazide diuretics gives a blood pressure lowering effect greater than that seen with either agent alone, and the additional effect of trandolapril is similar to the effect of monotherapy.

Heart Failure Post Myocardial Infarction or Left Ventricular Dysfunction Post Myocardial Infarction

The Trandolapril Cardiac Evaluation (TRACE) Trial was a Danish, 27-center, double-blind, placebo controlled, parallel-group study of the effect of trandolapril on all-cause mortality in stable patients with echocardiographic evidence of left ventricular dysfunction 3 to 7 days after a myocardial infarction. Subjects with residual ischemia or overt heart failure were included. Patients tolerant of a test dose of 1 mg trandolapril were randomized to placebo (n=873) or trandolapril (n=876) and followed for 24 months. Among patients randomized to trandolapril, who began treatment on 1 mg, 62% were successfully titrated to a target dose of 4 mg once daily over a period of weeks. The use of trandolapril was associated with a 16% reduction in the risk of all-cause mortality (p=0.042), largely cardiovascular mortality. Trandolapril was also associated with a 20% reduction in the risk of progression of heart failure (p=0.047), defined by a time-to-first-event analysis of death attributed to heart failure, hospitalization for heart failure, or requirement for open-label ACE inhibitor for the treatment of heart failure. There was no significant effect of treatment on other endpoints: subsequent hospitalization, incidence of recurrent myocardial infarction, exercise tolerance, ventricular function, ventricular dimensions, or NYHA class.

The population in TRACE was entirely Caucasian and had less usage than would be typical in a U.S. population of other post-infarction interventions: 42% thrombolysis, 16% beta-adrenergic blockade, and 6.7% PTCA or CABG during the entire period of follow-up. Blood pressure control, especially in the placebo group, was poor: 47 to 53% of patients randomized to placebo and 32 to 40% of patients randomized to trandolapril had blood pressures > 140/95 at 90-day follow-up visits.

INDICATIONS AND USAGE

Hypertension

MAVIK is indicated for the treatment of hypertension. It may be used alone or in combination with other antihypertensive medication such as hydrochlorothiazide.

In considering the use of MAVIK, it should be noted that in controlled trials ACE inhibitors (for which adequate data are available) cause a higher rate of angioedema in black than in non-black patients. (See **WARNINGS - Angioedema.**)

When using MAVIK, consideration should be given to the fact that another angiotensin converting enzyme inhibitor, captopril, has caused agranulocytosis, particularly in patients with renal impairment or collagen-vascular disease. Available data are insufficient to show that MAVIK does not have a similar risk. (See **WARNINGS.**)

Heart Failure Post Myocardial Infarction or Left-Ventricular Dysfunction Post Myocardial Infarction

MAVIK is indicated in stable patients who have evidence of left-ventricular systolic dysfunction (identified by wall motion abnormalities) or who are symptomatic from congestive heart failure within the first few days after sustaining acute myocardial infarction. Administration of trandolapril to Caucasian patients has been shown to decrease the risk of death (principally cardiovascular death) and to decrease the risk of heart failure-related hospitalization (see **CLINICAL PHARMACOLOGY - Heart Failure or Left-Ventricular Dysfunction Post Myocardial Infarction** for details of the survival trial).

CONTRAINDICATIONS

MAVIK is contraindicated in patients who are hypersensitive to this product and in patients with a history of angioedema related to previous treatment with an ACE inhibitor.

WARNINGS

Anaphylactoid and Possibly Related Reactions

Presumably because angiotensin converting enzyme inhibitors affect the metabolism of eicosanoids and polypeptides, including endogenous bradykinin, patients receiving ACE inhibitors, including MAVIK, may be subject to a variety of adverse reactions, some of them serious.

Anaphylactoid Reactions During Desensitization

Two patients undergoing desensitizing treatment with hymenoptera venom while receiving ACE inhibitors sustained life-threatening anaphylactoid reactions. In the same patients, these reactions did not occur when ACE inhibitors were temporarily withheld, but they reappeared when the ACE inhibitors were inadvertently readministered.

Anaphylactoid Reactions During Membrane Exposure

Anaphylactoid reactions have been reported in patients dialyzed with high-flux membranes and treated concomitantly with an ACE inhibitor. Anaphylactoid reactions have also been reported in patients undergoing low-density lipoprotein apheresis with dextran sulfate absorption.

Head and Neck Angioedema

Angioedema of the face, extremities, lips, tongue, glottis, and larynx has been reported in patients treated with ACE inhibitors including MAVIK. Symptoms suggestive of angioedema or facial edema occurred in 0.13% of MAVIK-treated patients. Two of the four cases were life-threatening and resolved without treatment or with medication (corticosteroids). Angioedema associated with laryngeal edema can be fatal. If laryngeal stridor or angioedema of the face, tongue or glottis occurs, treatment with MAVIK should be discontinued immediately, the patient treated in accordance with accepted medical care and carefully observed until the swelling disappears. In instances where swelling is confined to the face and lips, the condition generally resolves without treatment; antihistamines may be useful in relieving symptoms. **Where there is involvement of the tongue, glottis, or larynx, likely to cause airway obstruction, emergency therapy, including but not limited to subcutaneous epinephrine solution 1:1,000 (0.3 to 0.5 mL) should be promptly administered.** (See **PRECAUTIONS - Information for Patients** and **ADVERSE REACTIONS.**)

Intestinal Angioedema

Intestinal angioedema has been reported in patients treated with ACE inhibitors. These patients presented with abdominal pain (with or without nausea or vomiting); in some cases there was no prior history of facial angioedema and C-1 esterase levels were normal. The angioedema was diagnosed by procedures including abdominal CT scan or ultrasound, or at surgery, and symptoms resolved after stopping the ACE inhibitor. Intestinal angioedema should be included in the differential diagnosis of patients on ACE inhibitors presenting with abdominal pain.

Hypotension

MAVIK can cause symptomatic hypotension. Like other ACE inhibitors, MAVIK has only rarely been associated with symptomatic hypotension in uncomplicated hypertensive patients. Symptomatic hypotension is most likely to occur in patients who have been salt- or volume-depleted as a result of prolonged treatment with diuretics, dietary salt restriction, dialysis, diarrhea, or vomiting. Volume and/or salt depletion should be corrected before initiating treatment with MAVIK. (See **PRECAUTIONS - Drug Interactions**, and **ADVERSE REACTIONS**.) In controlled and uncontrolled studies, hypotension was reported as an adverse event in 0.6% of patients and led to discontinuations in 0.1% of patients.

In patients with concomitant congestive heart failure, with or without associated renal insufficiency, ACE inhibitor therapy may cause excessive hypotension, which may be associated with oliguria or azotemia, and rarely, with acute renal failure and death. In such patients, MAVIK therapy should be started at the recommended dose under close medical supervision. These patients should be followed closely during the first 2 weeks of treatment and, thereafter, whenever the dosage of MAVIK or diuretic is increased. (See **DOSAGE AND ADMINISTRATION**.) Care in avoiding hypotension should also be taken in patients with ischemic heart disease, aortic stenosis, or cerebrovascular disease.

If symptomatic hypotension occurs, the patient should be placed in the supine position and, if necessary, normal saline may be administered intravenously. A transient hypotensive response is not a contraindication to further doses; however, lower doses of MAVIK or reduced concomitant diuretic therapy should be considered.

Neutropenia/Agranulocytosis
Another ACE inhibitor, captopril, has been shown to cause agranulocytosis and bone marrow depression rarely in patients with uncomplicated hypertension, but more frequently in patients with renal impairment, especially if they also have a collagen-vascular disease such as systemic lupus erythematosus or scleroderma. Available data from clinical trials of trandolapril are insufficient to show that trandolapril does not cause agranulocytosis at similar rates. As with other ACE inhibitors, periodic monitoring of white blood cell counts in patients with collagen-vascular disease and/or renal disease should be considered.

Hepatic Failure
ACE inhibitors rarely have been associated with a syndrome of cholestatic jaundice, fulminant hepatic necrosis, and death. The mechanism of this syndrome is not understood. Patients receiving ACE inhibitors who develop jaundice should discontinue the ACE inhibitor and receive appropriate medical follow-up.

Fetal/Neonatal Morbidity and Mortality
ACE inhibitors can cause fetal and neonatal morbidity and death when administered to pregnant women. Several dozen cases have been reported in the world literature. When pregnancy is detected, ACE inhibitors should be discontinued as soon as possible.

The use of ACE inhibitors during the second and third trimesters of pregnancy has been associated with fetal and neonatal injury, including hypotension, neonatal skull hypoplasia, anuria, reversible or irreversible renal failure, and death. Oligohydramnios has also been reported, presumably resulting from decreased fetal renal function; oligohydramnios in this setting has been associated with fetal limb contractures, craniofacial deformation, and hypoplastic lung development. Prematurity, intrauterine growth retardation, and patent ductus arteriosus have also been reported, although it is not clear whether these occurrences were due to the ACE inhibitor exposure.

These adverse effects do not appear to have resulted from intrauterine ACE-inhibitor exposure that has been limited to the first trimester. Mothers whose embryos and fetuses are exposed to ACE inhibitors only during the first trimester should be so informed. Nonetheless, when patients become pregnant, physicians should make every effort to discontinue the use of trandolapril as soon as possible.

Rarely (probably less often than once in every thousand pregnancies), no alternative to ACE inhibitors will be found. In these rare cases, the mothers should be apprised of the potential hazards to their fetuses, and serial ultrasound examinations should be performed to assess the intra-amniotic environment.

If oligohydramnios is observed, trandolapril should be discontinued unless it is considered life-saving for the mother. Contraction stress testing (CST), a non-stress test (NST), or biophysical profiling (BPP) may be appropriate, depending upon the week of pregnancy.

Patients and physicians should be aware, however, that oligohydramnios may not appear until after the fetus has sustained irreversible injury.

Infants with histories of *in utero* exposure to ACE inhibitors should be closely observed for hypotension, oliguria, and hyperkalemia. If oliguria occurs, attention should be directed toward support of blood pressure and renal perfusion. Exchange transfusions or dialysis may be required as a means of reversing hypotension and/or substituting for disordered renal function.

Doses of 0.8 mg/kg/day (9.4 mg/m^2/day) in rabbits, 1000 mg/kg/day (7000 mg/m^2/day) in rats, and 25 mg/kg/day (295 mg/m^2/day) in cynomolgus monkeys did not produce teratogenic effects. These doses represent 10 and 3 times (rabbits), 1250 and 2564 times (rats), and 312 and 108 times (monkeys) the

maximum projected human dose of 4 mg based on body-weight and body-surface-area, respectively assuming a 50 kg woman.

PRECAUTIONS
General
Impaired Renal Function
As a consequence of inhibiting the renin-angiotensin-aldosterone system, changes in renal function may be anticipated in susceptible individuals. In patients with severe heart failure whose renal function may depend on the activity of the renin-angiotensin-aldosterone system, treatment with ACE inhibitors, including MAVIK® (trandolapril), may be associated with oliguria and/or progressive azotemia and rarely with acute renal failure and/or death.

In hypertensive patients with unilateral or bilateral renal artery stenosis, increases in blood urea nitrogen and serum creatinine have been observed in some patients following ACE inhibitor therapy. These increases were almost always reversible upon discontinuation of the ACE inhibitor and/or diuretic therapy. In such patients, renal function should be monitored during the first few weeks of therapy.

Some hypertensive patients with no apparent preexisting renal vascular disease have developed increases in blood urea and serum creatinine, usually minor and transient, especially when ACE inhibitors have been given concomitantly with a diuretic. This is more likely to occur in patients with preexisting renal impairment. Dosage reduction and/or discontinuation of any diuretic and/or the ACE inhibitor may be required. **Evaluation of hypertensive patients should always include assessment of renal function.** (See **DOSAGE AND ADMINISTRATION**.)

Hyperkalemia and Potassium-sparing Diuretics
In clinical trials, hyperkalemia (serum potassium > 6.00 mEq/L) occurred in approximately 0.4% of hypertensive patients receiving MAVIK. In most cases, elevated serum potassium levels were isolated values, which resolved despite continued therapy. None of these patients were discontinued from the trials because of hyperkalemia. Risk factors for the development of hyperkalemia include renal insufficiency, diabetes mellitus, and the concomitant use of potassium-sparing diuretics, potassium supplements, and/or potassium-containing salt substitutes, which should be used cautiously, if at all, with MAVIK. (See **PRECAUTIONS - Drug Interactions**.)

Cough
Presumably due to the inhibition of the degradation of endogenous bradykinin, persistent nonproductive cough has been reported with all ACE inhibitors, always resolving after discontinuation of therapy. ACE inhibitor-induced cough should be considered in the differential diagnosis of cough. In controlled trials of trandolapril, cough was present in 2% of trandolapril patients and 0% of patients given placebo. There was no evidence of a relationship to dose.

Surgery/Anesthesia
In patients undergoing major surgery or during anesthesia with agents that produce hypotension, MAVIK will block angiotensin II formation secondary to compensatory renin release. If hypotension occurs and is considered to be due to this mechanism, it can be corrected by volume expansion.

Information for Patients
Angioedema
Angioedema, including laryngeal edema, may occur at any time during treatment with ACE inhibitors, including MAVIK. Patients should be so advised and told to report immediately any signs or symptoms suggesting angioedema (swelling of face, extremities, eyes, lips, tongue, difficulty in swallowing or breathing) and to stop taking the drug until they have consulted with their physician. (See **WARNINGS** and **ADVERSE REACTIONS**.)

Symptomatic Hypotension
Patients should be cautioned that light-headedness can occur, especially during the first days of MAVIK therapy, and should be reported to a physician. If actual syncope occurs, patients should be told to stop taking the drug until they have consulted with their physician (see **WARNINGS**).

All patients should be cautioned that inadequate fluid intake, excessive perspiration, diarrhea, or vomiting, resulting in reduced fluid volume, may precipitate an excessive fall in blood pressure with the same consequences of light-headedness and possible syncope.

Patients planning to undergo any surgery and/or anesthesia should be told to inform their physician that they are taking an ACE inhibitor that has a long duration of action.

Hyperkalemia
Patients should be told not to use potassium supplements or salt substitutes containing potassium without consulting their physician. (See **PRECAUTIONS**.)

Neutropenia
Patients should be told to report promptly any indication of infection (e.g., sore throat, fever) which could be a sign of neutropenia.

Pregnancy
Female patients of childbearing age should be told about the consequences of second- and third-trimester exposure to ACE inhibitors, and they should also be told that these consequences do not appear to have resulted from intrauterine ACE-inhibitor exposure that has been limited to the first trimester. These patients should be asked to report pregnancies to their physicians as soon as possible.

NOTE: As with many other drugs, certain advice to patients being treated with MAVIK is warranted. This information is intended to aid in the safe and effective use of this medication. It is not a disclosure of all possible adverse or intended effects.

Drug Interactions
Concomitant Diuretic Therapy
As with other ACE inhibitors, patients on diuretics, especially those on recently instituted diuretic therapy, may experience an excessive reduction of blood pressure after initiation of therapy with MAVIK. The possibility of exacerbation of hypotensive effects with MAVIK may be minimized by either discontinuing the diuretic or cautiously increasing salt intake prior to initiation of treatment with MAVIK. If it is not possible to discontinue the diuretic, the starting dose of trandolapril should be reduced. (See **DOSAGE AND ADMINISTRATION**.)

Agents Increasing Serum Potassium
Trandolapril can attenuate potassium loss caused by thiazide diuretics and increase serum potassium when used alone. Use of potassium-sparing diuretics (spironolactone, triamterene, or amiloride), potassium supplements, or potassium-containing salt substitutes concomitantly with ACE inhibitors can increase the risk of hyperkalemia. If concomitant use of such agents is indicated, they should be used with caution and with appropriate monitoring of serum potassium. (See **PRECAUTIONS**.)

Lithium
Increased serum lithium levels and symptoms of lithium toxicity have been reported in patients receiving concomitant lithium and ACE inhibitor therapy. These drugs should be coadministered with caution, and frequent monitoring of serum lithium levels is recommended. If a diuretic is also used, the risk of lithium toxicity may be increased.

Gold
Nitritoid reactions (symptoms include facial flushing, nausea, vomiting and hypotension) have been reported rarely in patients on therapy with injectable gold (sodium aurothiomalate) and concomitant ACE inhibitor therapy including MAVIK.

Other
No clinically significant pharmacokinetic interaction has been found between trandolaprilat and food, cimetidine, digoxin, or furosemide.

The anticoagulant effect of warfarin was not significantly changed by trandolapril.

As with all other inhibitors of RAS, NSAIDs may reduce the antihypertensive effects of trandolapril. Blood pressure monitoring should be increased when any NSAID is added or discontinued in a patient treated with trandolapril.

The hypotensive effect of certain inhalation anesthetics may be enhanced by ACE inhibitors including trandolapril (See **PRECAUTIONS-Surgery/Anesthesia**.)

Carcinogenesis, Mutagenesis, Impairment of Fertility
Long-term studies were conducted with oral trandolapril administered by gavage to mice (78 weeks) and rats (104 and 106 weeks). No evidence of carcinogenic potential was seen in mice dosed up to 25 mg/kg/day (85 mg/m^2/day) or rats dosed up to 8 mg/kg/day (60 mg/m^2/day). These doses are 313 and 32 times (mice), and 100 and 23 times (rats) the maximum recommended human daily dose (MRHDD) of 4 mg based on body-weight and body-surface-area, respectively assuming a 50 kg individual. The genotoxic potential of trandolapril was evaluated in the microbial mutagenicity (Ames) test, the point mutation and chromosome aberration assays in Chinese hamster V79 cells, and the micronucleus test in mice. There was no evidence of mutagenic or clastogenic potential in these *in vitro* and *in vivo* assays.

Reproduction studies in rats did not show any impairment of fertility at doses up to 100 mg/kg/day (710 mg/m^2/day) of trandolapril, or 1250 and 260 times the MRHDD on the basis of body-weight and body-surface-area, respectively.

Pregnancy
Pregnancy Categories C (first trimester) and D (second and third trimesters)

(See WARNINGS - Fetal/Neonatal Morbidity and Mortality.)

Information on the Abbott Pharmaceutical Products listed on these pages is from the prescribing information in use as of June 1, 2010. For more information, please visit rxabbott.com or call 1-800-633-9110.

Nursing Mothers

Radiolabeled trandolapril or its metabolites are secreted in rat milk. MAVIK should not be administered to nursing mothers.

Geriatric Use

In placebo-controlled studies of MAVIK, 31.1% of patients were 60 years and older, 20.1% were 65 years and older, and 2.3% were 75 years and older. No overall differences in effectiveness or safety were observed between these patients and younger patients. (Greater sensitivity of some older individual patients cannot be ruled out).

Pediatric Use

The safety and effectiveness of MAVIK in pediatric patients have not been established.

ADVERSE REACTIONS

The safety experience in U.S. placebo-controlled trials included 1069 hypertensive patients, of whom 832 received MAVIK. Nearly 200 hypertensive patients received MAVIK for over one year in open-label trials. In controlled trials, withdrawals for adverse events were 2.1% on placebo and 1.4% on MAVIK. Adverse events considered at least possibly related to treatment occurring in 1% of MAVIK-treated patients and more common on MAVIK than placebo, pooled for all doses, are shown below, together with the frequency of discontinuation of treatment because of these events.

ADVERSE EVENTS IN PLACEBO-CONTROLLED HYPERTENSION TRIALS

| | Occurring at 1% or greater | |
	MAVIK (N=832) % Incidence (% Discontinuance)	PLACEBO (N=237) % Incidence (% Discontinuance)
Cough	1.9 (0.1)	0.4 (0.4)
Dizziness	1.3 (0.2)	0.4 (0.4)
Diarrhea	1.0 (0.0)	0.4 (0.0)

Headache and fatigue were all seen in more than 1% of MAVIK-treated patients but were more frequently seen on placebo. Adverse events were not usually persistent or difficult to manage.

Left Ventricular Dysfunction Post Myocardial Infarction

Adverse reactions related to MAVIK occurring at a rate greater than that observed in placebo-treated patients with left ventricular dysfunction, are shown below. The incidences represent the experiences from the TRACE study. The follow-up time was between 24 and 50 months for this study.

Percentage of Patients with Adverse Events Greater Than Placebo

| | Placebo-Controlled (TRACE) Mortality Study | |
Adverse Event	Trandolapril N=876	Placebo N=873
Cough	35	22
Dizziness	23	17
Hypotension	11	6.8
Elevated serum uric acid	15	13
Elevated BUN	9.0	7.6
PICA or CABG	7.3	6.1
Dyspepsia	6.4	6.0
Syncope	5.9	3.3
Hyperkalemia	5.3	2.8
Bradycardia	4.7	4.4
Hypocalcemia	4.7	3.9
Myalgia	4.7	3.1
Elevated creatinine	4.7	2.4
Gastritis	4.2	3.6
Cardiogenic shock	3.8	< 2
Intermittent claudication	3.8	< 2
Stroke	3.3	3.2
Asthenia	3.3	2.6

Clinical adverse experiences possibly or probably related or of uncertain relationship to therapy occurring in 0.3% to 1.0% (except as noted) of the patients treated with MAVIK (with or without concomitant calcium ion antagonist or diuretic) in controlled or uncontrolled trials (N=1134) and less frequent, clinically significant events seen in clinical trials or post-marketing experience include (listed by body system):

General Body Function
Chest pain, malaise, fever.

Cardiovascular
AV first degree block, bradycardia, edema, flushing, hypotension, palpitations.

Central Nervous System
Drowsiness, insomnia, paresthesia, vertigo.

Dermatologic
Pruritus, rash, pemphigus, alopecia, sweating.

Eye, Ear, Nose, Throat
Epistaxis, throat inflammation, upper respiratory tract infection.

Emotional, Mental, Sexual States
Anxiety, impotence, decreased libido.

Gastrointestinal
Abdominal distention, abdominal pain/cramps, constipation, dyspepsia, diarrhea, vomiting, nausea, dry mouth, pancreatitis.

Hemopoietic
Agranulocytosis, decreased leukocytes, decreased neutrophils.

Metabolism and Endocrine
Increased creatinine, increased potassium, increased liver enzymes including SGPT (ALT) and increased SGOT (AST).

Musculoskeletal System
Extremity pain, muscle cramps, gout.

Pulmonary
Dyspnea, bronchitis.

Angioedema
Angioedema has been reported in 4 (0.13%) patients receiving MAVIK in U.S. and foreign studies. Angioedema associated with laryngeal edema may be fatal. If angioedema of the face, extremities, lips, tongue, glottis, and/or larynx occurs, treatment with MAVIK should be discontinued and appropriate therapy instituted immediately. (See **WARNINGS**.)

Hypotension
In hypertensive patients, symptomatic hypotension occurred in 0.6% and near syncope occurred in 0.2%. Hypotension or syncope was a cause for discontinuation of therapy in 0.1% of hypertensive patients.

Fetal/Neonatal Morbidity and Mortality
(See **WARNINGS - Fetal Neonatal Morbidity and Mortality**.)

Cough
(See **PRECAUTIONS - Cough**.)

Clinical Laboratory Test Findings

Hematology
(See **WARNINGS**.) Low white blood cells, low neutrophils, low lymphocytes, thrombocytopenia.

Serum Electrolytes
Hyperkalemia (See **PRECAUTIONS**), hyponatremia.

Creatinine and Blood Urea Nitrogen
Increases in creatinine levels occurred in 1.1% of patients receiving MAVIK alone and 7.3% of patients treated with MAVIK, a calcium ion antagonist and a diuretic. Increases in blood urea nitrogen levels occurred in 0.6% of patients receiving MAVIK alone and 1.4% of patients receiving MAVIK, a calcium ion antagonist, and a diuretic. None of these increases required discontinuation of treatment. Increases in these laboratory values are more likely to occur in patients with renal insufficiency or those pretreated with a diuretic and, based on experience with other ACE inhibitors, would be expected to be especially likely in patients with renal artery stenosis. (See **PRECAUTIONS** and **WARNINGS**.)

Liver Function Tests
Occasional elevation of transaminases at the rate of 3× upper normals occurred in 0.8% of patients and persistent increase in bilirubin occurred in 0.2% of patients. Discontinuation for elevated liver enzymes occurred in 0.2% of patients.

Other
Another potentially important adverse experience, eosinophilic pneumonitis, has been attributed to other ACE inhibitors.

OVERDOSAGE

No data are available with respect to overdosage in humans. The oral LD_{50} of trandolapril in mice was 4875 mg/Kg in males and 3990 mg/Kg in females. In rats, an oral dose of 5000 mg/Kg caused low mortality (1 male out of 5; 0 females). In dogs, an oral dose of 1000 mg/Kg did not cause mortality and abnormal clinical signs were not observed. In humans the most likely clinical manifestation would be symptoms attributable to severe hypotension. Laboratory determinations of serum levels of trandolapril and its metabolites are not widely available, and such determinations have, in any event, no established role in the management of trandolapril overdose. No data are available to suggest that physiological maneuvers (e.g., maneuvers to change the pH of the urine) might accelerate elimination of trandolapril and its metabolites. Trandolaprilat is removed by hemodialysis. Angiotensin II could presumably serve as a specific antagonist antidote in the setting of trandolapril overdose, but angiotensin II is essentially unavailable outside of scattered research facilities. Because the hypotensive effect of trandolapril is achieved through vasodilation and effective hypovolemia, it is reasonable to treat trandolapril overdose by infusion of normal saline solution.

DOSAGE AND ADMINISTRATION

Hypertension

The recommended initial dosage of MAVIK for patients not receiving a diuretic is 1 mg once daily in non-black patients and 2 mg in black patients. Dosage should be adjusted according to the blood pressure response. Generally, dosage adjustments should be made at intervals of at least 1 week. Most patients have required dosages of 2 to 4 mg once daily. There is little clinical experience with doses above 8 mg. Patients inadequately treated with once-daily dosing at 4 mg may be treated with twice-daily dosing. If blood pressure is not adequately controlled with MAVIK monotherapy, a diuretic may be added.

In patients who are currently being treated with a diuretic, symptomatic hypotension occasionally can occur following the initial dose of MAVIK. To reduce the likelihood of hypotension, the diuretic should, if possible, be discontinued two to three days prior to beginning therapy with MAVIK. (See **WARNINGS**.) Then, if blood pressure is not controlled with MAVIK alone, diuretic therapy should be resumed. If the diuretic cannot be discontinued, an initial dose of 0.5 mg MAVIK should be used with careful medical supervision for several hours until blood pressure has stabilized. The dosage should subsequently be titrated (as described above) to the optimal response. (See **WARNINGS, PRECAUTIONS**, and **DRUG INTERACTIONS**.)

Concomitant administration of MAVIK with potassium supplements, potassium salt substitutes, or potassium sparing diuretics can lead to increases of serum potassium. (See **PRECAUTIONS**.)

Heart Failure Post Myocardial Infarction or Left-Ventricular Dysfunction Post Myocardial Infarction

The recommended starting dose is 1 mg, once daily. Following the initial dose, all patients should be titrated (as tolerated) toward a target dose of 4 mg, once daily. If a 4 mg dose is not tolerated, patients can continue therapy with the greatest tolerated dose.

Dosage Adjustment in Renal Impairment or Hepatic Cirrhosis

For patients with a creatinine clearance < 30 mL/min. or with hepatic cirrhosis, the recommended starting dose, based on clinical and pharmacokinetic data, is 0.5 mg daily. Patients should subsequently have their dosage titrated (as described above) to the optimal response.

HOW SUPPLIED

MAVIK® (trandolapril tablets) are supplied as follows:

1 mg tablet—Salmon colored, round shaped, scored, compressed tablets, with **Abbott "囗" logo** on one side and Abbo-Code identification letters FT on the other side. NDC 0074-2278-13 - bottles of 100 NDC 0074-2278-11 - unit dose packs of 100

2 mg tablet—Yellow colored, round shaped, compressed tablets, with **Abbott "囗" logo** on one side and Abbo-Code identification letters FX on the other side. NDC 0074-2279-13 - bottles of 100 NDC 0074-2279-11 - unit dose packs of 100

4 mg tablet—Rose colored, round shaped, compressed tablets, with **Abbott "囗" logo** on one side and Abbo-Code identification letters FZ on the other side. NDC 0074-2280-13 - bottles of 100 NDC 0074-2280-11 - unit dose packs of 100

Dispense in well-closed container with safety closure.

Storage

Store at controlled room temperature: 20-25°C (68-77°F) see USP.

Manufactured by
Halo Pharmaceutical Inc.
Whippany, N.J. 07981, U.S.A.

for

Abbott Laboratories
North Chicago, IL 60064, U.S.A.
Ref. 03-A246-Revised June, 2009
Shown in Product Identification Guide, page 303

MERIDIA®   © Ŗ

[mer-ID-dee-uh]
(sibutramine hydrochloride monohydrate)
Capsules

DESCRIPTION

MERIDIA® (sibutramine hydrochloride monohydrate) is an orally administered agent for the treatment of obesity. Chemically, the active ingredient is a racemic mixture of the (+) and (-) enantiomers of cyclobutanemethanamine, 1-(4-chlorophenyl)-N,N-dimethyl-α-(2-methylpropyl)-, hydrochloride, monohydrate, and has an empirical formula of $C_{17}H_{29}Cl_2NO$. Its molecular weight is 334.33.

The structural formula is shown below:

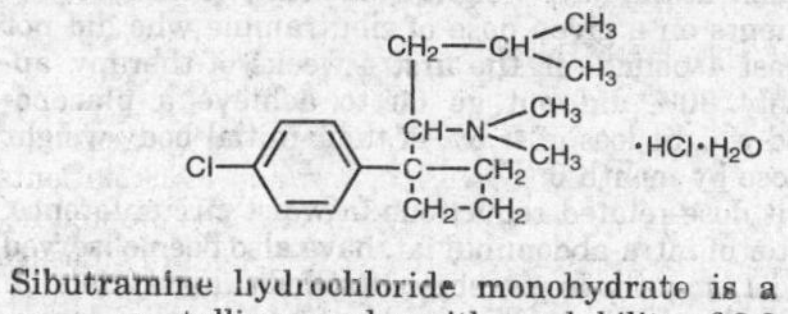

Sibutramine hydrochloride monohydrate is a white to cream crystalline powder with a solubility of 2.9 mg/mL in pH 5.2 water. Its octanol: water partition coefficient is 30.9 at pH 5.0.

Each MERIDIA capsule contains 5 mg, 10 mg, and 15 mg of sibutramine hydrochloride monohydrate. It also contains as inactive ingredients: lactose monohydrate, NF; microcrystalline cellulose, NF; colloidal silicon dioxide, NF; and magnesium stearate, NF in a hard-gelatin capsule [which contains titanium dioxide, USP; gelatin; FD&C Blue No. 2 (5- and 10-mg capsules only); D&C Yellow No. 10 (5- and 15-mg capsules only), and other inactive ingredients].

CLINICAL PHARMACOLOGY

Mode of Action

Sibutramine produces its therapeutic effects by norepinephrine, serotonin and dopamine reuptake inhibition. Sibutramine and its major pharmacologically active metabolites (M_1 and M_2) do not act via release of monoamines.

Pharmacodynamics

Sibutramine exerts its pharmacological actions predominantly via its secondary (M_1) and primary (M_2) amine metabolites. The parent compound, sibutramine, is a potent inhibitor of serotonin (5-hydroxytryptamine, 5-HT) and norepinephrine reuptake *in vivo*, but not *in vitro*. However, metabolites M_1 and M_2 inhibit the reuptake of these neurotransmitters both *in vitro* and *in vivo*.

In human brain tissue, M_1 and M_2 also inhibit dopamine reuptake *in vitro*, but with ~3-fold lower potency than for the reuptake inhibition of serotonin or norepinephrine.

Potencies of Sibutramine, M_1 and M_2 as *In Vitro* Inhibitors of Monoamine Reuptake in Human Brain Potency to Inhibit Monoamine Reuptake (K_i;nM)

	Serotonin	Norepinephrine	Dopamine
Sibutramine	298	5451	943
M_1	15	20	49
M_2	20	15	45

A study using plasma samples taken from sibutramine-treated volunteers showed monoamine reuptake inhibition of norepinephrine > serotonin > dopamine; maximum inhibitions were norepinephrine = 73%, serotonin = 54% and dopamine = 16%.

Sibutramine and its metabolites (M_1 and M_2) are not serotonin, norepinephrine or dopamine releasing agents. Following chronic administration of sibutramine to rats, no depletion of brain monoamines has been observed.

Sibutramine, M_1 and M_2 exhibit no evidence of anticholinergic or antihistaminergic actions. In addition, receptor binding profiles show that sibutramine, M_1 and M_2 have low affinity for serotonin (5-HT_1, 5-HT_{1A}, 5-HT_{1B}, 5-HT_{2A}, 5-HT_{2C}), norepinephrine (β, β_1, β_3, α_1 and α_2), dopamine (D_1 and D_2), benzodiazepine, and glutamate (NMDA) receptors. These compounds also lack monoamine oxidase inhibitory activity *in vitro* and *in vivo*.

Pharmacokinetics

Absorption

Sibutramine is rapidly absorbed from the GI tract (T_{max} of 1.2 hours) following oral administration and undergoes extensive first-pass metabolism in the liver (oral clearance of 1750 L/h and half-life of 1.1 h) to form the pharmacologically active mono- and di-desmethyl metabolites M_1 and M_2. Peak plasma concentrations of M_1 and M_2 are reached within 3 to 4 hours. On the basis of mass balance studies, on average, at least 77% of a single oral dose of sibutramine is absorbed. The absolute bioavailability of sibutramine has not been determined.

Distribution

Radiolabeled studies in animals indicated rapid and extensive distribution into tissues: highest concentrations of radiolabeled material were found in the eliminating organs, liver and kidney. *In vitro*, sibutramine, M_1 and M_2 are extensively bound (97%, 94% and 94%, respectively) to human plasma proteins at plasma concentrations seen following therapeutic doses.

Metabolism

Sibutramine is metabolized in the liver principally by the cytochrome P450 ($3A_4$) isoenzyme, to desmethyl metabolites, M_1 and M_2. These active metabolites are further metabolized by hydroxylation and conjugation to pharmacologically inactive metabolites, M_5 and M_6. Following oral administration of radiolabeled sibutramine, essentially all

Summary of Pharmacokinetic Parameters

Mean (% CV) and 95% Confidence Intervals of Pharmacokinetic Parameters (Dose = 15 mg)

Study Population	C_{max} (ng/mL)	T_{max} (h)	AUC† (ng*h/mL)	T½ (h)
Metabolite M_1				
Target Population:				
Obese Subjects	4.0 (42)	3.6 (28)	25.5 (63)	
(n = 18)	3.2-4.8	3.1-4.1	18.1-32.9	—
Special Population:				
Moderate Hepatic	2.2 (36)	3.3 (33)	18.7 (65)	
Impairment (n = 12)	1.8-2.7	2.7-3.9	11.9-25.5	—
Metabolite M_2				
Target Population:				
Obese Subjects	6.4 (28)	3.5 (17)	92.1 (26)	17.2 (58)
(n = 18)	5.6-7.2	3.2-3.8	81.2-103	12.5-21.8
Special Population:				
Moderate Hepatic	4.3 (37)	3.8 (34)	90.5 (27)	22.7 (30)
Impairment (n = 12)	3.4-5.2	3.1-4.5	76.9-104	18.9-26.5

† Calculated only up to 24 hr for M_1.

of the peak radiolabeled material in plasma was accounted for by unchanged sibutramine (3%), M_1 (6%), M_2 (12%), M_5 (52%), and M_6 (27%).

M_1 and M_2 plasma concentrations reached steady-state within four days of dosing and were approximately two-fold higher than following a single dose. The elimination half-lives of M_1 and M_2, 14 and 16 hours, respectively, were unchanged following repeated dosing.

Excretion

Approximately 85% (range 68-95%) of a single orally administered radiolabeled dose was excreted in urine and feces over a 15-day collection period with the majority of the dose (77%) excreted in the urine. Major metabolites in urine were M_5 and M_6; unchanged sibutramine, M_1, and M_2 were not detected. The primary route of excretion for M_1 and M_2 is hepatic metabolism and for M_5 and M_6 is renal excretion.

[See table above]

Effect of Food

Administration of a single 20 mg dose of sibutramine with a standard breakfast resulted in reduced peak M_1 and M_2 concentrations (by 27% and 32%, respectively) and delayed the time to peak by approximately three hours. However, the AUCs of M_1 and M_2 were not significantly altered.

Special Populations

Geriatric

Plasma concentrations of M_1 and M_2 were similar between elderly (ages 61 to 77 yr) and young (ages 19 to 30 yr) subjects following a single 15-mg oral sibutramine dose. Plasma concentrations of the inactive metabolites M_5 and M_6 were higher in the elderly; these differences are not likely to be of clinical significance. Sibutramine is contraindicated in patients over 65 years of age (see **CONTRAINDICATIONS**).

Pediatric

The safety and effectiveness of sibutramine in pediatric patients under 16 years old have not been established.

Gender

Pooled pharmacokinetic parameters from 54 young, healthy volunteers (37 males and 17 females) receiving a 15-mg oral dose of sibutramine showed the mean C_{max} and AUC of M_1 and M_2 to be slightly (≤ 19% and ≤ 36%, respectively) higher in females than males. Somewhat higher steady-state trough plasma levels were observed in female obese patients from a large clinical efficacy trial. However, these differences are not likely to be of clinical significance. Dosage adjustment based upon the gender of a patient is not necessary (see **DOSAGE AND ADMINISTRATION**).

Race

The relationship between race and steady-state trough M_1 and M_2 plasma concentrations was examined in a clinical trial in obese patients. A trend towards higher concentrations in Black patients over Caucasian patients was noted for M_1 and M_2. However, these differences are not considered to be of clinical significance.

Renal Insufficiency

The disposition of sibutramine metabolites (M_1, M_2, M_5 and M_6) following a single oral dose of sibutramine was studied in patients with varying degrees of renal function. Sibutramine itself was not measurable.

In patients with moderate and severe renal impairment, the AUC values of the active metabolite M_1 were 24 to 46% higher and the AUC values of M_2 were similar as compared to healthy subjects. Cross-study comparison showed that the patients with end-stage renal disease on dialysis had similar AUC values of M_1 but approximately half of the AUC values of M_2 measured in healthy subjects (CLcr ≥ 80 mL/min). The AUC values of inactive metabolites M_5 and M_6 increased 2-3 fold (range 1- to 7-fold) in patients with moderate impairment (30 mL/min < CLcr = 60 mL/min) and 8-11 fold (range 5- to 15-fold) in patients with severe impairment (CLcr ≤ 30 mL/min) as compared to healthy subjects. Cross-study comparison showed that the AUC values of M_5 and M_6 increased 22-33 fold in patients with end-stage renal disease on dialysis as compared to healthy subjects. Approximately 1% of the oral dose was recovered in the dialysate as a combination of M_5 and M_6 during the hemodialysis process, while M_1 and M_2 were not measurable in the dialysate.

Sibutramine should not be used in patients with severe renal impairment, including those with end-stage renal disease on dialysis.

Hepatic Insufficiency

In 12 patients with moderate hepatic impairment receiving a single 15-mg oral dose of sibutramine, the combined AUCs of M_1 and M_2 were increased by 24% compared to healthy subjects while M_5 and M_6 plasma concentrations were unchanged. The observed differences in M_1 and M_2 concentrations do not warrant dosage adjustment in patients with mild to moderate hepatic impairment. Sibutramine should not be used in patients with severe hepatic dysfunction.

Drug-Drug Interactions

In vitro studies indicated that the cytochrome P450 ($3A_4$)-mediated metabolism of sibutramine was inhibited by ketoconazole and to a lesser extent by erythromycin. Phase 1 clinical trials were conducted to assess the interactions of sibutramine with drugs that are substrates and/or inhibitors of various cytochrome P450 isozymes. The potential for studied interactions is described below.

Ketoconazole

Concomitant administration of 200 mg doses of ketoconazole twice daily and 20 mg sibutramine once daily for 7 days in 12 uncomplicated obese subjects resulted in moderate increases in AUC and C_{max} of 58% and 36% for M_1 and of 20% and 19% for M_2, respectively.

Erythromycin

The steady-state pharmacokinetics of sibutramine and metabolites M_1 and M_2 were evaluated in 12 uncomplicated obese subjects following concomitant administration of 500 mg of erythromycin three times daily and 20 mg of sibutramine once daily for 7 days. Concomitant erythromycin resulted in small increases in the AUC (less than 14%) for M_1 and M_2. A small reduction in C_{max} for M_1 (11%) and a slight increase in C_{max} for M_2 (10%) were observed.

Cimetidine

Concomitant administration of cimetidine 400 mg twice daily and sibutramine 15 mg once daily for 7 days in 12 volunteers resulted in small increases in combined (M_1 and M_2) plasma C_{max} (3.4%) and AUC (7.3%).

Simvastatin

Steady-state pharmacokinetics of sibutramine and metabolites M_1 and M_2 were evaluated in 27 healthy volunteers after the administration of simvastatin 20 mg once daily in the evening and sibutramine 15 mg once daily in the morning for 7 days. Simvastatin had no significant effect on plasma C_{max} and AUC of M_2 or M_1 and M_2 combined. The C_{max} (16%) and AUC (12%) of M_1 were slightly decreased. Simvastatin slightly decreased sibutramine C_{max} (14%) and AUC (21%). Sibutramine increased the AUC (7%) of the pharmacologically active moiety, simvastatin acid and reduced the C_{max} (25%) and AUC (15%) of inactive simvastatin.

Omeprazole

Steady-state pharmacokinetics of sibutramine and metabolites M_1 and M_2 were evaluated in 26 healthy volunteers

Information on the Abbott Pharmaceutical Products listed on these pages is from the prescribing information in use as of June 1, 2010. For more information, please visit rxabbott.com or call 1-800-633-9110.

Mean Weight Loss (lbs) in the Six-Month and One-Year Trials

Study/Patient Group	Placebo (n)	Sibutramine (mg) 5 (n)	10 (n)	15 (n)	20 (n)
Study 1					
All patients*	2.0 (142)	6.6 (148)	9.7 (148)	12.1 (150)	13.6 (145)
Completers**	2.9 (84)	8.1 (103)	12.1 (95)	15.4 (94)	18.0 (89)
Early responders***	8.5 (17)	13.0 (60)	16.0 (64)	18.2 (73)	20.1 (76)
Study 2					
All patients*	3.5 (157)		9.8 (154)	14.0 (152)	
Completers**	4.8 (76)		13.6 (80)	15.2 (93)	
Early responders***	10.7 (24)		18.2 (57)	18.8 (76)	
Study 3**					
All patients*	15.2 (78)		28.4 (81)		
Completers**	16.7 (48)		29.7 (60)		
Early responders***	21.5 (22)		33.0 (46)		

* Data for all patients who received study drug and who had any post-baseline measurement (last observation carried forward analysis).
** Data for patients who completed the entire 6-month (Study 1) or one-year period of dosing and have data recorded for the month 6 (Study 1) or month 12 visit.
*** Data for patients who lost at least 4 lbs in the first 4 weeks of treatment and completed the study.
**** Weight loss data shown describe changes in weight from the pre-VLCD; mean weight loss during the 4-week VLCD was 16.9 lbs for sibutramine and 16.3 lbs for placebo.

Combined Analysis (11 Studies) of Changes in Serum Lipids - LOCF

Category	TG % (n)	CHOL % (n)	LDL-C % (n)	HDL-C % (n)
All Placebo	0.53 (475)	-1.53 (475)	-0.09 (233)	-0.56 (248)
< 5% Weight Loss	4.52 (382)	-0.42 (382)	-0.70 (205)	-0.71 (217)
≥ 5% Weight Loss	-15.30 (92)	-6.23 (92)	-6.19 (27)	0.94 (30)
All Sibutramine	-8.75 (1164)	-2.21 (1165)	-1.85 (642)	4.13 (664)
< 5% Weight Loss	-0.54 (547)	0.17 (548)	-0.37 (320)	3.19 (331)
≥ 5% Weight Loss	-16.59 (612)	-4.87 (612)	-4.56 (317)	4.68 (328)

Baseline mean values:
Placebo: TG 187 mg/dL; CHOL 221 mg/dL; LDL-C 140 mg/dL; HDL-C 47 mg/dL
Sibutramine: TG 172 mg/dL; CHOL 215 mg/dL; LDL-C 140 mg/dL; HDL-C 47 mg/dL
TG: Triglycerides, CHOL: Cholesterol, LDL-C Low Density Lipoprotein-Cholesterol
HDL-C: High Density Lipoprotein-Cholesterol

after the co-administration of omeprazole 20 mg once daily and sibutramine 15 mg once daily for 7 days. Omeprazole slightly increased plasma C_{max} and AUC of M_1 and M_2 combined (approximately 15%). M_2 C_{max} and AUC were not significantly affected whereas M_1 C_{max} (30%) and AUC (40%) were modestly increased. Plasma C_{max} (57%) and AUC (67%) of unchanged sibutramine were moderately increased. Sibutramine had no significant effect on omeprazole pharmacokinetics.

Olanzapine
Steady-state pharmacokinetics of sibutramine and metabolites M_1 and M_2 were evaluated in 24 healthy volunteers after the co-administration of sibutramine 15 mg once daily with olanzapine 5 mg twice daily for 3 days and 10 mg once daily thereafter for 7 days. Olanzapine had no significant effect on plasma C_{max} and AUC of M_2 and M_1 and M_2 combined, or the AUC of M_1. Olanzapine slightly increased M_1 C_{max} (19%), and moderately increased sibutramine C_{max} (47%) and AUC (63%). Sibutramine had no significant effect on olanzapine pharmacokinetics.

Lorazepam
Steady-state pharmacokinetics of sibutramine and metabolites M_1 and M_2 after sibutramine 15 mg once daily for 11 days were compared in 25 healthy volunteers in the presence or absence of lorazepam 2 mg twice daily for 3 days plus one morning dose. Lorazepam had no significant effect on the pharmacokinetics of sibutramine metabolites M_1 and M_2. Sibutramine had no significant effect on lorazepam pharmacokinetics.

Drugs Highly Bound to Plasma Proteins
Although sibutramine and its active metabolites M_1 and M_2 are extensively bound to plasma proteins (≥94%), the low therapeutic concentrations and basic characteristics of these compounds make them unlikely to result in clinically significant protein binding interactions with other highly protein bound drugs such as warfarin and phenytoin. *In vitro* protein binding interaction studies have not been conducted.

CLINICAL STUDIES

Observational epidemiologic studies have established a relationship between obesity and the risks for cardiovascular disease, non-insulin dependent diabetes mellitus (NIDDM), certain forms of cancer, gallstones, certain respiratory disorders, and an increase in overall mortality. These studies suggest that weight loss, if maintained, may produce health benefits for some patients with chronic obesity who may also be at risk for other diseases.
The long-term effects of sibutramine on the morbidity and mortality associated with obesity have not been established. Weight loss was examined in 11 double-blind, placebo-controlled obesity trials (BMI range across all studies 27-43) with study durations of 12 to 52 weeks and doses ranging from 1 to 30 mg once daily. Weight was significantly reduced in a dose-related manner in sibutramine-treated patients compared to placebo over the dose range of 5 to 20 mg once daily. In two 12-month studies, maximal weight loss was achieved by 6 months and statistically significant weight loss was maintained over 12 months. The amount of placebo-subtracted weight loss achieved on sibutramine was consistent across studies.
Analysis of the data in three long-term (≥ 6 months) obesity trials indicates that patients who lose at least 4 pounds in the first 4 weeks of therapy with a given dose of sibutramine are most likely to achieve significant long-term weight loss on that dose of sibutramine. Approximately 60% of such patients went on to achieve a placebo-subtracted weight loss of ≥ 5% of their initial body weight by month 6. Conversely, of those patients on a given dose of sibutramine who did not lose at least 4 pounds in the first 4 weeks of therapy, approximately 80% did not go on to achieve a placebo-subtracted weight loss of ≥ 5% of their initial body weight on that dose by month 6.
Significant dose-related reductions in waist circumference, an indicator of intra-abdominal fat, have also been observed over 6 and 12 months in placebo-controlled clinical trials. In a 12-week placebo-controlled study of non-insulin dependent diabetes mellitus patients randomized to placebo or 15 mg per day of sibutramine, Dual Energy X-Ray Absorptiometry (DEXA) assessment of changes in body composition showed that total body fat mass decreased by 1.8 kg in the sibutramine group versus 0.2 kg in the placebo group (p < 0.001). Similarly, truncal (android) fat mass decreased by 0.6 kg in the sibutramine group versus 0.1 kg in the placebo group (p < 0.01). The changes in lean mass, fasting blood sugar, and HbA_1 were not statistically significantly different between the two groups.
Eleven double-blind, placebo-controlled obesity trials with study durations of 12 to 52 weeks have provided evidence that sibutramine does not adversely affect glycemia, serum lipid profiles, or serum uric acid in obese patients. Treatment with sibutramine (5 to 20 mg once daily) is associated with mean increases in blood pressure of 1 to 3 mm Hg and with mean increases in pulse rate of 4 to 5 beats per minute relative to placebo. These findings are similar in normotensives and in patients with hypertension controlled with medication. Those patients who lose significant (≥ 5% weight loss) amounts of weight on sibutramine tend to have smaller increases in blood pressure and pulse rate (see **WARNINGS**).
In Study 1, a 6-month, double-blind, placebo-controlled study in obese patients, Study 2, a 1-year, double-blind, placebo-controlled study in obese patients, and Study 3, a 1-year, double-blind, placebo-controlled study in obese patients who lost at least 6 kg on a 4-week very low calorie diet (VLCD), sibutramine produced significant reductions in weight, as shown below. In the two 1-year studies, maximal weight loss was achieved by 6 months and statistically significant weight loss was maintained over 12 months.
[See table above]
Maintenance of weight loss with sibutramine was examined in a 2-year, double-blind, placebo-controlled trial. After a 6-month run-in phase in which all patients received sibutramine 10 mg (mean weight loss, 26 lbs.), patients were randomized to sibutramine (10 to 20 mg, 352 patients) or placebo (115 patients). The mean weight loss from initial body weight to endpoint was 21 lbs. and 12 lbs. for sibutramine and placebo patients, respectively. A statistically significantly (p < 0.001) greater proportion of sibutramine treated patients, 75%, 62%, and 43%, maintained at least 80% of their initial weight loss at 12, 18, and 24 months, respectively, compared with the placebo group (38%, 23%, and 16%). Also 67%, 37%, 17%, and 9% of sibutramine treated patients compared with 49%, 19%, 5%, and 3% of placebo patients lost ≥ 5%, ≥ 10%, ≥ 15%, and ≥ 20%, respectively, of their initial body weight at endpoint. From endpoint to the post-study follow-up visit (about 1 month), weight regain was approximately 4 lbs for the sibutramine patients and approximately 2 lbs for the placebo patients.
Sibutramine induced weight loss has been accompanied by beneficial changes in serum lipids that are similar to those seen with nonpharmacologically-mediated weight loss. A combined, weighted analysis of the changes in serum lipids in 11 placebo-controlled obesity studies ranging in length from 12 to 52 weeks is shown below for the last observation carried forward (LOCF) analysis.
[See second table above]
Sibutramine induced weight loss has been accompanied by reductions in serum uric acid. Certain centrally-acting weight loss agents that cause release of serotonin from nerve terminals have been associated with cardiac valve dysfunction. The possible occurrence of cardiac valve disease was specifically investigated in two studies. In one study 2-D and color Doppler echocardiography were performed on 210 patients (mean age, 54 years) receiving sibutramine 15 mg or placebo daily for periods of 2 weeks to 16 months (mean duration of treatment, 7.6 months). In patients without a prior history of valvular heart disease, the incidence of valvular heart disease was 3/132 (2.3%) in the sibutramine treatment group (all three cases were mild aortic insufficiency) and 2/77 (2.6%) in the placebo treatment group (one case of mild aortic insufficiency and one case of severe aortic insufficiency). In another study, 25 patients underwent 2-D and color Doppler echocardiography before treatment with sibutramine and again after treatment with sibutramine 5 to 30 mg daily for three months; there were no cases of valvular heart disease.
The effect of sibutramine 15 mg once daily on measures of 24-hour blood pressure was evaluated in a 12-week placebo-controlled study. Twenty-six male and female, primarily Caucasian individuals with an average BMI of 34 kg/m² and

an average age of 39 years underwent 24-hour ambulatory blood pressure monitoring (ABPM). The mean changes from baseline to Week 12 in various measures of ABPM are shown in the following table.

Parameter mm Hg	Systolic			Diastolic		
	Placebo	Sibutramine 15 mg	Sibutramine 20 mg	Placebo	Sibutramine 15 mg	Sibutramine 20 mg
	n=12	n=14	n=16		n=12	n=16
Daytime	0.2	3.9	4.4	0.5	5.0	5.7
Nighttime	-0.3	4.1	6.4	-1.0	4.3	5.4
Early am	-0.9	9.4	5.3	-3.0	6.7	5.8
24-hour mean	-0.1	4.0	4.7	0.1	5.0	5.6

Normal diurnal variation of blood pressure was maintained.

INDICATIONS AND USAGE

MERIDIA® (sibutramine hydrochloride monohydrate) is indicated for the management of obesity, including weight loss and maintenance of weight loss, and should be used in conjunction with a reduced calorie diet. MERIDIA is recommended for obese patients with an initial body mass index ≥ 30 kg/m^2, or ≥ 27 kg/m^2 in the presence of other risk factors (e.g., diabetes, dyslipidemia, controlled hypertension).

Below is a chart of Body Mass Index (BMI) based on various heights and weights.

BMI is calculated by taking the patient's weight, in kg, and dividing by the patient's height, in meters, squared. Metric conversions are as follows: pounds ÷ 2.2 = kg; inches × 0.0254 = meters.

BMI	25	26	27	28	29	30	31	32	33	34	35	40
HEIGHT	WEIGHT (lbs)											
4'10"	119	124	129	134	138	143	149	153	158	163	167	191
4'11"	124	128	133	138	143	148	154	158	164	169	173	198
5'	128	133	138	143	148	153	159	164	169	175	179	204
5'1"	132	137	143	148	153	158	165	169	175	180	185	211
5'2"	136	142	147	153	158	164	170	175	181	186	191	218
5'3"	141	146	152	158	163	169	175	181	187	192	197	225
5'4"	145	151	157	163	169	174	181	187	193	199	204	232
5'5"	150	156	162	168	174	180	187	193	199	205	210	240
5'6"	155	161	167	173	179	186	192	199	205	211	216	247
5'7"	159	166	172	178	185	191	198	205	211	218	223	255
5'8"	164	171	177	184	190	197	204	211	218	224	230	262
5'9"	169	176	182	189	196	203	210	217	224	231	236	270
5'10"	174	181	188	195	202	207	216	223	230	237	243	278
5'11"	179	186	193	200	208	215	222	230	237	244	250	286
6'	184	191	199	206	213	221	228	236	244	251	258	294
6'1"	189	197	204	212	219	227	236	243	251	258	265	302
6'2"	194	202	210	218	225	233	241	250	258	265	272	311
6'3"	200	208	216	224	232	240	248	256	264	272	279	319

CONTRAINDICATIONS

MERIDIA is contraindicated in patients:

- with a history of coronary artery disease (e.g., angina, history of myocardial infarction), congestive heart failure, tachycardia, peripheral arterial occlusive disease, arrhythmia or cerebrovascular disease (stroke or transient ischemic attack (TIA)) (see **WARNINGS**).
- with inadequately controlled hypertension > 145/90 mm Hg (see **WARNINGS**).
- over 65 years of age.
- receiving monoamine oxidase inhibitors (MAOIs) (see **WARNINGS**).
- with hypersensitivity to sibutramine or any of the inactive ingredients of MERIDIA.
- who have a major eating disorder (anorexia nervosa or bulimia nervosa).
- taking other centrally acting weight loss drugs.

WARNINGS

Concomitant Cardiovascular Disease

Due to an increased risk of heart attack and stroke in patients with cardiovascular disease, MERIDIA should not be used in patients with a history of coronary artery disease, congestive heart failure, arrhythmias, or stroke.

Blood Pressure and Pulse

MERIDIA SUBSTANTIALLY INCREASES BLOOD PRESSURE AND/OR PULSE RATE IN SOME PATIENTS. REGULAR MONITORING OF BLOOD PRESSURE AND PULSE RATE IS REQUIRED WHEN PRESCRIBING MERIDIA.

In placebo-controlled obesity studies, sibutramine 5 to 20 mg once daily was associated with mean increases in systolic and diastolic blood pressure of approximately 1 to 3 mm Hg relative to placebo, and with mean increases in pulse rate relative to placebo of approximately 4 to 5 beats per minute. Larger increases were seen in some patients, particularly when therapy with sibutramine was initiated at the higher doses (see table below). In premarketing placebo-controlled obesity studies, 0.4% of patients treated with sibutramine were discontinued for hypertension (SBP $\geq$160 mm Hg or DBP $\geq$ 95 mm Hg), compared with 0.4% in the placebo group, and 0.4% of patients treated with sibutramine were discontinued for tachycardia (pulse rate $\geq$ 100 bpm), compared with 0.1% in the placebo group. **Blood pressure and pulse should be measured prior to starting therapy with MERIDIA and should be monitored at regular intervals thereafter.** For patients who experience a sustained increase in blood pressure or pulse rate while receiving MERIDIA, either dose reduction or discontinuation should be considered. MERIDIA should be given with caution to those patients with a history of hypertension (see **DOSAGE AND ADMINISTRATION**), and should not be given to patients with uncontrolled or poorly controlled hypertension.

Percent Outliers in Studies 1 and 2

Dose (mg)	% Outliers* SBP	DBP	Pulse
Placebo	9	7	12
5	6	20	16
10	12	15	28
15	13	17	24
20	14	22	37

* Outlier defined as increase from baseline of $\geq$ 15 mm Hg for three consecutive visits (SBP), $\geq$ 10 mm Hg for three consecutive visits (DBP), or pulse $\geq$ 10 bpm for three consecutive visits.

Potential Interaction With Monoamine Oxidase Inhibitors

MERIDIA is a norepinephrine, serotonin and dopamine reuptake inhibitor and should not be used concomitantly with MAOIs (see **PRECAUTIONS**, Drug Interactions subsection). There should be at least a 2-week interval after stopping MAOIs before commencing treatment with MERIDIA. Similarly, there should be at least a 2-week interval after stopping MERIDIA before starting treatment with MAOIs.

Serotonin Syndrome or Neuroleptic Malignant Syndrome (NMS)-Like Reactions

The development of a potentially life-threatening serotonin syndrome, or Neuroleptic Malignant Syndrome (NMS)-like reactions, has been reported with SNRIs and SSRIs alone, including MERIDIA treatment, but particularly with concomitant use of serotonergic drugs (including triptans), with drugs which impair metabolism of serotonin (including MAOIs), or with antipsychotics or other dopamine antagonists. Serotonin syndrome symptoms may include mental status changes (e.g., agitation, hallucinations, coma), autonomic instability (e.g., tachycardia, labile blood pressure, hyperthermia), neuromuscular aberrations (e.g., hyperreflexia, incoordination) and/or gastrointestinal symptoms [e.g., nausea, vomiting, diarrhea] (see **PRECAUTIONS, Drug Interactions**). Serotonin syndrome, in its most severe form, can resemble neuroleptic malignant syndrome, which includes hyperthermia, muscle rigidity, autonomic instability with possible rapid fluctuation of vital signs, and mental status changes. Patients should be monitored for the emergence of serotonin syndrome or NMS-like signs and symptoms.

Glaucoma

Because MERIDIA can cause mydriasis, it should be used with caution in patients with narrow angle glaucoma.

Miscellaneous

Organic causes of obesity (e.g., untreated hypothyroidism) should be excluded before prescribing MERIDIA.

PRECAUTIONS

Pulmonary Hypertension

Certain centrally-acting weight loss agents that cause release of serotonin from nerve terminals have been associated with pulmonary hypertension (PPH), a rare but lethal disease. In premarketing clinical studies, no cases of PPH have been reported with sibutramine capsules. Because of the low incidence of this disease in the underlying population, however, it is not known whether or not MERIDIA may cause this disease.

Seizures

During premarketing testing, seizures were reported in < 0.1% of sibutramine treated patients. MERIDIA should be used cautiously in patients with a history of seizures. It should be discontinued in any patient who develops seizures.

Bleeding

There have been reports of bleeding in patients taking sibutramine. While a causal relationship is unclear, caution is advised in patients predisposed to bleeding events and those taking concomitant medications known to affect hemostasis or platelet function.

Gallstones

Weight loss can precipitate or exacerbate gallstone formation.

Renal Impairment

MERIDIA should be used with caution in patients with mild to moderate renal impairment. MERIDIA should not be used in patients with severe renal impairment, including those with end stage renal disease on dialysis (see **Pharmacokinetics**-Special Populations-*Renal Insufficiency*).

Hepatic Dysfunction

Patients with severe hepatic dysfunction have not been systematically studied; MERIDIA should therefore not be used in such patients.

Interference With Cognitive and Motor Performance

Although sibutramine did not affect psychomotor or cognitive performance in healthy volunteers, any CNS active drug has the potential to impair judgment, thinking or motor skills.

Information For Patients

Physicians should instruct their patients to read the patient package insert before starting therapy with MERIDIA and to reread it each time the prescription is renewed.

Physicians should also discuss with their patients any part of the package insert that is relevant to them. In particular, the importance of keeping appointments for follow-up visits should be emphasized.

Patients should be advised to notify their physician if they develop a rash, hives, or other allergic reactions.

Patients should be advised to inform their physicians if they are taking, or plan to take, any prescription or over-the-counter drugs, especially weight-reducing agents, decongestants, antidepressants, cough suppressants, lithium, dihydroergotamine, sumatriptan (Imitrex®), or tryptophan, since there is a potential for interactions.

Patients should be reminded of the importance of having their blood pressure and pulse monitored at regular intervals.

Drug Interactions

CNS Active Drugs:

The use of MERIDIA® (sibutramine hydrochloride monohydrate) in combination with other CNS-active drugs, particularly serotonergic agents, has not been systematically evaluated. Consequently, caution is advised if the concomitant administration of MERIDIA with other centrally-acting drugs is indicated (see **CONTRAINDICATIONS** and **WARNINGS**).

In patients receiving monoamine oxidase inhibitors (MAOIs) (e.g., phenelzine, selegiline) in combination with serotonergic agents (e.g., fluoxetine, fluvoxamine, paroxetine, sertraline, venlafaxine), there have been reports of serious, sometimes fatal, reactions ("serotonin syndrome;" see below). Because sibutramine inhibits serotonin reuptake, MERIDIA should not be used concomitantly with a MAOI (see **CONTRAINDICATIONS**). At least 2 weeks should elapse between discontinuation of a MAOI and initiation of treatment with MERIDIA. Similarly, at least 2 weeks should elapse between discontinuation of MERIDIA and initiation of treatment with a MAOI.

The rare, but serious, constellation of symptoms termed "serotonin syndrome" has also been reported with the concomitant use of selective serotonin reuptake inhibitors and agents for migraine therapy, such as Imitrex® (sumatriptan succinate) and dihydroergotamine, certain opioids, such as dextromethorphan, meperidine, pentazocine and fentanyl, lithium, or tryptophan. Serotonin syndrome has also been reported with the concomitant use of two serotonin reuptake inhibitors. The syndrome requires immediate medical attention and may include one or more of the following symptoms: excitement, hypomania, restlessness, loss of consciousness, confusion, disorientation, anxiety, agitation, motor weakness, myoclonus, tremor, hemiballismus, hyperreflexia, ataxia, dysarthria, incoordination, hyperthermia, shivering, pupillary dilation, diaphoresis, emesis, and tachycardia.

Because sibutramine inhibits serotonin reuptake, in general, it should not be administered with other serotonergic agents such as those listed above. However, if such a combination is clinically indicated, appropriate observation of the patient is warranted.

Drugs That May Raise Blood Pressure and/or Heart Rate

Concomitant use of MERIDIA and other agents that may raise blood pressure or heart rate have not been evaluated. These include certain decongestants, cough, cold, and allergy medications that contain agents such as ephedrine, or pseudoephedrine. Caution should be used when prescribing MERIDIA to patients who use these medications.

Alcohol

In a double-blind, placebo-controlled, crossover study in 19 volunteers, administration of a single dose of ethanol (0.5 mL/kg) together with 20 mg of sibutramine resulted in no psychomotor interactions of clinical significance between alcohol and sibutramine. However, the concomitant use of MERIDIA and excess alcohol is not recommended.

Information on the Abbott Pharmaceutical Products listed on these pages is from the prescribing information in use as of June 1, 2010. For more information, please visit rxabbott.com or call 1-800-633-9110.

Oral Contraceptives

The suppression of ovulation by oral contraceptives was not inhibited by sibutramine. In a crossover study, 12 healthy female volunteers on oral steroid contraceptives received placebo in one period and 15 mg sibutramine in another period over the course of 8 weeks. No clinically significant systemic interaction was observed; therefore, no requirement for alternative contraceptive precautions are needed when patients taking oral contraceptives are concurrently prescribed sibutramine.

Carcinogenesis, Mutagenesis, Impairment of Fertility

Carcinogenicity

Sibutramine was administered in the diet to mice (1.25, 5 or 20 mg/kg/day) and rats (1, 3, or 9 mg/kg/day) for two years generating combined maximum plasma AUC's of the two major active metabolites equivalent to 0.4 and 16 times, respectively, those following a daily human dose of 15 mg. There was no evidence of carcinogenicity in mice or in female rats. In male rats there was a higher incidence of benign tumors of the testicular interstitial cells; such tumors are commonly seen in rats and are hormonally mediated. The relevance of these tumors to humans is not known.

Mutagenicity

Sibutramine was not mutagenic in the Ames test, *in vitro* Chinese hamster V79 cell mutation assay, *in vitro* clastogenicity assay in human lymphocytes or micronucleus assay in mice. Its two major active metabolites were found to have equivocal bacterial mutagenic activity in the Ames test. However, both metabolites gave consistently negative results in the *in vitro* Chinese hamster V79 cell mutation assay, *in vitro* clastogenicity assay in human lymphocytes, *in vitro* DNA-repair assay in HeLa cells, micronucleus assay in mice and *in vivo* unscheduled DNA-synthesis assay in rat hepatocytes.

Impairment of Fertility

In rats, there were no effects on fertility at doses generating combined plasma AUC's of the two major active metabolites up to 32 times those following a human dose of 15 mg. At 13 times the human combined AUC, there was maternal toxicity, and the dams' nest-building behavior was impaired, leading to a higher incidence of perinatal mortality; there was no effect at approximately 4 times the human combined AUC.

Pregnancy

Teratogenic Effects

Pregnancy Category C

Radiolabeled studies in animals indicated that tissue distribution was unaffected by pregnancy, with relatively low transfer to the fetus. In rats, there was no evidence of teratogenicity at doses of 1, 3, or 10 mg/kg/day generating combined plasma AUC's of the two major active metabolites up to approximately 32 times those following the human dose of 15 mg. In rabbits dosed at 3, 15, or 75 mg/kg/day, plasma AUC's greater than approximately 5 times those following the human dose of 15 mg caused maternal toxicity. At markedly toxic doses, Dutch Belted rabbits had a slightly higher than control incidence of pups with a broad short snout, short rounded pinnae, short tail and, in some, shorter thickened long bones in the limbs; at comparably high doses in New Zealand White rabbits, one study showed a slightly higher than control incidence of pups with cardiovascular anomalies while a second study showed a lower incidence than in the control group.

No adequate and well controlled studies with sibutramine have been conducted in pregnant women. The use of MERIDIA during pregnancy is not recommended. Women of childbearing potential should employ adequate contraception while taking MERIDIA. Patients should be advised to notify their physician if they become pregnant or intend to become pregnant while taking MERIDIA.

Nursing Mothers

It is not known whether sibutramine or its metabolites are excreted in human milk. MERIDIA is not recommended for use in nursing mothers. Patients should be advised to notify their physician if they are breast-feeding.

Pediatric Use

The efficacy of sibutramine in adolescents who are obese has not been adequately studied.

Sibutramine's mechanism of action inhibiting the reuptake of serotonin and norepinephrine is similar to the mechanism of action of some antidepressants. Pooled analyses of short-term placebo-controlled trials of antidepressants in children and adolescents with major depressive disorder (MDD), obsessive compulsive disorder (OCD), and other psychiatric disorders have revealed a greater risk of adverse events representing suicidal behavior or thinking during the first few months of treatment in those receiving antidepressants. The average risk of such events in patients receiving antidepressants was 4%, twice the placebo risk of 2%.

No placebo-controlled trials of sibutramine have been conducted in children or adolescents with MDD, OCD, or other psychiatric disorders. In a study of adolescents with obesity in which 368 patients were treated with sibutramine and 130 patients with placebo, one patient in the sibutramine group and one patient in the placebo group attempted suicide. Suicidal ideation was reported by 2 sibutramine-treated patients and none of the placebo patients. It is unknown if sibutramine increases the risk of suicidal behavior or thinking in pediatric patients.

The data are inadequate to recommend the use of sibutramine for the treatment of obesity in pediatric patients.

Geriatric Use

Clinical studies of sibutramine did not include sufficient numbers of patients over 65 years of age. Sibutramine is contraindicated in this group of patients (see **CONTRAINDICATIONS**). Pharmacokinetics in elderly patients are discussed in "CLINICAL PHARMACOLOGY."

ADVERSE REACTIONS

In placebo-controlled studies, 9% of patients treated with sibutramine (n = 2068) and 7% of patients treated with placebo (n = 884) withdrew for adverse events.

In placebo-controlled studies, the most common events were dry mouth, anorexia, insomnia, constipation and headache. Adverse events in these studies occurring in ≥ 1% of sibutramine treated patients and more frequently than in the placebo group are shown in the following table.

Obese Patients in Placebo-Controlled Studies

BODY SYSTEM Adverse Event	Sibutramine (n = 2068)	Placebo (n = 884)
	% Incidence	% Incidence
BODY AS A WHOLE:		
Headache	30.3	18.6
Back pain	8.2	5.5
Flu syndrome	8.2	5.8
Injury accident	5.9	4.1
Asthenia	5.9	5.3
Abdominal pain	4.5	3.6
Chest pain	1.8	1.2
Neck pain	1.6	1.1
Allergic reaction	1.5	0.8
CARDIOVASCULAR SYSTEM		
Tachycardia	2.6	0.6
Vasodilation	2.4	0.9
Migraine	2.4	2.0
Hypertension/increased blood pressure	2.1	0.9
Palpitation	2.0	0.8
DIGESTIVE SYSTEM		
Anorexia	13.0	3.5
Constipation	11.5	6.0
Increased appetite	8.7	2.7
Nausea	5.9	2.8
Dyspepsia	5.0	2.6
Gastritis	1.7	1.2
Vomiting	1.5	1.4
Rectal disorder	1.2	0.5
METABOLIC & NUTRITIONAL		
Thirst	1.7	0.9
Generalized edema	1.2	0.8
MUSCULOSKELETAL SYSTEM		
Arthralgia	5.9	5.0
Myalgia	1.9	1.1
Tenosynovitis	1.2	0.5
Joint disorder	1.1	0.6
NERVOUS SYSTEM		
Dry mouth	17.2	4.2
Insomnia	10.7	4.5
Dizziness	7.0	3.4
Nervousness	5.2	2.9
Anxiety	4.5	3.4
Depression	4.3	2.5
Paresthesia	2.0	0.5
Somnolence	1.7	0.9
CNS stimulation	1.5	0.5
Emotional lability	1.3	0.6
RESPIRATORY SYSTEM		
Rhinitis	10.2	7.1
Pharyngitis	10.0	8.4
Sinusitis	5.0	2.6
Cough increase	3.8	3.3
Laryngitis	1.3	0.9
SKIN & APPENDAGES		
Rash	3.8	2.5
Sweating	2.5	0.9
Herpes simplex	1.3	1.0
Acne	1.0	0.8
SPECIAL SENSES		
Taste perversion	2.2	0.8
Ear disorder	1.7	0.9
Ear pain	1.1	0.7
UROGENITAL SYSTEM		
Dysmenorrhea	3.5	1.4
Urinary tract infection	2.3	2.0
Vaginal monilia	1.2	0.5
Metrorrhagia	1.0	0.8

The following additional adverse events were reported in ≥ 1% of all patients who received sibutramine in controlled and uncontrolled premarketing studies.

Body as a Whole
fever.

Digestive System
diarrhea, flatulence, gastroenteritis, tooth disorder.

Metabolic and Nutritional
peripheral edema.

Musculoskeletal System
arthritis.

Nervous System
agitation, leg cramps, hypertonia, thinking abnormal.

Respiratory System
bronchitis, dyspnea.

Skin and Appendages
pruritus.

Special Senses
amblyopia.

Urogenital System
menstrual disorders.

Other Adverse Events

Clinical Studies

Seizures

Convulsions were reported as an adverse event in three of 2068 (0.1%) sibutramine treated patients and in none of 884 placebo-treated patients in placebo-controlled premarketing obesity studies. Two of the three patients with seizures had potentially predisposing factors (one had a prior history of epilepsy; one had a subsequent diagnosis of brain tumor). The incidence in all subjects who received sibutramine (three of 4,588 subjects) was less than 0.1%.

Ecchymosis/Bleeding Disorders

Ecchymosis (bruising) was observed in 0.7% of sibutramine treated patients and in 0.2% of placebo-treated patients in premarketing placebo-controlled obesity studies. One patient had prolonged bleeding of a small amount which occurred during minor facial surgery. Sibutramine may have an effect on platelet function due to its effect on serotonin uptake.

Interstitial Nephritis

Acute interstitial nephritis (confirmed by biopsy) was reported in one obese patient receiving sibutramine during premarketing studies. After discontinuation of the medication, dialysis and oral corticosteroids were administered; renal function normalized. The patient made a full recovery.

Altered Laboratory Findings

Abnormal liver function tests, including increases in AST, ALT, GGT, LDH, alkaline phosphatase and bilirubin, were reported as adverse events in 1.6% of sibutramine-treated obese patients in placebo-controlled trials compared with 0.8% of placebo patients. In these studies, potentially clinically significant values (total bilirubin ≥ 2 mg/dL; ALT, AST, GGT, LDH, or alkaline phosphatase ≥ 3 × upper limit of normal) occurred in 0% (alkaline phosphatase) to 0.6% (ALT) of the sibutramine treated patients and in none of the placebo-treated patients. Abnormal values tended to be sporadic, often diminished with continued treatment, and did not show a clear dose-response relationship.

Postmarketing Reports

Voluntary reports of adverse events temporally associated with the use of sibutramine are listed below. It is important to emphasize that although these events occurred during treatment with sibutramine, they may have no causal relationship with the drug. Obesity itself, concurrent disease states/risk factors, or weight reduction may be associated with an increased risk for some of these events.

Psychiatric

Cases of depression, psychosis, mania, suicidal ideation and suicide have been reported rarely in patients on sibutramine treatment. However, a relationship has not been established between these events and the use of sibutramine. If any of these events should occur during treatment with sibutramine, discontinuation should be considered.

Hypersensitivity

Allergic hypersensitivity reactions ranging from mild skin eruptions and urticaria to angioedema and anaphylaxis have been reported (see **CONTRAINDICATIONS** and **PRECAUTIONS-Information For Patients**, and other reports of allergic reactions listed below).

Other Postmarketing Reported Events:

Body as a Whole

anaphylactic shock, anaphylactoid reaction, chest pressure, chest tightness, facial edema, limb pain, sudden unexplained death.

Cardiovascular System
angina pectoris, atrial fibrillation, congestive heart failure, heart arrest, heart rate decreased, myocardial infarction, supraventricular tachycardia, syncope, torsade de pointes, vascular headache, ventricular tachycardia, ventricular extrasystoles, ventricular fibrillation.
Digestive System
cholecystitis, cholelithiasis, duodenal ulcer, eructation, gastrointestinal hemorrhage, increased salivation, intestinal obstruction, mouth ulcer, stomach ulcer, tongue edema.
Endocrine System
goiter, hyperthyroidism, hypothyroidism.
Hemic and Lymphatic System
anemia, leukopenia, lymphadenopathy, petechiae, thrombocytopenia.
Metabolic and Nutritional
hyperglycemia, hypoglycemia.
Musculoskeletal System
arthrosis, bursitis.
Nervous System
abnormal dreams, abnormal gait, amnesia, anger, cerebrovascular accident, concentration impaired, confusion, depression aggravated, Gilles de la Tourette's syndrome, hypesthesia, libido decreased, libido increased, mood changes, nightmares, short term memory loss, speech disorder, transient ischemic attack, tremor, twitch, vertigo.
Respiratory System
epistaxis, nasal congestion, respiratory disorder, yawn.
Skin and Appendages
alopecia, dermatitis, photosensitivity (skin), urticaria.
Special Senses
abnormal vision, blurred vision, dry eye, eye pain, increased intraocular pressure, otitis externa, otitis media, photosensitivity (eyes), tinnitus.
Urogenital System
abnormal ejaculation, hematuria, impotence, increased urinary frequency, micturition difficulty, urinary retention.

DRUG ABUSE AND DEPENDENCE

Controlled Substance

MERIDIA is controlled in Schedule IV of the Controlled Substances Act (CSA).

Abuse and Physical and Psychological Dependence

Physicians should carefully evaluate patients for history of drug abuse and follow such patients closely, observing them for signs of misuse or abuse (e.g., drug development of tolerance, incrementation of doses, drug seeking behavior).

OVERDOSAGE

Overdose Management

There is limited experience of overdose with sibutramine. The most frequently noted adverse events associated with overdose are tachycardia, hypertension, headache and dizziness. Treatment should consist of general measures employed in the management of overdosage: an airway should be established as needed; cardiac and vital sign monitoring is recommended; general symptomatic and supportive measures should be instituted. Cautious use of β-blockers may be indicated to control elevated blood pressure or tachycardia. The results from a study in patients with end-stage renal disease on dialysis showed that sibutramine metabolites were not eliminated to a significant degree with hemodialysis. (see **Pharmacokinetics**-Special Populations-*Renal Insufficiency*).

DOSAGE AND ADMINISTRATION

The recommended starting dose of MERIDIA is 10 mg administered once daily with or without food. If there is inadequate weight loss, the dose may be titrated after four weeks to a total of 15 mg once daily. The 5 mg dose should be reserved for patients who do not tolerate the 10 mg dose. Blood pressure and heart rate changes should be taken into account when making decisions regarding dose titration (see **WARNINGS** and **PRECAUTIONS**).

Doses above 15 mg daily are not recommended. In most of the clinical trials, MERIDIA was given in the morning.

Analysis of numerous variables has indicated that approximately 60% of patients who lose at least 4 pounds in the first 4 weeks of treatment with a given dose of MERIDIA in combination with a reduced-calorie diet lose at least 5% (placebo-subtracted) of their initial body weight by the end of 6 months to 1 year of treatment on that dose of MERIDIA. Conversely, approximately 80% of patients who do not lose at least 4 pounds in the first 4 weeks of treatment with a given dose of MERIDIA do not lose at least 5% (placebo-subtracted) of their initial body weight by the end of 6 months to 1 year of treatment on that dose. If a patient has not lost at least 4 pounds in the first 4 weeks of treatment, the physician should consider reevaluation of therapy which may include increasing the dose or discontinuation of MERIDIA.

The safety and effectiveness of MERIDIA, as demonstrated in double-blind, placebo-controlled trials, have not been determined beyond 2 years at this time.

HOW SUPPLIED

MERIDIA® (sibutramine hydrochloride monohydrate) Capsules contain 5 mg, 10 mg, or 15 mg sibutramine hydrochloride monohydrate and are supplied as follows:

5 mg, NDC 0074-2456-12, blue/yellow capsules imprinted with "MERIDIA" on the cap and "-5-" on the body, in bottles of 30 capsules.

10 mg, NDC 0074-2457-12, blue/white capsules imprinted with "MERIDIA" on the cap and "-10-" on the body, in bottles of 30 capsules.

15 mg, NDC 0074-2458-12, yellow/white capsules imprinted with "MERIDIA" on the cap and "-15-" on the body, in bottles of 30 capsules.

Storage

Store at 25°C (77°F); excursions permitted to 15°-30°C (59°-86°F) [see USP controlled room temperature]. Protect capsules from heat and moisture. Dispense in a tight, light-resistant container as defined in USP.

Manufactured for Abbott Laboratories, North Chicago, IL 60064, USA by KNOLL LLC B.V. Jayuya PR, 00664.

IMITREX is a registered trademark of Glaxo Group Limited.

Sibutramine is covered by US Patent Nos. 4,746,680; 4,929,629; and 5,436,272.

03-A336- Revised: January, 2010

©Abbott

MERIDIA®
(mer-ID-dee-uh)
(sibutramine hydrochloride monohydrate) Capsules Ⓒ**IV**
PATIENT INFORMATION

Read the Patient Information that comes with MERIDIA before you start using it and each time you get a refill. There may be new information. This leaflet does not take the place of talking with your healthcare provider about your medical condition or treatment.

What is the most important information I should know about MERIDIA?

Some people taking MERIDIA can have a large increase in blood pressure or heart rate (pulse). Do not take MERIDIA if your blood pressure is not well controlled. Contact your doctor if you experience an increase in blood pressure while taking MERIDIA.

Your doctor should check your blood pressure and heart rate before you start MERIDIA and continue checking it regularly while you are using MERIDIA. It is important to have regular check-ups while taking MERIDIA.

What is MERIDIA?

MERIDIA is a medicine that may help obese people, as determined by their doctor, lose weight and keep weight off. MERIDIA may help with weight loss because it affects areas of the brain that control hunger. You should use MERIDIA with a low calorie diet.

The use of MERIDIA for more than 2 years has not been studied.

MERIDIA has not been studied in children under 16 years of age.

Who should not take MERIDIA?

Do not take MERIDIA if you:

- **have, or have ever had, heart problems**, including:
  - a heart attack;
  - chest pain or heart disease caused by poor blood flow in the heart (e.g., angina);
  - heart failure;
  - a fast heart rate or uneven heart beat;
  - hardening of the arteries or other blood vessels;
  - poor circulation in the legs.
- **have, or have ever had, a stroke or stroke symptoms.**
- **have high blood pressure** (is above 145/90 mm Hg) that is not controlled by blood pressure medicines, or your blood pressure is above 145/90 mm Hg and you do not take blood pressure medicines.
- **are over age 65.**
- **are taking or have taken a medicine called a monoamine oxidase inhibitor (MAOI).** Ask your doctor or pharmacist if you are not sure if any of your medicines are MAOIs. Do not take MAOIs for at least 2 weeks before using MERIDIA. Do not take MAOIs for at least 2 weeks after stopping MERIDIA.
- **have an eating disorder called anorexia nervosa or bulimia nervosa.**
- **are taking weight loss medicines to control your appetite.**
- **are allergic to MERIDIA.** The active ingredient is sibutramine hydrochloride monohydrate. See the end of this leaflet for a complete list of ingredients in MERIDIA.

How should I take MERIDIA?

- Take MERIDIA exactly as prescribed. Your doctor may adjust your dose. Do not change your dose unless your doctor tells you to do so.
- You can take MERIDIA with or without food.
- If you miss a dose of MERIDIA, just skip it. Do not take an extra dose to make up for missed doses.
- If you take too much MERIDIA, call your doctor or Poison Control Center right away, or go to the emergency room.
- Tell your doctor if you do not lose at least 4 pounds in the first 4 weeks of taking MERIDIA and eating a low calorie diet. Your doctor may change your dose or stop MERIDIA. MERIDIA does not work for everyone.

What should I avoid while taking MERIDIA?

MERIDIA may not be the right medicine for you if you have certain medical conditions. Tell your doctor about all of your medical conditions, especially if you:

- **have, or have ever had, heart problems**, including:
  - a heart attack;
  - chest pain or heart disease caused by poor blood flow in the heart (e.g., angina);
  - heart failure;
  - a fast heart rate or uneven heart beat;
  - hardening of the arteries or other blood vessels;
  - poor circulation in the legs.
- **have high blood pressure.**
- **have, or have ever had, a stroke or stroke symptoms.**
- **have liver or kidney problems.**
- **have an eye problem called glaucoma.**
- **have a thyroid problem (hypothyroidism).**
- **have or had seizures (convulsions, fits).**
- **have bleeding problems.**
- **have or had gallstones.**
- **have depression.**
- **are over age 65.**
- **are under age 16.**
- **are pregnant or planning to become pregnant.** The effects of MERIDIA on your unborn baby are not known. If you can become pregnant, you should use birth control while taking MERIDIA. Tell your doctor right away if you get pregnant while taking MERIDIA.
- **are breastfeeding.** It is not known if MERIDIA passes into your milk. The effects of MERIDIA on your baby are not known. You should not breastfeed while taking MERIDIA.

Do not drive, operate heavy machinery or do other dangerous activities until you know how MERIDIA affects you.

Tell your doctor about all the medicines you take, including prescription and non-prescription medicines, vitamins, and herbal supplements. Taking MERIDIA and certain other medicines may affect each other and may cause serious and in some cases life-threatening side effects. Make sure you tell your doctor if you take:

- medicines called MAOIs, see "Who should not take MERIDIA?"
- other weight loss medicines
- cough and cold medicines
- migraine medicines
- depression medicines
- narcotic pain-killers
- lithium
- tryptophan
- medicines that increase bleeding
- antibiotic medicines

Know the medicines you take. Keep a list of them and show it to your doctor and pharmacist each time you get new medicine. They can tell you if it is okay to take MERIDIA with other medicines.

What are the possible side effects of MERIDIA?

Common side effects of MERIDIA include: dry mouth, headache, loss of appetite, trouble sleeping, and constipation.

The following serious side effects have been reported with MERIDIA:

- **a large increase in blood pressure or heart rate in some people.** See "What is the most important information I should know about MERIDIA?"
- **seizures**
- **bleeding**
- **a rare, but life-threatening problem called "serotonin syndrome."** It may occur when people take drugs that affect a brain chemical called serotonin along with MERIDIA. Do not take other medicines with MERIDIA unless your doctor has told you it is okay to do so. Get medical help right away if you have any of the following symptoms especially when taking other medicines with MERIDIA:
  - feel weak, restless, confused, or anxious
  - lose consciousness
  - have a fever, vomiting, sweating, shivering or shaking
  - have a fast heartbeat

Certain weight loss medicines have been associated with a rare, but life-threatening condition that affects the blood pressure in lungs (pulmonary hypertension). Because the

Information on the Abbott Pharmaceutical Products listed on these pages is from the prescribing information in use as of June 1, 2010. For more information, please visit rxabbott.com or call 1-800-633-9110.

condition is so rare it is not known if MERIDIA may cause this disease. If you experience new or worsening shortness of breath notify your doctor immediately.

Tell your doctor if you get a rash or hives while taking MERIDIA. You may be having an allergic reaction.

Tell your doctor if you get effects that bother you or that do not go away.

These are not all the side effects of MERIDIA. For more information, ask your doctor or pharmacist.

MERIDIA is a controlled substance (CIV). This means that MERIDIA can be a target for people who abuse prescription medicines. Keep your MERIDIA in a safe place. Selling or giving away MERIDIA is against the law.

How should I store MERIDIA?

- Store MERIDIA at room temperature between 59° to 86° F (15° to 30° C). Never leave it in a hot or moist place.
- Safely throw away MERIDIA that is out of date or no longer needed.
- Keep MERIDIA and all medicines out of reach of children. If your child accidentally takes MERIDIA, call their doctor or Poison Control Center right away, or take your child to the emergency room.

General information about MERIDIA.

Medicines are sometimes prescribed for conditions other than those described in patient information leaflets. Do not use MERIDIA for a condition for which it was not prescribed. Do not give MERIDIA to other people, even if they have the same symptoms you have. It may harm them and it is against the law.

This leaflet summarizes the most important information about MERIDIA. If you would like more information, talk to your doctor. You can also ask your doctor or pharmacist for information that is written for health professionals.

For more information call Abbott Laboratories at 1-800-633-9110 or visit www.Meridia.net.

What are the ingredients in MERIDIA?

Active Ingredient: sibutramine hydrochloride monohydrate Inactive Ingredients: lactose monohydrate, NF; microcrystalline cellulose, NF; colloidal silicon dioxide, NF; and magnesium stearate, NF in a hard-gelatin capsule [which contains titanium dioxide, USP; gelatin; FD&C Blue No. 2 (5- and 10-mg capsules only); D&C Yellow No. 10 (5- and 15-mg capsules only), and other inactive ingredients]. ©Abbott

Manufactured for Abbott Laboratories, North Chicago, IL 60064, USA by KNOLL LLC B.V. Jayuya, PR, 00664.

Ref. 03-A336-Revised January, 2010

Shown in Product Identification Guide, page 303

NIASPAN® TABLETS ℞
[*NEE-uh-span*]
(niacin extended-release)
tablet, film coated, extended release for oral use

HIGHLIGHTS OF PRESCRIBING INFORMATION

These highlights do not include all the information needed to use NIASPAN® safely and effectively. See full prescribing information for NIASPAN.

NIASPAN (niacin extended-release) tablet, film coated, extended release for oral use.

Initial U.S. Approval: 1997

————INDICATIONS AND USAGE————
NIASPAN contains extended-release niacin (nicotinic acid), and is indicated:

- To reduce elevated TC, LDL-C, Apo B and TG, and to increase HDL-C in patients with primary hyperlipidemia and mixed dyslipidemia. (1)
- *In combination with simvastatin or lovastatin:* to treat primary hyperlipidemia and mixed dyslipidemia when treatment with NIASPAN, simvastatin, or lovastatin monotherapy is considered inadequate. (1)
- To reduce the risk of recurrent nonfatal myocardial infarction in patients with a history of myocardial infarction and hyperlipidemia. (1)
- *In combination with a bile acid binding resin:*
  - Slows progression or promotes regression of atherosclerotic disease in patients with a history of coronary artery disease (CAD) and hyperlipidemia. (1)
  - As an adjunct to diet to reduce elevated TC and LDL-C in adult patients with primary hyperlipidemia. (1)
- To reduce TG in adult patients with severe hypertriglyceridemia. (1)

Limitations of use:
No incremental benefit of NIASPAN coadministered with simvastatin or lovastatin on cardiovascular morbidity and mortality over and above that demonstrated for niacin, simvastatin and lovastatin monotherapy, has been established. NIASPAN has not been studied in Fredrickson Type I and III dyslipidemias.

————DOSAGE AND ADMINISTRATION————
- NIASPAN should be taken at bedtime with a low-fat snack. (2)
- Dose range: 500 mg to 2000 mg once daily. (2)

- Therapy with NIASPAN must be initiated at 500 mg at bedtime in order to reduce the incidence and severity of side effects which may occur during early therapy and should not be increased by more than 500 mg in any four week period. (2)
- Maintenance dose: 1000 to 2000 mg once daily. (2)
- Doses greater than 2000 mg daily are not recommended. (2)
- Concomitant therapy with lovastatin: Initial dose of lovastatin is 20 mg once a day; combination therapy with NIASPAN and lovastatin should not exceed doses of 2000 mg and 40 mg daily, respectively. (2)
- Concomitant therapy with simvastatin: Initial dose of simvastatin is 20 mg once a day; combination therapy with NIASPAN and simvastatin should not exceed doses of 2000 mg and 40 mg daily, respectively. (2)

————DOSAGE FORMS AND STRENGTHS————
Unscored film-coated tablets for oral administration: 500, 750 and 1000 mg niacin extended-release. (3)

————CONTRAINDICATIONS————
- Active liver disease, which may include unexplained persistent elevations in hepatic transaminase levels. (4, 5.2)
- Active peptic ulcer disease. (4)
- Arterial bleeding. (4)
- Known hypersensitivity to product components. (4, 6.1)

————WARNINGS AND PRECAUTIONS————
- Severe hepatic toxicity has occurred in patients substituting sustained-release niacin for immediate-release niacin at equivalent doses. (5.2)
- Myopathy has been reported in patients taking NIASPAN. The risk for myopathy and rhabdomyolysis are increased when lovastatin or simvastatin are coadministered with NIASPAN, particularly in elderly patients and patients with diabetes, renal failure, or uncontrolled hypothyroidism. (5.1)
- Liver enzyme abnormalities and monitoring: Persistent elevations in hepatic transaminase can occur. Monitor liver enzymes before and during treatment. (5.2)
- Use with caution in patients with unstable angina or in the acute phase of an MI. (5)
- NIASPAN can increase serum glucose levels. Glucose levels should be closely monitored in diabetic or potentially diabetic patients particularly during the first few months of use or dose adjustment. (5.3)

————ADVERSE REACTIONS————
Most common adverse reactions (incidence >5% and greater than placebo) are flushing, diarrhea, nausea, vomiting, increased cough, and pruritus. (6.1)

Flushing of the skin may be reduced in frequency or severity by pretreatment with aspirin (up to the recommended dose of 325 mg taken 30 minutes prior to NIASPAN dose). (2)

To report SUSPECTED ADVERSE REACTIONS, contact Abbott Laboratories at 1-800-633-9110 or FDA at 1-800-FDA-1088 or www.fda.gov/medwatch.

————DRUG INTERACTIONS————
- Statins: Caution should be used when prescribing niacin with statins as these agents can increase risk of myopathy/rhabdomyolysis. (5.1, 7.1)
- Bile Acid Sequestrants: Bile acid sequestrants have a high niacin-binding capacity and should be taken at least 4-6 hours before NIASPAN administration. (7.2)

————USE IN SPECIFIC POPULATIONS————
- Renal impairment: NIASPAN should be used with caution in patients with renal impairment. (5, 8.6)
- Hepatic impairment: NIASPAN is contraindicated in active liver disease or significant or unexplained hepatic dysfunction or unexplained elevations of serum transaminases. (4, 5, 5.2, 8.7)

See 17 for PATIENT COUNSELING INFORMATION

Revised: 03/2010

————————————————————————————

————————————————————————————

FULL PRESCRIBING INFORMATION

1   INDICATIONS AND USAGE

Therapy with lipid-altering agents should be only one component of multiple risk factor intervention in individuals at significantly increased risk for atherosclerotic vascular disease due to hyperlipidemia. Niacin therapy is indicated as an adjunct to diet when the response to a diet restricted in saturated fat and cholesterol and other nonpharmacologic measures alone has been inadequate.

1. NIASPAN is indicated to reduce elevated TC, LDL-C, Apo B and TG levels, and to increase HDL-C in patients with primary hyperlipidemia (heterozygous familial and nonfamilial) and mixed dyslipidemia (Fredrickson Types IIa and IIb).
2. NIASPAN in combination with simvastatin or lovastatin is indicated for the treatment of primary hyperlipidemia (heterozygous familial and nonfamilial) and mixed dyslipidemia (Fredrickson Types IIa and IIb) when treatment with NIASPAN, simvastatin, or lovastatin monotherapy is considered inadequate.
3. In patients with a history of myocardial infarction and hyperlipidemia, niacin is indicated to reduce the risk of recurrent nonfatal myocardial infarction.
4. In patients with a history of coronary artery disease (CAD) and hyperlipidemia, niacin, in combination with a bile acid binding resin, is indicated to slow progression or promote regression of atherosclerotic disease.
5. NIASPAN in combination with a bile acid binding resin is indicated to reduce elevated TC and LDL-C levels in adult patients with primary hyperlipidemia (Type IIa).
6. Niacin is also indicated as adjunctive therapy for treatment of adult patients with severe hypertriglyceridemia (Types IV and V hyperlipidemia) who present a risk of pancreatitis and who do not respond adequately to a determined dietary effort to control them.

Limitations of Use

No incremental benefit of NIASPAN coadministered with simvastatin or lovastatin on cardiovascular morbidity and mortality over and above that demonstrated for niacin, simvastatin, or lovastatin monotherapy has been established. NIASPAN has not been studied in Fredrickson Type I and III dyslipidemias.

2   DOSAGE AND ADMINISTRATION

NIASPAN should be taken at bedtime, after a low-fat snack, and doses should be individualized according to patient response. Therapy with NIASPAN must be initiated at 500 mg at bedtime in order to reduce the incidence and severity of side effects which may occur during early therapy. The recommended dose escalation is shown in Table 1 below.

[See table 1 at top of next page]

Maintenance Dose

The daily dosage of NIASPAN should not be increased by more than 500 mg in any 4–week period. The recommended maintenance dose is 1000 mg (two 500 mg tablets or one 1000 mg tablet) to 2000 mg (two 1000 mg tablets or four 500 mg tablets) once daily at bedtime. Doses greater than 2000 mg daily are not recommended. Women may respond at lower NIASPAN doses than men [*see Clinical Studies (14.2)*].

Single-dose bioavailability studies have demonstrated that two of the 500 mg and one of the 1000 mg tablet strengths are interchangeable but three of the 500 mg and two of the 750 mg tablet strengths are not interchangeable.

If lipid response to NIASPAN alone is insufficient or if higher doses of NIASPAN are not well tolerated, some patients may benefit from combination therapy with a bile acid binding resin or statin *[see Drug Interactions (7.3), Concomitant Therapy* below and *Clinical Studies (14.3, 14.4)]*.

Flushing of the skin *[see Adverse Reactions (6.1)]* may be reduced in frequency or severity by pretreatment with aspirin (up to the recommended dose of 325 mg taken 30 minutes prior to NIASPAN dose). Tolerance to this flushing develops rapidly over the course of several weeks. Flushing, pruritus, and gastrointestinal distress are also greatly reduced by slowly increasing the dose of niacin and avoiding administration on an empty stomach. Concomitant alcoholic, hot drinks or spicy foods may increase the side effects of flushing and pruritus and should be avoided around the time of NIASPAN ingestion.

Equivalent doses of NIASPAN should not be substituted for sustained-release (modified-release, timed-release) niacin preparations or immediate-release (crystalline) niacin *[see Warnings and Precautions (5)]*. Patients previously receiving other niacin products should be started with the recommended NIASPAN titration schedule (see Table 1), and the dose should subsequently be individualized based on patient response.

If NIASPAN therapy is discontinued for an extended period, reinstitution of therapy should include a titration phase (see Table 1).

NIASPAN tablets should be taken whole and should not be broken, crushed or chewed before swallowing.

Concomitant Therapy

Concomitant Therapy with Lovastatin or Simvastatin

Patients already receiving a stable dose of lovastatin or simvastatin who require further TG-lowering or HDL-raising (e.g., to achieve NCEP non-HDL-C goals), may receive concomitant dosage titration with NIASPAN per NIASPAN recommended initial titration schedule *[see Dosage and Administration (2)]*. For patients already receiving a stable dose of NIASPAN who require further LDL-lowering (e.g., to achieve NCEP LDL-C goals), the usual recommended starting dose of lovastatin and simvastatin is 20 mg once a day. Dose adjustments should be made at intervals of 4 weeks or more. Combination therapy with NIASPAN and lovastatin or NIASPAN and simvastatin should not exceed doses of 2000 mg NIASPAN and 40 mg lovastatin or simvastatin daily.

Dosage in Patients with Renal or Hepatic Impairment

Use of NIASPAN in patients with renal or hepatic impairment has not been studied. NIASPAN is contraindicated in patients with significant or unexplained hepatic dysfunction. NIASPAN should be used with caution in patients with renal impairment *[see Warnings and Precautions (5)]*.

Table 1. Recommended Dosing

	Week(s)	Daily dose	NIASPAN Dosage
INITIAL TITRATION SCHEDULE	1 to 4	500 mg	1 NIASPAN 500 mg tablet at bedtime
	5 to 8	1000 mg	1 NIASPAN 1000 mg tablet or 2 NIASPAN 500 mg tablets at bedtime
	*	1500 mg	2 NIASPAN 750 mg tablets or 3 NIASPAN 500 mg tablets at bedtime
	*	2000 mg	2 NIASPAN 1000 mg tablets or 4 NIASPAN 500 mg tablets at bedtime

*After Week 8, titrate to patient response and tolerance. If response to 1000 mg daily is inadequate, increase dose to 1500 mg daily; may subsequently increase dose to 2000 mg daily. Daily dose should not be increased more than 500 mg in a 4-week period, and doses above 2000 mg daily are not recommended. Women may respond at lower doses than men.

3 DOSAGE FORMS AND STRENGTHS

- 500 mg unscored, medium-orange, film-coated, capsule-shaped tablets
- 750 mg unscored, medium-orange, film-coated, capsule-shaped tablets
- 1000 mg unscored, medium-orange, film-coated, capsule-shaped tablets

4 CONTRAINDICATIONS

NIASPAN is contraindicated in the following conditions:

- Active liver disease or unexplained persistent elevations in hepatic transaminases *[see Warnings and Precautions (5.2)]*
- Patients with active peptic ulcer disease
- Patients with arterial bleeding
- Hypersensitivity to niacin or any component of this medication *[see Adverse Reactions (6.1)]*

5 WARNINGS AND PRECAUTIONS

NIASPAN preparations should not be substituted for equivalent doses of immediate-release (crystalline) niacin. For patients switching from immediate-release niacin to NIASPAN, therapy with NIASPAN should be initiated with low doses (i.e., 500 mg at bedtime) and the NIASPAN dose should then be titrated to the desired therapeutic response *[see Dosage and Administration (2)]*.

Caution should also be used when NIASPAN is used in patients with unstable angina or in the acute phase of an MI, particularly when such patients are also receiving vasoactive drugs such as nitrates, calcium channel blockers, or adrenergic blocking agents.

Niacin is rapidly metabolized by the liver, and excreted through the kidneys. NIASPAN is contraindicated in patients with significant or unexplained hepatic impairment *[see Contraindications (4) and Warnings and Precautions (5.2)]* and should be used with caution in patients with renal impairment. Patients with a past history of jaundice, hepatobiliary disease, or peptic ulcer should be observed closely during NIASPAN therapy.

5.1 Skeletal Muscle

Cases of rhabdomyolysis have been associated with concomitant administration of lipid-altering doses (≥1 g/day) of niacin and statins. Physicians contemplating combined therapy with statins and NIASPAN should carefully weigh the potential benefits and risks and should carefully monitor patients for any signs and symptoms of muscle pain, tenderness, or weakness, particularly during the initial months of therapy and during any periods of upward dosage titration of either drug. Periodic serum creatine phosphokinase (CPK) and potassium determinations should be considered in such situations, but there is no assurance that such monitoring will prevent the occurrence of severe myopathy.

The risk for myopathy and rhabdomyolysis are increased when lovastatin or simvastatin are coadministered with NIASPAN, particularly in elderly patients and patients with diabetes, renal failure, or uncontrolled hypothyroidism.

5.2 Liver Dysfunction

Cases of severe hepatic toxicity, including fulminant hepatic necrosis, have occurred in patients who have substituted sustained-release (modified-release, timed-release) niacin products for immediate-release (crystalline) niacin at equivalent doses.

NIASPAN should be used with caution in patients who consume substantial quantities of alcohol and/or have a past history of liver disease. Active liver diseases or unexplained transaminase elevations are contraindications to the use of NIASPAN.

Niacin preparations have been associated with abnormal liver tests. In three placebo-controlled clinical trials involving titration to final daily NIASPAN doses ranging from 500 to 3000 mg, 245 patients received NIASPAN for a mean duration of 17 weeks. No patient with normal serum transaminase levels (AST, ALT) at baseline experienced elevations to more than 3 times the upper limit of normal (ULN) during treatment with NIASPAN. In these studies, fewer than 1% (2/245) of NIASPAN patients discontinued due to transaminase elevations greater than 2 times the ULN.

In three safety and efficacy studies with a combination tablet of NIASPAN and lovastatin involving titration to final daily doses (expressed as mg of niacin/mg of lovastatin) 500 mg/10 mg to 2500 mg/40 mg, ten of 1028 patients (1.0%) experienced reversible elevations in AST/ALT to more than 3 times the ULN. Three of ten elevations occurred at doses outside the recommended dosing limit of 2000 mg/40 mg; no patient receiving 1000 mg/20 mg had 3-fold elevations in AST/ALT.

Niacin extended-release and simvastatin can cause abnormal liver tests. In a simvastatin-controlled, 24 week study with a fixed dose combination of NIASPAN and simvastatin in 641 patients, there were no persistent increases (more than 3x the ULN) in serum transaminases. In three placebo-controlled clinical studies of extended-release niacin there were no patients with normal serum transaminase levels at baseline who experienced elevations to more than 3x the ULN. Persistent increases (more than 3x the ULN) in serum transaminases have occurred in approximately 1% of patients who received simvastatin in clinical studies. When drug treatment was interrupted or discontinued in these patients, the transaminases levels usually fell slowly to pretreatment levels. The increases were not associated with jaundice or other clinical signs or symptoms. There was no evidence of hypersensitivity.

In the placebo-controlled clinical trials and the long-term extension study, elevations in transaminases did not appear to be related to treatment duration; elevations in AST levels did appear to be dose related. Transaminase elevations were reversible upon discontinuation of NIASPAN.

Liver function tests should be performed on all patients during therapy with NIASPAN. Serum transaminase levels, including AST and ALT (SGOT and SGPT), should be monitored before treatment begins, every 6 to 12 weeks for the first year, and periodically thereafter (e.g., at approximately 6-month intervals). Special attention should be paid to patients who develop elevated serum transaminase levels, and in these patients, measurements should be repeated promptly and then performed more frequently. If the transaminase levels show evidence of progression, particularly if they rise to 3 times ULN and are persistent, or if they are associated with symptoms of nausea, fever, and/or malaise, the drug should be discontinued.

5.3 Laboratory Abnormalities

Increase in Blood Glucose: Niacin treatment can increase fasting blood glucose. Frequent monitoring of blood glucose should be performed to ascertain that the drug is producing no adverse effects. Diabetic patients may experience a dose-related increase in glucose intolerance. Diabetic or potentially diabetic patients should be observed closely during treatment with NIASPAN, particularly during the first few months of use or dose adjustment; adjustment of diet and/or hypoglycemic therapy may be necessary.

Reduction in platelet count: NIASPAN has been associated with small but statistically significant dose-related reductions in platelet count (mean of -11% with 2000 mg). Caution should be observed when NIASPAN is administered concomitantly with anticoagulants; platelet counts should be monitored closely in such patients.

Increase in Prothrombin Time (PT): NIASPAN has been associated with small but statistically significant increases in prothrombin time (mean of approximately +4%); accordingly, patients undergoing surgery should be carefully evaluated. Caution should be observed when NIASPAN is administered concomitantly with anticoagulants; prothrombin time should be monitored closely in such patients.

Increase in Uric Acid: Elevated uric acid levels have occurred with niacin therapy, therefore use with caution in patients predisposed to gout.

Decrease in Phosphorus: In placebo-controlled trials, NIASPAN has been associated with small but statistically significant, dose-related reductions in phosphorus levels (mean of -13% with 2000 mg). Although these reductions were transient, phosphorus levels should be monitored periodically in patients at risk for hypophosphatemia.

6 ADVERSE REACTIONS

Because clinical studies are conducted under widely varying conditions, adverse reaction rates observed in the clinical studies of a drug cannot be directly compared to rates in the clinical studies of another drug and may not reflect the rates observed in practice.

6.1 Clinical Studies Experience

In the placebo-controlled clinical trials database of 402 patients (age range 21-75 years, 33% women, 89% Caucasians, 7% Blacks, 3% Hispanics, 1% Asians) with a median treatment duration of 16 weeks, 16% of patients on NIASPAN and 4% of patients on placebo discontinued due to adverse reactions. The most common adverse reactions in the group of patients treated with NIASPAN that led to treatment discontinuation and occurred at a rate greater than placebo were flushing (6% vs. 0%), rash (2% vs. 0%), diarrhea (2% vs. 0%), nausea (1% vs. 0%), and vomiting (1% vs. 0%). The most commonly reported adverse reactions (incidence >5% and greater than placebo) in the NIASPAN controlled clinical trial database of 402 patients were flushing, diarrhea, nausea, vomiting, increased cough and pruritus.

In the placebo-controlled clinical trials, flushing episodes (i.e., warmth, redness, itching and/or tingling) were the most common treatment-emergent adverse reactions (reported by as many as 88% of patients) for NIASPAN. Spontaneous reports suggest that flushing may also be accompanied by symptoms of dizziness, tachycardia, palpitations, shortness of breath, sweating, burning sensation/skin burning sensation, chills, and/or edema, which in rare cases may lead to syncope. In pivotal studies, 6% (14/245) of NIASPAN patients discontinued due to flushing. In comparisons of immediate-release (IR) niacin and NIASPAN, although the proportion of patients who flushed was similar, fewer flushing episodes were reported by patients who received

Information on the Abbott Pharmaceutical Products listed on these pages is from the prescribing information in use as of June 1, 2010. For more information, please visit rxabbott.com or call 1-800-633-9110.

Table 2. Treatment-Emergent Adverse Reactions by Dose Level in ≥ 5% of Patients and at an Incidence Greater than Placebo; Regardless of Causality Assessment in Placebo-Controlled Clinical Trials

	Placebo-Controlled Studies NIASPAN Treatment@				
			Recommended Daily Maintenance Doses[†]		
	Placebo (n = 157) %	500 mg[‡] (n = 87) %	1000 mg (n = 110) %	1500 mg (n = 136) %	2000 mg (n = 95) %
Gastrointestinal Disorders					
Diarrhea	13	7	10	10	14
Nausea	7	5	6	4	11
Vomiting	4	0	2	4	9
Respiratory					
Cough, Increased	6	3	2	< 2	8
Skin and Subcutaneous Tissue Disorders					
Pruritus	2	8	0	3	0
Rash	0	5	5	5	0
Vascular Disorders					
Flushing&	19	68	69	63	55

Note: Percentages are calculated from the total number of patients in each column.
[†] Adverse reactions are reported at the initial dose where they occur.
@ Pooled results from placebo-controlled studies; for NIASPAN, n = 245 and median treatment duration = 16 weeks. Number of NIASPAN patients (n) are not additive across doses.
[‡] The 500 mg/day dose is outside the recommended daily maintenance dosing range [see Dosage and Administration (2)].
& 10 patients discontinued before receiving 500 mg, therefore they were not included.

Table 3. Lipid Response to NIASPAN Therapy

Treatment	n	Mean Percent Change from Baseline to Week 16*							
		TC	LDL-C	HDL-C	TC/HDL-C	TG	Lp(a)	Apo B	Apo A-I
NIASPAN 1000 mg at bedtime	41	-3	-5	+18	-17	-21	-13	-6	+9
NIASPAN 2000 mg at bedtime	41	-10	-14	+22	-25	-28	-27	-16	+8
Placebo	40	0	-1	+4	-3	0	0	+1	+3
NIASPAN 1500 mg at bedtime	76	-8	-12	+20	-20	-13	-15	-12	+8
Placebo	73	+2	+1	+2	+1	+12	+2	+1	+2

n = number of patients at baseline;
*Mean percent change from baseline for all NIASPAN doses was significantly different ($p < 0.05$) from placebo for all lipid parameters shown except Apo A-I at 2000 mg.

NIASPAN. Following 4 weeks of maintenance therapy at daily doses of 1500 mg, the incidence of flushing over the 4-week period averaged 8.6 events per patient for IR niacin versus 1.9 following NIASPAN.
Other adverse reactions occurring in ≥5% of patients treated with NIASPAN and at an incidence greater than placebo are shown in Table 2 below.
[See table above]
In general, the incidence of adverse events was higher in women compared to men.

6.2 Postmarketing Experience
Because the below reactions are reported voluntarily from a population of uncertain size, it is generally not possible to reliably estimate their frequency or establish a causal relationship to drug exposure.
The following additional adverse reactions have been identified during post-approval use of NIASPAN:
Hypersensitivity reactions, including anaphylaxis, angioedema, urticaria, flushing, dyspnea, tongue edema, larynx edema, face edema, peripheral edema, laryngismus, and vesiculobullous rash; maculopapular rash; dry skin; tachycardia; palpitations; atrial fibrillation; other cardiac arrhythmias; syncope; hypotension; postural hypotension; blurred vision; macular edema; peptic ulcers; eructation; flatulence; hepatitis; jaundice; decreased glucose tolerance; gout; myalgia; myopathy; dizziness; insomnia; asthenia; nervousness; paresthesia; dyspnea; sweating; burning sensation/skin burning sensation; skin discoloration, and migraine.
Clinical Laboratory Abnormalities
Chemistry: Elevations in serum transaminases [see Warnings and Precautions (5.2)], LDH, fasting glucose, uric acid, total bilirubin, amylase and creatine kinase, and reduction in phosphorus.
Hematology: Slight reductions in platelet counts and prolongation in prothrombin time [see Warnings and Precautions (5.3)].

7 DRUG INTERACTIONS
7.1 Statins
Caution should be used when prescribing niacin (≥1 gm/day) with statins as these drugs can increase risk of myopathy/rhabdomyolysis. Combination therapy with NIASPAN and lovastatin or NIASPAN and simvastatin should not ex-ceed doses of 2000 mg NIASPAN and 40 mg lovastatin or simvastatin daily. [see Warnings and Precautions (5) and Clinical Pharmacology (12.3)].

7.2 Bile Acid Sequestrants
An *in vitro* study results suggest that the bile acid-binding resins have high niacin binding capacity. Therefore, 4 to 6 hours, or as great an interval as possible, should elapse between the ingestion of bile acid-binding resins and the administration of NIASPAN [see Clinical Pharmacology (12.3)].

7.3 Aspirin
Concomitant aspirin may decrease the metabolic clearance of nicotinic acid. The clinical relevance of this finding is unclear.

7.4 Antihypertensive Therapy
Niacin may potentiate the effects of ganglionic blocking agents and vasoactive drugs resulting in postural hypotension.

7.5 Other
Vitamins or other nutritional supplements containing large doses of niacin or related compounds such as nicotinamide may potentiate the adverse effects of NIASPAN.

7.6 Laboratory Test Interactions
Niacin may produce false elevations in some fluorometric determinations of plasma or urinary catecholamines. Niacin may also give false-positive reactions with cupric sulfate solution (Benedict's reagent) in urine glucose tests.

8 USE IN SPECIFIC POPULATIONS
8.1 Pregnancy
Pregnancy Category C.
Animal reproduction studies have not been conducted with niacin or with NIASPAN. It is also not known whether niacin at doses typically used for lipid disorders can cause fetal harm when administered to pregnant women or whether it can affect reproductive capacity. If a woman receiving niacin for primary hyperlipidemia (Types IIa or IIb) becomes pregnant, the drug should be discontinued. If a woman being treated with niacin for hypertriglyceridemia (Types IV or V) conceives, the benefits and risks of continued therapy should be assessed on an individual basis.
All statins are contraindicated in pregnant and nursing women. When NIASPAN is administered with a statin in a woman of childbearing potential, refer to the pregnancy category and product labeling for the statin.

8.3 Nursing Mothers
Niacin is excreted into human milk but the actual infant dose or infant dose as a percent of the maternal dose is not known. Because of the potential for serious adverse reactions in nursing infants from lipid-altering doses of nicotinic acid, a decision should be made whether to discontinue nursing or to discontinue the drug, taking into account the importance of the drug to the mother. No studies have been conducted with NIASPAN in nursing mothers.

8.4 Pediatric Use
Safety and effectiveness of niacin therapy in pediatric patients (≤16 years) have not been established.

8.5 Geriatric Use
Of 979 patients in clinical studies of NIASPAN, 21% of the patients were age 65 and over. No overall differences in safety and effectiveness were observed between these patients and younger patients, and other reported clinical experience has not identified differences in responses between the elderly and younger patients, but greater sensitivity of some older individuals cannot be ruled out.

8.6 Renal Impairment
No studies have been performed in this population. NIASPAN should be used with caution in patients with renal impairment [see Warnings and Precautions (5)].

8.7 Hepatic Impairment
No studies have been performed in this population. NIASPAN should be used with caution in patients with a past history of liver disease and/or who consume substantial quantities of alcohol. Active liver disease, unexplained transaminase elevations and significant or unexplained hepatic dysfunction are contraindications to the use of NIASPAN [see Contraindications (4.0) and Warnings and Precautions (5.2)].

8.8 Gender
Data from the clinical trials suggest that women have a greater hypolipidemic response than men at equivalent doses of NIASPAN.

10 OVERDOSAGE
Supportive measures should be undertaken in the event of an overdose.

11 DESCRIPTION
NIASPAN (niacin tablet, film-coated extended-release), contains niacin, which at therapeutic doses is an antihyperlipidemic agent. Niacin (nicotinic acid, or 3-pyridinecarboxylic acid) is a white, crystalline powder, very soluble in water, with the following structural formula:

$C_6H_5NO_2$ M.W. = 123.11

NIASPAN is an unscored, medium-orange, film-coated tablet for oral administration and is available in three tablet strengths containing 500, 750, and 1000 mg niacin. NIASPAN tablets also contain the inactive ingredients hypromellose, povidone, stearic acid, and polyethylene glycol, and the following coloring agents: FD&C yellow #6/sunset yellow FCF Aluminum Lake, synthetic red and yellow iron oxides, and titanium dioxide.

12 CLINICAL PHARMACOLOGY
12.1 Mechanism of Action
The mechanism by which niacin alters lipid profiles has not been well defined. It may involve several actions including partial inhibition of release of free fatty acids from adipose tissue, and increased lipoprotein lipase activity, which may increase the rate of chylomicron triglyceride removal from plasma. Niacin decreases the rate of hepatic synthesis of VLDL and LDL, and does not appear to affect fecal excretion of fats, sterols, or bile acids.

12.2 Pharmacodynamics
Niacin functions in the body after conversion to nicotinamide adenine dinucleotide (NAD) in the NAD coenzyme system. Niacin (but not nicotinamide) in gram doses reduces total cholesterol (TC), low density lipoprotein cholesterol (LDL-C), and triglycerides (TG), and increases high-density lipoprotein cholesterol (HDL-C). The magnitude of individual lipid and lipoprotein responses may be influenced by the severity and type of underlying lipid abnormality. The increase in HDL-C is associated with an increase in apolipoprotein A-I (Apo A-I) and a shift in the distribution of HDL subfractions. These shifts include an increase in the HDL_2: HDL_3 ratio, and an elevation in lipoprotein A-I (Lp A-I, an HDL-C particle containing only Apo A-I). Niacin treatment also decreases serum levels of apolipoprotein B-100 (Apo B), the major protein component of the very low-density lipoprotein (VLDL) and LDL fractions, and of Lp(a), a variant form of LDL independently associated with coronary risk. In addition, preliminary reports suggest that niacin causes

favorable LDL particle size transformations, although the clinical relevance of this effect requires further investigation. The effect of niacin-induced changes in lipids/proteins on cardiovascular morbidity or mortality in individuals without preexisting coronary disease has not been established.

A variety of clinical studies have demonstrated that elevated levels of TC, LDL-C, and Apo B promote human atherosclerosis. Similarly, decreased levels of HDL-C are associated with the development of atherosclerosis. Epidemiological investigations have established that cardiovascular morbidity and mortality vary directly with the level of Total-C and LDL-C, and inversely with the level of HDL-C.

Like LDL, cholesterol-enriched triglyceride-rich lipoproteins, including VLDL, intermediate-density lipoprotein (IDL), and their remnants, can also promote atherosclerosis. Elevated plasma TG are frequently found in a triad with low HDL-C levels and small LDL particles, as well as in association with non-lipid metabolic risk factors for coronary heart disease (CHD). As such, total plasma TG has not consistently been shown to be an independent risk factor for CHD. Furthermore, the independent effect of raising HDL-C or lowering TG on the risk of coronary and cardiovascular morbidity and mortality has not been determined.

12.3 Pharmacokinetics

Absorption

Due to extensive and saturable first-pass metabolism, niacin concentrations in the general circulation are dose dependent and highly variable. Time to reach the maximum niacin plasma concentrations was about 5 hours following NIASPAN. To reduce the risk of gastrointestinal (GI) upset, administration of NIASPAN with a low-fat meal or snack is recommended.

Single-dose bioavailability studies have demonstrated that the 500 mg and 1000 mg tablet strengths are dosage form equivalent but the 500 mg and 750 mg tablet strengths are not dosage form equivalent.

Metabolism

The pharmacokinetic profile of niacin is complicated due to extensive first-pass metabolism that is dose-rate specific and, at the doses used to treat dyslipidemia, saturable. In humans, one pathway is through a simple conjugation step with glycine to form nicotinuric acid (NUA). NUA is then excreted in the urine, although there may be a small amount of reversible metabolism back to niacin. The other pathway results in the formation of nicotinamide adenine dinucleotide (NAD). It is unclear whether nicotinamide is formed as a precursor to, or following the synthesis of, NAD. Nicotinamide is further metabolized to at least N-methylnicotinamide (MNA) and nicotinamide-N-oxide (NNO). MNA is further metabolized to two other compounds, N-methyl-2-pyridone-5-carboxamide (2PY) and N-methyl-4-pyridone-5-carboxamide (4PY). The formation of 2PY appears to predominate over 4PY in humans. At the doses used to treat hyperlipidemia, these metabolic pathways are saturable, which explains the nonlinear relationship between niacin dose and plasma concentrations following multiple-dose NIASPAN administration.

Nicotinamide does not have hypolipidemic activity; the activity of the other metabolites is unknown.

Elimination

Following single and multiple doses, approximately 60 to 76% of the niacin dose administered as NIASPAN was recovered in urine as niacin and metabolites; up to 12% was recovered as unchanged niacin after multiple dosing. The ratio of metabolites recovered in the urine was dependent on the dose administered.

Pediatric Use

No pharmacokinetic studies have been performed in this population (≤16 years) *[see Use in Specific Populations (8.4)].*

Geriatric Use

No pharmacokinetic studies have been performed in this population (> 65 years) *[see Use in Specific Populations (8.5)].*

Renal Impairment

No pharmacokinetic studies have been performed in this population. NIASPAN should be used with caution in patients with renal disease *[see Warnings and Precautions (5)].*

Hepatic Impairment

No pharmacokinetic studies have been performed in this population. Active liver disease, unexplained transaminase elevations and significant or unexplained hepatic dysfunction are contraindications to the use of NIASPAN *[see Contraindications (4) and Warnings and Precautions (5.2)].*

Gender

Steady-state plasma concentrations of niacin and metabolites after administration of NIASPAN are generally higher in women than in men, with the magnitude of the difference varying with dose and metabolite. This gender differences

Table 4. Lipid Response in Dose-Escalation Study

| | | | | | Mean Percent Change from Baseline* | | | | |
Treatment	n	TC	LDL-C	HDL-C	TC/HDL-C	TG	Lp(a)	Apo B	Apo A-I
Placebo[‡]	44	-2	-1	+5	-7	-6	-5	-2	+4
NIASPAN	87								
500 mg at bedtime		-2	-3	+10	-10	-5	-3	-2	+5
1000 mg at bedtime		-5	-9	+15	-17	-11	-12	-7	+8
1500 mg at bedtime		-11	-14	+22	-26	-28	-20	-15	+10
2000 mg at bedtime		-12	-17	+26	-29	-35	-24	-16	+12

n = number of patients enrolled;
[‡] Placebo data shown are after 24 weeks of placebo treatment.
* For all NIASPAN doses except 500 mg, mean percent change from baseline was significantly different ($p < 0.05$) from placebo for all lipid parameters shown except Lp(a) and Apo A-I which were significantly different from placebo starting with 1500 mg and 2000 mg, respectively.

Table 5. Selected Lipid Response to NIASPAN in Placebo-Controlled Clinical Studies*

| | | Mean Baseline and Median Percent Change from Baseline (25th, 75th Percentiles) | | |
NIASPAN Dose	n	LDL-C	HDL-C	TG
1000 mg at bedtime	104			
Baseline (mg/dL)		218	45	172
Percent Change		-7 (-15, 0)	+14 (+7, +23)	-16 (-34, +3)
1500 mg at bedtime	120			
Baseline (mg/dL)		212	46	171
Percent Change		-13 (-21, -4)	+19 (+9, +31)	-25 (-45, -2)
2000 mg at bedtime	85			
Baseline (mg/dL)		220	44	160
Percent Change		-16 (-26, -7)	+22 (+15, +34)	-38 (-52, -14)

* Represents pooled analyses of results; minimum duration on therapy at each dose was 4 weeks.

Table 6. Effect of Gender on NIASPAN Dose Response

| | | Mean Percent Change from Baseline | | | | | | | |
| NIASPAN | n | LDL-C | | HDL-C | | TG | | Apo B | |
Dose	(M/F)	M	F	M	F	M	F	M	F
500 mg at bedtime	50/37	-2	-5	+11	+8	-3	-9	-1	-5
1000 mg at bedtime	76/52	-6*	-11*	+14	+20	-10	-20	-5*	-10*
1500 mg at bedtime	104/59	-12	-16	+19	+24	-17	-28	-13	-15
2000 mg at bedtime	75/53	-15	-18	+23	+26	-30	-36	-16	-16

n = number of male/female patients enrolled.
* Percent change significantly different between genders ($p < 0.05$).

Table 7. Lipid Response to NIASPAN in Patients with Low HDL-C

| | | | | | Mean Baseline and Mean Percent Change from Baseline* | | | | | |
	n	TC	LDL-C	HDL-C	TC/HDL-C	TG	Lp(a)[†]	Apo B[†]	Apo A-I[†]	Lp A-I[††]
Baseline (mg/dL)	88	190	120	31	6	194	8	106	105	32
Week 19 (% Change)	71	-3	0	+26	-22	-30	-20	-9	+11	+20

n = number of patients
* Mean percent change from baseline was significantly different ($p < 0.05$) for all lipid parameters shown except LDL-C.
[†] n = 72 at baseline and 69 at week 19.
[††] n = 30 at baseline and week 19.

observed in plasma levels of niacin and its metabolites may be due to gender-specific differences in metabolic rate or volume of distribution. Recovery of niacin and metabolites in urine, however, is generally similar for men and women, indicating that absorption is similar for both genders *[see Gender (8.8)].*

Drug interactions

Fluvastatin

Niacin did not affect fluvastatin pharmacokinetics *[see Drug Interactions (7.1)].*

Lovastatin

When NIASPAN 2000 mg and lovastatin 40 mg were coadministered, NIASPAN increased lovastatin C_{max} and AUC by 2% and 14%, respectively, and decreased lovastatin acid C_{max} and AUC by 22% and 2%, respectively. Lovastatin reduced NIASPAN bioavailability by 2-3% *[see Drug Interactions (7.1)].*

Simvastatin

When NIASPAN 2000 mg and simvastatin 40 mg were coadministered, NIASPAN increased simvastatin C_{max} and AUC by 1% and 9%, respectively, and simvastatin acid C_{max} and AUC by 2% and 18%, respectively. Simvastatin reduced NIASPAN bioavailability by 2% *[see Drug Interactions (7.1)].*

Bile Acid Sequestrants

An *in vitro* study was carried out investigating the niacin-binding capacity of colestipol and cholestyramine. About

---

Information on the Abbott Pharmaceutical Products listed on these pages is from the prescribing information in use as of June 1, 2010. For more information, please visit rxabbott.com or call 1-800-633-9110.

Table 8. LDL-C mean percent change from baseline

Week	Combination Tablet of NIASPAN and Lovastatin			NIASPAN			Lovastatin		
	n*	Dose (mg/mg)	LDL	n*	Dose (mg)	LDL	n*	Dose (mg)	LDL
Baseline	57	-	190.9 mg/dL	61	-	189.7 mg/dL	61	-	185.6 mg/dL
12	47	1000/20	-30%	46	1000	-3%	56	20	-29%
16	45	1000/40	-36%	44	1000	-6%	56	40	-31%
20	42	1500/40	-37%	43	1500	-12%	54	40	-34%
28	42	2000/40	-42%	41	2000	-14%	53	40	-32%

*n = number of patients remaining in trial at each time point

Table 9. HDL-C mean percent change from baseline

Week	Combination Tablet of NIASPAN and Lovastatin			NIASPAN			Lovastatin		
	n*	Dose (mg/mg)	HDL	n*	Dose (mg)	HDL	n*	Dose (mg)	HDL
Baseline	57	-	45 mg/dL	61	-	47 mg/dL	61	-	43 mg/dL
12	47	1000/20	+20%	46	1000	+14%	56	20	+3%
16	45	1000/40	+20%	44	1000	+15%	56	40	+5%
20	42	1500/40	+27%	43	1500	+22%	54	40	+6%
28	42	2000/40	+30%	41	2000	+24%	53	40	+6%

*n = number of patients remaining in trial at each time point

Table 10. TG median percent change from baseline

Week	Combination Tablet of NIASPAN and Lovastatin			NIASPAN			Lovastatin		
	n*	Dose (mg/mg)	TG	n*	Dose (mg)	TG	n*	Dose (mg)	TG
Baseline	57	-	174 mg/dL	61	-	186 mg/dL	61	-	171 mg/dL
12	47	1000/20	-32%	46	1000	-22%	56	20	-20%
16	45	1000/40	-39%	44	1000	-23%	56	40	-17%
20	42	1500/40	-44%	43	1500	-31%	54	40	-21%
28	42	2000/40	-44%	41	2000	-31%	53	40	-20%

*n = number of patients remaining in trial at each time point

Table 11. Lp(a) median percent change from baseline

Week	Combination Tablet of NIASPAN and Lovastatin			NIASPAN			Lovastatin		
	n*	Dose (mg/mg)	Lp(a)	n*	Dose (mg)	Lp(a)	n*	Dose (mg)	Lp(a)
Baseline	57	-	34 mg/dL	61	-	41 mg/dL	60	-	42 mg/dL
12	47	1000/20	-9%	46	1000	-8%	55	20	+8%
16	45	1000/40	-9%	44	1000	-12%	55	40	+8%
20	42	1500/40	-17%	43	1500	-22%	53	40	+6%
28	42	2000/40	-22%	41	2000	-32%	52	40	0%

*n = number of patients remaining in trial at each time point

98% of available niacin was bound to colestipol, with 10 to 30% binding to cholestyramine [see Drug Interactions (7.2)].

13 NONCLINICAL TOXICOLOGY
13.1 Carcinogenesis and Mutagenesis and Impairment of Fertility
Niacin administered to mice for a lifetime as a 1% solution in drinking water was not carcinogenic. The mice in this study received approximately 6 to 8 times a human dose of 3000 mg/day as determined on a mg/m² basis. Niacin was negative for mutagenicity in the Ames test. No studies on impairment of fertility have been performed. No studies have been conducted with NIASPAN regarding carcinogenesis, mutagenesis, or impairment of fertility.

14 CLINICAL STUDIES
14.1 Niacin Clinical Studies
The role of LDL-C in atherogenesis is supported by pathological observations, clinical studies, and many animal experiments. Observational epidemiological studies have clearly established that high TC or LDL-C and low HDL-C are risk factors for CHD. Additionally, elevated levels of Lp(a) have been shown to be independently associated with CHD risk.
Niacin's ability to reduce mortality and the risk of definite, nonfatal myocardial infarction (MI) has been assessed in

long-term studies. The Coronary Drug Project, completed in 1975, was designed to assess the safety and efficacy of niacin and other lipid-altering drugs in men 30 to 64 years old with a history of MI. Over an observation period of 5 years, niacin treatment was associated with a statistically significant reduction in nonfatal, recurrent MI. The incidence of definite, nonfatal MI was 8.9% for the 1,119 patients randomized to nicotinic acid versus 12.2% for the 2,789 patients who received placebo (p<0.004). Total mortality was similar in the two groups at 5 years (24.4% with nicotinic acid versus 25.4% with placebo; p=N.S.). At the time of a 15-year follow-up, there were 11% (69) fewer deaths in the niacin group compared to the placebo cohort (52.0% versus 58.2%; p=0.0004). However, mortality at 15 years was not an original endpoint of the Coronary Drug Project. In addition, patients had not received niacin for approximately 9 years, and confounding variables such as concomitant medication use and medical or surgical treatments were not controlled.
The Cholesterol-Lowering Atherosclerosis Study (CLAS) was a randomized, placebo-controlled, angiographic trial testing combined colestipol and niacin therapy in 162 nonsmoking males with previous coronary bypass surgery. The primary, per-subject cardiac endpoint was global coronary artery change score. After 2 years, 61% of patients in the

placebo cohort showed disease progression by global change score (n=82), compared with only 38.8% of drug-treated subjects (n=80), when both native arteries and grafts were considered (p<0.005); disease regression also occurred more frequently in the drug-treated group (16.2% versus 2.4%; p=0.002). In a follow-up to this trial in a subgroup of 103 patients treated for 4 years, again, significantly fewer patients in the drug-treated group demonstrated progression than in the placebo cohort (48% versus 85%, respectively; p<0.0001).
The Familial Atherosclerosis Treatment Study (FATS) in 146 men ages 62 and younger with Apo B levels ≥ 125 mg/dL, established coronary artery disease, and family histories of vascular disease, assessed change in severity of disease in the proximal coronary arteries by quantitative arteriography. Patients were given dietary counseling and randomized to treatment with either conventional therapy with double placebo (or placebo plus colestipol if the LDL-C was elevated); lovastatin plus colestipol; or niacin plus colestipol. In the conventional therapy group, 46% of patients had disease progression (and no regression) in at least one of nine proximal coronary segments; regression was the only change in 11%. In contrast, progression (as the only change) was seen in only 25% in the niacin plus colestipol group, while regression was observed in 39%. Though not an original endpoint of the trial, clinical events (death, MI, or revascularization for worsening angina) occurred in 10 of 52 patients who received conventional therapy, compared with 2 of 48 who received niacin plus colestipol.
The Harvard Atherosclerosis Reversibility Project (HARP) was a randomized placebo-controlled, 2.5-year study of the effect of a stepped-care antihyperlipidemic drug regimen on 91 patients (80 men and 11 women) with CHD and average baseline TC levels less than 250 mg/dL and ratios of TC to HDL-C greater than 4.0. Drug treatment consisted of an HMG-CoA reductase inhibitor administered alone as initial therapy followed by addition of varying dosages of either a slow-release nicotinic acid, cholestyramine, or gemfibrozil. Addition of nicotinic acid to the HMG-CoA reductase inhibitor resulted in further statistically significant mean reductions in TC, LDL-C, and TG, as well as a further increase in HDL-C in a majority of patients (40 of 44 patients). The ratios of TC to HDL-C and LDL-C to HDL-C were also significantly reduced by this combination drug regimen [see Warnings and Precautions (5.1)].

14.2 NIASPAN Clinical Studies
Placebo-Controlled Clinical Studies in Patients with Primary Hyperlipidemia and Mixed Dyslipidemia: In two randomized, double-blind, parallel, multi-center, placebo-controlled trials, NIASPAN dosed at 1000, 1500 or 2000 mg daily at bedtime with a low-fat snack for 16 weeks (including 4 weeks of dose escalation) favorably altered lipid profiles compared to placebo (Table 3). Women appeared to have a greater response than men at each NIASPAN dose level (see Gender Effect, below).
[See table 3 at top of page 500]
In a double-blind, multi-center, forced dose-escalation study, monthly 500 mg increases in NIASPAN dose resulted in incremental reductions of approximately 5% in LDL-C and Apo B levels in the daily dose range of 500 mg through 2000 mg (Table 4). Women again tended to have a greater response to NIASPAN than men (see Gender Effect, below).
[See table 4 on previous page]
Pooled results for major lipids from these three placebo-controlled studies are shown below (Table 5).
[See table 5 on previous page]
Gender Effect: Combined data from the three placebo-controlled NIASPAN studies in patients with primary hyperlipidemia and mixed dyslipidemia suggest that, at each NIASPAN dose level studied, changes in lipid concentrations are greater for women than for men (Table 6).
[See table 6 on previous page]
Other Patient Populations: In a double-blind, multi-center, 19-week study the lipid-altering effects of NIASPAN (forced titration to 2000 mg at bedtime) were compared to baseline in patients whose primary lipid abnormality was a low level of HDL-C (HDL-C ≤40 mg/dL, TG ≤400 mg/dL, and LDL-C ≤160, or <130 mg/dL in the presence of CHD). Results are shown below (Table 7).
[See table 7 on previous page]
At NIASPAN 2000 mg/day, median changes from baseline (25th, 75th percentiles) for LDL-C, HDL-C, and TG were -3% (-14, +12%), +27% (+13, +38%), and -33% (-50, -19%), respectively.

14.3 NIASPAN and Lovastatin Clinical Studies
Combination NIASPAN and Lovastatin Study: In a multi-center, randomized, double-blind, parallel, 28-week study, a combination tablet of NIASPAN and lovastatin was compared to each individual component in patients with Type IIa and IIb hyperlipidemia. Using a forced dose-escalation study design, patients received each dose for at least 4 weeks. Patients randomized to treatment with the combination tablet of NIASPAN and lovastatin initially received 500 mg/20 mg (expressed as mg of niacin/mg of lovastatin) once daily before bedtime. The dose was increased by 500 mg at 4-week intervals (based on the NIASPAN com-

Table 12. Non-HDL Treatment Response Following 24-Week Treatment Mean Percent Change from Simvastatin 20-mg Treated Baseline

Group A

Week		Combination Tablet of NIASPAN and Simvastatin 2000/20			Combination Tablet of NIASPAN and Simvastatin 1000/20			Simvastatin 20	
	n[a]	Dose (mg/mg)	Non-HDL[b]	n[a]	Dose (mg/mg)	Non-HDL[b]	n[a]	Dose (mg/mg)	Non-HDL[b]
Baseline	56	-	163.1 mg/dL	108	-	164.8 mg/dL	102	-	163.7 mg/dL
4	52	500/20	-12.9%	86	500/20	-12.8%	91	20	-8.3%
8	46	1000/20	-17.5%	91	1000/20	-15.5%	95	20	-8.3%
12	46	1500/20	-18.9%	90	1000/20	-14.8%	96	20	-6.4%
24	40	2000/20	-19.5%[†]	78	1000/20	-13.6%[†]	90	20	-5.0%
Dropouts by week 24:	28.6%			27.8%			11.8%		

[a] n=number of subjects with values in the analysis window at each timepoint
[b] The percent change from baseline is the model-based mean from a repeated measures mixed model with no imputation for missing data from study dropouts.
[†] significant vs. simvastatin 20 mg at the primary endpoint (Week 24), $p<0.05$

Table 13. Non-HDL Treatment Response Following 24-Week Treatment Mean Percent Change from Simvastatin 40-mg Treated Baseline

Group B

Week		Combination Tablet of NIASPAN and Simvastatin 2000/40			Combination Tablet of NIASPAN and Simvastatin 1000/40			Simvastatin 80	
	n[a]	Dose (mg/mg)	Non-HDL[b]	n[a]	Dose (mg/mg)	Non-HDL[b]	n[a]	Dose (mg/mg)	Non-HDL[b]
Baseline	98	-	144.4 mg/dL	111	-	141.2 mg/dL	113	-	134.5 mg/dL
4	96	500/40	-6.0%	108	500/40	-5.9%	110	80	-11.3%
8	93	1000/40	-15.5%	100	1000/40	-16.2%	104	80	-13.7%
12	90	1500/40	-18.4%	97	1000/40	-12.6%	100	80	-9.5%
24	80	2000/40	-7.6%[c]	82	1000/40	-6.7%[d]	90	80	-6.0%
Dropouts by week 24:	18.4%			26.1%			20.4%		

[a] n=number of subjects with values in the analysis window at each timepoint
[b] The percent change from baseline is the model-based mean from a repeated measures mixed model with no imputation for missing data from study dropouts.
[c] non-inferior to simvastatin 80 arm; 95% confidence interval of mean difference in non-HDL for the combination tablet of NIASPAN and simvastatin 2000/40 vs. simvastatin 80 is (-7.7%, 4.5%)
[d] non-inferior to simvastatin 80 arm; 95% confidence interval of mean difference in non-HDL for combination tablet of NIASPAN and simvastatin 1000/40 vs. combination tablet of NIASPAN and simvastatin 80 is (-6.6%, 5.3%)

Table 14. Mean Percent Change from Baseline to Week 24 in Lipoprotein Lipid Levels

	Treatment Group A					
TREATMENT	N	LDL-C	Total-C	HDL-C	TG[a]	Apo B
Baseline (mg/dL)*	266	120	207	43	209	102
Simvastatin 20 mg	102	-6.7%	-4.5%	7.8%	-15.3%	-5.6%
Combination Tablet of NIASPAN and Simvastatin 1000/20	108	-11.9%	-8.8%	20.7%	-26.5%	-13.2%
Combination Tablet of NIASPAN and Simvastatin 2000/20	56	-14.3%	-11.1%	29.0%	-38.0%	-18.5%

* either treatment naïve or after receiving simvastatin 20 mg
[a] medians are reported for TG

Table 15. Mean Percent Change from Baseline to Week 24 in Lipoprotein Lipid Levels

	Treatment Group B					
TREATMENT	N	LDL-C	Total-C	HDL-C	TG[a]	Apo B
Baseline (mg/dL)*	322	108	187	47	145	93
Simvastatin 80 mg	113	-11.4%	-6.2%	0.1%	0.3%	-7.5%
Combination Tablet of NIASPAN and Simvastatin 1000/40	111	-7.1%	-3.1%	15.4%	-22.8%	-7.7%
Combination Tablet of NIASPAN and Simvastatin 2000/40	98	-5.1	-1.6%	24.4%	-31.8%	-10.5%

* after receiving simvastatin 40 mg
[a] medians are reported for TG

ponent) to a maximum dose of 1000 mg/20 mg in one-half of the patients and 2000 mg/40 mg in the other half. The NIASPAN monotherapy group underwent a similar titration from 500 mg to 2000 mg. The patients randomized to lovastatin monotherapy received 20 mg for 12 weeks titrated to 40 mg for up to 16 weeks. Up to a third of the patients randomized to the combination tablet of NIASPAN and lovastatin or NIASPAN monotherapy discontinued prior to Week 28. Results from this study showed that com-

bination therapy decreased LDL-C, TG and Lp(a), and increased HDL-C in a dose-dependent fashion (Tables 8, 9, 10, and 11). Results from this study for LDL-C mean percent change from baseline (the primary efficacy variable) showed that:

1. LDL-lowering with the combination tablet of NIASPAN and lovastatin was significantly greater than that achieved with lovastatin 40 mg only after 28 weeks of titration to a dose of 2000 mg/40 mg ($p<0.0001$)

2. The combination tablet of NIASPAN and lovastatin at doses of 1000 mg/20 mg or higher achieved greater LDL-lowering than NIASPAN ($p<0.0001$)

The LDL-C results are summarized in Table 8.
[See table 8 on previous page]
Combination therapy achieved significantly greater HDL-raising compared to lovastatin and NIASPAN monotherapy at all doses (Table 9).
[See table 9 on previous page]
In addition, combination therapy achieved significantly greater TG lowering at doses of 1000 mg/20mg or greater compared to lovastatin and NIASPAN monotherapy (Table 10).
[See table 10 on previous page]
The Lp(a)-lowering effects of combination therapy and NIASPAN monotherapy were similar, and both were superior to lovastatin (Table 11). The independent effect of lowering Lp(a) with NIASPAN or combination therapy on the risk of coronary and cardiovascular morbidity and mortality has not been determined.
[See table 11 on previous page]

14.4 NIASPAN and Simvastatin Clinical Studies
In a double-blind, randomized, multicenter, multi-national, active-controlled, 24-week study, the lipid effects of a combination tablet of NIASPAN and simvastatin were compared to simvastatin 20 mg and 80 mg in 641 patients with type II hyperlipidemia or mixed dyslipidemia. Following a lipid qualification phase, patients were eligible to enter one of two treatment groups. In Group A, patients on simvastatin 20 mg monotherapy, with elevated non-HDL levels and LDL-C levels at goal per the NCEP guidelines, were randomized to one of three treatment arms: combination tablet of NIASPAN and simvastatin 1000/20 mg, combination tablet of NIASPAN and simvastatin 2000/20 mg, or simvastatin 20 mg. In Group B, patients on simvastatin 40 mg monotherapy, with elevated non-HDL levels per the NCEP guidelines regardless of attainment of LDL-C goals, were randomized to one of three treatment arms: combination tablet of NIASPAN and simvastatin 1000/40 mg, combination tablet of NIASPAN and simvastatin 2000/40 mg, or simvastatin 80 mg. Therapy was initiated at the 500 mg dose of combination tablet of NIASPAN and simvastatin and increased by 500 mg every four weeks. Thus patients were titrated to the 1000 mg dose of combination tablet of NIASPAN and simvastatin after four weeks and to the 2000 mg dose of combination tablet of NIASPAN and simvastatin after 12 weeks. All patients randomized to simvastatin monotherapy received 50 mg immediate-release niacin daily in an attempt to keep the study from becoming unblinded due to flushing in the combination tablet of NIASPAN and simvastatin groups. Patients were instructed to take one 325 mg aspirin or 200 mg ibuprofen 30 minutes prior to taking the double-blind medication to help minimize flushing effects.
In Group A, the primary efficacy analysis was a comparison of the mean percent change in non-HDL levels between the combination tablet of NIASPAN and simvastatin 2000/20 mg and simvastatin 20 mg groups, and if statistically significant, then a comparison was conducted between the combination tablet of NIASPAN and simvastatin 1000/20 mg and simvastatin 20 mg groups. In Group B, the primary efficacy analysis was a determination of whether the mean percent change in non-HDL in the combination tablet of NIASPAN and simvastatin 2000/40 mg group was non-inferior to the mean percent change in the simvastatin 80 mg group, and if so, whether the mean percent change in non-HDL in the combination tablet of NIASPAN and simvastatin 1000/40 mg group was non-inferior to the mean percent change in the simvastatin 80 mg group.
In Group A, the non-HDL-C lowering with combination tablet of NIASPAN and simvastatin 2000/20 and combination tablet of NIASPAN and simvastatin 1000/20 was statistically significantly greater than that achieved with simvastatin 20 mg after 24 weeks ($p<0.05$; Table 12). The completion rate after 24 weeks was 72% for the combination tablet of NIASPAN and simvastatin arms and 88% for the simvastatin 20 mg arm. In Group B, the non-HDL-C lowering with combination tablet of NIASPAN and simvastatin 2000/40 and combination tablet of NIASPAN and simvastatin 1000/40 was non-inferior to that achieved with simvastatin 80 mg after 24 weeks (Table 13). The completion rate after 24 weeks was 78% for the combination tablet of NIASPAN and simvastatin arms and 80% for the simvastatin 80 mg arm.
The combination tablet of NIASPAN and simvastatin was not superior to simvastatin in lowering LDL-C in either Group A or Group B. However, the combination tablet of

---

Information on the Abbott Pharmaceutical Products listed on these pages is from the prescribing information in use as of June 1, 2010. For more information, please visit rxabbott.com or call 1-800-633-9110.

NIASPAN and simvastatin was superior to simvastatin in both groups in lowering TG and raising HDL (Tables 14 and 15).

[See table 12 on previous page]
[See table 13 on previous page]
[See table 14 on previous page]
[See table 15 on previous page]

16 HOW SUPPLIED/STORAGE AND HANDLING

NIASPAN tablets are supplied as unscored, medium-orange, film-coated, capsule-shaped (containing 500 or 750 mg of niacin) or oval shaped (containing 1000 mg of niacin) tablets, in an extended-release formulation. Tablets are printed with the Abbott " ⊡ " logo and the tablet strength (500, 750 or 1000). Tablets are supplied in bottles of 90 as shown below.

500 mg tablets: bottles of 90 - NDC# 0074-3074-90
750 mg tablets: bottles of 90 - NDC# 0074-3079-90
1000 mg tablets: bottles of 90 - NDC# 0074-3080-90
Storage: Store at room temperature 20° to 25°C (68° to 77°F).

17 PATIENT COUNSELING INFORMATION

17.1 Patient Counseling

Patients should be advised to adhere to their National Cholesterol Education Program (NCEP) recommended diet, a regular exercise program, and periodic testing of a fasting lipid panel.

Patients should be advised to inform other healthcare professionals prescribing a new medication that they are taking NIASPAN.

The patient should be informed of the following:

Dosing Time
NIASPAN tablets should be taken at bedtime, after a low-fat snack. Administration on an empty stomach is not recommended.

Tablet Integrity
NIASPAN tablets should not be broken, crushed or chewed, but should be swallowed whole.

Dosing Interruption
If dosing is interrupted for any length of time, their physician should be contacted prior to restarting therapy; re-titration is recommended.

Muscle Pain
Notify their physician of any unexplained muscle pain, tenderness, or weakness promptly. They should discuss all medication, both prescription and over the counter, with their physician.

Flushing
Flushing (warmth, redness, itching and/or tingling of the skin) is a common side effect of niacin therapy that may subside after several weeks of consistent NIASPAN use. Flushing may vary in severity and is more likely to occur with initiation of therapy, or during dose increases. By dosing at bedtime, flushing will most likely occur during sleep. However, if awakened by flushing at night, the patient should get up slowly, especially if feeling dizzy, feeling faint, or taking blood pressure medications.

Use of Aspirin Medication
Taking aspirin approximately 30 minutes before dosing can minimize flushing.

Diet
Avoid ingestion of alcohol, hot beverages and spicy foods around the time of taking NIASPAN to minimize flushing.

Supplements
Notify their physician if they are taking vitamins or other nutritional supplements containing niacin or nicotinamide.

Dizziness
Notify their physician if symptoms of dizziness occur.

Diabetics
If diabetic, to notify their physician of changes in blood glucose.

Pregnancy
Discuss future pregnancy plans with your patients, and discuss when to stop NIASPAN if they are trying to conceive. Patients should be advised that if they become pregnant, they should stop taking NIASPAN and call their healthcare professional.

Breastfeeding
Women who are breastfeeding should be advised to not use NIASPAN. Patients, who have a lipid disorder and are breastfeeding, should be advised to discuss the options with their healthcare professional.

©2010 Abbott Laboratories
Manufactured for Abbott Laboratories, North Chicago, IL 60064, U.S.A.
500 mg NIASPAN tablets
by Norwich Pharmaceuticals, Inc., Norwich, NY 13815
or
500 mg, 750 mg and 1000 mg tablets
by Abbott Pharmaceuticals PR Ltd., Barceloneta, PR 00617
U.S. Patent Nos. 6,080,428; 6,129,930; 6,406,715 B1;

6,676,967; 6,746,691; 6,818,229; 7,011,848; 6,469,035 and other patents pending.
Ref. 03-A357-Revised March, 2010
Shown in Product Identification Guide, page 303

NIMBEX® INJECTION   ℞
[nĭm-bĕks]
(cisatracurium besylate)

This drug should be administered only by adequately trained individuals familiar with its actions, characteristics, and hazards.

DESCRIPTION

NIMBEX (cisatracurium besylate) is a nondepolarizing skeletal muscle relaxant for intravenous administration. Compared to other neuromuscular blocking agents, it is intermediate in its onset and duration of action. Cisatracurium besylate is one of 10 isomers of atracurium besylate and constitutes approximately 15% of that mixture. Cisatracurium besylate is [1R-[1α,2α(1′R*,2′R*)]]-2,2′-[1,5-pentanediylbis[oxy(3-oxo-3,1-propanediyl)]]bis[1-[(3,4-dimethoxyphenyl)methyl]-1,2,3,4-tetrahydro-6,7-dimethoxy-2-methylisoquinolinium] dibenzenesulfonate. The molecular formula of the cisatracurium parent bis-cation is $C_{53}H_{72}N_2O_{12}$ and the molecular weight is 929.2. The molecular formula of cisatracurium as the besylate salt is $C_{65}H_{82}N_2O_{18}S_2$ and the molecular weight is 1243.50. The structural formula of cisatracurium besylate is:

The log of the partition coefficient of cisatracurium besylate is -2.12 in a 1-octanol/distilled water system at 25°C.
NIMBEX Injection is a sterile, non-pyrogenic aqueous solution provided in 5 mL, 10 mL, and 20 mL vials. The pH is adjusted to 3.25 to 3.65 with benzenesulfonic acid. The 5 mL

and 10 mL vials each contain cisatracurium besylate, equivalent to 2 mg/mL cisatracurium. The 20 mL vial, **intended for ICU use only**, contains cisatracurium besylate, equivalent to 10 mg/mL cisatracurium. The 10 mL vial, intended for multiple-dose use, contains 0.9% benzyl alcohol as a preservative. The 5 mL and 20 mL vials are single-use vials and do not contain benzyl alcohol.
Cisatracurium besylate slowly loses potency with time at a rate of approximately 5% per year under refrigeration (5°C). NIMBEX should be refrigerated at 2° to 8°C (36° to 46°F) in the carton to preserve potency. The rate of loss in potency increases to approximately 5% per *month* at 25°C (77°F). Upon removal from refrigeration to room temperature storage conditions (25°C/77°F), use NIMBEX within 21 days, even if rerefrigerated.

CLINICAL PHARMACOLOGY

NIMBEX binds competitively to cholinergic receptors on the motor end-plate to antagonize the action of acetylcholine, resulting in block of neuromuscular transmission. This action is antagonized by acetylcholinesterase inhibitors such as neostigmine.

Pharmacodynamics
The neuromuscular blocking potency of NIMBEX is approximately threefold that of atracurium besylate. The time to maximum block is up to 2 minutes longer for equipotent doses of NIMBEX compared to atracurium besylate. The clinically effective duration of action and rate of spontaneous recovery from equipotent doses of NIMBEX and atracurium besylate are similar.
The average ED_{95} (dose required to produce 95% suppression of the adductor pollicis muscle twitch response to ulnar nerve stimulation) of cisatracurium is 0.05 mg/kg (range: 0.048 to 0.053) in adults receiving opioid/nitrous oxide/oxygen anesthesia. For comparison, the average ED_{95} for atracurium when also expressed as the parent bis-cation is 0.17 mg/kg under similar anesthetic conditions.
The pharmacodynamics of $2 \times ED_{95}$ to $8 \times ED_{95}$ doses of cisatracurium administered over 5 to 10 seconds during opioid/nitrous oxide/oxygen anesthesia are summarized in Table 1. When the dose is doubled, the clinically effective duration of block increases by approximately 25 minutes. Once recovery begins, the rate of recovery is independent of dose.

Table 1. Pharmacodynamic Dose Response* of NIMBEX During Opioid/Nitrous Oxide/Oxygen Anesthesia

Initial Dose of NIMBEX (mg/kg)	Time to 90% Block (min)	Time to Maximum Block (min)	Time to Spontaneous Recovery				
			5% Recovery (min)	25% Recovery† (min)	95% Recovery (min)	T_4:T_1 Ratio‡ ≥70% (min)	25%-75% Recovery Index (min)
Adults							
0.1 (2 × ED_{95}) (n§ = 98)	3.3 (1.0-8.7)	5.0 (1.2-17.2)	33 (15-51)	42 (22-63)	64 (25-93)	64 (32-91)	13 (5-30)
0.15 ‖ (3 × ED_{95}) (n = 39)	2.6 (1.0-4.4)	3.5 (1.6-6.8)	46 (28-65)	55 (44-74)	76 (60-103)	75 (63-98)	13 (11-16)
0.2 (4 × ED_{95}) (n = 30)	2.4 (1.5-4.5)	2.9 (1.9-5.2)	59 (31-103)	65 (43-103)	81 (53-114)	85 (55-114)	12 (2-30)
0.25 (5 × ED_{95}) (n = 15)	1.6 (0.8-3.3)	2.0 (1.2-3.7)	70 (58-85)	78 (66-86)	91 (76-109)	97 (82-113)	8 (5-12)
0.4 (8 × ED_{95}) (n = 15)	1.5 (1.3-1.8)	1.9 (1.4-2.3)	83 (37-103)	91 (59-107)	121 (110-134)	126 (115-137)	14 (10-18)
Infants (1-23 mos.)							
0.15** (n = 18-26)	1.5 (0.7-3.2)	2.0 (1.3-4.3)	36 (28-50)	43 (34-58)	64 (54-84)	59 (49-76)	11.3 (7.3-18.3)
Children (2-12 yr)							
0.08¶ (2 × ED_{95}) (n = 60)	2.2 (1.2-6.8)	3.3 (1.7-9.7)	22 (11-38)	29 (20-46)	52 (37-64)	50 (37-62)	11 (7-15)
0.1 (n = 16)	1.7 (1.3-2.7)	2.8 (1.8-6.7)	21 (13-31)	28 (21-38)	46 (37-58)	44 (36-58)	10 (7-12)
0.15** (n = 23-24)	2.1 (1.3-2.8)	3.0 (1.5-8.0)	29 (19-38)	36 (29-46)	55 (45-72)	54 (44-66)	10.6 (8.5-17.7)

* Values shown are medians of means from individual studies. Values in parentheses are ranges of individual patient values.
† Clinically effective duration of block.
‡ Train-of-four ratio.
§ n=the number of patients with Time to Maximum Block data.
‖ Propofol anesthesia.
¶ Halothane anesthesia.
** Thiopentone, alfentanil, N_2O/O_2 anesthesia.

Isoflurane or enflurane administered with nitrous oxide/oxygen to achieve 1.25 MAC [Minimum Alveolar Concentration] may prolong the clinically effective duration of action of initial and maintenance doses, and decrease the average infusion rate requirement of NIMBEX. The magnitude of these effects may depend on the duration of administration of the volatile agents. Fifteen to 30 minutes of exposure to 1.25 MAC isoflurane or enflurane had minimal effects on the duration of action of initial doses of NIMBEX and therefore, no adjustment to the initial dose should be necessary when NIMBEX is administered shortly after initiation of volatile agents. In long surgical procedures during enflurane or isoflurane anesthesia, less frequent maintenance dosing, lower maintenance doses, or reduced infusion rates of NIMBEX may be necessary. The average infusion rate requirement may be decreased by as much as 30% to 40%. The onset, duration of action, and recovery profiles of NIMBEX during propofol/oxygen or propofol/nitrous oxide/oxygen anesthesia are similar to those during opioid/nitrous oxide/oxygen anesthesia.

[See table 1 at bottom of previous page]

When administered during the induction of adequate anesthesia using propofol, nitrous oxide/oxygen, and co-induction agents (e.g., fentanyl and midazolam), GOOD or EXCELLENT conditions for tracheal intubation occurred in 96/102 (94%) patients in 1.5 to 2.0 minutes following 0.15 mg/kg cisatracurium and in 97/110 (88%) patients in 1.5 minutes following 0.2 mg/kg cisatracurium.

In one intubation study during thiopental anesthesia in which fentanyl and midazolam were administered two minutes prior to induction, intubation conditions were assessed at 120 seconds. Table 2 displays these results in this study of 51 patients.

Table 2. Study of Tracheal Intubation Comparing Two Doses of Cisatracurium (Thiopental Anesthesia)

Intubating Conditions at 120 seconds	$3 \times ED_{95}$ 0.15 mg/kg n = 26	$4 \times ED_{95}$ 0.20 mg/kg n = 25
Excellent and Good		
Proportion	23/26	24/25
Percent	88%	96%
95% CI	76,100	88,100
Excellent		
Proportion	8/26	15/26
Percent	31%	60%
Good		
Proportion	15/26	9/25
Percent	58%	36%

While GOOD or EXCELLENT intubation conditions were achieved in the majority of patients in this setting, EXCELLENT intubation conditions were more frequently achieved with the 0.2 mg/kg dose (60%) than the 0.15 mg/kg dose (31%) when intubation was attempted 2.0 minutes following cisatracurium.

A second study evaluated intubation conditions after 3 and $4 \times ED_{95}$ (0.15 mg/kg and 0.20 mg/kg) following induction with fentanyl and midazolam and either thiopental or propofol anesthesia. This study compared intubation conditions produced by these doses of cisatracurium after 1.5 minutes. Table 3 displays these results.

[See table 3 at top right]

EXCELLENT intubation conditions were more frequently observed with the 0.2 mg/kg dose when intubation was attempted 1.5 minutes following cisatracurium.

A third study in pediatric patients (ages 1 month to 12 years) evaluated intubation conditions at 120 seconds after 0.15 mg/kg NIMBEX following induction with either halothane (with halothane/nitrous oxide/oxygen maintenance) or thiopentone and fentanyl (with thiopentone/fentanyl nitrous oxide/oxygen maintenance). The results are summarized in Table 4.

[See table 4 at top right]

EXCELLENT or GOOD intubating conditions were produced 120 seconds following 0.15 mg/kg NIMBEX in 88/90 (98%) of patients induced with halothane and in 85/90 (94%) of patients induced with thiopentone and fentanyl. There were no patients for whom intubation was not possible, but there were 7/120 patients ages 1-12 years for whom intubating conditions were described as poor.

Repeated administration of maintenance doses or a continuous infusion of NIMBEX for up to 3 hours is not associated with development of tachyphylaxis or cumulative neuromuscular blocking effects. The time needed to recover from successive maintenance doses does not change with the number of doses administered as long as partial recovery is allowed to occur between doses. Maintenance doses can

Table 3. Study of Tracheal Intubation Comparing Three Doses of Cisatracurium (Thiopental or Propofol Anesthesia)

Intubating Conditions at 90 seconds	$3 \times ED_{95}$ 0.15 mg/kg Propofol n = 31	$3 \times ED_{95}$ 0.15 mg/kg Thiopental n = 31	$4 \times ED_{95}$ 0.20 mg/kg Propofol n = 30	$4 \times ED_{95}$ 0.20 mg/kg Thiopental n = 28
Excellent and Good				
Proportion	29/31	28/31	28/30	27/28
Percent	94%	90%	93%	96%
95% CI	85,100	80,100	84,100	90,100
Excellent				
Proportion	18/31	17/31	22/30	16/28
Percent	58%	55%	70%	57%
Good				
Proportion	11/31	11/31	6/30	11/28
Percent	35%	35%	20%	39%

Table 4. Study of Tracheal Intubation for Pediatrics Stratified by Age Group (0.15 mg/kg NIMBEX with Halothane or Thiopentone/Fentanyl Anesthesia)

Intubating Conditions at 120 seconds**	NIMBEX 0.15 mg/kg 1-11 mo. n = 30 Halothane Anesthesia	NIMBEX 0.15 mg/kg 1-11 mo. n = 30 Thiopentone/Fentanyl Anesthesia	NIMBEX 0.15 mg/kg 1-4 years n = 31 Halothane Anesthesia	NIMBEX 0.15 mg/kg 1-4 years n = 31 Thiopentone/Fentanyl Anesthesia	NIMBEX 0.15 mg/kg 5-12 years n = 30 Halothane Anesthesia	NIMBEX 0.15 mg/kg 5-12 years n = 30 Thiopentone/Fentanyl Anesthesia
Excellent and Good						
Proportion	30/30	30/30	29/30	26/30	29/30	29/30
Percent	100%	100%	97%	87%	97%	97%
Excellent						
Proportion	30/30	25/30	27/30	19/30	22/30	21/30
Percent	100%	83%	90%	63%	73%	70%
Good						
Proportion	0	5/30	2/30	7/30	7/30	8/30
Percent	0%	17%	7%	23%	23%	27%
Poor						
Proportion	0/30	0/30	1/30	4/30	1/30	1/30
Percent	0%	0%	3%	13%	3%	3%

** **Excellent:** Easy passage of the tube without coughing. Vocal cords relaxed and abducted.
Good: Passage of tube with slight coughing and/or bucking. Vocal cords relaxed and abducted.
Poor: Passage of tube with moderate coughing and/or bucking. Vocal cords moderately adducted. Response of patient requires adjustment of ventilation pressure and/or rate.

therefore be administered at relatively regular intervals with predictable results. The rate of spontaneous recovery of neuromuscular function after infusion is independent of the duration of infusion and comparable to the rate of recovery following initial doses (Table 1).

Long-term infusion (up to 6 days) of NIMBEX during mechanical ventilation in the ICU has been evaluated in two studies. In a randomized, double-blind study using presence of a single twitch during train-of-four (TOF) monitoring to regulate dosage, patients treated with NIMBEX (n = 19) recovered neuromuscular function ($T_4:T_1$ ratio $\geq$ 70%) following termination of infusion in approximately 55 minutes (range: 20 to 270) whereas those treated with vecuronium (n = 12) recovered in 178 minutes (range: 40 minutes to 33 hours). In another study comparing NIMBEX and atracurium, patients recovered neuromuscular function in approximately 50 minutes for both NIMBEX (range: 20 to 175; n = 34) and atracurium (range: 35 to 85; n = 15).

The neuromuscular block produced by NIMBEX is readily antagonized by anticholinesterase agents once recovery has started. As with other nondepolarizing neuromuscular blocking agents, the more profound the neuromuscular block at the time of reversal, the longer the time required for recovery of neuromuscular function.

In children (2 to 12 years) cisatracurium has a lower ED_{95} than in adults (0.04 mg/kg, halothane/nitrous oxide/oxygen anesthesia). At 0.1 mg/kg during opioid anesthesia, cisatracurium had a faster onset and shorter duration of action in children than in adults (Table 1). Recovery following reversal is faster in children than in adults.

At 0.15 mg/kg during opioid anesthesia, cisatracurium had a faster onset and longer clinically effective duration of action in infants aged 1-23 months compared to children aged 2-12 years (Table 1).

Studies were conducted during both opioid-based and halothane-based anesthesia in children aged 1-11 months, 1-4 years, and 5-12 years. Cisatracurium had a faster onset and longer duration of action in infants 1-11 months compared to children 1-4 years, who in turn have a faster onset

and longer duration of action for cisatracurium compared to children 5-12 years.

The mean time to onset of maximum T_1 suppression was generally faster for pediatric patients induced with halothane compared to thiopentone/fentanyl and the clinically effective duration (time to 25% recovery) was longer (by up to 15%) for pediatric patients under halothane anesthesia.

Hemodynamics Profile

The cardiovascular profile of NIMBEX allows it to be administered by rapid bolus at higher multiples of the ED_{95} than atracurium. NIMBEX has no dose-related effects on mean arterial blood pressure (MAP) or heart rate (HR) following doses ranging from 2 to $8 \times ED_{95}$ (> 0.1 to > 0.4 mg/kg), administered over 5 to 10 seconds, in healthy adult patients (Figure 1) or in patients with serious cardiovascular disease (Figure 2).

A total of 141 patients undergoing coronary artery bypass grafting (CABG) have been administered NIMBEX in three active controlled clinical trials and have received doses ranging from 2 to $8 \times ED_{95}$. While the hemodynamic profile was comparable in both the NIMBEX and active control groups, data for doses above 0.3 mg/kg in this population are limited.

Unlike atracurium, NIMBEX, at therapeutic doses of $2 \times ED_{95}$ to $8 \times ED_{95}$ (0.1 to 0.4 mg/kg), administered over 5 to 10 seconds, does not cause dose-related elevations in mean plasma histamine concentration.

[See figure 1 at top of next column]
[See figure 2 at top of next column]

No clinically significant changes in MAP or HR were observed following administration of doses up to 0.1 mg/kg NIMBEX over 5 to 10 seconds in 2- to 12-year-old children receiving either halothane/nitrous oxide/oxygen or opioid/

Information on the Abbott Pharmaceutical Products listed on these pages is from the prescribing information in use as of June 1, 2010. For more information, please visit rxabbott.com or call 1-800-633-9110.

Figure 1
Maximum Percent Change from Preinjection in Heart Rate (HR) and Mean Arterial Pressure (MAP) During First 5 Minutes after Initial 4 x ED₉₅ to 8 x ED₉₅ Doses of NIMBEX in Healthy Adult Patients Receiving Opioid/Nitrous Oxide/Oxygen Anesthesia (n = 44)

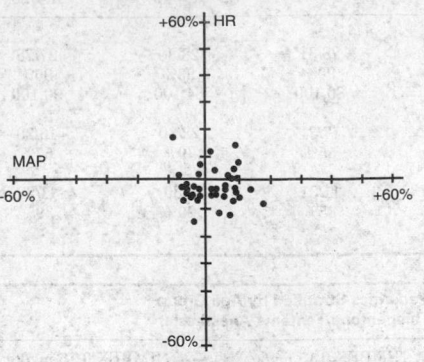

Figure 2
Percent Change from Preinjection in Heart Rate (HR) and Mean Arterial Pressure (MAP) 10 Minutes After an Initial 4 x ED₉₅ to 8 x ED₉₅ Dose of NIMBEX in Patients Undergoing CABG Surgery Receiving Oxygen/Fentanyl/Midazolam/Anesthesia (n = 54)

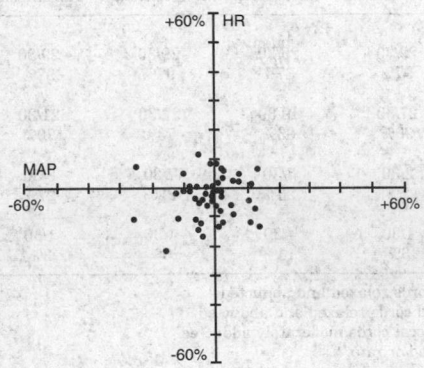

nitrous oxide/oxygen anesthesia. Doses of 0.15 mg/kg NIMBEX administered over 5 seconds were not consistently associated with changes in HR and MAP in pediatric patients aged 1 month to 12 years receiving opioid/nitrous oxide/oxygen or halothane/nitrous oxide/oxygen anesthesia.
[See figure 3 at top of next column]
[See figure 4 at top of third column]

Pharmacokinetics

General

The neuromuscular blocking activity of NIMBEX is due to parent drug. Cisatracurium plasma concentration-time data following IV bolus administration are best described by a two-compartment open model (with elimination from both compartments) with an elimination half-life ($t_{1/2}\beta$) of 22 minutes, a plasma clearance (CL) of 4.57 mL/min/kg, and a volume of distribution at steady state (V_{ss}) of 145 mL/kg. Cisatracurium undergoes organ-independent Hofmann elimination (a chemical process dependent on pH and temperature) to form the monoquaternary acrylate metabolite and laudanosine, neither of which has any neuromuscular blocking activity (see **Pharmacokinetics** - Metabolism section). Following administration of radiolabeled cisatracurium, 95% of the dose was recovered in the urine; less than 10% of the dose was excreted as unchanged parent drug. Laudanosine, a metabolite of cisatracurium (and atracurium) has been noted to cause transient hypotension and, in higher doses, cerebral excitatory effects when administered to several animal species. The relationship between CNS excitation and laudanosine concentrations in humans has not been established (see **PRECAUTIONS** - Long-term Use in the Intensive Care Unit). Because cisatracurium is three times more potent than atracurium and lower doses are required, the corresponding laudanosine concentrations following cisatracurium are one third of those that would be expected following an equipotent dose of atracurium (see **Pharmacokinetics** - Special Populations - Intensive Care Unit Patients).

Results from population pharmacokinetic/pharmacodynamic (PK/PD) analyses from 241 healthy surgical patients are summarized in Table 5.

Figure 3
Heart Rate and MAP Change at 1 Minute After the Initial Dose, By Age Group Treatment Group: NIMBEX 0:3 x ED₉₅ Opioid Intubation at 120 Sec.

1-11 Months

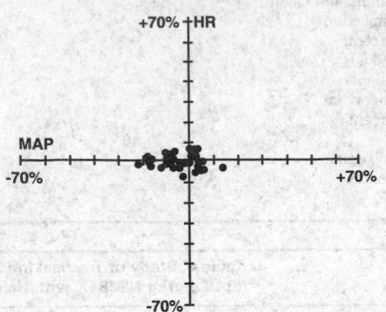

1-5 Years

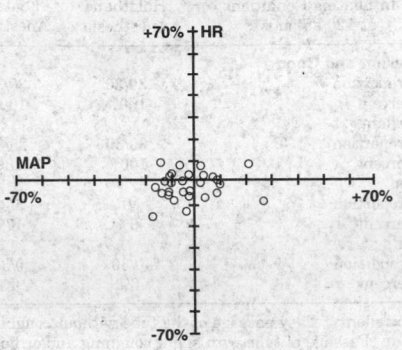

5-13 Years

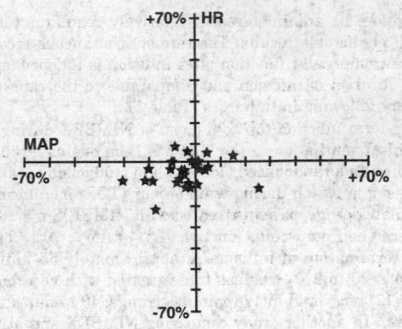

Table 5. Key Population PK/PD Parameter Estimates for Cisatracurium in Healthy Surgical Patients* Following 0.1 (2 × ED₉₅) to 0.4 mg/kg (8 × ED₉₅) NIMBEX

Parameter	Estimate†	Magnitude of Interpatient Variability (CV)‡
CL (mL/min/kg)	4.57	16%
V_{ss} (mL/kg)§	145	27%
k_{eo} (min-1)‖	0.0575	61%
EC_{50} (ng/mL)¶	141	52%

* Healthy male non-obese patients 19-64 years of age with creatinine clearance values greater than 70 mL/min who received cisatracurium during opioid anesthesia and had venous samples collected.
† The percent standard error of the mean (%SEM) ranged from 3% to 12% indicating good precision for the PK/PD estimates.
‡ Expressed as a coefficient of variation; the %SEM ranged from 20% to 35% indicating adequate precision for the estimates of interpatient variability.

Figure 4
Heart Rate and MAP Change at 1 Minute After the Initial Dose, By Age Group Treatment Group: NIMBEX H:3 x ED₉₅ Halothane Intubation at 120 Sec.

1-11 Months

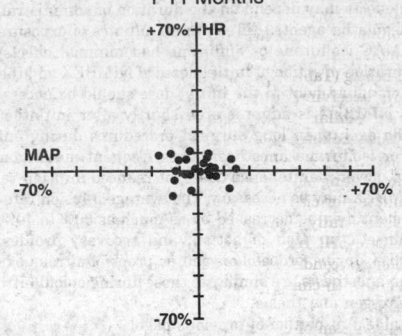

1-5 Years

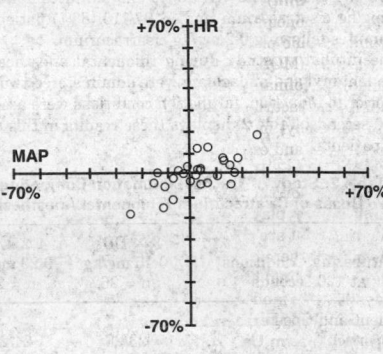

5-13 Years

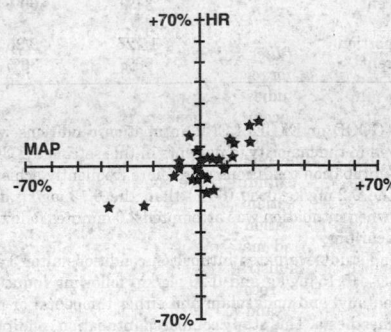

§ V_{ss} is the volume of distribution at steady state estimated using a two-compartment model with elimination from both compartments. V_{ss} is equal to the sum of the volume in the central compartment (V_c) and the volume in the peripheral compartment (V_p); interpatient variability could only be estimated for V_c.
‖ Rate constant describing the equilibration between plasma concentrations and neuromuscular block.
¶ Concentration required to produce 50% T_1 suppression; an index of patient sensitivity.

The magnitude of interpatient variability in CL was low (16%), as expected based on the importance of Hofmann elimination (see **Pharmacokinetics** - Elimination). The magnitudes of interpatient variability in CL and volume of distribution were low in comparison to those for k_{eo} and EC_{50}. This suggests that any alterations in the time course of cisatracurium-induced block are more likely to be due to variability in the pharmacodynamic parameters than in the pharmacokinetic parameters. Parameter estimates from the population pharmacokinetic analyses were supported by noncompartmental pharmacokinetic analyses on data from healthy patients and from special patient populations. Conventional pharmacokinetic analyses have shown that the pharmacokinetics of cisatracurium are proportional to dose between 0.1 (2 × ED_{95}) and 0.2 (4 × ED_{95}) mg/kg cisatracurium. In addition, population pharmacokinetic analyses revealed no statistically significant effect of initial dose on CL for doses between 0.1 (2 × ED_{95}) and 0.4 (8 × ED_{95}) mg/kg cisatracurium.

Distribution

The volume of distribution of cisatracurium is limited by its large molecular weight and high polarity. The V_{ss} was equal to 145 mL/kg (Table 4) in healthy 19- to 64-year-old surgical patients receiving opioid anesthesia. The V_{ss} was 21% larger in similar patients receiving inhalation anesthesia (see **Pharmacokinetics** - Special Populations - Other Patient Factors).

Protein Binding

The binding of cisatracurium to plasma proteins has not been successfully studied due to its rapid degradation at physiologic pH. Inhibition of degradation requires non-physiological conditions of temperature and pH which are associated with changes in protein binding.

Metabolism

The degradation of cisatracurium is largely independent of liver metabolism. Results from *in vitro* experiments suggest that cisatracurium undergoes Hofmann elimination (a pH and temperature-dependent chemical process) to form laudanosine (see **PRECAUTIONS - Long-term Use in the Intensive Care Unit**) and the monoquaternary acrylate metabolite. The monoquaternary acrylate undergoes hydrolysis by non-specific plasma esterases to form the monoquaternary alcohol (MQA) metabolite. The MQA metabolite can also undergo Hofmann elimination but at a much slower rate than cisatracurium. Laudanosine is further metabolized to desmethyl metabolites which are conjugated with glucuronic acid and excreted in the urine.

Organ-independent Hofmann elimination is the predominant pathway for the elimination of cisatracurium. The liver and kidney play a minor role in the elimination of cisatracurium but are primary pathways for the elimination of metabolites. Therefore, the $t_{1/2}\beta$ values of metabolites (including laudanosine) are longer in patients with kidney or liver dysfunction and metabolite concentrations may be higher after long-term administration (see **PRECAUTIONS - Long-term Use in the Intensive Care Unit**). Most importantly, C_{max} values of laudanosine are significantly lower in healthy surgical patients receiving infusions of NIMBEX than in patients receiving infusions of atracurium (mean ± SD C_{max}: 60 ± 52 and 342 ± 93 ng/mL, respectively).

Elimination

Clearance and Half-life

Mean CL values for cisatracurium ranged from 4.5 to 5.7 mL/min/kg in studies of healthy surgical patients. Compartmental pharmacokinetic modeling suggests that approximately 80% of the CL is accounted for by Hofmann elimination and the remaining 20% by renal and hepatic elimination. These findings are consistent with the low magnitude of interpatient variability in CL (16%) estimated as part of the population PK/PD analyses and with the recovery of parent and metabolites in urine. Following ^{14}C-cisatracurium administration to 6 healthy male patients, 95% of the dose was recovered in the urine (mostly as conjugated metabolites) and 4% in the feces; less than 10% of the dose was excreted as unchanged parent drug in the urine. In 12 healthy surgical patients receiving non-radiolabeled cisatracurium who had Foley catheters placed for surgical management, approximately 15% of the dose was excreted unchanged in the urine.

In studies of healthy surgical patients, mean $t_{1/2}\beta$ values of cisatracurium ranged from 22 to 29 minutes and were consistent with the $t_{1/2}\beta$ of cisatracurium *in vitro* (29 minutes). The mean ± SD $t_{1/2}\beta$ values of laudanosine were 3.1 ± 0.4 and 3.3 ± 2.1 hours in healthy surgical patients receiving NIMBEX (n = 10) or atracurium (n = 10), respectively. During IV infusions of NIMBEX, peak plasma concentrations (C_{max}) of laudanosine and the MQA metabolite are approximately 6% and 11% of the parent compound, respectively.

Special Populations

Geriatric Patients (≥65 years)

The results of conventional pharmacokinetic analysis from a study of 12 healthy elderly patients and 12 healthy young adult patients receiving a single IV dose of 0.1 mg/kg NIMBEX are summarized in Table 6. Plasma clearances of cisatracurium were not affected by age; however, the volumes of distribution were slightly larger in elderly patients than in young patients resulting in slightly longer $t_{1/2}\beta$ values for cisatracurium. The rate of equilibration between plasma cisatracurium concentrations and neuromuscular block was slower in elderly patients than in young patients (mean ± SD k_{eo}: 0.071 ± 0.036 and 0.105 ± 0.021 $minutes^{-1}$, respectively); there was no difference in the patient sensitivity to cisatracurium-induced block, as indicated by EC_{50} values (mean ± SD EC_{50}: 91 ± 22 and 89 ± 23 ng/mL, respectively). These changes were consistent with the 1-minute slower times to maximum block in elderly patients receiving 0.1 mg/kg NIMBEX, when compared to young patients receiving the same dose. The minor differences in PK/PD parameters of cisatracurium between elderly patients and young patients were not associated with clinically significant differences in the recovery profile of NIMBEX.

Table 6. Pharmacokinetic Parameters* of Cisatracurium in Healthy Elderly and Young Adult Patients Following 0.1 mg/kg (2 × ED_{95}) NIMBEX (Isoflurane/Nitrous Oxide/Oxygen Anesthesia)

Parameter	Healthy Elderly Patients	Healthy Young Adult Patients
Elimination Half-Life ($t_{½}\beta$, min)	25.8 ± 3.6†	22.1 ± 2.5
Volume of Distribution at Steady State‡ (mL/kg)	156 ± 17†	133 ± 15
Plasma Clearance (mL/min/kg)	5.7 ± 1.0	5.3 ± 0.9

* Values presented are mean ± SD.
† $P < 0.05$ for comparisons between healthy elderly and healthy young adult patients.
‡ Volume of distribution is underestimated because elimination from the peripheral compartment is ignored.

Patients with Hepatic Disease

Table 7 summarizes the conventional pharmacokinetic analysis from a study of NIMBEX in 13 patients with end-stage liver disease undergoing liver transplantation and 11 healthy adult patients undergoing elective surgery. The slightly larger volumes of distribution in liver transplant patients were associated with slightly higher plasma clearances of cisatracurium. The parallel changes in these parameters resulted in no difference in $t_{1/2}\beta$ values. There were no differences in k_{eo} or EC_{50} between patient groups. The times to maximum block were approximately one minute faster in liver transplant patients than in healthy adult patients receiving 0.1 mg/kg NIMBEX. These minor differences in pharmacokinetics were not associated with clinically significant differences in the recovery profile of NIMBEX.

The $t_{1/2}\beta$ values of metabolites are longer in patients with hepatic disease and concentrations may be higher after long-term administration (see **Pharmacokinetics** - Special Populations - Intensive Care Unit Patients).

Table 7. Pharmacokinetic Parameters* of Cisatracurium in Healthy Adult Patients and in Patients Undergoing Liver Transplantation Following 0.1 mg/kg (2 × ED_{95}) NIMBEX (Isoflurane/Nitrous Oxide/Oxygen Anesthesia)

Parameter	Liver Transplant Patients	Healthy Adult Patients
Elimination Half-Life ($t_{½}\beta$, min)	24.4 ± 2.9	23.5 ± 3.5
Volume of Distribution at Steady State‡ (mL/kg)	195 ± 38†	161 ± 23
Plasma Clearance (mL/min/kg)	6.6 ± 1.1†	5.7 ± 0.8

* Values presented are mean ± SD.
† $P < 0.05$ for comparisons between liver transplant patients and healthy adult patients.
‡ Volume of distribution is underestimated because elimination from the peripheral compartment is ignored.

Patients with Renal Dysfunction

Results from a conventional pharmacokinetic study of NIMBEX in 13 healthy adult patients and 15 patients with end-stage renal disease (ESRD) undergoing elective surgery are summarized in Table 8. The PK/PD parameters of cisatracurium were similar in healthy adult patients and ESRD patients. The times to 90% block were approximately one minute slower in ESRD patients following 0.1 mg/kg NIMBEX. There were no differences in the durations or rates of recovery of NIMBEX between ESRD and healthy adult patients.

The $t_{1/2}\beta$ values of metabolites are longer in patients with renal failure and concentrations may be higher after long-term administration (see **Pharmacokinetics** - Special Populations - *Intensive Care Unit Patients*).

Table 8. Pharmacokinetic Parameters* for Cisatracurium in Healthy Adult Patients and in Patients With End-Stage Renal Disease (ESRD) Receiving 0.1 mg/kg (2 × ED_{95}) NIMBEX (Opioid/Nitrous Oxide/Oxygen Anesthesia)

Parameter	Healthy Adult Patients	ESRD Patients
Elimination Half-Life ($t_{½}\beta$, min)	29.4 ± 4.1	32.3 ± 6.3
Volume of Distribution at Steady State† (mL/kg)	149 ± 35	160 ± 32
Plasma Clearance (mL/min/kg)	4.66 ± 0.86	4.26 ± 0.62

* Values presented are mean ± SD.
† Volume of distribution is underestimated because elimination from the peripheral compartment is ignored.

Population pharmacokinetic analyses revealed that patients with creatinine clearances ≤ 70 mL/min had a slower rate of equilibration between plasma concentrations and neuromuscular block than patients with normal renal function; this change was associated with a slightly slower (~ 40 seconds) predicted time to 90% T_1 suppression in patients with renal dysfunction following 0.1 mg/kg NIMBEX. There was no clinically significant alteration in the recovery profile of NIMBEX in patients with renal dysfunction. The recovery profile of NIMBEX is unchanged in the presence of renal or hepatic failure, which is consistent with predominantly organ-independent elimination.

Intensive Care Unit (ICU) Patients

The pharmacokinetics of cisatracurium, atracurium, and their metabolites were determined in six ICU patients receiving NIMBEX and in six ICU patients receiving atracurium and are presented in Table 9. The plasma clearances of cisatracurium and atracurium are similar. The volume of distribution was larger and the $t_{1/2}\beta$ was longer for cisatracurium than for atracurium. The relationships between plasma cisatracurium or atracurium concentrations and neuromuscular block have not been evaluated in ICU patients. The minor differences in pharmacokinetics were not associated with any differences in the recovery profiles of NIMBEX and atracurium in ICU patients.

[See table 9 at top of next page]

Plasma metabolite pharmacokinetics are listed in Table 9. Limited pharmacokinetic data are available for patients with liver/kidney dysfunction receiving NIMBEX. Data from studies of atracurium demonstrate that renal/hepatic failure in ICU patients produces little to no effect on its pharmacokinetics, but decreases the biotransformation and elimination of the metabolites. Following atracurium, $t_{1/2}\beta$ values for laudanosine were longer in ICU patients with renal failure than in ICU patients with normal renal function (15 and 6 hours, respectively). The $t_{1/2}\beta$ values of laudanosine were 39 ± 14 hours in ICU patients with liver failure receiving atracurium after an unsuccessful liver transplantation and 5 ± 2 hours in similar ICU patients after successful liver transplantation. Therefore, relative to ICU patients with normal renal and hepatic function receiving NIMBEX, metabolite concentrations (plasma and tissues) may be higher in ICU patients with renal or hepatic failure (see **PRECAUTIONS - Long-term Use in the Intensive Care Unit**). Consistent with the decreased infusion rate requirements for NIMBEX, metabolite concentrations were lower in patients receiving NIMBEX than in patients receiving atracurium besylate.

Pediatric Patients

The population PK/PD of cisatracurium were described in 20 healthy pediatric patients during halothane anesthesia, using the same model developed for healthy adult patients. The CL was higher in healthy pediatric patients (5.89 mL/min/kg) than in healthy adult patients (4.57 mL/min/kg) during opioid anesthesia. The rate of equilibration between plasma concentrations and neuromuscular block, as indicated by k_{eo}, was faster in healthy pediatric patients receiving halothane anesthesia (0.1330 $minutes^{-1}$) than in healthy adult patients receiving opioid anesthesia (0.0575 $minutes^{-1}$). The EC_{50} in healthy pediatric patients (125 ng/mL) was similar to the value in healthy adult patients (141 ng/mL) during opioid anesthesia. The minor differences in the PK/PD parameters of cisatracurium were associated with a faster time to onset and a shorter duration of cisatracurium-induced neuromuscular block in pediatric patients.

Information on the Abbott Pharmaceutical Products listed on these pages is from the prescribing information in use as of June 1, 2010. For more information, please visit rxabbott.com or call 1-800-633-9110.

Other Patient Factors

Population PK/PD analyses revealed that gender and obesity were associated with statistically significant effects on the pharmacokinetics and/or pharmacodynamics of cisatracurium; these factors were not associated with clinically significant alterations in the predicted onset or recovery profile of NIMBEX. The use of inhalation agents was associated with a 21% larger V_{ss}, a 78% larger k_{eo}, and a 15% lower EC_{50} for cisatracurium. These changes resulted in a slightly faster (~ 45 seconds) predicted time to 90% T_1 suppression in patients receiving 0.1 mg/kg cisatracurium during inhalation anesthesia than in patients receiving the same dose of cisatracurium during opioid anesthesia; however, there were no clinically significant differences in the predicted recovery profile of NIMBEX between patient groups.

Table 9. Parameter Estimates* for Cisatracurium, Atracurium, and Metabolites in ICU Patients After Long-Term (24-48 Hour) Administration of NIMBEX or Atracurium Besylate

	Parameter	Cisatracurium (n = 6)	Atracurium (n = 6)
Parent Compound	CL (mL/min/kg)	7.45 ± 1.02	7.49 ± 0.66†
	$t_{½}β$ (min)	26.8 ± 11.1	16.5 ± 6.0†
	Vβ (mL/kg)‡	280 ± 103	178 ± 71†
Laudanosine	C_{max} (ng/mL)	707 ± 360	2318 ± 1498
	$t_{½}β$ (hrs)	6.6 ± 4.1	8.4 ± 7.3
MQA metabolite	C_{max} (ng/mL)	152-181§	943 ± 333‖
	$t_{½}β$ (min)	26-31§	21-58§

* Presented as mean ± standard deviation.
† n = 5.
‡ Volume of distribution during the terminal elimination phase, an underestimate because elimination from the peripheral compartment is ignored.
§ n = 2, range presented.
‖ n = 3.

Individualization of Dosages

DOSES OF **NIMBEX** SHOULD BE INDIVIDUALIZED AND A PERIPHERAL NERVE STIMULATOR SHOULD BE USED TO MEASURE NEUROMUSCULAR FUNCTION DURING ADMINISTRATION OF **NIMBEX** IN ORDER TO MONITOR DRUG EFFECT, TO DETERMINE THE NEED FOR ADDITIONAL DOSES, AND TO CONFIRM RECOVERY FROM NEUROMUSCULAR BLOCK.

Based on the known action of NIMBEX and other neuromuscular blocking agents, the following factors should be considered when administering NIMBEX.

Renal and Hepatic Disease

See **PRECAUTIONS** section.

Long-Term Use in the Intensive Care Unit (ICU)

The long-term infusion (up to 6 days) of NIMBEX during mechanical ventilation in the ICU has been evaluated in two studies. Average infusion rates of approximately 3 mcg/kg/min (range: 0.5 to 10.2) were required to achieve adequate neuromuscular block. As with other neuromuscular blocking agents, these data indicate the presence of wide interpatient variability in dosage requirements. In addition, dosage requirements may increase or decrease with time (see **PRECAUTIONS**). Use of NIMBEX in the ICU for longer than 6 days has not been studied.

Drugs or Conditions Causing Potentiation of or Resistance to Neuromuscular Block

Persons with certain pre-existing conditions or receiving certain drugs may require individualization of dosing (see **PRECAUTIONS**).

Burns

Patients with burns have been shown to develop resistance to nondepolarizing neuromuscular blocking agents, and may require individualization of dosing (see **PRECAUTIONS**).

INDICATIONS AND USAGE

NIMBEX is an intermediate-onset/intermediate-duration neuromuscular blocking agent indicated for inpatients and outpatients as an adjunct to general anesthesia, to facilitate tracheal intubation, and to provide skeletal muscle relaxation during surgery or mechanical ventilation in the ICU.

CONTRAINDICATIONS

NIMBEX is contraindicated in patients known to have an allergic hypersensitivity to NIMBEX or other bis-benzylisoquinolinium agents. Use of NIMBEX from vials containing benzyl alcohol as a preservative is contraindicated in patients with a known hypersensitivity to benzyl alcohol.

WARNINGS

NIMBEX SHOULD BE ADMINISTERED IN CAREFULLY ADJUSTED DOSAGE BY OR UNDER THE SUPERVISION OF EXPERIENCED CLINICIANS WHO ARE FAMILIAR WITH THE DRUG'S ACTIONS AND THE POSSIBLE COMPLICATIONS OF ITS USE. THE DRUG SHOULD NOT BE ADMINISTERED UNLESS PERSONNEL AND FACILITIES FOR RESUSCITATION AND LIFE SUPPORT (TRACHEAL INTUBATION, ARTIFICIAL VENTILATION, OXYGEN THERAPY), AND AN ANTAGONIST OF **NIMBEX** ARE IMMEDIATELY AVAILABLE. IT IS RECOMMENDED THAT A PERIPHERAL NERVE STIMULATOR BE USED TO MEASURE NEUROMUSCULAR FUNCTION DURING THE ADMINISTRATION OF **NIMBEX** IN ORDER TO MONITOR DRUG EFFECT, DETERMINE THE NEED FOR ADDITIONAL DOSES, AND CONFIRM RECOVERY FROM NEUROMUSCULAR BLOCK.

NIMBEX HAS NO KNOWN EFFECT ON CONSCIOUSNESS, PAIN THRESHOLD, OR CEREBRATION. TO AVOID DISTRESS TO THE PATIENT, NEUROMUSCULAR BLOCK SHOULD NOT BE INDUCED BEFORE UNCONSCIOUSNESS.

NIMBEX Injection is acidic (pH 3.25 to 3.65) and may not be compatible with alkaline solutions having a pH greater than 8.5 (e.g., barbiturate solutions).

The 10 mL multiple-dose vials of NIMBEX contain benzyl alcohol. In newborn infants, benzyl alcohol has been associated with an increased incidence of neurological and other complications which are sometimes fatal. Single-use vials (5 mL and 20 mL) of NIMBEX do not contain benzyl alcohol (see **PRECAUTIONS - Pediatric Use**).

PRECAUTIONS

Because of its intermediate onset of action, NIMBEX is not recommended for rapid sequence endotracheal intubation.

Recommended doses of NIMBEX have no clinically significant effects on heart rate; therefore, NIMBEX will not counteract the bradycardia produced by many anesthetic agents or by vagal stimulation.

Neuromuscular blocking agents may have a profound effect in patients with neuromuscular diseases (e.g., myasthenia gravis and the myasthenic syndrome). In these and other conditions in which prolonged neuromuscular block is a possibility (e.g., carcinomatosis), the use of a peripheral nerve stimulator and a dose of not more than 0.02 mg/kg NIMBEX is recommended to assess the level of neuromuscular block and to monitor dosage requirements.

Patients with burns have been shown to develop resistance to nondepolarizing neuromuscular blocking agents, including atracurium. The extent of altered response depends upon the size of the burn and the time elapsed since the burn injury. NIMBEX has not been studied in patients with burns; however, based on its structural similarity to atracurium, the possibility of increased dosing requirements and shortened duration of action must be considered if NIMBEX is administered to burn patients.

Patients with hemiparesis or paraparesis also may demonstrate resistance to nondepolarizing muscle relaxants in the affected limbs. To avoid inaccurate dosing, neuromuscular monitoring should be performed on a non-paretic limb.

Acid-base and/or serum electrolyte abnormalities may potentiate or antagonize the action of neuromuscular blocking agents. No data are available to support the use of NIMBEX by intramuscular injection.

Renal and Hepatic Disease

No clinically significant alterations in the recovery profile were observed in patients with renal dysfunction or in patients with end-stage liver disease following a 0.1 mg/kg dose of cisatracurium. The onset time was approximately 1 minute faster in patients with end-stage liver disease and approximately 1 minute slower in patients with renal dysfunction than in healthy adult control patients.

Malignant Hyperthermia (MH)

In a study of MH-susceptible pigs, cisatracurium besylate (highest dose 2000 mcg/kg equivalent to 3 × ED_{95} in pigs and 40 × ED_{95} in humans) did not trigger MH. Cisatracurium besylate has not been studied in MH-susceptible patients. Because MH can develop in the absence of established triggering agents, the clinician should be prepared to recognize and treat MH in any patient undergoing general anesthesia.

Long-Term Use in the Intensive Care Unit (ICU)

Long-term infusion (up to 6 days) of NIMBEX during mechanical ventilation in the ICU has been safely used in two studies. Dosage requirements may increase or decrease with time (see **CLINICAL PHARMACOLOGY - Individualization of Doses**).

Little information is available on the plasma levels and clinical consequences of cisatracurium metabolites that may accumulate during days to weeks of cisatracurium administration in ICU patients. Laudanosine, a major, biologically active metabolite of atracurium and cisatracurium without neuromuscular blocking activity, produces transient hypotension and, in higher doses, cerebral excitatory effects (generalized muscle twitching and seizures) when administered to several species of animals. There have been rare spontaneous reports of seizures in ICU patients who have received atracurium or other agents. These patients usually had predisposing causes (such as cranial trauma, cerebral edema, hypoxic encephalopathy, viral encephalitis, uremia). There are insufficient data to determine whether or not laudanosine contributes to seizures in ICU patients. Consistent with the decreased infusion rate requirements for NIMBEX, laudanosine concentrations were lower in patients receiving NIMBEX than in patients receiving atracurium for up to 48 hours (see **Pharmacokinetics** - Special Populations - Intensive Care Unit Patients).

In a randomized, double-blind study using train-of-four nerve stimulator monitoring to maintain at least one visible twitch, evaluable patients treated with NIMBEX (n = 19) recovered neuromuscular function (T_4:T_1 ratio ≥ 70%) following termination of infusion in approximately 55 minutes (range: 20 to 270) whereas evaluable vecuronium-treated patients (n = 12) recovered in 178 minutes (range: 40 minutes to 33 hours). In another study comparing NIMBEX and atracurium, patients recovered neuromuscular function in approximately 50 minutes for both NIMBEX (range: 20 to 175; n = 34) and atracurium (range: 35 to 85; n = 15).

WHENEVER THE USE OF **NIMBEX** OR ANY OTHER NEUROMUSCULAR BLOCKING AGENT IN THE ICU IS CONTEMPLATED, IT IS RECOMMENDED THAT NEUROMUSCULAR FUNCTION BE MONITORED DURING ADMINISTRATION WITH A NERVE STIMULATOR. ADDITIONAL DOSES OF **NIMBEX** OR ANY OTHER NEUROMUSCULAR BLOCKING AGENT SHOULD NOT BE GIVEN BEFORE THERE IS A DEFINITE RESPONSE TO NERVE STIMULATION. IF NO RESPONSE IS ELICITED, INFUSION ADMINISTRATION SHOULD BE DISCONTINUED UNTIL A RESPONSE RETURNS.

The effects of hemofiltration, hemodialysis, and hemoperfusion on plasma levels of NIMBEX and its metabolites are unknown.

Drug Interactions

NIMBEX has been used safely following varying degrees of recovery from succinylcholine-induced neuromuscular block. Administration of 0.1 mg/kg (2 × ED_{95}) NIMBEX at 10% or 95% recovery following an intubating dose of succinylcholine (1 mg/kg) produced ≥ 95% neuromuscular block. The time to onset of maximum block following NIMBEX is approximately 2 minutes faster with prior administration of succinylcholine. Prior administration of succinylcholine had no effect on the duration of neuromuscular block following initial or maintenance bolus doses of NIMBEX. Infusion requirements of NIMBEX in patients administered succinylcholine prior to infusions of NIMBEX were comparable to or slightly greater than when succinylcholine was not administered.

The use of NIMBEX before succinylcholine to attenuate some of the side effects of succinylcholine has not been studied.

Although not studied systematically in clinical trials, no drug interactions were observed when vecuronium, pancuronium, or atracurium were administered following varying degrees of recovery from single doses or infusions of NIMBEX.

Isoflurane or enflurane administered with nitrous oxide/oxygen to achieve 1.25 MAC [Minimum Alveolar Concentration] may prolong the clinically effective duration of action of initial and maintenance doses of NIMBEX and decrease the required infusion rate of NIMBEX. The magnitude of these effects may depend on the duration of administration of the volatile agents. Fifteen to 30 minutes of exposure to 1.25 MAC isoflurane or enflurane had minimal effects on the duration of action of initial doses of NIMBEX and therefore, no adjustment to the initial dose should be necessary when NIMBEX is administered shortly after initiation of volatile agents. In long surgical procedures during enflurane or isoflurane anesthesia, less frequent maintenance dosing, lower maintenance doses, or reduced infusion rates of NIMBEX may be necessary. The average infusion rate requirement may be decreased by as much as 30% to 40%.

In clinical studies propofol had no effect on the duration of action or dosing requirements for NIMBEX.

Other drugs which may enhance the neuromuscular blocking action of nondepolarizing agents such as NIMBEX include certain antibiotics (e.g., aminoglycosides, tetracyclines, bacitracin, polymyxins, lincomycin, clindamycin, colistin, and sodium colistemethate), magnesium salts, lithium, local anesthetics, procainamide, and quinidine.

Resistance to the neuromuscular blocking action of nondepolarizing neuromuscular blocking agents has been demonstrated in patients chronically administered phenytoin or carbamazepine. While the effects of chronic phenytoin or carbamazepine therapy on the action of NIMBEX are unknown, slightly shorter durations of neuromuscular block may be anticipated and infusion rate requirements may be higher.

Drug/Laboratory Test Interactions

None known.

Carcinogenesis, Mutagenesis, Impairment of Fertility

Carcinogenesis and fertility studies have not been performed. Cisatracurium besylate was evaluated in a battery of four short-term mutagenicity tests. It was non-mutagenic in the Ames Salmonella assay, a rat bone marrow cytogenetic assay, and an *in vitro* human lymphocyte cytogenetics assay. As was the case with atracurium, the mouse lymphoma assay was positive both in the presence and absence of exogenous metabolic activation (rat liver S-9). In the absence of S-9, cisatracurium besylate was positive at *in vitro* cisatracurium concentrations of 40 mcg/mL and higher. The highest non-mutagenic concentration (30 mcg/mL) and incubation time (4 hours) resulted in an AUC approximately 120 times that noted in clinical studies and approximately 8.5 times the mean peak clinical concentration noted. In the presence of S-9, cisatracurium besylate was positive at a cisatracurium concentration of 300 mcg/mL but not at lower or higher concentrations.

Pregnancy

Teratogenic Effects

Pregnancy Category B

Teratology testing in nonventilated pregnant rats treated subcutaneously with maximum subparalyzing doses (4 mg/kg daily; equivalent to 8 × the human ED_{95} following a bolus dose of 0.2 mg/kg IV) and in ventilated rats treated intravenously with paralyzing doses of NIMBEX at 0.5 and 1.0 mg/kg; equivalent to 10 × and 20 × the human ED_{95} dose, respectively, revealed no maternal or fetal toxicity or teratogenic effects. There are no adequate and well-controlled studies of NIMBEX in pregnant women. Because animal studies are not always predictive of human response, NIMBEX should be used during pregnancy only if clearly needed.

Labor and Delivery

The use of NIMBEX during labor, vaginal delivery, or cesarean section has not been studied in humans and it is not known whether NIMBEX administered to the mother has effects on the fetus. Doses of 0.2 or 0.4 mg/kg cisatracurium given to female beagles undergoing cesarean section resulted in negligible levels of cisatracurium in umbilical vessel blood of neonates and no deleterious effects on the puppies. The action of neuromuscular blocking agents may be enhanced by magnesium salts administered for the management of toxemia of pregnancy.

Nursing Mothers

It is not known whether cisatracurium besylate is excreted in human milk. Because many drugs are excreted in human milk, caution should be exercised following administration of NIMBEX to a nursing woman.

Pediatric Use

NIMBEX has not been studied in pediatric patients below the age of 1 month (see **CLINICAL PHARMACOLOGY** and **DOSAGE AND ADMINISTRATION** for clinical experience and recommendations for use in children 1 month to 12 years of age). Intubation of the trachea in patients 1-4 years old was facilitated more reliably when NIMBEX was used in combination with Halothane than when opioids and nitrous oxide were used for induction of anesthesia.

Geriatric Use

Of the total number of subjects in clinical studies of NIMBEX, 57 were 65 and over, 63 were 70 and over, and 15 were 80 and over. The geriatric population included a subset of patients with significant cardiovascular disease (see **CLINICAL PHARMACOLOGY - Hemodynamics Profile** and Special Populations - Geriatric Patients subsections). No overall differences in safety or effectiveness were observed between these subjects and younger subjects, and other reported clinical experience has not identified differences in responses between elderly and younger subjects, but greater sensitivity of some older individuals to NIMBEX cannot be ruled out.

Minor differences in the pharmacokinetics of cisatracurium between elderly and young adult patients are not associated with clinically significant differences in the recovery profile of NIMBEX following a single 0.1 mg/kg dose; the time to maximum block is approximately 1 minute slower in elderly patients (see **CLINICAL PHARMACOLOGY - Pharmacokinetics**).

ADVERSE REACTIONS

Observed in Clinical Trials of Surgical Patients

Adverse experiences were uncommon among the 945 surgical patients who received NIMBEX in conjunction with other drugs in US and European clinical studies in the course of a wide variety of procedures in patients receiving opioid, propofol, or inhalation anesthesia. The following adverse experiences were judged by investigators during the clinical trials to have a possible causal relationship to administration of NIMBEX:

Incidence Greater than 1%:

None.

Incidence Less than 1%

Cardiovascular:

bradycardia (0.4%),

hypotension (0.2%),

flushing (0.2%).

Respiratory:

bronchospasm (0.2%).

Dermatological:

rash (0.1%).

Observed in Clinical Trials of Intensive Care Unit Patients

Adverse experiences were uncommon among the 68 ICU patients who received NIMBEX in conjunction with other drugs in US and European clinical studies. One patient experienced bronchospasm. In one of the two ICU studies, a randomized and double-blind study of ICU patients using TOF neuromuscular monitoring, there were two reports of prolonged recovery (167 and 270 minutes) among 28 patients administered NIMBEX and 13 reports of prolonged recovery (range: 90 minutes to 33 hours) among 30 patients administered vecuronium.

Observed During Clinical Practice

In addition to adverse events reported from clinical trials, the following events have been identified during post-approval use of cisatracurium besylate in conjunction with one or more anesthetic agents in clinical practice. Because they are reported voluntarily from a population of unknown size, estimates of frequency cannot be made. These events have been chosen for inclusion due to a combination of their seriousness, frequency of reporting, or potential causal connection to cisatracurium besylate.

General

Histamine release, hypersensitivity reactions including anaphylactic or anaphylactoid responses which, in rare instances, were severe. There are rare reports of wheezing, laryngospasm, bronchospasm, rash and itching following administration of NIMBEX in children. These reported adverse events were not serious and their etiology could not be established with certainty.

Musculoskeletal

Prolonged neuromuscular block, inadequate neuromuscular block, muscle weakness, and myopathy.

OVERDOSAGE

Overdosage with neuromuscular blocking agents may result in neuromuscular block beyond the time needed for surgery and anesthesia. The primary treatment is maintenance of a patent airway and controlled ventilation until recovery of normal neuromuscular function is assured. Once recovery from neuromuscular block begins, further recovery may be facilitated by administration of an anticholinesterase agent (e.g., neostigmine, edrophonium) in conjunction with an appropriate anticholinergic agent (see Antagonism of Neuromuscular Block below).

Antagonism of Neuromuscular Block

ANTAGONISTS (SUCH AS NEOSTIGMINE AND EDROPHONIUM) SHOULD NOT BE ADMINISTERED WHEN COMPLETE NEUROMUSCULAR BLOCK IS EVIDENT OR SUSPECTED. THE USE OF A PERIPHERAL NERVE STIMULATOR TO EVALUATE RECOVERY AND ANTAGONISM OF NEUROMUSCULAR BLOCK IS RECOMMENDED.

Administration of 0.04 to 0.07 mg/kg neostigmine at approximately 10% recovery from neuromuscular block (range: 0 to 15%) produced 95% recovery of the muscle twitch response and a T_4:T_1 ratio ≥ 70% in an average of 9 to 10 minutes. The times from 25% recovery of the muscle twitch response to a T_4:T_1 ratio ≥ 70% following these doses of neostigmine averaged 7 minutes. The mean 25% to 75% recovery index following reversal was 3 to 4 minutes.

Administration of 1.0 mg/kg edrophonium at approximately 25% recovery from neuromuscular block (range: 16% to 30%) produced 95% recovery and a T_4:T_1 ratio ≥ 70% in an average of 3 to 5 minutes.

Patients administered antagonists should be evaluated for evidence of adequate clinical recovery (e.g., 5-second head lift and grip strength). Ventilation must be supported until no longer required.

The onset of antagonism may be delayed in the presence of debilitation, cachexia, carcinomatosis, and the concomitant use of certain broad spectrum antibiotics, or anesthetic agents and other drugs which enhance neuromuscular block or separately cause respiratory depression (see **PRECAUTIONS - Drug Interactions**). Under such circumstances the management is the same as that of prolonged neuromuscular block (see **OVERDOSAGE**).

DOSAGE AND ADMINISTRATION

NIMBEX SHOULD ONLY BE ADMINISTERED INTRAVENOUSLY.

The dosage information provided below is intended as a guide only. Doses of NIMBEX should be individualized (see CLINICAL PHARMACOLOGY - Individualization of Dosages). The use of a peripheral nerve stimulator will permit the most advantageous use of NIMBEX, minimize the possibility of overdosage or underdosage, and assist in the evaluation of recovery.

Adults

Initial Doses

One of two intubating doses of NIMBEX may be chosen, based on the desired time to tracheal intubation and the anticipated length of surgery. In addition to the dose of neuromuscular blocking agent, the presence of co-induction agents (e.g., fentanyl and midazolam) and the depth of anesthesia are factors that can influence intubation conditions. Doses of 0.15 (3 × ED_{95}) and 0.20 (4 × ED_{95}) mg/kg NIMBEX, as components of a propofol/nitrous oxide/oxygen induction-intubation technique, may produce generally GOOD or EXCELLENT conditions for intubation in 2.0 and 1.5 minutes, respectively. Similar intubation conditions may be expected when these doses of NIMBEX are administered as components of a thiopental/nitrous oxide/oxygen induction-intubation technique. In two intubation studies using thiopental or propofol and midazolam and fentanyl as co-induction agents, EXCELLENT intubation conditions were most frequently achieved with the 0.2 mg/kg compared to 0.15 mg/kg dose of cisatracurium. The clinically effective durations of action for 0.15 and 0.20 mg/kg NIMBEX during propofol anesthesia are 55 minutes (range: 44 to 74 minutes) and 61 minutes (range: 41 to 81 minutes), respectively. Lower doses may result in a longer time for the development of satisfactory intubation conditions. Doses up to 8 × ED_{95} NIMBEX have been safely administered to healthy adult patients and patients with serious cardiovascular disease. These larger doses are associated with longer clinically effective durations of action (see **CLINICAL PHARMACOLOGY**).

Because slower times to onset of complete neuromuscular block were observed in elderly patients and patients with renal dysfunction, extending the interval between administration of NIMBEX and the intubation attempt for these patients may be required to achieve adequate intubation conditions.

A dose of 0.03 mg/kg NIMBEX is recommended for maintenance of neuromuscular block during prolonged surgical procedures. Maintenance doses of 0.03 mg/kg each sustain neuromuscular block for approximately 20 minutes. Maintenance dosing is generally required 40 to 50 minutes following an initial dose of 0.15 mg/kg NIMBEX and 50 to 60 minutes following an initial dose of 0.20 mg/kg NIMBEX, but the need for maintenance doses should be determined by clinical criteria. For shorter or longer durations of action, smaller or larger maintenance doses may be administered. Isoflurane or enflurane administered with nitrous oxide/oxygen to achieve 1.25 MAC (Minimum Alveolar Concentration) may prolong the clinically effective duration of action of initial and maintenance doses. The magnitude of these effects may depend on the duration of administration of the volatile agents. Fifteen to 30 minutes of exposure to 1.25 MAC isoflurane or enflurane had minimal effects on the duration of action of initial doses of NIMBEX and therefore, no adjustment to the initial dose should be necessary when NIMBEX is administered shortly after initiation of volatile agents. In long surgical procedures during enflurane or isoflurane anesthesia, less frequent maintenance dosing or lower maintenance doses of NIMBEX may be necessary. No adjustments to the initial dose of NIMBEX are required when used in patients receiving propofol anesthesia.

Children

Initial Doses

The recommended dose of NIMBEX for children 2 to 12 years of age is 0.10-0.15 mg/kg administered over 5 to 10 seconds during either halothane or opioid anesthesia. When administered during stable opioid/nitrous oxide/oxygen anesthesia, 0.10 mg/kg NIMBEX produces maximum neuromuscular block in an average of 2.8 minutes (range: 1.8 to 6.7 minutes) and clinically effective block for 28 minutes (range: 21 to 38 minutes). When administered during stable opioid/nitrous oxide/oxygen anesthesia, 0.15 mg/kg NIMBEX produces maximum neuromuscular block in about

Information on the Abbott Pharmaceutical Products listed on these pages is from the prescribing information in use as of June 1, 2010. For more information, please visit rxabbott.com or call 1-800-633-9110.

3.0 minutes (range: 1.5 to 8.0 minutes) and clinically effective block (time to 25% recovery) for 36 minutes (range: 29 to 46 minutes).

Infants
Initial Doses
The recommended dose of NIMBEX for intubation of infants 1 month to 23 months is 0.15 mg/kg administered over 5 to 10 seconds during either halothane or opioid anesthesia. When administered during stable opioid/nitrous oxide/oxygen anesthesia, 0.15 mg/kg NIMBEX produces maximum neuromuscular block in about 2.0 minutes (range: 1.3 to 3.4 minutes) and clinically effective block (time to 25% recovery) for about 43 minutes (range: 34 to 58 minutes).

Use by Continuous Infusion
Infusion in the Operating Room (OR)
After administration of an initial bolus dose of NIMBEX, a diluted solution of NIMBEX can be administered by continuous infusion to adults and children aged 2 or more years for maintenance of neuromuscular block during extended surgical procedures. Infusion of NIMBEX should be individualized for each patient. The rate of administration should be adjusted according to the patient's response as determined by peripheral nerve stimulation. Accurate dosing is best achieved using a precision infusion device.

Infusion of NIMBEX should be initiated only after early evidence of spontaneous recovery from the initial bolus dose. An initial infusion rate of 3 mcg/kg/min may be required to rapidly counteract the spontaneous recovery of neuromuscular function. Thereafter, a rate of 1 to 2 mcg/kg/min should be adequate to maintain continuous neuromuscular block in the range of 89% to 99% in most pediatric and adult patients under opioid/nitrous oxide/oxygen anesthesia.

Reduction of the infusion rate by up to 30% to 40% should be considered when NIMBEX is administered during stable isoflurane or enflurane anesthesia (administered with nitrous oxide/oxygen at the 1.25 MAC level). Greater reductions in the infusion rate of NIMBEX may be required with longer durations of administration of isoflurane or enflurane.

The rate of infusion of atracurium required to maintain adequate surgical relaxation in patients undergoing coronary artery bypass surgery with induced hypothermia (25° to 28°C) is approximately half the rate required during normothermia. Based on the structural similarity between NIMBEX and atracurium, a similar effect on the infusion rate of NIMBEX may be expected.

Spontaneous recovery from neuromuscular block following discontinuation of infusion of NIMBEX may be expected to proceed at a rate comparable to that following administration of a single bolus dose.

Infusion in the Intensive Care Unit (ICU)
The principles for infusion of NIMBEX in the OR are also applicable to use in the ICU. An infusion rate of approximately 3 mcg/kg/min (range: 0.5 to 10.2 mcg/kg/min) should provide adequate neuromuscular block in adult patients in the ICU. There may be wide interpatient variability in dosage requirements and these may increase or decrease with time (see **PRECAUTIONS - Long-Term Use in the Intensive Care Unit [ICU]**). Following recovery from neuromuscular block, readministration of a bolus dose may be necessary to quickly re-establish neuromuscular block prior to reinstitution of the infusion.

Infusion Rate Tables
The amount of infusion solution required per minute will depend upon the concentration of NIMBEX in the infusion solution, the desired dose of NIMBEX, and the patient's weight. The contribution of the infusion solution to the fluid requirements of the patient also must be considered. Tables 10 and 11 provide guidelines for delivery, in mL/hr (equivalent to microdrops/minute when 60 microdrops = 1 mL), of NIMBEX solutions in concentrations of 0.1 mg/mL (10 mg/100 mL) or 0.4 mg/mL (40 mg/100 mL).

Table 10. Infusion Rates of NIMBEX for Maintenance of Neuromuscular Block During Opioid/Nitrous Oxide/Oxygen Anesthesia for a Concentration of 0.1 mg/mL

Patient Weight (kg)	Drug Delivery Rate (mcg/kg/min) Infusion Delivery Rate (mL/hr)				
	1.0	1.5	2.0	3.0	5.0
10	6	9	12	18	30
45	27	41	54	81	135
70	42	63	84	126	210
100	60	90	120	180	300

Table 11. Infusion Rates of NIMBEX for Maintenance of Neuromuscular Block During Opioid/Nitrous Oxide/Oxygen Anesthesia for a Concentration of 0.4 mg/mL

Patient Weight (kg)	Drug Delivery Rate (mcg/kg/min) Infusion Delivery Rate (mL/hr)				
	1.0	1.5	2.0	3.0	5.0
10	1.5	2.3	3.0	4.5	7.5
45	6.8	10.1	13.5	20.3	33.8
70	10.5	15.8	21.0	31.5	52.5
100	15.0	22.5	30.0	45.0	75.0

NIMBEX Injection Compatibility and Admixtures
Y-site Administration
NIMBEX Injection is acidic (pH = 3.25 to 3.65) and may not be compatible with alkaline solution having a pH greater than 8.5 (e.g., barbiturate solutions).
Studies have shown that NIMBEX Injection is compatible with:
- 5% Dextrose Injection, USP
- 0.9% Sodium Chloride Injection, USP
- 5% Dextrose and 0.9% Sodium Chloride Injection, USP
- SUFENTA® (sufentanil citrate) Injection, diluted as directed
- ALFENTA® (alfentanil hydrochloride) Injection, diluted as directed
- SUBLIMAZE® (fentanyl citrate) Injection, diluted as directed
- VERSED® (midazolam hydrochloride) Injection, diluted as directed
- Droperidol Injection, diluted as directed

NIMBEX Injection is not compatible with DIPRIVAN® (propofol) Injection or TORADOL® (ketorolac) Injection for Y-site administration. Studies of other parenteral products have not been conducted.

Dilution Stability
NIMBEX Injection diluted in 5% Dextrose Injection, USP; 0.9% Sodium Chloride Injection, USP; or 5% Dextrose and 0.9% Sodium Chloride Injection, USP to 0.1 mg/mL may be stored either under refrigeration or at room temperature for 24 hours without significant loss of potency. Dilutions to 0.1 mg/mL or 0.2 mg/mL in 5% Dextrose and Lactated Ringer's Injection may be stored under refrigeration for 24 hours.
NIMBEX Injection should not be diluted in Lactated Ringer's Injection, USP due to chemical instability.

NOTE: Parenteral drug products should be inspected visually for particulate matter and discoloration prior to administration whenever solution and container permit. Solutions which are not clear, or contain visible particulates, should not be used. NIMBEX Injection is a colorless to slightly yellow or greenish-yellow solution.

HOW SUPPLIED
NIMBEX Injection, 2 mg cisatracurium per mL, is supplied in the following:

List No.	Container	Size
4378	Single-dose Vial	5 mL
4380	Multiple-dose Vial	10 mL

NOTE: 10 mL Multiple-dose Vials contain 0.9% w/v benzyl alcohol as a preservative (see **WARNINGS** concerning newborn infants).

NIMBEX Injection, 10 mg cisatracurium per mL is supplied in the following:

4382	Single-dose Vial	20 mL

Intended only for use in the ICU.

Storage
NIMBEX Injection should be refrigerated at 2° to 8°C (36° to 46°F) in the carton to preserve potency. Protect from light. DO NOT FREEZE. Upon removal from refrigeration to room temperature storage conditions (25°C/77°F), use NIMBEX Injection within 21 days even if rerefrigerated.
U.S. Patent No. 5,453,510
Registered trademark of GlaxoSmithKline, licensed for use by Abbott Laboratories.
Revised: May, 2008
EN-1795 (05/08)
Mfd By: Hospira, Inc.
Lake Forest, IL 60045 USA
For: Abbott Laboratories
North Chicago, IL 60064 USA

NORVIR® ℞
[nor - veer]
(ritonavir capsules) Soft Gelatin
(ritonavir oral solution)

> **WARNING**
> CO-ADMINISTRATION OF NORVIR WITH SEDATIVE HYPNOTICS, ANTIARRHYTHMICS, OR ERGOT ALKALOID PREPARATIONS MAY RESULT IN POTENTIALLY SERIOUS AND/OR LIFE-THREATENING ADVERSE EVENTS DUE TO POSSIBLE EFFECTS OF NORVIR ON THE HEPATIC METABOLISM OF CERTAIN DRUGS. SEE **CONTRAINDICATIONS** AND **PRECAUTIONS** SECTIONS.

DESCRIPTION
NORVIR (ritonavir) is an inhibitor of HIV protease with activity against the Human Immunodeficiency Virus (HIV). Ritonavir is chemically designated as 10-Hydroxy-2-methyl-5-(1-methylethyl)-1-[2-(1-methylethyl)-4-thiazolyl]-3,6-dioxo-8,11-bis(phenylmethyl)-2,4,7,12-tetraazatridecan-13-oic acid, 5-thiazolylmethyl ester, [5S-(5R*,8R*,10R*,11R*)]. Its molecular formula is $C_{37}H_{48}N_6O_5S_2$, and its molecular weight is 720.95. Ritonavir has the following structural formula:

Ritonavir is a white-to-light-tan powder. Ritonavir has a bitter metallic taste. It is freely soluble in methanol and ethanol, soluble in isopropanol and practically insoluble in water.
NORVIR soft gelatin capsules are available for oral administration in a strength of 100 mg ritonavir with the following inactive ingredients: Butylated hydroxytoluene, ethanol, gelatin, iron oxide, oleic acid, polyoxyl 35 castor oil, and titanium dioxide.
NORVIR oral solution is available for oral administration as 80 mg/mL of ritonavir in a peppermint and caramel flavored vehicle. Each 8-ounce bottle contains 19.2 grams of ritonavir. NORVIR oral solution also contains ethanol, water, polyoxyl 35 castor oil, propylene glycol, anhydrous citric acid to adjust pH, saccharin sodium, peppermint oil, creamy caramel flavoring, and FD&C Yellow No. 6.

CLINICAL PHARMACOLOGY
Microbiology
Mechanism of Action
Ritonavir is a peptidomimetic inhibitor of both the HIV-1 and HIV-2 proteases. Inhibition of HIV protease renders the enzyme incapable of processing the gag-pol polyprotein precursor which leads to production of non-infectious immature HIV particles.
Antiviral Activity In Vitro
The activity of ritonavir was assessed in vitro in acutely infected lymphoblastoid cell lines and in peripheral blood lymphocytes. The concentration of drug that inhibits 50% (EC_{50}) of viral replication ranged from 3.8 to 153 nM depending upon the HIV-1 isolate and the cells employed. The average EC_{50} for low passage clinical isolates was 22 nM (n = 13). In MT_4 cells, ritonavir demonstrated additive effects against HIV-1 in combination with either zidovudine (ZDV) or didanosine (ddI). Studies which measured cytotoxicity of ritonavir on several cell lines showed that > 20 μM was required to inhibit cellular growth by 50% resulting in an in vitro therapeutic index of at least 1000.
Resistance
HIV-1 isolates with reduced susceptibility to ritonavir have been selected in vitro. Genotypic analysis of these isolates showed mutations in the HIV protease gene at amino acid positions 84 (Ile to Val), 82 (Val to Phe), and 46 (Met to Ile). Phenotypic (n = 18) and genotypic (n = 44) changes in HIV isolates from selected patients treated with ritonavir were monitored in phase I/II trials over a period of 3 to 32 weeks. Mutations associated with the HIV viral protease in isolates obtained from 41 patients appeared to occur in a stepwise and ordered fashion; in sequence, these mutations were position 82 (Val to Ala/Phe), 54 (Ile to Val), 71 (Ala to Val/Thr), and 36 (Ile to Leu), followed by combinations of mutations at an additional 5 specific amino acid positions. Of 18 patients for whom both phenotypic and genotypic analysis were performed on free virus isolated from plasma, 12 showed reduced susceptibility to ritonavir in vitro. All 18 patients possessed one or more mutations in the viral protease gene. The 82 mutation appeared to be

necessary but not sufficient to confer phenotypic resistance. Phenotypic resistance was defined as a ≥ 5-fold decrease in viral sensitivity *in vitro* from baseline. The clinical relevance of phenotypic and genotypic changes associated with ritonavir therapy has not been established.

Cross-Resistance to Other Antiretrovirals

Among protease inhibitors variable cross-resistance has been recognized. Serial HIV isolates obtained from six patients during ritonavir therapy showed a decrease in ritonavir susceptibility *in vitro* but did not demonstrate a concordant decrease in susceptibility to saquinavir *in vitro* when compared to matched baseline isolates. However, isolates from two of these patients demonstrated decreased susceptibility to indinavir *in vitro* (8-fold). Isolates from 5 patients were also tested for cross-resistance to amprenavir and nelfinavir; isolates from 2 patients had a decrease in susceptibility to nelfinavir (12- to 14-fold), and none to amprenavir. Cross-resistance between ritonavir and reverse transcriptase inhibitors is unlikely because of the different enzyme targets involved. One ZDV-resistant HIV isolate tested *in vitro* retained full susceptibility to ritonavir.

Pharmacokinetics

The pharmacokinetics of ritonavir have been studied in healthy volunteers and HIV-infected patients ($CD_4 \geq 50$ cells/μL). See Table 1 for ritonavir pharmacokinetic characteristics.

Absorption

The absolute bioavailability of ritonavir has not been determined. After a 600 mg dose of oral solution, peak concentrations of ritonavir were achieved approximately 2 hours and 4 hours after dosing under fasting and non-fasting (514 KCal; 9% fat, 12% protein, and 79% carbohydrate) conditions, respectively.

Effect of Food on Oral Absorption

When the oral solution was given under non-fasting conditions, peak ritonavir concentrations decreased 23% and the extent of absorption decreased 7% relative to fasting conditions. Dilution of the oral solution, within one hour of administration, with 240 mL of chocolate milk, Advera® or Ensure® did not significantly affect the extent and rate of ritonavir absorption. After a single 600 mg dose under non-fasting conditions, in two separate studies, the soft gelatin capsule (n = 57) and oral solution (n = 18) formulations yielded mean ± SD areas under the plasma concentration-time curve (AUCs) of 121.7 ± 53.8 and 129.0 ± 39.3 μg•h/mL, respectively. Relative to fasting conditions, the extent of absorption of ritonavir from the soft gelatin capsule formulation was 13% higher when administered with a meal (615 KCal; 14.5% fat, 9% protein, and 76% carbohydrate).

Metabolism

Nearly all of the plasma radioactivity after a single oral 600 mg dose of ^{14}C-ritonavir oral solution (n = 5) was attributed to unchanged ritonavir. Five ritonavir metabolites have been identified in human urine and feces. The isopropylthiazole oxidation metabolite (M-2) is the major metabolite and has antiviral activity similar to that of parent drug; however, the concentrations of this metabolite in plasma are low. *In vitro* studies utilizing human liver microsomes have demonstrated that cytochrome P450 3A (CYP3A) is the major isoform involved in ritonavir metabolism, although CYP2D6 also contributes to the formation of M-2.

Elimination

In a study of five subjects receiving a 600 mg dose of ^{14}C-ritonavir oral solution, 11.3 ± 2.8% of the dose was excreted into the urine, with 3.5 ± 1.8% of the dose excreted as unchanged parent drug. In that study, 86.4 ± 2.9% of the dose was excreted in the feces with 33.8 ± 10.8% of the dose excreted as unchanged parent drug. Upon multiple dosing, ritonavir accumulation is less than predicted from a single dose possibly due to a time and dose-related increase in clearance.

Table 1. Ritonavir Pharmacokinetic Characteristics

Parameter	n	Values (Mean ± SD)
C_{max} SS[†]	10	11.2 ± 3.6 μg/mL
C_{trough} SS[†]	10	3.7 ± 2.6 μg/mL
$V_\beta/F^{\ddagger}$	91	0.41 ± 0.25 L/kg
$t_{1/2}$		3-5 h
CL/F SS[†]	10	8.8 ± 3.2 L/h
CL/F[‡]	91	4.6 ± 1.6 L/h
CL_R	62	< 0.1 L/h
RBC/Plasma Ratio		0.14
Percent Bound*		98 to 99%

† SS = steady state; patients taking ritonavir 600 mg q12h.

‡ Single ritonavir 600 mg dose.

* Primarily bound to human serum albumin and alpha-1 acid glycoprotein over the ritonavir concentration range of 0.01 to 30 μg/mL.

Table 2. Drug Interactions - Pharmacokinetic Parameters for Ritonavir in the Presence of the Co-administered Drug
(See PRECAUTIONS - Table 6 for Recommended Alterations in Dose or Regimen)

Co-administered Drug	Dose of Co-administered Drug (mg)	Dose of NORVIR (mg)	n	AUC % (95% CI)	C_{max} (95% CI)	C_{min} (95% CI)
Clarithromycin	500 q12h, 4 d	200 q8h, 4 d	22	↑ 12% (2, 23%)	↑ 15% (2, 28%)	↑ 14% (-3, 36%)
Didanosine	200 q12h, 4 d	600 q12h, 4 d	12	↔	↔	↔
Fluconazole	400 single dose, day 1; 200 daily, 4 d	200 q6h, 4 d	8	↑ 12% (5, 20%)	↑ 15% (7, 22%)	↑ 14% (0, 26%)
Fluoxetine	30 q12h, 8 d	600 single dose, 1 d	16	↑ 19% (7, 34%)	↔	ND
Ketoconazole	200 daily, 7 d	500 q12h, 10 d	12	↑ 18% (-3, 52%)	↑ 10% (-11, 36%)	ND
Rifampin	600 or 300 daily, 10 d	500 q12h, 20 d	7, 9*	↓ 35% (7, 55%)	↓ 25% (-5, 46%)	↓ 49% (-14, 91%)
Voriconazole	400 q12h, 1 d; then 200 q12h, 8 d	400 q12h, 9 d		↔	↔	ND
Zidovudine	200 q8h, 4 d	300 q6h, 4 d	10	↔	↔	↔

Table 3. Drug Interactions - Pharmacokinetic Parameters for Co-administered Drug in the Presence of NORVIR
(See PRECAUTIONS - Table 6 for Recommended Alterations in Dose or Regimen)

Co-administered Drug	Dose of Co-administered Drug (mg)	Dose of NORVIR (mg)	n	AUC % (95% CI)	C_{max} (95% CI)	C_{min} (95% CI)
Alprazolam	1, single dose	500 q12h, 10 d	12	↓ 12% (-5, 30%)	↓ 16% (5, 27%)	ND
Clarithromycin	500 q12h, 4 d	200 q8h, 4 d	22	↑ 77% (56, 103%)	↑ 31% (15, 51%)	↑ 2.8-fold (2.4, 3.3X)
14-OH clarithromycin metabolite				↓ 100%	↓ 99%	↓ 100%
Desipramine	100, single dose	500 q12h, 12 d	14	↑ 145% (103, 211%)	↑ 22% (12, 35%)	ND
2-OH desipramine metabolite				↓ 15% (3, 26%)	↓ 67% (62, 72%)	ND
Didanosine	200 q12h, 4 d	600 q12h, 4 d	12	↓ 13% (0, 23%)	↓ 16% (5, 26%)	↔
Ethinyl estradiol	50 μg single dose	500 q12h, 16 d	23	↓ 40% (31, 49%)	↓ 32% (24, 39%)	ND
Fluticasone propionate aqueous nasal spray	200 mcg qd, 7 d	100 mg q12h, 7 d	18	↑ approximately 350-fold[5]	↑ approximately 25-fold[5]	
Indinavir[1] Day 14 Day 15	400 q12h, 15 d	400 q12h, 15 d	10	↑ 6% (-14, 29%) ↓ 7% (-22, 28%)	↓ 51% (40, 61%) ↓ 62% (52, 70%)	↑ 4-fold (2.8, 6.8X) ↑ 4-fold (2.5, 6.5X)
Ketoconazole	200 daily, 7 d	500 q12h, 10 d	12	↑ 3.4-fold (2.8, 4.3X)	↑ 55% (40, 72%)	ND
Meperidine Normeperidine metabolite	50 oral single dose	500 q12h, 10 d	8 6	↓ 62% (59, 65%) ↑ 47% (-24, 345%)	↓ 59% (42, 72%) ↑ 87% (42, 147%)	ND ND
Methadone[2]	5, single dose	500 q12h, 15 d	11	↓ 36% (16, 52%)	↓ 38% (28, 46%)	ND

(Table continued on next page)

Effects on Electrocardiogram

QTcF interval was evaluated in a randomized, placebo and active (moxifloxacin 400 mg once-daily) controlled crossover study in 45 healthy adults, with 10 measurements over 12 hours on Day 3. The maximum mean (95% upper confidence bound) time-matched difference in QTcF from placebo after baseline correction was 5.5 (7.6) milliseconds (msec) for 400 mg twice-daily ritonavir. Ritonavir 400 mg twice daily resulted in Day 3 ritonavir exposure that was approximately 1.5 fold higher than observed with ritonavir 600 mg twice-daily dose at steady state.

PR interval prolongation was also noted in subjects receiving ritonavir in the same study on Day 3. The maximum mean (95% confidence interval) difference from placebo in the PR interval after baseline correction was 22 (25) msec for 400 mg twice-daily ritonavir (See **PRECAUTIONS – PR Interval Prolongation**).

Special Populations

Gender, Race and Age

No age-related pharmacokinetic differences have been observed in adult patients (18 to 63 years). Ritonavir pharmacokinetics have not been studied in older patients.

A study of ritonavir pharmacokinetics in healthy males and females showed no statistically significant differences in the pharmacokinetics of ritonavir. Pharmacokinetic differences due to race have not been identified.

Pediatric Patients

Steady-state pharmacokinetics were evaluated in 37 HIV-infected patients ages 2 to 14 years receiving doses ranging from 250 mg/m² twice-daily to 400 mg/m² twice-daily in PACTG Study 310, and in 41 HIV-infected patients ages 1 month to 2 years at doses of 350 and 450 mg/m² twice-daily in PACTG Study 345. Across dose groups, ritonavir steady-state oral clearance (CL/F/m²) was approximately 1.5 to 1.7 times faster in pediatric patients than in adult subjects. Ritonavir concentrations obtained after 350 to 400 mg/m² twice-daily in pediatric patients > 2 years were comparable

Information on the Abbott Pharmaceutical Products listed on these pages is from the prescribing information in use as of June 1, 2010. For more information, please visit rxabbott.com or call 1-800-633-9110.

Table 3 (cont.). Drug Interactions - Pharmacokinetic Parameters for Co-administered Drug in the Presence of NORVIR (See PRECAUTIONS - Table 6 for Recommended Alterations in Dose or Regimen)

Co-administered Drug	Dose of Co-administered Drug (mg)	Dose of NORVIR (mg)	n	AUC % (95% CI)	C_{max} (95% CI)	C_{min} (95% CI)
Rifabutin	150 daily, 16 d	500 q12h, 10 d	5	↑ 4-fold (2.8, 6.1X)	↑ 2.5-fold (1.9, 3.4X)	↑ 6-fold
25-O-desacetyl rifabutin metabolite			11*	↑ 38-fold (28, 56X)	↑ 16-fold (13, 20X)	(3.5, 18.3X) ↑ 181-fold (ND)
Sildenafil	100, single dose	500 BID, 8 d	28	↑ 11-fold	↑ 4-fold	ND
Sulfa-methoxazole[3]	800, single dose	500 q12h, 12 d	15	↓ 20% (16, 23%)	↔	ND
Tadalafil	20 mg, single dose	200 mg q12h		↑ 124%	↔	ND
Theophylline	3 mg/kg q8h, 15 d	500 q12h, 10 d	13, 11*	↓ 43% (42, 45%)	↓ 32% (29, 34%)	↓ 57% (55, 59%)
Trazodone	50 mg, single dose	200 mg q12h, 4 doses	10	↑ 2.4-fold	↑ 34%	
Trimethoprim[3]	160, single dose	500 q12h, 12 d	15	↑ 20% (3, 43%)	↔	ND
Vardenafil	5 mg	600 q12h,		↑ 49-fold	↑ 13-fold	ND
Voriconazole	400 q12h, 1 d; then 200 q12h, 8 d	400 q12h, 9 d		↓ 82%	↓ 66%	
Warfarin S-Warfarin R-Warfarin	5, single dose	400 q12h, 12d	12	↑ 9% (-17, 44%)[4] ↓ 33% (-38, -27%)[4]	↓ 9% (-16, -2%)[4] ↔	ND ND
Zidovudine	200 q8h, 4 d	300 q6h, 4 d	9	↓ 25% (15, 34%)	↓ 27% (4, 45%)	ND

[1] Ritonavir and indinavir were co-administered for 15 days; Day 14 doses were administered after a 15%-fat breakfast (757 Kcal) and 9%-fat evening snack (236 Kcal), and Day 15 doses were administered after a 15%-fat breakfast (757 Kcal) and 32%-fat dinner (815 Kcal). Indinavir C_{min} was also increased 4-fold. Effects were assessed relative to an indinavir 800 mg q8h regimen under fasting conditions.

[2] Effects were assessed on a dose-normalized comparison to a methadone 20 mg single dose.

[3] Sulfamethoxazole and trimethoprim taken as single combination tablet.

[4] 90% CI presented for R- and s-warfarin AUC and C_{max} ratios.

[5] This significant increase in plasma fluticasone propionate exposure resulted in a significant decrease (86%) in plasma cortisol AUC.

↑ Indicates increase.
↓ Indicates decrease.
↔ Indicates no change.
* Parallel group design; entries are subjects receiving combination and control regimens, respectively.

to those obtained in adults receiving 600 mg (approximately 330 mg/m^2) twice-daily. The following observations were seen regarding ritonavir concentrations after administration with 350 or 450 mg/m^2 twice-daily in children < 2 years of age. Higher ritonavir exposures were not evident with 450 mg/m^2 twice-daily compared to the 350 mg/m^2 twice-daily. Ritonavir trough concentrations were somewhat lower than those obtained in adults receiving 600 mg twice-daily. The area under the ritonavir plasma concentration-time curve and trough concentrations obtained after administration with 350 or 450 mg/m^2 twice-daily in children < 2 years were approximately 16% and 60% lower, respectively, than that obtained in adults receiving 600 mg twice-daily.

Renal Insufficiency
Ritonavir pharmacokinetics have not been studied in patients with renal insufficiency, however, since renal clearance is negligible, a decrease in total body clearance is not expected in patients with renal insufficiency.

Hepatic Insufficiency
Dose-normalized steady-state ritonavir concentrations in subjects with mild hepatic insufficiency (400 mg twice-daily, n = 6) were similar to those in control subjects dosed with 500 mg twice-daily. Dose-normalized steady-state ritonavir exposures in subjects with moderate hepatic impairment (400 mg twice-daily, n= 6) were about 40% lower than those in subjects with normal hepatic function (500 mg twice-daily, n = 6). Protein binding of ritonavir was not statistically significantly affected by mild or moderately impaired hepatic function. No dose adjustment is recommended in patients with mild or moderate hepatic impairment. However, health care providers should be aware of the potential for lower ritonavir concentrations in patients with moderate hepatic impairment and should monitor patient response carefully. Ritonavir has not been studied in patients with severe hepatic impairment.

Drug-Drug Interactions
See also **CONTRAINDICATIONS, WARNINGS,** and **PRECAUTIONS - Drug Interactions**.
Table 2 and Table 3 summarize the effects on AUC and C_{max}, with 95% confidence intervals (95% CI), of co-administration of ritonavir with a variety of drugs. For information about clinical recommendations see **PRECAUTIONS - Drug Interactions**.
[See table 2 at top of previous page]
[See table 3 on previous page and above]

INDICATIONS AND USAGE

NORVIR is indicated in combination with other antiretroviral agents for the treatment of HIV-infection. This indication is based on the results from a study in patients with advanced HIV disease that showed a reduction in both mortality and AIDS-defining clinical events for patients who received NORVIR either alone or in combination with nucleoside analogues. Median duration of follow-up in this study was 13.5 months.

Description of Clinical Studies
The activity of NORVIR as monotherapy or in combination with nucleoside reverse transcriptase inhibitors has been evaluated in 1446 patients enrolled in two double-blind, randomized trials.
Advanced Patients with Prior Antiretroviral Therapy
Study 247 was a randomized, double-blind trial (with open-label follow-up) conducted in HIV-infected patients with at least nine months of prior antiretroviral therapy and baseline CD$_4$ cell counts ≤ 100 cells/μL. NORVIR 600 mg twice-daily or placebo was added to each patient's baseline antiretroviral therapy regimen, which could have consisted of up to two approved antiretroviral agents. The study accrued 1090 patients, with mean baseline CD$_4$ cell count at study entry of 32 cells/μL. After the clinical benefit of NORVIR therapy was demonstrated, all patients were eligible to switch to open-label NORVIR for the duration of the follow-up period. Median duration of double-blind therapy

with NORVIR and placebo was 6 months. The median duration of follow-up through the end of the open-label phase was 13.5 months for patients randomized to NORVIR and 14 months for patients randomized to placebo.
The cumulative incidence of clinical disease progression or death during the double-blind phase of Study 247 was 26% for patients initially randomized to NORVIR compared to 42% for patients initially randomized to placebo. This difference in rates was statistically significant (see Figure 1).

Figure 1. Time to Disease Progression or Death During the Double-blind Phase of Study 247

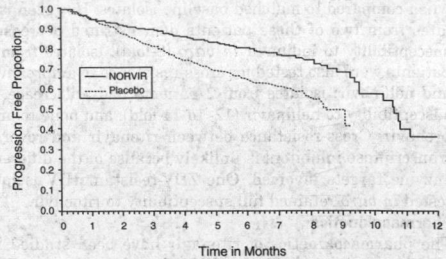

The cumulative mortality through the end of the open-label follow-up phase for patients enrolled in Study 247 was 18% for patients initially randomized to NORVIR compared to 26% for patients initially randomized to placebo. This difference in rates was statistically significant (see Figure 2). Since the analysis at the end of the open-label phase includes patients in the placebo arm who were switched from placebo to NORVIR therapy, the survival benefit of NORVIR cannot be precisely estimated.

Figure 2. Survival of Patients by Randomized Treatment Regimen in Study 247

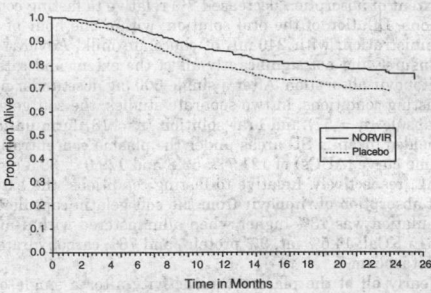

Figure 3 and Figure 4 summarize the mean change from baseline for CD$_4$ cell count and plasma HIV RNA (copies/mL), respectively, during the first 24 weeks for the double-blind phase of Study 247.

Figure 3. Mean Change from Baseline in CD$_4$ Cell Count (cells/μL) During the Double-blind Phase of Study 247

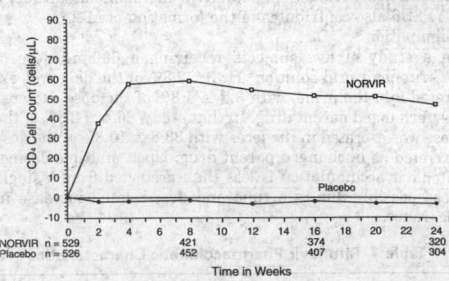

Figure 4. Mean Change from Baseline in HIV RNA (log copies/mL) During the Double-blind Phase of Study 247

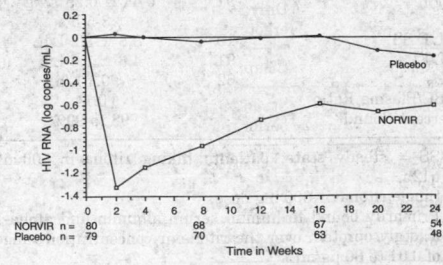

Patients Without Prior Antiretroviral Therapy

In Study 245, 356 antiretroviral-naive HIV-infected patients (mean baseline CD_4 = 364 cells/μL) were randomized to receive either NORVIR 600 mg twice-daily, zidovudine 200 mg three-times-daily, or a combination of these drugs. Figure 5 and Figure 6 summarize the mean change from baseline for CD_4 cell count and plasma HIV RNA (copies/mL), respectively, during the first 24 weeks for the double-blind phase of Study 245.

Figure 5. Mean Change from Baseline in CD_4 Cell Count (cells/μL) During Study 245

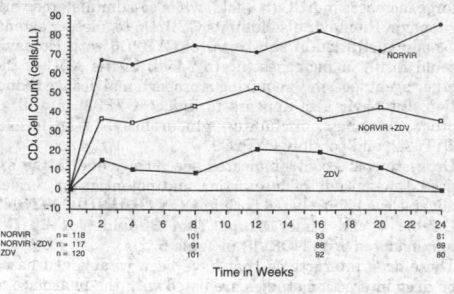

NORVIR	n = 118	101	88	81
NORVIR+ZDV	n = 117	91	88	69
ZDV	n = 120	101	92	80

Figure 6. Mean Change from Baseline in HIV RNA (log copies/mL) During Study 245

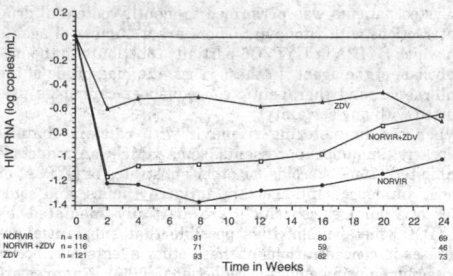

NORVIR	n = 118	91	80	69
NORVIR+ZDV	n = 116	71	59	46
ZDV	n = 121	93	82	73

CONTRAINDICATIONS

- When co-administering NORVIR with other protease inhibitors, see the full prescribing information for that protease inhibitor including contraindication information.
- NORVIR is contraindicated in patients with known hypersensitivity to ritonavir or any of its ingredients.
- Co-administration of NORVIR is contraindicated with the drugs listed in Table 4 (also see **PRECAUTIONS - Table 5. Drugs that Should Not be Co-administered with NORVIR**) because ritonavir mediated CYP3A inhibition can result in serious and/or life-threatening reactions. Voriconazole and St. John's Wort are exceptions in that co-administration of NORVIR and voriconazole results in a significant decrease in plasma concentrations of voriconazole, and co-administration of NORVIR with St. John's Wort may result in decreased ritonavir plasma concentrations.

Table 4. Drugs that are Contraindicated with NORVIR

Drug Class	Drugs Within Class That Are CONTRAINDICATED With NORVIR**
Alpha$_1$-adrenoreceptor antagonist	Alfuzosin HCL
Antiarrhythmics	Amiodarone, bepridil, flecainide, propafenone, quinidine
Antifungal	Voriconazole
Ergot Derivatives	Dihydroergotamine, ergonovine, ergotamine, methylergonovine
GI Motility Agent	Cisapride
Herbal Products	St. John's Wort (hypericum perforatum)
HMG-CoA Reductase Inhibitors:	Lovastatin, simvastatin
Neuroleptic	Pimozide

PDE5 enzyme inhibitor	Sildenafil* (Revatio®) only when used for the treatment of pulmonary arterial hypertension (PAH)
Sedative/hypnotics	Oral midazolam, triazolam

*see **WARNINGS - Drug Interactions** and **PRECAUTIONS – Table 6. Established and Other Potentially Significant Drug Interactions** for coadministration of sildenafil in patients with erectile dysfunction.

For additional information for these contraindicated drugs, see also **PRECAUTIONS – Table 5. Drugs that Should Not be Co-administered with NORVIR.

WARNINGS

ALERT: Find out about medicines that should NOT be taken with NORVIR. This statement is included on the product's bottle label.

When co-administering NORVIR with other protease inhibitors, see the full prescribing information for that protease inhibitor including **WARNINGS**.

Drug Interactions

See **CONTRAINDICATIONS** - Table 4 for a listing of drugs that are contraindicated with NORVIR due to potentially life-threatening adverse events, significant drug interactions, or loss of virologic activity. Also, see **PRECAUTIONS** – Table 5 and Table 6 for drugs that should not be co-administered with NORVIR and for a listing of drugs with established and other significant drug interactions.

Allergic Reactions

Allergic reactions including urticaria, mild skin eruptions, bronchospasm, and angioedema have been reported. Rare cases of anaphylaxis and Stevens-Johnson syndrome have also been reported.

Hepatic Reactions

Hepatic transaminase elevations exceeding 5 times the upper limit of normal, clinical hepatitis, and jaundice have occurred in patients receiving NORVIR alone or in combination with other antiretroviral drugs (see Table 8). There may be an increased risk for transaminase elevations in patients with underlying hepatitis B or C. Therefore, caution should be exercised when administering NORVIR to patients with pre-existing liver diseases, liver enzyme abnormalities, or hepatitis. Increased AST/ALT monitoring should be considered in these patients, especially during the first three months of NORVIR treatment.

There have been postmarketing reports of hepatic dysfunction, including some fatalities. These have generally occurred in patients taking multiple concomitant medications and/or with advanced AIDS.

Pancreatitis

Pancreatitis has been observed in patients receiving NORVIR therapy, including those who developed hypertriglyceridemia. In some cases fatalities have been observed. Patients with advanced HIV disease may be at increased risk of elevated triglycerides and pancreatitis.

Pancreatitis should be considered if clinical symptoms (nausea, vomiting, abdominal pain) or abnormalities in laboratory values (such as increased serum lipase or amylase values) suggestive of pancreatitis should occur. Patients who exhibit these signs or symptoms should be evaluated and NORVIR therapy should be discontinued if a diagnosis of pancreatitis is made.

Diabetes Mellitus/Hyperglycemia

New onset diabetes mellitus, exacerbation of pre-existing diabetes mellitus, and hyperglycemia have been reported during postmarketing surveillance in HIV-infected patients receiving protease inhibitor therapy. Some patients required either initiation or dose adjustments of insulin or oral hypoglycemic agents for treatment of these events. In some cases, diabetic ketoacidosis has occurred. In those patients who discontinued protease inhibitor therapy, hyperglycemia persisted in some cases. Because these events have been reported voluntarily during clinical practice, estimates of frequency cannot be made and a causal relationship between protease inhibitor therapy and these events has not been established.

PRECAUTIONS

When co-administering NORVIR with other protease inhibitors, see the full prescribing information for that protease inhibitor including **PRECAUTIONS**.

General

Ritonavir is principally metabolized by the liver. Therefore, caution should be exercised when administering this drug to patients with impaired hepatic function (see **WARNINGS** and **CLINICAL PHARMACOLOGY** - *Hepatic Insufficiency*).

Resistance/Cross-resistance

Varying degrees of cross-resistance among protease inhibitors have been observed. Continued administration of

ritonavir therapy following loss of viral suppression may increase the likelihood of cross-resistance to other protease inhibitors (see **Microbiology**).

Hemophilia

There have been reports of increased bleeding, including spontaneous skin hematomas and hemarthrosis, in patients with hemophilia type A and B treated with protease inhibitors. In some patients additional factor VIII was given. In more than half of the reported cases, treatment with protease inhibitors was continued or reintroduced. A causal relationship has not been established.

PR Interval Prolongation

Ritonavir prolongs the PR interval in some patients. Post marketing cases of second or third degree atrioventricular block have been reported in patients. NORVIR should be used with caution in patients with underlying structural heart disease, preexisting conduction system abnormalities, ischemic heart disease, cardiomyopathies, as these patients may be at increased risk for developing cardiac conduction abnormalities. The impact on the PR interval of co-administration of ritonavir with other drugs that prolong the PR interval (including calcium channel blockers, beta-adrenergic blockers, digoxin and atazanavir) has not been evaluated. As a result, co-administration of ritonavir with these drugs should be undertaken with caution, particularly with those drugs metabolized by CYP3A. Clinical monitoring is recommended. See **CLINICAL PHARMACOLOGY - Effects on Electrocardiogram**.

Fat Redistribution

Redistribution/accumulation of body fat including central obesity, dorsocervical fat enlargement (buffalo hump), peripheral wasting, facial wasting, breast enlargement, and "cushingoid appearance" have been observed in patients receiving antiretroviral therapy. The mechanism and long-term consequences of these events are currently unknown. A causal relationship has not been established.

Lipid Disorders

Treatment with NORVIR therapy alone or in combination with saquinavir has resulted in substantial increases in the concentration of total triglycerides and cholesterol. Triglyceride and cholesterol testing should be performed prior to initiating NORVIR therapy and at periodic intervals during therapy. Lipid disorders should be managed as clinically appropriate. See **PRECAUTIONS - Table 5** and **Table 6** for additional information on potential drug interactions with NORVIR and HMG CoA reductase inhibitors.

Immune Reconstitution Syndrome

Immune reconstitution syndrome has been reported in HIV-infected patients treated with combination antiretroviral therapy, including NORVIR. During the initial phase of combination antiretroviral treatment, patients whose immune system responds may develop an inflammatory response to indolent or residual opportunistic infections (such as *Mycobacterium avium* infection, cytomegalovirus, *Pneumocystis jiroveci* pneumonia, or tuberculosis), which may necessitate further evaluation and treatment.

Information For Patients

A statement to patients and health care providers is included on the product's bottle label: **ALERT: Find out about medicines that should NOT be taken with NORVIR.** A Patient Package Insert (PPI) for Norvir is available for patient information.

Patients should be informed that NORVIR is not a cure for HIV infection and that they may continue to acquire illnesses associated with advanced HIV infection, including opportunistic infections.

Patients should be told that the long-term effects of NORVIR are unknown at this time. They should be informed that NORVIR therapy has not been shown to reduce the risk of transmitting HIV to others through sexual contact or blood contamination.

Patients should be advised to take NORVIR with food, if possible.

Patients should be informed to take NORVIR every day as prescribed. Patients should not alter the dose or discontinue NORVIR without consulting their doctor. If a dose is missed, patients should take the next dose as soon as possible. However, if a dose is skipped, the patient should not double the next dose.

Patients should be informed that redistribution or accumulation of body fat may occur in patients receiving antiretroviral therapy and that the cause and long term health effects of these conditions are not known at this time.

NORVIR may interact with some drugs; therefore, patients should be advised to report to their doctor the use of any other prescription, non-prescription medication or herbal products, particularly St. John's wort.

Patients receiving PDE5 inhibitors for erectile dysfunction (e.g., sildenafil, tadalafil, or vardenafil) should be advised that they may be at an increased risk of associated adverse

Information on the Abbott Pharmaceutical Products listed on these pages is from the prescribing information in use as of June 1, 2010. For more information, please visit rxabbott.com or call 1-800-633-9110.

Table 6. Established and Other Potentially Significant Drug Interactions: Alteration in Dose or Regimen Recommended Based on Drug Interaction Studies or Predicted Interaction (see CLINICAL PHARMACOLOGY - Table 2 and Table 3 for Magnitude of Interaction)

Concomitant Drug Class: Drug Name	Effect on Concentration of Ritonavir or Concomitant Drug	Clinical Comment
HIV-Antiviral Agents		
HIV Protease Inhibitor: atazanavir	When co-administered with reduced doses of atazanavir and ritonavir $\uparrow$ atazanavir ($\uparrow$ AUC, $\uparrow$ C_{max}, $\uparrow$ C_{min})	Atazanavir plasma concentrations achieved with atazanavir 300 mg q.d and ritonavir 100 mg q.d. are higher than those achieved with atazanavir 400 mg q.d. See the complete prescribing information for Reyataz® (atazanavir) for details on co-administration of atazanavir 300 mg q.d, with ritonavir 100 mg q.d.
HIV Protease Inhibitor: darunavir	When co-administered with reduced doses of ritonavir $\uparrow$ darunavir ($\uparrow$ AUC, $\uparrow$ C_{max}, $\uparrow$ C_{min})	See the complete prescribing information for Prezista® (darunavir) for details on co-administration of darunavir 600 mg b.i.d. with ritonavir 100 mg b.i.d. or darunavir 800 mg q.d. with ritonavir 100 mg q.d.
HIV Protease Inhibitor: fosamprenavir	When co-administered with reduced doses of ritonavir $\uparrow$ amprenavir ($\uparrow$ AUC, $\uparrow$ C_{max}, $\uparrow$ C_{min})	See the complete prescribing information for Lexiva® (fosamprenavir) for details on co-administration of fosamprenavir 700 mg b.i.d. with ritonavir 100 mg b.i.d. fosamprenavir 1400 mg q.d. with ritonavir 200 mg q.d. or fosamprenavir 1400 mg q.d. with ritonavir 100 mg q.d.
HIV Protease Inhibitor: indinavir	When co-administered with reduced doses of indinavir and ritonavir $\uparrow$ indinavir ($\leftrightarrow$ AUC, $\downarrow$ C_{max}, $\uparrow$ C_{min})	Alterations in concentrations are noted when reduced doses of indinavir are co-administered with NORVIR. Appropriate doses for this combination, with respect to efficacy and safety, have not been established.
HIV Protease Inhibitor: saquinavir	When co-administered with reduced doses of ritonavir $\uparrow$ saquinavir ($\uparrow$ AUC, $\uparrow$ C_{max}, $\uparrow$ C_{min})	See the complete prescribing information for Invirase® (saquinavir) for details on co-administration of saquinavir 1000 mg b.i.d. with ritonavir 100 mg b.i.d. Saquinavir/ritonavir should not be given together with rifampin, due to the risk of severe hepatotoxicity (presenting as increased hepatic transaminases) if the three drugs are given together.
HIV Protease Inhibitor: tipranavir	When co-administered with reduced doses of ritonavir $\uparrow$ tipranavir ($\uparrow$ AUC, $\uparrow$ C_{max}, $\uparrow$ C_{min})	See the complete prescribing information for Aptivus® (tipranavir) for details on co-administration of tipranavir 500 mg b.i.d. with ritonavir 200 mg b.i.d. There have been reports of clinical hepatitis and hepatic decompensation including some fatalities. All patients should be followed closely with clinical and laboratory monitoring, especially those with chronic hepatitis B or C co-infection, as these patients have an increased risk of hepatotoxicity. Liver function tests should be performed prior to initiating therapy with tipranavir/ritonavir, and frequently throughout the duration of treatment.
Non-Nucleoside Reverse Transcriptase Inhibitor: delavirdine	$\uparrow$ ritonavir ($\uparrow$ AUC, $\uparrow$ C_{max}, $\uparrow$ C_{min})	Appropriate doses of this combination with respect to safety and efficacy have not been established.
HIV CCR5 – antagonist: maraviroc	$\uparrow$ maraviroc	Concurrent administration of maraviroc with ritonavir will increase plasma levels of maraviroc. For specific dosage adjustment recommendations, please refer to the complete prescribing information for Selzentry® (maraviroc).
Other Agents		
Analgesics, Narcotic: tramadol, propoxyphene		A dose decrease may be needed for these drugs when co-administered with ritonavir.
Anesthetic: meperidine	$\downarrow$ meperidine/ $\uparrow$ normeperidine (metabolite)	Dosage increase and long-term use of meperidine with ritonavir are not recommended due to the increased concentrations of the metabolite normeperidine which has both analgesic activity and CNS stimulant activity (e.g., seizures).
Antialcoholics: disulfiram/ metronidazole		Ritonavir formulations contain alcohol, which can produce disulfiram-like reactions when co-administered with disulfiram or other drugs that produce this reaction (e.g., metronidazole).

(Table continued on next page)

events including hypotension, visual changes, and sustained erection, and should promptly report any symptoms to their doctor. Concomitant use of sildenafil with NORVIR is contraindicated in patients with pulmonary arterial hypertension (PAH).

Patients receiving estrogen-based hormonal contraceptives should be instructed that additional or alternate contraceptive measures should be used during therapy with NORVIR.

Patients should be informed that NORVIR may produce changes in the electrocardiogram (e.g., PR prolongation). Patients should consult their physician if they experience symptoms such as dizziness, lightheadedness, abnormal heart rhythm, or loss of consciousness.

Laboratory Tests

Ritonavir has been shown to increase triglycerides, cholesterol, SGOT (AST), SGPT (ALT), GGT, CPK, and uric acid.

Appropriate laboratory testing should be performed prior to initiating NORVIR therapy and at periodic intervals or if any clinical signs or symptoms occur during therapy. For comprehensive information concerning laboratory test alterations associated with reverse transcriptase inhibitors, physicians should refer to the complete product information for each of these drugs.

Drug Interactions

Ritonavir has been found to be an inhibitor of cytochrome P450 3A (CYP3A) both *in vitro* and *in vivo* (Table 3). Agents that are extensively metabolized by CYP3A and have high first pass metabolism appear to be the most susceptible to large increases in AUC (> 3-fold) when co-administered with ritonavir. Ritonavir also inhibits CYP2D6 to a lesser extent. Co-administration of substrates of CYP2D6 with ritonavir could result in increases (up to 2-fold) in the AUC of the other agent, possibly requiring a proportional dosage reduction. Ritonavir also appears to induce CYP3A as well as other enzymes, including glucuronosyl transferase, CYP1A2, and possibly CYP2C9.

Drugs that are contraindicated specifically due to the expected magnitude of interaction and potential for serious adverse events are listed both in CONTRAINDICATIONS - Table 4 and under Drugs That Should Not Be Co-administered with NORVIR in Table 5.

Those drug interactions that have been established based on drug interaction studies are listed with the pharmacokinetic results in CLINICAL PHARMACOLOGY - Table 2 and Table 3. The clinical recommendations based on the results of these studies are listed in Table 6. Established and Other Potentially Significant Drug Interactions. A systematic review of over 200 medications prescribed to HIV-infected patients was performed to identify potential drug interactions with ritonavir.[2] There are a number of agents in which CYP3A or CYP2D6 partially contribute to the metabolism of the agent. In these cases, the magnitude of the interaction and therapeutic consequences cannot be predicted with any certainty.

When co-administering ritonavir with calcium channel blockers, immunosuppressants, some HMG-CoA reductase inhibitors, some steroids, or other substrates of CYP3A; or most antidepressants, certain antiarrhythmics, and some narcotic analgesics which are partially mediated by CYP2D6 metabolism, it is possible that substantial increases in concentrations of these other agents may occur, possibly requiring a dosage reduction (> 50%); examples are listed in Table 6. Established and Other Potentially Significant Drug Interactions.

When co-administering ritonavir with any agent having a narrow therapeutic margin, such as anticoagulants, anticonvulsants, and antiarrhythmics, special attention is warranted. With some agents, the metabolism may be induced, resulting in decreased concentrations (see Table 6. Established and Other Potentially Significant Drug Interactions).

Table 5. Drugs that Should Not be Co-administered with NORVIR

Drug Class: Drug Name	Clinical Comment
Alpha Adrenergic Antagonist: alfuzosin	CONTRAINDICATED due to potential for serious reactions such as hypotension.
Antiarrhythmics: amiodarone, bepridil, flecainide, propafenone, quinidine	CONTRAINDICATED due to potential for serious and/or life-threatening reactions such as cardiac arrhythmias.
Antifungal: voriconazole	CONTRAINDICATED due to significant decreases in voriconazole plasma concentrations and may lead to loss of antifungal response.
Ergot Derivatives: dihydroergotamine, ergonovine, ergotamine, methylergonovine	CONTRAINDICATED due to potential for serious and/or life-threatening reactions such as acute ergot toxicity characterized by vasospasm and ischemia of the extremities and other tissues including the central nervous system.
GI Motility Agent: cisapride	CONTRAINDICATED due to potential for serious and/or life-threatening reactions such as cardiac arrhythmias.
Herbal Products: St. John's wort (hypericum	CONTRAINDICATED as the combination may lead to loss of virologic response and possible

perforatum)	resistance to NORVIR or to the class of protease inhibitors.
HMG-CoA Reductase Inhibitors: lovastatin, simvastatin	CONTRAINDICATED due to potential for serious reactions such as risk of myopathy including rhabdomyolysis.
Neuroleptic: pimozide	CONTRAINDICATED due to the potential for serious and/or life-threatening reactions such as cardiac arrhythmias.
PDE5 enzyme inhibitor: Sildenafil* (Revatio®)	CONTRAINDICATED in the treatment of pulmonary arterial hypertension (PAH). A safe and effective dose has not been established when used with ritonavir. There is an increased potential for sildenafil-associated adverse events, including visual abnormalities, hypotension, prolonged erection, and syncope.
Sedative/hypnotics: oral midazolam, triazolam	CONTRAINDICATED due to potential for serious and/or life-threatening reactions such as prolonged or increased sedation or respiratory depression.

*see **WARNINGS - Drug Interactions** and **PRECAUTIONS - Table 6. Established and Other Potentially Significant Drug Interactions** for coadministration of sildenafil in patients with erectile dysfunction.

[See table 6 on pages 514 through 518]

Carcinogenesis and Mutagenesis

Carcinogenicity studies in mice and rats have been carried out on ritonavir. In male mice, at levels of 50, 100 or 200 mg/kg/day, there was a dose dependent increase in the incidence of both adenomas and combined adenomas and carcinomas in the liver. Based on AUC measurements, the exposure at the high dose was approximately 0.3-fold for males that of the exposure in humans with the recommended therapeutic dose (600 mg twice-daily). There were no carcinogenic effects seen in females at the dosages tested. The exposure at the high dose was approximately 0.6-fold for the females that of the exposure in humans. In rats dosed at levels of 7, 15 or 30 mg/kg/day there were no carcinogenic effects. In this study, the exposure at the high dose was approximately 6% that of the exposure in humans with the recommended therapeutic dose. Based on the exposures achieved in the animal studies, the significance of the observed effects is not known. However, ritonavir was found to be negative for mutagenic or clastogenic activity in a battery of in vitro and in vivo assays including the Ames bacterial reverse mutation assay using S. typhimurium and E. coli, the mouse lymphoma assay, the mouse micronucleus test and chromosomal aberration assays in human lymphocytes.

Pregnancy, Fertility, and Reproduction

Pregnancy Category B

There are no adequate and well-controlled studies in pregnant women. Because animal reproduction studies are not always predictive of human response, this drug should be used during pregnancy only if clearly needed.

Ritonavir produced no effects on fertility in rats at drug exposures approximately 40% (male) and 60% (female) of that achieved with the proposed therapeutic dose. Higher dosages were not feasible due to hepatic toxicity.

No treatment related malformations were observed when ritonavir was administered to pregnant rats or rabbits. Developmental toxicity observed in rats (early resorptions, decreased fetal body weight and ossification delays and developmental variations) occurred at a maternally toxic dosage at an exposure equivalent to approximately 30% of that achieved with the proposed therapeutic dose. A slight increase in the incidence of cryptorchidism was also noted in rats at an exposure approximately 22% of that achieved with the proposed therapeutic dose.

Developmental toxicity observed in rabbits (resorptions, decreased litter size and decreased fetal weights) also occurred at a maternally toxic dosage equivalent to 1.8 times the proposed therapeutic dose based on a body surface area conversion factor.

Antiretroviral Pregnancy Registry

To monitor maternal-fetal outcomes of pregnant women exposed to NORVIR, an Antiretroviral Pregnancy Registry has been established. Physicians are encouraged to register patients by calling 1-800-258-4263.

Nursing Mothers

The Centers for Disease Control and Prevention recommend that HIV-infected mothers not breast-feed their infants to avoid risking postnatal transmission of HIV. It is not known whether ritonavir is secreted in human milk. Because of both the potential for HIV transmission and the potential for serious adverse reactions in nursing infants, mothers should be instructed **not to breast-feed if they are receiving NORVIR.**

Pediatric Use

In HIV-infected patients age > 1 month to 21 years, the antiviral activity and adverse event profile seen during clinical trials and through postmarketing experience were similar to that for adult patients.

Geriatric Use

Clinical studies of NORVIR did not include sufficient numbers of subjects aged 65 and over to determine whether they respond differently from younger subjects. In general, dose selection for an elderly patient should be cautious, usually starting at the low end of the dosing range, reflecting the greater frequency of decreased hepatic, renal or cardiac function, and of concomitant disease or other drug therapy.

ADVERSE REACTIONS

When co-administering NORVIR with other protease inhibitors, see the full prescribing information for that protease inhibitor including **ADVERSE REACTIONS.**

Information on the Abbott Pharmaceutical Products listed on these pages is from the prescribing information in use as of June 1, 2010. For more information, please visit rxabbott.com or call 1-800-633-9110.

Table 6 (cont.). Established and Other Potentially Significant Drug Interactions: Alteration in Dose or Regimen Recommended Based on Drug Interaction Studies or Predicted Interaction (see CLINICAL PHARMACOLOGY - Table 2 and Table 3 for Magnitude of Interaction)

Concomitant Drug Class: Drug Name	Effect on Concentration of Ritonavir or Concomitant Drug	Clinical Comment
Other Agents (continued)		
Antiarrhythmics: disopyramide, lidocaine, mexilltine	↑ antiarrhythmics	Caution is warranted and therapeutic concentration monitoring is recommended for antiarrhythmics when co-administered with ritonavir, if available.
Anticancer Agents: vincristine, vinblastine	↑ anticancer agents	Concentrations of vincristine or vinblastine may be increased when co-administered with ritonavir resulting in the potential for increased adverse events usually associated with these anticancer agents. Consideration should be given to temporarily withholding the ritonavir containing antiretroviral regimen in patients who develop significant hematologic or gastrointestinal side effects when ritonavir is administered concurrently with vincristine or vinblastine. Clinicians should be aware that if the ritonavir containing regimen is withheld for a prolonged period, consideration should be given to altering the regimen to not include a CYP3A or P-gp inhibitor in order to control HIV-1 viral load.
Anticoagulant: warfarin	↓ R-warfarin ↓↑ S-warfarin	Initial frequent monitoring of the INR during ritonavir and warfarin co-administration is indicated.
Anticonvulsants: carbamazepine, clonazepam, ethosuximide	↑ anticonvulsants	Use with caution. A dose increase may be needed for these drugs when co-administered with ritonavir and therapeutic concentration monitoring is recommended for these anticonvulsants, if available.
Anticonvulsants: divalproex, lamotrigine, phenytoin	↓ anticonvulsants	Use with caution. A dose increase may be needed for these drugs when co-administered with ritonavir and therapeutic concentration monitoring is recommended for these anticonvulsants, if available.
Antidepressants: nefazodone, selective serotonin reuptake inhibitors (SSRIs), tricyclics	↑ antidepressants	A dose decrease may be needed for these drugs when co-administered with ritonavir.
Antidepressant: bupropion	↓ bupropion ↓ active metabolite, hydroxybupropion	Concurrent administration of bupropion with ritonavir may decrease plasma levels of both bupropion and its active metabolite (hydroxybupropion). Patients receiving ritonavir and bupropion concurrently should be monitored for an adequate clinical response to bupropion.
Antidepressant: desipramine	↑ desipramine	Dosage reduction and concentration monitoring of desipramine is recommended.
Antidepressant: trazodone	↑ trazodone	Concomitant use of trazodone and NORVIR increases plasma concentrations of trazodone. Adverse events of nausea, dizziness, hypotension and syncope have been observed following co-administration of trazodone and NORVIR. If trazodone is used with a CYP3A4 inhibitor such as ritonavir, the combination should be used with caution and a lower dose of trazodone should be considered.
Antiemetic: dronabinol	↑ dronabinol	A dose decrease of dronabinol may be needed when co-administered with ritonavir.
Antifungal: ketoconazole itraconazole voriconazole	↑ ketoconazole ↑ itraconazole ↓ voriconazole	High doses of ketoconazole or itraconazole (> 200 mg/day) are not recommended. Coadministration of voriconazole and ritonavir doses of 400 mg every 12 hours or greater is contraindicated. Coadministration of voriconazole and ritonavir 100 mg should be avoided, unless an assessment of the benefit/risk to the patient justifies the use of voriconazole.

(Table continued on next page)

Table 6 (cont.). Established and Other Potentially Significant Drug Interactions: Alteration in Dose or Regimen Recommended Based on Drug Interaction Studies or Predicted Interaction (see CLINICAL PHARMACOLOGY - Table 2 and Table 3 for Magnitude of Interaction)

Concomitant Drug Class: Drug Name	Effect on Concentration of Ritonavir or Concomitant Drug	Clinical Comment
	Other Agents (continued)	
Anti-gout: colchicine	↑ colchicine	Patients with renal or hepatic impairment should not be given colchicine with ritonavir. Treatment of gout flares co-administration of colchicine in patients on ritonavir: 0.6 mg (1 tablet) × 1 dose, followed by 0.3 mg (half tablet) 1 hour later. Dose to be repeated no earlier than 3 days. Prophylaxis of gout flares-co-administration of colchicine in patients on ritonavir: If the original colchicine regimen was 0.6 mg twice a day, the regimen should be adjusted to 0.3 mg once a day. If the original colchicine regimen was 0.6 mg once a day, the regimen should be adjusted to 0.3 mg once every other day. Treatment of familial Mediterranean fever (FMF)-co-administration of colchicine in patients on ritonavir: Maximum daily dose of 0.6 mg (may be given as 0.3 mg twice a day).
Anti-infective: clarithromycin	↑ clarithromycin	For patients with renal impairment the following dosage adjustments should be considered: • For patients with CL_{CR} 30 to 60 mL/min the dose of clarithromycin should be reduced by 50%. • For patients with CL_{CR} < 30 mL/min the dose of clarithromycin should be decreased by 75%. No dose adjustment for patients with normal renal function is necessary.
Antimycobacterial: rifabutin	↑ rifabutin and rifabutin metabolite	Dosage reduction of rifabutin by at least three-quarters of the usual dose of 300 mg/day is recommended (e.g., 150 mg every other day or three times a week). Further dosage reduction may be necessary.
Antimycobacterial: rifampin	↓ ritonavir	May lead to loss of virologic response. Alternate antimycobacterial agents such as rifabutin should be considered (see Antimycobacterial: rifabutin, for dose reduction recommendations).
Antiparasitic: atovaquone	↓ atovaquone	Clinical significance is unknown; however, increase in atovaquone dose may be needed.
Antiparasitic: quinine	↑ quinine	A dose decrease of quinine may be needed when co-administered with ritonavir.
β-Blockers: metoprolol, timolol	↑ Beta-Blockers	Caution is warranted and clinical monitoring of patients is recommended. A dose decrease may be needed for these drugs when co-administered with ritonavir.
Bronchodilator: theophylline	↓ theophylline	Increased dosage of theophylline may be required; therapeutic monitoring should be considered.
Calcium channel blockers: diltiazem, nifedipine, verapamil	↑ calcium channel blockers	Caution is warranted and clinical monitoring of patients is recommended. A dose decrease may be needed for these drugs when co-administered with ritonavir.
Digoxin	↑ digoxin	Concomitant administration of ritonavir with digoxin may increase digoxin levels. Caution should be exercised when coadministering ritonavir with digoxin, with appropriate monitoring of serum digoxin levels.
Endothelin receptor antagonists: bosentan	↑ bosentan	Co-administration of bosentan in patients on ritonavir: In patients who have been receiving ritonavir for at least 10 days, start bosentan at 62.5 mg once daily or every other day based upon individual tolerability. Co-administration of ritonavir in patients on bosentan: Discontinue use of bosentan at least 36 hours prior to initiation of ritonavir. After at least 10 days following the initiation of ritonavir, resume bosentan at 62.5 mg once daily or every other day based upon individual tolerability.
HMG-CoA Reductase Inhibitor: atorvastatin rosuvastatin	↑ atorvastatin ↑ rosuvastatin	Use the lowest possible dose of atorvastatin or rosuvastatin with careful monitoring or consider other HMG-CoA reductase inhibitors such as pravastatin or fluvastatin in combination with NORVIR.

(Table continued on next page)

Adults

The safety of NORVIR alone and in combination with nucleoside reverse transcriptase inhibitors was studied in 1270 adult patients. Table 7 lists treatment-emergent adverse events (at least possibly related and of at least moderate intensity) that occurred in 2% or greater of adult patients receiving NORVIR alone or in combination with nucleoside reverse transcriptase inhibitors in Study 245 or Study 247 and in combination with saquinavir in study 462. In that study, 141 protease inhibitor-naive, HIV-infected patients with mean baseline CD_4 of 300 cells/µL were randomized to one of four regimens of NORVIR + saquinavir, including NORVIR 400 mg twice-daily + saquinavir 400 mg twice-daily. Overall the most frequently reported clinical ad-

verse events, other than asthenia, among adult patients receiving NORVIR were gastrointestinal and neurological disturbances including nausea, diarrhea, vomiting, anorexia, abdominal pain, taste perversion, and circumoral and peripheral paresthesias. Similar adverse event profiles were reported in adult patients receiving ritonavir in other trials. [See table 7 on pages 518 and 519]

Adverse events occurring in less than 2% of adult patients receiving NORVIR in all phase II/phase III studies and considered at least possibly related or of unknown relationship to treatment and of at least moderate intensity are listed below by body system.

Body as a Whole
Abdomen enlarged, accidental injury, allergic reaction, back pain, cachexia, chest pain, chills, facial edema, facial pain, flu syndrome, hormone level altered, hypothermia, kidney pain, neck pain, neck rigidity, pelvic pain, photosensitivity reaction, and substernal chest pain.

Cardiovascular System
Cardiovascular disorder, cerebral ischemia, cerebral venous thrombosis, hypertension, hypotension, migraine, myocardial infarct, palpitation, peripheral vascular disorder, phlebitis, postural hypotension, tachycardia and vasospasm.

Digestive System
Abnormal stools, bloody diarrhea, cheilitis, cholestatic jaundice, colitis, dry mouth, dysphagia, eructation, esophageal ulcer, esophagitis, gastritis, gastroenteritis, gastrointestinal disorder, gastrointestinal hemorrhage, gingivitis, hepatic coma, hepatitis, hepatomegaly, hepatosplenomegaly, ileus, liver damage, melena, mouth ulcer, pancreatitis, pseudomembranous colitis, rectal disorder, rectal hemorrhage, sialadenitis, stomatitis, tenesmus, thirst, tongue edema, and ulcerative colitis.

Endocrine System
Adrenal cortex insufficiency and diabetes mellitus.

Hemic and Lymphatic System
Acute myeloblastic leukemia, anemia, ecchymosis, leukopenia, lymphadenopathy, lymphocytosis, myeloproliferative disorder, and thrombocytopenia.

Metabolic and Nutritional Disorders
Albuminuria, alcohol intolerance, avitaminosis, BUN increased, dehydration, edema, enzymatic abnormality, glycosuria, gout, hypercholesteremia, peripheral edema, and xanthomatosis.

Musculoskeletal System
Arthritis, arthrosis, bone disorder, bone pain, extraocular palsy, joint disorder, leg cramps, muscle cramps, muscle weakness, myositis, and twitching.

Nervous System
Abnormal dreams, abnormal gait, agitation, amnesia, aphasia, ataxia, coma, convulsion, dementia, depersonalization, diplopia, emotional lability, euphoria, grand mal convulsion, hallucinations, hyperesthesia, hyperkinesia, hypesthesia, incoordination, libido decreased, manic reaction, nervousness, neuralgia, neuropathy, paralysis, peripheral neuropathic pain, peripheral neuropathy, peripheral sensory neuropathy, personality disorder, sleep disorder, speech disorder, stupor, subdural hematoma, tremor, urinary retention, vertigo, and vestibular disorder.

Respiratory System
Asthma, bronchitis, dyspnea, epistaxis, hiccup, hypoventilation, increased cough, interstitial pneumonia, larynx edema, lung disorder, rhinitis, and sinusitis.

Skin and Appendages
Acne, contact dermatitis, dry skin, eczema, erythema multiforme, exfoliative dermatitis, folliculitis, fungal dermatitis, furunculosis, maculopapular rash, molluscum contagiosum, onychomycosis, pruritus, psoriasis, pustular rash, seborrhea, skin discoloration, skin disorder, skin hypertrophy, skin melanoma, urticaria, and vesiculobullous rash.

Special Senses
Abnormal electro-oculogram, abnormal electroretinogram, abnormal vision, amblyopia/blurred vision, blepharitis, conjunctivitis, ear pain, eye disorder, eye pain, hearing impairment, increased cerumen, iritis, parosmia, photophobia, taste loss, tinnitus, uveitis, visual field defect, and vitreous disorder.

Urogenital System
Acute kidney failure, breast pain, cystitis, dysuria, hematuria, impotence, kidney calculus, kidney failure, kidney function abnormal, kidney pain, menorrhagia, penis disorder, polyuria, urethritis, urinary frequency, urinary tract infection, and vaginitis.

Post-Marketing Experience
The following adverse events have been reported during post-marketing use of NORVIR. Because these reactions are reported voluntarily from a population of unknown size, it is not possible to reliably estimate their frequency or establish a causal relationship to NORVIR exposure.

Table 6 (cont.). Established and Other Potentially Significant Drug Interactions: Alteration in Dose or Regimen Recommended Based on Drug Interaction Studies or Predicted Interaction (see CLINICAL PHARMACOLOGY - Table 2 and Table 3 for Magnitude of Interaction)

Concomitant Drug Class: Drug Name	Effect on Concentration of Ritonavir or Concomitant Drug	Clinical Comment
Other Agents (continued)		
Immunosuppressants: cyclosporine, tacrolimus, sirolimus (rapamycin)	↑ immunosuppressants	Therapeutic concentration monitoring is recommended for immunosuppressant agents when co-administered with ritonavir.
Inhaled Steroid: Fluticasone	↑ fluticasone	Concomitant use of fluticasone propionate and NORVIR increases plasma concentrations of fluticasone propionate, resulting in significantly reduced serum cortisol concentrations. Co-administration of fluticasone propionate and NORVIR is not recommended unless the potential benefit to the patient outweighs the risk of systemic corticosteroid side effects.
Long-acting beta-adrenoceptor agonist: salmeterol	↑ salmeterol	Concurrent administration of salmeterol and ritonavir is not recommended. The combination may result in increased risk of cardiovascular adverse events associated with salmeterol, including QT prolongation, palpitations and sinus tachycardia.
Narcotic Analgesic: methadone	↓ methadone	Dosage increase of methadone may be considered.
Neuroleptics: perphenazine, risperidone, thioridazine	↑ neuroleptics	A dose decrease may be needed for these drugs when co-administered with ritonavir.
Oral Contraceptives or Patch Contraceptives: ethinyl estradiol	↓ ethinyl estradiol	A pharmacokinetic study demonstrated that the concomitant administration of ritonavir 500 mg q. 12h. and a fixed-combination oral contraceptive resulted in reductions of the ethinyl estradiol mean C_{max} and mean AUC by 32% and 40%, respectively. Alternate methods of contraception should be considered.
PDE5 Inhibitors: sildenafil, tadalafil, vardenafil	↑ sildenafil ↑ tadalafil ↑ vardenafil	Particular caution should be used when prescribing sildenafil, tadalafil or vardenafil in patients receiving ritonavir. Co-administration of ritonavir with these drugs is expected to substantially increase their concentrations and may result in an increase in PDE5 inhibitor associated adverse events, including hypotension, syncope, visual changes, and prolonged erection. Use of PDE5 inhibitors for pulmonary arterial hypertension (PAH): Sildenafil (Revatio®) is contraindicated when used for the treatment of pulmonary arterial hypertension (PAH) because a safe and effective dose has not been established when used with ritonavir (see CONTRAINDICATIONS and PRECAUTIONS - Drug Interactions, Table 5). The following dose adjustments are recommended for use of tadalafil (Adcirca™) with ritonavir: Co-administration of ADCIRCA in patients on ritonavir: In patients receiving ritonavir for at least one week, start ADCIRCA at 20 mg once daily. Increase to 40 mg once daily based upon individual tolerability. Co-administration of ritonavir in patients on ADCIRCA: Avoid use of ADCIRCA during in initiation of ritonavir. Stop ADCIRCA at least 24 hours prior to starting ritonavir. After at least one week following the initiation of ritonavir, resume ADCIRCA at 20 mg once daily. Increase to 40 mg once daily based upon individual tolerability. Use of PDE5 inhibitors for the treatment of erectile dysfunction: It is recommended not to exceed the following doses: • Sildenafil: 25 mg every 48 hours • Tadalafil: 10 mg every 72 hours • Vardenafil: 2.5 mg every 72 hours Use with increased monitoring for adverse events.

(Table continued on next page)

Body as a Whole
Dehydration, usually associated with gastrointestinal symptoms, and sometimes resulting in hypotension, syncope, or renal insufficiency has been reported. Syncope, orthostatic hypotension, and renal insufficiency have also been reported without known dehydration.

Co-administration of ritonavir with ergotamine or dihydroergotamine has been associated with acute ergot toxicity characterized by vasospasm and ischemia of the extremities and other tissues including the central nervous system.

Redistribution/accumulation of body fat has been reported (see PRECAUTIONS - Fat Redistribution).
Cardiovascular System
First-degree AV block, second-degree AV block, third-degree AV block, right bundle branch block have been reported (see PRECAUTIONS - PR Interval Prolongation).
Cardiac and neurologic events have been reported when ritonavir has been co-administered with disopyramide, mexiletine, nefazodone, fluoxetine, and beta blockers. The possibility of drug interaction cannot be excluded.

Endocrine System
Cushing's syndrome and adrenal suppression have been reported when ritonavir has been co-administered with fluticasone propionate.
Hemic and Lymphatic System
There have been reports of increased bleeding in patients with hemophilia A or B (see PRECAUTIONS - Hemophilia).
Nervous System
There have been postmarketing reports of seizure. Also, see *Cardiovascular System*.
Laboratory Abnormalities
Table 8 shows the percentage of adult patients who developed marked laboratory abnormalities.
[See table 8 at top of page 520]
Pediatrics
Treatment-Emergent Adverse Events
NORVIR has been studied in 265 pediatric patients > 1 month to 21 years of age. The adverse event profile observed during pediatric clinical trials was similar to that for adult patients.
Vomiting, diarrhea, and skin rash/allergy were the only drug-related clinical adverse events of moderate to severe intensity observed in ≥ 2% of pediatric patients enrolled in NORVIR clinical trials.
Laboratory Abnormalities
The following Grade 3-4 laboratory abnormalities occurred in > 3% of pediatric patients who received treatment with NORVIR either alone or in combination with reverse transcriptase inhibitors: neutropenia (9%), hyperamylasemia (7%), thrombocytopenia (5%), anemia (4%), and elevated AST (3%).

OVERDOSAGE
Acute Overdosage
Human Overdose Experience
Human experience of acute overdose with NORVIR is limited. One patient in clinical trials took NORVIR 1500 mg/day for two days. The patient reported paresthesias which resolved after the dose was decreased. A post-marketing case of renal failure with eosinophilia has been reported with ritonavir overdose.
The approximate lethal dose was found to be greater than 20 times the related human dose in rats and 10 times the related human dose in mice.
Management of Overdosage
NORVIR oral solution contains 43% alcohol by volume. Accidental ingestion of the product by a young child could result in significant alcohol-related toxicity and could approach the potential lethal dose of alcohol.
Treatment of overdose with NORVIR consists of general supportive measures including monitoring of vital signs and observation of the clinical status of the patient. There is no specific antidote for overdose with NORVIR. If indicated, elimination of unabsorbed drug should be achieved by emesis or gastric lavage; usual precautions should be observed to maintain the airway. Administration of activated charcoal may also be used to aid in removal of unabsorbed drug. Since ritonavir is extensively metabolized by the liver and is highly protein bound, dialysis is unlikely to be beneficial in significant removal of the drug. A Certified Poison Control Center should be consulted for up-to-date information on the management of overdose with NORVIR.

DOSAGE AND ADMINISTRATION
NORVIR is administered orally. It is recommended that NORVIR be taken with meals if possible. Patients may improve the taste of NORVIR oral solution by mixing with chocolate milk, Ensure®, or Advera® within one hour of dosing. The effects of antacids on the absorption of ritonavir have not been studied.
Adults
Recommended Dosage
The recommended dosage of ritonavir is 600 mg twice daily by mouth. Use of a dose titration schedule may help to reduce treatment-emergent adverse events while maintaining appropriate ritonavir plasma levels. Ritonavir should be started at no less than 300 mg twice daily and increased at 2 to 3 day intervals by 100 mg twice daily.
Dose modification for NORVIR
Dose reduction of NORVIR is necessary when used with other protease inhibitors: amprenavir, atazanavir, darunavir, fosamprenavir, saquinavir, and tipranavir. Prescribers should consult the full prescribing information and clinical study information of these protease inhibitors if they are co-administered with a reduced dose of ritonavir

Information on the Abbott Pharmaceutical Products listed on these pages is from the prescribing information in use as of June 1, 2010. For more information, please visit rxabbott.com or call 1-800-633-9110.

(See also, WARNINGS-Drug Interactions and Table 6, Established and Other Potentially Significant Drug Interactions.)

Pediatric Patients
Ritonavir should be used in combination with other antiretroviral agents (see **General Dosing Guidelines**). The recommended dosage of ritonavir in children > 1 month is 350 to 400 mg/m^2 twice daily by mouth and should not exceed 600 mg twice daily. Ritonavir should be started at 250 mg/m^2 and increased at 2 to 3 day intervals by 50 mg/m^2 twice daily. If patients do not tolerate 400 mg/m^2 twice daily due to adverse events, the highest tolerated dose may be used for maintenance therapy in combination with other antiretroviral agents, however, alternative therapy should be considered. When possible, dose should be administered using a calibrated dosing syringe.
[See second table at top of page 520]
Body surface area (BSA) can be calculated as follows:

$$BSA \ (m^2) = \sqrt{\frac{Ht \ (Cm) \ x \ Wt \ (kg)}{3600}}$$

General Dosing Guidelines
Patients should be aware that frequently observed adverse events, such as mild to moderate gastrointestinal disturbances and paraesthesias, may diminish as therapy is continued. In addition, patients initiating combination regimens with NORVIR and reverse transcriptase inhibitors may improve gastrointestinal tolerance by initiating NORVIR alone and subsequently adding reverse transcriptase inhibitors before completing two weeks of NORVIR monotherapy.

HOW SUPPLIED
NORVIR (ritonavir capsules) soft gelatin are white capsules imprinted with the corporate logo ⊐, 100 and the Abbo-Code DS, available in the following package size:
Bottles of 120 capsules each (**NDC** 0074-6633-22).
Bottles of 30 capsules each (**NDC** 0074-6633-30).
Recommended Storage
Store soft gelatin capsules in the refrigerator between 2°-8°C (36°-46°F) until dispensed. Refrigeration of NORVIR soft gelatin capsules by the patient is recommended, but not required if used within 30 days and stored below 25°C (77°F). Protect from light. Avoid exposure to excessive heat.
NORVIR (ritonavir oral solution) is an orange-colored liquid, supplied in amber-colored, multi-dose bottles containing 600 mg ritonavir per 7.5 mL marked dosage cup (80 mg/mL) in the following size:
240 mL bottles (**NDC** 0074-1940-63).
Recommended Storage
Store NORVIR oral solution at room temperature 20°-25°C (68°-77°F). Do not refrigerate. Shake well before each use. Use by product expiration date.
Product should be stored and dispensed in the original container.
Avoid exposure to excessive heat. Keep cap tightly closed.

REFERENCES
1. Sewester CS. Calculations. In: Drug Facts and Comparisons. St. Louis, MO: J.B. Lippincott Co; January, 1997: xix.
2. Bertz RJ and Granneman GR. Use of *in vitro* and *in vivo* data to estimate the likelihood of metabolic pharmacokinetic interactions. *Clin Pharmacokinet* 1997; 32(3): 210-258.
(Nos. 1940 and 6633)
Abbott Laboratories
North Chicago, IL 60064, U.S.A.
03-A358-R28-Rev. April, 2010

NORVIR®
(ritonavir capsules) Soft Gelatin
(ritonavir oral solution)
ALERT: Find out about medicines that should **NOT be taken with NORVIR.** Please also read the section "MEDICINES YOU SHOULD NOT TAKE WITH NORVIR."
Patient Information
NORVIR® (NOR - VEER)
Generic name: ritonavir (rit-ON-uh-veer)
Please read this leaflet carefully before you start taking NORVIR. Also, read it each time you get your NORVIR prescription refilled, just in case something has changed. Remember that this information does not take the place of careful discussions with your doctor when you start this medication and at check ups.
You should remain under a doctor's care when taking NORVIR and you should not change or stop treatment without first talking with your doctor.
You should tell your doctor about any medicine you are taking or planning to take because taking NORVIR with some medications can result in serious or life-threatening problems.
Talk to your doctor if you have any questions about NORVIR. Your doctor or pharmacist can also give you more information about NORVIR.

Table 6 (cont.). Established and Other Potentially Significant Drug Interactions: Alteration in Dose or Regimen Recommended Based on Drug Interaction Studies or Predicted Interaction (see CLINICAL PHARMACOLOGY - Table 2 and Table 3 for Magnitude of Interaction)

Concomitant Drug Class: Drug Name	Effect on Concentration of Ritonavir or Concomitant Drug	Clinical Comment
Other Agents (continued)		
Sedative/hypnotics: buspirone, clorazepate, diazepam, estazolam, flurazepam, zolpidem	↑ sedative/hypnotics	A dose decrease may be needed for these drugs when co-administered with ritonavir.
Sedative/hypnotics: Parenteral midazolam	↑ midazolam	Co-administration of oral midazolam with NORVIR is CONTRAINDICATED. Concomitant use of parenteral midazolam with NORVIR may increase plasma concentrations of midazolam. Co-administration should be done in a setting which ensures close clinical monitoring and appropriate medical management in case of respiratory depression and/or prolonged sedation. Dosage reduction for midazolam should be considered, especially if more than a single dose of midazolam is administered.
Steroids: dexamethasone, fluticasone, prednisone		A dose decrease may be needed for these drugs when co-administered with ritonavir.
Stimulant: methamphetamine	↑ methamphetamine	Use with caution. A dose decrease of methamphetamine may be needed when co-administered with ritonavir.

Table 7. Percentage of Patients with Treatment-emergent Adverse Events[1] of Moderate or Severe Intensity Occurring in ≥ 2% of Adult Patients Receiving NORVIR

Adverse Events	Study 245 Naive Patients[2]			Study 247 Advanced Patients[3]		Study 462 PI-Naive Patients[4]
	NORVIR +ZDV n = 116	NORVIR n = 117	ZDV n = 119	NORVIR n = 541	Placebo n = 545	NORVIR + Saquinavir n = 141
Body as a Whole						
Abdominal Pain	5.2	6.0	5.9	8.3	5.1	2.1
Asthenia	28.4	10.3	11.8	15.3	6.4	16.3
Fever	1.7	0.9	1.7	5.0	2.4	0.7
Headache	7.8	6.0	6.7	6.5	5.7	4.3
Malaise	5.2	1.7	3.4	0.7	0.2	2.8
Pain (unspecified)	0.9	1.7	0.8	2.2	1.8	4.3
Cardiovascular						
Syncope	0.9	1.7	0.8	0.6	0.0	2.1
Vasodilation	3.4	1.7	0.8	1.7	0.0	3.5
Digestive						
Anorexia	8.6	1.7	4.2	7.8	4.2	4.3
Constipation	3.4	0.0	0.8	0.2	0.4	1.4
Diarrhea	25.0	15.4	2.5	23.3	7.9	22.7
Dyspepsia	2.6	0.0	1.7	5.9	1.5	0.7
Fecal Incontinence	0.0	0.0	0.0	0.0	0.0	2.8
Flatulence	2.6	0.9	1.7	1.7	0.7	3.5
Local Throat Irritation	0.9	1.7	0.8	2.8	0.4	1.4
Nausea	46.6	25.6	26.1	29.8	8.4	18.4
Vomiting	23.3	13.7	12.6	17.4	4.4	7.1

(Table continued on next page)

What is NORVIR and How Does it work?
NORVIR is in a class of medicines called the HIV protease (PRO-tee-ase) inhibitors. NORVIR is used in combination with other anti-HIV medicines to treat people with human immunodeficiency virus (HIV) infection. NORVIR is for adults and for children age > 1 month and older.

HIV infection leads to the destruction of CD$_4$ (T) cells, which are important to the immune system. After a large number of CD$_4$ (T) cells have been destroyed, acquired immune deficiency syndrome (AIDS) develops.
NORVIR blocks HIV protease, a chemical which is needed for HIV to multiply. NORVIR reduces the amount of HIV

and helps to increase the number of CD_4 (T) cells in your blood. Patients who took NORVIR in clinical studies had significant reductions in both death and AIDS defining diseases; however NORVIR may not have these effects in all patients.

Does NORVIR Cure HIV or AIDS?
NORVIR does not cure HIV infection or AIDS. The long-term effects of NORVIR are not known at this time. People taking NORVIR may still get opportunistic infections or other conditions that happen with HIV infection. Some of these conditions are pneumonia, herpes virus infections, and *Mycobacterium avium* complex (MAC) infections.

Does NORVIR Reduce the Risk of Passing HIV to Others?
NORVIR does not reduce the risk of passing HIV to others through sexual contact or blood contamination. Continue to practice safe sex and do not use or share dirty needles.

How Should I Take NORVIR?
• You should stay under a doctor's care when taking NORVIR. Do not change your treatment or stop treatment without first talking with your doctor.
• It is very important that you take NORVIR every day exactly as your doctor prescribed it.
• The usual dose for adults is six 100 mg capsules or 7.5 mL of the oral solution twice a day (morning and night), in combination with other anti-HIV medicines.
• The dosing of NORVIR may be different for you than for other patients. Follow the directions from your doctor, exactly as written on the label.
• Children from > 1 month to 21 years of age can also take NORVIR. The child's doctor will decide the right dose based on the child's height and weight.
• Take NORVIR with food if possible.
• NORVIR Oral Solution is peppermint/caramel flavored. You can take it alone, or may improve the taste by mixing it with 8 ounces of chocolate milk, Ensure®, or Advera®. NORVIR Oral Solution should be taken within 1 hour if mixed with these items. Ask your doctor, nurse or pharmacist about other ways to improve the taste of NORVIR Oral Solution.
• Do not change or stop taking NORVIR without first talking with your health care provider.
• When your NORVIR supply starts to run low, get more from your doctor or pharmacy. This is very important because the amount of virus in your blood may increase if the medicine is stopped for even a short time. The virus may develop resistance to NORVIR and become harder to treat.
• Be sure to set up a schedule and follow it carefully.
• Only take medicine that has been prescribed specifically for you. Do not give NORVIR to others or take medicine prescribed for someone else.

What Should I Do if I Miss a Dose of NORVIR?
It is important that you do not miss any doses. If you miss a dose of NORVIR, take it as soon as possible and then take your next scheduled dose at its regular time. If it is almost time for your next dose, wait and take the next dose at the regular time. Do not double the next dose.

What Happens If I Take Too Much NORVIR?
If you think that you took more than the prescribed dose of this medicine, contact your local poison control center or emergency room immediately.
As with all prescription medicines, NORVIR should be kept out of the reach of young children. NORVIR liquid contains a large amount of alcohol. If a toddler or young child accidentally drinks more than the recommended dose of NORVIR, it could make him/her sick from too much alcohol. Contact your local poison control center or emergency room immediately if this happens.

Who Should Not Take NORVIR?
Together with your doctor, you need to decide whether NORVIR is right for you.
• Do not take NORVIR if you are taking certain medicines. These could cause serious side effects that could cause death. Before you take NORVIR, you must tell your doctor about all the medicines you are taking or are planning to take. These include other prescription and non-prescription medicines and herbal supplements.
For more information about medicines you should not take with NORVIR, please read the section "MEDICINES YOU SHOULD NOT TAKE WITH NORVIR."
• Do not take NORVIR if you have had a serious allergic reaction to NORVIR or any of its ingredients.

Can I Take NORVIR With Other Medications?*
NORVIR may interact with other medicines, including those you take without a prescription. You must tell your doctor about all the medicines you are taking or are planning to take.

MEDICINES YOU SHOULD NOT TAKE WITH NORVIR.
• *Do not take the following medicines with NORVIR because they can cause serious or life-threatening problems such as irregular heartbeat, breathing difficulties, or excessive sleepiness:*
  ◦ Cordarone® (amiodarone)

Table 7 (cont.). Percentage of Patients with Treatment-emergent Adverse Events[1] of Moderate or Severe Intensity Occurring in ≥ 2% of Adult Patients Receiving NORVIR

Adverse Events	Study 245 Naive Patients[2]			Study 247 Advanced Patients[3]		Study 462 PI-Naive Patients[4]
	NORVIR +ZDV n = 116	NORVIR n = 117	ZDV n = 119	NORVIR n = 541	Placebo n = 545	NORVIR + Saquinavir n = 141
Metabolic and Nutritional						
Weight Loss	0.0	0.0	0.0	2.4	1.7	0.0
Musculoskeletal						
Arthralgia	0.0	0.0	0.0	1.7	0.7	2.1
Myalgia	1.7	1.7	0.8	2.4	1.1	2.1
Nervous						
Anxiety	0.9	0.0	0.8	1.7	0.9	2.1
Circumoral Paresthesia	5.2	3.4	0.0	6.7	0.4	6.4
Confusion	0.0	0.9	0.0	0.6	0.6	2.1
Depression	1.7	1.7	2.5	1.7	0.7	7.1
Dizziness	5.2	2.6	3.4	3.9	1.1	8.5
Insomnia	3.4	2.6	0.8	2.0	1.8	2.8
Paresthesia	5.2	2.6	0.0	3.0	0.4	2.1
Peripheral Paresthesia	0.0	6.0	0.8	5.0	1.1	5.7
Somnolence	2.6	2.6	0.0	2.4	0.2	0.0
Thinking Abnormal	2.6	0.0	0.8	0.9	0.4	0.7
Respiratory						
Pharyngitis	0.9	2.6	0.0	0.4	0.4	1.4
Skin and Appendages						
Rash	0.9	0.0	0.8	3.5	1.5	0.7
Sweating	3.4	2.6	1.7	1.7	1.1	2.8
Special Senses						
Taste Perversion	17.2	11.1	8.4	7.0	2.2	5.0
Urogenital						
Nocturia	0.0	0.0	0.0	0.2	0.0	2.8

[1]Includes those adverse events at least possibly related to study drug or of unknown relationship and excludes concurrent HIV conditions.
[2]The median duration of treatment for patients randomized to regimens containing NORVIR in Study 245 was 9.1 months.
[3]The median duration of treatment for patients randomized to regimens containing NORVIR in Study 247 was 9.4 months.
[4]The median duration of treatment for patients in Study 462 was 48 weeks.

◦ Ergotamine, ergonovine, methylergonovine, and dihydroergotamine such as Cafergot®, Migranal®, D.H.E 45®, and others
◦ Halcion® (triazolam)
◦ Hismanal® (astemizole)
◦ Orap® (pimozide)
◦ Propulsid® (cisapride)
◦ Quinidine, also known as Quinaglute®, Cardioquin®, Quinidex®, and others
◦ Rythmol® (propafenone)
◦ Seldane® (terfenadine)
◦ Revatio® (sildenafil) only when used for the treatment of pulmonary arterial hypertension
◦ Tambocor® (flecainide)
◦ Uroxatral® (alfuzosin hydrochloride)
◦ Vascor® (bepridil)
◦ Versed® (midazolam)
◦ Vfend® (voriconazole)
• Do not take NORVIR with St. John's wort (hypericum perforatum), an herbal product sold as a dietary supplement or products containing St. John's wort. Talk with your doctor if you are taking or are planning to take St. John's wort. Taking St. John's wort may decrease NORVIR levels and lead to increased viral load and possible resistance to NORVIR or cross-resistance to other antiretroviral medicines.

• Do not take NORVIR with the cholesterol-lowering medicines Mevacor® (lovastatin) or Zocor® (simvastatin) because of possible serious reactions. There is also an increased risk of drug interactions between NORVIR and Lipitor® (atorvastatin); talk to your doctor before you take any of these cholesterol-lowering medicines with NORVIR.

Medicines That May Require Dosage Adjustments
It is possible that your doctor may need to increase or decrease the dose of other medicines when you are also taking NORVIR. Remember to tell your doctor all medicines you are taking or plan to take.
• The following medicines require dose reduction if taken with NORVIR:
If you are taking PDE5 inhibitors for erectile dysfunction including Viagra® (sildenafil), Cialis® (tadalafil), or Levitra® (vardenafil), your doctor may lower your dose of these medications. You should not use sildenafil (Revatio®) with NORVIR if you are being treated for pulmonary arte-

Information on the Abbott Pharmaceutical Products listed on these pages is from the prescribing information in use as of June 1, 2010. For more information, please visit rxabbott.com or call 1-800-633-9110.

rial hypertension. If you are taking Adcirca™ (tadalafil) for pulmonary arterial hypertension, your doctor may change your dose of this medicine.

Before you take Viagra®, Cialis® or Levitra® with NORVIR, talk to your doctor about possible drug interactions and side effects. If you take these medications with NORVIR you may be at risk of side effects such as low blood pressure, visual changes, and penile erection lasting more than 4 hours. If an erection lasts longer than 4 hours, you should get medical help immediately to avoid permanent damage to your penis. Your doctor can explain these symptoms to you.

- If you are taking Oral contraceptives ("the pill") or the contraceptive patch to prevent pregnancy, you should use a different type of contraception since NORVIR may reduce the effectiveness of oral or patch contraceptives.
- If you are taking Mycobutin® (rifabutin), your doctor will lower the dose of Mycobutin.
- If you are taking Colcrys® (colchicine), your doctor will tell you what dose to use.
- If you are taking Tracleer® (bosentan), your doctor will tell you what dose to use.
- **Other Special Considerations:**
  NORVIR oral solution contains alcohol. Talk with your doctor if you are taking or planning to take metronidazole or disulfiram. Severe nausea and vomiting can occur.
- **If you are taking both didanosine (Videx) and NORVIR:** Didanosine and NORVIR should be separated by at least 2.5 hours.
- Rifampin, also known as Rimactane®, Rifadin®, Rifater®, or Rifamate®, may reduce blood levels of NORVIR. Be sure to tell your doctor if you are taking rifampin.
- If you are taking or before you begin using inhaled Flonase® (fluticasone propionate), talk to your doctor about problems these two medicines may cause when taken together. Your doctor may choose not to keep you on inhaled Flonase®.
- Rifampin and saquinavir should not be taken with NORVIR. Be sure to tell your doctor if you are taking rifampin and saquinavir.
- If you are taking or before you begin using Serevent® (salmeterol) and NORVIR, talk to your doctor about problems these medicines may cause when taken together. Your doctor may choose not to keep you on Serevent® (salmeterol).
- If you are taking or before you begin using Advair® (salmeterol in combination with fluticasone propionate) and NORVIR, talk to your doctor about problems these two medicines may cause when taken together. Your doctor may choose not to keep you on Advair® (salmeterol in combination with fluticasone propionate).

What Are the Possible Side Effects of NORVIR?
- This list of side effects is **not** complete. If you have questions about side effects, ask your doctor, nurse, or pharmacist. You should report any new or continuing symptoms to your doctor right away. Your doctor may be able to help you manage these side effects.
- The most commonly reported side effects are: feeling weak/tired, nausea, vomiting, diarrhea, loss of appetite, abdominal pain, changes in taste, tingling feeling or numbness in hands or feet or around the lips, headache, and dizziness.
- Blood tests in patients taking NORVIR may show possible liver problems. People with liver disease such as Hepatitis B and Hepatitis C who take NORVIR may have worsening liver disease. Liver problems including rare cases of death have occurred in patients taking NORVIR. It is unclear if NORVIR caused these liver problems because some patients had other illnesses or were taking other medicines.
- Some patients taking NORVIR can develop serious problems with their pancreas (pancreatitis) which may cause death. Tell your doctor if you have nausea, vomiting, or abdominal pain. These may be signs of pancreatitis.
- Some patients have large increases in triglycerides and cholesterol. The long-term chance of getting complications such as heart attacks or stroke due to increases in triglycerides and cholesterol caused by protease inhibitors is not known at this time.
- Diabetes and high blood sugar (hyperglycemia) have occurred in patients taking protease inhibitors. Some patients had diabetes before starting protease inhibitors, others did not. Some patients need changes in their diabetes medication. Others needed new diabetes medication.
- Changes in body fat have been seen in some patients taking antiretroviral therapy. These changes may include increased amount of fat in the upper back and neck ("buffalo hump"), breast and around the trunk. Loss of fat from the legs, arms and face may also happen. The cause and long term health effects of these conditions are not known at this time.

Table 8. Percentage of Adult Patients, by Study and Treatment Group, with Chemistry and Hematology Abnormalities Occurring in > 3% of Patients Receiving NORVIR

Variable	Limit	Study 245 Naive Patients			Study 247 Advanced Patients		Study 462 PI-Naive Patients
		NORVIR +ZDV	NORVIR	ZDV	NORVIR	Placebo	NORVIR + Saquinavir
Chemistry	**High**						
Cholesterol	> 240 mg/dL	30.7	44.8	9.3	36.5	8.0	65.2
CPK	> 1000 IU/L	9.6	12.1	11.0	9.1	6.3	9.9
GGT	> 300 IU/L	1.8	5.2	1.7	19.6	11.3	9.2
SGOT (AST)	> 180 IU/L	5.3	9.5	2.5	6.4	7.0	7.8
SGPT (ALT)	> 215 IU/L	5.3	7.8	3.4	8.5	4.4	9.2
Triglycerides	> 800 mg/dL	9.6	17.2	3.4	33.6	9.4	23.4
Triglycerides	> 1500 mg/dL	1.8	2.6	-	12.6	0.4	11.3
Triglycerides Fasting	> 1500 mg/dL	1.5	1.3	-	9.9	0.3	-
Uric Acid	> 12 mg/dL	-	-	-	3.8	0.2	1.4
Hematology	**Low**						
Hematocrit	< 30%	2.6	-	0.8	17.3	22.0	0.7
Hemoglobin	< 8.0 g/dL	0.9	-	-	3.8	3.9	-
Neutrophils	≤ 0.5 × 10⁹/L	-	-	-	6.0	8.3	-
RBC	< 3.0 × 10¹²/L	1.8	-	5.9	18.6	24.4	-
WBC	< 2.5 × 10⁹/L	-	0.9	6.8	36.9	59.4	3.5

- Indicates no events reported.

Pediatric Dosage Guidelines[1]

Body Surface Area (m²)	Twice Daily Dose 250 mg/m²	Twice Daily Dose 300 mg/m²	Twice Daily Dose 350 mg/m²	Twice Daily Dose 400 mg/m²
0.20	0.6 mL (50 mg)	0.75 mL (60 mg)	0.9 mL (70 mg)	1.0 mL (80 mg)
0.25	0.8 mL (62.5 mg)	0.9 mL (75 mg)	1.1 mL (87.5 mg)	1.25 mL (100 mg)
0.50	1.6 mL (125 mg)	1.9 mL (150 mg)	2.2 mL (175 mg)	2.5 mL (200 mg)
0.75	2.3 mL (187.5 mg)	2.8 mL (225 mg)	3.3 mL (262.5 mg)	3.75 mL (300 mg)
1.00	3.1 mL (250 mg)	3.75 mL (300 mg)	4.4 mL (350 mg)	5 mL (400 mg)
1.25	3.9 mL (312.5 mg)	4.7 mL (375 mg)	5.5 mL (437.5 mg)	6.25 mL (500 mg)
1.50	4.7 mL (375 mg)	5.6 mL (450 mg)	6.6 mL (525 mg)	7.5 mL (600 mg)

- Some patients with hemophilia have increased bleeding with protease inhibitors.
- Allergic reactions ranging from mild to severe have occurred in patients taking NORVIR.
- Changes in the electrocardiogram (EKG). Consult your physician if you experience dizziness, lightheadedness, fainting spells or abnormal heart beat. Patients with heart defects or conduction defects should avoid NORVIR.

There have been other side effects noted in patients receiving NORVIR; however, these side effects may have been due to other medicines that patients were taking or to the illness itself. Some of these side effects can be serious. If you have questions about side effects, ask your doctor, nurse, or pharmacist. You should report any new or persistent symptoms to your doctor immediately.

What Should I Tell My Doctor Before Taking NORVIR?
- *If you are pregnant or planning to become pregnant:* The effects of NORVIR on pregnant women or their unborn babies are not known.
- *If you are breast-feeding:* Do not breast-feed if you are taking NORVIR. You should not breast-feed if you have HIV. If you are a woman who has or will have a baby, talk with your doctor about the best way to feed your baby. You should be aware that if your baby does not already have HIV, there is a chance that HIV can be transmitted through breast-feeding.
- *If you have liver problems:* If you have liver problems or are infected with Hepatitis B or Hepatitis C, you should tell your doctor before taking NORVIR.

- *If you have diabetes:* Some people taking protease inhibitors develop new or more serious diabetes or high blood sugar. Be sure to tell your doctor if you have diabetes or an increase in thirst and/or frequent urination.
- *If you have hemophilia:* Some people with hemophilia have had increased bleeding. It is not known whether the protease inhibitors caused these problems. Be sure to tell your doctor if you have hemophilia types A and B.

How Do I Store NORVIR?
- Keep NORVIR and all other medicines out of the reach of children.
- Store NORVIR Oral Solution at room temperature. Do not refrigerate NORVIR Oral Solution. Avoid exposing NORVIR Oral Solution to excessive heat or cold.
- Refrigeration of NORVIR soft gelatin capsules by the patient is recommended, but not required if used within 30 days and stored below 77°F (25°C). Avoid exposing NORVIR soft gelatin capsules to excessive heat or cold.
- Store NORVIR soft gelatin capsules and NORVIR Oral Solution in the original container.
- Shake NORVIR Oral Solution well before each use.
- Use NORVIR soft gelatin capsules and NORVIR Oral Solution by the expiration date on the bottle.

Do not keep medicine that is out of date or that you no longer need. Be sure that if you throw any medicine away, it is out of the reach of children.

General Advice About Prescription Medicines
Talk to your doctor or other health care provider if you have any questions or concerns about this medicine or your con-

dition. Medicines are sometimes prescribed for purposes other than those listed in a Patient Information Leaflet. Your doctor or pharmacist can give you information about this medicine that was written for health care professionals. Do not use this medicine for a condition for which it was not prescribed. Do not share this medicine with other people.

* The brands listed are trademarks of their respective owners and are not trademarks of Abbott Laboratories. The makers of these brands are not affiliated with and do not endorse Abbott Laboratories or its products.

Abbott Laboratories
North Chicago, IL 60064, U.S.A.
Ref. 03-A358-Revised April, 2010
Shown in Product Identification Guide, page 304

NORVIR®
[NOR-VEER]
(ritonavir)
Tablet for Oral use
NORVIR®
(ritonavir)
Solution for Oral use

HIGHLIGHTS OF PRESCRIBING INFORMATION
These highlights do not include all the information needed to use NORVIR safely and effectively. See full prescribing information for NORVIR.
NORVIR (ritonavir) Tablet for Oral use
NORVIR (ritonavir) Solution for Oral use
Initial U.S. Approval: 1996

> **WARNING:**
> **Co-administration of NORVIR with sedative hypnotics, antiarrhythmics, or ergot alkaloid preparations may result in potentially serious and/or life-threatening adverse events due to possible effects of NORVIR on the hepatic metabolism of certain drugs. (4, 5.1)**

―――――**INDICATIONS AND USAGE**―――――
NORVIR is an HIV protease inhibitor indicated in combination with other antiretroviral agents for the treatment of HIV-1 infection (1).

―――――**DOSAGE AND ADMINISTRATION**―――――
Take NORVIR with meals. (2)
See Full Prescribing Information for complete dosing guidelines.
Dose modification for NORVIR is necessary when used with other protease inhibitors. (2)
ADULT PATIENTS (2.1)
600 mg twice-daily with meals.
PEDIATRIC PATIENTS (2.2)
The recommended twice-daily dose for children greater than 1 month of age is based on body surface area and should not exceed 600 mg twice daily with meals.

―――――**DOSAGE FORMS AND STRENGTHS**―――――
• Tablet: 100 mg ritonavir (3)
• Oral solution: 80 mg ritonavir per milliliter (3)
―――――**CONTRAINDICATIONS**―――――
• NORVIR is contraindicated in patients with known hypersensitivity to ritonavir or any of its ingredients. (4)
• Co-administration with drugs highly dependent on CYP3A for clearance and for which elevated plasma concentrations may be associated with serious and/or life-threatening events. (4)
• Co-administration with drugs that significantly reduce ritonavir.

―――――**WARNINGS AND PRECAUTIONS**―――――
The following have been observed in patients receiving NORVIR:
• Drug Interactions: Consider drug-drug interaction potential to reduce risk of serious or life-threatening adverse reactions. (5.1)
• Hepatic Reactions: Fatalities have occurred. Monitor liver function before and during therapy, especially in patients with underlying hepatic disease, including hepatitis B and hepatitis C, or marked transaminase elevations. (5.2, 8.6)
• Pancreatitis: Fatalities have occurred; suspend therapy as clinically appropriate. (5.3)
• Allergic Reactions/Hypersensitivity: Allergic reactions have been reported and include anaphylaxis, Stevens-Johnson Syndrome, bronchospasm and angioedema. Discontinue treatment if severe reactions develop. (5.4, 6.3)
• PR interval prolongation may occur in some patients. Cases of second and third degree heart block have been reported. Use with caution with patients with preexisting conduction system disease, ischemic heart disease, cardiomyopathy, underlying structural heart disease or when administering with other drugs that may prolong the PR interval. (5.5, 12.3)
• Total cholesterol and triglycerides elevations: Monitor prior to therapy and periodically thereafter. (5.6)

• Patients may develop new onset or exacerbations of diabetes mellitus, hyperglycemia. (5.7)
• Patients may develop immune reconstitution syndrome. (5.8)
• Patients may develop redistribution/accumulation of body fat. (5.9)
• Hemophilia: Spontaneous bleeding may occur, and additional factor VIII may be required. (5.10)

―――――**ADVERSE REACTIONS**―――――
The most common adverse reactions (> 5% and of moderate to severe intensity) were abdominal pain, asthenia, headache, malaise, anorexia, diarrhea, dyspepsia, nausea, vomiting, paresthesia, circumoral paresthesia, peripheral paresthesia, dizziness, and taste perversion. (6.1)
To report SUSPECTED ADVERSE REACTIONS, contact Abbott Laboratories at 1-800-633-9110 or FDA at 1-800-FDA-1088 or www.fda.gov/medwatch.

―――――**DRUG INTERACTIONS**―――――
• Coadministration of NORVIR can alter the concentrations of other drugs. The potential for drug-drug interactions must be considered prior to and during therapy. (4, 5.1, 7, 12.3)

―――――**USE IN SPECIFIC POPULATIONS**―――――
• Pregnancy: Use during pregnancy only if the potential benefit justifies the potential risk. Antiretroviral Pregnancy Registry available. Register patients by calling 1–800–258–4263. (8.1)
• Nursing Mothers: Because of both the potential for HIV transmission and the potential for serious adverse reactions in nursing infants, mothers should be instructed *not* to breast-feed if they are receiving NORVIR. (8.3)

See 17 for PATIENT COUNSELING INFORMATION and the FDA-approved patient labeling
Revised: 04/2010

FULL PRESCRIBING INFORMATION: CONTENTS*
WARNING:
1 INDICATIONS AND USAGE
2 DOSAGE AND ADMINISTRATION
  2.1 Adult Patients
  2.2 Pediatric Patients
3 DOSAGE FORMS AND STRENGTHS
4 CONTRAINDICATIONS
5 WARNINGS AND PRECAUTIONS
  5.1 Drug Interactions
  5.2 Hepatic Reactions
  5.3 Pancreatitis
  5.4 Allergic Reactions/Hypersensitivity
  5.5 PR Interval Prolongation
  5.6 Lipid Disorders
  5.7 Diabetes Mellitus/Hyperglycemia
  5.8 Immune Reconstitution Syndrome
  5.9 Fat Redistribution
  5.10 Patients with Hemophilia
  5.11 Resistance/Cross-resistance
  5.12 Laboratory Tests
6 ADVERSE REACTIONS
  6.1 Adults — Clinical Trials Experience
  6.2 Pediatrics — Treatment-Emergent Adverse Events
  6.3 Postmarketing Experience
7 DRUG INTERACTIONS
  7.1 Potential for NORVIR to Affect Other Drugs
  7.2 Established and Other Potentially Significant Drug Interactions
8 USE IN SPECIFIC POPULATIONS
  8.1 Pregnancy
  8.3 Nursing Mothers
  8.4 Pediatric Use
  8.5 Geriatric Use
  8.6 Hepatic Impairment
10 OVERDOSAGE
  10.1 Acute Overdosage — Human Overdose Experience
  10.2 Management of Overdosage
11 DESCRIPTION
12 CLINICAL PHARMACOLOGY
  12.1 Mechanism of Action
  12.3 Pharmacokinetics
  12.4 Microbiology
13 NONCLINICAL TOXICOLOGY
  13.1 Carcinogenesis, Mutagenesis, Impairment of Fertility
14 CLINICAL STUDIES
  14.1 Advanced Patients with Prior Antiretroviral Therapy
  14.2 Patients without Prior Antiretroviral Therapy
15 REFERENCES
16 HOW SUPPLIED/STORAGE AND HANDLING
  16.1 NORVIR Tablets, 100 mg Ritonavir
  16.2 NORVIR Oral Solution, 80 mg/mL Ritonavir
17 PATIENT COUNSELING INFORMATION
* Sections or subsections omitted from the full prescribing information are not listed

---

FULL PRESCRIBING INFORMATION

> **WARNING:**
> **Co-administration of NORVIR with sedative hypnotics, antiarrhythmics, or ergot alkaloid preparations may result in potentially serious and/or life-threatening adverse events due to possible effects of NORVIR on the hepatic metabolism of certain drugs [see Contraindications (4) and Warnings and Precautions (5.1)].**

1 INDICATIONS AND USAGE
NORVIR is indicated in combination with other antiretroviral agents for the treatment of HIV-infection.

2 DOSAGE AND ADMINISTRATION
NORVIR is administered orally. NORVIR tablets should be swallowed whole, and not chewed, broken or crushed. Take NORVIR with meals. Patients may improve the taste of NORVIR oral solution by mixing with chocolate milk, Ensure®, or Advera® within one hour of dosing.
General Dosing Guidelines
Patients who take the 600 mg twice daily soft gel capsule NORVIR dose may experience more gastrointestinal side effects such as nausea, vomiting, abdominal pain or diarrhea when switching from the soft gel capsule to the tablet formulation because of greater maximum plasma concentration (C_{max}) achieved with the tablet formulation relative to the soft gel capsule [see Clinical Pharmacology (12.3)]. Patients should also be aware that these adverse events (gastrointestinal or paresthesias) may diminish as therapy is continued.
Dose Modification for NORVIR
Dose reduction of NORVIR is necessary when used with other protease inhibitors: amprenavir, atazanavir, darunavir, fosamprenavir, saquinavir, and tipranavir. Prescribers should consult the full prescribing information and clinical study information of these protease inhibitors if they are co-administered with a reduced dose of ritonavir [see Warnings and Precautions (5) and Table 5, Established and Other Potentially Significant Drug Interactions].

2.1 Adult Patients
Recommended Dosage for Treatment of HIV-1.
The recommended dosage of ritonavir is 600 mg twice daily by mouth to be taken with meals. Use of a dose titration schedule may help to reduce treatment-emergent adverse events while maintaining appropriate ritonavir plasma levels. Ritonavir should be started at no less than 300 mg twice daily and increased at 2 to 3 day intervals by 100 mg twice daily. The maximum dose of 600 mg twice daily should not be exceeded upon completion of the titration.
2.2 Pediatric Patients
Ritonavir should be used in combination with other antiretroviral agents [see Dosage and Administration (2)]. The recommended dosage of ritonavir in children > 1 month is 350 to 400 mg/m^2 twice daily by mouth to be taken with meals and should not exceed 600 mg twice daily. Ritonavir should be started at 250 mg/m^2 and increased at 2 to 3 day intervals by 50 mg/m^2 twice daily. If patients do not tolerate 400 mg/m^2 twice daily due to adverse events, the highest tolerated dose may be used for maintenance therapy in combination with other antiretroviral agents, however, alternative therapy should be considered. When possible, dose should be administered using a calibrated dosing syringe.
[See table 1 at top of next page]
Body surface area (BSA) can be calculated as follows[1]:

$$BSA\ (m^2) = \sqrt{\dfrac{Ht\ (Cm) \times Wt\ (kg)}{3600}}$$

3 DOSAGE FORMS AND STRENGTHS
• NORVIR Tablets
White film-coated ovaloid tablets debossed with the corporate Abbott ⊐ logo and the Abbo-Code NK providing 100 mg ritonavir.
• NORVIR Oral Solution
Orange-colored liquid containing 600 mg ritonavir per 7.5 mL marked dosage cup (80 mg/mL).

4 CONTRAINDICATIONS
• When co-administering NORVIR with other protease inhibitors, see the full prescribing information for that protease inhibitor including contraindication information.

Table 1. Pediatric Dosage Guidelines

Body Surface Area (m²)	Twice Daily Dose 250 mg/m²	Twice Daily Dose 300 mg/m²	Twice Daily Dose 350 mg/m²	Twice Daily Dose 400 mg/m²
0.20	0.6 mL (50 mg)	0.75 mL (60 mg)	0.9 mL (70 mg)	1.0 mL (80 mg)
0.25	0.8 mL (62.5 mg)	0.9 mL (75 mg)	1.1 mL (87.5 mg)	1.25 mL (100 mg)
0.50	1.6 mL (125 mg)	1.9 mL (150 mg)	2.2 mL (175 mg)	2.5 mL (200 mg)
0.75	2.3 mL (187.5 mg)	2.8 mL (225 mg)	3.3 mL (262.5 mg)	3.75 mL (300 mg)
1.00	3.1 mL (250 mg)	3.75 mL (300 mg)	4.4 mL (350 mg)	5 mL (400 mg)
1.25	3.9 mL (312.5 mg)	4.7 mL (375 mg)	5.5 mL (437.5 mg)	6.25 mL (500 mg)
1.50	4.7 mL (375 mg)	5.6 mL (450 mg)	6.6 mL (525 mg)	7.5 mL (600 mg)

Table 2. Drugs that are Contraindicated with NORVIR

Drug Class	Drugs Within Class That Are Contraindicated With NORVIR**	Clinical Comments:
Alpha₁-adrenoreceptor antagonist	Alfuzosin HCl	Potential for hypotension.
Antiarrhythmics	Amiodarone, bepridil, flecainide, propafenone, quinidine	Potential for cardiac arrhythmias.
Antifungal	Voriconazole	Coadministration of voriconazole with ritonavir 400 mg every 12 hours significantly decreases voriconazole plasma concentrations and may lead to loss of antifungal response. Voriconazole is contraindicated with ritonavir doses of 400 mg every 12 hours or greater [see Drug Interactions (7.2)].
Ergot Derivatives	Dihydroergotamine, ergonovine, ergotamine, methylergonovine	Potential for acute ergot toxicity characterized by vasospasm and ischemia of the extremities and other tissues including the central nervous system.
GI Motility Agent	Cisapride	Potential for cardiac arrhythmias.
Herbal Products	St. John's Wort (hypericum perforatum)	May lead to loss of virologic response and possible resistance to NORVIR or to the class of protease inhibitors.
HMG-CoA Reductase Inhibitors:	Lovastatin, simvastatin	Potential for myopathy including rhabdomyolysis.
Neuroleptic	Pimozide	Potential for cardiac arrhythmias.
PDE5 enzyme inhibitor	Sildenafil* (Revatio®) only when used for the treatment of pulmonary arterial hypertension (PAH)	A safe and effective dose has not been established when used with ritonavir. There is an increased potential for sildenafil-associated adverse events, including visual abnormalities, hypotension, prolonged erection, and syncope [see Drug Interactions (7)].
Sedative/hypnotics	Oral midazolam, triazolam	Prolonged or increased sedation or respiratory depression [see Drug Interactions (7.2)].

* see Drug Interactions (7), Table 5 for coadministration of sildenafil in patients with erectile dysfunction.
** For additional information for these contraindicated drugs, see also Drug Interactions (7), Table 5.

- NORVIR is contraindicated in patients with known hypersensitivity to ritonavir or any of its ingredients.
- Co-administration of NORVIR is contraindicated with the drugs listed in Table 2 because ritonavir mediated CYP3A inhibition can result in serious and/or life-threatening reactions. Voriconazole and St. John's Wort are exceptions in that co-administration of NORVIR and voriconazole results in a significant decrease in plasma concentrations of voriconazole, and co-administration of NORVIR with St. John's Wort may result in decreased ritonavir plasma concentrations.

[See table above]

5 WARNINGS AND PRECAUTIONS

When co-administering NORVIR with other protease inhibitors, see the full prescribing information for that protease inhibitor including important Warnings and Precautions.

5.1 Drug Interactions

See Table 2 for a listing of drugs that are contraindicated with NORVIR due to potentially life-threatening adverse events, significant drug interactions, or loss of virologic activity. Also, see Table 5 for a listing of drugs with established and other significant drug interactions [see Contraindications (4) and Drug Interactions (7)].

5.2 Hepatic Reactions

Hepatic transaminase elevations exceeding 5 times the upper limit of normal, clinical hepatitis, and jaundice have occurred in patients receiving NORVIR alone or in combination with other antiretroviral drugs (see Table 4). There may be an increased risk for transaminase elevations in patients with underlying hepatitis B or C. Therefore, caution should be exercised when administering NORVIR to patients with pre-existing liver diseases, liver enzyme abnormalities, or hepatitis. Increased AST/ALT monitoring should be considered in these patients, especially during the first three months of NORVIR treatment [see Use In Specific Populations (8.6)].

There have been postmarketing reports of hepatic dysfunction, including some fatalities. These have generally occurred in patients taking multiple concomitant medications and/or with advanced AIDS.

5.3 Pancreatitis

Pancreatitis has been observed in patients receiving NORVIR therapy, including those who developed hypertriglyceridemia. In some cases fatalities have been observed. Patients with advanced HIV disease may be at increased risk of elevated triglycerides and pancreatitis [see Warnings and Precautions (5.8)]. Pancreatitis should be considered if clinical symptoms (nausea, vomiting, abdominal pain) or abnormalities in laboratory values (such as increased serum lipase or amylase values) suggestive of pancreatitis should occur. Patients who exhibit these signs or symptoms should be evaluated and NORVIR therapy should be discontinued if a diagnosis of pancreatitis is made.

5.4 Allergic Reactions/Hypersensitivity

Allergic reactions including urticaria, mild skin eruptions, bronchospasm, and angioedema have been reported. Cases of anaphylaxis and Stevens-Johnson syndrome have also been reported. Discontinue treatment if severe reactions develop.

5.5 PR Interval Prolongation

Ritonavir prolongs the PR interval in some patients. Post marketing cases of second or third degree atrioventricular block have been reported in patients.

NORVIR should be used with caution in patients with underlying structural heart disease, preexisting conduction system abnormalities, ischemic heart disease, cardiomyopathies, as these patients may be at increased risk for developing cardiac conduction abnormalities.

The impact on the PR interval of co-administration of ritonavir with other drugs that prolong the PR interval (including calcium channel blockers, beta-adrenergic blockers, digoxin and atazanavir) has not been evaluated. As a result, co-administration of ritonavir with these drugs should be undertaken with caution, particularly with those drugs metabolized by CYP3A. Clinical monitoring is recommended. [see Clinical Pharmacology (12.3)].

5.6 Lipid Disorders

Treatment with NORVIR therapy alone or in combination with saquinavir has resulted in substantial increases in the concentration of total cholesterol and triglycerides [see Adverse Reactions (6.1)]. Triglyceride and cholesterol testing should be performed prior to initiating NORVIR therapy and at periodic intervals during therapy. Lipid disorders should be managed as clinically appropriate, taking into account any potential drug-drug interactions with NORVIR and HMG CoA reductase inhibitors [see Contraindications (4) and Drug Interactions (7)].

5.7 Diabetes Mellitus/Hyperglycemia

New onset diabetes mellitus, exacerbation of pre-existing diabetes mellitus, and hyperglycemia have been reported during postmarketing surveillance in HIV-infected patients receiving protease inhibitor therapy. Some patients required either initiation or dose adjustments of insulin or oral hypoglycemic agents for treatment of these events. In some cases, diabetic ketoacidosis has occurred. In those patients who discontinued protease inhibitor therapy, hyperglycemia persisted in some cases. Because these events have been reported voluntarily during clinical practice, estimates of frequency cannot be made and a causal relationship between protease inhibitor therapy and these events has not been established.

5.8 Immune Reconstitution Syndrome

Immune reconstitution syndrome has been reported in HIV-infected patients treated with combination antiretroviral therapy, including NORVIR. During the initial phase of combination antiretroviral treatment, patients whose immune system responds may develop an inflammatory response to indolent or residual opportunistic infections (such as Mycobacterium avium infection, cytomegalovirus, Pneumocystis jiroveci pneumonia, or tuberculosis), which may necessitate further evaluation and treatment.

5.9 Fat Redistribution

Redistribution/accumulation of body fat including central obesity, dorsocervical fat enlargement (buffalo hump), peripheral wasting, facial wasting, breast enlargement, and "cushingoid appearance" have been observed in patients receiving antiretroviral therapy. The mechanism and long-term consequences of these events are currently unknown. A causal relationship has not been established.

5.10 Patients with Hemophilia

There have been reports of increased bleeding, including spontaneous skin hematomas and hemarthrosis, in patients with hemophilia type A and B treated with protease inhibitors. In some patients additional factor VIII was given. In more than half of the reported cases, treatment with protease inhibitors was continued or reintroduced. A causal relationship between protease inhibitor therapy and these events has not been established.

5.11 Resistance/Cross-resistance

Varying degrees of cross-resistance among protease inhibitors have been observed. Continued administration of ritonavir 600 mg twice daily following loss of viral suppression may increase the likelihood of cross-resistance to other protease inhibitors [see Clinical Pharmacology (12.4)].

5.12 Laboratory Tests

Ritonavir has been shown to increase triglycerides, cholesterol, SGOT (AST), SGPT (ALT), GGT, CPK, and uric acid. Appropriate laboratory testing should be performed prior to

Table 3. Percentage of Patients with Treatment-emergent Adverse Events[1] of Moderate or Severe Intensity Occurring in ≥ 2% of Adult Patients Receiving NORVIR

Adverse Events	Study 245 Naive Patients[2]			Study 247 Advanced Patients[3]		Study 462 PI-Naive Patients[4]
	NORVIR + ZDV n = 116	NORVIR n = 117	ZDV n = 119	NORVIR n = 541	Placebo n = 545	NORVIR + Saquinavir n = 141
Body as a Whole						
Abdominal Pain	5.2	6.0	5.9	8.3	5.1	2.1
Asthenia	28.4	10.3	11.8	15.3	6.4	16.3
Fever	1.7	0.9	1.7	5.0	2.4	0.7
Headache	7.8	6.0	6.7	6.5	5.7	4.3
Malaise	5.2	1.7	3.4	0.7	0.2	2.8
Pain (unspecified)	0.9	1.7	0.8	2.2	1.8	4.3
Cardiovascular						
Syncope	0.9	1.7	0.8	0.6	0.0	2.1
Vasodilation	3.4	1.7	0.8	1.7	0.0	3.5
Digestive						
Anorexia	8.6	1.7	4.2	7.8	4.2	4.3
Constipation	3.4	0.0	0.8	0.2	0.4	1.4
Diarrhea	25.0	15.4	2.5	23.3	7.9	22.7
Dyspepsia	2.6	0.0	1.7	5.9	1.5	0.7
Fecal Incontinence	0.0	0.0	0.0	0.0	0.0	2.8
Flatulence	2.6	0.9	1.7	1.7	0.7	3.5
Local Throat Irritation	0.9	1.7	0.8	2.8	0.4	1.4
Nausea	46.6	25.6	26.1	29.8	8.4	18.4
Vomiting	23.3	13.7	12.6	17.4	4.4	7.1
Metabolic and Nutritional						
Weight Loss	0.0	0.0	0.0	2.4	1.7	0.0
Musculoskeletal						
Arthralgia	0.0	0.0	0.0	1.7	0.7	2.1
Myalgia	1.7	1.7	0.8	2.4	1.1	2.1
Nervous						
Anxiety	0.9	0.0	0.8	1.7	0.9	2.1
Circumoral Paresthesia	5.2	3.4	0.0	6.7	0.4	6.4
Confusion	0.0	0.9	0.0	0.6	0.6	2.1
Depression	1.7	1.7	2.5	1.7	0.7	7.1
Dizziness	5.2	2.6	3.4	3.9	1.1	8.5
Insomnia	3.4	2.6	0.8	2.0	1.8	2.8
Paresthesia	5.2	2.6	0.0	3.0	0.4	2.1
Peripheral Paresthesia	0.0	6.0	0.8	5.0	1.1	5.7
Somnolence	2.6	2.6	0.0	2.4	0.2	0.0
Thinking Abnormal	2.6	0.0	0.8	0.9	0.4	0.7

(Table continued on next page)

initiating NORVIR therapy and at periodic intervals or if any clinical signs or symptoms occur during therapy. For comprehensive information concerning laboratory test alterations associated with reverse transcriptase inhibitors, physicians should refer to the complete product information for each of these drugs.

6   ADVERSE REACTIONS
The following adverse reactions are discussed in greater detail in other sections of the labeling.

- Drug Interactions *[see Warnings and Precautions (5.1)]*
- Hepatotoxicity *[see Warnings and Precautions (5.2)]*
- Pancreatitis *[see Warnings and Precautions (5.3)]*
- Allergic Reactions/Hypersensitivity *[see Warnings and Precautions (5.4)]*

Because clinical trials are conducted under widely varying conditions, adverse reactions rates observed in the clinical trials of a drug cannot be directly compared to rates in the clinical trials of another drug and may not reflect the rates observed in practice.

When co-administering NORVIR with other protease inhibitors, see the full prescribing information for that protease inhibitor including adverse reactions.

6.1   Adults — Clinical Trials Experience
The safety of NORVIR alone and in combination with nucleoside reverse transcriptase inhibitors was studied in 1270 adult patients. Table 3 lists treatment-emergent adverse events (at least possibly related and of at least moderate intensity) that occurred in 2% or greater of adult patients receiving NORVIR alone or in combination with nucleoside reverse transcriptase inhibitors in Study 245 or Study 247 and in combination with saquinavir in study 462. In that study, 141 protease inhibitor-naive, HIV-infected patients with mean baseline CD_4 of 300 cells/µL were randomized to one of four regimens of NORVIR + saquinavir, including NORVIR 400 mg twice-daily + saquinavir 400 mg twice-daily. Overall the most frequently reported clinical adverse events, other than asthenia, among adult patients receiving NORVIR were gastrointestinal and neurological disturbances including nausea, diarrhea, vomiting, anorexia, abdominal pain, taste perversion, and circumoral and peripheral paresthesias. Similar adverse event profiles were reported in adult patients receiving ritonavir in other trials. [See table 3 at left and on next page]

Adverse events occurring in less than 2% of adult patients receiving NORVIR in all phase II/phase III studies and considered at least possibly related or of unknown relationship to treatment and of at least moderate intensity are listed below by body system.

Body as a Whole
Abdomen enlarged, accidental injury, allergic reaction, back pain, cachexia, chest pain, chills, facial edema, facial pain, flu syndrome, hormone level altered, hypothermia, kidney pain, neck pain, neck rigidity, pelvic pain, photosensitivity reaction, and substernal chest pain.

Cardiovascular System
Cardiovascular disorder, cerebral ischemia, cerebral venous thrombosis, hypertension, hypotension, migraine, myocardial infarct, palpitation, peripheral vascular disorder, phlebitis, postural hypotension, tachycardia and vasospasm.

Digestive System
Abnormal stools, bloody diarrhea, cheilitis, cholestatic jaundice, colitis, dry mouth, dysphagia, eructation, esophageal ulcer, esophagitis, gastritis, gastroenteritis, gastrointestinal disorder, gastrointestinal hemorrhage, gingivitis, hepatic coma, hepatitis, hepatomegaly, hepatosplenomegaly, ileus, liver damage, melena, mouth ulcer, pancreatitis, pseudomembranous colitis, rectal disorder, rectal hemorrhage, sialadenitis, stomatitis, tenesmus, thirst, tongue edema, and ulcerative colitis.

Endocrine System
Adrenal cortex insufficiency and diabetes mellitus.

Hemic and Lymphatic System
Acute mycloblastic leukemia, anemia, ecchymosis, leukopenia, lymphadenopathy, lymphocytosis, myeloproliferative disorder, and thrombocytopenia.

Metabolic and Nutritional Disorders
Albuminuria, alcohol intolerance, avitaminosis, BUN increased, dehydration, edema, enzymatic abnormality, glycosuria, gout, hypercholesteremia, peripheral edema, and xanthomatosis.

Musculoskeletal System
Arthritis, arthrosis, bone disorder, bone pain, extraocular palsy, joint disorder, leg cramps, muscle cramps, muscle weakness, myositis, and twitching.

Nervous System
Abnormal dreams, abnormal gait, agitation, amnesia, aphasia, ataxia, coma, convulsion, dementia, depersonalization, diplopia, emotional lability, euphoria, grand mal convulsion, hallucinations, hyperesthesia, hyperkinesia, hypesthesia, incoordination, libido decreased, manic reaction, nervousness, neuralgia, neuropathy, paralysis, peripheral neuropathic pain, peripheral neuropathy, peripheral sensory neuropathy, personality disorder, sleep disorder, speech disorder, stupor, subdural hematoma, tremor, urinary retention, vertigo, and vestibular disorder.

Respiratory System
Asthma, bronchitis, dyspnea, epistaxis, hiccup, hypoventilation, increased cough, interstitial pneumonia, larynx edema, lung disorder, rhinitis, and sinusitis.

Skin and Appendages
Acne, contact dermatitis, dry skin, eczema, erythema multiforme, exfoliative dermatitis, folliculitis, fungal dermati-

Information on the Abbott Pharmaceutical Products listed on these pages is from the prescribing information in use as of June 1, 2010. For more information, please visit rxabbott.com or call 1-800-633-9110.

Table 3 (cont.). Percentage of Patients with Treatment-emergent Adverse Events[1] of Moderate or Severe Intensity Occurring in ≥ 2% of Adult Patients Receiving NORVIR

Adverse Events	Study 245 Naive Patients[2]			Study 247 Advanced Patients[3]		Study 462 PI-Naive Patients[4]
	NORVIR + ZDV n = 116	NORVIR n = 117	ZDV n = 119	NORVIR n = 541	Placebo n = 545	NORVIR + Saquinavir n = 141
Respiratory						
Pharyngitis	0.9	2.6	0.0	0.4	0.4	1.4
Skin and Appendages						
Rash	0.9	0.0	0.8	3.5	1.5	0.7
Sweating	3.4	2.6	1.7	1.7	1.1	2.8
Special Senses						
Taste Perversion	17.2	11.1	8.4	7.0	2.2	5.0
Urogenital						
Nocturia	0.0	0.0	0.0	0.2	0.0	2.8

[1]Includes those adverse events at least possibly related to study drug or of unknown relationship and excludes concurrent HIV conditions.
[2]The median duration of treatment for patients randomized to regimens containing NORVIR in Study 245 was 9.1 months.
[3]The median duration of treatment for patients randomized to regimens containing NORVIR in Study 247 was 9.4 months.
[4]The median duration of treatment for patients in Study 462 was 48 weeks.

Table 4. Percentage of Adult Patients, by Study and Treatment Group, with Chemistry and Hematology Abnormalities Occurring in > 3% of Patients Receiving NORVIR

Variable	Limit	Study 245 Naive Patients			Study 247 Advanced Patients		Study 462 PI-Naive Patients
		NORVIR + ZDV	NORVIR	ZDV	NORVIR	Placebo	NORVIR + Saquinavir
Chemistry	**High**						
Cholesterol	> 240 mg/dL	30.7	44.8	9.3	36.5	8.0	65.2
CPK	> 1000 IU/L	9.6	12.1	11.0	9.1	6.3	9.9
GGT	> 300 IU/L	1.8	5.2	1.7	19.6	11.3	9.2
SGOT (AST)	> 180 IU/L	5.3	9.5	2.5	6.4	7.0	7.8
SGPT (ALT)	> 215 IU/L	5.3	7.8	3.4	8.5	4.4	9.2
Triglycerides	> 800 mg/dL	9.6	17.2	3.4	33.6	9.4	23.4
Triglycerides	> 1500 mg/dL	1.8	2.6	-	12.6	0.4	11.3
Triglycerides Fasting	> 1500 mg/dL	1.5	1.3	-	9.9	0.3	-
Uric Acid	> 12 mg/dL	-	-	-	3.8	0.2	1.4
Hematology	**Low**						
Hematocrit	< 30%	2.6	-	0.8	17.3	22.0	0.7
Hemoglobin	< 8.0 g/dL	0.9	-	-	3.8	3.9	-
Neutrophils	≤ 0.5 × 10⁹/L	-	-	-	6.0	8.3	-
RBC	< 3.0 × 10¹²/L	1.8	-	5.9	18.6	24.4	-
WBC	< 2.5 × 10⁹/L	-	0.9	6.8	36.9	59.4	3.5

- Indicates no events reported.

tis, furunculosis, maculopapular rash, molluscum contagiosum, onychomycosis, pruritus, psoriasis, pustular rash, seborrhea, skin discoloration, skin disorder, skin hypertrophy, skin melanoma, urticaria, and vesiculobullous rash.
Special Senses
Abnormal electro-oculogram, abnormal electroretinogram, abnormal vision, amblyopia/blurred vision, blepharitis, conjunctivitis, ear pain, eye disorder, eye pain, hearing impairment, increased cerumen, iritis, parosmia, photophobia, taste loss, tinnitus, uveitis, visual field defect, and vitreous disorder.

Urogenital System
Acute kidney failure, breast pain, cystitis, dysuria, hematuria, impotence, kidney calculus, kidney failure, kidney function abnormal, kidney pain, menorrhagia, penis disorder, polyuria, urethritis, urinary frequency, urinary tract infection, and vaginitis.
Laboratory Abnormalities
Table 4 shows the percentage of adult patients who developed marked laboratory abnormalities.
[See table 4 above]

6.2 Pediatrics — Treatment-Emergent Adverse Events
NORVIR has been studied in 265 pediatric patients > 1 month to 21 years of age. The adverse event profile observed during pediatric clinical trials was similar to that for adult patients.
Vomiting, diarrhea, and skin rash/allergy were the only drug-related clinical adverse events of moderate to severe intensity observed in ≥ 2% of pediatric patients enrolled in NORVIR clinical trials.
Laboratory Abnormalities
The following Grade 3-4 laboratory abnormalities occurred in > 3% of pediatric patients who received treatment with NORVIR either alone or in combination with reverse transcriptase inhibitors: neutropenia (9%), hyperamylasemia (7%), thrombocytopenia (5%), anemia (4%), and elevated AST (3%).

6.3 Postmarketing Experience
The following adverse events (not previously mentioned in the labeling) have been reported during post-marketing use of NORVIR. Because these reactions are reported voluntarily from a population of unknown size, it is not possible to reliably estimate their frequency or establish a causal relationship to NORVIR exposure.
Body as a Whole
Dehydration, usually associated with gastrointestinal symptoms, and sometimes resulting in hypotension, or renal insufficiency has been reported. Syncope, orthostatic hypotension, and renal insufficiency have also been reported without known dehydration.
Co-administration of ritonavir with ergotamine or dihydroergotamine has been associated with acute ergot toxicity characterized by vasospasm and ischemia of the extremities and other tissues including the central nervous system.
Cardiovascular System
First-degree AV block, second-degree AV block, third-degree AV block, right bundle branch block have been reported [see Warnings and Precautions (5.5)].
Cardiac and neurologic events have been reported when ritonavir has been co-administered with disopyramide, mexiletine, nefazodone, fluoxetine, and beta blockers. The possibility of drug interaction cannot be excluded.
Endocrine System
Cushing's syndrome and adrenal suppression have been reported when ritonavir has been co-administered with fluticasone propionate.
Nervous System
There have been postmarketing reports of seizure. Also, see Cardiovascular System.

7 DRUG INTERACTIONS
See also Contraindications (4), Clinical Pharmacology (12.3)
When co-administering NORVIR with other protease inhibitors (amprenavir, atazanavir, darunavir, fosamprenavir, saquinavir, and tipranavir), see the full prescribing information for that protease inhibitor including important information for drug interactions.

7.1 Potential for NORVIR to Affect Other Drugs
Ritonavir has been found to be an inhibitor of cytochrome P450 3A (CYP3A) and may increase plasma concentrations of agents that are primarily metabolized by CYP3A. Agents that are extensively metabolized by CYP3A and have high first pass metabolism appear to be the most susceptible to large increases in AUC (> 3-fold) when co-administered with ritonavir. Thus, co-administration of NORVIR with drugs highly dependent on CYP3A for clearance and for which elevated plasma concentrations are associated with serious and/or life-threatening events is contraindicated. Co-administration with other CYP3A substrates may require a dose adjustment or additional monitoring as shown in Table 5.
Ritonavir also inhibits CYP2D6 to a lesser extent. Co-administration of substrates of CYP2D6 with ritonavir could result in increases (up to 2-fold) in the AUC of the other agent, possibly requiring a proportional dosage reduction. Ritonavir also appears to induce CYP3A, CYP1A2, CYP2C9, CYP2C19, and CYP2B6 as well as other enzymes, including glucuronosyl transferase.

7.2 Established and Other Potentially Significant Drug Interactions
Table 5 provides a list of established or potentially clinically significant drug interactions. Alteration in dose or regimen may be recommended based on drug interaction studies or predicted interaction [see Clinical Pharmacology (12.3) for magnitude of interaction].
[See table 5 on pages 525 through 528]

8 USE IN SPECIFIC POPULATIONS
When co-administering NORVIR with other protease inhibitors, see the full prescribing information for the co-administered protease inhibitor including important information for use in special populations.

Table 5. Established and Other Potentially Significant Drug Interactions

Concomitant Drug Class: Drug Name	Effect on Concentration of Ritonavir or Concomitant Drug	Clinical Comment
HIV-Antiviral Agents		
HIV Protease Inhibitor: atazanavir	When co-administered with reduced doses of atazanavir and ritonavir ↑ atazanavir (↑ AUC, ↑ C_{max}, ↑ C_{min})	Atazanavir plasma concentrations achieved with atazanavir 300 mg q.d. and ritonavir 100 mg q.d. are higher than those achieved with atazanavir 400 mg q.d. See the complete prescribing information for Reyataz® (atazanavir) for details on co-administration of atazanavir 300 mg q.d. with ritonavir 100 mg q.d.
HIV Protease Inhibitor: darunavir	When co-administered with reduced doses of ritonavir ↑ darunavir (↑ AUC, ↑ C_{max}, ↑ C_{min})	See the complete prescribing information for Prezista® (darunavir) for details on co-administration of darunavir 600 mg b.i.d. with ritonavir 100 mg b.i.d. or darunavir 800 mg q.d. with ritonavir 100 mg q.d.
HIV Protease Inhibitor: fosamprenavir	When co-administered with reduced doses of ritonavir ↑ amprenavir (↑ AUC, ↑ C_{max}, ↑ C_{min})	See the complete prescribing information for Lexiva® (fosamprenavir) for details on co-administration of fosamprenavir 700 mg b.i.d. with ritonavir 100 mg b.i.d., fosamprenavir 1400 mg q.d. with ritonavir 200 mg q.d. or fosamprenavir 1400 mg q.d. with ritonavir 100 mg q.d.
HIV Protease Inhibitor: indinavir	When co-administered with reduced doses of indinavir and ritonavir ↑ indinavir (↔ AUC, ↓ C_{max}, ↑ C_{min})	Alterations in concentrations are noted when reduced doses of indinavir are co-administered with NORVIR. Appropriate doses for this combination, with respect to efficacy and safety, have not been established.
HIV Protease Inhibitor: saquinavir	When co-administered with reduced doses of ritonavir ↑ saquinavir (↑ AUC, ↑ C_{max}, ↑ C_{min})	See the complete prescribing information for Invirase® (saquinavir) for details on co-administration of saquinavir 1000 mg b.i.d with ritonavir 100 mg b.i.d. Saquinavir/ritonavir should not be given together with rifampin, due to the risk of severe hepatotoxicity (presenting as increased hepatic transaminases) if the three drugs are given together.
HIV Protease Inhibitor: tipranavir	When co-administered with reduced doses of ritonavir ↑ tipranavir (↑ AUC, ↑ C_{max}, ↑ C_{min})	See the complete prescribing information for Aptivus® (tipranavir) for details on co-administration of tipranavir 500 mg b.i.d. with ritonavir 200 mg b.i.d. There have been reports of clinical hepatitis and hepatic decompensation including some fatalities. All patients should be followed closely with clinical and laboratory monitoring, especially those with chronic hepatitis B or C co-infection, as these patients have an increased risk of hepatotoxicity. Liver function tests should be performed prior to initiating therapy with tipranavir/ritonavir, and frequently throughout the duration of treatment.
Non-Nucleoside Reverse Transcriptase Inhibitor: delavirdine	↑ ritonavir (↑ AUC, ↑ C_{max}, ↑ C_{min})	Appropriate doses of this combination with respect to safety and efficacy have not been established.
HIV CCR5 – antagonist: maraviroc	↑ maraviroc	Concurrent administration of maraviroc with ritonavir will increase plasma levels of maraviroc. For specific dosage adjustment recommendations, please refer to the complete prescribing information for Selzentry® (maraviroc).
Other Agents		
Analgesics, Narcotic: tramadol, propoxyphene		A dose decrease may be needed for these drugs when co-administered with ritonavir.
Anesthetic: meperidine	↓ meperidine/ ↑ normeperidine (metabolite)	Dosage increase and long-term use of meperidine with ritonavir are not recommended due to the increased concentrations of the metabolite normeperidine which has both analgesic activity and CNS stimulant activity (e.g., seizures).
Antialcoholics: disulfiram/metronidazole		Ritonavir formulations contain alcohol, which can produce disulfiram-like reactions when co-administered with disulfiram or other drugs that produce this reaction (e.g., metronidazole).
Antiarrhythmics: disopyramide, lidocaine, mexiletine	↑ antiarrhythmics	Caution is warranted and therapeutic concentration monitoring is recommended for antiarrhythmics when co-administered with ritonavir, if available.

(Table continued on next page)

8.1 Pregnancy

Pregnancy Category B
There are no adequate and well-controlled studies in pregnant women. Because animal reproduction studies are not always predictive of human response, this drug should be used during pregnancy only if clearly needed.

No treatment related malformations were observed when ritonavir was administered to pregnant rats or rabbits. Developmental toxicity observed in rats (early resorptions, decreased fetal body weight and ossification delays and developmental variations) occurred at a maternally toxic dosage at an exposure equivalent to approximately 30% of that achieved with the proposed therapeutic dose. A slight in-crease in the incidence of cryptorchidism was also noted in rats at an exposure approximately 22% of that achieved with the proposed therapeutic dose.

Developmental toxicity observed in rabbits (resorptions, decreased litter size and decreased fetal weights) also occurred at a maternally toxic dosage equivalent to 1.8 times the proposed therapeutic dose based on a body surface area conversion factor.

Antiretroviral Pregnancy Registry: To monitor maternal-fetal outcomes of pregnant women exposed to NORVIR, an Antiretroviral Pregnancy Registry has been established. Physicians are encouraged to register patients by calling 1-800-258-4263.

8.3 Nursing Mothers

The Centers for Disease Control and Prevention recommend that HIV-infected mothers not breast-feed their infants to avoid risking postnatal transmission of HIV. It is not known whether ritonavir is secreted in human milk. Because of both the potential for HIV transmission and the potential for serious adverse reactions in nursing infants, mothers should be instructed not to breast-feed if they are receiving NORVIR.

8.4 Pediatric Use

In HIV-infected patients age greater than 1 month to 21 years, the antiviral activity and adverse event profile seen during clinical trials and through postmarketing experience were similar to that for adult patients.

8.5 Geriatric Use

Clinical studies of NORVIR did not include sufficient numbers of subjects aged 65 and over to determine whether they respond differently from younger subjects. In general, dose selection for an elderly patient should be cautious, usually starting at the low end of the dosing range, reflecting the greater frequency of decreased hepatic, renal or cardiac function, and of concomitant disease or other drug therapy.

8.6 Hepatic Impairment

No dose adjustment of ritonavir is necessary for patients with either mild or moderate hepatic impairment. No pharmacokinetic or safety data are available regarding the use of ritonavir in subjects with severe hepatic impairment, therefore, ritonavir is not recommended for use in patients with severe hepatic impairment [see Clinical Pharmacology (12.3)].

10   OVERDOSAGE

10.1   Acute Overdosage — Human Overdose Experience

Human experience of acute overdose with NORVIR is limited. One patient in clinical trials took NORVIR 1500 mg/day for two days. The patient reported paresthesias which resolved after the dose was decreased. A post-marketing case of renal failure with eosinophilia has been reported with ritonavir overdose.

The approximate lethal dose was found to be greater than 20 times the related human dose in rats and 10 times the related human dose in mice.

10.2   Management of Overdosage

NORVIR oral solution contains 43% alcohol by volume. Accidental ingestion of the product by a young child could result in significant alcohol-related toxicity and could approach the potential lethal dose of alcohol.

Treatment of overdose with NORVIR consists of general supportive measures including monitoring of vital signs and observation of the clinical status of the patient. There is no specific antidote for overdose with NORVIR. If indicated, elimination of unabsorbed drug should be achieved by emesis or gastric lavage; usual precautions should be observed to maintain the airway. Administration of activated charcoal may also be used to aid in removal of unabsorbed drug. Since ritonavir is extensively metabolized by the liver and is highly protein bound, dialysis is unlikely to be beneficial in significant removal of the drug. A Certified Poison Control Center should be consulted for up-to-date information on the management of overdose with NORVIR.

11   DESCRIPTION

NORVIR (ritonavir) is an inhibitor of HIV protease with activity against the Human Immunodeficiency Virus (HIV). Ritonavir is chemically designated as 10-Hydroxy-2-methyl-5-(1-methylethyl)-1-   [2-(1-methylethyl)-4-thiazolyl]-3,6-dioxo-8,11-bis(phenylmethyl)-2,4,7,12- tetraazatridecan-13-oic acid, 5-thiazolylmethyl ester, [5S-(5R*,8R*,10R*,11R*)]. Its molecular formula is $C_{37}H_{48}N_6O_5S_2$, and its molecular weight is 720.95. Ritonavir has the following structural formula:

Ritonavir is a white-to-light-tan powder. Ritonavir has a bitter metallic taste. It is freely soluble in methanol and ethanol, soluble in isopropanol and practically insoluble in water.

NORVIR tablets are available for oral administration in a strength of 100 mg ritonavir with the following inactive ingredients: copovidone, anhydrous dibasic calcium phos-

Information on the Abbott Pharmaceutical Products listed on these pages is from the prescribing information in use as of June 1, 2010. For more information, please visit rxabbott.com or call 1-800-633-9110.

Table 5 (cont.). Established and Other Potentially Significant Drug Interactions

Concomitant Drug Class: Drug Name	Effect on Concentration of Ritonavir or Concomitant Drug	Clinical Comment
Other Agents (continued)		
Anticancer Agents: vincristine, vinblastine	↑ anticancer agents	Concentrations of vincristine or vinblastine may be increased when co-administered with ritonavir resulting in the potential for increased adverse events usually associated with these anticancer agents. Consideration should be given to temporarily withholding the ritonavir containing antiretroviral regimen in patients who develop significant hematologic or gastrointestinal side effects when ritonavir is administered concurrently with vincristine or vinblastine. Clinicians should be aware that if the ritonavir containing regimen is withheld for a prolonged period, consideration should be given to altering the regimen to not include a CYP3A or P-gp inhibitor in order to control HIV-1 viral load.
Anticoagulant: warfarin	↓ R-warfarin ↓ ↑ S-warfarin	Initial frequent monitoring of the INR during ritonavir and warfarin co-administration is indicated.
Anticonvulsants: carbamazepine, clonazepam, ethosuximide	↑anticonvulsants	Use with caution. A dose decrease may be needed for these drugs when co-administered with ritonavir and therapeutic concentration monitoring is recommended for these anticonvulsants, if available.
Anticonvulsants: divalproex, lamotrigine, phenytoin	↓ anticonvulsants	Use with caution. A dose increase may be needed for these drugs when co-administered with ritonavir and therapeutic concentration monitoring is recommended for these anticonvulsants, if available.
Antidepressants: nefazodone, selective serotonin reuptake inhibitors (SSRIs), tricyclics	↑ antidepressants	A dose decrease may be needed for these drugs when co-administered with ritonavir.
Antidepressant: bupropion	↓ bupropion ↓ active metabolite, hydroxybupropion	Concurrent administration of bupropion with ritonavir may decrease plasma levels of both bupropion and its active metabolite (hydroxybupropion). Patients receiving ritonavir and bupropion concurrently should be monitored for an adequate clinical response to bupropion.
Antidepressant: desipramine	↑ desipramine	Dosage reduction and concentration monitoring of desipramine is recommended.
Antidepressant: trazodone	↑ trazodone	Concomitant use of trazodone and NORVIR increases plasma concentrations of trazodone. Adverse events of nausea, dizziness, hypotension and syncope have been observed following co-administration of trazodone and NORVIR. If trazodone is used with a CYP3A4 inhibitor such as ritonavir, the combination should be used with caution and a lower dose of trazodone should be considered.
Antiemetic: dronabinol	↑ dronabinol	A dose decrease of dronabinol may be needed when co-administered with ritonavir.
Antifungal: ketoconazole itraconazole voriconazole	↑ ketoconazole ↑ itraconazole ↓ voriconazole	High doses of ketoconazole or itraconazole (> 200 mg/day) are not recommended. Coadministration of voriconazole and ritonavir doses of 400 mg every 12 hours or greater is contraindicated. Coadministration of voriconazole and ritonavir 100 mg should be avoided, unless an assessment of the benefit/risk to the patient justifies the use of voriconazole.
Anti-gout: colchicine	↑ colchicine	Patients with renal or hepatic impairment should not be given colchicine with ritonavir. Treatment of gout flares-co-administration of colchicine in patients on ritonavir: 0.6 mg (1 tablet) × 1 dose, followed by 0.3 mg (half tablet) 1 hour later. Dose to be repeated no earlier than 3 days. Prophylaxis of gout flares-co-administration of colchicine in patients on ritonavir: If the original colchicine regimen was 0.6 mg twice a day, the regimen should be adjusted to 0.3 mg once a day. If the original colchicine regimen was 0.6 mg once a day, the regimen should be adjusted to 0.3 mg once every other day. Treatment of familial Mediterranean fever (FMF)-co-administration of colchicine in patients on ritonavir: Maximum daily dose of 0.6 mg (may be given as 0.3 mg twice a day).

(Table continued on next page)

phate, sorbitan monolaurate, colloidal silicon dioxide, and sodium stearyl fumarate. The following are the ingredients in the film coating: hypromellose, titanium dioxide, polyethylene glycol 400, hydroxypropyl cellulose, talc, polyethylene glycol 3350, colloidal silicon dioxide, and polysorbate 80.

NORVIR oral solution is available for oral administration as 80 mg/mL of ritonavir in a peppermint and caramel flavored vehicle. Each 8-ounce bottle contains 19.2 grams of ritonavir. NORVIR oral solution also contains ethanol, water, polyoxyl 35 castor oil, propylene glycol, anhydrous citric acid to adjust pH, saccharin sodium, peppermint oil, creamy caramel flavoring, and FD&C Yellow No. 6.

12   CLINICAL PHARMACOLOGY

12.1   Mechanism of Action

Ritonavir is an antiviral drug [see Clinical Pharmacology (12.4)].

12.3   Pharmacokinetics

The pharmacokinetics of ritonavir have been studied in healthy volunteers and HIV-infected patients (CD$_4$ ≥ 50 cells/μL). See Table 6 for ritonavir pharmacokinetic characteristics.

Absorption

The absolute bioavailability of ritonavir has not been determined. After a 600 mg dose of oral solution, peak concentrations of ritonavir were achieved approximately 2 hours and 4 hours after dosing under fasting and non-fasting (514 KCal; 9% fat, 12% protein, and 79% carbohydrate) conditions, respectively.

NORVIR tablets are not bioequivalent to NORVIR capsules. Under moderate fat conditions (857 kcal; 31% fat, 13% protein, 56% carbohydrates), when a single 100 mg NORVIR dose was administered as a tablet compared with a capsule, AUC$_{(0-\infty)}$ met equivalence criteria but mean C$_{max}$ was increased by 26% (92.8% confidence intervals: ↑ 15-↑ 39%).

No information is available comparing NORVIR tablets to NORVIR capsules under fasting conditions.

Effect of Food on Oral Absorption

When the oral solution was given under non-fasting conditions, peak ritonavir concentrations decreased 23% and the extent of absorption decreased 7% relative to fasting conditions. Dilution of the oral solution, within one hour of administration, with 240 mL of chocolate milk, Advera® or Ensure® did not significantly affect the extent and rate of ritonavir absorption. Administration of a single 600 mg oral solution under non-fasting conditions yielded mean ± SD areas under the plasma concentration-time curve (AUCs) of 129.0 ± 39.3 mg•h/mL.

A food effect is observed for NORVIR tablets. Food decreased the bioavailability of the ritonavir tablets when a single 100 mg dose of NORVIR was administered. Under high fat conditions (907 kcal; 52% fat, 15% protein, 33% carbohydrates), a 23% decrease in mean AUC$_{(0-\infty)}$ [90% confidence intervals: ↓ 30%-↓ 15%], and a 23% decrease in mean C$_{max}$ [90% confidence intervals: ↓ 34%-↓ 11%]) was observed relative to fasting conditions. Under moderate fat conditions, a 21% decrease in mean AUC$_{(0-\infty)}$ [90% confidence intervals: ↓ 28%-↓ 13%], and a 22% decrease in mean C$_{max}$ [90% confidence intervals: ↓ 33%-↓ 9%]) was observed relative to fasting conditions.

However, the type of meal administered did not change ritonavir tablet bioavailability when high fat was compared to moderate fat meals.

Metabolism

Nearly all of the plasma radioactivity after a single oral 600 mg dose of ^{14}C-ritonavir oral solution (n = 5) was attributed to unchanged ritonavir. Five ritonavir metabolites have been identified in human urine and feces. The isopropylthiazole oxidation metabolite (M-2) is the major metabolite and has antiviral activity similar to that of parent drug; however, the concentrations of this metabolite in plasma are low. In vitro studies utilizing human liver microsomes have demonstrated that cytochrome P450 3A (CYP3A) is the major isoform involved in ritonavir metabolism, although CYP2D6 also contributes to the formation of M–2.

Elimination

In a study of five subjects receiving a 600 mg dose of ^{14}C-ritonavir oral solution, 11.3 ± 2.8% of the dose was excreted into the urine, with 3.5 ± 1.8% of the dose excreted as unchanged parent drug. In that study, 86.4 ± 2.9% of the dose was excreted in the feces with 33.8 ± 10.8% of the dose excreted as unchanged parent drug. Upon multiple dosing, ritonavir accumulation is less than predicted from a single dose possibly due to a time and dose-related increase in clearance.

Table 6. Ritonavir Pharmacokinetic Characteristics

Parameter	N	Values (Mean ± SD)
C$_{max}$ SS[†]	10	11.2 ± 3.6 μg/mL
C$_{trough}$ SS[†]	10	3.7 ± 2.6 μg/mL
V$_\beta$/F[‡]	91	0.41 ± 0.25 L/kg
t$_{1/2}$		3-5 h
CL/F SS[†]	10	8.8 ± 3.2 L/h

CL/F[‡]	91	4.6 ± 1.6 L/h
CL$_R$	62	< 0.1 L/h
RBC/Plasma Ratio		0.14
Percent Bound*		98 to 99%

† SS = steady state; patients taking ritonavir 600 mg q12h.
‡ Single ritonavir 600 mg dose.
* Primarily bound to human serum albumin and alpha-1 acid glycoprotein over the ritonavir concentration range of 0.01 to 30 µg/mL.

Effects on Electrocardiogram
QTcF interval was evaluated in a randomized, placebo and active (moxifloxacin 400 mg once-daily) controlled crossover study in 45 healthy adults, with 10 measurements over 12 hours on Day 3. The maximum mean (95% upper confidence bound) time-matched difference in QTcF from placebo after baseline correction was 5.5 (7.6) milliseconds (msec) for 400 mg twice-daily ritonavir. Ritonavir 400 mg twice daily resulted in Day 3 ritonavir exposure that was approximately 1.5 fold higher than observed with ritonavir 600 mg twice-daily dose at steady state.

PR interval prolongation was also noted in subjects receiving ritonavir in the same study on Day 3. The maximum mean (95% confidence interval) difference from placebo in the PR interval after baseline correction was 22 (25) msec for 400 mg twice-daily ritonavir [see Warnings and Precautions (5.6)].

Special Populations
Gender, Race and Age
No age-related pharmacokinetic differences have been observed in adult patients (18 to 63 years). Ritonavir pharmacokinetics have not been studied in older patients.
A study of ritonavir pharmacokinetics in healthy males and females showed no statistically significant differences in the pharmacokinetics of ritonavir. Pharmacokinetic differences due to race have not been identified.

Pediatric Patients
Steady-state pharmacokinetics were evaluated in 37 HIV-infected patients ages 2 to 14 years receiving doses ranging from 250 mg/m² twice-daily to 400 mg/m² twice-daily in PACTG Study 310, and in 41 HIV-infected patients ages 1 month to 2 years at doses of 350 and 450 mg/m² twice-daily in PACTG Study 345. Across dose groups, ritonavir steady-state oral clearance (CL/F/m²) was approximately 1.5 to 1.7 times faster in pediatric patients than in adult subjects. Ritonavir concentrations obtained after 350 to 400 mg/m² twice-daily in pediatric patients > 2 years were comparable to those obtained in adults receiving 600 mg (approximately 330 mg/m²) twice-daily. The following observations were seen regarding ritonavir concentrations after administration with 350 or 450 mg/m² twice-daily in children < 2 years of age. Higher ritonavir exposures were not evident with 450 mg/m² twice-daily compared to the 350 mg/m² twice-daily. Ritonavir trough concentrations were somewhat lower than those obtained in adults receiving 600 mg twice-daily. The area under the ritonavir plasma concentration time curve and trough concentrations obtained after administration with 350 or 450 mg/m² twice-daily in children < 2 years were approximately 16% and 60% lower, respectively, than that obtained in adults receiving 600 mg twice daily.

Renal Impairment
Ritonavir pharmacokinetics have not been studied in patients with renal impairment, however, since renal clearance is negligible, a decrease in total body clearance is not expected in patients with renal impairment.

Hepatic Impairment
Dose-normalized steady-state ritonavir concentrations in subjects with mild hepatic impairment (400 mg twice-daily, n = 6) were similar to those in control subjects dosed with 500 mg twice-daily. Dose-normalized steady-state ritonavir exposures in subjects with moderate hepatic impairment (400 mg twice-daily, n= 6) were about 40% lower than those in subjects with normal hepatic function (500 mg twice-daily, n = 6). Protein binding of ritonavir was not statistically significantly affected by mild or moderately impaired hepatic function. No dose adjustment is recommended in patients with mild or moderate hepatic impairment. However, health care providers should be aware of the potential for lower ritonavir concentrations in patients with moderate hepatic impairment and should monitor patient response carefully. Ritonavir has not been studied in patients with severe hepatic impairment.

Drug Interactions
[see also Contraindications (4) and Warnings and Precautions (5.1)]

Table 5 (cont.). Established and Other Potentially Significant Drug Interactions

Concomitant Drug Class: Drug Name	Effect on Concentration of Ritonavir or Concomitant Drug	Clinical Comment
Other Agents (continued)		
Anti-infective: clarithromycin	↑ clarithromycin	For patients with renal impairment the following dosage adjustments should be considered: • For patients with CL$_{CR}$ 30 to 60 mL/min the dose of clarithromycin should be reduced by 50%. • For patients with CL$_{CR}$ <30 mL/min the dose of clarithromycin should be decreased by 75%. No dose adjustment for patients with normal renal function is necessary.
Antimycobacterial: rifabutin	↑ rifabutin and rifabutin metabolite	Dosage reduction of rifabutin by at least three-quarters of the usual dose of 300 mg/day is recommended (e.g., 150 mg every other day or three times a week). Further dosage reduction may be necessary.
Antimycobacterial: rifampin	↓ ritonavir	May lead to loss of virologic response. Alternate antimycobacterial agents such as rifabutin should be considered (see Antimycobacterial: rifabutin, for dose reduction recommendations).
Antiparasitic: atovaquone	↓ atovaquone	Clinical significance is unknown; however, increase in atovaquone dose may be needed.
Antiparasitic: quinine	↑ quinine	A dose decrease of quinine may be needed when co-administered with ritonavir.
β-Blockers: metoprolol, timolol	↑ Beta-Blockers	Caution is warranted and clinical monitoring of patients is recommended. A dose decrease may be needed for these drugs when co-administered with ritonavir.
Bronchodilator: theophylline	↓ theophylline	Increased dosage of theophylline may be required; therapeutic monitoring should be considered.
Calcium channel blockers: diltiazem, nifedipine, verapamil	↑ calcium channel blockers	Caution is warranted and clinical monitoring of patients is recommended. A dose decrease may be needed for these drugs when co-administered with ritonavir.
Digoxin	↑ digoxin	Concomitant administration of ritonavir with digoxin may increase digoxin levels. Caution should be exercised when coadministering ritonavir with digoxin, with appropriate monitoring of serum digoxin levels.
Endothelin receptor antagonists: bosentan	↑ bosentan	Co-administration of bosentan in patients on ritonavir: In patients who have been receiving ritonavir for at least 10 days, start bosentan at 62.5 mg once daily or every other day based upon individual tolerability. Co-administration of ritonavir in patients on bosentan: Discontinue use of bosentan at least 36 hours prior to initiation of ritonavir. After at least 10 days following the initiation of ritonavir, resume bosentan at 62.5 mg once daily or every other day based upon individual tolerability.
HMG-CoA Reductase Inhibitor: atorvastatin rosuvastatin	↑ atorvastatin ↑ rosuvastatin	Use the lowest possible dose of atorvastatin or rosuvastatin with careful monitoring or consider other HMG-CoA reductase inhibitors such as pravastatin or fluvastatin in combination with NORVIR.
Immunosuppressants: cyclosporine, tacrolimus, sirolimus (rapamycin)	↑ immunosuppressants	Therapeutic concentration monitoring is recommended for immunosuppressant agents when co-administered with ritonavir.
Inhaled Steroid: Fluticasone	↑ fluticasone	Concomitant use of fluticasone propionate and NORVIR increases plasma concentrations of fluticasone propionate, resulting in significantly reduced serum cortisol concentrations. Co-administration of fluticasone propionate and NORVIR is not recommended unless the potential benefit to the patient outweighs the risk of systemic corticosteroid side effects.

(Table continued on next page)

Table 7 and Table 8 summarize the effects on AUC and Cmax, with 95% confidence intervals (95% CI), of co-administration of ritonavir with a variety of drugs. For information about clinical recommendations see Table 5 in *Drug Interactions (7)*.

[See table 7 at top of page 529]
[See table 8 at top of page 530]

12.4   Microbiology
Mechanism of Action
Ritonavir is a peptidomimetic inhibitor of the HIV-1 protease. Inhibition of HIV protease renders the enzyme incapable of processing the *gag-pol* polyprotein precursor which leads to production of non-infectious immature HIV particles.

Antiviral Activity in Cell Culture
The activity of ritonavir was assessed in acutely infected lymphoblastoid cell lines and in peripheral blood lympho-

---

Information on the Abbott Pharmaceutical Products listed on these pages is from the prescribing information in use as of June 1, 2010. For more information, please visit rxabbott.com or call 1-800-633-9110.

cytes. The concentration of drug that inhibits 50% (EC_{50}) of viral replication ranged from 3.8 to 153 nM depending upon the HIV-1 isolate and the cells employed. The average EC_{50} value for low passage clinical isolates was 22 nM (n = 13). In MT_4 cells, ritonavir demonstrated additive effects against HIV-1 in combination with either didanosine (ddI) or zidovudine (ZDV). Studies which measured cytotoxicity of ritonavir on several cell lines showed that > 20 μM was required to inhibit cellular growth by 50% resulting in a cell culture therapeutic index of at least 1000.

Resistance

HIV-1 isolates with reduced susceptibility to ritonavir have been selected in cell culture. Genotypic analysis of these isolates showed mutations in the HIV-1 protease gene leading to amino acid substitutions I84V, V82F, A71V, and M46I. Phenotypic (n = 18) and genotypic (n = 48) changes in HIV-1 isolates from selected patients treated with ritonavir were monitored in phase I/II trials over a period of 3 to 32 weeks. Substitutions associated with the HIV-1 viral protease in isolates obtained from 43 patients appeared to occur in a stepwise and ordered fashion at positions V82A/F/T/S, I54V, A71V/T, and I36L, followed by combinations of substitutions at an additional 5 specific amino acid positions (M46I/L, K20R, I84V, L33F and L90M). Of 18 patients for whom both phenotypic and genotypic analysis were performed on free virus isolated from plasma, 12 showed reduced susceptibility to ritonavir in cell culture. All 18 patients possessed one or more substitutions in the viral protease gene. The V82A/F substitution appeared to be necessary but not sufficient to confer phenotypic resistance. Phenotypic resistance was defined as a $\geq$ 5-fold decrease in viral sensitivity in cell culture from baseline.

Cross-Resistance to Other Antiretrovirals

Among protease inhibitors variable cross-resistance has been recognized. Serial HIV-1 isolates obtained from six patients during ritonavir therapy showed a decrease in ritonavir susceptibility in cell culture but did not demonstrate a concordant decrease in susceptibility to saquinavir in cell culture when compared to matched baseline isolates. However, isolates from two of these patients demonstrated decreased susceptibility to indinavir in cell culture (8-fold). Isolates from 5 patients were also tested for cross-resistance to amprenavir and nelfinavir; isolates from 3 patients had a decrease in susceptibility to nelfinavir (6- to 14-fold), and none to amprenavir. Cross-resistance between ritonavir and reverse transcriptase inhibitors is unlikely because of the different enzyme targets involved. One ZDV-resistant HIV-1 isolate tested in cell culture retained full susceptibility to ritonavir.

13 NONCLINICAL TOXICOLOGY

13.1 Carcinogenesis, Mutagenesis, Impairment of Fertility

Carcinogenicity studies in mice and rats have been carried out on ritonavir. In male mice, at levels of 50, 100 or 200 mg/kg/day, there was a dose dependent increase in the incidence of both adenomas and combined adenomas and carcinomas in the liver. Based on AUC measurements, the exposure at the high dose was approximately 0.3-fold for males that of the exposure in humans with the recommended therapeutic dose (600 mg twice-daily). There were no carcinogenic effects seen in females at the dosages tested. The exposure at the high dose was approximately 0.6-fold for the females that of the exposure in humans. In rats dosed at levels of 7, 15 or 30 mg/kg/day there were no carcinogenic effects. In this study, the exposure at the high dose was approximately 6% that of the exposure in humans with the recommended therapeutic dose. Based on the exposures achieved in the animal studies, the significance of the observed effects is not known. However, ritonavir was found to be negative for mutagenic or clastogenic activity in a battery of *in vitro* and *in vivo* assays including the Ames bacterial reverse mutation assay using *S. typhimurium* and *E. coli*, the mouse lymphoma assay, the mouse micronucleus test and chromosomal aberration assays in human lymphocytes.

Ritonavir produced no effects on fertility in rats at drug exposures approximately 40% (male) and 60% (female) of that achieved with the proposed therapeutic dose. Higher dosages were not feasible due to hepatic toxicity.

14 CLINICAL STUDIES

The activity of NORVIR as monotherapy or in combination with nucleoside reverse transcriptase inhibitors has been evaluated in 1446 patients enrolled in two double-blind, randomized trials.

14.1 Advanced Patients with Prior Antiretroviral Therapy

Study 247 was a randomized, double-blind trial (with open-label follow-up) conducted in HIV-infected patients with at least nine months of prior antiretroviral therapy and baseline CD_4 cell counts $\leq$100 cells/μL. NORVIR 600 mg twice-daily or placebo was added to each patient's baseline anti-

retroviral therapy regimen, which could have consisted of up to two approved antiretroviral agents. The study accrued 1090 patients, with mean baseline CD_4 cell count at study entry of 32 cells/μL. After the clinical benefit of NORVIR therapy was demonstrated, all patients were eligible to switch to open-label NORVIR for the duration of the follow-up period. Median duration of double-blind therapy with NORVIR and placebo was 6 months. The median duration of follow-up through the end of the open-label phase was 13.5 months for patients randomized to NORVIR and 14 months for patients randomized to placebo.

The cumulative incidence of clinical disease progression or death during the double-blind phase of Study 247 was 26% for patients initially randomized to NORVIR compared to 42% for patients initially randomized to placebo. This difference in rates was statistically significant (see Figure 1). [See figure at top of next column]

The cumulative mortality through the end of the open-label follow-up phase for patients enrolled in Study 247 was 18% for patients initially randomized to NORVIR compared to 26% for patients initially randomized to placebo. This difference in rates was statistically significant (see Figure 2).

Table 5 *(cont.)*. Established and Other Potentially Significant Drug Interactions

Concomitant Drug Class: Drug Name	Effect on Concentration of Ritonavir or Concomitant Drug	Clinical Comment
Other Agents (continued)		
Long-acting beta-adrenoceptor agonist: salmeterol	↑ salmeterol	Concurrent administration of salmeterol and ritonavir is not recommended. The combination may result in increased risk of cardiovascular adverse events associated with salmeterol, including QT prolongation, palpitations and sinus tachycardia.
Narcotic Analgesic: methadone	↓ methadone	Dosage increase of methadone may be considered.
Neuroleptics: perphenazine, risperidone, thioridazine	↑ neuroleptics	A dose decrease may be needed for these drugs when co-administered with ritonavir.
Oral Contraceptives or Patch Contraceptives: ethinyl estradiol	↓ ethinyl estradiol	A pharmacokinetic study demonstrated that the concomitant administration of ritonavir 500 mg q. 12h. and a fixed-combination oral contraceptive resulted in reductions of the ethinyl estradiol mean C_{max} and mean AUC by 32% and 40%, respectively. Alternate methods of contraception should be considered.
PDE5 Inhibitors: sildenafil, tadalafil, vardenafil	↑ sildenafil ↑ tadalafil ↑ vardenafil	Particular caution should be used when prescribing sildenafil, tadalafil or vardenafil in patients receiving ritonavir. Co-administration of ritonavir with these drugs is expected to substantially increase their concentrations and may result in an increase in PDE5 inhibitor associated adverse events, including hypotension, syncope, visual changes, and prolonged erection. Use of PDE5 inhibitors for pulmonary arterial hypertension (PAH): Sildenafil (Revatio®) is contraindicated when used for the treatment of pulmonary arterial hypertension (PAH) because a safe and effective dose has not been established when used with ritonavir *[see Contraindications (4)]*. The following dose adjustments are recommended for use of tadalafil (Adcirca™) with ritonavir: Co-administration of ADCIRCA in patients on ritonavir: In patients receiving ritonavir for at least one week, start ADCIRCA at 20 mg once daily. Increase to 40 mg once daily based upon individual tolerability. Co-administration of ritonavir in patients on ADCIRCA: Avoid use of ADCIRCA during the initiation of ritonavir. Stop ADCIRCA at least 24 hours prior to starting ritonavir. After at least one week following the initiation of ritonavir, resume ADCIRCA at 20 mg once daily. Increase to 40 mg once daily based upon individual tolerability. Use of PDE5 inhibitors for the treatment of erectile dysfunction: It is recommended not to exceed the following doses: • Sildenafil: 25 mg every 48 hours • Tadalafil: 10 mg every 72 hours • Vardenafil: 2.5 mg every 72 hours. Use with increased monitoring for adverse events.
Sedative/hypnotics: buspirone, clorazepate, diazepam, estazolam, flurazepam, zolpidem	↑ sedative/hypnotics	A dose decrease may be needed for these drugs when co-administered with ritonavir.
Sedative/hypnotics: Parenteral midazolam	↑ midazolam	Co-administration of oral midazolam with NORVIR is CONTRAINDICATED. Concomitant use of parenteral midazolam with NORVIR may increase plasma concentrations of midazolam. Co-administration should be done in a setting which ensures close clinical monitoring and appropriate medical management in case of respiratory depression and/or prolonged sedation. Dosage reduction for midazolam should be considered, especially if more than a single dose of midazolam is administered.
Steroids: dexamethasone, fluticasone, prednisone		A dose decrease may be needed for these drugs when co-administered with ritonavir.
Stimulant: methamphetamine	↑ methamphetamine	Use with caution. A dose decrease of methamphetamine may be needed when co-administered with ritonavir.

Table 7. Drug Interactions - Pharmacokinetic Parameters for Ritonavir in the Presence of the Co-administered Drug

Co-administered Drug	Dose of Co-administered Drug (mg)	Dose of NORVIR (mg)	N	AUC % (95% CI)	Cmax (95% CI)	Cmin (95% CI)
Clarithromycin	500 q12h, 4 d	200 q8h, 4 d	22	↑ 12% (2, 23%)	↑ 15% (2, 28%)	↑ 14% (-3, 36%)
Didanosine	200 q12h, 4 d	600 q12h, 4 d	12	↔	↔	↔
Fluconazole	400 single dose, day 1; 200 daily, 4 d	200 q6h, 4 d	8	↑ 12% (5, 20%)	↑ 15% (7, 22%)	↑ 14% (0, 26%)
Fluoxetine	30 q12h, 8 d	600 single dose, 1 d	16	↑ 19% (7, 34%)	↑ 15% (7, 22%)	ND
Ketoconazole	200 daily, 7 d	500 q12h, 10 d	12	↑ 18% (-3, 52%)	↑ 10% (-11, 36%)	ND
Rifampin	600 or 300 daily, 10 d	500 q12h, 20 d	7, 9*	↓ 35% (7, 55%)	↓ 25% (-5, 46%)	↓ 49% (-14, 91%)
Voriconazole	400 q12h, 1 d; then 200 q12h, 8 d	400 q12h, 9 d		↔	↔	ND
Zidovudine	200 q8h, 4 d	300 q6h, 4 d	10	↔	↔	↔

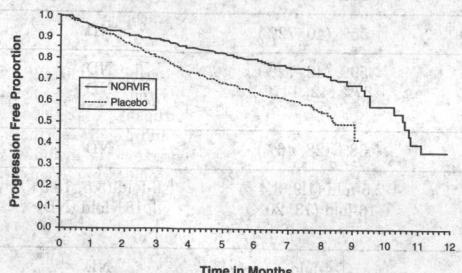

Figure 1. Time to Disease Progression or Death During the Double-blind Phase of Study 247

Since the analysis at the end of the open-label phase includes patients in the placebo arm who were switched from placebo to NORVIR therapy, the survival benefit of NORVIR cannot be precisely estimated.

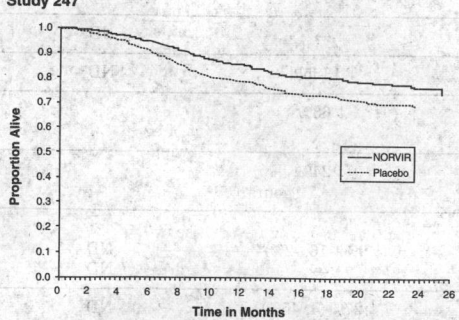

Figure 2. Survival of Patients by Randomized Regimen in Study 247

Figure 3 and Figure 4 summarize the mean change from baseline for CD4 cell count and plasma HIV RNA (copies/mL), respectively, during the first 24 weeks for the double-blind phase of Study 247.

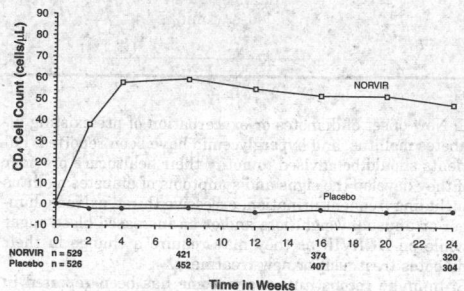

Figure 3. Mean Change from Baseline in CD4 Cell Count (cells/μL) During the Double-blind Phase of Study 247

[See figure at top of next column]

14.2   Patients without Prior Antiretroviral Therapy

In Study 245, 356 antiretroviral-naive HIV-infected patients (mean baseline CD4 = 364 cells/μL) were randomized to receive either NORVIR 600 mg twice-daily, zidovudine 200 mg three-times-daily, or a combination of these drugs. Figure 5 and Figure 6 summarize the mean change from baseline for CD4 cell count and plasma HIV RNA (copies/

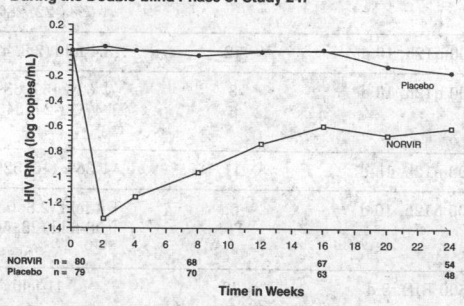

Figure 4. Mean Change from Baseline in HIV RNA (log copies/mL) During the Double-blind Phase of Study 247

mL), respectively, during the first 24 weeks for the double-blind phase of Study 245.

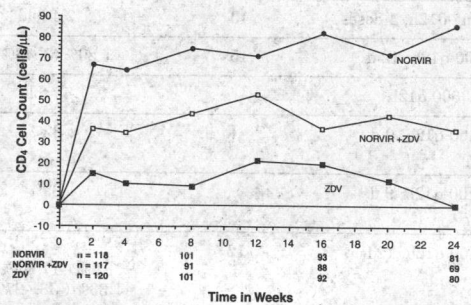

Figure 5. Mean Change from Baseline in CD4 Cell Count (cells/μL) During Study 245

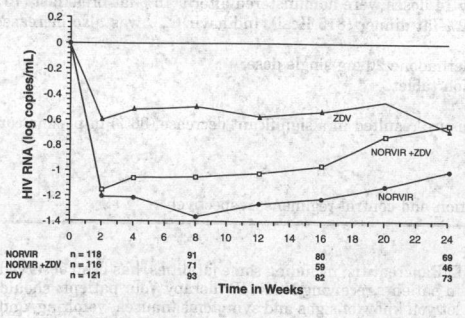

Figure 6. Mean Change from Baseline in HIV RNA (log copies/mL) During Study 245

15   REFERENCES

1. Sewester CS. Calculations. In: Drug Facts and Comparisons. St. Louis, MO: J.B. Lippincott Co; January, 1997: xix.

16   HOW SUPPLIED/STORAGE AND HANDLING

NORVIR (ritonavir) tablets and NORVIR (ritonavir) oral solution are available in the following strengths and package sizes:

16.1   NORVIR Tablets, 100 mg Ritonavir

NORVIR (ritonavir) tablets are white film-coated ovaloid tablets debossed with the corporate Abbott ☐ logo and the Abbo-Code NK.

Bottles of 30 tablets each (**NDC** 0074-3333-30).

Recommended Storage

Store NORVIR film-coated tablets at 20°-25°C (68°-77°F); excursions permitted to 15°-30°C (59°-86°F) [see USP controlled room temperature]. Dispense in original container or USP equivalent tight container (60 mL or less). For patient use: exposure of this product to high humidity outside the original or USP equivalent tight container (60 mL or less) for longer than 2 weeks is not recommended.

16.2   NORVIR Oral Solution, 80 mg/mL Ritonavir

NORVIR (ritonavir) oral solution is an orange-colored liquid, supplied in amber-colored, multi-dose bottles containing 600 mg ritonavir per 7.5 mL marked dosage cup (80 mg/mL).

240 mL bottles (**NDC** 0074-1940-63).

Recommended Storage

Store NORVIR oral solution at room temperature 20°-25°C (68°-77°F). Do not refrigerate. Shake well before each use. Use by product expiration date.

Product should be stored and dispensed in the original container.

Avoid exposure to excessive heat. Keep cap tightly closed.

17   PATIENT COUNSELING INFORMATION

See FDA-Approved Patient Labeling

Information For Patients

Patients or parents of patients should be informed that:

General Information

☐ They should pay special attention to accurate administration of their dose to minimize the risk of accidental overdose or underdose of NORVIR.

☐ They should inform their healthcare provider if their children's weight changes in order to make sure that the child's NORVIR dose is the correct one.

☐ Take NORVIR with meals.

☐ For adult patients taking NORVIR tablets, the maximum dose of 600 mg twice daily by mouth with meals should not be exceeded.

☐ Patients should remain under the care of a physician while using NORVIR. Patients should be advised to take NORVIR and other concomitant antiretroviral therapy every day as prescribed. NORVIR must always be used in combination with other antiretroviral drugs. Patients should not alter the dose or discontinue therapy without consulting with their doctor. If a dose of NORVIR is missed patients should take the dose as soon as possible and then return to their normal schedule. However, if a dose is skipped the patient should not double the next dose.

☐ NORVIR is not a cure for HIV-1 infection and that they may continue to develop opportunistic infections and other complications associated with HIV-1 disease. The long-term effects of NORVIR are unknown at this time. Patients should be told that there are currently no data demonstrating that therapy with NORVIR can reduce the risk of transmitting HIV-1 to others through sexual contact, sharing needles, or being exposed to their blood. For their health and the health of others, it is important that they always practice safer sex by using a latex or polyurethane condom or other barrier method to lower the chance of sexual contact with any body fluids such as semen, vaginal secretions, or blood. They should also be advised to never re-use or share needles.

☐ Sustained decreases in plasma HIV-1 RNA have been associated with a reduced risk of progression to AIDS and death.

Information on the Abbott Pharmaceutical Products listed on these pages is from the prescribing information in use as of June 1, 2010. For more information, please visit rxabbott.com or call 1-800-633-9110.

Table 8. Drug Interactions - Pharmacokinetic Parameters for Co-administered Drug in the Presence of NORVIR

Co-administered Drug	Dose of Co-administered Drug (mg)	Dose of NORVIR (mg)	N	AUC % (95% CI)	C$_{max}$ (95% CI)	C$_{min}$ (95% CI)
Alprazolam	1, single dose	500 q12h, 10 d	12	↓ 12% (-5, 30%)	↓ 16% (5, 27%)	ND
Clarithromycin 14-OH clarithromycin metabolite	500 q12h, 4 d	200 q8h, 4 d	22	↑ 77% (56, 103%) ↓ 100%	↑ 31% (15, 51%) ↓ 99%	↑ 2.8-fold (2.4, 3.3×) ↓ 100%
Desipramine 2-OH desipramine metabolite	100, single dose	500 q12h, 12 d	14	↑ 145% (103, 211%) ↓ 15% (3, 26%)	↑ 22% (12, 35%) ↓ 67% (62, 72%)	ND ND
Didanosine	200 q12h, 4 d	600 q12h, 4 d	12	↓ 13% (0, 23%)	↓ 16% (5, 26%)	↔
Ethinyl estradiol	50 μg single dose	500 q12h, 16 d	23	↓ 40% (31, 49%)	↓ 32% (24, 39%)	ND
Fluticasone propionate aqueous nasal spray	200 mcg qd, 7 d	100 mg q12h, 7 d	18	↑ approximately 350-fold[5]	↑ approximately 25-fold[5]	
Indinavir[1] Day 14 Day 15	400 q12h, 15 d	400 q12h, 15 d	10	↑ 6% (-14, 29%) ↓ 7% (-22, 28%)	↓ 51% (40, 61%) ↓ 62% (52, 70%)	↑ 4-fold (2.8, 6.8×) ↑ 4-fold (2.5, 6.5×)
Ketoconazole	200 daily, 7 d	500 q12h, 10 d	12	↑ 3.4-fold (2.8, 4.3×)	↑ 55% (40, 72%)	ND
Meperidine Normeperidine metabolite	50 oral single dose	500 q12h, 10 d	8 6	↓ 62% (59, 65%) ↑ 47% (-24, 345%)	↓ 59% (42, 72%) ↑ 87% (42, 147%)	ND ND
Methadone[2]	5, single dose	500 q12h, 15 d	11	↓ 36% (16, 52%)	↓ 38% (28, 46%)	ND
Rifabutin 25-O-desacetyl rifabutin metabolite	150 daily, 16 d	500 q12h, 10 d	5, 11*	↑ 4-fold (2.8, 6.1×) ↑ 38-fold (28, 56×)	↑ 2.5-fold (1.9, 3.4×) ↑ 16-fold (13, 20×)	↑ 6-fold (3.5, 18.3×) ↑ 181-fold (ND)
Sildenafil	100, single dose	500 BID, 8 d	28	↑ 11-fold	↑ 4-fold	ND
Sulfamethoxazole[3]	800, single dose	500 q12h, 12 d	15	↓ 20% (16, 23%)	↔	ND
Tadalafil	20 mg, single dose	200 mg q12h		↑ 124%	↔	ND
Theophylline	3 mg/kg q8h, 15 d	500 q12h, 10 d	13, 11*	↓ 43% (42, 45%)	↓ 32% (29, 34%)	↓ 57% (55, 59%)
Trazodone	50 mg, single dose	200 mg q12h, 4 doses	10	↑ 2.4-fold	↑ 34%	
Trimethoprim[3]	160, single dose	500 q12h, 12 d	15	↑ 20% (3, 43%)	↔	ND
Vardenafil	5 mg	600 q12h		↑ 49-fold	↑ 13-fold	ND
Voriconazole	400 q12h, 1 d; then 200 q12h, 8 d	400 q12h, 9 d		↓ 82%	↓ 66%	
	400 q12h, 1 d; then 200 q12h, 8 d	100 q12h, 9 d		↓ 39%	↓ 24%	
Warfarin S-Warfarin R-Warfarin	5, single dose	400 q12h, 12d	12	↑ 9% (-17, 44%)[4] ↓ 33% (-38, -27%)[4]	↓ 9% (-16, -2%)[4] ↔	ND ND
Zidovudine	200 q8h, 4 d	300 q6h, 4 d	9	↓ 25% (15, 34%)	↓ 27% (4, 45%)	ND

[1]Ritonavir and indinavir were co-administered for 15 days; Day 14 doses were administered after a 15%-fat breakfast (757 Kcal) and 9%-fat evening snack (236 Kcal), and Day 15 doses were administered after a 15%-fat breakfast (757 Kcal) and 32%-fat dinner (815 Kcal). Indinavir C$_{min}$ was also increased 4-fold. Effects were assessed relative to an indinavir 800 mg q8h regimen under fasting conditions.
[2]Effects were assessed on a dose-normalized comparison to a methadone 20 mg single dose.
[3]Sulfamethoxazole and trimethoprim taken as single combination tablet.
[4]90% CI presented for R- and S-warfarin AUC and C$_{max}$ ratios.
[5]This significant increase in plasma fluticasone propionate exposure resulted in a significant decrease (86%) in plasma cortisol AUC.
↑ Indicates increase.
↓ Indicates decrease.
↔ Indicates no change.
* Parallel group design; entries are subjects receiving combination and control regimens, respectively.

Drug Interactions
□ NORVIR may interact with some drugs; therefore, patients should be advised to report to their doctor the use of any other prescription, non-prescription medication or herbal products, particularly St. John's Wort.
□ If they are receiving estrogen-based hormonal contraceptives, additional or alternate contraceptive measures should be used during therapy with NORVIR.

Potential Adverse Effects
□ Pre-existing liver disease including Hepatitis B or C can worsen with use of NORVIR. This can be seen as worsening of transaminase elevations or hepatic decompensation. Patients should be advised that their liver function tests will need to be monitored closely especially during the first several months of NORVIR treatment and that they should notify their healthcare provider if they develop the signs and symptoms of worsening liver disease including loss of appetite, abdominal pain, jaundice, and itchy skin.

□ Pancreatitis, including some fatalities, has been observed in patients receiving NORVIR therapy. Your patients should let you know of signs and symptoms (nausea, vomiting, and abdominal pain) that might be suggestive of pancreatitis.
□ Skin rashes ranging in severity from mild to Stevens Johnson syndrome have been reported in patients receiving NORVIR. Patients should be advised to contact their healthcare provider if they develop a rash while taking NORVIR. The healthcare provider will determine if treatment should be continued or an alternative antiretroviral regimen used.
□ NORVIR may produce changes in the electrocardiogram (e.g., PR prolongation). Patients should consult their physician if they experience symptoms such as dizziness, lightheadedness, abnormal heart rhythm or loss of consciousness.
□ Treatment with NORVIR therapy can result in substantial increases in the concentration of total cholesterol and triglycerides.

□ New onset of diabetes or exacerbation of pre-existing diabetes mellitus, and hyperglycemia have been reported. Patients should be advised to notify their healthcare provider if they develop the signs and symptoms of diabetes mellitus including frequent urination, excessive thirst, extreme hunger or unusual weight loss and/or an increased blood sugar while on NORVIR as they may require a change in their diabetes treatment or new treatment.
□ Immune reconstitution syndrome has been reported in HIV-infected patients treated with combination antiretroviral therapy, including NORVIR.
□ Redistribution or accumulation of body fat may occur in patients receiving antiretroviral therapy and that the cause and long term health effects of these conditions are not known at this time.
□ Patients with hemophilia may experience increased bleeding when treated with protease inhibitors such as NORVIR.

☐ If they are receiving sildenafil, tadalafil, or vardenafil, they may be at an increased risk of associated adverse reactions including hypotension, visual changes, and sustained erection, and should promptly report any symptoms to their doctor. They should seek medical assistance immediately if they develop a sustained penile erection lasting more than 4 hours while taking NORVIR and a PDE 5 Inhibitor such as Viagra®, Cialis® or Levitra®. Concomitant use of Revatio® (sildenafil) with NORVIR is contraindicated in patients with pulmonary arterial hypertension (PAH).

☐ Continued NORVIR therapy at a dose of 600 mg twice daily following loss of viral suppression may increase the likelihood of cross-resistance to other protease inhibitors.

Abbott Laboratories
North Chicago, IL 60064, U.S.A.
Rev. 04/2010

FDA-Approved Patient Labeling

NORVIR®
(ritonavir) tablets
(ritonavir) oral solution

ALERT: Find out about medicines that should NOT be taken with NORVIR. Please also read the section "MEDICINES YOU SHOULD NOT TAKE WITH NORVIR."

Patient Information

NORVIR® (NOR - VEER)

Generic name: ritonavir (rit-ON-uh-veer)

Please read this leaflet carefully before you start taking NORVIR. Also, read it each time you get your NORVIR prescription refilled, just in case something has changed. Remember that this information does not take the place of careful discussions with your doctor when you start this medication and at check ups.

You should remain under a doctor's care when taking NORVIR and you should not change or stop treatment without first talking with your doctor.

You should tell your doctor about any medicine you are taking or planning to take because taking NORVIR with some medications can result in serious or life-threatening problems.

Talk to your doctor if you have any questions about NORVIR. Your doctor or pharmacist can also give you more information about NORVIR.

What is NORVIR and How Does It Work?

NORVIR is in a class of medicines called the HIV protease (PRO-tee-ase) inhibitors. NORVIR is used in combination with other anti-HIV medicines to treat people with human immunodeficiency virus (HIV) infection. NORVIR is for adults and for children age greater than 1 month and older. NORVIR can be used at the full dose on its own, or at lower doses with other protease inhibitors.

HIV infection leads to the destruction of CD_4 (T) cells, which are important to the immune system. After a large number of CD_4 (T) cells have been destroyed, acquired immune deficiency syndrome (AIDS) develops.

NORVIR blocks HIV protease, a chemical which is needed for HIV to multiply. When used with other HIV medicines, NORVIR may reduce the amount of HIV in your blood and increase the number of CD_4 (T) cells. Patients who took NORVIR in clinical studies had significant reductions in both death and AIDS defining diseases; however NORVIR may not have these effects in all patients.

Does NORVIR Cure HIV or AIDS?

NORVIR does not cure HIV infection or AIDS. The long-term effects of NORVIR are not known at this time. People taking NORVIR may still get opportunistic infections or other conditions that happen with HIV infection. Some of these conditions are pneumonia, herpes virus infections, and *Mycobacterium avium* complex (MAC) infections.

Does NORVIR Reduce the Risk of Passing HIV to Others?

NORVIR does not reduce the risk of passing HIV to others through sexual contact or blood contamination. Continue to practice safe sex and do not use or share dirty needles.

How Should I Take NORVIR?

- You should stay under a doctor's care when taking NORVIR. Do not change your treatment or stop treatment without first talking with your doctor.
- It is very important that you take NORVIR every day exactly as your doctor prescribed it.
- The usual dose for adults is six 100 mg tablets or 7.5 mL of the oral solution twice a day (morning and night), in combination with other anti-HIV medicines.
- The dosing of NORVIR may be different for you than for other patients. Follow the directions from your doctor, exactly as written on the label.
- Children from greater than 1 month to 18 years of age can also take NORVIR. The child's doctor will decide the right dose based on the child's height and weight.
- NORVIR tablets should be swallowed whole, and not chewed, broken, or crushed.
- Take NORVIR with meals.
- NORVIR Oral Solution is peppermint/caramel flavored. You can take it alone, or may improve the taste by mixing it with 8 ounces of chocolate milk, Ensure®, or Advera®. NORVIR Oral Solution should be taken within 1 hour if mixed with these items. Ask your doctor, nurse or pharmacist about other ways to improve the taste of NORVIR Oral Solution.
- If a young child drinks more than recommended dose of NORVIR oral solution, contact your local poison control center or emergency room right away.
- Talk with your doctor if you take or plan to take Flagyl® (metronidazole) or Antabuse® (disulfiram) with NORVIR oral solution. You can have severe nausea and vomiting if you take these medicines with NORVIR.
- Do not change or stop taking NORVIR without first talking with your health care provider.
- When your NORVIR supply starts to run low, get more from your doctor or pharmacy. This is very important because the amount of virus in your blood may increase if the medicine is stopped for even a short time. The virus may develop resistance to NORVIR and become harder to treat.
- Be sure to set up a schedule and follow it carefully.
- Only take medicine that has been prescribed specifically for you. Do not give NORVIR to others or take medicine prescribed for someone else.

What Should I Do if I Miss a Dose of NORVIR?

It is important that you do not miss any doses. If you miss a dose of NORVIR, take it as soon as possible and then take your next scheduled dose at its regular time. If it is almost time for your next dose, wait and take the next dose at the regular time. Do not double the next dose.

What Happens If I Take Too Much NORVIR?

If you think that you took more than the prescribed dose of this medicine, contact your local poison control center or emergency room immediately.

As with all prescription medicines, NORVIR should be kept out of the reach of young children. NORVIR liquid contains a large amount of alcohol. If a toddler or young child accidentally drinks more than the recommended dose of NORVIR, it could make him/her sick from too much alcohol. Contact your local poison control center or emergency room immediately if this happens.

Who Should Not Take NORVIR?

Together with your doctor, you need to decide whether NORVIR is right for you.

- Do not take NORVIR if you are taking certain medicines. These could cause serious side effects that could cause death. Before you take NORVIR, you must tell your doctor about all the medicines you are taking or are planning to take. These include other prescription and non-prescription medicines and herbal supplements.

For more information about medicines you should not take with NORVIR, please read the section "MEDICINES YOU SHOULD NOT TAKE WITH NORVIR."

- Do not take NORVIR if you have had a serious allergic reaction to NORVIR or any of its ingredients.

Can I Take NORVIR With Other Medications?*

NORVIR may interact with other medicines, including those you take without a prescription. You must tell your doctor about all the medicines you are taking or are planning to take.

MEDICINES YOU SHOULD NOT TAKE WITH NORVIR.

- *Do not take the following medicines with NORVIR because they can cause serious or life-threatening problems such as irregular heartbeat, breathing difficulties, or excessive sleepiness:*
  - Cordarone® (amiodarone)
  - Ergotamine, ergonovine, methylergonovine, and dihydroergotamine such as Cafergot®, Migranal®, D.H.E 45®, and others
  - Halcion® (triazolam)
  - Orap® (pimozide)
  - Propulsid® (cisapride)
  - Quinidine, also known as Quinaglute®, Cardioquin®, Quinidex®, and others
  - Revatio® (sildenafil) only when used for the treatment of pulmonary arterial hypertension
  - Rythmol® (propafenone)
  - Tambocor® (flecainide)
  - Uroxatral® (alfuzosin hydrochloride)
  - Vascor® (bepridil)
  - Versed® (oral midazolam)
  - Vfend® (voriconazole)
- Do not take NORVIR with St. John's Wort (hypericum perforatum), an herbal product sold as a dietary supplement or products containing St. John's Wort. Talk with your doctor if you are taking or are planning to take St. John's Wort. Taking St. John's Wort may decrease NORVIR levels and lead to increased viral load and possible resistance to NORVIR or cross-resistance to other antiretroviral medicines.
- Do not take NORVIR with the cholesterol-lowering medicines Mevacor® (lovastatin) or Zocor® (simvastatin) because of possible serious reactions. There is also an increased risk of drug interactions between NORVIR and Lipitor® (atorvastatin) and Crestor® (rosuvastatin); talk to your doctor before you take any of these cholesterol-lowering medicines with NORVIR.

Medicines That May Require Dosage Adjustments

It is possible that your doctor may need to increase or decrease the dose of other medicines when you are also taking NORVIR. Remember to tell your doctor all medicines you are taking or plan to take.

- The following medicines require dose reduction if taken with NORVIR:

If you are taking PDE5 inhibitors for erectile dysfunction including Viagra® (sildenafil), Cialis® (tadalafil), or Levitra® (vardenafil), your doctor may lower your dose of these medications. You should not use sildenafil (Revatio®) with NORVIR if you are being treated for pulmonary arterial hypertension. If you are taking Adcirca™ (tadalafil) for pulmonary arterial hypertension, your doctor may change your dose of this medicine.

Before you take Viagra®, Cialis® or Levitra® with NORVIR, talk to your doctor about possible drug interactions and side effects. If you take these medications with NORVIR you may be at risk of side effects such as low blood pressure, visual changes, and penile erection lasting more than 4 hours. If an erection lasts longer than 4 hours, you should get medical help immediately to avoid permanent damage to your penis. Your doctor can explain these symptoms to you.

- If you are taking Oral contraceptives ("the pill") or the contraceptive patch to prevent pregnancy, you should use a different type of contraception since NORVIR may reduce the effectiveness of oral or patch contraceptives.
- If you are taking Mycobutin® (rifabutin), your doctor will lower the dose of Mycobutin®.
- If you are taking Colcrys® (colchicine), your doctor will tell you what dose to use.
- If you are taking Tracleer® (bosentan), your doctor will tell you what dose to use.
- *Other Special Considerations:*

NORVIR oral solution contains alcohol. Talk with your doctor if you are taking or planning to take Flagyl® (metronidazole) or Antabuse® (disulfiram). Severe nausea and vomiting can occur.

- Rifampin, also known as Rimactane®, Rifadin®, Rifater®, or Rifamate®, may reduce blood levels of NORVIR. Be sure to tell your doctor if you are taking rifampin.
- Rifampin and saquinavir should not be taken with NORVIR. Be sure to tell your doctor if you are taking rifampin and saquinavir.
- If you are taking or before you begin using inhaled Flonase® (fluticasone propionate), talk to your doctor about problems these two medicines may cause when taken together. Your doctor may choose not to keep you on inhaled Flonase®.
- If you are taking or before you begin using Serevent® (salmeterol) and NORVIR, talk to your doctor about problems these medicines may cause when taken together. Your doctor may choose not to keep you on Serevent® (salmeterol).
- If you are taking or before you begin using Advair® (salmeterol in combination with fluticasone propionate) and NORVIR, talk to your doctor about problems these two medicines may cause when taken together. Your doctor may choose not to keep you on Advair® (salmeterol in combination with fluticasone propionate).

What Are the Possible Side Effects of NORVIR?

- This list of side effects is not complete. If you have questions about side effects, ask your doctor, nurse, or pharmacist. You should report any new or continuing symptoms to your doctor right away. Your doctor may be able to help you manage these side effects.
- The most commonly reported side effects are: feeling weak/tired, nausea, vomiting, diarrhea, loss of appetite, abdominal pain, changes in taste, tingling feeling or numbness in hands or feet or around the lips, headache, and dizziness.
- Blood tests in patients taking NORVIR may show possible liver problems. People with liver disease such as Hepatitis B and Hepatitis C who take NORVIR may have worsening liver disease. Liver problems including rare cases of death have occurred in patients taking NORVIR. It is unclear if NORVIR caused these liver problems because some patients had other illnesses or were taking other medicines. Tell your healthcare provider right away if you have any of these signs and symptoms of liver problems:
  - loss of appetite
  - yellow skin and whites of eyes (jaundice)

Information on the Abbott Pharmaceutical Products listed on these pages is from the prescribing information in use as of June 1, 2010. For more information, please visit rxabbott.com or call 1-800-633-9110.

  - dark-colored urine, pale colored stools and itchy skin
  - stomach area (abdominal) pain.
- Liver disease, such as hepatitis and worsening liver function, resulting in death, have occurred in patients taking Aptivus® (tipranavir) with NORVIR. Extra care should be taken if you also have chronic hepatitis B or hepatitis C.
- Some patients taking NORVIR can develop serious problems with their pancreas (pancreatitis) which may cause death. Tell your doctor if you have nausea, vomiting, or abdominal pain. These may be signs of pancreatitis.
- Some patients have large increases in triglycerides and cholesterol. The long-term chance of getting complications such as heart attacks or stroke due to increases in triglycerides and cholesterol caused by protease inhibitors is not known at this time.
- Diabetes and high blood sugar (hyperglycemia) have occurred in patients taking protease inhibitors. Some patients had diabetes before starting protease inhibitors, others did not. Some patients need changes in their diabetes medication. Others needed new diabetes medication.
- Changes in body fat have been seen in some patients taking antiretroviral therapy. These changes may include increased amount of fat in the upper back and neck ("buffalo hump"), breast and around the trunk. Loss of fat from the legs, arms and face may also happen. The cause and long term health effects of these conditions are not known at this time.
- Some patients with hemophilia have increased bleeding with protease inhibitors, including NORVIR.
- Allergic reactions ranging from hives, asthma, severe breathing issues and mild to severe skin reactions have occurred in patients taking NORVIR.
- Changes in the electrocardiogram (EKG). Consult your physician if you experience dizziness, lightheadedness, fainting spells or abnormal heart beat. Patients with heart defects or conduction defects should avoid NORVIR.

There have been other side effects noted in patients receiving NORVIR; however, these side effects may have been due to other medicines that patients were taking or to the illness itself. Some of these side effects can be serious. Let your doctor know about medications you are taking.

If you have questions about side effects, ask your doctor, nurse, or pharmacist. You should report any new or persistent symptoms to your doctor immediately.

What Should I Tell My Doctor Before Taking NORVIR?

- *If you are pregnant or planning to become pregnant:* It is not known if NORVIR can harm your unborn baby. You and your healthcare professional will need to decide if NORVIR is right for you. If you take NORVIR while you are pregnant, talk to your healthcare professional about how you can take part in the Antiretroviral Pregnancy Registry.
- *If you are breast-feeding:* Mothers should not breast-feed if they are taking NORVIR. It is not known whether ritonavir is passed to the baby through breast milk or whether the baby could experience side effects as a result. If you are HIV positive, you may pass HIV onto your baby. If you are a woman who has or will have a baby, talk with your doctor about the best way to feed your baby.
- *If you have liver problems:* If you have liver problems or are infected with Hepatitis B or Hepatitis C, you should tell your doctor before taking NORVIR.
- *If you have diabetes:* Some people taking protease inhibitors develop new or more serious diabetes or high blood sugar. Be sure to tell your doctor if you have diabetes or an increase in thirst and/or frequent urination.
- *If you have hemophilia:* Some people with hemophilia have had increased bleeding. It is not known whether the protease inhibitors caused these problems. Be sure to tell your doctor if you have hemophilia types A and B.

How Do I Store NORVIR?

- Keep NORVIR and all other medicines out of the reach of children.
- Store NORVIR Oral Solution at room temperature. Do not refrigerate NORVIR Oral Solution. Avoid exposing NORVIR Oral Solution to excessive heat or cold.
- Store NORVIR film-coated tablets at 20°-25°C (68°-77°F); excursions permitted to 15°-30°C (59°-86° F) [Room temperature]. For patient use: exposure of this product to high humidity outside the original or USP equivalent tight container (60 mL or less) for longer than 2 weeks is not recommended.
- Store NORVIR tablets and NORVIR Oral Solution in the original container or container given to you by the pharmacist.
- Shake NORVIR Oral Solution well before each use.
- Use NORVIR tablets and NORVIR Oral Solution by the expiration date on the bottle.

Do not keep medicine that is out of date or that you no longer need. Be sure that if you throw any medicine away, it is out of the reach of children.

General Advice About Prescription Medicines

Talk to your doctor or other health care provider if you have any questions or concerns about this medicine or your condition. Medicines are sometimes prescribed for purposes other than those listed in a Patient Information Leaflet. Your doctor or pharmacist can give you information about this medicine that was written for health care professionals. Do not use this medicine for a condition for which it was not prescribed. Do not share this medicine with other people.

* The brands listed are trademarks of their respective owners and are not trademarks of Abbott Laboratories. The makers of these brands are not affiliated with and do not endorse Abbott Laboratories or its products.

Abbott Laboratories
North Chicago, IL 60064, U.S.A.
Ref. 03-A359-Revised April, 2010

Shown in Product Identification Guide, page 304

OMNICEF® ℞

[omnē-sĕf]
(cefdinir) Capsules

OMNICEF®

(cefdinir) For Oral Suspension

To reduce the development of drug-resistant bacteria and maintain the effectiveness of OMNICEF and other antibacterial drugs, OMNICEF should be used only to treat or prevent infections that are proven or strongly suspected to be caused by bacteria.

DESCRIPTION

OMNICEF® (cefdinir) capsules and OMNICEF® (cefdinir) for oral suspension contain the active ingredient cefdinir, an extended-spectrum, semisynthetic cephalosporin, for oral administration. Chemically, cefdinir is [6R-[6α,7β (Z)]]-7-[[(2-amino-4-thiazolyl)(hydroxyimino)acetyl]amino]-3-ethenyl-8-oxo-5-thia-1-azabicyclo[4.2.0]oct-2-ene-2-carboxylic acid. Cefdinir is a white to slightly brownish-yellow solid. It is slightly soluble in dilute hydrochloric acid and sparingly soluble in 0.1 M pH 7.0 phosphate buffer. The empirical formula is $C_{14}H_{13}N_5O_5S_2$ and the molecular weight is 395.42. Cefdinir has the structural formula shown below:

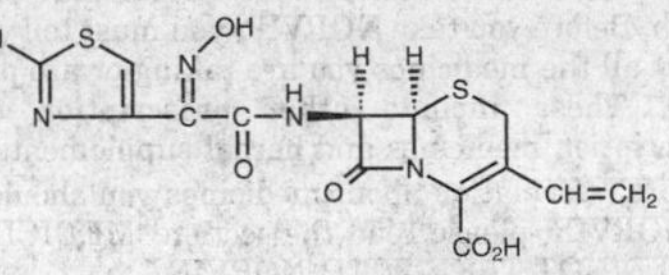

OMNICEF Capsules contain 300 mg cefdinir and the following inactive ingredients: carboxymethylcellulose calcium, NF; polyoxyl 40 stearate, NF; and magnesium stearate, NF. The capsule shells contain FD&C Blue #1; FD&C Red #40; D&C Red #28; titanium dioxide, NF; gelatin, NF; silicon dioxide, NF; and sodium lauryl sulfate, NF.

OMNICEF for Oral Suspension, after reconstitution, contains 125 mg cefdinir per 5 mL or 250 mg cefdinir per 5 mL and the following inactive ingredients: sucrose, NF; citric acid, USP; sodium citrate, USP; sodium benzoate, NF; xanthan gum, NF; guar gum, NF; artificial strawberry and cream flavors; silicon dioxide, NF; and magnesium stearate, NF.

CLINICAL PHARMACOLOGY

Pharmacokinetics and Drug Metabolism

Absorption

Oral Bioavailability

Maximal plasma cefdinir concentrations occur 2 to 4 hours postdose following capsule or suspension administration. Plasma cefdinir concentrations increase with dose, but the increases are less than dose-proportional from 300 mg (7 mg/kg) to 600 mg (14 mg/kg). Following administration of suspension to healthy adults, cefdinir bioavailability is 120% relative to capsules. Estimated bioavailability of cefdinir capsules is 21% following administration of a 300 mg capsule dose, and 16% following administration of a 600 mg capsule dose. Estimated absolute bioavailability of cefdinir suspension is 25%. Cefdinir oral suspension of 250 mg/5 mL strength was shown to be bioequivalent to the 125 mg/5 mL strength in healthy adults under fasting conditions.

Effect of Food

The C_{max} and AUC of cefdinir from the capsules are reduced by 16% and 10%, respectively, when given with a high-fat meal. In adults given the 250 mg/5 mL oral suspension with a high-fat meal, the C_{max} and AUC of cefdinir are reduced by 44% and 33%, respectively. The magnitude of these reductions is not likely to be clinically significant because the safety and efficacy studies of oral suspension in pediatric patients were conducted without regard to food intake. Therefore, cefdinir may be taken without regard to food.

Cefdinir Capsules

Cefdinir plasma concentrations and pharmacokinetic parameter values following administration of single 300- and 600-mg oral doses of cefdinir to adult subjects are presented in the following table:

Mean (±SD) Plasma Cefdinir Pharmacokinetic Parameter Values Following Administration of Capsules to Adult Subjects

Dose	C_{max} (μg/mL)	t_{max} (hr)	AUC (μg·hr/mL)
300 mg	1.60 (0.55)	2.9 (0.89)	7.05 (2.17)
600 mg	2.87 (1.01)	3.0 (0.66)	11.1 (3.87)

Cefdinir Suspension

Cefdinir plasma concentrations and pharmacokinetic parameter values following administration of single 7- and 14-mg/kg oral doses of cefdinir to pediatric subjects (age 6 months-12 years) are presented in the following table:

Mean (±SD) Plasma Cefdinir Pharmacokinetic Parameter Values Following Administration of Suspension to Pediatric Subjects

Dose	C_{max} (μg/mL)	t_{max} (hr)	AUC (μg·hr/mL)
7 mg/kg	2.30 (0.65)	2.2 (0.6)	8.31 (2.50)
14 mg/kg	3.86 (0.62)	1.8 (0.4)	13.4 (2.64)

Multiple Dosing

Cefdinir does not accumulate in plasma following once- or twice-daily administration to subjects with normal renal function.

Distribution

The mean volume of distribution (Vd_{area}) of cefdinir in adult subjects is 0.35 L/kg (±0.29); in pediatric subjects (age 6 months-12 years), cefdinir Vd_{area} is 0.67 L/kg (±0.38). Cefdinir is 60% to 70% bound to plasma proteins in both adult and pediatric subjects; binding is independent of concentration.

Skin Blister

In adult subjects, median (range) maximal blister fluid cefdinir concentrations of 0.65 (0.33-1.1) and 1.1 (0.49-1.9) μg/mL were observed 4 to 5 hours following administration of 300- and 600-mg doses, respectively. Mean (± SD) blister C_{max} and AUC (0-∞) values were 48% (± 13) and 91% (± 18) of corresponding plasma values.

Tonsil Tissue

In adult patients undergoing elective tonsillectomy, respective median tonsil tissue cefdinir concentrations 4 hours after administration of single 300- and 600-mg doses were 0.25 (0.22-0.46) and 0.36 (0.22-0.80) μg/g. Mean tonsil tissue concentrations were 24% (± 8) of corresponding plasma concentrations.

Sinus Tissue

In adult patients undergoing elective maxillary and ethmoid sinus surgery, respective median sinus tissue cefdinir concentrations 4 hours after administration of single 300- and 600-mg doses were < 0.12 (<0.12-0.46) and 0.21 (< 0.12-2.0) μg/g. Mean sinus tissue concentrations were 16% (± 20) of corresponding plasma concentrations.

Lung Tissue

In adult patients undergoing diagnostic bronchoscopy, respective median bronchial mucosa cefdinir concentrations 4 hours after administration of single 300- and 600-mg doses were 0.78 (<0.06-1.33) and 1.14 (<0.06-1.92) μg/mL, and were 31% (± 18) of corresponding plasma concentrations. Respective median epithelial lining fluid concentrations were 0.29 (<0.3-4.73) and 0.49 (<0.3-0.59) μg/mL, and were 35% (± 83) of corresponding plasma concentrations.

Middle Ear Fluid

In 14 pediatric patients with acute bacterial otitis media, respective median middle ear fluid cefdinir concentrations 3 hours after administration of single 7- and 14-mg/kg doses were 0.21 (<0.09-0.94) and 0.72 (0.14-1.42) μg/mL. Mean middle ear fluid concentrations were 15% (± 15) of corresponding plasma concentrations.

CSF

Data on cefdinir penetration into human cerebrospinal fluid are not available.

Metabolism and Excretion

Cefdinir is not appreciably metabolized. Activity is primarily due to parent drug. Cefdinir is eliminated principally via renal excretion with a mean plasma elimination half-life ($t_{1/2}$) of 1.7 (± 0.6) hours. In healthy subjects with normal renal function, renal clearance is 2.0 (± 1.0) mL/min/kg, and apparent oral clearance is 11.6 (± 6.0) and 15.5 (± 5.4) mL/min/kg following doses of 300- and 600-mg, respectively. Mean percent of dose recovered unchanged in the urine following 300- and 600-mg doses is 18.4% (± 6.4) and 11.6% (± 4.6), respectively. Cefdinir clearance is reduced in patients with renal dysfunction (see **Special Populations**: *Patients with Renal Insufficiency*).

Because renal excretion is the predominant pathway of elimination, dosage should be adjusted in patients with markedly compromised renal function or who are undergoing hemodialysis (see **DOSAGE AND ADMINISTRATION**).

Special Populations
Patients with Renal Insufficiency
Cefdinir pharmacokinetics were investigated in 21 adult subjects with varying degrees of renal function. Decreases in cefdinir elimination rate, apparent oral clearance (CL/F), and renal clearance were approximately proportional to the reduction in creatinine clearance (CL_{cr}). As a result, plasma cefdinir concentrations were higher and persisted longer in subjects with renal impairment than in those without renal impairment. In subjects with CL_{cr} between 30 and 60 mL/min, C_{max} and $t_{1/2}$ increased by approximately 2-fold and AUC by approximately 3-fold. In subjects with CL_{cr} <30 mL/min, C_{max} increased by approximately 2-fold, $t_{1/2}$ by approximately 5-fold, and AUC by approximately 6-fold. Dosage adjustment is recommended in patients with markedly compromised renal function (creatinine clearance < 30 mL/min; see **DOSAGE AND ADMINISTRATION**).

Hemodialysis
Cefdinir pharmacokinetics were studied in 8 adult subjects undergoing hemodialysis. Dialysis (4 hours duration) removed 63% of cefdinir from the body and reduced apparent elimination $t_{1/2}$ from 16 (±3.5) to 3.2 (±1.2) hours. Dosage adjustment is recommended in this patient population (see **DOSAGE AND ADMINISTRATION**).

Hepatic Disease
Because cefdinir is predominantly renally eliminated and not appreciably metabolized, studies in patients with hepatic impairment were not conducted. It is not expected that dosage adjustment will be required in this population.

Geriatric Patients
The effect of age on cefdinir pharmacokinetics after a single 300-mg dose was evaluated in 32 subjects 19 to 91 years of age. Systemic exposure to cefdinir was substantially increased in older subjects (N = 16), C_{max} by 44% and AUC by 86%. This increase was due to a reduction in cefdinir clearance. The apparent volume of distribution was also reduced, thus no appreciable alterations in apparent elimination $t_{1/2}$ were observed (elderly: 2.2 ± 0.6 hours vs young: 1.8 ± 0.4 hours). Since cefdinir clearance has been shown to be primarily related to changes in renal function rather than age, elderly patients do not require dosage adjustment unless they have markedly compromised renal function (creatinine clearance <30 mL/min, see *Patients with Renal Insufficiency*, above).

Gender and Race
The results of a meta-analysis of clinical pharmacokinetics (N = 217) indicated no significant impact of either gender or race on cefdinir pharmacokinetics.

Microbiology

As with other cephalosporins, bactericidal activity of cefdinir results from inhibition of cell wall synthesis. Cefdinir is stable in the presence of some, but not all, β-lactamase enzymes. As a result, many organisms resistant to penicillins and some cephalosporins are susceptible to cefdinir.

Cefdinir has been shown to be active against most strains of the following microorganisms, both *in vitro* and in clinical infections as described in **INDICATIONS AND USAGE**.
Aerobic Gram-Positive Microorganisms
Staphylococcus aureus (including β-lactamase producing strains)
NOTE: Cefdinir is inactive against methicillin-resistant staphylococci.
Streptococcus pneumoniae (penicillin-susceptible strains only)
Streptococcus pyogenes
Aerobic Gram-Negative Microorganisms
Haemophilus influenzae (including β-lactamase producing strains)
Haemophilus parainfluenzae (including β-lactamase producing strains)
Moraxella catarrhalis (including β-lactamase producing strains)
The following *in vitro* data are available, **but their clinical significance is unknown.**
Cefdinir exhibits *in vitro* minimum inhibitory concentrations (MICs) of 1 μg/mL or less against (≥ 90%) strains of the following microorganisms; however, the safety and effectiveness of cefdinir in treating clinical infections due to these microorganisms have not been established in adequate and well-controlled clinical trials.
Aerobic Gram-Positive Microorganisms
Staphylococcus epidermidis (methicillin-susceptible strains only)
Streptococcus agalactiae
Viridans group streptococci
NOTE: Cefdinir is inactive against *Enterococcus* and methicillin-resistant *Staphylococcus* species.
Aerobic Gram-Negative Microorganisms
Citrobacter diversus
Escherichia coli
Klebsiella pneumoniae
Proteus mirabilis
NOTE: Cefdinir is inactive against *Pseudomonas* and *Enterobacter* species.
Susceptibility Tests
Dilution Techniques
Quantitative methods are used to determine antimicrobial minimum inhibitory concentrations (MICs). These MICs provide estimates of the susceptibility of bacteria to antimicrobial compounds. The MICs should be determined using a standardized procedure. Standardized procedures are based on a dilution method[1] (broth or agar) or equivalent with standardized inoculum concentrations and standardized concentrations of cefdinir powder. The MIC values should be interpreted according to the following criteria:

For organisms other than *Haemophilus* spp. and *Streptococcus* spp:

MIC (μg/mL)	Interpretation
≤1	Susceptible (S)
2	Intermediate (I)
≥4	Resistant (R)

For *Haemophilus* spp:[a]

MIC (μg/mL)	Interpretation[b]
≤1	Susceptible (S)

[a] These interpretive standards are applicable only to broth microdilution susceptibility tests with *Haemophilus* spp. using *Haemophilus* Test Medium (HTM).[1]
[b] The current absence of data on resistant strains precludes defining any results other than "Susceptible." Strains yielding MIC results suggestive of a "nonsusceptible" category should be submitted to a reference laboratory for further testing.

For *Streptococcus* spp:
Streptococcus pneumoniae that are susceptible to penicillin (MIC ≤ 0.06 μg/mL), or streptococci other than *S. pneumoniae* that are susceptible to penicillin (MIC ≤ 0.12 μg/mL), can be considered susceptible to cefdinir. Testing of cefdinir against penicillin-intermediate or penicillin-resistant isolates is not recommended. Reliable interpretive criteria for cefdinir are not available.
A report of "Susceptible" indicates that the pathogen is likely to be inhibited if the antimicrobial compound in the blood reaches the concentration usually achievable. A report of "Intermediate" indicates that the result should be considered equivocal, and, if the microorganism is not fully susceptible to alternative, clinically feasible drugs, the test should be repeated. This category implies possible clinical applicability in body sites where the drug is physiologically concentrated or in situations where high dosage of drug can be used. This category also provides a buffer zone which prevents small uncontrolled technical factors from causing major discrepancies in interpretation. A report of "Resistant" indicates that the pathogen is not likely to be inhibited if the antimicrobial compound in the blood reaches the concentrations usually achievable; other therapy should be selected.
Standardized susceptibility test procedures require the use of laboratory control microorganisms to control the technical aspects of laboratory procedures. Standard cefdinir powder should provide the following MIC values:

Microorganism	MIC Range (μg/mL)
Escherichia coli ATCC 25922	0.12-0.5
Haemophilus influenzae ATCC 49766[c]	0.12-0.5
Staphylococcus aureus ATCC 29213	0.12-0.5

[c] This quality control range is applicable only to *H. influenzae* ATCC 49766 tested by a broth microdilution procedure using HTM.

Diffusion Techniques
Quantitative methods that require measurement of zone diameters also provide reproducible estimates of the susceptibility of bacteria to antimicrobial compounds. One such standardized procedure[2] requires the use of standardized inoculum concentrations. This procedure uses paper disks impregnated with 5-μg cefdinir to test the susceptibility of microorganisms to cefdinir.
Reports from the laboratory providing results of the standard single-disk susceptibility test with a 5-μg cefdinir disk should be interpreted according to the following criteria:

For organisms other than *Haemophilus* spp. and *Streptococcus* spp:[d]

Zone Diameter (mm)	Interpretation
≥20	Susceptible (S)
17-19	Intermediate (I)
≤16	Resistant (R)

[d] Because certain strains of *Citrobacter, Providencia,* and *Enterobacter* spp. have been reported to give false susceptible results with the cefdinir disk, strains of these genera should not be tested and reported with this disk.

For *Haemophilus* spp:[e]

Zone Diameter (mm)	Interpretation[f]
≥20	Susceptible (S)

[e] These zone diameter standards are applicable only to tests with *Haemophilus* spp. using HTM.[2]
[f] The current absence of data on resistant strains precludes defining any results other than "Susceptible." Strains yielding MIC results suggestive of a "nonsusceptible" category should be submitted to a reference laboratory for further testing.

For *Streptococcus* spp:
Isolates of *Streptococcus pneumoniae* should be tested against a 1-μg oxacillin disk. Isolates with oxacillin zone sizes ≥ 20 mm are susceptible to penicillin and can be considered susceptible to cefdinir. Streptococci other than *S. pneumoniae* should be tested with a 10-unit penicillin disk. Isolates with penicillin zone sizes ≥ 28 mm are susceptible to penicillin and can be considered susceptible to cefdinir. As with standardized dilution techniques, diffusion methods require the use of laboratory control microorganisms to control the technical aspects of laboratory procedures. For the diffusion technique, the 5-μg cefdinir disk should provide the following zone diameters in these laboratory quality control strains:

Organism	Zone Diameter (mm)
Escherichia coli ATCC 25922	24-28
Haemophilus influenzae ATCC 49766[g]	24-31
Staphylococcus aureus ATCC 25923	25-32

[g] This quality control range is applicable only to testing of *H. influenzae* ATCC 49766 using HTM.

INDICATIONS AND USAGE

To reduce the development of drug-resistant bacteria and maintain the effectiveness of OMNICEF and other antibacterial drugs, OMNICEF should be used only to treat or prevent infections that are proven or strongly suspected to be caused by susceptible bacteria. When culture and susceptibility information are available, they should be considered in selecting or modifying antibacterial therapy. In the absence of such data, local epidemiology and susceptibility patterns may contribute to the empiric selection of therapy.
OMNICEF (cefdinir) capsules and OMNICEF (cefdinir) for oral suspension are indicated for the treatment of patients with mild to moderate infections caused by susceptible strains of the designated microorganisms in the conditions listed below.

Adults and Adolescents

Community-Acquired Pneumonia
caused by *Haemophilus influenzae* (including β-lactamase producing strains), *Haemophilus parainfluenzae* (including

Information on the Abbott Pharmaceutical Products listed on these pages is from the prescribing information in use as of June 1, 2010. For more information, please visit rxabbott.com or call 1-800-633-9110.

β-lactamase producing strains), *Streptococcus pneumoniae* (penicillin-susceptible strains only), and *Moraxella catarrhalis* (including β-lactamase producing strains) (see **CLINICAL STUDIES**).

Acute Exacerbations of Chronic Bronchitis
caused by *Haemophilus influenzae* (including β-lactamase producing strains), *Haemophilus parainfluenzae* (including β-lactamase producing strains), *Streptococcus pneumoniae* (penicillin-susceptible strains only), and *Moraxella catarrhalis* (including β-lactamase producing strains).

Acute Maxillary Sinusitis
caused by *Haemophilus influenzae* (including β-lactamase producing strains), *Streptococcus pneumoniae* (penicillin-susceptible strains only), and *Moraxella catarrhalis* (including β-lactamase producing strains).

NOTE: For information on use in pediatric patients, see **Pediatric Use** and **DOSAGE AND ADMINISTRATION**.

Pharyngitis/Tonsillitis
caused by *Streptococcus pyogenes* (see **CLINICAL STUDIES**).

NOTE: Cefdinir is effective in the eradication of *S. pyogenes* from the oropharynx. Cefdinir has not, however, been studied for the prevention of rheumatic fever following *S. pyogenes* pharyngitis/tonsillitis. Only intramuscular penicillin has been demonstrated to be effective for the prevention of rheumatic fever.

Uncomplicated Skin and Skin Structure Infections
caused by *Staphylococcus aureus* (including β-lactamase producing strains) and *Streptococcus pyogenes*.

Pediatric Patients
Acute Bacterial Otitis Media caused by *Haemophilus influenzae* (including β-lactamase producing strains), *Streptococcus pneumoniae* (penicillin-susceptible strains only), and *Moraxella catarrhalis* (including β-lactamase producing strains).

Pharyngitis/Tonsillitis
caused by *Streptococcus pyogenes* (see **CLINICAL STUDIES**).

NOTE: Cefdinir is effective in the eradication of *S. pyogenes* from the oropharynx. Cefdinir has not, however, been studied for the prevention of rheumatic fever following *S. pyogenes* pharyngitis/tonsillitis. Only intramuscular penicillin has been demonstrated to be effective for the prevention of rheumatic fever.

Uncomplicated Skin and Skin Structure Infections
caused by *Staphylococcus aureus* (including β-lactamase producing strains) and *Streptococcus pyogenes*.

CONTRAINDICATIONS

OMNICEF (cefdinir) is contraindicated in patients with known allergy to the cephalosporin class of antibiotics.

WARNINGS

BEFORE THERAPY WITH OMNICEF (CEFDINIR) IS INSTITUTED, CAREFUL INQUIRY SHOULD BE MADE TO DETERMINE WHETHER THE PATIENT HAS HAD PREVIOUS HYPERSENSITIVITY REACTIONS TO CEFDINIR, OTHER CEPHALOSPORINS, PENICILLINS, OR OTHER DRUGS. IF CEFDINIR IS TO BE GIVEN TO PENICILLIN-SENSITIVE PATIENTS, CAUTION SHOULD BE EXERCISED BECAUSE CROSS-HYPERSENSITIVITY AMONG β-LACTAM ANTIBIOTICS HAS BEEN CLEARLY DOCUMENTED AND MAY OCCUR IN UP TO 10% OF PATIENTS WITH A HISTORY OF PENICILLIN ALLERGY. IF AN ALLERGIC REACTION TO CEFDINIR OCCURS, THE DRUG SHOULD BE DISCONTINUED. SERIOUS ACUTE HYPERSENSITIVITY REACTIONS MAY REQUIRE TREATMENT WITH EPINEPHRINE AND OTHER EMERGENCY MEASURES, INCLUDING OXYGEN, INTRAVENOUS FLUIDS, INTRAVENOUS ANTIHISTAMINES, CORTICOSTEROIDS, PRESSOR AMINES, AND AIRWAY MANAGEMENT, AS CLINICALLY INDICATED.

Clostridium difficile associated diarrhea (CDAD) has been reported with use of nearly all antibacterial agents, including OMNICEF, and may range in severity from mild diarrhea to fatal colitis. Treatment with antibacterial agents alters the normal flora of the colon leading to overgrowth of *C. difficile*.

C. difficile produces toxins A and B which contribute to the development of CDAD. Hypertoxin producing strains of *C. difficile* cause increased morbidity and mortality, as these infections can be refractory to antimicrobial therapy and may require colectomy. CDAD must be considered in all patients who present with diarrhea following antibiotic use. Careful medical history is necessary since CDAD has been reported to occur over two months after the administration of antibacterial agents.

If CDAD is suspected or confirmed, ongoing antibiotic use not directed against *C. difficile* may need to be discontinued. Appropriate fluid and electrolyte management, protein supplementation, antibiotic treatment of *C. difficile*, and surgical evaluation should be instituted as clinically indicated.

PRECAUTIONS
General
Prescribing OMNICEF in the absence of a proven or strongly suspected bacterial infection or a prophylactic in-

dication is unlikely to provide benefit to the patient and increases the risk of the development of drug-resistant bacteria.

As with other broad-spectrum antibiotics, prolonged treatment may result in the possible emergence and overgrowth of resistant organisms. Careful observation of the patient is essential. If superinfection occurs during therapy, appropriate alternative therapy should be administered.

Cefdinir, as with other broad-spectrum antimicrobials (antibiotics), should be prescribed with caution in individuals with a history of colitis.

In patients with transient or persistent renal insufficiency (creatinine clearance <30 mL/min), the total daily dose of OMNICEF should be reduced because high and prolonged plasma concentrations of cefdinir can result following recommended doses (see **DOSAGE AND ADMINISTRATION**).

Information for Patients
Patients should be counseled that antibacterial drugs including OMNICEF should only be used to treat bacterial infections. They do not treat viral infections (e.g., the common cold). When OMNICEF is prescribed to treat a bacterial infection, patients should be told that although it is common to feel better early in the course of therapy, the medication should be taken exactly as directed. Skipping doses or not completing the full course of therapy may (1) decrease the effectiveness of the immediate treatment and (2) increase the likelihood that bacteria will develop resistance and will not be treatable by OMNICEF or other antibacterial drugs in the future.

Antacids containing magnesium or aluminum interfere with the absorption of cefdinir. If this type of antacid is required during OMNICEF therapy, OMNICEF should be taken at least 2 hours before or after the antacid.

Iron supplements, including multivitamins that contain iron, interfere with the absorption of cefdinir. If iron supple-

ments are required during OMNICEF therapy, OMNICEF should be taken at least 2 hours before or after the supplement.

Iron-fortified infant formula does not significantly interfere with the absorption of cefdinir. Therefore, OMNICEF for Oral Suspension can be administered with iron-fortified infant formula.

Diabetic patients and caregivers should be aware that the oral suspension contains 2.86 g of sucrose per teaspoon.

Diarrhea is a common problem caused by antibiotics which usually ends when the antibiotic is discontinued. Sometimes after starting treatment with antibiotics, patients can develop watery and bloody stools (with or without stomach cramps and fever) even as late as two or more months after having taken the last dose of the antibiotic. If this occurs, patients should contact their physician as soon as possible.

Drug Interactions
Antacids (aluminum- or magnesium-containing)
Concomitant administration of 300-mg cefdinir capsules with 30 mL Maalox® TC suspension reduces the rate (C_{max}) and extent (AUC) of absorption by approximately 40%. Time to reach C_{max} is also prolonged by 1 hour. There are no significant effects on cefdinir pharmacokinetics if the antacid is administered 2 hours before or 2 hours after cefdinir. If antacids are required during OMNICEF therapy, OMNICEF should be taken at least 2 hours before or after the antacid.

Probenecid
As with other β-lactam antibiotics, probenecid inhibits the renal excretion of cefdinir, resulting in an approximate doubling in AUC, a 54% increase in peak cefdinir plasma levels, and a 50% prolongation in the apparent elimination $t_{1/2}$.

Iron Supplements and Foods Fortified With Iron
Concomitant administration of cefdinir with a therapeutic iron supplement containing 60 mg of elemental iron (as $FeSO_4$) or vitamins supplemented with 10 mg of elemental iron reduced extent of absorption by 80% and 31%, respec-

LABORATORY VALUE CHANGES OBSERVED WITH CEFDINIR CAPSULES US TRIALS IN ADULT AND ADOLESCENT PATIENTS (N = 3841)

Incidence ≥ 1%	↑ Urine leukocytes	2%
	↑ Urine protein	2%
	↑ Gamma-glutamyltransferase[a]	1%
	↓ Lymphocytes, ↑ Lymphocytes	1%, 0.2%
	↑ Microhematuria	1%
Incidence <1% but >0.1%	↑ Glucose[a]	0.9%
	↑ Urine glucose	0.9%
	↑ White blood cells, ↓ White blood cells	0.9%, 0.7%
	↑ Alanine aminotransferase (ALT)	0.7%
	↑ Eosinophils	0.7%
	↑ Urine specific gravity, ↓ Urine specific gravity[a]	0.6%, 0.2%
	↓ Bicarbonate[a]	0.6%
	↑ Phosphorus, ↓ Phosphorus[a]	0.6%, 0.3%
	↑ Aspartate aminotransferase (AST)	0.4%
	↑ Alkaline phosphatase	0.3%
	↑ Blood urea nitrogen (BUN)	0.3%
	↓ Hemoglobin	0.3%
	↑ Polymorphonuclear neutrophils (PMNs), ↓ PMNs	0.3%, 0.2%
	↑ Bilirubin	0.2%
	↑ Lactate dehydrogenase[a]	0.2%
	↑ Platelets	0.2%
	↑ Potassium[a]	0.2%
	↑ Urine pH[a]	0.2%

[a] N <3841 for these parameters

ADVERSE EVENTS ASSOCIATED WITH CEFDINIR SUSPENSION US TRIALS IN PEDIATRIC PATIENTS (N = 1783)[a]

Incidence ≥1%	Diarrhea	8%
	Rash	3%
	Vomiting	1%
Incidence <1% but >0.1%	Cutaneous moniliasis	0.9%
	Abdominal pain	0.8%
	Leukopenia[b]	0.3%
	Vaginal moniliasis	0.3% of girls
	Vaginitis	0.3% of girls
	Abnormal stools	0.2%
	Dyspepsia	0.2%
	Hyperkinesia	0.2%
	Increased AST[b]	0.2%
	Maculopapular rash	0.2%
	Nausea	0.2%

[a] 977 males, 806 females
[b] Laboratory changes were occasionally reported as adverse events.

tively. If iron supplements are required during OMNICEF therapy, OMNICEF should be taken at least 2 hours before or after the supplement.

The effect of foods highly fortified with elemental iron (primarily iron-fortified breakfast cereals) on cefdinir absorption has not been studied.

Concomitantly administered iron-fortified infant formula (2.2 mg elemental iron/6 oz) has no significant effect on cefdinir pharmacokinetics. Therefore, OMNICEF for Oral Suspension can be administered with iron-fortified infant formula.

There have been reports of reddish stools in patients receiving cefdinir. In many cases, patients were also receiving iron-containing products. The reddish color is due to the formation of a nonabsorbable complex between cefdinir or its breakdown products and iron in the gastrointestinal tract.

Drug/Laboratory Test Interactions

A false-positive reaction for ketones in the urine may occur with tests using nitroprusside, but not with those using nitroferricyanide. The administration of cefdinir may result in a false-positive reaction for glucose in urine using Clinitest®, Benedict's solution, or Fehling's solution. It is recommended that glucose tests based on enzymatic glucose oxidase reactions (such as Clinistix® or Tes-Tape®) be used. Cephalosporins are known to occasionally induce a positive direct Coombs' test.

Carcinogenesis, Mutagenesis, Impairment of Fertility

The carcinogenic potential of cefdinir has not been evaluated. No mutagenic effects were seen in the bacterial reverse mutation assay (Ames) or point mutation assay at the hypoxanthine-guanine phosphoribosyltransferase locus (HGPRT) in V79 Chinese hamster lung cells. No clastogenic effects were observed in vitro in the structural chromosome aberration assay in V79 Chinese hamster lung cells or in vivo in the micronucleus assay in mouse bone marrow. In rats, fertility and reproductive performance were not affected by cefdinir at oral doses up to 1000 mg/kg/day (70 times the human dose based on mg/kg/day, 11 times based on mg/m^2/day).

Pregnancy

Teratogenic Effects

Pregnancy Category B

Cefdinir was not teratogenic in rats at oral doses up to 1000 mg/kg/day (70 times the human dose based on mg/kg/day, 11 times based on mg/m^2/day) or in rabbits at oral doses up to 10 mg/kg/day (0.7 times the human dose based on mg/kg/day, 0.23 times based on mg/m^2/day). Maternal toxicity (decreased body weight gain) was observed in rabbits at the maximum tolerated dose of 10 mg/kg/day without adverse effects on offspring. Decreased body weight occurred in rat fetuses at ≥ 100 mg/kg/day, and in rat offspring at ≥32 mg/kg/day. No effects were observed on maternal reproductive parameters or offspring survival, development, behavior, or reproductive function.

There are, however, no adequate and well-controlled studies in pregnant women. Because animal reproduction studies are not always predictive of human response, this drug should be used during pregnancy only if clearly needed.

Labor and Delivery

Cefdinir has not been studied for use during labor and delivery.

Nursing Mothers

Following administration of single 600-mg doses, cefdinir was not detected in human breast milk.

Pediatric Use

Safety and efficacy in neonates and infants less than 6 months of age have not been established. Use of cefdinir for the treatment of acute maxillary sinusitis in pediatric patients (age 6 months through 12 years) is supported by evidence from adequate and well-controlled studies in adults and adolescents, the similar pathophysiology of acute sinusitis in adult and pediatric patients, and comparative pharmacokinetic data in the pediatric population.

Geriatric Use

Efficacy is comparable in geriatric patients and younger adults. While cefdinir has been well-tolerated in all age groups, in clinical trials geriatric patients experienced a lower rate of adverse events, including diarrhea, than younger adults. Dose adjustment in elderly patients is not necessary unless renal function is markedly compromised (see **DOSAGE AND ADMINISTRATION**).

ADVERSE EVENTS

Clinical Trials - OMNICEF Capsules (Adult and Adolescent Patients)

In clinical trials, 5093 adult and adolescent patients (3841 US and 1252 non-US) were treated with the recommended dose of cefdinir capsules (600 mg/day). Most adverse events were mild and self-limiting. No deaths or permanent disabilities were attributed to cefdinir. One hundred forty-seven of 5093 (3%) patients discontinued medication due to adverse events thought by the investigators to be possibly, probably, or definitely associated with cefdinir therapy. The discontinuations were primarily for gastrointestinal distur-

bances, usually diarrhea or nausea. Nineteen of 5093 (0.4%) patients were discontinued due to rash thought related to cefdinir administration.

In the US, the following adverse events were thought by investigators to be possibly, probably, or definitely related to cefdinir capsules in multiple-dose clinical trials (N = 3841 cefdinir-treated patients):

ADVERSE EVENTS ASSOCIATED WITH CEFDINIR CAPSULES
US TRIALS IN ADULT AND ADOLESCENT PATIENTS
(N = 3841)[a]

Incidence ≥1%	Diarrhea	15%
	Vaginal moniliasis	4% of women
	Nausea	3%
	Headache	2%
	Abdominal pain	1%
	Vaginitis	1% of women
Incidence <1% but >0.1%	Rash	0.9%
	Dyspepsia	0.7%
	Flatulence	0.7%
	Vomiting	0.7%
	Abnormal stools	0.3%
	Anorexia	0.3%
	Constipation	0.3%
	Dizziness	0.3%
	Dry mouth	0.3%
	Asthenia	0.2%
	Insomnia	0.2%
	Leukorrhea	0.2% of women
	Moniliasis	0.2%
	Pruritus	0.2%
	Somnolence	0.2%

[a] 1733 males, 2108 females

The following laboratory value changes of possible clinical significance, irrespective of relationship to therapy with cefdinir, were seen during clinical trials conducted in the US:

[See first table at top of previous page]

Clinical Trials - OMNICEF for Oral Suspension (Pediatric Patients)

In clinical trials, 2289 pediatric patients (1783 US and 506 non-US) were treated with the recommended dose of cefdinir suspension (14 mg/kg/day). Most adverse events were mild and self-limiting. No deaths or permanent disabilities were attributed to cefdinir. Forty of 2289 (2%) patients discontinued medication due to adverse events considered by the investigators to be possibly, probably, or definitely associated with cefdinir therapy. Discontinuations were primarily for gastrointestinal disturbances, usually diarrhea. Five of 2289 (0.2%) patients were discontinued due to rash thought related to cefdinir administration.

In the US, the following adverse events were thought by investigators to be possibly, probably, or definitely related to cefdinir suspension in multiple-dose clinical trials (N = 1783 cefdinir-treated patients):

[See second table at top of previous page]

NOTE: In both cefdinir- and control-treated patients, rates of diarrhea and rash were higher in the youngest pediatric patients. The incidence of diarrhea in cefdinir-treated patients ≤ 2 years of age was 17% (95/557) compared with 4%

(51/1226) in those >2 years old. The incidence of rash (primarily diaper rash in the younger patients) was 8% (43/557) in patients ≤ 2 years of age compared with 1% (8/1226) in those >2 years old.

The following laboratory value changes of possible clinical significance, irrespective of relationship to therapy with cefdinir, were seen during clinical trials conducted in the US:

[See table above]

Postmarketing Experience

The following adverse experiences and altered laboratory tests, regardless of their relationship to cefdinir, have been reported during extensive postmarketing experience, beginning with approval in Japan in 1991: shock, anaphylaxis with rare cases of fatality, facial and laryngeal edema, feeling of suffocation, serum sickness-like reactions, conjunctivitis, stomatitis, Stevens-Johnson syndrome, toxic epidermal necrolysis, exfoliative dermatitis, erythema multiforme, erythema nodosum, acute hepatitis, cholestasis, fulminant hepatitis, hepatic failure, jaundice, increased amylase, acute enterocolitis, bloody diarrhea, hemorrhagic colitis, melena, pseudomembranous colitis, pancytopenia, granulocytopenia, leukopenia, thrombocytopenia, idiopathic thrombocytopenic purpura, hemolytic anemia, acute respiratory failure, asthmatic attack, drug-induced pneumonia, eosinophilic pneumonia, idiopathic interstitial pneumonia, fever, acute renal failure, nephropathy, bleeding tendency, coagulation disorder, disseminated intravascular coagulation, upper GI bleed, peptic ulcer, ileus, loss of consciousness, allergic vasculitis, possible cefdinir-diclofenac interaction, cardiac failure, chest pain, myocardial infarction, hypertension, involuntary movements, and rhabdomyolysis.

Cephalosporin Class Adverse Events

The following adverse events and altered laboratory tests have been reported for cephalosporin-class antibiotics in general:

Allergic reactions, anaphylaxis, Stevens-Johnson syndrome, erythema multiforme, toxic epidermal necrolysis, renal dysfunction, toxic nephropathy, hepatic dysfunction including cholestasis, aplastic anemia, hemolytic anemia, hemorrhage, false-positive test for urinary glucose, neutropenia, pancytopenia, and agranulocytosis.

Pseudomembranous colitis symptoms may begin during or after antibiotic treatment (see **WARNINGS**).

Several cephalosporins have been implicated in triggering seizures, particularly in patients with renal impairment when the dosage was not reduced (see **DOSAGE AND ADMINISTRATION** and **OVERDOSAGE**). If seizures associated with drug therapy occur, the drug should be discontinued. Anticonvulsant therapy can be given if clinically indicated.

OVERDOSAGE

Information on cefdinir overdosage in humans is not available. In acute rodent toxicity studies, a single oral 5600-mg/kg dose produced no adverse effects. Toxic signs and symptoms following overdosage with other β-lactam antibiotics have included nausea, vomiting, epigastric distress, diarrhea, and convulsions. Hemodialysis removes cefdinir

LABORATORY VALUE CHANGES OF POSSIBLE CLINICAL SIGNIFICANCE OBSERVED WITH CEFDINIR SUSPENSION
US TRIALS IN PEDIATRIC PATIENTS
(N = 1783)

Incidence ≥1%	↑Lymphocytes, ↓Lymphocytes	2%, 0.8%
	↑Alkaline phosphatase	1%
	↓Bicarbonate[a]	1%
	↑Eosinophils	1%
	↑Lactate dehydrogenase	1%
	↑Platelets	1%
	↑PMNs, ↓PMNs	1%, 1%
	↑Urine protein	1%
Incidence <1% but >0.1%	↑Phosphorus, ↓Phosphorus	0.9%, 0.4%
	↑Urine pH	0.8%
	↓White blood cells, ↑White blood cells	0.7%, 0.3%
	↓Calcium[a]	0.5%
	↓Hemoglobin	0.5%
	↑Urine leukocytes	0.5%
	↑Monocytes	0.4%
	↑AST	0.3%
	↑Potassium[a]	0.3%
	↑Urine specific gravity, ↓Urine specific gravity	0.3%, 0.1%
	↓Hematocrit[a]	0.2%

[a] N = 1387 for these parameters

Information on the Abbott Pharmaceutical Products listed on these pages is from the prescribing information in use as of June 1, 2010. For more information, please visit rxabbott.com or call 1-800-633-9110.

Adults and Adolescents (Age 13 Years and Older)

Type of Infection	Dosage	Duration
Community-Acquired Pneumonia	300 mg q12h	10 days
Acute Exacerbations of Chronic Bronchitis	300 mg q12h	5 to 10 days
	or	
	600 mg q24h	10 days
Acute Maxillary Sinusitis	300 mg q12h	10 days
	or	
	600 mg q24h	10 days
Pharyngitis/Tonsillitis	300 mg q12h	5 to 10 days
	or	
	600 mg q24h	10 days
Uncomplicated Skin and Skin Structure Infections	300 mg q12h	10 days

Pediatric Patients (Age 6 Months Through 12 Years)

Type of Infection	Dosage	Duration
Acute Bacterial Otitis Media	7 mg/kg q12h	5 to 10 days
	or	
	14 mg/kg q24h	10 days
Acute Maxillary Sinusitis	7 mg/kg q12h	10 days
	or	
	14 mg/kg q24h	10 days
Pharyngitis/Tonsillitis	7 mg/kg q12h	5 to 10 days
	or	
	14 mg/kg q24h	10 days
Uncomplicated Skin and Skin Structure Infections	7 mg/kg q12h	10 days

OMNICEF FOR ORAL SUSPENSION PEDIATRIC DOSAGE CHART

Weight	125 mg/5 mL	250 mg/5 mL
9 kg/20 lbs	2.5 mL q12h or 5 mL q24h	Use 125 mg/5 mL product
18 kg/40 lbs	5 mL q12h or 10 mL q24h	2.5 mL q12h or 5 mL q24h
27 kg/60 lbs	7.5 mL q12h or 15 mL q24h	3.75 mL q12h or 7.5 mL q24h
36 kg/80 lbs	10 mL q12h or 20 mL q24h	5 mL q12h or 10 mL q24h
≥43 kg[a]/95 lbs	12 mL q12h or 24 mL q24h	6 mL q12h or 12 mL q24h

[a] Pediatric patients who weigh ≥43 kg should receive the maximum daily dose of 600 mg.

US Community-Acquired Pneumonia Study Cefdinir vs Cefaclor

	Cefdinir BID	Cefaclor TID	Outcome
Clinical Cure Rates	150/187 (80%)	147/186 (79%)	Cefdinir equivalent to control
Eradication Rates			
Overall	177/195 (91%)	184/200 (92%)	Cefdinir equivalent to control
S. pneumoniae	31/31 (100%)	35/35 (100%)	
H. influenzae	55/65 (85%)	60/72 (83%)	
M. catarrhalis	10/10 (100%)	11/11 (100%)	
H. parainfluenzae	81/89 (91%)	78/82 (95%)	

from the body. This may be useful in the event of a serious toxic reaction from overdosage, particularly if renal function is compromised.

DOSAGE AND ADMINISTRATION

(see **INDICATIONS AND USAGE** for Indicated Pathogens)

Capsules

The recommended dosage and duration of treatment for infections in adults and adolescents are described in the following chart; the total daily dose for all infections is 600 mg. Once-daily dosing for 10 days is as effective as BID dosing. Once-daily dosing has not been studied in pneumonia or skin infections; therefore, OMNICEF Capsules should be administered twice daily in these infections. OMNICEF Capsules may be taken without regard to meals.
[See first table above]

Powder for Oral Suspension

The recommended dosage and duration of treatment for infections in pediatric patients are described in the following chart; the total daily dose for all infections is 14 mg/kg, up to a maximum dose of 600 mg per day. Once-daily dosing for 10 days is as effective as BID dosing. Once-daily dosing has not been studied in skin infections; therefore, OMNICEF for Oral Suspension should be administered twice daily in this infection. OMNICEF for Oral Suspension may be administered without regard to meals.
[See second table above]
[See third table above]

Patients With Renal Insufficiency

For adult patients with creatinine clearance < 30 mL/min, the dose of cefdinir should be 300 mg given once daily.

Creatinine clearance is difficult to measure in outpatients. However, the following formula may be used to estimate creatinine clearance (CL_{cr}) in adult patients. For estimates to be valid, serum creatinine levels should reflect steady-state levels of renal function.

Males: $CL_{cr} = \dfrac{(weight)\,(140 - age)}{(72)(serum\ creatinine)}$

Females: $CL_{cr} = 0.85 \times above\ value$

where creatinine clearance is in mL/min, age is in years, weight is in kilograms, and serum creatinine is in mg/dL.[3] The following formula may be used to estimate creatinine clearance in pediatric patients:

$$CL_{cr} = K \times \frac{body\ length\ or\ height}{serum\ creatinine}$$

where K = 0.55 for pediatric patients older than 1 year[4] and 0.45 for infants (up to 1 year)[5].
In the above equation, creatinine clearance is in mL/min/1.73 m², body length or height is in centimeters, and serum creatinine is in mg/dL.
For pediatric patients with a creatinine clearance of < 30 mL/min/1.73 m², the dose of cefdinir should be 7 mg/kg (up to 300 mg) given once daily.

Patients on Hemodialysis

Hemodialysis removes cefdinir from the body. In patients maintained on chronic hemodialysis, the recommended initial dosage regimen is a 300-mg or 7-mg/kg dose every other

day. At the conclusion of each hemodialysis session, 300 mg (or 7 mg/kg) should be given. Subsequent doses (300 mg or 7 mg/kg) are then administered every other day.

Directions for Mixing Omnicef for Oral Suspension

Final Concentration	Final Volume (mL)	Amount of Water	Directions
125 mg/5 mL	60	38 mL	Tap bottle to loosen powder, then add water in 2 portions. Shake well after each aliquot.
	100	63 mL	
250 mg/5 mL	60	38 mL	Tap bottle to loosen powder, then add water in 2 portions. Shake well after each aliquot.
	100	63 mL	

After mixing, the suspension can be stored at room temperature (25°C/77°F). The container should be kept tightly closed, and the suspension should be shaken well before each administration. The suspension may be used for 10 days, after which any unused portion must be discarded.

HOW SUPPLIED

OMNICEF Capsules, containing 300 mg cefdinir, as lavender and turquoise capsules imprinted with the product name, are available as follows:
60 Capsules/Bottle **NDC** 0074-3769-60
OMNI-PAC™ carton of 3 unit-of-use, 5-day, 10-capsule blister cards **NDC** 0074-3769-30
OMNICEF for Oral Suspension is a cream-colored powder formulation that, when reconstituted as directed, contains 125 mg cefdinir/5 mL or 250 mg cefdinir/5 mL. The reconstituted suspensions have a cream color and strawberry flavor. The powder is available as follows:
125 mg/5 mL
60-mL bottles **NDC** 0074-3771-60
100-mL bottles **NDC** 0074-3771-13
250 mg/5 mL
60-mL bottles **NDC** 0074-6151-60
100-mL bottles **NDC** 0074-6151-13
Store the capsules and unsuspended powder at 25°C (77°F); excursions permitted to 15°-30°C (59°-86°F) [see USP Controlled Room Temperature]. Once reconstituted, the oral suspension can be stored at controlled room temperature for 10 days.

CLINICAL STUDIES

Community-Acquired Bacterial Pneumonia

In a controlled, double-blind study in adults and adolescents conducted in the US, cefdinir BID was compared with cefaclor 500 mg TID. Using strict evaluability and microbiologic/clinical response criteria 6 to 14 days posttherapy, the following clinical cure rates, presumptive microbiologic eradication rates, and statistical outcomes were obtained:
[See fourth table at left]
In a second controlled, investigator-blind study in adults and adolescents conducted primarily in Europe, cefdinir BID was compared with amoxicillin/clavulanate 500/125 mg TID. Using strict evaluability and clinical response criteria 6 to 14 days posttherapy, the following clinical cure rates, presumptive microbiologic eradication rates, and statistical outcomes were obtained:
[See first table at top of next page]

Streptococcal Pharyngitis/Tonsillitis

In four controlled studies conducted in the United States, cefdinir was compared with 10 days of penicillin in adult, adolescent, and pediatric patients. Two studies (one in adults and adolescents, the other in pediatric patients) compared 10 days of cefdinir QD or BID to penicillin 250 mg or 10 mg/kg QID. Using strict evaluability and microbiologic/clinical response criteria 5 to 10 days posttherapy, the following clinical cure rates, microbiologic eradication rates, and statistical outcomes were obtained:
[See second table at top of next page]
Two studies (one in adults and adolescents, the other in pediatric patients) compared 5 days of cefdinir BID to 10 days of penicillin 250 mg or 10 mg/kg QID. Using strict evaluability and microbiologic/clinical response criteria 4 to 10 days posttherapy, the following clinical cure rates, microbiologic eradication rates, and statistical outcomes were obtained:
[See third table at top of next page]

REFERENCES

1. National Committee for Clinical Laboratory Standards. Methods for Dilution Antimicrobial Susceptibility Tests for Bacteria That Grow Aerobically, 4th ed. Approved Standard, NCCLS Document M7-A4, Vol 17(2). NCCLS, Villanova, PA, Jan 1997.

European Community-Acquired Pneumonia Study Cefdinir vs Amoxicillin/Clavulanate

	Cefdinir BID	Amoxicillin/Clavulanate TID	Outcome
Clinical Cure Rates	83/104 (80%)	86/97 (89%)	Cefdinir not equivalent to control
Eradication Rates			
Overall	85/96 (89%)	84/90 (93%)	Cefdinir equivalent to control
S. pncumoniae	42/44 (95%)	43/44 (98%)	
H. influenzae	26/35 (74%)	21/26 (81%)	
M. catarrhalis	6/6 (100%)	8/8 (100%)	
H. parainfluenzae	11/11 (100%)	12/12 (100%)	

Pharyngitis/Tonsillitis Studies Cefdinir (10 days) vs Penicillin (10 days)

Study	Efficacy Parameter	Cefdinir QD	Cefdinir BID	Penicillin QID	Outcome
Adults/Adolescents	Eradication of *S. pyogenes*	192/210 (91%)	199/217 (92%)	181/217 (83%)	Cefdinir superior to control
	Clinical Cure Rates	199/210 (95%)	209/217 (96%)	193/217 (89%)	Cefdinir superior to control
Pediatric Patients	Eradication of *S. pyogenes*	215/228 (94%)	214/227 (94%)	159/227 (70%)	Cefdinir superior to control
	Clinical Cure Rates	222/228 (97%)	218/227 (96%)	196/227 (86%)	Cefdinir superior to control

Pharyngitis/Tonsillitis Studies Cefdinir (5 days) vs Penicillin (10 days)

Study	Efficacy Parameter	Cefdinir BID	Penicillin QID	Outcome
Adults/Adolescents	Eradication of *S. pyogenes*	193/218 (89%)	176/214 (82%)	Cefdinir equivalent to control
	Clinical Cure Rates	194/218 (89%)	181/214 (85%)	Cefdinir equivalent to control
Pediatric Patients	Eradication of *S. pyogenes*	176/196 (90%)	135/193 (70%)	Cefdinir superior to control
	Clinical Cure Rates	179/196 (91%)	173/193 (90%)	Cefdinir equivalent to control

2. National Committee for Clinical Laboratory Standards. Performance Standards for Antimicrobial Disk Susceptibility Tests, 6th ed. Approved Standard, NCCLS Document M2-A6, Vol 17(1). NCCLS, Villanova, PA, Jan 1997.
3. Cockcroft DW, Gault MH. Prediction of creatinine clearance from serum creatinine. Nephron 1976;16:31-41.
4. Schwartz GJ, Haycock GB, Edelmann CM, Spitzer A. A simple estimate of glomerular filtration rate in children derived from body length and plasma creatinine. Pediatrics 1976;58:259-63.
5. Schwartz GJ, Feld LG, Langford DJ. A simple estimate of glomerular filtration rate in full-term infants during the first year of life. J Pediatrics 1984;104:849-54.

Ref: 03-A038/03-A037
Rev. July, 2007
TM - Trademark
©2007 Abbott Laboratories
Manufactured by:
CEPH International Corporation
Carolina, Puerto Rico 00986
For:
Abbott Laboratories
North Chicago, IL 60064
Under License of:
Astellas Pharma Inc.
Tokyo, Japan
Please check the Abbott website, www.rxabbott.com, or call (800) 633-9110 for full prescribing information.
Shown in Product Identification Guide, page 304

SIMCOR® ℞
[sĭm-kŏr]
(simvastatin/niacin extended-release)
Tablet, Film Coated, Extended Release For Oral Use

HIGHLIGHTS OF PRESCRIBING INFORMATION
These highlights do not include all the information needed to use SIMCOR safely and effectively. See full prescribing information for SIMCOR.
SIMCOR (simvastatin/niacin extended-release) tablet, film coated, extended release for oral use
Initial U.S. Approval: 2008

INDICATIONS AND USAGE

SIMCOR is a combination of simvastatin, an HMG-Co-A reductase inhibitor, and extended-release niacin (Niaspan), nicotinic acid. SIMCOR is indicated to:
• Reduce elevated total—C, LDL-C, Apo B, non-HDL-C, TG, or to increase HDL-C in patients with primary hypercholesterolemia and mixed dyslipidemia when treatment with simvastatin monotherapy or niacin extended-release monotherapy is considered inadequate. (1.1)
• Reduce TG in patients with hypertriglyceridemia (Fredrickson type IV hyperlipidemia) when treatment with simvastatin monotherapy or niacin extended-release monotherapy is considered inadequate. (1.1)
Limitations of use:
No incremental benefit of SIMCOR on cardiovascular morbidity and mortality over and above that demonstrated for simvastatin monotherapy and niacin monotherapy has been established. (1.1)

DOSAGE AND ADMINISTRATION

• SIMCOR should be taken at bedtime with a low-fat snack. (2)
• Dose range: 500/20 mg to 2000/40 mg once daily. (2)
• Initial dose for patients naïve to or switching from immediate-release niacin: 500/20 mg once daily. (2)
• The initial dose for patients already receiving niacin extended-release should not exceed 2000/40 mg once daily. (2)
• Maintenance dose: 1000/20 mg to 2000/40 mg once daily. (2)
• Doses greater than 2000/40 mg daily are not recommended. (2)

DOSAGE FORMS AND STRENGTHS

• Unscored film-coated tablets:
500 mg niacin extended-release/20 mg simvastatin (3)
750 mg niacin extended-release/20 mg simvastatin (3)
1000 mg niacin extended-release/20 mg simvastatin (3)

CONTRAINDICATIONS

• Active liver disease, which may include unexplained persistent elevations in hepatic transaminase levels (4, 5.2)
• Active peptic ulcer disease (4)
• Arterial bleeding (4)
• Women who are pregnant or may become pregnant (4, 8.1)
• Nursing mothers (4, 8.3)

• Known hypersensitivity to product components (4, 6.1)

WARNINGS AND PRECAUTIONS

• Skeletal muscle effects (e.g., myopathy and rhabdomyolysis): Risks increase with higher doses, advanced age (≥ 65), hypothyroidism, renal impairment, and concomitant use of cyclosporine, danazol, gemfibrozil, amiodarone, and verapamil and potent CYP3A4 inhibitors. (5.1)
• Liver enzyme abnormalities and monitoring: Persistent elevations in hepatic transaminase can occur. Monitor liver enzymes before and during treatment. (5.2)
• Severe hepatic toxicity has occurred in patients substituting sustained-release niacin for immediate-release niacin at equivalent doses. If switching from other niacin preparations, initiate with lowest SIMCOR dose; niacin extended-release can be converted at equivalent doses. (5.2)
• Niacin extended-release can increase serum glucose levels. Glucose levels should be closely monitored in diabetic or potentially diabetic patients particularly during the first few months of use. (5.3)

ADVERSE REACTIONS

The most common (incidence > 3%) adverse reactions with SIMCOR are flushing, headache, back pain, diarrhea, nausea, and pruritus. (6.1)
To report SUSPECTED ADVERSE REACTIONS, contact Abbott Laboratories at 1-800-633-9110 or FDA at 1-800-FDA-1088 or www.fda.gov/medwatch

DRUG INTERACTIONS

• Potent inhibitors of CYP3A4: Combination increases simvastatin exposure. SIMCOR should not be used with potent inhibitors of CYP3A4. (7.1)
• Cyclosporine: Combination with SIMCOR should be avoided. (7.2)
• Danazol: Combination with SIMCOR should be avoided. (7.2)
• Amiodarone: Combination with SIMCOR should be limited to the 20 mg once daily dose of simvastatin. (7.3)
• Verapamil: Combination with SIMCOR should be limited to the 20 mg once daily dose of simvastatin. (7.3)
• Gemfibrozil: Combination with SIMCOR should be avoided. (7.4)
• Fenofibrate: Combination with SIMCOR should be avoided. (7.4)
• Coumarin anticoagulants: Combination prolongs INR. Achieve stable INR prior to starting SIMCOR. Monitor INR frequently until stable upon initiation or alteration of SIMCOR therapy. (7.7)

USE IN SPECIFIC POPULATIONS

• Severe renal impairment (not on dialysis): SIMCOR should be used with extreme caution. (8.7)
See 17 for PATIENT COUNSELING INFORMATION
Revised: 02/2008

FULL PRESCRIBING INFORMATION: CONTENTS*

Information on the Abbott Pharmaceutical Products listed on these pages is from the prescribing information in use as of June 1, 2010. For more information, please visit rxabbott.com or call 1-800-633-9110.

FULL PRESCRIBING INFORMATION

1 INDICATIONS AND USAGE

Therapy with lipid-altering agents should be only one component of multiple risk factor intervention in individuals at significantly increased risk for atherosclerotic vascular disease due to hypercholesterolemia. Drug therapy is indicated as an adjunct to diet when the response to a diet restricted in saturated fat and cholesterol and other nonpharmacologic measures alone has been inadequate.

1.1 Patients with Hypercholesterolemia Requiring Modifications of Lipid Profiles

SIMCOR

SIMCOR is indicated to reduce total-C, LDL-C, Apo B, non-HDL-C, or TG, or to increase HDL-C in patients with primary hypercholesterolemia and mixed dyslipidemia (Fredrickson type IIa and IIb) when treatment with simvastatin monotherapy or niacin extended-release monotherapy is considered inadequate.

SIMCOR is indicated to reduce TG in patients with hypertriglyceridemia (Fredrickson type IV hyperlipidemia) when treatment with simvastatin monotherapy or niacin extended-release monotherapy is considered inadequate.

Limitations of use

No incremental benefit of SIMCOR on cardiovascular morbidity and mortality over and above that demonstrated for simvastatin monotherapy and niacin monotherapy has been established.

2 DOSAGE AND ADMINISTRATION

SIMCOR should be taken as a single daily dose at bedtime, with a low fat snack. Patients not currently on niacin extended-release and patients currently on niacin products other than niacin extended-release should start SIMCOR at a single 500/20 mg tablet daily at bedtime *[See Warnings and Precautions (5.2)]*. The dose of niacin extended-release should not be increased by more than 500 mg daily every 4 weeks - see Table 1. The recommended maintenance dose for SIMCOR is 1000/20 mg to 2000/40 mg (two 1000/20 tablets) once daily depending on patient tolerability and lipid levels. The efficacy and safety of doses of SIMCOR greater than 2000/40 mg daily have not been studied and are therefore not recommended. If SIMCOR therapy is discontinued for an extended period of time (> 7 days), re-titration as tolerated is recommended. SIMCOR tablets should be taken whole and should not be broken, crushed, or chewed before swallowing.

Table 1. Recommended niacin extended-release dosing

	Week(s)	Daily dose of niacin extended-release
Initial Titration Schedule	1 to 4	500 mg
	5 to 8	1000 mg
	*	1500 mg
	*	2000 mg

* After Week 8, titrate to patient response and tolerance. If response to 1000 mg daily is inadequate, increase dose to 1500 mg daily; may subsequently increase dose to 2000 mg daily. Daily dose should not be increased more than 500 mg in a 4-week period, and doses above 2000 mg daily are not recommended.

Due to the increased risk of hepatotoxicity with other modified-release (sustained-release or time-release) niacin preparations or immediate-release (crystalline) niacin, SIMCOR should only be substituted for equivalent doses of niacin extended-release (NIASPAN).

Flushing *[See Adverse Reactions (6.1)]* may be reduced in frequency or severity by pretreatment with aspirin or other non-steroidal anti-inflammatory drugs (approximately 30 minutes prior to SIMCOR dose). Flushing, pruritus, and gastrointestinal distress are also reduced by gradually increasing the dose of niacin (refer to Table 1) and avoiding administration on an empty stomach.

3 DOSAGE FORMS AND STRENGTHS

SIMCOR tablets are formulated for oral administration in the following strength combinations:

Table 2. SIMCOR Tablet Strengths

	500mg/ 20mg	750mg/ 20mg	1000mg/ 20mg
Niacin extended-release equivalent (mg)	500	750	1000
simvastatin equivalent (mg)	20	20	20

- 500 mg/20 mg blue unscored tablets debossed with 021 on one side and KOS on the other
- 750 mg/20 mg blue unscored tablets debossed with 022 on one side and KOS on the other
- 1000 mg/20 mg blue unscored tablets debossed with 023 on one side and KOS on the other

4 CONTRAINDICATIONS

SIMCOR is contraindicated in the following conditions:
- Active liver disease, which may include unexplained persistent elevations in hepatic transaminase levels *[See Warnings and Precautions (5.2)]*
- Patients with active peptic ulcer disease
- Patients with arterial bleeding
- Women who are pregnant or may become pregnant. SIMCOR may cause fetal harm when administered to a pregnant woman. Serum cholesterol and triglycerides increase during normal pregnancy, and cholesterol or cholesterol derivatives are essential for fetal development. Atherosclerosis is a chronic process and discontinuation of lipid-lowering drugs during pregnancy should have little impact on long-term outcomes of primary hypercholesterolemia therapy. There are no adequate and well-controlled studies of SIMCOR use during pregnancy; however in rare reports congenital anomalies were observed following intrauterine exposure to HMG-CoA reductase inhibitors. In rat and rabbit animal reproduction studies, simvastatin revealed no evidence of teratogenicity. There are no animal reproductive studies conducted with niacin. If SIMCOR is used during pregnancy or if the patient becomes pregnant while taking this drug, the patient should be apprised of the potential hazard to the fetus. *[See Use In Specific Populations (8.1)]*
- Nursing mothers. SIMCOR contains simvastatin and nicotinic acid. Nicotinic acid is excreted into human milk and it is not known whether simvastatin is excreted into human milk; however a small amount of another drug in this class does pass into breast milk. Because of the potential for serious adverse reactions in nursing infants, women who require SIMCOR treatment should not breastfeed their infants. *[See Use In Specific Populations (8.3)]*
- Patients with a known hypersensitivity to any component of this product. Hypersensitivity reactions including one of more of the following adverse reactions have been reported for simvastatin and/or niacin extended-release: anaphylaxis, angioedema, urticaria, fever, dyspnea, tongue edema, larynx edema, face edema, peripheral edema, laryngismus, and flushing. *[See Adverse Reactions (6.1)]*

5 WARNINGS AND PRECAUTIONS

SIMCOR should not be substituted for equivalent doses of immediate-release (crystalline) niacin. For patients switching from immediate-release niacin to SIMCOR, therapy with SIMCOR should be initiated at 500/20 mg and appropriately titrated to the desired therapeutic response. Doses of SIMCOR greater than 2000/40 mg are not recommended.

5.1 Myopathy/Rhabdomyolysis

Simvastatin

Simvastatin, like other inhibitors of HMG-CoA reductase, occasionally causes myopathy manifested as muscle pain, tenderness or weakness with creatine kinase (CK) above ten times the upper limit of normal (ULN). Myopathy sometimes takes the form of rhabdomyolysis with or without acute renal failure secondary to myoglobinuria, and rare fatalities have occurred. The risk of myopathy is increased by high levels of HMG-CoA reductase inhibitory activity in plasma.

As with other HMG-CoA reductase inhibitors, the risk of myopathy/rhabdomyolysis is dose related. In a clinical trial database in which 41,050 patients were treated with simvastatin with 24,747 (approximately 60%) treated for at least 4 years, the incidence of myopathy was approximately 0.02%, 0.08%, and 0.53% at 20, 40, and 80 mg/day, respectively. In these trials, patients were carefully monitored and some interacting medicinal products were excluded.

Potent inhibitors of CYP3A4: The risk of myopathy appears to be increased by high levels of HMG-CoA reductase inhibitory activity in plasma. Simvastatin is metabolized by the cytochrome P450 isoform 3A4. Certain drugs which share this metabolic pathway can raise the plasma levels of simvastatin and may increase the risk of myopathy. These include cyclosporine, itraconazole, ketoconazole, and other antifungal azoles, the macrolide antibiotics erythromycin and clarithromycin, and the ketolide antibiotic telithromycin, HIV protease inhibitors, the antidepressant nefazodone, or large quantities of grapefruit juice (> 1 quart daily). The risk of myopathy/rhabdomyolysis is increased by concomitant use of simvastatin and, therefore, SIMCOR with the following:

Potent inhibitors of cytochrome P-450 isoform, 3A4 (CYP 3A4):
  Itraconazole, ketoconazole, and other antifungal azoles
  Macrolide antibiotics erythromycin, clarithromycin, and telithromycin
  HIV protease inhibitors
  Antidepressant nefazodone
  Grapefruit juice in large quantities (> 1 quart daily)

The use of SIMCOR concomitantly with these potent CYP3A4 inhibitors should be avoided. *[See Drug Interactions (7.1)]*

Cyclosporine or Danazol: Simvastatin dose should not exceed 10 mg daily in combination with cyclosporine or danazol. Therefore, the combined use of SIMCOR with cyclosporine or danazol should be avoided. *[See Drug Interactions (7.2)]*

Gemfibrozil: Simvastatin dose should not exceed 10 mg daily when concomitantly used with gemfibrozil. Therefore, the combined use of SIMCOR with gemfibrozil should be avoided. *[See Drug Interactions (7.4)]*

Other Fibrates: Combined use of SIMCOR with drugs that cause myopathy/rhabdomyolysis when given alone, such as fibrates, should be avoided. *[See Drug Interactions (7.4)]*

Amiodarone or Verapamil: The dose of the simvastatin component of SIMCOR should not exceed 20 mg in patients receiving amiodarone or verapamil concomitantly. The combined use of the simvastatin at doses higher than 20 mg daily with amiodarone or verapamil should be avoided unless the clinical benefit is likely to outweigh the increased risk of myopathy. *[See Drug Interactions (7.3)]*

SIMCOR

Myopathy and/or rhabdomyolysis have been reported when simvastatin is used in combination with lipid-altering doses (≥ 1 gram/day) of niacin. Physicians contemplating the use of SIMCOR, a combination of simvastatin and niacin, should weigh the potential benefits and risks, and should carefully monitor for any signs and symptoms of muscle pain, tenderness, or weakness, particularly during the initial month of treatment or during any period of upward dosage titration of either drug. Periodic determination of serum creatine kinase (CK) determinations may be considered in such situations, but there is no assurance that such monitoring will prevent myopathy.

Patients starting therapy with SIMCOR should be advised of the risk of myopathy, and told to report promptly unexplained muscle pain, tenderness, or weakness. A CK level above 10 times ULN in a patient with unexplained muscle symptoms indicates myopathy. SIMCOR therapy should be discontinued if myopathy is diagnosed or suspected.

In patients with complicated medical histories predisposing to rhabdomyolysis, such as renal insufficiency, dose escalation requires caution. Also, as there are no known adverse consequences of brief interruption of therapy, treatment with SIMCOR should be stopped for a few days before elective major surgery and when any major acute medical or surgical condition supervenes (e.g., sepsis, hypotension, dehydration, major surgery, trauma, severe metabolic, endocrine, and electrolyte disorders, or uncontrolled seizures).

5.2 Liver Dysfunction

Cases of severe hepatic toxicity, including fulminant hepatic necrosis, have occurred in patients who have substituted sustained-release (modified-release, timed-release) niacin products for immediate-release (crystalline) niacin at equivalent doses. Patients previously receiving niacin products other than niacin extended-release should be started on SIMCOR at the lowest recommended starting dose. *[See Dosage and Administration (2)]*

SIMCOR should be used with caution in patients who consume substantial quantities of alcohol and/or have a past history of liver disease. Active liver disease or unexplained transaminase elevations are contraindications to the use of SIMCOR. *[See Contraindications (4)]*

Niacin extended-release and simvastatin can cause abnormal liver tests. In a simvastatin-controlled, 24 week study with SIMCOR in 641 patients, there were no persistent increases (to more than 3× the ULN) in serum transaminases. In three placebo-controlled clinical studies of extended-release niacin there were no patients with normal serum transaminases levels at baseline who experienced elevations to more than 3× the ULN. Persistent increases (to more than 3× the ULN) in serum transaminases have occurred in approximately 1% of patients who received simvastatin in clinical studies. When drug treatment was interrupted or discontinued in these patients, the transaminases levels usually fell slowly to pretreatment levels. The increases were not associated with jaundice or other clinical signs or symptoms. There was no evidence of hypersensitivity.

Liver function tests should be performed on all patients during therapy with SIMCOR. It is recommended that liver function tests be performed before treatment begins, every 12 weeks for the first 6 months, and periodically thereafter (e.g., at approximately 6-month intervals). Patients who develop increased transaminase levels should be monitored with a second liver function evaluation to confirm the finding and be followed thereafter with frequent liver function tests until the abnormality returns to normal. Should an increase in transaminase levels of more than 3× ULN persist, or if transaminase elevations are associated with symptoms of nausea, fever, and/or malaise, withdrawal of SIMCOR therapy is recommended.

5.3 Laboratory Abnormalities

Increase in Blood Glucose: Niacin treatment can increase fasting blood glucose. In a simvastatin-controlled, 24-week study with SIMCOR the change from baseline in glycosylated hemoglobin levels was 0.2% for SIMCOR-treated patients and 0.2% for simvastatin-treated patients. Diabetic or potentially diabetic patients should be observed closely during treatment with SIMCOR, particularly during the first few months of therapy. Adjustment of diet and/or hypoglycemic therapy or discontinuation of SIMCOR may be necessary.

Reduction in platelet count: Niacin can reduce platelet count. In a simvastatin-controlled, 24-week study with SIMCOR the mean percent change from baseline for patients treated with 2000/40 mg daily was -5.6%.

Increase in Prothrombin Time (PT): Niacin can cause small increases in PT. In a simvastatin-controlled, 24-week study with SIMCOR this effect was not seen.

Increase in Uric Acid: Elevated uric acid levels have occurred with niacin therapy. In a simvastatin-controlled, 24-week study with SIMCOR this effect was not seen. Nevertheless, in patients predisposed to gout, SIMCOR therapy should be used with caution.

Decrease in Phosphorus: Small dose-related reductions in phosphorous levels were seen in clinical studies with niacin. In a simvastatin-controlled, 24-week study with SIMCOR this effect was not seen.

6 ADVERSE REACTIONS

Overview

In a controlled clinical study, 14% of patients randomized to SIMCOR discontinued therapy due to an adverse event. Flushing episodes (i.e., warmth, redness, itching and/or tingling) were the most common treatment-emergent adverse reactions, occurring in up to 59% of patients treated with SIMCOR. Spontaneous reports with niacin extended-release and clinical studies of SIMCOR suggest that flushing may be accompanied by symptoms of dizziness or syncope, tachycardia, palpitations, shortness of breath, sweating, chills, and/or edema.

6.1 Clinical Studies Experience

SIMCOR

Because clinical studies are conducted under widely varying conditions, adverse reaction rates observed in the clinical studies of a drug cannot be directly compared to rates in the clinical studies of another drug and may not reflect the rates observed in practice.

The safety data described below reflect exposure to SIMCOR in 403 patients in a controlled study for a period of 6 months.

Flushing: Flushing (warmth, redness, itching and/or tingling) occurred in up to 59% of patients treated with SIMCOR. Flushing resulted in study discontinuation for 6.0% of patients.

More Common Adverse Reactions: In addition to flushing, adverse reactions occurring in ≥ 3% of patients (irrespective of investigator causality) treated with SIMCOR are shown in Table 3 below:

Table 3. Adverse Reactions Occurring in ≥ 3% of Patients in a Controlled Clinical Trial

Adverse Event	SIMCOR overall*	Simvastatin overall**
Total Number of Patients	N=403	N=238
Headache	18 (4.5%)	11 (4.6%)
Pruritus	13 (3.2%)	0 (0.0%)
Nausea	13 (3.2%)	10 (4.2%)
Back Pain	13 (3.2%)	5 (2.1%)
Diarrhea	12 (3.0%)	7 (2.9%)

* SIMCOR overall included all doses from 500/20 mg to 2000/40 mg

** Simvastatin overall included 20 mg, 40 mg, and 80 mg doses

Simvastatin

In pre-marketing controlled clinical studies and their open extensions (2,423 patients with mean duration of follow-up of approximately 18 months) 1.4% of patients discontinued due to adverse reactions. The most commonly reported adverse reactions (incidence > 1%) in simvastatin controlled clinical trials were: headache (3.5%), abdominal pain (3.5%), constipation (2.3%), upper respiratory infection (2.1%), diarrhea (1.9%), and flatulence (1.9%).

Niacin Extended-Release

In placebo-controlled clinical trials (n=245), flushing episodes were the most common treatment-emergent adverse events (up to 88% of patients) for niacin extended-release. Other adverse events occurring in 5% or greater of patients treated with niacin extended-release are headache (9%), diarrhea (7%), nausea (5%), rhinitis (5%), and dyspepsia (4%) at a maintenance dose of 1000mg daily.

Clinical Laboratory Abnormalities:

SIMCOR

Chemistry

Elevations in serum transaminases *[See Warnings and Precautions (5.2)]*, CK, fasting glucose, uric acid, alkaline phosphatase, LDH, amylase, γ-glutamyl transpeptidase, bilirubin, and reductions in phosphorus, and abnormal thyroid function tests.

Hematology

Reductions in platelet counts and prolongation of PT. *[See Warnings and Precautions (5.3)]*

Postmarketing Experience

Because the below reactions are reported voluntarily from a population of uncertain size, it is generally not possible to reliably estimate their frequency or establish a causal relationship to drug exposure.

Simvastatin

The following additional adverse reactions have been identified during postapproval use of simvastatin. Hypersensitivity reaction including one or more of the following features: anaphylaxis, angioedema, lupus erythematous-like syndrome, vasculitis, purpura, thrombocytopenia, leucopenia, hemolytic anemia, positive ANA, ESR increase, eosinophilia, arthritis, photosensitivity, chills, toxic epidermal necrolysis, erythema multiforme, Stevens-Johnson syndrome, urticaria, fever, dyspnea, and arthralgia; pancreatitis, hepatitis, hepatic failure, pruritus, cataracts, polymyositis, dermatomyositis, polymyalgia rheumatica, global amnesia, tendon rupture, peripheral neuropathy, memory impairment.

NIASPAN

The following additional adverse reactions have been identified during post-approval use of NIASPAN. Hypersensitivity reaction including one or more of the following features: anaphylaxis, angioedema, urticaria, flushing, dyspnea, tongue edema, larynx edema, face edema, peripheral edema, laryngismus, vesiculobullous rash, palpitations, syncope, hypotension, orthostasis, decreased glucose tolerance, gout, hepatitis, skin discoloration, rhabdomyolysis, amblyopia, and insomnia.

7 DRUG INTERACTIONS

No drug interaction studies were conducted with SIMCOR. However, the following interactions have been noted with the individual components of SIMCOR:

Simvastatin

7.1 CYP3A4 Inhibitors

Simvastatin, like several other inhibitors of HMG-CoA reductase, is a substrate of CYP3A4. Simvastatin is metabolized by CYP3A4 but has no CYP3A4 inhibitory activity; therefore it is not expected to affect the plasma concentrations of other drugs metabolized by CYP3A4.

Potent inhibitors of CYP3A4 include:
Itraconazole, ketoconazole, and other antifungal azoles,
Macrolide antibiotics erythromycin, clarithromycin, and telithromycin,
HIV protease inhibitors,
Antidepressant nefazodone,
Grapefruit juice in large quantities (> 1 quart daily).

Potent inhibitors of CYP3A4 increase the risk of myopathy by reducing the elimination of simvastatin. Hence when simvastatin is used with a potent inhibitor of CYP3A4, elevated plasma levels of HMG-CoA reductase inhibitory activity can increase the risk of myopathy and rhabdomyolysis, particularly with higher doses of simvastatin. *[See Warnings and Precautions (5.1)]*

Serious skeletal muscle disorder, e.g., rhabdomyolysis, have been reported during concomitant therapy of simvastatin or other HMG-CoA reductase inhibitors with cyclosporine, danazol, itraconazole, ketoconazole, gemfibrozil, niacin, erythromycin, clarithromycin, telithromycin, nefazodone or HIV protease inhibitors.

Concomitant use of drugs labeled as potent inhibitors of CYP3A4 should be avoided unless the benefits of combined therapy outweigh the increased risk. If treatment with itraconazole, ketoconazole, erythromycin, clarithromycin or telithromycin is unavoidable, therapy with SIMCOR should be suspended during the course of treatment.

7.2 Cyclosporine or Danazol

Although the mechanism is not fully understood, cyclosporine has been shown to increase the area under the curve (AUC) of HMG-CoA reductase inhibitors. The increase in AUC for simvastatin acid is presumably due, in part, to inhibition of CYP3A4. The risk of myopathy/rhabdomyolysis is increased by concomitant administration of cyclosporine or danazol particularly with higher doses of simvastatin. *[See Warnings and Precautions (5.1)]*

7.3 Amiodarone or Verapamil

The risk of myopathy/rhabdomyolysis is increased by concomitant administration of amiodarone or verapamil with higher doses of simvastatin. *[See Warnings and Precautions (5.1)]*

7.4 Gemfibrozil and other Fibrates

Coadministration of gemfibrozil (600 mg twice daily for 3 days) with simvastatin (40 mg daily) resulted in clinically significant increases in simvastatin acid AUC (185%) and peak plasma concentration (C_{max}, 112%), possibly due to inhibition of simvastatin acid glucuronidation by gemfibrozil. The increase in simvastatin exposure increases the risk of myopathy when coadministred with gemfibrozil. The combined use of SIMCOR with gemfibrozil should be avoided *[See Warnings and Precautions (5.1)]*. The risk of myopathy also increases to a lesser extent when simvastatin is used in combination with other fibrates. Coadministration of 160 mg fenofibrate daily with 80 mg simvastatin daily for 7 days had no effect on plasma AUC (and C_{max}) of either total HMG-CoA reductase inhibitory activity or fenofibric acid; there was a modest reduction (approximately 35%) of simvastatin acid which was not considered clinically significant.

7.5 Propranolol

In healthy male volunteers there was a significant decrease in mean C_{max}, but no change in AUC, for simvastatin total and active inhibitors with concomitant administration of single doses of simvastatin and propranolol. The clinical relevance of this finding is unclear. The pharmacokinetics of the enantiomers of propranolol were not affected.

7.6 Digoxin

Concomitant administration of a single dose of digoxin in healthy male volunteers receiving simvastatin resulted in a slight elevation (less than 0.3 ng/mL) in digoxin concentrations in plasma (as measured by a radioimmunoassay) compared to concomitant administration of placebo and digoxin. Patients taking digoxin should be monitored appropriately when SIMCOR is initiated.

7.7 Coumarin Anticoagulants

In normal volunteers and hypercholesterolemic patients, simvastatin 20–40 mg/day modestly potentiated the effect of coumarin anticoagulants since the prothrombin time, reported as International Normalized Ratio (INR), increased from a baseline of 1.7 to 1.8 and from 2.6 to 3.4 in the volunteers and patients, respectively. With other reductase inhibitors, clinically evident bleeding and/or increased prothrombin time has been reported in a few patients taking coumarin anticoagulants concomitantly. In such patients, prothrombin time should be determined before starting SIMCOR and frequently enough during early therapy to ensure that no significant alteration of prothrombin time occurs. Once a stable prothrombin time has been documented, prothrombin times can be monitored at the intervals usu-

Information on the Abbott Pharmaceutical Products listed on these pages is from the prescribing information in use as of June 1, 2010. For more information, please visit rxabbott.com or call 1-800-633-9110.

ally recommended for patients on coumarin anticoagulants. If the dose of SIMCOR is changed or discontinued, the same procedure should be repeated.

Niacin

7.8 Aspirin

Concomitant use of aspirin may decrease the metabolic clearance of niacin. The clinical relevance of this finding is unclear.

7.9 Antihypertensive Therapy

Niacin may potentiate the effects of ganglionic blocking agents and vasoactive drugs resulting in postural hypotension.

7.10 Bile Acid Sequestrants

An *in vitro* study was carried out investigating the niacin-binding capacity of colestipol and cholestyramine. About 98% of available niacin was bound to colestipol, with 10 to 30% binding to cholestyramine. These results suggest that 4 to 6 hours, or as great an interval as possible, should elapse between the ingestion of bile acid-binding resins and the administration of SIMCOR.

7.11 Other

Nutritional supplements containing large doses of niacin or related compounds may potentiate the adverse effects of SIMCOR.

8 USE IN SPECIFIC POPULATIONS

8.1 Pregnancy

Pregnancy Category X – *[See Contraindications (4)]*

SIMCOR is contraindicated in women who are or may become pregnant. Lipid lowering drugs offer no benefit during pregnancy, because cholesterol and cholesterol derivatives are needed for normal fetal development. Serum cholesterol and triglycerides increase during normal pregnancy. Atherosclerosis is a chronic process, and discontinuation of lipid-lowering drugs during pregnancy should have little impact on long-term outcomes of primary hypercholesterolemia therapy. There are no adequate and well-controlled studies of SIMCOR use during pregnancy; however, there are rare reports of congenital anomalies in infants exposed to HMG-CoA reductase inhibitors *in utero*. Animal reproduction studies of simvastatin in rats and rabbits showed no evidence of teratogenicity. SIMCOR may cause fetal harm when administered to a pregnant woman. If SIMCOR is used during pregnancy or if the patient becomes pregnant while taking this drug, the patient should be apprised of the potential hazard to the fetus.

SIMCOR contains simvastatin (a HMG-CoA reductase inhibitor) and niacin (nicotinic acid). There are rare reports of congenital anomalies following intrauterine exposure to HMG-CoA reductase inhibitors. In a review of approximately 100 prospectively followed pregnancies in women exposed to simvastatin or another structurally related HMG-CoA reductase inhibitor, the incidences of congenital anomalies, spontaneous abortions, and fetal deaths/stillbirths did not exceed those expected in the general population. However, the study was only able to exclude a 3- to 4-fold increased risk of congenital anomalies over the background rate. In 89% of these cases, drug treatment was initiated prior to pregnancy and was discontinued during the first trimester when pregnancy was identified. It is not known whether niacin at doses used for lipid disorders can cause fetal harm when administered to a pregnant woman. Simvastatin was not teratogenic in rats or rabbits at doses that resulted in 3 times the human exposure based on mg/m^2 surface area. However, in studies with another structurally-related HMG-CoA reductase inhibitor, skeletal malformations were observed in rats and mice. Animal reproduction studies have not been conducted with niacin.

Women of childbearing potential, who require SIMCOR treatment for a lipid disorder, should use effective contraception. Patients trying to conceive should contact their prescriber to discuss stopping SIMCOR treatment. If pregnancy occurs, SIMCOR should be immediately discontinued.

8.3 Nursing Mothers

It is not known whether simvastatin is excreted into human milk; however, a small amount of another drug in this class does pass into breast milk. Niacin is excreted into human milk but the actual infant dose or infant dose as a percent of the maternal dose is not known. Because of the potential for serious adverse reactions in nursing infants, nursing mothers who require SIMCOR treatment should not breastfeed their infants. A decision should be made whether to discontinue nursing or discontinue drug, taking into account the importance of the drug to the mother. *[see Contraindications (4)].*

8.4 Pediatric Use

The safety and effectiveness of SIMCOR in pediatric patients have not been established.

8.5 Geriatric Use

There were 281 (30.8%) patients aged 65 years and older treated with SIMCOR in Phase III clinical studies. No overall differences in safety and effectiveness were observed between these patients and younger patients, but greater sensitivity of some older individuals cannot be ruled out. A pharmacokinetic study with simvastatin showed the mean plasma level of HMG-CoA reductase inhibitory activity to be approximately 45% higher in elderly patients between 70–78 years of age compared with patients between 18–30 years of age.

8.6 Gender

Data from the clinical trials suggest that women have a greater hypolipidemic response than men at equivalent doses of niacin extended-release. No consistent gender differences in efficacy and safety were observed in SIMCOR studies.

8.7 Renal Impairment

No pharmacokinetic studies have been conducted in patients with renal impairment for SIMCOR. Caution should be exercised when SIMCOR is administered to patients with renal disease. For patients with severe renal insufficiency, SIMCOR should not be started unless the patient has already tolerated treatment with simvastatin at a dose of 10 mg or higher. Caution should be exercised when SIMCOR is administered to these patients and they should be closely monitored.

8.8 Hepatic Impairment

No pharmacokinetic studies have been conducted in patients with hepatic insufficiency for SIMCOR. *[See Warnings and Precautions (5.2)]*

10 OVERDOSAGE

Supportive measures should be taken in the event of an overdose. The dialyzability of niacin, or of simvastatin and its metabolites, is not known.

A few cases of overdosage with simvastatin have been reported; the maximum dose taken was 3.6 g. All patients recovered without sequelae.

11 DESCRIPTION

SIMCOR tablets contain niacin extended-release (NIASPAN) and simvastatin in combination. Simvastatin, an inhibitor of HMG-CoA reductase, and niacin are both lipid-altering agents.

Niacin Extended-Release

Niacin is nicotinic acid, or 3-pyridinecarboxylic acid. Niacin is a white, nonhygroscopic crystalline powder that is very soluble in water, boiling ethanol, and propylene glycol. It is insoluble in ethyl ether. The empirical formula of niacin is $C_6H_5NO_2$ and its molecular weight is 123.11. Niacin has the following structural formula:

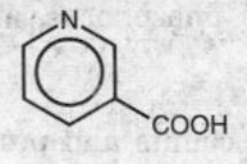

Simvastatin

Simvastatin is butanoic acid, 2,2-dimethyl-,1,2,3,7,8,8a-hexahydro-3-7-dimethyl-8-[2-(tetrahydro-4-hydroxy-6-oxo-2H-pyran-2-yl)-ethyl]-1-naphthalenyl ester, [1S-[1α,3α,7β,8β(2S*4S*),-8aβ]]. Simvastatin is a white to off-white, nonhygroscopic, crystalline powder that is practically insoluble in water and freely soluble in chloroform, methanol, and ethanol. The empirical formula of simvastatin is $C_{25}H_{38}O_5$ and its molecular weight is 418.57. Simvastatin has the following structural formula:

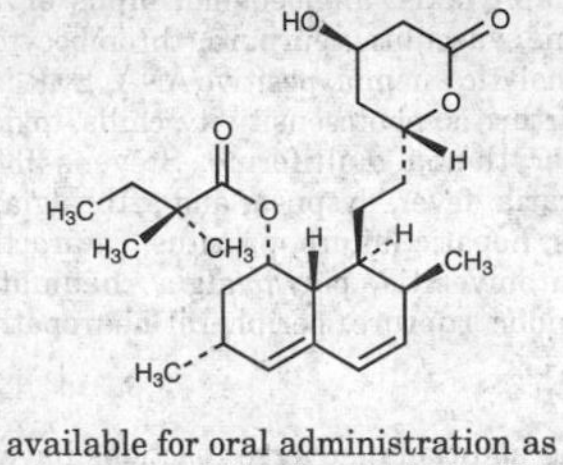

SIMCOR is available for oral administration as tablets containing 500 mg of extended-release niacin (NIASPAN) and 20 mg simvastatin (SIMCOR 500/20), 750 mg of extended-release niacin (NIASPAN) and 20 mg simvastatin (SIMCOR 750/20), and 1000 mg of extended-release niacin (NIASPAN) and 20 mg simvastatin (SIMCOR 1000/20). Each tablet contains the following inactive ingredients: hypromellose, povidone, stearic acid, polyethylene glycol, butylated hydroxyanisole, a blue Opadry® color coat (FD&C Blue #2, hypromellose, lactose monohydrate, titanium dioxide, triacetin), and a clear Opadry® coat (hypromellose, polyethylene glycol).

12 CLINICAL PHARMACOLOGY

12.1 Mechanism of Action

Niacin

Niacin functions in the body after conversion to nicotinamide adenine dinucleotide (NAD) in the NAD coenzyme system. The mechanism by which niacin alters lipid profiles is not completely understood and may involve several actions, including partial inhibition of release of free fatty acids from adipose tissue, and increased lipoprotein lipase activity (which may increase the rate of chylomicron triglyceride removal from plasma). Niacin decreases the rate of hepatic synthesis of VLDL-C and LDL-C, and does not appear to affect fecal excretion of fats, sterols, or bile acids.

Simvastatin

Simvastatin is a prodrug and is hydrolyzed to its active β-hydroxyacid form, simvastatin acid, after administration. Simvastatin is a specific inhibitor of 3-hydroxy-3-methylglutaryl-coenzyme A (HMG-CoA) reductase, the enzyme that catalyzes the conversion of HMG-CoA to mevalonate, an early and rate-limiting step in the biosynthetic pathway for cholesterol. In addition, simvastatin reduces VLDL and TG and increases HDL-C.

12.2 Pharmacodynamics

A variety of clinical studies have demonstrated that elevated levels of Total-C, LDL-C, and Apo B promote human atherosclerosis. Similarly, decreased levels of HDL-C are associated with the development of atherosclerosis. Epidemiological investigations have established that cardiovascular morbidity and mortality vary directly with the level of Total-C and LDL-C, and inversely with the level of HDL-C. Like LDL, cholesterol-enriched triglyceride-rich lipoproteins, including VLDL, intermediate-density lipoprotein (IDL), and their remnants, can also promote atherosclerosis. Elevated plasma TG are frequently found in a triad with low HDL-C levels and small LDL particles, as well as in association with non-lipid metabolic risk factors for coronary heart disease (CHD). As such, total plasma TG has not consistently been shown to be an independent risk factor for CHD. Furthermore, the independent effect of raising HDL-C or lowering TG on the risk of coronary and cardiovascular morbidity and mortality has not been determined.

SIMCOR

SIMCOR reduces total-C, LDL-C, non-HDL-C, Apo B, TG, and Lp(a) levels and increases HDL-C in patients with primary type II hyperlipidemia (heterozygous familial and nonfamilial), mixed dyslipidemia, or hypertriglyceridemia.

Niacin

Niacin (but not nicotinamide) in gram doses reduces LDL-C, Apo B, Lp(a), TG, and Total-C, and increases HDL-C. The magnitude of individual lipid and lipoprotein responses may be influenced by the severity and type of underlying lipid abnormality. The increase in HDL-C is associated with an increase in apolipoprotein A-I (Apo A-I) and a shift in the distribution of HDL subfractions. These shifts include an increase in the HDL2:HDL3 ratio, and an elevation in lipoprotein A-I (Lp A-I, an HDL-C particle containing only Apo A-I). Niacin treatment also decreases serum levels of apolipoprotein B-100 (Apo B), the major protein component of the very low-density lipoprotein (VLDL) and LDL fractions, and of Lp(a), a variant form of LDL independently associated with coronary risk. In addition, preliminary reports suggest that niacin causes favorable LDL particle size transformations, although the clinical relevance of this effect requires further investigation.

Simvastatin

Simvastatin reduces elevated total-C, LDL-C, Apo B, and TG, and increases HDL-C in patients with primary heterozygous familial and nonfamilial hypercholesterolemia and mixed dyslipidemia. Simvastatin reduces total-C and LDL-C in patients with homozygous familial hypercholesterolemia. Simvastatin decreases VLDL, total-C/HDL-C ratio, and LDL-C/HDL-C ratio.

12.3 Pharmacokinetics

Absorption and Bioavailability

SIMCOR

The relative bioavailability of niacin (Nicotinuric acid, NUA, C_{max} and total urinary excretion as the surrogate), simvastatin, and simvastatin acid was evaluated under a light snack conditions in healthy volunteers (n=42), following administration of two 1000/20 mg SIMCOR tablets. Niacin exposure (C_{max} and AUC) after SIMCOR was similar to that of a niacin extended-release formulation. However, simvastatin and simvastatin acid AUC after SIMCOR increased by 23% and 41%, respectively, compared to those of a simvastatin immediate release formulation. The mean time to C_{max} (T_{max}) for niacin ranged from 4.6 to 4.9 hours and simvastatin from 1.9 to 2.0 hours. Following administration of 2 × 1000/20 mg SIMCOR, the mean C_{max}, T_{max} and $AUC_{(0-t)}$ for simvastatin acid, active metabolite of simvastatin, were 3.29 ng/mL, 6.56 hours and 30.81 ng•hr/mL respectively.

Bioequivalence has not been evaluated among different SIMCOR dosage strengths. Therefore, dosage strengths of SIMCOR should not be considered exchangeable.

Niacin

Due to extensive and saturable first-pass metabolism, niacin concentrations in the general circulation are dose dependent and highly variable. Peak steady-state niacin concentrations were 0.6, 4.9, and 15.5 mcg/mL after doses of 1000, 1500, and 2000 mg NIASPAN once daily (given as two 500 mg, two 750 mg, and two 1000 mg tablets, respectively).

To reduce the risk of gastrointestinal upset, administration of niacin extended-release with a low-fat meal or snack is recommended.

Simvastatin
Since simvastatin undergoes extensive first-pass extraction in the liver, the availability of the drug to the general circulation is low (<5%). Peak plasma concentrations of both active and total inhibitors were attained within 1.3 to 2.4 hours postdose. Following an oral dose of ^{14}C-labeled simvastatin in man, plasma concentration of total radioactivity (simvastatin plus ^{14}C-metabolites) peaked at 4 hours and declined rapidly to about 10% of peak by 12 hours postdose. Relative to the fasting state, the plasma profile of inhibitors was not affected when simvastatin was administered immediately before an American Heart Association recommended low-fat meal.

Metabolism
SIMCOR
Following administration of SIMCOR, niacin and simvastatin undergo rapid and extensive first-pass metabolism as described in the following niacin and simvastatin sections. Following administration of 2 × 1000/20 mg SIMCOR in healthy volunteers, 10.2%, 10.7%, and 29.5% of the administered niacin dose was recovered in urine as niacin metabolites, nicotinuric acid (NUA), N-methylnicotinamide (MNA), and N-methyl-2-pyridone-5-carboxamide (2PY), respectively. Following administration of 2 × 1000/20 mg SIMCOR, the mean C_{max}, T_{max}, and $AUC_{(0-t)}$ for the simvastatin metabolite, simvastatin acid were 3.29 ng/mL, 6.56 hours, and 30.81 ng•hr/mL respectively.

Niacin
Niacin undergoes rapid and extensive first-pass metabolism that is dose-rate specific and, at the doses used to treat dyslipidemia, saturable. In humans, one pathway is through a simple conjugation step with glycine to form NUA. NUA is then excreted, although there may be a small amount of reversible metabolism back to niacin. The other pathway results in the formation of nicotinamide adenine dinucleotide (NAD). It is unclear whether nicotinamide is formed as a precursor to, or following the synthesis of, NAD. Nicotinamide is further metabolized to at least MNA and nicotinamide-N-oxide NNO. MNA is further metabolized to two other compounds, 2PY and N-methyl-4-pyridone-5-carboxamide (4PY). The formation of 2PY appears to predominate over 4PY in humans.

Simvastatin
Simvastatin is a substrate of CYP3A4. Simvastatin is a lactone that is readily hydrolyzed *in vivo* to the corresponding β-hydroxyacid, a potent inhibitor of HMG-CoA reductase. The major active metabolites of simvastatin present in human plasma are the β-hydroxyacid of simvastatin and its 6'-hydroxy, 6'-hydroxymethyl, and 6'-exomethylene derivatives.

Elimination
SIMCOR
Following 2 × 1000/20 mg SIMCOR administration, approximately 54% of the niacin dose administered was recovered in urine in 96 hours as niacin and metabolites of which 3.6% was recovered as niacin.
After SIMCOR administration, the mean terminal plasma half-life for simvastatin was 4.2 to 4.9 hours and for simvastatin acid was 4.6 to 5.0 hours.

Niacin
Niacin and its metabolites are rapidly eliminated in the urine. Following single and multiple doses of 1500 to 2000 mg niacin, approximately 53 to 77% of the niacin dose administered as NIASPAN was recovered in urine as niacin and metabolites; up to 7.7% of the dose was recovered in urine as unchanged niacin after multiple dosing with 2 × 1000 mg NIASPAN. The ratio of metabolites recovered in the urine was dependent on the dose administered.

Simvastatin
Simvastatin is excreted in urine, based on studies in humans. Following an oral dose of ^{14}C-labeled simvastatin in man, 13% of the dose was excreted in urine and 60% in feces.

Special Populations
A pharmacokinetic study with simvastatin showed the mean plasma level of HMG-CoA reductase inhibitory activity to be approximately 45% higher in elderly patients between 70–78 years of age compared with patients between 18–30 years of age.
Steady-state plasma concentrations of niacin and metabolites after administration of niacin extended-release are generally higher in women than in men, with the magnitude of the difference varying with dose and metabolite. Recovery of niacin and metabolites in urine, however, is generally similar for men and women, indicating that absorption is similar for both genders. The gender differences observed in plasma levels of niacin and its metabolites may be due to gender-specific differences in metabolic rate or volume of distribution.

Pharmacokinetic studies with a statin having a similar principal route of elimination to that of simvastatin have suggested that for a given dose level, higher systemic exposure may be achieved in patients with severe renal insufficiency (as measured by creatinine clearance).

13 NONCLINICAL TOXICOLOGY
13.1 Carcinogenesis, Mutagenesis, Impairment of Fertility
No studies have been conducted with SIMCOR regarding carcinogenesis, mutagenesis, or impairment of fertility.
Niacin
Niacin, administered to mice for a lifetime as a 1% solution in drinking water, was not carcinogenic. The mice in this study received approximately 6 to 8 times a human dose of 3000 mg/day as determined on a mg/m² basis. Niacin was negative for mutagenicity in the Ames test. No studies on impairment of fertility have been performed.
Simvastatin
In a 72-week carcinogenicity study, mice were administered daily doses of simvastatin of 25, 100, and 400 mg/kg body weight, which resulted in mean plasma drug levels approximately 1, 4, and 8 times higher than the mean human plasma drug level, respectively (as total inhibitory activity based on AUC) after an 80-mg oral dose. Liver carcinomas were significantly increased in high-dose females and mid- and high-dose males with a maximum incidence of 90% in males. The incidence of adenomas of the liver was significantly increased in mid- and high-dose females. Drug treatment also significantly increased the incidence of lung adenomas in mid- and high-dose males and females. Adenomas of the Harderian gland (a gland of the eye of rodents) were significantly higher in high-dose mice than in controls. No evidence of a tumorigenic effect was observed at 25 mg/kg/day.
In a separate 92-week carcinogenicity study in mice at doses up to 25 mg/kg/day, no evidence of a tumorigenic effect was observed (mean plasma drug levels were 1 times higher than humans given 80 mg simvastatin as measured by AUC). In a two-year study in rats at 25 mg/kg/day, there was a statistically significant increase in the incidence of thyroid follicular adenomas in female rats exposed to approximately 11 times higher levels of simvastatin than in humans given 80 mg simvastatin (as measured by AUC). A second two-year rat carcinogenicity study with doses of 50 and 100 mg/kg/day produced hepatocellular adenomas and carcinomas (in female rats at both doses and in males at 100 mg/kg/day). Thyroid follicular cell adenomas were increased in males and females at both doses; thyroid follicular cell carcinomas were increased in females at 100 mg/kg/day. The increased incidence of thyroid neoplasms appears to be consistent with findings from other HMG-CoA reductase inhibitors. These treatment levels represented plasma drug levels (AUC) of approximately 7 and 15 times (males) and 22 and 25 times (females) the mean human plasma drug exposure after an 80 milligram daily dose. No evidence of mutagenicity was observed in a microbial mutagenicity (Ames) test with or without rat or mouse liver metabolic activation. In addition, no evidence of damage to genetic material was noted in an *in vitro* alkaline elution assay using rat hepatocytes, a V-79 mammalian cell forward mutation study, an *in vitro* chromosome aberration study in CHO cells, or an *in vivo* chromosomal aberration assay in mouse bone marrow. There was decreased fertility in male rats treated with simvastatin for 34 weeks at 25 mg/kg body weight (4 times the maximum human exposure level, based on AUC, in patients receiving 80 mg/day); however, this effect was not observed during a subsequent fertility study in which simvastatin was administered at this same dose level to male rats for 11 weeks (the entire cycle of spermatogenesis including epididymal maturation). No microscopic changes were observed in the testes of rats from either study. At 180 mg/kg/day, (which produces exposure levels 22 times higher than those in humans taking 80 mg/day based on surface area, mg/m²), seminiferous tubule degeneration (necrosis and loss of spermatogenic epithelium) was observed. In dogs, there was drug-related testicular atrophy, decreased spermatogenesis, spermatocytic degeneration and giant cell formation at 10 mg/kg/day, (approximately 2 times the human exposure, based on AUC, at 80 mg/day). The clinical significance of these findings is unclear.
13.2 Animal Toxicology and/or Pharmacology
SIMCOR
No animal toxicology or pharmacology studies were done with SIMCOR.
Niacin
No animal toxicology or pharmacology studies were done with niacin extended-release.
Simvastatin
Optic nerve degeneration was seen in clinically normal dogs treated with simvastatin for 14 weeks at 180 mg/kg/day, a dose that produced mean plasma drug levels about 12 times

higher than the mean plasma drug level in humans taking 80 mg/day. A chemically similar drug in this class also produced optic nerve degeneration (Wallerian degeneration of retinogeniculate fibers) in clinically normal dogs in a dose-dependent fashion starting at 60 mg/kg/day, a dose that produced mean plasma drug levels about 30 times higher than the mean plasma drug level in humans taking the highest recommended dose (as measured by total enzyme inhibitory activity). This same drug also produced vestibulocochlear Wallerian-like degeneration and retinal ganglion cell chromatolysis in dogs treated for 14 weeks at 180 mg/kg/day, a dose that resulted in a mean plasma drug level similar to that seen with the 60 mg/kg/day dose.
Central Nervous System (CNS) vascular lesions, characterized by perivascular hemorrhage and edema, mononuclear cell infiltration of perivascular spaces, perivascular fibrin deposits and necrosis of small vessels were seen in dogs treated with simvastatin at a dose of 360 mg/kg/day, a dose that produced mean plasma drug levels that were about 14 times higher than the mean plasma drug levels in humans taking 80 mg/day. Similar CNS vascular lesions have been observed with several other drugs of this class.
There were cataracts in female rats after two years of simvastatin treatment with 50 and 100 mg/kg/day (22 and 25 times the human AUC at 80 mg/day, respectively) and in dogs after three months at 90 mg/kg/day (19 times) and at two years at 50 mg/kg/day (5 times).
Reproductive Toxicology Studies
Simvastatin was not teratogenic in rats at doses of 25 mg/kg/day or in rabbits at doses up to 10 mg/kg/day. These doses resulted in 3 times (rat) or 3 times (rabbit) the human exposure based on mg/m² surface area. However, in studies with another structurally-related HMG-CoA reductase inhibitor, skeletal malformations were observed in rats and mice.

14 CLINICAL STUDIES
14.1 Modifications of Lipid Profiles
SIMCOR
In a double-blind, randomized, multicenter, multi-national, active-controlled, 24-week study, the lipid effects of SIMCOR were compared to simvastatin 20 mg and 80 mg in 641 patients with type II hyperlipidemia or mixed dyslipidemia. Following a lipid qualification phase, patients were eligible to enter one of two treatment groups. In Group A, patients on simvastatin 20 mg monotherapy, with elevated non-HDL levels and LDL-C levels at goal per the NCEP guidelines, were randomized to one of three treatment arms: SIMCOR 1000/20 mg, SIMCOR 2000/20 mg, or simvastatin 20 mg. In Group B, patients on simvastatin 40 mg monotherapy, with elevated non-HDL levels per the NCEP guidelines regardless of attainment of LDL-C goals, were randomized to one of three treatment arms: SIMCOR 1000/40 mg, SIMCOR 2000/40 mg, or simvastatin 80 mg. Therapy was initiated at the 500 mg dose of SIMCOR and increased by 500 mg every four weeks. Thus patients were titrated to the 1000 mg dose of SIMCOR after four weeks and to the 2000 mg dose of SIMCOR after 12 weeks. All patients randomized to simvastatin monotherapy received 50 mg immediate-release niacin daily in an attempt to keep the study from becoming unblinded due to flushing in the SIMCOR groups. Patients were instructed to take one 325 mg aspirin or 200 mg ibuprofen 30 minutes prior to taking the double-blind medication to help minimize flushing effects.
In Group A, the primary efficacy analysis was a comparison of the mean percent change in non-HDL levels between the SIMCOR 2000/20 mg and simvastatin 20 mg groups, and if statistically significant, then a comparison was conducted between the SIMCOR 1000/20 mg and simvastatin 20 mg groups. In Group B, the primary efficacy analysis was a determination of whether the mean percent change in non-HDL in the SIMCOR 2000/40 mg group was non-inferior to the mean percent change in the simvastatin 80 mg group, and if so, whether the mean percent change in non-HDL in the SIMCOR 1000/40 mg group was non-inferior to the mean percent change in the simvastatin 80 mg group.
In Group A, the non-HDL-C lowering with SIMCOR 2000/20 and SIMCOR 1000/20 was statistically significantly greater than that achieved with simvastatin 20 mg after 24 weeks (p<0.05; Table 4). The completion rate after 24 weeks was 72% for the SIMCOR arms and 88% for the simvastatin 20 mg arm. In Group B, the non-HDL-C lowering with SIMCOR 2000/40 and SIMCOR 1000/40 was non-inferior to that achieved with simvastatin 80 mg after 24 weeks (Table 5). The completion rate after 24 weeks was 78% for the SIMCOR arms and 80% for the simvastatin 80 mg arm.
SIMCOR was not superior to simvastatin in lowering

Information on the Abbott Pharmaceutical Products listed on these pages is from the prescribing information in use as of June 1, 2010. For more information, please visit rxabbott.com or call 1-800-633-9110.

Table 4. Non-HDL Treatment Response Following 24-Week Treatment Mean Percent Change from Simvastatin 20-mg Treated Baseline

		Group A							
		Simcor 2000/20			Simcor 1000/20			Simvastatin 20	
Week	n[a]	dose (mg/mg)	non-HDL[b]	n[a]	Dose (mg/mg)	non-HDL[b]	n[a]	Dose (mg/mg)	non-HDL[b]
Baseline	56	—	163.1 mg/dL	108	—	164.8 mg/dL	102	—	163.7 mg/dL
4	52	500/20	-12.9%	86	500/20	-12.8%	91	20	-8.3%
8	46	1000/20	-17.5%	91	1000/20	-15.5%	95	20	-8.3%
12	46	1500/20	-18.9%	90	1000/20	-14.8%	96	20	-6.4%
24	40	2000/20	-19.5%[†]	78	1000/20	-13.6%[†]	90	20	-5.0%
Dropouts by week 24:	28.6%			27.8%			11.8%		

[a] n=number of subjects with values in the analysis window at each timepoint
[b] The percent change from baseline is the model-based mean from a repeated measures mixed model with no imputation for missing data from study dropouts.
[†] significant vs. simvastatin 20 mg at the primary endpoint (Week 24), $p<0.05$

Table 5. Non-HDL Treatment Response Following 24-Week Treatment Mean Percent Change from Simvastatin 40-mg Treated Baseline

		Group B							
		Simcor 2000/40			Simcor 1000/40			Simvastatin 80	
Week	n[a]	dose (mg/mg)	non-HDL[b]	n[a]	Dose (mg/mg)	non-HDL[b]	n[a]	Dose (mg/mg)	non-HDL[b]
Baseline	98	—	144.4 mg/dL	111	—	141.2 mg/dL	113	—	134.5 mg/dL
4	96	500/40	-6.0%	108	500/40	-5.9%	110	80	-11.3%
8	93	1000/40	-15.5%	100	1000/40	-16.2%	104	80	-13.7%
12	90	1500/40	-18.4%	97	1000/40	-12.6%	100	80	-9.5%
24	80	2000/40	-7.6%[c]	82	1000/40	-6.7%[d]	90	80	-6.0%
Dropouts by week 24:	18.4%			26.1%			20.4%		

[a] n=number of subjects with values in the analysis window at each timepoint
[b] The percent change from baseline is the model-based mean from a repeated measures mixed model with no imputation for missing data from study dropouts.
[c] non-inferior to Simvastatin 80 arm; 95% confidence interval of mean difference in non-HDL for Simcor 2000/40 vs. Simvastatin 80 is (-7.7%, 4.5%)
[d] non-inferior to Simvastatin 80 arm; 95% confidence interval of mean difference in non-HDL for Simcor 1000/40 vs. Simvastatin 80 is (-6.6%, 5.3%)

Table 6. Mean Percent Change from Baseline to Week 24 in Lipoprotein Lipid Levels

		Treatment Group A				
TREATMENT	N	LDL-C	Total-C	HDL-C	TG[a]	Apo B
Baseline (mg/dL)*	266	120	207	43	209	102
Simvastatin 20 mg	102	-6.7%	-4.5%	7.8%	-15.3%	-5.6%
SIMCOR 1000/20	108	-11.9%	-8.8%	20.7%	-26.5%	-13.2%
SIMCOR 2000/20	56	-14.3%	-11.1%	29.0%	-38.0%	-18.5%

* either treatment naïve or after receiving simvastatin 20 mg
[a] medians are reported for TG

Table 7. Mean Percent Change from Baseline to Week 24 in Lipoprotein Lipid Levels

		Treatment Group B				
TREATMENT	N	LDL-C	Total-C	HDL-C	TG[a]	Apo B
Baseline (mg/dL)*	322	108	187	47	145	93
Simvastatin 80 mg	113	-11.4%	-6.2%	0.1%	0.3%	-7.5%
SIMCOR 1000/40	111	-7.1%	-3.1%	15.4%	-22.8%	-7.7%
SIMCOR 2000/40	98	-5.1%	-1.6%	24.4%	-31.8%	-10.5%

* after receiving simvastatin 40 mg
[a] medians are reported for TG

LDL-C in either Group A or Group B. However, SIMCOR was superior to simvastatin in both groups in lowering TG and raising HDL (Tables 6 and 7).

[See table 4 above]
[See table 5 above]
[See table 6 above]
[See table 7 above]

Limitations of use

No incremental benefit of SIMCOR on cardiovascular morbidity and mortality over and above that demonstrated for simvastatin monotherapy and niacin monotherapy has been established.

16   HOW SUPPLIED/STORAGE AND HANDLING

SIMCOR tablets are available as blue, unscored, tablets, packaged in bottles of 90 tablets. Each tablet has "KOS" debossed on one side and a code number specific to the tablet strength on the other. Please see the table below:

SIMCOR Tablet Strength	Debossed ID	NDC Number
500mg/20mg	KOS/021	0074-3312-90
750mg/20mg	KOS/022	0074-3315-90
1000mg/20mg	KOS/023	0074-3316-90

Storage: Store at controlled room temperature 20°–25°C (68°–77°F).

17   PATIENT COUNSELING INFORMATION

The patient should be informed of the following:

17.1   Dosing Time
SIMCOR tablets should be taken at bedtime, after a low-fat snack. Administration on an empty stomach is not recommended.

17.2   Tablet Integrity
SIMCOR tablets should not be broken, crushed or chewed, but should be swallowed whole.

17.3   Dosing Interruption
If dosing is interrupted for any length of time, their physician should be contacted prior to re-starting therapy; re-titration is recommended.

17.4   Muscle Pain
To notify their physician of any unexplained muscle pain, tenderness, or weakness promptly. The risk of this occurring is increased when taking certain types of medication or consuming larger quantities of grapefruit juice. They should discuss all medication, both prescription and over the counter, with their physician.

17.5   Flushing
Flushing is a common side effect of niacin therapy that may subside after several weeks of consistent SIMCOR use. Flushing may vary in severity and is more likely to occur with initiation of therapy, or during dose increases. By dosing at bedtime, flushing will most likely occur during sleep. However, if awakened by flushing at night, the patient should get up slowly, especially if feeling dizzy, feeling faint, or taking blood pressure medications.

17.6   Use of Aspirin or other Non-Inflammatory Medication
Taking aspirin or non-steroidal anti-inflammatory medications (e.g., ibuprofen) approximately 30 minutes before dosing can minimize flushing.

17.7   Diet
To avoid ingestion of alcohol, hot beverages and spicy foods around the time of taking SIMCOR to minimize flushing.

17.8   Supplements
To notify their physician if they are taking vitamins or other nutritional supplements containing niacin or nicotinamide.

17.9   Dizziness
To notify their physician if symptoms of dizziness occur.

17.10   Diabetics
If diabetic, to notify their physician of changes in blood glucose.

17.11   Pregnancy
Women of childbearing age should use an effective method of birth control to prevent pregnancy while using SIMCOR. Discuss future pregnancy plans with your healthcare professional, and discuss when to stop SIMCOR if you are trying to conceive. If you are pregnant, stop SIMCOR and call your healthcare professional.

17.12   Breastfeeding
Women who are breastfeeding should not use SIMCOR. If you have a lipid disorder and are breastfeeding, speak with your healthcare professionals about your lipid disorder and whether or not you should breastfeed your infant.

03-A138-R2
Rev.: August, 2008
Manufactured for:
Abbott Laboratories
North Chicago, IL 60064, U.S.A.
Shown in Product Identification Guide, page 304

SYNTHROID®   ℞
[sĭn-thrŏĭd]
(levothyroxine sodium tablets, USP)

DESCRIPTION

SYNTHROID® (levothyroxine sodium tablets, USP) contain synthetic crystalline L-3,3′,5,5′-tetraiodothyronine sodium salt [levothyroxine (T$_4$) sodium]. Synthetic T$_4$ is identical to that produced in the human thyroid gland. Levothyroxine (T$_4$) sodium has an empirical formula of $C_{15}H_{10}I_4N\ NaO_4 \bullet$

H_2O, molecular weight of 798.86 g/mol (anhydrous), and structural formula as shown:

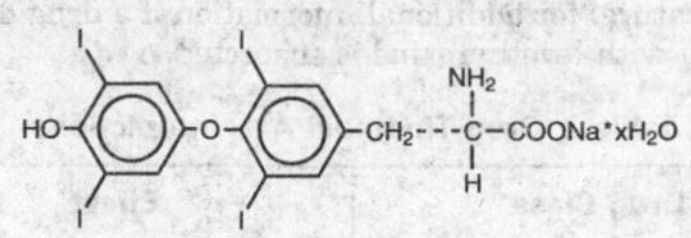

Inactive Ingredients: acacia, confectioner's sugar (contains corn starch), lactose monohydrate, magnesium stearate, povidone, and talc. The following are the color additives by tablet strength:

Strength (mcg)	Color additive(s)
25	FD&C Yellow No. 6 Aluminum Lake
50	None
75	FD&C Red No. 40 Aluminum Lake, FD&C Blue No. 2 Aluminum Lake
88	FD&C Blue No. 1 Aluminum Lake, FD&C Yellow No. 6 Aluminum Lake, D&C Yellow No. 10 Aluminum Lake
100	D&C Yellow No. 10 Aluminum Lake, FD&C Yellow No. 6 Aluminum Lake
112	D&C Red No. 27 & 30 Aluminum Lake
125	FD&C Yellow No. 6 Aluminum Lake, FD&C Red No. 40 Aluminum Lake, FD&C Blue No. 1 Aluminum Lake
137	FD&C Blue No. 1 Aluminum Lake
150	FD&C Blue No. 2 Aluminum Lake
175	FD&C Blue No. 1 Aluminum Lake, D&C Red No. 27 & 30 Aluminum Lake
200	FD&C Red No. 40 Aluminum Lake
300	D&C Yellow No. 10 Aluminum Lake, FD&C Yellow No. 6 Aluminum Lake, FD&C Blue No. 1 Aluminum Lake

Meets USP Dissolution Test 3

CLINICAL PHARMACOLOGY

Thyroid hormone synthesis and secretion is regulated by the hypothalamic-pituitary-thyroid axis. Thyrotropin-releasing hormone (TRH) released from the hypothalamus stimulates secretion of thyrotropin-stimulating hormone, TSH, from the anterior pituitary. TSH, in turn, is the physiologic stimulus for the synthesis and secretion of thyroid hormones, L-thyroxine (T_4) and L-triiodothyronine (T_3), by the thyroid gland. Circulating serum T_3 and T_4 levels exert a feedback effect on both TRH and TSH secretion. When serum T_3 and T_4 levels increase, TRH and TSH secretion decrease. When thyroid hormone levels decrease, TRH and TSH secretion increase.

The mechanisms by which thyroid hormones exert their physiologic actions are not completely understood, but it is thought that their principal effects are exerted through control of DNA transcription and protein synthesis. T_3 and T_4 diffuse into the cell nucleus and bind to thyroid receptor proteins attached to DNA. This hormone nuclear receptor complex activates gene transcription and synthesis of messenger RNA and cytoplasmic proteins.

Thyroid hormones regulate multiple metabolic processes and play an essential role in normal growth and development, and normal maturation of the central nervous system and bone. The metabolic actions of thyroid hormones include augmentation of cellular respiration and thermogenesis, as well as metabolism of proteins, carbohydrates and lipids. The protein anabolic effects of thyroid hormones are essential to normal growth and development.

The physiological actions of thyroid hormones are produced predominantly by T_3, the majority of which (approximately 80%) is derived from T_4 by deiodination in peripheral tissues.

Levothyroxine, at doses individualized according to patient response, is effective as replacement or supplemental therapy in hypothyroidism of any etiology, except transient hypothyroidism during the recovery phase of subacute thyroiditis.

Levothyroxine is also effective in the suppression of pituitary TSH secretion in the treatment or prevention of various types of euthyroid goiters, including thyroid nodules, Hashimoto's thyroiditis, multinodular goiter and, as adjunctive therapy in the management of thyrotropin-dependent well-differentiated thyroid cancer (see **INDICATIONS AND USAGE, PRECAUTIONS**, and **DOSAGE AND ADMINISTRATION**).

Pharmacokinetics

Absorption

Absorption of orally administered T_4 from the gastrointestinal (GI) tract ranges from 40% to 80%. The majority of the levothyroxine dose is absorbed from the jejunum and upper ileum. The relative bioavailability of SYNTHROID tablets, compared to an equal nominal dose of oral levothyroxine sodium solution, is approximately 93%. T_4 absorption is increased by fasting, and decreased in malabsorption syndromes and by certain foods such as soybean infant formula. Dietary fiber decreases bioavailability of T_4. Absorption may also decrease with age. In addition, many drugs and foods affect T_4 absorption (see **PRECAUTIONS - Drug Interactions** and **Drug-Food Interactions**).

Table 1. Pharmacokinetic Parameters of Thyroid Hormones in Euthyroid Patients

Hormone	Ratio in Thyroglobulin	Biologic Potency	$t_{1/2}$ (days)	Protein Binding (%)[2]
Levothyroxine (T_4)	10-20	1	6-7[1]	99.96
Liothyronine (T_3)	1	4	≤ 2	99.5

[1] 3 to 4 days in hyperthyroidism, 9 to 10 days in hypothyroidism
[2] Includes TBG, TBPA, and TBA

Distribution

Circulating thyroid hormones are greater than 99% bound to plasma proteins, including thyroxine-binding globulin (TBG), thyroxine-binding prealbumin (TBPA), and albumin (TBA), whose capacities and affinities vary for each hormone. The higher affinity of both TBG and TBPA for T_4 partially explains the higher serum levels, slower metabolic clearance, and longer half-life of T_4 compared to T_3. Protein-bound thyroid hormones exist in reverse equilibrium with small amounts of free hormone. Only unbound hormone is metabolically active. Many drugs and physiologic conditions affect the binding of thyroid hormones to serum proteins (see **PRECAUTIONS - Drug Interactions** and **Drug-Laboratory Test Interactions**). Thyroid hormones do not readily cross the placental barrier (see **PRECAUTIONS - Pregnancy**).

Metabolism

T_4 is slowly eliminated (see **Table 1**). The major pathway of thyroid hormone metabolism is through sequential deiodination. Approximately eighty-percent of circulating T_3 is derived from peripheral T_4 by monodeiodination. The liver is the major site of degradation for both T_4 and T_3, with T_4 deiodination also occurring at a number of additional sites, including the kidney and other tissues. Approximately 80% of the daily dose of T_4 is deiodinated to yield equal amounts of T_3 and reverse T_3 (rT_3). T_3 and rT_3 are further deiodinated to diiodothyronine. Thyroid hormones are also metabolized via conjugation with glucuronides and sulfates and excreted directly into the bile and gut where they undergo enterohepatic recirculation.

Elimination

Thyroid hormones are primarily eliminated by the kidneys. A portion of the conjugated hormone reaches the colon unchanged and is eliminated in the feces. Approximately 20% of T_4 is eliminated in the stool. Urinary excretion of T_4 decreases with age.

[See table 1 above]

INDICATIONS AND USAGE

Levothyroxine sodium is used for the following indications:

Hypothyroidism

As replacement or supplemental therapy in congenital or acquired hypothyroidism of any etiology, except transient hypothyroidism during the recovery phase of subacute thyroiditis. Specific indications include: primary (thyroidal), secondary (pituitary), and tertiary (hypothalamic) hypothyroidism and subclinical hypothyroidism. Primary hypothyroidism may result from functional deficiency, primary atrophy, partial or total congenital absence of the thyroid gland, or from the effects of surgery, radiation, or drugs, with or without the presence of goiter.

Pituitary TSH Suppression

In the treatment or prevention of various types of euthyroid goiters (see **WARNINGS** and **PRECAUTIONS**), including thyroid nodules (see **WARNINGS** and **PRECAUTIONS**), subacute or chronic lymphocytic thyroiditis (Hashimoto's thyroiditis), multinodular goiter (see **WARNINGS** and **PRECAUTIONS**) and, as an adjunct to surgery and radioiodine therapy in the management of thyrotropin-dependent well-differentiated thyroid cancer.

CONTRAINDICATIONS

Levothyroxine is contraindicated in patients with untreated subclinical (suppressed serum TSH level with normal T_3 and T_4 levels) or overt thyrotoxicosis of any etiology and in patients with acute myocardial infarction. Levothyroxine is contraindicated in patients with uncorrected adrenal insufficiency since thyroid hormones may precipitate an acute adrenal crisis by increasing the metabolic clearance of glucocorticoids (see **PRECAUTIONS**). SYNTHROID is contraindicated in patients with hypersensitivity to any of the inactive ingredients in SYNTHROID tablets (See **DESCRIPTION - Inactive Ingredients**).

WARNINGS

BOXED WARNING

WARNING: Thyroid hormones, including SYNTHROID, either alone or with other therapeutic agents, should not be used for the treatment of obesity or for weight loss. In euthyroid patients, doses within the range of daily hormonal requirements are ineffective for weight reduction. Larger doses may produce serious or even life threatening manifestations of toxicity, particularly when given in association with sympathomimetic amines such as those used for their anorectic effects.

Levothyroxine sodium should not be used in the treatment of male or female infertility unless this condition is associated with hypothyroidism.

In patients with nontoxic diffuse goiter or nodular thyroid disease, particularly the elderly or those with underlying cardiovascular disease, levothyroxine sodium therapy is contraindicated if the serum TSH level is already suppressed due to the risk of precipitating overt thyrotoxicosis (see **CONTRAINDICATIONS**). If the serum TSH level is not suppressed, SYNTHROID should be used with caution in conjunction with careful monitoring of thyroid function for evidence of hyperthyroidism and clinical monitoring for potential associated adverse cardiovascular signs and symptoms of hyperthyroidism.

PRECAUTIONS

General

Levothyroxine has a narrow therapeutic index. Regardless of the indication for use, careful dosage titration is necessary to avoid the consequences of over- or under-treatment. These consequences include, among others, effects on growth and development, cardiovascular function, bone metabolism, reproductive function, cognitive function, emotional state, gastrointestinal function, and on glucose and lipid metabolism. Many drugs interact with levothyroxine sodium necessitating adjustments in dosing to maintain therapeutic response (see **Drug Interactions**).

Effects on Bone Mineral Density

In women, long-term levothyroxine sodium therapy has been associated with increased bone resorption, thereby decreasing bone mineral density, especially in post-menopausal women on greater than replacement doses or in women who are receiving suppressive doses of levothyroxine sodium. The increased bone resorption may be associated with increased serum levels and urinary excretion of calcium and phosphorus, elevations in bone alkaline phosphatase and suppressed serum parathyroid hormone levels. Therefore, it is recommended that patients receiving levothyroxine sodium be given the minimum dose necessary to achieve the desired clinical and biochemical response.

Patients with Underlying Cardiovascular Disease

Exercise caution when administering levothyroxine to patients with cardiovascular disorders and to the elderly in whom there is an increased risk of occult cardiac disease. In these patients, levothyroxine therapy should be initiated at lower doses than those recommended in younger individuals or in patients without cardiac disease (see **WARNINGS, PRECAUTIONS - Geriatric Use**, and **DOSAGE AND ADMINISTRATION**). If cardiac symptoms develop or worsen, the levothyroxine dose should be reduced or withheld for one week and then cautiously restarted at a lower dose. Overtreatment with levothyroxine sodium may have adverse cardiovascular effects such as an increase in heart rate, cardiac wall thickness, and cardiac contractility and may precipitate angina or arrhythmias. Patients with coronary artery disease who are receiving levothyroxine therapy should be monitored closely during surgical procedures, since the possibility of precipitating cardiac arrhythmias may be greater in those treated with levothyroxine. Con-

Information on the Abbott Pharmaceutical Products listed on these pages is from the prescribing information in use as of June 1, 2010. For more information, please visit rxabbott.com or call 1-800-633-9110.

comitant administration of levothyroxine and sympathomimetic agents to patients with coronary artery disease may precipitate coronary insufficiency.

Patients with Nontoxic Diffuse Goiter or Nodular Thyroid Disease

Exercise caution when administering levothyroxine to patients with nontoxic diffuse goiter or nodular thyroid disease in order to prevent precipitation of thyrotoxicosis (see **WARNINGS**). If the serum TSH is already suppressed, levothyroxine sodium should not be administered (see **CONTRAINDICATIONS**).

Associated Endocrine Disorders

Hypothalamic/pituitary hormone deficiencies

In patients with secondary or tertiary hypothyroidism, additional hypothalamic/pituitary hormone deficiencies should be considered, and, if diagnosed, treated (see **PRECAUTIONS - Autoimmune polyglandular syndrome** for adrenal insufficiency).

Autoimmune polyglandular syndrome

Occasionally, chronic autoimmune thyroiditis may occur in association with other autoimmune disorders such as adrenal insufficiency, pernicious anemia, and insulin-dependent diabetes mellitus. Patients with concomitant adrenal insufficiency should be treated with replacement glucocorticoids prior to initiation of treatment with levothyroxine sodium. Failure to do so may precipitate an acute adrenal crisis when thyroid hormone therapy is initiated, due to increased metabolic clearance of glucocorticoids by thyroid hormone. Patients with diabetes mellitus may require upward adjustments of their antidiabetic therapeutic regimens when treated with levothyroxine (see **PRECAUTIONS - Drug Interactions**).

Other Associated Medical Conditions

Infants with congenital hypothyroidism appear to be at increased risk for other congenital anomalies, with cardiovascular anomalies (pulmonary stenosis, atrial septal defect, and ventricular septal defect) being the most common association.

Information for Patients

Patients should be informed of the following information to aid in the safe and effective use of SYNTHROID:

1. Notify your physician if you are allergic to any foods or medicines, are pregnant or intend to become pregnant, are breast-feeding or are taking any other medications, including prescription and over-the-counter preparations.
2. Notify your physician of any other medical conditions you may have, particularly heart disease, diabetes, clotting disorders, and adrenal or pituitary gland problems. Your dose of medications used to control these other conditions may need to be adjusted while you are taking SYNTHROID. If you have diabetes, monitor your blood and/or urinary glucose levels as directed by your physician and immediately report any changes to your physician. If you are taking anticoagulants (blood thinners), your clotting status should be checked frequently.
3. Use SYNTHROID only as prescribed by your physician. Do not discontinue or change the amount you take or how often you take it, unless directed to do so by your physician.
4. The levothyroxine in SYNTHROID is intended to replace a hormone that is normally produced by your thyroid gland. Generally, replacement therapy is to be taken for life, except in cases of transient hypothyroidism, which is usually associated with an inflammation of the thyroid gland (thyroiditis).
5. Take SYNTHROID as a single dose, preferably on an empty stomach, one-half to one hour before breakfast. Levothyroxine absorption is increased on an empty stomach.
6. It may take several weeks before you notice an improvement in your symptoms.
7. Notify your physician if you experience any of the following symptoms: rapid or irregular heartbeat, chest pain, shortness of breath, leg cramps, headache, nervousness, irritability, sleeplessness, tremors, change in appetite, weight gain or loss, vomiting, diarrhea, excessive sweating, heat intolerance, fever, changes in menstrual periods, hives or skin rash, or any other unusual medical event.
8. Notify your physician if you become pregnant while taking SYNTHROID. It is likely that your dose of SYNTHROID will need to be increased while you are pregnant.
9. Notify your physician or dentist that you are taking SYNTHROID prior to any surgery.
10. Partial hair loss may occur rarely during the first few months of SYNTHROID therapy, but this is usually temporary.
11. SYNTHROID should not be used as a primary or adjunctive therapy in a weight control program.
12. Keep SYNTHROID out of the reach of children. Store SYNTHROID away from heat, moisture, and light.

13. Agents such as iron and calcium supplements and antacids can decrease the absorption of levothyroxine sodium tablets. Therefore, levothyroxine sodium tablets should not be administered within 4 hours of these agents.

Laboratory Tests

General

The diagnosis of hypothyroidism is confirmed by measuring TSH levels using a sensitive assay (second generation assay sensitivity ≤ 0.1 mIU/L or third generation assay sensitivity ≤ 0.01 mIU/L) and measurement of free-T_4.

The adequacy of therapy is determined by periodic assessment of appropriate laboratory tests and clinical evaluation. The choice of laboratory tests depends on various factors including the etiology of the underlying thyroid disease, the presence of concomitant medical conditions, including pregnancy, and the use of concomitant medications (see **PRECAUTIONS - Drug Interactions** and **Drug-Laboratory Test Interactions**). Persistent clinical and laboratory evidence of hypothyroidism despite an apparent adequate replacement dose of SYNTHROID may be evidence of inadequate absorption, poor compliance, drug interactions, or decreased T_4 potency of the drug product.

Adults

In adult patients with primary (thyroidal) hypothyroidism, serum TSH levels (using a sensitive assay) alone may be used to monitor therapy. The frequency of TSH monitoring during levothyroxine dose titration depends on the clinical situation but it is generally recommended at 6-8 week intervals until normalization. For patients who have recently initiated levothyroxine therapy and whose serum TSH has normalized or in patients who have had their dosage or brand of levothyroxine changed, the serum TSH concentration should be measured after 8-12 weeks. When the optimum replacement dose has been attained, clinical (physical examination) and biochemical monitoring may be performed every 6-12 months, depending on the clinical situation, and whenever there is a change in the patient's status. It is recommended that a physical examination and a serum TSH measurement be performed at least annually in patients receiving SYNTHROID (see **WARNINGS, PRECAUTIONS**, and **DOSAGE AND ADMINISTRATION**).

Pediatrics

In patients with congenital hypothyroidism, the adequacy of replacement therapy should be assessed by measuring both serum TSH (using a sensitive assay) and total- or free-T_4. During the first three years of life, the serum total- or free-T_4 should be maintained at all times in the upper half of the normal range. While the aim of therapy is to also normalize the serum TSH level, this is not always possible in a small percentage of patients, particularly in the first few months of therapy. TSH may not normalize due to a resetting of the pituitary-thyroid feedback threshold as a result of *in utero* hypothyroidism. Failure of the serum T_4 to increase into the upper half of the normal range within 2 weeks of initiation of SYNTHROID therapy and/or of the serum TSH to decrease below 20 mU/L within 4 weeks should alert the physician to the possibility that the child is not receiving adequate therapy. Careful inquiry should then be made regarding compliance, dose of medication administered, and method of administration prior to raising the dose of SYNTHROID.

The recommended frequency of monitoring of TSH and total or free T_4 in children is as follows: at 2 and 4 weeks after the initiation of treatment; every 1-2 months during the first year of life; every 2-3 months between 1 and 3 years of age; and every 3 to 12 months thereafter until growth is completed. More frequent intervals of monitoring may be necessary if poor compliance is suspected or abnormal values are obtained. It is recommended that TSH and T_4 levels, and a physical examination, if indicated, be performed 2 weeks after any change in SYNTHROID dosage. Routine clinical examination, including assessment of mental and physical growth and development, and bone maturation, should be performed at regular intervals (see **PRECAUTIONS - Pediatric Use** and **DOSAGE AND ADMINISTRATION**).

Secondary (Pituitary) and Tertiary (Hypothalamic) Hypothyroidism

Adequacy of therapy should be assessed by measuring serum free-T_4 levels, which should be maintained in the upper half of the normal range in these patients.

Drug Interactions

Many drugs affect thyroid hormone pharmacokinetics and metabolism (e.g., absorption, synthesis, secretion, catabolism, protein binding, and target tissue response) and may alter the therapeutic response to SYNTHROID. In addition, thyroid hormones and thyroid status have varied effects on the pharmacokinetics and actions of other drugs. A listing of drug-thyroidal axis interactions is contained in Table 2.

The list of drug-thyroidal axis interactions in Table 2 may not be comprehensive due to the introduction of new drugs that interact with the thyroidal axis or the discovery of previously unknown interactions. The prescriber should be

aware of this fact and should consult appropriate reference sources (e.g., package inserts of newly approved drugs, medical literature) for additional information if a drug-drug interaction with levothyroxine is suspected.

Table 2. Drug-Thyroidal Axis Interactions

Drug or Drug Class	Effect
Drugs that may reduce TSH secretion – the reduction is not sustained; therefore, hypothyroidism does not occur	
Dopamine/Dopamine Agonists Glucocorticoids Octreotide	Use of these agents may result in a transient reduction in TSH secretion when administered at the following doses: Dopamine (≥ 1 mcg/kg/min); Glucocorticoids (hydrocortisone ≥ 100 mg/day or equivalent); Octreotide (> 100 mcg/day).
Drugs that alter thyroid hormone secretion	
Drugs that may decrease thyroid hormone secretion, which may result in hypothyroidism	
Aminoglutethimide Amiodarone Iodide (including iodine-containing radiographic contrast agents) Lithium Methimazole Propylthiouracil (PTU) Sulfonamides Tolbutamide	Long-term lithium therapy can result in goiter in up to 50% of patients, and either subclinical or overt hypothyroidism, each in up to 20% of patients. The fetus, neonate, elderly and euthyroid patients with underlying thyroid disease (e.g., Hashimoto's thyroiditis or with Grave's disease previously treated with radioiodine or surgery) are among those individuals who are particularly susceptible to iodine-induced hypothyroidism. Oral cholecystographic agents and amiodarone are slowly excreted, producing more prolonged hypothyroidism than parenterally administered iodinated contrast agents. Long-term aminoglutethimide therapy may minimally decrease T_4 and T_3 levels and increase TSH, although all values remain within normal limits in most patients.
Drugs that may increase thyroid hormone secretion, which may result in hyperthyroidism	
Amiodarone Iodide (including iodine-containing radiographic contrast agents)	Iodide and drugs that contain pharmacologic amounts of iodide may cause hyperthyroidism in euthyroid patients with Grave's disease previously treated with antithyroid drugs or in euthyroid patients with thyroid autonomy (e.g., multinodular goiter or hyperfunctioning thyroid adenoma). Hyperthyroidism may develop over several weeks and may persist for several months after therapy discontinuation. Amiodarone may induce hyperthyroidism by causing thyroiditis.
Drugs that may decrease T_4 absorption, which may result in hypothyroidism	
Antacids - Aluminum & Magnesium Hydroxides - Simethicone Bile Acid Sequestrants - Cholestyramine - Colestipol Calcium Carbonate	Concurrent use may reduce the efficacy of levothyroxine by binding and delaying or preventing absorption, potentially resulting in hypothyroidism. Calcium carbonate may form an insoluble chelate with

| Cation Exchange Resins
- Kayexalate
Ferrous Sulfate
Orlistat
Sucralfate | levothyroxine, and ferrous sulfate likely forms a ferric-thyroxine complex. Administer levothyroxine at least 4 hours apart from these agents. Patients treated concomitantly with orlistat and levothyroxine should be monitored for changes in thyroid function. |

Drugs that may alter T_4 and T_3 serum transport - but FT_4 concentration remains normal; and therefore, the patient remains euthyroid

Drugs that may increase serum TBG concentration	Drugs that may decrease serum TBG concentration

Clofibrate
Estrogen-containing
  oral contraceptives
Estrogens (oral)
Heroin / Methadone
5-Fluorouracil
Mitotane
Tamoxifen
	Androgens/Anabolic
	  Steroids
	Asparaginase
	Glucocorticoids
	Slow-Release Nicotinic Acid

Drugs that may cause protein-binding site displacement

| Furosemide (> 80 mg IV)
Heparin
Hydantoins
NonSteroidal
Anti-Inflammatory Drugs
- Fenamates
- Phenylbutazone
Salicylates (> 2 g/day) | Administration of these agents with levothyroxine results in an initial transient increase in FT_4. Continued administration results in a decrease in serum T_4 and normal FT_4 and TSH concentrations and, therefore, patients are clinically euthyroid. Salicylates inhibit binding of T_4 and T_3 to TBG and transthyretin. An initial increase in serum FT_4 is followed by return of FT_4 to normal levels with sustained therapeutic serum salicylate concentrations, although total-T_4 levels may decrease by as much as 30%. |

Drugs that may alter T_4 and T_3 metabolism

Drugs that may increase hepatic metabolism, which may result in hypothyroidism

| Carbamazepine
Hydantoins
Phenobarbital
Rifampin | Stimulation of hepatic microsomal drug-metabolizing enzyme activity may cause increased hepatic degradation of levothyroxine, resulting in increased levothyroxine requirements. Phenytoin and carbamazepine reduce serum protein binding of levothyroxine, and total- and free-T_4 may be reduced by 20% to 40%, but most patients have normal serum TSH levels and are clinically euthyroid. |

Drugs that may decrease T_4 5'-deiodinase activity

| Amiodarone
Beta-adrenergic
  antagonists
- (e.g., Propranolol
  > 160 mg/day)
Glucocorticoids
- (e.g., Dexamethasone
  ≥ 4 mg/day)
Propylthiouracil (PTU) | Administration of these enzyme inhibitors decreases the peripheral conversion of T_4 to T_3, leading to decreased T_3 levels. However, serum T_4 levels are usually normal but may occasionally be slightly increased. In patients |

treated with large doses of propranolol (> 160 mg/day), T_3 and T_4 levels change slightly, TSH levels remain normal, and patients are clinically euthyroid. It should be noted that actions of particular beta-adrenergic antagonists may be impaired when the hypothyroid patient is converted to the euthyroid state. Short-term administration of large doses of glucocorticoids may decrease serum T_3 concentrations by 30% with minimal change in serum T_4 levels. However, long-term glucocorticoid therapy may result in slightly decreased T_3 and T_4 levels due to decreased TBG production (see above).

Miscellaneous

Anticoagulants (oral) - Coumarin Derivatives - Indandione Derivatives	Thyroid hormones appear to increase the catabolism of vitamin K-dependent clotting factors, thereby increasing the anticoagulant activity of oral anticoagulants. Concomitant use of these agents impairs the compensatory increases in clotting factor synthesis. Prothrombin time should be carefully monitored in patients taking levothyroxine and oral anticoagulants and the dose of anticoagulant therapy adjusted accordingly.
Antidepressants - Tricyclics (e.g., Amitriptyline) - Tetracyclics (e.g., Maprotiline) - Selective Serotonin Reuptake Inhibitors (SSRIs; e.g., Sertraline)	Concurrent use of tri/tetracyclic antidepressants and levothyroxine may increase the therapeutic and toxic effects of both drugs, possibly due to increased receptor sensitivity to catecholamines. Toxic effects may include increased risk of cardiac arrhythmias and CNS stimulation; onset of action of tricyclics may be accelerated. Administration of sertraline in patients stabilized on levothyroxine may result in increased levothyroxine requirements.
Antidiabetic Agents - Biguanides - Meglitinides - Sulfonylureas - Thiazolidinediones - Insulin	Addition of levothyroxine to antidiabetic or insulin therapy may result in increased antidiabetic agent or insulin requirements. Careful monitoring of diabetic control is recommended, especially when thyroid therapy is started, changed, or discontinued.
Cardiac Glycosides	Serum digitalis glycoside levels may be reduced in hyperthyroidism or when the hypothyroid patient is converted to the euthyroid state. Therapeutic effect of digitalis glycosides may be reduced.
Cytokines - Interferon-α - Interleukin-2	Therapy with interferon-α has been associated with the development of

antithyroid microsomal antibodies in 20% of patients and some have transient hypothyroidism, hyperthyroidism, or both. Patients who have antithyroid antibodies before treatment are at higher risk for thyroid dysfunction during treatment. Interleukin-2 has been associated with transient painless thyroiditis in 20% of patients. Interferon-β and -γ have not been reported to cause thyroid dysfunction.

Growth Hormones - Somatrem - Somatropin	Excessive use of thyroid hormones with growth hormones may accelerate epiphyseal closure. However, untreated hypothyroidism may interfere with growth response to growth hormone.
Ketamine	Concurrent use may produce marked hypertension and tachycardia; cautious administration to patients receiving thyroid hormone therapy is recommended.
Methylxanthine Bronchodilators - (e.g., Theophylline)	Decreased theophylline clearance may occur in hypothyroid patients; clearance returns to normal when the euthyroid state is achieved.
Radiographic Agents	Thyroid hormones may reduce the uptake of ^{123}I, ^{131}I, and ^{99m}Tc.
Sympathomimetics	Concurrent use may increase the effects of sympathomimetics or thyroid hormone. Thyroid hormones may increase the risk of coronary insufficiency when sympathomimetic agents are administered to patients with coronary artery disease.

Chloral Hydrate
Diazepam
Ethionamide
Lovastatin
Metoclopramide
6-Mercaptopurine
Nitroprusside
Para-aminosalicylate
  sodium
Perphenazine
Resorcinol (excessive
  topical use)
Thiazide Diuretics
	These agents have been associated with thyroid hormone and/or TSH level alterations by various mechanisms.

Oral anticoagulants
Levothyroxine increases the response to oral anticoagulant therapy. Therefore, a decrease in the dose of anticoagulant may be warranted with correction of the hypothyroid state or when the SYNTHROID dose is increased. Prothrombin time should be closely monitored to permit appropriate and timely dosage adjustments (see **Table 2**).

Digitalis glycosides
The therapeutic effects of digitalis glycosides may be reduced by levothyroxine. Serum digitalis glycoside levels may be decreased when a hypothyroid patient becomes euthyroid, necessitating an increase in the dose of digitalis glycosides (see **Table 2**).

Information on the Abbott Pharmaceutical Products listed on these pages is from the prescribing information in use as of June 1, 2010. For more information, please visit rxabbott.com or call 1-800-633-9110.

Drug-Food Interactions

Consumption of certain foods may affect levothyroxine absorption thereby necessitating adjustments in dosing. Soybean flour (infant formula), cotton seed meal, walnuts, and dietary fiber may bind and decrease the absorption of levothyroxine sodium from the GI tract.

Drug-Laboratory Test Interactions

Changes in TBG concentration must be considered when interpreting T_4 and T_3 values, which necessitates measurement and evaluation of unbound (free) hormone and/or determination of the free T_4 index (FT_4I). Pregnancy, infectious hepatitis, estrogens, estrogen-containing oral contraceptives, and acute intermittent porphyria increase TBG concentrations. Decreases in TBG concentrations are observed in nephrosis, severe hypoproteinemia, severe liver disease, acromegaly, and after androgen or corticosteroid therapy (see also **Table 2**). Familial hyper- or hypothyroxine binding globulinemias have been described, with the incidence of TBG deficiency approximating 1 in 9000.

Carcinogenesis, Mutagenesis, and Impairment of Fertility

Animal studies have not been performed to evaluate the carcinogenic potential, mutagenic potential or effects on fertility of levothyroxine. The synthetic T_4 in SYNTHROID is identical to that produced naturally by the human thyroid gland. Although there has been a reported association between prolonged thyroid hormone therapy and breast cancer, this has not been confirmed. Patients receiving SYNTHROID for appropriate clinical indications should be titrated to the lowest effective replacement dose.

Pregnancy

Category A

Studies in women taking levothyroxine sodium during pregnancy have not shown an increased risk of congenital abnormalities. Therefore, the possibility of fetal harm appears remote. SYNTHROID should not be discontinued during pregnancy and hypothyroidism diagnosed during pregnancy should be promptly treated.

Hypothyroidism during pregnancy is associated with a higher rate of complications, including spontaneous abortion, pre-eclampsia, stillbirth and premature delivery. Maternal hypothyroidism may have an adverse effect on fetal and childhood growth and development. During pregnancy, serum T_4 levels may decrease and serum TSH levels increase to values outside the normal range. Since elevations in serum TSH may occur as early as 4 weeks gestation, pregnant women taking SYNTHROID should have their TSH measured during each trimester. An elevated serum TSH level should be corrected by an increase in the dose of SYNTHROID. Since postpartum TSH levels are similar to preconception values, the SYNTHROID dosage should return to the pre-pregnancy dose immediately after delivery. A serum TSH level should be obtained 6-8 weeks postpartum.

Thyroid hormones cross the placental barrier to some extent as evidenced by levels in cord blood of athyreotic fetuses being approximately one-third maternal levels. Transfer of thyroid hormone from the mother to the fetus, however, may not be adequate to prevent *in utero* hypothyroidism.

Nursing Mothers

Although thyroid hormones are excreted only minimally in human milk, caution should be exercised when SYNTHROID is administered to a nursing woman. However, adequate replacement doses of levothyroxine are generally needed to maintain normal lactation.

Pediatric Use

General

The goal of treatment in pediatric patients with hypothyroidism is to achieve and maintain normal intellectual and physical growth and development.

The initial dose of levothyroxine varies with age and body weight (see **DOSAGE AND ADMINISTRATION - Table 3**). Dosing adjustments are based on an assessment of the individual patient's clinical and laboratory parameters (see **PRECAUTIONS - Laboratory Tests**).

In children in whom a diagnosis of permanent hypothyroidism has not been established, it is recommended that levothyroxine administration be discontinued for a 30-day trial period, but only after the child is at least 3 years of age. Serum T_4 and TSH levels should then be obtained. If the T_4 is low and the TSH high, the diagnosis of permanent hypothyroidism is established, and levothyroxine therapy should be reinstituted. If the T_4 and TSH levels are normal, euthyroidism may be assumed and, therefore, the hypothyroidism can be considered to have been transient. In this instance, however, the physician should carefully monitor the child and repeat the thyroid function tests if any signs or symptoms of hypothyroidism develop. In this setting, the clinician should have a high index of suspicion of relapse. If the results of the levothyroxine withdrawal test are inconclusive, careful follow-up and subsequent testing will be necessary.

Since some more severely affected children may become clinically hypothyroid when treatment is discontinued for 30 days, an alternate approach is to reduce the replacement dose of levothyroxine by half during the 30-day trial period. If, after 30 days, the serum TSH is elevated above 20 mU/L, the diagnosis of permanent hypothyroidism is confirmed, and full replacement therapy should be resumed. However, if the serum TSH has not risen to greater than 20 mU/L, levothyroxine treatment should be discontinued for another 30-day trial period followed by repeat serum T_4 and TSH testing.

The presence of concomitant medical conditions should be considered in certain clinical circumstances and, if present, appropriately treated (see **PRECAUTIONS**).

Congenital Hypothyroidism (see **PRECAUTIONS - Laboratory Tests** and **DOSAGE AND ADMINISTRATION**)

Rapid restoration of normal serum T_4 concentrations is essential for preventing the adverse effects of congenital hypothyroidism on intellectual development as well as on overall physical growth and maturation. Therefore, SYNTHROID therapy should be initiated immediately upon diagnosis and is generally continued for life.

During the first 2 weeks of SYNTHROID therapy, infants should be closely monitored for cardiac overload, arrhythmias, and aspiration from avid suckling.

The patient should be monitored closely to avoid undertreatment or overtreatment. Undertreatment may have deleterious effects on intellectual development and linear growth. Overtreatment has been associated with craniosynostosis in infants, and may adversely affect the tempo of brain maturation and accelerate the bone age with resultant premature closure of the epiphyses and compromised adult stature.

Acquired Hypothyroidism in Pediatric Patients

The patient should be monitored closely to avoid undertreatment and overtreatment. Undertreatment may result in poor school performance due to impaired concentration and slowed mentation and in reduced adult height. Overtreatment may accelerate the bone age and result in premature epiphyseal closure and compromised adult stature.

Treated children may manifest a period of catch-up growth, which may be adequate in some cases to normalize adult height. In children with severe or prolonged hypothyroidism, catch-up growth may not be adequate to normalize adult height.

Geriatric Use

Because of the increased prevalence of cardiovascular disease among the elderly, levothyroxine therapy should not be initiated at the full replacement dose (see **WARNINGS, PRECAUTIONS**, and **DOSAGE AND ADMINISTRATION**).

ADVERSE REACTIONS

Adverse reactions associated with levothyroxine therapy are primarily those of hyperthyroidism due to therapeutic overdosage (see **PRECAUTIONS** and **OVERDOSAGE**). They include the following:

General

fatigue, increased appetite, weight loss, heat intolerance, fever, excessive sweating;

Central nervous system

headache, hyperactivity, nervousness, anxiety, irritability, emotional lability, insomnia;

Musculoskeletal

tremors, muscle weakness;

Cardiovascular

palpitations, tachycardia, arrhythmias, increased pulse and blood pressure, heart failure, angina, myocardial infarction, cardiac arrest;

Respiratory

dyspnea;

Gastrointestinal

diarrhea, vomiting, abdominal cramps and elevations in liver function tests;

Dermatologic

hair loss, flushing;

Endocrine

decreased bone mineral density;

Reproductive

menstrual irregularities, impaired fertility.

Pseudotumor cerebri and slipped capital femoral epiphysis have been reported in children receiving levothyroxine therapy. Overtreatment may result in craniosynostosis in infants and premature closure of the epiphyses in children with resultant compromised adult height.

Seizures have been reported rarely with the institution of levothyroxine therapy.

Inadequate levothyroxine dosage will produce or fail to ameliorate the signs and symptoms of hypothyroidism.

Hypersensitivity reactions to inactive ingredients have occurred in patients treated with thyroid hormone products. These include urticaria, pruritus, skin rash, flushing, angioedema, various GI symptoms (abdominal pain, nausea, vomiting and diarrhea), fever, arthralgia, serum sickness and wheezing. Hypersensitivity to levothyroxine itself is not known to occur.

OVERDOSAGE

The signs and symptoms of overdosage are those of hyperthyroidism (see **PRECAUTIONS** and **ADVERSE REACTIONS**). In addition, confusion and disorientation may occur. Cerebral embolism, shock, coma, and death have been reported. Seizures have occurred in a child ingesting 18 mg of levothyroxine. Symptoms may not necessarily be evident or may not appear until several days after ingestion of levothyroxine sodium.

Treatment of Overdosage

Levothyroxine sodium should be reduced in dose or temporarily discontinued if signs or symptoms of overdosage occur.

Acute Massive Overdosage

This may be a life-threatening emergency, therefore, symptomatic and supportive therapy should be instituted immediately. If not contraindicated (e.g., by seizures, coma, or loss of the gag reflex), the stomach should be emptied by emesis or gastric lavage to decrease gastrointestinal absorption. Activated charcoal or cholestyramine may also be used to decrease absorption. Central and peripheral increased sympathetic activity may be treated by administering β-receptor antagonists, e.g., propranolol, provided there are no medical contraindications to their use. Provide respiratory support as needed; control congestive heart failure and arrhythmia; control fever, hypoglycemia, and fluid loss as necessary. Large doses of antithyroid drugs (e.g., methimazole or propylthiouracil) followed in one to two hours by large doses of iodine may be given to inhibit synthesis and release of thyroid hormones. Glucocorticoids may be given to inhibit the conversion of T_4 to T_3. Plasmapheresis, charcoal hemoperfusion and exchange transfusion have been reserved for cases in which continued clinical deterioration occurs despite conventional therapy. Because T_4 is highly protein bound, very little drug will be removed by dialysis.

DOSAGE AND ADMINISTRATION

General Principles

The goal of replacement therapy is to achieve and maintain a clinical and biochemical euthyroid state. The goal of suppressive therapy is to inhibit growth and/or function of abnormal thyroid tissue. The dose of SYNTHROID that is adequate to achieve these goals depends on a variety of factors including the patient's age, body weight, cardiovascular status, concomitant medical conditions, including pregnancy, concomitant medications, and the specific nature of the condition being treated (see **WARNINGS** and **PRECAUTIONS**). Hence, the following recommendations serve only as dosing guidelines. Dosing must be individualized and adjustments made based on periodic assessment of the patient's clinical response and laboratory parameters (see **PRECAUTIONS - Laboratory Tests**).

SYNTHROID is administered as a single daily dose, preferably one-half to one-hour before breakfast. SYNTHROID should be taken at least 4 hours apart from drugs that are known to interfere with its absorption (see **PRECAUTIONS - Drug Interactions**).

Due to the long half-life of levothyroxine, the peak therapeutic effect at a given dose of levothyroxine sodium may not be attained for 4-6 weeks.

Caution should be exercised when administering SYNTHROID to patients with underlying cardiovascular disease, to the elderly, and to those with concomitant adrenal insufficiency (see **PRECAUTIONS**).

Specific Patient Populations

Hypothyroidism in Adults and in Children in Whom Growth and Puberty are Complete (see **WARNINGS** and **PRECAUTIONS - Laboratory Tests**)

Therapy may begin at full replacement doses in otherwise healthy individuals less than 50 years old and in those older than 50 years who have been recently treated for hyperthyroidism or who have been hypothyroid for only a short time (such as a few months). The average full replacement dose of levothyroxine sodium is approximately 1.7 mcg/kg/day (e.g., **100-125 mcg/day** for a 70 kg adult). Older patients may require less than 1 mcg/kg/day. Levothyroxine sodium doses greater than 200 mcg/day are seldom required. An inadequate response to daily doses ≥ 300 mcg/day is rare and may indicate poor compliance, malabsorption, and/or drug interactions.

For most patients older than 50 years or for patients under 50 years of age with underlying cardiac disease, an initial starting dose of **25-50 mcg/day** of levothyroxine sodium is recommended, with gradual increments in dose at 6-8 week intervals, as needed. The recommended starting dose of levothyroxine sodium in elderly patients with cardiac disease is **12.5-25 mcg/day**, with gradual dose increments at 4-6 week intervals. The levothyroxine sodium dose is generally adjusted in 12.5-25 mcg increments until the patient with primary hypothyroidism is clinically euthyroid and the serum TSH has normalized.

In patients with severe hypothyroidism, the recommended initial levothyroxine sodium dose is **12.5-25 mcg/day** with

Strength (mcg)	Color	NDC # for bottles of 100	NDC # for bottles of 1000	NDC # for unit dose cartons of 100
25	orange	0074-4341-13	0074-4341-19	—
50	white	0074-4552-13	0074-4552-19	0074-4552-11
75	violet	0074-5182-13	0074-5182-19	0074-5182-11
88	olive	0074-6594-13	0074-6594-19	—
100	yellow	0074-6624-13	0074-6624-19	0074-6624-11
112	rose	0074-9296-13	0074-9296-19	—
125	brown	0074-7068-13	0074 7068 19	0074-7068-11
137	turquoise	0074-3727-13	0074-3727-19	—
150	blue	0074-7069-13	0074-7069-19	0074-7069-11
175	lilac	0074-7070-13	0074-7070-19	—
200	pink	0074-7148-13	0074-7148-19	0074-7148-11
300	green	0074-7149-13	0074-7149-19	—

increases of 25 mcg/day every 2-4 weeks, accompanied by clinical and laboratory assessment, until the TSH level is normalized.

In patients with secondary (pituitary) or tertiary (hypothalamic) hypothyroidism, the levothyroxine sodium dose should be titrated until the patient is clinically euthyroid and the serum free-T$_4$ level is restored to the upper half of the normal range.

Pediatric Dosage - Congenital or Acquired Hypothyroidism (see **PRECAUTIONS - Laboratory Tests**)

General Principles
In general, levothyroxine therapy should be instituted at full replacement doses as soon as possible. Delays in diagnosis and institution of therapy may have deleterious effects on the child's intellectual and physical growth and development.

Undertreatment and overtreatment should be avoided (see **PRECAUTIONS - Pediatric Use**).

SYNTHROID may be administered to infants and children who cannot swallow intact tablets by crushing the tablet and suspending the freshly crushed tablet in a small amount (5-10 mL or 1-2 teaspoons) of water. This suspension can be administered by spoon or by dropper. **DO NOT STORE THE SUSPENSION.** Foods that decrease absorption of levothyroxine, such as soybean infant formula, should not be used for administering levothyroxine sodium tablets (see **PRECAUTIONS - Drug-Food Interactions**).

Newborns
The recommended starting dose of levothyroxine sodium in newborn infants is **10-15 mcg/kg/day**. A lower starting dose (e.g., 25 mcg/day) should be considered in infants at risk for cardiac failure, and the dose should be increased in 4-6 weeks as needed based on clinical and laboratory response to treatment. In infants with very low (< 5 mcg/dL) or undetectable serum T$_4$ concentrations, the recommended initial starting dose is **50 mcg/day** of levothyroxine sodium.

Infants and Children
Levothyroxine therapy is usually initiated at full replacement doses, with the recommended dose per body weight decreasing with age (see **Table 3**). However, in children with chronic or severe hypothyroidism, an initial dose of **25 mcg/day** of levothyroxine sodium is recommended with increments of 25 mcg every 2-4 weeks until the desired effect is achieved.

Hyperactivity in an older child can be minimized if the starting dose is one-fourth of the recommended full replacement dose, and the dose is then increased on a weekly basis by an amount equal to one-fourth the full-recommended replacement dose until the full recommended replacement dose is reached.

Table 3. Levothyroxine Sodium Dosing Guidelines for Pediatric Hypothyroidism

AGE	Daily Dose Per Kg Body Weight[a]
0-3 months	10-15 mcg/kg/day
3-6 months	8-10 mcg/kg/day
6-12 months	6-8 mcg/kg/day
1-5 years	5-6 mcg/kg/day
6-12 years	4-5 mcg/kg/day
> 12 years but growth and puberty incomplete	2-3 mcg/kg/day
Growth and puberty complete	1.7 mcg/kg/day

[a] The dose should be adjusted based on clinical response and laboratory parameters (see **PRECAUTIONS - Laboratory Tests** and **Pediatric Use**).

Pregnancy
Pregnancy may increase levothyroxine requirements (see **PREGNANCY**).

Subclinical Hypothyroidism
If this condition is treated, a lower levothyroxine sodium dose (e.g., **1 mcg/kg/day**) than that used for full replacement may be adequate to normalize the serum TSH level.

Patients who are not treated should be monitored yearly for changes in clinical status and thyroid laboratory parameters.

TSH Suppression in Well-differentiated Thyroid Cancer and Thyroid Nodules
The target level for TSH suppression in these conditions has not been established with controlled studies. In addition, the efficacy of TSH suppression for benign nodular disease is controversial. Therefore, the dose of SYNTHROID used for TSH suppression should be individualized based on the specific disease and the patient being treated.

In the treatment of well-differentiated (papillary and follicular) thyroid cancer, levothyroxine is used as an adjunct to surgery and radioiodine therapy. Generally, TSH is suppressed to < 0.1 mU/L, and this usually requires a levothyroxine sodium dose of **greater than 2 mcg/kg/day**. However, in patients with high-risk tumors, the target level for TSH suppression may be < 0.01 mU/L.

In the treatment of benign nodules and nontoxic multinodular goiter, TSH is generally suppressed to a higher target (e.g., 0.1 to either 0.5 or 1.0 mU/L) than that used for the treatment of thyroid cancer. Levothyroxine sodium is contraindicated if the serum TSH is already suppressed due to the risk of precipitating overt thyrotoxicosis (see **CONTRAINDICATIONS - WARNINGS** and **PRECAUTIONS**).

Myxedema Coma
Myxedema coma is a life-threatening emergency characterized by poor circulation and hypometabolism, and may result in unpredictable absorption of levothyroxine sodium from the gastrointestinal tract. Therefore, oral thyroid hormone drug products are not recommended to treat this condition. Thyroid hormone products formulated for intravenous administration should be administered.

HOW SUPPLIED
SYNTHROID® **(levothyroxine sodium tablets, USP)** are round, color coded, scored and debossed with "SYNTHROID" on one side and potency on the other side. They are supplied as follows:
[See table above]

Storage Conditions
Store at 25°C (77°F); excursions permitted to 15°-30°C (59°-86°F) [see USP Controlled Room Temperature]. SYNTHROID tablets should be protected from light and moisture.
(Nos. 4341, 4552, 5182, 6594, 6624, 9296, 7068, 3727, 7069, 7070, 7148, 7149)
Abbott Laboratories,
North Chicago, IL 60064, U.S.A.
Ref. 03-A295-Revised August, 2009
Shown in Product Identification Guide, page 304

TARKA®   ℞
(trandolapril/verapamil hydrochloride ER tablets)

> **USE IN PREGNANCY**
> **When used in pregnancy during the second and third trimesters, ACE inhibitors can cause injury and even death to the developing fetus.** When pregnancy is detected, TARKA® should be discontinued as soon as possible. **See WARNINGS - Fetal/Neonatal Morbidity and Mortality.**

DESCRIPTION
TARKA® (trandolapril/verapamil hydrochloride ER) combines a slow release formulation of a calcium channel blocker, verapamil hydrochloride, and an immediate release formulation of an angiotensin converting enzyme inhibitor, trandolapril.

Verapamil Component
Verapamil hydrochloride is chemically described as benzeneacetonitrile, α[3-[[2-(3,4-dimethoxyphenyl)ethyl]methylamino]propyl]-3,4-dimethoxy-α-(1-methylethyl) hy-

drochloride. Its empirical formula is $C_{27}H_{38}N_2O_4$ HCl and its structural formula is:

Verapamil hydrochloride is an almost white crystalline powder, with a molecular weight of 491.08. It is soluble in water, chloroform, and methanol. It is practically free of odor, with a bitter taste.

Trandolapril Component
Trandolapril is the ethyl ester prodrug of a nonsulfhydryl angiotensin converting enzyme (ACE) inhibitor, trandolaprilat. It is chemically described as (2S,3aR,7aS)-1-[(S)-N-[(S)-Carboxy-3-phenylpropyl]alanyl]hexahydro-2-indolinecarboxylic acid, 1-ethyl ester. Its empirical formula is $C_{24}H_{34}N_2O_5$ and its structural formula is:

Trandolapril is a colorless, crystalline substance with a molecular weight of 430.54. It is soluble (>100 mg/mL) in chloroform, dichloromethane, and methanol.

TARKA tablets are formulated for oral administration, containing verapamil hydrochloride as a controlled release formulation and trandolapril as an immediate release formulation. The tablet strengths are trandolapril 2 mg/verapamil hydrochloride ER 180 mg, trandolapril 1 mg/verapamil hydrochloride ER 240 mg, trandolapril 2 mg/verapamil hydrochloride ER 240 mg, and trandolapril 4 mg/verapamil hydrochloride ER 240 mg. The tablets also contain the following ingredients: corn starch, dioctyl sodium sulfosuccinate, ethanol, hydroxypropyl cellulose, hypromellose, lactose, magnesium stearate, microcrystalline cellulose, polyethylene glycol, povidone, purified water, silicon dioxide, sodium alginate, sodium stearyl fumarate, synthetic iron oxides, talc, and titanium dioxide.

CLINICAL PHARMACOLOGY
Verapamil hydrochloride and trandolapril have been used individually and in combination for the treatment of hypertension. For the four dosing strengths, the antihypertensive effect of the combination is approximately additive to the individual components.

Verapamil Component
Verapamil is a calcium channel blocker that exerts its pharmacologic effects by modulating the influx of ionic calcium across the cell membrane of the arterial smooth muscle as well as in conductile and contractile myocardial cells. Verapamil exerts antihypertensive effects by decreasing systemic vascular resistance, usually without orthostatic decreases in blood pressure or reflex tachycardia. During isometric or dynamic exercise, verapamil does not alter systolic cardiac function in patients with normal ventricular function. Verapamil does not alter total serum calcium levels.

Trandolapril Component
Trandolapril is de-esterified to its diacid metabolite, trandolaprilat. Both inhibit angiotensin-converting enzyme (ACE) in human subjects and in animals. Trandolaprilat is about 8 times more potent than trandolapril. ACE is a peptidyl dipeptidase that catalyzes the conversion of angiotensin I to the vasoconstrictor, angiotensin II. Angiotensin II also stimulates aldosterone secretion by the adrenal cortex. Inhibition of ACE results in decreased plasma angiotensin II, which leads to decreased vasopressor activity and to decreased aldosterone secretion. The latter decrease may result in a small increase of serum potassium. In controlled clinical trials, treatment with TARKA resulted in mean increases in potassium of 0.1 mEq/L (see **PRECAUTIONS**). Removal of angiotensin II negative feedback on renin secretion leads to increased plasma renin activity (PRA).

ACE is identical to kininase II, an enzyme that degrades bradykinin. Whether increased levels of bradykinin, a potent vasodepressor peptide, play a role in the therapeutic effect of TARKA remains to be elucidated.

While the mechanism through which trandolapril lowers blood pressure is believed to be primarily suppression of the renin-angiotensin-aldosterone system, trandolapril has an antihypertensive effect even in patients with low renin hypertension. Trandolapril is an effective antihypertensive in all races studied. Both black patients (usually a predominantly low renin group) and non-black patients respond to 2 to 4 mg of trandolapril.

Pharmacokinetics and Metabolism

TARKA

Following a single oral dose of TARKA in healthy subjects, peak plasma concentrations are reached within 0.5-2 hours for trandolapril and within 4-15 hours for verapamil. Peak plasma concentrations of the active desmethyl metabolite of verapamil, norverapamil, are reached within 5-15 hours. Cleavage of the ester group converts trandolapril to its active diacid metabolite, trandolaprilat, which reaches peak plasma concentrations within 2-12 hours. The pharmacokinetics of trandolapril and trandolaprilat are not altered when trandolapril is administered in combination with verapamil, compared to monotherapy. The AUC and C_{max} for both verapamil and norverapamil are increased when 240 mg of controlled release verapamil is administered concomitantly with 4 mg trandolapril. The increase in C_{max} is 54 and 30% and the AUC is increased by 65 and 32% for verapamil and norverapamil, respectively. Administration of TARKA 4/240 (4 mg trandolapril and 240 mg verapamil hydrochloride ER) with a high-fat meal does not alter the bioavailability of trandolapril whereas verapamil peak concentrations and area under the curve (AUC) decrease 37% and 28%, respectively. Food thus decreases verapamil bioavailability and the time to peak plasma concentration for both verapamil and norverapamil are delayed by approximately 7 hours. Both optical isomers of verapamil are similarly affected.

Trandolaprilat has an effective elimination half-life of approximately 10 hours but like all ACE inhibitors, it has a prolonged terminal elimination half-life. The terminal half-life of verapamil is 6-11 hours. Steady-state plasma concentrations of the two components are achieved after about a week of once-daily dosing of TARKA. At steady-state, plasma concentrations of verapamil and trandolaprilat are up to two-fold higher than those observed after a single oral TARKA dose.

The pharmacokinetics of verapamil and trandolaprilat are significantly different in the elderly (≥65 years) than in younger subjects. The bioavailability of verapamil and norverapamil are increased by 87% and 77%, respectively, and that of trandolapril by approximately 35% in the elderly. AUCs are approximately 80% and 35% higher, respectively.

Verapamil Component

With the immediate release formulation, more than 90% of the orally administered dose is absorbed with peak plasma concentrations of verapamil observed 1 to 2 hours after dosing. A delayed rate but similar extent of absorption is observed for the sustained release formulation when compared to the immediate release formulation. Because of the rapid biotransformation of verapamil during its first pass through the portal circulation, absolute bioavailability ranges from 20% to 35%. A nonlinear correlation exists between verapamil dose and plasma concentrations.

In early dose titration with verapamil, a relationship exists between plasma concentrations of verapamil and prolongation of the PR interval. However, during chronic administration, this relationship may disappear. No relationship has been established between the plasma concentration of verapamil and reduction in blood pressure.

In healthy subjects, orally administered verapamil undergoes extensive metabolism in the liver. Twelve metabolites have been identified in plasma; all except norverapamil are present in trace amounts only. Approximately 70% of an administered dose is excreted as metabolites in the urine and 16% or more in the feces within 5 days. Urinary excretion of unchanged drug is about 3% to 4% of the dose. Verapamil is approximately 90% bound to plasma proteins.

In patients with hepatic insufficiency, verapamil clearance is decreased about 30% and the elimination half-life is prolonged up to 14 to 16 hours (see **PRECAUTIONS**). In patients with liver dysfunction, a dosage adjustment may be required. In the elderly (≥65 years), verapamil clearance is reduced resulting in increases in elimination half-life.

Trandolapril Component

Following oral administration of trandolapril, the absolute bioavailability of trandolapril is approximately 10% as trandolapril and 10% as trandolaprilat. Plasma concentrations of trandolaprilat but not trandolapril increase in proportion with dose. Plasma concentrations of trandolaprilat decline in a triphasic manner. The more prolonged terminal elimination phase probably represents a small fraction of dose saturably bound to ACE.

After an oral radiolabeled dose of trandolapril, excretion of trandolapril and metabolites account for 33% of the dose in the urine and about 66% in the feces. Less than 1% of the dose is excreted in the urine as unchanged drug. Serum protein binding of trandolapril is about 80%, and is independent of concentration. Binding of trandolaprilat is concentration-dependent, varying from 65% at 1000 ng/mL to 94% at 0.1 ng/mL, indicating saturation of binding with increasing concentration.

Compared to normal subjects, the plasma concentrations of trandolapril and trandolaprilat are approximately 2-fold greater and renal clearance is reduced by about 85% in patients with creatinine clearance below 30 mL/min and in patients on hemodialysis. Dosage adjustment is recommended in renally impaired patients. (See **DOSAGE AND ADMINISTRATION**).

Following oral administration in patients with mild to moderate alcoholic cirrhosis, plasma concentrations of trandolapril and trandolaprilat were, respectively, 9-fold and 2-fold greater than in normal subjects, but inhibition of ACE activity was not affected. Lower doses should be considered in patients with hepatic insufficiency (see **DOSAGE AND ADMINISTRATION**).

Pharmacodynamics

TARKA

Verapamil does not interfere with ACE inhibition by trandolapril. Trandolapril does not alter the effect of verapamil on intra-cardiac conduction.

Verapamil Component

Verapamil dilates the main coronary arteries and coronary arterioles, both in normal and ischemic regions, and is a potent inhibitor of coronary artery spasm. This property increases myocardial oxygen delivery in patients with coronary artery spasm, and is responsible for the effectiveness of verapamil in vasospastic (Prinzmetal's or variant) as well as unstable angina at rest.

Verapamil regularly reduces the total systemic resistance (afterload) by dilating peripheral arterioles. By decreasing the influx of calcium, verapamil prolongs the effective refractory period within the AV node and slows AV conduction in a rate-related manner.

Normal sinus rhythm is usually not affected, but in patients with sick sinus syndrome, verapamil may interfere with sinus node impulse generation and may induce sinus arrest or sinoatrial block. Atrioventricular block can occur in patients without preexisting conduction defects (see **WARNINGS**).

Verapamil does not alter the normal atrial action potential or intraventricular conduction time, but depresses amplitude, velocity of depolarization and conduction in depressed atrial fibers. Verapamil may shorten the antegrade effective refractory period of accessory bypass tracts. Acceleration of ventricular rate and/or ventricular fibrillation has been reported in patients with atrial flutter or atrial fibrillation and a coexisting accessory AV pathway following administration of verapamil (see **WARNINGS**).

Hemodynamics and Myocardial Metabolism: Verapamil reduces afterload and myocardial contractility. Improved left ventricular diastolic function in patients with idiopathic hypertrophic subaortic stenosis (IHSS) and those with coronary heart disease has also been observed with verapamil therapy. In most patients, including those with organic cardiac disease, the negative inotropic action of verapamil is countered by a reduction of afterload and cardiac index is usually not reduced. However, in patients with severe left ventricular dysfunction (e.g., pulmonary wedge pressure about 20 mmHg or ejection fraction less than 30%), or in patients taking beta-adrenergic blocking agents or other cardio-depressant drugs, deterioration of ventricular function may occur (see **Drug Interactions**).

Pulmonary Function: Verapamil does not induce bronchoconstriction and hence, does not impair ventilatory function.

Trandolapril Component

After a single 2 mg dose of trandolapril, inhibition of ACE activity reaches a maximum (70-85%) at 4 hours with about 1% decline at 24 hours. Eight days after dosing, ACE inhibition is still 40%.

Four placebo-controlled dose response studies were conducted using once daily oral dosing of trandolapril in doses from 0.25 to 16 mg per day in 827 black and non-black patients with mild to moderate hypertension. The minimal effective once daily dose was 1.0 mg in non-black patients and 2.0 mg in black patients. Further decreases in trough supine diastolic blood pressure were obtained in non-black patients with higher doses, and no further response was seen with doses above 4 mg (up to 16 mg). The antihypertensive effect diminished somewhat at the end of the dosing interval.

During chronic therapy, the maximum reduction in blood pressure with any dose is achieved within one week. Following 6 weeks of monotherapy in placebo-controlled trials in patients with mild to moderate hypertension, once daily doses of 2 to 4 mg lowered supine or standing systolic/diastolic blood pressure 24 hours after dosing by an average 7-10/4-5 mmHg below placebo responses in non-black patients. Once daily doses of 2 to 4 mg lowered blood pressures 4-6/3-4 mmHg below placebo responses in black patients.

CLINICAL STUDIES

In controlled clinical trials, once daily doses of TARKA, trandolapril 4 mg/verapamil HCl ER 240 mg or trandolapril 2 mg/verapamil HCl ER 180 mg, decreased placebo-corrected seated pressure (systolic/diastolic) 24 hours after dosing by about 7-12/6-8 mmHg. Each of the components of TARKA added to the antihypertensive effect. Treatment effects were consistent across age groups (<65, ≥65 years), and gender (male, female).

Blood pressure reductions were significantly greater for the TARKA 4/240 combination than for either of the components used alone.

The antihypertensive effects of TARKA have continued during therapy for at least 1 year.

INDICATIONS AND USAGE

TARKA is indicated for the treatment of hypertension.

This fixed combination drug is not indicated for the initial therapy of hypertension (see DOSAGE and ADMINISTRATION).

In using TARKA, consideration should be given to the fact that an angiotensin converting enzyme inhibitor, captopril, has caused agranulocytosis, particularly in patients with renal impairment or collagen vascular disease, and that available data are insufficient to show that trandolapril does not have similar risk (see **WARNINGS - Neutropenia/Agranulocytosis**).

CONTRAINDICATIONS

TARKA is contraindicated in patients who are hypersensitive to any ACE inhibitor or verapamil.

Because of the verapamil component, TARKA is contraindicated in:

1. Severe left ventricular dysfunction (see **WARNINGS**).
2. Hypotension (systolic pressure less than 90 mmHg) or cardiogenic shock.
3. Sick sinus syndrome (except in patients with a functioning artificial ventricular pacemaker).
4. Second- or third-degree AV block (except in patients with a functioning artificial ventricular pacemaker).
5. Patients with atrial flutter or atrial fibrillation and an accessory bypass tract (e.g. Wolff-Parkinson-White, Lown-Ganong-Levine syndromes) (see **WARNINGS**).

Because of the trandolapril component, TARKA is contraindicated in patients with a history of angioedema related to previous treatment with an angiotensin converting enzyme (ACE) inhibitor.

WARNINGS

Heart Failure

Verapamil Component

Verapamil has a negative inotropic effect which, in most patients, is compensated by its afterload reduction (decreased systemic vascular resistance) properties without a net impairment of ventricular performance. In clinical experience with 4,954 patients, 87 (1.8%) developed congestive heart failure or pulmonary edema. Verapamil should be avoided in patients with severe left ventricular dysfunction (e.g., ejection fraction less than 30%, pulmonary wedge pressure above 20 mmHg, or severe symptoms of cardiac failure) and in patients with any degree of ventricular dysfunction if they are receiving a beta adrenergic blocker (see **Drug Interactions**). Patients with milder ventricular dysfunction should, if possible, be controlled with optimum doses of digitalis and/or diuretics before verapamil treatment (Note interactions with digoxin under: **PRECAUTIONS**).

Trandolapril Component

Trandolapril, as an ACE inhibitor, may cause excessive hypotension in patients with congestive heart failure (see **WARNINGS - Hypotension**).

Hypotension

Verapamil Component

Occasionally, the pharmacologic action of verapamil may produce a decrease in blood pressure below normal levels which may result in dizziness or symptomatic hypotension.

Trandolapril Component

Trandolapril can cause symptomatic hypotension. Like other ACE inhibitors, trandolapril has only rarely been associated with symptomatic hypotension in uncomplicated hypertensive patients. Symptomatic hypotension is most likely to occur in patients who are salt- or volume-depleted as a result of prolonged treatment with diuretics, dietary salt restriction, dialysis, diarrhea, or vomiting. Volume and/or salt depletion should be corrected before initiating treatment with trandolapril (see **PRECAUTIONS - Drug Interactions** and **ADVERSE REACTIONS**).

In controlled studies, hypotension was observed in 0.6% of patients receiving any combination of trandolapril and verapamil HCl ER.

In patients with concomitant congestive heart failure, with or without associated renal insufficiency, ACE inhibitor therapy may cause excessive hypotension, which may be associated with oliguria or azotemia, and, rarely, with acute renal failure and death (see **DOSAGE AND ADMINISTRATION**).

If symptomatic hypotension occurs, the patient should be placed in the supine position and, if necessary, normal saline may be administered intravenously. A transient hypotensive response is not a contraindication to further doses; however, lower doses of verapamil HCl ER and/or trandolapril or reduced concomitant diuretic therapy should be considered.

Elevated Liver Enzymes/Hepatic Failure
Verapamil Component
Elevations of transaminases with and without concomitant elevations in alkaline phosphatase and bilirubin have been reported. Such elevations have sometimes been transient and may disappear even in the face of continued verapamil treatment. Several cases of hepatocellular injury related to verapamil have been proven by rechallenge; half of these had clinical symptoms (malaise, fever, and/or right upper quadrant pain) in addition to elevations of SGOT, SGPT, and alkaline phosphatase.
Trandolapril Component
ACE inhibitors rarely have been associated with a syndrome of cholestatic jaundice, fulminant hepatic necrosis, and death. The mechanism of this syndrome is not understood. Patients receiving ACE inhibitors who develop jaundice should discontinue the ACE inhibitor and receive appropriate medical follow-up.
Liver abnormalities were noted in 3.2% of patients taking any of several combinations of trandolapril/verapamil doses. Periodic monitoring of liver function in patients taking TARKA is therefore prudent.

Accessory Bypass Tract (Wolff-Parkinson-White or Lown-Ganong-Levine Syndromes)
Verapamil Component
Some patients with paroxysmal and/or chronic atrial fibrillation or atrial flutter and a coexisting accessory AV pathway have developed increased antegrade conduction across the accessory pathway bypassing the AV node, producing a very rapid ventricular response or ventricular fibrillation after receiving intravenous verapamil (or digitalis). Although a risk of this occurring with oral verapamil has not been established, such patients receiving oral verapamil may be at risk and its use in these patients is contraindicated (see **CONTRAINDICATIONS**).
Treatment is usually DC-cardioversion. Cardioversion has been used safely and effectively after oral verapamil.

Atrioventricular Block
Verapamil Component
The effect of verapamil on AV conduction and the SA node may lead to asymptomatic first-degree AV block and transient bradycardia, sometimes accompanied by nodal escape rhythms. PR interval prolongation is correlated with verapamil plasma concentrations, especially during the early titration phases of therapy. Higher degrees of AV block, however, were infrequently (0.8%) observed. Marked first-degree block or progressive development to second- or third-degree AV block requires a reduction in dosage or, in rare instances, discontinuation of verapamil HCl and institution of appropriate therapy depending upon the clinical situation.

Patients with Hypertrophic Cardiomyopathy (IHSS)
Verapamil Component
In 120 patients with hypertrophic cardiomyopathy (most of them refractory or intolerant to propranolol) who received therapy with verapamil at doses up to 720 mg/day, a variety of serious adverse effects were seen. Three patients died in pulmonary edema; all had severe left ventricular outflow obstruction and a past history of left ventricular dysfunction. Eight other patients had pulmonary edema and/or severe hypotension; abnormally high (over 20 mmHg) capillary wedge pressure and a marked left ventricular outflow obstruction were present in most of these patients. Sinus bradycardia occurred in 11% of the patients, second-degree AV block in 4% and sinus arrest in 2%. It must be appreciated that this group of patients had a serious disease with a high mortality rate. Most adverse effects responded well to dose reduction and only rarely did verapamil have to be discontinued.

Anaphylactoid and Possibly Related Reactions
Presumably because angiotensin-converting enzyme inhibitors affect the metabolism of eicosanoids and polypeptides, including endogenous bradykinin, patients receiving ACE inhibitors, including trandolapril may be subject to a variety of adverse reactions, some of them serious.
Angioedema
Angioedema of the face, extremities, lips, tongue, glottis, and larynx has been reported in patients treated with ACE inhibitors including trandolapril. Symptoms suggestive of angioedema or facial edema occurred in 0.13% of trandolapril-treated patients. Two of the four cases were life-threatening and resolved without treatment or with medication (corticosteroids). Angioedema associated with laryngeal edema can be fatal. If laryngeal stridor or angio-

edema of the face, tongue or glottis occurs, treatment with TARKA should be discontinued immediately, the patient treated in accordance with accepted medical care and carefully observed until the swelling disappears. In instances where swelling is confined to the face and lips, the condition generally resolves without treatment; antihistamines may be useful in relieving symptoms. **Where there is involvement of the tongue, glottis, or larynx, likely to cause airway obstruction, emergency therapy, including but not limited to subcutaneous epinephrine solution 1:1,000 (0.3 to 0.5 mL) should be promptly administered** (see **PRECAUTIONS - Information for Patients and ADVERSE REACTIONS**).
Anaphylactoid Reactions During Desensitization
Two patients undergoing desensitizing treatment with hymenoptera venom while receiving ACE inhibitors sustained life-threatening anaphylactoid reactions. In the same patients, these reactions did not occur when ACE inhibitors were temporarily withheld, but they reappeared when the ACE inhibitors were inadvertently readministered.
Anaphylactoid Reactions During Membrane Exposure
Anaphylactoid reactions have been reported in patients dialyzed with high-flux membranes and treated concomitantly with an ACE inhibitor. Anaphylactoid reactions have also been reported in patients undergoing low-density lipoprotein apheresis with dextran sulfate absorption.
Neutropenia/Agranulocytosis
Trandolapril Component
Another ACE inhibitor, captopril, has been shown to cause agranulocytosis and bone marrow depression rarely in patients with uncomplicated hypertension, but more frequently in patients with renal impairment, especially if they also have a collagen-vascular disease such as systemic lupus erythematosus or scleroderma. Available data from clinical trials of trandolapril or TARKA are insufficient to show that trandolapril does not cause agranulocytosis at similar rates. As with other ACE inhibitors, periodic monitoring of white blood cell counts in patients with collagen-vascular disease and/or renal disease should be considered.
Fetal/Neonatal Morbidity and Mortality
Trandolapril Component
ACE inhibitors can cause fetal and neonatal morbidity and death when administered to pregnant women. Several dozen cases have been reported in the world literature. When pregnancy is detected, ACE inhibitors should be discontinued as soon as possible.
The use of ACE inhibitors during the second and third trimesters of pregnancy has been associated with fetal and neonatal injury, including hypotension, neonatal skull hypoplasia, anuria, reversible or irreversible renal failure, and death. Oligohydramnios has also been reported, presumably resulting from decreased fetal renal function; oligohydramnios in this setting has been associated with fetal limb contractures, craniofacial deformation, and hypoplastic lung development. Prematurity, intrauterine growth retardation, and patent ductus arteriosus have also been reported, although it is not clear whether these occurrences were due to the ACE-inhibitor exposure.
These adverse effects do not appear to have resulted from intrauterine ACE-inhibitor exposure that has been limited to the first trimester. Mothers whose embryos and fetuses are exposed to ACE inhibitors only during the first trimester should be so informed. Nonetheless, when patients become pregnant, physicians should make every effort to discontinue the use of TARKA as soon as possible.
Rarely (probably less often than once in every thousand pregnancies), no alternative to ACE inhibitors will be found. In these rare cases, the mothers should be apprised of the potential hazards to their fetuses, and serial ultrasound examinations should be performed to assess the intra-amniotic environment.
If oligohydramnios is observed, TARKA should be discontinued unless it is considered life-saving for the mother. Contraction stress testing (CST), a non-stress test (NST), or biophysical profiling (BPP) may be appropriate, depending upon the week of pregnancy. Patients and physicians should be aware, however, that oligohydramnios may not appear until after the fetus has sustained irreversible injury.
Infants with histories of in utero exposure to ACE inhibitors should be closely observed for hypotension, oliguria, and hyperkalemia. If oliguria occurs, attention should be directed toward support of blood pressure and renal perfusion. Exchange transfusion or dialysis may be required as a means of reversing hypotension and/or substituting for disordered renal function.
Trandolapril in doses of 0.8 mg/kg/day in rabbits, 100.0 mg/kg/day in rats, and 25 mg/kg/day in cynomolgus monkeys (10, 1,250, and 312 times the maximum projected human dose, respectively, assuming a 50 kg woman) did not produce teratogenic effects.

PRECAUTIONS
Use in Patients with Impaired Hepatic Function
TARKA has not been evaluated in subjects with impaired hepatic function.

Verapamil Component
Since verapamil is highly metabolized by the liver, it should be administered cautiously to patients with impaired hepatic function. Severe liver dysfunction prolongs the elimination half-life of immediate release verapamil to about 14 to 16 hours; hence, approximately 30% of the dose given to patients with normal liver function should be administered to these patients.
Careful monitoring for abnormal prolongation of the PR interval or other signs of excessive pharmacologic effects (see **OVERDOSAGE**) should be carried out.
Trandolapril Component
Trandolapril and trandolaprilat concentrations increase in patients with impaired liver function.
Use in Patients with Impaired Renal Function
TARKA has not been evaluated in patients with impaired renal function.
Verapamil Component
About 70% of an administered dose of verapamil is excreted as metabolites in the urine. Verapamil is not removed by hemodialysis. Until further data are available, verapamil should be administered cautiously to patients with impaired renal function. These patients should be carefully monitored for abnormal prolongation of the PR interval or other signs of overdosage (see **OVERDOSAGE**).
Trandolapril Component
As a consequence of inhibiting the renin-angiotensin-aldosterone system, changes in renal function may be anticipated in susceptible individuals. In patients with severe heart failure whose renal function may depend on the activity of the renin-angiotensin-aldosterone system, treatment with ACE inhibitors, including trandolapril, may be associated with oliguria and/or progressive azotemia and rarely with acute renal failure and/or death.
In hypertensive patients with unilateral or bilateral renal artery stenosis, increases in blood urea nitrogen and serum creatinine have been observed in some patients following ACE inhibitor therapy. These increases were almost always reversible upon discontinuation of the ACE inhibitor and/or diuretic therapy. In such patients, renal function should be monitored during the first few weeks of therapy.
Some hypertensive patients with no apparent pre-existing renal vascular disease have developed increases in blood urea and serum creatinine, usually minor and transient, especially when ACE inhibitors have been given concomitantly with a diuretic. This is more likely to occur in patients with pre-existing renal impairment. Dosage reduction and/or discontinuation of any diuretic and/or the ACE inhibitor may be required.
Evaluation of hypertensive patients should always include assessment of renal function (see DOSAGE AND ADMINISTRATION).
Use in Patients with Attenuated (Decreased) Neuromuscular Transmission
Verapamil Component
It has been reported that verapamil decreases neuromuscular transmission in patients with Duchenne's muscular dystrophy, and that verapamil prolongs recovery from the neuromuscular blocking agent vecuronium. It may be necessary to decrease the dosage of verapamil when it is administered to patients with attenuated neuromuscular transmission. (See **PRECAUTIONS - Surgery/Anesthesia**.)
Hyperkalemia and Potassium-sparing Diuretics
Trandolapril Component
In clinical trials, hyperkalemia (serum potassium > 6.00 mEq/L) occurred in approximately 0.4 percent of hypertensive patients receiving trandolapril and in 0.8% of patients receiving a dose of trandolapril (0.5-8 mg) in combination with a dose of verapamil SR (120-240 mg). In most cases, elevated serum potassium levels were isolated values, which resolved despite continued therapy. None of these patients were discontinued from the trials because of hyperkalemia. Risk factors for the development of hyperkalemia include renal insufficiency, diabetes mellitus, and the concomitant use of potassium-sparing diuretics, potassium supplements, and/or potassium-containing salt substitutes, which should be used cautiously, if at all, with trandolapril (see **PRECAUTIONS - Drug Interactions**).
Cough
Presumably due to the inhibition of the degradation of endogenous bradykinin, persistent nonproductive cough has been reported with all ACE inhibitors, always resolving after discontinuation of therapy. ACE inhibitor-induced cough should be considered in the differential diagnosis of cough.

Information on the Abbott Pharmaceutical Products listed on these pages is from the prescribing information in use as of June 1, 2010. For more information, please visit rxabbott.com or call 1-800-633-9110.

In controlled trials of trandolapril, cough was present in 2% of trandolapril patients and 0% of patients given placebo. There was no evidence of a relationship to dose.

Surgery/anesthesia

Trandolapril Component

In patients undergoing major surgery or during anesthesia with agents that produce hypotension, trandolapril will block angiotensin II formation secondary to compensatory renin release. If hypotension occurs and is considered to be due to this mechanism, it can be corrected by volume expansion. (See **PRECAUTIONS - Use in Patients with Attenuated (Decreased) Neuromuscular Transmission**.)

Drug Interactions

Digitalis

Clinical use of verapamil in digitalized patients has shown the combination to be well tolerated if digoxin doses are properly adjusted. Chronic verapamil treatment can increase serum digoxin levels by 50 to 75% during the first week of therapy, and this can result in digoxin toxicity. In patients with hepatic cirrhosis, the influence of verapamil on digoxin kinetics is magnified. Verapamil may reduce total body clearance and extrarenal clearance of digitoxin by 27% and 29%, respectively. Maintenance digoxin doses should be reduced when verapamil is administered, and the patient should be carefully monitored to avoid over- or under-digitalization. Whenever overdigitalization is suspected, the daily dose of digoxin should be reduced or temporarily discontinued. Upon discontinuation of any verapamil-containing regime including TARKA® (trandolapril/verapamil hydrochloride ER), the patient should be reassessed to avoid underdigitalization. Neither trandolapril nor its metabolites have been found to interact with digoxin.

Lithium

Increased sensitivity to the effects of lithium (neurotoxicity) has been reported during concomitant verapamil-lithium therapy with either no change or an increase in serum lithium levels. Increased serum lithium levels and symptoms of lithium toxicity have been reported in patients receiving concomitant lithium and ACE inhibitor therapy. TARKA and lithium should be coadministered with caution, and frequent monitoring of serum lithium levels is recommended. If a diuretic is also used, the risk of lithium toxicity may be increased.

Clarithromycin

Hypotension, bradyarrhythmias, and lactic acidosis have been observed in patients receiving concurrent clarithromycin.

Erythromycin

Hypotension, bradyarrhythmias, and lactic acidosis have been observed in patients receiving concurrent erythromycin ethylsuccinate.

Cimetidine

The interaction between cimetidine and chronically administered verapamil has not been studied. Variable results on clearance have been obtained in acute studies of healthy volunteers; clearance of verapamil was either reduced or unchanged. Neither trandolapril nor its metabolites have been found to interact with cimetidine.

Beta Blockers

Verapamil Component

Concomitant therapy with beta-adrenergic blockers and verapamil may result in additive negative effects on heart rate, atrioventricular conduction, and/or cardiac contractility. The use of verapamil in combination with a beta-blocker should be used only with caution, and close monitoring.

Asymptomatic bradycardia (36 beats/min) with a wandering atrial pacemaker has been observed in a patient receiving concomitant timolol (a beta-adrenergic blocker) eyedrops and oral verapamil.

Antiarrhythmic Agents

Verapamil Component

Disopyramide

Data on possible interactions between verapamil and disopyramide phosphate are not available. Therefore, disopyramide should not be administered within 48 hours before or 24 hours after verapamil administration.

Flecainide

A study of healthy volunteers showed that the concomitant administration of flecainide and verapamil may have additive effects on myocardial contractility, AV conduction, and repolarization. Concomitant therapy with flecainide and verapamil may result in additive negative inotropic effect and prolongation of atrioventricular conduction.

Quinidine

In a small number of patients with hypertrophic cardiomyopathy (IHSS), concomitant use of verapamil and quinidine resulted in significant hypotension. Until further data are obtained, combined therapy of verapamil and quinidine in patients with hypertrophic cardiomyopathy should probably be avoided.

The electrophysiological effects of quinidine and verapamil on AV conduction were studied in 8 patients. Verapamil sig-

nificantly counteracted the effects of quinidine on AV conduction. There has been a report of increased quinidine levels during verapamil therapy.

Nitrates

Verapamil has been given concomitantly with short- and long-acting nitrates without any undesirable drug interactions. The pharmacologic profile of both drugs and the clinical experience suggest beneficial interactions.

Other

Verapamil Component

Carbamazepine

Verapamil may increase carbamazepine concentrations during combined therapy. This may produce carbamazepine side effects such as diplopia, headache, ataxia, or dizziness.

Rifampin

Therapy with rifampin may markedly reduce oral verapamil bioavailability.

Phenobarbital

Phenobarbital therapy may increase verapamil clearance.

Cyclosporin

Verapamil therapy may increase serum levels of cyclosporin.

Theophylline

Verapamil therapy may inhibit the clearance and increase the plasma levels of theophylline.

Inhalation Anesthetics

Animal experiments have shown that inhalation anesthetics depress cardiovascular activity by decreasing the inward movement of calcium ions. When used concomitantly, inhalation anesthetics and calcium antagonists, such as verapamil, should be titrated carefully to avoid excessive cardiovascular depression.

Neuromuscular Blocking Agents

Clinical data and animal studies suggest that verapamil may potentiate the activity of neuromuscular blocking agents (curare-like and depolarizing). It may be necessary to decrease the dose of verapamil and/or the dose of the neuromuscular blocking agent when the drugs are used concomitantly.

Concomitant Diuretic Therapy

Trandolapril Component

As with other ACE inhibitors, patients on diuretics, especially those on recently instituted diuretic therapy, may occasionally experience an excessive reduction of blood pressure after initiation of therapy with TARKA. The possibility of exacerbation of hypotensive effects with TARKA may be minimized by either discontinuing the diuretic or cautiously increasing salt intake prior to initiation of treatment with TARKA. If it is not possible to discontinue the diuretic, the starting dose of TARKA should be reduced (see **DOSAGE AND ADMINISTRATION**).

Agents Increasing Serum Potassium

Trandolapril can attenuate potassium loss caused by thiazide diuretics and increase serum potassium when used alone. Use of potassium-sparing diuretics (spironolactone, triamterene, or amiloride), potassium supplements, or potassium-containing salt substitutes concomitantly with ACE inhibitors can increase the risk of hyperkalemia. If concomitant use of such agents is indicated, they should be used with caution and with appropriate monitoring of serum potassium. (See **PRECAUTIONS**.)

Gold

Nitritoid reactions (symptoms include facial flushing, nausea, vomiting and hypotension) have been reported rarely in patients on therapy with injectable gold (sodium aurothiomalate) and concomitant ACE inhibitor therapy including TARKA.

Other

Trandolapril Component

Neither trandolapril nor its metabolites have been found to interact with furosemide or nifedipine. The anticoagulant effect of warfarin was not significantly changed by trandolapril.

Carcinogenesis, Mutagenesis, Impairment of Fertility

Verapamil Component

An 18-month toxicity study in rats, at a low multiple (6 fold) of the maximum recommended human dose, and not the maximum tolerated dose, did not suggest a tumorigenic potential. There was no evidence of a carcinogenic potential of verapamil administered in the diet of rats for two years at doses of 10, 35, and 120 mg/kg per day or approximately 1×, 3.5×, and 12×, respectively, the maximum recommended human daily dose (480 mg per day or 9.6 mg/kg/day). Verapamil was not mutagenic in the Ames test in 5 test strains at 3 mg per plate, with or without metabolic activation.

Studies in female rats at daily dietary doses up to 5.5 times (55 mg/kg/day) the maximum recommended human dose did not show impaired fertility. Effects on male fertility have not been determined.

Long-term studies were conducted with oral trandolapril administered by gavage to mice (78 weeks) and rats (104 and 106 weeks). No evidence of carcinogenic potential was seen in mice dosed up to 25 mg/kg/day (85 mg/m²/day) or

rats dosed up to 8 mg/kg/day (60 mg/m²/day). These doses are 313 and 32 times (mice), and 100 and 23 times (rats) the maximum recommended human daily dose (MRHDD) of 4 mg based on body-weight and body-surface-area, respectively assuming a 50 kg individual. The genotoxic potential of trandolapril was evaluated in the microbial mutagenicity (Ames) test, the point mutation and chromosome aberration assays in Chinese hamster V79 cells, and the micronucleus test in mice. There was no evidence of mutagenic or clastogenic potential in these *in vitro* and *in vivo* assays. Reproduction studies in rats did not show any impairment of fertility at doses up to 100 mg/kg/day (710 mg/m²/day) of trandolapril, or 1250 and 260 times the MRHDD on the basis of body-weight and body-surface-area, respectively.

Pregnancy

Pregnancy Categories C (first trimester) and D (second and third trimesters). See WARNINGS - Fetal/Neonatal Morbidity and Mortality.

Nursing Mothers

Verapamil is excreted in human milk. Radiolabeled trandolapril or its metabolites are secreted in rat milk. TARKA should not be administered to nursing mothers.

Geriatric Use

In placebo-controlled studies, where 23% of patients receiving TARKA were 65 years and older, and 2.4% were 75 years and older, no overall differences in effectiveness or safety were observed between these patients and younger patients. However, greater sensitivity of some older individual patients cannot be ruled out.

Pediatric Use

The safety and effectiveness of TARKA in children below the age of 18 have not been established.

Animal Pharmacology and/or Animal Toxicology

In chronic animal toxicology studies, verapamil caused lenticular and/or suture line changes at 30 mg/kg/day or greater and frank cataracts at 62.5 mg/kg/day or greater in the beagle dog but not the rat. Development of cataracts due to verapamil has not been reported in man.

ADVERSE REACTIONS

TARKA has been evaluated in over 1,957 subjects and patients. Of these, 541 patients, including 23% elderly patients, participated in U.S. controlled clinical trials, and 251 were studied in foreign controlled clinical trials. In clinical trials with TARKA, no adverse experiences peculiar to this combination drug have been observed. Adverse experiences that have occurred have been limited to those that have been previously reported with verapamil or trandolapril. TARKA has been evaluated for long-term safety in 272 patients treated for 1 year or more. Adverse experiences were usually mild and transient.

Discontinuation of therapy because of adverse events in U.S. placebo-controlled hypertension studies was required in 2.6% and 1.9% of patients treated with TARKA and placebo, respectively.

Adverse experiences occurring in 1% or more of the 541 patients in placebo-controlled hypertension trials who were treated with a range of trandolapril (0.5-8 mg) and verapamil (120-240 mg) combinations are shown below.

[See table at top of next page]

Other clinical adverse experiences possibly, probably, or definitely related to drug treatment occurring in 0.3% or more of patients treated with trandolapril/verapamil combinations with or without concomitant diuretic in controlled or uncontrolled trials (N = 990) and less frequent, clinically significant events (in italics) include the following:

Cardiovascular

Angina, *AV block second degree, bundle branch block*, edema, flushing, hypotension, *myocardial infarction*, palpitations, premature ventricular contractions, nonspecific ST-T changes, near syncope, tachycardia.

Central Nervous System

drowsiness, *hypesthesia, insomnia, loss of balance, paresthesia, vertigo*.

Dermatologic

pruritus, rash.

Emotional, Mental, Sexual States

anxiety, impotence, *abnormal mentation*.

Eye, Ear, Nose, Throat

epistaxis, tinnitus, upper respiratory tract infection, *blurred vision*.

Gastrointestinal

diarrhea, dyspepsia, dry mouth, nausea.

General Body Function

chest pain, malaise, weakness.

Genitourinary

endometriosis, hematuria, nocturia, polyuria, proteinuria.

Hemopoietic

decreased leukocytes, *decreased neutrophils*.

Musculoskeletal System

arthralgias/myalgias, *gout (increased uric acid)*.

Pulmonary

dyspnea.

Angioedema

Angioedema has been reported in 3 (0.15%) patients receiving TARKA in U.S. and foreign studies (N = 1,957). Angioedema associated with laryngeal edema may be fatal. If angioedema of the face, extremities, lips, tongue, glottis, and/or larynx occurs, treatment with TARKA should be discontinued and appropriate therapy instituted immediately (see **WARNINGS**).

Hypotension

(See **WARNINGS**.) In hypertensive patients, hypotension occurred in 0.6% and near syncope occurred in 0.1%. Hypotension or syncope was a cause for discontinuation of therapy in 0.4% of hypertensive patients.

Treatment of Acute Cardiovascular Adverse Reactions

The frequency of cardiovascular adverse reactions which require therapy is rare, hence, experience with their treatment is limited. Whenever severe hypotension or complete AV block occur following oral administration of TARKA (verapamil component), the appropriate emergency measures should be applied immediately, e.g., intravenously administered isoproterenol HCl, levarterenol bitartrate, atropine (all in the usual doses), or calcium gluconate (10% solution). In patients with hypertrophic cardiomyopathy (IHSS), alpha-adrenergic agents (phenylephrine, metaraminol bitartrate or methoxamine) should be used to maintain blood pressure, and isoproterenol and levarterenol should be avoided. If further support is necessary, inotropic agents (dopamine or dobutamine) may be administered. Actual treatment and dosage should depend on the severity and the clinical situation and the judgment and experience of the treating physician.

Fetal/Neonatal Morbidity and Mortality

See **WARNINGS - Fetal Neonatal Morbidity and Mortality**.

Other adverse experiences (in addition to those in table and listed above) that have been reported with the individual components are listed below.

Verapamil Component

Cardiovascular

(See **WARNINGS**.) CHF/pulmonary edema, AV block 3°, atrioventricular dissociation, claudication, purpura (vasculitis), syncope.

Digestive System

gingival hyperplasia. Reversible, (upon discontinuation of verapamil) nonobstructive, paralytic ileus has been infrequently reported in association with the use of verapamil.

Hemic and Lymphatic

ecchymosis or bruising.

Nervous System

cerebrovascular accident, confusion, psychotic symptoms, shakiness, somnolence.

Skin

exanthema, hair loss, hyperkeratosis, maculae, sweating, urticaria, Stevens-Johnson syndrome, erythema multiform.

Urogenital

gynecomastia, galactorrhea/hyperprolactinemia, increased urination, spotty menstruation.

Trandolapril Component

Emotional, Mental, Sexual States

decreased libido.

Gastrointestinal

pancreatitis.

Clinical Laboratory Test Findings

Hematology

(See **WARNINGS**.) Low white blood cells, low neutrophils, low lymphocytes, low platelets.

Serum Electrolytes

Hyperkalemia (see **PRECAUTIONS**), hyponatremia.

Renal Function Tests

Increases in creatinine and blood urea nitrogen levels occurred in 1.1 percent and 0.3 percent, respectively, of patients receiving TARKA with or without hydrochlorothiazide therapy. None of these increases required discontinuation of treatment. Increases in these laboratory values are more likely to occur in patients with renal insufficiency or those pretreated with a diuretic and, based on experience with other ACE inhibitors, would be expected to be especially likely in patients with renal artery stenosis. (See **PRECAUTIONS** and **WARNINGS**.)

Liver Function Tests

Elevations of liver enzymes (SGOT, SGPT, LDH, and alkaline phosphatase) and/or serum bilirubin occurred. Discontinuation for elevated liver enzymes occurred in 0.9 percent of patients. (See **WARNINGS**.)

OVERDOSAGE

No specific information is available on the treatment of overdosage with TARKA.

Verapamil Component

Overdose with verapamil may lead to pronounced hypotension, bradycardia, and conduction system abnormalities (e.g., junctional rhythm with AV dissociation and high degree AV block, including asystole). Other symptoms secondary to hypoperfusion (e.g., metabolic acidosis, hyperglycemia, hyperkalemia, renal dysfunction, and convulsions) may be evident.

Treat all verapamil overdoses as serious and maintain observation for at least 48 hours, preferably under continuous hospital care. Delayed pharmacodynamic consequences may occur with the sustained release formulation. Verapamil is known to decrease gastrointestinal transit time. In cases of overdose, tablets of ISOPTIN SR have occasionally been reported to form concretions within the stomach or intestines. These concretions have not been visible on plain radiographs of the abdomen, and no medical means of gastrointestinal emptying is of proven efficacy in removing them. Endoscopy might reasonably be considered in cases of overdose when symptoms are unusually prolonged. Verapamil cannot be removed by hemodialysis.

Treatment of overdosage should be supportive. Beta adrenergic stimulation or parenteral administration of calcium solutions may increase calcium ion flux across the slow channel, and have been used effectively in treatment of deliberate overdosage with verapamil. The following measures may be considered:

Bradycardia and Conduction System Abnormalities

Atropine, isoproterenol, and cardiac pacing.

Hypotension

Intravenous fluids, vasopressors (e.g., dopamine, dobutamine), calcium solutions (e.g., 10% calcium chloride solution).

Cardiac Failures

Inotropic agents (e.g., isoproterenol, dopamine, dobutamine), diuretics. Asystole should be handled by the usual measures including cardiopulmonary resuscitation.

Trandolapril Component

The oral LD$_{50}$ of trandolapril in mice was 4875 mg/kg in males and 3990 mg/kg in females. In rats, an oral dose of 5000 mg/kg caused low mortality (1 male out of 5; 0 females). In dogs, an oral dose of 1000 mg/kg did not cause mortality and abnormal clinical signs were not observed.

In humans, the most likely clinical manifestation would be symptoms attributable to severe hypotension. Laboratory determinations of serum levels of trandolapril and its metabolites are not widely available, and such determinations have, in any event, no established role in the management of trandolapril overdose. No data are available to suggest that physiological maneuvers (e.g., maneuvers to change pH of the urine) might accelerate elimination of trandolapril and its metabolites. It is not known if trandolapril or trandolaprilat can be usefully removed from the body by hemodialysis.

Angiotensin II could presumably serve as a specific antagonist antidote in the setting of trandolapril overdose, but angiotensin II is essentially unavailable outside of scattered research facilities. Because the hypotensive effect of trandolapril is achieved through vasodilation and effective hypovolemia, it is reasonable to treat trandolapril overdose by infusion of normal saline solution.

DOSAGE AND ADMINISTRATION

The recommended usual dosage range of trandolapril for hypertension is 1 to 4 mg per day administered in a single dose or two divided doses. The recommended usual dosage range of Isoptin-SR for hypertension is 120 to 480 mg per day administered in a single dose or two divided doses.

The hazards (see **WARNINGS**) of trandolapril are generally independent of dose; those of verapamil are a mixture of dose-dependent phenomena (primarily dizziness, AV block, constipation) and dose-independent phenomena, the former much more common than the latter. Therapy with any combination of trandolapril and verapamil will thus be associated with both sets of dose-independent hazards. The dose-dependent side effects of verapamil have not been shown to be decreased by the addition of trandolapril nor visa versa. Rarely, the dose-independent hazards of trandolapril are serious. To minimize dose-independent hazards, it is usually appropriate to begin therapy with TARKA only after a patient has either (a) failed to achieve the desired antihypertensive effect with one or the other monotherapy at its respective maximally recommended dose and shortest dosing interval, or (b) the dose of one or the other monotherapy cannot be increased further because of dose-limiting side effects.

Clinical trials with TARKA have explored only once-a-day doses. The antihypertensive effect and or adverse effects of adding 4 mg of trandolapril once-a-day to a dose of 240 mg Isoptin-SR administered twice-a-day has not been studied, nor have the effects of adding as little of 180 mg Isoptin-SR to 2 mg trandolapril administered twice-a-day been evaluated. Over the dose range of Isoptin-SR 120 to 240 mg once-a-day and trandolapril 0.5 to 8 mg once-a-day, the effects of the combination increase with increasing doses of either component.

Replacement Therapy

For convenience, patients receiving trandolapril (up to 8 mg) and verapamil (up to 240 mg) in separate tablets, administered once-a-day, may instead wish to receive tablets of TARKA containing the same component doses.

TARKA should be administered with food.

HOW SUPPLIED

TARKA 2/180 mg tablets are supplied as pink, oval, film-coated tablets containing 2 mg trandolapril in an immediate release form and 180 mg verapamil hydrochloride in a sustained release form. The tablet is embossed with a triangle and 182 on one side and plain on the other side.

NDC 0074-3287-13 - bottles of 100

TARKA 1/240 mg tablets are supplied as white, oval, film-coated tablets containing 1 mg trandolapril in an immediate release form and 240 mg verapamil hydrochloride in a sustained release form. The tablet is embossed with a triangle and 241 on one side and plain on the other side.

NDC 0074-3288-13 - bottles of 100

TARKA 2/240 mg tablets are supplied as gold, oval, film-coated tablets containing 2 mg trandolapril in an immediate release form and 240 mg verapamil hydrochloride in a sustained release form. The tablet is embossed with a triangle and 242 on one side and plain on the other side.

NDC 0074-3289-13 - bottles of 100

TARKA 4/240 mg tablets are supplied as reddish-brown, oval, film-coated tablets containing 4 mg trandolapril in an immediate release form and 240 mg verapamil

Information on the Abbott Pharmaceutical Products listed on these pages is from the prescribing information in use as of June 1, 2010. For more information, please visit rxabbott.com or call 1-800-633-9110.

ADVERSE EVENTS OCCURRING IN ≥ 1% OF TARKA® PATIENTS IN U.S. PLACEBO-CONTROLLED TRIALS

	TARKA (N = 541) % Incidence (% Discontinuance)	PLACEBO (N = 206) % Incidence (% Discontinuance)
AV Block First Degree	3.9 (0.2)	0.5 (0.0)
Bradycardia	1.8 (0.0)	0.0 (0.0)
Bronchitis	1.5 (0.0)	0.5 (0.0)
Chest Pain	2.2 (0.0)	1.0 (0.0)
Constipation	3.3 (0.0)	1.0 (0.0)
Cough	4.6 (0.0)	2.4 (0.0)
Diarrhea	1.5 (0.2)	1.0 (0.0)
Dizziness	3.1 (0.0)	1.9 (0.5)
Dyspnea	1.3 (0.4)	0.0 (0.0)
Edema	1.3 (0.0)	2.4 (0.0)
Fatigue	2.8 (0.4)	2.4 (0.0)
Headache(s)+	8.9 (0.0)	9.7 (0.5)
Increased Liver Enzymes*	2.8 (0.2)	1.0 (0.0)
Nausea	1.5 (0.2)	0.5 (0.0)
Pain Extremity(ies)	1.1 (0.2)	0.5 (0.0)
Pain Back+	2.2 (0.0)	2.4 (0.0)
Pain Joint(s)	1.7 (0.0)	1.0 (0.0)
Upper Respiratory Tract Infection(s)+	5.4 (0.0)	7.8 (0.0)
Upper Respiratory Tract Congestion+	2.4 (0.0)	3.4 (0.0)

* Also includes increase in SGPT, SGOT, Alkaline Phosphatase
+ Incidence of adverse events is higher in Placebo group than TARKA patients

hydrochloride in a sustained release form. The tablet is embossed with a triangle and 244 on one side and plain on the other side.

NDC 0074-3290-13 - bottles of 100

Dispense in well-closed container with safety closure.

Storage

Store at 15°-25°C (59°-77°F) see USP.

Abbott Laboratories
North Chicago, IL 60064, U.S.A.
Ref: 03-A208
Revised: 02/2009

Shown in Product Identification Guide, page 304

TEVETEN® ℞
[*tĕ-vĕ-tĕn*]
(eprosartan mesylate)
Rx Only

PRESCRIBING INFORMATION

> **USE IN PREGNANCY**
> **When used in pregnancy during the second and third trimesters, drugs that act directly on the renin-angiotensin system can cause injury and even death to the developing fetus.** When pregnancy is detected, TEVETEN® should be discontinued as soon as possible. See **WARNINGS: Fetal/Neonatal Morbidity and Mortality.**

DESCRIPTION

TEVETEN® (eprosartan mesylate) is a non-biphenyl non-tetrazole angiotensin II receptor (AT_1) antagonist. A selective non-peptide molecule, TEVETEN® is chemically described as the monomethanesulfonate of (*E*)-2-butyl-1-(*p*-carboxybenzyl)-α-2-thienylmethylimidazole-5-acrylic acid.

Its empirical formula is $C_{23}H_{24}N_2O_4S \cdot CH_4O_3S$ and molecular weight is 520.625. Its structural formula is:

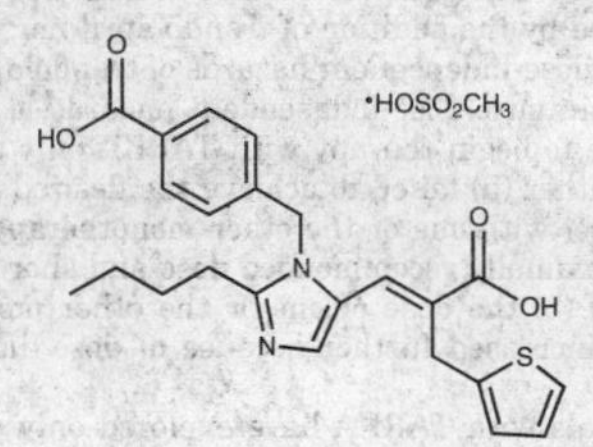

Eprosartan mesylate is a white to off-white free-flowing crystalline powder that is insoluble in water, freely soluble in ethanol, and melts between 248°C and 250°C.

TEVETEN® is available as aqueous film-coated tablets containing eprosartan mesylate equivalent to 400 mg or 600 mg eprosartan zwitterion (pink, oval, non-scored tablets or white, non-scored, capsule-shaped tablets, respectively).

Inactive Ingredients

The 400 mg tablet contains the following: croscarmellose sodium, hypromellose, iron oxide red, iron oxide yellow, lactose monohydrate, magnesium stearate, microcrystalline cellulose, polyethylene glycol, polysorbate 80, pregelatinized starch, and titanium dioxide. The 600 mg tablet contains crospovidone, hypromellose, lactose monohydrate, magnesium stearate, microcrystalline cellulose, polyethylene glycol, polysorbate 80, pregelatinized starch, and titanium dioxide.

CLINICAL PHARMACOLOGY

Mechanism of Action

Angiotensin II (formed from angiotensin I in a reaction catalyzed by angiotensin-converting enzyme [kininase II]), a potent vasoconstrictor, is the principal pressor agent of the renin-angiotensin system. Angiotensin II also stimulates aldosterone synthesis and secretion by the adrenal cortex, cardiac contraction, renal resorption of sodium, activity of the sympathetic nervous system, and smooth muscle cell growth. Eprosartan blocks the vasoconstrictor and aldosterone-secreting effects of angiotensin II by selectively blocking the binding of angiotensin II to the AT_1 receptor found in many tissues (e.g., vascular smooth muscle, adrenal gland). There is also an AT_2 receptor found in many tissues but it is not known to be associated with cardiovascular homeostasis. Eprosartan does not exhibit any partial agonist activity at the AT_1 receptor. Its affinity for the AT_1 receptor is 1,000 times greater than for the AT_2 receptor. *In vitro* binding studies indicate that eprosartan is a reversible, competitive inhibitor of the AT_1 receptor.

Blockade of the AT_1 receptor removes the negative feedback of angiotensin II on renin secretion, but the resulting increased plasma renin activity and circulating angiotensin II do not overcome the effect of eprosartan on blood pressure.

TEVETEN® does not inhibit kininase II, the enzyme that converts angiotensin I to angiotensin II and degrades bradykinin; whether this has clinical relevance is not known. It does not bind to or block other hormone receptors or ion channels known to be important in cardiovascular regulation.

Pharmacokinetics

General

Absolute bioavailability following a single 300 mg oral dose of eprosartan is approximately 13%. Eprosartan plasma concentrations peak at 1 to 2 hours after an oral dose in the fasted state. Administering eprosartan with food delays absorption, and causes variable changes (<25%) in C_{max} and AUC values which do not appear clinically important. Plasma concentrations of eprosartan increase in a slightly less than dose-proportional manner over the 100 mg to 800 mg dose range. The mean terminal elimination half-life of eprosartan following multiple oral doses of 600 mg was approximately 20 hours. Eprosartan does not significantly accumulate with chronic use.

Metabolism and Excretion

Eprosartan is eliminated by biliary and renal excretion, primarily as unchanged compound. Less than 2% of an oral dose is excreted in the urine as a glucuronide. There are no active metabolites following oral and intravenous dosing with [^{14}C] eprosartan in human subjects. Eprosartan was the only drug-related compound found in the plasma and feces. Following intravenous [^{14}C] eprosartan, about 61% of the material is recovered in the feces and about 37% in the urine. Following an oral dose of [^{14}C] eprosartan, about 90% is recovered in the feces and about 7% in the urine. Approximately 20% of the radioactivity excreted in the urine was an acyl glucuronide of eprosartan with the remaining 80% being unchanged eprosartan.

Distribution

Plasma protein binding of eprosartan is high (approximately 98%) and constant over the concentration range achieved with therapeutic doses.

The pooled population pharmacokinetic analysis from two Phase 3 trials of 299 men and 172 women with mild to moderate hypertension (aged 20 to 93 years) showed that eprosartan exhibited a population mean oral clearance (CL/F) for an average 60-year-old patient of 48.5 L/hr. The population mean steady-state volume of distribution (Vss/F) was 308 L. Eprosartan pharmacokinetics were not influenced by weight, race, gender or severity of hypertension at baseline. Oral clearance was shown to be a linear function of age with CL/F decreasing 0.62 L/hr for every year increase.

Special Populations

Pediatric

Eprosartan pharmacokinetics have not been investigated in patients younger than 18 years of age.

Geriatric

Following single oral dose administration of eprosartan to healthy elderly men (aged 68 to 78 years), AUC, C_{max}, and T_{max} eprosartan values increased, on average by approximately twofold, compared to healthy young men (aged 20 to 39 years) who received the same dose. The extent of plasma protein binding was not influenced by age.

Gender

There was no difference in the pharmacokinetics and plasma protein binding between men and women following single oral dose administration of eprosartan.

Race

A pooled population pharmacokinetic analysis of 442 Caucasian and 29 non-Caucasian hypertensive patients showed that oral clearance and steady-state volume of distribution were not influenced by race.

Renal Insufficiency

Following administration of 600 mg once daily, there was a 70-90% increase in AUC, and a 30-50% increase in C_{max} in moderate or severe renal impairment. The unbound eprosartan fractions increased by 35% and 59% in patients with moderate and severe renal impairment, respectively. No initial dosing adjustment is generally necessary in patients with moderate or severe renal impairment, with maximum dose not exceeding 600 mg daily. Eprosartan was poorly removed by hemodialysis (CL_{HD}<1 L/hr) (see **DOSAGE AND ADMINISTRATION).**

Hepatic Insufficiency

Eprosartan AUC (but not C_{max}) values increased, on average, by approximately 40% in men with decreased hepatic function compared to healthy men after a single 100 mg oral dose of eprosartan. Hepatic disease was defined as a documented clinical history of chronic hepatic abnormality diagnosed by liver biopsy, liver/spleen scan or clinical laboratory tests. The extent of eprosartan plasma protein binding was not influenced by hepatic dysfunction. No dosage adjustment is necessary for patients with hepatic impairment (see **DOSAGE AND ADMINISTRATION).**

Drug Interactions

Concomitant administration of eprosartan and digoxin had no effect on single oral-dose digoxin pharmacokinetics. Concomitant administration of eprosartan and warfarin had no effect on steady-state prothrombin time ratios (INR) in healthy volunteers. Concomitant administration of eprosartan and glyburide in diabetic patients did not affect 24-hour plasma glucose profiles. Eprosartan pharmacokinetics were not affected by concomitant administration of ranitidine. Eprosartan did not inhibit human cytochrome P450 enzymes CYP1A, 2A6, 2C9/8, 2C19, 2D6, 2E and 3A *in vitro*. Eprosartan is not metabolized by the cytochrome P450 system; eprosartan steady-state concentrations were not affected by concomitant administration of ketoconazole or fluconazole, potent inhibitors of CYP3A and 2C9, respectively.

Pharmacodynamics and Clinical Effects

Eprosartan inhibits the pharmacologic effects of angiotensin II infusions in healthy adult men. Single oral doses of eprosartan from 10 mg to 400 mg have been shown to inhibit the vasopressor, renal vasoconstrictive and aldosterone secretory effects of infused angiotensin II with complete inhibition evident at doses of 350 mg and above. Eprosartan inhibits the pressor effects of angiotensin II infusions. A single oral dose of 350 mg of eprosartan inhibits pressor effects by approximately 100% at peak, with approximately 30% inhibition persisting for 24 hours. The absence of angiotensin II AT_1 agonist activity has been demonstrated in healthy adult men. In hypertensive patients treated chronically with eprosartan, there was a twofold rise in angiotensin II plasma concentration and a twofold rise in plasma renin activity, while plasma aldosterone levels remained unchanged. Serum potassium levels also remained unchanged in these patients.

Achievement of maximal blood pressure response to a given dose in most patients may take 2 to 3 weeks of treatment. Onset of blood pressure reduction is seen within 1 to 2 hours of dosing with few instances of orthostatic hypotension. Blood pressure control is maintained with once- or twice-daily dosing over a 24-hour period. Discontinuing treatment with eprosartan does not lead to a rapid rebound increase in blood pressure.

There was no change in mean heart rate in patients treated with eprosartan in controlled clinical trials.

Eprosartan increases mean effective renal plasma flow (ERPF) in salt-replete and salt-restricted normal subjects. A dose-related increase in ERPF of 25% to 30% occurred in salt-restricted normal subjects, with the effect plateauing between the 200 mg and 400 mg doses. There was no change in ERPF in hypertensive patients and patients with renal insufficiency on normal salt diets. Eprosartan did not reduce glomerular filtration rate in patients with renal insufficiency or in patients with hypertension, after 7 days and 28 days of dosing, respectively. In hypertensive patients and patients with chronic renal insufficiency, eprosartan did not change fractional excretion of sodium and potassium.

Eprosartan (1200 mg once daily for 7 days or 300 mg twice daily for 28 days) had no effect on the excretion of uric acid in healthy men, patients with essential hypertension or those with varying degrees of renal insufficiency.

There were no effects on mean levels of fasting triglycerides, total cholesterol, HDL cholesterol, LDL cholesterol or fasting glucose.

Clinical Trials

The safety and efficacy of TEVETEN® have been evaluated in controlled clinical trials worldwide that enrolled predominantly hypertensive patients with sitting DBP ranging from 95 mmHg to ≤115 mmHg.

There is also some experience with use of eprosartan together with other anti-hypertensive drugs in more severe hypertension.

The antihypertensive effects of TEVETEN® were demonstrated principally in five placebo-controlled trials (4 to 13 weeks' duration) including dosages of 400 mg to 1200 mg given once daily (two studies), 25 mg to 400 mg twice daily (two studies), and one study comparing total daily doses of 400 mg to 800 mg given once daily or twice daily. The five studies included 1,111 patients randomized to eprosartan and 395 patients randomized to placebo. The studies showed dose-related antihypertensive responses.

At study endpoint, patients treated with TEVETEN® at doses of 600 mg to 1200 mg given once daily experienced significant decreases in sitting systolic and diastolic blood pressure at trough, with differences from placebo of approximately 5-10/3-6 mmHg. Limited experience is available with the dose of 1200 mg administered once daily. In a direct comparison of 200 mg to 400 mg b.i.d. with 400 mg to 800 mg q.d. of TEVETEN®, effects at trough were similar. Patients treated with TEVETEN® at doses of 200 mg to 400 mg given twice daily experienced significant decreases in sitting systolic and diastolic blood pressure at trough, with differences from placebo of approximately 7-10/4-6 mmHg.

Peak (1 to 3 hours) effects were uniformly, but moderately, larger than trough effects with b.i.d. dosing, with the trough-to-peak ratio for diastolic blood pressure 65% to 80%. In the once-daily dose-response study, trough-to-peak responses of ≤50% were observed at some doses (including 1200 mg), suggesting attenuation of effect at the end of the dosing interval.

The antihypertensive effect of TEVETEN® was similar in men and women, but was somewhat smaller in patients over 65. There were too few black subjects to determine whether their response was similar to Caucasians. In general, blacks (usually a low renin population) have had smaller responses to ACE inhibitors and angiotensin II inhibitors than Caucasian populations.

Angiotensin-converting enzyme (ACE) inhibitor-induced cough (a dry, persistent cough) can lead to discontinuation of ACE inhibitor therapy. In one study, patients who had previously coughed while taking an ACE inhibitor were treated with eprosartan, an ACE inhibitor (enalapril) or placebo for six weeks. The incidence of dry, persistent cough was 2.2% on eprosartan, 4.4% on placebo, and 20.5% on the ACE inhibitor; p=0.008 for the comparison of eprosartan with enalapril. In a second study comparing the incidence of cough in 259 patients treated with eprosartan to 261 patients treated with the ACE inhibitor enalapril, the incidence of dry, persistent cough in eprosartan-treated patients (1.5%) was significantly lower (p=0.018) than that observed in patients treated with the ACE inhibitor (5.4%). In addition, analysis of overall data from six double-blind clinical trials involving 1,554 patients showed an incidence of spontaneously reported cough in patients treated with eprosartan of 3.5%, similar to placebo (2.6%).

INDICATIONS AND USAGE

TEVETEN® is indicated for the treatment of hypertension. It may be used alone or in combination with other antihypertensives such as diuretics and calcium channel blockers.

CONTRAINDICATIONS

TEVETEN® is contraindicated in patients who are hypersensitive to this product or any of its components.

WARNINGS

Fetal/Neonatal Morbidity and Mortality

Drugs that act directly on the renin-angiotensin system can cause fetal and neonatal morbidity and death when administered to pregnant women. Several dozen cases have been reported in the world literature in patients who were taking angiotensin-converting enzyme inhibitors. When pregnancy is detected, TEVETEN® should be discontinued as soon as possible.

The use of drugs that act directly on the renin-angiotensin system during the second and third trimesters of pregnancy has been associated with fetal and neonatal injury, including hypotension, neonatal skull hypoplasia, anuria, reversible or irreversible renal failure, and death. Oligohydramnios has also been reported, presumably resulting from decreased fetal renal function; oligohydramnios in this setting has been associated with fetal limb contractures, craniofacial deformation, and hypoplastic lung development. Prematurity, intrauterine growth retardation, and patent ductus arteriosus have also been reported, although it is not clear whether these occurrences were due to exposure to the drug.

These adverse effects do not appear to have resulted from intrauterine drug exposure that has been limited to the first trimester. Mothers whose embryos and fetuses are exposed to an angiotensin II receptor antagonist only during the first trimester should be so informed. Nonetheless, when patients become pregnant, physicians should advise the patient to discontinue the use of eprosartan as soon as possible.

Rarely (probably less often than once in every thousand pregnancies), no alternative to a drug acting on the renin-angiotensin system will be found. In these rare cases, the mothers should be apprised of the potential hazards to their fetuses, and serial ultrasound examinations should be performed to assess the intra-amniotic environment.

If oligohydramnios is observed, TEVETEN® should be discontinued unless it is considered life-saving for the mother. Contraction stress testing (CST), a nonstress test (NST) or biophysical profiling (BPP) may be appropriate, depending upon the week of pregnancy. Patients and physicians should be aware, however, that oligohydramnios may not appear until after the fetus has sustained irreversible injury.

Infants with histories of *in utero* exposure to an angiotensin II receptor antagonist should be closely observed for hypotension, oliguria, and hyperkalemia. If oliguria occurs, attention should be directed toward support of blood pressure and renal perfusion. Exchange transfusion or dialysis may be required as means of reversing hypotension and/or substituting for disordered renal function.

Eprosartan mesylate has been shown to produce maternal and fetal toxicities (maternal and fetal mortality, low maternal body weight and food consumption, resorptions, abortions and litter loss) in pregnant rabbits given oral doses as low as 10 mg eprosartan/kg/day. No maternal or fetal adverse effects were observed at 3 mg/kg/day; this oral dose yielded a systemic exposure (AUC) to unbound eprosartan 0.8 times that achieved in humans given 400 mg b.i.d. No adverse effects on *in utero* or postnatal development and maturation of offspring were observed when eprosartan

mesylate was administered to pregnant rats at oral doses up to 1000 mg eprosartan/kg/day (the 1000 mg eprosartan/kg/day dose in non-pregnant rats yielded systemic exposure to unbound eprosartan approximately 0.6 times the exposure achieved in humans given 400 mg b.i.d.).

Hypotension in Volume- and/or Salt-Depleted Patients

In patients with an activated renin-angiotensin system, such as volume- and/or salt-depleted patients (e.g., those being treated with diuretics), symptomatic hypotension may occur. These conditions should be corrected prior to administration of TEVETEN®, or the treatment should start under close medical supervision. If hypotension occurs, the patient should be placed in the supine position and, if necessary, given an intravenous infusion of normal saline. A transient hypotensive response is not a contraindication to further treatment, which usually can be continued without difficulty once the blood pressure has stabilized.

PRECAUTIONS

Risk of Renal Impairment

As a consequence of inhibiting the renin-angiotensin-aldosterone system, changes in renal function have been reported in susceptible individuals treated with angiotensin II antagonists; in some patients, these changes in renal function were reversible upon discontinuation of therapy. In patients whose renal function may depend on the activity of the renin-angiotensin-aldosterone system (e.g., patients with severe congestive heart failure), treatment with angiotensin-converting enzyme inhibitors and angiotensin II receptor antagonists has been associated with oliguria and/or progressive azotemia and (rarely) with acute renal failure and/or death. TEVETEN® would be expected to behave similarly.

In studies of ACE inhibitors in patients with unilateral or bilateral renal artery stenosis, increases in serum creatinine or BUN have been reported. Similar effects have been reported with angiotensin II antagonists; in some patients, these effects were reversible upon discontinuation of therapy.

Information for Patients

Pregnancy

Female patients of childbearing age should be told about the consequences of second- and third-trimester exposure to drugs that act on the renin-angiotensin system, and they should also be told that these consequences do not appear to have resulted from intrauterine drug exposure that has been limited to the first trimester. These patients should be asked to report pregnancies to their physicians as soon as possible so that treatment may be discontinued under medical supervision.

Drug Interactions

Eprosartan has been shown to have no effect on the pharmacokinetics of digoxin and the pharmacodynamics of warfarin and glyburide. Thus, no dosing adjustments are necessary during concomitant use with these agents. Because eprosartan is not metabolized by the cytochrome P450 system, inhibitors of CYP450 enzyme would not be expected to affect its metabolism, and ketoconazole and fluconazole, potent inhibitors of CYP3A and 2C9, respectively, have been shown to have no effect on eprosartan pharmacokinetics. Ranitidine also has no effect on eprosartan pharmacokinetics.

Eprosartan (up to 400 mg b.i.d. or 800 mg q.d.) doses have been safely used concomitantly with a thiazide diuretic (hydrochlorothiazide). Eprosartan doses of up to 300 mg b.i.d. have been safely used concomitantly with sustained-release calcium channel blockers (sustained-release nifedipine) with no clinically significant adverse interactions.

Carcinogenesis, Mutagenesis, Impairment of Fertility

Eprosartan mesylate was not carcinogenic in dietary restricted rats or *ad libitum* fed mice dosed at 600 mg and 2000 mg eprosartan/kg/day, respectively, for up to 2 years. In male and female rats, the systemic exposure (AUC) to unbound eprosartan at the dose evaluated was only approximately 20% of the exposure achieved in humans given 400 mg b.i.d. In mice, the systemic exposure (AUC) to unbound eprosartan was approximately 25 times the exposure achieved in humans given 400 mg b.i.d.

Eprosartan mesylate was not mutagenic *in vitro* in bacteria or mammalian cells (mouse lymphoma assay). Eprosartan mesylate also did not cause structural chromosomal damage *in vivo* (mouse micronucleus assay). In human peripheral lymphocytes *in vitro*, eprosartan mesylate was equivocal for clastogenicity with metabolic activation, and was negative without metabolic activation. In the same assay, eprosartan mesylate was positive for polyploidy with metabolic activation and equivocal for polyploidy without metabolic activation.

Eprosartan mesylate had no adverse effects on the reproductive performance of male or female rats at oral doses up to 1000 mg eprosartan/kg/day. This dose provided systemic exposure (AUC) to unbound eprosartan approximately 0.6 times the exposure achieved in humans given 400 mg b.i.d.

Pregnancy

Pregnancy Category C (first trimester) and D (second and third trimesters): See WARNINGS: Fetal/Neonatal Morbidity and Mortality.

Nursing Mothers

Eprosartan is excreted in animal milk; it is not known whether eprosartan is excreted in human milk. Because many drugs are excreted in human milk and because of the potential for serious adverse reactions in nursing infants from eprosartan, a decision should be made whether to discontinue nursing or to discontinue the drug, taking into account the importance of the drug to the mother.

Pediatric Use

Safety and effectiveness in pediatric patients have not been established.

Geriatric Use

Of the total number of patients receiving TEVETEN® in clinical studies, 29% (681 of 2,334) were 65 years and over, while 5% (124 of 2,334) were 75 years and over. Based on the pooled data from randomized trials, the decrease in diastolic blood pressure and systolic blood pressure with TEVETEN® was slightly less in patients ≥65 years of age compared to younger patients. In a study of only patients over the age of 65, TEVETEN® at 200 mg twice daily (and increased optionally up to 300 mg twice daily) decreased diastolic blood pressure on average by 3 mmHg (placebo corrected). Adverse experiences were similar in younger and older patients.

ADVERSE REACTIONS

TEVETEN® has been evaluated for safety in more than 3,300 healthy volunteers and patients worldwide, including more than 1,460 patients treated for more than 6 months, and more than 980 patients treated for 1 year or longer. TEVETEN® was well tolerated at doses up to 1200 mg daily. Most adverse events were of mild or moderate severity and did not require discontinuation of therapy. The overall incidence of adverse experiences and the incidences of specific adverse events reported with eprosartan were similar to placebo.

Adverse experiences were similar in patients regardless of age, gender, or race. Adverse experiences were not dose-related.

In placebo-controlled clinical trials, about 4% of 1,202 patients treated with TEVETEN® discontinued therapy due to clinical adverse experiences, compared to 6.5% of 352 patients given placebo.

Adverse Events Occurring at an Incidence of 1% or More Among Eprosartan-treated Patients

The following table lists adverse events that occurred at an incidence of 1% or more among eprosartan-treated patients who participated in placebo-controlled trials of 8 to 13 weeks' duration, using doses of 25 mg to 400 mg twice daily, and 400 mg to 1200 mg once daily. The overall incidence of adverse events reported with TEVETEN® (54.4%) was similar to placebo (52.8%).

Table 1. Adverse Events Reported by ≥1% of Patients Receiving TEVETEN® (eprosartan mesylate) and Were More Frequent on Eprosartan than Placebo

Event	Eprosartan (n=1,202) %	Placebo (n=352) %
Body as a Whole		
Infection viral	2	1
Injury	2	1
Fatigue	2	1
Gastrointestinal		
Abdominal pain	2	1
Metabolic and Nutritional		
Hypertriglyceridemia	1	0
Musculoskeletal		
Arthralgia	2	1
Nervous System		
Depression	1	0
Respiratory		
Upper respiratory tract infection	8	5
Rhinitis	4	3
Pharyngitis	4	3

Information on the Abbott Pharmaceutical Products listed on these pages is from the prescribing information in use as of June 1, 2010. For more information, please visit rxabbott.com or call 1-800-633-9110.

Coughing	4	3
Urogenital		
Urinary tract infection	1	0

The following adverse events were also reported at a rate of 1% or greater in patients treated with eprosartan, but were as, or more, frequent in the placebo group: headache, myalgia, dizziness, sinusitis, diarrhea, bronchitis, dependent edema, dyspepsia, and chest pain.

Facial edema was reported in 5 patients receiving eprosartan. Angioedema has been reported with other angiotensin II antagonists.

Rare cases of rhabdomyolysis have been reported in patients receiving angiotensin II receptor blockers.

In addition to the adverse events above, potentially important events that occurred in at least two patients/subjects exposed to eprosartan or other adverse events that occurred in <1% of patients in clinical studies are listed below. It cannot be determined whether events were causally related to eprosartan:

Body as a Whole: alcohol intolerance, asthenia, substernal chest pain, peripheral edema, fatigue, fever, hot flushes, influenza-like symptoms, malaise, rigors, pain;

Cardiovascular: angina pectoris, bradycardia, abnormal ECG, specific abnormal ECG, extrasystoles, atrial fibrillation, hypotension (including orthostatic hypotension), tachycardia, palpitations;

Gastrointestinal: anorexia, constipation, dry mouth, esophagitis, flatulence, gastritis, gastroenteritis, gingivitis, nausea, periodontitis, toothache, vomiting;

Hematologic: anemia, purpura;

Liver and Biliary: increased SGOT, increased SGPT;

Metabolic and Nutritional: increased creatine phosphokinase, diabetes mellitus, glycosuria, gout, hypercholesterolemia, hyperglycemia, hyperkalemia, hypokalemia, hyponatremia;

Musculoskeletal: arthritis, aggravated arthritis, arthrosis, skeletal pain, tendinitis, back pain;

Nervous System/Psychiatric: anxiety, ataxia, insomnia, migraine, neuritis, nervousness, paresthesia, somnolence, tremor, vertigo;

Resistance Mechanism: herpes simplex, otitis externa, otitis media, upper respiratory tract infection;

Respiratory: asthma, epistaxis;

Skin and Appendages: eczema, furunculosis, pruritus, rash, maculopapular rash, increased sweating;

Special Senses: conjunctivitis, abnormal vision, xerophthalmia, tinnitus;

Urinary: albuminuria, cystitis, hematuria, micturition frequency, polyuria, renal calculus, urinary incontinence;

Vascular: leg cramps, peripheral ischemia.

Laboratory Test Findings
In placebo-controlled studies, clinically important changes in standard laboratory parameters were rarely associated with administration of TEVETEN®. Patients were rarely withdrawn from TEVETEN® because of laboratory test results.

Creatinine, Blood Urea Nitrogen

Minor elevations in creatinine and in BUN occurred in 0.6% and 1.3%, respectively, of patients taking TEVETEN® and 0.9% and 0.3%, respectively, of patients given placebo in controlled clinical trials. Two patients were withdrawn from clinical trials for elevations in serum creatinine and BUN, and three additional patients were withdrawn for increases in serum creatinine.

Liver Function Tests

Minor elevations of ALAT, ASAT, and alkaline phosphatase occurred for comparable percentages of patients taking TEVETEN® or placebo in controlled clinical trials. An elevated ALAT of >3.5 × ULN occurred in 0.1% of patients taking TEVETEN® (one patient) and in no patient given placebo in controlled clinical trials. Four patients were withdrawn from clinical trials for an elevation in liver function tests.

Hemoglobin

A greater than 20% decrease in hemoglobin was observed in 0.1% of patients taking TEVETEN® (one patient) and in no patient given placebo in controlled clinical trials. Two patients were withdrawn from clinical trials for anemia.

Leukopenia

A WBC count of $\leq 3.0 \times 10^3/mm^3$ occurred in 0.3% of patients taking TEVETEN® and in 0.3% of patients given placebo in controlled clinical trials. One patient was withdrawn from clinical trials for leukopenia.

Neutropenia

A neutrophil count of $\leq 1.5 \times 10^3/mm^3$ occurred in 1.3% of patients taking TEVETEN® and in 1.4% of patients given placebo in controlled clinical trials. No patient was withdrawn from any clinical trial for neutropenia.

Thrombocytopenia

A platelet count of $\leq 100 \times 10^9/L$ occurred in 0.3% of patients taking TEVETEN® (one patient) and in no patient given placebo in controlled clinical trials. Four patients receiving TEVETEN® in clinical trials were withdrawn for thrombocytopenia. In one case, thrombocytopenia was present prior to dosing with TEVETEN®.

Serum Potassium

A potassium value of ≥ 5.6 mmol/L occurred in 0.9% of patients taking TEVETEN® and 0.3% of patients given placebo in controlled clinical trials. One patient was withdrawn from clinical trials for hyperkalemia and three for hypokalemia.

OVERDOSAGE
Limited data are available regarding overdosage. Appropriate symptomatic and supportive therapy should be given if overdosage should occur. There was no mortality in rats and mice receiving oral doses of up to 3000 mg eprosartan/kg and in dogs receiving oral doses of up to 1000 mg eprosartan/kg.

DOSAGE AND ADMINISTRATION
The usual recommended starting dose of TEVETEN® is 600 mg once daily when used as monotherapy in patients who are not volume-depleted (see **WARNINGS, Hypotension in Volume- and/or Salt-Depleted Patients**). TEVETEN® can be administered once or twice daily with total daily doses ranging from 400 mg to 800 mg. There is limited experience with doses beyond 800 mg/day.

If the antihypertensive effect measured at trough using once-daily dosing is inadequate, a twice-a-day regimen at the same total daily dose or an increase in dose may give a more satisfactory response. Achievement of maximum blood pressure reduction in most patients may take 2 to 3 weeks. TEVETEN® may be used in combination with other antihypertensive agents such as thiazide diuretics or calcium channel blockers if additional blood-pressure-lowering effect is required. Discontinuation of treatment with eprosartan does not lead to a rapid rebound increase in blood pressure.

Elderly, Hepatically Impaired or Renally Impaired Patients

No initial dosing adjustment is generally necessary for elderly or hepatically impaired patients or those with renal impairment. No initial dosing adjustment is generally necessary in patients with moderate and severe renal impairment, with maximum dose not exceeding 600 mg daily. TEVETEN® may be taken with or without food.

HOW SUPPLIED
TEVETEN® is available as aqueous film-coated tablets as follows:

400 mg pink, non-scored, oval tablets, debossed with "SOLVAY" on one side and "5044" on the other.
NDC 0074-3025-11 (bottles of 100)
600 mg white, non-scored, capsule-shaped tablets, debossed with "SOLVAY" on one side and "5046" on the other.
NDC 0074-3040-11 (bottles of 100)

STORAGE
Store at controlled room temperature 20 - 25°C (68 - 77°F) [see USP controlled room temperature].
Teveten 400 mg Tablets are
Manufactured by:
Solvay Pharmaceuticals, BV
81121 AA Olst, The Netherlands
Olst, The Netherlands 81121
Teveten 600 mg Tablets are
Manufactured by:
Solvay Pharmaceuticals, SAS
01400 Châtillon-sur-Chalaronne, France
©2007 Abbott Laboratories
Manufactured for:
Abbott Laboratories
North Chicago, IL 60064 U.S.A.
Please check the Abbott website, www.rxabbott.com, or call (800) 633-9110 for full prescribing information.
Ref: 107899
Rev. August, 2007

Shown in Product Identification Guide, page 304

TEVETEN® HCT   ℞
[tĕ-vĕ-tĕn]
(eprosartan mesylate/hydrochlorothiazide)
600/12.5mg and 600/25mg Tablets
Rx only

PRESCRIBING INFORMATION

USE IN PREGNANCY
When used in pregnancy during the second and third trimesters, drugs that act directly on the renin-angiotensin system can cause injury and even death to the developing fetus. When pregnancy is detected,

TEVETEN® HCT Tablets should be discontinued as soon as possible. See **WARNINGS: Fetal/Neonatal Morbidity and Mortality.**

DESCRIPTION
TEVETEN® HCT 600/12.5 mg and TEVETEN® HCT 600/25 mg (eprosartan mesylate-hydrochlorothiazide) combine an angiotensin II receptor (AT₁ subtype) antagonist and a diuretic, hydrochlorothiazide. TEVETEN® (eprosartan mesylate) is a non-biphenyl non-tetrazole angiotensin II receptor (AT₁) antagonist. A selective non-peptide molecule, TEVETEN® is chemically described as the monomethanesulfonate of (E)-2-butyl-1-(p-carboxybenzyl)-α-2-thienylmethylimidazole-5-acrylic acid. Its empirical formula is $C_{23}H_{24}N_2O_4S \cdot CH_4O_3S$ and molecular weight is 520.625. Its structural formula is:

Eprosartan mesylate is a white to off-white free-flowing crystalline powder that is insoluble in water, freely soluble in ethanol, and melts between 248°C and 250°C. Hydrochlorothiazide is 6-chloro-3,4-dihydro-2 H 1,2,4-benzothiadiazine-7-sulfonamide 1,1-dioxide. Its empirical formula is $C_7H_8ClN_3O_4S_2$ and its structural formula is:

Hydrochlorothiazide is a white, or practically white, crystalline powder with a molecular weight of 297.74, which is slightly soluble in water, but freely soluble in sodium hydroxide solution. TEVETEN® HCT is available for oral administration in film-coated, non-scored, capsule-shaped tablet combinations of eprosartan mesylate and hydrochlorothiazide. TEVETEN® HCT 600/12.5 mg contains 735.8 mg of eprosartan mesylate (equivalent to 600 mg eprosartan) and 12.5 mg hydrochlorothiazide in a butterscotch-colored tablet. TEVETEN® HCT 600/25 mg contains 735.8 mg of eprosartan mesylate (equivalent to 600 mg eprosartan) and 25 mg hydrochlorothiazide in a brick-red tablet. Inactive ingredients of both tablets: microcrystalline cellulose, lactose monohydrate, pregelatinized starch, crospovidone, magnesium stearate, and purified water. Ingredients of the OPADRY® 85F27320 butterscotch film coating: polyethylene glycol 3350, talc, polyvinyl alcohol, titanium dioxide, iron oxide black, and iron oxide yellow. Ingredients of the OPADRY® II 85F24297 pink film coating: polyethylene glycol 3350, titanium dioxide, talc, polyvinyl alcohol, iron oxide red, and iron oxide yellow.

CLINICAL PHARMACOLOGY
Mechanism of Action
Eprosartan: Angiotensin II (formed from angiotensin I in a reaction catalyzed by angiotensin-converting enzyme [kininase II]), a potent vasoconstrictor, is the principal pressor agent of the renin-angiotensin system. Angiotensin II also stimulates aldosterone synthesis and secretion by the adrenal cortex, cardiac contraction, renal resorption of sodium, activity of the sympathetic nervous system, and smooth muscle cell growth. Eprosartan blocks the vasoconstrictor and aldosterone-secreting effects of angiotensin II by selectively blocking the binding of angiotensin II to the AT₁ receptor found in many tissues (e.g., vascular smooth muscle, adrenal gland). There is also an AT₂ receptor found in many tissues but it is not known to be associated with cardiovascular homeostasis. Eprosartan does not exhibit any partial agonist activity at the AT₁ receptor. Its affinity for the AT₁ receptor is 1,000 times greater than for the AT₂ receptor. In vitro binding studies indicate that eprosartan is a reversible, competitive inhibitor of the AT₁ receptor. Blockade of the AT₁ receptor removes the negative feedback of angiotensin II on renin secretion, but the resulting increased plasma renin activity and circulating angiotensin II do not overcome the effect of eprosartan on blood pressure. TEVETEN® HCT does not inhibit kininase II, the enzyme that converts angiotensin I to angiotensin II and degrades bradykinin; whether this has clinical relevance is not known. It does not bind to or block other hormone receptors or ion channels known to be important in cardiovascular regulation.

Hydrochlorothiazide: Hydrochlorothiazide is a thiazide diuretic. Thiazides affect the renal tubular mechanisms of electrolyte reabsorption, directly increasing excretion of sodium and chloride in approximately equivalent amounts. Indirectly, the diuretic action of hydrochlorothiazide reduces plasma volume, with consequent increases in plasma renin activity, increases in aldosterone secretion, increases in urinary potassium loss, and decreases in serum potassium. The renin-aldosterone link is mediated by angiotensin II, so coadministration of an angiotensin II receptor antagonist tends to reverse the potassium loss associated with these diuretics. The mechanism of the antihypertensive effect of thiazides is unknown.

Pharmacokinetics

General

Eprosartan: Absolute bioavailability following a single 300-mg oral dose of eprosartan is approximately 13%. Eprosartan plasma concentrations peak at 1 to 2 hours after an oral dose in the fasted state. Administering eprosartan with food delays absorption, and causes variable changes (<25%) in C_{max} and AUC values which do not appear clinically important. Plasma concentrations of eprosartan increase in a slightly less than dose-proportional manner over the 100 mg to 800 mg dose range. The mean terminal elimination half-life of eprosartan following multiple oral doses of 600 mg was approximately 20 hours. Eprosartan does not significantly accumulate with chronic use.

Hydrochlorothiazide: When hydrochlorothiazide plasma levels have been followed for at least 24 hours, the plasma half-life has been observed to vary between 5.6 and 14.8 hours.

Metabolism and Excretion

Eprosartan: Eprosartan is eliminated by biliary and renal excretion, primarily as unchanged compound. Less than 2% of an oral dose is excreted in the urine as a glucuronide. There are no active metabolites following oral and intravenous dosing with $[^{14}C]$ eprosartan in human subjects. Eprosartan was the only drug-related compound found in the plasma and feces. Following intravenous $[^{14}C]$ eprosartan, about 61% of the material is recovered in the feces and about 37% in the urine. Following an oral dose of $[^{14}C]$ eprosartan, about 90% is recovered in the feces and about 7% in the urine. Approximately 20% of the radioactivity excreted in the urine was an acyl glucuronide of eprosartan with the remaining 80% being unchanged eprosartan. Eprosartan is not metabolized by cytochrome P450 enzymes.

Hydrochlorothiazide: Hydrochlorothiazide is not metabolized but is eliminated rapidly by the kidney. At least 61% of the oral dose is eliminated unchanged within 24 hours.

Distribution

Eprosartan: Plasma protein binding of eprosartan is high (approximately 98%) and constant over the concentration range achieved with therapeutic doses. The pooled population pharmacokinetic analysis from two Phase 3 trials of 299 men and 172 women with mild to moderate hypertension (aged 20 to 93 years) showed that eprosartan exhibited a population mean oral clearance (CL/F) for an average 60-year-old patient of 48.5 L/hr. The population mean steady-state volume of distribution (Vss/F) was 308 L. Eprosartan pharmacokinetics were not influenced by weight, race, gender or severity of hypertension at baseline. Oral clearance was shown to be a linear function of age with CL/F decreasing 0.62 L/hr for every year increase.

Hydrochlorothiazide: Hydrochlorothiazide crosses the placental but not the blood-brain barrier and it is excreted in breast milk.

Special Populations

Pediatric: Eprosartan pharmacokinetics have not been investigated in patients younger than 18 years of age.

Geriatric: Following single oral dose administration of eprosartan to healthy elderly men, (aged 68 to 78 years), AUC, C_{max}, and T_{max} eprosartan values increased, on average, by approximately twofold, compared to healthy young men (aged 20 to 38 years) who received the same dose. The extent of plasma protein binding is not influenced by age.

Gender: There was no difference in the pharmacokinetics and plasma protein binding between men and women following single oral dose administration of eprosartan.

Race: A pooled population pharmacokinetic analysis of 442 Caucasian and 29 non-Caucasian hypertensive patients showed that oral clearance and steady-state volume of distribution were not influenced by race.

Renal Insufficiency: Following administration of 600 mg once daily, there was a 70-90% increase in AUC, and a 30-50% increase in C_{max} in moderate or severe renal impairment. The unbound eprosartan fractions increased by 35% and 59% in patients with moderate and severe renal impairment, respectively. No initial dosing adjustment is generally necessary in patients with moderate or severe renal impairment, with maximum dose not exceeding 600 mg daily. Eprosartan was poorly removed by hemodialysis (CL_{HD}<1L/hr) (see **DOSAGE AND ADMINISTRATION**).

Hepatic Insufficiency: Eprosartan AUC (but not C_{max}) values increased, on average, by approximately 40% in men with decreased hepatic function compared to healthy men after a single 100 mg oral dose of eprosartan. The extent of eprosartan plasma protein binding was not influenced by hepatic dysfunction. No dosage adjustment is necessary for patients with hepatic impairment.

Drug Interactions

Eprosartan: Concomitant administration of eprosartan with digoxin had no effect on a single oral-dose digoxin pharmacokinetics. Concomitant administration of eprosartan and warfarin had no effect on steady-state prothrombin time ratios (INR) in healthy volunteers. Concomitant administration of eprosartan and glyburide in diabetic patients did not affect 24-hour plasma glucose profiles. Eprosartan pharmacokinetics were not affected by concomitant administration of ranitidine. Eprosartan did not inhibit human cytochrome P450 enzymes CYP1A, 2A6, 2C9/8, 2C19, 2D6, 2E, and 3A *in vitro*. Eprosartan steady-state plasma concentrations were not affected by concomitant administration of ketoconazole or fluconazole, potent inhibitors of CYP3A and 2C9, respectively.

Eprosartan-Hydrochlorothiazide: There is no pharmacokinetic interaction between 600 mg eprosartan and 12.5 mg hydrochlorothiazide.

Pharmacodynamics and Clinical Effects

Eprosartan: Eprosartan inhibits the pharmacologic effects of angiotensin II infusions in healthy adult men. Single oral doses of eprosartan from 10 mg to 400 mg have been shown to inhibit the vasopressor, renal vasoconstrictive and aldosterone secretory effects of infused angiotensin II with complete inhibition evident at doses of 350 mg and above. Eprosartan inhibits the pressor effects of angiotensin II infusions. A single oral dose of 350 mg of eprosartan inhibits pressor effects by approximately 100% at peak, with approximately 30% inhibition persisting for 24 hours. The absence of angiotensin II AT_1 agonist activity has been demonstrated in healthy adult men. In hypertensive patients treated chronically with eprosartan, there was a twofold rise in angiotensin II plasma concentration and a twofold rise in plasma renin activity, while plasma aldosterone levels remained unchanged. Serum potassium levels also remained unchanged in these patients. Achievement of maximal blood pressure response to a given dose in most patients may take 2 to 3 weeks of treatment. Onset of blood pressure reduction is seen within 1 to 2 hours of dosing with few instances of orthostatic hypotension. Blood pressure control is maintained with once- or twice-daily dosing over a 24-hour period. Discontinuing treatment with eprosartan does not lead to a rapid rebound increase in blood pressure. There was no change in mean heart rate in patients treated with eprosartan in controlled clinical trials. Eprosartan increases mean effective renal plasma flow (ERPF) in salt-replete and salt-restricted normal subjects. A dose-related increase in ERPF of 25% to 30% occurred in salt-restricted normal subjects, with the effect plateauing between 200 mg and 400 mg doses. There was no change in ERPF in hypertensive patients and patients with renal insufficiency on normal salt diets. Eprosartan did not reduce glomerular filtration rate in patients with renal insufficiency or in patients with hypertension, after 7 days and 28 days of dosing, respectively. In hypertensive patients and patients with chronic renal insufficiency, eprosartan did not change fractional excretion of sodium and potassium. Eprosartan (1200 mg once daily for 7 days or 300 mg twice daily for 28 days) had no effect on the excretion of uric acid in healthy men, patients with essential hypertension or those with varying degrees of renal insufficiency. There were no effects on mean levels of fasting triglycerides, total cholesterol, HDL cholesterol, LDL cholesterol or fasting glucose.

Clinical Trials

Eprosartan Mesylate: The safety and efficacy of TEVETEN® has been evaluated in controlled clinical trials worldwide that enrolled predominantly hypertensive patients with sitting DBP ranging from 95 mmHg to ≤115 mmHg. There is also some experience with use of eprosartan together with other antihypertensive drugs in more severe hypertension. The antihypertensive effects of TEVETEN® were demonstrated principally in five placebo-controlled trials (4 to 13 weeks' duration) including dosages of 400 mg to 1200 mg given once daily (two studies), 25 mg to 400 mg twice daily (two studies), and one study comparing total daily doses of 400 mg to 800 mg given once daily or twice daily. The five studies included 1,111 patients randomized to eprosartan and 395 patients randomized to placebo. The studies showed dose-related antihypertensive responses. At study endpoint, patients treated with TEVETEN® at doses of 600 mg to 1200 mg given once daily experienced significant decreases in sitting systolic and diastolic blood pressure at trough, with differences from placebo of approximately 5-10/3-6 mmHg. Limited experience is available with the dose of 1200 mg administered once daily. In a direct comparison of 200 mg to 400 mg b.i.d. with 400 mg to 800 mg q.d. of TEVETEN®, effects at trough were similar. Patients treated with TEVETEN® at doses of 200 mg to 400 mg given twice daily experienced significant decreases in sitting systolic and diastolic blood pressure at trough, with differences from placebo of approximately 7-10/4-6 mmHg. Peak (1 to 3 hours) effects were uniformly, but moderately, larger than trough effects with b.i.d. dosing, with the trough-to-peak ratio for diastolic blood pressure 65% to 80%. In the once-daily dose-response study, trough-to-peak responses of ≤50% were observed at some doses (including 1200 mg), suggesting attenuation of effect at the end of the dosing interval. The antihypertensive effect of TEVETEN® was similar in men and women, but was somewhat smaller in patients over 65. There were too few black subjects to determine whether their response was similar to Caucasians. In general, blacks (usually a low renin population) have had smaller responses to ACE inhibitors and angiotensin II inhibitors than Caucasian populations. Angiotensin-converting enzyme (ACE) inhibitor-induced cough (a dry, persistent cough) can lead to discontinuation of ACE inhibitor therapy. In one study, patients who had previously coughed while taking an ACE inhibitor were treated with eprosartan, an ACE inhibitor (enalapril) or placebo for six weeks. The incidence of dry, persistent cough was 2.2% on eprosartan, 4.4% on placebo, and 20.5% on the ACE inhibitor; p=0.008 for the comparison of eprosartan with enalapril. In a second study comparing the incidence of cough in 259 patients treated with eprosartan to 261 patients treated with the ACE inhibitor enalapril, the incidence of dry, persistent cough in eprosartan-treated patients (1.5%) was significantly lower (p=0.018) than that observed in patients treated with the ACE inhibitor (5.4%). In addition, analysis of overall data from six double-blind clinical trials involving 1,554 patients showed an incidence of spontaneously reported cough in patients treated with eprosartan of 3.5%, similar to placebo (2.6%).

Hydrochlorothiazide: After oral administration of hydrochlorothiazide, diuresis begins within 2 hours, peaks in about 4 hours, and lasts about 6 to 12 hours.

Eprosartan Mesylate – Hydrochlorothiazide: Four adequate and well-controlled studies were conducted to assess the antihypertensive effectiveness of TEVETEN® HCT (eprosartan mesylate/hydrochlorothiazide) in 1457 patients with mild-to-moderate essential hypertension. In a 2×2 factorial study with 112-119 hypertensive patients per arm, the mean baseline- and placebo-subtracted reductions in blood pressure at 8 weeks were 3.6/2.1 mmHg on eprosartan 600 mg, 5.6/1.9 mmHg on hydrochlorothiazide 12.5 mg, and 10.0/5.0 mmHg on the combination.

INDICATIONS AND USAGE

TEVETEN® HCT is indicated for the treatment of hypertension. It may be used alone or in combination with other antihypertensives such as calcium channel blockers. This fixed dose combination is not indicated for initial therapy (see **DOSAGE AND ADMINISTRATION**).

CONTRAINDICATIONS

TEVETEN® HCT is contraindicated in patients who are hypersensitive to this product or any of its components. Because of the hydrochlorothiazide component, this product is contraindicated in patients with anuria or hypersensitivity to other sulfonamide-derived drugs.

WARNINGS

Fetal/Neonatal Morbidity and Mortality

Drugs that act directly on the renin-angiotensin system can cause fetal and neonatal morbidity and death when administered to pregnant women. Several dozen cases have been reported in the world literature in patients who were taking angiotensin-converting enzyme inhibitors. When pregnancy is detected, TEVETEN® HCT should be discontinued as soon as possible. The use of drugs that act directly on the renin-angiotensin system during the second and third trimesters of pregnancy has been associated with fetal and neonatal injury, including hypotension, neonatal skull hypoplasia, anuria, reversible or irreversible renal failure, and death. Oligohydramnios has also been reported, presumably resulting from decreased fetal renal function; oligohydramnios in this setting has been associated with fetal limb contractures, craniofacial deformation, and hypoplastic lung development. Prematurity, intrauterine growth retardation, and patent ductus arteriosus have also been reported, although it is not clear whether these occurrences were due to exposure to the drug. These adverse effects do not appear to have resulted from intrauterine drug exposure that has been limited to the first trimester. Mothers whose embryos and fetuses are exposed to an angiotensin II receptor antagonist only during the first trimester should be so informed. Nonetheless, when patients become pregnant, physicians should advise the patient to discontinue the use of eprosartan as soon as possible. Rarely (probably less often than once in every thousand pregnancies), no alternative to

Information on the Abbott Pharmaceutical Products listed on these pages is from the prescribing information in use as of June 1, 2010. For more information, please visit rxabbott.com or call 1-800-633-9110.

a drug acting on the renin-angiotensin system will be found. In these rare cases, the mothers should be apprised of the potential hazards to their fetuses, and serial ultrasound examinations should be performed to assess the intra-amniotic environment. If oligohydramnios is observed, TEVETEN® HCT should be discontinued unless it is considered life-saving for the mother. Contraction stress testing (CST), a nonstress test (NST) or biophysical profiling (BPP) may be appropriate, depending upon the week of pregnancy. Patients and physicians should be aware, however, that oligohydramnios may not appear until after the fetus has sustained irreversible injury. Infants with histories of *in utero* exposure to an angiotensin II receptor antagonist should be closely observed for hypotension, oliguria, and hyperkalemia. If oliguria occurs, attention should be directed toward support of blood pressure and renal perfusion. Exchange transfusion or dialysis may be required as means of reversing hypotension and/or substituting for disordered renal function. Eprosartan mesylate, alone or in combination with hydrochlorothiazide, has been shown to produce maternal and fetal toxicities (maternal and fetal mortality, low maternal body weight and food consumption, resorptions, abortions and litter loss) in pregnant rabbits given oral doses as low as 10 mg eprosartan/kg/day and 3 mg hydrochlorothiazide/kg/day. No maternal or fetal adverse effects were observed in rabbits at 3 mg eprosartan/kg/day alone or in combination with 1 mg/kg/day of hydrochlorothiazide; this oral dose yielded a systemic exposure (AUC) to unbound eprosartan approximately equal to the human systemic exposure achieved with the dose of eprosartan mesylate contained in the maximum recommended human dose of TEVETEN® HCT (600 mg eprosartan/day). No adverse effects on *in utero* or postnatal development and maturation of offspring were observed when eprosartan mesylate was administered to pregnant rats at oral doses up to 1000 mg eprosartan/kg/day (the 1000 mg eprosartan/kg/day dose in non-pregnant rats yielded systemic exposure to unbound eprosartan approximately 0.8 times the exposure achieved in humans given 600 mg/day). Thiazides cross the placental barrier and appear in cord blood. There is a risk of fetal or neonatal jaundice, thrombocytopenia, and possibly other adverse reactions that have occurred in adults.

Hypotension in Volume- and/or Salt-Depleted Patients
In patients with an activated renin-angiotensin system, such as volume- and/or salt-depleted patients (e.g., those being treated with diuretics), symptomatic hypotension may occur. These conditions should be corrected prior to administration of TEVETEN® HCT, or the treatment should start under close medical supervision. If hypotension occurs, the patient should be placed in the supine position and, if necessary, given an intravenous infusion of normal saline. A transient hypotensive response is not a contraindication to further treatment, which usually can be continued without difficulty once the blood pressure has stabilized.

Hydrochlorothiazide
Impaired Hepatic Function: Thiazides should be used with caution in patients with impaired hepatic function or progressive liver disease, since minor alterations of fluid and electrolyte balance may precipitate hepatic coma.

Hypersensitivity Reactions: Hypersensitivity reactions to hydrochlorothiazide may occur in patients with or without a history of allergy or bronchial asthma, but are more likely in patients with such a history.

Systemic Lupus Erythematosus: Thiazide diuretics have been reported to cause exacerbation or activation of systemic lupus erythematosus.

Lithium Interaction: Lithium generally should not be given with thiazides (see **PRECAUTIONS, Drug Interactions, Hydrochlorothiazide,** *Lithium*).

PRECAUTIONS
General
Hyperuricemia may occur or frank gout may be precipitated in certain patients receiving thiazide therapy. Thiazides have been shown to increase the urinary excretion of magnesium; this may result in hypomagnesemia. Thiazides may decrease urinary calcium excretion. Thiazides may cause intermittent and slight elevation of serum calcium in the absence of known disorders of calcium metabolism. Marked hypercalcemia may be evidence of hidden hyperparathyroidism. Thiazides should be discontinued before carrying out tests for parathyroid function. In diabetic patients, dosage adjustment of insulin or oral hypoglycemic agents may be required. Hyperglycemia may occur with thiazide diuretics. Thus, latent diabetes mellitus may become manifest during thiazide therapy. The antihypertensive effects of hydrochlorothiazide may be enhanced in postsympathectomy patients.

Electrolyte Imbalance
Periodic determination of serum electrolytes to detect possible electrolyte imbalance should be performed at appropriate intervals. All patients receiving thiazide therapy should be observed for clinical signs of fluid or electrolyte imbal-

ance: hyponatremia, hypochloremic alkalosis, and hypokalemia. Serum and urine electrolyte determinations are particularly important when the patient is vomiting excessively or receiving parenteral fluids. Warning signs or symptoms of fluid and electrolyte imbalance, irrespective of cause, include: dryness of mouth, thirst, weakness, lethargy, drowsiness, restlessness, confusion, seizures, muscle pains or cramps, muscular fatigue, hypotension, oliguria, tachycardia, and gastrointestinal disturbances such as nausea and vomiting. Hypokalemia may develop, especially with brisk diuresis, when severe cirrhosis is present, or after prolonged therapy. Interference with adequate oral electrolyte intake will also contribute to hypokalemia. Hypokalemia may cause cardiac arrhythmia and may also sensitize or exaggerate the response of the heart to the toxic effects of digitalis (e.g., increased ventricular irritability). Although any chloride deficit is generally mild and usually does not require specific treatment except under extraordinary circumstances (as in liver disease or renal disease), chloride replacement may be required in the treatment of metabolic alkalosis. Dilutional hyponatremia may occur in edematous patients in hot weather; appropriate therapy is water restriction, rather than administration of salt except in rare instances when the hyponatremia is life-threatening. In actual salt depletion, appropriate replacement is the therapy of choice.

Risk of Renal Impairment
As a consequence of inhibiting the renin-angiotensin-aldosterone system, changes in renal function have been reported in susceptible individuals treated with angiotensin II antagonists; in some patients, these changes in renal function were reversible upon discontinuation of therapy. In patients whose renal function may depend on the activity of the renin-angiotensin-aldosterone system (e.g., patients with severe congestive heart failure), treatment with angiotensin-converting enzyme inhibitors and angiotensin II receptor antagonists has been associated with oliguria and/or progressive azotemia and (rarely) with acute renal failure and/or death. TEVETEN® HCT would be expected to behave similarly. In studies of ACE inhibitors in patients with unilateral or bilateral renal artery stenosis, increases in serum creatinine or BUN have been reported. Similar effects have been reported with angiotensin II antagonists; in some patients, these effects were reversible upon discontinuation of therapy. Thiazides should be used with caution in severe renal disease. In patients with renal disease, thiazides may precipitate azotemia. Cumulative effects of the drug may develop in patients with impaired renal function. If progressive renal impairment becomes evident, consider withholding or discontinuing diuretic therapy.

Information for Patients
Pregnancy: Female patients of childbearing age should be told about the consequences of second- and third-trimester exposure to drugs that act on the renin-angiotensin system, and they should also be told that these consequences do not appear to have resulted from intrauterine drug exposure that has been limited to the first trimester. These patients should be asked to report pregnancies to their physicians as soon as possible so that treatment may be discontinued under medical supervision.

Symptomatic Hypotension: A patient receiving TEVETEN® HCT should be cautioned that lightheadedness can occur, especially during the first days of therapy, and that it should be reported to the prescribing physician. The patient should be told that if syncope occurs, TEVETEN® HCT should be discontinued until the physician has been consulted. All patients should be cautioned that inadequate fluid intake, excessive perspiration, diarrhea, or vomiting can lead to an excessive fall in blood pressure, with the same consequences of lightheadedness and possible syncope.

Potassium Supplements: A patient receiving TEVETEN® HCT should be told not to use potassium supplements or salt substitutes containing potassium without consulting the prescribing physician (see **PRECAUTIONS, Drug Interactions, Eprosartan Mesylate**).

Drug Interactions
Eprosartan Mesylate: Eprosartan has been shown to have no effect on the pharmacokinetics of digoxin and the pharmacodynamics of warfarin and glyburide. Thus, no dosing adjustments are necessary during concomitant use with these agents. Because eprosartan is not metabolized by the cytochrome P450 system, inhibitors of CYP450 enzyme would not be expected to affect its metabolism, and ketoconazole and fluconazole, potent inhibitors of CYP3A and 2C9, respectively, have been shown to have no effect on eprosartan pharmacokinetics. Ranitidine also has no effect on eprosartan pharmacokinetics. Eprosartan (up to 400 mg b.i.d. or 800 mg q.d.) doses have been safely used concomitantly with a thiazide diuretic (hydrochlorothiazide). Eprosartan doses of up to 300 mg b.i.d. have been safely used concomitantly with sustained-release calcium channel blockers (sustained-release nifedipine) with no clinically significant adverse interactions. As with other drugs that

block angiotensin II or its effects, concomitant use of potassium-sparing diuretics (e.g., spironolactone, triamterene, amiloride), potassium supplements or salt substitutes containing potassium may lead to increases in serum potassium (see **PRECAUTIONS, Information for Patients, Potassium Supplements**).

Hydrochlorothiazide: When administered concurrently the following drugs may interact with thiazide diuretics: *Alcohol, barbiturates, or narcotics* – potentiation of orthostatic hypotension may occur. *Antidiabetic drug (oral agents and insulin)* – dosage adjustment of the antidiabetic drug may be required. *Other antihypertensive drugs* – additive effect or potentiation. *Cholestyramine and colestipol resins* – Absorption of hydrochlorothiazide is impaired in the presence of anionic exchange resins. Single doses of either cholestyramine or colestipol resins bind the hydrochlorothiazide and reduce its absorption from the gastrointestinal tract by up to 85% and 43%, respectively. *Corticosteroids, ACTH* – intensified electrolyte depletion, particularly hypokalemia. *Pressor amines (e.g., norepinephrine)* – possible decreased response to pressor amines but not sufficient to preclude their use. *Skeletal muscle relaxants, nondepolarizing (e.g., tubocurarine)* – possible increased responsiveness to the muscle relaxant. *Lithium* – should not generally be given with diuretics. Diuretic agents reduce the renal clearance of lithium and add a high risk of lithium toxicity. Refer to the package insert for lithium preparations before use of such preparations with TEVETEN® HCT. *Nonsteroidal Anti-Inflammatory Drugs* – in some patients, the administration of a nonsteroidal anti-inflammatory agent can reduce the diuretic, natriuretic, and antihypertensive effects of loop, potassium-sparing and thiazide diuretics. Therefore, when TEVETEN® HCT and nonsteroidal anti-inflammatory agents are used concomitantly, the patient should be observed closely to determine if the desired effect of the diuretic is obtained.

Carcinogenesis, Mutagenesis, Impairment of Fertility
No carcinogenicity studies have been conducted with eprosartan mesylate in combination with hydrochlorothiazide. Eprosartan mesylate was not carcinogenic in dietary restricted rats or *ad libitum* fed mice dosed at 600 mg and 2000 mg eprosartan/kg/day, respectively, for up to 2 years. In male and female rats, the systemic exposure (AUC) to unbound eprosartan at the dose evaluated was only approximately 25% of the exposure achieved in humans given TEVETEN® HCT. In mice, the systemic exposure (AUC) to unbound eprosartan was approximately 35 times the exposure achieved in humans given TEVETEN® HCT. Two-year feeding studies in mice and rats conducted under the auspices of the National Toxicology Program (NTP) uncovered no evidence of a carcinogenic potential of hydrochlorothiazide in female mice (at doses of up to approximately 600 mg/kg/day) or in male and female rats (at doses of up to approximately 100 mg/kg/day). The NTP, however, found equivocal evidence for hepatocarcinogenicity in male mice. Eprosartan mesylate was not mutagenic *in vitro* in mammalian cells (mouse lymphoma assay). Eprosartan mesylate alone or in combination with hydrochlorothiazide was not mutagenic *in vitro* in bacteria (Ames test) and did not cause structural chromosomal damage *in vivo* (mouse micronucleus assay). In human peripheral lymphocytes *in vitro*, eprosartan mesylate in combination with hydrochlorothiazide was positive for clastogenicity with and without metabolic activation. In the same assay, eprosartan mesylate alone was associated with polyploidy but there was only equivocal evidence of structural chromosomal damage. Hydrochlorothiazide was not genotoxic *in vitro* in the Ames test and in the Chinese Hamster Ovary (CHO) test for chromosomal aberrations, or *in vivo* in assays using mouse germinal cell chromosomes, Chinese hamster bone marrow chromosomes, and the *Drosophila* sex-linked recessive lethal trait gene. Positive test results were obtained in the *in vitro* CHO Sister Chromatid Exchange (clastogenicity) and Mouse Lymphoma Cell (mutagenicity) assays and in the *Aspergillus nidulans* non-disjunction assay. No fertility studies have been conducted with eprosartan mesylate in combination with hydrochlorothiazide. Eprosartan mesylate had no adverse effects on the reproductive performance of male or female rats at oral doses up to 1000 mg eprosartan/kg/day. Hydrochlorothiazide had no adverse effects on the fertility of mice and rats of either sex in studies wherein these species were exposed, via their diet, to doses of up to 100 and 4 mg/kg/day, respectively, prior to conception and throughout gestation.

Pregnancy
Pregnancy Category C (first trimester) and D (second and third trimesters): See *WARNINGS: Fetal/Neonatal Morbidity and Mortality.*

Nursing Mothers
Eprosartan is excreted in animal milk; it is not known whether eprosartan is excreted in human milk. Because many drugs are excreted in human milk and because of the potential for serious adverse reactions in nursing infants

from eprosartan, a decision should be made whether to discontinue nursing or to discontinue the drug, taking into account the importance of the drug to the mother. Thiazides appear in human milk. Because of the potential for adverse effects on the nursing infant, a decision should be made whether to discontinue nursing or discontinue the drug, taking into account the importance of the drug to the mother.

Pediatric Use

Safety and effectiveness in pediatric patients have not been established.

Geriatric Use

In the controlled clinical trials where patients received eprosartan/hydrochlorothiazide combination therapy, 15% to 33% of the patients were 65 years of age or greater. There was no difference in the effect of TEVETEN® HCT 600/12.5 mg treatment according to age. However, following single oral dose administration of eprosartan to healthy elderly men, (aged 68 to 78 years), AUC, C_{max}, and T_{max} eprosartan values increased, on average, by approximately twofold, compared to healthy young men (aged 20 to 38 years) who received the same dose. (See **Pharmacokinetics, Special Populations.**)

ADVERSE REACTIONS

TEVETEN® HCT 600/12.5 mg has been evaluated for safety in 268 patients in double-blind, controlled clinical trials. Most of these patients were treated with TEVETEN® HCT 600/12.5 mg for 29 to 60 days. Eprosartan/hydrochlorothiazide combination therapy has been evaluated for safety in 890 patients in open-label, long-term clinical trials. Approximately 50% of these patients were treated with eprosartan/hydrochlorothiazide for over 2 years. Eprosartan/hydrochlorothiazide combination therapy was well tolerated. Most adverse events were of mild or moderate severity and did not require discontinuation of therapy. Adverse experiences were similar in patients regardless of age, gender, or race. In the controlled clinical trials, about 3% of the 268 patients treated with TEVETEN® HCT 600/12.5 mg discontinued therapy due to clinical adverse experiences.

Adverse Events Occurring at an Incidence of Greater Than 3% Among TEVETEN® HCT Treated Patients

The following table lists adverse events that occurred at an incidence of >3% among TEVETEN® HCT 600/12.5 mg- or monotherapy-treated patients who participated in the controlled clinical trials. Of the 268 patients who received TEVETEN® HCT 600/12.5 mg during the double-blind treatment period in the controlled trials, 110 patients were reported to have adverse events.

[See table 1 at top right]

Table 1 Incidence of Adverse Events >3% During the Double-Blind Treatment Period by Preferred Term and Treatment Grouping: Controlled Studies

	Placebo (N=246)	Eprosartan 600 mg (N=275)	HCTZ 12.5 mg (N=117)	HCTZ 25 mg (N=52)	Eprosartan 600 mg/HCTZ 12.5 mg (N=268)
Preferred Term	n (%)	n (%)	n (%)	n (%)	n (%)
Dizziness	4 (1.6)	5 (1.8)	2 (1.7)	2 (3.8)	11 (4.1)
Headache	22 (8.9)	10 (3.6)	4 (3.4)	3 (5.8)	9 (3.4)
Back pain	6 (2.4)	7 (2.5)	2 (1.7)	2 (3.8)	7 (2.6)
Fatigue	6 (2.4)	5 (1.8)	1 (0.9)	2 (3.8)	5 (1.9)
Myalgia	8 (3.3)	2 (0.7)	3 (2.6)	0 (0.0)	1 (0.4)
Upper Respiratory Tract Infection	8 (3.3)	2 (0.7)	0 (0.0)	2 (3.8)	1 (0.4)
Sinusitis	4 (1.6)	1 (0.4)	0 (0.0)	2 (3.8)	0 (0.0)
Viral Infection	4 (1.6)	0 (0.0)	2 (1.7)	2 (3.8)	0 (0.0)

The adverse events reported in over 600 patients that received TEVETEN®/hydrochlorothiazide combination therapy for at least 1 year in the open-label, long-term clinical trials were comparable to those reported in the controlled trials.

Eprosartan Mesylate: In addition to the adverse events above, potentially important adverse events that are included in the current labeling for TEVETEN® monotherapy are listed below. Most of these adverse events occurred in <1% of patients, or were as frequent or more frequent in the placebo group. It is not known if these events were related to eprosartan usage: ***Body as a Whole:*** alcohol intolerance, asthenia, substernal chest pain, dependent edema, peripheral edema, facial edema, fatigue, fever, hot flushes, influenza-like symptoms, injury, malaise, pain, rigors, viral infection; ***Cardiovascular:*** angina pectoris, bradycardia, abnormal ECG, specific abnormal ECG, extrasystoles, atrial fibrillation, hypotension (including orthostatic hypotension), tachycardia, palpitations; ***Gastrointestinal:*** abdominal pain, anorexia, constipation, diarrhea, dry mouth, dyspepsia, esophagitis, flatulence, gastritis, gastroenteritis, gingivitis, nausea, periodontitis, toothache, vomiting; ***Hematologic:*** anemia, purpura; ***Liver and Biliary:*** increased SGOT, increased SGPT; ***Metabolic and Nutritional:*** increased creatine phosphokinase, diabetes mellitus, glycosuria, gout, hypercholesterolemia, hyperglycemia, hyperkalemia, hypokalemia, hyponatremia, hypertriglyceridemia; ***Musculoskeletal:*** arthralgia, arthritis, aggravated arthritis, arthrosis, skeletal pain, tendinitis; ***Nervous System/Psychiatric:*** anxiety, ataxia, depression, dizziness, insomnia, migraine, neuritis, nervousness, paresthesia, somnolence, tremor, vertigo; ***Resistance Mechanism:*** herpes simplex, otitis externa, otitis media, upper respiratory tract infection; ***Respiratory:*** asthma, bronchitis, coughing, epistaxis, pharyngitis, rhinitis; ***Skin and Appendages:*** eczema, furunculosis, pruritus, rash, maculopapular rash, increased sweating; ***Special Senses:*** conjunctivitis, abnormal vision, xerophthalmia, tinnitus; ***Urinary:*** albuminuria, cystitis, hematuria, micturition frequency, polyuria, renal calculus, urinary incontinence, urinary tract infection; ***Vascular:*** leg cramps, peripheral ischemia.

Hydrochlorothiazide: Other adverse events that have been reported for hydrochlorothiazide, without regard to causality, are listed below: ***Body as a Whole:*** weakness; ***Cardiovascular:*** hypotension (including orthostatic hypotension); ***Digestive:*** pancreatitis, jaundice (intrahepatic cholestatic jaundice), diarrhea, vomiting, sialadenitis, cramping, constipation, gastric irritation, nausea, anorexia; ***Hematologic:*** aplastic anemia, agranulocytosis, leukopenia, hemolytic anemia, thrombocytopenia; ***Hypersensitivity:*** anaphylactic reactions, necrotizing angiitis (vasculitis and cutaneous vasculitis), respiratory distress including pneumonitis, and pulmonary edema, photosensitivity, fever, urticaria, rash, purpura; ***Metabolic:*** electrolyte imbalance including hyponatremia, hypokalemia, and hypochloremic alkalosis, hyperglycemia, glycosuria, hyperuricemia; ***Musculoskeletal:*** muscle spasm; ***Nervous System/Psychiatric:*** vertigo, paresthesias, restlessness; ***Renal:*** renal failure, renal dysfunction, interstitial nephritis, azotemia; ***Skin:*** erythema multiform, including Stevens-Johnson syndrome, exfoliative dermatitis, including toxic epidermal necrolysis, alopecia; ***Special Senses:*** transient blurred vision, xanthopsia; ***Urogenital:*** impotence.

Laboratory Test Findings

In placebo-controlled studies, clinically important changes in standard laboratory parameters were rarely associated with administration of TEVETEN®. Patients were rarely withdrawn from TEVETEN® because of laboratory test results. Laboratory test findings that have been reported for TEVETEN® are listed below: ***Creatinine, Blood Urea Nitrogen:*** Minor elevations in creatinine and in BUN occurred in 0.6% and 1.3%, respectively, of patients taking TEVETEN® and 0.9% and 0.3%, respectively, of patients given placebo in controlled clinical trials. Two patients were withdrawn from clinical trials for elevations in serum creatinine and BUN, and three additional patients were withdrawn for increases in serum creatinine. ***Liver Function Tests:*** Minor elevations of ALAT, ASAT, and alkaline phosphatase occurred for comparable percentages of patients taking TEVETEN® or placebo in controlled clinical trials. An elevated ALAT of $>3.5 \times$ ULN occurred in 0.1% of patients taking TEVETEN® (one patient) and in no patient given placebo in controlled clinical trials. Four patients were withdrawn from clinical trials for an elevation in liver function tests. ***Hemoglobin:*** A greater than 20% decrease in hemoglobin was observed in 0.1% of patients taking TEVETEN® (one patient) and in no patient given placebo in controlled clinical trials. Two patients were withdrawn from clinical trials for anemia. ***Leukopenia:*** A WBC count of $\leq 3.0 \times 10^3/mm^3$ occurred in 0.3% of patients taking TEVETEN® and in 0.3% of patients given placebo in controlled clinical trials. One patient was withdrawn from clinical trials for leukopenia. ***Neutropenia:*** A neutrophil count of $\leq 1.5 \times 10^3/mm^3$ occurred in 1.3% of patients taking TEVETEN® and in 1.4% of patients given placebo in controlled clinical trials. No patient was withdrawn from any clinical trials for neutropenia. ***Thrombocytopenia:*** A platelet count of $\leq 100 \times 10^9/L$ occurred in 0.3% of patients taking TEVETEN® (one patient) and in no patient given placebo in controlled clinical trials. Four patients receiving TEVETEN® in clinical trials were withdrawn for thrombocytopenia. In one case, thrombocytopenia was present prior to dosing with TEVETEN®. ***Serum Potassium:*** A potassium value of ≥ 5.6 mmol/L occurred in 0.9% of patients taking TEVETEN® and 0.3% of patients given placebo in controlled clinical trials. One patient was withdrawn from clinical trials for hyperkalemia and three for hypokalemia.

Additional Information

Among the adverse events reported for patients receiving either TEVETEN® monotherapy or TEVETEN®/hydrochlorothiazide combination therapy in the TEVETEN® HCT clinical trials, some adverse events are not included in the current labeling for either TEVETEN® or hydrochlorothiazide monotherapy. The adverse events which are not currently included in the labeling for TEVETEN® or hydrochlorothiazide monotherapy include the following: angioedema, bilirubinemia, blood urea nitrogen increased, edema periorbital, eosinophilia, and NPN increased. The majority of these adverse events were reported in the open-label, long-term trials and were reported in small numbers of patients receiving TEVETEN® alone or TEVETEN® in combination with hydrochlorothiazide. All of these adverse events were either not reported in patients receiving TEVETEN® monotherapy or combination therapy with hydrochlorothiazide during the double-blind period of the controlled trials, or were reported at an incidence of ≤1% or in only one patient per treatment group in the controlled trials. The overall safety profile of the TEVETEN®/hydrochlorothiazide combination treatment is as expected based on the safety profile of each of the components and what is generally known about the patient population.

OVERDOSAGE

Eprosartan Mesylate: Limited data are available regarding overdosage. Appropriate symptomatic and supportive therapy should be given if overdosage should occur. There was no mortality in rats and mice receiving oral doses of up to 3000 mg eprosartan/kg and in dogs receiving oral doses of up to 1000 mg eprosartan/kg.

Hydrochlorothiazide: The most common signs and symptoms observed are those caused by electrolyte depletion (hypokalemia, hypochloremia, and hyponatremia) and dehydration resulting from excessive diuresis. If digitalis has also been administered, hypokalemia may accentuate cardiac arrhythmias. The degree to which hydrochlorothiazide is removed by hemodialysis has not been established. The oral LD_{50} of hydrochlorothiazide is greater than 10 g/kg in both mice and rats.

DOSAGE AND ADMINISTRATION

The usual recommended starting dose of eprosartan is 600 mg once daily when used as monotherapy in patients who are not volume-depleted (see **WARNINGS, Hypotension in Volume- and/or Salt-Depleted Patients**). Eprosartan can be administered once or twice daily and total daily doses ranging from 400 mg to 800 mg. There is limited experience with doses beyond 800 mg/day. If the antihypertensive effect measured at trough using once-daily monotherapy dosing is inadequate, a twice-a-day regimen at the same total daily dose or an increase in dose may give a more satisfactory response. Achievement of maximum blood pressure reduction in most patients may take 2 to 3 weeks. Hydrochlorothiazide is effective in doses of 12.5 mg to 50 mg once daily. To minimize dose-independent side effects, it is usually appropriate to begin combination therapy only after a patient has failed to achieve the desired effect with monotherapy. The side effects (see **WARNINGS**) of eprosartan are generally rare and apparently independent of dose; those of hydrochlorothiazide are a mixture of dose-dependent (primarily hypokalemia) and dose-independent (e.g., pancreatitis) phenomena, the former much more common than the latter. Therapy with any combination of eprosartan and hydrochlorothiazide will be associated with both sets of dose-independent side effects.

Replacement Therapy:

TEVETEN® HCT may be substituted for the individual components. The usual recommended dose of TEVETEN® HCT is 600 mg/12.5 mg once daily when used as combination therapy in patients who are not volume-depleted (see **WARNINGS, Hypotension in Volume-and/or Salt-Depleted Patients**). If the antihypertensive effect measured at trough using TEVETEN® HCT 600/12.5 mg is inadequate, patients may be titrated to TEVETEN® HCT 600/25 mg once daily. Higher doses have not been studied in combination. Achievement of maximum blood pressure reduction in most patients may take 2 to 3 weeks. If the patient under treatment with TEVETEN® HCT requires ad-

Information on the Abbott Pharmaceutical Products listed on these pages is from the prescribing information in use as of June 1, 2010. For more information, please visit rxabbott.com or call 1-800-633-9110.

Eprosartan (mg)	HCTZ (mg)	Color	NDC
600	12.5	Butterscotch	0074-3015-11
600	25	Brick red	0074-3020-11

ditional blood pressure control at trough, or to maintain a twice a day dosing schedule of monotherapy, 300 mg TEVETEN® may be added as evening dose. TEVETEN® HCT may be used in combination with other antihypertensive agents such as calcium channel blockers if additional blood-pressure-lowering effect is required. Discontinuation of treatment with eprosartan does not lead to a rapid rebound increase in blood pressure.

Elderly, Hepatically Impaired or Renally Impaired Patients: No initial dosing adjustment is generally necessary for elderly or hepatically impaired patients or those with renal impairment. No initial dosing adjustment is generally necessary in patients with moderate and severe renal impairment with maximum dose not exceeding 600 mg daily. TEVETEN® HCT may be taken with or without food.

HOW SUPPLIED

TEVETEN® HCT is available as film-coated, capsule-shaped tablets, debossed with "SOLVAY" on one side and "5147" or "5150" on the other, supplied as bottles of 100 tablets as follows:

[See table above]

STORAGE

Store at controlled room temperature 20° to 25°C (68° to 77°F) [see USP Controlled Room Temperature].

Manufactured by:
Solvay Pharmaceuticals
01400 Châtillon-sur-Chalaronne, France
Manufactured for:
Abbott Laboratories
North Chicago, IL 60064 U.S.A.
Ref: 108536
Revised: October, 2008

Shown in Product Identification Guide, page 304

TRICOR® ℞

[tri cōr]
48 mg and 145 mg
(fenofibrate tablets)

DESCRIPTION

TRICOR (fenofibrate tablets), is a lipid regulating agent available as tablets for oral administration. Each tablet contains 48 mg or 145 mg of fenofibrate. The chemical name for fenofibrate is 2-[4-(4-chlorobenzoyl) phenoxy]-2-methyl-propanoic acid, 1-methylethyl ester with the following structural formula:

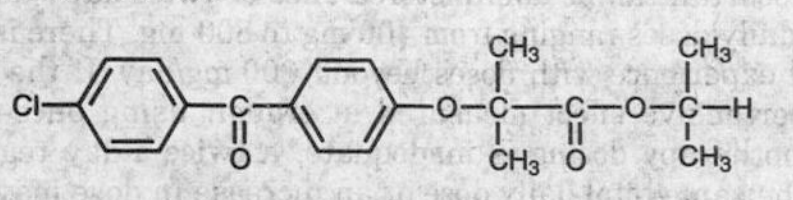

The empirical formula is $C_{20}H_{21}O_4Cl$ and the molecular weight is 360.83; fenofibrate is insoluble in water. The melting point is 79-82°C. Fenofibrate is a white solid which is stable under ordinary conditions.

Inactive Ingredients

Each tablet contains hypromellose 2910 (3 cps), docusate sodium, sucrose, sodium lauryl sulfate, lactose monohydrate, silicified microcrystalline cellulose, crospovidone, and magnesium stearate.

In addition, individual tablets contain:

48 mg tablets

polyvinyl alcohol, titanium dioxide, talc, soybean lecithin, xanthan gum, D&C Yellow #10 aluminum lake, FD&C Yellow #6 /sunset yellow FCF aluminum lake, FD&C Blue #2 /indigo carmine aluminum lake.

145 mg tablets

polyvinyl alcohol, titanium dioxide, talc, soybean lecithin, xanthan gum.

CLINICAL PHARMACOLOGY

A variety of clinical studies have demonstrated that elevated levels of total cholesterol (total-C), low density lipoprotein cholesterol (LDL-C), and apolipoprotein B (apo B), an LDL membrane complex, are associated with human atherosclerosis. Similarly, decreased levels of high density lipoprotein cholesterol (HDL-C) and its transport complex, apolipoprotein A (apo AI and apo AII) are associated with the development of atherosclerosis. Epidemiologic investigations have established that cardiovascular morbidity and mortality vary directly with the level of total-C, LDL-C, and triglycerides, and inversely with the level of HDL-C. The independent effect of raising HDL-C or lowering triglycerides (TG) on the risk of cardiovascular morbidity and mortality has not been determined.

Fenofibric acid, the active metabolite of fenofibrate, produces reductions in total cholesterol, LDL cholesterol, apolipoprotein B, total triglycerides and triglyceride rich lipoprotein (VLDL) in treated patients. In addition, treatment with fenofibrate results in increases in high density lipoprotein (HDL) and apoproteins apoAI and apoAII.

The effects of fenofibric acid seen in clinical practice have been explained *in vivo* in transgenic mice and *in vitro* in human hepatocyte cultures by the activation of peroxisome proliferator activated receptor α (PPARα). Through this mechanism, fenofibrate increases lipolysis and elimination of triglyceride-rich particles from plasma by activating lipoprotein lipase and reducing production of apoprotein C-III (an inhibitor of lipoprotein lipase activity).

The resulting fall in triglycerides produces an alteration in the size and composition of LDL from small, dense particles (which are thought to be atherogenic due to their susceptibility to oxidation), to large buoyant particles. These larger particles have a greater affinity for cholesterol receptors and are catabolized rapidly. Activation of PPARα also induces an increase in the synthesis of apoproteins A-I, A-II and HDL-cholesterol.

Fenofibrate also reduces serum uric acid levels in hyperuricemic and normal individuals by increasing the urinary excretion of uric acid.

Pharmacokinetics/Metabolism

Plasma concentrations of fenofibric acid after administration of three 48 mg or one 145 mg tablets are equivalent under fed conditions to one 200 mg capsule.

Absorption

The absolute bioavailability of fenofibrate cannot be determined as the compound is virtually insoluble in aqueous media suitable for injection. However, fenofibrate is well absorbed from the gastrointestinal tract. Following oral administration in healthy volunteers, approximately 60% of a single dose of radiolabelled fenofibrate appeared in urine, primarily as fenofibric acid and its glucuronate conjugate, and 25% was excreted in the feces. Peak plasma levels of fenofibric acid occur within 6 to 8 hours after administration.

Exposure to fenofibric acid in plasma, as measured by C_{max} and AUC, is not significantly different when a single 145 mg dose of fenofibrate is administered under fasting or nonfasting conditions.

Distribution

Upon multiple dosing of fenofibrate, fenofibric acid steady state is achieved within 9 days. Plasma concentrations of fenofibric acid at steady state are approximately double those following a single dose. Serum protein binding was approximately 99% in normal and hyperlipidemic subjects.

Metabolism

Following oral administration, fenofibrate is rapidly hydrolyzed by esterases to the active metabolite, fenofibric acid; no unchanged fenofibrate is detected in plasma.

Fenofibric acid is primarily conjugated with glucuronic acid and then excreted in urine. A small amount of fenofibric acid is reduced at the carbonyl moiety to a benzhydrol metabolite which is, in turn, conjugated with glucuronic acid and excreted in urine.

In vivo metabolism data indicate that neither fenofibrate nor fenofibric acid undergo oxidative metabolism (e.g., cytochrome P450) to a significant extent.

Excretion

After absorption, fenofibrate is mainly excreted in the urine in the form of metabolites, primarily fenofibric acid and fenofibric acid glucuronide. After administration of radiolabelled fenofibrate, approximately 60% of the dose appeared in the urine and 25% was excreted in the feces.

Fenofibric acid is eliminated with a half-life of 20 hours, allowing once daily administration in a clinical setting.

Special Populations

Geriatrics

In elderly volunteers 77-87 years of age, the oral clearance of fenofibric acid following a single oral dose of fenofibrate was 1.2 L/h, which compares to 1.1 L/h in young adults. This indicates that a similar dosage regimen can be used in the elderly, without increasing accumulation of the drug or metabolites.

Pediatrics

TRICOR has not been investigated in adequate and well-controlled trials in pediatric patients.

Gender

No pharmacokinetic difference between males and females has been observed for fenofibrate.

Race

The influence of race on the pharmacokinetics of fenofibrate has not been studied, however fenofibrate is not metabolized by enzymes known for exhibiting inter-ethnic variability. Therefore, inter-ethnic pharmacokinetic differences are very unlikely.

Renal Insufficiency

The pharmacokinetics of fenofibric acid was examined in patients with mild, moderate, and severe renal impairment. Patients with severe renal impairment (creatinine clearance [CrCl] ≤ 30 mL/min) showed 2.7-fold increase in exposure for fenofibric acid and increased accumulation of fenofibric acid during chronic dosing compared to that of healthy subjects. Patients with mild to moderate renal impairment (CrCl 30-80 mL/min) had similar exposure but an increase in the half-life for fenofibric acid compared to that of healthy subjects. Based on these findings, the use of TRICOR should be avoided in patients who have severe renal impairment and dose reduction is required in patients having mild to moderate renal impairment.

Hepatic Insufficiency

No pharmacokinetic studies have been conducted in patients having hepatic insufficiency.

Drug-drug Interactions

In vitro studies using human liver microsomes indicate that fenofibrate and fenofibric acid are not inhibitors of cytochrome (CYP) P450 isoforms CYP3A4, CYP2D6, CYP2E1, or CYP1A2. They are weak inhibitors of CYP2C8, CYP2C19 and CYP2A6, and mild-to-moderate inhibitors of CYP2C9 at therapeutic concentrations.

Potentiation of coumarin-type anticoagulants has been observed with prolongation of the prothrombin time/INR.

Bile acid sequestrants have been shown to bind other drugs given concurrently. Therefore, fenofibrate should be taken at least 1 hour before or 4-6 hours after a bile acid binding resin to avoid impeding its absorption. (See **WARNINGS** and **PRECAUTIONS**).

Concomitant administration of fenofibrate (equivalent to TRICOR 145 mg) with pravastatin (40 mg) once daily for 10 days has been shown to increase the mean C_{max} and AUC values for pravastatin by 36% (range from 69% decrease to 321% increase) and 28% (range from 54% decrease to 128% increase), respectively, and for 3α-hydroxy-iso-pravastatin by 55% (range from 32% decrease to 314% increase) and 39% (range from 24% decrease to 261% increase), respectively in 23 healthy adults.

Concomitant administration of a single dose of fenofibrate (equivalent to 145 mg TRICOR) and a single dose of fluvastatin (40 mg) resulted in a small increase (approximately 15-16%) in exposure to (+)3R,5S-fluvastatin, the active enantiomer of fluvastatin.

A single dose of either pravastatin or fluvastatin had no clinically important effect on the pharmacokinetics of fenofibric acid.

Concomitant administration of fenofibrate (equivalent to TRICOR 145 mg) with atorvastatin (20 mg) once daily for 10 days resulted in approximately 17% decrease (range from 67% decrease to 44% increase) in atorvastatin AUC values in 22 healthy males. The atorvastatin C_{max} values were not significantly affected by fenofibrate. The pharmacokinetics of fenofibric acid were not significantly affected by atorvastatin.

Concomitant administration of fenofibrate (equivalent to TRICOR 145 mg) once daily for 10 days with glimepiride (1 mg tablet) single dose simultaneously with the last dose of fenofibrate resulted in a 35% increase in mean AUC of glimepiride in healthy subjects. Glimepiride C_{max} was not significantly affected by fenofibrate co-administration. There was no statistically significant effect of multiple doses of fenofibrate on glucose nadir or AUC with the baseline glucose concentration as the covariate after glimepiride administration in healthy volunteers. However, glucose concentrations at 24 hours remained statistically significantly lower after pretreatment with fenofibrate than with glimepiride alone. Glimepiride had no significant effect on the pharmacokinetics of fenofibric acid.

Concomitant administration of fenofibrate (54 mg) and metformin (850 mg) three times a day for 10 days resulted in no significant changes in the pharmacokinetics of fenofibric acid and metformin when compared with the two drugs administered alone in healthy subjects.

Concomitant administration of fenofibrate (equivalent to TRICOR 145 mg) once daily for 14 days with rosiglitazone tablet (rosiglitazone maleate) (8 mg) once daily for 5 days, Day 10 through Day 14, resulted in no significant changes in the pharmacokinetics of fenofibric acid and rosiglitazone when compared with the two drugs administered alone in healthy subjects.

Concomitant administration of fenofibrate (145 mg TRICOR) with ezetimibe (10 mg) once daily for 10 days to 18 healthy adults resulted in increases in total ezetimibe AUC, C_{max} and C_{min} of approximately 43%, 33% and 56%, respectively, and increases in ezetimibe glucuronide AUC, C_{max} and C_{min} of approximately 49%, 34% and 62%, respectively. The pharmacokinetics of fenofibric acid were not significantly affected by ezetimibe and the multiple-dose pharmacokinetics of free (unconjugated) ezetimibe were not significantly affected by fenofibrate.

Clinical Trials

Hypercholesterolemia (Heterozygous Familial and Nonfamilial) and Mixed Dyslipidemia (Fredrickson Types IIa and IIb)

The effects of fenofibrate at a dose equivalent to 145 mg TRICOR (fenofibrate tablets) per day were assessed from four randomized, placebo-controlled, double-blind, parallel-group studies including patients with the following mean baseline lipid values: total-C 306.9 mg/dL; LDL-C 213.8 mg/dL; HDL-C 52.3 mg/dL; and triglycerides 191.0 mg/dL. TRICOR therapy lowered LDL-C, Total-C, and the LDL-C/HDL-C ratio. TRICOR therapy also lowered triglycerides and raised HDL-C (see Table 1).

[See table 1 at right]

In a subset of the subjects, measurements of apo B were conducted. TRICOR treatment significantly reduced apo B from baseline to endpoint as compared with placebo (-25.1% vs. 2.4%, p < 0.0001, n=213 and 143 respectively).

Hypertriglyceridemia (Fredrickson Type IV and V)

The effects of fenofibrate on serum triglycerides were studied in two randomized, double-blind, placebo-controlled clinical trials[1] of 147 hypertriglyceridemic patients (Fredrickson Types IV and V). Patients were treated for eight weeks under protocols that differed only in that one entered patients with baseline triglyceride (TG) levels of 500 to 1500 mg/dL, and the other TG levels of 350 to 500 mg/dL. In patients with hypertriglyceridemia and normal cholesterolemia with or without hyperchylomicronemia (Type IV/V hyperlipidemia), treatment with fenofibrate at dosages equivalent to TRICOR 145 mg per day decreased primarily very low density lipoprotein (VLDL) triglycerides and VLDL cholesterol. Treatment of patients with Type IV hyperlipoproteinemia and elevated triglycerides often results in an increase of low density lipoprotein (LDL) cholesterol (see Table 2).

[See table 2 at right]

The effect of TRICOR on cardiovascular morbidity and mortality has not been determined.

INDICATIONS AND USAGE

Treatment of Hypercholesterolemia

TRICOR is indicated as adjunctive therapy to diet to reduce elevated LDL-C, Total-C, Triglycerides and Apo B, and to increase HDL-C in adult patients with primary hypercholesterolemia or mixed dyslipidemia (Fredrickson Types IIa and IIb). Lipid-altering agents should be used in addition to a diet restricted in saturated fat and cholesterol when response to diet and non-pharmacological interventions alone has been inadequate (see National Cholesterol Education Program [NCEP] Treatment Guidelines, below).

Treatment of Hypertriglyceridemia

TRICOR is also indicated as adjunctive therapy to diet for treatment of adult patients with hypertriglyceridemia (Fredrickson Types IV and V hyperlipidemia). Improving glycemic control in diabetic patients showing fasting chylomicronemia will usually reduce fasting triglycerides and eliminate chylomicronemia thereby obviating the need for pharmacologic intervention.

Markedly elevated levels of serum triglycerides (e.g. > 2,000 mg/dL) may increase the risk of developing pancreatitis. The effect of TRICOR therapy on reducing this risk has not been adequately studied.

Drug therapy is not indicated for patients with Type I hyperlipoproteinemia, who have elevations of chylomicrons and plasma triglycerides, but who have normal levels of very low density lipoprotein (VLDL). Inspection of plasma refrigerated for 14 hours is helpful in distinguishing Types I, IV and V hyperlipoproteinemia[2].

The initial treatment for dyslipidemia is dietary therapy specific for the type of lipoprotein abnormality. Excess body weight and excess alcoholic intake may be important factors in hypertriglyceridemia and should be addressed prior to any drug therapy. Physical exercise can be an important ancillary measure. Diseases contributory to hyperlipidemia, such as hypothyroidism or diabetes mellitus should be looked for and adequately treated. Estrogen therapy, thiazide diuretics and beta-blockers, are sometimes associated with massive rises in plasma triglycerides, especially in subjects with familial hypertriglyceridemia. In such cases, discontinuation of the specific etiologic agent may obviate the need for specific drug therapy of hypertriglyceridemia. The use of drugs should be considered only when reasonable attempts have been made to obtain satisfactory results with non-drug methods. If the decision is made to use drugs, the patient should be instructed that this does not reduce the importance of adhering to diet. (See WARNINGS and PRECAUTIONS).

Table 1. Mean Percent Change in Lipid Parameters at End of Treatment[†]

Treatment Group	Total-C	LDL-C	HDL-C	TG
Pooled Cohort				
Mean baseline lipid values (n=646)	306.9 mg/dL	213.8 mg/dL	52.3 mg/dL	191.0 mg/dL
All FEN (n=361)	-18.7%*	-20.6%*	+11.0%*	-28.9%*
Placebo (n=285)	-0.4%	-2.2%	+0.7%	+7.7%
Baseline LDL-C > 160 mg/dL and TG < 150 mg/dL (Type IIa)				
Mean baseline lipid values (n=334)	307.7 mg/dL	227.7 mg/dL	58.1 mg/dL	101.7 mg/dL
All FEN (n=193)	-22.4%*	-31.4%*	+9.8%*	-23.5%*
Placebo (n=141)	+0.2%	-2.2%	+2.6%	+11.7%
Baseline LDL-C > 160 mg/dL and TG ≥ 150 mg/dL (Type IIb)				
Mean baseline lipid values (n=242)	312.8 mg/dL	219.8 mg/dL	46.7 mg/dL	231.9 mg/dL
All FEN (n=126)	-16.8%*	-20.1%*	+14.6%*	-35.9%*
Placebo (n=116)	-3.0%	-6.6%	+2.3%	+0.9%

† Duration of study treatment was 3 to 6 months.
* p = < 0.05 vs. Placebo

Table 2. Effects of TRICOR in Patients With Fredrickson Type IV/V Hyperlipidemia

Study 1	Placebo				TRICOR			
Baseline TG levels 350 to 499 mg/dL	N	Baseline (Mean)	Endpoint (Mean)	% Change (Mean)	N	Baseline (Mean)	Endpoint (Mean)	% Change (Mean)
Triglycerides	28	449	450	-0.5	27	432	223	-46.2*
VLDL Triglycerides	19	367	350	2.7	19	350	178	-44.1*
Total Cholesterol	28	255	261	2.8	27	252	227	-9.1*
HDL Cholesterol	28	35	36	4	27	34	40	19.6*
LDL Cholesterol	28	120	129	12	27	128	137	14.5
VLDL Cholesterol	27	99	99	5.8	27	92	46	-44.7*

Study 2	Placebo				TRICOR			
Baseline TG levels 500 to 1500 mg/dL	N	Baseline (Mean)	Endpoint (Mean)	% Change (Mean)	N	Baseline (Mean)	Endpoint (Mean)	% Change (Mean)
Triglycerides	44	710	750	7.2	48	726	308	-54.5*
VLDL Triglycerides	29	537	571	18.7	33	543	205	-50.6*
Total Cholesterol	44	272	271	0.4	48	261	223	-13.8*
HDL Cholesterol	44	27	28	5.0	48	30	36	22.9*
LDL Cholesterol	42	100	90	-4.2	45	103	131	45.0*
VLDL Cholesterol	42	137	142	11.0	45	126	54	-49.4*

* =p < 0.05 vs. Placebo

Fredrickson Classification of Hyperlipoproteinemias

Type	Lipoprotein Elevated	Lipid Elevation Major	Minor
I (rare)	chylomicrons	TG	↑ ↔C
IIa	LDL	C	-
IIb	LDL, VLDL	C	TG
III (rare)	IDL	C, TG	-
IV	VLDL	TG	↑ ↔C
V (rare)	chylomicrons, VLDL	TG	↑ ↔C

C = cholesterol
TG = triglycerides
LDL = low density lipoprotein
VLDL = very low density lipoprotein
IDL = intermediate density lipoprotein

[See table at top of next page]

After the LDL-C goal has been achieved, if the TG is still ≥ 200 mg/dL, non HDL-C (total-C minus HDL-C) becomes a secondary target of therapy. Non-HDL-C goals are set 30 mg/dL higher than LDL-C goals for each risk category.

CONTRAINDICATIONS

TRICOR is contraindicated in patients who exhibit hypersensitivity to fenofibrate.

TRICOR is contraindicated in patients with hepatic or severe renal dysfunction, including primary biliary cirrhosis, and patients with unexplained persistent liver function abnormality.

TRICOR is contraindicated in patients with preexisting gallbladder disease (see WARNINGS).

WARNINGS

Liver Function

Fenofibrate at doses equivalent to 96 mg to 145 mg TRICOR per day has been associated with increases in serum transaminases [AST (SGOT) or ALT (SGPT)]. In a pooled analysis of 10 placebo-controlled trials, increases to > 3 times the upper limit of normal occurred in 5.3% of patients taking fenofibrate versus 1.1% of patients treated with placebo. When transaminase determinations were followed either after discontinuation of treatment or during continued treatment, a return to normal limits was usually observed. The incidence of increases in transaminases related to fenofibrate therapy appear to be dose related. In an 8-week dose-ranging study, the incidence of ALT or AST elevations to at least three times the upper limit of normal was 13% in patients receiving dosages equivalent to 96 mg to 145 mg TRICOR per day and was 0% in those receiving dosages equivalent to 48 mg or less TRICOR per day, or placebo. Hepatocellular, chronic active and cholestatic hepatitis associated with fenofibrate therapy have been reported after exposures of weeks to several years. In extremely rare cases, cirrhosis has been reported in association with chronic active hepatitis.

Regular periodic monitoring of liver function, including serum ALT (SGPT) should be performed for the duration of therapy with TRICOR, and therapy discontinued if enzyme levels persist above three times the normal limit.

Cholelithiasis

Fenofibrate, like clofibrate and gemfibrozil, may increase cholesterol excretion into the bile, leading to cholelithiasis. If cholelithiasis is suspected, gallbladder studies are indicated. TRICOR therapy should be discontinued if gallstones are found.

Concomitant Oral Anticoagulants

Caution should be exercised when anticoagulants are given in conjunction with TRICOR because of the potentiation of coumarin-type anticoagulants in prolonging the prothrombin time/INR. The dosage of the anticoagulant should be reduced to maintain the prothrombin time/INR at the desired level to prevent bleeding complications. Frequent prothrombin time/INR determinations are advisable until it has been definitely determined that the prothrombin time/INR has stabilized.

Concomitant HMG-CoA Reductase Inhibitors

The combined use of TRICOR and HMG-CoA reductase inhibitors should be avoided unless the benefit of further al-

Information on the Abbott Pharmaceutical Products listed on these pages is from the prescribing information in use as of June 1, 2010. For more information, please visit rxabbott.com or call 1-800-633-9110.

terations in lipid levels is likely to outweigh the increased risk of this drug combination.
Concomitant administration of fenofibrate (equivalent to TRICOR 145 mg) and pravastatin (40 mg) once daily for 10 days increased the mean C_{max} and AUC values for pravastatin by 36% (range from 69% decrease to 321% increase) and 28% (range from 54% decrease to 128% increase), respectively, and for 3α-hydroxy-iso-pravastatin by 55% (range from 32% decrease to 314% increase) and 39% (range from 24% decrease to 261% increase), respectively. (See also **CLINICAL PHARMACOLOGY, Drug-drug Interactions**).
The combined use of fibric acid derivatives and HMG-CoA reductase inhibitors has been associated, in the absence of a marked pharmacokinetic interaction, in numerous case reports, with rhabdomyolysis, markedly elevated creatine kinase (CK) levels and myoglobinuria, leading in a high proportion of cases to acute renal failure.
The use of fibrates alone, including TRICOR, may occasionally be associated with myositis, myopathy, or rhabdomyolysis. Patients receiving TRICOR and complaining of muscle pain, tenderness, or weakness should have prompt medical evaluation for myopathy, including serum creatine kinase level determination. If myopathy/myositis is suspected or diagnosed, TRICOR therapy should be stopped.

Mortality

The effect of TRICOR on coronary heart disease morbidity and mortality and non-cardiovascular mortality has not been established.

Other Considerations

The Fenofibrate Intervention and Event Lowering in Diabetes (FIELD) study was a 5-year randomized, placebo-controlled study of 9795 patients with type 2 diabetes mellitus treated with fenofibrate. Fenofibrate demonstrated a non-significant 11% relative reduction in the primary outcome of coronary heart disease events (hazard ratio [HR] 0.89, 95% CI 0.75-1.05, p=0.16) and a significant 11% reduction in the secondary outcome of total cardiovascular disease events (HR 0.89 [0.80-0.99], p=0.04). There was a non-significant 11% (HR 1.11 [0.95, 1.29], p=0.18) and 19% (HR 1.19 [0.90, 1.57], p=0.22) increase in total and coronary heart disease mortality, respectively, with fenofibrate as compared to placebo.
In the Coronary Drug Project, a large study of post myocardial infarction of patients treated for 5 years with clofibrate, there was no difference in mortality seen between the clofibrate group and the placebo group. There was however, a difference in the rate of cholelithiasis and cholecystitis requiring surgery between the two groups (3.0% vs. 1.8%).
Because of chemical, pharmacological, and clinical similarities between TRICOR (fenofibrate tablets), Atromid-S (clofibrate), and Lopid (gemfibrozil), the adverse findings in 4 large randomized, placebo-controlled clinical studies with these other fibrate drugs may also apply to TRICOR.
In a study conducted by the World Health Organization (WHO), 5000 subjects without known coronary artery disease were treated with placebo or clofibrate for 5 years and followed for an additional one year. There was a statistically significant, higher age – adjusted all-cause mortality in the clofibrate group compared with the placebo group (5.70% vs. 3.96%, p = < 0.01). Excess mortality was due to a 33% increase in non-cardiovascular causes, including malignancy, post-cholecystectomy complications, and pancreatitis. This appeared to confirm the higher risk of gallbladder disease seen in clofibrate-treated patients studied in the Coronary Drug Project.
The Helsinki Heart Study was a large (n=4081) study of middle-aged men without a history of coronary artery disease. Subjects received either placebo or gemfibrozil for 5 years, with a 3.5 year open extension afterward. Total mortality was numerically higher in the gemfibrozil randomization group but did not achieve statistical significance (p = 0.19, 95% confidence interval for relative risk G:P = .91-1.64). Although cancer deaths trended higher in the gemfibrozil group (p = 0.11), cancers (excluding basal cell carcinoma) were diagnosed with equal frequency in both study groups. Due to the limited size of the study, the relative risk of death from any cause was not shown to be different than that seen in the 9 year follow-up data from World Health Organization study (RR=1.29). Similarly, the numerical excess of gallbladder surgeries in the gemfibrozil group did not differ statistically from that observed in the WHO study.
A secondary prevention component of the Helsinki Heart Study enrolled middle-aged men excluded from the primary prevention study because of known or suspected coronary heart disease. Subjects received gemfibrozil or placebo for 5 years. Although cardiac deaths trended higher in the gemfibrozil group, this was not statistically significant (hazard ratio 2.2, 95% confidence interval: 0.94-5.05). The rate of gallbladder surgery was not statistically significant between study groups, but did trend higher in the gemfibrozil group, (1.9% vs. 0.3%, p = 0.07). There was a statistically significant difference in the number of appendectomies in the gemfibrozil group (6/311 vs. 0/317, p = 0.029).

NCEP Treatment Guidelines: LDL-C Goals and Cutpoints for Therapeutic Lifestyle Changes and Drug Therapy in Different Risk Categories

Risk Category	LDL Goal (mg/dL)	LDL Level at Which to Initiate Therapeutic Lifestyle Changes (mg/dL)	LDL Level at Which to Consider Drug Therapy (mg/dL)
CHD† or CHD risk equivalents (10-year risk > 20%)	< 100	≥ 100	≥ 130 (100-129: drug optional)††
2+ Risk Factors (10-year risk ≤ 20%)	< 130	≥ 130	10-year risk 10%-20%: ≥ 130 10-year risk < 10%: ≥ 160
0-1 Risk Factor†††	< 160	≥ 160	≥ 190 (160-189: LDL-lowering drug optional)

† CHD = coronary heart disease
†† Some authorities recommend use of LDL-lowering drugs in this category if an LDL-C level of < 100 mg/dL cannot be achieved by therapeutic lifestyle changes. Others prefer use of drugs that primarily modify triglycerides and HDL-C, e.g., nicotinic acid or fibrate. Clinical judgment also may call for deferring drug therapy in this subcategory.
††† Almost all people with 0-1 risk factor have 10-year risk < 10%; thus, 10-year risk assessment in people with 0-1 risk factor is not necessary.

PRECAUTIONS

Initial Therapy

Laboratory studies should be done to ascertain that the lipid levels are consistently abnormal before instituting TRICOR therapy. Every attempt should be made to control serum lipids with appropriate diet, exercise, weight loss in obese patients, and control of any medical problems such as diabetes mellitus and hypothyroidism that are contributing to the lipid abnormalities. Medications known to exacerbate hypertriglyceridemia (beta blockers, thiazides, estrogens) should be discontinued or changed if possible prior to consideration of triglyceride-lowering drug therapy.

Continued Therapy

Periodic determination of serum lipids should be obtained during initial therapy in order to establish the lowest effective dose of TRICOR. Therapy should be withdrawn in patients who do not have an adequate response after two months of treatment with the maximum recommended dose of 145 mg per day.

Pancreatitis

Pancreatitis has been reported in patients taking fenofibrate, gemfibrozil, and clofibrate. This occurrence may represent a failure of efficacy in patients with severe hypertriglyceridemia, a direct drug effect, or a secondary phenomenon mediated through biliary tract stone or sludge formation with obstruction of the common bile duct.

Hypersensitivity Reactions

Acute hypersensitivity reactions including severe skin rashes requiring patient hospitalization and treatment with steroids have occurred very rarely during treatment with fenofibrate, including rare spontaneous reports of Stevens-Johnson syndrome, and toxic epidermal necrolysis. Urticaria was seen in 1.1 vs. 0%, and rash in 1.4 vs. 0.8% of fenofibrate and placebo patients respectively in controlled trials.

Hematologic Changes

Mild to moderate hemoglobin, hematocrit, and white blood cell decreases have been observed in patients following initiation of fenofibrate therapy. However, these levels stabilize during long-term administration. Extremely rare spontaneous reports of thrombocytopenia and agranulocytosis have been received during post-marketing surveillance outside of the U.S. Periodic blood counts are recommended during the first 12 months of TRICOR administration.

Skeletal Muscle

The use of fibrates alone, including TRICOR, may occasionally be associated with myopathy. Treatment with drugs of the fibrate class has been associated on rare occasions with rhabdomyolysis, usually in patients with impaired renal function. Myopathy should be considered in any patient with diffuse myalgias, muscle tenderness or weakness, and/or marked elevations of creatine phosphokinase levels. Patients should be advised to report promptly unexplained muscle pain, tenderness or weakness, particularly if accompanied by malaise or fever. CPK levels should be assessed in patients reporting these symptoms, and fenofibrate therapy should be discontinued if markedly elevated CPK levels occur or myopathy is diagnosed.

Venothromboembolic Disease

In the FIELD trial, pulmonary embolus (PE) and deep vein thrombosis (DVT) were observed at higher rates in the fenofibrate- than the placebo-treated group. Of 9,795 patients enrolled in FIELD, there were 4,900 in the placebo group and 4,895 in the fenofibrate group. For DVT, there were 48 events (1%) in the placebo group and 67 (1%) in the fenofibrate group (p = 0.074); and for PE, there were 32 (0.7%) events in the placebo group and 53 (1%) in the fenofibrate group (p = 0.022).
In the Coronary Drug Project, a higher proportion of the clofibrate group experienced definite or suspected fatal or nonfatal pulmonary embolism or thrombophlebitis than the placebo group (5.2% vs. 3.3% at five years; p < 0.01).

Serum Creatinine

Elevations in serum creatinine have been reported in patients on fenofibrate. These elevations tend to return to baseline following discontinuation of fenofibrate. The clinical significance of these observations is unknown.

Drug Interactions

Oral Anticoagulants

CAUTION SHOULD BE EXERCISED WHEN COUMARIN ANTICOAGULANTS ARE GIVEN IN CONJUNCTION WITH TRICOR. THE DOSAGE OF THE ANTICOAGULANTS SHOULD BE REDUCED TO MAINTAIN THE PROTHROMBIN TIME/INR AT THE DESIRED LEVEL TO PREVENT BLEEDING COMPLICATIONS. FREQUENT PROTHROMBIN TIME/INR DETERMINATIONS ARE ADVISABLE UNTIL IT HAS BEEN DEFINITELY DETERMINED THAT THE PROTHROMBIN TIME/INR HAS STABILIZED.

HMG-CoA Reductase Inhibitors

The combined use of TRICOR and HMG-CoA reductase inhibitors should be avoided unless the benefit of further alterations in lipid levels is likely to outweigh the increased risk of this drug combination (see **WARNINGS**).

Resins

Since bile acid sequestrants may bind other drugs given concurrently, patients should take TRICOR at least 1 hour before or 4-6 hours after a bile acid binding resin to avoid impeding its absorption.

Cyclosporine

Because cyclosporine can produce nephrotoxicity with decreases in creatinine clearance and rises in serum creatinine, and because renal excretion is the primary elimination route of fibrate drugs including TRICOR, there is a risk that an interaction will lead to deterioration. The benefits and risks of using TRICOR (fenofibrate tablets) with immunosuppressants and other potentially nephrotoxic agents should be carefully considered, and the lowest effective dose employed.

Carcinogenesis, Mutagenesis, Impairment of Fertility

Two dietary carcinogenicity studies have been conducted in rats with fenofibrate. In the first 24-month study, rats were dosed with fenofibrate at 10, 45, and 200 mg/kg/day, approximately 0.3, 1, and 6 times the maximum recommended human dose (MRHD), based on body surface area comparisons (mg/m^2). At a dose of 200 mg/kg/day (at 6 times the MRHD), the incidence of liver carcinomas was significantly increased in both sexes. A statistically significant increase in pancreatic carcinomas was observed in males at 1 and 6 times the MRHD; an increase in pancreatic adenomas and benign testicular interstitial cell tumors was observed at 6 times the MRHD in males. In a second 24-month rat carcinogenicity study in a different strain of rats, doses of 10 and 60 mg/kg/day (0.3 and 2 times the MRHD) produced significant increases in the incidence of pancreatic acinar adenomas in both sexes and increases in testicular interstitial cell tumors in males at 2 times the MRHD.
A 117-week carcinogenicity study was conducted in rats comparing three drugs: fenofibrate 10 and 60 mg/kg/day (0.3 and 2 times the MRHD), clofibrate (400 mg/kg/day; 2 times the human dose), and gemfibrozil (250 mg/kg/day; 2 times the human dose, based on mg/m^2 surface area). Fenofibrate increased pancreatic acinar adenomas in both sexes. Clofibrate increased hepatocellular carcinoma and

pancreatic acinar adenomas in males and hepatic neoplastic nodules in females. Gemfibrozil increased hepatic neoplastic nodules in males and females, while all three drugs increased testicular interstitial cell tumors in males.

In a 21-month study in mice, fenofibrate 10, 45, and 200 mg/kg/day (approximately 0.2, 1, and 3 times the MRHD on the basis of mg/m² surface area) significantly increased the liver carcinomas in both sexes at 3 times the MRHD. In a second 18-month study at 10, 60, and 200 mg/kg/day, fenofibrate significantly increased the liver carcinomas in male mice and liver adenomas in female mice at 3 times the MRHD.

Electron microscopy studies have demonstrated peroxisomal proliferation following fenofibrate administration to the rat. An adequate study to test for peroxisome proliferation in humans has not been done, but changes in peroxisome morphology and numbers have been observed in humans after treatment with other members of the fibrate class when liver biopsies were compared before and after treatment in the same individual.

Fenofibrate has been demonstrated to be devoid of mutagenic potential in the following tests: Ames, mouse lymphoma, chromosomal aberration and unscheduled DNA synthesis in primary rat hepatocytes.

In fertility studies rats were given oral dietary doses of fenofibrate, males received 61 days prior to mating and females 15 days prior to mating through weaning which resulted in no adverse effect on fertility at doses up to 300 mg/kg/day (~10 times the MRHD, based on mg/m² surface area comparisons).

Pregnancy

Pregnancy Category C

Safety in pregnant women has not been established. There are no adequate and well controlled studies of fenofibrate in pregnant women. Fenofibrate should be used during pregnancy only if the potential benefit justifies the potential risk to the fetus.

In female rats given oral dietary doses of 15, 75, and 300 mg/kg/day of fenofibrate from 15 days prior to mating through weaning, maternal toxicity was observed at 0.3 times the MRHD, based on body surface area comparisons; mg/m².

In pregnant rats given oral dietary doses of 14, 127, and 361 mg/kg/day from gestation day 6-15 during the period of organogenesis, adverse developmental findings were not observed at 14 mg/kg/day (less than 1 times the MRHD, based on body surface area comparisons; mg/m²). At higher multiples of human doses evidence of maternal toxicity was observed.

In pregnant rabbits given oral gavage doses of 15, 150, and 300 mg/kg/day from gestation day 6-18 during the period of organogenesis and allowed to deliver, aborted litters were observed at 150 mg/kg/day (10 times the MRHD, based on body surface area comparisons: mg/m²). No developmental findings were observed at 15 mg/kg/day (at less than 1 times the MRHD, based on body surface area comparisons; mg/m²).

In pregnant rats given oral dietary doses of 15, 75, and 300 mg/kg/day from gestation day 15 through lactation day 21 (weaning), maternal toxicity was observed at less than 1 times the MRHD, based on body surface area comparisons; mg/m².

Nursing Mothers

It is not known whether fenofibrate is excreted into milk. Because many drugs are excreted in human milk and because of the potential for serious adverse reactions in nursing infants from fenofibrate, a decision should be made whether to discontinue nursing or administration of fenofibrate taking into account the importance of the drug to the lactating woman.

Pediatric Use

Safety and efficacy in pediatric patients have not been established.

Geriatric Use

Fenofibric acid is known to be substantially excreted by the kidney, and the risk of adverse reactions to this drug may be greater in patients with impaired renal function. Fenofibric acid exposure is not influenced by age. However, elderly patients have a higher incidence of renal impairment, such that dose selection for the elderly should be made on the basis of renal function (see **CLINICAL PHARMACOLOGY, Special Populations,** Renal Insufficiency). Elderly patients with normal renal function should require no dose modifications.

ADVERSE REACTIONS

Adverse events reported by 2% or more of patients treated with fenofibrate during the double-blind, placebo-controlled trials, regardless of causality, are listed in the table below. Adverse events led to discontinuation of treatment in 5.0% of patients treated with fenofibrate and in 3.0% treated with placebo. Increases in liver function tests were the most frequent events, causing discontinuation of fenofibrate treatment in 1.6% of patients in double-blind trials.

BODY SYSTEM Adverse Event	Fenofibrate* (N=439)	Placebo (N=365)
BODY AS A WHOLE		
Abdominal Pain	4.6%	4.4%
Back Pain	3.4%	2.5%
Headache	3.2%	2.7%
Asthenia	2.1%	3.0%
Flu Syndrome	2.1%	2.7%
DIGESTIVE		
Liver Function Tests Abnormal	7.5%**	1.4%
Diarrhea	2.3%	4.1%
Nausea	2.3%	1.9%
Constipation	2.1%	1.4%
METABOLIC AND NUTRITIONAL DISORDERS		
SGPT Increased	3.0%	1.6%
Creatine Phosphokinase Increased	3.0%	1.4%
SGOT Increased	3.4%**	0.5%
RESPIRATORY		
Respiratory Disorder	6.2%	5.5%
Rhinitis	2.3%	1.1%

* Dosage equivalent to 145 mg TRICOR.
**Significantly different from Placebo.

[See table above]

Additional adverse events reported during post-marketing surveillance or by three or more patients in placebo-controlled trials or reported in other controlled or open trials, regardless of causality are listed below.

Body as a Whole

Accidental injury, allergic reaction, chest pain, cyst, fever, hernia, infection, malaise and pain (unspecified).

Cardiovascular System

Angina pectoris, arrhythmia, atrial fibrillation, cardiovascular disorder, coronary artery disorder, electrocardiogram abnormal, extrasystoles, hypertension, hypotension, migraine, myocardial infarct, palpitation, peripheral vascular disorder, phlebitis, tachycardia, varicose vein, vascular disorder, vasodilatation, venous thromboembolic events (deep vein thrombosis, pulmonary embolus) and ventricular extrasystoles.

Digestive System

Anorexia, cholecystitis, cholelithiasis, colitis, diarrhea, duodenal ulcer, dyspepsia, eructation, esophagitis, flatulence, gastritis, gastroenteritis, gastrointestinal disorder, increased appetite, jaundice, liver fatty deposit, nausea, pancreatitis, peptic ulcer, rectal disorder, rectal hemorrhage, tooth disorder and vomiting.

Endocrine System

Diabetes mellitus.

Hemic and Lymphatic System

Anemia, ecchymosis, eosinophilia, leukopenia, lymphadenopathy, and thrombocytopenia.

Laboratory Investigations

Alkaline phosphatase increased, bilirubin increased, blood urea nitrogen increased, serum creatinine increased, gamma glutamyl transpeptidase increased, lactate dehydrogenase increased, SGOT and SGPT increased.

Metabolic and Nutritional Disorders

Edema, gout, hyperuricemia, hypoglycemia, peripheral edema, weight gain, and weight loss.

Musculoskeletal System

Arthralgia, arthritis, arthrosis, bursitis, joint disorder, leg cramps, myalgia, myasthenia, myositis, rhabdomyolysis and tenosynovitis.

Nervous System

Anxiety or nervousness, depression, dizziness, dry mouth, hypertonia, insomnia, libido decreased, neuralgia, paresthesia, somnolence and vertigo.

Respiratory System

Allergic pulmonary alveolitis, asthma, bronchitis, cough increased, dyspnea, laryngitis, pharyngitis, pneumonia and sinusitis.

Skin and Appendages

Acne, alopecia, contact dermatitis, eczema, fungal dermatitis, herpes simplex, herpes zoster, maculopapular rash, nail disorder, photosensitivity reaction, pruritus, rash, sweating, skin disorder, skin ulcer and urticaria.

Special Senses

Abnormal vision, amblyopia, cataract specified, conjunctivitis, ear pain, eye disorder, otitis media and refraction disorder.

Urogenital System

Abnormal kidney function, cystitis, dysuria, gynecomastia, prostatic disorder, unintended pregnancy, urinary frequency, urolithiasis and vaginal moniliasis.

OVERDOSAGE

There is no specific treatment for overdose with TRICOR. General supportive care of the patient is indicated, including monitoring of vital signs and observation of clinical status, should an overdose occur. If indicated, elimination of unabsorbed drug should be achieved by emesis or gastric lavage; usual precautions should be observed to maintain the airway. Because fenofibrate is highly bound to plasma proteins, hemodialysis should not be considered.

DOSAGE AND ADMINISTRATION

Patients should be placed on an appropriate lipid-lowering diet before receiving TRICOR, and should continue this diet during treatment with TRICOR. TRICOR tablets can be given without regard to meals.

For the treatment of adult patients with primary hypercholesterolemia or mixed hyperlipidemia, the initial dose of TRICOR is 145 mg per day.

For adult patients with hypertriglyceridemia, the initial dose is 48 to 145 mg per day. Dosage should be individualized according to patient response, and should be adjusted if necessary following repeat lipid determinations at 4 to 8 week intervals. The maximum dose is 145 mg per day.

Treatment with TRICOR should be initiated at a dose of 48 mg/day in patients having mild to moderately impaired renal function, and increased only after evaluation of the effects on renal function and lipid levels at this dose.

Lipid levels should be monitored periodically and consideration should be given to reducing the dosage of TRICOR if lipid levels fall significantly below the targeted range.

HOW SUPPLIED

TRICOR® (fenofibrate tablets) is available in two strengths:

48 mg yellow tablets, imprinted with **"Abbott "A" logo"** and Abbo-Code identification letters "FI", available in bottles of 90 (**NDC** 0074-6122-90).

145 mg white tablets, imprinted with **"Abbott "A" logo"** and Abbo-Code identification letters "FO", available in bottles of 90 (**NDC** 0074-6123-90).

Storage

Store at 25°C (77°F); excursions permitted to 15-30°C (59-86°F) [see USP Controlled Room Temperature]. Keep out of the reach of children. Protect from moisture.

REFERENCES

1. GOLDBERG AC, et al. Fenofibrate for the Treatment of Type IV and V Hyperlipoproteinemias: A Double-Blind, Placebo-Controlled Multicenter US Study. Clinical Therapeutics, 11, pp. 69-83, 1989.

2. NIKKILA EA. Familial Lipoprotein Lipase Deficiency and Related Disorders of Chylomicron Metabolism. In Stanbury J.B., et al. (eds.): The Metabolic Basis of Inherited Disease, 5th edition, McGraw-Hill, 1983, Chap. 30, pp. 622-642.

3. BROWN WV, et al. Effects of Fenofibrate on Plasma Lipids: Double-Blind, Multicenter Study In Patients with Type IIA or IIB Hyperlipidemia. Arteriosclerosis. 6, pp. 670-678, 1986.

Manufactured for Abbott Laboratories, North Chicago, IL 60064, U.S.A.

by Fournier Laboratories Ireland Limited, Anngrove, Carigtwohill Co. Cork, Ireland

03-A196-R5

Rev. December, 2008

Shown in Product Identification Guide, page 304

TRILIPIX®
[*try-lip-iks*]
(fenofibric acid)
Capsule, Delayed Release for Oral use

HIGHLIGHTS OF PRESCRIBING INFORMATION
These highlights do not include all the information needed to use Trilipix safely and effectively. See full prescribing information for Trilipix.
Trilipix (fenofibric acid) Capsule, Delayed Release for Oral use
Initial U.S. Approval: 2008

――――――――INDICATIONS AND USAGE――――――――
Trilipix is a peroxisome proliferator receptor alpha (PPARα) activator indicated:
- In combination with a statin to reduce TG and increase HDL-C in patients with mixed dyslipidemia and CHD or a CHD risk equivalent who are on optimal statin therapy to achieve their LDL-C goal (1.1).
- As monotherapy to reduce TG in patients with severe hypertriglyceridemia (1.2).
- As monotherapy to reduce elevated LDL-C, Total-C, TG and Apo B, and to increase HDL-C in patients with primary hyperlipidemia or mixed dyslipidemia (1.3).
Limitations of use: No incremental benefit of Trilipix on cardiovascular morbidity and mortality over and above that demonstrated for statin monotherapy has been established. General Considerations For Treatment: Fenofibrate at a dose equivalent to 135 mg of Trilipix was not shown to reduce coronary heart disease morbidity and mortality in a large, randomized controlled trial of patients with type 2 diabetes mellitus.

――――――――DOSAGE AND ADMINISTRATION――――――――
- Mixed dyslipidemia: 135 mg once daily (2.2).
- Hypertriglyceridemia: 45 to 135 mg once daily (2.3).
- Renally impaired patients: 45 mg once daily (2.5).
- Maximum dose: 135 mg once daily (2.1).
- May be taken without regard to food (2.1).
- May be taken at the same time as a statin (2.2).
- Co-administration with the maximum dose of a statin has not been evaluated in clinical studies and should be avoided unless the benefits are expected to outweigh the risks (2.2).

――――――――DOSAGE FORMS AND STRENGTHS――――――――
Oral Delayed Release Capsules: 45 mg and 135 mg (3).

――――――――CONTRAINDICATIONS――――――――
- Severe renal dysfunction, including patients receiving dialysis (4, 12.3).
- Active liver disease (4, 5.3).
- Gallbladder disease (4, 5.4).
- Nursing mothers (4, 8.3).

――――――――WARNINGS AND PRECAUTIONS――――――――
- Myopathy and rhabdomyolysis have been reported in patients taking fenofibrate. The risks for myopathy and rhabdomyolysis are increased when fibrates are co-administered with a statin (with a significantly higher rate observed for gemfibrozil), particularly in elderly patients and patients with diabetes, renal failure, or hypothyroidism (5.1).
- Trilipix can increase serum transaminases. Liver tests should be monitored periodically (5.3).
- Trilipix can reversibly increase serum creatinine levels (5.2). Renal function should be monitored periodically in patients with renal insufficiency (8.6).
- Trilipix increases cholesterol excretion into the bile, leading to risk of cholelithiasis. If cholelithiasis is suspected, gallbladder studies are indicated (5.4).
- Exercise caution in concomitant treatment with oral coumarin anticoagulants. Adjust the dosage of coumarin anticoagulant to maintain the prothrombin time/INR at the desired level to prevent bleeding complications (5.5).

――――――――ADVERSE REACTIONS――――――――
The most common adverse events (≥ 3% of patients receiving Trilipix or Trilipix co-administered with statins) are headache, back pain, nasopharyngitis, nausea, myalgia, diarrhea, and upper respiratory tract infection (6.1).
To report SUSPECTED ADVERSE REACTIONS, contact Abbott Laboratories at 1-800-633-9110 or FDA at 1-800-FDA-1088 or www.fda.gov/medwatch

――――――――DRUG INTERACTIONS――――――――
- Coumarin Anticoagulants: (7.1).
- Bile Acid Resins: (7.2).
- Cyclosporine: (7.3).

――――――――USE IN SPECIFIC POPULATIONS――――――――
- Geriatric Use: Dose selection for the elderly should be made on the basis of renal function (8.5).
- Renal Impairment: Trilipix should be avoided in patients with severe renal impairment. Dose adjustment is required in patients with mild to moderate renal impairment (8.6).
- The use of Trilipix has not been evaluated in patients with hepatic impairment (8.7).

See 17 for PATIENT COUNSELING INFORMATION and the FDA-approved Medication Guide

Revised: 12/2008

FULL PRESCRIBING INFORMATION: CONTENTS*

FULL PRESCRIBING INFORMATION

1　INDICATIONS AND USAGE
1.1　Co-administration Therapy with Statins for the Treatment of Mixed Dyslipidemia
Trilipix is indicated as an adjunct to diet in combination with a statin to reduce TG and increase HDL-C in patients with mixed dyslipidemia and CHD or a CHD risk equivalent who are on optimal statin therapy to achieve their LDL-C goal.
CHD risk equivalents comprise:
- Other clinical forms of atherosclerotic disease (peripheral arterial disease, abdominal aortic aneurysm, and symptomatic carotid artery disease);
- Diabetes;
- Multiple risk factors that confer a 10-year risk for CHD > 20%

1.2　Treatment of Severe Hypertriglyceridemia
Trilipix is indicated as adjunctive therapy to diet to reduce TG in patients with severe hypertriglyceridemia. Improving glycemic control in diabetic patients showing fasting chylomicronemia will usually obviate the need for pharmacological intervention. Markedly elevated levels of serum triglycerides (e.g. > 2,000 mg/dL) may increase the risk of developing pancreatitis. The effect of Trilipix therapy on reducing this risk has not been adequately studied.

1.3　Treatment of Primary Hyperlipidemia or Mixed Dyslipidemia
Trilipix is indicated as adjunctive therapy to diet to reduce elevated LDL-C, Total-C, TG, and Apo B, and to increase HDL-C in patients with primary hyperlipidemia or mixed dyslipidemia.
1.4　Important Limitations of Use
No incremental benefit of Trilipix on cardiovascular morbidity and mortality over and above that demonstrated for statin monotherapy has been established.
1.5　General Considerations for Treatment
Fenofibrate at a dose equivalent to 135 mg of Trilipix was not shown to reduce coronary heart disease morbidity and mortality in a large, randomized controlled trial of patients with type 2 diabetes mellitus.
Laboratory studies should be performed to establish that lipid levels are abnormal before instituting Trilipix therapy. Every reasonable attempt should be made to control serum lipids with non-drug methods including appropriate diet, exercise, weight loss in obese patients, and control of any medical problems such as diabetes mellitus and hypothyroidism that may be contributing to the lipid abnormalities. Medications known to exacerbate hypertriglyceridemia (beta-blockers, thiazides, estrogens) should be discontinued or changed if possible, and excessive alcohol intake should be addressed before triglyceride-lowering drug therapy is considered. If the decision is made to use lipid-altering drugs, the patient should be instructed that this does not reduce the importance of adhering to diet.
Drug therapy is not indicated for patients who have elevations of chylomicrons and plasma triglycerides, but who have normal levels of VLDL.

2　DOSAGE AND ADMINISTRATION
2.1　General Considerations
Patients should be placed on an appropriate lipid-lowering diet before receiving Trilipix as monotherapy or co-administered with a statin [see DOSAGE and ADMINISTRATION (2.2, 2.3 and 2.4)], and should continue this diet during treatment. Trilipix delayed release capsules can be taken without regard to meals. Serum lipids should be monitored periodically. The maximum dose is 135 mg once daily.
2.2　Co-administration Therapy with Statins for the Treatment of Mixed Dyslipidemia
Trilipix 135 mg may be co-administered with an HMG-CoA reductase inhibitor (statin) in patients with mixed dyslipidemia. For convenience, the daily dose of Trilipix may be taken at the same time as a statin, according to the dosing recommendations for each medication. Co-administration with the maximum dose of a statin has not been evaluated in clinical studies and should be avoided unless the benefits are expected to outweigh the risks.
2.3　Severe Hypertriglyceridemia
The initial dose of Trilipix is 45 to 135 mg once daily. Dosage should be individualized according to patient response, and should be adjusted if necessary following repeat lipid determinations at 4 to 8 week intervals. The maximum dose is 135 mg once daily.
2.4　Primary Hyperlipidemia or Mixed Dyslipidemia
The dose of Trilipix is 135 mg once daily.
2.5　Impaired Renal Function
Treatment with Trilipix should be initiated at a dose of 45 mg once daily in patients with mild to moderate renal impairment and should only be increased after evaluation of the effects on renal function and lipid levels at this dose. The use of Trilipix should be avoided in patients with severely impaired renal function.
2.6　Elderly Patients
Dose selection for the elderly should be made on the basis of renal function [see USE IN SPECIFIC POPULATIONS (8.5)].

3　DOSAGE FORMS AND STRENGTHS
- 45 mg choline fenofibrate delayed release capsules with a reddish-brown cap imprinted in white ink the Abbott "A" logo and a yellow body imprinted in black ink the number "45".
- 135 mg choline fenofibrate delayed release capsules with a blue cap imprinted in white ink the Abbott "A" logo and a yellow body imprinted in black ink the number "135".

4　CONTRAINDICATIONS
Trilipix is contraindicated in:
- patients with severe renal impairment, including those receiving dialysis.
- patients with active liver disease, including those with primary biliary cirrhosis and unexplained persistent liver function abnormalities.
- patients with preexisting gallbladder disease.
- nursing mothers.
- patients with hypersensitivity to fenofibric acid, choline fenofibrate or fenofibrate [see WARNINGS and PRECAUTIONS (5.7)].
When Trilipix is co-administered with a statin, refer to the Contraindications section of the respective statin labeling.

5　WARNINGS AND PRECAUTIONS
5.1　Skeletal Muscle
Fibrate and statin monotherapy increase the risk of myositis or myopathy, and have been associated with rhabdomyolysis. Data from observational studies suggest that the

risk for rhabdomyolysis is increased when fibrates are co-administered with a statin (with a significantly higher rate observed for gemfibrozil). Refer to the respective statin labeling for important drug-drug interactions that increase statin levels and could increase this risk. The risk for serious muscle toxicity appears to be increased in elderly patients and in patients with diabetes, renal failure, or hypothyroidism.

Myalgia was reported in 3.3% of patients treated with Trilipix monotherapy and 3.1% to 3.5% of patients treated with Trilipix co-administered with statins compared to 4.7% to 6.1% of patients treated with statin monotherapy. Increases in creatine phosphokinase (CPK) to > 5 times upper limit of normal occurred in no patients treated with Trilipix monotherapy and 0.2% to 1.2% of patients treated with Trilipix co-administered with statins compared to 0.4% to 1.3% of patients treated with statin monotherapy.

Myopathy should be considered in any patient with diffuse myalgias, muscle tenderness or weakness, and/or marked elevations of CPK levels. Patients should promptly report unexplained muscle pain, tenderness or weakness, particularly if accompanied by malaise or fever. CPK levels should be assessed in patients reporting these symptoms, and Trilipix and statin therapy should be discontinued if markedly elevated CPK levels occur or myopathy or myositis is diagnosed.

5.2 Serum Creatinine

Reversible elevations in serum creatinine have been reported in patients receiving Trilipix as monotherapy or co-administered with statins as well as patients receiving fenofibrate. In the pooled analysis of three double-blind controlled studies of Trilipix administered as monotherapy or in combination with statins, increases in creatinine to > 2 mg/dL occurred in 0.8% of patients treated with Trilipix monotherapy and 1.1% to 1.3% of patients treated with Trilipix co-administered with statins compared to 0% to 0.4% of patients treated with statin monotherapy. Elevations in serum creatinine were generally stable over time with no evidence for continued increases in serum creatinine with long-term therapy and tended to return to baseline following discontinuation of treatment. The clinical significance of these observations is unknown. Monitoring renal function in patients with renal impairment taking Trilipix is suggested. Renal monitoring should be considered for patients at risk for renal insufficiency, such as the elderly and those with diabetes.

5.3 Liver Function

Trilipix at a dose of 135 mg once daily administered as monotherapy or co-administered with low to moderate doses of statins has been associated with increases in serum transaminases [AST (SGOT) or ALT (SGPT)]. In a pooled analysis of three double-blind controlled studies of Trilipix administered as monotherapy or in combination with statins, increases to > 3 times the upper limit of normal on two consecutive occasions in ALT and AST occurred in 1.9% and 0.2%, respectively, of patients receiving Trilipix monotherapy and in 1.3% and 0.4%, respectively, of patients receiving Trilipix co-administered with statins. Increases to > 3 times the upper limit of normal in ALT and AST occurred in no patients receiving low- to moderate-dose statin monotherapy. Increases to > 3 times the upper limit of normal in ALT and AST occurred in 0.8% and 0.4%, respectively in patients receiving high-dose statin monotherapy. In a long-term study of Trilipix co-administered with statins for up to 52 weeks, increases of > 3 times the upper limit of normal on two consecutive occasions of ALT and AST occurred in 1.2% and 0.5% of patients, respectively. When transaminase determinations were followed either after discontinuation of treatment or during continued treatment, a return to normal limits was usually observed. Increases in ALT and/or AST were not accompanied by increases in bilirubin or clinically significant increases in alkaline phosphatase.

In a pooled analysis of 10 placebo-controlled trials of fenofibrate, increases to > 3 times the upper limit of normal in ALT occurred in 5.3% of patients taking fenofibrate versus 1.1% of patients treated with placebo. The incidence of increases in transaminases observed with fenofibrate therapy may be dose related. In an 8-week dose-ranging study of fenofibrate in hypertriglyceridemia, the incidence of ALT or AST elevations ≥ 3 times the upper limit of normal was 13% in patients receiving dosages equivalent to 90 mg to 135 mg Trilipix once daily and was 0% in those receiving dosages equivalent to 45 mg Trilipix once daily or less, or placebo. Hepatocellular, chronic active, and cholestatic hepatitis observed with fenofibrate therapy have been reported after exposures of weeks to several years. In extremely rare cases, cirrhosis has been reported in association with chronic active hepatitis.

Regular monitoring of liver function, including serum ALT (SGPT) should be performed for the duration of therapy with Trilipix, and therapy discontinued if enzyme levels persist above 3 times the upper limit of normal.

Table 1. Treatment-Emergent Adverse Events Reported in ≥ 3% of Patients Receiving Trilipix or Trilipix Co-Administered with a Statin During Double-Blind Controlled Studies [Number (%)]

Adverse Event	Trilipix (N = 490)	Low-Dose Statin (N = 493)	Trilipix + Low-Dose Statin (N = 490)	Moderate-Dose Statin (N = 491)	Trilipix + Moderate-Dose Statin (N = 489)	High-Dose Statin (N = 245)
Gastrointestinal Disorders						
Constipation	16 (3.3)	11 (2.2)	16 (3.3)	13 (2.6)	15 (3.1)	6 (2.4)
Diarrhea	19 (3.9)	16 (3.2)	15 (3.1)	24 (4.9)	18 (3.7)	17 (6.9)
Dyspepsia	18 (3.7)	13 (2.6)	13 (2.7)	17 (3.5)	23 (4.7)	6 (2.4)
Nausea	21 (4.3)	18 (3.7)	17 (3.5)	22 (4.5)	27 (5.5)	10 (4.1)
General Disorders and Administration Site Conditions						
Fatigue	10 (2.0)	13 (2.6)	13 (2.7)	13 (2.6)	16 (3.3)	5 (2.0)
Pain	17 (3.5)	9 (1.8)	16 (3.3)	8 (1.6)	7 (1.4)	8 (3.3)
Infections and Infestations						
Nasopharyngitis	17 (3.5)	29 (5.9)	23 (4.7)	16 (3.3)	21 (4.3)	9 (3.7)
Sinusitis	16 (3.3)	4 (0.8)	14 (2.9)	8 (1.6)	17 (3.5)	4 (1.6)
Upper Respiratory Tract Infection	26 (5.3)	13 (2.6)	18 (3.7)	23 (4.7)	23 (4.7)	7 (2.9)
Investigations						
ALT Increased	6 (1.2)	2 (0.4)	15 (3.1)	2 (0.4)	12 (2.5)	4 (1.6)
Musculoskeletal and Connective Tissue Disorders						
Arthralgia	19 (3.9)	22 (4.5)	21 (4.3)	21 (4.3)	17 (3.5)	12 (4.9)
Back Pain	31 (6.3)	31 (6.3)	30 (6.1)	32 (6.5)	20 (4.1)	8 (3.3)
Muscle Spasms	8 (1.6)	18 (3.7)	12 (2.4)	24 (4.9)	15 (3.1)	6 (2.4)
Myalgia	16 (3.3)	24 (4.9)	17 (3.5)	23 (4.7)	15 (3.1)	15 (6.1)
Pain in Extremity	22 (4.5)	24 (4.9)	14 (2.9)	21 (4.3)	13 (2.7)	9 (3.7)
Nervous System Disorders						
Dizziness	20 (4.1)	8 (1.6)	19 (3.9)	11 (2.2)	16 (3.3)	2 (0.8)
Headache	62 (12.7)	64 (13.0)	64 (13.1)	82 (16.7)	58 (11.9)	32 (13.1)

Low-dose statin = rosuvastatin 10 mg, simvastatin 20 mg, or atorvastatin 20 mg
Moderate-dose statin = rosuvastatin 20 mg, simvastatin 40 mg, or atorvastatin 40 mg
High-dose statin = rosuvastatin 40 mg, simvastatin 80 mg, or atorvastatin 80 mg

5.4 Cholelithiasis

Trilipix, like fenofibrate, clofibrate, and gemfibrozil, may increase cholesterol excretion into the bile, potentially leading to cholelithiasis. If cholelithiasis is suspected, gallbladder studies are indicated. Trilipix therapy should be discontinued if gallstones are found.

5.5 Concomitant Oral Anticoagulants

Caution should be exercised when Trilipix is given in conjunction with oral coumarin anticoagulants. Trilipix may potentiate the anticoagulant effects of these agents resulting in prolongation of the prothrombin time/INR. Frequent monitoring of prothrombin time/INR and dose adjustment of the oral anticoagulant are recommended until the prothrombin time/INR has stabilized in order to prevent bleeding complications.

5.6 Pancreatitis

Pancreatitis has been reported in patients taking drugs of the fibrate class, including Trilipix. This occurrence may represent a failure of efficacy in patients with severe hypertriglyceridemia, a direct drug effect, or a secondary phenomenon mediated through biliary tract stone or sludge formation with obstruction of the common bile duct.

5.7 Hypersensitivity Reactions

Acute hypersensitivity reactions including severe skin rashes requiring patient hospitalization and treatment with steroids have occurred very rarely during treatment with fenofibrate, including rare spontaneous reports of Stevens-Johnson Syndrome and toxic epidermal necrolysis.

5.8 Hematological Changes

Mild to moderate hemoglobin, hematocrit, and white blood cell decreases have been observed in patients following initiation of Trilipix and fenofibrate therapy. Extremely rare spontaneous reports of thrombocytopenia and agranulocytosis have been received with fenofibrate therapy.

5.9 Mortality and Coronary Heart Disease Morbidity

The effect of Trilipix on coronary heart disease morbidity and mortality and non-cardiovascular mortality has not been established. Because of similarities between Trilipix and fenofibrate, clofibrate, and gemfibrozil, the findings in the following large randomized, placebo-controlled clinical studies with these fibrate drugs may also apply to Trilipix. The Fenofibrate Intervention and Event Lowering in Diabetes (FIELD) study was a 5-year randomized, placebo-controlled study of 9795 patients with type 2 diabetes mellitus treated with fenofibrate. Fenofibrate demonstrated a non-significant 11% relative reduction in the primary outcome of coronary heart disease events (hazard ratio [HR] 0.89, 95% CI 0.75–1.05, p = 0.16) and a significant 11% reduction in the secondary outcome of total cardiovascular disease events (HR 0.89 [0.80–0.99], p = 0.04). There was a non-significant 11% (HR 1.11 [0.95, 1.29], p = 0.18) and 19% (HR 1.19 [0.90, 1.57], p = 0.22) increase in total and coronary heart disease mortality, respectively, with fenofibrate as compared to placebo.

In the Coronary Drug Project, a large study of post-myocardial infarction patients treated for 5 years with clofibrate, there was no difference in mortality seen between the clofibrate group and the placebo group. There was, however, a difference in the rate of cholelithiasis and cholecystitis requiring surgery between the two groups (3.0% vs. 1.8%).

In a study conducted by the World Health Organization (WHO), 5000 subjects without known coronary artery disease were treated with placebo or clofibrate for 5 years and followed for an additional one year. There was a statistically significant, higher age-adjusted all-cause mortality in the clofibrate group compared with the placebo group (5.70% vs. 3.96%, p = < 0.01). Excess mortality was due to a 33% increase in non-cardiovascular causes, including malignancy, post-cholecystectomy complications, and pancreatitis. This appeared to confirm the higher risk of gallbladder disease seen in clofibrate-treated patients studied in the Coronary Drug Project.

The Helsinki Heart Study was a large (N = 4081) study of middle-aged men without a history of coronary artery disease. Subjects received either placebo or gemfibrozil for 5 years, with a 3.5 year open extension afterward. Total mortality was numerically higher in the gemfibrozil randomization group but did not achieve statistical significance (p = 0.19, 95% confidence interval for relative risk G:P = 0.91–1.64). Although cancer deaths trended higher in the gemfibrozil group (p = 0.11), cancers (excluding basal cell carcinoma) were diagnosed with equal frequency in both study groups. Due to the limited size of the study, the relative risk of death from any cause was not shown to be different than that seen in the 9 year follow-up data from WHO study (RR = 1.29). A secondary prevention component of the Helsinki Heart Study enrolled middle-aged men excluded from the primary prevention study because of known or suspected coronary heart disease. Subjects received gemfibrozil or placebo for 5 years. Although cardiac deaths trended higher in the gemfibrozil group, this was not statistically significant (hazard ratio 2.2, 95% confidence interval: 0.94–5.05).

5.10 Venothromboembolic Disease

In the FIELD trial, pulmonary embolus (PE) and deep vein thrombosis (DVT) were observed at higher rates in the fenofibrate- than the placebo-treated group. Of 9,795 patients enrolled in FIELD, there were 4,900 in the placebo group and 4,895 in the fenofibrate group. For DVT, there were 48 events (1%) in the placebo group and 67 (1%) in the

---

Information on the Abbott Pharmaceutical Products listed on these pages is from the prescribing information in use as of June 1, 2010. For more information, please visit rxabbott.com or call 1-800-633-9110.

fenofibrate group (p = 0.074); and for PE, there were 32 (0.7%) events in the placebo group and 53 (1%) in the fenofibrate group (p = 0.022).

In the Coronary Drug Project, a higher proportion of the clofibrate group experienced definite or suspected fatal or nonfatal PE or thrombophlebitis than the placebo group (5.2% vs. 3.3% at five years; p < 0.01).

6 ADVERSE REACTIONS

6.1 Clinical Studies Experience

Because clinical studies are conducted under widely varying conditions, adverse event rates observed in the clinical studies of a drug cannot be directly compared to rates in the clinical studies of another drug.

Trilipix (fenofibric acid)

Monotherapy

Treatment-emergent adverse events reported in 3% or more of patients treated with Trilipix during the randomized controlled trials are listed in Table 1 below.

Co-Administration Therapy with Statins (Double-blind Controlled Trials)

Treatment-emergent adverse events reported in 3% or more of patients treated with Trilipix co-administered with statins during the randomized controlled trials are listed in Table 1 below.

[See table at top of previous page]

Co-Administration Therapy with Statins (Long-Term Exposure for up to 64 Weeks)

Patients successfully completing any one of the three double-blind, controlled studies were eligible to participate in a 52-week long-term extension study where they received Trilipix co-administered with the moderate dose statin. A total of 2201 patients received at least one dose of Trilipix co-administered with a statin in the double-blind controlled study or the long-term extension study for up to a total of 64 weeks of treatment. Additional treatment-emergent adverse events (not listed in Table 1 above) reported in 3% or more of patients receiving Trilipix co-administered with a statin in either the double-blind controlled studies or the long-term extension study are provided below.

Infections and Infestations

Bronchitis, influenza, and urinary tract infection.

Investigations

AST increased, blood CPK increased, and hepatic enzyme increased.

Musculoskeletal and Connective Tissue Disorders

Musculoskeletal pain.

Psychiatric Disorders

Insomnia.

Respiratory, Thoracic, and Mediastinal Disorders

Cough and pharyngolaryngeal pain.

Vascular Disorders

Hypertension.

Fenofibrate

Fenofibric acid is the active metabolite of fenofibrate. Adverse events reported by 2% or more of patients treated with fenofibrate and greater than placebo during double-blind, placebo-controlled trials are listed in Table 2. Adverse events led to discontinuation of treatment in 5.0% of patients treated with fenofibrate and in 3.0% treated with placebo. Increases in liver tests were the most frequent events, causing discontinuation of fenofibrate treatment in 1.6% of patients in double-blind trials.

Table 2. Adverse Events Reported by 2% or More of Patients Treated with Fenofibrate and Greater than Placebo During the Double-Blind, Placebo-Controlled Trials

BODY SYSTEM Adverse Event	Fenofibrate* (N = 439)	Placebo (N = 365)
BODY AS A WHOLE		
Abdominal Pain	4.6%	4.4%
Back Pain	3.4%	2.5%
Headache	3.2%	2.7%
DIGESTIVE		
Nausea	2.3%	1.9%
Constipation	2.1%	1.4%
INVESTIGATIONS		
Abnormal Liver Tests	7.5%	1.4%
Increased AST	3.4%	0.5%
Increased ALT	3.0%	1.6%
Increased Creatine Phosphokinase	3.0%	1.4%
RESPIRATORY		
Respiratory Disorder	6.2%	5.5%
Rhinitis	2.3%	1.1%

*Dosage equivalent to 135 mg Trilipix

The following adverse events have been identified during postapproval use of fenofibrate: myalgia, rhabdomyolysis, increased creatine phosphokinase, pancreatitis, increased alanine aminotransaminase, increased aspartate aminotransaminase, renal failure, muscle spasms, acute renal failure, hepatitis, cirrhosis, nausea, abdominal pain, anemia, headache, arthralgia, and asthenia. Because these events are reported voluntarily from a population of uncertain size, it is not always possible to reliably estimate their frequency or establish a casual relationship to drug exposure.

7 DRUG INTERACTIONS

7.1 Oral Anticoagulants

Caution should be exercised when oral coumarin anticoagulants are given in conjunction with Trilipix *[see WARNINGS AND PRECAUTIONS (5.5)]*.

7.2 Bile Acid Resins

Since bile acid resins may bind other drugs given concurrently, patients should take Trilipix at least 1 hour before or 4–6 hours after a bile acid resin to avoid impeding its absorption.

7.3 Cyclosporine

Because cyclosporine can produce nephrotoxicity with decreases in creatinine clearance and rises in serum creatinine, and because renal excretion is the primary elimination route of drugs of the fibrate class including Trilipix, there is a risk that an interaction will lead to decline of renal function. The benefits and risks of using Trilipix with immunosuppressants and other potentially nephrotoxic agents should be carefully considered, and the lowest effective dose employed.

8 USE IN SPECIFIC POPULATIONS

8.1 Pregnancy

Pregnancy Category: C

The safety of Trilipix in pregnant women has not been established. There are no adequate and well controlled studies of Trilipix in pregnant women. Trilipix should be used during pregnancy only if the potential benefit justifies the potential risk to the fetus.

When Trilipix is administered with a statin in a woman of childbearing potential, refer to pregnancy category and product labeling for the statin *[see Precautions, Pregnancy]*. All statins are contraindicated in pregnant women.

In pregnant rats given oral dietary doses of 14, 127, and 361 mg/kg/day from gestation day 6–15 during the period of organogenesis, adverse developmental findings were not observed at 14 mg/kg/day (less than 1 times the maximum recommended human dose [MRHD], based on body surface area comparisons; mg/m^2). At higher multiples of human doses evidence of maternal toxicity was observed.

In pregnant rabbits given oral gavage doses of 15, 150, and 300 mg/kg/day from gestation day 6–18 during the period of organogenesis and allowed to deliver, aborted litters were observed at 150 mg/kg/day (10 times the MRHD, based on body surface area comparisons; mg/m^2). No developmental findings were observed at 15 mg/kg/day (at less than 1 times the MRHD, based on body surface area comparisons; mg/m^2).

In pregnant rats given oral dietary doses of 15, 75, and 300 mg/kg/day from gestation day 15 through lactation day 21 (weaning), maternal toxicity was observed at less than 1 times the MRHD, based on body surface area comparisons; mg/m^2.

8.3 Nursing Mothers

Trilipix should not be used in nursing mothers. A decision should be made whether to discontinue nursing or to discontinue the drug.

8.4 Pediatric Use

The safety and effectiveness of Trilipix monotherapy or co-administration with a statin in pediatric patients have not been established.

8.5 Geriatric Use

Trilipix is substantially excreted by the kidney as fenofibric acid and fenofibric acid glucuronide, and the risk of adverse reactions to this drug may be greater in patients with impaired renal function. Since elderly patients have a higher incidence of renal impairment, the dose selection for the elderly should be made on the basis of renal function *[see CLINICAL PHARMACOLOGY (12.3)]*. Consider monitoring renal function in elderly patients taking Trilipix.

8.6 Renal Impairment

The use of Trilipix should be avoided in patients who have severe renal impairment. Dose reduction is required in patients with mild to moderate renal impairment *[see CLINICAL PHARMACOLOGY (12.3) and DOSAGE AND ADMINISTRATION (2.5)]*. Monitoring renal function in patients with renal impairment is recommended.

8.7 Hepatic Impairment

The use of Trilipix has not been evaluated in subjects with hepatic impairment *[see CONTRAINDICATIONS (4) and CLINICAL PHARMACOLOGY (12.3)]*.

10 OVERDOSAGE

There is no specific treatment for overdose with Trilipix. General supportive care of the patient is indicated, including monitoring of vital signs and observation of clinical status, should an overdose occur. If indicated, elimination of unabsorbed drug should be achieved by emesis or gastric lavage; usual precautions should be observed to maintain the airway. Because Trilipix is highly bound to plasma proteins, hemodialysis should not be considered.

11 DESCRIPTION

Trilipix (fenofibric acid) is a lipid regulating agent available as delayed release capsules for oral administration. Each delayed release capsule contains choline fenofibrate, equivalent to 45 mg or 135 mg of fenofibric acid. The chemical name for choline fenofibrate is ethanaminium, 2-hydroxy-N,N,N-trimethyl, 2-[4-(4-chlorobenzoyl)phenoxy] -2-methylpropanoate (1:1) with the following structural formula:

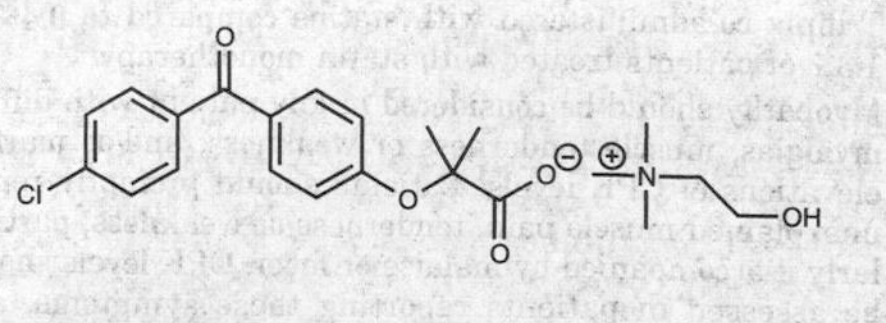

The empirical formula is $C_{22}H_{28}ClNO_5$ and the molecular weight is 421.91. Choline fenofibrate is freely soluble in water. The melting point is approximately 210°C. Choline fenofibrate is a white to yellow powder, which is stable under ordinary conditions.

Each delayed release capsule contains enteric coated mini-tablets comprised of choline fenofibrate and the following inactive ingredients: hypromellose, povidone, water, hydroxylpropyl cellulose, colloidal silicon dioxide, sodium stearyl fumarate, methacrylic acid copolymer, talc, triethyl citrate. The capsule shell of the 45 mg capsule contains the following inactive ingredients: gelatin, titanium dioxide, yellow iron oxide, black iron oxide, and red iron oxide. The capsule shell of the 135 mg capsule contains the following inactive ingredients: gelatin, titanium dioxide, yellow iron oxide, and FD&C Blue #2.

12 CLINICAL PHARMACOLOGY

12.1 Mechanism of Action

The active moiety of Trilipix is fenofibric acid. The pharmacological effects of fenofibric acid in both animals and humans have been extensively studied through oral administration of fenofibrate.

The lipid-modifying effects of fenofibric acid seen in clinical practice have been explained *in vivo* in transgenic mice and *in vitro* in human hepatocyte cultures by the activation of peroxisome proliferator activated receptor α (PPARα). Through this mechanism, fenofibric acid increases lipolysis and elimination of triglyceride-rich particles from plasma by activating lipoprotein lipase and reducing production of Apo CIII (an inhibitor of lipoprotein lipase activity).

The resulting decrease in TG produces an alteration in the size and composition of LDL from small, dense particles (which are thought to be atherogenic due to their susceptibility to oxidation), to large buoyant particles. These larger particles have a greater affinity for cholesterol receptors and are catabolized rapidly. Activation of PPARα also induces an increase in the synthesis of HDL-C and Apo AI and AII.

12.2 Pharmacodynamics

Elevated levels of Total-C, LDL-C, and Apo B, and decreased levels of HDL-C and its transport complex, Apo AI and Apo AII, are risk factors for human atherosclerosis. Epidemiologic studies have established that cardiovascular morbidity and mortality vary directly with the levels of Total-C, LDL-C, and TG, and inversely with the level of HDL-C. The independent effect of raising HDL-C or lowering TG on the risk of cardiovascular morbidity and mortality has not been determined.

12.3 Pharmacokinetics

Trilipix contains fenofibric acid, which is the only circulating pharmacologically active moiety in plasma after oral administration of Trilipix. Fenofibric acid is also the circulating pharmacologically active moiety in plasma after oral administration of fenofibrate, the ester of fenofibric acid.

Plasma concentrations of fenofibric acid after administration of one 135 mg Trilipix delayed release capsule are equivalent to those after one 200 mg capsule of micronized fenofibrate administered under fed conditions.

Absorption

Fenofibric acid is well absorbed throughout the gastrointestinal tract. The absolute bioavailability of fenofibric acid is approximately 81%.

Peak plasma levels of fenofibric acid occur within 4 to 5 hours after a single dose administration of Trilipix capsule under fasting conditions.

Fenofibric acid exposure in plasma, as measured by C_{max} and AUC, is not significantly different when a single 135 mg dose of Trilipix is administered under fasting or nonfasting conditions.

Distribution
Upon multiple dosing of Trilipix, fenofibric acid levels reach steady state within 8 days. Plasma concentrations of fenofibric acid at steady state are approximately slightly more than double those following a single dose. Serum protein binding is approximately 99% in normal and dyslipidemic subjects.

Metabolism
Fenofibric acid is primarily conjugated with glucuronic acid and then excreted in urine. A small amount of fenofibric acid is reduced at the carbonyl moiety to a benzhydrol metabolite which is, in turn, conjugated with glucuronic acid and excreted in urine.

In vivo metabolism data after fenofibrate administration indicate that fenofibric acid does not undergo oxidative metabolism (e.g., cytochrome P450) to a significant extent.

Excretion
After absorption, Trilipix is primarily excreted in the urine in the form of fenofibric acid and fenofibric acid glucuronide. Fenofibric acid is eliminated with a half-life of approximately 20 hours, allowing once daily administration of Trilipix.

Specific Populations
Geriatrics
In five elderly volunteers 77 to 87 years of age, the oral clearance of fenofibric acid following a single oral dose of fenofibrate was 1.2 L/h, which compares to 1.1 L/h in young adults. This indicates that an equivalent dose of Trilipix can be used in elderly subjects with normal renal function, without increasing accumulation of the drug or metabolites *[see USE IN SPECIFIC POPULATIONS (8.5)]*.

Pediatrics
Trilipix has not been investigated in adequate and well-controlled trials in pediatric patients.

Gender
No pharmacokinetic difference between males and females has been observed for Trilipix.

Race
The influence of race on the pharmacokinetics of Trilipix has not been studied.

Renal Impairment
The pharmacokinetics of fenofibric acid was examined in patients with mild, moderate, and severe renal impairment. Patients with severe renal impairment (creatinine clearance [CrCl] < 30 mL/min showed a 2.7-fold increase in exposure for fenofibric acid and increased accumulation of fenofibric acid during chronic dosing compared to that of healthy subjects. Patients with mild to moderate renal impairment (CrCl 30–80 mL/min) had similar exposure but an increase in the half-life for fenofibric acid compared to that of healthy subjects. Based on these findings, the use of Trilipix should be avoided in patients who have severe renal impairment and dose reduction is required in patients having mild to moderate renal impairment.

Hepatic Impairment
No pharmacokinetic studies have been conducted in patients with hepatic impairment.

Drug-drug Interactions
In vitro studies using human liver microsomes indicate that fenofibric acid is not an inhibitor of cytochrome (CYP) P450 isoforms CYP3A4, CYP2D6, CYP2E1, or CYP1A2. It is a weak inhibitor of CYP2C8, CYP2C19, and CYP2A6, and mild-to-moderate inhibitor of CYP2C9 at therapeutic concentrations.

Table 3 describes the effects of co-administered drugs on fenofibric acid systemic exposure. Table 4 describes the effects of co-administered fenofibric acid on other drugs.

[See table 3 at top right]

[See table 4 at top of next page]

13 NONCLINICAL TOXICOLOGY

13.1 Carcinogenesis, Mutagenesis, Impairment of Fertility

Trilipix (fenofibric acid)
No carcinogenicity and fertility studies have been conducted with choline fenofibrate or fenofibric acid. However, because fenofibrate is rapidly converted to its active metabolite, fenofibric acid, either during or immediately following absorption both in animals and humans, studies conducted with fenofibrate are relevant for the assessment of the toxicity profile of fenofibric acid. A similar toxicity spectrum is expected after treatment with either Trilipix or fenofibrate.

Fenofibrate
Two dietary carcinogenicity studies have been conducted in rats with fenofibrate. In the first 24-month study, rats were dosed with fenofibrate at 10, 45, and 200 mg/kg/day, approximately 0.3, 1, and 6 times the maximum recommended human dose (MRHD), based on body surface area comparisons (mg/m^2). At a dose of 200 mg/kg/day (6 times the MRHD), the incidence of liver carcinomas was significantly increased in both sexes. A statistically significant increase in pancreatic carcinomas was observed in males at 1 and 6 times the

---

Table 3. Effects of Co-Administered Drugs on Fenofibric Acid Systemic Exposure from Trilipix or Fenofibrate Administration

Co-Administered Drug	Dosage Regimen of Co-Administered Drug	Dosage Regimen of Trilipix or Fenofibrate	Changes in Fenofibric Acid Exposure	
			AUC	C$_{max}$
No dosing adjustment required for Trilipix with the following co-administered drugs				
Lipid-lowering agents				
Rosuvastatin	40 mg QD for 10 days	Trilipix 135 mg QD for 10 days	↓2%	↓2%
Atorvastatin	20 mg QD for 10 days	Fenofibrate 160 mg[1] QD for 10 days	↓2%	↓4%
Pravastatin	40 mg as a single dose	Fenofibrate 3 × 67 mg[2] as a single dose	↓1%	↓2%
Fluvastatin	40 mg as a single dose	Fenofibrate 160 mg[1] as a single dose	↓2%	↓10%
Simvastatin	80 mg QD for 7 days	Fenofibrate 160 mg[1] QD for 7 days	↓5%	↓11%
Ezetimibe	10 mg QD for 10 days	Fenofibrate 145 mg[1] QD for 10 days	0%	↑3%
Anti-diabetic agents				
Glimepiride	1 mg as a single dose	Fenofibrate 145 mg[1] QD for 10 days	↑1%	↓1%
Metformin	850 mg TID for 10 days	Fenofibrate 54 mg[1] TID for 10 days	↓9%	↓6%
Rosiglitazone	8 mg QD for 5 days	Fenofibrate 145 mg[1] QD for 14 days	↑10%	↑3%
Gastrointestinal agents				
Omeprazole	40 mg QD for 5 days	Trilipix 135 mg as a single dose fasting	↑6%	↑17%
Omeprazole	40 mg QD for 5 days	Trilipix 135 mg as a single dose with food	↑4%	↓2%

[1] TriCor (fenofibrate) oral tablet
[2] TriCor (fenofibrate) oral micronized capsule

MRHD; an increase in pancreatic adenomas and benign testicular interstitial cell tumors was observed at 6 times the MRHD in males.

A 117-week carcinogenicity study was conducted in rats comparing three drugs: fenofibrate 10 and 60 mg/kg/day (0.3 and 2 times the MRHD), clofibrate (400 mg/kg/day; 2 times the human dose), and gemfibrozil (250 mg/kg/day; 2 times the human dose, based on mg/m^2 surface area). Fenofibrate increased pancreatic acinar adenomas in both sexes and testicular interstitial cell tumors in males at 2 times the MRHD. Clofibrate increased hepatocellular carcinoma and pancreatic acinar adenomas in males and hepatic neoplastic nodules in females. Gemfibrozil increased hepatic neoplastic nodules in males and females, while all three drugs increased testicular interstitial cell tumors in males.

In an 80-week study in mice, fenofibrate 10, 45, and 200 mg/kg/day (approximately 0.2, 1, and 3 times the MRHD on the basis of mg/m^2 surface area) significantly increased the liver carcinomas in both sexes at 3 times the MRHD. In a second 93-week study at 10, 60, and 200 mg/kg/day, fenofibrate significantly increased the liver carcinomas in male and female mice at 3 times the MRHD.

Electron microscopy studies have demonstrated peroxisomal proliferation following fenofibrate administration to the rat. An adequate study to test for peroxisome proliferation in humans has not been done, but changes in peroxisome morphology and numbers have been observed in humans after treatment with other members of the fibrate class when liver biopsies were compared before and after treatment in the same individual.

Fenofibrate has been demonstrated to be devoid of mutagenic potential in the following tests: Ames, and micronucleus *in vivo*/rat. In addition, fenofibric acid, has been demonstrated to be devoid of mutagenic potential in the following tests: Ames, mouse lymphoma, chromosomal aberration and sister chromatid exchange in human lymphocytes, and unscheduled DNA synthesis in primary rat hepatocytes.

In a fertility study, rats were given oral dietary doses of fenofibrate. Males received doses for 61 days prior to mating and females for 15 days prior to mating through weaning, which resulted in no adverse effect on fertility at doses up to 300 mg/kg/day (~10 times the MRHD, based on mg/m^2 surface area comparisons).

14 CLINICAL STUDIES

14.1 Co-Administration Therapy with Statins
Efficacy and safety of Trilipix co-administered with statins were assessed in three 12-week, double-blind, controlled Phase 3 studies and one 52-week, long-term, open-label extension study in 2698 patients with mixed dyslipidemia. Patients were required to meet the following fasting lipid entry criteria: TG ≥ 150 mg/dL, and HDL-C < 40 mg/dL (males) and < 50 mg/dL (females), and LDL-C ≥ 130 mg/dL. The three multicenter, randomized, double-blind, controlled studies had similar designs, differing primarily in the statin used for combination therapy/monotherapy. Each study compared the effects of 135 mg Trilipix co-administered with either a low dose or a moderate dose of statin with

---

Trilipix monotherapy and statin monotherapy at the corresponding dose on CHD lipid risk factors. A smaller group of patients received a high dose of statin monotherapy. In study 1, patients received Trilipix co-administered with 10 mg or 20 mg rosuvastatin. In study 2, patients received Trilipix co-administered with 20 mg or 40 mg simvastatin. In study 3, patients received Trilipix co-administered with 20 mg or 40 mg atorvastatin.

Patients were enrolled for a total of approximately 22 weeks, consisting of a 6-week diet run-in/washout period, a 12-week treatment period, and a 30-day safety follow up period. Patients who completed the 12-week treatment period were eligible to participate in the 52-week long-term extension study. Of the 2698 randomized and treated subjects in the controlled studies, 51.6% were female and 48.4% were male; 92.6% of all subjects were White, 4.7% were Black, and 2.8% were of other races. Hispanics comprised 9.9% of the study population. Mean age was 54.9 years.

The primary efficacy endpoints for all three studies were mean percent changes from baseline to final value in HDL-C, TG, and LDL-C. For each statin dose co-administered with Trilipix, there were three primary comparisons. For HDL-C and TG, Trilipix co-administered with each statin dose was compared with statin monotherapy at the corresponding dose. For LDL-C, Trilipix co-administered with each statin dose was compared with Trilipix monotherapy. In order to declare combination therapy successful for a particular statin dose, all three primary comparisons were required to demonstrate superiority of the combination therapy over the corresponding monotherapy. The primary efficacy results were consistent in the three studies and were confirmed by the pooled analysis of the three studies. The results from the individual studies and the pooled analysis demonstrated that Trilipix co-administered with low-dose statins and moderate-dose statins was superior to the corresponding monotherapy. Statistically significant differences were observed for all three primary efficacy comparisons for both doses of combination therapy in all three double-blind, controlled studies as well as the pooled analysis.

In the pooled analysis, Trilipix co-administered with both low-dose statins and moderate-dose statins resulted in mean percent increases (18.1% and 17.5%) in HDL-C and mean percent decreases (-43.9% and -42.0%) in TG that were significantly greater than the corresponding dose of statin monotherapy (7.4% and 8.7% for HDL-C; -16.8% and -23.7% for TG). In addition, both doses of combination therapy resulted in mean percent decreases (-33.1% and -34.6%) in LDL-C that were significantly greater than Trilipix monotherapy (-5.1%). The results of the pooled analysis are described in Table 5.

[See table 5 at top of next page]

Information on the Abbott Pharmaceutical Products listed on these pages is from the prescribing information in use as of June 1, 2010. For more information, please visit rxabbott.com or call 1-800-633-9110.

Secondary efficacy endpoints in all three double-blind, controlled studies were percent changes in non-HDL-C (Trilipix co-administered with statin compared to Trilipix monotherapy and corresponding statin monotherapy), and percent changes in VLDL-C, Total-C, and Apo B (Trilipix co-administered with statin compared to corresponding statin monotherapy). Co-administration of Trilipix with statins resulted in the following changes in secondary parameters (Table 6).

[See table 6 at bottom of next page]

A total of 1895 patients who completed 12 weeks of treatment in the double-blind, controlled studies were treated in the 52-week, long-term extension study. Patients received Trilipix co-administered with the moderate-dose of the statin that had been used in the double-blind, controlled study in which they were enrolled. Whether combination therapy was initiated during the double-blind, controlled studies or introduced during the long-term extension study, the treatment effect of combination therapy was observed within four weeks, and was sustained over the duration of treatment in the long-term study. A total of 568 patients completed 52 weeks of treatment with Trilipix co-administered with statins. Mean 52-week values and mean percent change from baseline (at time of enrollment in randomized controlled trials) were 91.7 mg/dL (-38.2%) for LDL-C, 47.3 mg/dL (+24.0%) for HDL-C, 135.5 mg/dL (-47.6%) for TG, 117.9 mg/dL (-45.7%) for non-HDL-C, 26.2 mg/dL (-53.1%) for VLDL-C, 165.2 mg/dL (-35.4%) for Total-C, and 81.4 mg/dL (-43.6%) for Apo B.

14.2 Hypertriglyceridemia

The effects of fenofibrate on serum triglycerides were studied in two randomized, double-blind, placebo-controlled clinical trials of 147 hypertriglyceridemic patients. Patients were treated for eight weeks under protocols that differed only in that one entered patients with baseline TG levels of 500 to 1500 mg/dL, and the other TG levels of 350 to 500 mg/dL. In patients with hypertriglyceridemia and normal cholesterolemia with or without hyperchylomicronemia, treatment with fenofibrate at dosages equivalent to 135 mg once daily of Trilipix decreased primarily VLDL-TG and VLDL-C. Treatment of patients with elevated TG often results in an increase of LDL-C (Table 7).

[See table 7 at bottom of next page]

14.3 Primary Hypercholesterolemia (Heterozygous Familial and Nonfamilial) and Mixed Dyslipidemia

The effects of fenofibrate at a dose equivalent to Trilipix 135 mg once daily were assessed from four randomized, placebo-controlled, double-blind, parallel-group studies including patients with the following mean baseline lipid values: Total-C 306.9 mg/dL; LDL-C 213.8 mg/dL; HDL-C 52.3 mg/dL; and triglycerides 191.0 mg/dL. Fenofibrate therapy lowered LDL-C, Total-C, and the LDL-C/HDL-C ratio. Fenofibrate therapy also lowered triglycerides and raised HDL-C (Table 8).

[See table 8 at bottom of next page]

In a subset of the subjects, measurements of Apo B were conducted. Fenofibrate treatment significantly reduced Apo B from baseline to endpoint as compared with placebo (-25.1% vs. 2.4%; p < 0.0001, n = 213 and 143, respectively).

16 HOW SUPPLIED/STORAGE AND HANDLING

Trilipix (fenofibric acid) delayed release capsules are supplied in two dose strengths as follows:

• Trilipix 45 mg fenofibric acid delayed release capsules have a reddish-brown cap imprinted in white ink the Abbott "A" logo and a yellow body imprinted in black ink the number "45". Each hard gelatin capsule contains enteric coated white to off white bi-convex round mini-tablets. The delayed release capsules are available in bottles of 90 (NDC 0074-9642-90).

• Trilipix 135 mg fenofibric acid delayed release capsules have a blue cap imprinted in white ink the Abbott "A" logo and a yellow body imprinted in black ink the number "135". Each hard gelatin capsule contains enteric coated white to off white bi-convex round mini-tablets. The delayed release capsules are available in bottles of 90 (NDC 0074-9189-90).

Storage and Handling

Store Trilipix 45 and 135 mg delayed release capsules at 25°C (77°F); excursions permitted to 15°–30°C (59° to 86°F) [See USP controlled room temperature]. Keep out of the reach of children. Protect from moisture.

17 PATIENT COUNSELING INFORMATION

See Medication Guide (17.2)

17.1 Patient Counseling

Patients should be advised:

• of the potential benefits and risks of Trilipix.

• to read the Medication Guide before starting Trilipix therapy and to reread it each time the prescription is renewed.

• of medications that should not be taken in combination with Trilipix.

Table 4. Effects of Trilipix or Fenofibrate Co-Administration on Systemic Exposure of Other Drugs

Dosage Regimen of Trilipix or Fenofibrate	Dosage Regimen of Co-Administered Drug	Change in Co-Administered Drug Exposure		
		Analyte	AUC	C_{max}
No dosing adjustments required for these co-administered drugs with Trilipix				
Lipid-lowering agents				
Trilipix 135 mg QD for 10 days	Rosuvastatin, 40 mg QD for 10 days	Rosuvastatin	↑6%	↑20%
Fenofibrate 160 mg[1] QD for 10 days	Atorvastatin, 20 mg QD for 10 days	Atorvastatin	↓17%	0%
Fenofibrate 3 × 67 mg[2] as a single dose	Pravastatin, 40 mg as a single dose	Pravastatin 3α-Hydroxyl-iso-pravastatin	↑13% ↑26%	↑13% ↑29%
Fenofibrate 160 mg[1] QD for 10 days	Pravastatin, 40 mg QD for 10 days	Pravastatin 3α-Hydroxyl-iso-pravastatin	↑28% ↑39%	↑36% ↑55%
Fenofibrate 160 mg[1] as a single dose	Fluvastatin, 40 mg as a single dose	(+)-3R, 5S-Fluvastatin	↑15%	↑16%
Fenofibrate 160 mg[1] QD for 7 days	Simvastatin, 80 mg QD for 7 days	Simvastatin acid Simvastatin Active HMG-CoA Inhibitors Total HMG-CoA Inhibitors	↓36% ↓11% ↓12% ↓8%	↓11% ↓17% ↓1% ↓10%
Fenofibrate 145 mg[1] QD for 10 days	Ezetimibe, 10 mg QD for 10 days	Total Ezetimibe Free Ezetimibe Ezetimibe Glucuronide	↑43% ↑3% ↑49%	↑33% ↑11% ↑34%
Anti-diabetic agents				
Fenofibrate 145 mg[1] QD for 10 days	Glimepiride, 1 mg as a single dose	Glimepiride	↑35%	↑18%
Fenofibrate 54 mg[1] TID for 10 days	Metformin, 850 mg TID for 10 days	Metformin	↑3%	↑6%
Fenofibrate 145 mg[1] QD for 14 days	Rosiglitazone, 8 mg QD for 5 days	Rosiglitazone	↑6%	↓1%

[1] TriCor (fenofibrate) oral tablet
[2] TriCor (fenofibrate) oral micronized capsule

Table 5. Mean Percent Change from Baseline to the Final Value in HDL-C, TG, and LDL-C (Pooled Double-Blind, Controlled Studies)

	Trilipix	Low-Dose Statin	Trilipix + Low-Dose Statin	Between-group Δ (p-value)	Moderate-Dose Statin	Trilipix + Moderate-Dose Statin	Between-group Δ (p-value)	High-Dose Statin
HDL-C (mg/dL)	(N = 420)	(N = 455)	(N = 423)		(N = 430)	(N = 422)		(N = 217)
BL mean	38.4	38.4	38.2		38.4	38.1		38.0
Mean % Δ	16.3%	7.4%	18.1%	10.7%[a] (< 0.001)	8.7%	17.5%	8.8%[a] (< 0.001)	7.9%
TG (mg/dL)	(N = 459)	(N = 477)	(N = 470)		(N = 472)	(N = 462)		(N = 235)
BL mean	280.7	286.1	282.1		287.9	286.1		282.5
Mean % Δ	-31.0%	-16.8%	-43.9%	-27.2%[a] (< 0.001)	-23.7%	-42.0%	-18.3%[a] (< 0.001)	-28.1%
LDL-C (mg/dL)	(N = 427)	(N = 463)	(N = 436)		(N = 439)	(N = 434)		(N = 225)
BL mean	158.4	153.8	155.7		158.0	156.4		156.1
Mean % Δ	-5.1%	-33.9%	-33.1%	-28.0%[b] (< 0.001)	-40.6%	-34.6%	-29.5%[b] (< 0.001)	-47.1%

[a] Combination therapy vs. corresponding statin monotherapy
[b] Combination therapy vs. Trilipix monotherapy
Low-dose statin = rosuvastatin 10 mg, simvastatin 20 mg, or atorvastatin 20 mg
Moderate-dose statin = rosuvastatin 20 mg, simvastatin 40 mg, or atorvastatin 40 mg
High-dose statin = rosuvastatin 40 mg, simvastatin 80 mg, or atorvastatin 80 mg
BL = Baseline
% Δ = Percent change from baseline to final value

• to continue to follow an appropriate lipid-modifying diet while taking Trilipix.

• to take Trilipix once daily, without regard to food, at the prescribed dose, swallowing each capsule whole. If Trilipix is co-administered with a statin, they may be taken together.

• to return for routine monitoring.

• to inform their physician of all medications, supplements, and herbal preparations they are taking and any change to their medical condition. Patients should also be advised to inform their physicians prescribing a new medication that they are taking Trilipix.

• to inform their physician of any muscle pain, tenderness, or weakness; onset of abdominal pain; or any other new symptoms.

©Abbott

03-A199-R2
Revised: December, 2008
Manufactured for Abbott Laboratories, North Chicago, IL 60064, U.S.A. by Fournier Laboratories Ireland Limited, Anngrove, Carrigtwohill Co. Cork, Ireland, or Abbott Pharmaceutical PR Ltd., Barceloneta, PR 00617.

17.2 Medication Guide

MEDICATION GUIDE

Trilipix

(try-lip-iks)

(fenofibric acid, delayed release capsules)

Read this Medication Guide before you start taking Trilipix and each time you get a refill. There may be new information. This information does not take the place of talking to your healthcare provider about your medical condition or your treatment.

What is the most important information I should know about Trilipix?

Trilipix can be used with other cholesterol-lowering medicines called statins. Statins include:

- atorvastatin (Lipitor, Caduet)
- fluvastatin (Lescol, Lescol XL)
- lovastatin (Altoprev, Mevacor, Advicor)
- pravastatin (Pravachol)
- rosuvastatin (Crestor)
- simvastatin (Zocor, Simcor, Vytorin)

Statins can cause muscle pain, tenderness or weakness, which may be symptoms of a rare but serious muscle condition called rhabdomyolysis. In some cases rhabdomyolysis can cause kidney damage and death. The risk of rhabdomyolysis may be higher when Trilipix is given with statins. If you take a statin, tell your healthcare provider.

Other medicines or large amounts of grapefruit juice (more than a quart) may raise the levels of statins in your body, and could then raise the risk of muscle problems. Tell your healthcare provider if you are taking any medicines listed below.

- Heart medicine
- Stomach medicine
- Antibiotic
- Anti-fungal
- Cholesterol-lowering medicine
- Hormones
- HIV/AIDS medicine
- Antidepressant
- Immunosuppressant
- Anti-seizure medicine

Ask your healthcare provider or pharmacist for a list of these medicines, if you are not sure.

Tell your healthcare provider if you drink grapefruit juice.

What is Trilipix?

Trilipix is a prescription medicine used to treat cholesterol in the blood by lowering the total amount of triglycerides and LDL (bad) cholesterol, and increasing the HDL (good) cholesterol. You should be on a low fat and low cholesterol diet while you take Trilipix.

The safety and effectiveness of Trilipix in children is not known.

Who should not take Trilipix?

Do not take Trilipix if you:

- are allergic to fenofibric acid, or any of the ingredients in Trilipix. See the end of this Medication Guide for a list of all the ingredients in Trilipix.
- have severe kidney disease.
- have liver disease.
- have gallbladder disease.
- are a nursing mother.

Talk to your healthcare provider before you take Trilipix if you have any of these conditions.

What should I tell my healthcare provider before taking Trilipix?

Before taking Trilipix, tell your healthcare provider about all your medical conditions, including if you:

- are allergic to any medicines.
- have ever had kidney problems.
- have ever had liver problems.
- have ever had gallbladder problems.
- are pregnant or if you plan to become pregnant. It is not known if Trilipix will harm your unborn baby.
- are breastfeeding or plan to breastfeed. It is not known if Trilipix passes into your breast milk. You and your healthcare provider should decide if you will take Trilipix or breastfeed. You should not do both.

Tell your healthcare provider about all the medicines you take, including prescription and non-prescription medicines, vitamins and herbal supplements.

Using Trilipix with certain other medicines can affect the way these medicines work and other medicines may affect how Trilipix works. In some cases, using Trilipix with other medicines can cause serious side effects.

Know all the medicines you take. Keep a list of them and show it to your healthcare provider when you get a new medicine.

It is especially important to tell your healthcare provider if you take any of the medicines mentioned in, "What is the most important information I should know about Trilipix?"or any of the medicines listed below:

- **anticoagulants**, also known as blood thinners (warfarin, Coumadin)
- **bile acid resins**
- **cyclosporine**

Ask your healthcare provider if you are not sure if your medicine is one of these.

How should I take Trilipix?

- You should be on a low fat and low cholesterol diet while you take Trilipix.
- Take Trilipix one time each day as prescribed by your healthcare provider.
- Take Trilipix with or without food.
- Swallow Trilipix capsules whole. Do not break, crush, dissolve, or chew Trilipix capsules before swallowing. If you cannot swallow Trilipix capsules whole, tell your healthcare provider, you may need a different medicine.
- If you take a medicine called a statin, you can take Trilipix and your statin at the same time of day.
- If you miss a dose of Trilipix, take it as soon as you remember. If it is almost time for your next dose, just skip the missed dose. Take the next dose at your regular time. If you are not sure about your dosing, call your healthcare provider. **Do not take more than one dose of Trilipix a day unless your healthcare provider tells you to.**
- If you take too much Trilipix, contact your healthcare provider or your local emergency department.
- Do not change your dose or stop Trilipix unless your healthcare provider tells you to.

Table 6. Percent Change from Baseline to the Final Value in Non-HDL-C, VLDL-C, Total-C, and Apo B (Pooled Double-Blind, Controlled Studies)

Secondary Endpoints	Trilipix	Low-Dose Statin	Trilipix + Low-Dose Statin	Between-group Δ	Moderate-Dose Statin	Trilipix + Moderate-Dose Statin	Between-group Δ	High-Dose Statin
Non HDL-C								
(mg/dL)	(N = 420)	(N = 454)	(N = 422)		(N = 431)	(N = 420)		(N = 217)
BL mean	222.5	217.6	219.9		222.4	218.9		220.2
Mean % Δ	-17.3%	-34.9%	-40.4%	-23.1%[a] -5.5%[b]	-42.4%	-42.0%	-24.8%[a] 0.4%[b]	-47.3%
VLDL-C								
(mg/dL)	(N = 449)	(N = 463)	(N = 455)		(N = 458)	(N = 449)		(N = 232)
BL mean	65.0	66.0	65.5		67.8	64.5		66.1
Mean % Δ	-34.2%	-32.1%	-50.0%	-18.0%[b]	-38.9%	-51.2%	-12.3%[b]	-42.1%
Total-C								
(mg/dL)	(N = 459)	(N = 477)	(N = 469)		(N = 472)	(N = 462)		(N = 235)
BL mean	260.9	257.0	258.6		261.3	257.3		258.8
Mean % Δ	-12.4%	-28.7%	-31.5%	-2.8%[b]	-34.7%	-33.3%	1.4%[b]	-39.5%
Apo B								
(mg/dL)	(N = 455)	(N = 470)	(N = 465)		(N = 468)	(N = 455)		(N = 229)
BL mean	146.2	145.0	146.1		147.1	145.0		146.0
Mean % Δ	-15.6%	-31.1%	-36.3%	-5.2%[b]	-36.9%	-36.7%	0.2%[b]	-42.4%

[a] Trilipix + statin vs. Trilipix monotherapy
[b] Trilipix + statin vs. corresponding statin monotherapy
Low-dose statin = rosuvastatin 10 mg, simvastatin 20 mg, or atorvastatin 20 mg
Moderate-dose statin = rosuvastatin 20 mg, simvastatin 40 mg, or atorvastatin 40 mg
High-dose statin = rosuvastatin 40 mg, simvastatin 80 mg, or atorvastatin 80 mg
BL = Baseline
% Δ = Percent change from baseline to final value

Table 7. Effects of Fenofibrate in Patients With Hypertriglyceridemia

Study 1	Placebo					Fenofibrate			
Baseline TG levels 350 to 499 mg/dL	N	Baseline Mean (mg/dL)	Endpoint Mean (mg/dL)	Mean % Change		N	Baseline Mean (mg/dL)	Endpoint Mean (mg/dL)	Mean % Change
Triglycerides	28	449	450	-0.5		27	432	223	-46.2*
VLDL Triglycerides	19	367	350	2.7		19	350	178	-44.1*
Total Cholesterol	28	255	261	2.8		27	252	227	-9.1*
HDL Cholesterol	28	35	36	4		27	34	40	19.6*
LDL Cholesterol	28	120	129	12		27	128	137	14.5
VLDL Cholesterol	27	99	99	5.8		27	92	46	-44.7*
Study 2	**Placebo**					**Fenofibrate**			
Baseline TG levels 500 to 1500 mg/dL	N	Baseline Mean (mg/dL)	Endpoint Mean (mg/dL)	Mean % Change		N	Baseline Mean (mg/dL)	Endpoint Mean (mg/dL)	Mean % Change
Triglycerides	44	710	750	7.2		48	726	308	-54.5*
VLDL Triglycerides	29	537	571	18.7		33	543	205	-50.6*
Total Cholesterol	44	272	271	0.4		48	261	223	-13.8*
HDL Cholesterol	44	27	28	5.0		48	30	36	22.9*
LDL Cholesterol	42	100	90	-4.2		45	103	131	45.0*
VLDL Cholesterol	42	137	142	11.0		45	126	54	-49.4*

* = p < 0.05 vs. Placebo

Table 8. Mean Percent Change in Lipid Parameters at End of Treatment[†]

Treatment Group	Total-C (mg/dL)	LDL-C (mg/dL)	HDL-C (mg/dL)	TG (mg/dL)
Pooled Cohort				
Mean baseline lipid values (n = 646)	306.9	213.8	52.3	191.0
All Fenofibrate (n = 361)	-18.7%*	-20.6%*	+11.0%*	-28.9%*
Placebo (n = 285)	-0.4%	-2.2%	+0.7%	+7.7%
Baseline LDL-C > 160 mg/dL and TG < 150 mg/dL				
Mean baseline lipid values (n = 334)	307.7	227.7	58.1	101.7
All Fenofibrate (n = 193)	-22.4%*	-31.4%*	+9.8%*	-23.5%*
Placebo (n = 141)	+0.2%	-2.2%	+2.6%	+11.7%
Baseline LDL-C > 160 mg/dL and TG ≥ 150 mg/dL				
Mean baseline lipid values (n = 242)	312.8	219.8	46.7	231.9
All Fenofibrate (n = 126)	-16.8%*	-20.1%*	+14.6%*	-35.9%*
Placebo (n = 116)	-3.0%	-6.6%	+2.3%	+0.9%

[†] Duration of study treatment was 3 to 6 months
* p = < 0.05 vs. Placebo

Information on the Abbott Pharmaceutical Products listed on these pages is from the prescribing information as of June 1, 2010. For more information, please visit rxabbott.com or call 1-800-633-9110.

- Your healthcare provider may do blood tests before you start taking Trilipix and during treatment. See your healthcare provider regularly to check your cholesterol and triglyceride levels and to check for side effects.

What are the possible side effects with Trilipix?
Trilipix may cause serious side effects, including:
- **muscle pain, tenderness, or weakness.** See "What is the most important information that I should know about Trilipix?"
- **tiredness and fever.**
- **abdominal pain, nausea, or vomiting.** These may be signs of inflammation (swelling) of the gallbladder or pancreas.

Call your healthcare provider right away if you have any of these serious side effects.
The most common side effects with Trilipix include:
- headache
- heartburn (indigestion)
- nausea
- muscle aches
- increases in muscle or liver enzymes that are measured by blood tests

Tell your healthcare provider if you have any side effect that bothers you or that does not go away. These are not all the possible side effects of Trilipix. For more information, ask your healthcare provider or pharmacist.

Call your doctor for medical advice about side effects. You may report side effects to FDA at 1-800-FDA-1088.

How do I store Trilipix?
- Store Trilipix between 59° to 86° F (15° to 30° C).
- Protect Trilipix from moisture.

Keep Trilipix and all medicines out of the reach of children.

General information about the safe and effective use of Trilipix
Medicines are sometimes prescribed for conditions that are not mentioned in the Medication Guide. Do not use Trilipix for a condition for which it was not prescribed. Do not give Trilipix to other people, even if they have the same condition you have. It may harm them.

This Medication Guide summarizes the most important information about Trilipix. If you would like more information, talk to your healthcare provider. You can also ask your pharmacist or healthcare provider for information that is written for health professionals.

For more information go to www.Trilipix.com or call 1-800-633-9110.

What are the ingredients in Trilipix?
Active Ingredient: Fenofibric acid
Inactive Ingredients: Hypromellose, povidone, water, hydroxylpropyl cellulose, colloidal silicon dioxide, sodium stearyl fumarate, methacrylic acid copolymer, talc, triethyl citrate, gelatin, titanium dioxide, and yellow iron oxide. Additionally, the 45 mg capsule shell contains black iron oxide and red iron oxide, and the 135 mg capsule shell contains FD&C Blue #2.

©Abbott
03-A199-R2
Revised: December, 2008
Manufactured for Abbott Laboratories, North Chicago, IL 60064, U.S.A. by Fournier Laboratories Ireland Limited, Anngrove, Carrigtwohill Co. Cork, Ireland, or Abbott Pharmaceutical PR Ltd., Barceloneta, PR 00617.
This Medication Guide has been approved by the U.S. Food and Drug Administration.

Shown in Product Identification Guide, page 304

ULTANE® ℞
[ul-tān]
(sevoflurane)
volatile liquid for inhalation

DESCRIPTION
ULTANE (sevoflurane), volatile liquid for inhalation, a nonflammable and nonexplosive liquid administered by vaporization, is a halogenated general inhalation anesthetic drug. Sevoflurane is fluoromethyl 2,2,2,-trifluoro-1-(trifluoromethyl) ethyl ether and its structural formula is:

$$\begin{array}{c} F_3C \\ | \\ H-C-OCH_2F \\ | \\ F_3C \end{array}$$

Sevoflurane, Physical Constants are:

Molecular weight	200.05
Boiling point at 760 mm Hg	58.6°C
Specific gravity at 20°C	1.520-1.525
Vapor pressure in mm Hg	157 mm Hg at 20°C
	197 mm Hg at 25°C
	317 mm Hg at 36°C

Distribution Partition Coefficients at 37°C:

Blood/Gas	0.63-0.69
Water/Gas	0.36
Olive Oil/Gas	47-54
Brain/Gas	1.15

Mean Component/Gas Partition Coefficients at 25°C for Polymers Used Commonly in Medical Applications:

Conductive rubber	14.0
Butyl rubber	7.7
Polyvinylchloride	17.4
Polyethylene	1.3

Sevoflurane is nonflammable and nonexplosive as defined by the requirements of International Electrotechnical Commission 601-2-13.

Sevoflurane is a clear, colorless, liquid containing no additives. Sevoflurane is not corrosive to stainless steel, brass, aluminum, nickel-plated brass, chrome-plated brass or copper beryllium. Sevoflurane is nonpungent. It is miscible with ethanol, ether, chloroform, and benzene, and it is slightly soluble in water. Sevoflurane is stable when stored under normal room lighting conditions according to instructions. No discernible degradation of sevoflurane occurs in the presence of strong acids or heat. When in contact with alkaline CO_2 absorbents (e.g. Baralyme® and to a lesser extent soda lime) within the anesthesia machine, sevoflurane can undergo degradation under certain conditions. Degradation of sevoflurane is minimal, and degradants are either undetectable or present in non-toxic amounts when used as directed with fresh absorbents. Sevoflurane degradation and subsequent degradant formation are enhanced by increasing absorbent temperature increased sevoflurane concentration, decreased fresh gas flow and desiccated CO_2 absorbents (especially with potassium hydroxide containing absorbents e.g. Baralyme).

Sevoflurane alkaline degradation occurs by two pathways. The first results from the loss of hydrogen fluoride with the formation of pentafluoroisopropenyl fluoromethyl ether, (PIFE, $C_4H_2F_6O$), also known as Compound A, and trace amounts of pentafluoromethoxy isopropyl fluoromethyl ether, (PMFE, $C_5H_6F_6O$), also known as Compound B. The second pathway for degradation of sevoflurane, which occurs primarily in the presence of desiccated CO_2 absorbents, is discussed later.

In the first pathway, the defluorination pathway, the production of degradants in the anesthesia circuit results from the extraction of the acidic proton in the presence of a strong base (KOH and/or NaOH) forming an alkene (Compound A) from sevoflurane similar to formation of 2-bromo-2-chloro-1,1-difluoro ethylene (BCDFE) from halothane. Laboratory simulations have shown that the concentration of these degradants is inversely correlated with the fresh gas flow rate (See Figure 1).

Figure 1. Fresh Gas Flow Rate versus Compound A Levels in a Circle Absorber System

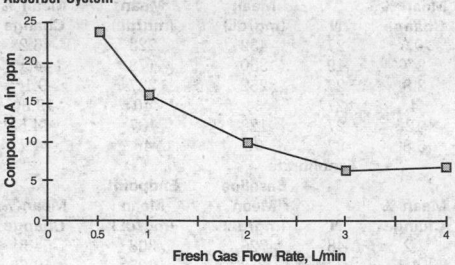

Since the reaction of carbon dioxide with absorbents is exothermic, the temperature increase will be determined by quantities of CO_2 absorbed, which in turn will depend on fresh gas flow in the anesthesia circle system, metabolic status of the patient, and ventilation. The relationship of temperature produced by varying levels of CO_2 and Compound A production is illustrated in the following *in vitro* simulation where CO_2 was added to a circle absorber system.

Figure 2. Carbon Dioxide Flow Versus Compound A and Maximum Temperature

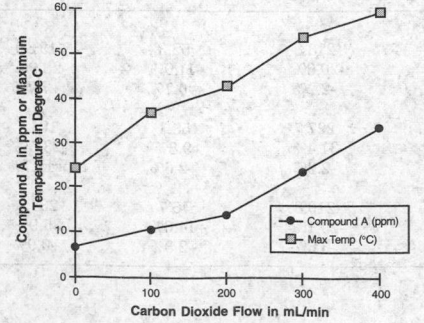

Compound A concentration in a circle absorber system increases as a function of increasing CO_2 absorbent temperature and composition (Baralyme producing higher levels than soda lime), increased body temperature, and increased minute ventilation, and decreasing fresh gas flow rates. It has been reported that the concentration of Compound A increases significantly with prolonged dehydration of Baralyme. Compound A exposure in patients also has been shown to rise with increased sevoflurane concentrations and duration of anesthesia. In a clinical study in which sevoflurane was administered to patients under low flow conditions for ≥ 2 hours at flow rates of 1 Liter/minute, Compound A levels were measured in an effort to determine the relationship between MAC hours and Compound A levels produced. The relationship between Compound A levels and sevoflurane exposure are shown in Figure 2a.

Figure 2a. ppm•hr versus MAC•hr at Flow Rate of 1 L/min

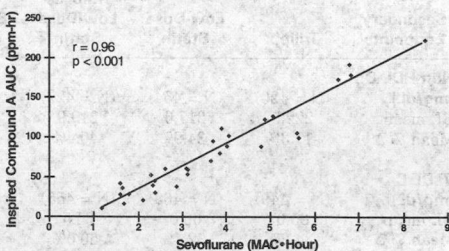

Compound A has been shown to be nephrotoxic in rats after exposures that have varied in duration from one to three hours. No histopathologic change was seen at a concentration of up to 270 ppm for one hour. Sporadic single cell necrosis of proximal tubule cells has been reported at a concentration of 114 ppm after a 3-hour exposure to Compound A in rats. The LC_{50} reported at 1 hour is 1050-1090 ppm (male-female) and, at 3 hours, 350-490 ppm (male-female).

An experiment was performed comparing sevoflurane plus 75 or 100 ppm Compound A with an active control to evaluate the potential nephrotoxicity of Compound A in non-human primates. A single 8-hour exposure of Sevoflurane in the presence of Compound A produced single-cell renal tubular degeneration and single-cell necrosis in cynomolgus monkeys. These changes are consistent with the increased urinary protein, glucose level and enzymic activity noted on days one and three on the clinical pathology evaluation. This nephrotoxicity produced by Compound A is dose and duration of exposure dependent.

At a fresh gas flow rate of 1 L/min, mean maximum concentrations of Compound A in the anesthesia circuit in clinical settings are approximately 20 ppm (0.002%) with soda lime and 30 ppm (0.003%) with Baralyme in adult patients; mean maximum concentrations in pediatric patients with soda lime are about half those found in adults. The highest concentration observed in a single patient with Baralyme was 61 ppm (0.0061%) and 32 ppm (0.0032%) with soda lime. The levels of Compound A at which toxicity occurs in humans is not known.

The second pathway for degradation of sevoflurane occurs primarily in the presence of desiccated CO_2 absorbents and leads to the dissociation of sevoflurane into hexafluoroisopropanol (HFIP) and formaldehyde. HFIP is inactive, nongenotoxic, rapidly glucuronidated and cleared by the liver. Formaldehyde is present during normal metabolic processes. Upon exposure to a highly desiccated absorbent, formaldehyde can further degrade into methanol and formate. Formate can contribute to the formation of carbon monoxide in the presence of high temperature that can be associated with desiccated Baralyme®. Methanol can react with Compound A to form the methoxy addition product Compound B. Compound B can undergo further HF elimination to form Compounds C, D, and E.

Sevoflurane degradants were observed in the respiratory circuit of an experimental anesthesia machine using desiccated CO_2 absorbents and maximum sevoflurane concentrations (8%) for extended periods of time (> 2 hours). Concentrations of formaldehyde observed with desiccated soda lime in this experimental anesthesia respiratory circuit were consistent with levels that could potentially result in respiratory irritation. Although KOH containing CO_2 absorbents are no longer commercially available, in the laboratory experiments, exposure of sevoflurane to the desiccated KOH containing CO_2 absorbent, Baralyme, resulted in the detection of substantially greater degradant levels.

CLINICAL PHARMACOLOGY
Sevoflurane is an inhalational anesthetic agent for use in induction and maintenance of general anesthesia. Minimum alveolar concentration (MAC) of sevoflurane in oxygen for a 40-year-old adult is 2.1%. The MAC of sevoflurane decreases with age (see **DOSAGE AND ADMINISTRATION** for details).

Pharmacokinetics

Uptake and Distribution

Solubility

Because of the low solubility of sevoflurane in blood (blood/gas partition coefficient @ 37°C = 0.63-0.69), a minimal amount of sevoflurane is required to be dissolved in the blood before the alveolar partial pressure is in equilibrium with the arterial partial pressure. Therefore there is a rapid rate of increase in the alveolar (end-tidal) concentration (F_A) toward the inspired concentration (F_I) during induction.

Induction of Anesthesia

In a study in which seven healthy male volunteers were administered 70% N_2O/30%O_2 for 30 minutes followed by 1.0% sevoflurane and 0.6% isoflurane for another 30 minutes the F_A/F_I ratio was greater for sevoflurane than isoflurane at all time points. The time for the concentration in the alveoli to reach 50% of the inspired concentration was 4-8 minutes for isoflurane and approximately 1 minute for sevoflurane. F_A/F_I data from this study were compared with F_A/F_I data of other halogenated anesthetic agents from another study. When all data were normalized to isoflurane, the uptake and distribution of sevoflurane was shown to be faster than isoflurane and halothane, but slower than desflurane. The results are depicted in Figure 3.

Recovery from Anesthesia

The low solubility of sevoflurane facilitates rapid elimination via the lungs. The rate of elimination is quantified as the rate of change of the alveolar (end-tidal) concentration following termination of anesthesia (F_A), relative to the last alveolar concentration (Fa_O) measured immediately before discontinuance of the anesthetic. In the healthy volunteer study described above, rate of elimination of sevoflurane was similar compared with desflurane, but faster compared with either halothane or isoflurane. These results are depicted in Figure 4.

Figure 3. Ratio of Concentration of Anesthetic in Alveolar Gas to Inspired Gas

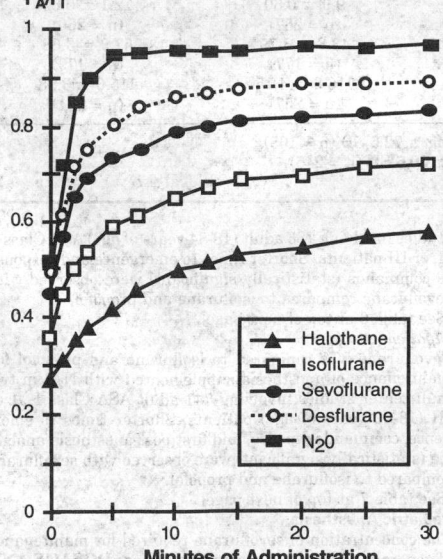

[See figure at top of next column]
Yasuda N, Lockhart S, Eger EI II, et al: Comparison of kinetics of sevoflurane and isoflurane in humans. Anesth Analg 72:316, 1991.

Protein Binding

The effects of sevoflurane on the displacement of drugs from serum and tissue proteins have not been investigated. Other fluorinated volatile anesthetics have been shown to displace drugs from serum and tissue proteins *in vitro*. The clinical significance of this is unknown. Clinical studies have shown no untoward effects when sevoflurane is administered to patients taking drugs that are highly bound and have a small volume of distribution (e.g., phenytoin).

Metabolism

Sevoflurane is metabolized by cytochrome P450 2E1, to hexafluoroisopropanol (HFIP) with release of inorganic fluoride and CO_2. Once formed HFIP is rapidly conjugated with glucuronic acid and eliminated as a urinary metabolite. No other metabolic pathways for sevoflurane have been identified. *In vivo* metabolism studies suggest that approximately 5% of the sevoflurane dose may be metabolized. Cytochrome P450 2E1 is the principal isoform identified for sevoflurane metabolism and this may be induced by chronic exposure to isoniazid and ethanol. This is similar to the me-

Table 1. Fluoride Ion Estimates in Special Populations Following Administration of Sevoflurane

	n	Age (yr)	Duration (hr)	Dose (MAC·hr)	C_{max} (µM)
PEDIATRIC PATIENTS					
Anesthetic					
Sevoflurane-O_2	76	0-11	0.8	1.1	12.6
Sevoflurane-O_2	40	1-11	2.2	3.0	16.0
Sevoflurane/N_2O	25	5-13	1.9	2.4	21.3
Sevoflurane/N_2O	42	0-18	2.4	2.2	18.4
Sevoflurane/N_2O	40	1-11	2.0	2.6	15.5
ELDERLY	33	65-93	2.6	1.4	25.6
RENAL	21	29-83	2.5	1.0	26.1
HEPATIC	8	42-79	3.6	2.2	30.6
OBESE	35	24-73	3.0	1.7	38.0

n = number of patients studied.

Figure 4. Concentration of Anesthetic in Alveolar Gas Following Termination of Anesthesia

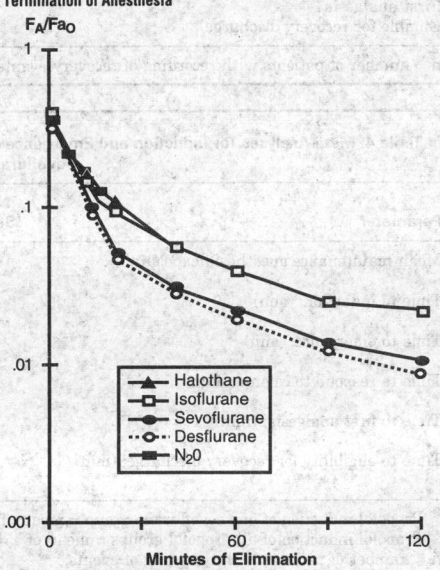

tabolism of isoflurane and enflurane and is distinct from that of methoxyflurane which is metabolized via a variety of cytochrome P450 isoforms. The metabolism of sevoflurane is not inducible by barbiturates. As shown in Figure 5, inorganic fluoride concentrations peak within 2 hours of the end of sevoflurane anesthesia and return to baseline concentrations within 48 hours post-anesthesia in the majority of cases (67%). The rapid and extensive pulmonary elimination of sevoflurane minimizes the amount of anesthetic available for metabolism.

Figure 5. Serum Inorganic Fluoride Concentrations for Sevoflurane and Other Volatile Anesthetics

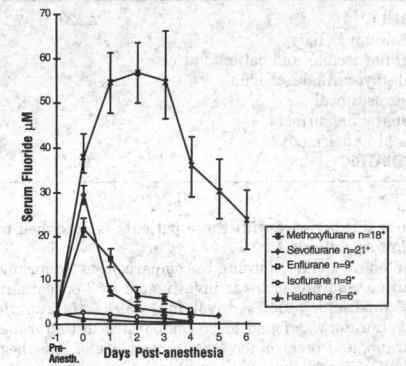

Cousins M.J., Greenstein L.R., Hitt B.A., et al: Metabolism and renal effects of enflurane in man. Anesthesiology 44:44; 1976* and Sevo-93-044+.

Legend:

Pre-Anesth. = Pre-anesthesia

Elimination

Up to 3.5% of the sevoflurane dose appears in the urine as inorganic fluoride. Studies on fluoride indicate that up to 50% of fluoride clearance is nonrenal (via fluoride being taken up into bone).

Pharmacokinetics of Fluoride Ion

Fluoride ion concentrations are influenced by the duration of anesthesia, the concentration of sevoflurane adminis-

tered, and the composition of the anesthetic gas mixture. In studies where anesthesia was maintained purely with sevoflurane for periods ranging from 1 to 6 hours, peak fluoride concentrations ranged between 12 µM and 90 µM. As shown in Figure 6, peak concentrations occur within 2 hours of the end of anesthesia and are less than 25 µM (475 ng/mL) for the majority of the population after 10 hours. The half-life is in the range of 15-23 hours.

It has been reported that following administration of methoxyflurane, serum inorganic fluoride concentrations > 50 µM were correlated with the development of vasopressin-resistant, polyuric, renal failure. In clinical trials with sevoflurane, there were no reports of toxicity associated with elevated fluoride ion levels.

Figure 6. Fluoride Ion Concentrations Following Administration of Sevoflurane (mean MAC = 1.27, mean duration = 2.06 hr) Mean Fluoride Ion Concentrations (n = 48)

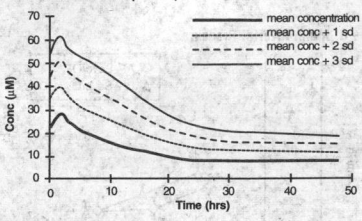

Fluoride Concentrations After Repeat Exposure and in Special Populations

Fluoride concentrations have been measured after single, extended, and repeat exposure to sevoflurane in normal surgical and special patient populations, and pharmacokinetic parameters were determined.

Compared with healthy individuals, the fluoride ion half-life was prolonged in patients with renal impairment, but not in the elderly. A study in 8 patients with hepatic impairment suggests a slight prolongation of the half-life. The mean half-life in patients with renal impairment averaged approximately 33 hours (range 21-61 hours) as compared to a mean of approximately 21 hours (range 10-48 hours) in normal healthy individuals. The mean half-life in the elderly (greater than 65 years) approximated 24 hours (range 18-72 hours). The mean half-life in individuals with hepatic impairment was 23 hours (range 16-47 hours). Mean maximal fluoride values (C_{max}) determined in individual studies of special populations are displayed below.

[See table above]

Pharmacodynamics

Changes in the depth of sevoflurane anesthesia rapidly follow changes in the inspired concentration.

In the sevoflurane clinical program, the following recovery variables were evaluated:

1. Time to events measured from the end of study drug:
- Time to removal of the endotracheal tube (extubation time)
- Time required for the patient to open his/her eyes on verbal command (emergence time)
- Time to respond to simple command (e.g., squeeze my hand) or demonstrates purposeful movement (response to command time, orientation time)

2. Recovery of cognitive function and motor coordination was evaluated based on:
- psychomotor performance tests (Digit Symbol Substitution Test [DSST], Treiger Dot Test)
- the results of subjective (Visual Analog Scale [VAS]) and objective (objective pain-discomfort scale [OPDS]) measurements

Information on the Abbott Pharmaceutical Products listed on these pages is from the prescribing information in use as of June 1, 2010. For more information, please visit rxabbott.com or call 1-800-633-9110.

- time to administration of the first post-anesthesia analgesic medication
- assessments of post-anesthesia patient status

3. Other recovery times were:
- time to achieve an Aldrete Score of ≥ 8
- time required for the patient to be eligible for discharge from the recovery area, per standard criteria at site
- time when the patient was eligible for discharge from the hospital
- time when the patient was able to sit up or stand without dizziness

Some of these variables are summarized as follows:
[See table 2 at right]
[See table 3 at right]
[See table 4 at right]

Cardiovascular Effects

Sevoflurane was studied in 14 healthy volunteers (18-35 years old) comparing sevoflurane-O_2 (Sevo/O_2) to sevoflurane-N_2O/O_2 (Sevo/N_2O/O_2) during 7 hours of anesthesia. During controlled ventilation, hemodynamic parameters measured are shown in Figures 7-10:

Figure 7. Heart Rate

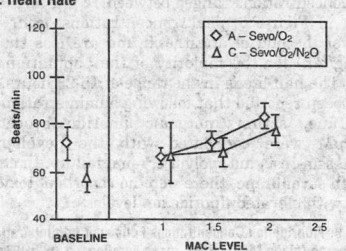

Figure 8. Mean Arterial Pressure

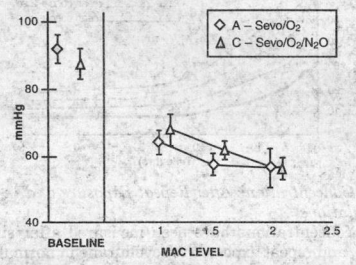

Figure 9. Systemic Vascular Resistance

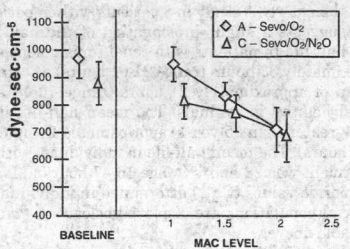

Figure 10. Cardiac Index

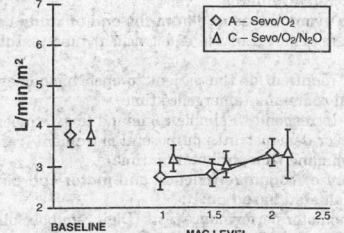

Sevoflurane is a dose-related cardiac depressant. Sevoflurane does not produce increases in heart rate at doses less than 2 MAC.

A study investigating the epinephrine induced arrhythmogenic effect of sevoflurane versus isoflurane in adult patients undergoing transsphenoidal hypophysectomy demonstrated that the threshold dose of epinephrine (i.e., the dose at which the first sign of arrhythmia was observed) producing multiple ventricular arrhythmias was 5 mcg/kg with

Table 2. Induction and Recovery Variables for Evaluable Pediatric Patients in Two Comparative Studies: Sevoflurane versus Halothane

Time to End-Point (min)	Sevoflurane Mean ± SEM	Halothane Mean ± SEM
Induction	2.0 ± 0.2 (n = 294)	2.7 ± 0.2 (n = 252)
Emergence	11.3 ± 0.7 (n = 293)	15.8 ± 0.8 (n = 252)
Response to command	13.7 ± 1.0 (n = 271)	19.3 ± 1.1 (n = 230)
First analgesia	52.2 ± 8.5 (n = 216)	67.6 ± 10.6 (n = 150)
Eligible for recovery discharge	76.5 ± 2.0 (n = 292)	81.1 ± 1.9 (n = 246)

n = number of patients with recording of events.

Table 3. Recovery Variables for Evaluable Adult Patients in Two Comparative Studies: Sevoflurane versus Isoflurane

Time to Parameter: (min)	Sevoflurane Mean ± SEM	Isoflurane Mean ± SEM
Emergence	7.7 ± 0.3 (n = 395)	9.1 ± 0.3 (n = 348)
Response to command	8.1 ± 0.3 (n = 395)	9.7 ± 0.3 (n = 345)
First analgesia	42.7 ± 3.0 (n = 269)	52.9 ± 4.2 (n = 228)
Eligible for recovery discharge	87.6 ± 5.3 (n = 244)	79.1 ± 5.2 (n = 252)

n = number of patients with recording of recovery events.

Table 4. Meta-Analyses for Induction and Emergence Variables for Evaluable Adult Patients in Comparative Studies: Sevoflurane versus Propofol

Parameter	No. of Studies	Sevoflurane Mean ± SEM	Propofol Mean ± SEM
Mean maintenance anesthesia exposure	3	1.0 MAC•hr. ± 0.8 (n = 259)	7.2 mg/kg/hr ± 2.6 (n = 258)
Time to induction: (min)	1	3.1 ± 0.18* (n = 93)	2.2 ± 0.18** (n = 93)
Time to emergence: (min)	3	8.6 ± 0.57 (n = 255)	11.0 ± 0.57 (n = 260)
Time to respond to command: (min)	3	9.9 ± 0.60 (n = 257)	12.1 ± 0.60 (n = 260)
Time to first analgesia: (min)	3	43.8 ± 3.79 (n = 177)	57.9 ± 3.68 (n = 179)
Time to eligibility for recovery discharge: (min)	3	116.0 ± 4.15 (n = 257)	115.6 ± 3.98 (n = 261)

* Propofol induction of one sevoflurane group = mean of 178.8 mg ± 72.5 SD (n = 165)
**Propofol induction of all propofol groups = mean of 170.2 mg ± 60.6 SD (n = 245)
n = number of patients with recording of events.

both sevoflurane and isoflurane. Consequently, the interaction of sevoflurane with epinephrine appears to be equal to that seen with isoflurane.

Clinical Trials

Sevoflurane was administered to a total of 3185 patients prior to sevoflurane NDA submission. The types of patients are summarized as follows:

Table 5. Patients Receiving Sevoflurane in Clinical Trials

Type of Patients	Number Studied
ADULT	2223
Cesarean Delivery	29
Cardiovascular and patients at risk of myocardial ischemia	246
Neurosurgical	22
Hepatic impairment	8
Renal impairment	35
PEDIATRIC	962

Clinical experience with these patients is described below.

Adult Anesthesia

The efficacy of sevoflurane in comparison to isoflurane, enflurane, and propofol was investigated in 3 outpatient and 25 inpatient studies involving 3591 adult patients. Sevoflurane was found to be comparable to isoflurane, enflurane, and propofol for the maintenance of anesthesia in adult patients. Patients administered sevoflurane showed shorter times (statistically significant) to some recovery events (extubation, response to command, and orientation) than patients who received isoflurane or propofol.

Mask Induction

Sevoflurane has a nonpungent odor and does not cause respiratory irritability. Sevoflurane is suitable for mask induction in adults. In 196 patients, mask induction was smooth and rapid, with complications occurring with the following frequencies: cough, 6%; breathholding, 6%; agitation, 6%; laryngospasm, 5%.

Ambulatory Surgery

Sevoflurane was compared to isoflurane and propofol for maintenance of anesthesia supplemented with N_2O in two

studies involving 786 adult (18-84 years of age) ASA Class I, II, or III patients. Shorter times to emergence and response to commands (statistically significant) were observed with sevoflurane compared to isoflurane and propofol.
[See table 6 at top of next page]

Inpatient Surgery

Sevoflurane was compared to isoflurane and propofol for maintenance of anesthesia supplemented with N_2O in two multicenter studies involving 741 adult ASA Class I, II or III (18-92 years of age) patients. Shorter times to emergence, command response, and first post-anesthesia analgesia (statistically significant) were observed with sevoflurane compared to isoflurane and propofol.
[See table 7 at top of next page]

Pediatric Anesthesia

The concentration of sevoflurane required for maintenance of general anesthesia is age-dependent (see **DOSAGE AND ADMINISTRATION**). Sevoflurane or halothane was used to anesthetize 1620 pediatric patients aged 1 day to 18 years, and ASA physical status I or II (948 sevoflurane, 672 halothane). In one study involving 90 infants and children, there were no clinically significant decreases in heart rate compared to awake values at 1 MAC. Systolic blood pressure decreased 15-20% in comparison to awake values following administration of 1 MAC sevoflurane; however, clinically significant hypotension requiring immediate intervention did not occur. Overall incidences of bradycardia [more than 20 beats/min lower than normal (80 beats/min)] in comparative studies was 3% for sevoflurane and 7% for halothane. Patients who received sevoflurane had slightly faster emergence times (12 vs. 19 minutes), and a higher incidence of post-anesthesia agitation (14% vs. 10%). Sevoflurane (n = 91) was compared to halothane (n = 89) in a single-center study for elective repair or palliation of congenital heart disease. The patients ranged in age from 9 days to 11.8 years with an ASA physical status of II, III, and IV (18%, 68%, and 13% respectively). No significant differences were demonstrated between treatment groups with respect to the primary outcome measures: cardiovascular decompensation and severe arterial desaturation. Adverse event data was limited to the study outcome variables collected during surgery and before institution of cardiopulmonary bypass.

Table 6. Recovery Parameters in Two Outpatient Surgery Studies: Least Squares Mean ± SEM

	Sevoflurane/N$_2$O	Isoflurane/N$_2$O	Sevoflurane/N$_2$O	Propofol/N$_2$O
Mean Maintenance	0.64 ± 0.03	0.66 ± 0.03	0.8 ± 0.5	7.3 ± 2.3
Anesthesia	MAC•hr.	MAC•hr.	MAC•hr.	mg/kg/hr.
Exposure ± SD	(n = 245)	(n = 249)	(n = 166)	(n = 166)
Time to Emergence	8.2 ± 0.4	9.3 ± 0.3	8.3 ± 0.7	10.4 ± 0.7
(min)	(n = 246)	(n = 251)	(n = 137)	(n = 142)
Time to Respond to	8.5 ± 0.4	9.8 ± 0.4	9.1 ± 0.7	11.5 ± 0.7
Commands (min)	(n = 246)	(n = 248)	(n = 139)	(n = 143)
Time to First Analgesia	45.9 ± 4.7	59.1 ± 6.0	46.1 ± 5.4	60.0 ± 4.7
(min)	(n = 160)	(n = 252)	(n = 83)	(n = 88)
Time to Eligibility for Discharge	87.6 ± 5.3	79.1 ± 5.2	103.1 ± 3.8	105.1 ± 3.7
from Recovery Area (min)	(n = 244)	(n = 252)	(n = 139)	(n = 143)

n = number of patients with recording of recovery events.

Table 7. Recovery Parameters in Two Inpatient Surgery Studies: Least Squares Mean ± SEM

	Sevoflurane/N$_2$O	Isoflurane/N$_2$O	Sevoflurane/N$_2$O	Propofol/N$_2$O
Mean Maintenance	1.27 MAC•hr.	1.58 MAC•hr.	1.43 MAC•hr.	7.0 mg/kg/hr
Anesthesia	± 0.05	± 0.06	± 0.94	± 2.9
Exposure ± SD	(n = 271)	(n = 282)	(n = 93)	(n = 92)
Time to Emergence	11.0 ± 0.6	16.4 ± 0.6	8.8 ± 1.2	13.2 ± 1.2
(min)	(n = 270)	(n = 281)	(n = 92)	(n = 92)
Time to Respond to	12.8 ± 0.7	18.4 ± 0.7	11.0 ± 1.20	14.4 ± 1.21
Commands (min)	(n = 270)	(n = 281)	(n = 92)	(n = 91)
Time to First Analgesia	46.1 ± 3.0	55.4 ± 3.2	37.8 ± 3.3	49.2 ± 3.3
(min)	(n = 233)	(n = 242)	(n = 82)	(n = 79)
Time to Eligibility for Discharge	139.2 ± 15.6	165.9 ± 16.3	148.4 ± 8.9	141.4 ± 8.9
from Recovery Area (min)	(n = 268)	(n = 282)	(n = 92)	(n = 92)

n = number of patients with recording of recovery events.

Mask Induction

Sevoflurane has a nonpungent odor and is suitable for mask induction in pediatric patients. In controlled pediatric studies in which mask induction was performed, the incidence of induction events is shown below (see **ADVERSE REACTIONS**).

Table 8. Incidence of Pediatric Induction Events

	Sevoflurane (n = 836)	Halothane (n = 660)
Agitation	14%	11%
Cough	6%	10%
Breathholding	5%	6%
Secretions	3%	3%
Laryngospasm	2%	2%
Bronchospasm	< 1%	0%

n = number of patients.

Ambulatory Surgery

Sevoflurane (n = 518) was compared to halothane (n = 382) for the maintenance of anesthesia in pediatric outpatients. All patients received N$_2$O and many received fentanyl, midazolam, bupivacaine, or lidocaine. The time to eligibility for discharge from post-anesthesia care units was similar between agents (see **CLINICAL PHARMACOLOGY** and **ADVERSE REACTIONS**).

Cardiovascular Surgery

Coronary Artery Bypass Graft (CABG) Surgery

Sevoflurane was compared to isoflurane as an adjunct with opioids in a multicenter study of 273 patients undergoing CABG surgery. Anesthesia was induced with midazolam (0.1-0.3 mg/kg); vecuronium (0.1-0.2 mg/kg), and fentanyl (5-15 mcg/kg). Both isoflurane and sevoflurane were administered at loss of consciousness in doses of 1.0 MAC and titrated until the beginning of cardiopulmonary bypass to a maximum of 2.0 MAC. The total dose of fentanyl did not exceed 25 mcg/kg. The average MAC dose was 0.49 for sevoflurane and 0.53 for isoflurane. There were no significant differences in hemodynamics, cardioactive drug use, or ischemia incidence between the two groups. Outcome was also equivalent. In this small multicenter study, sevoflurane appears to be as effective and as safe as isoflurane for supplementation of opioid anesthesia for coronary bypass grafting.

Non-Cardiac Surgery Patients at Risk for Myocardial Ischemia

Sevoflurane-N$_2$O was compared to isoflurane-N$_2$O for maintenance of anesthesia in a multicenter study in 214 patients, age 40-87 years who were at mild-to-moderate risk for myocardial ischemia and were undergoing elective noncardiac surgery. Forty-six percent (46%) of the operations were cardiovascular, with the remainder evenly divided between gastrointestinal and musculoskeletal and small numbers of other surgical procedures. The average duration of surgery was less than 2 hours. Anesthesia induction usually was performed with thiopental (2-5 mg/kg) and fentanyl (1-5 mcg/kg). Vecuronium (0.1-0.2 mg/kg) was also administered to facilitate intubation, muscle relaxation or immobility during surgery. The average MAC dose was 0.49 for both anesthetics. There was no significant difference between the anesthetic regimens for intraoperative hemodynamics, cardioactive drug use, or ischemic incidents, although only 83 patients in the sevoflurane group and 85 patients in the isoflurane group were successfully monitored for ischemia. The outcome was also equivalent in terms of adverse events, death, and postoperative myocardial infarction. Within the limits of this small multicenter study in patients at mild-to-moderate risk for myocardial ischemia, sevoflurane was a satisfactory equivalent to isoflurane in providing supplemental inhalation anesthesia to intravenous drugs.

Cesarean Section

Sevoflurane (n = 29) was compared to isoflurane (n = 27) in ASA Class I or II patients for the maintenance of anesthesia during cesarean section. Newborn evaluations and recovery events were recorded. With both anesthetics, Apgar scores averaged 8 and 9 at 1 and 5 minutes, respectively. Use of sevoflurane as part of general anesthesia for elective cesarean section produced no untoward effects in mother or neonate. Sevoflurane and isoflurane demonstrated equivalent recovery characteristics. There was no difference between sevoflurane and isoflurane with regard to the effect on the newborn, as assessed by Apgar Score and Neurological and Adaptive Capacity Score (average = 29.5). The safety of sevoflurane in labor and vaginal delivery has not been evaluated.

Neurosurgery

Three studies compared sevoflurane to isoflurane for maintenance of anesthesia during neurosurgical procedures. In a study of 20 patients, there was no difference between sevoflurane and isoflurane with regard to recovery from anesthesia. In 2 studies, a total of 22 patients with intracranial pressure (ICP) monitors received either sevoflurane or isoflurane. There was no difference between sevoflurane and isoflurane with regard to ICP response to inhalation of 0.5, 1.0, and 1.5 MAC inspired concentrations of volatile agent during N$_2$O-O$_2$-fentanyl anesthesia. During progressive hyperventilation from PaCO$_2$ = 40 to PaCO$_2$ = 30, ICP response to hypocarbia was preserved with sevoflurane at both 0.5 and 1.0 MAC concentrations. In patients at risk for elevations of ICP, sevoflurane should be administered cautiously in conjunction with ICP-reducing maneuvers such as hyperventilation.

Hepatic Impairment

A multicenter study (2 sites) compared the safety of sevoflurane and isoflurane in 16 patients with mild-to-moderate hepatic impairment utilizing the lidocaine MEGX assay for assessment of hepatocellular function. All patients received intravenous propofol (1-3 mg/kg) or thiopental (2-7 mg/kg) for induction and succinylcholine, vecuronium, or atracurium for intubation. Sevoflurane or isoflurane was administered in either 100% O$_2$ or up to 70% N$_2$O/O$_2$. Neither drug adversely affected hepatic function. No serum inorganic fluoride level exceeded 45 µM/L, but sevoflurane patients had prolonged terminal disposition of fluoride, as evidenced by longer inorganic fluoride half-life than patients with normal hepatic function (23 hours vs. 10-48 hours).

Renal Impairment

Sevoflurane was evaluated in renally impaired patients with baseline serum creatinine > 1.5 mg/dL. Fourteen patients who received sevoflurane were compared with 12 patients who received isoflurane. In another study, 21 patients who received sevoflurane were compared with 20 patients who received enflurane. Creatinine levels increased in 7% of patients who received sevoflurane, 8% of patients who received isoflurane, and 10% of patients who received enflurane. Because of the small number of patients with renal insufficiency (baseline serum creatinine greater than 1.5 mg/dL) studied, the safety of sevoflurane administration in this group has not yet been fully established. Therefore, sevoflurane should be used with caution in patients with renal insufficiency (see **WARNINGS**).

INDICATIONS AND USAGE

Sevoflurane is indicated for induction and maintenance of general anesthesia in adult and pediatric patients for inpatient and outpatient surgery.

Sevoflurane should be administered only by persons trained in the administration of general anesthesia. Facilities for maintenance of a patent airway, artificial ventilation, oxygen enrichment, and circulatory resuscitation must be immediately available. Since level of anesthesia may be altered rapidly, only vaporizers producing predictable concentrations of sevoflurane should be used.

CONTRAINDICATIONS

Sevoflurane can cause malignant hyperthermia. It should not be used in patients with known sensitivity to sevoflurane or to other halogenated agents nor in patients with known or suspected susceptibility to malignant hyperthermia.

WARNINGS

Although data from controlled clinical studies at low flow rates are limited, findings taken from patient and animal studies suggest that there is a potential for renal injury which is presumed due to Compound A. Animal and human studies demonstrate that sevoflurane administered for more than 2 MAC•hours and at fresh gas flow rates of < 2 L/min may be associated with proteinuria and glycosuria.

While a level of Compound A exposure at which clinical nephrotoxicity might be expected to occur has not been established, it is prudent to consider all of the factors leading to Compound A exposure in humans, especially duration of exposure, fresh gas flow rate, and concentration of sevoflurane. During sevoflurane anesthesia the clinician should adjust inspired concentration and fresh gas flow rate to minimize exposure to Compound A. To minimize exposure to Compound A, sevoflurane exposure should not exceed 2 MAC•hours at flow rates of 1 to < 2 L/min. Fresh gas flow rates < 1 L/min are not recommended.

Because clinical experience in administering sevoflurane to patients with renal insufficiency (creatinine > 1.5 mg/dL) is limited, its safety in these patients has not been established.

Sevoflurane may be associated with glycosuria and proteinuria when used for long procedures at low flow rates. The safety of low flow sevoflurane on renal function was evaluated in patients with normal preoperative renal function. One study compared sevoflurane (N = 98) to an active control (N = 90) administered for ≥ 2 hours at a fresh gas flow rate of ≤ 1 Liter/minute. Per study defined criteria (Hou et al.) one patient in the sevoflurane group developed elevations of creatinine, in addition to glycosuria and proteinuria. This patient received sevoflurane at fresh gas flow rates of ≤ 800 mL/minute. Using these same criteria, there were no patients in the active control group who developed treatment emergent elevations in serum creatinine.

Sevoflurane may present an increased risk in patients with known sensitivity to volatile halogenated anesthetic agents. KOH containing CO$_2$ absorbents are not recommended for use with sevoflurane.

Malignant Hyperthermia

In susceptible individuals, potent inhalation anesthetic agents, including sevoflurane, may trigger a skeletal muscle hypermetabolic state leading to high oxygen demand and the clinical syndrome known as malignant hyperthermia. In clinical trials, one case of malignant hyperthermia was reported. In genetically susceptible pigs, sevoflurane induced malignant hyperthermia. The clinical syndrome is signaled by hypercapnia, and may include muscle rigidity, tachycardia, tachypnea, cyanosis, arrhythmias, and/or unstable blood pressure. Some of these nonspecific signs may also appear during light anesthesia, acute hypoxia, hypercapnia, and hypovolemia.

Treatment of malignant hyperthermia includes discontinuation of triggering agents, administration of intravenous dantrolene sodium, and application of supportive therapy. (Consult prescribing information for dantrolene sodium intravenous for additional information on patient management.) Renal failure may appear later, and urine flow should be monitored and sustained if possible.

Perioperative Hyperkalemia

Use of inhaled anesthetic agents has been associated with rare increases in serum potassium levels that have resulted in cardiac arrhythmias and death in pediatric patients during the postoperative period. Patients with latent as well as overt neuromuscular disease, particularly Duchenne muscular dystrophy, appear to be most vulnerable. Concomitant use of succinylcholine has been associated with most, but not all, of these cases. These patients also experienced significant elevations in serum creatine kinase levels and, in some cases, changes in urine consistent with myoglobinuria. Despite the similarity in presentation to malignant hyperthermia, none of these patients exhibited signs or symptoms of muscle rigidity or hypermetabolic state. Early and aggressive intervention to treat the hyperkalemia and resistant arrhythmias is recommended; as is subsequent evaluation for latent neuromuscular disease.

PRECAUTIONS

During the maintenance of anesthesia, increasing the concentration of sevoflurane produces dose-dependent decreases in blood pressure. Due to sevoflurane's insolubility in blood, these hemodynamic changes may occur more rapidly than with other volatile anesthetics. Excessive decreases in blood pressure or respiratory depression may be related to depth of anesthesia and may be corrected by decreasing the inspired concentration of sevoflurane.

Rare cases of seizures have been reported in association with sevoflurane use (see **PRECAUTIONS - Pediatric Use** and **ADVERSE REACTIONS**).

The recovery from general anesthesia should be assessed carefully before a patient is discharged from the post-anesthesia care unit.

Drug Interactions

In clinical trials, no significant adverse reactions occurred with other drugs commonly used in the perioperative period, including: central nervous system depressants, autonomic drugs, skeletal muscle relaxants, anti-infective agents, hormones and synthetic substitutes, blood derivatives, and cardiovascular drugs.

Intravenous Anesthetics

Sevoflurane administration is compatible with barbiturates, propofol, and other commonly used intravenous anesthetics.

Benzodiazepines and Opioids

Benzodiazepines and opioids would be expected to decrease the MAC of sevoflurane in the same manner as with other inhalational anesthetics. Sevoflurane administration is compatible with benzodiazepines and opioids as commonly used in surgical practice.

Nitrous Oxide

As with other halogenated volatile anesthetics, the anesthetic requirement for sevoflurane is decreased when administered in combination with nitrous oxide. Using 50% N_2O, the MAC equivalent dose requirement is reduced approximately 50% in adults, and approximately 25% in pediatric patients (see **DOSAGE AND ADMINISTRATION**).

Neuromuscular Blocking Agents

As is the case with other volatile anesthetics, sevoflurane increases both the intensity and duration of neuromuscular blockade induced by nondepolarizing muscle relaxants. When used to supplement alfentanil-N_2O anesthesia, sevoflurane and isoflurane equally potentiate neuromuscular block induced with pancuronium, vecuronium or atracurium. Therefore, during sevoflurane anesthesia, the dosage adjustments for these muscle relaxants are similar to those required with isoflurane.

Potentiation of neuromuscular blocking agents requires equilibration of muscle with delivered partial pressure of sevoflurane. Reduced doses of neuromuscular blocking agents during induction of anesthesia may result in delayed onset of conditions suitable for endotracheal intubation or inadequate muscle relaxation.

Among available nondepolarizing agents, only vecuronium, pancuronium and atracurium interactions have been studied during sevoflurane anesthesia. In the absence of specific guidelines:

1. For endotracheal intubation, do not reduce the dose of nondepolarizing muscle relaxants.
2. During maintenance of anesthesia, the required dose of nondepolarizing muscle relaxants is likely to be reduced compared to that during N_2O/opioid anesthesia. Administration of supplemental doses of muscle relaxants should be guided by the response to nerve stimulation.

The effect of sevoflurane on the duration of depolarizing neuromuscular blockade induced by succinylcholine has not been studied.

Hepatic Function

Results of evaluations of laboratory parameters (e.g., ALT, AST, alkaline phosphatase, and total bilirubin, etc.), as well as investigator-reported incidence of adverse events relating to liver function, demonstrate that sevoflurane can be administered to patients with normal or mild-to-moderately impaired hepatic function. However, patients with severe hepatic dysfunction were not investigated.

Occasional cases of transient changes in postoperative hepatic function tests were reported with both sevoflurane and reference agents. Sevoflurane was found to be comparable to isoflurane with regard to these changes in hepatic function.

Very rare cases of mild, moderate and severe post-operative hepatic dysfunction or hepatitis with or without jaundice have been reported from postmarketing experiences. Clinical judgement should be exercised when sevoflurane is used in patients with underlying hepatic conditions or under treatment with drugs known to cause hepatic dysfunction (see **ADVERSE REACTIONS**).

Desiccated CO_2 Absorbents

An exothermic reaction occurs when sevoflurane is exposed to CO_2 absorbents. This reaction is increased when the CO_2 absorbent becomes desiccated, such as after an extended period of dry gas flow through the CO_2 absorbent canisters. Rare cases of extreme heat, smoke, and/or spontaneous fire in the anesthesia breathing circuit have been reported during sevoflurane use in conjunction with the use of desiccated CO_2 absorbent, specifically those containing potassium hydroxide (e.g. Baralyme). KOH containing CO_2 absorbents are not recommended for use with sevoflurane. An unusually delayed rise or unexpected decline of inspired sevoflurane concentration compared to the vaporizer setting may be associated with excessive heating of the CO_2 absorbent and chemical breakdown of sevoflurane.

As with other inhalational anesthetics, degradation and production of degradation products can occur when sevoflurane is exposed to desiccated absorbents. When a clinician suspects that the CO_2 absorbent may be desiccated, it should be replaced. The color indicator of most CO_2 absorbents may not change upon desiccation. Therefore, the lack of significant color change should not be taken as an assurance of adequate hydration. CO_2 absorbents should be replaced routinely regardless of the state of the color indicator.

Carcinogenesis, Mutagenesis, Impairment of Fertility

Studies on carcinogenesis have not been performed for either sevoflurane or Compound A. No mutagenic effect of sevoflurane was noted in the Ames test, mouse micronucleus test, mouse lymphoma mutagenicity assay, human lymphocyte culture assay, mammalian cell transformation assay, ^{32}P DNA adduct assay, and no chromosomal aberrations were induced in cultured mammalian cells.

Similarly, no mutagenic effect of Compound A was noted in the Ames test, the Chinese hamster chromosomal aberration assay and the *in vivo* mouse micronucleus assay. However, positive responses were observed in the human lymphocyte chromosome aberration assay. These responses were seen only at high concentrations and in the absence of metabolic activation (human S-9).

Pregnancy Category B

Reproduction studies have been performed in rats and rabbits at doses up to 1 MAC (minimum alveolar concentration) without CO_2 absorbent and have revealed no evidence of impaired fertility or harm to the fetus due to sevoflurane at 0.3 MAC, the highest nontoxic dose. Developmental and reproductive toxicity studies of sevoflurane in animals in the presence of strong alkalies (i.e., degradation of sevoflurane and production of Compound A) have not been conducted. There are no adequate and well-controlled studies in pregnant women. Because animal reproduction studies are not always predictive of human response, sevoflurane should be used during pregnancy only if clearly needed.

Labor and Delivery

Sevoflurane has been used as part of general anesthesia for elective cesarean section in 29 women. There were no untoward effects in mother or neonate (see **PHARMACODYNAMICS - Clinical Trials**). The safety of sevoflurane in labor and delivery has not been demonstrated.

Nursing Mothers

The concentrations of sevoflurane in milk are probably of no clinical importance 24 hours after anesthesia. Because of rapid washout, sevoflurane concentrations in milk are predicted to be below those found with many other volatile anesthetics.

Geriatric Use

MAC decreases with increasing age. The average concentration of sevoflurane to achieve MAC in an 80 year old is approximately 50% of that required in a 20 year old.

Pediatric Use

Induction and maintenance of general anesthesia with sevoflurane have been established in controlled clinical trials in pediatric patients aged 1 to 18 years (see **PHARMACODYNAMICS - Clinical Trials** and **ADVERSE REACTIONS**). Sevoflurane has a nonpungent odor and is suitable for mask induction in pediatric patients.

The concentration of sevoflurane required for maintenance of general anesthesia is age dependent. When used in combination with nitrous oxide, the MAC equivalent dose of sevoflurane should be reduced in pediatric patients. MAC in premature infants has not been determined (see **PRECAUTIONS - Drug Interactions** and **DOSAGE AND ADMINISTRATION** for recommendations in pediatric patients 1 day of age and older).

The use of sevoflurane has been associated with seizures (see **PRECAUTIONS** and **ADVERSE REACTIONS**). The majority of these have occurred in children and young adults starting from 2 months of age, most of whom had no predisposing risk factors. Clinical judgement should be exercised when using sevoflurane in patients who may be at risk for seizures.

ADVERSE REACTIONS

Adverse events are derived from controlled clinical trials conducted in the United States, Canada, and Europe. The reference drugs were isoflurane, enflurane, and propofol in adults and halothane in pediatric patients. The studies were conducted using a variety of premedications, other anesthetics, and surgical procedures of varying length. Most adverse events reported were mild and transient, and may reflect the surgical procedures, patient characteristics (including disease) and/or medications administered.

Of the 5182 patients enrolled in the clinical trials, 2906 were exposed to sevoflurane, including 118 adults and 507 pediatric patients who underwent mask induction. Each patient was counted once for each type of adverse event. Adverse events reported in patients in clinical trials and considered to be possibly or probably related to sevoflurane are presented within each body system in order of decreasing frequency in the following listings. One case of malignant hyperthermia was reported in pre-registration clinical trials.

Adverse Events During the Induction Period (from Onset of Anesthesia by Mask Induction to Surgical Incision) Incidence > 1%

Adult Patients (N = 118)

Cardiovascular

Bradycardia 5%, Hypotension 4%, Tachycardia 2%

Nervous System

Agitation 7%

Respiratory System

Laryngospasm 8%, Airway obstruction 8%, Breathholding 5%, Cough Increased 5%

Pediatric Patients (N = 507)

Cardiovascular

Tachycardia 6%, Hypotension 4%

Nervous System

Agitation 15%

Respiratory System

Breathholding 5%, Cough Increased 5%, Laryngospasm 3%, Apnea 2%

Digestive System

Increased salivation 2%

Adverse Events During Maintenance and Emergence Periods, Incidence > 1% (N = 2906)

Body as a whole

Fever 1%, Shivering 6%, Hypothermia 1%, Movement 1%, Headache 1%

Cardiovascular

Hypotension 11%, Hypertension 2%, Bradycardia 5%, Tachycardia 2%

Nervous System

Somnolence 9%, Agitation 9%, Dizziness 4%, Increased salivation 4%

Digestive System

Nausea 25%, Vomiting 18%

Respiratory System

Cough increased 11%, Breathholding 2%, Laryngospasm 2%

Adverse Events, All Patients in Clinical Trials (N = 2906), All Anesthetic Periods, Incidence < 1% (Reported in 3 or More Patients)

Body as a whole

Asthenia, Pain

Cardiovascular

Arrhythmia, Ventricular Extrasystoles, Supraventricular Extrasystoles, Complete AV Block, Bigeminy, Hemorrhage, Inverted T Wave, Atrial Fibrillation, Atrial Arrhythmia, Second Degree AV Block, Syncope, S-T Depressed

Nervous System

Crying, Nervousness, Confusion, Hypertonia, Dry Mouth, Insomnia

Respiratory System
Sputum Increased, Apnea, Hypoxia, Wheezing, Bronchospasm, Hyperventilation, Pharyngitis, Hiccup, Hypoventilation, Dyspnea, Stridor
Metabolism and Nutrition
Increases in LDH, AST, ALT, BUN, Alkaline Phosphatase, Creatinine, Bilirubinemia, Glycosuria, Fluorosis, Albuminuria, Hypophosphatemia, Acidosis, Hyperglycemia
Hemic and Lymphatic System
Leucocytosis, Thrombocytopenia
Skin and Special Senses
Amblyopia, Pruritus, Taste Perversion, Rash, Conjunctivitis
Urogenital
Urination Impaired, Urine Abnormality, Urinary Retention, Oliguria
See **WARNINGS** for information regarding malignant hyperthermia.

Post-Marketing Adverse Events
The following adverse events have been identified during post-approval use of Ultane (sevoflurane USP). Due to the spontaneous nature of these reports, the actual incidence and relationship of Ultane to these events cannot be established with certainty.

CNS
Seizures—Post-marketing reports indicate that sevoflurane use has been associated with seizures. The majority of cases were in children and young adults, most of whom had no medical history of seizures. Several cases reported no concomitant medications, and at least one case was confirmed by EEG. Although many cases were single seizures that resolved spontaneously or after treatment, cases of multiple seizures have also been reported. Seizures have occurred during, or soon after sevoflurane induction, during emergence, and during post-operative recovery up to a day following anesthesia.

Cardiac
Cardiac arrest

Hepatic
• Cases of mild, moderate and severe post-operative hepatic dysfunction or hepatitis with or without jaundice have been reported. Histological evidence was not provided for any of the reported hepatitis cases. In most of these cases, patients had underlying hepatic conditions or were under treatment with drugs known to cause hepatic dysfunction. Most of the reported events were transient and resolved spontaneously (see **PRECAUTIONS**).
• Hepatic necrosis
• Hepatic failure

Other
• Malignant hyperthermia (see **CONTRAINDICATIONS** and **WARNINGS**)
• Allergic reactions, such as rash, urticaria, pruritus, bronchospasm, anaphylactic or anaphylactoid reactions (see **CONTRAINDICATIONS**)

Laboratory Findings
• Transient elevations in glucose, liver function tests, and white blood cell count may occur as with use of other anesthetic agents.

OVERDOSAGE

In the event of overdosage, or what may appear to be overdosage, the following action should be taken: discontinue administration of sevoflurane, maintain a patent airway, initiate assisted or controlled ventilation with oxygen, and maintain adequate cardiovascular function.

DOSAGE AND ADMINISTRATION

The concentration of sevoflurane being delivered from a vaporizer during anesthesia should be known. This may be accomplished by using a vaporizer calibrated specifically for sevoflurane. The administration of general anesthesia must be individualized based on the patient's response.

Replacement of Desiccated CO₂ Absorbents
When a clinician suspects that the CO_2 absorbent may be desiccated, it should be replaced. The exothermic reaction that occurs with sevoflurane and CO_2 absorbents is increased when the CO_2 absorbent becomes desiccated, such as after an extended period of dry gas flow through the CO_2 absorbent canisters (see **PRECAUTIONS**).

Pre-anesthetic Medication
No specific premedication is either indicated or contraindicated with sevoflurane. The decision as to whether or not to premedicate and the choice of premedication is left to the discretion of the anesthesiologist.

Induction
Sevoflurane has a nonpungent odor and does not cause respiratory irritability; it is suitable for mask induction in pediatrics and adults.

Maintenance
Surgical levels of anesthesia can usually be achieved with concentrations of 0.5-3% sevoflurane with or without the concomitant use of nitrous oxide. Sevoflurane can be administered with any type of anesthesia circuit.

Table 9. MAC Values for Adults and Pediatric Patients According to Age

Age of Patient (years)	Sevoflurane in Oxygen	Sevoflurane in 65% N₂O/35% O₂
0-1 months #	3.3%	
1-< 6 months	3.0%	
6 months-< 3 years	2.8%	2.0%@
3-12	2.5%	
25	2.6%	1.4%
40	2.1%	1.1%
60	1.7%	0.9%
80	1.4%	0.7%

Neonates are full-term gestational age. MAC in premature infants has not been determined.
@ In 1 - < 3 year old pediatric patients, 60% N₂O/40% O₂ was used.

HOW SUPPLIED

ULTANE (sevoflurane), Volatile Liquid for Inhalation, is packaged in amber colored bottles containing 250 mL sevoflurane, List 4456, NDC # 0074-4456-04 (plastic).

SAFETY AND HANDLING
Occupational Caution
There is no specific work exposure limit established for sevoflurane. However, the National Institute for Occupational Safety and Health has recommended an 8 hour time-weighted average limit of 2 ppm for halogenated anesthetic agents in general (0.5 ppm when coupled with exposure to N_2O).

Storage
Store at controlled room temperature, 15°-30°C (59°-86°F). See USP.
Product of Japan
Product inquiries should be directed to Abbott Laboratories, North Chicago, IL 60064, USA
Manufactured by:
Abbott Laboratories, North Chicago, IL 60064, USA under license from Maruishi Pharmaceutical Company LTD. 2-3-5, Fushimi-machi, Chuo-Ku, Osaka, Japan.
©Abbott 2009
Ref. 03-A280-R3-Revised July, 2009

VICODIN® ⓒ ℞
(hydrocodone bitartrate and acetaminophen tablets, USP)
5 mg/500 mg

DESCRIPTION

Hydrocodone bitartrate and acetaminophen is supplied in tablet form for oral administration.
Hydrocodone bitartrate is an opioid analgesic and antitussive and occurs as fine, white crystals or as a crystalline powder. It is affected by light. The chemical name is: 4,5α-epoxy-3-methoxy-17-methylmorphinan-6-one tartrate (1:1) hydrate (2:5). It has the following structural formula:

$C_{18}H_{21}NO_3 \cdot C_4H_6O_6 \cdot 2\frac{1}{2}H_2O$ M.W. 494.50

Acetaminophen, 4'-hydroxyacetanilide, a slightly bitter, white, odorless, crystalline powder, is a non-opiate, non-salicylate analgesic and antipyretic. It has the following structural formula:

$C_8H_9NO_2$ M.W. 151.16

Each VICODIN tablet contains:
Hydrocodone Bitartrate   5 mg
Acetaminophen   500 mg
In addition each tablet contains the following inactive ingredients: colloidal silicon dioxide, starch, croscarmellose sodium, dibasic calcium phosphate, magnesium stearate, microcrystalline cellulose, povidone, and stearic acid.

Meets USP Dissolution Test 2.

CLINICAL PHARMACOLOGY

Hydrocodone is a semisynthetic narcotic analgesic and antitussive with multiple actions qualitatively similar to those of codeine. Most of these involve the central nervous system and smooth muscle. The precise mechanism of action of hydrocodone and other opiates is not known, although it is believed to relate to the existence of opiate receptors in the central nervous system. In addition to analgesia, narcotics may produce drowsiness, changes in mood and mental clouding.
The analgesic action of acetaminophen involves peripheral influences, but the specific mechanism is as yet undetermined. Antipyretic activity is mediated through hypothalamic heat regulating centers. Acetaminophen inhibits prostaglandin synthetase. Therapeutic doses of acetaminophen have negligible effects on the cardiovascular or respiratory systems; however, toxic doses may cause circulatory failure and rapid, shallow breathing.

Pharmacokinetics
The behavior of the individual components is described below.

Hydrocodone
Following a 10 mg oral dose of hydrocodone administered to five adult male subjects, the mean peak concentration was 23.6 ± 5.2 ng/mL. Maximum serum levels were achieved at 1.3 ± 0.3 hours and the half-life was determined to be 3.8 ± 0.3 hours. Hydrocodone exhibits a complex pattern of metabolism including O-demethylation, N-demethylation and 6-keto reduction to the corresponding 6-α- and 6-β-hydroxy-metabolites. See **OVERDOSAGE** for toxicity information.

Acetaminophen
Acetaminophen is rapidly absorbed from the gastrointestinal tract and is distributed throughout most body tissues. The plasma half-life is 1.25 to 3 hours, but may be increased by liver damage and following overdosage. Elimination of acetaminophen is principally by liver metabolism (conjugation) and subsequent renal excretion of metabolites. Approximately 85% of an oral dose appears in the urine within 24 hours of administration, most as the glucuronide conjugate, with small amounts of other conjugates and unchanged drug. See **OVERDOSAGE** for toxicity information.

INDICATIONS AND USAGE

VICODIN tablets are indicated for the relief of moderate to moderately severe pain.

CONTRAINDICATIONS

This product should not be administered to patients who have previously exhibited hypersensitivity to hydrocodone or acetaminophen.
Patients known to be hypersensitive to other opioids may exhibit cross-sensitivity to hydrocodone.

WARNINGS

Respiratory Depression
At high doses or in sensitive patients, hydrocodone may produce dose-related respiratory depression by acting directly on the brain stem respiratory center. Hydrocodone also affects the center that controls respiratory rhythm, and may produce irregular and periodic breathing.

Head Injury and Increased Intracranial Pressure
The respiratory depressant effects of narcotics and their capacity to elevate cerebrospinal fluid pressure may be markedly exaggerated in the presence of head injury, other intracranial lesions or a preexisting increase in intracranial pressure. Furthermore, narcotics produce adverse reactions which may obscure the clinical course of patients with head injuries.

Acute Abdominal Conditions
The administration of narcotics may obscure the diagnosis or clinical course of patients with acute abdominal conditions.

Misuse, Abuse, and Diversion of Opioids
VICODIN tablets contains hydrocodone an opioid agonist, and is a Schedule III controlled substance. Opioid agonists have the potential for being abused and are sought by abusers and people with addiction disorders, and are subject to diversion.
VICODIN tablets can be abused in a manner similar to other opioid agonists, legal or illicit. This should be considered when prescribing or dispensing VICODIN tablets in situations where the physician or pharmacist is concerned about an increased risk of misuse, abuse or diversion (see **DRUG ABUSE AND DEPENDENCE**).

Information on the Abbott Pharmaceutical Products listed on these pages is from the prescribing information in use as of June 1, 2010. For more information, please visit rxabbott.com or call 1-800-633-9110.

PRECAUTIONS

General

Special Risk Patients

As with any narcotic analgesic agent, VICODIN Tablets should be used with caution in elderly or debilitated patients and those with severe impairment of hepatic or renal function, hypothyroidism, Addison's disease, prostatic hypertrophy or urethral stricture. The usual precautions should be observed and the possibility of respiratory depression should be kept in mind.

Cough Reflex

Hydrocodone suppresses the cough reflex; as with all narcotics, caution should be exercised when VICODIN Tablets are used postoperatively and in patients with pulmonary disease.

Information for Patients

Hydrocodone, like all narcotics, may impair the mental and/or physical abilities required for the performance of potentially hazardous tasks such as driving a car or operating machinery; patients should be cautioned accordingly. Alcohol and other CNS depressants may produce an additive CNS depression, when taken with this combination product, and should be avoided.

Hydrocodone may be habit forming. Patients should take the drug only for as long as it is prescribed, in the amounts prescribed, and no more frequently than prescribed.

Laboratory Tests

In patients with severe hepatic or renal disease, effects of therapy should be monitored with serial liver and/or renal function tests.

Drug Interactions

Patients receiving other narcotic analgesics, antihistamines, antipsychotics, antianxiety agents, or other CNS depressants (including alcohol) concomitantly with VICODIN Tablets may exhibit an additive CNS depression. When combined therapy is contemplated, the dose of one or both agents should be reduced.

The use of MAO inhibitors or tricyclic antidepressants with hydrocodone preparations may increase the effect of either the antidepressant or hydrocodone.

Drug/Laboratory Test Interactions

Acetaminophen may produce false-positive test results for urinary 5-hydroxyindoleacetic acid.

Carcinogenesis, Mutagenesis, Impairment of Fertility

No adequate studies have been conducted in animals to determine whether hydrocodone or acetaminophen have a potential for carcinogenesis, mutagenesis, or impairment of fertility.

Pregnancy

Teratogenic Effects

Pregnancy Category C

There are no adequate and well-controlled studies in pregnant women. VICODIN Tablets should be used during pregnancy only if the potential benefit justifies the potential risk to the fetus.

Nonteratogenic Effects

Babies born to mothers who have been taking opioids regularly prior to delivery will be physically dependent. The withdrawal signs include irritability and excessive crying, tremors, hyperactive reflexes, increased respiratory rate, increased stools, sneezing, yawning, vomiting, and fever. The intensity of the syndrome does not always correlate with the duration of maternal opioid use or dose. There is no consensus on the best method of managing withdrawal.

Labor and Delivery

As with all narcotics, administration of VICODIN Tablets to the mother shortly before delivery may result in some degree of respiratory depression in the newborn, especially if higher doses are used.

Nursing Mothers

Acetaminophen is excreted in breast milk in small amounts, but the significance of its effects on nursing infants is not known. It is not known whether hydrocodone is excreted in human milk. Because many drugs are excreted in human milk and because of the potential for serious adverse reactions in nursing infants from hydrocodone and acetaminophen, a decision should be made whether to discontinue nursing or to discontinue the drug, taking into account the importance of the drug to the mother.

Pediatric Use

Safety and effectiveness in the pediatric population have not been established.

Geriatric Use

Clinical studies of VICODIN (hydrocodone bitartrate 5 mg and acetaminophen 500 mg) did not include sufficient numbers of subjects aged 65 and over to determine whether they respond differently from younger subjects. Other reported clinical experience has not identified differences in responses between the elderly and younger patients. In general, dose selection for an elderly patient should be cautious, usually starting at the low end of the dosing range, reflecting the greater frequency of decreased hepatic, renal, or cardiac function, and of concomitant disease or other drug therapy.

Hydrocodone and the major metabolites of acetaminophen are known to be substantially excreted by the kidney. Thus the risk of toxic reactions may be greater in patients with impaired renal function due to accumulation of the parent compound and/or metabolites in the plasma. Because elderly patients are more likely to have decreased renal function, care should be taken in dose selection, and it may be useful to monitor renal function.

Hydrocodone may cause confusion and over-sedation in the elderly; elderly patients generally should be started on low doses of hydrocodone bitartrate and acetaminophen tablets and observed closely.

ADVERSE REACTIONS

The most frequently reported adverse reactions include: lightheadedness, dizziness, sedation, nausea and vomiting. These effects seem to be more prominent in ambulatory than in nonambulatory patients and some of these adverse reactions may be alleviated if the patient lies down.

Other adverse reactions include:

Central Nervous System

Drowsiness, mental clouding, lethargy, impairment of mental and physical performance, anxiety, fear, dysphoria, psychic dependence, mood changes.

Gastrointestinal System

Prolonged administration of VICODIN Tablets may produce constipation.

Genitourinary System

Ureteral spasm, spasm of vesical sphincters and urinary retention have been reported with opiates.

Respiratory Depression

Hydrocodone bitartrate may produce dose-related respiratory depression by acting directly on the brain stem respiratory center (see **OVERDOSAGE**).

Special Senses

Cases of hearing impairment or permanent loss have been reported predominantly in patients with chronic overdose.

Dermatological

Skin rash, pruritus.

The following adverse drug events may be borne in mind as potential effects of acetaminophen: allergic reactions, rash, thrombocytopenia, agranulocytosis.

Potential effects of high dosage are listed in the **OVERDOSAGE** section.

DRUG ABUSE AND DEPENDENCE

Misuse, Abuse, and Diversion of Opioids

VICODIN® (hydrocodone bitartrate and acetaminophen, 5 mg/500 mg) contains hydrocodone, an opioid agonist, and is a Schedule III controlled substance. VICODIN, and other opioids used in analgesia can be abused and are subject to criminal diversion.

Addiction is a primary, chronic, neurobiologic disease, with genetic, psychosocial, and environmental factors influencing its development and manifestations. It is characterized by behaviors that include one or more of the following: impaired control over drug use, compulsive use, continued use despite harm, and craving. Drug addiction is a treatable disease utilizing a multidisciplinary approach, but relapse is common.

"Drug seeking" behavior is very common in addicts and drug abusers. Drug-seeking tactics include emergency calls or visits near the end of office hours, refusal to undergo appropriate examination, testing or referral, repeated "loss" of prescriptions, tampering with prescriptions and reluctance to provide prior medical records or contact information for other treating physician(s). "Doctor shopping" to obtain additional prescriptions is common among drug abusers and people suffering from untreated addiction.

Abuse and addiction are separate and distinct from physical dependence and tolerance. Physical dependence usually assumes clinically significant dimensions only after several weeks of continued opioid use, although a mild degree of physical dependence may develop after a few days of opioid therapy. Tolerance, in which increasingly large doses are required in order to produce the same degree of analgesia, is manifested initially by a shortened duration of analgesic effect, and subsequently by decreases in the intensity of analgesia. The rate of development of tolerance varies among patients. Physicians should be aware that abuse of opioids can occur in the absence of true addiction and is characterized by misuse for non-medical purposes, often in combination with other psychoactive substances. VICODIN, like other opioids, may be diverted for non-medical use. Record-keeping of prescribing information, including quantity, frequency, and renewal requests is strongly advised.

Proper assessment of the patient, proper prescribing practices, periodic re-evaluation of therapy, and proper dispensing and storage are appropriate measures that help to limit abuse of opioid drugs.

OVERDOSAGE

Following an acute overdosage, toxicity may result from hydrocodone or acetaminophen.

Signs and Symptoms

Hydrocodone

Serious overdose with hydrocodone is characterized by respiratory depression (a decrease in respiratory rate and/or tidal volume, Cheyne-Stokes respiration, cyanosis), extreme somnolence progressing to stupor or coma, skeletal muscle flaccidity, cold and clammy skin, and sometimes bradycardia and hypotension. In severe overdosage, apnea, circulatory collapse, cardiac arrest and death may occur.

Acetaminophen

In acetaminophen overdosage: dose-dependent, potentially fatal hepatic necrosis is the most serious adverse effect. Renal tubular necrosis, hypoglycemic coma, and thrombocytopenia may also occur.

Early symptoms following a potentially hepatotoxic overdose may include: nausea, vomiting, diaphoresis and general malaise. Clinical and laboratory evidence of hepatic toxicity may not be apparent until 48 to 72 hours post-ingestion.

In adults, hepatic toxicity has rarely been reported with acute overdoses of less than 10 grams and fatalities with less than 15 grams.

Treatment

A single or multiple overdose with hydrocodone and acetaminophen is a potentially lethal polydrug overdose, and consultation with a regional poison control center is recommended.

Immediate treatment includes support of cardiorespiratory function and measures to reduce drug absorption. Vomiting should be induced mechanically, or with syrup of ipecac, if the patient is alert (adequate pharyngeal and laryngeal reflexes). Oral activated charcoal (1 g/kg) should follow gastric emptying. The first dose should be accompanied by an appropriate cathartic. If repeated doses are used, the cathartic might be included with alternate doses as required. Hypotension is usually hypovolemic and should respond to fluids. Vasopressors and other supportive measures should be employed as indicated. A cuffed endo-tracheal tube should be inserted before gastric lavage of the unconscious patient and, when necessary, to provide assisted respiration.

Meticulous attention should be given to maintaining adequate pulmonary ventilation. In severe cases of intoxication, peritoneal dialysis, or preferably hemodialysis may be considered. If hypoprothrombinemia occurs due to acetaminophen overdose, vitamin K should be administered intravenously.

Naloxone, an opioid antagonist, can reverse respiratory depression and coma associated with opioid overdose. Naloxone hydrochloride 0.4 mg to 2 mg is given parenterally. Since the duration of action of hydrocodone may exceed that of the naloxone, the patient should be kept under continuous surveillance and repeated doses of the antagonist should be administered as needed to maintain adequate respiration. An opioid antagonist should not be administered in the absence of clinically significant respiratory or cardiovascular depression.

If the dose of acetaminophen may have exceeded 140 mg/kg, acetylcysteine should be administered as early as possible. Serum acetaminophen levels should be obtained, since levels four or more hours following ingestion help predict acetaminophen toxicity. Do not await acetaminophen assay results before initiating treatment. Hepatic enzymes should be obtained initially, and repeated at 24-hour intervals. Methemoglobinemia over 30% should be treated with methylene blue by slow intravenous administration.

The toxic dose for adults for acetaminophen is 10 g.

DOSAGE AND ADMINISTRATION

Dosage should be adjusted according to the severity of the pain and the response of the patient. However, it should be kept in mind that tolerance to hydrocodone can develop with continued use and that the incidence of untoward effects is dose related.

The usual adult dosage is one or two tablets every four to six hours as needed for pain. The total daily dosage should not exceed 8 tablets.

HOW SUPPLIED

VICODIN is supplied as white, capsule-shaped tablets containing 5 mg hydrocodone bitartrate and 500 mg acetaminophen, bisected on one side and debossed with "VICODIN" on the other.

Bottles of 100-NDC 0074-1949-14.

Bottles of 500-NDC 0074-1949-54.

Hospital Unit Dose Package-100 tablets (4 × 25 tablets)-NDC 0074-1949-12.

Storage

Store at 25°C (77°F); excursions permitted to 15°-30°C (59°-86°F). [See USP Controlled Room Temperature].

Dispense in a tight, light-resistant container as defined in the USP.

A Schedule Ⓒⓘⓘⓘ controlled drug substance.

Manufactured for
Abbott Laboratories
North Chicago, IL 60064, U.S.A.
by Halo Pharmaceutical Inc.
Whippany, NJ 07981 U.S.A.
Ref: 03-A187
Revised: December, 2008

VICODIN ES®   Ⓒ Ⱳ
(hydrocodone bitartrate and
acetaminophen tablets, USP)
7.5 mg/750 mg

DESCRIPTION

Hydrocodone bitartrate and acetaminophen is supplied in tablet form for oral administration.
Hydrocodone bitartrate is an opioid analgesic and antitussive and occurs as fine, white crystals or as a crystalline powder. It is affected by light. The chemical name is: 4,5α-epoxy-3-methoxy-17-methylmorphinan-6-one tartrate (1:1) hydrate (2:5). It has the following structural formula:

$C_{18}H_{21}NO_3 \cdot C_4H_6O_6 \cdot 2\frac{1}{2}H_2O$ M.W.=494.50

Acetaminophen, 4'-hydroxyacetanilide, a slightly bitter, white, odorless, crystalline powder, is a non-opiate, non-salicylate analgesic and antipyretic. It has the following structural formula:

$C_8H_9NO_2$ M.W.151.16

Each VICODIN ES Tablet contains:
Hydrocodone Bitartrate   7.5 mg
Acetaminophen   750 mg
In addition each tablet contains the following inactive ingredients: Colloidal silicon dioxide, pregelatinized starch, magnesium stearate, croscarmellose sodium povidone, and stearic acid.
Meets USP Dissolution Test 2.

CLINICAL PHARMACOLOGY

Hydrocodone is a semisynthetic narcotic analgesic and antitussive with multiple actions qualitatively similar to those of codeine. Most of these involve the central nervous system and smooth muscle. The precise mechanism of action of hydrocodone and other opiates is not known, although it is believed to relate to the existence of opiate receptors in the central nervous system. In addition to analgesia, narcotics may produce drowsiness, changes in mood and mental clouding.
The analgesic action of acetaminophen involves peripheral influences, but the specific mechanism is as yet undetermined. Antipyretic activity is mediated through hypothalmic heat regulating centers. Acetaminophen inhibits prostaglandin synthetase. Therapeutic doses of acetaminophen have negligible effects on the cardiovascular or respiratory systems; however, toxic doses may cause circulatory failure and rapid, shallow breathing.

Pharmacokinetics
The behavior of the individual components is described below.

Hydrocodone
Following a 10 mg oral dose of hydrocodone administered to five adult male subjects, the mean peak concentration was 23.6 ± 5.2 ng/mL. Maximum serum levels were achieved at 1.3 ± 0.3 hours and the half-life was determined to be 3.8 ± 0.3 hours. Hydrocodone exhibits a complex pattern of metabolism including O-demethylation, N-demethylation and 6-keto reduction to the corresponding 6-α- and 6-β-hydroxy-metabolites. See **OVERDOSAGE** for toxicity information.

Acetaminophen
Acetaminophen is rapidly absorbed from the gastrointestinal tract and is distributed throughout most body tissues. The plasma half-life is 1.25 to 3 hours, but may be increased by liver damage and following overdosage. Elimination of acetaminophen is principally by liver metabolism (conjuga-

tion) and subsequent renal excretion of metabolites. Approximately 85% of an oral dose appears in the urine within 24 hours of administration, most as the glucuronide conjugate, with small amounts of other conjugates and unchanged drug. See **OVERDOSAGE** for toxicity information.

INDICATIONS AND USAGE

VICODIN ES Tablets are indicated for the relief of moderate to moderately severe pain.

CONTRAINDICATIONS

This product should not be administered to patients who have previously exhibited hypersensitivity to hydrocodone or acetaminophen.
Patients known to be hypersensitive to other opioids may exhibit cross-sensitivity to hydrocodone.

WARNINGS
Respiratory Depression
At high doses or in sensitive patients, hydrocodone may produce dose-related respiratory depression by acting directly on the brain stem respiratory center. Hydrocodone also affects the center that controls respiratory rhythm, and may produce irregular and periodic breathing.

Head Injury and Increased Intracranial Pressure
The respiratory depressant effects of narcotics and their capacity to elevate cerebrospinal fluid pressure may be markedly exaggerated in the presence of head injury, other intracranial lesions or a preexisting increase in intracranial pressure. Furthermore, narcotics produce adverse reactions, which may obscure the clinical course of patients with head injuries.

Acute Abdominal Conditions
The administration of narcotics may obscure the diagnosis or clinical course of patients with acute abdominal conditions.

Misuse Abuse and Diversion of Opioids
VICODIN ES contains hydrocodone an opioid agonist, and is a Schedule III controlled substance. Opioid agonists have the potential for being abused and are sought by abusers and people with addiction disorders, and are subject to diversion.
VICODIN ES can be abused in a manner similar to other opioid agonists, legal or illicit. This should be considered when prescribing or dispensing VICODIN ES in situations where the physician or pharmacist is concerned about an increased risk of misuse, abuse or diversion (see **DRUG ABUSE AND DEPENDENCE**).

PRECAUTIONS
General
Special Risk Patients
As with any narcotic analgesic agent, VICODIN ES Tablets should be used with caution in elderly or debilitated patients and those with severe impairment of hepatic or renal function, hypothyroidism, Addison's disease, prostatic hypertrophy or urethral stricture. The usual precautions should be observed and the possibility of respiratory depression should be kept in mind.
Cough Reflex
Hydrocodone suppresses the cough reflex; as with all narcotics, caution should be exercised when VICODIN ES Tablets are used postoperatively and in patients with pulmonary disease.

Information for Patients
Hydrocodone, like all narcotics, may impair the mental and/or physical abilities required for the performance of potentially hazardous tasks such as driving a car or operating machinery; patients should be cautioned accordingly.
Alcohol and other CNS depressants may produce an additive CNS depression, when taken with this combination product, and should be avoided.
Hydrocodone may be habit forming. Patients should take the drug only for as long as it is prescribed, in the amounts prescribed, and no more frequently than prescribed.

Laboratory Tests
In patients with severe hepatic or renal disease, effects of therapy should be monitored with serial liver and/or renal function tests.

Drug Interactions
Patients receiving other narcotic analgesics, antihistamines, antipsychotics, antianxiety agents, or other CNS depressants (including alcohol) concomitantly with VICODIN ES Tablets may exhibit an additive CNS depression. When combined therapy is contemplated, the dose of one or both agents should be reduced.
The use of MAO inhibitors or tricyclic antidepressants with hydrocodone preparations may increase the effect of either the antidepressant or hydrocodone.

Drug/Laboratory Test Interactions
Acetaminophen may produce false-positive test results for urinary 5-hydroxyindoleacetic acid.

Carcinogenesis, Mutagenesis, Impairment of Fertility
No adequate studies have been conducted in animals to determine whether hydrocodone or acetaminophen have a potential for carcinogenesis, mutagenesis, or impairment of fertility.

Pregnancy
Teratogenic Effects
Pregnancy Category C
There are no adequate and well-controlled studies in pregnant women. VICODIN ES Tablets should be used during pregnancy only if the potential benefit justifies the potential risk to the fetus.
Nonteratogenic Effects
Babies born to mothers who have been taking opioids regularly prior to delivery will be physically dependent. The withdrawal signs include irritability and excessive crying, tremors, hyperactive reflexes, increased respiratory rate, increased stools, sneezing, yawning, vomiting, and fever. The intensity of the syndrome does not always correlate with the duration of maternal opioid use or dose. There is no consensus on the best method of managing withdrawal.

Labor and Delivery
As with all narcotics, administration of VICODIN ES Tablets to the mother shortly before delivery may result in some degree of respiratory depression in the newborn, especially if higher doses are used.

Nursing Mothers
Acetaminophen is excreted in breast milk in small amounts, but the significance of its effects on nursing infants is not known. It is not known whether hydrocodone is excreted in human milk. Because many drugs are excreted in human milk and because of the potential for serious adverse reactions in nursing infants from hydrocodone and acetaminophen, a decision should be made whether to discontinue nursing or to discontinue the drug, taking into account the importance of the drug to the mother.

Pediatric Use
Safety and effectiveness in the pediatric population have not been established.

Geriatric Use
Clinical studies of VICODIN ES® (hydrocodone bitartrate 7.5 mg and acetaminophen 750 mg) did not include sufficient numbers of subjects aged 65 and over to determine whether they respond differently from younger subjects. Other reported clinical experience has not identified differences in responses between the elderly and younger patients. In general, dose selection for an elderly patient should be cautious, usually starting at the low end of the dosing range, reflecting the greater frequency of decreased hepatic, renal, or cardiac function, and of concomitant disease or other drug therapy.
Hydrocodone and the major metabolites of acetaminophen are known to be substantially excreted by the kidney. Thus the risk of toxic reactions may be greater in patients with impaired renal function due to accumulation of the parent compound and/or metabolites in the plasma. Because elderly patients are more likely to have decreased renal function, care should be taken in dose selection, and it may be useful to monitor renal function.
Hydrocodone may cause confusion and over-sedation in the elderly; elderly patients generally should be started on low doses of hydrocodone bitartrate and acetaminophen tablets and observed closely.

ADVERSE REACTIONS
The most frequently reported adverse reactions include: lightheadedness, dizziness, sedation, nausea and vomiting. These effects seem to be more prominent in ambulatory than in nonambulatory patients and some of these adverse reactions may be alleviated if the patient lies down.
Other adverse reactions include:

Central Nervous System
Drowsiness, mental clouding, lethargy, impairment of mental and physical performance, anxiety, fear, dysphoria, psychic dependence, mood changes.

Gastrointestinal System
Prolonged administration of VICODIN ES Tablets may produce constipation.

Genitourinary System
Ureteral spasm, spasm of vesical sphincters and urinary retention have been reported with opiates.

Respiratory Depression
Hydrocodone bitartrate may produce dose-related respiratory depression by acting directly on the brain stem respiratory center (see **OVERDOSAGE**).

Special Senses
Cases of hearing impairment or permanent loss have been reported predominantly in patients with chronic overdose.

Information on the Abbott Pharmaceutical Products listed on these pages is from the prescribing information in use as of June 1, 2010. For more information, please visit rxabbott.com or call 1-800-633-9110.

Dermatological
Skin rash, pruritus.
The following adverse drug events may be borne in mind as potential effects of acetaminophen: allergic reactions, rash, thrombocytopenia, agranulocytosis.
Potential effects of high dosage are listed in the **OVER-DOSAGE** section.

DRUG ABUSE AND DEPENDENCE
Misuse, Abuse, and Diversion of Opioids
VICODIN ES® (hydrocodone bitartrate 7.5 mg and acetaminophen 750 mg) contains hydrocodone, an opioid agonist, and is a Schedule III controlled substance. VICODIN ES, and other opioids used in analgesia can be abused and are subject to criminal diversion.
Addiction is a primary, chronic, neurobiologic disease, with genetic, psychosocial, and environmental factors influencing its development and manifestations. It is characterized by behaviors that include one or more of the following: impaired control over drug use, compulsive use, continued use despite harm, and craving. Drug addiction is a treatable disease utilizing a multidisciplinary approach, but relapse is common.
"Drug seeking" behavior is very common in addicts and drug abusers. Drug-seeking tactics include emergency calls or visits near the end of office hours, refusal to undergo appropriate examination, testing or referral, repeated "loss" of prescriptions, tampering with prescriptions and reluctance to provide prior medical records or contact information for other treating physician(s). "Doctor shopping" to obtain additional prescriptions is common among drug abusers and people suffering from untreated addiction.
Abuse and addiction are separate and distinct from physical dependence and tolerance. Physical dependence usually assumes clinically significant dimensions only after several weeks of continued opioid use, although a mild degree of physical dependence may develop after a few days of opioid therapy. Tolerance, in which increasingly large doses are required in order to produce the same degree of analgesia, is manifested initially by a shortened duration of analgesic effect, and subsequently by decreases in the intensity of analgesia. The rate of development of tolerance varies among patients. Physicians should be aware that abuse of opioids can occur in the absence of true addiction and is characterized by misuse for non-medical purposes, often in combination with other psychoactive substances. VICODIN ES, like other opioids, may be diverted for non-medical use. Record-keeping of prescribing information, including quantity, frequency, and renewal requests is strongly advised.
Proper assessment of the patient, proper prescribing practices, periodic re-evaluation of therapy, and proper dispensing and storage are appropriate measures that help to limit abuse of opioid drugs.

OVERDOSAGE
Following an acute overdosage, toxicity may result from hydrocodone or acetaminophen.
Signs and Symptoms
Hydrocodone
Serious overdose with hydrocodone is characterized by respiratory depression (a decrease in respiratory rate and/or tidal volume, Cheyne-Stokes respiration, cyanosis), extreme somnolence progressing to stupor or coma, skeletal muscle flaccidity, cold and clammy skin, and sometimes bradycardia and hypotension. In severe overdosage, apnea, circulatory collapse, cardiac arrest and death may occur.
Acetaminophen
In acetaminophen overdosage: dose-dependent, potentially fatal hepatic necrosis is the most serious adverse effect. Renal tubular necrosis, hypoglycemic coma, and thrombocytopenia may also occur.
Early symptoms following a potentially hepatotoxic overdose may include: nausea, vomiting, diaphoresis and general malaise. Clinical and laboratory evidence of hepatic toxicity may not be apparent until 48 to 72 hours post-ingestion.
In adults, hepatic toxicity has rarely been reported with acute overdoses of less than 10 grams and fatalities with less than 15 grams.
Treatment
A single or multiple overdose with hydrocodone and acetaminophen is a potentially lethal polydrug overdose, and consultation with a regional poison control center is recommended.
Immediate treatment includes support of cardiorespiratory function and measures to reduce drug absorption. Vomiting should be induced mechanically, or with syrup of ipecac, if the patient is alert (adequate pharyngeal and laryngeal reflexes). Oral activated charcoal (1 g/kg) should follow gastric emptying. The first dose should be accompanied by an appropriate cathartic. If repeated doses are used, the cathartic might be included with alternate doses as required. Hypotension is usually hypovolemic and should respond to fluids. Vasopressors and other supportive measures should be em-

ployed as indicated. A cuffed endo-tracheal tube should be inserted before gastric lavage of the unconscious patient and, when necessary, to provide assisted respiration.
Meticulous attention should be given to maintaining adequate pulmonary ventilation. In severe cases of intoxication, peritoneal dialysis, or preferably hemodialysis may be considered. If hypoprothrombinemia occurs due to acetaminophen overdose, vitamin K should be administered intravenously.
Naloxone, an opioid antagonist, can reverse respiratory depression and coma associated with opioid overdose. Naloxone hydrochloride 0.4 mg to 2 mg is given parenterally. Since the duration of action of hydrocodone may exceed that of the naloxone, the patient should be kept under continuous surveillance and repeated doses of the antagonist should be administered as needed to maintain adequate respiration. An opioid antagonist should not be administered in the absence of clinically significant respiratory or cardiovascular depression.
If the dose of acetaminophen may have exceeded 140 mg/kg, acetylcysteine should be administered as early as possible. Serum acetaminophen levels should be obtained, since levels four or more hours following ingestion help predict acetaminophen toxicity. Do not await acetaminophen assay results before initiating treatment. Hepatic enzymes should be obtained initially, and repeated at 24-hour intervals. Methemoglobinemia over 30% should be treated with methylene blue by slow intravenous administration.
The toxic dose for adults for acetaminophen is 10 g.

DOSAGE AND ADMINISTRATION
Dosage should be adjusted according to the severity of the pain and the response of the patient. However, it should be kept in mind that tolerance to hydrocodone can develop with continued use and that the incidence of untoward effects is dose related. The usual adult dosage is one tablet every four to six hours as needed for pain. The total daily dosage should not exceed 5 tablets.

HOW SUPPLIED
White, oval-shaped, faceted edged tablet bisected on one side and imprinted with "VICODIN ES" on the other side.
Bottles of 100-NDC #0074-1973-14
Bottles of 500-NDC #0074-1973-54
Hospital Unit Dosage Package-100 tablets (4 × 25 tablets)-NDC #0074-1973-12
Storage
Store at 25°C (77°F); excursions permitted to 15°-30°C (59°-86°F). [See USP Controlled Room Temperature].
Dispense in a tight, light-resistant container as defined in the USP.
A Schedule Ⓒ Controlled Drug Substance.
©Abbott
Manufactured for
Abbott Laboratories
North Chicago, IL 60064, U.S.A.
by Halo Pharmaceutical Inc.
Whippany, NJ 07981 U.S.A.
Ref: 03-A189
Revised: December 2008
Shown in Product Identification Guide, page 304

VICODIN HP® Ⓒ ℞
[*vīkō-dĭn*]
(hydrocodone bitartrate and acetaminophen tablets, USP)
10 mg/660 mg

DESCRIPTION
Hydrocodone bitartrate and acetaminophen is supplied in tablet form for oral administration.
Hydrocodone bitartrate is an opioid analgesic and antitussive and occurs as fine, white crystals or as a crystalline powder. It is affected by light. The chemical name is 4,5α-epoxy-3-methoxy-17-methylmorphinan-6-one tartrate (1:1) hydrate (2:5). It has the following structural formula:

$C_{18}H_{21}NO_3 \cdot C_4H_6O_6 \cdot 2\frac{1}{2}H_2O$ M.W.=494.50

Acetaminophen, 4'-hydroxyacetanilide, a slightly bitter, white, odorless, crystalline powder, is a non-opiate, non-salicylate analgesic and antipyretic. It has the following structural formula:

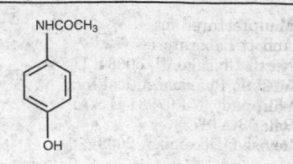

$C_8H_9NO_2$ M.W. = 151.17

Each VICODIN HP Tablet contains:
Hydrocodone Bitartrate .... 10 mg
Acetaminophen .... 660 mg
In addition each tablet contains the following inactive ingredients: colloidal silicon dioxide, croscarmellose sodium, magnesium stearate, microcrystalline cellulose, povidone, pregelatinized starch, and stearic acid.
Meets USP Dissolution Test 2.

CLINICAL PHARMACOLOGY
Hydrocodone is a semisynthetic narcotic analgesic and antitussive with multiple actions qualitatively similar to those of codeine. Most of these involve the central nervous system and smooth muscle. The precise mechanism of action of hydrocodone and other opiates is not known, although it is believed to relate to the existence of opiate receptors in the central nervous system. In addition to analgesia, narcotics may produce drowsiness, changes in mood and mental clouding.
The analgesic action of acetaminophen involves peripheral influences, but the specific mechanism is as yet undetermined. Antipyretic activity is mediated through hypothalamic heat regulating centers. Acetaminophen inhibits prostaglandin synthetase. Therapeutic doses of acetaminophen have negligible effects on the cardiovascular or respiratory systems; however, toxic doses may cause circulatory failure and rapid, shallow breathing.
Pharmacokinetics
The behavior of the individual components is described below.
Hydrocodone
Following a 10 mg oral dose of hydrocodone administered to five adult male subjects, the mean peak concentration was 23.6 ± 5.2 ng/mL. Maximum serum levels were achieved at 1.3 ± 0.3 hours and the half-life was determined to be 3.8 ± 0.3 hours. Hydrocodone exhibits a complex pattern of metabolism including O-demethylation, N-demethylation and 6-keto reduction to the corresponding 6-α- and 6-β-hydroxy-metabolites. See **OVERDOSAGE** for toxicity information.
Acetaminophen
Acetaminophen is rapidly absorbed from the gastrointestinal tract and is distributed throughout most body tissues. The plasma half-life is 1.25 to 3 hours, but may be increased by liver damage and following overdosage. Elimination of acetaminophen is principally by liver metabolism (conjugation) and subsequent renal excretion of metabolites. Approximately 85% of an oral dose appears in the urine within 24 hours of administration, most as the glucuronide conjugate, with small amounts of other conjugates and unchanged drug. See **OVERDOSAGE** for toxicity information.

INDICATIONS AND USAGE
VICODIN HP Tablets are indicated for the relief of moderate to moderately severe pain.

CONTRAINDICATIONS
This product should not be administered to patients who have previously exhibited hypersensitivity to hydrocodone or acetaminophen.
Patients known to be hypersensitive to other opioids may exhibit cross-sensitivity to hydrocodone.

WARNINGS
Respiratory Depression
At high doses or in sensitive patients, hydrocodone may produce dose-related respiratory depression by acting directly on the brain stem respiratory center. Hydrocodone also affects the center that controls respiratory rhythm, and may produce irregular and periodic breathing.
Head Injury and Increased Intracranial Pressure
The respiratory depressant effects of narcotics and their capacity to elevate cerebrospinal fluid pressure may be markedly exaggerated in the presence of head injury, other intracranial lesions or a preexisting increase in intracranial pressure. Furthermore, narcotics produce adverse reactions which may obscure the clinical course of patients with head injuries.
Acute Abdominal Conditions
The administration of narcotics may obscure the diagnosis or clinical course of patients with acute abdominal conditions.
Misuse Abuse and Diversion of Opioids
VICODIN HP contains hydrocodone an opioid agonist, and is a Schedule III controlled substance. Opioid agonists have

the potential for being abused and are sought by abusers and people with addiction disorders, and are subject to diversion.

VICODIN HP can be abused in a manner similar to other opioid agonists, legal or illicit. This should be considered when prescribing or dispensing VICODIN HP in situations where the physician or pharmacist is concerned about an increased risk of misuse, abuse or diversion (see **DRUG ABUSE AND DEPENDENCE**).

PRECAUTIONS
General
Special Risk Patients
As with any narcotic analgesic agent, VICODIN HP Tablets should be used with caution in elderly or debilitated patients, and those with severe impairment of hepatic or renal function, hypothyroidism, Addison's disease, prostatic hypertrophy or urethral stricture. The usual precautions should be observed and the possibility of respiratory depression should be kept in mind.
Cough Reflex
Hydrocodone suppresses the cough reflex; as with all narcotics, caution should be exercised when VICODIN HP Tablets are used postoperatively and in patients with pulmonary disease.
Information for Patients
Hydrocodone, like all narcotics, may impair the mental and/or physical abilities required for the performance of potentially hazardous tasks such as driving a car or operating machinery; patients should be cautioned accordingly. Alcohol and other CNS depressants may produce an additive CNS depression, when taken with this combination product, and should be avoided.

Hydrocodone may be habit forming. Patients should take the drug only for as long as it is prescribed, in the amounts prescribed, and no more frequently than prescribed.
Laboratory Tests
In patients with severe hepatic or renal disease, effects of therapy should be monitored with serial liver and/or renal function tests.
Drug Interactions
Patients receiving narcotics, antihistamines, antipsychotics, antianxiety agents, or other CNS depressants (including alcohol) concomitantly with VICODIN HP Tablets may exhibit an additive CNS depression. When combined therapy is contemplated, the dose of one or both agents should be reduced.

The use of MAO inhibitors or tricyclic antidepressants with hydrocodone preparations may increase the effect of either the antidepressant or hydrocodone.
Drug/Laboratory Test Interactions
Acetaminophen may produce false-positive test results for urinary 5-hydroxyindoleacetic acid.
Carcinogenesis, Mutagenesis, Impairment of Fertility
No adequate studies have been conducted in animals to determine whether hydrocodone or acetaminophen have a potential for carcinogenesis, mutagenesis, or impairment of fertility.
Pregnancy
Teratogenic Effects
Pregnancy Category C
There are no adequate and well-controlled studies in pregnant women. VICODIN HP Tablets should be used during pregnancy only if the potential benefit justifies the potential risk to the fetus.
Nonteratogenic Effects
Babies born to mothers who have been taking opioids regularly prior to delivery will be physically dependent. The withdrawal signs include irritability and excessive crying, tremors, hyperactive reflexes, increased respiratory rate, increased stools, sneezing, yawning, vomiting, and fever. The intensity of the syndrome does not always correlate with the duration of maternal opioid use or dose. There is no consensus on the best method of managing withdrawal.
Labor and Delivery
As with all narcotics, administration of VICODIN HP Tablets to the mother shortly before delivery may result in some degree of respiratory depression in the newborn, especially if higher doses are used.
Nursing Mothers
Acetaminophen is excreted in breast milk in small amounts, but the significance of its effects on nursing infants is not known. It is not known whether hydrocodone is excreted in human milk. Because many drugs are excreted in human milk and because of the potential for serious adverse reactions in nursing infants from hydrocodone and acetaminophen, a decision should be made whether to discontinue nursing or to discontinue the drug, taking into account the importance of the drug to the mother.
Pediatric Use
Safety and effectiveness in the pediatric population have not been established.

Geriatric Use
Clinical studies of VICODIN HP® (hydrocodone bitartrate and acetaminophen 10 mg/660 mg) did not include sufficient numbers of subjects aged 65 and over to determine whether they respond differently from younger subjects. Other reported clinical experience has not identified differences in responses between the elderly and younger patients. In general, dose selection for an elderly patient should be cautious, usually starting at the low end of the dosing range, reflecting the greater frequency of decreased hepatic, renal, or cardiac function, and of concomitant disease or other drug therapy.

Hydrocodone and the major metabolites of acetaminophen are known to be substantially excreted by the kidney. Thus the risk of toxic reactions may be greater in patients with impaired renal function due to accumulation of the parent compound and/or metabolites in the plasma. Because elderly patients are more likely to have decreased renal function, care should be taken in dose selection, and it may be useful to monitor renal function.

Hydrocodone may cause confusion and over-sedation in the elderly; elderly patients generally should be started on low doses of hydrocodone bitartrate and acetaminophen tablets and observed closely.

ADVERSE REACTIONS
The most frequently reported adverse reactions are light-headedness, dizziness, sedation, nausea and vomiting. These effects seem to be more prominent in ambulatory than in nonambulatory patients, and some of these adverse reactions may be alleviated if the patient lies down.
Other adverse reactions include:
Central Nervous System
Drowsiness, mental clouding, lethargy, impairment of mental and physical performance, anxiety, fear, dysphoria, psychic dependence, mood changes.
Gastrointestinal System
Prolonged administration of VICODIN HP Tablets may produce constipation.
Genitourinary System
Ureteral spasm, spasm of vesical sphincters and urinary retention have been reported with opiates.
Respiratory Depression
Hydrocodone bitartrate may produce dose-related respiratory depression by acting directly on the brain stem respiratory centers (see **OVERDOSAGE**).
Special Senses
Cases of hearing impairment or permanent loss have been reported predominantly in patients with chronic overdose.
Dermatological
Skin rash, pruritus.
The following adverse drug events may be borne in mind as potential effects of acetaminophen: allergic reactions, rash, thrombocytopenia, agranulocytosis.
Potential effects of high dosage are listed in the **OVERDOSAGE** section.

DRUG ABUSE AND DEPENDENCE
Misuse, Abuse, and Diversion of Opioids
VICODIN HP® (hydrocodone bitartrate and acetaminophen, 10 mg/660 mg) contains hydrocodone, an opioid agonist, and is a Schedule III controlled substance. VICODIN HP, and other opioids used in analgesia can be abused and are subject to criminal diversion.

Addiction is a primary, chronic, neurobiologic disease, with genetic, psychosocial, and environmental factors influencing its development and manifestations. It is characterized by behaviors that include one or more of the following: impaired control over drug use, compulsive use, continued use despite harm, and craving. Drug addiction is a treatable disease utilizing a multidisciplinary approach, but relapse is common.

"Drug seeking" behavior is very common in addicts and drug abusers. Drug-seeking tactics include emergency calls or visits near the end of office hours, refusal to undergo appropriate examination, testing or referral, repeated "loss" of prescriptions, tampering with prescriptions and reluctance to provide prior medical records or contact information for other treating physician(s). "Doctor shopping" to obtain additional prescriptions is common among drug abusers and people suffering from untreated addiction.

Abuse and addiction are separate and distinct from physical dependence and tolerance. Physical dependence usually assumes clinically significant dimensions only after several weeks of continued opioid use, although a mild degree of physical dependence may develop after a few days of opioid therapy. Tolerance, in which increasingly large doses are required in order to produce the same degree of analgesia, is manifested initially by a shortened duration of analgesic effect, and subsequently by decreases in the intensity of analgesia. The rate of development of tolerance varies among patients. Physicians should be aware that abuse of opioids can occur in the absence of true addiction and is characterized by misuse for non-medical purposes, often in combination with other psychoactive substances. VICODIN HP, like

other opioids, may be diverted for non-medical use. Record-keeping of prescribing information, including quantity, frequency, and renewal requests is strongly advised.

Proper assessment of the patient, proper prescribing practices, periodic re-evaluation of therapy, and proper dispensing and storage are appropriate measures that help to limit abuse of opioid drugs.

OVERDOSAGE
Following an acute overdosage, toxicity may result from hydrocodone or acetaminophen.
Signs and Symptoms
Hydrocodone
Serious overdose with hydrocodone is characterized by respiratory depression (a decrease in respiratory rate and/or tidal volume, Cheyne-Stokes respiration, cyanosis), extreme somnolence progressing to stupor or coma, skeletal muscle flaccidity, cold and clammy skin, and sometimes bradycardia and hypotension. In severe overdosage, apnea, circulatory collapse, cardiac arrest and death may occur.
Acetaminophen
In acetaminophen overdosage: dose-dependent, potentially fatal hepatic necrosis is the most serious adverse effect. Renal tubular necrosis, hypoglycemic coma, and thrombocytopenia may also occur.

Early symptoms following a potentially hepatotoxic overdose may include: nausea, vomiting, diaphoresis and general malaise. Clinical and laboratory evidence of hepatic toxicity may not be apparent until 48 to 72 hours post-ingestion.

In adults, hepatic toxicity has rarely been reported with acute overdoses of less than 10 grams, or fatalities with less than 15 grams.
Treatment
A single or multiple overdose with hydrocodone and acetaminophen is a potentially lethal polydrug overdose, and consultation with a regional poison control center is recommended.

Immediate treatment includes support of cardiorespiratory function and measures to reduce drug absorption. Vomiting should be induced mechanically, or with syrup of ipecac, if the patient is alert (adequate pharyngeal and laryngeal reflexes). Oral activated charcoal (1 g/kg) should follow gastric emptying. The first dose should be accompanied by an appropriate cathartic. If repeated doses are used, the cathartic might be included with alternate doses as required. Hypotension is usually hypovolemic and should respond to fluids. Vasopressors and other supportive measures should be employed as indicated. A cuffed endo-tracheal tube should be inserted before gastric lavage of the unconscious patient and, when necessary, to provide assisted respiration.

Meticulous attention should be given to maintaining adequate pulmonary ventilation. In severe cases of intoxication, peritoneal dialysis, or preferably hemodialysis may be considered. If hypoprothrombinemia occurs due to acetaminophen overdose, vitamin K should be administered intravenously.

Naloxone, an opioid antagonist, can reverse respiratory depression and coma associated with opioid overdose. Naloxone hydrochloride 0.4 mg to 2 mg is given parenterally. Since the duration of action of hydrocodone may exceed that of the naloxone, the patient should be kept under continuous surveillance and repeated doses of the antagonist should be administered as needed to maintain adequate respiration. An opioid antagonist should not be administered in the absence of clinically significant respiratory or cardiovascular depression.

If the dose of acetaminophen may have exceeded 140 mg/kg, acetylcysteine should be administered as early as possible. Serum acetaminophen levels should be obtained, since levels four or more hours following ingestion help predict acetaminophen toxicity. Do not await acetaminophen assay results before initiating treatment. Hepatic enzymes should be obtained initially, and repeated at 24-hour intervals.

Methemoglobinemia over 30% should be treated with methylene blue by slow intravenous administration.

The toxic dose for adults for acetaminophen is 10 g.

DOSAGE AND ADMINISTRATION
Dosage should be adjusted according to severity of pain and the response of the patient. However, it should be kept in mind that tolerance to hydrocodone can develop with continued use and that the incidence of untoward effects is dose related.

The usual adult dosage is one tablet every four to six hours as needed for pain. The total daily dosage should not exceed 6 tablets.

Information on the Abbott Pharmaceutical Products listed on these pages is from the prescribing information in use as of June 1, 2010. For more information, please visit rxabbott.com or call 1-800-633-9110.

HOW SUPPLIED

VICODIN HP® (hydrocodone bitartrate and acetaminophen, 10 mg/660 mg) is supplied as a white, oval-shaped, tablet bisected on one side and debossed with "VICODIN HP" on the other side.

Bottles of 100-NDC #0074-2274-14

Bottles of 500-NDC #0074-2274-54

Storage

Store at 25°C (77°F); excursions permitted to 15°-30°C (59°-86°F). [see USP Controlled Room Temperature]. Dispense in a tight, light-resistant container as defined in the USP.

A Schedule CIII Controlled Drug Substance.

©Abbott

Manufactured for

Abbott Laboratories

North Chicago, IL 60064, U.S.A.

by Halo Pharmaceutical Inc.

Whippany, NJ 07981 U.S.A.

Ref: 03-A188

Revised: December, 2008

Shown in Product Identification Guide, page 304

VICOPROFEN® CIII ℞

(hydrocodone bitartrate and ibuprofen tablets)
7.5 mg/200 mg

DESCRIPTION

Each VICOPROFEN tablet contains:

Hydrocodone Bitartrate, USP 7.5 mg

Ibuprofen, USP 200 mg

VICOPROFEN is supplied in a fixed combination tablet form for oral administration. VICOPROFEN combines the opioid analgesic agent, hydrocodone bitartrate, with the nonsteroidal anti-inflammatory (NSAID) agent, ibuprofen. Hydrocodone bitartrate is a semisynthetic and centrally acting opioid analgesic. Its chemical name is: 4,5 α-epoxy-3-methoxy-17-methylmorphinan-6-one tartrate (1:1) hydrate (2:5). Its chemical formula is: $C_{18}H_{21}NO_3 \bullet C_4H_6O_6 \bullet 2\frac{1}{2}H_2O$, and the molecular weight is 494.50. Its structural formula is:

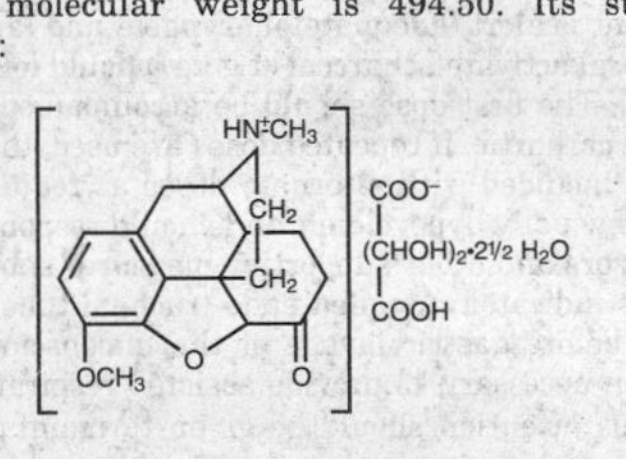

Ibuprofen is a nonsteroidal anti-inflammatory agent [nonselective COX inhibitor] with analgesic and antipyretic properties. Its chemical name is: (±)-2-(*p*-isobutylphenyl) propionic acid. Its chemical formula is: $C_{13}H_{18}O_2$, and the molecular weight is: 206.29. Its structural formula is:

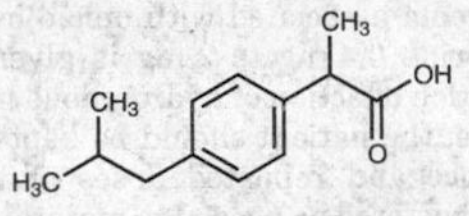

Inactive ingredients in VICOPROFEN tablets include: colloidal silicon dioxide, corn starch, croscarmellose sodium, hypromellose, magnesium stearate, microcrystalline cellulose, polyethylene glycol, polysorbate 80, propylene glycol and titanium dioxide.

CLINICAL PHARMACOLOGY

Hydrocodone Component

Hydrocodone is a semisynthetic opioid analgesic and antitussive with multiple actions qualitatively similar to those of codeine. Most of these involve the central nervous system and smooth muscle. The precise mechanism of action of hydrocodone and other opioids is not known, although it is believed to relate to the existence of opiate receptors in the central nervous system. In addition to analgesia, opioids may produce drowsiness, changes in mood, and mental clouding.

Ibuprofen Component

Ibuprofen is a non-steroidal anti-inflammatory agent that possesses analgesic and antipyretic activities. Its mode of action, like that of other NSAIDs, is not completely understood, but may be related to inhibition of cyclooxygenase activity and prostaglandin synthesis. Ibuprofen is a peripherally acting analgesic. Ibuprofen does not have any known effects on opiate receptors.

Pharmacokinetics

Absorption

After oral dosing with the VICOPROFEN tablet, a peak hydrocodone plasma level of 27 ng/mL is achieved at 1.7 hours, and a peak ibuprofen plasma level of 30 mcg/mL is achieved at 1.8 hours. The effect of food on the absorption of either component from the VICOPROFEN tablet has not been established.

Distribution

Ibuprofen is highly protein-bound (99%) like most other non-steroidal anti-inflammatory agents. Although the extent of protein binding of hydrocodone in human plasma has not been definitely determined, structural similarities to related opioid analgesics suggest that hydrocodone is not extensively protein bound. As most agents in the 5-ring morphinan group of semi-synthetic opioids bind plasma protein to a similar degree (range 19% [hydromorphone] to 45% [oxycodone]), hydrocodone is expected to fall within this range.

Metabolism

Hydrocodone exhibits a complex pattern of metabolism, including *O*-demethylation, *N*-demethylation, and 6-keto reduction to the corresponding 6-α-and 6-β-hydroxy metabolites. Hydromorphone, a potent opioid, is formed from the *O*-demethylation of hydrocodone and contributes to the total analgesic effect of hydrocodone. The *O*- and *N*-demethylation processes are mediated by separate P-450 isoenzymes: CYP2D6 and CYP3A4, respectively.

Ibuprofen is present in this product as a racemate, and following absorption it undergoes interconversion in the plasma from the R-isomer to the S-isomer. Both the R- and S-isomers are metabolized to two primary metabolites: (+)-2-4′-(2hydroxy-2-methyl-propyl) phenyl propionic acid and (+)-2-4′-(2carboxypropyl) phenyl propionic acid, both of which circulate in the plasma at low levels relative to the parent.

Elimination

Hydrocodone and its metabolites are eliminated primarily in the kidneys, with a mean plasma half-life of 4.5 hours. Ibuprofen is excreted in the urine, 50% to 60% as metabolites and approximately 15% as unchanged drug and conjugate. The plasma half-life is 2.2 hours.

Special Populations

No significant pharmacokinetic differences based on age or gender have been demonstrated. The pharmacokinetics of hydrocodone and ibuprofen from VICOPROFEN has not been evaluated in children.

Renal Impairment

The effect of renal insufficiency on the pharmacokinetics of the VICOPROFEN dosage form has not been determined.

CLINICAL STUDIES

In single-dose studies of post surgical pain (abdominal, gynecological, orthopedic), 940 patients were studied at doses of one or two tablets. VICOPROFEN produced greater efficacy than placebo and each of its individual components given at the same dose. No advantage was demonstrated for the two-tablet dose.

INDICATIONS AND USAGE

Carefully consider the potential benefits and risks of VICOPROFEN and other treatment options before deciding to use VICOPROFEN. Use the lowest effective dose for the shortest duration consistent with individual patient treatment goals (see **WARNINGS**).

VICOPROFEN tablets are indicated for the short-term (generally less than 10 days) management of acute pain. VICOPROFEN is not indicated for the treatment of such conditions as osteoarthritis or rheumatoid arthritis.

CONTRAINDICATIONS

VICOPROFEN is contraindicated in patients with known hypersensitivity to hydrocodone or ibuprofen. Patients known to be hypersensitive to other opioids may exhibit cross-sensitivity to hydrocodone.

VICOPROFEN should not be given to patients who have experienced asthma, urticaria, or allergic-type reactions after taking aspirin or other NSAIDs. Severe, rarely fatal, anaphylactic-like reactions to NSAIDs have been reported in such patients (see **WARNINGS – Anaphylactoid Reactions**, and **PRECAUTIONS - Preexisting Asthma**).

VICOPROFEN is contraindicated for the treatment of perioperative pain in the setting of coronary artery bypass graft (CABG) surgery (see **WARNINGS**).

WARNINGS

CARDIOVASCULAR EFFECTS

Cardiovascular Thrombotic Events

Clinical trials of several COX-2 selective and nonselective NSAIDs of up to three years duration have shown an increased risk of serious cardiovascular (CV) thrombotic events, myocardial infarction, and stroke, which can be fatal. All NSAIDs, both COX-2 selective and nonselective, may have a similar risk. Patients with known CV disease or risk factors for CV disease may be at greater risk. To minimize the potential risk for an adverse CV event in patients treated with an NSAID, the lowest effective dose should be used for the shortest duration possible. Physicians and patients should remain alert for the development of such events, even in the absence of previous CV symptoms. Patients should be informed about the signs and/or symptoms of serious CV events and the steps to take if they occur.

There is no consistent evidence that concurrent use of aspirin mitigates the increased risk of serious CV thrombotic events associated with NSAID use. The concurrent use of aspirin and an NSAID does increase the risk of serious GI events (see **GI WARNINGS**).

Two large, controlled, clinical trials of a COX-2 selective NSAID for the treatment of pain in the first 10-14 days following CABG surgery found an increased incidence of myocardial infarction and stroke (see **CONTRAINDICATIONS**).

Hypertension

NSAID-containing products, including VICOPROFEN, can lead to onset of new hypertension or worsening of preexisting hypertension, either of which may contribute to the increased incidence of CV events. Patients taking thiazides or loop diuretics may have impaired response to these therapies when taking NSAIDs. NSAID-containing products, including VICOPROFEN, should be used with caution in patients with hypertension. Blood pressure (BP) should be monitored closely during the initiation of NSAID treatment and throughout the course of therapy.

Congestive Heart Failure and Edema

Fluid retention and edema have been observed in some patients taking NSAIDs. VICOPROFEN should be used with caution in patients with fluid retention or heart failure.

Misuse Abuse and Diversion of Opioids

VICOPROFEN contains hydrocodone an opioid agonist, and is a Schedule III controlled substance. Opioid agonists have the potential for being abused and are sought by abusers and people with addiction disorders, and are subject to diversion.

VICOPROFEN can be abused in a manner similar to other opioid agonists, legal or illicit. This should be considered when prescribing or dispensing VICOPROFEN in situations where the physician or pharmacist is concerned about an increased risk of misuse, abuse or diversion (see **DRUG ABUSE AND DEPENDENCE**).

Respiratory Depression

At high doses or in opioid-sensitive patients, hydrocodone may produce dose-related respiratory depression by acting directly on the brain stem respiratory centers. Hydrocodone also affects the center that controls respiratory rhythm, and may produce irregular and periodic breathing.

Head Injury and Increased Intracranial Pressure

The respiratory depressant effects of opioids and their capacity to elevate cerebrospinal fluid pressure may be markedly exaggerated in the presence of head injury, intracranial lesions or a pre-existing increase in intracranial pressure. Furthermore, opioids produce adverse reactions, which may obscure the clinical course of patients with head injuries.

Acute Abdominal Conditions

The administration of opioids may obscure the diagnosis or clinical course of patients with acute abdominal conditions.

Gastrointestinal (GI) Effects - Risk of GI Ulceration, Bleeding and Perforation

NSAIDs, including VICOPROFEN, can cause serious gastrointestinal (GI) adverse events including inflammation, bleeding, ulceration, and perforation of the stomach, small intestine, or large intestine, which can be fatal. These serious adverse events can occur at any time, with or without warning symptoms, in patients treated with NSAIDs. Only one in five patients who develops a serious upper GI adverse event on NSAID therapy, is symptomatic. Upper GI ulcers, gross bleeding, or perforation caused by NSAIDs occur in approximately 1% of patients treated for 3-6 months, and in about 2-4% of patients treated for one year. These trends continue with longer duration of use, increasing the likelihood of developing a serious GI event at some time during the course of therapy. However, even short-term therapy is not without risk.

NSAIDs should be prescribed with extreme caution in those with a prior history of ulcer disease or gastrointestinal bleeding. Patients with a *prior history of peptic ulcer disease and/or gastrointestinal bleeding who* use NSAIDs have a greater than 10-fold increased risk for developing a GI bleed compared to patients with neither of these risk factors. Other factors that increase the risk for GI bleeding in patients treated with NSAIDs include concomitant use of oral corticosteroids or anticoagulants, longer duration of NSAID therapy, smoking, use of alcohol, older age, and poor general health status. Most spontaneous reports of fatal GI events are in elderly or debilitated patients and therefore, special care should be taken in treating this population.

To minimize the potential risk for an adverse GI event in patients treated with an NSAID, the lowest effective dose should be used for the shortest possible duration. Patients and physicians should remain alert for signs and symptoms of GI ulceration and bleeding during NSAID therapy and promptly initiate additional evaluation and treatment if a serious GI adverse event is suspected. This should include discontinuation of the NSAID until a serious GI adverse event is ruled out. For high-risk patients, alternate therapies that do not involve NSAIDs should be considered.

Renal Effects
Long-term administration of NSAIDs has resulted in renal papillary necrosis and other renal injury. Renal toxicity has also been seen in patients in whom renal prostaglandins have a compensatory role in the maintenance of renal perfusion. In these patients, administration of a nonsteroidal anti-inflammatory drug may cause a dose-dependent reduction in prostaglandin formation and, secondarily, in renal blood flow, which may precipitate overt renal decompensation. Patients at greatest risk of this reaction are those with impaired renal function, heart failure, liver dysfunction, those taking diuretics and ACE inhibitors, and the elderly. Discontinuation of NSAID therapy is usually followed by recovery to the pretreatment state.

Advanced Renal Disease
No information is available from controlled clinical studies regarding the use of VICOPROFEN in patients with advanced renal disease. Therefore, treatment with VICOPROFEN is not recommended in patients with advanced renal disease. If VICOPROFEN therapy must be initiated, close monitoring of the patient's renal function is advisable.

Anaphylactoid Reactions
As with other NSAID-containing products, anaphylactoid reactions may occur in patients without known prior exposure to VICOPROFEN. VICOPROFEN should not be given to patients with the aspirin triad. This symptom complex typically occurs in asthmatic patients who experience rhinitis with or without nasal polyps, or who exhibit severe, potentially fatal bronchospasm after taking aspirin or other NSAIDs. Fatal reactions to NSAIDs have been reported in such patients (see **CONTRAINDICATIONS** and **PRECAUTIONS** - Pre-existing Asthma). Emergency help should be sought in cases where an anaphylactoid reaction occurs.

Skin Reactions
Products containing NSAIDs, including VICOPROFEN, can cause serious skin adverse events such as exfoliative dermatitis, Stevens-Johnson Syndrome (SJS), and toxic epidermal necrolysis (TEN), which can be fatal. These serious events may occur without warning. Patients should be informed about the signs and symptoms of serious skin manifestations and use of the drug should be discontinued at the first appearance of skin rash or any other sign of hypersensitivity.

Pregnancy
As with other NSAID-containing products, VICOPROFEN should be avoided in late pregnancy because it may cause premature closure of the ductus arteriosus.

PRECAUTIONS
General
VICOPROFEN cannot be expected to substitute for corticosteroids or to treat corticosteroid insufficiency. Abrupt discontinuation of corticosteroids may lead to disease exacerbation. Patients on prolonged corticosteroid therapy should have their therapy tapered slowly if a decision is made to discontinue corticosteroids.

The pharmacological activity of VICOPROFEN in reducing fever and inflammation may diminish the utility of these diagnostic signs in detecting complications of presumed noninfectious, painful conditions.

Special Risk Patients
As with any opioid analgesic agent, VICOPROFEN tablets should be used with caution in elderly or debilitated patients, and those with severe impairment of hepatic or renal function, hypothyroidism, Addison's disease, prostatic hypertrophy or urethral stricture. The usual precautions should be observed and the possibility of respiratory depression should be kept in mind.

Cough Reflex
Hydrocodone suppresses the cough reflex; as with opioids, caution should be exercised when VICOPROFEN is used postoperatively and in patients with pulmonary disease.

Hepatic Effects
Borderline elevations of one or more liver enzymes may occur in up to 15% of patients taking NSAIDs including ibuprofen as found in VICOPROFEN. These laboratory abnormalities may progress, may remain essentially unchanged, or may be transient with continued therapy. Notable elevations of SGPT (ALT) or SGOT (AST) (approximately three or more times the upper limit of normal) have been reported in approximately 1% of patients in clinical trials with NSAIDs. In addition, rare cases of severe hepatic reactions, including jaundice and fatal fulminant hepatitis, liver necrosis and hepatic failure, some of them with fatal outcomes have been reported.

A patient with symptoms and/or signs suggesting liver dysfunction, or in whom an abnormal liver test has occurred, should be evaluated for evidence of the development of more severe hepatic reactions while on VICOPROFEN therapy. If

clinical signs and symptoms consistent with liver disease develop, or if systemic manifestations occur (e.g., eosinophilia, rash, etc.), VICOPROFEN should be discontinued.

Hematological Effects
Anemia is sometimes seen in patients receiving NSAIDs including ibuprofen as found in VICOPROFEN. This may be due to fluid retention, occult or gross GI blood loss, or an incompletely described effect upon erythropoiesis. Patients on long-term treatment with NSAIDs including ibuprofen, should have their hemoglobin or hematocrit checked if they exhibit any signs or symptoms of anemia.

NSAIDs inhibit platelet aggregation and have been shown to prolong bleeding time in some patients. Unlike aspirin, their effect on platelet function is quantitatively less, of shorter duration, and reversible. Patients receiving VICOPROFEN who may be adversely affected by alterations in platelet function, such as those with coagulation disorders or patients receiving anticoagulants, should be carefully monitored.

Pre-existing Asthma
Patients with asthma may have aspirin-sensitive asthma. The use of aspirin in patients with aspirin-sensitive asthma has been associated with severe bronchospasm, which may be fatal. Since cross-reactivity between aspirin and other NSAIDs has been reported in such aspirin-sensitive patients, VICOPROFEN should not be administered to patients with this form of aspirin sensitivity and should be used with caution in patients with pre-existing asthma.

Aseptic Meningitis
Aseptic meningitis with fever and coma has been observed on rare occasions in patients on ibuprofen therapy as found in VICOPROFEN. Although it is probably more likely to occur in patients with systemic lupus erythematosus and related connective tissue diseases, it has been reported in patients who do not have an underlying chronic disease. If signs or symptoms of meningitis develop in a patient on VICOPROFEN, the possibility of its being related to ibuprofen should be considered.

Information for Patients
Patients should be informed of the following information before initiating therapy with an NSAID and periodically during the course of ongoing therapy. Patients should also be encouraged to read the NSAID Medication Guide that accompanies each prescription dispensed.

1. VICOPROFEN® (hydrocodone bitartrate 7.5 mg and ibuprofen 200 mg), like other opioid-containing analgesics, may impair mental and/or physical abilities required for the performance of potentially hazardous tasks such as driving a car or operating machinery; patients should be cautioned accordingly.

2. Alcohol and other CNS depressants may produce an additive CNS depression, when taken with this combination product, and should be avoided.

3. VICOPROFEN can be abused in a manner similar to other opioid agonists, legal or illicit. VICOPROFEN may be habit-forming. Patients should take the drug only for as long as it is prescribed, in the amounts prescribed, and no more frequently than prescribed.

4. VICOPROFEN, like other NSAID-containing products, may cause serious CV side effects, such as MI or stroke, which may result in hospitalization and even death. Although serious CV events can occur without warning symptoms, patients should be alert for the signs and symptoms of chest pain, shortness of breath, weakness, slurring of speech, and should ask for medical advice when observing any indicative sign or symptoms. Patients should be apprised of the importance of this follow-up (see **WARNINGS, Cardiovascular Effects**).

5. VICOPROFEN, like other NSAID-containing products, can cause GI discomfort and serious GI side effects, such as ulcers and bleeding, which may result in hospitalization and even death. Although serious GI tract ulcerations and bleeding can occur without warning symptoms, patients should be alert for the signs and symptoms of ulcerations and bleeding, and should ask for medical advice when observing any indicative sign or symptoms including epigastric pain, dyspepsia, melena, and hematemesis. Patients should be apprised of the importance of this follow-up (see **WARNINGS, Gastrointestinal Effects: Risk of Ulceration, Bleeding, and Perforation**).

6. VICOPROFEN, like other NSAID-containing products, can cause serious skin side effects such as exfoliative dermatitis, SJS, and TEN, which may result in hospitalizations and even death. Although serious skin reactions may occur without warning, patients should be alert for the signs and symptoms of skin rash and blisters, fever, or other signs of hypersensitivity such as itching, and should ask for medical advice when observing any indicative signs or symptoms. Patients should be advised to stop the drug immediately if they develop any type of rash and contact their physicians as soon as possible.

7. Patients should promptly report signs or symptoms of unexplained weight gain or edema to their physicians.

8. Patients should be informed of the warning signs and symptoms of hepatotoxicity (e.g., nausea, fatigue, lethargy, pruritus, jaundice, right upper quadrant tenderness, and "flu-like" symptoms). If these occur, patients should be instructed to stop therapy and seek immediate medical therapy.

9. Patients should be informed of the signs of an anaphylactoid reaction (e.g., difficulty breathing, swelling of the face or throat). If these occur, patients should be instructed to seek immediate emergency help (see **WARNINGS**).

10. In late pregnancy, as with other NSAIDs, VICOPROFEN should be avoided because it may cause premature closure of the ductus arteriosus.

11. Patients should be instructed to report any signs of blurred vision or other eye symptoms.

Laboratory Tests
Because serious GI tract ulcerations and bleeding can occur without warning symptoms, physicians should monitor for signs or symptoms of GI bleeding. Patients on long-term treatment with NSAIDs should have their CBC and a chemistry profile checked periodically. If clinical signs and symptoms consistent with liver or renal disease develop, systemic manifestations occur (e.g., eosinophilia, rash, etc.) or if abnormal liver tests persist or worsen, VICOPROFEN should be discontinued.

Drug Interactions
ACE-inhibitors
Reports suggest that NSAIDs may diminish the antihypertensive effect of ACE-inhibitors. This interaction should be given consideration in patients taking VICOPROFEN concomitantly with ACE-inhibitors.

Anticholinergics
The concurrent use of anticholinergics with hydrocodone preparations may produce paralytic ileus.

Antidepressants
The use of Monoamine Oxidase Inhibitors (MAOIs) or tricyclic antidepressants with VICOPROFEN may increase the effect of either the antidepressant or hydrocodone.

MAOIs have been reported to intensify the effects of at least one opioid drug causing anxiety, confusion and significant depression of respiration or coma. The use of hydrocodone is not recommended for patients taking MAOIs or within 14 days of stopping such treatment.

Aspirin
When VICOPROFEN is administered with aspirin, the protein binding of aspirin is reduced, although the clearance of free VICOPROFEN is not altered. The clinical significance of this interaction is not known; however, as with other NSAID-containing products, concomitant administration of VICOPROFEN and aspirin is not generally recommended because of the potential of increased adverse effects.

CNS Depressants
Patients receiving other opioids, antihistamines, antipsychotics, antianxiety agents, or other CNS depressants (including alcohol) concomitantly with VICOPROFEN may exhibit an additive CNS depression. When combined therapy is contemplated, the dose of one or both agents should be reduced.

Diuretics
Ibuprofen has been shown to reduce the natriuretic effect of furosemide and thiazides in some patients. This response has been attributed to inhibition of renal prostaglandin synthesis. During concomitant therapy with VICOPROFEN the patient should be observed closely for signs of renal failure (see **WARNINGS** - Renal Effects), as well as diuretic efficacy.

Lithium
Ibuprofen has been shown to elevate plasma lithium concentration and reduce renal lithium clearance. The mean minimum lithium concentration increased 15% and the renal clearance was decreased by approximately 20%. This effect has been attributed to inhibition of renal prostaglandin synthesis by ibuprofen. Thus, when VICOPROFEN and lithium are administered concurrently, patients should be observed for signs of lithium toxicity.

Methotrexate
Ibuprofen, as well as other NSAIDs, has been reported to competitively inhibit methotrexate accumulation in rabbit kidney slices. This may indicate that ibuprofen could enhance the toxicity of methotrexate. Caution should be used when VICOPROFEN is administered concomitantly with methotrexate.

Information on the Abbott Pharmaceutical Products listed on these pages is from the prescribing information in use as of June 1, 2010. For more information, please visit rxabbott.com or call 1-800-633-9110.

Mixed Agonist/Antagonist Opioid Analgesics
Agonist/antagonist analgesics (i.e., pentazocine, nalbuphine, butorphanol and buprenorphine) should be administered with caution to patients who have received or are receiving a course of therapy with a pure opioid agonist analgesic such as hydrocodone. In this situation, mixed agonist/antagonist analgesics may reduce the analgesic effect of hydrocodone and/or may precipitate withdrawal symptoms in these patients.

Neuromuscular Blocking Agents
Hydrocodone, as well as other opioid analgesics, may enhance the neuromuscular blocking action of skeletal muscle relaxants and produce an increased degree of respiratory depression.

Warfarin
The effects of warfarin and NSAIDs on GI bleeding are synergistic, such that users of both drugs together have a risk of serious GI bleeding higher than users of either drug alone.

Carcinogenicity, Mutagenicity, and Impairment of Fertility
The carcinogenic and mutagenic potential of VICOPROFEN has not been investigated. The ability of VICOPROFEN to impair fertility has not been assessed.

Pregnancy
Pregnancy Category C.
Teratogenic Effects
Reproductive studies conducted in rats and rabbits have not demonstrated evidence of developmental abnormalities. VICOPROFEN, administered to rabbits at 95 mg/kg (5.72 and 1.9 times the maximum clinical dose based on body weight and surface area, respectively), a maternally toxic dose, resulted in an increase in the percentage of litters and fetuses with any major abnormality and an increase in the number of litters and fetuses with one or more nonossified metacarpals (a minor abnormality). VICOPROFEN, administered to rats at 166 mg/kg (10.0 and 1.66 times the maximum clinical dose based on body weight and surface area, respectively), a maternally toxic dose, did not result in any reproductive toxicity. However, animal reproduction studies are not always predictive of human response. There are no adequate and well-controlled studies in pregnant women. VICOPROFEN should be used during pregnancy only if the potential benefit justifies the potential risk to the fetus.
Nonteratogenic Effects
Because of the known effects of nonsteroidal antiinflammatory drugs on the fetal cardiovascular system (closure of the ductus arteriosus), use during pregnancy (particularly late pregnancy) should be avoided. Babies born to mothers who have been taking opioids regularly prior to delivery will be physically dependent. The withdrawal signs include irritability and excessive crying, tremors, hyperactive reflexes, increased respiratory rate, increased stools, sneezing, yawning, vomiting, and fever. The intensity of the syndrome does not always correlate with the duration of maternal opioid use or dose. There is no consensus on the best method of managing withdrawal.

Labor and Delivery
As with other drugs known to inhibit prostaglandin synthesis, an increased incidence of dystocia and delayed parturition occurred in rats. Administration of VICOPROFEN is not recommended during labor and delivery. The effects of VICOPROFEN on labor and delivery in pregnant women are unknown.

Nursing Mothers
It is not known whether hydrocodone is excreted in human milk. In limited studies, an assay capable of detecting 1 mcg/mL did not demonstrate ibuprofen in the milk of lactating mothers. However, because of the limited nature of the studies, and because of the potential for serious adverse reactions in nursing infants from VICOPROFEN, a decision should be made whether to discontinue nursing or to discontinue the drug, taking into account the importance of the drug to the mother.

Pediatric Use
The safety and effectiveness of VICOPROFEN in pediatric patients below the age of 16 have not been established.

Geriatric Use
In controlled clinical trials there was no difference in tolerability between patients < 65 years of age and those ≥ 65, apart from an increased tendency of the elderly to develop constipation. However, because the elderly may be more sensitive to the renal and gastrointestinal effects of nonsteroidal anti-inflammatory agents as well as possible increased risk of respiratory depression with opioids, extra caution and reduced dosages should be used when treating the elderly with VICOPROFEN.

ADVERSE REACTIONS
VICOPROFEN was administered to approximately 300 pain patients in a safety study that employed dosages and a duration of treatment sufficient to encompass the recommended usage (see **DOSAGE AND ADMINISTRATION**). Adverse event rates generally increased with increasing daily dose. The event rates reported below are from approx-

imately 150 patients who were in a group that received one tablet of VICOPROFEN an average of three to four times daily. The overall incidence rates of adverse experiences in the trials were fairly similar for this patient group and those who received the comparison treatment, acetaminophen 600 mg with codeine 60 mg.
The following lists adverse events that occurred with an incidence of 1% or greater in clinical trials of VICOPROFEN, without regard to the causal relationship of the events to the drug. To distinguish different rates of occurrence in clinical studies, the adverse events are listed as follows:
name of adverse event = less than 3%
*adverse events marked with an asterisk * = 3% to 9%*
adverse event rates over 9% are in parentheses

Body as a Whole
Abdominal pain*; Asthenia*; Fever; Flu syndrome; Headache (27%); Infection*; Pain.

Cardiovascular
Palpitations; Vasodilation.

Central Nervous System
Anxiety*; Confusion; Dizziness (14%); Hypertonia; Insomnia*; Nervousness*; Paresthesia; Somnolence (22%); Thinking abnormalities.

Digestive
Anorexia; Constipation (22%); Diarrhea*; Dry mouth*; Dyspepsia (12%); Flatulence*; Gastritis; Melena; Mouth ulcers; Nausea (21%); Thirst; Vomiting*.

Metabolic and Nutritional Disorders
Edema*.

Respiratory
Dyspnea; Hiccups; Pharyngitis; Rhinitis.

Skin and Appendages
Pruritus*; Sweating*.

Special Senses
Tinnitus.

Urogenital
Urinary frequency.

Incidence less than 1%
Body as a Whole
Allergic reaction.
Cardiovascular
Arrhythmia; Hypotension; Tachycardia.
Central Nervous System
Agitation; Abnormal dreams; Decreased libido; Depression; Euphoria; Mood changes; Neuralgia; Slurred speech; Tremor, Vertigo.
Digestive
Chalky stool; "Clenching teeth"; Dysphagia; Esophageal spasm; Esophagitis; Gastroenteritis; Glossitis; Liver enzyme elevation.
Metabolic and Nutritional
Weight decrease.
Musculoskeletal
Arthralgia; Myalgia.
Respiratory
Asthma; Bronchitis; Hoarseness; Increased cough; Pulmonary congestion; Pneumonia; Shallow breathing; Sinusitis.
Skin and Appendages
Rash; Urticaria.
Special Senses
Altered vision; Bad taste; Dry eyes.
Urogenital
Cystitis; Glycosuria; Impotence; Urinary incontinence; Urinary retention.

DRUG ABUSE AND DEPENDENCE
Misuse Abuse and Diversion of Opioids
VICOPROFEN contains hydrocodone, an opioid agonist, and is a Schedule III controlled substance. VICOPROFEN, and other opioids used in analgesia can be abused and are subject to criminal diversion.
Addiction is a primary, chronic, neurobiologic disease, with genetic, psychosocial, and environmental factors influencing its development and manifestations. It is characterized by behaviors that include one or more of the following: impaired control over drug use, compulsive use, continued use despite harm, and craving. Drug addiction is a treatable disease utilizing a multidisciplinary approach, but relapse is common.
"Drug seeking" behavior is very common in addicts and drug abusers. Drug-seeking tactics include emergency calls or visits near the end of office hours, refusal to undergo appropriate examination, testing or referral, repeated "loss" of prescriptions, tampering with prescriptions and reluctance to provide prior medical records or contact information for other treating physician(s). "Doctor shopping" to obtain additional prescriptions is common among drug abusers and people suffering from untreated addiction.
Abuse and addiction are separate and distinct from physical dependence and tolerance. Physical dependence usually assumes clinically significant dimensions only after several weeks of continued opioid use, although a mild degree of physical dependence may develop after a few days of opioid therapy. Tolerance, in which increasingly large doses are re-

quired in order to produce the same degree of analgesia, is manifested initially by a shortened duration of analgesic effect, and subsequently by decreases in the intensity of analgesia. The rate of development of tolerance varies among patients. Physicians should be aware that abuse of opioids can occur in the absence of true addiction and is characterized by misuse for non-medical purposes, often in combination with other psychoactive substances. VICOPROFEN, like other opioids, may be diverted for non-medical use. Record-keeping of prescribing information, including quantity, frequency, and renewal requests is strongly advised. Proper assessment of the patient, proper prescribing practices, periodic re-evaluation of therapy, and proper dispensing and storage are appropriate measures that help to limit abuse of opioid drugs.

OVERDOSAGE
Following an acute overdosage, toxicity may result from hydrocodone and/or ibuprofen.
Signs and Symptoms
Hydrocodone Component
Serious overdose with hydrocodone is characterized by respiratory depression (a decrease in respiratory rate and/or tidal volume, Cheyne-Stokes respiration, cyanosis) extreme somnolence progressing to stupor or coma, skeletal muscle flaccidity, cold and clammy skin, and sometimes bradycardia and hypotension. In severe overdosage, apnea, circulatory collapse, cardiac arrest and death may occur.
Ibuprofen Component
Symptoms include gastrointestinal irritation with erosion and hemorrhage or perforation, kidney damage, liver damage, heart damage, hemolytic anemia, agranulocytosis, thrombocytopenia, aplastic anemia, and meningitis. Other symptoms may include headache, dizziness, tinnitus, confusion, blurred vision, mental disturbances, skin rash, stomatitis, edema, reduced retinal sensitivity, corneal deposits, and hyperkalemia.
Treatment
Primary attention should be given to the re-establishment of adequate respiratory exchange through provision of a patent airway and the institution of assisted or controlled ventilation. Naloxone, a narcotic antagonist, can reverse respiratory depression and coma associated with opioid overdose or unusual sensitivity to opioids, including hydrocodone. Therefore, an appropriate dose of naloxone hydrochloride should be administered intravenously with simultaneous efforts at respiratory resuscitation. Since the duration of action of hydrocodone may exceed that of the naloxone, the patient should be kept under continuous surveillance and repeated doses of the antagonist should be administered as needed to maintain adequate respiration. Supportive measures should be employed as indicated. Gastric emptying may be useful in removing unabsorbed drug. In cases where consciousness is impaired it may be inadvisable to perform gastric lavage. If gastric lavage is performed, little drug will likely be recovered if more than an hour has elapsed since ingestion. Ibuprofen is acidic and is excreted in the urine; therefore, it may be beneficial to administer alkali and induce diuresis. In addition to supportive measures the use of oral activated charcoal may help to reduce the absorption and reabsorption of ibuprofen. Dialysis is not likely to be effective for removal of ibuprofen because it is very highly bound to plasma proteins.

DOSAGE AND ADMINISTRATION
Carefully consider the potential benefits and risks of VICOPROFEN and other treatment options before deciding to use VICOPROFEN. Use the lowest effective dose for the shortest duration consistent with individual patient treatment goals (see **WARNINGS**).
After observing the response to initial therapy with VICOPROFEN, the dose and frequency should be adjusted to suit an individual patient's needs.
For the short-term (generally less than 10 days) management of acute pain, the recommended dose of VICOPROFEN is one tablet every 4 to 6 hours, as necessary. Dosage should not exceed 5 tablets in a 24-hour period. It should be kept in mind that tolerance to hydrocodone can develop with continued use and that the incidence of untoward effects is dose related.
The lowest effective dose or the longest dosing interval should be sought for each patient (see **WARNINGS**), especially in the elderly. After observing the initial response to therapy with VICOPROFEN, the dose and frequency of dosing should be adjusted to suit the individual patient's need, without exceeding the total daily dose recommended.

HOW SUPPLIED
VICOPROFEN tablets are available as:
White film-coated round convex tablets, engraved with "VP" over **Abbott "A"** logo on one side and plain on the other side.
Bottles of 100-NDC 0074-2277-14
Bottles of 500-NDC 0074-2277-54
Hospital Unit Dosage Package-100 tablets
(4 × 25 tablets)-NDC 0074-2277-12

Storage

Store at 25°C (77°F); excursions permitted to 15°-30°C (59°-86°F). [See USP Controlled Room Temperature].
Dispense in a tight, light-resistant container.
A Schedule CS-III Controlled Substance.
© Abbott
Manufactured by Halo Pharmaceutical Inc.
Whippany, NJ 07981 U.S.A.
for Abbott Laboratories
North Chicago, IL 60064 U.S.A.
Rev. 10/2009

MEDICATION GUIDE

for
Non-Steroidal Anti-Inflammatory Drugs (NSAIDs)
(See the end of this Medication Guide for a list of prescription NSAID medicines.)

What is the most important information I should know about medicines called Non-Steroidal Anti-Inflammatory Drugs (NSAIDs)?
NSAID medicines may increase the chance of a heart attack or stroke that can lead to death.
This chance increases:
• with longer use of NSAID medicines
• in people who have heart disease
NSAID medicines should never be used right before or after a heart surgery called a "coronary artery bypass graft (CABG)."
NSAID medicines can cause ulcers and bleeding in the stomach and intestines at any time during treatment. Ulcers and bleeding:
• can happen without warning symptoms
• may cause death
The chance of a person getting an ulcer or bleeding increases with:
• taking medicines called "corticosteroids" and "anticoagulants"
• longer use
• smoking
• drinking alcohol
• older age
• having poor health
NSAID medicines should only be used:
• exactly as prescribed
• at the lowest dose possible for your treatment
• for the shortest time needed
What are Non-Steroidal Anti-Inflammatory Drugs (NSAIDs)?
NSAID medicines are used to treat pain and redness, swelling, and heat (inflammation) from medical conditions such as:
• different types of arthritis
• menstrual cramps and other types of short-term pain
Who should not take a Non-Steroidal Anti-Inflammatory Drug (NSAID)?
Do not take an NSAID medicine:
• if you had an asthma attack, hives, or other allergic reaction with aspirin or any other NSAID medicine
• for pain right before or after heart bypass surgery
Tell your healthcare provider:
• about all your medical conditions.
• about all of the medicines you take. NSAIDs and some other medicines can interact with each other and cause serious side effects. **Keep a list of your medicines to show to your healthcare provider and pharmacist.**
• if you are pregnant. NSAID medicines should not be used by pregnant women late in their pregnancy.
• if you are breastfeeding. **Talk to your doctor.**
What are the possible side effects of Non-Steroidal Anti-Inflammatory Drugs (NSAIDs)?

Serious side effects include:	Other side effects include:
• heart attack	• stomach pain
• stroke	• constipation
• high blood pressure	• diarrhea
• heart failure from body swelling (fluid retention)	• gas
• kidney problems including kidney failure	• heartburn
• bleeding and ulcers in the stomach and intestine	• nausea
• low red blood cells (anemia)	• vomiting
• life-threatening skin reactions	• dizziness
• life-threatening allergic reactions	
• liver problems including liver failure	
• asthma attacks in people who have asthma	

Get emergency help right away if you have any of the following symptoms:
• shortness of breath or trouble breathing
• chest pain
• weakness in one part or side of your body
• slurred speech
• swelling of the face or throat
Stop your NSAID medicine and call your healthcare provider right away if you have any of the following symptoms:
• nausea
• more tired or weaker than usual
• itching
• your skin or eyes look yellow
• stomach pain
• flu-like symptoms
• vomit blood
• there is blood in your bowel movement or it is black and sticky like tar
• unusual weight gain
• skin rash or blisters with fever
• swelling of the arms and legs, hands and feet
These are not all the side effects with NSAID medicines. Talk to your healthcare provider or pharmacist for more information about NSAID medicines. Call your doctor for medical advice about side effects. You may report side effects to FDA at 1–800–FDA-1088.
Other information about Non-Steroidal Anti-Inflammatory Drugs (NSAIDs)
• Aspirin is an NSAID medicine but it does not increase the chance of a heart attack. Aspirin can cause bleeding in the brain, stomach, and intestines. Aspirin can also cause ulcers in the stomach and intestines.
• Some of these NSAID medicines are sold in lower doses without a prescription (over the counter). Talk to your healthcare provider before using over the counter NSAIDs for more than 10 days.
NSAID medicines that need a prescription

Generic Name	Tradename
Celecoxib	Celebrex
Diclofenac	Cataflam, Voltaren, Arthrotec (combined with misoprostol)
Diflunisal	Dolobid
Etodolac	Lodine, Lodine XL
Fenoprofen	Nalfon, Nalfon 200
Flurbirofen	Ansaid
Ibuprofen	Motrin, Tab-Profen, Vicoprofen* (combined with hydrocodone), Combunox (combined with oxycodone)
Indomethacin	Indocin, Indocin SR, Indo-Lemmon, Indomethagan
Ketoprofen	Oruvail
Ketorolac	Toradol
Mefenamic Acid	Ponstel
Meloxicam	Mobic
Nabumetone	Relafen
Naproxen	Naprosyn, Anaprox, Anaprox DS, EC-Naproxyn, Naprelan, Naprapac (copackaged with lansoprazole)
Oxaprozin	Daypro
Piroxicam	Feldene
Sulindac	Clinoril
Tolmetin	Tolectin, Tolectin DS, Tolectin 600

* Vicoprofen contains the same dose of ibuprofen as over-the-counter (OTC) NSAIDs, and is usually used for less than 10 days to treat pain. The OTC NSAID label warns that long term continuous use may increase the risk of heart attack or stroke.

Manufactured by Halo Pharmaceutical Inc.
Whippany, NJ 07981 U.S.A.
for Abbott Laboratories
North Chicago, IL 60064 U.S.A.
Ref. 03-A253-Revised October, 2009

This Medication Guide has been approved by the U.S. Food and Drug Administration.
Shown in Product Identification Guide, page 304

ZEMPLAR®

[zĕm-plər]
(paricalcitol)
Capsules   ℞

HIGHLIGHTS OF PRESCRIBING INFORMATION
These highlights do not include all the information needed to use ZEMPLAR safely and effectively. See full prescribing information for ZEMPLAR.
ZEMPLAR (paricalcitol) capsules
Initial U.S. Approval: 1998

———————**RECENT MAJOR CHANGES**———————
Indications and Usage (1.2) 6/2009
Dosage and Administration (2.2) 6/2009
———————**INDICATIONS AND USAGE**———————
Zemplar is a vitamin D analog indicated for the prevention and treatment of secondary hyperparathyroidism associated with
• Chronic kidney disease (CKD) Stages 3 and 4 (1.1).
• CKD Stage 5 in patients on hemodialysis (HD) or peritoneal dialysis (PD) (1.2).
———————**DOSAGE AND ADMINISTRATION**———————
• CKD Stages 3 and 4: Zemplar Capsules may be administered once daily or every other day, three times a week (2.1).
• CKD Stage 5: Zemplar Capsules are dosed every other day, three times a week (2.2). To minimize the risk of hypercalcemia patients should be treated only after their baseline serum calcium has been reduced to 9.5 mg/dL or lower.
[See first table at top of next page]
[See second table at top of next page]
———————**DOSAGE FORMS AND STRENGTHS**———————
Capsules: 1 mcg, 2 mcg, and 4 mcg (3).
———————**CONTRAINDICATIONS**———————
Evidence of hypercalcemia or vitamin D toxicity (4).
———————**WARNINGS AND PRECAUTIONS**———————
• Hypercalcemia: Excessive administration of Zemplar Capsules can cause over suppression of PTH, hypercalcemia, hypercalciuria, hyperphosphatemia, and adynamic bone disease. Pharmacologic doses of vitamin D and its derivatives should be withheld during Zemplar treatment (5.1).
• Digitalis toxicity: Potentiated by hypercalcemia of any cause. Use caution when Zemplar Capsules are prescribed concomitantly with digitalis compounds (5.2).
• Laboratory tests: Monitor serum calcium, serum phosphorus, and serum or plasma iPTH during initial dosing or following any dose adjustment (5.3).
• Aluminum overload and toxicity: Avoid excessive use of aluminum containing compounds (5.4).
———————**ADVERSE REACTIONS**———————
The most common adverse reactions (> 5% and more frequent than placebo) include diarrhea, infection, hypertension, and dizziness.
To report SUSPECTED ADVERSE REACTIONS, contact Abbott Laboratories at 1-800-633-9110 or FDA at 1-800-FDA-1088 or www.fda.gov/medwatch
———————**DRUG INTERACTIONS**———————
Strong CYP3A inhibitors (e.g. ketoconazole) will increase the exposure of paricalcitol. Use with caution (7).
See 17 for PATIENT COUNSELING INFORMATION
                                            Revised: 06/2010

FULL PRESCRIBING INFORMATION: CONTENTS*
1 **INDICATIONS AND USAGE**
   1.1 Chronic Kidney Disease Stages 3 and 4
   1.2 Chronic Kidney Disease Stage 5
2 **DOSAGE AND ADMINISTRATION**
   2.1 Chronic Kidney Disease Stages 3 and 4
   2.2 Chronic Kidney Disease Stage 5
3 **DOSAGE FORMS AND STRENGTHS**
4 **CONTRAINDICATIONS**
5 **WARNINGS AND PRECAUTIONS**
   5.1 Hypercalcemia
   5.2 Digitalis Toxicity
   5.3 Laboratory Tests
   5.4 Aluminum Overload and Toxicity
6 **ADVERSE REACTIONS**
   6.1 Clinical Trials Experience
   6.2 Postmarketing Experience
7 **DRUG INTERACTIONS**

8   USE IN SPECIFIC POPULATIONS
8.1   Pregnancy
8.3   Nursing Mothers
8.4   Pediatric Use
8.5   Geriatric Use
10   OVERDOSAGE
11   DESCRIPTION
12   CLINICAL PHARMACOLOGY
12.1   Mechanism of Action
12.2   Pharmacodynamics
12.3   Pharmacokinetics
13   NONCLINICAL TOXICOLOGY
13.1   Carcinogenesis, Mutagenesis and Impairment of Fertility
14   CLINICAL STUDIES
14.1   Chronic Kidney Disease Stages 3 and 4
14.2   Chronic Kidney Disease Stage 5
16   HOW SUPPLIED/STORAGE AND HANDLING
17   PATIENT COUNSELING INFORMATION
* Sections or subsections omitted from the full prescribing information are not listed

---

FULL PRESCRIBING INFORMATION

1   INDICATIONS AND USAGE
1.1   Chronic Kidney Disease Stages 3 and 4
Zemplar Capsules are indicated for the prevention and treatment of secondary hyperparathyroidism associated with Chronic Kidney Disease (CKD) Stages 3 and 4.
1.2   Chronic Kidney Disease Stage 5
Zemplar Capsules are indicated for the prevention and treatment of secondary hyperparathyroidism associated with CKD Stage 5 in patients on hemodialysis (HD) or peritoneal dialysis (PD).

2   DOSAGE AND ADMINISTRATION
2.1   Chronic Kidney Disease Stages 3 and 4
Zemplar Capsules may be administered daily or three times a week. When dosing three times weekly, the dose should be administered not more frequently than every other day. The total weekly doses for both daily and three times a week dosage regimens are similar [see Clinical Studies (14.1)]. Zemplar Capsules may be taken without regard to food. No dosing adjustment is required in patients with mild and moderate hepatic impairment.

Initial Dose
The initial dose of Zemplar Capsules for CKD Stages 3 and 4 patients is based on baseline intact parathyroid hormone (iPTH) levels.

Baseline iPTH Level	Daily Dose	Three Times a Week Dose*
≤ 500 pg/mL	1 mcg	2 mcg
> 500 pg/mL	2 mcg	4 mcg

*To be administered not more often than every other day

Dose Titration
Dosing must be individualized and based on serum or plasma iPTH levels, with monitoring of serum calcium and serum phosphorus. The following is a suggested approach to dose titration.

iPTH Level Relative to Baseline	Zemplar Capsule Dose	Dose Adjustment at 2 to 4 Week Intervals	
		Daily Dosage	Three Times a Week Dosage*
The same, increased or decreased by < 30%	Increase dose by	1 mcg	2 mcg
Decreased by ≥ 30% and ≤ 60%	Maintain dose	-	-
Decreased by > 60% or iPTH < 60 pg/mL	Decrease dose by	1 mcg	2 mcg

*To be administered not more often than every other day

If a patient is taking the lowest dose, 1 mcg, on the daily regimen and a dose reduction is needed, the dose can be decreased to 1 mcg three times a week. If a further dose reduction is required, the drug should be withheld as needed and restarted at a lower dosing frequency. If a patient is on a calcium-based phosphate binder, the phosphate-binder dose may be decreased or withheld, or the patient may be switched to a non-calcium-based phosphate binder. If hypercalcemia or an elevated Ca × P is observed, the dose of Zemplar should be reduced or withheld until these parameters are normalized.

Serum calcium and phosphorus levels should be closely monitored after initiation of Zemplar Capsules, during dose titration periods and during co-administration with strong CYP3A inhibitors [see Warnings and Precautions (5.3), Drug Interactions (7) and Clinical Pharmacology (12.3)].

2.2   Chronic Kidney Disease Stage 5
Zemplar Capsules are to be administered three times a week, not more frequently than every other day.
Zemplar Capsules may be taken without regard to food. No dosing adjustment is required in patients with mild and moderate hepatic impairment.

Initial Dose
The initial dose of Zemplar Capsules in micrograms is based on a baseline iPTH level (pg/mL)/80. To minimize the risk of hypercalcemia patients should be treated only after their baseline serum calcium has been adjusted to 9.5 mg/dL or lower [see Clinical Pharmacology (12.2) and Clinical Studies (14.2)].

Dose Titration
Subsequent dosing should be individualized and based on iPTH, serum calcium and phosphorus levels. A suggested dose titration of Zemplar Capsules is based on the following formula:
Titration dose (micrograms) = most recent iPTH level (pg/mL)/80
Serum calcium and phosphorus levels should be closely monitored after initiation, during dose titration periods, and with co-administration of strong P450 3A inhibitors. If an elevated serum calcium or elevated Ca × P is observed and the patient is on a calcium-based phosphate binder, the binder dose may be decreased or withheld, or the patient may be switched to a non-calcium-based phosphate binder. If serum calcium or Ca × P are elevated, the dose should be decreased by 2 to 4 micrograms lower than that calculated by the most recent iPTH/80. If further adjustment is required, the dose of paricalcitol capsules should be reduced or withheld until these parameters are normalized.
As iPTH approaches the target range, small, individualized dose adjustments may be necessary in order to achieve a stable iPTH. In situations where monitoring of iPTH, Ca or P occurs less frequently than once per week, a more modest initial and dose titration ratio (e.g., iPTH/100) may be warranted.

3   DOSAGE FORMS AND STRENGTHS
Zemplar Capsules are available as 1 mcg, 2 mcg, and 4 mcg soft gelatin capsules.
- 1 mcg: oval, gray capsule imprinted with Abbott ⧉ logo and "ZA"
- 2 mcg: oval, orange-brown capsule imprinted with Abbott ⧉ logo and "ZF"
- 4 mcg: oval, gold capsule imprinted with Abbott ⧉ logo and "ZK"

Initial Dosage

CKD Stages 3, 4		CKD Stage 5
Baseline intact parathyroid (iPTH) Level	Starting Dose	
≤ 500 pg/mL	1 mcg daily or 2 mcg three times a week (e.g. every other day)	Dose in micrograms is based on baseline iPTH level (pg/mL)/80.
> 500 pg/mL	2 mcg daily or 4 mcg three times a week (e.g. every other day)	Dose three times a week (e.g. every other day).

Dose Titration

CKD Stages 3, 4		CKD Stage 5
iPTH Level Relative to Baseline	Dosing Recommendation	
Decreased by < 30%	Increase dose by 1 mcg daily or 2 mcg three times a week (e.g. every other day)	Dose in micrograms is based on most recent iPTH level (pg/mL)/80 with adjustments based on serum calcium and phosphorous levels.
Decreased by ≥ 30% and ≤ 60%	Maintain dose	Dose three times a week (e.g. every other day).
Decreased by > 60% or iPTH < 60 pg/mL	Decrease dose by 1 mcg daily or 2 mcg three times a week (e.g. every other day)	

4   CONTRAINDICATIONS
Zemplar Capsules should not be given to patients with evidence of
- hypercalcemia or
- vitamin D toxicity [see Warnings and Precautions (5.1)].

5   WARNINGS AND PRECAUTIONS
Excessive administration of vitamin D compounds, including Zemplar Capsules, can cause over suppression of PTH, hypercalcemia, hypercalciuria, hyperphosphatemia, and adynamic bone disease.
5.1   Hypercalcemia
Progressive hypercalcemia due to overdosage of vitamin D and its metabolites may be so severe as to require emergency attention. Acute hypercalcemia may exacerbate tendencies for cardiac arrhythmias and seizures and may potentiate the action of digitalis. Chronic hypercalcemia can lead to generalized vascular calcification and other soft-tissue calcification. High intake of calcium and phosphate concomitant with vitamin D compounds may lead to serum abnormalities requiring more frequent patient monitoring and individualized dose titration. Patients also should be informed about the symptoms of elevated calcium, which include feeling tired, difficulty thinking clearly, loss of appetite, nausea, vomiting, constipation, increased thirst, increased urination and weight loss.
Pharmacologic doses of vitamin D and its derivatives should be withheld during Zemplar treatment to avoid hypercalcemia.
5.2   Digitalis Toxicity
Digitalis toxicity is potentiated by hypercalcemia of any cause. Use caution when Zemplar Capsules are prescribed concomitantly with digitalis compounds.
5.3   Laboratory Tests
During the initial dosing or following any dose adjustment of medication, serum calcium, serum phosphorus, and serum or plasma iPTH should be monitored at least every two weeks for 3 months, then monthly for 3 months, and every 3 months thereafter.
5.4   Aluminum Overload and Toxicity
To prevent aluminum toxicity, the regular administration of aluminum should be avoided and the dialysate concentration of aluminum should be maintained at < 10 mcg/L.

6   ADVERSE REACTIONS
Because clinical studies are conducted under widely varying conditions, adverse reaction rates observed in the clinical studies of a drug cannot be directly compared to rates in the clinical studies of another drug and may not reflect the rates observed in practice.
6.1   Clinical Trials Experience
CKD Stages 3 and 4
The safety of Zemplar Capsules has been evaluated in three 24-week (approximately six-month), double-blind, placebo-controlled, multicenter clinical studies involving 220 CKD Stages 3 and 4 patients. Six percent (6%) of Zemplar Capsules treated patients and 4% of placebo treated patients discontinued from clinical studies due to an adverse event. All reported adverse events occurring in at least 2% in either treatment group and more common in the Zemplar group are presented in Table 1.

Table 1. Treatment-Emergent Adverse Events by Body System Occurring in ≥ 2% of Subjects in the Zemplar-Treated Group of Three, Double-Blind, Placebo-Controlled, Phase 3, CKD Stages 3 and 4 Studies; All Treated Patients

Body System[a] COSTART V Term	Number (%) of Subjects			
	Zemplar Capsules (n = 107)		Placebo (n = 113)	
Overall	88	(82%)	86	(76%)
Body as a Whole				
Pain	8	(7.5%)	7	(6.2%)
Viral Infection	8	(7.5%)	8	(7.1%)
Allergic Reaction	6	(5.6%)	2	(1.8%)
Headache	5	(4.7%)	5	(4.4%)
Abdominal Pain	4	(3.7%)	2	(1.8%)
Back Pain	4	(3.7%)	1	(0.9%)
Infection	4	(3.7%)	4	(3.5%)
Asthenia	3	(2.8%)	2	(1.8%)
Chest Pain	3	(2.8%)	1	(0.9%)
Fever	3	(2.8%)	1	(0.9%)
Infection Fungal	3	(2.8%)	0	(0.0%)
Cardiovascular				
Hypertension	7	(6.5%)	4	(3.5%)
Hypotension	5	(4.7%)	3	(2.7%)
Syncope	3	(2.8%)	1	(0.9%)
Digestive				
Diarrhea	7	(6.5%)	5	(4.4%)
Nausea	6	(5.6%)	4	(3.5%)
Vomiting	6	(5.6%)	5	(4.4%)
Constipation	4	(3.7%)	4	(3.5%)
Gastroenteritis	3	(2.8%)	3	(2.7%)
Metabolic and Nutritional Disorders				
Edema	7	(6.5%)	5	(4.4%)
Dehydration	3	(2.8%)	1	(0.9%)
Musculoskeletal				
Arthritis	5	(4.7%)	1	(0.9%)
Leg Cramps	3	(2.8%)	0	(0.0%)
Nervous				
Dizziness	5	(4.7%)	5	(4.4%)
Vertigo	5	(4.7%)	0	(0.0%)
Depression	3	(2.8%)	0	(0.0%)
Respiratory				
Rhinitis	5	(4.7%)	4	(3.5%)
Bronchitis	3	(2.8%)	1	(0.9%)
Cough Increased	3	(2.8%)	2	(1.8%)
Sinusitis	3	(2.8%)	1	(0.9%)
Skin and Appendages				
Rash	6	(5.6%)	3	(2.7%)
Pruritus	3	(2.8%)	3	(2.7%)
Skin Ulcer	3	(2.8%)	0	(0.0%)
Urogenital System				
Urinary Tract Infection	3	(2.8%)	1	(0.9%)

a. Includes only events more common in the Zemplar treatment group.

CKD Stage 5

The safety of Zemplar Capsules has been evaluated in one 12-week, double-blind, placebo-controlled, multicenter clinical study involving 88 CKD Stage 5 patients. Sixty-one patients received Zemplar Capsules and 27 patients received placebo.

The proportion of patients who terminated prematurely from the study due to adverse events was 7% for Zemplar Capsules treated patients and 7% for placebo patients. Adverse events occurring in the Zemplar Capsules group at a frequency of 2% or greater and more frequently than in the placebo group are as follows:

Table 2. Treatment-Emergent Adverse Events by Body System Occurring in ≥ 2% of Subjects in the Zemplar-Treated Group, Double-Blind, Placebo-Controlled, Phase 3, CKD Stage 5 Study; All Treated Patients

Body System[a] COSTART V Term	Number (%) of Subjects			
	Zemplar Capsules (n = 61)		Placebo (n = 27)	
Overall	43	(70%)	19	(70%)
Body as a Whole				
Infection	9	(14.8%)	3	(11.1%)
Asthenia	3	(4.9%)	0	(0.0%)
Peritonitis	3	(4.9%)	0	(0.0%)
Headache	2	(3.3%)	0	(0.0%)
Digestive				
Diarrhea	7	(11.5%)	3	(11.1%)
Constipation	3	(4.9%)	0	(0.0%)
Nausea and Vomiting	3	(4.9%)	0	(0.0%)
Dyspepsia	2	(3.3%)	0	(0.0%)
Hemic and Lymphatic System				
Hypervolemia	3	(4.9%)	0	(0.0%)
Ecchymosis	2	(3.3%)	0	(0.0%)
Metabolic and Nutritional Disorders				
Hypoglycemia	2	(3.3%)	0	(0.0%)
Peripheral Edema	2	(3.3%)	0	(0.0%)
Uremia	2	(3.3%)	0	(0.0%)
Nervous				
Dizziness	4	(6.6%)	0	(0.0%)
Insomnia	3	(4.9%)	0	(0.0%)
Anxiety	2	(3.3%)	0	(0.0%)
Respiratory				
Sinusitis	2	(3.3%)	0	(0.0%)
Urogenital System				
Urinary Tract Infection	2	(3.3%)	0	(0.0%)

a. Includes only events more common in the Zemplar treatment group.

6.2 Postmarketing Experience

Taste perversion, such as metallic taste, and allergic reactions, such as rash, urticaria, pruritus, and angioedema (including laryngeal edema) have been reported with the active ingredient in Zemplar capsules.

7 DRUG INTERACTIONS

Since paricalcitol is partially metabolized by CYP3A, exposure of paricalcitol will increase while dosing paricalcitol with strong CYP3A inhibitors including ketoconazole, atazanavir, clarithromycin, indinavir, itraconazole, nefazodone, nelfinavir, ritonavir, saquinavir, telithromycin or voriconazole. Dose adjustment of Zemplar Capsules may be required, and iPTH and serum calcium concentrations should be closely monitored if a patient initiates or discontinues therapy with a strong CYP3A4 inhibitor [see *Clinical Pharmacology (12.3)*].

Drugs that impair intestinal absorption of fat-soluble vitamins, such as cholestyramine, may interfere with the absorption of Zemplar Capsules.

8 USE IN SPECIFIC POPULATIONS

8.1 Pregnancy

Pregnancy Category C.

Paricalcitol has been shown to cause minimal decreases in fetal viability (5%) when administered daily to rabbits at a dose 0.5 times a human dose of 14 mcg or 0.24 mcg/kg (based on body surface area, mcg/m^2), and when administered to rats at a dose two times the 0.24 mcg/kg human dose (based on body surface area, mcg/m^2). At the highest dose tested, 20 mcg/kg administered three times per week in rats (13 times the 14 mcg human dose based on surface area, mcg/m^2), there was a significant increase in the mortality of newborn rats at doses that were maternally toxic and are known to produce hypercalcemia in rats. No other effects on offspring development were observed.

Paricalcitol was not teratogenic at the doses tested.

Paricalcitol (20 mcg/kg) has been shown to cross the placental barrier in rats. There are no adequate and well-controlled clinical studies in pregnant women. Zemplar Capsules should be used during pregnancy only if the potential benefit to the mother justifies the potential risk to the fetus.

8.3 Nursing Mothers

Studies in rats have shown that paricalcitol is present in the milk. It is not known whether paricalcitol is excreted in human milk. In the nursing patient, a decision should be made whether to discontinue nursing or to discontinue the drug, taking into account the importance of the drug to the mother.

8.4 Pediatric Use

Safety and efficacy of Zemplar Capsules in pediatric patients have not been established.

8.5 Geriatric Use

Of the total number (n = 220) of CKD Stages 3 and 4 patients in clinical studies of Zemplar Capsules, 49% were age 65 and over, while 17% were age 75 and over. Of the total number (n = 88) of CKD Stage 5 patients in the pivotal study of Zemplar Capsules, 28% were age 65 and over, while 6% were age 75 and over. No overall differences in safety and effectiveness were observed between these patients and younger patients, and other reported clinical experience has not identified differences in responses between the elderly and younger patients, but greater sensitivity of some older individuals cannot be ruled out.

10 OVERDOSAGE

Excessive administration of Zemplar Capsules can cause hypercalcemia, hypercalciuria, and hyperphosphatemia, and over suppression of PTH [see *Warnings and Precautions (5.1)*].

Treatment of Overdosage

The treatment of acute overdosage of Zemplar Capsules should consist of general supportive measures. If drug ingestion is discovered within a relatively short time, induction of emesis or gastric lavage may be of benefit in preventing further absorption. If the drug has passed through the stomach, the administration of mineral oil may promote its fecal elimination. Serial serum electrolyte determinations (especially calcium), rate of urinary calcium excretion, and assessment of electrocardiographic abnormalities due to hypercalcemia should be obtained. Such monitoring is critical in patients receiving digitalis. Discontinuation of supplemental calcium and institution of a low-calcium diet are also indicated in accidental overdosage. Due to the relatively short duration of the pharmacological action of paricalcitol, further measures are probably unnecessary. If

Information on the Abbott Pharmaceutical Products listed on these pages is from the prescribing information in use as of June 1, 2010. For more information, please visit rxabbott.com or call 1-800-633-9110.

persistent and markedly elevated serum calcium levels occur, there are a variety of therapeutic alternatives that may be considered depending on the patient's underlying condition. These include the use of drugs such as phosphates and corticosteroids, as well as measures to induce an appropriate forced diuresis.

11 DESCRIPTION

Paricalcitol, USP, the active ingredient in Zemplar Capsules, is a synthetically manufactured, metabolically active vitamin D analog of calcitriol with modifications to the side chain (D_2) and the A (19-nor) ring. Zemplar is indicated for the prevention and treatment of secondary hyperparathyroidism in chronic kidney disease. Zemplar is available as soft gelatin capsules for oral administration containing 1 microgram, 2 micrograms or 4 micrograms of paricalcitol. Each capsule also contains medium chain triglycerides, alcohol, and butylated hydroxytoluene. The medium chain triglycerides are fractionated from coconut oil or palm kernel oil. The capsule shell is composed of gelatin, glycerin, titanium dioxide, iron oxide red (2 microgram capsules only), iron oxide yellow (2 microgram and 4 microgram capsules), iron oxide black (1 microgram capsules only), and water.

Paricalcitol is a white, crystalline powder with the empirical formula of $C_{27}H_{44}O_3$, which corresponds to a molecular weight of 416.64. Paricalcitol is chemically designated as 19-nor-1α,3β,25-trihydroxy-9,10-secoergosta-5(Z),7(E),22(E)-triene and has the following structural formula:

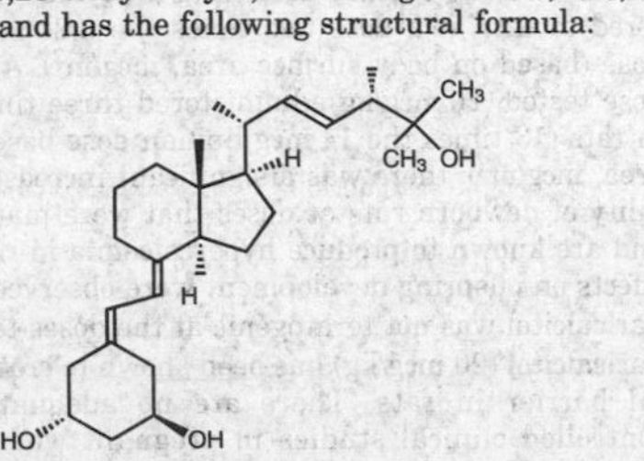

12 CLINICAL PHARMACOLOGY

Secondary hyperparathyroidism is characterized by an elevation in parathyroid hormone (PTH) associated with inadequate levels of active vitamin D hormone. The source of vitamin D in the body is from synthesis in the skin as vitamin D_3 and from dietary intake as either vitamin D_2 or D_3. Both vitamin D_2 and D_3 require two sequential hydroxylations in the liver and the kidney to bind to and to activate the vitamin D receptor (VDR). The endogenous VDR activator, calcitriol [1,25$(OH)_2D_3$], is a hormone that binds to VDRs that are present in the parathyroid gland, intestine, kidney, and bone to maintain parathyroid function and calcium and phosphorus homeostasis, and to VDRs found in many other tissues, including prostate, endothelium and immune cells. VDR activation is essential for the proper formation and maintenance of normal bone. In the diseased kidney, the activation of vitamin D is diminished, resulting in a rise of PTH, subsequently leading to secondary hyperparathyroidism and disturbances in the calcium and phosphorus homeostasis. Decreased levels of 1,25$(OH)_2D_3$ have been observed in early stages of chronic kidney disease. The decreased levels of 1,25$(OH)_2D_3$ and resultant elevated PTH levels, both of which often precede abnormalities in serum calcium and phosphorus, affect bone turnover rate and may result in renal osteodystrophy.

12.1 Mechanism of Action

Paricalcitol is a synthetic, biologically active vitamin D_2 analog of calcitriol. Preclinical and *in vitro* studies have demonstrated that paricalcitol's biological actions are mediated through binding of the VDR, which results in the selective activation of vitamin D responsive pathways. Vitamin D and paricalcitol have been shown to reduce parathyroid hormone levels by inhibiting PTH synthesis and secretion.

12.2 Pharmacodynamics

Paricalcitol decreases serum intact parathyroid hormone (iPTH) and increases serum calcium and serum phosphorous in both HD and PD patients. This observed relationship was quantified using a mathematical model for HD and PD patient populations separately. Computer-based simulations of 100 trials in HD or PD patients (N = 100) using these relationships predict slightly lower efficacy (at least two consecutive ≥ 30% reductions from baseline iPTH) with lower hypercalcemia rates (at least two consecutive serum calcium ≥ 10.5 mg/dL) for lower iPTH-based dosing regimens. Further lowering of hypercalcemia rates was predicted if the treatment with paricalcitol is initiated in patients with lower serum calcium levels at screening.

Based on these simulations, a dosing regimen of iPTH/80 with a screening serum calcium ≤ 9.5 mg/dL, approximately 76.5% (95% CI: 75.6%–77.3%) of HD patients are predicted to achieve at least two consecutive weekly ≥ 30% reductions from baseline iPTH over a duration of 12 weeks. The predicted incidence of hypercalcemia is 0.8% (95% CI: 0.7%–1.0%). In PD patients, with this dosing regimen, approximately 83.3% (95% CI: 82.6%–84.0%) of patients are predicted to achieve at least two consecutive weekly ≥ 30% reductions from baseline iPTH. The predicted incidence of hypercalcemia is 12.4% (95% CI: 11.7%-13.0%) [*see Clinical Studies (14.2) and Dosage and Administration (2.2)*].

12.3 Pharmacokinetics

Absorption

The mean absolute bioavailability of Zemplar Capsules under low-fat fed condition ranged from 72% to 86% in healthy subjects, CKD Stage 5 patients on HD, and CKD Stage 5 patients on PD. A food effect study in healthy subjects indicated that the C_{max} and $AUC_{0-\infty}$ were unchanged when paricalcitol was administered with a high fat meal compared to fasting. Food delayed T_{max} by about 2 hours. The $AUC_{0-\infty}$ of paricalcitol increased proportionally over the dose range of 0.06 to 0.48 mcg/kg in healthy subjects.

Distribution

Paricalcitol is extensively bound to plasma proteins (≥ 99.8%). The mean apparent volume of distribution following a 0.24 mcg/kg dose of paricalcitol in healthy subjects was 34 L. The mean apparent volume of distribution following a 4 mcg dose of paricalcitol in CKD Stage 3 and a 3 mcg dose in CKD Stage 4 patients is between 44 and 46 L.

Metabolism

After oral administration of a 0.48 mcg/kg dose of ^{3}H-paricalcitol, parent drug was extensively metabolized, with only about 2% of the dose eliminated unchanged in the feces, and no parent drug was found in the urine. Several metabolites were detected in both the urine and feces. Most of the systemic exposure was from the parent drug. Two minor metabolites, relative to paricalcitol, were detected in human plasma. One metabolite was identified as 24(R)-hydroxy paricalcitol, while the other metabolite was unidentified. The 24(R)-hydroxy paricalcitol is less active than paricalcitol in an *in vivo* rat model of PTH suppression.

In vitro data suggest that paricalcitol is metabolized by multiple hepatic and non-hepatic enzymes, including mitochondrial CYP24, as well as CYP3A4 and UGT1A4. The identified metabolites include the product of 24(R)-hydroxylation, 24,26- and 24,28-dihydroxylation and direct glucuronidation.

Elimination

Paricalcitol is eliminated primarily via hepatobiliary excretion; approximately 70% of the radiolabeled dose is recovered in the feces and 18% is recovered in the urine. While the mean elimination half-life of paricalcitol is 4 to 6 hours in healthy subjects, the mean elimination half-life of paricalcitol in CKD Stages 3, 4, and 5 (on HD and PD) patients ranged from 14 to 20 hours.

[See table below]

Specific Populations

Geriatric

The pharmacokinetics of paricalcitol has not been investigated in geriatric patients greater than 65 years [*see Use in Specific Populations (8.5)*].

Table 3. Paricalcitol Capsule Pharmacokinetic Characteristics in CKD Stages 3, 4, and 5 Patients

Pharmacokinetic Parameters	CKD Stage 3 n = 15*	CKD Stage 4 n = 14*	CKD Stage 5 HD** n = 14	CKD Stage 5 PD** n = 8
C_{max} (ng/mL)	0.11 ± 0.04	0.06 ± 0.01	0.575 ± 0.17	0.413 ± 0.06
$AUC_{0-\infty}$ (ng•h/mL)	2.42 ± 0.61	2.13 ± 0.73	11.67 ± 3.23	13.41 ± 5.48
CL/F (L/h)	1.77 ± 0.50	1.52 ± 0.36	1.82 ± 0.75	1.76 ± 0.77
V/F (L)	43.7 ± 14.4	46.4 ± 12.4	38 ± 16.4	48.7 ± 15.6
$t_{1/2}$	16.8 ± 2.65	19.7 ± 7.2	13.9 ± 5.1	17.7 ± 9.6

* Four mcg paricalcitol capsules were given to CKD Stage 3 patients; three mcg paricalcitol capsules were given to CKD Stage 4 patients.

**CKD Stage 5 HD and PD patients received a 0.24 mcg/kg dose of paricalcitol as capsules.

Pediatric

The pharmacokinetics of paricalcitol has not been investigated in patients less than 18 years of age.

Gender

The pharmacokinetics of paricalcitol following single doses over the 0.06 to 0.48 mcg/kg dose range was gender independent.

Hepatic Impairment

The disposition of paricalcitol (0.24 mcg/kg) was compared in patients with mild (n = 5) and moderate (n = 5) hepatic impairment (as indicated by the Child-Pugh method) and subjects with normal hepatic function (n = 10). The pharmacokinetics of unbound paricalcitol was similar across the range of hepatic function evaluated in this study. No dosing adjustment is required in patients with mild and moderate hepatic impairment. The influence of severe hepatic impairment on the pharmacokinetics of paricalcitol has not been evaluated.

Renal Impairment

Following administration of Zemplar Capsules, the pharmacokinetic profile of paricalcitol for CKD Stage 5 on HD or PD was comparable to that in CKD 3 or 4 patients. Therefore, no special dosing adjustments are required other than those recommended in the Dosage and Administration section [*see Dosage and Administration (2)*].

Drug Interactions

An *in vitro* study indicates that paricalcitol is neither an inhibitor of CYP1A2, CYP2A6, CYP2B6, CYP2C8, CYP2C9, CYP2C19, CYP2D6, CYP2E1 or CYP3A nor an inducer of CYP2B6, CYP2C9 or CYP3A. Hence, paricalcitol is neither expected to inhibit nor induce the clearance of drugs metabolized by these enzymes.

Omeprazole

The effect of omeprazole (40 mg capsule) on paricalcitol (four 4 mcg capsules) pharmacokinetics was investigated in a single dose, crossover study in healthy subjects. The pharmacokinetics of paricalcitol was not affected when omeprazole was administered approximately 2 hours prior to the paricalcitol dose.

Ketoconazole

The effect of multiple doses of ketoconazole administered as 200 mg BID for 5 days on the pharmacokinetics of paricalcitol (4 mcg capsule) has been studied in healthy subjects. The C_{max} of paricalcitol was minimally affected, but $AUC_{0-\infty}$ approximately doubled in the presence of ketoconazole. The mean half-life of paricalcitol was 17.0 hours in the presence of ketoconazole as compared to 9.8 hours, when paricalcitol was administered alone [*see Drug Interactions (7)*].

Cholestyramine

Cholestyramine has been reported to reduce intestinal absorption of fat-soluble vitamins; therefore, it may impair intestinal absorption of paricalcitol.

Mineral Oil

The use of mineral oil or other substances that may affect absorption of fat may influence the absorption of paricalcitol.

13 NONCLINICAL TOXICOLOGY

13.1 Carcinogenesis, Mutagenesis and Impairment of Fertility

In a 104-week carcinogenicity study in CD-1 mice, an increased incidence of uterine leiomyoma and leiomyosarcoma was observed at subcutaneous doses of 1, 3, 10 mcg/kg given three times weekly (2 to 15 times the AUC at a human dose of 14 mcg, equivalent to 0.24 mcg/kg based on AUC). The incidence rate of uterine leiomyoma was significantly different than the control group at the highest dose of 10 mcg/kg. In a 104-week carcinogenicity study in rats, there was an increased incidence of benign adrenal pheochromocytoma at subcutaneous doses of 0.15, 0.5, 1.5 mcg/kg (< 1 to 7 times the exposure following a human dose of 14 mcg, equivalent to 0.24 mcg/kg based on AUC). The increased incidence of pheochromocytomas in rats may be related to the alteration of calcium homeostasis by paricalcitol. Paricalcitol did not exhibit genetic toxicity *in vitro* with or without metabolic activation in the microbial mutagenesis assay (Ames Assay), mouse lymphoma mutagenesis assay (L5178Y), or a human lymphocyte cell chromosomal aberration assay. There was also no evidence of genetic toxicity in an *in vivo* mouse micronucleus assay. Paricalcitol had no effect on fertility (male or female) in rats at intravenous doses up to 20 mcg/kg/dose (equivalent to 13 times a human dose of 14 mcg based on surface area, mcg/m^2).

14 CLINICAL STUDIES

14.1 Chronic Kidney Disease Stages 3 and 4

The safety and efficacy of Zemplar Capsules were evaluated in three, 24-week, double blind, placebo-controlled, randomized, multicenter, Phase 3 clinical studies in CKD Stages 3 and 4 patients. Two studies used an identical three times a week dosing design, and one study used a daily dosing design. A total of 107 patients received Zemplar Capsules and 113 patients received placebo. The mean age of the patients was 63 years, 68% were male, 71% were Caucasian, and

26% were African-American. The average baseline iPTH was 274 pg/mL (range: 145-856 pg/mL). The average duration of CKD prior to study entry was 5.7 years. At study entry 22% were receiving calcium based phosphate binders and/or calcium supplements. Baseline 25-hydroxyvitamin D levels were not measured.

The initial dose of Zemplar Capsules was based on baseline iPTH. If iPTH was ≤ 500 pg/mL, Zemplar Capsules were administered 1 mcg daily or 2 mcg three times a week, not more than every other day. If iPTH was > 500 pg/mL, Zemplar Capsules were administered 2 mcg daily or 4 mcg three times a week, not more than every other day. The dose was increased by 1 mcg daily or 2 mcg three times a week every 2 to 4 weeks until iPTH levels were reduced by at least 30% from baseline. The overall average weekly dose of Zemplar Capsules was 9.6 mcg/week in the daily regimen and 9.5 mcg/week in the three times a week regimen.

In the clinical studies, doses were titrated for any of the following reasons: if iPTH fell to < 60 pg/mL, or decreased > 60% from baseline, the dose was reduced or temporarily withheld; if iPTH decreased < 30% from baseline and serum calcium was ≤ 10.3 mg/dL and serum phosphorus was ≤ 5.5 mg/dL, the dose was increased; and if iPTH decreased between 30 to 60% from baseline and serum calcium and phosphorus were ≤ 10.3 mg/dL and ≤ 5.5 mg/dL, respectively, the dose was maintained. Additionally, if serum calcium was between 10.4 to 11.0 mg/dL, the dose was reduced irrespective of iPTH, and the dose was withheld if serum calcium was > 11.0 mg/dL. If serum phosphorus was > 5.5 mg/dL, dietary counseling was provided, and phosphate binders could have been initiated or increased. If the elevation persisted, the Zemplar Capsules dose was decreased. Seventy-seven percent (77%) of the Zemplar Capsules treated patients and 82% of the placebo treated patients completed the 24-week treatment. The primary efficacy endpoint of at least two consecutive ≥ 30% reductions from baseline iPTH was achieved by 91% of Zemplar Capsules treated patients and 13% of placebo treated patients (p < 0.001). The proportion of Zemplar Capsules treated patients achieving two consecutive ≥ 30% reductions was similar between the daily and the three times a week regimens (daily: 30/33, 91%; three times a week: 62/68, 91%).

The incidence of hypercalcemia (defined as two consecutive serum calcium values > 10.5 mg/dL), hyperphosphatemia and elevated Ca × P product in Zemplar Capsules treated patients was similar to placebo. There were no treatment related adverse events associated with hypercalcemia or hyperphosphatemia in the Zemplar Capsules group. No increases in urinary calcium or phosphorous were detected in Zemplar Capsules treated patients compared to placebo.

The pattern of change in the mean values for serum iPTH during the studies is shown in Figure 1.

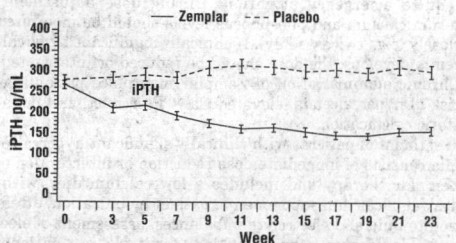

Figure 1. Mean Values for Serum iPTH Over Time in the Three Double-Blind, Placebo-Controlled, Phase 3, CKD Stages 3 and 4 Studies Combined

The mean changes from baseline to final treatment visit in serum iPTH, calcium, phosphorus, calcium-phosphorus product (Ca × P), and bone-specific alkaline phosphatase are shown in Table 4.

Table 4. Mean Changes from Baseline to Final Treatment Visit in Serum iPTH, Bone Specific Alkaline Phosphatase, Calcium, Phosphorus, and Calcium × Phosphorus Product in Three Combined Double-Blind, Placebo-Controlled, Phase 3, CKD Stages 3 and 4 Studies

	Zemplar Capsules	Placebo
iPTH (pg/mL)	n = 104	n = 110
Mean Baseline Value	266	279
Mean Final Treatment Value	162	315
Mean Change from Baseline (SE)	-104 (9.2)	+35 (9.0)

Bone Specific Alkaline Phosphatase (mcg/L)	n = 101	n = 107
Mean Baseline	17.1	18.8
Mean Final Treatment Value	9.2	17.4
Mean Change from Baseline (SE)	-7.9 (0.76)	-1.4 (0.74)
Calcium (mg/dL)	n = 104	n = 110
Mean Baseline	9.3	9.4
Mean Final Treatment Value	9.5	9.3
Mean Change from Baseline (SE)	+0.2 (0.04)	-0.1 (0.04)
Phosphorus (mg/dL)	n = 104	n = 110
Mean Baseline	4.0	4.0
Mean Final Treatment Value	4.3	4.3
Mean Change from Baseline (SE)	+0.3 (0.08)	+0.3 (0.08)
Calcium × Phosphorus Product (mg²/dL²)	n = 104	n = 110
Mean Baseline	36.7	36.9
Mean Final Treatment Value	40.7	39.7
Mean Change from Baseline (SE)	+4.0 (0.74)	+2.9 (0.72)

14.2 Chronic Kidney Disease Stage 5

The safety and efficacy of Zemplar Capsules were evaluated in a Phase 3, 12-week, double blind, placebo-controlled, randomized, multicenter study in patients with CKD Stage 5 on HD or PD. The study used a three times a week dosing design. A total of 61 patients received Zemplar Capsules and 27 patients received placebo. The mean age of the patients was 57 years, 67% were male, 50% were Caucasian, 45% were African-American, and 53% were diabetic. The average baseline iPTH was 701 pg/mL (range: 216-1933 pg/mL). The average time since first dialysis across all subjects was 3.3 years.

The initial dose of Zemplar Capsules was based on baseline iPTH/60. Subsequent dose adjustments were based on iPTH/60 as well as primary chemistry results that were measured once a week. Starting at Treatment Week 2, study drug was maintained, increased or decreased weekly based on the results of the previous week's calculation of iPTH/60. Zemplar Capsules were administered three times a week, not more than every other day.

The proportion of patients achieving at least two consecutive weekly ≥ 30% reductions from baseline iPTH was 88% of Zemplar Capsules treated patients and 13% of the placebo treated patients. The proportion of patients achieving at least two consecutive weekly ≥ 30% reductions from baseline iPTH was similar for HD and PD patients.

The incidence of hypercalcemia (defined as two consecutive serum calcium values > 10.5 mg/dL) in patients treated with Zemplar Capsules was 6.6% as compared to 0% for patients given placebo. In PD patients the incidence of hypercalcemia in patients treated with Zemplar Capsules was 21% as compared to 0% for patients given placebo. The patterns of change in the mean values for serum iPTH are shown in Figure 2. The rate of hypercalcemia with Zemplar Capsules may be reduced with a lower dosing regimen based on the iPTH/80 formula as shown by computer simulations. The hypercalcemia rate can be further predicted to decrease, if the treatment is initiated in only those with baseline serum calcium ≤ 9.5 mg/dL [see Clinical Pharmacology (12.2) and Dosage and Administration (2.2)]. [See figure at top of next column]

16   HOW SUPPLIED/STORAGE AND HANDLING

Zemplar Capsules are available as 1 mcg, 2 mcg, and 4 mcg capsules.

The 1 mcg capsule is an oval, gray, soft gelatin capsule imprinted with **Abbott** ⊐ logo and ZA, and is available in the following package size:
Bottles of 30 (NDC 0074-4317-30)
The 2 mcg capsule is an oval, orange-brown, soft gelatin capsule imprinted with **Abbott** ⊐ logo and ZF, and is available in the following package size:

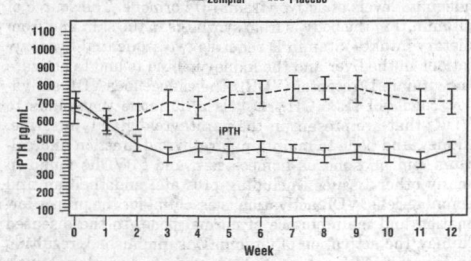

Figure 2. Mean Values for Serum iPTH Over Time in a Phase 3, Double-Blind, Placebo-Controlled CKD Stage 5 Study

Bottles of 30 (NDC 0074-4314-30)
The 4 mcg capsule is an oval, gold soft gelatin capsule imprinted with **Abbott** ⊐ logo and ZK, and is available in the following package size:
Bottles of 30 (NDC 0074-4315-30)

Storage
Store Zemplar Capsules at 25°C (77°F). Excursions permitted between 15°-30°C (59°-86°F). See USP Controlled Room Temperature.

17   PATIENT COUNSELING INFORMATION
Patients should be advised:
• of the most common adverse reactions with use of Zemplar Capsules, which include diarrhea, infection, hypertension and dizziness.
• to adhere to instructions regarding diet and phosphorus restriction.
• to contact a health care provider if you develop symptoms of elevated calcium, (e.g. feeling tired, difficulty thinking clearly, loss of appetite, nausea, vomiting, constipation, increased thirst, increased urination and weight loss).
• to return to the physician's office for routine monitoring. More frequent monitoring is necessary during the initiation of therapy, following dose changes or when potentially interacting medications are started or discontinued.
• to inform their physician of all medications, including prescription and nonprescription drugs, supplements, and herbal preparations they are taking and any change to their medical condition. Patients should also be advised to inform their physicians prescribing a new medication that they are taking Zemplar Capsules.

© Abbott
Abbott Laboratories
North Chicago, IL 60064, U.S.A.
Ref: 03-A330- Revised June 2010
Shown in Product Identification Guide, page 304

ZEMPLAR®   ℞
[zĕm-plər]
(paricalcitol) Injection
Fliptop Vial

DESCRIPTION
Paricalcitol, USP, the active ingredient in Zemplar Injection, is a synthetically manufactured analog of calcitriol, the metabolically active form of vitamin D indicated for the prevention and treatment of secondary hyperparathyroidism associated with chronic kidney disease (CKD) Stage 5. Zemplar is available as a sterile, clear, colorless, aqueous solution for intravenous injection. Each mL contains paricalcitol, 2 mcg or 5 mcg; propylene glycol, 30% (v/v); and alcohol, 20% (v/v).

Paricalcitol is a white powder chemically designated as 19-nor-1α,3β,25-trihydroxy-9,10-secoergosta-5(Z),7(E),22(E)-triene and has the following structural formula:

Molecular formula is $C_{27}H_{44}O_3$.
Molecular weight is 416.64.

CLINICAL PHARMACOLOGY

Secondary hyperparathyroidism is characterized by an elevation in parathyroid hormone (PTH) associated with inadequate levels of active vitamin D hormone. The source of vitamin D in the body is from synthesis in the skin and from dietary intake. Vitamin D requires two sequential hydroxylations in the liver and the kidney to bind to and to activate the vitamin D receptor (VDR). The endogenous VDR activator, calcitriol $[1,25(OH)_2 D_3]$, is a hormone that binds to VDRs that are present in the parathyroid gland, intestine, kidney, and bone to maintain parathyroid function and calcium and phosphorus homeostasis, and to VDRs found in many other tissues, including prostate, endothelium and immune cells. VDR activation is essential for the proper formation and maintenance of normal bone. In the diseased kidney, the activation of vitamin D is diminished, resulting in a rise of PTH, subsequently leading to secondary hyperparathyroidism, and disturbances in the calcium and phosphorus homeostasis.[1] The decreased levels of $1,25(OH)_2D_3$ and resultant elevated PTH levels, both of which often precede abnormalities in serum calcium and phosphorus, affect bone turnover rate and may result in renal osteodystrophy.

Mechanism of Action

Paricalcitol is a synthetic, biologically active vitamin D analog of calcitriol with modifications to the side chain (D_2) and the A (19-nor) ring. Preclinical and *in vitro* studies have demonstrated that paricalcitol's biological actions are mediated through binding of the VDR, which results in the selective activation of vitamin D responsive pathways. Vitamin D and paricalcitol have been shown to reduce parathyroid hormone levels by inhibiting PTH synthesis and secretion.

Pharmacokinetics

Within two hours after administering Zemplar intravenous doses ranging from 0.04 to 0.24 mcg/kg, concentrations of paricalcitol decreased rapidly; thereafter, concentrations of paricalcitol declined log-linearly. No accumulation of paricalcitol was observed with multiple dosing.

Distribution

Paricalcitol is extensively bound to plasma proteins ($\geq$99.8%). In healthy subjects, the steady state volume of distribution is approximately 23.8 L. The mean apparent volume of distribution following a 0.24 mcg/kg dose of paricalcitol in CKD Stage 5 subjects requiring hemodialysis (HD) and peritoneal dialysis (PD) is between 31 and 35 L.

Metabolism

After IV administration of a 0.48 mcg/kg dose of ^{3}H-paricalcitol, parent drug was extensively metabolized, with only about 2% of the dose eliminated unchanged in the feces and no parent drug found in the urine. Several metabolites were detected in both the urine and feces. Most of the systemic exposure was from the parent drug. Two minor metabolites, relative to paricalcitol, were detected in human plasma. One metabolite was identified as 24(R)-hydroxy paricalcitol, while the other metabolite was unidentified. The 24(R)-hydroxy paricalcitol is less active than paricalcitol in an *in vivo* rat model of PTH suppression. *In vitro* data suggest that paricalcitol is metabolized by multiple hepatic and non-hepatic enzymes, including mitochondrial CYP24, as well as CYP3A4 and UGT1A4. The identified metabolites include the product of 24(R)-hydroxylation (present at low levels in plasma), as well as 24,26- and 24,28-dihydroxylation and direct glucuronidation.

Elimination

Paricalcitol is excreted primarily by hepatobiliary excretion. Approximately 63% of the radioactivity was eliminated in the feces and 19% was recovered in the urine in healthy subjects. In healthy subjects, the mean elimination half-life of paricalcitol is about five to seven hours over the studied dose range of 0.04 to 0.16 mcg/kg. The pharmacokinetics of paricalcitol has been studied in CKD Stage 5 subjects requiring hemodialysis (HD) and peritoneal dialysis (PD). The mean elimination half-life of paricalcitol after administration of 0.24 mcg/kg paricalcitol IV bolus dose in CKD Stage 5 HD and PD patients is 13.9 and 15.4 hours, respectively (Table 1).

Table 1 Mean ± SD Paricalcitol Pharmacokinetic Parameters in CKD Stage 5 Subjects Following Single 0.24 mcg/kg IV Bolus Dose

	CKD Stage 5-HD (n=14)	CKD Stage 5-PD (n=8)
C_{max} (ng/mL)	1.680 ± 0.511	1.832 ± 0.315
$AUC_{0-\infty}$ (ng•h/mL)	14.51 ± 4.12	16.01 ± 5.98
β (1/h)	0.050 ± 0.023	0.045 ± 0.026
$t_{1/2}$ (h) [†]	13.9 ± 7.3	15.4 ± 10.5
CL (L/h)	1.49 ± 0.60	1.54 ± 0.95
Vd_β (L)	30.8 ± 7.5	34.9 ± 9.5

[†] harmonic mean ± pseudo standard deviation, HD: hemodialysis, PD: peritoneal dialysis

The degree of accumulation was consistent with the half-life and dosing frequency.

Special Populations

Geriatric

The pharmacokinetics of paricalcitol have not been investigated in geriatric patients greater than 65 years.

Pediatrics

The pharmacokinetics of paricalcitol have not been investigated in patients less than 18 years of age.

Gender

The pharmacokinetics of paricalcitol were gender independent.

Hepatic Impairment

The disposition of paricalcitol (0.24 mcg/kg) was compared in patients with mild (n=5) and moderate (n=5) hepatic impairment (as indicated by the Child-Pugh method) and subjects with normal hepatic function (n=10). The pharmacokinetics of unbound paricalcitol were similar across the range of hepatic function evaluated in this study. No dosing adjustment is required in patients with mild and moderate hepatic impairment. The influence of severe hepatic impairment on the pharmacokinetics of paricalcitol has not been evaluated.

Renal Impairment

The pharmacokinetics of paricalcitol have been studied in CKD Stage 5 subjects requiring hemodialysis (HD) and peritoneal dialysis (PD). Hemodialysis procedure has essentially no effect on paricalcitol elimination. However, compared to healthy subjects, CKD Stage 5 subjects showed a decreased CL and increased half-life (see **Pharmacokinetics - Elimination**).

Drug Interactions

An *in vitro* study indicates that paricalcitol is not an inhibitor of CYP1A2, CYP2A6, CYP2B6, CYP2C8, CYP2C9, CYP2C19, CYP2D6, CYP2E1, or CYP3A at concentrations up to 50 nM (21 ng/mL) (approximately 20-fold greater than that obtained after highest tested dose). In fresh primary cultured hepatocytes, the induction observed at paricalcitol concentrations up to 50 nM was less than two-fold for CYP2B6, CYP2C9 or CYP3A, where the positive controls rendered a six- to nineteen-fold induction. Hence, paricalcitol is not expected to inhibit or induce the clearance of drugs metabolized by these enzymes.

Drug interactions with paricalcitol injection have not been studied.

Omeprazole

The pharmacokinetic interaction between paricalcitol capsule (16 mcg) and omeprazole (40 mg; oral) was investigated in a single dose, crossover study in healthy subjects. The pharmacokinetics of paricalcitol were unaffected when omeprazole was administered approximately 2 hours prior to the paricalcitol dose.

Ketoconazole

Although no data are available for the drug interaction between paricalcitol injection and ketoconazole, the effect of multiple doses of ketoconazole administered as 200 mg BID for 5 days on the pharmacokinetics of paricalcitol capsule has been studied in healthy subjects. The C_{max} of paricalcitol was minimally affected, but $AUC_{0-\infty}$ approximately doubled in the presence of ketoconazole. The mean

half-life of paricalcitol was 17.0 hours in the presence of ketoconazole as compared to 9.8 hours, when paricalcitol was administered alone (See **PRECAUTIONS**).

CLINICAL STUDIES

In three 12-week, placebo-controlled, phase 3 studies in chronic kidney disease Stage 5 patients on dialysis, the dose of Zemplar was started at 0.04 mcg/kg 3 times per week. The dose was increased by 0.04 mcg/kg every 2 weeks until intact parathyroid hormone (iPTH) levels were decreased at least 30% from baseline or a fifth escalation brought the dose to 0.24 mcg/kg, or iPTH fell to less than 100 pg/mL, or the Ca × P product was greater than 75 within any 2 week period, or serum calcium became greater than 11.5 mg/dL at any time.

Patients treated with Zemplar achieved a mean iPTH reduction of 30% within 6 weeks. In these studies, there was no significant difference in the incidence of hypercalcemia or hyperphosphatemia between Zemplar and placebo-treated patients. The results from these studies are as follows:
[See table at bottom left]

A long-term, open-label safety study of 164 CKD Stage 5 patients (mean dose of 7.5 mcg three times per week), demonstrated that mean serum Ca, P, and Ca × P remained within clinically appropriate ranges with PTH reduction (mean decrease of 319 pg/mL at 13 months).

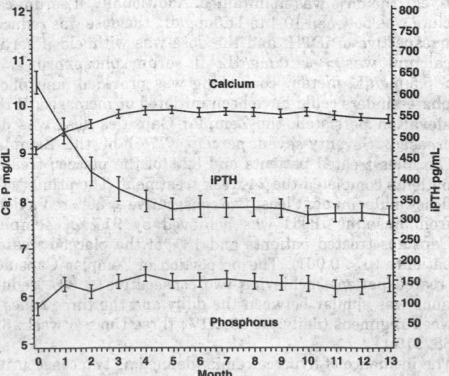

INDICATIONS AND USAGE

Zemplar is indicated for the prevention and treatment of secondary hyperparathyroidism associated with chronic kidney disease Stage 5.

CONTRAINDICATIONS

Zemplar should not be given to patients with evidence of vitamin D toxicity, hypercalcemia, or hypersensitivity to any ingredient in this product (see **WARNINGS**).

WARNINGS

Acute overdose of Zemplar may cause hypercalcemia, and require emergency attention. During dose adjustment, serum calcium and phosphorus levels should be monitored closely (e.g., twice weekly). If clinically significant hypercalcemia develops, the dose should be reduced or interrupted. Chronic administration of Zemplar may place patients at risk of hypercalcemia, elevated Ca × P product, and metastatic calcification.

Treatment of patients with clinically significant hypercalcemia consists of immediate dose reduction or interruption of Zemplar therapy and includes a low calcium diet, withdrawal of calcium supplements, patient mobilization, attention to fluid and electrolyte imbalances, assessment of electrocardiographic abnormalities (critical in patients receiving digitalis), hemodialysis or peritoneal dialysis against a calcium-free dialysate, as warranted. Serum calcium levels should be monitored frequently until normocalcemia ensues.

Phosphate or vitamin D-related compounds should not be taken concomitantly with Zemplar.

PRECAUTIONS

General

Digitalis toxicity is potentiated by hypercalcemia of any cause, so caution should be applied when digitalis compounds are prescribed concomitantly with Zemplar. Adynamic bone lesions may develop if PTH levels are suppressed to abnormal levels.

Information for the Patient

The patient should be instructed that, to ensure effectiveness of Zemplar therapy, it is important to adhere to a dietary regimen of calcium supplementation and phosphorus restriction. Appropriate types of phosphate-binding compounds may be needed to control serum phosphorus levels in patients with chronic kidney disease (CKD) Stage 5, but excessive use of aluminum containing compounds should be avoided. Patients should also be carefully informed about the symptoms of elevated calcium (see **ADVERSE REACTIONS**).

	Group (No. of Pts.)	Baseline Mean (Range)	Mean (SE) Change From Baseline to Final Evaluation
PTH (pg/mL)	Zemplar (n = 40)	783 (291–2076)	-379 (43.7)
	placebo (n = 38)	745 (320–1671)	-69.6 (44.8)
Alkaline Phosphatase (U/L)	Zemplar (n = 31)	150 (40–600)	-41.5 (10.6)
	placebo (n = 34)	169 (56–911)	+2.6 (10.1)
Calcium (mg/dL)	Zemplar (n = 40)	9.3 (7.2–10.4)	+0.47 (0.1)
	placebo (n = 38)	9.1 (7.8–10.7)	+0.02 (0.1)
Phosphorus (mg/dL)	Zemplar (n = 40)	5.8 (3.7–10.2)	+0.47 (0.3)
	placebo (n = 38)	6.0 (2.8–8.8)	-0.47 (0.3)
Calcium × Phosphorus Product	Zemplar (n = 40)	54 (32–106)	+7.9 (2.2)
	placebo (n = 38)	54 (26–77)	-3.9 (2.3)

Laboratory Tests
During the initial phase of medication, serum calcium and phosphorus should be determined frequently (e.g., twice weekly). Once dosage has been established, serum calcium and phosphorus should be measured at least monthly. Measurements of serum or plasma PTH are recommended every 3 months. An intact PTH (iPTH) assay is recommended for reliable detection of biologically active PTH in patients with CKD Stage 5. During dose adjustment of Zemplar, laboratory tests may be required more frequently.

Drug Interactions
Paricalcitol is not expected to inhibit the clearance of drugs metabolized by cytochrome P450 enzymes CYP1A2, CYP2A6, CYP2B6, CYP2C8, CYP2C9, CYP2C19, CYP2D6, CYP2E1, or CYP3A nor induce the clearance of drug metabolized by CYP2B6, CYP2C9 or CYP3A.
Specific interaction studies were not performed with Zemplar Injection.
A multiple dose drug-drug interaction study with ketoconazole and paricalcitol capsule demonstrated that ketoconazole approximately doubled paricalcitol $AUC_{0-\infty}$ (see **CLINICAL PHARMACOLOGY**). Since paricalcitol is partially metabolized by CYP3A and ketoconazole is known to be a strong inhibitor of cytochrome P450 3A enzyme, care should be taken while dosing paricalcitol with ketoconazole and other strong P450 3A inhibitors including atazanavir, clarithromycin, indinavir, itraconazole, nefazodone, nelfinavir, ritonavir, saquinavir, telithromycin or voriconazole.
Digitalis toxicity is potentiated by hypercalcemia of any cause, so caution should be applied when digitalis compounds are prescribed concomitantly with Zemplar.

Carcinogenesis, Mutagenesis, Impairment of Fertility
In a 104-week carcinogenicity study in CD-1 mice, an increased incidence of uterine leiomyoma and leiomyosarcoma was observed at subcutaneous doses of 1, 3, 10 mcg/kg (2 to 15 times the AUC at a human dose of 14 mcg, equivalent to 0.24 mcg/kg based on AUC). The incidence rate of uterine leiomyoma was significantly different than the control group at the highest dose of 10 mcg/kg.
In a 104-week carcinogenicity study in rats, there was an increased incidence of benign adrenal pheochromocytoma at subcutaneous doses of 0.15, 0.5, 1.5 mcg/kg (< 1 to 7 times the exposure following a human dose of 14 mcg, equivalent to 0.24 mcg/kg based on AUC). The increased incidence of pheochromocytomas in rats may be related to the alteration of calcium homeostasis by paricalcitol.
Paricalcitol did not exhibit genetic toxicity *in vitro* with or without metabolic activation in the microbial mutagenesis assay (Ames Assay), mouse lymphoma mutagenesis assay (L5178Y), or a human lymphocyte cell chromosomal aberration assay. There was also no evidence of genetic toxicity in an *in vivo* mouse micronucleus assay. Zemplar had no effect on fertility (male or female) in rats at intravenous doses up to 20 mcg/kg/dose [equivalent to 13 times the highest recommended human dose (0.24 mcg/kg) based on surface area, mg/m^2].

Pregnancy
Pregnancy Category C
Paricalcitol has been shown to cause minimal decreases in fetal viability (5%) when administered daily to rabbits at a dose 0.5 times the 0.24 mcg/kg human dose (based on surface area, mg/m^2) and when administered to rats at a dose 2 times the 0.24 mcg/kg human dose (based on plasma levels of exposure). At the highest dose tested (20 mcg/kg 3 times per week in rats, 13 times the 0.24 mcg/kg human dose based on surface area), there was a significant increase of the mortality of newborn rats at doses that were maternally toxic (hypercalcemia). No other effects on offspring development were observed. Paricalcitol was not teratogenic at the doses tested.
There are no adequate and well-controlled studies in pregnant women. Zemplar should be used during pregnancy only if the potential benefit to the mother justifies the potential risk to the fetus.

Nursing Mothers
Studies in rats have shown that paricalcitol is present in the milk. It is not known whether paricalcitol is excreted in human milk. In the nursing patient, a decision should be made whether to discontinue nursing or to discontinue the drug, taking into account the importance of the drug to the mother.

Pediatric Use
The safety and effectiveness of Zemplar were examined in a 12-week randomized, double-blind, placebo-controlled study of 29 pediatric patients, aged 5-19 years, with end-stage renal disease on hemodialysis and nearly all had received some form of vitamin D prior to the study. Seventy-six percent of the patients were male, 52% were Caucasian and 45% were African-American. The initial dose of Zemplar was 0.04 mcg/kg 3 times per week based on baseline iPTH level of less than 500 pg/mL, or 0.08 mcg/kg 3 times a week, based on baseline iPTH level of ≥ 500 pg/mL, respectively. The dose of Zemplar was adjusted in 0.04 mcg/kg increments based on the levels of serum iPTH, calcium and Ca × P. The mean baseline levels of iPTH were 841 pg/mL for the 15 Zemplar-treated patients and 740 pg/mL for the 14 placebo-treated subjects. The mean dose of Zemplar administered was 4.6 mcg (range: 0.8 mcg–9.6 mcg). Ten of the 15 (67%) Zemplar-treated patients and 2 of the 14 (14%) placebo-treated patients completed the trial. Ten of the placebo patients (71%) were discontinued due to excessive elevations in iPTH levels as defined by 2 consecutive iPTH levels > 700 pg/mL and greater than baseline after 4 weeks of treatment.
In the primary efficacy analysis, 9 of 15 (60%) subjects in the Zemplar group had 2 consecutive 30% decreases from baseline iPTH compared with 3 of 14 (21%) patients in the placebo group (95% CI for the difference between groups −1%, 63%). Twenty-three percent of Zemplar vs. 31% of placebo patients had at least one serum calcium level > 10.3 mg/dL, and 40% vs. 14% of Zemplar vs. placebo subjects had at least one Ca × P ion product > 72 $(mg/dL)^2$. The overall percentage of serum calcium measurements > 10.3 mg/dL was 7% in the Zemplar group and 7% in the placebo group; the overall percentage of patients with Ca × P product > 72 $(mg/dL)^2$ was 8% in the Zemplar group and 7% in the placebo group. No subjects in either the Zemplar group or placebo group developed hypercalcemia (defined as at least one calcium value > 11.2 mg/dL) during the study.

Geriatric Use
Of the 40 patients receiving Zemplar in the three phase 3 placebo-controlled CKD Stage 5 studies, 10 patients were 65 years or over. In these studies, no overall differences in efficacy or safety were observed between patients 65 years or older and younger patients.

ADVERSE REACTIONS

Zemplar has been evaluated for safety in clinical studies in 454 CKD Stage 5 patients. In four, placebo-controlled, double-blind, multicenter studies, discontinuation of therapy due to any adverse event occurred in 6.5% of 62 patients treated with Zemplar (dosage titrated as tolerated, see **CLINICAL PHARMACOLOGY - Clinical Studies**) and 2.0% of 51 patients treated with placebo for 1 to 3 months. Adverse events occurring with greater frequency in the Zemplar group at a frequency of 2% or greater, regardless of causality, are presented in the following table:

Adverse Event Incidence Rates for All Treated Patients In All Placebo-Controlled Studies

Adverse Event	Zemplar (n = 62) %	Placebo (n = 51) %
Overall	71	78
Body as a Whole		
Chills	5	0
Feeling unwell	3	0
Fever	5	2
Flu	5	4
Sepsis	5	2
Cardiovascular System		
Palpitation	3	0
Digestive System		
Dry mouth	3	2
Gastrointestinal bleeding	5	2
Nausea	13	8
Vomiting	8	4
Metabolic and Nutritional Disorders		
Edema	7	0
Nervous System		
Light-headedness	5	2
Respiratory System		
Pneumonia	5	0

A patient who reported the same medical term more than once was counted only once for that medical term.
Safety parameters (changes in mean Ca, P, Ca × P) in an open-label safety study up to 13 months in duration support the long-term safety of Zemplar in this patient population.
Potential adverse events of Zemplar Injection are, in general, similar to those encountered with excessive vitamin D intake. Signs and symptoms of vitamin D intoxication associated with hypercalcemia include:

Early
Weakness, headache, somnolence, nausea, vomiting, dry mouth, constipation, muscle pain, bone pain, and metallic taste.

Late
Anorexia, weight loss, conjunctivitis (calcific), pancreatitis, photophobia, rhinorrhea, pruritus, hyperthermia, decreased libido, elevated BUN, hypercholesterolemia, elevated AST and ALT, ectopic calcification, hypertension, cardiac arrhythmias, somnolence, death, and rarely, overt psychosis.

Adverse Events During Post-marketing Experience
Taste perversion, such as metallic taste, and allergic reactions, such as rash, urticaria, pruritus, and angioedema (including laryngeal edema) have been reported.

OVERDOSAGE

Overdosage of Zemplar may lead to hypercalcemia, hypercalciuria, hyperphosphatemia, and over suppression of PTH. (see **WARNINGS**).

Treatment of Overdosage and Hypercalcemia
The treatment of acute overdosage should consist of general supportive measures. Serial serum electrolyte determinations (especially calcium), rate of urinary calcium excretion, and assessment of electrocardiographic abnormalities due to hypercalcemia should be obtained. Such monitoring is critical in patients receiving digitalis. Discontinuation of supplemental calcium and institution of a low calcium diet are also indicated in acute overdosage.
General treatment of hypercalcemia due to overdosage consists of immediate suspension of Zemplar therapy, institution of a low calcium diet, and withdrawal of calcium supplements. Serum calcium levels should be determined at least weekly until normocalcemia ensues. When serum calcium levels have returned to within normal limits, Zemplar may be reinitiated at a lower dose. If persistent and markedly elevated serum calcium levels occur, there are a variety of therapeutic alternatives that may be considered. These include the use of drugs such as phosphates and corticosteroids as well as measures to induce diuresis. Also, one may consider dialysis against a calcium-free dialysate.

DOSAGE AND ADMINISTRATION

The currently accepted target range for iPTH levels in CKD Stage 5 patients is no more than 1.5 to 3 times the non-uremic upper limit of normal.
The recommended initial dose of Zemplar is 0.04 mcg/kg to 0.1 mcg/kg (2.8–7 mcg) administered as a bolus dose no more frequently than every other day at any time during dialysis.
If a satisfactory response is not observed, the dose may be increased by 2 to 4 mcg at 2- to 4-week intervals. During any dose adjustment period, serum calcium and phosphorus levels should be monitored more frequently, and if an elevated calcium level or a Ca × P product greater than 75 is noted, the drug dosage should be immediately reduced or interrupted until these parameters are normalized. Then, Zemplar should be reinitiated at a lower dose. If a patient is on a calcium-based phosphate binder, the dose may be decreased or withheld, or the patient may be switched to a non-calcium-based phosphate binder. Zemplar doses may need to be decreased as the PTH levels decrease in response to therapy. Thus, incremental dosing must be individualized.
The following table is a suggested approach in dose titration:

Suggested Dosing Guidelines

PTH Level	Zemplar Dose
the same or increasing	increase
decreasing by < 30%	increase
decreasing by ≥ 30%, < 60%	maintain
decreasing by > 60%	decrease
one and one-half to three times upper limit of normal	maintain

The influence of mild to moderately impaired hepatic function on paricalcitol pharmacokinetics is sufficiently small that no dosing adjustment is required.
Parenteral drug products should be inspected visually for particulate matter and discoloration prior to administration whenever solution and container permit.
Discard unused portion.

HOW SUPPLIED

Zemplar Injection is available as 2 mcg/mL (**NDC** 0074-4637-01) and 5 mcg/mL (**NDC** 0074-1658-01 and **NDC** 0074-1658-02).

Information on the Abbott Pharmaceutical Products listed on these pages is from the prescribing information in use as of June 1, 2010. For more information, please visit rxabbott.com or call 1-800-633-9110.

List No.	Volume/Container	Concentration	Total Content
4637-01	1 mL/Fliptop Vial	2 mcg/mL	2 mcg
1658-01	1 mL/Fliptop Vial	5 mcg/mL	5 mcg
1658-02	2 mL/Fliptop Vial	5 mcg/mL	10 mcg

Store at 25°C (77°F). Excursions permitted between 15°-30°C (59°-86°F).
U.S. patents: 5,246,925; 5,587,497; 6,136,799; 6,361,758

REFERENCES

1. K/DOQI Clinical Practice Guidelines for Bone Metabolism and Disease in Chronic Kidney Disease. Am J Kidney Dis 2003; Volume 42(4): Supplement 3.

© Abbott
Manufactured by
Hospira, Inc.
Lake Forest, IL 60045 USA
For
Abbott Laboratories
North Chicago, IL 60064, U.S.A.
Ref. EN-2198-Revised August, 2009

Adolor Corporation
**700 PENNSYLVANIA DRIVE
EXTON, PA 19341**

Direct Inquiries to:
1-866-4ADOLOR (1-866-423-6567)

ENTEREG®   ℞
[ĕnt-ĕr-ĕg]
(alvimopan)
Capsules

HIGHLIGHTS OF PRESCRIBING INFORMATION
These highlights do not include all the information needed to use ENTEREG safely and effectively. See full prescribing information for ENTEREG.
ENTEREG® (alvimopan) Capsules
Initial U.S. Approval: 2008

> **WARNING: FOR SHORT-TERM HOSPITAL USE ONLY**
> ENTEREG is available only for short-term (15 doses) use in hospitalized patients. Only hospitals that have registered in and met all of the requirements for the ENTEREG Access Support and Education (E.A.S.E.™) program may use ENTEREG.

INDICATIONS AND USAGE
ENTEREG is a peripherally acting μ-opioid receptor antagonist indicated to accelerate the time to upper and lower gastrointestinal recovery following partial large or small bowel resection surgery with primary anastomosis. (1)

DOSAGE AND ADMINISTRATION
12 mg administered 30 minutes to 5 hours prior to surgery followed by 12 mg twice daily for up to 7 days for a maximum of 15 doses. (2.1)

DOSAGE FORMS AND STRENGTHS
Capsules: 12 mg (3)

CONTRAINDICATIONS
Therapeutic doses of opioids for more than 7 consecutive days prior to ENTEREG (4)

WARNINGS AND PRECAUTIONS
- A higher number of myocardial infarctions was reported in patients treated with alvimopan 0.5 mg twice daily compared with placebo in a 12-month study in patients treated with opioids for chronic pain, although a causal relationship has not been established. (5.1)
- Patients recently exposed to opioids are expected to be more sensitive to the effects of ENTEREG and therefore may experience abdominal pain, nausea and vomiting, and diarrhea. (5.3)
- Not recommended in patients with severe hepatic impairment. (5.4)
- Not recommended in patients with end stage renal disease. (5.5)

ADVERSE REACTIONS
Most common adverse reactions (incidence ≥3% and ≥1% placebo) in patients undergoing bowel resection were anemia, dyspepsia, hypokalemia, back pain, and urinary retention. (6.1)
To report SUSPECTED ADVERSE REACTIONS, contact Adolor Corporation at 1-866-4ADOLOR (1-866-423-6567) or FDA at 1-800-FDA-1088 or www.fda.gov/medwatch.

USE IN SPECIFIC POPULATIONS
- Hepatic impairment: Patients with mild-to-moderate hepatic impairment do not require dosage adjustment, but they should be monitored for adverse effects. ENTEREG is not recommended for patients with severe hepatic impairment. (8.6)
- Renal impairment: Alvimopan has not been studied in patients with end stage renal disease. ENTEREG is not recommended for use in these patients. Dosage adjustment is not required in patients with mild to severe renal impairment but they should be monitored for adverse effects. (8.7)

See 17 for PATIENT COUNSELING INFORMATION
Revised: 11/2009

FULL PRESCRIBING INFORMATION: CONTENTS*
WARNING: FOR SHORT-TERM HOSPITAL USE ONLY

* Sections or subsections omitted from the full prescribing information are not listed

FULL PRESCRIBING INFORMATION

> **WARNING: FOR SHORT-TERM HOSPITAL USE ONLY**
> ENTEREG is available only for short-term (15 doses) use in hospitalized patients. Only hospitals that have registered in and met all of the requirements for the ENTEREG Access Support and Education (E.A.S.E.) program may use ENTEREG. *[see Warnings and Precautions (5.1 and 5.2)]*

1   INDICATIONS AND USAGE
ENTEREG is indicated to accelerate the time to upper and lower gastrointestinal recovery following partial large or small bowel resection surgery with primary anastomosis.

2   DOSAGE AND ADMINISTRATION
2.1   Usual Dosage in Adults
For hospital use only. The recommended adult dosage of ENTEREG is 12 mg administered 30 minutes to 5 hours prior to surgery followed by 12 mg twice daily beginning the day after surgery for a maximum of 7 days or until dis-

charge. Patients should not receive more than 15 doses of ENTEREG.

2.2   Special Populations
Geriatric Use: No dosage adjustment is necessary in elderly patients *[see Use in Specific Populations (8.5)]*.
Hepatic Impairment: No dosage adjustment is necessary in patients with mild-to-moderate hepatic impairment (Child-Pugh Class A and B). ENTEREG is not recommended for use in patients with severe hepatic impairment (Child-Pugh Class C) *[see Use in Specific Populations (8.6) and Clinical Pharmacology (12.3)]*.
Renal Impairment: No dosage adjustment is necessary in patients with mild-to-severe renal impairment, but they should be monitored for adverse effects. ENTEREG is not recommended for use in patients with end-stage renal disease *[see Use in Specific Populations (8.7) and Clinical Pharmacology (12.3)]*.
Race: No dosage adjustment is necessary in Black, Hispanic and Japanese patients, however, due to observed 2-fold greater ENTEREG plasma concentrations in healthy male Japanese subjects, Japanese patients should be monitored for possible adverse effects. *[see Use in Specific Populations (8.8) and Clinical Pharmacology (12.3)]*

3   DOSAGE FORMS AND STRENGTHS
12 mg blue, hard gelatin capsules with "ADL2698" printed on both the body and the cap of the capsule.

4   CONTRAINDICATIONS
ENTEREG is contraindicated in patients who have taken therapeutic doses of opioids for more than 7 consecutive days immediately prior to taking ENTEREG.

5   WARNINGS AND PRECAUTIONS
5.1   Myocardial Infarction in a 12 Month Study in Patients treated with Opioids for Chronic Pain
There were more reports of myocardial infarctions in patients treated with alvimopan 0.5 mg twice daily compared with placebo-treated patients in a 12-month study of patients treated with opioids for chronic pain. In this study, the majority of myocardial infarctions occurred between 1 and 4 months after initiation of treatment. This imbalance has not been observed in other studies of alvimopan, including studies in patients undergoing bowel resection surgery who received alvimopan 12 mg twice daily for up to 7 days. A causal relationship with alvimopan has not been established.

5.2   Distribution Program for ENTEREG
ENTEREG is available only to hospitals that enroll in the E.A.S.E. program. To enroll in the E.A.S.E. program, the hospital must acknowledge that:
- hospital staff who prescribe, dispense, or administer ENTEREG have been provided the educational materials on the need to limit use of ENTEREG to short-term, in-patient use;
- patients will not receive more than 15 doses of alvimopan; and
- ENTEREG will not be dispensed to patients after they have been discharged from the hospital.

Contact the E.A.S.E. program at 1-866-4ADOLOR (1-866-423-6567).

5.3   Opioid Tolerance and Gastrointestinal-Related Adverse Effects
Patients recently exposed to opioids are expected to be more sensitive to the effects of μ-opioid receptor antagonists, such as ENTEREG. Since ENTEREG acts peripherally, clinical signs and symptoms of increased sensitivity would likely be limited to the gastrointestinal tract (e.g., abdominal pain, nausea and vomiting, diarrhea). Patients receiving more than 3 doses of an opioid within the week prior to surgery were not studied in the postoperative ileus clinical trials; therefore, ENTEREG 12 mg capsules should be administered with caution to these patients.

5.4   Severe Hepatic Impairment
In patients with severe hepatic impairment, there is a potential for 10-fold higher plasma levels of drug *[see Clinical Pharmacology (12.3)]*. There are no studies of ENTEREG in patients with severe hepatic impairment undergoing bowel resection. Because of the limited data available, ENTEREG is not recommended for use in patients with severe hepatic impairment.

5.5   End-Stage Renal Disease
No studies have been conducted with end-stage renal disease. ENTEREG is not recommended for use in these patients.

5.6   Bowel Obstruction
Use of ENTEREG in patients undergoing surgery for correction of complete bowel obstruction is not recommended.

6   ADVERSE REACTIONS
6.1   Clinical Trials Experience
Because clinical trials are conducted under widely varying conditions, adverse reaction rates observed in the clinical

trials of a drug cannot be directly compared to rates in the clinical trials of another drug and may not reflect the rates observed in clinical practice. The adverse event information from clinical trials does, however, provide a basis for identifying the adverse events that appear to be related to drug use and for approximating rates.

The data described below reflect exposure to ENTEREG in 1,650 patients in 9 placebo-controlled studies worldwide. The population was 19 to 97 years old, 68% were female, and 83% were Caucasian; 61% were undergoing bowel resection surgery. The first dose of ENTEREG was administered 30 minutes to 5 hours before the scheduled start of surgery and then twice daily until hospital discharge (or for a maximum of 7 days of postoperative treatment).

Table 1 presents treatment-emergent adverse reactions reported in ≥3% patients treated with ENTEREG and for which the rate for ENTEREG was ≥1% than placebo. Treatment-emergent adverse reactions are those events occurring after the first dose of study medication treatment and within 7 days of the last dose of study medication or those events present at baseline that increased in severity after the start of study medication treatment.

[See table above]

Table 1. Treatment-Emergent Adverse Reactions That Were Reported in ≥3% of Either Bowel Resection Patients Treated With ENTEREG or All Surgical Patients Treated With ENTEREG and for Which the Rate for ENTEREG Was ≥1% Than Placebo

System Organ Class	Bowel Resection Patients		All Surgical Patients	
	Placebo (n = 986) %	ENTEREG (n = 999) %	Placebo (n = 1,365) %	ENTEREG (n = 1,650) %
Blood and lymphatic system disorders				
Anemia	4.2	5.2	5.4	5.4
Gastrointestinal disorders				
Constipation	3.9	4.0	7.6	9.7
Dyspepsia	4.6	7.0	4.8	5.9
Flatulence	4.5	3.1	7.7	8.7
Metabolism and nutrition disorders				
Hypokalemia	8.5	9.5	7.5	6.9
Musculoskeletal and connective tissue disorders				
Back Pain	1.7	3.3	2.6	3.4
Renal and urinary disorders				
Urinary retention	2.1	3.2	2.3	3.5

7 DRUG INTERACTIONS

7.1 Potential for Drugs to Affect Alvimopan Pharmacokinetics

Based on *in vitro* data, alvimopan is not a substrate of CYP enzymes. Therefore, concomitant administration of ENTEREG with inducers or inhibitors of CYP enzymes is unlikely to alter the metabolism of alvimopan. No clinical studies have been performed to assess the effect of concomitant administration of inducers or inhibitors of cytochrome P450 enzymes on alvimopan pharmacokinetics.

In vitro studies suggest that alvimopan and its 'metabolite' are substrates for p-glycoprotein. A population PK analysis did not reveal any evidence that alvimopan or 'metabolite' pharmacokinetics were influenced by concomitant medications that are mild-to-moderate p-glycoprotein inhibitors. No clinical studies of concomitant administration of alvimopan and strong inhibitors of p-glycoprotein (e.g., verapamil, cyclosporine, amiodarone, itraconazole, quinine, spirinolactone, quinidine, diltiazem, bepridil) have been conducted.

A population PK analysis suggests that the pharmacokinetics of alvimopan were not affected by concomitant administration of acid blockers or antibiotics. However, plasma concentrations of the 'metabolite' were lower in patients receiving acid blockers or preoperative oral antibiotics (49% and 81%, respectively). Because the 'metabolite' is not required for efficacy, no dosage adjustments are necessary in these patients.

7.2 Potential for Alvimopan to Affect the Pharmacokinetics of Other Drugs

Alvimopan and its 'metabolite' are not inhibitors of CYP 1A2, 2C9, 2C19, 3A4, 2D6, and 2E1 *in vitro* at concentrations far in excess of those observed clinically. Alvimopan and its 'metabolite' are not inducers of CYP 1A2, 2B6, 2C9, 2C19 and 3A4. *In vitro* studies also suggest that alvimopan and its 'metabolite' are not inhibitors of p-glycoprotein. These *in vitro* findings suggest that ENTEREG is unlikely to alter the pharmacokinetics of coadministered drugs through inhibition or induction of CYP enzymes or inhibition of p-glycoprotein.

Coadministration of alvimopan does not appear to alter the pharmacokinetics of morphine and its metabolite, morphine-6-glucuronide, to a clinically significant degree when morphine is administered intravenously. Dosage adjustment for intravenously administered morphine is not necessary when it is coadministered with alvimopan.

8 USE IN SPECIFIC POPULATIONS

8.1 Pregnancy
Teratogenic Effects: Pregnancy Category B
Reproduction studies have been performed in pregnant rats at about 68 to 136 times the recommended human oral dose based on the body surface area and intravenous doses of about 3.4 to 6.8 times the recommended human oral dose based on the body surface area and in pregnant rabbits at intravenous doses at about 5 to 10 times the recommended human oral dose based on the body surface area and have revealed no evidence of impaired fertility or harm to the fetus due to alvimopan. There are, however, no adequate and well-controlled studies in pregnant women. Because animal reproduction studies are not always predictive of human response, this drug should be used during pregnancy only if clearly needed.

8.3 Nursing Mothers
Alvimopan and its 'metabolite' are detected in the milk of lactating rats. It is not known whether alvimopan is excreted in human milk. Because many drugs are excreted in human milk, caution should be exercised when ENTEREG is administered to a nursing woman.

8.4 Pediatric Use
Safety and effectiveness in pediatric patients have not been established.

8.5 Geriatric Use
Of the total number of patients in 5 clinical efficacy studies treated with ENTEREG or placebo, 45% were 65 years of age and over, while 18% were 75 years of age and over. No overall differences in safety or effectiveness were observed between these patients and younger patients, and other reported clinical experience has not identified differences in responses between the elderly and younger patients, but greater sensitivity of some older individuals cannot be ruled out. No dosage adjustment based on increased age is required [see Clinical Pharmacology (12.3)].

8.6 Hepatic Impairment
Although there is a potential for higher plasma levels of drug in patients with mild-to-moderate hepatic impairment [see Clinical Pharmacology (12.3)], dosage adjustment in these patients is not required. Patients with mild-to-moderate hepatic impairment should be closely monitored for possible adverse effects (e.g., diarrhea, gastrointestinal pain, cramping) that could indicate high drug or 'metabolite' levels, and ENTEREG should be discontinued if adverse events occur. ENTEREG is not recommended for use in patients with severe hepatic impairment [see Dosage and Administration (2.2), Warnings and Precautions (5.4), and Clinical Pharmacology (12.3)].

8.7 Renal Impairment
Alvimopan has not been studied in patients with end-stage renal disease and ENTEREG is not recommended for use in these patients. Patients with mild-to-severe renal impairment do not require dosage adjustment, but they should be monitored for adverse effects. [see Dosage and Administration (2.2) and Clinical Pharmacology (12.3)]. Patients with severe impairment should be closely monitored for possible adverse effects (e.g., diarrhea, gastrointestinal pain, cramping) that could indicate high drug or 'metabolite' levels, and ENTEREG should be discontinued if adverse events occur.

8.8 Race
No dosage adjustment is necessary in Black, Hispanic and Japanese patients. However, the exposure of ENTEREG in Japanese male healthy volunteers was approximately 2-fold greater than in Caucasian subjects. Japanese patients should be closely monitored for possible adverse effects (e.g., diarrhea, gastrointestinal pain, cramping) that could indicate high drug or 'metabolite' levels, and ENTEREG should be discontinued if adverse events occur.
[see Dosage and Administration (2.2) and Clinical Pharmacology (12.3)].

9 DRUG ABUSE AND DEPENDENCE

ENTEREG has no known potential for abuse or dependence.

10 OVERDOSAGE

There is no specific antidote for overdosage with ENTEREG. Patients should be managed with appropriate supportive therapy. Single doses up to 120 mg and multiple doses up to 48 mg for 7 days have been administered to normal, healthy subjects in clinical studies. In these studies, alvimopan was well tolerated with no discontinuations due to adverse events and no reported serious adverse events or deaths.

11 DESCRIPTION

ENTEREG Capsules contain alvimopan, a peripherally-acting μ-opioid receptor (PAM-OR) antagonist. Chemically, alvimopan is the single stereoisomer [[2(S)-[[4(R)-(3-hydroxyphenyl)-3(R),4-dimethyl-1-piperidinyl]methyl]-1-oxo-3-phenylpropyl]amino]acetic acid dihydrate. It has the following structural formula:

Alvimopan is a white to light beige powder with a molecular weight of 460.6, and the empirical formula is $C_{25}H_{32}N_2O_4 \cdot 2H_2O$. It has a solubility of <0.1 mg/mL in water or buffered solutions between pH 3.0 and 9.0, 1 to 5 mg/mL in buffered solutions at pH 1.2, and 10 to 25 mg/mL in aqueous 0.1 N sodium hydroxide. At physiological pH, alvimopan is zwitterionic, a property that contributes to its low solubility.

ENTEREG Capsules for oral administration contain 12 mg of alvimopan on an anhydrous basis suspended in the inactive ingredient polyethylene glycol.

12 CLINICAL PHARMACOLOGY

12.1 Mechanism of Action
Alvimopan is a selective antagonist of the cloned human μ-opioid receptor with a Ki of 0.4 nM (0.2 ng/mL) and no measurable opioid-agonist effects in standard pharmacologic assays. The dissociation of [³H]-alvimopan from the human μ-opioid receptor is slower than that of other opioid ligands, consistent with its higher affinity for the receptor. At concentrations of 1 to 10 μM, alvimopan demonstrated no activity at any of over 70 non-opioid receptors, enzymes, and ion channels.

Postoperative ileus is the impairment of gastrointestinal motility after intra-abdominal surgery or other non-abdominal surgeries. Postoperative ileus affects all segments of the gastrointestinal tract and may last from 5 to 6 days, or even longer. This may potentially delay gastrointestinal recovery and hospital discharge until its resolution. It is characterized by abdominal distention and bloating, nausea, vomiting, pain, accumulation of gas and fluids in the bowel, and delayed passage of flatus and defecation. Postoperative ileus is the result of a multifactorial process that includes inhibitory sympathetic input, release of hormones, neurotransmitters, and other mediators (e.g., endogenous opioids). A component of postoperative ileus also results from an inflammatory reaction and the effects of opioid analgesics. Morphine and other μ-opioid receptor agonists are universally used for the treatment of acute postsurgical pain; however, they are known to have an inhibitory effect on gastrointestinal motility and may prolong the duration of postoperative ileus.

Following oral administration, alvimopan antagonizes the peripheral effects of opioids on gastrointestinal motility and secretion by competitively binding to gastrointestinal tract μ-opioid receptors. The antagonism produced by alvimopan at opioid receptors is evident in isolated guinea pig ileum preparations where alvimopan competitively antagonizes the effects of morphine on contractility. Alvimopan achieves this selective gastrointestinal opioid antagonism without reversing the central analgesic effects of μ-opioid agonists.

12.2 Pharmacodynamics

In exploratory studies in healthy volunteers, alvimopan 3 mg three times daily appeared to reduce the delay in gastrointestinal transit produced by morphine 30 mg twice daily as measured by radio-opaque markers.

In a study designed to evaluate potential effects on cardiac conduction, alvimopan did not cause clinically significant QTc prolongation at doses up to 24 mg twice daily for 7 days. The potential for QTc effects at higher doses has not been studied.

12.3 Pharmacokinetics

Following oral administration of alvimopan, an amide hydrolysis compound is present in the systemic circulation, which is considered a product exclusively of intestinal flora metabolism. This compound is referred to as the 'metabolite'. It is also a μ-opioid receptor antagonist with a Ki of 0.8 nM (0.3 ng/mL).

Absorption: Following oral administration of ENTEREG Capsules in healthy volunteers, plasma alvimopan concentration peaked at approximately 2 hours postdose. No significant accumulation in alvimopan concentration was observed following twice daily (BID) dosing. The mean peak plasma concentration was 10.98 (±6.43) ng/mL and mean AUC_{0-12h} was 40.2 (±22.5) ng•h/mL after dosing of alvimopan at 12 mg BID for 5 days. The absolute bioavailability was estimated to be 6% (range, 1% to 19%). Plasma concentrations of alvimopan increased approximately proportionally with increasing doses between 6 and 18 mg, but less than proportionally from 18 to 24 mg.

There was a delay in the appearance of the 'metabolite', which had a median T_{max} of 36 hours following administration of a single dose of alvimopan. Concentrations of the 'metabolite' were highly variable between subjects and within a subject. The 'metabolite' accumulated after multiple doses of ENTEREG. The mean C_{max} for the 'metabolite' after alvimopan 12 mg twice daily for 5 days was 35.73±35.29 ng/mL.

Concentrations of alvimopan and its 'metabolite' are higher (~1.9-fold and ~1.4-fold, respectively) in POI patients than in healthy volunteers.

Food Effects: A high-fat meal decreased the extent and rate of alvimopan absorption. The C_{max} and AUC were decreased by approximately 38% and 21%, respectively, and the T_{max} was prolonged by approximately 1 hour. The clinical significance of this decreased bioavailability is unknown. In POI clinical trials, the preoperative dose of ENTEREG was administered in a fasting state. Subsequent doses were given without regard to meals.

Distribution: The steady state volume of distribution of alvimopan was estimated to be 30±10 L. Plasma protein binding of alvimopan and its 'metabolite' was independent of concentration over ranges observed clinically and averaged 80% and 94%, respectively. Both alvimopan and the 'metabolite' were bound to albumin and not to alpha-1 acid glycoprotein.

Metabolism and Elimination: The average plasma clearance for alvimopan was 402 (±89) mL/min. Renal excretion accounted for approximately 35% of total clearance. There was no evidence that hepatic metabolism was a significant route for alvimopan elimination. Biliary secretion was considered the primary pathway for alvimopan elimination. Unabsorbed drug and unchanged alvimopan resulting from biliary excretion were then hydrolyzed to its 'metabolite' by gut microflora. The 'metabolite' was eliminated in the feces and in the urine as unchanged 'metabolite', the glucuronide conjugate of the 'metabolite', and other minor metabolites. The mean terminal phase half-life of alvimopan after multiple oral doses of ENTEREG ranged from 10 to 17 hours. The terminal half-life of the 'metabolite' ranged 10 to 18 hours.

Special Populations:

Age: The pharmacokinetics of alvimopan, but not its 'metabolite', were related to age, but this effect was not clinically significant and does not warrant dosage adjustment based on increased age.

Race: The pharmacokinetic characteristics of alvimopan were not affected by Hispanic or black race. Plasma 'metabolite' concentrations were lower in black and in Hispanic patients (by 43% and 82%, respectively) than in Caucasian patients following alvimopan administration. These changes are not considered to be clinically significant in surgical patients. Japanese male healthy volunteers had an approximately 2-fold increase in plasma alvimopan concentrations, but no change in metabolite pharmacokinetics. The pharmacokinetics of alvimopan have not been studied in subjects of other East Asian ancestry. Dosage adjustment in Japanese patients is not required [see Use in Specific Populations (8.8)].

Table 2. GI2 Recovery (Hours) in Bowel Resection Patients

Study No.	ENTEREG 12-mg Mean	Placebo Mean	Treatment Difference Mean	Hazard Ratio (95% CI)
1	92.0	111.8	19.8	1.533 (1.293, 1.816)
2	105.9	132.0	26.1	1.625 (1.256, 2.102)
3	116.4	130.3	14.0	1.365 (1.057, 1.764)
4	106.7	119.9	13.2	1.400 (1.035, 1.894)
5	98.8	109.5	10.7	1.299 (1.070, 1.575)

Gender: There was no effect of gender on the pharmacokinetics of alvimopan or the 'metabolite'.

Hepatic Impairment: Exposure to alvimopan following a single 12-mg dose tended to be higher (1.5 to 2 fold, on average) in patients with mild or moderate hepatic impairment (as defined by Child-Pugh Class A and B, n = 8 each) compared with healthy controls (n = 4). There were no consistent effects on the C_{max} or half-life of alvimopan in patients with hepatic impairment. However, two of 16 patients with mild to moderate impairment had longer than expected half-lives of alvimopan indicating that some accumulation may occur upon multiple dosing. The C_{max} of the 'metabolite' tended to be more variable in patients with mild or moderate hepatic impairment than in matched normal subjects. A study of 3 patients with severe hepatic impairment (Child-Pugh Class C), indicated similar alvimopan exposure in 2 patients and an approximately 10-fold increase in C_{max} and exposure in 1 patient with severe hepatic impairment when compared with healthy control volunteers [see Warnings and Precautions (5.4) and Use in Specific Populations (8.6)].

Renal Impairment: There was no relationship between renal function (i.e., creatinine clearance [CrCl]) and plasma alvimopan pharmacokinetics (C_{max}, AUC, or half-life) in patients with mild (CrCl 51-80 mL/min), moderate (CrCl 31-50 mL/min), or severe (CrCl <30 mL/min) renal impairment (n = 6 each). Renal clearance of alvimopan was related to renal function; however, because renal clearance was only a small fraction (35%) of the total clearance, renal impairment had a small effect on the apparent oral clearance of alvimopan. The half-lives of alvimopan were comparable in the mild, moderate and control renal impairment groups but longer in the severe renal impairment group. Exposure to the 'metabolite' tended to be 2- to 5-fold higher in patients with moderate or severe renal impairment compared to patients with mild renal impairment or control subjects. Thus, there may be accumulation of alvimopan and 'metabolite' in patients with severe renal impairment receiving multiple doses of ENTEREG. Patients with end-stage renal disease were not studied [see Warnings and Precautions (5.5) and Use in Specific Populations (8.7)].

Crohn's Disease: There was no relationship between disease activity in patients with Crohn's disease (measured as Crohn's Disease Activity Index or bowel movement frequency) and alvimopan pharmacokinetics (AUC or C_{max}). Patients with active or quiescent Crohn's disease had increased variability in alvimopan pharmacokinetics and exposure tended to be 2-fold higher in patients with quiescent disease than in those with active disease or normal subjects. Concentrations of the 'metabolite' were lower in patients with Crohn's disease.

13 NONCLINICAL TOXICOLOGY

13.1 Carcinogenesis, Mutagenesis, Impairment of Fertility

Two year carcinogenicity studies have been conducted with alvimopan in CD-1 mice at oral doses up to 4000 mg/kg/day and in Sprague Dawley rats at oral doses up to 500 mg/kg/day. Oral administration of alvimopan for 104 weeks produced significant increases in the incidences of fibroma, fibrosarcoma and sarcoma in the skin/subcutis, and osteoma/osteosarcoma in bones of female mice at 4000 mg/kg/day (about 674 times the recommended human dose based on body surface area). In rats, oral administration of alvimopan for 104 weeks did not produce any tumor up to 500 mg/kg/day (about 166 times the recommended human dose based on body surface area).

Alvimopan was not genotoxic in the Ames test, the mouse lymphoma cell (L5178Y/TK$^{+/-}$) forward mutation test, the Chinese Hamster Ovary (CHO) cell chromosome aberration test or the mouse micronucleus test. The pharmacologically active 'metabolite' ADL 08-0011 was negative in the Ames test, chromosome aberration test in CHO cells and mouse micronucleus test.

Alvimopan at intravenous doses up to 10 mg/kg/day (about 3.4 to 6.8 times the recommended human oral dose based on the body surface area) was found to have no adverse effect on fertility and reproductive performance of male and female rats.

13.2 Animal Toxicology and/or Pharmacology

A single oral dose of 500 mg/kg of alvimopan was not lethal to mice and rats.

Reproduction studies have been performed in pregnant rats at oral doses up to 200 mg/kg/day (about 68 to 136 times the recommended human oral dose based on the body surface area) and intravenous doses up to 10 mg/kg/day (about 3.4 to 6.8 times the recommended human oral dose based on the body surface area) and in pregnant rabbits at intravenous doses up to 15 mg/kg/day (about 5 to 10 times the recommended human oral dose based on the body surface area) and have revealed no evidence of impaired fertility or harm to the fetus due to alvimopan.

14 CLINICAL STUDIES

14.1 Postoperative Ileus

The efficacy of ENTEREG in the management of postoperative ileus was evaluated in 5 multicenter, randomized, double-blind, parallel-group, placebo-controlled studies: 4 US studies (Studies 1-4) and 1 non-US study (Study 5). Patients 18 years of age or older undergoing partial large or small bowel resection surgery with primary anastomosis or total abdominal hysterectomy under general anesthesia were randomly assigned to receive oral doses of ENTEREG 12 mg or matching placebo. The initial dose was administered at least 30 minutes and up to 5 hours prior to the scheduled start of surgery for most patients, and subsequent doses were administered twice daily beginning on the first postoperative day and continued until hospital discharge or a maximum of 7 days. There were no limitations on the type of general anesthesia used, but intrathecal or epidural opioids or anesthetics were prohibited.

All patients in the US studies were scheduled to receive intravenous patient-controlled opioid analgesia. In the non-US study, patients were scheduled to receive opioids either by intravenous patient-controlled opioid analgesia or bolus parenteral administration (intravenous or intramuscular). In all studies, there was no restriction on the type of opioid used or the duration of intravenous patient-controlled opioid analgesia. A standardized accelerated postoperative care pathway was implemented: early nasogastric tube removal (end of surgery); early ambulation (day following surgery); early diet advancement (liquids offered the day following surgery) and solids by the second day following surgery, as tolerated.

Patients who received more than 3 doses of an opioid (regardless of route) during the 7 days prior to surgery and patients with complete bowel obstruction or who were scheduled for a total colectomy, colostomy, or ileostomy were excluded.

The primary endpoint for all studies was time to achieve resolution of postoperative ileus, a clinically defined composite measure of both upper and lower gastrointestinal recovery. Although both 2-component (GI2: toleration of solid food and first bowel movement) and 3-component (GI3: toleration of solid food and either first flatus or bowel movement) endpoints were used in all studies, GI2 is presented as it represents the most objective and clinically relevant measure of treatment response in the bowel resection population. The time from the end of surgery to when the discharge order was written represented the length of hospital stay. In the 5 studies, 1,081 patients received placebo (157 for total abdominal hysterectomy) and 1,096 patients received ENTEREG (143 for total abdominal hysterectomy). The efficacy of ENTEREG following total abdominal hysterectomy has not been established. Therefore, the following data are presented for the bowel resection population only. Bowel Resection: A total of 1,877 patients underwent bowel resection. The average age was 61 years with equal proportions of males and females, and 88% were Caucasian. The most common indications for surgery were colon or rectal cancer and diverticular disease. In the non-US study (Study 5), average daily postoperative opioid consumption was approximately 50% lower and the use of non-opioid analgesics substantially higher, as compared with the US studies (Studies 1-4) for both treatment groups. During the first 48 hours postoperatively, the use of non-opioid analgesics was 69% compared with 4% for the non-US and US studies, respectively. In each of the 5 studies, ENTEREG accelerated the time to recovery of gastrointestinal function, as measured by the composite endpoint GI2, and time to discharge order written as compared with placebo. Hazard ratios greater than 1 indicate a higher probability of achieving the event during the study period with treatment with ENTEREG than with placebo. Table 2 provides the Hazard Ratios, Kaplan Meier means and the mean treatment differences (hours) in gastrointestinal recovery between ENTEREG and placebo.

[See table 2 at top of previous page]

Gastrointestinal recovery began after approximately 48 hours post surgery. The proportion of patients receiving ENTEREG who achieved GI2 was higher at all times throughout the study observation period compared with those receiving placebo (Figure 1).

Figure 1. Time to GI2 Based on the Combined Data from Five Studies

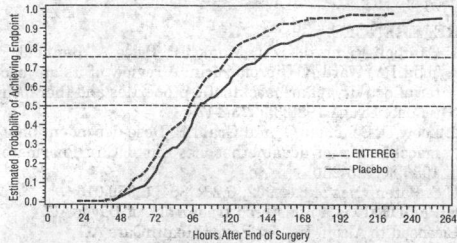

Across studies 1-4, patients receiving ENTEREG had their discharge order written approximately 13 to 21 hours sooner compared to patients receiving placebo.
ENTEREG did not reverse opioid analgesia as measured by visual analog scale pain intensity scores and/or amount of postoperative opioids administered across all 5 studies.
There were no gender-, age-, or race-related differences in treatment effect.
The incidence of anastomotic leak was low and comparable in patients receiving either ENTEREG or placebo (0.8% and 1.1%, respectively).

16   HOW SUPPLIED/STORAGE AND HANDLING

ENTEREG Capsules, 12 mg, are blue, hard-gelatin capsules printed with "ADL2698" on both the body and the cap of the capsule. ENTEREG Capsules are available in unit-dose packs of 30 capsules (30 doses) (NDC 11227-010-30) for hospital use only.
Store at 25°C (77°F); excursions permitted to 15-30°C (59-86°F) [see USP Controlled Room Temperature.]

17   PATIENT COUNSELING INFORMATION

17.1   Recent Use of Opioids

Patients should be informed that they must disclose long-term or intermittent opioid pain therapy, including any use of opioids in the week prior to receiving ENTEREG. They should understand that recent use of opioids may make them more susceptible to adverse reactions to ENTEREG, primarily those limited to the gastrointestinal tract (e.g., abdominal pain, nausea and vomiting, diarrhea).

17.2   Hospital Use Only

Patients should be informed that ENTEREG is for hospital use only for no more than 7 days after their bowel resection surgery.

17.3   Most Common Side Effects

Patients should be informed that the most common side effects with ENTEREG in patients undergoing bowel resection are constipation, dyspepsia, and flatulence.
Manufactured for Adolor Corporation
Exton, PA 19341-1127
Distributed by GlaxoSmithKline
Research Triangle Park, NC 27709
US Patent Nos. 5,250,542; 5,434,171; 6,469,030
©2008, Adolor Corporation. All rights reserved.
Shown in Product Identification Guide, page 304

Alcon Laboratories, Inc.
AND ITS AFFILIATES
CORPORATE HEADQUARTERS
6201 SOUTH FREEWAY
FORT WORTH, TX 76134

Address Inquiries to:
6201 South Freeway
Fort Worth, TX 76134
(800) 757-9195
Outside the U.S. call (817) 568-6725
medinfo@alconlabs.com

OPHTHALMIC PRODUCTS

For information on Alcon ophthalmic products, consult the *PDR For Ophthalmic Medicines*. See a complete listing of products in the Manufacturers' Index section of this book. For information, literature, samples or service items contact Alcon at the phone numbers listed above.

CIPRODEX®   ℞
[sĭ-prō-dĕks]
(ciprofloxacin 0.3% and dexamethasone 0.1%)
Sterile Otic Suspension

DESCRIPTION

CIPRODEX® (ciprofloxacin 0.3% and dexamethasone 0.1%) Sterile Otic Suspension contains the synthetic broad-spectrum antibacterial agent, ciprofloxacin hydrochloride, combined with the anti-inflammatory corticosteroid, dexamethasone, in a sterile, preserved suspension for otic use. Each mL of CIPRODEX® Otic contains ciprofloxacin hydrochloride (equivalent to 3 mg ciprofloxacin base), 1 mg dexamethasone, and 0.1 mg benzalkonium chloride as a preservative. The inactive ingredients are boric acid, sodium chloride, hydroxyethyl cellulose, tyloxapol, acetic acid, sodium acetate, edetate disodium, and purified water. Sodium hydroxide or hydrochloric acid may be added for adjustment of pH.
Ciprofloxacin, a fluoroquinolone is available as the monohydrochloride monohydrate salt of 1-cyclopropyl-6-fluoro-1,4-dihydro-4-oxo-7-(1-piperazinyl)-3-quinolinecarboxylic acid. The empirical formula is $C_{17}H_{18}FN_3O_3 \cdot HCl \cdot H_2O$.
Dexamethasone, 9-fluoro-11(beta),17, 21-trihydroxy-16(alpha)-methylpregna-1, 4-diene-3,20-dione, is an anti-inflammatory corticosteroid. The empirical formula is $C_{22}H_{29}FO_5$.

CLINICAL PHARMACOLOGY

Pharmacokinetics: Following a single bilateral 4-drop (total dose = 0.28 mL, 0.84 mg ciprofloxacin, 0.28 mg dexamethasone) topical otic dose of CIPRODEX® Otic to pediatric patients after tympanostomy tube insertion, measurable plasma concentrations of ciprofloxacin and dexamethasone were observed at 6 hours following administration in 2 of 9 patients and 5 of 9 patients, respectively.
Mean ± SD peak plasma concentrations of ciprofloxacin were 1.39 ± 0.880 ng/mL (n=9). Peak plasma concentrations ranged from 0.543 ng/mL to 3.45 ng/mL and were on average approximately 0.1% of peak plasma concentrations achieved with an oral dose of 250-mg[1]. Peak plasma concentrations of ciprofloxacin were observed within 15 minutes to 2 hours post dose application.
Mean ± SD peak plasma concentrations of dexamethasone were 1.14 ± 1.54 ng/mL (n=9). Peak plasma concentrations ranged from 0.135 ng/mL to 5.10 ng/mL and were on average approximately 14% of peak concentrations reported in the literature following an oral 0.5-mg tablet dose[2]. Peak plasma concentrations of dexamethasone were observed within 15 minutes to 2 hours post dose application.
Dexamethasone has been added to aid in the resolution of the inflammatory response accompanying bacterial infection (such as otorrhea in pediatric patients with AOM with tympanostomy tubes).
Microbiology: Ciprofloxacin has *in vitro* activity against a wide range of gram-positive and gram-negative microorganisms. The bactericidal action of ciprofloxacin results from interference with the enzyme, DNA gyrase, which is needed for the synthesis of bacterial DNA. Cross-resistance has been observed between ciprofloxacin and other fluoroquinolones. There is generally no cross-resistance between ciprofloxacin and other classes of antibacterial agents such as beta-lactams or aminoglycosides.
Ciprofloxacin has been shown to be active against most isolates of the following microorganisms, both *in vitro* and clinically in otic infections as described in the INDICATIONS AND USAGE section.
Aerobic and facultative gram-positive microorganisms
Staphylococcus aureus
Streptococcus pneumoniae

Aerobic and facultative gram-negative microorganisms
Haemophilus influenzae
Moraxella catarrhalis
Pseudomonas aeruginosa

INDICATIONS AND USAGE

CIPRODEX® Otic is indicated for the treatment of infections caused by susceptible isolates of the designated microorganisms in the specific conditions listed below:
Acute Otitis Media in pediatric patients (age 6 months and older) with tympanostomy tubes due to *Staphylococcus aureus, Streptococcus pneumoniae, Haemophilus influenzae, Moraxella catarrhalis,* and *Pseudomonas aeruginosa*.
Acute Otitis Externa in pediatric (age 6 months and older), adult and elderly patients due to *Staphylococcus aureus* and *Pseudomonas aeruginosa*.

CONTRAINDICATIONS

CIPRODEX® Otic is contraindicated in patients with a history of hypersensitivity to ciprofloxacin, to other quinolones, or to any of the components in this medication. Use of this product is contraindicated in viral infections of the external canal including herpes simplex infections.

WARNINGS

FOR OTIC USE ONLY
(This product is not approved for ophthalmic use.)
NOT FOR INJECTION
CIPRODEX® Otic should be discontinued at the first appearance of a skin rash or any other sign of hypersensitivity. Serious and occasionally fatal hypersensitivity (anaphylactic) reactions, some following the first dose, have been reported in patients receiving systemic quinolones. Serious acute hypersensitivity reactions may require immediate emergency treatment.

PRECAUTIONS

General: As with other antibacterial preparations, use of this product may result in overgrowth of nonsusceptible organisms, including yeast and fungi. If the infection is not improved after one week of treatment, cultures should be obtained to guide further treatment. If otorrhea persists after a full course of therapy, or if two or more episodes of otorrhea occur within six months, further evaluation is recommended to exclude an underlying condition such as cholesteatoma, foreign body, or a tumor.
The systemic administration of quinolones, including ciprofloxacin at doses much higher than given or absorbed by the otic route, has led to lesions or erosions of the cartilage in weight-bearing joints and other signs of arthropathy in immature animals of various species.
Guinea pigs dosed in the middle ear with CIPRODEX® Otic for one month exhibited no drug-related structural or functional changes of the cochlear hair cells and no lesions in the ossicles. CIPRODEX® Otic was also shown to lack dermal sensitizing potential in the guinea pig when tested according to the method of Buehler.
No signs of local irritation were found when CIPRODEX® Otic was applied topically in the rabbit eye.
Information for Patients
For otic use only. (This product is not approved for use in the eye.) Warm the bottle in your hand for one to two minutes prior to use and shake well immediately before using.
Avoid contaminating the tip with material from the ear, fingers, or other sources.
Protect from light.
If rash or allergic reaction occurs, discontinue use immediately and contact your physician.
It is very important to use the ear drops for as long as the doctor has instructed, **even if the symptoms improve.** Discard unused portion after therapy is completed.
Acute Otitis Media in pediatric patients with tympanostomy tubes Prior to administration of CIPRODEX® Otic in patients (6 months and older) with acute otitis media through tympanostomy tubes, the suspension should be warmed by holding the bottle in the hand for one or two minutes to avoid dizziness which may result from the instillation of a cold suspension. The patient should lie with the affected ear upward, and then the drops should be instilled. The tragus should then be pumped 5 times by pushing inward to facilitate penetration of the drops into the middle ear. This position should be maintained for 60 seconds. Repeat, if necessary, for the opposite ear (see **DOSAGE AND ADMINISTRATION**).
Acute Otitis Externa
Prior to administration of CIPRODEX® Otic in patients with acute otitis externa, the suspension should be warmed by holding the bottle in the hand for one or two minutes to avoid dizziness which may result from the instillation of a cold suspension. The patient should lie with the affected ear upward, and then the drops should be instilled. This position should be maintained for 60 seconds to facilitate penetration of the drops into the ear canal. Repeat, if necessary, for the opposite ear (see **DOSAGE AND ADMINISTRATION**).

Drug Interactions
Specific drug interaction studies have not been conducted with CIPRODEX Otic.

Carcinogenesis, Mutagenesis, Impairment of Fertility
Long-term carcinogenicity studies in mice and rats have been completed for ciprofloxacin. After daily oral doses of 750 mg/kg (mice) and 250 mg/kg (rats) were administered for up to 2 years, there was no evidence that ciprofloxacin had any carcinogenic or tumorigenic effects in these species. No long term studies of CIPRODEX® Otic have been performed to evaluate carcinogenic potential.
Eight *in vitro* mutagenicity tests have been conducted with ciprofloxacin, and the test results are listed below:
Salmonella/Microsome Test (Negative)
E. coli DNA Repair Assay (Negative)
Mouse Lymphoma Cell Forward Mutation Assay (Positive)
Chinese Hamster V_{79} Cell HGPRT Test (Negative)
Syrian Hamster Embryo Cell Transformation Assay (Negative)
Saccharomyces cerevisiae Point Mutation Assay (Negative)
Saccharomyces cerevisiae Mitotic Crossover and Gene Conversion Assay (Negative)
Rat Hepatocyte DNA Repair Assay (Positive)
Thus, 2 of the 8 tests were positive, but results of the following 3 *in vivo* test systems gave negative results:
Rat Hepatocyte DNA Repair Assay
Micronucleus Test (Mice)
Dominant Lethal Test (Mice)
Fertility studies performed in rats at oral doses of ciprofloxacin up to 100 mg/kg/day revealed no evidence of impairment. This would be over 100 times the maximum recommended clinical dose of ototopical ciprofloxacin based upon body surface area, assuming total absorption of ciprofloxacin from the ear of a patient treated with CIPRODEX® Otic twice per day according to label directions.
Long term studies have not been performed to evaluate the carcinogenic potential of topical otic dexamethasone. Dexamethasone has been tested for *in vitro* and *in vivo* genotoxic potential and shown to be positive in the following assays; chromosomal aberrations, sister-chromatid exchange in human lymphocytes and micronuclei and sister-chromatid exchanges in mouse bone marrow. However, the Ames/Salmonella assay, both with and without S9 mix, did not show any increase in His+ revertants.
The effect of dexamethasone on fertility has not been investigated following topical otic application. However, the lowest toxic dose of dexamethasone identified following topical dermal application was 1.802 mg/kg in a 26-week study in male rats and resulted in changes to the testes, epididymis, sperm duct, prostate, seminal vessicle, Cowper's gland and accessory glands. The relevance of this study for short term topical otic use is unknown.

Pregnancy
Teratogenic Effects. Pregnancy Category C:
Reproduction studies have been performed in rats and mice using oral doses of up to 100 mg/kg and IV doses up to 30 mg/kg and have revealed no evidence of harm to the fetus as a result of ciprofloxacin. In rabbits, ciprofloxacin (30 and 100 mg/kg orally) produced gastrointestinal disturbances resulting in maternal weight loss and an increased incidence of abortion, but no teratogenicity was observed at either dose. After intravenous administration of doses up to 20 mg/kg, no maternal toxicity was produced in the rabbit, and no embryotoxicity or teratogenicity was observed.
Corticosteroids are generally teratogenic in laboratory animals when administered systemically at relatively low dosage levels. The more potent corticosteroids have been shown to be teratogenic after dermal application in laboratory animals.
Animal reproduction studies have not been conducted with CIPRODEX® Otic. No adequate and well controlled studies have been performed in pregnant women. Caution should be exercised when CIPRODEX® Otic is used by a pregnant woman.

Nursing Mothers:
Ciprofloxacin and corticosteroids, as a class, appear in milk following oral administration. Dexamethasone in breast milk could suppress growth, interfere with endogenous corticosteroid production, or cause other untoward effects. It is not known whether topical otic administration of ciprofloxacin or dexamethasone could result in sufficient systemic absorption to produce detectable quantities in human milk. Because of the potential for unwanted effects in nursing infants, a decision should be made whether to discontinue nursing or to discontinue the drug, taking into account the importance of the drug to the mother.

Pediatric Use:
The safety and efficacy of CIPRODEX® Otic have been established in pediatric patients 6 months and older (937 patients) in adequate and well-controlled clinical trials. Although no data are available on patients less than age 6 months, there are no known safety concerns or differences

in the disease process in this population that would preclude use of this product. (See **DOSAGE AND ADMINISTRATION**.)
No clinically relevant changes in hearing function were observed in 69 pediatric patients (age 4 to 12 years) treated with CIPRODEX Otic and tested for audiometric parameters.

ADVERSE REACTIONS
In Phases II and III clinical trials, a total of 937 patients were treated with CIPRODEX® Otic. This included 400 patients with acute otitis media with tympanostomy tubes and 537 patients with acute otitis externa. The reported treatment-related adverse events are listed below:

Acute Otitis Media in pediatric patients with tympanostomy tubes
The following treatment-related adverse events occurred in 0.5% or more of the patients with non-intact tympanic membranes.

Adverse Event	Incidence (N=400)
Ear discomfort	3.0%
Ear pain	2.3%
Ear precipitate (residue)	0.5%
Irritability	0.5%
Taste perversion	0.5%

The following treatment-related adverse events were each reported in a single patient: tympanostomy tube blockage; ear pruritus; tinnitus; oral moniliasis; crying; dizziness; and erythema.

Acute Otitis Externa
The following treatment-related adverse events occurred in 0.4% or more of the patients with intact tympanic membranes.

Adverse Event	Incidence (N=537)
Ear pruritus	1.5%
Ear debris	0.6%
Superimposed ear infection	0.6%
Ear congestion	0.4%
Ear pain	0.4%
Erythema	0.4%

The following treatment-related adverse events were each reported in a single patient: ear discomfort; decreased hearing; and ear disorder (tingling).

DOSAGE AND ADMINISTRATION

CIPRODEX® OTIC SHOULD BE SHAKEN WELL IMMEDIATELY BEFORE USE
CIPRODEX® Otic contains 3 mg/mL (3000 µg/mL) ciprofloxacin and 1 mg/mL dexamethasone.
Acute Otitis Media in pediatric patients with tympanostomy tubes: The recommended dosage regimen for the treatment of acute otitis media in pediatric patients (age 6 months and older) through tympanostomy tubes is:
Four drops (0.14 mL, 0.42 mg ciprofloxacin, 0.14 mg dexamethasone) instilled into the affected ear twice daily for seven days. The suspension should be warmed by holding the bottle in the hand for one or two minutes to avoid dizziness, which may result from the instillation of a cold suspension. The patient should lie with the affected ear upward, and then the drops should be instilled. The tragus should then be pumped 5 times by pushing inward to facilitate penetration of the drops into the middle ear. This position should be maintained for 60 seconds. Repeat, if necessary, for the opposite ear. Discard unused portion after therapy is completed.
Acute Otitis Externa: The recommended dosage regimen for the treatment of acute otitis externa is: For patients (age 6 months and older): Four drops (0.14 mL, 0.42 mg ciprofloxacin, 0.14 mg dexamethasone) instilled into the affected ear twice daily for seven days. The suspension should be warmed by holding the bottle in the hand for one or two minutes to avoid dizziness, which may result from the instillation of a cold suspension. The patient should lie with the affected ear upward, and then the drops should be instilled. This position should be maintained for 60 seconds to facilitate penetration of the drops into the ear canal. Repeat, if necessary, for the opposite ear. Discard unused portion after therapy is completed.

HOW SUPPLIED
CIPRODEX® (ciprofloxacin 0.3% and dexamethasone 0.1%) Sterile Otic Suspension is supplied as follows: 7.5 mL fill in a DROP-TAINER® system. The DROP-TAINER® system consists of a natural polyethylene bottle and natural plug, with a white polypropylene closure. Tamper evidence is provided with a shrink band around the closure and neck area of the package.
NDC 0065-8533-02, 7.5 mL fill
Storage:
Store at controlled room temperature, 15°C to 30°C (59°F to 86°F). Avoid freezing. Protect from light.

CLINICAL STUDIES
In a randomized, multicenter, controlled clinical trial, CIPRODEX® Otic dosed 2 times per day for 7 days demonstrated clinical cures in the per protocol analysis in 86% of AOMT patients compared to 79% for ofloxacin solution, 0.3%, dosed 2 times per day for 10 days. Among culture positive patients, clinical cures were 90% for CIPRODEX® Otic compared to 79% for ofloxacin solution, 0.3%. Microbiological eradication rates for these patients in the same clinical trial were 91% for CIPRODEX® Otic compared to 82% for ofloxacin solution, 0.3%. In 2 randomized multicenter, controlled clinical trials, CIPRODEX® Otic dosed 2 times per day for 7 days demonstrated clinical cures in 87% and 94% of per protocol evaluable AOE patients, respectively, compared to 84% and 89%, respectively, for otic suspension containing neomycin 0.35%, polymyxin B 10,000 IU/mL, and hydrocortisone 1.0% (neo/poly/HC). Among culture positive patients clinical cures were 86% and 92% for CIPRODEX® Otic compared to 84% and 89%, respectively, for neo/poly/HC. Microbiological eradication rates for these patients in the same clinical trials were 86% and 92% for CIPRODEX® Otic compared to 85% and 85%, respectively, for neo/poly/HC.

REFERENCES
1. Campoli-Richards DM, Monk JP, Price A, Benfield P, Todd PA, Ward A. Ciprofloxacin: A review of its antibacterial activity, pharmacokinetic properties and therapeutic use. Drugs 1988;35:373-447.
2. Loew D, Schuster O, and Graul E. Dose-dependent pharmacokinetics of dexamethasone. Eur J Clin Pharmacol 1986;30:225-230.
U.S. Patent Nos. 4,844,902; 6,284,804; 6,359,016
CIPRODEX® is a registered trademark of Bayer AG.
Licensed to Alcon, Inc. by Bayer HealthCare AG
Manufactured by Alcon Laboratories, Inc.
Rx Only
©2003, 2004 Alcon, Inc.
Revision date: 17 July 2003

PATADAY™   ℞
(olopatadine hydrochloride ophthalmic solution) 0.2%

DESCRIPTION
PATADAY™ (olopatadine hydrochloride ophthalmic solution) 0.2% is a sterile ophthalmic solution containing olopatadine for topical administration to the eyes. Olopatadine hydrochloride is a white, crystalline, water-soluble powder with a molecular weight of 373.88 and a molecular formula of $C_{21}H_{23}NO_3$ • HCl.
Chemical Name: 11-[(Z)-3-(Dimethylamino) propylidene]-6-11-dihydrodibenz[b,e] oxepin-2-acetic acid, hydrochloride.
Each mL of PATADAY™ solution contains: **Active:** 2.22 mg olopatadine hydrochloride equivalent to 2 mg olopatadine.
Inactives: povidone; dibasic sodium phosphate; sodium chloride; edetate disodium; benzalkonium chloride 0.01% **(preservative)** hydrochloric acid / sodium hydroxide (adjust pH); and purified water.
It has a pH of approximately 7 and an osmolality of approximately 300 mOsm/kg.

CLINICAL PHARMACOLOGY
Olopatadine is a relatively selective histamine H_1 antagonist and an inhibitor of the release of histamine from the mast cells. Decreased chemotaxis and inhibition of eosinophil activation has also been demonstrated. Olopatadine is devoid of effects on alpha-adrenergic, dopaminergic, and muscarinic type 1 and 2 receptors.
Systemic bioavailability data upon topical ocular administration of PATADAY™ solution are not available. Following topical ocular administration of olopatadine 0.15% ophthalmic solution in man, olopatadine was shown to have a low systemic exposure. Two studies in normal volunteers (totaling 24 subjects) dosed bilaterally with olopatadine 0.15% ophthalmic solution once every 12 hours for 2 weeks demonstrated plasma concentrations to be generally below the quantitation limit of the assay (< 0.5 ng/mL). Samples in which olopatadine was quantifiable were typically found within 2 hours of dosing and ranged from 0.5 to 1.3 ng/mL. The elimination half-life in plasma following oral dosing was 8 to 12 hours, and elimination was predominantly

through renal excretion. Approximately 60–70% of the dose was recovered in the urine as parent drug. Two metabolites, the mono-desmethyl and the N-oxide, were detected at low concentrations in the urine.

CLINICAL STUDIES

Results from clinical studies of up to 12 weeks duration demonstrate that PATADAY™ solution when dosed once a day is effective in the treatment of ocular itching associated with allergic conjunctivitis.

INDICATIONS AND USAGE

PATADAY™ solution is indicated for the treatment of ocular itching associated with allergic conjunctivitis.

CONTRAINDICATIONS

Hypersensitivity to any components of this product.

WARNINGS

For topical ocular use only. Not for injection or oral use.

PRECAUTIONS

Information for Patients

As with any eye drop, to prevent contaminating the dropper tip and solution, care should be taken not to touch the eyelids or surrounding areas with the dropper tip of the bottle. Keep bottle tightly closed when not in use. Patients should be advised not to wear a contact lens if their eye is red. PATADAY™ (olopatadine hydrochloride ophthalmic solution) 0.2% should not be used to treat contact lens related irritation. The preservative in PATADAY™ solution, benzalkonium chloride, may be absorbed by soft contact lenses. Patients who wear soft contact lenses and **whose eyes are not red**, should be instructed to wait at least ten minutes after instilling PATADAY™ (olopatadine hydrochloride ophthalmic solution) 0.2% before they insert their contact lenses.

Carcinogenesis, Mutagenesis, Impairment of Fertility

Olopatadine administered orally was not carcinogenic in mice and rats in doses up to 500 mg/kg/day and 200 mg/kg/day, respectively. Based on a 40 μL drop size and a 50 kg person, these doses were approximately 150,000 and 50,000 times higher than the maximum recommended ocular human dose (MROHD). No mutagenic potential was observed when olopatadine was tested in an *in vitro* bacterial reverse mutation (Ames) test, an *in vitro* mammalian chromosome aberration assay or an *in vivo* mouse micronucleus test. Olopatadine administered to male and female rats at oral doses of approximately 100,000 times MROHD level resulted in a slight decrease in the fertility index and reduced implantation rate; no effects on reproductive function were observed at doses of approximately 15,000 times the MROHD level.

Pregnancy:

Teratogenic effects: Pregnancy Category C

Olopatadine was found not to be teratogenic in rats and rabbits. However, rats treated at 600 mg/kg/day, or 150,000 times the MROHD and rabbits treated at 400 mg/kg/day, or approximately 100,000 times the MROHD, during organogenesis showed a decrease in live fetuses. In addition, rats treated with 600 mg/kg/day of olopatadine during organogenesis showed a decrease in fetal weight. Further, rats treated with 600 mg/kg/day of olopatadine during late gestation through the lactation period showed a decrease in neonatal survival and body weight.

There are, however, no adequate and well-controlled studies in pregnant women. Because animal studies are not always predictive of human responses, this drug should be used in pregnant women only if the potential benefit to the mother justifies the potential risk to the embryo or fetus.

Nursing Mothers:

Olopatadine has been identified in the milk of nursing rats following oral administration. It is not known whether topical ocular administration could result in sufficient systemic absorption to produce detectable quantities in the human breast milk. Nevertheless, caution should be exercised when PATADAY™ (olopatadine hydrochloride ophthalmic solution) 0.2% is administered to a nursing mother.

Pediatric Use:

Safety and effectiveness in pediatric patients below the age of 3 years have not been established.

Geriatric Use:

No overall differences in safety and effectiveness have been observed between elderly and younger patients.

ADVERSE REACTIONS

Symptoms similar to cold syndrome and pharyngitis were reported at an incidence of approximately 10%.

The following adverse experiences have been reported in 5% or less of patients:

Ocular: blurred vision, burning or stinging, conjunctivitis, dry eye, foreign body sensation, hyperemia, hypersensitivity, keratitis, lid edema, pain and ocular pruritus.

Non-ocular: asthenia, back pain, flu syndrome, headache, increased cough, infection, nausea, rhinitis, sinusitis and taste perversion.

Some of these events were similar to the underlying disease being studied.

DOSAGE AND ADMINISTRATION

The recommended dose is one drop in each affected eye once a day.

HOW SUPPLIED

PATADAY™ (olopatadine hydrochloride ophthalmic solution) 0.2% is supplied in a white, oval, low density polyethylene DROP-TAINER® dispenser with a natural low density polyethylene dispensing plug and a white polypropylene cap. Tamper evidence is provided with a shrink band around the closure and neck area of the package.

NDC 0065-0272-25   2.5 mL fill in 4 mL oval bottle

Storage:

Store at 2°C to 25°C (36°F to 77°F)

U.S. Patents Nos. 5,116,863; 5,641,805; 6,995,186

Rx Only

ALCON LABORATORIES, INC.
Fort Worth, Texas 76134 USA
© 2006-2008 Alcon, Inc.

PATANASE®   ℞

[pat-uh-nase]

(olopatadine hydrochloride)

Nasal Spray

HIGHLIGHTS OF PRESCRIBING INFORMATION

These highlights do not include all the information needed to use PATANASE® Nasal Spray safely and effectively. See full prescribing information for PATANASE Nasal Spray.

PATANASE (olopatadine hydrochloride) Nasal Spray

Initial U.S. Approval: 1996

———————INDICATIONS AND USAGE———————

PATANASE Nasal Spray is an H_1 receptor antagonist indicated for the relief of the symptoms of seasonal allergic rhinitis in adults and children 6 years of age and older. (1)

———————DOSAGE AND ADMINISTRATION———————

For intranasal use only.

Recommended dosages:

• Adults and adolescents ≥12 years: Two sprays per nostril twice daily. (2.1)

• Children 6 to 11 years: One spray per nostril twice daily. (2.2)

Priming Information: Prime PATANASE Nasal Spray before initial use and when PATANASE Nasal Spray has not been used for more than 7 days. (2.3)

———————DOSAGE FORMS AND STRENGTHS———————

Nasal spray 0.6%: 665 mcg of olopatadine hydrochloride in each 100-microliter spray. (3)

Supplied as a 30.5 g bottle containing 240 sprays.

———————CONTRAINDICATIONS———————

None. (4)

———————WARNINGS AND PRECAUTIONS———————

• Epistaxis, nasal ulceration, and nasal septal perforation. Monitor patients periodically for signs of adverse effects on the nasal mucosa. Discontinue if ulcerations or perforations occur. Avoid use in patients with nasal disease other than allergic rhinitis (5.1).

• Avoid engaging in hazardous occupations requiring complete mental alertness and coordination such as driving or operating machinery when taking PATANASE Nasal Spray (5.2).

• Avoid concurrent use of alcohol or other central nervous system depressants with PATANASE Nasal Spray (5.2).

———————ADVERSE REACTIONS———————

The most common (>1%) adverse reactions included bitter taste, headache, epistaxis, pharyngolaryngeal pain, postnasal drip, cough, and urinary tract infection in patients 12 years of age and older and epistaxis, headache, upper respiratory tract infection, bitter taste, pyrexia, and rash in patients 6 to 11 years of age (6.1).

To report SUSPECTED ADVERSE REACTIONS, contact Alcon Laboratories, Inc. at 1-800-757-9195 or FDA at 1-800-FDA-1088 or www.fda.gov/medwatch.

See 17 for PATIENT COUNSELING INFORMATION and FDA-approved patient labeling.

Revised: 2009

FULL PRESCRIBING INFORMATION

1   INDICATIONS AND USAGE

1.1   Seasonal Allergic Rhinitis: PATANASE Nasal Spray is an H_1 receptor antagonist indicated for the relief of the symptoms of seasonal allergic rhinitis in adults and children 6 years of age and older.

2   DOSAGE AND ADMINISTRATION

Administer PATANASE Nasal Spray by the intranasal route only.

2.1   Adults and Adolescents 12 years of age and older: The recommended dosage is two sprays per nostril twice daily.

2.2   Children 6 to 11 years of age: The recommended dosage is one spray per nostril twice daily.

2.3   Administration Information

Priming: Before initial use, prime PATANASE Nasal Spray by releasing 5 sprays or until a fine mist appears. When PATANASE Nasal Spray has not been used for more than 7 days, re-prime by releasing 2 sprays. Avoid spraying PATANASE Nasal Spray into the eyes.

3   DOSAGE FORMS AND STRENGTHS

PATANASE Nasal Spray is a nasal spray solution supplied in a white plastic bottle with a metered-dose manual spray pump, a white nasal applicator, and a blue overcap.

Each spray (100 microliters) delivers 665 mcg of olopatadine hydrochloride.

4   CONTRAINDICATIONS

None.

5   WARNINGS AND PRECAUTIONS

5.1   Local Nasal Effects

Epistaxis and Nasal Ulceration: In placebo (vehicle nasal spray)-controlled clinical trials of 2 weeks to 12 months duration, epistaxis and nasal ulcerations were reported [see *Adverse Reactions (6)*].

Nasal Septal Perforation:

Two placebo (vehicle nasal spray)-controlled long term (12 months) safety trials were conducted. In the first safety trial, patients were treated with an investigational formulation of PATANASE Nasal Spray containing povidone (not the commercially marketed formulation) or a vehicle nasal spray containing povidone. Nasal septal perforations were reported in one patient treated with the investigational formulation of PATANASE Nasal Spray and 2 patients treated with the vehicle nasal spray. In the second safety trial with PATANASE Nasal Spray, which does not contain povidone, there were no reports of nasal septal perforation [see *Adverse Reactions (6)*].

Before starting PATANASE Nasal Spray, conduct a nasal examination to ensure that patients are free of nasal disease other than allergic rhinitis. Perform nasal examinations periodically for signs of adverse effects on the nasal mucosa and consider stopping PATANASE Nasal Spray if patients develop nasal ulcerations.

5.2   Activities Requiring Mental Alertness

In clinical trials, the occurrence of somnolence has been reported in some patients taking PATANASE Nasal Spray [see *Adverse Reactions (6)*]. Patients should be cautioned against engaging in hazardous occupations requiring complete mental alertness and motor coordination such as driving or operating machinery after administration of PATANASE Nasal Spray. Concurrent use of PATANASE Nasal Spray with alcohol or other central nervous system depressants should be avoided because additional reductions in alertness and additional impairment of central nervous system performance may occur.

6 ADVERSE REACTIONS

Use of PATANASE Nasal Spray has been associated with epistaxis, nasal ulcerations, and somnolence [*see Warnings and Precautions (5.1 and 5.2)*].

6.1 Clinical Trials Experience

The safety data described below reflect exposure to PATANASE Nasal Spray in 2,427 patients with seasonal or perennial allergic rhinitis in 9 controlled clinical trials of 2 weeks to 12 months duration.

The safety data from adults and adolescents are based upon 5 placebo (vehicle nasal spray)-controlled clinical trials in which 1,491 patients with seasonal or perennial allergic rhinitis (513 males and 978 females) 12 years of age and older were treated with PATANASE Nasal Spray two sprays per nostril twice daily. There were 1,180 patients (PATANASE Nasal Spray, 587; vehicle nasal spray, 593) that participated in 3 efficacy and safety trials of 2 weeks duration. There were 1,814 patients (PATANASE Nasal Spray, 904; vehicle nasal spray, 910) that participated in 2 long-term clinical trials of 1 year duration. The racial distribution of adult and adolescent patients receiving PATANASE Nasal Spray was 76% white, 8% black, 12% Hispanic and 3% other. The incidence of discontinuation due to adverse reactions in these controlled clinical trials was comparable for PATANASE Nasal Spray and vehicle nasal spray. Overall, 3.9% of the 1,491 adult and adolescent patients across all 5 studies treated with PATANASE Nasal Spray and 3.2% of the 1,503 patients treated with vehicle nasal spray discontinued due to adverse reactions.

The safety data from pediatric patients 6-11 years of age are based upon 3 clinical trials in which 870 children with seasonal allergic rhinitis (376 females and 494 males) were treated with PATANASE Nasal Spray 1 or 2 sprays per nostril twice daily for 2 weeks. The racial distribution of pediatric patients receiving PATANASE Nasal Spray was 68.6% white, 16.6% black, and 14.8% other. The incidence of discontinuation due to adverse reactions in these controlled clinical trials was comparable for PATANASE Nasal Spray and vehicle nasal spray.

Overall, 1.4% of the 870 pediatric patients across all 3 studies treated with PATANASE Nasal Spray and 1.3% of the 872 pediatric patients treated with vehicle nasal spray discontinued due to adverse reactions. Safety information for pediatric patients 2 to 5 years of age is obtained from one vehicle-controlled study of 2 weeks duration [*See Pediatric Use (8.4)*].

Because clinical trials are conducted under widely varying conditions, adverse reaction rates observed in the clinical trials of a drug cannot be directly compared to rates in the clinical trials of another drug and may not reflect the rates observed in practice.

Adults and Adolescents 12 Years of Age and Older in Short-Term (2-week) Trials:

There were 1,180 patients 12 years of age and older (PATANASE Nasal Spray, 587; vehicle nasal spray, 593) that participated in 3 efficacy and safety trials of 2 weeks duration. Table 1 presents the most common adverse reactions (0.9% or greater in patients treated with PATANASE Nasal Spray) that occurred more frequently in patients treated with PATANASE Nasal Spray compared with vehicle nasal spray in the 3 clinical trials of 2 weeks duration.

Table 1: Adverse Reactions Occurring at an Incidence of 0.9% or Greater in Controlled Clinical Trials of 2 Weeks Duration with PATANASE Nasal Spray in Adolescent and Adult Patients 12 Years of Age and Older with Seasonal Allergic Rhinitis

Adverse Reaction	Adult and Adolescent Patients 12 Years and Older	
	PATANASE Nasal Spray N = 587	Vehicle Nasal Spray N = 593
Bitter taste	75 (12.8%)	5 (0.8%)
Headache	26 (4.4%)	24 (4.0%)
Epistaxis	19 (3.2%)	10 (1.7%)
Pharyngolaryngeal Pain	13 (2.2%)	8 (1.3%)
Post-nasal drip	9 (1.5%)	5 (0.8%)
Cough	8 (1.4%)	3 (0.5%)
Urinary tract infection	7 (1.2%)	3 (0.5%)
CPK elevation	5 (0.9%)	2 (0.3%)
Dry mouth	5 (0.9%)	1 (0.2%)
Fatigue	5 (0.9%)	4 (0.7%)
Influenza	5 (0.9%)	1 (0.2%)
Nasopharyngitis	5 (0.9%)	4 (0.7%)
Somnolence	5 (0.9%)	2 (0.3%)
Throat irritation	5 (0.9%)	0 (0.0%)

There were no differences in the incidence of adverse reactions based on gender or race. Clinical trials did not include sufficient numbers of patients 65 years of age and older to determine whether they respond differently from younger subjects.

Pediatric Patients 6 to 11 Years of Age: There were 1,742 pediatric patients 6 to 11 years of age (Olopatadine nasal spray, 870; vehicle nasal spray, 872) with seasonal allergic rhinitis that participated in 3 clinical trials of 2 weeks duration. Two of the studies used the investigational formulation of olopatadine nasal spray, and one of the studies used PATANASE Nasal Spray. One study evaluated the safety of PATANASE Nasal Spray at doses of 1 and 2 sprays per nostril twice daily in 1188 patients, in which 298 were exposed to PATANASE 1 spray, 296 were exposed to PATANASE 2 sprays, 297 were exposed to vehicle 1 spray, and 297 were exposed to vehicle 2 sprays twice daily for 2 weeks. Table 2 presents the most common adverse reactions (greater than 1.0% in pediatric patients 6-11 years of age treated with PATANASE Nasal Spray 1 spray/nostril) that occurred more frequently with PATANASE Nasal Spray compared with vehicle nasal spray.

[See table above]

Table 2. Adverse Reactions Occurring at an Incidence of Greater than 1.0% in a Controlled Clinical Trial of 2 Weeks Duration with PATANASE Nasal Spray in Pediatric Patients 6-11 Years of Age With Seasonal Allergic Rhinitis

Adverse Reaction	Pediatric Patients 6 to 11 Years of Age	
	PATANASE Nasal Spray 1 spray per nostril N = 298	Vehicle Nasal Spray 1 spray per nostril N = 297
Epistaxis	17 (5.7%)	11 (3.7%)
Headache	13 (4.4%)	11 (3.7%)
Upper respiratory tract infection	8 (2.6%)	0
Bitter taste	3 (1.0%)	0
Pyrexia	4 (1.3%)	3 (1.0%)
Rash	4 (1.3%)	0

There were no differences in the incidence of adverse reactions based on gender, race, or ethnicity.

The safety of PATANASE Nasal Spray at a dose of 1 spray per nostril twice daily was evaluated in one 2-week vehicle-controlled study in 132 patients (PATANASE Nasal Spray, 66; vehicle nasal spray. 66) 2 to 5 years of age with allergic rhinitis [*see Pediatric Use (8.4)*].

Long-Term (12-month) Safety Trials:

In a 12-month, placebo (vehicle nasal spray)-controlled, safety trial, 890 patients 12 years of age and older with perennial allergic rhinitis were randomized to treatment with PATANASE Nasal Spray 2 sprays per nostril twice daily (445 patients) or vehicle nasal spray (445 patients). In the PATANASE and vehicle nasal spray groups, 72% and 74% of patients, respectively, completed the trial. Overall, 7% and 5%, respectively, discontinued study participation due to an adverse event. The most frequently reported adverse reaction was epistaxis, which occurred in 25% of patients treated with PATANASE Nasal Spray and 28% in patients treated with vehicle nasal spray. Epistaxis resulted in discontinuation of 0.9% of patients treated with PATANASE Nasal Spray and 0.2% of patients treated with vehicle nasal spray. Nasal ulcerations occurred in 10% of patients treated with PATANASE Nasal Spray and 9% of patients treated with vehicle nasal spray. Nasal ulcerations resulted in discontinuation of 0.4% of patients treated with PATANASE Nasal Spray and 0.2% patients treated with vehicle nasal spray. There were no patients with nasal septal perforation in either treatment group. Somnolence was reported in 1 patient treated with PATANASE Nasal Spray and 1 patient treated with vehicle nasal spray. Weight increase was reported in 6 patients treated with PATANASE Nasal Spray and 1 patient treated with vehicle nasal spray. Depression or worsening of depression occurred in 9 patients treated with PATANASE Nasal Spray and in 5 patients treated with vehicle nasal spray. Three patients, two of whom had pre-existing histories of depression, who received PATANASE Nasal Spray were hospitalized for depression compared to none who received vehicle nasal spray.

In a second 12-month, placebo (vehicle nasal spray)-controlled, safety trial, 459 patients 12 years of age and older with perennial allergic rhinitis were treated with 2 sprays per nostril of an investigational formulation of PATANASE Nasal Spray containing povidone (not the commercially marketed formulation) and 465 patients were treated with 2 sprays of a vehicle nasal spray containing povidone. Nasal septal perforations were reported in one patient treated with the investigational formulation of PATANASE Nasal Spray and 2 patients treated with the vehicle nasal spray. Epistaxis was reported in 19% of patients treated with the investigational formulation of PATANASE Nasal Spray and 12% of patients treated with vehicle nasal spray. Somnolence was reported in 3 patients treated with the investigational formulation of PATANASE Nasal Spray compared to 1 patient treated with vehicle nasal spray. Fatigue was reported in 5 patients treated with the investigational formulation of PATANASE Nasal Spray compared to 1 patient treated with vehicle nasal spray.

There were no long-term clinical trials in children below 12 years of age.

6.2 Post-Marketing Experience

The post-marketing adverse events reported post-approval are consistent with the adverse events reported during clinical trials. Because post-marketing adverse events are reported voluntarily from a population of uncertain size, it is not always possible to reliably estimate their frequency or establish a causal relationship to drug exposure.

7 DRUG INTERACTIONS

Formal drug-drug interaction studies were not conducted for PATANASE Nasal Spray. Drug interactions with inhibitors of liver enzymes are not anticipated because olopatadine is eliminated predominantly by renal excretion. Drug interactions involving P450 inhibition and plasma protein binding are also not expected. [*See Clinical Pharmacology (12.3)*].

8 USE IN SPECIFIC POPULATIONS

8.1 Pregnancy

Pregnancy Category C:

No adequate and well-controlled studies in pregnant women have been conducted. Animal reproductive studies in rats and rabbits revealed treatment-related effects on fetuses or pups. Because animal studies are not always predictive of human responses, PATANASE Nasal Spray should be used in pregnant women only if the potential benefit to the mother justifies the potential risk to the embryo or fetus.

A decrease in the number of live fetuses was observed in rabbits and rats at the oral olopatadine doses approximately 88 times and 100 times the maximum recommended human dose (MRHD) and above, respectively, for adults on a mg/m^2 basis. In rats, viability and body weights of pups were reduced on day 4 post partum at the oral dose approximately 100 times the MRHD for adults on a mg/m^2 basis, but no effect on viability was observed at the dose approximately 35 times the MRHD for adults on a mg/m^2 basis.

8.3 Nursing Mothers

Olopatadine has been identified in the milk of nursing rats following oral administration. It is not known whether topical nasal administration could result in sufficient systemic absorption to produce detectable quantities in human breast milk. PATANASE Nasal Spray should be used by nursing mothers only if the potential benefit to the patient outweighs the potential risks to the infant.

8.4 Pediatric Use

The safety and effectiveness of PATANASE Nasal Spray has not been established for patients under 6 years of age. The safety of olopatadine nasal spray was evaluated in 3 vehicle-controlled 2-week studies in 870 patients 6 to 11 years of age [*see Adverse Reactions (6.1)*]. Doses studied included 1 and 2 sprays per nostril twice daily. One of these studies evaluated the safety of PATANASE Nasal Spray at doses of 1 and 2 sprays per nostril twice daily in 1188 patients, of which, 298 patients were exposed to PATANASE 1 spray and 297 patients were exposed to vehicle 1 spray. In this study, the incidence of epistaxis with PATANASE Nasal Spray treatment was 5.7%, compared to 3.2% seen in adult and adolescent studies. This study also evaluated the effectiveness of PATANASE Nasal Spray in patients 6 through 11 years of age with seasonal allergic rhinitis [*see Clinical Studies (14.1)*].

The safety of PATANASE Nasal Spray at a dose of 1 spray per nostril twice daily was evaluated in one 2-week vehicle-controlled study in 132 children ages 2 to 5 years of age with allergic rhinitis. In this trial, 66 patients (28 females and 38 males) were exposed to PATANASE Nasal Spray. The racial distribution of patients receiving PATANASE Nasal Spray was 66.7% white, 27.3% black, and 6.4% other. Two patients exposed to vehicle nasal spray discontinued due to an adverse reaction (1 patient with pneumonia and 1 patient with rhinitis) compared to no patients exposed to PATANASE Nasal Spray. The most common (greater than 1.0%) adverse events reported were diarrhea (9.1%), epistaxis (6.1%), rhinorrhea (4.5%), bitter taste (3.0%) and wheezing (3.0%). Diarrhea was reported less frequently (< 1%) in the 6 to 11 year old age group.

The incidence of epistaxis was higher in the pediatric population (5.7% in 6-11 year old patients and 6.1% in 2-5 year old patients) compared to the adult and adolescent population (3.2%).

8.5 Geriatric Use

Clinical studies of PATANASE Nasal Spray did not include sufficient numbers of patients aged 65 years and older to determine whether they respond differently from younger patients. Other reported clinical experience has not identified differences in responses between the elderly and younger patients. In general, dose selection for an elderly patient should be cautious, reflecting the greater frequency of decreased hepatic, renal, or cardiac function and of concomitant disease or other drug therapy.

10 OVERDOSAGE

There have been no reported overdosages with PATANASE Nasal Spray.

Acute overdosage with this dosage form is unlikely due to the configuration of the primary container closure system. However, symptoms of antihistamine overdose may include drowsiness in adults and, initially, agitation and restlessness, followed by drowsiness in children. There is no known specific antidote to PATANASE Nasal Spray. Should overdose occur, symptomatic or supportive treatment is recommended, taking into account any concomitantly ingested medications.

No mortality was observed in rats at an intranasal dose of 3.6 mg/kg (approximately 6 times the MRHD for adults and adolescents ≥12 years of age and 7 times the MRHD for children 6-11 years of age on a mg/m^2 basis), or in dogs at an oral dose of 5 g/kg (approximately 28,000 times the MRHD for adults and adolescents ≥12 years of age and 33,000 the MRHD for children 6-11 years of age on a mg/m^2 basis). The oral median lethal dose (MLD) in mice and rats were 1,490 mg/kg and 3,870 mg/kg respectively (approximately 1,200 times and 6,500 times the MRHD for adults and adolescents ≥12 years of age and 1,500 times and 7,700 times the MRHD for children 6-11 years of age, on a mg/m2 basis, respectively).

For additional information about overdose treatment, call a poison control center (1-800-222-1222).

11 DESCRIPTION

PATANASE (olopatadine hydrochloride) Nasal Spray, 665 micrograms (mcg) is a metered-spray solution for intranasal administration. Olopatadine hydrochloride, the active component of PATANASE Nasal Spray, is a white, water-soluble crystalline powder. The chemical name for olopatadine hydrochloride is (Z)-11-[3-(dimethylamino)propylidene]-6,11-dihydrodibenz[b,e]oxepin-2-acetic acid hydrochloride. It has a molecular weight of 373.88, and its molecular formula is $C_{21}H_{23}NO_3$ • HCl with the following chemical structure:

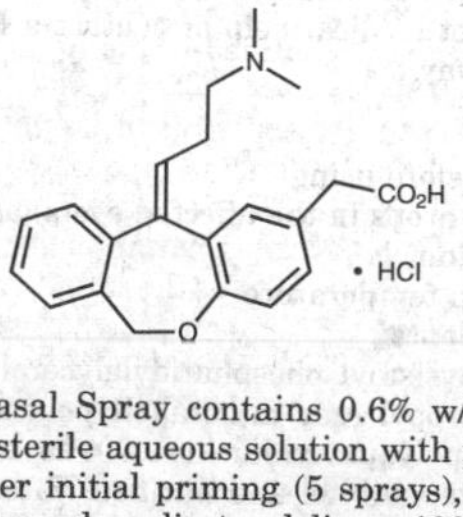

PATANASE Nasal Spray contains 0.6% w/v olopatadine (base) in a nonsterile aqueous solution with pH of approximately 3.7. After initial priming (5 sprays), each metered spray from the nasal applicator delivers 100 microliters of the aqueous solution containing 665 mcg of olopatadine hydrochloride, which is equivalent to 600 mcg of olopatadine (base) [*see Dosage and Administration*]. PATANASE Nasal Spray also contains benzalkonium chloride (0.01%), dibasic sodium phosphate, edetate disodium, sodium chloride, hydrochloric acid and/or sodium hydroxide (to adjust pH), and purified water.

12 CLINICAL PHARMACOLOGY

12.1 Mechanism of Action

Olopatadine is a histamine H_1-receptor antagonist. The antihistaminic activity of olopatadine has been documented in isolated tissues, animal models, and humans.

12.2 Pharmacodynamics

Cardiac effects: In a placebo-controlled cardiovascular safety study, 32 healthy volunteers received 20 mg oral solution of olopatadine twice daily for 14 days (8-fold greater daily dose than the recommended daily nasal dose). The mean QTcF (QT corrected by Fridericia's correction method for heart rate) change from baseline was -2.7 msec and -3.8 msec for olopatadine, and placebo, respectively. In this study, 8 subjects treated with olopatadine had a QTcF change from baseline of 30–60 msec, 1 subject had a QTcF change from baseline greater than 60 msec, and no subjects had QTcF values greater than 500 msec. Eight subjects treated with placebo had a QTcF change from baseline of 30–60 msec, no subjects had a QTcF change from baseline greater than 60 msec, and no subjects had QTcF values greater than 500 msec. In a 12-month study in 429 perennial allergic rhinitis patients treated with PATANASE Nasal Spray 2 sprays per nostril twice daily, no evidence of any effect of olopatadine hydrochloride on QT prolongation was observed.

12.3 Pharmacokinetics

The pharmacokinetic properties of olopatadine were studied after administration by the nasal, oral, intravenous, and topical ocular routes. Olopatadine exhibited linear pharmacokinetics across the routes studied over a large dose range.

Absorption:

Healthy Subjects: Olopatadine was absorbed with individual peak plasma concentrations observed between 30 minutes and 1 hour after twice daily intranasal administration of PATANASE Nasal Spray. The mean (± SD) steady-state peak plasma concentration (C_{max}) of olopatadine was 16.0 ± 8.99 ng/mL. Systemic exposure as indexed by area under the curve (AUC_{0-12}) averaged 66.0 ± 26.8 ng•h/mL. The average absolute bioavailability of intranasal olopatadine is 57%. The mean accumulation ratio following multiple intranasal administration of PATANASE Nasal Spray was about 1.3.

Seasonal Allergic Rhinitis (SAR) Patients: Systemic exposure of olopatadine in SAR patients after twice daily intranasal administration of PATANASE Nasal Spray was comparable to that observed in healthy subjects. Olopatadine was absorbed with peak plasma concentrations observed between 15 minutes and 2 hours. The mean steady-state C_{max} was 23.3 ± 6.2 ng/mL and AUC_{0-12} averaged 78.0 ± 13.9 ng•h/mL.

Distribution: The protein binding of olopatadine was moderate at approximately 55% in human serum, and independent of drug concentration over the range of 0.1 to 1000 ng/mL. Olopatadine was bound predominately to human serum albumin.

Metabolism: Olopatadine is not extensively metabolized. Based on plasma metabolite profiles following oral administration of [^{14}C] olopatadine, at least six minor metabolites circulate in human plasma. Olopatadine accounts for 77% of peak plasma total radioactivity and all metabolites amounted to <6% combined. Two of these have been identified as the olopatadine N-oxide and N-desmethyl olopatadine. In *in vitro* studies with cDNA-expressed human cytochrome P450 isoenzymes (CYP) and flavin-containing monooxygenases (FMO), N-desmethyl olopatadine (Ml) formation was catalyzed mainly by CYP3A4, while olopatadine N-oxide (M3) was primarily catalyzed by FMO1 and FMO3. Olopatadine at concentrations up to 33,900 ng/mL did not inhibit the *in vitro* metabolism of specific substrates for CYP1A2, CYP2C9, CYP2C19, CYP2D6, CYP2E1 and CYP3A4. The potential for olopatadine and its metabolites to act as inducers of CYP enzymes has not been evaluated.

Elimination: The plasma elimination half-life of olopatadine is 8 to 12 hours. Olopatadine is mainly eliminated through urinary excretion. Approximately 70% of a [^{14}C] olopatadine hydrochloride oral dose was recovered in urine with 17% in the feces. Of the drug-related material recovered within the first 24 hours in the urine, 86% was unchanged olopatadine with the balance comprised of olopatadine N-oxide and N-desmethyl olopatadine.

Special Population:

Hepatic Impairment: No specific pharmacokinetic study examining the effect of hepatic impairment was conducted. Since metabolism of olopatadine is a minor route of elimination, no adjustment of the dosing regimen of PATANASE Nasal Spray is warranted in patients with hepatic impairment.

Renal Impairment: The mean C_{max} values for olopatadine following single intranasal doses were not markedly different between healthy subjects (18.1 ng/mL) and patients with mild, moderate and severe renal impairment (range 15.5 to 21.6 ng/mL). Mean plasma AUC_{0-12} was two-fold higher in patients with severe impairment (creatinine clearance <30 mL/min/1.73 m^2). In these patients, peak steady-state plasma concentrations of olopatadine are approximately 10-fold lower than those observed after higher 20 mg oral doses, twice daily, which were well-tolerated. These findings indicate that no adjustment of the dosing regimen of PATANASE Nasal Spray is warranted in patients with renal impairment.

Gender: The mean systemic exposure (C_{max} and AUC_{0-12}) in female SAR patients following multiple administration of olopatadine was 40% and 27% higher, respectively than those values observed in male SAR patients.

Race: The effects of race on olopatadine pharmacokinetics have not been adequately investigated.

Age: Pediatric Patients 6 to 11 Years of Age: The systemic pharmacokinetics of olopatadine, olopatadine N-oxide and Ndesmethyl olopatadine in patients 6 through 11 years of age were characterized using data from 42 pediatric patients administered PATANASE Nasal Spray, one spray per nostril twice daily for a minimum of 14 days. The mean C_{max} (15.4 ± 7.3 ng/mL) of olopatadine was approximately 2-fold less than was comparable to that observed in adults (78.0 ± 13.9 ng•h/mL). The C_{max} and AUC_{0-12} of olopatadine N-oxide were comparable to that observed in adults. The C_{max} and AUC_{0-12} of N-desmethyl olopatadine are approximately 18% and 37% higher than that observed in adults, respectively.

Pediatric Patients 2 to 5 Years of Age: The systemic pharmacokinetics of olopatadine, olopatadine N-oxide, and N-desmethyl olopatadine were characterized using population pharmacokinetic methods applied to sparse data (approximately 5 samples per patient) obtained from 66 pediatric patients (2 to less than 6 years of age) administered one-half the recommended adult dose (1 spray per nostril) of PATANASE Nasal Spray twice daily for a minimum of 14 days. The mean C_{max} and AUC_{0-12} of olopatadine were 13.4 ± 4.6 ng/mL and 75.0± 26.4 ng*hr/mL respectively. The mean C_{max} and AUC_{0-12} of olopatdine N-oxide and N-desmethyl olopatadine were similar to that of patients 6 to 11 years of age.

Drug Interaction Studies

Drug interactions with inhibitors of liver enzymes are not anticipated because olopatadine is eliminated predominantly by renal excretion. Olopatadine did not inhibit the *in vitro* metabolism of specific substrates for CYP1A2, CYP2C9, CYP2C19, CYP2D6, CYP2E1 and CYP3A4. Based on these data, drug interactions involving P450 inhibition are not expected. Due to the modest protein binding of olopatadine (55%), drug interactions through displacement from plasma proteins are also not expected.

13 NONCLINICAL TOXICOLOGY

13.1 Carcinogenesis, Mutagenesis, Impairment of Fertility

Olopatadine administered orally was not carcinogenic in mice and rats at doses of up to 500 mg/kg/day and 200 mg/kg/day, respectively (approximately 420 and 340 times the MRHD for adults and adolescents ≥12 years of age and 500 and 400 times the MRHD for children 6-11 years of age by intranasal administration on a mg/m^2 basis, respectively).

There was no evidence of genotoxicity when olopatadine was tested in an *in vitro* bacteria reverse mutation test (Ames), an *in vitro* mammalian chromosome aberration assay or an *in vivo* mouse micronucleus test.

Olopatadine administered orally to male and female rats at dose of 400 mg/kg/day, (approximately 680 times the MRHD for adults on a mg/m^2 basis) resulted in a decrease in the fertility index and reduced implantation rate. No effects on fertility were observed at dose of 50 mg/kg/day (approximately 85 times the MRHD for adults on a mg/m^2 basis).

13.2 Animal Toxicology

Reproductive Toxicology Studies

Olopatadine was not teratogenic in rabbits and rats at oral doses of up to 400 or 600 mg/kg/day, respectively (approximately 1,400 and 1,000 times the MRHD for adults on a mg/m^2 basis, respectively). However, a decrease in the number of live fetuses was observed in rabbits at the oral olopatadine doses of 25 mg/kg (approximately 88 times the MRHD for adults on a mg/m^2 basis) and above, and in rats at oral doses of 60 mg/kg (approximately 100 times the MRHD for adults on a mg/m^2 basis) and above. In rats, viability and body weights of pups were reduced on day 4 post partum at the oral doses of 60 mg/kg (approximately 100 times the MRHD for adults on a mg/m^2 basis) and above, but no effect on viability was observed at the dose of 20 mg/kg (approximately 35 times the MRHD for adults on a mg/m^2 basis).

Table 3: Mean Reflective Total Nasal Symptom Score (rTNSS) in Adult and Adolescent Patients with Seasonal Allergic Rhinitis

	Treatment	N	Baseline	Change from Baseline	Difference from Placebo		
					Estimate	95% CI	p-value
Study 1	PATANASE Nasal Spray 0.6%	183	8.71	-3.63	-0.96	(-1.42, -0.51)	<0.0001
	PATANASE Nasal Spray 0.4%	188	8.90	-3.38	-0.71	(-1.17, -0.26)	0.0023
	Vehicle Nasal Spray	191	8.75	-2.67			
Study 2	PATANASE Nasal Spray 0.6%	220	9.17	-2.90	-0.98	(-1.37, -0.59)	<0.0001
	PATANASE Nasal Spray 0.4%	228	9.26	-2.63	-0.72	(-1.11, -0.33)	0.0003
	Vehicle Nasal Spray	223	9.07	-1.92			

Table 4: Mean Reflective Total Nasal Symptom Score (rTNSS) in Pediatric Patients 6-11 Years of Age with Seasonal Allergic Rhinitis

Treatment	N	Baseline	Change from Baseline	Difference from Placebo		
				Estimate	95% CI	p-value
PATANASE Nasal Spray 0.6%, 1 spray per nostril twice daily	294	8.99	-2.24	-0.55	(-0.90, -0.19)	0.0015
Vehicle Nasal Spray, 1 spray per nostril twice daily	294	9.09	-1.70			

14 CLINICAL STUDIES

14.1 Seasonal Allergic Rhinitis

Adult and Adolescent Patients 12 Years of Age and Older:
The efficacy and safety of PATANASE Nasal Spray were evaluated in three randomized, double blind, parallel group, multicenter, placebo (vehicle nasal spray)-controlled clinical trials of 2 weeks duration in adult and adolescent patients, 12 years of age and older with symptoms of seasonal allergic rhinitis. The three clinical trials were conducted in the United States and included 1,598 patients (556 males, and 1,042 females) 12 years of age and older. In these three trials 587 patients were treated with PATANASE Nasal Spray 0.6%, 418 patients were treated with PATANASE Nasal Spray 0.4%, and 593 patients were treated with vehicle nasal spray. Assessment of efficacy was based on patient recording of 4 individual nasal symptoms (nasal congestion, rhinorrhea, itchy nose, and sneezing) on a 0 to 3 categorical severity scale (0 = absent, 1 = mild, 2 = moderate, 3 = severe) as reflective or instantaneous scores. Reflective scoring required patients to record symptom severity over the previous 12 hours; the instantaneous scoring required patients to record symptom severity at the time of recording. The primary efficacy endpoint was the difference from placebo in the percent change from baseline in the average of morning and evening reflective total nasal symptom score (rTNSS) averaged for the 2-week treatment period. In all 3 trials, patients treated with PATANASE Nasal Spray, two sprays per nostril, twice-daily, exhibited statistically significantly greater decreases in rTNSS compared to vehicle nasal spray. Results for the rTNSS from two representative trials are shown in Table 3.
[See table above]
Itchy eyes and watery eyes were evaluated as secondary endpoints but eye redness was not evaluated. In two of the studies, patients treated with PATANASE Nasal Spray had significantly greater decreases in reflective symptom scores for itchy eyes and watery eyes, compared to vehicle nasal spray.
In the 2-week seasonal allergy trials, onset of action was also evaluated by instantaneous TNSS assessments twice-daily after the first dose of study medication. In these trials, onset of action was seen after 1 day of dosing. Onset of action was evaluated in three environmental exposure unit studies with single doses of PATANASE Nasal Spray. In these studies, patients with seasonal allergic rhinitis were exposed to high levels of pollen in the environmental exposure unit and then treated with either PATANASE Nasal Spray or vehicle nasal spray, two sprays in each nostril, after which they self-reported their allergy symptoms hourly as instantaneous scores for the subsequent 12 hours.

PATANASE Nasal Spray 0.6% was found to have an onset of action of 30 minutes after dosing in the environmental exposure unit.

Pediatric Patients 6 to 11 Years of Age:
There were 3 clinical trials of 2 weeks duration with olopatadine nasal spray in patients 6 to 11 years of age with seasonal allergic rhinitis. Efficacy of Patanase Nasal Spray was evaluated in 2 of the 3 trials. One of the 2 trials that showed efficacy was a randomized, double blind, parallel group, multicenter, placebo (vehicle nasal spray)-controlled clinical trial of 2 weeks duration including 1,188 children ages 6 to < 12 years with seasonal allergic rhinitis. Assessment of efficacy was based on patient/caregiver recording of 4 individual nasal symptoms (nasal congestion, rhinorrhea, itchy nose, and sneezing) on a 0 to 3 categorical severity scale (0 = absent, 1 = mild, 2 = moderate, 3 = severe) as reflective or instantaneous scores. Reflective scoring captured symptom severity over the previous 12 hours; the instantaneous scoring captured symptom severity at the time of recording. The primary efficacy endpoint was the difference from placebo in the percent change from baseline in the average of patient/caregiver-reported morning and evening reflective total nasal symptom score (rTNSS) averaged for the 2-week treatment period. Patients treated with PATANASE Nasal Spray, 1 or 2 sprays per nostril twice daily, had statistically significantly greater decreases in rTNSS compared to vehicle nasal spray. Results for rTNSS are shown in Table 4.
[See table 4 above]
Itchy eyes and watery eyes were evaluated as secondary endpoints in the same study but eye redness was not evaluated. Patients treated with PATANASE Nasal Spray had significantly greater decreases in reflective symptom scores for itchy eyes and watery eyes, compared to vehicle nasal spray.

16 HOW SUPPLIED/STORAGE AND HANDLING

16.1 How Supplied

PATANASE Nasal Spray, 665 mcg is supplied in a white plastic bottle with a metered-dose manual spray pump, a white nasal applicator and a blue overcap in a box of 1 (NDC 0065-0332-30). Each trade size bottle contains 30.5 g of clear, colorless liquid and will provide 240 metered sprays. After priming [see Dosage and Administration (2)], each spray delivers a fine mist containing 665 mcg of olopatadine hydrochloride in 100 microliters of formulation through the nozzle.
Before initial use, prime PATANASE Nasal Spray by releasing 5 sprays or until a fine mist appears. After periods of non-use greater than 7 days, re-prime PATANASE Nasal Spray by releasing 2 sprays. The correct amount of medication cannot be assured before the initial priming and after 240 sprays have been used, even though the bottle is not completely empty. The nasal device should be discarded after 240 sprays (enough for 30 days of dosing) have been used.
Net content 30.5 g, 240 sprays: NDC 0065-0332-30 (trade size)

16.2 Storage

Store at 4° to 25°C (39° to 77°F). Rx Only.

17 PATIENT COUNSELING INFORMATION

See FDA-approved Patient Labeling accompanying the product.

17.1 Local Nasal Effects and Other Common Adverse Reactions

Patients should be informed that treatment with PATANASE Nasal Spray may lead to adverse reactions, which include epistaxis and nasal ulcerations. [see Warnings and Precautions (5.1)] Other common adverse reactions reported with use of PATANASE Nasal Spray include bitter taste, headache, and pharyngolaryngeal pain, [see Adverse Reactions (6)].

17.2 Activities Requiring Mental Alertness

Somnolence has been reported in some patients taking PATANASE Nasal Spray. Patients should be cautioned against engaging in hazardous occupations requiring complete mental alertness and motor coordination such as driving or operating machinery after administration of PATANASE Nasal Spray [see Warnings and Precautions (5.2)].

17.3 Concurrent Use of Alcohol and other Central Nervous System Depressants

Concurrent use of PATANASE Nasal Spray with alcohol or other central nervous system depressants should be avoided because additional reductions in alertness and additional impairment of central nervous system performance may occur [see Warnings and Precautions (5.2)].

17.4 Keep Spray Out of Eyes

Patients should be informed to avoid spraying PATANASE Nasal Spray in their eyes.
U.S. Pat. No. 5,116,863
Revised: April 2010
Mfd for:
ALCON LABORATORIES, INC.
Fort Worth, Texas 76134 USA
Mfd by:
ALCON CUSI, S.A.
08320 El Masnou-Barcelona
Spain
© 2009, 2010 Alcon, Inc.
Alcon®
6-15-332

SYSTANE® BALANCE LUBRICANT EYE DROPS   OTC

DRUG FACTS

Active Ingredients	**Purpose**
Propylene Glycol 0.6%	Lubricant

USES

☐ For the temporary relief of burning and irritation due to dryness of the eye

WARNINGS

For external use only.
Do not use
☐ if this product changes color
☐ if you are sensitive to any ingredient in this product
When using this product
☐ do not touch tip of container to any surface to avoid contamination
☐ replace cap after each use
Stop use and ask a doctor if
☐ you feel eye pain
☐ changes in vision occur
☐ redness or irritation of the eye(s) gets worse, persists or lasts more than 72 hours
Keep out of reach of children.
If swallowed, get medical help or contact a Poison Control Center right away.

DIRECTIONS

☐ Shake well before using.
☐ Instill 1 or 2 drops in the affected eye(s) as needed.
Other Information
☐ Store at room temperature.
Inactive Ingredients:
Boric acid, dimyristoyl phosphatidylglycerol, edetate disodium, hydroxypropyl guar, mineral oil, polyoxyl 40 stearate, POLYQUAD® (polyquaternium-1) 0.001% preservative, sorbitan tristearate, sorbitol and purified water. May contain hydrochloric acid and/or sodium hydroxide to adjust pH.

Questions:
In the U.S. call **1-800-757-9195**
www.systane.com
MedInfo@AlconLabs.com

SYSTANE ® BALANCE Lubricant Eye Drops has the proven power to restore the natural tear's lipid layer to treat dryness and provide long lasting relief.

U.S. Patent Nos. 5,278,151; 5,294,607; 5,578,586; 6,583,124; 6,838,449; 6,849,253

©2010 Alcon, Inc.

Alcon Laboratories, Inc.
Fort Worth, TX 76134 USA

SYSTANE® ULTRA LUBRICANT Eye Drops — OTC

DRUG FACTS

Active Ingredients	***Purpose***
Polyethylene Glycol 400 0.4%	Lubricant
Propylene Glycol 0.3%	Lubricant

USES

- For the temporary relief of burning and irritation due to dryness of the eye

WARNINGS

For external use only.

Do not use

- if this product changes color or becomes cloudy
- if you are sensitive to any ingredient in this product

When using this product

- do not touch tip of container to any surface to avoid contamination
- replace cap after each use

Stop use and ask a doctor if

- you feel eye pain
- changes in vision occur
- redness or irritation of the eye(s) gets worse, persists or lasts more than 72 hours

Keep out of reach of children.

If swallowed, get medical help or contact a Poison Control Center right away.

DIRECTIONS

- Shake well before using.
- Instill 1 or 2 drops in the affected eye(s) as needed.

Other Information

- Store at room temperature.

Inactive Ingredients:

Aminomethylpropanol, boric acid, hydroxypropyl guar, POLYQUAD® (polyquaternium-1) 0.001% preservative, potassium chloride, purified water, sodium chloride, sorbitol. May contain hydrochloric acid and/or sodium hydroxide to adjust pH.

Questions:
In the U.S. call **1-800-757-9195**
www.systane.com

TAMPER EVIDENT: For your protection, this bottle has an imprinted seal around the neck. Do not use if seal is damaged or missing at time of purchase.

Open your eyes to a breakthrough in comfort with SYSTANE® ULTRA Lubricant Eye Drops. SYSTANE® ULTRA elevates the science of dry eye therapy to a new level. From first blink, eyes feel lubricated and refreshed. Feel the difference in dry eye relief with SYSTANE® ULTRA.

U.S. Patent Nos. 6,403,609, 6,583,124 and 6,838,449.

©2008-2009 Alcon, Inc.

Alcon Laboratories, Inc.
Fort Worth, TX 76134 USA

TRAVATAN Z® — ℞

[tra-va-tan]
(travoprost ophthalmic solution) 0.004%
Sterile

DESCRIPTION

Travoprost is a synthetic prostaglandin $F_{2\alpha}$ analogue. Its chemical name is [1R-[1α(Z),2β(1E,3R*),3α,5α]]-7-[3,5-Dihydroxy-2-[3-hydroxy-4-[3-(trifluoromethyl)phenoxy]-1-butenyl]cyclopentyl]-5-heptenoic acid, 1-methylethylester. It has a molecular formula of $C_{26}H_{35}F_3O_6$ and a molecular weight of 500.55.

Travoprost is a clear, colorless to slightly yellow oil that is very soluble in acetonitrile, methanol, octanol, and chloroform. It is practically insoluble in water.

TRAVATAN Z® ophthalmic solution is supplied as sterile, buffered aqueous solution of travoprost with a pH of approximately 5.7 and an osmolality of approximately 290 mOsmol/kg. Each mL of TRAVATAN Z® contains: Active: travoprost 0.004%. Inactives: polyoxyl 40 hydrogenated castor oil, *sof*Zia® (boric acid, propylene glycol, sorbitol, zinc chloride), sodium hydroxide and/or hydrochloric acid to adjust pH, and purified water, USP. Preserved in the bottle with an ionic buffered system, *sof*Zia®.

CLINICAL PHARMACOLOGY

Mechanism of Action

Travoprost free acid is a selective FP prostanoid receptor agonist which is believed to reduce intraocular pressure by increasing trabecular meshwork and uveoscleral outflow. The exact mechanism of action is unknown at this time.

Pharmacokinetics/Pharmacodynamics

Absorption:

Travoprost is absorbed through the cornea and is hydrolyzed to the active free acid. Data from four multiple dose pharmacokinetic studies (totaling 107 subjects) have shown that plasma concentrations of the free acid are below 0.01 ng/mL (the quantitation limit of the assay) in two-thirds of the subjects. In those individuals with quantifiable plasma concentrations (N = 38), the mean plasma C_{max} was 0.018 ± 007 ng/mL (ranged 0.01 to 0.052 ng/mL) and was reached within 30 minutes. From these studies, travoprost is estimated to have a plasma half-life of 45 minutes. There was no difference in plasma concentrations between Days 1 and 7, indicating that there was no significant accumulation.

Metabolism:

Travoprost, an isopropyl ester prodrug, is hydrolyzed by esterases in the cornea to its biologically active free acid. Systemically, travoprost free acid is metabolized to inactive metabolites via beta-oxidation of the α(carboxylic acid) chain to give the 1,2-dinor and 1,2,3,4-tetranor analogs, via oxidation of the 15-hydroxyl moiety, as well as via reduction of the 13,14 double bond.

Elimination:

The elimination of travoprost free acid from plasma was rapid and levels were generally below the limit of quantification within one hour after dosing. The terminal elimination half-life of travoprost free acid was estimated from fourteen subjects and ranged from 17 minutes to 86 minutes with the mean half-life of 45 minutes. Less than 2% of the topical ocular dose of travoprost was excreted in the urine within 4 hours as the travoprost free acid.

Clinical Studies

In clinical studies, patients with open-angle glaucoma or ocular hypertension and baseline pressure of 25–27 mm Hg, who were treated with TRAVATAN® (travoprost ophthalmic solution) or TRAVATAN Z® (travoprost ophthalmic solution) dosed once-daily in the evening demonstrated 7–8 mm Hg reduction in intraocular pressure. In subgroup analysis of this study, mean IOP reduction in black patients was up to 1.8 mm Hg greater than in non-black patients. It is not known at this time whether this difference is attributed to race or to heavily pigmented irides.

In a multi-center, randomized, controlled trial, patients with mean baseline intraocular pressure of 24–26 mm Hg on TIMOPTIC* 0.5% BID who were treated with travoprost 0.004% dosed QD adjunctively to TIMOPTIC* 0.5% BID demonstrated 6–7 mm Hg reductions in intraocular pressure.

Travoprost ophthalmic solution, 0.004% has been studied in patients with hepatic impairment and also in patients with renal impairment. No clinically relevant changes in hematology, blood chemistry, or urinalysis laboratory data were observed in these patients.

INDICATIONS AND USAGE

TRAVATAN Z® ophthalmic solution is indicated for the reduction of elevated intraocular pressure in patients with open-angle glaucoma or ocular hypertension who are intolerant of other intraocular pressure lowering medications or insufficiently responsive (failed to achieve target IOP determined after multiple measurements over time) to another intraocular pressure lowering medication.

CONTRAINDICATIONS

TRAVATAN Z® is contraindicated in patients with hypersensitivity to travoprost or any other ingredients in this product.

WARNINGS

Prostaglandin analogues, including travoprost ophthalmic solution, 0.004% have been reported to cause changes to pigmented tissues. The most frequently reported changes have been increased pigmentation of the iris and periorbital tissue (eyelid) and increased pigmentation and growth of eyelashes. These changes may be permanent.

Prostaglandin analogues, including travoprost ophthalmic solution, 0.004% may gradually change eye color, increasing the amount of brown pigmentation in the iris by increasing the number of melanosomes (pigment granules) in melanocytes. The long term effects on the melanocytes and the consequences of potential injury to the melanocytes and/or deposition of pigment granules to other areas of the eye are currently unknown. The change in iris color occurs slowly and may not be noticeable for months to years. Patients should be informed of the possibility of iris color change.

Eyelid skin darkening has been reported in association with the use of prostaglandin analogues, including travoprost ophthalmic solution, 0.004%.

Prostaglandin analogues, including travoprost ophthalmic solution, 0.004% may gradually change eyelashes in the treated eye; these changes include increased length, thickness, pigmentation, and/or number of lashes.

Patients who are expected to receive treatment in only one eye should be informed about the potential for increased brown pigmentation of the iris, periorbital and/or eyelid tissue, and eyelashes in the treated eye and thus heterochromia between the eyes. They should also be advised of the potential for a disparity between the eyes in length, thickness, and/or number of eyelashes.

PRECAUTIONS

General

There have been reports of bacterial keratitis associated with the use of multiple-dose containers of topical ophthalmic products. These containers had been inadvertently contaminated by patients who, in most cases, had a concurrent corneal disease or a disruption of the epithelial surface (see **Information for Patients**).

Patients may slowly develop increased brown pigmentation of the iris. This change may not be noticeable for months to years (see **WARNINGS**). Iris pigmentation changes may be more noticeable in patients with mixed colored irides, i.e., blue-brown, grey-brown, yellow-brown, and green-brown; however, it has also been observed in patients with brown eyes. The color change is believed to be due to increased melanin content in the stromal melanocytes of the iris. The exact mechanism of action is unknown at this time. Typically the brown pigmentation around the pupil spreads concentrically towards the periphery in affected eyes, but the entire iris or parts of it may become more brownish. Until more information about increased brown pigmentation is available, patients should be examined regularly and, depending on the situation, treatment may be stopped if increased pigmentation ensues.

TRAVATAN Z® ophthalmic solution should be used with caution in patients with a history of intraocular inflammation (iritis/uveitis) and should generally not be used in patients with active intraocular inflammation.

Macular edema, including cystoid macular edema, has been reported during treatment with prostaglandin $F_{2\alpha}$ analogues. These reports have mainly occurred in aphakic patients, pseudophakic patients with a torn posterior lens capsule, or in patients with known risk factors for macular edema. TRAVATAN Z® should be used with caution in these patients.

TRAVATAN Z® has not been evaluated for the treatment of angle closure, inflammatory or neovascular glaucoma.

Information for Patients

Patients should be advised concerning all the information contained in the Warnings and Precautions sections. Patients should also be instructed to avoid allowing the tip of the dispensing container to contact the eye or surrounding structures because this could cause the tip to become contaminated by common bacteria known to cause ocular infections. Serious damage to the eye and subsequent loss of vision may result from using contaminated solutions.

Patients also should be advised that if they develop an intercurrent ocular condition (e.g., trauma, or infection) or have ocular surgery, they should immediately seek their physician's advice concerning the continued use of the multi-dose container.

Patients should be advised that if they develop any ocular reactions, particularly conjunctivitis and lid reactions, they should immediately seek their physician's advice.

If more than one topical ophthalmic drug is being used, the drugs should be administered at least five (5) minutes apart.

Carcinogenesis, Mutagenesis, Impairment of Fertility

Two-year carcinogenicity studies in mice and rats at subcutaneous doses of 10, 30, or 100 μg/kg/day did not show any evidence of carcinogenic potential. However, at 100 μg/kg/day, male rats were only treated for 82 weeks, and the maximum tolerated dose (MTD) was not reached in the mouse study. The high dose (100 μg/kg) corresponds to exposure levels over 400 times the human exposure at the maximum recommended human ocular dose (MRHOD) of 0.04 μg/kg, based on plasma active drug levels.

Travoprost was not mutagenic in the Ames test, mouse micronucleus test and rat chromosome aberration assay. A slight increase in the mutant frequency was observed in one of two mouse lymphoma assays in the presence of rat S-9 activation enzymes.

Travoprost did not affect mating or fertility indices in male or female rats at subcutaneous doses up to 10 μg/kg/day [250 times the maximum recommended human ocular dose of 0.04 μg/kg/day on a μg/kg basis (MRHOD)]. At 10 μg/kg/

day, the mean number of corpora lutea was reduced, and the post-implantation losses were increased. These effects were not observed at 3 µg/kg/day (75 times the MRHOD).

Pregnancy: Teratogenic Effects

Pregnancy Category: C

Travoprost was teratogenic in rats, at an intravenous (IV) dose up to 10 µg/kg/day (250 times the MRHOD), evidenced by an increase in the incidence of skeletal malformations as well as external and visceral malformations, such as fused sternebrae, domed head and hydrocephaly.

Travoprost was not teratogenic in rats at IV doses up to 3 µg/kg/day (75 times the MRHOD), or in mice at subcutaneous doses up to 1.0 µg/kg/day (25 times the MRHOD). Travoprost produced an increase in post-implantation losses and a decrease in fetal viability in rats at IV doses > 3 µg/kg/day (75 times the MRHOD) and in mice at subcutaneous doses > 0.3 µg/kg/day (7.5 times the MRHOD). In the off-spring of female rats that received travoprost subcutaneously from Day 7 of pregnancy to lactation Day 21 at the doses of ≥ 0.12 µg/kg/day (3 times the MRHOD), the incidence of postnatal mortality was increased, and neonatal body weight gain was decreased. Neonatal development was also affected, evidenced by delayed eye opening, pinna detachment and preputial separation, and by decreased motor activity.

There are no adequate and well-controlled studies in pregnant women. TRAVATAN Z® should be used during pregnancy only if the potential benefit justifies the potential risk to the fetus.

Nursing Mothers

A study in lactating rats demonstrated that radiolabeled travoprost and/or its metabolites were excreted in milk. It is not known whether this drug or its metabolites are excreted in human milk. Because many drugs are excreted in human milk, caution should be exercised when TRAVATAN Z® ophthalmic solution is administered to a nursing woman.

Pediatric Use

Safety and effectiveness in pediatric patients have not been established.

Geriatric Use

No overall differences in safety or effectiveness have been observed between elderly and other adult patients.

ADVERSE REACTIONS

The most common adverse event observed in controlled clinical studies with TRAVATAN® (travoprost ophthalmic solution) 0.004% and TRAVATAN Z® (travoprost ophthalmic solution) 0.004% was ocular hyperemia which was reported in 30 to 50% of patients. Up to 3% of patients discontinued therapy due to subconjunctival hyperemia.

Ocular adverse events reported at an incidence of 5 to 10% in these clinical studies included decreased visual acuity, eye discomfort, foreign body sensation, pain and pruritus.

Ocular adverse events reported at an incidence of 1 to 4% in clinical studies with TRAVATAN® or TRAVATAN Z® included abnormal vision, blepharitis, blurred vision, cataract, cells, conjunctivitis, corneal staining, dry eye, eye disorder, flare, iris discoloration, keratitis, lid margin crusting, photophobia, subconjunctival hemorrhage, and tearing.

Nonocular adverse events reported at an incidence of 1 to 5% in these clinical studies were accidental injury, allergy, angina pectoris, anxiety, arthritis, back pain, bradycardia, bronchitis, chest pain, cold/flu syndrome, depression, dyspepsia, gastrointestinal disorder, headache, hypercholesterolemia, hypertension, hypotension, infection, pain, prostate disorder, sinusitis, urinary incontinence, and urinary tract infection.

DOSAGE AND ADMINISTRATION

The recommended dosage is one drop in the affected eye(s) once-daily in the evening. The dosage of TRAVATAN Z® ophthalmic solution should not exceed once-daily since it has been shown that more frequent administration of travoprost may decrease the intraocular pressure lowering effect.

Reduction of intraocular pressure starts approximately 2 hours after administration of travoprost. The maximum effect is observed 12 hours after administration and is maintained throughout the day.

TRAVATAN Z® may be used concomitantly with other topical ophthalmic drug products to lower intraocular pressure. If more than one topical ophthalmic drug is being used, the drugs should be administered at least five (5) minutes apart.

HOW SUPPLIED

TRAVATAN Z® (travoprost ophthalmic solution) 0.004% is a sterile, isotonic, buffered, preserved, aqueous solution of travoprost (0.04 mg/mL) supplied in Alcon's oval DROP-TAINER® package system.

TRAVATAN Z® is supplied as a 2.5 mL solution in a 4 mL and a 5 mL solution in a 7.5 mL natural polypropylene dispenser bottle with a natural polypropylene dropper tip and a turquoise polypropylene overcap. Tamper evidence is provided with a shrink band around the closure and neck area of the package.

2.5 mL fill in 4 mL bottle	NDC 0065-0260-25
5 mL fill in 7.5 mL bottle	NDC 0065-0260-05

Storage: Store at 2° - 25°C (36° - 77°F).

Rx Only

U.S. Patent Nos. 5,889,052 and 6,235,781

---

* TIMOPTIC is the registered trademark of Merck & Co., Inc.

Alcon®

ALCON LABORATORIES, INC.
Fort Worth, Texas 76134 USA
© 2005-2007 Alcon, Inc.

VIGAMOX®   ℞

[*vi-ga-mox*]
(moxifloxacin hydrochloride ophthalmic solution)
0.5% as base

DESCRIPTION

VIGAMOX® (moxifloxacin HCl ophthalmic solution) 0.5% is a sterile ophthalmic solution. It is an 8-methoxy fluoroquinolone anti-infective for topical ophthalmic use.

Chemical Name: 1-Cyclopropyl-6-fluoro-1,4-dihydro-8-methoxy-7-[(4aS,7aS)-octahydro-6H-pyrrolol[3,4-b]pyridin-6-yl]-4-oxo-3-quinolinecarboxylic acid, monohydrochloride.

Moxifloxacin hydrochloride is a slightly yellow to yellow crystalline powder. Each mL of VIGAMOX® solution contains 5.45 mg moxifloxacin hydrochloride equivalent to 5 mg moxifloxacin base.

Contains:

Active: Moxifloxacin 0.5% (5 mg/mL); **Inactives:** Boric acid, sodium chloride, and purified water. May also contain hydrochloric acid/sodium hydroxide to adjust pH to approximately 6.8.

VIGAMOX® solution is an isotonic solution with an osmolality of approximately 290 mOsm/kg.

CLINICAL PHARMACOLOGY

Pharmacokinetics: Plasma concentrations of moxifloxacin were measured in healthy adult male and female subjects who received bilateral topical ocular doses of VIGAMOX® solution 3 times a day. The mean steady-state C_{max} (2.7 ng/mL) and estimated daily exposure AUC (45 ng·hr/mL) values were 1,600 and 1,000 times lower than the mean C_{max} and AUC reported after therapeutic 400 mg oral doses of moxifloxacin. The plasma half-life of moxifloxacin was estimated to be 13 hours.

Microbiology

Moxifloxacin is an 8-methoxy fluoroquinolone with a diazabicyclononyl ring at the C7 position. The antibacterial action of moxifloxacin results from inhibition of the topoisomerase II (DNA gyrase) and topoisomerase IV. DNA gyrase is an essential enzyme that is involved in the replication, transcription and repair of bacterial DNA. Topoisomerase IV is an enzyme known to play a key role in the partitioning of the chromosomal DNA during bacterial cell division.

The mechanism of action for quinolones, including moxifloxacin, is different from that of macrolides, aminoglycosides, or tetracyclines. Therefore, moxifloxacin may be active against pathogens that are resistant to these antibiotics and these antibiotics may be active against pathogens that are resistant to moxifloxacin. There is no cross-resistance between moxifloxacin and the aforementioned classes of antibiotics. Cross resistance has been observed between systemic moxifloxacin and some other quinolones.

In vitro resistance to moxifloxacin develops via multiple-step mutations. Resistance to moxifloxacin occurs *in vitro* at a general frequency of between 1.8×10^{-9} to $< 1 \times 10^{-11}$ for Gram-positive bacteria.

Moxifloxacin has been shown to be active against most strains of the following microorganisms, both *in vitro* and in clinical infections as described in the INDICATIONS AND USAGE section:

Aerobic Gram-positive microorganisms:

Corynebacterium species*
*Micrococcusluteus**
Staphylococcus aureus
Staphylococcus epidermidis
Staphylococcus haemolyticus
Staphylococcus hominis
*Staphylococcus warneri**
Streptococcus pneumoniae
Streptococcus viridans group

Aerobic Gram-negative microorganisms:

*Acinetobacter lwoffii**
Haemophilus influenzae
*Haemophilus parainfluenzae**

Other microorganisms:

Chlamydia trachomatis

*Efficacy for this organism was studied in fewer than 10 infections.

The following *in vitro* data are also available, but their clinical significance in ophthalmic infections is unknown. The safety and effectiveness of VIGAMOX® solution in treating ophthalmological infections due to these microorganisms have not been established in adequate and well-controlled trials.

The following organisms are considered susceptible when evaluated using systemic breakpoints. However, a correlation between the in vitro systemic breakpoint and ophthalmological efficacy has not been established. The list of organisms is provided as guidance only in assessing the potential treatment of conjunctival infections. Moxifloxacin exhibits *in vitro* minimal inhibitory concentrations (MICs) of 2 µg/ml or less (systemic susceptible breakpoint) against most (≥ 90%) of strains of the following ocular pathogens.

Aerobic Gram-positive microorganisms:

Listeria monocytogenes
Staphylococcus saprophyticus
Streptococcus agalactiae
Streptococcus mitis
Streptococcus pyogenes
Streptococcus Group C, G and F

Aerobic Gram-negative microorganisms:

Acinetobacter baumannii
Acinetobacter calcoaceticus
Citrobacter freundii
Citrobacter koseri
Enterobacter aerogenes
Enterobacter cloacae
Escherichia coli
Klebsiella oxytoca
Klebsiella pneumoniae
Moraxella catarrhalis
Morganella morganii
Neisseria gonorrhoeae
Proteus mirabilis
Proteus vulgaris
Pseudomonas stutzeri

Anaerobic microorganisms:

Clostridium perfringens
Fusobacterium species
Prevotella species
Propionibacterium acnes

Other microorganisms:

Chlamydia pneumoniae
Legionella pneumophila
Mycobacterium avium
Mycobacterium marinum
Mycoplasma pneumoniae

Clinical Studies:

In two randomized, double-masked, multicenter, controlled clinical trials in which patients were dosed 3 times a day for 4 days, VIGAMOX® solution produced clinical cures on day 5–6 in 66% to 69% of patients treated for bacterial conjunctivitis. Microbiological success rates for the eradication of the baseline pathogens ranged from 84% to 94%. Please note that microbiologic eradication does not always correlate with clinical outcome in anti-infective trials.

INDICATIONS AND USAGE

VIGAMOX® solution is indicated for the treatment of bacterial conjunctivitis caused by susceptible strains of the following organisms:

Aerobic Gram-positive microorganisms:

Corynebacterium species*
*Micrococcus luteus**
Staphylococcus aureus
Staphylococcus epidermidis
Staphylococcus haemolyticus
Staphylococcus hominis
*Staphylococcus warneri**
Streptococcus pneumoniae
Streptococcus viridans group

Aerobic Gram-negative microorganisms:

*Acinetobacter lwoffii**
Haemophilus influenzae
*Haemophilus parainfluenzae**

Other microorganisms:

Chlamydia trachomatis

*Efficacy for this organism was studied in fewer than 10 infections.

CONTRAINDICATIONS

VIGAMOX® solution is contraindicated in patients with a history of hypersensitivity to moxifloxacin, to other quinolones, or to any of the components in this medication.

WARNINGS

NOT FOR INJECTION.

VIGAMOX® solution should not be injected subconjunctivally, nor should it be introduced directly into the anterior chamber of the eye.

In patients receiving systemically administered quinolones, including moxifloxacin, serious and occasionally fatal hypersensitivity (anaphylactic) reactions have been reported, some following the first dose. Some reactions were accompanied by cardiovascular collapse, loss of consciousness, angioedema (including laryngeal, pharyngeal or facial edema), airway obstruction, dyspnea, urticaria, and itching. If an allergic reaction to moxifloxacin occurs, discontinue use of the drug. Serious acute hypersensitivity reactions may require immediate emergency treatment. Oxygen and airway management should be administered as clinically indicated.

PRECAUTIONS

General: As with other anti-infectives, prolonged use may result in overgrowth of non-susceptible organisms, including fungi. If superinfection occurs, discontinue use and institute alternative therapy. Whenever clinical judgment dictates, the patient should be examined with the aid of magnification, such as slit-lamp biomicroscopy, and, where appropriate, fluorescein staining. Patients should be advised not to wear contact lenses if they have signs and symptoms of bacterial conjunctivitis.

Information for Patients: Avoid contaminating the applicator tip with material from the eye, fingers or other source. Systemically administered quinolones including moxifloxacin have been associated with hypersensitivity reactions, even following a single dose. Discontinue use immediately and contact your physician at the first sign of a rash or allergic reaction.

Drug Interactions: Drug-drug interaction studies have not been conducted with VIGAMOX® solution. *In vitro* studies indicate that moxifloxacin does not inhibit CYP3A4, CYP2D6, CYP2C9, CYP2C19, or CYP1A2 indicating that moxifloxacin is unlikely to alter the pharmacokinetics of drugs metabolized by these cytochrome P450 isozymes.

Carcinogenesis, Mutagenesis, Impairment of Fertility: Long-term studies in animals to determine the carcinogenic potential of moxifloxacin have not been performed. However, in an accelerated study with initiators and promoters, moxifloxacin was not carcinogenic in rats following up to 38 weeks of oral dosing at 500 mg/kg/day (approximately 21,700 times the highest recommended total daily human ophthalmic dose for a 50 kg person, on a mg/kg basis). Moxifloxacin was not mutagenic in four bacterial strains used in the Ames *Salmonella* reversion assay. As with other quinolones, the positive response observed with moxifloxacin in strain TA 102 using the same assay may be due to the inhibition of DNA gyrase. Moxifloxacin was not mutagenic in the CHO/HGPRT mammalian cell gene mutation assay. An equivocal result was obtained in the same assay when v79 cells were used. Moxifloxacin was clastogenic in the v79 chromosome aberration assay, but it did not induce unscheduled DNA synthesis in cultured rat hepatocytes. There was no evidence of genotoxicity *in vivo* in a micronucleus test or a dominant lethal test in mice.

Moxifloxacin had no effect on fertility in male and female rats at oral doses as high as 500 mg/kg/day, approximately 21,700 times the highest recommended total daily human ophthalmic dose. At 500 mg/kg orally there were slight effects on sperm morphology (head-tail separation) in male rats and on the estrous cycle in female rats.

Pregnancy: Teratogenic Effects.

Pregnancy Category C: Moxifloxacin was not teratogenic when administered to pregnant rats during organogenesis at oral doses as high as 500 mg/kg/day (approximately 21,700 times the highest recommended total daily human ophthalmic dose); however, decreased fetal body weights and slightly delayed fetal skeletal development were observed. There was no evidence of teratogenicity when pregnant Cynomolgus monkeys were given oral doses as high as 100 mg/kg/day (approximately 4,300 times the highest recommended total daily human ophthalmic dose). An increased incidence of smaller fetuses was observed at 100 mg/kg/day.

Since there are no adequate and well-controlled studies in pregnant women, VIGAMOX® solution should be used during pregnancy only if the potential benefit justifies the potential risk to the fetus.

Nursing Mothers: Moxifloxacin has not been measured in human milk, although it can be presumed to be excreted in human milk. Caution should be exercised when VIGAMOX® solution is administered to a nursing mother.

Pediatric Use: The safety and effectiveness of VIGAMOX® solution in infants below 1 year of age have not been established. There is no evidence that the ophthalmic administration of VIGAMOX® solution has any effect on weight bearing joints, even though oral administration of some quinolones has been shown to cause arthropathy in immature animals.

Geriatric Use: No overall differences in safety and effectiveness have been observed between elderly and younger patients.

ADVERSE REACTIONS

The most frequently reported ocular adverse events were conjunctivitis, decreased visual acuity, dry eye, keratitis, ocular discomfort, ocular hyperemia, ocular pain, ocular pruritus, subconjunctival hemorrhage, and tearing. These events occurred in approximately 1-6% of patients. Nonocular adverse events reported at a rate of 1-4% were fever, increased cough, infection, otitis media, pharyngitis, rash, and rhinitis.

DOSAGE AND ADMINISTRATION

Instill one drop in the affected eye 3 times a day for 7 days.

HOW SUPPLIED

VIGAMOX® solution is supplied as a sterile ophthalmic solution in Alcon's DROP-TAINER® dispensing system consisting of a natural low density polyethylene bottle and dispensing plug and tan polypropylene closure. Tamper evidence is provided with a shrink band around the closure and neck area of the package.

3 mL in 4 mL bottle - **NDC** 0065-4013-03

Storage: Store at 2°C-25°C (36°F-77°F).

Rx Only

Manufactured by
Alcon Laboratories, Inc.
Fort Worth, Texas 76134 USA

Licensed to Alcon, Inc. by Bayer HealthCare AG.

U.S. PAT. NO. 4,990,517; 5,607,942; 6,716,830.

© 2003-2006, 2008 Alcon, Inc.

Allergan, Inc.

2525 DUPONT DRIVE
P.O. BOX 19534
IRVINE, CA 92623-9534

Direct Inquiries to:
(714) 246-4500

OPHTHALMIC PRODUCTS

For information on Allergan, Inc., prescription, OTC, and ophthalmic products, consult the *Physicians' Desk Reference® for Ophthalmology*. For literature, service items, or sample material, contact Allergan directly. See a complete listing of products in the Manufacturers' Index section of this book.

ACZONE®
(dapsone)
Gel, 5%

℞

HIGHLIGHTS OF PRESCRIBING INFORMATION

These highlights do not include all the information needed to use ACZONE® safely and effectively. See full prescribing information for ACZONE®.

ACZONE® (dapsone) Gel, 5%
For topical use only
Initial U.S. Approval: 1955

—————INDICATIONS AND USAGE—————

ACZONE® Gel is indicated for the topical treatment of acne vulgaris (1).

—————DOSAGE AND ADMINISTRATION—————

- Apply twice daily (2).
- Apply approximately a pea-sized amount of ACZONE® Gel, 5%, in a thin layer to the acne affected area (2).
- If there is no improvement after 12 weeks, treatment with ACZONE® Gel, 5%, should be reassessed (2).

For topical use only. Not for oral, ophthalmic, or intravaginal use (2).

—————DOSAGE FORMS AND STRENGTHS—————

ACZONE® (dapsone) Gel, 5%, is supplied in the following size tubes:
- Professional Sample: 3 gram laminate tube (3).
- Commercially: 30 and 60 gram laminate tubes (3).

—————CONTRAINDICATIONS—————

None.

—————WARNINGS AND PRECAUTIONS—————

Hematological Effects: Some subjects with G6PD deficiency using ACZONE® Gel developed laboratory changes suggestive of mild hemolysis. (5.1) (8.6)

The following are seen with oral dapsone treatment:
- Hematological Effects (5.1).
- Peripheral Neuropathy (5.2).
- Skin Reactions (5.3).

—————ADVERSE REACTIONS—————

Most common adverse reactions (incidence ≥ 10%) are oiliness/peeling, dryness and erythema at the application site (6).

To report SUSPECTED ADVERSE REACTIONS, contact Allergan at 1-800-433-8871 or FDA at 1-800-FDA-1088 or *www.fda.gov/medwatch*.

—————DRUG INTERACTIONS—————

- Trimethoprim/sulfamethoxazole (TMP/SMX) increases the level of dapsone and its metabolites. (7.1)
- Topical benzoyl peroxide used at the same time as ACZONE® may result in temporary local yellow or orange skin discoloration. (7.2)

—————USE IN SPECIFIC POPULATIONS—————

G6PD Deficiency (8.6).

See 17 for PATIENT COUNSELING INFORMATION and FDA-approved patient labeling.

Revised: 03/2009

FULL PRESCRIBING INFORMATION: CONTENTS*

*Sections or subsections omitted from the full prescribing information are not listed.

FULL PRESCRIBING INFORMATION

1 INDICATIONS AND USAGE

ACZONE® Gel, 5%, is indicated for the topical treatment of acne vulgaris.

2 DOSAGE AND ADMINISTRATION

For topical use only. Not for oral, ophthalmic, or intravaginal use.

After the skin is gently washed and patted dry, apply approximately a pea-sized amount of ACZONE® Gel, 5%, in a thin layer to the acne affected areas twice daily. Rub in ACZONE® Gel, 5%, gently and completely. ACZONE® Gel, 5%, is gritty with visible drug substance particles. Wash hands after application of ACZONE® Gel, 5%.

If there is no improvement after 12 weeks, treatment with ACZONE® Gel, 5%, should be reassessed.

3 DOSAGE FORMS AND STRENGTHS

ACZONE® (dapsone) Gel, 5%, is supplied in the following size tubes:
- Professional Sample: 3 gram laminate tube
- Commercially: 30 and 60 gram laminate tubes

4 CONTRAINDICATIONS

None.

5 WARNINGS AND PRECAUTIONS
5.1 Hematological Effects

Oral dapsone treatment has produced dose-related hemolysis and hemolytic anemia. Individuals with glucose-6-phosphate dehydrogenase (G6PD) deficiency are more prone to hemolysis with the use of certain drugs. G6PD deficiency is most prevalent in populations of African, South Asian, Middle Eastern and Mediterranean ancestry.

There was no evidence of clinically relevant hemolysis or anemia in patients treated with ACZONE® Gel, 5%, including patients who were G6PD deficient. Some subjects with G6PD deficiency using ACZONE® Gel developed laboratory changes suggestive of mild hemolysis.

If signs and symptoms suggestive of hemolytic anemia occur, ACZONE® Gel, 5% should be discontinued. ACZONE® Gel, 5% should not be used in patients who are taking oral dapsone or antimalarial medications because of the potential for hemolytic reactions. Combination of

ACZONE® Gel, 5%, with trimethoprim/sulfamethoxazole (TMP/SMX) may increase the likelihood of hemolysis in patients with G6PD deficiency.

5.2 Peripheral Neuropathy

Peripheral neuropathy (motor loss and muscle weakness) has been reported with oral dapsone treatment. No events of peripheral neuropathy were observed in clinical trials with topical ACZONE® Gel, 5% treatment.

5.3 Skin

Skin reactions (toxic epidermal necrolysis, erythema multiforme, morbilliform and scarlatiniform reactions, bullous and exfoliative dermatitis, erythema nodosum, and urticaria) have been reported with oral dapsone treatment. These types of skin reactions were not observed in clinical trials with topical ACZONE® Gel, 5% treatment.

6 ADVERSE REACTIONS

6.1 Clinical Studies Experience

Because clinical trials are conducted under prescribed conditions, adverse reaction rates observed in the clinical trials of a drug cannot be directly compared to rates in the clinical trials of another drug and may not reflect the rates observed in practice.

Serious adverse reactions reported in patients treated with ACZONE® Gel, 5%, during clinical trials included but were not limited to the following:

- Nervous system/Psychiatric – Suicide attempt, tonic clonic movements.
- Gastrointestinal – Abdominal pain, severe vomiting, pancreatitis.
- Other – Severe pharyngitis

In the clinical trials, a total of 12 out of 4032 patients were reported to have depression (3 of 1660 treated with vehicle and 9 of 2372 treated with ACZONE® Gel, 5%). Psychosis was reported in 2 of 2372 patients treated with ACZONE® Gel, 5%, and in 0 of 1660 patients treated with vehicle. Combined contact sensitization/irritation studies with ACZONE® Gel, 5%, in 253 healthy subjects resulted in at least 3 subjects with moderate erythema. ACZONE® Gel, 5%, did not induce phototoxicity or photoallergy in human dermal safety studies.

ACZONE® Gel, 5%, was evaluated for 12 weeks in four controlled studies for local cutaneous events in 1819 patients. The most common events reported from these studies include oiliness/peeling, dryness, and erythema. These data are shown by severity in Table 1 below.

[See table at top right]

The adverse reactions occurring in at least 1% of patients in either arm in the four vehicle controlled studies are presented in Table 2.

Table 2–Adverse Reactions Occurring in at least 1% of Patients

	ACZONE® N=1819	Vehicle N=1660
Application Site Reaction NOS	18%	20%
Application Site Dryness	16%	17%
Application Site Erythema	13%	14%
Application Site Burning	1%	2%
Application Site Pruritus	1%	1%
Pyrexia	1%	1%
Nasopharyngitis	5%	6%
Upper Respiratory Tract Inf. NOS	3%	3%
Sinusitis NOS	2%	1%
Influenza	1%	1%
Pharyngitis	2%	2%
Cough	2%	2%
Joint Sprain	1%	1%
Headache NOS	4%	4%

NOS = Not otherwise specified

One patient treated with ACZONE® Gel in the clinical trials had facial swelling which led to discontinuation of medication.

In addition, 486 patients were evaluated in a 12 month safety study. The adverse event profile in this study was consistent with that observed in the vehicle-controlled studies.

Table 1–Application Site Adverse Reactions by Maximum Severity

Application Site Event	ACZONE® (N=1819)			Vehicle (N=1660)		
	Mild	Moderate	Severe	Mild	Moderate	Severe
Erythema	9%	5%	<1%	9%	6%	<1%
Dryness	14%	3%	<1%	14%	4%	<1%
Oiliness/Peeling	13%	6%	<1%	15%	6%	<1%

Table 3–Mean Hemoglobin, Bilirubin, and Reticulocyte Levels in Acne Subjects with G6PD Deficiency in ACZONE®/Vehicle Cross-Over Study

		ACZONE®		Vehicle	
		N	Mean	N	Mean
Hemoglobin (g/dL)	Pre-treatment	53	13.44	56	13.36
	2 weeks	53	13.12	55	13.34
	12 weeks	50	13.42	50	13.37
Bilirubin (mg/dL)	Pre-treatment	54	0.58	56	0.55
	2 weeks	53	0.65	55	0.56
	12 weeks	50	0.61	50	0.62
Reticulocytes (%)	Pre-treatment	53	1.30	55	1.34
	2 weeks	53	1.51	55	1.34
	12 weeks	50	1.48	50	1.41

6.2 Experience with Oral Use of Dapsone

Although not observed in the clinical trials with ACZONE® Gel (topical dapsone) serious adverse reactions have been reported with oral use of dapsone, including agranulocytosis, hemolytic anemia, peripheral neuropathy (motor loss and muscle weakness), and skin reactions (toxic epidermal necrolysis, erythema multiforme, morbilliform and scarlatiniform reactions, bullous and exfoliative dermatitis, erythema nodosum, and urticaria).

7 DRUG INTERACTIONS

7.1 Trimethoprim-Sulfomethoxazole

A drug-drug interaction study evaluated the effect of the use of ACZONE® Gel, 5%, in combination with double strength (160 mg/800 mg) trimethoprim-sulfamethoxazole (TMP/SMX). During co-administration, systemic levels of TMP and SMX were essentially unchanged. However, levels of dapsone and its metabolites increased in the presence of TMP/SMX. Systemic exposure (AUC_{0-12}) of dapsone and N-acetyl-dapsone (NAD) were increased by about 40% and 20% respectively in presence of TMP/SMX. Notably, systemic exposure (AUC_{0-12}) of dapsone hydroxylamine (DHA) was more than doubled in the presence of TMP/SMX. Exposure from the proposed topical dose is about 1% of that from the 100 mg oral dose, even when co-administered with TMP/SMX.

7.2 Topical Benzoyl Peroxide

Topical application of ACZONE® Gel followed by benzoyl peroxide in subjects with acne vulgaris resulted in a temporary local yellow or orange discoloration of the skin and facial hair (reported by 7 out of 95 subjects in a clinical study) with resolution in 4 to 57 days.

7.3 Drug Interactions with Oral Dapsone

Certain concomitant medications (such as rifampin, anticonvulsants, St. John's wort) may increase the formation of dapsone hydroxylamine, a metabolite of dapsone associated with hemolysis. With oral dapsone treatment, folic acid antagonists such as pyrimethamine have been noted to possibly increase the likelihood of hematologic reactions.

8 USE IN SPECIFIC POPULATIONS

8.1 Pregnancy

Teratogenic Effects: Pregnancy Category C

There are no adequate and well controlled studies in pregnant women. Dapsone has been shown to have an embryocidal effect in rats and rabbits when administered orally in doses of 75 mg/kg/day and 150 mg/kg/day (approximately 800 and 500 times the systemic exposure observed in human females as a result of use of the maximum recommended topical dose, based on AUC comparisons), respectively. These effects were probably secondary to maternal toxicity. ACZONE® Gel, 5%, should be used during pregnancy only if the potential benefit justifies the potential risk to the fetus.

8.3 Nursing Mothers

Although systemic absorption of dapsone following topical application of ACZONE® Gel, 5%, is minimal relative to oral dapsone administration, it is known that dapsone is excreted in human milk. Because of the potential for oral dapsone to cause adverse reactions in nursing infants, a decision should be made whether to discontinue nursing or to discontinue ACZONE® Gel, 5%, taking into account the importance of the drug to the mother.

8.4 Pediatric Use

Safety and efficacy was evaluated in 1169 children aged 12-17 years old treated with ACZONE® Gel, 5%, in the clinical studies. The adverse event rate for ACZONE® Gel, 5%, was similar to the vehicle control group. Safety and efficacy was not studied in pediatric patients less than 12 years of age, therefore ACZONE® Gel, 5%, is not recommended for use in this age group.

8.5 Geriatric Use

Clinical studies of ACZONE® Gel, 5%, did not include sufficient number of patients aged 65 and over to determine whether they respond differently from younger patients.

8.6 G6PD Deficiency

ACZONE® Gel, 5% and vehicle were evaluated in a randomized, double-blind, cross-over design clinical study of 64 patients with G6PD deficiency and acne vulgaris. Subjects were Black (88%), Asian (6%), Hispanic (2%) or of other racial origin (5%). Blood samples were taken at Baseline, Week 2, and Week 12 during both vehicle and ACZONE® Gel, 5% treatment periods. There were 56 out of 64 subjects who had a Week 2 blood draw and applied at least 50% of treatment applications. Table 3 contains results from testing of relevant hematology parameters for these two treatment periods. ACZONE® Gel was associated with a 0.32 g/dL drop in hemoglobin after two weeks of treatment, but hemoglobin levels generally returned to baseline levels at Week 12.

[See table 3 above]

There were no changes from baseline in haptoglobin or lactate dehydrogenase during ACZONE® or vehicle treatment at either the 2-week or 12-week time point.

The proportion of subjects who experienced decreases in hemoglobin ≥1 g/dL was similar between ACZONE® Gel, 5% and vehicle treatment (8 of 58 subjects had such decreases during ACZONE® treatment compared to 7 of 56 subjects during vehicle treatment among subjects with at least one on-treatment hemoglobin assessment). Subgroups based on gender, race, or G6PD enzyme activity did not display any differences in laboratory results from the overall study group. There was no evidence of clinically significant hemolytic anemia in this study. Some of these subjects developed laboratory changes suggestive of mild hemolysis.

10 OVERDOSAGE

ACZONE® Gel, 5%, is not for oral use. If oral ingestion occurs, medical advice should be sought.

11 DESCRIPTION

ACZONE® Gel, 5%, contains dapsone, a sulfone, in an aqueous gel base for topical dermatologic use. ACZONE® Gel, 5% is a gritty translucent material with visible drug substance particles. Chemically, dapsone has an empirical formula of $C_{12}H_{12}N_2O_2S$. It is a white, odorless crystalline powder that has a molecular weight of 248. Dapsone's chemical name is 4,4'-diaminodiphenylsulfone and its structural formula is:

$$NH_2 - \langle \text{} \rangle - SO_2 - \langle \text{} \rangle - NH_2$$

Each gram of ACZONE® Gel, 5%, contains 50 mg of dapsone, USP, in a gel of carbomer 980; diethylene glycol monoethyl ether, NF; methylparaben, NF; sodium hydroxide, NF; and purified water, USP.

12 CLINICAL PHARMACOLOGY

12.1 Mechanism of Action

The mechanism of action of dapsone gel in treating acne vulgaris is not known.

12.3 Pharmacokinetics

An open-label study compared the pharmacokinetics of dapsone after ACZONE® Gel, 5%, (110 ± 60 mg/day) was applied twice daily (~BSA 22.5%) for 14 days (n=18) with a single 100 mg dose of oral dapsone administered to a subgroup of patients (n=10) in a crossover design. On Day 14 the mean dapsone $AUC_{0-24 h}$ was 415 ± 224 ng•h/mL for ACZONE® Gel, 5%, whereas following a single 100 mg dose of oral dapsone the $AUC_{0-infinity}$ was 52,641 ± 36,223 ng•h/mL. Exposure after the oral dose of 100 mg dapsone was approximately 100 times greater than after the topical ACZONE® Gel, 5% dose, twice a day.

In a long-term safety study of ACZONE® Gel, 5% treatment, periodic blood samples were collected up to 12 months to determine systemic exposure of dapsone and its metabolites in approximately 500 patients. Based on the measurable dapsone concentrations from 408 patients (M=192, F=216), obtained at month 3, neither gender, nor race appeared to affect the pharmacokinetics of dapsone. Similarly, dapsone exposures were approximately the same between the age groups of 12-15 years (N=155) and those greater than or equal to 16 years (N=253). There was no evidence of increasing systemic exposure to dapsone over the study year in these patients.

12.4 Microbiology

In Vivo Activity: No microbiology or immunology studies were conducted during dapsone gel clinical trials.

Drug Resistance: No dapsone resistance studies were conducted during dapsone gel clinical trials. Because no microbiology studies were done, there are no data available as to whether dapsone treatment may have resulted in decreased susceptibility of Propionibacterium acnes, an organism associated with acne, to other antimicrobials that may be used to treat acne. Therapeutic resistance to dapsone has been reported for Mycobacterium leprae, when patients have been treated with oral dapsone.

13 NONCLINICAL TOXICOLOGY

13.1 Carcinogenesis, Mutagenesis, Impairment of Fertility

Dapsone was not mutagenic in a bacterial reverse mutation assay (Ames test) using S. typhimurium and E. coli, with and without metabolic activation and was negative in a micronucleus assay conducted in mice. Dapsone increased both numerical and structural aberrations in a chromosome aberration assay conducted with Chinese hamster ovary (CHO) cells.

Dapsone was not carcinogenic to rats when orally administered to females for 92 weeks or males for 100 weeks at dose levels up to 15 mg/kg/day (approximately 160 times the systemic exposure observed in human males and 300 times the systemic exposure observed in human females as a result of use of the maximum recommended topical dose, based on AUC comparisons).

No evidence of potential to induce carcinogenicity was obtained in a dermal study in which dapsone gel was topically applied to Tg.AC transgenic mice for approximately 26 weeks. Dapsone concentrations of 3%, 5%, and 10% were evaluated; 3% material was judged to be the maximum tolerated dosage.

ACZONE® Gel, 5%, did not increase the rate of formation of ultra violet light-induced skin tumors when topically applied to hairless mice in a 12-month photocarcinogenicity study.

The effects of dapsone on fertility and general reproduction performance were assessed in male and female rats following oral (gavage) dosing. Dapsone reduced sperm motility at dosages of 3 mg/kg/day or greater (approximately 17 times the systemic exposure observed in human males as a result of use of the maximum recommended topical dose, based on AUC comparisons). The mean numbers of embryo implantations and viable embryos were significantly reduced in untreated females mated with males that had been dosed at 12 mg/kg/day or greater (approximately 70 times the systemic exposure observed in human males as a result of use of the maximum recommended topical dose, based on AUC comparisons), presumably due to reduced numbers or effectiveness of sperm, indicating impairment of fertility. Dapsone had no effect on male fertility at dosages of 2 mg/kg/day or less (approximately 13 times the systemic exposure observed in human males as a result of use of the maximum recommended topical dose, based on AUC comparisons). When administered to female rats at a dosage of 75 mg/kg/day (approximately 800 times the systemic exposure observed in human females as a result of use of the maximum recommended topical dose, based on AUC comparisons) for 15 days prior to mating and for 17 days thereafter, dapsone reduced the mean number of implantations, increased the mean early resorption rate, and reduced the mean litter size. These effects were probably secondary to maternal toxicity.

Dapsone was assessed for effects on perinatal/postnatal pup development and postnatal maternal behavior and function in a study in which dapsone was orally administered to female rats daily beginning on the seventh day of gestation and continuing until the twenty-seventh day postpartum. Maternal toxicity (decreased body weight and food consumption) and developmental effects (increase in stillborn pups and decreased pup weight) were seen at a dapsone dose of 30 mg/kg/day (approximately 500 times the systemic exposure observed in human females as a result of use of the maximum recommended topical dose, based on AUC comparisons). No effects were observed on the viability, physical development, behavior, learning ability, or reproductive function of surviving pups.

14 CLINICAL STUDIES

Two randomized, double-blind, vehicle-controlled, clinical studies were conducted to evaluate ACZONE® Gel, 5%, for the treatment of patients with acne vulgaris (N=1475 and 1525). The studies were designed to enroll patients 12 years of age and older with 20 to 50 inflammatory and 20 to 100 non-inflammatory lesions at baseline. In these studies patients applied either ACZONE® Gel, 5%, or vehicle control twice daily for up to 12 weeks. Efficacy was evaluated in terms of success on the Global Acne Assessment Score (no or minimal acne) and in the percent reduction in inflammatory, non-inflammatory, and total lesions.

The Global Acne Assessment Score was a 5-point scale as follows:

0   None: no evidence of facial acne vulgaris

1   Minimal: few non-inflammatory lesions (comedones) are present; a few inflammatory lesions (papules/pustules) may be present

2   Mild: several to many non-inflammatory lesions (comedones) are present; a few inflammatory lesions (papules/pustules) are present

3   Moderate: many non-inflammatory (comedones) and inflammatory lesions (papules/pustules) are present; no nodulo-cystic lesions are allowed

4   Severe: significant degree of inflammatory disease; papules/pustules are a predominant feature; a few nodulo-cystic lesions may be present; comedones may be present.

The success rates on the Global Acne Assessment Score (no or minimal acne) at Week 12 are presented in Table 4.

[See table 4 above]

Table 5 presents the mean percent reduction in inflammatory, non-inflammatory, and total lesions from baseline to Week 12.

[See table 5 above]

The clinical studies enrolled about equal proportions of male and female subjects. Female patients tended to have greater percent reductions in lesions and greater success on the Global Acne Assessment Score than males. The breakdown by race in the clinical studies was about 73% Caucasian, 14% Black, 9% Hispanic, and 2% Asian. Efficacy results were similar across the racial subgroups.

16 HOW SUPPLIED/STORAGE AND HANDLING

ACZONE® (dapsone) Gel, 5%, is supplied in the following size tubes:

Professional Sample
5% NDC 0023-3670-03
3 gram laminate tube
Commercially Available as:
5% NDC 0023-3670-30
30 gram laminate tube
5% NDC 0023-3670-60
60 gram laminate tube

Table 4 - Success (No or Minimal Acne) on the Global Acne Assessment Score at Week 12

	Study 1*		Study 2*	
	ACZONE® N=699	Vehicle N=687	ACZONE® N=729	Vehicle N=738
Subjects with No or Minimal Acne	291 (42%)	223 (32%)	253 (35%)	206 (28%)

*Analysis excludes subjects classified with minimal acne at baseline

Table 5 - Percent Reduction in Lesions from Baseline to Week 12

	Study 1		Study 2	
	ACZONE® N=745	Vehicle N=740	ACZONE® N=761	Vehicle N=764
Inflammatory	46%	42%	48%	40%
Non-Inflammatory	31%	24%	30%	21%
Total	38%	32%	37%	29%

KEEP OUT OF THE REACH OF CHILDREN LESS THAN 12 YEARS OLD.

Storage conditions:

Store at controlled room temperature, 20-25° C (68-76° F), excursions permitted to 15-30° C (59-86° F). Protect from freezing.

17 PATIENT COUNSELING INFORMATION

See FDA Approved-Patient Labeling (17.2)

17.1 Information for Patients

1. Patients should use ACZONE® Gel, 5%, as directed by the physician. ACZONE® Gel, 5%, is for external topical use only. ACZONE® Gel, 5%, is not for oral, ophthalmic or intravaginal use.

2. Patients should not use this medication for any disorder other than that for which it was prescribed.

3. Patients should report any signs of adverse reactions to their physician.

4. Protect ACZONE® Gel, 5%, from freezing.

5. See Patient Labeling for additional information on safety, efficacy, general use, and storage of ACZONE® Gel, 5%.

17.2 FDA-Approved Patient Labeling

ACZONE® (dapsone) Gel 5%

Read this important information before you start using ACZONE® (AK-zōn) Gel and each time you refill your prescription. There may be new information that you need to know. This summary is not meant to take the place of your doctor's advice. If you have any questions or want more information about ACZONE® Gel, ask your doctor or pharmacist.

What is ACZONE® Gel?

ACZONE® Gel is a prescription medicine used on your skin (topical) to treat acne in people 12 years and older.

ACZONE® Gel has not been studied in children under 12 years of age.

Who should not use ACZONE® Gel?

Do not use ACZONE® Gel if you are allergic to any of the ingredients in ACZONE® Gel or if you are younger than 12 years of age.

Active ingredient: dapsone.

Inactive ingredients: Carbomer 980, diethylene glycol monoethyl ether (DGME), methylparaben, sodium hydroxide, and purified water.

What should I tell my doctor before using ACZONE® Gel?

Tell your doctor about all of your medical conditions, including if you:

• **are pregnant or planning to become pregnant.** It is not known if ACZONE® Gel may harm your unborn baby. You and your doctor will need to decide if ACZONE® is right for you.

• **are breastfeeding.** ACZONE® Gel passes into your milk and may harm your baby. You should choose either to use ACZONE® Gel, or breastfeed, but not both. Talk to your doctor about the best way to feed your baby while using ACZONE® Gel.

• have glucose-6-phosphate dehydrogenase deficiency.

Tell your doctor about all the medicines you are taking including prescription and nonprescription medicines, vitamins and herbal supplements. Especially, tell your doctor if you are using any other medicines applied to the skin, such as acne medicines with benzoyl peroxide.

How do I use ACZONE® Gel?

• Use ACZONE® Gel exactly as prescribed by your doctor. ACZONE® Gel is usually used on your affected skin twice a day, once in the morning and once in the evening.

- Wash the areas of your skin where you will apply ACZONE® Gel. Gently pat your skin dry with a clean towel.
- Apply a thin layer of ACZONE® Gel to the areas of your skin that have acne. A pea-sized amount of ACZONE® Gel will usually be enough.
- Rub the medicine in gently and completely
- Make sure to put the cap back on the ACZONE® Gel tube. Close it tightly.
- Wash your hands after applying ACZONE® Gel.
- Keep ACZONE® Gel away from your mouth and eyes. Do not swallow ACZONE® Gel. If you swallow ACZONE® Gel, call your doctor or poison control center right away.
- If your acne does not get better after using ACZONE® Gel for 12 weeks, talk to your doctor about other treatments for acne.

What are the possible side effects of ACZONE® Gel?

Like all medicines, ACZONE® Gel can cause some side effects. The most common side effects of ACZONE® Gel are dryness, redness, oiliness and peeling of the skin being treated.

When the active ingredient of ACZONE® Gel (called dapsone) is taken orally as a pill, it has been related to the abnormal breakdown of red blood cells (hemolytic anemia). If you have glucose-6-phoshate dehydrogenase deficiency, you may have a greater risk for lowering your hemoglobin level. However, using ACZONE® Gel on the skin is not expected to put enough dapsone in the blood to cause clinical symptoms of hemolytic anemia. You are advised to be alert for signs and symptoms suggestive of this type of anemia (sudden onset of: back pain, breathlessness, tiredness/weakness with daily activities, dark-brown urine, high fever and yellow or pale skin). If you experience these signs and symptoms, stop use and call your doctor immediately.

Use of benzoyl peroxide together with ACZONE® Gel at the same time may cause your skin to temporarily turn yellow or orange at the site of application.

This is not a complete list of all the possible side effects. Call your doctor if you have any side effects that do not go away or bother you. If you have any questions, ask your doctor or pharmacist.

How should I store ACZONE® Gel?

Store ACZONE® Gel at room temperature 68 to 76°F. Do not freeze ACZONE® Gel.

Keep ACZONE® Gel out of the reach of children less than 12 years of age.

Where can I find more information about ACZONE® Gel?

If you have any questions or want more information about ACZONE® Gel, ask your doctor or pharmacist. Your doctor or pharmacist can also give you a copy of the ACZONE® Gel Package Insert written for health professionals. Ask them to explain anything you do not understand.

You may call 1-800-433-8871 or visit www.allergan.com to obtain more information about ACZONE® Gel.

ACZONE® (dapsone) Gel, 5%

Manufactured for: Allergan, Inc., Irvine, CA 92612, U.S.A.
Manufactured by: TOLMAR Inc., Fort Collins, CO 80526, U.S.A.
© 2009 Allergan, Inc., Irvine, CA 92612, U.S.A.
® marks owned by Allergan, Inc.
U.S. Patents 5,863,560; 6,060,085; and 6,620,435
72062US11A   44426 Rev 1 2/09
Shown in Product Identification Guide, page 304

ALPHAGAN® P   ℞
(brimonidine tartrate ophthalmic solution)
0.1% and 0.15%
Sterile

DESCRIPTION

ALPHAGAN® P (brimonidine tartrate ophthalmic solution) is a relatively selective alpha-2 adrenergic agonist for ophthalmic use. The chemical name of brimonidine tartrate is 5-Bromo-6-(2-imidazolidinylideneamino)quinoxaline L-tartrate. It is an off-white to pale yellow powder. It has a molecular weight of 442.24 as the tartrate salt, and is both soluble in water (0.6 mg/mL) and in the product vehicle (1.4 mg/mL) at pH 7.7. The structural formula is:

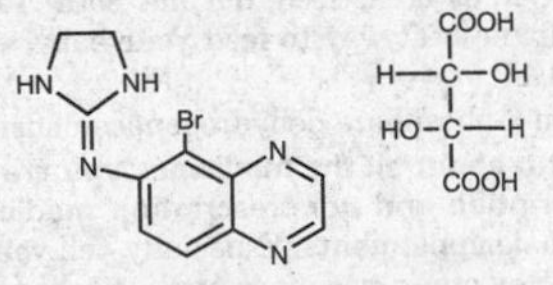

Formula: $C_{11}H_{10}BrN_5 \cdot C_4H_6O_6$ CAS Number: 70359-46-5
In solution, ALPHAGAN® P (brimonidine tartrate ophthalmic solution) has a clear, greenish-yellow color. It has an osmolality of 250-350 mOsmol/kg and a pH of 7.4-8.0 (0.1%) or 6.6-7.4 (0.15%).

Each mL of ALPHAGAN® P contains:
Active ingredient: brimonidine tartrate 0.1% (1.0 mg/mL) or 0.15% (1.5 mg/mL)
Inactives: sodium carboxymethylcellulose; sodium borate; boric acid; sodium chloride; potassium chloride; calcium chloride; magnesium chloride; PURITE® 0.005% (0.05 mg/mL) as a preservative; purified water; with hydrochloric acid and/or sodium hydroxide to adjust pH.

CLINICAL PHARMACOLOGY

Mechanism of Action

ALPHAGAN® P is an alpha adrenergic receptor agonist. It has a peak ocular hypotensive effect occurring at two hours post-dosing. Fluorophotometric studies in animals and humans suggest that brimonidine tartrate has a dual mechanism of action by reducing aqueous humor production and increasing uveoscleral outflow.

Pharmacokinetics

After ocular administration of either a 0.1% or 0.2% solution, plasma concentrations peaked within 0.5 to 2.5 hours and declined with a systemic half-life of approximately 2 hours.

In humans, systemic metabolism of brimonidine is extensive. It is metabolized primarily by the liver. Urinary excretion is the major route of elimination of the drug and its metabolites. Approximately 87% of an orally-administered radioactive dose was eliminated within 120 hours, with 74% found in the urine.

Clinical Evaluations

Elevated IOP presents a major risk factor in glaucomatous field loss. The higher the level of IOP, the greater the likelihood of optic nerve damage and visual field loss. Brimonidine tartrate has the action of lowering intraocular pressure with minimal effect on cardiovascular and pulmonary parameters.

Clinical studies were conducted to evaluate the safety, efficacy, and acceptability of ALPHAGAN® P (brimonidine tartrate ophthalmic solution) 0.15% compared with ALPHAGAN® administered three-times-daily in patients with open-angle glaucoma or ocular hypertension. Those results indicated that ALPHAGAN® P (brimonidine tartrate ophthalmic solution) 0.15% is comparable in IOP lowering effect to ALPHAGAN® (brimonidine tartrate ophthalmic solution) 0.2%, and effectively lowers IOP in patients with open-angle glaucoma or ocular hypertension by approximately 2-6 mmHg.

A clinical study was conducted to evaluate the safety, efficacy, and acceptability of ALPHAGAN® P (brimonidine tartrate ophthalmic solution) 0.1% compared with ALPHAGAN® administered three-times-daily in patients with open-angle glaucoma or ocular hypertension. Those results indicated that ALPHAGAN® P (brimonidine tartrate ophthalmic solution) 0.1% is equivalent in IOP lowering effect to ALPHAGAN® (brimonidine tartrate ophthalmic solution) 0.2%, and effectively lowers IOP in patients with open-angle glaucoma or ocular hypertension by approximately 2-6 mmHg.

INDICATIONS AND USAGE

ALPHAGAN® P is indicated for the lowering of intraocular pressure in patients with open-angle glaucoma or ocular hypertension.

CONTRAINDICATIONS

ALPHAGAN® P is contraindicated in patients with hypersensitivity to brimonidine tartrate or any component of this medication. It is also contraindicated in patients receiving monoamine oxidase (MAO) inhibitor therapy.

PRECAUTIONS

General

Although brimonidine tartrate ophthalmic solution had minimal effect on the blood pressure of patients in clinical studies, caution should be exercised in treating patients with severe cardiovascular disease.

ALPHAGAN® P has not been studied in patients with hepatic or renal impairment; caution should be used in treating such patients.

ALPHAGAN® P should be used with caution in patients with depression, cerebral or coronary insufficiency, Raynaud's phenomenon, orthostatic hypotension, or thromboangiitis obliterans. Patients prescribed IOP-lowering medication should be routinely monitored for IOP.

Information for Patients

As with other drugs in this class, ALPHAGAN® P may cause fatigue and/or drowsiness in some patients. Patients who engage in hazardous activities should be cautioned of the potential for a decrease in mental alertness.

Drug Interactions

Although specific drug interaction studies have not been conducted with ALPHAGAN® P, the possibility of an additive or potentiating effect with CNS depressants (alcohol, barbiturates, opiates, sedatives, or anesthetics) should be considered. Alpha-agonists, as a class, may reduce pulse

---

and blood pressure. Caution in using concomitant drugs such as anti-hypertensives and/or cardiac glycosides is advised.

Tricyclic antidepressants have been reported to blunt the hypotensive effect of systemic clonidine. It is not known whether the concurrent use of these agents with ALPHAGAN® P in humans can lead to resulting interference with the IOP lowering effect. No data on the level of circulating catecholamines after ALPHAGAN® P administration are available. Caution, however, is advised in patients taking tricyclic antidepressants which can affect the metabolism and uptake of circulating amines.

Carcinogenesis, Mutagenesis, and Impairment of Fertility

No compound-related carcinogenic effects were observed in either mice or rats following a 21-month and 24-month study, respectively. In these studies, dietary administration of brimonidine tartrate at doses up to 2.5 mg/kg/day in mice and 1.0 mg/kg/day in rats achieved 150 and 120 times or 90 and 80 times, respectively, the plasma drug concentration (C_{max}) estimated in humans treated with one drop of ALPHAGAN® P 0.1% or 0.15% into both eyes 3 times per day.

Brimonidine tartrate was not mutagenic or cytogenic in a series of *in vitro* and *in vivo* studies including the Ames test, chromosomal aberration assay in Chinese Hamster Ovary (CHO) cells, a host-mediated assay and cytogenic studies in mice, and dominant lethal assay.

Pregnancy: Teratogenic effects: Pregnancy Category B. Reproductive studies performed in rats and rabbits with oral doses of 0.66 mg base/kg revealed no evidence of impaired fertility or harm to the fetus due to ALPHAGAN® P. Dosing at this level produced an exposure in rats and rabbits that is 190 and 100 times or 120 and 60 times higher, respectively, than the exposure seen in humans following multiple ophthalmic doses of ALPHAGAN® P 0.1% or 0.15%. There are no adequate and well-controlled studies in pregnant women. In animal studies, brimonidine crossed the placenta and entered the fetal circulation to a limited extent. ALPHAGAN® P should be used during pregnancy only if the potential benefit to the mother justifies the potential risk to the fetus.

Nursing Mothers

It is not known whether this drug is excreted in human milk; although in animal studies brimonidine tartrate was excreted in breast milk. A decision should be made whether to discontinue nursing or to discontinue the drug, taking into account the importance of the drug to the mother.

Pediatric Use

In a well-controlled clinical study conducted in pediatric glaucoma patients (ages 2 to 7 years) the most commonly observed adverse events with brimonidine tartrate ophthalmic solution 0.2% dosed three times daily were somnolence (50%-83% in patients ages 2 to 6 years) and decreased alertness. In pediatric patients 7 years of age or older (>20kg), somnolence appears to occur less frequently (25%). Approximately 16% of patients on brimonidine tartrate ophthalmic solution discontinued from the study due to somnolence.

The safety and effectiveness of brimonidine tartrate ophthalmic solution have not been studied in pediatric patients below the age of 2 years. Brimonidine tartrate ophthalmic solution is not recommended for use in pediatric patients under the age of 2 years. (Also refer to Adverse Reactions section.)

Geriatric Use

No overall differences in safety or effectiveness have been observed between elderly and other adult patients.

ADVERSE REACTIONS

Adverse events occurring in approximately 10-20% of the subjects receiving brimonidine ophthalmic solution (0.1-0.2%) included: allergic conjunctivitis, conjunctival hyperemia, and eye pruritus. Adverse events occurring in approximately 5-9% included: burning sensation, conjunctival folliculosis, hypertension, ocular allergic reaction, oral dryness, and visual disturbance.

Adverse events occurring in approximately 1-4% of the subjects receiving brimonidine ophthalmic solution (0.1-0.2%) included: allergic reaction, asthenia, blepharitis, blepharoconjunctivitis, blurred vision, bronchitis, cataract, conjunctival edema, conjunctival hemorrhage, conjunctivitis, cough, dizziness, dyspepsia, dyspnea, epiphora, eye discharge, eye dryness, eye irritation, eye pain, eyelid edema, eyelid erythema, fatigue, flu syndrome, follicular conjunctivitis, foreign body sensation, gastrointestinal disorder, headache, hypercholesterolemia, hypotension, infection (primarily colds and respiratory infections), insomnia, keratitis, lid disorder, pharyngitis, photophobia, rash, rhinitis, sinus infection, sinusitis, somnolence, stinging, superficial punctate keratopathy, tearing, visual field defect, vitreous detachment, vitreous disorder, vitreous floaters, and worsened visual acuity.

The following events were reported in less than 1% of subjects: corneal erosion, hordeolum, nasal dryness, and taste perversion.

The following events have been identified during postmarketing use of brimonidine tartrate ophthalmic solutions in clinical practice. Because they are reported voluntarily from a population of unknown size, estimates of frequency

---

cannot be made. The events, which have been chosen for inclusion due to either their seriousness, frequency of reporting, possible causal connection to brimonidine tartrate ophthalmic solutions, or a combination of these factors, include: bradycardia; depression; iritis; keratoconjunctivitis sicca; miosis; nausea; skin reactions (including erythema, eyelid pruritus, rash, and vasodilation) and tachycardia. Apnea; bradycardia; hypotension; hypothermia; hypotonia; and somnolence have been reported in infants receiving brimonidine tartrate ophthalmic solutions.

OVERDOSAGE

No information is available on overdosage in humans. Treatment of an oral overdose includes supportive and symptomatic therapy; a patent airway should be maintained.

DOSAGE AND ADMINISTRATION

The recommended dose is one drop of ALPHAGAN® P in the affected eye(s) three times daily, approximately 8 hours apart.

ALPHAGAN® P ophthalmic solution may be used concomitantly with other topical ophthalmic drug products to lower intraocular pressure. If more than one topical ophthalmic product is being used, the products should be administered at least 5 minutes apart.

HOW SUPPLIED

ALPHAGAN® P is supplied sterile in opaque teal LDPE plastic bottles and droppers with purple high impact polystyrene (HIPS) caps as follows:

0.1%

5 mL in 10 mL bottle	NDC 0023-9321-05
10 mL in 10 mL bottle	NDC 0023-9321-10
15 mL in 15 mL bottle	NDC 0023-9321-15

0.15%

5 mL in 10 mL bottle	NDC 0023-9177-05
10 mL in 10 mL bottle	NDC 0023-9177-10
15 mL in 15 mL bottle	NDC 0023-9177-15

NOTE: Store at 15°-25° C (59°-77° F).
Rx Only
Revised: 05/2010
© 2010 Allergan, Inc.
Irvine, CA 92612, U.S.A.
® marks owned by Allergan, Inc.
U.S. Patents 5,424,078; 6,562,873; 6,627,210; 6,641,834; and 6,673,337

71816US12B

Shown in Product Identification Guide, page 304

BOTOX®
[Boe-tox]
(onabotulinumtoxinA)   ℞

HIGHLIGHTS OF PRESCRIBING INFORMATION
These highlights do not include all the information needed to use BOTOX® safely and effectively. See full prescribing information for BOTOX.
BOTOX (onabotulinumtoxinA)
Initial U.S. Approval: 1989

WARNING: Distant Spread of Toxin Effect
See full prescribing information for complete boxed warning.
The effects of **BOTOX** and all botulinum toxin products may spread from the area of injection to produce symptoms consistent with botulinum toxin effects. These symptoms have been reported hours to weeks after injection. Swallowing and breathing difficulties can be life threatening and there have been reports of death. The risk of symptoms is probably greatest in children treated for spasticity but symptoms can also occur in adults, particularly in those patients who have underlying conditions that would predispose them to these symptoms.

———RECENT MAJOR CHANGES———
- Indications and Usage, Upper Limb Spasticity (1.1) 3/2010
- Dosage and Administration, Upper Limb Spasticity (2.2) 3/2010
- Warnings and Precautions (5.3, 5.6, 5.9) 3/2010

———INDICATIONS AND USAGE———
BOTOX is an acetylcholine release inhibitor and a neuromuscular blocking agent indicated for the treatment of:
- Upper limb spasticity in adult patients (1.1)
- Cervical dystonia in adult patients, to reduce the severity of abnormal head position and neck pain (1.2)
- Severe axillary hyperhidrosis that is inadequately managed by topical agents in adult patients (1.3)
- Blepharospasm associated with dystonia in patients ≥12 years of age (1.4)
- Strabismus in patients ≥12 years of age (1.4)

Important limitations:
- Safety and effectiveness of **BOTOX** have not been established for the treatment of upper limb spasticity in pediatric patients, and for the treatment of lower limb spasticity in adult and pediatric patients.
- Safety and effectiveness of **BOTOX** for hyperhidrosis in body areas other than axillary have not been established.

———DOSAGE AND ADMINISTRATION———
- Indication specific dosage and administration recommendations should be followed; Do not exceed a total dose of 360 Units administered every 12 to 16 weeks or at longer intervals (2)
- See Preparation and Dilution Technique for instructions on **BOTOX** reconstitution, storage, and preparation before injection (2.1)
- Upper Limb Spasticity: Select dose based on muscles affected, severity of muscle activity, prior response to treatment, and adverse event history; Electromyographic guidance recommended (2.2)
- Cervical Dystonia: Base dosing on the patient's head and neck position, localization of pain, muscle hypertrophy, patient response, and adverse event history; use lower initial dose in botulinum toxin naïve patients (2.3)
- Axillary Hyperhidrosis: 50 Units per axilla (2.4)
- Blepharospasm: 1.25 Units-2.5 Units into each of 3 sites per affected eye (2.5)
- Strabismus: 1.25 Units-2.5 Units initially in any one muscle (2.6)

———DOSAGE FORMS AND STRENGTHS———
Single-use, sterile 100 Units or 200 Units vacuum-dried powder for reconstitution only with sterile, non-preserved 0.9% Sodium Chloride Injection USP prior to injection (3)

———CONTRAINDICATIONS———
- Hypersensitivity to any botulinum toxin preparation or to any of the components in the formulation (4.1, 5.3, 6.2)
- Infection at the proposed injection site (4.2)

———WARNINGS AND PRECAUTIONS———
- Potency Units of **BOTOX** not interchangeable with other preparations of botulinum toxin products (5.1, 11)
- Spread of toxin effects; swallowing and breathing difficulties can lead to death (5.2)
- Immediate medical attention may be required in cases of respiratory, speech or swallowing difficulties (5.2, 5.4)
- Concomitant neuromuscular disorder may exacerbate clinical effects of treatment (5.5)
- Use with caution in patients with compromised respiratory function (5.4, 5.6)
- Corneal exposure and ulceration (5.7)
- Retrobulbar hemorrhages and compromised retinal circulation (5.8)
- Bronchitis and upper respiratory tract infections in patients treated for upper limb spasticity (5.9)

———ADVERSE REACTIONS———
In controlled studies, the most commonly observed adverse reactions (≥ 5% and > placebo) were:
- Spasticity: pain in extremity (6.1)
- Cervical Dystonia: dysphagia, upper respiratory infection, neck pain, headache, increased cough, flu syndrome, back pain, rhinitis (6.1)
- Axillary Hyperhidrosis: injection site pain and hemorrhage, non-axillary sweating, pharyngitis, flu syndrome (6.1)

To report SUSPECTED ADVERSE REACTIONS, contact Allergan at 1-800-433-8871 or FDA at 1-800-FDA-1088 or www.fda.gov/medwatch.

———DRUG INTERACTIONS———
- Patients receiving concomitant treatment of **BOTOX** and aminoglycosides or other agents interfering with neuromuscular transmission (e.g., curare-like agents), or muscle relaxants, should be observed closely because the effect of **BOTOX** may be potentiated (7)

———USE IN SPECIFIC POPULATIONS———
- Pregnancy: Based on animal data, may cause fetal harm (8.1)
- Pediatric Use: Safety and efficacy are not established in patients under 18 years of age for the treatment of upper limb spasticity and axillary hyperhidrosis, in patients under 16 years of age for the treatment of cervical dystonia, and in patients under 12 years of age for the treatment of blepharospasm and strabismus (8.4)

See 17 for PATIENT COUNSELING INFORMATION and Medication Guide

Revised: 08/2010

FULL PRESCRIBING INFORMATION

Distant Spread of Toxin Effect
Postmarketing reports indicate that the effects of BOTOX and all botulinum toxin products may spread from the area of injection to produce symptoms consistent with botulinum toxin effects. These may include asthenia, generalized muscle weakness, diplopia, ptosis, dysphagia, dysphonia, dysarthria, urinary incontinence and breathing difficulties. These symptoms have been reported hours to weeks after injection. Swallowing and breathing difficulties can be life threatening and there have been reports of death. The risk of symptoms is probably greatest in children treated for spasticity but symptoms can also occur in adults treated for spasticity and other conditions, particularly in those patients who have underlying conditions that would predispose them to these symptoms. In unapproved uses, including spasticity in children, and in approved indications, cases of spread of effect have been reported at doses comparable to those used to treat cervical dystonia and at lower doses.

1   INDICATIONS AND USAGE

1.1   Upper Limb Spasticity
BOTOX (onabotulinumtoxinA) for injection is indicated for the treatment of upper limb spasticity in adult patients, to decrease the severity of increased muscle tone in elbow flexors (biceps), wrist flexors (flexor carpi radialis and flexor carpi ulnaris) and finger flexors (flexor digitorum profundus and flexor digitorum sublimis).

Important limitations
Safety and effectiveness of **BOTOX** have not been established for the treatment of other upper limb muscle groups, or for the treatment of lower limb spasticity. Safety and effectiveness of **BOTOX** have not been established for the treatment of spasticity in pediatric patients under age 18 years. **BOTOX** has not been shown to improve upper extremity functional abilities, or range of motion at a joint affected by a fixed contracture. Treatment with **BOTOX** is not intended to substitute for usual standard of care rehabilitation regimens.

1.2 Cervical Dystonia
BOTOX is indicated for the treatment of adults with cervical dystonia, to reduce the severity of abnormal head position and neck pain associated with cervical dystonia.

1.3 Primary Axillary Hyperhidrosis
BOTOX is indicated for the treatment of severe primary axillary hyperhidrosis that is inadequately managed with topical agents.
Important limitations
The safety and effectiveness of **BOTOX** for hyperhidrosis in other body areas have not been established. Weakness of hand muscles and blepharoptosis may occur in patients who receive **BOTOX** for palmar hyperhidrosis and facial hyperhidrosis, respectively. Patients should be evaluated for potential causes of secondary hyperhidrosis (e.g., hyperthyroidism) to avoid symptomatic treatment of hyperhidrosis without the diagnosis and/or treatment of the underlying disease.
Safety and effectiveness of **BOTOX** have not been established for the treatment of axillary hyperhidrosis in pediatric patients under age 18.

1.4 Blepharospasm and Strabismus
BOTOX is indicated for the treatment of strabismus and blepharospasm associated with dystonia, including benign essential blepharospasm or VII nerve disorders in patients 12 years of age and above.

2 DOSAGE AND ADMINISTRATION
The potency Units of **BOTOX** (onabotulinumtoxinA) for injection are specific to the preparation and assay method utilized. They are not interchangeable with other preparations of botulinum toxin products and, therefore, units of biological activity of **BOTOX** cannot be compared to nor converted into units of any other botulinum toxin products assessed with any other specific assay method *[see Warnings and Precautions (5.1) and Description (11)]*.
Injection specific dosage and administration recommendations should be followed. In treating adult patients for one or more indications, the maximum cumulative dose should generally not exceed 360 Units, in a 3 month interval.
The safe and effective use of **BOTOX** depends upon proper storage of the product, selection of the correct dose, and proper reconstitution and administration techniques. Physicians administering **BOTOX** must understand the relevant neuromuscular and/or orbital anatomy of the area involved and any alterations to the anatomy due to prior surgical procedures. An understanding of standard electromyographic techniques is also required for treatment of strabismus and of upper limb spasticity, and may be useful for the treatment of cervical dystonia.
Use caution when **BOTOX** treatment is used in the presence of inflammation at the proposed injection site(s) or when excessive weakness or atrophy is present in the target muscle(s).

2.1 Preparation and Dilution Technique
BOTOX is supplied in single-use 100 Units and 200 Units per vial. Prior to injection, reconstitute each vacuum-dried vial of **BOTOX** with sterile, non-preserved 0.9% Sodium Chloride Injection USP. Draw up the proper amount of diluent in the appropriate size syringe (Dilution Table), and slowly inject the diluent into the vial. Discard the vial if a vacuum does not pull the diluent into the vial. Gently mix **BOTOX** with the saline by rotating the vial. Record the date and time of reconstitution on the space on the label. **BOTOX** should be administered within 24 hours after reconstitution. During this time period, reconstituted **BOTOX** should be stored in a refrigerator (2° to 8°C).
[See table below]

Dilution Table: 0.9% Sodium Chloride Injection Dilution Instructions for 100 Unit and 200 Unit BOTOX Vials

Diluent* Added to **100 Unit** Vial	Resulting Dose Units per 0.1 mL	Diluent* Added to **200 Unit** Vial	Resulting Dose Units per 0.1 mL
1 mL	10 Units	1 mL	20 Units
2 mL	5 Units	2 mL	10 Units
4 mL	2.5 Units	4 mL	5 Units
8 mL	1.25 Units	8 mL	2.5 Units
		10 mL	2 Units

*0.9% Sodium Chloride Injection Only

Note: These dilutions are calculated for an injection volume of 0.1 mL. A decrease or increase in the **BOTOX** dose is also possible by administering a smaller or larger injection volume - from 0.05 mL (50% decrease in dose) to 0.15 mL (50% increase in dose).
An injection of **BOTOX** is prepared by drawing into an appropriately sized sterile syringe an amount of the properly reconstituted toxin slightly greater than the intended dose. Air bubbles in the syringe barrel are expelled and the syringe is attached to an appropriate injection needle. Patency of the needle should be confirmed. A new, sterile, needle and syringe should be used to enter the vial on each occasion for removal of **BOTOX**.
Reconstituted **BOTOX** should be clear, colorless, and free of particulate matter. Parenteral drug products should be inspected visually for particulate matter and discoloration prior to administration and whenever the solution and the container permit.

2.2 Upper Limb Spasticity
Dosing in initial and sequential treatment sessions should be tailored to the individual based on the size, number and location of muscles involved, severity of spasticity, the presence of local muscle weakness, the patient's response to previous treatment, or adverse event history with **BOTOX**. In clinical trials, doses ranging from 75 Units to 360 Units were divided among selected muscles at a given treatment session.
Following are recommended dose ranges per muscle:

	Total Dosage (Number of Sites)
Biceps Brachii	100 Units-200 Units divided in 4 sites
Flexor Carpi Radialis	12.5 Units-50 Units in 1 site
Flexor Carpi Ulnaris	12.5 Units-50 Units in 1 site
Flexor Digitorum Profundus	30 Units-50 Units in 1 site
Flexor Digitorum Sublimis	30 Units-50 Units in 1 site

The recommended dilution is 200 Units/4 mL or 100 Units/2 mL with 0.9% non-preserved sterile saline (see Dilution Table). The lowest recommended starting dose should be used, and no more than 50 Units per site should generally be administered. An appropriately sized needle (e.g., 25-30 gauge) may be used for superficial muscles, and a longer 22 gauge needle may be used for deeper musculature. Localization of the involved muscles with electromyographic guidance or nerve stimulation techniques is recommended.
Repeat **BOTOX** treatment may be administered when the effect of a previous injection has diminished, but generally no sooner than 12 weeks after the previous injection. The degree and pattern of muscle spasticity at the time of re-injection may necessitate alterations in the dose of **BOTOX** and muscles to be injected.

2.3 Cervical Dystonia
The phase 3 study enrolled patients who had extended histories of receiving and tolerating **BOTOX** injections, with prior individualized adjustment of dose. The mean **BOTOX** dose administered to patients in the phase 3 study was 236 Units (25th to 75th percentile range of 198 Units to 300 Units). The **BOTOX** dose was divided among the affected muscles *[see Clinical Studies (14.2)]*. Dosing in initial and sequential treatment sessions should be tailored to the individual patient based on the patient's head and neck position, localization of pain, muscle hypertrophy, patient response, and adverse event history. The initial dose for a patient without prior use of **BOTOX** should be at a lower dose, with subsequent dosing adjusted based on individual response. Limiting the total dose injected into the sternocleidomastoid muscle to 100 Units or less may decrease the occurrence of dysphagia *[see Warnings and Precautions (5.2, 5.4, 5.5)]*.
The recommended dilution is 200 Units/2 mL, 200 Units/4 mL, 100 Units/1 mL, or 100 Units/2 mL with 0.9% non-preserved sterile saline, depending on volume and number of injection sites desired to achieve treatment objectives (see Dilution Table). In general, no more than 50 Units per site should be administered. An appropriately sized needle (e.g., 25-30 gauge) may be used for superficial muscles, and a longer 22 gauge needle may be used for deeper musculature. Localization of the involved muscles with electromyographic guidance may be useful.
Clinical improvement generally begins within the first two weeks after injection with maximum clinical benefit at approximately six weeks post-injection. In the phase 3 study most subjects were observed to have returned to pre-treatment status by 3 months post-treatment.

2.4 Primary Axillary Hyperhidrosis
The recommended dose is 50 Units per axilla. The hyperhidrotic area to be injected should be defined using standard staining techniques, e.g., Minor's Iodine-Starch Test. The recommended dilution is 100 Units/4 mL with 0.9% preservative-free sterile saline (see Dilution Table). Using a 30 gauge needle, 50 Units of **BOTOX** (2 mL) is injected intradermally in 0.1 to 0.2 mL aliquots to each axilla evenly distributed in multiple sites (10-15) approximately 1-2 cm apart.
Repeat injections for hyperhidrosis should be administered when the clinical effect of a previous injection diminishes.
Instructions for the Minor's Iodine-Starch Test Procedure:
Patients should shave underarms and abstain from use of over-the-counter deodorants or antiperspirants for 24 hours prior to the test. Patient should be resting comfortably without exercise, hot drinks, etc. for approximately 30 minutes prior to the test. Dry the underarm area and then immediately paint it with iodine solution. Allow the area to dry, then lightly sprinkle the area with starch powder. Gently blow off any excess starch powder. The hyperhidrotic area will develop a deep blue-black color over approximately 10 minutes.
Each injection site has a ring of effect of up to approximately 2 cm in diameter. To minimize the area of no effect, the injection sites should be evenly spaced as shown in Figure 1:

Figure 1:

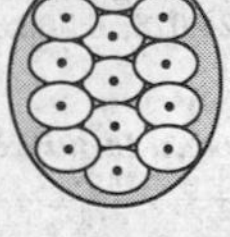

Each dose is injected to a depth of approximately 2 mm and at a 45° angle to the skin surface, with the bevel side up to minimize leakage and to ensure the injections remain intradermal. If injection sites are marked in ink, do not inject **BOTOX** directly through the ink mark to avoid a permanent tattoo effect.

2.5 Blepharospasm
For blepharospasm, reconstituted **BOTOX** is injected using a sterile, 27-30 gauge needle without electromyographic guidance. The initial recommended dose is 1.25 Units -2.5 Units (0.05 mL to 0.1 mL volume at each site) injected into the medial and lateral pre-tarsal orbicularis oculi of the upper lid and into the lateral pre-tarsal orbicularis oculi of the lower lid. Avoiding injection near the levator palpebrae superioris may reduce the complication of ptosis. Avoiding medial lower lid injections, and thereby reducing diffusion into the inferior oblique, may reduce the complication of diplopia. Ecchymosis occurs easily in the soft eyelid tissues. This can be prevented by applying pressure at the injection site immediately after the injection.
The recommended dilution to achieve 1.25 Units is 100 Units/8 mL; for 2.5 Units it is 100 Units/4 mL (see Dilution Table).
In general, the initial effect of the injections is seen within three days and reaches a peak at one to two weeks post-treatment. Each treatment lasts approximately three months, following which the procedure can be repeated. At repeat treatment sessions, the dose may be increased up to two-fold if the response from the initial treatment is considered insufficient- usually defined as an effect that does not last longer than two months. However, there appears to be little benefit obtainable from injecting more than 5 Units per site. Some tolerance may be found when **BOTOX** is used in treating blepharospasm if treatments are given any more frequently than every three months, and is rare to have the effect be permanent.
The cumulative dose of **BOTOX** treatment for blepharospasm in a 30-day period should not exceed 200 Units.

2.6 Strabismus
BOTOX is intended for injection into extraocular muscles utilizing the electrical activity recorded from the tip of the injection needle as a guide to placement within the target muscle. Injection without surgical exposure or

electromyographic guidance should not be attempted. Physicians should be familiar with electromyographic technique.

To prepare the eye for **BOTOX** injection, it is recommended that several drops of a local anesthetic and an ocular decongestant be given several minutes prior to injection.

Note: The volume of **BOTOX** injected for treatment of strabismus should be between 0.05-0.15 mL per muscle.

The initial listed doses of the reconstituted **BOTOX** *[see Dosage and Administration (2.1)]* typically create paralysis of the injected muscles beginning one to two days after injection and increasing in intensity during the first week. The paralysis lasts for 2-6 weeks and gradually resolves over a similar time period. Overcorrections lasting over six months have been rare. About one half of patients will require subsequent doses because of inadequate paralytic response of the muscle to the initial dose, or because of mechanical factors such as large deviations or restrictions, or because of the lack of binocular motor fusion to stabilize the alignment.

I. Initial doses in Units. Use the lower listed doses for treatment of small deviations. Use the larger doses only for large deviations.
   A. For vertical muscles, and for horizontal strabismus of less than 20 prism diopters: 1.25 Units-2.5 Units in any one muscle.
   B. For horizontal strabismus of 20 prism diopters to 50 prism diopters: 2.5 Units-5 Units in any one muscle.
   C. For persistent VI nerve palsy of one month or longer duration: 1.25 Units-2.5 Units in the medial rectus muscle.

II. Subsequent doses for residual or recurrent strabismus.
   A. It is recommended that patients be re-examined 7-14 days after each injection to assess the effect of that dose.
   B. Patients experiencing adequate paralysis of the target muscle that require subsequent injections should receive a dose comparable to the initial dose.
   C. Subsequent doses for patients experiencing incomplete paralysis of the target muscle may be increased up to two-fold compared to the previously administered dose.
   D. Subsequent injections should not be administered until the effects of the previous dose have dissipated as evidenced by substantial function in the injected and adjacent muscles.
   E. The maximum recommended dose as a single injection for any one muscle is 25 Units.

The recommended dilution to achieve 1.25 Units is 100 Units/8 mL; for 2.5 Units it is 100 Units/4 mL (see Dilution Table).

3 DOSAGE FORMS AND STRENGTHS

Single-use, sterile 100 Units or 200 Units vacuum-dried powder for reconstitution only with sterile, non-preserved 0.9% Sodium Chloride Injection USP prior to injection *[see Dosage and Administration (2.1)]*.

4 CONTRAINDICATIONS

4.1 Known Hypersensitivity to Botulinum Toxin

BOTOX is contraindicated in patients who are hypersensitive to any botulinum toxin preparation or to any of the components in the formulation *[see Warnings and Precautions (5.3)]*.

4.2 Infection at the Injection Site(s)

BOTOX is contraindicated in the presence of infection at the proposed injection site(s).

5 WARNINGS AND PRECAUTIONS

5.1 Lack of Interchangeability between Botulinum Toxin Products

The potency Units of BOTOX are specific to the preparation and assay method utilized. They are not interchangeable with other preparations of botulinum toxin products and, therefore, units of biological activity of BOTOX cannot be compared to nor converted into units of any other botulinum toxin products assessed with any other specific assay method *[see Description (11)]*.

5.2 Spread of Toxin Effect

Postmarketing safety data from **BOTOX** and other approved botulinum toxins suggest that botulinum toxin effects may, in some cases, be observed beyond the site of local injection. The symptoms are consistent with the mechanism of action of botulinum toxin and may include asthenia, generalized muscle weakness, diplopia, ptosis, dysphagia, dysphonia, dysarthria, urinary incontinence, and breathing difficulties. These symptoms have been reported hours to weeks after injection. Swallowing and breathing difficulties can be life threatening and there have been reports of death related to spread of toxin effects. The risk of the symptoms is probably greatest in children treated for spasticity but symptoms can also occur in adults treated for spasticity and other conditions, and particularly in those patients who have underlying conditions that would predispose them to these symptoms. In unapproved uses, including spasticity in children, and in approved indications, symptoms consistent with spread of toxin effect have been reported at doses comparable to or lower than doses used to treat cervical dystonia.

No definitive serious adverse event reports of distant spread of toxin effect associated with dermatologic use of **BOTOX/BOTOX Cosmetic** at the labeled dose of 20 Units (for glabellar lines) or 100 Units (for severe primary axillary hyperhidrosis) have been reported.

No definitive serious adverse event reports of distant spread of toxin effect associated with **BOTOX** for blepharospasm at the recommended dose (30 Units and below) or for strabismus at the labeled doses have been reported.

5.3 Hypersensitivity Reactions

Serious and/or immediate hypersensitivity reactions have been reported. These reactions include anaphylaxis, serum sickness, urticaria, soft tissue edema, and dyspnea. If such a reaction occurs, further injection of **BOTOX** should be discontinued and appropriate medical therapy immediately instituted. One fatal case of anaphylaxis has been reported in which lidocaine was used as the diluent, and consequently the causal agent cannot be reliably determined.

5.4 Dysphagia and Breathing Difficulties in Treatment of Cervical Dystonia>

Treatment with **BOTOX** and other botulinum toxin products can result in swallowing or breathing difficulties. Patients with pre-existing swallowing or breathing difficulties may be more susceptible to these complications. In most cases, this is a consequence of weakening of muscles in the area of injection that are involved in breathing or swallowing. When distant effects occur, additional respiratory muscles may be involved *[see Warnings and Precautions (5.2)]*.

Deaths as a complication of severe dysphagia have been reported after treatment with botulinum toxin. Dysphagia may persist for several months, and require use of a feeding tube to maintain adequate nutrition and hydration. Aspiration may result from severe dysphagia and is a particular risk when treating patients in whom swallowing or respiratory function is already compromised.

Treatment of cervical dystonia with botulinum toxins may weaken neck muscles that serve as accessory muscles of ventilation. This may result in a critical loss of breathing capacity in patients with respiratory disorders who may have become dependent upon these accessory muscles. There have been postmarketing reports of serious breathing difficulties, including respiratory failure, in cervical dystonia patients.

Patients with smaller neck muscle mass and patients who require bilateral injections into the sternocleidomastoid muscle have been reported to be at greater risk for dysphagia. Limiting the dose injected into the sternocleidomastoid muscle may reduce the occurrence of dysphagia. Injections into the levator scapulae may be associated with an increased risk of upper respiratory infection and dysphagia.

Patients treated with botulinum toxin may require immediate medical attention should they develop problems with swallowing, speech or respiratory disorders. These reactions can occur within hours to weeks after injection with botulinum toxin *[see Warnings and Precautions (5.2) and Adverse Reactions (6.1)]*.

5.5 Pre-Existing Neuromuscular Disorders

Individuals with peripheral motor neuropathic diseases, amyotrophic lateral sclerosis or neuromuscular junction disorders (e.g., myasthenia gravis or Lambert-Eaton syndrome) should be monitored particularly closely when given botulinum toxin. Patients with neuromuscular disorders may be at increased risk of clinically significant effects including severe dysphagia and respiratory compromise from typical doses of **BOTOX** *[see Adverse Reactions (6.1)]*.

5.6 Pulmonary Effects of BOTOX in Patients with Compromised Respiratory Status Treated for Spasticity

Patients with compromised respiratory status treated with **BOTOX** for upper limb spasticity should be monitored closely. In a double-blind, placebo-controlled, parallel group study in patients with stable reduced pulmonary function (defined as FEV1 40-80% of predicted value and FEV1/FVC ≤ 0.75), the event rate in change of Forced Vital Capacity ≥15% or ≥20% was generally greater in patients treated with **BOTOX** than in patients treated with placebo (see Table 1).

[See table 1 above]

Table 1: Event rate per patient treatment cycle among patients with reduced lung function who experienced at least a 15% or 20% decrease in forced vital capacity from baseline at Week 1, 6, 12 post-injection with up to two treatment cycles with BOTOX or placebo

	BOTOX 360 Units		BOTOX 240 Units		Placebo	
	≥15%	≥20%	≥15%	≥20%	≥15%	≥20%
Week 1	4%	0%	3%	0%	7%	3%
Week 6	7%	4%	4%	2%	2%	2%
Week 12	10%	5%	2%	1%	4%	1%

Differences from placebo were not statistically significant

In patients with reduced lung function, upper respiratory tract infections were also reported more frequently as adverse reactions in patients treated with **BOTOX** *[see Warnings and Precautions (5.9)]*.

5.7 Corneal Exposure and Ulceration in Patients Treated with BOTOX for Blepharospasm

Reduced blinking from **BOTOX** injection of the orbicularis muscle can lead to corneal exposure, persistent epithelial defect, and corneal ulceration, especially in patients with VII nerve disorders. Vigorous treatment of any epithelial defect should be employed. This may require protective drops, ointment, therapeutic soft contact lenses, or closure of the eye by patching or other means.

5.8 Retrobulbar Hemorrhages in Patients Treated with BOTOX for Strabismus

During the administration of **BOTOX** for the treatment of strabismus, retrobulbar hemorrhages sufficient to compromise retinal circulation have occurred. It is recommended that appropriate instruments to decompress the orbit be accessible.

5.9 Bronchitis and Upper Respiratory Tract Infections in Patients Treated for Spasticity

Bronchitis was reported more frequently as an adverse reaction in patients treated for upper limb spasticity with **BOTOX** (3% at 251 Units-360 Units total dose), compared to placebo (1%). In patients with reduced lung function treated for upper limb spasticity, upper respiratory tract infections were also reported more frequently as adverse reactions in patients treated with **BOTOX** (11% at 360 Units total dose; 8% at 240 Units total dose) compared to placebo (6%).

5.10 Human Albumin and Transmission of Viral Diseases

This product contains albumin, a derivative of human blood. Based on effective donor screening and product manufacturing processes, it carries an extremely remote risk for transmission of viral diseases. A theoretical risk for transmission of Creutzfeldt-Jakob disease (CJD) is also considered extremely remote. No cases of transmission of viral diseases or CJD have ever been reported for albumin.

6 ADVERSE REACTIONS

The following adverse reactions to **BOTOX** (onabotulinumtoxinA) for injection are discussed in greater detail in other sections of the labeling:

- Spread of Toxin Effects *[see Warnings and Precautions (5.2)]*
- Hypersensitivity *[see Contraindications (4.1) and Warnings and Precautions (5.3)]*
- Dysphagia and Breathing Difficulties in Treatment of Cervical Dystonia *[see Warnings and Precautions (5.4)]*
- Bronchitis and Upper Respiratory Tract Infections in Patients Treated for Spasticity *[see Warnings and Precautions (5.9)]*

6.1 Clinical Studies Experience

Because clinical trials are conducted under widely varying conditions, the adverse reaction rates observed cannot be directly compared to rates in other trials and may not reflect the rates observed in clinical practice.

BOTOX and **BOTOX Cosmetic** contain the same active ingredient in the same formulation, but with different labeled Indications and Usage. Therefore, adverse events observed with the use of **BOTOX Cosmetic** also have the potential to be observed with the use of **BOTOX** and vice-versa.

In general, adverse events occur within the first week following injection of **BOTOX** and while generally transient, may have a duration of several months or longer. Localized pain, infection, inflammation, tenderness, swelling, erythema, and/or bleeding/bruising may be associated with the injection. Needle-related pain and/or anxiety may result in vasovagal responses (including e.g., syncope, hypotension), which may require appropriate medical therapy.

Local weakness of the injected muscle(s) represents the expected pharmacological action of botulinum toxin. However, weakness of nearby muscles may also occur due to spread of toxin *[see Warnings and Precautions (5.2)]*.

Upper Limb Spasticity

Table 2 below lists the adverse reactions reported by ≥ 2% of **BOTOX**-treated patients and more frequent than in placebo-treated patients in double-blind, placebo-controlled clinical trials.

[See table 2 below]

Cervical Dystonia

In cervical dystonia patients evaluated for safety in double-blind and open-label studies following injection of **BOTOX**, the most frequently reported adverse reactions were dysphagia (19%), upper respiratory infection (12%), neck pain (11%), and headache (11%).

Other events reported in 2-10% of patients in any one study in decreasing order of incidence include: increased cough, flu syndrome, back pain, rhinitis, dizziness, hypertonia, soreness at injection site, asthenia, oral dryness, speech disorder, fever, nausea, and drowsiness. Stiffness, numbness, diplopia, ptosis, and dyspnea have been reported.

Dysphagia and symptomatic general weakness may be attributable to an extension of the pharmacology of **BOTOX** resulting from the spread of the toxin outside the injected muscles *[see Warnings and Precautions (5.2, 5.4)]*.

The most common severe adverse event associated with the use of **BOTOX** injection in patients with cervical dystonia is dysphagia with about 20% of these cases also reporting dyspnea *[see Warnings and Precautions (5.2, 5.4)]*. Most dysphagia is reported as mild or moderate in severity. However, it may be associated with more severe signs and symptoms *[see Warnings and Precautions (5.4)]*.

Additionally, reports in the literature include a case of a female patient who developed brachial plexopathy two days after injection of 120 Units of **BOTOX** for the treatment of cervical dystonia, and reports of dysphonia in patients who have been treated for cervical dystonia.

Primary Axillary Hyperhidrosis

The most frequently reported adverse events (3-10% of adult patients) following injection of **BOTOX** in double-blind studies included injection site pain and hemorrhage, non-axillary sweating, infection, pharyngitis, flu syndrome, headache, fever, neck or back pain, pruritus, and anxiety.

The data reflect 346 patients exposed to **BOTOX** 50 Units and 110 patients exposed to **BOTOX** 75 Units in each axilla.

Blepharospasm

In a study of blepharospasm patients who received an average dose per eye of 33 Units (injected at 3 to 5 sites) of the currently manufactured **BOTOX**, the most frequently reported treatment-related adverse reactions were ptosis (21%), superficial punctate keratitis (6%), and eye dryness (6%).

Other events reported in prior clinical studies in decreasing order of incidence include: irritation, tearing, lagophthalmos, photophobia, ectropion, keratitis, diplopia, entropion, diffuse skin rash, and local swelling of the eyelid skin lasting for several days following eyelid injection.

In two cases of VII nerve disorder, reduced blinking from **BOTOX** injection of the orbicularis muscle led to serious corneal exposure, persistent epithelial defect, corneal ulceration and a case of corneal perforation. Focal facial paralysis, syncope, and exacerbation of myasthenia gravis have also been reported after treatment of blepharospasm.

Strabismus

Extraocular muscles adjacent to the injection site can be affected, causing vertical deviation, especially with higher doses of **BOTOX**. The incidence rates of these adverse effects in 2058 adults who received a total of 3650 injections for horizontal strabismus was 17%.

The incidence of ptosis has been reported to be dependent on the location of the injected muscles, 1% after inferior rectus injections, 16% after horizontal rectus injections and 38% after superior rectus injections.

In a series of 5587 injections, retrobulbar hemorrhage occurred in 0.3% of cases.

6.2 Post-Marketing Experience

There have been spontaneous reports of death, sometimes associated with dysphagia, pneumonia, and/or other significant debility or anaphylaxis, after treatment with botulinum toxin *[see Warnings and Precautions (5.3, 5.4)]*.

There have also been reports of adverse events involving the cardiovascular system, including arrhythmia and myocardial infarction, some with fatal outcomes. Some of these patients had risk factors including cardiovascular disease. The exact relationship of these events to the botulinum toxin injection has not been established.

New onset or recurrent seizures have also been reported, typically in patients who are predisposed to experiencing these events. The exact relationship of these events to the botulinum toxin injection has not been established.

The following events, not already addressed elsewhere in the package insert, have been reported since the drug has been marketed: abdominal pain; anorexia; brachial plexopathy; diarrhea; facial palsy; facial paresis; hyperhidrosis; hypoacusis; hypoaesthesia; localized numbness; malaise; myalgia; paresthesia; pyrexia; radiculopathy; skin rash (including erythema multiforme, and psoriasiform eruption); tinnitus; vertigo; visual disturbances; and vomiting.

Because these events are reported voluntarily from a population of uncertain size, it is not always possible to reliably estimate their frequency or establish a causal relationship to botulinum toxin.

6.3 Immunogenicity

As with all therapeutic proteins, there is a potential for immunogenicity. Formation of neutralizing antibodies to botulinum toxin type A may reduce the effectiveness of **BOTOX** treatment by inactivating the biological activity of the toxin.

In a long term, open-label study evaluating 326 cervical dystonia patients treated for an average of 9 treatment sessions with the current formulation of **BOTOX**, 4 (1.2%) patients had positive antibody tests. All 4 of these patients responded to **BOTOX** therapy at the time of the positive antibody test. However, 3 of these patients developed clinical resistance after subsequent treatment, while the fourth patient continued to respond to **BOTOX** therapy for the remainder of the study.

One patient among the 445 hyperhidrosis patients (0.2%) and two patients among the 380 adult upper limb spasticity patients (0.5%) with analyzed specimens showed the presence of neutralizing antibodies.

The data reflect the patients whose test results were considered positive or negative for neutralizing activity to **BOTOX** in a mouse protection assay. The results of these tests are highly dependent on the sensitivity and specificity of the assay. For these reasons, comparison of the incidence of neutralizing activity to **BOTOX** with the incidence reported to other products may be misleading.

The critical factors for neutralizing antibody formation have not been well characterized. The results from some studies suggest that **BOTOX** injections at more frequent intervals or at higher doses may lead to greater incidence of antibody formation. The potential for antibody formation may be minimized by injecting with the lowest effective dose given at the longest feasible intervals between injections.

Table 2: Adverse Reactions Reported by ≥ 2% of BOTOX-treated Patients and More Frequent than in Placebo-treated Patients in Adult Spasticity Double-blind, Placebo-controlled Clinical Trials

Adverse Reactions by Body System	BOTOX 251 Units-360 Units (N=115)	BOTOX 150 Units-250 Units (N=188)	BOTOX <150 Units (N=54)	Placebo (N=182)
Gastrointestinal disorder				
Nausea	3 (3%)	3 (2%)	1 (2%)	1 (1%)
General disorders and administration site conditions				
Fatigue	4 (3%)	4 (2%)	1 (2%)	0
Infections and infestations				
Bronchitis	4 (3%)	4 (2%)	0	2 (1%)
Musculoskeletal and connective tissue disorders				
Pain in extremity	7 (6%)	10 (5%)	5 (9%)	8 (4%)
Muscular weakness	0	7 (4%)	1 (2%)	2 (1%)

7 DRUG INTERACTIONS

No formal drug interaction studies have been conducted with **BOTOX** (onabotulinumtoxinA) for injection.

Co-administration of **BOTOX** and aminoglycosides or other agents interfering with neuromuscular transmission (e.g., curare-like compounds) should only be performed with caution as the effect of the toxin may be potentiated.

Use of anticholinergic drugs after administration of **BOTOX** may potentiate systemic anticholinergic effects.

The effect of administering different botulinum neurotoxin products at the same time or within several months of each other is unknown. Excessive neuromuscular weakness may be exacerbated by administration of another botulinum toxin prior to the resolution of the effects of a previously administered botulinum toxin.

Excessive weakness may also be exaggerated by administration of a muscle relaxant before or after administration of **BOTOX**.

8 USE IN SPECIFIC POPULATIONS

8.1 Pregnancy

Pregnancy Category C.

There are no adequate and well-controlled studies in pregnant women. **BOTOX** should be used during pregnancy only if the potential benefit justifies the potential risk to the fetus.

When **BOTOX** (4, 8, or 16 Units/kg) was administered intramuscularly to pregnant mice or rats two times during the period of organogenesis (on gestation days 5 and 13), reductions in fetal body weight and decreased fetal skeletal ossification were observed at the two highest doses. The no-effect dose for developmental toxicity in these studies (4 Units/kg) is approximately 1½ times the average high human dose for upper limb spasticity of 360 Units on a body weight basis (Units/kg).

When **BOTOX** was administered intramuscularly to pregnant rats (0.125, 0.25, 0.5, 1, 4, or 8 Units/kg) or rabbits (0.063, 0.125, 0.25, or 0.5 Units/kg) daily during the period of organogenesis (total of 12 doses in rats, 13 doses in rabbits), reduced fetal body weights and decreased fetal skeletal ossification were observed at the two highest doses in rats and at the highest dose in rabbits. These doses were also associated with significant maternal toxicity, including abortions, early deliveries, and maternal death. The developmental no-effect doses in these studies of 1 Unit/kg in rats and 0.25 Units/kg in rabbits are less than the average high human dose based on Units/kg.

When pregnant rats received single intramuscular injections (1, 4, or 16 Units/kg) at three different periods of development (prior to implantation, implantation, or organogenesis), no adverse effects on fetal development were observed. The developmental no-effect level for a single maternal dose in rats (16 Units/kg) is approximately 3 times the average high human dose based on Units/kg.

8.3 Nursing Mothers

It is not known whether **BOTOX** is excreted in human milk. Because many drugs are excreted in human milk, caution should be exercised when **BOTOX** is administered to a nursing woman.

8.4 Pediatric Use

Spasticity

Safety and effectiveness of **BOTOX** for the treatment of spasticity have not been established in patients below the age of 18 years.

Cervical Dystonia

Safety and effectiveness in pediatric patients below the age of 16 years have not been established.

Blepharospasm and Strabismus

Safety and effectiveness in pediatric patients below the age of 12 years have not been established.

Axillary Hyperhidrosis

Safety and effectiveness in pediatric patients below the age of 18 years have not been established.

8.5 Geriatric Use

Clinical studies of **BOTOX** did not include sufficient numbers of subjects aged 65 and over to determine whether they respond differently from younger subjects. Other reported clinical experience has not identified differences in responses between the elderly and younger patients. There were too few patients over the age of 75 to enable any comparisons. In general, dose selection for an elderly patient should be cautious, usually starting at the low end of the dosing range, reflecting the greater frequency of decreased hepatic, renal, or cardiac function, and of concomitant disease or other drug therapy.

10 OVERDOSAGE

Excessive doses of **BOTOX** (onabotulinumtoxinA) for injection may be expected to produce neuromuscular weakness with a variety of symptoms. Respiratory support may be required where excessive doses cause paralysis of respiratory muscles. In the event of overdose, the patient should be medically monitored for symptoms of excessive muscle weakness or muscle paralysis *[see Boxed Warning and Warnings and Precautions (5.2, 5.4)]*. Symptomatic treatment may be necessary.

Symptoms of overdose are likely not to be present immediately following injection. Should accidental injection or oral ingestion occur, the person should be medically supervised for several weeks for signs and symptoms of excessive muscle weakness or paralysis.

In the event of overdose, antitoxin raised against botulinum toxin is available from the Centers for Disease Control and Prevention (CDC) in Atlanta, GA. However, the antitoxin will not reverse any botulinum toxin-induced effects already apparent by the time of antitoxin administration. In the event of suspected or actual cases of botulinum toxin poisoning, please contact your local or state Health Department to process a request for antitoxin through the CDC. If you do not receive a response within 30 minutes, please contact the CDC directly at 1-770-488-7100. More information can be obtained at http://www.cdc.gov/mmwr/preview/mmwrhtml/mm5232a8.htm.

11 DESCRIPTION

BOTOX (onabotulinumtoxinA) for injection is a sterile, vacuum-dried purified botulinum toxin type A, produced from fermentation of Hall strain Clostridium botulinum type A, and intended for intramuscular and intradermal use. It is purified from the culture solution by dialysis and a series of acid precipitations to a complex consisting of the neurotoxin, and several accessory proteins. The complex is dissolved in sterile sodium chloride solution containing Albumin Human and is sterile filtered (0.2 microns) prior to filling and vacuum-drying.

One Unit of **BOTOX** corresponds to the calculated median intraperitoneal lethal dose (LD_{50}) in mice. The method utilized for performing the assay is specific to Allergan's product, **BOTOX**. Due to specific details of this assay such as the vehicle, dilution scheme, and laboratory protocols for the various mouse LD_{50} assays, Units of biological activity of **BOTOX** cannot be compared to nor converted into Units of any other botulinum toxin or any toxin assessed with any other specific assay method. Therefore, differences in species sensitivities to different botulinum neurotoxin serotypes preclude extrapolation of animal-dose activity relationships to human dose estimates. The specific activity of **BOTOX** is approximately 20 Units/nanogram of neurotoxin protein complex.

Each vial of **BOTOX** contains either 100 Units of Clostridium botulinum type A neurotoxin complex, 0.5 mg of Albumin Human, and 0.9 mg of sodium chloride; or 200 Units of Clostridium botulinum type A neurotoxin complex, 1 mg of Albumin Human, and 1.8 mg of sodium chloride in a sterile, vacuum-dried form without a preservative.

12 CLINICAL PHARMACOLOGY
12.1 Mechanism of Action
BOTOX blocks neuromuscular transmission by binding to acceptor sites on motor or sympathetic nerve terminals, entering the nerve terminals, and inhibiting the release of acetylcholine. This inhibition occurs as the neurotoxin cleaves SNAP-25, a protein integral to the successful docking and release of acetylcholine from vesicles situated within nerve endings. When injected intramuscularly at therapeutic doses, **BOTOX** produces partial chemical denervation of the muscle resulting in a localized reduction in muscle activity. In addition, the muscle may atrophy, axonal sprouting may occur, and extrajunctional acetylcholine receptors may develop. There is evidence that reinnervation of the muscle may occur, thus slowly reversing muscle denervation produced by **BOTOX**. When injected intradermally, **BOTOX** produces temporary chemical denervation of the sweat gland resulting in local reduction in sweating.

12.3 Pharmacokinetics
Using currently available analytical technology, it is not possible to detect **BOTOX** in the peripheral blood following intramuscular injection at the recommended doses.

13 NONCLINICAL TOXICOLOGY
13.1 Carcinogenesis, Mutagenesis, Impairment of Fertility
Carcinogenesis
Long term studies in animals have not been performed to evaluate the carcinogenic potential of **BOTOX**.
Mutagenesis
BOTOX was negative in a battery of in vitro (microbial reverse mutation assay, mammalian cell mutation assay, and chromosomal aberration assay) and in vivo (micronucleus assay) genetic toxicologic assays.
Impairment of Fertility
In fertility studies of **BOTOX** (4, 8, or 16 Units/kg) in which either male or female rats were injected intramuscularly prior to mating and on the day of mating (3 doses, 2 weeks apart for males, 2 doses, 2 weeks apart for females) to

untreated animals, reduced fertility was observed in males at the intermediate and high doses and in females at the high dose. The no-effect doses for reproductive toxicity (4 Units/kg in males, 8 Units/kg in females) are approximately equal to the average high human dose for upper limb spasticity of 360 Units on a body weight basis (Units/kg).

14 CLINICAL STUDIES
14.1 Upper Limb Spasticity
The efficacy and safety of **BOTOX** for the treatment of upper limb spasticity were evaluated in three randomized, multi-center, double-blind, placebo-controlled studies.
Study 1 included 126 patients (64 **BOTOX** and 62 placebo) with upper limb spasticity (Ashworth score of at least 3 for wrist flexor tone and at least 2 for finger flexor tone) who were at least 6 months post-stroke. **BOTOX** (a total dose of 200 Units to 240 Units) and placebo were injected intramuscularly (IM) into the flexor digitorum profundus, flexor digitorum sublimis, flexor carpi radialis, flexor carpi ulnaris, and if necessary into the adductor pollicis and flexor pollicis longus (see Table 3). Use of an EMG/nerve stimulator was recommended to assist in proper muscle localization for injection. Patients were followed for 12 weeks.
[See table 3 above]
Study 2 compared 3 doses of **BOTOX** with placebo and included 91 patients [**BOTOX** 360 Units (N=21), **BOTOX** 180

The primary efficacy variable was wrist flexors muscle tone at week 6, as measured by the Ashworth score. The Ashworth Scale is a clinical measure of the force required to move an extremity around a joint, with a reduction in score clinically representing a reduction in the force needed to move a joint (i.e., improvement in spasticity).
Possible scores range from 0 to 4:
0 = No increase in muscle tone (none)
1 = Slight increase in muscle tone, giving a 'catch' when the limb was moved in flexion or extension (mild)
2 = More marked increase in muscle tone but affected limb is easily flexed (moderate)
3 = Considerable increase in muscle tone - passive movement difficult (severe)
4 = Limb rigid in flexion or extension (very severe).
Key secondary endpoints included Physician Global Assessment, finger flexors muscle tone, and thumb flexors tone at Week 6. The Physician Global Assessment evaluated the response to treatment in terms of how the patient was doing in his/her life using a scale from -4 = very marked worsening to +4 = very marked improvement. Study 1 results on the primary endpoint and the key secondary endpoints are shown in Table 4.
[See table 4 above]

Table 3: Study Medication Dose and Injection Sites in Study 1

Muscles Injected	Volume (mL)	BOTOX (Units)	Number of Injection Sites
Wrist			
Flexor Carpi Radialis	1	50	1
Flexor Carpi Ulnaris	1	50	1
Finger			1
Flexor Digitorum Profundus	1	50	
Flexor Digitorum Sublimis	1	50	1
Thumb			
Adductor Pollicis[a]	0.4	20	1
Flexor Pollicis Longus[a]	0.4	20	1

[a] injected only if spasticity is present in this muscle

Table 4: Primary and Key Secondary Endpoints by Muscle Group at Week 6 in Study 1

	BOTOX (N=64)	Placebo (N=62)
Median Change from Baseline in Wrist Flexor Muscle Tone on the Ashworth Scale[†a]	-2.0*	0.0
Median Change from Baseline in Finger Flexor Muscle Tone on the Ashworth Scale[††b]	-1.0*	0.0
Median Change from Baseline in Thumb Flexor Muscle Tone on the Ashworth Scale[††c]	-1.0	-1.0
Median Physician Global Assessment of Response to Treatment[††]	2.0*	0.0

[†] Primary endpoint at Week 6
[††] Secondary endpoints at Week 6
[*] Significantly different from placebo (p≤0.05)
[a] **BOTOX** injected into both the flexor carpi radialis and ulnaris muscles
[b] **BOTOX** injected into the flexor digitorum profundus and flexor digitorum sublimis muscles
[c] **BOTOX** injected into the adductor pollicis and flexor pollicis longus muscles

Table 5: Study Medication Dose and Injection Sites in Study 2 and Study 3

Muscles Injected	Total Dose BOTOX low dose (90 Units)	BOTOX mid dose (180 Units)	BOTOX high dose (360 Units)	Volume (mL) per site	Injection Sites (n)
Wrist					
Flexor Carpi Ulnaris	10 Units	20 Units	40 Units	0.4	1
Flexor Carpi Radialis	15 Units	30 Units	60 Units	0.6	1
Finger					
Flexor Digitorum Profundus	7.5 Units	15 Units	30 Units	0.3	1
Flexor Digitorum Sublimis	7.5 Units	15 Units	30 Units	0.3	1
Elbow					
Biceps Brachii	50 Units	100 Units	200 Units	0.5	4

Table 6: Primary and Key Secondary Endpoints by Muscle Group and BOTOX Dose at Week 6 in Study 2

	BOTOX low dose (90 Units) (N=21)	BOTOX mid dose (180 Units) (N=23)	BOTOX high dose (360 Units) (N=21)	Placebo (N=26)
Median Change from Baseline in Wrist Flexor Muscle Tone on the Ashworth Scale[†b]	-1.5*	-1.0*	-1.5*	-1.0
Median Change from Baseline in Finger Flexor Muscle Tone on the Ashworth Scale[††c]	-0.5	-0.5	-1.0	-0.5
Median Change from Baseline in Elbow Flexor Muscle Tone on the Ashworth Scale[††d]	-0.5	-1.0*	-0.5[a]	-0.5
Median Physician Global Assessment of Response to Treatment	1.0*	1.0*	1.0*	0.0

[†] Primary endpoint at Week 6
[††] Secondary endpoints at Week 6
* Significantly different from placebo (p≤0.05)
[a] p=0.053
[b] Total dose of BOTOX injected into both the flexor carpi radialis and ulnaris muscles
[c] Total dose of BOTOX injected into the flexor digitorum profundus and flexor digitorum sublimis muscles
[d] Dose of BOTOX injected into biceps brachii muscle

Table 7: Primary and Key Secondary Endpoints by Muscle Group and BOTOX Dose at Week 4 in Study 3

	BOTOX low dose (90 Units) (N=23)	BOTOX mid dose (180 Units) (N=21)	BOTOX high dose (360 Units) (N=22)	Placebo (N=19)
Median Change from Baseline in Wrist Flexor Muscle Tone on the Ashworth Scale[†b]	-1.0	-1.0	-1.5*	-0.5
Median Change from Baseline in Finger Flexor Muscle Tone on the Ashworth Scale[††c]	-1.0	-1.0	-1.0*	-0.5
Median Change from Baseline in Elbow Flexor Muscle Tone on the Ashworth Scale[††d]	-0.5	-0.5	-1.0*	-0.5

[†] Primary endpoint at Week 4
[††] Secondary endpoints at Week 4
* Significantly different from placebo (p≤0.05)
[b] Total dose of BOTOX injected into both the flexor carpi radialis and ulnaris muscles
[c] Total dose of BOTOX injected into the flexor digitorum profundus and flexor digitorum sublimis muscles
[d] Dose of BOTOX injected into biceps brachii muscle

Table 8: Efficacy Outcomes of the Phase 3 Cervical Dystonia Study (Group Means)

	Placebo (N=82)	BOTOX (N=88)	95% CI on Difference
Baseline CDSS	9.3	9.2	
Change in CDSS at Week 6	-0.3	-1.3	(-2.3, 0.3)[a,b]
% Patients with Any Improvement on Physician Global Assessment	31%	51%	(5%, 34%)[a]
Pain Intensity Baseline	1.8	1.8	
Change in Pain Intensity at Week 6	-0.1	-0.4	(-0.7, -0.2)[c]
Pain Frequency Baseline	1.9	1.8	
Change in Pain Frequency at Week 6	-0.0	-0.3	(-0.5, -0.0)[c]

[a] Confidence intervals are constructed from the analysis of covariance table with treatment and investigational site as main effects, and baseline CDSS as a covariate.
[b] These values represent the prospectively planned method for missing data imputation and statistical test. Sensitivity analyses indicated that the 95% confidence interval excluded the value of no difference between groups and the p-value was less than 0.05. These analyses included several alternative missing data imputation methods and non-parametric statistical tests.
[c] Confidence intervals are based on the t-distribution.

Units (N=23), BOTOX 90 Units (N=21), and placebo (N=26)] with upper limb spasticity (expanded Ashworth score of at least 2 for elbow flexor tone and at least 3 for wrist flexor tone) who were at least 6 weeks post-stroke. BOTOX and placebo were injected with EMG guidance into the flexor digitorum profundus, flexor digitorum sublimis, flexor carpi radialis, flexor carpi ulnaris, and biceps brachii (see Table 5).

[See table 5 on previous page]
The primary efficacy variable in Study 2 was the wrist flexor tone at Week 6 as measured by the expanded Ashworth Scale. The expanded Ashworth Scale uses the same scoring system as the Ashworth Scale, but allows for half-point increments.
Key secondary endpoints in Study 2 included Physician Global Assessment, finger flexors muscle tone, and elbow flexors muscle tone at Week 6. Study 2 results on the primary endpoint and the key secondary endpoints at Week 6 are shown in Table 6.
[See table 6 at left]
Study 3 compared 3 doses of BOTOX with placebo and enrolled 88 patients [BOTOX 360 Units (N=23), BOTOX 180 Units (N=23), BOTOX 90 Units (N=23), and placebo (N=19)] with upper limb spasticity (expanded Ashworth score of at least 2 for elbow flexor tone and at least 3 for wrist flexor tone and/or finger flexor tone) who were at least 6 weeks post-stroke. BOTOX and placebo were injected with EMG guidance into the flexor digitorum profundus, flexor digitorum sublimis, flexor carpi radialis, flexor carpi ulnaris, and biceps brachii (see Table 5).
The primary efficacy variable in Study 3 was wrist and elbow flexor tone as measured by the expanded Ashworth score. A key secondary endpoint was assessment of finger flexors muscle tone. Study 3 results on the primary endpoint at Week 4 are shown in Table 7.
[See table 7 at left]

14.2 Cervical Dystonia

A phase 3 randomized, multi-center, double-blind, placebo-controlled study of the treatment of cervical dystonia was conducted. This study enrolled adult patients with cervical dystonia and a history of having received BOTOX in an open label manner with perceived good response and tolerable side effects. Patients were excluded if they had previously received surgical or other denervation treatment for their symptoms or had a known history of neuromuscular disorder. Subjects participated in an open label enrichment period where they received their previously employed dose of BOTOX. Only patients who were again perceived as showing a response were advanced to the randomized evaluation period. The muscles in which the blinded study agent injections were to be administered were determined on an individual patient basis.
There were 214 subjects evaluated for the open label period, of which 170 progressed into the randomized, blinded treatment period (88 in the BOTOX group, 82 in the placebo group). Patient evaluations continued for at least 10 weeks post-injection. The primary outcome for the study was a dual endpoint, requiring evidence of both a change in the Cervical Dystonia Severity Scale (CDSS) and an increase in the percentage of patients showing any improvement on the Physician Global Assessment Scale at 6 weeks after the injection session. The CDSS quantifies the severity of abnormal head positioning and was newly devised for this study. CDSS allots 1 point for each 5 degrees (or part thereof) of head deviation in each of the three planes of head movement (range of scores up to theoretical maximum of 54). The Physician Global Assessment Scale is a 9 category scale scoring the physician's evaluation of the patients' status compared to baseline, ranging from −4 to +4 (very marked worsening to complete improvement), with 0 indicating no change from baseline and +1 slight improvement. Pain is also an important symptom of cervical dystonia and was evaluated by separate assessments of pain frequency and severity on scales of 0 (no pain) to 4 (constant in frequency or extremely severe in intensity). Study results on the primary endpoints and the pain-related secondary endpoints are shown in Table 8.
[See table 8 at left]
Exploratory analyses of this study suggested that the majority of patients who had shown a beneficial response by week 6 had returned to their baseline status by 3 months after treatment. Exploratory analyses of subsets by patient sex and age suggest that both sexes receive benefit, although female patients may receive somewhat greater amounts than male patients. There is a consistent treatment-associated effect between subsets greater than and less than age 65. There were too few non-Caucasian patients enrolled to draw any conclusions regarding relative efficacy in racial subsets.
There were several randomized studies conducted prior to the phase 3 study, which were supportive but not adequately designed to assess or quantitatively estimate the efficacy of BOTOX.
In the phase 3 study the median total BOTOX dose in patients randomized to receive BOTOX (N=88) was 236 Units, with 25th to 75th percentile ranges of 198 Units to 300 Units. Of these 88 patients, most received injections to 3 or 4 muscles; 38 received injections to 3 muscles, 28 to 4 muscles, 5 to 5 muscles, and 5 to 2 muscles. The dose was divided amongst the affected muscles in quantities shown in Table 9. The total dose and muscles selected were tailored to meet individual patient needs.
[See table 9 at top of next page]

14.3 Primary Axillary Hyperhidrosis

The efficacy and safety of BOTOX for the treatment of primary axillary hyperhidrosis were evaluated in two randomized, multi-center, double-blind, placebo-controlled studies. Study 1 included adult patients with persistent primary axillary hyperhidrosis who scored 3 or 4 on a Hyperhidrosis Disease Severity Scale (HDSS) and who produced at least 50 mg of sweat in each axilla at rest over 5 minutes. HDSS is a 4-point scale with 1 = "underarm sweating is never noticeable and never interferes with my daily activities"; to 4 = "underarm sweating is intolerable and always interferes with my daily activities". A total of 322 patients were randomized in a 1:1:1 ratio to treatment in both axillae with either 50 Units of **BOTOX**, 75 Units of **BOTOX**, or placebo. Patients were evaluated at 4-week intervals. Patients who responded to the first injection were re-injected when they reported a re-increase in HDSS score to 3 or 4 and produced at least 50 mg sweat in each axilla by gravimetric measurement, but no sooner than 8 weeks after the initial injection.

Study responders were defined as patients who showed at least a 2-grade improvement from baseline value on the HDSS 4 weeks after both of the first two treatment sessions or had a sustained response after their first treatment session and did not receive re-treatment during the study. Spontaneous resting axillary sweat production was assessed by weighing a filter paper held in the axilla over a period of 5 minutes (gravimetric measurement). Sweat production responders were those patients who demonstrated a reduction in axillary sweating from baseline of at least 50% at week 4.

In the three study groups the percentage of patients with baseline HDSS score of 3 ranged from 50% to 54% and from 46% to 50% for a score of 4. The median amount of sweat production (averaged for each axilla) was 102 mg, 123 mg, and 114 mg for the placebo, 50 Units and 75 Units groups respectively.

The percentage of responders based on at least a 2-grade decrease from baseline in HDSS or based on a >50% decrease from baseline in axillary sweat production was greater in both **BOTOX** groups than in the placebo group (p<0.001), but was not significantly different between the two **BOTOX** doses (see Table 10).

Duration of response was calculated as the number of days between injection and the date of the first visit at which patients returned to 3 or 4 on the HDSS scale. The median duration of response following the first treatment in **BOTOX**-treated patients with either dose was 201 days. Among those who received a second **BOTOX** injection, the median duration of response was similar to that observed after the first treatment.

In study 2, 320 adults with bilateral axillary primary hyperhidrosis were randomized to receive either 50 Units of **BOTOX** (n=242) or placebo (n=78). Treatment responders were defined as subjects showing at least a 50% reduction from baseline in axillary sweating measured by gravimetric measurement at 4 weeks. At week 4 post-injection, the percentages of responders were 91% (219/242) in the **BOTOX** group and 36% (28/78) in the placebo group, p<0.001. The difference in percentage of responders between **BOTOX** and placebo was 55% (95% CI=43.3, 65.9). [See table 10 at right]

14.4 Blepharospasm

Botulinum toxin has been investigated for use in patients with blepharospasm in several studies. In an open label, historically controlled study, 27 patients with essential blepharospasm were injected with 2 Units of **BOTOX** at each of six sites on each side. Twenty-five of the 27 patients treated with botulinum toxin reported improvement within 48 hours. One patient was controlled with a higher dosage at 13 weeks post initial injection and one patient reported mild improvement but remained functionally impaired.

In another study, 12 patients with blepharospasm were evaluated in a double-blind, placebo-controlled study. Patients receiving botulinum toxin (n=8) improved compared with the placebo group (n=4). The effects of the treatment lasted a mean of 12 weeks.

One thousand six hundred eighty-four patients with blepharospasm who were evaluated in an open label trial showed clinical improvement as evaluated by measured eyelid

force and clinically observed intensity of lid spasm, lasting an average of 12 weeks prior to the need for re-treatment.

14.5 Strabismus

Six hundred seventy-seven patients with strabismus treated with one or more injections of **BOTOX** were evaluated in an open label trial. Fifty-five percent of these patients improved to an alignment of 10 prism diopters or less when evaluated six months or more following injection.

16 HOW SUPPLIED/STORAGE AND HANDLING

BOTOX is supplied in a single-use vial in the following sizes:
100 Units   NDC 0023-1145-01
200 Units   NDC 0023-3921-02

Vials of **BOTOX** have a holographic film on the vial label that contains the name "Allergan" within horizontal lines of rainbow color. In order to see the hologram, rotate the vial back and forth between your fingers under a desk lamp or fluorescent light source. (Note: the holographic film on the label is absent in the date/lot area.) If you do not see the

Table 9: Number of Patients Treated per Muscle and Fraction of Total Dose Injected into Involved Muscles

Muscle	Number of Patients Treated in this Muscle (N=88)	Mean % Dose per Muscle	Mid-Range of % Dose per Muscle*
Splenius capitis/cervicis	83	38	25-50
Sternocleidomastoid	77	25	17-31
Levator scapulae	52	20	16-25
Trapezius	49	29	18-33
Semispinalis	16	21	13-25
Scalene	15	15	6-21
Longissimus	8	29	17-41

*The mid-range of dose is calculated as the 25th to 75th percentiles.

Table 10: Study 1 - Study Outcomes

Treatment Response	BOTOX 50 Units (N=104)	BOTOX 75 Units (N=110)	Placebo (N=108)	BOTOX 50-placebo (95% CI)	BOTOX 75-placebo (95% CI)
HDSS Score change ≥2% (n)[a]	55% (57)	49% (54)	6% (6)	49.3% (38.8, 59.7)	43% (33.2, 53.8)
>50% decrease in axillary sweat production % (n)	81% (84)	86% (94)	41% (44)	40% (28.1, 52.0)	45% (33.3, 56.1)

[a] Patients who showed at least a 2-grade improvement from baseline value on the HDSS 4 weeks after both of the first two treatment sessions or had a sustained response after their first treatment session and did not receive re-treatment during the study.

lines of rainbow color or the name "Allergan", do not use the product and contact Allergan for additional information at 1-800-890-4345 from 7:00 AM to 3:00 PM Pacific Time.

Storage

Unopened vials of **BOTOX** should be stored in a refrigerator (2° to 8°C) for up to 36 months for the 100 Unit vial or up to 24 months for the 200 Unit vial. Do not use after the expiration date on the vial. Administer **BOTOX** within 24 hours of reconstitution; during this period reconstituted **BOTOX** should be stored in a refrigerator (2° to 8°C). Reconstituted **BOTOX** should be clear, colorless, and free of particulate matter.

All vials, including expired vials, or equipment used with the drug should be disposed of carefully, as is done with all medical waste.

Rx Only

17 PATIENT COUNSELING INFORMATION

Provide a copy of the Medication Guide and review the contents with the patient.

17.1 Swallowing, Speaking or Breathing Difficulties, or Other Unusual Symptoms

Patients should be advised to inform their doctor or pharmacist if they develop any unusual symptoms (including difficulty with swallowing, speaking, or breathing), or if any existing symptom worsens [see Boxed Warning and Warnings and Precautions (5.2, 5.4)].

17.2 Ability to Operate Machinery or Vehicles

Patients should be counseled that if loss of strength, muscle weakness, blurred vision, or drooping eyelids occur, they should avoid driving a car or engaging in other potentially hazardous activities.

17.3 Medication Guide

MEDICATION GUIDE
BOTOX®
BOTOX® Cosmetic
(Boe-tox)
(onabotulinumtoxinA)
for Injection

Read the Medication Guide that comes with **BOTOX** or **BOTOX Cosmetic** before you start using it and each time it is given to you. There may be new information. This information does not take the place of talking with your doctor about your medical condition or your treatment. You should share this information with your family members and caregivers.

What is the most important information I should know about BOTOX and BOTOX Cosmetic?

BOTOX and BOTOX Cosmetic may cause serious side effects that can be life threatening. Call your doctor or get medical help right away if you have any of these problems after treatment with BOTOX or BOTOX Cosmetic:

• **Problems swallowing, speaking, or breathing. These problems can happen hours to weeks after an injection**

of **BOTOX or BOTOX Cosmetic** usually because the muscles that you use to breathe and swallow can become weak after the injection. Death can happen as a complication if you have severe problems with swallowing or breathing after treatment with **BOTOX or BOTOX Cosmetic**.

• People with certain breathing problems may need to use muscles in their neck to help them breathe. These patients may be at greater risk for serious breathing problems with **BOTOX or BOTOX Cosmetic**.

• Swallowing problems may last for several months. People who cannot swallow well may need a feeding tube to receive food and water. If swallowing problems are severe, food or liquids may go into your lungs. People who already have swallowing or breathing problems before receiving **BOTOX or BOTOX Cosmetic** have the highest risk of getting these problems.

• **Spread of toxin effects**. In some cases, the effect of botulinum toxin may affect areas of the body away from the injection site and cause symptoms of a serious condition called botulism. The symptoms of botulism include:

  • loss of strength and muscle weakness all over the body
  • double vision
  • blurred vision and drooping eyelids
  • hoarseness or change or loss of voice (dysphonia)
  • trouble saying words clearly (dysarthria)
  • loss of bladder control
  • trouble breathing
  • trouble swallowing

These symptoms can happen hours to weeks after you receive an injection of **BOTOX or BOTOX Cosmetic**.

These problems could make it unsafe for you to drive a car or do other dangerous activities. See "What should I avoid while receiving **BOTOX or BOTOX Cosmetic**?"

There has not been a confirmed serious case of spread of toxin effect away from the injection site when **BOTOX** has been used at the recommended dose to treat severe underarm sweating, blepharospasm, or strabismus, or when **BOTOX Cosmetic** has been used at the recommended dose to treat frown lines.

What are BOTOX and BOTOX Cosmetic?

BOTOX is a prescription medicine that is injected into muscles and used:

• to treat increased muscle stiffness in elbow, wrist, and finger muscles in adults with upper limb spasticity.
• to treat the abnormal head position and neck pain that happens with cervical dystonia (CD) in adults.
• to treat certain types of eye muscle problems (strabismus) or abnormal spasm of the eyelids (blepharospasm) in people 12 years and older.

BOTOX is also injected into the skin to treat the symptoms of severe underarm sweating (severe primary axillary hyperhidrosis) when medicines used on the skin (topical) do not work well enough.

BOTOX Cosmetic is a prescription medicine that is injected into muscles and used to improve the look of moderate to severe frown lines between the eyebrows (glabellar lines) in adults younger than 65 years of age for a short period of time (temporary).

It is not known whether BOTOX is safe or effective in children younger than:

- 18 years of age for treatment of spasticity
- 16 years of age for treatment of cervical dystonia
- 18 years of age for treatment of hyperhidrosis
- 12 years of age for treatment of strabismus or blepharospasm

BOTOX Cosmetic is not recommended for use in children younger than 18 years of age.

It is not known whether BOTOX and BOTOX Cosmetic are safe or effective for other types of muscle spasms or for severe sweating anywhere other than your armpits.

Who should not take BOTOX or BOTOX Cosmetic?

Do not take BOTOX or BOTOX Cosmetic if you:

- are allergic to any of the ingredients in BOTOX or BOTOX Cosmetic. See the end of this Medication Guide for a list of ingredients in BOTOX and BOTOX Cosmetic.
- had an allergic reaction to any other botulinum toxin product such as Myobloc® or Dysport®
- have a skin infection at the planned injection site

What should I tell my doctor before taking BOTOX or BOTOX Cosmetic?

Tell your doctor about all your medical conditions, including if you have:

- a disease that affects your muscles and nerves (such as amyotrophic lateral sclerosis [ALS or Lou Gehrig's disease], myasthenia gravis or Lambert-Eaton syndrome). See "What is the most important information I should know about BOTOX and BOTOX Cosmetic?"
- allergies to any botulinum toxin product
- had any side effect from any botulinum toxin product in the past
- a breathing problem, such as asthma or emphysema
- swallowing problems
- bleeding problems
- plans to have surgery
- had surgery on your face
- weakness of your forehead muscles, such as trouble raising your eyebrows
- drooping eyelids
- any other change in the way your face normally looks
- are pregnant or plan to become pregnant. It is not known if BOTOX or BOTOX Cosmetic can harm your unborn baby.
- are breast-feeding or plan to breastfeed. It is not known if BOTOX or BOTOX Cosmetic passes into breast milk.

Tell your doctor about all the medicines you take, including prescription and nonprescription medicines, vitamins and herbal products. Using BOTOX or BOTOX Cosmetic with certain other medicines may cause serious side effects. **Do not start any new medicines until you have told your doctor that you have received BOTOX or BOTOX Cosmetic in the past.**

Especially tell your doctor if you:

- have received any other botulinum toxin product in the last four months
- have received injections of botulinum toxin, such as Myobloc® (rimabotulinumtoxinB) or Dysport® (abobotulinumtoxinA) in the past. Be sure your doctor knows exactly which product you received.
- have recently received an antibiotic by injection
- take muscle relaxants
- take an allergy or cold medicine
- take a sleep medicine

Ask your doctor if you are not sure if your medicine is one that is listed above.

Know the medicines you take. Keep a list of your medicines with you to show your doctor and pharmacist each time you get a new medicine.

How should I take BOTOX or BOTOX Cosmetic?

- BOTOX or BOTOX Cosmetic is an injection that your doctor will give you.
- BOTOX is injected into your affected muscles or skin.
- BOTOX Cosmetic is injected into your affected muscles.
- Your doctor may change your dose of BOTOX or BOTOX Cosmetic, until you and your doctor find the best dose for you.

What should I avoid while taking BOTOX or BOTOX Cosmetic?

BOTOX and BOTOX Cosmetic may cause loss of strength or general muscle weakness, or vision problems within hours to weeks of taking BOTOX or BOTOX Cosmetic. If this happens, do not drive a car, operate machinery, or do other dangerous activities. See "What is the most important information I should know about BOTOX and BOTOX Cosmetic?"

What are the possible side effects of BOTOX and BOTOX Cosmetic?

BOTOX and BOTOX Cosmetic can cause serious side effects. See "What is the most important information I should know about BOTOX and BOTOX Cosmetic?"

Other side effects of BOTOX and BOTOX Cosmetic include:

- dry mouth
- discomfort or pain at the injection site
- tiredness
- headache
- neck pain
- eye problems: double vision, blurred vision, decreased eyesight, drooping eyelids, swelling of your eyelids, and dry eyes.
- allergic reactions. Symptoms of an allergic reaction to BOTOX or BOTOX Cosmetic may include: itching, rash, red itchy welts, wheezing, asthma symptoms, or dizziness or feeling faint. Tell your doctor or get medical help right away if you are wheezing or have asthma symptoms, or if you become dizzy or faint.

Tell your doctor if you have any side effect that bothers you or that does not go away.

These are not all the possible side effects of BOTOX and BOTOX Cosmetic. For more information, ask your doctor or pharmacist.

Call your doctor for medical advice about side effects. You may report side effects to FDA at 1-800-FDA-1088.

General information about BOTOX and BOTOX Cosmetic:

Medicines are sometimes prescribed for purposes other than those listed in a Medication Guide.

This Medication Guide summarizes the most important information about BOTOX and BOTOX Cosmetic. If you would like more information, talk with your doctor. You can ask your doctor or pharmacist for information about BOTOX and BOTOX Cosmetic that is written for healthcare professionals. For more information about BOTOX and BOTOX Cosmetic call Allergan at 1-800-433-8871 or go to www.botox.com.

What are the ingredients in BOTOX and BOTOX Cosmetic?

Active ingredient: botulinum toxin type A

Inactive ingredients: human albumin and sodium chloride

Issued: 03/2010

This Medication Guide has been approved by the U.S. Food and Drug Administration.

Manufactured by: Allergan Pharmaceuticals Ireland a subsidiary of: Allergan, Inc.

2525 Dupont Dr.
Irvine, CA 92612
© 2010 Allergan, Inc.
® mark owned by Allergan, Inc.
Myobloc® is a registered trademark of Solstice Neurosciences, Inc.
Dysport® is a registered trademark of Ipsen Biopharm Limited Company.
71580US10B
72284US11B

COMBIGAN®
(brimonidine tartrate/timolol maleate ophthalmic solution)

℞

Highlights Of Prescribing Information

These highlights do not include all the information needed to use COMBIGAN® safely and effectively. See full prescribing information for COMBIGAN®.

COMBIGAN® (brimonidine tartrate/timolol maleate ophthalmic solution) 0.2%/0.5%
Initial U.S. Approval: 2007

———INDICATIONS AND USAGE———

COMBIGAN® is an alpha adrenergic receptor agonist with a beta adrenergic receptor inhibitor indicated for the reduction of elevated intraocular pressure (IOP) in patients with glaucoma or ocular hypertension who require adjunctive or replacement therapy due to inadequately controlled IOP; the IOP-lowering of COMBIGAN® dosed twice a day was slightly less than that seen with the concomitant administration of timolol maleate ophthalmic solution, 0.5% dosed twice a day and brimonidine tartrate ophthalmic solution, 0.2% dosed three times per day. (1)

———DOSAGE AND ADMINISTRATION———

- One drop in the affected eye(s), twice daily approximately 12 hours apart. (2)

———DOSAGE FORMS AND STRENGTHS———

- Solution containing 2 mg/mL brimonidine tartrate and 5 mg/mL timolol. (3)

———CONTRAINDICATIONS———

- Bronchial asthma, a history of bronchial asthma, severe chronic obstructive pulmonary disease. (4, 5.1, 5.3)

- Sinus bradycardia, second or third degree atrioventricular block, overt cardiac failure, cardiogenic shock. (4, 5.2)
- Hypersensitivity to any component of this product. (4)

———WARNINGS AND PRECAUTIONS———

- Potentiation of respiratory reactions including asthma (5.1)
- Cardiac Failure (5.2)
- Obstructive Pulmonary Disease (5.3)
- Potentiation of vascular insufficiency (5.4)
- Increased reactivity to allergens (5.5)
- Potentiation of muscle weakness (5.6)
- Masking of hypoglycemic symptoms in patients with diabetes mellitus (5.7)
- Masking of thyrotoxicosis (5.8)

———ADVERSE REACTIONS———

Most common adverse reactions occurring in approximately 5 to 15% of patients included allergic conjunctivitis, conjunctival folliculosis, conjunctival hyperemia, eye pruritus, ocular burning, and stinging. (6.1)

To report SUSPECTED ADVERSE REACTIONS, contact Allergan at 800-433-8871 or the FDA at 800-FDA-1088 or www.fda.gov/medwatch.

———DRUG INTERACTIONS———

- Antihypertensives/cardiac glycosides may lower blood pressure. (7.1)
- Concomitant use with systemic beta-blockers may potentiate systemic beta-blockade. (7.2)
- Oral or intravenous calcium antagonists may cause atrioventricular conduction disturbances, left ventricular failure, and hypotension. (7.3)
- Catecholamine-depleting drugs may have additive effects and produce hypotension and/or marked bradycardia. (7.4)
- Use with CNS depressants may result in an additive or potentiating effect. (7.5)
- Digitalis and calcium antagonists may have additive effects in prolonging atrioventricular conduction time. (7.6)
- CYP2D6 inhibitors may potentiate systemic beta-blockade. (7.7)
- Tricyclic antidepressants may potentially blunt the hypotensive effect of systemic clonidine. (7.8)
- Monoamine oxidase inhibitors may result in increased hypotension. (7.9)

———USE IN SPECIFIC POPULATIONS———

- Not for use in children below the age of 2 years. (8.4)

See 17 for PATIENT COUNSELING INFORMATION
Revised: 06/2008

14 CLINICAL STUDIES
16 HOW SUPPLIED/STORAGE AND HANDLING
17 PATIENT COUNSELING INFORMATION
*Sections or subsections omitted from the full prescribing information are not listed.

FULL PRESCRIBING INFORMATION

1 INDICATIONS AND USAGE

COMBIGAN® (brimonidine tartrate/timolol maleate ophthalmic solution) 0.2%/0.5% is an alpha adrenergic receptor agonist with a beta adrenergic receptor inhibitor indicated for the reduction of elevated intraocular pressure (IOP) in patients with glaucoma or ocular hypertension who require adjunctive or replacement therapy due to inadequately controlled IOP; the IOP-lowering of **COMBIGAN®** dosed twice a day was slightly less than that seen with the concomitant administration of 0.5% timolol maleate ophthalmic solution dosed twice a day and 0.2% brimonidine tartrate ophthalmic solution dosed three times per day.

2 DOSAGE AND ADMINISTRATION

The recommended dose is one drop of **COMBIGAN®** in the affected eye(s) twice daily approximately 12 hours apart. If more than one topical ophthalmic product is to be used, the different products should be instilled at least 5 minutes apart.

3 DOSAGE FORMS AND STRENGTHS

Solution containing 2 mg/mL brimonidine tartrate and 5 mg/mL timolol (6.8 mg/mL timolol maleate).

4 CONTRAINDICATIONS

Asthma, COPD

COMBIGAN® is contraindicated in patients with bronchial asthma; a history of bronchial asthma; severe chronic obstructive pulmonary disease (see **WARNINGS AND PRECAUTIONS**, 5.1, 5.3).

Sinus bradycardia, AV block, Cardiac failure, Cardiogenic shock

COMBIGAN® is contraindicated in patients with sinus bradycardia; second or third degree atrioventricular block; overt cardiac failure (see **WARNINGS AND PRECAUTIONS**, 5.2); cardiogenic shock.

Hypersensitivity reactions

Local hypersensitivity reactions have occurred following the use of different components of **COMBIGAN®**. **COMBIGAN®** is contraindicated in patients who have exhibited a hypersensitivity reaction to any component of this medication in the past.

5 WARNINGS AND PRECAUTIONS

5.1 Potentiation of respiratory reactions including asthma

COMBIGAN® contains timolol maleate; and although administered topically can be absorbed systemically. Therefore, the same types of adverse reactions found with systemic administration of beta-adrenergic blocking agents may occur with topical administration. For example, severe respiratory reactions including death due to bronchospasm in patients with asthma have been reported following systemic or ophthalmic administration of timolol maleate (see **CONTRAINDICATIONS**, 4).

5.2 Cardiac Failure

Sympathetic stimulation may be essential for support of the circulation in individuals with diminished myocardial contractility, and its inhibition by beta-adrenergic receptor blockade may precipitate more severe failure.

In patients without a history of cardiac failure, continued depression of the myocardium with beta-blocking agents over a period of time can, in some cases, lead to cardiac failure. At the first sign or symptom of cardiac failure, **COMBIGAN®** should be discontinued (see also **CONTRAINDICATIONS**, 4).

5.3 Obstructive Pulmonary Disease

Patients with chronic obstructive pulmonary disease (e.g., chronic bronchitis, emphysema) of mild or moderate severity, bronchospastic disease, or a history of bronchospastic disease (other than bronchial asthma or a history of bronchial asthma, in which **COMBIGAN®** is contraindicated (see **CONTRAINDICATIONS**, 4)) should, in general, not receive beta-blocking agents, including **COMBIGAN®**.

5.4 Potentiation of vascular insufficiency

COMBIGAN® may potentiate syndromes associated with vascular insufficiency. **COMBIGAN®** should be used with caution in patients with depression, cerebral or coronary insufficiency, Raynaud's phenomenon, orthostatic hypotension, or thromboangiitis obliterans.

5.5 Increased reactivity to allergens

While taking beta-blockers, patients with a history of atopy or a history of severe anaphylactic reactions to a variety of allergens may be more reactive to repeated accidental, diagnostic, or therapeutic challenge with such allergens. Such patients may be unresponsive to the usual doses of epinephrine used to treat anaphylactic reactions.

5.6 Potentiation of muscle weakness

Beta-adrenergic blockade has been reported to potentiate muscle weakness consistent with certain myasthenic symptoms (e.g., diplopia, ptosis, and generalized weakness). Timolol has been reported rarely to increase muscle weakness in some patients with myasthenia gravis or myasthenic symptoms.

5.7 Masking of hypoglycemic symptoms in patients with diabetes mellitus

Beta-adrenergic blocking agents should be administered with caution in patients subject to spontaneous hypoglycemia or to diabetic patients (especially those with labile diabetes) who are receiving insulin or oral hypoglycemic agents. Beta-adrenergic receptor blocking agents may mask the signs and symptoms of acute hypoglycemia.

5.8 Masking of thyrotoxicosis

Beta-adrenergic blocking agents may mask certain clinical signs (e.g., tachycardia) of hyperthyroidism. Patients suspected of developing thyrotoxicosis should be managed carefully to avoid abrupt withdrawal of beta-adrenergic blocking agents that might precipitate a thyroid storm.

5.9 Contamination of topical ophthalmic products after use

There have been reports of bacterial keratitis associated with the use of multiple dose containers of topical ophthalmic products. These containers had been inadvertently contaminated by patients who, in most cases, had a concurrent corneal disease or a disruption of the ocular epithelial surface (see **PATIENT COUNSELING INFORMATION**, 17).

5.10 Impairment of beta-adrenergically mediated reflexes during surgery

The necessity or desirability of withdrawal of beta-adrenergic blocking agents prior to major surgery is controversial. Beta-adrenergic receptor blockade impairs the ability of the heart to respond to beta-adrenergically mediated reflex stimuli. This may augment the risk of general anesthesia in surgical procedures. Some patients receiving beta-adrenergic receptor blocking agents have experienced protracted severe hypotension during anesthesia. Difficulty in restarting and maintaining the heartbeat has also been reported. For these reasons, in patients undergoing elective surgery, some authorities recommend gradual withdrawal of beta-adrenergic receptor blocking agents.

If necessary during surgery, the effects of beta-adrenergic blocking agents may be reversed by sufficient doses of adrenergic agonists.

6 ADVERSE REACTIONS

6.1 Clinical Studies Experience

Because clinical studies are conducted under widely varying conditions, adverse reaction rates observed in the clinical studies of a drug cannot be directly compared to rates in the clinical studies of another drug and may not reflect the rates observed in practice.

COMBIGAN®

In clinical trials of 12 months duration with **COMBIGAN®**, the most frequent reactions associated with its use occurring in approximately 5% to 15% of the patients included: allergic conjunctivitis, conjunctival folliculosis, conjunctival hyperemia, eye pruritus, ocular burning, and stinging. The following adverse reactions were reported in 1% to 5% of patients: asthenia, blepharitis, corneal erosion, depression, epiphora, eye discharge, eye dryness, eye irritation, eye pain, eyelid edema, eyelid erythema, eyelid pruritus, foreign body sensation, headache, hypertension, oral dryness, somnolence, superficial punctate keratitis, and visual disturbance.

Other adverse reactions that have been reported with the individual components are listed below.

Brimonidine Tartrate (0.1%-0.2%)

Abnormal taste, allergic reaction, blepharoconjunctivitis, blurred vision, bronchitis, cataract, conjunctival edema, conjunctival hemorrhage, conjunctivitis, cough, dizziness, dyspepsia, dyspnea, fatigue, flu syndrome, follicular conjunctivitis, gastrointestinal disorder, hypercholesterolemia, hypotension, infection (primarily colds and respiratory infections), hordeolum, insomnia, keratitis, lid disorder, nasal dryness, ocular allergic reaction, pharyngitis, photophobia, rash, rhinitis, sinus infection, sinusitis, taste perversion, tearing, visual field defect, vitreous detachment, vitreous disorder, vitreous floaters, and worsened visual acuity.

Timolol (Ocular Administration)

Body as a whole: chest pain; *Cardiovascular*: Arrhythmia, bradycardia, cardiac arrest, cardiac failure, cerebral ischemia, cerebral vascular accident, claudication, cold hands and feet, edema, heart block, palpitation, pulmonary edema, Raynaud's phenomenon, syncope, and worsening of angina pectoris; *Digestive*: Anorexia, diarrhea, nausea; *Immunologic*: Systemic lupus erythematosus; *Nervous System/Psychiatric*: Increase in signs and symptoms of myasthenia gravis, insomnia, nightmares, paresthesia, behavioral changes and psychic disturbances including confusion, hallucinations, anxiety, disorientation, nervousness, and memory loss; *Skin*: Alopecia, psoriasiform rash or exacerbation of psoriasis; *Hypersensitivity*: Signs and symptoms of systemic allergic reactions, including anaphylaxis, angioedema, urticaria, and generalized and localized rash; *Respiratory*: Bronchospasm (predominantly in patients with preexisting bronchospastic disease), dyspnea, nasal congestion, respiratory failure; *Endocrine*: Masked symptoms of hypoglycemia in diabetes patients (see **WARNINGS AND PRECAUTIONS**, 5.7); *Special Senses*: diplopia, choroidal detachment following filtration surgery, cystoid macular edema, decreased corneal sensitivity, pseudopemphigoid, ptosis, refractive changes, tinnitus; *Urogenital*: Decreased libido, impotence, Peyronie's disease, retroperitoneal fibrosis.

6.2 Postmarketing Experience

Brimonidine

The following reactions have been identified during postmarketing use of brimonidine tartrate ophthalmic solutions in clinical practice. Because they are reported voluntarily from a population of unknown size, estimates of frequency cannot be made. The reactions, which have been chosen for inclusion due to either their seriousness, frequency of reporting, possible causal connection to brimonidine tartrate ophthalmic solutions, or a combination of these factors, include: bradycardia, depression, iritis, keratoconjunctivitis sicca, miosis, nausea, skin reactions (including erythema, eyelid pruritus, rash, and vasodilation), and tachycardia. Apnea, bradycardia, hypotension, hypothermia, hypotonia, and somnolence have been reported in infants receiving brimonidine tartrate ophthalmic solutions.

Oral Timolol/Oral Beta-blockers

The following additional adverse reactions have been reported in clinical experience with ORAL timolol maleate or other ORAL beta-blocking agents and may be considered potential effects of ophthalmic timolol maleate: *Allergic*: Erythematous rash, fever combined with aching and sore throat, laryngospasm with respiratory distress; *Body as a whole*: Decreased exercise tolerance, extremity pain, weight loss; *Cardiovascular*: Vasodilatation, worsening of arterial insufficiency; *Digestive*: Gastrointestinal pain, hepatomegaly, ischemic colitis, mesenteric arterial thrombosis, vomiting; *Hematologic*: Agranulocytosis, nonthrombocytopenic purpura, thrombocytopenic purpura; *Endocrine*: Hyperglycemia, hypoglycemia; *Skin*: Increased pigmentation, pruritus, skin irritation, sweating; *Musculoskeletal*: Arthralgia; *Nervous System/Psychiatric*: An acute reversible syndrome characterized by disorientation for time and place, decreased performance on neuropsychometrics, diminished concentration, emotional lability, local weakness, reversible mental depression progressing to catatonia, slightly clouded sensorium, vertigo; *Respiratory*: Bronchial obstruction, rales; *Urogenital*: Urination difficulties.

7 DRUG INTERACTIONS

7.1 Antihypertensives/Cardiac Glycosides

Because **COMBIGAN®** may reduce blood pressure, caution in using drugs such as antihypertensives and/or cardiac glycosides with **COMBIGAN®** is advised.

7.2 Beta-adrenergic Blocking Agents

Patients who are receiving a beta-adrenergic blocking agent orally and **COMBIGAN®** should be observed for potential additive effects of beta-blockade, both systemic and on intraocular pressure. The concomitant use of two topical beta-adrenergic blocking agents is not recommended.

7.3 Calcium Antagonists

Caution should be used in the co-administration of beta-adrenergic blocking agents, such as **COMBIGAN®**, and oral or intravenous calcium antagonists because of possible atrioventricular conduction disturbances, left ventricular failure, and hypotension. In patients with impaired cardiac function, co-administration should be avoided.

7.4 Catecholamine-depleting Drugs

Close observation of the patient is recommended when a beta blocker is administered to patients receiving catecholamine-depleting drugs such as reserpine, because of possible additive effects and the production of hypotension and/or marked bradycardia, which may result in vertigo, syncope, or postural hypotension.

7.5 CNS Depressants

Although specific drug interaction studies have not been conducted with **COMBIGAN®**, the possibility of an additive or potentiating effect with CNS depressants (alcohol, barbiturates, opiates, sedatives, or anesthetics) should be considered.

7.6 Digitalis and Calcium Antagonists

The concomitant use of beta-adrenergic blocking agents with digitalis and calcium antagonists may have additive effects in prolonging atrioventricular conduction time.

7.7 CYP2D6 Inhibitors

Potentiated systemic beta-blockade (e.g., decreased heart rate, depression) has been reported during combined treatment with CYP2D6 inhibitors (e.g., quinidine, SSRIs) and timolol.

7.8 Tricyclic Antidepressants

Tricyclic antidepressants have been reported to blunt the hypotensive effect of systemic clonidine. It is not known whether the concurrent use of these agents with **COMBIGAN®** in humans can lead to resulting interference with the IOP lowering effect. Caution, however, is advised in patients taking tricyclic antidepressants which can affect the metabolism and uptake of circulating amines.

7.9 Monoamine oxidase inhibitors

Monoamine oxidase (MAO) inhibitors may theoretically interfere with the metabolism of brimonidine and potentially result in an increased systemic side-effect such as hypotension. Caution is advised in patients taking MAO inhibitors which can affect the metabolism and uptake of circulating amines.

8 USE IN SPECIFIC POPULATIONS

8.1 Pregnancy

Pregnancy Category C: Teratogenicity studies have been performed in animals.

Brimonidine tartrate was not teratogenic when given orally during gestation days 6 through 15 in rats and days 6 through 18 in rabbits. The highest doses of brimonidine tartrate in rats (1.65 mg/kg/day) and rabbits (3.33 mg/kg/day) achieved AUC exposure values 580 and 37-fold higher, respectively, than similar values estimated in humans treated with **COMBIGAN®**, 1 drop in both eyes twice daily.

Teratogenicity studies with timolol in mice, rats, and rabbits at oral doses up to 50 mg/ kg/day [4,200 times the maximum recommended human ocular dose of 0.012 mg/kg/day on a mg/kg basis (MRHOD)] demonstrated no evidence of fetal malformations. Although delayed fetal ossification was observed at this dose in rats, there were no adverse effects on postnatal development of offspring. Doses of 1,000 mg/kg/day (83,000 times the MRHOD) were maternotoxic in mice and resulted in an increased number of fetal resorptions. Increased fetal resorptions were also seen in rabbits at doses 8,300 times the MRHOD without apparent maternotoxicity.

There are no adequate and well-controlled studies in pregnant women; however, in animal studies, brimonidine crossed the placenta and entered into the fetal circulation to a limited extent. Because animal reproduction studies are not always predictive of human response, **COMBIGAN®** should be used during pregnancy only if the potential benefit to the mother justifies the potential risk to the fetus.

8.3 Nursing Mothers

Timolol has been detected in human milk following oral and ophthalmic drug administration. It is not known whether brimonidine tartrate is excreted in human milk, although in animal studies, brimonidine tartrate has been shown to be excreted in breast milk. Because of the potential for serious adverse reactions from **COMBIGAN®** in nursing infants, a decision should be made whether to discontinue nursing or to discontinue the drug, taking into account the importance of the drug to the mother.

8.4 Pediatric Use

COMBIGAN® is not recommended for use in children under the age of 2 years. During post-marketing surveillance, apnea, bradycardia, hypotension, hypothermia, hypotonia, and somnolence have been reported in infants receiving brimonidine. The safety and effectiveness of brimonidine tartrate and timolol maleate have not been studied in children below the age of two years.

The safety and effectiveness of **COMBIGAN®** have been established in the age groups 2–16 years of age. Use of **COMBIGAN®** in these age groups is supported by evidence from adequate and well-controlled studies of **COMBIGAN®** in adults with additional data from a study of the concomitant use of brimonidine tartrate ophthalmic solution 0.2% and timolol maleate ophthalmic solution in pediatric glaucoma patients (ages 2 to 7 years). In this study, brimonidine tartrate ophthalmic solution 0.2% was dosed three times a day as adjunctive therapy to beta-blockers. The most commonly observed adverse reactions were somnolence (50%-83% in patients 2 to 6 years) and decreased alertness. In pediatric patients 7 years of age or older (>20 kg), somnolence appears to occur less frequently (25%). Approximately 16% of patients on brimonidine tartrate ophthalmic solution discontinued from the study due to somnolence.

8.5 Geriatric Use

No overall differences in safety or effectiveness have been observed between elderly and other adult patients.

10 OVERDOSAGE

No information is available on overdosage with **COMBIGAN®** in humans. There have been reports of inadvertent overdosage with timolol ophthalmic solution resulting in systemic effects similar to those seen with systemic beta-adrenergic blocking agents such as dizziness, headache, shortness of breath, bradycardia, bronchospasm, and cardiac arrest. Treatment of an oral overdose includes supportive and symptomatic therapy; a patent airway should be maintained.

11 DESCRIPTION

COMBIGAN® (brimonidine tartrate/timolol maleate ophthalmic solution) 0.2%/0.5%, sterile, is a relatively selective alpha-2 adrenergic receptor agonist with a non-selective beta-adrenergic receptor inhibitor (topical intraocular pressure lowering agent).

The structural formulae are:

Brimonidine tartrate:

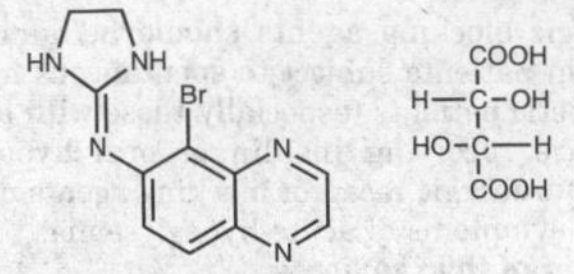

5-bromo-6-(2-imidazolidinylideneamino) quinoxaline L-tartrate; MW= 442.24

Timolol maleate:

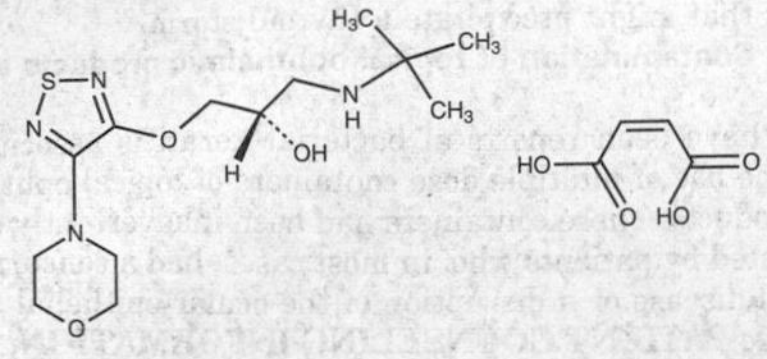

(-)-1-(*tert*-butylamino)-3-[(4-morpholino-1,2,5-thiadiazol-3-yl)-oxy]-2-propanol maleate (1:1) (salt); MW= 432.50 as the maleate salt

In solution, **COMBIGAN®** (brimonidine tartrate/timolol maleate ophthalmic solution) 0.2%/0.5% has a clear, greenish-yellow color. It has an osmolality of 260-330 mOsmol/kg and a pH during its shelf life of 6.5-7.3.

Brimonidine tartrate appears as an off-white, or white to pale-yellow powder and is soluble in both water (1.5 mg/mL) and in the product vehicle (3.0 mg/mL) at pH 7.2. Timolol maleate appears as a white, odorless, crystalline powder and is soluble in water, methanol, and alcohol.

Each mL of **COMBIGAN®** contains the active ingredients brimonidine tartrate 0.2% and timolol 0.5% with the inactive ingredients benzalkonium chloride 0.005%; sodium phosphate, monobasic; sodium phosphate, dibasic; purified water; and hydrochloric acid and/or sodium hydroxide to adjust pH.

12 CLINICAL PHARMACOLOGY

12.1 Mechanism of Action

COMBIGAN® is comprised of two components: brimonidine tartrate and timolol. Each of these two components decreases elevated intraocular pressure, whether or not associated with glaucoma. Elevated intraocular pressure is a major risk factor in the pathogenesis of optic nerve damage and glaucomatous visual field loss. The higher the level of intraocular pressure, the greater the likelihood of glaucomatous field loss and optic nerve damage.

COMBIGAN® is a selective alpha-2 adrenergic receptor agonist with a non-selective beta-adrenergic receptor inhibitor. Both brimonidine and timolol have a rapid onset of action, with peak ocular hypotensive effect seen at two hours post-dosing for brimonidine and one to two hours for timolol.

Fluorophotometric studies in animals and humans suggest that brimonidine tartrate has a dual mechanism of action by reducing aqueous humor production and increasing non-pressure dependent uveoscleral outflow.

Timolol maleate is a $beta_1$ and $beta_2$ adrenergic receptor inhibitor that does not have significant intrinsic sympathomimetic, direct myocardial depressant, or local anesthetic (membrane-stabilizing) activity.

12.3 Pharmacokinetics

Absorption

Systemic absorption of brimonidine and timolol was assessed in healthy volunteers and patients following topical dosing with **COMBIGAN®**. Normal volunteers dosed with one drop of **COMBIGAN®** twice daily in both eyes for seven days showed peak plasma brimonidine and timolol concentrations of 30 pg/mL and 400 pg/mL, respectively. Plasma concentrations of brimonidine peaked at 1 to 4 hours after ocular dosing. Peak plasma concentrations of timolol occurred approximately 1 to 3 hours post-dose. In a crossover study of **COMBIGAN®**, brimonidine tartrate 0.2%, and timolol 0.5% administered twice daily for 7 days in healthy volunteers, the mean brimonidine area-under-the-plasma-concentration-time curve (AUC) for **COMBIGAN®** was 128 ± 61 pg•hr/mL versus 141 ± 106 pg•hr/mL for the respective monotherapy treatments; mean C_{max} values of brimonidine were comparable following **COMBIGAN®** treatment versus monotherapy (32.7 ± 15.0 pg/mL versus 34.7 ± 22.6 pg/mL, respectively). Mean timolol AUC for **COMBIGAN®** was similar to that of the respective monotherapy treatment (2919 ± 1679 pg•hr/mL versus 2909 ± 1231 pg•hr/mL, respectively); mean C_{max} of timolol was approximately 20% lower following **COMBIGAN®** treatment versus monotherapy.

In a parallel study in patients dosed twice daily with **COMBIGAN®**, twice daily with timolol 0.5%, or three times daily with brimonidine tartrate 0.2%, one-hour post dose plasma concentrations of timolol and brimonidine were approximately 30-40% lower with **COMBIGAN®** than their respective monotherapy values. The lower plasma brimonidine concentrations with **COMBIGAN®** appears to be due to twice-daily dosing for **COMBIGAN®** versus three-times dosing with brimonidine tartrate 0.2%.

Distribution

The protein binding of timolol is approximately 60%. The protein binding of brimonidine has not been studied.

Metabolism

In humans, brimonidine is extensively metabolized by the liver. Timolol is partially metabolized by the liver.

Excretion

In the crossover study in healthy volunteers, the plasma concentration of brimonidine declined with a systemic half-life of approximately 3 hours. The apparent systemic half-life of timolol was about 7 hours after ocular administration.

Urinary excretion is the major route of elimination of brimonidine and its metabolites. Approximately 87% of an orally-administered radioactive dose of brimonidine was eliminated within 120 hours, with 74% found in the urine. Unchanged timolol and its metabolites are excreted by the kidney.

Special Populations

COMBIGAN® has not been studied in patients with hepatic impairment.

COMBIGAN® has not been studied in patients with renal impairment.

A study of patients with renal failure showed that timolol was not readily removed by dialysis. The effect of dialysis on brimonidine pharmacokinetics in patients with renal failure is not known.

Following oral administration of timolol maleate, the plasma half-life of timolol is essentially unchanged in patients with moderate renal insufficiency.

13 NONCLINICAL TOXICOLOGY

13.1 Carcinogenesis, Mutagenesis, and Impairment of Fertility

With brimonidine tartrate, no compound-related carcinogenic effects were observed in either mice or rats following a 21-month and 24-month study, respectively. In these studies, dietary administration of brimonidine tartrate at doses up to 2.5 mg/kg/day in mice and 1 mg/kg/day in rats achieved 150 and 210 times, respectively, the plasma C_{max} drug concentration in humans treated with one drop **COMBIGAN®** into both eyes twice daily, the recommended daily human dose.

In a two-year study of timolol maleate administered orally to rats, there was a statistically significant increase in the incidence of adrenal pheochromocytomas in male rats administered 300 mg/kg/day [approximately 25,000 times the maximum recommended human ocular dose of 0.012 mg/kg/day on a mg/kg basis (MRHOD)]. Similar differences were not observed in rats administered oral doses equivalent to approximately 8,300 times the daily dose of **COMBIGAN®** in humans.

In a lifetime oral study of timolol maleate in mice, there were statistically significant increases in the incidence of benign and malignant pulmonary tumors, benign uterine polyps and mammary adenocarcinomas in female mice at 500 mg/kg/day, (approximately 42,000 times the MRHOD), but not at 5 or 50 mg/kg/day (approximately 420 to 4,200 times higher, respectively, than the MRHOD). In a subsequent study in female mice, in which post-mortem examinations were limited to the uterus and the lungs, a statistically significant increase in the incidence of pulmonary tumors was again observed at 500 mg/kg/day.

The increased occurrence of mammary adenocarcinomas was associated with elevations in serum prolactin which occurred in female mice administered oral timolol at 500 mg/kg/day, but not at doses of 5 or 50 mg/kg/day. An increased incidence of mammary adenocarcinomas in rodents has been associated with administration of several other therapeutic agents that elevate serum prolactin, but no correlation between serum prolactin levels and mammary tumors has been established in humans. Furthermore, in adult human female subjects who received oral dosages of up to 60 mg of timolol maleate (the maximum recommended human oral dosage), there were no clinically meaningful changes in serum prolactin.

Brimonidine tartrate was not mutagenic or clastogenic in a series of in vitro and in vivo studies including the Ames bacterial reversion test, chromosomal aberration assay in Chinese Hamster Ovary (CHO) cells, and three in vivo studies in CD-1 mice: a host-mediated assay, cytogenetic study, and dominant lethal assay.

Timolol maleate was devoid of mutagenic potential when tested in vivo (mouse) in the micronucleus test and cytogenetic assay (doses up to 800 mg/kg) and in vitro in a neoplastic cell transformation assay (up to 100 mcg/mL). In Ames tests the highest concentrations of timolol employed, 5,000 or 10,000 mcg/plate, were associated with statistically significant elevations of revertants observed with tester strain TA100 (in seven replicate assays), but not in the remaining three strains. In the assays with tester strain TA100, no consistent dose response relationship was observed, and the ratio of test to control revertants did not reach 2. A ratio of 2 is usually considered the criterion for a positive Ames test.

Reproduction and fertility studies in rats with timolol maleate and in rats with brimonidine tartrate demonstrated no adverse effect on male or female fertility at doses up to approximately 100 times the systemic exposure following the maximum recommended human ophthalmic dose of **COMBIGAN®**.

14 CLINICAL STUDIES

Clinical studies were conducted to compare the IOP-lowering effect over the course of the day of **COMBIGAN®** administered twice a day (BID) to individually-administered brimonidine tartrate ophthalmic solution, 0.2% administered three times per day (TID) and timolol maleate ophthalmic solution, 0.5% BID in patients with glaucoma or ocular hypertension. **COMBIGAN®** BID provided an additional 1 to 3 mm Hg decrease in IOP over brimonidine treatment TID and an additional 1 to 2 mm Hg decrease over timolol treatment BID during the first 7 hours post dosing. However, the IOP-lowering of **COMBIGAN®** BID was less (approximately 1-2 mm Hg) than that seen with the concomitant administration of 0.5% timolol BID and 0.2% brimonidine tartrate TID.

COMBIGAN® administered BID had a favorable safety profile versus concurrently administered brimonidine TID and timolol BID in the self-reported level of severity of sleepiness for patients over age 40.

16 HOW SUPPLIED/STORAGE AND HANDLING

COMBIGAN® is supplied sterile, in white opaque plastic LDPE bottles and tips, with blue high impact polystyrene (HIPS) caps as follows:

5 mL in 10 mL bottle NDC 0023-9211-05
10 mL in 10 mL bottle NDC 0023-9211-10

Storage:

Store between 15° to 25°C (59° to 77°F). Protect from light.

17 PATIENT COUNSELING INFORMATION

Patients with bronchial asthma, a history of bronchial asthma, severe chronic obstructive pulmonary disease, sinus bradycardia, second or third degree atrioventricular block, or cardiac failure should be advised not to take this product (see **CONTRAINDICATIONS**, 4).

Patients should be instructed that ocular solutions, if handled improperly or if the tip of the dispensing container contacts the eye or surrounding structures, can become contaminated by common bacteria known to cause ocular infections. Serious damage to the eye and subsequent loss of vision may result from using contaminated solutions (see **WARNINGS AND PRECAUTIONS**, 5.9).

Patients also should be advised that if they have ocular surgery or develop an intercurrent ocular condition (e.g., trauma or infection), they should immediately seek their physician's advice concerning the continued use of the present multidose container.

If more than one topical ophthalmic drug is being used, the drugs should be administered at least five minutes apart.

Patients should be advised that **COMBIGAN®** contains benzalkonium chloride which may be absorbed by soft contact lenses. Contact lenses should be removed prior to administration of the solution. Lenses may be reinserted 15 minutes following administration of **COMBIGAN®**.

As with other similar medications, **COMBIGAN®** may cause fatigue and/or drowsiness in some patients. Patients who engage in hazardous activities should be cautioned of the potential for a decrease in mental alertness.

Irvine, CA 92612, U.S.A.
® mark owned by Allergan, Inc.
U.S. Patents 6,248,741; 6,194,415; 6,465,464; and 7,030,149
72060US10X

Shown in Product Identification Guide, page 305

LUMIGAN® ℞
(bimatoprost ophthalmic solution) 0.03%

DESCRIPTION

LUMIGAN® (bimatoprost ophthalmic solution) 0.03% is a synthetic prostamide analog with ocular hypotensive activity. Its chemical name is (Z)-7-[(1R,2R,3R,5S)-3,5-Dihydroxy-2-[1E,3S)-3-hydroxy-5-phenyl-1-pentenyl]cyclopentyl]-5-N-ethylheptenamide, and its molecular weight is 415.58. Its molecular formula is $C_{25}H_{37}NO_4$. Its chemical structure is:

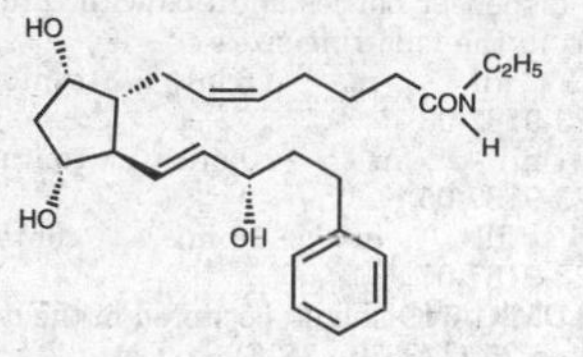

Bimatoprost is a powder, which is very soluble in ethyl alcohol and methyl alcohol and slightly soluble in water. **LUMIGAN®** is a clear, isotonic, colorless, sterile ophthalmic solution with an osmolality of approximately 290 mOsmol/kg.

Contains: Active: bimatoprost 0.3 mg/mL; **Preservative:** Benzalkonium chloride 0.05 mg/mL; **Inactives:** Sodium chloride; sodium phosphate, dibasic; citric acid; and purified water. Sodium hydroxide and/or hydrochloric acid may be added to adjust pH. The pH during its shelf life ranges from 6.8-7.8.

CLINICAL PHARMACOLOGY

Mechanism of Action: Bimatoprost is a prostamide, a synthetic structural analog of prostaglandin with ocular hypotensive activity. It selectively mimics the effects of naturally occurring substances, prostamides. Bimatoprost is believed to lower intraocular pressure (IOP) in humans by increasing outflow of aqueous humor through both the trabecular meshwork and uveoscleral routes. Elevated IOP presents a major risk factor for glaucomatous field loss. The higher the level of IOP, the greater the likelihood of optic nerve damage and visual field loss.

Pharmacokinetics

Absorption: After one drop of bimatoprost ophthalmic solution 0.03% was administered once daily to both eyes of 15 healthy subjects for two weeks, blood concentrations peaked within 10 minutes after dosing and were below the lower limit of detection (0.025 ng/mL) in most subjects within 1.5 hours after dosing. Mean C_{max} and AUC_{0-24hr} values were similar on days 7 and 14 at approximately 0.08 ng/mL and 0.09 ng•hr/mL, respectively, indicating that steady state was reached during the first week of ocular dosing. There was no significant systemic drug accumulation over time.

Distribution: Bimatoprost is moderately distributed into body tissues with a steady-state volume of distribution of 0.67 L/kg. In human blood, bimatoprost resides mainly in the plasma. Approximately 12% of bimatoprost remains unbound in human plasma.

Metabolism: Bimatoprost is the major circulating species in the blood once it reaches the systemic circulation following ocular dosing. Bimatoprost then undergoes oxidation, N-deethylation and glucuronidation to form a diverse variety of metabolites.

Elimination: Following an intravenous dose of radiolabeled bimatoprost (3.12 µg/kg) to six healthy subjects, the maximum blood concentration of unchanged drug was 12.2 ng/mL and decreased rapidly with an elimination half-life of approximately 45 minutes. The total blood clearance of bimatoprost was 1.5 L/hr/kg. Up to 67% of the administered dose was excreted in the urine while 25% of the dose was recovered in the feces.

Clinical Studies:

In clinical studies of patients with open angle glaucoma or ocular hypertension with a mean baseline IOP of 26 mmHg, the IOP-lowering effect of **LUMIGAN®** (bimatoprost ophthalmic solution) 0.03% once daily (in the evening) was 7-8 mmHg.

Results of dosing for up to five years with products in this drug class showed that the onset of noticeable increased iris pigmentation occurred within the first year of treatment for the majority of the patients who developed noticeable iris pigmentation. Patients continued to show sign of increasing iris pigmentation throughout the five years of the study. Observation of increased iris pigmentation did not affect the incidence, nature or severity of adverse events (other than increased iris pigmentation) recorded in the study. IOP reduction was similar regardless of the development of increased iris pigmentation during the study.

In patients with a history of liver disease or abnormal ALT, AST and/or bilirubin at baseline, **LUMIGAN®** had no adverse effect on liver function over 48 months.

INDICATIONS AND USAGE

LUMIGAN® (bimatoprost ophthalmic solution) 0.03% is indicated for the reduction of elevated intraocular pressure in patients with open angle glaucoma or ocular hypertension.

CONTRAINDICATIONS

LUMIGAN® (bimatoprost ophthalmic solution) 0.03% is contraindicated in patients with hypersensitivity to bimatoprost or any other ingredient in this product.

WARNINGS

LUMIGAN® (bimatoprost ophthalmic solution) 0.03% has been reported to cause changes to pigmented tissues. The most frequently reported changes have been increased pigmentation of the iris, periorbital tissue (eyelid) and eyelashes, and growth of eyelashes. Pigmentation is expected to increase as long as **LUMIGAN®** is administered. After discontinuation of **LUMIGAN®** pigmentation of the iris is likely to be permanent while pigmentation of the periorbital tissue and eyelash changes have been reported to be reversible in some patients. Patients who receive treatment should be informed of the possibility of increased pigmentation. The effects of increased pigmentation beyond 5 years are not known.

PRECAUTIONS

General: LUMIGAN® (bimatoprost ophthalmic solution) 0.03% may gradually increase the pigmentation of the iris. The eye color change is due to increased melanin content in the stromal melanocytes of the iris rather than to an increase in the number of melanocytes. This change may not be noticeable for several months to years (see WARNINGS). Typically, the brown pigmentation around the pupil spreads concentrically towards the periphery of the iris and the entire iris or parts of the iris become more brownish. Neither nevi nor freckles of the iris appear to be affected by treatment. While treatment with **LUMIGAN®** can be continued in patients who develop noticeably increased iris pigmentation, these patients should be examined regularly.

During clinical trials, the increase in brown iris pigment has not been shown to progress further upon discontinuation of treatment, but the resultant color change may be permanent.

Eyelid skin darkening, which may be reversible upon discontinuation of the treatment has been reported in association with the use of **LUMIGAN®**.

LUMIGAN® may gradually change eyelashes and vellus hair in the treated eye; these changes include increased length, thickness and number of lashes. Eyelash changes are usually reversible upon discontinuation of treatment.

LUMIGAN® (bimatoprost ophthalmic solution) 0.03% should be used with caution in patients with active intraocular inflammation (e.g., uveitis).

Macular edema, including cystoid macular edema, has been reported during treatment with bimatoprost ophthalmic solution. **LUMIGAN®** should be used with caution in aphakic patients, in pseudophakic patients with a torn posterior lens capsule, or in patients with known risk factors for macular edema.

LUMIGAN® has not been evaluated for the treatment of angle closure, inflammatory or neovascular glaucoma.

There have been reports of bacterial keratitis associated with the use of multiple-dose containers of topical ophthalmic products. These containers had been inadvertently contaminated by patients who, in most cases, had a concurrent corneal disease or a disruption of the ocular epithelial surface (see **PRECAUTIONS,** Information for Patients).

Contact lenses should be removed prior to instillation of **LUMIGAN®** and may be reinserted 15 minutes following its administration (see **PRECAUTIONS,** Information for Patients).

Information for Patients: (see WARNINGS and PRECAUTIONS): Patients should be advised about the potential for increased brown pigmentation of the iris, which may be permanent. Patients should also be informed about the possibility of eyelid skin darkening, which may be reversible after discontinuation of **LUMIGAN®**.

Patients should also be informed of the possibility of eyelash and vellus hair changes in the treated eye during treatment with **LUMIGAN®**. These changes may result in a disparity between eyes in length, thickness, pigmentation, number of eyelashes or vellus hairs, and/or direction of eyelash growth. Eyelash changes are usually reversible upon discontinuation of treatment.

Patients should be instructed to avoid allowing the tip of the dispensing container to contact the eye, surrounding structures, fingers, or any other surface in order to avoid contamination of the solution by common bacteria known to cause ocular infections. Serious damage to the eye and subsequent loss of vision may result from using contaminated solutions.

Patients should also be advised that if they develop an intercurrent ocular condition (e.g., trauma or infection) or have ocular surgery, they should immediately seek their physician's advice concerning the continued use of the multidose container.

Patients should be advised that if they develop any ocular reactions, particularly conjunctivitis and eyelid reactions, they should immediately seek their physician's advice.

Patients should be advised that **LUMIGAN®** contains benzalkonium chloride, which may be absorbed by soft contact lenses. Contact lenses should be removed prior to instillation of **LUMIGAN®** and may be reinserted 15 minutes following its administration.

If more than one topical ophthalmic drug is being used, the drugs should be administered at least five (5) minutes between applications.

Carcinogenesis, Mutagenesis, Impairment of fertility: Bimatoprost was not carcinogenic in either mice or rats when administered by oral gavage at doses of up to 2 mg/kg/day and 1mg/kg/day respectively (approximately 192 times and 291 times the recommended human exposure based on blood AUC levels respectively) for 104 weeks.

Bimatoprost was not mutagenic or clastogenic in the Ames test, in the mouse lymphoma test, or in the *in vivo* mouse micronucleus tests.

Bimatoprost did not impair fertility in male or female rats up to doses of 0.6 mg/kg/day (approximately 103 times the recommended human exposure based on blood AUC levels).

Pregnancy: Teratogenic effects: *Pregnancy Category C.* In embryo/fetal developmental studies in pregnant mice and rats, abortion was observed at oral doses of bimatoprost which achieved at least 33 or 97 times, respectively, the intended human exposure based on blood AUC levels.

At doses 41 times the intended human exposure based on blood AUC levels, the gestation length was reduced in the dams, the incidence of dead fetuses, late resorptions, peri- and postnatal pup mortality was increased, and pup body weights were reduced.

There are no adequate and well-controlled studies of **LUMIGAN®** administration in pregnant women. Because animal reproductive studies are not always predictive of human response, **LUMIGAN®** should be administered during pregnancy only if the potential benefit justifies the potential risk to the fetus.

Nursing mothers: It is not known whether **LUMIGAN®** is excreted in human milk, although in animal studies, bimatoprost has been shown to be excreted in breast milk. Because many drugs are excreted in human milk, caution should be exercised when **LUMIGAN®** is administered to a nursing woman.

Pediatric Use: Safety and effectiveness in pediatric patients have not been established.

Geriatric Use: No overall clinical differences in safety or effectiveness have been observed between elderly and other adult patients.

ADVERSE REACTIONS

In clinical trials, the most frequent events associated with the use of **LUMIGAN®** (bimatoprost ophthalmic solution) 0.03% occurring in approximately 15% to 45% of patients, in descending order of incidence, included conjunctival hyperemia, growth of eyelashes, and ocular pruritus. Approximately 3% of patients discontinued therapy due to conjunctival hyperemia.

Ocular adverse events occurring in approximately 3 to 10% of patients, in descending order of incidence, included ocular dryness, visual disturbance, ocular burning, foreign body sensation, eye pain, pigmentation of the periocular skin, blepharitis, cataract, superficial punctate keratitis, eyelid erythema, ocular irritation, and eyelash darkening. The following ocular adverse events reported in approximately 1 to 3% of patients, in descending order of incidence, included: eye discharge, tearing, photophobia, allergic conjunctivitis, asthenopia, increases in iris pigmentation, and conjunctival edema. In less than 1% of patients, intraocular inflammation was reported as iritis.

Systemic adverse events reported in approximately 10% of patients were infections (primarily colds and upper respiratory tract infections). The following systemic adverse events reported in approximately 1 to 5% of patients, in descending order of incidence, included headaches, abnormal liver function tests, asthenia and hirsutism.

OVERDOSAGE

No information is available on overdosage in humans. If overdose with **LUMIGAN®** (bimatoprost ophthalmic solution) 0.03% occurs, treatment should be symptomatic.

In oral (by gavage) mouse and rat studies, doses up to 100 mg/kg/day did not produce any toxicity. This dose expressed as mg/m^2 is at least 70 times higher than the accidental dose of one bottle of **LUMIGAN®** for a 10 kg child.

DOSAGE AND ADMINISTRATION

The recommended dosage is one drop in the affected eye(s) once daily in the evening. The dosage of **LUMIGAN®** (bimatoprost ophthalmic solution) 0.03% should not exceed once daily since it has been shown that more frequent administration may decrease the intraocular pressure lowering effect.

Reduction of the intraocular pressure starts approximately 4 hours after the first administration with maximum effect reached within approximately 8 to 12 hours.

LUMIGAN® may be used concomitantly with other topical ophthalmic drug products to lower intraocular pressure. If more than one topical ophthalmic drug is being used, the drugs should be administered at least five (5) minutes apart.

HOW SUPPLIED

LUMIGAN® (bimatoprost ophthalmic solution) 0.03% is supplied sterile in opaque white low density polyethylene ophthalmic dispenser bottles and tips with turquoise polystyrene caps in the following sizes:

2.5 mL fill in 5 mL container - NDC 0023-9187-03

5 mL fill in 10 mL container - NDC 0023-9187-05

7.5 mL fill in 10 mL container - NDC 0023-9187-07

Storage: **LUMIGAN®** should be stored in the original container at 2° to 25°C (36° to 77°F).

Rx only

Revised September 2006

Irvine, CA 92612
® marks owned by Allergan, Inc.
U.S. Patents 5,688,819 and 6,403,649
71669US11T

Shown in Product Identification Guide, page 305

RESTASIS® ℞

(cyclosporine ophthalmic emulsion) 0.05%
Sterile, Preservative-Free

DESCRIPTION

RESTASIS® (cyclosporine ophthalmic emulsion) 0.05% contains a topical immunomodulator with anti-inflammatory effects. Cyclosporine's chemical name is Cyclo[[(*E*)-(2*S*,3*R*,4*R*)-3-hydroxy-4-methyl-2-(methylamino)-6-octenoyl]-L-2-aminobutyryl-*N*-methylglycyl-*N*-methyl-L-leucyl-L-valyl-*N*-methyl-L-leucyl-L-alanyl-D-alanyl-*N*-methyl-L-leucyl-*N*-methyl-L-leucyl-*N*-methyl-L-valyl] and it has the following structure:

Structural Formula

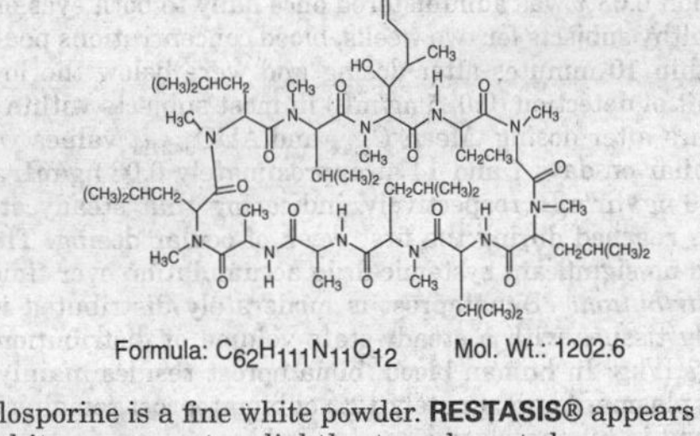

Formula: $C_{62}H_{111}N_{11}O_{12}$ Mol. Wt.: 1202.6

Cyclosporine is a fine white powder. **RESTASIS®** appears as a white opaque to slightly translucent homogeneous emulsion. It has an osmolality of 230 to 320 mOsmol/kg and a pH of 6.5-8.0. Each mL of **RESTASIS®** ophthalmic emulsion contains: **Active:** cyclosporine 0.05%. **Inactives:** glycerin; castor oil; polysorbate 80; carbomer copolymer type A; purified water; and sodium hydroxide to adjust pH.

CLINICAL PHARMACOLOGY

Mechanism of Action

Cyclosporine is an immunosuppressive agent when administered systemically.

In patients whose tear production is presumed to be suppressed due to ocular inflammation associated with keratoconjunctivitis sicca, cyclosporine emulsion is thought to act as a partial immunomodulator. The exact mechanism of action is not known.

Pharmacokinetics

Blood cyclosporin A concentrations were measured using a specific high pressure liquid chromatography-mass spectrometry assay. Blood concentrations of cyclosporine, in all the samples collected, after topical administration of **RESTASIS®** 0.05%, BID, in humans for up to 12 months, were below the quantitation limit of 0.1 ng/mL. There was no detectable drug accumulation in blood during 12 months of treatment with **RESTASIS®** ophthalmic emulsion.

Clinical Evaluations

Four multicenter, randomized, adequate and well-controlled clinical studies were performed in approximately 1200 patients with moderate to severe keratoconjunctivitis sicca. **RESTASIS®** demonstrated statistically significant increases in Schirmer wetting of 10 mm versus vehicle at six months in patients whose tear production was presumed to be suppressed due to ocular inflammation. This effect was seen in approximately 15% of **RESTASIS®** ophthalmic emulsion treated patients versus approximately 5% of vehicle treated patients. Increased tear production was not seen in patients currently taking topical anti-inflammatory drugs or using punctal plugs.

No increase in bacterial or fungal ocular infections was reported following administration of **RESTASIS®**.

INDICATIONS AND USAGE

RESTASIS® ophthalmic emulsion is indicated to increase tear production in patients whose tear production is presumed to be suppressed due to ocular inflammation associated with keratoconjunctivitis sicca. Increased tear production was not seen in patients currently taking topical anti-inflammatory drugs or using punctal plugs.

CONTRAINDICATIONS

RESTASIS® is contraindicated in patients with active ocular infections and in patients with known or suspected hypersensitivity to any of the ingredients in the formulation.

WARNING

RESTASIS® ophthalmic emulsion has not been studied in patients with a history of herpes keratitis.

PRECAUTIONS

General: For ophthalmic use only.

Information for Patients

The emulsion from one individual single-use vial is to be used immediately after opening for administration to one or both eyes, and the remaining contents should be discarded immediately after administration.

Do not allow the tip of the vial to touch the eye or any surface, as this may contaminate the emulsion.

RESTASIS® should not be administered while wearing contact lenses. Patients with decreased tear production typically should not wear contact lenses. If contact lenses are worn, they should be removed prior to the administration of the emulsion. Lenses may be reinserted 15 minutes following administration of **RESTASIS®** ophthalmic emulsion.

Carcinogenesis, Mutagenesis, and Impairment of Fertility

Systemic carcinogenicity studies were carried out in male and female mice and rats. In the 78-week oral (diet) mouse study, at doses of 1, 4, and 16 mg/kg/day, evidence of a statistically significant trend was found for lymphocytic lymphomas in females, and the incidence of hepatocellular carcinomas in mid-dose males significantly exceeded the control value.

In the 24-month oral (diet) rat study, conducted at 0.5, 2, and 8 mg/kg/day, pancreatic islet cell adenomas significantly exceeded the control rate in the low dose level. The hepatocellular carcinomas and pancreatic islet cell adenomas were not dose related. The low doses in mice and rats are approximately 1000 and 500 times greater, respectively, than the daily human dose of one drop (28 µL) of 0.05% **RESTASIS®** BID into each eye of a 60 kg person (0.001 mg/kg/day), assuming that the entire dose is absorbed.

Cyclosporine has not been found mutagenic/genotoxic in the Ames Test, the V79-HGPRT Test, the micronucleus test in mice and Chinese hamsters, the chromosome-aberration tests in Chinese hamster bone-marrow, the mouse dominant lethal assay, and the DNA-repair test in sperm from treated mice. A study analyzing sister chromatid exchange (SCE) induction by cyclosporine using human lymphocytes *in vitro* gave indication of a positive effect (i.e., induction of SCE).

No impairment in fertility was demonstrated in studies in male and female rats receiving oral doses of cyclosporine up to 15 mg/kg/day (approximately 15,000 times the human daily dose of 0.001 mg/kg/day) for 9 weeks (male) and 2 weeks (female) prior to mating.

Pregnancy-Teratogenic Effects

Pregnancy category C.

Teratogenic Effects: No evidence of teratogenicity was observed in rats or rabbits receiving oral doses of cyclosporine up to 300 mg/kg/day during organogenesis. These doses in rats and rabbits are approximately 300,000 times greater than the daily human dose of one drop (28 µL) 0.05% **RESTASIS®** BID into each eye of a 60 kg person (0.001 mg/kg/day), assuming that the entire dose is absorbed.

Non-Teratogenic Effects: Adverse effects were seen in reproduction studies in rats and rabbits only at dose levels toxic to dams. At toxic doses (rats at 30 mg/kg/day and rabbits at 100 mg/kg/day), cyclosporine oral solution, USP, was embryo- and fetotoxic as indicated by increased pre- and postnatal mortality and reduced fetal weight together with related skeletal retardations. These doses are 30,000 and 100,000 times greater, respectively than the daily human dose of one drop (28 µL) of 0.05% **RESTASIS®** BID into each eye of a 60 kg person (0.001 mg/kg/day), assuming that the entire dose is absorbed. No evidence of embryofetal toxicity was observed in rats or rabbits receiving cyclosporine at oral doses up to 17 mg/kg/day or 30 mg/kg/day, respectively, during organogenesis. These doses in rats and rabbits are approximately 17,000 and 30,000 times greater, respectively, than the daily human dose.

Offspring of rats receiving a 45 mg/kg/day oral dose of cyclosporine from Day 15 of pregnancy until Day 21 postpartum, a maternally toxic level, exhibited an increase in postnatal mortality; this dose is 45,000 times greater than the daily human topical dose, 0.001 mg/kg/day, assuming that the entire dose is absorbed. No adverse events were observed at oral doses up to 15 mg/kg/day (15,000 times greater than the daily human dose).

There are no adequate and well-controlled studies of **RESTASIS®** in pregnant women. **RESTASIS®** should be administered to a pregnant woman only if clearly needed.

Nursing Mothers

Cyclosporine is known to be excreted in human milk following systemic administration but excretion in human milk after topical treatment has not been investigated. Although blood concentrations are undetectable after topical administration of **RESTASIS®** ophthalmic emulsion, caution should be exercised when **RESTASIS®** is administered to a nursing woman.

Pediatric Use

The safety and efficacy of **RESTASIS®** ophthalmic emulsion have not been established in pediatric patients below the age of 16.

Geriatric Use

No overall difference in safety or effectiveness has been observed between elderly and younger patients.

ADVERSE REACTIONS

The most common adverse event following the use of **RESTASIS®** was ocular burning (17%).

Other events reported in 1% to 5% of patients included conjunctival hyperemia, discharge, epiphora, eye pain, foreign body sensation, pruritus, stinging, and visual disturbance (most often blurring).

DOSAGE AND ADMINISTRATION

Invert the unit dose vial a few times to obtain a uniform, white, opaque emulsion before using. Instill one drop of **RESTASIS®** ophthalmic emulsion twice a day in each eye approximately 12 hours apart. **RESTASIS®** can be used concomitantly with artificial tears, allowing a 15 minute interval between products. Discard vial immediately after use.

HOW SUPPLIED

RESTASIS® ophthalmic emulsion is packaged in single use vials. Each vial contains 0.4 mL fill in a 0.9 mL LDPE vial; 30 vials are packaged in a polypropylene tray with an aluminum peelable lid. The entire contents of each tray (30 vials) must be dispensed intact. **RESTASIS®** is also provided in a 60 count (2 × 30) package (one month supply) that must be dispensed intact.

30 Vials 0.4 mL each - NDC 0023-9163-30

60 (2 × 30) Vials 0.4 mL each - NDC 0023-9163-60

Storage: Store **RESTASIS®** ophthalmic emulsion at 15-25° C (59-77° F).

KEEP OUT OF THE REACH OF CHILDREN.

Rx Only

Revised: 02/2010

© 2010 Allergan, Inc.

Irvine, CA 92612, U.S.A.

® marks owned by Allergan, Inc.

U.S. Patent 5,474,979

Made in the U.S.A.

71876US14B

Shown in Product Identification Guide, page 305

SANCTURA XR®   ℞

(trospium chloride extended release capsules)

HIGHLIGHTS OF PRESCRIBING INFORMATION

These highlights do not include all the information needed to use SANCTURA XR® safely and effectively. See full prescribing information for SANCTURA XR®.

SANCTURA XR® (trospium chloride extended release capsules)

Initial U.S. Approval: May 2004

————————**INDICATIONS AND USAGE**————————

SANCTURA XR® is an anticholinergic indicated for the treatment of overactive bladder (OAB) with symptoms of urge urinary incontinence, urgency, and urinary frequency. (1)

————————**DOSAGE AND ADMINISTRATION**————————

The recommended dosage of **SANCTURA XR®** is one 60 mg capsule daily in the morning.

SANCTURA XR® should be dosed with water on an empty stomach, at least one hour before a meal. (2)

SANCTURA XR® is not recommended for use in patients with severe renal impairment (creatinine clearance < 30 mL/minute). (2)

————————**DOSAGE FORMS AND STRENGTHS**————————

• 60 mg capsules (white opaque body and orange opaque cap, printed with SAN 60) (3)

————————**CONTRAINDICATIONS**————————

SANCTURA XR® is contraindicated in patients with urinary retention, gastric retention, or uncontrolled narrow-angle glaucoma, and in patients who are at risk for these conditions. (4)

————————**WARNINGS AND PRECAUTIONS**————————

SANCTURA XR® should be administered with caution to patients with clinically significant bladder outflow obstruction or gastrointestinal obstructive disorders due to risk of urinary or gastric retention. (5.1, 5.2)

In patients with narrow angle glaucoma **SANCTURA XR®** should be used only with careful monitoring. (5.3)

SANCTURA XR® is not recommended for use in patients with severe renal impairment (creatinine clearance < 30 mL/minute). (5.4)

Alcohol should not be consumed within 2 hours of **SANCTURA XR®** administration. (5.5)

————————**ADVERSE REACTIONS**————————

The most common adverse reactions with **SANCTURA XR®** were dry mouth (10.7%) and constipation (8.5%). (6.1)

To report SUSPECTED ADVERSE REACTIONS, contact Allergan, Inc. at 1-800-433-8871 or FDA at 1-800-FDA-1088 or www.fda.gov/medwatch.

————————**DRUG INTERACTIONS**————————

Trospium is metabolized by ester hydrolysis and excreted by the kidneys through a combination of tubular secretion and glomerular filtration. (7)

Based on *in vitro* data, no clinically relevant metabolic drug-drug interactions are anticipated with **SANCTURA XR®**. (7)

Some drugs which are actively secreted by the kidney may interact with **SANCTURA XR®** by competing for renal tubular secretion. (7)

• Concomitant use with digoxin did not affect the pharmacokinetics of either drug (7.1)

• Exposure to trospium on average was comparable in the presence of and without antacid, however, some individuals demonstrated increases or decreases in trospium exposure in the presence of antacid. The clinical relevance of these findings is not known. (7.2)

• The oral bioavailability was reduced following a high fat-content meal (7.3)

————————**USE IN SPECIFIC POPULATIONS**————————

• PREGNANCY CATEGORY C

• In post-parturition animal studies trospium chloride was excreted to a limited extent into the milk (8.3)

• The safety and effectiveness of **SANCTURA XR®** in pediatric patients have not been established. (8.4)

• **SANCTURA XR®** is not recommended for use in patients with severe renal impairment (8.6)

• Caution is advised when **SANCTURA XR®** is used in patients with moderate to severe hepatic impairment (8.7)

See 17 for PATIENT COUNSELING INFORMATION and FDA-approved patient labeling

Revised: 09/2009

FULL PRESCRIBING INFORMATION: CONTENTS*

1   INDICATIONS AND USAGE

2   DOSAGE AND ADMINISTRATION

3   DOSAGE FORMS AND STRENGTHS

4   CONTRAINDICATIONS

5   WARNINGS AND PRECAUTIONS

    5.1   Risk of Urinary Retention

    5.2   Decreased Gastrointestinal Motility

    5.3   Controlled Narrow-angle Glaucoma

    5.4   Patients with Severe Renal Impairment

    5.5   Alcohol Interaction

6   ADVERSE REACTIONS

    6.1   Adverse Reactions in Clinical Trials

    6.2   Post-marketing Experience

7   DRUG INTERACTIONS

    7.1   Digoxin

    7.2   Antacid

    7.3   Food Interaction

8   USE IN SPECIFIC POPULATIONS

    8.1   Pregnancy

    8.2   Labor and Delivery

    8.3   Nursing Mothers

    8.4   Pediatric Use

    8.5   Geriatric Use

    8.6   Renal Impairment

    8.7   Hepatic Impairment

10   OVERDOSAGE

11   DESCRIPTION

12   CLINICAL PHARMACOLOGY

    12.1   Mechanism of Action

    12.2   Pharmacodynamics

    12.3   Pharmacokinetics

13   NONCLINICAL TOXICOLOGY

    13.1   Carcinogenesis, Mutagenesis, Impairment of Fertility

14   CLINICAL STUDIES

16   HOW SUPPLIED/STORAGE AND HANDLING

17   PATIENT COUNSELING INFORMATION

* Sections or subsections omitted from the full prescribing information are not listed

FULL PRESCRIBING INFORMATION

1   INDICATIONS AND USAGE

SANCTURA XR® is indicated for the treatment of overactive bladder (OAB) with symptoms of urge urinary incontinence, urgency, and urinary frequency.

2   DOSAGE AND ADMINISTRATION

The recommended dosage of **SANCTURA XR®** is one 60 mg capsule daily in the morning. **SANCTURA XR®** capsules should be dosed with water on an empty stomach, at least one hour before a meal.

SANCTURA XR® is not recommended for use in patients with severe renal impairment (creatinine clearance < 30 mL/minute) (see *Warnings and Precautions (5)*, *Use in Specific Populations (8)*, and *Clinical Pharmacology (12)*).

3   DOSAGE FORMS AND STRENGTHS

SANCTURA XR® is supplied as 60 mg capsules (white opaque body and orange opaque cap, printed with SAN 60).

4   CONTRAINDICATIONS

SANCTURA XR® is contraindicated in patients with urinary retention, gastric retention, or uncontrolled narrow-angle glaucoma and in patients who are at risk for these conditions. **SANCTURA XR®** is also contraindicated in patients who have demonstrated hypersensitivity to the drug or any of its ingredients.

5   WARNINGS AND PRECAUTIONS

5.1   Risk of Urinary Retention

SANCTURA XR® capsules should be administered with caution to patients with clinically significant bladder outflow obstruction because of the risk of urinary retention (see *Contraindications (4)*).

5.2   Decreased Gastrointestinal Motility

SANCTURA XR® should be administered with caution to patients with gastrointestinal obstructive disorders because of the risk of gastric retention. **SANCTURA XR®**, like other antimuscarinic agents, may decrease gastrointestinal motility and should be used with caution in patients with conditions such as ulcerative colitis, intestinal atony and myasthenia gravis (see *Contraindications (4)*).

5.3   Controlled Narrow-angle Glaucoma

In patients being treated for narrow-angle glaucoma, **SANCTURA XR®** should only be used if the potential benefits outweigh the risks, and in that circumstance only with careful monitoring (see *Contraindications (4)*).

5.4   Patients with Severe Renal Impairment

SANCTURA XR® is not recommended for use in patients with severe renal impairment (creatinine clearance < 30 mL/minute) (see *Dosage and Administration (2)*, *Use in Specific Populations (8)*, and *Clinical Pharmacology (12)*).

5.5   Alcohol Interaction

Alcohol should not be consumed within 2 hours of **SANCTURA XR®** administration. In addition, patients should be informed that alcohol may enhance the drowsiness caused by anticholinergic agents.

6   ADVERSE REACTIONS

6.1   Adverse Reactions in Clinical Trials

The data described below reflect exposure to **SANCTURA XR®** capsules in 578 patients for 12 weeks in two Phase 3 double-blind, placebo controlled trials (n = 1165). These studies included overactive bladder patients of ages 21 to 90 years, of which 86% were female and 85% were Caucasian. Patients received 60 mg daily doses of **SANCTURA XR®**. Patients in these studies were eligible to continue treatment with **SANCTURA XR®** 60 mg for up to one year. From both these controlled trials combined, 769 and 238 patients received treatment with **SANCTURA XR®** for at least 24 and 52 weeks, respectively.

There were 157 (27.2%) **SANCTURA XR®** patients and 98 (16.7%) placebo patients who experienced one or more double-blind treatment-emergent adverse events (TEAEs) that were assessed by the investigator as at least possibly related to study medication. The most common TEAEs were dry mouth and constipation which, when reported, commonly occurred early in treatment (often within the first week). In the two Phase 3 studies, constipation, dry mouth, and urinary retention led to discontinuation in 1%, 0.7%, and 0.5% of patients treated with **SANCTURA XR®** 60 mg daily, respectively. In the placebo group, there were no discontinuations due to dry mouth or urinary retention and one due to constipation.

The incidence of serious adverse events was similar among patients receiving **SANCTURA XR®** and patients receiving placebo. No treatment-emergent serious adverse events in either treatment group were judged by the investigators as being possibly related to the study medication.

Table 1 lists those treatment-emergent adverse events from the trials that were assessed by the investigator as possibly related to study medication, reported in at least 1% of **SANCTURA XR®** patients, and were more common for the **SANCTURA XR®** group than for placebo.

Table 1: Incidence of treatment-emergent adverse events reported in at least 1% of patients judged by the investigator as at least possibly related to treatment and more common for the SANCTURA XR® group than for placebo.

MedDRA Preferred term	Number of patients (%)	
	Placebo N = 587	SANCTURA XR® N = 578
Dry Mouth	22 (3.7)	62 (10.7)
Constipation	9 (1.5)	49 (8.5)
Dry eye	1 (0.2)	9 (1.6)
Flatulence	3 (0.5)	9 (1.6)
Nausea	2 (0.3)	8 (1.4)
Abdominal Pain	2 (0.3)	8 (1.4)
Dyspepsia	4 (0.7)	7 (1.2)
Urinary tract infection	5 (0.9)	7 (1.2)
Constipation aggravated	3 (0.5)	7 (1.2)
Abdominal distension	2 (0.3)	6 (1.0)
Nasal dryness	0 (0.0)	6 (1.0)

Additional adverse events reported in less than 1% of SANCTURA XR®-treated patients and more common for SANCTURA XR® than placebo, judged by the investigator at least possibly related to treatment were: vision blurred, feces hard, back pain, somnolence, urinary retention, and dry skin.

Table 2 lists all treatment-emergent adverse events for the trials reported in at least 2% of all SANCTURA XR® patients and more common for the SANCTURA XR® group than for placebo without regard to the investigator's judgment on drug relatedness.

Table 2: Incidence of treatment-emergent adverse events reported in at least 2% of patients regardless of reported relationship to treatment and more common for the SANCTURA XR® group than for placebo.

MedDRA Preferred term	Number of patients (%)	
	Placebo N = 587	SANCTURA XR® N = 578
Dry Mouth	22 (3.7)	64 (11.1)
Constipation	10 (1.7)	52 (9.0)
Urinary tract infection	29 (4.9)	42 (7.3)
Nasopharyngitis	10 (1.7)	17 (2.9)
Influenza	9 (1.5)	13 (2.2)

Additional adverse events reported in less than 2% of SANCTURA XR®-treated patients and twice as frequent for SANCTURA XR® compared to placebo, regardless of reported relationship to treatment were: tachycardia, dry eyes, abdominal pain, dyspepsia, abdominal distension, constipation aggravated, nasal dryness, and rash.

In the open-label treatment phase, the most common TEAEs reported in the 769 patients with at least 6 months exposure to SANCTURA XR® were: constipation, and dry mouth. Urinary tract infection and rash was also reported in several patients, including one of each judged by the investigator to be possibly related to treatment. Several adverse events were reported as severe in the open-label treatment phase, including one urinary tract infection, two urinary retention events, and one aggravated constipation.

Electrophysiology

The effect of 20 mg BID and up to 100 mg BID of an immediate-release formulation of trospium chloride on QT interval was evaluated in a single-blind, randomized, placebo and active (moxifloxacin 400 mg daily) controlled, 5-day parallel trial in 170 male and female healthy volunteer subjects aged 18 to 45 years. The QT interval was measured over a 24-hour period at steady state. Trospium chloride was not associated with an increase in individual corrected (QTcI) or Fridericia corrected (QTcF) QT interval at any time during steady state measurement, while moxifloxacin was associated with a 6.4 msec increase in QTcF. In this study, asymptomatic, non-specific T-wave inversions were observed more often in subjects receiving trospium chloride than in subjects receiving moxifloxacin or placebo following five days of treatment. The clinical significance of T-wave inversion in this study is unknown. This finding was not observed during routine safety monitoring in overactive bladder patients from 2 placebo-controlled clinical trials in 591 patients treated with 20 mg BID of immediate-release trospium chloride, nor was it observed in 2 placebo-controlled clinical trials in 578 patients treated with SANCTURA XR® capsules.

Also in this study, the immediate-release formulation of trospium chloride was associated with an increase in heart rate that correlated with increasing plasma concentration, with a mean elevation in heart rate compared to placebo of 9 beats per minute for the 20 mg dose and of 18 beats per minute for the 100 mg dose. In the two Phase 3 SANCTURA XR® trials the mean increase in heart rate compared to placebo was approximately 3 beats per minute in both studies.

6.2   Post-marketing Experience

The following adverse reactions have been identified during European and US postapproval use of trospium chloride 20 mg BID. Reported events have included: Gastrointestinal – gastritis; Cardiovascular – palpitations, supraventricular tachycardia, chest pain, syncope, "hypertensive crisis"; Immunological – Stevens-Johnson syndrome, anaphylactic reaction; Nervous System – vision abnormal, hallucinations and delirium; Musculoskeletal – rhabdomyolysis; General – rash.

7   DRUG INTERACTIONS

Trospium is metabolized by ester hydrolysis and excreted by the kidneys through a combination of tubular secretion and glomerular filtration. Based on *in vitro* data, no clinically relevant metabolic drug-drug interactions are anticipated with SANCTURA XR®. However, some drugs which are actively secreted by the kidney may interact with SANCTURA XR® by competing for renal tubular secretion.

The concomitant use of SANCTURA XR® with other antimuscarinic agents that produce dry mouth and constipation and other anticholinergic effects may increase the frequency and/or severity of such effects. SANCTURA XR® capsules may potentially alter the absorption of some concomitantly administered drugs due to anticholinergic effects on GI motility.

7.1   Digoxin

Concomitant use of trospium chloride 20mg BID and digoxin did not affect the pharmacokinetics of either drug.

7.2   Antacid

A drug interaction study was conducted to evaluate the effect of an antacid containing aluminum hydroxide and magnesium carbonate on the PK of SANCTURA XR® (n =11). While the systemic exposure of trospium on average was comparable with and without antacid, 5 individuals demonstrated either an increase or decrease in trospium exposure, in presence of antacid. The clinical relevance of these findings is not known.

7.3   Food Interaction

Administration of SANCTURA XR® immediately after a high fat-content meal reduced the oral bioavailability of trospium chloride by 35% for $AUC_{(0-Tlast)}$ and by 60% for C_{max}. It is therefore recommended that SANCTURA XR® be taken on an empty stomach at least one hour before a meal.

8   USE IN SPECIFIC POPULATIONS

8.1   Pregnancy

Pregnancy Category C: Trospium chloride was not teratogenic at statistically significant levels in rats or rabbits at doses up to 200 mg/kg/day (approximately 16 and 32 times the maximum expected clinical dose, respectively). However, in rabbits, one fetus in each of the low, medium and high dose groups (1, 1, and 32 times, respectively) demonstrated multiple malformations, including umbilical hernia and skeletal malformations. At 200 mg/kg/day trospium chloride, maternal toxicity was observed in rats and rabbits. At 20 mg/kg/day in rats and rabbits, no maternal or fetal toxicity was observed (approximately equivalent to the expected clinical dose via AUC). No developmental toxicity was observed in rats up to 200 mg/kg/day. There are no adequate and well-controlled studies in pregnant women. SANCTURA XR® should be used during pregnancy only if the potential benefit justifies the potential risk.

8.2   Labor and Delivery

The effect of SANCTURA XR® capsules on labor and delivery is unknown.

8.3   Nursing Mothers

Trospium chloride (2 mg/kg PO and 50 µg/kg IV) was excreted, to a limited extent (<1%), into the milk of lactating rats (primarily parent compound). It is not known whether this drug is excreted into human milk. Because many drugs are excreted into human milk, SANCTURA XR® should be used during lactation only if the potential benefit justifies the potential risk.

8.4   Pediatric Use

The safety and effectiveness of SANCTURA XR® in pediatric patients have not been established.

8.5   Geriatric Use

Of 1165 patients in Phase 3 clinical studies of SANCTURA XR®, 37% (n=428) were ages 65 and over, while 12% (n=143) were ages 75 and over.

No overall differences in effectiveness were observed between those subjects aged 65 and over and younger subjects. In SANCTURA XR® subjects ages 65 and over compared to younger subjects, the following adverse reactions were reported at a higher incidence: dry mouth, constipation, abdominal pain, dyspepsia, urinary tract infection and urinary retention. In subjects ages 75 and over, three reported a fall and in one of them a relationship to the event could not be excluded.

8.6   Renal Impairment

Severe renal impairment (creatinine clearance < 30 mL/minute) may significantly alter the disposition of SANCTURA XR®. In a study of immediate-release trospium chloride, 4.5-fold and 2-fold increases in mean AUC and C_{max}, respectively, were detected in patients with severe renal impairment. Use of SANCTURA XR® is not recommended in patients with severe renal impairment (see *Clinical Pharmacology (12)*). The pharmacokinetics of trospium chloride have not been studied in people with moderate or mild renal impairment (CLcr ranging from 30-80 mL/min). Trospium is known to be substantially excreted by the kidney, and the risk of adverse reactions may be greater in patients with impaired renal function.

8.7   Hepatic Impairment

There is no information regarding the effect of moderate to severe hepatic impairment on exposure to SANCTURA XR®. Caution is advised when administering SANCTURA XR® to patients with moderate to severe hepatic impairment.

10   OVERDOSAGE

Overdosage with antimuscarinic agents, including SANCTURA XR®, can result in severe antimuscarinic effects. Supportive treatment should be provided according to symptoms. In the event of overdosage, ECG monitoring is recommended.

11   DESCRIPTION

SANCTURA XR® is an extended-release formulation of trospium chloride, a quaternary ammonium compound with the chemical name of spiro[8-azoniabicyclo[3,2,1]octane-8,1'-pyrrolidinium]-3-[(hydroxydiphenyl-acetyl)-oxy]chloride(1α,3β,5α)-(9Cl). The empirical formula of trospium chloride is $C_{25}H_{30}ClNO_3$ and its molecular weight is 427.97. The structural formula of trospium chloride is represented below:

Trospium chloride is a fine, colorless to slightly yellow, crystalline solid. The compound's solubility in water is approximately 1 g/2 mL.

SANCTURA XR® capsules contain 60 mg of trospium chloride to be given orally. Each capsule also contains the following inactive ingredients: sugar spheres, methacrylic acid copolymer, ethyl cellulose, hydroxypropyl methylcellulose, triethyl citrate, talc, and *Opadry*® white.

12   CLINICAL PHARMACOLOGY

12.1   Mechanism of Action

Trospium chloride is an antispasmodic, antimuscarinic agent.

Trospium chloride antagonizes the effect of acetylcholine on muscarinic receptors in cholinergically innervated organs including the bladder. Its parasympatholytic action reduces the tonus of smooth muscle in the bladder.

In vitro receptor binding studies have demonstrated the selectivity of trospium chloride for muscarinic over nicotinic receptors, and similar affinity for the M_2 and M_3 muscarinic receptor subtypes. M_2 and M_3 receptors are found in the bladder and may play a role in the pathogenesis of overactive bladder.

12.2 Pharmacodynamics

Placebo-controlled studies assessing the impact on urodynamic variables of an immediate-release formulation of trospium chloride were conducted in patients with conditions characterized by involuntary detrusor contractions. The results demonstrated that trospium chloride increases maximum cystometric bladder capacity and volume at first detrusor contraction.

12.3 Pharmacokinetics

Absorption: Mean absolute bioavailability of a 20 mg immediate-release dose is 9.6% (range 4.0-16.1%). Following a single 60 mg dose of **SANCTURA XR®**, peak plasma concentration (C_{max}) of 2.0 ng/mL occurred 5.0 hours post dose. By contrast, following a single 20 mg dose of an immediate-release formulation of trospium chloride, C_{max} was 2.7 ng/mL.

A summary of mean (± standard deviation) pharmacokinetic parameters for a single dose of 60 mg **SANCTURA XR®** is provided in Table 3.

[See table 3 at right]

The mean sample concentration-time (+ standard deviation) profile for **SANCTURA XR®** is shown in Figure 1.

Figure 1: Mean (+SD) Concentration-Time Profile for a Single 60 mg Oral Dose of SANCTURA XR® in Healthy Volunteers

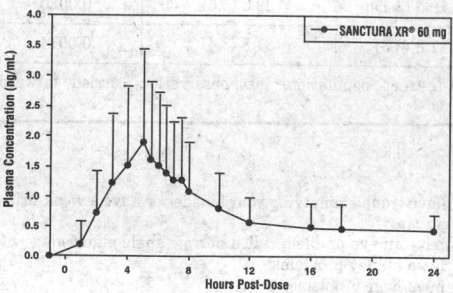

Administration of **SANCTURA XR®** capsules immediately after a high (50%) fat-content meal reduced the oral bioavailability of trospium chloride by 35% for $AUC_{(0-Tlast)}$ and by 60% for C_{max}. Other pharmacokinetic parameters such as T_{max} and $t_{1/2}$ were unchanged in the presence of food. Coadministration with antacid had inconsistent effects on the oral bioavailability of **SANCTURA XR®**.

Distribution: Protein binding ranged from 48 to 78%, depending upon the assessment method used, when a range of concentration levels of trospium chloride (0.5-100 µg/L) were incubated *in vitro* with human serum.

The ratio of ³H-trospium chloride in plasma to whole blood was 1.6:1. This ratio indicates that the majority of ³H-trospium chloride is distributed in plasma.

Trospium chloride is widely distributed, with an apparent volume of distribution >600 L.

Metabolism: The metabolic pathway of trospium in humans has not been fully defined. Of the dose absorbed following oral administration, metabolites account for approximately 40% of the excreted dose. The major metabolic pathway of trospium is hypothesized as ester hydrolysis with subsequent conjugation of benzylic acid to form azoniaspironortropanol with glucuronic acid. Cytochrome P450 does not contribute significantly to the elimination of trospium. Data taken from *in vitro* studies of human liver microsomes, investigating the inhibitory effect of trospium on seven cytochrome P450 isoenzyme substrates (CYP1A2, 2A6, 2C9, 2C19, 2D6, 2E1, and 3A4), suggest a lack of inhibition at clinically relevant concentrations.

Excretion: The plasma half-life for trospium following oral administration of **SANCTURA XR®** is approximately 35 hours. After oral administration of ¹⁴C-labeled trospium chloride, a majority of the dose (85.2%) was recovered in feces and a smaller amount (5.8% of the dose) was recovered in urine. Of the radioactivity excreted into the urine, 60% was unchanged trospium.

The mean renal clearance for trospium (29.07 L/hour) is 4-fold higher than average glomerular filtration rate, indicating that active tubular secretion is a major route of elimination. There may be competition for elimination with other compounds that are also renally eliminated (see *Drug Interactions (7)*).

Pharmacokinetics in Specific Populations

Age: In a phase 3 clinical trial of **SANCTURA XR®**, the observed plasma trospium concentrations were similar in older (≥ 65 years) and younger (< 65 years) OAB patients.

Pediatric: The pharmacokinetics of **SANCTURA XR®** were not evaluated in pediatric patients.

Race: Pharmacokinetic differences due to race have not been studied.

Gender: Gender differences in pharmacokinetics of **SANCTURA XR®** have not been formally assessed. Data from healthy subjects suggests lower exposure in males compared to females.

Hepatic: There is no information regarding the effect of moderate to severe hepatic impairment on exposure to **SANCTURA XR®**.

Renal Impairment: The pharmacokinetics of **SANCTURA XR®** in patients with severe renal impairment has not been evaluated.

In a study of an immediate-release formulation of trospium chloride, 4.5-fold and 2-fold increases in mean $AUC_{(0-\infty)}$ and C_{max}, respectively, were detected in patients with severe renal impairment (creatinine clearance < 30 mL/minute), compared with healthy subjects, along with the appearance of an additional elimination phase with a long half-life (~33 hours vs. 18 hours). Use of **SANCTURA XR®** is not recommended in patients with severe renal impairment (see *Dosage and Administration (2)*). The pharmacokinetics of trospium chloride have not been studied in people with mild or moderate renal impairment (CLcr ranging from 30-80 mL/min).

13 NONCLINICAL TOXICOLOGY

13.1 Carcinogenesis, Mutagenesis, Impairment of Fertility

Carcinogenicity studies with trospium chloride were conducted in mice and rats for 78 weeks and 104 weeks, respectively, at maximally tolerated doses. No evidence of a carcinogenic effect was found in either mice or rats administered up to 200 mg/kg/day (approximately 1 and 16 times the expected clinical exposure levels, respectively, via AUC). Trospium chloride was not mutagenic nor genotoxic in tests *in vitro* in bacteria (Ames test) and mammalian cells (L5178Y mouse lymphoma and CHO cells) or *in vivo* in the mouse micronucleus test.

No evidence of impaired fertility was observed in rats administered doses up to 200 mg/kg/day (about 16 times the expected clinical exposure via AUC).

14 CLINICAL STUDIES

SANCTURA XR® was evaluated for the treatment of patients with overactive bladder who had symptoms of urinary frequency, urgency and urge urinary incontinence in two 12-week, randomized, double-blind, placebo-controlled studies. For both studies, entry criteria required the presence of urge incontinence (predominance of urge), at least one incontinence episode per day, and 10 or more micturitions (voids) per day (assessed by 3-day urinary diary). Medical history and data from the baseline urinary diary confirmed the diagnosis. Approximately 88% of the patients enrolled completed the 12-week studies. The mean age was 60 years, and the majority of patients were female (84%) and Caucasian (86%).

The co-primary endpoints in the trials were the mean change from baseline to Week 12 in number of voids/24 hours (reductions in urinary frequency) and the mean change from baseline to Week 12 in number of incontinence episodes/24 hours. Secondary endpoints included mean change from baseline to Week 12 in volume per void.

Study 1 included 592 patients in both **SANCTURA XR®** 60 mg and placebo groups. As illustrated in Table 4 and Figures 2 and 3, **SANCTURA XR®** demonstrated statistically significantly (p<0.01) greater reductions in the urinary frequency and incontinence episodes, and increases in void volume when compared to placebo starting at Week 1 and maintained through Weeks 4 and 12.

[See table 4 above]

Table 3: Mean (±SD) Pharmacokinetic Parameter Estimates for a Single 60 mg Oral Dose of SANCTURA XR® in Healthy Volunteers

Treatment	AUC$_{(0-24)}$ (ng•h/mL)	C$_{max}$ (ng/mL)	T$_{max}$ [a] (h)	t$_{1/2}$ [b] (h)
SANCTURA XR® 60 mg	18.0 ± 13.4	2.0 ± 1.5	5.0 (3.0-7.5)	36 ± 22

[a] T$_{max}$ expressed as median (range).
[b] t$_{1/2}$ was determined following multiple (10) doses.

Table 4: Mean (SE) Change from Baseline in Urinary Frequency, Urge Incontinence Episodes and Void Volume in Study 1

Efficacy Endpoint [a]	Week	Placebo	SANCTURA XR®	P-Value
Urinary frequency / 24 hours		(N = 300)	(N = 292)	
Mean Baseline	0	12.7 (0.2)	12.8 (0.2)	
Mean Change from Baseline	1	-1.2 (0.1)	-1.7 (0.1)	0.0092
	4	-1.6 (0.2)	-2.4 (0.2)	<0.0001
	12	-2.0 (0.2)	-2.8 (0.2)	<0.0001
Urge incontinence episodes / week		(N = 300)	(N = 292)	
Mean Baseline	0	29.0 (1.3)	28.8 (1.3)	
Mean Change from Baseline	1	-8.7 (1.0)	-13.0 (0.9)	0.0003
	4	-12.2 (1.1)	-16.5 (1.2)	0.0054
	12	-13.5 (1.1)	-17.3 (1.2)	0.0024
Urinary volume / void (mL)		(N = 300)	(N = 290)	
Mean Baseline	0	155.9 (3.0)	151.0 (2.9)	
Mean Change from Baseline	1	12.1 (2.1)	21.6 (2.8)	0.0036
	4	17.2 (2.5)	30.0 (3.1)	0.0007
	12	18.9 (2.8)	29.8 (3.2)	0.0039

[a] treatment differences assessed by rank ANOVA for intent-to-treat population, last observation carried forward (ITT:LOCF) data set

Figure 2: Mean Change from Baseline in Urinary Frequency/24 hours by Visit: Study 1

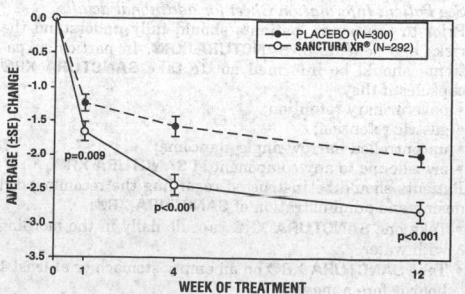

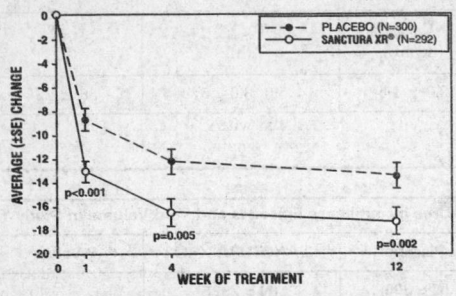

Figure 3: Mean Change from Baseline in Incontinence Episodes/ Week by Visit: Study 1

Study 2 included 543 patients in both **SANCTURA XR®** 60 mg and placebo groups and was identical in design to Study 1. As illustrated in Table 5 and Figures 4 and 5, **SANCTURA XR®** capsules demonstrated statistically significantly (p<0.01) greater reductions in urinary frequency and incontinence episodes, and increases in void volume when compared to placebo at Weeks 4 and 12. However, at Week 1, statistically significant reductions were seen in urinary incontinence episodes and volume void only.
[See table 5 at right]

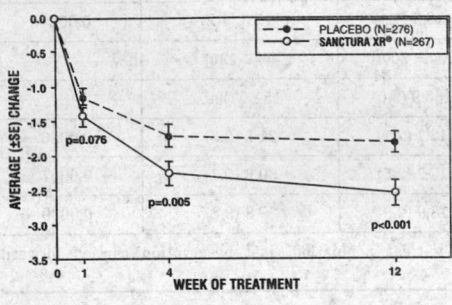

Figure 4: Mean Change from Baseline in Urinary Frequency/24 hours by Visit: Study 2

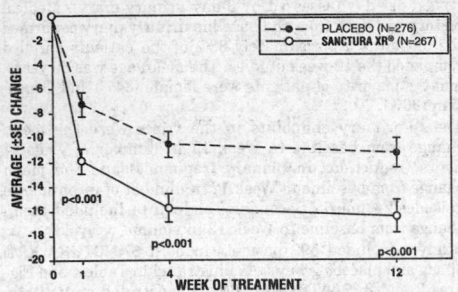

Figure 5: Mean Change from Baseline in Incontinence Episodes/ Week by Visit: Study 2

16   HOW SUPPLIED/STORAGE AND HANDLING

SANCTURA XR® is supplied as 60 mg capsules (white opaque body and orange opaque cap, printed with SAN 60): 60 mg capsule, 30 count, HDPE bottle: NDC 0023-9350-30 Store at controlled room temperature 20° to 25°C (68° to 77°F). Excursion permitted at 15° to 30°C (see USP).

17   PATIENT COUNSELING INFORMATION

See Patient Information Sheet for additional details
Prior to treatment, patients should fully understand the risks and benefits of **SANCTURA XR®**. In particular, patients should be informed not to take **SANCTURA XR®** capsules if they:
• have urinary retention;
• gastric retention;
• uncontrolled narrow-angle glaucoma;
• are allergic to any component of **SANCTURA XR®**
Patients should be instructed regarding the recommended dosing and administration of **SANCTURA XR®**:
• Take one **SANCTURA XR®** capsule daily in the morning with water.
• Take **SANCTURA XR®** on an empty stomach or at least 1 hour before a meal.

Table 5: Mean (SE) Change from Baseline in Urinary Frequency, Urge Incontinence Episodes and Void Volume in Study 2

Efficacy Endpoint [a]	Week	Placebo	SANCTURA XR®	P-Value
Urinary frequency / 24 hours		**(N = 276)**	**(N = 267)**	
Mean Baseline	0	12.9 (0.2)	12.8 (0.2)	
Mean Change from Baseline	1	-1.2 (0.2)	-1.4 (0.2)	0.0759
	4	-1.7 (0.2)	-2.3 (0.2)	0.0047
	12	-1.8 (0.2)	-2.5 (0.2)	0.0009
Urge incontinence episodes / week		**(N = 276)**	**(N = 267)**	
Mean Baseline	0	28.3 (1.4)	28.2 (1.2)	
Mean Change from Baseline	1	-7.3 (1.0)	-11.9 (1.0)	<0.0001
	4	-10.6 (1.1)	-15.8 (1.1)	<0.0001
	12	-11.3 (1.2)	-16.4 (1.3)	<0.0001
Urinary volume / void (mL)		**(N = 276)**	**(N = 266)**	
Mean Baseline	0	151.8 (2.8)	149.6 (2.9)	
Mean Change from Baseline	1	11.9 (2.5)	24.1 (2.4)	<0.0001
	4	19.6 (3.1)	29.3 (3.0)	0.0020
	12	17.8 (3.3)	31.5 (3.4)	0.0014

[a] treatment differences assessed by rank ANOVA for intent-to-treat population, last observation carried forward (ITT:LOCF) data set

---

• Use of alcoholic beverages within 2 hours of dosing with **SANCTURA XR®** is not recommended.
Patients should be informed that the most common side effects with **SANCTURA XR®** are dry mouth and constipation and that other less common side effects include trouble emptying the bladder, blurred vision, and heat prostration. Patients should be informed that alcohol may enhance the drowsiness caused by anticholinergic agents.
Manufactured for:
Allergan, Inc.
Irvine, CA 92612, U.S.A.
Manufactured by:
Catalent Pharma Solutions, Inc.
Somerset, NJ 08873, U.S.A.
© 2009 Allergan, Inc.
Irvine, CA 92612, U.S.A.
® mark owned by Allergan, Inc.
Opadry is a registered trademark of BPSI Holdings, Inc.

Patient Information
SANCTURA XR® [SANK-TOUR-AH EKS-AHR]
(trospium chloride extended release capsules)
Read the Patient Information that comes with **SANCTURA XR®** before you start taking it and each time you get a refill. There may be new information. This leaflet does not take the place of talking with your doctor about your medical condition or your treatment.

What is SANCTURA XR®?
SANCTURA XR® is a prescription medicine used to treat adults with overactive bladder who have the following symptoms:
• a strong need to urinate right away;
• leaking or wetting accidents due to a strong need to urinate right away;
• a need to urinate often.

Who should not take SANCTURA XR®?
Do not take **SANCTURA XR®** if you:
• have trouble emptying your bladder;
• have delayed or slow emptying of your stomach;
• have an eye problem called "uncontrolled narrow-angle glaucoma";
• are allergic to **SANCTURA XR®** or any of its ingredients. See the end of this leaflet for a complete list of ingredients.
SANCTURA XR® has not been studied in children under the age of 18 years.

What should I tell my doctor before starting SANCTURA XR®?
Tell your doctor about all of your medical conditions including if you:
• have any stomach or intestinal problems or problems with constipation;

• have trouble emptying your bladder or have a weak urine stream;
• have an eye problem called narrow-angle glaucoma;
• have kidney problems;
• have liver problems;
• are pregnant or planning to become pregnant. It is not known if **SANCTURA XR®** can harm your unborn baby.
• are breastfeeding. It is not known if **SANCTURA XR®** passes into breast milk and if it can harm your baby. You should talk to your doctor about the best way to feed your baby if you are taking **SANCTURA XR®**.
Tell your doctor about all the medicines you take including prescription and nonprescription medicines, vitamins and herbal supplements. **SANCTURA XR®** and certain other medicines can interact and make some side effects worse. **SANCTURA XR®** can affect how other medicines are handled by the body.
Know all the medicines you take. Keep a list of them with you to show your doctor and pharmacist each time you get a new medicine.

How should I take SANCTURA XR®?
Take **SANCTURA XR®** exactly as prescribed.
• Take one **SANCTURA XR®** capsule daily in the morning with water.
• Take **SANCTURA XR®** on an empty stomach or at least 1 hour before a meal.
• Do not take alcohol within 2 hours of taking **SANCTURA XR®**.
• If you take too much **SANCTURA XR®**, call your local Poison Control Center or go to an emergency room right away.

What are the possible side effects of SANCTURA XR®?
The most common side effects with **SANCTURA XR®** are:
• dry mouth;
• constipation.
SANCTURA XR® may cause other less common side effects, including:
• trouble emptying the bladder;
• blurred vision;
• heat prostration. Due to decreased sweating, heat prostration can occur when drugs such as **SANCTURA XR®** are used in a hot environment. Tell your doctor if you have any side effects that bother you or that do not go away.
These are not all possible side effects of **SANCTURA XR®**. For more information, ask your doctor, healthcare professional or pharmacist.

How should I store SANCTURA XR®?
• **SANCTURA XR®** and all other medicines out of the reach of children.
• Store **SANCTURA XR®** at room temperature, 68° to 77°F (20° to 25°C).
• Safely dispose of **SANCTURA XR®** capsules that are out of date or that you no longer need.

General information about SANCTURA XR®

Medicines are sometimes prescribed for conditions that are not mentioned in patient information leaflets. Do not use **SANCTURA XR®** for a condition for which it was not prescribed. Do not give **SANCTURA XR®** to other people, even if they have the same symptoms you have. It may harm them.

This leaflet summarizes the most important information about **SANCTURA XR®**. If you would like more information, talk with your doctor. You can ask your doctor or pharmacist for information about **SANCTURA XR®** that is written for health professionals. You can also call Allergan's product information department at 1-800-433-8871.

What are the ingredients in SANCTURA XR®?

Active Ingredient: trospium chloride.

Inactive Ingredients: sugar spheres, methacrylic acid copolymer, ethyl cellulose, hydroxypropyl methylcellulose, triethyl citrate, talc, and *Opadry®* white.

750-04191R2
71966US13A

Amgen
ONE AMGEN CENTER DRIVE
THOUSAND OAKS, CA 91320-1799

**For Product Inquiries and
Adverse Event Reporting Contact:**
Amgen Medical Information
(800) 772-6436
FAX: (866) 292-6436
www.amgen.com
Sales and Ordering:
Amgen Trade Operations
(800) 282-6436
FAX: (866) 292-6436

ARANESP®

[ără-nŭsp]
(darbepoetin alfa)
For Injection

℞

WARNINGS: INCREASED MORTALITY, SERIOUS CARDIOVASCULAR EVENTS, THROMBOEMBOLIC EVENTS, STROKE AND INCREASED RISK OF TUMOR PROGRESSION OR RECURRENCE

Chronic Renal Failure:

- In clinical studies, patients experienced greater risks for death, serious cardiovascular events, and stroke when administered erythropoiesis-stimulating agents (ESAs) to target hemoglobin levels of 13 g/dL and above.
- Individualize dosing to achieve and maintain hemoglobin levels within the range of 10 to 12 g/dL.

Cancer:

- ESAs shortened overall survival and/or increased the risk of tumor progression or recurrence in some clinical studies in patients with breast, non-small cell lung, head and neck, lymphoid, and cervical cancers (see WARNINGS: Table 1).
- To decrease these risks, as well as the risk of serious cardio- and thrombovascular events, use the lowest dose needed to avoid red blood cell transfusion.
- Because of these risks, prescribers and hospitals must enroll in and comply with the ESA APPRISE Oncology Program to prescribe and/or dispense Aranesp® to patients with cancer. To enroll in the ESA APPRISE Oncology Program, visit www.esa-apprise.com or call 1-866-284-8089 for further assistance.
- Use ESAs only for treatment of anemia due to concomitant myelosuppressive chemotherapy.
- ESAs are not indicated for patients receiving myelosuppressive therapy when the anticipated outcome is cure.
- Discontinue following the completion of a chemotherapy course.

(See WARNINGS: Increased Mortality, Serious Cardiovascular Events, Thromboembolic Events, and Stroke, WARNINGS: Increased Mortality and/or Increased Risk of Tumor Progression or Recurrence, INDICATIONS AND USAGE and DOSAGE AND ADMINISTRATION.)

DESCRIPTION

Aranesp® is an erythropoiesis stimulating protein, closely related to erythropoietin, that is produced in Chinese hamster ovary (CHO) cells by recombinant DNA technology. Aranesp® is a 165–amino acid protein that differs from recombinant human erythropoietin in containing 5 N–linked oligosaccharide chains, whereas recombinant human erythropoietin contains 3 chains.[1] The two additional N-glycosylation sites result from amino acid substitutions in the erythropoietin peptide backbone. The additional carbohydrate chains increase the approximate molecular weight of the glycoprotein from 30,000 to 37,000 daltons. Aranesp® is formulated as a sterile, colorless, preservative-free protein solution for intravenous or subcutaneous administration.

Single-dose vials are available containing 25, 40, 60, 100, 150, 200, 300, or 500 mcg of Aranesp®.

Single-dose prefilled syringes and prefilled SureClick™ autoinjectors are available containing 25, 40, 60, 100, 150, 200, 300, or 500 mcg of Aranesp®. Each prefilled syringe is equipped with a needle guard that covers the needle during disposal.

Single-dose vials, prefilled syringes and autoinjectors are available in two formulations that contain excipients as follows:

- **Polysorbate solution** Each 1 mL contains 0.05 mg polysorbate 80, and is formulated at pH 6.2 ± 0.2 with 2.12 mg sodium phosphate monobasic monohydrate, 0.66 mg sodium phosphate dibasic anhydrous, and 8.18 mg sodium chloride in Water for Injection, USP (to 1 mL).
- **Albumin solution** Each 1 mL contains 2.5 mg albumin (human), and is formulated at pH 6.0 ± 0.3 with 2.23 mg sodium phosphate monobasic monohydrate, 0.53 mg sodium phosphate dibasic anhydrous, and 8.18 mg sodium chloride in Water for Injection, USP (to 1 mL).

CLINICAL PHARMACOLOGY

Mechanism of Action

Aranesp® stimulates erythropoiesis by the same mechanism as endogenous erythropoietin. A primary growth factor for erythroid development, erythropoietin is produced in the kidney and released into the bloodstream in response to hypoxia. In responding to hypoxia, erythropoietin interacts with progenitor stem cells to increase red blood cell (RBC) production. Production of endogenous erythropoietin is impaired in patients with chronic renal failure (CRF), and erythropoietin deficiency is the primary cause of their anemia. Increased hemoglobin levels are not generally observed until 2 to 6 weeks after initiating treatment with Aranesp® (see **DOSAGE AND ADMINISTRATION**). In patients with cancer receiving concomitant chemotherapy, the etiology of anemia is multifactorial.

Pharmacokinetics

Adult Patients

The pharmacokinetics of Aranesp® were studied in patients with CRF receiving or not receiving dialysis and cancer patients receiving chemotherapy.

Following intravenous administration in CRF patients receiving dialysis, Aranesp® serum concentration-time profiles were biphasic, with a distribution half-life of approximately 1.4 hours and a mean terminal half-life of 21 hours. The terminal half-life of Aranesp® was approximately 3-fold longer than that of Epoetin alfa when administered intravenously.

Following subcutaneous administration of Aranesp® to CRF patients (receiving or not receiving dialysis), absorption was slow and peak concentrations occurred at 48 hours (range: 12 to 72 hours). In CRF patients receiving dialysis, the average half-life was 46 hours (range: 12 to 89 hours), and in CRF patients not receiving dialysis, the average half-life was 70 hours (range: 35 to 139 hours). Aranesp® apparent clearance was approximately 1.4 times faster on average in patients receiving dialysis compared to patients not receiving dialysis. The bioavailability of Aranesp® in CRF patients receiving dialysis after subcutaneous administration was 37% (range: 30% to 50%).

Following the first subcutaneous dose of 6.75 mcg/kg (equivalent to 500 mcg for a 74-kg patient) in patients with cancer, the mean terminal half-life was 74 hours (range: 24 to 144 hours). Peak concentrations were observed at 90 hours (range: 71 to 123 hours) after a dose of 2.25 mcg/kg, and 71 hours (range: 28 to 120 hours) after a dose of 6.75 mcg/kg. When administered on a once every 3 week schedule, 48-hour post-dose Aranesp® levels after the fourth dose were similar to those after the first dose.

Over the dose range of 0.45 to 4.5 mcg/kg Aranesp® administered intravenously or subcutaneously on a once weekly schedule and 4.5 to 15 mcg/kg administered subcutaneously on a once every 3 week schedule, systemic exposure was approximately proportional to dose. No evidence of accumulation was observed beyond an expected < 2-fold increase in blood levels when compared to the initial dose.

Pediatric Patients

Aranesp® pharmacokinetics were studied in 12 pediatric CRF patients (age 3-16 years) receiving or not receiving dialysis. Following a single intravenous or subcutaneous Aranesp® dose, Cmax and half-life were similar to those obtained in adult CRF patients on dialysis. Following a single subcutaneous dose, the average bioavailability was 54% (range: 32% to 70%), which was higher than that obtained in adult CRF patients on dialysis.

CLINICAL STUDIES

Throughout this section of the package insert, the Aranesp® study numbers associated with the nephrology and cancer clinical programs are designated with the letters "N" and "C", respectively.

Chronic Renal Failure Patients

The safety and effectiveness of Aranesp® have been assessed in a number of multicenter studies. Two studies evaluated the safety and efficacy of Aranesp® for the correction of anemia in adult patients with CRF, and three studies (2 in adults and 1 in pediatric patients) assessed the ability of Aranesp® to maintain hemoglobin concentrations in patients with CRF who had been receiving other recombinant erythropoietins.

De Novo Use of Aranesp®

Once Weekly Aranesp® Starting Dose

In two open-label studies, Aranesp® or Epoetin alfa was administered for the correction of anemia in CRF patients who had not been receiving prior treatment with exogenous erythropoietin. Study N1 evaluated CRF patients receiving dialysis; Study N2 evaluated patients not requiring dialysis. In both studies, the starting dose of Aranesp® was 0.45 mcg/kg administered once weekly. The starting dose of Epoetin alfa was 50 Units/kg 3 times weekly in Study N1 and 50 Units/kg twice weekly in Study N2. When necessary, dosage adjustments were instituted to maintain hemoglobin in the study target range of 11 to 13 g/dL. (Note: The recommended hemoglobin target is lower than the target range of these studies. See **DOSAGE AND ADMINISTRATION** for recommended clinical hemoglobin target.) The primary efficacy endpoint was the proportion of patients who experienced at least a 1 g/dL increase in hemoglobin concentration to a level of at least 11 g/dL by 20 weeks (Study N1) or 24 weeks (Study N2). The studies were designed to assess the safety and effectiveness of Aranesp® but not to support conclusions regarding comparisons between the two products. In Study N1, the hemoglobin target was achieved by 72% (95% CI: 62%, 81%) of the 90 patients treated with Aranesp® and 84% (95% CI: 66%, 95%) of the 31 patients treated with Epoetin alfa. The mean increase in hemoglobin over the initial 4 weeks of Aranesp® treatment was 1.1 g/dL (95% CI: 0.82 g/dL, 1.37 g/dL).

In Study N2, the primary efficacy endpoint was achieved by 93% (95% CI: 87%, 97%) of the 129 patients treated with Aranesp® and 92% (95% CI: 78%, 98%) of the 37 patients treated with Epoetin alfa. The mean increase in hemoglobin from baseline through the initial 4 weeks of Aranesp® treatment was 1.38 g/dL (95% CI: 1.21 g/dL, 1.55 g/dL).

Once Every 2 Week Aranesp® Starting Dose

In two single arm studies (N3 and N4), Aranesp® was administered for the correction of anemia in CRF patients not receiving dialysis. In both studies, the starting dose of Aranesp® was 0.75 mcg/kg administered once every 2 weeks.

In Study N3 (study duration of 18 weeks), the hemoglobin goal (hemoglobin concentration ≥ 11 g/dL) was achieved by 92% (95% CI: 86%, 96%) of the 128 patients treated with Aranesp®.

In Study N4 (study duration of 24 weeks), the hemoglobin goal (hemoglobin concentration of 11-13 g/dL) was achieved by 85% (95% CI: 77%, 93%) of the 75 patients treated with Aranesp®.

Conversion From Other Recombinant Erythropoietins

Two adult studies (N5 and N6) and one pediatric study (N7) were conducted in patients with CRF who had been receiving other recombinant erythropoietins. The studies compared the abilities of Aranesp® and other erythropoietins to maintain hemoglobin concentrations within a study target range of 9 to 13 g/dL in adults and 10 to 12.5 g/dL in pediatric patients. (Note: The recommended hemoglobin target is lower than the target range of these studies. See **DOSAGE AND ADMINISTRATION** for recommended clinical hemoglobin target.) CRF patients who had been receiving stable doses of other recombinant erythropoietins were randomized to Aranesp®, or to continue with their prior erythropoietin at the previous dose and schedule. For patients randomized to Aranesp®, the initial weekly dose was determined on the basis of the previous total weekly dose of recombinant erythropoietin.

Adult Patients

Study N5 was a double-blind study conducted in North America, in which 169 hemodialysis patients were randomized to treatment with Aranesp® and 338 patients continued on Epoetin alfa. Study N6 was an open-label study conducted in Europe and Australia in which 347 patients were randomized to treatment with Aranesp® and 175 patients were randomized to continue on Epoetin alfa or Epoetin beta. Of the 347 patients randomized to Aranesp®, 92% were receiving hemodialysis and 8% were receiving peritoneal dialysis.

In Study N5, a median weekly dose of 0.53 mcg/kg Aranesp® (25th, 75th percentiles: 0.30, 0.93 mcg/kg) was required to maintain hemoglobin in the study target range. In Study N6, a median weekly dose of 0.41 mcg/kg Aranesp® (25th, 75th percentiles: 0.26, 0.65 mcg/kg) was required to maintain hemoglobin in the study target range.

Pediatric Patients

Study N7 was an open-label, randomized study, conducted in the United States in pediatric patients from 1 to 18 years of age with CRF receiving or not receiving dialysis. Patients that were stable on Epoetin alfa were randomized to receive either darbepoetin alfa (n = 82) administered once weekly (subcutaneously or intravenously) or to continue receiving Epoetin alfa (n = 42) at the current dose, schedule, and route of administration. A median weekly dose of 0.41 mcg/kg Aranesp® (25th, 75th percentiles: 0.25, 0.82 mcg/kg) was required to maintain hemoglobin in the study target range.

Cancer Patients Receiving Chemotherapy

Efficacy in patients with anemia due to concomitant chemotherapy was demonstrated based on reduction in the requirement for RBC transfusions.

Once Weekly Dosing

The safety and effectiveness of Aranesp® in reducing the requirement for RBC transfusions in patients undergoing chemotherapy was assessed in a randomized, placebo-controlled, double-blind, multinational study (C1). This study was conducted in anemic (Hgb ≤ 11 g/dL) patients with advanced, small cell or non-small cell lung cancer, who received a platinum-containing chemotherapy regimen. Patients were randomized to receive Aranesp® 2.25 mcg/kg (n = 156) or placebo (n = 158) administered as a single weekly SC injection for up to 12 weeks. The dose was escalated to 4.5 mcg/kg/week at week 6, in subjects with an inadequate response to treatment, defined as less than 1 g/dL hemoglobin increase. There were 67 patients in the Aranesp® arm who had their dose increased from 2.25 to 4.5 mcg/kg/week, at any time during the treatment period. Efficacy was determined by a reduction in the proportion of patients who were transfused over the 12-week treatment period. A significantly lower proportion of patients in the Aranesp® arm, 26% (95% CI: 20%, 33%) required transfusion compared to 60% (95% CI: 52%, 68%) in the placebo arm (Kaplan-Meier estimate of proportion; p < 0.001 by Cochran-Mantel-Haenszel test). Of the 67 patients who received a dose increase, 28% had a 2 g/dL increase in hemoglobin over baseline, generally occurring between weeks 8 to 13. Of the 89 patients who did not receive a dose increase, 69% had a 2 g/dL increase in hemoglobin over baseline, generally occurring between weeks 6 to 13. On-study deaths occurred in 14% (22/156) of patients treated with Aranesp® and 12% (19/158) of the placebo-treated patients.

Once Every 3 Week Dosing

The safety and effectiveness of once every 3 week Aranesp® therapy in reducing the requirement for red blood cell (RBC) transfusions in patients undergoing chemotherapy was assessed in a randomized, double-blind, multinational study (C2). This study was conducted in anemic (Hgb < 11 g/dL) patients with non-myeloid malignancies receiving multicycle chemotherapy. Patients were randomized to receive Aranesp® at 500 mcg once every 3 weeks (n = 353) or 2.25 mcg/kg (n = 352) administered weekly as a subcutaneous injection for up to 15 weeks. In both groups, the dose was reduced by 40% of the previous dose (e.g., for first dose reduction, to 300 mcg in the once every 3 week group and 1.35 mcg/kg in the once weekly group) if hemoglobin increased by more than 1 g/dL in a 14-day period. Study drug was withheld if hemoglobin exceeded 13 g/dL. In the once every 3 week group, 254 patients (72%) required dose reductions (median time to first reduction at 6 weeks). In the once weekly group, 263 patients (75%) required dose reductions (median time to first reduction at 5 weeks).

Efficacy was determined by a comparison of the Kaplan-Meier estimates of the proportion of patients who received at least one RBC transfusion between day 29 and the end of treatment. Three hundred thirty-five patients in the once every 3 week group and 337 patients in the once weekly group remained on study through or beyond day 29 and were evaluated for efficacy. Twenty-seven percent (95% CI: 22%, 32%) of patients in the once every 3 week group and 34% (95% CI: 29%, 39%) in the weekly group required a RBC transfusion. The observed difference in the transfusion

rates (once every 3 week-once weekly) was -6.7% (95% CI: -13.8%, 0.4%).

Lack of Efficacy in Improving Survival

Study C3 was conducted in patients required to have a hemoglobin concentration ≥ 9 g/dL and ≤ 13 g/dL with previously untreated extensive-stage small cell lung cancer (SCLC) receiving platinum and etoposide chemotherapy. Randomization was stratified by region (Western Europe, Australia/North America, and rest of world), Eastern Cooperative Oncology Group (ECOG) performance status (0 or 1 vs. 2), and lactate dehydrogenase (below vs. above the upper limit of normal). Patients were randomized to receive Aranesp® (n = 298) at a dose of 300 mcg once weekly for the first 4 weeks, followed by 300 mcg once every 3 weeks for the remainder of the treatment period or placebo (n = 298). This study was designed to detect a prolongation in overall survival (from a median of 9 months to a median of 12 months). For the final analysis, there was no evidence of improved survival (p = 0.43, log-rank test).

INDICATIONS AND USAGE

Anemia With Chronic Renal Failure

Aranesp® is indicated for the treatment of anemia associated with chronic renal failure, including patients on dialysis and patients not on dialysis.

Anemia With Non-Myeloid Malignancies Due to Chemotherapy

Aranesp® is indicated for the treatment of anemia due to the effect of concomitantly administered chemotherapy based on studies that have shown a reduction in the need for RBC transfusions in patients with metastatic, non-myeloid malignancies. Studies to determine whether Aranesp® increases mortality or decreases progression-free/recurrence-free survival are ongoing.

- Aranesp® is not indicated for use in patients receiving hormonal agents, therapeutic biologic products, or radiotherapy unless receiving concomitant myelosuppressive chemotherapy.
- Aranesp® is not indicated for patients receiving myelosuppressive therapy when the anticipated outcome is cure due to the absence of studies that adequately characterize the impact of Aranesp® on progression-free and overall survival (see WARNINGS: Increased Mortality and/or Increased Risk of Tumor Progression or Recurrence).
- Aranesp® use has not been demonstrated in controlled clinical trials to improve symptoms of anemia, quality of life, fatigue, or patient well-being.

CONTRAINDICATIONS

Aranesp® is contraindicated in patients with:
- uncontrolled hypertension
- known hypersensitivity to the active substance or any of the excipients

WARNINGS

Increased Mortality, Serious Cardiovascular Events, Thromboembolic Events, and Stroke

Patients with chronic renal failure experienced greater risks for death, serious cardiovascular events, and stroke when administered erythropoiesis-stimulating agents (ESAs) to target hemoglobin levels of 13 g/dL and above in clinical studies. Patients with chronic renal failure and an insufficient hemoglobin response to ESA therapy may be at even greater risk for cardiovascular events and mortality than other patients. Aranesp® and other ESAs increased the risks for death and serious cardiovascular events in controlled clinical trials of patients with cancer. These events included myocardial infarction, stroke, congestive heart failure, and hemodialysis vascular access thrombosis. A rate of hemoglobin rise of > 1 g/dL over 2 weeks may contribute to these risks.

In a randomized prospective trial, 1432 anemic chronic renal failure patients who were not undergoing dialysis were assigned to Epoetin alfa (rHuEPO) treatment targeting a maintenance hemoglobin concentration of 13.5 g/dL or 11.3 g/dL. A major cardiovascular event (death, myocardial infarction, stroke, or hospitalization for congestive heart failure) occurred among 125 (18%) of the 715 patients in the higher hemoglobin group compared to 97 (14%) among the 717 patients in the lower hemoglobin group [Hazard Ratio (HR) 1.3, 95% CI: 1.0, 1.7, p = 0.03].[2]

In a randomized, double-blind, placebo-controlled study of 4038 patients, there was an increased risk of stroke when Aranesp® was administered to patients with anemia, type 2 diabetes, and CRF who were not on dialysis. Patients were randomized to Aranesp® treatment targeted to a hemoglobin level of 13 g/dL or to placebo. Placebo patients received Aranesp® only if their hemoglobin levels were less than 9 g/dL. A total of 101 patients receiving Aranesp® experienced stroke compared to 53 patients receiving placebo (5% vs. 2.6%; HR 1.92, 95% CI: 1.38, 2.68; p < 0.001).

Increased risk for serious cardiovascular events was also reported from a randomized, prospective trial of 1265 hemodialysis patients with clinically evident cardiac disease (ischemic heart disease or congestive heart failure). In this trial, patients were assigned to Epoetin alfa treatment targeted to a maintenance hemoglobin of either 14 ± 1 g/dL or 10 ± 1 g/dL.[3] Higher mortality (35% vs. 29%) was observed in the 634 patients randomized to a target hemoglobin of 14 g/dL than in the 631 patients assigned a target hemoglobin of 10 g/dL. The reason for the increased mortality observed in this study is unknown; however, the incidence of nonfatal myocardial infarction, vascular access thrombosis, and other thrombotic events was also higher in the group randomized to a target hemoglobin of 14 g/dL.

An increased incidence of thrombotic events has also been observed in patients with cancer treated with erythropoietic agents. In patients with cancer who received Aranesp®, pulmonary emboli, thrombophlebitis, and thrombosis occurred more frequently than in placebo controls (see ADVERSE REACTIONS: Cancer Patients Receiving Chemotherapy, Table 5).

In a randomized controlled study (referred to as Cancer Study 1 - the 'BEST' study) with another ESA in 939 women with metastatic breast cancer receiving chemotherapy, patients received either weekly Epoetin alfa or placebo for up to a year. This study was designed to show that survival was superior when an ESA was administered to prevent anemia (maintain hemoglobin levels between 12 and 14 g/dL or hematocrit between 36% and 42%). The study was terminated prematurely when interim results demonstrated that a higher mortality at 4 months (8.7% vs. 3.4%) and a higher rate of fatal thrombotic events (1.1% vs. 0.2%) in the first 4 months of the study were observed among patients treated with Epoetin alfa. Based on Kaplan-Meier estimates, at the time of study termination, the 12-month survival was lower in the Epoetin alfa group than in the placebo group (70% vs. 76%; HR 1.37, 95% CI: 1.07, 1.75, p = 0.012).[4]

A systematic review of 57 randomized controlled trials (including Cancer Studies 1 and 5 - the 'BEST' and 'ENHANCE' studies) evaluating 9353 patients with cancer compared ESAs plus RBC transfusion with RBC transfusion alone for prophylaxis or treatment of anemia in cancer patients with or without concurrent antineoplastic therapy. An increased relative risk (RR) of thromboembolic events (RR 1.67, 95% CI: 1.35, 2.06; 35 trials and 6769 patients) was observed in ESA-treated patients. An overall survival hazard ratio of 1.08 (95% CI: 0.99, 1.18; 42 trials and 8167 patients) was observed in ESA-treated patients.[5]

An increased incidence of deep vein thrombosis (DVT) in patients receiving Epoetin alfa undergoing surgical orthopedic procedures has been observed. In a randomized controlled study (referred to as the 'SPINE' study), 681 adult patients, not receiving prophylactic anticoagulation and undergoing spinal surgery, received Epoetin alfa and standard of care (SOC) treatment, or SOC treatment alone. Preliminary analysis showed a higher incidence of DVT, determined by either Color Flow Duplex Imaging or by clinical symptoms, in the Epoetin alfa group [16 patients (4.7%) compared to the SOC group [7 patients (2.1%)]. In addition, 12 patients in the Epoetin alfa group and 7 patients in the SOC group had other thrombotic vascular events.

Increased mortality was observed in a randomized placebo-controlled study of Epoetin alfa in adult patients who were undergoing coronary artery bypass surgery (7 deaths in 126 patients randomized to Epoetin alfa versus no deaths among 56 patients receiving placebo). Four of these deaths occurred during the period of study drug administration and all four deaths were associated with thrombotic events. Aranesp® is not approved for reduction in allogeneic RBC transfusions in patients scheduled for surgical procedures.

Increased Mortality and/or Increased Risk of Tumor Progression or Recurrence

Erythropoiesis-stimulating agents resulted in decreased locoregional control/progression-free survival and/or overall survival (see Table 1). These findings were observed in studies of patients with advanced head and neck cancer receiving radiation therapy (Cancer Studies 5 and 6), in patients receiving chemotherapy for metastatic breast cancer (Cancer Study 1) or lymphoid malignancy (Cancer Study 2), and in patients with non-small cell lung cancer or various malignancies who were not receiving chemotherapy or radiotherapy (Cancer Studies 7 and 8).

[See table 1 at top of next page]

Decreased overall survival:

Cancer Study 1 (the 'BEST' study) was previously described (see WARNINGS: Increased Mortality, Serious Cardiovascular Events, Thromboembolic Events, and Stroke). Mortality at 4 months (8.7% vs. 3.4%) was significantly higher in the Epoetin alfa arm. The most common investigator-attributed cause of death within the first 4 months was disease progression; 28 of 41 deaths in the Epoetin alfa arm and 13 of 16 deaths in the placebo arm were attributed to disease progression. Investigator assessed time to tumor progression was not different between the two groups. Survival at 12 months was significantly lower in the Epoetin alfa arm (70% vs. 76%, HR 1.37, 95% CI: 1.07, 1.75; p = 0.012).[4]

Cancer Study 2 was a Phase 3, double-blind, randomized (Aranesp® vs. placebo) study conducted in 344 anemic patients with lymphoid malignancy receiving chemotherapy. With a median follow-up of 29 months, overall mortality rates were significantly higher among patients randomized to Aranesp® as compared to placebo (HR 1.36, 95% CI: 1.02, 1.82).

Cancer Study 7 was a Phase 3, multicenter, randomized (Epoetin alfa vs. placebo), double-blind study, in which patients with advanced non-small cell lung cancer receiving only palliative radiotherapy or no active therapy were treated with Epoetin alfa to achieve and maintain hemoglobin levels between 12 and 14 g/dL. Following an interim analysis of 70 of 300 patients planned, a significant difference in survival in favor of the patients on the placebo arm of the trial was observed (median survival 63 vs. 129 days; HR 1.84; p = 0.04).

Cancer Study 8 was a Phase 3, double-blind, randomized (Aranesp® vs. placebo), 16-week study in 989 anemic patients with active malignant disease, neither receiving nor planning to receive chemotherapy or radiation therapy. There was no evidence of a statistically significant reduction in proportion of patients receiving RBC transfusions. The median survival was shorter in the Aranesp® treatment group (8 months) compared with the placebo group (10.8 months); HR 1.30, 95% CI: 1.07, 1.57.

Decreased progression-free survival and overall survival:
Cancer Study 3 (the 'PREPARE' study) was a randomized controlled study in which Aranesp® was administered to prevent anemia conducted in 733 women receiving neoadjuvant breast cancer treatment. After a median follow-up of approximately 3 years the survival rate (86% vs. 90%, HR 1.42, 95% CI: 0.93, 2.18) and relapse-free survival rate lower (72% vs. 78%, HR 1.33, 95% CI: 0.99, 1.79) in the Aranesp®-treated arm compared to the control arm.

Cancer Study 4 (protocol GOG 191) was a randomized controlled study that enrolled 114 of a planned 460 cervical cancer patients receiving chemotherapy and radiotherapy. Patients were randomized to receive Epoetin alfa to maintain hemoglobin between 12 and 14 g/dL or to transfusion support as needed. The study was terminated prematurely due to an increase in thromboembolic events in Epoetin alfa-treated patients compared to control (19% vs. 9%). Both local recurrence (21% vs. 20%) and distant recurrence (12% vs. 7%) were more frequent in Epoetin alfa-treated patients compared to control. Progression-free survival at 3 years was lower in the Epoetin alfa-treated group compared to control (59% vs. 62%, HR 1.06, 95% CI: 0.58, 1.91). Overall survival at 3 years was lower in the Epoetin alfa-treated group compared to control (61% vs. 71%, HR 1.28, 95% CI: 0.68, 2.42).

Cancer Study 5 (the 'ENHANCE' study) was a randomized controlled study in 351 head and neck cancer patients where Epoetin beta or placebo was administered to achieve target hemoglobins of 14 and 15 g/dL for women and men, respectively. Locoregional progression-free survival was significantly shorter in patients receiving Epoetin beta (HR 1.62, 95% CI: 1.22, 2.14, p = 0.0008) with a median of 406 days Epoetin beta vs. 745 days placebo. Overall survival was significantly shorter in patients receiving Epoetin beta (HR 1.39, 95% CI: 1.05, 1.84; p = 0.02).

Decreased locoregional control:
Cancer Study 6 (DAHANCA 10) was conducted in 522 patients with primary squamous cell carcinoma of the head and neck receiving radiation therapy randomized to Aranesp® with radiotherapy or radiotherapy alone. An interim analysis on 484 patients demonstrated that locoregional control at 5 years was significantly shorter in patients receiving Aranesp® (RR 1.44, 95% CI: 1.06, 1.96; p = 0.02). Overall survival was shorter in patients receiving Aranesp® (RR 1.28, 95% CI: 0.98, 1.68; p = 0.08).

ESA APPRISE Oncology Program
Prescribers and hospitals must enroll in and comply with the ESA APPRISE Oncology Program to prescribe and/or dispense Aranesp® to patients with cancer. To enroll, visit www.esa-apprise.com or call 1-866-284-8089 for further assistance. Additionally, prescribers and patients must provide written acknowledgment of a discussion of the risks associated with Aranesp®.

Hypertension
Patients with uncontrolled hypertension should not be treated with Aranesp®; blood pressure should be controlled

Table 1: Randomized, Controlled Trials with Decreased Survival and/or Decreased Locoregional Control

Study/Tumor/(n)	Hemoglobin Target	Achieved Hemoglobin (Median Q1,Q3)	Primary Endpoint	Adverse Outcome for ESA-containing Arm
Chemotherapy				
Cancer Study 1 Metastatic breast cancer (n=939)	12-14 g/dL	12.9 g/dL 12.2, 13.3 g/dL	12-month overall survival	Decreased 12-month survival
Cancer Study 2 Lymphoid malignancy (n=344)	13-15 g/dL (M) 13-14 g/dL (F)	11.0 g/dL 9.8, 12.1 g/dL	Proportion of patients achieving a hemoglobin response	Decreased overall survival
Cancer Study 3 Early breast cancer (n=733)	12.5-13 g/dL	13.1 g/dL 12.5, 13.7 g/dL	Relapse-free and overall survival	Decreased 3 yr. relapse-free and overall survival
Cancer Study 4 Cervical Cancer (n=114)	12-14 g/dL	12.7 g/dL 12.1, 13.3 g/dL	Progression-free and overall survival and locoregional control	Decreased 3 yr. progression-free and overall survival and locoregional control
Radiotherapy Alone				
Cancer Study 5 Head and neck cancer (n=351)	≥15 g/dL (M) ≥14 g/dL (F)	Not available	Locoregional progression-free survival	Decreased 5-year locoregional progression-free survival Decreased overall survival
Cancer Study 6 Head and neck cancer (n=522)	14-15.5 g/dL	Not available	Locoregional disease control	Decreased locoregional disease control
No Chemotherapy or Radiotherapy				
Cancer Study 7 Non-small cell lung cancer (n=70)	12-14 g/dL	Not available	Quality of life	Decreased overall survival
Cancer Study 8 Non-myeloid malignancy (n=989)	12-13 g/dL	10.6 g/dL 9.4, 11.8 g/dL	RBC transfusions	Decreased overall survival

adequately before initiation of therapy. Blood pressure may rise during treatment of anemia with Aranesp® or Epoetin alfa. In Aranesp® clinical trials, approximately 40% of patients with CRF required initiation or intensification of antihypertensive therapy during the early phase of treatment when the hemoglobin was increasing. Hypertensive encephalopathy and seizures have been observed in patients with CRF treated with Aranesp® or Epoetin alfa.

Special care should be taken to closely monitor and control blood pressure in patients treated with Aranesp®. During Aranesp® therapy, patients should be advised of the importance of compliance with antihypertensive therapy and dietary restrictions. If blood pressure is difficult to control by pharmacologic or dietary measures, the dose of Aranesp® should be reduced or withheld (see **DOSAGE AND ADMINISTRATION**). A clinically significant decrease in hemoglobin may not be observed for several weeks.

Seizures
Seizures have occurred in patients with CRF participating in clinical trials of Aranesp® and Epoetin alfa. During the first several months of therapy, blood pressure and the presence of premonitory neurologic symptoms should be monitored closely. While the relationship between seizures and the rate of rise of hemoglobin is uncertain, it is recommended that the dose of Aranesp® be decreased if the hemoglobin increase exceeds 1 g/dL in any 2–week period.

Pure Red Cell Aplasia
Cases of pure red cell aplasia (PRCA) and of severe anemia, with or without other cytopenias, associated with neutralizing antibodies to erythropoietin have been reported in patients treated with Aranesp®. This has been reported predominantly in patients with CRF receiving ESAs by subcutaneous administration. PRCA has also been reported in patients receiving ESAs while undergoing treatment for hepatitis C with interferon and ribavirin. Any patient who develops a sudden loss of response to Aranesp®, accompanied by severe anemia and low reticulocyte count, should be evaluated for the etiology of loss of effect, including the presence of neutralizing antibodies to erythropoietin (see **PRECAUTIONS: Lack or Loss of Response to Aranesp®**). If anti-erythropoietin antibody-associated anemia is suspected, withhold Aranesp® and other ESAs. Contact Amgen (1-800-77AMGEN) to perform assays for binding and neutralizing antibodies. Aranesp® should be permanently discontinued in patients with antibody-mediated anemia. Patients should not be switched to other ESAs as antibodies may cross-react (see **ADVERSE REACTIONS: Immunogenicity**).

Albumin (Human)
Aranesp® is supplied in two formulations with different excipients, one containing polysorbate 80 and another containing albumin (human), a derivative of human blood (see **DESCRIPTION**). Based on effective donor screening and product manufacturing processes, Aranesp® formulated with albumin carries an extremely remote risk for transmission of viral diseases. A theoretical risk for transmission of Creutzfeldt-Jakob disease (CJD) also is considered extremely remote. No cases of transmission of viral diseases or CJD have ever been identified for albumin.

PRECAUTIONS
General
The safety and efficacy of Aranesp® therapy have not been established in patients with underlying hematologic diseases (e.g., hemolytic anemia, sickle cell anemia, thalassemia, porphyria).

The needle cover of the prefilled syringe contains dry natural rubber (a derivative of latex), which may cause allergic reactions in individuals sensitive to latex.

Lack or Loss of Response to Aranesp®
A lack of response or failure to maintain a hemoglobin response with Aranesp® doses within the recommended dosing range should prompt a search for causative factors. Deficiencies of folic acid, iron, or vitamin B_{12} should be excluded or corrected. Depending on the clinical setting, intercurrent infections, inflammatory or malignant processes, osteofibrosis cystica, occult blood loss, hemolysis, severe aluminum toxicity, and bone marrow fibrosis may compromise an erythropoietic response. In the absence of another etiology, the patient should be evaluated for evidence of PRCA and sera should be tested for the presence of antibodies to erythropoietin (see **WARNINGS: Pure Red Cell Aplasia**).
See **DOSAGE AND ADMINISTRATION:** *Chronic Renal Failure Patients*, *Dose Adjustment* for management of patients with an insufficient hemoglobin response to Aranesp® therapy.

Hematology

Sufficient time should be allowed to determine a patient's responsiveness to a dosage of Aranesp® before adjusting the dose. Because of the time required for erythropoiesis and the RBC half-life, an interval of 2 to 6 weeks may occur between the time of a dose adjustment (initiation, increase, decrease, or discontinuation) and a significant change in hemoglobin.

In order to prevent the hemoglobin from exceeding the recommended target range (10 to 12 g/dL) or rising too rapidly (greater than 1 g/dL in 2 weeks), the guidelines for dose and frequency of dose adjustments should be followed (see **WARNINGS** and **DOSAGE AND ADMINISTRATION**).

Allergic Reactions

There have been rare reports of potentially serious allergic reactions, including skin rash and urticaria, associated with Aranesp®. Symptoms have recurred with rechallenge, suggesting a causal relationship exists in some instances. If a serious allergic or anaphylactic reaction occurs, Aranesp® should be immediately and permanently discontinued and appropriate therapy should be administered.

Patients with CRF Not Requiring Dialysis

Patients with CRF not yet requiring dialysis may require lower maintenance doses of Aranesp® than patients receiving dialysis. Though CRF patients not on dialysis generally receive less frequent monitoring of blood pressure and laboratory parameters than dialysis patients, CRF patients not on dialysis may be more responsive to the effects of Aranesp®, and require judicious monitoring of blood pressure and hemoglobin. Renal function and fluid and electrolyte balance should also be closely monitored.

Patients Transitioning to Dialysis

During the transition period onto dialysis, hemoglobin and blood pressure should be monitored carefully and patients may need to have their maintenance doses adjusted to maintain hemoglobin levels within the range of 10 to 12 g/dL (see **DOSAGE AND ADMINISTRATION: Maintenance Dose**).

Dialysis Management

Therapy with Aranesp® results in an increase in RBCs and a decrease in plasma volume, which could reduce dialysis efficiency; patients who are marginally dialyzed may require adjustments in their dialysis prescription.

Laboratory Tests

After initiation of Aranesp® therapy, the hemoglobin should be determined weekly until it has stabilized and the maintenance dose has been established (see **DOSAGE AND ADMINISTRATION**). After a dose adjustment, the hemoglobin should be determined weekly for at least 4 weeks, until it has been determined that the hemoglobin has stabilized in response to the dose change. The hemoglobin should then be monitored at regular intervals.

In order to ensure effective erythropoiesis, iron status should be evaluated for all patients before and during treatment, as the majority of patients will eventually require supplemental iron therapy. Supplemental iron therapy is recommended for all patients whose serum ferritin is below 100 mcg/L or whose serum transferrin saturation is below 20%.

Information for Patients

Patients should be informed of the increased risks of mortality, serious cardiovascular events, thromboembolic events, and increased risk of tumor progression or recurrence (see **WARNINGS**). Patients should be informed of the possible side effects of Aranesp® and be instructed to report them to the prescribing physician. Patients should be informed of the signs and symptoms of allergic drug reactions and be advised of appropriate actions. Patients should be counseled on the importance of compliance with their Aranesp® treatment, dietary and dialysis prescriptions, and the importance of judicious monitoring of blood pressure and hemoglobin concentration should be stressed.

In those rare cases where it is determined that a patient can safely and effectively administer Aranesp® at home, appropriate instruction on the proper use of Aranesp® should be provided for patients and their caregivers. Patients should be instructed to read the Aranesp® Medication Guide and Patient Instructions for Use and should be informed that the Medication Guide is not a disclosure of all possible side effects. Patients and caregivers should also be cautioned against the reuse of needles, syringes, prefilled SureClick™ autoinjectors, or drug product, and be thoroughly instructed in their proper disposal. A puncture-resistant container for the disposal of used syringes, autoinjectors, and needles should be made available to the patient. Patients should be informed that the needle cover on the prefilled syringe contains dry natural rubber (a derivative of latex), which should not be handled by persons sensitive to latex.

Drug Interactions

No formal drug interaction studies of Aranesp® have been performed.

Carcinogenesis, Mutagenesis, and Impairment of Fertility

Carcinogenicity: The carcinogenic potential of Aranesp® has not been evaluated in long-term animal studies.

Aranesp® did not alter the proliferative response of non-hematological cells in vitro or in vivo. In toxicity studies of approximately 6 months duration in rats and dogs, no tumorigenic or unexpected mitogenic responses were observed in any tissue type. Using a panel of human tissues, the in vitro tissue binding profile of Aranesp® was identical to Epoetin alfa. Neither molecule bound to human tissues other than those expressing the erythropoietin receptor.

Mutagenicity: Aranesp® was negative in the in vitro bacterial and CHO cell assays to detect mutagenicity and in the in vivo mouse micronucleus assay to detect clastogenicity.

Impairment of Fertility: When administered intravenously to male and female rats prior to and during mating, reproductive performance, fertility, and sperm assessment parameters were not affected at any doses evaluated (up to 10 mcg/kg/dose, administered 3 times weekly). An increase in post implantation fetal loss was seen at doses equal to or greater than 0.5 mcg/kg/dose, administered 3 times weekly.

Pregnancy Category C

When Aranesp® was administered intravenously to rats and rabbits during gestation, no evidence of a direct embryotoxic, fetotoxic, or teratogenic outcome was observed at doses up to 20 mcg/kg/day. The only adverse effect observed was a slight reduction in fetal weight, which occurred at doses causing exaggerated pharmacological effects in the dams (1 mcg/kg/day and higher). No deleterious effects on uterine implantation were seen in either species. No significant placental transfer of Aranesp® was observed in rats. An increase in post implantation fetal loss was observed in studies assessing fertility (see **PRECAUTIONS: Carcinogenesis, Mutagenesis, and Impairment of Fertility: Impairment of Fertility**).

Intravenous injection of Aranesp® to female rats every other day from day 6 of gestation through day 23 of lactation at doses of 2.5 mcg/kg/dose and higher resulted in offspring (F1 generation) with decreased body weights, which correlated with a low incidence of deaths, as well as delayed eye opening and delayed preputial separation. No adverse effects were seen in the F2 offspring.

There are no adequate and well-controlled studies in pregnant women. Aranesp® should be used during pregnancy only if the potential benefit justifies the potential risk to the fetus.

Nursing Mothers

It is not known whether Aranesp® is excreted in human milk. Because many drugs are excreted in human milk, caution should be exercised when Aranesp® is administered to a nursing woman.

Pediatric Use

Pediatric CRF Patients

A study of the conversion from Epoetin alfa to Aranesp® among pediatric CRF patients over 1 year of age showed similar safety and efficacy to the findings from adult conversion studies (see **CLINICAL PHARMACOLOGY** and **CLINICAL STUDIES**). Safety and efficacy in the initial treatment of anemic pediatric CRF patients or in the conversion from another erythropoietin to Aranesp® in pediatric CRF patients less than 1 year of age have not been established.

Pediatric Cancer Patients

The safety and efficacy of Aranesp® in pediatric cancer patients have not been established.

Geriatric Use

Of the 1801 CRF patients in clinical studies of Aranesp®, 44% were age 65 and over, while 17% were age 75 and over. Of the 873 cancer patients in clinical studies receiving Aranesp® and concomitant chemotherapy, 45% were age 65 and over, while 14% were age 75 and over. No overall differences in safety or efficacy were observed between older and younger patients.

ADVERSE REACTIONS

General

Because clinical trials are conducted under widely varying conditions, adverse reaction rates observed in the clinical trials of Aranesp® cannot be directly compared to rates in the clinical trials of other drugs and may not reflect the rates observed in practice.

Immunogenicity

As with all therapeutic proteins, there is a potential for immunogenicity. Neutralizing antibodies to erythropoietin, in association with PRCA or severe anemia (with or without other cytopenias), have been reported in patients receiving Aranesp® (see **WARNINGS: Pure Red Cell Aplasia**) during post-marketing experience.

In clinical studies, the percentage of patients with antibodies to Aranesp® was examined using the BIAcore assay. Sera from 1501 CRF patients and 1159 cancer patients were tested. At baseline, prior to Aranesp® treatment, binding antibodies were detected in 59 (4%) of CRF patients and 36 (3%) of cancer patients. While receiving Aranesp® therapy (range 22-177 weeks), a follow-up sample was taken. One additional CRF patient and eight additional cancer patients developed antibodies capable of binding Aranesp®. None of

the patients had antibodies capable of neutralizing the activity of Aranesp® or endogenous erythropoietin at baseline or at end of study. No clinical sequelae consistent with PRCA were associated with the presence of these antibodies.

The incidence of antibody formation is highly dependent on the sensitivity and specificity of the assay. Additionally, the observed incidence of antibody (including neutralizing antibody) positivity in an assay may be influenced by several factors including assay methodology, sample handling, timing of sample collection, concomitant medications, and underlying disease. For these reasons, comparison of the incidence of antibodies across products within this class (erythropoietic proteins) may be misleading.

Chronic Renal Failure Patients

Adult Patients

In all studies, the most frequently reported serious adverse events with Aranesp® were infection, congestive heart failure, angina pectoris/cardiac chest pain, thrombosis vascular access, and cardiac arrhythmia/cardiac arrest. The most frequently reported adverse events resulting in clinical intervention (e.g., discontinuation of Aranesp®, adjustment in dosage, or the need for concomitant medication to treat an adverse reaction symptom) were infection, hypertension, hypotension, and muscle spasm. See **WARNINGS: Increased Mortality, Serious Cardiovascular Events, Thromboembolic Events, and Stroke** and **Hypertension**.

The data described below reflect exposure to Aranesp® in 1801 CRF patients, including 675 exposed for at least 6 months, of whom 185 were exposed for greater than 1 year. Aranesp® was evaluated in active-controlled (n = 823) and uncontrolled studies (n = 978). These data include a pooled analysis of CRF patients not on dialysis and dialysis patients who were studied for the correction of anemia and maintenance of hemoglobin.

The population encompassed an age range from 18 to 94 years. Fifty-five percent of the patients were male. The percentages of Caucasian, Black, Asian, and Hispanic patients were 80%, 13%, 3%, and 2%, respectively. The median weekly dose of Aranesp® for patients who received either once weekly or once every 2 week administration was 0.44 mcg/kg (25th, 75th percentiles: 0.30, 0.64 mcg/kg).

Some of the adverse events reported are typically associated with CRF, or recognized complications of dialysis, and may not necessarily be attributable to Aranesp® therapy. No important differences in adverse event rates between treatment groups were observed in controlled studies in which patients received Aranesp® or other recombinant erythropoietins.

The data in Table 2 reflect those adverse events occurring in at least 5% of patients treated with Aranesp®.

Table 2. Adverse Events Occurring in ≥ 5% of CRF Patients

Event	Patients Treated with Aranesp® (n = 1801)
APPLICATION SITE	
Injection Site Pain	6%
BODY AS A WHOLE	
Peripheral Edema	10%
Fatigue	9%
Fever	7%
Death	6%
Chest Pain, Unspecified	7%
Fluid Overload	6%
Access Infection	6%
Influenza-like Symptoms	6%
Access Hemorrhage	7%
Asthenia	5%
CARDIOVASCULAR	
Hypertension	20%
Hypotension	20%
Cardiac Arrhythmias/Cardiac Arrest	8%
Angina Pectoris/Cardiac Chest Pain	8%
Thrombosis Vascular Access	6%
Congestive Heart Failure	5%

CNS/PNS	
Headache	15%
Dizziness	7%
GASTROINTESTINAL	
Diarrhea	14%
Vomiting	14%
Nausea	11%
Abdominal Pain	10%
Constipation	5%
MUSCULO-SKELETAL	
Muscle Spasm	17%
Arthralgia	9%
Limb Pain	8%
Back Pain	7%
RESISTANCE MECHANISM	
Infection*	24%
RESPIRATORY	
Upper Respiratory Infection	15%
Dyspnea	10%
Cough	9%
Bronchitis	5%
SKIN AND APPENDAGES	
Pruritus	6%

*Infection includes sepsis, bacteremia, pneumonia, peritonitis, and abscess.

The incidence rates for other clinically significant events are shown in Table 3.

Table 3. Percent Incidence of Other Clinically Significant Events in CRF Patients

Event	Patients Treated with Aranesp® (n = 1801)
Acute Myocardial Infarction	2%
Stroke	2%
Seizure	1%
Transient Ischemic Attack	≤1%

Pediatric Patients
In Study N7, Aranesp® was administered to 81 pediatric CRF patients who had stable hemoglobin concentrations while previously receiving Epoetin alfa (see **CLINICAL STUDIES**). In this study, the most frequently reported serious adverse events with Aranesp® were catheter sepsis, fever, catheter related infection, chronic renal failure, and vascular access complication. The most commonly reported adverse events were fever, headache, nasopharyngitis, hypertension, hypotension, injection site pain, cough, peritonitis, and vomiting. Aranesp® administration was discontinued because of injection site pain in two patients and moderate hypertension in a third patient.
Studies have not evaluated the effects of Aranesp® when administered to pediatric patients as the initial treatment for the anemia associated with CRF.
Thrombotic Events
Vascular access thrombosis in hemodialysis patients occurred in clinical trials at an annualized rate of 0.22 events per patient year of Aranesp® therapy. Rates of thrombotic events (e.g., vascular access thrombosis, venous thrombosis, and pulmonary emboli) with Aranesp® therapy were similar to those observed with other recombinant erythropoietins in these trials; the median duration of exposure was 12 weeks.
Cancer Patients Receiving Chemotherapy
The incidence data described below reflect the exposure to Aranesp® in 873 cancer patients including patients exposed to Aranesp® once weekly (547, 63%), once every 2 weeks (128, 16%), and once every 3 weeks (198, 23%). Aranesp® was evaluated in seven studies that were active-controlled and/or placebo-controlled studies of up to 6 months duration. The Aranesp®-treated patient demographics were as follows: median age of 63 years (range of 20 to 91 years); 40% male; 88% Caucasian, 5% Hispanic, 4% Black, and 3% Asian. Over 90% of patients had locally advanced or meta-

static cancer, with the remainder having early stage disease. Patients with solid tumors (e.g., lung, breast, colon, ovarian cancers) and lymphoproliferative malignancies (e.g., lymphoma, multiple myeloma) were enrolled in the clinical studies. All of the 873 Aranesp®-treated subjects also received concomitant cyclic chemotherapy.
The most frequently reported serious adverse events included death (10%), fever (4%), pneumonia (3%), dehydration (3%), vomiting (2%), and dyspnea (2%). The most commonly reported adverse events were fatigue, edema, nausea, vomiting, diarrhea, fever, and dyspnea (see **Table 4**). Except for those events listed in Tables 4 and 5, the incidence of adverse events in clinical studies occurred at a similar rate compared with patients who received placebo and were generally consistent with the underlying disease and its treatment with chemotherapy. The most frequently reported reasons for discontinuation of Aranesp® were progressive disease, death, discontinuation of the chemotherapy, asthenia, dyspnea, pneumonia, and gastrointestinal hemorrhage. No important differences in adverse event rates between treatment groups were observed in controlled studies in which patients received Aranesp® or other recombinant erythropoietins.

Table 4. Adverse Events Occurring in ≥ 5% of Patients Receiving Chemotherapy

Event	Aranesp® (n = 873)	Placebo (n = 221)
BODY AS A WHOLE		
Fatigue	33%	30%
Edema	21%	10%
Fever	19%	16%
CNS/PNS		
Dizziness	14%	8%
Headache	12%	9%
GASTROINTESTINAL		
Diarrhea	22%	12%
Constipation	18%	17%
METABOLIC/NUTRITION		
Dehydration	5%	3%
MUSCULO-SKELETAL		
Arthralgia	13%	6%
Myalgia	8%	5%
SKIN AND APPENDAGES		
Rash	7%	3%

Table 5. Incidence of Other Clinically Significant Adverse Events in Patients Receiving Chemotherapy

Event	All Aranesp® (n = 873)	Placebo (n = 221)
Hypertension	3.7%	3.2%
Seizures/Convulsions*	0.6%	0.5%
Thrombotic Events	6.2%	4.1%
Pulmonary Embolism	1.3%	0.0%
Thrombosis†	5.6%	4.1%

*Seizures/Convulsions include the preferred terms: Convulsions, Convulsions Grand Mal, and Convulsions Local.
†Thrombosis includes: Thrombophlebitis, Thrombophlebitis Deep, Thrombosis Venous, Thrombosis Venous Deep, Thromboembolism, and Thrombosis.

In a randomized controlled trial of Aranesp® 500 mcg once every 3 weeks (n = 353) and Aranesp® 2.25 mcg/kg once weekly (n = 352), the incidences of all adverse events and of serious adverse events were similar between the two groups.
Thrombotic and Cardiovascular Events
Overall, the incidence of thrombotic events was 6.2% for Aranesp® and 4.1% for placebo. However, the following events were reported more frequently in Aranesp®-treated patients than in placebo controls: pulmonary embolism, thromboembolism, thrombosis, and thrombophlebitis (deep and/or superficial). In addition, edema of any type was more frequently reported in Aranesp®-treated patients (21%) than in patients who received placebo (10%).

OVERDOSAGE
The expected manifestations of Aranesp® overdosage include signs and symptoms associated with an excessive

and/or rapid increase in hemoglobin concentration, including any of the cardiovascular events described in **WARNINGS** and listed in **ADVERSE REACTIONS**. Patients receiving an overdosage of Aranesp® should be monitored closely for cardiovascular events and hematologic abnormalities. Polycythemia should be managed acutely with phlebotomy, as clinically indicated. Following resolution of the effects due to Aranesp® overdosage, reintroduction of Aranesp® therapy should be accompanied by close monitoring for evidence of rapid increases in hemoglobin concentration (> 1 g/dL in any 2-week period). In patients with an excessive hematopoietic response, reduce the Aranesp® dose in accordance with the recommendations described in **DOSAGE AND ADMINISTRATION**.

DOSAGE AND ADMINISTRATION
IMPORTANT: See BOXED WARNINGS and WARNINGS: Increased Mortality, Serious Cardiovascular Events, Thromboembolic Events, and Stroke.
Aranesp® is supplied in vials or in prefilled syringes with UltraSafe® Needle Guards*. Following administration of Aranesp® from the prefilled syringe, the UltraSafe® Needle Guard should be activated to prevent accidental needle sticks.
Aranesp® is also supplied in prefilled SureClick™ autoinjectors containing the same dosage strengths as the prefilled syringes. Because the autoinjectors are designed to deliver the full content, autoinjectors should only be used for patients who need the full dose. If the required dose is not available in an autoinjector, prefilled syringes, or vials should be used to administer the required dose. Autoinjectors are for subcutaneous administration only.
Chronic Renal Failure Patients
Aranesp® may be administered either intravenously or subcutaneously as a single weekly injection. *In patients on hemodialysis, the intravenous route is recommended.* The dose should be started and slowly adjusted as described below based on hemoglobin levels. If a patient fails to respond or maintain a response, this should be evaluated (see **WARNINGS: Pure Red Cell Aplasia, PRECAUTIONS: Lack or Loss of Response to Aranesp® and PRECAUTIONS: Laboratory Tests**). When Aranesp® therapy is initiated or adjusted, the hemoglobin should be followed weekly until stabilized and monitored at least monthly thereafter. During therapy, hematological parameters should be monitored regularly. Doses must be individualized to ensure that hemoglobin is maintained at an appropriate level for each patient.
For patients who respond to Aranesp® with a rapid increase in hemoglobin (e.g., more than 1 g/dL in any 2-week period), the dose of Aranesp® should be reduced.
Individualize dosing to achieve and maintain hemoglobin levels within the range of 10 to 12 g/dL.
Starting Dose
Correction of Anemia
The initial dose by subcutaneous or intravenous administration is 0.45 mcg/kg body weight, as a single injection once weekly. Alternatively, in patients not receiving dialysis, an initial dose of 0.75 mcg/kg may be administered subcutaneously as a single injection once every 2 weeks. If hemoglobin excursions outside the recommended range occur, the Aranesp® dose should be adjusted as described below.
The use of Aranesp® in pediatric CRF patients as the initial treatment to correct anemia has not been studied.
Maintenance Dose
The dose should be individualized to maintain hemoglobin levels within the range of 10 to 12 g/dL (see **Dose Adjustment**). If hemoglobin excursions outside the recommended range occur, the Aranesp® dose should be adjusted as described below. For many patients, the appropriate maintenance dose will be lower than the starting dose. CRF patients not on dialysis, in particular, may require lower maintenance doses. In the maintenance phase, Aranesp® may continue to be administered as a single injection once weekly or once every 2 weeks.
Dose Adjustment
The dose should be adjusted for each patient to achieve and maintain hemoglobin levels within the range of 10 to 12 g/dL. If hemoglobin excursions outside the recommended range occur, the Aranesp® dose should be adjusted as described below. Increases in dose should not be made more frequently than once a month.
If the hemoglobin is increasing and approaching 12 g/dL, the dose should be reduced by approximately 25%. If the hemoglobin continues to increase, doses should be temporarily withheld until the hemoglobin begins to decrease, at which point therapy should be reinitiated at a dose approximately 25% below the previous dose. If the hemoglobin increases by more than 1 g/dL in a 2-week period, the dose should be decreased by approximately 25%.
If the increase in hemoglobin is less than 1 g/dL over 4 weeks and iron stores are adequate (see **PRECAUTIONS: Laboratory Tests**), the dose of Aranesp® may be increased

by approximately 25% of the previous dose. Further increases may be made at 4-week intervals until the specified hemoglobin is obtained.

For patients whose hemoglobin does not attain a level within the range of 10 to 12 g/dL despite the use of appropriate Aranesp® dose titrations over a 12-week period:

- do not administer higher Aranesp® doses and use the lowest dose that will maintain a hemoglobin level sufficient to avoid the need for recurrent RBC transfusions,
- evaluate and treat for other causes of anemia (see **PRECAUTIONS: Lack or Loss of Response to Aranesp®**), and
- thereafter, hemoglobin should continue to be monitored and if responsiveness improves, Aranesp® dose adjustments should be made as described above; discontinue Aranesp® if responsiveness does not improve and the patient needs recurrent RBC transfusions.

Conversion From Epoetin alfa to Aranesp®
The starting weekly dose of Aranesp® for adults and pediatric patients should be estimated on the basis of the weekly Epoetin alfa dose at the time of substitution (see **Table 6**). For pediatric patients receiving a weekly Epoetin alfa dose of < 1500 units/week, the available data are insufficient to determine an Aranesp® conversion dose. Because of variability, doses should be titrated to achieve and maintain hemoglobin levels within the range of 10 to 12 g/dL. Due to the longer serum half-life, Aranesp® should be administered less frequently than Epoetin alfa. Aranesp® should be administered once a week if a patient was receiving Epoetin alfa 2 to 3 times weekly. Aranesp® should be administered once every 2 weeks if a patient was receiving Epoetin alfa once per week. The route of administration (intravenous or subcutaneous) should be maintained.

Table 6. Estimated Aranesp® Starting Doses (mcg/week) for Patients Based on Previous Epoetin alfa Dose (Units/week)

Previous Weekly Epoetin alfa Dose (Units/week)	Weekly Aranesp® Dose (mcg/week)	
	Adult	Pediatric
< 1,500	6.25	See text*
1,500 to 2,499	6.25	6.25
2,500 to 4,999	12.5	10
5,000 to 10,999	25	20
11,000 to 17,999	40	40
18,000 to 33,999	60	60
34,000 to 89,999	100	100
≥ 90,000	200	200

*For pediatric patients receiving a weekly Epoetin alfa dose of < 1,500 units/week, the available data are insufficient to determine an Aranesp® conversion dose.

Cancer Patients Receiving Chemotherapy
Only prescribers enrolled in the ESA APPRISE Oncology Program may prescribe and/or dispense Aranesp® (see **WARNINGS: ESA APPRISE Oncology Program**).
For pediatric patients, see **PRECAUTIONS: Pediatric Use**. The recommended starting dose for Aranesp® administered weekly is 2.25 mcg/kg as a subcutaneous injection.
The recommended starting dose for Aranesp® administered once every 3 weeks is 500 mcg as a subcutaneous injection. Therapy should not be initiated at hemoglobin levels ≥ 10 g/dL. For both dosing schedules, the dose should be adjusted for each patient to maintain the lowest hemoglobin level sufficient to avoid RBC transfusion. If the rate of hemoglobin increase is more than 1 g/dL per 2-week period or

when the hemoglobin reaches a level needed to avoid transfusion, the dose should be reduced by 40% of the previous dose. If the hemoglobin exceeds a level needed to avoid transfusion, Aranesp® should be temporarily withheld until the hemoglobin approaches a level where transfusions may be required. At this point, therapy should be reinitiated at a dose 40% below the previous dose.
For patients receiving weekly administration, if there is less than a 1 g/dL increase in hemoglobin after 6 weeks of therapy, the dose of Aranesp® should be increased up to 4.5 mcg/kg.
Discontinue Aranesp® if after 8 weeks of therapy there is no response as measured by hemoglobin levels or if transfusions are still required.
Discontinue Aranesp® following the completion of a chemotherapy course (see **BOXED WARNINGS: Cancer**).

Preparation and Administration of Aranesp®
Do not shake Aranesp® or leave vials, syringes, or prefilled SureClick™ autoinjectors exposed to light. After removing the vials, prefilled syringes, or autoinjectors from the refrigerator, protect from room light until administration. Vigorous shaking or exposure to light may denature Aranesp®, causing it to become biologically inactive. Always store vials, prefilled syringes, or autoinjectors of Aranesp® in their carton until use.
Parenteral drug products should be inspected visually for particulate matter and discoloration prior to administration. Do not use any vials, prefilled syringes, or autoinjectors exhibiting particulate matter or discoloration.
Do not dilute Aranesp®.
Do not administer Aranesp® in conjunction with other drug solutions.
Aranesp® contains no preservatives. Discard any unused portion. **Do not pool unused portions from the vials or prefilled syringes. Do not use the vial, prefilled syringe, or autoinjector more than one time.**
Following administration of Aranesp® from the prefilled syringe, activate the UltraSafe® Needle Guard. Place your hands behind the needle, grasp the guard with one hand, and slide the guard forward until the needle is completely covered and the guard clicks into place. NOTE: If an audible click is not heard, the needle guard may not be completely activated.
The prefilled SureClick™ autoinjector is designed to deliver the full dose. The completion of the injection is signaled by an audible click. Removal of the autoinjector from the injection site automatically extends a needle cover.
The autoinjectors, the syringes used with vials, and the entire prefilled syringe with activated needle guard should be disposed of in a puncture-proof container.
See the accompanying "Patient Instructions for Use" insert for complete instructions on the preparation and administration of Aranesp® for patients, including injection site selection.

HOW SUPPLIED

Aranesp® is available in single-dose vials in two solutions, an albumin solution and a polysorbate solution. The words "Albumin Free" appear on the polysorbate container labels and the package main panels as well as other panels as space permits. Aranesp® single-dose prefilled syringes and prefilled SureClick™ autoinjectors are available in albumin and polysorbate solutions. Both prefilled syringes and autoinjectors are supplied with a 27-gauge, ½-inch needle.
Each prefilled syringe is equipped with an UltraSafe® Needle Guard that is manually activated to cover the needle during disposal. The needle cover of the prefilled syringe contains dry natural rubber (a derivative of latex). The autoinjector has a needle cover that automatically extends as the autoinjector is removed from the injection site after completion of the injection.
Aranesp® is available in the following packages:
[See table at left]

Single-dose Vial, Polysorbate Solution

1 Vial/Pack, 4 Packs/Case	4 Vials/Pack, 4 Packs/Case	4 Vials/Pack, 10 Packs/Case
200 mcg/1 mL (NDC 55513-006-01)	200 mcg/1 mL (NDC 55513-006-04)	25 mcg/1 mL (NDC 55513-002-04)
300 mcg/1 mL (NDC 55513-110-01)	300 mcg/1 mL (NDC 55513-110-04)	40 mcg/1 mL (NDC 55513-003-04)
500 mcg/1 mL (NDC 55513-008-01)		60 mcg/1 mL (NDC 55513-004-04)
		100 mcg/1 mL (NDC 55513-005-04)
		150 mcg/0.75 mL (NDC 55513-053-04)

Single-dose Vial, Albumin Solution

1 Vial/Pack, 4 Packs/Case	4 Vials/Pack, 4 Packs/Case	4 Vials/Pack, 10 Packs/Case
200 mcg/1 mL (NDC 55513-014-01)	200 mcg/1 mL (NDC 55513-014-04)	25 mcg/1 mL (NDC 55513-010-04)
300 mcg/1 mL (NDC 55513-015-01)	300 mcg/1 mL (NDC 55513-015-04)	40 mcg/1 mL (NDC 55513-011-04)
500 mcg/1 mL (NDC 55513-016-01)		60 mcg/1 mL (NDC 55513-012-04)
		100 mcg/1 mL (NDC 55513-013-04)
		150 mcg/0.75 mL (NDC 55513-054-04)

Single-dose Prefilled Syringe (SingleJect®) with a 27-gauge, ½-inch needle with an UltraSafe® Needle Guard, Polysorbate Solution

1 Syringe/Pack, 4 Packs/Case	4 Syringes/Pack, 4 Packs/Case	4 Syringes/Pack, 10 Packs/Case
200 mcg/0.4 mL (NDC 55513-028-01)	200 mcg/0.4 mL (NDC 55513-028-04)	25 mcg/0.42 mL (NDC 55513-057-04)
300 mcg/0.6 mL (NDC 55513-111-01)	300 mcg/0.6 mL (NDC 55513-111-04)	40 mcg/0.4 mL (NDC 55513-021-04)
500 mcg/1 mL (NDC 55513-032-01)		60 mcg/0.3 mL (NDC 55513-023-04)
		100 mcg/0.5 mL (NDC 55513-025-04)
		150 mcg/0.3 mL (NDC 55513-027-04)

Single-dose Prefilled Syringe (SingleJect®) with a 27-gauge, ½-inch needle with an UltraSafe® Needle Guard, Albumin Solution

1 Syringe/Pack, 4 Packs/Case	4 Syringes/Pack, 4 Packs/Case	4 Syringes/Pack, 10 Packs/Case
200 mcg/0.4 mL (NDC 55513-044-01)	200 mcg/0.4 mL (NDC 55513-044-04)	25 mcg/0.42 mL (NDC 55513-058-04)
300 mcg/0.6 mL (NDC 55513-046-01)	300 mcg/0.6 mL (NDC 55513-046-04)	40 mcg/0.4 mL (NDC 55513-037-04)
500 mcg/1 mL (NDC 55513-048-01)		60 mcg/0.3 mL (NDC 55513-039-04)
		100 mcg/0.5 mL (NDC 55513-041-04)
		150 mcg/0.3 mL (NDC 55513-043-04)

Single-dose Prefilled SureClick™ Autoinjector with a 27-gauge, ½-inch needle, Polysorbate Solution

1 Autoinjector/Pack
25 mcg/0.42 mL (NDC 55513-090-01)
40 mcg/0.4 mL (NDC 55513-091-01)
60 mcg/0.3 mL (NDC 55513-092-01)
100 mcg/0.5 mL (NDC 55513-093-01)
150 mcg/0.3 mL (NDC 55513-094-01)
200 mcg/0.4 mL (NDC 55513-095-01)
300 mcg/0.6 mL (NDC 55513-096-01)
500 mcg/1 mL (NDC 55513-097-01)

Single-dose Prefilled SureClick™ Autoinjector with a 27-gauge, ½-inch needle, Albumin Solution

1 Autoinjector/Pack
25 mcg/0.42 mL
(NDC 55513-080-01)
40 mcg/0.4 mL
(NDC 55513-081-01)
60 mcg/0.3 mL
(NDC 55513-082-01)
100 mcg/0.5 mL
(NDC 55513-083-01)
150 mcg/0.3 mL
(NDC 55513-084-01)
200 mcg/0.4 mL
(NDC 55513-085-01)
300 mcg/0.6 mL
(NDC 55513-086-01)
500 mcg/1 mL
(NDC 55513-087-01)

Storage
Store at 2° to 8°C (36° to 46°F). Do not freeze or shake. Protect from light.

REFERENCES

1. Egrie JC, Browne JK. Development and characterization of novel erythropoiesis stimulating protein (NESP). *Br J Cancer*. 2001;84 (suppl 1):3-10.
2. Singh AK, Szczech L, Tang KL, et al. Correction of Anemia with Epoetin Alfa in Chronic Kidney Disease. *N Engl J Med*. 2006; 355: 2085-98.
3. Besarab A, Bolton WK, Browne JK, et al. The effects of normal as compared with low hematocrit values in patients with cardiac disease who are receiving hemodialysis and epoetin. *N Engl J Med*. 1998; 339:584-590.
4. Leyland-Jones B, Semiglazov V, Pawlicki M, et al. Maintaining Normal Hemoglobin Levels With Epoetin Alfa in Mainly Nonanemic Patients With Metastatic Breast Cancer Receiving First-Line Chemotherapy: A Survival Study. *JCO*. 2005; 23(25): 1-13.
5. Bohlius J, Wilson J, Seidenfeld J, et al. Recombinant Human Erythropoietins and Cancer Patients: Updated Meta-Analysis of 57 Studies Including 9353 Patients. *J Natl Cancer Inst*. 2006; 98: 708-14.

Rx only
This product's label may have been revised after this insert was used in production. For further product information and the current package insert, please visit www.amgen.com or call our medical information department toll-free at 1-800-77AMGEN (1-800-772-6436). This product, the process of its manufacture, or its use, may be covered by one or more US Patents, including US Patent No. 7,217,689.

Manufactured by:
Amgen Manufacturing, Limited, a subsidiary of Amgen Inc.
One Amgen Center Drive
Thousand Oaks, CA 91320-1799
©2001-2010 Amgen Inc. All rights reserved.
* UltraSafe® is a registered trademark of Safety Syringes, Inc.
1xxxxxx - v24
Revised: 05/2010

MEDICATION GUIDE

Aranesp® (Air-uh-nesp)
(darbepoetin alfa)

Read this Medication Guide before you start Aranesp, each time you refill your prescription, and if you are told by your healthcare provider that there is new information about Aranesp. This Medication Guide does not take the place of talking to your healthcare provider about your medical condition or your treatment. Talk with your healthcare provider regularly about the use of Aranesp and ask if there is new information about Aranesp.

What is the most important information I should know about Aranesp?

Using Aranesp can lead to death or other serious side effects.

Patients with cancer:

Your healthcare provider has received special training through the ESA APPRISE Oncology Program in order to prescribe Aranesp. Before you can begin to receive Aranesp, you must sign the ESA APPRISE Oncology Patient and Healthcare Professional (HCP) Acknowledgement Form to document that your healthcare provider discussed the risks of Aranesp with you. When you sign this form, you are stating that you are aware of the risks associated with use of Aranesp.

These risks include that your tumor may grow faster and you may die sooner when Aranesp is used experimentally to try to raise your hemoglobin beyond the amount needed to

avoid red blood cell transfusion or if you are not getting strong doses of chemotherapy. It is not known whether these risks exist when Aranesp is given according to the FDA-approved directions for use.
You should discuss with your doctor:
• Why Aranesp treatment is being prescribed.
• What are the chances you will get red blood cell transfusions if you do not take Aranesp.
• What are the chances you will get red blood cell transfusions even if you take Aranesp.
• How taking Aranesp may affect the success of your cancer treatment.
If you decide to take Aranesp, your healthcare provider should prescribe the smallest dose of Aranesp to lower the chance of getting red blood cell transfusions.
• After you have finished your chemotherapy course, Aranesp treatment should be stopped.
• Aranesp does not improve the symptoms of anemia (lower than normal number of red blood cells), quality of life, fatigue, or well-being for patients with cancer.

All patients, including patients with cancer or chronic kidney failure:
• You may get serious heart problems such as heart attack, stroke, heart failure, and may die sooner if you are treated with Aranesp to a hemoglobin level above 12 g/dL.
• You may get blood clots at any time while taking Aranesp. If you are receiving Aranesp and you are going to have surgery, talk to your healthcare provider about whether or not you need to take a blood thinner to lessen the chance of blood clots during or following surgery. Clots can form in blood vessels (veins), especially in your leg (deep venous thrombosis or DVT). Pieces of a blood clot may travel to the lungs and block the blood circulation in the lungs (pulmonary embolus).
Call your healthcare provider or get medical help right away if you have any of these symptoms of blood clots:
• Chest pain
• Trouble breathing or shortness of breath
• Pain in your legs, with or without swelling
• A cool or pale arm or leg
• Sudden confusion, trouble speaking, or trouble understanding others' speech
• Sudden numbness or weakness in your face, arm, or leg, especially on one side of your body
• Sudden trouble seeing
• Sudden trouble walking, dizziness, loss of balance or coordination
• Loss of consciousness (fainting)
• Hemodialysis vascular access stops working. If you are a patient with chronic kidney failure and have a hemodialysis vascular access, blood clots may form in this access.
Also see "**What are the possible side effects of Aranesp?**" below.

What is Aranesp?
Aranesp is a man-made form of the protein human erythropoietin that is given to patients to lessen the need for red blood cell transfusions. Aranesp stimulates your bone marrow to make more red blood cells. Having more red blood cells raises your hemoglobin level. If your hemoglobin level stays too high or if your hemoglobin goes up too quickly, this may lead to serious health problems which may result in death. These serious health problems may happen even if you take Aranesp and do not have an increase in your hemoglobin level.
Aranesp may be used to treat a lower than normal number of red blood cells (anemia) if it is caused by:
• Chronic kidney failure (you may or may not be on dialysis)
• Chemotherapy that is used to treat some types of cancer
Aranesp should not be used for treatment of anemia:
• If you have cancer and you are not receiving chemotherapy that may cause anemia
• If your cancer has a high chance of being cured

Who should not take Aranesp?
Do not take Aranesp if you:
• Have cancer and have not been counseled by your healthcare provider regarding the risks of Aranesp and signed the ESA APPRISE Oncology Program Patient and Healthcare Professional (HCP) Acknowledgement Form before you begin to receive Aranesp.
• Have high blood pressure that is not controlled (uncontrolled hypertension).
• Have been told by your healthcare provider that you have or have ever had a type of anemia called Pure Red Cell Aplasia (PRCA) that starts after treatment with Aranesp or other erythropoietin medicines.
• Have allergies to any of the ingredients in Aranesp. See the end of this Medication Guide for a complete list of ingredients in Aranesp.

What should I tell my healthcare provider before taking Aranesp?
Aranesp may not be right for you. **Tell your healthcare provider about all your health conditions,** including if you:
• Have heart disease.

• Have high blood pressure.
• Have had a seizure (convulsion) or stroke.
• Are pregnant or planning to become pregnant. It is not known if Aranesp may harm your unborn baby. Talk to your healthcare provider about possible pregnancy and birth control choices that are right for you.
• Are breast-feeding or planning to breast-feed. It is not known if Aranesp passes into breast milk.
Tell your healthcare provider about all the medicines you take, including prescription and nonprescription medicines, vitamins, and herbal supplements.
Know the medicines you take. Keep a list of your medicines with you and show it to your healthcare provider when you get a new medicine.

How should I take Aranesp?
Patients with cancer:
Before you begin to receive Aranesp, your healthcare provider will:
• Ask you to review this Aranesp Medication Guide
• Explain the risks of Aranesp and answer all your questions about Aranesp
• Have you sign the ESA APPRISE Oncology Program Patient and Healthcare Professional (HCP) Acknowledgement Form

All patients:
• Continue to follow your healthcare provider's instructions for diet, dialysis, and medicines, including medicines for high blood pressure, while taking Aranesp.
• Have your blood pressure checked as instructed by your healthcare provider.
• If you or your caregiver has been trained to give Aranesp shots (injections) at home:
  • Be sure that you read, understand, and follow the "Patient Instructions for Use" that come with Aranesp.
  • Take Aranesp exactly as your healthcare provider tells you to. Do not change the dose of Aranesp unless told to do so by your healthcare provider.
  • Your healthcare provider will show you how much Aranesp to use, how to inject it, how often it should be injected, and how to safely throw away the used vial, syringes, and needles.
• If you miss a dose of Aranesp, call your healthcare provider right away and ask what to do.
• If you take more than the prescribed amount of Aranesp, call your healthcare provider right away.

What are the possible side effects of Aranesp?
Aranesp may cause serious side effects. See "**What is the most important information I should know about Aranesp?**"
Other side effects of Aranesp, which may also be serious, include:
• **High blood pressure in patients with chronic kidney failure.** Your blood pressure may go up or be difficult to control with blood pressure medicine while taking Aranesp. This can happen even if you have never had high blood pressure before. Your healthcare provider should check your blood pressure often. If your blood pressure does go up, your healthcare provider may prescribe new or more blood pressure medicine.
• **Seizures.** If you have any seizures while taking Aranesp, get medical help right away and tell your healthcare provider.
• **Antibodies to Aranesp.** Your body may make antibodies to Aranesp. These antibodies can block or lessen your body's ability to make red blood cells and cause you to have severe anemia. Call your healthcare provider if you have unusual tiredness, lack of energy, dizziness, or fainting. You may need to stop taking Aranesp.
• **Serious allergic reactions.** Serious allergic reactions can cause a rash over your whole body, shortness of breath, wheezing, dizziness and fainting because of a drop in blood pressure, swelling around your mouth or eyes, fast pulse, or sweating. If you have a serious allergic reaction, stop using Aranesp and call your healthcare provider or get medical help right away.
The needle cover on the prefilled syringe contains a material that is like latex. If you know you are allergic to latex, talk to your healthcare provider before using Aranesp.
Common side effects of Aranesp include:
• Swelling in cancer patients
• Rash
• Injection site pain
These are not all of the possible side effects of Aranesp. Your healthcare provider can give you a more complete list. Tell your healthcare provider about any side effects that bother you or that do not go away.
Call your doctor for medical advice about side effects. You may report side effects to FDA at 1-800-FDA-1088.

How should I store Aranesp?
• Do not shake Aranesp.
• Protect Aranesp from light.
• Store Aranesp in the refrigerator between 36°F to 46°F (2°C to 8°C).
• **Do not freeze.** Do not use Aranesp that has been frozen.

Keep Aranesp and all medicines out of the reach of children.

General information about Aranesp

Medicines are sometimes prescribed for purposes other than those listed in a Medication Guide. Use Aranesp only for the condition for which it has been prescribed. Do not give Aranesp to other people even if they have the same symptoms that you have. It may harm them.

This Medication Guide summarizes the most important information about Aranesp. If you would like more information about Aranesp, talk with your healthcare provider. You can ask your healthcare provider or pharmacist for information about Aranesp that is written for healthcare professionals. For more information, go to the following website: www.aranesp.com or call 1-800-77-AMGEN.

What are the ingredients in Aranesp?

Active Ingredient: darbepoetin alfa

Inactive Ingredients:

- polysorbate solution: polysorbate 80, sodium phosphate monobasic monohydrate, sodium phosphate dibasic anhydrous, and sodium chloride in Water for Injection, USP.
- albumin solution: albumin (human), sodium phosphate monobasic monohydrate, sodium phosphate dibasic anhydrous, and sodium chloride in Water for Injection, USP.

Manufactured by:

Amgen Manufacturing, Limited, a subsidiary of Amgen Inc.
One Amgen Center Drive
Thousand Oaks, CA 91320-1799
© 2001-2010 Amgen Inc. All rights reserved.
1xxxxxx - v2
Revised: 02/2010
This Medication Guide has been approved by the U.S. Food and Drug Administration.

PATIENT INSTRUCTIONS FOR USE

Aranesp® (Air-uh-nesp)
(darbepoetin alfa)
Single-dose Vial

Use these instructions if you or your caregiver has been trained to give Aranesp injections at home. Do not try to give yourself per the injection unless you have received training from your healthcare provider. If you are not sure about giving the injection or if you have questions, ask your healthcare provider for help.

Before reading these instructions for use, read the Medication Guide that comes with Aranesp for the most important information you need to know.

When you receive your Aranesp vial and syringes make sure that:

- The name Aranesp appears on the carton and vial label.
- The expiration date on the vial label has not passed. Do not use a vial of Aranesp after the expiration date on the label.
- The dose strength of the Aranesp vial (number of micrograms [mcg] in the colored square on the package and on the vial label) is the same as your healthcare provider prescribed.
- The Aranesp liquid in the vial is clear and colorless. Do not use Aranesp if the liquid in the vial looks discolored or cloudy, or if the liquid has lumps, flakes, or particles.
- The Aranesp vial has a color cap on the top of the vial. Do not use a vial of Aranesp if the color cap on the top of the vial has been removed or is missing.
- Use only the type of disposable syringe and needle that your healthcare provider has prescribed.
- Do not shake Aranesp. If shaking has occurred, the solution in the vial may look foamy and should not be used.
- Do not freeze Aranesp. Do not use a vial of Aranesp that has been frozen.
- Keep Aranesp away from light.

How should I prepare for an injection of Aranesp?

- Always keep an extra syringe and needle on hand.
- Follow your healthcare provider's instructions on how to measure your dose of Aranesp. This dose will be measured in mcg per milliliter (mL) or cc (1 mL is the same as 1 cc). Use a syringe that is marked in tenths of mL (for example, 0.2 mL or 0.2 cc). Using the wrong syringe can lead to a mistake in your dose and you could inject too much or too little Aranesp.

Only use disposable syringes and needles. Use the syringes and needles only one time and then throw them away as instructed by your healthcare provider.

Important: Follow these instructions exactly to help avoid infections.

Preparing the dose:

1. Remove the vial of Aranesp from the refrigerator. During this time, protect the solution from light.
2. Do not use a vial of Aranesp more than one time.
3. Do not shake Aranesp.
4. Gather the other supplies you will need for your injection (vial, syringe, alcohol wipes, cotton ball, and a puncture-proof container for throwing away the syringe and needle). See Figure 1.

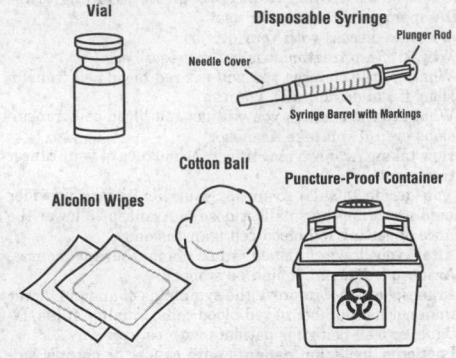

Figure 1

5. Check the date on the Aranesp vial to be sure that the drug has not expired.
6. Wash your hands well with soap and water before preparing the medicine. See Figure 2.

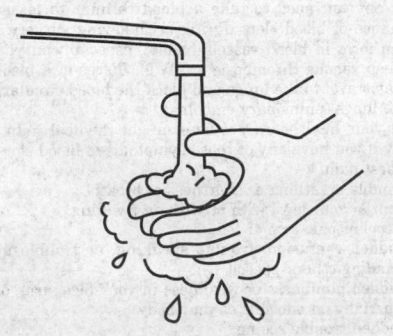

Figure 2

7. Flip off the protective color cap on the top of the vial. Do not remove the grey rubber stopper. Wipe the top of the grey rubber stopper with an alcohol wipe. See Figures 3 and 4.

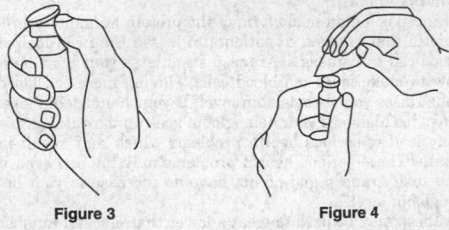

Figure 3   **Figure 4**

8. Check the package containing the syringe. If the package has been opened or damaged, do not use that syringe. Throw away the syringe in the puncture-proof disposable container. If the syringe package is undamaged, open the package and remove the syringe.
9. Using a syringe and needle that has been recommended by your healthcare provider, carefully remove the needle cover. See Figure 5. Then draw air into the syringe by pulling back on the plunger. The amount of air drawn into the syringe should be equal to the amount (mL or cc) of the Aranesp dose prescribed by your healthcare provider. See Figure 6.

Pull Straight Off

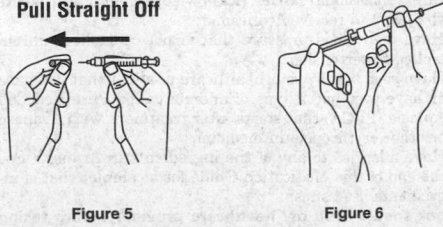

Figure 5   **Figure 6**

10. With the vial on a flat work surface, insert the needle straight down through the grey rubber stopper of the Aranesp vial. See Figure 7.

11. Push the plunger of the syringe down to inject the air from the syringe into the vial of Aranesp. The air injected into the vial will allow Aranesp to be easily withdrawn into the syringe. See Figure 7.

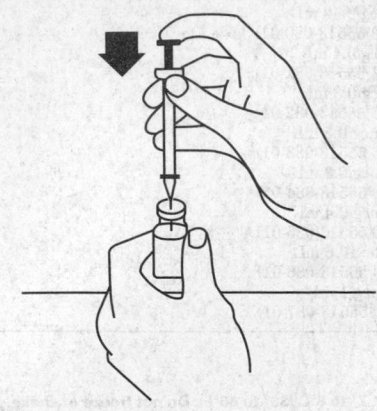

Figure 7

12. Keep the needle inside the vial. Turn the vial and syringe upside down. Be sure the tip of the needle is in the Aranesp liquid. Keep the vial upside down. Slowly pull back on the plunger to fill the syringe with Aranesp liquid to the number (mL or cc) that matches the dose your healthcare provider prescribed. See Figure 8.

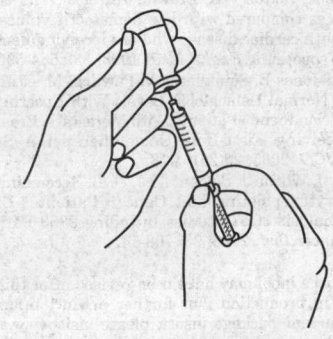

Figure 8

13. Keep the needle in the vial. Check for air bubbles in the syringe. A small amount of air is harmless. Too large an air bubble will give you the wrong Aranesp dose. To remove air bubbles, gently tap the syringe with your fingers until the air bubbles rise to the top of the syringe. Slowly push the plunger up to force the air bubbles out of the syringe. Keep the tip of the needle in the Aranesp liquid. Pull the plunger back to the number on the syringe that matches your dose. Check again for air bubbles. If there are still air bubbles, repeat the steps above to remove them. See Figures 9 and 10.

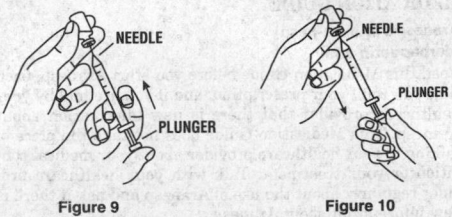

Figure 9   **Figure 10**

14. Double-check that you have the correct dose in the syringe. Lay the vial down on its side with the needle still in it until after you have selected and prepared a site for injection.

Selecting and preparing the injection site:

Aranesp can be injected into your body using two different ways (routes) as described below. Follow your healthcare provider's instructions about how you should inject Aranesp. In patients on hemodialysis, the intravenous (IV) route is recommended.

1. Subcutaneous Route:

- Aranesp can be injected directly into a layer of fat under your skin. This is called a subcutaneous injection. When giving subcutaneous injections, follow your healthcare provider's instructions about changing the site for each injection. You may wish to write down the site where you have injected.

- Do not inject Aranesp into an area that is tender, red, bruised, hard, or has scars or stretch marks. Recommended sites for injection are shown in Figure 11 below, including:
  - The outer area of the upper arms
  - The abdomen (except for the 2-inch area around the navel)
  - The front of the middle thighs
  - The upper outer area of the buttocks

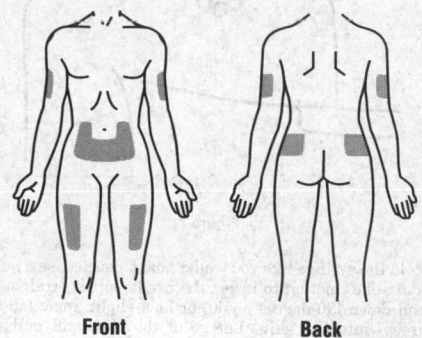

Front　　　　**Back**

Figure 11

- Clean the skin with an alcohol wipe where the injection is to be made. Be careful not to touch the skin that has been wiped clean. See Figure 12.

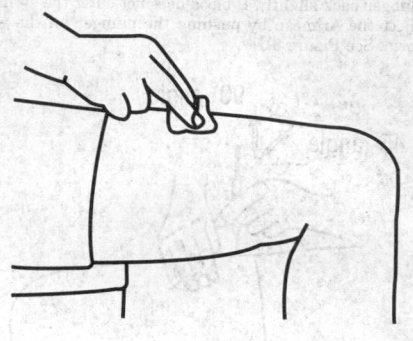

Figure 12

- Double-check that the correct amount of Aranesp is in the syringe.
- Remove the prepared syringe and needle from the vial of Aranesp and hold it in the hand that you will use to inject the medicine.
- Use the other hand to pinch a fold of skin at the cleaned injection site. Do not touch the cleaned area of skin. See Figure 13.

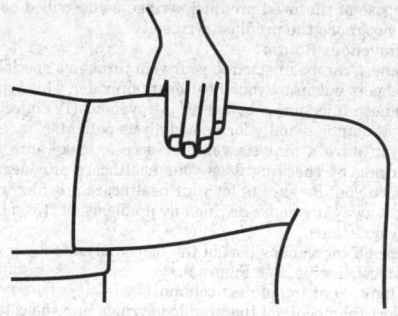

Figure 13

- Hold the syringe like you would hold a pencil. Use a quick "dart-like" motion to insert the needle either straight up and down (90-degree angle) or at a slight angle (45 degrees) into the skin. Let go of the skin and pull the plunger back slightly. If blood comes into the syringe, do not inject Aranesp since the needle may have entered a blood vessel; instead, withdraw the syringe, discard it in the puncture-proof container. Prepare a new syringe of Aranesp using the instructions above. Clean a new area of skin. In this new area of clean skin, again insert a new

needle (as you did before), and again pull the plunger back slightly. If blood does not enter the syringe, inject the Aranesp by pushing the plunger all the way down. See Figure 14.

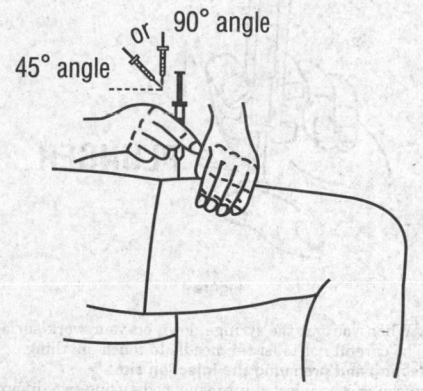

Figure 14

- Pull the needle out of the skin and press a cotton ball or gauze over the injection site and hold it there for several seconds. Do not recap the needle.
- Dispose of the used syringe and needle as described below. Do not reuse syringes and needles.

2. Intravenous Route:

- Aranesp can be injected in your vein through a special access port put in by your healthcare provider. This type of Aranesp injection is called an intravenous (IV) injection. This route is usually for hemodialysis patients.
- If you have a dialysis vascular access, make sure it is working by checking it as your healthcare provider has shown you. Be sure to let your healthcare provider know right away if you are having any problems, or if you have any questions.
- Wipe off the venous port of the hemodialysis tubing with an alcohol wipe. See Figure 15.

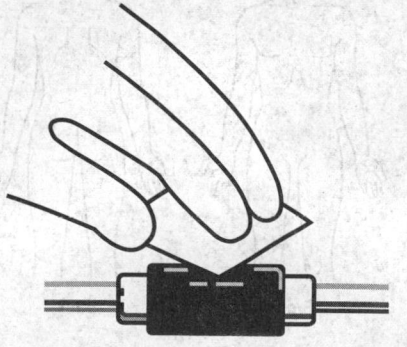

Figure 15

- Insert the needle of the syringe into the cleaned venous port and push the plunger all the way down to inject all the Aranesp. See Figure 16.

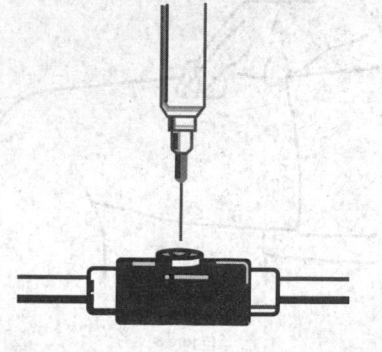

Figure 16

- Remove the syringe from the venous port. Do not recap the needle.
- Dispose of the used syringe and needle as described below.

How should I dispose of syringes and needles?

Do not reuse disposable syringes and needles. Throw away syringes and needles as instructed by your healthcare provider by following these steps:

- Do not throw the needle, syringe, or disposable container in the household trash or recycle.
- Do not put the needle cover back on the needle.
- Place all used needles and syringes in a puncture-proof disposable container with a lid. Do not use glass or clear plastic containers, or any container that will be recycled or returned to a store.
- Keep the container out of the reach of children.
- When the container is full, tape around the cap or lid to make sure the cap or lid does not come off. Throw away the puncture-proof disposable container as instructed by your healthcare provider. There may be special state and local laws for disposing of used needles and syringes. **Do not throw the disposable container in the household trash. Do not recycle.**

Manufactured by:
Amgen Manufacturing, Limited, a subsidiary of Amgen Inc.
One Amgen Center Drive
Thousand Oaks, CA 91320-1799
©2001-2008 Amgen Inc. All rights reserved.
1xxxxxx - v1
Revised: 08/2008

PATIENT INSTRUCTIONS FOR USE

Aranesp® (Air-uh-nesp)
(darbepoetin alfa)
Single-Dose Prefilled Syringe (SingleJect®)

Use these instructions if you or your caregiver has been trained to give Aranesp injections at home. Do not give yourself the injection unless you have received training from your healthcare provider. If you are not sure about giving the injection or if you have questions, ask your healthcare provider for help.

Before reading these instructions, read the Medication Guide that comes with Aranesp for the most important information you need to know.

When you receive your Aranesp prefilled syringe make sure that:

- The name Aranesp appears on the carton and prefilled syringe label.
- The expiration date on the prefilled syringe label has not passed. Do not use a prefilled syringe of Aranesp after the expiration date on the label.
- The dose strength of the Aranesp prefilled syringe (number of micrograms [mcg] in the colored square on the package and on the prefilled syringe label) is the same as your healthcare provider prescribed.
- The Aranesp liquid in the prefilled syringe is clear and colorless. Do not use Aranesp if the liquid in the prefilled syringe looks discolored or cloudy, or if the liquid looks like it has lumps, flakes, or particles.
- Do not use Aranesp in a prefilled syringe if the grey cover on the needle is off, or the needle guard (yellow sleeve on the syringe) has been pulled to extend over the needle (activated).
- Do not shake Aranesp. Shaking could cause Aranesp not to work. If you shake Aranesp the solution may look foamy and it should not be used.
- Do not freeze Aranesp. Do not use an Aranesp prefilled syringe that has been frozen.
- Keep Aranesp away from light.

How should I prepare for an injection of Aranesp?

- Follow your healthcare provider's instructions on how to measure your dose of Aranesp. This dose will be measured in mcg per milliliter (mL) or cc (1 mL is the same as 1 cc). Use a syringe that is marked in tenths of mL (for example, 0.2 mL or 0.2 cc).

Use the prefilled syringe only one time and throw it away as instructed by your healthcare provider.

Important: Follow these instructions exactly to help avoid infections.

Preparing the dose:

1. Remove one prefilled syringe from the refrigerator. During this time, protect the prefilled syringe from light. Keep the prefilled syringe in its wrapper until you are ready to prepare your dose. Do not leave the prefilled syringe in light.
2. Use each Aranesp prefilled syringe only one time.
3. Do not shake Aranesp.
4. Gather the other supplies you will need for your injection (prefilled syringe with a transparent [clear] yellow plastic needle guard attached, alcohol wipes, cotton ball, and a puncture-proof container for throwing away the prefilled syringe). See Figure 1.

[See figure 1 at top of next column]

5. Check the date on the label on your Aranesp prefilled syringe to be sure that the drug has not expired.

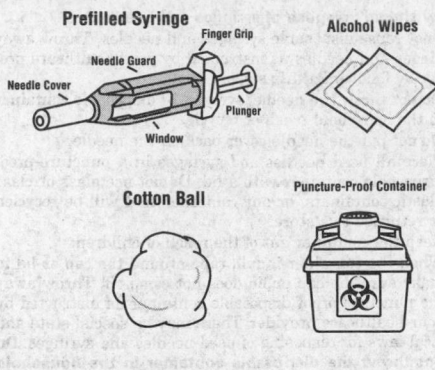

Figure 1

6. Wash your hands well with soap and water before preparing the medicine. See Figure 2.

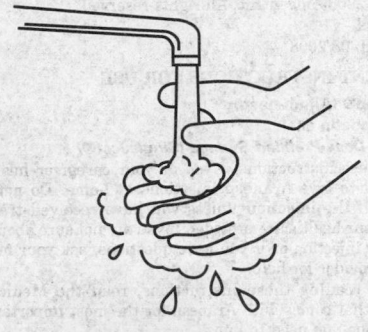

Figure 2

7. Open the package and remove the syringe from the tray. Check to see that the needle cover is on and the yellow needle guard is covering the barrel of the syringe. If the needle guard is covering the needle, then it has already been activated. **Do not** use that syringe. Throw away the syringe in the puncture-proof disposable container. Use a new syringe. **Do not** slide the needle guard over the needle cover before injection. This will "activate" or lock the needle guard.

8. Hold the syringe with the needle pointing up to prevent the Aranesp from leaking out of the needle. Carefully pull the needle cover straight off. See Figure 3.

Pull Straight Off

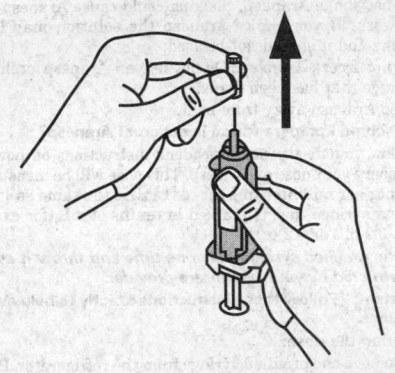

Figure 3

9. Check the syringe for air bubbles. If there are air bubbles, gently tap the syringe with your fingers until the air bubbles rise to the top of the syringe. Slowly push the plunger up to force the air bubbles out of the syringe. See Figure 4.
[See figure 4 at top of next column]

10. Keep holding the syringe up. Slowly push the plunger to the line on the syringe that matches the dose your healthcare provider has prescribed.

11. Check again to make sure that you have the correct dose in the syringe.

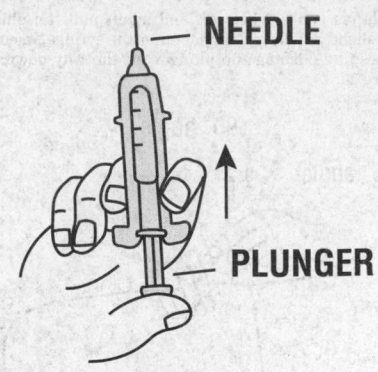

Figure 4

12. When you put the syringe down on your work surface, be careful not to let the needle to touch anything.

Selecting and preparing the injection site:
Aranesp can be injected into your body using two different ways (routes) as described below. Follow your healthcare provider's instructions about how you should inject Aranesp. In patients on hemodialysis, the intravenous (IV) route is recommended.

1. Subcutaneous Route:
• Aranesp can be injected directly into a layer of fat under your skin. This is called a subcutaneous injection. When giving subcutaneous injections, follow your healthcare provider's instructions about changing the site for each injection. You may wish to write down the site where you have injected.
• Do not inject Aranesp into an area that is tender, red, bruised, hard, or has scars or stretch marks. Recommended sites for injection are shown in Figure 5 below, including:
  • The outer area of the upper arms
  • The abdomen (except for the 2-inch area around the navel)
  • The front of the middle thighs
  • The upper outer area of your buttocks

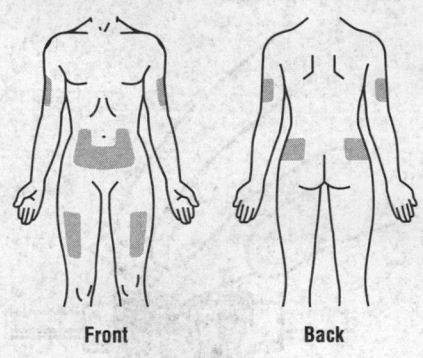

Front   **Back**

Figure 5

• Clean the skin with an alcohol wipe where the injection is to be made. Be careful not to touch the skin that has been wiped clean. See Figure 6.

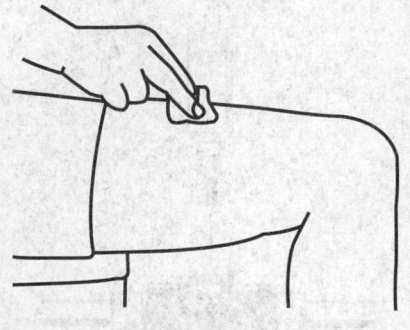

Figure 6

• Hold the prefilled syringe in the hand that you will use to inject the medicine.
• Use the other hand to pinch a fold of skin at the cleaned injection site. Do not touch the cleaned area of skin. See

Figure 7. Note: Hold the syringe barrel through the two needle guard windows when giving the injection.

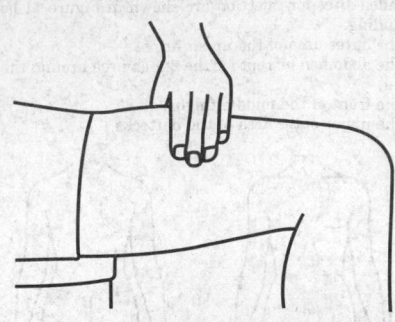

Figure 7

• Hold the syringe like you would hold a pencil. Use a quick "dart-like" motion to insert the needle either straight up and down (90-degree angle) or at a slight angle (45 degrees) into the skin. Let go of the skin and pull the plunger back slightly. If blood comes into the syringe, do not inject Aranesp since the needle may have entered a blood vessel; instead, withdraw the syringe, discard it in the puncture-proof container. Prepare a new prefilled syringe of Aranesp using the instructions above. Clean a new area of skin. In this new area of clean skin, again insert the needle (as you did before), and again pull the plunger back slightly. If blood does not enter the syringe, inject the Aranesp by pushing the plunger all the way down. See Figure 8.

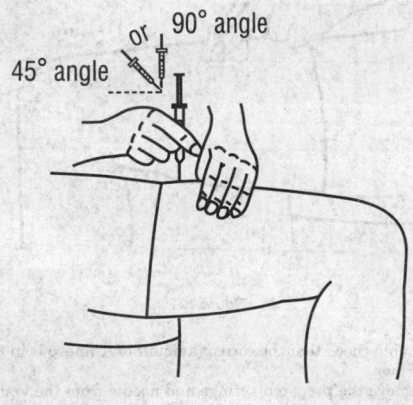

Figure 8

• Pull the needle out of the skin and press a cotton ball or gauze over the injection site and hold it there for several seconds. Do not recap the needle.
• Dispose of the used prefilled syringe as described below. Do not reuse the prefilled syringe.

2. Intravenous Route:
• Aranesp can be injected in your vein through a special access port put in by your healthcare provider. This type of Aranesp injection is called an intravenous (IV) injection. This route is usually for hemodialysis patients.
• If you have a dialysis vascular access, make sure it is working by checking it as your healthcare provider has shown you. Be sure to let your healthcare provider know right away if you are having any problems, or if you have any questions.
• Wipe off the venous port of the hemodialysis tubing with an alcohol wipe. See Figure 9.
[See figure 9 at top of next column]
• Insert the needle of the prefilled syringe into the cleaned venous port and push the plunger all the way down to inject all the Aranesp. See Figure 10.
[See figure 10 at top of next column]
• Remove the prefilled syringe from the venous port. Do not recap the needle.
• Dispose of the used prefilled syringe as described below. Do not reuse the prefilled syringe.

Activation of the needle guard on used prefilled syringes
After injecting Aranesp from the prefilled syringe, do not recap the needle. Keep your hands behind the needle at all times. To activate the needle guard, hold the finger grip of the syringe with one hand and grasp the needle guard with your free hand. Slide the needle guard completely over the needle until the needle guard clicks into place. See Figures

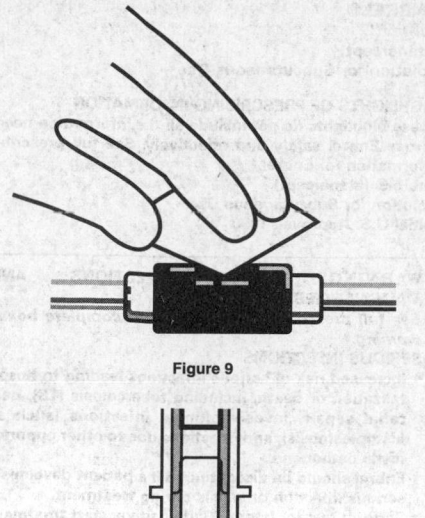

Figure 9

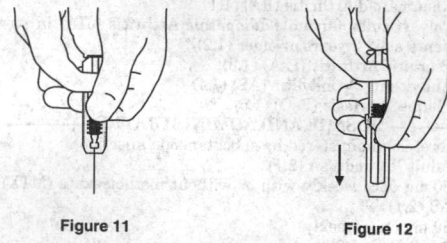

Figure 10

11 and 12. **NOTE: If an audible click is not heard, the needle guard may not be completely activated.**

Figure 11   **Figure 12**

How should I dispose of the prefilled syringe?

Do not reuse the prefilled syringe. Throw away the prefilled syringe with the activated needle guard as directed by your healthcare provider by following these steps:

- Do not throw the prefilled syringe or disposable container in the household trash or recycle.
- Do not put the needle cover back on the needle.
- Place the used prefilled syringe in a puncture-proof disposable container with a lid. Do not use glass or clear plastic containers, or any container that will be recycled or returned to a store.
- Keep the container out of the reach of children.
- When the container is full, tape around the cap or lid to make sure the cap or lid does not come off. Throw away the puncture-proof disposable container as instructed by your healthcare provider. There may be special state and local laws for disposing of used prefilled syringes. **Do not throw the disposable container in the household trash. Do not recycle.**

Manufactured by:
Amgen Manufacturing, Limited, a subsidiary of Amgen Inc.
One Amgen Center Drive
Thousand Oaks, CA 91320-1799
©2001-2008 Amgen Inc. All rights reserved.
1xxxxxx - v1
Revised: 08/2008

PATIENT INSTRUCTIONS FOR USE

Aranesp® (Air-uh-nesp)
(darbepoetin alfa)
Single-Use Prefilled SureClick™ Autoinjector
Use these instructions if you or your caregiver has been trained to give Aranesp injections at home. Do not give

yourself the injection unless you have received training from your healthcare provider. If you are not sure about giving the injection or if you have questions, ask your healthcare provider for help.

Before reading these instructions for use, read the Medication Guide that comes with Aranesp for the most important information you need to know.

How should I take Aranesp?

This section explains how to give yourself an injection of Aranesp using the single-use prefilled SureClick™ autoinjector. You will give the injection into the tissue just under your skin. This is called a subcutaneous injection.

To give yourself a subcutaneous injection, you need:
- A new, single-use Aranesp prefilled SureClick™ autoinjector
- Alcohol or sterile wipe
- A puncture-proof container so you can safely throw away the used autoinjector

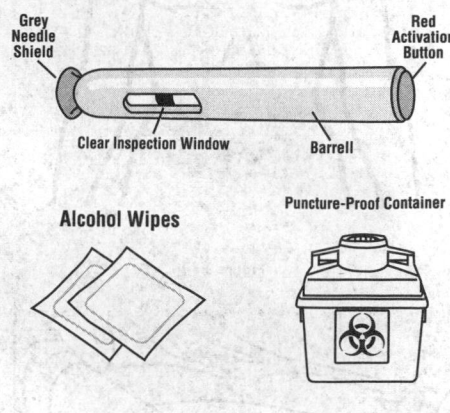

Figure 1

Important: Follow these instructions exactly to help avoid infections.

1. Take your autoinjector out of the refrigerator. Keep the autoinjector in the box until you are ready to use it.
   - **Do not shake your autoinjector.** Shaking could cause Aranesp not to work. If you shake your Aranesp prefilled SureClick™ autoinjector, the solution may look foamy and it should not be used.
   - **Do not freeze your autoinjector. Do not use an autoinjector that has been frozen.**
   - Do not leave your autoinjector in bright light. Do not use an autoinjector that has been left in light.
2. Check that your single-use Aranesp prefilled Sure-Click™ autoinjector is the correct dose that your healthcare provider has prescribed.
3. Do not use your autoinjector after the expiration date on the carton and on the autoinjector label.
4. Remove the autoinjector from the box. During this time, protect the solution from light.
5. **Do not** warm your single-use Aranesp prefilled Sure-Click™ autoinjector (for example, do not warm it in a microwave or in hot water).
6. **Do not** remove the grey needle shield from the autoinjector until you are ready to inject.
7. **Do not** put the grey needle shield back into the autoinjector.
8. Look at Aranesp through the inspection window. It should be clear and colorless. **Do not inject Aranesp if it looks discolored, cloudy, or has lumps, flakes, or particles.**
9. Wash your hands well.
10. Find a comfortable, well-lit place and put your supplies (autoinjector, alcohol or sterile wipe, and puncture-proof container) where you can reach them.

On what part of my body should I give my injection?

Inject your single-use Aranesp prefilled SureClick™ autoinjector into:
- The front center of your thighs
- The back of your upper arms, only if someone else is injecting you

The abdomen may be used if your healthcare provider tells you it is alright.
[See figure 2 at top of next column]
Change the site for each injection to avoid soreness at any one site.
- Do not inject into areas where the skin is tender, bruised, red, or hard.
- Avoid areas with scars or stretch marks.

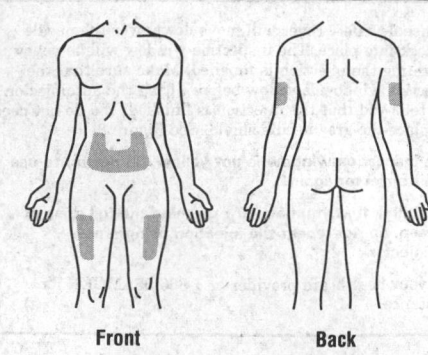

Front   **Back**

Figure 2

Sometimes a problem may develop at the injection site. If there is a lump, swelling, or bruising at the injection site that does not go away, talk to your healthcare provider.

How do I give an injection into my thigh or the back of my arm?

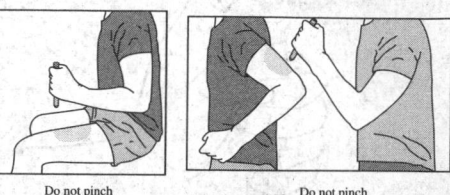

Do not pinch   Do not pinch

Figure 3

1. Wipe the injection site with a new alcohol or sterile wipe and allow your skin to dry. **Do not touch this area again before giving the injection.**
2. Pick up your single-use Aranesp prefilled SureClick™ autoinjector in one hand and remove the grey needle shield by pulling it straight off. Do not twist it off and do not recap the grey needle shield, as either of these may damage the needle inside the autoinjector. Your single-use Aranesp prefilled SureClick™ autoinjector has a cover that will protect you from needlesticks or an accidental loss of medicine by bumping or touching. See Figure 4.

Pull straight off

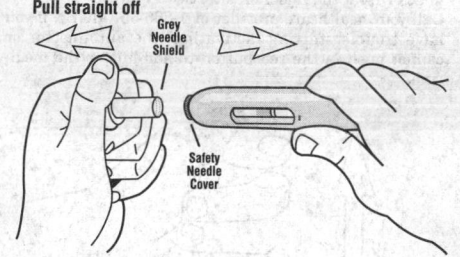

Figure 4

3. **Without** pressing the red activation button, place the open end of the autoinjector on the injection site straight up and down at a right angle (90°) to your skin. Push the safety needle cover firmly against your skin to unlock it. **Keep holding the autoinjector firmly against your skin.** See Figure 5.

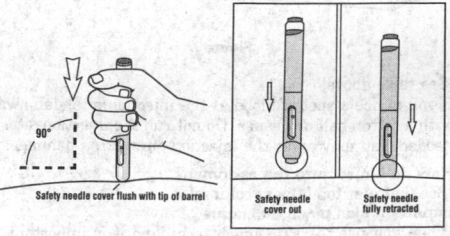

Figure 5

4. To start the injection: (1) press the red button; you will hear the first click, and then (2) right away, release your thumb. This starts the injection. **Do not lift** the autoinjector off of your skin. See Figure 6.
[See figure 6 at top of next column]
5. **Wait until you hear the second click.** After you hear the second click, lift the autoinjector straight up from the in-

The needle safety cover will move down over the needle and lock into place. The inspection window will be yellow, confirming the injection is finished. Make sure that the inspection window is yellow before lifting the autoinjector. This tells you that the injection is finished. You do not need to replace the grey needle shield. See Figure 8.

If the inspection window is not yellow, do not try to use the autoinjector again.

If you think that you have not received the full dose of Aranesp, do not repeat the injection using a new autoinjector.

Call your healthcare provider or 1-866-55AMGEN for assistance.

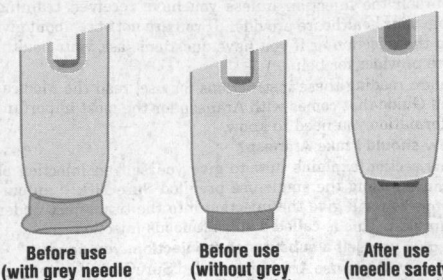

Before use (with grey needle shield)   Before use (without grey needle shield)   After use (needle safety cover down)

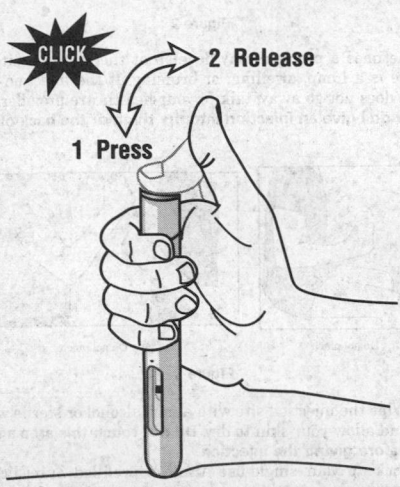

Figure 6

jection site. Your injection is finished. The safety needle cover on the autoinjector will automatically extend to cover the needle. If you did not remove your thumb from the red button, your will not hear the second "click." If this happens, slowly count to 15 before lifting the autoinjector from the injection site. See Figure 7.

Call your healthcare provider or 1-866-55AMGEN if you have trouble starting (activating) the autoinjector or cannot push in the red button to administer the medicine.

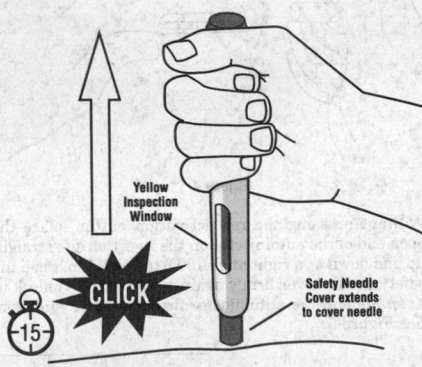

Figure 7

[See table above]
If you notice a spot of blood at the injection site, dab away with a cotton ball or tissues. Do not rub the injection site. If needed, you may cover the injection site with a bandage.

How do I inject into the abdomen?
[See figure at top of next column]
Important skin pinch technique
When you use the skin pinch technique it is important to create a firm site for the injection.
- Choose a site at least 2 inches away from the belly button (navel).
- Pinch the skin of the abdomen **firmly** between the thumb and fingers. Creatie a space at least 2 inches wide (twice the width of the tip of the autoinjector). Keep a firm skin pinch for the whole injection. See Figure 10.
[See figure 10 at top of next column]
- Follow steps 1-5 above.

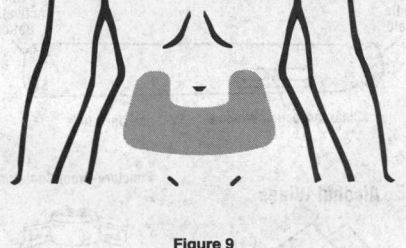

Figure 9

Pinch
Figure 10

Remember
If you have any problems, ask your healthcare provider for help and advice.

How do I dispose of used autoinjectors?
Do not reuse the Aranesp prefilled SureClick™ autoinjector.
Do not put the grey needle shield back into the autoinjector. Throw away the used autoinjector as instructed by your healthcare provider or by following these steps:
- Do not throw the used autoinjector in the household trash or recycle.
- Place the used autoinjector in a puncture-proof disposable container with a lid. Do not use glass or clear plastic containers, or any container that will be recycled or returned to a store.
- Keep the container out of the reach of children.
- When the container is full, tape around the cap or lid to make sure the cap or lid does not come off. Throw away the puncture-proof disposable container as instructed by your healthcare provider. There may be special state and local laws for disposing of used needles and syringes. **Do not throw the disposable container in the household trash. Do not recycle.**

Keep Aranesp out of reach of children.
Manufactured by:
Amgen Manufacturing, Limited, a subsidiary of Amgen Inc.
One Amgen Center Drive
Thousand Oaks, CA 91320-1799
©2001-2008 Amgen Inc. All rights reserved.
1xxxxxx - v1
Revised: 08/2008
Shown in Product Identification Guide, page 305

ENBREL®   ℞
[ən-brél]
(etanercept)
Solution for Subcutaneous Use

HIGHLIGHTS OF PRESCRIBING INFORMATION
These highlights do not include all the information needed to use Enbrel safely and effectively. See full prescribing information for Enbrel.
Enbrel® (etanercept)
Solution for Subcutaneous Use
Initial U.S. Approval: 1998

WARNINGS: SERIOUS INFECTIONS AND MALIGNANCIES
See full prescribing information for complete boxed warning.
SERIOUS INFECTIONS
- Increased risk of serious infections leading to hospitalization or death, including tuberculosis (TB), bacterial sepsis, invasive fungal infections (such as histoplasmosis), and infections due to other opportunistic pathogens.
- Enbrel should be discontinued if a patient develops a serious infection or sepsis during treatment.
- Perform test for latent TB; if positive, start treatment for TB prior to starting Enbrel.
- Monitor all patients for active TB during treatment, even if initial latent TB test is negative. (5.1)
MALIGNANCIES
- Lymphoma and other malignancies, some fatal, have been reported in children and adolescent patients treated with TNF blockers, including Enbrel. (5.3)

RECENT MAJOR CHANGES

Boxed Warning, Malignancies	11/2009
Warnings and Precautions, (5.3)	
Malignancies (5.3)	11/2009

INDICATIONS AND USAGE
Enbrel is a tumor necrosis factor (TNF) blocker indicated for the treatment of:
- Rheumatoid Arthritis (RA) (1.1)
- Polyarticular Juvenile Idiopathic Arthritis (JIA) in patients aged 2 years or older (1.2)
- Psoriatic Arthritis (PsA) (1.3)
- Ankylosing Spondylitis (AS) (1.4)
- Plaque Psoriasis (PsO) (1.5)

DOSAGE AND ADMINISTRATION
Enbrel is administered by subcutaneous injection.
- Adult RA and PsA (2.1)
  50 mg once weekly with or without methotrexate (MTX)
- AS (2.1)
  50 mg once weekly
- Adult PsO (2.2)
  50 mg twice weekly for 3 months, followed by 50 mg once weekly
- JIA (2.3)
  0.8 mg/kg weekly, with a maximum of 50 mg per week

DOSAGE FORMS AND STRENGTHS
- 50 mg Single-use Prefilled Syringe (3)
  0.98 mL of a 50 mg/mL solution of etanercept
- 50 mg Single-use Prefilled SureClick® Autoinjector (3)
  0.98 mL of a 50 mg/mL solution of etanercept
- 25 mg Single-use Prefilled Syringe (3)
  0.51 mL of a 50 mg/mL solution of etanercept
- 25 mg Multiple-use Vial (3)
  25 mg of etanercept

CONTRAINDICATIONS
- Sepsis (4)

WARNINGS AND PRECAUTIONS
- Do not start Enbrel during an active infection. If an infection develops, monitor carefully and stop Enbrel if infection becomes serious. (5.1)
- Demyelinating disease, exacerbation or new onset, may occur. (5.2)
- Cases of lymphoma have been observed in patients receiving TNF-blocking agents. (5.3)
- Congestive heart failure, worsening or new onset, may occur. (5.4)
- Advise patients to seek immediate medical attention if symptoms of pancytopenia or aplastic anemia develop, and consider stopping Enbrel. (5.5)
- Monitor hepatitis B virus carriers for reactivation during and several months after therapy. If reactivation occurs, consider stopping Enbrel and beginning anti viral therapy. (5.6)
- Anaphylaxis or serious allergic reactions may occur. (5.7)
- Stop Enbrel if lupus-like syndrome or autoimmune hepatitis develops. (5.9)

---ADVERSE REACTIONS---

Most common adverse reactions (incidence > 5%): infections and injection site reactions. (6.1)

To report SUSPECTED ADVERSE REACTIONS, contact Amgen Inc. at 1-800-77-AMGEN (1-800-772-6437) or FDA at 1-800-FDA-1088 or www.fda.gov/medwatch

---DRUG INTERACTIONS---

• Live vaccines—should not be given with Enbrel (5.8, 7.1)
• Anakinra—increased risk of serious infection (5.12, 7.2)
• Abatacept—increased risk of serious adverse events, including infections (5.12, 7.2)
• Cyclophosphamide—use with Enbrel is not recommended (7.3)

---USE IN SPECIFIC POPULATIONS---

• Pregnancy registry available (8.1)

See 17 for PATIENT COUNSELING INFORMATION and Medication Guide

Revised: 06/2010

FULL PRESCRIBING INFORMATION: CONTENTS*

MEDICATION GUIDE
PATIENT INSTRUCTIONS FOR USE
ENBREL® (EN-BREL)
(ETANERCEPT)
SINGLE-USE PREFILLED SYRINGE
PATIENT INSTRUCTIONS FOR USE
ENBREL® (EN-BREL)
(ETANERCEPT)
MULTIPLE-USE VIAL
PATIENT INSTRUCTIONS FOR USE
ENBREL® (EN-BREL)
(ETANERCEPT)
SINGLE-USE PREFILLED SURECLICK™ AUTOINJECTOR

* Sections or subsections omitted from the full prescribing information are not listed

FULL PRESCRIBING INFORMATION

WARNINGS:
SERIOUS INFECTIONS
SERIOUS INFECTIONS

Patients treated with Enbrel are at increased risk for developing serious infections that may lead to hospitalization or death *[see Warnings and Precautions (5.1) and Adverse Reactions (6)]*. Most patients who developed these infections were taking concomitant immunosuppressants such as methotrexate or corticosteroids.

Enbrel should be discontinued if a patient develops a serious infection or sepsis.

Reported infections include:

• Active tuberculosis, including reactivation of latent tuberculosis. Patients with tuberculosis have frequently presented with disseminated or extrapulmonary disease. Patients should be tested for latent tuberculosis before Enbrel use and during therapy. Treatment for latent infection should be initiated prior to Enbrel use.

• Invasive fungal infections, including histoplasmosis, coccidioidomycosis, candidiasis, aspergillosis, blastomycosis, and pneumocystosis. Patients with histoplasmosis or other invasive fungal infections may present with disseminated, rather than localized, disease. Antigen and antibody testing for histoplasmosis may be negative in some patients with active infection. Empiric anti-fungal therapy should be considered in patients at risk for invasive fungal infections who develop severe systemic illness.

• Bacterial, viral, and other infections due to opportunistic pathogens.

The risks and benefits of treatment with Enbrel should be carefully considered prior to initiating therapy in patients with chronic or recurrent infection.

Patients should be closely monitored for the development of signs and symptoms of infection during and after treatment with Enbrel, including the possible development of tuberculosis in patients who tested negative for latent tuberculosis infection prior to initiating therapy.

MALIGNANCIES

Lymphoma and other malignancies, some fatal, have been reported in children and adolescent patients treated with TNF blockers, including Enbrel.

---

1 INDICATIONS AND USAGE

1.1 Rheumatoid Arthritis

Enbrel is indicated for reducing signs and symptoms, inducing major clinical response, inhibiting the progression of structural damage, and improving physical function in patients with moderately to severely active rheumatoid arthritis (RA). Enbrel can be initiated in combination with methotrexate (MTX) or used alone.

1.2 Polyarticular Juvenile Idiopathic Arthritis

Enbrel is indicated for reducing signs and symptoms of moderately to severely active polyarticular juvenile idiopathic arthritis (JIA) in patients ages 2 and older.

1.3 Psoriatic Arthritis

Enbrel is indicated for reducing signs and symptoms, inhibiting the progression of structural damage of active arthritis, and improving physical function in patients with psoriatic arthritis (PsA). Enbrel can be used in combination with methotrexate (MTX) in patients who do not respond adequately to MTX alone.

1.4 Ankylosing Spondylitis

Enbrel is indicated for reducing signs and symptoms in patients with active ankylosing spondylitis (AS).

1.5 Plaque Psoriasis

Enbrel is indicated for the treatment of adult patients (18 years or older) with chronic moderate to severe plaque psoriasis (PsO) who are candidates for systemic therapy or phototherapy.

---

2 DOSAGE AND ADMINISTRATION

Table 1. Dosing and Administration for Adult Patients

Patient Population	Recommended Dosage Strength and Frequency
Adult RA, AS, and PsA Patients	50 mg weekly
Adult PsO Patients	Starting Dose: 50 mg twice weekly for 3 months Maintenance Dose: 50 mg once weekly

See the Enbrel (etanercept) "Patient Instructions for Use" insert for detailed information on injection site selection and dose administration.

2.1 Adult Rheumatoid Arthritis, Ankylosing Spondylitis, and Psoriatic Arthritis Patients

MTX, glucocorticoids, salicylates, nonsteroidal antiinflammatory drugs (NSAIDs), or analgesics may be continued during treatment with Enbrel.

Based on a study of 50 mg Enbrel twice weekly in patients with RA that suggested higher incidence of adverse reactions but similar ACR response rates, doses higher than 50 mg per week are not recommended.

2.2 Adult Plaque Psoriasis Patients

In addition to the 50 mg twice weekly recommended starting dose, starting doses of 25 mg or 50 mg per week were shown to be efficacious. The proportion of responders were related to Enbrel dosage *[see Clinical Studies (14.5)]*.

2.3 JIA Patients

Table 2. Dosing and Administration for Juvenile Idiopathic Arthritis

Pediatric Patients Weight	Recommended Dose
63 kg (138 pounds) or more	50 mg weekly
Less than 63 kg (138 pounds)	0.8 mg/kg weekly

In JIA patients, glucocorticoids, NSAIDs, or analgesics may be continued during treatment with Enbrel. Higher doses of Enbrel have not been studied in pediatric patients.

2.4 Preparation of Enbrel

Enbrel is intended for use under the guidance and supervision of a physician. Patients may self-inject when deemed appropriate and if they receive medical follow-up, as necessary. Patients should not self-administer until they receive proper training in how to prepare and administer the correct dose.

The Enbrel (etanercept) "Patient Instructions for Use" insert for each presentation contains more detailed instructions on the preparation of Enbrel.

Preparation of Enbrel Using the Single-use Prefilled Syringe or Single-use Prefilled SureClick Autoinjector

Before injection, Enbrel may be allowed to reach room temperature (approximately 15 to 30 minutes). DO NOT remove the needle cover while allowing the prefilled syringe to reach room temperature.

Parenteral drug products should be inspected visually for particulate matter and discoloration prior to administration. There may be small white particles of protein in the solution. This is not unusual for proteinaceous solutions. The solution should not be used if discolored or cloudy, or if foreign particulate matter is present.

When using the Enbrel single-use prefilled syringe, check to see if the amount of liquid in the prefilled syringe falls between the two purple fill level indicator lines on the syringe. If the syringe does not have the right amount of liquid, DO NOT USE THAT SYRINGE.

Preparation of Enbrel Using the Multiple-use Vial

Enbrel should be reconstituted aseptically with 1 mL of the supplied Sterile Bacteriostatic Water for Injection, USP (0.9% benzyl alcohol), giving a solution of 1.0 mL containing 25 mg of Enbrel.

A vial adapter is supplied for use when reconstituting the lyophilized powder. However, the vial adapter should not be used if multiple doses are going to be withdrawn from the vial. If the vial will be used for multiple doses, a 25-gauge needle should be used for reconstituting and withdrawing Enbrel, and the supplied "Mixing Date:" sticker should be attached to the vial and the date of reconstitution entered. Reconstituted solution must be used within 14 days. Discard reconstituted solution after 14 days because product stability and sterility cannot be assured after 14 days.

If using the vial adapter, twist the vial adapter onto the diluent syringe. Then, place the vial adapter over the Enbrel vial and insert the vial adapter into the vial stopper. Push down on the plunger to inject the diluent into the Enbrel vial. If using a 25-gauge needle to reconstitute and withdraw Enbrel, the diluent should be injected very slowly into the Enbrel vial. It is normal for some foaming to occur. Keeping the diluent syringe in place, gently swirl the contents of the Enbrel vial during dissolution. To avoid excessive foaming, do not shake or vigorously agitate.

Generally, dissolution of Enbrel takes less than 10 minutes. Do not use the solution if discolored or cloudy, or if particulate matter remains.

Withdraw the correct dose of reconstituted solution into the syringe. Some foam or bubbles may remain in the vial. Remove the syringe from the vial adapter or remove the 25-gauge needle from the syringe. Attach a 27-gauge needle to inject Enbrel.

The contents of one vial of Enbrel solution should not be mixed with, or transferred into, the contents of another vial of Enbrel. No other medications should be added to solutions containing Enbrel and do not reconstitute Enbrel with other diluents. Do not filter reconstituted solution during preparation or administration.

3   DOSAGE FORMS AND STRENGTHS

50 mg Single-use Prefilled Syringe
0.98 mL of a 50 mg/mL solution of etanercept
50 mg Single-use Prefilled SureClick Autoinjector
0.98 mL of a 50 mg/mL solution of etanercept
25 mg Single-use Prefilled Syringe
0.51 mL of a 50 mg/mL solution of etanercept
25 mg Multiple-use Vial
25 mg of etanercept

4   CONTRAINDICATIONS

Enbrel should not be administered to patients with sepsis.

5   WARNINGS AND PRECAUTIONS

5.1   Infections

Serious and sometimes fatal infections due to bacterial, mycobacterial, invasive fungal, viral, or other opportunistic pathogens have been reported in patients receiving TNF-blocking agents. Among opportunistic infections, tuberculosis, histoplasmosis, aspergillosis, candidiasis, coccidioidomycosis, listeriosis, and pneumocystosis were the most commonly reported. Patients have frequently presented with disseminated rather than localized disease, and are often taking concomitant immunosuppressants such as methotrexate or corticosteroids with Enbrel.

Treatment with Enbrel should not be initiated in patients with an active infection, including clinically important localized infections. The risks and benefits of treatment should be considered prior to initiating therapy in patients:

- With chronic or recurrent infection;
- Who have been exposed to tuberculosis;
- Who have resided or traveled in areas of endemic tuberculosis or endemic mycoses, such as histoplasmosis, coccidioidomycosis, or blastomycosis; or
- With underlying conditions that may predispose them to infection, such as advanced or poorly controlled diabetes *[see Adverse Reactions (6.1)]*.

Patients should be closely monitored for the development of signs and symptoms of infection during and after treatment with Enbrel.

Enbrel should be discontinued if a patient develops a serious infection or sepsis. A patient who develops a new infection during treatment with Enbrel should be closely monitored, undergo a prompt and complete diagnostic workup appropriate for an immunocompromised patient, and appropriate antimicrobial therapy should be initiated.

Tuberculosis

Cases of reactivation of tuberculosis or new tuberculosis infections have been observed in patients receiving Enbrel, including patients who have previously received treatment for latent or active tuberculosis. Data from clinical trials and preclinical studies suggest that the risk of reactivation of latent tuberculosis infection is lower with Enbrel than with TNF-blocking monoclonal antibodies. Nonetheless, postmarketing cases of tuberculosis reactivation have been reported for TNF blockers, including Enbrel. Tuberculosis has developed in patients who tested negative for latent tuberculosis prior to initiation of therapy. Patients should be evaluated for tuberculosis risk factors and tested for latent infection prior to initiating Enbrel and periodically during therapy. Tests for latent tuberculosis infection may be falsely negative while on therapy with Enbrel.

Treatment of latent tuberculosis infection prior to therapy with TNF-blocking agents has been shown to reduce the risk of tuberculosis reactivation during therapy. Induration of 5 mm or greater with tuberculin skin testing should be considered a positive test result when assessing if treatment for latent tuberculosis is needed prior to initiating Enbrel, even for patients previously vaccinated with Bacille Calmette-Guerin (BCG).

Anti-tuberculosis therapy should also be considered prior to initiation of Enbrel in patients with a past history of latent or active tuberculosis in whom an adequate course of treatment cannot be confirmed, and for patients with a negative

test for latent tuberculosis but having risk factors for tuberculosis infection. Consultation with a physician with expertise in the treatment of tuberculosis is recommended to aid in the decision whether initiating anti-tuberculosis therapy is appropriate for an individual patient.

Tuberculosis should be strongly considered in patients who develop a new infection during Enbrel treatment, especially in patients who have previously or recently traveled to countries with a high prevalence of tuberculosis, or who have had close contact with a person with active tuberculosis.

Invasive Fungal Infections

Cases of serious and sometimes fatal fungal infections, including histoplasmosis, have been reported with TNF blockers, including Enbrel. For patients who reside or travel in regions where mycoses are endemic, invasive fungal infection should be suspected if they develop a serious systemic illness. Appropriate empiric antifungal therapy should be considered while a diagnostic workup is being performed. Antigen and antibody testing for histoplasmosis may be negative in some patients with active infection. When feasible, the decision to administer empiric antifungal therapy in these patients should be made in consultation with a physician with expertise in the diagnosis and treatment of invasive fungal infections and should take into account both the risk for severe fungal infection and the risks of antifungal therapy. In 38 Enbrel clinical trials and 4 cohort studies in all approved indications representing 27,169 patient-years of exposure (17,696 patients) from the United States and Canada, no histoplasmosis infections were reported among patients treated with Enbrel.

5.2   Neurologic Events

Treatment with TNF-blocking agents, including Enbrel, has been associated with rare (< 0.1%) cases of new onset or exacerbation of central nervous system demyelinating disorders, some presenting with mental status changes and some associated with permanent disability. Cases of transverse myelitis, optic neuritis, multiple sclerosis, and new onset or exacerbation of seizure disorders have been reported in postmarketing experience with Enbrel therapy. Prescribers should exercise caution in considering the use of Enbrel in patients with preexisting or recent-onset central nervous system demyelinating disorders *[see Adverse Reactions (6.2)]*.

5.3   Malignancies

Lymphomas

In the controlled portions of clinical trials of TNF blocking agents, more cases of lymphoma have been observed among patients receiving a TNF blocker compared to control patients. During the controlled portions of Enbrel trials in adult patients with RA, AS, and PsA, 2 lymphomas were observed among 3306 Enbrel-treated patients versus 0 among 1521 control patients (duration of controlled treatment ranged from 3 to 36 months).

Among 6543 adult rheumatology (RA, PsA, AS) patients treated with Enbrel in controlled and uncontrolled portions of clinical trials, representing approximately 12,845 patient-years of therapy, the observed rate of lymphoma was 0.10 cases per 100 patient-years. This was 3-fold higher than the rate of lymphoma expected in the general US population based on the Surveillance, Epidemiology, and End Results (SEER) Database. An increased rate of lymphoma up to several-fold has been reported in the RA patient population, and may be further increased in patients with more severe disease activity.

Among 4410 adult PsO patients treated with Enbrel in clinical trials up to 36 months, representing approximately 4278 patient-years of therapy, the observed rate of lymphoma was 0.05 cases per 100 patient-years, which is comparable to the rate in the general population. No cases were observed in Enbrel- or placebo-treated patients during the controlled portions of these trials.

Leukemia

Cases of acute and chronic leukemia have been reported in association with postmarketing TNF-blocker use in rheumatoid arthritis and other indications. Even in the absence of TNF-blocker therapy, patients with rheumatoid arthritis may be at higher risk (approximately 2-fold) than the general population for the development of leukemia.

During the controlled portions of Enbrel trials, 2 cases of leukemia were observed among 5445 (0.06 cases per 100 patient-years) Enbrel-treated patients versus 0 among 2890 (0%) control patients (duration of controlled treatment ranged from 3 to 48 months).

Among 15,401 patients treated with Enbrel in controlled and open portions of clinical trials representing approximately 23,325 patient-years of therapy, the observed rate of leukemia was 0.03 cases per 100 patient-years.

Other Malignancies

Information is available from 10,953 adult patients with 17,123 patient-years and 696 pediatric patients with 1282 patient-years of experience across 45 Enbrel clinical studies.

For malignancies other than lymphoma and non-melanoma skin cancer, there was no difference in exposure-adjusted rates between the Enbrel and control arms in the controlled portions of clinical studies for all indications. Analysis of the malignancy rate in combined controlled and uncontrolled portions of studies has demonstrated that types and rates are similar to what is expected in the general US population based on the SEER database and suggests no increase in rates over time. Whether treatment with Enbrel might influence the development and course of malignancies in adults is unknown.

Non-melanoma skin cancer (NMSC)

Non-melanoma skin cancer has been reported in patients treated with TNF antagonists including etanercept. Among 3306 adult rheumatology (RA, PsA, AS) patients treated with Enbrel in controlled clinical trials representing approximately 2669 patient-years of therapy, the observed rate of NMSC was 0.41 cases per 100 patient-years vs 0.37 cases per 100 patient-years among 1521 control-treated patients representing 1077 patient-years. Among 1245 adult psoriasis patients treated with Enbrel in controlled clinical trials, representing approximately 283 patient-years of therapy, the observed rate of NMSC was 3.54 cases per 100 patient-years vs 1.28 cases per 100 patient-years among 720 control-treated patients representing 156 patient-years. Periodic skin examinations should be considered for all patients at increased risk for NMSC.

Pediatric Patients

Malignancies, some fatal, have been reported among children, adolescents, and young adults who received treatment with TNF-blocking agents (initiation of therapy at ≤ 18 years of age), including Enbrel. Approximately half the cases were lymphomas, including Hodgkin's and non-Hodgkin's lymphoma. The other cases represented a variety of different malignancies and included rare malignancies usually associated with immunosuppression and malignancies that are not usually observed in children and adolescents. The malignancies occurred after a median of 30 months of therapy (range 1 to 84 months). Most of the patients were receiving concomitant immunosuppressants. These cases were reported postmarketing and are derived from a variety of sources, including registries and spontaneous postmarketing reports.

In clinical trials of 696 patients representing 1282 patient-years of therapy, no malignancies, including lymphoma or NMSC, have been reported.

Postmarketing Use

In global postmarketing adult and pediatric use, lymphoma and other malignancies have been reported.

5.4   Patients With Heart Failure

Two clinical trials evaluating the use of Enbrel in the treatment of heart failure were terminated early due to lack of efficacy. One of these studies suggested higher mortality in Enbrel-treated patients compared to placebo *[see Adverse Reactions (6.2)]*. There have been postmarketing reports of worsening of congestive heart failure (CHF), with and without identifiable precipitating factors, in patients taking Enbrel. There have also been rare (< 0.1%) reports of new onset CHF, including CHF in patients without known pre-existing cardiovascular disease. Some of these patients have been under 50 years of age. Physicians should exercise caution when using Enbrel in patients who also have heart failure, and monitor patients carefully.

5.5   Hematologic Events

Rare (< 0.1%) reports of pancytopenia, including very rare (< 0.01%) reports of aplastic anemia, some with a fatal outcome, have been reported in patients treated with Enbrel. The causal relationship to Enbrel therapy remains unclear. Although no high-risk group has been identified, caution should be exercised in patients being treated with Enbrel who have a previous history of significant hematologic abnormalities. All patients should be advised to seek immediate medical attention if they develop signs and symptoms suggestive of blood dyscrasias or infection (eg, persistent fever, bruising, bleeding, pallor) while on Enbrel. Discontinuation of Enbrel therapy should be considered in patients with confirmed significant hematologic abnormalities.

Two percent of patients treated concurrently with Enbrel and anakinra developed neutropenia (ANC < 1 × 10⁹/L). While neutropenic, one patient developed cellulitis that resolved with antibiotic therapy.

5.6   Hepatitis B Virus Reactivation

Use of TNF-blocking agents has been associated with reactivation of hepatitis B virus (HBV), including very rare cases (< 0.01%) with Enbrel, in patients who are chronic carriers of this virus. In some instances, HBV reactivation occurring in conjunction with TNF-blocker therapy has been fatal. The majority of these reports have occurred in patients concomitantly receiving other medications that suppress the immune system, which may also contribute to HBV reactivation. Patients at risk for HBV infection should be evaluated for prior evidence of HBV infection before initiating TNF-blocker therapy. Prescribers should exercise caution in prescribing TNF blockers for patients identified as carriers of HBV. Adequate data are not available on the safety or efficacy of treating patients who are carriers of HBV with anti viral therapy in conjunction with TNF-blocker therapy to prevent HBV reactivation. Patients who are carriers of HBV and require treatment with Enbrel should be closely monitored for clinical and laboratory signs of active HBV infection throughout therapy and for several months following termination of therapy. In patients who develop HBV reactivation, consideration should be given to stopping Enbrel and initiating anti viral therapy with appropriate supportive treatment. The safety of resuming Enbrel therapy after HBV reactivation is controlled is not known. Therefore, prescribers should weigh the risks and benefits when considering resumption of therapy in this situation.

5.7 Allergic Reactions

Allergic reactions associated with administration of Enbrel during clinical trials have been reported in < 2% of patients. If an anaphylactic reaction or other serious allergic reaction occurs, administration of Enbrel should be discontinued immediately and appropriate therapy initiated.

Caution: The needle cap on the prefilled syringe and on the SureClick autoinjector contains dry natural rubber (a derivative of latex) that may cause allergic reactions in individuals sensitive to latex.

5.8 Immunizations

Live vaccines should not be given concurrently with Enbrel. It is recommended that pediatric patients, if possible, be brought up-to-date with all immunizations in agreement with current immunization guidelines prior to initiating Enbrel therapy *[see Drug Interactions (7.1)]*.

5.9 Autoimmunity

Treatment with Enbrel may result in the formation of autoantibodies *[see Adverse Reactions (6.1)]* and, rarely (< 0.1%), in the development of a lupus-like syndrome or autoimmune hepatitis *[see Adverse Reactions (6.2)]*, which may resolve following withdrawal of Enbrel. If a patient develops symptoms and findings suggestive of a lupus-like syndrome or autoimmune hepatitis following treatment with Enbrel, treatment should be discontinued and the patient should be carefully evaluated.

5.10 Immunosuppression

TNF mediates inflammation and modulates cellular immune responses. TNF-blocking agents, including Enbrel, affect host defenses against infections. In a study of 49 patients with RA treated with Enbrel, there was no evidence of depression of delayed-type hypersensitivity, depression of immunoglobulin levels, or change in enumeration of effector cell populations *[see Warnings and Precautions (5.1, 5.3), Adverse Reactions (6.1)]*.

5.11 Use in Wegener's Granulomatosis Patients

The use of Enbrel in patients with Wegener's granulomatosis receiving immunosuppressive agents is not recommended. In a study of patients with Wegener's granulomatosis, the addition of Enbrel to standard therapy (including cyclophosphamide) was associated with a higher incidence of non cutaneous solid malignancies and was not associated with improved clinical outcomes when compared with standard therapy alone *[see Drug Interactions (7.3)]*.

5.12 Use with Anakinra or Abatacept

Use of Enbrel with anakinra or abatacept is not recommended *[see Drug Interactions (7.2)]*.

5.13 Use in Patients with Moderate to Severe Alcoholic Hepatitis

In a study of 48 hospitalized patients treated with Enbrel or placebo for moderate to severe alcoholic hepatitis, the mortality rate in patients treated with Enbrel was similar to patients treated with placebo at 1 month but significantly higher after 6 months. Physicians should use caution when using Enbrel in patients with moderate to severe alcoholic hepatitis.

6 ADVERSE REACTIONS

Across clinical studies and postmarketing experience, the most serious adverse reactions with Enbrel were infections, neurologic events, CHF, and hematologic events *[see Warnings and Precautions (5)]*. The most common adverse reactions with Enbrel were infections and injection site reactions.

6.1 Clinical Studies Experience

Adverse Reactions in Adult Patients With Rheumatoid Arthritis, Psoriatic Arthritis, Ankylosing Spondylitis, or Plaque Psoriasis

The data described below reflect exposure to Enbrel in 2219 adult patients with RA followed for up to 80 months, in 182 patients with PsA for up to 24 months, in 138 patients with AS for up to 6 months, and in 1204 adult patients with PsO for up to 18 months.

In controlled trials, the proportion of Enbrel-treated patients who discontinued treatment due to adverse events was approximately 4% in the indications studied.

Because clinical trials are conducted under widely varying conditions, adverse reactions rates observed in the clinical trials of a drug cannot be directly compared to rates in the clinical trials of another drug and may not predict the rates observed in clinical practice.

Table 3. Percent of Adult RA Patients Experiencing Adverse Reactions in Controlled Clinical Trials

	Placebo Controlled* (Studies I, II, and a Phase 2 Study)		Active Controlled† (Study III)	
	Placebo (N = 152)	**Enbrel‡** (N = 349)	**MTX** (N = 217)	**Enbrel‡** (N = 415)
Reaction	**Percent of Patients**		**Percent of Patients**	
Infection§ (total)	39	50	86	81
Upper Respiratory Infections¶	30	38	70	65
Non-upper Respiratory Infections	15	21	59	54
Injection Site Reactions	11	37	18	43
Diarrhea	9	8	16	16
Rash	2	3	19	13
Pruritus	1	2	5	5
Pyrexia	-	3	4	2
Urticaria	1	-	4	2
Hypersensitivity	-	-	1	1

* Includes data from the 6-month study in which patients received concurrent MTX therapy in both arms.
† Study duration of 2 years.
‡ Any dose.
§ Includes bacterial, viral, and fungal infections.
¶ Most frequent Upper Respiratory Infections were upper respiratory tract infection, sinusitis, and influenza.

Infections

Infections, including viral, bacterial, and fungal infections, have been observed in adult and pediatric patients. Infections have been noted in all body systems and have been reported in patients receiving Enbrel alone or in combination with other immunosuppressive agents.

In controlled portions of trials, the types and severity of infection were similar between Enbrel and the respective control group (placebo or MTX for RA and PsA patients) in RA, PsA, AS, and PsO patients. Rates of infections in RA and PsO patients are provided in Table 3 and Table 4, respectively. Infections consisted primarily of upper respiratory tract infection, sinusitis, and influenza.

In controlled portions of trials in RA, PsA, AS, and PsO, the rates of serious infection were similar (0.8% in placebo, 3.6% in MTX, and 1.4% in Enbrel/Enbrel + MTX-treated groups). In clinical trials in rheumatologic indications, serious infections experienced by patients have included, but are not limited to, pneumonia, cellulitis, septic arthritis, bronchitis, gastroenteritis, pyelonephritis, sepsis, abscess, and osteomyelitis. In clinical trials in PsO, serious infections experienced by patients have included, but are not limited to, pneumonia, cellulitis, gastroenteritis, abscess, and osteomyelitis. The rate of serious infections was not increased in open-label extension trials and was similar to that observed in Enbrel- and placebo-treated patients from controlled trials.

In 66 global clinical trials of 17,505 patients (21,015 patient-years of therapy), tuberculosis was observed in approximately 0.02% of patients. In 17,696 patients (27,169 patient-years of therapy) from 38 clinical trials and 4 cohort studies in the US and Canada, tuberculosis was observed in approximately 0.006% of patients. These studies include reports of pulmonary and extrapulmonary tuberculosis *[see Warnings and Precautions (5.1)]*.

Injection Site Reactions

In placebo-controlled trials in rheumatologic indications, approximately 37% of patients treated with Enbrel developed injection site reactions. In controlled trials in patients with PsO, 15% of patients treated with Enbrel developed injection site reactions during the first 3 months of treatment. All injection site reactions were described as mild to moderate (erythema, itching, pain, swelling, bleeding, bruising) and generally did not necessitate drug discontinuation. Injection site reactions generally occurred in the first month and subsequently decreased in frequency. The mean duration of injection site reactions was 3 to 5 days. Seven percent of patients experienced redness at a previous injection site when subsequent injections were given.

Immunogenicity

Patients with RA, PsA, AS, or PsO were tested at multiple time points for antibodies to etanercept. Antibodies to the TNF receptor portion or other protein components of the Enbrel drug product were detected at least once in sera of approximately 6% of adult patients with RA, PsA, AS, or PsO. These antibodies were all non-neutralizing. Results from JIA patients were similar to those seen in adult RA patients treated with Enbrel.

In PsO studies that evaluated the exposure of etanercept for up to 120 weeks, the percentage of patients testing positive at the assessed time points of 24, 48, 72, and 96 weeks ranged from 3.6%-8.7% and were all non-neutralizing. The percentage of patients testing positive increased with an increase in the duration of study; however, the clinical significance of this finding is unknown. No apparent correlation of antibody development to clinical response or adverse events was observed. The immunogenicity data of Enbrel beyond 120 weeks of exposure are unknown.

The data reflect the percentage of patients whose test results were considered positive for antibodies to etanercept in an ELISA assay, and are highly dependent on the sensitivity and specificity of the assay. Additionally, the observed incidence of any antibody positivity in an assay is highly dependent on several factors, including assay sensitivity and specificity, assay methodology, sample handling, timing of sample collection, concomitant medications, and underlying disease. For these reasons, comparison of the incidence of antibodies to etanercept with the incidence of antibodies to other products may be misleading.

Autoantibodies

Patients with RA had serum samples tested for autoantibodies at multiple time points. In RA Studies I and II, the percentage of patients evaluated for antinuclear antibodies (ANA) who developed new positive ANA (titer ≥ 1:40) was higher in patients treated with Enbrel (11%) than in placebo-treated patients (5%). The percentage of patients who developed new positive anti-double-stranded DNA antibodies was also higher by radioimmunoassay (15% of patients treated with Enbrel compared to 4% of placebo-treated patients) and by *Crithidia luciliae* assay (3% of patients treated with Enbrel compared to none of placebo-treated patients). The proportion of patients treated with Enbrel who developed anticardiolipin antibodies was similarly increased compared to placebo-treated patients. In RA Study III, no pattern of increased autoantibody development was seen in Enbrel patients compared to MTX patients *[see Autoimmunity (5.9)]*.

Other Adverse Reactions

Table 3 summarizes adverse reactions reported in adult RA patients. The types of adverse reactions seen in patients with PsA or AS were similar to the types of adverse reactions seen in patients with RA.

[See table 3 above]

In placebo-controlled PsO trials, the percentages of patients reporting adverse reactions in the 50 mg twice a week dose group were similar to those observed in the 25 mg twice a week dose group or placebo group.

Table 4 summarizes adverse reactions reported in adult PsO patients from Studies I and II.

Table 4. Percent of Adult PsO Patients Experiencing Adverse Reactions in Placebo-Controlled Portions of Clinical Trials (Studies I & II)

	Placebo (N = 359)	**Enbrel*** (N = 876)
Reaction	**Percent of Patients**	
Infection† (total)	28	27
Non-upper Respiratory Infections	14	12
Upper Respiratory Infections‡	17	17
Injection Site Reactions	6	15
Diarrhea	2	3
Rash	1	1
Pruritus	2	1
Urticaria	-	1
Hypersensitivity	-	1
Pyrexia	1	-

* Includes 25 mg SC QW, 25 mg SC BIW, 50 mg SC QW, and 50 mg SC BIW doses.
† Includes bacterial, viral, and fungal infections.
‡ Most frequent Upper Respiratory Infections were upper respiratory tract infection, nasopharyngitis, and sinusitis.

Adverse Reactions in Pediatric Patients

In general, the adverse reactions in pediatric patients were similar in frequency and type as those seen in adult patients [see Warnings and Precautions (5), Adverse Reactions (6), Clinical Studies (14.2)]. The types of infections reported in pediatric patients were generally mild and consistent with those commonly seen in the general pediatric population. Two JIA patients developed varicella infection and signs and symptoms of aseptic meningitis, which resolved without sequelae.

In open-label clinical studies of children with JIA, adverse reactions reported in those ages 2 to 4 years were similar to adverse reactions reported in older children.

6.2   Postmarketing Experience

Adverse reactions have been reported during post approval use of Enbrel in adults and pediatric patients. Because these reactions are reported voluntarily from a population of uncertain size, it is not always possible to reliably estimate their frequency or establish a causal relationship to Enbrel exposure.

Adverse reactions are listed by body system below:

Blood and lymphatic system disorders:	pancytopenia, anemia, leukopenia, neutropenia, thrombocytopenia, lymphadenopathy, aplastic anemia [see Warnings and Precautions (5.5)]
Cardiac disorders:	congestive heart failure [see Warnings and Precautions (5.4)]
General disorders:	angioedema, chest pain
Hepatobiliary disorders:	autoimmune hepatitis, elevated transaminases
Immune disorders:	macrophage activation syndrome
Musculoskeletal and connective tissue disorders:	lupus-like syndrome
Neoplasms benign, malignant and unspecified:	Non-melanoma skin cancers [see Warnings and Precautions (5.3)]
Nervous system disorders:	convulsions, multiple sclerosis, demyelination, optic neuritis, transverse myelitis, paresthesias [see Warnings and Precautions (5.2)]
Ocular disorders:	uveitis
Respiratory, thoracic, and mediastinal disorders:	interstitial lung disease
Skin and subcutaneous tissue disorders:	cutaneous lupus erythematous, cutaneous vasculitis (including leukocytoclastic vasculitis), erythema multiforme, Stevens-Johnson syndrome, toxic epidermal necrolysis, subcutaneous nodule new or worsening psoriasis (all sub-types including pustular and palmoplantar)

Opportunistic infections, including atypical mycobacterial infection, herpes zoster, aspergillosis, and *Pneumocystis jiroveci* pneumonia, and protozoal infections have also been reported in postmarketing use.

7   DRUG INTERACTIONS

Specific drug interaction studies have not been conducted with Enbrel.

7.1   Vaccines

Most PsA patients receiving Enbrel were able to mount effective B-cell immune responses to pneumococcal polysaccharide vaccine, but titers in aggregate were moderately lower and fewer patients had 2-fold rises in titers compared to patients not receiving Enbrel. The clinical significance of this is unknown. Patients receiving Enbrel may receive concurrent vaccinations, except for live vaccines. No data are available on the secondary transmission of infection by live vaccines in patients receiving Enbrel.

Patients with a significant exposure to varicella virus should temporarily discontinue Enbrel therapy and be considered for prophylactic treatment with varicella zoster immune globulin [see Warnings and Precautions (5.8, 5.10)].

Table 5. Contents of Enbrel

Presentation	Active Ingredient Content	Inactive Ingredients Content
Enbrel 50 mg prefilled syringe and SureClick autoinjector	0.98 mL of a 50 mg/mL solution of etanercept	1% sucrose 100 mM sodium chloride 25 mM L-arginine hydrochloride 25 mM sodium phosphate
Enbrel 25 mg prefilled syringe	0.51 mL of a 50 mg/mL solution of etanercept	1% sucrose 100 mM sodium chloride 25 mM L-arginine hydrochloride 25 mM sodium phosphate
Enbrel 25 mg multiple-use vial	25 mg etanercept	40 mg mannitol 10 mg sucrose 1.2 mg tromethamine

7.2   Immune-Modulating Biologic Products

In a study in which patients with active RA were treated for up to 24 weeks with concurrent Enbrel and anakinra therapy, a 7% rate of serious infections was observed, which was higher than that observed with Enbrel alone (0%) [see Warnings and Precautions (5.12)] and did not result in higher ACR response rates compared to Enbrel alone. The most common infections consisted of bacterial pneumonia (4 cases) and cellulitis (4 cases). One patient with pulmonary fibrosis and pneumonia died due to respiratory failure. Two percent of patients treated concurrently with Enbrel and anakinra developed neutropenia (ANC < 1 × 10^9/L).

In clinical studies, concurrent administration of abatacept and Enbrel resulted in increased incidences of serious adverse events, including infections, and did not demonstrate increased clinical benefit [see Warnings and Precautions (5.12)].

7.3   Cyclophosphamide

The use of Enbrel in patients receiving concurrent cyclophosphamide therapy is not recommended [see Warnings and Precautions (5.11)].

7.4   Sulfasalazine

Patients in a clinical study who were on established therapy with sulfasalazine, to which Enbrel was added, were noted to develop a mild decrease in mean neutrophil counts in comparison to groups treated with either Enbrel or sulfasalazine alone. The clinical significance of this observation is unknown.

8   USE IN SPECIFIC POPULATIONS

8.1   Pregnancy

Pregnancy Category B. Developmental toxicity studies have been performed in rats and rabbits at doses ranging from 60- to 100-fold higher than the human dose and have revealed no evidence of harm to the fetus due to Enbrel. There are, however, no studies in pregnant women. Because animal reproduction studies are not always predictive of human response, this drug should be used during pregnancy only if clearly needed.

Pregnancy Registry: To monitor outcomes of pregnant women exposed to Enbrel, a pregnancy registry has been established. Physicians are encouraged to register patients by calling 1-877-311-8972.

8.3   Nursing Mothers

It is not known whether Enbrel is excreted in human milk or absorbed systemically after ingestion. Because many drugs and immunoglobulins are excreted in human milk, and because of the potential for serious adverse reactions in nursing infants from Enbrel, a decision should be made whether to discontinue nursing or to discontinue the drug.

8.4   Pediatric Use

Enbrel is indicated for treatment of polyarticular JIA in patients ages 2 years and older [see Indications and Usage (1.2), Dosage and Administrations (2.3), Warnings and Precautions (5.8), Adverse Reactions (6), Clinical Studies (14.2)].

Enbrel has not been studied in children < 2 years of age with JIA.

The safety and efficacy of Enbrel in pediatric patients with PsO have not been studied.

8.5   Geriatric Use

A total of 480 RA patients ages 65 years or older have been studied in clinical trials. In PsO randomized clinical trials, a total of 138 out of 1965 subjects treated with Enbrel or placebo were age 65 or older. No overall differences in safety or effectiveness were observed between these patients and younger patients, but the number of geriatric PsO subjects is too small to determine whether they respond differently from younger subjects. Because there is a higher incidence of infections in the elderly population in general, caution should be used in treating the elderly.

8.6   Use in Diabetics

There have been reports of hypoglycemia following initiation of Enbrel therapy in patients receiving medication for diabetes, necessitating a reduction in anti-diabetic medication in some of these patients.

10   OVERDOSAGE

Toxicology studies have been performed in monkeys at doses up to 30 times the human dose with no evidence of dose-limiting toxicities. No dose-limiting toxicities have been observed during clinical trials of Enbrel. Single IV doses up to 60 mg/m^2 (approximately twice the recommended dose) have been administered to healthy volunteers in an endotoxemia study without evidence of dose-limiting toxicities.

11   DESCRIPTION

Enbrel (etanercept) is a dimeric fusion protein consisting of the extracellular ligand-binding portion of the human 75 kilodalton (p75) tumor necrosis factor receptor (TNFR) linked to the Fc portion of human IgG1. The Fc component of etanercept contains the C_H2 domain, the C_H3 domain and hinge region, but not the C_H1 domain of IgG1. Etanercept is produced by recombinant DNA technology in a Chinese hamster ovary (CHO) mammalian cell expression system. It consists of 934 amino acids and has an apparent molecular weight of approximately 150 kilodaltons.

The solution of Enbrel in the single-use prefilled syringe and the single-use prefilled SureClick autoinjector is clear and colorless, sterile, preservative-free, and is formulated at pH 6.3 ± 0.2.

Enbrel is also supplied in a multiple-use vial as a sterile, white, preservative-free, lyophilized powder. Reconstitution with 1 mL of the supplied Sterile Bacteriostatic Water for Injection, USP (containing 0.9% benzyl alcohol) yields a multiple-use, clear, and colorless solution with a pH of 7.4 ± 0.3.

[See table 5 above]

12   CLINICAL PHARMACOLOGY

12.1   Mechanism of Action

TNF is a naturally occurring cytokine that is involved in normal inflammatory and immune responses. It plays an important role in the inflammatory processes of RA, polyarticular JIA, PsA, and AS and the resulting joint pathology. In addition, TNF plays a role in the inflammatory process of PsO. Elevated levels of TNF are found in involved tissues and fluids of patients with RA, JIA, PsA, AS, and PsO.

Two distinct receptors for TNF (TNFRs), a 55 kilodalton protein (p55) and a 75 kilodalton protein (p75), exist naturally as monomeric molecules on cell surfaces and in soluble forms. Biological activity of TNF is dependent upon binding to either cell surface TNFR.

Etanercept is a dimeric soluble form of the p75 TNF receptor that can bind TNF molecules. Etanercept inhibits binding of TNF-α and TNF-β (lymphotoxin alpha [LT-α]) to cell surface TNFRs, rendering TNF biologically inactive. In *in vitro* studies, large complexes of etanercept with TNF-α were not detected and cells expressing transmembrane TNF (that binds Enbrel) are not lysed in the presence or absence of complement.

12.2   Pharmacodynamics

Etanercept can modulate biological responses that are induced or regulated by TNF, including expression of adhesion molecules responsible for leukocyte migration (eg, E-selectin, and to a lesser extent, intercellular adhesion molecule-1 [ICAM-1]), serum levels of cytokines (eg, IL-6), and serum levels of matrix metalloproteinase-3 (MMP-3 or stromelysin). Etanercept has been shown to affect several animal models of inflammation, including murine collagen-induced arthritis.

12.3   Pharmacokinetics

After administration of 25 mg of Enbrel by a single subcutaneous (SC) injection to 25 patients with RA, a mean ±

Table 6. ACR Responses in Placebo- and Active-Controlled Trials (Percent of Patients)

	Placebo Controlled				Active Controlled	
	Study I		Study II		Study III	
	Placebo	Enbrel*	MTX/Placebo	MTX/Enbrel*	MTX	Enbrel*
Response	N = 80	N = 78	N = 30	N = 59	N = 217	N = 207
ACR 20						
Month 3	23%	62%[†]	33%	66%[†]	56%	62%
Month 6	11%	59%[†]	27%	71%[†]	58%	65%
Month 12	NA	NA	NA	NA	65%	72%
ACR 50						
Month 3	8%	41%[†]	0%	42%[†]	24%	29%
Month 6	5%	40%[†]	3%	39%[†]	32%	40%
Month 12	NA	NA	NA	NA	43%	49%
ACR 70						
Month 3	4%	15%[†]	0%	15%[†]	7%	13%[‡]
Month 6	1%	15%[†]	0%	15%[†]	14%	21%[‡]
Month 12	NA	NA	NA	NA	22%	25%

* 25 mg Enbrel SC twice weekly
† $p < 0.01$, Enbrel vs. placebo
‡ $p < 0.05$, Enbrel vs. MTX

standard deviation half-life of 102 ± 30 hours was observed with a clearance of 160 ± 80 mL/hr. A maximum serum concentration (Cmax) of 1.1 ± 0.6 mcg/mL and time to Cmax of 69 ± 34 hours was observed in these patients following a single 25 mg dose. After 6 months of twice weekly 25 mg doses in these same RA patients, the mean Cmax was 2.4 ± 1.0 mcg/mL (N = 23). Patients exhibited a 2- to 7-fold increase in peak serum concentrations and approximately 4-fold increase in $AUC_{0-72\ hr}$ (range 1- to 17-fold) with repeated dosing. Serum concentrations in patients with RA have not been measured for periods of dosing that exceed 6 months. The pharmacokinetic parameters in patients with PsO were similar to those seen in patients with RA.

In another study, serum concentration profiles at steady state were comparable among patients with RA treated with 50 mg Enbrel once weekly and those treated with 25 mg Enbrel twice weekly. The mean ($\pm$ standard deviation) Cmax, Cmin, and partial AUC were 2.4 ± 1.5 mcg/mL, 1.2 ± 0.7 mcg/mL, and 297 ± 166 mcg•h/mL, respectively, for patients treated with 50 mg Enbrel once weekly (N = 21); and 2.6 ± 1.2 mcg/mL, 1.4 ± 0.7 mcg/mL, and 316 ± 135 mcg•h/mL for patients treated with 25 mg Enbrel twice weekly (N = 16).

Patients with JIA (ages 4 to 17 years) were administered 0.4 mg/kg of Enbrel twice weekly (up to a maximum dose of 50 mg per week) for up to 18 weeks. The mean serum concentration after repeated SC dosing was 2.1 mcg/mL, with a range of 0.7 to 4.3 mcg/mL. Limited data suggest that the clearance of etanercept is reduced slightly in children ages 4 to 8 years. Population pharmacokinetic analyses predict that the pharmacokinetic differences between the regimens of 0.4 mg/kg twice weekly and 0.8 mg/kg once weekly in JIA patients are of the same magnitude as the differences observed between twice weekly and weekly regimens in adult RA patients.

In clinical studies with Enbrel, pharmacokinetic parameters were not different between men and women and did not vary with age in adult patients. The pharmacokinetics of etanercept were unaltered by concomitant MTX in RA patients. No formal pharmacokinetic studies have been conducted to examine the effects of renal or hepatic impairment on etanercept disposition.

13 NONCLINICAL TOXICOLOGY

13.1 Carcinogenesis, Mutagenesis, Impairment of Fertility

Long-term animal studies have not been conducted to evaluate the carcinogenic potential of Enbrel or its effect on fertility. Mutagenesis studies were conducted in vitro and in vivo, and no evidence of mutagenic activity was observed.

14 CLINICAL STUDIES

14.1 Adult Rheumatoid Arthritis

The safety and efficacy of Enbrel were assessed in four randomized, double-blind, controlled studies. The results of all four trials were expressed in percentage of patients with improvement in RA using American College of Rheumatology (ACR) response criteria.

Study I evaluated 234 patients with active RA who were ≥ 18 years old, had failed therapy with at least one but no more than four DMARDs (eg, hydroxychloroquine, oral or injectable gold, MTX, azathioprine, D-penicillamine, sulfasalazine), and had ≥ 12 tender joints, ≥ 10 swollen joints, and either erythrocyte sedimentation rate (ESR) ≥ 28 mm/hr, C-reactive protein (CRP) > 2.0 mg/dL, or morning stiffness for ≥ 45 minutes. Doses of 10 mg or 25 mg Enbrel or placebo were administered SC twice a week for 6 consecutive months.

Study II evaluated 89 patients and had similar inclusion criteria to Study I except that subjects in Study II had additionally received MTX for at least 6 months with a stable dose (12.5 to 25 mg/week) for at least 4 weeks and they had at least 6 tender or painful joints. Subjects in Study II received a dose of 25 mg Enbrel or placebo SC twice a week for 6 months in addition to their stable MTX dose.

Study III compared the efficacy of Enbrel to MTX in patients with active RA. This study evaluated 632 patients who were ≥ 18 years old with early (≤ 3 years disease duration) active RA, had never received treatment with MTX, and had ≥ 12 tender joints, ≥ 10 swollen joints, and either ESR ≥ 28 mm/hr, CRP > 2.0 mg/dL, or morning stiffness for ≥ 45 minutes. Doses of 10 mg or 25 mg Enbrel were administered SC twice a week for 12 consecutive months. The study was unblinded after all patients had completed at least 12 months (and a median of 17.3 months) of therapy. The majority of patients remained in the study on the treatment to which they were randomized through 2 years, after which they entered an extension study and received open-label 25 mg Enbrel. MTX tablets (escalated from 7.5 mg/week to a maximum of 20 mg/week over the first 8 weeks of the trial) or placebo tablets were given once a week on the same day as the injection of placebo or Enbrel doses, respectively.

Study IV evaluated 682 adult patients with active RA of 6 months to 20 years duration (mean of 7 years) who had an inadequate response to at least one DMARD other than MTX. Forty-three percent of patients had previously received MTX for a mean of 2 years prior to the trial at a mean dose of 12.9 mg. Patients were excluded from this study if MTX had been discontinued for lack of efficacy or for safety considerations. The patient baseline characteristics were similar to those of patients in Study I. Patients were randomized to MTX alone (7.5 to 20 mg weekly, dose escalated as described for Study III; median dose 20 mg), Enbrel alone (25 mg twice weekly), or the combination of Enbrel and MTX initiated concurrently (at the same doses as above). The study evaluated ACR response, Sharp radiographic score, and safety.

Clinical Response

A higher percentage of patients treated with Enbrel and Enbrel in combination with MTX achieved ACR 20, ACR 50, and ACR 70 responses and Major Clinical Responses than in the comparison groups. The results of Studies I, II, and III are summarized in Table 6. The results of Study IV are summarized in Table 7.
[See table 6 at left]

Table 7. Study IV Clinical Efficacy Results: Comparison of MTX vs Enbrel vs Enbrel in Combination with MTX in Patients With Rheumatoid Arthritis of 6 Months to 20 Years Duration (Percent of Patients)

Endpoint	MTX (N = 228)	Enbrel) (N = 223)	Enbrel/MTX (N = 231)
ACR N*,†			
Month 12	40%	47%	63%[‡]
ACR 20			
Month 12	59%	66%	75%[‡]
ACR 50			
Month 12	36%	43%	63%[‡]
ACR 70			
Month 12	17%	22%	40%[‡]
Major Clinical Response§	6%	10%	24%[‡]

* Values are medians.
† ACR N is the percent improvement based on the same core variables used in defining ACR 20, ACR 50, and ACR 70.
‡ $p < 0.05$ for comparisons of Enbrel/MTX vs Enbrel alone or MTX alone.
§ Major clinical response is achieving an ACR 70 response for a continuous 6-month period.

The time course for ACR 20 response rates for patients receiving placebo or 25 mg Enbrel in Studies I and II is summarized in Figure 1. The time course of responses to Enbrel in Study III was similar.

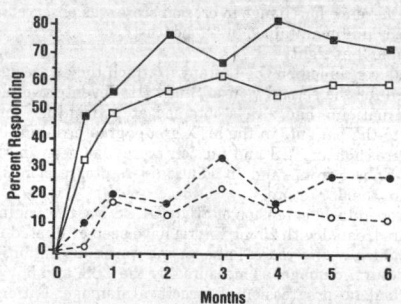

Legend:
--o-- Placebo, Study I (placebo alone)
--●-- Placebo, Study II (placebo + MTX)
--□-- 25 mg Enbrel, Study I (Enbrel alone)
--■-- 25 mg Enbrel, Study II (Enbrel + MTX)

Figure 1: Time Course of ACR 20 Responses

Among patients receiving Enbrel, the clinical responses generally appeared within 1 to 2 weeks after initiation of therapy and nearly always occurred by 3 months. A dose response was seen in Studies I and III: 25 mg Enbrel was more effective than 10 mg (10 mg was not evaluated in Study II). Enbrel was significantly better than placebo in all components of the ACR criteria as well as other measures of RA disease activity not included in the ACR response criteria, such as morning stiffness.

In Study III, ACR response rates and improvement in all the individual ACR response criteria were maintained through 24 months of Enbrel therapy. Over the 2-year study, 23% of Enbrel patients achieved a major clinical response, defined as maintenance of an ACR 70 response over a 6-month period.

The results of the components of the ACR response criteria for Study I are shown in Table 8. Similar results were observed for Enbrel-treated patients in Studies II and III.
[See table 8 at top of next page]

After discontinuation of Enbrel, symptoms of arthritis generally returned within a month. Reintroduction of treatment with Enbrel after discontinuations of up to 18 months resulted in the same magnitudes of response as patients who received Enbrel without interruption of therapy, based on results of open-label studies.

Continued durable responses were seen for over 60 months in open-label extension treatment trials when patients received Enbrel without interruption. A substantial number of patients who initially received concomitant MTX or corticosteroids were able to reduce their doses or discontinue these concomitant therapies while maintaining their clinical responses.

Physical Function Response

In Studies I, II, and III, physical function and disability were assessed using the Health Assessment Questionnaire (HAQ). Additionally, in Study III, patients were administered the SF-36 Health Survey. In Studies I and II, patients treated with 25 mg Enbrel twice weekly showed greater improvement from baseline in the HAQ score beginning in month 1 through month 6 in comparison to placebo ($p < 0.001$) for the HAQ disability domain (where 0 = none and 3 = severe). In Study I, the mean improvement in the HAQ score from baseline to month 6 was 0.6 (from 1.6 to 1.0) for the 25 mg Enbrel group and 0 (from 1.7 to 1.7) for the placebo group. In Study II, the mean improvement from baseline to month 6 was 0.6 (from 1.5 to 0.9) for the Enbrel/MTX group and 0.2 (from 1.3 to 1.2) for the placebo/MTX group. In Study III, the mean improvement in the HAQ score from baseline to month 6 was 0.7 (from 1.5 to 0.7) for 25 mg Enbrel twice weekly. All subdomains of the HAQ in Studies I and III were improved in patients treated with Enbrel.

In Study III, patients treated with 25 mg Enbrel twice weekly showed greater improvement from baseline in SF-36 physical component summary score compared to Enbrel 10 mg twice weekly and no worsening in the SF-36 mental component summary score. In open-label Enbrel studies, improvements in physical function and disability measures have been maintained for up to 4 years.

In Study IV, median HAQ scores improved from baseline levels of 1.8, 1.8, and 1.8 to 1.1, 1.0, and 0.6 at 12 months in the MTX, Enbrel, and Enbrel/MTX combination treatment groups, respectively (combination versus both MTX and Enbrel, $p < 0.01$). Twenty-nine percent of patients in the MTX alone treatment group had an improvement of HAQ of at least 1 unit versus 40% and 51% in the Enbrel alone and the Enbrel/MTX combination treatment groups, respectively.

Radiographic Response

In Study III, structural joint damage was assessed radiographically and expressed as change in Total Sharp Score (TSS) and its components, the erosion score and joint space narrowing (JSN) score. Radiographs of hands/wrists and forefeet were obtained at baseline, 6 months, 12 months, and 24 months and scored by readers who were unaware of treatment group. The results are shown in Table 9. A significant difference for change in erosion score was observed at 6 months and maintained at 12 months.

[See table 9 at right]

Patients continued on the therapy to which they were randomized for the second year of Study III. Seventy-two percent of patients had x-rays obtained at 24 months. Compared to the patients in the MTX group, greater inhibition of progression in TSS and erosion score was seen in the 25 mg Enbrel group, and, in addition, less progression was noted in the JSN score.

In the open-label extension of Study III, 48% of the original patients treated with 25 mg Enbrel have been evaluated radiographically at 5 years. Patients had continued inhibition of structural damage, as measured by the TSS, and 55% of them had no progression of structural damage. Patients originally treated with MTX had further reduction in radiographic progression once they began treatment with Enbrel. In Study IV, less radiographic progression (TSS) was observed with Enbrel in combination with MTX compared with Enbrel alone or MTX alone at month 12 (Table 10). In the MTX treatment group, 55% of patients experienced no radiographic progression (TSS change ≤ 0.0) at 12 months compared to 63% and 76% in the Enbrel alone and the Enbrel/MTX combination treatment groups, respectively.

[See table 10 at right]

Once Weekly Dosing

The safety and efficacy of 50 mg Enbrel (two 25 mg SC injections) administered once weekly were evaluated in a double-blind, placebo-controlled study of 420 patients with active RA. Fifty-three patients received placebo, 214 patients received 50 mg Enbrel once weekly, and 153 patients received 25 mg Enbrel twice weekly. The safety and efficacy profiles of the two Enbrel treatment groups were similar.

14.2 Polyarticular Juvenile Idiopathic Arthritis (JIA)

The safety and efficacy of Enbrel were assessed in a 2-part study in 69 children with polyarticular JIA who had a variety of JIA onset types. Patients ages 2 to 17 years with moderately to severely active polyarticular JIA refractory to or intolerant of MTX were enrolled; patients remained on a stable dose of a single nonsteroidal anti-inflammatory drug and/or prednisone (≤ 0.2 mg/kg/day or 10 mg maximum). In part 1, all patients received 0.4 mg/kg (maximum 25 mg per dose) Enbrel SC twice weekly. In part 2, patients with a

Table 8. Components of ACR Response in Study I

Parameter (median)	Placebo N = 80		ENBREL* N = 78	
	Baseline	3 Months	Baseline	3 Months[†]
Number of tender joints[‡]	34.0	29.5	31.2	10.0[§]
Number of swollen joints[¶]	24.0	22.0	23.5	12.6[§]
Physician global assessment[#]	7.0	6.5	7.0	3.0[§]
Patient global assessment[#]	7.0	7.0	7.0	3.0[§]
Pain[#]	6.9	6.6	6.9	2.4[§]
Disability index[Þ]	1.7	1.8	1.6	1.0[§]
ESR (mm/hr)	31.0	32.0	28.0	15.5[§]
CRP (mg/dL)	2.8	3.9	3.5	0.9[§]

* 25 mg Enbrel SC twice weekly.
† Results at 6 months showed similar improvement.
‡ Scale 0-71.
§ $p < 0.01$, Enbrel vs. placebo, based on mean percent change from baseline.
¶ Scale 0-68.
# Visual analog scale; 0 = best; 10 = worst.
Þ Health Assessment Questionnaire: 0 = best; 3 = worst; includes eight categories: dressing and grooming, arising, eating, walking, hygiene, reach, grip, and activities.

Table 9. Mean Radiographic Change Over 6 and 12 Months in Study III

		MTX	25 mg Enbrel	MTX/Enbrel (95% Confidence Interval*)	P Value
12 Months	Total Sharp Score	1.59	1.00	0.59 (-0.12, 1.30)	0.1
	Erosion Score	1.03	0.47	0.56 (0.11, 1.00)	0.002
	JSN Score	0.56	0.52	0.04 (-0.39, 0.46)	0.5
6 Months	Total Sharp Score	1.06	0.57	0.49 (0.06, 0.91)	0.001
	Erosion Score	0.68	0.30	0.38 (0.09, 0.66)	0.001
	JSN Score	0.38	0.27	0.11 (-0.14, 0.35)	0.6

*95% confidence intervals for the differences in change scores between MTX and Enbrel

Table 10. Mean Radiographic Change in Study IV at 12 Months (95% Confidence Interval)

	MTX (N = 212)*	Enbrel (N = 212)*	Enbrel/MTX (N = 218)*
Total Sharp Score (TSS)	2.80 (1.08, 4.51)	0.52[†] (-0.10, 1.15)	-0.54[‡,§] (-1.00, -0.07)
Erosion Score (ES)	1.68 (0.61, 2.74)	0.21[†] (-0.20, 0.61)	-0.30[‡] (-0.65, 0.04)
Joint Space Narrowing (JSN) Score	1.12 (0.34, 1.90)	0.32 (0.00, 0.63)	-0.23[‡,§] (-0.45, -0.02)

* Analyzed radiographic ITT population.
† $p < 0.05$ for comparison of Enbrel vs MTX.
‡ $p < 0.05$ for comparison of Enbrel/MTX vs MTX.
§ $p < 0.05$ for comparison of Enbrel/MTX vs Enbrel.

clinical response at day 90 were randomized to remain on Enbrel or receive placebo for 4 months and assessed for disease flare. Responses were measured using the JIA Definition of Improvement (DOI), defined as ≥ 30% improvement in at least three of six and ≥ 30% worsening in no more than one of the six JIA core set criteria, including active joint count, limitation of motion, physician and patient/parent global assessments, functional assessment, and ESR. Disease flare was defined as a ≥ 30% worsening in three of the six JIA core set criteria and ≥ 30% improvement in not more than one of the six JIA core set criteria and a minimum of two active joints.

In part 1 of the study, 51 of 69 (74%) patients demonstrated a clinical response and entered part 2. In part 2, 6 of 25 (24%) patients remaining on Enbrel experienced a disease flare compared to 20 of 26 (77%) patients receiving placebo (p = 0.007). From the start of part 2, the median time to flare was ≥ 116 days for patients who received Enbrel and 28 days for patients who received placebo. Each component of the JIA core set criteria worsened in the arm that received placebo and remained stable or improved in the arm

that continued on Enbrel. The data suggested the possibility of a higher flare rate among those patients with a higher baseline ESR. Of patients who demonstrated a clinical response at 90 days and entered part 2 of the study, some of the patients remaining on Enbrel continued to improve from month 3 through month 7, while those who received placebo did not improve.

The majority of JIA patients who developed a disease flare in part 2 and reintroduced Enbrel treatment up to 4 months after discontinuation re-responded to Enbrel therapy in open-label studies. Most of the responding patients who continued Enbrel therapy without interruption have maintained responses for up to 48 months.

Studies have not been done in patients with polyarticular JIA to assess the effects of continued Enbrel therapy in patients who do not respond within 3 months of initiating Enbrel therapy, or to assess the combination of Enbrel with MTX.

14.3 Psoriatic Arthritis

The safety and efficacy of Enbrel were assessed in a randomized, double-blind, placebo-controlled study in 205 patients with PsA. Patients were between 18 and 70 years of age and had active PsA (≥ 3 swollen joints and ≥ 3 tender joints) in one or more of the following forms: (1) distal interphalangeal (DIP) involvement (N = 104); (2) polyarticular arthritis (absence of rheumatoid nodules and presence of psoriasis; N = 173); (3) arthritis mutilans (N = 3); (4) asymmetric psoriatic arthritis (N = 81); or (5) ankylosing spondylitis-like (N = 7). Patients also had plaque psoriasis with a qualifying target lesion ≥ 2 cm in diameter. Patients on MTX therapy at enrollment (stable for ≥ 2 months) could continue at a stable dose of < 25 mg/week MTX. Doses of 25 mg Enbrel or placebo were administered SC twice a week during the initial 6-month double-blind period of the study. Patients continued to receive blinded therapy in an up to 6-month maintenance period until all patients had completed the controlled period. Following this, patients received open-label 25 mg Enbrel twice a week in a 12-month extension period.

Compared to placebo, treatment with Enbrel resulted in significant improvements in measures of disease activity (Table 11).

[See table 11 at right]

Among patients with PsA who received Enbrel, the clinical responses were apparent at the time of the first visit (4 weeks) and were maintained through 6 months of therapy. Responses were similar in patients who were or were not receiving concomitant MTX therapy at baseline. At 6 months, the ACR 20/50/70 responses were achieved by 50%, 37%, and 9%, respectively, of patients receiving Enbrel, compared to 13%, 4%, and 1%, respectively, of patients receiving placebo. Similar responses were seen in patients with each of the subtypes of PsA, although few patients were enrolled with the arthritis mutilans and ankylosing spondylitis-like subtypes. The results of this study were similar to those seen in an earlier single-center, randomized, placebo-controlled study of 60 patients with PsA.

The skin lesions of psoriasis were also improved with Enbrel, relative to placebo, as measured by percentages of patients achieving improvements in the Psoriasis Area and Severity Index (PASI). Responses increased over time, and at 6 months, the proportions of patients achieving a 50% or 75% improvement in the PASI were 47% and 23%, respectively, in the Enbrel group (N = 66), compared to 18% and 3%, respectively, in the placebo group (N = 62). Responses were similar in patients who were or were not receiving concomitant MTX therapy at baseline.

Radiographic Response

Radiographic changes were also assessed in the PsA study. Radiographs of hands and wrists were obtained at baseline and months 6, 12, and 24. A modified Total Sharp Score (TSS), which included distal interphalangeal joints (ie, not identical to the modified TSS used for RA) was used by readers blinded to treatment group to assess the radiographs. Some radiographic features specific to PsA (eg, pencil-and-cup deformity, joint space widening, gross osteolysis, and ankylosis) were included in the scoring system, but others (eg, phalangeal tuft resorption, juxta-articular and shaft periostitis) were not.

Most patients showed little or no change in the modified TSS during this 24-month study (median change of 0 in both patients who initially received Enbrel or placebo). More placebo-treated patients experienced larger magnitudes of radiographic worsening (increased TSS) compared to Enbrel treatment during the controlled period of the study. At 12 months, in an exploratory analysis, 12% (12 of 104) of placebo patients compared to none of the 101 Enbrel-treated patients had increases of 3 points or more in TSS. Inhibition of radiographic progression was maintained in patients who continued on Enbrel during the second year. Of the patients with 1-year and 2-year x-rays, 3% (2 of 71) had increases of 3 points or more in TSS at 1 and 2 years.

Physical Function Response

In the PsA study, physical function and disability were assessed using the HAQ Disability Index (HAQ-DI) and the SF-36 Health Survey. Patients treated with 25 mg Enbrel twice weekly showed greater improvement from baseline in the HAQ-DI score (mean decreases of 54% at both months 3 and 6) in comparison to placebo (mean decreases of 6% at both months 3 and 6) (p < 0.001). At months 3 and 6, patients treated with Enbrel showed greater improvement from baseline in the SF-36 physical component summary score compared to patients treated with placebo, and no worsening in the SF-36 mental component summary score. Improvements in physical function and disability measures were maintained for up to 2 years through the open-label portion of the study.

14.4 Ankylosing Spondylitis

The safety and efficacy of Enbrel were assessed in a randomized, double-blind, placebo-controlled study in 277 patients with active AS. Patients were between 18 and 70 years of age and had AS as defined by the modified New York Criteria for Ankylosing Spondylitis. Patients were to have evidence of active disease based on values of ≥ 30 on a 0-100 unit Visual Analog Scale (VAS) for the average of

Table 11. Components of Disease Activity in Psoriatic Arthritis

Parameter (median)	Placebo N = 104		Enbrel* N = 101	
	Baseline	6 Months	Baseline	6 Months
Number of tender joints†	17.0	13.0	18.0	5.0
Number of swollen joints‡	12.5	9.5	13.0	5.0
Physician global assessment§	3.0	3.0	3.0	1.0
Patient global assessment§	3.0	3.0	3.0	1.0
Morning stiffness (minutes)	60	60	60	15
Pain§	3.0	3.0	3.0	1.0
Disability index¶	1.0	0.9	1.1	0.3
CRP (mg/dL)#	1.1	1.1	1.6	0.2

* p < 0.001 for all comparisons between Enbrel and placebo at 6 months.
† Scale 0-78.
‡ Scale 0-76.
§ Likert scale: 0 = best; 5 = worst.
¶ Health Assessment Questionnaire: 0 = best; 3 = worst; includes eight categories: dressing and grooming, arising, eating, walking, hygiene, reach, grip, and activities.
# Normal range: 0-0.79 mg/dL.

Table 12. Components of Ankylosing Spondylitis Disease Activity

Mean values at time points	Placebo N = 139		Enbrel* N = 138	
	Baseline	6 Months	Baseline	6 Months
ASAS response criteria				
Patient global assessment†	63	56	63	36
Back pain‡	62	56	60	34
BASFI§	56	55	52	36
Inflammation¶	64	57	61	33
Acute phase reactants				
CRP (mg/dL)#	2.0	1.9	1.9	0.6
Spinal mobility (cm):				
Modified Schober's test	3.0	2.9	3.1	3.3
Chest expansion	3.2	3.0	3.3	3.9
Occiput-to-wall measurement	5.3	6.0	5.6	4.5

* p < 0.0015 for all comparisons between Enbrel and placebo at 6 months. P values for continuous endpoints were based on percent change from baseline.
† Measured on a Visual Analog Scale (VAS) with 0 = "none" and 100 = "severe."
‡ Average of total nocturnal and back pain scores, measured on a VAS scale with 0 = "no pain" and 100 = "most severe pain."
§ Bath Ankylosing Spondylitis Functional Index (BASFI), average of 10 questions.
¶ Inflammation represented by the average of the last 2 questions on the 6-question Bath Ankylosing Spondylitis Disease Activity Index (BASDAI).
# C-reactive protein (CRP) normal range: 0-1.0 mg/dL.

morning stiffness duration and intensity, and two of the following three other parameters: a) patient global assessment, b) average of nocturnal and total back pain, and c) the average score on the Bath Ankylosing Spondylitis Functional Index (BASFI). Patients with complete ankylosis of the spine were excluded from study participation. Patients taking hydroxychloroquine, sulfasalazine, methotrexate, or prednisone (≤ 10 mg/day) could continue these drugs at stable doses for the duration of the study. Doses of 25 mg Enbrel or placebo were administered SC twice a week for 6 months.

The primary measure of efficacy was a 20% improvement in the Assessment in Ankylosing Spondylitis (ASAS) response criteria Compared to placebo, treatment with Enbrel resulted in improvements in the ASAS and other measures of disease activity (Figure 2 and Table 12).

[See figure 2 at right]

At 12 weeks, the ASAS 20/50/70 responses were achieved by 60%, 45%, and 29%, respectively, of patients receiving Enbrel, compared to 27%, 13%, and 7%, respectively, of patients receiving placebo (p ≤ 0.0001, Enbrel vs placebo). Similar responses were seen at week 24. Responses were

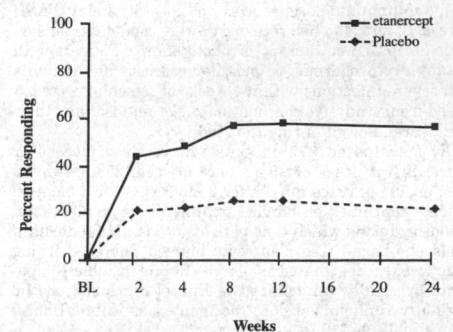

Figure 2. ASAS 20 Responses in Ankylosing Spondylitis

similar between those patients receiving concomitant therapies at baseline and those who were not. The results of this

Table 13. Study I Outcomes at 3 and 6 Months

	Placebo/Enbrel 25 mg BIW (N = 168)	Enbrel/Enbrel		
		25 mg QW (N = 169)	25 mg BIW (N = 167)	50 mg BIW (N = 168)
3 Months				
PASI 75 n (%)	6 (4%)	23 (14%)*	53 (32%)†	79 (47%)†
Difference (95% CI)		10% (4, 16)	28% (21, 36)	43% (35, 52)
sPGA, "clear" or "minimal" n (%)	8 (5%)	36 (21%)†	53 (32%)†	79 (47%)†
Difference (95% CI)		17% (10, 24)	27% (19, 35)	42% (34, 50)
PASI 50 n (%)	24 (14%)	62 (37%)†	90 (54%)†	119 (71%)†
Difference (95% CI)		22% (13, 31)	40% (30, 49)	57% (48, 65)
6 Months				
PASI 75 n (%)	55 (33%)	36 (21%)	68 (41%)	90 (54%)

* p = 0.001 compared with placebo.
† p < 0.0001 compared with placebo.

Table 14. Study II Outcomes at 3 Months

	Placebo (N = 204)	Enbrel	
		25 mg BIW (N = 204)	50 mg BIW (N = 203)
PASI 75 n (%)	6 (3%)	66 (32%)*	94 (46%)*
Difference (95% CI)		29% (23, 36)	43% (36, 51)
sPGA "clear" or "minimal" n (%)	7 (3%)	75 (37%)*	109 (54%)*
Difference (95% CI)		34% (26, 41)	50% (43, 58)
PASI 50 n (%)	18 (9%)	124 (61%)*	147 (72%)*
Difference (95% CI)		52% (44, 60)	64% (56, 71)

*p < 0.0001 compared with placebo.

50 mg single-use prefilled syringe	Carton of 4	NDC 58406-435-04
50 mg single-use prefilled SureClick autoinjector	Carton of 4	NDC 58406-445-04
25 mg single-use prefilled syringe	Carton of 4	NDC 58406-455-04

25 mg multiple-use vial	Carton of 4	NDC 58406-425-34

study were similar to those seen in a single-center, randomized, placebo-controlled study of 40 patients and a multicenter, randomized, placebo-controlled study of 84 patients with AS.
[See table 12 on previous page]

14.5   Plaque Psoriasis
The safety and efficacy of Enbrel were assessed in two randomized, double-blind, placebo-controlled studies in adults with chronic stable PsO involving ≥ 10% of the body surface area, a minimum Psoriasis Area and Severity Index (PASI) score of 10 and who had received or were candidates for systemic antipsoriatic therapy or phototherapy. Patients with guttate, erythrodermic, or pustular psoriasis and patients with severe infections within 4 weeks of screening were excluded from study. No concomitant major antipsoriatic therapies were allowed during the study.
Study I evaluated 672 patients who received placebo or Enbrel SC at doses of 25 mg once a week, 25 mg twice a week or 50 mg twice a week for 3 months. After 3 months, patients continued on blinded treatments for an additional 3 months during which time patients originally randomized to placebo began treatment with blinded Enbrel at 25 mg twice weekly (designated as placebo/Enbrel in Table 13); patients originally randomized to Enbrel continued on the originally randomized dose (designated as Enbrel/Enbrel groups in Table 13).
Study II evaluated 611 patients who received placebo or Enbrel SC at doses of 25 mg or 50 mg twice a week for 3 months. After 3 months of randomized, blinded treatment, patients in all three arms began receiving open-label Enbrel at 25 mg twice weekly for 9 additional months.

Response to treatment in both studies was assessed after 3 months of therapy and was defined as the proportion of patients who achieved a reduction in PASI score of at least 75% from baseline. The PASI is a composite score that takes into consideration both the fraction of body surface area affected and the nature and severity of psoriatic changes within the affected regions (induration, erythema, and scaling).
Other evaluated outcomes included the proportion of patients who achieved a score of "clear" or "minimal" by the Static Physician Global Assessment (sPGA) and the proportion of patients with a reduction of PASI of at least 50% from baseline. The sPGA is a 6-category scale ranging from "5 = severe" to "0 = none" indicating the physician's overall assessment of the PsO severity focusing on induration, erythema, and scaling. Treatment success of "clear" or "minimal" consisted of none or minimal elevation in plaque, up to faint red coloration in erythema, and none or minimal fine scale over < 5% of the plaque.
Patients in all treatment groups and in both studies had a median baseline PASI score ranging from 15 to 17, and the percentage of patients with baseline sPGA classifications ranged from 54% to 66% for moderate, 17% to 26% for marked, and 1% to 5% for severe. Across all treatment groups, the percentage of patients who previously received systemic therapy for PsO ranged from 61% to 65% in Study I and 71% to 75% in Study II, and those who previously received phototherapy ranged from 44% to 50% in Study I and 72% to 73% in Study II.
More patients randomized to Enbrel than placebo achieved at least a 75% reduction from baseline PASI score (PASI 75)

with a dose response relationship across doses of 25 mg once a week, 25 mg twice a week and 50 mg twice a week (Tables 13 and 14). The individual components of the PASI (induration, erythema, and scaling) contributed comparably to the overall treatment-associated improvement in PASI.
[See table 13 at left]
[See table 14 at left]
Among PASI 75 achievers in both studies, the median time to PASI 50 and PASI 75 was approximately 1 month and approximately 2 months, respectively, after the start of therapy with either 25 or 50 mg twice a week.
In Study I, patients who achieved PASI 75 at month 6 were entered into a study drug withdrawal and retreatment period. Following withdrawal of study drug, these patients had a median duration of PASI 75 of between 1 and 2 months.
In Study I, among patients who were PASI 75 responders at 3 months, retreatment with their original blinded Enbrel dose after discontinuation of up to 5 months resulted in a similar proportion of responders as in the initial double-blind portion of the study.
In Study II, most patients initially randomized to 50 mg twice a week continued in the study after month 3 and had their Enbrel dose decreased to 25 mg twice a week. Of the 91 patients who were PASI 75 responders at month 3, 70 (77%) maintained their PASI 75 response at month 6.

15   REFERENCES
1. National Cancer Institute. Surveillance, Epidemiology, and End Results Database (SEER) Program. SEER Incidence Crude Rates, 13 Registries, 1992-2002.

16   HOW SUPPLIED/STORAGE AND HANDLING
Administration of one 50 mg Enbrel prefilled syringe or one Enbrel SureClick autoinjector provides a dose equivalent to two 25 mg Enbrel prefilled syringes or two multiple-use vials of lyophilized Enbrel, when vials are reconstituted and administered as recommended.
16.1   Enbrel Single-use Prefilled Syringe and Enbrel Single-use Prefilled SureClick Autoinjector
Each Enbrel single-use prefilled syringe and Enbrel single-use prefilled SureClick autoinjector contains 50 mg/mL of etanercept in a single-dose syringe with a 27-gauge, ½-inch needle.
[See third table at top left]
Do not use Enbrel beyond the expiration date stamped on the carton or barrel label. Enbrel must be refrigerated at 2° to 8°C (36° to 46°F). DO NOT FREEZE. Keep the product in the original carton to protect from light until the time of use. Do not shake.
16.2   Enbrel Multiple-use Vial (Recommended for Weight-based Dosing)
Enbrel multiple-use vial is supplied in a carton containing four dose trays. Each dose tray contains one 25 mg vial of etanercept, one diluent syringe (1 mL Sterile Bacteriostatic Water for Injection, USP, containing 0.9% benzyl alcohol), one 27-gauge ½-inch needle, one vial adapter, one plunger, and two alcohol swabs. Each carton contains four "Mixing Date:" stickers.
[See fourth table at left]
Do not use a dose tray beyond the expiration date stamped on the dose tray label. The dose tray containing Enbrel (sterile powder) must be refrigerated at 2° to 8°C (36° to 46°F). DO NOT FREEZE.

17   PATIENT COUNSELING INFORMATION
See Medication Guide
Patients or their caregivers should be provided the Enbrel "Medication Guide" and provided an opportunity to read it and ask questions prior to initiation of therapy. The healthcare provider should ask the patient questions to determine any risk factors for treatment. Patients developing signs and symptoms of infection should seek medical evaluation immediately.
17.1   Patient Counseling
Patients should be advised of the potential benefits and risks of Enbrel. Physicians should instruct their patients to read the Patient Package Insert before starting Enbrel therapy and to reread each time the prescription is renewed.
Infections
Inform patients that Enbrel may lower the ability of their immune system to fight infections. Advise patients of the importance of contacting their doctor if they develop any symptoms of infection, tuberculosis, or reactivation of hepatitis B virus infections.
Other Medical Conditions
Advise patients to report any signs of new or worsening medical conditions, such as central nervous system demyelinating disorders, heart failure, or autoimmune disorders such as lupus-like syndrome or autoimmune hepatitis. Counsel about the risk of lymphoma and other malignancies while receiving Enbrel. Advise patients to report any symptoms suggestive of a pancytopenia, such as bruising, bleeding, persistent fever, or pallor.
Allergic Reactions
Advise patients to seek immediate medical attention if they experience any symptoms of severe allergic reactions. Advise latex-sensitive patients that the needle cap of the pre-

filled syringe and SureClick autoinjector contains dry natural rubber (a derivative of latex), which should not be handled by persons sensitive to latex.

17.2 Administration of Enbrel

If a patient or caregiver is to administer Enbrel, the patient or caregiver should be instructed in injection techniques and how to measure and administer the correct dose [see the Enbrel (etanercept) "Patient Instructions for Use" insert]. The first injection should be performed under the supervision of a qualified healthcare professional. The patient's or caregiver's ability to inject subcutaneously should be assessed. Patients and caregivers should be instructed in the technique, as well as proper syringe and needle disposal, and be cautioned against reuse of needles and syringes.

A puncture-resistant container for disposal of needles, syringes, and autoinjectors should be used. If the product is intended for multiple use, additional syringes, needles, and alcohol swabs will be required.

Enbrel® (etanercept)
Manufactured by:
Immunex Corporation
Thousand Oaks, CA 91320-1799
U.S. License Number 1132
Marketed by Amgen Inc. and Pfizer Inc.
Patents covering methods, vectors, and/or host cells for making the product or methods for using the product:
US Patent Nos. 5,395,760; 5,605,690, Re. 36,755.
© 1998-2010 Immunex Corporation. All rights reserved.
1XXXXXX - v39
Issue Date: 06/2010

Medication Guide

Enbrel® (en-brel)
(etanercept)
Read the Medication Guide that comes with Enbrel before you start using it and each time you get a refill. There may be new information. This Medication Guide does not take the place of talking with your doctor about your medical condition or treatment. It is important to remain under your doctor's care while using Enbrel.

Enbrel is a prescription medicine called a Tumor Necrosis Factor (TNF) blocker that affects your immune system.

What is the most important information I should know about Enbrel?
Enbrel may cause serious side effects, including:

1. Risk of infection
Enbrel can lower the ability of your immune system to fight infections. Some people have serious infections while taking Enbrel. These infections include tuberculosis (TB), and infections caused by viruses, fungi, or bacteria that spread throughout their body. Some people have died from these infections.

• Your doctor should test you for TB before starting Enbrel.
• Your doctor should monitor you closely for symptoms of TB during treatment with Enbrel even if you tested negative for TB.
• Your doctor should check you for symptoms of any type of infection before, during, and after your treatment with Enbrel.

You should not start taking Enbrel if you have any kind of infection unless your doctor says it is okay.

2. Risk of cancer
• There have been cases of unusual cancers in children and teenage patients who started using TNF-blocking agents at less than 18 years of age.
• For children, teenagers, and adults taking TNF-blocker medicines, including Enbrel, the chances of getting lymphoma or other cancers may increase.
• People with rheumatoid arthritis or psoriasis, especially those with very active disease, may be more likely to get lymphoma.

Before starting Enbrel, be sure to talk to your doctor:
Enbrel may not be right for you. Before starting Enbrel, tell your doctor about all of your medical conditions, including:

Infections—tell your doctor if you:
• have an infection. (See **"What is the most important information I should know about Enbrel?"**)
• are being treated for an infection.
• think you have an infection.
• have symptoms of an infection such as fever, sweats or chills, cough or flu-like symptoms, shortness of breath, blood in your phlegm, weight loss, muscle aches, warm, red, or painful areas on your skin, sores on your body, diarrhea or stomach pain, burning when you urinate or urinating more often than normal, and feel very tired.
• have any open cuts on your body.
• get a lot of infections or have infections that keep coming back.
• have diabetes, HIV, or a weak immune system. People with these conditions have a higher chance for infections.
• have TB, or have been in close contact with someone with TB.

• were born in, lived in, or traveled to countries where there is a risk for getting TB. Ask your doctor if you are not sure.
• live, have lived in, or traveled to certain parts of the country (such as the Ohio and Mississippi River valleys, or the Southwest) where there is a greater risk for getting certain kinds of fungal infections (histoplasmosis, coccidioidomycosis, blastomycosis). These infections may happen or become more severe if you use Enbrel. Ask your doctor if you do not know if you live or have lived in an area where these infections are common.
• have or have had hepatitis B.

Also, BEFORE starting Enbrel, tell your doctor:
• **About all the medicines you take including prescription and nonprescription medicines, vitamins and herbal supplements including:**
  ◦ **Orencia® (abatacept) or Kineret® (anakinra).** You have a higher chance for serious infections when taking Enbrel with Orencia or Kineret.
  ◦ **Cyclophosphamide (Cytoxan®).** You may have a higher chance for getting certain cancers when taking Enbrel with cyclophosphamide.
  ◦ **Anti-diabetic Medicines.** If you have diabetes and are taking medication to control your diabetes, your doctor may decide you need less anti-diabetic medicine while taking Enbrel.

Keep a list of all your medications with you to show your doctor and pharmacist each time you get a new medicine. Ask your doctor if you are not sure if your medicine is one listed above.

Other important medical information you should tell your doctor BEFORE starting Enbrel, includes if you:
• have or had a nervous system problem such as multiple sclerosis.
• have or had heart failure.
• are scheduled to have surgery.
• have recently received or are scheduled to receive a vaccine.
  ◦ all vaccines should be brought up-to-date before starting Enbrel.
  ◦ people taking Enbrel should not receive live vaccines.
  ◦ ask your doctor if you are not sure if you received a live vaccine.
• are allergic to rubber or latex.
  ◦ the needle covers on the single-use prefilled syringes and the single-use prefilled SureClick autoinjectors contains dry natural rubber.
• have been around someone with varicella zoster (chicken pox).
• are pregnant or plan to become pregnant. It is not known if Enbrel will harm your unborn baby.
  ◦ **Pregnancy Registry:** Amgen has a registry for pregnant women who take Enbrel. The purpose of this registry is to check the health of the pregnant mother and her child. Talk to your doctor if you are pregnant and contact the registry at 1-877-311-8972.
• are breastfeeding or plan to breastfeed. It is not known if Enbrel passes into your breast milk. You and your doctor should decide if you will take Enbrel or breast feed. You should not do both.

See the section "What are the possible side effects of Enbrel?" below for more information.

What is Enbrel?
Enbrel is a prescription medicine called a Tumor Necrosis Factor (TNF) blocker.
Enbrel is used to treat:
• **moderately to severely active rheumatoid arthritis (RA).** Enbrel can be used alone or with a medicine called methotrexate.
• **psoriatic arthritis.** Enbrel can be used alone or with methotrexate.
• **ankylosing spondylitis (AS).**
• **chronic moderate to severe plaque psoriasis in adults ages 18 years and older**
• **moderately to severely active polyarticular juvenile idiopathic arthritis (JIA) in children ages 2 years and older.**
You may continue to use other medicines that help treat your condition while taking Enbrel, such as nonsteroidal anti-inflammatory drugs (NSAIDs) and prescription steroids, as recommended by your doctor.
Enbrel can help reduce joint damage and the signs and symptoms of the above mentioned diseases. People with these diseases have too much of a protein called tumor necrosis factor (TNF), which is made by your immune system. Enbrel can reduce the effect of TNF in the body and block the damage that too much TNF can cause, but it can also lower the ability of your immune system to fight infections. See "What is the most important information I should know about Enbrel?" and "What are the possible side effects of Enbrel?"

Who should not use Enbrel
Do not use Enbrel if you:
• have an infection that has spread through your body (sepsis).

How should I use Enbrel
• Enbrel is given as an injection under the skin (subcutaneous or SC).
• If your doctor decides that you or a caregiver can give the injections of Enbrel at home, you or your caregiver should receive training on the right way to prepare and inject Enbrel. Do not try to inject Enbrel until you have been shown the right way by your doctor or nurse.
• Enbrel is available in the forms listed below. Your doctor will prescribe the type that is best for you.
  ◦ Single-use Prefilled Syringe
  ◦ Single-use Prefilled SureClick Autoinjector
  ◦ Multiple-use Vial
• See the detailed "Patient Instructions for Use" with this Medication Guide for instructions about the right way to store, prepare, and give your Enbrel injections at home.
• Your doctor will tell you how often you should use Enbrel. Do not miss any doses of Enbrel. If you forget to use Enbrel, inject your dose as soon as you remember. Then, take your next dose at your regular(ly) scheduled time. In case you are not sure when to inject Enbrel, call your doctor or pharmacist. **Do not use Enbrel more often than as directed by your doctor.**
• Your child's dose of Enbrel depends on his or her weight. Your child's doctor will tell you which form of Enbrel to use and how much to give your child.

What are the possible side effects of Enbrel?
Enbrel can cause serious side effects, including:
See "What is the most important information I should know about Enbrel?"
• **Infections.** Enbrel can make you more likely to get infections or make any infection that you have worse. Call your doctor right away if you have any symptoms of an infection. See "Before starting Enbrel, be sure to talk to your doctor" for a list of symptoms of infection.
• **Hepatitis B infection** in people who carry the virus in their blood. If you are a carrier of the hepatitis B virus (a virus that affects the liver), the virus can become active while you use Enbrel. Your doctor may do a blood test before you start treatment with Enbrel and while you use Enbrel.
• **Nervous system problems.** Rarely, people who use TNF-blocker medicines have developed nervous system problems such as multiple sclerosis, seizures, or inflammation of the nerves of the eyes. Tell your doctor right away if you get any of these symptoms: numbness or tingling in any part of your body, vision changes, weakness in your arms and legs, and dizziness.
• **Blood problems.** Low blood counts have been seen with other TNF-blocker medicines. Your body may not make enough of the blood cells that help fight infections or help stop bleeding. Symptoms include fever, bruising or bleeding very easily, or looking pale.
• **Heart failure** including new heart failure or worsening of heart failure you already have. New or worse heart failure can happen in people who use TNF-blocker medicines like Enbrel. If you have heart failure your condition should be watched closely while you take Enbrel. Call your doctor right away if you get new or worsening symptoms of heart failure while taking Enbrel, such as shortness of breath or swelling of your lower legs or feet.
• **Psoriasis.** Some people using Enbrel developed new psoriasis or worsening of psoriasis they already had. Tell your doctor if you develop red scaly patches or raised bumps that may be filled with pus. Your doctor may decide to stop your treatment with Enbrel.
• **Allergic reactions.** Allergic reactions can happen to people who use TNF-blocker medicines. Call your doctor right away if you have any symptoms of an allergic reaction. Symptoms of an allergic reaction include a severe rash, a swollen face, or trouble breathing.
• **Autoimmune reactions, including:**
  ◦ **Lupus-like syndrome.** Symptoms include a rash on your face and arms that gets worse in the sun. Tell your doctor if you have this symptom. Symptoms may go away when you stop using Enbrel.
  ◦ **Autoimmune hepatitis.** Liver problems can happen in people who use TNF-blocker medicines, including Enbrel. These problems can lead to liver failure and death. Call your doctor right away if you have any of these symptoms: feel very tired, skin or eyes look yellow, poor appetite or vomiting, pain on the right side of your stomach (abdomen).

Common side effects of Enbrel include:
• **Injection site reactions** such as redness, swelling, itching, or pain. These symptoms usually go away within 3 to 5 days. If you have pain, redness, or swelling around the injection site that doesn't go away or gets worse, call your doctor.

- **Upper respiratory infections** (sinus infections).
- **Headache.**

These are not all the side effects with Enbrel. Tell your doctor about any side effect that bothers you or does not go away.

Call your doctor for medical advice about side effects. You may report side effects to FDA at 1-800-FDA-1088.

How should I store Enbrel?

- Store Enbrel in the refrigerator at 36° to 46°F (2° to 8°C).
- **Do not freeze.**
- **Do not shake.**
- Keep Enbrel in the original carton to protect from light.
- Keep Enbrel and all medicines out of the reach of children.

General Information about Enbrel

Medicines are sometimes prescribed for purposes not mentioned in a Medication Guide. Do not use Enbrel for a condition for which it was not prescribed. Do not give Enbrel to other people, even if they have the same condition. It may harm them.

This Medication Guide summarizes the most important information about Enbrel. If you would like more information, talk with your doctor. You can ask your doctor or pharmacist for information about Enbrel that was written for healthcare professionals. For more information call, 1-888-4Enbrel (1-888-436-2735).

What are the ingredients in Enbrel?

Single-use Prefilled Syringe and the Single-use Prefilled SureClick Autoinjector:

Active Ingredient: etanercept

Inactive Ingredients: sucrose, sodium chloride, L-arginine hydrochloride and sodium phosphate

Multiple-use Vial:

Active Ingredient: etanercept

Inactive Ingredients: mannitol, sucrose, tromethamine

Manufactured by:

Immunex Corporation,
Thousand Oaks, CA 91320-1799
Marketed by Amgen Inc. and Pfizer Inc.
© 1998-2010 Immunex Corporation. All rights reserved.
1XXXXXX - v4
Issue Date: 06/2010
Printed in the USA
This Medication Guide has been approved by the US Food and Drug Administration.

Patient Instructions for Use

ENBREL® (en-brel)
(etanercept)
Single-use Prefilled Syringe

How do I prepare and give an injection with ENBREL® Single-use Prefilled Syringe?

There are 2 types of ENBREL® single-use prefilled syringes:

- The 50 mg single-use prefilled syringe that contains one 50 mg dose of ENBREL®.
- The 25 mg single-use prefilled syringe that contains one 25 mg dose of ENBREL®.

Your doctor will tell you which one to use.

A 50 mg dose can be given as one injection using a 50 mg single-use prefilled syringe or as two injections using 25 mg single-use prefilled syringes. Your doctor will tell you whether the two injections with 25 mg single-use prefilled syringes should be given on the same day once a week or on two different days (3 or 4 days apart) in the same week.

Children must weigh at least 138 pounds to use the ENBREL® 50 mg single-use prefilled syringe. Children who weigh less than 138 pounds should use a different form of ENBREL®. The ENBREL® 25 mg single-use prefilled syringe should not be used in pediatric patients weighing less than 68 pounds.

IMPORTANT: The needle cover on the single-use prefilled syringe contains latex. Tell your doctor if you are allergic to latex.

STEP 1: Setting for an Injection

1. Select a clean, well-lit, flat work surface, such as a table.
2. Take the ENBREL® carton containing the prefilled syringes out of the refrigerator and place it on your flat work surface. Remove one prefilled syringe and place it on your work surface. Do not shake the prefilled syringe of ENBREL®. Place the carton containing any remaining prefilled syringes back into the refrigerator (2° to 8°C [36° to 46°F]). If you have any questions about storage, contact your doctor, nurse, or pharmacist for further instructions.
3. Check the expiration date on the prefilled syringe. If the expiration date has passed, do not use the prefilled syringe and contact your pharmacist or call 1-888-4ENBREL (1-888-436-2735) for assistance.
4. Wait 15 to 30 minutes to allow the ENBREL® in the prefilled syringe to reach room temperature. DO NOT remove the needle cover while allowing it to reach room temperature. DO NOT warm ENBREL® in any other way (for example, do not warm it in a microwave or in hot water).

5. Hold the prefilled syringe with the covered needle pointing down. If bubbles are seen in the syringe, very gently tap the prefilled syringe to allow any bubbles to rise to the top of the syringe. Turn the syringe so that the purple horizontal lines on the barrel are directly facing you. Check to see if the amount of liquid in the syringe falls between the purple lines. The top of the liquid may be curved. If the syringe does not have the right amount of liquid, DO NOT USE THAT SYRINGE. Contact your pharmacist or call 1-888-4ENBREL (1-888-436-2735) for assistance.

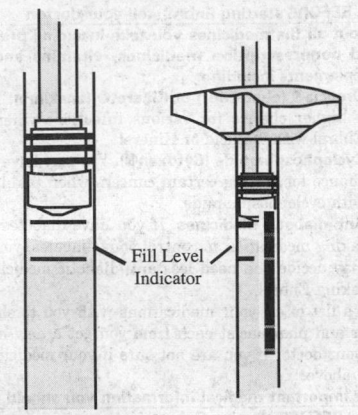

Fill Level Indicator

6. Assemble the additional supplies you will need for your injection. These include an alcohol swab, a cotton ball or gauze, and a puncture-resistant disposal container.
7. Wash your hands with soap and warm water.
8. Make sure the solution in the prefilled syringe is clear and colorless. You may notice small white particles in the solution. These particles are formed from ENBREL® and this is acceptable. However, **do not inject the solution if it is cloudy or discolored, or contains large or colored particles**—contact your pharmacist or call 1-888-4ENBREL (1-888-436-2735) for assistance.

STEP 2: Choosing and Preparing an Injection Site

1. Three recommended injection sites for ENBREL® using a prefilled syringe include: (1) the front of the middle thighs; (2) the abdomen, except for the two-inch area right around the navel; and, (3) the outer area of the upper arms.

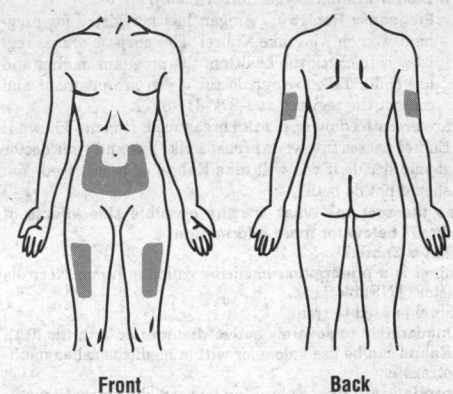

Front   Back

2. Rotate the site for each injection. Do not inject into areas where the skin is tender, bruised, red, or hard. Avoid areas with scars or stretch marks.
3. If you have psoriasis, you should try not to inject directly into any raised, thick, red, or scaly skin patches ("psoriasis skin lesions").
4. To prepare the area of skin where ENBREL® is to be injected, wipe the injection site with an alcohol swab. **Do not touch this area again before giving the injection.**

STEP 3: Injecting ENBREL® Using a Prefilled Syringe

1. Pick up the prefilled syringe from your flat work surface. Hold the barrel of the prefilled syringe with one hand and pull the needle cover straight off.

When you remove the needle cover, there may be a drop of liquid at the end of the needle; this is normal. Do not touch the needle or allow it to touch any surface. Do not touch or bump the plunger. Doing so could cause the liquid to leak out.

2. Holding the syringe with the needle pointing up, check the syringe for air bubbles. If there are bubbles, gently tap the syringe with your finger until the air bubbles rise to the top of the syringe. Slowly push the plunger up to force the air bubbles out of the syringe.
3. Holding the syringe in one hand like a pencil, use the other hand to gently pinch a fold of skin at the cleaned injection site and hold it firmly.
4. Insert the needle at a slight angle (45 degrees) to the skin. With a quick, "dart-like" motion, insert the needle into the skin.

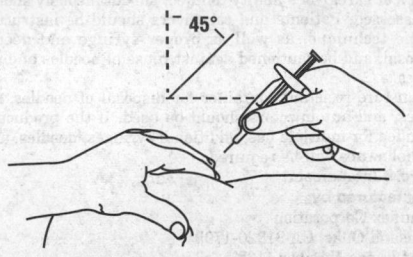

45°

5. After the needle is inserted, let go of the skin. Pull the plunger back slightly. If blood comes into the syringe, do not inject ENBREL® because the needle has entered a blood vessel. Withdraw the needle and discard it in a puncture-resistant container. Repeat the steps to prepare for an injection using a new prefilled syringe of ENBREL®. Do not use the same prefilled syringe.
6. If no blood appears in the syringe, slowly push the plunger all the way down to inject ENBREL®.
7. When the syringe is empty, pull the needle out of the skin, being careful to keep it at the same angle as inserted. There may be a little bleeding at the injection site. You can press a cotton ball or gauze over the injection site for 10 seconds. Do not rub the injection site. If needed, you may cover the injection site with a bandage.

STEP 4: Disposing of Supplies

The syringe should **NEVER** be reused. **NEVER** recap a needle.

Dispose of the used syringe as instructed by your healthcare provider, or by following these steps:

- Do not throw the used syringe in the household trash or recycle.
- Place the used syringe in a hard plastic disposal container with a screw-on cap or a metal container with a plastic lid, such as a coffee can, labeled "used syringes." If a metal container is used, cut a small hole in the plastic lid and tape the lid to the metal container. If a hard plastic container is used, always screw the cap on tightly after each use. Do not use glass or clear plastic containers. Puncture-resistant containers may also be purchased at your local pharmacy.
- When the container is full, tape around the cap or lid to make sure the cap or lid does not come off.
- You should always check first with your healthcare provider for instructions on how to properly dispose of a filled disposal container. There may be special state and local laws for disposing of used needles and syringes. **Do not throw the disposal container in household trash. Do not recycle.**
- **Always** keep the container out of the reach of children.

A healthcare provider familiar with ENBREL® should answer all questions. A toll-free information service is also available: 1-888-4ENBREL (1-888-436-2735).

Manufactured by:

Immunex Corporation,
Thousand Oaks, CA 91320-1799
Marketed by Amgen Inc. and Wyeth Pharmaceuticals
© 1998–2008 Immunex Corporation. All rights reserved.
1XXXXXX- v1
Issue Date: 06/2008

Patient Instructions for Use

ENBREL® (en-brel)
(etanercept)
Multiple-use Vial

How do I prepare and give an injection with ENBREL® Multiple-use Vial?

A multiple-use vial contains 25 mg of ENBREL®.

STEP 1: Setting up for an Injection

1. Select a clean, well-lit, flat work surface, such as a table.
2. Take the ENBREL dose tray out of the refrigerator and place it on your flat work surface.
3. Check the expiration date on the dose tray. If the expiration date has passed, do not use the dose tray. Also check to make sure the dose tray has seven items as pictured below:
   - One prefilled diluent syringe containing 1 mL of diluent (liquid) with attached adapter and twist-off cap
   - One plunger
   - One ENBREL® vial
   - One 27-gauge ½ inch needle in hard plastic cover

○ One vial adapter
○ Two alcohol swabs

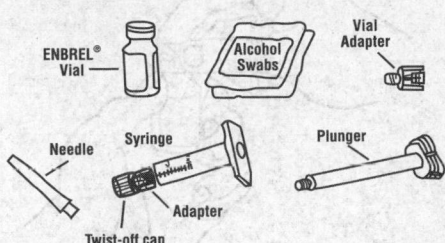

If the expiration date has passed, the seven items are not included in the dose tray or if any item looks damaged, contact your pharmacist or call 1-888-4ENBREL (1-888-436-2735) for assistance.

4. Wash your hands with soap and warm water.
5. Peel the paper seal off the dose tray and remove all items.
6. Inspect the volume of diluent in the syringe with the twist-off cap pointing down. Use the unit markings on the side of the syringe to make sure there is at least 1 mL of liquid in the syringe. If the level of liquid is below the 1 mL mark, do not use. Call 1-888-4ENBREL (1-888-436-2735) for assistance.

STEP 2: Preparing the ENBREL® Solution

There are two methods for preparing the ENBREL® solution. For some children, one vial of ENBREL® solution can be used for more than one dose. The free-hand method should be used for children on ENBREL® who are using one vial of ENBREL® solution for more than one dose. **You should not use the vial adapter method if you will be using the vial more than once.** Ask your healthcare provider if you have questions about which method to use.

• **The Vial Adapter Method**

Adult patients and larger children on ENBREL® may use the vial adapter device to assist with mixing the powder with the liquid and withdrawing ENBREL®, and then use a 27-gauge needle to inject the dose. **This method should not be used for children using multiple doses from the same vial of ENBREL®.** The instructions for using the vial adapter method are in STEP 2A.

• **The Free-Hand Method**

In the free-hand method, a 25-gauge needle is used to assist with mixing the powder with the liquid and withdrawing ENBREL®, and a 27-gauge needle is used to inject the dose. Obtain 25-gauge needles from your healthcare provider. Instructions for using the free-hand method are in STEP 2B. The instructions for preparing additional doses from the same vial of ENBREL® solution are in STEP 3. For each additional dose, you will need two new needles (one 25-gauge needle to withdraw the solution and one 27-gauge needle for injection) and one new empty syringe (1 mL). **NEVER REUSE A SYRINGE OR NEEDLE.**

If you are using the vial of ENBREL® for more than one dose, you should write the date you mixed the powder and liquid in the area marked "Mixing Date:" on the sticker supplied with these instructions, and attach the sticker to the ENBREL® vial.

After you have withdrawn the dose of ENBREL® that you need, store the ENBREL® vial (in the dose tray) in the refrigerator at 36° to 46°F (2° to 8°C) as soon as possible, but always within 4 hours of mixing the solution.

The ENBREL® solution must be used within 14 days of the mixing date. You should discard the ENBREL® vial and any remaining solution if it is not used within 14 days. Do not mix any remaining liquid in one vial of ENBREL® solution with another.

STEP 2A: Vial Adapter Method

1. Remove the pink plastic cap from the ENBREL® vial. Do not remove the gray stopper or silver metal ring around the top of the ENBREL® vial.

Plastic Cap

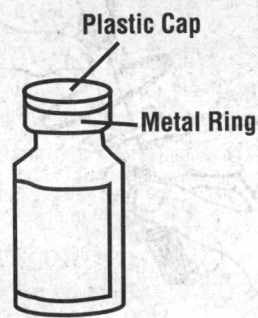

Metal Ring

[See figure at top of next column]

2. Place the ENBREL® vial on your flat work surface or turn your dose tray upside down and place your

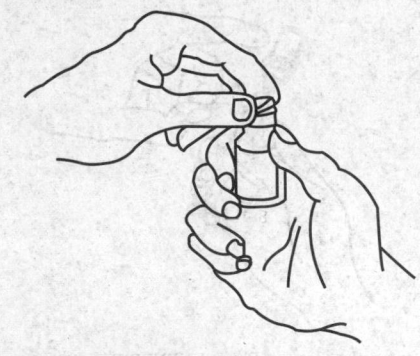

ENBREL® vial in the round space marked "V". Use one alcohol swab to clean the gray stopper on the ENBREL® vial. Do not touch the gray stopper with your hands.

3. Open the wrapper that contains the 27-gauge needle by peeling apart the tabs and set the needle aside for later use.

27-Gauge Needle

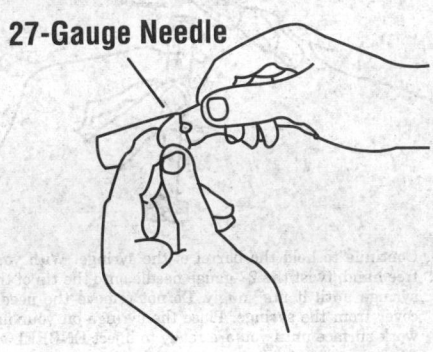

4. Open the wrapper that contains the vial adapter by peeling apart the tabs and set the vial adapter aside for later use. Do not touch the vial adapter's twist-on end or the spike inside.

Vial Adapter

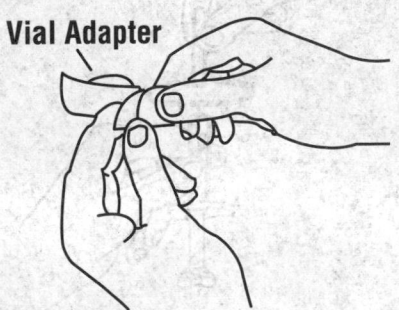

5. Slide the plunger into the flange end of the syringe.

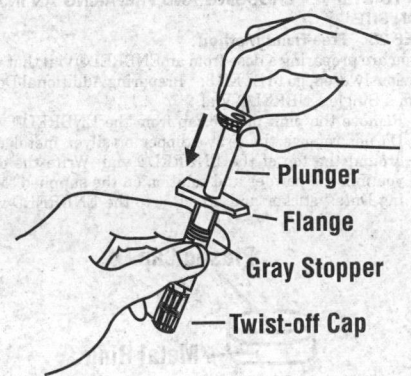

— **Plunger**
— **Flange**
— **Gray Stopper**
— **Twist-off Cap**

6. Attach the plunger to the gray rubber stopper in the syringe by turning the plunger clockwise until a slight resistance is felt.

[See figure at top of next column]

7. Remove the twist-off cap from the prefilled diluent syringe by turning counter-clockwise. Do not bump or touch the plunger. Doing so could cause the liquid to leak out. You may see a drop of liquid when removing

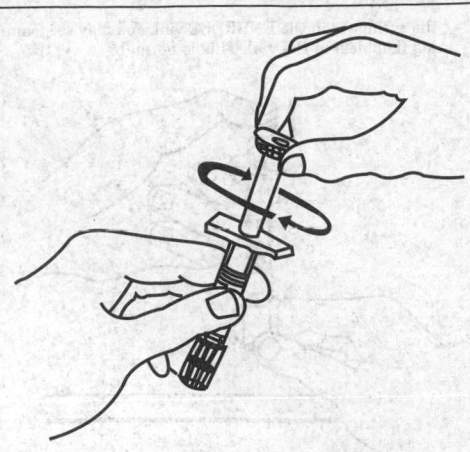

the cap. This is normal. Place the cap on your flat work surface. Do not touch the syringe tip.

Twist-off Cap

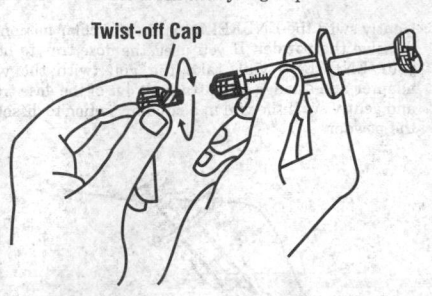

8. Once the twist-off cap is removed, pick up the vial adapter with your free hand. Twist the vial adapter onto the syringe until a slight resistance is felt. Do not over-tighten.

Vial Adapter

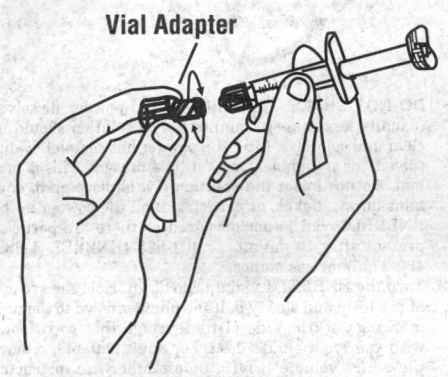

9. Hold the ENBREL® vial upright on your flat work surface. Grasp the sides of the vial adapter and place it over the top of the ENBREL® vial. Do not bump or touch the plunger. Doing so could cause the liquid to leak out. Insert the vial adapter into the gray stopper on the ENBREL® vial. The plastic spike inside the vial adapter should puncture the gray stopper. The vial adapter should fit snugly.

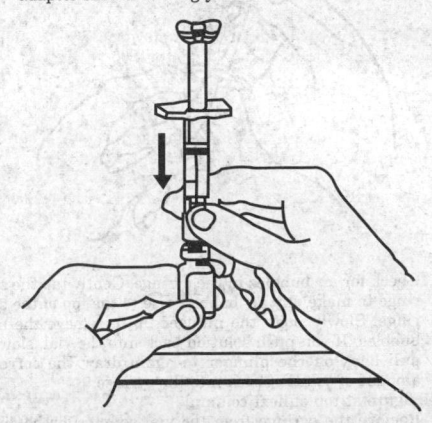

10. Hold the ENBREL® vial upright on your flat work surface and push the plunger down until all the liquid from

the syringe is in the ENBREL® vial. You may see foaming (bubbles) in the vial. This is normal.

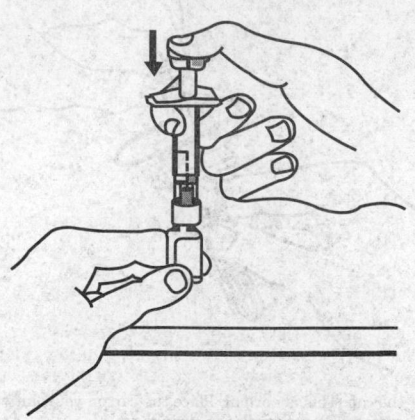

11. Gently swirl the ENBREL® vial in a circular motion to dissolve the powder. If you used the dose tray to hold your ENBREL® vial, take the vial (with the vial adapter and syringe still attached) out of the dose tray, and gently swirl the vial in a circular motion to dissolve the powder.

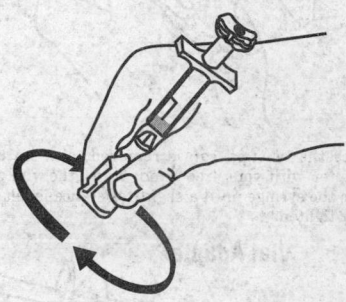

DO NOT SHAKE. Wait until all the powder dissolves (usually less than 10 minutes). The solution should be clear and colorless. After the powder has completely dissolved, foam (bubbles) may still be present. This is normal. **Do not inject the solution if it is discolored, contains lumps, flakes, or particles.** If all the powder in the ENBREL® vial is not dissolved or there are particles present after 10 minutes, call 1-888-4ENBREL (1-888-436-2735) for assistance.

12. Turn the ENBREL® vial upside down. Hold the syringe at eye level and slowly pull the plunger down to the unit markings on the side of the syringe that correspond with your/your child's dose. For adult patients, remove the entire volume (1 mL), unless otherwise instructed by your doctor. Be careful not to pull the plunger completely out of the syringe. Some white foam may remain in the ENBREL® vial. This is normal.

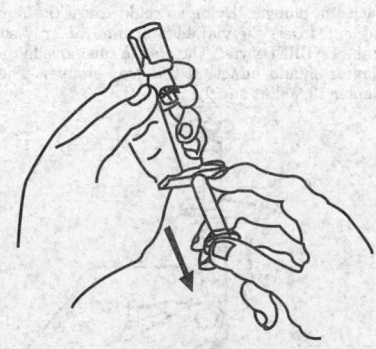

13. Check for air bubbles in the syringe. Gently tap the syringe to make any air bubbles rise to the top of the syringe. Slowly push the plunger up to remove the air bubbles. If you push solution back into the vial, slowly pull back on the plunger to again draw the correct amount of solution back into the syringe.

[See figure at top of next column]

14. Remove the syringe from the vial adapter, by holding the vial adapter with one hand and turning the syringe counterclockwise with your other hand. Do not touch or

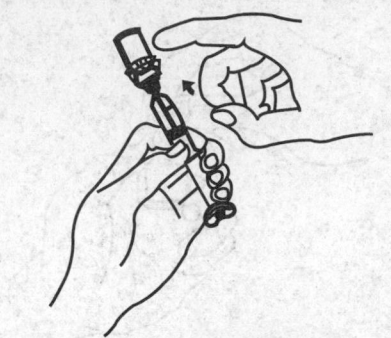

bump the plunger. Place the ENBREL® vial with the vial adapter on your flat work surface.

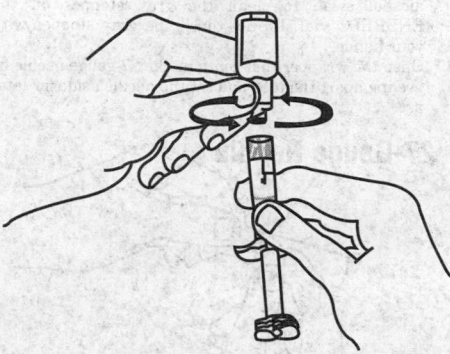

15. Continue to hold the barrel of the syringe. With your free hand, twist the 27-gauge needle onto the tip of the syringe until it fits snugly. Do not remove the needle cover from the syringe. Place the syringe on your flat work surface until you are ready to inject ENBREL®.

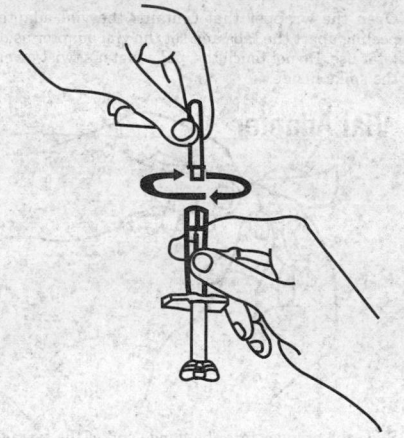

GO TO STEP 4: CHOOSING AND PREPARING AN INJECTION SITE.

STEP 2B: Free-Hand Method

If you are preparing a dose from an ENBREL® vial that was previously used, go to STEP 3: Preparing Additional Doses from a Single ENBREL® Vial.

1. Remove the pink plastic cap from the ENBREL® vial. Do not remove the gray stopper or silver metal ring around the top of the ENBREL® vial. Write the date you mix the powder and solution on the supplied "Mixing Date:" sticker and attach it to the ENBREL® vial.

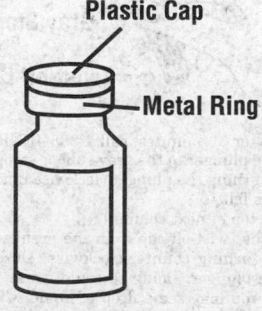

Plastic Cap

Metal Ring

2. Place the ENBREL® vial on your flat work surface. Use one alcohol swab to clean the gray stopper on the ENBREL® vial. Do not touch the gray stopper with your hands.

3. Open the wrapper that contains the 25-gauge needle by peeling apart the tabs and set the needle aside for later use. The 25-gauge needle will be used to mix the liquid with the powder and for withdrawing ENBREL® from the vial.

25-Gauge Needle

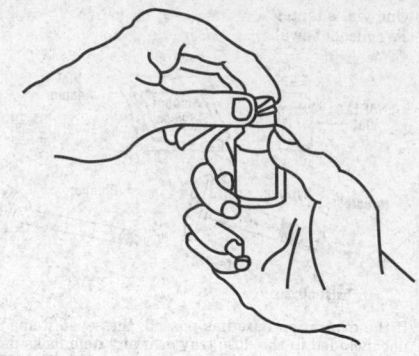

4. Slide the plunger into the flange end of the syringe.

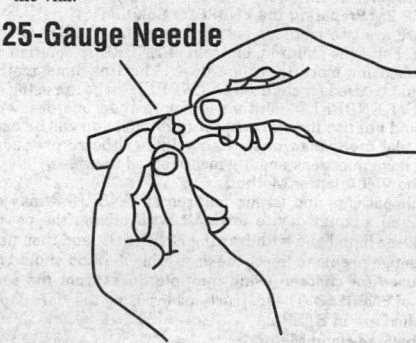

Plunger

Flange

Gray Stopper

Twist-off Cap

5. Attach the plunger to the gray rubber stopper in the syringe by turning the plunger clockwise until a slight resistance is felt.

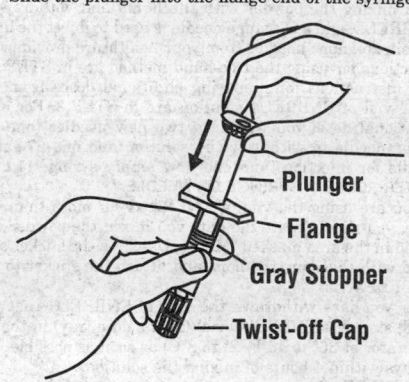

6. Remove the twist-off cap from the prefilled diluent syringe by turning counter-clockwise. Do not touch or bump the plunger. Doing so could cause the liquid to

leak out. You may see a drop of liquid when removing the cap. This is normal. Place the cap on your flat work surface. Do not touch the syringe tip.

Twist-off Cap

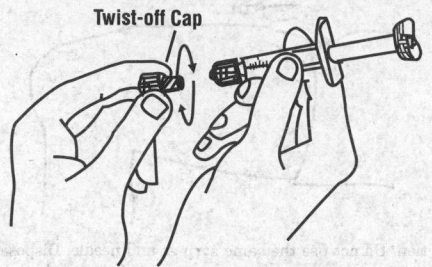

7. Continue to hold the barrel of the syringe. With your free hand, twist the 25-gauge needle onto the tip of the syringe until it fits snugly. Place the syringe on your flat work surface.

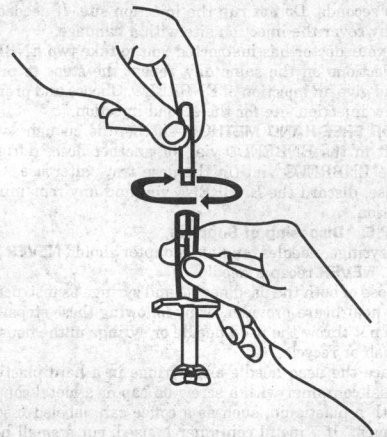

8. Open the wrapper that contains the 27-gauge needle by peeling apart the tabs and set the needle aside for later use. The 27-gauge needle will be used to inject the dose.

27-Gauge Needle

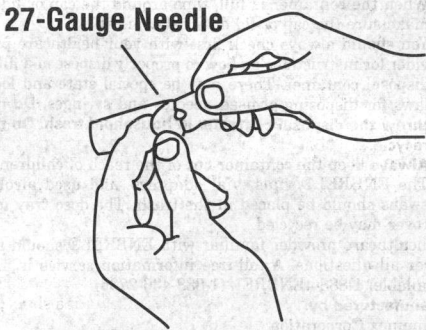

9. Pick up the syringe from your flat work surface. Hold the barrel of the syringe with one hand, and pull the needle cover straight off. Do not touch the needle or allow it to touch any surface. Do not touch or bump the plunger. Doing so could cause the liquid to leak out.

Pull Straight Off

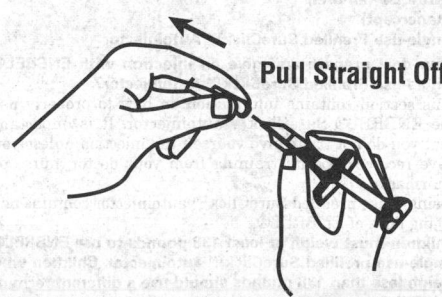

10. Place the needle cover (open side up) in the round space marked "N" in the ENBREL® dose tray.

Needle Cover

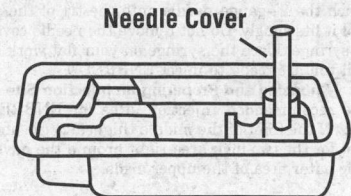

11. Place the ENBREL® vial on your flat work surface. Hold the syringe with the needle facing up, and gently pull back on the plunger to pull a small amount of air into the syringe. Then, insert the needle straight down through the center ring of the gray stopper (see illustrations). You should feel a slight resistance and then a "pop" as the needle goes through the center of the stopper. Look for the needle tip inside the open stopper window. If the needle is not correctly lined up with the center of the stopper, you will feel constant resistance as it goes through the stopper and no "pop". The needle may enter at an angle and bend, break or prevent you from adding diluent into the ENBREL® vial.

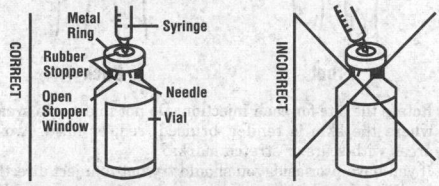

12. Push the plunger down VERY SLOWLY until all liquid from the syringe is in the ENBREL® vial. Adding the liquid too fast will cause foaming (bubbles).

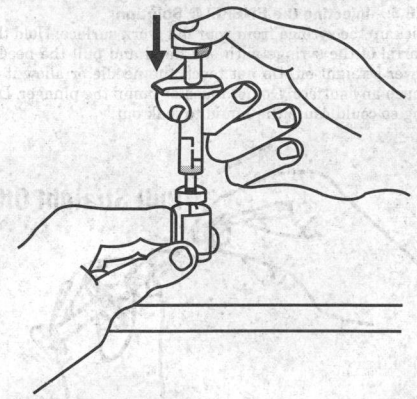

13. Leave the syringe in place. Gently swirl the ENBREL® vial in a circular motion to dissolve the powder.

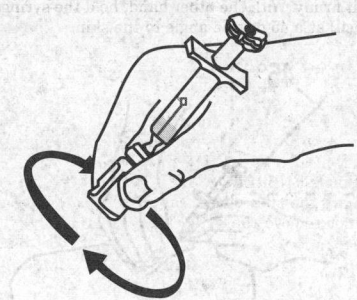

DO NOT SHAKE. Wait until all the powder dissolves (usually less than 10 minutes). The solution should be clear and colorless. After the powder has completely dissolved, foam (bubbles) may still be present. This is normal. **Do not inject the solution if it is discolored, contains lumps, flakes, or particles.** If all the powder in the ENBREL® vial is not dissolved or there are particles present after 10 minutes, call 1-888-4ENBREL (1-888-436-2735) for assistance.

14. With the needle in the ENBREL® vial, turn the vial upside down. Hold the syringe at eye level and slowly pull the plunger down to the unit markings on the side of the syringe that correspond with the correct dose. Make sure to keep the tip of the needle in the solution. Some white foam may remain in the ENBREL® vial. This is normal.

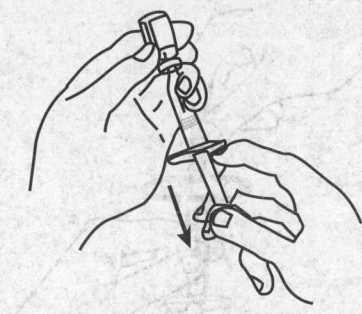

15. With the needle still inserted in the ENBREL® vial, check for air bubbles in the syringe. Gently tap the syringe to make any air bubbles rise to the top of the syringe. Slowly push the plunger up to remove the air bubbles. If you push solution back into the vial, slowly pull back on the plunger to draw the correct amount of solution back into the syringe.

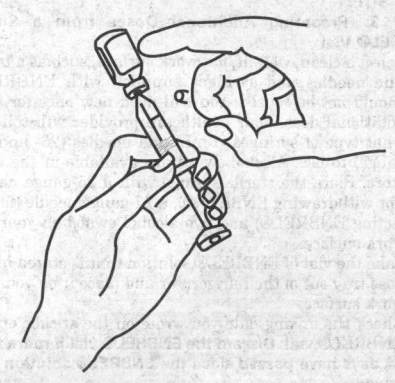

16. Remove the syringe and needle from the ENBREL® vial. Keep the needle attached to the syringe and insert the 25-gauge needle straight down into the needle cover in the ENBREL® dose tray.

Needle Cover

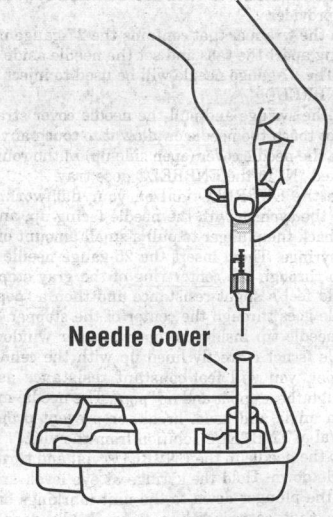

You should hear a "snap" when the needle is secure in the needle cover. Once the needle is secure in the needle cover, untwist the 25-gauge needle from the syringe and dispose of the needle in your SHARPS container.

17. Twist the 27-gauge needle onto the syringe until it fits snugly. Do not remove the needle cover from the syringe. Place the syringe on your flat work surface until you are ready to inject ENBREL®.

[See figure at top of next column]

18. If there is enough solution left in the ENBREL® vial for another dose, write the date you mixed the powder and liquid in the area marked "Mixing Date:" on the sticker supplied with these instructions, and attach the sticker to the ENBREL® vial. Refrigerate the ENBREL® vial (in the dose tray) after use. Prepare additional doses from the ENBREL® vial as described in STEP 3. Otherwise, discard the ENBREL® vial and any remaining solution.

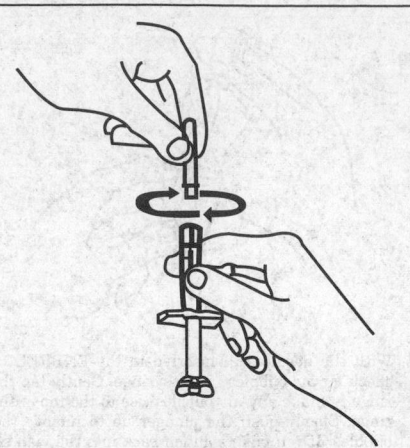

GO TO STEP 4: CHOOSING AND PREPARING AN INJECTION SITE.

STEP 3: Preparing Additional Doses from a Single ENBREL® Vial

1. Select a clean, well-lit, flat work surface, such as a table.
2. The needles and syringes supplied with ENBREL® should not be reused. You will need new ones for each additional dose. Your healthcare provider will tell you what type of syringes (1 mL) and needles (25- and 27-gauge) to use. Alcohol swabs are available at the drug store. Place the sterile syringe with a 25-gauge needle (for withdrawing ENBREL®), a 27-gauge needle (for injecting ENBREL®) and two alcohol swabs on your flat work surface.
3. Take the vial of ENBREL® solution that is stored in the dose tray out of the refrigerator and place it on your flat work surface.
4. Check the mixing date you wrote on the sticker on the ENBREL® vial. **Discard the ENBREL® vial if more than 14 days have passed since the ENBREL® solution was mixed.**
5. Wash your hands with soap and warm water.
6. Use one alcohol swab to clean the gray stopper on the ENBREL® vial. Do not touch the stopper with your hands.
7. If the syringe and the 25-gauge needle are not pre-assembled, assemble them as instructed by your health-care provider.
8. Open the wrapper that contains the 27-gauge needle by peeling apart the tabs and set the needle aside for later use. The 27-gauge needle will be used to inject the dose of ENBREL®.
9. Hold the syringe and pull the needle cover straight off. Do not touch the needle or allow it to touch any surface. Place the needle cover (open side up) in the round space marked "N" in the ENBREL® dose tray.
10. Place the ENBREL® vial on your flat work surface. Hold the syringe with the needle facing up, and gently pull back the plunger to pull a small amount of air into the syringe. Then, insert the 25-gauge needle straight down through the center ring of the gray stopper. You should feel a slight resistance and then a "pop" as the needle goes through the center of the stopper. Look for the needle tip inside the open stopper window. If the needle is not correctly lined up with the center of the stopper, you will feel constant resistance as it goes through the stopper and no "pop". The needle may enter at an angle and bend, break, or prevent proper withdrawal of ENBREL® solution from the vial.
11. Keep the needle in the ENBREL® vial and turn the vial upside down. Hold the syringe at eye level, and slowly pull the plunger down to the unit markings on the syringe that correspond to your child's dose. As the amount of solution in the ENBREL® vial drops, you may need to pull the needle back just enough to keep the tip of the needle in the solution.
12. With the needle still inserted in the ENBREL® vial, check for air bubbles in the syringe. Gently tap the syringe to make any air bubbles rise to the top of the syringe. Slowly push the plunger up to remove the air bubbles. If you push solution back into the ENBREL® vial, slowly pull back on the plunger to again draw the correct amount of solution back into the syringe.
13. Remove the syringe and needle from the ENBREL® vial. Keep the needle attached to the syringe and insert the 25-gauge needle straight down into the needle cover in the ENBREL® dose tray. You should hear a "snap" when the needle is secure in the needle cover. Once the needle is secure in the needle cover, remove the 25-gauge needle from the syringe and dispose of the needle in a puncture-resistant container.

14. Attach the 27-gauge needle onto the tip of the syringe until it fits snugly. Do not remove the needle cover from the syringe. Place the syringe on your flat work surface until you are ready to inject ENBREL®.

STEP 4: Choosing and Preparing an Injection Site

1. Three recommended injection sites for ENBREL® include: (1) the front of the middle thighs; (2) the abdomen, except for the two-inch area right around the navel; and, (3) the outer area of the upper arms.

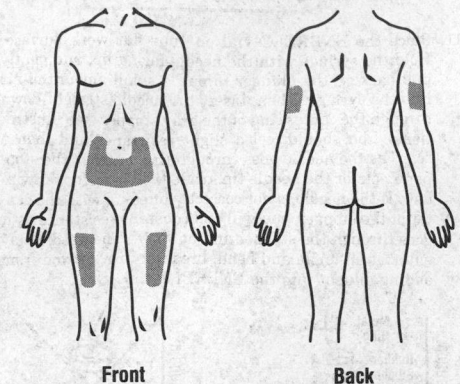

Front   **Back**

2. Rotate the site for each injection. Do not inject into areas where the skin is tender, bruised, red, or hard. Avoid areas with scars or stretch marks.
3. If you have psoriasis, you should try not to inject directly into any raised, thick, red, or scaly skin patches or lesions.
4. To prepare the area of skin where ENBREL® is to be injected, wipe the injection site with a new alcohol swab. **Do not touch this area again before giving the injection.**

STEP 5: Injecting the ENBREL® Solution

1. Pick up the syringe from your flat work surface. Hold the barrel of the syringe with one hand and pull the needle cover straight off. Do not touch the needle or allow it to touch any surface. Do not touch or bump the plunger. Doing so could cause the liquid to leak out.

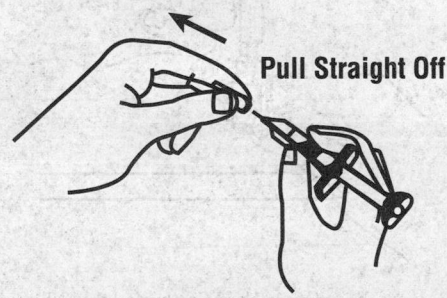

Pull Straight Off

2. With one hand, gently pinch the cleaned area of skin and hold it firmly. With the other hand, hold the syringe (like a pencil) at a 45-degree angle to the skin.

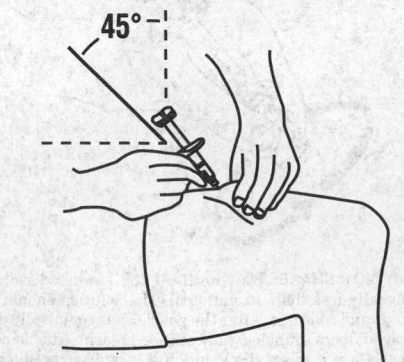

45°

3. With a quick, "dart-like" motion, push the needle into the skin.
4. After the needle is inserted, let go of the skin. Pull the plunger back slightly. If no blood appears in the syringe, slowly push the plunger all the way down to inject ENBREL®.
[See figure at top of next column]
    If blood comes into the syringe, do not inject ENBREL® because the needle has entered a blood vessel. Withdraw the needle and repeat the steps to prepare for an injec-

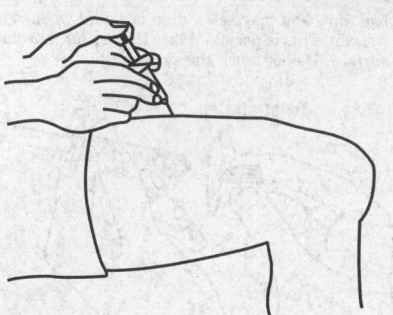

tion. Do not use the same syringe and needle. Dispose of the used needle and syringe in a puncture-resistant container.
5. When the syringe is empty, pull the needle out of the skin, being careful to keep it at the same angle as inserted.
6. There may be a little bleeding at the injection site. You can press a cotton ball or gauze over the injection site for 10 seconds. Do not rub the injection site. If needed, you may cover the injection site with a bandage.
7. If your doctor has instructed you to take two ENBREL® injections on the same day, repeat the steps to prepare and give an injection of ENBREL®. Choose and prepare a new injection site for the second injection.
8. **FOR FREE-HAND METHOD**—If there is enough solution left in the ENBREL® vial for another dose, refrigerate the ENBREL® vial (in the dose tray) after use. Otherwise, discard the ENBREL® vial and any remaining solution.

STEP 6: Disposing of Supplies

The syringe, needles, and vial adapter should **NEVER** be reused. **NEVER** recap a needle.
Dispose of both the used needle and syringe as instructed by your healthcare provider, or by following these steps:
- Do not throw the used needle or syringe in the household trash or recycle.
- Place the used needle and syringe in a hard plastic disposal container with a screw-on cap or a metal container with a plastic lid, such as a coffee can, labeled "used syringes." If a metal container is used, cut a small hole in the plastic lid and tape the lid to the metal container. If a hard plastic container is used, always screw the cap on tightly after each use. Do not use glass or clear plastic containers. Puncture-resistant containers may also be purchased at your local pharmacy.
- When the container is full, tape around the cap or lid to make sure the cap or lid does not come off.
- You should always check first with your healthcare provider for instructions on how to properly dispose of a filled disposal container. There may be special state and local laws for disposing of used needles and syringes. **Do not throw the disposal container in household trash. Do not recycle.**
- **Always** keep the container out of the reach of children.
- The ENBREL® vials, vial adapters, and used alcohol swabs should be placed in the trash. The dose tray and cover may be recycled.

A healthcare provider familiar with ENBREL® should answer all questions. A toll-free information service is also available: 1-888-4ENBREL (1-888-436-2735).

Manufactured by:
Immunex Corporation,
Thousand Oaks, CA 91320-1799
Marketed by Amgen Inc. and Wyeth Pharmaceuticals
©1998–2008 Immunex Corporation. All rights reserved.
1XXXXXX – v1
Issue Date: 06/2008

Patient Instructions for Use
ENBREL® (en-brel)
(etanercept)
Single-use Prefilled SureClick™ Autoinjector

How do I prepare and give an injection with ENBREL® Single-use Prefilled SureClick™ Autoinjector?
This section contains information on how to properly use the ENBREL® SureClick™ autoinjector. It is important that you do not try to give yourself the injection unless you have received special training from your doctor, nurse or pharmacist.
A single-use prefilled SureClick™ autoinjector contains one 50 mg dose of ENBREL®.
Children must weigh at least 138 pounds to use ENBREL® single-use prefilled SureClick™ autoinjector. Children who weigh less than 138 pounds should use a different form of ENBREL®.
IMPORTANT: The needle cap on the single-use prefilled SureClick™ autoinjector contains latex. Tell your doctor if you are allergic to latex.

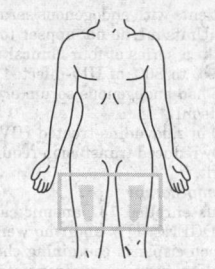

The **front of the thigh** is the preferred injection site.

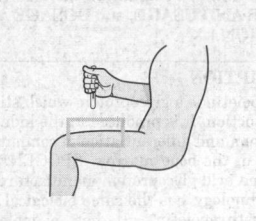

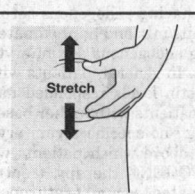

Stretch technique

Make sure the skin under and around the prefilled autoinjector is firm and taut to provide enough resistance to fully retract the safety guard and unlock the prefilled autoinjector.

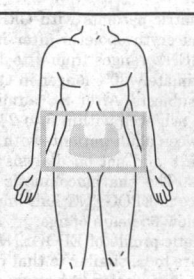

You can use the **abdomen**, except for the two-inch area right around the navel. Stretch the skin at the injection site to create a firm and taut surface.

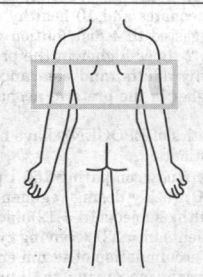

If someone else is giving you the injection, they can also use the **outer area of the upper arms**. For the upper arms, it is recommended to stretch the skin at the injection site to create a firm and taut surface.

Equipment
- A new ENBREL® SureClick™ autoinjector, and
- Alcohol wipes or similar
- Cotton ball or gauze
- Puncture resistant disposable container

Preparing for an ENBREL® Injection
- Find a comfortable, well-lit, clean surface and put all the equipment you need within reach.
- Remove one single-use prefilled ENBREL® SureClick™ autoinjector from the carton. Do not shake the autoinjector. Place the carton containing any remaining autoinjectors back into the refrigerator (2° to 8°C [36° to 46°F]). **Do not freeze.** If you have any questions about storage, contact your doctor, nurse, or pharmacist for further instructions.
- Check the expiration date on the autoinjector label. Do not use if the date has passed the last day of the month shown.
- Make sure the solution in the autoinjector is clear and colorless by looking through the inspection window. You may notice small white particles in solution. These particles are formed from ENBREL® and this is acceptable. However, **do not inject the solution if it is cloudy or discolored, or contains large or colored particles**—contact your pharmacist or call 1-888-4ENBREL (1-888-436-2735) for assistance.
- For a more comfortable injection, wait 15 to 30 minutes to allow the autoinjector to reach room temperature. **Do not** remove the white needle cap while allowing it to reach room temperature. Do not warm ENBREL® in any other way (for example, do not warm it in a microwave or in hot water).
- Wash your hands thoroughly.

- **Do not** remove the white needle cap from the autoinjector until you are ready to inject.

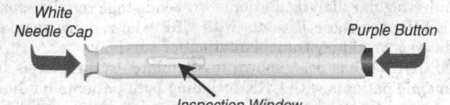

White Needle Cap · Purple Button · Inspection Window

Choosing and Preparing an Injection Site
Choose an Injection Site
The injection site must be firm for the autoinjector to work properly. The preferred injection site for ENBREL® using a prefilled SureClick™ autoinjector is the front of the thigh.
- **Rotate Injection Location**
  Rotate the site for each injection. Do not inject into areas where the skin is tender, bruised, red, or hard. Avoid areas with stretch marks.
- **Patients with Psoriasis**
  If you have psoriasis, you should try not to inject directly into any raised, thick, red, or scaly skin patches or lesions.

Instructions for Preferred Injection Site
[See first table above]

Instructions for Alternate Injection sites
When using alternate injection sites, it is particularly important to create enough firmness on the site to be able to successfully complete the injection.

[See second table above]

[See third table above]

Prepare the site
To prepare the area of skin where ENBREL® is to be injected, wipe the injection site with an alcohol swab. **Do not touch this area again before giving the injection.**

Injecting ENBREL® Using a Single-use Prefilled SureClick™ Autoinjector
1. Pull off the white needle cap.

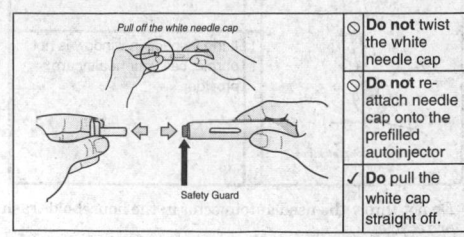

⊘	**Do not** twist the white needle cap
⊘	**Do not** re-attach needle cap onto the prefilled autoinjector
✓	**Do** pull the white cap straight off.

2. Do not touch the purple button. Press prefilled autoinjector onto skin to unlock safety guard.

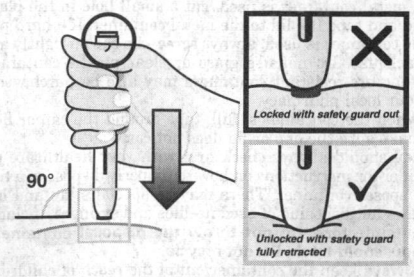

Locked with safety guard out

Unlocked with safety guard fully retracted

⊘	**Do not** press the purple button until the safety guard is fully retracted.
✓	**Do** keep enough downward pressure to fully retract the purple safety guard and to keep the purple button unlocked.
✓	**Do** hold the prefilled autoinjector at a right angle (90°) at the injection site.

3. Briefly press and release purple button.

release button

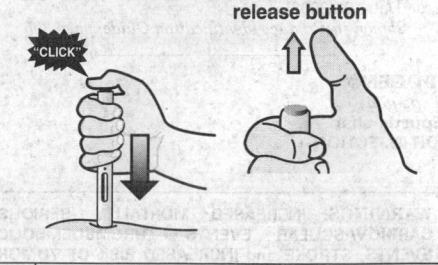

"CLICK"

✓	**Do** maintain pressure on the skin during the injection

4. Count slowly to 15 seconds for injection to end.

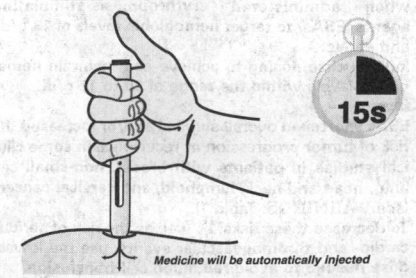

15s

Medicine will be automatically injected

⊘	**Do not** move the prefilled autoinjector during the injection.
✓	**Do** wait for the injection to finish before releasing pressure.
✓	You might hear a second click as the purple button pops back up.

After the Injection
- Check window to confirm delivery of full dose.
- There may be a little bleeding at the injection site. You can press a cotton ball or gauze over the injection site.
- Do not rub the injection site. If needed, you may cover the injection site with a bandage.

[See figure at top of next column]

Remember
If you have any problems, please call 1-888-4ENBREL (1-888-436-2735) for assistance.

Disposing of Supplies
The SureClick™ autoinjector should **NEVER** be reused. Dispose of the used autoinjector as instructed by your healthcare provider, or by following these steps:

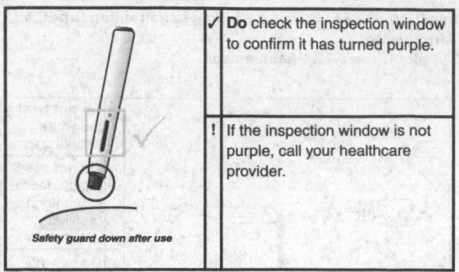

✓	**Do** check the inspection window to confirm it has turned purple.
!	If the inspection window is not purple, call your healthcare provider.

Safety guard down after use

- Do not throw the used autoinjector in the household trash or recycle.
- Place the used autoinjector in a hard plastic disposal container with a screw-on cap or a metal container with a plastic lid, such as a coffee can, labeled "used syringes." If a metal container is used, cut a small hole in the plastic lid and tape the lid to the metal container. If a hard plastic container is used, always screw the cap on tightly after each use. Do not use glass or clear plastic containers. Puncture-resistant containers may also be purchased at your local pharmacy.
- When the container is full, tape around the cap or lid to make sure the cap or lid does not come off.
- You should always check first with your healthcare provider for instructions on how to properly dispose of a filled disposal container. There may be special state and local laws for disposing of used needles and syringes, including autoinjectors. **Do not throw the disposal container in household trash. Do not recycle.**
- **Always** keep the container out of the reach of children.

A healthcare provider familiar with ENBREL® should answer all questions. A toll-free information service is also available: 1-888-4ENBREL (1-888-436-2735).

Manufactured by:
Immunex Corporation,
Thousand Oaks, CA 91320-1799
Marketed by Amgen Inc. and Wyeth Pharmaceuticals
©1998-2008 Immunex Corporation. All rights reserved.
1XXXXXX- v1
Issue Date: 06/2008
Shown in Product Identification Guide, page 305

EPOGEN®
[ĕ' pə-gĕn]
(Epoetin alfa)
FOR INJECTION

℞

WARNINGS: INCREASED MORTALITY, SERIOUS CARDIOVASCULAR EVENTS, THROMBOEMBOLIC EVENTS, STROKE and INCREASED RISK OF TUMOR PROGRESSION OR RECURRENCE

Chronic Renal Failure:
- **In clinical studies, patients experienced greater risks for death, serious cardiovascular events, and stroke when administered erythropoiesis-stimulating agents (ESAs) to target hemoglobin levels of 13 g/dL and above.**
- **Individualize dosing to achieve and maintain hemoglobin levels within the range of 10 to 12 g/dL.**

Cancer:
- **ESAs shortened overall survival and/or increased the risk of tumor progression or recurrence in some clinical studies in patients with breast, non-small cell lung, head and neck, lymphoid, and cervical cancers (see WARNINGS: Table 1).**
- **To decrease these risks, as well as the risk of serious cardio- and thrombovascular events, use the lowest dose needed to avoid red blood cell transfusion.**
- **Because of these risks, prescribers and hospitals must enroll in and comply with the ESA APPRISE Oncology Program to prescribe and/or dispense EPOGEN® to patients with cancer. To enroll in the ESA APPRISE Oncology Program, visit www.esa-apprise.com or call 1-866-284-8089 for further assistance.**
- **Use ESAs only for treatment of anemia due to concomitant myelosuppressive chemotherapy.**
- **ESAs are not indicated for patients receiving myelosuppressive therapy when the anticipated outcome is cure.**
- **Discontinue following the completion of a chemotherapy course.**

Perisurgery: **EPOGEN® increased the rate of deep venous thromboses in patients not receiving prophylactic anticoagulation. Consider deep venous thrombosis prophylaxis.**

(See WARNINGS: Increased Mortality, Serious Cardiovascular Events, Thromboembolic Events and Stroke, WARNINGS: Increased Mortality and/or Increased

Risk of Tumor Progression or Recurrence, **INDICATIONS AND USAGE, and DOSAGE AND ADMINISTRATION.)**

DESCRIPTION

Erythropoietin is a glycoprotein which stimulates red blood cell production. It is produced in the kidney and stimulates the division and differentiation of committed erythroid progenitors in the bone marrow. EPOGEN® (Epoetin alfa), a 165 amino acid glycoprotein manufactured by recombinant DNA technology, has the same biological effects as endogenous erythropoietin.[1] It has a molecular weight of 30,400 daltons and is produced by mammalian cells into which the human erythropoietin gene has been introduced. The product contains the identical amino acid sequence of isolated natural erythropoietin.

EPOGEN® is formulated as a sterile, colorless liquid in an isotonic sodium chloride/sodium citrate buffered solution or a sodium chloride/sodium phosphate buffered solution for intravenous (IV) or subcutaneous (SC) administration.

Single-dose, Preservative-free Vial: Each 1 mL of solution contains 2000, 3000, 4000 or 10,000 Units of Epoetin alfa, 2.5 mg Albumin (Human), 5.8 mg sodium citrate, 5.8 mg sodium chloride, and 0.06 mg citric acid in Water for Injection, USP (pH 6.9 ± 0.3). This formulation contains no preservative.

Single-dose, Preservative-free Vial: 1 mL (40,000 Units/mL). Each 1 mL of solution contains 40,000 Units of Epoetin alfa, 2.5 mg Albumin (Human), 1.2 mg sodium phosphate monobasic monohydrate, 1.8 mg sodium phosphate dibasic anhydrate, 0.7 mg sodium citrate, 5.8 mg sodium chloride, and 6.8 mcg citric acid in Water for Injection, USP (pH 6.9 ± 0.3). This formulation contains no preservative.

Multidose, Preserved Vial: 2 mL (20,000 Units, 10,000 Units/mL). Each 1 mL of solution contains 10,000 Units of Epoetin alfa, 2.5 mg Albumin (Human), 1.3 mg sodium citrate, 8.2 mg sodium chloride, 0.11 mg citric acid, and 1% benzyl alcohol as preservative in Water for Injection, USP (pH 6.1 ± 0.3).

Multidose, Preserved Vial: 1 mL (20,000 Units/mL). Each 1 mL of solution contains 20,000 Units of Epoetin alfa, 2.5 mg Albumin (Human), 1.3 mg sodium citrate, 8.2 mg sodium chloride, 0.11 mg citric acid, and 1% benzyl alcohol as preservative in Water for Injection, USP (pH 6.1 ± 0.3).

CLINICAL PHARMACOLOGY
Chronic Renal Failure Patients

Endogenous production of erythropoietin is normally regulated by the level of tissue oxygenation. Hypoxia and anemia generally increase the production of erythropoietin, which in turn stimulates erythropoiesis.[2] In normal subjects, plasma erythropoietin levels range from 0.01 to 0.03 Units/mL and increase up to 100- to 1000-fold during hypoxia or anemia.[2] In contrast, in patients with chronic renal failure (CRF), production of erythropoietin is impaired, and this erythropoietin deficiency is the primary cause of their anemia.[3,4]

Chronic renal failure is the clinical situation in which there is a progressive and usually irreversible decline in kidney function. Such patients may manifest the sequelae of renal dysfunction, including anemia, but do not necessarily require regular dialysis. Patients with end-stage renal disease (ESRD) are those patients with CRF who require regular dialysis or kidney transplantation for survival.

EPOGEN® has been shown to stimulate erythropoiesis in anemic patients with CRF, including both patients on dialysis and those who do not require regular dialysis.[4-12] The first evidence of a response to the three times weekly (TIW) administration of EPOGEN® is an increase in the reticulocyte count within 10 days, followed by increases in the red cell count, hemoglobin, and hematocrit, usually within 2 to 6 weeks.[4,5] Because of the length of time required for erythropoiesis — several days for erythroid progenitors to mature and be released into the circulation — a clinically significant increase in hematocrit is usually not observed in less than 2 weeks and may require up to 6 weeks in some patients. Once the hematocrit reaches the suggested target range (30% to 36%), that level can be sustained by EPOGEN® therapy in the absence of iron deficiency and concurrent illnesses.

The rate of hematocrit increase varies between patients and is dependent upon the dose of EPOGEN®, within a therapeutic range of approximately 50 to 300 Units/kg TIW.[4] A greater biologic response is not observed at doses exceeding 300 Units/kg TIW.[6] Other factors affecting the rate and extent of response include availability of iron stores, the baseline hematocrit, and the presence of concurrent medical problems.

Zidovudine-treated HIV-infected Patients

Responsiveness to EPOGEN® in HIV-infected patients is dependent upon the endogenous serum erythropoietin level prior to treatment. Patients with endogenous serum erythropoietin levels ≤ 500 mUnits/mL, and who are receiving a dose of zidovudine ≤ 4200 mg/week, may respond to

EPOGEN® therapy. Patients with endogenous serum erythropoietin levels > 500 mUnits/mL do not appear to respond to EPOGEN® therapy. In a series of four clinical trials involving 255 patients, 60% to 80% of HIV-infected patients treated with zidovudine had endogenous serum erythropoietin levels ≤ 500 mUnits/mL.

Response to EPOGEN® in zidovudine-treated HIV-infected patients is manifested by reduced transfusion requirements and increased hematocrit.

Cancer Patients on Chemotherapy

A series of clinical trials enrolled 131 anemic cancer patients who received EPOGEN® TIW and who were receiving cyclic cisplatin- or non cisplatin-containing chemotherapy. Endogenous baseline serum erythropoietin levels varied among patients in these trials with approximately 75% (n = 83/110) having endogenous serum erythropoietin levels ≤ 132 mUnits/mL, and approximately 4% (n = 4/110) of patients having endogenous serum erythropoietin levels > 500 mUnits/mL. In general, patients with lower baseline serum erythropoietin levels responded more vigorously to EPOGEN® than patients with higher baseline erythropoietin levels. Although no specific serum erythropoietin level can be stipulated above which patients would be unlikely to respond to EPOGEN® therapy, treatment of patients with grossly elevated serum erythropoietin levels (eg, > 200 mUnits/mL) is not recommended.

Pharmacokinetics

In adult and pediatric patients with CRF, the elimination half-life of plasma erythropoietin after intravenously administered EPOGEN® ranges from 4 to 13 hours.[13-15] The half-life is approximately 20% longer in CRF patients than that in healthy subjects. After SC administration, peak plasma levels are achieved within 5 to 24 hours. The half-life is similar between adult patients with serum creatinine level greater than 3 and not on dialysis and those maintained on dialysis. The pharmacokinetic data indicate no apparent difference in EPOGEN® half-life among adult patients above or below 65 years of age.

The pharmacokinetic profile of EPOGEN® in children and adolescents appears to be similar to that of adults. Limited data are available in neonates.[16] A study of 7 preterm very low birth weight neonates and 10 healthy adults given IV erythropoietin suggested that distribution volume was approximately 1.5 to 2 times higher in the preterm neonates than in the healthy adults, and clearance was approximately 3 times higher in the preterm neonates than in the healthy adults.[39]

The pharmacokinetics of EPOGEN® have not been studied in HIV-infected patients.

A pharmacokinetic study comparing 150 Units/kg SC TIW to 40,000 Units SC weekly dosing regimen was conducted for 4 weeks in healthy subjects (n = 12) and for 6 weeks in anemic cancer patients (n = 32) receiving cyclic chemotherapy. There was no accumulation of serum erythropoietin after the 2 dosing regimens during the study period. The 40,000 Units weekly regimen had a higher C_{max} (3- to 7-fold), longer T_{max} (2- to 3-fold), higher AUC_{0-168h} (2- to 3-fold) of erythropoietin and lower clearance (50%) than the 150 Units/kg TIW regimen. In anemic cancer patients, the average $t_{1/2}$ was similar (40 hours with range of 16 to 67 hours) after both dosing regimens. After the 150 Units/kg TIW dosing, the values of T_{max} and clearance are similar (13.3 ± 12.4 vs. 14.2 ± 6.7 hours, and 20.2 ± 15.9 vs. 23.6 ± 9.5 mL/h/kg) between Week 1 when patients were receiving chemotherapy (n = 14) and Week 3 when patients were not receiving chemotherapy (n = 4). Differences were observed after the 40,000 Units weekly dosing with longer T_{max} (38 ± 18 hours) and lower clearance (9.2 ± 4.7 mL/h/kg) during Week 1 when patients were receiving chemotherapy (n = 18) compared with those (22 ± 4.5 hours, 13.9 ± 7.6 mL/h/kg) during Week 3 when patients were not receiving chemotherapy (n = 7).

The bioequivalence between the 10,000 Units/mL citrate-buffered Epoetin alfa formulation and the 40,000 Units/mL phosphate-buffered Epoetin alfa formulation has been demonstrated after SC administration of single 750 Units/kg doses to healthy subjects.

INDICATIONS AND USAGE
Treatment of Anemia of Chronic Renal Failure Patients

EPOGEN® is indicated for the treatment of anemia associated with CRF, including patients on dialysis and patients not on dialysis. EPOGEN® is indicated to elevate or maintain the red blood cell level (as manifested by the hematocrit or hemoglobin determinations) and to decrease the need for transfusions in these patients.

Non-dialysis patients with symptomatic anemia considered for therapy should have a hemoglobin less than 10 g/dL.

EPOGEN® is not intended for patients who require immediate correction of severe anemia. EPOGEN® may obviate the need for maintenance transfusions but is not a substitute for emergency transfusion.

Prior to initiation of therapy, the patient's iron stores should be evaluated. Transferrin saturation should be at least 20%

and ferritin at least 100 ng/mL. Blood pressure should be adequately controlled prior to initiation of EPOGEN® therapy, and must be closely monitored and controlled during therapy.

Treatment of Anemia in Zidovudine-treated HIV-infected Patients

EPOGEN® is indicated for the treatment of anemia related to therapy with zidovudine in HIV-infected patients. EPOGEN® is indicated to elevate or maintain the red blood cell level (as manifested by the hematocrit or hemoglobin determinations) and to decrease the need for transfusions in these patients. EPOGEN® is not indicated for the treatment of anemia in HIV-infected patients due to other factors such as iron or folate deficiencies, hemolysis, or gastrointestinal bleeding, which should be managed appropriately.

EPOGEN® use has not been demonstrated in controlled clinical trials to improve symptoms of anemia, quality of life, fatigue, or patient well-being.

EPOGEN®, at a dose of 100 Units/kg TIW, is effective in decreasing the transfusion requirement and increasing the red blood cell level of anemic, HIV-infected patients treated with zidovudine, when the endogenous serum erythropoietin level is ≤ 500 mUnits/mL and when patients are receiving a dose of zidovudine ≤ 4200 mg/week.

Treatment of Anemia in Cancer Patients on Chemotherapy

EPOGEN® is indicated for the treatment of anemia due to the effect of concomitantly administered chemotherapy based on studies that have shown a reduction in the need for RBC transfusions in patients with metastatic, non-myeloid malignancies receiving chemotherapy for a minimum of 2 months. Studies to determine whether EPOGEN® increases mortality or decreases progression-free/recurrence-free survival are ongoing.

- EPOGEN® is not indicated for use in patients receiving hormonal agents, therapeutic biologic products, or radiotherapy unless receiving concomitant myelosuppressive chemotherapy.
- EPOGEN® is not indicated for patients receiving myelosuppressive therapy when the anticipated outcome is cure due to the absence of studies that adequately characterize the impact of EPOGEN® on progression-free and overall survival (see WARNINGS: Increased Mortality and/or Increased Risk of Tumor Progression or Recurrence).
- EPOGEN® is not indicated for the treatment of anemia in cancer patients due to other factors such as iron or folate deficiencies, hemolysis, or gastrointestinal bleeding (see PRECAUTIONS: Lack or Loss of Response).
- EPOGEN® use has not been demonstrated in controlled clinical trials to improve symptoms of anemia, quality of life, fatigue, or patient well-being.

Reduction of Allogeneic Blood Transfusion in Surgery Patients

EPOGEN® is indicated for the treatment of anemic patients (hemoglobin > 10 to ≤ 13 g/dL) who are at high risk for perioperative blood loss from elective, noncardiac, nonvascular surgery to reduce the need for allogeneic blood transfusions.[17-19] EPOGEN® is not indicated for anemic patients who are willing to donate autologous blood (see BOXED WARNINGS and DOSAGE AND ADMINISTRATION).

CLINICAL EXPERIENCE: RESPONSE TO EPOGEN®

Chronic Renal Failure Patients

When dosed with EPOGEN®, patients responded with an increase in hematocrit.[5] After 3 months on study, more than 95% of patients were transfusion-independent.

In the presence of adequate iron stores (see IRON EVALUATION), the time to reach the target hematocrit is a function of the baseline hematocrit and the rate of hematocrit rise.

The rate of increase in hematocrit is dependent upon the dose of EPOGEN® administered and individual patient variation. In clinical trials at starting doses of 50 to 150 Units/kg TIW, adult patients responded with an average rate of hematocrit rise of:

Starting Dose (TIW IV)	Hematocrit Increase Points/Day	Points/2 Weeks
50 Units/kg	0.11	1.5
100 Units/kg	0.18	2.5
150 Units/kg	0.25	3.5

In a 26 week, double-blind, placebo-controlled trial, 118 anemic dialysis patients with an average hemoglobin of approximately 7 g/dL were randomized to either EPOGEN® or placebo. By the end of the study, average hemoglobin increased to approximately 11 g/dL in the EPOGEN®-treated patients and remained unchanged in patients receiving placebo. EPOGEN®-treated patients experienced improvements in exercise tolerance and patient-reported physical functioning at month 2 that was maintained throughout the study.

Adult Patients on Dialysis: Thirteen clinical studies were conducted, involving IV administration to a total of 1010 anemic patients on dialysis for 986 patient-years of EPOGEN® therapy. In the three largest of these clinical trials, the median maintenance dose necessary to maintain the hematocrit between 30% to 36% was approximately 75 Units/kg TIW. In the US multicenter phase 3 study, approximately 65% of the patients required doses of 100 Units/kg TIW, or less, to maintain their hematocrit at approximately 35%. Almost 10% of patients required a dose of 25 Units/kg, or less, and approximately 10% required a dose of more than 200 Units/kg TIW to maintain their hematocrit at this level.

A multicenter unit dose study was also conducted in 119 patients receiving peritoneal dialysis who self-administered EPOGEN® subcutaneously for approximately 109 patient-years of experience. Patients responded to EPOGEN® administered SC in a manner similar to patients receiving IV administration.[20]

Pediatric Patients on Dialysis: One hundred twenty-eight children from 2 months to 19 years of age with CRF requiring dialysis were enrolled in 4 clinical studies of EPOGEN®. The largest study was a placebo-controlled, randomized trial in 113 children with anemia (hematocrit ≤ 27%) undergoing peritoneal dialysis or hemodialysis. The initial dose of EPOGEN® was 50 Units/kg IV or SC TIW. The dose of study drug was titrated to achieve either a hematocrit of 30% to 36% or an absolute increase in hematocrit of 6 percentage points over baseline.

At the end of the initial 12 weeks, a statistically significant rise in mean hematocrit (9.4% vs 0.9%) was observed only in the EPOGEN® arm. The proportion of children achieving a hematocrit of 30%, or an increase in hematocrit of 6 percentage points over baseline, at any time during the first 12 weeks was higher in the EPOGEN® arm (96% vs 58%). Within 12 weeks of initiating EPOGEN® therapy, 92.3% of the pediatric patients were transfusion-independent as compared to 65.4% who received placebo. Among patients who received 36 weeks of EPOGEN®, hemodialysis patients required a higher median maintenance dose (167 Units/kg/week [n = 28] vs 76 Units/kg/week [n = 36]) and took longer to achieve a hematocrit of 30% to 36% (median time to response 69 days vs 32 days) than patients undergoing peritoneal dialysis.

Patients With CRF Not Requiring Dialysis

Four clinical trials were conducted in patients with CRF not on dialysis involving 181 patients treated with EPOGEN® for approximately 67 patient-years of experience. These patients responded to EPOGEN® therapy in a manner similar to that observed in patients on dialysis. Patients with CRF not on dialysis demonstrated a dose-dependent and sustained increase in hematocrit when EPOGEN® was administered by either an IV or SC route, with similar rates of rise of hematocrit when EPOGEN® was administered by either route. Moreover, EPOGEN® doses of 75 to 150 Units/kg per week have been shown to maintain hematocrits of 36% to 38% for up to 6 months.[21-22]

Zidovudine-treated HIV-infected Patients

Efficacy in HIV-infected patients with anemia related to therapy with zidovudine was demonstrated based on reduction in the requirement for RBC transfusions.

EPOGEN® has been studied in four placebo-controlled trials enrolling 297 anemic (hematocrit < 30%) HIV-infected (AIDS) patients receiving concomitant therapy with zidovudine (all patients were treated with Epoetin alfa manufactured by Amgen Inc). In the subgroup of patients (89/125 EPOGEN® and 88/130 placebo) with prestudy endogenous serum erythropoietin levels ≤ 500 mUnits/mL, EPOGEN® reduced the mean cumulative number of units of blood transfused per patient by approximately 40% as compared to the placebo group.[24] Among those patients who required transfusions at baseline, 43% of patients treated with EPOGEN® versus 18% of placebo-treated patients were transfusion-independent during the second and third months of therapy. EPOGEN® therapy also resulted in significant increases in hematocrit in comparison to placebo. When examining the results according to the weekly dose of zidovudine received during month 3 of therapy, there was a statistically significant ($p < 0.003$) reduction in transfusion requirements in patients treated with EPOGEN® (n = 51) compared to placebo treated patients (n = 54) whose mean weekly zidovudine dose was ≤ 4200 mg/week.[23]

Approximately 17% of the patients with endogenous serum erythropoietin levels ≤ 500 mUnits/mL receiving EPOGEN® in doses from 100 to 200 Units/kg TIW achieved a hematocrit of 38% without administration of transfusions or significant reduction in zidovudine dose. In the subgroup of patients whose prestudy endogenous serum erythropoietin levels were > 500 mUnits/mL, EPOGEN® therapy did not reduce transfusion requirements or increase hematocrit, compared to the corresponding responses in placebo-treated patients.

In a 6 month open-label EPOGEN® study, patients responded with decreased transfusion requirements and sustained increases in hematocrit and hemoglobin with doses of EPOGEN® up to 300 Units/kg TIW.[23-25]

Responsiveness to EPOGEN® therapy may be blunted by intercurrent infectious/inflammatory episodes and by an increase in zidovudine dosage. Consequently, the dose of EPOGEN® must be titrated based on these factors to maintain the desired erythropoietic response.

Cancer Patients on Chemotherapy

Adult Patients

Efficacy in patients with anemia due to concomitant chemotherapy was demonstrated based on reduction in the requirement for RBC transfusions.

Three-Times Weekly (TIW) Dosing

EPOGEN® administered TIW has been studied in a series of six placebo-controlled, double-blind trials that enrolled 131 anemic cancer patients receiving EPOGEN® or matching placebo. Across all studies, 72 patients were treated with concomitant non cisplatin-containing chemotherapy regimens and 59 patients were treated with concomitant cisplatin-containing chemotherapy regimens. Patients were randomized to EPOGEN® 150 Units/kg or placebo subcutaneously TIW for 12 weeks in each study.

The results of the pooled data from these six studies are shown in the table below. Because of the length of time required for erythropoiesis and red cell maturation, the efficacy of EPOGEN® (reduction in proportion of patients requiring transfusions) is not manifested until 2 to 6 weeks after initiation of EPOGEN®.

[See table above]

Proportion of Patients Transfused During Chemotherapy (Efficacy Population*)

Chemotherapy Regimen	On Study† EPOGEN®	On Study† Placebo	During Months 2 and 3‡ EPOGEN®	During Months 2 and 3‡ Placebo
Regimens without cisplatin	44% (15/34)	44% (16/36)	21% (6/29)	33% (11/33)
Regimens containing cisplatin	50% (14/28)	63% (19/30)	23% (5/22)§	56% (14/25)
Combined	47% (29/62)	53% (35/66)	22% (11/51)§	43% (25/58)

*Limited to patients remaining on study at least 15 days (1 patient excluded from EPOGEN®, 2 patients excluded from placebo).
†Includes all transfusions from day 1 through the end of study.
‡Limited to patients remaining on study beyond week 6 and includes only transfusions during weeks 5-12.
§Unadjusted 2-sided $p < 0.05$

Intensity of chemotherapy in the above trials was not directly assessed, however the degree and timing of neutropenia was comparable across all trials. Available evidence suggests that patients with lymphoid and solid cancers respond similarly to EPOGEN® therapy, and that patients with or without tumor infiltration of the bone marrow respond similarly to EPOGEN® therapy.

Weekly (QW) Dosing

EPOGEN® was also studied in a placebo-controlled, double-blind trial utilizing weekly dosing in a total of 344 anemic cancer patients. In this trial, 61 (35 placebo arm and 26 in the EPOGEN® arm) patients were treated with concomitant cisplatin containing regimens and 283 patients received concomitant chemotherapy regimens that did not contain cisplatinum. Patients were randomized to EPOGEN® 40,000 Units weekly (n = 174) or placebo (n = 170) SC for a planned treatment period of 16 weeks. If hemoglobin had not increased by > 1 g/dL after 4 weeks of therapy or the patient received RBC transfusion during the first 4 weeks of therapy, study drug was increased to 60,000 Units weekly. Forty-three percent of patients in the Epoetin alfa group required an increase in EPOGEN® dose to 60,000 Units weekly.[23]

Results demonstrated that EPOGEN® therapy reduced the proportion of patients transfused in day 29 through week 16 of the study as compared to placebo. Twenty-five patients (14%) in the EPOGEN® group received transfusions compared to 48 patients (28%) in the placebo group ($p = 0.0010$) between day 29 and week 16 or the last day on study.

Comparable intensity of chemotherapy for patients enrolled in the two study arms was suggested by similarities in mean dose and frequency of administration for the 10 most commonly administered chemotherapy agents, and similarity in the incidence of changes in chemotherapy during the trial in the two arms.

Pediatric Patients

The safety and effectiveness of EPOGEN® were evaluated in a randomized, double-blind, placebo-controlled, multicenter study in anemic patients ages 5 to 18 receiving chemotherapy for the treatment of various childhood malignancies. Two hundred twenty-two patients were randomized (1:1) to EPOGEN® or placebo. EPOGEN® was administered at 600 Units/kg (maximum 40,000 Units) intravenously once per week for 16 weeks. If hemoglobin had not increased by 1g/dL after the first 4-5 weeks of therapy, EPOGEN® was increased to 900 Units/kg (maximum 60,000 Units). Among the EPOGEN®-treated patients 60% required dose escalation to 900 Units/kg/week.

The effect of EPOGEN® on transfusion requirements is shown in the table below:

Percentage of Patients Transfused:

On Study*		After 28 Days Post-Randomization	
EPOGEN® (n=111)	Placebo (n=111)	EPOGEN® (n=111)	Placebo (n=111)
65% (72)	77% (86)	51% (57)†	69% (77)

*Includes all transfusions from day 1 through the end of study

†Adjusted 2 sided $p < 0.05$

There was no evidence of an improvement in health-related quality of life, including no evidence of an effect on fatigue, energy or strength, in patients receiving EPOGEN® as compared to those receiving placebo.

Surgery Patients

EPOGEN® has been studied in a placebo-controlled, double-blind trial enrolling 316 patients scheduled for major, elective orthopedic hip or knee surgery who were expected to require ≥ 2 units of blood and who were not able or willing to participate in an autologous blood donation program. Based on previous studies which demonstrated that pretreatment hemoglobin is a predictor of risk of receiving transfusion,[19,26] patients were stratified into one of three groups based on their pretreatment hemoglobin [≤ 10 (n = 2), > 10 to ≤ 13 (n = 96), and > 13 to ≤ 15 g/dL (n = 218)] and then randomly assigned to receive 300 Units/kg EPOGEN®, 100 Units/kg EPOGEN® or placebo by SC injection for 10 days before surgery, on the day of surgery, and for 4 days after surgery.[17] All patients received oral iron and a low-dose post-operative warfarin regimen.[17]

Treatment with EPOGEN® 300 Units/kg significantly (p = 0.024) reduced the risk of allogeneic transfusion in patients with a pretreatment hemoglobin of > 10 to ≤ 13; 5/31 (16%) of EPOGEN® 300 Units/kg, 6/26 (23%) of EPOGEN® 100 Units/kg, and 13/29 (45%) of placebo-treated patients were transfused.[17] There was no significant difference in the number of patients transfused between EPOGEN® (9% 300 Units/kg, 6% 100 Units/kg) and placebo (13%) in the > 13 to ≤ 15 g/dL hemoglobin stratum. There were too few patients in the ≤ 10 g/dL group to determine if EPOGEN® is useful in this hemoglobin strata. In the > 10 to ≤ 13 g/dL pretreatment stratum, the mean number of units transfused per EPOGEN®-treated patient (0.45 units blood for 300 Units/kg, 0.42 units blood for 100 Units/kg) was less than the mean transfused per placebo-treated patient (1.14 units) (overall p = 0.028). In addition, mean hemoglobin, hematocrit, and reticulocyte counts increased significantly during the presurgery period in patients treated with EPOGEN®.[17]

EPOGEN® was also studied in an open-label, parallel-group trial enrolling 145 subjects with a pretreatment hemoglobin level of ≥ 10 to ≤ 13 g/dL who were scheduled for major orthopedic hip or knee surgery and who were not participating in an autologous program.[18] Subjects were randomly assigned to receive one of two SC dosing regimens of EPOGEN® (600 Units/kg once weekly for 3 weeks prior to surgery and on the day of surgery, or 300 Units/kg once daily for 10 days prior to surgery, on the day of surgery and for 4 days after surgery). All subjects received oral iron and appropriate pharmacologic anticoagulation therapy.

From pretreatment to presurgery, the mean increase in hemoglobin in the 600 Units/kg weekly group (1.44 g/dL) was greater than observed in the 300 Units/kg daily group.[18] The mean increase in absolute reticulocyte count was smaller in the weekly group ($0.11 \times 10^6/mm^3$) compared to the daily group ($0.17 \times 10^6/mm^3$). Mean hemoglobin levels were similar for the two treatment groups throughout the postsurgical period.

The erythropoietic response observed in both treatment groups resulted in similar transfusion rates [11/69 (16%) in the 600 Units/kg weekly group and 14/71 (20%) in the 300 Units/kg daily group].[18] The mean number of units transfused per subject was approximately 0.3 units in both treatment groups.

CONTRAINDICATIONS

EPOGEN® is contraindicated in patients with:

1. Uncontrolled hypertension.
2. Known hypersensitivity to mammalian cell-derived products.
3. Known hypersensitivity to Albumin (Human).

WARNINGS

Pediatrics

Risk in Premature Infants

The multidose preserved formulation contains benzyl alcohol. Benzyl alcohol has been reported to be associated with an increased incidence of neurological and other complications in premature infants which are sometimes fatal.

Adults

Increased Mortality, Serious Cardiovascular Events, Thromboembolic Events, and Stroke

Patients with chronic renal failure experienced greater risks for death, serious cardiovascular events, and stroke when administered erythropoiesis-stimulating agents (ESAs) to target hemoglobin levels of 13 g/dL and above in clinical studies. Patients with chronic renal failure and an insufficient hemoglobin response to ESA therapy may be at even greater risk for cardiovascular events and mortality than other patients. EPOGEN® and other ESAs increased the risks for death and serious cardiovascular events in controlled clinical trials of patients with cancer. These events included myocardial infarction, stroke, congestive heart failure, and hemodialysis vascular access thrombosis. A rate of hemoglobin rise of > 1 g/dL over 2 weeks may contribute to these risks.

In a randomized prospective trial, 1432 anemic chronic renal failure patients who were not undergoing dialysis were assigned to Epoetin alfa (rHuEPO) treatment targeting a maintenance hemoglobin concentration of 13.5 g/dL or 11.3 g/dL. A major cardiovascular event (death, myocardial infarction, stroke, or hospitalization for congestive heart failure) occurred among 125 (18%) of the 715 patients in the higher hemoglobin group compared to 97 (14%) among the 717 patients in the lower hemoglobin group (HR 1.3, 95% CI: 1.0, 1.7, p = 0.03).[40]

In a randomized, double-blind, placebo-controlled study of 4038 patients, there was an increased risk of stroke when darbepoetin alfa was administered to patients with anemia, type 2 diabetes, and CRF who were not on dialysis. Patients were randomized to darbepoetin alfa treatment targeted to a hemoglobin level of 13 g/dL or to placebo. Placebo patients received darbepoetin alfa only if their hemoglobin levels were less than 9 g/dL. A total of 101 patients receiving darbepoetin alfa experienced stroke compared to 53 patients receiving placebo (5% vs. 2.6%; HR 1.92, 95% CI: 1.38, 2.68; p < 0.001).

Increased risk for serious cardiovascular events was also reported from a randomized, prospective trial of 1265 hemodialysis patients with clinically evident cardiac disease (ischemic heart disease or congestive heart failure). In this trial, patients were assigned to EPOGEN® treatment targeted to a maintenance hematocrit of either 42 ± 3% or 30 ± 3%.[37] Increased mortality was observed in 634 patients randomized to a target hematocrit of 42% [221 deaths (35% mortality)] compared to 631 patients targeted to remain at a hematocrit of 30% [185 deaths (29% mortality)]. The reason for the increased mortality observed in this study is unknown, however, the incidence of non-fatal myocardial infarctions (3.1% vs. 2.3%), vascular access thromboses (39% vs. 29%), and all other thrombotic events (22% vs. 18%) were also higher in the group randomized to achieve a hematocrit of 42%. An increased incidence of thrombotic events has also been observed in patients with cancer treated with erythropoietic agents.

In a randomized controlled study (referred to as Cancer Study 1 - the 'BEST' study) with another ESA in 939 women with metastatic breast cancer receiving chemotherapy, patients received either weekly Epoetin alfa or placebo for up to a year. This study was designed to show that survival was superior when an ESA was administered to prevent anemia (maintain hemoglobin levels between 12 and 14 g/dL or hematocrit between 36% and 42%). The study was terminated prematurely when interim results demonstrated that a higher mortality at 4 months (8.7% vs. 3.4%) and a higher rate of fatal thrombotic events (1.1% vs. 0.2%) in the first 4 months of the study were observed among patients treated with Epoetin alfa. Based on Kaplan-Meier estimates, at the time of study termination, the 12-month survival was lower in the Epoetin alfa group than in the placebo group (70% vs. 76%; HR 1.37, 95% CI: 1.07, 1.75; p = 0.012).[43]

A systematic review of 57 randomized controlled trials (including Cancer Studies 1 and 5 - the 'BEST' and 'ENHANCE' studies) evaluating 9353 patients with cancer compared ESAs plus red blood cell transfusion with red blood cell transfusion alone for prophylaxis or treatment of anemia in cancer patients with or without concurrent antineoplastic therapy. An increased relative risk of thromboembolic events (RR 1.67, 95% CI: 1.35, 2.06; 35 trials and 6769 patients) was observed in ESA-treated patients. An overall survival hazard ratio of 1.08 (95% CI: 0.99, 1.18; 42 trials and 8167 patients) was observed in ESA-treated patients.[41]

An increased incidence of deep vein thrombosis (DVT) in patients receiving Epoetin alfa undergoing surgical orthopedic procedures has been observed (see ADVERSE REACTIONS, Surgery Patients: Thrombotic/Vascular Events). In a randomized controlled study (referred to as the 'SPINE' study), 681 adult patients, not receiving prophylactic anticoagulation and undergoing spinal surgery, received either 4 doses of 600 U/kg Epoetin alfa (7, 14, and 21 days before surgery, and the day of surgery) and standard of care (SOC) treatment, or SOC treatment alone. Preliminary analysis showed a higher incidence of DVT, determined by either Color Flow Duplex Imaging or by clinical symptoms, in the Epoetin alfa group [16 patients (4.7%)] compared to the SOC group [7 patients (2.1%)]. In addition, 12 patients in the Epoetin alfa group and 7 patients in the SOC group had other thrombotic vascular events. Deep venous thrombosis prophylaxis should be strongly considered when ESAs are used for the reduction of allogeneic RBC transfusions in surgical patients (see BOXED WARNINGS and DOSAGE AND ADMINISTRATION).

Increased mortality was also observed in a randomized placebo-controlled study of EPOGEN® in adult patients who were undergoing coronary artery bypass surgery (7 deaths in 126 patients randomized to EPOGEN® versus no deaths among 56 patients receiving placebo). Four of these deaths occurred during the period of study drug administration and all four deaths were associated with thrombotic events.[42] ESAs are not approved for reduction of allogeneic red blood cell transfusions in patients scheduled for cardiac surgery.

Increased Mortality and/or Increased Risk of Tumor Progression or Recurrence

Erythropoiesis-stimulating agents resulted in decreased locoregional control/progression-free survival and/or overall survival (see Table 1). These findings were observed in studies of patients with advanced head and neck cancer receiving radiation therapy (Cancer Studies 5 and 6), in patients receiving chemotherapy for metastatic breast cancer (Cancer Study 1) or lymphoid malignancy (Cancer Study 2), and in patients with non-small cell lung cancer or various malignancies who were not receiving chemotherapy or radiotherapy (Cancer Studies 7 and 8).

[See table 1 at top right of next page]

Decreased overall survival:

Cancer Study 1 (the 'BEST' study) was previously described (see **WARNINGS: Increased Mortality, Serious Cardiovascular Events, Thromboembolic Events, and Stroke**). Mortality at 4 months (8.7% vs. 3.4%) was significantly higher in the Epoetin alfa arm. The most common investigator-attributed cause of death within the first 4 months was disease progression; 28 of 41 deaths in the Epoetin alfa arm and 13 of 16 deaths in the placebo arm were attributed to disease progression. Investigator assessed time to tumor progression was not different between the two groups. Survival at 12 months was significantly lower in the Epoetin alfa arm (70% vs. 76%, HR 1.37, 95% CI: 1.07, 1.75; p = 0.012).[43]

Cancer Study 2 was a Phase 3, double-blind, randomized (darbepoetin alfa vs. placebo) study conducted in 344 anemic patients with lymphoid malignancy receiving chemotherapy. With a median follow-up of 29 months, overall mortality rates were significantly higher among patients randomized to darbepoetin alfa as compared to placebo (HR 1.36, 95% CI: 1.02, 1.82).

Cancer Study 7 was a Phase 3, multicenter, randomized (Epoetin alfa vs. placebo), double-blind study, in which patients with advanced non-small cell lung cancer receiving only palliative radiotherapy or no active therapy were treated with Epoetin alfa to achieve and maintain hemoglobin levels between 12 and 14 g/dL. Following an interim analysis of 70 of 300 patients planned, a significant difference in survival in favor of the patients on the placebo arm of the trial was observed (median survival 63 vs. 129 days; HR 1.84; p = 0.04).

Cancer Study 8 was a Phase 3, double-blind, randomized (darbepoetin alfa vs. placebo), 16-week study in 989 anemic patients with active malignant disease, neither receiving nor planning to receive chemotherapy or radiation therapy. There was no evidence of a statistically significant reduction in proportion of patients receiving RBC transfusions. The median survival was shorter in the darbepoetin alfa treatment group (8 months) compared with the placebo group (10.8 months); HR 1.30, 95% CI: 1.07, 1.57.

Decreased progression-free survival and overall survival:

Cancer Study 3 (the 'PREPARE' study) was a randomized controlled study in which darbepoetin alfa was administered to prevent anemia conducted in 733 women receiving neo-adjuvant breast cancer treatment. After a median follow-up of approximately 3 years, the survival rate (86% vs. 90%, HR 1.42, 95% CI: 0.93, 2.18) and relapse-free survival rate (72% vs. 78%, HR 1.33, 95% CI: 0.99, 1.79) were lower in the darbepoetin alfa-treated arm compared to the control arm.

Cancer Study 4 (protocol GOG 191) was a randomized controlled study that enrolled 114 of a planned 460 cervical cancer patients receiving chemotherapy and radiotherapy. Patients were randomized to receive Epoetin alfa to maintain hemoglobin between 12 and 14 g/dL or to transfusion support as needed. The study was terminated prematurely due to an increase in thromboembolic events in Epoetin alfa-treated patients compared to control (19% vs. 9%). Both local recurrence (21% vs. 20%) and distant recurrence (12% vs. 7%) were more frequent in Epoetin alfa-treated patients compared to control. Progression-free survival at 3 years was lower in the Epoetin alfa-treated group compared to control (59% vs. 62%, HR 1.06, 95% CI: 0.58, 1.91). Overall survival at 3 years lower in the Epoetin alfa-treated group compared to control (61% vs. 71%, HR 1.28, 95% CI: 0.68, 2.42).

Cancer Study 5 (the 'ENHANCE' study) was a randomized controlled study in 351 head and neck cancer patients where Epoetin beta or placebo was administered to achieve target hemoglobin of 14 and 15 g/dL for women and men, respectively. Locoregional progression-free survival was significantly shorter in patients receiving Epoetin beta (HR 1.62, 95% CI: 1.22, 2.14; p = 0.0008) with a median of 406 days Epoetin beta vs. 745 days placebo. Overall survival was significantly shorter in patients receiving Epoetin beta (HR 1.39, 95% CI: 1.05, 1.84; p = 0.02).[38]

Decreased locoregional control:
Cancer Study 6 (DAHANCA 10) was conducted in 522 patients with primary squamous cell carcinoma of the head and neck receiving radiation therapy randomized to darbepoetin alfa with radiotherapy or radiotherapy alone. An interim analysis on 484 patients demonstrated that locoregional control at 5 years was significantly shorter in patients receiving darbepoetin alfa (RR 1.44, 95% CI: 1.06, 1.96; p = 0.02). Overall survival was shorter in patients receiving darbepoetin alfa (RR 1.28, 95% CI: 0.98, 1.68; p = 0.08).

ESA APPRISE Oncology Program
Prescribers and hospitals must enroll in and comply with the ESA APPRISE Oncology Program to prescribe and/or dispense EPOGEN® to patients with cancer. To enroll, visit www.esa-apprise.com or call 1-866-284-8089 for further assistance. Additionally, prescribers and patients must provide written acknowledgement of a discussion of the risks associated with EPOGEN®.

Pure Red Cell Aplasia
Cases of pure red cell aplasia (PRCA) and of severe anemia, with or without other cytopenias, associated with neutralizing antibodies to erythropoietin have been reported in patients treated with EPOGEN®. This has been reported predominantly in patients with CRF receiving ESAs by subcutaneous administration. PRCA has also been reported in patients receiving ESAs while undergoing treatment for hepatitis C with interferon and ribavirin. Any patient who develops a sudden loss of response to EPOGEN®, accompanied by severe anemia and low reticulocyte count, should be evaluated for the etiology of loss of effect, including the presence of neutralizing antibodies to erythropoietin (see PRECAUTIONS: Lack or Loss of Response). If anti-erythropoietin antibody-associated anemia is suspected, withhold EPOGEN® and other ESAs. Contact Amgen (1-800-77AMGEN) to perform assays for binding and neutralizing antibodies. EPOGEN® should be permanently discontinued in patients with antibody-mediated anemia. Patients should not be switched to other ESAs as antibodies may cross-react (see ADVERSE REACTIONS: Immunogenicity).

Albumin (Human)
EPOGEN® contains albumin, a derivative of human blood. Based on effective donor screening and product manufacturing processes, it carries an extremely remote risk for transmission of viral diseases. A theoretical risk for transmission of Creutzfeldt-Jakob disease (CJD) also is considered extremely remote. No cases of transmission of viral diseases or CJD have ever been identified for albumin.

Chronic Renal Failure Patients
Hypertension: Patients with uncontrolled hypertension should not be treated with EPOGEN®; blood pressure should be controlled adequately before initiation of therapy. Although there do not appear to be any direct pressor effects of EPOGEN®, blood pressure may rise during EPOGEN® therapy. During the early phase of treatment when the hematocrit is increasing, approximately 25% of patients on dialysis may require initiation of, or increases in, antihypertensive therapy. Hypertensive encephalopathy and seizures

have been observed in patients with CRF treated with EPOGEN®.

Special care should be taken to closely monitor and aggressively control blood pressure in patients treated with EPOGEN®. Patients should be advised as to the importance of compliance with antihypertensive therapy and dietary restrictions. If blood pressure is difficult to control by initiation of appropriate measures, the hemoglobin may be reduced by decreasing or withholding the dose of EPOGEN®. A clinically significant decrease in hemoglobin may not be observed for several weeks.

It is recommended that the dose of EPOGEN® be decreased if the hemoglobin increase exceeds 1 g/dL in any 2-week period, because of the possible association of excessive rate of rise of hemoglobin with an exacerbation of hypertension. In CRF patients on hemodialysis with clinically evident ischemic heart disease or congestive heart failure, the dose of EPOGEN® should be carefully adjusted to achieve and maintain hemoglobin levels between 10-12 g/dL (see WARNINGS: Increased Mortality, Serious Cardiovascular Events, Thromboembolic Events, and Stroke, and DOSAGE AND ADMINISTRATION: Chronic Renal Failure Patients).

Seizures: Seizures have occurred in patients with CRF participating in EPOGEN® clinical trials.

In adult patients on dialysis, there was a higher incidence of seizures during the first 90 days of therapy (occurring in approximately 2.5% of patients) as compared with later timepoints.

Given the potential for an increased risk of seizures during the first 90 days of therapy, blood pressure and the presence of premonitory neurologic symptoms should be monitored closely. Patients should be cautioned to avoid potentially hazardous activities such as driving or operating heavy machinery during this period.

While the relationship between seizures and the rate of rise of hemoglobin is uncertain, it is recommended that the dose of EPOGEN® be decreased if the hemoglobin increase exceeds 1 g/dL in any 2-week period.

Thrombotic Events: During hemodialysis, patients treated with EPOGEN® may require increased anticoagu-

lation with heparin to prevent clotting of the artificial kidney (see ADVERSE REACTIONS for more information about thrombotic events).

Other thrombotic events (eg, myocardial infarction, cerebrovascular accident, transient ischemic attack) have occurred in clinical trials at an annualized rate of less than 0.04 events per patient year of EPOGEN® therapy. These trials were conducted in adult patients with CRF (whether on dialysis or not) in whom the target hematocrit was 32% to 40%. However, the risk of thrombotic events, including vascular access thrombosis, was significantly increased in adult patients with ischemic heart disease or congestive heart failure receiving EPOGEN® therapy with the goal of reaching a normal hematocrit (42%) as compared to a target hematocrit of 30%. Patients with pre-existing cardiovascular disease should be monitored closely.

Zidovudine-treated HIV-infected Patients
In contrast to CRF patients, EPOGEN® therapy has not been linked to exacerbation of hypertension, seizures, and thrombotic events in HIV-infected patients. However, the clinical data do not rule out an increased risk for serious cardiovascular events.

PRECAUTIONS
The parenteral administration of any biologic product should be attended by appropriate precautions in case allergic or other untoward reactions occur (see CONTRAINDICATIONS). In clinical trials, while transient rashes were occasionally observed concurrently with EPOGEN® therapy, no serious allergic or anaphylactic reactions were reported (see ADVERSE REACTIONS for more information regarding allergic reactions).

The safety and efficacy of EPOGEN® therapy have not been established in patients with a known history of a seizure disorder or underlying hematologic disease (eg, sickle cell anemia, myelodysplastic syndromes, or hypercoagulable disorders).

In some female patients, menses have resumed following EPOGEN® therapy; the possibility of pregnancy should be discussed and the need for contraception evaluated.

Table 1: Randomized, Controlled Trials with Decreased Survival and/or Decreased Locoregional Control

Study / Tumor / (n)	Hemoglobin Target	Achieved Hemoglobin (Median Q1,Q3)	Primary Endpoint	Adverse Outcome for ESA-containing Arm
Chemotherapy				
Cancer Study 1 Metastatic breast cancer (n=939)	12-14 g/dL	12.9 g/dL 12.2, 13.3 g/dL	12-month overall survival	Decreased 12-month survival
Cancer Study 2 Lymphoid malignancy (n=344)	13-15 g/dL (M) 13-14 g/dL (F)	11.0 g/dL 9.8, 12.1 g/dL	Proportion of patients achieving a hemoglobin response	Decreased overall survival
Cancer Study 3 Early breast cancer (n=733)	12.5-13 g/dL	13.1 g/dL 12.5, 13.7 g/dL	Relapse-free and overall survival	Decreased 3 yr. relapse-free and overall survival
Cancer Study 4 Cervical Cancer (n=114)	12-14 g/dL	12.7 g/dL 12.1, 13.3 g/dL	Progression-free and overall survival and locoregional control	Decreased 3 yr. progression-free and overall survival and locoregional control
Radiotherapy Alone				
Cancer Study 5 Head and neck cancer (n=351)	≥15 g/dL (M) ≥14 g/dL (F)	Not available	Locoregional progression-free survival	Decreased 5-year locoregional progression-free survival Decreased overall survival
Cancer Study 6 Head and neck cancer (n=522)	14-15.5 g/dL	Not available	Locoregional disease control	Decreased locoregional disease control
No Chemotherapy or Radiotherapy				
Cancer Study 7 Non-small cell lung cancer (n=70)	12-14 g/dL	Not available	Quality of life	Decreased overall survival
Cancer Study 8 Non-myeloid malignancy (n=989)	12-13 g/dL	10.6 g/dL 9.4, 11.8 g/dL	RBC transfusions	Decreased overall survival

Hematology

Exacerbation of porphyria has been observed rarely in patients with CRF treated with EPOGEN®. However, EPOGEN® has not caused increased urinary excretion of porphyrin metabolites in normal volunteers, even in the presence of a rapid erythropoietic response. Nevertheless, EPOGEN® should be used with caution in patients with known porphyria.

In preclinical studies in dogs and rats, but not in monkeys, EPOGEN® therapy was associated with subclinical bone marrow fibrosis. Bone marrow fibrosis is a known complication of CRF in humans and may be related to secondary hyperparathyroidism or unknown factors. The incidence of bone marrow fibrosis was not increased in a study of adult patients on dialysis who were treated with EPOGEN® for 12 to 19 months, compared to the incidence of bone marrow fibrosis in a matched group of patients who had not been treated with EPOGEN®.

Hemoglobin in CRF patients should be measured twice a week; zidovudine-treated HIV-infected and cancer patients should have hemoglobin measured once a week until hemoglobin has been stabilized, and measured periodically thereafter.

Lack or Loss of Response

If the patient fails to respond or to maintain a response to doses within the recommended dosing range, the following etiologies should be considered and evaluated:

1. Iron deficiency: Virtually all patients will eventually require supplemental iron therapy (see IRON EVALUATION).
2. Underlying infectious, inflammatory, or malignant processes.
3. Occult blood loss.
4. Underlying hematologic diseases (ie, thalassemia, refractory anemia, or other myelodysplastic disorders).
5. Vitamin deficiencies: Folic acid or vitamin B_{12}.
6. Hemolysis.
7. Aluminum intoxication.
8. Osteitis fibrosa cystica.
9. Pure Red Cell Aplasia (PRCA) or anti-erythropoietin antibody-associated anemia: In the absence of another etiology, the patient should be evaluated for evidence of PRCA and sera should be tested for the presence of antibodies to erythropoietin (see WARNINGS: Pure Red Cell Aplasia).

See DOSAGE AND ADMINISTRATION: Chronic Renal Failure Patients for management of patients with an insufficient hemoglobin response to EPOGEN® therapy.

Iron Evaluation

During EPOGEN® therapy, absolute or functional iron deficiency may develop. Functional iron deficiency, with normal ferritin levels but low transferrin saturation, is presumably due to the inability to mobilize iron stores rapidly enough to support increased erythropoiesis. Transferrin saturation should be at least 20% and ferritin should be at least 100 ng/mL.

Prior to and during EPOGEN® therapy, the patient's iron status, including transferrin saturation (serum iron divided by iron binding capacity) and serum ferritin, should be evaluated. Virtually all patients will eventually require supplemental iron to increase or maintain transferrin saturation to levels which will adequately support erythropoiesis stimulated by EPOGEN®. All surgery patients being treated with EPOGEN® should receive adequate iron supplementation throughout the course of therapy in order to support erythropoiesis and avoid depletion of iron stores.

Drug Interaction

No evidence of interaction of EPOGEN® with other drugs was observed in the course of clinical trials.

Carcinogenesis, Mutagenesis, and Impairment of Fertility

Carcinogenic potential of EPOGEN® has not been evaluated. EPOGEN® does not induce bacterial gene mutation (Ames Test), chromosomal aberrations in mammalian cells, micronuclei in mice, or gene mutation at the HGPRT locus. In female rats treated IV with EPOGEN®, there was a trend for slightly increased fetal wastage at doses of 100 and 500 Units/kg.

Pregnancy Category C

EPOGEN® has been shown to have adverse effects in rats when given in doses 5 times the human dose. There are no adequate and well-controlled studies in pregnant women. EPOGEN® should be used during pregnancy only if potential benefit justifies the potential risk to the fetus.

In studies in female rats, there were decreases in body weight gain, delays in appearance of abdominal hair, delayed eyelid opening, delayed ossification, and decreases in the number of caudal vertebrae in the F1 fetuses of the 500 Units/kg group. In female rats treated IV, there was a trend for slightly increased fetal wastage at doses of 100 and 500 Units/kg. EPOGEN® has not shown any adverse effect at doses as high as 500 Units/kg in pregnant rabbits (from day 6 to 18 of gestation).

Nursing Mothers

Postnatal observations of the live offspring (F1 generation) of female rats treated with EPOGEN® during gestation and lactation revealed no effect of EPOGEN® at doses of up to 500 Units/kg. There were, however, decreases in body weight gain, delays in appearance of abdominal hair, eyelid opening, and decreases in the number of caudal vertebrae in the F1 fetuses of the 500 Units/kg group. There were no EPOGEN®-related effects on the F2 generation fetuses.

It is not known whether EPOGEN® is excreted in human milk. Because many drugs are excreted in human milk, caution should be exercised when EPOGEN® is administered to a nursing woman.

Pediatric Use

See WARNINGS: Pediatrics.

Pediatric Patients on Dialysis: EPOGEN® is indicated in infants (1 month to 2 years), children (2 years to 12 years), and adolescents (12 years to 16 years) for the treatment of anemia associated with CRF requiring dialysis. Safety and effectiveness in pediatric patients less than 1 month old have not been established (see CLINICAL EXPERIENCE: CHRONIC RENAL FAILURE, PEDIATRIC PATIENTS ON DIALYSIS). The safety data from these studies show that there is no increased risk to pediatric CRF patients on dialysis when compared to the safety profile of EPOGEN® in adult CRF patients (see ADVERSE REACTIONS and WARNINGS). Published literature[27-30] provides supportive evidence of the safety and effectiveness of EPOGEN® in pediatric CRF patients on dialysis.

Pediatric Patients Not Requiring Dialysis: Published literature[30,31] has reported the use of EPOGEN® in 133 pediatric patients with anemia associated with CRF not requiring dialysis, ages 3 months to 20 years, treated with 50 to 250 Units/kg SC or IV, QW to TIW. Dose-dependent increases in hemoglobin and hematocrit were observed with reductions in transfusion requirements.

Pediatric HIV-infected Patients: Published literature[32,33] has reported the use of EPOGEN® in 20 zidovudine-treated anemic HIV-infected pediatric patients ages 8 months to 17 years, treated with 50 to 400 Units/kg SC or IV, 2 to 3 times per week. Increases in hemoglobin levels and in reticulocyte counts, and decreases in or elimination of blood transfusions were observed.

Pediatric Cancer Patients on Chemotherapy: The safety and effectiveness of EPOGEN® were evaluated in a randomized, double-blind, placebo-controlled, multicenter study (see CLINICAL EXPERIENCE, Weekly (QW) Dosing, Pediatric Patients).

Geriatric Use

Among 1051 patients enrolled in the 5 clinical trials of EPOGEN® for reduction of allogeneic blood transfusions in patients undergoing elective surgery 745 received EPOGEN® and 306 received placebo. Of the 745 patients who received EPOGEN®, 432 (58%) were aged 65 and over, while 175 (23%) were 75 and over. No overall differences in safety or effectiveness were observed between geriatric and younger patients. The dose requirements for EPOGEN® in geriatric and younger patients within the 4 trials using the TIW schedule were similar. Insufficient numbers of patients were enrolled in the study using the weekly dosing regimen to determine whether the dosing requirements differ for this schedule.

Of the 882 patients enrolled in the 3 studies of chronic renal failure patients on dialysis, 757 received EPOGEN® and 125 received placebo. Of the 757 patients who received EPOGEN®, 361 (47%) were aged 65 and over, while 100 (13%) were 75 and over. No differences in safety or effectiveness were observed between geriatric and younger patients. Dose selection and adjustment for an elderly patient should be individualized to achieve and maintain the target hematocrit (See DOSAGE AND ADMINISTRATION).

Insufficient numbers of patients age 65 or older were enrolled in clinical studies of EPOGEN® for the treatment of anemia associated with pre-dialysis chronic renal failure, cancer chemotherapy, and Zidovudine-treatment of HIV infection to determine whether they respond differently from younger subjects.

Information for Patients

Patients should be informed of the increased risks of mortality, serious cardiovascular events, thromboembolic events, and increased risk of tumor progression or recurrence (see WARNINGS). In those situations in which the physician determines that a patient or their caregiver can safely and effectively administer EPOGEN® at home, instruction as to the proper dosage and administration should be provided. Patients should be instructed to read the EPOGEN® Medication Guide and Patient Instructions for Use and should be informed that the Medication Guide is not a disclosure of all possible side effects. Patients should be informed of the possible side effects of EPOGEN® and of the signs and symptoms of allergic drug reaction and advised of appropriate actions. If home use is prescribed for a patient, the patient should be thoroughly instructed in the importance of proper disposal and cautioned against the re-

use of needles, syringes, or drug product. A puncture-resistant container should be available for the disposal of used syringes and needles, and guidance provided on disposal of the full container.

Chronic Renal Failure Patients

Patients with CRF Not Requiring Dialysis

Blood pressure and hemoglobin should be monitored no less frequently than for patients maintained on dialysis. Renal function and fluid and electrolyte balance should be closely monitored.

Hematology

Sufficient time should be allowed to determine a patient's responsiveness to a dosage of EPOGEN® before adjusting the dose. Because of the time required for erythropoiesis and the red cell half-life, an interval of 2 to 6 weeks may occur between the time of a dose adjustment (initiation, increase, decrease, or discontinuation) and a significant change in hemoglobin.

For patients who respond to EPOGEN® with a rapid increase in hemoglobin (eg, more than 1 g/dL in any 2-week period), the dose of EPOGEN® should be reduced because of the possible association of excessive rate of rise of hemoglobin with an exacerbation of hypertension.

The elevated bleeding time characteristic of CRF decreases toward normal after correction of anemia in adult patients treated with EPOGEN®. Reduction of bleeding time also occurs after correction of anemia by transfusion.

Laboratory Monitoring

The hemoglobin should be determined twice a week until it has stabilized in the suggested hemoglobin range and the maintenance dose has been established. After any dose adjustment, the hemoglobin should also be determined twice weekly for at least 2 to 6 weeks until it has been determined that the hemoglobin has stabilized in response to the dose change. The hemoglobin should then be monitored at regular intervals.

A complete blood count with differential and platelet count should be performed regularly. During clinical trials, modest increases were seen in platelets and white blood cell counts. While these changes were statistically significant, they were not clinically significant and the values remained within normal ranges.

In patients with CRF, serum chemistry values (including blood urea nitrogen [BUN], uric acid, creatinine, phosphorus, and potassium) should be monitored regularly. During clinical trials in adult patients on dialysis, modest increases were seen in BUN, creatinine, phosphorus, and potassium. In some adult patients with CRF not on dialysis treated with EPOGEN®, modest increases in serum uric acid and phosphorus were observed. While changes were statistically significant, the values remained within the ranges normally seen in patients with CRF.

Diet

The importance of compliance with dietary and dialysis prescriptions should be reinforced. In particular, hyperkalemia is not uncommon in patients with CRF. In US studies in patients on dialysis, hyperkalemia has occurred at an annualized rate of approximately 0.11 episodes per patient-year of EPOGEN® therapy, often in association with poor compliance to medication, diet, and/or dialysis.

Dialysis Management

Therapy with EPOGEN® results in an increase in hematocrit and a decrease in plasma volume which could affect dialysis efficiency. In studies to date, the resulting increase in hematocrit did not appear to adversely affect dialyzer function[8,9] or the efficiency of high flux hemodialysis.[10] During hemodialysis, patients treated with EPOGEN® may require increased anticoagulation with heparin to prevent clotting of the artificial kidney.

Patients who are marginally dialyzed may require adjustments in their dialysis prescription. As with all patients on dialysis, the serum chemistry values (including BUN, creatinine, phosphorus, and potassium) in patients treated with EPOGEN® should be monitored regularly to assure the adequacy of the dialysis prescription.

Renal Function

In adult patients with CRF not on dialysis, renal function and fluid and electrolyte balance should be closely monitored. In patients with CRF not on dialysis, placebo-controlled studies of progression of renal dysfunction over periods of greater than 1 year have not been completed. In shorter term trials in adult patients with CRF not on dialysis, changes in creatinine and creatinine clearance were not significantly different in patients treated with EPOGEN® compared with placebo-treated patients. Analysis of the slope of 1/serum creatinine versus time plots in these patients indicates no significant change in the slope after the initiation of EPOGEN® therapy.

Zidovudine-treated HIV-infected Patients

Hypertension

Exacerbation of hypertension has not been observed in zidovudine-treated HIV-infected patients treated with EPOGEN®. However, EPOGEN® should be withheld in these patients if pre-existing hypertension is uncontrolled, and should not be started until blood pressure is controlled. In double-blind studies, a single seizure has been experienced by a patient treated with EPOGEN®.[23]

Cancer Patients on Chemotherapy

Hypertension

Hypertension, associated with a significant increase in hemoglobin, has been noted rarely in patients treated with EPOGEN®. Nevertheless, blood pressure in patients treated with EPOGEN® should be monitored carefully, particularly in patients with an underlying history of hypertension or cardiovascular disease.

Seizures

In double-blind, placebo-controlled trials, 3.2% (n = 2/63) of patients treated with EPOGEN® TIW and 2.9% (n = 2/68) of placebo-treated patients had seizures. Seizures in 1.6% (n = 1/63) of patients treated with EPOGEN® TIW occurred in the context of a significant increase in blood pressure and hematocrit from baseline values. However, both patients treated with EPOGEN® also had underlying CNS pathology which may have been related to seizure activity.

In a placebo-controlled, double-blind trial utilizing weekly dosing with EPOGEN®, 1.2% (n = 2/168) of safety-evaluable patients treated with EPOGEN® and 1% (n = 1/165) of placebo-treated patients had seizures. Seizures in the patients treated with weekly EPOGEN® occurred in the context of a significant increase in hemoglobin from baseline values however significant increases in blood pressure were not seen. These patients may have had other CNS pathology.

Thrombotic Events

In double-blind, placebo-controlled trials, 3.2% (n = 2/63) of patients treated with EPOGEN® TIW and 11.8% (n = 8/68) of placebo-treated patients had thrombotic events (eg, pulmonary embolism, cerebrovascular accident), (see WARNINGS: Increased Mortality, Serious Cardiovascular Events, Thromboembolic Events, and Stroke).

In a placebo-controlled, double-blind trial utilizing weekly dosing with EPOGEN®, 6.0% (n = 10/168) of safety-evaluable patients treated with EPOGEN® and 3.6% (n = 6/165) (p = 0.444) of placebo-treated patients had clinically significant thrombotic events (deep vein thrombosis requiring anticoagulant therapy, embolic event including pulmonary embolism, myocardial infarction, cerebral ischemia, left ventricular failure and thrombotic microangiopathy). A definitive relationship between the rate of hemoglobin increase and the occurrence of clinically significant thrombotic events could not be evaluated due to the limited schedule of hemoglobin measurements in this study.

The safety and efficacy of EPOGEN® were evaluated in a randomized, double-blind, placebo-controlled, multicenter study that enrolled 222 anemic patients ages 5 to 18 receiving treatment for a variety of childhood malignancies. Due to the study design (small sample size and the heterogeneity of the underlying malignancies and of anti-neoplastic treatments employed), a determination of the effect of EPOGEN® on the incidence of thrombotic events could not be performed. In the EPOGEN® arm, the overall incidence of thrombotic events was 10.8% and the incidence of serious or life-threatening events was 7.2%.

Surgery Patients

Hypertension

Blood pressure may rise in the perioperative period in patients being treated with EPOGEN®. Therefore, blood pressure should be monitored carefully.

ADVERSE REACTIONS

Immunogenicity

As with all therapeutic proteins, there is the potential for immunogenicity. Neutralizing antibodies to erythropoietin, in association with PRCA or severe anemia (with or without other cytopenias), have been reported in patients receiving EPOGEN® (see WARNINGS: Pure Red Cell Aplasia) during post-marketing experience.

There has been no systematic assessment of immune responses, i.e., the incidence of either binding or neutralizing antibodies to EPOGEN®, in controlled clinical trials.

Where reported, the incidence of antibody formation is highly dependent on the sensitivity and specificity of the assay. Additionally, the observed incidence of antibody (including neutralizing antibody) positivity in an assay may be influenced by several factors including assay methodology, sample handling, timing of sample collection, concomitant medications, and underlying disease. For these reasons, comparison of the incidence of antibodies across products within this class (erythropoietic proteins) may be misleading.

Chronic Renal Failure Patients

In double-blind, placebo-controlled studies involving over 300 patients with CRF, the events reported in greater than 5% of patients treated with EPOGEN® during the blinded phase were:

Percent of Patients Reporting Event

Event	Patients Treated With EPOGEN® (n = 200)	Placebo-treated Patients (n = 135)
Hypertension	24%	19%
Headache	16%	12%
Arthralgias	11%	6%
Nausea	11%	9%
Edema	9%	10%
Fatigue	9%	14%
Diarrhea	9%	6%
Vomiting	8%	5%
Chest Pain	7%	9%
Skin Reaction (Administration Site)	7%	12%
Asthenia	7%	12%
Dizziness	7%	13%
Clotted Access	7%	2%

Significant adverse events of concern in patients with CRF treated in double-blind, placebo-controlled trials occurred in the following percent of patients during the blinded phase of the studies:

Seizure	1.1%	1.1%
CVA/TIA	0.4%	0.6%
MI	0.4%	1.1%
Death	0%	1.7%

In the US EPOGEN® studies in adult patients on dialysis (over 567 patients), the incidence (number of events per patient-year) of the most frequently reported adverse events were: hypertension (0.75), headache (0.40), tachycardia (0.31), nausea/vomiting (0.26), clotted vascular access (0.25), shortness of breath (0.14), hyperkalemia (0.11), and diarrhea (0.11). Other reported events occurred at a rate of less than 0.10 events per patient per year.

Events reported to have occurred within several hours of administration of EPOGEN® were rare, mild, and transient, and included injection site stinging in dialysis patients and flu-like symptoms such as arthralgias and myalgias.

In all studies analyzed to date, EPOGEN® administration was generally well-tolerated, irrespective of the route of administration.

Pediatric CRF Patients: In pediatric patients with CRF on dialysis, the pattern of most adverse events was similar to that found in adults. Additional adverse events reported during the double-blind phase in >10% of pediatric patients in either treatment group were: abdominal pain, dialysis access complications including access infections and peritonitis in those receiving peritoneal dialysis, fever, upper respiratory infection, cough, pharyngitis, and constipation. The rates are similar between the treatment groups for each event.

Hypertension: Increases in blood pressure have been reported in clinical trials, often during the first 90 days of therapy. On occasion, hypertensive encephalopathy and seizures have been observed in patients with CRF treated with EPOGEN®. When data from all patients in the US phase 3 multicenter trial were analyzed, there was an apparent trend of more reports of hypertensive adverse events in patients on dialysis with a faster rate of rise of hematocrit (greater than 4 hematocrit points in any 2-week period). However, in a double-blind, placebo-controlled trial, hypertensive adverse events were not reported at an increased rate in the group treated with EPOGEN® (150 Units/kg TIW) relative to the placebo group.

Seizures: There have been 47 seizures in 1010 patients on dialysis treated with EPOGEN® in clinical trials, with an exposure of 986 patient-years for a rate of approximately 0.048 events per patient-year. However, there appeared to be a higher rate of seizures during the first 90 days of therapy (occurring in approximately 2.5% of patients) when compared to subsequent 90-day periods. The baseline incidence of seizures in the untreated dialysis population is difficult to determine; it appears to be in the range of 5% to 10% per patient-year.[34-36]

Thrombotic Events: In clinical trials where the maintenance hematocrit was 35 ± 3% on EPOGEN®, clotting of the vascular access (A-V shunt) has occurred at an annualized rate of about 0.25 events per patient-year, and other thrombotic events (eg, myocardial infarction, cerebral vascular accident, transient ischemic attack, and pulmonary embolism) occurred at a rate of 0.04 events per patient-year. In a separate study of 1111 untreated dialysis patients, clotting of the vascular access occurred at a rate of 0.50 events per patient-year. However, in CRF patients on hemodialysis who also had clinically evident ischemic heart disease or congestive heart failure, the risk of A-V shunt thrombosis

was higher (39% vs 29%, p < 0.001), and myocardial infarctions, vascular ischemic events, and venous thrombosis were increased, in patients targeted to a hematocrit of 42 ± 3% compared to those maintained at 30 ± 3% (see WARNINGS).

In patients treated with commercial EPOGEN®, there have been rare reports of serious or unusual thromboembolic events including migratory thrombophlebitis, microvascular thrombosis, pulmonary embolus, and thrombosis of the retinal artery, and temporal and renal veins. A causal relationship has not been established.

Allergic Reactions: There have been no reports of serious allergic reactions or anaphylaxis associated with EPOGEN® administration during clinical trials. Skin rashes and urticaria have been observed rarely and when reported have generally been mild and transient in nature. There have been rare reports of potentially serious allergic reactions including urticaria with associated respiratory symptoms or circumoral edema, or urticaria alone. Most reactions occurred in situations where a causal relationship could not be established. Symptoms recurred with rechallenge in a few instances, suggesting that allergic reactivity may occasionally be associated with EPOGEN® therapy. If an anaphylactoid reaction occurs, EPOGEN® should be immediately discontinued and appropriate therapy initiated.

Zidovudine-treated HIV-infected Patients

In double-blind, placebo-controlled studies of 3 months duration involving approximately 300 zidovudine-treated HIV-infected patients, adverse events with an incidence of ≥ 10% in either patients treated with EPOGEN® or placebo-treated patients were:

Percent of Patients Reporting Event

Event	Patients Treated With EPOGEN® (n = 144)	Placebo-treated Patients (n = 153)
Pyrexia	38%	29%
Fatigue	25%	31%
Headache	19%	14%
Cough	18%	14%
Diarrhea	16%	18%
Rash	16%	8%
Congestion, Respiratory	15%	10%
Nausea	15%	12%
Shortness of Breath	14%	13%
Asthenia	11%	14%
Skin Reaction, Medication Site	10%	7%
Dizziness	9%	10%

In the 297 patients studied, EPOGEN® was not associated with significant increases in opportunistic infections or mortality.[23] In 71 patients from this group treated with EPOGEN® at 150 Units/kg TIW, serum p24 antigen levels did not appear to increase.[25] Preliminary data showed no enhancement of HIV replication in infected cell lines in vitro.[23]

Peripheral white blood cell and platelet counts are unchanged following EPOGEN® therapy.

Allergic Reactions: Two zidovudine-treated HIV-infected patients had urticarial reactions within 48 hours of their first exposure to study medication. One patient was treated with EPOGEN® and one was treated with placebo (EPOGEN® vehicle alone). Both patients had positive immediate skin tests against their study medication with a negative saline control. The basis for this apparent pre-existing hypersensitivity to components of the EPOGEN® formulation is unknown, but may be related to HIV-induced immunosuppression or prior exposure to blood products.

Seizures: In double-blind and open-label trials of EPOGEN® in zidovudine-treated HIV-infected patients, 10 patients have experienced seizures.[23] In general, these seizures appear to be related to underlying pathology such as meningitis or cerebral neoplasms, not EPOGEN® therapy.

Cancer Patients on Chemotherapy

In double-blind, placebo-controlled studies of up to 3 months duration involving 131 cancer patients, adverse events with an incidence > 10% in either patients treated with EPOGEN® or placebo-treated patients were as indicated below:

Percent of Patients Reporting Event

Event	Patients Treated With EPOGEN® (n=63)	Placebo-treated Patients (n=68)
Pyrexia	29%	19%
Diarrhea	21%*	7%

Percent of Patients Reporting Event

Event	Patients Treated With EPOGEN® 300 U/kg (n = 112)*	Patients Treated With EPOGEN® 100 U/kg (n = 101)*	Placebo-treated Patients (n = 103)*	Patients Treated With EPOGEN® 600 U/kg (n = 73)†	Patients Treated With EPOGEN® 300 U/kg (n = 72)†
Pyrexia	51%	50%	60%	47%	42%
Nausea	48%	43%	45%	45%	58%
Constipation	43%	42%	43%	51%	53%
Skin Reaction, Medication Site	25%	19%	22%	26%	29%
Vomiting	22%	12%	14%	21%	29%
Skin Pain	18%	18%	17%	5%	4%
Pruritus	16%	16%	14%	14%	22%
Insomnia	13%	16%	13%	21%	18%
Headache	13%	11%	9%	10%	19%
Dizziness	12%	9%	12%	11%	21%
Urinary Tract Infection	12%	3%	11%	11%	8%
Hypertension	10%	11%	10%	5%	10%
Diarrhea	10%	7%	12%	10%	6%
Deep Venous Thrombosis	10%	3%	5%	0%‡	0%‡
Dyspepsia	9%	11%	6%	7%	8%
Anxiety	7%	2%	11%	11%	4%
Edema	6%	11%	8%	11%	7%

* Study including patients undergoing orthopedic surgery treated with EPOGEN® or placebo for 15 days
† Study including patients undergoing orthopedic surgery treated with EPOGEN® 600 Units/kg weekly × 4 or 300 Units/kg daily × 15
‡ Determined by clinical symptoms

Nausea	17%*	32%
Vomiting	17%	15%
Edema	17%*	1%
Asthenia	13%	16%
Fatigue	13%	15%
Shortness of Breath	13%	9%
Parasthesia	11%	6%
Upper Respiratory Infection	11%	4%
Dizziness	5%	12%
Trunk Pain	3%*	16%

*Statistically significant

Although some statistically significant differences between patients being treated with EPOGEN® and placebo-treated patients were noted, the overall safety profile of EPOGEN® appeared to be consistent with the disease process of advanced cancer. During double-blind and subsequent open-label therapy in which patients (n = 72 for total exposure to EPOGEN®) were treated for up to 32 weeks with doses as high as 927 Units/kg, the adverse experience profile of EPOGEN® was consistent with the progression of advanced cancer.

Three hundred thirty-three (333) cancer patients enrolled in a placebo-controlled double-blind trial utilizing Weekly dosing with EPOGEN® for up to 4 months were evaluable for adverse events. The incidence of adverse events was similar in both the treatment and placebo arms.

Surgery Patients
Adverse events with an incidence of ≥ 10% are shown in the following table:
[See first table above]

Thrombotic/Vascular Events: In three double-blind, placebo-controlled orthopedic surgery studies, the rate of deep venous thrombosis (DVT) was similar among Epoetin alfa and placebo-treated patients in the recommended population of patients with a pretreatment hemoglobin of > 10 g/dL to ≤ 13 g/dL.[17,19,26] However, in 2 of 3 orthopedic surgery studies the overall rate (all pretreatment hemoglobin groups combined) of DVTs detected by postoperative ultrasonography and/or surveillance venography was higher in the group treated with Epoetin alfa than in the placebo-treated group (11% vs. 6%). This finding was attributable to the difference in DVT rates observed in the subgroup of patients with pretreatment hemoglobin > 13 g/dL.

In the orthopedic surgery study of patients with pretreatment hemoglobin of > 10 g/dL to ≤ 13 g/dL which compared two dosing regimens (600 Units/kg weekly × 4 and 300 Units/kg daily × 15), 4 subjects in the 600 Units/kg weekly EPOGEN® group (5%) and no subjects in the 300 Units/kg daily group had a thrombotic vascular event during the study period.[18]

In a study examining the use of Epoetin alfa in 182 patients scheduled for coronary artery bypass graft surgery, 23% of patients treated with Epoetin alfa and 29% treated with placebo experienced thrombotic/vascular events. There were 4 deaths among the Epoetin alfa-treated patients that were associated with a thrombotic/vascular event (see WARNINGS).

OVERDOSAGE
The expected manifestations of EPOGEN® overdosage include signs and symptoms associated with an excessive and/or rapid increase in hemoglobin concentration, including any of the cardiovascular events described in WARNINGS and listed in ADVERSE REACTIONS. Patients receiving an overdosage of EPOGEN® should be monitored closely for cardiovascular events and hematologic abnormalities. Polycythemia should be managed acutely with phlebotomy as clinically indicated. Following resolution of the effects due to EPOGEN® overdosage, reintroduction of EPOGEN® therapy should be accompanied by close monitoring for evidence of rapid increases in hemoglobin concentration (>1 gm/dL per 14 days). In patients with an excessive hematopoietic response, reduce the EPOGEN® dose in accordance with the recommendations described in DOSAGE AND ADMINISTRATION.

DOSAGE AND ADMINISTRATION
IMPORTANT: See BOXED WARNINGS and WARNINGS: Increased Mortality, Serious Cardiovascular Events, Thromboembolic Events, and Stroke.
Chronic Renal Failure Patients
The recommended range for the starting dose of EPOGEN® is 50 to 100 Units/kg TIW for adult patients. The recommended starting dose for pediatric CRF patients on dialysis is 50 Units/kg TIW. Individualize dosing to achieve and maintain hemoglobin levels between 10-12 g/dL. The dose of EPOGEN® should be reduced as the hemoglobin approaches 12 g/dL or increases by more than 1 g/dL in any 2-week period. If hemoglobin excursions outside the recommended range occur, the EPOGEN® dose should be adjusted as described below.
EPOGEN® may be given either as an IV or SC injection. *In patients on hemodialysis, the IV route is recommended* (see WARNINGS: Pure Red Cell Aplasia). While the administration of EPOGEN® is independent of the dialysis procedure, EPOGEN® may be administered into the venous line at the end of the dialysis procedure to obviate the need for additional venous access. In adult patients with CRF not on dialysis, EPOGEN® may be given either as an IV or SC injection.
Patients who have been judged competent by their physicians to self-administer EPOGEN® without medical or other supervision may give themselves either an IV or SC injection. The table below provides general therapeutic guidelines for patients with CRF:
Individually titrate to achieve and maintain hemoglobin levels between 10 to 12 g/dL.

Starting Dose:

Adults	50 to 100 Units/kg TIW; IV or SC
Pediatric Patients	50 Units/kg TIW; IV or SC

Increase Dose by 25% If:	1. Hemoglobin is < 10 g/dL and has not increased by 1 g/dL after 4 weeks of therapy or 2. Hemoglobin decreases below 10 g/dL
Reduce Dose by 25% When:	1. Hemoglobin approaches 12 g/dL or, 2. Hemoglobin increases > 1 g/dL in any 2-week period

During therapy, hematological parameters should be monitored regularly. Doses must be individualized to ensure that hemoglobin is maintained at an appropriate level for each patient.
For patients whose hemoglobin does not attain a level within the range of 10 to 12 g/dL despite the use of appropriate EPOGEN® dose titrations over a 12-week period:
• do not administer higher EPOGEN® doses and use the lowest dose that will maintain a hemoglobin level sufficient to avoid the need for recurrent RBC transfusions,
• evaluate and treat for other causes of anemia (see PRECAUTIONS: Lack or Loss of Response), and
• thereafter, hemoglobin should continue to be monitored and if responsiveness improves, EPOGEN® dose adjustments should be made as described above; discontinue EPOGEN® if responsiveness does not improve and the patient needs recurrent RBC transfusions.
Pretherapy Iron Evaluation: Prior to and during EPOGEN® therapy, the patient's iron stores, including transferrin saturation (serum iron divided by iron binding capacity) and serum ferritin, should be evaluated. Transferrin saturation should be at least 20%, and ferritin should be at least 100 ng/mL. Virtually all patients will eventually require supplemental iron to increase or maintain transferrin saturation to levels that will adequately support erythropoiesis stimulated by EPOGEN®.
Dose Adjustment: The dose should be adjusted for each patient to achieve and maintain hemoglobin levels between 10 to 12 g/dL.
Increases in dose should not be made more frequently than once a month. If the hemoglobin is increasing and approaching 12 g/dL, the dose should be reduced by approximately 25%. If the hemoglobin continues to increase, dose should be temporarily withheld until the hemoglobin begins to decrease, at which point therapy should be reinitiated at a dose approximately 25% below the previous dose. If the hemoglobin increases by more than 1 g/dL in a 2-week period, the dose should be decreased by approximately 25%.
If the increase in the hemoglobin is less than 1 g/dL over 4 weeks and iron stores are adequate (see PRECAUTIONS: Laboratory Monitoring), the dose of EPOGEN® may be increased by approximately 25% of the previous dose. Further increases may be made at 4-week intervals until the specified hemoglobin is obtained.
Maintenance Dose: The maintenance dose must be individualized for each patient on dialysis. In the US Phase 3 multicenter trial in patients on hemodialysis, the median maintenance dose was 75 Units/kg TIW, with a range from 12.5 to 525 Units/kg TIW. Almost 10% of the patients required doses of 25 Units/kg, or less, and approximately 10% of the patients required more than 200 Units/kg TIW to maintain their hematocrit in the suggested target range. In pediatric hemodialysis and peritoneal dialysis patients, the median maintenance dose was 167 Units/kg/week (49 to 447 Units/kg per week) and 76 Units/kg per week (24 to 323 Units/kg/week) administered in divided doses (TIW or BIW), respectively to achieve the target range of 30% to 36%.
If the transferrin saturation is greater than 20%, the dose of EPOGEN® may be increased. Such dose increases should not be made more frequently than once a month, unless clinically indicated, as the response time of the hemoglobin to a dose increase can be 2 to 6 weeks. Hemoglobin should be measured twice weekly for 2 to 6 weeks following dose increases. In adult patients with CRF not on dialysis, the dose should also be individualized to maintain hemoglobin levels between 10 to 12 g/dL. EPOGEN® doses of 75 to 150 Units/kg/week have been shown to maintain hematocrits of 36% to 38% for up to 6 months.
Lack or Loss of Response: If a patient fails to respond or maintain a response, an evaluation for causative factors should be undertaken (see WARNINGS: Pure Red Cell Aplasia, PRECAUTIONS: Lack or Loss of Response, and PRECAUTIONS: Iron Evaluation). If the transferrin saturation is less than 20%, supplemental iron should be administered.
Zidovudine-treated HIV-infected Patients
Prior to beginning EPOGEN®, it is recommended that the endogenous serum erythropoietin level be determined (prior to transfusion). Available evidence suggests that patients

receiving zidovudine with endogenous serum erythropoietin levels > 500 mUnits/mL are unlikely to respond to therapy with EPOGEN®.

In zidovudine-treated HIV-infected patients the dosage of EPOGEN® should be titrated for each patient to achieve and maintain the lowest hemoglobin level sufficient to avoid the need for blood transfusion and not to exceed the upper safety limit of 12 g/dL.

Starting Dose: For adult patients with serum erythropoietin levels ≤ 500 mUnits/mL who are receiving a dose of zidovudine ≤ 4200 mg/week, the recommended starting dose of EPOGEN® is 100 Units/kg as an IV or SC injection TIW for 8 weeks. For pediatric patients, see PRECAUTIONS: PEDIATRIC USE.

Increase Dose: During the dose adjustment phase of therapy, the hemoglobin should be monitored weekly. If the response is not satisfactory in terms of reducing transfusion requirements or increasing hemoglobin after 8 weeks of therapy, the dose of EPOGEN® can be increased by 50 to 100 Units/kg TIW. Response should be evaluated every 4 to 8 weeks thereafter and the dose adjusted accordingly by 50 to 100 Units/kg increments TIW. If patients have not responded satisfactorily to an EPOGEN® dose of 300 Units/kg TIW, it is unlikely that they will respond to higher doses of EPOGEN®.

Maintenance Dose: After attainment of the desired response (ie, reduced transfusion requirements or increased hemoglobin), the dose of EPOGEN® should be titrated to maintain the response based on factors such as variations in zidovudine dose and the presence of intercurrent infectious or inflammatory episodes. If the hemoglobin exceeds the upper safety limit of 12 g/dL, the dose should be discontinued until the hemoglobin drops below 11 g/dL. The dose should be reduced by 25% when treatment is resumed and then titrated to maintain the desired hemoglobin.

Cancer Patients on Chemotherapy

Only prescribers enrolled in the ESA APPRISE Oncology Program may prescribe and/or dispense EPOGEN® (see **WARNINGS: ESA APPRISE Oncology Program**).

Although no specific serum erythropoietin level has been established which predicts which patients would be unlikely to respond to EPOGEN® therapy, treatment of patients with grossly elevated serum erythropoietin levels (eg, > 200 mUnits/mL) is not recommended. Therapy should not be initiated at hemoglobin levels ≥ 10 g/dL. The hemoglobin should be monitored on a weekly basis in patients receiving EPOGEN® therapy until hemoglobin becomes stable. The dose of EPOGEN® should be titrated for each patient to achieve and maintain the lowest hemoglobin level sufficient to avoid the need for blood transfusion (see recommended Dose Modifications, below).

Recommended Dose: The initial recommended dose of EPOGEN® in adults is 150 Units/kg SC TIW or 40,000 Units SC Weekly. The initial recommended dose of EPOGEN® in pediatric patients is 600 Units/kg IV weekly. Discontinue EPOGEN® following the completion of a chemotherapy course (see BOXED WARNINGS: *Cancer*).

Dose Modification

TIW Dosing

Starting Dose:

Adults	150 Units/kg SC TIW
Reduce Dose by 25% when:	Hemoglobin reaches a level needed to avoid transfusion or increases > 1 g/dL in any 2-week period.
Withhold Dose if:	Hemoglobin exceeds a level needed to avoid transfusion. Restart at 25% below the previous dose when the hemoglobin approaches a level where transfusions may be required.
Increase Dose to 300 Units/kg TIW if:	Response is not satisfactory (no reduction in transfusion requirements or rise in hemoglobin) after 4 weeks to achieve and maintain the lowest hemoglobin level sufficient to avoid the need for RBC transfusion.

Discontinue:	If after 8 weeks of therapy there is no response as measured by hemoglobin levels or if transfusions are still required.

Weekly Dosing

Starting Dose:

Adults	40,000 Units SC
Pediatrics	600 Units/kg IV (maximum 40,000 Units)
Reduce Dose by 25% when:	Hemoglobin reaches a level needed to avoid transfusion or increases > 1 g/dL in any 2-weeks.
Withhold Dose if:	Hemoglobin exceeds a level needed to avoid transfusion and restart at 25% below the previous dose when the hemoglobin approaches a level where transfusions may be required.
Increase Dose if: For Adults: 60,000 Units SC Weekly	Response is not satisfactory (no increase in hemoglobin by ≥ 1 g/dL after 4 weeks of therapy, in the absence of a RBC transfusion) to achieve and maintain the lowest hemoglobin level sufficient to avoid the need for RBC transfusion.
For Pediatrics: 900 Units/kg IV (maximum 60,000 Units) if:	
Discontinue:	If after 8 weeks of therapy there is no response as measured by hemoglobin levels or if transfusions are still required.

Surgery Patients

Prior to initiating treatment with EPOGEN® a hemoglobin should be obtained to establish that it is > 10 to ≤ 13 g/dL.[17] The recommended dose of EPOGEN® is 300 Units/kg/day subcutaneously for 10 days before surgery, on the day of surgery, and for 4 days after surgery.

An alternate dose schedule is 600 Units/kg EPOGEN® subcutaneously in once weekly doses (21, 14, and 7 days before surgery) plus a fourth dose on the day of surgery.[18]

All patients should receive adequate iron supplementation. Iron supplementation should be initiated no later than the beginning of treatment with EPOGEN® and should continue throughout the course of therapy. Deep venous thrombosis prophylaxis should be strongly considered (see BOXED WARNINGS).

PREPARATION AND ADMINISTRATION OF EPOGEN®

1. Do not shake. It is not necessary to shake EPOGEN®. Prolonged vigorous shaking may denature any glycoprotein, rendering it biologically inactive.

2. Protect the solution from light. Parenteral drug products should be inspected visually for particulate matter and discoloration prior to administration. Do not use any vials exhibiting particulate matter or discoloration.

3. Using aseptic techniques, attach a sterile needle to a sterile syringe. Remove the flip top from the vial containing EPOGEN®, and wipe the septum with a disinfectant. Insert the needle into the vial, and withdraw into the syringe an appropriate volume of solution.

4. **Single-dose:** 1 mL vial contains no preservative. Use one dose per vial; do not re-enter the vial. Discard unused portions.
   Multidose: 1 mL and 2 mL vials contain preservative. Store at 2° to 8° C after initial entry and between doses. Discard 21 days after initial entry.

5. Do not dilute or administer in conjunction with other drug solutions. However, at the time of SC administration, preservative-free EPOGEN® from single-use vials may be admixed in a syringe with bacteriostatic 0.9% sodium chloride injection, USP, with benzyl alcohol 0.9% (bacteriostatic saline) at a 1:1 ratio using aseptic technique. The benzyl alcohol in the bacteriostatic saline acts as a local anesthetic which may ameliorate SC injection

site discomfort. Admixing is not necessary when using the multidose vials of EPOGEN® containing benzyl alcohol.

HOW SUPPLIED

EPOGEN®, containing Epoetin alfa, is available in the following packages:

1 mL **Single-dose, Preservative-free** Solution
2000 Units/mL (NDC 55513-126-10)
3000 Units/mL (NDC 55513-267-10)
4000 Units/mL (NDC 55513-148-10)
10,000 Units/mL (NDC 55513-144-10)
40,000 Units/mL (NDC 55513-823-10)
Supplied in dispensing packs containing 10 single-dose vials.

2 mL **Multidose, Preserved** Solution
10,000 Units/mL (NDC 55513-283-10)
1 mL **Multidose, Preserved** Solution
20,000 Units/mL (NDC 55513-478-10)
Supplied in dispensing packs containing 10 multidose vials.

STORAGE

Store at 2° to 8° C (36° to 46° F). Do not freeze or shake. Protect from light.

REFERENCES

1. Egrie JC, Strickland TW, Lane J, et al. Characterization and Biological Effects of Recombinant Human Erythropoietin. *Immunobiol.* 1986;72:213-224.

2. Graber SE, Krantz SB. Erythropoietin and the Control of Red Cell Production. *Ann Rev Med.* 1978;29:51-66.

3. Eschbach JW, Adamson JW. Anemia of End-Stage Renal Disease (ESRD). *Kidney Intl.* 1985;28:1-5.

4. Eschbach JW, Egrie JC, Downing MR, et al. Correction of the Anemia of End-Stage Renal Disease with Recombinant Human Erythropoietin. *NEJM.* 1987;316:73-78.

5. Eschbach JW, Abdulhadi MH, Browne JK, et al. Recombinant Human Erythropoietin in Anemic Patients with End-Stage Renal Disease. *Ann Intern Med.* 1989;111:992-1000.

6. Eschbach JW, Egrie JC, Downing MR, et al. The Use of Recombinant Human Erythropoietin (r-HuEPO): Effect in End-Stage Renal Disease (ESRD). In: Friedman, Beyer, DeSanto, Giordano, eds. *Prevention of Chronic Uremia.* Philadelphia, PA: Field and Wood Inc; 1989: 148-155.

7. Egrie JC, Eschbach JW, McGuire T, Adamson JW. Pharmacokinetics of Recombinant Human Erythropoietin (rHuEPO) Administered to Hemodialysis (HD) Patients. *Kidney Intl.* 1988;33:262.

8. Paganini E, Garcia J, Ellis P, et al. Clinical Sequelae of Correction of Anemia with Recombinant Human Erythropoietin (r-HuEPO); Urea Kinetics, Dialyzer Function and Reuse. *Am J Kid Dis.* 1988;11:16.

9. Delano BG, Lundin AP, Golansky R, et al. Dialyzer Urea and Creatinine Clearances Not Significantly Changed in rHuEPO Treated Maintenance Hemodialysis (MD) Patients. *Kidney Intl.* 1988;33:219.

10. Stivelman J, Van Wyck D, Ogden D. Use of Recombinant Erythropoietin (r-HuEPO) with High Flux Dialysis (HFD) Does Not Worsen Azotemia or Shorten Access Survival. *Kidney Intl.* 1988;33:239.

11. Lim VS, DeGowin RL, Zavala D, et al. Recombinant Human Erythropoietin Treatment in Pre-Dialysis Patients: A Double-Blind Placebo Controlled Trial. *Ann Int Med.* 1989;110:108-114.

12. Stone WJ, Graber SE, Krantz SB, et al. Treatment of the Anemia of Pre-Dialysis Patients with Recombinant Human Erythropoietin: A Randomized, Placebo-Controlled Trial. *Am J Med Sci.* 1988;296:171-179.

13. Braun A, Ding R, Seidel C, Fies T, Kurtz A, Scharer K. Pharmacokinetics of recombinant human erythropoietin applied subcutaneously to children with chronic renal failure. *Pediatr Nephrol.* 1993;7:61-64.

14. Geva P, Sherwood JB. Pharmacokinetics of recombinant human erythropoietin (rHuEPO) in pediatric patients on chronic cycling peritoneal dialysis (CCPD). *Blood.* 1991;78 (Suppl 1):91a.

15. Jabs K, Grant JR, Harmon W, *et al.* Pharmacokinetics of Epoetin alfa (rHuEPO) in pediatric hemodialysis (HD) patients. *J Am Soc Nephrol.* 1991;2:380.

16. Kling PJ, Widness JA, Guillery EN, Veng-Pedersen P, Peters C, DeAlarcon PA. Pharmacokinetics and pharmacodynamics of erythropoietin during therapy in an infant with renal failure. *J Pediatr.* 1992;121:822-825.

17. deAndrade JR and Jove M. Baseline Hemoglobin as a Predictor of Risk of Transfusion and Response to Epoetin alfa in Orthoperdic Surgery Patients. *Am. J. of Orthoped.* 1996;25 (8):533-542.

18. Goldberg MA and McCutchen JW. A Safety and Efficacy Comparison Study of Two Dosing Regimens of Epoetin alfa in Patients Undergoing Major Orthopedic Surgery. *Am. J. of Orthoped.* 1996;25 (8):544-552.

19. Faris PM and Ritter MA. The Effects of Recombinant Human Erythropoietin on Perioperative Transfusion

Requirements in Patients Having a Major Orthopedic Operation. *J. Bone and Joint surgery*. 1996;78-A:62-72.

20. Amgen Inc., data on file.

21. Eschbach JW, Kelly MR, Haley NR, et al. Treatment of the Anemia of Progressive Renal Failure with Recombinant Human Erythropoietin. *NEJM*. 1989;321:158-163.

22. The US Recombinant Human Erythropoietin Predialysis Study Group. Double-Blind, Placebo-Controlled Study of the Therapeutic Use of Recombinant Human Erythropoietin for Anemia Associated with Chronic Renal Failure in Predialysis Patients. *Am J Kid Dis*. 1991;18:50-59.

23. Ortho Biologics, Inc., data on file.

24. Danna RP, Rudnick SA, Abels RI. Erythropoietin Therapy for the Anemia Associated with AIDS and AIDS Therapy and Cancer. In: MB Garnick, ed. *Erythropoietin in Clinical Applications - An International Perspective*. New York, NY: Marcel Dekker; 1990:301-324.

25. Fischl M, Galpin JE, Levine JD, et al. Recombinant Human Erythropoietin for Patients with AIDS Treated with Zidovudine. *NEJM*. 1990;322:1488-1493.

26. Laupacis A. Effectiveness of Perioperative Recombinant Human Eyrthropoietin in Elective Hip Replacement. *Lancet*. 1993;341:1228-1232.

27. Campos A, Garin EH. Therapy of renal anemia in children and adolescents with recombinant human erythropoietin (rHuEPO). *Clin Pediatr* (Phila). 1992;31:94-99.

28. Montini G, Zacchello G, Baraldi E, et al. Benefits and risks of anemia correction with recombinant human erythropoietin in children maintained by hemodialysis. *J Pediatr*. 1990;117:556-560.

29. Offner G, Hoyer PF, Latta K, Winkler L, Brodehl J, Scigalla P. One year's experience with recombinant erythropoietin in children undergoing continuous ambulatory or cycling peritoneal dialysis. *Pediatr Nephrol*. 1990;4:498-500.

30. Muller-Wiefel DE, Scigalla P. Specific problems of renal anemia in childhood. *Contrib Nephrol*. 1988;66:71-84.

31. Scharer K, Klare B, Dressel P, Gretz N. Treatment of renal anemia by subcutaneous erythropoietin in children with preterminal chronic renal failure. *Acta Paediatr*. 1993;82:953-958.

32. Mueller BU, Jacobsen RN, Jarosinski P, et al. Erythropoietin for zidovudine-associated anemia in children with HIV infection. *Pediatr AIDS and HIV Infect: Fetus to Adolesc*. 1994;5:169-173.

33. Zuccotti GV, Plebani A, Biasucci G, et al. Granulocyte-colony stimulating factor and erythropoietin therapy in children with human immunodeficiency virus infection. *J Int Med Res*. 1996;24:115-121.

34. Raskin NH, Fishman RA. Neurologic Disorders in Renal Failure (First of Two Parts). *NEJM*. 1976;294:143-148.

35. Raskin NH and Fishman RA. Neurologic Disorders in Renal Failure (Second of Two Parts). *NEJM*. 1976;294:204-210.

36. Messing RO, Simon RP. Seizures as a Manifestation of Systemic Disease. *Neurologic Clinics*. 1986;4:563-584.

37. Besarab A, Bolton WK, Browne JK, et al. The effects of normal as compared with low hematocrit values in patients with cardiac disease who are receiving hemodialysis and epoetin. *NEJM*. 1998;339:584-90.

38. Henke, M, Laszig, R, Rübe, C., et al. Erythropoietin to treat head and neck cancer patients with anaemia undergoing radiotherapy: randomized, double-blind, placebo-controlled trial. *The Lancet*. 2003; 362: 1255-1260.

39. Widness JA, Veng-Pedersen P, Peters C, Pereira LM, Schmidt RL, Lowe SL. Erythropoietin Pharmacokinetics in Premature Infants: Developmental, Nonlinearity, and Treatment Effects. *JAppl Physiol*. 1996;80 (1): 140-148.

40. Singh AK, Szczech L, Tang KL, et al. Correction of Anemia with Epoetin Alfa in Chronic Kidney Disease, *N Engl j Med*. 2006; 355:2085-98.

41. Bohlius J, Wilson J, Seidenfeld J, et at. Recombinant HumanErythropoietins and Cancer Patients: Updated Meta-Analysis of 57 Studies Including 9353 Patients. *J Natl Cancer Inst*. 2006; 98:708-14.

42. D'Ambra MN, Gray RJ, Hillman R, et al. Effect of Recombinant Human Erythropoietin on Transfusion Risk in Coronary Bypass Patients. *Ann Thorac Surg*. 1997; 64: 1686-93.

43. Leyland-Jones B, Semiglazov V, Pawlicki M, et al. Maintaining Normal Hemoglobin Levels With Epoetin Alfa in Mainly Nonanemic Patients With Metastatic Breast Cancer Receiving First-Line Chemotherapy: A Survival Study. *JCO*. 2005; 23(25): 1-13.

This product's label may have been revised after this insert was used in production. For further product information and the current package insert, please visit www.amgen.com or call our medical information department toll-free at 1-800-77AMGEN (1-800-772-6436).

Manufactured by:
Amgen Manufacturing, Limited, a subsidiary of Amgen Inc.
One Amgen Center Drive
Thousand Oaks, CA 91320-1799
©1989-2010 Amgen Inc. All rights reserved.
1xxxxxx – v24
Revised: 02/2010

MEDICATION GUIDE

Epogen® (Ee-po-jen)
(epoetin alfa)

Read this Medication Guide before you start Epogen, each time you refill your prescription, and if you are told by your healthcare provider that there is new information about Epogen. This Medication Guide does not take the place of talking to your healthcare provider about your medical condition or your treatment. Talk with your healthcare provider regularly about the use of Epogen and ask if there is new information about Epogen.

What is the most important information I should know about Epogen?

Using Epogen can lead to death or other serious side effects.

Patients with cancer:

Your healthcare provider has received special training through the ESA APPRISE Oncology Program in order to prescribe Epogen. Before you can begin to receive Epogen, you must sign the ESA APPRISE Oncology Patient and Healthcare Professional (HCP) Acknowledgement Form to document that your healthcare provider discussed the risks of Epogen with you. When you sign this form, you are stating that you are aware of the risks associated with use of Epogen.

These risks include that your tumor may grow faster and you may die sooner when Epogen is used experimentally to try to raise your hemoglobin beyond the amount needed to avoid red blood cell transfusion or if you are not getting strong doses of chemotherapy. It is not known whether these risks exist when Epogen is given according to the FDA-approved directions for use.

You should discuss with your doctor:
• Why Epogen treatment is being prescribed.
• What are the chances you will get red blood cell transfusions if you do not take Epogen.
• What are the chances you will get red blood cell transfusions even if you take Epogen.
• How taking Epogen may affect the success of your cancer treatment.

If you decide to take Epogen, your healthcare provider should prescribe the smallest dose of Epogen to lower the chance of getting red blood cell transfusions.
• After you have finished your chemotherapy course, Epogen treatment should be stopped.
• Epogen does not improve the symptoms of anemia (lower than normal number of red blood cells), quality of life, fatigue, or well-being for patients with cancer.

All patients, including patients with cancer or chronic kidney failure:

• You may get serious heart problems such as heart attack, stroke, heart failure, and may die sooner if you are treated with Epogen to a hemoglobin level above 12 g/dL.
• You may get blood clots at any time while taking Epogen. If you are receiving Epogen and you are going to have surgery, talk to your healthcare provider about whether or not you need to take a blood thinner to lessen the chance of blood clots during or following surgery. Clots can form in blood vessels (veins), especially in your leg (deep venous thrombosis or DVT). Pieces of a blood clot may travel to the lungs and block the blood circulation in the lungs (pulmonary embolus).

Call your healthcare provider or get medical help right away if you have any of these symptoms of blood clots:
• Chest pain
• Trouble breathing or shortness of breath
• Pain in your legs, with or without swelling
• A cool or pale arm or leg
• Sudden confusion, trouble speaking, or trouble understanding others' speech
• Sudden numbness or weakness in your face, arm, or leg, especially on one side of your body
• Sudden trouble seeing
• Sudden trouble walking, dizziness, loss of balance or coordination
• Loss of consciousness (fainting)
• Hemodialysis vascular access stops working. If you are a patient with chronic kidney failure and have a hemodialysis vascular access, blood clots may form in this access.

Also see "**What are the possible side effects of Epogen?**" below.

What is Epogen?

Epogen is a man-made form of the protein human erythropoietin that is given to patients to lessen the need for red blood cell transfusions. Epogen stimulates your bone marrow to make more red blood cells. Having more red blood cells raises your hemoglobin level. If your hemoglobin level stays too high or if your hemoglobin goes up too quickly, this may lead to serious health problems which may result in death. These serious health problems may happen even if you take Epogen and do not have an increase in your hemoglobin level.

Epogen may be used to treat a lower than normal number of red blood cells (anemia) if it is caused by:
• Chronic kidney failure (you may or may not be on dialysis)
• Chemotherapy that is used for at least two months to treat some types of cancer
• A medicine called zidovudine (AZT) used to treat HIV infection

Epogen may also be used if you are scheduled for certain surgeries with a lot of blood loss to reduce the chance you will need red blood cell transfusions.

Epogen should not be used for treatment of anemia:
• In place of emergency treatment (red blood cell transfusions)
• If you have cancer and you are not receiving chemotherapy that may cause anemia
• If your cancer has a high chance of being cured

Epogen should not be used if you are scheduled for certain surgeries and you are able and willing to donate blood prior to surgery.

Who should not take Epogen?

Do not take Epogen if you:
• Have cancer and have not been counseled by your healthcare provider regarding the risks of Epogen and signed the ESA APPRISE Oncology Program Patient and Healthcare Professional (HCP) Acknowledgement Form before you begin to receive Epogen.
• Have high blood pressure that is not controlled (uncontrolled hypertension).
• Have been told by your healthcare provider that you have or have ever had a type of anemia called Pure Red Cell Aplasia (PRCA) that starts after treatment with Epogen or other erythropoietin medicines.
• Have allergies to any of the ingredients in Epogen. See the end of this Medication Guide for a complete list of ingredients in Epogen.

Do not give Epogen from multidose vials to premature babies.

What should I tell my healthcare provider before taking Epogen?

Epogen may not be right for you. **Tell your healthcare provider about all your health conditions**, including if you:
• Have heart disease.
• Have high blood pressure.
• Have had a seizure (convulsion) or stroke.
• Are pregnant or planning to become pregnant. It is not known if Epogen may harm your unborn baby. Talk with your healthcare provider about possible pregnancy and birth control choices that are right for you.
• Are breast-feeding or planning to breast-feed. It is not known if Epogen passes into breast milk.

Tell your healthcare provider about all the medicines you take, including prescription and nonprescription medicines, vitamins, and herbal supplements.

Know the medicines you take. Keep a list of your medicines with you and show it to your healthcare provider when you get a new medicine.

How should I take Epogen?

Patients with cancer:

Before you begin to receive Epogen, your healthcare provider will:
• Ask you to review this Epogen Medication Guide
• Explain the risks of Epogen and answer all your questions about Epogen
• Have you sign the ESA APPRISE Oncology Program Patient and Healthcare Professional (HCP) Acknowledgement Form

All patients:

• Continue to follow your healthcare provider's instructions for diet, dialysis, and medicines, including medicines for high blood pressure, while taking Epogen.
• Have your blood pressure checked as instructed by your healthcare provider.
• If you or your caregiver has been trained to give Epogen shots (injections) at home:
  • Be sure that you read, understand, and follow the "Patient Instructions for Use" that come with Epogen.
  • Take Epogen exactly as your healthcare provider tells you to. Do not change the dose of Epogen unless told to do so by your healthcare provider.
  • Your healthcare provider will show you how much Epogen to use, how to inject it, how often it should be injected, and how to safely throw away the used vial, syringes, and needles.
  • If you miss a dose of Epogen, call your healthcare provider right away and ask what to do.
  • If you take more than the prescribed amount of Epogen, call your healthcare provider right away.

What are the possible side effects of Epogen?

Epogen may cause serious side effects. See "**What is the most important information I should know about Epogen?**" Other side effects of Epogen, which may also be serious, include:

- **High blood pressure in patients with chronic kidney failure.** Your blood pressure may go up or be difficult to control with blood pressure medicine while taking Epogen. This can happen even if you have never had high blood pressure before. Your healthcare provider should check your blood pressure often. If your blood pressure does go up, your healthcare provider may prescribe new or more blood pressure medicine.
- **Seizures.** If you have any seizures while taking Epogen, get medical help right away and tell your healthcare provider.
- **Antibodies to Epogen.** Your body may make antibodies to Epogen. These antibodies can block or lessen your body's ability to make red blood cells and cause you to have severe anemia. Call your healthcare provider if you have unusual tiredness, lack of energy, dizziness, or fainting. You may need to stop taking Epogen.
- **Serious allergic reactions.** Serious allergic reactions can cause a rash over your whole body, shortness of breath, wheezing, dizziness and fainting because of a drop in blood pressure, swelling around your mouth or eyes, fast pulse, or sweating. If you have a serious allergic reaction, stop using Epogen and call your healthcare provider or get medical help right away.
- **Dangers of giving Epogen to premature babies.** Epogen from multi-dose vials contain benzyl alcohol. Do not give Epogen from multidose vials to premature babies because it can cause death and brain damage.

Common side effects of Epogen include:
- Rash
- Swelling in your legs and arms
- Injection site reaction, including irritation and pain

These are not all of the possible side effects of Epogen. Your healthcare provider can give you a more complete list. Tell your healthcare provider about any side effects that bother you or that do not go away.

Call your doctor for medical advice about side effects. You may report side effects to FDA at 1-800-FDA-1088.

How should I store Epogen?

- Store Epogen in the refrigerator between 36°F to 46°F (2°C to 8°C).
- **Do not freeze.** Do not use a vial of Epogen that has been frozen.
- Keep away from direct light.
- Do not shake Epogen.
- Throw away multidose vials of Epogen after 21 days from the first day that you put a needle into the vial.
- Single use vials of Epogen should be used only one time. Throw the vial away after use even if there is medicine left in the vial.

Keep Epogen and all medicines out of the reach of children.

General information about Epogen

Medicines are sometimes prescribed for purposes other than those listed in a Medication Guide. Use Epogen only for the condition for which it has been prescribed. Do not give Epogen to other people even if they have the same symptoms that you may have. It may harm them.

This Medication Guide summarizes the most important information about Epogen. If you would like more information about Epogen, talk to your healthcare provider. You can ask your healthcare provider or pharmacist for information about Epogen that is written for healthcare professionals. For more information, go to the following website: www.epogen.com or call 1-800-77-AMGEN.

What are the ingredients in Epogen?

Active Ingredient: epoetin alfa

Inactive Ingredients: All formulations include albumin (human), sodium citrate, sodium chloride, and citric acid in Water for Injection. Multidose vials contain benzyl alcohol. Certain formulations also contain sodium phosphate monobasic monohydrate and sodium phosphate dibasic anhydrate.

Manufactured by:
Amgen Manufacturing, Limited, a subsidiary of Amgen Inc.
One Amgen Center Drive
Thousand Oaks, CA 91320-1799
© 1989-2010 Amgen Inc. All rights reserved.
1xxxxxx- v2
Revised: 02/2010
This Medication Guide has been approved by the U.S. Food and Drug Administration.

PATIENT INSTRUCTIONS FOR USE

Epogen® (Ee-po-jen)
(epoetin alfa)

Use these instructions if you or your caregiver has been trained to give Epogen injections at home. Do not give yourself the injection unless you have received training from your healthcare provider. If you are not sure about giving the injection or you have questions, ask your healthcare provider for help.

Before reading these instructions for use, read the Medication Guide that comes with Epogen for the most important information you need to know.

When you receive your Epogen vial and syringes make sure that:

- The name Epogen appears on the carton and vial label.
- The expiration date on the vial label has not passed. Do not use a vial of Epogen after the expiration date on the label.
- The dose strength of the Epogen vial (number of Units per mL on the vial label) is the same as your healthcare provider prescribed.
- You understand what the dose strength of Epogen means. Epogen vials come in several dose strengths. For example, the dose strength may be described as 10,000 Units/mL on the vial label. This strength means that 10,000 Units of medicine are contained in each 1 mL (milliliter) of liquid. Your healthcare provider may also refer to a mL as a "cc." One mL is the same as one "cc."
- The Epogen liquid in the vial is clear and colorless. Do not use Epogen if the liquid in the vial looks discolored or cloudy, or if the liquid has lumps, flakes, or particles.
- The Epogen vial has a color cap on the top of the vial. Do not use a vial of Epogen if the color cap on the top of the vial has been removed or is missing.
- Use only the type of disposable syringe and needle that your healthcare provider has prescribed.
- Do not shake Epogen. If shaking has occurred, the solution in the vial may look foamy and should not be used.
- Do not freeze Epogen. Do not use a vial of Epogen that has been frozen.
- Keep Epogen away from light.

How should I prepare for an injection of Epogen?

- Always keep an extra syringe and needle on hand.
- Follow your healthcare provider's instructions on how to measure your dose of Epogen. This dose will be measured in Units per mL or cc (1 mL is the same as 1 cc). Use a syringe that is marked in tenths of mL (for example, 0.2 mL or 0.2 cc). Using the wrong syringe can lead to a mistake in your dose and you could inject too much or too little Epogen.

Only use disposable syringes and needles. Use the syringes and needles only one time and then throw them away as instructed by your healthcare provider.

What do I need to know about the different types of Epogen vials?

Epogen comes in two different types of vials.
- Single-Use Vials
- Multidose-Use Vials

Single-Use Vials

If you have been prescribed Epogen vials for single use:
- Single-Use vials of Epogen come in several different strengths (Units per mL). For example, the vial label may say the strength is 2,000 Units/mL, which means the vial contains 2,000 Units of medicine in 1 mL. Injecting 1 mL of this strength means you will receive 2,000 Units of Epogen.
- Double-check to be sure you are using a vial that contains the correct strength of Epogen.
- The Single-Use Vials cannot be used more than one time and any unused medicine in the vial should be thrown away as directed by your healthcare provider.

Multidose-Use Vials

If you have been prescribed Epogen vials for use multiple times:
- Multidose vials of Epogen may be used to inject more than one dose of Epogen, as prescribed by your healthcare provider.
- Multidose vials of Epogen come in 1 mL and 2 mL vials.
  - 1 mL vials contain 20,000 Units of Epogen in 1 mL of liquid (this means each vial contains a total of 20,000 Units of Epogen).
  - 2 mL vials contain 10,000 Units of Epogen in each 1 mL of liquid, and since the vials contain a total of 2 mL of liquid, each vial contains a total of 20,000 Units of Epogen.
- After removing a dose from the vial, store the vial in the refrigerator (but not the freezer). Do not store the vial for more than 21 days.
- If the vial is stored for more than 21 days, or when a vial no longer contains a full dose of medicine, throw the vial away as directed by your healthcare provider.

Important: Follow these instructions exactly to help avoid infections.

Preparing the dose:
1. Remove the vial of Epogen from the refrigerator. During this time, protect the solution from light.
2. Do not use a Single-Use vial of Epogen more than one time.
3. Do not shake Epogen.
4. Gather the other supplies you will need for your injection (vial, syringe, alcohol wipes, cotton ball, and a puncture-proof container for throwing away the syringe and needle). See Figure 1.

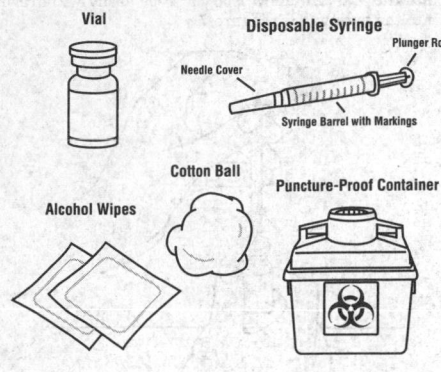

Figure 1

5. Check the date on the Epogen vial to be sure that the drug has not expired.
6. Wash your hands well with soap and water before preparing the medicine. See Figure 2.

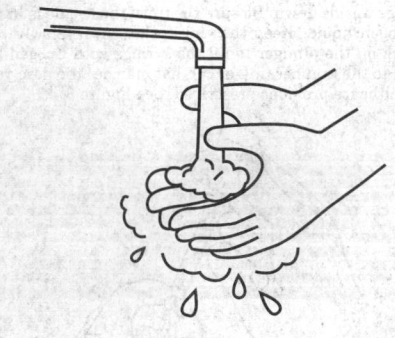

Figure 2

7. Flip off the protective color cap on the top of the vial. Do not remove the grey rubber stopper. Wipe the top of the grey rubber stopper with an alcohol wipe. See Figures 3 and 4.

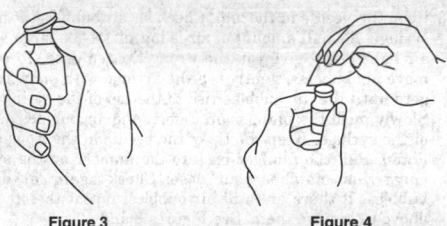

Figure 3   **Figure 4**

8. Check the package containing the syringe. If the package has been opened or damaged, do not use that syringe. Throw away the syringe in the puncture-proof disposable container. If the syringe package is undamaged, open the package and remove the syringe.
9. Using a syringe and needle that has been recommended by your healthcare provider, carefully remove the needle cover. See Figure 5. Then draw air into the syringe by pulling back on the plunger. The amount of air drawn into the syringe should be equal to the amount (mL or cc) of the Epogen dose prescribed by your healthcare provider. See Figure 6.

Pull Straight Off

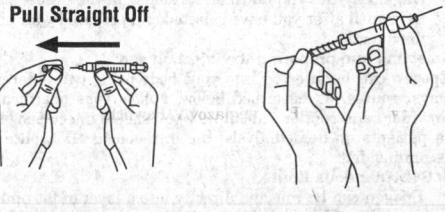

Figure 5   **Figure 6**

10. With the vial on a flat work surface, insert the needle straight down through the grey rubber stopper of the Epogen vial. See Figure 7.

11. Push the plunger of the syringe down to inject the air from the syringe into the vial of Epogen. The air injected into the vial will allow Epogen to be easily withdrawn into the syringe. See Figure 7.

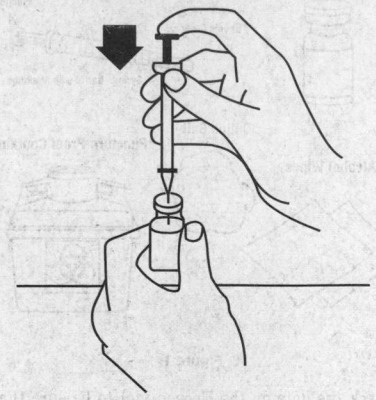

Figure 7

12. Keep the needle inside the vial. Turn the vial and syringe upside down. Be sure the tip of the needle is in the Epogen liquid. Keep the vial upside down. Slowly pull back on the plunger to fill the syringe with Epogen liquid to the number (mL or cc) that matches the dose your healthcare provider prescribed. See Figure 8.

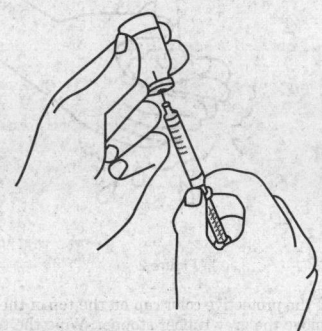

Figure 8

13. Keep the needle in the vial. Check for air bubbles in the syringe. A small amount of air is harmless. Too large an air bubble will give you the wrong Epogen dose. To remove air bubbles, gently tap the syringe with your fingers until the air bubbles rise to the top of the syringe. Slowly push the plunger up to force the air bubbles out of the syringe. Keep the tip of the needle in the Epogen liquid. Pull the plunger back to the number on the syringe that matches your dose. Check again for air bubbles. If there are still air bubbles, repeat the steps above to remove them. See Figures 9 and 10.

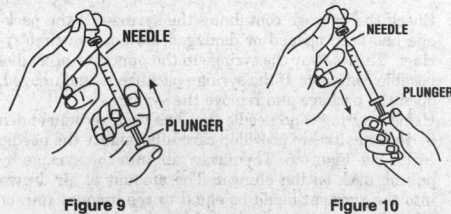

Figure 9   **Figure 10**

14. Double-check that you have the correct dose in the syringe. Lay the vial down on its side with the needle still in it until after you have selected and prepared your site for injection.

Selecting and preparing the injection site:
Epogen can be injected into your body using two different ways (routes) as described below. Follow your healthcare provider's instructions about how you should inject Epogen. In patients on hemodialysis, the intravenous (IV) route is recommended.

1. Subcutaneous Route:
• Epogen can be injected directly into a layer of fat under your skin. This is called a subcutaneous injection. When giving subcutaneous injections, follow your healthcare provider's instructions about changing the site for each injection. You may wish to write down the site where you have injected.

• Do not inject Epogen into an area that is tender, red, bruised, hard, or has scars or stretch marks. Recommended sites for injection are presented in Figure 11 below, including:
  • The outer area of the upper arms
  • The abdomen (except for the 2-inch area around the navel)
  • The front of the middle thighs
  • The upper outer area of the buttocks

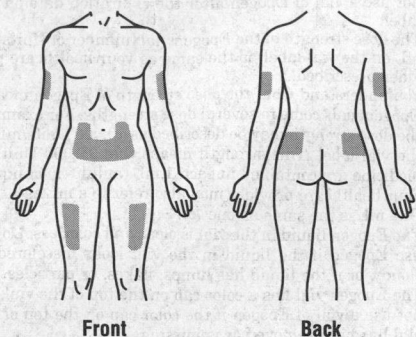

Front   **Back**

Figure 11

• Clean the skin with an alcohol wipe where the injection is to be made. Be careful not to touch the skin that has been wiped clean. See Figure 12.

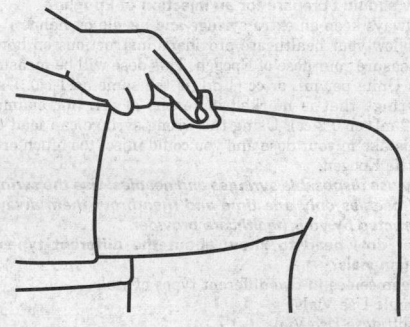

Figure 12

• Double-check that the correct amount of Epogen is in the syringe.
• Remove the prepared syringe and needle from the vial of Epogen and hold it in the hand that you will use to inject the medicine.
• Use the other hand to pinch a fold of skin at the cleaned injection site. Do not touch the cleaned area of skin. See Figure 13.

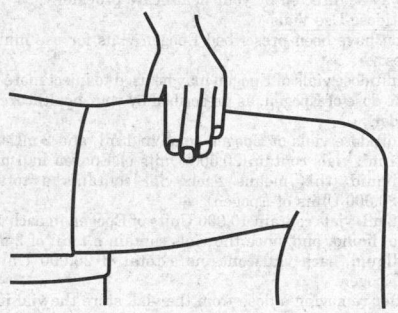

Figure 13

• Hold the syringe like you would hold a pencil. Use a quick "dart-like" motion to insert the needle either straight up and down (90-degree angle) or at a slight angle (45 degrees) into the skin. Let go of the skin and pull the plunger back slightly. If blood comes into the syringe, do not inject Epogen since the needle may have entered a blood vessel; instead, withdraw the syringe, discard it in the puncture-proof container. Prepare a new syringe of Epogen using the instructions above. Clean a new area of skin. In this new area of clean skin, again

insert a new needle (as you did before), and again pull the plunger back slightly. If blood does not enter the syringe, inject the Epogen by pushing the plunger all the way down. See Figure 14.

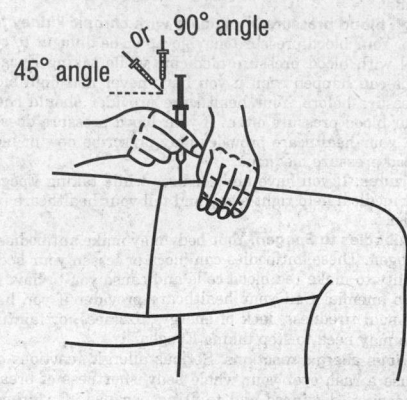

Figure 14

• Pull the needle out of the skin and press a cotton ball or gauze over the injection site and hold it there for several seconds. Do not recap the needle.
• Dispose of the used syringe and needle as described below. Do not reuse syringes and needles.

2. Intravenous Route:
• Epogen can be injected in your vein through a special access port put in by your healthcare provider. This type of Epogen injection is called an intravenous (IV) injection. This route is usually for hemodialysis patients.
• If you have a dialysis vascular access, make sure it is working by checking it as your healthcare provider has shown you. Be sure to let your healthcare provider know right away if you are having any problems, or if you have any questions.
• Wipe off the venous port of the hemodialysis tubing with an alcohol wipe. See Figure 15.

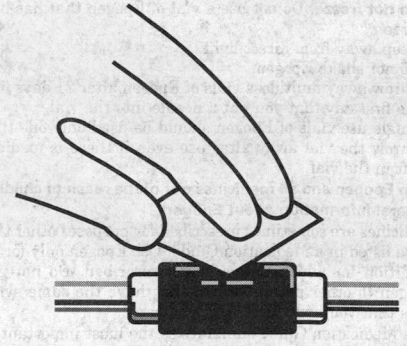

Figure 15

• Insert the needle of the syringe into the cleaned venous port and push the plunger all the way down to inject all the Epogen. See Figure 16.

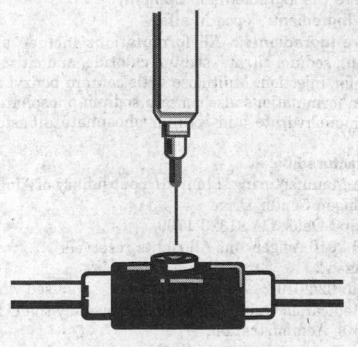

Figure 16

• Remove the syringe from the venous port. Do not recap the needle.
• Dispose of the used syringe and needle as described below.

IMPORTANT NOTICE: Updated drug information is sent bi-monthly via the PDR® Update Insert. For *monthly* email updates, register at PDR.net.

How should I dispose of syringes and needles?

Do not reuse disposable syringes and needles. Throw away syringes and needles as instructed by your healthcare provider by following these steps:

- Do not throw the needle, syringe, or disposable container in the household trash or recycle.
- Do not put the needle cover back on the needle.
- Place all used needles and syringes in a puncture-proof disposable container with a lid. Do not use glass or clear plastic containers, or any container that will be recycled or returned to a store.
- Keep the container out of the reach of children.
- When the container is full, tape around the cap or lid to make sure the cap or lid does not come off. Throw away the puncture-proof disposable container as instructed by your healthcare provider. There may be special state and local laws for disposing of used needles and syringes. **Do not throw the disposable container in the household trash. Do not recycle.**

Manufactured by:

Amgen Manufacturing, Limited, a subsidiary of Amgen Inc.
One Amgen Center Drive
Thousand Oaks, California 91320-1799
© 1989-2008 Amgen Inc. All rights reserved.
1xxxxxx - v1
Revised: 08/2008

Shown in Product Identification Guide, page 305

NEULASTA®   ℞

[nū lăs-tă]
(pegfilgrastim)
injection, for subcutaneous use

HIGHLIGHTS OF PRESCRIBING INFORMATION

These highlights do not include all the information needed to use Neulasta safely and effectively. See full prescribing information for Neulasta.
Neulasta® (pegfilgrastim)
injection, for subcutaneous use
Initial U.S. Approval: 2002

──────INDICATIONS AND USAGE──────

Neulasta is a leukocyte growth factor indicated to decrease the incidence of infection, as manifested by febrile neutropenia, in patients with non-myeloid malignancies receiving myelosuppressive anti-cancer drugs associated with a clinically significant incidence of febrile neutropenia. (1)
Neulasta is not indicated for the mobilization of peripheral blood progenitor cells for hematopoietic stem cell transplantation.

──────DOSAGE AND ADMINISTRATION──────

- 6 mg administered subcutaneously once per chemotherapy cycle. (2)
- Do not administer between 14 days before and 24 hours after administration of cytotoxic chemotherapy. (2)

──────DOSAGE FORMS AND STRENGTHS──────

6 mg per 0.6 mL in single use prefilled syringe. (3)

──────CONTRAINDICATIONS──────

Do not administer Neulasta to patients with a history of serious allergic reactions to pegfilgrastim or filgrastim. (4)

──────WARNINGS AND PRECAUTIONS──────

- Fatal splenic rupture can occur. Evaluate for splenomegaly or splenic rupture in patients with left upper abdominal or shoulder pain. (5.1)
- Acute respiratory distress syndrome (ARDS) can occur. Evaluate for ARDS in patients who develop fever, lung infiltrates, or respiratory distress. Discontinue Neulasta in patients with ARDS. (5.2)
- Serious allergic reactions, including anaphylaxis, can occur. Permanently discontinue Neulasta in patients with serious allergic reactions. (5.3)
- Severe and sometimes fatal sickle cell crises can occur. (5.4)

──────ADVERSE REACTIONS──────

Most common adverse reactions (≥ 5% difference in incidence) in placebo controlled clinical trials are bone pain and pain in extremity. (6)
To report SUSPECTED ADVERSE REACTIONS, contact Amgen Inc. at 1-800-77-AMGEN (1-800-772-6436) or FDA at 1-800-FDA-1088 or www.fda.gov/medwatch

──────USE IN SPECIFIC POPULATIONS──────

- Pregnancy: Based on animal data, may cause fetal harm. Physicians are encouraged to enroll pregnant patients in Amgen's Pregnancy Surveillance Program by calling 1-800-772-6436 (1-800-77-AMGEN). (8.1)
- Nursing Mothers: Caution should be exercised when administered to a nursing woman.(8.3)
- Pediatric Use: The safety and effectiveness of Neulasta have not been established. (8.4)
- Geriatric Use: No overall differences in safety or effectiveness were observed in patients age 65 and older. (8.5)
- Renal Impairment: No dose adjustment required. (8.6)

See 17 for PATIENT COUNSELING INFORMATION and FDA-approved patient labeling

Revised: 02/2010

FULL PRESCRIBING INFORMATION: CONTENTS*

FULL PRESCRIBING INFORMATION

1   INDICATIONS AND USAGE

Neulasta is indicated to decrease the incidence of infection, as manifested by febrile neutropenia, in patients with non-myeloid malignancies receiving myelosuppressive anti-cancer drugs associated with a clinically significant incidence of febrile neutropenia *[see Clinical Studies (14)]*.
Neulasta is not indicated for the mobilization of peripheral blood progenitor cells for hematopoietic stem cell transplantation.

2   DOSAGE AND ADMINISTRATION

The recommended dosage of Neulasta is a single subcutaneous injection of 6 mg administered once per chemotherapy cycle in adults. Do not administer Neulasta between 14 days before and 24 hours after administration of cytotoxic chemotherapy.
Visually inspect parenteral drug products for particulate matter and discoloration prior to administration, whenever solution and container permit. Do not administer Neulasta if discoloration or particulates are observed.
NOTE: The needle cover on the single-use prefilled syringe contains dry natural rubber (latex); persons with latex allergies should not administer this product.

3   DOSAGE FORMS AND STRENGTHS

6 mg per 0.6 mL in single use prefilled syringe. (3)

4   CONTRAINDICATIONS

Do not administer Neulasta to patients with a history of serious allergic reactions to pegfilgrastim or filgrastim.

5   WARNINGS AND PRECAUTIONS

5.1   Splenic Rupture

Splenic rupture, including fatal cases, can occur following the administration of Neulasta. Evaluate for an enlarged spleen or splenic rupture in patients who report left upper abdominal or shoulder pain after receiving Neulasta.

5.2   Acute Respiratory Distress Syndrome

Acute respiratory distress syndrome (ARDS) can occur in patients receiving Neulasta. Evaluate patients who develop fever and lung infiltrates or respiratory distress after receiving Neulasta, for ARDS. Discontinue Neulasta in patients with ARDS.

5.3   Serious Allergic Reactions

Serious allergic reactions, including anaphylaxis, can occur in patients receiving Neulasta. The majority of reported events occurred upon initial exposure. Allergic reactions, including anaphylaxis, can recur within days after the discontinuation of initial anti-allergic treatment. Permanently discontinue Neulasta in patients with serious allergic reactions. Do not administer Neulasta to patients with a history of serious allergic reactions to pegfilgrastim or filgrastim.

5.4   Use in Patients with Sickle Cell Disorders

Severe sickle cell crises can occur in patients with sickle cell disorders receiving Neulasta. Severe and sometimes fatal sickle cell crises can occur in patients with sickle cell disorders receiving filgrastim, the parent compound of pegfilgrastim.

5.5   Potential for Tumor Growth Stimulatory Effects on Malignant Cells

The granulocyte-colony stimulating factor (G-CSF) receptor through which pegfilgrastim and filgrastim act has been found on tumor cell lines. The possibility that pegfilgrastim acts as a growth factor for any tumor type, including myeloid malignancies and myelodysplasia, diseases for which pegfilgrastim is not approved, cannot be excluded.

6   ADVERSE REACTIONS

The following serious adverse reactions are discussed in greater detail in other sections of the labeling:

- Splenic Rupture *[See Warnings and Precautions (5.1)]*
- Acute Respiratory Distress Syndrome *[See Warnings and Precautions (5.2)]*
- Serious Allergic Reactions *[See Warnings and Precautions (5.3)]*
- Use in Patients with Sickle Cell Disorders *[See Warnings and Precautions (5.4)]*
- Potential for Tumor Growth Stimulatory Effects on Malignant Cells *[See Warnings and Precautions (5.5)]*

The most common adverse reactions occurring in ≥ 5% of patients and with a between-group difference of ≥ 5% higher in the pegfilgrastim arm in placebo controlled clinical trials are bone pain and pain in extremity.

6.1   Clinical Trials Experience

Because clinical trials are conducted under widely varying conditions, adverse reaction rates observed in the clinical trials of a drug cannot be directly compared with rates in the clinical trials of another drug and may not reflect the rates observed in clinical practice. Neulasta clinical trials safety data are based upon 932 patients receiving Neulasta in seven randomized clinical trials. The population was 21 to 88 years of age and 92% female. The ethnicity was 75% Caucasian, 18% Hispanic, 5% Black, and 1% Asian. Patients with breast (n = 823), lung and thoracic tumors (n = 53) and lymphoma (n = 56) received Neulasta after nonmyeloablative cytotoxic chemotherapy. Most patients received a single 100 mcg/kg (n = 259) or a single 6 mg (n = 546) dose per chemotherapy cycle over 4 cycles.

The following adverse reaction data in Table 1 are from a randomized, double-blind, placebo-controlled study in patients with metastatic or non-metastatic breast cancer receiving docetaxel 100 mg/m^2 every 21 days (Study 3). A total of 928 patients were randomized to receive either 6 mg Neulasta (n = 467) or placebo (n = 461). The patients were 21 to 88 years of age and 99% female. The ethnicity was 66% Caucasian, 31% Hispanic, 2% Black, and <1% Asian, Native American or other.

Bone pain and pain in extremity occurred at a higher incidence in Neulasta-treated patients as compared with placebo-treated patients.

Table 1. Adverse Reactions With ≥ 5% Higher Incidence in Neulasta Patients Compared to Placebo in Study 3

System Organ Class Preferred Term	Placebo (N= 461)	Neulasta 6 mg SC on Day 2 (N= 467)
Musculoskeletal and connective tissue disorders		
Bone pain	26%	31%
Pain in extremity	4%	9%

Leukocytosis
In clinical studies, leukocytosis (WBC counts > 100 × 10^9/L) was observed in less than 1% of 932 patients with non-myeloid malignancies receiving Neulasta. No complications attributable to leukocytosis were reported in clinical studies.

6.2   Immunogenicity

As with all therapeutic proteins, there is a potential for immunogenicity. Binding antibodies to pegfilgrastim were detected using a BIAcore assay. The approximate limit of detection for this assay is 500 ng/mL. Pre-existing binding antibodies were detected in approximately 6% (51/849) of patients with metastatic breast cancer. Four of 521 pegfilgrastim-treated subjects who were negative at baseline developed binding antibodies to pegfilgrastim following treatment. None of these 4 patients had evidence of neutralizing antibodies detected using a cell-based bioassay.

The detection of antibody formation is highly dependent on the sensitivity and specificity of the assay, and the observed incidence of antibody positivity in an assay may be influenced by several factors, including assay methodology, sample handling, timing of sample collection, concomitant medications, and underlying disease. For these reasons, comparison of the incidence of antibodies to Neulasta with the incidence of antibodies to other products may be misleading.

6.3 Postmarketing Experience

The following adverse reactions have been identified during post approval use of Neulasta. Because these reactions are reported voluntarily from a population of uncertain size, it is not always possible to reliably estimate their frequency or establish a causal relationship to drug exposure. Decisions to include these reactions in labeling are typically based on one or more of the following factors: (1) seriousness of the reaction, (2) reported frequency of the reaction, or (3) strength of causal relationship to Neulasta.

Gastro-intestinal disorders: Splenic rupture *[See Warnings and Precautions (5.1)]*

Blood and lymphatic system disorder: Sickle cell crisis *[See Warnings and Precautions (5.4)]*

Respiratory, thoracic, and mediastinal disorder: ARDS *[See Warnings and Precautions (5.2)]*

General disorders and administration site conditions: Injection site reactions

Skin and subcutaneous tissue disorders: Allergic reactions/hypersensitivity, including anaphylaxis, skin rash, and urticaria, Sweet's syndrome, generalized erythema and flushing *[See Warnings and Precautions (5.3)]*

7 DRUG INTERACTIONS

No formal drug interaction studies between Neulasta and other drugs have been performed. Increased hematopoietic activity of the bone marrow in response to growth factor therapy may result in transiently positive bone-imaging changes. Consider these findings when interpreting bone-imaging results.

8 USE IN SPECIFIC POPULATIONS

8.1 Pregnancy

Pregnancy Category C

There are no adequate and well-controlled studies in pregnant women. Pegfilgrastim was embryotoxic and increased pregnancy loss in pregnant rabbits that received cumulative doses approximately 4 times the recommended human dose (based on body surface area). Signs of maternal toxicity occurred at these doses. Neulasta should be used during pregnancy only if the potential benefit to the mother justifies the potential risk to the fetus.

In animal reproduction studies, when pregnant rabbits received pegfilgrastim at cumulative doses approximately 4 times the recommended human dose (based on body surface area), increased embryolethality and spontaneous abortions occurred. Signs of maternal toxicity (reductions in body weight gain/food consumption) and decreased fetal weights occurred at maternal doses approximately equivalent to the recommended human dose (based on body surface area). There were no structural anomalies observed in rabbit offspring at any dose tested. No evidence of reproductive/developmental toxicity occurred in the offspring of pregnant rats that received cumulative doses of pegfilgrastim approximately 10 times the recommended human dose (based on body surface area) *[see Nonclinical Toxicology (13.3)]*.

Women who become pregnant during Neulasta treatment are encouraged to enroll in Amgen's Pregnancy Surveillance Program. Patients or their physicians should call 1-800-77-AMGEN (1-800-772-6436) to enroll.

8.3 Nursing Mothers

It is not known whether pegfilgrastim is secreted in human milk. Other recombinant G-CSF products are poorly secreted in breast milk and G-CSF is not orally absorbed by neonates. Caution should be exercised when administered to a nursing woman.

8.4 Pediatric Use

Safety and effectiveness of Neulasta in pediatric patients have not been established. The adverse reaction profile and pharmacokinetics of pegfilgrastim were studied in 37 pediatric patients with sarcoma. The mean (± standard deviation [SD]) systemic exposure (AUC_{0-inf}) of pegfilgrastim after subcutaneous administration at 100 mcg/kg was 22.0 (± 13.1) mcg•hr/mL in the 6 to 11 years age group (n = 10), 29.3 (± 23.2) mcg•hr/mL in the 12 to 21 years age group (n = 13), and 47.9 (± 22.5) mcg•hr/mL in the youngest age group (0 to 5 years, n = 11). The terminal elimination half-lives of the corresponding age groups were 20.2 (± 11.3) hours, 21.2 (± 16.0) hours, and 30.1 (± 38.2) hours, respectively. The most common adverse reaction was bone pain.

8.5 Geriatric Use

Of the 932 patients with cancer who received Neulasta in clinical studies, 139 (15%) were age 65 and over, and 18 (2%) were age 75 and over. No overall differences in safety or effectiveness were observed between patients age 65 and older and younger patients.

8.6 Renal Impairment

In a study of 30 subjects with varying degrees of renal dysfunction, including end stage renal disease, renal dysfunction had no effect on the pharmacokinetics of pegfilgrastim. Therefore, pegfilgrastim dose adjustment in patients with renal dysfunction is not necessary *[Clinical Pharmacology (12.3)]*.

10 OVERDOSAGE

The maximum amount of Neulasta that can be safely administered in single or multiple doses has not been determined. Single subcutaneous doses of 300 mcg/kg have been administered to 8 healthy volunteers and 3 patients with non-small cell lung cancer without serious adverse effects. These patients experienced a mean maximum absolute neutrophil count (ANC) of 55×10^9/L, with a corresponding mean maximum WBC of 67×10^9/L. The absolute maximum ANC observed was 96×10^9/L with a corresponding absolute maximum WBC observed of 120×10^9/L. The duration of leukocytosis ranged from 6 to 13 days. The effectiveness of leukapheresis in the management of symptomatic individuals with Neulasta-induced leukocytosis has not been studied.

11 DESCRIPTION

Neulasta (pegfilgrastim) is a covalent conjugate of recombinant methionyl human G-CSF (filgrastim) and monomethoxypolyethylene glycol. Filgrastim is a water-soluble 175 amino acid protein with a molecular weight of approximately 19 kilodaltons (kD). Filgrastim is obtained from the bacterial fermentation of a strain of *E coli* transformed with a genetically engineered plasmid containing the human G-CSF gene. To produce pegfilgrastim, a 20 kD monomethoxypolyethylene glycol molecule is covalently bound to the N-terminal methionyl residue of filgrastim. The average molecular weight of pegfilgrastim is approximately 39 kD. Neulasta is supplied in 0.6 mL prefilled syringes for subcutaneous injection. Each syringe contains 6 mg pegfilgrastim (based on protein weight) in a sterile, clear, colorless, preservative-free solution (pH 4.0) containing acetate (0.35 mg), polysorbate 20 (0.02 mg), sodium (0.02 mg), and sorbitol (30 mg) in Water for Injection, USP.

12 CLINICAL PHARMACOLOGY

12.1 Mechanism of Action

Pegfilgrastim is a colony-stimulating factor that acts on hematopoietic cells by binding to specific cell surface receptors, thereby stimulating proliferation, differentiation, commitment, and end cell functional activation.

12.3 Pharmacokinetics

The pharmacokinetics of pegfilgrastim were studied in 379 patients with cancer. The pharmacokinetics of pegfilgrastim were nonlinear and clearance decreased with increases in dose. Neutrophil receptor binding is an important component of the clearance of pegfilgrastim, and serum clearance is directly related to the number of neutrophils. In addition to numbers of neutrophils, body weight appeared to be a factor. Patients with higher body weights experienced higher systemic exposure to pegfilgrastim after receiving a dose normalized for body weight. A large variability in the pharmacokinetics of pegfilgrastim was observed. The half-life of Neulasta ranged from 15 to 80 hours after subcutaneous injection.

No gender-related differences were observed in the pharmacokinetics of pegfilgrastim, and no differences were observed in the pharmacokinetics of geriatric patients (≥ 65 years of age) compared with younger patients (< 65 years of age) *[see Use in Specific Populations (8.5)]*. The pharmacokinetics of pegfilgrastim were studied in pediatric patients with sarcoma *[see Use in Specific Populations (8.4)]*. Renal dysfunction had no effect on the pharmacokinetics of pegfilgrastim. *[see Use in Specific Populations (8.6)]*. The pharmacokinetic profile in patients with hepatic insufficiency has not been assessed.

13 NONCLINICAL TOXICOLOGY

13.1 Carcinogenesis, Mutagenesis, Impairment of Fertility

No carcinogenicity or mutagenesis studies have been performed with pegfilgrastim.

Pegfilgrastim did not affect reproductive performance or fertility in male or female rats at cumulative weekly doses approximately 6 to 9 times higher than the recommended human dose (based on body surface area).

13.3 Reproductive and Developmental Toxicology

Pregnant rabbits were dosed with pegfilgrastim subcutaneously every other day during the period of organogenesis. At cumulative doses ranging from the approximate human dose to approximately 4 times the recommended human dose (based on body surface area), treated rabbits exhibited decreased maternal food consumption, maternal weight loss, as well as reduced fetal body weights and delayed ossification of the fetal skull; however, no structural anomalies were observed in the offspring from either study. Increased incidences of post-implantation losses and spontaneous abortions (more than half the pregnancies) were observed at cumulative doses approximately 4 times the recommended human dose, which were not seen when pregnant rabbits were exposed to the recommended human dose.

Three studies were conducted in pregnant rats dosed with pegfilgrastim at cumulative doses up to approximately 10 times the recommended human dose at the following stages of gestation: during the period of organogenesis, from mating through the first half of pregnancy, and from the first

trimester through delivery and lactation. No evidence of fetal loss or structural malformations was observed in any study. Cumulative doses equivalent to approximately 3 and 10 times the recommended human dose resulted in transient evidence of wavy ribs in fetuses of treated mothers (detected at the end of gestation but no longer present in pups evaluated at the end of lactation).

14 CLINICAL STUDIES

Neulasta was evaluated in three randomized, double blind, controlled studies. Studies 1 and 2 were active-controlled studies that employed doxorubicin 60 mg/m² and docetaxel 75 mg/m² administered every 21 days for up to 4 cycles for the treatment of metastatic breast cancer. Study 1 investigated the utility of a fixed dose of Neulasta. Study 2 employed a weight-adjusted dose. In the absence of growth factor support, similar chemotherapy regimens have been reported to result in a 100% incidence of severe neutropenia (ANC < 0.5×10^9/L) with a mean duration of 5 to 7 days and a 30% to 40% incidence of febrile neutropenia. Based on the correlation between the duration of severe neutropenia and the incidence of febrile neutropenia found in studies with filgrastim, duration of severe neutropenia was chosen as the primary endpoint in both studies, and the efficacy of Neulasta was demonstrated by establishing comparability to filgrastim-treated patients in the mean days of severe neutropenia.

In Study 1, 157 patients were randomized to receive a single subcutaneous injection of Neulasta (6 mg) on day 2 of each chemotherapy cycle or daily subcutaneous filgrastim (5 mcg/kg/day) beginning on day 2 of each chemotherapy cycle. In Study 2, 310 patients were randomized to receive a single subcutaneous injection of Neulasta (100 mcg/kg) on day 2 or daily subcutaneous filgrastim (5 mcg/kg/day) beginning on day 2 of each chemotherapy cycle.

Both studies met the major efficacy outcome measure of demonstrating that the mean days of severe neutropenia of Neulasta-treated patients did not exceed that of filgrastim-treated patients by more than 1 day in cycle 1 of chemotherapy. The mean days of cycle 1 severe neutropenia in Study 1 were 1.8 days in the Neulasta arm compared to 1.6 days in the filgrastim arm [difference in means 0.2 (95% CI -0.2, 0.6)] and in Study 2 were 1.7 days in the Neulasta arm compared to 1.6 days in the Filgrastim arm [difference in means 0.1 (95% CI -0.2, 0.4)].

A secondary endpoint in both studies was days of severe neutropenia in cycles 2 through 4 with results similar to those for cycle 1. Study 3 was a randomized, double-blind, placebo-controlled study that employed docetaxel 100 mg/m² administered every 21 days for up to 4 cycles for the treatment of metastatic or non-metastatic breast cancer. In this study, 928 patients were randomized to receive a single subcutaneous injection of Neulasta (6 mg) or placebo on day 2 of each chemotherapy cycle. Study 3 met the major trial outcome measure of demonstrating that the incidence of febrile neutropenia (defined as temperature ≥ 38.2°C and ANC ≤ 0.5×10^9/L) was lower for Neulasta-treated patients as compared to placebo-treated patients (1% versus 17%, respectively, p < 0.001). The incidence of hospitalizations (1% versus 14%) and IV anti-infective use (2% versus 10%) for the treatment of febrile neutropenia was also lower in the Neulasta-treated patients compared to the placebo-treated patients.

16 HOW SUPPLIED/STORAGE AND HANDLING

Neulasta is supplied in a prefilled single use syringe containing 6 mg pegfilgrastim, supplied with a 27-gauge, 1/2-inch needle with an UltraSafe® Needle Guard.

The needle cover of the prefilled syringe contains dry natural rubber (a derivative of latex).

Neulasta is provided in a dispensing pack containing one syringe (NDC 55513-190-01).

Store refrigerated between 2° to 8°C (36° to 46°F) in the carton to protect from light. Do not shake. Discard syringes stored at room temperature for more than 48 hours. Avoid freezing; if frozen, thaw in the refrigerator before administration. Discard syringe if frozen more than once.

17 PATIENT COUNSELING INFORMATION

Advise patients of the following risks:
• Splenic rupture
• Acute Respiratory Distress Syndrome
• Serious allergic reactions
• Sickle cell crisis
Have patients immediately contact their healthcare provider and report:
• Left upper quadrant or shoulder pain
• Shortness of breath
• Signs or symptoms of sickle cell crisis
• Signs or symptoms of infection
• Flushing, dizziness, or rash
Neulasta® (pegfilgrastim)

Manufactured by:
Amgen Inc.
One Amgen Center Drive
Thousand Oaks, California 91320-1799

This product, its production, and/or its use may be covered by one or more US Patents, including US Patent Nos. 5,824,784; 5,582,823; 5,580,755, as well as other patents or patents pending.

www.neulasta.com
1-800-77-AMGEN (1-800-772-6436)
1xxxxx
v11.0

FDA APPROVED PATIENT LABELING

Neulasta®

Pegfilgrastim

This patient package insert provides information and instructions for people who will be receiving Neulasta or their caregivers. This patient package insert does not tell you everything about Neulasta. You should discuss any questions you have about treatment with Neulasta with your doctor.

What is Neulasta?

Neulasta is a man-made form of granulocyte colony-stimulating factor (G-CSF), which is made using the bacteria *E coli.* G-CSF is a substance produced by the body. It stimulates the growth of neutrophils (**nu**-tro-fils), a type of white blood cell important in the body's fight against infection.

Who should not take Neulasta?

Do not take Neulasta if you have had:
• A serious allergic reaction to Neulasta® (pegfilgrastim) or to Neupogen® (filgrastim).

What important information do I need to know about receiving Neulasta?

Occasionally pain and redness may occur at the injection site. If there is a lump, swelling, or bruising at the injection site that does not go away, talk to the doctor.

Neulasta should only be injected on the day the doctor has determined and should not be injected until approximately 24 hours after receiving chemotherapy.

The needle cover on the single-use prefilled syringe contains dry natural rubber (latex), which should not be handled by persons sensitive to this substance.

What should I tell my healthcare provider before taking Neulasta?

If you have a sickle cell disorder, make sure that your doctor knows about it before using Neulasta. If you have a sickle cell crisis after getting Neulasta, tell your doctor right away. If you have any questions, talk to your doctor.

What are possible serious side effects of Neulasta?

• **Spleen Rupture.** Your spleen may become enlarged and can rupture while taking Neulasta. A ruptured spleen can cause death. The spleen is located in the upper left section of your stomach area. Call your doctor right away if you have pain in the left upper stomach area or left shoulder tip area. This pain could mean your spleen is enlarged or ruptured.

• **A serious lung problem called Acute Respiratory Distress Syndrome (ARDS).** Call your doctor or seek emergency care right away if you have shortness of breath, trouble breathing, or a fast rate of breathing.

• **Serious Allergic Reactions.** Neulasta can cause serious allergic reactions. These reactions can cause shortness of breath, wheezing, dizziness, swelling around the mouth or eyes, fast pulse, sweating, and hives. If you start to have any of these symptoms, call your doctor or seek emergency care right away. If you have an allergic reaction during the injection of Neulasta, stop the injection. Call your doctor right away.

• **Sickle Cell Crises.** You may have a serious sickle cell crisis if you have a sickle cell disorder and take Neulasta. Serious and sometimes fatal sickle cell crises can occur in patients with sickle cell disorders receiving filgrastim, a medicine similar to Neulasta (pegfilgrastim). Call your doctor right away if you have symptoms of sickle cell crisis such as pain or difficulty breathing.

What are the most common side effects of Neulasta?

The most common side effect you may experience is aching in the bones and muscles. If this happens, it can usually be relieved with a non aspirin pain reliever, such as acetaminophen.

What about pregnancy or breastfeeding?

Neulasta has not been studied in pregnant women, and its effects on unborn babies are not known. If you take Neulasta while you are pregnant, it is possible that small amounts of it may get into your baby's blood. It is not known if Neulasta can get into human breast milk. If you are pregnant, plan to become pregnant, think you may be pregnant, or are breastfeeding, you should tell your doctor before using Neulasta. If you become pregnant during Neulasta treatment, you are encouraged to enroll in Amgen's Pregnancy Surveillance Program. You should call 1-800-77-AMGEN (1-800-772-6436) to enroll.

HOW TO PREPARE AND GIVE A NEULASTA INJECTION

Neulasta is provided in a prefilled syringe. **Neulasta should be stored in its carton to protect from light until use.** If you are giving someone else Neulasta injections, it is important that you know how to inject Neulasta. Before getting your Neulasta injection, always check to see that:

• The name Neulasta appears on the carton and prefilled syringe label.

• The expiration date on the prefilled syringe has not passed. **You should not use a prefilled syringe after the date on the label.**

• The Neulasta liquid should always be clear and colorless. Do not use Neulasta if the contents of the prefilled syringe appear discolored or cloudy, or if the prefilled syringe appears to contain lumps, flakes, or particles.

IMPORTANT: TO HELP AVOID POSSIBLE INFECTION, YOU SHOULD FOLLOW THESE INSTRUCTIONS.

Setting up for an injection

Note: The needle cover on the single-use prefilled syringe contains dry natural rubber (latex), which should not be handled by persons sensitive to this substance.

1. Find a clean, flat working surface, such as a table.

2. Remove the carton containing the prefilled syringe of Neulasta from the refrigerator. Allow Neulasta to reach room temperature (this takes about 30 minutes). Remove the syringe from the carton before injection. Each prefilled syringe should be used only once. DO NOT SHAKE THE PREFILLED SYRINGE. Shaking may damage Neulasta. If the prefilled syringe has been shaken vigorously, the solution may appear foamy and it should not be used.

3. Assemble the supplies you will need for an injection:
• Neulasta prefilled syringe with transparent (clear) plastic blue needle guard attached

Prefilled Syringe

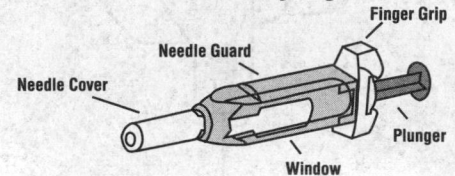

Alcohol Swab

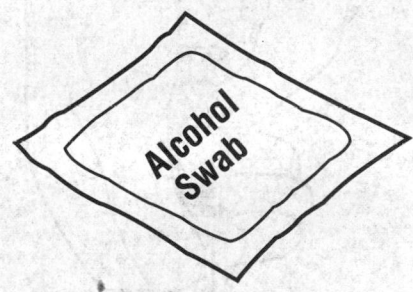

• An alcohol swab and a cotton ball or gauze

Cotton Ball

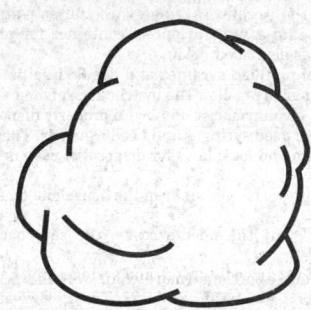

• Puncture-proof disposal container

4. Wash your hands with soap and warm water.

[See figure at top of next column]

HOW TO PREPARE FOR INJECTION OF NEULASTA

5. Remove the syringe from the package and the tray. Check to see that the plastic blue needle guard is covering the barrel of the glass syringe. DO NOT push the

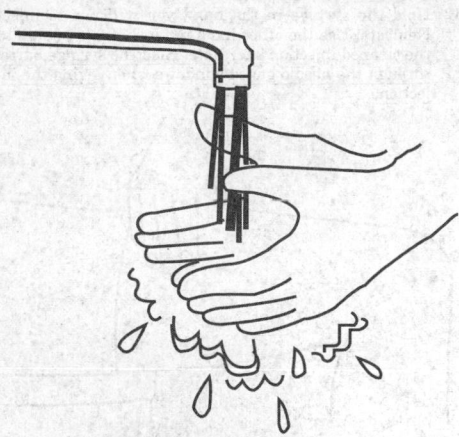

blue needle guard over the needle cover before injection. This may activate or lock the needle guard. If the blue needle guard is covering the needle that means it has been activated. Do NOT use that syringe. Dispose of that syringe in the puncture-proof disposal container. Use a new syringe. **Do not activate the needle guard prior to injection.**

6. Hold the syringe barrel through the needle guard windows with the needle pointing up. Holding the syringe with the needle pointing up helps to prevent medicine from leaking out of the needle. Carefully pull the needle cover straight off.

7. Check the syringe for air bubbles. If there are air bubbles, gently tap the syringe with your fingers until the air bubbles rise to the top of the syringe. Slowly push the plunger up to force the air bubbles out of the syringe.

8. Gently place the prefilled syringe with the window flat on your clean working surface so that the needle does not touch anything.

Selecting and preparing the injection site

9. Choose an injection site. Four recommended injection sites for Neulasta are:
• The outer area of the upper arms
• The abdomen, except for the two-inch area around the navel
• The front of the middle thighs
• The upper outer areas of the buttocks

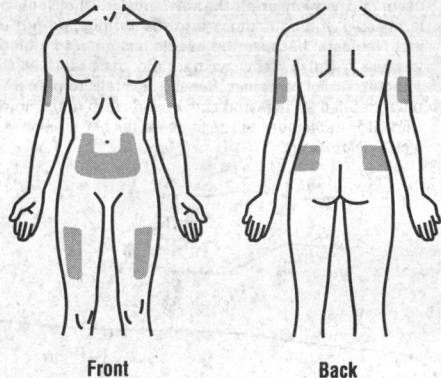

Front   Back

10. Clean the injection site with an alcohol swab.

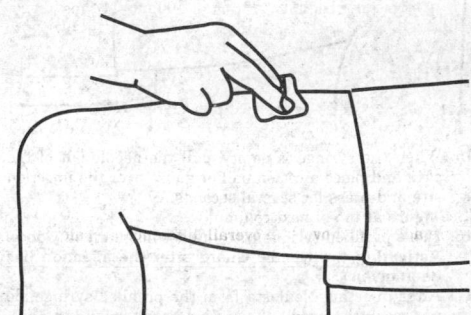

Injecting the dose of Neulasta

11. Pick up the prefilled syringe from your clean, flat working surface by grabbing the sides of the needle guard with your thumb and forefinger.

12. Hold the syringe in the hand you will use to inject Neulasta. Use the other hand to pinch a fold of skin at the cleaned injection site. Note: Hold the syringe barrel through the needle guard windows when giving the injection.

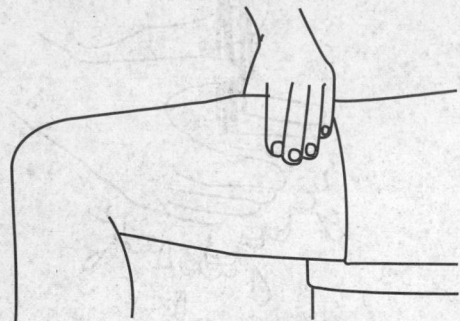

13. Holding the syringe like a pencil, use a quick "dart-like" motion to insert the needle either straight up and down (90 degree angle) or at a slight angle (45 degrees) into the skin.

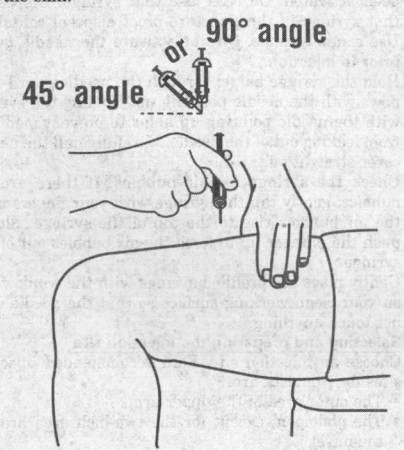

90° angle

45° angle or

14. After the needle is inserted, let go of the skin. Pull the plunger back slightly. If no blood appears, slowly push down on the plunger all the way, until all the Neulasta is injected. **If blood comes into the syringe, do not inject Neulasta, because the needle has entered a blood vessel.** Withdraw the syringe and discard it in the puncture-proof container. Repeat the steps to prepare a new prefilled syringe and choose and clean a new injection site. Remember to check again for blood before injecting Neulasta.

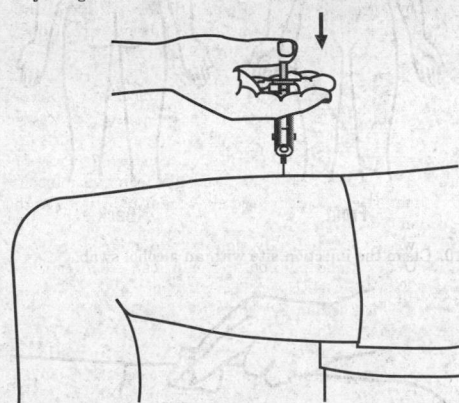

15. When the syringe is empty, pull the needle out of the skin and place a cotton ball or gauze over the injection site and press for several seconds.
[See figure at top of next column]

16. Use a prefilled syringe with the needle guard only once.

Activating the Needle Guard after the injection has been given

17. After injecting Neulasta from the prefilled syringe, do not recap the needle. Keep your hands behind the needle at all times. While holding the clear plastic finger grip of the syringe with one hand, grasp the blue needle guard with your free hand and slide the blue needle guard over the needle until the needle is completely covered and the needle guard clicks into place. **NOTE: If an**

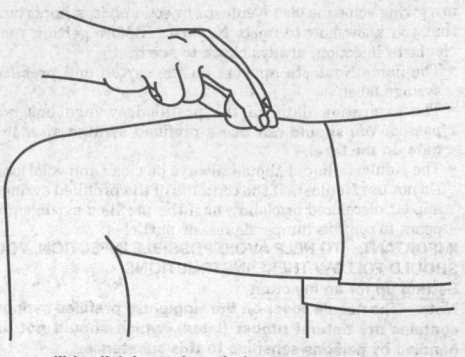

audible click is not heard, the needle guard may not be completely activated.

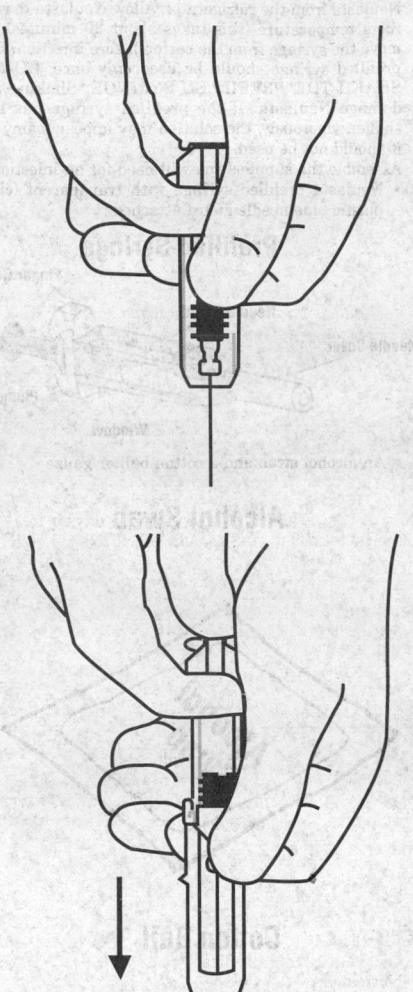

18. Place the prefilled syringe with the activated needle guard into a puncture-proof container for proper disposal as described below.

Disposal of prefilled syringes and needle guards
You should always follow the instructions given by your doctor, nurse, or pharmacist on how to properly dispose of containers with used syringes and needle guards. There may be special state and local laws for disposal of used needles and syringes.
• Do not throw the container in the household trash. Do not recycle.
• DO NOT put the needle cover (the cap) back on the needle.
• Place all used needle covers and syringes in a hard plastic container with a screw-on cap or in a metal container with a plastic lid, such as a coffee can, labeled "used syringes." If a metal container is used, cut a small hole in the plastic lid and tape the lid to the metal container. If a hard plastic container is used, always screw the cap on tightly after each use.
• Do not use glass or clear plastic containers.
• When the container is full, tape around the cap or lid to make sure the cap or lid does not come off.

• **Always** keep the container out of the reach of children.
How should Neulasta be stored?
Neulasta should be stored in the refrigerator at 2° to 8°C (36° to 46°F), but not in the freezer. Neulasta should be protected from light, so you should keep it in its carton until you are ready to use it. Avoid shaking Neulasta. If Neulasta is accidentally frozen, allow it to thaw in the refrigerator before injecting. However, if it is frozen a second time, do not use. Neulasta can be left out at room temperature for up to 48 hours. Do not leave Neulasta in direct sunlight. For all questions about storage, contact your doctor, nurse, or pharmacist.
What are the ingredients in Neulasta?
Each syringe contains pegfilgrastim in a sterile, clear, colorless, preservative-free solution containing acetate, sorbitol, polysorbate 20, and sodium.
Neulasta® (pegfilgrastim)
Manufactured by:
Amgen Inc.
One Amgen Center Drive
Thousand Oaks, California 91320-1799
This product, its production, and/or its use may be covered by one or more US Patents, including US Patent Nos. 5,824,784; 5,582,823; 5,580,755, as well as other patents or patents pending.
© 2010 Amgen Inc. All rights reserved.
www.neulasta.com
1-800-77-AMGEN (1-800-772-6436)
1xxxxx
v 8.0
Shown in Product Identification Guide, page 305

NEUPOGEN®   ℞
[nūe´pō-jĕn]
(Filgrastim)

DESCRIPTION
Filgrastim is a human granulocyte colony-stimulating factor (G-CSF), produced by recombinant DNA technology. NEUPOGEN® is the Amgen Inc. trademark for Filgrastim, which has been selected as the name for recombinant methionyl human granulocyte colony-stimulating factor (r-metHuG-CSF).
NEUPOGEN® is a 175 amino acid protein manufactured by recombinant DNA technology.[1] NEUPOGEN® is produced by *Escherichia coli (E coli)* bacteria into which has been inserted the human granulocyte colony-stimulating factor gene. NEUPOGEN® has a molecular weight of 18,800 daltons. The protein has an amino acid sequence that is identical to the natural sequence predicted from human DNA sequence analysis, except for the addition of an N-terminal methionine necessary for expression in *E coli*. Because NEUPOGEN® is produced in *E coli*, the product is nonglycosylated and thus differs from G-CSF isolated from a human cell.
NEUPOGEN® is a sterile, clear, colorless, preservative-free liquid for parenteral administration containing Filgrastim at a specific activity of $1.0 \pm 0.6 \times 10^8$ U/mg (as measured by a cell mitogenesis assay). The product is available in single use vials and prefilled syringes. The single use vials contain either 300 mcg or 480 mcg Filgrastim at a fill volume of 1.0 mL or 1.6 mL, respectively. The single use prefilled syringes contain either 300 mcg or 480 mcg Filgrastim at a fill volume of 0.5 mL or 0.8 mL, respectively. See table below for product composition of each single use vial or prefilled syringe.
[See table at top of next page]

CLINICAL PHARMACOLOGY
Colony-stimulating Factors
Colony-stimulating factors are glycoproteins which act on hematopoietic cells by binding to specific cell surface receptors and stimulating proliferation, differentiation commitment, and some end-cell functional activation.
Endogenous G-CSF is a lineage specific colony-stimulating factor which is produced by monocytes, fibroblasts, and endothelial cells. G-CSF regulates the production of neutrophils within the bone marrow and affects neutrophil progenitor proliferation,[2,3] differentiation,[2,4] and selected end-cell functional activation (including enhanced phagocytic ability,[5] priming of the cellular metabolism associated with respiratory burst,[6] antibody dependent killing,[7] and the increased expression of some functions associated with cell surface antigens[8]). G-CSF is not species specific and has been shown to have minimal direct in vivo or in vitro effects on the production of hematopoietic cell types other than the neutrophil lineage.
Preclinical Experience
Filgrastim was administered to monkeys, dogs, hamsters, rats, and mice as part of a preclinical toxicology program which included single-dose acute, repeated-dose subacute, subchronic, and chronic studies. Single-dose administration of Filgrastim by the oral, intravenous (IV), subcutaneous (SC), or intraperitoneal (IP) routes resulted in no significant

toxicity in mice, rats, hamsters, or monkeys. Although no deaths were observed in mice, rats, or monkeys at dose levels up to 3450 mcg/kg or in hamsters using single doses up to approximately 860 mcg/kg, deaths were observed in a subchronic (13-week) study in monkeys. In this study, evidence of neurological symptoms was seen in monkeys treated with doses of Filgrastim greater than 1150 mcg/kg/day for up to 18 days. Deaths were seen in 5 of the 8 treated animals and were associated with 15- to 28-fold increases in peripheral leukocyte counts, and neutrophil-infiltrated hemorrhagic foci were seen in both the cerebrum and cerebellum. In contrast, no monkeys died following 13 weeks of daily IV administration of Filgrastim at a dose level of 115 mcg/kg. In an ensuing 52-week study, one 115 mcg/kg dosed female monkey died after 18 weeks of daily IV administration of Filgrastim. Death was attributed to cardiopulmonary insufficiency.

In subacute, repeated-dose studies, changes observed were attributable to the expected pharmacological actions of Filgrastim (ie, dose-dependent increases in white cell counts, increased circulating segmented neutrophils, and increased myeloid:erythroid ratio in bone marrow). In all species, histopathologic examination of the liver and spleen revealed evidence of ongoing extramedullary granulopoiesis; increased spleen weights were seen in all species and appeared to be dose-related. A dose-dependent increase in serum alkaline phosphatase was observed in rats, and may reflect increased activity of osteoblasts and osteoclasts. Changes in serum chemistry values were reversible following discontinuation of treatment.

In rats treated at doses of 1150 mcg/kg/day for 4 weeks (5 of 32 animals) and for 13 weeks at doses of 100 mcg/kg/day (4 of 32 animals) and 500 mcg/kg/day (6 of 32 animals), articular swelling of the hind legs was observed. Some degree of hind leg dysfunction was also observed; however, symptoms reversed following cessation of dosing. In rats, osteoclasis and osteoanagenesis were found in the femur, humerus, coccyx, and hind legs (where they were accompanied by synovitis) after IV treatment for 4 weeks (115 to 1150 mcg/kg/day), and in the sternum after IV treatment for 13 weeks (115 to 575 mcg/kg/day). These effects reversed to normal within 4 to 5 weeks following cessation of treatment. In the 52-week chronic, repeated-dose studies performed in rats (IP injection up to 57.5 mcg/kg/day), and cynomolgus monkeys (IV injection of up to 115 mcg/kg/day), changes observed were similar to those noted in the subacute studies. Expected pharmacological actions of Filgrastim included dose-dependent increases in white cell counts, increased circulating segmented neutrophils and alkaline phosphatase levels, and increased myeloid:erythroid ratios in the bone marrow. Decreases in platelet counts were also noted in primates. In no animals tested were hemorrhagic complications observed. Rats displayed dose-related swelling of the hind limb, accompanied by some degree of hind limb dysfunction; osteopathy was noted microscopically. Enlarged spleens (both species) and livers (monkeys), reflective of ongoing extramedullary granulopoiesis, as well as myeloid hyperplasia of the bone marrow, were observed in a dose-dependent manner.

Pharmacologic Effects of NEUPOGEN®

In phase 1 studies involving 96 patients with various nonmyeloid malignancies, NEUPOGEN® administration resulted in a dose-dependent increase in circulating neutrophil counts over the dose range of 1 to 70 mcg/kg/day.[9-11] This increase in neutrophil counts was observed whether NEUPOGEN® was administered IV (1 to 70 mcg/kg twice daily),[9] SC (1 to 3 mcg/kg once daily),[11] or by continuous SC infusion (3 to 11 mcg/kg/day).[10] With discontinuation of NEUPOGEN® therapy, neutrophil counts returned to baseline, in most cases within 4 days. Isolated neutrophils displayed normal phagocytic (measured by zymosan-stimulated chemoluminescence) and chemotactic (measured by migration under agarose using N-formyl-methionyl-leucyl-phenylalanine [fMLP] as the chemotaxin) activity in vitro.

The absolute monocyte count was reported to increase in a dose-dependent manner in most patients receiving NEUPOGEN®; however, the percentage of monocytes in the differential count remained within the normal range. In all studies to date, absolute counts of both eosinophils and basophils did not change and were within the normal range following administration of NEUPOGEN®. Increases in lymphocyte counts following NEUPOGEN® administration have been reported in some normal subjects and cancer patients.

White blood cell (WBC) differentials obtained during clinical trials have demonstrated a shift towards earlier granulocyte progenitor cells (left shift), including the appearance of promyelocytes and myeloblasts, usually during neutrophil recovery following the chemotherapy-induced nadir. In addition, Dohle bodies, increased granulocyte granulation, and hypersegmented neutrophils have been observed. Such changes were transient and were not associated with clinical sequelae, nor were they necessarily associated with infection.

	300 mcg/ 1.0 mL Vial	480 mcg/ 1.6 mL Vial	300 mcg/ 0.5 mL Syringe	480 mcg/ 0.8 mL Syringe
Filgrastim	300 mcg	480 mcg	300 mcg	480 mcg
Acetate	0.59 mg	0.94 mg	0.295 mg	0.472 mg
Sorbitol	50.0 mg	80.0 mg	25.0 mg	40.0 mg
Polysorbate 80	0.04 mg	0.064 mg	0.02 mg	0.032 mg
Sodium	0.035 mg	0.056 mg	0.0175 mg	0.028 mg
Water for Injection USP q.s. ad	1.0 mL	1.6 mL	0.5 mL	0.8 mL

Pharmacokinetics

Absorption and clearance of NEUPOGEN® follows first-order pharmacokinetic modeling without apparent concentration dependence. A positive linear correlation occurred between the parenteral dose and both the serum concentration and area under the concentration-time curves. Continuous IV infusion of 20 mcg/kg of NEUPOGEN® over 24 hours resulted in mean and median serum concentrations of approximately 48 and 56 ng/mL, respectively. Subcutaneous administration of 3.45 mcg/kg and 11.5 mcg/kg resulted in maximum serum concentrations of 4 and 49 ng/mL, respectively, within 2 to 8 hours. The volume of distribution averaged 150 mL/kg in both normal subjects and cancer patients. The elimination half-life, in both normal subjects and cancer patients, was approximately 3.5 hours. Clearance rates of NEUPOGEN® were approximately 0.5 to 0.7 mL/minute/kg. Single parenteral doses or daily IV doses, over a 14-day period, resulted in comparable half-lives. The half-lives were similar for IV administration (231 minutes, following doses of 34.5 mcg/kg) and for SC administration (210 minutes, following NEUPOGEN® doses of 3.45 mcg/kg). Continuous 24-hour IV infusions of 20 mcg/kg over an 11- to 20-day period produced steady-state serum concentrations of NEUPOGEN® with no evidence of drug accumulation over the time period investigated.

Pharmacokinetic data in geriatric patients ($\geq$ 65 years) are not available.

CLINICAL EXPERIENCE

Cancer Patients Receiving Myelosuppressive Chemotherapy

NEUPOGEN® has been shown to be safe and effective in accelerating the recovery of neutrophil counts following a variety of chemotherapy regimens. In a phase 3 clinical trial in small cell lung cancer, patients received SC administration of NEUPOGEN® (4 to 8 mcg/kg/day, days 4 to 17) or placebo. In this study, the benefits of NEUPOGEN® therapy were shown to be prevention of infection as manifested by febrile neutropenia, decreased hospitalization, and decreased IV antibiotic usage. No difference in survival or disease progression was demonstrated.

In the phase 3, randomized, double-blind, placebo-controlled trial conducted in patients with small cell lung cancer, patients were randomized to receive NEUPOGEN® (n = 99) or placebo (n = 111) starting on day 4, after receiving standard dose chemotherapy with cyclophosphamide, doxorubicin, and etoposide. A total of 210 patients were evaluated for efficacy and 207 evaluated for safety. Treatment with NEUPOGEN® resulted in a clinically and statistically significant reduction in the incidence of infection, as manifested by febrile neutropenia; the incidence of at least one infection over all cycles of chemotherapy was 76% (84/111) for placebo-treated patients, versus 40% (40/99) for NEUPOGEN®-treated patients (p < 0.001). The following secondary analyses were also performed. The requirements for in-patient hospitalization and antibiotic use were also significantly decreased during the first cycle of chemotherapy; incidence of hospitalization was 69% (77/111) for placebo-treated patients in cycle 1, versus 52% (51/99) for NEUPOGEN®-treated patients (p = 0.032). The incidence of IV antibiotic usage was 60% (67/111) for placebo-treated patients in cycle 1, versus 38% (38/99) for NEUPOGEN®-treated patients (p = 0.003). The incidence, severity, and duration of severe neutropenia (absolute neutrophil count [ANC] < 500/mm^3) following chemotherapy were all significantly reduced. The incidence of severe neutropenia in cycle 1 was 84% (83/99) for patients receiving NEUPOGEN® versus 96% (106/110) for patients receiving placebo (p = 0.004). Over all cycles, patients randomized to NEUPOGEN® had a 57% (286/500 cycles) rate of severe neutropenia versus 77% (416/543 cycles) for patients randomized to placebo. The median duration of severe neutropenia in cycle 1 was reduced from 6 days (range 0 to 10 days) for patients receiving placebo to 2 days (range 0 to 9 days) for patients receiving NEUPOGEN® (p < 0.001). The mean duration of neutropenia in cycle 1 was 5.64 ± 2.27 days for patients receiving placebo versus 2.44 ± 1.90 days for patients receiving NEUPOGEN®. Over all cycles, the median duration of neutropenia was 3 days for patients randomized to placebo versus 1 day for patients randomized to NEUPOGEN®. The median severity of neutropenia (as measured by ANC nadir) was 72/mm^3 (range 0/mm^3 to 7912/mm^3) in cycle 1 for patients receiving NEUPOGEN® versus 38/mm^3 (range 0/mm^3 to 9520/mm^3) for patients receiving placebo (p = 0.012). The mean severity of neutropenia in cycle 1 was 496/mm^3 ± 1382/mm^3 for patients receiving NEUPOGEN® versus 204/mm^3 ± 953/mm^3 for patients receiving placebo. Over all cycles, the ANC nadir for patients randomized to NEUPOGEN® was 403/mm^3, versus 161/mm^3 for patients randomized to placebo. Administration of NEUPOGEN® resulted in an earlier ANC nadir following chemotherapy than was experienced by patients receiving placebo (day 10 vs day 12). NEUPOGEN® was well tolerated when given SC daily at doses of 4 to 8 mcg/kg for up to 14 consecutive days following each cycle of chemotherapy (see ADVERSE REACTIONS).

Several other phase 1/2 studies, which did not directly measure the incidence of infection, but which did measure increases in neutrophils, support the efficacy of NEUPOGEN®. The regimens are presented to provide some background on the clinical experience with NEUPOGEN®. No claim regarding the safety or efficacy of the chemotherapy regimens is made. The effects of NEUPOGEN® on tumor growth or on the anti-tumor activity of the chemotherapy were not assessed. The doses of NEUPOGEN® used in these studies are considerably greater than those found to be effective in the phase 3 study described above. Such phase 1/2 studies are summarized in the following table. [See table at top of next page]

Patients With Acute Myeloid Leukemia Receiving Induction or Consolidation Chemotherapy

In a randomized, double-blind, placebo-controlled, multicenter, phase 3 clinical trial, 521 patients (median age 54, range 16 to 89 years) were treated for de novo acute myeloid leukemia (AML). Following a standard induction chemotherapy regimen comprising daunorubicin, cytosine arabinoside, and etoposide[15] (DAV 3+7+5), patients received either NEUPOGEN® at 5 mcg/kg/day or placebo, SC, from 24 hours after the last dose of chemotherapy until neutrophil recovery (ANC 1000/mm^3 for 3 consecutive days or 10,000/mm^3 for 1 day) or for a maximum of 35 days.

Treatment with NEUPOGEN® significantly reduced the median time to ANC recovery and the median duration of fever, antibiotic use, and hospitalization following induction chemotherapy. In the NEUPOGEN®-treated group, the median time from initiation of chemotherapy to ANC recovery (ANC $\geq$ 500/mm^3) was 20 days (vs 25 days in the control group, p = 0.0001), the median duration of fever was reduced by 1.5 days (p = 0.009), and there were statistically significant reductions in the durations of IV antibiotic use and hospitalization. During consolidation therapy (DAV 2+5+5), patients treated with NEUPOGEN® also experienced significant reductions in the incidence of severe neutropenia, time to neutrophil recovery, the incidence and duration of fever, and the durations of IV antibiotic use and hospitalization. Patients treated with a further course of standard (DAV 2+5+5) or high-dose cytosine arabinoside consolidation also experienced significant reductions in the duration of neutropenia.

There were no statistically significant differences between NEUPOGEN® and placebo groups in complete remission rate (69% NEUPOGEN® vs 68% placebo, p = 0.77), disease-free survival (median 342 days NEUPOGEN® [n = 178], 322 days placebo [n = 177], p = 0.99), time to progression of all randomized patients (median 165 days NEUPOGEN®, 186 days placebo, p = 0.87), or overall survival (median 380 days NEUPOGEN®, 425 days placebo, p = 0.83).

Cancer Patients Receiving Bone Marrow Transplant

In two separate randomized, controlled trials, patients with Hodgkin's disease (HD) and non-Hodgkin's lymphoma (NHL) were treated with myeloablative chemotherapy and autologous bone marrow transplantation (ABMT). In one study (n = 54), NEUPOGEN® was administered at doses of 10 or 30 mcg/kg/day; a third treatment group in this study received no NEUPOGEN®. A statistically significant reduction in the median number of days of severe neutropenia (ANC < 500/mm^3) occurred in the NEUPOGEN®-treated group versus the control group (23 days in the control group, 11 days in the 10 mcg/kg/day group, and 14 days in the 30 mcg/kg/day group [11 days in the combined treatment groups, p = 0.004]). In the second study (n = 44, 43

Type of Malignancy	Regimen	Chemotherapy Dose	No. Pts.	Trial Phase	NEUPOGEN® Daily Dosage*
Small Cell Lung Cancer	Cyclophosphamide	1 g/m²/day	210	3	4–8 mcg/kg SC days 4–17
	Doxorubicin	50 mg/m²/day			
	Etoposide	120 mg/m²/day × 3 q 21 days			
Small Cell Lung Cancer[11]	Ifosfamide	5 g/m²/day	12	1/2	5.75–46 mcg/kg IV days 4–17
	Doxorubicin	50 mg/m²/day			
	Etoposide	120 mg/m²/day × 3			
	Mesna	8 g/m²/day q 21 days			
Urothelial Cancer[12]	Methotrexate	30 mg/m²/day × 2	40	1/2	3.45–69 mcg/kg IV days 4–11
	Vinblastine	3 mg/m²/day × 2			
	Doxorubicin	30 mg/m²/day			
	Cisplatin	70 mg/m²/day q 28 days			
Various Nonmyeloid Malignancies[13]	Cyclophosphamide	2.5 g/m²/day × 2	18	1/2	23–69 mcg/kg[†] IV days 8–28
	Etoposide	500 mg/m²/day × 3			
	Cisplatin	50 mg/m²/day × 3 q 28 days			
Breast/Ovarian Cancer[14]	Doxorubicin[‡]	75 mg/m²	21	2	11.5 mcg/kg IV days 2–9
		100 mg/m²			
		125 mg/m²			5.75 mcg/kg IV days 10–12
		150 mg/m² q 14 days			
Neuroblastoma	Cyclophosphamide	150 mg/m² × 7	12	2	5.45–17.25 mcg/kg SC days 6–19
	Doxorubicin	35 mg/m²			
	Cisplatin	90 mg/m² q 28 days (cycles 1,3,5) [§]			

*NEUPOGEN® doses were those that accelerated neutrophil production. Doses which provided no additional acceleration beyond that achieved at the next lower dose are not reported.
†Lowest dose(s) tested in the study.
‡Patients received doxorubicin at either 75, 100, 125, or 150 mg/m².
§Cycles 2,6 = cyclophosphamide 150 mg/m² × 7 and etoposide 280 mg/m² × 3.
Cycle 4 = cisplatin 90 mg/m² × 1 and etoposide 280 mg/m² × 3.

patients evaluable), NEUPOGEN® was administered at doses of 10 or 20 mcg/kg/day; a third treatment group in this study received no NEUPOGEN®. A statistically significant reduction in the median number of days of severe neutropenia occurred in the NEUPOGEN®-treated group versus the control group (21.5 days in the control group and 10 days in both treatment groups, p < 0.001). The number of days of febrile neutropenia was also reduced significantly in this study (13.5 days in the control group, 5 days in the 10 mcg/kg/day group, and 5.5 days in the 20 mcg/kg/day group [5 days in the combined treatment groups, p < 0.0001]). Reductions in the number of days of hospitalization and antibiotic use were also seen, although these reductions were not statistically significant. There were no effects on red blood cell or platelet levels.

In a randomized, placebo-controlled trial, 70 patients with myeloid and nonmyeloid malignancies were treated with myeloablative therapy and allogeneic bone marrow transplant followed by 300 mcg/m²/day of a Filgrastim product. A statistically significant reduction in the median number of days of severe neutropenia occurred in the treated group versus the control group (19 days in the control group and 15 days in the treatment group, p < 0.001) and time to recovery of ANC to ≥ 500/mm³ (21 days in the control group and 16 days in the treatment group, p < 0.001).

In three nonrandomized studies (n = 119), patients received ABMT and treatment with NEUPOGEN®. One study (n = 45) involved patients with breast cancer and malignant melanoma. A second study (n = 39) involved patients with HD. The third study (n = 35) involved patients with NHL, acute lymphoblastic leukemia (ALL), and germ cell tumor. In these studies, the recovery of the ANC to ≥ 500/mm³ ranged from a median of 11.5 to 13 days.

None of the conditioning regimens used in the ABMT studies included radiation therapy.

While these studies were not designed to compare survival, this information was collected and evaluated. The overall survival and disease progression of patients receiving NEUPOGEN® in these studies were similar to those observed in the respective control groups and to historical data.

Peripheral Blood Progenitor Cell Collection and Therapy in Cancer Patients

All patients in the Amgen-sponsored trials received a similar mobilization/collection regimen: NEUPOGEN® was administered for 6 to 7 days, with an apheresis procedure on days 5, 6, and 7 (except for a limited number of patients receiving apheresis on days 4, 6, and 8). In a non-Amgen-sponsored study, patients underwent mobilization to a target number of mononuclear cells (MNC), with apheresis starting on day 5. There are no data on the mobilization of peripheral blood progenitor cells (PBPC) after days 4 to 5 that are not confounded by leukapheresis.

Mobilization: Mobilization of PBPC was studied in 50 heavily pretreated patients (median number of prior cycles = 9.5) with NHL, HD, or ALL (Amgen study 1). CFU-GM was used as the marker for engraftable PBPC. The median CFU-GM level on each day of mobilization was determined from the data available (CFU-GM assays were not obtained on all patients on each day of mobilization). These data are presented below.

The data from Amgen study 1 were supported by data from Amgen study 2 in which 22 pretreated breast cancer patients (median number of prior cycles = 3) were studied. Both the CFU-GM and CD34⁺ cells reached a maximum on day 5 at > 10-fold over baseline and then remained elevated with leukapheresis.

[See table below]

In three studies of patients with prior exposure to chemotherapy, the median CFU-GM yield in the leukapheresis product ranged from 20.9 to 32.7 × 10⁴/kg body weight (n = 105). In two of these studies where CD34⁺ yields in the leukapheresis product were also determined, the median CD34⁺ yields were 3.11 and 2.80 × 10⁶/kg, respectively (n = 56). In an additional study of 18 chemotherapy-naive patients, the median CFU-GM yield was 123.4 × 10⁴/kg.

Engraftment: Engraftment following NEUPOGEN®-mobilized PBPC is summarized for 101 patients in the following table. In all studies, a Cox regression model showed that the total number of CFU-GM and/or CD34⁺ cells collected was a significant predictor of time to platelet recovery.

In a randomized, unblinded study of patients with HD or NHL undergoing myeloablative chemotherapy (Amgen study 3), 27 patients received NEUPOGEN®-mobilized PBPC followed by NEUPOGEN® and 31 patients received ABMT followed by NEUPOGEN®. Patients randomized to the NEUPOGEN®-mobilized PBPC group compared to the ABMT group had significantly fewer days of platelet transfusions (median 6 vs 10 days), a significantly shorter time to a sustained platelet count > 20,000/mm³ (median 16 vs 23 days), a significantly shorter time to recovery of a sustained ANC ≥ 500/mm³ (median 11 vs 14 days), significantly fewer days of red blood cell transfusions (median 2 vs 3 days) and a significantly shorter duration of posttransplant hospitalization.

[See first table at top of next page]

Three of the 101 patients (3%) did not achieve the criteria for engraftment as defined by a platelet count ≥ 20,000/mm³ by day 28. In clinical trials of NEUPOGEN® for the mobilization of PBPC, NEUPOGEN® was administered to patients at 5 to 24 mcg/kg/day after reinfusion of the collected cells until a sustainable ANC (≥ 500/mm³) was reached. The rate of engraftment of these cells in the absence of NEUPOGEN® posttransplantation has not been studied.

Patients With Severe Chronic Neutropenia

Severe chronic neutropenia (SCN) (idiopathic, cyclic, and congenital) is characterized by a selective decrease in the number of circulating neutrophils and an enhanced susceptibility to bacterial infections.

The daily administration of NEUPOGEN® has been shown to be safe and effective in causing a sustained increase in the neutrophil count and a decrease in infectious morbidity in children and adults with the clinical syndrome of SCN.[16]

In the phase 3 trial, summarized in the following table, daily treatment with NEUPOGEN® resulted in significant beneficial changes in the incidence and duration of infection, fever, antibiotic use, and oropharyngeal ulcers. In this trial, 120 patients with a median age of 12 years (range 1 to 76 years) were treated.

[See second table on next page]

The incidence for each of these 5 clinical parameters was lower in the NEUPOGEN® arm compared to the control arm for cohorts in each of the 3 major diagnostic categories. All 3 diagnostic groups showed favorable trends in favor of treatment. An analysis of variance showed no significant interaction between treatment and diagnosis, suggesting that efficacy did not differ substantially in the different diseases. Although NEUPOGEN® substantially reduced neutropenia in all patient groups, in patients with cyclic neutropenia, cycling persisted but the period of neutropenia was shortened to 1 day.

As a result of the lower incidence and duration of infections, there was also a lower number of episodes of hospitalization (28 hospitalizations in 62 patients in the treated group vs 44 hospitalizations in 60 patients in the control group over a 4-month period [p = 0.0034]). Patients treated with NEUPOGEN® also reported a lower number of episodes of diarrhea, nausea, fatigue, and sore throat.

Progenitor Cell Levels in Peripheral Blood by Mobilization Day

	Overall Study 1 CFU-GM/mL		Study 2 CFU-GM/mL		Study 2 CD34⁺ (× 10⁴/mL)	
	No. Samples	Median (25%–75%)	No. Samples	Median (25%–75%)	No. Samples	Median (25%–75%)
Day 1	11	18 (13–62)	20	42 (15–151)	20	0.13 (0.02–0.66)
Day 2	7	22 (3–61)	n/a*	n/a*	n/a*	n/a*
Day 3	10	138 (39–364)	n/a*	n/a*	n/a*	n/a*
Day 4	18	365 (158–864)	18	576 (108–1819)	17	2.11 (0.58–3.93)
Day 5	36	781 (391–1608)	21	960 (72–1677)	22	3.16 (1.08–6.11)
Day 6	46	505 (199–1397)	22	756 (70–3486)	22	2.67 (1.09–4.40)
Day 7	37	333 (111–938)	22	597 (118–2009)	21	2.64 (0.78–4.22)
Day 8	15	383 (94–815)		51 (10–746)	12	1.61 (0.38–4.31)

*n/a = not available

In the phase 3 trial, untreated patients had a median ANC of 210/mm^3 (range 0 to 1550/mm^3). NEUPOGEN® therapy was adjusted to maintain the median ANC between 1500 and 10,000/mm^3. Overall, the response to NEUPOGEN® was observed in 1 to 2 weeks. The median ANC after 5 months of NEUPOGEN® therapy for all patients was 7460/mm^3 (range 30 to 30,880/mm^3). NEUPOGEN® dosing requirements were generally higher for patients with congenital neutropenia (2.3 to 40 mcg/kg/day) than for patients with idiopathic (0.6 to 11.5 mcg/kg/day) or cyclic (0.5 to 6 mcg/kg/day) neutropenia.

		Amgen-sponsored Study 1 N = 13	Amgen-sponsored Study 2 N = 22	Amgen-sponsored Study 3 N = 27	Non-Amgen-sponsored Study N = 39
Median PBPC/kg Collected	MNC	9.5 × 10^8	9.5 × 10^8	8.1 × 10^8	10.3 × 10^8
	CD34$^+$	n/a*	3.1 × 10^6	2.8 × 10^6	6.2 × 10^6
	CFU-GM	63.9 × 10^4	25.3 × 10^4	32.6 × 10^4	n/a*
Days to ANC ≥ 500/mm^3	Median	9	10	11	10
	Range	8–10	8–15	9–38	7–40
Days to Plt. ≥ 20,000/mm^3	Median	10	12.5	16	15.5
	Range	7–16	10–30	8–52	7–63

*n/a = not available

Overall Significant Changes in Clinical Endpoints Median Incidence* (events) or Duration (days) per 28-day Period

	Control Patients†	NEUPOGEN®-treated Patients	p-value
Incidence of Infection	0.50	0.20	< 0.001
Incidence of Fever	0.25	0.20	< 0.001
Duration of Fever	0.63	0.20	0.005
Incidence of Oropharyngeal Ulcers	0.26	0.00	< 0.001
Incidence of Antibiotic Use	0.49	0.20	< 0.001

* Incidence values were calculated for each patient, and are defined as the total number of events experienced divided by the number of 28-day periods of exposure (on-study). Median incidence values were then reported for each patient group.
†Control patients were observed for a 4-month period.

INDICATIONS AND USAGE

Cancer Patients Receiving Myelosuppressive Chemotherapy

NEUPOGEN® is indicated to decrease the incidence of infection, as manifested by febrile neutropenia, in patients with nonmyeloid malignancies receiving myelosuppressive anti-cancer drugs associated with a significant incidence of severe neutropenia with fever (see **CLINICAL EXPERIENCE**). A complete blood count (CBC) and platelet count should be obtained prior to chemotherapy, and twice per week (see **LABORATORY MONITORING**) during NEUPOGEN® therapy to avoid leukocytosis and to monitor the neutrophil count. In phase 3 clinical studies, NEUPOGEN® therapy was discontinued when the ANC was ≥ 10,000/mm^3 after the expected chemotherapy-induced nadir.

Patients With Acute Myeloid Leukemia Receiving Induction or Consolidation Chemotherapy

NEUPOGEN® is indicated for reducing the time to neutrophil recovery and the duration of fever, following induction or consolidation chemotherapy treatment of adults with AML.

Cancer Patients Receiving Bone Marrow Transplant

NEUPOGEN® is indicated to reduce the duration of neutropenia and neutropenia-related clinical sequelae, eg, febrile neutropenia, in patients with nonmyeloid malignancies undergoing myeloablative chemotherapy followed by marrow transplantation (see **CLINICAL EXPERIENCE**). It is recommended that CBCs and platelet counts be obtained at a minimum of 3 times per week (see **LABORATORY MONITORING**) following marrow infusion to monitor the recovery of marrow reconstitution.

Patients Undergoing Peripheral Blood Progenitor Cell Collection and Therapy

NEUPOGEN® is indicated for the mobilization of hematopoietic progenitor cells into the peripheral blood for collection by leukapheresis. Mobilization allows for the collection of increased numbers of progenitor cells capable of engraftment compared with collection by leukapheresis without mobilization or bone marrow harvest. After myeloablative chemotherapy, the transplantation of an increased number of progenitor cells can lead to more rapid engraftment, which may result in a decreased need for supportive care (see **CLINICAL EXPERIENCE**).

Patients With Severe Chronic Neutropenia

NEUPOGEN® is indicated for chronic administration to reduce the incidence and duration of sequelae of neutropenia (eg, fever, infections, oropharyngeal ulcers) in symptomatic patients with congenital neutropenia, cyclic neutropenia, or idiopathic neutropenia (see **CLINICAL EXPERIENCE**). It is essential that serial CBCs with differential and platelet counts, and an evaluation of bone marrow morphology and karyotype be performed prior to initiation of NEUPOGEN® therapy (see **WARNINGS**). The use of NEUPOGEN® prior to confirmation of SCN may impair diagnostic efforts and may thus impair or delay evaluation and treatment of an underlying condition, other than SCN, causing the neutropenia.

CONTRAINDICATIONS

NEUPOGEN® is contraindicated in patients with known hypersensitivity to *E coli*-derived proteins, Filgrastim, or any component of the product.

WARNINGS

Allergic Reactions

Allergic-type reactions occurring on initial or subsequent treatment have been reported in < 1 in 4000 patients treated with NEUPOGEN®. These have generally been characterized by systemic symptoms involving at least 2 body systems, most often skin (rash, urticaria, facial edema), respiratory (wheezing, dyspnea), and cardiovascular (hypotension, tachycardia). Some reactions occurred on initial exposure. Reactions tended to occur within the first 30 minutes after administration and appeared to occur more frequently in patients receiving NEUPOGEN® IV. Rapid resolution of symptoms occurred in most cases after administration of antihistamines, steroids, bronchodilators, and/or epinephrine. Symptoms recurred in more than half the patients who were rechallenged.

SPLENIC RUPTURE

SPLENIC RUPTURE, INCLUDING FATAL CASES, HAS BEEN REPORTED FOLLOWING THE ADMINISTRATION OF NEUPOGEN®. INDIVIDUALS RECEIVING NEUPOGEN® WHO REPORT LEFT UPPER ABDOMINAL AND/OR SHOULDER TIP PAIN SHOULD BE EVALUATED FOR AN ENLARGED SPLEEN OR SPLENIC RUPTURE.

Acute Respiratory Distress Syndrome (ARDS)

Acute respiratory distress syndrome (ARDS) has been reported in patients receiving NEUPOGEN®, and is postulated to be secondary to an influx of neutrophils to sites of inflammation in the lungs. Patients receiving NEUPOGEN® who develop fever, lung infiltrates, or respiratory distress should be evaluated for the possibility of ARDS. In the event that ARDS occurs, NEUPOGEN® should be withheld until resolution of ARDS or discontinued. Patients should receive appropriate medical management for this condition.

Alveolar Hemorrhage and Hemoptysis

Alveolar hemorrhage manifesting as pulmonary infiltrates and hemoptysis requiring hospitalization has been reported in healthy donors undergoing peripheral blood progenitor cell (PBPC) mobilization. Hemoptysis resolved with discontinuation of NEUPOGEN®. The use of NEUPOGEN® for PBPC mobilization in healthy donors is not an approved indication.

Sickle Cell Disorders

Severe sickle cell crises, in some cases resulting in death, have been associated with the use of NEUPOGEN® in patients with sickle cell disorders. Only physicians qualified by specialized training or experience in the treatment of patients with sickle cell disorders should prescribe NEUPOGEN® for such patients, and only after careful consideration of the potential risks and benefits.

Patients With Severe Chronic Neutropenia

The safety and efficacy of NEUPOGEN® in the treatment of neutropenia due to other hematopoietic disorders (eg, myelodysplastic syndrome [MDS]) have not been established. Care should be taken to confirm the diagnosis of SCN before initiating NEUPOGEN® therapy.

MDS and AML have been reported to occur in the natural history of congenital neutropenia without cytokine therapy.[17] Cytogenetic abnormalities, transformation to MDS, and AML have also been observed in patients treated with NEUPOGEN® for SCN. Based on available data including a postmarketing surveillance study, the risk of developing MDS and AML appears to be confined to the subset of patients with congenital neutropenia (see **ADVERSE REACTIONS**). Abnormal cytogenetics and MDS have been associated with the eventual development of myeloid leukemia. The effect of NEUPOGEN® on the development of abnormal cytogenetics and the effect of continued NEUPOGEN® administration in patients with abnormal cytogenetics or MDS are unknown. If a patient with SCN develops abnormal cytogenetics or myelodysplasia, the risks and benefits of continuing NEUPOGEN® should be carefully considered.

PRECAUTIONS

General

Simultaneous Use With Chemotherapy and Radiation Therapy

The safety and efficacy of NEUPOGEN® given simultaneously with cytotoxic chemotherapy have not been established. Because of the potential sensitivity of rapidly dividing myeloid cells to cytotoxic chemotherapy, do not use NEUPOGEN® in the period 24 hours before through 24 hours after the administration of cytotoxic chemotherapy (see **DOSAGE AND ADMINISTRATION**).

The efficacy of NEUPOGEN® has not been evaluated in patients receiving chemotherapy associated with delayed myelosuppression (eg, nitrosoureas) or with mitomycin C or with myelosuppressive doses of antimetabolites such as 5-fluorouracil.

The safety and efficacy of NEUPOGEN® have not been evaluated in patients receiving concurrent radiation therapy. Simultaneous use of NEUPOGEN® with chemotherapy and radiation therapy should be avoided.

Potential Effect on Malignant Cells

NEUPOGEN® is a growth factor that primarily stimulates neutrophils. However, the possibility that NEUPOGEN® can act as a growth factor for any tumor type cannot be excluded. In a randomized study evaluating the effects of NEUPOGEN® versus placebo in patients undergoing remission induction for AML, there was no significant difference in remission rate, disease-free, or overall survival (see **CLINICAL EXPERIENCE**).

The safety of NEUPOGEN® in chronic myeloid leukemia (CML) and myelodysplasia has not been established.

When NEUPOGEN® is used to mobilize PBPC, tumor cells may be released from the marrow and subsequently collected in the leukapheresis product. The effect of reinfusion of tumor cells has not been well studied, and the limited data available are inconclusive.

Leukocytosis

Cancer Patients Receiving Myelosuppressive Chemotherapy

White blood cell counts of 100,000/mm^3 or greater were observed in approximately 2% of patients receiving NEUPOGEN® at doses above 5 mcg/kg/day. There were no reports of adverse events associated with this degree of leukocytosis. In order to avoid the potential complications of excessive leukocytosis, a CBC is recommended twice per week during NEUPOGEN® therapy (see **LABORATORY MONITORING**).

Premature Discontinuation of NEUPOGEN® Therapy

Cancer Patients Receiving Myelosuppressive Chemotherapy

A transient increase in neutrophil counts is typically seen 1 to 2 days after initiation of NEUPOGEN® therapy. However, for a sustained therapeutic response, NEUPOGEN® therapy should be continued following chemotherapy until the post nadir ANC reaches 10,000/mm^3. Therefore, the premature discontinuation of NEUPOGEN® therapy, prior to the time of recovery from the expected neutrophil nadir, is generally not recommended (see **DOSAGE AND ADMINISTRATION**).

Immunogenicity

As with all therapeutic proteins, there is a potential for immunogenicity. The incidence of antibody development in patients receiving NEUPOGEN® has not been adequately determined. While available data suggest that a small proportion of patients developed binding antibodies to Filgrastim, the nature and specificity of these antibodies has not been adequately studied. In clinical studies comparing NEUPOGEN® and Neulasta®, the incidence of antibodies binding to NEUPOGEN® was 3% (11/333). In these 11 patients, no evidence of a neutralizing response was observed using a cell-based bioassay. The detection of antibody formation is highly dependent on the sensitivity and specificity of the assay, and the observed incidence of antibody positivity in an assay may be influenced by several factors including timing of sampling, sample handling, concomitant medications, and underlying disease. Therefore, comparison of the incidence of antibodies to NEUPOGEN® with the incidence of antibodies to other products may be misleading. Cytopenias resulting from an antibody response to exogenous growth factors have been reported on rare occasions in patients treated with other recombinant growth factors. There is a theoretical possibility that an antibody directed against Filgrastim may cross-react with endogenous G-CSF, resulting in immune-mediated neutropenia; however, this has not been reported in clinical studies or in post-marketing experience. Patients who develop hypersensitivity to Filgrastim (NEUPOGEN®) may have allergic or hypersensitivity reactions to other E coli-derived proteins.

Cutaneous Vasculitis
Cutaneous vasculitis has been reported in patients treated with NEUPOGEN®. In most cases, the severity of cutaneous vasculitis was moderate or severe. Most of the reports involved patients with SCN receiving long-term NEUPOGEN® therapy. Symptoms of vasculitis generally developed simultaneously with an increase in the ANC and abated when the ANC decreased. Many patients were able to continue NEUPOGEN® at a reduced dose.

Information for Patients and Caregivers
Patients should be referred to the "Information for Patients and Caregivers" labeling included with the package insert in each dispensing pack of NEUPOGEN® vials or NEUPOGEN® prefilled syringes. The "Information for Patients and Caregivers" labeling provides information about neutrophils and neutropenia and the safety and efficacy of NEUPOGEN®. It is not intended to be a disclosure of all known or possible effects.

Laboratory Monitoring
Cancer Patients Receiving Myelosuppressive Chemotherapy
A CBC and platelet count should be obtained prior to chemotherapy, and at regular intervals (twice per week) during NEUPOGEN® therapy. Following cytotoxic chemotherapy, the neutrophil nadir occurred earlier during cycles when NEUPOGEN® was administered, and WBC differentials demonstrated a left shift, including the appearance of promyelocytes and myeloblasts. In addition, the duration of severe neutropenia was reduced, and was followed by an accelerated recovery in the neutrophil counts.

Cancer Patients Receiving Bone Marrow Transplant
Frequent CBCs and platelet counts are recommended (at least 3 times per week) following marrow transplantation.

Patients With Severe Chronic Neutropenia
During the initial 4 weeks of NEUPOGEN® therapy and during the 2 weeks following any dose adjustment, a CBC with differential and platelet count should be performed twice weekly. Once a patient is clinically stable, a CBC with differential and platelet count should be performed monthly during the first year of treatment. Thereafter, if clinically stable, routine monitoring with regular CBCs (ie, as clinically indicated but at least quarterly) is recommended. Additionally, for those patients with congenital neutropenia, annual bone marrow and cytogenetic evaluations should be performed throughout the duration of treatment (see WARNINGS, ADVERSE REACTIONS).
In clinical trials, the following laboratory results were observed:
• Cyclic fluctuations in the neutrophil counts were frequently observed in patients with congenital or idiopathic neutropenia after initiation of NEUPOGEN® therapy.
• Platelet counts were generally at the upper limits of normal prior to NEUPOGEN® therapy. With NEUPOGEN® therapy, platelet counts decreased but usually remained within normal limits (see ADVERSE REACTIONS).
• Early myeloid forms were noted in peripheral blood in most patients, including the appearance of metamyelocytes and myelocytes. Promyelocytes and myeloblasts were noted in some patients.
• Relative increases were occasionally noted in the number of circulating eosinophils and basophils. No consistent increases were observed with NEUPOGEN® therapy.
• As in other trials, increases were observed in serum uric acid, lactic dehydrogenase, and serum alkaline phosphatase.

Drug Interaction
Drug interactions between NEUPOGEN® and other drugs have not been fully evaluated. Drugs which may potentiate the release of neutrophils, such as lithium, should be used with caution.
Increased hematopoietic activity of the bone marrow in response to growth factor therapy has been associated with transient positive bone imaging changes. This should be considered when interpreting bone-imaging results.

Carcinogenesis, Mutagenesis, Impairment of Fertility
The carcinogenic potential of NEUPOGEN® has not been studied. NEUPOGEN® failed to induce bacterial gene mu-

tations in either the presence or absence of a drug metabolizing enzyme system. NEUPOGEN® had no observed effect on the fertility of male or female rats, or on gestation at doses up to 500 mcg/kg.

Pregnancy Category C
NEUPOGEN® has been shown to have adverse effects in pregnant rabbits when given in doses 2 to 10 times the human dose. Since there are no adequate and well-controlled studies in pregnant women, the effect, if any, of NEUPOGEN® on the developing fetus or the reproductive capacity of the mother is unknown. However, the scientific literature describes transplacental passage of NEUPOGEN® when administered to pregnant rats during the latter part of gestation[18] and apparent transplacental passage of NEUPOGEN® when administered to pregnant humans by ≤ 30 hours prior to preterm delivery (≤ 30 weeks gestation).[19] NEUPOGEN® should be used during pregnancy only if the potential benefit justifies the potential risk to the fetus.
In rabbits, increased abortion and embryolethality were observed in animals treated with NEUPOGEN® at 80 mcg/kg/day. NEUPOGEN® administered to pregnant rabbits at doses of 80 mcg/kg/day during the period of organogenesis was associated with increased fetal resorption, genitourinary bleeding, developmental abnormalities, decreased body weight, live births, and food consumption. External abnormalities were not observed in the fetuses of dams treated at 80 mcg/kg/day. Reproductive studies in pregnant rats have shown that NEUPOGEN® was not associated with lethal, teratogenic, or behavioral effects on fetuses when administered by daily IV injection during the period of organogenesis at dose levels up to 575 mcg/kg/day.
In Segment III studies in rats, offspring of dams treated at > 20 mcg/kg/day exhibited a delay in external differentiation (detachment of auricles and descent of testes) and slight growth retardation, possibly due to lower body weight of females during rearing and nursing. Offspring of dams treated at 100 mcg/kg/day exhibited decreased body weights at birth, and a slightly reduced 4-day survival rate.
Women who become pregnant during Neupogen treatment are encouraged to enroll in Amgen's Pregnancy Surveillance Program. Patients or their physicians should call 1-800-77-AMGEN (1-800-772-6436) to enroll.

Nursing Mothers
It is not known whether NEUPOGEN® is excreted in human milk. Because many drugs are excreted in human milk, caution should be exercised if NEUPOGEN® is administered to a nursing woman.

Pediatric Use
In a phase 3 study to assess the safety and efficacy of NEUPOGEN® in the treatment of SCN, 120 patients with a median age of 12 years were studied. Of the 120 patients, 12 were infants (1 month to 2 years of age), 47 were children (2 to 12 years of age), and 9 were adolescents (12 to 16 years of age). Additional information is available from a SCN postmarketing surveillance study, which includes long-term follow-up of patients in the clinical studies and information from additional patients who entered directly into the postmarketing surveillance study. Of the 531 patients in the surveillance study as of 31 December 1997, 32 were infants, 200 were children, and 68 were adolescents (see CLINICAL EXPERIENCE, INDICATIONS AND USAGE, LABORATORY MONITORING, DOSAGE AND ADMINISTRATION).
Pediatric patients with congenital types of neutropenia (Kostmann's syndrome, congenital agranulocytosis, or Schwachman-Diamond syndrome) have developed cytogenetic abnormalities and have undergone transformation to MDS and AML while receiving chronic NEUPOGEN® treatment. The relationship of these events to NEUPOGEN® administration is unknown (see WARNINGS, ADVERSE REACTIONS).
Long-term follow-up data from the postmarketing surveillance study suggest that height and weight are not adversely affected in patients who received up to 5 years of NEUPOGEN® treatment. Limited data from patients who were followed in the phase 3 study for 1.5 years did not suggest alterations in sexual maturation or endocrine function. The safety and efficacy in neonates and patients with autoimmune neutropenia of infancy have not been established.
In the cancer setting, 12 pediatric patients with neuroblastoma have received up to 6 cycles of cyclophosphamide, cisplatin, doxorubicin, and etoposide chemotherapy concurrently with NEUPOGEN®; in this population, NEUPOGEN® was well tolerated. There was one report of palpable splenomegaly associated with NEUPOGEN® therapy; however, the only consistently reported adverse event was musculoskeletal pain, which is no different from the experience in the adult population.

Geriatric Use
Among 855 subjects enrolled in 3 randomized, placebo-controlled trials of NEUPOGEN® use following myelosuppressive chemotherapy, there were 232 subjects age 65 or older, and 22 subjects age 75 or older. No overall differences

in safety or effectiveness were observed between these subjects and younger subjects, and other clinical experience has not identified differences in the responses between elderly and younger patients.
Clinical studies of NEUPOGEN® in other approved indications (ie, bone marrow transplant recipients, PBPC mobilization, and SCN) did not include sufficient numbers of subjects aged 65 and older to determine whether elderly subjects respond differently from younger subjects.

ADVERSE REACTIONS
Clinical Trial Experience
Cancer Patients Receiving Myelosuppressive Chemotherapy
In clinical trials involving over 350 patients receiving NEUPOGEN® following nonmyeloablative cytotoxic chemotherapy, most adverse experiences were the sequelae of the underlying malignancy or cytotoxic chemotherapy. In all phase 2 and 3 trials, medullary bone pain, reported in 24% of patients, was the only consistently observed adverse reaction attributed to NEUPOGEN® therapy. This bone pain was generally reported to be of mild-to-moderate severity, and could be controlled in most patients with non-narcotic analgesics; infrequently, bone pain was severe enough to require narcotic analgesics. Bone pain was reported more frequently in patients treated with higher doses (20 to 100 mcg/kg/day) administered IV, and less frequently in patients treated with lower SC doses of NEUPOGEN® (3 to 10 mcg/kg/day).
In the randomized, double-blind, placebo-controlled trial of NEUPOGEN® therapy following combination chemotherapy in patients (n = 207) with small cell lung cancer, the following adverse events were reported during blinded cycles of study medication (placebo or NEUPOGEN® at 4 to 8 mcg/kg/day). Events are reported as exposure-adjusted since patients remained on double-blind NEUPOGEN® a median of 3 cycles versus 1 cycle for placebo.

Event	% of Blinded Cycles With Events NEUPOGEN® N = 384 Patient Cycles	Placebo N = 257 Patient Cycles
Nausea/Vomiting	57	64
Skeletal Pain	22	11
Alopecia	18	27
Diarrhea	14	23
Neutropenic Fever	13	35
Mucositis	12	20
Fever	12	11
Fatigue	11	16
Anorexia	9	11
Dyspnea	9	11
Headache	7	9
Cough	6	8
Skin Rash	6	9
Chest Pain	5	6
Generalized Weakness	4	7
Sore Throat	4	9
Stomatitis	5	10
Constipation	5	10
Pain (Unspecified)	2	7

In this study, there were no serious, life-threatening, or fatal adverse reactions attributed to NEUPOGEN® therapy. Specifically, there were no reports of flu-like symptoms, pleuritis, pericarditis, or other major systemic reactions to NEUPOGEN®.
Spontaneously reversible elevations in uric acid, lactate dehydrogenase, and alkaline phosphatase occurred in 27% to 58% of 98 patients receiving blinded NEUPOGEN® therapy following cytotoxic chemotherapy; increases were generally mild-to-moderate. Transient decreases in blood pressure (< 90/60 mmHg), which did not require clinical treatment, were reported in 7 of 176 patients in phase 3 clinical studies following administration of NEUPOGEN®. Cardiac events (myocardial infarctions, arrhythmias) have been reported in 11 of 375 cancer patients receiving NEUPOGEN® in clinical studies; the relationship to NEUPOGEN® therapy is unknown. No evidence of interaction of NEUPOGEN® with other drugs was observed in the course of clinical trials (see PRECAUTIONS).
There has been no evidence for the development of antibodies or of a blunted or diminished response to NEUPOGEN® in treated patients, including those receiving NEUPOGEN® daily for almost 2 years.

Patients With Acute Myeloid Leukemia
In a randomized phase 3 clinical trial, 259 patients received NEUPOGEN® and 262 patients received placebo postchemotherapy. Overall, the frequency of all reported adverse events was similar in both the NEUPOGEN® and placebo groups (83% vs 82% in Induction 1; 61% vs 64% in Consolidation 1). Adverse events reported more frequently in

the NEUPOGEN®-treated group included: petechiae (17% vs 14%), epistaxis (9% vs 5%), and transfusion reactions (10% vs 5%). There were no significant differences in the frequency of these events.

There were a similar number of deaths in each treatment group during induction (25 NEUPOGEN® vs 27 placebo). The primary causes of death included infection (9 vs 18), persistent leukemia (7 vs 5), and hemorrhage (6 vs 3). Of the hemorrhagic deaths, 5 cerebral hemorrhages were reported in the NEUPOGEN® group and 1 in the placebo group. Other serious nonfatal hemorrhagic events were reported in the respiratory tract (4 vs 1), skin (4 vs 4), gastrointestinal tract (2 vs 2), urinary tract (1 vs 1), ocular (1 vs 0), and other nonspecific sites (2 vs 1). While 19 (7%) patients in the NEUPOGEN® group and 5 (2%) patients in the placebo group experienced severe or fatal hemorrhagic events, overall, hemorrhagic adverse events were reported at a similar frequency in both groups (40% vs 38%). The time to transfusion-independent platelet recovery and the number of days of platelet transfusions were similar in both groups.

Cancer Patients Receiving Bone Marrow Transplant
In clinical trials, the reported adverse effects were those typically seen in patients receiving intensive chemotherapy followed by bone marrow transplant (BMT). The most common events reported in both control and treatment groups included stomatitis, nausea, and vomiting, generally of mild-to-moderate severity and were considered unrelated to NEUPOGEN®. In the randomized studies of BMT involving 167 patients who received study drug, the following events occurred more frequently in patients treated with Filgrastim than in controls: nausea (10% vs 4%), vomiting (7% vs 3%), hypertension (4% vs 0%), rash (12% vs 10%), and peritonitis (2% vs 0%). None of these events were reported by the investigator to be related to NEUPOGEN®. One event of erythema nodosum was reported moderate in severity and possibly related to NEUPOGEN®.

Generally, adverse events observed in nonrandomized studies were similar to those seen in randomized studies, occurred in a minority of patients, and were of mild-to-moderate severity. In one study (n = 45), 3 serious adverse events reported by the investigator were considered possibly related to NEUPOGEN®. These included 2 events of renal insufficiency and 1 event of capillary leak syndrome. The relationship of these events to NEUPOGEN® remains unclear since they occurred in patients with culture-proven infection with clinical sepsis who were receiving potentially nephrotoxic antibacterial and antifungal therapy.

Cancer Patients Undergoing Peripheral Blood Progenitor Cell Collection and Therapy
In clinical trials, 126 patients received NEUPOGEN® for PBPC mobilization. In this setting, NEUPOGEN® was generally well tolerated. Adverse events related to NEUPOGEN® consisted primarily of mild-to-moderate musculoskeletal symptoms, reported in 44% of patients. These symptoms were predominantly events of medullary bone pain (33%). Headache was reported related to NEUPOGEN® in 7% of patients. Transient increases in alkaline phosphatase related to NEUPOGEN® were reported in 21% of the patients who had serum chemistries measured; most were mild-to-moderate.

All patients had increases in neutrophil counts during mobilization, consistent with the biological effects of NEUPOGEN®. Two patients had a WBC count > 100,000/mm³. No sequelae were associated with any grade of leukocytosis.

Sixty-five percent of patients had mild-to-moderate anemia and 97% of patients had decreases in platelet counts; 5 patients (out of 126) had decreased platelet counts to < 50,000/mm³. Anemia and thrombocytopenia have been reported to be related to leukapheresis; however, the possibility that NEUPOGEN® mobilization may contribute to anemia or thrombocytopenia has not been ruled out.

Patients With Severe Chronic Neutropenia
Mild-to-moderate bone pain was reported in approximately 33% of patients in clinical trials. This symptom was readily controlled with non-narcotic analgesics. Generalized musculoskeletal pain was also noted in higher frequency in patients treated with NEUPOGEN®. Palpable splenomegaly was observed in approximately 30% of patients. Abdominal or flank pain was seen infrequently, and thrombocytopenia (< 50,000/mm³) was noted in 12% of patients with palpable spleens. Fewer than 3% of all patients underwent splenectomy, and most of these had a prestudy history of splenomegaly. Fewer than 6% of patients had thrombocytopenia (< 50,000/mm³) during NEUPOGEN® therapy, most of whom had a pre-existing history of thrombocytopenia. In most cases, thrombocytopenia was managed by NEUPOGEN® dose reduction or interruption. An additional 5% of patients had platelet counts between 50,000 and 100,000/mm³. There were no associated serious hemorrhagic sequelae in these patients. Epistaxis was noted in 15% of patients treated with NEUPOGEN®, but was associated with thrombocytopenia in 2% of patients. Anemia was reported in approximately 10% of patients, but in most

cases appeared to be related to frequent diagnostic phlebotomy, chronic illness, or concomitant medications. Other adverse events infrequently observed and possibly related to NEUPOGEN® therapy were: injection site reaction, rash, hepatomegaly, arthralgia, osteoporosis, cutaneous vasculitis, hematuria/proteinuria, alopecia, and exacerbation of some pre-existing skin disorders (eg, psoriasis).

Cytogenetic abnormalities, transformation to MDS, and AML have been observed in patients treated with NEUPOGEN® for SCN (see **WARNINGS, PRECAUTIONS: Pediatric Use**). As of 31 December 1997, data were available from a postmarketing surveillance study of 531 SCN patients with an average follow-up of 4.0 years. Based on analysis of these data, the risk of developing MDS and AML appears to be confined to the subset of patients with congenital neutropenia. A life-table analysis of these data revealed that the cumulative risk of developing leukemia or MDS by the end of the 8th year of NEUPOGEN® treatment in a patient with congenital neutropenia was 16.5% (95% C.I. = 9.8%, 23.3%); this represents an annual rate of approximately 2%. Cytogenetic abnormalities, most commonly involving chromosome 7, have been reported in patients treated with NEUPOGEN® who had previously documented normal cytogenetics. It is unknown whether the development of cytogenetic abnormalities, MDS, or AML is related to chronic daily NEUPOGEN® administration or to the natural history of congenital neutropenia. It is also unknown if the rate of conversion in patients who have not received NEUPOGEN® is different from that of patients who have received NEUPOGEN®. Routine monitoring through regular CBCs is recommended for all SCN patients. Additionally, annual bone marrow and cytogenetic evaluations are recommended in all patients with congenital neutropenia (see **LABORATORY MONITORING**).

Postmarketing Experience
The following adverse reactions have been identified during postapproval of NEUPOGEN®. Because these reactions are reported voluntarily from a population of uncertain size, it is not always possible to reliably estimate their frequency or establish a causal relationship to drug exposure.
- splenic rupture (see **WARNINGS: Splenic Rupture**)
- acute respiratory distress syndrome (ARDS) (see **WARNINGS: Acute Respiratory Distress Syndrome**)
- alveolar hemorrhage and hemoptysis (see **WARNINGS: Alveolar Hemorrhage and Hemoptysis**)
- sickle cell crisis (see **WARNINGS: Sickle Cell Disorders**)
- cutaneous vasculitis (see **PRECAUTIONS: Cutaneous Vasculitis**)
- Sweet's syndrome (acute febrile neutrophilic dermatosis)

OVERDOSAGE
In cancer patients receiving NEUPOGEN® as an adjunct to myelosuppressive chemotherapy, it is recommended, to avoid the potential risks of excessive leukocytosis, that NEUPOGEN® therapy be discontinued if the ANC surpasses 10,000/mm³ after the chemotherapy-induced ANC nadir has occurred. Doses of NEUPOGEN® that increase the ANC beyond 10,000/mm³ may not result in any additional clinical benefit.

The maximum tolerated dose of NEUPOGEN® has not been determined. Efficacy was demonstrated at doses of 4 to 8 mcg/kg/day in the phase 3 study of nonmyeloablative chemotherapy. Patients in the BMT studies received up to 138 mcg/kg/day without toxic effects, although there was a flattening of the dose response curve above daily doses of greater than 10 mcg/kg/day.

In NEUPOGEN® clinical trials of cancer patients receiving myelosuppressive chemotherapy, WBC counts > 100,000/mm³ have been reported in less than 5% of patients, but were not associated with any reported adverse clinical effects.

In cancer patients receiving myelosuppressive chemotherapy, discontinuation of NEUPOGEN® therapy usually results in a 50% decrease in circulating neutrophils within 1 to 2 days, with a return to pretreatment levels in 1 to 7 days.

DOSAGE AND ADMINISTRATION
NEUPOGEN® is supplied in either vials or in prefilled syringes with UltraSafe® Needle Guards. Following administration of NEUPOGEN® from the prefilled syringe, the UltraSafe® Needle Guard should be activated to prevent accidental needle sticks. To activate the UltraSafe® Needle Guard, place your hands behind the needle, grasp the guard with one hand, and slide the guard forward until the needle is completely covered and the guard clicks into place. **NOTE: If an audible click is not heard, the needle guard may not be completely activated.** The prefilled syringe should be disposed of by placing the entire prefilled syringe with guard activated into an approved puncture-proof container.

Cancer Patients Receiving Myelosuppressive Chemotherapy
The recommended starting dose of NEUPOGEN® is 5 mcg/kg/day, administered as a single daily injection by SC bolus

injection, by short IV infusion (15 to 30 minutes), or by continuous SC or continuous IV infusion. A CBC and platelet count should be obtained before instituting NEUPOGEN® therapy, and monitored twice weekly during therapy. Doses may be increased in increments of 5 mcg/kg for each chemotherapy cycle, according to the duration and severity of the ANC nadir.

NEUPOGEN® should be administered no earlier than 24 hours after the administration of cytotoxic chemotherapy. NEUPOGEN® should not be administered in the period 24 hours before the administration of chemotherapy (see **PRECAUTIONS**). NEUPOGEN® should be administered daily for up to 2 weeks, until the ANC has reached 10,000/mm³ following the expected chemotherapy-induced neutrophil nadir. The duration of NEUPOGEN® therapy needed to attenuate chemotherapy-induced neutropenia may be dependent on the myelosuppressive potential of the chemotherapy regimen employed. NEUPOGEN® therapy should be discontinued if the ANC surpasses 10,000/mm³ after the expected chemotherapy-induced neutrophil nadir (see **PRECAUTIONS**). In phase 3 trials, efficacy was observed at doses of 4 to 8 mcg/kg/day.

Cancer Patients Receiving Bone Marrow Transplant
The recommended dose of NEUPOGEN® following BMT is 10 mcg/kg/day given as an IV infusion of 4 or 24 hours, or as a continuous 24-hour SC infusion. For patients receiving BMT, the first dose of NEUPOGEN® should be administered at least 24 hours after cytotoxic chemotherapy and at least 24 hours after bone marrow infusion.

During the period of neutrophil recovery, the daily dose of NEUPOGEN® should be titrated against the neutrophil response as follows:

Absolute Neutrophil Count	NEUPOGEN® Dose Adjustment
When ANC > 1000/mm³ for 3 consecutive days then:	Reduce to 5 mcg/kg/day*
If ANC remains > 1000/mm³ for 3 more consecutive days then:	Discontinue NEUPOGEN®
If ANC decreases to < 1000/mm³	Resume at 5 mcg/kg/day

* If ANC decreases to < 1000/mm³ at any time during the 5 mcg/kg/day administration, NEUPOGEN® should be increased to 10 mcg/kg/day, and the above steps should then be followed.

Peripheral Blood Progenitor Cell Collection and Therapy in Cancer Patients
The recommended dose of NEUPOGEN® for the mobilization of PBPC is 10 mcg/kg/day SC, either as a bolus or a continuous infusion. It is recommended that NEUPOGEN® be given for at least 4 days before the first leukapheresis procedure and continued until the last leukapheresis. Although the optimal duration of NEUPOGEN® administration and leukapheresis schedule have not been established, administration of NEUPOGEN® for 6 to 7 days with leukaphereses on days 5, 6, and 7 was found to be safe and effective (see **CLINICAL EXPERIENCE** for schedules used in clinical trials). Neutrophil counts should be monitored after 4 days of NEUPOGEN®, and NEUPOGEN® dose modification should be considered for those patients who develop a WBC count > 100,000/mm³.

In all clinical trials of NEUPOGEN® for the mobilization of PBPC, NEUPOGEN® was also administered after reinfusion of the collected cells (see **CLINICAL EXPERIENCE**).

Patients With Severe Chronic Neutropenia
NEUPOGEN® should be administered to those patients in whom a diagnosis of congenital, cyclic, or idiopathic neutropenia has been definitively confirmed. Other diseases associated with neutropenia should be ruled out.

Starting Dose:
Congenital Neutropenia: The recommended daily starting dose is 6 mcg/kg BID SC every day.
Idiopathic or Cyclic Neutropenia: The recommended daily starting dose is 5 mcg/kg as a single injection SC every day.
Dose Adjustments:
Chronic daily administration is required to maintain clinical benefit. Absolute neutrophil count should not be used as the sole indication of efficacy. The dose should be individually adjusted based on the patients' clinical course as well as ANC. In the SCN postmarketing surveillance study, the reported median daily doses of NEUPOGEN® were: 6.0 mcg/kg (congenital neutropenia), 2.1 mcg/kg (cyclic neutropenia), and 1.2 mcg/kg (idiopathic neutropenia). In rare instances, patients with congenital neutropenia have required doses of NEUPOGEN® ≥ 100 mcg/kg/day.

Dilution
If required, NEUPOGEN® may be diluted in 5% dextrose. NEUPOGEN® diluted to concentrations between 5 and

15 mcg/mL should be protected from adsorption to plastic materials by the addition of Albumin (Human) to a final concentration of 2 mg/mL. When diluted in 5% dextrose or 5% dextrose plus Albumin (Human), NEUPOGEN® is compatible with glass bottles, PVC and polyolefin IV bags, and polypropylene syringes.

Dilution of NEUPOGEN® to a final concentration of less than 5 mcg/mL is not recommended at any time. **Do not dilute with saline at any time; product may precipitate.**

Storage

NEUPOGEN® should be stored in the refrigerator at 2° to 8°C (36° to 46°F). Avoid shaking. Prior to injection, NEUPOGEN® may be allowed to reach room temperature for a maximum of 24 hours. Any vial or prefilled syringe left at room temperature for greater than 24 hours should be discarded. Parenteral drug products should be inspected visually for particulate matter and discoloration prior to administration, whenever solution and container permit; if particulates or discoloration are observed, the container should not be used.

HOW SUPPLIED

NEUPOGEN®: Use only one dose per vial; do not re-enter the vial. Discard unused portions. Do not save unused drug for later administration.

Use only one dose per prefilled syringe. Discard unused portions. Do not save unused drug for later administration.

Vials

Single-dose, preservative-free vials containing 300 mcg (1 mL) of Filgrastim (300 mcg/mL). Dispensing packs of 10 (NDC 55513-530-10).

Single-dose, preservative-free vials containing 480 mcg (1.6 mL) of Filgrastim (300 mcg/mL). Dispensing packs of 10 (NDC 55513-546-10).

Prefilled Syringes (SingleJect®)

Single-dose, preservative-free, prefilled syringes with 27 gauge, ½ inch needles with an UltraSafe® Needle Guard, containing 300 mcg (0.5 mL) of Filgrastim (600 mcg/mL). Dispensing packs of 10 (NDC 55513-924-10).

Single-dose, preservative-free, prefilled syringes with 27 gauge, ½ inch needles with an UltraSafe® Needle Guard, containing 480 mcg (0.8 mL) of Filgrastim (600 mcg/mL). Dispensing packs of 10 (NDC 55513-209-10).

The needle cover of the prefilled syringe contains dry natural rubber (a derivative of latex).

NEUPOGEN® should be stored at 2° to 8°C (36° to 46°F). Avoid shaking.

REFERENCES

1. Zsebo KM, Cohen AM, Murdock DC, et al. Recombinant human granulocyte colony-stimulating factor: Molecular and biological characterization. *Immunobiol.* 1986; 172:175-184.
2. Welte K, Bonilla MA, Gillio AP, et al. Recombinant human G-CSF: Effects on hematopoiesis in normal and cyclophosphamide treated primates. *J Exp Med.* 1987; 165:941-948.
3. Duhrsen U, Villeval JL, Boyd J, et al. Effects of recombinant human granulocyte colony-stimulating factor on hematopoietic progenitor cells in cancer patients. *Blood.* 1988;72:2074-2081.
4. Souza LM, Boone TC, Gabrilove J, et al. Recombinant human granulocyte colony-stimulating factor: Effects on normal and leukemic myeloid cells. *Science.* 1986;232: 61-65.
5. Weisbart RH, Kacena A, Schuh A, Golde DW. GM-CSF induces human neutrophil IgA-mediated phagocytosis by an IgA Fc receptor activation mechanism. *Nature.* 1988;332:647-648.
6. Kitagawa S, Yuo A, Souza LM, Saito M, Miura Y, Takaku F. Recombinant human granulocyte colony-stimulating factor enhances superoxide release in human granulocytes stimulated by chemotactic peptide. *Biochem Biophys Res Commun.* 1987;1443:1146.
7. Glaspy JA, Baldwin GC, Robertson PA, et al. Therapy for neutropenia in hairy cell leukemia with recombinant human granulocyte colony-stimulating factor. *Ann Int Med.* 1988;109:789-795.
8. Yuo A, Kitagawa S, Ohsaka A, et al. Recombinant human granulocyte colony-stimulating factor as an activator of human granulocytes: Potentiation of responses triggered by receptor-mediated agonists and stimulation of C3bi receptor expression and adherence. *Blood.* 1989;74:2144-2149.
9. Gabrilove JL, Jakubowski A, Fain K, et al. Phase I study of granulocyte colony-stimulating factor in patients with transitional cell carcinoma of the urothelium. *J Clin Invest.* 1988;82:1454-1461.
10. Morstyn G, Souza L, Keech J, et al. Effect of granulocyte colony-stimulating factor on neutropenia induced by cytotoxic chemotherapy. *Lancet.* 1988;1:667-672.
11. Bronchud MH, Scarffe JH, Thatcher N, et al. Phase I/II study of recombinant human granulocyte colony-

stimulating factor in patients receiving intensive chemotherapy for small cell lung cancer. *Br J Cancer.* 1987;56:809-813.
12. Gabrilove JL, Jakubowski A, Scher H, et al. Effect of granulocyte colony-stimulating factor on neutropenia and associated morbidity due to chemotherapy for transitional cell carcinoma of the urothelium. *N Engl J Med.* 1988;318:1414-1422.
13. Neidhart J, Mangalik A, Kohler W, et al. Granulocyte colony-stimulating factor stimulates recovery of granulocytes in patients receiving dose-intensive chemotherapy without bone-marrow transplantation. *J Clin Oncol.* 1989;7:1685-1691.
14. Bronchud MH, Howell A, Crowther D, et al. The use of granulocyte colony-stimulating factor to increase the intensity of treatment with doxorubicin in patients with advanced breast and ovarian cancer. *Br J Cancer.* 1989;60:121-128.
15. Heil G, Hoelzer D, Sanz MA, et al. A randomized, double-blind, placebo-controlled, phase III study of Filgrastim in remission induction and consolidation therapy for adults with de novo Acute Myeloid Leukemia. *Blood.* 1997;90:4710-4718.
16. Dale DC, Bonilla MA, Davis MW, et al. A randomized controlled phase III trial of recombinant human granulocyte colony-stimulating factor (Filgrastim) for treatment of severe chronic neutropenia. *Blood.* 1993;81: 2496-2502.
17. Schroeder TM and Kurth R. Spontaneous chromosomal breakage and high incidence of leukemia in inherited disease. *Blood.* 1971;37:96-112.
18. Medlock ES, Kaplan DL, Cecchini M, Ulich TR, del Castillo J, Andresen J. Granulocyte colony-stimulating factor crosses the placenta and stimulates fetal rat granulopoiesis. *Blood.* 1993;81:916-922.
19. Calhoun DA, Rosa C, Christensen RD. Transplacental passage of recombinant human granulocyte colony-stimulating factor in women with an imminent preterm delivery. *Am J Obstet Gynecol.* 1996;174:1306-1311.

This product and its use are covered by the following US Patent Nos.: 5,582,823; 5,580,755.

Manufactured by:
Amgen Manufacturing, Limited, a subsidiary of Amgen Inc.
One Amgen Center Drive
Thousand Oaks, California 91320-1799
1xxxxxx
v.21 - Issue Date: 03/2010

NEUPOGEN®
(FILGRASTIM)
INFORMATION FOR PATIENTS AND CAREGIVERS

This patient package insert provides information and instructions for people who will be receiving NEUPOGEN® and their caregivers. This patient package insert does not tell you everything about NEUPOGEN®. You should discuss any questions you have about treatment with NEUPOGEN® with your doctor.

What is NEUPOGEN®?

NEUPOGEN® is a man-made form of granulocyte colony-stimulating factor (G-CSF), which is made using the bacteria *E coli*. G-CSF is a substance naturally produced by the body. It stimulates the growth of neutrophils (nu-tro-fils), a type of white blood cell important in the body's fight against infection.

What is NEUPOGEN® used for?

NEUPOGEN® is used to treat neutropenia (nu-tro-**peen**-ee-ah), a condition where the body makes too few neutrophils. Neutropenia may be a long-standing condition where your body does not make enough neutrophils, or it may be caused by drugs used to treat cancer. In some cases, your body may make enough neutrophils, but as part of your treatment for cancer, your doctor may want to increase the number of certain blood cells (CD34 cells) and collect them. The cells are collected using a process called apheresis (ay-fer-**ree**-sis). These collected cells are given back to you after you receive very high doses of treatment for cancer to make your blood counts get back to normal more quickly.

How does NEUPOGEN® work?

NEUPOGEN® works by helping your body make more neutrophils. To make sure NEUPOGEN® is working, your doctor will ask that you have regular blood tests to count the number of neutrophils you have. It is important that you follow your doctor's instructions about getting these tests.

Who should not take NEUPOGEN®?

Do not take NEUPOGEN® if you are:
• Allergic to NEUPOGEN® (Filgrastim) or any of its ingredients. See the end of this leaflet for a list of ingredients in NEUPOGEN®.

• Allergic to other medicines made using the bacteria *E coli*. Ask your doctor if you are not sure.

What important information do I need to know about taking NEUPOGEN®?

NEUPOGEN® may reduce your chance of getting an infection, but does not prevent all infections. An infection can still happen during the short time when your/your child's neutrophil levels are low. You must be alert and look for some of the common signs or symptoms of infection, such as fever, chills, rash, sore throat, diarrhea, or redness, swelling, or pain around a cut or sore. If you/your child has any of these signs or symptoms during treatment with NEUPOGEN®, tell your doctor or nurse immediately.

There is a possibility that you could have a reaction at an injection site. If there is a lump, swelling, or bruising at an injection site that does not go away, call your doctor.

If you have a sickle cell disorder, make sure that you tell your doctor before you start taking NEUPOGEN®. If you have a sickle cell crisis after getting NEUPOGEN®, tell your doctor right away.

Make sure your doctor knows about all medicines, and herbal or vitamin supplements you are taking before starting NEUPOGEN®. If you are taking lithium you may need more frequent blood tests.

If you/your child are receiving NEUPOGEN® because you are also receiving chemotherapy, the last dose of NEUPOGEN® should be injected at least 24 hours before your next dose of chemotherapy.

There is more information about NEUPOGEN® in the Physician Package Insert. If you have any questions, you should talk to your doctor.

What are possible serious side effects of NEUPOGEN®?

• **Spleen Rupture.** Your spleen may become enlarged and can rupture while taking NEUPOGEN®. A ruptured spleen can cause death. The spleen is located in the upper left section of your stomach area. Call your doctor right away if you or your child has pain in the left upper stomach area or left shoulder tip area. This pain could mean your or your child's spleen is enlarged or ruptured.

• **Serious Allergic Reactions.** NEUPOGEN® can cause serious allergic reactions. These reactions can cause a rash over the whole body, shortness of breath, wheezing, dizziness, swelling around the mouth or eyes, fast pulse, and sweating. If you or your child starts to have any of these symptoms, stop using NEUPOGEN® and call your doctor or seek emergency care right away. If you or your child has an allergic reaction during the injection of NEUPOGEN®, stop the injection right away.

• **A serious lung problem called acute respiratory distress syndrome (ARDS).** Call your doctor or seek emergency care right away if you or your child has shortness of breath, trouble breathing or a fast rate of breathing.

What are the most common side effects of NEUPOGEN®?

The most common side effect you/your child may experience is aching in the bones and muscles. This aching can usually be relieved by taking a non-aspirin pain reliever such as acetaminophen.

Some people experience redness, swelling, or itching at the site of injection. This may be an allergy to the ingredients in NEUPOGEN®, or it may be a local reaction. If you are giving an injection to a child, look for signs of redness, swelling, or itching at the site of injection because they may not be able to tell you they are experiencing a reaction. If you notice any signs of a local reaction, call your doctor.

What about pregnancy or breastfeeding?

NEUPOGEN® has not been studied in pregnant women, and its effects on unborn babies are not known. If you take NEUPOGEN® while you are pregnant, it is possible that small amounts of it may get into your baby's blood. It is not known if NEUPOGEN® can get into human breast milk.

If you are pregnant, plan to become pregnant, think you may be pregnant, or are breast feeding, you should tell your doctor before using NEUPOGEN®.

How to prepare and give a NEUPOGEN® injection

NEUPOGEN® should be injected at the same time each day. If you miss a dose contact your doctor or nurse.

You must always use the correct dose of NEUPOGEN®. Too little NEUPOGEN® may not protect you against infections, and too much NEUPOGEN® may cause too many neutrophils to be in your blood. Your doctor will determine your/your child's correct dose based on your/your child's body weight.

If you are giving someone else NEUPOGEN® injections, it is important that you know how to inject NEUPOGEN®, how much to inject, and how often to inject NEUPOGEN®. NEUPOGEN® is available as a liquid in vials or in prefilled syringes. When you receive your NEUPOGEN®, always check to see that:

• The name NEUPOGEN® appears on the package and vial or prefilled syringe label.

- The expiration date on the vial or prefilled syringe label has not passed. **You should not use a vial or prefilled syringe after the date on the label.**
- The strength of the NEUPOGEN® (number of micrograms in the colored dot on the package containing the vial or prefilled syringe) is the same as your doctor prescribed.
- The NEUPOGEN® liquid in the vial or in the prefilled syringe is clear and colorless. **Do not use NEUPOGEN®** if the contents of the vial or prefilled syringe appear discolored or cloudy, or if the vial or prefilled syringe appears to contain lumps, flakes, or particles.

If you are using vials of NEUPOGEN® only use the syringe that your doctor prescribes.

Your doctor or nurse will give you instructions on how to measure the correct dose of NEUPOGEN®. This dose will be measured in milliliters. You should only use a syringe that is marked in tenths of milliliters, or mL (for example, 0.2 mL). The doctor or nurse may refer to an mL as a cc (1 mL = 1 cc). If you do not use the correct syringe, you or your child could receive too much or too little NEUPOGEN®.

Only use disposable syringes and needles. Use the syringes only once and dispose of them as instructed by your doctor or nurse.

IMPORTANT: TO HELP AVOID POSSIBLE INFECTION, YOU SHOULD FOLLOW THESE INSTRUCTIONS.

Setting up for an injection
1. Find a clean flat working surface, such as a table.
2. Remove the vial or prefilled syringe of NEUPOGEN® from the refrigerator. Allow NEUPOGEN® to reach room temperature (this takes about 30 minutes). Vials or prefilled syringes should be used only once. DO NOT SHAKE THE VIAL OR PREFILLED SYRINGE. Shaking may damage the NEUPOGEN®. If the vial or prefilled syringe has been shaken vigorously, the solution may appear foamy and it should not be used.
3. Assemble the supplies you will need for an injection:
   - NEUPOGEN® vial <u>and</u> disposable syringe and needle

Vial

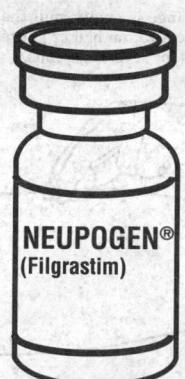

- Or NEUPOGEN® prefilled syringe with transparent (clear) plastic orange needle guard attached

Prefilled Syringe

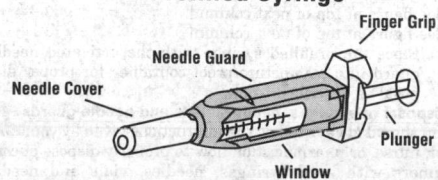

- two alcohol swabs and one cotton ball or gauze pad

Alcohol Swabs

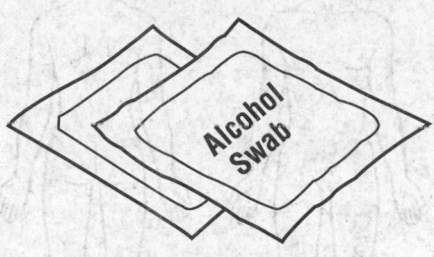

Cotton Ball

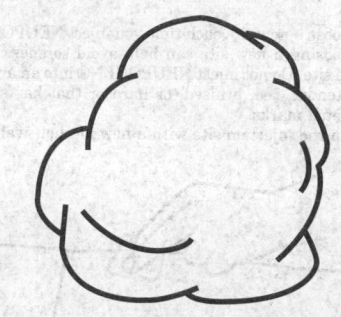

- puncture-proof disposal container
4. Wash your hands with soap and warm water.

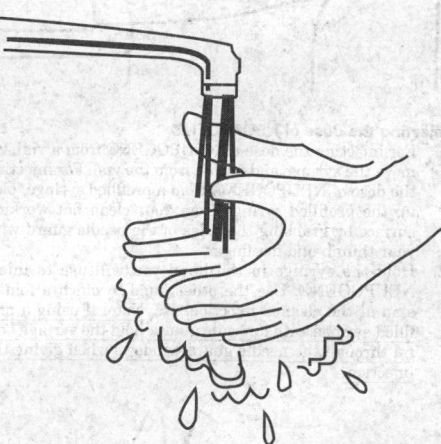

HOW TO PREPARE THE DOSE OF NEUPOGEN® IN VIALS OR PREFILLED SYRINGES

If you are using NEUPOGEN® in a vial, follow the instructions in Section A. If you are using NEUPOGEN® in a prefilled syringe, go to Section B.

Section A. Preparing the dose of NEUPOGEN® in a vial
1. Take the cap off the vial. Clean the rubber stopper with one alcohol swab.
[See figure at top of next column]
[See figure at top of next column]
2. Check the package containing the syringe. If the package has been opened or damaged, do not use that syringe. Dispose of that syringe in the puncture-proof disposal container. If the syringe package is undamaged, open the package and remove the syringe.
3. Pull the needle cover straight off the syringe. Then, pull back the plunger and draw air into the syringe. The amount of air drawn into the syringe should be the same amount (mL or cc) as the dose of NEUPOGEN® that your doctor prescribed.
[See figure at top of next column]
4. Keep the vial on your flat working surface and insert the needle straight down through the rubber stopper. Do not put the needle through the rubber stopper more than once.
5. Push the plunger of the syringe down and inject the air from the syringe into the vial of NEUPOGEN®.
[See figure at top of next page]

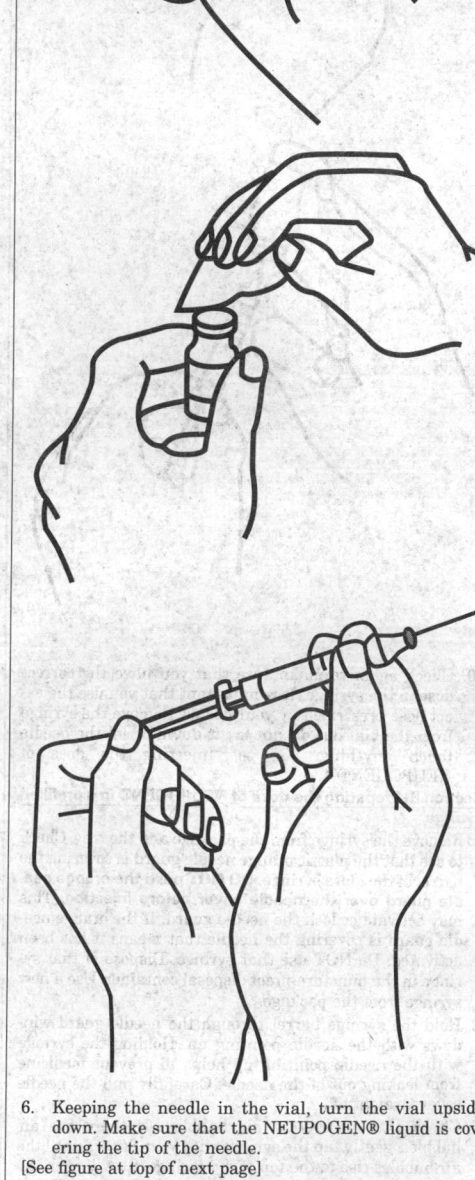

6. Keeping the needle in the vial, turn the vial upside down. Make sure that the NEUPOGEN® liquid is covering the tip of the needle.
[See figure at top of next page]
7. Keeping the vial upside down, slowly pull back on the plunger to fill the syringe with NEUPOGEN® liquid to the number (mL or cc) that matches the dose your doctor prescribed.
8. Keeping the needle in the vial, check for air bubbles in the syringe. If there are air bubbles, gently tap the syringe with your fingers until the air bubbles rise to the top of the syringe. Then slowly push the plunger up to force the air bubbles out of the syringe.
9. Keeping the tip of the needle in the liquid, once again pull the plunger back to the number on the syringe that matches your dose. Check again for air bubbles. The air in the syringe will not hurt you, but too large an air bubble can reduce your dose of NEUPOGEN®. If there are still air bubbles, repeat the steps above to remove them.

Needle Cover

Plunger

Syringe Barrel with Markings

Disposable Syringe

Finger Grip

Needle Guard

Needle Cover

Plunger

Window

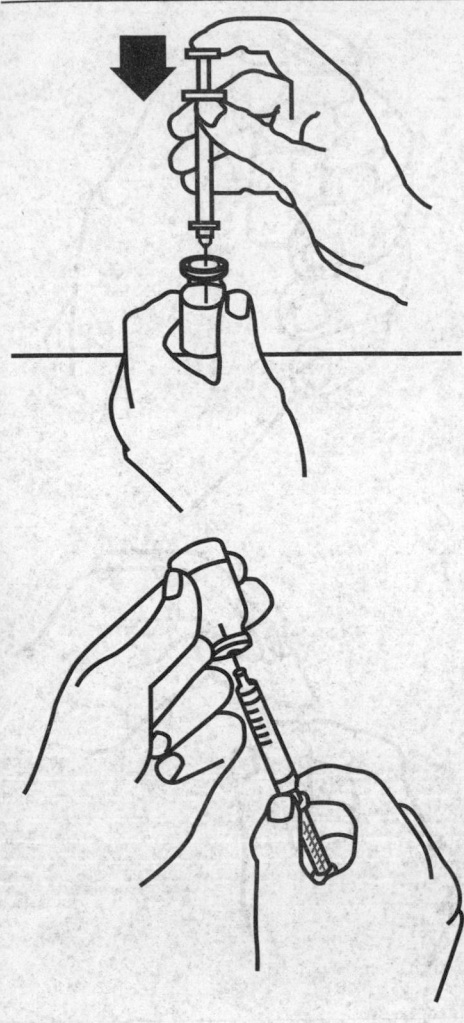

10. Check again to make sure that you have the correct dose in the syringe. It is important that you use the exact dose prescribed by your doctor. Remove the syringe from the vial but **do not lay it down** or let the needle touch anything. (Go to "Injecting the dose of NEUPOGEN®").

Section B. Preparing the dose of NEUPOGEN® in a prefilled syringe

1. Remove the syringe from the package and the tray. Check to see that the plastic orange needle guard is covering the barrel of the glass syringe. **DO NOT push the orange needle guard over the needle cover before injection.** This may activate or lock the needle guard. If the orange needle guard is covering the needle that means it has been activated. Do NOT use that syringe. Dispose of that syringe in the puncture-proof disposal container. Use a new syringe from the package.
2. Hold the syringe barrel through the needle guard windows with the needle pointing up. Holding the syringe with the needle pointing up helps to prevent medicine from leaking out of the needle. Carefully pull the needle cover straight off.
3. Check the syringe for air bubbles. If there are air bubbles, gently tap the syringe with your fingers until the air bubbles rise to the top of the syringe. Slowly push the plunger up to force the air bubbles out of the syringe.
4. Push the plunger up to the number (mL) on the syringe that matches the dose of NEUPOGEN® that your doctor prescribed.
5. Check again to make sure the correct dose of NEUPOGEN® is in the syringe.
6. Gently place the prefilled syringe with the window flat on your clean working surface so that the needle does not touch anything.

Selecting and preparing the injection site

1. Choose an injection site. Four recommended injection sites for NEUPOGEN® are:
   • The outer area of your upper arms
   • The abdomen, except for the two inch area around your navel

• The front of your middle thighs
• The upper outer areas of your buttocks

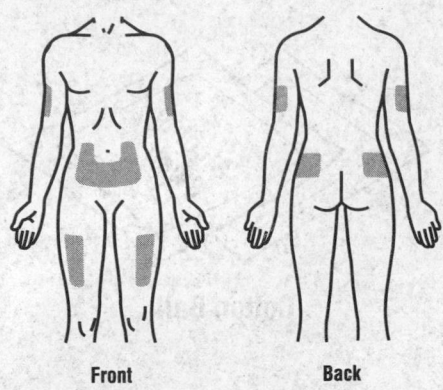

Front   **Back**

Choose a new site each time you inject NEUPOGEN®. Choosing a new site can help avoid soreness at any one site. Do not inject NEUPOGEN® into an area that is tender, red, bruised, or hard or that has scars or stretch marks.
2. Clean the injection site with a new alcohol swab.

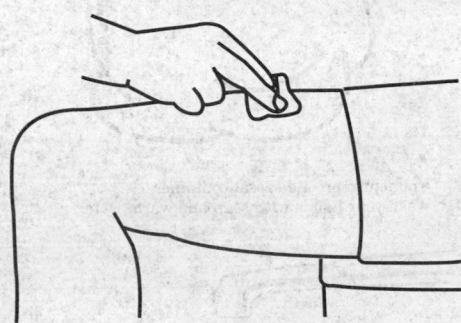

Injecting the dose of NEUPOGEN®

1. For injecting the dose of NEUPOGEN® from a vial, remove the syringe and needle from the vial. For injecting the dose of NEUPOGEN® from a prefilled syringe, pick up the prefilled syringe from your clean flat working surface by grabbing the sides of the needle guard with your thumb and forefinger.
2. Hold the syringe in the hand you will use to inject NEUPOGEN®. Use the other hand to pinch a fold of skin at the cleaned injection site. Note: If using a prefilled syringe with a needle guard, hold the syringe barrel through the needle guard windows when giving the injection.

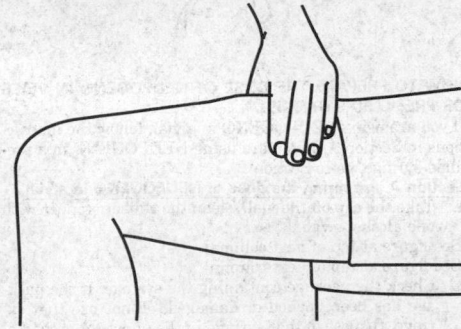

3. Holding the syringe like a pencil, use a quick "dart-like" motion to insert the needle either straight up and down (90 degree angle) or at a slight angle (45 degrees) into the skin.
[See figure at top of next column]
4. After the needle is inserted, let go of the skin. Pull the plunger back slightly. If no blood appears, slowly push down on the plunger all the way, until all the NEUPOGEN® is injected. **If blood comes into the syringe, do not inject NEUPOGEN®, because the needle has entered a blood vessel.** Withdraw the syringe and discard it in the puncture-proof container. Repeat the steps to prepare a new syringe (or get a new prefilled syringe) and choose and clean a new injection site. Re-

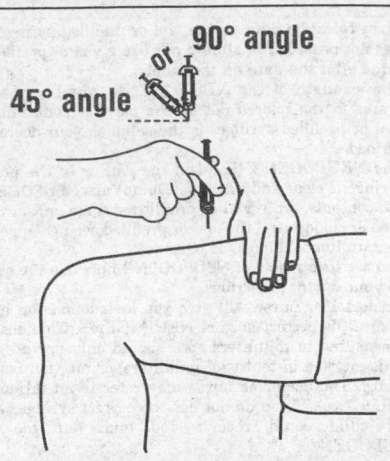

45° angle or **90° angle**

member to check again for blood before injecting NEUPOGEN®.

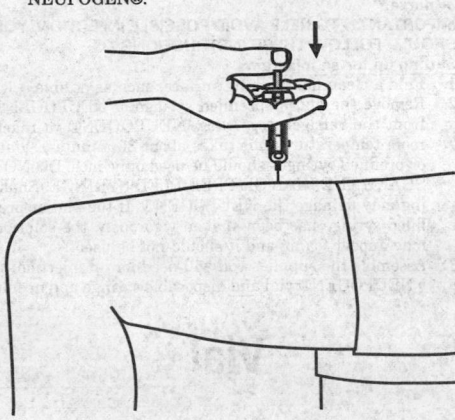

5. When the syringe is empty, pull the needle out of the skin and place a cotton ball or gauze over the injection site and press for several seconds.

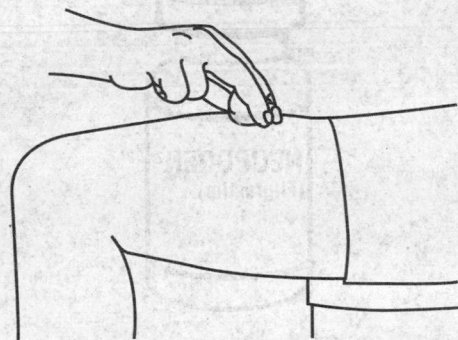

6. Use a prefilled syringe with the needle guard or a syringe and vial only once. If you are using a syringe, DO NOT put the needle cover (the cap) back on the needle. Discard the vial with any remaining NEUPOGEN® liquid.

Activating the Needle Guard for the prefilled syringe after the injection has been given

1. After injecting NEUPOGEN® from the prefilled syringe, do not recap the needle. Keep your hands behind the needle at all times. While holding the clear plastic finger grip of the syringe with one hand, grasp the orange needle guard with your free hand and slide the orange needle guard over the needle until the needle is completely covered and the needle guard clicks into place. **NOTE: If an audible click is not heard, the needle guard may not be completely activated.**
[See figure at top of next column]
[See figure at top of next column]
2. Place the prefilled syringe with the activated needle guard into a puncture-proof container for proper disposal as described below.

Disposal of syringes, needles, vials and needle guards
You should always follow the instructions given by your doctor, nurse, or pharmacist on how to properly dispose of containers with used syringes, needles, vials and needle guards. There may be special state and local laws for disposal of used needles and syringes.

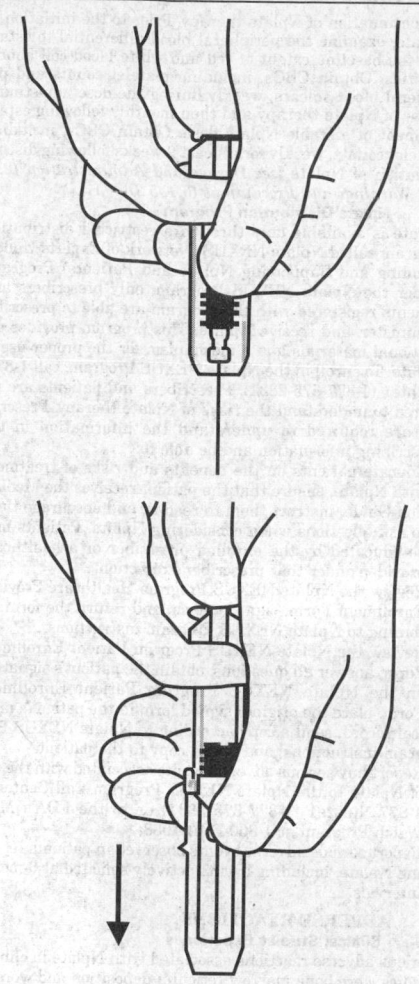

- Place all used needles, needle covers, syringes, and vials (empty or unused contents) into a "Sharps" container given to you by your doctor or pharmacist or in a hard-plastic container with a screw-on cap, or a metal container with a plastic lid, such as a coffee can, labeled "used syringes." If a metal container is used, cut a small hole in the plastic lid and tape the lid to the metal container. If a hard-plastic container is used, always screw the cap on tightly after each use.
- Do not use glass or clear plastic containers.
- When the container is full, tape around the cap or lid to make sure the cap or lid does not come off. **Do not throw the container in the household trash. Do not recycle.**
- **Always** keep the container out of the reach of children.

How should NEUPOGEN® be stored?
NEUPOGEN® should be stored in the refrigerator at 2° to 8°C (36° to 46°F), but not in the freezer. Avoid shaking NEUPOGEN®. If NEUPOGEN® is accidentally frozen, allow it to thaw in the refrigerator before giving the next dose. However, if it is frozen a second time, do not use it and contact your doctor or nurse for further instructions. NEUPOGEN® can be left out at room temperature for up to 24 hours. Do not leave NEUPOGEN® in direct sunlight. If you have any questions about storage or how to carry NEUPOGEN® when you travel, contact your doctor, nurse, or pharmacist.

What are the ingredients in NEUPOGEN®?
Each syringe and vial contains Filgrastim in a sterile, clear, colorless, preservative-free solution containing acetate, sorbitol, polysorbate 80, and sodium.
The needle cover on the single-use prefilled syringe contains dry natural rubber (latex), which should not be handled by persons sensitive to this substance.

Manufactured by:
Amgen Manufacturing, Limited,
a subsidiary of Amgen Inc.
One Amgen Center Drive
Thousand Oaks, California 91320-1799 U.S.A.
3xxxxxx
© 1991-2007 Amgen Inc. All rights reserved.
v8.1 - Issue Date: 09/2007
Shown in Product Identification Guide, page 305

NPLATE
[N-plāt]
(romiplostim)
injection, powder, lyophilized, for solution for subcutaneous use

Rx

HIGHLIGHTS OF PRESCRIBING INFORMATION
These highlights do not include all the information needed to use NPLATE safely and effectively. See full prescribing information for NPLATE.
NPLATE (romiplostim) injection, powder, lyophilized, for solution for subcutaneous use
Initial U.S. Approval: 2008

——INDICATIONS AND USAGE——
Nplate is a thrombopoietin receptor agonist indicated for the treatment of thrombocytopenia in patients with chronic immune (idiopathic) thrombocytopenic purpura (ITP) who have had an insufficient response to corticosteroids, immunoglobulins, or splenectomy.
Nplate should be used only in patients with ITP whose degree of thrombocytopenia and clinical condition increase the risk for bleeding. Nplate should not be used in an attempt to normalize platelet counts. (1)

——DOSAGE AND ADMINISTRATION——
- Initial dose of 1 mcg/kg once weekly as a subcutaneous injection. (2.1)
- Adjust weekly dose by increments of 1 mcg/kg to achieve and maintain a platelet count $\geq 50 \times 10^9$/L as necessary to reduce the risk for bleeding. (2.1)
- Do not exceed the maximum weekly dose of 10 mcg/kg. Do not dose if platelet count is $> 400 \times 10^9$/L. (2.1)
- Discontinue Nplate if platelet count does not increase after 4 weeks at the maximum dose. (2.1)
- Do not shake during reconstitution; protect reconstituted Nplate from light; administer reconstituted Nplate within 24 hours. (2.2)
- The injection volume may be very small. Use a syringe with gradations to 0.01 mL. (2.2)
- Discard any unused portion of the single-use vial. (2.2)

——DOSAGE FORMS AND STRENGTHS——
- 250 mcg or 500 mcg of deliverable romiplostim in single-use vials (3)

——CONTRAINDICATIONS——
- None (4)

——WARNINGS AND PRECAUTIONS——
- Nplate increases the risk for reticulin deposition within the bone marrow; clinical studies have not ruled out the possibility that reticulin and other fiber deposition may result in bone marrow fibrosis with cytopenias. Monitor peripheral blood for signs of marrow fibrosis. (5.1)
- Discontinuation of Nplate may result in worsened thrombocytopenia than was present prior to Nplate therapy. Monitor complete blood counts (CBCs), including platelet counts, for at least 2 weeks following Nplate discontinuation. (5.2)
- Excessive Nplate doses may increase platelet counts to a level that produces thrombotic/thromboembolic complications. (5.3)
- Assess patients for the formation of neutralizing antibodies if platelet counts importantly decrease following an initial Nplate response. (5.4)
- Nplate may increase the risk for hematological malignancies, especially in patients with myelodysplastic syndrome. (5.5)
- Monitor CBCs, including platelet counts and peripheral blood smears, weekly until a stable Nplate dose has been achieved. Thereafter, monitor CBCs, including platelet counts and peripheral blood smears, at least monthly. (5.6)
- Nplate is available only through a restricted distribution program called the Nplate NEXUS (Network of Experts Understanding and Supporting Nplate and Patients) Program. Under the Nplate NEXUS Program, only prescribers and patients registered with the program are able to prescribe, administer, and receive product. To enroll in the Nplate NEXUS Program, call 1-877-Nplate1 (1-877-675-2831). (5.7)

——ADVERSE REACTIONS——
The most common adverse reactions ($\geq 5\%$ higher patient incidence in Nplate versus placebo) are arthralgia, dizziness, insomnia, myalgia, pain in extremity, abdominal pain, shoulder pain, dyspepsia, and paresthesia. Headache was the most commonly reported adverse reaction that did not occur at $\geq 5\%$ higher patient incidence in Nplate versus placebo. (6.1)

To report SUSPECTED ADVERSE REACTIONS, contact Amgen, Inc. at 1-877-Nplate1 (1-877-675-2831) or FDA at 1-800-FDA-1088 or www.fda.gov/medwatch

——USE IN SPECIFIC POPULATIONS——
- Pregnancy: Based on animal data, Nplate may cause fetal harm. Enroll pregnant patients in the Nplate pregnancy registry by calling 1-877-Nplate1 (1-877-675-2831). (8.1)

- Nursing Mothers: A decision should be made to discontinue Nplate or nursing, taking into account the importance of Nplate to the mother. (8.3)

See 17 for PATIENT COUNSELING INFORMATION and Medication Guide

Revised: 09/2008

FULL PRESCRIBING INFORMATION

1. INDICATIONS AND USAGE

Nplate is indicated for the treatment of thrombocytopenia in patients with chronic immune (idiopathic) thrombocytopenic purpura (ITP) who have had an insufficient response to corticosteroids, immunoglobulins or splenectomy. Nplate should be used only in patients with ITP whose degree of thrombocytopenia and clinical condition increases the risk for bleeding. Nplate should not be used in an attempt to normalize platelet counts.

2. DOSAGE AND ADMINISTRATION

Only prescribers enrolled in the Nplate NEXUS (Network of Experts Understanding and Supporting Nplate and Patients) Program may prescribe Nplate [*see Warnings and Precautions (5.7)*]. Nplate must be administered by the enrolled prescribers or healthcare providers under their direction.

2.1 Recommended Dosage Regimen
Monitor complete blood counts (CBCs), including platelet counts and peripheral blood smears, prior to initiation of Nplate and throughout Nplate therapy. Monitor CBCs, including platelet counts, for at least 2 weeks following discontinuation of Nplate [*see Warnings and Precautions (5.6)*]. Use the lowest dose of Nplate to achieve and maintain a platelet count $\geq 50 \times 10^9$/L as necessary to reduce the risk for bleeding. Administer Nplate as a weekly subcutaneous injection with dose adjustments based upon the platelet count response. Nplate should not be used in an attempt to normalize platelet counts [*see Warnings and Precautions (5.3)*].
The prescribed Nplate dose may consist of a very small volume (eg, 0.15 mL). Administer Nplate only with a syringe that contains 0.01 mL graduations.

Table 1. Reconstitution of Nplate Single-Use Vials

Nplate Single-Use Vials	Total Vial Content of Romiplostim		Sterile Water for Injection*		Deliverable Product and Volume	Final Concentration
250 mcg	375 mcg	add	0.72 mL	=	250 mcg/0.5 in mL	500 mcg/mL
500 mcg	625 mcg	add	1.2 mL	=	500 mcg/1m in	500 mcg/mL

*Use preservative-free Sterile Water for Injection.

Initial Dose

The initial dose for Nplate is 1 mcg/kg based on actual body weight.

Dose Adjustments

Use the actual body weight at initiation of therapy, then adjust the weekly dose of Nplate by increments of 1 mcg/kg until the patient achieves a platelet count $\geq 50 \times 10^9$/L as necessary to reduce the risk for bleeding; do not exceed a maximum weekly dose of 10 mcg/kg. In clinical studies, most patients who responded to Nplate achieved and maintained platelet counts $\geq 50 \times 10^9$/L with a median dose of 2 mcg/kg.

During Nplate therapy, assess CBCs, including platelet count and peripheral blood smears, weekly until a stable platelet count ($\geq 50 \times 10^9$/L for at least 4 weeks without dose adjustment) has been achieved. Obtain CBCs, including platelet counts and peripheral blood smears, monthly thereafter.

Adjust the dose as follows:

- If the platelet count is < 50×10^9/L, increase the dose by 1 mcg/kg.
- If platelet count is > 200×10^9/L for 2 consecutive weeks, reduce the dose by 1 mcg/kg.
- If platelet count is > 400×10^9/L, do not dose. Continue to assess the platelet count weekly. After the platelet count has fallen to < 200×10^9/L, resume Nplate at a dose reduced by 1 mcg/kg.

Discontinuation

Discontinue Nplate if the platelet count does not increase to a level sufficient to avoid clinically important bleeding after 4 weeks of Nplate therapy at the maximum weekly dose of 10 mcg/kg [see Warnings and Precautions (5.4)]. Obtain CBCs, including platelet counts, weekly for at least 2 weeks following discontinuation of Nplate [see Warnings and Precautions (5.6)].

2.2 Preparation and Administration

Nplate is supplied in single-use vials as a sterile, preservative-free, white lyophilized powder that must be reconstituted as outlined in Table 1 and administered using a syringe with 0.01 mL graduations. Using aseptic technique, reconstitute Nplate with preservative-free Sterile Water for Injection, USP as described in Table 1. Do not use bacteriostatic water for injection.

[See table above]

Gently swirl and invert the vial to reconstitute. Avoid excess or vigorous agitation: **DO NOT SHAKE**. Generally, dissolution of Nplate takes less than 2 minutes. The reconstituted Nplate solution should be clear and colorless. Visually inspect the reconstituted solution for particulate matter and/or discoloration. Do not administer Nplate if particulate matter and/or discoloration is observed.

Reconstituted Nplate can be kept at room temperature (25°C/77°F) or refrigerated at 2° to 8°C (36° to 46°F) for up to 24 hours prior to administration. Protect the reconstituted product from light.

To determine the injection volume to be administered, first identify the patient's total dose in micrograms (mcg) using the dosing information in section 2.1. For example, a 75 kg patient initiating therapy at 1 mcg/kg will begin with a dose of 75 mcg. Next, calculate the volume of Nplate solution that is given to the patient by dividing the microgram dose by the concentration of the reconstituted Nplate solution (500 mcg/mL). For this patient example, the 75 mcg dose is divided by 500 mcg/mL, resulting in an injection volume of 0.15 mL.

As the injection volume may be very small, use a syringe with graduations to 0.01 mL.

Discard any unused portion. Do not pool unused portions from the vials. Do not administer more than one dose from a vial.

2.3 Use of Nplate With Concomitant Medical ITP Therapies

Nplate may be used with other medical ITP therapies such as corticosteroids, danazol, azathioprine, intravenous immunoglobulin (IVIG), and anti-D immunoglobulin. If the patient's platelet count is $\geq 50 \times 10^9$/L, medical ITP therapies may be reduced or discontinued [Clinical Studies (14.1)].

3. DOSAGE FORMS AND STRENGTHS

Single-use vials contain 250 or 500 mcg of deliverable romiplostim as a sterile, lyophilized, solid white powder.

4. CONTRAINDICATIONS

None

5. WARNINGS AND PRECAUTIONS

5.1 Bone Marrow Reticulin Formation and Risk for Bone Marrow Fibrosis

Nplate administration increases the risk for development or progression of reticulin fiber deposition within the bone marrow. In clinical studies, Nplate was discontinued in four of the 271 patients because of bone marrow reticulin deposition. Six additional patients had reticulin observed upon bone marrow biopsy. All 10 patients with bone marrow reticulin deposition had received Nplate doses ≥ 5 mcg/kg and six received doses ≥ 10 mcg/kg. Progression to marrow fibrosis with cytopenias was not reported in the controlled clinical studies. In the extension study, one patient with ITP and hemolytic anemia developed marrow fibrosis with collagen during Nplate therapy. Clinical studies have not excluded a risk of bone marrow fibrosis with cytopenias.

Prior to initiation of Nplate, examine the peripheral blood smear closely to establish a baseline level of cellular morphologic abnormalities. Following identification of a stable Nplate dose, examine peripheral blood smears and CBCs monthly for new or worsening morphological abnormalities (eg, teardrop and nucleated red blood cells, immature white blood cells) or cytopenia(s). If the patient develops new or worsening morphological abnormalities or cytopenia(s), discontinue treatment with Nplate and consider a bone marrow biopsy, including staining for fibrosis [see Adverse Reactions (6.1)].

5.2 Worsened Thrombocytopenia After Cessation of Nplate

Discontinuation of Nplate may result in thrombocytopenia of greater severity than was present prior to Nplate therapy. This worsened thrombocytopenia may increase the patient's risk of bleeding, particularly if Nplate is discontinued while the patient is on anticoagulants or antiplatelet agents. In clinical studies of patients with chronic ITP who had Nplate discontinued, four of 57 patients developed thrombocytopenia of greater severity than was present prior to Nplate therapy. This worsened thrombocytopenia resolved within 14 days. Following discontinuation of Nplate, obtain weekly CBCs, including platelet counts, for at least 2 weeks and consider alternative treatments for worsening thrombocytopenia, according to current treatment guidelines [see Adverse Reactions (6.1)].

5.3 Thrombotic/Thromboembolic Complications

Thrombotic/thromboembolic complications may result from excessive increases in platelet counts. Excessive doses of Nplate or medication errors that result in excessive Nplate doses may increase platelet counts to a level that produces thrombotic/thromboembolic complications. In controlled clinical studies, the incidence of thrombotic/thromboembolic complications was similar between Nplate and placebo. To minimize the risk for thrombotic/thromboembolic complications, do not use Nplate in an attempt to normalize platelet counts. Follow the dose adjustment guidelines to achieve and maintain a platelet count of $\geq 50 \times 10^9$/L [see Dosage and Administration (2.1)].

5.4 Lack or Loss of Response to Nplate

Hyporesponsiveness or failure to maintain a platelet response with Nplate should prompt a search for causative factors, including neutralizing antibodies to Nplate or bone marrow fibrosis [see Warnings and Precautions (5.1) and Adverse Reactions (6.2)]. To detect antibody formation, submit blood samples to Amgen (1-800-772-6436). Amgen will assay these samples for antibodies to Nplate and thrombopoietin (TPO). Discontinue Nplate if the platelet count does not increase to a level sufficient to avoid clinically important bleeding after 4 weeks at the highest weekly dose of 10 mcg/kg.

5.5 Malignancies and Progression of Malignancies

Nplate stimulation of the TPO receptor on the surface of hematopoietic cells may increase the risk for hematologic malignancies. In controlled clinical studies among patients with chronic ITP, the incidence of hematologic malignancy was low and similar between Nplate and placebo. In a separate single-arm clinical study of 44 patients with myelodysplastic syndrome (MDS), 11 patients were reported as having possible disease progression, among whom four patients had confirmation of acute myelogenous leukemia (AML) during follow-up. Nplate is not indicated for the treatment of thrombocytopenia due to MDS or any cause of thrombocytopenia other than chronic ITP.

5.6 Laboratory Monitoring

Monitor CBCs, including platelet counts and peripheral blood smears, prior to initiation, throughout, and following discontinuation of Nplate therapy. Prior to the initiation of Nplate, examine the peripheral blood differential to establish the baseline extent of red and white blood cell abnormalities. Obtain CBCs, including platelet counts and peripheral blood smears, weekly during the dose adjustment phase of Nplate therapy and then monthly following establishment of a stable Nplate dose. Obtain CBCs, including platelet counts, weekly for at least 2 weeks following discontinuation of Nplate [see Dosage and Administration (2.1) and Warnings and Precautions (5.1, 5.2)].

5.7 Nplate Distribution Program

Nplate is available only through a restricted distribution program called Nplate NEXUS (Network of Experts Understanding and Supporting Nplate and Patients) Program. Under the Nplate NEXUS Program, only prescribers and patients registered with the program are able to prescribe, administer, and receive Nplate. This program provides educational materials and a mechanism for the proper use of Nplate. To enroll in the Nplate NEXUS Program, call 1-877-Nplate1 (1-877-675-2831). Prescribers and patients are required to understand the risks of Nplate therapy. Prescribers are required to understand the information in the prescribing information and be able to:

- Educate patients on the benefits and risks of treatment with Nplate, ensure that the patient receives the Medication Guide, instruct them to read it, and encourage them to ask questions when considering Nplate. Patients may be educated by the enrolled prescriber or a healthcare provider under that prescriber's direction.
- Review the Nplate NEXUS Program Healthcare Provider Enrollment Form, sign the form, and return the form according to Nplate NEXUS Program instructions.
- Review the Nplate NEXUS Program Patient Enrollment Form, answer all questions, obtain the patient's signature on the Nplate NEXUS Program Patient Enrollment Form, place the original signed form in the patient's medical record, send a copy according to Nplate NEXUS Program instructions, and give a copy to the patient.
- Report any serious adverse events associated with the use of Nplate to the Nplate NEXUS Program Call Center at 1-877-Nplate1 (1-877-675-2831) or to the FDA's MedWatch Program at 1-800-FDA-1088.
- Report serious adverse events observed in patients receiving Nplate, including events actively solicited at 6-month intervals.

6. ADVERSE REACTIONS

6.1 Clinical Studies Experience

Serious adverse reactions associated with Nplate in clinical studies were bone marrow reticulin deposition and worsening thrombocytopenia after Nplate discontinuation [see Warnings and Precautions (5.1, 5.2)].

The data described below reflect Nplate exposure to 271 patients with chronic ITP, aged 18 to 88, of whom 62% were female. Nplate was studied in two randomized, placebo-controlled, double-blind studies that were identical in design, with the exception that Study 1 evaluated nonsplenectomized patients with ITP and Study 2 evaluated splenectomized patients with ITP. Data are also reported from an open-label, single-arm study in which patients received Nplate over an extended period of time. Overall, Nplate was administered to 114 patients for at least 52 weeks and 53 patients for at least 96 weeks.

Because clinical studies are conducted under widely varying conditions, adverse reaction rates observed in the clinical trials of a drug cannot be directly compared to rates in the clinical trials of another drug and may not reflect the rates observed in practice.

In the placebo-controlled studies, headache was the most commonly reported adverse drug reaction, occurring in 35% of patients receiving Nplate and 32% of patients receiving placebo. Headaches were usually of mild or moderate severity. Table 2 presents adverse drug reactions from Studies 1 and 2 with a $\geq 5\%$ higher patient incidence in Nplate versus placebo. The majority of these adverse drug reactions were mild to moderate in severity.

Table 2. Adverse Drug Reactions Identified in Two Placebo-Controlled Studies

Preferred Term	Nplate (n = 84)	Placebo (n = 41)
Arthralgia	26%	20%
Dizziness	17%	0%
Insomnia	16%	7%
Myalgia	14%	2%
Pain in extremity	13%	5%
Abdominal Pain	11%	0%

Shoulder Pain	8%	0%
Dyspepsia	7%	0%
Paresthesia	6%	0%

Among 142 patients with chronic ITP who received Nplate in the single-arm extension study, the incidence rates of the adverse reactions occurred in a pattern similar to those reported in the placebo-controlled clinical studies.

6.2   Immunogenicity
As with all therapeutic proteins, patients may develop antibodies to the therapeutic protein. Patients were screened for immunogenicity to romiplostim using a BIAcore-based biosensor immunoassay. This assay is capable of detecting both high- and low-affinity binding antibodies that bind to romiplostim and cross-react with TPO. The samples from patients that tested positive for binding antibodies were further evaluated for neutralizing capacity using a cell-based bioassay.

In clinical studies, the incidence of preexisting antibodies to romiplostim was 8% (17/225) and the incidence of binding antibody development during Nplate treatment was 10% (23/225). The incidence of preexisting antibodies to endogenous TPO was 5% (12/225) and the incidence of binding antibody development to endogenous TPO during Nplate treatment was 5% (12/225). Of the patients with positive antibodies to romiplostim or to TPO, one (0.4%) patient had neutralizing activity to romiplostim and none had neutralizing activity to TPO. No correlation was observed between antibody activity and clinical effectiveness or safety.

Immunogenicity assay results are highly dependent on the sensitivity and specificity of the assay used in detection and may be influenced by several factors, including sample handling, concomitant medications, and underlying disease. For these reasons, comparison of incidence of antibodies to romiplostim with the incidence of antibodies to other products may be misleading.

7.   DRUG INTERACTIONS
No formal drug interaction studies of Nplate have been performed.

8.   USE IN SPECIFIC POPULATIONS
8.1   Pregnancy
Pregnancy Category C
There are no adequate and well-controlled studies of Nplate use in pregnant women. In animal reproduction and developmental toxicity studies, romiplostim crossed the placenta, and adverse fetal effects included thrombocytosis, postimplantation loss, and an increase in pup mortality. Nplate should be used during pregnancy only if the potential benefit to the mother justifies the potential risk to the fetus.
Pregnancy Registry: A pregnancy registry has been established to collect information about the effects of Nplate use during pregnancy. Physicians are encouraged to register pregnant patients, or pregnant women may enroll themselves in the Nplate pregnancy registry by calling 1-877-Nplate1 (1-877-675-2831).

In rat and rabbit developmental toxicity studies no evidence of fetal harm was observed at romiplostim doses up to 11 times (rats) and 82 times (rabbit) the maximum human dose (MHD) based on systemic exposure. In mice at doses 5 times the MHD, reductions in maternal body weight and increased postimplantation loss occurred.

In a prenatal and postnatal development study in rats, at doses 11 times the MHD, there was an increase in perinatal pup mortality. Romiplostim crossed the placental barrier in rats and increased fetal platelet counts at clinically equivalent and higher doses.

8.3   Nursing Mothers
It is not known whether Nplate is excreted in human milk; however, human IgG is excreted in human milk. Published data suggest that breast milk antibodies do not enter the neonatal and infant circulation in substantial amounts. Because many drugs are excreted in human milk and because of the potential for serious adverse reactions in nursing infants from Nplate, a decision should be made whether to discontinue nursing or to discontinue Nplate, taking into account the importance of Nplate to the mother and the known benefits of nursing.

8.4   Pediatric Use
The safety and effectiveness in pediatric patients (<18 years) have not been established.

8.5   Geriatric Use
Of the 271 patients who received Nplate in ITP clinical studies, 55 (20%) were age 65 and over, and 27 (10%) were 75 and over. No overall differences in safety or efficacy have been observed between older and younger patients in the placebo-controlled studies, but greater sensitivity of some older individuals cannot be ruled out. In general, dose adjustment for an elderly patient should be cautious, reflect-

Table 3: Results from Placebo-Controlled Studies*

Outcomes	Study 1 Nonsplenectomized Patients		Study 2 Splenectomized Patients	
	Nplate (n = 41)	Placebo (n = 21)	Nplate (n = 42)	Placebo (n = 21)
Platelet Responses and Rescue Therapy				
Durable Platelet Response, n (%)	25 (61%)	1 (5%)	16 (38%)	0 (0%)
Overall Platelet Response, n (%)	36 (88%)	3 (14%)	33 (79%)	0 (0%)
Number of Weeks With Platelet Counts $\geq 50 \times 10^9$/L, average	15	1	12	0
Requiring Rescue Therapy, n (%)	8 (20%)	13 (62%)	11 (26%)	12 (57%)
Reduction/Discontinuation of Baseline Concurrent ITP Medical Therapy				
Receiving Therapy at Baseline	(n = 11)	(n = 10)	(n = 12)	(n = 6)
Patients Who Had > 25% Dose Reduction in Concurrent Therapy, n (%)	4/11 (36%)	2/10 (20%)	4/12 (33%)	1/6 (17%)
Patients Who Discontinued Baseline Therapy, n (%)[†]	4/11 (36%)	3/10 (30%)	8/12 (67%)	0/6 (0%)

*All P values < 0.05 for platelet response and rescue therapy comparisons between Nplate and placebo.
[†]For multiple concomitant baseline therapies, all therapies were discontinued.

ing the greater frequency of decreased hepatic, renal, or cardiac function, and of concomitant disease or other drug therapy.
8.6   Renal Impairment
No clinical studies were conducted in patients with renal impairment. Use Nplate with caution in this population.
8.7   Hepatic Impairment
No clinical studies were conducted in patients with hepatic impairment. Use Nplate with caution in this population.

10.   OVERDOSAGE
In the event of overdose, platelet counts may increase excessively and result in thrombotic/thromboembolic complications. In this case, discontinue Nplate and monitor platelet counts. Reinitiate treatment with Nplate in accordance with dosing and administration recommendations [see *Dosage and Administration (2.2)*].

11.   DESCRIPTION
Romiplostim, a member of the TPO mimetic class, is an Fc-peptide fusion protein (peptibody) that activates intracellular transcriptional pathways leading to increased platelet production via the TPO receptor (also known as cMpl). The peptibody molecule contains two identical single-chain subunits, each consisting of human immunoglobulin IgG1 Fc domain, covalently linked at the C-terminus to a peptide containing two thrombopoietin receptor-binding domains. Romiplostim has no amino acid sequence homology to endogenous TPO. Romiplostim is produced by recombinant DNA technology in *Escherichia coli (E coli)*.
Nplate is supplied as a sterile, preservative-free, lyophilized, solid white powder for subcutaneous injection. Two vial presentations are available, which contain a sufficient amount of active ingredient to provide either 250 mcg or 500 mcg of deliverable romiplostim, respectively. Each single-use 250 mcg vial of Nplate contains the following: 375 mcg romiplostim, 30 mg mannitol, 15 mg sucrose, 1.2 mg L-histidine, 0.03 mg polysorbate 20, and sufficient HCl to adjust the pH to a target of 5.0. Each single-use 500 mcg vial of Nplate contains the following: 625 mcg romiplostim, 50 mg mannitol, 25 mg sucrose, 1.9 mg L-histidine, 0.05 mg polysorbate 20, and sufficient HCl to adjust the pH to a target of 5.0 [see *Dosage and Administration (2.2)*].

12.   CLINICAL PHARMACOLOGY
12.1   Mechanism Of Action
Nplate increases platelet production through binding and activation of the TPO receptor, a mechanism analogous to endogenous TPO.
12.2   Pharmacodynamics
In clinical studies, treatment with Nplate resulted in dose-dependent increases in platelet counts. After a single subcutaneous dose of 1 to 10 mcg/kg Nplate in patients with chronic ITP, the peak platelet count was 1.3 to 14.9 times greater than the baseline platelet count over a 2- to 3-week period. The platelet counts were above 50×10^9/L for seven out of eight patients with chronic ITP who received six weekly doses of Nplate at 1 mcg/kg.
12.3   Pharmacokinetics
In the long-term extension study in patients with ITP receiving weekly treatment of Nplate subcutaneously, the pharmacokinetics of romiplostim over the dose range of 3 to 15 mcg/kg indicated that peak serum concentrations of

romiplostim were observed about 7 to 50 hours post dose (median: 14 hours) with half-life values ranging from 1 to 34 days (median: 3.5 days). The serum concentrations varied among patients and did not correlate with the dose administered. The elimination of serum romiplostim is in part dependent on the TPO receptor on platelets. As a result, for a given dose, patients with high platelet counts are associated with low serum concentrations and vice versa. In another ITP clinical study, no accumulation in serum concentrations was observed (n = 4) after six weekly doses of Nplate (3 mcg/kg). The accumulation at higher doses of romiplostim is unknown.

13.   NONCLINICAL TOXICOLOGY
13.1   Carcinogenesis, Mutagenesis, Impairment Of Fertility
The carcinogenic potential of romiplostim has not been evaluated. The mutagenic potential of romiplostim has not been evaluated. Romiplostim had no effect on the fertility of rats at doses up to 37 times the MHD based on systemic exposure.
13.2   Animal Toxicology and/or Pharmacology
In a 4-week repeat-dose toxicity study in which rats were dosed subcutaneously three times per week, romiplostim caused extramedullary hematopoiesis, bone hyperostosis and marrow fibrosis at clinically equivalent and higher doses. In this study, these findings were not observed in animals after a 4-week post treatment recovery period. Studies of long-term treatment with romiplostim in rats have not been conducted; therefore, it is not known if the fibrosis of the bone marrow is reversible in rats after long-term treatment.

14.   CLINICAL STUDIES
14.1   Chronic ITP
The safety and efficacy of Nplate were assessed in two double-blind, placebo-controlled clinical studies and in an open-label extension study.
Studies 1 and 2
In Studies 1 and 2, patients with chronic ITP who had completed at least one prior treatment and had a platelet count of $\leq 30 \times 10^9$/L prior to study entry were randomized (2:1) to 24 weeks of Nplate (1 mcg/kg subcutaneous [SC]) or placebo. Prior ITP treatments in both study groups included corticosteroids, immunoglobulins, rituximab, cytotoxic therapies, danazol, and azathioprine. Patients already receiving ITP medical therapies at a constant dosing schedule were allowed to continue receiving these medical treatments throughout the studies. Rescue therapies (ie, corticosteroids, IVIG, platelet transfusions, and anti-D immunoglobulin) were permitted for bleeding, wet purpura, or if the patient was at immediate risk for hemorrhage. Patients received single weekly SC injections of Nplate, with individual dose adjustments to maintain platelet counts (50 × 10^9/L to 200 × 10^9/L).
Study 1 evaluated patients who had not undergone a splenectomy. The patients had been diagnosed with ITP for approximately 2 years and had received a median of three prior ITP treatments. Overall, the median platelet count was 19×10^9/L at study entry. During the study, the median weekly Nplate dose was 2 mcg/kg (25th–75th percentile: 1–3 mcg/kg).
Study 2 evaluated patients who had undergone a splenectomy. The patients had been diagnosed with ITP for

approximately 8 years and had received a median of six prior ITP treatments. Overall, the median platelet count was 14×10^9/L at study entry. During the study, the median weekly Nplate dose was 3 mcg/kg (25th–75th percentile: 2–7 mcg/kg).

Study 1 and 2 outcomes are shown in Table 3. A durable platelet response was the achievement of a weekly platelet count $\geq 50 \times 10^9$/L for any 6 of the last 8 weeks of the 24-week treatment period in the absence of rescue medication at any time. A transient platelet response was the achievement of any weekly platelet counts $\geq 50 \times 10^9$/L for any 4 weeks during the treatment period without a durable platelet response. An overall platelet response was the achievement of either a durable or a transient platelet response. Platelet responses were excluded for 8 weeks after receiving rescue medications.

[See table at top of previous page]

In Studies 1 and 2, nine patients reported a serious bleeding event [five (6%) Nplate, four (10%) placebo]. Bleeding events that were grade 2 severity or higher occurred in 15% of patients treated with Nplate and 34% of patients treated with placebo.

Extension Study

Patients who had participated in either Study 1 or Study 2 were withdrawn from study medications. If platelet counts subsequently decreased to $\leq 50 \times 10^9$/L, the patients were allowed to receive Nplate in an open-label extension study with weekly dosing based on platelet counts. Following Nplate discontinuation in Studies 1 and 2, seven patients maintained platelet counts of $\geq 50 \times 10^9$/L. Among 100 patients who subsequently entered the extension study, platelet counts were increased and sustained regardless of whether they had received Nplate or placebo in the prior placebo-controlled studies. The majority of patients reached a median platelet count of 50×10^9/L after receiving one to three doses of Nplate, and these platelet counts were maintained throughout the remainder of the study with a median duration of Nplate treatment of 60 weeks and a maximum duration of 96 weeks.

16. HOW SUPPLIED/STORAGE AND HANDLING

Nplate is supplied in single-use vials containing 250 mcg (NDC 55513-221-01) and 500 mcg (NDC 55513-222-01) **deliverable romiplostim**.

Store Nplate vials in their carton to protect from light until time of use. Keep Nplate vials refrigerated at 2° to 8°C (36° to 46°F). Do not freeze.

17. PATIENT COUNSELING INFORMATION

See FDA-Approved Medication Guide.

17.1 Information for Patients

Prior to treatment, patients should fully understand the risks and benefits of Nplate. Inform patients that the risks associated with long-term administration of Nplate are unknown and that they must enroll in the Nplate NEXUS Program, which provides for the proper use of Nplate in ITP patients.

Inform patients of the following risks and considerations for Nplate:

- Nplate can only be administered by a healthcare provider who is enrolled in the Nplate NEXUS Program or a healthcare provider under their direction.
- Nplate therapy is administered to achieve and maintain a platelet count $\geq 50 \times 10^9$/L as necessary to reduce the risk for bleeding; Nplate is not used to normalize platelet counts.
- Following discontinuation of Nplate, thrombocytopenia and risk of bleeding may develop that is worse than that experienced prior to the Nplate therapy.
- Nplate therapy increases the risk of reticulin fiber formation within the bone marrow, and further fiber formation may progress to marrow fibrosis. Detection of peripheral blood cell abnormalities may necessitate a bone marrow examination.
- Too much Nplate may result in excessive platelet counts and a risk for thrombotic/thromboembolic complications.
- Nplate stimulates certain bone marrow cells to make platelets and may increase the risk for progression of underlying MDS or hematological malignancies.
- Platelet counts and CBCs, including peripheral blood smears, must be performed weekly until a stable Nplate dose has been achieved; thereafter, platelet counts and CBCs, including peripheral blood smears, must be performed monthly while taking Nplate.
- Patients must be closely monitored with weekly platelet counts and CBCs for at least 2 weeks following Nplate discontinuation.
- Even with Nplate therapy, patients should continue to avoid situations or medications that may increase the risk for bleeding.

17.2 FDA-Approved Medication Guide

Nplate™ (romiplostim)

Manufactured by:

Amgen Inc.
One Amgen Center Drive
Thousand Oaks, California 91320-1799

This product, its production, and/or its use may be covered by one or more U.S. Patents, including U.S. Patent Nos. 6,835,809 and 7,189,827, as well as other patents or patents pending.

© 2008 Amgen Inc. All rights reserved.

www.Nplate.com
1-877-Nplate1 (1-877-675-2831)
3xxxxxx
v1

MEDICATION GUIDE

Nplate™ (N-plāt)
(romiplostim)

Read this Medication Guide before you start Nplate and before each Nplate injection. There may be new information. This Medication Guide does not take the place of talking to your healthcare provider about your medical condition or your treatment.

What is the most important information I should know about Nplate?

Nplate can cause uncommon but serious side effects:

- **Bone marrow changes (increased reticulin and possible bone marrow fibrosis).** Long-term use of Nplate may cause changes in your bone marrow. These changes may lead to abnormal blood cells or your body making less blood cells. The mild form of these bone marrow changes is called "increased reticulin." It is not known if this may progress to a more severe form called "fibrosis." The mild form may cause no problems while the severe form may cause life-threatening blood problems. Signs of bone marrow changes may show up as abnormalities in your blood tests. Your healthcare provider will decide if abnormal blood tests mean that you should have bone marrow tests or if you should stop taking Nplate.
- **Worsening low blood platelet count (thrombocytopenia) and risk of bleeding shortly after stopping Nplate.** When you stop receiving Nplate, your low blood platelet count (thrombocytopenia) may become worse than before you started receiving Nplate. These effects are most likely to happen shortly after stopping Nplate and may last about 2 weeks. The lower platelet counts during this time period may increase your risk of bleeding, especially if you are taking a blood thinner or other medicine that affects platelets. Your healthcare provider will check your blood platelet counts for at least two weeks after you stop taking Nplate. Call your healthcare provider right away to report any bruising or bleeding.
- **High platelet counts and higher chance for blood clots.** You have a higher chance of getting a blood clot if your platelet count is too high during treatment with Nplate. You may have severe complications or die from some forms of blood clots, such as clots that spread to the lungs or that cause heart attacks or strokes. Your healthcare provider will check your blood platelet counts and change your dose or stop Nplate if your platelet counts get too high.
- **Worsening of blood cancers.** Nplate is not for use in patients with blood cancer or a precancerous condition called myelodysplastic syndrome (MDS). If you have one of these conditions, Nplate may worsen your cancer or condition and may cause you to die sooner.

When you are being treated with Nplate, your healthcare provider will closely monitor your Nplate dose and blood tests, including platelet counts.

- Nplate is available only after you and your healthcare provider agree to join a program that is intended to help in the safe use of Nplate. This program is called the "Nplate NEXUS Program."
- Only a healthcare provider can inject a dose of Nplate. Injection of too much Nplate may cause a dangerous increase in your blood platelet count and serious side effects.
- During Nplate therapy, your healthcare provider may change your Nplate dose, depending upon the change in your blood platelet count. You must have blood platelet counts done before you start Nplate, during Nplate therapy, and after Nplate therapy is stopped.
- Nplate is used to try to keep your platelet count about 50,000 per microliter in order to lower the risk for bleeding. Nplate is not used to make your platelet count normal.

See "What are the possible side effects of Nplate?" for other side effects of Nplate.

What is Nplate?

Nplate is a man-made protein medicine used to treat low blood platelet counts in adults with chronic immune (idiopathic) thrombocytopenic purpura (ITP), when other medicine to treat your ITP is not the best choice for you or surgery to remove the spleen has not worked well enough.

Nplate is only:

- Prescribed by healthcare providers who are enrolled in the Nplate NEXUS Program.
- Given to patients who are enrolled in the Nplate NEXUS Program.
- Given by the enrolled healthcare provider or a provider under their direction. You may not give Nplate injections to yourself.

It is not known if Nplate works or if it is safe in people under the age of 18.

Nplate is for treatment of certain people with low blood platelet counts caused by chronic ITP, not low platelet counts caused by other conditions or diseases.

What should I tell my doctor before taking Nplate?

Tell your doctor about all your medical conditions, including if you:

- Have had surgery to remove your spleen (splenectomy).
- Have a bone marrow problem, including a blood cancer or MDS.
- Have or had a blood clot.
- Have bleeding problems.
- Are pregnant, think you may be pregnant, or plan to get pregnant. It is not known if Nplate will harm an unborn baby.

  Pregnancy Registry: There is a registry for women who become pregnant during treatment with Nplate. If you become pregnant, consider this registry. The purpose of the registry is to collect safety information about the health of you and your baby. Contact the registry as soon as you become aware of the pregnancy, or ask your healthcare provider to contact the registry for you. You or your healthcare provider can get information and enroll in the registry by calling 1-877-Nplate1 (1-877-675-2831).
- Are breast-feeding or plan to breast-feed. It is not known if Nplate passes into your breast milk. You and your healthcare provider should decide whether you will take Nplate or breast-feed. You should not do both.

Tell your healthcare provider about all the medicines you take, including prescription and nonprescription medicines, vitamins, and herbal products. Know the medicines you take. Keep a list of them and show it to your healthcare provider and pharmacist when you get a new medicine.

How should I take Nplate?

To receive Nplate, you must first talk with your healthcare provider and understand the benefits and risks of Nplate. You must agree to and follow all of the instructions in the Nplate NEXUS Program.

Before you can begin to receive Nplate, your healthcare provider will:

- Explain the Nplate NEXUS Program to you.
- Answer all of your questions about Nplate and the Nplate NEXUS Program.
- Make sure you read the Nplate Medication Guide.
- Have you sign the Nplate NEXUS Patient Enrollment Form.

Nplate is given by your healthcare provider as a subcutaneous (SC) injection under the skin one time each week.

Your healthcare provider will check your platelet count every week and change your dose of Nplate as needed. This will continue until your healthcare provider decides that your dose of Nplate can stay the same. After that, you will need to have blood tests every month. When you stop receiving Nplate, you will need blood tests for at least 2 weeks to check if your platelet count drops too low.

Tell your healthcare provider about any bruising or bleeding that occurs while you are receiving Nplate.

If you miss a scheduled dose of Nplate, call your healthcare provider to arrange for your next dose as soon as possible.

What should I avoid while receiving Nplate?

Avoid situations that may increase your risk of bleeding, such as missing a scheduled dose of Nplate. You should arrange for your next dose as soon as possible. Call your doctor or the Nplate NEXUS Program at 1-877-Nplate1 (1-877-675-2831).

What are the possible side effects of Nplate?

Nplate may cause serious side effects. See **"What is the most important information I should know about Nplate?"**

The most common side effects of Nplate are:

- Headache
- Joint pain
- Dizziness
- Trouble sleeping
- Muscle tenderness or weakness
- Pain in hands and feet
- Abdominal pain
- Shoulder pain
- Indigestion
- Tingling or numbness in hands and feet

These are not all the possible side effects of Nplate. Tell your healthcare provider if you have any side effect that bothers you or that does not go away. For more information, ask your healthcare provider or pharmacist.

Call your doctor for medical advice about side effects. You may report side effects to the Nplate NEXUS Program at 1-877-Nplate1 (1-877-675-2831) or FDA at 1-800-FDA-1088.

General information about the safe and effective use of Nplate
This Medication Guide summarizes the most important information about Nplate. If you would like more information, talk with your healthcare provider. You can ask your healthcare provider or pharmacist for information about Nplate that is written for health professionals.
What are the ingredients in Nplate?
Active ingredient: romiplostim
Inactive ingredients: L-histidine, sucrose, mannitol, polysorbate-20 and dilute hydrochloric acid
Nplate™ (romiplostim)
Manufactured by:
Amgen Inc..
One Amgen Center Drive
Thousand Oaks, California 91320-1799
This product, its production, and/or its use may be covered by one or more U.S. Patents, including U.S. Patent Nos. 6,835,809 and 7,189,827, as well as other patents or patents pending.
© 2008 Amgen Inc. All rights reserved.
www.Nplate.com
1-877-Nplate1 (1-877-675-2831)
3xxxxxx
v1 Issue Date: 08/2008
This Medication Guide has been approved by the U.S. Food and Drug Administration.
Revised: 09/2008 Distributed by: Amgen, Inc.
Shown in Product Identification Guide, page 306

PROLIA™ ℞
[PRŌ-lee-a]
(denosumab)
Injection, for subcutaneous use

HIGHLIGHTS OF PRESCRIBING INFORMATION
These highlights do not include all the information needed to use Prolia safely and effectively. See full prescribing information for Prolia.
Prolia™ (denosumab)
Injection, for subcutaneous use
Initial U.S. Approval: 2010

INDICATIONS AND USAGE

Prolia is a RANK ligand (RANKL) inhibitor indicated for:
- Treatment of postmenopausal women with osteoporosis at high risk for fracture (1.1)

DOSAGE AND ADMINISTRATION

- Prolia should be administered by a healthcare professional (2.1)
- Administer 60 mg every 6 months as a subcutaneous injection in the upper arm, upper thigh, or abdomen (2.1)
- Instruct patients to take calcium 1000 mg daily and at least 400 IU vitamin D daily (2.1)

DOSAGE FORMS AND STRENGTHS

- Single-use prefilled syringe containing 60 mg in a 1 mL solution (3)
- Single-use vial containing 60 mg in a 1 mL solution (3)

CONTRAINDICATIONS

- Hypocalcemia (4.1, 5.1)

WARNINGS AND PRECAUTIONS

- Hypocalcemia: Must be corrected before initiating Prolia. May worsen especially in patients with renal impairment. Adequately supplement patients with calcium and vitamin D (5.1)
- Serious infections including skin infections: May occur, including those leading to hospitalization. Advise patients to seek prompt medical attention if they develop signs or symptoms of infection, including cellulitis (5.2)
- Dermatologic reactions: Dermatitis, rashes, and eczema have been reported. Consider discontinuing Prolia if severe symptoms develop (5.3)
- Osteonecrosis of the jaw: Has been reported with Prolia. Monitor for symptoms (5.4)
- Suppression of bone turnover: Significant suppression has been demonstrated. Monitor for consequences of bone oversuppression (5.5)

ADVERSE REACTIONS

Most common adverse reactions (> 5% and more common than placebo): back pain, pain in extremity, hypercholesterolemia, musculoskeletal pain, and cystitis. Pancreatitis has been reported in clinical trials (6.1).
To report SUSPECTED ADVERSE REACTIONS, contact Amgen Inc. at 1-800-77-AMGEN (1-800-772-6436) or FDA at 1-800-FDA-1088 or www.fda.gov/medwatch.

USE IN SPECIFIC POPULATIONS

- Pregnancy: Based on animal data, may cause fetal harm. Pregnancy Surveillance Program available (8.1)
- Nursing mothers: May impair mammary gland development and lactation. Discontinue drug or nursing (8.3)
- Pediatric patients: Safety and efficacy not established (8.4)
- Renal impairment: No dose adjustment is necessary in patients with renal impairment. Patients with creatinine clearance < 30 mL/min or receiving dialysis are at risk for hypocalcemia. Supplement with calcium and vitamin D and consider monitoring serum calcium (8.6)

See 17 for PATIENT COUNSELING INFORMATION and Medication Guide

Revised: 06/2010

FULL PRESCRIBING INFORMATION: CONTENTS*
1 INDICATIONS AND USAGE
1.1 Treatment of Postmenopausal Women with Osteoporosis at High Risk for Fracture
2 DOSAGE AND ADMINISTRATION
2.1 Recommended Dosage
2.2 Preparation and Administration
3 DOSAGE FORMS AND STRENGTHS
4 CONTRAINDICATIONS
4.1 Hypocalcemia
5 WARNINGS AND PRECAUTIONS
5.1 Hypocalcemia and Mineral Metabolism
5.2 Serious Infections
5.3 Dermatologic Adverse Reactions
5.4 Osteonecrosis of the Jaw
5.5 Suppression of Bone Turnover
6 ADVERSE REACTIONS
6.1 Clinical Trials Experience
7 DRUG INTERACTIONS
8 USE IN SPECIFIC POPULATIONS
8.1 Pregnancy
8.3 Nursing Mothers
8.4 Pediatric Use
8.5 Geriatric Use
8.6 Renal Impairment
8.7 Hepatic Impairment
10 OVERDOSAGE
11 DESCRIPTION
12 CLINICAL PHARMACOLOGY
12.1 Mechanism of Action
12.2 Pharmacodynamics
12.3 Pharmacokinetics
13 NONCLINICAL TOXICOLOGY
13.1 Carcinogenesis, Mutagenesis, Impairment of Fertility
13.2 Animal Toxicology and/or Pharmacology
14 CLINICAL STUDIES
14.1 Postmenopausal Women with Osteoporosis
16 HOW SUPPLIED/STORAGE AND HANDLING
17 PATIENT COUNSELING INFORMATION
17.1 Hypocalcemia
17.2 Serious Infections
17.3 Dermatologic Reactions
17.4 Osteonecrosis of the Jaw
17.5 Schedule of Administration
MEDICATION GUIDE
*** Sections or subsections omitted from the full prescribing information are not listed**

FULL PRESCRIBING INFORMATION

1 INDICATIONS AND USAGE

1.1 Treatment of Postmenopausal Women with Osteoporosis at High Risk for Fracture

Prolia is indicated for the treatment of postmenopausal women with osteoporosis at high risk for fracture, as defined by factors such as a history of osteoporotic fracture, or multiple risk factors for fracture; or patients who have failed or are intolerant to other available osteoporosis therapy. In postmenopausal women with osteoporosis, Prolia reduces the incidence of vertebral, nonvertebral and hip fractures *[see Clinical Studies (14.1)]*.

2 DOSAGE AND ADMINISTRATION

2.1 Recommended Dosage

Prolia should be administered by a healthcare professional.
The recommended dose of Prolia is 60 mg administered as a single subcutaneous injection once every 6 months. Administer Prolia via subcutaneous injection in the upper arm, the upper thigh, or the abdomen. All patients should receive calcium 1000 mg daily and at least 400 IU vitamin D daily *[see Warnings and Precautions (5.1)]*.
If a dose of Prolia is missed, administer the injection as soon as the patient is available. Thereafter, schedule injections every 6 months from the date of the last injection.

2.2 Preparation and Administration

Visually inspect Prolia for particulate matter and discoloration prior to administration whenever solution and container permit. Prolia is a clear, colorless to pale yellow solution that may contain trace amounts of translucent to white proteinaceous particles. Do not use if the solution is discolored or cloudy or if the solution contains many particles or foreign particulate matter.
Latex Allergy: People sensitive to latex should not handle the grey needle cap on the single-use prefilled syringe, which contains dry natural rubber (a derivative of latex).
Prior to administration, Prolia may be removed from the refrigerator and brought to room temperature (up to 25°C/77°F) by standing in the original container. This generally takes 15 to 30 minutes. Do not warm Prolia in any other way *[see How Supplied/Storage and Handling (16)]*.
Instructions for Prefilled Syringe with Needle Safety Guard
IMPORTANT: In order to minimize accidental needlesticks, the Prolia single-use prefilled syringe will have a green safety guard; manually activate the safety guard after the injection is given.
DO NOT slide the green safety guard forward over the needle before administering the injection – it will lock in place and prevent injection.

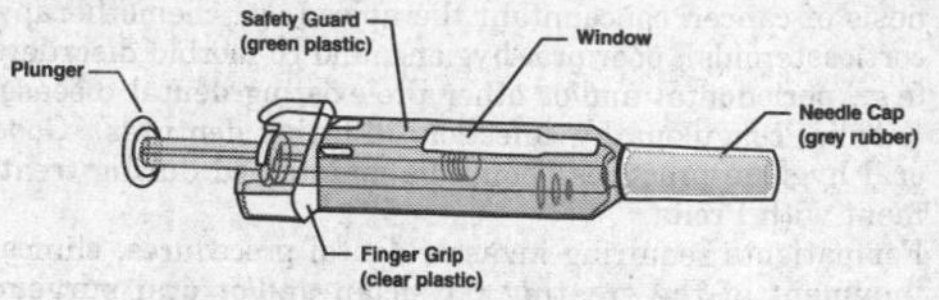

Activate the green safety guard (slide over the needle) after the injection.
The grey needle cap on the single use prefilled syringe contains dry natural rubber (a derivative of latex); people sensitive to latex should not handle the cap.
[See table at top of next page]
Immediately dispose of the syringe and needle cap in the nearest sharps container. **DO NOT** put the needle cap back on the used syringe.
Instructions for Single-use Vial
For administration of Prolia from the single-use vial, use a 27-gauge needle to withdraw and inject the 1 mL dose. Do not re-enter the vial. Discard vial and any liquid remaining in the vial.

3 DOSAGE FORMS AND STRENGTHS

- 1 mL of a 60 mg/mL solution in a single-use prefilled syringe
- 1 mL of a 60 mg/mL solution in a single-use vial

4 CONTRAINDICATIONS

4.1 Hypocalcemia

Pre-existing hypocalcemia must be corrected prior to initiating therapy with Prolia *[see Warnings and Precautions (5.1)]*.

5 WARNINGS AND PRECAUTIONS

5.1 Hypocalcemia and Mineral Metabolism

Hypocalcemia may be exacerbated by the use of Prolia. Pre-existing hypocalcemia must be corrected prior to initiating therapy with Prolia. In patients predisposed to hypocalcemia and disturbances of mineral metabolism (e.g. history of hypoparathyroidism, thyroid surgery, parathyroid surgery, malabsorption syndromes, excision of small intestine, severe renal impairment [creatinine clearance < 30 mL/min] or receiving dialysis), clinical monitoring of calcium and mineral levels (phosphorus and magnesium) is highly recommended.
Hypocalcemia following Prolia administration is a significant risk in patients with severe renal impairment [creatinine clearance < 30 mL/min], or receiving dialysis. Instruct all patients with severe renal impairment, including those receiving dialysis, about the symptoms of hypocalcemia and the importance of maintaining calcium levels with adequate calcium and vitamin D supplementation.
Adequately supplement all patients with calcium and vitamin D *[see Dosage and Administration (2.1), Contraindications (4.1), Adverse Reactions (6.1), and Patient Counseling Information (17.1)]*.

5.2 Serious Infections

In a clinical trial of over 7800 women with postmenopausal osteoporosis, serious infections leading to hospitalization were reported more frequently in the Prolia group than in the placebo group *[see Adverse Reactions (6.1)]*. Serious skin infections, as well as infections of the abdomen, urinary tract, and ear, were more frequent in patients treated with Prolia. Endocarditis was also reported more frequently in Prolia-treated subjects. The incidence of opportunistic infections was balanced between placebo and Prolia groups, and the overall incidence of infections was similar between the treatment groups. Advise patients to seek prompt medical attention if they develop signs or symptoms of severe infection, including cellulitis.
Patients on concomitant immunosuppressant agents or with impaired immune systems may be at increased risk for serious infections. Consider the benefit-risk profile in such patients before treating with Prolia. In patients who develop serious infections while on Prolia, prescribers should assess the need for continued Prolia therapy.

5.3 Dermatologic Adverse Reactions

In a large clinical trial of over 7800 women with postmenopausal osteoporosis, epidermal and dermal adverse events such as dermatitis, eczema, and rashes occurred at a significantly higher rate in the Prolia group compared to the placebo group. Most of these events were not specific to the injection site *[see Adverse Reactions (6.1)]*. Consider discontinuing Prolia if severe symptoms develop.

5.4 Osteonecrosis of the Jaw

Osteonecrosis of the jaw (ONJ), which can occur spontaneously, is generally associated with tooth extraction and/or local infection with delayed healing. ONJ has been reported in patients receiving denosumab *[see Adverse Reactions (6.1)]*. A routine oral exam should be performed by the prescriber prior to initiation of Prolia treatment. A dental examination with appropriate preventive dentistry should be considered prior to treatment with Prolia in patients with risk factors for ONJ such as invasive dental procedures (e.g., tooth extraction, dental implants, oral surgery), diagnosis of cancer, concomitant therapies (e.g., chemotherapy, corticosteroids), poor oral hygiene, and co-morbid disorders (e.g., periodontal and/or other pre-existing dental disease, anemia, coagulopathy, infection, ill-fitting dentures). Good oral hygiene practices should be maintained during treatment with Prolia.

For patients requiring invasive dental procedures, clinical judgment of the treating physician and/or oral surgeon should guide the management plan of each patient based on individual benefit-risk assessment.

Patients who are suspected of having or who develop ONJ while on Prolia should receive care by a dentist or an oral surgeon. In these patients, extensive dental surgery to treat ONJ may exacerbate the condition. Discontinuation of Prolia therapy should be considered based on individual benefit-risk assessment.

5.5 Suppression of Bone Turnover

In clinical trials in women with postmenopausal osteoporosis, treatment with Prolia resulted in significant suppression of bone remodeling as evidenced by markers of bone turnover and bone histomorphometry *[see Clinical Pharmacology (12.2), Clinical Studies (14.1)]*. The significance of these findings and the effect of long-term treatment with Prolia are unknown. The long-term consequences of the degree of suppression of bone remodeling observed with Prolia may contribute to adverse outcomes such as osteonecrosis of the jaw, atypical fractures, and delayed fracture healing. Monitor patients for these consequences.

6 ADVERSE REACTIONS

The following serious adverse reactions are discussed below and also elsewhere in the labeling:
- Hypocalcemia *[see Warnings and Precautions (5.1)]*
- Serious Infections *[see Warnings and Precautions (5.2)]*
- Dermatologic Adverse Reactions *[see Warnings and Precautions (5.3)]*
- Osteonecrosis of the Jaw *[see Warnings and Precautions (5.4)]*

The most common adverse reactions reported with Prolia are back pain, pain in extremity, musculoskeletal pain, hypercholesterolemia, and cystitis.

The most common adverse reactions leading to discontinuation of Prolia are breast cancer, back pain, and constipation.

The Prolia Postmarketing Active Safety Surveillance Program is available to collect information from prescribers on specific adverse events. Please see www.proliasafety.com or call 1-800-772-6436 for more information about this program.

6.1 Clinical Trials Experience

Because clinical studies are conducted under widely varying conditions, adverse reaction rates observed in the clinical studies of a drug cannot be directly compared to rates in the clinical studies of another drug and may not reflect the rates observed in clinical practice.

Treatment of postmenopausal women with osteoporosis
The safety of Prolia in the treatment of postmenopausal osteoporosis was assessed in a 3-year, randomized, double-blind, placebo-controlled, multinational study of 7808 postmenopausal women aged 60 to 91 years. A total of 3876 women were exposed to placebo and 3886 women were exposed to Prolia administered subcutaneously once every 6 months as a single 60 mg dose. All women were instructed to take at least 1000 mg of calcium and 400 IU of vitamin D supplementation per day.

The incidence of all-cause mortality was 2.3% (n = 90) in the placebo group and 1.8% (n = 70) in the Prolia group. The incidence of nonfatal serious adverse events was 24.2% in the placebo group and 25.0% in the Prolia group. The percentage of patients who withdrew from the study due to adverse events was 2.1% and 2.4% for the placebo and Prolia groups, respectively.

Adverse reactions reported in ≥ 2% of postmenopausal women with osteoporosis and more frequently in the Prolia-treated women than in the placebo-treated women are shown in the table below.

[See table 1 at bottom of next page]

Hypocalcemia
Decreases in serum calcium levels to less than 8.5 mg/dL were reported in 0.4% women in the placebo group and 1.7% women in the Prolia group at the month 1 visit. The nadir in serum calcium level occurs at approximately day 10 after Prolia dosing in subjects with normal renal function.

Step 1: Remove Grey Needle Cap

Remove needle cap.

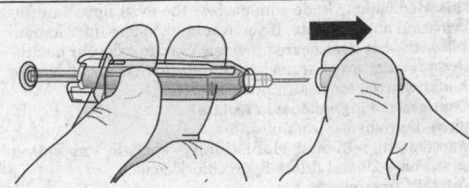

Step 2: Administer Injection

Insert needle and inject all the liquid.

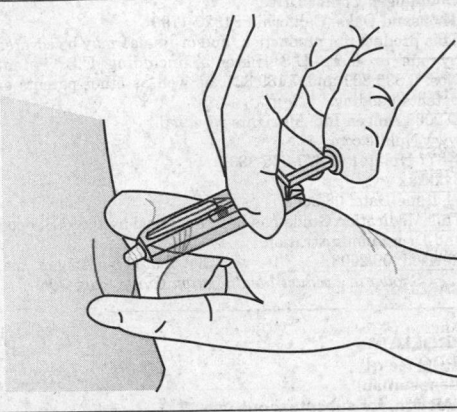

DO NOT put grey needle cap back on needle.
Step 3: Immediately Slide Green Safety Guard Over Needle
With the *needle pointing away from you…*
Hold the prefilled syringe by the clear plastic finger grip with one hand. Then, with the other hand, grasp the green safety guard by its base and gently slide it towards the needle until the green safety guard locks securely in place and/or you hear a "click." **DO NOT** grip the green safety guard too firmly – it will move easily if you hold and slide it gently.

Hold clear finger grip.

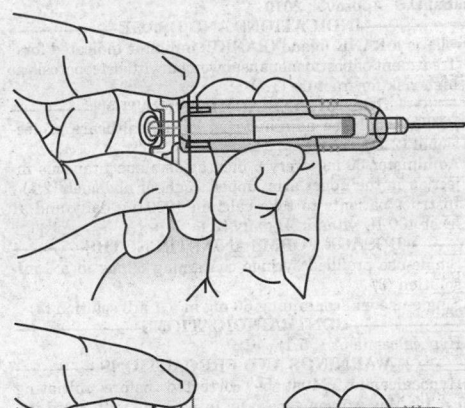

Gently slide green safety guard over needle and lock securely in place. Do not grip green safety guard too firmly when sliding over needle.

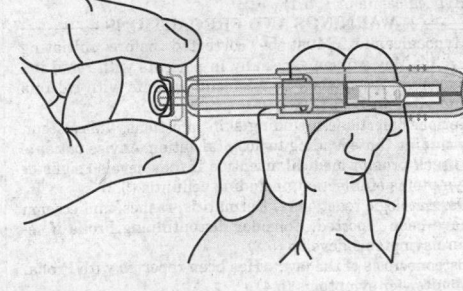

In clinical studies, subjects with impaired renal function were more likely to have greater reductions in serum calcium levels compared to subjects with normal renal function. In a study of 55 patients with varying degrees of renal function, serum calcium levels < 7.5 mg/dL or symptomatic hypocalcemia were observed in 5 subjects. These included no subjects in the normal renal function group, 10% of subjects in the CrCL 50 to 80 mL/min group, 29% of subjects in the CrCL <30 mL/min group, and 29% of subjects in the hemodialysis group. These subjects did not receive calcium and vitamin D supplementation. In a study of 4,550 postmenopausal women with osteoporosis, the mean change from baseline in serum calcium level 10 days after Prolia dosing was -5.5% in subjects with creatinine clearance < 30 mL/min vs. -3.1% in subjects with CrCL ≥ 30 mL/min.

Serious Infections
Receptor activator of nuclear factor kappa-B ligand (RANKL) is expressed on activated T and B lymphocytes and in lymph nodes. Therefore, a RANKL inhibitor such as Prolia may increase the risk of infection.

In the clinical study of 7808 postmenopausal women with osteoporosis, the incidence of infections resulting in death was 0.2% in both placebo and Prolia treatment groups. However, the incidence of nonfatal serious infections was 3.3% in the placebo group and 4.0% in the Prolia group. Hospitalizations due to serious infections in the abdomen (0.7% placebo vs. 0.9% Prolia), urinary tract (0.5% placebo vs. 0.7% Prolia), and ear (0.0% placebo vs. 0.1% Prolia) were reported. Endocarditis was reported in no placebo patients and 3 patients receiving Prolia.

Skin infections, including erysipelas and cellulitis, leading to hospitalization were reported more frequently in patients treated with Prolia (< 0.1% placebo vs. 0.4% Prolia).
There was no imbalance in the reporting of opportunistic infections.

Dermatologic Reactions
A significantly higher number of patients treated with Prolia developed epidermal and dermal adverse events (such as dermatitis, eczema and rashes), with these events reported in 8.2% of placebo and 10.8% of Prolia group (p < 0.0001). Most of these events were not specific to the injection site [see Warnings and Precautions (5.3)].

Osteonecrosis of the Jaw
ONJ has been reported in the osteoporosis clinical trial program in patients treated with Prolia [see Warnings and Precautions (5.4)].

Pancreatitis
Pancreatitis was reported in 4 patients (0.1%) in the placebo and 8 patients (0.2%) in the Prolia groups. Of these reports, one subject in the placebo group and all 8 subjects in the Prolia group had serious events including one death in the Prolia group. Several patients had a prior history of pancreatitis. The time from product administration to event occurrence was variable.

New Malignancies
The overall incidence of new malignancies was 4.3% in the placebo and 4.8% in the Prolia groups. New malignancies related to breast (0.7% placebo vs. 0.9% Prolia), reproductive (0.2% placebo vs. 0.5% Prolia) and gastrointestinal systems (0.6% placebo vs. 0.9% Prolia) were reported. A causal relationship to drug exposure has not been established.

Immunogenicity
Denosumab is a human monoclonal antibody. As with all therapeutic proteins, there is potential for immunogenicity. Using an electrochemiluminescent bridging immunoassay, less than 1% (55 out of 8113) of patients treated with Prolia for up to 5 years tested positive for binding antibodies (including pre-existing, transient, and developing antibodies). None of the patients tested positive for neutralizing antibodies, as was assessed using a chemiluminescent cell-based in vitro biological assay. No evidence of altered pharmacokinetic profile, toxicity profile, or clinical response was associated with binding antibody development.

The incidence of antibody formation is highly dependent on the sensitivity and specificity of the assay. Additionally, the observed incidence of a positive antibody (including neutralizing antibody) test result may be influenced by several factors, including assay methodology, sample handling, timing of sample collection, concomitant medications, and underlying disease. For these reasons, comparison of antibodies to denosumab with the incidence of antibodies to other products may be misleading.

7   DRUG INTERACTIONS
No drug-drug interaction studies have been conducted with Prolia.

8   USE IN SPECIFIC POPULATIONS
8.1   Pregnancy
Pregnancy Category C
There are no adequate and well-controlled studies of Prolia in pregnant women. In genetically engineered mice in which RANK ligand (RANKL) was turned off by gene removal (a "knockout mouse"), absence of RANKL (the target of denosumab) caused fetal lymph node agenesis and led to postnatal impairment of dentition and bone growth. Pregnant RANKL knockout mice also showed altered maturation of the maternal mammary gland, leading to impaired lactation postpartum [see Use in Specific Populations (8.3)]. Prolia is approved only for use in postmenopausal women. Prolia should be used during pregnancy only if the potential benefit justifies the potential risk to the fetus. Women who become pregnant during Prolia treatment are encouraged to enroll in Amgen's Pregnancy Surveillance Program. Patients or their physicians should call 1-800-77-AMGEN (1-800-772-6436) to enroll.

In an embryofetal developmental study, cynomolgus monkeys received subcutaneous denosumab weekly during organogenesis at doses up to 13-fold higher than the recommended human dose of 60 mg administered once every 6 months based on body weight (mg/kg). No evidence of maternal toxicity or fetal harm was observed. However, this study only assessed fetal toxicity during a period equivalent to the first trimester and fetal lymph nodes were not examined. Monoclonal antibodies are transported across the placenta in a linear fashion as pregnancy progresses, with the largest amount transferred during the third trimester. Potential adverse developmental effects resulting from exposures during the second and third trimesters have not been assessed in animals [see Nonclinical Toxicology (13.2)].

8.3   Nursing Mothers
It is not known whether Prolia is excreted into human milk. Because many drugs are excreted in human milk and because of the potential for serious adverse reactions in nursing infants from Prolia, a decision should be made whether to discontinue nursing or discontinue the drug, taking into account the importance of the drug to the mother.

Maternal exposure to Prolia during pregnancy may impair mammary gland development and lactation based on animal studies in pregnant mice lacking the RANK/RANKL signaling pathway that have shown altered maturation of the maternal mammary gland, leading to impaired lactation postpartum [see Nonclinical Toxicology (13.2)].

8.4   Pediatric Use
Prolia is not recommended in pediatric patients. The safety and effectiveness of Prolia in pediatric patients have not been established.

Treatment with Prolia may impair bone growth in children with open growth plates and may inhibit eruption of dentition. In neonatal rats, inhibition of RANKL (the target of Prolia therapy) with a construct of osteoprotegerin bound to Fc (OPG-Fc) at doses ≤10 mg/kg was associated with inhibition of bone growth and tooth eruption. Adolescent primates dosed with denosumab at 10 and 50 times (10 and 50 mg/kg dose) higher than the recommended human dose of 60 mg administered once every 6 months, based on body weight (mg/kg), had abnormal growth plates [see Nonclinical Toxicology (13.2)].

8.5   Geriatric Use
Of the total number of patients in clinical studies of Prolia, 9943 patients (76%) were ≥ 65 years old, while 3576 (27%) were ≥ 75 years old. No overall differences in safety or efficacy were observed between these patients and younger patients and other reported clinical experience has not identi-

Table 1. Adverse Reactions Occurring in ≥ 2% of Patients with Osteoporosis and More Frequently than in Placebo-treated Patients

SYSTEM ORGAN CLASS Preferred Term	Prolia (N = 3886) n (%)	Placebo (N = 3876) n (%)
BLOOD AND LYMPHATIC SYSTEM DISORDERS		
Anemia	129 (3.3)	107 (2.8)
CARDIAC DISORDERS		
Angina pectoris	101 (2.6)	87 (2.2)
Atrial fibrillation	79 (2.0)	77 (2.0)
EAR AND LABYRINTH DISORDERS		
Vertigo	195 (5.0)	187 (4.8)
GASTROINTESTINAL DISORDERS		
Abdominal pain upper	129 (3.3)	111 (2.9)
Flatulence	84 (2.2)	53 (1.4)
Gastroesophageal reflux disease	80 (2.1)	66 (1.7)
GENERAL DISORDERS AND ADMINISTRATION SITE CONDITIONS		
Edema peripheral	189 (4.9)	155 (4.0)
Asthenia	90 (2.3)	73 (1.9)
INFECTIONS AND INFESTATIONS		
Cystitis	228 (5.9)	225 (5.8)
Upper respiratory tract infection	190 (4.9)	167 (4.3)
Pneumonia	152 (3.9)	150 (3.9)
Pharyngitis	91 (2.3)	78 (2.0)
Herpes zoster	79 (2.0)	72 (1.9)
METABOLISM AND NUTRITION DISORDERS		
Hypercholesterolemia	280 (7.2)	236 (6.1)
MUSCULOSKELETAL AND CONNECTIVE TISSUE DISORDERS		
Back pain	1347 (34.7)	1340 (34.6)
Pain in extremity	453 (11.7)	430 (11.1)
Musculoskeletal pain	297 (7.6)	291 (7.5)
Bone pain	142 (3.7)	117 (3.0)
Myalgia	114 (2.9)	94 (2.4)
Spinal osteoarthritis	82 (2.1)	64 (1.7)
NERVOUS SYSTEM DISORDERS		
Sciatica	178 (4.6)	149 (3.8)
PSYCHIATRIC DISORDERS		
Insomnia	126 (3.2)	122 (3.1)
SKIN AND SUBCUTANEOUS TISSUE DISORDERS		
Rash	96 (2.5)	79 (2.0)
Pruritus	87 (2.2)	82 (2.1)

Table 2. The Effect of Prolia on the Incidence of New Vertebral Fractures

	Proportion of Women With Fracture (%)*		Absolute Risk Reduction (%)[†] (95% CI)	Relative Risk Reduction (%)[†] (95% CI)
	Placebo N = 3691 (%)	Prolia N = 3702 (%)		
0-1 Year	2.2	0.9	1.4 (0.8, 1.9)	61 (42, 74)
0-2 Years	5.0	1.4	3.5 (2.7, 4.3)	71 (61, 79)
0-3 Years	7.2	2.3	4.8 (3.9, 5.8)	68 (59, 74)

*Event rates based on crude rates in each interval
†Absolute risk reduction and relative risk reduction based on Mantel-Haenszel method adjusting for age group variable

fied differences in responses between the elderly and younger patients, but greater sensitivity of some older individuals cannot be ruled out.

8.6   Renal Impairment
No dose adjustment is necessary in patients with renal impairment.
In clinical studies, patients with severe renal impairment (creatinine clearance < 30 mL/min) or receiving dialysis were at greater risk of developing hypocalcemia. Consider the benefit-risk profile when administering Prolia to patients with severe renal impairment or receiving dialysis. Clinical monitoring of calcium and mineral levels (phosphorus and magnesium) is highly recommended. Adequate intake of calcium and vitamin D is important in patients with severe renal impairment or receiving dialysis [see Warnings and Precautions (5.1), Adverse Reactions (6.1), and Clinical Pharmacology (12.3)].

8.7   Hepatic Impairment
No clinical studies have been conducted to evaluate the effect of hepatic impairment on the pharmacokinetics of Prolia.

10   OVERDOSAGE
There is no experience with overdosage with Prolia.

11   DESCRIPTION
Prolia (denosumab) is a human IgG2 monoclonal antibody with affinity and specificity for human RANKL (receptor activator of nuclear factor kappa-B ligand). Denosumab has an approximate molecular weight of 147 kDa and is produced in genetically engineered mammalian (Chinese hamster ovary) cells.
Prolia is a sterile, preservative-free, clear, colorless to pale yellow solution.
Each 1 mL single-use prefilled syringe of Prolia contains 60 mg denosumab (60 mg/mL solution), 4.7% sorbitol, 17 mM acetate, 0.01% polysorbate 20, Water for Injection (USP), and sodium hydroxide to a pH of 5.2.
Each 1 mL single-use vial of Prolia contains 60 mg denosumab (60 mg/mL solution), 4.7% sorbitol, 17 mM acetate, Water for Injection, (USP), and sodium hydroxide to a pH of 5.2.

12   CLINICAL PHARMACOLOGY
12.1   Mechanism of Action
Prolia binds to RANKL, a transmembrane or soluble protein essential for the formation, function, and survival of osteoclasts, the cells responsible for bone resorption. Prolia prevents RANKL from activating its receptor, RANK, on the surface of osteoclasts and their precursors. Prevention of the RANKL/RANK interaction inhibits osteoclast formation, function, and survival, thereby decreasing bone resorption and increasing bone mass and strength in both cortical and trabecular bone.

12.2   Pharmacodynamics
In clinical studies, treatment with 60 mg of Prolia resulted in reduction in the bone resorption marker serum type 1 C-telopeptide (CTX) by approximately 85% by 3 days, with maximal reductions occurring by 1 month. CTX levels were below the limit of assay quantitation (0.049 ng/mL) in 39-68% of subjects 1-3 months after dosing of Prolia. At the end of each dosing interval, CTX reductions were partially attenuated from a maximal reduction of ≥ 87% to ≥ 45% (range: 45% to 80%), as serum denosumab levels diminished, reflecting the reversibility of the effects of Prolia on bone remodeling. These effects were sustained with continued treatment. Upon reinitiation, the degree of inhibition of CTX by Prolia was similar to that observed in patients initiating Prolia treatment.
Consistent with the physiological coupling of bone formation and resorption in skeletal remodeling, subsequent reductions in bone formation markers (i.e., osteocalcin and procollagen type 1 N-terminal peptide [P1NP]), were observed starting 1 month after the first dose of Prolia. After discontinuation of Prolia therapy, markers of bone resorption increased to levels 40-60% above pretreatment values but returned to baseline levels within 12 months.

12.3   Pharmacokinetics
In a study conducted in healthy male and female volunteers (n = 73, age range: 18 to 64 years) following a single subcutaneously administered Prolia dose of 60 mg after fasting (at least for 12 hours), the mean maximum denosumab concentration (C_{max}) was 6.75 mcg/mL (standard deviation [SD] = 1.89 mcg/mL). The median time to maximum denosumab concentration (T_{max}) was 10 days (range: 3 to 21 days). After C_{max}, serum denosumab concentrations declined over a period of 4 to 5 months with a mean half-life of 25.4 days (SD = 8.5 days; n = 46). The mean area-under-the-concentration-time curve up to 16 weeks ($AUC_{0-16\ weeks}$) of denosumab was 316 mcg•day/mL (SD = 101 mcg•day/mL).
No accumulation or change in denosumab pharmacokinetics with time was observed upon multiple dosing of 60 mg subcutaneously administered once every 6 months.
Prolia pharmacokinetics were not affected by the formation of binding antibodies.
A population pharmacokinetic analysis was performed to evaluate the effects of demographic characteristics. This analysis showed no notable differences in pharmacokinetics with age (in postmenopausal women), race, or body weight (36 to 140 kg).
Drug Interactions
No drug-drug interaction studies have been conducted with Prolia.
Specific Populations
Gender: Mean serum denosumab concentration-time profiles observed in a study conducted in healthy men ≥ 50 years were similar to those observed in a study conducted in postmenopausal women using the same dose regimen.
Age: The pharmacokinetics of denosumab was not affected by age across all populations studied whose ages ranged from 28-87 years.
Race: The pharmacokinetics of denosumab was not affected by race.
Renal Impairment: In a study of 55 patients with varying degrees of renal function, including patients on dialysis, the degree of renal impairment had no effect on the pharmacokinetics of denosumab; thus, dose adjustment for renal impairment is not necessary.
Hepatic Impairment: No clinical studies have been conducted to evaluate the effect of hepatic impairment on the pharmacokinetics of denosumab.

13   NONCLINICAL TOXICOLOGY
13.1   Carcinogenesis, Mutagenesis, Impairment of Fertility
Carcinogenicity
The carcinogenic potential of denosumab has not been evaluated in long-term animal studies.
Mutagenicity
The genotoxic potential of denosumab has not been evaluated.
Impairment of Fertility
Denosumab had no effect on female fertility or male reproductive organs in monkeys at doses that were 13- to 50-fold higher than the recommended human dose of 60 mg administered once every 6 months, based on body weight (mg/kg).

13.2   Animal Toxicology and/or Pharmacology
Prolia is an inhibitor of osteoclastic bone resorption via inhibition of RANKL.
In ovariectomized monkeys, once-monthly treatment with denosumab suppressed bone turnover and increased bone mineral density (BMD) and strength of cancellous and cortical bone at doses 50-fold higher than the recommended human dose of 60 mg administered once every 6 months, based on body weight (mg/kg). Bone tissue was normal with no evidence of mineralization defects, accumulation of osteoid, or woven bone.
Adolescent primates treated with denosumab at doses > 10 times (10 and 50 mg/kg dose) higher than the recommended human dose of 60 mg administered once every 6 months, based on mg/kg, had abnormal growth plates, considered to be consistent with the pharmacological activity of denosumab [see Use in Specific Populations (8.4)].

Because the biological activity of denosumab in animals is specific to nonhuman primates, evaluation of genetically engineered ("knockout") mice or use of other biological inhibitors of the RANK/RANKL pathway, namely OPG-Fc, provided additional information on the pharmacodynamic properties of denosumab. RANK/RANKL knockout mice exhibited absence of lymph node formation, as well as an absence of lactation due to inhibition of mammary gland maturation (lobulo-alveolar gland development during pregnancy). Neonatal RANK/RANKL knockout mice exhibited reduced bone growth and lack of tooth eruption. A corroborative study in 2-week-old rats given the RANKL inhibitor OPG-Fc also showed reduced bone growth, altered growth plates, and impaired tooth eruption. These changes were partially reversible in this model when dosing with the RANKL inhibitors was discontinued [see Use in Specific Populations (8.1, 8.4)].

14   CLINICAL STUDIES
14.1   Postmenopausal Women with Osteoporosis
The efficacy and safety of Prolia in the treatment of postmenopausal osteoporosis was demonstrated in a 3-year, randomized, double-blind, placebo-controlled, trial. Enrolled women had a baseline BMD T-score between -2.5 and -4.0 at either the lumbar spine or total hip. Women with other diseases (such as rheumatoid arthritis, osteogenesis imperfecta, and Paget's disease) or on therapies that affect bone were excluded from this study. The 7808 enrolled women were aged 60 to 91 years with a mean age of 72 years. Overall, the mean baseline lumbar spine BMD T-score was -2.8 and 23% of women had a vertebral fracture at baseline. Women were randomized to receive SC injections of either placebo (N = 3906) or Prolia 60 mg (N = 3902) once every 6 months. All women received at least 1000 mg calcium and 400 IU vitamin D supplementation daily.
The primary efficacy variable was the incidence of new morphometric (radiologically-diagnosed) vertebral fractures at 3 years. Vertebral fractures were diagnosed based on lateral spine radiographs (T4-L4) using a semiquantitative scoring method. Secondary efficacy variables included the incidence of hip fracture and nonvertebral fracture, assessed at 3 years.
Effect on Vertebral Fractures
Prolia significantly reduced the incidence of new morphometric vertebral fractures at 1, 2, and 3 years (p < 0.0001), as shown in Table 2. The incidence of new vertebral fractures at year 3 was 7.2% in the placebo-treated women compared to 2.3% for the Prolia-treated women. The absolute risk reduction was 4.8% and relative risk reduction was 68% for new morphometric vertebral fractures at year 3.
[See table 2 at top left]
Prolia was effective in reducing the risk for new morphometric vertebral fractures regardless of age, baseline rate of bone turnover, baseline BMD, baseline history of fracture, or prior use of a drug for osteoporosis.
Effect on Hip Fractures
The incidence of hip fracture was 1.2% for placebo-treated women compared to 0.7% for Prolia-treated women at year 3. The age-adjusted absolute risk reduction of hip fractures was 0.3% with a relative risk reduction of 40% at 3 years (p = 0.04) (Figure 1).

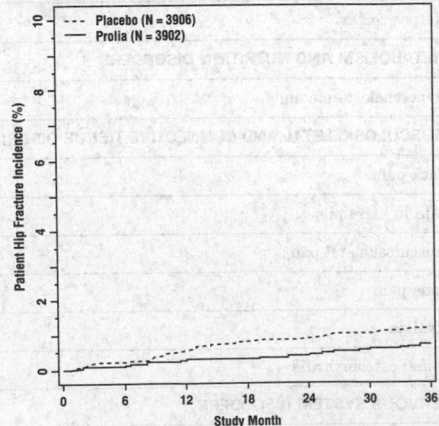

N = number of subjects randomized

Figure 1. Cumulative Incidence of Hip Fractures Over 3 Years

Effect on Nonvertebral Fractures
Treatment with Prolia resulted in a significant reduction in the incidence of nonvertebral fractures (Table 3).
[See table 3 at top of next page]
Effect on Bone Mineral Density (BMD)
Treatment with Prolia significantly increased BMD at all anatomic sites measured at 3 years. The treatment differ-

ences in BMD at 3 years were 8.8% at the lumbar spine, 6.4% at the total hip, and 5.2% at the femoral neck. Consistent effects on BMD were observed at the lumbar spine, regardless of baseline age, race, weight/body mass index (BMI), baseline BMD, and level of bone turnover.

After Prolia discontinuation, BMD returned to approximately baseline levels within 12 months.

Bone Histology and Histomorphometry

A total of 115 transiliac crest bone biopsy specimens were obtained from 92 postmenopausal women with osteoporosis at either month 24 and/or month 36 (53 specimens in Prolia group, 62 specimens in placebo group). Of the biopsies obtained, 115 (100%) were adequate for qualitative histology and 7 (6%) were adequate for full quantitative histomorphometry assessment.

Qualitative histology assessments showed normal architecture and quality with no evidence of mineralization defects, woven bone, or marrow fibrosis in patients treated with Prolia.

The presence of double tetracycline labeling in a biopsy specimen provides an indication of active bone remodeling, while the absence of tetracycline label suggests suppressed bone formation. In subjects treated with Prolia, 35% had no tetracycline label present at the month 24 biopsy and 38% had no tetracycline label present at the month 36 biopsy, while 100% of placebo-treated patients had double label present at both time points. When compared to placebo, treatment with Prolia resulted in virtually absent activation frequency and markedly reduced bone formation rates. However, the long-term consequences of this degree of suppression of bone remodeling are unknown.

16 HOW SUPPLIED/STORAGE AND HANDLING

Prolia is supplied in a single-use prefilled syringe with a safety guard or in a single-use vial. The grey needle cap on the single-use prefilled syringe contains dry natural rubber (a derivative of latex).

60 mg/1 mL in a single-use prefilled syringe	1 per carton	NDC 55513-710-01
60 mg/1 mL in a single-use vial	1 per carton	NDC 55513-720-01

Store Prolia in a refrigerator at 2°C to 8°C (36°F to 46°F) in the original carton. Do not freeze. Prior to administration, Prolia may be allowed to reach room temperature (up to 25°C/77°F) in the original container. Once removed from the refrigerator, Prolia must not be exposed to temperatures above 25°C/77°F and must be used within 14 days. If not used within the 14 days, Prolia should be discarded. Do not use Prolia after the expiry date printed on the label.
Protect Prolia from direct light and heat.
Avoid vigorous shaking of Prolia.

17 PATIENT COUNSELING INFORMATION

See Medication Guide.

17.1 Hypocalcemia

Adequately supplement patients with calcium and vitamin D and instruct them on the importance of maintaining serum calcium levels while receiving Prolia *[see Warnings and Precautions (5.1) and Use in Specific Populations (8.6)].* Advise patients to seek prompt medical attention if they develop signs or symptoms of hypocalcemia.

17.2 Serious Infections

Advise patients to seek prompt medical attention if they develop signs or symptoms of infections, including cellulitis *[see Warnings and Precautions (5.2)].*

17.3 Dermatologic Reactions

Advise patients to seek prompt medical attention if they develop signs or symptoms of dermatological reactions (dermatitis, rashes, and eczema) *[see Warnings and Precautions (5.3)].*

17.4 Osteonecrosis of the Jaw

Advise patients to maintain good oral hygiene during treatment with Prolia and to inform their dentist prior to dental procedures that they are receiving Prolia. Patients should inform their physician or dentist if they experience persistent pain and/or slow healing of the mouth or jaw after dental surgery *[see Warnings and Precautions (5.4)].*

17.5 Schedule of Administration

If a dose of Prolia is missed, administer the injection as soon as convenient. Thereafter, schedule injections every 6 months from the date of the last injection.

Manufactured by:
Amgen Manufacturing Limited, a subsidiary of Amgen Inc.
One Amgen Center Drive
Thousand Oaks, California 91320-1799
This product, its production, and/or its use may be covered by one or more US Patents, including US Patent Nos. 6,740,522; 7,097,834; 7,364,736; and 7,411,050, as well as other patents or patents pending.
© 2010 Amgen Inc. All rights reserved.
1xxxxxx - v1

Table 3. The Effect of Prolia on the Incidence of Nonvertebral Fractures at Year 3

	Proportion of Women With Fracture (%)*		Absolute Risk Reduction (%) (95% CI)	Relative Risk Reduction (%) (95% CI)
	Placebo N = 3906 (%)	Prolia N = 3902 (%)		
Nonvertebral fracture†	8.0	6.5	1.5 (0.3, 2.7)	20 (5, 33)‡

*Event rates based on Kaplan-Meier estimates at 3 years.
†Excluding those of the vertebrae (cervical, thoracic, and lumbar), skull, facial, mandible, metacarpus, and finger and toe phalanges.
‡p-value = 0.01.

MEDICATION GUIDE

Prolia™ (PRÓ-lee-a)
(denosumab)
Injection

Read the Medication Guide that comes with Prolia before you start taking it and each time you get a refill. There may be new information. This Medication Guide does not take the place of talking with your doctor about your medical condition or treatment. Talk to your doctor if you have any questions about Prolia.

What is the most important information I should know about Prolia?

Prolia can cause serious side effects including:

1. **Low calcium levels in your blood (hypocalcemia).**
Prolia may lower the calcium levels in your blood. If you have low blood calcium before you start receiving Prolia, it may get worse during treatment. Your low blood calcium must be treated before you receive Prolia. Most people with low blood calcium levels do not have symptoms, but some people may have symptoms. Call your doctor right away if you have symptoms of low blood calcium such as:
   • Spasms, twitches, or cramps in your muscles
   • Numbness or tingling in your fingers, toes, or around your mouth
Your doctor may prescribe calcium and vitamin D to help prevent low calcium levels in your blood while you take Prolia. Take calcium and vitamin D as your doctor tells you to.

2. **Serious infections.**
Serious infections in your skin, lower stomach area (abdomen), bladder, or ear may happen if you take Prolia. Inflammation of the inner lining of the heart (endocarditis) due to an infection also may happen more often in people who take Prolia. You may need to go to the hospital for treatment if you develop an infection.
Prolia is a medicine that may affect your immune system. People who have weakened immune system or take medicines that affect the immune system may have an increased risk for developing serious infections.
Call your doctor right away if you have any of the following symptoms of infection:
   • Fever or chills
   • Skin that looks red or swollen and is hot or tender to touch
   • Severe abdominal pain
   • Frequent or urgent need to urinate or burning feeling when you urinate

3. **Skin problems.**
Skin problems such as inflammation of your skin (dermatitis), rash, and eczema may happen if you take Prolia. Call your doctor if you have any of the following symptoms of skin problems that do not go away or get worse:
   • Redness
   • Itching
   • Small bumps or patches (rash)
   • Your skin is dry or feels like leather
   • Blisters that ooze or become crusty
   • Skin peeling

4. **Severe jaw bone problems (osteonecrosis).**
Severe jaw bone problems may happen when you take Prolia. Your doctor should examine your mouth before you start Prolia. Your doctor may tell you to see your dentist before you start Prolia. It is important for you to practice good mouth care during treatment with Prolia.

Call your doctor right away if you have any of these side effects.

What is Prolia?
Prolia is a prescription medicine used to treat osteoporosis (thinning and weakening of bone) in women after menopause ("change of life") who
   • Have an increased risk for fractures (broken bones).
   • Cannot use another osteoporosis medicine or other osteoporosis medicines did not work well.

Who should not receive Prolia?
Do not take Prolia if you have been told by your doctor that your blood calcium level is too low.

What should I tell my doctor before receiving Prolia?
Before taking Prolia, tell your doctor if you:
   • Have low blood calcium.
   • Cannot take daily calcium and vitamin D.
   • Had parathyroid or thyroid surgery (glands located in your neck).
   • Have been told you have trouble absorbing minerals in your stomach or intestines (malabsorption syndrome).
   • Have kidney problems or are on kidney dialysis.
   • Plan to have dental surgery or teeth removed.
   • Are pregnant or plan to become pregnant. Prolia may harm your unborn baby. Tell your doctor right away if you become pregnant while taking Prolia.
   Pregnancy Surveillance Program: Prolia is not intended for use in pregnant women. If you become pregnant while taking Prolia, talk to your doctor about enrolling with Amgen's Pregnancy Surveillance Program or call 1-800-772-6436 (1-800-77- AMGEN). The purpose of this program is to collect information about women who have become pregnant while taking Prolia.
   • Are breast-feeding or plan to breast-feed. It is not known if Prolia passes into your breast milk. You and your doctor should decide if you will take Prolia or breast-feed. You should not do both.

Tell your doctor about all the medicines you take, including prescription and nonprescription drugs, vitamins, and herbal supplements.
Know the medicines you take. Keep a list of medicines with you to show to your doctor or pharmacist when you get a new medicine.

How will I receive Prolia?
   • Prolia is an injection that will be given to you by a healthcare professional. Prolia is injected under your skin (subcutaneous).
   • You will receive Prolia 1 time every 6 months.
   • You should take calcium and vitamin D as your doctor tells you to while you receive Prolia.
   • If you miss a dose of Prolia, you should receive your injection as soon as you can.
   • Take good care of your teeth and gums while you receive Prolia. Brush and floss your teeth regularly.
   • Tell your dentist that you are receiving Prolia before you have dental work.

What are the possible side effects of Prolia?
Prolia may cause serious side effects.
   • See "What is the most important information I should know about Prolia?"
   • **Long-term effects on bone:** It is not known if the use of Prolia over a long period of time may cause slow healing of broken bones or unusual fractures.
The most common side effects of Prolia are:
   • Back pain
   • Pain in your arms and legs
   • High cholesterol
   • Muscle pain
   • Bladder infection
These are not all the possible side effects of Prolia. For more information, ask your doctor or pharmacist.
Call your doctor for medical advice about side effects. You may report side effects to FDA at 1-800-FDA-1088.

How should I handle Prolia if I need to pick it up from a pharmacy?
   • Keep Prolia in a refrigerator at 36°F to 46°F (2°C to 8°C) in the original carton.
   • Do not freeze Prolia.
   • When you remove Prolia from the refrigerator, Prolia must be kept at room temperature [up to 77°F (25°C)] in the original carton and must be used within 14 days.
   • Do not keep Prolia at temperatures above 77°F (25°C). Warm temperatures will affect how Prolia works.
   • Do not shake Prolia.
   • Keep Prolia in the original carton to protect from light.

Keep Prolia and all medicines out of reach of children.

General information about Prolia

Do not give Prolia to other people even if they have the same symptoms that you have. It may harm them.

This Medication Guide summarizes the most important information about Prolia. If you would like more information, talk with your doctor. You can ask your doctor or pharmacist for information about Prolia that is written for health professionals.

For more information, go to www.Prolia.com or call Amgen at 1-800-772-6436.

What are the ingredients in Prolia?

Active ingredient: denosumab

Inactive ingredients: sorbitol, acetate, polysorbate 20 (prefilled syringe only), Water for Injection (USP), and sodium hydroxide

What is osteoporosis?

Osteoporosis is a disease in which the bones become thin and weak, increasing the chance of having a broken bone. Osteoporosis usually causes no symptoms until a fracture happens. The most common fractures are in the spine (backbone). They can shorten height, even without causing pain. Over time, the spine can become curved or deformed and the body bent over. Fractures from osteoporosis can also happen in almost any bone in the body, for example: the wrist, rib, or hip. Once you have had a fracture, the chance for more fractures greatly increases.

The following risk factors increase your chance of getting fractures from osteoporosis:

- Past broken bones from osteoporosis
- Very low bone mineral density (BMD)
- Frequent falls
- Limited movement, such as using a wheelchair
- Medical conditions likely to cause bone loss, such as some kinds of arthritis
- Taking steroid medicines called glucocorticoids, such as prednisone
- Other medicines that may cause bone loss, for example: seizure medicines (such as phenytoin), blood thinners (such as heparin), high doses of vitamin A

What can I do to treat osteoporosis?

There are many steps you can take to treat osteoporosis. Taking Prolia, along with calcium and vitamin D, may be one option for you.

Amgen Manufacturing Limited, a subsidiary of Amgen Inc.
One Amgen Center Drive
Thousand Oaks, California 91320-1799

This Medication Guide has been approved by the US Food and Drug Administration.

1xxxxxx - v1
Issued: 06/2010

Shown in Product Identification Guide, page 306

SENSIPAR® ℞
[sĕn-sĭ-par]
(cinacalcet)
Tablets

DESCRIPTION

Sensipar® (cinacalcet) is a calcimimetic agent that increases the sensitivity of the calcium-sensing receptor to activation by extracellular calcium. Its empirical formula is $C_{22}H_{22}F_3N \bullet HCl$ with a molecular weight of 393.9 g/mol (hydrochloride salt) and 357.4 g/mol (free base). It has one chiral center having an R-absolute configuration. The R-enantiomer is the more potent enantiomer and has been shown to be responsible for pharmacodynamic activity.

Cinacalcet is a white to off-white, crystalline solid that is soluble in methanol or 95% ethanol and slightly soluble in water.

Sensipar® tablets are formulated as light-green, film-coated, oval-shaped tablets for oral administration in strengths of 30 mg, 60 mg, and 90 mg of cinacalcet as the free base equivalent (33 mg, 66 mg, and 99 mg as the hydrochloride salt, respectively).

Cinacalcet is described chemically as N-[1-(R)-(-)-(1-naphthyl)ethyl]-3-[3-(trifluoromethyl)phenyl]-1-aminopropane hydrochloride and has the following structural formula:

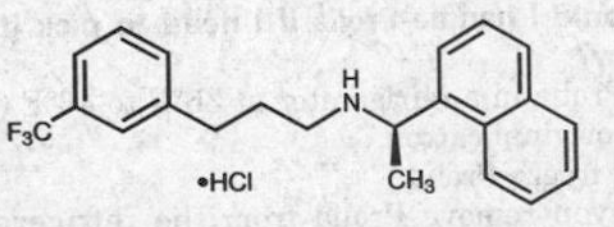

Inactive Ingredients: Sensipar® tablets are comprised of the active ingredient, and the following inactive ingredients: pre-gelatinized starch, microcrystalline cellulose, povidone, crospovidone, colloidal silicon dioxide, and magnesium stearate. Tablets are coated with color (Opadry® II green), clear film-coat (Opadry® clear) and carnauba wax.

CLINICAL PHARMACOLOGY

Mechanism of Action

Secondary hyperparathyroidism (HPT) in patients with chronic kidney disease (CKD) is a progressive disease, associated with increases in parathyroid hormone (PTH) levels and derangements in calcium and phosphorus metabolism. Increased PTH stimulates osteoclastic activity resulting in cortical bone resorption and marrow fibrosis. The goals of treatment of secondary hyperparathyroidism are to lower levels of PTH, calcium, and phosphorus in the blood, in order to prevent progressive bone disease and the systemic consequences of disordered mineral metabolism. In CKD patients on dialysis with uncontrolled secondary HPT, reductions in PTH are associated with a favorable impact on bone-specific alkaline phosphatase (BALP), bone turnover and bone fibrosis.

The calcium-sensing receptor on the surface of the chief cell of the parathyroid gland is the principal regulator of PTH secretion. Sensipar® directly lowers PTH levels by increasing the sensitivity of the calcium-sensing receptor to extracellular calcium. The reduction in PTH is associated with a concomitant decrease in serum calcium levels.

Pharmacokinetics

Absorption and Distribution: After oral administration of cinacalcet, maximum plasma concentration (C_{max}) is achieved in approximately 2 to 6 hours. A food-effect study in healthy volunteers indicated that the C_{max} and area under the curve ($AUC_{(0\text{-}inf)}$) were increased 82% and 68%, respectively, when cinacalcet was administered with a high-fat meal compared to fasting. C_{max} and $AUC_{(0\text{-}inf)}$ of cinacalcet were increased 65% and 50%, respectively, when cinacalcet was administered with a low-fat meal compared to fasting.

After absorption, cinacalcet concentrations decline in a biphasic fashion with a terminal half-life of 30 to 40 hours. Steady-state drug levels are achieved within 7 days. The mean accumulation ratio is approximately 2 with once-daily oral administration. The median accumulation ratio is approximately 2 to 5 with twice-daily oral administration. The AUC and C_{max} of cinacalcet increase proportionally over the dose range of 30 to 180 mg once daily. The pharmacokinetic profile of cinacalcet does not change over time with once-daily dosing of 30 to 180 mg. The volume of distribution is high (approximately 1000 L), indicating extensive distribution. Cinacalcet is approximately 93 to 97% bound to plasma protein(s). The ratio of blood cinacalcet concentration to plasma cinacalcet concentration is 0.80 at a blood cinacalcet concentration of 10 ng/mL.

Metabolism and Excretion: Cinacalcet is metabolized by multiple enzymes, primarily CYP3A4, CYP2D6 and CYP1A2. After administration of a 75 mg radiolabeled dose to healthy volunteers, cinacalcet was rapidly and extensively metabolized via: 1) oxidative N-dealkylation to hydrocinnamic acid and hydroxy-hydrocinnamic acid, which are further metabolized via β-oxidation and glycine conjugation; the oxidative N-dealkylation process also generates metabolites that contain the naphthalene ring; and 2) oxidation of the naphthalene ring on the parent drug to form dihydrodiols, which are further conjugated with glucuronic acid. The plasma concentrations of the major circulating metabolites including the cinnamic acid derivatives and glucuronidated dihydrodiols markedly exceed parent drug concentrations. The hydrocinnamic acid metabolite was shown to be inactive at concentrations up to 10 μM in a cell-based assay measuring calcium-receptor activation. The glucuronide conjugates formed after cinacalcet oxidation were shown to have a potency approximately 0.003 times that of cinacalcet in a cell-based assay measuring a calcimimetic response. Renal excretion of metabolites was the primary route of elimination of radioactivity. Approximately 80% of the dose was recovered in the urine and 15% in the feces.

Special Populations

Hepatic Insufficiency: The disposition of a 50 mg cinacalcet single dose was compared in patients with hepatic impairment and subjects with normal hepatic function. Cinacalcet exposure, $AUC_{(0\text{-}inf)}$, was comparable between healthy volunteers and patients with mild hepatic impairment. However, in patients with moderate and severe hepatic impairment (as indicated by the Child-Pugh method), cinacalcet exposures as defined by the $AUC_{(0\text{-}inf)}$ were 2.4 and 4.2 times higher, respectively, than that in normals. The mean half-life of cinacalcet is prolonged by 33% and 70% in patients with moderate and severe hepatic impairment, respectively. Protein binding of cinacalcet is not affected by impaired hepatic function. See PRECAUTIONS and DOSAGE AND ADMINISTRATION.

Renal Insufficiency: The pharmacokinetic profile of a 75 mg Sensipar® single dose in patients with mild, moderate, and severe renal insufficiency, and those on hemodialysis or peritoneal dialysis is comparable to that in healthy volunteers.

Geriatric Patients: The pharmacokinetic profile of Sensipar® in geriatric patients (age ≥ 65, n = 12) is similar to that for patients who are < 65 years of age (n = 268).

Pediatric Patients: The pharmacokinetics of Sensipar® have not been studied in patients < 18 years of age.

Drug Interactions

An in vitro study indicates that cinacalcet is a strong inhibitor of CYP2D6, but not of CYP1A2, CYP2C9, CYP2C19, and CYP3A4. In vitro induction studies indicate that cinacalcet is not an inducer of CYP450 enzymes.

Ketoconazole: Cinacalcet $AUC_{(0\text{-}inf)}$ and C_{max} increased 2.3 and 2.2 times, respectively, when a single 90 mg cinacalcet dose on Day 5 was administered to subjects treated with 200 mg ketoconazole twice daily for 7 days compared to 90 mg cinacalcet given alone (see DOSAGE AND ADMINISTRATION).

Calcium Carbonate: No significant pharmacokinetic interaction was observed when a single dose of 1500 mg calcium carbonate was coadministered with 100 mg cinacalcet.

Pantoprazole: No significant pharmacokinetic interaction was observed when cinacalcet 90 mg was administered to subjects treated with 80 mg pantoprazole daily for 3 days.

Sevelamer HCl: No significant pharmacokinetic interaction was observed when 2400 mg sevelamer HCl was coadministered with 90 mg cinacalcet tablet (subjects subsequently received 2400 mg sevelamer HCl two more times on Day 1 and three more times on Day 2).

Desipramine: The effect of cinacalcet (90 mg) on the pharmacokinetics of desipramine (50 mg) has been studied in healthy subjects who were CYP2D6 extensive metabolizers. The AUC and C_{max} of desipramine increased by 3.6 (296.5-446.7%) and 1.75 (157.5-194.9%) fold, respectively, in the presence of cinacalcet. This indicates that cinacalcet is a strong in vivo inhibitor of CYP2D6 and can increase the blood concentrations of drugs metabolized by CYP2D6.

Amitriptyline: Concurrent administration of 25 mg or 100 mg cinacalcet with 50 mg amitriptyline increased amitriptyline exposure and nortriptyline (active metabolite) exposure by approximately 20% in CYP2D6 extensive metabolizers.

Warfarin: R- and S-warfarin pharmacokinetics and warfarin pharmacodynamics were not affected in subjects treated with warfarin 25 mg who received cinacalcet 30 mg twice daily. The lack of effect of cinacalcet on the pharmacokinetics of R- and S-warfarin and the absence of auto-induction upon multiple dosing in patients indicates that cinacalcet is not an inducer of CYP2C9 in humans.

Midazolam: There were no significant differences in the pharmacokinetics of midazolam, a CYP3A4 and CYP3A5 substrate, in subjects receiving 90 mg cinacalcet once daily for 5 days and a single dose of 2 mg midazolam on day 5 as compared to those of subjects receiving 2 mg midazolam alone. This suggests that cinacalcet would not affect the pharmacokinetics of drugs predominantly metabolized by CYP3A4 and CYP3A5.

Pharmacodynamics

Reduction in intact PTH (iPTH) levels correlated with cinacalcet concentrations in CKD patients. The nadir in iPTH level occurs approximately 2 to 6 hours post dose, corresponding with the C_{max} of cinacalcet. After steady state is reached, serum calcium concentrations remain constant over the dosing interval in CKD patients.

CLINICAL STUDIES

Secondary Hyperparathyroidism in Patients with Chronic Kidney Disease on Dialysis

Three 6-month, multicenter, randomized, double-blind, placebo-controlled clinical studies of similar design were conducted in CKD patients on dialysis. A total of 665 patients were randomized to Sensipar® and 471 patients to placebo. The mean age of the patients was 54 years, 62% were male, and 52% Caucasian. The average baseline iPTH level by the Nichols intact immunoradiometric assay (IRMA) was 712 pg/mL, with 26% of the patients having a baseline iPTH level > 800 pg/mL. The mean baseline Ca × P ion product was 61 mg^2/dL^2. The average duration of dialysis prior to study enrollment was 67 months. Ninety-six percent of patients were on hemodialysis and 4% peritoneal dialysis. At study entry, 66% of the patients were receiving vitamin D sterols and 93% were receiving phosphate binders. Sensipar® (or placebo) was initiated at a dose of 30 mg once daily and titrated every 3 or 4 weeks to a maximum dose of 180 mg once daily to achieve an iPTH of ≤ 250 pg/mL. The dose was not increased if a patient had any of the following: iPTH ≤ 200 pg/mL, serum calcium < 7.8 mg/dL, or any symptoms of hypocalcemia. If a patient experienced symptoms of hypocalcemia or had a serum calcium < 8.4 mg/dL, calcium supplements and/or calcium-based phosphate binders could be increased. If these measures were insufficient, the vitamin D dose could be increased. Approximately 70% of the Sensipar® patients and 80% of the placebo patients completed the 6-month studies. In the primary efficacy analysis, 40% of Sensipar® patients and 5% of placebo patients achieved an iPTH ≤ 250 pg/mL (p<0.001) (Table 1, Figure 1). Secondary efficacy parameters also improved in patients treated with Sensipar®. These studies showed that Sensipar® reduced PTH while lowering Ca × P, calcium and phosphorus levels (Table 1, Figure 2). The median dose of Sensipar® at the completion of the studies was 90 mg. Patients with milder disease typically required lower doses.

Similar results were observed when either the iPTH or bio-intact PTH (biPTH) assay was used to measure PTH levels in CKD patients on dialysis; treatment with cinacalcet did not alter the relationship between iPTH and biPTH. [See table 1 at right]

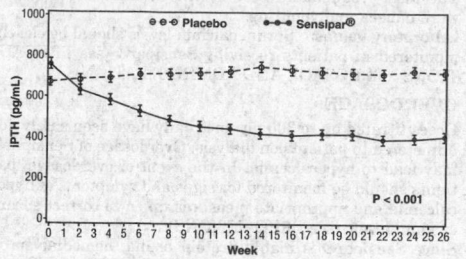

Figure 1. Mean (SE) iPTH Values (Pooled Phase 3 Studies)

Data are presented for patients who completed the studies; Placebo (N = 342), Sensipar® (N = 439).

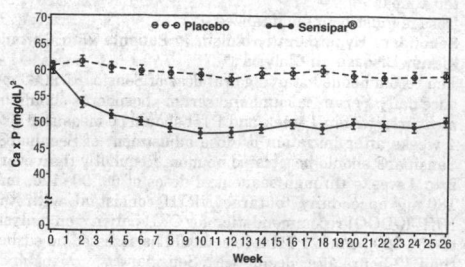

Figure 2. Mean (SE) Ca x P Values (Pooled Phase 3 Studies)

Data are presented for patients who completed the studies; Placebo (N = 342), Sensipar® (N = 439).

Reductions in iPTH and Ca × P were maintained for up to 12 months of treatment. Sensipar® decreased iPTH and Ca × P levels regardless of disease severity (i.e., baseline iPTH value), duration of dialysis, and whether or not vitamin D sterols were administered. Approximately 60% of patients with mild (iPTH ≥ 300 to ≤ 500 pg/mL), 41% with moderate (iPTH > 500 to 800 pg/mL), and 11% with severe (iPTH > 800 pg/mL) secondary HPT achieved a mean iPTH value of 250 pg/mL. Plasma iPTH levels were measured using the Nichols IRMA.

Parathyroid Carcinoma

Ten patients with parathyroid carcinoma were enrolled in an open-label study. The study consisted of 2 phases, a dose-titration phase and a maintenance phase.

The range of exposure was 2 to 16 weeks in the titration phase (n = 10) and 16 to 48 weeks (n = 3) for the maintenance phase. Baseline mean (SD) serum calcium was 14.7 (1.8) mg/dL. The range of change from baseline to last measurement was −7.5 to 2.7 mg/dL during the titration phase and −7.4 to 0.9 mg/dL during the maintenance phase (Figure 3). No patients maintained a serum calcium level within the normal range. The doses ranged from 70 mg twice daily to 90 mg four times daily for patients in the maintenance phase.

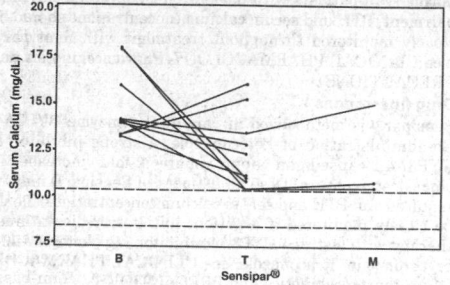

Figure 3. Serum Calcium Values in Parathyroid Carcinoma Patients Receiving Sensipar® at Baseline, Titration and Maintenance Phase

Solid lines represent individual patient data
B = baseline; T = last value in titration phase; M = last value in maintenance phase
Reference lines (dashed) show the normal range for serum calcium values

INDICATIONS AND USAGE

Sensipar® is indicated for the treatment of secondary hyperparathyroidism in patients with Chronic Kidney Disease on dialysis.

Table 1. Effects of Sensipar® on iPTH, Ca × P, Serum Calcium, and Serum Phosphorus in 6-month Phase 3 Studies (Patients on Dialysis)

		Study 1 Placebo (N = 205)	Study 1 Sensipar® (N = 205)	Study 2 Placebo (N = 165)	Study 2 Sensipar® (N = 166)	Study 3 Placebo (N = 101)	Study 3 Sensipar® (N = 294)
iPTH							
Baseline (pg/mL):	Median	535	537	556	547	670	703
	Mean (SD)	651 (398)	636 (341)	630 (317)	652 (372)	832 (486)	848 (685)
Evaluation Phase (pg/mL)		563	275	592	238	737	339
Median Percent Change		+3.8	-48.3	+8.4	-54.1	+2.3	-48.2
Patients Achieving Primary Endpoint (iPTH ≤ 250 pg/mL) (%)*		4%	41%[†]	7%	46%[†]	6%	35%[†]
Patients Achieving ≥ 30% Reduction in iPTH (%)*		11%	61%	12%	68%	10%	59%
Patients Achieving iPTH ≤ 250 pg/mL and Ca × P < 55 mg²/dL² (%)		1%	32%	5%	35%	5%	28%
Ca × P							
Baseline (mg²/dL²)		62	61	61	61	61	59
Evaluation Phase (mg²/dL²)		59	52	59	47	57	48
Median Percent Change		-2.0	-14.9	-3.1	-19.7	-4.8	-15.7
Calcium							
Baseline (mg/dL)		9.8	9.8	9.9	10.0	9.9	9.8
Evaluation Phase (mg/dL)		9.9	9.1	9.9	9.1	10.0	9.1
Median Percent Change		+0.5	-5.5	+0.1	-7.4	+0.3	-6.0
Phosphorus							
Baseline (mg/dL)		6.3	6.1	6.1	6.0	6.1	6.0
Evaluation Phase (mg/dL)		6.0	5.6	5.9	5.1	5.6	5.3
Median Percent Change		-1.0	-9.0	-2.4	-12.4	-5.6	-8.6

* iPTH value based on averaging over the evaluation phase (defined as weeks 13 to 26 in studies 1 and 2 and weeks 17 to 26 in study 3)
Values shown are medians unless indicated otherwise
[†]p < 0.001 compared to placebo; p-values presented for primary endpoint only

Sensipar® is indicated for the treatment of hypercalcemia in patients with parathyroid carcinoma.

CONTRAINDICATIONS

Sensipar® is contraindicated in patients with hypersensitivity to any component(s) of this product.

WARNINGS

Seizures

In three clinical studies of CKD patients on dialysis, 5% of the patients in both the Sensipar® and placebo groups reported a history of seizure disorder at baseline. During the trials, seizures (primarily generalized or tonic-clonic) were observed in 1.4% (9/656) of Sensipar®-treated patients and 0.4% (2/470) of placebo-treated patients. Five of the nine Sensipar®-treated patients had a history of a seizure disorder and two were receiving anti-seizure medication at the time of their seizure. Both placebo-treated patients had a history of seizure disorder and were receiving anti-seizure medication at the time of their seizure. While the basis for the reported difference in seizure rate is not clear, the threshold for seizures is lowered by significant reductions in serum calcium levels. Therefore, serum calcium levels should be closely monitored in patients receiving Sensipar®, particularly in patients with a history of a seizure disorder (see PRECAUTIONS, Hypocalcemia).

Hypotension and/or Worsening Heart Failure

In postmarketing safety surveillance, isolated, idiosyncratic cases of hypotension, worsening heart failure, and/or arrhythmia have been reported in patients with impaired cardiac function, in which a causal relationship to Sensipar® could not be completely excluded and which may be mediated by reductions in serum calcium levels. Clinical trial data showed hypotension occurred in 7% of Sensipar®-treated patients and 12% of placebo-treated patients, heart failure occurred in 2% of both Sensipar®- and placebo-treated patients.

PRECAUTIONS

General

Hypocalcemia

Sensipar® lowers serum calcium, and therefore patients should be carefully monitored for the occurrence of hypocalcemia. Potential manifestations of hypocalcemia include paresthesias, myalgias, cramping, tetany, and convulsions. Sensipar® treatment should not be initiated if serum calcium is less than the lower limit of the normal range (8.4 mg/dL). Serum calcium should be measured within 1 week after initiation or dose adjustment of Sensipar®. Once the maintenance dose has been established, serum calcium should be measured approximately monthly (see DOSAGE AND ADMINISTRATION).

If serum calcium falls below 8.4 mg/dL but remains above 7.5 mg/dL, or if symptoms of hypocalcemia occur, calcium-containing phosphate binders and/or vitamin D sterols can be used to raise serum calcium. If serum calcium falls below 7.5 mg/dL, or if symptoms of hypocalcemia persist and the

dose of vitamin D cannot be increased, withhold administration of Sensipar® until serum calcium levels reach 8.0 mg/dL, and/or symptoms of hypocalcemia have resolved. Treatment should be re-initiated using the next lowest dose of Sensipar® (see DOSAGE AND ADMINISTRATION).

In the 26-week studies of patients with CKD on dialysis, 66% of patients receiving Sensipar® compared with 25% of patients receiving placebo developed at least one serum calcium value < 8.4 mg/dL. Less than 1% of patients in each group permanently discontinued study drug due to hypocalcemia.

Sensipar® is not indicated for CKD patients not on dialysis. In CKD patients with secondary HPT not on dialysis, the long-term safety and efficacy of Sensipar® have not been established. Clinical studies indicate that Sensipar®-treated CKD patients not on dialysis have an increased risk for hypocalcemia compared to Sensipar®-treated CKD patients on dialysis, which may be due to lower baseline calcium levels. In a phase 3 study of 32 weeks duration and including 404 subjects (302 cinacalcet, 102 placebo), in which the median dose for cinacalcet was 60 mg at the completion of the study, 80% of Sensipar®-treated patients experienced at least one serum calcium value < 8.4 mg/dL compared to 5% of patients receiving placebo.

Adynamic Bone Disease

Adynamic bone disease may develop if iPTH levels are suppressed below 100 pg/mL. One clinical study evaluated bone histomorphometry in patients treated with Sensipar® for one year. Three patients with mild hyperparathyroid bone disease at the beginning of the study developed adynamic bone disease during treatment with Sensipar®. Two of these patients had iPTH levels below 100 pg/mL at multiple time points during the study. In the three 6-month, phase 3 studies conducted in CKD patients on dialysis, 11% of patients treated with Sensipar® had mean iPTH values below 100 pg/mL during the efficacy-assessment phase. If iPTH levels decrease below the NKF-K/DOQI recommended target range (150-300 pg/mL)[1] in patients treated with Sensipar®, the dose of Sensipar® and/or vitamin D sterols should be reduced or therapy discontinued.

Hepatic Insufficiency

Cinacalcet exposure as assessed by $AUC_{(0-inf)}$ in patients with moderate and severe hepatic impairment (as indicated by the Child-Pugh method) were 2.4 and 4.2 times higher, respectively, than that in normals. Patients with moderate and severe hepatic impairment should be monitored throughout treatment with Sensipar® (see CLINICAL PHARMACOLOGY, Pharmacokinetics and DOSAGE AND ADMINISTRATION).

Information for Patients

It is recommended that Sensipar® be taken with food or shortly after a meal. Tablets should be taken whole and should not be divided.

Laboratory Tests

Patients with CKD on Dialysis with Secondary Hyperparathyroidism

Serum calcium and serum phosphorus should be measured within 1 week and iPTH should be measured 1 to 4 weeks after initiation or dose adjustment of Sensipar®. Once the maintenance dose has been established, serum calcium and serum phosphorus should be measured approximately monthly, and PTH every 1 to 3 months (see DOSAGE AND ADMINISTRATION). All iPTH measurements during the Sensipar® trials were obtained using the Nichols IRMA.

In patients with end-stage renal disease, testosterone levels are often below the normal range. In a placebo-controlled trial in patients with CKD on dialysis, there were reductions in total and free testosterone in male patients following six months of treatment with Sensipar®. Levels of total testosterone decreased by a median of 15.8% in the Sensipar®-treated patients and by 0.6% in the placebo-treated patients. Levels of free testosterone decreased by a median of 31.3% in the Sensipar®-treated patients and by 16.3% in the placebo-treated patients. The clinical significance of these reductions in serum testosterone is unknown.

Patients with Parathyroid Carcinoma
Serum calcium should be measured within 1 week after initiation or dose adjustment of Sensipar®. Once maintenance dose levels have been established, serum calcium should be measured every 2 months (see DOSAGE AND ADMINISTRATION).

Drug Interactions and/or Drug/Laboratory Test Interactions
See CLINICAL PHARMACOLOGY, Pharmacokinetics and Drug Interactions.

Effect of Sensipar® on other drugs:
Drugs metabolized by cytochrome P450 2D6 (CYP2D6): Sensipar® is a strong in vitro, as well as in vivo, inhibitor of CYP2D6. Therefore, dose adjustments of concomitant medications that are predominantly metabolized by CYP2D6 (eg, metoprolol and carvedilol) and particularly those with a narrow therapeutic index (eg, flecainide, vinblastine, thioridazine and most tricyclic antidepressants) may be required.

Desipramine: Concurrent administration of cinacalcet (90 mg) with desipramine (50 mg) increased the exposure of desipramine by 3.6 fold in CYP2D6 extensive metabolizers.

Amitriptyline: Concurrent administration of 25 mg or 100 mg cinacalcet with 50 mg amitriptyline increased amitriptyline exposure and nortriptyline (active metabolite) exposure by approximately 20% in CYP2D6 extensive metabolizers.

Midazolam: There were no significant differences in the pharmacokinetics of midazolam, a CYP3A4 and CYP3A5 substrate, in subjects receiving 90 mg cinacalcet once daily for 5 days and a single dose of 2 mg midazolam on day 5 as compared to those of subjects receiving 2 mg midazolam alone. This suggests that cinacalcet would not affect the pharmacokinetics of drugs predominantly metabolized by CYP3A4 and CYP3A5.

Effect of other drugs on Sensipar®:
Sensipar® is metabolized by multiple cytochrome P450 enzymes, primarily CYP3A4, CYP2D6, and CYP1A2.

Ketoconazole: Sensipar® is metabolized in part by CYP3A4. Co-administration of ketoconazole, a strong inhibitor of CYP3A4, increased cinacalcet exposure following a single 90 mg dose of Sensipar® by 2.3 fold. Dose adjustment of Sensipar® may be required and PTH and serum calcium concentrations should be closely monitored if a patient initiates or discontinues therapy with a strong CYP3A4 inhibitor (e.g., ketoconazole, erythromycin, itraconazole; see DOSAGE AND ADMINISTRATION).

Carcinogenesis, Mutagenesis, and Impairment of Fertility
Carcinogenicity: Standard lifetime dietary carcinogenicity bioassays were conducted in mice and rats. Mice were given dietary doses of 15, 50, 125 mg/kg/day in males and 30, 70, 200 mg/kg/day in females (exposures up to 2 times those resulting with a human oral dose of 180 mg/day based on AUC comparison). Rats were given dietary doses of 5, 15, 35 mg/kg/day in males and 5, 20, 35 mg/kg/day in females (exposures up to 2 times those resulting with a human oral dose of 180 mg/day based on AUC comparison). No increased incidence of tumors was observed following treatment with cinacalcet.

Mutagenicity: Cinacalcet was not genotoxic in the Ames bacterial mutagenicity assay or in the Chinese Hamster Ovary (CHO) cell HGPRT forward mutation assay and CHO cell chromosomal aberration assay, with and without metabolic activation or in the in vivo mouse micronucleus assay.

Impairment of Fertility: Female rats were given oral gavage doses of 5, 25, 75 mg/kg/day beginning 2 weeks before mating and continuing through gestation day 7. Male rats were given oral doses 4 weeks prior to mating, during mating (3 weeks) and 2 weeks post-mating. No effects were observed in male or female fertility at 5 and 25 mg/kg/day (exposures up to 3 times those resulting with a human oral dose of 180 mg/day based on AUC comparison). At 75 mg/kg/day, there were slight adverse effects (slight decreases in body weight and food consumption) in males and females.

Pregnancy Category C
In pregnant female rats given oral gavage doses of 2, 25, 50 mg/kg/day during gestation no teratogenicity was observed at doses up to 50 mg/kg/day (exposure 4 times those

resulting with a human oral dose of 180 mg/day based on AUC comparison). Decreased fetal body weights were observed at all doses (less than 1 to 4 times a human oral dose of 180 mg/day based on AUC comparison) in conjunction with maternal toxicity (decreased food consumption and body weight gain).

In pregnant female rabbits given oral gavage doses of 2, 12, 25 mg/kg/day during gestation no adverse fetal effects were observed (exposures less than with a human oral dose of 180 mg/day based on AUC comparisons). Reductions in maternal food consumption and body weight gain were seen at doses of 12 and 25 mg/kg/day.

In pregnant rats given oral gavage doses of 5, 15, 25 mg/kg/day during gestation through lactation no adverse fetal or pup (post-weaning) effects were observed at 5 mg/kg/day (exposures less than with a human therapeutic dose of 180 mg/day based on AUC comparisons). Higher doses of 15 and 25 mg/kg/day (exposures 2-3 times a human oral dose of 180 mg/day based on AUC comparisons) were accompanied by maternal signs of hypocalcemia (periparturient mortality and early postnatal pup loss), and reductions in postnatal maternal and pup body-weight gain. Sensipar® has been shown to cross the placental barrier in rabbits.

There are no adequate and well-controlled studies in pregnant women. Sensipar® should be used during pregnancy only if the potential benefit justifies the potential risk to the fetus.

Lactating Women
Studies in rats have shown that Sensipar® is excreted in the milk with a high milk-to-plasma ratio. It is not known whether this drug is excreted in human milk. Considering these data in rats and because many drugs are excreted in human milk and because of the potential for clinically significant adverse reactions in infants from Sensipar®, a decision should be made whether to discontinue nursing or to discontinue the drug, taking into account the importance of the drug to the lactating woman.

Pediatric Use
The safety and efficacy of Sensipar® in pediatric patients have not been established.

Geriatric Use
Of the 1136 patients enrolled in the Sensipar® phase 3 clinical program, 26% were ≥ 65 years old, and 9% were ≥ 75 years old. No differences in the safety and efficacy of Sensipar® were observed in patients greater or less than 65 years of age (see DOSAGE AND ADMINISTRATION, Geriatric Patients).

ADVERSE EVENTS
Secondary Hyperparathyroidism in Patients with Chronic Kidney Disease on Dialysis
In 3 double-blind placebo-controlled clinical trials, 1126 CKD patients on dialysis received study drug (656 Sensipar®, 470 placebo) for up to 6 months. The most frequently reported adverse events (incidence of at least 5% in the Sensipar® group and greater than placebo) are provided in Table 2. The most frequently reported events in the Sensipar® group were nausea, vomiting, and diarrhea.

Table 2. Adverse Event Incidence (≥ 5%) in Patients on Dialysis

Event*	Placebo (n = 470) (%)	Sensipar® (n = 656) (%)
Nausea	19	31
Vomiting	15	27
Diarrhea	20	21
Myalgia	14	15
Dizziness	8	10
Hypertension	5	7
Asthenia	4	7
Anorexia	4	6
Pain Chest, Non-Cardiac	4	6
Access Infection	4	5

*Included are events that were reported at a greater incidence in the Sensipar® group than in the placebo group.

The incidence of serious adverse events (29% vs. 31%) was similar in the Sensipar® and placebo groups, respectively.
12-Month Experience with Sensipar®: Two hundred and sixty-six patients from 2 phase 3 studies continued to receive Sensipar® or placebo treatment in a 6-month double-blind extension study (12-month total treatment duration). The incidence and nature of adverse events in this study were similar in the two treatment groups, and comparable to those observed in the phase 3 studies.
Postmarketing Experience with Sensipar®: Rash, hypersensitivity reactions (including angioedema and urticaria), diarrhea and myalgia have been identified as adverse reactions during post-approval use of Sensipar®. Isolated, idio-

syncratic cases of hypotension, worsening heart failure, and/or arrhythmia have been reported in Sensipar®-treated patients with impaired cardiac function in postmarketing safety surveillance. Because these reactions are reported voluntarily from a population of uncertain size, it is not always possible to reliably estimate their frequency or establish a causal relationship to drug exposure.

Parathyroid Carcinoma
The most frequent adverse events in this patient group were nausea and vomiting.
Laboratory values: Serum calcium levels should be closely monitored in patients receiving Sensipar® (see PRECAUTIONS and DOSAGE AND ADMINISTRATION).

OVERDOSAGE
Doses titrated up to 300 mg once daily have been safely administered to patients on dialysis. Overdosage of Sensipar® may lead to hypocalcemia. In the event of overdosage, patients should be monitored for signs and symptoms of hypocalcemia and appropriate measures taken to correct serum calcium levels (see PRECAUTIONS).
Since Sensipar® is highly protein bound, hemodialysis is not an effective treatment for overdosage of Sensipar®.

DOSAGE AND ADMINISTRATION
Sensipar® tablets should be taken whole and should not be divided. Sensipar® should be taken with food or shortly after a meal.
Dosage must be individualized.
Secondary Hyperparathyroidism in Patients with Chronic Kidney Disease on Dialysis
The recommended starting oral dose of Sensipar® is 30 mg once daily. Serum calcium and serum phosphorus should be measured within 1 week and PTH should be measured 1 to 4 weeks after initiation or dose adjustment of Sensipar®. Sensipar® should be titrated no more frequently than every 2 to 4 weeks through sequential doses of 60, 90, 120, and 180 mg once daily to target iPTH consistent with the NKF-K/DOQI recommendation for CKD patients on dialysis of 150-300 pg/mL. PTH levels should be assessed no earlier than 12 hours after dosing with Sensipar®.
Sensipar® can be used alone or in combination with vitamin D sterols and/or phosphate binders.
During dose titration, serum calcium levels should be monitored frequently and if levels decrease below the normal range, appropriate steps should be taken to increase serum calcium levels, such as by providing supplemental calcium, initiating or increasing the dose of calcium-based phosphate binder, initiating or increasing the dose of vitamin D sterols, or temporarily withholding treatment with Sensipar® (see PRECAUTIONS).
Parathyroid Carcinoma
The recommended starting oral dose of Sensipar® is 30 mg twice daily.
The dosage of Sensipar® should be titrated every 2 to 4 weeks through sequential doses of 30 mg twice daily, 60 mg twice daily, 90 mg twice daily, and 90 mg three or four times daily as necessary to normalize serum calcium levels.
Special Populations
Geriatric patients: Age does not alter the pharmacokinetics of Sensipar®; no dosage adjustment is required for geriatric patients.
Patients with renal impairment: Renal impairment does not alter the pharmacokinetics of Sensipar®; no dosage adjustment is necessary for renal impairment.
Patients with hepatic impairment: Cinacalcet exposures, as assessed by $AUC_{(0-inf)}$, in patients with moderate and severe hepatic impairment (as indicated by the Child-Pugh method) were 2.4 and 4.2 times higher, respectively, than in normals. In patients with moderate and severe hepatic impairment, PTH and serum calcium concentrations should be closely monitored throughout treatment with Sensipar® (see CLINICAL PHARMACOLOGY, Pharmacokinetics and PRECAUTIONS).
Drug Interactions
Sensipar® is metabolized in part by the enzyme CYP3A4. Co-administration of ketoconazole, a strong inhibitor of CYP3A4, caused an approximate 2-fold increase in cinacalcet exposure. Dose adjustment of Sensipar® may be required and PTH and serum calcium concentrations should be closely monitored if a patient initiates or discontinues therapy with a strong CYP3A4 inhibitor (e.g., ketoconazole, erythromycin, itraconazole; see CLINICAL PHARMACOLOGY, Pharmacokinetics and PRECAUTIONS).

HOW SUPPLIED
Sensipar® 30 mg tablets are formulated as light-green, film-coated, oval-shaped tablets marked with "AMG" on one side and "30" on the opposite side, packaged in bottles of 30 tablets. (NDC 55513-073-30)
Sensipar® 60 mg tablets are formulated as light-green, film-coated, oval-shaped tablets marked with "AMG" on one side and "60" on the opposite side, packaged in bottles of 30 tablets. (NDC 55513-074-30)

Sensipar® 90 mg tablets are formulated as light-green, film-coated, oval-shaped tablets marked with "AMG" on one side and "90" on the opposite side, packaged in bottles of 30 tablets. (NDC 55513-075-30)

Storage
Store at 25°C (77°F); excursions permitted to 15-30°C (59-86°F). [See USP controlled room temperature].

Rx Only
This product, or its use, may be covered by one or more US Patents including US Patent Nos. 6313146, 6211244, 6031003 and 6011068, in addition to others, including patents pending.

REFERENCES
1. National Kidney Foundation: K/DOQI clinical practice guidelines: bone metabolism and disease in chronic kidney disease. American Journal of Kidney Disease 4 2:S1-S201, 2003
Manufactured for: Amgen
Amgen Inc.
One Amgen Center Drive
Thousand Oaks, CA 91320-1799
1xxxxxx
©2004-2010 Amgen Inc. All rights reserved.
v6 - Issue Date 02/2010
Shown in Product Identification Guide, page 306

VECTIBIX®
[veks-ti-biks]
(panitumumab)
Injection for intravenous infusion   ℞

HIGHLIGHTS OF PRESCRIBING INFORMATION
These highlights do not include all the information needed to use Vectibix safely and effectively. See full prescribing information for Vectibix.
Vectibix® (panitumumab)
Injection for intravenous infusion
Initial U.S. Approval: 2006

WARNING: DERMATOLOGIC TOXICITY and INFUSION REACTIONS
See full prescribing information for complete boxed warning.
- Dermatologic toxicities were reported in 89% of patients and were severe in 12% of patients receiving monotherapy. (2.1, 5.1, 6.1)
- Severe infusion reactions occurred in approximately 1% of patients. Fatal infusion reactions occurred in postmarketing experience. (2.1, 5.2, 6.1, 6.3)

---**RECENT MAJOR CHANGES**---

Indications and Usage: Colorectal Cancer (1)	07/2009
Warnings and Precautions: Increased Toxicity With Combination Chemotherapy (5.3)	07/2009
Boxed Warnings	05/2010
Dosage and Administration: Recommended Dose and Dose Modifications (2.1)	05/2010
Warnings and Precautions: Infusion Reactions (5.2)	05/2010

---**INDICATIONS AND USAGE**---

- Vectibix is an epidermal growth factor receptor antagonist indicated as a single agent for the treatment of metastatic colorectal carcinoma with disease progression on or following fluoropyrimidine, oxaliplatin, and irinotecan chemotherapy regimens. Approval is based on progression-free survival; no data demonstrate an improvement in disease-related symptoms or increased survival with Vectibix. (1)
- Retrospective subset analyses of metastatic colorectal cancer trials have not shown a treatment benefit for Vectibix in patients whose tumors had KRAS mutations in codon 12 or 13. Use of Vectibix is not recommended for the treatment of colorectal cancer with these mutations. (1, 12.1, 14)

---**DOSAGE AND ADMINISTRATION**---

- Administer at 6 mg/kg every 14 days as an intravenous infusion over 60 minutes (≤1000 mg) or 90 minutes (>1000 mg). (2)
- Infusion reactions: Reduce infusion rate by 50% for mild reactions; terminate the infusion for severe infusion reactions. Depending on the severity and/or persistence of the reaction, permanently discontinue Vectibix. (2.1)
- Dermatologic toxicities: Withhold for severe or intolerable toxicity; may resume at 50% of dose if toxicity improves. (2.1)

---**DOSAGE FORMS AND STRENGTHS**---

- Single-use vials (20 mg/mL): 100 mg/5 mL, 200 mg/10 mL, 400 mg/20 mL (3)

---**CONTRAINDICATIONS**---
None. (4)

---**WARNINGS AND PRECAUTIONS**---
- Dermatologic Toxicity: Withhold or discontinue Vectibix and monitor for inflammatory or infectious sequelae in patients with severe dermatologic toxicities. Limit sun exposure. (5.1, 5.6)
- Infusion Reactions: Terminate the infusion for severe infusion reactions. (5.2)
- Increased Toxicity With Combination Chemotherapy: Vectibix is not indicated for use in combination with chemotherapy. (5.3)
- Pulmonary Fibrosis: Discontinue Vectibix in patients developing interstitial lung disease, pneumonitis, or lung infiltrates. (5.4)
- Electrolyte Depletion/Monitoring: Monitor electrolytes during and for 8 weeks after completion of Vectibix therapy and institute appropriate treatment. (5.5)

---**ADVERSE REACTIONS**---
Most common adverse reactions (≥ 20%) are skin toxicities (i.e., erythema, dermatitis acneiform, pruritus, exfoliation, rash, and fissures), paronychia, hypomagnesemia, fatigue, abdominal pain, nausea, diarrhea, and constipation. (6)
To report SUSPECTED ADVERSE REACTIONS, contact Amgen Inc. at 1-800-77-AMGEN (1-800-772-6436) or FDA at 1-800-FDA-1088 or www.fda.gov/medwatch

---**USE IN SPECIFIC POPULATIONS**---
- Pregnancy: Based on animal data, may cause fetal harm. (8.1)
Physicians are encouraged to enroll pregnant patients in Amgen's Pregnancy Surveillance Program by calling 1-800-772-6436 (1-800-77-AMGEN). (8.1)
- Nursing Mothers: Discontinue nursing or discontinue drug, taking into account the importance of the drug to the mother. (8.3)

See 17 for PATIENT COUNSELING INFORMATION
Revised: 05/2010

FULL PRESCRIBING INFORMATION: CONTENTS*
WARNING: DERMATOLOGIC TOXICITY AND INFUSION REACTIONS

FULL PRESCRIBING INFORMATION

WARNING: DERMATOLOGIC TOXICITY AND INFUSION REACTIONS
Dermatologic Toxicity: Dermatologic toxicities occurred in 89% of patients and were severe (NCI-CTC grade 3 and higher) in 12% of patients receiving Vectibix monotherapy *[see Dosage and Administration (2.1), Warnings and Precautions (5.1), and Adverse Reactions (6.1)]*.
Infusion Reactions: Severe infusion reactions occurred in approximately 1% of patients. Fatal infusion reactions occurred in postmarketing experience *[see Dosage and Administration (2.1), Warnings and Precautions (5.2), and Adverse Reactions (6.1, 6.3)]*.

1   INDICATIONS AND USAGE
Vectibix is indicated as a single agent for the treatment of epidermal growth factor receptor (EGFR)-expressing, metastatic colorectal carcinoma (mCRC) with disease progression on or following fluoropyrimidine-, oxaliplatin-, and irinotecan-containing chemotherapy regimens *[see Clinical Studies (14)]*.
The effectiveness of Vectibix as a single agent for the treatment of EGFR-expressing, metastatic colorectal carcinoma is based on progression-free survival *[see Clinical Studies (14)]*. Currently, no data demonstrate an improvement in disease-related symptoms or increased survival with Vectibix.
Retrospective subset analyses of metastatic colorectal cancer trials have not shown a treatment benefit for Vectibix in patients whose tumors had KRAS mutations in codon 12 or 13. Use of Vectibix is not recommended for the treatment of colorectal cancer with these mutations *[see Clinical Studies (14) and Clinical Pharmacology (12.1)]*.

2   DOSAGE AND ADMINISTRATION
2.1   Recommended Dose and Dose Modifications
The recommended dose of Vectibix is 6 mg/kg, administered as an intravenous infusion over 60 minutes, every 14 days. Doses higher than 1000 mg should be administered over 90 minutes *[see Dosage and Administration (2.2)]*.
Appropriate medical resources for the treatment of severe infusion reactions should be available during Vectibix infusions.
Dose Modifications for Infusion Reactions [see Boxed Warning, Warnings and Precautions (5.2), and Adverse Reactions (6.1, 6.3)]
- Reduce infusion rate by 50% in patients experiencing a mild or moderate (grade 1 or 2) infusion reaction for the duration of that infusion.
- Terminate the infusion in patients experiencing severe infusion reactions. Depending on the severity and/or persistence of the reaction, permanently discontinue Vectibix.
Dose Modifications for Dermatologic Toxicity [see Boxed Warning, Warnings and Precautions (5.1), and Adverse Reactions (6.1)]
- Withhold Vectibix for dermatologic toxicities that are grade 3 or higher or are considered intolerable. If toxicity does not improve to ≤ grade 2 within 1 month, permanently discontinue Vectibix.
- If dermatologic toxicity improves to ≤ grade 2, and the patient is symptomatically improved after withholding no more than two doses of Vectibix, treatment may be resumed at 50% of the original dose.
- If toxicities recur, permanently discontinue Vectibix.
- If toxicities do not recur, subsequent doses of Vectibix may be increased by increments of 25% of the original dose until the recommended dose of 6 mg/kg is reached.

2.2   Preparation and Administration
Do not administer Vectibix as an intravenous push or bolus.
Preparation
Prepare the solution for infusion, using aseptic technique, as follows:
- Parenteral drug products should be inspected visually for particulate matter and discoloration prior to administration. Although Vectibix should be colorless, the solution may contain a small amount of visible translucent-to-white, amorphous, proteinaceous, panitumumab particulates (which will be removed by filtration; see below). Do not shake. Do not administer Vectibix if discoloration is observed.
- Withdraw the necessary amount of Vectibix for a dose of 6 mg/kg.
- Dilute to a total volume of 100 mL with 0.9% sodium chloride injection, USP. Doses higher than 1000 mg should be diluted to 150 mL with 0.9% sodium chloride injection, USP. Do not exceed a final concentration of 10 mg/mL.
- Mix diluted solution by gentle inversion. Do not shake.
Administration
- Administer using a low-protein-binding 0.2 μm or 0.22 μm in-line filter.
- Vectibix must be administered via infusion pump.
- Flush line before and after Vectibix administration with 0.9% sodium chloride injection, USP, to avoid mixing with other drug products or intravenous solutions. Do not mix Vectibix with, or administer as an infusion with, other medicinal products. Do not add other medications to solutions containing panitumumab.

- Infuse over 60 minutes through a peripheral intravenous line or indwelling intravenous catheter. Doses higher than 1000 mg should be infused over 90 minutes.

Use the diluted infusion solution of Vectibix within 6 hours of preparation if stored at room temperature, or within 24 hours of dilution if stored at 2° to 8°C (36° to 46°F). DO NOT FREEZE.

Discard any unused portion remaining in the vial.

3 DOSAGE FORMS AND STRENGTHS

100 mg of panitumumab in 5 mL (20 mg/mL) single-use vial.
200 mg of panitumumab in 10 mL (20 mg/mL) single-use vial.
400 mg of panitumumab in 20 mL (20 mg/mL) single-use vial.

4 CONTRAINDICATIONS

None.

5 WARNINGS AND PRECAUTIONS

5.1 Dermatologic Toxicity

In Study 1, dermatologic toxicities occurred in 90% of patients and were severe (NCI-CTC grade 3 and higher) in 16% of patients with mCRC receiving Vectibix. The clinical manifestations included, but were not limited to, dermatitis acneiform, pruritus, erythema, rash, skin exfoliation, paronychia, dry skin, and skin fissures. Subsequent to the development of severe dermatologic toxicities, infectious complications, including sepsis, septic death, and abscesses requiring incisions and drainage were reported. Withhold Vectibix for severe or life-threatening dermatologic toxicity [see Boxed Warning, Adverse Reactions (6.1) and Dosage and Administration (2.1)].

5.2 Infusion Reactions

In Study 1, 4% of patients experienced infusion reactions and in 1% of patients, these reactions were graded as severe (NCI-CTC grade 3-4).

Infusion reactions, manifesting as anaphylactoid reactions, bronchospasm, and hypotension, can occur following Vectibix administration [see Boxed Warning, and Adverse Reactions (6.1, 6.3)]. In clinical studies, severe infusion reactions occurred with the administration of Vectibix in approximately 1% of patients. Fatal infusion reactions occurred in postmarketing experience. Terminate the infusion for severe infusion reactions [see Dosage and Administration (2.1)].

5.3 Increased Toxicity With Combination Chemotherapy

Vectibix is not indicated for use in combination with chemotherapy. In an interim analysis of Study 2, the addition of Vectibix to the combination of bevacizumab and chemotherapy resulted in decreased overall survival and increased incidence of NCI-CTC grade 3-5 (87% vs 72%) adverse reactions [see Clinical Studies (14)]. NCI-CTC grade 3-4 adverse drug reactions occurring at a higher rate in Vectibix-treated patients included rash/dermatitis acneiform (26% vs 1%), diarrhea (23% vs 12%), dehydration (16% vs 5%), primarily occurring in patients with diarrhea, hypokalemia (10% vs 4%), stomatitis/mucositis (4% vs < 1%), and hypomagnesemia (4% vs 0). NCI-CTC grade 3-5 pulmonary embolism occurred at a higher rate in Vectibix-treated patients (7% vs 4%) and included fatal events in three (< 1%) Vectibix-treated patients.

As a result of the toxicities experienced, patients randomized to Vectibix, bevacizumab, and chemotherapy received a lower mean relative dose intensity of each chemotherapeutic agent (oxaliplatin, irinotecan, bolus 5-FU, and/or infusional 5-FU) over the first 24 weeks on study, compared with those randomized to bevacizumab and chemotherapy.

In a single-arm study of 19 patients receiving Vectibix in combination with IFL, the incidence of NCI-CTC grade 3-4 diarrhea was 58%; in addition, grade 5 diarrhea occurred in one patient. In a single-arm study of 24 patients receiving Vectibix plus FOLFIRI, the incidence of NCI-CTC grade 3 diarrhea was 25%.

Severe diarrhea and dehydration, which may lead to acute renal failure and other complications, have been observed in patients treated with Vectibix in combination with chemotherapy.

5.4 Pulmonary Fibrosis

Pulmonary fibrosis occurred in less than 1% (2/1467) of patients enrolled in clinical studies of Vectibix. Following the initial fatality described below, patients with a history of interstitial pneumonitis, pulmonary fibrosis, evidence of interstitial pneumonitis, or pulmonary fibrosis were excluded from clinical studies. Therefore, the estimated risk in a general population that may include such patients is uncertain.

One case occurred in a patient with underlying idiopathic pulmonary fibrosis who received Vectibix in combination with chemotherapy and resulted in death from worsening pulmonary fibrosis after four doses of Vectibix. The second case was characterized by cough and wheezing 8 days following the initial dose, exertional dyspnea on the day of the seventh dose, and persistent symptoms and CT evidence of pulmonary fibrosis following the 11th dose of Vectibix as monotherapy. An additional patient died with bilateral pulmonary infiltrates of uncertain etiology with hypoxia after 23 doses of Vectibix in combination with chemotherapy. Permanently discontinue Vectibix therapy in patients developing interstitial lung disease, pneumonitis, or lung infiltrates.

5.5 Electrolyte Depletion/Monitoring

In Study 1, median magnesium levels decreased by 0.1 mmol/L in the Vectibix arm; hypomagnesemia (NCI-CTC grade 3 or 4) requiring oral or intravenous electrolyte repletion occurred in 2% of patients. Hypomagnesemia occurred 6 weeks or longer after the initiation of Vectibix. In some patients, both hypomagnesemia and hypocalcemia occurred. Patients' electrolytes should be periodically monitored during and for 8 weeks after the completion of Vectibix therapy. Institute appropriate treatment, e.g., oral or intravenous electrolyte repletion, as needed.

5.6 Photosensitivity

Exposure to sunlight can exacerbate dermatologic toxicity. Advise patients to wear sunscreen and hats and limit sun exposure while receiving Vectibix.

5.7 EGF Receptor Testing

Detection of EGFR protein expression is necessary for selection of patients appropriate for Vectibix therapy because these are the only patients studied and for whom benefit has been shown [see Indications and Usage (1) and Clinical Studies (14)]. Patients with colorectal cancer enrolled in Study 1 were required to have immunohistochemical evidence of EGFR expression using the Dako EGFR pharmDx® test kit.

Assessment for EGFR expression should be performed by laboratories with demonstrated proficiency in the specific technology being utilized. Improper assay performance, including use of suboptimally fixed tissue, failure to utilize specific reagents, deviation from specific assay instructions, and failure to include appropriate controls for assay validation can lead to unreliable results. Refer to the package insert for the Dako EGFR pharmDx® test kit, or other test kits approved by FDA, for identification of patients eligible for treatment with Vectibix and for full instructions on assay performance.

6 ADVERSE REACTIONS

The following adverse reactions are discussed in greater detail in other sections of the label:
- Dermatologic Toxicity [see Boxed Warning, Dosage and Administration (2.1), and Warnings and Precautions (5.1)]
- Infusion Reactions [see Boxed Warning, Dosage and Administration (2.1), and Warnings and Precautions (5.2)]
- Increased Toxicity With Combination Chemotherapy [see Warnings and Precautions (5.3)]
- Pulmonary Fibrosis [see Warnings and Precautions (5.4)]
- Electrolyte Depletion/Monitoring [see Warnings and Precautions (5.5)]
- Photosensitivity [see Warnings and Precautions (5.6)]

The most common adverse events of Vectibix are skin rash with variable presentations, hypomagnesemia, paronychia, fatigue, abdominal pain, nausea, and diarrhea, including diarrhea resulting in dehydration.

The most serious adverse events of Vectibix are pulmonary fibrosis, pulmonary embolism, severe dermatologic toxicity complicated by infectious sequelae and septic death, infusion reactions, abdominal pain, hypomagnesemia, nausea, vomiting, and constipation. Adverse reactions requiring discontinuation of Vectibix were infusion reactions, severe skin toxicity, paronychia, and pulmonary fibrosis.

6.1 Clinical Trials Experience

Because clinical trials are conducted under widely varying conditions, adverse reaction rates in the clinical trials of a drug cannot be directly compared to rates in clinical trials of another drug and may not reflect the rates observed in practice. The adverse reaction information from clinical studies does, however, provide a basis for identifying the adverse events that appear to be related to drug use and for approximating rates.

Safety data are available from 15 clinical trials in which 1467 patients received Vectibix; of these, 1293 received Vectibix monotherapy and 174 received Vectibix in combination with chemotherapy [see Warnings and Precautions (5.3)].

The data described in Table 1 and in other sections below, except where noted, reflect exposure to Vectibix administered as a single agent at the recommended dose and schedule (6 mg/kg every 2 weeks) in 229 patients with mCRC enrolled in Study 1, a randomized, controlled trial. The median number of doses was five (range: one to 26 doses), and 71% of patients received eight or fewer doses. The population had a median age of 62 years (range: 27 to 82 years), 63% were male, and 99% were white with < 1% black, < 1% Hispanic, and 0% other.

[See table 1 at left]

Table 1. Per-Patient Incidence of Adverse Reactions Occurring in ≥ 5% of Patients With a Between-Group Difference of ≥ 5% (Study 1)

Body System	Patients Treated With Vectibix Plus BSC (n = 229)		Best Supportive Care (BSC) Alone (n = 234)	
	All Grades (%)	Grade 3-4 (%)	All Grades (%)	Grade 3-4 (%)
Body as a Whole				
Fatigue	26	4	15	3
General Deterioration	11	8	4	3
Digestive				
Abdominal Pain	25	7	17	5
Nausea	23	1	16	< 1
Diarrhea	21	2	11	0
Constipation	21	3	9	1
Vomiting	19	2	12	1
Stomatitis	7	0	1	0
Mucosal Inflammation	6	< 1	1	0
Metabolic/Nutritional				
Hypomagnesemia (Lab)	38	4	2	0
Peripheral Edema	12	1	6	< 1
Respiratory				
Cough	14	< 1	7	0
Skin/Appendages				
All Skin/Integument Toxicity	90	16	9	0
Skin	90	14	6	0
Erythema	65	5	1	0
Dermatitis Acneiform	57	7	1	0
Pruritus	57	2	2	0
Nail	29	2	0	0
Paronychia	25	2	0	0
Skin Exfoliation	25	2	0	0
Rash	22	1	1	0
Skin Fissures	20	1	< 1	0
Eye	15	< 1	2	0
Acne	13	1	0	0
Dry Skin	10	0	0	0
Other Nail Disorder	9	0	0	0
Hair	9	0	1	0
Growth of Eyelashes	6	0	0	0

* Version 2.0 of the NCI-CTC was used for grading toxicities. Skin toxicity was coded based on a modification of the NCI-CTCAE, version 3.0.

Dermatologic, Mucosal, and Ocular Toxicity

In Study 1, dermatologic toxicities occurred in 90% of patients receiving Vectibix. Skin toxicity was severe (NCI-CTC grade 3 and higher) in 16% of patients. Ocular toxicities occurred in 15% of patients and included, but were not limited to conjunctivitis (4%), ocular hyperemia (3%), increased lacrimation (2%), and eye/eyelid irritation (1%). Stomatitis (7%) and oral mucositis (6%) were reported. One patient experienced an NCI-CTC grade 3 event of mucosal inflammation. The incidence of paronychia was 25% and was severe in 2% of patients. Nail disorders occurred in 9% of patients *[see Warnings and Precautions (5.1)]*.

Median time to the development of dermatologic, nail, or ocular toxicity was 14 days after the first dose of Vectibix; the median time to most severe skin/ocular toxicity was 15 days after the first dose of Vectibix; and the median time to resolution after the last dose of Vectibix was 84 days. Severe toxicity necessitated dose interruption in 11% of Vectibix-treated patients *[see Dosage and Administration (2.1)]*.

Subsequent to the development of severe dermatologic toxicities, infectious complications, including sepsis, septic death, and abscesses requiring incisions and drainage, were reported.

Infusion Reactions

Infusional toxicity was defined as any event within 24 hours of an infusion during the clinical study described as allergic reaction or anaphylactoid reaction, or any event occurring on the first day of dosing described as allergic reaction, anaphylactoid reaction, fever, chills, or dyspnea. Vital signs and temperature were measured within 30 minutes prior to initiation and upon completion of the Vectibix infusion. The use of premedication was not standardized in the clinical trials. Thus, the utility of premedication in preventing the first or subsequent episodes of infusional toxicity is unknown. Across several clinical trials of Vectibix monotherapy, 3% (43/1336) experienced infusion reactions of which approximately 1% (6/1336) were severe (NCI-CTC grade 3–4). In one patient, Vectibix was permanently discontinued for a serious infusion reaction *[see Dosage and Administration (2.1)]*.

6.2 Immunogenicity

As with all therapeutic proteins, there is potential for immunogenicity. The immunogenicity of Vectibix has been evaluated using two different screening immunoassays for the detection of anti-panitumumab antibodies: an acid dissociation bridging enzyme-linked immunosorbent assay (ELISA) (detecting high-affinity antibodies) and a Biacore® biosensor immunoassay (detecting both high- and low-affinity antibodies). The incidence of binding antibodies to panitumumab (excluding predose and transient positive patients), as detected by the acid dissociation ELISA, was 3/613 (< 1%) and as detected by the Biacore® assay was 28/613 (4.6%).

For patients whose sera tested positive in screening immunoassays, an in vitro biological assay was performed to detect neutralizing antibodies. Excluding predose and transient positive patients, 10/613 patients (1.6%) with postdose samples and 3/356 (0.8%) of the patients with follow-up samples tested positive for neutralizing antibodies.

No evidence of altered pharmacokinetic profile or toxicity profile was found between patients who developed antibodies to panitumumab as detected by screening immunoassays and those who did not.

The incidence of antibody formation is highly dependent on the sensitivity and specificity of the assay. Additionally, the observed incidence of antibody (including neutralizing antibody) positivity in an assay may be influenced by several factors, including assay methodology, sample handling, timing of sample collection, concomitant medications, and underlying disease. For these reasons, comparison of the incidence of antibodies to panitumumab with the incidence of antibodies to other products may be misleading.

6.3 Postmarketing Experience

The following adverse reaction has been identified during post-approval use of panitumumab. Because these reactions are reported in a population of uncertain size, it is not always possible to reliably estimate their frequency or establish a causal relationship to drug exposure.

- Angioedema *[see Boxed Warning, Dosage and Administration (2.1), and Warnings and Precautions (5.2)]*
- Anaphylaxis *[see Boxed Warning, Dosage and Administration (2.1), and Warnings and Precautions (5.2)]*

7 DRUG INTERACTIONS

No formal drug-drug interaction studies have been conducted with Vectibix.

8 USE IN SPECIFIC POPULATIONS

8.1 Pregnancy

Pregnancy Category C. There are no studies of Vectibix in pregnant women. Reproduction studies in cynomolgus monkeys treated with 1.25 to 5 times the recommended human dose of panitumumab resulted in significant embryolethality and abortions; however, no other evidence of teratogenesis was noted in offspring *[see Reproductive and Developmental Toxicology (13.3)]*. Vectibix should be used during pregnancy only if the potential benefit justifies the potential risk to the fetus.

Based on animal models, EGFR is involved in prenatal development and may be essential for normal organogenesis, proliferation, and differentiation in the developing embryo. Human IgG is known to cross the placental barrier; therefore, panitumumab may be transmitted from the mother to the developing fetus, and has the potential to cause fetal harm when administered to pregnant women.

Women who become pregnant during Vectibix treatment are encouraged to enroll in Amgen's Pregnancy Surveillance Program. Patients or their physicians should call 1-800-772-6436 (1-800-77-AMGEN) to enroll.

8.3 Nursing Mothers

It is not known whether panitumumab is excreted into human milk; however, human IgG is excreted into human milk. Published data suggest that breast milk antibodies do not enter the neonatal and infant circulation in substantial amounts. Because many drugs are excreted into human milk and because of the potential for serious adverse reactions in nursing infants from Vectibix, a decision should be made whether to discontinue nursing or to discontinue the drug, taking into account the importance of the drug to the mother. If nursing is interrupted, based on the mean half-life of panitumumab, nursing should not be resumed earlier than 2 months following the last dose of Vectibix *[see Clinical Pharmacology (12.3)]*.

8.4 Pediatric Use

The safety and effectiveness of Vectibix have not been established in pediatric patients. The pharmacokinetic profile of Vectibix has not been studied in pediatric patients.

8.5 Geriatric Use

Of 229 patients with mCRC who received Vectibix in Study 1, 96 (42%) were ≥ age 65. Although the clinical study did not include a sufficient number of geriatric patients to determine whether they respond differently from younger patients, there were no apparent differences in safety and effectiveness between these patients and younger patients.

10 OVERDOSAGE

Doses up to approximately twice the recommended therapeutic dose (12 mg/kg) resulted in adverse reactions of skin toxicity, diarrhea, dehydration, and fatigue.

11 DESCRIPTION

Vectibix (panitumumab) is a recombinant, human IgG2 kappa monoclonal antibody that binds specifically to the human epidermal growth factor receptor (EGFR). Panitumumab has an approximate molecular weight of 147 kDa. Panitumumab is produced in genetically engineered mammalian (Chinese hamster ovary) cells.

Vectibix is a sterile, colorless, pH 5.6 to 6.0 liquid for intravenous (IV) infusion, which may contain a small amount of visible translucent-to-white, amorphous, proteinaceous, panitumumab particulates. Each single-use 5 mL vial contains 100 mg of panitumumab, 29 mg sodium chloride, 34 mg sodium acetate, and Water for Injection, USP. Each single-use 10 mL vial contains 200 mg of panitumumab, 58 mg sodium chloride, 68 mg sodium acetate, and Water for Injection, USP. Each single-use 20 mL vial contains 400 mg of panitumumab, 117 mg sodium chloride, 136 mg sodium acetate, and Water for Injection, USP.

12 CLINICAL PHARMACOLOGY

12.1 Mechanism of Action

The EGFR is a transmembrane glycoprotein that is a member of a subfamily of type I receptor tyrosine kinases, including EGFR, HER2, HER3, and HER4. EGFR is constitutively expressed in normal epithelial tissues, including the skin and hair follicle. EGFR is over-expressed in certain human cancers, including colon and rectum cancers. Interaction of EGFR with its normal ligands (e.g., EGF, transforming growth factor-alpha) leads to phosphorylation and activation of a series of intracellular proteins, which in turn regulate transcription of genes involved with cellular growth and survival, motility, and proliferation. Signal transduction through the EGFR results in activation of the wild-type KRAS protein. However, in cells with activating *KRAS* somatic mutations, the mutant KRAS protein is continuously active and appears independent of EGFR regulation.

Panitumumab binds specifically to EGFR on both normal and tumor cells, and competitively inhibits the binding of ligands for EGFR. Nonclinical studies show that binding of panitumumab to the EGFR prevents ligand-induced receptor autophosphorylation and activation of receptor-associated kinases, resulting in inhibition of cell growth, induction of apoptosis, decreased proinflammatory cytokine and vascular growth factor production, and internalization of the EGFR. *In vitro* assays and *in vivo* animal studies demonstrate that panitumumab inhibits the growth and survival of selected human tumor cell lines expressing EGFR.

12.3 Pharmacokinetics

Panitumumab administered as a single agent exhibits nonlinear pharmacokinetics.

Following single-dose administrations of panitumumab as 1-hour infusions, the area under the concentration-time curve (AUC) increased in a greater than dose-proportional manner, and clearance (CL) of panitumumab decreased from 30.6 to 4.6 mL/day/kg as the dose increased from 0.75 to 9 mg/kg. However, at doses above 2 mg/kg, the AUC of panitumumab increased in an approximately dose-proportional manner.

Following the recommended dose regimen (6 mg/kg given once every 2 weeks as a 1-hour infusion), panitumumab concentrations reached steady-state levels by the third infusion with mean (± SD) peak and trough concentrations of 213 ± 59 and 39 ± 14 mcg/mL, respectively. The mean (± SD) $AUC_{0\text{-tau}}$ and CL were 1306 ± 374 mcg•day/mL and 4.9 ± 1.4 mL/kg/day, respectively. The elimination half-life was approximately 7.5 days (range: 3.6 to 10.9 days).

A population pharmacokinetic analysis was performed to explore the potential effects of selected covariates on panitumumab pharmacokinetics. Results suggest that age (21-88 years), gender, race (15% non-white), mild-to-moderate renal dysfunction, mild-to-moderate hepatic dysfunction, and EGFR membrane-staining intensity (1+, 2+, 3+) in tumor cells had no apparent impact on the pharmacokinetics of panitumumab.

No formal pharmacokinetic studies of panitumumab have been conducted in patients with renal or hepatic impairment.

13 NONCLINICAL TOXICOLOGY

13.1 Carcinogenesis, Mutagenesis, Impairment of Fertility

No carcinogenicity or mutagenicity studies of panitumumab have been conducted. It is not known if panitumumab can impair fertility in humans. Prolonged menstrual cycles and/or amenorrhea occurred in normally cycling, female cynomolgus monkeys treated weekly with 1.25 to 5 times the recommended human dose of panitumumab (based on body weight). Menstrual cycle irregularities in panitumumab-treated female monkeys were accompanied by both a decrease and delay in peak progesterone and 17β-estradiol levels. Normal menstrual cycling resumed in most animals after discontinuation of panitumumab treatment. A no-effect level for menstrual cycle irregularities and serum hormone levels was not identified. The effects of panitumumab on male fertility have not been studied. However, no adverse effects were observed microscopically in reproductive organs from male cynomolgus monkeys treated for 26 weeks with panitumumab at doses of up to approximately 5-fold the recommended human dose (based on body weight).

13.2 Animal Toxicology and/or Pharmacology

Weekly administration of panitumumab to cynomolgus monkeys for 4 to 26 weeks resulted in dermatologic findings, including dermatitis, pustule formation and exfoliative rash, and deaths secondary to bacterial infection and sepsis at doses of 1.25 to 5-fold higher (based on body weight) than the recommended human dose.

13.3 Reproductive and Developmental Toxicology

Pregnant cynomolgus monkeys were treated weekly with panitumumab during the period of organogenesis (gestation day [GD] 20-50). While no panitumumab was detected in serum of neonates from panitumumab-treated dams, anti-panitumumab antibody titers were present in 14 of 27 offspring delivered at GD 100. There were no fetal malformations or other evidence of teratogenesis noted in the offspring. However, significant increases in embryolethality and abortions occurred at doses of approximately 1.25 to 5 times the recommended human dose (based on body weight).

14 CLINICAL STUDIES

Vectibix Monotherapy

The safety and efficacy of Vectibix were studied in Study 1, an open-label, multinational, randomized, controlled trial of 463 patients with EGFR-expressing, metastatic carcinoma of the colon or rectum (mCRC). Patients were required to have progressed on or following treatment with a regimen(s) containing a fluoropyrimidine, oxaliplatin, and irinotecan; progression was confirmed by an independent review committee (IRC) for 75% of the patients. All patients were required to have EGFR expression defined as at least 1+ membrane staining in ≥ 1% of tumor cells by the Dako EGFR pharmDx® test kit. Patients were randomized 1:1 to receive panitumumab at a dose of 6 mg/kg given once every 2 weeks plus best supportive care (BSC) (n = 231) or BSC alone (n = 232) until investigator-determined disease progression. Randomization was stratified based on ECOG performance status (0–1 vs 2) and geographic region (western Europe, eastern/central Europe, or other). Upon investigator-determined disease progression, patients in the

BSC-alone arm were eligible to receive panitumumab and were followed until disease progression was confirmed by the IRC. The analyses of progression-free survival (PFS), objective response, and response duration were based on events confirmed by the IRC that was masked to treatment assignment.

Among the 463 patients, 63% were male, the median age was 62 years, 40% were 65 years or older, 99% were white, 86% had a baseline ECOG performance status of 0 or 1, and 67% had colon cancer. The median number of prior therapies for metastatic disease was 2.4. The membrane-staining intensity for EGFR was 3+ in 19%, 2+ in 51%, and 1+ in 30% of patients' tumors. The percentage of tumor cells with EGFR membrane staining in the following categories of > 35%, > 20%-35%, 10%-20%, and 1%-< 10% was 38%, 8%, 31%, and 22%, respectively.

Based upon IRC determination of disease progression, a statistically significant prolongation in PFS was observed in patients receiving Vectibix compared to those receiving BSC alone. The mean PFS was 96 days in the Vectibix arm and 60 days in the BSC-alone arm. Results are presented in Figure 1 below.

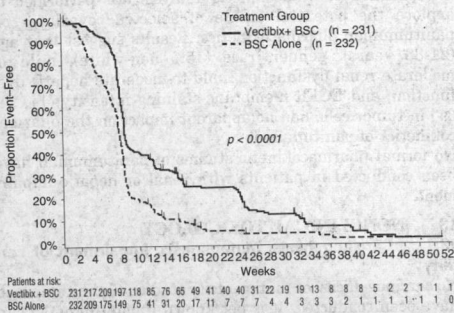

Treatment Group
— Vectibix+ BSC (n = 231)
---- BSC Alone (n = 232)

$p < 0.0001$

Patients at risk:
Vectibix + BSC 231 217 209 197 118 85 76 65 49 41 40 31 22 19 19 13 8 8 3 2 1 1 1 1 1 0
BSC Alone 232 209 175 149 75 41 31 20 17 11 7 7 7 4 4 3 2 1 1 1 1 1 1 1 1 1 0

Figure 1. Kaplan-Meier Plot of Progression-Free Survival Time as Determined by the IRC

In a series of sensitivity analyses, including one adjusting for potential ascertainment bias, i.e., assessment for progressive disease at a nonstudy specified time point, PFS was still significantly prolonged among patients receiving Vectibix as compared to patients receiving BSC alone.

Of the 232 patients randomized to BSC alone, 75% of patients crossed over to receive Vectibix following investigator determination of disease progression; the median time to cross over was 8.4 weeks (0.3–26.4 weeks). Partial responses were identified by the IRC in 19 patients randomized to Vectibix, for an overall response of 8% (95% CI: 5.0%, 12.6%). No patient in the control arm had an objective response identified by the IRC. The median duration of response was 17 weeks (95% CI: 16 weeks, 25 weeks). There was no difference in overall survival between the study arms.

Vectibix in Combination With Bevacizumab and Chemotherapy

Vectibix shortened PFS, decreased survival time, and increased toxicity when given in combination with bevacizumab and chemotherapy in Study 2, a randomized, open-label, multicenter trial in the first-line treatment of metastatic colorectal cancer. Patients (n = 1053) were randomized 1:1 to Vectibix at a dose of 6 mg/kg given once every 2 weeks, in combination with bevacizumab and an oxaliplatin- or irinotecan-based 5-fluorouracil-containing chemotherapy regimen, or to bevacizumab and chemotherapy alone. Randomization was stratified by type of regimen (oxaliplatin- or irinotecan-based); 86% of patients received an oxaliplatin-based regimen and 14% received an irinotecan-based regimen.

The major study objective was comparison of PFS in the oxaliplatin stratum as determined by an independent central review. An interim analysis based on 257 PFS events in the oxaliplatin stratum demonstrated shorter PFS in patients receiving Vectibix, bevacizumab, and chemotherapy compared to those receiving bevacizumab and chemotherapy alone (median PFS were 8.8 months and 10.5 months; hazard ratio 1.44 [95% CI: 1.12, 1.85], p-value = 0.0024, Cox model with randomization factors as covariates). An unplanned analysis of overall survival after 155 deaths (both strata combined), conducted at the time of the interim analysis of PFS, yielded an adjusted hazard ratio of 1.55 [95% CI: 1.12, 2.14], comparing patients receiving Vectibix, bevacizumab, and chemotherapy (92 deaths) to those receiving bevacizumab and chemotherapy alone (63 deaths) [see Warnings and Precautions (5.3)].

Lack of Efficacy of Anti-EGFR Monoclonal Antibodies in Patients With mCRC Containing KRAS Mutations

Retrospective analyses as presented in Table 2 across seven randomized clinical trials suggest that anti-EGFR-directed monoclonal antibodies are not effective for the treatment of patients with mCRC containing KRAS mutations. In these trials, patients received standard of care (i.e., BSC or chemotherapy) and were randomized to receive either an anti-EGFR antibody (cetuximab or panitumumab) or no additional therapy. In all studies, investigational tests were used to detect KRAS mutations in codon 12 or 13. The percentage of study populations for which KRAS status was assessed ranged from 23% to 92% [see Clinical Pharmacology (12.1)].

[See table 2 at bottom]

16 HOW SUPPLIED/STORAGE AND HANDLING

Vectibix is supplied as a sterile, colorless, preservative-free solution containing 20 mg/mL Vectibix (panitumumab) in a single-use vial.

Vectibix is provided as one vial per carton.

Each 5 mL single-use vial contains 100 mg of panitumumab in 5 mL (20 mg/mL) (NDC 55513-954-01).

Each 10 mL single-use vial contains 200 mg of panitumumab in 10 mL (20 mg/mL) (NDC 55513-955-01).

Each 20 mL single-use vial contains 400 mg of panitumumab in 20 mL (20 mg/mL) (NDC 55513-956-01).

Store vials in the original carton under refrigeration at 2° to 8°C (36° to 46°F) until time of use. Protect from direct sunlight. DO NOT FREEZE. Since Vectibix does not contain preservatives, any unused portion remaining in the vial must be discarded.

The diluted infusion solution of Vectibix should be used within 6 hours of preparation if stored at room temperature, or within 24 hours of dilution if stored at 2° to 8°C (36° to 46°F). DO NOT FREEZE.

17 PATIENT COUNSELING INFORMATION

Advise patients to contact a healthcare professional for any of the following:
- Skin and ocular/visual changes [see Boxed Warning, and Warnings and Precautions (5.1)],
- Signs and symptoms of infusion reactions, including fever, chills, or breathing problems [see Boxed Warning, Dosage and Administration (2.1), Warnings and Precautions (5.2), and Adverse Reactions (6.1, 6.3)]
- Diarrhea and dehydration [see Warnings and Precautions (5.3)]
- Persistent or recurrent coughing, wheezing, dyspnea, or new onset facial swelling [see Warnings and Precautions (5.4), and Adverse Reactions (6.1)]
- Pregnancy or nursing [see Use in Specific Populations (8.1, 8.3)]

Advise patients of the need for:
- Periodic monitoring of electrolytes [see Warnings and Precautions (5.5)]
- Limitation of sun exposure (use sunscreen, wear hats) while receiving Vectibix and for 2 months after the last dose of Vectibix therapy [see Warnings and Precautions (5.6)]
- Adequate contraception in both males and females while receiving Vectibix and for 6 months after the last dose of Vectibix therapy [see Use in Specific Populations (8.1, 8.3)]

Vectibix® (panitumumab)

Manufactured by:
Amgen Inc.
One Amgen Center Drive
Thousand Oaks, CA 91320-1799 USA

This product, its production, and/or its use may be covered by one or more US Patents, including US Patent No. 6,235,883, as well as other patents or patents pending.

© 2006-2010 Amgen Inc. All rights reserved.

1xxxxxx - v9

Table 2. Retrospective Analyses of Treatment Effect in the Subset of Patients With mCRC Containing KRAS Mutations Enrolled in Randomized Clinical Trials

Population (n: ITT*)	Treatment	Number of Patients with KRAS Results (% ITT)	Number of Patients with KRAS mutant (mAb†/control)	Effect of mAb on Endpoints: KRAS mutant‡
1st line treatment mCRC (n = 1198)	FOLFIRI ± cetuximab	540 (45%)	105/87	PFS†: no difference OS†: no difference ORR†: decreased
1st line treatment mCRC (n =337)	FOLFOX-4 ± cetuximab	233 (69%)	52/47	ORR: decreased PFS: decreased OS: no difference
Study 2: 1st line treatment mCRC (n = 1053)	oxaliplatin or irinotecan-based chemotherapy, bevacizumab ± Vectibix	oxaliplatin 664 (81%)	135/125	PFS: decreased OS: no difference ORR: increased
		irinotecan 201 (87%)	47/39	ORR: decreased PFS: decreased OS: decreased
1st line treatment mCRC (n = 736)	bevacizumab, capecitabine, oxaliplatin ± cetuximab	528 (72%)	98/108	PFS: decreased OS: decreased ORR: decreased
2nd line treatment mCRC (n = 1298)	irinotecan ± cetuximab	300 (23%)	49/59	OS: decreased PFS: no difference ORR: increased
3rd line treatment mCRC (n = 572)	BSC ± cetuximab	394 (69%)	81/83	OS: no difference PFS: no difference ORR: increased
Study 1: 3rd line treatment mCRC (n = 463)	BSC ± Vectibix	427 (92%)	84/100	PFS: no difference OS: no difference ORR: no difference

* ITT: intent-to-treat
† mAb: monoclonal antibody; PFS: progression-free-survival; ORR: overall response rate; OS: overall survival
‡ Results from the primary efficacy endpoint are in bold. A given endpoint is designated as "decreased" if there was a numerically smaller result and as "increased" if there was a numerically higher result in the mAb group than in the control group.

Amylin Pharmaceuticals, Inc.
9360 TOWNE CENTRE DRIVE
SAN DIEGO, CA 92121

Direct inquries to:
Ph: 858-552-2200
Fax: 858-552-2212

BYETTA®   ℞
[bye-A-tuh]
(exenatide)
Injection

HIGHLIGHTS OF PRESCRIBING INFORMATION
These highlights do not include all the information needed to use BYETTA safely and effectively. See full prescribing information for BYETTA.
BYETTA® (exenatide) Injection
Initial U.S. Approval: 2005

——RECENT MAJOR CHANGES——

Warnings and Precautions 10/2009
Pancreatitis (5.1)
Renal Impairment (5.3)
Macrovascular Outcomes (5.7)

———INDICATIONS AND USAGE———

BYETTA is a glucagon-like peptide-1 (GLP-1) receptor agonist indicated as an adjunct to diet and exercise to improve glycemic control in adults with type 2 diabetes mellitus.

Important Limitations of Use

- BYETTA is not a substitute for insulin. BYETTA should not be used in patients with type 1 diabetes or for the treatment of diabetic ketoacidosis (1.2).
- The concurrent use of BYETTA with insulin has not been studied and cannot be recommended (1.2).
- BYETTA has not been studied in patients with a history of pancreatitis. Consider other antidiabetic therapies in patients with a history of pancreatitis (1.2).

———DOSAGE AND ADMINISTRATION———

- Inject subcutaneously within 60 minutes prior to morning and evening meals (or before the two main meals of the day, approximately 6 hours or more apart) (2.1).
- Initiate at 5 mcg per dose twice daily; increase to 10 mcg twice daily after 1 month based on clinical response (2.1).

———DOSAGE FORMS AND STRENGTHS———

BYETTA is supplied as 250 mcg/mL exenatide in:

- 5 mcg per dose, 60 doses, 1.2 mL prefilled pen
- 10 mcg per dose, 60 doses, 2.4 mL prefilled pen

———CONTRAINDICATIONS———

- History of severe hypersensitivity to exenatide or any product components (4.1).

———WARNINGS AND PRECAUTIONS———

- Pancreatitis: Postmarketing reports, including fatal and non-fatal hemorrhagic or necrotizing pancreatitis. *Discontinue BYETTA promptly. BYETTA should not be restarted.* Consider other antidiabetic therapies in patients with a history of pancreatitis (5.1).
- Hypoglycemia: Increased risk when BYETTA is used in combination with a sulfonylurea. Consider reducing the sulfonylurea dose (5.2).
- Renal Impairment: Postmarketing reports, sometimes requiring hemodialysis and kidney transplantation. BYETTA should *not* be used in patients with severe renal impairment or end-stage renal disease and should be used with caution in patients with renal transplantation. Caution should be applied when initiating BYETTA or escalating the dose of BYETTA in patients with moderate renal failure (5.3).
- Severe Gastrointestinal Disease: Use of BYETTA is not recommended in patients with severe gastrointestinal disease (e.g., gastroparesis) (5.4).
- Hypersensitivity: Postmarketing reports of hypersensitivity reactions (e.g. anaphylaxis and angioedema). The patient should discontinue BYETTA and other suspect medications and promptly seek medical advice (5.6).
- There have been no clinical studies establishing conclusive evidence of macrovascular risk reduction with BYETTA or any other antidiabetic drug (5.7).

———ADVERSE REACTIONS———

- Most common (≥5%) and occurring more frequently than placebo in clinical trials: nausea, hypoglycemia, vomiting, diarrhea, feeling jittery, dizziness, headache, dyspepsia. Nausea usually decreases over time (5.2; 6).
- Postmarketing reports of increased international normalized ratio (INR) with concomitant use of warfarin, sometimes with bleeding (6.2).

To report SUSPECTED ADVERSE REACTIONS contact Amylin Pharmaceuticals, Inc. and Eli Lilly and Company at 1-800-868-1190 and www.byetta.com or FDA at 1-800-FDA-1088 or www.fda.gov/medwatch

———DRUG INTERACTIONS———

- Warfarin: Postmarketing reports of increased INR sometimes associated with bleeding. Monitor INR frequently until stable upon initiation or alteration of BYETTA therapy (7.2).

———USE IN SPECIFIC POPULATIONS———

- Pregnancy: Based on animal data, BYETTA may cause fetal harm. BYETTA should be used during pregnancy only if the potential benefit justifies the potential risk to the fetus. To report drug exposure during pregnancy call 1-800-633-9081 (8.1).
- Nursing Mothers: Caution should be exercised when BYETTA is administered to a nursing woman (8.3).

See 17 for PATIENT COUNSELING INFORMATION and FDA-approved patient labeling.

Revised: 10/2009

———————————————————————

FULL PRESCRIBING INFORMATION

1   INDICATIONS AND USAGE

1.1   Type 2 Diabetes Mellitus

BYETTA is indicated as an adjunct to diet and exercise to improve glycemic control in adults with type 2 diabetes mellitus.

1.2   Important Limitations of Use

BYETTA is not a substitute for insulin. BYETTA should not be used in patients with type 1 diabetes or for the treatment of diabetic ketoacidosis, as it would not be effective in these settings.

The concurrent use of BYETTA with insulin has not been studied and cannot be recommended.

Based on postmarketing data BYETTA has been associated with acute pancreatitis, including fatal and non-fatal hemorrhagic or necrotizing pancreatitis. BYETTA has not been studied in patients with a history of pancreatitis. It is unknown whether patients with a history of pancreatitis are at increased risk for pancreatitis while using BYETTA. Other antidiabetic therapies should be considered in patients with a history of pancreatitis.

2   DOSAGE AND ADMINISTRATION

2.1   Recommended Dosing

BYETTA should be initiated at 5 mcg administered twice daily at any time within the 60-minute period before the morning and evening meals (or before the two main meals of the day, approximately 6 hours or more apart). BYETTA should not be administered after a meal. Based on clinical response, the dose of BYETTA can be increased to 10 mcg twice daily after 1 month of therapy. Initiation with 5 mcg reduces the incidence and severity of gastrointestinal side effects. Each dose should be administered as a subcutaneous (SC) injection in the thigh, abdomen, or upper arm. No data are available on the safety or efficacy of intravenous or intramuscular injection of BYETTA.

Use BYETTA only if it is clear, colorless and contains no particles.

3   DOSAGE FORMS AND STRENGTHS

BYETTA is supplied as a sterile solution for subcutaneous injection containing 250 mcg/mL exenatide in the following packages:

- 5 mcg per dose, 60 doses, 1.2 mL prefilled pen
- 10 mcg per dose, 60 doses, 2.4 mL prefilled pen

4   CONTRAINDICATIONS

4.1   Hypersensitivity

BYETTA is contraindicated in patients with prior severe hypersensitivity reactions to exenatide or to any of the product components.

5   WARNINGS AND PRECAUTIONS

5.1   Acute Pancreatitis

Based on postmarketing data BYETTA has been associated with acute pancreatitis, including fatal and non-fatal hemorrhagic or necrotizing pancreatitis. After initiation of BYETTA, and after dose increases, observe patients carefully for signs and symptoms of pancreatitis (including persistent severe abdominal pain, sometimes radiating to the back, which may or may not be accompanied by vomiting). If pancreatitis is suspected, BYETTA should promptly be discontinued and appropriate management should be initiated. If pancreatitis is confirmed, BYETTA should not be restarted. Consider antidiabetic therapies other than BYETTA in patients with a history of pancreatitis.

5.2   Hypoglycemia

The risk of hypoglycemia is increased when BYETTA is used in combination with a sulfonylurea (hypoglycemia can also occur when other antidiabetic agents are used in combination with a sulfonylurea). Therefore, patients receiving BYETTA and a sulfonylurea may require a lower dose of the sulfonylurea to reduce the risk of hypoglycemia. It is also possible that the use of BYETTA with other glucose-independent insulin secretagogues (e.g. meglitinides) could increase the risk of hypoglycemia.

For additional information on glucose dependent effects see *Mechanism of Action (12.1)*.

5.3   Renal Impairment

BYETTA should not be used in patients with severe renal impairment (creatinine clearance < 30 mL/min) or end-stage renal disease and should be used with caution in patients with renal transplantation [see Use in Specific Populations (8.6)]. In patients with end-stage renal disease receiving dialysis, single doses of BYETTA 5 mcg were not well-tolerated due to gastrointestinal side effects. Because BYETTA may induce nausea and vomiting with transient hypovolemia, treatment may worsen renal function. Caution should be applied when initiating or escalating doses of BYETTA from 5 mcg to 10 mcg in patients with renal impairment (creatinine clearance 30 to 50 mL/min).

There have been postmarketing reports of altered renal function, including increased serum creatinine, renal impairment, worsened chronic renal failure and acute renal failure, sometimes requiring hemodialysis or kidney transplantation. Some of these events occurred in patients receiving one or more pharmacologic agents known to affect renal function or hydration status, such as angiotensin converting enzyme inhibitors, nonsteroidal anti-inflammatory drugs, or diuretics. Some events occurred in patients who had been experiencing nausea, vomiting, or diarrhea, with or without dehydration. Reversibility of altered renal function has been observed in many cases with supportive treatment and discontinuation of potentially causative agents, including BYETTA. Exenatide has not been found to be directly nephrotoxic in preclinical or clinical studies.

5.4   Gastrointestinal Disease

BYETTA has not been studied in patients with severe gastrointestinal disease, including gastroparesis. Because BYETTA is commonly associated with gastrointestinal adverse reactions, including nausea, vomiting, and diarrhea, the use of BYETTA is not recommended in patients with severe gastrointestinal disease.

5.5   Immunogenicity

Patients may develop antibodies to exenatide following treatment with BYETTA, consistent with the potentially immunogenic properties of protein and peptide pharmaceuticals. In a small proportion of patients, the formation of antibodies to exenatide at high titers could result in failure to achieve adequate improvement in glycemic control. If there is worsening glycemic control or failure to achieve targeted glycemic control, alternative antidiabetic therapy should be considered [see Adverse Reactions (6.1)].

5.6   Hypersensitivity

There have been postmarketing reports of serious hypersensitivity reactions (e.g. anaphylaxis and angioedema) in patients treated with BYETTA. If a hypersensitivity reaction occurs, the patient should discontinue BYETTA and other suspect medications and promptly seek medical advice [see Adverse Reactions (6.2)].

5.7   Macrovascular Outcomes

There have been no clinical studies establishing conclusive evidence of macrovascular risk reduction with BYETTA or any other antidiabetic drug.

6   ADVERSE REACTIONS

6.1   Clinical Trial Experience

Because clinical trials are conducted under widely varying conditions, adverse reaction rates observed in the clinical

Table 1: Incidence (%) and Rate of Hypoglycemia When BYETTA was Used as Monotherapy or With Concomitant Antidiabetic Therapy in Five Placebo-Controlled Clinical Trials*

	BYETTA		
	Placebo twice daily	5 mcg twice daily	10 mcg twice daily
Monotherapy (24 Weeks)			
N	77	77	78
% Overall	1.3%	5.2%	3.8%
Rate (episodes/patient-year)	0.03	0.21	0.52
% Severe	0.0%	0.0%	0.0%
With Metformin (30 Weeks)			
N	113	110	113
% Overall	5.3%	4.5%	5.3%
Rate (episodes/patient-year)	0.12	0.13	0.12
% Severe	0.0%	0.0%	0.0%
With a Sulfonylurea (30 Weeks)			
N	123	125	129
% Overall	3.3%	14.4%	35.7%
Rate (episodes/patient-year)	0.07	0.64	1.61
% Severe	0.0%	0.0%	0.0%
With Metformin and a Sulfonylurea (30 Weeks)			
N	247	245	241
% Overall	12.6%	19.2%	27.8%
Rate (episodes/patient-year)	0.58	0.78	1.71
% Severe	0.0%	0.4%	0.0%
With a Thiazolidinedione (16 Weeks)			
N	112	Dose not studied	121
% Overall	7.1%	Dose not studied	10.7%
Rate (episodes/patient-years)	0.56	Dose not studied	0.98
% Severe	0.0%	Dose not studied	0.0%

* For the 30-week trials, a hypoglycemia episode was recorded if the patient reported symptoms consistent with hypoglycemia and was recorded as severe if the subject required the assistance of another person to treat the event. For the other trials, a hypoglycemic episode was recorded if a patient reported signs or symptoms of hypoglycemia or had a blood glucose value consistent with hypoglycemia regardless of associated symptoms or treatment and was recorded as severe if the subject required the assistance of another person to treat the event. The requirement for assistance had to be accompanied by a blood glucose measurement of <50 mg/dL or prompt recovery after administration of oral carbohydrate.
N = The number of Intent-to-Treat subjects in each treatment group.

trials of a drug cannot be directly compared to rates in the clinical trials of another drug and may not reflect the rates observed in practice.
Hypoglycemia
Table 1 summarizes the incidence and rate of hypoglycemia with BYETTA in five placebo-controlled clinical trials.
[See table above]
Immunogenicity
In the 30-week controlled trials of BYETTA add-on to metformin and/or sulfonylurea, 38% of patients had low titer antibodies to exenatide at 30 weeks. For this group, the level of glycemic control (hemoglobin A1c [HbA$_{1c}$]) was generally comparable to that observed in those without antibody titers. An additional 6% of patients had higher titer antibodies at 30 weeks. In about half of this 6% (3% of the total patients given BYETTA in the 30-week controlled studies), the glycemic response to BYETTA was attenuated; the remainder had a glycemic response comparable to that of patients without antibodies.
In the 16-week trial of BYETTA add-on to thiazolidinediones, with or without metformin, 9% of patients had higher titer antibodies at 16 weeks. In the 24-week trial of BYETTA used as monotherapy, 3% of patients had higher titer antibodies at 24 weeks. Compared with patients who did not develop antibodies to BYETTA, on average the glycemic response in patients with higher titer antibodies was attenuated [see Warnings and Precautions (5.5)].

Other Adverse Reactions
Monotherapy
For the 24-week placebo-controlled study of BYETTA used as a monotherapy, Table 2 summarizes adverse reactions (excluding hypoglycemia) occurring with an incidence ≥2% and occurring more frequently in BYETTA-treated patients compared with placebo-treated patients.

Table 2: Treatment-Emergent Adverse Reactions ≥2% Incidence With BYETTA Used as Monotherapy (Excluding Hypoglycemia)*

Monotherapy	Placebo BID N = 77 %	All BYETTA BID N = 155 %
Nausea	0	8
Vomiting	0	4
Dyspepsia	0	3

* In a 24-week placebo-controlled trial.
BID = twice daily.

Adverse reactions reported in ≥1.0 to <2.0% of patients receiving BYETTA and reported more frequently than with

placebo included decreased appetite, diarrhea, and dizziness. The most frequently reported adverse reaction associated with BYETTA, nausea, occurred in a dose-dependent fashion.
Two of the 155 patients treated with BYETTA withdrew due to adverse reactions of headache and nausea. No placebo-treated patients withdrew due to adverse reactions.
Combination Therapy
Add-on to metformin and/or sulfonylurea
In the three 30-week controlled trials of BYETTA add-on to metformin and/or sulfonylurea, adverse reactions (excluding hypoglycemia) with an incidence ≥2% and occurring more frequently in BYETTA-treated patients compared with placebo-treated patients [see Warnings and Precautions (5.2)] are summarized in Table 3.

Table 3: Treatment-Emergent Adverse Reactions ≥2% Incidence and Greater Incidence With BYETTA Treatment Used With Metformin and/or a Sulfonylurea (Excluding Hypoglycemia)*

	Placebo BID N = 483 %	All BYETTA BID N = 963 %
Nausea	18	44
Vomiting	4	13
Diarrhea	6	13
Feeling Jittery	4	9
Dizziness	6	9
Headache	6	9
Dyspepsia	3	6
Asthenia	2	4
Gastroesophageal Reflux Disease	1	3
Hyperhidrosis	1	3

* In three 30-week placebo-controlled clinical trials.
BID = twice daily.

Adverse reactions reported in ≥1.0 to <2.0% of patients receiving BYETTA and reported more frequently than with placebo included decreased appetite. Nausea was the most frequently reported adverse reaction and occurred in a dose-dependent fashion. With continued therapy, the frequency and severity decreased over time in most of the patients who initially experienced nausea. Patients in the long-term uncontrolled open-label extension studies at 52 weeks reported no new types of adverse reactions than those observed in the 30-week controlled trials.
The most common adverse reactions leading to withdrawal for BYETTA-treated patients were nausea (3% of patients) and vomiting (1%). For placebo-treated patients, <1% withdrew due to nausea and none due to vomiting.
Add-on to thiazolidinedione with or without metformin
For the 16-week placebo-controlled study of BYETTA add-on to a thiazolidinedione, with or without metformin, Table 4 summarizes the adverse reactions (excluding hypoglycemia) with an incidence of ≥2% and occurring more frequently in BYETTA-treated patients compared with placebo-treated patients.

Table 4: Treatment-Emergent Adverse Reactions ≥2% Incidence With BYETTA Used With a Thiazolidinedione, With or Without Metformin (Excluding Hypoglycemia)*

With a TZD or TZD/MET	Placebo N = 112 %	All BYETTA BID N = 121 %
Nausea	15	40
Vomiting	1	13
Dyspepsia	1	7
Diarrhea	3	6
Gastroesophageal Reflux Disease	0	3

* In a 16-week placebo-controlled clinical trial.
BID = twice daily.

Adverse reactions reported in ≥1.0 to <2.0% of patients receiving BYETTA and reported more frequently than with placebo included decreased appetite. Chills (n = 4) and injection-site reactions (n = 2) occurred only in BYETTA-treated patients. The two patients who reported an injection-site reaction had high titers of antibodies to exenatide. Two serious adverse events (chest pain and chronic hypersensitivity pneumonitis) were reported in the BYETTA arm. No serious adverse events were reported in the placebo arm.

The most common adverse reactions leading to withdrawal for BYETTA-treated patients were nausea (9%) and vomiting (5%). For placebo-treated patients, <1% withdrew due to nausea.

6.2 Post-Marketing Experience
The following additional adverse reactions have been reported during post-approval use of BYETTA. Because these events are reported voluntarily from a population of uncertain size, it is generally not possible to reliably estimate their frequency or establish a causal relationship to drug exposure.

Allergy/Hypersensitivity: injection-site reactions, generalized pruritus and/or urticaria, macular or papular rash, angioedema, anaphylactic reaction [see Warnings and Precautions (5.6)].

Drug Interactions: International normalized ratio (INR) increased with concomitant warfarin use sometimes associated with bleeding [see Drug Interactions (7.2)].

Gastrointestinal: nausea, vomiting, and/or diarrhea resulting in dehydration; abdominal distension, abdominal pain, eructation, constipation, flatulence, acute pancreatitis, hemorrhagic and necrotizing pancreatitis sometimes resulting in death [see Limitations of Use (1.2) and Warnings and Precautions (5.1)].

Neurologic: dysgeusia; somnolence

Renal and Urinary Disorders: altered renal function, including increased serum creatinine, renal impairment, worsened chronic renal failure or acute renal failure (sometimes requiring hemodialysis), kidney transplant and kidney transplant dysfunction [see Warnings and Precautions (5.3)].

7 DRUG INTERACTIONS
7.1 Orally Administered Drugs
The effect of BYETTA to slow gastric emptying can reduce the extent and rate of absorption of orally administered drugs. BYETTA should be used with caution in patients receiving oral medications that have narrow therapeutic index or require rapid gastrointestinal absorption [see Adverse Reactions (6.2)]. For oral medications that are dependent on threshold concentrations for efficacy, such as contraceptives and antibiotics, patients should be advised to take those drugs at least 1 hour before BYETTA injection. If such drugs are to be administered with food, patients should be advised to take them with a meal or snack when BYETTA is not administered [see Clinical Pharmacology (12.3)].

7.2 Warfarin
There are postmarketing reports of increased INR sometimes associated with bleeding, with concomitant use of warfarin and BYETTA [see Adverse Reactions (6.2)]. In a drug interaction study, BYETTA did not have a significant effect on INR [see Clinical Pharmacology (12.3)]. In patients taking warfarin, prothrombin time should be monitored more frequently after initiation or alteration of BYETTA therapy. Once a stable prothrombin time has been documented, prothrombin times can be monitored at the intervals usually recommended for patients on warfarin.

8 USE IN SPECIFIC POPULATIONS
8.1 Pregnancy
Pregnancy Category C
There are no adequate and well-controlled studies of BYETTA use in pregnant women. In animal studies, exenatide caused cleft palate, irregular skeletal ossification and an increased number of neonatal deaths. BYETTA should be used during pregnancy only if the potential benefit justifies the potential risk to the fetus.

Female mice given SC doses of 6, 68, or 760 mcg/kg/day beginning 2 weeks prior to and throughout mating until gestation day 7 had no adverse fetal effects. At the maximal dose, 760 mcg/kg/day, systemic exposures were up to 390 times the human exposure resulting from the maximum recommended dose of 20 mcg/day, based on AUC [see Nonclinical Toxicology (13.3)].

In developmental toxicity studies, pregnant animals received exenatide subcutaneously during organogenesis. Specifically, fetuses from pregnant rabbits given SC doses of 0.2, 2, 22, 156, or 260 mcg/kg/day from gestation day 6 through 18 experienced irregular skeletal ossifications from exposures 12 times the human exposure resulting from the maximum recommended dose of 20 mcg/day, based on AUC. Moreover, fetuses from pregnant mice given SC doses of 6, 68, 460, or 760 mcg/kg/day from gestation day 6 through 15 demonstrated reduced fetal and neonatal growth, cleft palate and skeletal effects at systemic exposure 3 times the hu-

man exposure resulting from the maximum recommended dose of 20 mcg/day, based on AUC [see Nonclinical Toxicology (13.3)].

Lactating mice given SC doses of 6, 68, or 760 mcg/kg/day from gestation day 6 through lactation day 20 (weaning), experienced an increased number of neonatal deaths. Deaths were observed on postpartum days 2-4 in dams given 6 mcg/kg/day, a systemic exposure 3 times the human exposure resulting from the maximum recommended dose of 20 mcg/day, based on AUC [see Nonclinical Toxicology (13.3)].

Pregnancy Registry
Amylin Pharmaceuticals, Inc. maintains a Pregnancy Registry to monitor pregnancy outcomes of women exposed to exenatide during pregnancy. Physicians are encouraged to register patients by calling 1-800-633-9081.

8.3 Nursing Mothers
It is not known whether exenatide is excreted in human milk. However, exenatide is present at low concentrations (less than or equal to 2.5% of the concentration in maternal plasma following subcutaneous dosing) in the milk of lactating mice. Many drugs are excreted in human milk and because of the potential for clinically significant adverse reactions in nursing infants from exenatide, a decision should be made whether to discontinue nursing or discontinue the drug, taking into account these potential risks against the glycemic benefits to the lactating woman. Caution should be exercised when BYETTA is administered to a nursing woman.

8.4 Pediatric Use
Safety and effectiveness of BYETTA have not been established in pediatric patients.

8.5 Geriatric Use
Population pharmacokinetic analysis of patients ranging from 22 to 73 years of age suggests that age does not influence the pharmacokinetic properties of exenatide [see Clinical Pharmacology (12.3)]. BYETTA was studied in 282 patients 65 years of age or older and in 16 patients 75 years of age or older. No differences in safety or effectiveness were observed between these patients and younger patients. Because elderly patients are more likely to have decreased renal function, care should be taken in dose selection in the elderly based on renal function.

8.6 Renal Impairment
BYETTA is not recommended for use in patients with end-stage renal disease or severe renal impairment (creatinine clearance < 30 mL/min) and should be used with caution in patients with renal transplantation. No dosage adjustment of BYETTA is required in patients with mild renal impairment (creatinine clearance 50 to 80 mL/min). Caution should be applied when initiating or escalating doses of BYETTA from 5 mcg to 10 mcg in patients with moderate renal impairment (creatinine clearance 30 to 50 mL/min) [see Clinical Pharmacology (12.3)].

8.7 Hepatic Impairment
No pharmacokinetic study has been performed in patients with a diagnosis of acute or chronic hepatic impairment. Because exenatide is cleared primarily by the kidney, hepatic dysfunction is not expected to affect blood concentrations of exenatide [see Clinical Pharmacology (12.3)].

10 OVERDOSAGE
In a clinical study of BYETTA, three patients with type 2 diabetes each experienced a single overdose of 100 mcg SC (10 times the maximum recommended dose). Effects of the overdoses included severe nausea, severe vomiting, and rapidly declining blood glucose concentrations. One of the three patients experienced severe hypoglycemia requiring parenteral glucose administration. The three patients recovered without complication. In the event of overdose, appropriate supportive treatment should be initiated according to the patient's clinical signs and symptoms.

11 DESCRIPTION
BYETTA (exenatide) is a synthetic peptide that was originally identified in the lizard Heloderma suspectum. Exenatide differs in chemical structure and pharmacological action from insulin, sulfonylureas (including D-phenylalanine derivatives and meglitinides), biguanides, thiazolidinediones, alpha-glucosidase inhibitors, amylinomimetics and dipeptidyl peptidase-4 inhibitors.

Exenatide is a 39-amino acid peptide amide. Exenatide has the empirical formula $C_{184}H_{282}N_{50}O_{60}S$ and molecular weight of 4186.6 Daltons. The amino acid sequence for exenatide is shown below.

H-His-Gly-Glu-Gly-Thr-Phe-Thr-Ser-Asp-Leu-Ser-Lys-Gln-Met-Glu-Glu-Glu-Ala-Val-Arg-Leu-Phe-Ile-Glu-Trp-Leu-Lys-Asn-Gly-Gly-Pro-Ser-Ser-Gly-Ala-Pro-Pro-Pro-Ser-NH_2

BYETTA is supplied for SC injection as a sterile, preserved isotonic solution in a glass cartridge that has been assembled in a pen-injector (pen). Each milliliter (mL) contains 250 micrograms (mcg) synthetic exenatide, 2.2 mg metacresol as an antimicrobial preservative, mannitol as a tonicity-adjusting agent, and glacial acetic acid and sodium acetate

trihydrate in water for injection as a buffering solution at pH 4.5. Two prefilled pens are available to deliver unit doses of 5 mcg or 10 mcg. Each prefilled pen will deliver 60 doses to provide for 30 days of twice daily administration (BID).

12 CLINICAL PHARMACOLOGY
12.1 Mechanism of Action
Incretins, such as glucagon-like peptide-1 (GLP-1), enhance glucose-dependent insulin secretion and exhibit other antihyperglycemic actions following their release into the circulation from the gut. BYETTA is a GLP-1 receptor agonist that enhances glucose-dependent insulin secretion by the pancreatic beta-cell, suppresses inappropriately elevated glucagon secretion, and slows gastric emptying.

The amino acid sequence of exenatide partially overlaps that of human GLP-1. Exenatide has been shown to bind and activate the human GLP-1 receptor in vitro. This leads to an increase in both glucose-dependent synthesis of insulin, and in vivo secretion of insulin from pancreatic beta cells, by mechanisms involving cyclic AMP and/or other intracellular signaling pathways. Exenatide promotes insulin release from pancreatic beta cells in the presence of elevated glucose concentrations.

BYETTA improves glycemic control by reducing fasting and postprandial glucose concentrations in patients with type 2 diabetes through the actions described below.

Glucose-dependent insulin secretion: BYETTA has acute effects on pancreatic beta-cell responsiveness to glucose leading to insulin release predominantly in the presence of elevated glucose concentrations. This insulin secretion subsides as blood glucose concentrations decrease and approach euglycemia. However, BYETTA does not impair the normal glucagon response to hypoglycemia.

First-phase insulin response: In healthy individuals, robust insulin secretion occurs during the first 10 minutes following intravenous (IV) glucose administration. This secretion, known as the "first-phase insulin response," is characteristically absent in patients with type 2 diabetes. The loss of the first-phase insulin response is an early beta-cell defect in type 2 diabetes. Administration of BYETTA at therapeutic plasma concentrations restored first-phase insulin response to an IV bolus of glucose in patients with type 2 diabetes (Figure 1). Both first-phase insulin secretion and second-phase insulin secretion were significantly increased in patients with type 2 diabetes treated with BYETTA compared with saline (p <0.001 for both).

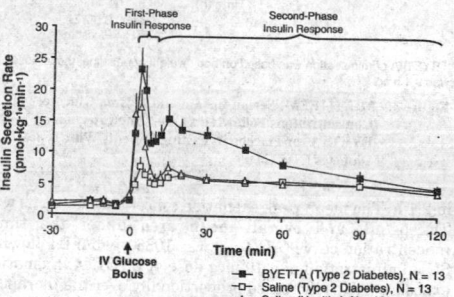

Patients received an IV infusion of insulin for 6.5 h (discontinued at time [t] = -30 min) to normalize plasma glucose concentrations and a continuous IV infusion of either BYETTA or saline for 5 h beginning 3 h prior to an IV bolus of glucose (0.3 g/kg over 30 sec) at t = 0 min.

Figure 1: Mean (+SEM) Insulin Secretion Rate During Infusion of BYETTA or Saline in Patients With Type 2 Diabetes and During Infusion of Saline in Healthy Subjects

Glucagon secretion: In patients with type 2 diabetes, BYETTA moderates glucagon secretion and lowers serum glucagon concentrations during periods of hyperglycemia. Lower glucagon concentrations lead to decreased hepatic glucose output and decreased insulin demand.

Gastric emptying: BYETTA slows gastric emptying, thereby reducing the rate at which meal-derived glucose appears in the circulation.

Food intake: In both animals and humans, administration of exenatide has been shown to reduce food intake.

12.2 Pharmacodynamics
Postprandial Glucose
In patients with type 2 diabetes, BYETTA reduces postprandial plasma glucose concentrations (Figure 2).
[See figure at top of next column]
Fasting Glucose
In a single-dose crossover study in patients with type 2 diabetes and fasting hyperglycemia, immediate insulin release followed injection of BYETTA. Plasma glucose concentrations were significantly reduced with BYETTA compared with placebo (Figure 3).
[See figure at top of next column]
12.3 Pharmacokinetics
Absorption
Following SC administration to patients with type 2 diabetes, exenatide reaches median peak plasma concentrations

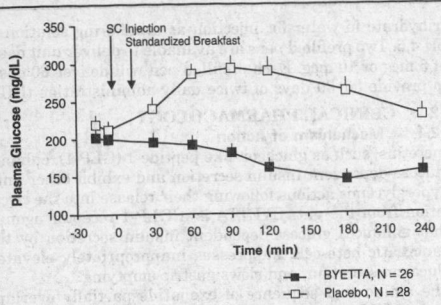

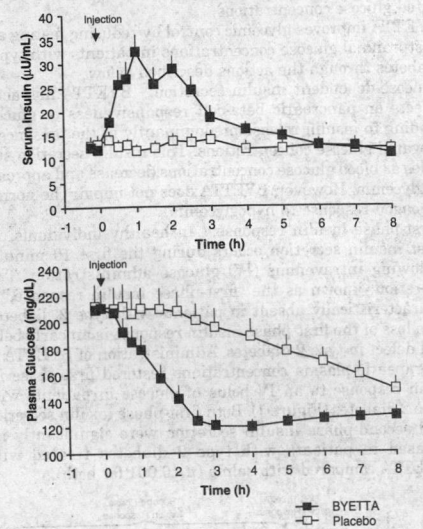

Figure 2: Mean (+SEM) Postprandial Plasma Glucose Concentrations on Day 1 of BYETTA[a] Treatment in Patients With Type 2 Diabetes Treated With Metformin, a Sulfonylurea, or Both (N = 54)

[a]Mean dose (7.8 mcg based on body weight) was administered by subcutaneous (SC) injection.

Figure 3: Mean (+SEM) Serum Insulin and Plasma Glucose Concentrations Following a One-Time Injection of BYETTA[a] or Placebo in Fasting Patients With Type 2 Diabetes (N = 12)

[a] BYETTA administration was based on body weight at baseline, mean dose was 9.1 mcg.

Table 5: Results of 24-Week Placebo-Controlled Trial of BYETTA Used as Monotherapy

	Placebo BID	BYETTA 5 mcg BID	BYETTA 10 mcg* BID
Intent-to-Treat Population (N)	77	77	78
HbA$_{1c}$ (%), Mean			
Baseline	7.8	7.9	7.8
Change at Week 24[†]	-0.2	-0.7	-0.9
Difference from placebo[†] (95% CI)		-0.5 [-0.9, -0.2][‡]	-0.7 [-1.0, -0.3][‡]
Proportion Achieving HbA$_{1c}$ <7%	38%	48%	53%
Body Weight (kg), Mean			
Baseline	86.1	85.1	86.2
Change at Week 24[†]	-1.5	-2.7	-2.9
Difference from placebo[†] (95% CI)		-1.3 [-2.3, -0.2]	-1.5 [-2.5, -0.4]
Fasting Serum Glucose[§] (mg/dL), Mean			
Baseline	159	166	155
Change at Week 24[†]	-5	-17	-19
Difference from placebo[†] (95% CI)		-12 [-23.2, -1.3]	-14 [-24.5, -2.5]

* BYETTA 5 mcg twice daily (BID) for 1 month followed by 10 mcg BID for 5 months before the morning and evening meals.
[†] Least squares means are adjusted for screening HbA$_{1c}$ strata and baseline value of the dependent variable.
[‡] p <0.01, treatment vs. placebo.
[§] Measured using the hexokinase-based glucose method.
BID = twice daily.

in 2.1 h. The mean peak exenatide concentration (C$_{max}$) was 211 pg/mL and overall mean area under the time-concentration curve (AUC$_{0-inf}$) was 1036 pg•h/mL following SC administration of a 10-mcg dose of BYETTA. Exenatide exposure (AUC) increased proportionally over the therapeutic dose range of 5 mcg to 10 mcg. The C$_{max}$ values increased less than proportionally over the same range. Similar exposure is achieved with SC administration of BYETTA in the abdomen, thigh, or upper arm.

Distribution
The mean apparent volume of distribution of exenatide following SC administration of a single dose of BYETTA is 28.3 L.

Metabolism and Elimination
Nonclinical studies have shown that exenatide is predominantly eliminated by glomerular filtration with subsequent proteolytic degradation. The mean apparent clearance of exenatide in humans is 9.1 L/h and the mean terminal half-life is 2.4 h. These pharmacokinetic characteristics of exenatide are independent of the dose. In most individuals, exenatide concentrations are measurable for approximately 10 h post-dose.

Drug Interactions
Acetaminophen
When 1000 mg acetaminophen elixir was given with 10 mcg BYETTA (0 h) and 1 hour, 2 hours, and 4 hours after BYETTA injection, acetaminophen AUCs were decreased by 21%, 23%, 24%, and 14%, respectively; C$_{max}$ was decreased by 37%, 56%, 54%, and 41%, respectively; T$_{max}$ was increased from 0.6 hour in the control period to 0.9 hour, 4.2 hours, 3.3 hours, and 1.6 hours, respectively. Acetaminophen AUC, C$_{max}$ and T$_{max}$ were not significantly changed when acetaminophen was given 1 hour before BYETTA injection.

Digoxin
Administration of repeated doses of BYETTA (10 mcg BID) 30 minutes before oral digoxin (0.25 mg QD) decreased the C$_{max}$ of digoxin by 17% and delayed the T$_{max}$ of digoxin by approximately 2.5 hours; however, the overall steady-state pharmacokinetic exposure (e.g., AUC) of digoxin was not changed.

Lovastatin
Administration of BYETTA (10 mcg BID) 30 minutes before a single oral dose of lovastatin (40 mg) decreased the AUC and C$_{max}$ of lovastatin by approximately 40% and 28%, respectively, and delayed the T$_{max}$ by about 4 hours compared with lovastatin administered alone. In the 30-week controlled clinical trials of BYETTA, the use of BYETTA in patients already receiving HMG CoA reductase inhibitors was not associated with consistent changes in lipid profiles compared to baseline.

Lisinopril
In patients with mild to moderate hypertension stabilized on lisinopril (5 to 20 mg/day), BYETTA (10 mcg BID) did not alter steady-state C$_{max}$ or AUC of lisinopril. Lisinopril steady-state T$_{max}$ was delayed by 2 hours. There were no changes in 24-h mean systolic and diastolic blood pressure.

Oral Contraceptives
The effect of BYETTA (10 mcg BID) on single and on multiple doses of a combination oral contraceptive (35 mcg ethinyl estradiol plus 150 mcg levonorgestrel) was studied in healthy female subjects. Repeated daily doses of the oral contraceptive (OC) given 30 minutes after BYETTA administration decreased the C$_{max}$ of ethinyl estradiol and levonorgestrel by 45% and 27%, respectively and delayed the T$_{max}$ of ethinyl estradiol and levonorgestrel by 3.0 hours and 3.5 hours, respectively, as compared to the oral contraceptive administered alone. Administration of repeated daily doses of the OC one hour prior to BYETTA administration decreased the mean C$_{max}$ of ethinyl estradiol by 15% but the mean C$_{max}$ of levonorgestrel was not significantly changed as compared to when the OC was given alone. BYETTA did not alter the mean trough concentrations of levonorgestrel after repeated daily dosing of the oral contraceptive for both regimens. However, the mean trough concentration of ethinyl estradiol was increased by 20% when the OC was administered 30 minutes after BYETTA administration injection as compared to when the OC was given alone. The effect of BYETTA on OC pharmacokinetics is confounded by the possible food effect on OC in this study. Therefore, OC products should be administered at least one hour prior to BYETTA injection.

Warfarin
Administration of warfarin (25 mg) 35 minutes after repeated doses of BYETTA (5 mcg BID on days 1-2 and 10 mcg BID on days 3-9) in healthy volunteers delayed warfarin T$_{max}$ by approximately 2 hours. No clinically relevant effects on C$_{max}$ or AUC of S- and R-enantiomers of warfarin were observed. BYETTA did not significantly alter the pharmacodynamic properties (e.g., international normalized ratio) of warfarin [see Drug Interactions (7.2)].

Specific Populations
Renal Impairment
Pharmacokinetics of exenatide was studied in subjects with normal, mild, or moderate renal impairment and subjects with end stage renal disease. In subjects with mild to moderate renal impairment (creatinine clearance 30 to 80 mL/min), exenatide exposure was similar to that of subjects with normal renal function. However, in subjects with end-stage renal disease receiving dialysis, mean exenatide exposure increased by 3.37-fold compared to that of subjects with normal renal function. [see Use in Specific Populations (8.6)].

Hepatic Impairment
No pharmacokinetic study has been performed in patients with a diagnosis of acute or chronic hepatic impairment [see Use in Specific Populations (8.7)].

Age
Population pharmacokinetic analysis of patients ranging from 22 to 73 years of age suggests that age does not influence the pharmacokinetic properties of exenatide [see Use in Specific Population (8.5)].

Gender
Population pharmacokinetic analysis of male and female patients suggests that gender does not influence the distribution and elimination of exenatide.

Race
Population pharmacokinetic analysis of samples from Caucasian, Hispanic, Asian, and Black patients suggests that race has no significant influence on the pharmacokinetics of exenatide.

Body Mass Index
Population pharmacokinetic analysis of patients with body mass indices (BMI) ≥30 kg/m^2 and <30 kg/m^2 suggests that BMI has no significant effect on the pharmacokinetics of exenatide.

13   NONCLINICAL TOXICOLOGY
13.1   Carcinogenesis, Mutagenesis, Impairment of Fertility
A 104-week carcinogenicity study was conducted in male and female rats at doses of 18, 70, or 250 mcg/kg/day administered by bolus SC injection. Benign thyroid C-cell adenomas were observed in female rats at all exenatide doses. The incidences in female rats were 8% and 5% in the two control groups and 14%, 11%, and 23% in the low-, medium-, and high-dose groups with systemic exposures of 5, 22, and 130 times, respectively, the human exposure resulting from the maximum recommended dose of 20 mcg/day, based on plasma area under the curve (AUC).
In a 104-week carcinogenicity study in mice at doses of 18, 70, or 250 mcg/kg/day administered by bolus SC injection, no evidence of tumors was observed at doses up to 250 mcg/

Table 6: Results of 30-Week and 16-Week Placebo-Controlled Trials of BYETTA Used in Combination with Oral Antidiabetic Agents

	Placebo BID	BYETTA 5 mcg BID	BYETTA 10 mcg* BID
In Combination With Metformin (30 Weeks)			
Intent-to-Treat Population (N)	113	110	113
HbA$_{1c}$ (%), Mean			
Baseline	8.2	8.3	8.2
Change at Week 30[†]	-0.0	-0.5	-0.9
Difference from placebo[†] (95% CI)		-0.5 [-0.7, -0.2][‡]	-0.9 [-1.1, -0.6][‡]
Proportion Achieving HbA$_{1c}$ <7%	12%	32%	40%
Body Weight (kg), Mean			
Baseline	99.9	100.0	100.9
Change at Week 30[†]	-0.2	-1.3	-2.6
Difference from placebo[†] (95% CI)		-1.1 [-2.2, -0.0]	-2.4 [-3.5, -1.3]
Fasting Plasma Glucose[§] (mg/dL), Mean			
Baseline	169	176	168
Change at Week 30[†]	+14	-5	-10
Difference from placebo[†] (95% CI)		-20 [-32, -7]	-24 [-37, -12]
In Combination With a Sulfonylurea (30 Weeks)			
Intent-to-Treat Population (N)	123	125	129
HbA$_{1c}$ (%), Mean			
Baseline	8.7	8.5	8.6
Change at Week 30[†]	+0.1	-0.5	-0.9
Difference from placebo[†] (95% CI)		-0.6 [-0.9, -0.3][‡]	-1.0 [-1.3, -0.7][‡]
Proportion Achieving HbA$_{1c}$ <7%	10%	25%	36%
Body Weight (kg), Mean			
Baseline	99.1	94.9	95.2
Change at Week 30[†]	-0.8	-1.1	-1.6
Difference from placebo[†] (95% CI)		-0.3 [-1.1, 0.6]	-0.9 [-1.7, -0.0]
Fasting Plasma Glucose[§] (mg/dL), Mean			
Baseline	194	180	178
Change at Week 30[†]	+6	-5	-11
Difference from placebo[†] (95% CI)		-11 [-25, 3]	-17 [-30, -3]

(Table continued on next page)

kg/day, a systemic exposure up to 95 times the human exposure resulting from the maximum recommended dose of 20 mcg/day, based on AUC.

Exenatide was not mutagenic or clastogenic, with or without metabolic activation, in the Ames bacterial mutagenicity assay or chromosomal aberration assay in Chinese hamster ovary cells. Exenatide was negative in the in vivo mouse micronucleus assay.

In mouse fertility studies with SC doses of 6, 68 or 760 mcg/kg/day, males were treated for 4 weeks prior to and throughout mating, and females were treated 2 weeks prior to mating and throughout mating until gestation day 7. No adverse effect on fertility was observed at 760 mcg/kg/day, a systemic exposure 390 times the human exposure resulting from the maximum recommended dose of 20 mcg/day, based on AUC.

13.3 Reproductive and Developmental Toxicology

In female mice given SC doses of 6, 68, or 760 mcg/kg/day beginning 2 weeks prior to and throughout mating until gestation day 7, there were no adverse fetal effects at doses up to 760 mcg/kg/day, systemic exposures up to 390 times the human exposure resulting from the maximum recommended dose of 20 mcg/day, based on AUC.

In pregnant mice given SC doses of 6, 68, 460, or 760 mcg/kg/day from gestation day 6 through 15 (organogenesis), cleft palate (some with holes) and irregular fetal skeletal ossification of rib and skull bones were observed at 6 mcg/kg/day, a systemic exposure 3 times the human exposure resulting from the maximum recommended dose of 20 mcg/day, based on AUC.

In pregnant rabbits given SC doses of 0.2, 2, 22, 156, or 260 mcg/kg/day from gestation day 6 through 18 (organogenesis), irregular fetal skeletal ossifications were observed at 2 mcg/kg/day, a systemic exposure 12 times the human exposure resulting from the maximum recommended dose of 20 mcg/day, based on AUC.

In pregnant mice given SC doses of 6, 68, or 760 mcg/kg/day from gestation day 6 through lactation day 20 (weaning), an increased number of neonatal deaths was observed on postpartum days 2-4 in dams given 6 mcg/kg/day, a systemic exposure 3 times the human exposure resulting from the maximum recommended dose of 20 mcg/day, based on AUC.

14 CLINICAL STUDIES

BYETTA has been studied as monotherapy and in combination with metformin, a sulfonylurea, a thiazolidinedione, a combination of metformin and a sulfonylurea, or a combination of metformin and a thiazolidinedione.

14.1 Monotherapy

In a randomized, double-blind, placebo-controlled trial of 24 weeks duration, BYETTA 5 mcg BID (n = 77), BYETTA 10 mcg BID (n = 78), or placebo BID (n = 77) was used as monotherapy in patients with entry HbA$_{1c}$ ranging from 6.5-10%. All patients assigned to BYETTA initially received 5 mcg BID for 4 weeks. After 4 weeks, those patients either continued to receive BYETTA 5 mcg BID or had their dose increased to 10 mcg BID. Patients assigned to placebo received placebo BID throughout the trial. BYETTA or placebo was injected subcutaneously before the morning and evening meals. The majority of patients (68%) were Caucasian, 26% were West Asian, 3% were Hispanic, 3% were Black, and 0.4% were East Asian.

The primary endpoint was the change in HbA$_{1c}$ from baseline to Week 24 (or the last value at time of early discontinuation). Compared to placebo, BYETTA 5 mcg BID and 10 mcg BID resulted in statistically significant reductions in HbA$_{1c}$ from baseline at Week 24 (Table 5).

[See table 5 at top of previous page]

On average, there were no adverse effects of exenatide on blood pressure or lipids.

14.2 Combination Therapy

Three 30-week, double-blind, placebo-controlled trials were conducted to evaluate the safety and efficacy of BYETTA in patients with type 2 diabetes whose glycemic control was inadequate with metformin alone, a sulfonylurea alone, or metformin in combination with a sulfonylurea. In addition, a 16-week, placebo-controlled trial was conducted where BYETTA was added to existing thiazolidinedione (pioglitazone or rosiglitazone) treatment, with or without metformin, in patients with type 2 diabetes with inadequate glycemic control.

In the 30-week trials, after a 4-week placebo lead-in period, patients were randomly assigned to receive BYETTA 5 mcg BID, BYETTA 10 mcg BID, or placebo BID before the morning and evening meals, in addition to their existing oral antidiabetic agent. All patients assigned to BYETTA initially received 5 mcg BID for 4 weeks. After 4 weeks, those patients either continued to receive BYETTA 5 mcg BID or had their dose increased to 10 mcg BID. Patients assigned to placebo received placebo BID throughout the study. A total of 1446 patients were randomized in the three 30-week trials: 991 (69%) were Caucasian, 224 (16%) were Hispanic, and 174 (12%) were Black. Mean HbA$_{1c}$ values at baseline for the trials ranged from 8.2% to 8.7%.

In the placebo-controlled trial of 16 weeks duration, BYETTA (n = 121) or placebo (n = 112) was added to existing thiazolidinedione (pioglitazone or rosiglitazone) treatment, with or without metformin. Randomization to BYETTA or placebo was stratified based on whether the patients were receiving metformin. BYETTA treatment was initiated at a dose of 5 mcg BID for 4 weeks then increased to 10 mcg BID for 12 more weeks. Patients assigned to placebo received placebo BID throughout the study. BYETTA or placebo was injected subcutaneously before the morning and evening meals. In this trial, 79% of patients were taking a thiazolidinedione and metformin and 21% were taking a thiazolidinedione alone. The majority of patients (84%) were Caucasian, 8% were Hispanic and 3% were Black. The mean baseline HbA$_{1c}$ values were 7.9% for BYETTA and placebo. The primary endpoint in each study was the mean change in HbA$_{1c}$ from baseline to study end (or early discontinuation). Table 6 summarizes the study results for the 30-week and 16-week clinical trials.

[See table 6 at left and on next page]

HbA$_{1c}$

The addition of BYETTA to a regimen of metformin, a sulfonylurea, or both, resulted in statistically significant reductions from baseline in HbA$_{1c}$ compared with patients receiving placebo added to these agents in the three controlled trials (Table 6).

In the 16-week trial of BYETTA add-on to thiazolidinediones, with or without metformin, BYETTA resulted in statistically significant reductions from baseline in HbA$_{1c}$ compared with patients receiving placebo (Table 6).

Postprandial Glucose

Postprandial glucose was measured after a mixed meal tolerance test in 9.5% of patients participating in the 30-week add-on to metformin, add-on to sulfonylurea, and add-on to metformin in combination with sulfonylurea clinical trials. In this pooled subset of patients, BYETTA reduced postprandial plasma glucose concentrations in a dose-dependent manner. The mean (SD) change in 2-h postprandial glucose concentration following administration of BYETTA at Week 30 relative to baseline was -63 (65) mg/dL for 5 mcg BID (n=42), -71 (73) mg/dL for 10 mcg BID (n=52), and +11 (69) mg/dL for placebo BID (n=44).

16 HOW SUPPLIED/STORAGE AND HANDLING

16.1 How Supplied

BYETTA is supplied as a sterile solution for subcutaneous injection containing 250 mcg/mL exenatide.

The following packages are available:

5 mcg per dose, 60 doses, 1.2 mL prefilled pen, NDC 66780-210-07

10 mcg per dose, 60 doses, 2.4 mL prefilled pen, NDC 66780-212-01

Table 6 (cont.): Results of 30-Week and 16-Week Placebo-Controlled Trials of BYETTA Used in Combination with Oral Antidiabetic Agents

	Placebo BID	BYETTA 5 mcg BID	BYETTA 10 mcg* BID
	In Combination With Metformin (30 Weeks)		
	In Combination With Metformin and a Sulfonylurea (30 Weeks)		
Intent-to-Treat Population (N)	247	245	241
HbA$_{1c}$ (%), Mean			
Baseline	8.5	8.5	8.5
Change at Week 30[†]	+0.1	-0.7	-0.9
Difference from placebo[†] (95% CI)		-0.8 [-1.0, -0.6][‡]	-1.0 [-1.2, -0.8][‡]
Proportion Achieving HbA$_{1c}$ <7%	8%	25%	31%
Body Weight (kg), Mean			
Baseline	99.1	96.9	98.4
Change at Week 30[†]	-0.9	-1.6	-1.6
Difference from placebo[†] (95% CI)		-0.7 [-1.2, -0.2]	-0.7 [-1.3, -0.2]
Fasting Plasma Glucose[§] (mg/dL), Mean			
Baseline	181	182	178
Change at Week 30[†]	+13	-11	-12
Difference from placebo[†] (95% CI)		-24 [-33, -15]	-25 [-34, -16]
	In Combination With a Thiazolidinedione or a Thiazolidinedione plus Metformin (16 Weeks)		
Intent-to-Treat Population (N)	112	Dose not studied	121
HbA$_{1c}$ (%), Mean			
Baseline	7.9	Dose not studied	7.9
Change at Week 16[†]	+0.1	Dose not studied	-0.7
Difference from placebo[†] (95% CI)		Dose not studied	-0.9 [-1.1, -0.7][‡]
Proportion Achieving HbA$_{1c}$ <7%	15%	Dose not studied	51%
Body Weight (kg), Mean			
Baseline	96.8	Dose not studied	97.5
Change at Week 16[†]	-0.0	Dose not studied	-1.5
Difference from placebo[†] (95% CI)		Dose not studied	-1.5 [-2.2, -0.7]
Fasting Plasma Glucose[§] (mg/dL), Mean			
Baseline	159	Dose not studied	164
Change at Week 16[†]	+4	Dose not studied	-21
Difference from placebo[†] (95% CI)		Dose not studied	-25 [-33, -16]

* BYETTA 5 mcg twice daily for 1 month followed by 10 mcg BID for 6 months for the 30-week trials or 10 mcg BID for 3 months in the 16-week trial before the morning and evening meals.
[†] Least squares means are adjusted for baseline HbA$_{1c}$ strata or value, investigator site, baseline value of the dependent variable (if applicable), and background antihyperglycemic therapy (if applicable).
[‡] p <0.01, treatment vs. placebo.
[§] Measured using the hexokinase-based glucose method.
BID = twice daily.

16.2 Storage and Handling
Prior to first use, BYETTA must be stored refrigerated at 36°F to 46°F (2°C to 8°C). After first use, BYETTA can be kept at a temperature not to exceed 77°F (25°C). Do not freeze. Do not use BYETTA if it has been frozen. BYETTA should be protected from light. The pen should be discarded 30 days after first use, even if some drug remains in the pen. BYETTA should not be used past the expiration date. **BYETTA pens are not to be shared with other patients.**

17 PATIENT COUNSELING INFORMATION
Patients should be advised that BYETTA pens are never to be shared with another patient.
Patients should be informed of the potential risks and benefits of BYETTA and of alternative modes of therapy. Patients should also be fully informed about self-management practices, including the importance of proper storage of BYETTA, injection technique, timing of dosage of BYETTA

and concomitant oral drugs, adherence to meal planning, regular physical activity, periodic blood glucose monitoring and HbA$_{1c}$ testing, recognition and management of hypoglycemia and hyperglycemia, and assessment for diabetes complications.
Patients should be advised to inform their physicians if they are pregnant or intend to become pregnant.
Each dose of BYETTA should be administered as a SC injection in the thigh, abdomen, or upper arm at any time within the 60-minute period **before** the morning and evening meals (or before the two main meals of the day, approximately 6 hours or more apart). BYETTA **should not** be administered after a meal. If a dose is missed, the treatment regimen should be resumed as prescribed with the next scheduled dose.
The risk of hypoglycemia is increased when BYETTA is used in combination with an agent that induces hypoglycemia, such as a sulfonylurea. The symptoms, treatment, and

conditions that predispose to development of hypoglycemia should be explained to the patient. While the patient's usual instructions for hypoglycemia management do not need to be changed, these instructions should be reviewed and reinforced when initiating BYETTA therapy, particularly when concomitantly administered with a sulfonylurea [see Warnings and Precautions (5.2)].
Patients should be advised that treatment with BYETTA may result in a reduction in appetite, food intake, and/or body weight, and that there is no need to modify the dosing regimen due to such effects. Treatment with BYETTA may also result in nausea, particularly upon initiation of therapy [see Adverse Reactions (6)].
Patients should be informed that persistent severe abdominal pain that may radiate to the back and which may or may not be accompanied by vomiting, is the hallmark symptom of acute pancreatitis. Patients should be instructed to promptly discontinue BYETTA and contact their physician if persistent severe abdominal pain occurs [see Warnings and Precautions (5.1)].
Patients treated with BYETTA should be informed of the potential risk for worsening renal function and informed about associated signs and symptoms of renal dysfunction, as well as the possibility of dialysis as a medical intervention if renal failure occurs [see Warnings and Precautions (5.3)].
Patients should be informed that serious hypersensitivity reactions have been reported during postmarketing use of BYETTA. If symptoms of hypersensitivity reactions occur, patients must stop taking BYETTA and seek medical advice promptly [see Warnings and Precautions (5.6)].
The patient should read the Medication Guide and the Pen User Manual before starting BYETTA therapy and review them each time the prescription is refilled. The patient should be instructed on proper use and storage of the pen, emphasizing how and when to set up a new pen and noting that only one setup step is necessary at initial use. The patient should be advised not to share the pen and needles.
Patients should be informed that pen needles are not included with the pen and must be purchased separately. Patients should be advised which needle length and gauge should be used.
Manufactured for Amylin Pharmaceuticals, Inc., San Diego, CA 92121
Marketed by Amylin Pharmaceuticals, Inc. and Eli Lilly and Company
1-800-868-1190
http://www.BYETTA.com
Literature Revised October 2009
BYETTA is a registered trademark of Amylin Pharmaceuticals, Inc.
© 2005, 2009 Amylin Pharmaceuticals, Inc. All rights reserved.   822011-DD
Shown in Product Identification Guide, page 306

SYMLIN®   ℞
(pramlintide acetate)
injection
PRESCRIBING INFORMATION
Rx only

> **WARNING**
> **SYMLIN is used with insulin and has been associated with an increased risk of insulin-induced severe hypoglycemia, particularly in patients with type 1 diabetes. When severe hypoglycemia associated with SYMLIN use occurs, it is seen within 3 hours following a SYMLIN injection. If severe hypoglycemia occurs while operating a motor vehicle, heavy machinery, or while engaging in other high-risk activities, serious injuries may occur. Appropriate patient selection, careful patient instruction, and insulin dose adjustments are critical elements for reducing this risk.**

DESCRIPTION
SYMLIN® (pramlintide acetate) injection is an antihyperglycemic drug for use in patients with diabetes treated with insulin. Pramlintide is a synthetic analog of human amylin, a naturally occurring neuroendocrine hormone synthesized by pancreatic beta cells that contributes to glucose control during the postprandial period. Pramlintide is provided as an acetate salt of the synthetic 37-amino acid polypeptide, which differs in amino acid sequence from human amylin by replacement with proline at positions 25 (alanine), 28 (serine), and 29 (serine).

The structural formula of pramlintide acetate is as shown:

Lys-Cys-Asn-Thr-Ala-Thr-Cys-Ala-Thr-Gln-Arg-Leu-Ala-Asn-Phe-Leu-Val-His-Ser-Ser-Asn-Asn-Phe-Gly-Pro-Ile-Leu-Pro-Pro-Thr-Asn-Val-Gly-Ser-Asn-Thr-Tyr-NH₂ acetate (salt) with a disulfide bridge between the two Cys residues.

Pramlintide acetate is a white powder that has a molecular formula of $C_{171}H_{267}N_{51}O_{53}S_2 \bullet \times C_2H_4O_2$ ($3 \le \times \le 8$); the molecular weight is 3949.4. Pramlintide acetate is soluble in water.

SYMLIN is formulated as a clear, isotonic, sterile solution for subcutaneous (SC) administration. The disposable multidose SymlinPen® pen-injector contains 1000 mcg/mL of pramlintide (as acetate); SYMLIN vials contain 600 mcg/mL of pramlintide (as acetate). Both formulations contain 2.25 mg/mL of metacresol as a preservative, D-mannitol as a tonicity modifier, and acetic acid and sodium acetate as pH modifiers. SYMLIN has a pH of approximately 4.0.

CLINICAL PHARMACOLOGY

Amylin Physiology
Amylin is co-located with insulin in secretory granules and co-secreted with insulin by pancreatic beta cells in response to food intake. Amylin and insulin show similar fasting and postprandial patterns in healthy individuals (**Figure 1**).

Figure 1:   Secretion Profile of Amylin and Insulin in Healthy Adults

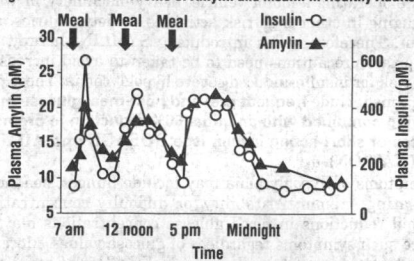

Amylin affects the rate of postprandial glucose appearance through a variety of mechanisms. Amylin slows gastric emptying (i.e., the rate at which food is released from the stomach to the small intestine) without altering the overall absorption of nutrients. In addition, amylin suppresses glucagon secretion (not normalized by insulin alone), which leads to suppression of endogenous glucose output from the liver. Amylin also regulates food intake due to centrally-mediated modulation of appetite.

In patients with insulin-using type 2 or type 1 diabetes, the pancreatic beta cells are dysfunctional or damaged, resulting in reduced secretion of both insulin and amylin in response to food.

Mechanism of Action
SYMLIN, by acting as an amylinomimetic agent, has the following effects: 1) modulation of gastric emptying; 2) prevention of the postprandial rise in plasma glucagon; and 3) satiety leading to decreased caloric intake and potential weight loss.

Gastric Emptying. The gastric-emptying rate is an important determinant of the postprandial rise in plasma glucose. SYMLIN slows the rate at which food is released from the stomach to the small intestine following a meal and, thus, it reduces the initial postprandial increase in plasma glucose. This effect lasts for approximately 3 hours following SYMLIN administration. SYMLIN does not alter the net absorption of ingested carbohydrate or other nutrients.

Postprandial Glucagon Secretion. In patients with diabetes, glucagon concentrations are abnormally elevated during the postprandial period, contributing to hyperglycemia. SYMLIN has been shown to decrease postprandial glucagon concentrations in insulin-using patients with diabetes.

Satiety. SYMLIN administered prior to a meal has been shown to reduce total caloric intake. This effect appears to be independent of the nausea that can accompany SYMLIN treatment.

Pharmacokinetics
Absorption. The absolute bioavailability of a single SC dose of SYMLIN is approximately 30 to 40%. Subcutaneous administration of different doses of SYMLIN into the abdominal area or thigh of healthy subjects resulted in dose-proportionate maximum plasma concentrations (C_{max}) and overall exposure (expressed as area under the plasma concentration curve or (AUC)) (**Table 1**).

Table 1:   Mean Pharmacokinetic Parameters Following Administration of Single SC Doses of SYMLIN

SC Dose (mcg)	$AUC_{(0-\infty)}$ (pmol*min/L)	C_{max} (pmol/L)	T_{max} (min)	Elimination $t_{1/2}$ (min)
30	3750	39	21	55
60	6778	79	20	49
90	8507	102	19	51
120	11970	147	21	48

Injection of SYMLIN into th arm showed higher exposure with greater variability, compared with exposure after injection of SYMLIN into the abdominal area or thigh. There was no strong correlation between the degree of adiposity as assessed by BMI or skin fold thickness measurements and relative bioavailability. Injections administered with 6.0-mm and 12.7-mm needles yielded similar bioavailability.

Distribution. SYMLIN does not extensively bind to blood cells or albumin (approximately 40% of the drug is unbound in plasma), and thus SYMLIN's pharmacokinetics should be insensitive to changes in binding sites.

Metabolism and Elimination. In healthy subjects, the half-life of SYMLIN is approximately 48 minutes. SYMLIN is metabolized primarily by the kidneys. Des-lys[1] pramlintide (2–37 pramlintide), the primary metabolite, has a similar half-life and is biologically active both *in vitro* and *in vivo* in rats. AUC values are relatively constant with repeat dosing, indicating no bioaccumulation.

Special Populations
Renal Insufficiency: Patients with moderate or severe renal impairment (Cl_{Cr} >20 to ≤50 mL/min) did not show increased SYMLIN exposure or reduced SYMLIN clearance, compared to subjects with normal renal function. No studies have been done in dialysis patients.

Hepatic Insufficiency: Pharmacokinetic studies have not been conducted in patients with hepatic insufficiency. However, based on the large degree of renal metabolism (see Metabolism and Elimination), hepatic dysfunction is not expected to affect blood concentrations of SYMLIN.

Geriatric: Pharmacokinetic studies have not been conducted in the geriatric population. SYMLIN should only be used in patients known to fully understand and adhere to proper insulin adjustments and glucose monitoring. No consistent age-related differences in the activity of SYMLIN have been observed in the geriatric population (n=539 for patients 65 years of age or older in the clinical trials).

Pediatric: SYMLIN has not been evaluated in the pediatric population.

Gender: No study has been conducted to evaluate possible gender effects on SYMLIN pharmacokinetics. However, no consistent gender-related differences in the activity of SYMLIN have been observed in the clinical trials (n=2799 for male and n=2085 for female).

Race/Ethnicity: No study has been conducted to evaluate the effect of ethnicity on SYMLIN pharmacokinetics. However, no consistent differences in the activity of SYMLIN have been observed among patients of differing race/ethnicity in the clinical trials (n=4257 for white, n=229 for black, n=337 for Hispanic, and n=61 for other ethnic origins).

Drug Interactions: The effect of SYMLIN (120 mcg) on acetaminophen (1000 mg) pharmacokinetics as a marker of gastric-emptying was evaluated in patients with type 2 diabetes (n=24). SYMLIN did not significantly alter the AUC of acetaminophen. However, SYMLIN decreased acetaminophen C_{max} (about 29% with simultaneous co-administration) and increased the time to maximum plasma concentration or t_{max} (ranging from 48 to 72 minutes) dependent on the time of acetaminophen administration relative to SYMLIN injection. SYMLIN did not significantly affect acetaminophen t_{max} when acetaminophen was administered 1 to 2 hours before SYMLIN injection. However, the t_{max} of acetaminophen was significantly increased when acetaminophen was administered simultaneously with or up to 2 hours following SYMLIN injection (see PRECAUTIONS, Drug Interactions).

Pharmacodynamics
In clinical studies in patients with insulin-using type 2 and type 1 diabetes, SYMLIN administration resulted in a reduction in mean postprandial glucose concentrations, reduced glucose fluctuations, and reduced food intake. SYMLIN doses differ for insulin-using type 2 and type 1 patients (see DOSAGE AND ADMINISTRATION).

Reduction in Postprandial Glucose Concentrations. SYMLIN administered subcutaneously immediately prior to a meal reduced plasma glucose concentrations following the meal when used with regular insulin and rapid-acting insulin analogs (**Figure 2**). **This reduction in postprandial glucose decreased the amount of short-acting insulin required and limited glucose fluctuations based upon 24-hour glucose monitoring.** When rapid-acting analog insulins were used, plasma glucose concentrations tended to rise during the interval between 150 minutes following SYMLIN injection and the next meal (see DOSAGE and ADMINISTRATION).

Figure 2:   Postprandial Plasma Glucose Profiles in Patients With Type 2 and Type 1 Diabetes Receiving SYMLIN and/or Insulin

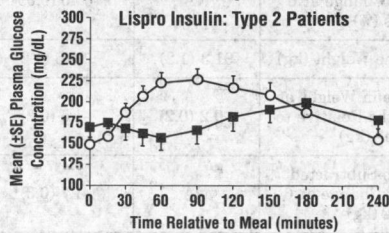

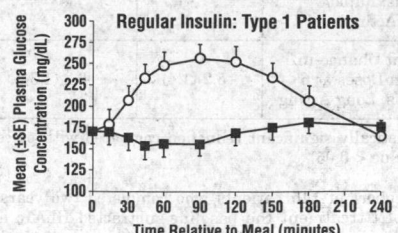

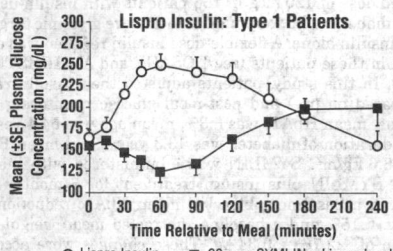

Reduced Food Intake. A single, subcutaneous dose of SYMLIN 120 mcg (type 2) or 30 mcg (type 1) administered 1 hour prior to an unlimited buffet meal was associated with reductions in total caloric intake (placebo-subtracted mean changes of ~23% and 21%, respectively), which occurred without decreases in meal duration.

CLINICAL STUDIES
A total of 5325 patients and healthy volunteers received SYMLIN in clinical studies. This includes 1688 with type 2 diabetes and 2375 with type 1 diabetes in short- and long-term controlled clinical trials, long-term uncontrolled clinical trials, and an open-label study in the clinical practice setting.

Clinical Studies in Type 2 Diabetes
The efficacy of a range of SYMLIN doses was evaluated in several placebo-controlled and open-label clinical trials in insulin-using patients with type 2 diabetes. Based on results obtained in these studies, the recommended dose of SYMLIN for patients with insulin-using type 2 diabetes is 120 mcg administered immediately prior to major meals.

Two, long-term (26 to 52 week), randomized, double-blind, placebo-controlled studies of SYMLIN were conducted in patients with type 2 diabetes using fixed dose insulin to isolate the SYMLIN effect. Demographic and baseline characteristics for the 871 SYMLIN-treated patients are as follows: mean baseline HbA1c ranged from 9.0 to 9.4%, mean age was 56.4 to 59.1 years, mean duration of diabetes ranged from 11.5 to 14.4 years, and mean BMI ranged from 30.1 to 34.4 kg/m². In both of these studies, SYMLIN or placebo was added to the participants' existing diabetes therapies, which included insulin with or without a sulfonylurea agent and/or metformin.

Table 2 summarizes the composite results across both studies for patients assigned to the 120-mcg dose after 6 months of treatment.

Table 2:   Mean (SE) Change in HbA1c, Weight, and Insulin at 6 Months in the Double-Blind, Placebo-Controlled Studies in Patients With Insulin-Using Type 2 Diabetes

Variable	Placebo	SYMLIN (120 mcg)
Baseline HbA1c (%)	9.3 (0.08)	9.1 (0.06)
Change in HbA1c at 6 Months Relative to Baseline (%)	-0.17 (0.07)	-0.57 (0.06)*

Placebo-Subtracted HbA1c Change at 6 Months (%)	NA	-0.40 (0.09)*
Baseline Weight (kg)	91.3 (1.2)	92.5 (1.2)
Change in Weight at 6 Months Relative to Baseline (kg)	+0.2 (0.2)	-1.5 (0.2)*
Placebo-Subtracted Weight Change at 6 Months (kg)	NA	-1.7 (0.3)*
Percent Change in Insulin Doses at 6 Months: Rapid/ Short-Acting	+6.5 (2.7)	-3.0 (1.6)*
Percent Change in Insulin Doses at 6 Months: Long-Acting	+5.2 (1.4)	-0.2 (1.3)*

*Statistically significant reduction compared with placebo (p-value < 0.05).

In a cohort of 145 patients who completed two years of SYMLIN treatment the baseline-subtracted HbA1c and weight reductions were: -0.40% and -0.36 kg, respectively.

Open-Label Study in the Clinical Practice Setting. An open-label study of SYMLIN was conducted at the recommended dose of 120 mcg in 166 patients with insulin-using type 2 diabetes who were unable to achieve glycemic targets using insulin alone. A flexible-dose insulin regimen was employed in these patients (see DOSAGE and ADMINISTRATION). In this study, patients adjusted their insulin regimen based on pre- and post-meal glucose monitoring. At baseline, mean HbA1c was 8.3%, mean age was 54.4 years, mean duration of diabetes was 13.3 years, and mean BMI was 38.6 kg/m². SYMLIN was administered with major meals. SYMLIN plus insulin treatment for 6 months resulted in a baseline-subtracted mean HbA1c reduction of -0.56 ± 0.15% and a baseline-subtracted mean weight reduction of -2.76 ± 0.34 kg. These changes were accomplished with reductions in doses of total, short-acting, and long-acting insulin (-6.4 ± 2.66, -10.3 ± 4.84, and -4.20 ± 2.42%, respectively).

Clinical Studies in Type 1 Diabetes
The efficacy of a range of SYMLIN doses was evaluated in several placebo-controlled and open-label clinical trials conducted in patients with type 1 diabetes. Based on results obtained in these studies, the recommended dose of SYMLIN for patients with type 1 diabetes is 30 mcg or 60 mcg administered immediately prior to major meals.
Three, long-term (26 to 52 week), randomized, double-blind, placebo-controlled studies of SYMLIN were conducted in patients with type 1 diabetes (N=1717). Two of these studies allowed only minimal insulin adjustments in order to isolate the SYMLIN effect; in the third study, insulin adjustments were made according to standard medical practice. Demographic and baseline characteristics for the 1179 SYMLIN-treated patients were as follows: mean baseline HbA1c range was 8.7 to 9.0%, mean age range was 37.3 to 41.9 years, mean duration of diabetes range was 15.5 to 19.2 years, and mean BMI range was 25.0 to 26.8 kg/m². SYMLIN or placebo was added to existing insulin therapies. **Table 3** summarizes the composite results across these studies for patients assigned to the 30 or 60 mcg dose after 6 months of treatment.

Table 3:   Mean (SE) Change in HbA1c, Weight, and Insulin at 6 Months in the Double-Blind, Placebo-Controlled Studies in Patients With Type 1 Diabetes

Variable	Placebo	SYMLIN (30 or 60 mcg)
Baseline HbA1c (%)	9.0 (0.06)	8.9 (0.04)
Change in HbA1c at 6 Months Relative to Baseline (%)	-0.10 (0.05)	-0.43 (0.04)*
Placebo-Subtracted HbA1c Change at 6 Months (%)	NA	-0.33 (0.06)*
Baseline Weight (kg)	75.1 (0.6)	76.1 (0.5)
Change in Weight at 6 Months Relative to Baseline (kg)	+0.6 (0.1)	-1.1 (0.1)*
Placebo-Subtracted Weight Change at 6 Months (kg)	NA	-1.7 (0.1)*
Percent Change in Insulin Doses at 6 Months: Rapid/ Short-Acting	+1.7 (3.3)	-3.6 (2.9)
Percent Change in Insulin Doses at 6 Months: Long-Acting	+2.5 (1.9)	+1.9 (1.3)

*Statistically significant reduction compared with placebo (p-value < 0.05).

In a cohort of 73 patients who completed two years of SYMLIN treatment the baseline-subtracted HbA1c and weight changes were: -0.35% and 0.60 kg, respectively.
SYMLIN Dose-Titration Trial. A dose-titration study of SYMLIN was conducted in patients with type 1 diabetes. Patients with relatively good baseline glycemic control (mean HbA1c = 8.1%) were randomized to receive either insulin plus placebo or insulin plus SYMLIN. Other baseline and demographics characteristics were: mean age of 41 years, mean duration of diabetes of 20 years, mean BMI of 28 kg/m². SYMLIN was initiated at a dose of 15 mcg and titrated upward at weekly intervals by 15-mcg increments to doses of 30 mcg or 60 mcg, based on whether patients experienced nausea. Once a tolerated dose of either 30 mcg or 60 mcg was reached, the SYMLIN dose was maintained for the remainder of the study (SYMLIN was administered before major meals). During SYMLIN titration, the insulin dose (mostly the short/rapid-acting insulin) was reduced by 30-50% in order to reduce the occurrence of hypoglycemia. Once a tolerated SYMLIN dose was reached, insulin dose adjustments were made according to standard clinical practice, based on pre- and post-meal blood glucose monitoring. By 6 months of treatment, patients treated with SYMLIN and insulin and patients treated with insulin and placebo had equivalent reductions in mean HbA1c (-0.47 ± 0.07% vs. -0.49 ± 0.07%, respectively); patients on SYMLIN lost weight (-1.33 ± 0.31 kg relative to baseline and -2.6 kg relative to placebo plus insulin-treated patients). SYMLIN-treated patients used less total insulin (-11.7% relative to baseline) and less short/rapid-acting insulin (-22.8% relative to baseline.

Open-Label Study in the Clinical Practice Setting. An open-label study of SYMLIN was conducted in patients with type 1 diabetes who were unable to achieve glycemic targets using insulin alone. A flexible-dose insulin regimen was employed in these patients after SYMLIN titration was completed (see DOSAGE and ADMINISTRATION). In this study, patients adjusted their insulin regimen based on pre- and post-meal glucose monitoring. At baseline, mean HbA1c was 8.0%, mean age was 42.7 years, mean duration of diabetes was 21.2 years, and mean BMI was 28.6 kg/m². SYMLIN daily dosage was 30 mcg or 60 mcg with major meals.
SYMLIN plus insulin reduced HbA1c and body weight from baseline at 6 months by a mean of 0.18% and 3.0 kg, respectively. These changes in glycemic control and body weight were achieved with reductions in doses of total, short-acting, and long-acting insulin (-12.0 ± 1.36, -21.7 ± 2.81, and -0.4 ± 1.59%, respectively).

INDICATIONS AND USAGE
SYMLIN is given at mealtimes and is indicated for:
• Type 1 diabetes, as an adjunct treatment in patients who use mealtime insulin therapy and who have failed to achieve desired glucose control despite optimal insulin therapy.
• Type 2 diabetes, as an adjunct treatment in patients who use mealtime insulin therapy and who have failed to achieve desired glucose control despite optimal insulin therapy, with or without a concurrent sulfonylurea agent and/or metformin.

CONTRAINDICATIONS
SYMLIN is contraindicated in patients with any of the following:
• a known hypersensitivity to SYMLIN or any of its components, including metacresol;
• a confirmed diagnosis of gastroparesis;
• hypoglycemia unawareness.

WARNINGS
Patient Selection
Proper patient selection is critical to safe and effective use of SYMLIN. Before initiation of therapy, the patient's HbA1c, recent blood glucose monitoring data, history of insulin-induced hypoglycemia, current insulin regimen, and body weight should be reviewed. SYMLIN therapy should only be considered in patients with insulin-using type 2 or type 1 diabetes who fulfill the following criteria:

• have failed to achieve adequate glycemic control despite individualized insulin management;
• are receiving ongoing care under the guidance of a health-care professional skilled in the use of insulin and supported by the services of diabetes educator(s).
Patients meeting any of the following criteria should NOT be considered for SYMLIN therapy:
• poor compliance with current insulin regimen;
• poor compliance with prescribed self-blood glucose monitoring;
• have an HbA1c >9%;
• recurrent severe hypoglycemia requiring assistance during the past 6 months;
• presence of hypoglycemia unawareness;
• confirmed diagnosis of gastroparesis;
• require the use of drugs that stimulate gastrointestinal motility;
• pediatric patients.
Hypoglycemia. SYMLIN alone does not cause hypoglycemia. However, SYMLIN is indicated to be co-administered with insulin therapy and in this setting SYMLIN increases the risk of insulin-induced severe hypoglycemia, particularly in patients with type 1 diabetes. Severe hypoglycemia associated with SYMLIN occurs within the first 3 hours following a SYMLIN injection. If severe hypoglycemia occurs while operating a motor vehicle, heavy machinery, or while engaging in other high-risk activities, serious injuries may occur. Therefore, when introducing SYMLIN therapy, appropriate precautions need to be taken to avoid increasing the risk for insulin-induced severe hypoglycemia. These precautions include **frequent pre- and post-meal glucose monitoring combined with an initial 50% reduction in pre-meal doses of short-acting insulin (see DOSAGE and ADMINISTRATION).**
Symptoms of hypoglycemia may include hunger, headache, sweating, tremor, irritability, or difficulty concentrating. Rapid reductions in blood glucose concentrations may induce such symptoms regardless of glucose values. More severe symptoms of hypoglycemia include loss of consciousness, coma, or seizure.
Early warning symptoms of hypoglycemia may be different or less pronounced under certain conditions, such as long duration of diabetes; diabetic nerve disease; use of medications such as beta-blockers, clonidine, guanethidine, or reserpine; or intensified diabetes control.
The addition of any antihyperglycemic agent such as SYMLIN to an existing regimen of one or more antihyperglycemic agents (e.g., insulin, sulfonylurea), or other agents that can increase the risk of hypoglycemia may necessitate further insulin dose adjustments and particularly close monitoring of blood glucose.
The following are examples of substances that may increase the blood glucose-lowering effect and susceptibility to hypoglycemia: oral anti-diabetic products, ACE inhibitors, disopyramide, fibrates, fluoxetine, MAO inhibitors, pentoxifylline, propoxyphene, salicylates, and sulfonamide antibiotics.
Clinical studies employing a controlled hypoglycemic challenge have demonstrated that SYMLIN does not alter the counter-regulatory hormonal response to insulin-induced hypoglycemia. Likewise, in SYMLIN-treated patients, the perception of hypoglycemic symptoms was not altered with plasma glucose concentrations as low as 45 mg/dL.

PRECAUTIONS
General
Hypoglycemia (See WARNINGS).
SYMLIN should be prescribed with caution to persons with visual or dexterity impairment.
Information for Patients: Healthcare providers should inform patients of the potential risks and advantages of SYMLIN therapy. Healthcare providers should also inform patients about self-management practices including glucose monitoring, proper injection technique, timing of dosing, and proper storage of SYMLIN. In addition, reinforce the importance of adherence to meal planning, physical activity, recognition and management of hypoglycemia and hyperglycemia, and assessment of diabetes complications. Refer patients to the SYMLIN Medication Guide and Patient Instructions for Use for additional information.
Instruct patients on handling of special situations such as intercurrent conditions (illness or stress), an inadequate or omitted insulin dose, inadvertent administration of increased insulin or SYMLIN dose, inadequate food intake or missed meals.
SYMLIN and insulin should always be administered as separate injections and never be mixed.
Women with diabetes should be advised to inform their healthcare professional if they are pregnant or contemplating pregnancy.
Renal Impairment: The dosing requirements for SYMLIN are not altered in patients with moderate or severe renal impairment (Cl$_{Cr}$ >20 to ≤50 mL/min). No studies have

been done in dialysis patients (see CLINICAL PHARMACOLOGY; Special Populations).

Hepatic Impairment: Studies have not been performed in patients with hepatic impairment. However, hepatic dysfunction is not expected to affect blood concentrations of SYMLIN (see CLINICAL PHARMACOLOGY; Special Populations).

Allergy:

Local allergy. Patients may experience redness, swelling, or itching at the site of injection. These minor reactions usually resolve in a few days to a few weeks. In some instances, these reactions may be related to factors other than SYMLIN, such as irritants in a skin cleansing agent or improper injection technique.

Systemic Allergy. In controlled clinical trials up to 12 months, potential systemic allergic reactions were reported in 65 (5%) of type 2 patients and 59 (5%) of type 1 SYMLIN-treated patients. Similar reactions were reported by 18 (4%) and 28 (5%) of placebo-treated type 2 and type 1 patients, respectively. No patient receiving SYMLIN was withdrawn from a trial due to a potential systemic allergic reaction.

Drug Interactions

Due to its effects on gastric emptying, SYMLIN therapy should not be considered for patients taking drugs that alter gastrointestinal motility (e.g., anticholinergic agents such as atropine) and agents that slow the intestinal absorption of nutrients (e.g., α-glucosidase inhibitors). Patients using these drugs have not been studied in clinical trials.

SYMLIN has the potential to delay the absorption of concomitantly administered oral medications. When the rapid onset of a concomitant orally administered agent is a critical determinant of effectiveness (such as analgesics), the agent should be administered at least 1 hour prior to or 2 hours after SYMLIN injection.

In clinical trials, the concomitant use of sulfonylureas or biguanides did not alter the adverse event profile of SYMLIN. No formal interaction studies have been performed to assess the effect of SYMLIN on the kinetics of oral antidiabetic agents.

Mixing SYMLIN and Insulin

The pharmacokinetic parameters of SYMLIN were altered when mixed with regular, NPH, and 70/30 premixed formulations of recombinant human insulin immediately prior to injection. **Thus, SYMLIN and insulin should not be mixed and must be administered separately.**

Carcinogenesis, Mutagenesis, Impairment of Fertility

Carcinogenesis. A two-year carcinogenicity study was conducted in CD-1 mice with doses of 0.2, 0.5, and 1.2 mg/kg/day of SYMLIN (32, 67, and 159 times the exposure resulting from the maximum recommended human dose based on area under the plasma concentration curve or AUC, respectively). No drug-induced tumors were observed. A two-year carcinogenicity study was conducted in Sprague-Dawley rats with doses of 0.04, 0.2, and 0.5 mg/kg/day of SYMLIN (3, 9, and 25 times the exposure resulting from the maximum recommended human dose based on AUC, respectively). No drug-induced tumors were observed in any organ.

Mutagenesis. SYMLIN was not mutagenic in the Ames test and did not increase chromosomal aberration in the human lymphocytes assay. SYMLIN was not clastogenic in the *in vivo* mouse micronucleus test or in the chromosomal aberration assay utilizing Chinese hamster ovary cells.

Impairment of Fertility. Administration of 0.3, 1, or 3 mg/kg/day of SYMLIN (8, 17, and 82 times the exposure resulting from the maximum recommended human dose based on body surface area) had no significant effects on fertility in male or female rats. The highest dose of 3 mg/kg/day resulted in dystocia in 8/12 female rats secondary to significant decreases in serum calcium levels.

Pregnancy

Teratogenic Effects: Pregnancy Category C. No adequate and well-controlled studies have been conducted in pregnant women. Studies in perfused human placenta indicate that SYMLIN has low potential to cross the maternal/fetal placental barrier. Embryofetal toxicity studies with SYMLIN have been performed in rats and rabbits. Increases in congenital abnormalities (neural tube defect, cleft palate, exencephaly) were observed in fetuses of rats treated during organogenesis with 0.3 and 1.0 mg/kg/day (10 and 47 times the exposure resulting from the maximum recommended human dose based on AUC, respectively). Administration of doses up to 0.3 mg/kg/day SYMLIN (9 times maximum recommended dose based on AUC) to pregnant rabbits had no adverse effects in embryofetal development; however, animal reproduction studies are not always predictive of human response. SYMLIN should be used during pregnancy only if it is determined by the healthcare professional that the potential benefit justifies the potential risk to the fetus.

Nursing Mothers

It is unknown whether SYMLIN is excreted in human milk. Many drugs, including peptide drugs, are excreted in human milk. Therefore, SYMLIN should be administered to nursing women only if it is determined by the healthcare professional that the potential benefit outweighs the potential risk to the infant.

Pediatric Use

Safety and effectiveness of SYMLIN in pediatric patients have not been established.

Geriatric Use

SYMLIN has been studied in patients ranging in age from 15 to 84 years of age, including 539 patients 65 years of age or older. The change in HbA1c values and hypoglycemia frequencies did not differ by age, but greater sensitivity in some older individuals cannot be ruled out. Thus, both SYMLIN and insulin regimens should be carefully managed to obviate an increased risk of severe hypoglycemia.

ADVERSE REACTIONS

Adverse events (excluding hypoglycemia, discussed below) commonly associated with SYMLIN when co-administered with a fixed dose of insulin in the long-term, placebo-controlled trials in insulin-using type 2 patients and type 1 patients are presented in **Table 4** and **Table 5**, respectively. The same adverse events were also shown in the open-label clinical practice study, which employed flexible insulin dosing.

Table 4: Treatment-Emergent Adverse Events Occurring With ≥5% Incidence and Greater Incidence With SYMLIN Compared With Placebo in Long-Term, Placebo-Controlled Trials. Incidence of the Same Events in the Open-Label Clinical Practice Study (Patients With Insulin-Using Type 2 Diabetes, 120 mcg)

	Long-Term, Placebo-Controlled Studies		Open-Label, Clinical Practice Study
	Placebo + Insulin (n(%)) (N=284)	SYMLIN + Insulin (n(%)) (N=292)	SYMLIN + Insulin (n(%)) (N=166)
Nausea	34 (12)	81 (28)	53 (30)
Headache	19 (7)	39 (13)	8 (5)
Anorexia	5 (2)	27 (9)	1 (<1)
Vomiting	12 (4)	24 (8)	13 (7)
Abdominal Pain	19 (7)	23 (8)	3 (2)
Fatigue	11 (4)	20 (7)	5 (3)
Dizziness	11 (4)	17 (6)	3 (2)
Coughing	12 (4)	18 (6)	4 (2)
Pharyngitis	7 (2)	15 (5)	6 (3)

Table 6: Incidence and Event Rate of Severe Hypoglycemia in Long-Term, Placebo-Controlled and Open-Label, Clinical Practice Studies in Patients With Insulin-Using Type 2 Diabetes

	Long-Term, Placebo-Controlled Studies (No Insulin Dose-Reduction During Initiation)				Open-Label, Clinical Practice Study (Insulin Dose-Reduction During Initiation)	
	Placebo + Insulin		SYMLIN + Insulin		SYMLIN + Insulin	
Severe Hypoglycemia	0–3 Months (n=284)	>3–6 Months (n=251)	0–3 Months (n=292)	>3–6 Months (n=255)	0–3 Months (n=166)	>3–6 Months (n=150)
Patient-Ascertained*						
Event Rate (event rate/patient year)	0.24	0.13	0.45	0.39	0.05	0.03
Incidence (%)	2.1	2.4	8.2	4.7	0.6	0.7
Medically Assisted**						
Event Rate (event rate/patient year)	0.06	0.07	0.09	0.02	0.05	0.03
Incidence (%)	0.7	1.2	1.7	0.4	0.6	0.7

* Patient-ascertained severe hypoglycemia: Requiring the assistance of another individual (including aid in ingestion of oral carbohydrate); and/or requiring the administration of glucagon injection, intravenous glucose, or other medical intervention.

**Medically assisted severe hypoglycemia: Requiring glucagon, IV glucose, hospitalization, paramedic assistance, emergency room visit, and/or assessed as an SAE by the investigator.

Table 5: Treatment-Emergent Adverse Events Occurring With ≥5% Incidence and Greater Incidence With SYMLIN Compared to Placebo in Long-Term, Placebo-Controlled Studies. Incidence of the Same Events in the Open-Label Clinical Practice Study (Patients With Type 1 Diabetes, 30 or 60 mcg)

	Long-Term, Placebo-Controlled Studies		Open-Label, Clinical Practice Study
	Placebo + Insulin (n(%)) (N=538)	SYMLIN + Insulin (n(%)) (N=716)	SYMLIN + Insulin (n(%)) (N=265)
Nausea	92 (17)	342 (48)	98 (37)
Anorexia	12 (2)	122 (17)	0 (0)
Inflicted Injury	55 (10)	97 (14)	20 (8)
Vomiting	36 (7)	82 (11)	18 (7)
Arthralgia	27 (5)	51 (7)	6 (2)
Fatigue	22 (4)	51 (7)	12 (4.5)
Allergic Reaction	28 (5)	41 (6)	1 (< 1)
Dizziness	21 (4)	34 (5)	5 (2)

Most adverse events were gastrointestinal in nature. In patients with type 2 or type 1 diabetes, the incidence of nausea was higher at the beginning of SYMLIN treatment and decreased with time in most patients. The incidence and severity of nausea are reduced when SYMLIN is gradually titrated to the recommended doses (see DOSAGE and ADMINISTRATION).

Severe Hypoglycemia

SYMLIN alone (without the concomitant administration of insulin) does not cause hypoglycemia. However, SYMLIN is indicated as an adjunct treatment in patients who use mealtime insulin therapy and co-administration of SYMLIN with insulin can increase the risk of insulin-induced hypoglycemia, particularly in patients with type 1 diabetes (see Boxed Warning). The incidence of severe hypoglycemia during the SYMLIN clinical development program is summarized in **Table 6** and **Table 7.**

[See table 6 above]

[See table 7 at top of next page]

Post Marketing Experience

Since market introduction of SYMLIN, the following adverse reactions have been reported. Because these events

Table 7: Incidence and Event Rate of Severe Hypoglycemia in Long-Term, Placebo-Controlled and Open-Label, Clinical Practice Studies in Patients With Type 1 Diabetes

Severe Hypoglycemia	Long-Term, Placebo-Controlled Studies (No Insulin Dose-Reduction During Initiation)				Open-Label, Clinical Practice Study (Insulin Dose-Reduction During Initiation)	
	Placebo + Insulin		SYMLIN + Insulin		SYMLIN + Insulin	
	0–3 Months (n=538)	>3–6 Months (n=470)	0–3 Months (n=716)	>3–6 Months (n=576)	0–3 Months (n=265)	>3–6 Months (n=213)
Patient-Ascertained*						
Event Rate (event rate/patient year)	1.33	1.06	1.55	0.82	0.29	0.16
Incidence (%)	10.8	8.7	16.8	11.1	5.7	3.8
Medically Assisted**						
Event Rate (event rate/patient year)	0.19	0.24	0.50	0.27	0.10	0.04
Incidence (%)	3.3	4.3	7.3	5.2	2.3	0.9

* Patient-ascertained severe hypoglycemia: Requiring the assistance of another individual (including aid in ingestion of oral carbohydrate); and/or requiring the administration of glucagon injection, intravenous glucose, or other medical intervention.

**Medically assisted severe hypoglycemia: Requiring glucagon, IV glucose, hospitalization, paramedic assistance, emergency room visit, and/or assessed as an SAE by the investigator.

Table 9: Storage Conditions

Dosage Form	Unopened (not in use) Refrigerated	Open (in use) Refrigerated or Temperature Up To 86°F (30°C)
1.5 mL pen-injector 2.7 mL pen-injector 5 mL vial	Until Expiration Date	Use Within 30 Days

are reported voluntarily from a population of uncertain size, it is not always possible to reliably estimate their frequency or establish a causal relationship to drug exposure.
General: Injection site reactions.

OVERDOSAGE

Single 10 mg doses of SYMLIN (83 times the maximum dose of 120 mcg) were administered to three healthy volunteers. Severe nausea was reported in all three individuals and was associated with vomiting, diarrhea, vasodilatation, and dizziness. No hypoglycemia was reported. SYMLIN has a short half-life and in the case of overdose, supportive measures are indicated.

DOSAGE AND ADMINISTRATION

SYMLIN dosage differs depending on whether the patient has type 2 or type 1 diabetes (see below). When initiating therapy with SYMLIN, initial insulin dose reduction is required in all patients (both type 2 and type 1) to reduce the risk of insulin-induced hypoglycemia. As this reduction in insulin can lead to glucose elevations, patients should be monitored at regular intervals to assess SYMLIN tolerability and the effect on blood glucose, so that **individualized** insulin adjustments can be initiated. If SYMLIN therapy is discontinued for any reason (e.g., surgery or illnesses), the same initiation protocol should be followed when SYMLIN therapy is re-instituted (see below).

Initiation of SYMLIN therapy
Patients With Insulin-Using Type 2 Diabetes
In patients with insulin-using type 2 diabetes, SYMLIN should be initiated at a dose of 60 mcg and increased to a dose of 120 mcg as tolerated.
Patients should be instructed to:
- Initiate SYMLIN at 60 mcg subcutaneously, immediately prior to major meals;
- Reduce preprandial, rapid-acting or short-acting insulin dosages, including fixed-mix insulins (70/30) by **50%;**
- Monitor blood glucose frequently, including pre- and post-meals and at bedtime;
- Increase the SYMLIN dose to 120 mcg when no clinically significant nausea has occurred for 3–7 days. **SYMLIN dose adjustments should be made only as directed by the healthcare professional.** If significant nausea persists at the 120 mcg dose, the SYMLIN dose should be decreased to 60 mcg;
- Adjust insulin doses to optimize glycemic control once the target dose of SYMLIN is achieved and nausea (if experienced) has subsided. **Insulin dose adjustments should be made only as directed by the healthcare professional;**
- Contact a healthcare professional skilled in the use of in-

sulin to review SYMLIN and insulin dose adjustments at least once a week until a target dose of SYMLIN is achieved, SYMLIN is well-tolerated, and blood glucose concentrations are stable.

Patients With Type 1 Diabetes
In patients with type 1 diabetes, SYMLIN should be initiated at a dose of 15 mcg and titrated at 15-mcg increments to a maintenance dose of 30 mcg or 60 mcg as tolerated.
Patients should be instructed to:
- Initiate SYMLIN at a starting dose of 15 mcg subcutaneously, immediately prior to major meals;
- Reduce preprandial, rapid-acting or short-acting insulin dosages, including fixed-mix insulins (e.g., 70/30) by **50%;**
- Monitor blood glucose frequently, including pre- and post-meals and at bedtime;
- Increase the SYMLIN dose to the next increment (30 mcg, 45 mcg, or 60 mcg) when no clinically significant nausea has occurred for at least 3 days. **SYMLIN dose adjustments should be made only as directed by the healthcare professional.** If significant nausea persists at the 45 or 60 mcg dose level, the SYMLIN dose should be decreased to 30 mcg. If the 30 mcg dose is not tolerated, discontinuation of SYMLIN therapy should be considered;
- Adjust insulin doses to optimize glycemic control once the target dose of SYMLIN is achieved and nausea (if experienced) has subsided. **Insulin dose adjustments should be made only as directed by the healthcare professional;**
- Contact a healthcare professional skilled in the use of insulin to review SYMLIN and insulin dose adjustments at least once a week until a target dose of SYMLIN is achieved, SYMLIN is well-tolerated, and blood glucose concentrations are stable.

Once Target Dose of SYMLIN is Achieved in Type 2 or Type 1 Patients
After a maintenance dose of SYMLIN is achieved, both insulin-using patients with type 2 diabetes and patients with type 1 diabetes should be instructed to:
- Adjust insulin doses to optimize glycemic control once the target dose of SYMLIN is achieved and nausea (if experienced) has subsided. **Insulin dose adjustments should be made only as directed by a healthcare professional;**
- Contact a healthcare professional in the event of recurrent nausea or hypoglycemia. An increased frequency of mild to moderate hypoglycemia should be viewed as a warning sign of increased risk for severe hypoglycemia.

Administration
SYMLIN should be administered subcutaneously immediately prior to each major meal (≥250 kcal or containing ≥30 g of carbohydrate).

SYMLIN should be at room temperature before injecting to reduce potential injection site reactions. Each SYMLIN dose should be administered subcutaneously into the abdomen or thigh (administration into the arm is not recommended because of variable absorption). Injection sites should be rotated so that the same site is not used repeatedly. The injection site selected should also be distinct from the site chosen for any concomitant insulin injection.
- **SYMLIN and insulin should always be administered as separate injections.**
- **SYMLIN should not be mixed with any type of insulin.**
- **If a SYMLIN dose is missed, wait until the next scheduled dose and administer the usual amount.**

SymlinPen® pen-injector
The SymlinPen® pen-injector is available in two presentations:
- SymlinPen® 60 pen-injector for doses of 15 mcg, 30 mcg, 45 mcg and 60 mcg.
- SymlinPen® 120 pen-injector for doses of 60 mcg and 120 mcg.
See the accompanying Patient Instructions for Use for instructions for using the SymlinPen® pen-injector.
The patient should be advised:
- to confirm they are using the correct pen-injector that will deliver their prescribed dose;
- on proper use of the pen-injector, emphasizing how and when to set up a new pen-injector;
- **not to transfer SYMLIN from the pen-injector to a syringe. Doing so could result in a higher dose than intended, because SYMLIN in the pen-injector is a higher concentration than SYMLIN in the SYMLIN vial;**
- not to share the pen-injector and needles with others;
- that needles are not included with the pen-injector and must be purchased separately;
- which needle length and gauge should be used;
- to use a new needle for each injection.

SYMLIN vials
To administer SYMLIN from vials, use a U-100 insulin syringe (preferably a 0.3 mL [0.3 cc] size) for optimal accuracy. If using a syringe calibrated for use with U-100 insulin, use the chart below (**Table 8**) to measure the microgram dosage in unit increments.

Table 8: Conversion of SYMLIN Dose to Insulin Unit Equivalents

Dosage Prescribed (mcg)	Increment Using a U-100 Syringe (Units)	Volume (cc or mL)
15	2½	0.025
30	5	0.05
45	7½	0.075
60	10	0.1
120	20	0.2

Always use separate, new syringes and needles to give SYMLIN and insulin injections.
Discontinuation of Therapy
SYMLIN therapy should be discontinued if any of the following occur:
- Recurrent unexplained hypoglycemia that requires medical assistance;
- Persistent clinically significant nausea;
- Noncompliance with self-monitoring of blood glucose concentrations;
- Noncompliance with insulin dose adjustments;
- Noncompliance with scheduled healthcare professional contacts or recommended clinic visits.

Preparation and Handling
SYMLIN should be inspected visually for particulate matter or discoloration prior to administration whenever the solution and the container permit.

HOW SUPPLIED

SYMLIN is supplied as a sterile injection in the following dosage forms:
- 1.5 mL disposable multidose SymlinPen® 60 pen-injector containing 1000 mcg/mL pramlintide (as acetate).
- 2.7 mL disposable multidose SymlinPen® 120 pen-injector containing 1000 mcg/mL pramlintide (as acetate).
- 5 mL vial, containing 600 mcg/mL pramlintide (as acetate), for use with an insulin syringe.
To administer SYMLIN from vials, use a U-100 insulin syringe (preferably a 0.3 mL [0.3 cc] size). If using a syringe calibrated for use with U-100 insulin, use the chart (**Table 8**) in the DOSAGE AND ADMINISTRATION section to measure the microgram dosage in unit increments.
Do not mix SYMLIN with insulin.

SYMLIN Injection is available in the following package sizes:

- SymlinPen® 60 pen-injector, containing 1000 mcg/mL pramlintide (as acetate) 2×1.5 mL disposable multidose pen-injector
(NDC 66780-115-02)
- SymlinPen® 120 pen-injector, containing 1000 mcg/mL pramlintide (as acetate) 2×2.7 mL disposable multidose pen-injector
(NDC 66780-121-02)
- 5 mL vial, containing 600 mcg/mL pramlintide (as acetate), for use with an insulin syringe
(NDC 66780-110-01)

STORAGE
SYMLIN pen-injectors and vials not in use: Refrigerate (36°F to 46°F; 2°C to 8°C), and protect from light. Do not freeze. Do not use if product has been frozen. Unused SYMLIN (opened or unopened) should not be used after the expiration (EXP) date printed on the carton and the label.
SYMLIN pen-injectors and vials in use: After first use, refrigerate or keep at a temperature not greater than 86°F (30°C) for 30 days. Use within 30 days, whether or not refrigerated.
Storage conditions are summarized in **Table 9.**
[See table 9 on previous page]
The SymlinPen® pen-injectors and SYMLIN vials are manufactured for:
Amylin Pharmaceuticals, Inc.
San Diego, CA 92121 USA
1-800-349 8919
http://www.SYMLIN.com
Rx only
The SYMLIN mark, SYMLIN design mark, and SymlinPen are registered trademarks of Amylin Pharmaceuticals, Inc. Copyright © 2005–2008, Amylin Pharmaceuticals, Inc. All rights reserved.
Literature Revised July 2008   812003-CC
01-05-1341-D
Shown in Product Identification Guide, page 306

AstraZeneca LP
WILMINGTON, DE 19850-5437

For Product Full Prescribing Information, Business Information, Medical Information, Adverse Drug Experiences, and Customer Service:
Information Center
1-800-236-9933
For Product Ordering:
Trade Customer Service
1-800-842-9920
For Product Full Prescribing Information:
Internet: www.astrazeneca-us.com

NEXIUM®   Rx
[nex-e-um]
(esomeprazole magnesium)
DELAYED-RELEASE CAPSULES
NEXIUM
(esomeprazole magnesium)
FOR DELAYED-RELEASE ORAL SUSPENSION

HIGHLIGHTS OF PRESCRIBING INFORMATION
These highlights do not include all the information needed to use NEXIUM safely and effectively. See full prescribing information for NEXIUM.
NEXIUM (esomeprazole magnesium) DELAYED-RELEASE CAPSULES
NEXIUM (esomeprazole magnesium) FOR DELAYED-RELEASE ORAL SUSPENSION
Initial U.S. Approval: 1989 (omeprazole)
————INDICATIONS AND USAGE————
NEXIUM is a proton pump inhibitor indicated for the following:
- Treatment of gastroesophageal reflux disease (GERD) (1.1)
- Risk reduction of NSAID-associated gastric ulcer (1.2)
- *H. pylori* eradication to reduce the risk of duodenal ulcer recurrence (1.3)
- Pathological hypersecretory conditions including Zollinger-Ellison syndrome (1.4)
————DOSAGE AND ADMINISTRATION————

Indication	Dose	Frequency
Gastroesophageal Reflux Disease (GERD)		
Adults	20 mg or 40 mg	Once daily for 4 to 8 weeks
12 to17 years	20 mg or 40 mg	Once daily for up to 8 weeks
1 to 11 years	10 mg or 20 mg	Once daily for up to 8 weeks
Risk Reduction of NSAID-Associated Gastric Ulcer		
	20 mg or 40 mg	Once daily for up to 6 months
H. pylori Eradication (Triple Therapy):		
NEXIUM	40 mg	Once daily for 10 days
Amoxicillin	1000 mg	Twice daily for 10 days
Clarithromycin	500 mg	Twice daily for 10 days
Pathological Hypersecretory Conditions	40 mg	Twice daily

•

See full prescribing information for administration options (2)
————DOSAGE FORMS AND STRENGTHS————
- NEXIUM Delayed-Release Capsules, 20 mg and 40 mg (3)
- NEXIUM For Delayed-Release Oral Suspension, 10 mg, 20 mg, and 40 mg (3)
————CONTRAINDICATIONS————
Patients with known hypersensitivity to any component of the formulation or to substituted benzimidazoles (angioedema and anaphylaxis have occurred) (4)
————WARNINGS AND PRECAUTIONS————
- Symptomatic response does not preclude the presence of gastric malignancy (5.1)
- Atrophic gastritis has been noted with long-term omeprazole therapy (5.2)
- Triple therapy for *H. pylori* – there are risks due to the antibiotics; see separate prescribing information for individual antibiotics (5.3, 5.4)
————ADVERSE REACTIONS————
Most common adverse reactions:
Adult (≥ 18 years) use (incidence ≥ 1%):
- Headache, diarrhea, nausea, flatulence, abdominal pain, constipation, and dry mouth (6.1)
Pediatric (1-17 years) use (incidence ≥ 1–2%):
- Headache, diarrhea, abdominal pain, nausea, and somnolence (6.1)
To report SUSPECTED ADVERSE REACTIONS, contact AstraZeneca at 1-800-236-9933 or FDA at 1-800-FDA-1088 or www.fda.gov/medwatch
————DRUG INTERACTIONS————
- May affect plasma levels of antiretroviral drugs – use with atazanavir and nelfinavir is not recommended; if saquinavir is used with NEXIUM, monitor for toxicity and consider saquinavir dose reduction (7.1)
- May interfere with drugs for which gastric pH affects bioavailability (e.g., ketoconazole, iron salts, and digoxin) (7.2)
- Combined inhibitor of CYP 2C19 and 3A4 may raise esomeprazole levels (7.3)
- May increase systemic exposure of cilostazol and an active metabolite. Consider dose reduction (7.3)
————USE IN SPECIFIC POPULATIONS————
- Severe liver impairment – do not exceed dose of 20 mg (2)
See 17 for PATIENT COUNSELING INFORMATION and FDA-APPROVED PATIENT LABELING
                                    Revised: 03/2010

FULL PRESCRIBING INFORMATION

1   INDICATIONS AND USAGE
1.1   Treatment of Gastroesophageal Reflux Disease (GERD)
Healing of Erosive Esophagitis
NEXIUM is indicated for the short-term treatment (4 to 8 weeks) in the healing and symptomatic resolution of diagnostically confirmed erosive esophagitis. For those patients who have not healed after 4 to 8 weeks of treatment, an additional 4 to 8 week course of NEXIUM may be considered.
Maintenance of Healing of Erosive Esophagitis
NEXIUM is indicated to maintain symptom resolution and healing of erosive esophagitis. Controlled studies do not extend beyond 6 months.
Symptomatic Gastroesophageal Reflux Disease
NEXIUM is indicated for short-term treatment (4 to 8 weeks) of heartburn and other symptoms associated with GERD in adults and children 1 year or older.
1.2   Risk Reduction of NSAID-Associated Gastric Ulcer
NEXIUM is indicated for the reduction in the occurrence of gastric ulcers associated with continuous NSAID therapy in patients at risk for developing gastric ulcers. Patients are considered to be at risk due to their age (≥ 60) and/or documented history of gastric ulcers. Controlled studies do not extend beyond 6 months.
1.3   *H. pylori* Eradication to Reduce the Risk of Duodenal Ulcer Recurrence
Triple Therapy (NEXIUM plus amoxicillin and clarithromycin): NEXIUM, in combination with amoxicillin and clarithromycin, is indicated for the treatment of patients with *H. pylori* infection and duodenal ulcer disease (active or history of within the past 5 years) to eradicate *H. pylori*. Eradication of *H. pylori* has been shown to reduce the risk of duodenal ulcer recurrence [*see Clinical Studies (14) and Dosage and Administration. (2)*].
In patients who fail therapy, susceptibility testing should be done. If resistance to clarithromycin is demonstrated or susceptibility testing is not possible, alternative antimicrobial therapy should be instituted [*see Clinical Pharmacology (12.4) and the clarithromycin package insert, Clinical Pharmacology, Microbiology*].
1.4   Pathological Hypersecretory Conditions Including Zollinger-Ellison Syndrome
NEXIUM is indicated for the long-term treatment of pathological hypersecretory conditions, including Zollinger-Ellison Syndrome.

2   DOSAGE AND ADMINISTRATION
NEXIUM is supplied as delayed-release capsules for oral administration or in packets for preparation of delayed-release oral suspensions. The recommended dosages are outlined in the table below. NEXIUM should be taken at least one hour before meals.
The duration of proton pump inhibitor administration should be based on available safety and efficacy data specific to the defined indication and dosing frequency, as described in the Prescribing Information, and individual patient med-

Table 1

Recommended Dosage Schedule of NEXIUM

Indication	Dose	Frequency
Gastroesophageal Reflux Disease (GERD)		
Healing of Erosive Esophagitis	20 mg or 40 mg	Once Daily for 4 to 8 Weeks*
Maintenance of Healing of Erosive Esophagitis	20 mg	Once Daily†
Symptomatic Gastroesophageal Reflux Disease	20 mg	Once Daily for 4 Weeks‡
Pediatric GERD		
12 to 17 Year Olds Short-term Treatment of GERD	20 mg or 40 mg	Once Daily for up to 8 Weeks
1 to 11 Year Olds§ Short-term Treatment of Symptomatic GERD	10 mg	Once Daily for up to 8 Weeks
Healing of Erosive Esophagitis		
weight < 20 kg	10 mg	Once Daily for 8 Weeks
weight ≥ 20 kg	10 mg or 20 mg	Once Daily for 8 Weeks
Risk Reduction of NSAID-Associated Gastric Ulcer	20 mg or 40 mg	Once Daily for up to 6 months†
***H. pylori* Eradication to Reduce the Risk of Duodenal Ulcer Recurrence**		
Triple Therapy:		
NEXIUM	40 mg	Once Daily for 10 Days
Amoxicillin	1000 mg	Twice Daily for 10 Days
Clarithromycin	500 mg	Twice Daily for 10 Days
Pathological Hypersecretory Conditions Including Zollinger-Ellison Syndrome	40 mg¶	#Twice Daily

* [*See Clinical Studies (14.1)*] The majority of patients are healed within 4 to 8 weeks. For patients who do not heal after 4 to 8 weeks, an additional 4 to 8 weeks of treatment may be considered.
† Controlled studies did not extend beyond six months.
‡ If symptoms do not resolve completely after 4 weeks, an additional 4 weeks of treatment may be considered.
§ Doses over 1 mg/kg/day have not been studied.
¶ The dosage of NEXIUM in patients with pathological hypersecretory conditions varies with the individual patient. Dosage regimens should be adjusted to individual patient needs.
# Doses up to 240 mg daily have been administered [see *Drug Interactions (7)*].

ical needs. Proton pump inhibitor treatment should only be initiated and continued if the benefits outweigh the risks of treatment.
[See table above]
Please refer to amoxicillin and clarithromycin full prescribing information for Contraindications, Warnings and dosing in elderly and renally-impaired patients.
Special Populations
Geriatric
No dosage adjustment is necessary [see *Clinical Pharmacology (12.3)*].
Renal Insufficiency
No dosage adjustment is necessary [see *Clinical Pharmacology (12.3)*].
Hepatic Insufficiency
In patients with mild to moderate liver impairment (Child Pugh Classes A and B), no dosage adjustment is necessary. For patients with severe liver impairment (Child Pugh Class C), a dose of 20 mg of NEXIUM should not be exceeded [see *Clinical Pharmacology (12.3)*].
Gender
No dosage adjustment is necessary [see *Clinical Pharmacology (12.3)*].
Administration Options
Directions for use specific to the route and available methods of administration for each of these dosage forms are presented below.

Table 2

Administration Options
(See text following table for additional instructions)

Type	Route	Options
Delayed-Release Capsule	Oral	Capsule can be swallowed whole. -or- Capsule can be opened and mixed with applesauce.
Delayed-Release Capsule	Nasogastric Tube	Capsule can be opened and the intact granules emptied into a syringe and delivered through the nasogastric tube.
For Delayed-Release Oral Suspension	Oral	Mix contents of packet with 1 tablespoon (15 mL) of water, leave 2 to 3 minutes to thicken, stir and drink within 30 minutes.
For Delayed-Release Oral Suspension	Nasogastric or Gastric Tube	Add 15 mL of water to a syringe and then add contents of packet. Shake the syringe; leave 2 to 3 minutes to thicken. Shake the syringe and inject through the nasogastric or gastric tube within 30 minutes.

NEXIUM Delayed-Release Capsules
NEXIUM Delayed-Release Capsules should be swallowed whole.
Alternatively, for patients who have difficulty swallowing capsules, one tablespoon of applesauce can be added to an empty bowl and the NEXIUM Delayed-Release Capsule can be opened, and the granules inside the capsule carefully emptied onto the applesauce. The granules should be mixed with the applesauce and then swallowed immediately. The applesauce used should not be hot and should be soft enough to be swallowed without chewing. The granules should not be chewed or crushed. The granules/applesauce mixture should not be stored for future use.
For patients who have a nasogastric tube in place, NEXIUM Delayed-Release Capsules can be opened and the intact granules emptied into a 60 mL catheter tipped syringe and mixed with 50 mL of water. It is important to only use a catheter tipped syringe when administering NEXIUM through a nasogastric tube. Replace the plunger and shake the syringe vigorously for 15 seconds. Hold the syringe with the tip up and check for granules remaining in the tip. Attach the syringe to a nasogastric tube and deliver the contents of the syringe through the nasogastric tube into the stomach. After administering the granules, the nasogastric tube should be flushed with additional water. Do not administer the granules if they have dissolved or disintegrated. The suspension must be used immediately after preparation.
NEXIUM For Delayed-Release Oral Suspension
NEXIUM For Delayed-Release Oral Suspension should be administered as follows:
• Empty the contents of a 10 mg, 20 mg, or 40 mg packet into a container containing 1 tablespoon (15 mL) of water.
• Stir.
• Leave 2 to 3 minutes to thicken.
• Stir and drink within 30 minutes.
• If any material remains after drinking, add more water, stir, and drink immediately.
For patients who have a nasogastric or gastric tube in place, NEXIUM For Delayed-Release Oral Suspension can be administered as follows:
• Add 15 mL of water to a catheter tipped syringe and then add the contents of a 10 mg, 20 mg, or 40 mg NEXIUM packet. It is important to only use a catheter tipped syringe when administering NEXIUM through a nasogastric tube or gastric tube.
• Immediately shake the syringe and leave 2 to 3 minutes to thicken.
• Shake the syringe and inject through the nasogastric or gastric tube, French size 6 or larger, into the stomach within 30 minutes.
• Refill the syringe with 15 mL of water.
• Shake and flush any remaining contents from the nasogastric or gastric tube into the stomach.

3 DOSAGE FORMS AND STRENGTHS
NEXIUM Delayed-Release Capsules, 20 mg—opaque, hard gelatin, amethyst colored capsules with two radial bars in yellow on the cap and NEXIUM 20 mg in yellow on the body. NEXIUM Delayed-Release Capsules, 40 mg—opaque, hard gelatin, amethyst colored capsules with three radial bars in yellow on the cap and NEXIUM 40 mg in yellow on the body. NEXIUM For Delayed-Release Oral Suspension, 10 mg, 20 mg or 40 mg—unit dose packet containing a fine yellow powder, consisting of white to pale brownish esomeprazole granules and pale yellow inactive granules.

4 CONTRAINDICATIONS
NEXIUM is contraindicated in patients with known hypersensitivity to any component of the formulation [see *Description (11)*] or to substituted benzimidazoles. Hypersensitivity reactions, e.g., angioedema and anaphylactic shock, have been reported with NEXIUM use.

5 WARNINGS AND PRECAUTIONS
5.1 Concurrent Gastric Malignancy
Symptomatic response to therapy with NEXIUM does not preclude the presence of gastric malignancy.
5.2 Atrophic Gastritis
Atrophic gastritis has been noted occasionally in gastric corpus biopsies from patients treated long-term with omeprazole, of which esomeprazole is an enantiomer.
5.3 Risks of Amoxicillin (as Part of *H. pylori* Triple Therapy)
[*See Warnings and Precautions in the prescribing information for amoxicillin for complete information.*]
Serious and occasionally fatal hypersensitivity (anaphylactic) reactions have been reported in patients on penicillin therapy. These reactions are more apt to occur in individuals with a history of penicillin hypersensitivity and/or a history of sensitivity to multiple allergens.
There have been well documented reports of individuals with a history of penicillin hypersensitivity reactions that have experienced severe hypersensitivity reactions when treated with a cephalosporin. Before initiating therapy with any penicillin, careful inquiry should be made concerning previous hypersensitivity reactions to penicillins, cephalosporins, and other allergens. If an allergic reaction occurs, amoxicillin should be discontinued and the appropriate therapy instituted.
Serious anaphylactic reactions require immediate emergency treatment with epinephrine. Oxygen, intravenous steroids, and airway management, including intubation, should also be administered as indicated.
Pseudomembranous colitis has been reported with nearly all antibacterial agents, including clarithromycin and amoxicillin, and may range in severity from mild to life threatening. Therefore, it is important to consider this diagnosis

in patients who present with diarrhea subsequent to the administration of antibacterial agents.

Treatment with antibacterial agents alters the normal flora of the colon and may permit overgrowth of clostridia. Studies indicate that a toxin produced by *Clostridium difficile* is a primary cause of "antibiotic-associated colitis".

After the diagnosis of pseudomembranous colitis has been established, therapeutic measures should be initiated. Mild cases of pseudomembranous colitis usually respond to discontinuation of the drug alone. In moderate to severe cases, consideration should be given to management with fluids and electrolytes, protein supplementation, and treatment with an antibacterial drug clinically effective against *Clostridium difficile* colitis.

5.4 Risks of Clarithromycin (as Part of *H. pylori* Triple Therapy)

[*See Warnings and Precautions in the prescribing information for clarithromycin for complete information.*]

Clarithromycin should not be used in pregnant women except in clinical circumstances where no alternative therapy is appropriate. If pregnancy occurs while taking clarithromycin, the patient should be apprised of the potential hazard to the fetus.

Concomitant administration of clarithromycin with cisapride, pimozide, astemizole, terfenadine, ergotamine, or dihydroergotamine is contraindicated.

6 ADVERSE REACTIONS
6.1 Clinical Trials Experience

Because clinical trials are conducted under widely varying conditions, adverse reaction rates observed in the clinical trials of a drug cannot be directly compared to rates in the clinical trials of another drug and may not reflect the rates observed in practice.

The safety of NEXIUM was evaluated in over 15,000 patients (aged 18 to 84 years) in clinical trials worldwide including over 8,500 patients in the United States and over 6,500 patients in Europe and Canada. Over 2,900 patients were treated in long-term studies for up to 6-12 months. In general, NEXIUM was well tolerated in both short and long-term clinical trials.

The safety of NEXIUM was evaluated in 316 pediatric and adolescent patients aged 1 to 17 years in four clinical trials for the treatment of symptomatic GERD [*see Clinical Studies (14.2)*]. In 109 pediatric patients aged 1 to 11 years, the most frequently reported (at least 1%) treatment-related adverse reactions in these patients were diarrhea (2.8%), headache (1.9%) and somnolence (1.9%). In 149 pediatric patients aged 12 to 17 years the most frequently reported (at least 2%) treatment-related adverse reactions in these patients were headache (8.1%), abdominal pain (2.7%), diarrhea (2%), and nausea (2%). No new safety concerns were identified in pediatric patients.

The safety in the treatment of healing of erosive esophagitis was assessed in four randomized comparative clinical trials, which included 1,240 patients on NEXIUM 20 mg, 2,434 patients on NEXIUM 40 mg, and 3,008 patients on omeprazole 20 mg daily. The most frequently occurring adverse reactions (≥1%) in all three groups were headache (5.5, 5.0, and 3.8, respectively) and diarrhea (no difference among the three groups). Nausea, flatulence, abdominal pain, constipation, and dry mouth occurred at similar rates among patients taking NEXIUM or omeprazole.

Additional adverse reactions that were reported as possibly or probably related to NEXIUM with an incidence < 1% are listed below by body system:

Body as a Whole: abdomen enlarged, allergic reaction, asthenia, back pain, chest pain, substernal chest pain, facial edema, peripheral edema, hot flushes, fatigue, fever, flu-like disorder, generalized edema, leg edema, malaise, pain, rigors;

Cardiovascular: flushing, hypertension, tachycardia;

Endocrine: goiter;

Gastrointestinal: bowel irregularity, constipation aggravated, dyspepsia, dysphagia, dysplasia GI, epigastric pain, eructation, esophageal disorder, frequent stools, gastroenteritis, GI hemorrhage, GI symptoms not otherwise specified, hiccup, melena, mouth disorder, pharynx disorder, rectal disorder, serum gastrin increased, tongue disorder, tongue edema, ulcerative stomatitis, vomiting;

Hearing: earache, tinnitus;

Hematologic: anemia, anemia hypochromic, cervical lymphadenopathy, epistaxis, leukocytosis, leukopenia, thrombocytopenia;

Hepatic: bilirubinemia, hepatic function abnormal, SGOT increased, SGPT increased;

Metabolic/Nutritional: glycosuria, hyperuricemia, hyponatremia, increased alkaline phosphatase, thirst, vitamin B12 deficiency, weight increase, weight decrease;

Musculoskeletal: arthralgia, arthritis aggravated, arthropathy, cramps, fibromyalgia syndrome, hernia, polymyalgia rheumatica;

Nervous System/Psychiatric: anorexia, apathy, appetite increased, confusion, depression aggravated, dizziness, hypertonia, nervousness, hypoesthesia, impotence, insomnia, migraine, migraine aggravated, paresthesia, sleep disorder, somnolence, tremor, vertigo, visual field defect;

Reproductive: dysmenorrhea, menstrual disorder, vaginitis;

Respiratory: asthma aggravated, coughing, dyspnea, larynx edema, pharyngitis, rhinitis, sinusitis;

Skin and Appendages: acne, angioedema, dermatitis, pruritus, pruritus ani, rash, rash erythematous, rash maculopapular, skin inflammation, sweating increased, urticaria;

Special Senses: otitis media, parosmia, taste loss, taste perversion;

Urogenital: abnormal urine, albuminuria, cystitis, dysuria, fungal infection, hematuria, micturition frequency, moniliasis, genital moniliasis, polyuria;

Visual: conjunctivitis, vision abnormal.

The following potentially clinically significant laboratory changes in clinical trials, irrespective of relationship to NEXIUM, were reported in ≤ 1% of patients: increased creatinine, uric acid, total bilirubin, alkaline phosphatase, ALT, AST, hemoglobin, white blood cell count, platelets, serum gastrin, potassium, sodium, thyroxine and thyroid stimulating hormone [*see Clinical Pharmacology (12) for further information on thyroid effects*]. Decreases were seen in hemoglobin, white blood cell count, platelets, potassium, sodium, and thyroxine.

Endoscopic findings that were reported as adverse reactions include: duodenitis, esophagitis, esophageal stricture, esophageal ulceration, esophageal varices, gastric ulcer, gastritis, hernia, benign polyps or nodules, Barrett's esophagus, and mucosal discoloration.

The incidence of treatment-related adverse reactions during 6-month maintenance treatment was similar to placebo. There were no differences in types of related adverse reactions seen during maintenance treatment up to 12 months compared to short-term treatment.

Two placebo-controlled studies were conducted in 710 patients for the treatment of symptomatic gastroesophageal reflux disease. The most common adverse reactions that were reported as possibly or probably related to NEXIUM were diarrhea (4.3%), headache (3.8%), and abdominal pain (3.8%).

6.2 Combination Treatment with Amoxicillin and Clarithromycin

In clinical trials using combination therapy with NEXIUM plus amoxicillin and clarithromycin, no additional adverse reactions specific to these drug combinations were observed. Adverse reactions that occurred were limited to those observed when using NEXIUM, amoxicillin, or clarithromycin alone.

The most frequently reported drug-related adverse reactions for patients who received triple therapy for 10 days were diarrhea (9.2%), taste perversion (6.6%), and abdominal pain (3.7%). No treatment-emergent adverse reactions were observed at higher rates with triple therapy than were observed with NEXIUM alone.

For more information on adverse reactions with amoxicillin or clarithromycin, refer to their package inserts, Adverse Reactions sections.

In clinical trials using combination therapy with NEXIUM plus amoxicillin and clarithromycin, no additional increased laboratory abnormalities particular to these drug combinations were observed.

For more information on laboratory changes with amoxicillin or clarithromycin, refer to their package inserts, Adverse Reactions section.

6.3 Postmarketing Experience

The following adverse reactions have been identified during post-approval use of NEXIUM. Because these reactions are reported voluntarily from a population of uncertain size, it is not always possible to reliably estimate their frequency or establish a causal relationship to drug exposure. These reports are listed below by body system:

Blood And Lymphatic: agranulocytosis, pancytopenia;

Eye: blurred vision;

Gastrointestinal: pancreatitis; stomatitis;

Hepatobiliary: hepatic failure, hepatitis with or without jaundice;

Immune System: anaphylactic reaction/shock;

Infections and Infestations: GI candidiasis;

Musculoskeletal and Connective Tissue: muscular weakness, myalgia;

Nervous System: hepatic encephalopathy, taste disturbance;

Psychiatric: aggression, agitation, depression, hallucination;

Renal and Urinary: interstitial nephritis;

Reproductive System and Breast: gynecomastia;

Respiratory, Thoracic, and Mediastinal: bronchospasm;

Skin and Subcutaneous Tissue: alopecia, erythema multiforme, hyperhidrosis, photosensitivity, Stevens-Johnson syndrome, toxic epidermal necrolysis (some fatal).

7 DRUG INTERACTIONS
7.1 Interference with Antiretroviral Therapy

Concomitant use of atazanavir and nelfinavir with proton pump inhibitors is not recommended. Co-administration of atazanavir with proton pump inhibitors is expected to substantially decrease atazanavir plasma concentrations and may result in a loss of therapeutic effect and the development of drug resistance. Co-administration of saquinavir with proton pump inhibitors is expected to increase saquinavir concentrations, which may increase toxicity and require dose reduction.

Omeprazole, of which esomeprazole is an enantiomer, has been reported to interact with some antiretroviral drugs. The clinical importance and the mechanisms behind these interactions are not always known. Increased gastric pH during omeprazole treatment may change the absorption of the antiretroviral drug. Other possible interaction mechanisms are via CYP 2C19.

Reduced concentrations of atazanavir and nelfinavir

For some antiretroviral drugs, such as atazanavir and nelfinavir, decreased serum levels have been reported when given together with omeprazole. Following multiple doses of nelfinavir (1250 mg, twice daily) and omeprazole (40 mg daily), AUC was decreased by 36% and 92%, C_{max} by 37% and 89% and C_{min} by 39% and 75% respectively for nelfinavir and M8. Following multiple doses of atazanavir (400 mg, daily) and omeprazole (40 mg, daily, 2 hr before atazanavir), AUC was decreased by 94%, C_{max} by 96%, and C_{min} by 95%. Concomitant administration with omeprazole and drugs such as atazanavir and nelfinavir is therefore not recommended.

Increased concentrations of saquinavir

For other antiretroviral drugs, such as saquinavir, elevated serum levels have been reported, with an increase in AUC by 82%, in C_{max} by 75%, and in C_{min} by 106%, following multiple dosing of saquinavir/ritonavir (1000/100 mg) twice daily for 15 days with omeprazole 40 mg daily co-administered days 11 to 15. Therefore, clinical and laboratory monitoring for saquinavir toxicity is recommended during concurrent use with NEXIUM. Dose reduction of saquinavir should be considered from the safety perspective for individual patients.

There are also some antiretroviral drugs of which unchanged serum levels have been reported when given with omeprazole.

7.2 Drugs for Which Gastric pH Can Affect Bioavailability

Esomeprazole inhibits gastric acid secretion. Therefore, esomeprazole may interfere with the absorption of drugs where gastric pH is an important determinant of bioavailability (e.g., ketoconazole, atazanavir, iron salts, and digoxin).

7.3 Effects on Hepatic Metabolism/Cytochrome P-450 Pathways

Esomeprazole is extensively metabolized in the liver by CYP 2C19 and CYP 3A4. *In vitro* and in vivo studies have shown that esomeprazole is not likely to inhibit CYPs 1A2, 2A6, 2C9, 2D6, 2E1, and 3A4. No clinically relevant interactions with drugs metabolized by these CYP enzymes would be expected. Drug interaction studies have shown that esomeprazole does not have any clinically significant interactions with phenytoin, warfarin, quinidine, clarithromycin, or amoxicillin.

However, post-marketing reports of changes in prothrombin measures have been received among patients on concomitant warfarin and esomeprazole therapy. Increases in INR and prothrombin time may lead to abnormal bleeding and even death. Patients treated with proton pump inhibitors and warfarin concomitantly may need to be monitored for increases in INR and prothrombin time.

Esomeprazole may potentially interfere with CYP 2C19, the major esomeprazole metabolizing enzyme. Coadministration of esomeprazole 30 mg and diazepam, a CYP 2C19 substrate, resulted in a 45% decrease in clearance of diazepam.

Concomitant administration of esomeprazole and a combined inhibitor of CYP 2C19 and CYP 3A4, such as voriconazole, may result in more than doubling of the esomeprazole exposure. Dose adjustment of esomeprazole is not normally required. However, in patients with Zollinger-Ellison's Syndrome, who may require higher doses up to 240 mg/day, dose adjustment may be considered.

Omeprazole acts as an inhibitor of CYP 2C19. Omeprazole, given in doses of 40 mg daily for one week to 20 healthy subjects in cross-over study, increased Cmax and AUC of cilostazol by 18% and 26% respectively. Cmax and AUC of one of its active metabolites, 3,4-dihydrocilostazol, which has 4-7 times the activity of cilostazol, were increased by 29% and 69% respectively. Co-administration of cilostazol with esomeprazole is expected to increase concentrations of cilostazol and its above mentioned active metabolite. Therefore a dose reduction of cilostazol from 100 mg b.i.d. to 50 mg b.i.d. should be considered.

7.4 Combination Therapy with Clarithromycin

Co-administration of esomeprazole, clarithromycin, and amoxicillin has resulted in increases in the plasma levels of esomeprazole and 14-hydroxyclarithromycin [*see Clinical Pharmacology (12.4)*].

Concomitant administration of clarithromycin with cisapride, pimozide, astemizole, terfenadine, ergotamine, or dihydroergotamine is contraindicated [*see prescribing information for clarithromycin*].

8 USE IN SPECIFIC POPULATIONS

8.1 Pregnancy

Pregnancy Category B

Reproductive studies in rats and rabbits with NEXIUM (esomeprazole) and multiple cohort studies in pregnant women with omeprazole use during the first trimester do not show an increased risk of congenital anomalies or adverse pregnancy outcomes. There are, however, no adequate and well controlled studies of NEXIUM use in pregnancy. Because animal reproduction studies are not always predictive of human response, this drug should be used during pregnancy only if clearly needed.

Esomeprazole is the s-isomer of omeprazole. In four population-based cohort studies that included 1226 women exposed during the first trimester of pregnancy to omeprazole there was no increased risk of congenital anomalies.

Reproductive studies with esomeprazole have been performed in rats at doses up to 57 times the human dose and in rabbits at doses up to 35 times the human dose and have revealed no evidence of impaired fertility or harm to the fetus. See Animal Toxicology and/or Pharmacology (13.2).

Reproductive studies conducted with omeprazole on rats at oral doses up to 56 times the human dose and in rabbits at doses up to 56 times the human dose did not show any evidence of teratogenicity. In pregnant rabbits, omeprazole at doses about 5.5 to 56 times the human dose produced dose-related increases in embryo-lethality, fetal resorptions, and pregnancy loss. In rats treated with omeprazole at doses about 5.6 to 56 times the human dose, dose-related embryo/fetal toxicity and postnatal developmental toxicity occurred in offspring.

8.3 Nursing Mothers

Omeprazole concentrations have been measured in breast milk of one woman taking omeprazole 20 mg per day. However, the excretion of esomeprazole in milk has not been studied. It is not known whether this drug is excreted in human milk. Because many drugs are excreted in human milk and because of the potential for tumorigenicity shown for NEXIUM in rat carcinogenicity studies, a decision should be made whether to discontinue nursing or to discontinue the drug, taking into account the importance of the drug to the mother.

8.4 Pediatric Use

The safety and effectiveness of NEXIUM have been established in pediatric patients 1 to 17 years of age for short-term treatment (up to eight weeks) of GERD. However, effectiveness has not been demonstrated in patients less than 1 year of age.

1 to 17 years of age

Use of NEXIUM in pediatric and adolescent patients 1 to 17 years of age for short-term treatment (up to eight weeks) of GERD is supported by: a) extrapolation of results, already included in the currently approved labeling, from adequate and well-controlled studies that supported the approval of NEXIUM for adults, and b) safety and pharmacokinetic studies performed in pediatric and adolescent patients [*see Clinical Pharmacology (12.3), Dosage and Administration (2), Adverse Reactions (6.1), and Clinical Studies, (14.3)*]. The safety and effectiveness of NEXIUM for other pediatric uses have not been established.

Neonates to less than one year of age

There was no statistically significant difference between NEXIUM and placebo in the rate of discontinuation in a multicenter, randomized, double-blind, controlled, treatment-withdrawal study of patients ages 1 to 11 months, inclusive. Patients were enrolled if they had either a clinical diagnosis of suspected GERD, symptomatic GERD, or endoscopically proven GERD. All patients received NEXIUM Delayed-Release Oral Suspension once daily during a two-week, open-label phase of the study. There were 80 patients who attained a pre-specified level of symptom improvement and who entered the double-blind phase, in which they were randomized in equal proportions to receive NEXIUM or placebo for the next four weeks. Efficacy was assessed by observing the time from randomization to study discontinuation due to symptom worsening during the four-week, treatment-withdrawal phase.

The following pharmacokinetic and pharmacodynamic information was obtained in pediatric patients with GERD aged birth to less than one year of age. In neonates (< 1 month old) given NEXIUM 0.5 mg/kg once daily, the percent time with intragastric pH > 4 over the 24-hour dosing period increased from 44% at baseline to 83% on Day 7. In infants (1 to 11 months old, inclusive) given NEXIUM 1.0 mg/kg once daily, the percent time with intragastric pH > 4 increased from 29% at baseline to 69% on Day 7, which is similar to the pharmacodynamic effect in adults [*see Clinical Pharmacology (12.2)*]. Apparent clearance (CL/F) increases with age in pediatric patients from birth to 2 years of age.

Because NEXIUM was not shown to be effective in the randomized, placebo-controlled study for this age group, the use of NEXIUM in patients less than 1 year of age is not indicated.

8.5 Geriatric Use

Of the total number of patients who received NEXIUM in clinical trials, 1459 were 65 to 74 years of age and 354 patients were ≥ 75 years of age.

No overall differences in safety and efficacy were observed between the elderly and younger individuals, and other reported clinical experience has not identified differences in responses between the elderly and younger patients, but greater sensitivity of some older individuals cannot be ruled out.

10 OVERDOSAGE

A single oral dose of esomeprazole at 510 mg/kg (about 103 times the human dose on a body surface area basis), was lethal to rats. The major signs of acute toxicity were reduced motor activity, changes in respiratory frequency, tremor, ataxia, and intermittent clonic convulsions.

The symptoms described in connection with deliberate NEXIUM overdose (limited experience of doses in excess of 240 mg/day) are transient. Single doses of 80 mg of esomeprazole were uneventful. Reports of overdosage with omeprazole in humans may also be relevant. Doses ranged up to 2,400 mg (120 times the usual recommended clinical dose). Manifestations were variable, but included confusion, drowsiness, blurred vision, tachycardia, nausea, diaphoresis, flushing, headache, dry mouth, and other adverse reactions similar to those seen in normal clinical experience (see omeprazole package insert - *Adverse Reactions*). No specific antidote for esomeprazole is known. Since esomeprazole is extensively protein bound, it is not expected to be removed by dialysis. In the event of overdosage, treatment should be symptomatic and supportive.

As with the management of any overdose, the possibility of multiple drug ingestion should be considered. For current information on treatment of any drug overdose contact a Poison Control Center at 1–800–222–1222.

11 DESCRIPTION

The active ingredient in NEXIUM® (esomeprazole magnesium) Delayed-Release Capsules and NEXIUM (esomeprazole magnesium) For Delayed-Release Oral Suspension is bis(5-methoxy-2-[(S)-[(4-methoxy-3,5-dimethyl-2-pyridinyl)methyl]sulfinyl]-1*H*-benzimidazole-1-yl) magnesium trihydrate. Esomeprazole is the S-isomer of omeprazole, which is a mixture of the S- and R-isomers. (Initial U.S. approval of esomeprazole magnesium: 2001). Its molecular formula is $(C_{17}H_{18}N_3O_3S)_2Mg \times 3\ H_2O$ with molecular weight of 767.2 as a trihydrate and 713.1 on an anhydrous basis. The structural formula is:

Figure 1

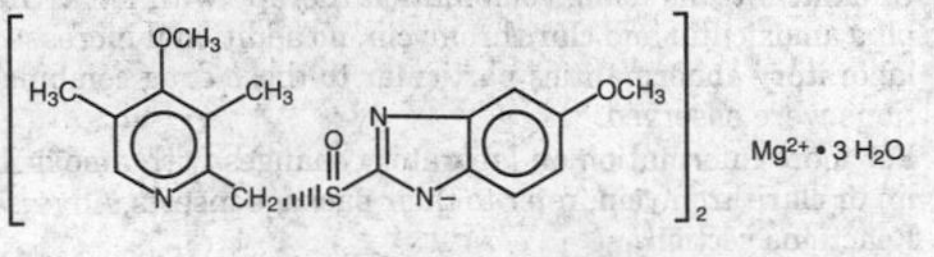

The magnesium salt is a white to slightly colored crystalline powder. It contains 3 moles of water of solvation and is slightly soluble in water. The stability of esomeprazole magnesium is a function of pH; it rapidly degrades in acidic media, but it has acceptable stability under alkaline conditions. At pH 6.8 (buffer), the half-life of the magnesium salt is about 19 hours at 25°C and about 8 hours at 37°C.

NEXIUM is supplied in delayed-release capsules and in packets for a delayed-release oral suspension. Each delayed-release capsule contains 20 mg, or 40 mg of esomeprazole (present as 22.3 mg, or 44.5 mg esomeprazole magnesium trihydrate) in the form of enteric-coated granules with the following inactive ingredients: glyceryl monostearate 40-55, hydroxypropyl cellulose, hypromellose, magnesium stearate, methacrylic acid copolymer type C, polysorbate 80, sugar spheres, talc, and triethyl citrate. The capsule shells have the following inactive ingredients: gelatin, FD&C Blue #1, FD&C Red #40, D&C Red #28, titanium dioxide, shellac, ethyl alcohol, isopropyl alcohol, n-butyl alcohol, propylene glycol, sodium hydroxide, polyvinyl pyrrolidone, and D&C Yellow #10.

Each packet of NEXIUM For Delayed-Release Oral Suspension contains 10 mg, 20 mg, or 40 mg of esomeprazole, in the form of the same enteric-coated granules used in NEXIUM Delayed-Release Capsules, and also inactive granules. The inactive granules are composed of the following ingredients: dextrose, xanthan gum, crospovidone, citric acid, iron oxide, and hydroxypropyl cellulose. The esomeprazole granules and inactive granules are constituted with water to form a suspension and are given by oral, nasogastric, or gastric administration.

12 CLINICAL PHARMACOLOGY

12.1 Mechanism of Action

Esomeprazole is a proton pump inhibitor that suppresses gastric acid secretion by specific inhibition of the H^+/K^+-ATPase in the gastric parietal cell. The S- and R-isomers of omeprazole are protonated and converted in the acidic compartment of the parietal cell forming the active inhibitor, the achiral sulphenamide. By acting specifically on the proton pump, esomeprazole blocks the final step in acid production, thus reducing gastric acidity. This effect is dose-related up to a daily dose of 20 to 40 mg and leads to inhibition of gastric acid secretion.

12.2 Pharmacodynamics

Antisecretory Activity

The effect of NEXIUM on intragastric pH was determined in patients with symptomatic gastroesophageal reflux disease in two separate studies. In the first study of 36 patients, NEXIUM 40 mg and 20 mg capsules were administered over 5 days. The results are shown in the following table:

Table 3

Effect on Intragastric pH on Day 5 (N=36)

Parameter	NEXIUM 40 mg	NEXIUM 20 mg
% Time Gastric pH >4* (Hours)	70%† (16.8 h)	53% (12.7 h)
Coefficient of variation	26%	37%
Median 24 Hour pH	4.9†	4.1
Coefficient of variation	16%	27%

* Gastric pH was measured over a 24-hour period
† p< 0.01 NEXIUM 40 mg vs NEXIUM 20 mg

In a second study, the effect on intragastric pH of NEXIUM 40 mg administered once daily over a five day period was similar to the first study, (% time with pH > 4 was 68% or 16.3 hours).

Serum Gastrin Effects

The effect of NEXIUM on serum gastrin concentrations was evaluated in approximately 2,700 patients in clinical trials up to 8 weeks and in over 1,300 patients for up to 6 to 12 months. The mean fasting gastrin level increased in a dose-related manner. This increase reached a plateau within two to three months of therapy and returned to baseline levels within four weeks after discontinuation of therapy.

Enterochromaffin-like (ECL) Cell Effects

In 24-month carcinogenicity studies of omeprazole in rats, a dose-related significant occurrence of gastric ECL cell carcinoid tumors and ECL cell hyperplasia was observed in both male and female animals [*see Nonclinical Toxicology (13.1)*]. Carcinoid tumors have also been observed in rats subjected to fundectomy or long-term treatment with other proton pump inhibitors or high doses of H_2-receptor antagonists.

Human gastric biopsy specimens have been obtained from more than 3,000 patients treated with omeprazole in long-term clinical trials. The incidence of ECL cell hyperplasia in these studies increased with time; however, no case of ECL cell carcinoids, dysplasia, or neoplasia has been found in these patients.

In over 1,000 patients treated with NEXIUM (10, 20 or 40 mg/day) up to 6 to 12 months, the prevalence of ECL cell hyperplasia increased with time and dose. No patient developed ECL cell carcinoids, dysplasia, or neoplasia in the gastric mucosa.

Endocrine Effects

NEXIUM had no effect on thyroid function when given in oral doses of 20 or 40 mg for 4 weeks. Other effects of NEXIUM on the endocrine system were assessed using omeprazole studies. Omeprazole given in oral doses of 30 or 40 mg for 2 to 4 weeks had no effect on carbohydrate metabolism, circulating levels of parathyroid hormone, cortisol, estradiol, testosterone, prolactin, cholecystokinin, or secretin.

12.3 Pharmacokinetics

Absorption

NEXIUM Delayed-Release Capsules and NEXIUM For Delayed-Release Oral Suspension contain a bioequivalent enteric-coated granule formulation of esomeprazole magnesium. Bioequivalency is based on a single dose (40 mg) study in 94 healthy male and female volunteers under fasting condition. After oral administration peak plasma levels (C_{max}) occur at approximately 1.5 hours (T_{max}). The C_{max} increases proportionally when the dose is increased, and there is a three-fold increase in the area under the plasma concentration-time curve (AUC) from 20 to 40 mg. At repeated once-daily dosing with 40 mg, the systemic bioavailability is approximately 90% compared to 64% after a single dose of 40 mg. The mean exposure (AUC) to esomeprazole increases from 4.32 μmol*hr/L on Day 1 to 11.2 μmol*hr/L on Day 5 after 40 mg once daily dosing. The AUC after administration of a single 40 mg dose of NEXIUM is decreased by 43% to 53% after food intake compared to fasting conditions. NEXIUM should be taken at least one hour before meals.

The pharmacokinetic profile of NEXIUM was determined in 36 patients with symptomatic gastroesophageal reflux disease following repeated once daily administration of 20 mg and 40 mg capsules of NEXIUM over a period of five days. The results are shown in the following table:

Table 4

Pharmacokinetic Parameters of NEXIUM on Day 5 Following Oral Dosing for 5 days

Parameter* (CV)	NEXIUM 40 mg	NEXIUM 20 mg
AUC (μmol*h/L)	12.6 (42%)	4.2 (59%)
C_{max} (μmol/L)	4.7 (37%)	2.1 (45%)
T_{max} (h)	1.6	1.6
$t_{1/2}$ (h)	1.5	1.2

* Values represent the geometric mean, except the T_{max}, which is the arithmetic mean; CV = Coefficient of variation

Distribution
Esomeprazole is 97% bound to plasma proteins. Plasma protein binding is constant over the concentration range of 2 to 20 μmol/L. The apparent volume of distribution at steady state in healthy volunteers is approximately 16 L.

Metabolism
Esomeprazole is extensively metabolized in the liver by the cytochrome P450 (CYP) enzyme system. The metabolites of esomeprazole lack antisecretory activity. The major part of esomeprazole's metabolism is dependent upon the CYP 2C19 isoenzyme, which forms the hydroxy and desmethyl metabolites. The remaining amount is dependent on CYP 3A4 which forms the sulphone metabolite. CYP 2C19 isoenzyme exhibits polymorphism in the metabolism of esomeprazole, since some 3% of Caucasians and 15 to 20% of Asians lack CYP 2C19 and are termed Poor Metabolizers. At steady state, the ratio of AUC in Poor Metabolizers to AUC in the rest of the population (Extensive Metabolizers) is approximately 2.

Following administration of equimolar doses, the S- and R-isomers are metabolized differently by the liver, resulting in higher plasma levels of the S- than of the R-isomer.

Excretion
The plasma elimination half-life of esomeprazole is approximately 1 to 1.5 hours. Less than 1% of parent drug is excreted in the urine. Approximately 80% of an oral dose of esomeprazole is excreted as inactive metabolites in the urine, and the remainder is found as inactive metabolites in the feces.

Pharmacokinetics: Combination Therapy with Antimicrobials
Esomeprazole magnesium 40 mg once daily was given in combination with clarithromycin 500 mg twice daily and amoxicillin 1000 mg twice daily for 7 days to 17 healthy male and female subjects. The mean steady state AUC and C_{max} of esomeprazole increased by 70% and 18%, respectively, during triple combination therapy compared to treatment with esomeprazole alone. The observed increase in esomeprazole exposure during co-administration with clarithromycin and amoxicillin is not expected to produce significant safety concerns.

The pharmacokinetic parameters for clarithromycin and amoxicillin were similar during triple combination therapy and administration of each drug alone. However, the mean AUC and C_{max} for 14-hydroxyclarithromycin increased by 19% and 22%, respectively, during triple combination therapy compared to treatment with clarithromycin alone. This increase in exposure to 14-hydroxyclarithromycin is not considered to be clinically significant.

Special Populations
Geriatric
The AUC and C_{max} values were slightly higher (25% and 18%, respectively) in the elderly as compared to younger subjects at steady state. Dosage adjustment based on age is not necessary.

Pediatric
1 to 11 Years of Age
The pharmacokinetics of esomeprazole were studied in pediatric patients with GERD aged 1 to 11 years. Following once daily dosing for 5 days, the total exposure (AUC) for

the 10 mg dose in patients aged 6 to 11 years was similar to that seen with the 20 mg dose in adults and adolescents aged 12 to 17 years. The total exposure for the 10 mg dose in patients aged 1 to 5 years was approximately 30% higher than the 10 mg dose in patients aged 6 to 11 years. The total exposure for the 20 mg dose in patients aged 6 to 11 years was higher than that observed with the 20 mg dose in 12 to 17 year-olds and adults, but lower than that observed with the 40 mg dose in 12 to 17 year-olds and adults.

Table 5

Summary of PK Parameters in 1 to 11 Year Olds with GERD Following 5 Days of Once-Daily Oral Esomeprazole Treatment

Parameter	1 to 5 Year Olds 10 mg (N=8)	6 to 11 Year Olds 10 mg (N=7)	6 to 11 Year Olds 20 mg (N=6)
AUC (μmol*h/L)*	4.83	3.70	6.28
C_{max} (μmol/L)*	2.98	1.77	3.73
t_{max} (h)†	1.44	1.79	1.75
$t_{1/2\lambda z}$ (h)*	0.74	0.88	0.73
Cl/F (L/h)*	5.99	7.84	9.22

* Geometric mean:
† arithmetic mean

12 to 17 Years of Age
The pharmacokinetics of NEXIUM were studied in 28 adolescent patients with GERD aged 12 to 17 years inclusive, in a single center study. Patients were randomized to receive NEXIUM 20 mg or 40 mg once daily for 8 days. Mean C_{max} and AUC values of esomeprazole were not affected by body weight or age; and more than dose-proportional increases in mean C_{max} and AUC values were observed between the two dose groups in the study. Overall, NEXIUM pharmacokinetics in adolescent patients aged 12 to 17 years were similar to those observed in adult patients with symptomatic GERD.

Table 6

Comparison of PK Parameters in 12 to 17 Year Olds with GERD and Adults with Symptomatic GERD Following the Repeated Daily Oral Dose Administration of Esomeprazole*

Parameter	12 to 17 Year Olds (N=28) 20 mg	12 to 17 Year Olds (N=28) 40 mg	Adults (N=36) 20 mg	Adults (N=36) 40 mg
AUC (μmol*h/L)	3.65	13.86	4.2	12.6
C_{max} (μmol/L)	1.45	5.13	2.1	4.7
t_{max} (h)	2.00	1.75	1.6	1.6
$t_{1/2\lambda z}$ (h)	0.82	1.22	1.2	1.5

Data presented are geometric means for AUC, C_{max} and $t_{1/2\lambda z}$, and median value for t_{max}.

* Duration of treatment for 12 to 17 year olds and adults were 8 days and 5 days, respectively. Data were obtained from two independent studies.

Gender
The AUC and C_{max} values were slightly higher (13%) in females than in males at steady state. Dosage adjustment based on gender is not necessary.

Hepatic Insufficiency
The steady state pharmacokinetics of esomeprazole obtained after administration of 40 mg once daily to 4 patients each with mild (Child Pugh A), moderate (Child Pugh

Table 7

Clarithromycin Susceptibility Test Results and Clinical/Bacteriological Outcomes* for Triple Therapy - (Esomeprazole magnesium 40 mg once daily/amoxicillin 1000 mg twice daily/clarithromycin 500 mg twice daily for 10 days)

Clarithromycin Pretreatment Results	H. pylori negative (Eradicated)	H. pylori positive (Not Eradicated) Post-treatment susceptibility results S†	I†	R†	No MIC
Susceptible† 182	162	4	0	2	14
Intermediate† 1	1	0	0	0	0
Resistant† 29	13	1	0	13	2

* Includes only patients with pretreatment and post-treatment clarithromycin susceptibility test results
† Susceptible (S) MIC ≤ 0.25 mcg/mL, Intermediate (I) MIC = 0.5 mcg/mL, Resistant (R) MIC ≥ 1.0 mcg/mL

Class B), and severe (Child Pugh Class C) liver insufficiency were compared to those obtained in 36 male and female GERD patients with normal liver function. In patients with mild and moderate hepatic insufficiency, the AUCs were within the range that could be expected in patients with normal liver function. In patients with severe hepatic insufficiency the AUCs were 2 to 3 times higher than in the patients with normal liver function. No dosage adjustment is recommended for patients with mild to moderate hepatic insufficiency (Child Pugh Classes A and B). However, in patients with severe hepatic insufficiency (Child Pugh Class C) a dose of 20 mg once daily should not be exceeded [see Dosage and Administration (2)].

Renal Insufficiency
The pharmacokinetics of NEXIUM in patients with renal impairment are not expected to be altered relative to healthy volunteers as less than 1% of esomeprazole is excreted unchanged in urine.

Other pharmacokinetic observations
Coadministration of oral contraceptives, diazepam, phenytoin, or quinidine did not seem to change the pharmacokinetic profile of esomeprazole.

Studies evaluating concomitant administration of esomeprazole and either naproxen (non-selective NSAID) or rofecoxib (COX-2 selective NSAID) did not identify any clinically relevant changes in the pharmacokinetic profiles of esomeprazole or these NSAIDs.

12.4 Microbiology
NEXIUM, amoxicillin, and clarithromycin triple therapy has been shown to be active against most strains of Helicobacter pylori (H. pylori) in vitro and in clinical infections as described in the Clinical Studies (14) and Indications and Usage (1) sections.

Helicobacter pylori: Susceptibility testing of H. pylori isolates was performed for amoxicillin and clarithromycin using agar dilution methodology, and minimum inhibitory concentrations (MICs) were determined.

Pretreatment Resistance: Clarithromycin pretreatment resistance rate (MIC ≥ 1 mcg/mL) to H. pylori was 15% (66/445) at baseline in all treatment groups combined. A total of > 99% (394/395) of patients had H. pylori isolates that were considered to be susceptible (MIC ≤ 0.25 mcg/mL) to amoxicillin at baseline. One patient had a baseline H. pylori isolate with an amoxicillin MIC = 0.5 mcg/mL.

Clarithromycin Susceptibility Test Results and Clinical/Bacteriologic Outcomes: The baseline H. pylori clarithromycin susceptibility results and the H. pylori eradication results at the Day 38 visit are shown in the table below:
[See table 7 above]

Patients not eradicated of H. pylori following NEXIUM/amoxicillin/clarithromycin triple therapy will likely have clarithromycin resistant H. pylori isolates. Therefore, clarithromycin susceptibility testing should be done, when possible. Patients with clarithromycin resistant H. pylori should not be re-treated with a clarithromycin-containing regimen.

Amoxicillin Susceptibility Test Results and Clinical/Bacteriological Outcomes:
In the NEXIUM/amoxicillin/clarithromycin clinical trials, 83% (176/212) of the patients in the NEXIUM/amoxicillin/clarithromycin treatment group who had pretreatment amoxicillin susceptible MICs (≤ 0.25 mcg/mL) were eradicated of H. pylori, and 17% (36/212) were not eradicated of H. pylori. Of the 36 patients who were not eradicated of H. pylori on triple therapy, 16 had no post-treatment susceptibility test results and 20 had post-treatment H. pylori isolates with amoxicillin susceptible MICs. Fifteen of the patients who were not eradicated of H. pylori on triple therapy also had post-treatment H. pylori isolates with clarithromycin resistant MICs. There were no patients with H. pylori isolates who developed treatment emergent resistance to amoxicillin.

Susceptibility Test for Helicobacter pylori: The reference methodology for susceptibility testing of H. pylori is agar dilution MICs. One to three microliters of an inoculum equivalent to a No.2 McFarland standard (1×10^7 - 1×10^8 CFU/mL for *H. pylori*) are inoculated directly onto freshly prepared antimicrobial containing Mueller-Hinton agar plates with 5% aged defibrinated sheep blood ($\geq$ 2 weeks old). The agar dilution plates are incubated at 35°C in a microaerobic environment produced by a gas generating system suitable for *Campylobacter*. After 3 days of incubation, the MICs are recorded as the lowest concentration of antimicrobial agent required to inhibit growth of the organism. The clarithromycin and amoxicillin MIC values should be interpreted according to the following criteria:

Table 8

Clarithromycin MIC (mcg/mL)*	Interpretation
≤ 0.25	Susceptible (S)
0.5	Intermediate (I)
≥1.0	Resistant (R)
Amoxicillin MIC (mcg/mL)*†	Interpretation
≤ 0.25	Susceptible (S)

* These are breakpoints for the agar dilution methodology and they should not be used to interpret results obtained using alternative methods.
† There were not enough organisms with MICs > 0.25 mcg/mL to determine a resistance breakpoint.

Standardized susceptibility test procedures require the use of laboratory control microorganisms to control the technical aspects of the laboratory procedures. Standard clarithromycin and amoxicillin powders should provide the following MIC values:

Table 9

Microorganism	Antimicrobial Agent	MIC (mcg/mL)*
H. pylori ATCC 43504	Clarithromycin	0.016–0.12 (mcg/mL)
H. pylori ATCC 43504	Amoxicillin	0.016–0.12 (mcg/mL)

*These are quality control ranges for the agar dilution methodology and they should not be used to control test results obtained using alternative methods.

Effects on Gastrointestinal Microbial Ecology: Decreased gastric acidity due to any means, including proton pump inhibitors, increases gastric counts of bacteria normally present in the gastrointestinal tract. Treatment with proton pump inhibitors may lead to slightly increased risk of gastrointestinal infections such as *Salmonella* and *Campylobacter* and possibly *Clostridium difficile* in hospitalized patients.

13 NONCLINICAL TOXICOLOGY
13.1 Carcinogenesis, Mutagenesis, Impairment of Fertility

The carcinogenic potential of NEXIUM was assessed using studies of omeprazole, of which esomeprazole is an enantiomer. In two 24-month oral carcinogenicity studies in rats, omeprazole at daily doses of 1.7, 3.4, 13.8, 44, and 141 mg/kg/day (about 0.7 to 57 times the human dose of 20 mg/day expressed on a body surface area basis) produced gastric ECL cell carcinoids in a dose-related manner in both male and female rats; the incidence of this effect was markedly higher in female rats, which had higher blood levels of omeprazole. Gastric carcinoids seldom occur in the untreated rat. In addition, ECL cell hyperplasia was present in all treated groups of both sexes. In one of these studies, female rats were treated with 13.8 mg omeprazole/kg/day (about 5.6 times the human dose on a body surface area basis) for 1 year, then followed for an additional year without the drug. No carcinoids were seen in these rats. An increased incidence of treatment-related ECL cell hyperplasia was observed at the end of 1 year (94% treated vs. 10% controls). By the second year the difference between treated and control rats was much smaller (46% vs. 26%) but still showed more hyperplasia in the treated group. Gastric adenocarcinoma was seen in one rat (2%). No similar tumor was seen in male or female rats treated for 2 years. For this strain of rat no similar tumor has been noted historically, but a finding involving only one tumor is difficult to interpret. A 78-week mouse carcinogenicity study of omeprazole did not show increased tumor occurrence, but the study was not conclusive.

Esomeprazole was negative in the Ames mutation test, in the *in vivo* rat bone marrow cell chromosome aberration test, and the *in vivo* mouse micronucleus test. Esomeprazole, however, was positive in the *in vitro* human lymphocyte chromosome aberration test. Omeprazole was positive in the *in vitro* human lymphocyte chromosome aberration test, the *in vivo* mouse bone marrow cell chromosome aberration test, and the *in vivo* mouse micronucleus test.

The potential effects of esomeprazole on fertility and reproductive performance were assessed using omeprazole studies. Omeprazole at oral doses up to 138 mg/kg/day in rats (about 56 times the human dose on a body surface area basis) was found to have no effect on reproductive performance of parental animals.

13.2. Animal Toxicology and/or Pharmacology

Reproductive Toxicology Studies
Reproductive studies have been performed in rats at oral doses up to 280 mg/kg/day (about 57 times the human dose on a body surface area basis) and in rabbits at oral doses up to 86 mg/kg/day (about 35 times the human dose on a body surface area basis) and have revealed no evidence of impaired fertility or harm to the fetus due to esomeprazole. Reproductive studies conducted with omeprazole in rats at oral doses up to 138 mg/kg/day (about 56 times the human dose on a body surface area basis) and in rabbits at doses up to 69 mg/kg/day (about 56 times the human dose on a body surface area basis) did not disclose any evidence for a teratogenic potential of omeprazole. In rabbits, omeprazole in a dose range of 6.9 to 69.1 mg/kg/day (about 5.5 to 56 times the human dose on a body surface area basis) produced dose-related increases in embryo-lethality, fetal resorptions, and pregnancy disruptions. In rats, dose-related embryo/fetal toxicity and postnatal developmental toxicity were observed in offspring resulting from parents treated with omeprazole at 13.8 to 138.0 mg/kg/day (about 5.6 to 56 times the human dose on a body surface area basis).

14 CLINICAL STUDIES
14.1 Healing of Erosive Esophagitis
The healing rates of NEXIUM 40 mg, NEXIUM 20 mg, and omeprazole 20 mg (the approved dose for this indication) were evaluated in patients with endoscopically diagnosed erosive esophagitis in four multicenter, double-blind, randomized studies. The healing rates at Weeks 4 and 8 were evaluated and are shown in the table below:
[See table 10 above]
In these same studies of patients with erosive esophagitis, sustained heartburn resolution and time to sustained heartburn resolution were evaluated and are shown in the table below:
[See table 11 above]
In these four studies, the range of median days to the start of sustained resolution (defined as 7 consecutive days with no heartburn) was 5 days for NEXIUM 40 mg, 7 to 8 days for NEXIUM 20 mg and 7 to 9 days for omeprazole 20 mg. There are no comparisons of 40 mg of NEXIUM with 40 mg of omeprazole in clinical trials assessing either healing or symptomatic relief of erosive esophagitis.
Long-Term Maintenance of Healing of Erosive Esophagitis
Two multicenter, randomized, double-blind placebo-controlled 4-arm trials were conducted in patients with endoscopically confirmed, healed erosive esophagitis to evaluate NEXIUM 40 mg (n=174), 20 mg (n=180), 10 mg (n=168) or placebo (n=171) once daily over six months of treatment. No additional clinical benefit was seen with NEXIUM 40 mg over NEXIUM 20 mg.
The percentages of patients that maintained healing of erosive esophagitis at the various time points are shown in the figures below:

Table 10

			Erosive Esophagitis Healing Rate (Life-Table Analysis)		
Study	No. of Patients	Treatment Groups	Week 4	Week 8	Significance Level*
1	588	NEXIUM 20 mg	68.7%	90.6%	N.S.†
	588	Omeprazole 20 mg	69.5%	88.3%	
2	654	NEXIUM 40 mg	75.9%	94.1%	p < 0.001
	656	NEXIUM 20 mg	70.5%	89.9%	p < 0.05
	650	Omeprazole 20 mg	64.7%	86.9%	
3	576	NEXIUM 40 mg	71.5%	92.2%	N.S.†
	572	Omeprazole 20 mg	68.6%	89.8%	
4	1216	NEXIUM 40 mg	81.7%	93.7%	p < 0.001
	1209	Omeprazole 20 mg	68.7%	84.2%	

* log-rank test vs omeprazole 20 mg
† N.S. = not significant (p > 0.05)

Table 11

			Sustained Resolution* of Heartburn (Erosive Esophagitis Patients)		
			Cumulative Percent† with Sustained Resolution		
Study	No. of Patients	Treatment Groups	Day 14	Day 28	Significance Level‡
1	573	NEXIUM 20 mg	64.3%	72.7%	N.S.§
	555	Omeprazole 20 mg	64.1%	70.9%	
2	621	NEXIUM 40 mg	64.8%	74.2%	p < 0.001
	620	NEXIUM 20 mg	62.9%	70.1%	N.S.§
	626	Omeprazole 20 mg	56.5%	66.6%	
3	568	NEXIUM 40 mg	65.4%	73.9%	N.S.§
	551	Omeprazole 20 mg	65.5%	73.1%	
4	1187	NEXIUM 40 mg	67.6%	75.1%	p < 0.001
	1188	Omeprazole 20 mg	62.5%	70.8%	

* Defined as 7 consecutive days with no heartburn reported in daily patient diary.
† Defined as the cumulative proportion of patients who have reached the start of sustained resolution
‡ log-rank test vs omeprazole 20 mg
§ N.S. = not significant (p > 0.05)

Figure 2
Maintenance of Healing Rates by Month (Study 177)

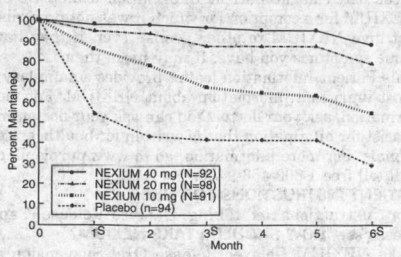

s= scheduled visit

Figure 3
Maintenance of Healing Rates by Month (Study 178)

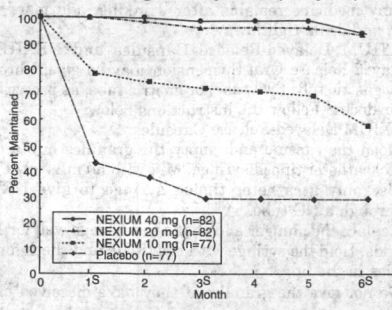

s= scheduled visit

Patients remained in remission significantly longer and the number of recurrences of erosive esophagitis were significantly less in patients treated with NEXIUM compared to placebo.

In both studies, the proportion of patients on NEXIUM who remained in remission and were free of heartburn and other GERD symptoms was well differentiated from placebo.

In a third multicenter open label study of 808 patients treated for 12 months with NEXIUM 40 mg, the percentage of patients that maintained healing of erosive esophagitis was 93.7% for six months and 89.4% for one year.

14.2 Symptomatic Gastroesophageal Reflux Disease (GERD)

Two multicenter, randomized, double-blind, placebo-controlled studies were conducted in a total of 717 patients comparing four weeks of treatment with NEXIUM 20 mg or 40 mg once daily versus placebo for resolution of GERD symptoms. Patients had ≥ 6-month history of heartburn episodes, no erosive esophagitis by endoscopy, and heartburn on at least four of the seven days immediately preceding randomization.

The percentage of patients that were symptom-free of heartburn was significantly higher in the NEXIUM groups compared to placebo at all follow-up visits (Weeks 1, 2, and 4).

No additional clinical benefit was seen with NEXIUM 40 mg over NEXIUM 20 mg.

The percent of patients symptom-free of heartburn by day are shown in the figures below:

Figure 4
Percent of Patients Symptom-Free of Heartburn by Day (Study 225)

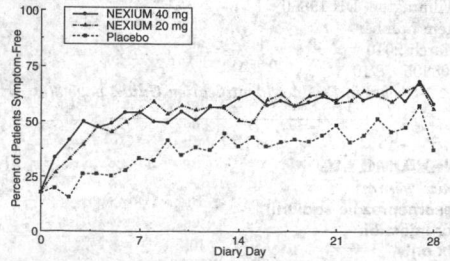

[See figure at top of next column]
In three European symptomatic GERD trials, NEXIUM 20 mg and 40 mg and omeprazole 20 mg were evaluated. No significant treatment related differences were seen.

Figure 5
Percent of Patients Symptom-Free of Heartburn by Day (Study 226)

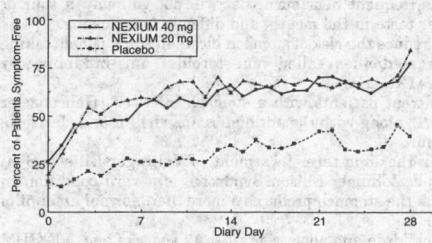

14.3 Pediatric Gastroesophageal Reflux Disease (GERD)
1 to 11 Years of Age
In a multicenter, parallel-group study, 109 pediatric patients with a history of endoscopically-proven GERD (1 to 11 years of age; 53 female; 89 Caucasian, 19 Black, 1 Other) were treated with NEXIUM once daily for up to 8 weeks to evaluate safety and tolerability. Dosing by patient weight was as follows:

weight < 20 kg: once daily treatment with NEXIUM 5 mg or 10 mg

weight ≥ 20 kg: once daily treatment with NEXIUM 10 mg or 20 mg

Patients were endoscopically characterized as to the presence or absence of erosive esophagitis.

Of the 109 patients, 53 had erosive esophagitis at baseline (51 had mild, 1 moderate, and 1 severe esophagitis). Although most of the patients who had a follow up endoscopy at the end of 8 weeks of treatment healed, spontaneous healing cannot be ruled out because these patients had low grade erosive esophagitis prior to treatment, and the trial did not include a concomitant control.
12 to 17 Years of Age
In a multicenter, randomized, double-blind, parallel-group study, 149 adolescent patients (12 to 17 years of age; 89 female; 124 Caucasian, 15 Black, 10 Other) with clinically diagnosed GERD were treated with either NEXIUM 20 mg or NEXIUM 40 mg once daily for up to 8 weeks to evaluate safety and tolerability. Patients were not endoscopically characterized as to the presence or absence of erosive esophagitis.

14.4 Risk Reduction of NSAID-Associated Gastric Ulcer
Two multicenter, double-blind, placebo-controlled studies were conducted in patients at risk of developing gastric and/or duodenal ulcers associated with continuous use of non-selective and COX-2 selective NSAIDs. A total of 1429 patients were randomized across the 2 studies. Patients ranged in age from 19 to 89 (median age 66.0 years) with 70.7% female, 29.3% male, 82.9% Caucasian, 5.5% Black, 3.7% Asian, and 8.0% Others. At baseline, the patients in these studies were endoscopically confirmed not to have ulcers but were determined to be at risk for ulcer occurrence due to their age (≥60 years) and/or history of a documented gastric or duodenal ulcer within the past 5 years. Patients receiving NSAIDs and treated with NEXIUM 20 mg or 40 mg once-a-day experienced significant reduction in gastric ulcer occurrences relative to placebo treatment at 26 weeks. No additional benefit was seen with NEXIUM 40 mg over NEXIUM 20 mg. These studies did not demonstrate significant reduction in the development of NSAID-associated duodenal ulcer due to the low incidence.

Table 12
Cumulative percentage of patients without gastric ulcers at 26 weeks:

Study	No. of Patients	Treatment Group	% of Patients Remaining Gastric Ulcer Free*
1	191	NEXIUM 20 mg	95.4
	194	NEXIUM 40 mg	96.7
	184	Placebo	88.2
2	267	NEXIUM 20 mg	94.7
	271	NEXIUM 40 mg	95.3
	257	Placebo	83.3

*%= Life Table Estimate. Significant difference from placebo (p<0.01).

14.5 *Helicobacter pylori (H.pylori)* Eradication in Patients with Duodenal Ulcer Disease
Triple Therapy (NEXIUM/amoxicillin/clarithromycin):
Two multicenter, randomized, double-blind studies were conducted using a 10 day treatment regimen. The first

study (191) compared NEXIUM 40 mg once daily in combination with amoxicillin 1000 mg twice daily and clarithromycin 500 mg twice daily to NEXIUM 40 mg once daily plus clarithromycin 500 mg twice daily. The second study (193) compared NEXIUM 40 mg once daily in combination with amoxicillin 1000 mg twice daily and clarithromycin 500 mg twice daily to NEXIUM 40 mg once daily. *H. pylori* eradication rates, defined as at least two negative tests and no positive tests from CLOtest®, histology and/or culture, at 4 weeks post-therapy were significantly higher in the NEXIUM plus amoxicillin and clarithromycin group than in the NEXIUM plus clarithromycin or NEXIUM alone group. The results are shown in the following table:

Table 13
H. pylori Eradication Rates at 4 Weeks after 10 Day Treatment Regimen % of Patients Cured [95% Confidence Interval] (Number of Patients)

Study	Treatment Group	Per-Protocol*	Intent-to-Treat[†]
191	NEXIUM plus amoxicillin and clarithromycin	84%[‡] [78, 89] (n=196)	77%[‡] [71, 82] (n=233)
	NEXIUM plus clarithromycin	55% [48, 62] (n=187)	52% [45, 59] (n=215)
193	NEXIUM plus amoxicillin and clarithromycin	85%[§] [74, 93] (n=67)	78%[§] [67, 87] (n=74)
	NEXIUM	5% [0, 23] (n=22)	4% [0, 21] (n=24)

* Patients were included in the analysis if they had *H. pylori* infection documented at baseline, had at least one endoscopically verified duodenal ulcer ≥ 0.5 cm in diameter at baseline or had a documented history of duodenal ulcer disease within the past 5 years, and were not protocol violators. Patients who dropped out of the study due to an adverse reaction related to the study drug were included in the analysis as not *H. pylori* eradicated.
† Patients were included in the analysis if they had documented *H. pylori* infection at baseline, had at least one documented duodenal ulcer at baseline, or had a documented history of duodenal ulcer disease, and took at least one dose of study medication. All dropouts were included as not *H. pylori* eradicated.
‡ p < 0.05 compared to NEXIUM plus clarithromycin
§ p < 0.05 compared to NEXIUM alone

The percentage of patients with a healed baseline duodenal ulcer by 4 weeks after the 10 day treatment regimen in the NEXIUM plus amoxicillin and clarithromycin group was 75% (n=156) and 57% (n=60) respectively, in the 191 and 193 studies (per-protocol analysis).

14.6 Pathological Hypersecretory Conditions Including Zollinger-Ellison Syndrome
In a multicenter, open-label dose-escalation study of 21 patients (15 males and 6 females, 18 Caucasian and 3 Black, mean age of 55.5 years) with pathological hypersecretory conditions, such as Zollinger-Ellison Syndrome, NEXIUM significantly inhibited gastric acid secretion. Initial dose was 40 mg twice daily in 19/21 patients and 80 mg twice daily in 2/21 patients. Total daily doses ranging from 80 mg to 240 mg for 12 months maintained gastric acid output below the target levels of 10 mEq/h in patients without prior gastric acid-reducing surgery and below 5 mEq/hr in patients with prior gastric acid-reducing surgery. At the Month 12 final visit, 18/20 (90%) patients had Basal Acid Output (BAO) under satisfactory control (median BAO = 0.17 mmol/hr). Of the 18 patients evaluated with a starting dose of 40 mg twice daily, 13 (72%) had their BAO controlled with the original dosing regimen at the final visit.

Table 14
Adequate Acid Suppression at Final Visit by Dose Regimen

NEXIUM dose at the Month 12 visit	BAO under adequate control at the Month 12 visit (N=20)*
40 mg twice daily	13/15
80 mg twice daily	4/4
80 mg three times daily	1/1

* One patient was not evaluated.

15 REFERENCES

1. National Committee for Clinical Laboratory Standards. Methods for Dilution Antimicrobial Susceptibility Tests for Bacteria That Grow Aerobically. Fifth Edition: Approved Standard NCCLS Document M7-A5, Vol. 20, no. 2, NCCLS, Wayne, PA, January 2000.

16 HOW SUPPLIED/STORAGE AND HANDLING

NEXIUM Delayed-Release Capsules, 20 mg, are opaque, hard gelatin, amethyst colored capsules with two radial bars in yellow on the cap and NEXIUM 20 mg in yellow on the body. They are supplied as follows:
NDC 0186-5020-31 unit of use bottles of 30
NDC 0186-5022-28 unit dose packages of 100
NDC 0186-5020-54 bottles of 90
NDC 0186-5020-82 bottles of 1000
NEXIUM Delayed-Release Capsules, 40 mg, are opaque, hard gelatin, amethyst colored capsules with three radial bars in yellow on the cap and NEXIUM 40 mg in yellow on the body. They are supplied as follows:
NDC 0186-5040-31 unit of use bottles of 30
NDC 0186-5042-28 unit dose packages of 100
NDC 0186-5040-54 bottles of 90
NDC 0186-5040-82 bottles of 1000
NEXIUM For Delayed-Release Oral Suspension is supplied as a unit dose packet containing a fine yellow powder, consisting of white to pale brownish esomeprazole granules and pale yellow inactive granules. NEXIUM unit dose packets are supplied as follows:
NDC 0186-4010–01 unit dose packages of 30: 10 mg packets
NDC 0186-4020–01 unit dose packages of 30: 20 mg packets
NDC 0186-4040–01 unit dose packages of 30: 40 mg packets
Store at 25°C (77°F); excursions permitted to 15 to 30°C (59 to 86°F). [See USP Controlled Room Temperature]. Keep NEXIUM Delayed-Release Capsules container tightly closed. Dispense in a tight container if the NEXIUM Delayed-Release Capsules product package is subdivided.
NEXIUM and the color purple as applied to the capsule are registered trademarks of the AstraZeneca group of companies.
©AstraZeneca 2010

17 PATIENT COUNSELING INFORMATION

See FDA-Approved Patient Labeling
• Advise patients to let you know if they are taking, or begin taking, other medications, because NEXIUM can interfere with antiretroviral drugs and drugs that are affected by gastric pH changes [see Drug Interactions (7.1)].
• Let patients know that antacids may be used while taking NEXIUM.
• Advise patients to take NEXIUM at least one hour before a meal.
• For patients who are prescribed NEXIUM Delayed-Release Capsules, advise them not to chew or crush the capsules.
• Advise patients that, if they open NEXIUM Delayed-Release Capsules to mix the granules with food, the granules should only be mixed with applesauce. Use with other foods has not been evaluated and is not recommended.
• For patients who are advised to open the NEXIUM Delayed-Release Capsules before taking them or who are prescribed NEXIUM For Delayed-Release Oral Suspension, instruct them in the proper technique for administration [see Dosage and Administration (2)] and tell them to follow the dosing instructions in the PATIENT INFORMATION insert included in the package.
Distributed by:
AstraZeneca LP
Wilmington, DE 19850

FDA-APPROVED PATIENT LABELING

NEXIUM® (nex-e-um) (esomeprazole magnesium)
Delayed-Release Capsules and Delayed-Release Oral Suspension
Read the Patient Information that comes with NEXIUM before you start taking it and each time you get a refill. There may be new information. This leaflet does not take the place of talking with your doctor about your medical condition or your treatment.
If you have any questions about NEXIUM, ask your doctor.
WHAT IS NEXIUM?
NEXIUM is a prescription medicine called a proton pump inhibitor (PPI).
NEXIUM is used in adults:
• to treat the symptoms of gastroesophageal reflux disease (GERD). NEXIUM may also be prescribed to heal acid-related damage to the lining of the esophagus (erosive esophagitis), and to help continue this healing.

GERD is a chronic condition (lasts a long time) that occurs when acid from the stomach backs up into the esophagus (food pipe) causing symptoms, such as heartburn, or damage to the lining of the esophagus. Common symptoms include frequent heartburn that will not go away, a sour or bitter taste in the mouth, and difficulty swallowing.
• to reduce the risk of stomach ulcers in some people taking pain medicines called non-steroidal anti-inflammatory drugs (NSAIDs).
• to treat patients with a stomach infection (Helicobacter pylori), along with the antibiotics amoxicillin and clarithromycin.
• for the long-term treatment of Zollinger-Ellison Syndrome. Zollinger-Ellison Syndrome is a rare condition in which the stomach produces a more than normal amount of acid.
For children and adolescents 1 to 17 years of age, NEXIUM may be prescribed for short-term treatment of GERD.
NEXIUM is not recommended for children under the age of 1 year.
WHO SHOULD NOT TAKE NEXIUM?
Do not take NEXIUM if you:
• are allergic to any of the ingredients in NEXIUM. See the end of this leaflet for a complete list of ingredients in NEXIUM.
• are allergic to any other Proton Pump Inhibitor (PPI) medicine.
WHAT SHOULD I TELL MY DOCTOR BEFORE TAKING NEXIUM?
Tell your doctor about all your medical conditions, including if you:
• have liver problems
• are pregnant, think you may be pregnant, or are planning to become pregnant.
• are breastfeeding or planning to breastfeed. Talk with your doctor about the best way to feed your baby if you take NEXIUM.
Tell your doctor about all of the medicines you take including prescription and non-prescription drugs, vitamins and herbal supplements. NEXIUM may affect how other medicines work, and other medicines may affect how NEXIUM works. Especially tell your doctor if you take:
• warfarin (COUMADIN)
• ketoconazole (NIZORAL)
• voriconazole (VFEND)
• atazanavir (REYATAZ)
• nelfinavir (VIRACEPT)
• saquinavir (FORTOVASE)
• products that contain iron
• digoxin (LANOXIN, LANOXICAPS)
HOW SHOULD I TAKE NEXIUM?
• Take NEXIUM exactly as prescribed by your doctor.
• Do not change your dose or stop NEXIUM without talking to your doctor.
• Take NEXIUM at least 1 hour before a meal.
• Swallow NEXIUM capsules whole. **Never chew or crush NEXIUM.**
• If you have difficulty swallowing NEXIUM capsules, you may open the capsule and empty the contents into a tablespoon of applesauce. Be sure to swallow the applesauce right away. Do not store it for later use.
• If you forget to take a dose of NEXIUM, take it as soon as you remember. If it is almost time for your next dose, do not take the missed dose. Take the next dose on time. Do not take a double dose to make up for a missed dose.
• If you take too much NEXIUM, tell your doctor right away.
• See the "Patient Instructions for Use" at the end of this leaflet for instructions how to take NEXIUM Delayed-Release Oral Suspension, and how to mix and give NEXIUM Delayed-Release Capsules and NEXIUM For Delayed-Release Oral Suspension, through a nasogastric tube or gastric tube.
WHAT ARE THE POSSIBLE SIDE EFFECTS OF NEXIUM?
The most common side effects with NEXIUM may include:
• Headache
• Diarrhea
• Nausea
• Gas
• Abdominal pain
• Constipation
• Dry mouth
• Drowsiness
Tell your doctor about any side effects that bother you or that do not go away. These are not all the possible side effects with NEXIUM. Talk with your doctor or pharmacist if you have any questions about side effects.
HOW SHOULD I STORE NEXIUM?
• Store NEXIUM at room temperature between 59°F to 86°F (15°C to 30°C).
• Keep the container of NEXIUM closed tightly.
Keep NEXIUM and all medicines out of the reach of children.

GENERAL ADVICE
Medicines are sometimes prescribed for purposes other than those listed in the Patient Information leaflet. Do not use NEXIUM for a condition for which it was not prescribed. Do not give NEXIUM to other people, even if they have the same symptoms you have. It may harm them.
This Patient Information leaflet provides a summary of the most important information about NEXIUM. For more information, ask your doctor. You can ask your doctor or pharmacist for information that is written for healthcare professionals. For more information, go to www.purplepill.com or call toll free 1-800-463-9486.
PATIENT INSTRUCTIONS FOR USE
For instructions on taking Delayed-Release Capsules, please see "HOW SHOULD I TAKE NEXIUM?"
Take NEXIUM Delayed-Release Oral Suspension as follows:
• Empty the contents of a packet into a container with 1 tablespoon (15 mL) of water
• Stir.
• Leave 2 to 3 minutes to thicken
• Stir and drink within 30 minutes.
If any medicine remains after drinking, add more water, stir, and drink right away.
NEXIUM Delayed-Release Capsules and NEXIUM for Delayed-Release Oral Suspension may be given through a nasogastric tube (NG tube) or gastric tube, as prescribed by your doctor. Follow the instructions below:
NEXIUM Delayed-Release Capsules:
• Open the capsule and empty the granules into a 60 mL (cc) catheter tipped syringe. Mix with 50 mL (cc) of water. Use only a catheter tipped syringe to give NEXIUM through a NG tube.
• Replace the plunger and shake the syringe well for 15 seconds. Hold the syringe with the tip up and check for granules in the tip.
• Do not give the granules if they have dissolved or have broken into pieces.
• Attach the syringe to the NG tube and give the medicine in the syringe through the NG tube into the stomach.
• After giving the granules, flush the NG tube with more water.
NEXIUM For Delayed-Release Oral Suspension:
• Add 15 mL of water to a catheter tipped syringe and then add the contents of a NEXIUM packet (as instructed by your doctor). Use only a catheter tipped syringe to give NEXIUM through a NG tube or gastric tube.
• Shake the syringe right away and then leave it for 2 to 3 minutes to thicken.
• Shake the syringe and give the medicine through the NG or gastric tube (French size 6 or larger) into the stomach within 30 minutes.
• Refill the syringe with 15 mL (cc) of water.
• Shake and flush any remaining contents from the NG tube or gastric tube into the stomach.
WHAT ARE THE INGREDIENTS IN NEXIUM?
Active ingredient: esomeprazole magnesium trihydrate
Inactive ingredients in NEXIUM Delayed-Release Capsules (including the capsule shells): glyceryl monostearate 40-55, hydroxypropyl cellulose, hypromellose, magnesium stearate, methacrylic acid copolymer type C, polysorbate 80, sugar spheres, talc, triethyl citrate, gelatin, FD&C Blue #1, FD&C Red #40, D&C Red #28, titanium dioxide, shellac, ethyl alcohol, isopropyl alcohol, n-butyl alcohol, propylene glycol, sodium hydroxide, polyvinyl pyrrolidone, and D&C Yellow #10.
Inactive granules in NEXIUM Delayed-Release Oral Suspension: dextrose, xanthan gum, crospovidone, citric acid, iron oxide, and hydroxypropyl cellulose.
NEXIUM is a registered trademark of the AstraZeneca group of companies.
©2008 AstraZeneca Pharmaceuticals LP. All rights reserved.
AstraZeneca Pharmaceuticals LP
Wilmington, DE 19850
Item number
March 2010
308305 8/10

Shown in Product Identification Guide, page 306

NEXIUM® I.V.   ℞

[něx' sē-um]
(esomeprazole sodium)
for Injection
Rx only

DESCRIPTION
The active ingredient in NEXIUM® I.V. (esomeprazole sodium) for Injection is (S)-5-methoxy-2[((4-methoxy-3,5-dimethyl-2-pyridinyl)-methyl]sulfinyl]-1 H-benzimidazole

sodium a compound that inhibits gastric acid secretion. Esomeprazole is the S-isomer of omeprazole, which is a mixture of the S- and R-isomers. Its empirical formula is $C_{17}H_{18}N_3O_3SNa$ with molecular weight of 367.4 g/mol (sodium salt) and 345.4 g/mol (parent compound). Esomeprazole sodium is very soluble in water and freely soluble in ethanol (95%). The structural formula is:

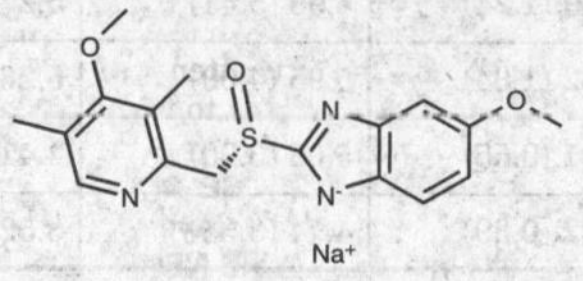

NEXIUM I.V. for Injection is supplied as a sterile, freeze-dried, white to off-white, porous cake or powder in a 5 mL vial, intended for intravenous administration after reconstitution with 0.9% Sodium Chloride Injection, USP; Lactated Ringer's Injection, USP or 5% Dextrose Injection, USP. NEXIUM I.V. for Injection contains esomeprazole sodium 21.3 mg or 42.5 mg equivalent to esomeprazole 20 mg or 40 mg, edetate disodium 1.5 mg and sodium hydroxide q.s. for pH adjustment. The pH of reconstituted solution of NEXIUM I.V. for Injection depends on the reconstitution volume and is in the pH range of 9 to 11. The stability of esomeprazole sodium in aqueous solution is strongly pH dependent. The rate of degradation increases with decreasing pH.

CLINICAL PHARMACOLOGY

Pharmacokinetics

Absorption

The pharmacokinetic profile of NEXIUM I.V. for Injection 20 mg and 40 mg was determined in 24 healthy volunteers for the 20 mg dose and 38 healthy volunteers for the 40 mg dose following once daily administration of 20 mg and 40 mg of NEXIUM I.V. for Injection by constant rate over 30 minutes for five days. The results are shown in the following table:

Pharmacokinetic Parameters of NEXIUM Following I.V. Dosing for 5 days

Parameter	NEXIUM I.V. 20 mg	NEXIUM I.V. 40 mg
AUC (μmol*h/L)	5.11 (3.96:6.61)	16.21 (14.46:18.16)
C_{max} (μmol/L)	3.86 (3.16:4.72)	7.51 (6.93:8.13)
$t_{1/2}$ (h)	1.05 (0.90:1.22)	1.41 (1.30:1.52)

*Values represent the geometric mean (95% CI)

Distribution

Esomeprazole is 97% bound to plasma proteins. Plasma protein binding is constant over the concentration range of 2-20 μmol/L. The apparent volume of distribution at steady state in healthy volunteers is approximately 16 L.

Metabolism

Esomeprazole is extensively metabolized in the liver by the cytochrome P450 (CYP) enzyme system. The metabolites of esomeprazole lack antisecretory activity. The major part of esomeprazole's metabolism is dependent upon the CYP2C19 isoenzyme, which forms the hydroxy and desmethyl metabolites. The remaining amount is dependent on CYP3A4 which forms the sulphone metabolite. CYP2C19 isoenzyme exhibits polymorphism in the metabolism of esomeprazole, since some 3% of Caucasians and 15-20% of Asians lack CYP2C19 and are termed Poor Metabolizers. At steady state, the ratio of AUC in Poor Metabolizers to AUC in the rest of the population (Extensive metabolizers) is approximately 2.

Following administration of equimolar doses, the S- and R-isomers are metabolized differently by the liver, resulting in higher plasma levels of the S- than of the R-isomer.

Excretion

Esomeprazole is excreted as metabolites primarily in urine but also in feces. Less than 1% of parent drug is excreted in the urine. Esomeprazole is completely eliminated from plasma and there is no accumulation during once daily administration. The plasma elimination half-life of intravenous esomeprazole is approximately 1.1 to 1.4 hours and is prolonged with increasing dose of intravenous esomeprazole.

Special Populations

Investigation of age, gender, race, renal, and hepatic impairment and metabolizer status have been made previously with oral esomeprazole. The pharmacokinetics of esomeprazole is not expected to be affected differently by intrinsic or extrinsic factors after intravenous administration compared to oral administration. The same recommendations for dose adjustment in special populations are suggested for intravenous esomeprazole as for oral esomeprazole.

Geriatric

In oral studies, the AUC and C_{max} values were slightly higher (25% and 18%, respectively) in the elderly as compared to younger subjects at steady state. Dosage adjustment based on age is not necessary.

Pediatric

The pharmacokinetics of esomeprazole sodium have not been studied in patients < 18 years of age.

Gender

In oral studies, the AUC and C_{max} values were slightly higher (13%) in females than in males at steady state. Similar differences have been seen for intravenous administration of esomeprazole. Dosage adjustment based on gender is not necessary.

Hepatic Insufficiency

In oral studies, the steady state pharmacokinetics of esomeprazole obtained after administration of 40 mg once daily to 4 patients each with mild (Child Pugh Class A), moderate (Child Pugh Class B), and severe (Child Pugh Class C) liver insufficiency were compared to those obtained in 36 male and female GERD patients with normal liver function. In patients with mild and moderate hepatic insufficiency, the AUCs were within the range that could be expected in patients with normal liver function. In patients with severe hepatic insufficiency the AUCs were 2 to 3 times higher than in the patients with normal liver function. No dosage adjustment is recommended for patients with mild to moderate hepatic insufficiency (Child Pugh Classes A and B). However, in patients with severe hepatic insufficiency (Child Pugh Class C) a dose of 20 mg once daily should not be exceeded (See DOSAGE AND ADMINISTRATION).

Renal Insufficiency

The pharmacokinetics of esomeprazole in patients with renal impairment are not expected to be altered relative to healthy volunteers as less than 1% of esomeprazole is excreted unchanged in urine.

Pharmacodynamics

Mechanism of Action

Esomeprazole is a proton pump inhibitor that suppresses gastric acid secretion by specific inhibition of the H^+/K^+-ATPase in the gastric parietal cell. The S- and R-isomers of omeprazole are protonated and converted in the acidic compartment of the parietal cell forming the active inhibitor, the achiral sulphenamide. By acting specifically on the proton pump, esomeprazole blocks the final step in acid production, thus reducing gastric acidity. This effect is dose-related up to a daily dose of 20 to 40 mg and leads to inhibition of gastric acid secretion.

Antisecretory Activity

The effect of intravenous esomeprazole on intragastric pH was determined in two separate studies. In the first study, 20 mg of NEXIUM I.V. for Injection was administered intravenously once daily at constant rate over 30 minutes for 5 days. Twenty-two healthy subjects were included in the study. In the second study, 40 mg of NEXIUM I.V. for Injection was administered intravenously once daily at constant rate over 30 minutes for 5 days. Thirty-eight healthy subjects were included in the study.

Effect of NEXIUM I.V. for Injection on Intragastric pH on Day 5

	Esomeprazole 20 mg	Esomeprazole 40 mg
	(n=22)	(n=38)
% Time Gastric	49.5	66.2
PH>4 (95% CI)*	41.9-57.2	62.4-70.0

*Gastric pH was measured over a 24-hour period

Serum Gastrin Effects

In oral studies, the effect of NEXIUM on serum gastrin concentrations was evaluated in approximately 2,700 patients in clinical trials up to 8 weeks and in over 1,300 patients for up to 6-12 months. The mean fasting gastrin level increased in a dose-related manner. This increase reached a plateau within two to three months of therapy and returned to baseline levels within four weeks after discontinuation of therapy.

Enterochromaffin-like (ECL) Cell Effects

There are no data available on the effects of intravenous esomeprazole on ECL cells.

In 24-month carcinogenicity studies of oral omeprazole in rats, a dose-related significant occurrence of gastric ECL cell carcinoid tumors and ECL cell hyperplasia was observed in both male and female animals (see **PRECAUTIONS, Carcinogenesis, Mutagenesis, Impairment of Fertility**). Carcinoid tumors have also been observed in rats subjected to fundectomy or long-term treatment with other proton pump inhibitors or high doses of H_2-receptor antagonists.

Human gastric biopsy specimens have been obtained from more than 3,000 patients treated orally with omeprazole in long-term clinical trials. The incidence of ECL cell hyperplasia in these studies increased with time; however, no case of ECL cell carcinoids, dysplasia, or neoplasia has been found in these patients.

In over 1,000 patients treated with NEXIUM (10, 20 or 40 mg/day) up to 6-12 months, the prevalence of ECL cell hyperplasia increased with time and dose. No patient developed ECL cell carcinoids, dysplasia, or neoplasia in the gastric mucosa.

Endocrine Effects

NEXIUM had no effect on thyroid function when given in oral doses of 20 or 40 mg for 4 weeks. Other effects of NEXIUM on the endocrine system were assessed using omeprazole studies. Omeprazole given in oral doses of 30 or 40 mg for 2 to 4 weeks had no effect on carbohydrate metabolism, circulating levels of parathyroid hormone, cortisol, estradiol, testosterone, prolactin, cholecystokinin or secretin.

Effects on Gastrointestinal Microbial Ecology

Decreased gastric acidity due to any means including proton pump inhibitors, increases gastric counts of bacteria normally present in the gastrointestinal tract. Treatment with proton pump inhibitors may lead to slightly increased risk of gastrointestinal infections such as *Salmonella* and *Campylobacter* and possibly *Clostridium difficile* in hospitalized patients.

Clinical Studies

Acid Suppression in Gastroesophageal Reflux Disease (GERD)

Four multicenter, open-label, two-period crossover studies were conducted to compare the pharmacodynamic efficacy of the intravenous formulation of esomeprazole (20 mg and 40 mg) to that of NEXIUM delayed-release capsules at corresponding doses in patients with symptoms of GERD, with or without erosive esophagitis. The patients (n=206, 18 to 72 years old; 112 female; 110 Caucasian, 50 Black, 10 Oriental, and 36 Other Race) were randomized to receive either 20 or 40 mg of intravenous or oral esomeprazole once daily for 10 days (Period 1), and then were switched in Period 2 to the other formulation for 10 days, matching their respective dose level from Period 1. The intravenous formulation was administered as a 3-minute injection in two of the studies, and as a 15-minute infusion in the other two studies. Basal acid output (BAO) and maximal acid output (MAO) were determined 22-24 hours post-dose on Period 1, Day 11; on Period 2, Day 3; and on Period 2, Day 11. BAO and MAO were estimated from 1-hour continuous collections of gastric contents prior to and following (respectively) subcutaneous injection of 6.0 μg/kg of pentagastrin.

In these studies, after 10 days of once daily administration, the intravenous dosage forms of NEXIUM 20 mg and 40 mg were similar to the corresponding oral dosage forms in their ability to suppress BAO and MAO in these GERD patients (see table below).

There were no major changes in acid suppression when switching between intravenous and oral dosage forms.

[See table at top of next page]

INDICATIONS AND USAGE

NEXIUM I.V. for Injection is indicated for the short-term treatment (up to 10 days) of GERD patients with a history of erosive esophagitis as an alternative to oral therapy in patients when therapy with NEXIUM Delayed-Release Capsules is not possible or appropriate.

When oral therapy is possible or appropriate, intravenous therapy with NEXIUM I.V. for Injection should be discontinued and the therapy should be continued orally.

CONTRAINDICATIONS

NEXIUM is contraindicated in patients with known hypersensitivity to any component of the formulation or to substituted benzimidazoles.

PRECAUTIONS

General

Symptomatic response to therapy with NEXIUM does not preclude the presence of gastric malignancy.

Atrophic gastritis has been noted occasionally in gastric corpus biopsies from patients treated long-term with omeprazole, of which NEXIUM is an enantiomer.

Treatment with NEXIUM I.V. for Injection should be discontinued as soon as the patient is able to resume treatment with NEXIUM Delayed-Release Capsules.

Drug Interactions

Esomeprazole is extensively metabolized in the liver by CYP2C19 and CYP3A4.

In vitro and *in vivo* studies have shown that esomeprazole is not likely to inhibit CYPs 1A2, 2A6, 2C9, 2D6, 2E1 and 3A4.

No clinically relevant interactions with drugs metabolized by these CYP enzymes would be expected. Drug interaction studies have shown that esomeprazole does not have any clinically significant interactions with phenytoin, warfarin, quinidine, clarithromycin or amoxicillin. Post-marketing reports of changes in prothrombin measures have been received among patients on concomitant warfarin and esomeprazole therapy. Increases in INR and prothrombin time may lead to abnormal bleeding and even death. Patients treated with proton pump inhibitors and warfarin concomitantly may need to be monitored for increases in INR and prothrombin time.
Esomeprazole may potentially interfere with CYP2C19, the major esomeprazole metabolizing enzyme. Coadministration of esomeprazole 30 mg and diazepam, a CYP2C19 substrate, resulted in a 45% decrease in clearance of diazepam. Increased plasma levels of diazepam were observed 12 hours after dosing and onwards. However, at that time, the plasma levels of diazepam were below the therapeutic interval, and thus this interaction is unlikely to be of clinical relevance.
Concomitant administration of esomeprazole and a combined inhibitor of CYP2C19 and CYP3A4, such as voriconazole, may result in more than doubling of the esomeprazole exposure. Dose adjustment of esomeprazole is not normally required for the recommended doses. However, in patients who may require higher doses, dose adjustment may be considered.
Omeprazole acts as an inhibitor of CYP 2C19. Omeprazole, given in doses of 40 mg daily for one week to 20 healthy subjects in cross-over study, increased C_{max} and AUC of cilostazol by 18% and 26% respectively. C_{max} and AUC of one of its active metabolites, 3,4-dihydro-cilostazol, which has 4-7 times the activity of cilostazol, were increased by 29% and 69% respectively. Co-administration of cilostazol with esomeprazole is expected to increase concentrations of cilostazol and its above mentioned active metabolite. Therefore a dose reduction of cilostazol from 100 mg b.i.d. to 50 mg b.i.d. should be considered.
Coadministration of oral contraceptives, diazepam, phenytoin, or quinidine did not seem to change the pharmacokinetic profile of esomeprazole.

Antiretroviral Agents

Concomitant use of atazanavir and nelfinavir with proton pump inhibitors is not recommended. Co-administration of atazanavir with proton pump inhibitors is expected to substantially decrease atazanavir plasma concentrations and thereby reduce its therapeutic effect.
Omeprazole has been reported to interact with some antiretroviral drugs. The clinical importance and the mechanisms behind these interactions are not always known. Increased gastric pH during omeprazole treatment may change the absorption of the antiretroviral drug. Other possible interaction mechanisms are via CYP2C19. For some antiretroviral drugs, such as atazanavir and nelfinavir, decreased serum levels have been reported when given together with omeprazole. Following multiple doses of nelfinavir (1250 mg, bid) and omeprazole (40 mg qd), AUC was decreased by 36% and 92%, C_{max} by 37% and 89% and C_{min} by 39% and 75% respectively for nelfinavir and M8. Following multiple doses of atazanavir (400 mg, qd) and omeprazole (40 mg, qd, 2 hr before atazanavir), AUC was decreased by 94%, C_{max} by 96%, and C_{min} by 95%. Concomitant administration with omeprazole and drugs such as atazanavir and nelfinavir is therefore not recommended. For other antiretroviral drugs, such as saquinavir, elevated serum levels have been reported with an increase in AUC by 82%, in C_{max} by 75% and in C_{min} by 106% following multiple dosing of saquinavir/ritonavir (1000/100 mg) bid for 15 days with omeprazole 40 mg qd coadministered days 11 to 15. Therefore, clinical and laboratory monitoring for saquinavir toxicity is recommended during concurrent use with NEXIUM. Dose reduction of saquinavir should be considered from the safety perspective for individual patients. There are also some antiretroviral drugs of which unchanged serum levels have been reported when given with omeprazole.
Studies evaluating concomitant administration of esomeprazole and either naproxen (non-selective NSAID) or rofecoxib (COX-2 selective NSAID) did not identify any clinically relevant changes in the pharmacokinetic profiles of esomeprazole or these NSAIDs.
Esomeprazole inhibits gastric acid secretion. Therefore, esomeprazole may interfere with the absorption of drugs where gastric pH is an important determinant of bioavailability (eg, ketoconazole, iron salts and digoxin).

Carcinogenesis, Mutagenesis, Impairment of Fertility

The carcinogenic potential of esomeprazole was assessed using omeprazole studies. In two 24-month oral carcinogenicity studies in rats, omeprazole at daily doses of 1.7, 3.4, 13.8, 44.0 and 140.8 mg/kg/day (about 0.7 to 57 times the human dose of 20 mg/day expressed on a body surface area basis) produced gastric ECL cell carcinoids in a dose-related manner in both male and female rats; the incidence of this effect was markedly higher in female rats, which had higher blood levels of omeprazole. Gastric carcinoids seldom occur in the untreated rat. In addition, ECL cell hyperplasia was present in all treated groups of both sexes. In one of these studies, female rats were treated with 13.8 mg omeprazole/kg/day (about 5.6 times the human dose on a body surface area basis) for 1 year, then followed for an additional year without the drug. No carcinoids were seen in these rats. An increased incidence of treatment-related ECL cell hyperplasia was observed at the end of 1 year (94% treated vs 10% controls). By the second year the difference between treated and control rats was much smaller (46% vs 26%) but still showed more hyperplasia in the treated group. Gastric adenocarcinoma was seen in one rat (2%). No similar tumor was seen in male or female rats treated for 2 years. For this strain of rat no similar tumor has been noted historically, but a finding involving only one tumor is difficult to interpret. A 78-week oral mouse carcinogenicity study of omeprazole did not show increased tumor occurrence, but the study was not conclusive.

Mean (SD) BAO and MAO measured 22-24 hours post-dose following once daily oral and intravenous administration of esomeprazole for 10 days in GERD patients with or without a history of erosive esophagitis

Study	Dose in mg	Intravenous Administration Method	BAO in mmol H^+/h		MAO in mmol H+/h	
			Intravenous	Oral	Intravenous	Oral
1 (N=42)	20	3-minute injection	0.71 (1.24)	0.69 (1.24)	5.96 (5.41)	5.27 (5.39)
2 (N=44)	20	15-minute infusion	0.78 (1.38)	0.82 (1.34)	5.95 (4.00)	5.26 (4.12)
3 (N=50)	40	3-minute injection	0.36 (0.61)	0.31 (0.55)	5.06 (3.90)	4.41 (3.11)
4 (N=47)	40	15-minute infusion	0.36 (0.79)	0.22 (0.39)	4.74 (3.65)	3.52 (2.86)

Esomeprazole was negative in the Ames mutation test, in the *in vivo* rat bone marrow cell chromosome aberration test, and the *in vivo* mouse micronucleus test. Esomeprazole, however, was positive in the *in vitro* human lymphocyte chromosome aberration test. Omeprazole was positive in the *in vitro* human lymphocyte chromosome aberration test, the *in vivo* mouse bone marrow cell chromosome aberration test, and the *in vivo* mouse micronucleus test.
The potential effects of esomeprazole on fertility and reproductive performance were assessed using omeprazole studies. Omeprazole at oral doses up to 138 mg/kg/day in rats (about 56 times the human dose on a body surface area basis) was found to have no effect on reproductive performance of parental animals.

Pregnancy

Teratogenic Effects. Pregnancy Category B

Teratology studies have been performed in rats at oral doses up to 280 mg/kg/day (about 57 times the human dose on a body surface area basis) and in rabbits at oral doses up to 86 mg/kg/day (about 35 times the human dose on a body surface area basis) and have revealed no evidence of impaired fertility or harm to the fetus due to esomeprazole. There are, however, no adequate and well-controlled studies in pregnant women. Because animal reproduction studies are not always predictive of human response, this drug should be used during pregnancy only if clearly needed.
Teratology studies conducted with omeprazole in rats at oral doses up to 138 mg/kg/day (about 56 times the human dose on a body surface area basis) and in rabbits at doses up to 69 mg/kg/day (about 56 times the human dose on a body surface area basis) did not disclose any evidence for a teratogenic potential of omeprazole. In rabbits, omeprazole in a dose range of 6.9 to 69.1 mg/kg/day (about 5.5 to 56 times the human dose on a body surface area basis) produced dose-related increases in embryo-lethality, fetal resorptions, and pregnancy disruptions. In rats, dose-related embryo/fetal toxicity and postnatal developmental toxicity were observed in offspring resulting from parents treated with omeprazole at 13.8 to 138.0 mg/kg/day (about 5.6 to 56 times the human doses on a body surface area basis). There are no adequate and well-controlled studies in pregnant women. Sporadic reports have been received of congenital abnormalities occurring in infants born to women who have received omeprazole during pregnancy.

Nursing Mothers

The excretion of esomeprazole in milk has not been studied. However, omeprazole concentrations have been measured in breast milk of a woman following oral administration of 20 mg. Because esomeprazole is likely to be excreted in human milk, because of the potential for serious adverse reactions in nursing infants from esomeprazole, and because of the potential for tumorigenicity shown for omeprazole in rat carcinogenicity studies, a decision should be made whether to discontinue nursing or to discontinue the drug, taking into account the importance of the drug to the mother.

Pediatric Use

Safety and effectiveness in pediatric patients have not been established.

Geriatric Use

Of the total number of patients who received oral NEXIUM in clinical trials, 1,459 were 65 to 74 years of age and 354 patients were ≥ 75 years of age.
No overall differences in safety and efficacy were observed between the elderly and younger individuals, and other reported clinical experience has not identified differences in responses between the elderly and younger patients, but greater sensitivity of some older individuals cannot be ruled out.

ADVERSE REACTIONS

Safety Experience with Intravenous NEXIUM

The safety of intravenous esomeprazole is based on results from clinical trials conducted in three different populations including patients having symptomatic GERD with or without a history of erosive esophagitis (n=206), patients with erosive esophagitis (n=246) and healthy subjects (n=204).
Adverse experiences occurring in >1% of patients treated with intravenous esomeprazole (n=359) in trials irrespective of the relationship to NEXIUM are listed below by body system:
Skin and appendages disorders: pruritus (1.1%); ***Central and peripheral nervous system disorders:*** dizziness (2.5%), headache (10.9%); ***Gastrointestinal system disorders:*** abdominal pain (5.8%), constipation (2.5%), diarrhea (3.9%), dyspepsia (6.4%), flatulence (10.3%), mouth dry (3.9%), nausea (6.4%); ***Respiratory system disorders:*** respiratory infection (1.1%), sinusitis (1.7%); ***Body as a whole – general disorders:*** AE associated with test procedure (23.1%); and ***Application site disorders:*** application site reaction (1.7%) (including mild focal erythema and pruritus at IV insertion site).
Intravenous treatment with esomeprazole 20 and 40 mg administered as an injection or as an infusion was found to have a safety profile similar to that of oral administration of esomeprazole 20 and 40 mg.

Safety Experience with Oral NEXIUM

The safety of oral NEXIUM was evaluated in over 15,000 patients (aged 18-84 years) in clinical trials worldwide including over 8,500 patients in the United States and over 6,500 patients in Europe and Canada. Over 2,900 patients were treated in long-term studies for up to 6-12 months.
The safety in the treatment of healing of erosive esophagitis was assessed in four randomized comparative clinical trials, which included 1,240 patients on NEXIUM 20 mg, 2,434 patients on NEXIUM 40 mg, and 3,008 patients on omeprazole 20 mg daily. The most frequently occurring adverse events (≥1%) in all three groups was headache (5.5, 5.0, and 3.8, respectively) and diarrhea (no difference among the three groups). Nausea, flatulence, abdominal pain, constipation, and dry mouth occurred at similar rates among patients taking NEXIUM or omeprazole.
Additional adverse events that were reported as possibly or probably related to NEXIUM with an incidence < 1% are listed below by body system:
Body as a Whole: abdomen enlarged, allergic reaction, asthenia, back pain, chest pain, chest pain substernal, facial edema, peripheral edema, hot flushes, fatigue, fever, flu-like disorder, generalized edema, leg edema, malaise, pain, rigors; ***Cardiovascular:*** flushing, hypertension, tachycardia; ***Endocrine:*** goiter; ***Gastrointestinal:*** bowel irregularity, constipation aggravated, dyspepsia, dysphagia, dysplasia GI, epigastric pain, eructation, esophageal disorder, frequent stools, gastroenteritis, GI hemorrhage, GI symptoms not otherwise specified, hiccup, melena, mouth disorder, pharynx disorder, rectal disorder, serum gastrin increased, tongue disorder, tongue edema, ulcerative stomatitis, vomiting; ***Hearing:*** earache, tinnitus; ***Hematologic:*** anemia, anemia hypochromic, cervical lymphoadenopathy, epistaxis, leukocytosis, leukopenia, thrombocytopenia; ***Hepatic:*** bilirubinemia, hepatic function abnormal, SGOT increased, SGPT increased; ***Metabolic/Nutritional:*** glycosuria, hyperuricemia, hyponatremia, increased alkaline phosphatase, thirst, vitamin B12 deficiency, weight increase, weight decrease; ***Musculoskeletal:*** arthralgia, arthritis aggravated, arthropathy, cramps, fibromyalgia syndrome, hernia, polymyalgia rheumatica; ***Nervous System/Psychiatric:*** an-

orexia, apathy, appetite increased, confusion, depression aggravated, dizziness, hypertonia, nervousness, hypoesthesia, impotence, insomnia, migraine, migraine aggravated, paresthesia, sleep disorder, somnolence, tremor, vertigo, visual field defect; ***Reproductive:*** dysmenorrhea, menstrual disorder, vaginitis; ***Respiratory:*** asthma aggravated, coughing, dyspnea, larynx edema, pharyngitis, rhinitis, sinusitis; ***Skin and Appendages:*** acne, angioedema, dermatitis, pruritus, pruritus ani, rash, rash erythematous, rash maculopapular, skin inflammation, sweating increased, urticaria; ***Special Senses:*** otitis media, parosmia, taste loss, taste perversion; ***Urogenital:*** abnormal urine, albuminuria, cystitis, dysuria, fungal infection, hematuria, micturition frequency, moniliasis, genital moniliasis, polyuria; ***Visual:*** conjunctivitis, vision abnormal.

Endoscopic findings that were reported as adverse events include: duodenitis, esophagitis, esophageal stricture, esophageal ulceration, esophageal varices, gastric ulcer, gastritis, hernia, benign polyps or nodules, Barrett's esophagus, and mucosal discoloration.

The incidence of treatment-related adverse events during 6-month maintenance treatment was similar to placebo. There were no differences in types of related adverse events seen during maintenance treatment up to 12 months compared to short-term treatment.

Two placebo-controlled studies were conducted in 710 patients for the treatment of symptomatic gastroesophageal reflux disease. The most common adverse events that were reported as possibly or probably related to NEXIUM were diarrhea (4.3%), headache (3.8%), and abdominal pain (3.8%).

Postmarketing Reports—There have been spontaneous reports of adverse events with postmarketing use of esomeprazole. These reports occurred rarely and are listed below by body system:

Blood And Lymphatic System Disorders: agranulocytosis, pancytopenia; ***Eye Disorders:*** blurred vision; ***Gastrointestinal Disorders:*** pancreatitis; stomatitis; ***Hepatobiliary Disorders:*** hepatic failure, hepatitis with or without jaundice; ***Immune System Disorders:*** anaphylactic reaction/shock; ***Infections and Infestations:*** GI candidiasis; ***Musculoskeletal And Connective Tissue Disorders:*** muscular weakness, myalgia; ***Nervous System Disorders:*** hepatic encephalopathy, taste disturbance; ***Psychiatric Disorders:*** aggression, agitation, depression, hallucination; ***Renal and Urinary Disorders:*** interstitial nephritis; ***Reproductive System and Breast Disorders:*** gynecomastia; ***Respiratory, Thoracic and Mediastinal Disorders:*** bronchospasm; ***Skin and Subcutaneous Tissue Disorders:*** alopecia, erythema multiforme, hyperhidrosis, photosensitivity, Stevens-Johnson syndrome, toxic epidermal necrolysis (TEN, some fatal).

Other adverse events not observed with NEXIUM, but occurring with omeprazole can be found in the omeprazole package insert, **ADVERSE REACTIONS** section.

Laboratory Events

The following potentially clinically significant laboratory changes in clinical trials, irrespective of relationship to NEXIUM, were reported in ≤ 1% of patients: increased creatinine, uric acid, total bilirubin, alkaline phosphatase, ALT, AST, hemoglobin, white blood cell count, platelets, serum gastrin, potassium, sodium, thyroxine and thyroid stimulating hormone (see **CLINICAL PHARMACOLOGY,** *Endocrine Effects* for further information on thyroid effects). Decreases were seen in hemoglobin, white blood cell count, platelets, potassium, sodium, and thyroxine.

OVERDOSAGE

The minimum lethal dose of esomeprazole sodium in rats after bolus administration was 310 mg/kg (about 62 times the human dose on a body surface area basis). The major signs of acute toxicity were reduced motor activity, changes in respiratory frequency, tremor, ataxia and intermittent clonic convulsions.

The symptoms described in connection with deliberate NEXIUM overdose (limited experience of doses in excess of 240 mg/day) are transient. Single doses of 80 mg of esomeprazole were uneventful. Reports of overdosage with omeprazole in humans may also be relevant. Doses ranged up to 2,400 mg (120 times the usual recommended clinical dose). Manifestations were variable, but included confusion, drowsiness, blurred vision, tachycardia, nausea, diaphoresis, flushing, headache, dry mouth, and other adverse reactions similar to those seen in normal clinical experience (see omeprazole package insert - **ADVERSE REACTIONS**). No specific antidote for esomeprazole is known. Since esomeprazole is extensively protein bound, it is not expected to be removed by dialysis. In the event of overdosage, treatment should be symptomatic and supportive.

As with the management of any overdose, the possibility of multiple drug ingestion should be considered. For current information on treatment of any drug overdose, a certified Regional Poison Control Center should be contacted. Telephone numbers are listed in the Physicians' Desk Reference (PDR) or local telephone book.

DOSAGE AND ADMINISTRATION

GERD with a history of Erosive Esophagitis

The recommended adult dose is either 20 or 40 mg esomeprazole given once daily by intravenous injection (no less than 3 minutes) or intravenous infusion (10 to 30 minutes).

NEXIUM I.V. for Injection should not be administered concomitantly with any other medications through the same intravenous site and or tubing. The intravenous line should always be flushed with either 0.9% Sodium Chloride Injection, USP, Lactated Ringer's Injection, USP or 5% Dextrose Injection, USP both prior to and after administration of NEXIUM I.V. for Injection.

Treatment with NEXIUM I.V. for Injection should be discontinued as soon as the patient is able to resume treatment with NEXIUM Delayed-Release Capsules.

Safety and efficacy of NEXIUM I.V. for Injection as a treatment of GERD patients with a history of erosive esophagitis for more than 10 days have not been demonstrated (see INDICATIONS AND USAGE).

Special Populations

Geriatric:

No dosage adjustment is necessary. (See **CLINICAL PHARMACOLOGY, Pharmacokinetics.**)

Renal Insufficiency:

No dosage adjustment is necessary. (See **CLINICAL PHARMACOLOGY, Pharmacokinetics.**)

Hepatic Insufficiency:

No dosage adjustment is necessary in patients with mild to moderate liver impairment (Child Pugh Classes A and B). For patients with severe liver impairment (Child Pugh Class C), a dose of 20 mg of NEXIUM should not be exceeded (See **CLINICAL PHARMACOLOGY, Pharmacokinetics.**)

Gender:

No dosage adjustment is necessary. (See **CLINICAL PHARMACOLOGY, Pharmacokinetics.**)

Preparations for use:

Intravenous Injection (20 or 40 mg) over no less than 3 minutes

The freeze-dried powder should be reconstituted with 5 mL of 0.9% Sodium Chloride Injection, USP. Withdraw 5 mL of the reconstituted solution and administer as an intravenous injection over no less than 3 minutes.

The reconstituted solution should be stored at room temperature up to 30°C (86°F) and administered within 12 hours after reconstitution. No refrigeration is required.

Intravenous Infusion (20 or 40 mg) over 10 to 30 minutes

A solution for intravenous infusion is prepared by first reconstituting the contents of one vial with 5 mL of 0.9% Sodium Chloride Injection, USP, Lactated Ringer's Injection, USP or 5% Dextrose Injection, USP and further diluting the resulting solution to a final volume of 50 mL. The solution (admixture) should be administered as an intravenous infusion over a period of 10 to 30 minutes.

The admixture should be stored at room temperature up to 30°C (86°F) and should be administered within the designated time period as listed in the Table below. No refrigeration is required.

Diluent	Administer within:
0.9% Sodium Chloride Injection, USP	12 hours
Lactated Ringer's Injection, USP	12 hours
5% Dextrose Injection, USP	6 hours

NEXIUM I.V. for Injection should not be administered concomitantly with any other medications through the same intravenous site and or tubing. The intravenous line should always be flushed with either 0.9% Sodium Chloride Injection, USP, Lactated Ringer's Injection, USP or 5% Dextrose Injection, USP both prior to and after administration of NEXIUM I.V. for Injection.

Parenteral drug products should be inspected visually for particulate matter and discoloration prior to administration, whenever solution and container permit.

HOW SUPPLIED

NEXIUM I.V. for Injection is supplied as a freeze-dried powder containing 20 mg or 40 mg of esomeprazole per single-use vial.

NDC 0186-6020-01 one carton containing 10 vials of NEXIUM I.V. for Injection (each vial contains 20 mg of esomeprazole).

NDC 0186-6040-01 one carton containing 10 vials of NEXIUM I.V. for Injection (each vial contains 40 mg of esomeprazole).

Storage

Store at 25°C (77°F); excursions permitted to 15°-30°C (59°-86°F). [See USP Controlled Room Temperature]. Protect from light. Store in carton until time of use.

NEXIUM is a registered trademark of the AstraZeneca group of companies

©AstraZeneca 2005, 2006, 2007, 2008

AstraZeneca LP
Wilmington, DE 19850
Rev. March 2010
308306 8/10

Shown in Product Identification Guide, page 306

PULMICORT FLEXHALER™ ℞

[*pŭl-mĭ-cōrt*]
(budesonide inhalation powder)
90 MCG, 180 MCG

HIGHLIGHTS OF PRESCRIBING INFORMATION

These highlights do not include all the information needed to use PULMICORT FLEXHALER™ safely and effectively. See full prescribing information for PULMICORT FLEXHALER™.

PULMICORT FLEXHALER™ 90 MCG, 180 MCG (BUDESONIDE INHALATION POWDER)
U.S. Approval: 2006

INDICATIONS AND USAGE

PULMICORT FLEXHALER is a corticosteroid indicated for:

• Maintenance treatment of asthma as prophylactic therapy in adult and pediatric patients six years of age or older. (1.1)

Important Limitations:

• Not indicated for the relief of acute bronchospasm. (1.1)

DOSAGE AND ADMINISTRATION

For oral inhalation only.

Patients 18 Years of Age and Older: For patients 18 years of age and older, the recommended starting dosage is 360 mcg twice daily. In some adult patients, a starting dose of 180 mcg twice daily may be adequate. The maximum dosage should not exceed 720 mcg twice daily. (2.1)

Patients 6 to 17 Years of Age: The recommended starting dosage is 180 mcg twice daily. In some pediatric patients, a starting dose of 360 mcg twice daily may be appropriate. The maximum dosage should not exceed 360 mcg twice daily. (2.1)

DOSAGE FORMS AND STRENGTHS

FLEXHALER device containing budesonide (90 mcg or 180 mcg) as an inhalation powder. (3)

CONTRAINDICATIONS

• Primary treatment of status asthmaticus or other acute episodes of asthma where intensive measures are required. (4)

• Severe hypersensitivity to milk proteins and any of the ingredients in PULMICORT FLEXHALER. (4)

WARNINGS AND PRECAUTIONS

• Localized infections: *Candida albicans* infection of the mouth and throat may occur. Monitor patients periodically for signs of adverse effects on the oral cavity. Advise patients to rinse the mouth following inhalation. (5.1)

• Deterioration of asthma or acute episodes: PULMICORT FLEXHALER should not be used for relief of acute symptoms. Patients require immediate re-evaluation during rapidly deteriorating asthma. (5.2)

• Hypersensitivity reactions: Anaphylaxis, rash, contact dermatitis, urticaria, angioedema, and bronchospasm have been reported with use of PULMICORT FLEXHALER. Discontinue PULMICORT FLEXHALER if such reactions occur. (5.3)

• Immunosuppression: Potential worsening of infections (e.g., existing tuberculosis, fungal, bacterial, viral, or parasitic infection; or ocular herpes simplex). Use with caution in patients with these infections. More serious or even fatal course of chickenpox or measles can occur in susceptible patients. (5.4)

• Transferring patients from systemic corticosteroids: Risk of impaired adrenal function when transferring from oral steroids. Taper patients slowly from systemic corticosteroids if transferring to PULMICORT FLEXHALER. (5.5)

• Hypercorticism and adrenal suppression: May occur with very high dosages or at the regular dosage in susceptible individuals. If such changes occur, reduce PULMICORT FLEXHALER slowly. (5.6)

• Reduction in bone mineral density with long term administration. Monitor patients with major risk factors for decreased bone mineral content. (5.8)

• Effects on growth: Monitor growth of pediatric patients. (5.9)

• Glaucoma and cataracts: Close monitoring is warranted. (5.10)

• Paradoxical bronchospasm: Discontinue PULMICORT FLEXHALER and institute alternative therapy if paradoxical bronchospasm occurs. (5.11)

• Eosinophilic conditions and Churg-Strauss: Be alert to eosinophilic conditions. (5.12)

---------------ADVERSE REACTIONS---------------

Most common adverse reactions (incidence ≥1%): nasopharyngitis, nasal congestion, pharyngitis, rhinitis allergic, viral upper respiratory tract infection, nausea, viral gastroenteritis, otitis media, oral candidiasis. (6.1)

To report SUSPECTED ADVERSE REACTIONS, contact AstraZeneca at 1-800-236-9933 or FDA at 1-800-FDA-1088 or www.fda.gov/medwatch

---------------DRUG INTERACTIONS---------------

• Strong cytochrome P450 3A4 inhibitors (e.g., ritonavir): Use with caution. May cause increased systemic corticosteroid effects. (7.1)

See 17 for PATIENT COUNSELING INFORMATION and FDA-approved patient labeling

Revised: 07/2010

FULL PRESCRIBING INFORMATION

1 INDICATIONS AND USAGE

1.1 Treatment of Asthma

PULMICORT FLEXHALER is indicated for the maintenance treatment of asthma as prophylactic therapy in patients six years of age or older.
Important Limitations of Use:
• PULMICORT FLEXHALER is NOT indicated for the relief of acute bronchospasm.

2 DOSAGE AND ADMINISTRATION

PULMICORT FLEXHALER should be administered twice daily by the orally inhaled route only. After inhalation, the patient should rinse the mouth with water without swallowing [see Patient Counseling Information (17.1)].
Patients should be instructed to prime PULMICORT FLEXHALER prior to its initial use, and instructed to inhale deeply and forcefully each time the device is used.
The safety and efficacy of PULMICORT FLEXHALER when administered in excess of recommended doses have not been established.
After asthma stability has been achieved, it is desirable to titrate to the lowest effective dosage to reduce the possibility of side effects. For patients who do not respond adequately to the starting dose after 1-2 weeks of therapy with PULMICORT FLEXHALER, increasing the dose may provide additional asthma control.

2.1 Asthma

If asthma symptoms arise in the period between doses, an inhaled, short-acting beta₂-agonist should be taken for immediate relief.
Patients 18 Years of Age and Older: For patients 18 years of age and older, the recommended starting dosage is 360 mcg twice daily. In some adult patients, a starting dose of 180 mcg twice daily may be adequate. The maximum dosage should not exceed 720 mcg twice daily.
Patients 6 to 17 Years of Age: The recommended starting dosage is 180 mcg twice daily. In some pediatric patients, a starting dose of 360 mcg twice daily may be appropriate. The maximum dosage should not exceed 360 mcg twice daily.
For all patients, it is desirable to titrate to the lowest effective dose after adequate asthma stability is achieved.
Improvement in asthma control following inhaled administration of budesonide can occur within 24 hours of initiation of treatment, although maximum benefit may not be achieved for 1 to 2 weeks, or longer. Individual patients will experience a variable onset and degree of symptom relief.
If a previously effective dosage regimen of PULMICORT FLEXHALER fails to provide adequate control of asthma, the therapeutic regimen should be re-evaluated and additional therapeutic options (e.g. replacing the lower strength of PULMICORT FLEXHALER with the higher strength or initiating oral corticosteroids) should be considered.

3 DOSAGE FORMS AND STRENGTHS

PULMICORT FLEXHALER is available as a dry powder for inhalation containing budesonide in the following 2 strengths: 90 mcg and 180 mcg. Each inhaler contains 60 or 120 actuations.

4 CONTRAINDICATIONS

The use of PULMICORT FLEXHALER is contraindicated in the following conditions:
• Primary treatment of status asthmaticus or other acute episodes of asthma where intensive measures are required.
• Severe hypersensitivity to milk proteins or any ingredients of PULMICORT FLEXHALER [see Warnings and Precautions (5.3), Description (11)].

5 WARNINGS AND PRECAUTIONS

5.1 Local Effects

In clinical studies, the development of localized infections of the mouth and pharynx with *Candida albicans* has occurred in patients treated with PULMICORT FLEXHALER. When such an infection develops, it should be treated with appropriate local or systemic (i.e. oral antifungal) therapy while treatment with PULMICORT FLEXHALER continues, but at times, therapy with PULMICORT FLEXHALER may need to be interrupted. Patients should rinse the mouth after inhalation of PULMICORT FLEXHALER.

5.2 Deterioration of Asthma or Acute Episodes

PULMICORT FLEXHALER is not a bronchodilator and is not indicated for the rapid relief of bronchospasm or other acute episodes of asthma. Patients should be instructed to contact their physician immediately if episodes of asthma not responsive to their usual doses of bronchodilators occur during the course of treatment with PULMICORT FLEXHALER. During such episodes, patients may require therapy with oral corticosteroids.
An inhaled short acting beta₂-agonist, not PULMICORT FLEXHALER, should be used to relieve acute symptoms such as shortness of breath. When prescribing PULMICORT FLEXHALER, the physician must also provide the patient with an inhaled, short-acting beta₂-agonist (e.g. albuterol) for treatment of acute symptoms, despite regular twice-daily (morning and evening) use of PULMICORT FLEXHALER.

5.3 Hypersensitivity Reactions Including Anaphylaxis

Hypersensitivity reactions including anaphylaxis, rash, contact dermatitis, urticaria, angioedema, and bronchospasm have been reported with use of PULMICORT

FLEXHALER. Discontinue PULMICORT FLEXHALER if such reactions occur [see Contraindications (4) and Adverse Reactions (6)].
PULMICORT FLEXHALER contains small amounts of lactose, which contains trace levels of milk proteins. It is possible that cough, wheezing, or bronchospasm may occur in patients who have a severe milk protein allergy [see Contraindications (4) and Adverse Reactions, Post-marketing Experience (6.2)].

5.4 Immunosuppression

Patients who are on drugs that suppress the immune system are more susceptible to infection than healthy individuals. Chicken pox and measles, for example, can have a more serious or even fatal course in susceptible children or adults using corticosteroids. In children or adults who have not had these diseases or been properly immunized, particular care should be taken to avoid exposure. How the dose, route, and duration of corticosteroid administration affects the risk of developing a disseminated infection is not known. The contribution of the underlying disease and/or prior corticosteroid treatment to the risk is also not known. If exposed to chicken pox, therapy with varicella zoster immune globulin (VZIG) or pooled intravenous immunoglobulin (IVIG), as appropriate, may be indicated. If exposed to measles, prophylaxis with pooled intramuscular immunoglobulin (IG) may be indicated. (See the respective package inserts for complete VZIG and IG prescribing information.) If chicken pox develops, treatment with antiviral agents may be considered. The immune responsiveness to varicella vaccine was evaluated in pediatric patients with asthma ages 12 months to 8 years with budesonide inhalation suspension.
An open-label, nonrandomized clinical study examined the immune responsiveness to varicella vaccine in 243 asthma patients 12 months to 8 years of age who were treated with budesonide inhalation suspension 0.25 mg to 1 mg daily (n=151) or non-corticosteroid asthma therapy (n=92) (i.e., beta₂-agonists, leukotriene receptor antagonists, cromones). The percentage of patients developing a seroprotective antibody titer of ≥5.0 (gpELISA value) in response to the vaccination was similar in patients treated with budesonide inhalation suspension (85%), compared to patients treated with non-corticosteroid asthma therapy (90%). No patient treated with budesonide inhalation suspension developed chicken pox as a result of vaccination.
Inhaled corticosteroids should be used with caution, if at all, in patients with active or quiescent tuberculosis infection of the respiratory tract, untreated systemic fungal, bacterial, viral or parasitic infections, or ocular herpes simplex.

5.5 Transferring Patients from Systemic Corticosteroid Therapy

Particular care is needed for patients who are transferred from systemically active corticosteroids to PULMICORT FLEXHALER because deaths due to adrenal insufficiency have occurred in asthmatic patients during and after transfer from systemic corticosteroids to less systemically available inhaled corticosteroids. After withdrawal from systemic corticosteroids, a number of months are required for recovery of hypothalamic-pituitary-adrenal (HPA) function. Patients who have been previously maintained on 20 mg or more per day of prednisone (or its equivalent) may be most susceptible, particularly when their systemic corticosteroids have been almost completely withdrawn.
During this period of HPA suppression, patients may exhibit signs and symptoms of adrenal insufficiency when exposed to trauma, surgery, or infection (particularly gastroenteritis) or other conditions associated with severe electrolyte loss. Although PULMICORT FLEXHALER may provide control of asthma symptoms during these episodes, in recommended doses it supplies less than normal physiological amounts of glucocorticoid systemically and does NOT provide the mineralocorticoid activity that is necessary for coping with these emergencies.
During periods of stress or a severe asthma attack, patients who have been withdrawn from systemic corticosteroids should be instructed to resume oral corticosteroids (in large doses) immediately and to contact their physicians for further instruction. These patients should also be instructed to carry a medical identification card indicating that they may need supplementary systemic corticosteroids during periods of stress or a severe asthma attack.
Patients requiring oral corticosteroids should be weaned slowly from systemic corticosteroid use after transferring to PULMICORT FLEXHALER. Prednisone reduction can be accomplished by reducing the daily prednisone dose by 2.5 mg on a weekly basis during therapy with PULMICORT FLEXHALER. Lung function (mean forced expiratory volume in 1 second [FEV₁] or morning peak expiratory flow [PEF]), beta-agonist use, and asthma symptoms should be carefully monitored during withdrawal of oral corticosteroids. In addition to monitoring asthma signs and symptoms, patients should be observed for signs and symptoms of adrenal insufficiency such as fatigue, lassitude, weakness, nausea and vomiting, and hypotension.

Transfer of patients from systemic corticosteroid therapy to PULMICORT FLEXHALER may unmask allergic conditions previously suppressed by the systemic corticosteroid therapy, (e.g., rhinitis, conjunctivitis, eczema, arthritis, eosinophilic conditions). Some patients may experience symptoms of systemically active corticosteroid withdrawal (e.g., joint and/or muscular pain, lassitude, depression) despite maintenance or even improvement of respiratory function.

5.6 Hypercorticism and Adrenal Suppression

PULMICORT FLEXHALER will often help control asthma symptoms with less suppression of HPA function than therapeutically equivalent oral doses of prednisone. Since budesonide is absorbed into the circulation and can be systemically active at higher doses, the beneficial effects of PULMICORT FLEXHALER in minimizing HPA dysfunction may be expected only when recommended dosages are not exceeded and individual patients are titrated to the lowest effective dose. Since individual sensitivity to effects on cortisol production exists, physicians should consider this information when prescribing PULMICORT FLEXHALER.

Because of the possibility of systemic absorption of inhaled corticosteroids, patients treated with PULMICORT FLEXHALER should be observed carefully for any evidence of systemic corticosteroid effects. Particular care should be taken in observing patients postoperatively or during periods of stress for evidence of inadequate adrenal response.

It is possible that systemic corticosteroid effects such as hypercorticism and adrenal suppression (including adrenal crisis) may appear in a small number of patients, particularly when budesonide is administered at higher than recommended doses over prolonged periods of time. If such effects occur, the dosage of PULMICORT FLEXHALER should be reduced slowly, consistent with accepted procedures for reducing systemic corticosteroids and for management of asthma symptoms.

5.7 Interactions with Strong Cytochrome P450 3A4 Inhibitors

Caution should be exercised when considering the co-administration of PULMICORT FLEXHALER with ketoconazole, and other known strong CYP3A4 inhibitors (e.g. ritonavir, atazanavir, clarithromycin, indinavir, itraconazole, nefazodone, nelfinavir, saquinavir, telithromycin) because adverse effects related to increased systemic exposure to budesonide may occur [ee *Drug Interactions (7.1), Clinical Pharmacology (12.3)*].

5.8 Reduction in Bone Mineral Density

Decreases in bone mineral density (BMD) have been observed with long-term administration of products containing inhaled corticosteroids. The clinical significance of small changes in BMD with regard to long-term consequences such as fracture is unknown. Patients with major risk factors for decreased bone mineral content, such as prolonged immobilization, family history of osteoporosis, post menopausal status, tobacco use, advance age, poor nutrition, or chronic use of drugs that can reduce bone mass (e.g, anticonvulsants, oral corticosteroids) should be monitored and treated with established standards of care.

5.9 Effect on Growth

Orally inhaled corticosteroids, including budesonide, may cause a reduction in growth velocity when administered to pediatric patients. Monitor the growth of pediatric patients receiving PULMICORT FLEXHALER routinely (e.g., via stadiometry). To minimize the systemic effects of orally inhaled corticosteroids, including PULMICORT FLEXHALER, titrate each patient's dose to the lowest dosage that effectively controls his/her symptoms [see *Dosage and Administration (2.1), Use in Specific Populations (8.4)*].

5.10 Glaucoma and Cataracts

Glaucoma, increased intraocular pressure, and cataracts have been reported following the long-term administration of inhaled corticosteroids, including budesonide. Therefore, close monitoring is warranted in patients with a change in vision or with a history of increased intraocular pressure, glaucoma, and/or cataracts.

5.11 Paradoxical Bronchospasm and Upper Airway Symptoms

As with other inhaled asthma medications, PULMICORT FLEXHALER can produce paradoxical bronchospasm, which may be life threatening. If paradoxical bronchospasm occurs following dosing with PULMICORT FLEXHALER, it should be treated immediately with an inhaled, short-acting beta$_2$-bronchodilator. PULMICORT FLEXHALER should be discontinued immediately, and alternative therapy should be instituted.

5.12 Eosinophilic Conditions and Churg-Strauss Syndrome

In rare cases, patients on inhaled corticosteroids may present with systemic eosinophilic conditions. Some of these patients have clinical features of vasculitis consistent with Churg-Strauss syndrome, a condition that is often treated with systemic corticosteroid therapy. These events usually, but not always, have been associated with the reduction and/or withdrawal of oral corticosteroid therapy following the introduction of inhaled corticosteroids. Physicians should be alert to eosinophilia, vasculitic rash, worsening pulmonary symptoms, cardiac complications, and/or neuropathy presenting in their patients. A causal relationship between budesonide and these underlying conditions has not been established.

6 ADVERSE REACTIONS

Systemic and inhaled corticosteroid use may result in the following:

- *Candida albicans* infection [see *Warnings and Precautions (5.1)*]
- Hypersensitivity Including Anaphylaxis [see *Warnings and Precautions (5.3)*]
- Immunosuppression [see *Warnings and Precautions (5.4)*]
- Hypercorticism and Adrenal Suppression [see *Warnings and Precautions (5.6)*]
- Reduction in Bone Mineral Density [see *Warnings and Precautions (5.8)*]
- Growth Effects [see *Warnings and Precautions (5.9) and Use in Specific Populations (8.4)*]
- Glaucoma and Cataracts [see *Warnings and Precautions (5.10)*]
- Eosinophilic conditions and Churg-Strauss [see *Warnings and Precautions (5.12)*]

6.1 Clinical Trials Experience

Because clinical trials are conducted under widely varying conditions, adverse reaction rates observed in the clinical trials of a drug cannot be directly compared to rates in the clinical trials of another drug and may not reflect the rates observed in practice.

PULMICORT FLEXHALER

Patients 6 years and older

The incidence of common adverse reactions in Table 1 is based upon pooled data reported in patients treated with PULMICORT FLEXHALER 180 or 90 mcg in two double-blind, placebo-controlled clinical trials in which 226 patients (106 females and 120 males) with mild to moderate asthma, previously receiving bronchodilators, inhaled corticosteroids, or both, were treated with PULMICORT FLEXHALER, administered as 360 mcg twice daily for 12 weeks. In these trials, the patients on PULMICORT FLEXHALER had a mean age of 28 years (range 6-80 years) and were predominantly Caucasian (59.7%) and Asian (31.4%). Table 1 includes all adverse reactions (regardless of investigator causality assessment) that occurred at a rate of ≥1% in the PULMICORT FLEXHALER group and more commonly than the placebo group.

Table 1 - Adverse Reactions occurring at an incidence of ≥1% and more commonly than placebo in the PULMICORT FLEXHALER group: pooled data from two 12-week, double-blind, placebo-controlled clinical asthma trials in patients 6 years and older

Adverse Event	PULMICORT FLEXHALER 360 mcg twice daily N=226 %	Placebo N=230 %
Nasopharyngitis	9.3	8.3
Nasal congestion	2.7	0.4
Pharyngitis	2.7	1.7
Rhinitis allergic	2.2	1.3
Viral upper respiratory tract infection	2.2	1.3
Nausea	1.8	0.9
Viral gastroenteritis	1.8	0.4
Otitis media	1.3	0.9
Oral candidiasis	1.3	0.4
Average exposure duration (days)	76.2	68.2

Long-Term Safety in Patients 6 years of age and older

Non-placebo controlled long-term studies in children (at doses up to 360 mcg daily), and adolescent and adult subjects (at doses up to 720 mcg daily), treated for up to one year with PULMICORT FLEXHALER, revealed a similar pattern and incidence of adverse events.

PULMICORT TURBUHALER; a different PULMICORT DPI

The following adverse reactions occurred in placebo-controlled clinical trials with similar or lower doses with inhaled budesonide via a different PULMICORT dry powder inhaler with an incidence of ≥1% in the budesonide group and were more common than in the placebo group:

≥3%: respiratory infection, sinusitis, headache, pain, back pain, fever.

≥1-3%: neck pain, syncope, abdominal pain, dry mouth, vomiting, weight gain, fracture, myalgia, hypertonia, migraine, ecchymosis, insomnia, infection, taste perversion, voice alteration.

Higher doses of inhaled budesonide (800 mcg twice daily) via a different PULMICORT dry powder inhaler resulted in an increased incidence of voice alteration, flu syndrome, dyspepsia, gastroenteritis, nausea, and back pain, compared with doses of 400 mcg twice daily.

In a 20-week trial in adult asthmatics who previously required oral corticosteroids, the incidence of adverse reactions was evaluated with 400 mcg twice daily (N=53) and 800 mcg twice daily (N=53) of inhaled budesonide via a different PULMICORT dry powder inhaler and compared with placebo (N=53). In considering these data, the increased average duration of exposure for inhaled budesonide patients (78 days for inhaled budesonide vs. 41 days for placebo) should be taken into account. Adverse reactions, regardless of investigator causality assessment, reported in more than five patients in the budesonide group and which occurred more commonly than the placebo group in decreasing order of frequency include: respiratory infection, sinusitis, headache, oral candidiasis, pain, asthenia, dyspepsia, arthralgia, cough increased, nausea and rhinitis.

6.2 Post-marketing Experience

The following adverse reactions have been reported during post-approval use of PULMICORT FLEXHALER. Because these reactions are reported voluntarily from a population of uncertain size, it is not always possible to reliably estimate their frequency or establish a causal relationship to drug exposure.

Immune system disorders: immediate and delayed hypersensitivity reactions including anaphylactic reaction, angioedema, bronchospasm, rash, contact dermatitis, urticaria, and cough, wheezing or bronchospasm in patients with severe milk protein hypersensitivity [see *Warnings and Precautions (5.3) and Containdications (4)*]

Endocrine disorders: symptoms of hypocorticism and hypercorticism [see *Warnings and Precautions (5.6)*]

Eye disorders: cataracts, glaucoma, increased intraocular pressure [see *Warnings and Precautions (5.10)*]

Psychiatric disorders: psychiatric symptoms including psychosis, depression, aggressive reactions, irritability, nervousness, restlessness, and anxiety

Respiratory, thoracic, and mediastinal disorders: throat irritation

Skin and subcutaneous tissue disorders: skin bruising

7 DRUG INTERACTIONS

7.1 Inhibitors of Cytochrome P4503A4

The main route of metabolism of corticosteroids, including budesonide, is via cytochrome P450 (CYP) isoenzyme 3A4 (CYP3A4). After oral administration of ketoconazole, a strong inhibitor of CYP3A4, the mean plasma concentration of orally administered budesonide increased. Concomitant administration of CYP3A4 may inhibit the metabolism of, and increase the systemic exposure to, budesonide. Caution should be exercised when considering the co-administration of PULMICORT FLEXHALER with long-term ketoconazole and other known strong CYP3A4 inhibitors (e.g., ritonavir, atazanavir, clarithromycin, indinavir, itraconazole, nefazodone, nelfinavir, saquinavir, telithromycin) [see *Warnings and Precautions (5.7)*].

8 USE IN SPECIFIC POPULATIONS

8.1 Pregnancy

Teratogenic Effects: Pregnancy Category B

Studies of pregnant women, have not shown that inhaled budesonide increases the risk of abnormalities when administered during pregnancy. The results from a large population-based prospective cohort epidemiological study reviewing data from three Swedish registries covering approximately 99% of the pregnancies from 1995-1997 (i.e., Swedish Medical Birth Registry; Registry of Congenital Malformations; Child Cardiology Registry) indicate no increased risk for congenital malformations from the use of inhaled budesonide during early pregnancy. Congenital malformations were studied in 2014 infants born to mothers reporting the use of inhaled budesonide for asthma in early pregnancy (usually 10-12 weeks after the last menstrual period), the period when most major organ malformations occur. The rate of recorded congenital malformations was similar compared to the general population rate (3.8% vs. 3.5%, respectively). In addition, after exposure to inhaled budesonide, the number of infants born with orofacial clefts was similar to the expected number in the normal population (4 children vs. 3.3, respectively).

These same data were utilized in a second study bringing the total to 2534 infants whose mothers were exposed to inhaled budesonide. In this study, the rate of congenital malformations among infants whose mothers were exposed to

inhaled budesonide during early pregnancy was not different from the rate for all newborn babies during the same period (3.6%).
Despite the animal findings, it would appear that the possibility of fetal harm is remote if the drug is used during pregnancy. Nevertheless, because the studies in humans cannot rule out the possibility of harm, PULMICORT FLEXHALER should be used during pregnancy only if clearly needed.
As with other glucocorticoids, budesonide produced fetal loss, decreased pup weight, and skeletal abnormalities at a subcutaneous dose in rabbits that was approximately 0.3 times the maximum recommended daily inhalation dose in adults on a mcg/m^2 basis and at a subcutaneous dose in rats that was approximately 3 times the maximum recommended daily inhalation dose in adults on a mcg/m^2 basis. No teratogenic or embryocidal effects were observed in rats when budesonide was administered by inhalation at doses up to approximately equivalent to the maximum recommended daily inhalation dose in adults on a mcg/m^2 basis.
Experience with oral corticosteroids since their introduction in pharmacologic as opposed to physiologic doses suggests that rodents are more prone to teratogenic effects from corticosteroids than humans.
Nonteratogenic Effects
Hypoadrenalism may occur in infants born of mothers receiving corticosteroids during pregnancy. Such infants should be carefully observed.

8.3 Nursing Mothers
Budesonide, like other corticosteroids, is secreted in human milk. Data with budesonide delivered via dry powder inhaler indicates that the total daily oral dose of budesonide available in breast milk to the infant is approximately 0.3% to 1% of the dose inhaled by the mother [see *Clinical Pharmacology, Pharmacokinetics, Special Populations, Nursing Mothers (12.3)*]. No studies have been conducted in breastfeeding women specifically with PULMICORT FLEXHALER; however, the dose of budesonide available to the infant in breast milk, as a percentage of the maternal dose, would be expected to be similar. PULMICORT FLEXHALER should be used in nursing women only if clinically appropriate. Prescribers should weigh the known benefits of breastfeeding for the mother and the infant against the potential risks of minimal budesonide exposure in the infant. Dosing considerations include prescription or titration to the lowest clinically effective dose and use of PULMICORT FLEXHALER immediately after breastfeeding to maximize the time interval between dosing and breastfeeding to minimize infant exposure. However, in general, PULMICORT FLEXHALER use should not delay or interfere with infant feeding.

8.4 Pediatric Use
In a 12-week pivotal study, 204 patients 6 to 17 years of age were treated with PULMICORT FLEXHALER twice daily [see *Clinical Studies (14.1)*]. Efficacy results in this age group were similar to those observed in patients 18 years and older. There were no obvious differences in the type or frequency of adverse events reported in this age group compared with patients 18 years of age and older. The safety and effectiveness of PULMICORT FLEXHALER in asthma patients below 6 years of age have not been established.
Controlled clinical studies have shown that orally inhaled corticosteroids, including budesonide, may cause a reduction in growth velocity in pediatric patients. This effect has been observed in the absence of laboratory evidence of hypothalamic-pituitary-adrenal (HPA) axis suppression, suggesting that growth velocity is a more sensitive indicator of systemic corticosteroid exposure in pediatric patients than some commonly used tests of HPA-axis function. The long-term effects of this reduction in growth velocity associated with orally inhaled corticosteroids including the impact on final adult height are unknown. The potential for "catch up" growth following discontinuation of treatment with orally inhaled corticosteroids has not been adequately studied.
In a study of asthmatic children 5-12 years of age, those treated with inhaled budesonide via a different PULMICORT dry powder inhaler 200 mcg twice daily (n=311) had a 1.1-centimeter reduction in growth compared with those receiving placebo (n=418) at the end of one year; the difference between these two treatment groups did not increase further over three years of additional treatment. By the end of four years, children treated with a different PULMICORT dry powder inhaler and children treated with placebo had similar growth velocities. Conclusions drawn from this study may be confounded by the unequal use of corticosteroids in the treatment groups and inclusion of data from patients attaining puberty during the course of the study.
The administration of inhaled budesonide via a different PULMICORT dry-powder inhaler in doses up to 800 mcg/day (mean daily dose 445 mcg/day) or via a pressurized metered-dose inhaler in doses up to 1200 mcg/day (mean daily dose 620 mcg/day) to 216 pediatric patients (age 3 to 11 years) for 2 to 6 years had no significant effect on statural growth compared with non-corticosteroid therapy in 62 matched control patients. However, the long-term effect of inhaled budesonide on growth is not fully known.
The growth of pediatric patients receiving orally inhaled corticosteroids, including PULMICORT FLEXHALER, should be monitored (eg, via stadiometry). If a child or adolescent on any corticosteroid appears to have growth suppression, the possibility that he/she is particularly sensitive to this effect should be considered. The potential growth effects of prolonged treatment should be weighed against clinical benefits obtained. To minimize the systemic effects of inhaled corticosteroids, including PULMICORT FLEXHALER, each patient should be titrated to the lowest dose that effectively controls his/her asthma [see *Dosage and Administration (2)*].

8.5 Geriatric Use
Of the total number of patients in controlled clinical studies receiving inhaled budesonide, 153 (n=11 treated with PULMICORT FLEXHALER) were 65 years of age or older and one was age 75 years or older. No overall differences in safety were observed between these patients and younger patients. Clinical studies did not include sufficient numbers of patients aged 65 years and over to determine differences in efficacy between elderly and younger patients. Other reported clinical or medical surveillance experience has not identified differences in responses between the elderly and younger patients. In general, dose selection for an elderly patient should be cautious, usually starting at the low end of the dosing range, reflecting the greater frequency of decreased hepatic, renal, or cardiac function, and of concomitant disease or other drug therapy.

8.6 Hepatic Impairment
Formal pharmacokinetic studies using PULMICORT FLEXHALER have not been conducted in patients with hepatic impairment. However, since budesonide is predominantly cleared by hepatic metabolism, impairment of liver function may lead to accumulation of budesonide in the plasma. Therefore, patients with hepatic disease should be closely monitored.

10 OVERDOSAGE
The potential for acute toxic effects following overdose of PULMICORT FLEXHALER is low. If used at excessive doses for prolonged periods, systemic corticosteroid effects such as hypercorticism may occur [see *Warnings and Precautions, Hypercorticism and Adrenal Suppression (5.6)*]. Another budesonide-containing dry powder inhaler at 3200 mcg daily administered for 6 weeks caused a significant reduction (27%) in the plasma cortisol response to a 6-hour infusion of ACTH compared with placebo (+1%). The corresponding effect of 10 mg prednisone daily was a 35% reduction in the plasma cortisol response to ACTH.
The minimal inhalation lethal dose in mice was 100 mg/kg (approximately 280 times the maximum recommended daily inhalation dose in adults and approximately 330 times the maximum recommended daily inhalation dose in children 6 to 17 years of age on a mcg/m^2 basis). There were no deaths following the administration of an inhalation dose of 68 mg/kg in rats (approximately 380 times the maximum recommended daily inhalation dose in adults and approximately 450 times the maximum recommended daily inhalation dose in children 6 to 17 years of age on a mcg/m^2 basis). The minimal oral lethal dose was 200 mg/kg in mice (approximately 560 times the maximum recommended daily inhalation dose in adults and approximately 670 times the maximum recommended daily inhalation dose in children 6 to 17 years of age on a mcg/m^2 basis) and less than 100 mg/kg in rats (approximately 560 times the maximum recommended daily inhalation dose in adults and approximately 670 times the maximum recommended daily inhalation dose in children 6 to 17 years of age based on a mcg/m^2 basis).
Post-marketing experience showed that acute overdose of inhaled budesonide commonly remained asymptomatic. The use of excessive doses (up to 6400 mcg daily) for prolonged periods showed systemic corticosteroid effects such as hypercorticism.

11 DESCRIPTION
Budesonide, the active component of PULMICORT FLEXHALER, is a corticosteroid designated chemically as (RS)-11β, 16α, 17,21-Tetrahydroxypregna-1,4-diene-3,20-dione cyclic 16,17-acetal with butyraldehyde. Budesonide is provided as a mixture of two epimers (22R and 22S). The empirical formula of budesonide is $C_{25}H_{34}O_6$ and its molecular weight is 430.5. Its structural formula is:
[See chemical structure at top of next column]
Budesonide is a white to off-white, tasteless, odorless powder that is practically insoluble in water and in heptane, sparingly soluble in ethanol, and freely soluble in chloroform. Its partition coefficient between octanol and water at pH 7.4 is $1.6 \times 10_3$.

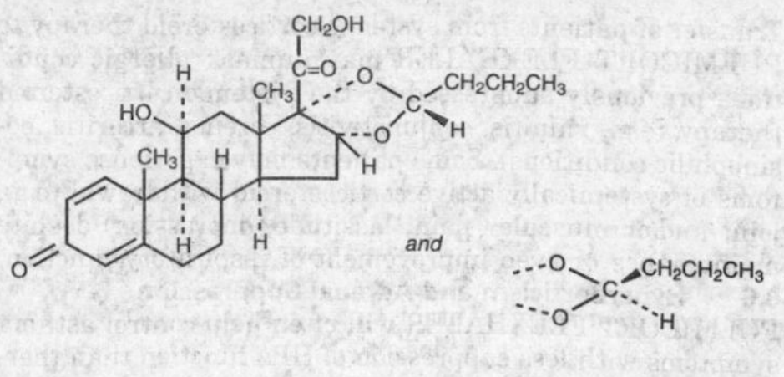

PULMICORT FLEXHALER is an inhalation-driven multidose dry powder inhaler containing a formulation of 1 mg per actuation of micronized budesonide and micronized lactose monohydrate which contains trace levels of milk proteins [see *Contraindications (4) and Post-marketing Experience (6.2)*]. Each actuation of PULMICORT FLEXHALER 180 mcg delivers 160 mcg budesonide from the mouthpiece and each actuation of PULMICORT FLEXHALER 90 mcg delivers 80 mcg budesonide from the mouthpiece (based on *in vitro* testing at 60 L/min for 2 sec). Each PULMICORT FLEXHALER 180 mcg contains 120 actuations and each PULMICORT FLEXHALER 90 mcg contains 60 actuations.
In vitro testing has shown that the dose delivery for PULMICORT FLEXHALER is dependent on airflow through the device, as evidenced by a decrease in the fine particle dose at a flow rate of 30 L/min to a value that is approximately 40-50% of that produced at 60 L/min. At a flow rate of 40 L/min, the fine particle dose is approximately 70% of that produced at 60 L/min. Patient factors such as inspiratory flow rates will also affect the dose delivered to the lungs of patients in actual use [see *Patient Information and Instructions for Use (17.11)*]. In asthmatic children age 6 to 17 (N=516, FEV_1 2.29 [0.97–4.28]) peak inspiratory flow (PIF) through PULMICORT FLEXHALER was 72.5 [19.1–103.6] L/min). Inspiratory flows were not measured in the adult pivotal study. Patients should be carefully instructed on the use of this drug product to assure optimal dose delivery.

12 CLINICAL PHARMACOLOGY
12.1 Mechanism of Action
Budesonide is an anti-inflammatory corticosteroid that exhibits potent glucocorticoid activity and weak mineralocorticoid activity. In standard *in vitro* and animal models, budesonide has approximately a 200-fold higher affinity for the glucocorticoid receptor and a 1000-fold higher topical anti-inflammatory potency than cortisol (rat croton oil ear edema assay). As a measure of systemic activity, budesonide is 40 times more potent than cortisol when administered subcutaneously and 25 times more potent when administered orally in the rat thymus involution assay. The clinical significance of this is unknown.
The activity of PULMICORT FLEXHALER is due to the parent drug, budesonide. In glucocorticoid receptor affinity studies, the 22R form was two times as active as the 22S epimer. *In vitro* studies indicated that the two forms of budesonide do not interconvert.
The precise mechanism of corticosteroid actions on inflammation in asthma is not known. Inflammation is an important component in the pathogenesis of asthma. Corticosteroids have a wide range of inhibitory activities against multiple cell types (e.g., mast cells, eosinophils, neutrophils, macrophages, and lymphocytes) and mediators (e.g., histamine, eicosanoids, leukotrienes, and cytokines) involved in allergic and non-allergic-mediated inflammation. These anti-inflammatory actions of corticosteroids may contribute to their efficacy in asthma.
Studies in asthmatic patients have shown a favorable ratio between topical anti-inflammatory activity and systemic corticosteroid effects over a wide range of doses of inhaled budesonide. This is explained by a combination of a relatively high local anti-inflammatory effect, extensive first pass hepatic degradation of orally absorbed drug (85-95%), and the low potency of formed metabolites (see below).

12.2 Pharmacodynamics
To confirm that systemic absorption is not a significant factor in the clinical efficacy of inhaled budesonide, a clinical study in patients with asthma was performed comparing 400 mcg budesonide administered via a pressurized metered-dose inhaler with a tube spacer to 1400 mcg of oral budesonide and placebo. The study demonstrated the efficacy of inhaled budesonide but not orally administered budesonide, even though systemic budesonide exposure was comparable for both treatments, indicating that the inhaled treatment is working locally in the lung. Thus, the therapeutic effect of conventional doses of orally inhaled budesonide are largely explained by its direct action on the respiratory tract.
Inhaled budesonide has been shown to decrease airway reactivity in various challenge models, including histamine, methacholine, sodium metabisulfite, and adenosine monophosphate in patients with hyperreactive airways. The clinical relevance of these models is not certain.

Pre-treatment with inhaled budesonide 1600 mcg daily (800 mcg twice daily) for 2 weeks reduced the acute (early-phase reaction) and delayed (late-phase reaction) decrease in FEV_1 following inhaled allergen challenge.

HPA Axis effects: The effects of inhaled budesonide on the hypothalamic-pituitary-adrenal (HPA) axis were studied in 905 adults and 404 pediatric patients with asthma. For most patients, the ability to increase cortisol production in response to stress, as assessed by cosyntropin (ACTH) stimulation test, remained intact with inhaled budesonide treatment at recommended doses. For adult patients treated with 100, 200, 400, or 800 mcg twice daily for 12 weeks, 4%, 2%, 6%, and 13% respectively, had an abnormal stimulated cortisol response (peak cortisol <14.5 mcg/dL assessed by liquid chromatography following short-cosyntropin test) as compared with 8% of patients treated with placebo. Similar results were obtained in pediatric patients. In another study in adults, doses of 400, 800 and 1600 mcg of inhaled budesonide twice daily for 6 weeks were examined; 1600 mcg twice daily (twice the maximum recommended dose) resulted in a 27% reduction in stimulated cortisol (6-hour ACTH infusion) while 10 mg prednisone resulted in a 35% reduction. In this study, no patient taking doses of 400 and 800 mcg twice daily met the criterion for an abnormal stimulated cortisol response (peak cortisol <14.5 mcg/dL assessed by liquid chromatography) following ACTH infusion. An open-label, long-term follow-up of 1133 patients for up to 52 weeks confirmed the minimal effect on the HPA axis (both basal and stimulated plasma cortisol) of inhaled budesonide when administered at doses ranging from 100 to 800 mcg twice daily. In patients who had previously been oral steroid-dependent, use of inhaled budesonide at doses ranging from 100 to 800 mcg twice daily was associated with higher stimulated cortisol response compared with baseline following 1 year of therapy.

12.3 Pharmacokinetics

Absorption

After oral administration of budesonide, peak plasma concentration was achieved in about 1 to 2 hours and the absolute systemic availability was 6-13%. In contrast, most of budesonide delivered to the lungs is systemically absorbed. In healthy subjects, 34% of the metered dose was deposited in the lungs (as assessed by plasma concentration method and using a different budesonide containing dry-powder inhaler) with an absolute systemic availability of 39% of the metered dose. Peak steady-state plasma concentrations of budesonide delivered from PULMICORT FLEXHALER in adults with asthma (n=39) occurred at approximately 10 minutes post-dose and averaged 0.6 and 1.6 nmol/L at doses of 180 mcg once daily and 360 mcg twice daily, respectively. In asthmatic patients, budesonide showed a linear increase in AUC and C_{max} with increasing dose after both a single dose and repeated dosing of inhaled budesonide.

Distribution

The volume of distribution of budesonide was approximately 3 L/kg. It was 85-90% bound to plasma proteins. Protein binding was constant over the concentration range (1-100 nmol/L) achieved with, and exceeding, recommended doses of PULMICORT FLEXHALER. Budesonide showed little or no binding to corticosteroid binding globulin. Budesonide rapidly equilibrated with red blood cells in a concentration independent manner with a blood/plasma ratio of about 0.8.

Metabolism

In vitro studies with human liver homogenates have shown that budesonide is rapidly and extensively metabolized. Two major metabolites formed via cytochrome P450 (CYP) isoenzyme 3A4 (CYP3A4) catalyzed biotransformation have been isolated and identified as 16α-hydroxyprednisolone and 6β-hydroxybudesonide. The corticosteroid activity of each of these two metabolites is less than 1% of that of the parent compound. No qualitative differences between the *in vitro* and *in vivo* metabolic patterns have been detected. Negligible metabolic inactivation was observed in human lung and serum preparations.

Excretion/Elimination

The 22R form of budesonide was preferentially cleared by the liver with systemic clearance of 1.4 L/min vs. 1.0 L/min for the 22S form. The terminal half-life, 2 to 3 hours, was the same for both epimers and was independent of dose. Budesonide was excreted in urine and feces in the form of metabolites. Approximately 60% of an intravenous radiolabeled dose was recovered in the urine. No unchanged budesonide was detected in the urine.

Special Populations

No clinically relevant pharmacokinetic differences have been identified due to race, sex, or advanced age.

Geriatric

The pharmacokinetics of PULMICORT FLEXHALER in geriatric patients have not been specifically studied.

Pediatric

Following intravenous dosing in pediatric patients age 10-14 years, plasma half-life was shorter than in adults (1.5 hours vs. 2.0 hours in adults). In the same population following inhalation of budesonide via a pressurized metered-dose inhaler, absolute systemic availability was similar to that in adults.

Peak steady-state plasma concentrations of budesonide delivered via PULMICORT FLEXHALER in children and adolescents with asthma (n=14) occurred at approximately 15 to 30 minutes post-dose and averaged 0.4 and 1.5 nmol/L at doses of 180 mcg once daily and 360 mcg twice daily, respectively.

Nursing Mothers

The disposition of budesonide when delivered by inhalation from a dry powder inhaler at doses of 200 or 400 mcg twice daily for at least 3 months was studied in eight lactating women with asthma from 1 to 6 months postpartum. Systemic exposure to budesonide in these women appears to be comparable to that in non-lactating women with asthma from other studies. Breast milk obtained over eight hours post-dose revealed that the maximum concentration of budesonide for the 400 and 800 mcg doses was 0.39 and 0.78 nmol/L, respectively, and occurred within 45 minutes after dosing. The estimated oral daily dose of budesonide from breast milk to the infant is approximately 0.007 and 0.014 mcg/kg/day for the two dose regimens used in this study, which represents approximately 0.3% to 1% of the dose inhaled by the mother. Budesonide levels in plasma samples obtained from five infants at about 90 minutes after breastfeeding (and about 140 minutes after drug administration to the mother) were below quantifiable levels (<0.02 nmol/L in four infants and <0.04 nmol/L in one infant) [see *Use In Specific Populations, Nursing Mothers (8.3)*].

Renal or Hepatic Insufficiency

There are no data regarding the specific use of PULMICORT FLEXHALER in patients with hepatic or renal impairment. Reduced liver function may affect the elimination of corticosteroids. The pharmacokinetics of budesonide were affected by compromised liver function as evidenced by a doubled systemic availability after oral ingestion. The intravenous pharmacokinetics of budesonide were, however, similar in cirrhotic patients and in healthy subjects.

Drug-Drug Interactions

Inhibitors of cytochrome P450 enzymes

Ketoconazole: Ketoconazole, a strong inhibitor of cytochrome P450 (CYP) isoenzyme 3A4 (CYP3A4), the main metabolic enzyme for corticosteroids, increased plasma levels of orally ingested budesonide [see *Warnings and Precautions (5.7) and Drug Interactions (7.1)*].

Cimetidine: At recommended doses, cimetidine, a nonspecific inhibitor of CYP enzymes, had a slight but clinically insignificant effect on the pharmacokinetics of oral budesonide.

13 NONCLINICAL TOXICOLOGY

13.1 Carcinogenesis, Mutagenesis, Impairment of Fertility

In a 104-week oral study in Sprague-Dawley rats, a statistically significant increase in the incidence of gliomas was observed in male rats receiving an oral dose of 50 mcg/kg/day (approximately 0.3 times the maximum recommended daily inhalation dose in adults and children 6 to 17 years of age respectively, on a mcg/m^2 basis). No tumorigenicity was seen in male rats at oral doses up to 25 mcg/kg (approximately 0.1 and 0.2 times, respectively, the maximum recommended daily inhalation dose in adults and children 6 to 17 years of age, on a mcg/m^2 basis) and in female rats at oral doses up to 50 mc/kg (approximately 0.3 times the maximum recommended daily inhalation doses in adults and children 6 to 17 years of age, respectively, on a mcg/m^2 basis). In two additional two-year studies in male Fischer and Sprague-Dawley rats, budesonide caused no gliomas at an oral dose of 50 mcg/kg (approximately 0.3 times the maximum recommended daily inhalation dose in adults and children 6 to 17 years of age, respectively, on a mcg/m^2 basis). However, in the male Sprague-Dawley rats, budesonide caused a statistically significant increase in the incidence of hepatocellular tumors at an oral dose of 50 mcg/kg (approximately 0.3 times the maximum recommended daily inhalation doses in adults and children 6 to 17 years of age on a mcg/m^2 basis). The concurrent reference corticosteroids (prednisone and triamcinolone acetonide) in these two studies showed similar findings.

There was no evidence of a carcinogenic effect when budesonide was administered orally for 91 weeks to mice at doses up to 200 mcg/kg/day (approximately 0.6 and 0.7 times, respectively the maximum recommended daily inhalation dose in adults and children 6 to 17 years of age on a mcg/m^2 basis). Budesonide was not mutagenic or clastogenic in six different test systems: Ames *Salmonella*/microsome plate test, mouse micronucleus test, mouse lymphoma test, chromosome aberration test in human lymphocytes, sex-linked recessive lethal test in *Drosophila melanogaster*, and DNA repair analysis in rat hepatocyte culture.

In rats, budesonide had no effect on fertility at subcutaneous doses up to 80 mcg/kg (approximately 0.5 times the maximum recommended daily inhalation dose in adults on a mcg/m^2 basis).

At a subcutaneous dose of 20 mcg/kg/day (approximately 0.1 times the maximum recommended daily inhalation dose in adults on a mcg/m^2 basis), decreases in maternal body weight gain, prenatal viability, and viability of the young at birth and during lactation were observed. No such effects were noted at 5 mcg/kg (approximately 0.03 times the maximum recommended daily inhalation dose in adults on a mcg/m^2 basis).

13.2 Animal Toxicology

Reproductive Toxicology Studies

As with other corticosteroids, budesonide was teratogenic and embryocidal in rabbits and rats. Budesonide produced fetal loss, decreased pup weights, and skeletal abnormalities at a subcutaneous dose of 25 mcg/kg in rabbits (approximately 0.3 times the maximum recommended daily inhalation dose in adults on a mcg/m^2 basis) and at a subcutaneous dose of 500 mcg/kg in rats (approximately 3 times the maximum recommended daily inhalation dose in adults on a mcg/m^2 basis). No teratogenic or embryocidal effects were observed in rats when budesonide was administered by inhalation at doses up to 250 mcg/kg (approximately equivalent to the maximum recommended daily inhalation dose in adults on a mcg/m^2 basis).

14 CLINICAL STUDIES

14.1 Asthma

The safety and efficacy of PULMICORT FLEXHALER were evaluated in two 12-week, double-blind, randomized, parallel-group, placebo-controlled clinical studies conducted at sites in the United States and Asia involving 1137 patients aged 6 to 80 years with mild to moderate asthma. Study 1 evaluated PULMICORT FLEXHALER 180 mcg, PULMICORT TURBUHALER 200 mcg, and placebo, each administered as 1 inhalation once daily or 2 inhalations twice daily in patients 18 years of age and older with mild to moderate asthma previously treated with inhaled corticosteroids. The delivered dose of PULMICORT FLEXHALER 180 mcg and PULMICORT TURBUHALER 200 mcg are the same; each delivers 160 mcg from the mouthpiece. Study 2 evaluated PULMICORT FLEXHALER 90 mcg, 2 inhalations once daily or 4 inhalations twice daily, PULMICORT TURBUHALER 200 mcg, 1 inhalation once daily or 2 inhalations twice daily, and placebo in pediatric patients aged 6 to 17 years with mild to moderate asthma. Both of the studies had a 2-week placebo treatment run-in period followed by a 12-week randomized treatment period. The primary endpoint was the difference between baseline and the mean of the treatment-period FEV_1 (adults) or FEV_1 % predicted (children).

Patients ≥ 18 years of age and older (Study 1)

This study enrolled 621 patients aged ≥18 to 80 years with mild-to-moderate asthma (mean baseline % predicted FEV_1 64.3%) whose symptoms were previously controlled on inhaled corticosteroids. Mean change from baseline in FEV_1 in the PULMICORT FLEXHALER 180 mcg, 2 inhalations twice-daily group was 0.28 liters, as compared to 0.10 liters in the placebo group (p<0.001). Secondary endpoints of morning and evening peak expiratory flow rate, daytime asthma symptom severity, nighttime asthma symptom severity, daily rescue medication use, and the percentage of patients who met predefined asthma related withdrawal criteria showed differences from baseline favoring PULMICORT FLEXHALER over placebo (p<0.001).

12-Week Trial in Adult Patients with Mild Moderate Asthma (Study 1) Mean Change from Baseline in FEV_1 (L)

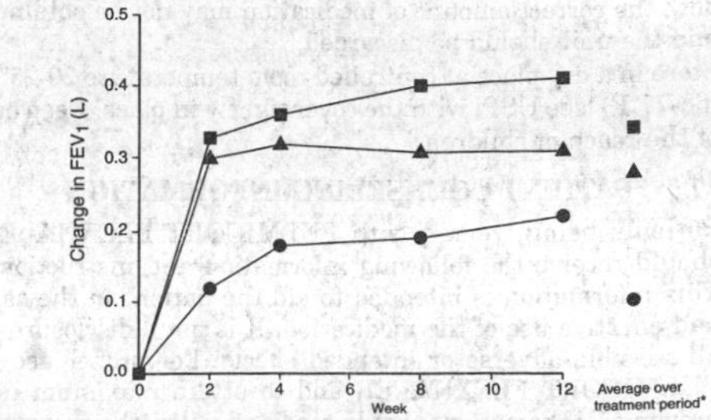

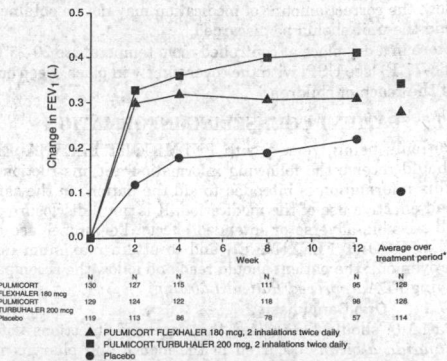

	N	N	N	N	N	N
PULMICORT FLEXHALER 180 mcg	130	127	115	111	95	128
PULMICORT TURBUHALER 200 mcg	129	124	122	118	98	128
Placebo	119	113	86	78	57	114

▲ PULMICORT FLEXHALER 180 mcg, 2 inhalations twice daily
■ PULMICORT TURBUHALER 200 mcg, 2 inhalations twice daily
● Placebo

* Average over treatment period; values are adjusted treatment means for the average difference during the treatment period using last observation carried forward (primary endpoint).
Comparison of PULMICORT FLEXHALER 180 mcg, 2 inhalations twice daily vs placebo for Average over treatment period: p<0.001
One inhalation of PULMICORT FLEXHALER 180 mcg and one inhalation of PULMICORT TURBUHALER 200 mcg result in the same delivered dose of 160 mcg.

Footnote: PULMICORT TURBUHALER; a different PULMICORT DPI. Statistical model is analysis of covariance with treatment and region (US/Asia) as factors and the baseline value as the covariate.

Patients 6 to 17 years of age (Study 2)

This study enrolled 516 patients aged 6 to 17 years with mild asthma (mean baseline % predicted FEV_1 84.9%). The study population included patients previously treated with inhaled corticosteroids for no more than 30 days before the study began (4%) and patients who were naïve to inhaled corticosteroids (96%). Mean change from baseline in % predicted FEV_1 during the 12-week treatment period in the PULMICORT FLEXHALER 90 mcg, 4 inhalations twice daily treatment group was 5.6 compared with 0.2 in the placebo group (p<0.001). Secondary endpoints of morning and evening PEF showed differences from baseline favoring PULMICORT FLEXHALER over placebo (p<0.001).

12-Week Trial in Pediatric Patients With Mild Asthma (Study 2)
Mean Change from Baseline in Percent Predicted FEV_1

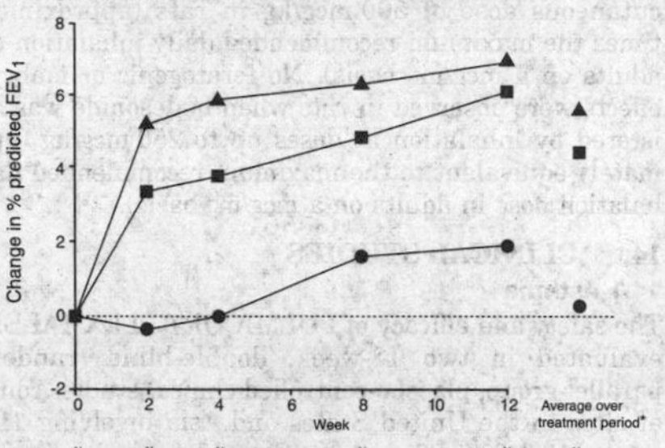

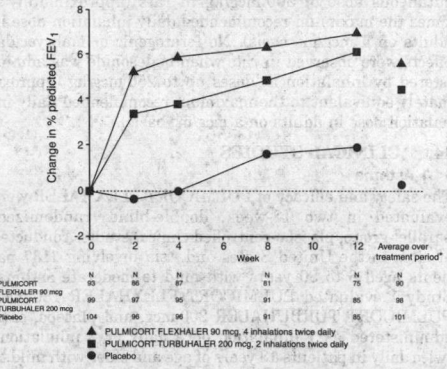

	N (0)	N (2)	N (4)	N (8)	N (12)	N (Average)
PULMICORT FLEXHALER 90 mcg	93	86	87	81	75	90
PULMICORT TURBUHALER 200 mcg	99	97	95	91	85	98
Placebo	104	96	96	91	85	101

▲ PULMICORT FLEXHALER 90 mcg, 4 inhalations twice daily
■ PULMICORT TURBUHALER 200 mcg, 2 inhalations twice daily
● Placebo

* Average over treatment period: values are adjusted treatment means for the average difference during the treatment period using last observation carried forward (primary endpoint).
Comparison of PULMICORT FLEXHALER 90 mcg, 4 inhalations twice daily vs placebo for Average over treatment period: p<0.001
Two inhalations of PULMICORT FLEXHALER 90 mcg and one inhalation of PULMICORT TURBUHALER 200 mcg result in the same delivered dose of 160 mcg.

Footnote: PULMICORT TURBUHALER; a different PULMICORT DPI. Statistical model is analysis of covariance with treatment and region (US/Asia) as factors and the baseline value as the covariate.

16 HOW SUPPLIED/STORAGE AND HANDLING

PULMICORT FLEXHALER is available as a dry powder for inhalation containing budesonide in the following 2 strengths: 90 mcg and 180 mcg. Each dosage strength contains 60 or 120 actuations per device. 180 mcg/dose (NDC 0186-0916-12) with a target fill weight of 225 mg (range 200-250), and 90 mcg/dose, 60 dose (NDC 0186-0917-06) with a target fill weight of 165 mg (range 140-190).

PULMICORT FLEXHALER consists of a number of assembled plastic details, the main parts being the dosing mechanism, the storage unit for drug substance, and the mouthpiece. The inhaler is protected by a white outer tubular cover screwed onto the inhaler. The body of the inhaler is white and the turning grip is brown. The PULMICORT FLEXHALER inhaler cannot be refilled and should be discarded when empty.

The number in the middle of the dose indicator window shows how many doses are left in the inhaler. The inhaler is empty when the number zero ("0") on the red background reaches the middle of the window. If the unit is used beyond the point at which the zero reaches the middle of the window, the correct amount of medication may not be obtained and the unit should be discarded.

Store in a dry place at controlled room temperature 20-25°C (68-77°F) [see USP] with the cover tightly in place. Keep out of the reach of children.

17 PATIENT COUNSELING INFORMATION

Patients being treated with PULMICORT FLEXHALER should receive the following information and instructions. This information is intended to aid the patient in the safe and effective use of the medication. It is not a disclosure of all possible adverse or intended effects. For proper use of PULMICORT FLEXHALER and to attain maximum improvement, the patient should read and follow the accompanying *FDA Approved Patient Labeling*.

17.1 Oral Candidiasis

Patients should be advised that localized infections with *Candida albicans* occurred in the mouth and pharynx in some patients. If oropharyngeal candidiasis develops, it should be treated with appropriate local or systemic (i.e. oral) antifungal therapy while still continuing therapy with PULMICORT FLEXHALER, but at times therapy with PULMICORT FLEXHALER may need to be temporarily interrupted under close medical supervision. Rinsing the mouth after inhalation is advised. [see *Warnings and Precautions (5.1)*]

17.2 Not for Acute Symptoms

PULMICORT FLEXHALER is not meant to relieve acute asthma symptoms and extra doses should not be used for that purpose. Acute symptoms should be treated with an inhaled, short-acting beta$_2$-agonist such as albuterol (The physician should provide that patient with such medication and instruct the patient in how it should be used.)

Patients should be instructed to notify their physician immediately if they experience any of the following:

- Decreasing effectiveness of inhaled, short-acting beta$_2$-agonists
- Need for more inhalations than usual of inhaled, short-acting beta$_2$-agonists
- Significant decrease in lung function as outlined by the physician

Patients should not stop therapy with PULMICORT FLEXHALER without physician/provider guidance since symptoms may recur after discontinuation. [see *Warnings and Precautions (5.1)*]

17.3 Hypersensitivity including Anaphylaxis

Hypersensitivity reactions including anaphylaxis, rash, contact dermatitis, urticaria, angioedema, and bronchospasm have been reported with use of PULMICORT FLEXHALER. Discontinue PULMICORT FLEXHALER if such reactions occur [see *Contraindications (4), Warnings and Precautions (5.3), and Adverse Reactions (6)*].

PULMICORT FLEXHALER contains small amounts of lactose, which contains trace levels of milk proteins. It is possible that cough, wheezing, or bronchospasm may occur in patients who have a severe milk protein allergy [see *Contraindications (4)*].

17.4 Immunosuppression

Patients who are on immunosuppressant doses of corticosteroids should be warned to avoid exposure to chickenpox or measles and, if exposed, to consult their physician without delay. Patients should be informed of potential worsening of existing tuberculosis, fungal, bacterial, viral, or parasitic infections, or ocular herpes simplex [see *Warnings and Precautions (5.4)*].

17.5 Hypercorticism and Adrenal Suppression

Patients should be advised that PULMICORT FLEXHALER may cause systemic corticosteroid effects of hypercorticism and adrenal suppression. Additionally, patients should be instructed that deaths due to adrenal insufficiency have occurred during and after transfer from systemic corticosteroids. Patients should taper slowly from systemic corticosteroids if transferring to PULMICORT FLEXHALER [see *Warnings and Precautions (5.5, 5.6)*].

17.6 Reduction in Bone Mineral Density

Patients who are at an increased risk for decreased BMD should be advised that the use of corticosteroids may pose an additional risk [see *Warnings and Precautions (5.8)*].

17.7 Reduced Growth Velocity

Patients should be informed that orally inhaled corticosteroids, including budesonide inhalation powder, may cause a reduction in growth velocity when administered to pediatric patients. Physicians should closely follow the growth of children and adolescents taking corticosteroids by any route [see *Warnings and Precautions (5.9)*].

17.8 Ocular Effects

Long-term use of inhaled corticosteroids may increase the risk of some eye problems (cataracts or glaucoma); regular eye examinations should be considered [see *Warnings and Precautions (5.10)*].

17.9 Use Daily

Patients should be advised to use PULMICORT FLEXHALER at regular intervals, since its effectiveness depends on regular use. Maximum benefit may not be achieved for 1 to 2 weeks or longer after starting treatment. If symptoms do not improve in that time frame or if the condition worsens, patients should be instructed to contact their physician.

17.10 How to Use Pulmicort Flexhaler

Patients should be carefully instructed on the use of this drug product to assure optimal dose delivery. The patient may not sense the presence of any medication entering their lungs when inhaling from PULMICORT FLEXHALER. This lack of sensation does not mean that they did not get the medication. They should not repeat their inhalation even if they did not feel the medication when inhaling [see *Patient Information*].

17.11 FDA–Approved Patient Labeling

Patient Information

PULMICORT FLEXHALER™ (bew DEH so nide) 180 mcg
(budesonide inhalation powder, 180 mcg)

PULMICORT FLEXHALER™ 90 mcg
(budesonide inhalation powder, 90 mcg)

Important Note: This medicine is to only be inhaled through the mouth (by oral inhalation only).

Read the Patient Information that comes with PULMICORT FLEXHALER before you start using it and each time you get a refill. There may be new information. This leaflet does not take the place of talking to your healthcare provider about your medical condition or treatment.

What is PULMICORT FLEXHALER?

PULMICORT FLEXHALER is an inhaled corticosteroid medicine. PULMICORT FLEXHALER is used for long-term (maintenance) treatment of asthma and to prevent asthma symptoms in adults and children 6 years of age and older. Inhaled corticosteroids help to decrease inflammation in the lungs. Inflammation in the lungs can lead to asthma symptoms.

PULMICORT FLEXHALER helps reduce inflammation and helps keep the airways open to reduce asthma symptoms.

PULMICORT FLEXHALER does not treat the symptoms of a sudden asthma attack. Always have a short-acting beta$_2$-agonist medicine (rescue inhaler) with you to treat sudden symptoms. If you do not have an inhaled, short-acting bronchodilator, call your healthcare provider to have one prescribed for you.

It is not known if PULMICORT FLEXHALER is safe and effective in children younger than 6 years of age.

Who should not use PULMICORT FLEXHALER?

Do not use PULMICORT FLEXHALER:

- to treat sudden severe symptoms of asthma.
- if you have a severe allergy to milk proteins. PULMICORT FLEXHALER contains a small amount of lactose (milk sugar). People with severe allergies to milk protein may have symptoms of an allergic reaction with PULMICORT FLEXHALER including: cough, wheezing, trouble breathing or feeling like your throat is closing.

What should I tell my healthcare provider before using PULMICORT FLEXHALER?

Before using PULMICORT FLEXHALER, tell your healthcare provider if you:

- have any allergies. See the section "Who should not use PULMICORT FLEXHALER". There is a complete list of ingredients in PULMICORT FLEXHALER at the end of this leaflet.
- have or had chicken pox or measles, or have recently been near anyone with chicken pox or measles.
- have or had tuberculosis of your respiratory tract.
- have certain kinds of serious infections that have not been treated, including:
- fungal infections
- bacterial infections
- viral infections
- parasitic infections
- herpes simplex infection of the eye (ocular herpes simplex)

PULMICORT FLEXHALER may not be right for people who have or had any of these types of infections.

- have liver problems
- have decreased bone mineral density.
  You are at risk for decreased bone mineral density if you:
  - are inactive for a long period of time
  - have a family history of osteoporosis
  - are a woman going through menopause or are past menopause ("the change of life")
  - smoke or use tobacco
  - do not eat well (poor nutrition)
  - are elderly
  - take bone thinning medicines (such as anticonvulsant medicines or corticosteroids) for a long time.
- have eye problems such as increased pressure in the eye, glaucoma, or cataracts
- are planning to have surgery
- are pregnant or plan to become pregnant. It is not known if PULMICORT FLEXHALER may harm your unborn baby
- are breast-feeding or plan to breast-feed. PULMICORT FLEXHALER can pass into breast milk. You and your healthcare provider should decide if you will use PULMICORT FLEXHALER or breast-feed

Tell your healthcare provider about all the medicines you take, including prescription and non-prescription medicines, vitamins, and herbal supplements. Using PULMICORT FLEXHALER with certain other medicines may affect each other causing side effects. Especially tell your healthcare provider if you take:

- a corticosteroid medicine
- anti-seizure medicine (anticonvulsants)
- medicines that suppress your immune system (immunosuppressant)
- ketoconazale (Nizoral), other medicines that affect how your liver works.

Ask your healthcare provider or pharmacist if you are not sure if your medicine is one listed above.

Know the medicines you take. Keep a list of them and show it to your healthcare provider and pharmacist when you get a new medicine.

How should I use PULMICORT FLEXHALER?

Use PULMICORT FLEXHALER exactly as prescribed by your healthcare provider. You must use PULMICORT FLEXHALER regularly for it to work.

- PULMICORT FLEXHALER comes in two strengths. Your healthcare provider has prescribed the strength that is best for you.
- Be sure you know the difference between PULMICORT FLEXHALER and any other inhaled medicines that are prescribed for you, including what you use them for (prescribed use) and what they look like.

Do not stop using PULMICORT FLEXHALER, even if your symptoms get better. Your healthcare provider will change your medicines as needed.

- Do not change or stop any medicines used to control or treat your breathing problems, unless your healthcare provider tells you to.
- Rinse your mouth with water and spit the water out after each dose of PULMICORT FLEXHALER. Do not swallow the water. This will lessen the chance of getting a fungal infection (thrush) in the mouth.
- If you miss a dose, just take your next regularly scheduled dose when it is due. **Do not use PULMICORT FLEXHALER more often or use more puffs than you have been prescribed.**
- Make sure you always have a short-acting beta$_2$-agonist medicine with you. Use your short acting beta$_2$-agonist medicine if you have breathing problems between doses of PULMICORT FLEXHALER or if a sudden asthma attack happens. Call your healthcare provider right away if:
  - your short-acting rescue medicine does not work as well for relieving asthma symptoms.
  - you need to use your short-acting rescue medicines more often than usual.
  - your breathing problems worsen with PULMICORT FLEXHALER.

If you use another inhaled medicine by mouth to treat your asthma, talk with your healthcare provider for instructions about when to use the other medicine and when to use your PULMICORT FLEXHALER.

- If you have used corticosteroid medicines for a long time and the dose is now being lowered or stopped, you should carry a medical alert card. The medical alert card should state that you may need increased corticosteroids during times of stress or during an asthma attack that does not get better with bronchodilator medicines.
- Your healthcare provider may check your breathing, do blood tests and eye exams during treatment with PULMICORT FLEXHALER.

Be sure to read, understand and follow the detailed Patient Instructions for Use at the end of this leaflet. These Instructions for Use tell you how to prime and use your PULMICORT FLEXHALER the right way.

What are the possible side effects of PULMICORT FLEXHALER?

PULMICORT FLEXHALER can cause serious side effects, including:

- **thrush (candida), a fungal infection in your mouth and throat.** Tell your healthcare provider if you have any redness or white colored patches in your mouth or throat.
- **worsening of asthma or sudden asthma attacks.**
- **allergic reactions.** Tell your healthcare provider or get medical help right away if you have:
  - skin rash, redness or swelling
  - severe itching
  - swelling of the face, mouth, and tongue
  - trouble breathing or swallowing
  - chest pain
  - anxiety (feeling of doom)
- **Immune system effects and a higher chance of infections.** You are more likely to get infections if you take medicines that weaken your immune system. Avoid contact with people who have contagious diseases such as chicken pox or measles while using PULMICORT FLEXHALER. Symptoms of infection may include: fever, pain, aches, chills, feeling tired, nausea and vomiting. Tell your healthcare provider about any signs of infection while you are using PULMICORT FLEXHALER.
- **Adrenal insufficiency.** Adrenal insufficiency is a condition in which the adrenal glands do not make enough steroid hormones. Symptoms of adrenal insufficiency include: tiredness, weakness, nausea and vomiting and low blood pressure.
- **Decrease in bone mineral density.** Your healthcare provider should check you for this during treatment with PULMICORT FLEXHALER.
- **Slowed or delayed growth problems in children.** A child's growth should be checked regularly while using PULMICORT FLEXHALER.
- **Eye problems, including glaucoma and cataracts.** You should have regular eye exams while using PULMICORT FLEXHALER.

- **Increased wheezing right after taking PULMICORT FLEXHALER. Always have a short-acting beta$_2$-agonist medicine (rescue inhaler) with you to treat sudden wheezing.**

Call your healthcare provider or get medical help right away if you have symptoms of any of the serious side effects listed above.

Common side effects reported by patients using PULMICORT FLEXHALER include:

- sore nose and throat
- stuffy nose
- runny nose
- nausea
- hay fever
- viral infections of the upper respiratory tract
- viral irritation and inflammation of the stomach and intestine (gastroenteritis). Symptoms may include stomach area pain, diarrhea, nausea and vomiting, loss of appetite, headaches, and weakness.
- ear infections

Tell your healthcare provider about any side effect that bothers you or that does not go away.

These are not all of the side effects of PULMICORT FLEXHALER. Ask your healthcare provider or pharmacist for more information.

Call your healthcare provider for medical advice about side effects. You may report side effects to AstraZeneca at 1-800-236-9933 or FDA at 1-800-FDA-1088 or www.fda.gov/medwatch.

How should I store PULMICORT FLEXHALER?

Store PULMICORT FLEXHALER at 68° to 77°F (20° to 25°C).

- Keep PULMICORT FLEXHALER dry.
- Keep your PULMICORT FLEXHALER with the cover tightly in place when not in use.

Keep your PULMICORT FLEXHALER and all medicines out of the reach of children.

General Information about PULMICORT FLEXHALER

Medicines are sometimes prescribed for conditions that are not mentioned in Patient Information Leaflets. Do not use PULMICORT FLEXHALER for a condition for which it was not prescribed. Do not give PULMICORT FLEXHALER to other people, even if they have the same symptoms that you have. It may harm them.

This Patient Information leaflet summarizes the most important information about PULMICORT FLEXHALER. If you would like more information, talk with your healthcare provider. You can ask your pharmacist or healthcare provider for information about PULMICORT FLEXHALER that is written for health professionals.

For more information, go to pulmicortflexhaler.com or call 1-800-236-9933.

What are the ingredients in PULMICORT FLEXHALER?

Active ingredient: budesonide

Inactive ingredient: lactose

Patient Instructions for Use

How to use your PULMICORT FLEXHALER

Parts of your PULMICORT FLEXHALER

Figure 1

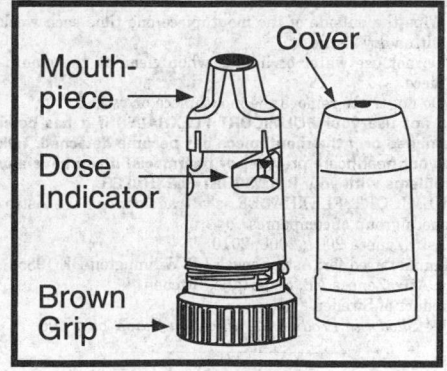

Priming PULMICORT FLEXHALER:

Before you use a new PULMICORT FLEXHALER for the first time, you must prime it.

To prime your PULMICORT FLEXHALER, follow the steps below:

1. Hold the inhaler by the brown grip so that the white cover points upward (upright position). With the other hand, turn the white cover and lift it off (see Figure 2).
2. Continue to hold your PULMICORT FLEXHALER upright as shown in Figure 1. Use your other hand to hold the inhaler in the middle. Do not hold the inhaler at the top of the mouthpiece.
3. Twist the brown grip as far as it will go in one direction and then fully back again in the other direction until it

stops (it does not matter which way you turn it first). You will hear a "click" during one of the twisting movements (see Figures 3 and 4).

4. Repeat Step 3. Your PULMICORT FLEXHALER is now primed. You are ready to load your first dose.

You do not have to prime your PULMICORT FLEXHALER again after this even if you do not use it for a long period of time.

1 Loading a dose

1. Hold your PULMICORT FLEXHALER upright as described above. With your other hand, twist the white cover and lift it off (see Figure 2).

Figure 2

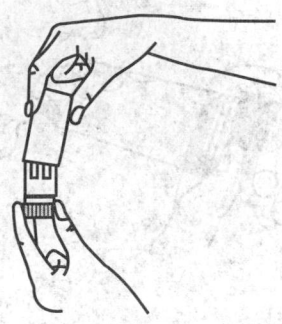

2. Continue to hold your PULMICORT FLEXHALER upright to be sure that the right dose of medicine is loaded.
3. Use your other hand to hold the inhaler in the middle. Do not hold the mouthpiece when you load the inhaler.
4. Twist the brown grip fully in one direction as far as it will go. Twist it fully back again in the other direction as far as it will go (it does not matter which way you turn it first) [see Figure 3].

Figure 3

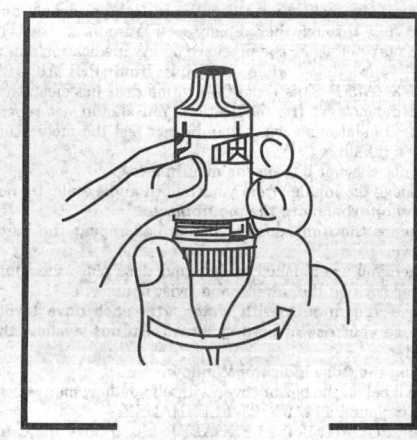

Twist

- You will hear a "click" during one of the twisting movements (see Figure 4).

Figure 4

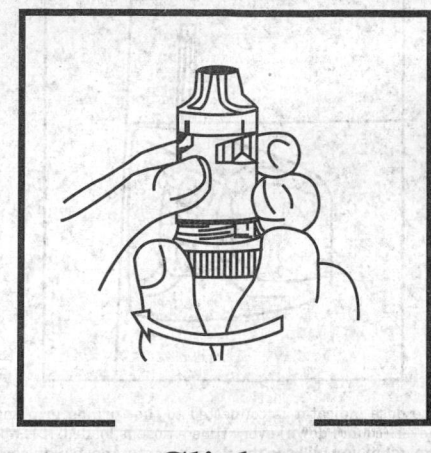

Click

- PULMICORT FLEXHALER will only give one dose at a time, no matter how often you click the brown grip, but the dose indicator will continue to move (advance). This means that if you continue to move the brown grip, it is possible for the indicator to show fewer doses or zero doses even if more doses are left in the inhaler.
- **Do not shake the inhaler after loading it.**

Figure 5
2 Inhaling a dose

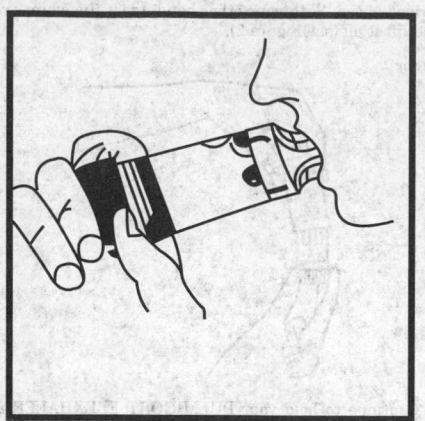

Inhale

1. Turn your head away from the inhaler and breathe out (exhale). If you accidentally blow into your inhaler after loading a dose, follow the instructions for loading a new dose.
2. Place the mouthpiece in your mouth and close your lips around the mouthpiece. Breathe in (inhale) deeply and forcefully through the inhaler (see Figure 5).
3. You may not sense the presence of any medication entering your lungs when inhaling from PULMICORT FLEXHALER. This lack of sensation does not mean that you did not get the medication. You should not repeat your inhalations even if you did not feel the medication when inhaling.
4. Do not chew or bite on the mouthpiece.
5. Remove the inhaler from your mouth and exhale. **Do not blow or exhale into the mouthpiece.**
6. If more than one dose is prescribed repeat the steps above.
7. When you are finished taking your dose place the white cover back on the inhaler and twist shut.
8. **Rinse your mouth with water after each dose to decrease your risk of getting thrush. Do not swallow the water.**

Reading the Dose Indicator Window
- The label on the box or cover will tell you how many doses are in your PULMICORT FLEXHALER.
- Your PULMICORT FLEXHALER has a dose indicator window just below the mouthpiece. The dose indicator tells you about how many doses are left in the inhaler. Look at the middle of the window to find out about how many doses are left in your inhaler (see Figure 6).

Figure 6

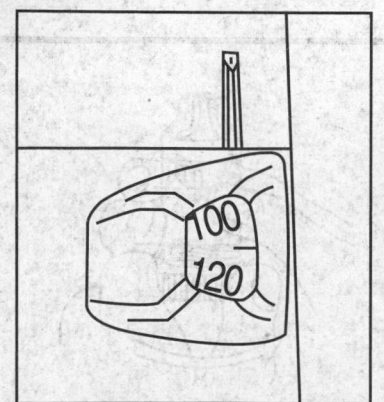

- The dose indicator is connected to the turning grip and moves (counts down) every time a dose is loaded. **It is not likely that you will see the dose indicator move with each dose.** You can usually see the indicator move each time you use about 5 doses.

- The dose indicator starts with either the number 60 or 120 when full, depending on the strength of the inhaler. The indicator is marked in intervals of 10 doses. Markings are either with numbers or dashes (alternating), counting down to "0".

60 Dose Inhaler	120 Dose Inhaler	
20	80	Dose indicator starts at 60 or
-	-	120 depending on strength
40	100	(90 mcg or 180 mcg) of the
-	-	inhaler and counts down to 0.
60	120	

- The dose indicator will tell you about how many doses are left in your PULMICORT FLEXHALER.
- **If you complete the instructions for loading the dose more than one time before you inhale the dose, you will only receive one dose.** The dose indicator will move a small amount but it is not likely that you will see the dose indicator move with each dose.
- **Your inhaler is empty when the number 0 on the red background reaches the middle of the dose indicator window. Throw away this inhaler. The inhaler may not give you the right amount of medicine, even though it may not feel completely empty and may seem like it continues to work (see Figure 7).**

Figure 7

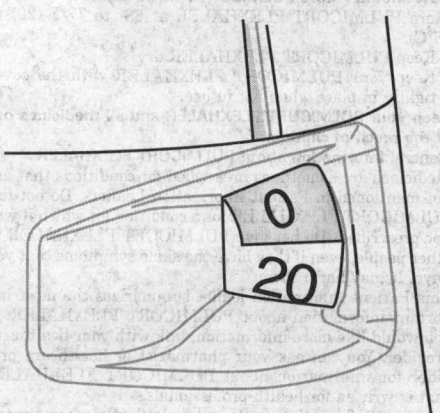

- **Do not put your PULMICORT FLEXHALER in water (do not immerse it) to find out if it is empty. Check the dose indicator window to see how many doses are left.**
- Refill your PULMICORT FLEXHALER prescription before your medicine runs out. You will get a new inhaler each time you refill your prescription.

Cleaning your PULMICORT FLEXHALER
- Keep your PULMICORT FLEXHALER clean and dry at all times. Do not immerse it in water.
- Wipe the outside of the mouthpiece one time each week with a dry tissue.
- Do not use water or liquids when cleaning the mouthpiece.
- Do not try to remove the mouthpiece or twist it.

Do not use your PULMICORT FLEXHALER if it has been damaged or if the mouthpiece has become detached. Talk to your healthcare provider or pharmacist if you have any problems with your PULMICORT FLEXHALER.

PULMICORT FLEXHALER is a trademark of the AstraZeneca group of companies.
©AstraZeneca 2007, 2008, 2010
Manufactured for: AstraZeneca LP, Wilmington DE 19850
By: AstraZeneca AB, Södertälje, Sweden
Product of Sweden

Shown in Product Identification Guide, page 306

SYMBICORT® 80/4.5
[sym-bi-cort]
(budesonide 80 mcg and formoterol fumarate dihydrate 4.5 mcg)
Inhalation Aerosol
SYMBICORT® 160/4.5
(budesonide 160 mcg and formoterol fumarate dihydrate 4.5 mcg)
Inhalation Aerosol
FOR ORAL INHALATION   ℞

HIGHLIGHTS OF PRESCRIBING INFORMATION
These highlights do not include all the information needed to use SYMBICORT safely and effectively. See full prescribing information for SYMBICORT.

SYMBICORT® 80/4.5
(budesonide 80 mcg and formoterol fumarate dihydrate 4.5 mcg) Inhalation Aerosol
SYMBICORT® 160/4.5
(budesonide 160 mcg and formoterol fumarate dihydrate 4.5 mcg) Inhalation Aerosol
FOR ORAL INHALATION
Initial U.S. Approval: 2006

> **WARNING: ASTHMA-RELATED DEATH**
> *(See full prescribing information for complete boxed warning.)*
> - **Long-acting beta$_2$-adrenergic agonists (LABA), such as formoterol one of the active ingredients in SYMBICORT, increase the risk of asthma-related death. A placebo-controlled study with another LABA (salmeterol) showed an increase in asthma-related deaths in patients receiving salmeterol. This finding with salmeterol is considered a class effect of LABAs, including formoterol. Currently available data are inadequate to determine whether concurrent use of an inhaled corticosteroids or other long-term asthma control drugs mitigates the increased risk of asthma-related death from LABA. Available data from controlled clinical trials suggest that LABA may increase the risk of asthma-related hospitalization in pediatric and adolescent patients. (5.1)**
> - **When treating patients with asthma, prescribe SYMBICORT only for patients not adequately controlled on a long-term asthma-control medication, such as an inhaled corticosteroid or whose disease severity clearly warrants initiation of treatment with both an inhaled corticosteroid and LABA. Once asthma control is achieved and maintained, assess the patient at regular intervals and step down therapy (e.g. discontinue SYMBICORT) if possible without loss of asthma control, and maintain the patient on a long-term asthma control medication, such as an inhaled corticosteroid. Do not use SYMBICORT for patients whose asthma is adequately controlled on low or medium dose inhaled corticosteroids. (1.1, 5.1)**

———RECENT MAJOR CHANGES———
Boxed Warning May 2010
Indications and Usage, Treatment of Asthma (1.1) May 2010
Dosage and Administration, Asthma (2.1) May 2010
Warnings and Precautions, Asthma-Related Death (5.1) May 2010

———INDICATIONS AND USAGE———
SYMBICORT is a combination product containing a corticosteroid and a long-acting beta$_2$-adrenergic agonist indicated for:
- Treatment of asthma in patients 12 years of age and older. (1.1)
- Maintenance treatment of airflow obstruction in patients with chronic obstructive pulmonary disease (COPD) including chronic bronchitis and emphysema. (1.2)

Important limitations:
- Not indicated for the relief of acute bronchospasm. (1.1, 1.2)

———DOSAGE AND ADMINISTRATION———
For oral inhalation only.
- Treatment of asthma in patients >12 years: 2 inhalations twice daily of SYMBICORT 80/4.5 or 160/4.5. Starting dosage is based on asthma severity. (2.1)
- Maintenance treatment of airflow obstruction in COPD: 2 inhalations of SYMBICORT 160/4.5 twice daily (2.2)

———DOSAGE FORMS AND STRENGTHS———
Metered-dose inhaler containing a combination of budesonide (80 or 160 mcg) and formoterol (4.5 mcg) as an inhalation aerosol (3)

———CONTRAINDICATIONS———
- Primary treatment of status asthmaticus or acute episodes of asthma or COPD requiring intensive measures. (4)
- Hypersensitivity to any of the ingredients in SYMBICORT (4)

———WARNINGS AND PRECAUTIONS———
- Asthma-related death: Long-acting beta$_2$-adrenergic agonists increase the risk. Prescribe only for recommended patient populations. (5.1)
- Deterioration of disease and acute episodes: Do not initiate in acutely deteriorating asthma or to treat acute symptoms. (5.2)
- Use with additional long-acting beta$_2$-agonist: Do not use in combination because of risk of overdose. (5.3)
- Localized infections: *Candida albicans* infection of the mouth and throat may occur. Monitor patients periodically for signs of adverse effects on the oral cavity. Advise patients to rinse the mouth following inhalation. (5.4)

- Pneumonia: Increased risk in patients with COPD. Monitor patients for signs and symptoms of pneumonia and other potential lung infections. (5.5)
- Immunosuppression: Potential worsening of infections (e.g., existing tuberculosis, fungal, bacterial, viral, or parasitic infection; or ocular herpes simplex). Use with caution in patients with these infections. More serious or even fatal course of chickenpox or measles can occur in susceptible patients. (5.6)
- Transferring patients from systemic corticosteroids: Risk of impaired adrenal function when transferring from oral steroids. Taper patients slowly from systemic corticosteroids if transferring to SYMBICORT. (5.7)
- Hypercorticism and adrenal suppression: May occur with very high dosages or at the regular dosage in susceptible individuals. If such changes occur, discontinue SYMBICORT slowly. (5.8)
- Strong cytochrome P450 3A4 inhibitors (e.g., ritonavir): Risk of increased systemic corticosteroid effects. Exercise caution when used with SYMBICORT. (5.9)
- Paradoxical bronchospasm: Discontinue SYMBICORT and institute alternative therapy if paradoxical bronchospasm occurs. (5.10)
- Patients with cardiovascular or central nervous system disorders: Use with caution because of beta-adrenergic stimulation. (5.12)
- Decreases in bone mineral density: Assess bone mineral density initially and periodically thereafter. (5.13)
- Effects on growth: Monitor growth of pediatric patients. (5.14)
- Glaucoma and cataracts: Close monitoring is warranted. (5.15)
- Metabolic effects: Be alert to eosinophilic conditions, hypokalemia, and hyperglycemia. (5.16, 5.18)
- Coexisting conditions: Use with caution in patients with convulsive disorders, thyrotoxicosis, diabetes mellitus, and ketoacidosis. (5.17)

―――――ADVERSE REACTIONS―――――

Most common adverse reactions (incidence ≥ 3%) are:
- Asthma: nasopharyngitis, headache, upper respiratory tract infection, pharygolaryngeal pain, sinusitis, influenza, back pain, nasal congestion, stomach discomfort, vomiting, and oral candidiasis. (6.1)
- COPD: nasopharyngitis, oral candidiasis, bronchitis, sinusitis, upper respiratory tract infections. (6.2)

To report SUSPECTED ADVERSE REACTIONS, contact AstraZeneca at 1-800-236-9933 or FDA at 1-800-FDA-1088 or www.fda.gov/medwatch.

―――――DRUG INTERACTIONS―――――

- Strong cytochrome P450 3A4 inhibitors (e.g., ritonavir): Use with caution. May cause increased systemic corticosteroid effects.
- Monoamine oxidase inhibitors and tricyclic antidepressants: Use with extreme caution. May potentiate effect of formoterol on vascular system. (7.2)
- Beta-blockers: Use with caution. May block bronchodilatory effects of beta-agonists and produce severe bronchospasm. (7.3)
- Diuretics: Use with caution. Electrocardiographic changes and/or hypokalemia associated with nonpotassium-sparing diuretics may worsen with concomitant beta-agonists. (7.4)

―――――USE IN SPECIFIC POPULATIONS―――――

Hepatic impairment: Monitor patients for signs of increased drug exposure. (8)

See 17 for PATIENT COUNSELING INFORMATION and Medication Guide

Revised: 06/2010

FULL PRESCRIBING INFORMATION: CONTENTS*
WARNING: ASTHMA-RELATED DEATH

* Sections or subsections omitted from the full prescribing information are not listed

FULL PRESCRIBING INFORMATION

―――――――――――――――――――――――――――――

WARNING: ASTHMA-RELATED DEATH
Long-acting beta₂-adrenergic agonists (LABA), such as formoterol one of the active ingredients in SYMBICORT, increase the risk of asthma-related death. Data from a large placebo-controlled U.S. study that compared the safety of another long-acting beta₂-adrenergic agonist (salmeterol) or placebo added to usual asthma therapy showed an increase in asthma-related deaths in patients receiving salmeterol. This finding with salmeterol is considered a class effect of the LABA, including formoterol. Currently available data are inadequate to determine whether concurrent use of inhaled corticosteroids or other long-term asthma control drugs mitigates the increased risk of asthma-related death from LABA. Available data from controlled clinical trials suggest that LABA increase the risk of asthma-related hospitalization in pediatric and adolescent patients. Therefore, when treating patients with asthma, SYMBICORT should be used for patients not adequately controlled on a long-term asthma control medication, such as an inhaled corticosteroid or whose disease severity clearly warrants initiation of treatment with both an inhaled corticosteroid and LABA. Once asthma control is achieved and maintained, assess the patient at regular intervals and step down therapy (e.g., discontinue SYMBICORT) if possible without loss of asthma control and maintain the patient on a long-term asthma control medication, such as an inhaled corticosteroid. Do not use SYMBICORT for patients whose asthma is adequately controlled on low or medium dose inhaled corticosteroids [see Warnings and Precautions (5.1)].

1 INDICATIONS AND USAGE

1.1 Treatment of Asthma

SYMBICORT is indicated for the treatment of asthma in patients 12 years of age and older.

Long-acting beta₂-adrenergic agonists, such as formoterol one of the active ingredients in SYMBICORT, increase the risk of asthma-related death. Available data from controlled clinical trials suggest that LABA increase the risk of asthma-related hospitalization in pediatric and adolescent patients [see Warnings and Precautions (5.1)]. Therefore, when treating patients with asthma, SYMBICORT should only be used for patients not adequately controlled on a long-term asthma-control medication such as an inhaled corticosteroid or whose disease severity clearly warrants initiation of treatment with both an inhaled corticosteroid and LABA. Once asthma control is achieved and maintained, assess the patient at regular intervals and step down therapy (e.g. discontinue SYMBICORT) if possible without loss of asthma control, and maintain the patient on a long-term asthma control medication, such as inhaled corticosteroid. Do not use SYMBICORT for patients whose asthma is adequately controlled on low or medium dose inhaled corticosteroids.

Important Limitations of Use:
- SYMBICORT is NOT indicated for the relief of acute bronchospasm.

1.2 Maintenance Treatment of Chronic Obstructive Pulmonary Disease (COPD)

SYMBICORT 160/4.5 is indicated for the twice daily maintenance treatment of airflow obstruction in patients with chronic obstructive pulmonary disease (COPD) including chronic bronchitis and emphysema. SYMBICORT 160/4.5 is the only approved dosage for the treatment of airflow obstruction in COPD.

Important Limitations of Use: SYMBICORT is not indicated for the relief of acute bronchospasm.

2 DOSAGE AND ADMINISTRATION

SYMBICORT should be administered twice daily every day by the orally inhaled route only. After inhalation, the patient should rinse the mouth with water without swallowing. [see Patient Counseling Information (17.4)]

Prime SYMBICORT before using for the first time by releasing two test sprays into the air away from the face, shaking well for 5 seconds before each spray. In cases where the inhaler has not been used for more than 7 days or when it has been dropped, prime the inhaler again by shaking well before each spray and releasing two test sprays into the air away from the face.

More frequent administration or a higher number of inhalations (more than 2 inhalations twice daily) of the prescribed strength of SYMBICORT is not recommended as some patients are more likely to experience adverse effects with higher doses of formoterol. Patients using SYMBICORT should not use additional long-acting beta₂-agonists for any reason. [See Warnings and Precautions (5.3, 5.12)]

2.1 Asthma

If asthma symptoms arise in the period between doses, an inhaled, short-acting beta₂-agonist should be taken for immediate relief.

Adult and Adolescent Patients 12 Years of Age and Older: For patients 12 years of age and older, the dosage is 2 inhalations twice daily (morning and evening, approximately 12 hours apart).

The recommended starting dosages for SYMBICORT for patients 12 years of age and older are based upon patients' asthma severity.

The maximum recommended dosage is SYMBICORT 160/4.5 mcg twice daily.

Improvement in asthma control following inhaled administration of SYMBICORT can occur within 15 minutes of beginning treatment, although maximum benefit may not be achieved for 2 weeks or longer after beginning treatment. Individual patients will experience a variable time to onset and degree of symptom relief.

For patients who do not respond adequately to the starting dose after 1-2 weeks of therapy with SYMBICORT 80/4.5, replacement with SYMBICORT 160/4.5 may provide additional asthma control.

If a previously effective dosage regimen of SYMBICORT fails to provide adequate control of asthma, the therapeutic regimen should be re-evaluated and additional therapeutic options, (e.g., replacing the lower strength of SYMBICORT with the higher strength, adding additional inhaled corticosteroid, or initiating oral corticosteroids) should be considered.

2.2 Chronic Obstructive Pulmonary Disease (COPD)

For patients with COPD the recommended dose is SYMBICORT 160/4.5, two inhalations twice daily.

If shortness of breath occurs in the period between doses, an inhaled, short-acting beta₂-agonist should be taken for immediate relief.

3 DOSAGE FORMS AND STRENGTHS

SYMBICORT is available as a metered-dose inhaler containing a combination of budesonide (80 or 160 mcg) and formoterol (4.5 mcg) as an inhalation aerosol in the following two strengths: 80/4.5 and 160/4.5. Each dosage strength contains 60 or 120 actuations per/canister. Each strength of SYMBICORT is supplied with a red plastic actuator with a gray dust cap.

4 CONTRAINDICATIONS

The use of SYMBICORT is contraindicated in the following conditions:

• Primary treatment of status asthmaticus or other acute episodes of asthma or COPD where intensive measures are required.
• Hypersensitivity to any of the ingredients in SYMBICORT.

5 WARNINGS AND PRECAUTIONS

5.1 Asthma-Related Death

Long-acting beta$_2$-adrenergic agonists, such as formoterol, one of the active ingredients in SYMBICORT, increase the risk of asthma-related death. Currently available data are inadequate to determine whether concurrent use of inhaled corticosteroids or other long-term asthma control drugs mitigates the increased risk of asthma-related death from LABA. Available data from controlled clinical trials suggest that LABA increase the risk of asthma-related hospitalization in pediatric and adolescent patients. Therefore, when treating patients with asthma, SYMBICORT should only be used for patients not adequately controlled on a long-term asthma-control medication, such as an inhaled corticosteroid or whose disease severity clearly warrants initiation of treatment with both an inhaled corticosteroid and LABA. Once asthma control is achieved and maintained, assess the patient at regular intervals and step down therapy (e.g. discontinue SYMBICORT) if possible without loss of asthma control, and maintain the patient on a long-term asthma control medication, such as an inhaled corticosteroid. Do not use SYMBICORT for patients whose asthma is adequately controlled on low or medium dose inhaled corticosteroids.

A 28-week, placebo controlled US study comparing the safety of salmeterol with placebo, each added to usual asthma therapy, showed an increase in asthma-related deaths in patients receiving salmeterol (13/13,176 in patients treated with salmeterol vs 3/13,179 in patients treated with placebo; RR 4.37, 95% CI 1.25, 15.34). This finding with salmeterol is considered a class effect of the LABA, including formoterol, one of the active ingredients in SYMBICORT. No study adequate to determine whether the rate of asthma-related death is increased with SYMBICORT has been conducted.

Clinical studies with formoterol suggested a higher incidence of serious asthma exacerbations in patients who received formoterol than in those who received placebo. The sizes of these studies were not adequate to precisely quantify the differences in serious asthma exacerbation rates between treatment groups.

5.2 Deterioration of Disease and Acute Episodes

SYMBICORT should not be initiated in patients during rapidly deteriorating or potentially life-threatening episodes of asthma or COPD. SYMBICORT has not been studied in patients with acutely deteriorating asthma or COPD. The initiation of SYMBICORT in this setting is not appropriate.

Increasing use of inhaled, short-acting beta$_2$-agonists is a marker of deteriorating asthma. In this situation, the patient requires immediate re-evaluation with reassessment of the treatment regimen, giving special consideration to the possible need for replacing the current strength of SYMBICORT with a higher strength, adding additional inhaled corticosteroid, or initiating systemic corticosteroids. Patients should not use more than 2 inhalations twice daily (morning and evening) of SYMBICORT.

SYMBICORT should not be used for the relief of acute symptoms, i.e., as rescue therapy for the treatment of acute episodes of bronchospasm. An inhaled, short-acting beta$_2$-agonist, not SYMBICORT, should be used to relieve acute symptoms such as shortness of breath. When prescribing SYMBICORT, the physician must also provide the patient with an inhaled, short-acting beta$_2$-agonist (e.g., albuterol) for treatment of acute symptoms, despite regular twice-daily (morning and evening) use of SYMBICORT.

When beginning treatment with SYMBICORT, patients who have been taking oral or inhaled, short-acting beta$_2$-agonists on a regular basis (e.g., 4 times a day) should be instructed to discontinue the regular use of these drugs.

5.3 Excessive Use of SYMBICORT and Use with Other Long-Acting Beta$_2$-Agonists

As with other inhaled drugs containing beta$_2$-adrenergic agents, SYMBICORT should not be used more often than recommended, at higher doses than recommended, or in conjunction with other medications containing long-acting beta$_2$-agonists, as an overdose may result. Clinically significant cardiovascular effects and fatalities have been reported in association with excessive use of inhaled sympathomimetic drugs. Patients using SYMBICORT should not use an additional long-acting beta$_2$-agonist (e.g., salmeterol, formoterol fumarate, arformoterol tartrate) for any reason, including prevention of exercise-induced bronchospasm (EIB) or the treatment of asthma or COPD.

5.4 Local Effects

In clinical studies, the development of localized infections of the mouth and pharynx with *Candida albicans* has occurred in patients treated with SYMBICORT. When such an infection develops, it should be treated with appropriate local or systemic (i.e., oral antifungal) therapy while treatment with SYMBICORT continues, but at times therapy with SYMBICORT may need to be interrupted. Patients should rinse the mouth after inhalation of SYMBICORT.

5.5 Pneumonia and Other Lower Respiratory Tract Infections

Physicians should remain vigilant for the possible development of pneumonia in patients with COPD as the clinical features of pneumonia and exacerbations frequently overlap. Lower respiratory tract infections, including pneumonia, have been reported following the inhaled administration of corticosteroids.

In a 6 month study of 1,704 patients with COPD, there was a higher incidence of lung infections other than pneumonia (e.g., bronchitis, viral lower respiratory tract infections, etc.) in patients receiving SYMBICORT 160/4.5 (7.6%) than in those receiving SYMBICORT 80/4.5 (3.2%), formoterol 4.5 mcg (4.6%) or placebo (3.3%). Pneumonia did not occur with greater incidence in the SYMBICORT 160/4.5 group (1.1 %) compared with placebo (1.3%). In a 12-month study of 1,964 patients with COPD, there was also a higher incidence of lung infections other than pneumonia in patients receiving SYMBICORT 160/4.5 (8.1%) than in those receiving SYMBICORT 80/4.5 (6.9%), formoterol 4.5 mcg (7.1%) or placebo (6.2%). Similar to the 6 month study, pneumonia did not occur with greater incidence in the SYMBICORT 160/4.5 group (4.0%) compared with placebo (5.0%).

5.6 Immunosuppression

Patients who are on drugs that suppress the immune system are more susceptible to infection than healthy individuals. Chicken pox and measles, for example, can have a more serious or even fatal course in susceptible children or adults using corticosteroids. In such children or adults who have not had these diseases or been properly immunized, particular care should be taken to avoid exposure. How the dose, route, and duration of corticosteroid administration affects the risk of developing a disseminated infection is not known. The contribution of the underlying disease and/or prior corticosteroid treatment to the risk is also not known. If exposed, therapy with varicella zoster immune globulin (VZIG) or pooled intravenous immunoglobulin (IVIG), as appropriate, may be indicated. If exposed to measles, prophylaxis with pooled intramuscular immunoglobulin (IG) may be indicated. (See the respective package inserts for complete VZIG and IG prescribing information.) If chicken pox develops, treatment with antiviral agents may be considered. The immune responsiveness to varicella vaccine was evaluated in pediatric patients with asthma ages 12 months to 8 years with budesonide inhalation suspension. An open-label, nonrandomized clinical study examined the immune responsiveness to varicella vaccine in 243 asthma patients 12 months to 8 years of age who were treated with budesonide inhalation suspension 0.25 mg to 1 mg daily (n=151) or noncorticosteroid asthma therapy (n=92) (i.e., beta$_2$-agonists, leukotriene receptor antagonists, cromones). The percentage of patients developing a seroprotective antibody titer of ≥5.0 (gpELISA value) in response to the vaccination was similar in patients treated with budesonide inhalation suspension (85%), compared to patients treated with noncorticosteroid asthma therapy (90%). No patient treated with budesonide inhalation suspension developed chicken pox as a result of vaccination.

Inhaled corticosteroids should be used with caution, if at all, in patients with active or quiescent tuberculosis infections of the respiratory tract; untreated systemic fungal, bacterial, viral, or parasitic infections; or ocular herpes simplex.

5.7 Transferring Patients From Systemic Corticosteroid Therapy

Particular care is needed for patients who have been transferred from systemically active corticosteroids to inhaled corticosteroids because deaths due to adrenal insufficiency have occurred in patients with asthma during and after transfer from systemic corticosteroids to less systemically available inhaled corticosteroids. After withdrawal from systemic corticosteroids, a number of months are required for recovery of hypothalamic-pituitary-adrenal (HPA) function.

Patients who have been previously maintained on 20 mg or more per day of prednisone (or its equivalent) may be most susceptible, particularly when their systemic corticosteroids have been almost completely withdrawn. During this period of HPA suppression, patients may exhibit signs and symptoms of adrenal insufficiency when exposed to trauma, surgery, or infection (particularly gastroenteritis) or other conditions associated with severe electrolyte loss. Although SYMBICORT may provide control of asthma symptoms during these episodes, in recommended doses it supplies less than normal physiological amounts of glucocorticoid systemically and does NOT provide the mineralocorticoid activity that is necessary for coping with these emergencies.

During periods of stress or a severe asthma attack, patients who have been withdrawn from systemic corticosteroids should be instructed to resume oral corticosteroids (in large doses) immediately and to contact their physicians for further instruction. These patients should also be instructed to carry a warning card indicating that they may need supplementary systemic corticosteroids during periods of stress or a severe asthma attack.

Patients requiring oral corticosteroids should be weaned slowly from systemic corticosteroid use after transferring to SYMBICORT. Prednisone reduction can be accomplished by reducing the daily prednisone dose by 2.5 mg on a weekly basis during therapy with SYMBICORT. Lung function (mean forced expiratory volume in 1 second [FEV$_1$] or morning peak expiratory flow [PEF], beta-agonist use, and asthma symptoms should be carefully monitored during withdrawal of oral corticosteroids. In addition to monitoring asthma signs and symptoms, patients should be observed for signs and symptoms of adrenal insufficiency, such as fatigue, lassitude, weakness, nausea and vomiting, and hypotension.

Transfer of patients from systemic corticosteroid therapy to inhaled corticosteroids or SYMBICORT may unmask conditions previously suppressed by the systemic corticosteroid therapy (e.g., rhinitis, conjunctivitis, eczema, arthritis, eosinophilic conditions). Some patients may experience symptoms of systemically active corticosteroid withdrawal (e.g., joint and/or muscular pain, lassitude, depression) despite maintenance or even improvement of respiratory function.

5.8 Hypercorticism and Adrenal Suppression

Budesonide, a component of SYMBICORT, will often help control asthma symptoms with less suppression of HPA function than therapeutically equivalent oral doses of prednisone. Since budesonide is absorbed into the circulation and can be systemically active at higher doses, the beneficial effects of SYMBICORT in minimizing HPA dysfunction may be expected only when recommended dosages are not exceeded and individual patients are titrated to the lowest effective dose.

Because of the possibility of systemic absorption of inhaled corticosteroids, patients treated with SYMBICORT should be observed carefully for any evidence of systemic corticosteroid effects. Particular care should be taken in observing patients postoperatively or during periods of stress for evidence of inadequate adrenal response.

It is possible that systemic corticosteroid effects such as hypercorticism and adrenal suppression (including adrenal crisis) may appear in a small number of patients, particularly when budesonide is administered at higher than recommended doses over prolonged periods of time. If such effects occur, the dosage of SYMBICORT should be reduced slowly, consistent with accepted procedures for reducing systemic corticosteroids and for management of asthma symptoms.

5.9 Drug Interactions With Strong Cytochrome P450 3A4 Inhibitors

Caution should be exercised when considering the coadministration of SYMBICORT with ketoconazole, and other known strong CYP3A4 inhibitors (e.g., ritonavir, atazanavir, clarithromycin, indinavir, itraconazole, nefazodone, nelfinavir, saquinavir, telithromycin) because adverse effects related to increased systemic exposure to budesonide may occur *[see Drug Interactions (7.1), Clinical Pharmacology (12.3)]*

5.10 Paradoxical Bronchospasm and Upper Airway Symptoms

As with other inhaled medications, SYMBICORT can produce paradoxical bronchospasm, which may be life threatening. If paradoxical bronchospasm occurs following dosing with SYMBICORT, it should be treated immediately with an inhaled, short-acting bronchodilator, SYMBICORT should be discontinued immediately, and alternative therapy should be instituted.

5.11 Immediate Hypersensitivity Reactions

Immediate hypersensitivity reactions may occur after administration of SYMBICORT, as demonstrated by cases of urticaria, angioedema, rash, and bronchospasm.

5.12 Cardiovascular and Central Nervous System Effects

Excessive beta-adrenergic stimulation has been associated with seizures, angina, hypertension or hypotension, tachycardia with rates up to 200 beats/min, arrhythmias, nervousness, headache, tremor, palpitation, nausea, dizziness, fatigue, malaise, and insomnia *[see Overdosage (10)]*. Therefore, SYMBICORT, like all products containing sympathomimetic amines, should be used with caution in patients with cardiovascular disorders, especially coronary insufficiency, cardiac arrhythmias, and hypertension.

Formoterol, a component of SYMBICORT, can produce a clinically significant cardiovascular effect in some patients as measured by pulse rate, blood pressure, and/or symptoms. Although such effects are uncommon after administration of formoterol at recommended doses, if they occur, the drug may need to be discontinued. In addition, beta-agonists have been reported to produce ECG changes, such as flattening of the T wave, prolongation of the QTc interval, and ST segment depression. The clinical significance of these findings is unknown. Fatalities have been reported in association with excessive use of inhaled sympathomimetic drugs.

5.13 Reduction in Bone Mineral Density

Decreases in bone mineral density (BMD) have been observed with long-term administration of products containing inhaled corticosteroids. The clinical significance of small changes in BMD with regard to long-term consequences such as fracture is unknown. Patients with major risk factors for decreased bone mineral content, such as prolonged immobilization, family history of osteoporosis, post menopausal status, tobacco use, advanced age, poor nutrition, or chronic use of drugs that can reduce bone mass (e.g., anticonvulsants, oral corticosteroids) should be monitored and treated with established standards of care. Since patients with COPD often have multiple risk factors for reduced BMD, assessment of BMD is recommended prior to initiating SYMBICORT and periodically thereafter. If significant reductions in BMD are seen and SYMBICORT is still considered medically important for that patient's COPD therapy, use of medication to treat or prevent osteoporosis should be strongly considered.

Effects of treatment with SYMBICORT 160/4.5, SYMBICORT 80/4.5, formoterol 4.5, or placebo on BMD was evaluated in a subset of 326 patients (females and males 41 to 88 years of age) with COPD in the 12-month study. BMD evaluations of the hip and lumbar spine regions were conducted at baseline and 52 weeks using dual energy x-ray absorptiometry (DEXA) scans. Mean changes in BMD from baseline to end of treatment were small (mean changes ranged from -0.01-0.01 g/cm²). ANCOVA results for total spine and total hip BMD based on the end of treatment time point showed that all geometric LS Mean ratios for the pairwise treatment group comparisons were close to 1, indicating that overall, bone mineral density for total hip and total spine regions for the 12 month time point were stable over the entire treatment period.

5.14 Effect on Growth

Orally inhaled corticosteroids may cause a reduction in growth velocity when administered to pediatric patients. Monitor the growth of pediatric patients receiving SYMBICORT routinely (e.g., via stadiometry). To minimize the systemic effects of orally inhaled corticosteroids, including SYMBICORT, titrate each patient's dose to the lowest dosage that effectively controls his/her symptoms. *[See Dosage and Administration (2.1), Use in Specific Populations (8.4).]*

5.15 Glaucoma and Cataracts

Glaucoma, increased intraocular pressure, and cataracts have been reported in patients with asthma and COPD following the long-term administration of inhaled corticosteroids, including budesonide, a component of SYMBICORT. Therefore, close monitoring is warranted in patients with a change in vision or with history of increased intraocular pressure, glaucoma, and/or cataracts.

Effects of treatment with SYMBICORT 160/4.5, SYMBICORT 80/4.5, formoterol 4.5, or placebo on development of cataracts or glaucoma were evaluated in a subset of 461 patients with COPD in the 12-month study. Ophthalmic examinations were conducted at baseline, 24 weeks, and 52 weeks. There were 26 subjects (6%) with an increase in posterior subcapsular score from baseline to maximum value (>0.7) during the randomized treatment period. Changes in posterior subcapsular scores of >0.7 from baseline to treatment maximum occurred in 11 patients (9.0%) in the SYMBICORT 160/4.5 group, 4 patients (3.8%) in the SYMBICORT 80/4.5 group, 5 patients (4.2%) in the formoterol group, and 6 patients (5.2%) in the placebo group.

5.16 Eosinophilic Conditions and Churg-Strauss Syndrome

In rare cases, patients on inhaled corticosteroids may present with systemic eosinophilic conditions. Some of these patients have clinical features of vasculitis consistent with Churg-Strauss syndrome, a condition that is often treated with systemic corticosteroid therapy. These events usually, but not always, have been associated with the reduction and/or withdrawal of oral corticosteroid therapy following the introduction of inhaled corticosteroids. Physicians should be alert to eosinophilia, vasculitic rash, worsening pulmonary symptoms, cardiac complications, and/or neu-

Table 1 Adverse-reactions occurring at an incidence of ≥ 3% and more commonly than placebo in the SYMBICORT groups: pooled data from three 12-week, double-blind, placebo-controlled clinical asthma trials in patients 12 years and older

Treatment*	SYMBICORT		Budesonide		Formoterol	Placebo
Adverse Event	80/4.5 mcg N = 277 %	160/4.5 mcg N = 124 %	80 mcg N = 121 %	160 mcg N = 109 %	4.5 mcg N = 237 %	N = 400 %
Nasopharyngitis	10.5	9.7	14.0	11.0	10.1	9.0
Headache	6.5	11.3	11.6	12.8	8.9	6.5
Upper respiratory tract infection	7.6	10.5	8.3	9.2	7.6	7.8
Pharyngolaryngeal pain	6.1	8.9	5.0	7.3	3.0	4.8
Sinusitis	5.8	4.8	5.8	2.8	6.3	4.8
Influenza	3.2	2.4	6.6	0.9	3.0	1.3
Back pain	3.2	1.6	2.5	5.5	2.1	0.8
Nasal congestion	2.5	3.2	2.5	3.7	1.3	1.0
Stomach discomfort	1.1	6.5	2.5	4.6	1.3	1.8
Vomiting	1.4	3.2	0.8	2.8	1.7	1.0
Oral Candidiasis	1.4	3.2	0	0	0	0.8
Average Duration of Exposure (days)	**77.7**	**73.8**	**77.0**	**71.4**	**62.4**	**55.9**

*All treatments were administered as two inhalations twice daily.

ropathy presenting in their patients. A causal relationship between budesonide and these underlying conditions has not been established.

5.17 Coexisting Conditions

SYMBICORT, like all medications containing sympathomimetic amines, should be used with caution in patients with convulsive disorders or thyrotoxicosis and in those who are unusually responsive to sympathomimetic amines. Doses of the related beta₂-adrenoceptor agonist albuterol, when administered intravenously, have been reported to aggravate preexisting diabetes mellitus and ketoacidosis.

5.18 Hypokalemia and Hyperglycemia

Beta-adrenergic agonist medications may produce significant hypokalemia in some patients, possibly through intracellular shunting, which has the potential to produce adverse cardiovascular effects *[see Clinical Pharmacology (12.2)]*. The decrease in serum potassium is usually transient, not requiring supplementation. Clinically significant changes in blood glucose and/or serum potassium were seen infrequently during clinical studies with SYMBICORT at recommended doses.

6 ADVERSE REACTIONS

Long-acting beta₂-adrenergic agonists, such as formoterol one of the active ingredients in SYMBICORT, increase the risk of asthma-related death. Currently available data are inadequate to determine whether concurrent use of inhaled corticosteroids or other long-term asthma control drugs mitigates the increased risk of asthma-related death from LABA. Available data from controlled clinical trials suggest that LABA increase the risk of asthma-related hospitalization in pediatric and adolescent patients. Data from a large placebo-controlled US study that compared the safety of another long-acting beta₂-adrenergic agonist (salmeterol) or placebo added to usual asthma therapy showed an increase in asthma-related deaths in patients receiving salmeterol. *[see Warnings and Precautions (5.1)].*

Systemic and inhaled corticosteroid use may result in the following:

- Candida albicans infection [see *Warnings and Precautions (5.4)*]
- Pneumonia or lower respiratory tract infections in patients with COPD [see *Warnings and Precautions (5.5)*]
- Immunosuppression [see *Warnings and Precautions (5.6)*]
- Hypercorticism and adrenal suppression [see *Warnings and Precautions (5.8)*]
- Growth effects in pediatric patients [see *Warnings and Precautions (5.14)*]
- Glaucoma and cataracts [see *Warnings and Precautions (5.15)*]

Because clinical trials are conducted under widely varying conditions, adverse reaction rates observed in the clinical trials of a drug cannot be directly compared to rates in the clinical trials of another drug and may not reflect the rates observed in practice.

6.1 Clinical Trials Experience in Asthma Patients 12 years and older

The overall safety data in adults and adolescents are based upon 10 active- and placebo-controlled clinical trials in which 3393 patients ages 12 years and older (2052 females and 1341 males) with asthma of varying severity were treated with SYMBICORT 80/4.5 or 160/4.5 mcg taken two inhalations once or twice daily for 12 to 52 weeks. In these trials, the patients on SYMBICORT had a mean age of 38 years and were predominantly Caucasian (82%).

The incidence of common adverse events in Table 1 below is based upon pooled data from three 12-week, double-blind, placebo-controlled clinical studies in which 401 adult and adolescent patients (148 males and 253 females) age 12 years and older were treated with two inhalations of SYMBICORT 80/4.5 or SYMBICORT 160/4.5 twice daily. The SYMBICORT group was composed of mostly Caucasian (84%) patients with a mean age of 38 years, and a mean percent predicted FEV₁ at baseline of 76 and 68 for the 80/4.5 mcg and 160/4.5 mcg treatment groups, respectively. Control arms for comparison included two inhalations of budesonide HFA metered dose inhaler (MDI) 80 or 160 mcg, formoterol dry powder inhaler (DPI) 4.5 mcg, or placebo (MDI and DPI) twice daily. Table 1 includes all adverse events that occurred at an incidence of ≥ 3% in any one SYMBICORT group and more commonly than in the placebo group with twice-daily dosing. In considering these data, the increased average duration of patient exposure for SYMBICORT patients should be taken into account, as incidences are not adjusted for an imbalance of treatment duration.

[See table 1 above]

Long-term safety - asthma clinical trials in patients 12 years and older

Long-term safety studies in adolescent and adult patients 12 years of age and older, treated for up to 1 year at doses up to 1280/36 mcg/day (640/18 mcg twice daily), revealed neither clinically important changes in the incidence nor new types of adverse events emerging after longer periods of treatment. Similarly, no significant or unexpected patterns of abnormalities were observed for up to 1 year in safety measures including chemistry, hematology, ECG, Holter monitor, and HPA-axis assessments.

6.2 Clinical Trials Experience in Chronic Obstructive Pulmonary Disease

The incidence of common adverse events in Table 2 below is based upon pooled data from two double-blind, placebo-controlled clinical trials (6 and 12 months in duration) in which 771 adult COPD patients (496 males and 275 females) 40 years of age and older were treated with SYMBICORT 160/4.5, two inhalations twice daily. Of these patients 651 were treated for 6 months and 366 were treated for 12 months. The SYMBICORT group was composed of mostly Caucasian (93%) patients with a mean age of 63 years, and a mean percent predicted FEV₁ at baseline

Table 2 Adverse reactions occurring at an incidence of ≥ 3% and more commonly than placebo in the SYMBICORT group: pooled data from two double-blind, placebo-controlled clinical COPD trials

Treatment* Adverse Event	SYMBICORT 160/4.5 mcg N=771 %	Budesonide 160 mcg N=275 %	Formoterol 4.5 mcg N=779 %	Placebo N=781 %
Nasopharyngitis	7.3	3.3	5.8	4.9
Oral candidiasis	6.0	4.4	1.2	1.8
Bronchitis	5.4	4.7	4.5	3.5
Sinusitis	3.5	1.5	3.1	1.8
Upper respiratory tract infection viral	3.5	1.8	3.6	2.7
Average Duration of Exposure (days)	**255.2**	**157.1**	**240.3**	**223.7**

*All treatments were administered as two inhalations twice daily

of 33%. Control arms for comparison included two inhalations of budesonide HFA (MDI) 160 mcg, formoterol (DPI) 4.5 mcg or placebo (MDI and DPI) twice daily. Table 2 includes all adverse events that occurred at an incidence of ≥ 3% in the SYMBICORT group and more commonly than in the placebo group. In considering these data, the increased average duration of patient exposure to SYMBICORT should be taken into account, as incidences are not adjusted for an imbalance of treatment duration. [See table above]

Lung infections other than pneumonia (mostly bronchitis) occurred in a greater percentage of subjects treated with SYMBICORT 160/4.5 compared with placebo (7.9% vs. 5.1%, respectively). There were no clinically important or unexpected patterns of abnormalities observed for up to 1 year in chemistry, haematology, ECG, ECG (Holter) monitoring, HPA-axis, bone mineral density and ophthalmology assessments.

6.3 Postmarketing Experience

The following adverse reactions have been reported during post-approval use of SYMBICORT. Because these reactions are reported voluntarily from a population of uncertain size, it is not always possible to reliably estimate their frequency or establish a causal relationship to drug exposure. Some of these adverse reactions may also have been observed in clinical studies with SYMBICORT.

Cardiac disorders: angina pectoris, tachycardia, atrial and ventricular tachyarrhythmias, atrial fibrillation, extrasystoles, palpitations

Endocrine disorders: hypercorticism, growth velocity reduction in pediatric patients

Eye disorders: cataract, glaucoma, increased intraocular pressure

Gastrointestinal disorders: oropharyngeal candidiasis, nausea

Immune system disorders: immediate and delayed hypersensitivity reactions, such as anaphylactic reaction, angioedema, bronchospasm, urticaria, exanthema, dermatitis, pruritus

Metabolic and nutrition disorders: hyperglycemia, hypokalemia

Musculoskeletal, connective tissue, and bone disorders: muscle cramps

Nervous system disorders: tremor, dizziness

Psychiatric disorders: behavior disturbances, sleep disturbances, nervousness, agitation, depression, restlessness

Respiratory, thoracic, and mediastinal disorders: dysphonia, cough, throat irritation

Skin and subcutaneous tissue disorders: skin bruising

Vascular disorders: hypotension, hypertension

7 DRUG INTERACTIONS

In clinical studies, concurrent administration of SYMBICORT and other drugs, such as short-acting beta$_2$-agonists, intranasal corticosteroids, and antihistamines/decongestants has not resulted in an increased frequency of adverse reactions. No formal drug interaction studies have been performed with SYMBICORT.

7.1 Inhibitors of Cytochrome P4503A4

The main route of metabolism of corticosteroids, including budesonide, a component of SYMBICORT, is via cytochrome P450 (CYP) isoenzyme 3A4 (CYP3A4). After oral administration of ketoconazole, a strong inhibitor of CYP3A4, the mean plasma concentration of orally administered budesonide increased. Concomitant administration of CYP3A4 may inhibit the metabolism of, and increase the systemic exposure to, budesonide. Caution should be exercised when considering the coadministration of SYMBICORT with long-term ketoconazole and other known strong CYP3A4 inhibitors (e.g., ritonavir, atazanavir, clarithromycin, indinavir, itraconazole, nefazodone, nelfinavir, saquinavir, telithromycin) [*see Warnings and Precautions (5.9)*].

7.2 Monoamine Oxidase Inhibitors and Tricyclic Antidepressants

SYMBICORT should be administered with caution to patients being treated with monoamine oxidase inhibitors or

tricyclic antidepressants, or within 2 weeks of discontinuation of such agents, because the action of formoterol, a component of SYMBICORT, on the vascular system may be potentiated by these agents. In clinical trials with SYMBICORT, a limited number of COPD and asthma patients received tricyclic antidepressants, and, therefore, no clinically meaningful conclusions on adverse events can be made.

7.3 Beta-Adrenergic Receptor Blocking Agents

Beta-blockers (including eye drops) may not only block the pulmonary effect of beta-agonists, such as formoterol, a component of SYMBICORT, but may produce severe bronchospasm in patients with asthma. Therefore, patients with asthma should not normally be treated with beta-blockers. However, under certain circumstances, there may be no acceptable alternatives to the use of beta-adrenergic blocking agents in patients with asthma. In this setting, cardioselective beta-blockers could be considered, although they should be administered with caution.

7.4 Diuretics

The ECG changes and/or hypokalemia that may result from the administration of non–potassium-sparing diuretics (such as loop or thiazide diuretics) can be acutely worsened by beta-agonists, especially when the recommended dose of the beta-agonist is exceeded. Although the clinical significance of these effects is not known, caution is advised in the coadministration of SYMBICORT with non-potassium-sparing diuretics.

8 USE IN SPECIFIC POPULATIONS

8.1 Pregnancy

Teratogenic Effects: Pregnancy Category C.

There are no adequate and well-controlled studies of SYMBICORT in pregnant women. SYMBICORT was teratogenic and embryocidal in rats. Budesonide alone was teratogenic and embryocidal in rats and rabbits, but not in humans at therapeutic doses. Formoterol fumarate alone was teratogenic in rats and rabbits. Formoterol fumarate was also embryocidal, increased pup loss at birth and during lactation, and decreased pup weight in rats. SYMBICORT should be used during pregnancy only if the potential benefit justifies the potential risk to the fetus.

SYMBICORT

In a reproduction study in rats, budesonide combined with formoterol fumarate by the inhalation route at doses approximately 1/7 and 1/3, respectively, the maximum recommended human daily inhalation dose on a mg/m^2 basis produced umbilical hernia. No teratogenic or embryocidal effects were detected with budesonide combined with formoterol fumarate by the inhalation route at doses approximately 1/32 and 1/16, respectively, the maximum recommended human daily inhalation dose on a mg/m^2 basis.

Budesonide

Studies of pregnant women have not shown that inhaled budesonide increases the risk of abnormalities when administered during pregnancy. The results from a large population-based prospective cohort epidemiological study reviewing data from three Swedish registries covering approximately 99% of the pregnancies from 1995-1997 (ie, Swedish Medical Birth Registry; Registry of Congenital Malformations; Child Cardiology Registry) indicate no increased risk for congenital malformations from the use of inhaled budesonide during early pregnancy. Congenital malformations were studied in 2014 infants born to mothers reporting the use of inhaled budesonide for asthma in early pregnancy (usually 10-12 weeks after the last menstrual period), the period when most major organ malformations occur. The rate of recorded congenital malformations was similar compared to the general population rate (3.8% vs 3.5%, respectively). In addition, after exposure to inhaled budesonide, the number of infants born with orofacial clefts was similar to the expected number in the normal population (4 children vs 3.3, respectively).

These same data were utilized in a second study bringing the total to 2534 infants whose mothers were exposed to inhaled budesonide. In this study, the rate of congenital malformations among infants whose mothers were exposed to

inhaled budesonide during early pregnancy was not different from the rate for all newborn babies during the same period (3.6%).

Budesonide produced fetal loss, decreased pup weight, and skeletal abnormalities at subcutaneous doses in rabbits less than the maximum recommended human daily inhalation dose on a mcg/m^2 basis and in rats at doses approximately 6 times the maximum recommended human daily inhalation dose on a mcg/m^2 basis. In another study in rats, no teratogenic or embryocidal effects were seen at inhalation doses up to 3 times the maximum recommended human daily inhalation dose on a mcg/m^2 basis.

Experience with oral corticosteroids since their introduction in pharmacologic as opposed to physiologic doses suggests that rodents are more prone to teratogenic effects from corticosteroids than humans.

Formoterol

Formoterol fumarate has been shown to be teratogenic, embryocidal, to increase pup loss at birth and during lactation, and to decrease pup weights in rats when given at oral doses 1400 times and greater the maximum recommended human daily inhalation dose on a mcg/m^2 basis. Umbilical hernia was observed in rat fetuses at oral doses 1400 times and greater the maximum recommended human daily inhalation dose on a mcg/m^2 basis. Brachygnathia was observed in rat fetuses at an oral dose 7000 times the maximum recommended human daily inhalation dose on a mcg/m^2 basis. Pregnancy was prolonged at an oral dose 7000 times the maximum recommended human daily inhalation dose on a mcg/m^2 basis. In another study in rats, no teratogenic effects were seen at inhalation doses up to 500 times the maximum recommended human daily inhalation dose on a mcg/m^2 basis.

Subcapsular cysts on the liver were observed in rabbit fetuses at an oral dose 54,000 times the maximum recommended human daily inhalation dose on a mcg/m^2 basis. No teratogenic effects were observed at oral doses up to 3200 times the maximum recommended human daily inhalation dose on a mcg/m^2 basis.

Nonteratogenic Effects

Hypoadrenalism may occur in infants born of mothers receiving corticosteroids during pregnancy. Such infants should be carefully observed.

8.2 Labor and Delivery

There are no well-controlled human studies that have investigated the effects of SYMBICORT on preterm labor or labor at term. Because of the potential for beta-agonist interference with uterine contractility, use of SYMBICORT for management of asthma during labor should be restricted to those patients in whom the benefits clearly outweigh the risks.

8.3 Nursing Mothers

Since there are no data from controlled trials on the use of SYMBICORT by nursing mothers, a decision should be made whether to discontinue nursing or to discontinue SYMBICORT, taking into account the importance of SYMBICORT to the mother.

Budesonide, like other corticosteroids, is secreted in human milk. Data with budesonide delivered via dry powder inhaler indicates that the total daily oral dose of budesonide available in breast milk to the infant is approximately 0.3% to 1% of the dose inhaled by the mother [*see Clinical Pharmacology, Pharmacokinetics (12.3)*]. For SYMBICORT, the dose of budesonide available to the infant in breast milk, as a percentage of the maternal dose, would be expected to be similar.

In reproductive studies in rats, formoterol was excreted in the milk. It is not known whether formoterol is excreted in human milk.

8.4 Pediatric Use

Safety and effectiveness of SYMBICORT in asthma patients 12 years of age and older have been established in studies up to 12 months. In the two 12-week, double-blind, placebo-controlled US pivotal studies 25 patients 12 to 17 years of age were treated with SYMBICORT twice daily [*see Clinical Studies (14.1)*]. Efficacy results in this age group were similar to those observed in patients 18 years and older. There were no obvious differences in the type or frequency of adverse events reported in this age group compared with patients 18 years of age and older.

The safety and effectiveness of SYMBICORT in asthma patients 6 to <12 years of age has not been established.

Overall 1447 asthma patients 6 to <12 years of age participated in placebo- and active-controlled SYMBICORT studies. Of these 1447 patients, 539 received SYMBICORT twice daily. The overall safety profile of these patients was similar to that observed in patients ≥12 years of age who also received SYMBICORT twice daily in studies of similar design. Controlled clinical studies have shown that orally inhaled corticosteroids including budesonide, a component of SYMBICORT, may cause a reduction in growth velocity in pediatric patients. This effect has been observed in the absence of laboratory evidence of HPA-axis suppression, suggesting that growth velocity is a more sensitive indicator of systemic corticosteroid exposure in pediatric patients than some commonly used tests of HPA-axis function. The long-term effect of this reduction in growth velocity associated with orally inhaled corticosteroids, including the impact on final height are unknown. The potential for "catch-up" growth following discontinuation of treatment with orally inhaled corticosteroids has not been adequately studied.

In a study of asthmatic children 5-12 years of age, those treated with budesonide DPI 200 mcg twice daily (n=311) had a 1.1 centimeter reduction in growth compared with those receiving placebo (n=418) at the end of one year; the difference between these two treatment groups did not increase further over three years of additional treatment. By the end of 4 years, children treated with budesonide DPI and children treated with placebo had similar growth velocities. Conclusions drawn from this study may be confounded by the unequal use of corticosteroids in the treatment groups and inclusion of data from patients attaining puberty during the course of the study.

The growth of pediatric patients receiving orally inhaled corticosteroids, including SYMBICORT, should be monitored. If a child or adolescent on any corticosteroid appears to have growth suppression, the possibility that he/she is particularly sensitive to this effect should be considered. The potential growth effects of prolonged treatment should be weighed against the clinical benefits obtained. To minimize the systemic effects of orally inhaled corticosteroids, including SYMBICORT, each patient should be titrated to the lowest strength that effectively controls his/her asthma [*see Dosage and Administration (2)*].

8.5 Geriatric Use

Of the total number of patients in asthma clinical studies treated with SYMBICORT twice daily, 149 were 65 years of age or older, of whom 25 were 75 years of age or older.

In the COPD studies of 6 to 12 months duration, 349 patients treated with SYMBICORT 160/4.5 twice daily were 65 years old and above and of those, 73 patients were 75 years of age and older. No overall differences in safety or effectiveness were observed between these patients and younger patients, and other reported clinical experience has not identified differences in responses between the elderly and younger patients.

As with other products containing beta$_2$-agonists, special caution should be observed when using SYMBICORT in geriatric patients who have concomitant cardiovascular disease that could be adversely affected by beta$_2$-agonists.

Based on available data for SYMBICORT or its active components, no adjustment of dosage of SYMBICORT in geriatric patients is warranted.

8.6 Hepatic Impairment

Formal pharmacokinetic studies using SYMBICORT have not been conducted in patients with hepatic impairment. However, since both budesonide and formoterol fumarate are predominantly cleared by hepatic metabolism, impairment of liver function may lead to accumulation of budesonide and formoterol fumarate in plasma. Therefore, patients with hepatic disease should be closely monitored.

8.7 Renal Impairment

Formal pharmacokinetic studies using SYMBICORT have not been conducted in patients with renal impairment.

10 OVERDOSAGE

SYMBICORT

SYMBICORT contains both budesonide and formoterol; therefore, the risks associated with overdosage for the individual components described below apply to SYMBICORT.

In pharmacokinetic studies, single doses of 960/54 mcg (12 actuations of SYMBICORT 80/4.5) and 1280/36 mcg (8 actuations of 160/4.5), were administered to patients with COPD. A total of 1920/54 mcg (12 actuations of SYMBICORT 160/4.5) was administered as a single dose to both healthy subjects and patients with asthma. In a long-term active-controlled safety study in asthma patients, SYMBICORT 160/4.5 was administered for up to 12 months at doses up to twice the highest recommended daily dose. There were no clinically significant adverse reactions observed in any of these studies.

Clinical signs in dogs that received a single inhalation dose of SYMBICORT (a combination of budesonide and formoterol) in a dry powder included tremor, mucosal redness, nasal catarrh, redness of intact skin, abdominal respiration, vomiting, and salivation; in the rat, the only clinical sign observed was increased respiratory rate in the first hour after dosing. No deaths occurred in rats given a combination of budesonide and formoterol at acute inhalation doses of 97 and 3 mg/kg, respectively (approximately 1200 and 1350 times the maximum recommended human daily inhalation dose on a mcg/m^2 basis). No deaths occurred in dogs given a combination of budesonide and formoterol at the acute inhalation doses of 732 and 22 mcg/kg, respectively (approximately 30 times the maximum recommended human daily inhalation dose of budesonide and formoterol on a mcg/m^2 basis).

Budesonide

The potential for acute toxic effects following overdose of budesonide is low. If used at excessive doses for prolonged periods, systemic corticosteroid effects such as hypercorticism may occur [*see Warnings and Precautions (5)*]. Budesonide at five times the highest recommended dose (3200 mcg daily) administered to humans for 6 weeks caused a significant reduction (27%) in the plasma cortisol response to a 6-hour infusion of ACTH compared with placebo (+1%). The corresponding effect of 10 mg prednisone daily was a 35% reduction in the plasma cortisol response to ACTH.

In mice, the minimal inhalation lethal dose was 100 mg/kg (approximately 600 times the maximum recommended human daily inhalation dose on a mcg/m^2 basis). In rats, there were no deaths following the administration of an inhalation dose of 68 mg/kg (approximately 900 times the maximum recommended human daily inhalation dose on a mcg/m^2 basis). The minimal oral lethal dose in mice was 200 mg/kg (approximately 1300 times the maximum recommended human daily inhalation dose on a mcg/m^2 basis) and less than 100 mg/kg in rats (approximately 1300 times the maximum recommended human daily inhalation dose on a mcg/m^2 basis).

Formoterol

An overdose of formoterol would likely lead to an exaggeration of effects that are typical for beta$_2$-agonists: seizures, angina, hypertension, hypotension, tachycardia, atrial and ventricular tachyarrhythmias, nervousness, headache, tremor, palpitations, muscle cramps, nausea, dizziness, sleep disturbances, metabolic acidosis, hyperglycemia, hypokalemia. As with all sympathomimetic medications, cardiac arrest and even death may be associated with abuse of formoterol. No clinically significant adverse reactions were seen when formoterol was delivered to adult patients with acute bronchoconstriction at a dose of 90 mcg/day over 3 hours or to stable asthmatics 3 times a day at a total dose of 54 mcg/day for 3 days.

Treatment of formoterol overdosage consists of discontinuation of the medication together with institution of appropriate symptomatic and/or supportive therapy. The judicious use of a cardioselective beta-receptor blocker may be considered, bearing in mind that such medication can produce bronchospasm. There is insufficient evidence to determine if dialysis is beneficial for overdosage of formoterol. Cardiac monitoring is recommended in cases of overdosage.

No deaths were seen in mice given formoterol at an inhalation dose of 276 mg/kg (more than 62,200 times the maximum recommended human daily inhalation dose on a mcg/m^2 basis). In rats, the minimum lethal inhalation dose was 40 mg/kg (approximately 18,000 times the maximum recommended human daily inhalation dose on a mcg/m^2 basis). No deaths were seen in mice that received an oral dose of 2000 mg/kg (more than 450,000 times the maximum recommended human daily inhalation dose on a mcg/m^2 basis). Maximum nonlethal oral doses were 252 mg/kg in young rats and 1500 mg/kg in adult rats (approximately 114,000 times and 675,000 times the maximum recommended human inhalation dose on a mcg/m^2 basis).

11 DESCRIPTION

SYMBICORT 80/4.5 and SYMBICORT 160/4.5 each contain micronized budesonide and micronized formoterol fumarate dihydrate for oral inhalation only.

Each SYMBICORT 80/4.5 and SYMBICORT 160/4.5 canister is formulated as a hydrofluoroalkane (HFA 227; 1,1,1,2,3,3,3-heptafluoropropane)-propelled pressurized metered dose inhaler containing either 60 or 120 actuations [*see Dosage Forms and Strengths (3) and How Supplied/ Storage and Handling (16)*]. After priming, each actuation meters either 91/5.1 mcg or 181/5.1 mcg from the valve and delivers either 80/4.5 mcg, or 160/4.5 mcg (budesonide micronized/formoterol fumarate dihydrate micronized) from the actuator. The actual amount of drug delivered to the lung may depend on patient factors, such as the coordination between actuation of the device and inspiration through the delivery system. SYMBICORT also contains povidone K25 USP as a suspending agent and polyethylene glycol 1000 NF as a lubricant.

SYMBICORT should be primed before using for the first time by releasing two test sprays into the air away from the face, shaking well for 5 seconds before each spray. In cases where the inhaler has not been used for more than 7 days or when it has been dropped, prime the inhaler again by shaking well for 5 seconds before each spray and releasing two test sprays into the air away from the face.

One active component of SYMBICORT is budesonide, a corticosteroid designated chemically as (RS)-11β, 16α, 17,21-Tetrahydroxypregna-1,4-diene-3,20-dione cyclic 16,17-acetal with butyraldehyde. Budesonide is provided as a mixture of two epimers (22R and 22S). The empirical formula of budesonide is $C_{25}H_{34}O_6$ and its molecular weight is 430.5. Its structural formula is:

[See chemical structure at top of next column]

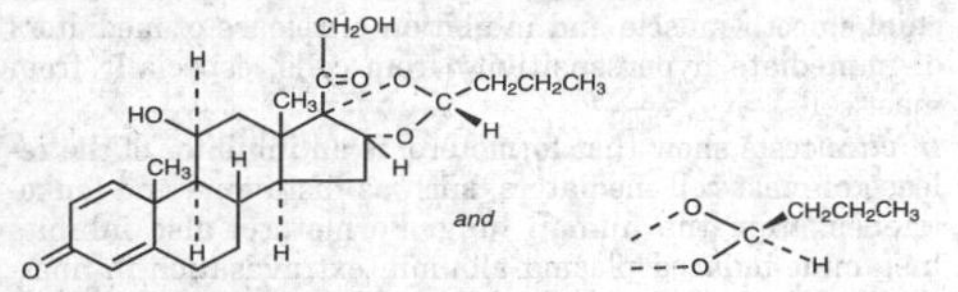

Budesonide is a white to off-white, tasteless, odorless powder which is practically insoluble in water and in heptane, sparingly soluble in ethanol, and freely soluble in chloroform. Its partition coefficient between octanol and water at pH 7.4 is 1.6×10^3.

The other active component of SYMBICORT is formoterol fumarate dihydrate, a selective beta$_2$-agonist designated chemically as (R*,R*)-(±)-N-[2-hydroxy-5-[1-hydroxy-2-[[2-(4-methoxyphenyl)-1-methylethyl]amino]ethyl]phenyl]formamide, (E)-2-butendioate(2:1), dihydrate. The empirical formula of formoterol is $C_{42}H_{56}N_4O_{14}$ and its molecular weight is 840.9. Its structural formula is:

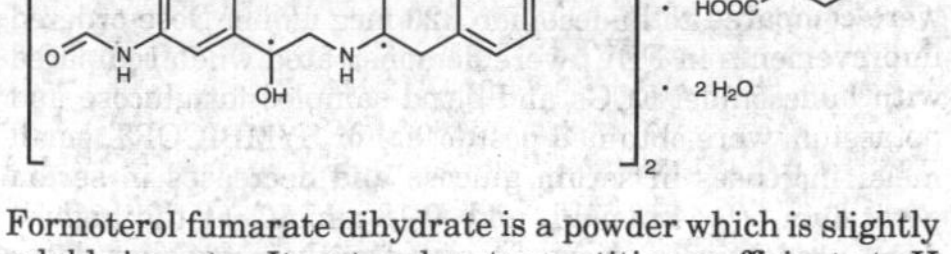

Formoterol fumarate dihydrate is a powder which is slightly soluble in water. Its octanol-water partition coefficient at pH 7.4 is 2.6. The pKa of formoterol fumarate dihydrate at 25°C is 7.9 for the phenolic group and 9.2 for the amino group.

12 CLINICAL PHARMACOLOGY

12.1 Mechanism of Action

SYMBICORT

SYMBICORT contains both budesonide and formoterol; therefore, the mechanisms of action described below for the individual components apply to SYMBICORT. These drugs represent two classes of medications (a synthetic corticosteroid and a long-acting selective beta$_2$-adrenoceptor agonist) that have different effects on clinical, physiological, and inflammatory indices of Chronic Obstructive Pulmonary Disease (COPD) and asthma.

Budesonide

Budesonide is an anti-inflammatory corticosteroid that exhibits potent glucocorticoid activity and weak mineralocorticoid activity. In standard *in vitro* and animal models, budesonide has approximately a 200-fold higher affinity for the glucocorticoid receptor and a 1000-fold higher topical anti-inflammatory potency than cortisol (rat croton oil ear edema assay). As a measure of systemic activity, budesonide is 40 times more potent than cortisol when administered subcutaneously and 25 times more potent when administered orally in the rat thymus involution assay.

In glucocorticoid receptor affinity studies, the 22R form of budesonide was two times as active as the 22S epimer. *In vitro* studies indicated that the two forms of budesonide do not interconvert.

Inflammation is an important component in the pathogenesis of COPD and asthma. Corticosteroids have a wide range of inhibitory activities against multiple cell types (eg, mast cells, eosinophils, neutrophils, macrophages, and lymphocytes) and mediators (eg, histamine, eicosanoids, leukotrienes, and cytokines) involved in allergic and non–allergic-mediated inflammation. These anti-inflammatory actions of corticosteroids may contribute to their efficacy in COPD and asthma.

Studies in asthmatic patients have shown a favorable ratio between topical anti-inflammatory activity and systemic corticosteroid effects over a wide range of doses of budesonide. This is explained by a combination of a relatively high local anti-inflammatory effect, extensive first pass hepatic degradation of orally absorbed drug (85%-95%), and the low potency of formed metabolites.

Formoterol

Formoterol fumarate is a long-acting selective beta$_2$-adrenergic agonist (beta$_2$-agonist) with a rapid onset of action. Inhaled formoterol fumarate acts locally in the lung as a bronchodilator. *In vitro* studies have shown that formoterol has more than 200-fold greater agonist activity at beta$_2$-receptors than at beta$_1$-receptors. The *in vitro* binding selectivity to beta$_2$- over beta$_1$-adrenoceptors is higher for formoterol than for albuterol (5 times), whereas salmeterol has a higher (3 times) beta $_2$-selectivity ratio than formoterol.

Although beta$_2$-receptors are the predominant adrenergic receptors in bronchial smooth muscle and beta$_1$-receptors are the predominant receptors in the heart, there are also beta$_2$-receptors in the human heart comprising 10% to 50% of the total beta-adrenergic receptors. The precise function of these receptors has not been established, but they raise the possibility that even highly selective beta$_2$-agonists may have cardiac effects.

The pharmacologic effects of beta$_2$-adrenoceptor agonist drugs, including formoterol, are at least in part attributable to stimulation of intracellular adenyl cyclase, the enzyme that catalyzes the conversion of adenosine triphosphate (ATP) to cyclic-3′, 5′-adenosine monophosphate (cyclic AMP). Increased cyclic AMP levels cause relaxation of bronchial smooth muscle and inhibition of release of mediators of immediate hypersensitivity from cells, especially from mast cells.

In vitro tests show that formoterol is an inhibitor of the release of mast cell mediators, such as histamine and leukotrienes, from the human lung. Formoterol also inhibits histamine-induced plasma albumin extravasation in anesthetized guinea pigs and inhibits allergen-induced eosinophil influx in dogs with airway hyper-responsiveness. The relevance of these *in vitro* and animal findings to humans is unknown.

12.2 Pharmacodynamics

Asthma

Cardiovascular effects: In a single-dose cross-over study involving 201 patients with persistent asthma, single-dose treatments of 4.5, 9, and 18 mcg of formoterol in combination with 320 mcg of budesonide delivered via SYMBICORT were compared to budesonide 320 mcg alone. Dose-ordered improvements in FEV_1 were demonstrated when compared with budesonide. ECGs and blood samples for glucose and potassium were obtained postdose. For SYMBICORT, small mean increases in serum glucose and decreases in serum potassium (+0.44 mmol/L and -0.18 mmol/L at the highest dose, respectively) were observed with increasing doses of formoterol, compared to budesonide. In ECGs, SYMBICORT produced small dose-related mean increases in heart rate (approximately 3 bpm at the highest dose), and QTc intervals (3-6 msec) compared to budesonide alone. No subject had a QT or QTc value ≥500 msec.

In the United States, five 12-week, active- and placebo-controlled studies evaluated 2152 patients aged 12 years and older with asthma. Systemic pharmacodynamic effects of formoterol (heart/pulse rate, blood pressure, QTc interval, potassium, and glucose) were similar in patients treated with SYMBICORT, compared with patients treated with formoterol dry inhalation powder 4.5 mcg, two inhalations twice daily. No patient had a QT or QTc value ≥500 msec during treatment.

In three placebo-controlled studies in adolescents and adults with asthma, aged 12 years and older, a total of 1232 patients (553 patients in the SYMBICORT group) had evaluable continuous 24-hour electrocardiographic monitoring. Overall, there were no important differences in the occurrence of ventricular or supraventricular ectopy and no evidence of increased risk for clinically significant dysrhythmia in the SYMBICORT group compared to placebo.

HPA axis effects: Overall, no clinically important effects on HPA axis, as measured by 24-hour urinary cortisol, were observed for SYMBICORT treated adult or adolescent patients at doses up to 640/18 mcg/day compared to budesonide.

Chronic Obstructive Pulmonary Disease:

Cardiovascular effects: In 2 clinical studies, 6 months and 12 months in duration including 3668 COPD patients, no clinically important differences were seen in pulse rate, blood pressure, potassium, and glucose between SYMBICORT, the individual components of SYMBICORT, and placebo. *[see Clinical Studies (14.2)]*.

ECGs recorded at multiple clinic visits on treatment in both studies showed no clinically important differences for heart rate, PR interval, QRS duration, heart rate, signs of cardiac ischemia or arrhythmias between SYMBICORT 160/4.5 the monoproducts and placebo, all administered as two inhalations twice daily. Based on ECGs, 6 patients treated with SYMBICORT 160/4.5, 6 patients treated with formoterol 4.5, and 6 patients in the placebo group experienced atrial fibrillation or flutter that was not present at baseline. There were no cases of nonsustained ventricular tachycardia in the SYMBICORT 160/4.5, formoterol 4.5, or placebo groups.

In the 12-month study, 520 patients had evaluable continuous 24-hour ECG (Holter) monitoring prior to the first dose and after approximately 1 and 4 months on treatment. No clinically important differences in ventricular or supraventricular arrhythmias, ventricular or supraventricular ectopic beats, or heart rate were observed among the groups treated with SYMBICORT 160/4.5, formoterol or placebo taken as two inhalations twice daily. Based on ECG (Holter) monitoring, one patient on SYMBICORT 160/4.5, no patients on formoterol 4.5, and three patients in the placebo group experienced atrial fibrillation or flutter that was not present at baseline.

HPA axis effects: Twenty-four hour urinary cortisol measurements were collected in a pooled subset (n=616) of patients from two COPD studies. The data indicated approximately 30% lower mean 24-hour urinary free cortisol values following chronic administration (> 6 months) of SYMBICORT relative to placebo. SYMBICORT appeared to exhibit comparable cortisol suppression to budesonide 160 mcg alone or coadministration of budesonide 160 mcg and formoterol 4.5 mcg. For patients treated with SYMBICORT or placebo for up to 12 months, the percentage of patients who shifted from normal to low for this measure were generally comparable.

Other Budesonide Products

To confirm that systemic absorption is not a significant factor in the clinical efficacy of inhaled budesonide, a clinical study in patients with asthma was performed comparing 400 mcg budesonide administered via a pressurized metered dose inhaler with a tube spacer to 1400 mcg of oral budesonide and placebo. The study demonstrated the efficacy of inhaled budesonide but not orally ingested budesonide, despite comparable systemic levels. Thus, the therapeutic effect of conventional doses of orally inhaled budesonide are largely explained by its direct action on the respiratory tract.

Inhaled budesonide has been shown to decrease airway reactivity to various challenge models, including histamine, methacholine, sodium metabisulfite, and adenosine monophosphate in patients with hyperreactive airways. The clinical relevance of these models is not certain.

Pretreatment with inhaled budesonide, 1600 mcg daily (800 mcg twice daily) for 2 weeks reduced the acute (early-phase reaction) and delayed (late-phase reaction) decrease in FEV_1 following inhaled allergen challenge.

The systemic effects of inhaled corticosteroids are related to the systemic exposure to such drugs. Pharmacokinetic studies have demonstrated that in both adults and children with asthma the systemic exposure to budesonide is lower with SYMBICORT compared with inhaled budesonide administered at the same delivered dose via a dry powder inhaler *[see Clinical Pharmacology, Pharmacokinetics, SYMBICORT (12.3)]*. Therefore, the systemic effects (HPA axis and growth) of budesonide delivered from SYMBICORT would be expected to be no greater than what is reported for inhaled budesonide when administered at comparable doses via the dry powder inhaler *[see Use in Specific Populations, Pediatric Use (8.4)]*.

HPA Axis Effects: The effects of inhaled budesonide administered via a dry powder inhaler on the hypothalamic-pituitary-adrenal (HPA) axis were studied in 905 adults and 404 pediatric patients with asthma. For most patients, the ability to increase cortisol production in response to stress, as assessed by cosyntropin (ACTH) stimulation test, remained intact with budesonide treatment at recommended doses. For adult patients treated with 100, 200, 400, or 800 mcg twice daily for 12 weeks, 4%, 2%, 6%, and 13%, respectively, had an abnormal stimulated cortisol response (peak cortisol <14.5 mcg/dL assessed by liquid chromatography following short-cosyntropin test) as compared to 8% of patients treated with placebo. Similar results were obtained in pediatric patients. In another study in adults, doses of 400, 800, and 1600 mcg of inhaled budesonide twice daily for 6 weeks were examined; 1600 mcg twice daily (twice the maximum recommended dose) resulted in a 27% reduction in stimulated cortisol (6-hour ACTH infusion) while 10-mg prednisone resulted in a 35% reduction. In this study, no patient on budesonide at doses of 400 and 800 mcg twice daily met the criterion for an abnormal stimulated-cortisol response (peak cortisol <14.5 mcg/dL assessed by liquid chromatography) following ACTH infusion. An open-label, long-term follow-up of 1133 patients for up to 52 weeks confirmed the minimal effect on the HPA axis (both basal- and stimulated-plasma cortisol) of budesonide when administered at recommended doses. In patients who had previously been oral-steroid–dependent, use of budesonide in recommended doses was associated with higher stimulated-cortisol response compared to baseline following 1 year of therapy.

Other Formoterol Products

While the pharmacodynamic effect is via stimulation of beta-adrenergic receptors, excessive activation of these receptors commonly leads to skeletal muscle tremor and cramps, insomnia, tachycardia, decreases in plasma potassium, and increases in plasma glucose. Inhaled formoterol, like other $beta_2$-adrenergic agonist drugs, can produce dose-related cardiovascular effects and effects on blood glucose and/or serum potassium *[see Warnings and Precautions (5)]*. For SYMBICORT, these effects are detailed in the *Clinical Pharmacology, Pharmacodynamics, SYMBICORT (12.2)* section.

Use of long-acting $beta_2$-adrenergic agonist drugs can result in tolerance to bronchoprotective and bronchodilatory effects.

Rebound bronchial hyperresponsiveness after cessation of chronic long-acting beta-agonist therapy has not been observed.

12.3 Pharmacokinetics

SYMBICORT

Absorption: *Budesonide: Healthy Subjects:* Orally inhaled budesonide is rapidly absorbed in the lungs and peak concentration is typically reached within 20 minutes. After oral administration of budesonide peak plasma concentration was achieved in about 1 to 2 hours and the absolute systemic availability was 6%-13% due to extensive first pass metabolism. In contrast, most of the budesonide delivered to the lungs was systemically absorbed. In healthy subjects, 34% of the metered dose was deposited in the lung (as assessed by plasma concentration method and using a budesonide-containing dry powder inhaler) with an absolute systemic availability of 39% of the metered dose.

Following administration of SYMBICORT 160/4.5 mcg, two or four inhalations twice daily) for 5 days in healthy subjects, plasma concentration of budesonide generally increased in proportion to dose. The accumulation index for the group that received two inhalations twice daily was 1.32 for budesonide.

Asthma Patients: In a single-dose study, higher than recommended doses of SYMBICORT (12 inhalations of SYMBICORT 160/4.5 mcg) were administered to patients with moderate asthma. Peak budesonide plasma concentration of 4.5 nmol/L occurred at 20 minutes following dosing. This study demonstrated that the total systemic exposure to budesonide from SYMBICORT was approximately 30% lower than from inhaled budesonide via a dry powder inhaler (DPI) at the same delivered dose. Following administration of SYMBICORT, the half-life of the budesonide component was 4.7 hours.

In a repeat dose study, the highest recommended dose of SYMBICORT (160/4.5 mcg, two inhalations twice daily) was administered to patients with moderate asthma and healthy subjects for 1 week. Peak budesonide plasma concentration of 1.2 nmol/L occurred at 21 minutes in asthma patients. Peak budesonide plasma concentration was 27% lower in asthma patients compared to that in healthy subjects. However, the total systemic exposure of budesonide was comparable to that in asthma patients.

Peak steady-state plasma concentrations of budesonide administered by DPI in adults with asthma averaged 0.6 and 1.6 nmol/L at doses of 180 mcg and 360 mcg twice daily, respectively. In asthmatic patients, budesonide showed a linear increase in AUC and C_{max} with increasing dose after both single and repeated dosing of inhaled budesonide.

COPD Patients: In a single-dose study, 12 inhalations of SYMBICORT 80/4.5 mcg (total dose 960/54 mcg) were administered to patients with COPD. Mean budesonide peak plasma concentration of 3.3 nmol/L occurred at 30 minutes following dosing. Budesonide systemic exposure was comparable between SYMBICORT pMDI and coadministration of budesonide via a metered-dose inhaler and formoterol via a dry powder inhaler (budesonide 960 mcg and formoterol 54 mcg). In the same study, an open-label group of moderate asthma patients also received the same higher dose of SYMBICORT. For budesonide, COPD patients exhibited 12% greater AUC and 10% lower C_{max} compared to asthma patients.

In the 6 month pivotal clinical study, steady-state pharmacokinetic data of budesonide was obtained in a subset of COPD patients with treatment arms of SYMBICORT pMDI 160/4.5 mcg, SYMBICORT pMDI 80/4.5 mcg, budesonide 160 mcg, budesonide 160 mcg and formoterol 4.5 mcg given together, all administered as two inhalations twice daily. Budesonide systemic exposure (AUC and C_{max}) increased proportionally with doses from 80 mcg to 160 mcg and was generally similar between the 3 treatment groups receiving the same dose of budesonide (SYMBICORT pMDI 160/4.5 mcg, budesonide 160 mcg, budesonide 160 mcg and formoterol 4.5 mcg administered together).

Formoterol:

Inhaled formoterol is rapidly absorbed; peak plasma concentrations are typically reached at the first plasma sampling time, within 5-10 minutes after dosing. As with many drug products for oral inhalation, it is likely that the majority of the inhaled formoterol delivered is swallowed and then absorbed from the gastrointestinal tract.

Healthy Subjects: Following administration of SYMBICORT (160/4.5 mcg, two or four inhalations twice daily) for 5 days in healthy subjects, plasma concentration of formoterol generally increased in proportion to dose. The accumulation index for the group that received two inhalations twice daily was 1.77 for formoterol.

Asthma patients: In a single-dose study, higher than recommended doses of SYMBICORT (12 inhalations of SYMBICORT 160/4.5 mcg) were administered to patients with moderate asthma. Peak plasma concentration for formoterol of 136 pmol occurred at 10 minutes following dosing. Approximately 8% of the delivered dose of formoterol was recovered in the urine as unchanged drug.

In a repeat dose study, the highest recommended dose of SYMBICORT (160/4.5 mcg, two inhalations twice daily) was administered to patients with moderate asthma and healthy subjects for 1 week. Peak formoterol plasma concentration of 28 pmol/L occurred at 10 minutes in asthma patients. Peak formoterol plasma concentration was about 42% lower in asthma patients compared to that in healthy subjects. However, the total systemic exposure of formoterol was comparable to that in asthma patients.

COPD patients: Following single-dose administration of 12 inhalations of SYMBICORT 80/4.5, mean peak formoterol plasma concentration of 167 pmol/L was rapidly achieved at 15 minutes after dosing. Formoterol exposure was slightly greater (~16-18%) from SYMBICORT pMDI compared to coadministration of budesonide via a metered-dose inhaler and formoterol via a dry powder inhaler (total dose of budesonide 960 mcg and formoterol 54 mcg). In the same study, an open label group of moderate asthma patients received the same dose of SYMBICORT. COPD patients exhibited 12-15% greater AUC and C_{max} for formoterol compared to asthma patients.

In the 6 month pivotal clinical study, steady-state pharmacokinetic data of formoterol was obtained in a subset of COPD patients with treatment arms of SYMBICORT pMDI 160/4.5 mcg, SYMBICORT pMDI 80/4.5 mcg, formoterol 4.5 mcg, budesonide 160 mcg and formoterol 4.5 mcg given together, all administered as two inhalations twice daily. The systemic exposure of formoterol as evidenced by AUC, was about 30% and 16% higher from SYMBICORT pMDI compared to formoterol alone treatment arm and coadministration of individual components of budesonide and formoterol treatment arm, respectively.

Distribution: *Budesonide:* The volume of distribution of budesonide was approximately 3 L/kg. It was 85%-90% bound to plasma proteins. Protein binding was constant over the concentration range (1-100 nmol/L) achieved with, and exceeding, recommended inhaled doses. Budesonide showed little or no binding to corticosteroid binding globulin. Budesonide rapidly equilibrated with red blood cells in a concentration independent manner with a blood plasma ratio of about 0.8.

Formoterol: Over the concentration range of 10-500 nmol/L, plasma protein binding for the RR and SS enantiomers of formoterol was 46% and 58%, respectively. The concentrations of formoterol used to assess the plasma protein binding were higher than those achieved in plasma following inhalation of a single 54 mcg dose.

Metabolism: *Budesonide: In vitro* studies with human liver homogenates have shown that budesonide was rapidly and extensively metabolized. Two major metabolites formed via cytochrome P450 (CYP) isoenzyme 3A4 (CYP3A4) catalyzed biotransformation have been isolated and identified as 16α-hydroxyprednisolone and 6ß-hydroxybudesonide. The corticosteroid activity of each of these two metabolites was less than 1% of that of the parent compound. No qualitative differences between the *in vitro* and *in vivo* metabolic patterns were detected. Negligible metabolic inactivation was observed in human lung and serum preparations.

Formoterol: The primary metabolism of formoterol is by direct glucuronidation and by O-demethylation followed by conjugation to inactive metabolites. Secondary metabolic pathways include deformylation and sulfate conjugation. CYP2D6 and CYP2C have been identified as being primarily responsible for O-demethylation.

Elimination: *Budesonide:* Budesonide was excreted in urine and feces in the form of metabolites. Approximately 60% of an intravenous radiolabeled dose was recovered in the urine.

No unchanged budesonide was detected in the urine. The 22R form of budesonide was preferentially cleared by the liver with systemic clearance of 1.4 L/min vs 1.0 L/min for the 22S form. The terminal half-life, 2 to 3 hours, was the same for both epimers and was independent of dose.

Formoterol: The excretion of formoterol was studied in four healthy subjects following simultaneous administration of radiolabeled formoterol via the oral and IV routes. In that study, 62% of the radiolabeled formoterol was excreted in the urine while 24% was eliminated in the feces.

Special Populations

Geriatric

The pharmacokinetics of SYMBICORT in geriatric patients have not been specifically studied.

Pediatric

Plasma concentrations of budesonide were measured following administration of four inhalations of SYMBICORT 160/4.5 mcg in a single-dose study in pediatric patients with asthma, 6-11 years of age. Urine was collected for determination of formoterol excretion. Peak budesonide concentrations of 1.4 nmol/L occurred at 20 minutes post-dose. Approximately 3.5% of the delivered formoterol dose was recovered in the urine as unchanged formoterol. This study also demonstrated that the total systemic exposure to budesonide from SYMBICORT was approximately 30% lower than from inhaled budesonide via a dry powder inhaler that was also evaluated at the same delivered dose.

Gender/Race

Specific studies to examine the effects of gender and race on the pharmacokinetics of SYMBICORT have not been conducted. Population PK analysis of the SYMBICORT data indicates that gender does not affect the pharmacokinetics of budesonide and formoterol. No conclusions can be drawn on the effect of race due to the low number of non-Caucasians evaluated for PK.

Nursing Mothers

The disposition of budesonide when delivered by inhalation from a dry powder inhaler at doses of 200 or 400 mcg twice daily for at least 3 months was studied in eight lactating women with asthma from 1 to 6 months postpartum. Systemic exposure to budesonide in these women appears to be comparable to that in non-lactating women with asthma from other studies. Breast milk obtained over eight hours post-dose revealed that the maximum concentration of budesonide for the 400 and 800 mcg total daily doses was 0.39 and 0.78 nmol/L, respectively, and occurred within 45 minutes after dosing. The estimated oral daily dose of budesonide from breast milk to the infant is approximately 0.007 and 0.014 mcg/kg/day for the two dose regimens used in this study, which represents approximately 0.3% to 1% of the dose inhaled by the mother. Budesonide levels in plasma samples obtained from five infants at about 90 minutes after breastfeeding (and about 140 minutes after drug administration to the mother) were below quantifiable levels (<0.02 nmol/L in four infants and <0.04 nmol/L in one infant) *[see Use in Specific Populations, Nursing Mothers (8.3)]*.

Renal or Hepatic Insufficiency

There are no data regarding the specific use of SYMBICORT in patients with hepatic or renal impairment. Reduced liver function may affect the elimination of corticosteroids. Budesonide pharmacokinetics was affected by compromised liver function as evidenced by a doubled systemic availability after oral ingestion. The intravenous budesonide pharmacokinetics was, however, similar in cirrhotic patients and in healthy subjects. Specific data with formoterol is not available, but because formoterol is primarily eliminated via hepatic metabolism, an increased exposure can be expected in patients with severe liver impairment.

Drug-Drug Interactions

A single-dose crossover study was conducted to compare the pharmacokinetics of eight inhalations of the following: budesonide, formoterol, and budesonide plus formoterol administered concurrently. The results of the study indicated that there was no evidence of a pharmacokinetic interaction between the two components of SYMBICORT.

Inhibitors of cytochrome P450 enzymes

Ketoconazole: Ketoconazole, a strong inhibitor of cytochrome P450 (CYP) isoenzyme 3A4 (CYP3A4), the main metabolic enzyme for corticosteroids, increased plasma levels of orally ingested budesonide.

Cimetidine: At recommended doses, cimetidine, a nonspecific inhibitor of CYP enzymes, had a slight but clinically insignificant effect on the pharmacokinetics of oral budesonide.

Specific drug-drug interaction studies with formoterol have not been performed.

13 NONCLINICAL TOXICOLOGY

13.1 Carcinogenesis, Mutagenesis, Impairment of Fertility

Budesonide

Long-term studies were conducted in rats and mice using oral administration to evaluate the carcinogenic potential of budesonide.

In a 2-year study in Sprague-Dawley rats, budesonide caused a statistically significant increase in the incidence of gliomas in male rats at an oral dose of 50 mcg/kg (less than the maximum recommended human daily inhalation dose on a mcg/m^2 basis). No tumorigenicity was seen in male and female rats at respective oral doses up to 25 and 50 mcg/kg (less than the maximum recommended human daily inhalation dose on a mcg/m^2 basis). In two additional 2-year studies in male Fischer and Sprague-Dawley rats, budesonide caused no gliomas at an oral dose of 50 mcg/kg (less than the maximum recommended human daily inhalation dose on a mcg/m^2 basis). However, in the male Sprague-Dawley rats, budesonide caused a statistically significant increase in the incidence of hepatocellular tumors at an oral dose of 50 mcg/kg (less than the maximum recommended human daily inhalation dose on a mcg/m^2 basis). The concurrent reference corticosteroids (prednisolone and triamcinolone acetonide) in these two studies showed similar findings.

In a 91-week study in mice, budesonide caused no treatment-related carcinogenicity at oral doses up to 200 mcg/kg (approximately equal to the maximum recommended human daily inhalation dose on a mcg/m^2 basis).

Budesonide was not mutagenic or clastogenic in six different test systems: Ames *Salmonella*/microsome plate test, mouse micronucleus test, mouse lymphoma test, chromosome aberration test in human lymphocytes, sex-linked recessive lethal test in *Drosophila melanogaster*, and DNA repair analysis in rat hepatocyte culture.

In rats, budesonide had no effect on fertility at subcutaneous doses up to 80 mcg/kg (approximately equal to the maximum recommended human daily inhalation dose on a mcg/m^2 basis). However, it caused a decrease in prenatal viability and viability in the pups at birth and during lactation, along with a decrease in maternal body-weight gain, at subcutaneous doses of 20 mcg/kg and above (less than the maximum recommended human daily inhalation dose on a mcg/m^2 basis). No such effects were noted at 5 mcg/kg (less than the maximum recommended human daily inhalation dose on a mcg/m^2 basis).

Formoterol

Long-term studies were conducted in mice using oral administration and rats using inhalation administration to evaluate the carcinogenic potential of formoterol fumarate.

In a 24-month carcinogenicity study in CD-1 mice, formoterol at oral doses of 0.1 mg/kg and above (approximately 20 times the maximum recommended human daily inhalation dose on a mcg/m^2 basis) caused a dose-related increase in the incidence of uterine leiomyomas.

In a 24-month carcinogenicity study in Sprague-Dawley rats, an increased incidence of mesovarian leiomyoma and uterine leiomyosarcoma were observed at the inhaled dose of 130 mcg/kg (approximately 60 times the maximum recommended human daily inhalation dose on a mcg/m^2 basis). No tumors were seen at 22 mcg/kg (approximately 10 times the maximum recommended human daily inhalation dose on a mcg/m^2 basis).

Other beta-agonist drugs have similarly demonstrated increases in leiomyomas of the genital tract in female rodents. The relevance of these findings to human use is unknown.

Formoterol was not mutagenic or clastogenic in Ames *Salmonella*/microsome plate test, mouse lymphoma test, chromosome aberration test in human lymphocytes, and rat micronucleus test.

A reduction in fertility and/or reproductive performance was identified in male rats treated with formoterol at an oral dose of 15 mg/kg (approximately 7000 times the maximum recommended human daily inhalation dose on a mcg/m^2 basis). In a separate study with male rats treated with an oral dose of 15 mg/kg (approximately 7000 times the maximum recommended human daily inhalation dose on a mcg/m^2 basis), there were findings of testicular tubular atrophy and spermatic debris in the testes and oligospermia in the epididymides. No such effect was seen at 3 mg/kg (approximately 1400 times the maximum recommended human daily inhalation dose on a mcg/m^2 basis). No effect on fertility was detected in female rats at doses up to 15 mg/kg (approximately 7000 times the maximum recommended human daily inhalation dose on a mcg/m^2 basis).

13.2 Animal Toxicology and/or Pharmacology

Preclinical: Studies in laboratory animals (minipigs, rodents, and dogs) have demonstrated the occurrence of cardiac arrhythmias and sudden death (with histologic evidence of myocardial necrosis) when beta-agonists and methylxanthines are administered concurrently. The clinical significance of these findings is unknown.

Reproductive Toxicology Studies:

SYMBICORT

SYMBICORT has been shown to be teratogenic and embryocidal in rats when given at inhalation doses of 12/0.66 mcg/kg (budesonide/formoterol) and above (less than the maximum recommended human daily inhalation dose on a mcg/m^2 basis). Umbilical hernia, a malformation, was observed for fetuses at doses of 12/0.66 mcg/kg and above (less than the maximum recommended human daily inhalation dose on a mcg/m^2 basis). No teratogenic or embryocidal effects were detected at 2.5/0.14 mcg/kg (less than the maximum recommended human daily inhalation dose on a mcg/m^2 basis).

Budesonide

As with other corticosteroids, budesonide has been shown to be teratogenic and embryocidal in rabbits and rats. Budesonide produced fetal loss, decreased pup weight, and skeletal abnormalities at subcutaneous doses of 25 mcg/kg/day in rabbits (less than the maximum recommended human daily inhalation dose on a mcg/m^2 basis) and 500 mcg/kg/day in rats (approximately 6 times the maximum recommended human daily inhalation dose on a mcg/m^2 basis). In another study in rats, no teratogenic or embryocidal effects were seen at inhalation doses up to 250 mcg/kg/day (approximately 3 times the maximum recommended human daily inhalation dose on a mcg/m^2 basis).

Formoterol

Formoterol fumarate has been shown to be teratogenic, embryocidal, to increase pup loss at birth and during lactation, and to decrease pup weights in rats when given at oral doses of 3 mg/kg/day and above (approximately 1400 times the maximum recommended human daily inhalation dose on a mcg/m^2 basis). Umbilical hernia, a malformation, was observed in rat fetuses at oral doses of 3 mg/kg/day and above (approximately 1400 times the maximum recommended human daily inhalation dose on a mcg/m^2 basis). Brachygnathia, a skeletal malformation, was observed in rat fetuses at an oral dose of 15 mg/kg/day (approximately 7000 times the maximum recommended human daily inhalation dose on a mcg/m^2 basis). Pregnancy was prolonged at an oral dose of 15 mg/kg/day (approximately 7000 times the maximum recommended human daily inhalation dose on a mcg/m^2 basis). In another study in rats, no teratogenic ef-

Table 3 The number and percentage of patients withdrawing due to or meeting predefined criteria for worsening asthma (Study 1)

	Symbicort 160/4.5 mcg n=124	Budesonide 160 mcg plus Formoterol 4.5 mcg n=115	Budesonide 160 mcg n=109	Formoterol 4.5 mcg n=123	Placebo n=125
Patients withdrawn due to predefined asthma event*	13 (10.5)	13 (11.3)	22 (20.2)	44 (35.8)	62 (49.6)
Patients with a predefined asthma event*†	37 (29.8)	24 (20.9)	48 (44.0)	68 (55.3)	84 (67.2)
Decrease in FEV₁	4 (3.2)	8 (7.0)	7 (6.4)	15 (12.2)	14 (11.2)
Rescue medication use	2 (1.6)	0	3 (2.8)	3 (2.4)	7 (5.6)
Decrease in AM PEF	2 (1.6)	5 (4.3)	5 (4.6)	17 (13.8)	15 (12.0)
Nighttime awakenings‡	24 (19.4)	11 (9.6)	29 (26.6)	32 (26.0)	49 (39.2)
Clinical exacerbation	7 (5.6)	6 (5.2)	5 (4.6)	17 (3.8)	16 (12.8)

*These criteria were assessed on a daily basis irrespective of the timing of the clinic visit, with the exception of FEV_1, which was assessed at each clinic visit.
†Individual criteria are shown for patients meeting any predefined asthma event, regardless of withdrawal status.
‡For the criterion of nighttime awakening due to asthma, patients were allowed to remain in the study at the discretion of the investigator if none of the other criteria were met.

Table 4 Mean values for selected secondary efficacy variables (Study 1)

Efficacy Variable	SYMBICORT 160/4.5 mcg (n*=124)	Budesonide 160 mcg plus Formoterol 4.5 mcg (n*=115)	Budesonide 160 mcg (n*=109)	Formoterol 4.5 mcg (n*=123)	Placebo (n*=125)
AM PEF (L/min) Baseline	341	338	342	339	355
Change from Baseline	35	28	9	-9	-18
PM PEF (L/min) Baseline	351	348	357	354	369
Change from Baseline	34	26	7	-7	-18
Albuterol rescue use Baseline	2.1	2.3	2.7	2.5	2.4
Change from Baseline	-1.0	-1.5	-0.8	-0.3	0.8
Average symptom score/day (0–3 scale) Baseline	0.99	1.03	1.04	1.04	1.08
Change from Baseline	-0.28	-0.32	-0.14	-0.05	0.10

*Number of patients (n) varies slightly due to the number of patients for whom data were available for each variable. Results shown are based on last available data for each variable.

Table 5 The number and percentage of patients withdrawing due to or meeting predefined criteria for worsening asthma (Study 2)

	SYMBICORT 80/4.5 mcg (n=123)	Budesonide 80 mcg (n=121)	Formoterol 4.5 mcg (n=114)	Placebo (n=122)
Patients withdrawn due to predefined asthma event*	9 (7.3)	8 (6.6)	21 (18.4)	40 (32.8)
Patients with a predefined asthma event*†	23 (18.7)	26 (21.5)	48 (42.1)	69 (56.6)
Decrease in FEV₁	3 (2.4)	3 (2.5)	11 (9.6)	9 (7.4)
Rescue medication use	1 (0.8)	3 (2.5)	1 (0.9)	3 (2.5)
Decrease in AM PEF	3 (2.4)	1 (0.8)	8 (7.0)	14 (11.5)
Nighttime awakening‡	17 (13.8)	20 (16.5)	31 (27.2)	52 (42.6)
Clinical exacerbation	1 (0.8)	3 (2.5)	5 (4.4)	20 (16.4)

*These criteria were assessed on a daily basis irrespective of the timing of the clinic visit, with the exception of FEV_1, which was assessed at each clinic visit.
†Individual criteria are shown for patients meeting any predefined asthma event, regardless of withdrawal status.
‡For the criterion of nighttime awakening due to asthma, patients were allowed to remain in the study at the discretion of the investigator if none of the other criteria were met.

fects were seen at inhalation doses up to 1.2 mg/kg/day (approximately 500 times the maximum recommended human daily inhalation dose on a mcg/m² basis).

Formoterol fumarate has been shown to be teratogenic in rabbits when given at an oral dose of 60 mg/kg (approximately 54,000 times the maximum recommended human daily inhalation dose on a mcg/m² basis). Subcapsular cysts on the liver were observed in rabbit fetuses at an oral dose of 60 mg/kg (approximately 54,000 times the maximum recommended human daily inhalation dose on a mcg/m² basis). No teratogenic effects were observed at oral doses up to 3.5 mg/kg (approximately 3200 times the maximum recommended human daily inhalation dose on a mcg/m² basis).

14 CLINICAL STUDIES

14.1 Asthma

SYMBICORT has been studied in patients with asthma 12 years of age and older. In two clinical studies comparing SYMBICORT with the individual components, improvements in most efficacy end points were greater with SYMBICORT than with the use of either budesonide or formoterol alone. In addition, one clinical study showed similar results between SYMBICORT and the concurrent use of budesonide and formoterol at corresponding doses from separate inhalers.

The safety and efficacy of SYMBICORT were demonstrated in two randomized, double-blind, placebo-controlled US clinical studies involving 1076 patients 12 years of age and older. Fixed SYMBICORT dosages of 160/9 mcg, and 320/9 mcg twice daily (each dose administered as two inhalations of the 80/4.5 and 160/4.5 mcg strengths, respectively) were compared with the monocomponents (budesonide and formoterol) and placebo to provide information about appropriate dosing to cover a range of asthma severity.

Study 1: Clinical Study with SYMBICORT 160/4.5

This 12-week study evaluated 596 patients 12 years of age and older by comparing SYMBICORT 160/4.5 mcg, the free combination of budesonide 160 mcg plus formoterol 4.5 mcg in separate inhalers, budesonide 160 mcg, formoterol 4.5 mcg, and placebo; each administered as two inhalations twice daily. The study included a 2-week run-in period with budesonide 80 mcg, two inhalations twice daily. Most patients had moderate to severe asthma and were using moderate to high doses of inhaled corticosteroids prior to study

entry. Randomization was stratified by previous inhaled corticosteroid treatment (71.6% on moderate- and 28.4% on high-dose inhaled corticosteroid). Mean percent predicted FEV_1 at baseline was 68.1% and was similar across treatment groups. The coprimary efficacy end points were 12-hour-average postdose FEV_1 at week 2, and predose FEV_1 averaged over the course of the study. The study also required that patients who satisfied a predefined asthma-worsening criterion be withdrawn. The predefined asthma-worsening criteria were a clinically important decrease in FEV_1 or peak expiratory flow (PEF), increase in rescue albuterol use, nighttime awakening due to asthma, emergency intervention or hospitalization due to asthma, or requirement for asthma medication not allowed by the protocol. For the criterion of nighttime awakening due to asthma, patients were allowed to remain in the study at the discretion of the investigator if none of the other asthma-worsening criteria were met. The percentage of patients withdrawing due to or meeting predefined criteria for worsening asthma is shown in Table 3.
[See table 3 at left]

Mean percent change from baseline in FEV_1 measured immediately prior to dosing (predose) over 12 weeks is displayed in Figure 1. Because this study used predefined withdrawal criteria for worsening asthma, which caused a differential withdrawal rate in the treatment groups, predose FEV_1 results at the last available study visit (end of treatment, EOT) are also provided. Patients receiving SYMBICORT 160/4.5 mcg had significantly greater mean improvements from baseline in predose FEV_1 at the end of treatment (0.19 L, 9.4%), compared with budesonide 160 mcg (0.10 L, 4.9%), formoterol 4.5 mcg (-0.12 L, -4.8%), and placebo (-0.17 L, -6.9%).

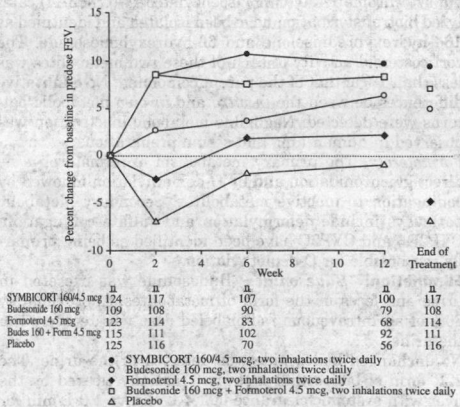

Figure 1 - Mean Percent Change From Baseline in Predose FEV₁ Over 12 Weeks (Study 1)

The effect of SYMBICORT 160/4.5 mcg two inhalations twice daily on selected secondary efficacy variables, including morning and evening PEF, albuterol rescue use, and asthma symptoms over 24 hours on a 0-3 scale is shown in Table 4.
[See table 4 at top left]

The subjective impact of asthma on patients' health-related quality of life was evaluated through the use of the standardized Asthma Quality of Life Questionnaire (AQLQ(S)) (based on a 7-point scale where 1 = maximum impairment and 7 = no impairment). Patients receiving SYMBICORT 160/4.5 had clinically meaningful improvement in overall asthma-specific quality of life, as defined by a mean difference between treatment groups of >0.5 points in change from baseline in overall AQLQ score (difference in AQLQ score of 0.70 [95% CI 0.47, 0.93], compared to placebo).

Study 2: Clinical Study with SYMBICORT 80/4.5

This 12-week study was similar in design to Study 1, and included 480 patients 12 years of age and older. This study compared SYMBICORT 80/4.5 mcg, budesonide 80 mcg, formoterol 4.5 mcg, and placebo; administered as two inhalations twice daily. The study included a 2-week placebo run-in period. Most patients had mild to moderate asthma and were using low to moderate doses of inhaled corticosteroids prior to study entry. Mean percent predicted FEV_1 at baseline was 71.3% and was similar across treatment groups. Efficacy variables and end points were identical to those in Study 1.

The percentage of patients withdrawing due to or meeting predefined criteria for worsening asthma is shown in Table 5. The method of assessment and criteria used were identical to that in Study 1.
[See table 5 above]

Mean percent change from baseline in predose FEV_1 over 12 weeks is displayed in Figure 2.

Figure 2 - Mean Percent Change From Baseline in Predose FEV₁ Over 12 Weeks (Study 2)

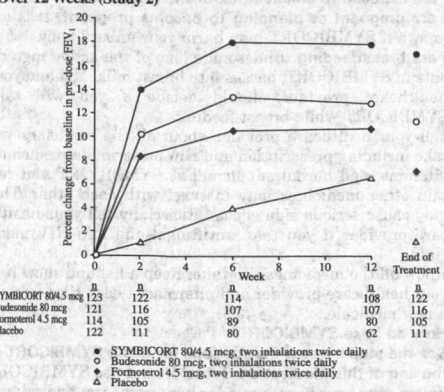

	n	n	n	n	n
SYMBICORT 80/4.5 mcg	123	122	114	108	122
Budesonide 80 mcg	121	116	107	107	116
Formoterol 4.5 mcg	114	105	89	80	105
Placebo	122	111	80	62	111

- ● SYMBICORT 80/4.5 mcg, two inhalations twice daily
- ○ Budesonide 80 mcg, two inhalations twice daily
- ◆ Formoterol 4.5 mcg, two inhalations twice daily
- △ Placebo

Efficacy results for other secondary end points, including quality of life, were similar to those observed in Study 1.

Onset and Duration of Action and Progression of Improvement in Asthma Control

The onset of action and progression of improvement in asthma control were evaluated in the two pivotal clinical studies. The median time to onset of clinically significant bronchodilation (>15% improvement in FEV₁) was seen within 15 minutes. Maximum improvement in FEV₁ occurred within 3 hours, and clinically significant improvement was maintained over 12 hours. Figures 3 and 4 show the percent change from baseline in postdose FEV₁ over 12 hours on the day of randomization and on the last day of treatment for Study 1.

Reduction in asthma symptoms and in albuterol rescue use, as well as improvement in morning and evening PEF, occurred within 1 day of the first dose of SYMBICORT; improvement in these variables was maintained over the 12 weeks of therapy.

Following the initial dose of SYMBICORT, FEV₁ improved markedly during the first 2 weeks of treatment, continued to show improvement at the Week 6 assessment, and was maintained through Week 12 for both studies.

No diminution in the 12-hour bronchodilator effect was observed with either SYMBICORT 80/4.5 mcg or SYMBICORT 160/4.5 mcg, as assessed by FEV₁, following 12 weeks of therapy or at the last available visit.

FEV₁ data from Study 1 evaluating SYMBICORT 160/4.5 mcg is displayed in Figures 3 and 4.

Figure 3 - Mean Percent Change From Baseline in FEV₁ on Day of Randomization (Study 1)

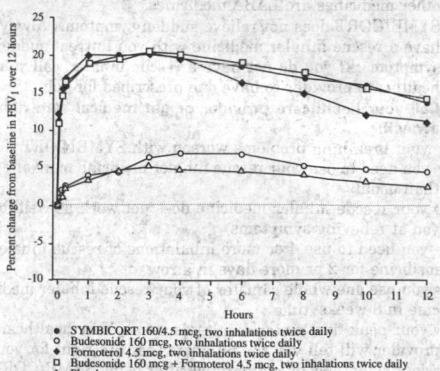

- ● SYMBICORT 160/4.5 mcg, two inhalations twice daily
- ○ Budesonide 160 mcg, two inhalations twice daily
- ◆ Formoterol 4.5 mcg, two inhalations twice daily
- □ Budesonide 160 mcg + Formoterol 4.5 mcg, two inhalations twice daily
- △ Placebo

[See figure at top of next column]

14.2   Chronic Obstructive Pulmonary Disease (COPD)

The efficacy of SYMBICORT 80/4.5 and SYMBICORT 160/4.5 in the maintenance treatment of airflow obstruction in COPD patients was evaluated in two randomized, double-blind, placebo-controlled multinational studies, conducted over 6 months (Study 1) and 12 months (Study 2), in a total of 3668 patients (2416 males and 1252 females). The majority of patients (93%) were Caucasian. All patients were required to be at least 40 years of age, with a FEV₁ of less than or equal to 50% predicted, a clinical diagnosis of COPD with symptoms for at least 2 years, and a smoking history of at least 10 pack years, prior to entering the trial. The mean prebronchodilator FEV₁ at baseline of the patients enrolled in the study was 34% predicted. Forty-eight percent of the patients enrolled were on inhaled corticosteroids and 52.7% of patients were on short-acting anticholinergic bronchodilators during run-in. On randomization, inhaled corticosteroids were discontinued, and ipratropium bromide was allowed at a stable dose for those patients previously treated with short-acting anticholinergic bronchodilators. The co-primary efficacy variables in both studies were the change from baseline in average pre-dose and 1-hour post-dose FEV₁ over the treatment period. The results of both studies 1 and 2 are described below.

Study 1

This was a 6-month, placebo-controlled study of 1704 COPD patients (mean % predicted FEV₁ at baseline ranging from 33.5%-34.7%) conducted to demonstrate the efficacy and safety of SYMBICORT in the treatment of airflow obstruction in COPD. The patients were randomized to one of the following treatment groups: SYMBICORT 160/4.5 (n=277), SYMBICORT 80/4.5 (n=281), budesonide 160 mcg + formoterol 4.5 mcg (n=287), budesonide 160 mcg (n=275), formoterol 4.5 mcg (n=284), or placebo (n=300). Patients receiving SYMBICORT 160/4.5 mcg, two inhalations twice daily, had significantly greater mean improvements from baseline in pre-dose FEV₁ averaged over the treatment period [0.08 L, 10.7%] compared with formoterol 4.5 mcg [0.04 L, 6.9%] and placebo [0.01 L, 2.2%] (See Figure 5). Patients receiving SYMBICORT 80/4.5 mcg, two inhalations twice daily, did not have significantly greater improvement from baseline in the pre-dose FEV₁ averaged over the treatment period compared with formoterol 4.5 mcg.

Figure 5 Mean Percent Change From Baseline in Pre-dose FEV₁ Over 6 months (Study 1)

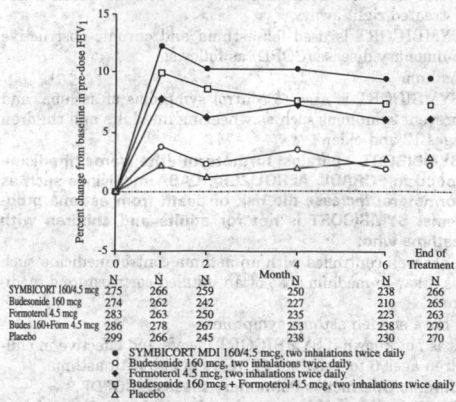

	N	N	N	N	N
SYMBICORT 160/4.5 mcg	275	266	259	250	238	266
Budesonide 160 mcg	274	262	242	227	210	265
Formoterol 4.5 mcg	283	263	250	235	223	263
Budes 160+Form 4.5 mcg	286	278	267	253	238	279
Placebo	299	266	245	238	230	270

- ● SYMBICORT MDI 160/4.5 mcg, two inhalations twice daily
- ○ Budesonide 160 mcg, two inhalations twice daily
- ◆ Formoterol 4.5 mcg, two inhalations twice daily
- □ Budesonide 160 mcg + Formoterol 4.5 mcg, two inhalations twice daily
- △ Placebo

Patients receiving SYMBICORT 160/4.5 mcg, two inhalations twice daily, had significantly greater mean improvements from baseline in 1-hour post-dose FEV₁ averaged over the treatment period [0.20 L, 22.6%], compared with budesonide 160 mcg [0.03 L, 4.9%] and placebo [0.03 L, 4.1%] (See Figure 6).

[See figure at top of next column]

Study 2

This was a 12-month, placebo-controlled study of 1964 COPD patients (mean % predicted FEV₁ at baseline ranging from 33.7%-35.5%) conducted to demonstrate the efficacy and safety of SYMBICORT in the treatment of airflow obstruction in COPD. The patients were randomized to one of the following treatment groups: SYMBICORT 160/4.5 (n=494), SYMBICORT 80/4.5 (n=494), formoterol 4.5 mcg (n=495), or placebo (n=481). Patients receiving SYMBICORT 160/4.5 mcg, two inhalations twice daily, had significantly greater improvements from baseline in mean pre-dose FEV₁ averaged over the treatment period [0.10 L, 10.8%] compared with formoterol 4.5 mcg [0.06 L, 7.2%] and placebo [0.01 L, 2.8%]. Patients receiving SYMBICORT 80/4.5 mcg, two inhalations twice daily, did not have significantly greater improvements from baseline in the mean pre-dose FEV₁ averaged over the treatment period com-

Figure 4 - Mean Percent Change From Baseline in FEV₁ At End of Treatment (Study 1)

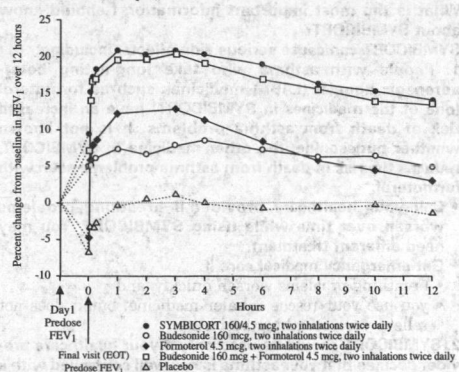

- Day1 Predose FEV₁
- Final visit (EOT) Predose FEV₁

- ● SYMBICORT 160/4.5 mcg, two inhalations twice daily
- □ Budesonide 160 mcg, two inhalations twice daily
- ◆ Formoterol 4.5 mcg, two inhalations twice daily
- ○ Budesonide 160 mcg + Formoterol 4.5 mcg, two inhalations twice daily
- △ Placebo

pared to formoterol. Patients receiving SYMBICORT 160/4.5 mcg, two inhalations twice daily, also had significantly greater mean improvements from baseline in 1-hour post-dose FEV₁ averaged over the treatment period [0.21 L, 24.0%] compared with placebo [0.02 L, 5.2%].

Serial FEV₁ measures over 12 hours were obtained in a subset of patients in Study 1 (n=99) and Study 2 (n=121). The median time to onset of bronchodilation, defined as an FEV₁ increase of 15% or greater from baseline, occurred at 5 minutes post-dose. Maximum improvement (calculated as the average change from baseline at each timepoint) in FEV₁ occurred at approximately 2 hours post-dose.

In both Studies 1 and 2, improvements in secondary endpoints of morning and evening peak expiratory flow and reduction in rescue medication use were supportive of the efficacy of SYMBICORT 160/4.5.

Figure 6 Mean Percent Change From Baseline in 1-hour Post-dose FEV₁ Over 6 months (Study 1)

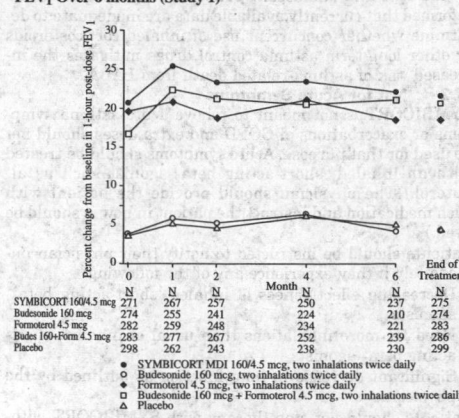

	N	N	N	N	N
SYMBICORT 160/4.5 mcg	271	267	257	250	237	275
Budesonide 160 mcg	255	241	224	224	210	274
Formoterol 4.5 mcg	282	259	248	234	221	283
Budes 160+Form 4.5 mcg	283	277	267	252	239	286
Placebo	298	262	243	230	230	299

- ● SYMBICORT MDI 160/4.5 mcg, two inhalations twice daily
- ○ Budesonide 160 mcg, two inhalations twice daily
- ◆ Formoterol 4.5 mcg, two inhalations twice daily
- □ Budesonide 160 mcg + Formoterol 4.5 mcg, two inhalations twice daily
- △ Placebo

16   HOW SUPPLIED/STORAGE AND HANDLING

SYMBICORT is available in two strengths and is supplied in the following package sizes:

Dosage Forms and Strengths

Package Size	NDC
SYMBICORT 80/4.5, 120 inhalations	0186-0372-20
SYMBICORT 80/4.5, 60 inhalations (institutional pack)	0186-0372-28
SYMBICORT 160/4.5, 120 inhalations	0186-0370-20
SYMBICORT 160/4.5, 60 inhalations (institutional pack)	0186-0370-28

Each strength is supplied as a pressurized aluminium canister with an attached counting device, a red plastic actuator body with a white mouthpiece, and attached gray dust cap. Each 120 inhalation canister has a net fill weight of 10.2 grams and each 60 inhalation canister has a net fill weight of 6.9 grams (SYMBICORT 80/4.5) or 6 grams (SYMBICORT 160/4.5). Each canister is packaged in a foil overwrap pouch with desiccant sachet and placed into a carton. Each carton contains one canister and a Medication Guide.

The SYMBICORT canister should only be used with the SYMBICORT actuator, and the SYMBICORT actuator should not be used with any other inhalation drug product. The correct amount of medication in each inhalation cannot be ensured after the labeled number of inhalations from the canister have been used, even though the inhaler may not feel completely empty and may continue to operate. The inhaler should be discarded when the labeled number of inhalations have been used or within 3 months after removal from the foil pouch. Never immerse the canister into water to determine the amount remaining in the canister ("float test").

Store at controlled room temperature 20°C to 25°C (68°F to 77°F) [see USP]. Store the inhaler with the mouthpiece down.

For best results, the canister should be at room temperature before use. Shake well for 5 seconds before using.

Keep out of the reach of children.

CONTENTS UNDER PRESSURE.

Do not puncture or incinerate. Do not store near heat or open flame. Exposure to temperatures over 120°F may cause bursting. Never throw container into fire or incinerator.

17   PATIENT COUNSELING INFORMATION

See Medication Guide (17.6)

17.1   Asthma-Related Death

Patients with asthma should be informed that formoterol fumarate dihydrate, one of the active ingredients in SYMBICORT, increases the risk of asthma-related death and may increase the risk of asthma-related hospitalization in pediatric and adolescent patients. They should also be informed that currently available data are inadequate to determine whether concurrent use of inhaled corticosteroids or other long-term asthma control drugs mitigates the increased risk of asthma-related death from LABA.

17.2 Not for Acute Symptoms

SYMBICORT is not meant to relieve acute asthma symptoms or exacerbations of COPD and extra doses should not be used for that purpose. Acute symptoms should be treated with an inhaled, short-acting beta$_2$-agonist such as albuterol. (The physician should provide the patient with such medication and instruct the patient in how it should be used.)

Patients should be instructed to notify their physician immediately if they experience any of the following:

• Decreasing effectiveness of inhaled, short-acting beta$_2$-agonists

• Need for more inhalations than usual of inhaled, short-acting beta$_2$-agonists

• Significant decrease in lung function as outlined by the physician

Patients should not stop therapy with SYMBICORT without physician/provider guidance since symptoms may recur after discontinuation.

17.3 Do Not Use Additional Long-Acting Beta$_2$-Agonists

When patients are prescribed SYMBICORT, other long-acting beta$_2$-agonists for asthma and COPD should not be used.

17.4 Risks Associated With Corticosteroid Therapy

Local Effects: Patients should be advised that localized infections with *Candida albicans* occurred in the mouth and pharynx in some patients. If oropharyngeal candidiasis develops, it should be treated with appropriate local or systemic (i.e., oral) antifungal therapy while still continuing therapy with SYMBICORT, but at times therapy with SYMBICORT may need to be temporarily interrupted under close medical supervision. Rinsing the mouth after inhalation is advised.

Pneumonia: Patients with COPD have a higher risk of pneumonia and should be instructed to contact their healthcare provider if they develop symptoms of pneumonia.

Immunosuppression: Patients who are on immunosuppressant doses of corticosteroids should be warned to avoid exposure to chicken pox or measles and, if exposed, to consult their physician without delay. Patients should be informed of potential worsening of existing tuberculosis, fungal, bacterial, viral, or parasitic infections, or ocular herpes simplex.

Hypercorticism and Adrenal Suppression: Patients should be advised that SYMBICORT may cause systemic corticosteroid effects of hypercorticism and adrenal suppression. Additionally, patients should be instructed that deaths due to adrenal insufficiency have occurred during and after transfer from systemic corticosteroids. Patients should taper slowly from systemic corticosteroids if transferring to SYMBICORT.

Reduction in Bone Mineral Density: Patients who are at an increased risk for decreased BMD should be advised that the use of corticosteroids may pose an additional risk.

Reduced Growth Velocity: Patients should be informed that orally inhaled corticosteroids, component of SYMBICORT, may cause a reduction in growth velocity when administered to pediatric patients. Physicians should closely follow the growth of children and adolescents taking corticosteroids by any route.

Ocular Effects: Long-term use of inhaled corticosteroids may increase the risk of some eye problems (cataracts or glaucoma); regular eye examinations should be considered.

17.5 Risks Associated With Beta-Agonist Therapy

Patients should be informed of adverse effects associated with beta$_2$-agonists, such as palpitations, chest pain, rapid heart rate, tremor, or nervousness.

SYMBICORT is a trademark of the AstraZeneca group of companies.

©AstraZeneca 2008, 2009, 2010

Manufactured for: AstraZeneca LP, Wilmington, DE 19850

By: AstraZeneca Dunkerque Production, Dunkerque, France

Product of France

31152–07

Rev. 06/10

17.6 MEDICATION GUIDE

SYMBICORT 80/4.5
(budesonide 80 mcg and formoterol fumarate dihydrate 4.5 mcg) Inhalation Aerosol

SYMBICORT 160/4.5
(budesonide 160 mcg and formoterol fumarate dihydrate 4.5 mcg) Inhalation Aerosol

Read the Medication Guide that comes with SYMBICORT before you start using it and each time you get a refill. There may be new information. This Medication Guide does not take the place of talking to your healthcare provider about your medical condition or treatment.

What is the most important information I should know about SYMBICORT?

SYMBICORT can cause serious side effects, including:

1. People with asthma who take long-acting beta$_2$-adrenegic agonist (LABA) medicines such as formoterol (one of the medicines in SYMBICORT) have an increased risk of death from asthma problems. It is not known whether budesonide, the other medicine in SYMBICORT, reduces the risk of death from asthma problems seen with formoterol.

• **Call your healthcare provider if breathing problems worsen over time while using SYMBICORT. You may need different treatment.**

• **Get emergency medical care if:**
  • breathing problems worsen quickly, and
  • you use your rescue inhaler medicine, but it does not relieve your breathing problems.

2. SYMBICORT should be used only if your healthcare provider decides that your asthma is not well controlled with a long-term asthma-control medicine, such as an inhaled corticosteroid.

3. When your asthma is well controlled, your healthcare provider may tell you to stop taking SYMBICORT. Your healthcare provider will decide if you can stop SYMBICORT without loss of asthma control. Your healthcare provider may prescribe a different long-term asthma-control medicine for you, such as an inhaled corticosteroid.

4. Children and adolescents who take LABA medicines may have an increased risk of being hospitalized for asthma problems.

What is SYMBICORT?

SYMBICORT combines an inhaled corticosteroid medicine, budesonide (the same medicine found in PULMICORT FLEXHALER), and a long-acting beta$_2$-agonist medicine (LABA), formoterol (the same medicine found in FORADIL AEROLIZER).

• Inhaled corticosteroids help to decrease inflammation in the lungs. Inflammation in the lungs can lead to asthma symptoms.

• LABA medicines are used in patients with chronic obstructive pulmonary disease (COPD) and asthma. LABA medicines help the muscles around the airways in your lungs stay relaxed to prevent asthma symptoms, such as wheezing and shortness of breath. These symptoms can happen when the muscles around the airways tighten. This makes it hard to breathe. In severe cases, wheezing can stop your breathing and may lead to death if not treated right away.

SYMBICORT is used for asthma and chronic obstructive pulmonary disease (COPD) as follows:

Asthma

SYMBICORT is used to control symptoms of asthma, and prevent symptoms such as wheezing in adults and children ages 12 and older.

SYMBICORT contains formoterol (the same medicine found in FORADIL AEROLIZER). LABA medicines such as formoterol increase the risk of death from asthma problems. SYMBICORT is not for adults and children with asthma who:

○ are well controlled with an asthma-control medicine such as a low to medium dose of an inhaled corticosteroid medicine

○ have sudden asthma symptoms

It is not known if SYMBICORT is safe and effective in children ages 6 to less than 12 years of age with asthma.

Chronic Obstructive Pulmonary Disease (COPD)

COPD is a chronic lung disease that includes chronic bronchitis, emphysema, or both. SYMBICORT 160/4.5 mcg is used long term, 2 times each day to help improve lung function for better breathing in adults with COPD.

Who should not use SYMBICORT?

Do not use SYMBICORT:

• to treat sudden severe symptoms of asthma or COPD.

• if you are allergic to any of the ingredients in SYMBICORT. See the end of the Medication Guide for a list of ingredients in SYMBICORT.

What should I tell my healthcare provider before using SYMBICORT?

Tell your healthcare provider about all of your health conditions, including if you:

○ have heart problems

○ have high blood pressure

○ have seizures

○ have thyroid problems

○ have diabetes

○ have liver problems

○ have osteoporosis

○ have an immune system problem

○ have eye problems such as increased pressure in the eye, glaucoma, or cataracts

○ are allergic to any medicines

○ are exposed to chicken pox or measles

○ are pregnant or planning to become pregnant. It is not known if SYMBICORT may harm your unborn baby.

○ are breastfeeding. Budesonide, one of the active ingredients in SYMBICORT, passes into breast milk. You and your healthcare provider should decide if you will take SYMBICORT while breast-feeding.

Tell your healthcare provider about all the medicines you take including prescription and non-prescription medicines, vitamins, and herbal supplements. SYMBICORT and certain other medicines may interact with each other. This may cause serious side effects. Especially tell your healthcare provider if you take antifungal and anti-HIV medicines.

Know all the medicines you take. Keep a list and show it to your healthcare provider and pharmacist each time you get a new medicine.

How do I use SYMBICORT?

See the step-by-step instructions for using SYMBICORT at the end of this Medication Guide. Do not use SYMBICORT unless your healthcare provider has taught you and you understand everything. Ask your healthcare provider or pharmacist if you have any questions.

• Use SYMBICORT exactly as prescribed. **Do not use SYMBICORT more often than prescribed.** SYMBICORT comes in 2 strengths. Your healthcare provider has prescribed the strength that is best for you. Note the differences between SYMBICORT and your other inhaled medications, including the differences in prescribed use and physical appearance.

• SYMBICORT should be taken every day as 2 puffs in the morning and 2 puffs in the evening.

• If you miss a dose of SYMBICORT, you should take your next dose at the same time you normally do. Do not take SYMBICORT more often or use more puffs than you have been prescribed.

• Rinse your mouth with water and spit the water out after each dose (2 puffs) of SYMBICORT. Do not swallow the water. This will help to lessen the chance of getting a fungus infection (thrush) in the mouth and throat.

• Do not spray SYMBICORT in your eyes. If you accidentally get SYMBICORT in your eyes, rinse your eyes with water, and if redness or irritation persists, consult your healthcare provider.

• Do not change or stop any medicines used to control or treat your breathing problems. Your healthcare provider will change your medicines as needed.

• **While you are using SYMBICORT 2 times each day, do not use other medicines that contain a long-acting beta$_2$-agonist (LABA) for any reason. Ask your healthcare provider or pharmacist if any of your other medicine are LABA medicines.**

• Ask your healthcare provider or pharmacist if any of your other medicines are LABA medicines.

• SYMBICORT does not relieve sudden symptoms. Always have a rescue inhaler medicine with you to treat sudden symptoms. If you do not have a rescue inhaler, call your healthcare provider to have one prescribed for you.

• **Call your healthcare provider or get medical care right away if:**

  ○ your breathing problems worsen with SYMBICORT

  ○ you need to use your rescue inhaler medicine more often than usual

  ○ your rescue inhaler medicine does not work as well for you at relieving symptoms

  ○ you need to use 4 or more inhalations of rescue inhaler medicine for 2 or more days in a row

  ○ you use one whole canister of your rescue inhaler medicine in 8 weeks' time

  ○ your peak flow meter results decrease. Your healthcare provider will tell you the numbers that are right for you.

  ○ your symptoms do not improve after using SYMBICORT regularly for 1 week.

What are the possible side effects with SYMBICORT?

SYMBICORT can cause serious side effects

• See "What is the most important information I should know about SYMBICORT?"

• **Pneumonia and other lower respiratory tract infections.** People with COPD have a higher chance of getting pneumonia and other lung infections. Inhaled corticosteroids may increase the chance of getting pneumonia. Call your healthcare provider if you notice any of these symptoms:

  • increase in mucus (sputum) production
  • change in mucus color
  • fever
  • chills
  • increased cough
  • increased breathing problems

• **Serious allergic reactions including rash, hives, swelling of the face, mouth, and tongue, and breathing problems.** Call your healthcare provider or get emergency medical care if you get any symptoms of a serious allergic reaction.

- **Immune system effects and a higher chance for infections.** Tell your healthcare provider about any signs of infection such as:
- fever
- pain
- body aches
- chills
- feeling tired
- nausea
- vomiting
- **Adrenal insufficiency.** Adrenal insufficiency is a condition in which the adrenal glands do not make enough steroid hormones. This can happen when you stop taking oral corticosteroid medicines and start inhaled corticosteroid medicine.
- **Using too much of a LABA medicine may cause:** chest pain, increased blood pressure, a fast and irregular heartbeat, headache, tremor, and nervousness.
- **Increased wheezing right after taking SYMBICORT.** Always have a rescue inhaler with you to treat sudden wheezing.
- **Eye problems including glaucoma and cataracts.** You should have regular eye exams while using SYMBICORT.
- **Lower bone mineral density.** This can happen in people who have a high chance for low bone mineral density (osteoporosis). Your healthcare provider should check you for this during treatment with SYMBICORT.
- **Slowed growth in children.** A child's growth should be checked regularly while using SYMBICORT.
- **Swelling of your blood vessels.** This can happen in people with asthma. Tell your healthcare provider right away if you have:
- a feeling of pins and needles or numbness of your arms or legs
- flu like symptoms
- rash
- pain and swelling of the sinuses
- Decreases in blood potassium levels (hypokalemia)
- Increases in blood sugar levels (hyperglycemia)

Common side effects of SYMBICORT include:

Patients with asthma:
- throat irritation
- headache
  upper respiratory tract infection
- throat pain
- inflammation of mucous membranes of the sinuses (sinusitis)
- flu
- back pain
- nasal congestion
- stomach discomfort
- vomiting
- thrush in the mouth and throat

Patients with COPD:
- throat irritation
- thrush in the mouth and throat
- lower respiratory tract infections, mostly infections and/or inflammation of the mucous membranes of the bronchial tubes (bronchitis)
- inflammation of mucous membranes in the sinuses (sinusitis)
- upper respiratory tract infection

Tell your healthcare provider about any side effect that bothers you or that does not go away.

These are not all the side effects of SYMBICORT. Ask your healthcare provider or pharmacist for more information.

Call your doctor for medical advice about side effects. You may report side effects to the FDA at 1-800-FDA-1088. You may also report side effects to ASTRAZENECA at 1-800-236-9933.

How do I store SYMBICORT?
- Store SYMBICORT at room temperature between 68°F to 77°F (20°C to 25°C).
- Store with the mouthpiece down.
- The contents of your SYMBICORT canister are under pressure. Do not puncture or throw the canister into a fire or incinerator. Do not use or store it near heat or open flame. Storage above 120°F may cause the canister to burst.
- Throw away SYMBICORT when the counter reaches zero ("0") or 3 months after you take SYMBICORT out of its foil pouch, whichever comes first.
- **Keep SYMBICORT and all medicines out of the reach of children.**

General Information about SYMBICORT
Medicines are sometimes prescribed for purposes other than those listed in a Medication Guide. Do not use SYMBICORT for a condition for which it was not prescribed. Do not give your SYMBICORT to other people, even if they have the same condition. It may harm them.

This Medication Guide summarizes the most important information about SYMBICORT. If you would like more infor-

mation, talk with your healthcare provider or pharmacist. You can ask your healthcare provider or pharmacist for information about SYMBICORT that was written for healthcare professionals. For more information, call 1-800-236-9933 or go to www.MySymbicort.com.

What are the ingredients in SYMBICORT?
Active ingredient: micronized budesonide and micronized formoterol fumarate dihydrate Inactive ingredients: hydrofluoroalkane (HFA 227), povidone K25 USP, and polyethylene glycol 1000 NF

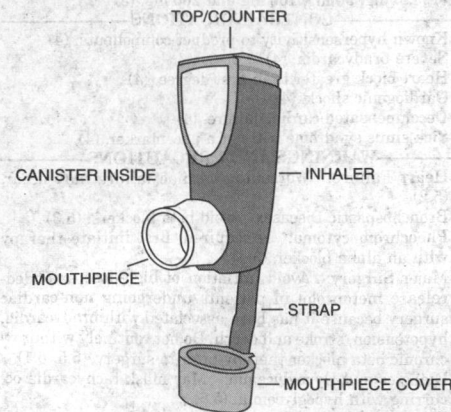

Figure 1

Upright Position
How to Use SYMBICORT
Follow the instructions below for using SYMBICORT. You will breathe-in (inhale) the medicine. If you have any questions, ask your doctor or pharmacist.

Preparing your inhaler for use
1. Take your SYMBICORT out of the moisture-protective foil pouch before you use it for the first time and throw the foil away. Write the date that you open the foil pouch on the box.
2. A counter is attached to the top of the metal canister. The counter will count down each time you release a puff of SYMBICORT. The arrow points to the number of inhalations (puffs) left in the canister. The counter will stop counting at zero ("0").
3. Use the SYMBICORT canister only with the red SYMBICORT inhaler supplied with the product. Parts of the SYMBICORT inhaler should not be used with parts from any other inhalation product.
4. Shake your SYMBICORT inhaler well for 5 seconds right before each use. Remove the mouthpiece cover. Check the mouthpiece for foreign objects before use.
5. **Priming** Before you use SYMBICORT for the first time, you will need to prime it. To prime SYMBICORT, hold it in the upright position. See figure 1 above. Shake the SYMBICORT inhaler well for 5 seconds. Hold your SYMBICORT inhaler facing away from you and then release a test spray. Then shake it again for 5 seconds and release a second test spray. Your SYMBICORT inhaler is now primed and ready for use. After you have primed the SYMBICORT inhaler for the first time, the counter will read either 120 or 60, depending on which size was provided to you.

If you do not use your SYMBICORT inhaler for more than 7 days or if you drop it, you will need to prime again. Ways to hold the SYMBICORT inhaler for use

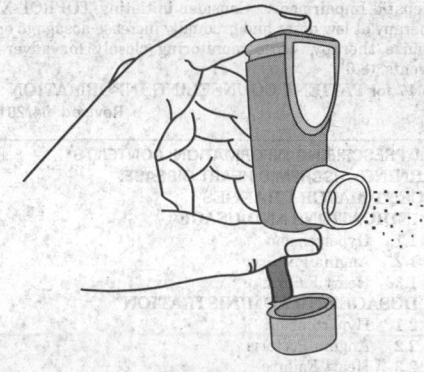

Figure 2

OR

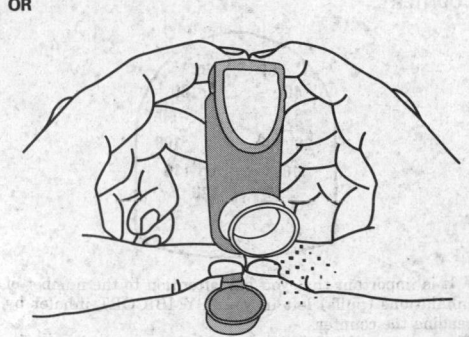

Figure 3

Using your SYMBICORT inhaler
6. Shake your SYMBICORT inhaler well for 5 seconds. Remove the mouthpiece cover. Check the mouthpiece for foreign objects.
7. Breathe out fully (exhale). Hold the SYMBICORT inhaler up to your mouth. Place the white mouthpiece fully into your mouth and close your lips around it. Make sure that the SYMBICORT inhaler is upright and that the opening of the mouthpiece is pointing towards the back of your throat (see Figure 4).

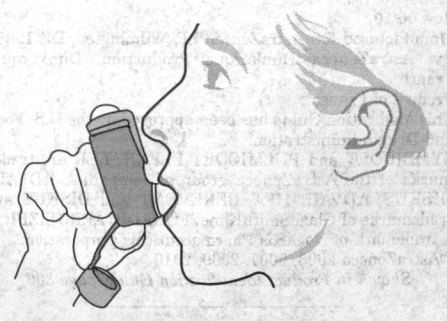

Figure 4

8. Breathe in (inhale) deeply and slowly through your mouth. Press down firmly and fully on the top of the counter on the SYMBICORT inhaler to release the medicine (see Figures 2 and 3).
9. Continue to breathe in (inhale) and hold your breath for about 10 seconds, or for as long as is comfortable. Before you breathe out (exhale), release your finger from the top of the counter. Keep the SYMBICORT inhaler upright and remove from your mouth.
10. Shake the SYMBICORT inhaler again for 5 seconds and repeat steps 7 to 9.

After using your SYMBICORT inhaler
11. Replace the mouthpiece cover after use.
12. After you finish taking SYMBICORT (two puffs), rinse your mouth with water. Spit out the water. Do not swallow it.

Reading the counter
- The arrow on the counter on the top of the SYMBICORT inhaler points to the number of inhalations (puffs) left in your inhaler.
COUNTER

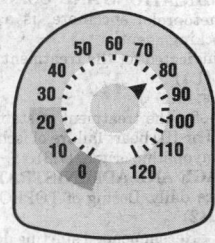

- The counter will count down each time you release a puff of medicine (either when preparing your SYMBICORT inhaler for use or when taking the medicine).
- When the arrow on the counter approaches 20, you will notice the beginning of a yellow area letting you know that it is time to call your healthcare provider for a refill.

COUNTER

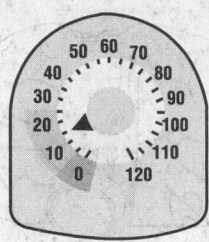

- It is important that you pay attention to the number of inhalations (puffs) left in your SYMBICORT inhaler by reading the counter.

Throw away SYMBICORT when the counter shows zero ("0"). Your SYMBICORT inhaler may not feel empty and it may continue to operate, but you will not get the right amount of medicine if you keep using it. Use a new SYMBICORT inhaler and follow the instructions for priming (instruction 5 above).

How to clean your SYMBICORT inhaler

Clean the white mouthpiece of your SYMBICORT inhaler every 7 days. To clean the mouthpiece:

- Remove the grey mouthpiece cover
- Wipe the inside and outside of the white mouthpiece opening with a clean, dry cloth
- Replace the mouthpiece cover
- **Do not put the SYMBICORT inhaler into water**
- Do not try to take apart your **SYMBICORT** inhaler

31154–05
Rev. 06/10
Manufactured for: AstraZeneca LP, Wilmington, DE 19850
By: AstraZeneca Dunkerque Production, Dunkerque, France
Product of France
This Medication Guide has been approved by the U.S. Food and Drug Administration.
SYMBICORT and PULMICORT FLEXHALER are trademarks of the AstraZeneca group of companies. ADVAIR DISKUS, ADVAIR HFA, SEREVENT and DISKUS are trademarks of GlaxoSmithKline. FORADIL AEROLIZER is a trademark of Novartis Pharmaceuticals Corporation.
©AstraZeneca 2006, 2007, 2009, 2010

Shown in Product Identification Guide, page 306

TOPROL-XL® ℞
[tō′prōl]
(metoprolol succinate)
Tablet, Extended-Release for Oral Use

HIGHLIGHTS OF PRESCRIBING INFORMATION
These highlights do not include all the information needed to use TOPROL-XL® safely and effectively. See full prescribing information for TOPROL-XL.
TOPROL-XL (metoprolol succinate) Tablet, Extended-Release for Oral Use
Initial U.S. Approval: 1992

> **WARNING: ISCHEMIC HEART DISEASE**
> *(See Full Prescribing Information for complete boxed warning)*
> **Following abrupt cessation of therapy with beta-blocking agents, exacerbations of angina pectoris and myocardial infarction have occurred. Warn patients against interruption or discontinuation of therapy without the physician's advice. (5.1)**

————RECENT MAJOR CHANGES————
Major Surgery (5.5) January 2010
————INDICATIONS AND USAGE————
TOPROL-XL, metoprolol succinate, is a beta₁-selective adrenoceptor blocking agent.
TOPROL-XL is indicated for the treatment of:
- Hypertension. (1.1)
- Angina Pectoris. (1.2)
- Heart Failure—for the treatment of stable, symptomatic (NYHA Class II or III) heart failure of ischemic, hypertensive, or cardiomyopathic origin. (1.3)

————DOSAGE AND ADMINISTRATION————
- Administer once daily. Dosing of TOPROL-XL should be individualized. (2)
- Heart Failure: Recommended starting dose is 12.5 mg or 25 mg doubled every two weeks to the highest dose tolerated or up to 200 mg. (2.3)
- Hypertension: Usual initial dosage is 25 to 100 mg once daily. The dosage may be increased at weekly (or longer) intervals until optimum blood pressure reduction is achieved. Dosages above 400 mg per day have not been studied. (2.1)

- Angina Pectoris: Usual initial dosage is 100 mg once daily. Gradually increase the dosage at weekly intervals until optimum clinical response has been obtained or there is an unacceptable bradycardia. Dosages above 400 mg per day have not been studied. (2.2)
- Switching from immediate-release metoprolol to TOPROL-XL: use the same total daily dose of TOPROL-XL. (2)

————DOSAGE FORMS AND STRENGTHS————
TOPROL-XL Extended Release Tablets (metoprolol succinate): 25 mg, 50 mg, 100 mg and 200 mg. (3)

————CONTRAINDICATIONS————
- Known hypersensitivity to product components. (4)
- Severe bradycardia. (4)
- Heart block greater than first degree. (4)
- Cardiogenic shock. (4)
- Decompensated cardiac failure. (4)
- Sick sinus syndrome without a pacemarker. (4)

————WARNINGS AND PRECAUTIONS————
- Heart Failure: Worsening cardiac failure may occur. (5.2)
- Bronchospastic Disease: Avoid beta blockers. (5.3)
- Pheochromocytoma: If required, first initiate therapy with an alpha blocker. (5.4)
- Major Surgery: Avoid initiation of high-dose extended-release metoprolol in patients undergoing non-cardiac surgery because it has been associated with bradycardia, hypotension, stroke and death. Do not routinely withdraw chronic beta blocker therapy prior to surgery. (5.5, 6.1)
- Diabetes and Hypoglycemia: May mask tachycardia occurring with hypoglycemia. (5.6)
- Patients with Hepatic Impairment: (5.7)
- Thyrotoxicosis: Abrupt withdrawal in patients with thyrotoxicosis might precipitate a thyroid storm. (5.8)
- Anaphylactic Reactions: Patients may be unresponsive to the usual doses of epinephrine used to treat allergic reaction. (5.9)
- Peripheral Vascular Disease: Can aggravate symptoms of arterial insufficiency. (5.10)
- Calcium Channel Blockers: Because of significant inotropic and chronotropic effects in patients treated with beta-blockers and calcium channel blockers of the verapamil and diltiazem type, caution should be exercised in patients treated with these agents concomitantly. (5.11)

————ADVERSE REACTIONS————
Most common adverse reactions: tiredness, dizziness, depression, shortness of breath, bradycardia, hypotension, diarrhea, pruritus, rash. (6.1)
To report SUSPECTED ADVERSE REACTIONS, contact AstraZeneca at 1-800-236-9933 or FDA at 1-800-FDA-1088 or www.fda.gov/medwatch.

————DRUG INTERACTIONS————
- Catecholamine-depleting drugs may have an additive effect when given with beta-blocking agents. (7.1)
- CYP2D6 Inhibitors are likely to increase metoprolol concentration. (7.2)
- Concomitant use of glycosides, clonidine, and diltiazem and verapamil with beta-blockers can increase the risk of bradycardia. (7.3)
- Beta-blockers including metoprolol, may exacerbate the rebound hypertension that can follow the withdrawal of clonidine. (7.3)

————USE IN SPECIFIC POPULATIONS————
- Pregnancy: There are no adequate and well-controlled studies in pregnant women. Use this drug during pregnancy only if clearly needed. (8.1)
- Nursing Mothers: Consider possible infant exposure. (8.3)
- Pediatrics: Safety and effectiveness have not been established in patients < 6 years of age. (8.4)
- Geriatrics: No notable difference in efficacy or safety vs. younger patients. (8.5)
- Hepatic Impairment: Consider initiating TOPROL-XL therapy at low doses and gradually increase dosage to optimize therapy, while monitoring closely for adverse events. (8.6)

See 17 for PATIENT COUNSELING INFORMATION
Revised: 04/2010

FULL PRESCRIBING INFORMATION: CONTENTS*
WARNING: ISCHEMIC HEART DISEASE:
RECENT MAJOR CHANGES

FULL PRESCRIBING INFORMATION

> **WARNING: ISCHEMIC HEART DISEASE:**
> Following abrupt cessation of therapy with certain beta-blocking agents, exacerbations of angina pectoris and, in some cases, myocardial infarction have occurred. When discontinuing chronically administered TOPROL-XL, particularly in patients with ischemic heart disease, the dosage should be gradually reduced over a period of 1-2 weeks and the patient should be carefully monitored. If angina markedly worsens or acute coronary insufficiency develops, TOPROL-XL administration should be reinstated promptly, at least temporarily, and other measures appropriate for the management of unstable angina should be taken. Warn patients against interruption or discontinuation of therapy without the physician's advice. Because coronary artery disease is common and may be unrecognized, it may be prudent not to discontinue TOPROL-XL therapy abruptly even in patients treated only for hypertension (5.1).

1   INDICATIONS AND USAGE

1.1   Hypertension
TOPROL-XL is indicated for the treatment of hypertension. It may be used alone or in combination with other antihypertensive agents *[see Dosage and Administration (2)]*.

1.2   Angina Pectoris
TOPROL-XL is indicated in the long-term treatment of angina pectoris, to reduce angina attacks and to improve exercise tolerance.

1.3   Heart Failure
TOPROL-XL is indicated for the treatment of stable, symptomatic (NYHA Class II or III) heart failure of ischemic, hypertensive, or cardiomyopathic origin. It was studied in patients already receiving ACE inhibitors, diuretics, and, in the majority of cases, digitalis. In this population, TOPROL-XL decreased the rate of mortality plus hospitalization, largely through a reduction in cardiovascular mortality and hospitalizations for heart failure.

2   DOSAGE AND ADMINISTRATION
TOPROL-XL is an extended-release tablet intended for once daily administration. For treatment of hypertension and angina, when switching from immediate-release metoprolol to

TOPROL-XL, use the same total daily dose of TOPROL-XL. Individualize the dosage of TOPROL-XL. Titration may be needed in some patients.

TOPROL-XL tablets are scored and can be divided; however, do not crush or chew the whole or half tablet.

2.1 Hypertension

Adults: The usual initial dosage is 25 to 100 mg daily in a single dose. The dosage may be increased at weekly (or longer) intervals until optimum blood pressure reduction is achieved. In general, the maximum effect of any given dosage level will be apparent after 1 week of therapy. Dosages above 400 mg per day have not been studied.

Pediatric Hypertensive Patients ≥ 6 Years of age: A pediatric clinical hypertension study in patients 6 to 16 years of age did not meet its primary endpoint (dose response for reduction in SBP); however some other endpoints demonstrated effectiveness [see Use in Specific Populations (8.4)]. If selected for treatment, the recommended starting dose of TOPROL-XL is 1.0 mg/kg once daily, but the maximum initial dose should not exceed 50 mg once daily. Dosage should be adjusted according to blood pressure response. Doses above 2.0 mg/kg (or in excess of 200 mg) once daily have not been studied in pediatric patients [see Clinical Pharmacology (12.3)].

TOPROL-XL is not recommended in pediatric patients < 6 years of age [see Use in Specific Populations (8.4)].

2.2 Angina Pectoris

Individualize the dosage of TOPROL-XL. The usual initial dosage is 100 mg daily, given in a single dose. Gradually increase the dosage at weekly intervals until optimum clinical response has been obtained or there is a pronounced slowing of the heart rate. Dosages above 400 mg per day have not been studied. If treatment is to be discontinued, reduce the dosage gradually over a period of 1-2 weeks [see Warnings and Precautions (5)].

2.3 Heart Failure

Dosage must be individualized and closely monitored during up-titration. Prior to initiation of TOPROL-XL, stabilize the dose of other heart failure drug therapy. The recommended starting dose of TOPROL-XL is 25 mg once daily for two weeks in patients with NYHA Class II heart failure and 12.5 mg once daily in patients with more severe heart failure. Double the dose every two weeks to the highest dosage level tolerated by the patient or up to 200 mg of TOPROL-XL. Initial difficulty with titration should not preclude later attempts to introduce TOPROL-XL. If patients experience symptomatic bradycardia, reduce the dose of TOPROL-XL. If transient worsening of heart failure occurs, consider treating with increased doses of diuretics, lowering the dose of TOPROL-XL or temporarily discontinuing it. The dose of TOPROL-XL should not be increased until symptoms of worsening heart failure have been stabilized.

3 DOSAGE FORMS AND STRENGTHS

25 mg tablets White, oval, biconvex, film-coated scored tablet engraved with "A/β".

50 mg tablets: White, round, biconvex, film-coated scored tablet engraved with "A/mo".

100 mg tablets: White, round, biconvex, film-coated scored tablet engraved with "A/ms".

200 mg tablets: White, oval, biconvex, film-coated scored tablet engraved with "A/my".

4 CONTRAINDICATIONS

TOPROL-XL is contraindicated in severe bradycardia, second or third degree heart block, cardiogenic shock, decompensated cardiac failure, sick sinus syndrome (unless a permanent pacemaker is in place), and in patients who are hypersensitive to any component of this product.

5 WARNINGS AND PRECAUTIONS

5.1 Ischemic Heart Disease

Following abrupt cessation of therapy with certain beta-blocking agents, exacerbations of angina pectoris and, in some cases, myocardial infarction have occurred. When discontinuing chronically administered TOPROL-XL, particularly in patients with ischemic heart disease, gradually reduce the dosage over a period of 1-2 weeks and monitor the patient. If angina markedly worsens or acute coronary ischemia develops, promptly reinstate TOPROL-XL, and take measures appropriate for the management of unstable angina. Warn patients not to interrupt therapy without their physician's advice. Because coronary artery disease is common and may be unrecognized, avoid abruptly discontinuing TOPROL-XL in patients treated only for hypertension.

5.2 Heart Failure

Worsening cardiac failure may occur during up-titration of TOPROL-XL. If such symptoms occur, increase diuretics and restore clinical stability before advancing the dose of TOPROL-XL [see Dosage and Administration (2)]. It may be necessary to lower the dose of TOPROL-XL or temporarily discontinue it. Such episodes do not preclude subsequent successful titration of TOPROL-XL.

5.3 Bronchospastic Disease

PATIENTS WITH BRONCHOSPASTIC DISEASES SHOULD, IN GENERAL, NOT RECEIVE BETA-BLOCKERS. Because of its relative beta$_1$ cardio-selectivity, however, TOPROL-XL may be used in patients with bronchospastic disease who do not respond to, or cannot tolerate, other antihypertensive treatment. Because beta$_1$-selectivity is not absolute, use the lowest possible dose of TOPROL-XL. Bronchodilators, including beta$_2$-agonists, should be readily available or administered concomitantly [see Dosage and Administration (2)].

5.4 Pheochromocytoma

If TOPROL-XL is used in the setting of pheochromocytoma, it should be given in combination with an alpha blocker, and only after the alpha blocker has been initiated. Administration of beta-blockers alone in the setting of pheochromocytoma has been associated with a paradoxical increase in blood pressure due to the attenuation of beta-mediated vasodilatation in skeletal muscle.

5.5 Major Surgery

Avoid initiation of a high-dose regimen of extended-release metoprolol in patients undergoing non-cardiac surgery, since such use in patients with cardiovascular risk factors has been associated with bradycardia, hypotension, stroke and death.

Chronically administered beta-blocking therapy should not be routinely withdrawn prior to major surgery, however, the impaired ability of the heart to respond to reflex adrenergic stimuli may augment the risks of general anesthesia and surgical procedures.

5.6 Diabetes and Hypoglycemia

Beta-blockers may mask tachycardia occurring with hypoglycemia, but other manifestations such as dizziness and sweating may not be significantly affected.

5.7 Hepatic Impairment

Consider initiating TOPROL-XL therapy at doses lower than those recommended for a given indication; gradually increase dosage to optimize therapy, while monitoring closely for adverse events.

5.8 Thyrotoxicosis

Beta-adrenergic blockade may mask certain clinical signs of hyperthyroidism, such as tachycardia. Abrupt withdrawal of beta-blockade may precipitate a thyroid storm.

5.9 Anaphylactic Reaction

While taking beta-blockers, patients with a history of severe anaphylactic reactions to a variety of allergens may be more reactive to repeated challenge and may be unresponsive to the usual doses of epinephrine used to treat an allergic reaction.

5.10 Peripheral Vascular Disease

Beta-blockers can precipitate or aggravate symptoms of arterial insufficiency in patients with peripheral vascular disease.

5.11 Calcium Channel Blockers

Because of significant inotropic and chronotropic effects in patients treated with beta-blockers and calcium channel blockers of the verapamil and diltiazem type, caution should be exercised in patients treated with these agents concomitantly.

6 ADVERSE REACTIONS

The following adverse reactions are described elsewhere in labeling:

- Worsening angina or myocardial infarction. [see Warnings and Precautions (5)]
- Worsening heart failure. [see Warnings and Precautions (5)]
- Worsening AV block. [see Contraindications (4)]

6.1 Clinical Trials Experience

Because clinical trials are conducted under widely varying conditions, adverse reaction rates observed in the clinical trials of a drug cannot be directly compared to rates in the clinical trials of another drug and may not reflect the rates observed in practice. The adverse reaction information from clinical trials does, however, provide a basis for identifying the adverse events that appear to be related to drug use and for approximating rates.

Hypertension and Angina: Most adverse reactions have been mild and transient. The most common (>2%) adverse reactions are tiredness, dizziness, depression, diarrhea, shortness of breath, bradycardia, and rash.

Heart Failure: In the MERIT-HF study comparing TOPROL-XL in daily doses up to 200 mg (mean dose 159 mg once-daily; n=1990) to placebo (n=2001), 10.3% of TOPROL-XL patients discontinued for adverse reactions vs. 12.2% of placebo patients.

The table below lists adverse reactions in the MERIT-HF study that occurred at an incidence of ≥ 1% in the TOPROL-XL group and greater than placebo by more than 0.5%, regardless of the assessment of causality.

Adverse Reactions Occurring in the MERIT-HF Study at an Incidence ≥ 1 % in the TOPROL-XL Group and Greater Than Placebo by More Than 0.5 %

	TOPROL-XL n=1990 % of patients	Placebo n=2001 % of patients
Dizziness/vertigo	1.8	1.0
Bradycardia	1.5	0.4
Accident and/or injury	1.4	0.8

Post-operative Adverse Events: In a randomized, double-blind, placebo-controlled trial of 8351 patients with or at risk for atherosclerotic disease undergoing non-vascular surgery and who were not taking beta-blocker therapy, TOPROL-XL 100 mg was started 2 to 4 hours prior to surgery then continued for 30 days at 200 mg per day. TOPROL-XL use was associated with a higher incidence of bradycardia (6.6% vs 2.4%; HR, 2.74; 95% CI 2.19, 3.43), hypotension (15% vs. 9.7%; HR 1.55; 95% CI 1.37, 1.74), stroke (1.0% vs 0.5%; HR 2.17; 95% CI 1.26, 3.74) and death (3.1% vs 2.3%; HR 1.33; 95% CI 1.03, 1.74) compared to placebo.

6.2 Post-Marketing Experience

The following adverse reactions have been identified during post-approval use of TOPROL-XL or immediate-release metoprolol. Because these reactions are reported voluntarily from a population of uncertain size, it is not always possible to reliably estimate their frequency or establish a causal relationship to drug exposure.

Cardiovascular: Cold extremities, arterial insufficiency (usually of the Raynaud type), palpitations, peripheral edema, syncope, chest pain and hypotension.

Respiratory: Wheezing (bronchospasm), dyspnea.

Central Nervous System: Confusion, short-term memory loss, headache, somnolence, nightmares, insomnia, anxiety/nervousness, hallucinations, paresthesia.

Gastrointestinal: Nausea, dry mouth, constipation, flatulence, heartburn, hepatitis, vomiting.

Hypersensitive Reactions: Pruritus.

Miscellaneous: Musculoskeletal pain, arthralgia, blurred vision, decreased libido, male impotence, tinnitus, reversible alopecia, agranulocytosis, dry eyes, worsening of psoriasis, Peyronie's disease, sweating, photosensitivity, taste disturbance.

Potential Adverse Reactions: In addition, there are adverse reactions not listed above that have been reported with other beta-adrenergic blocking agents and should be considered potential adverse reactions to TOPROL-XL.

Central Nervous System: Reversible mental depression progressing to catatonia; an acute reversible syndrome characterized by disorientation for time and place, short-term memory loss, emotional lability, clouded sensorium, and decreased performance on neuropsychometrics.

Hematologic: Agranulocytosis, nonthrombocytopenic purpura, thrombocytopenic purpura.

Hypersensitive Reactions: Laryngospasm, respiratory distress.

6.3 Laboratory Test Findings

Clinical laboratory findings may include elevated levels of serum transaminase, alkaline phosphatase, and lactate dehydrogenase.

7 DRUG INTERACTIONS

7.1 Catecholamine Depleting Drugs

Catecholamine depleting drugs (eg, reserpine, monoamine oxidase (MAO) inhibitors) may have an additive effect when given with beta-blocking agents. Observe patients treated with TOPROL-XL plus a catecholamine depletor for evidence of hypotension or marked bradycardia, which may produce vertigo, syncope, or postural hypotension.

7.2 CYP2D6 Inhibitors

Drugs that inhibit CYP2D6 such as quinidine, fluoxetine, paroxetine, and propafenone are likely to increase metoprolol concentration. In healthy subjects with CYP2D6 extensive metabolizer phenotype, coadministration of quinidine 100 mg and immediate-release metoprolol 200 mg tripled the concentration of S-metoprolol and doubled the metoprolol elimination half-life. In four patients with cardiovascular disease, coadministration of propafenone 150 mg t.i.d. with immediate-release metoprolol 50 mg t.i.d. resulted in two- to five-fold increases in the steady-state concentration of metoprolol. These increases in plasma concentration would decrease the cardioselectivity of metoprolol.

7.3 Digitalis, Clonidine, and Calcium Channel Blockers

Digitalis glycosides, clonidine, diltiazem and verapamil slow atrioventricular conduction and decrease heart rate. Concomitant use with beta blockers can increase the risk of bradycardia.

If clonidine and a beta blocker, such as metoprolol are coadministered, withdraw the beta-blocker several days before the gradual withdrawal of clonidine because beta-blockers may exacerbate the rebound hypertension that can follow the withdrawal of clonidine. If replacing clonidine by beta-blocker therapy, delay the introduction of beta-blockers for several days after clonidine administration has stopped *[see Warnings and Precautions (5.11)]*.

8 USE IN SPECIFIC POPULATIONS

8.1 Pregnancy

Pregnancy Category C

Metoprolol tartrate has been shown to increase post-implantation loss and decrease neonatal survival in rats at doses up to 22 times, on a mg/m^2 basis, the daily dose of 200 mg in a 60-kg patient. Distribution studies in mice confirm exposure of the fetus when metoprolol tartrate is administered to the pregnant animal. These studies have revealed no evidence of impaired fertility or teratogenicity. There are no adequate and well-controlled studies in pregnant women. Because animal reproduction studies are not always predictive of human response, use this drug during pregnancy only if clearly needed.

8.3 Nursing Mothers

Metoprolol is excreted in breast milk in very small quantities. An infant consuming 1 liter of breast milk daily would receive a dose of less than 1 mg of the drug. Consider possible infant exposure when TOPROL-XL is administered to a nursing woman.

8.4 Pediatric Use

One hundred forty-four hypertensive pediatric patients aged 6 to 16 years were randomized to placebo or to one of three dose levels of TOPROL-XL (0.2, 1.0 or 2.0 mg/kg once daily) and followed for 4 weeks. The study did not meet its primary endpoint (dose response for reduction in SBP). Some pre-specified secondary endpoints demonstrated effectiveness including:

- Dose-response for reduction in DBP,
- 1.0 mg/kg vs. placebo for change in SBP, and
- 2.0 mg/kg vs. placebo for change in SBP and DBP.

The mean placebo corrected reductions in SBP ranged from 3 to 6 mmHg, and DBP from 1 to 5 mmHg. Mean reduction in heart rate ranged from 5 to 7 bpm but considerably greater reductions were seen in some individuals *[see Dosage and Administration (2.1)]*.

No clinically relevant differences in the adverse event profile were observed for pediatric patients aged 6 to 16 years as compared with adult patients.

Safety and effectiveness of TOPROL-XL have not been established in patients < 6 years of age.

8.5 Geriatric Use

Clinical studies of TOPROL-XL in hypertension did not include sufficient numbers of subjects aged 65 and over to determine whether they respond differently from younger subjects. Other reported clinical experience in hypertensive patients has not identified differences in responses between elderly and younger patients.

Of the 1,990 patients with heart failure randomized to TOPROL-XL in the MERIT-HF trial, 50% (990) were 65 years of age and older and 12% (238) were 75 years of age and older. There were no notable differences in efficacy or the rate of adverse reactions between older and younger patients.

In general, use a low initial starting dose in elderly patients given their greater frequency of decreased hepatic, renal, or cardiac function, and of concomitant disease or other drug therapy.

8.6 Hepatic Impairment

No studies have been performed with TOPROL-XL in patients with hepatic impairment. Because TOPROL-XL is metabolized by the liver, metoprolol blood levels are likely to increase substantially with poor hepatic function. Therefore, initiate therapy at doses lower than those recommended for a given indication; and increase doses gradually in patients with impaired hepatic function.

8.7 Renal Impairment

The systemic availability and half-life of metoprolol in patients with renal failure do not differ to a clinically significant degree from those in normal subjects. No reduction in dosage is needed in patients with chronic renal failure *[see Clinical Pharmacology (12.3)]*.

10 OVERDOSAGE

Signs and Symptoms — Overdosage of TOPROL-XL may lead to severe bradycardia, hypotension, and cardiogenic shock. Clinical presentation can also include: atrioventricular block, heart failure, bronchospasm, hypoxia, impairment of consciousness/coma, nausea and vomiting.

Treatment–Consider treating the patient with intensive care. Patients with myocardial infarction or heart failure may be prone to significant hemodynamic instability. Seek consultation with a regional poison control center and a medical toxicologist as needed. Beta-blocker overdose may result in significant resistance to resuscitation with adrenergic agents, including beta-agonists. On the basis of the pharmacologic actions of metoprolol, employ the following measures.

There is very limited experience with the use of hemodialysis to remove metoprolol, however metoprolol is not highly protein bound.

Bradycardia: Administer intravenous atropine; repeat to effect. If the response is inadequate, consider intravenous isoproterenol or other positive chronotropic agents. Evaluate the need for transvenous pacemaker insertion.

Hypotension: Treat underlying bradycardia. Consider intravenous vasopressor infusion, such as dopamine or norepinephrine.

Bronchospasm: Administer a $beta_2$-agonist, including albuterol inhalation, or an oral theophylline derivative.

Cardiac Failure: Administer diuretics or digoxin for congestive heart failure. For cardiogenic shock, consider IV dobutamine, isoproterenol, or glucagon.

11 DESCRIPTION

TOPROL-XL, metoprolol succinate, is a $beta_1$-selective (cardioselective) adrenoceptor blocking agent, for oral administration, available as extended release tablets. TOPROL-XL has been formulated to provide a controlled and predictable release of metoprolol for once-daily administration. The tablets comprise a multiple unit system containing metoprolol succinate in a multitude of controlled release pellets. Each pellet acts as a separate drug delivery unit and is designed to deliver metoprolol continuously over the dosage interval. The tablets contain 23.75, 47.5, 95 and 190 mg of metoprolol succinate equivalent to 25, 50, 100 and 200 mg of metoprolol tartrate, USP, respectively. Its chemical name is (±)1- (isopropylamino)-3-[p-(2-methoxyethyl) phenoxy]-2-propanol succinate (2:1) (salt). Its structural formula is:

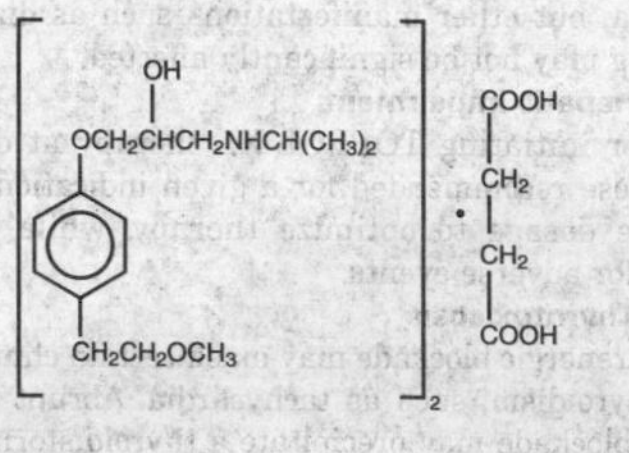

Metoprolol succinate is a white crystalline powder with a molecular weight of 652.8. It is freely soluble in water; soluble in methanol; sparingly soluble in ethanol; slightly soluble in dichloromethane and 2-propanol; practically insoluble in ethyl-acetate, acetone, diethylether and heptane. Inactive ingredients: silicon dioxide, cellulose compounds, sodium stearyl fumarate, polyethylene glycol, titanium dioxide, paraffin.

12 CLINICAL PHARMACOLOGY

12.1 Mechanism of Action

Hypertension: The mechanism of the antihypertensive effects of beta-blocking agents has not been elucidated. However, several possible mechanisms have been proposed: (1) competitive antagonism of catecholamines at peripheral (especially cardiac) adrenergic neuron sites, leading to decreased cardiac output; (2) a central effect leading to reduced sympathetic outflow to the periphery; and (3) suppression of renin activity.

Heart Failure: The precise mechanism for the beneficial effects of beta-blockers in heart failure has not been elucidated.

12.2 Pharmacodynamics

Clinical pharmacology studies have confirmed the beta-blocking activity of metoprolol in man, as shown by (1) reduction in heart rate and cardiac output at rest and upon exercise, (2) reduction of systolic blood pressure upon exercise, (3) inhibition of isoproterenol-induced tachycardia, and (4) reduction of reflex orthostatic tachycardia.

Metoprolol is a $beta_1$-selective (cardioselective) adrenergic receptor blocking agent. This preferential effect is not absolute, however, and at higher plasma concentrations, metoprolol also inhibits $beta_2$-adrenoreceptors, chiefly located in the bronchial and vascular musculature. Metoprolol has no intrinsic sympathomimetic activity, and membrane-stabilizing activity is detectable only at plasma concentrations much greater than required for beta-blockade. Animal and human experiments indicate that metoprolol slows the sinus rate and decreases AV nodal conduction.

The relative $beta_1$-selectivity of metoprolol has been confirmed by the following: (1) In normal subjects, metoprolol is unable to reverse the $beta_2$-mediated vasodilating effects of epinephrine. This contrasts with the effect of nonselective beta-blockers, which completely reverse the vasodilating effects of epinephrine. (2) In asthmatic patients, metoprolol reduces FEV_1 and FVC significantly less than a nonselective beta-blocker, propranolol, at equivalent $beta_1$-receptor blocking doses.

The relationship between plasma metoprolol levels and reduction in exercise heart rate is independent of the pharmaceutical formulation. Using an E_{max} model, the maximum effect is a 30% reduction in exercise heart rate, which is attributed to $beta_1$-blockade. $Beta_1$-blocking effects in the range of 30-80% of the maximal effect (approximately 8-23% reduction in exercise heart rate) correspond to metoprolol plasma concentrations from 30-540 nmol/L. The relative $beta_1$-selectivity of metoprolol diminishes and blockade of $beta_2$-adrenoceptors increases at plasma concentration above 300 nmol/L.

Although beta-adrenergic receptor blockade is useful in the treatment of angina, hypertension, and heart failure there are situations in which sympathetic stimulation is vital. In patients with severely damaged hearts, adequate ventricular function may depend on sympathetic drive. In the presence of AV block, beta-blockade may prevent the necessary facilitating effect of sympathetic activity on conduction. $Beta_2$-adrenergic blockade results in passive bronchial constriction by interfering with endogenous adrenergic bronchodilator activity in patients subject to bronchospasm and may also interfere with exogenous bronchodilators in such patients.

In other studies, treatment with TOPROL-XL produced an improvement in left ventricular ejection fraction. TOPROL-XL was also shown to delay the increase in left ventricular end-systolic and end-diastolic volumes after 6 months of treatment.

12.3 Pharmacokinetics

Adults: In man, absorption of metoprolol is rapid and complete. Plasma levels following oral administration of conventional metoprolol tablets, however, approximate 50% of levels following intravenous administration, indicating about 50% first-pass metabolism. Metoprolol crosses the blood-brain barrier and has been reported in the CSF in a concentration 78% of the simultaneous plasma concentration.

Plasma levels achieved are highly variable after oral administration. Only a small fraction of the drug (about 12%) is bound to human serum albumin. Metoprolol is a racemic mixture of R- and S- enantiomers, and is primarily metabolized by CYP2D6. When administered orally, it exhibits stereoselective metabolism that is dependent on oxidation phenotype. Elimination is mainly by biotransformation in the liver, and the plasma half-life ranges from approximately 3 to 7 hours. Less than 5% of an oral dose of metoprolol is recovered unchanged in the urine; the rest is excreted by the kidneys as metabolites that appear to have no beta-blocking activity.

Following intravenous administration of metoprolol, the urinary recovery of unchanged drug is approximately 10%. The systemic availability and half-life of metoprolol in patients with renal failure do not differ to a clinically significant degree from those in normal subjects. Consequently, no reduction in metoprolol succinate dosage is usually needed in patients with chronic renal failure.

Metoprolol is metabolized predominantly by CYP2D6, an enzyme that is absent in about 8% of Caucasians (poor metabolizers) and about 2% of most other populations. CYP2D6 can be inhibited by a number of drugs. Poor metabolizers and extensive metabolizers who concomitantly use CYP2D6 inhibiting drugs will have increased (several-fold) metoprolol blood levels, decreasing metoprolol's cardioselectivity *[see Drug Interactions (7.2)]*.

In comparison to conventional metoprolol, the plasma metoprolol levels following administration of TOPROL-XL are characterized by lower peaks, longer time to peak and significantly lower peak to trough variation. The peak plasma levels following once-daily administration of TOPROL-XL average one-fourth to one-half the peak plasma levels obtained following a corresponding dose of conventional metoprolol, administered once daily or in divided doses. At steady state the average bioavailability of metoprolol following administration of TOPROL-XL, across the dosage range of 50 to 400 mg once daily, was 77% relative to the corresponding single or divided doses of conventional metoprolol. Nevertheless, over the 24-hour dosing interval, β_1-blockade is comparable and dose-related *[see Clinical Pharmacology (12)]*. The bioavailability of metoprolol shows a dose-related, although not directly proportional, increase with dose and is not significantly affected by food following TOPROL-XL administration.

Pediatrics: The pharmacokinetic profile of TOPROL-XL was studied in 120 pediatric hypertensive patients (6-17 years of age) receiving doses ranging from 12.5 to 200 mg once daily. The pharmacokinetics of metoprolol were similar to those described previously in adults. Age, gender, race, and ideal body weight had no significant effects on metoprolol pharmacokinetics. Metoprolol apparent oral clearance (CL/F) increased linearly with body weight. Metoprolol pharmacokinetics have not been investigated in patients < 6 years of age.

13 NONCLINICAL TOXICOLOGY

13.1 Carcinogenesis, Mutagenesis, Impairment of Fertility

Long-term studies in animals have been conducted to evaluate the carcinogenic potential of metoprolol tartrate. In

2-year studies in rats at three oral dosage levels of up to 800 mg/kg/day (41 times, on a mg/m^2 basis, the daily dose of 200 mg for a 60-kg patient), there was no increase in the development of spontaneously occurring benign or malignant neoplasms of any type. The only histologic changes that appeared to be drug related were an increased incidence of generally mild focal accumulation of foamy macrophages in pulmonary alveoli and a slight increase in biliary hyperplasia. In a 21-month study in Swiss albino mice at three oral dosage levels of up to 750 mg/kg/day (18 times, on a mg/m^2 basis, the daily dose of 200 mg for a 60-kg pa tient), benign lung tumors (small adenomas) occurred more frequently in female mice receiving the highest dose than in untreated control animals. There was no increase in malignant or total (benign plus malignant) lung tumors, nor in the overall incidence of tumors or malignant tumors. This 21-month study was repeated in CD-1 mice, and no statistically or biologically significant differences were observed between treated and control mice of either sex for any type of tumor.

All genotoxicity tests performed on metoprolol tartrate (a dominant lethal study in mice, chromosome studies in somatic cells, a *Salmonella*/mammalian-microsome mutagenicity test, and a nucleus anomaly test in somatic interphase nuclei) and metoprolol succinate (a *Salmonella*/mammalian-microsome mutagenicity test) were negative. No evidence of impaired fertility due to metoprolol tartrate was observed in a study performed in rats at doses up to 22 times, on a mg/m^2 basis, the daily dose of 200 mg in a 60-kg patient.

14   CLINICAL STUDIES

In five controlled studies in normal healthy subjects, the same daily doses of TOPROL-XL and immediate-release metoprolol were compared in terms of the extent and duration of beta$_1$-blockade produced. Both formulations were given in a dose range equivalent to 100-400 mg of immediate-release metoprolol per day. In these studies, TOPROL-XL was administered once a day and immediate-release metoprolol was administered once to four times a day. A sixth controlled study compared the beta$_1$-blocking effects of a 50 mg daily dose of the two formulations. In each study, beta$_1$-blockade was expressed as the percent change from baseline in exercise heart rate following standardized submaximal exercise tolerance tests at steady state. TOPROL-XL administered once a day, and immediate-release metoprolol administered once to four times a day, provided comparable total beta$_1$-blockade over 24 hours (area under the beta$_1$-blockade versus time curve) in the dose range 100-400 mg. At a dosage of 50 mg once daily, TOPROL-XL produced significantly higher total beta$_1$-blockade over 24 hours than immediate-release metoprolol. For TOPROL-XL, the percent reduction in exercise heart rate was relatively stable throughout the entire dosage interval and the level of beta$_1$-blockade increased with increasing doses from 50 to 300 mg daily. The effects at peak/trough (ie, at 24-hours post-dosing) were: 14/9, 16/10, 24/14, 27/22 and 27/20% reduction in exercise heart rate for doses of 50, 100, 200, 300 and 400 mg TOPROL-XL once a day, respectively. In contrast to TOPROL-XL, immediate-release metoprolol given at a dose of 50-100 mg once a day produced a significantly larger peak effect on exercise tachycardia, but the effect was not evident at 24 hours. To match the peak to trough ratio obtained with TOPROL-XL over the dosing range of 200 to 400 mg, a t.i.d. to q.i.d. divided dosing regimen was required for immediate-release metoprolol. A controlled cross-over study in heart failure patients compared the plasma concentrations and beta$_1$-blocking effects of 50 mg immediate-release metoprolol administered t.i.d., 100 mg and 200 mg TOPROL-XL once daily. A 50 mg dose of immediate-release metoprolol t.i.d. produced a peak plasma level of metoprolol similar to the peak level observed with 200 mg of TOPROL-XL. A 200 mg dose of TOPROL-XL produced a larger effect on suppression of exercise-induced and Holter-monitored heart rate over 24 hours compared to 50 mg t.i.d. of immediate-release metoprolol.

In a double-blind study, 1092 patients with mild-to-moderate hypertension were randomized to once daily TOPROL-XL (25, 100, or 400 mg), PLENDIL® (felodipine extended-release tablets), the combination, or placebo. After 9 weeks, TOPROL-XL alone decreased sitting blood pressure by 6-8/4-7 mmHg (placebo-corrected change from baseline) at 24 hours post-dose. The combination of TOPROL-XL with PLENDIL has greater effects on blood pressure.

In controlled clinical studies, an immediate-release dosage form of metoprolol was an effective antihypertensive agent when used alone or as concomitant therapy with thiazide-type diuretics at dosages of 100-450 mg daily. TOPROL-XL, in dosages of 100 to 400 mg once daily, produces similar β$_1$-blockade as conventional metoprolol tablets administered two to four times daily. TOPROL-XL administered at a dose of 50 mg once daily lowered blood pressure 24-hours post-dosing in placebo-controlled studies. In controlled, comparative, clinical studies, immediate-release

metoprolol appeared comparable as an antihypertensive agent to propranolol, methyldopa, and thiazide-type diuretics, and affected both supine and standing blood pressure. Because of variable plasma levels attained with a given dose and lack of a consistent relationship of antihypertensive activity to drug plasma concentration, selection of proper dosage requires individual titration.

14.1   Angina Pectoris

By blocking catecholamine-induced increases in heart rate, in velocity and extent of myocardial contraction, and in blood pressure, metoprolol reduces the oxygen requirements of the heart at any given level of effort, thus making it useful in the long-term management of angina pectoris.

In controlled clinical trials, an immediate-release formulation of metoprolol has been shown to be an effective anti-anginal agent, reducing the number of angina attacks and increasing exercise tolerance. The dosage used in these studies ranged from 100 to 400 mg daily. TOPROL-XL, in dosages of 100 to 400 mg once daily, has been shown to possess beta-blockade similar to conventional metoprolol tablets administered two to four times daily.

14.2   Heart Failure

MERIT-HF was a double-blind, placebo-controlled study of TOPROL-XL conducted in 14 countries including the US. It randomized 3991 patients (1990 to TOPROL-XL) with ejection fraction ≤0.40 and NYHA Class II-IV heart failure at-

Clinical Endpoints in the MERIT-HF Study

Clinical Endpoint	Number of Patients		Relative Risk (95% CI)	Risk Reduction With TOPROL-XL	Nominal P-value
	Placebo n=2001	TOPROL-XL n=1990			
All-cause mortality plus all-cause hospitalization*	767	641	0.81 (0.73-0.90)	19%	0.00012
All-cause mortality	217	145	0.66 (0.53-0.81)	34%	0.00009
All-cause mortality plus heart failure hospitalization*	439	311	0.69 (0.60-0.80)	31%	0.0000008
Cardiovascular mortality	203	128	0.62 (0.50-0.78)	38%	0.000022
Sudden death	132	79	0.59 (0.45-0.78)	41%	0.0002
Death due to worsening heart failure	58	30	0.51 (0.33-0.79)	49%	0.0023
Hospitalizations due to worsening heart failure†	451	317	N/A	N/A	0.0000076
Cardiovascular hospitalization†	773	649	N/A	N/A	0.00028

* Time to first event
† Comparison of treatment groups examines the number of hospitalizations (Wilcoxon test); relative risk and risk reduction are not applicable.

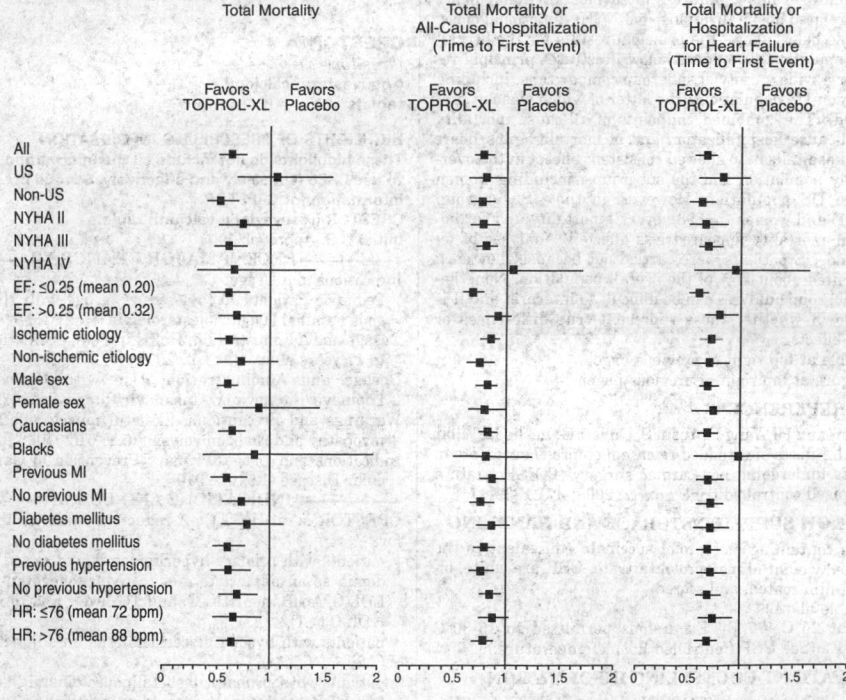

Results for Subgroups in MERIT-HF

Relative risk and 95% confidence interval

US = United States; NYHA = New York Heart Association; EF = ejection fraction; MI = myocardial infarction; HR = heart rate.

Tablet	Shape	Engraving	Bottle of 100 NDC 0186-	Unit Dose Packages of 100 NDC 0186-
25 mg	Oval	A/β	1088-05	1088-39
50 mg	Round	A/mo	1090-05	1090-39
100 mg	Round	A/ms	1092-05	1092-39
200 mg	Oval	A/my	1094-05	N/A

tributable to ischemia, hypertension, or cardiomyopathy. The protocol excluded patients with contraindications to beta-blocker use, those expected to undergo heart surgery, and those within 28 days of myocardial infarction or unstable angina. The primary endpoints of the trial were (1) all-cause mortality plus all-cause hospitalization (time to first event) and (2) all-cause mortality. Patients were stabilized on optimal concomitant therapy for heart failure, including diuretics, ACE inhibitors, cardiac glycosides, and nitrates. At randomization, 41% of patients were NYHA Class II; 55% NYHA Class III; 65% of patients had heart failure attributed to ischemic heart disease; 44% had a history of hypertension; 25% had diabetes mellitus; 48% had a history of myocardial infarction. Among patients in the trial, 90% were on diuretics, 89% were on ACE inhibitors, 64% were on digitalis, 27% were on a lipid-lowering agent, 37% were on an oral anticoagulant, and the mean ejection fraction was 0.28. The mean duration of follow-up was one year. At the end of the study, the mean daily dose of TOPROL-XL was 159 mg.

The trial was terminated early for a statistically significant reduction in all-cause mortality (34%, nominal p= 0.00009). The risk of all-cause mortality plus all-cause hospitalization was reduced by 19% (p= 0.00012). The trial also showed improvements in heart failure-related mortality and heart failure-related hospitalizations, and NYHA functional class. The table below shows the principal results for the overall study population. The figure below illustrates principal results for a wide variety of subgroup comparisons. US vs. non-US populations (the latter of which was not prespecified). The combined endpoints of all-cause mortality plus all-cause hospitalization and of mortality plus heart failure hospitalization showed consistent effects in the overall study population and the subgroups, including women and the US population. However, in the US subgroup (n=1071) and women (n=898), overall mortality and cardiovascular mortality appeared less affected. Analyses of female and US patients were carried out because they each represented about 25% of the overall population. Nonetheless, subgroup analyses can be difficult to interpret and it is not known whether these represent true differences or chance effects.

[See table at top right of previous page]
[See figure at top right of previous page]

15 REFERENCES

1. Devereaux PJ, Yang H, Yusuf S, Guyatt G, Leslie K, Villar JC et al. Effects of extended-release metoprolol succinate in patients undergoing non-cardiac surgery (POISE trial): a randomised controlled trial. *Lancet.* 2008; 371:1839-47.

16 HOW SUPPLIED/STORAGE AND HANDLING

Tablets containing metoprolol succinate equivalent to the indicated weight of metoprolol tartrate, USP, are white, biconvex, film-coated, and scored.
[See table above]
Store at 25°C (77°F). Excursions permitted to 15-30°C (59-86°F). (See USP Controlled Room Temperature.)

17 PATIENT COUNSELING INFORMATION

Advise patients to take TOPROL-XL regularly and continuously, as directed, preferably with or immediately following meals. If a dose is missed, the patient should take only the next scheduled dose (without doubling it). Patients should not interrupt or discontinue TOPROL-XL without consulting the physician.

Advise patients (1) to avoid operating automobiles and machinery or engaging in other tasks requiring alertness until the patient's response to therapy with TOPROL-XL has been determined; (2) to contact the physician if any difficulty in breathing occurs; (3) to inform the physician or dentist before any type of surgery that he or she is taking TOPROL-XL.

Heart failure patients should be advised to consult their physician if they experience signs or symptoms of worsening heart failure such as weight gain or increasing shortness of breath.

TOPROL-XL and PLENDIL are trademarks of the AstraZeneca group of companies.

© AstraZeneca 2010
Distributed by: AstraZeneca LP
Wilmington, DE 19850
35556—01
Rev. 04/2010
Shown in Product Identification Guide, page 306

AstraZeneca Pharmaceuticals LP
WILMINGTON, DE 19850-5437

For Product Full Prescribing Information, Business Information, Medical Information, Adverse Drug Experiences, and Customer Service:
Information Center
1-800-236-9933
For Product Ordering:
Trade Customer Service
1-800-842-9920
For Product Full Prescribing Information:
Internet: www.astrazeneca-us.com

CRESTOR®
[krĕs-tōr]
(rosuvastatin calcium)
tablets

HIGHLIGHTS OF PRESCRIBING INFORMATION
These highlights do not include all the information needed to use CRESTOR safely and effectively. See full prescribing information for CRESTOR.
CRESTOR (rosuvastatin calcium) tablets
Initial U.S. Approval: 2003

―――――RECENT MAJOR CHANGES―――――
Indications and Usage,
Pediatric Patients 10 to 17 years of age with Heterozygous Familial Hypercholesterolemia (HeFH) (1.1) 10/2009
Dosage and Administration, HeFH in Pediatric Patients (10 to 17 years of age) (2.2) 10/2009
Dosage and Administration, Use with Cyclosporine, Lopinavir/Ritonavir or Atazanavir/Ritonavir (2.5) 01/2010
Warnings and Precautions, Skeletal muscle effects (e.g., myopathy and rhabdomyolysis) (5.1) 01/2010
Indications and Usage, Primary Prevention of Cardiovascular Disease (1.6) 02/2010

―――――INDICATIONS AND USAGE―――――
CRESTOR is an HMG Co-A reductase inhibitor indicated for:
• patients with primary hyperlipidemia and mixed dyslipidemia as an adjunct to diet to reduce elevated total-C, LDL-C, ApoB, nonHDL-C, and TG levels and to increase HDL-C (1.1)
• patients with hypertriglyceridemia as an adjunct to diet (1.2)
• patients with primary dysbetalipoproteinemia (Type III hyperlipoproteinemia) as an adjunct to diet (1.3)
• patients with homozygous familial hypercholesterolemia (HoFH) to reduce LDL-C, total-C, and ApoB (1.4)
• slowing the progression of atherosclerosis as part of a treatment strategy to lower total-C and LDL-C as an adjunct to diet (1.5)
• pediatric patients 10 to 17 years of age with heterozygous familial hypercholesterolemia (HeFH) to reduce elevated total-C, LDL-C and ApoB after failing an adequate trial of diet therapy (1.1)
• risk reduction of MI, stroke, and arterial revascularization procedures in patients without clinically evident CHD, but with multiple risk factors (1.6)
Limitations of use (1.7):
• CRESTOR has not been studied in Fredrickson Type I and V dyslipidemias.

―――――DOSAGE AND ADMINISTRATION―――――
• CRESTOR can be taken with or without food, at any time of day. (2.1)

• Dose range: 5-40 mg once daily. Use 40 mg dose only for patients not reaching LDL-C goal with 20 mg. (2.1)
• HoFH: Starting dose 20 mg. (2.3)
• In pediatric patients 10 to 17 years of age with HeFH, the usual dose range is 5-20 mg/day; doses greater than 20 mg have not been studied in this patient population. (2.2)

―――――DOSAGE FORMS AND STRENGTHS―――――
Tablets: 5 mg, 10 mg, 20 mg, and 40 mg (3)

―――――CONTRAINDICATIONS―――――
• Known hypersensitivity to product components (4)
• Active liver disease, which may include unexplained persistent elevations in hepatic transaminase levels (4)
• Women who are pregnant or may become pregnant (4, 8.1)
• Nursing mothers (4, 8.3)

―――――WARNINGS AND PRECAUTIONS―――――
• Skeletal muscle effects (e.g., myopathy and rhabdomyolysis): Risks increase with use of 40 mg dose, advanced age (≥65), hypothyroidism, renal impairment, and combination use with cyclosporine, lopinavir/ritonavir, atazanavir/ritonavir, or certain other lipid-lowering drugs. Advise patients to promptly report unexplained muscle pain, tenderness, or weakness and discontinue CRESTOR if signs or symptoms appear (5.1)
• Liver enzyme abnormalities and monitoring: Persistent elevations in hepatic transaminases can occur. Monitor liver enzymes before and during treatment. (5.2)

―――――ADVERSE REACTIONS―――――
Most frequent adverse reactions (rate ≥ 2%) are headache, myalgia, abdominal pain, asthenia, and nausea. (6.1)
To report SUSPECTED ADVERSE REACTIONS, contact AstraZeneca at 1-800-236-9933 or FDA at 1-800-FDA-1088 or www.fda.gov/medwatch

―――――DRUG INTERACTIONS―――――
• Cyclosporine: Combination increases rosuvastatin exposure. Limit CRESTOR dose to 5 mg once daily. (2.5, 7.1)
• Gemfibrozil: Combination should be avoided. If used together, limit CRESTOR dose to 10 mg once daily. (2.6, 5.1, 7.2)
• Lopinavir/Ritonavir or atazanavir/ritonavir: Combination increases rosuvastatin exposure. Limit CRESTOR dose to 10 mg once daily. (2.5, 5.1, 7.3)
• Coumarin anticoagulants: Combination prolongs INR. Achieve stable INR prior to starting CRESTOR. Monitor INR frequently until stable upon initiation or alteration of CRESTOR therapy. (5.3, 7.4)
• Concomitant lipid-lowering therapies: Use with fibrates and niacin products may increase the risk of skeletal muscle effects. (2.6, 5.1, 7.5, 7.6)

―――――USE IN SPECIFIC POPULATIONS―――――
• Severe renal impairment (not on hemodialysis): Starting dose is 5 mg, not to exceed 10 mg. (2.7, 5.1, 8.6)
• Asian population: Consider 5 mg starting dose. (2.4, 8.8)
See 17 for PATIENT COUNSELING INFORMATION
Revised: 06/2010

FULL PRESCRIBING INFORMATION: CONTENTS*

* Sections or subsections omitted from the full prescribing information are not listed

---

FULL PRESCRIBING INFORMATION

1   INDICATIONS AND USAGE

1.1   Hyperlipidemia and Mixed Dyslipidemia

CRESTOR is indicated as adjunctive therapy to diet to reduce elevated Total-C, LDL-C, ApoB, nonHDL-C, and triglycerides and to increase HDL-C in adult patients with primary hyperlipidemia or mixed dyslipidemia. Lipid-altering agents should be used in addition to a diet restricted in saturated fat and cholesterol when response to diet and nonpharmacological interventions alone has been inadequate.

Pediatric Patients 10 to 17 years of age with Heterozygous Familial Hypercholesterolemia (HeFH)

Adjunct to diet to reduce Total-C, LDL-C and ApoB levels in adolescent boys and girls, who are at least one year postmenarche, 10-17 years of age with heterozygous familial hypercholesterolemia if after an adequate trial of diet therapy the following findings are present: LDL-C > 190 mg/dL or > 160 mg/dL and there is a positive family history of premature cardiovascular disease (CVD) or two or more other CVD risk factors.

1.2   Hypertriglyceridemia

CRESTOR is indicated as adjunctive therapy to diet for the treatment of adult patients with hypertriglyceridemia.

1.3   Primary Dysbetalipoproteinemia (Type III Hyperlipoproteinemia)

CRESTOR is indicated as an adjunct to diet for the treatment of patients with primary dysbetalipoproteinemia (Type III Hyperlipoproteinemia).

1.4   Homozygous Familial Hypercholesterolemia

CRESTOR is indicated as adjunctive therapy to other lipid-lowering treatments (e.g., LDL apheresis) or alone if such treatments are unavailable to reduce LDL-C, Total-C, and ApoB in adult patients with homozygous familial hypercholesterolemia.

1.5   Slowing of the Progression of Atherosclerosis

CRESTOR is indicated as adjunctive therapy to diet to slow the progression of atherosclerosis in adult patients as part of a treatment strategy to lower Total-C and LDL-C to target levels.

1.6   Primary Prevention of Cardiovascular Disease

In individuals without clinically evident coronary heart disease but with an increased risk of cardiovascular disease based on age ≥ 50 years old in men and ≥ 60 years old in women, hsCRP ≥ 2 mg/L, and the presence of at least one additional cardiovascular disease risk factor such as hypertension, low HDL-C, smoking, or a family history of premature coronary heart disease, CRESTOR is indicated to:
• reduce the risk of stroke
• reduce the risk of myocardial infarction
• reduce the risk of arterial revascularization procedures

1.7   Limitations of Use

CRESTOR has not been studied in Fredrickson Type I and V dyslipidemias.

2   DOSAGE AND ADMINISTRATION

2.1   General Dosing Information

The dose range for CRESTOR is 5 to 40 mg orally once daily. The usual starting dose is 10-20 mg.

CRESTOR can be administered as a single dose at any time of day, with or without food.

When initiating CRESTOR therapy or switching from another HMG-CoA reductase inhibitor therapy, the appropriate CRESTOR starting dose should first be utilized, and only then titrated according to the patient's response and individualized goal of therapy.

After initiation or upon titration of CRESTOR, lipid levels should be analyzed within 2 to 4 weeks and the dosage adjusted accordingly.

The 40 mg dose of CRESTOR should be used only for those patients who have not achieved their LDL-C goal utilizing the 20 mg dose [see Warnings and Precautions (5.1)].

2.2   Heterozygous Familial Hypercholesterolemia in Pediatric Patients (10 to 17 years of age)

The usual dose range of CRESTOR is 5-20 mg/day; the maximum recommended dose is 20 mg/day (doses greater than 20 mg have not been studied in this patient population). Doses should be individualized according to the recommended goal of therapy [see Clinical Pharmacology (12) and Indications and Usage (1.2)]. Adjustments should be made at intervals of 4 weeks or more.

2.3   Homozygous Familial Hypercholesterolemia

The recommended starting dose of CRESTOR is 20 mg once daily. Response to therapy should be estimated from preapheresis LDL-C levels.

2.4   Dosage in Asian Patients

Initiation of CRESTOR therapy with 5 mg once daily should be considered for Asian patients [see Use in Specific Populations (8.8) and Clinical Pharmacology (12.3)].

2.5   Use with Cyclosporine, Lopinavir/Ritonavir or Atazanavir/Ritonavir

In patients taking cyclosporine, the dose of CRESTOR should be limited to 5 mg once daily [see Warnings and Precautions (5.1) and Drug Interactions (7.1)]. In patients taking a combination of lopinavir and ritonavir or atazanavir and ritonavir, the dose of CRESTOR should be limited to 10 mg once daily [see Warnings and Precautions (5.1) and Drug Interactions (7.3)].

2.6   Concomitant Lipid-Lowering Therapy

The risk of skeletal muscle effects may be enhanced when CRESTOR is used in combination with niacin or fenofibrate; a reduction in CRESTOR dosage should be considered in this setting [see Warnings and Precautions (5.1) and Drug Interactions (7.5, 7.6)].

Combination therapy with gemfibrozil should be avoided because of an increase in CRESTOR exposure with concomitant use; if CRESTOR is used in combination with gemfibrozil, the dose of CRESTOR should be limited to 10 mg once daily [see Warnings and Precautions (5.1) and Drug Interactions (7.2)].

2.7   Dosage in Patients With Severe Renal Impairment

For patients with severe renal impairment (CL_{cr} <30 mL/min/1.73 m^2) not on hemodialysis, dosing of CRESTOR should be started at 5 mg once daily and not exceed 10 mg once daily [see Use in Specific Populations (8.6) and Clinical Pharmacology (12.3)].

3   DOSAGE FORMS AND STRENGTHS

5 mg: Yellow, round, biconvex, coated tablets. Debossed "CRESTOR" and "5" on one side of the tablet.

10 mg: Pink, round, biconvex, coated tablets. Debossed "CRESTOR" and "10" on one side of the tablet.

20 mg: Pink, round, biconvex, coated tablets. Debossed "CRESTOR" and "20" on one side of the tablet.

40 mg: Pink, oval, biconvex, coated tablets. Debossed "CRESTOR" on one side and "40" on the other side of the tablet.

4   CONTRAINDICATIONS

CRESTOR is contraindicated in the following conditions:
• Patients with a known hypersensitivity to any component of this product. Hypersensitivity reactions including rash, pruritus, urticaria and angioedema have been reported with CRESTOR [see Adverse Reactions (6.1)].
• Patients with active liver disease, which may include unexplained persistent elevations of hepatic transaminase levels [see Warnings and Precautions (5.2)].
• Women who are pregnant or may become pregnant. Because HMG-CoA reductase inhibitors decrease cholesterol synthesis and possibly the synthesis of other biologically active substances derived from cholesterol, CRESTOR may cause fetal harm when administered to pregnant women. Additionally, there is no apparent benefit to therapy during pregnancy, and safety in pregnant women has not been established. If the patient becomes pregnant while taking this drug, the patient should be apprised of the potential hazard to the fetus and the lack of known clinical benefit with continued use during pregnancy [see Use in Specific Populations (8.1) and Nonclinical Toxicology (13.2)].
• Nursing mothers. Because another drug in this class passes into breast milk, and because HMG-CoA reductase inhibitors have the potential to cause serious adverse re-

actions in nursing infants, women who require CRESTOR treatment should be advised not to nurse their infants [see Use in Specific Populations (8.3)].

5   WARNINGS AND PRECAUTIONS

5.1   Skeletal Muscle Effects

Cases of myopathy and rhabdomyolysis with acute renal failure secondary to myoglobinuria have been reported with HMG-CoA reductase inhibitors, including CRESTOR. These risks can occur at any dose level, but are increased at the highest dose (40 mg).

CRESTOR should be prescribed with caution in patients with predisposing factors for myopathy (e.g., age ≥ 65 years, inadequately treated hypothyroidism, renal impairment).

The risk of myopathy during treatment with CRESTOR may be increased with concurrent administration of some other lipid-lowering therapies (fibrates or niacin), gemfibrozil, cyclosporine, lopinavir/ritonavir, or atazanavir/ritonavir [see Dosage and Administration (2) and Drug Interactions (7)].

CRESTOR therapy should be discontinued if markedly elevated creatinine kinase levels occur or myopathy is diagnosed or suspected. CRESTOR therapy should also be temporarily withheld in any patient with an acute, serious condition suggestive of myopathy or predisposing to the development of renal failure secondary to rhabdomyolysis (e.g., sepsis, hypotension, dehydration, major surgery, trauma, severe metabolic, endocrine, and electrolyte disorders, or uncontrolled seizures). All patients should be advised to promptly report unexplained muscle pain, tenderness, or weakness, particularly if accompanied by malaise or fever.

5.2   Liver Enzyme Abnormalities and Monitoring

It is recommended that liver enzyme tests be performed before and at 12 weeks following both the initiation of therapy and any elevation of dose, and periodically (e.g., semiannually) thereafter.

Increases in serum transaminases [AST (SGOT) or ALT (SGPT)] have been reported with HMG-CoA reductase inhibitors, including CRESTOR. In most cases, the elevations were transient and resolved or improved on continued therapy or after a brief interruption in therapy. There were two cases of jaundice, for which a relationship to CRESTOR therapy could not be determined, which resolved after discontinuation of therapy. There were no cases of liver failure or irreversible liver disease in these trials.

In a pooled analysis of placebo-controlled trials, increases in serum transaminases to >3 times the upper limit of normal occurred in 1.1% of patients taking CRESTOR versus 0.5% of patients treated with placebo.

Patients who develop increased transaminase levels should be monitored until the abnormalities have resolved. Should an increase in ALT or AST of >3 times ULN persist, reduction of dose or withdrawal of CRESTOR is recommended. CRESTOR should be used with caution in patients who consume substantial quantities of alcohol and/or have a history of chronic liver disease [see Clinical Pharmacology (12.3)]. Active liver disease, which may include unexplained persistent transaminase elevations, is a contraindication to the use of CRESTOR [see Contraindications (4)].

5.3   Concomitant Coumarin Anticoagulants

Caution should be exercised when anticoagulants are given in conjunction with CRESTOR because of its potentiation of the effect of coumarin-type anticoagulants in prolonging the prothrombin time/INR. In patients taking coumarin anticoagulants and CRESTOR concomitantly, INR should be determined before starting CRESTOR and frequently enough during early therapy to ensure that no significant alteration of INR occurs [see Drug Interactions (7.4)].

5.4   Proteinuria and Hematuria

In the CRESTOR clinical trial program, dipstick-positive proteinuria and microscopic hematuria were observed among CRESTOR treated patients. These findings were more frequent in patients taking CRESTOR 40 mg, when compared to lower doses of CRESTOR or comparator HMG-CoA reductase inhibitors, though it was generally transient and was not associated with worsening renal function. Although the clinical significance of this finding is unknown, a dose reduction should be considered for patients on CRESTOR therapy with unexplained persistent proteinuria and/or hematuria during routine urinalysis testing.

5.5   Endocrine Effects

Increases in HbA1c and fasting serum glucose levels have been reported with HMG-CoA reductase inhibitors, including CRESTOR [see Adverse Reactions (6.1)].

Although clinical studies have shown that CRESTOR alone does not reduce basal plasma cortisol concentration or impair adrenal reserve, caution should be exercised if CRESTOR is administered concomitantly with drugs that may decrease the levels or activity of endogenous steroid hormones such as ketoconazole, spironolactone, and cimetidine.

6   ADVERSE REACTIONS

The following serious adverse reactions are discussed in greater detail in other sections of the label:

- Rhabdomyolysis with myoglobinuria and acute renal failure and myopathy (including myositis) [see Warnings and Precautions (5.1)]
- Liver enzyme abnormalities [see Warnings and Precautions (5.2)]

In the CRESTOR controlled clinical trials database (placebo or active-controlled) of 5394 patients with a mean treatment duration of 15 weeks, 1.4% of patients discontinued due to adverse reactions. The most common adverse reactions that led to treatment discontinuation were:
- myalgia
- abdominal pain
- nausea

The most commonly reported adverse reactions (incidence ≥ 2%) in the CRESTOR controlled clinical trial database of 5394 patients were:
- headache
- myalgia
- abdominal pain
- asthenia
- nausea

6.1   Clinical Studies Experience

Because clinical studies are conducted under widely varying conditions, adverse reaction rates observed in the clinical studies of a drug cannot be directly compared to rates in the clinical studies of another drug and may not reflect the rates observed in clinical practice.

Adverse reactions reported in ≥ 2% of patients in placebo-controlled clinical studies and at a rate greater than placebo are shown in Table 1. These studies had a treatment duration of up to 12 weeks.

[See table above]

Other adverse reactions reported in clinical studies were abdominal pain, dizziness, hypersensitivity (including rash, pruritus, urticaria, and angioedema) and pancreatitis. The following laboratory abnormalities have also been reported: dipstick-positive proteinuria and microscopic hematuria [see Warnings and Precautions (5.4)]; elevated creatine phosphokinase, transaminases, glucose, glutamyl transpeptidase, alkaline phosphatase, and bilirubin; and thyroid function abnormalities.

In the METEOR study, involving 981 participants treated with rosuvastatin 40 mg (n=700) or placebo (n=281) with a mean treatment duration of 1.7 years, 5.6% of subjects treated with CRESTOR versus 2.8% of placebo-treated subjects discontinued due to adverse reactions. The most common adverse reactions that led to treatment discontinuation were: myalgia, hepatic enzyme increased, headache, and nausea [see Clinical Studies (14.7)].

Adverse reactions reported in ≥ 2% of patients and at a rate greater than placebo are shown in Table 2.

Table 2. Adverse Reactions* Reported by ≥ 2% of Patients Treated with CRESTOR and > Placebo in the METEOR Trial (% of Patients)

Adverse Reactions	CRESTOR 40 mg N=700	Placebo N=281
Myalgia	12.7	12.1
Arthralgia	10.1	7.1
Headache	6.4	5.3
Dizziness	4.0	2.8
Increased CPK	2.6	0.7
Abdominal pain	2.4	1.8
†ALT >3× ULN	2.2	0.7

* Adverse reactions by MedDRA preferred term.
† Frequency recorded as abnormal laboratory value.

In the JUPITER study, 17,802 participants were treated with rosuvastatin 20 mg (n=8901) or placebo (n=8901) for a mean duration of 2 years. A higher percentage of rosuvastatin-treated patients versus placebo-treated patients, 6.6% and 6.2%, respectively, discontinued study medication due to an adverse event, irrespective of treatment causality. Myalgia was the most common adverse reaction that led to treatment discontinuation.

In JUPITER, there was a significantly higher frequency of diabetes mellitus reported in patients taking rosuvastatin (2.8%) versus patients taking placebo (2.3%). Mean HbA1c was significantly increased by 0.1% in rosuvastatin-treated patients compared to placebo-treated patients. The number of patients with a HbA1c > 6.5% at the end of the trial was significantly higher in rosuvastatin-treated versus placebo-treated patients [see Warnings and Precautions (5.5) and Clinical Studies (14.8)].

Table 1. Adverse Reactions* Reported by ≥ 2% of Patients Treated with CRESTOR and > Placebo in Placebo-Controlled Trials (% of Patients)

Adverse Reactions	CRESTOR 5 mg N=291	CRESTOR 10 mg N=283	CRESTOR 20 mg N=64	CRESTOR 40 mg N=106	Total CRESTOR 5 mg–40 mg N=744	Placebo N=382
Headache	5.5	4.9	3.1	8.5	5.5	5.0
Nausea	3.8	3.5	6.3	0	3.4	3.1
Myalgia	3.1	2.1	6.3	1.9	2.8	1.3
Asthenia	2.4	3.2	4.7	0.9	2.7	2.6
Constipation	2.1	2.1	4.7	2.8	2.4	2.4

* Adverse reactions by COSTART preferred term.

Adverse reactions reported in ≥ 2% of patients and at a rate greater than placebo are shown in Table 3.

Table 3. Adverse Reactions* Reported by ≥ 2% of Patients Treated with CRESTOR and > Placebo in the JUPITER Trial (% of Patients)

Adverse Reactions	CRESTOR 20 mg N=8901	Placebo N=8901
Myalgia	7.6	6.6
Arthralgia	3.8	3.2
Constipation	3.3	3.0
Nausea	2.4	2.3

* Treatment-emergent adverse reactions by MedDRA preferred term.

6.2   Pediatric patients 10 to 17 years of age

In a 12-week controlled study in boys and postmenarchal girls, the safety and tolerability profile of CRESTOR 5 to 20 mg daily was generally similar to that of placebo [see Clinical Studies (14.6) and Use in Special Populations, Pediatric Use (8.4)].

However, elevations in serum creatine phosphokinase (CK) > 10 × ULN were observed more frequently in rosuvastatin compared with placebo-treated children. Four of 130 (3%) children treated with rosuvastatin (2 treated with 10 mg and 2 treated with 20 mg) had increased CK >10 × ULN, compared to 0 of 46 children on placebo.

6.3   Postmarketing Experience

The following adverse reactions have been identified during postapproval use of CRESTOR: arthralgia, hepatic failure, hepatitis, jaundice, memory loss, depression, and sleep disorders (including insomnia and nightmares). Because these reactions are reported voluntarily from a population of uncertain size, it is not always possible to reliably estimate their frequency or establish a causal relationship to drug exposure.

7   DRUG INTERACTIONS

7.1   Cyclosporine

Cyclosporine significantly increased rosuvastatin exposure. Therefore, in patients taking cyclosporine, therapy should be limited to CRESTOR 5 mg once daily [see Dosage and Administration (2.5), Warnings and Precautions (5.1), and Clinical Pharmacology (12.3)].

7.2   Gemfibrozil

Gemfibrozil significantly increased rosuvastatin exposure. Therefore, combination therapy with CRESTOR and gemfibrozil should be avoided. If used, do not exceed CRESTOR 10 mg once daily [see Dosage and Administration (2.6) and Clinical Pharmacology (12.3)].

7.3   Protease Inhibitors

Coadministration of rosuvastatin with certain protease inhibitors given in combination with ritonavir has differing effects on rosuvastatin exposure. The protease inhibitor combinations lopinavir/ritonavir and atazanavir/ritonavir increase rosuvastatin exposure (AUC) up to threefold [see Table 3–Clinical Pharmacology (12.3)]. For these combinations the dose of CRESTOR should be limited to 10 mg. The combinations of tipranavir/ritonavir or fosamprenavir/ritonavir produce little or no change in rosuvastatin exposure. Caution should be exercised when rosuvastatin is coadministered with protease inhibitors given in combination with ritonavir [see Dosage and Administration (2.5), Warnings and Precautions (5.1) and Clinical Pharmacology (12.3)].

7.4   Coumarin Anticoagulants

CRESTOR significantly increased INR in patients receiving coumarin anticoagulants. Therefore, caution should be exercised when coumarin anticoagulants are given in conjunction with CRESTOR. In patients taking coumarin anticoagulants and CRESTOR concomitantly, INR should be determined before starting CRESTOR and frequently enough during early therapy to ensure that no significant alteration of INR occurs [see Warnings and Precautions (5.3) and Clinical Pharmacology (12.3)].

7.5   Niacin

The risk of skeletal muscle effects may be enhanced when CRESTOR is used in combination with niacin; a reduction in CRESTOR dosage should be considered in this setting [see Warnings and Precautions (5.1)].

7.6   Fenofibrate

When CRESTOR was coadministered with fenofibrate no clinically significant increase in the AUC of rosuvastatin or fenofibrate, was observed. The benefit of further alterations in lipid levels by the combined use of CRESTOR with fibrates should be carefully weighed against the potential risks of this combination [see Warnings and Precautions (5.1) and Clinical Pharmacology (12.3)].

8   USE IN SPECIFIC POPULATIONS

8.1   Pregnancy

Teratogenic effects: Pregnancy Category X.

CRESTOR is contraindicated in women who are or may become pregnant. Serum cholesterol and triglycerides increase during normal pregnancy, and cholesterol products are essential for fetal development. Atherosclerosis is a chronic process and discontinuation of lipid-lowering drugs during pregnancy should have little impact on long-term outcomes of primary hyperlipidemia therapy [see Contraindications (4)].

There are no adequate and well-controlled studies of CRESTOR in pregnant women. There have been rare reports of congenital anomalies following intrauterine exposure to HMG-CoA reductase inhibitors. In a review of about 100 prospectively followed pregnancies in women exposed to other HMG-CoA reductase inhibitors, the incidences of congenital anomalies, spontaneous abortions, and fetal deaths/stillbirths did not exceed the rate expected in the general population. However, this study was only able to exclude a three-to-fourfold increased risk of congenital anomalies over background incidence. In 89% of these cases, drug treatment started before pregnancy and stopped during the first trimester when pregnancy was identified.

Rosuvastatin crosses the placenta in rats and rabbits. In rats, CRESTOR was not teratogenic at systemic exposures equivalent to a human therapeutic dose of 40 mg/day. At 10-12 times the human dose of 40 mg/day, there was decreased pup survival, decreased fetal body weight among female pups, and delayed ossification. In rabbits, pup viability decreased and maternal mortality increased at doses equivalent to the human dose of 40 mg/day [see Nonclinical Toxicology (13.2)].

CRESTOR may cause fetal harm when administered to a pregnant woman. If the patient becomes pregnant while taking CRESTOR, the patient should be apprised of the potential risks to the fetus and the lack of known clinical benefit with continued use during pregnancy.

8.3   Nursing Mothers

It is not known whether rosuvastatin is excreted in human milk, but a small amount of another drug in this class does pass into breast milk. In rats, breast milk concentrations of rosuvastatin are three times higher than plasma levels; however, animal breast milk drug levels may not accurately reflect human breast milk levels. Because another drug in this class passes into human milk and because HMG-CoA reductase inhibitors have a potential to cause serious adverse reactions in nursing infants, women who require CRESTOR treatment should be advised not to nurse their infants [see Contraindications (4)].

8.4   Pediatric Use

The safety and effectiveness of CRESTOR in patients 10 to 17 years of age with heterozygous familial hypercholesterolemia were evaluated in a controlled clinical trial of 12 weeks duration followed by 40 weeks of open-label exposure. Patients treated with 5 mg, 10 mg and 20 mg daily CRESTOR had an adverse experience profile generally similar to that of patients treated with placebo [see *Adverse Reactions* (6.2)]. Although not all adverse reactions identified in the adult population have been observed in clinical trials of children and adolescent patients, the same warnings and precautions for adults should be considered for children and adolescents. There was no detectable effect of CRESTOR on growth, weight, BMI (body mass index), or sexual maturation [see *Clinical Studies* (14.5)] in pediatric patients (10 to 17 years of age). Adolescent females should be counseled on appropriate contraceptive methods while on CRESTOR therapy [see *Use in Specific Populations* (8.1)]. CRESTOR has not been studied in controlled clinical trials involving prepubertal patients or patients younger than 10 years of age. Doses of CRESTOR greater than 20 mg have not been studied in the pediatric population.

In children and adolescents with homozygous familial hypercholesterolemia experience is limited to eight patients (aged 8 years and above).

In a pharmacokinetic study, 18 patients (9 boys and 9 girls) 10 to 17 years of age with heterozygous FH received single and multiple oral doses of CRESTOR. Both C_{max} and AUC of rosuvastatin were similar to values observed in adult subjects administered the same doses.

8.5 Geriatric Use
Of the 10,275 patients in clinical studies with CRESTOR, 3159 (31%) were 65 years and older, and 698 (6.8%) were 75 years and older. No overall differences in safety or effectiveness were observed between these subjects and younger subjects, and other reported clinical experience has not identified differences in responses between the elderly and younger patients, but greater sensitivity of some older individuals cannot be ruled out.

Elderly patients are at higher risk of myopathy and CRESTOR should be prescribed with caution in the elderly [see *Warnings and Precautions* (5.1) and *Clinical Pharmacology* (12.3)].

8.6 Renal Impairment
Rosuvastatin exposure is not influenced by mild to moderate renal impairment ($CL_{cr} \geq 30$ mL/min/1.73 m^2); however, exposure to rosuvastatin is increased to a clinically significant extent in patients with severe renal impairment who are not receiving hemodialysis. CRESTOR dosing should be adjusted in patients with severe renal impairment ($CL_{cr} < 30$ mL/min/1.73 m^2) not requiring hemodialysis [see *Dosage and Administration* (2.7), *Warnings and Precautions* (5.1) and *Clinical Pharmacology* (12.3)].

8.7 Hepatic Impairment
CRESTOR is contraindicated in patients with active liver disease, which may include unexplained persistent elevations of hepatic transaminase levels. Chronic alcohol liver disease is known to increase rosuvastatin exposure; CRESTOR should be used with caution in these patients [see *Contraindications* (4), *Warning and Precautions* (5.2), and *Clinical Pharmacology* (12.3)].

8.8 Asian Patients
Pharmacokinetic studies have demonstrated an approximate 2-fold increase in median exposure to rosuvastatin in Asian subjects when compared with Caucasian controls. CRESTOR dosage should be adjusted in Asian patients [see *Dosage and Administration* (2.4) and *Clinical Pharmacology* (12.3)].

10 OVERDOSAGE
There is no specific treatment in the event of overdose. In the event of overdose, the patient should be treated symptomatically and supportive measures instituted as required. Hemodialysis does not significantly enhance clearance of rosuvastatin.

11 DESCRIPTION
CRESTOR (rosuvastatin calcium) is a synthetic lipid-lowering agent for oral administration.

The chemical name for rosuvastatin calcium is bis[(E)-7-[4-(4-fluorophenyl)-6-isopropyl-2-[methyl (methylsulfonyl) amino] pyrimidin-5-yl](3R,5S)-3,5-dihydroxyhept-6-enoic acid] calcium salt with the following structural formula:

Table 4. Effect of Coadministered Drugs on Rosuvastatin Systemic Exposure

Coadministered drug and dosing regimen	Rosuvastatin		
	Dose (mg)*	Change in AUC[†]	Change in C$_{max}$[†]
Cyclosporine – stable dose required (75 mg–200 mg BID)	10 mg QD for 10 days	↑ 7-fold[‡]	↑ 11-fold[‡]
Gemfibrozil 600 mg BID for 7 days	80 mg	↑ 1.9-fold[‡]	↑ 2.2-fold[‡]
Lopinavir/ritonavir combination 400 mg/100 mg BID for 10 days	20 mg QD for 7 days	↑ 2-fold[‡]	↑ 5-fold[‡]
Atazanavir/ritonavir combination 300 mg/100 mg QD for 7 days	10 mg	↑ 3-fold[‡]	↑ 7-fold[‡]
Tipranavir/ritonavir combination 500 mg/200mg BID for 11 days	10 mg	↑ 26%	↑ 2-fold
Fosamprenavir/ritonavir 700 mg/100 mg BID for 7 days	10 mg	↑ 8%	↑ 45%
Fenofibrate 67 mg TID for 7 days	10 mg	↑ 7%	↑ 21%
Aluminum & magnesium hydroxide combination antacid Administered simultaneously Administered 2 hours apart	40 mg 40 mg	↓ 54%[‡] ↓ 22%	↓ 50%[‡] ↓ 16%
Erythromycin 500 mg QID for 7 days	80 mg	↓ 20%	↓ 31%
Ketoconazole 200 mg BID for 7 days	80 mg	↑ 2%	↓ 5%
Itraconazole 200 mg QD for 5 days	10 mg 80 mg	↑ 39% ↑ 28%	↑ 36% ↑ 15%
Fluconazole 200 mg QD for 11 days	80 mg	↑ 14%	↑ 9%

* Single dose unless otherwise noted
† Mean ratio (with/without coadministered drug and no change = 1-fold) or % change (with/without coadministered drug and no change = 0%); symbols of ↑ and ↓ indicate the exposure increase and decrease, respectively.
‡ Clinically Significant [see *Dosage and Administration* (2) and *Warnings and Precautions* (5)]

The empirical formula for rosuvastatin calcium is $(C_{22}H_{27}FN_3O_6S)_2Ca$ and the molecular weight is 1001.14. Rosuvastatin calcium is a white amorphous powder that is sparingly soluble in water and methanol, and slightly soluble in ethanol. Rosuvastatin calcium is a hydrophilic compound with a partition coefficient (octanol/water) of 0.13 at pH of 7.0.

Inactive Ingredients: Each tablet contains: microcrystalline cellulose NF, lactose monohydrate NF, tribasic calcium phosphate NF, crospovidone NF, magnesium stearate NF, hypromellose NF, triacetin NF, titanium dioxide USP, yellow ferric oxide, and red ferric oxide NF.

12 CLINICAL PHARMACOLOGY
12.1 Mechanism of Action
CRESTOR is a selective and competitive inhibitor of HMG-CoA reductase, the rate-limiting enzyme that converts 3-hydroxy-3-methylglutaryl coenzyme A to mevalonate, a precursor of cholesterol. *In vivo* studies in animals, and *in vitro* studies in cultured animal and human cells have shown rosuvastatin to have a high uptake into, and selectivity for, action in the liver, the target organ for cholesterol lowering. In *in vivo* and *in vitro* studies, rosuvastatin produces its lipid-modifying effects in two ways. First, it increases the number of hepatic LDL receptors on the cell-surface to enhance uptake and catabolism of LDL. Second, rosuvastatin inhibits hepatic synthesis of VLDL, which reduces the total number of VLDL and LDL particles.

12.3 Pharmacokinetics
- *Absorption:* In clinical pharmacology studies in man, peak plasma concentrations of rosuvastatin were reached 3 to 5 hours following oral dosing. Both C_{max} and AUC increased in approximate proportion to CRESTOR dose. The absolute bioavailability of rosuvastatin is approximately 20%.
  Administration of CRESTOR with food did not affect the AUC of rosuvastatin.
  The AUC of rosuvastatin does not differ following evening or morning drug administration.
- *Distribution:* Mean volume of distribution at steady-state of rosuvastatin is approximately 134 liters. Rosuvastatin is 88% bound to plasma proteins, mostly albumin. This binding is reversible and independent of plasma concentrations.
- *Metabolism:* Rosuvastatin is not extensively metabolized; approximately 10% of a radiolabeled dose is recovered as metabolite. The major metabolite is N-desmethyl rosuvastatin, which is formed principally by cytochrome P450 2C9, and *in vitro* studies have demonstrated that N-desmethyl rosuvastatin has approximately one-sixth to one-half the HMG-CoA reductase inhibitory activity of the parent compound. Overall, greater than 90% of active plasma HMG-CoA reductase inhibitory activity is accounted for by the parent compound.
- *Excretion:* Following oral administration, rosuvastatin and its metabolites are primarily excreted in the feces (90%). The elimination half-life ($t_{1/2}$) of rosuvastatin is approximately 19 hours.
  After an intravenous dose, approximately 28% of total body clearance was via the renal route, and 72% by the hepatic route.
- *Race:* A population pharmacokinetic analysis revealed no clinically relevant differences in pharmacokinetics among Caucasian, Hispanic, and Black or Afro-Caribbean groups. However, pharmacokinetic studies, including one conducted in the US, have demonstrated an approximate 2-fold elevation in median exposure (AUC and C_{max}) in Asian subjects when compared with a Caucasian control group.
- *Gender:* There were no differences in plasma concentrations of rosuvastatin between men and women.
- *Geriatric:* There were no differences in plasma concentrations of rosuvastatin between the nonelderly and elderly populations (age ≥65 years).
- *Renal Impairment:* Mild to moderate renal impairment ($CL_{cr} \geq 30$ mL/min/1.73 m^2) had no influence on plasma concentrations of rosuvastatin. However, plasma concentrations of rosuvastatin increased to a clinically significant extent (about 3-fold) in patients with severe renal impairment ($CL_{cr} < 30$ mL/min/1.73 m^2) not receiving hemodialysis compared with healthy subjects ($CL_{cr} > 80$ mL/min/1.73 m^2).
- *Hemodialysis:* Steady-state concentrations of rosuvastatin in patients on chronic hemodialysis were approximately 50% greater compared with healthy volunteer subjects with normal renal function.
- *Hepatic Impairment:* In patients with chronic alcohol liver disease, plasma concentrations of rosuvastatin were modestly increased.
  In patients with Child-Pugh A disease, C_{max} and AUC were increased by 60% and 5%, respectively, as compared with patients with normal liver function. In patients with Child-Pugh B disease, C_{max} and AUC were increased 100% and 21%, respectively, compared with patients with normal liver function.

Drug-Drug Interactions:
Cytochrome P450 3A4
Rosuvastatin clearance is not dependent on metabolism by cytochrome P450 3A4 to a clinically significant extent.
[See table 4 above]
[See table 5 at top of next page]

Table 5. Effect of Rosuvastatin Coadministration on Systemic Exposure To Other Drugs

Rosuvastatin Dosage Regimen	Coadministered Drug		
	Name and Dose	Change in AUC	Change in C_{max}
40 mg QD for 10 days	Warfarin* 25 mg single dose	R-Warfarin ↑ 4% S-Warfarin ↑ 6%	R-Warfarin ↓ 1% S-Warfarin 0%
40 mg QD for 12 days	Digoxin 0.5 mg single dose	↑ 4%	↑ 4%
40 mg QD for 28 days	Oral Contraceptive (ethinyl estradiol 0.035 mg & norgestrel 0.180, 0.215 and 0.250 mg) QD for 21 Days	EE ↑ 26% NG ↑ 34%	EE ↑ 25% NG ↑ 23%

EE = ethinyl estradiol, NG = norgestrel

*Clinically significant pharmacodynamic effects [see *Warnings and Precautions* (5.4)]

Table 6. Dose-Response in Patients With Hyperlipidemia (Adjusted Mean % Change From Baseline at Week 6)

Dose	N	Total-C	LDL-C	Non-HDL-C	ApoB	TG	HDL-C
Placebo	13	-5	-7	-7	-3	-3	3
CRESTOR 5 mg	17	-33	-45	-44	-38	-35	13
CRESTOR 10 mg	17	-36	-52	-48	-42	-10	14
CRESTOR 20 mg	17	-40	-55	-51	-46	-23	8
CRESTOR 40 mg	18	-46	-63	-60	-54	-28	10

Table 7. Percent Change in LDL-C From Baseline to Week 6 (LS Mean*) by Treatment Group (sample sizes ranging from 156–167 patients per group)

Treatment	Treatment Daily Dose			
	10 mg	20 mg	40 mg	80 mg
CRESTOR	-46[†]	-52[‡]	-55[§]	—
Atorvastatin	-37	-43	-48	-51
Simvastatin	-28	-35	-39	-46
Pravastatin	-20	-24	-30	—

* Corresponding standard errors are approximately 1.00
† CRESTOR 10 mg reduced LDL-C significantly more than atorvastatin 10 mg; pravastatin 10 mg, 20 mg, and 40 mg; simvastatin 10 mg, 20 mg, and 40 mg. (p<0.002)
‡ CRESTOR 20 mg reduced LDL-C significantly more than atorvastatin 20 mg and 40 mg; pravastatin 20 mg and 40 mg; simvastatin 20 mg, 40 mg, and 80 mg. (p<0.002)
§ CRESTOR 40 mg reduced LDL-C significantly more than atorvastatin 40 mg; pravastatin 40 mg; simvastatin 40 mg, and 80 mg. (p<0.002)

Table 8. Mean LDL-C Percentage Change from Baseline

		CRESTOR (n=435) LS Mean* (95% CI)	Atorvastatin (n=187) LS Mean* (95% CI)
Week 6	20 mg	-47% (-49%, -46%)	-38% (-40%, -36%)
Week 12	40 mg	-55% (-57%, -54%)	-47% (-49%, -45%)
Week 18	80 mg	NA	-52% (-54%, -50%)

*LS Means are least square means adjusted for baseline LDL-C

13 NONCLINICAL TOXICOLOGY

13.1 Carcinogenesis, Mutagenesis, Impairment of Fertility

In a 104-week carcinogenicity study in rats at dose levels of 2, 20, 60, or 80 mg/kg/day by oral gavage, the incidence of uterine stromal polyps was significantly increased in females at 80 mg/kg/day at systemic exposure 20 times the human exposure at 40 mg/day based on AUC. Increased incidence of polyps was not seen at lower doses.

In a 107-week carcinogenicity study in mice given 10, 60, 200 mg/kg/day by oral gavage, an increased incidence of hepatocellular adenoma/carcinoma was observed at 200 mg/kg/day at systemic exposures 20 times the human exposure at 40 mg/day based on AUC. An increased incidence of hepatocellular tumors was not seen at lower doses.

Rosuvastatin was not mutagenic or clastogenic with or without metabolic activation in the Ames test with *Salmonella typhimurium* and *Escherichia coli*, the mouse lymphoma assay, and the chromosomal aberration assay in Chinese hamster lung cells. Rosuvastatin was negative in the *in vivo* mouse micronucleus test.

In rat fertility studies with oral gavage doses of 5, 15, 50 mg/kg/day, males were treated for 9 weeks prior to and throughout mating and females were treated 2 weeks prior to mating and throughout mating until gestation day 7. No adverse effect on fertility was observed at 50 mg/kg/day (systemic exposures up to 10 times the human exposure at 40 mg/day based on AUC). In testicles of dogs treated with rosuvastatin at 30 mg/kg/day for one month, spermatidic giant cells were seen. Spermatidic giant cells were observed in monkeys after 6-month treatment at 30 mg/kg/day in addition to vacuolation of seminiferous tubular epithelium. Exposures in the dog were 20 times and in the monkey 10 times the human exposure at 40 mg/day based on body surface area. Similar findings have been seen with other drugs in this class.

13.2 Animal Toxicology and/or Pharmacology

Embryo-fetal Development

Rosuvastatin crosses the placenta and is found in fetal tissue and amniotic fluid at 3% and 20%, respectively, of the maternal plasma concentration following a single 25 mg/kg oral gavage dose on gestation day 16 in rats. A higher fetal tissue distribution (25% maternal plasma concentration) was observed in rabbits after a single oral gavage dose of 1 mg/kg on gestation day 18.

In female rats given oral gavage doses of 5, 15, 50 mg/kg/day rosuvastatin before mating and continuing through day 7 postcoitus results in decreased fetal body weight (female pups) and delayed ossification at the high dose (systemic exposures 10 times the human exposure at 40 mg/day based on AUC).

In pregnant rats given oral gavage doses of 2, 10, 50 mg/kg/day from gestation day 7 through lactation day 21 (weaning), decreased pup survival occurred in groups given 50 mg/kg/day, systemic exposures ≥ 12 times the human exposure at 40 mg/day based on body surface area.

In pregnant rabbits given oral gavage doses of 0.3, 1, 3 mg/kg/day from gestation day 6 to lactation day 18 (weaning), exposures equivalent to the human exposure at 40 mg/day based on body surface area, decreased fetal viability and maternal mortality was observed.

Rosuvastatin was not teratogenic in rats at ≤ 25 mg/kg/day or in rabbits ≤ 3 mg/kg/day (systemic exposures equivalent to the human exposure at 40 mg/day based on AUC or body surface area, respectively).

Central Nervous System Toxicity

CNS vascular lesions, characterized by perivascular hemorrhages, edema, and mononuclear cell infiltration of perivascular spaces, have been observed in dogs treated with several other members of this drug class. A chemically similar drug in this class produced dose-dependent optic nerve degeneration (Wallerian degeneration of retinogeniculate fibers) in dogs, at a dose that produced plasma drug levels about 30 times higher than the mean drug level in humans taking the highest recommended dose. Edema, hemorrhage, and partial necrosis in the interstitium of the choroid plexus was observed in a female dog sacrificed moribund at day 24 at 90 mg/kg/day by oral gavage (systemic exposures 100 times the human exposure at 40 mg/day based on AUC). Corneal opacity was seen in dogs treated for 52 weeks at 6 mg/kg/day by oral gavage (systemic exposures 20 times the human exposure at 40 mg/day based on AUC). Cataracts were seen in dogs treated for 12 weeks by oral gavage at 30 mg/kg/day (systemic exposures 60 times the human exposure at 40 mg/day based on AUC). Retinal dysplasia and retinal loss were seen in dogs treated for 4 weeks by oral gavage at 90 mg/kg/day (systemic exposures 100 times the human exposure at 40 mg/day based on AUC). Doses ≤30 mg/kg/day (systemic exposures ≤60 times the human exposure at 40 mg/day based on AUC) did not reveal retinal findings during treatment for up to one year.

14 CLINICAL STUDIES

14.1 Hyperlipidemia and Mixed Dyslipidemia

CRESTOR reduces Total-C, LDL-C, ApoB, nonHDL-C, and TG, and increases HDL-C, in adult patients with hyperlipidemia and mixed dyslipidemia.

Dose-Ranging Study: In a multicenter, double-blind, placebo-controlled, dose-ranging study in patients with hyperlipidemia CRESTOR given as a single daily dose for 6 weeks significantly reduced Total-C, LDL-C, nonHDL-C, and ApoB, across the dose range (Table 6).

[See table 6 at left]

Active-Controlled Study: CRESTOR was compared with the HMG-CoA reductase inhibitors atorvastatin, simvastatin, and pravastatin in a multicenter, open-label, dose-ranging study of 2240 patients with hyperlipidemia or mixed dyslipidemia. After randomization, patients were treated for 6 weeks with a single daily dose of either CRESTOR, atorvastatin, simvastatin, or pravastatin (Figure 1 and Table 7).

[See figure at top of next column]

[See table 7 at left]

14.2 Heterozygous Familial Hypercholesterolemia

Active-Controlled Study: In a study of patients with heterozygous FH (baseline mean LDL of 291), patients were randomized to CRESTOR 20 mg or atorvastatin 20 mg. The dose was increased by 6-week intervals. Significant LDL-C reductions from baseline were seen at each dose in both treatment groups (Table 8).

[See table 8 at left]

14.3 Hypertriglyceridemia

Dose-Response Study: In a double-blind, placebo-controlled dose-response study in patients with baseline TG

Figure 1. Percent LDL-C Change by Dose of CRESTOR, Atorvastatin, Simvastatin, and Pravastatin at Week 6 in Patients with Hyperlipidemia or Mixed Dyslipidemia

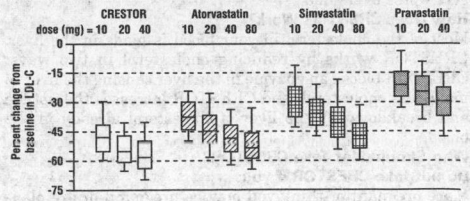

Box plots are a representation of the 25th, 50th, and 75th percentile values, with whiskers representing the 10th and 90th percentile values. Mean baseline LDL-C: 189 mg/dL

levels from 273 to 817 mg/dL, CRESTOR given as a single daily dose (5 to 40 mg) over 6 weeks significantly reduced serum TG levels (Table 9).

[See table 9 at right]

14.4   Primary Dysbetalipoproteinemia (Type III Hyperlipoproteinemia)

In a randomized, multicenter, double-blind crossover study, 32 patients (27 with ε2/ε2 and 4 with apo E mutation [Arg145Cys] with primary dysbetalipoproteinemia (Type III Hyperlipoproteinemia) entered a 6-week dietary lead-in period on the NCEP Therapeutic Lifestyle Change (TLC) diet. Following dietary lead-in, patients were randomized to a sequence of treatments in conjunction with the TLC diet for 6 weeks each: rosuvastatin 10 mg followed by rosuvastatin 20 mg or rosuvastatin 20 mg followed by rosuvastatin 10 mg. CRESTOR reduced nonHDL-C (primary end point) and circulating remnant lipoprotein levels. Results are shown in the table below.

[See table 10 at right]

14.5   Homozygous Familial Hypercholesterolemia

Dose-Titration Study: In an open-label, forced-titration study, homozygous FH patients (n=40, 8-63 years) were evaluated for their response to CRESTOR 20 to 40 mg titrated at a 6-week interval. In the overall population, the mean LDL-C reduction from baseline was 22%. About one-third of the patients benefited from increasing their dose from 20 mg to 40 mg with further LDL lowering of greater than 6%. In the 27 patients with at least a 15% reduction in LDL-C, the mean LDL-C reduction was 30% (median 28% reduction). Among 13 patients with an LDL-C reduction of <15%, 3 had no change or an increase in LDL-C. Reductions in LDL-C of 15% or greater were observed in 3 of 5 patients with known receptor negative status.

14.6   Pediatric Patients with Heterozygous Familial Hypercholesterolemia

In a double-blind, randomized, multicenter, placebo-controlled, 12-week study, 176 (97 male and 79 female) children and adolescents with heterozygous familial hypercholesterolemia were randomized to rosuvastatin 5, 10 or 20 mg or placebo daily. Patients ranged in age from 10 to 17 years (median age of 14 years) with approximately 30% of the patients 10 to 13 years and approximately 17%, 18%, 40%, and 25% at Tanner stages II, III, IV, and V, respectively. Females were at least 1 year postmenarche. Mean LDL-C at baseline was 233 mg/dL (range of 129 to 399). The 12-week double-blind phase was followed by a 40-week open-label dose-titration phase, where all patients (n=173) received 5 mg, 10 mg or 20 mg rosuvastatin daily.

Rosuvastatin significantly reduced LDL-C (primary end point), total cholesterol and ApoB levels at each dose compared to placebo. Results are shown in Table 11 below.

[See table 11 at right]

At the end of the 12-week, double-blind treatment period, the percentage of patients achieving the LDL-C goal of less than 110 mg/dL (2.8 mmol/L) was 0% for placebo, 12% for rosuvastatin 5 mg, 41% for rosuvastatin 10 mg and 41% for rosuvastatin 20 mg. For the 40-week, open-label phase, 71% of the patients were titrated to the maximum dose of 20 mg and 41% of patients achieved the LDL-C goal of 110 mg/dL.

The long-term efficacy of rosuvastatin therapy initiated in childhood to reduce morbidity and mortality in adulthood has not been established.

14.7   Slowing of the Progression of Atherosclerosis

In the *Measuring Effects on Intima Media Thickness: an Evaluation Of Rosuvastatin 40 mg (METEOR)* study, the effect of therapy with CRESTOR on carotid atherosclerosis was assessed by B-mode ultrasonography in patients with elevated LDL-C, at low risk (Framingham risk <10% over ten years) for symptomatic coronary artery disease and with subclinical atherosclerosis as evidenced by carotid intimal-medial thickness (cIMT). In this double-blind, placebo-controlled clinical study 984 patients were randomized (of whom 876 were analyzed) in a 5:2 ratio to CRESTOR 40 mg

Table 9. Dose-Response in Patients With Primary Hypertriglyceridemia Over 6 Weeks Dosing Median (Min, Max) Percent Change From Baseline

Dose	Placebo (n=26)	CRESTOR 5 mg (n=25)	CRESTOR 10 mg (n=23)	CRESTOR 20 mg (n=27)	CRESTOR 40 mg (n=25)
Triglycerides	1 (-40, 72)	-21 (-58, 38)	-37 (-65, 5)	-37 (-72, 11)	-43 (-80, -7)
nonHDL-C	2 (-13, 19)	-29 (-43, -8)	-49 (-59, -20)	-43 (-74, 12)	-51 (-62, -6)
VLDL-C	2 (-36, 53)	-25 (-62, 49)	-48 (-72, 14)	-49 (-83, 20)	-56 (-83, 10)
Total-C	1 (-13, 17)	-24 (-40, -4)	-40 (-51, -14)	-34 (-61, -11)	-40 (-51, -4)
LDL-C	5 (-30, 52)	-28 (-71, 2)	-45 (-59, 7)	-31 (-66, 34)	-43 (-61, -3)
HDL-C	-3 (-25, 18)	3 (-38, 33)	8 (-8, 24)	22 (-5, 50)	17 (-14, 63)

Table 10. Lipid-modifying Effects of Rosuvastatin 10 mg and 20 mg in Primary Dysbetalipoproteinemia (Type III hyperlipoproteinemia) after Six weeks by Median Percent Change (95% CI) from Baseline (N=32)

	Median at Baseline (mg/dL)	Median percent change from baseline (95% CI) CRESTOR 10 mg	Median percent change from baseline (95% CI) CRESTOR 20 mg
Total-C	342.5	-43.3 (-46.9, -37.5)	-47.6 (-51.6, -42.8)
Triglycerides	503.5	-40.1 (-44.9, -33.6)	-43.0 (-52.5, -33.1)
NonHDL-C	294.5	-48.2 (-56.7, -45.6)	-56.4 (-61.4, -48.5)
VLDL-C + IDL-C	209.5	-46.8 (-53.7, -39.4)	-56.2 (-67.7, -43.7)
LDL-C	112.5	-54.4 (-59.1, -47.3)	-57.3 (-59.4, -52.1)
HDL-C	35.5	10.2 (1.9, 12.3)	11.2 (8.3, 20.5)
RLP-C	82.0	-56.4 (-67.1, -49.0)	-64.9 (-74.0, -56.6)
Apo-E	16.0	-42.9 (-46.3, -33.3)	-42.5 (-47.1, -35.6)

Table 11–Lipid-modifying effects of rosuvastatin in pediatric patients 10 to 17 years of age with heterozygous familial hypercholesterolemia (least-squares mean percent change from baseline to week 12)

Dose (mg)	N	LDL-C	HDL-C	Total-C	TG*	ApoB
Placebo	46	-1%	+7%	0%	-7%	-2%
5	42	-38%	+4%[†]	-30%	-13%[†]	-32%
10	44	-45%	+11%[†]	-34%	-15%[†]	-38%
20	44	-50%	+9%[†]	-39%	16%[†]	-41%

* Median percent change
† Difference from placebo not statistically significant

or placebo once daily. Ultrasonograms of the carotid walls were used to determine the annualized rate of change per patient from baseline to two years in mean maximum cIMT of 12 measured segments. The estimated difference in the rate of change in the maximum cIMT analyzed over all 12 carotid artery sites between patients treated with CRESTOR and placebo-treated patients was -0.0145 mm/year (95% CI -0.0196, -0.0093; p<0.0001).

The annualized rate of change from baseline for the placebo group was +0.0131 mm/year (p<0.0001). The annualized rate of change from baseline for the group treated with CRESTOR was -0.0014 mm/year (p=0.32).

At an individual patient level in the group treated with CRESTOR, 52.1% of patients demonstrated an absence of disease progression (defined as a negative annualized rate of change), compared to 37.7% of patients in the placebo group.

14.8   Primary Prevention of Cardiovascular Disease

In the *Justification for the Use of Statins in Primary Prevention: An Intervention Trial Evaluating Rosuvastatin (JUPITER)* study, the effect of CRESTOR (rosuvastatin calcium) on the occurrence of major cardiovascular (CV) disease events was assessed in 17,802 men (≥50 years) and women (≥60 years) who had no clinically evident cardiovascular disease, LDL-C levels <130 mg/dL (3.3 mmol/l) and hs-CRP levels ≥2 mg/L. The study population had an esti-

mated baseline coronary heart disease risk of 11.6% over 10 years based on the Framingham risk criteria and included a high percentage of patients with additional risk factors such as hypertension (58%), low HDL-C levels (23%), cigarette smoking (16%), or a family history of premature CHD (12%). Study participants had a median baseline LDL-C of 108 mg/dL and hsCRP of 4.3 mg/L. Study participants were randomly assigned to placebo (n=8901) or rosuvastatin 20 mg once daily (n=8901) and were followed for a mean duration of 2 years. The JUPITER study was stopped early by the Data Safety Monitoring Board due to meeting predefined stopping rules for efficacy in rosuvastatin-treated subjects.

The primary end point was a composite end point consisting of the time-to-first occurrence of any of the following major CV events: CV death, nonfatal myocardial infarction, nonfatal stroke, hospitalization for unstable angina or an arterial revascularization procedure.

Rosuvastatin significantly reduced the risk of major CV events (252 events in the placebo group vs. 142 events in the rosuvastatin group) with a statistically significant (p<0.001) relative risk reduction of 44% and absolute risk reduction of 1.2% (see Figure 2). The risk reduction for the primary end point was consistent across the following predefined subgroups: age, sex, race, smoking status, family history of premature CHD, body mass index, LDL-C, HDL-C, and hsCRP levels.

Figure 2. Time to first occurence of major cardiovascular events in JUPITER

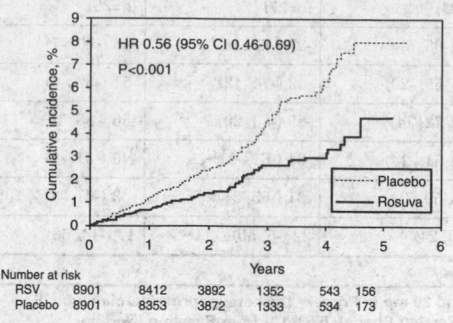

HR 0.56 (95% CI 0.46-0.69)
P<0.001

Number at risk						
RSV	8901	8412	3892	1352	543	156
Placebo	8901	8353	3872	1333	534	173

The individual components of the primary end point are presented in Figure 3. Rosuvastatin significantly reduced the risk of nonfatal myocardial infarction, nonfatal stroke, and arterial revascularization procedures. There were no significant treatment differences between the rosuvastatin and placebo groups due to cardiovascular causes or hospitalizations for unstable angina.

Rosuvastatin significantly reduced the risk of myocardial infarction (6 fatal events and 62 nonfatal events in placebo-treated subjects vs. 9 fatal events and 22 nonfatal events in rosuvastatin-treated subjects) and the risk of stroke (6 fatal events and 58 nonfatal events in placebo-treated subjects vs. 3 fatal events and 30 nonfatal events in rosuvastatin-treated subjects).

In a post-hoc subgroup analysis of JUPITER subjects (n=1405; rosuvastatin=725, placebo=680) with a hsCRP ≥2 mg/L and no other traditional risk factors (smoking, BP ≥140/90 or taking antihypertensives, low HDL-C) other than age, after adjustment for high HDL-C, there was no significant treatment benefit with rosuvastatin treatment. [See figure 3 below]

At one year, rosuvastatin increased HDL-C and reduced LDL-C, hsCRP, total cholesterol and serum triglyceride levels (p<0.001 for all versus placebo).

16 HOW SUPPLIED/STORAGE AND HANDLING

CRESTOR® (rosuvastatin calcium) Tablets are supplied as:
- NDC 0310-0755-90: 5 mg. Yellow, round, biconvex, coated tablets. Debossed "CRESTOR" and "5" on one side; bottle of 90 tablets
- NDC 0310-0751-90: 10 mg. Pink, round, biconvex, coated tablets. Debossed "CRESTOR" and "10" on one side; bottle of 90 tablets
- NDC 0310-0751-39: 10 mg. Pink, round, biconvex, coated tablets. Debossed "CRESTOR" and "10" on one side; unit dose packages of 100
- NDC 0310-0752-90: 20 mg. Pink, round, biconvex, coated tablets. Debossed "CRESTOR" and "20" on one side; bottles of 90
- NDC 0310-0752-39: 20 mg. Pink, round, biconvex, coated tablets. Debossed "CRESTOR" and "20"on one side; unit dose packages of 100
- NDC 0310-0754-30: 40 mg. Pink, oval, biconvex, coated tablets. Debossed "CRESTOR" on one side and "40" on the other side; bottles of 30

Storage

Store at controlled room temperature, 20-25°C (68-77°F) [see USP Controlled Room Temperature]. Protect from moisture.

17 PATIENT COUNSELING INFORMATION
17.1 Skeletal Muscle Effects
Patients should be advised to report promptly unexplained muscle pain, tenderness, or weakness, particularly if accompanied by malaise or fever.
17.2 Concomitant Use of Antacids
When taking CRESTOR with an aluminum and magnesium hydroxide combination antacid, the antacid should be taken at least 2 hours after CRESTOR administration.
17.3 Pregnancy
If the patient becomes pregnant while taking this drug, the patient should be apprised of the potential hazard to the fetus and the lack of known clinical benefit with continued use during pregnancy.
17.4 Liver Enzymes
It is recommended that liver enzymes be checked before and at 12 weeks following both the initiation of therapy and any elevation of dose, and periodically (e.g., semiannually) thereafter.

CRESTOR is a trademark of the AstraZeneca group of companies.

© AstraZeneca 2003, 2005, 2007, 2008, 2009, 2010
Licensed from SHIONOGI & CO., LTD., Osaka, Japan
Distributed by:
AstraZeneca Pharmaceuticals LP
Wilmington, DE 19850
ASTRAZENECA
Rev. June 2010

PATIENT INFORMATION
CRESTOR® (*rosuvastatin calcium*) Tablets
(Kres-tor)
Read this information carefully before you start taking CRESTOR. Each time you refill your prescription for CRESTOR, read the patient information, as there may be new information. This summary does not include everything there is to know about CRESTOR and does not take the place of talking with your health care professional about your medical condition or treatment.

If you have any questions about CRESTOR, ask your health care professional. Only your health care professional can tell you if CRESTOR is right for you.

What is CRESTOR?
CRESTOR is a prescription medicine that belongs to a group of cholesterol-lowering medicines called statins. Along with diet, CRESTOR lowers "bad" cholesterol (LDL-C), increases "good" cholesterol (HDL-C). If bad cholesterol levels are left untreated, fatty deposits (plaque) can build up in the walls of the blood vessels. This plaque buildup over time, can lead to narrowing of these vessels. This is one of the most common causes of heart disease. By lowering bad cholesterol in your blood, CRESTOR can slow this plaque buildup in the walls of blood vessels. CRESTOR has been proven to reduce the risk of heart attacks and strokes in older adults without known heart disease.

What is Cholesterol?
Cholesterol is a fatty substance, also called a lipid, normally found in your bloodstream. Your body needs a certain amount of cholesterol to function properly. But high cholesterol can lead to health problems. LDL-C is called bad cholesterol because if you have too much in your bloodstream, it can become a danger to your health and can lead to potentially serious conditions. HDL-C is known as good cholesterol because it may help remove excess cholesterol.

Common health factors such as diabetes, high blood pressure, smoking, obesity, family history of early heart disease, and age can make controlling your cholesterol even more important.

What is Atherosclerosis?
Atherosclerosis is the progressive buildup of plaque in the arteries over time. One major cause is high levels of LDL-C. Other health factors, such as family history, diabetes, high

blood pressure, or if you smoke, or are overweight, may also play a role in the formation of plaque in arteries. Often this plaque starts building up in arteries in early adulthood and gets worse over time.

How Does CRESTOR Work?
Most of the cholesterol in your blood is made in the liver. CRESTOR works by reducing cholesterol in two ways: CRESTOR blocks an enzyme in the liver causing the liver to make less cholesterol, and CRESTOR increases the uptake and breakdown by the liver of cholesterol already in the blood.

Who Should Not Take CRESTOR?
Do not take CRESTOR if you:
- are pregnant or think you may be pregnant, or are planning to become pregnant. CRESTOR may harm your unborn baby. If you become pregnant, stop taking CRESTOR and call your health care professional right away
- are breast-feeding. CRESTOR can pass into your breast milk and may harm your baby
- have liver problems
- have had an allergic reaction to CRESTOR or are allergic to any of its ingredients. The active ingredient is rosuvastatin calcium. The inactive ingredients are: microcrystalline cellulose, lactose monohydrate, tribasic calcium phosphate, crospovidone, magnesium stearate, hypromellose, triacetin, titanium dioxide, yellow ferric oxide, and red ferric oxide

The safety and effectiveness of CRESTOR have not been established in pediatric patients under the age of 10.

What should I tell my health care professional before taking CRESTOR?
Tell your health care professional if you:
- have a history of muscle pain or weakness
- are pregnant or think you may be pregnant, or are planning to become pregnant
- are breast-feeding
- drink more than 2 glasses of alcohol daily
- have liver problems
- have kidney problems
- have thyroid problems
- are Asian or of Asian descent

Tell your health care professional about all medicines you take or plan to take, including prescription and nonprescription medicines, vitamins, and herbal supplements. Some medicines may interact with CRESTOR, causing side effects. It is particularly important to tell your health care professional if you are taking or plan to take medicines for:
-your immune system
-cholesterol/triglycerides
-blood thinning
-HIV/AIDS
-preventing pregnancy

Know all of the medicines you take and what they look like. It's always a good idea to check that you have the right prescription before you leave the pharmacy and before you take any medicine. Keep a list of your medicines with you to show your health care professional.

If you need to go to the hospital or have surgery, tell all of your health care professionals about all medicines that you are taking.

How Should I Take CRESTOR?
Take CRESTOR exactly as prescribed by your health care professional. Do not change your dose or stop CRESTOR without talking to your health care professional, even if you are feeling well.

Your health care professional may do blood tests to check your cholesterol levels before and during your treatment with CRESTOR. Your dose of CRESTOR may be changed based on these blood tests results.

CRESTOR can be taken at any time of day, with or without food.

Swallow the tablets whole.

Your health care professional may start you on a cholesterol lowering diet before giving you CRESTOR. Stay on this diet when you take CRESTOR.

Wait at least 2 hours after taking CRESTOR to take an antacid that contains a combination of aluminum and magnesium hydroxide.

If you miss a dose of CRESTOR, take it as soon as you remember. However, **do not take 2 doses of CRESTOR within 12 hours of each other.**

If you take too much CRESTOR or overdose, call your health care professional or a Poison Control Center right away or go to the nearest emergency room.

What Should I Avoid While Taking CRESTOR?
Talk to your health care professional before you start any new medicines. This includes prescription and nonprescription medicines, vitamins, and herbal supplements. CRESTOR and certain other medicines can interact, causing serious side effects.

Talk to your health care professional if you are pregnant or plan to become pregnant. Do not use CRESTOR if you are pregnant, trying to become pregnant or suspect that you are

Figure 3. Major CV events by treatment group in JUPITER

End point	Rosuva 20 mg (n=8901) n (rate+)	Placebo 20 mg (n=8901) n (rate+)	HR (95% CI)	P value	Hazard Ratio (—95%—)
Primary end point (MCE)	142 (7.6)	252 (13.6)	0.56 (0.46, 0.69)	<0.001	
Cardiovascular death++	35 (1.9)	44 (2.4)	0.80 (0.51, 1.24)	0.315	
Nonfatal Stroke	30 (1.6)	58 (3.1)	0.52 (0.33, 0.80)	0.003	
Nonfatal MI	22 (1.2)	62 (3.3)	0.35 (0.22, 0.58)	<0.001	
Hospitalized unstable Angina	16 (0.9)	27 (1.5)	0.59 (0.32, 1.10)	0.093	
Arterial revascularization	71 (3.8)	131 (7.1)	0.54 (0.41, 0.72)	<0.001	

+ event rate/1000-patient years
++ Cardiovascular death included fatal MI, fatal stroke, sudden death, and other adjudicated causes of CV death

pregnant. If you become pregnant while taking CRESTOR, stop taking it and contact your health care professional immediately.

What are the Possible Side Effects of CRESTOR?
CRESTOR can cause side effects in some people.
Serious side effects may include:
Muscle Problems. Call your health care professional right away if you experience unexplained muscle pain, tenderness, or weakness especially with fever. This may be an early sign of a rare muscle problem that could lead to serious kidney problems. The risk of muscle problems is greater in people who are 65 years of age or older, or who already have thyroid or kidney problems. The chance of muscle problems may be increased if you are taking certain other medicines with CRESTOR.
Liver problems. Your health care professional should do blood tests before you start taking CRESTOR and during treatment to check for signs of possible liver problems.
The most common side effects may include:
Headache, muscle aches and pains, abdominal pain, weakness, and nausea.
This is not a complete list of side effects of CRESTOR. Talk to your health care professional for a complete list or if you have side effects that bother you or that do not go away.

How Do I Store CRESTOR?
Store CRESTOR at room temperature, 68 to 77°F (20 to 25°C) and in a dry place.
If your health care professional tells you to stop treatment or if your medicine is out of date, throw the medicine away.
Keep CRESTOR and all medicines in a secure place and out of the reach of children.

What are the Ingredients in CRESTOR?

Active Ingredient: rosuvastatin calcium
Inactive Ingredients: microcrystalline cellulose NF, lactose monohydrate NF, tribasic calcium phosphate NF, crospovidone NF, magnesium stearate NF, hypromellose NF, triacetin NF, titanium dioxide USP, yellow ferric oxide, and red ferric oxide NF.

General Information About CRESTOR
It is important to take CRESTOR as prescribed and to discuss any health changes you experience while taking CRESTOR with your health care professional. Do not use CRESTOR for a condition for which it was not prescribed. Do not give CRESTOR to other people, even if they have the same medical condition you have. It may harm them.
This leaflet summarizes important information about CRESTOR. If you would like more information about CRESTOR, ask your health care professional. You can also go to the CRESTOR website at www.crestor.com or call 1-800-CRESTOR.
CRESTOR is a trademark of the AstraZeneca group of companies.
© AstraZeneca 2003, 2005, 2007, 2008, 2009, 2010
Licensed from SHIONOGI & CO., LTD., Osaka, Japan
Distributed by:
AstraZeneca Pharmaceuticals LP
Wilmington, DE 19850
ASTRAZENECA
Rev. June 2010
Shown in Product Identification Guide, page 306

SEROQUEL®   ℞
[SER-oh-kwell]
(quetiapine fumarate)
Tablets

HIGHLIGHTS OF PRESCRIBING INFORMATION
These highlights do not include all the information needed to use SEROQUEL safely and effectively. See full prescribing information for SEROQUEL.
SEROQUEL® (quetiapine fumarate) Tablets
Initial U.S. Approval: 1997

WARNING: INCREASED MORTALITY IN ELDERLY PATIENTS WITH DEMENTIA-RELATED PSYCHOSIS
See full prescribing information for complete boxed warning.
• Antipsychotic drugs are associated with an increased risk of death (5.1)
• Quetiapine is not approved for elderly patients with Dementia-Related Psychosis (5.1)

WARNING: SUICIDALITY AND ANTIDEPRESSANT DRUGS
See full prescribing information for complete boxed warning.
• Increased risk of suicidal thinking and behavior in children, adolescents and young adults taking antidepressants for major depressive disorder and other psychiatric disorders (5.2)

Indication	Dosing Instructions*	Recommended Dose/Dose Range
Schizophrenia-Adults (2.1)	Day 1: 25 mg twice daily. Increase in increments of 25 mg-50 mg divided two or three times on Days 2 and 3 to range of 300-400 mg by Day 4. Further adjustments can be made in increments of 25–50 mg twice a day, in intervals of not less than 2 days.	150-750 mg/day
Schizophrenia-Adolescents (13-17 years) (2.1)	Day 1: 25 mg twice daily. Day 2: Twice daily dosing totaling 100 mg. Day 3: Twice daily dosing totaling 200 mg. Day 4: Twice daily dosing totaling 300 mg. Day 5: Twice daily dosing totaling 400 mg. Further adjustments should be in increments no greater than 100 mg/day within the recommended dose range of 400-800 mg/day. Based on response and tolerability, may be administered three times daily.	400-800 mg/day
Bipolar Mania-Adults Monotherapy or as an adjunct to lithium or divalproex (2.2)	Day 1: Twice daily dosing totaling 100 mg. Day 2: Twice daily dosing totaling 200 mg. Day 3: Twice daily dosing totaling 300 mg. Day 4: Twice daily dosing totaling 400 mg. Further dosage adjustments up to 800 mg/day by Day 6 should be in increments of no greater than 200 mg/day.	400-800 mg/day
Bipolar Mania-Children and Adolescents (10 to 17 years), Monotherapy	Day 1: 25 mg twice daily. Day 2: Twice daily dosing totaling 100 mg. Day 3: Twice daily dosing totaling 200 mg. Day 4: Twice daily dosing totaling 300 mg. Day 5: Twice daily dosing totaling 400 mg. Further adjustments should be in increments no greater than 100 mg/day within the recommended dose range of 400-600 mg/day. Based on response and tolerability, may be administered three times daily.	400-600 mg/day
Bipolar Depression-Adults	Administer once daily at bedtime Day 1: 50 mg. Day 2: 100 mg. Day 3: 200 mg. Day 4: 300 mg.	300 mg/day
Bipolar I Disorder Maintenance Therapy-Adults	Administer twice daily totaling 400-800 mg/day as adjunct to lithium or divalproex. Generally, in the maintenance phase, patients continued on the same dose on which they were stabilized.	

*After initial dosing, adjustments can be made upwards or downwards, if necessary, within the dose range depending upon the clinical response and tolerance of the patient.

───────RECENT MAJOR CHANGES───────
BOXED WARNING: Suicidality and Antidepressant Drugs, 12/2009
Indications and Usage, Schizophrenia (1.1), 12/2009
Indications and Usage, Bipolar Disorder (1.2), 12/2009
Indications and Usage, Special Considerations in Treating Pediatric Patients with Schizophrenia and Bipolar I Disorder (1.3), 12/2009
Dosage and Administration, Schizophrenia, Adolescents (2.1), 12/2009
Dosage and Administration, Bipolar Mania, Children and Adolescents (2.2), 12/2009
Warnings and Precautions, Hyperglycemia (5.4), 12/2009
Warnings and Precautions, Hyperlipidemia (5.5), 12/2009
Warnings and Precautions, Weight Gain (5.6), 12/2009
Warnings and Precautions, Increases in Blood Pressure in Children and Adolescents (5.9), 12/2009
Warnings and Precautions, Use in Patients with Concomitant Illness (5.21), 01/2010
Warnings and Precautions, Withdrawal (5.22), 05/2010

───────INDICATIONS AND USAGE───────
SEROQUEL is an atypical antipsychotic agent indicated for the:
Treatment of schizophrenia (1.1)
• Adults: Efficacy was established in three 6–week clinical trials in patients with schizophrenia (14.1)
• Adolescents (ages 13–17): Efficacy was established in one 6–week trial in patients with schizophrenia (14.1)
Acute treatment of manic episodes associated with bipolar I disorder, both as monotherapy and as an adjunct to lithium or divalproex (1.2)
• Adults: Efficacy was established in two 12–week monotherapy trials and in one 3–week adjunctive trial in patients with manic episodes associated with bipolar I disorder (14.2)
• Children and Adolescents (ages 10–17): Efficacy was established in one 3–week monotherapy trial in patients with manic episodes with bipolar I disorder (14.2)
Acute treatment of depressive episodes associated with bipolar disorder (1.2)
• Adults: Efficacy was established in two 8–week trials in patients with bipolar I or II disorder (14.2)

Maintenance treatment of bipolar disorder as an adjunct to lithium or divalproex (1.2)
• Adults: Efficacy was established in two maintenance trials in adults (14.2)
───────DOSAGE AND ADMINISTRATION───────
SEROQUEL can be taken with or without food.
[See table above]
───────DOSAGE FORMS AND STRENGTHS───────
25 mg, 50 mg, 100 mg, 200 mg, 300 mg, and 400 mg (3)
───────CONTRAINDICATIONS───────
none (4)

───────WARNINGS AND PRECAUTIONS───────
• **Increased Mortality in Elderly Patients with Dementia-Related Psychosis:** Atypical antipsychotic drugs, including quetiapine, are associated with an increased risk of death; causes of death are variable. (5.1)
• **Suicidality and Antidepressant Drugs:** Increased the risk of suicidal thinking and behavior in children, adolescents and young adults taking antidepressants for major depressive disorder and other psychiatric disorders. (5.2)
• **Neuroleptic Malignant Syndrome (NMS):** Manage with immediate discontinuation and close monitoring. (5.3)
• **Hyperglycemia and Diabetes Mellitus (DM):** Ketoacidosis, hyperosmolar coma and death have been reported in patients treated with atypical antipsychotics, including quetiapine. Any patient treated with atypical antipsychotics should be monitored for symptoms of hyperglycemia including polydipsia, polyuria, polyphagia, and weakness. When starting treatment, patients with diabetes or risk factors for diabetes should undergo blood glucose testing before and during treatment. (5.4)
• **Hyperlipidemia:** Undesirable alterations in lipids have been observed. Increases in total cholesterol, LDL-cholesterol and triglycerides and decreases in HDL-cholesterol have been reported in clinical trials. Appropriate clinical monitoring is recommended, including fasting blood lipid testing at the beginning of, and periodically during treatment. (5.5)
• **Weight Gain:** Patients should receive regular monitoring of weight. (5.6)
• **Tardive Dyskinesia** Discontinue if clinically appropriate. (5.7)

- **Orthostatic Hypotension:** Associated dizziness, tachycardia and syncope may occur especially during the initial dose titration period. (5.8)
- **Increased Blood Pressure in Children and Adolescents:** Blood pressure should be measured at the beginning of, and periodically during treatment in children and adolescents. (5.9)
- **Leukopenia, Neutropenia and Agranulocytosis** have been reported with atypical antipsychotics including SEROQUEL. Patients with a pre-existing low white cell count (WBC) or a history of leukopenia/neutropenia should have complete blood count (CBC) monitored frequently during the first few months of treatment and should discontinue SEROQUEL at the first sign of a decline in WBC in absence of other causative factors. (5.10)
- **Cataracts:** Lens changes have been observed in patients during long-term quetiapine treatment. Lens examination is recommended when starting treatment and at 6-month intervals during chronic treatment. (5.11)
- **Suicide:** The possibility of a suicide attempt is inherent in schizophrenia and bipolar disorder, and close supervision of high risk patients should accompany drug therapy. (5.20)
- See Full Prescribing Information for additional **WARNINGS and PRECAUTIONS.**

ADVERSE REACTIONS

Most common adverse reactions (incidence ≥5% and twice placebo): Adults: somnolence, dry mouth, dizziness, constipation, asthenia, abdominal pain, postural hypotension, pharyngitis, weight gain, lethargy, ALT increased, dyspepsia. (6.1)

Children and Adolescents: somnolence, dizziness, fatigue, increased appetite, nausea, vomiting, dry mouth, tachycardia, weight increased. (6.1)

To report SUSPECTED ADVERSE REACTIONS, contact AstraZeneca at 1-800-236-9933 or FDA at 1-800-FDA-1088 or www.fda.gov/medwatch.

DRUG INTERACTIONS

- **P450 3A Inhibitors:** May decrease the clearance of quetiapine. Lower doses of quetiapine may be required. (7.1)
- **Hepatic Enzyme Inducers:** May increase the clearance of quetiapine. Higher doses of quetiapine may be required with phenytoin or other inducers. (7.1)
- **Centrally Acting Drugs:** Caution should be used when quetiapine is used in combination with other CNS acting drugs. (7)
- **Antihypertensive Agents:** Quetiapine may add to the hypotensive effects of these agents. (7)
- **Levodopa and Dopamine Agents:** Quetiapine may antagonize the effect of these drugs. (7)
- **Drugs known to cause electrolyte imbalance or increase QT interval:** Caution should be used when quetiapine is used concomitantly with these drugs. (7)
- **Interference with Urine Drug Screens:** False positive urine drug screens for methadone or tricyclic antidepressants (TCAs) in patients taking quetiapine have been reported. (7)

USE IN SPECIFIC POPULATIONS

- **Geriatric Use:** Consider a lower starting dose (50 mg/day), slower titration, and careful monitoring during the initial dosing period. (8.5)
- **Hepatic Impairment:** Lower starting doses (25 mg/day) and slower titration may be needed. (2.3, 12.3)
- **Pregnancy and Nursing Mothers:** Quetiapine should be used only if the potential benefit justifies the potential risk. (8.1) Breastfeeding is not recommended. (8.3)
- **Pediatric Use:** Safety and effectiveness has only been established for schizophrenia in adolescent patients 13 to 17 years of age and in bipolar mania in children and adolescent patients 10 to 17 years of age. (8.4)

See 17 for **PATIENT COUNSELING INFORMATION and Medication Guide**

Revised: 05/2010

FULL PRESCRIBING INFORMATION: CONTENTS*
WARNING: INCREASED MORTALITY IN ELDERLY PATIENTS WITH DEMENTIA-RELATED PSYCHOSIS
SUICIDALITY AND ANTIDEPRESSANT DRUGS
RECENT MAJOR CHANGES

* Sections or subsections omitted from the full prescribing information are not listed

FULL PRESCRIBING INFORMATION

WARNING: INCREASED MORTALITY IN ELDERLY PATIENTS WITH DEMENTIA-RELATED PSYCHOSIS
Elderly patients with dementia-related psychosis treated with antipsychotic drugs are at an increased risk of death. Analyses of seventeen placebo-controlled trials (modal duration of 10 weeks) largely in patients taking atypical antipsychotic drugs, revealed a risk of death in drug-treated patients of between 1.6 to 1.7 times the risk of death in placebo-treated patients. Over the course of a typical 10-week controlled trial, the rate of death in drug-treated patients was about 4.5%, compared to a rate of about 2.6% in the placebo group. Although the causes of death were varied, most of the deaths appeared to be either cardiovascular (e.g., heart failure, sudden death) or infectious (e.g., pneumonia) in nature. Observational studies suggest that, similar to atypical antipsychotic drugs, treatment with conventional antipsychotic drugs may increase mortality. The extent to which the findings of increased mortality in observational studies may be attributed to the antipsychotic drug as opposed to some characteristic(s) of the patients is not clear. **SEROQUEL (quetiapine) is not approved for the treatment of patients with dementia-related psychosis** [*see Warnings and Precautions (5.1)*].

SUICIDALITY AND ANTIDEPRESSANT DRUGS
Antidepressants increased the risk compared to placebo of suicidal thinking and behavior (suicidality) in children, adolescents, and young adults in short-term studies of major depressive disorder (MDD) and other psychiatric disorders. Anyone considering the use of SEROQUEL or any other antidepressant in a child, adolescent, or young adult must balance this risk with the clinical need. Short-term studies did not show an increase in the risk of suicidality with antidepressants compared to placebo in adults beyond age 24; there was a reduction in risk with antidepressants compared to placebo in adults aged 65 and older. Depression and certain other psychiatric disorders are themselves associated with increases in the risk of suicide. Patients of all ages who are started on antidepressant therapy should be monitored appropriately and observed closely for clinical worsening, suicidality, or unusual changes in behavior. Families and caregivers should be advised of the need for close observation and communication with the prescriber. **SEROQUEL is not approved for use in patients under ten years of age** [*see Warnings and Precautions (5.2)*].

1   INDICATIONS AND USAGE

1.1   Schizophrenia

SEROQUEL is indicated for the treatment of schizophrenia. The efficacy of SEROQUEL in schizophrenia was established in three 6-week trials in adults and one 6-week trial in adolescents (13–17 years). The effectiveness of SEROQUEL for the maintenance treatment of schizophrenia has not been systematically evaluated in controlled clinical trials [see Clinical Studies (14.1)]

1.2   Bipolar Disorder

SEROQUEL is indicated for the acute treatment of manic episodes associated with bipolar I disorder, both as monotherapy and as an adjunct to lithium or divalproex. Efficacy was established in two 12-week monotherapy trials in adults, in one 3-week adjunctive trial in adults, and in one 3-week monotherapy trial in pediatric patients (10-17 years) [*see Clinical Studies (14.2)*].

SEROQUEL is indicated as monotherapy for the acute treatment of depressive episodes associated with bipolar disorder. Efficacy was established in two 8-week monotherapy trials in adult patients with bipolar I and bipolar II disorder [*see Clinical Studies (14.2)*].

SEROQUEL is indicated for the maintenance treatment of bipolar I disorder, as an adjunct to lithium or divalproex. Efficacy was established in two maintenance trials in adults. The effectiveness of SEROQUEL as monotherapy for the maintenance treatment of bipolar disorder has not been systematically evaluated in controlled clinical trials [*see Clinical Studies (14.2)*].

1.3   Special Considerations in Treating Pediatric Schizophrenia and Bipolar I Disorder

Pediatric schizophrenia and bipolar I disorder are serious mental disorders, however, diagnosis can be challenging. For pediatric schizophrenia, symptom profiles can be variable, and for bipolar I disorder, patients may have variable patterns of periodicity of manic or mixed symptoms. It is recommended that medication therapy for pediatric schizophrenia and bipolar I disorder be initiated only after a thorough diagnostic evaluation has been performed and careful consideration given to the risks associated with medication treatment. Medication treatment for both pediatric schizophrenia and bipolar I disorder is indicated as part of a total treatment program that often includes psychological, educational and social interventions.

2   DOSAGE AND ADMINISTRATION

SEROQUEL can be taken with or without food.

2.1   Schizophrenia

Adults

Dose Selection—SEROQUEL should generally be administered with an initial dose of 25 mg twice daily, with increases in total daily dose of 25 mg 50 mg divided in two or three doses on the second and third day, as tolerated, to a total dose range of 300 mg to 400 mg daily by the fourth day. Further dosage adjustments, if indicated, should generally occur at intervals of not less than 2 days, as steady-state for SEROQUEL would not be achieved for approximately 1-2 days in the typical patient. When dosage adjustments are necessary, dose increments/decrements of 25 mg 50 mg divided twice daily are recommended. Most efficacy data with SEROQUEL were obtained using three times daily dosing regimens, but in one controlled trial 225 mg given twice per day was also effective.

Efficacy in schizophrenia was demonstrated in a dose range of 150 mg/day to 750 mg/day in the clinical trials supporting the effectiveness of SEROQUEL. In a dose response study, doses above 300 mg/day were not demonstrated to be more efficacious than the 300 mg/day dose. In other studies, however, doses in the range of 400 mg/day 500 mg/day appeared to be needed. The safety of doses above 800 mg/day has not been evaluated in clinical trials.

Maintenance Treatment—The effectiveness of SEROQUEL for longer than 6 weeks has not been evaluated in controlled clinical trials. While there is no body of evidence available to answer the question of how long the patient treated with SEROQUEL should be maintained, it is generally recommended that responding patients be continued beyond the acute response, but at the lowest dose needed to maintain remission. Patients should be periodically reassessed to determine the need for maintenance treatment.

Adolescents (13-17 years)

Dose Selection—SEROQUEL should be administered twice daily. However, based on response and tolerability SEROQUEL may be administered three times daily where needed.

The total daily dose for the initial five days of therapy is 50 mg (Day 1), 100 mg (Day 2), 200 mg (Day 3), 300 mg (Day 4) and 400 mg (Day 5). After Day 5, the dose should be adjusted within the recommended dose range of 400 mg/day to 800 mg/day based on response and tolerability. Dosage adjustments should be in increments of no greater than 100 mg/day. Efficacy was demonstrated with SEROQUEL at both 400 mg and 800 mg; however, no additional benefit was seen in the 800 mg group.

Maintenance Treatment—The effectiveness of SEROQUEL for longer than 6 weeks has not been evaluated in controlled clinical trials. While there is no body of evidence available to answer the question of how long the patient treated with SEROQUEL should be maintained, it is generally recommended that responding patients be continued beyond the acute response, but at the lowest dose needed to maintain remission. Patients should be periodically reassessed to determine the need for maintenance treatment.

2.2   Bipolar Disorder

Adults

Acute Treatment of Manic Episodes in Bipolar I Disorder

Dose Selection—When used as monotherapy or adjunct therapy (with lithium or divalproex), SEROQUEL should be initiated in twice daily doses totaling 100 mg/day on Day 1, increased to 400 mg/day on Day 4 in increments of up to 100 mg/day in twice daily divided doses. Further dosage adjustments up to 800 mg/day by Day 6 should be in increments of no greater than 200 mg/day. Data indicate that the majority of patients responded between 400 mg/day to 800 mg/day. The safety of doses above 800 mg/day has not been evaluated in clinical trials.

Acute Treatment of Depressive Episodes in Bipolar Disorder

Dose Selection—SEROQUEL should be administered once daily at bedtime to reach 300 mg/day by Day 4.

Recommended Dosing Schedule

Day	Day 1	Day 2	Day 3	Day 4
SEROQUEL	50 mg	100 mg	200 mg	300 mg

In these clinical trials supporting effectiveness, the dosing schedule was 50 mg, 100 mg, 200 mg and 300 mg/day for Days 1-4 respectively. Patients receiving 600 mg increased to 400 mg on Day 5 and 600 mg on Day 8 (Week 1). Antidepressant efficacy was demonstrated with SEROQUEL at both 300 mg and 600 mg; however, no additional benefit was seen in the 600 mg group.

Maintenance Treatment of Bipolar I Disorder

Maintenance of efficacy in bipolar I disorder was demonstrated with SEROQUEL (administered twice daily totaling 400 to 800 mg per day) as adjunct therapy to lithium or divalproex. Generally, in the maintenance phase, patients continued on the same dose on which they were stabilized during the stabilization phase [see Clinical Studies (14.2)].

Children and Adolescents (10 to 17 years)

Acute Treatment of Manic Episodes in Bipolar I Disorder

Dose Selection—SEROQUEL should be administered twice daily. However, based on response and tolerability SEROQUEL may be administered three times daily where needed.

The total daily dose for the initial five days of therapy is 50 mg (Day 1), 100 mg (Day 2), 200 mg (Day 3), 300 mg (Day 4) and 400 mg (Day 5). After Day 5, the dose should be adjusted within the recommended dose range of 400 to 600 mg/day based on response and tolerability. Dosage adjustments should be in increments of no greater than 100 mg/day. Efficacy was demonstrated with SEROQUEL at both 400 mg and 600 mg; however, no additional benefit was seen in the 600 mg group.

Maintenance Treatment of Bipolar I Disorder

The effectiveness of SEROQUEL for longer than 3 weeks has not been evaluated in controlled clinical trials of children and adolescents. While there is no body of evidence available to answer the question of how long the patient

treated with SEROQUEL should be maintained, it is generally recommended that responding patients be continued beyond the acute response, but at the lowest dose needed to maintain remission. Patients should be periodically reassessed to determine the need for maintenance treatment.

2.3   Dosing in Special Populations

Consideration should be given to a slower rate of dose titration and a lower target dose in the elderly and in patients who are debilitated or who have a predisposition to hypotensive reactions [see Clinical Pharmacology (12)]. When indicated, dose escalation should be performed with caution in these patients.

Patients with hepatic impairment should be started on 25 mg/day. The dose should be increased daily in increments of 25 mg/day–50 mg/day to an effective dose, depending on the clinical response and tolerability of the patient.

2.4   Reinitiation of Treatment in Patients Previously Discontinued

Although there are no data to specifically address reinitiation of treatment, it is recommended that when restarting patients who have had an interval of less than one week off SEROQUEL, titration of SEROQUEL is not required and the maintenance dose may be reinitiated. When restarting therapy of patients who have been off SEROQUEL for more than one week, the initial titration schedule should be followed.

2.5   Switching from Antipsychotics

There are no systematically collected data to specifically address switching patients with schizophrenia from antipsychotics to SEROQUEL, or concerning concomitant administration with antipsychotics. While immediate discontinuation of the previous antipsychotic treatment may be acceptable for some patients with schizophrenia, more gradual discontinuation may be most appropriate for others. In all cases, the period of overlapping antipsychotic administration should be minimized. When switching patients with schizophrenia from depot antipsychotics, if medically appropriate, initiate SEROQUEL therapy in place of the next scheduled injection. The need for continuing existing EPS medication should be re-evaluated periodically.

3   DOSAGE FORMS AND STRENGTHS

25 mg tablets
50 mg tablets
100 mg tablets
200 mg tablets
300 mg tablets
400 mg tablets

4   CONTRAINDICATIONS

None known

5   WARNINGS AND PRECAUTIONS

5.1   Increased Mortality in Elderly Patients with Dementia-Related Psychosis

Elderly patients with dementia-related psychosis treated with antipsychotic drugs are at an increased risk of death. SEROQUEL (quetiapine fumarate) is not approved for the treatment of patients with dementia-related psychosis [see Boxed Warning].

5.2   Clinical Worsening and Suicide Risk

Patients with major depressive disorder (MDD), both adult and pediatric, may experience worsening of their depression and/or the emergence of suicidal ideation and behavior (suicidality) or unusual changes in behavior, whether or not they are taking antidepressant medications, and this risk may persist until significant remission occurs. Suicide is a known risk of depression and certain other psychiatric disorders, and these disorders themselves are the strongest predictors of suicide. There has been a long-standing concern, however, that antidepressants may have a role in inducing worsening of depression and the emergence of suicidality in certain patients during the early phases of treatment. Pooled analyses of short-term placebo-controlled trials of antidepressant drugs (SSRIs and others) showed that these drugs increase the risk of suicidal thinking and behavior (suicidality) in children, adolescents, and young adults (ages 18-24) with major depressive disorder (MDD) and other psychiatric disorders. Short-term studies did not show an increase in the risk of suicidality with antidepressants compared to placebo in adults beyond age 24; there was a reduction with antidepressants compared to placebo in adults aged 65 and older.

The pooled analyses of placebo-controlled trials in children and adolescents with MDD, obsessive compulsive disorder (OCD), or other psychiatric disorders included a total of 24 short-term trials of 9 antidepressant drugs in over 4400 patients. The pooled analyses of placebo-controlled trials in adults with MDD or other psychiatric disorders included a total of 295 short-term trials (median duration of 2 months) of 11 antidepressant drugs in over 77,000 patients. There was considerable variation in risk of suicidality among drugs, but a tendency toward an increase in the younger patients for almost all drugs studied. There were differences in absolute risk of suicidality across the different indica-

tions, with the highest incidence in MDD. The risk differences (drug vs. placebo), however, were relatively stable within age strata and across indications. These risk differences (drug-placebo difference in the number of cases of suicidality per 1000 patients treated) are provided in Table 1.

Table 1

Age Range	Drug-Placebo Difference in Number of Cases of Suicidality per 1000 Patients Treated
	Increases Compared to Placebo
<18	14 additional cases
18–24	5 additional cases
	Decreases Compared to Placebo
25–64	1 fewer case
≥65	6 fewer cases

No suicides occurred in any of the pediatric trials. There were suicides in the adult trials, but the number was not sufficient to reach any conclusion about drug effect on suicide.

It is unknown whether the suicidality risk extends to longer-term use, i.e., beyond several months. However, there is substantial evidence from placebo-controlled maintenance trials in adults with depression that the use of antidepressants can delay the recurrence of depression.

All patients being treated with antidepressants for any indication should be monitored appropriately and observed closely for clinical worsening, suicidality, and unusual changes in behavior, especially during the initial few months of a course of drug therapy, or at times of dose changes, either increases or decreases.

The following symptoms, anxiety, agitation, panic attacks, insomnia, irritability, hostility, aggressiveness, impulsivity, akathisia (psychomotor restlessness), hypomania, and mania, have been reported in adult and pediatric patients being treated with antidepressants for major depressive disorder as well as for other indications, both psychiatric and nonpsychiatric. Although a causal link between the emergence of such symptoms and either the worsening of depression and/or the emergence of suicidal impulses has not been established, there is concern that such symptoms may represent precursors to emerging suicidality.

Consideration should be given to changing the therapeutic regimen, including possibly discontinuing the medication, in patients whose depression is persistently worse, or who are experiencing emergent suicidality or symptoms that might be precursors to worsening depression or suicidality, especially if these symptoms are severe, abrupt in onset, or were not part of the patient's presenting symptoms.

Families and caregivers of patients being treated with antidepressants for major depressive disorder or other indications, both psychiatric and nonpsychiatric, should be alerted about the need to monitor patients for the emergence of agitation, irritability, unusual changes in behavior, and the other symptoms described above, as well as the emergence of suicidality, and to report such symptoms immediately to healthcare providers. Such monitoring should include daily observation by families and caregivers. Prescriptions for SEROQUEL should be written for the smallest quantity of tablets consistent with good patient management, in order to reduce the risk of overdose.

Screening Patients for Bipolar Disorder: A major depressive episode may be the initial presentation of bipolar disorder. It is generally believed (though not established in controlled trials) that treating such an episode with an antidepressant alone may increase the likelihood of precipitation of a mixed/manic episode in patients at risk for bipolar disorder. Whether any of the symptoms described above represent such a conversion is unknown. However, prior to initiating treatment with an antidepressant, patients with depressive symptoms should be adequately screened to determine if they are at risk for bipolar disorder; such screening should include a detailed psychiatric history, including a family history of suicide, bipolar disorder, and depression. It should be noted that SEROQUEL is approved for use in treating adult bipolar depression.

5.3   Neuroleptic Malignant Syndrome (NMS)

A potentially fatal symptom complex sometimes referred to as Neuroleptic Malignant Syndrome (NMS) has been reported in association with administration of antipsychotic drugs, including SEROQUEL. Rare cases of NMS have been reported with SEROQUEL. Clinical manifestations of NMS are hyperpyrexia, muscle rigidity, altered mental status, and evidence of autonomic instability (irregular pulse or blood pressure, tachycardia, diaphoresis, and cardiac dysrhythmia). Additional signs may include elevated creatine phosphokinase, myoglobinuria (rhabdomyolysis) and acute renal failure.

The diagnostic evaluation of patients with this syndrome is complicated. In arriving at a diagnosis, it is important to exclude cases where the clinical presentation includes both

Table 2: Fasting Glucose—Proportion of Patients Shifting to ≥ 126 mg/dL in Short-Term (≤ 12 weeks) Placebo-Controlled Studies

Laboratory Analyte	Category Change (At Least Once) from Baseline	Treatment Arm	N	Patients n (%)
Fasting Glucose	Normal to High (<100 mg/dL to ≥ 126 mg/dL)	Quetiapine	2907	71 (2.4%)
		Placebo	1346	19 (1.4%)
	Borderline to High (≥ 100 mg/dL and < 126 mg/dL to ≥ 126 mg/dL)	Quetiapine	572	67 (11.7%)
		Placebo	279	33 (11.8%)

Table 3: Percentage of Adult Patients with Shifts in Total Cholesterol, Triglycerides, LDL-Cholesterol and HDL-Cholesterol from Baseline to Clinically Significant Levels by Indication

Laboratory Analyte	Indication	Treatment Arm	N	Patients n (%)
Total Cholesterol ≥ 240 mg/dL	Schizophrenia*	SEROQUEL	137	24 (18%)
		Placebo	92	6 (7%)
	Bipolar Depression†	SEROQUEL	463	41 (9%)
		Placebo	250	15 (6%)
Triglycerides ≥200 mg/dL	Schizophrenia*	SEROQUEL	120	26 (22%)
		Placebo	70	11 (16%)
	Bipolar Depression†	SEROQUEL	436	59 (14%)
		Placebo	232	20 (9%)
LDL-Cholesterol ≥ 160 mg/dL	Schizophrenia*	SEROQUEL	na‡	na‡
		Placebo	na‡	na‡
	Bipolar Depression†	SEROQUEL	465	29 (6%)
		Placebo	256	12 (5%)
HDL-Cholesterol ≤ 40 mg/dL	Schizophrenia*	SEROQUEL	na‡	na‡
		Placebo	na‡	na‡
	Bipolar Depression†	SEROQUEL	393	56 (14%)
		Placebo	214	29 (14%)

* 6 weeks duration
† 8 weeks duration
‡ Parameters not measured in the SEROQUEL registration studies for schizophrenia. Lipid parameters also were not measured in the bipolar mania registration studies.

Table 4: Percentage of Children and Adolescents with Shifts in Total Cholesterol, Triglycerides, LDL-Cholesterol and HDL-Cholesterol from Baseline to Clinically Significant Levels

Laboratory Analyte	Indication	Treatment Arm	N	Patients n (%)
Total Cholesterol ≥ 200 mg/dL	Schizophrenia*	SEROQUEL	107	13 (12%)
		Placebo	56	1 (2%)
	Bipolar Mania†	SEROQUEL	159	16 (10%)
		Placebo	66	2 (3%)
Triglycerides ≥150 mg/dL	Schizophrenia*	SEROQUEL	103	17 (17%)
		Placebo	51	4 (8%)
	Bipolar Mania†	SEROQUEL	149	32 (22%)
		Placebo	60	8 (13%)
LDL-Cholesterol ≥ 130 mg/dL	Schizophrenia*	SEROQUEL	112	4 (4%)
		Placebo	60	1 (2%)
	Bipolar Mania†	SEROQUEL	169	13 (8%)
		Placebo	74	4 (5%)
HDL-Cholesterol ≤ 40 mg/dL	Schizophrenia*	SEROQUEL	104	16 (15%)
		Placebo	54	10 (19%)
	Bipolar Mania†	SEROQUEL	154	16 (10%)
		Placebo	61	4 (7%)

* 13-17 years, 6 weeks duration
† 10-17 years, 3 weeks duration

serious medical illness (e.g., pneumonia, systemic infection, etc.) and untreated or inadequately treated extrapyramidal signs and symptoms (EPS). Other important considerations in the differential diagnosis include central anticholinergic toxicity, heat stroke, drug fever and primary central nervous system (CNS) pathology.

The management of NMS should include: 1) immediate discontinuation of antipsychotic drugs and other drugs not essential to concurrent therapy; 2) intensive symptomatic treatment and medical monitoring; and 3) treatment of any concomitant serious medical problems for which specific treatments are available. There is no general agreement about specific pharmacological treatment regimens for NMS.

If a patient requires antipsychotic drug treatment after recovery from NMS, the potential reintroduction of drug therapy should be carefully considered. The patient should be carefully monitored since recurrences of NMS have been reported.

5.4 Hyperglycemia and Diabetes Mellitus
Hyperglycemia, in some cases extreme and associated with ketoacidosis or hyperosmolar coma or death, has been reported in patients treated with atypical antipsychotics, including quetiapine. Assessment of the relationship between atypical antipsychotic use and glucose abnormalities is complicated by the possibility of an increased background risk of diabetes mellitus in patients with schizophrenia and the increasing incidence of diabetes mellitus in the general population. Given these confounders, the relationship between atypical antipsychotic use and hyperglycemia-related adverse reactions is not completely understood. However, epidemiological studies suggest an increased risk of treatment-emergent hyperglycemia-related adverse reactions in patients treated with the atypical antipsychotics. Precise risk estimates for hyperglycemia-related adverse reactions in patients treated with atypical antipsychotics are not available.

Patients with an established diagnosis of diabetes mellitus who are started on atypical antipsychotics should be monitored regularly for worsening of glucose control. Patients with risk factors for diabetes mellitus (e.g., obesity, family history of diabetes) who are starting treatment with atypical antipsychotics should undergo fasting blood glucose testing at the beginning of treatment and periodically during treatment.

Any patient treated with atypical antipsychotics should be monitored for symptoms of hyperglycemia including polydipsia, polyuria, polyphagia, and weakness. Patients who develop symptoms of hyperglycemia during treatment with atypical antipsychotics should undergo fasting blood glucose testing. In some cases, hyperglycemia has resolved when the atypical antipsychotic was discontinued; however, some patients required continuation of anti-diabetic treatment despite discontinuation of the suspect drug.

Adults:
[See table 2 at left]
In a 24-week trial (active-controlled, 115 patients treated with SEROQUEL) designed to evaluate glycemic status with oral glucose tolerance testing of all patients, at week 24 the incidence of a treatment-emergent post-glucose challenge glucose level ≥ 200 mg/dL was 1.7% and the incidence of a fasting treatment-emergent blood glucose level ≥ 126 mg/dL was 2.6%. The mean change in fasting glucose from baseline was 3.2 mg/dL and mean change in 2 hour glucose from baseline was -1.8 mg/dL for quetiapine.

In 2 long-term placebo-controlled randomized withdrawal clinical trials for bipolar maintenance, mean exposure of 213 days for SEROQUEL (646 patients) and 152 days for placebo (680 patients), the mean change in glucose from baseline was +5.0 mg/dL for SEROQUEL and –0.05 mg/dL for placebo. The exposure-adjusted rate of any increased blood glucose level (≥ 126 mg/dL) for patients more than 8 hours since a meal (however, some patients may not have been precluded from calorie intake from fluids during fasting period) was 18.0 per 100 patient years for SEROQUEL (10.7% of patients; n=556) and 9.5 for placebo per 100 patient years (4.6% of patients; n=581).

Children and Adolescents: In a placebo-controlled SEROQUEL monotherapy study of adolescent patients (13–17 years of age) with schizophrenia (6 weeks duration), the mean change in fasting glucose levels for SEROQUEL (n=138) compared to placebo (n=67) was –0.75 mg/dL versus –1.70 mg/dL. In a placebo-controlled SEROQUEL monotherapy study of children and adolescent patients (10–17 years of age) with bipolar mania (3 weeks duration), the mean change in fasting glucose level for SEROQUEL (n=170) compared to placebo (n=81) was 3.62 mg/dL versus –1.17 mg/dL. No patient in either study with a baseline normal fasting glucose level (<100 mg/dL) or a baseline borderline fasting glucose level (≥100 mg/dL and <126 mg/dL) had a treatment-emergent blood glucose level of ≥126 mg/dL.

5.5 Hyperlipidemia
Adults: Undesirable alterations in lipids have been observed with quetiapine use. Clinical monitoring, including baseline and periodic follow-up lipid evaluations in patients using quetiapine is recommended.

Table 3 shows the percentage of adult patients with changes in total cholesterol, triglycerides, LDL-cholesterol and HDL-cholesterol from baseline by indication in clinical trials with SEROQUEL.
[See table 3 at left]

Children and Adolescents: Table 4 shows the percentage of children and adolescents with changes in total cholesterol, triglycerides, LDL-cholesterol and HDL-cholesterol from baseline in clinical trials with SEROQUEL.
[See table 4 at left]

5.6 Weight Gain
Increases in weight have been observed in clinical trials. Patients receiving quetiapine should receive regular monitoring of weight [see Patient Counseling Information (17)].
Adults: In clinical trials with SEROQUEL the following increases in weight have been reported.
[See table 5 at top of next page]
Children and Adolescents: In two clinical trials with SEROQUEL, one in bipolar mania and one in schizophrenia, reported increases in weight are included in the table below.
[See table 6 at top of next page]
The mean change in body weight in the schizophrenia trial was 2.0 kg in the SEROQUEL group and -0.4 kg in the placebo group and in the bipolar mania trial it was 1.7 kg in the SEROQUEL group and 0.4 kg in the placebo group.

In an open-label study that enrolled patients from the above two pediatric trials, 63% of patients (241/380) completed 26 weeks of therapy with SEROQUEL. After 26 weeks of treatment, the mean increase in body weight was 4.4 kg. Forty-five percent of the patients gained ≥ 7% of their body weight, not adjusted for normal growth. In order to adjust for normal growth over 26 weeks an increase of at least 0.5 standard deviation from baseline in BMI was used as a measure of a clinically significant change; 18.3% of patients on SEROQUEL met this criterion after 26 weeks of treatment.

When treating pediatric patients with SEROQUEL for any indication, weight gain should be assessed against that expected for normal growth.

5.7 Tardive Dyskinesia
A syndrome of potentially irreversible, involuntary, dyskinetic movements may develop in patients treated with antipsychotic drugs, including quetiapine. Although the prevalence of the syndrome appears to be highest among the

elderly, especially elderly women, it is impossible to rely upon prevalence estimates to predict, at the inception of antipsychotic treatment, which patients are likely to develop the syndrome. Whether antipsychotic drug products differ in their potential to cause tardive dyskinesia is unknown.

The risk of developing tardive dyskinesia and the likelihood that it will become irreversible are believed to increase as the duration of treatment and the total cumulative dose of antipsychotic drugs administered to the patient increase. However, the syndrome can develop, although much less commonly, after relatively brief treatment periods at low doses or may even arise after discontinuation of treatment.

There is no known treatment for established cases of tardive dyskinesia, although the syndrome may remit, partially or completely, if antipsychotic treatment is withdrawn. Antipsychotic treatment, itself, however, may suppress (or partially suppress) the signs and symptoms of the syndrome and thereby may possibly mask the underlying process. The effect that symptomatic suppression has upon the long-term course of the syndrome is unknown.

Given these considerations, SEROQUEL should be prescribed in a manner that is most likely to minimize the occurrence of tardive dyskinesia. Chronic antipsychotic treatment should generally be reserved for patients who appear to suffer from a chronic illness that (1) is known to respond to antipsychotic drugs, and (2) for whom alternative, equally effective, but potentially less harmful treatments are not available or appropriate. In patients who do require chronic treatment, the smallest dose and the shortest duration of treatment producing a satisfactory clinical response should be sought. The need for continued treatment should be reassessed periodically.

If signs and symptoms of tardive dyskinesia appear in a patient on SEROQUEL, drug discontinuation should be considered. However, some patients may require treatment with SEROQUEL despite the presence of the syndrome.

5.8 Orthostatic Hypotension

Quetiapine may induce orthostatic hypotension associated with dizziness, tachycardia and, in some patients, syncope, especially during the initial dose-titration period, probably reflecting its α1-adrenergic antagonist properties. Syncope was reported in 1% (28/3265) of the patients treated with SEROQUEL, compared with 0.2% (2/954) on placebo and about 0.4% (2/527) on active control drugs. Orthostatic hypotension, dizziness, and syncope may lead to falls.

SEROQUEL should be used with particular caution in patients with known cardiovascular disease (history of myocardial infarction or ischemic heart disease, heart failure or conduction abnormalities), cerebrovascular disease or conditions which would predispose patients to hypotension (dehydration, hypovolemia and treatment with antihypertensive medications) [*see Adverse Reactions* (6.2)]. The risk of orthostatic hypotension and syncope may be minimized by limiting the initial dose to 25 mg twice daily [*see Dosage and Administration* (2)]. If hypotension occurs during titration to the target dose, a return to the previous dose in the titration schedule is appropriate.

5.9 Increases in Blood Pressure in Children and Adolescents

In placebo-controlled trials in children and adolescents with schizophrenia (6-week duration) or bipolar mania (3-week duration), the incidence of increases at any time in systolic blood pressure (≥20 mmHg) was 15.2% (51/335) for SEROQUEL and 5.5% (9/163) for placebo; the incidence of increases at any time in diastolic blood pressure (≥10 mmHg) was 40.6% (136/335) for SEROQUEL and 24.5% (40/163) for placebo. In the 26-week open-label clinical trial, one child with a reported history of hypertension experienced a hypertensive crisis. Blood pressure in children and adolescents should be measured at the beginning of, and periodically during treatment.

5.10 Leukopenia, Neutropenia and Agranulocytosis

In clinical trial and postmarketing experience, events of leukopenia/neutropenia have been reported temporally related to atypical antipsychotic agents, including SEROQUEL. Agranulocytosis (including fatal cases) has also been reported.

Possible risk factors for leukopenia/neutropenia include pre-existing low white cell count (WBC) and history of drug induced leukopenia/neutropenia. Patients with a pre-existing low WBC or a history of drug induced leukopenia/neutropenia should have their complete blood count (CBC) monitored frequently during the first few months of therapy and should discontinue SEROQUEL at the first sign of a decline in WBC in absence of other causative factors.

Patients with neutropenia should be carefully monitored for fever or other symptoms or signs of infection and treated promptly if such symptoms or signs occur. Patients with severe neutropenia (absolute neutrophil count <1000/mm^3) should discontinue SEROQUEL and have their WBC followed until recovery [*see Adverse Reactions* (6.2)].

5.11 Cataracts

The development of cataracts was observed in association with quetiapine treatment in chronic dog studies [*see Nonclinical Toxicology, Animal Toxicology* (13.2)]. Lens changes have also been observed in adults, children and adolescents during long-term SEROQUEL treatment, but a causal relationship to SEROQUEL use has not been established. Nevertheless, the possibility of lenticular changes cannot be excluded at this time. Therefore, examination of the lens by methods adequate to detect cataract formation, such as slit lamp exam or other appropriately sensitive methods, is recommended at initiation of treatment or shortly thereafter, and at 6-month intervals during chronic treatment.

Table 5: Proportion of Patients with Weight Gain ≥7% of Body Weight (Adults)

Vital Sign	Indication	Treatment Arm	N	Patients n (%)
Weight Gain ≥7% of Body Weight	Schizophrenia*	SEROQUEL	391	89 (23%)
		Placebo	206	11 (6%)
	Bipolar Mania (monotherapy)†	SEROQUEL	209	44 (21%)
		Placebo	198	13 (7%)
	Bipolar Mania (adjunct therapy)‡	SEROQUEL	196	25 (13%)
		Placebo	203	8 (4%)
	Bipolar Depression§	SEROQUEL	554	47 (8%)
		Placebo	295	7 (2%)

* up to 6 weeks duration
† up to 12 weeks duration
‡ up to 3 weeks duration
§ up to 8 weeks duration

Table 6: Proportion of Patients with Weight Gain ≥7% of Body Weight (Children and Adolescents)

Vital Sign	Indication	Treatment Arm	N	Patients n (%)
Weight Gain ≥7% of Body Weight	Schizophrenia*	SEROQUEL	111	23 (21%)
		Placebo	44	3 (7%)
	Bipolar Mania†	SEROQUEL	157	18 (12%)
		Placebo	68	0 (0%)

*: 6 weeks duration
†: 3 weeks duration

5.12 Seizures

During clinical trials, seizures occurred in 0.5% (20/3490) of patients treated with SEROQUEL compared to 0.2% (2/954) on placebo and 0.7% (4/527) on active control drugs. As with other antipsychotics, SEROQUEL should be used cautiously in patients with a history of seizures or with conditions that potentially lower the seizure threshold, e.g., Alzheimer's dementia. Conditions that lower the seizure threshold may be more prevalent in a population of 65 years or older.

5.13 Hypothyroidism

Adults: Clinical trials with SEROQUEL demonstrated a dose-related decrease in total and free thyroxine (T4) of approximately 20% at the higher end of the therapeutic dose range and was maximal in the first two to four weeks of treatment and maintained without adaptation or progression during more chronic therapy. Generally, these changes were of no clinical significance and thyroid stimulating hormone (TSH) was unchanged in most patients and levels of thyroid binding globulin (TBG) were unchanged. In nearly all cases, cessation of SEROQUEL treatment was associated with a reversal of the effects on total and free T4, irrespective of the duration of treatment. About 0.7% (26/3489) of SEROQUEL patients did experience TSH increases in monotherapy studies. Six of the patients with TSH increases needed replacement thyroid treatment. In the mania adjunct studies, where SEROQUEL was added to lithium or divalproex, 12% (24/196) of SEROQUEL treated patients compared to 7% (15/203) of placebo-treated patients had elevated TSH levels. Of the SEROQUEL treated patients with elevated TSH levels, 3 had simultaneous low free T4 levels.

Children and Adolescents: In acute placebo-controlled trials in children and adolescent patients with schizophrenia (6-week duration) or bipolar mania (3-week duration), the incidence of shifts to potentially clinically important thyroid function values at any time for SEROQUEL treated patients and placebo-treated patients for elevated TSH was 2.9% (8/280) vs. 0.7% (1/138), respectively and for decreased total thyroxine was 2.8% (8/289) vs. 0% (0/145, respectively). Of the SEROQUEL treated patients with elevated TSH levels, 1 had simultaneous low free T4 level at end of treatment.

5.14 Hyperprolactinemia

Adults: During clinical trials with quetiapine, the incidence of shifts in prolactin levels to a clinically significant value occurred in 3.6% (158/4416) of patients treated with quetiapine compared to 2.6% (51/1968) on placebo.

Children and Adolescents: In acute placebo-controlled trials in children and adolescent patients with bipolar mania (3-week duration) or schizophrenia (6-week duration), the incidence of shifts in prolactin levels to a clinically significant value (>20 μg/L males; > 26 μg/L females at any time) was 13.4% (18/134) for SEROQUEL compared to 4% (3/75) for placebo in males and 8.7% (9/104) for SEROQUEL compared to 0% (0/39) for placebo in females.

Like other drugs that antagonize dopamine D2 receptors, SEROQUEL elevates prolactin levels in some patients and the elevation may persist during chronic administration. Hyperprolactinemia, regardless of etiology, may suppress hypothalamic GnRH, resulting in reduced pituitary gonadotrophin secretion. This, in turn, may inhibit reproductive function by impairing gonadal steroidogenesis in both female and male patients. Galactorrhea, amenorrhea, gynecomastia, and impotence have been reported in patients receiving prolactin-elevating compounds. Long-standing hyperprolactinemia when associated with hypogonadism may lead to decreased bone density in both female and male subjects.

Tissue culture experiments indicate that approximately one-third of human breast cancers are prolactin dependent *in vitro*, a factor of potential importance if the prescription of these drugs is considered in a patient with previously detected breast cancer. As is common with compounds which increase prolactin release, mammary gland and pancreatic islet cell neoplasia (mammary adenocarcinomas, pituitary and pancreatic adenomas) was observed in carcinogenicity studies conducted in mice and rats. Neither clinical studies nor epidemiologic studies conducted to date have shown an association between chronic administration of this class of drugs and tumorigenesis in humans, but the available evidence is too limited to be conclusive [*see Carcinogenesis, Mutagenesis, Impairment of Fertility* (13.1)].

5.15 Transaminase Elevations

Asymptomatic, transient and reversible elevations in serum transaminases (primarily ALT) have been reported. In schizophrenia trials in adults, the proportions of patients with transaminase elevations of > 3 times the upper limits of the normal reference range in a pool of 3- to 6-week placebo-controlled trials were approximately 6% (29/483) for SEROQUEL compared to 1% (3/194)for placebo. In acute bipolar mania trials in adults, the proportions of patients with transaminase elevations of > 3 times the upper limits of the normal reference range in a pool of 3- to 12-week placebo-controlled trials were approximately 1% for both SEROQUEL (3/560) and placebo (3/294). These hepatic enzyme elevations usually occurred within the first 3 weeks of drug treatment and promptly returned to pre-study levels with ongoing treatment with SEROQUEL. In bipolar depression trials, the proportions of patients with transaminase elevations of > 3 times the upper limits of the normal reference range in two 8-week placebo-controlled trials was 1% (5/698) for SEROQUEL and 2% (6/347) for placebo.

5.16 Potential for Cognitive and Motor Impairment

Somnolence was a commonly reported adverse event reported in patients treated with SEROQUEL especially during the 3-5 day period of initial dose-titration. In schizophrenia trials, somnolence was reported in 18% (89/510) of patients on SEROQUEL compared to 11% (22/206) of placebo patients. In acute bipolar mania trials using SEROQUEL as monotherapy, somnolence was reported in 16% (34/209) of patients on SEROQUEL compared to 4% of placebo patients. In acute bipolar mania trials using SEROQUEL as adjunct therapy, somnolence was reported in 34% (66/196) of patients on SEROQUEL compared to 9% (19/203) of placebo patients. In bipolar depression trials, somnolence was reported in 57% (398/698) of patients on SEROQUEL compared to 15% (51/347) of placebo patients. Since SEROQUEL has the potential to impair judgment, thinking, or motor skills, patients should be cautioned about performing activities requiring mental alertness, such as operating a motor vehicle (including automobiles) or operating hazardous machinery until they are reasonably certain that SEROQUEL therapy does not affect them adversely. Somnolence may lead to falls.

5.17 Priapism
One case of priapism in a patient receiving SEROQUEL has been reported prior to market introduction. While a causal relationship to use of SEROQUEL has not been established, other drugs with alpha-adrenergic blocking effects have been reported to induce priapism, and it is possible that SEROQUEL may share this capacity. Severe priapism may require surgical intervention.

5.18 Body Temperature Regulation
Although not reported with SEROQUEL, disruption of the body's ability to reduce core body temperature has been attributed to antipsychotic agents. Appropriate care is advised when prescribing SEROQUEL for patients who will be experiencing conditions which may contribute to an elevation in core body temperature, e.g., exercising strenuously, exposure to extreme heat, receiving concomitant medication with anticholinergic activity, or being subject to dehydration.

5.19 Dysphagia
Esophageal dysmotility and aspiration have been associated with antipsychotic drug use. Aspiration pneumonia is a common cause of morbidity and mortality in elderly patients, in particular those with advanced Alzheimer's dementia. SEROQUEL and other antipsychotic drugs should be used cautiously in patients at risk for aspiration pneumonia.

5.20 Suicide
The possibility of a suicide attempt is inherent in bipolar disorder and schizophrenia; close supervision of high risk patients should accompany drug therapy. Prescriptions for SEROQUEL should be written for the smallest quantity of tablets consistent with good patient management in order to reduce the risk of overdose.

In two 8-week clinical studies in patients with bipolar depression (N=1048), the incidence of treatment-emergent suicidal ideation or suicide attempt was low and similar to placebo (SEROQUEL 300 mg, 6/350, 1.7%; SEROQUEL 600 mg, 9/348, 2.6%; Placebo, 7/347, 2.0%).

5.21 Use in Patients with Concomitant Illness
Clinical experience with SEROQUEL in patients with certain concomitant systemic illnesses is limited [see *Pharmacokinetics* (12.3)].

SEROQUEL has not been evaluated or used to any appreciable extent in patients with a recent history of myocardial infarction or unstable heart disease. Patients with these diagnoses were excluded from premarketing clinical studies. Because of the risk of orthostatic hypotension with SEROQUEL, caution should be observed in cardiac patients [see *Warnings and Precautions* (5.8)].

In clinical trials quetiapine was not associated with a persistent increase in absolute QT intervals. However, in post marketing experience there were cases reported of QT prolongation in patients who overdosed on quetiapine [see *Overdosage* (10.1)], in patients with concomitant illness, and in patients taking medicines known to cause electrolyte imbalance or increase QT interval [see *Drug Interactions* (7)]. Caution should be exercised when quetiapine is prescribed in patients with cardiovascular disease or family history of QT prolongation. Also caution should be exercised when quetiapine is prescribed with medicines known to cause electrolyte imbalance or increase QT interval or with concomitant neuroleptics, especially for patients with increased risk of QT prolongation, i.e., the elderly, patients with congenital long QT syndrome, congestive heart failure, heart hypertrophy, hypokalemia, or hypomagnesemia.

5.22 Withdrawal
Acute withdrawal symptoms, such as insomnia, nausea, and vomiting, have been described after abrupt cessation of atypical antipsychotic drugs, including SEROQUEL. In short-term placebo-controlled, monotherapy clinical trials with SEROQUEL XR that included a discontinuation phase which evaluated discontinuation symptoms, the aggregated incidence of patients experiencing one or more discontinuation symptoms after abrupt cessation was 12.1% (241/1993) for SEROQUEL XR and 6.7% (71/1065) for placebo. The incidence of the individual adverse events (i.e., insomnia, nausea, headache, diarrhea, vomiting, dizziness and irritability) did not exceed 5.3% in any treatment group and usually resolved after 1 week post-discontinuation. Gradual withdrawal is advised.

6 ADVERSE REACTIONS
6.1 Clinical Study Experience
Adults
Because clinical studies are conducted under widely varying conditions, adverse reaction rates observed in the clinical studies of a drug cannot be directly compared to rates in the clinical studies of another drug and may not reflect the rates observed in practice.

The information below is derived from a clinical trial database for SEROQUEL consisting of over 4300 patients. This database includes 698 patients exposed to SEROQUEL for the treatment of bipolar depression, 405 patients exposed to SEROQUEL for the treatment of acute bipolar mania (monotherapy and adjunct therapy), 646 patients exposed to SEROQUEL for the maintenance treatment of bipolar I disorder as adjunct therapy, and approximately 2600 patients and/or normal subjects exposed to 1 or more doses of SEROQUEL for the treatment of schizophrenia.

Of these approximately 4300 subjects, approximately 4000 (2300 in schizophrenia, 405 in acute bipolar mania, 698 in bipolar depression, and 646 for the maintenance treatment of bipolar I disorder) were patients who participated in multiple dose effectiveness trials, and their experience corresponded to approximately 2400 patient-years. The conditions and duration of treatment with SEROQUEL varied greatly and included (in overlapping categories) open-label and double-blind phases of studies, inpatients and outpatients, fixed-dose and dose-titration studies, and short-term or longer-term exposure. Adverse reactions were assessed by collecting adverse events, results of physical examinations, vital signs, weights, laboratory analyses, ECGs, and results of ophthalmologic examinations.

Adverse reactions during exposure were obtained by general inquiry and recorded by clinical investigators using terminology of their own choosing. Consequently, it is not possible to provide a meaningful estimate of the proportion of individuals experiencing adverse reactions without first grouping similar types of reactions into a smaller number of standardized reaction categories.

In the tables and tabulations that follow, standard COSTART terminology has been used to classify reported adverse reactions for schizophrenia and bipolar mania. MedDRA terminology has been used to classify reported adverse reactions for bipolar depression.

The stated frequencies of adverse reactions represent the proportion of individuals who experienced, at least once, a treatment-emergent adverse reaction of the type listed. A reaction was considered treatment emergent if it occurred for the first time or worsened while receiving therapy following baseline evaluation.

Incidence of Adverse Reactions in Short-Term, Placebo-Controlled Trials in Adults
Adverse Reactions Associated with Discontinuation of Treatment in Short-Term, Placebo-Controlled Trials:
Schizophrenia: Overall, there was little difference in the incidence of discontinuation due to adverse reactions (4% for SEROQUEL vs. 3% for placebo) in a pool of controlled trials. However, discontinuations due to somnolence (0.8% SEROQUEL vs. 0% placebo) and hypotension (0.4% SEROQUEL vs. 0% placebo) were considered to be drug related [see *Warnings and Precautions* (5.8 and 5.16)].
Bipolar Disorder:
Mania: Overall, discontinuations due to adverse reactions were 5.7% for SEROQUEL vs. 5.1% for placebo in monotherapy and 3.6% for SEROQUEL vs. 5.9% for placebo in adjunct therapy.
Depression: Overall, discontinuations due to adverse reactions were 12.3% for SEROQUEL 300 mg vs. 19.0% for SEROQUEL 600 mg and 5.2% for placebo.
Commonly Observed Adverse Reactions in Short-Term, Placebo-Controlled Trials:
In the acute therapy of schizophrenia (up to 6 weeks) and bipolar mania (up to 12 weeks) trials, the most commonly observed adverse reactions associated with the use of SEROQUEL monotherapy (incidence of 5% or greater) and observed at a rate on SEROQUEL at least twice that of placebo were somnolence (18%), dizziness (11%), dry mouth (9%), constipation (8%), ALT increased (5%), weight gain (5%), and dyspepsia (5%).
Adverse Reactions Occurring at an Incidence of 1% or More Among SEROQUEL Treated Patients in Short-Term, Placebo-Controlled Trials:
The prescriber should be aware that the figures in the tables and tabulations cannot be used to predict the incidence of side effects in the course of usual medical practice where patient characteristics and other factors differ from those that prevailed in the clinical trials. Similarly, the cited frequencies cannot be compared with figures obtained from other clinical investigations involving different treatments, uses, and investigators. The cited figures, however, do provide the prescribing physician with some basis for estimating the relative contribution of drug and nondrug factors to the side effect incidence in the population studied.

Table 7 enumerates the incidence, rounded to the nearest percent, of treatment-emergent adverse reactions that occurred during acute therapy of schizophrenia (up to 6 weeks) and bipolar mania (up to 12 weeks) in 1% or more of patients treated with SEROQUEL (doses ranging from 75 to 800 mg/day) where the incidence in patients treated with SEROQUEL was greater than the incidence in placebo-treated patients.

Table 7: Treatment-Emergent Adverse Reaction Incidence in 3- to 12-Week Placebo-Controlled Clinical Trials for the Treatment of Schizophrenia and Bipolar Mania (Monotherapy)*

Body System/ Preferred Term	SEROQUEL (n=719)	PLACEBO (n=404)
Body as a Whole		
Headache	21%	14%
Pain	7%	5%
Asthenia	5%	3%
Abdominal Pain	4%	1%
Back Pain	3%	1%
Fever	2%	1%
Cardiovascular		
Tachycardia	6%	4%
Postural Hypotension	4%	1%
Digestive		
Dry Mouth	9%	3%
Constipation	8%	3%
Vomiting	6%	5%
Dyspepsia	5%	1%
Gastroenteritis	2%	0%
Gamma Glutamyl Transpeptidase Increased	1%	0%
Metabolic and Nutritional		
Weight Gain	5%	1%
ALT Increased	5%	1%
AST Increased	3%	1%
Nervous		
Agitation	20%	17%
Somnolence	18%	8%
Dizziness	11%	5%
Anxiety	4%	3%
Respiratory		
Pharyngitis	4%	3%
Rhinitis	3%	1%
Skin and Appendages		
Rash	4%	2%
Special Senses		
Amblyopia	2%	1%

* Reactions for which the SEROQUEL incidence was equal to or less than placebo are not listed in the table, but included the following: accidental injury, akathisia, chest pain, cough increased, depression, diarrhea, extrapyramidal syndrome, hostility, hypertension, hypertonia, hypotension, increased appetite, infection, insomnia, leukopenia, malaise, nausea, nervousness, paresthesia, peripheral edema, sweating, tremor, and weight loss.

In the acute adjunct therapy of bipolar mania (up to 3 weeks) studies, the most commonly observed adverse reactions associated with the use of SEROQUEL (incidence of 5% or greater) and observed at a rate on SEROQUEL at least twice that of placebo were somnolence (34%), dry mouth (19%), asthenia (10%), constipation (10%), abdominal pain (7%), postural hypotension (7%), pharyngitis (6%), and weight gain (6%).
Table 8 enumerates the incidence, rounded to the nearest percent, of treatment-emergent adverse reactions that occurred during therapy (up to 3 weeks) of acute mania in 1% or more of patients treated with SEROQUEL (doses ranging from 100 to 800 mg/day) used as adjunct therapy to lithium and divalproex where the incidence in patients treated with SEROQUEL was greater than the incidence in placebo-treated patients.

Table 8: Treatment-Emergent Adverse Reaction Incidence in 3-Week Placebo-Controlled Clinical Trials for the Treatment of Bipolar Mania (Adjunct Therapy)*

Body System/ Preferred Term	SEROQUEL (n=196)	PLACEBO (n=203)
Body as a Whole		
Headache	17%	13%
Asthenia	10%	4%
Abdominal Pain	7%	3%
Back Pain	5%	3%
Hormone Level Altered	3%	0%
Heaviness	2%	1%
Infection	2%	1%
Fever	2%	1%
Neck Rigidity	1%	0%

Cardiovascular		
Postural Hypotension	7%	2%
Hypotension	3%	1%
Hypertension	2%	1%
Tachycardia	2%	1%
Hemorrhage	1%	0%
Digestive		
Dry Mouth	19%	3%
Constipation	10%	5%
Dyspepsia	4%	3%
Increased Appetite	2%	1%
Flatulence	1%	0%
Gastrointestinal Disorder	1%	0%
Endocrine		
Hypothyroidism	2%	1%
Hemic and Lymphatic		
Lymphadenopathy	1%	0%
Metabolic and Nutritional		
Weight Gain	6%	3%
Peripheral Edema	4%	2%
Musculoskeletal		
Twitching	4%	1%
Joint Disorder	1%	0%
Nervous		
Somnolence	34%	9%
Dizziness	9%	6%
Tremor	8%	7%
Agitation	6%	4%
Hypertonia	4%	3%
Depression	3%	2%
Speech Disorder	3%	1%
Incoordination	2%	1%
Thinking Abnormal	2%	0%
Anxiety	2%	0%
Ataxia	2%	0%
Respiratory		
Pharyngitis	6%	3%
Rhinitis	4%	2%
Sinusitis	2%	1%
Skin and Appendages		
Sweating	2%	1%
Special Senses		
Amblyopia	3%	2%
Ear Disorder	1%	0%
Ear Pain	1%	0%
Urogenital		
Urinary Tract Infection	2%	1%
Female Lactation	1%	0%
Impotence	1%	0%
Urinary Tract Disorder	1%	0%

* Reactions for which the SEROQUEL incidence was equal to or less than placebo are not listed in the table, but included the following: akathisia, diarrhea, insomnia, nausea, accidental injury, chest pain, face edema, flu syndrome, electrocardiogram abnormal, vomiting, gastritis, SGPT increased, weight loss, nervousness, paresthesia, extrapyramidal syndrome, confusion, cough increased, rash and urinary incontinence.

In bipolar depression studies (up to 8 weeks), the most commonly observed treatment emergent adverse reactions associated with the use of SEROQUEL (incidence of 5% or greater) and observed at a rate on SEROQUEL at least twice that of placebo were somnolence, (57%) dry mouth (44%), dizziness (18%), constipation (10%), and lethargy (5%).

Table 9 enumerates the incidence, rounded to the nearest percent, of treatment-emergent adverse reactions that occurred during therapy (up to 8 weeks) of bipolar depression in 1% or more of patients treated with SEROQUEL (doses of 300 and 600 mg/day) where the incidence in patients treated with SEROQUEL was greater than the incidence in placebo-treated patients.

Table 9: Treatment-Emergent Adverse Reaction Incidence in 8-Week Placebo-Controlled Clinical Trials for the Treatment of Bipolar Depression*

Body System/ Preferred Term	SEROQUEL (n=698)	PLACEBO (n=347)
Cardiac Disorders		
Palpitations	4%	1%
Tachycardia	1%	0%
Eye Disorders		
Vision Blurred	4%	2%
Gastrointestinal Disorders		
Dry Mouth	44%	13%
Constipation	10%	4%
Dyspepsia	7%	4%
Vomiting	5%	4%
Gastroesophageal Reflux Disease	2%	1%
Dysphagia	2%	0%
General Disorders and Administrative Site Conditions		
Fatigue	10%	8%
Asthenia	2%	1%
Injury, Poisoning and Procedural Complications		
Injury	1%	0%
Investigations		
Weight increased	4%	1%
Metabolic and Nutritional Disorders		
Increased Appetite	5%	3%
Musculoskeletal and Connective Tissue Disorders		
Arthralgia	3%	2%
Pain in Extremity	2%	1%
Nervous System Disorders		
Somnolence†	57%	15%
Dizziness	18%	7%
Lethargy	5%	2%
Akathisia	4%	1%
Extrapyramidal Disorder	3%	1%
Paraesthesia	3%	2%
Dysarthria	3%	0%
Hypersomnia	3%	0%
Tremor	2%	1%
Restless Legs Syndrome	2%	0%
Balance Disorder	2%	1%
Hypoaesthesia	2%	1%
Dystonia	1%	0%
Dizziness, postural	1%	0%
Dyskinesia	1%	0%
Dysgeusia	1%	0%
Psychiatric disorders		
Irritability	3%	1%
Abnormal Dreams	2%	1%
Confusional State	1%	0%
Respiratory, Thoracic, and Mediastinal Disorders		
Nasal Congestion	5%	3%
Cough	3%	1%
Sinus Congestion	2%	1%
Vascular Disorders		
Orthostatic Hypotension	4%	3%
Hypertension	1%	0%

* Reactions for which the SEROQUEL incidence was equal to or less than placebo are not listed in the table, but included the following: nausea, upper respiratory tract infection, headache, tinnitus, diarrhea, flatulence, toothache, stomach discomt, abdominal pain, pyrexia, peripheral edema, nasopharyngitis, influenza, bronchitis, viral gastroenteritis, accidental overdose, decreased appetite, back pain, muscle twitching, myalgia, muscle cramp, headache, insomnia, anxiety, nightmare, libido decreased, suicidal ideation, pollakiuria, dyspnoea, pharyngolaryngeal pain, night sweats and hot flush.
† Somnolence combines adverse reaction terms somnolence and sedation.

Explorations for interactions on the basis of gender, age, and race did not reveal any clinically meaningful differences in the adverse reaction occurrence on the basis of these demographic factors.

Dose Dependency of Adverse Reactions in Short-Term, Placebo-Controlled Trials

Dose-related Adverse Reactions: Spontaneously elicited adverse reaction data from a study of schizophrenia compar-

Table 10: Adverse experiences potentially associated with EPS in a short-term, placebo-controlled multiple fixed-dose Phase III schizophrenia trial (6 weeks duration)

Preferred Term	Placebo (N=51)		SEROQUEL 75 mg/day (N=53)		SEROQUEL 150 mg/day (N=48)		SEROQUEL 300 mg/day (N=52)		SEROQUEL 600 mg/day (N=51)		SEROQUEL 750 mg/day (N=54)	
	n	%	n	%	n	%	n	%	n	%	n	%
Dystonic event*	4	7.8	2	3.8	2	4.2	0	0.0	2	3.9	3	5.6
Parkinsonism†	4	7.8	2	3.8	0	0.0	1	1.9	1	2.0	1	1.9
Akathisia‡	4	7.8	1	1.9	1	2.1	0	0.0	0	0.0	1	1.9
Dyskinetic event§	0	0.0	2	3.8	0	0.0	0	0.0	1	2.0	0	0.0
Other extrapyramidal event¶	4	7.8	2	3.8	0	0.0	3	5.8	3	5.9	1	1.9

* Patients with the following terms were counted in this category: nuchal rigidity, hypertonia, dystonia, muscle ridgidity
† Patients with the following terms were counted in this category: cogwheel rigidity, tremor
‡ Patients with the following terms were counted in this category: akathisia
§ Patients with the following terms were counted in this category: tardive dyskinesia, dyskinesia, choreoathetosis
¶ Patients with the following terms were counted in this category: restlessness, extrapyramidal disorder

ing five fixed doses of SEROQUEL (75 mg, 150 mg, 300 mg, 600 mg, and 750 mg/day) to placebo were explored for dose-relatedness of adverse reactions. Logistic regression analyses revealed a positive dose response (p<0.05) for the following adverse reactions: dyspepsia, abdominal pain, and weight gain.

Adverse Reactions in clinical trials with quetiapine and not listed elsewhere in the label:
The following adverse reactions have also been reported with quetiapine: nightmares, hypersensitivity and elevations in serum creatine phosphokinase (not associated with NMS).
Extrapyramidal Symptoms:
Dystonia
Class Effect: Symptoms of dystonia, prolonged abnormal contractions of muscle groups, may occur in susceptible individuals during the first few days of treatment. Dystonic symptoms include: spasm of the neck muscles, sometimes progressing to tightness of the throat, swallowing difficulty, difficulty breathing, and/or protrusion of the tongue. While these symptoms can occur at low doses, they occur more frequently and with greater severity with high potency and at higher doses of first generation antipsychotic drugs. An elevated risk of acute dystonia is observed in males and younger age groups.
Adults: Data from one 6-week clinical trial of schizophrenia comparing five fixed doses of SEROQUEL (75, 150, 300, 600, 750 mg/day) provided evidence for the lack of treatment-emergent extrapyramidal symptoms (EPS) and dose-relatedness for EPS associated with SEROQUEL treatment. Three methods were used to measure EPS: (1) Simpson-Angus total score (mean change from baseline) which evaluates Parkinsonism and akathisia, (2) incidence of spontaneous complaints of EPS (akathisia, akinesia, cogwheel rigidity, extrapyramidal syndrome, hypertonia, hypokinesia, neck rigidity, and tremor), and (3) use of anticholinergic medications to treat emergent EPS.
[See table above]
Parkinsonism incidence rates as measured by the Simpson-Angus total score for placebo and the five fixed doses (75, 150, 300, 600, 750 mg/day) were: -0.6; -1.0; -1.2; -1.6; -1.8 and -1.8. The rate of anticholinergic medication use to treat emergent EPS for placebo and the five fixed doses was: 14%; 11%; 10%; 8%; 12% and 11%.
In six additional placebo-controlled clinical trials (3 in acute mania and 3 in schizophrenia) using variable doses of SEROQUEL, there were no differences between the SEROQUEL and placebo treatment groups in the incidence of EPS, as assessed by Simpson-Angus total scores, spontaneous complaints of EPS and the use of concomitant anticholinergic medications to treat EPS.
In two placebo-controlled clinical trials for the treatment of bipolar depression using 300 mg and 600 mg of SEROQUEL, the incidence of adverse reactions potentially related to EPS was 12% in both dose groups and 6% in the placebo group. In these studies, the incidence of the individual adverse reactions (akathisia, extrapyramidal disorder, tremor, dyskinesia, dystonia, restlessness, muscle contractions involuntary, psychomotor hyperactivity and muscle rigidity) were generally low and did not exceed 4% in any treatment group.
The 3 treatment groups were similar in mean change in SAS total score and BARS Global Assessment score at the end of treatment. The use of concomitant anticholinergic medications was infrequent and similar across the three treatment groups.
Children and Adolescents:
The information below is derived from a clinical trial database for SEROQUEL consisting of over 1000 pediatric pa-

tients. This database includes 677 patients exposed to SEROQUEL for the treatment of schizophrenia and 393 patients exposed to SEROQUEL for the treatment of acute bipolar mania.

Incidence of Adverse Reactions in Short-Term, Placebo-Controlled Trials in Children and Adolescents

Adolescents 13 to 17 years of age with Schizophrenia

The following findings were based on a 6-week placebo-controlled trial in which quetiapine was administered in either doses of 400 or 800 mg/day.

Adverse Reactions Associated with Discontinuation of Treatment

The incidence of discontinuation due to adverse reactions for quetiapine-treated and placebo-treated patients was 8.2% and 2.7%, respectively. The adverse event leading to discontinuation in 1% or more of patients on SEROQUEL and at a greater incidence than placebo was somnolence (2.7% and 0% for placebo).

Commonly Observed Adverse Reactions

In therapy for schizophrenia (up to 6 weeks), the most commonly observed adverse reactions associated with the use of quetiapine in adolescents (incidence of 5% or greater and quetiapine incidence at least twice that for placebo) were somnolence (34%), dizziness (12%), dry mouth (7%), tachycardia (7%).

Table 11 enumerates the incidence, rounded to the nearest percent, of treatment-emergent adverse reactions that occurred during therapy (up to 6 weeks) of schizophrenia in 5% or more of patients treated with SEROQUEL (doses of 400 or 800 mg/day) where the incidence in patients treated with SEROQUEL was at least twice the incidence in placebo-treated patients.

Adverse events that were potentially dose-related with higher frequency in the 800 mg group compared to the 400 mg group included dizziness (8.2% vs. 14.9%), dry mouth (4.1% vs. 9.5%), and tachycardia (5.5% vs. 8.1%).

Table 11: Treatment-Emergent Adverse Reaction Incidence in a 6-Week Placebo-Controlled Clinical Trial for the Treatment of Schizophrenia in Adolescent Patients

Body System/ Preferred Term	SEROQUEL (n=147)	PLACEBO (n=75)
Central Nervous Disorders		
Solmnolence*	34%	11%
Digestive		
Dry Mouth	7%	1%
Cardiovascular Disorders		
Tachycardia	7%	0%
Nervous System Disorder		
Dizziness	12%	5%

*Somnolence combines adverse event terms somnolence and sedation

Children and Adolescents 10 to 17 years of age with Bipolar Mania

The following findings were based on a 3-week placebo-controlled trial in which quetiapine was administered in either doses of 400 or 600 mg/day.

Adverse Reactions Associated with Discontinuation of Treatment

The incidence of discontinuation due to adverse reactions for quetiapine-treated and placebo-treated patients was 11.4% and 4.4%, respectively. The adverse events leading to discontinuation in 1% or more of patients on SEROQUEL and at a greater incidence than placebo were somnolence (4.1% vs. 1.1%), fatigue (2.1% vs. 0), irritability (1.6% vs. 0) and syncope (1% vs. 0).

Commonly Observed Adverse Reactions

In bipolar mania therapy (up to 3 weeks) the most commonly observed adverse reactions associated with the use of quetiapine in children and adolescents (incidence of 5% or greater and quetiapine incidence at least twice that for placebo) were somnolence (53%), dizziness (18%), fatigue (11%), increased appetite (9%), nausea (8%), vomiting (8%), tachycardia (7%), dry mouth (7%), and weight increased (6%).

Table 12 enumerates the incidence, rounded to the nearest percent, of treatment-emergent adverse reactions that occurred during therapy (up to 3 weeks) of bipolar mania in 5% or more of patients treated with SEROQUEL (doses of 400 or 600 mg/day) where the incidence in patients treated with SEROQUEL was at least twice the incidence in placebo-treated patients.

Adverse events that were potentially dose-related with higher frequency in the 600 mg group compared to the 400 mg group included somnolence (49% vs. 57%), nausea (6.3% vs. 10.2%) and tachycardia (5.3% vs. 8.2%).

Table 12: Treatment-Emergent Adverse Reaction Incidence in a 3-Week Placebo-Controlled Clinical Trial for the Treatment of Bipolar Mania in Children and Adolescent Patients

Body System/ Preferred Term	SEROQUEL (n=193)	PLACEBO (n=90)
Nervous System Disorders		
Somnolence*	53%	14%
Dizziness	18%	2%
Fatigue	11%	4%
Metabolism and Nutrition Disorders		
Increased Appetite	9%	1%
Weight Increased	6%	0%
Gastrointestinal Disorders		
Nausea	8%	4%
Vomiting	8%	3%
Dry Mouth	7%	0%
Cardiac Disorders		
Tachycardia	7%	0%

*Somnolence combines adverse event terms somnolence and sedation

Adverse Reactions in Schizophrenia and Bipolar Mania Clinical Trials

Commonly Observed Adverse Reactions

In acute therapy for schizophrenia and bipolar mania (up to 6 weeks in schizophrenia and up to 3 weeks in bipolar mania) the most commonly observed adverse reactions associated with the use of quetiapine in children and adolescents (incidence of 5% or greater and quetiapine incidence at least twice that for placebo) were somnolence (47%), dizziness (15%), fatigue (9%), increased appetite (8%), dry mouth (7%), tachycardia (7%), and weight increased (5%).

Table 13 enumerates the pooled incidence of adverse reactions that occurred during acute therapy of children and adolescents (up to 6 weeks in schizophrenia and up to 3 weeks in bipolar Mania). The table includes only those reactions that occurred in 1% or more of patients treated with quetiapine (doses of 400, 600, or 800 mg/day) and for which the incidence in patients treated with quetiapine was greater than the incidence in patients treated with placebo.

Table 13: Adverse Reactions (incidence ≥ 1% and greater than placebo) in Short-Term, Placebo-Controlled Trials of Children and Adolescents (10 to 17 years of age) with Bipolar Mania or Schizophrenia*

Body System/ Preferred Term	SEROQUEL (n=340)	PLACEBO (n=165)
Central/Nervous System Disorders		
Somnolence†	47%	15%
Dizziness	15%	4%
Fatigue	9%	4%
Irritability	4%	1%
Tremor	3%	2%
Akathisia	2%	1%
Syncope	2%	0%
Lethargy	1%	0%
Metabolism and Nutrition Disorders		
Increased Appetite	8%	2%
Weight Increased	5%	1%
Digestive		
Dry Mouth	7%	1%
Cardiovascular Disorders		
Tachycardia	8%	0%
Musculoskeletal and Connective Tissue Disorders		
Arthralgia	3%	1%
Back Pain	2%	1%
Musculoskeletal Stiffness	2%	1%
Respiratory, Thoracic and Mediastinal Disorder		
Nasal Congestion	3%	2%
Gastrointestinal Disorder		
Vomiting	7%	6%
Stomach Discomfort	2%	1%
Skin and Subcutaneous Disorders		
Acne	2%	1%
General Disorders and Administration Site Conditions		
Pyrexia	2%	1%
Asthenia	2%	1%
Psychiatric Disorders		
Aggression	2%	1%
Restlessness	1%	0%
Eye Disorders		
Vision Blurred	2%	1%

Infections and Infestations

Tooth Abscess	1%	0%

* Threshold criteria were applied before rounding to the nearest integer

† Somnolence combines adverse event terms somnolence and sedation

Extrapyramidal Symptoms:

In a short-term placebo-controlled monotherapy trial in adolescent patients with schizophrenia (6-week duration), the aggregated incidence of extrapyramidal symptoms was 12.9% for SEROQUEL and 5.3% for placebo, though the incidence of the individual adverse events (akathisia, tremor, extrapyramidal disorder, hypokinesia, restlessness, psychomotor hyperactivity, muscle rigidity, dyskinesia) did not exceed 4.1% in any treatment group. In a short-term placebo-controlled monotherapy trial in children and adolescent patients with bipolar mania (3-week duration), the aggregated incidence of extrapyramidal symptoms was 3.6% for SEROQUEL and 1.1% for placebo.

Table 14 below presents a listing of patients with AEs potentially associated with EPS in the short-term placebo-controlled monotherapy trial in adolescent patients with schizophrenia (6-week duration).

[See table 14 at top of next page]

Table 15 below presents a listing of patients with Adverse Experiences potentially associated with EPS in a short-term placebo-controlled monotherapy trial in children and adolescent patients with bipolar mania (3-week duration).

[See table 15 on next page]

Adverse Reactions in Long-Term Open-Label Trial

The adverse reactions reported in a 26-week, open-label trial with SEROQUEL in 5% or greater of the children and adolescent patients with schizophrenia or bipolar mania were somnolence (30%), headache (19%), vomiting (11%), increased weight (13%), insomnia (8%), nausea (10%), fatigue (8%), dizziness (9%), increased appetite (7%), upper respiratory tract infection (7%), agitation (5%), tachycardia (5%), and irritability (5%).

Other Adverse Reactions Observed During the Pre-Marketing Evaluation of SEROQUEL

Following is a list of COSTART terms that reflect treatment-emergent adverse reactions as defined in the introduction to the ADVERSE REACTIONS section reported by patients treated with SEROQUEL at multiple doses ≥ 75 mg/day during any phase of a trial within the premarketing database of approximately 2200 patients treated for schizophrenia. All reported reactions are included except those already listed in the tables or elsewhere in labeling, those reactions for which a drug cause was remote, and those reaction terms which were so general as to be uninformative. It is important to emphasize that, although the reactions reported occurred during treatment with SEROQUEL, they were not necessarily caused by it.

Reactions are further categorized by body system and listed in order of decreasing frequency according to the following definitions: frequent adverse reactions are those occurring in at least 1/100 patients (only those not already listed in the tabulated results from placebo-controlled trials appear in this listing); infrequent adverse reactions are those occurring in 1/100 to 1/1000 patients; rare reactions are those occurring in fewer than 1/1000 patients.

Nervous System: **Infrequent:** abnormal dreams, dyskinesia, thinking abnormal, tardive dyskinesia, vertigo, involuntary movements, confusion, amnesia, psychosis, hallucinations, hyperkinesia, libido increased[1], urinary retention, incoordination, paranoid reaction, abnormal gait, myoclonus, delusions, manic reaction, apathy, ataxia, depersonalization, stupor, bruxism, catatonic reaction, hemiplegia; *Rare:* aphasia, buccoglossal syndrome, choreoathetosis, delirium, emotional lability, euphoria, libido decreased*, neuralgia, stuttering, subdural hematoma.

Body as a Whole: **Frequent:** flu syndrome; **Infrequent:** neck pain, pelvic pain[1], suicide attempt, malaise, photosensitivity reaction, chills, face edema, moniliasis; *Rare:* abdomen enlarged.

Digestive System: **Frequent:** anorexia; **Infrequent:** increased salivation, increased appetite, gamma glutamyl transpeptidase increased, gingivitis, dysphagia, flatulence, gastroenteritis, gastritis, hemorrhoids, stomatitis, thirst, tooth caries, fecal incontinence, gastroesophageal reflux, gum hemorrhage, mouth ulceration, rectal hemorrhage, tongue edema; *Rare:* glossitis, hematemesis, intestinal obstruction, melena, pancreatitis.

Cardiovascular System: **Infrequent:** vasodilatation, QT interval prolonged, migraine, bradycardia, cerebral ischemia, irregular pulse, T wave abnormality, bundle branch block, cerebrovascular accident, deep thrombophlebitis, T wave inversion; *Rare:* angina pectoris, atrial fibrillation, AV block first degree, congestive heart failure, ST elevated, thrombophlebitis, T wave flattening, ST abnormality, increased QRS duration.

Respiratory System: ***Frequent:*** cough increased, dyspnea; ***Infrequent:*** pneumonia, epistaxis, asthma; ***Rare:*** hiccup, hyperventilation.
Metabolic and Nutritional System: ***Infrequent:*** weight loss, alkaline phosphatase increased, hyperlipemia, alcohol intolerance, dehydration, hyperglycemia, creatinine increased, hypoglycemia; ***Rare:*** glycosuria, gout, hand edema, hypokalemia, water intoxication. •
Skin and Appendages System: **Infrequent:** pruritus, acne, eczema, contact dermatitis, maculopapular rash, seborrhea, skin ulcer; ***Rare:*** exfoliative dermatitis, psoriasis, skin discoloration.
Urogenital System: ***Infrequent:*** dysmenorrhea[1], vaginitis[1], urinary incontinence, metrorrhagia[1], impotence[1], dysuria, vaginal moniliasis[1], abnormal ejaculation[1], cystitis, urinary frequency, amenorrhea[1], female lactation[1], leukorrhea[1], vaginal hemorrhage[1], vulvovaginitis[1] orchitis[1]; ***Rare:*** gynecomastia[1], nocturia, polyuria, acute kidney failure.
Special Senses: ***Infrequent:*** conjunctivitis, abnormal vision, dry eyes, tinnitus, taste perversion, blepharitis, eye pain; ***Rare:*** abnormality of accommodation, deafness, glaucoma.
Musculoskeletal System: ***Infrequent:*** pathological fracture, myasthenia, twitching, arthralgia, arthritis, leg cramps, bone pain. Hemic and Lymphatic System: ***Infrequent:*** leukocytosis, anemia, ecchymosis, eosinophilia, hypochromic anemia; lymphadenopathy, cyanosis; ***Rare:*** hemolysis, thrombocytopenia.
Endocrine System: ***Infrequent:*** hypothyroidism, diabetes mellitus; ***Rare:*** hyperthyroidism.

1 Adjusted for gender

6.2 Vital Signs and Laboratory Values

Hyperglycemia, hyperlipidemia, weight gain and orthostatic hypotension have been reported with quetiapine. Increases in blood pressure have also been reported with quetiapine in children and adolescents [see *Warnings and Precautions* (5.4, 5.5, 5.6 and 5.9)].

Neutrophil Counts
In placebo-controlled monotherapy clinical trials involving 3368 patients on quetiapine fumarate and 1515 on placebo, the incidence of at least one occurrence of neutrophil count $<1.0 \times 10^9/L$ among patients with a normal baseline neutrophil count and at least one available follow up laboratory measurement was 0.3% (10/2967) in patients treated with quetiapine fumarate, compared to 0.1% (2/1349) in patients treated with placebo. Patients with a pre-existing low WBC or a history of drug induced leukopenia/neutropenia should have their complete blood count (CBC) monitored frequently during the first few months of therapy and should discontinue SEROQUEL at the first sign of a decline in WBC in absence of other causative factors [see *Warnings and Precautions* (5.10)].

Decreased Hemoglobin
In short-term placebo-controlled trials, decreases in hemoglobin to ≤ 13 g/dL males, ≤ 12 g/dL females on at least one occasion occurred in 8.3% (594/7155) of quetiapine-treated patients compared to 6.2% (219/3536) of patients treated with placebo. In a database of controlled and uncontrolled clinical trials, decreases in hemoglobin to ≤ 13 g/dL males, ≤ 12 g/dL females on at least one occasion occurred in 11% (2277/20729) of quetiapine-treated patients.

ECG Changes
Adults: Between-group comparisons for pooled placebo-controlled trials revealed no statistically significant SEROQUEL/placebo differences in the proportions of patients experiencing potentially important changes in ECG parameters, including QT, QTc, and PR intervals. However, the proportions of patients meeting the criteria for tachycardia were compared in four 3- to 6-week placebo-controlled clinical trials for the treatment of schizophrenia revealing a 1% (4/399) incidence for SEROQUEL compared to 0.6% (1/156) incidence for placebo. In acute (monotherapy) bipolar mania trials the proportions of patients meeting the criteria for tachycardia was 0.5% (1/192) for SEROQUEL compared to 0% (0/178) incidence for placebo. In acute bipolar mania (adjunct) trials the proportions of patients meeting the same criteria was 0.6% (1/166) for SEROQUEL compared to 0% (0/171) incidence for placebo. In bipolar depression trials, no patients had heart rate increases to > 120 beats per minute. SEROQUEL use was associated with a mean increase in heart rate, assessed by ECG, of 7 beats per minute compared to a mean increase of 1 beat per minute among placebo patients. This slight tendency in adults to tachycardia may be related to SEROQUEL's potential for inducing orthostatic changes [see *Warnings and Precautions* (5.8)].
Children and Adolescents: In the acute (6 week) schizophrenia trial in adolescents, potentially clinically significant increases in heart rate (> 110 bpm) occurred in 5.2% (3/73) of patients receiving SEROQUEL 400 mg and 8.5% (5/74) of patients receiving SEROQUEL 800 mg compared to 0% (0/75) of patients receiving placebo. Mean increases in heart rate were 3.8 bpm and 11.2 bpm for SEROQUEL 400 mg and 800 mg groups, respectively, compared to a decrease of 3.3 bpm in the placebo group [see Warnings and Precautions (5.8)].
In the acute (3 week) bipolar mania trial in children and adolescents, potentially clinically significant increases in heart rate (> 110 bpm) occurred in 1.1% (1/95) of patients receiving SEROQUEL 400 mg and 2.4% (2/98) of patients receiving SEROQUEL 600 mg compared to 0% (0/98) of patients receiving placebo. Mean increases in heart rate were 12.8 bpm and 13.4 bpm for SEROQUEL 400 mg and 600 mg groups, respectively, compared to a decrease of 1.7 bpm in the placebo group [see *Warnings and Precautions* (5.8)].

Table 14: Adverse experiences potentially associated with EPS in the short-term placebo-controlled monotherapy trial in adolescent patients with schizophrenia (6-week duration)

Preferred Term	Placebo (N=75)		SEROQUEL 400 mg/day (N=73)		SEROQUEL 800 mg/day (N=74)		All SEROQUEL (N=147)	
	n	%	n	%	n	%	n	%
Dystonic event*	0	0.0	2	2.7	0	0.0	2	1.4
Parkinsonism†	2	2.7	4	5.5	4	5.4	8	5.4
Akathisia‡	3	4.0	3	4.1	4	5.4	7	4.8
Dyskinetic event§	0	0.0	2	2.7	0	0.0	2	1.4
Other extrapyramidal event¶	0	0.0	2	2.7	2	2.7	4	2.7

* Patients with the following terms were counted in this category: nuchal rigidity, hypertonia, dystonia, muscle rigidity
† Patients with the following terms were counted in this category: cogwheel rigidity, tremor
‡ Patients with the following terms were counted in this category: akathisia
§ Patients with the following terms were counted in this category: tardive dyskinesia, dyskinesia, choreoathetosis
¶ Patients with the following terms were counted in this category: restlessness, extrapyramidal disorder

Table 15: Adverse experiences potentially associated with EPS in a short-term placebo-controlled monotherapy trial in children and adolescent patients with bipolar mania (3-week duration)

Preferred Term*	Placebo (N=90)		SEROQUEL 400 mg/day (N=95)		SEROQUEL 600 mg/day (N=98)		All SEROQUEL (N=193)	
	n	%	n	%	n	%	n	%
Parkinsonism†	1	1.1	2	2.1	1	1.0	3	1.6
Akathisia‡	0	0.0	1	1.0	1	1.0	2	1.0
Other extrapyramidal event§	0	0.0	1	1.1	1	1.0	2	1.0

* There were no adverse experiences with the preferred term of dystonic or dyskinetic events.
† Patients with the following terms were counted in this category: cogwheel rigidity, tremor
‡ Patients with the following terms were countedin this category: akathisia
§ Patients with the following terms were counted in this category: restlessness, extrapyramidal disorder

6.3 Post Marketing Experience

The following adverse reactions were identified during post approval of SEROQUEL. Because these reactions are reported voluntarily from a population of uncertain size, it is not always possible to reliably estimate their frequency or establish a causal relationship to drug exposure.
Adverse reactions reported since market introduction which were temporally related to SEROQUEL therapy include: anaphylactic reaction and galactorrhea.
Other adverse reactions reported since market introduction, which were temporally related to SEROQUEL therapy, but not necessarily causally related, include the following: agranulocytosis, cardiomyopathy, hyponatremia, myocarditis, rhabdomyolysis, syndrome of inappropriate antidiuretic hormone secretion (SIADH), Stevens-Johnson syndrome (SJS), and decreased platelets.
In post-marketing clinical trials, elevations in total cholesterol (predominantly LDL cholesterol) have been reported.

7 DRUG INTERACTIONS

The risks of using SEROQUEL in combination with other drugs have not been extensively evaluated in systematic studies. Given the primary CNS effects of SEROQUEL, caution should be used when it is taken in combination with other centrally acting drugs. SEROQUEL potentiated the cognitive and motor effects of alcohol in a clinical trial in subjects with selected psychotic disorders, and alcoholic beverages should be avoided while taking SEROQUEL.
Because of its potential for inducing hypotension, SEROQUEL may enhance the effects of certain antihypertensive agents.
SEROQUEL may antagonize the effects of levodopa and dopamine agonists.
Caution should be exercised when quetiapine is used concomitantly with drugs known to cause electrolyte imbalance or to increase QT interval [*see Warnings and Precautions* (5.21)].
There have been reports of false positive results in urine enzyme immunoassays for methadone and tricyclic antidepressants in patients who have taken quetiapine. If false positive results are suspected, confirmation by an appropriate chromatographic technique is recommended.

7.1 The Effect of Other Drugs on Quetiapine

Phenytoin: Coadministration of quetiapine (250 mg three times daily) and phenytoin (100 mg three times daily) increased the mean oral clearance of quetiapine by 5-fold. Increased doses of SEROQUEL may be required to maintain control of symptoms of schizophrenia in patients receiving quetiapine and phenytoin, or other hepatic enzyme inducers (e.g., carbamazepine, barbiturates, rifampin, glucocorticoids). Caution should be taken if phenytoin is withdrawn and replaced with a non-inducer (e.g., valproate) [see *Dosage and Administration* (2)].
Divalproex: Coadministration of quetiapine (150 mg twice daily) and divalproex (500 mg twice daily) increased the mean maximum plasma concentration of quetiapine at steady state by 17% without affecting the extent of absorption or mean oral clearance.
Thioridazine: Thioridazine (200 mg twice daily) increased the oral clearance of quetiapine (300 mg twice daily) by 65%.
Cimetidine: Administration of multiple daily doses of cimetidine (400 mg three times daily for 4 days) resulted in a 20% decrease in the mean oral clearance of quetiapine (150 mg three times daily). Dosage adjustment for quetiapine is not required when it is given with cimetidine.
P450 3A Inhibitors: Coadministration of ketoconazole (200 mg once daily for 4 days), a potent inhibitor of cytochrome P450 3A, reduced oral clearance of quetiapine by 84%, resulting in a 335% increase in maximum plasma concentration of quetiapine. Caution (reduced dosage) is indicated when SEROQUEL is administered with ketoconazole and other inhibitors of cytochrome P450 3A (e.g., itraconazole, fluconazole, erythromycin, and protease inhibitors).
Fluoxetine, Imipramine, Haloperidol, and Risperidone: Coadministration of fluoxetine (60 mg once daily), imipramine (75 mg twice daily), haloperidol (7.5 mg twice daily), or risperidone (3 mg twice daily) with quetiapine (300 mg twice daily) did not alter the steady-state pharmacokinetics of quetiapine.

7.2 Effect of Quetiapine on Other Drugs

Lorazepam: The mean oral clearance of lorazepam (2 mg, single dose) was reduced by 20% in the presence of quetiapine administered as 250 mg three times daily dosing.
Divalproex: The mean maximum concentration and extent of absorption of total and free valproic acid at steady state were decreased by 10 to 12% when divalproex (500 mg twice daily) was administered with quetiapine (150 mg twice daily). The mean oral clearance of total valproic acid (administered as divalproex 500 mg twice daily) was increased by 11% in the presence of quetiapine (150 mg twice daily). The changes were not significant.
Lithium: Concomitant administration of quetiapine (250 mg three times daily) with lithium had no effect on any of the steady-state pharmacokinetic parameters of lithium.

Antipyrine: Administration of multiple daily doses up to 750 mg/day (on a three times daily schedule) of quetiapine to subjects with selected psychotic disorders had no clinically relevant effect on the clearance of antipyrine or urinary recovery of antipyrine metabolites. These results indicate that quetiapine does not significantly induce hepatic enzymes responsible for cytochrome P450 mediated metabolism of antipyrine.

8 USE IN SPECIFIC POPULATIONS

8.1 Pregnancy

Pregnancy Category C:

The teratogenic potential of quetiapine was studied in Wistar rats and Dutch Belted rabbits dosed during the period of organogenesis. No evidence of a teratogenic effect was detected in rats at doses of 25 to 200 mg/kg or 0.3 to 2.4 times the maximum human dose on a mg/m^2 basis or in rabbits at 25 to 100 mg/kg or 0.6 to 2.4 times the maximum human dose on a mg/m^2 basis. There was, however, evidence of embryo/fetal toxicity. Delays in skeletal ossification were detected in rat fetuses at doses of 50 and 200 mg/kg (0.6 and 2.4 times the maximum human dose on a mg/m^2 basis) and in rabbits at 50 and 100 mg/kg (1.2 and 2.4 times the maximum human dose on a mg/m^2 basis). Fetal body weight was reduced in rat fetuses at 200 mg/kg and rabbit fetuses at 100 mg/kg (2.4 times the maximum human dose on a mg/m^2 basis for both species). There was an increased incidence of a minor soft tissue anomaly (carpal/tarsal flexure) in rabbit fetuses at a dose of 100 mg/kg (2.4 times the maximum human dose on a mg/m^2 basis). Evidence of maternal toxicity (i.e., decreases in body weight gain and/or death) was observed at the high dose in the rat study and at all doses in the rabbit study. In a peri/postnatal reproductive study in rats, no drug-related effects were observed at doses of 1, 10, and 20 mg/kg or 0.01, 0.12, and 0.24 times the maximum human dose on a mg/m^2 basis. However, in a preliminary peri/postnatal study, there were increases in fetal and pup death, and decreases in mean litter weight at 150 mg/kg, or 3.0 times the maximum human dose on a mg/m^2 basis.

There are no adequate and well-controlled studies in pregnant women and quetiapine should be used during pregnancy only if the potential benefit justifies the potential risk to the fetus.

8.2 Labor and Delivery

The effect of SEROQUEL on labor and delivery in humans is unknown.

8.3 Nursing Mothers

SEROQUEL was excreted in milk of treated animals during lactation. It is not known if SEROQUEL is excreted in human milk. It is recommended that women receiving SEROQUEL should not breast feed.

8.4 Pediatric Use

In general, the adverse reactions observed in children and adolescents during the clinical trials were similar to those in the adult population with few exceptions. Increases in systolic and diastolic blood pressure occurred in children and adolescents and did not occur in adults. Orthostatic hypotension occurred more frequently in adults (4-7%) compared to children and adolescents (< 1%).

Schizophrenia

The efficacy and safety of SEROQUEL in the treatment of schizophrenia in adolescents aged 13 to 17 years were demonstrated in one 6–week, double-blind, placebo-controlled trial [*see Indications and Usage* (1.1), *Dosage and Administration* (2.1), *Adverse Reactions* (6.1), *and Clinical Studies* (14.1)].

Safety and effectiveness of SEROQUEL in pediatric patients less than 13 years of age with schizophrenia have not been established.

Maintenance

The safety and effectiveness of SEROQUEL in the maintenance treatment of bipolar disorder has not been established in pediatric patients less than 18 years of age. The safety and effectiveness of SEROQUEL in the maintenance treatment of schizophrenia has not been established in any patient population, including pediatric patients.

Bipolar Mania

The efficacy and safety of SEROQUEL in the treatment of mania in children and adolescents ages 10 to 17 years with Bipolar I disorder was demonstrated in a 3-week, double-blind, placebo controlled, multicenter trial [*see Indications and Usage* (1.2), *Dosage and Administration* (2.2), *Adverse Reactions* (6.1), *and Clinical Studies* (14.2)].

Safety and effectiveness of SEROQUEL in pediatric patients less than 10 years of age with bipolar mania have not been established.

Bipolar Depression

Safety and effectiveness of SEROQUEL in pediatric patients less than 18 years of age with bipolar depression have not been established.

Some differences in the pharmacokinetics of quetiapine were noted between children/adolescents (10 to 17 years of age) and adults. When adjusted for weight, the AUC and C_{max} of quetiapine were 41% and 39% lower, respectively, in children and adolescents compared to adults. The pharmacokinetics of the active metabolite, norquetiapine, were similar between children/adolescents and adults after adjusting for weight [*see Clinical Pharmacology* (12.3)].

8.5 Geriatric Use

Of the approximately 3700 patients in clinical studies with SEROQUEL, 7% (232) were 65 years of age or over. In general, there was no indication of any different tolerability of SEROQUEL in the elderly compared to younger adults. Nevertheless, the presence of factors that might decrease pharmacokinetic clearance, increase the pharmacodynamic response to SEROQUEL, or cause poorer tolerance or orthostasis, should lead to consideration of a lower starting dose, slower titration, and careful monitoring during the initial dosing period in the elderly. The mean plasma clearance of SEROQUEL was reduced by 30% to 50% in elderly patients when compared to younger patients [*see Clinical Pharmacology* (12) *and Dosage and Administration* (2)].

9 DRUG ABUSE AND DEPENDENCE

9.1 Controlled Substance

SEROQUEL is not a controlled substance.

9.2 Abuse

SEROQUEL has not been systematically studied, in animals or humans, for its potential for abuse, tolerance or physical dependence. While the clinical trials did not reveal any tendency for any drug-seeking behavior, these observations were not systematic and it is not possible to predict on the basis of this limited experience the extent to which a CNS-active drug will be misused, diverted, and/or abused once marketed. Consequently, patients should be evaluated carefully for a history of drug abuse, and such patients should be observed closely for signs of misuse or abuse of SEROQUEL, e.g., development of tolerance, increases in dose, drug-seeking behavior.

10 OVERDOSAGE

10.1 Human Experience

In clinical trials, survival has been reported in acute overdoses of up to 30 grams of quetiapine. Most patients who overdosed experienced no adverse reactions or recovered fully from the reported reactions. Death has been reported in a clinical trial following an overdose of 13.6 grams of quetiapine alone. In general, reported signs and symptoms were those resulting from an exaggeration of the drugs known pharmacological effects, ie, drowsiness and sedation, tachycardia and hypotension. Patients with pre-existing severe cardiovascular disease may be at an increased risk of the effects of overdose [see *Warnings and Precautions* (5)]. One case, involving an estimated overdose of 9600 mg, was associated with hypokalemia and first degree heart block. In post-marketing experience, there were cases reported of QT prolongation with overdose. There were also very rare reports of overdose of SEROQUEL alone resulting in death or coma.

10.2 Management of Overdosage

In case of acute overdosage, establish and maintain an airway and ensure adequate oxygenation and ventilation. Gastric lavage (after intubation, if patient is unconscious) and administration of activated charcoal together with a laxative should be considered. The possibility of obtundation, seizure or dystonic reaction of the head and neck following overdose may create a risk of aspiration with induced emesis. Cardiovascular monitoring should commence immediately and should include continuous electrocardiographic monitoring to detect possible arrhythmias. If antiarrhythmic therapy is administered, disopyramide, procainamide and quinidine carry a theoretical hazard of additive QT-prolonging effects when administered in patients with acute overdosage of SEROQUEL. Similarly it is reasonable to expect that the alpha-adrenergic-blocking properties of bretylium might be additive to those of quetiapine, resulting in problematic hypotension.

There is no specific antidote to SEROQUEL. Therefore, appropriate supportive measures should be instituted. The possibility of multiple drug involvement should be considered. Hypotension and circulatory collapse should be treated with appropriate measures such as intravenous fluids and/or sympathomimetic agents (epinephrine and dopamine should not be used, since beta stimulation may worsen hypotension in the setting of quetiapine-induced alpha blockade). In cases of severe extrapyramidal symptoms, anticholinergic medication should be administered. Close medical supervision and monitoring should continue until the patient recovers.

11 DESCRIPTION

SEROQUEL® (quetiapine fumarate) is a psychotropic agent belonging to a chemical class, the dibenzothiazepine derivatives. The chemical designation is 2-[2-(4-dibenzo [*b,f*] [1,4]thiazepin-11-yl-1-piperazinyl)ethoxy]-ethanol fumarate (2:1) (salt). It is present in tablets as the fumarate salt. All doses and tablet strengths are expressed as milligrams of base, not as fumarate salt. Its molecular formula is $C_{42}H_{50}N_6O_4S_2 \bullet C_4H_4O_4$ and it has a molecular weight of 883.11 (fumarate salt). The structural formula is:

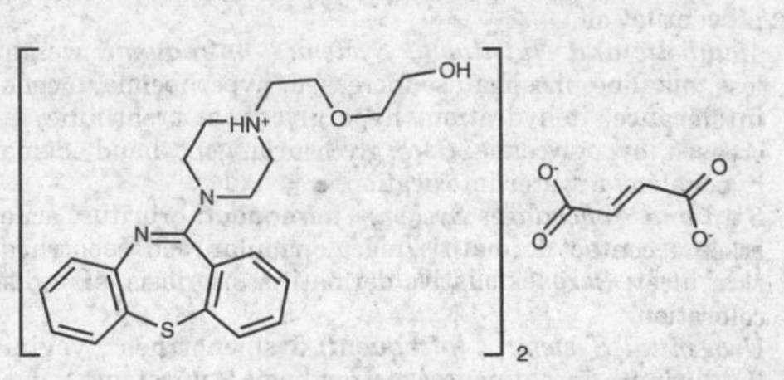

Quetiapine fumarate is a white to off-white crystalline powder which is moderately soluble in water.

SEROQUEL is supplied for oral administration as 25 mg (round, peach), 50 mg (round, white), 100 mg (round, yellow), 200 mg (round, white), 300 mg (capsule-shaped, white), and 400 mg (capsule-shaped, yellow) tablets.

Inactive ingredients are povidone, dibasic dicalcium phosphate dihydrate, microcrystalline cellulose, sodium starch glycolate, lactose monohydrate, magnesium stearate, hypromellose, polyethylene glycol and titanium dioxide.

The 25 mg tablets contain red ferric oxide and yellow ferric oxide and the 100 mg and 400 mg tablets contain only yellow ferric oxide.

12 CLINICAL PHARMACOLOGY

12.1 Mechanism of Action

The mechanism of action of SEROQUEL, as with other drugs having efficacy in the treatment of schizophrenia and bipolar disorder, is unknown. However, it has been proposed that the efficacy of SEROQUEL in schizophrenia and its mood stabilizing properties in bipolar depression and mania are mediated through a combination of dopamine type 2 (D_2) and serotonin type 2 ($5HT_2$) antagonism. Antagonism at receptors other than dopamine and $5HT_2$ with similar receptor affinities may explain some of the other effects of SEROQUEL.

SEROQUEL's antagonism of histamine H_1 receptors may explain the somnolence observed with this drug.

SEROQUEL's antagonism of adrenergic α_1 receptors may explain the orthostatic hypotension observed with this drug.

12.2 Pharmacodynamics

SEROQUEL is an antagonist at multiple neurotransmitter receptors in the brain: serotonin $5HT_{1A}$ and $5HT_2$ (IC_{50s}=717 & 148nM, respectively), dopamine D_1 and D_2 (IC_{50s}=1268 & 329nM, respectively), histamine H_1 (IC_{50}=30nM), and adrenergic α_1 and α_2 receptors (IC_{50s}=94 & 271nM, respectively). SEROQUEL has no appreciable affinity at cholinergic muscarinic and benzodiazepine receptors (IC_{50s}>5000 nM).

12.3 Pharmacokinetics

Adults

Quetiapine fumarate activity is primarily due to the parent drug. The multiple-dose pharmacokinetics of quetiapine are dose-proportional within the proposed clinical dose range, and quetiapine accumulation is predictable upon multiple dosing. Elimination of quetiapine is mainly via hepatic metabolism with a mean terminal half-life of about 6 hours within the proposed clinical dose range. Steady-state concentrations are expected to be achieved within two days of dosing. Quetiapine is unlikely to interfere with the metabolism of drugs metabolized by cytochrome P450 enzymes.

Children and Adolescents

At steady-state the pharmacokinetics of the parent compound, in children and adolescents (10-17 years of age), were similar to adults. However, when adjusted for dose and weight, AUC and C_{max} of the parent compound were 41% and 39% lower, respectively, in children and adolescents than in adults. For the active metabolite, norquetiapine, AUC and C_{max} were 45% and 31% higher, respectively, in children and adolescents than in adults. When adjusted for dose and weight, the pharmacokinetics of the metabolite, norquetiapine, was similar between children and adolescents and adults [see Use in Specific Populations (8.4)].

Absorption

Quetiapine fumarate is rapidly absorbed after oral administration, reaching peak plasma concentrations in 1.5 hours. The tablet formulation is 100% bioavailable relative to solution. The bioavailability of quetiapine is marginally affected by administration with food, with C_{max} and AUC values increased by 25% and 15%, respectively.

Distribution

Quetiapine is widely distributed throughout the body with an apparent volume of distribution of 10±4 L/kg. It is 83% bound to plasma proteins at therapeutic concentrations. *In vitro*, quetiapine did not affect the binding of warfarin or diazepam to human serum albumin. In turn, neither warfarin nor diazepam altered the binding of quetiapine.

Metabolism and Elimination

Following a single oral dose of ^{14}C-quetiapine, less than 1% of the administered dose was excreted as unchanged drug, indicating that quetiapine is highly metabolized. Approximately 73% and 20% of the dose was recovered in the urine and feces, respectively.

Quetiapine is extensively metabolized by the liver. The major metabolic pathways are sulfoxidation to the sulfoxide metabolite and oxidation to the parent acid metabolite; both metabolites are pharmacologically inactive. *In vitro* studies using human liver microsomes revealed that the cytochrome P450 3A4 isoenzyme is involved in the metabolism of quetiapine to its major, but inactive, sulfoxide metabolite and in the metabolism of its active metabolite N-desalkyl quetiapine.

Age
Oral clearance of quetiapine was reduced by 40% in elderly patients ($\geq$ 65 years, n=9) compared to young patients (n=12), and dosing adjustment may be necessary [see *Dosage and Administration* (2)].

Gender
There is no gender effect on the pharmacokinetics of quetiapine.

Race
There is no race effect on the pharmacokinetics of quetiapine.

Smoking
Smoking has no effect on the oral clearance of quetiapine.

Renal Insufficiency
Patients with severe renal impairment (Clcr=10-30 mL/min/1.73 m^2, n=8) had a 25% lower mean oral clearance than normal subjects (Clcr > 80 mL/min/1.73 m^2, n=8), but plasma quetiapine concentrations in the subjects with renal insufficiency were within the range of concentrations seen in normal subjects receiving the same dose. Dosage adjustment is therefore not needed in these patients.

Hepatic Insufficiency
Hepatically impaired patients (n=8) had a 30% lower mean oral clearance of quetiapine than normal subjects. In two of the 8 hepatically impaired patients, AUC and C$_{max}$ were 3 times higher than those observed typically in healthy subjects. Since quetiapine is extensively metabolized by the liver, higher plasma levels are expected in the hepatically impaired population, and dosage adjustment may be needed [see *Dosage and Administration* (2)].

Drug-Drug Interactions
In vitro enzyme inhibition data suggest that quetiapine and 9 of its metabolites would have little inhibitory effect on *in vivo* metabolism mediated by cytochromes P450 1A2, 2C9, 2C19, 2D6 and 3A4.

Quetiapine oral clearance is increased by the prototype cytochrome P450 3A4 inducer, phenytoin, and decreased by the prototype cytochrome P450 3A4 inhibitor, ketoconazole. Dose adjustment of quetiapine will be necessary if it is co-administered with phenytoin or ketoconazole [see *Drug Interactions* (7.1)].

Quetiapine oral clearance is not inhibited by the non-specific enzyme inhibitor, cimetidine.

Quetiapine at doses of 750 mg/day did not affect the single dose pharmacokinetics of antipyrine, lithium or lorazepam [see *Drug Interactions* (7.2)].

13 NONCLINICAL TOXICOLOGY

13.1 Carcinogenesis, Mutagenesis, Impairment of Fertility

Carcinogenesis
Carcinogenicity studies were conducted in C57BL mice and Wistar rats. Quetiapine was administered in the diet to mice at doses of 20, 75, 250, and 750 mg/kg and to rats by gavage at doses of 25, 75, and 250 mg/kg for two years. These doses are equivalent to 0.1, 0.5, 1.5, and 4.5 times the maximum human dose (800 mg/day) on a mg/m^2 basis (mice) or 0.3, 0.9, and 3.0 times the maximum human dose on a mg/m^2 basis (rats). There were statistically significant increases in thyroid gland follicular adenomas in male mice at doses of 250 and 750 mg/kg or 1.5 and 4.5 times the maximum human dose on a mg/m^2 basis and in male rats at a dose of 250 mg/kg or 3.0 times the maximum human dose on a mg/m^2 basis. Mammary gland adenocarcinomas were statistically significantly increased in female rats at all doses tested (25, 75, and 250 mg/kg or 0.3, 0.9, and 3.0 times the maximum recommended human dose on a mg/m^2 basis).

Thyroid follicular cell adenomas may have resulted from chronic stimulation of the thyroid gland by thyroid stimulating hormone (TSH) resulting from enhanced metabolism and clearance of thyroxine by rodent liver. Changes in TSH, thyroxine, and thyroxine clearance consistent with this mechanism were observed in subchronic toxicity studies in rat and mouse and in a 1-year toxicity study in rat; however, the results of these studies were not definitive. The relevance of the increases in thyroid follicular cell adenomas to human risk, through whatever mechanism, is unknown.

Antipsychotic drugs have been shown to chronically elevate prolactin levels in rodents. Serum measurements in a 1-year toxicity study showed that quetiapine increased median serum prolactin levels a maximum of 32- and 13-fold in male and female rats, respectively. Increases in mammary neoplasms have been found in rodents after chronic administration of other antipsychotic drugs and are considered to be prolactin-mediated. The relevance of this increased incidence of prolactin-mediated mammary gland tumors in rats to human risk is unknown [see *Warnings and Precautions* (5.14)].

Mutagenesis
The mutagenic potential of quetiapine was tested in six *in vitro* bacterial gene mutation assays and in an *in vitro* mammalian gene mutation assay in Chinese Hamster Ovary cells. However, sufficiently high concentrations of quetiapine may not have been used for all tester strains. Quetiapine did produce a reproducible increase in mutations in one *Salmonella typhimurium* tester strain in the presence of metabolic activation. No evidence of clastogenic potential was obtained in an *in vitro* chromosomal aberration assay in cultured human lymphocytes or in the *in vivo* micronucleus assay in rats.

Impairment of Fertility
Quetiapine decreased mating and fertility in male Sprague-Dawley rats at oral doses of 50 and 150 mg/kg or 0.6 and 1.8 times the maximum human dose on a mg/m^2 basis. Drug-related effects included increases in interval to mate and in the number of matings required for successful impregnation. These effects continued to be observed at 150 mg/kg even after a two-week period without treatment. The no-effect dose for impaired mating and fertility in male rats was 25 mg/kg, or 0.3 times the maximum human dose on a mg/m^2 basis. Quetiapine adversely affected mating and fertility in female Sprague-Dawley rats at an oral dose of 50 mg/kg, or 0.6 times the maximum human dose on a mg/m^2 basis. Drug-related effects included decreases in matings and in matings resulting in pregnancy, and an increase in the interval to mate. An increase in irregular estrus cycles was observed at doses of 10 and 50 mg/kg, or 0.1 and 0.6 times the maximum human dose on a mg/m^2 basis. The no-effect dose in female rats was 1 mg/kg, or 0.01 times the maximum human dose on a mg/m^2 basis.

13.2 Animal Toxicology

Quetiapine caused a dose-related increase in pigment deposition in thyroid gland in rat toxicity studies which were 4 weeks in duration or longer and in a mouse 2–year carcinogenicity study. Doses were 10-250 mg/kg in rats, 75-750 mg/kg in mice; these doses are 0.1-3.0, and 0.1-4.5 times the maximum recommended human dose (on a mg/m^2 basis), respectively. Pigment deposition was shown to be irreversible in rats. The identity of the pigment could not be determined, but was found to be co-localized with quetiapine in thyroid gland follicular epithelial cells. The functional effects and the relevance of this finding to human risk are unknown.

In dogs receiving quetiapine for 6 or 12 months, but not for 1 month, focal triangular cataracts occurred at the junction of posterior sutures in the outer cortex of the lens at a dose of 100 mg/kg, or 4 times the maximum recommended human dose on a mg/m^2 basis. This finding may be due to inhibition of cholesterol biosynthesis by quetiapine. Quetiapine caused a dose-related reduction in plasma cholesterol levels in repeat-dose dog and monkey studies; however, there was no correlation between plasma cholesterol and the presence of cataracts in individual dogs. The appearance of delta–8–cholestanol in plasma is consistent with inhibition of a late stage in cholesterol biosynthesis in these species. There also was a 25% reduction in cholesterol content of the outer cortex of the lens observed in a special study in quetiapine treated female dogs. Drug-related cataracts have not been seen in any other species; however, in a 1-year study in monkeys, a striated appearance of the anterior lens surface was detected in 2/7 females at a dose of 225 mg/kg or 5.5 times the maximum recommended human dose on a mg/m^2 basis.

14 CLINICAL STUDIES

14.1 Schizophrenia

Adults
The efficacy of SEROQUEL in the treatment of schizophrenia was established in 3 short-term (6-week) controlled trials of inpatients with schizophrenia who met DSM III-R criteria for schizophrenia. Although a single fixed dose haloperidol arm was included as a comparative treatment in one of the three trials, this single haloperidol dose group was inadequate to provide a reliable and valid comparison of SEROQUEL and haloperidol.

Several instruments were used for assessing psychiatric signs and symptoms in these studies, among them the Brief Psychiatric Rating Scale (BPRS), a multi-item inventory of general psychopathology traditionally used to evaluate the effects of drug treatment in schizophrenia. The BPRS psychosis cluster (conceptual disorganization, hallucinatory behavior, suspiciousness, and unusual thought content) is considered a particularly useful subset for assessing actively psychotic schizophrenic patients. A second traditional assessment, the Clinical Global Impression (CGI), reflects the impression of a skilled observer, fully familiar with the manifestations of schizophrenia, about the overall clinical state of the patient.

The results of the trials follow:
1. In a 6-week, placebo-controlled trial (n=361) involving 5 fixed doses of SEROQUEL (75 mg/day, 150 mg/day, 300 mg/day, 600 mg/day and 750 mg/day given in divided doses three times per day), the 4 highest doses of SEROQUEL were generally superior to placebo on the BPRS total score, the BPRS psychosis cluster and the CGI severity score, with the maximal effect seen at 300 mg/day, and the effects of doses of 150 mg/day to 750 mg/day were generally indistinguishable.
2. In a 6-week, placebo-controlled trial (n=286) involving titration of SEROQUEL in high (up to 750 mg/day given in divided doses three times per day) and low (up to 250 mg/day given in divided doses three times per day) doses, only the high dose SEROQUEL group (mean dose, 500 mg/day) was superior to placebo on the BPRS total score, the BPRS psychosis cluster, and the CGI severity score.
3. In a 6-week dose and dose regimen comparison trial (n=618) involving two fixed doses of SEROQUEL (450 mg/day given in divided doses both twice daily and three times daily and 50 mg/day given in divided doses twice daily), only the 450 mg/day (225 mg twice daily) dose group was superior to the 50 mg/day (25 mg given twice daily) SEROQUEL dose group on the BPRS total score, the BPRS psychosis cluster, and the CGI severity score.

Examination of population subsets (race, gender, and age) did not reveal any differential responsiveness on the basis of race or gender, with an apparently greater effect in patients under the age of 40 years compared to those older than 40. The clinical significance of this finding is unknown.

Adolescents (ages 13-17)
The efficacy of SEROQUEL in the treatment of schizophrenia in adolescents (13–17 years of age) was demonstrated in a 6–week, double-blind, placebo-controlled trial. Patients who met DSM-IV diagnostic criteria for schizophrenia were randomized into one of three treatment groups: SEROQUEL 400 mg/day (n = 73), SEROQUEL 800 mg/day (n = 74), or placebo (n = 75). Study medication was initiated at 50 mg/day and on day 2 increased to 100 mg/per day (divided and given two or three times per day). Subsequently, the dose was titrated to the target dose of 400 mg/day or 800 mg/day using increments of 100 mg/day, divided and given two or three times daily. The primary efficacy variable was the mean change from baseline in total Positive and Negative Syndrome Scale (PANSS).

SEROQUEL at 400 mg/day and 800 mg/day was superior to placebo in the reduction of PANSS total score.

14.2 Bipolar Disorder

Manic Episodes

Adults
The efficacy of SEROQUEL in the acute treatment of manic episodes was established in 3 placebo-controlled trials in patients who met DSM-IV criteria for bipolar I disorder with manic episodes. These trials included patients with or without psychotic features and excluded patients with rapid cycling and mixed episodes. Of these trials, 2 were monotherapy (12 weeks) and 1 was adjunct therapy (3 weeks) to either lithium or divalproex. Key outcomes in these trials were change from baseline in the Young Mania Rating Scale (YMRS) score at 3 and 12 weeks for monotherapy and at 3 weeks for adjunct therapy. Adjunct therapy is defined as the simultaneous initiation or subsequent administration of SEROQUEL with lithium or divalproex.

The primary rating instrument used for assessing manic symptoms in these trials was YMRS, an 11-item clinician-rated scale traditionally used to assess the degree of manic symptomatology (irritability, disruptive/aggressive behavior, sleep, elevated mood, speech, increased activity, sexual interest, language/thought disorder, thought content, appearance, and insight) in a range from 0 (no manic features) to 60 (maximum score).

The results of the trials follow:

Monotherapy
The efficacy of SEROQUEL in the acute treatment of bipolar mania was established in 2 placebo-controlled trials. In two 12-week trials (n=300, n=299) comparing SEROQUEL to placebo, SEROQUEL was superior to placebo in the reduction of the YMRS total score at weeks 3 and 12. The majority of patients in these trials taking SEROQUEL were dosed in a range between 400 mg/day and 800 mg per day.

Adjunct Therapy
In this 3-week placebo-controlled trial, 170 patients with bipolar mania (YMRS $\geq$ 20) were randomized to receive SEROQUEL or placebo as adjunct treatment to lithium or divalproex. Patients may or may not have received an adequate treatment course of lithium or divalproex prior to randomization. SEROQUEL was superior to placebo when added to lithium or divalproex alone in the reduction of YMRS total score.

The majority of patients in this trial taking SEROQUEL were dosed in a range between 400 mg/day and 800 mg per day. In a similarly designed trial (n=200), SEROQUEL was associated with an improvement in YMRS scores but did not demonstrate superiority to placebo, possibly due to a higher placebo effect.

Children and Adolescents (ages 10-17)
The efficacy of SEROQUEL in the acute treatment of manic episodes associated with bipolar I disorder in children and adolescents (10 to 17 years of age) was demonstrated in a 3-week, double-blind, placebo-controlled, multicenter trial. Patients who met DSM-IV diagnostic criteria for a manic episode were randomized into one of three treatment groups: SEROQUEL 400 mg/day (n = 95), SEROQUEL 600 mg/day (n = 98), or placebo (n = 91). Study medication was initiated at 50 mg/day and on day 2 increased to 100 mg/day (divided doses given two or three times daily). Subsequently, the dose was titrated to a target dose of 400 mg/day or 600 mg/day using increments of 100 mg/day, given in divided doses two or three times daily. The primary efficacy variable was the mean change from baseline in total YMRS score.

SEROQUEL 400 mg/day and 600 mg/day were superior to placebo in the reduction of YMRS total score.

Depressive Episodes
Adults
The efficacy of SEROQUEL for the acute treatment of depressive episodes associated with bipolar disorder was established in 2 identically designed 8-week, randomized, double-blind, placebo-controlled studies (N=1045). These studies included patients with either bipolar I or II disorder and those with or without a rapid cycling course. Patients randomized to SEROQUEL were administered fixed doses of either 300 mg or 600 mg once daily.

The primary rating instrument used to assess depressive symptoms in these studies was the Montgomery-Asberg Depression Rating Scale (MADRS), a 10-item clinician-rated scale with scores ranging from 0 to 60. The primary endpoint in both studies was the change from baseline in MADRS score at week 8. In both studies, SEROQUEL was superior to placebo in reduction of MADRS score. Improvement in symptoms, as measured by change in MADRS score relative to placebo, was seen in both studies at Day 8 (week 1) and onwards. In these studies, no additional benefit was seen with the 600 mg dose. For the 300 mg dose group, statistically significant improvements over placebo were seen in overall quality of life and satisfaction related to various areas of functioning, as measured using the Q-LES-Q(SF).

Maintenance Treatment as an Adjunct to Lithium or Divalproex
The efficacy of SEROQUEL in the maintenance treatment of bipolar I disorder was established in 2 placebo-controlled trials in patients (n=1326) who met DSM-IV criteria for bipolar I disorder. The trials included patients whose most recent episode was manic, depressed, or mixed, with or without psychotic features. In the open-label phase, patients were required to be stable on SEROQUEL plus lithium or divalproex for at least 12 weeks in order to be randomized. On average, patients were stabilized for 15 weeks. In the randomization phase, patients continued treatment with lithium or divalproex and were randomized to receive either SEROQUEL (administered twice daily totaling 400 mg/day to 800 mg/day) or placebo. Approximately 50% of the patients had discontinued from the SEROQUEL group by day 280 and 50% of the placebo group had discontinued by day 117 of double-blind treatment. The primary endpoint in these studies was time to recurrence of a mood event (manic, mixed or depressed episode). A mood event was defined as medication initiation or hospitalization for a mood episode; YMRS score ≥ 20 or MADRS score ≥ 20 at 2 consecutive assessments; or study discontinuation due to a mood event.

In both studies, SEROQUEL was superior to placebo in increasing the time to recurrence of any mood event. The treatment effect was present for increasing time to recurrence of both manic and depressed episodes. The effect of SEROQUEL was independent of any specific subgroup (assigned mood stabilizer, sex, age, race, most recent bipolar episode, or rapid cycling course).

16   HOW SUPPLIED/STORAGE AND HANDLING
25 mg Tablets (NDC 0310-0275) peach, round, biconvex, film coated tablets, identified with 'SEROQUEL' and '25' on one side and plain on the other side, are supplied in bottles of 100 tablets and 1000 tablets, and hospital unit dose packages of 100 tablets.

50 mg Tablets (NDC 0310-0278) white, round, biconvex, film coated tablets, identified with 'SEROQUEL' and '50' on one side and plain on the other side, are supplied in bottles of 100 tablets and 1000 tablets, and hospital unit dose packages of 100 tablets.

100 mg Tablets (NDC 0310-0271) yellow, round, biconvex film coated tablets, identified with 'SEROQUEL' and '100'

on one side and plain on the other side, are supplied in bottles of 100 tablets, and hospital unit dose packages of 100 tablets.

200 mg Tablets (NDC 0310-0272) white, round, biconvex, film coated tablets, identified with 'SEROQUEL' and '200' on one side and plain on the other side, are supplied in bottles of 100 tablets, and hospital unit dose packages of 100 tablets.

300 mg Tablets (NDC 0310-0274) white, capsule-shaped, biconvex, film coated tablets, intagliated with 'SEROQUEL' on one side and '300' on the other side, are supplied in bottles of 60 tablets, and hospital unit dose packages of 100 tablets.

400 mg Tablets (NDC 0310-0279) yellow, capsule-shaped, biconvex, film coated tablets, intagliated with 'SEROQUEL' on one side and '400' on the other side, are supplied in bottles of 100 tablets, and hospital unit dose packages of 100 tablets.

Store at 25°C (77°F); excursions permitted to 15-30°C (59-86°F) [See USP].

17   PATIENT COUNSELING INFORMATION
[see Medication Guide]
Prescribers or other health professionals should inform patients, their families, and their caregivers about the benefits and risks associated with treatment with SEROQUEL and should counsel them in its appropriate use. A patient Medication Guide about "Antidepressant Medicines, Depression and other Serious Mental Illness, and Suicidal Thoughts or Actions" is available for SEROQUEL. The prescriber or health professional should instruct patients, their families, and their caregivers to read the Medication Guide and should assist them in understanding its contents. Patients should be given the opportunity to discuss the contents of the Medication Guide and to obtain answers to any questions they may have. The complete text of the Medication Guide is reprinted at the end of this document.

Patients should be advised of the following issues and asked to alert their prescriber if these occur while taking SEROQUEL.

Increased Mortality in Elderly Patients with Dementia-Related Psychosis
Patients and caregivers should be advised that elderly patients with dementia-related psychosis treated with atypical antipsychotic drugs are at increased risk of death compared with placebo. Quetiapine is not approved for elderly patients with dementia-related psychosis [see Warnings and Precautions (5.1)].

Clinical Worsening and Suicide Risk
Patients, their families, and their caregivers should be encouraged to be alert to the emergence of anxiety, agitation, panic attacks, insomnia, irritability, hostility, aggressiveness, impulsivity, akathisia (psychomotor restlessness), hypomania, mania, other unusual changes in behavior, worsening of depression, and suicidal ideation, especially early during antidepressant treatment and when the dose is adjusted up or down. Families and caregivers of patients should be advised to look for the emergence of such symptoms on a day-to-day basis, since changes may be abrupt. Such symptoms should be reported to the patient's prescriber or health professional, especially if they are severe, abrupt in onset, or were not part of the patient's presenting symptoms. Symptoms such as these may be associated with an increased risk for suicidal thinking and behavior and indicate a need for very close monitoring and possibly changes in the medication [see Warnings and Precautions (5.2)].

Neuroleptic Malignant Syndrome (NMS)
Patients should be advised to report to their physician any signs or symptoms that may be related to NMS. These may include muscle stiffness and high fever [see Warnings and Precautions (5.3)].

Hyperglycemia and Diabetes Mellitus
Patients should be aware of the symptoms of hyperglycemia (high blood sugar) and diabetes mellitus. Patients who are diagnosed with diabetes, those with risk factors for diabetes, or those that develop these symptoms during treatment should have their blood glucose monitored at the beginning of and periodically during treatment [see Warnings and Precautions (5.4)].

Hyperlipidemia
Patients should be advised that elevations in total cholesterol, LDL cholesterol and triglycerides and decreases in HDL-cholesterol may occur. Patients should have their lipid profile monitored at the beginning of and periodically during treatment [see Warnings and Precautions (5.5)].

Weight Gain
Patients should be advised that they may experience weight gain. Patients should have their weight monitored regularly [see Warnings and Precautions (5.6)].

Orthostatic Hypotension
Patients should be advised of the risk of orthostatic hypotension (symptoms include feeling dizzy or lightheaded upon standing, which may lead to falls), especially during

the period of initial dose titration, and also at times of re-initiating treatment or increases in dose [see Warnings and Precautions (5.8)].

Increased Blood Pressure in Children and Adolescents
Blood pressure should be measured at the beginning of, and periodically during, treatment [see Warnings and Precautions (5.9)].

Leukopenia/Neutropenia
Patients with a pre-existing low WBC or a history of drug induced leukopenia/neutropenia should be advised that they should have their CBC monitored while taking SEROQUEL [see Warnings and Precautions (5.10)].

Interference with Cognitive and Motor Performance
Patients should be advised of the risk of somnolence or sedation (which may lead to falls), especially during the period of initial dose titration. Patients should be cautioned about performing any activity requiring mental alertness, such as operating a motor vehicle (including automobiles) or operating machinery, until they are reasonably certain quetiapine therapy does not affect them adversely. Patients should limit consumption of alcohol during treatment with quetiapine [see Warnings and Precautions (5.16)].

Heat Exposure and Dehydration
Patients should be advised regarding appropriate care in avoiding overheating and dehydration [see Warnings and Precautions (5.18)].

Concomitant Medication
As with other medications, patients should be advised to notify their physicians if they are taking, or plan to take, any prescription or over-the-counter drugs [see Warnings and Precautions (5.21)].

Pregnancy and Nursing
Patients should be advised to notify their physician if they become pregnant or intend to become pregnant during therapy. Patients should be advised not to breast feed if they are taking quetiapine [see Use in Specific Populations (8.1) and (8.3)].

Need for Comprehensive Treatment Program
SEROQUEL is indicated as an integral part of a total treatment program for adolescents with schizophrenia and pediatric bipolar disorder that may include other measures (psychological, educational, and social). Effectiveness and safety of SEROQUEL have not been established in pediatric patients less than 13 years of age for schizophrenia or less than 10 years of age for bipolar mania. Appropriate educational placement is essential and psychosocial intervention is often helpful. The decision to prescribe atypical antipsychotic medication will depend upon the physician's assessment of the chronicity and severity of the patient's symptoms.

SPL MEDGUIDE SECTION

Medication Guide
SEROQUEL (SER-oh-kwell)
(quetiapine fumarate)
Tablets
Read this Medication Guide before you start taking SEROQUEL and each time you get a refill. There may be new information. This Medication Guide does not take the place of talking to your healthcare provider about your medical condition or treatment.

What is the most important information I should know about SEROQUEL?
Serious side effects may happen when you take SEROQUEL, including
- **Risk of death in the elderly with dementia:** Medicines like SEROQUEL can raise the risk of death in elderly people who have lost touch with reality due to confusion and memory loss (dementia). SEROQUEL is not approved for treating psychosis in the elderly with dementia.
- **Risk of suicidal thoughts or actions:** Antidepressant medicines, depression and other serious mental illnesses, and suicidal thoughts or actions:
1. Antidepressant medicines may increase suicidal thoughts or actions in some children, teenagers, and young adults within the first few months of treatment.
2. Depression and other serious mental illnesses are the most important causes of suicidal thoughts and actions. Some people may have a particularly high risk of having suicidal thoughts or actions. These include people who have (or have a family history of) depression, bipolar illness (also called manic-depressive illness), or suicidal thoughts or actions.
3. How can I watch for and try to prevent suicidal thoughts and actions in myself or a family member?
   - Pay close attention to any changes, especially sudden changes, in mood, behaviors, thoughts, or feelings. This is very important when an antidepressant medicine is started or when the dose is changed.
   - Call the healthcare provider right away to report new or sudden changes in mood, behavior, thoughts, or feelings.
   - Keep all follow-up visits with the healthcare provider as scheduled. Call the healthcare provider between vis-

its as needed, especially if you have concerns about symptoms.

Call a healthcare provider right away if you or your family member has any of the following symptoms, especially if they are new, worse, or worry you:

- thoughts about suicide or dying
- attempts to commit suicide
- new or worse depression
- new or worse anxiety
- feeling very agitated or restless
- panic attacks
- trouble sleeping (insomnia)
- new or worse irritability
- acting aggressive, being angry, or violent
- acting on dangerous impulses
- an extreme increase in activity and talking (mania)
- other unusual changes in behavior or mood

What else do I need to know about antidepressant medicines?

- **Never stop an antidepressant medicine without first talking to a healthcare provider.** Stopping an antidepressant medicine suddenly can cause other symptoms.
- **Antidepressants are medicines used to treat depression and other illnesses.** It is important to discuss all the risks of treating depression and also the risks of not treating it. Patients and their families or other caregivers should discuss all treatment choices with the healthcare provider, not just the use of antidepressants.
- **Antidepressant medicines have other side effects.** Talk to the healthcare provider about the side effects of the medicine prescribed for you or your family member.
- **Antidepressant medicines can interact with other medicines.** Know all of the medicines that you or your family member take. Keep a list of all medicines to show the healthcare provider. Do not start new medicines without first checking with your healthcare provider.
- **Not all antidepressant medicines prescribed for children are FDA approved for use in children.** Talk to your child's healthcare provider for more information.

What is SEROQUEL?

- SEROQUEL is a prescription medicine used to treat schizophrenia in people age 13 or older.
- SEROQUEL is a prescription medicine used to treat bipolar disorder, including:
  - depressive episodes associated with bipolar disorder in adults
  - manic episodes associated with bipolar I disorder alone or with lithium or divalproex in adults
  - long-term treatment of bipolar I disorder with lithium or divalproex in adults
- SEROQUEL is used to treat manic episodes associated with bipolar I disorder in children ages 10 to 17 years. SEROQUEL has not been studied in patients younger than 10 years of age.

What should I tell my healthcare provider before taking SEROQUEL?

Before taking SEROQUEL, tell your healthcare provider if you have or have had:

- diabetes or high blood sugar in you or your family: your healthcare provider should check your blood sugar before you start SEROQUEL and also during therapy
- high levels of total cholesterol, triglycerides or LDL-cholesterol or low levels of HDL-cholesterol
- low or high blood pressure
- low white blood cell count
- cataracts
- seizures
- abnormal thyroid tests
- high prolactin levels
- heart problems
- liver problems
- any other medical condition
- pregnancy or plans to become pregnant. It is not known if SEROQUEL will harm your unborn baby
- breast-feeding or plans to breast-feed. It is not known if SEROQUEL will pass into your breast milk. You and your healthcare provider should decide if you will take SEROQUEL or breast-feed. You should not do both.

Tell the healthcare provider about all the medicines that you take or recently have taken including prescription medicines, non-prescription medicines, herbal supplements and vitamins.

SEROQUEL and other medicines may affect each other causing serious side effects. SEROQUEL may affect the way other medicines work, and other medicines may affect how SEROQUEL works.

Especially tell your healthcare provider if you take or plan to take medicines for:

- depression
- high blood pressure
- Parkinson's disease
- trouble sleeping

Also tell your healthcare provider if you take or plan to take any of these medicines:

- phenytoin, divalproex or carbamazepine (for epilepsy)
- barbiturates (to help you sleep)
- rifampin (for tuberculosis)
- glucocorticoids (steroids for inflammation)
- thioridazine (an antipsychotic)
- ketoconazole, fluconazole or itraconazole (for fungal infections)
- erythromycin (an antibiotic)
- protease inhibitors (for HIV)

This is not a complete list of medicines that can affect or be affected by SEROQUEL. Your doctor can tell you if it is safe to take SEROQUEL with your other medicines. Do not start or stop any medicines while taking SEROQUEL without talking to your healthcare provider first. Know the medicines you take. Keep a list of your medicines to show your healthcare provider and pharmacist when you get a new medicine.

Tell your healthcare provider if you are having a urine drug screen because SEROQUEL may affect your test results. Tell those giving the test that you are taking SEROQUEL.

How should I take SEROQUEL?

- Take SEROQUEL exactly as your healthcare provider tells you to take it. Do not change the dose yourself.
- Take SEROQUEL by mouth, with or without food.
- If you feel you need to stop SEROQUEL, talk with your healthcare provider first.

If you suddenly stop taking SEROQUEL, you may experience side effects such as trouble sleeping or trouble staying asleep (insomnia), nausea, and vomiting.

- If you miss a dose, take it as soon as you remember. If it is close to the next dose, skip the missed dose. Just take the next dose at your regular time. Do not take 2 doses at the same time unless your healthcare provider tells you to. If you are not sure about your dosing, call your healthcare provider.
- If you take too much SEROQUEL, call your healthcare provider or poison control center at 1-800-222-1222 right away or go to the nearest hospital emergency room.

What should I avoid while taking SEROQUEL?

Do not drive, operate machinery, or do other dangerous activities until you know how SEROQUEL affects you. SEROQUEL may make you drowsy.

- Avoid getting over-heated or dehydrated.
  - Do not over-exercise.
  - In hot weather, stay inside in a cool place if possible.
  - Stay out of the sun. Do not wear too much or heavy clothing.
  - Drink plenty of water.
- Do not drink alcohol while taking SEROQUEL. It may make some side effects of SEROQUEL worse.

What are possible side effects of SEROQUEL?

Serious side effects have been reported with SEROQUEL including:

Also, see "What is the most important information I should know about SEROQUEL?" at the beginning of this Medication Guide

- **Neuroleptic malignant syndrome (NMS):** Tell your healthcare provider right away if you have some or all of the following symptoms: high fever, stiff muscles, confusion, sweating, changes in pulse, heart rate, and blood pressure. These may be symptoms of a rare and serious condition that can lead to death. Stop SEROQUEL and call your healthcare provider right away.
- **High blood sugar (hyperglycemia):** Increases in blood sugar can happen in some people who take SEROQUEL. Extremely high blood sugar can lead to coma or death. If you have diabetes or risk factors for diabetes (such as being overweight or a family history of diabetes) your healthcare provider should check your blood sugar before you start SEROQUEL and during therapy.

Call your healthcare provider if you have any of these symptoms of high blood sugar while taking SEROQUEL:

- feel very thirsty
- need to urinate more than usual
- feel very hungry
- feel weak or tired
- feel sick to your stomach
- feel confused, or your breath smells fruity
- **High cholesterol and triglyceride levels in the blood (fat in the blood):** Increases in total cholesterol, triglycerides and LDL (bad) cholesterol and decreases in HDL (good) cholesterol have been reported in clinical trials with SEROQUEL. You may not have any symptoms, so your healthcare provider should do blood tests to check your cholesterol and triglyceride levels before you start taking SEROQUEL and during therapy.
- **Increase in weight (weight gain):** Weight gain has been seen in patients who take SEROQUEL so you and your healthcare provider should check your weight regularly.
- **Tardive dyskinesia:** Tell your healthcare provider about any movements you cannot control in your face, tongue, or other body parts. These may be signs of a serious condi-

tion. Tardive dyskinesia may not go away, even if you stop taking SEROQUEL. Tardive dyskinesia may also start after you stop taking SEROQUEL.

- **Orthostatic hypotension (decreased blood pressure):** lightheadedness or fainting caused by a sudden change in heart rate and blood pressure when rising too quickly from a sitting or lying position.
- **Increases in blood pressure:** reported in children and teenagers. Your healthcare provider should check blood pressure in children and adolescents before starting SEROQUEL and during therapy.
- **Low white blood cell count**
- **Cataracts**
- **Seizures**
- **Abnormal thyroid tests:** Your healthcare provider may do blood tests to check your thyroid hormone level.
- **Increases in prolactin levels:** Your healthcare provider may do blood tests to check your prolactin levels.
- **Increases in liver enzymes:** Your healthcare provider may do blood tests to check your liver enzyme levels.
- **Long lasting and painful erection**
- **Difficulty swallowing**

Common possible side effects with SEROQUEL include:

Adults:

- drowsiness
- dry mouth
- dizziness
- weakness
- weight gain
- abdominal pain
- constipation
- sore throat
- sluggishness
- upset stomach
- weight gain
- a sudden drop in blood pressure upon standing
- adnormal liver tests

Children and Adolescents:

- drowsiness
- fatigue
- nausea
- dry mouth
- weight gain
- dizziness
- increased appetite
- vomiting
- rapid heart rate

These are not all the possible side effects of SEROQUEL. For more information, ask your healthcare provider or pharmacist.

Call your healthcare provider for medical advice about side effects. You may report side effects to FDA at 1-800-FDA-1088.

How should I store SEROQUEL?

- Store SEROQUEL at room temperature, between 59°F to 86°F (15°C to 30°C).
- Keep SEROQUEL and all medicines out of the reach of children.

General information about SEROQUEL

Do not take SEROQUEL unless your healthcare provider has prescribed it for you for your condition. Do not share SEROQUEL with other people, even if they have the same condition. It may harm them.

This Medication Guide provides a summary of important information about SEROQUEL. For more information about SEROQUEL, talk with your healthcare provider or pharmacist or call 1-800-236-9933. You can ask your healthcare provider for information about SEROQUEL that is written for health professionals.

What are the ingredients in SEROQUEL?

Active ingredient: quetiapine fumarate

Inactive ingredients: povidone, dibasic dicalcium phosphate dihydrate, microcrystalline cellulose, sodium starch glycolate, lactose monohydrate, magnesium stearate, hypromellose, polyethylene glycol, and titanium dioxide. The 25 mg tablets contain red and yellow ferric oxide. The 100 mg and 400 mg tablets contain only yellow ferric oxide

The symptoms of Schizophrenia include:

- Having lost touch with reality (psychosis)
- Seeing things that are not there or hearing voices (hallucinations)
- Believing things that are not true (delusions)
- Being suspicious (paranoia).

The symptoms of Bipolar Disorder include:

- General symptoms of bipolar disorder include extreme mood swings, along with other specific symptoms and behaviors. These mood swings, or "episodes," include manic (highs) and depressive (lows)
- Common symptoms of a manic episode include feeling extremely happy, being very irritable, restless, talking too fast and too much, and having more energy and needing less sleep than usual
- Common symptoms of a depressive episode include feelings of sadness or emptiness, increased tearfulness, a loss

of interest in activities you once enjoyed, loss of energy, difficulty concentrating or making decisions, feelings of worthlessness or guilt, changes in sleep or appetite.
• Thoughts of death or suicide.

This Medication Guide has been approved by the U.S. Food and Drug Administration.
SEROQUEL is a trademark of the AstraZeneca group of companies.
©AstraZeneca 2010
Distributed by:
AstraZeneca Pharmaceuticals LP
Wilmington, DE 19850
SIC 35534–03
Rev. 05/10
Shown in Product Identification Guide, page 306

SEROQUEL XR®   ℞
[SER-oh-kwell]
(quetiapine fumarate)
Extended-Release Tablets

HIGHLIGHTS OF PRESCRIBING INFORMATION
These highlights do not include all the information needed to use SEROQUEL XR safely and effectively. See full prescribing information for SEROQUEL XR.
SEROQUEL XR® *(quetiapine fumarate) Extended-Release Tablets*
Initial U.S. Approval: 1997

WARNING: INCREASED MORTALITY IN ELDERLY PATIENTS WITH DEMENTIA-RELATED PSYCHOSIS
See full prescribing information for complete boxed warning.
• **Antipsychotic drugs are associated with an increased risk of death. (5.1)**
• **Quetiapine is not approved for elderly patients with Dementia-Related Psychosis. (5.1)**
WARNING: SUICIDALITY AND ANTIDEPRESSANT DRUGS *See full prescribing information for complete boxed warning.*
• **Increased risk of suicidal thinking and behavior in children, adolescents and young adults taking antidepressants for major depressive disorder and other psychiatric disorders. (5.2)**

RECENT MAJOR CHANGES
Indications and Usage, Schizophrenia (1.1), 12/2009
Indications and Usage, Bipolar Disorder (1.2), 12/2009
Indications and Usage, Major Depressive Disorder (MDD), Adjunctive Treatment with Antidepressants (1.3), 12/2009
Dosage and Administration, Schizophrenia (2.1), 12/2009
Dosage and Administration, Bipolar Disorder (2.2), 12/2009
Dosage and Administration, Major Depressive Disorder (MDD), Adjunctive Treatment with Antidepressants (2.3), 12/2009
Warnings and Precautions, Hyperglycemia (5.4), 12/2009
Warnings and Precautions, Hyperlipidemia (5.5), 12/2009
Warnings and Precautions, Weight Gain (5.6), 12/2009
Warnings and Precautions, Increases in Blood Pressure (Children and Adolescents) (5.9), 12/2009
Warnings and Precautions, Potential for Cognitive and Motor Impairment (5.16), 12/2009
Warnings and Precautions, Suicide (5.20), 12/2009
Warnings and Precautions, Use in Patients with Concomitant Illness (5.21), 01/2010
Warnings and Precautions, Withdrawal (5.22), 05/2010

INDICATIONS AND USAGE
SEROQUEL XR is an atypical antipsychotic indicated for the:
Treatment of schizophrenia (1.1)
• Adults: Efficacy was established with SEROQUEL XR in one 6-week and one maintenance trial in patients with schizophrenia as well as in three 6-week trials with SEROQUEL in patients with schizophrenia (14.1)
Acute treatment of manic or mixed episodes associated with bipolar I disorder, both as monotherapy and as an adjunct to lithium or divalproex (1.2)
• Adults: Efficacy was established with SEROQUEL XR in one 3-week trial in patients with manic or mixed episodes associated with bipolar I disorder as well as two 12-week monotherapy trials and one 3-week adjunctive trial with SEROQUEL in patients with manic episodes associated with bipolar I disorder (14.2)
Acute treatment of depressive episodes associated with bipolar disorder (1.2)
• Adults: Efficacy was established with SEROQUEL XR in one 8-week trial in patients with bipolar I or II disorder as well as two 8-week trials with SEROQUEL in patients with bipolar I or II disorder (14.2)
Maintenance treatment of bipolar I disorder as an adjunct to lithium or divalproex (1.2)
• Adults: Efficacy was established with SEROQUEL in two maintenance trials in patients with bipolar I disorder (14.2)
Adjunctive treatment of major depressive disorder (MDD) (1.3)
• Adults: Efficacy as an adjunct to antidepressants was established in two 6-week trials in patients with MDD who had an inadequate response to an antidepressant alone (14.3)

DOSAGE AND ADMINISTRATION
SEROQUEL XR Tablets should be swallowed whole and not split, chewed or crushed. SEROQUEL XR should be taken without food or with a light meal (approx. 300 calories). SEROQUEL XR should be administered once daily, preferably in the evening.
[See table below]

DOSAGE FORMS AND STRENGTHS
Extended-Release Tablets: 50 mg, 150 mg, 200 mg, 300 mg, and 400 mg

CONTRAINDICATIONS
None (4)

WARNINGS AND PRECAUTIONS
• **Increased Mortality in Elderly Patients with Dementia-Related Psychosis:** Antipsychotic drugs, including quetiapine, are associated with an increased risk of death; causes of death are variable. (5.1)
• **Suicidality and Antidepressant Drugs:** Increased the risk of suicidal thinking and behavior in children, adolescents and young adults taking antidepressants for major depressive disorder and other psychiatric disorders (5.2)
• **Neuroleptic Malignant Syndrome (NMS):** Manage with immediate discontinuation and close monitoring. (5.3)
• **Hyperglycemia and Diabetes Mellitus (DM):** Ketoacidosis, hyperosmolar coma and death have been reported in patients treated with atypical antipsychotics, including quetiapine. Any patient treated with atypical antipsychotics should be monitored for symptoms of hyperglycemia including polydipsia, polyuria, polyphagia, and weakness. When starting treatment, patients with diabetes or risk factors for diabetes should undergo blood glucose testing before and during treatment. (5.4)
• **Hyperlipidemia:** Undesirable alterations in lipids have been observed. Increases in total cholesterol, LDL-cholesterol and triglycerides and decreases in HDL-cholesterol have been reported in clinical trials. Appropriate clinical monitoring is recommended, including fasting

blood lipid testing at the beginning of, and periodically, during treatment. (5.5)
• **Weight Gain:** Patients should receive regular monitoring of weight. (5.6)
• **Tardive Dyskinesia:** Discontinue if clinically appropriate. (5.7)
• **Orthostatic Hypotension:** Associated dizziness, tachycardia and syncope may occur especially during the initial dose titration period. Use in caution in patients with known cardiovascular or cerebrovascular disease. (5.8)
• **Increased Blood Pressure in Children and Adolescents:** Blood pressure should be measured at the beginning of, and periodically during treatment in children and adolescents. SEROQUEL XR has not been evaluated in pediatric patients. (5.9)
• **Leukopenia, Neutropenia and Agranulocytosis:** have been reported with atypical antipsychotics including SEROQUEL XR. Patients with a pre-existing low white cell count (WBC) or a history of leukopenia/neutropenia should have complete blood count (CBC) monitored frequently during the first few months of treatment and should discontinue SEROQUEL XR at the first sign of a decline in WBC in absence of other causative factors. (5.10)
• **Cataracts:** Lens changes have been observed in patients during long-term quetiapine treatment. Lens examination is recommended when starting treatment and at 6-month intervals during chronic treatment. (5.11)
• **Suicide:** The possibility of a suicide attempt is inherent in schizophrenia, bipolar disorder and depression and close supervision of high risk patients should accompany drug therapy. (5.20)
• See Full Prescribing Information for additional **WARNINGS and PRECAUTIONS.**

ADVERSE REACTIONS
Most common adverse reactions (incidence ≥5% and twice placebo) in decreasing frequency are: somnolence, dry mouth, constipation, dizziness, increased appetite, dyspepsia, weight gain, fatigue, dysarthria, and nasal congestion. (6.1)
To report SUSPECTED ADVERSE REACTIONS, contact AstraZeneca at 1-800-236-9933 or FDA at 1-800-FDA-1088 or www.fda.gov/medwatch.

DRUG INTERACTIONS
• **P450 3A Inhibitors:** May decrease the clearance of quetiapine. Lower doses of quetiapine may be required. (7.1)
• **Hepatic Enzyme Inducers:** May increase the clearance of quetiapine. Higher doses of quetiapine may be required with phenytoin or other inducers. (7.1)
• **Centrally Acting Drugs:** Caution should be used when quetiapine is used in combination with other CNS acting drugs. (7)
• **Antihypertensive Agents:** Quetiapine may add to the hypotensive effects of these agents. (7)
• **Levodopa and Dopamine Agents:** Quetiapine may antagonize the effect of these drugs. (7)
• **Drugs known to cause electrolyte imbalance or increase QT interval:** Caution should be used when quetiapine is used concomitantly with these drugs. (7)
• **Interference with Urine Drug Screens:** False positive urine drug screens for methadone or tricyclic antidepressants (TCAs) in patients taking quetiapine have been reported. (7)

USE IN SPECIFIC POPULATIONS
• **Geriatric Use:** Consider a lower starting dose (50 mg/day), slower titration, and careful monitoring during the initial dosing period in the elderly. (2.3 and 8.5)
• **Hepatic Impairment:** Lower starting doses (50 mg/day) and slower titration may be needed. (2.3, 8.7, 12.3)
• **Pregnancy:** Limited human data. Based on animal data, may cause fetal harm. (8.1)
• **Nursing Mothers:** Caution should be exercised when administered to a nursing woman. (8.3)
• **Pediatric Use:** Safety and effectiveness have not been established. (8.4)
See 17 for PATIENT COUNSELING INFORMATION and Medication Guide

           Revised: 05/2010

FULL PRESCRIBING INFORMATION: CONTENTS*
WARNING: INCREASED MORTALITY IN ELDERLY PATIENTS WITH DEMENTIA-RELATED PSYCHOSIS
RECENT MAJOR CHANGES
1 INDICATIONS AND USAGE
    1.1 Schizophrenia
    1.2 Bipolar Disorder
    1.3 Adjunctive Treatment of Major Depressive Disorder (MDD)
2 DOSAGE AND ADMINISTRATION
    2.1 Schizophrenia
    2.2 Bipolar Disorder
    2.3 Major Depressive Disorder, Adjunctive Therapy with Antidepressants
    2.4 Dosing in Special Populations

Indication	Dosing Instructions*	Recommended Dose/Dose Range
Schizophrenia-(2.1)	Day 1: 300 mg/day	400-800 mg/day
	Dose increases can be made at intervals as short as 1 day and in increments of up to 300 mg/day.	
Schizophrenia Maintenance (Monotherapy) (2.1)	400 mg/day to 800 mg/day	400-800 mg/day
Bipolar Mania- Acute monotherapy or as an adjunct to lithium or divalproex (2.2)	Day 1: 300 mg. Day 2: 600 mg. Day 3: between 400 mg and 800 mg	400-800 mg/day
Depressive Episodes Associated with Bipolar Disorder (2.2)	Day 1: 50 mg Day 2: 100 mg Day 3: 200 mg Day 4: 300 mg	300 mg/day
Bipolar I Disorder- Maintenance Treatment as an adjunct to lithium or divalproex (2.2)	400 mg/day to 800 mg/day	400-800 mg/day
Major Depressive Disorder, Adjunctive Therapy with Antidepressants (2.3)	Day 1 and 2: 50 mg Day 3 and 4: 150 mg	150-300 mg/day

*After initial dosing, adjustments can be made upwards or downwards, if necessary, within the dose range depending upon the clinical response and tolerance of the patient.

FULL PRESCRIBING INFORMATION

> **WARNING: INCREASED MORTALITY IN ELDERLY PATIENTS WITH DEMENTIA-RELATED PSYCHOSIS**
> Elderly patients with dementia-related psychosis treated with antipsychotic drugs are at an increased risk of death. Analyses of seventeen placebo-controlled trials (modal duration of 10 weeks) largely in patients taking atypical antipsychotic drugs, revealed a risk of death in drug-treated patients of between 1.6 to 1.7 times the risk of death in placebo-treated patients. Over the course of a typical 10-week controlled trial, the rate of death in drug-treated patients was about 4.5%, compared to a rate of about 2.6% in the placebo group. Although the causes of death were varied, most of the deaths appeared to be either cardiovascular (e.g., heart failure, sudden death) or infectious (e.g., pneumonia) in nature. Observational studies suggest that, similar to atypical antipsychotic drugs, treatment with conventional antipsychotic drugs may increase mortality. The extent to which the findings of increased mortality in observational studies may be attributed to the antipsychotic drug as opposed to some characteristic(s) of the patients is not clear. SEROQUEL XR is not approved for the treatment of patients with dementia-related psychosis [see Warnings and Precautions (5.1)].
>
> **SUICIDALITY AND ANTIDEPRESSANT DRUGS**
> Antidepressants increased the risk compared to placebo of suicidal thinking and behavior (suicidality) in children, adolescents, and young adults in short-term studies of major depressive disorder (MDD) and other psychiatric disorders. Anyone considering the use of SEROQUEL XR or any other antidepressant in a child, adolescent, or young adult must balance this risk with the clinical need. Short-term studies did not show an increase in the risk of suicidality with antidepressants compared to placebo in adults beyond age 24; there was a reduction in risk with antidepressants compared to placebo in adults aged 65 and older. Depression and certain other psychiatric disorders are themselves associated with increases in the risk of suicide. Patients of all ages who are started on antidepressant therapy should be monitored appropriately and observed closely for clinical worsening, suicidality, or unusual changes in behavior. Families and caregivers should be advised of the need for close observation and communication with the prescriber. SEROQUEL XR is not approved for use in pediatric patients [see Warnings and Precautions (5.2)].

1 INDICATIONS AND USAGE

1.1 Schizophrenia

SEROQUEL XR is indicated for the treatment of schizophrenia. The efficacy of SEROQUEL XR in schizophrenia was established in one 6-week and one maintenance trial in adults with schizophrenia as well by extrapolation from three 6-week trials in adults with schizophrenia treated with SEROQUEL [see Clinical Studies (14.1)].

1.2 Bipolar Disorder

SEROQUEL XR is indicated for the acute treatment of manic or mixed episodes associated with bipolar I disorder, both as monotherapy and as an adjunct to lithium or divalproex. The efficacy of SEROQUEL XR in manic or mixed episodes of bipolar I disorder was established in one 3-week trial in adults with manic or mixed episodes associated with bipolar I disorder as well by extrapolation from two 12-week monotherapy and one 3-week adjunctive trial in adults with manic episodes associated with bipolar I disorder treated with SEROQUEL [see Clinical Studies (14.2)].

SEROQUEL XR is indicated for the acute treatment of depressive episodes associated with bipolar disorder. The efficacy of SEROQUEL XR was established in one 8-week trial in adults with bipolar I or II disorder as well as extrapolation from two 8-week trials in adults with bipolar I or II disorder treated with SEROQUEL [see Clinical Studies (14.2)].

SEROQUEL XR is indicated for the maintenance treatment of bipolar I disorder, as an adjunct to lithium or divalproex. Efficacy was extrapolated from two maintenance trials in adults with bipolar I disorder treated with SEROQUEL. The effectiveness of monotherapy for the maintenance treatment of bipolar disorder has not been systematically evaluated in controlled clinical trials [see Clinical Studies (14.2)].

1.3 Adjunctive Treatment of Major Depressive Disorder (MDD)

SEROQUEL XR is indicated for use as adjunctive therapy to antidepressants for the treatment of MDD. The efficacy of SEROQUEL XR as adjunctive therapy to antidepressants in MDD was established in two 6-week trials in adults with MDD who had an inadequate response to antidepressant treatment [see Clinical Studies (14.3)].

2 DOSAGE AND ADMINISTRATION

SEROQUEL XR tablets should be swallowed whole and not split, chewed or crushed.

It is recommended that SEROQUEL XR be taken without food or with a light meal (approximately 300 calories) [see Clinical Pharmacology (12.3)].

2.1 Schizophrenia

Dose Selection—SEROQUEL XR should be administered once daily, preferably in the evening. The recommended initial dose is 300 mg/day. Patients should be titrated within a dose range of 400 mg/day–800 mg/day depending on the response and tolerance of the individual patient [see Clinical Studies (14.1)]. Dose increases can be made at intervals as short as 1 day and in increments of up to 300 mg/day. The safety of doses above 800 mg/day has not been evaluated in clinical trials.

Maintenance Treatment—A maintenance trial in adult patients with schizophrenia treated with SEROQUEL XR has shown this drug to be effective in delaying time to relapse in patients who were stabilized on SEROQUEL XR at doses of 400 mg/day to 800 mg/day for 16 weeks. Patients should be periodically reassessed to determine the need for maintenance treatment and the appropriate dose for such treatment [see Clinical Studies (14.1)].

2.2 Bipolar Disorder

Bipolar Mania

Usual Dose for Acute Monotherapy or Adjunct Therapy (with lithium or divalproex)

Dose Selection—When used as monotherapy or adjunct therapy (with lithium or divalproex), SEROQUEL XR should be administered once daily in the evening starting with 300 mg on Day 1 and 600 mg on Day 2. SEROQUEL XR can be adjusted between 400 mg and 800 mg beginning on Day 3 depending on the response and tolerance of the individual patient.

Recommended Dosing Schedule

Day	Day 1	Day 2	Day 3
SEROQUEL XR	300 mg	600 mg	400 mg to 800 mg

Depressive Episodes Associated with Bipolar Disorder

Usual Dose—SEROQUEL XR should be administered once daily in the evening to reach 300 mg/day by Day 4.

Recommended Dosing Schedule

Day	Day 1	Day 2	Day 3	Day 4
SEROQUEL XR	50 mg	100 mg	200 mg	300 mg

Maintenance Treatment for Bipolar I Disorder

Maintenance Treatment—Maintenance of efficacy in bipolar I disorder was demonstrated with SEROQUEL (administered twice daily totaling 400 mg/day to 800 mg/day) as adjunct therapy to lithium or divalproex. Generally, in the maintenance phase, patients continued on the same dose on which they were stabilized during the stabilization phase. Patients should be periodically reassessed to determine the need for maintenance treatment and the appropriate dose for such treatment [see Clinical Studies (14.2)].

2.3 Major Depressive Disorder, Adjunctive Therapy with Antidepressants

Dose Selection—SEROQUEL XR in a dose range of 150 mg/day to 300 mg/day was demonstrated to be effective as adjunctive therapy to antidepressants. Begin with 50 mg once daily in the evening. On Day 3, the dose can be increased to 150 mg once daily in the evening. There were dose-dependent increases in adverse reactions in the recommended dose range of 150 mg/day to 300 mg/day. Doses above 300 mg/day were not studied [see Clinical Studies (14.3)].

2.4 Dosing in Special Populations

Consideration should be given to a slower rate of dose titration and a lower target dose in the elderly and in patients who are debilitated or who have a predisposition to hypotensive reactions [see Use in Specific Populations (8.5, 8.7) and Clinical Pharmacology (12)]. When indicated, dose escalation should be performed with caution in these patients.

Elderly patients should be started on SEROQUEL XR 50 mg/day and the dose can be increased in increments of 50 mg/day depending on the response and tolerance of the individual patient.

Patients with hepatic impairment should be started on SEROQUEL XR 50 mg/day. The dose can be increased daily in increments of 50 mg/day to an effective dose, depending on the clinical response and tolerance of the patient.

The elimination of quetiapine was enhanced in the presence of phenytoin. Higher maintenance doses of quetiapine may be required when it is coadministered with phenytoin and other enzyme inducers such as carbamazepine and phenobarbital [see Drug Interactions (7.1)].

2.5 Re-initiation of Treatment in Patients Previously Discontinued

Although there are no data to specifically address reinitiation of treatment, it is recommended that when restarting therapy of patients who have been off SEROQUEL XR for more than one week, the initial dosing schedule should be followed. When restarting patients who have been off SEROQUEL XR for less than one week, gradual dose escalation may not be required and the maintenance dose may be reinitiated.

2.6 Switching Patients from SEROQUEL Tablets to SEROQUEL XR Tablets

Patients who are currently being treated with SEROQUEL (immediate release formulation) may be switched to SEROQUEL XR at the equivalent total daily dose taken once daily. Individual dosage adjustments may be necessary.

2.7 Switching from Antipsychotics

There are no systematically collected data to specifically address switching patients from other antipsychotics to SEROQUEL XR, or concerning concomitant administration with other antipsychotics. While immediate discontinuation of the previous antipsychotic treatment may be acceptable for some patients, more gradual discontinuation may be most appropriate for others. In all cases, the period of overlapping antipsychotic administration should be minimized. When switching patients from depot antipsychotics, if medically appropriate, initiate SEROQUEL XR therapy in place of the next scheduled injection. The need for continuing existing extrapyramidal syndrome medication should be re-evaluated periodically.

3   DOSAGE FORMS AND STRENGTHS

50 mg extended-release tablets
150 mg extended-release tablets
200 mg extended-release tablets
300 mg extended-release tablets
400 mg extended-release tablets

4   CONTRAINDICATIONS

None

5   WARNINGS AND PRECAUTIONS

5.1   Increased Mortality in Elderly Patients with Dementia-Related Psychosis

Elderly patients with dementia-related psychosis treated with antipsychotic drugs are at an increased risk of death compared to placebo. SEROQUEL XR (quetiapine fumarate) is not approved for the treatment of patients with dementia-related psychosis [see Boxed Warning].

5.2   Clinical Worsening and Suicide Risk

Patients with major depressive disorder (MDD), both adult and pediatric, may experience worsening of their depression and/or the emergence of suicidal ideation and behavior (suicidality) or unusual changes in behavior, whether or not they are taking antidepressant medications, and this risk may persist until significant remission occurs. Suicide is a known risk of depression and certain other psychiatric disorders, and these disorders themselves are the strongest predictors of suicide. There has been a long-standing concern, however, that antidepressants may have a role in inducing worsening of depression and the emergence of suicidality in certain patients during the early phases of treatment. Pooled analyses of short-term placebo-controlled trials of antidepressant drugs (SSRIs and others) showed that these drugs increase the risk of suicidal thinking and behavior (suicidality) in children, adolescents, and young adults (ages 18-24) with major depressive disorder (MDD) and other psychiatric disorders. Short-term studies did not show an increase in the risk of suicidality with antidepressants compared to placebo in adults beyond age 24; there was a reduction with antidepressants compared to placebo in adults aged 65 and older.

The pooled analyses of placebo-controlled trials in children and adolescents with MDD, obsessive compulsive disorder (OCD), or other psychiatric disorders included a total of 24 short-term trials of 9 antidepressant drugs in over 4400 patients. The pooled analyses of placebo-controlled trials in adults with MDD or other psychiatric disorders included a total of 295 short-term trials (median duration of 2 months) of 11 antidepressant drugs in over 77,000 patients. There was considerable variation in risk of suicidality among drugs, but a tendency toward an increase in the younger patients for almost all drugs studied. There were differences in absolute risk of suicidality across the different indications, with the highest incidence in MDD. The risk differences (drug vs. placebo), however, were relatively stable within age strata and across indications. These risk differences (drug-placebo difference in the number of cases of suicidality per 1000 patients treated) are provided in Table 1.

Table 1

Age Range	Drug-Placebo Difference in Number of Cases of Suicidality per 1000 Patients Treated
	Increases Compared to Placebo
<18	14 additional cases
18–24	5 additional cases
	Decreases Compared to Placebo
25–64	1 fewer case
≥65	6 fewer cases

No suicides occurred in any of the pediatric trials. There were suicides in the adult trials, but the number was not sufficient to reach any conclusion about drug effect on suicide.

It is unknown whether the suicidality risk extends to longer-term use, i.e., beyond several months. However, there is substantial evidence from placebo-controlled maintenance trials in adults with depression that the use of antidepressants can delay the recurrence of depression.

Table 2: Fasting Glucose—Proportion of Patients Shifting to ≥ 126 mg/dL in short-term (≤ 12 weeks) Placebo Controlled Studies

Laboratory Analyte	Category Change (At Least Once) from Baseline	Treatment Arm	N	Patients n (%)
Fasting Glucose	Normal to High (<100 mg/dL to ≥ 126 mg/dL)	Quetiapine	2907	71 (2.4%)
		Placebo	1346	19 (1.4%)
	Borderline to High (≥ 100 mg/dL and <126 mg/dL to ≥ 126 mg/dL)	Quetiapine	572	67 (11.7%)
		Placebo	279	33 (11.8%)

All patients being treated with antidepressants for any indication should be monitored appropriately and observed closely for clinical worsening, suicidality, and unusual changes in behavior, especially during the initial few months of a course of drug therapy, or at times of dose changes, either increases or decreases.

The following symptoms, anxiety, agitation, panic attacks, insomnia, irritability, hostility, aggressiveness, impulsivity, akathisia (psychomotor restlessness), hypomania, and mania, have been reported in adult and pediatric patients being treated with antidepressants for major depressive disorder as well as for other indications, both psychiatric and nonpsychiatric. Although a causal link between the emergence of such symptoms and either the worsening of depression and/or the emergence of suicidal impulses has not been established, there is concern that such symptoms may represent precursors to emerging suicidality.

Consideration should be given to changing the therapeutic regimen, including possibly discontinuing the medication, in patients whose depression is persistently worse, or who are experiencing emergent suicidality or symptoms that might be precursors to worsening depression or suicidality, especially if these symptoms are severe, abrupt in onset, or were not part of the patient's presenting symptoms.

Families and caregivers of patients being treated with antidepressants for major depressive disorder or other indications, both psychiatric and nonpsychiatric, should be alerted about the need to monitor patients for the emergence of agitation, irritability, unusual changes in behavior, and the other symptoms described above, as well as the emergence of suicidality, and to report such symptoms immediately to healthcare providers. Such monitoring should include daily observation by families and caregivers. Prescriptions for SEROQUEL XR should be written for the smallest quantity of tablets consistent with good patient management, in order to reduce the risk of overdose.

Screening Patients for Bipolar Disorder: A major depressive episode may be the initial presentation of bipolar disorder. It is generally believed (though not established in controlled trials) that treating such an episode with an antidepressant alone may increase the likelihood of precipitation of a mixed/manic episode in patients at risk for bipolar disorder. Whether any of the symptoms described above represent such a conversion is unknown. However, prior to initiating treatment with an antidepressant, patients with depressive symptoms should be adequately screened to determine if they are at risk for bipolar disorder; such screening should include a detailed psychiatric history, including a family history of suicide, bipolar disorder, and depression.

5.3   Neuroleptic Malignant Syndrome (NMS)

A potentially fatal symptom complex sometimes referred to as Neuroleptic Malignant Syndrome (NMS) has been reported in association with administration of antipsychotic drugs, including quetiapine. Rare cases of NMS have been reported with quetiapine. Clinical manifestations of NMS are hyperpyrexia, muscle rigidity, altered mental status, and evidence of autonomic instability (irregular pulse or blood pressure, tachycardia, diaphoresis, and cardiac dysrhythmia). Additional signs may include elevated creatine phosphokinase, myoglobinuria (rhabdomyolysis) and acute renal failure.

The diagnostic evaluation of patients with this syndrome is complicated. In arriving at a diagnosis, it is important to exclude cases where the clinical presentation includes both serious medical illness (eg, pneumonia, systemic infection, etc.) and untreated or inadequately treated extrapyramidal signs and symptoms (EPS). Other important considerations in the differential diagnosis include central anticholinergic toxicity, heat stroke, drug fever and primary central nervous system (CNS) pathology.

The management of NMS should include: 1) immediate discontinuation of antipsychotic drugs and other drugs not essential to concurrent therapy; 2) intensive symptomatic treatment and medical monitoring; and 3) treatment of any concomitant serious medical problems for which specific treatments are available. There is no general agreement about specific pharmacological treatment regimens for NMS.

If a patient requires antipsychotic drug treatment after recovery from NMS, the potential reintroduction of drug therapy should be carefully considered. The patient should be carefully monitored since recurrences of NMS have been reported.

5.4   Hyperglycemia and Diabetes Mellitus

Hyperglycemia, in some cases extreme and associated with ketoacidosis or hyperosmolar coma or death, has been reported in patients treated with atypical antipsychotics, including quetiapine. Assessment of the relationship between atypical antipsychotic use and glucose abnormalities is complicated by the possibility of an increased background risk of diabetes mellitus in patients with schizophrenia and the increasing incidence of diabetes mellitus in the general population. Given these confounders, the relationship between atypical antipsychotic use and hyperglycemia-related adverse reactions is not completely understood. However, epidemiological studies suggest an increased risk of treatment-emergent hyperglycemia-related adverse reactions in patients treated with the atypical antipsychotics. Precise risk estimates for hyperglycemia-related adverse reactions in patients treated with atypical antipsychotics are not available.

Patients with an established diagnosis of diabetes mellitus who are started on atypical antipsychotics should be monitored regularly for worsening of glucose control. Patients with risk factors for diabetes mellitus (eg, obesity, family history of diabetes) who are starting treatment with atypical antipsychotics should undergo fasting blood glucose testing at the beginning of treatment and periodically during treatment. Any patient treated with atypical antipsychotics should be monitored for symptoms of hyperglycemia including polydipsia, polyuria, polyphagia, and weakness. Patients who develop symptoms of hyperglycemia during treatment with atypical antipsychotics should undergo fasting blood glucose testing. In some cases, hyperglycemia has resolved when the atypical antipsychotic was discontinued; however, some patients required continuation of antidiabetic treatment despite discontinuation of the suspect drug.

[See table 2 above]

Adults:

In a 24-week trial (active-controlled, 115 patients treated with SEROQUEL) designed to evaluate glycemic status with oral glucose tolerance testing of all patients, at week 24 the incidence of a treatment-emergent post-glucose challenge glucose level ≥ 200 mg/dL was 1.7% and the incidence of a fasting treatment-emergent blood glucose level ≥ 126 mg/dL was 2.6%. The mean change in fasting glucose from baseline was 3.2 mg/dL and mean change in 2 hour glucose from baseline was -1.8 mg/dL for quetiapine.

In 2 long-term placebo-controlled randomized withdrawal clinical trials for bipolar maintenance, mean exposure of 213 days for SEROQUEL (646 patients) and 152 days for placebo (680 patients), the mean change in glucose from baseline was +5.0 mg/dL for quetiapine and –0.05 mg/dL for placebo. The exposure-adjusted rate of any increased blood glucose level (≥ 126 mg/dL) for patients more than 8 hours since a meal (however, some patients may not have been precluded from calorie intake from fluids during fasting period) was 18.0 per 100 patient years for SEROQUEL (10.7% of patients; n=556) and 9.5 for placebo per 100 patient years (4.6% of patients; n=581).

Table 3 shows the percentage of patients with shifts in blood glucose to ≥ 126 mg/dL from normal baseline in MDD adjunct therapy trials by dose.

Table 3: Percentage of Patients with Shifts from Normal Baseline in Blood Glucose to ≥ 126 mg/dL (assumed fasting) in MDD Adjunct Therapy Trials by Dose

Laboratory Analyte	Treatment Arm	N	Patients n (%)
Blood Glucose ≥ 126 mg/dL	Placebo	277	17 (6%)
	SEROQUEL XR 150 mg	280	19 (7%)
	SEROQUEL XR 300 mg	269	32 (12%)

Children and Adolescents: Safety and effectiveness of SEROQUEL XR have not been established in pediatric patients and SEROQUEL XR is not approved for patients under the age of 18 years. In a placebo-controlled SEROQUEL monotherapy study of adolescent patients (13–17 years of age) with schizophrenia (6 weeks duration), the mean change in fasting glucose levels for SEROQUEL (n=138) compared to placebo (n=67) was –0.75 mg/dL versus –1.70 mg/dL. In a placebo-controlled SEROQUEL monotherapy study of children and adolescent patients (10–17 years of age) with bipolar mania (3 weeks duration), the mean change in fasting glucose level for SEROQUEL (n=170) compared to placebo (n=81) was 3.62 mg/dL versus –1.17 mg/dL. No patient in either study with a baseline normal fasting glucose level (<100 mg/dL) or a baseline borderline fasting glucose level (≥100 mg/dL and <126 mg/dL) had a treatment-emergent blood glucose level of ≥126 mg/dL.

5.5 Hyperlipidemia

Adults: Undesirable alterations in lipids have been observed with quetiapine use. Clinical monitoring, including baseline and periodic follow-up lipid evaluations in patients using quetiapine is recommended.

Table 4 shows the percentage of patients with changes in cholesterol and triglycerides from baseline by indication in clinical trials with SEROQUEL XR.

[See table 4 at right]

In SEROQUEL clinical trials for schizophrenia, the percentage of patients with shifts in cholesterol and triglycerides from baseline to clinically significant levels were 18% (placebo: 7%) and 22% (placebo: 16%). HDL-cholesterol and LDL-cholesterol parameters were not measured in these studies. In SEROQUEL clinical trials for bipolar depression, the following percentage of patients had shifts from baseline to clinically significant levels for the four lipid parameters measured: total cholesterol 9% (placebo: 6%); triglycerides 14% (placebo: 9%); LDL-cholesterol 6% (placebo: 5%) and HDLcholesterol 14% (placebo: 14%). Lipid parameters were not measured in the bipolar mania studies.

Table 5 shows the percentage of patients in MDD adjunctive therapy trials with clinically significant shifts in total-cholesterol, triglycerides, LDL-cholesterol and HDL-cholesterol from baseline by dose.

[See table 5 at right]

Children and Adolescents:
Safety and effectiveness of SEROQUEL XR have not been established in pediatric patients, and SEROQUEL XR is not approved for patients under the age of 18 years.

Table 6 shows the percentage of children and adolescents with shifts in total cholesterol, triglycerides, LDL-cholesterol and HDL-cholesterol from baseline to clinically significant levels by indication in clinical trials with SEROQUEL.

[See table 6 at top of next page]

5.6 Weight Gain

Increases in weight have been observed in clinical trials. Patients receiving quetiapine should receive regular monitoring of weight [*see Patient Counseling Information* (17)].
Adults: Table 7 shows the percentage of adult patients with weight gain of ≥ 7% of body weight by indication.

[See table 7 on next page]

In schizophrenia trials, the proportions of patients meeting a weight gain criterion of ≥ 7% of body weight were compared in a pool of four 3- to 6-week placebo-controlled clinical trials, revealing a statistically significant greater incidence of weight gain for SEROQUEL (23%) compared to placebo (6%).

Table 8 shows the percentage of adult patients with weight gain of ≥ 7% of body weight for MDD by dose.

Table 8: Percentage of Patients with Weight Gain ≥ 7% of Body Weight in MDD Adjunctive Therapy Trials by Dose (Adults)

Vital sign	Treatment Arm	N	Patients n (%)
Weight Gain ≥7% of Body weight in MDD Adjunctive Therapy	Placebo	302	5 (2%)
	SEROQUEL XR 150 mg	309	10 (3%)
	SEROQUEL XR 300 mg	307	22 (7%)

Children and Adolescents: Safety and effectiveness of SEROQUEL XR have not been established in pediatric patients and SEROQUEL XR is not approved for patients under the age of 18 years. In two clinical trials with SEROQUEL, one in bipolar mania and one in schizophrenia, reported increases in weight are included in table 9 below.

Table 9 shows the percentage of patients with weight gain ≥ 7% of body weight in clinical trials with SEROQUEL.

Table 4: Percentage of Adult Patients with Shifts in Total Cholesterol, Triglycerides, LDL-Cholesterol and HDL-Cholesterol from Baseline to Clinically Significant Levels by Indication

Laboratory Analyte	Indication	Treatment Arm	N	Patients n (%)
Total Cholesterol ≥240 mg/dL	Schizophrenia*	SEROQUEL XR	718	67 (9%)
		Placebo	232	21 (9%)
	Bipolar Depression†	SEROQUEL XR	85	6 (7%)
		Placebo	106	3 (3%)
	Bipolar Mania‡	SEROQUEL XR	128	9 (7%)
		Placebo	134	5 (4%)
	Major Depressive Disorder (Adjunct Therapy)§	SEROQUEL XR	420	67 (16%)
		Placebo	213	15 (7%)
Triglycerides ≥200 mg/dL	Schizophrenia*	SEROQUEL XR	659	118 (18%)
		Placebo	214	11 (5%)
	Bipolar Depression†	SEROQUEL XR	84	7 (8%)
		Placebo	93	7 (8%)
	Bipolar Mania‡	SEROQUEL XR	102	15 (15%)
		Placebo	125	8 (6%)
	Major Depressive Disorder (Adjunct Therapy)§	SEROQUEL XR	458	75 (16%)
		Placebo	223	18 (8%)
LDL-Cholesterol ≥ 160 mg/dL	Schizophrenia*	SEROQUEL XR	691	47 (7%)
		Placebo	227	17 (8%)
	Bipolar Depression†	SEROQUEL XR	86	3 (4%)
		Placebo	104	2 (2%)
	Bipolar Mania‡	SEROQUEL XR	125	5 (4%)
		Placebo	135	2 (2%)
	Major Depressive Disorder (Adjunct Therapy)§	SEROQUEL XR	457	51 (11%)
		Placebo	219	21 (10%)
HDL-Cholesterol ≤ 40 mg/dL	Schizophrenia*	SEROQUEL XR	600	87 (15%)
		Placebo	195	23 (12%)
	Bipolar Depression†	SEROQUEL XR	78	7 (9%)
		Placebo	83	6 (7%)
	Bipolar Mania‡	SEROQUEL XR	100	19 (19%)
		Placebo	115	15 (13%)
	Major Depressive Disorder (Adjunct Therapy)§	SEROQUEL XR	470	34 (7%)
		Placebo	230	19 (8%)

* 6 weeks duration
† 8 weeks duration
‡ 3 weeks duration
§ 6 weeks duration

Table 5: Percentage of Patients with Shifts in Total Cholesterol, Triglycerides, LDL-Cholesterol and HDL-Cholesterol from Baseline to Clinically Significant Levels in MDD Adjunctive Therapy Trials by Dose

Laboratory Analyte	Treatment Arm*	N	Patients n (%)
Cholesterol ≥ 240 mg/dL	Placebo	213	15 (7%)
	SEROQUEL XR 150 mg	223	41 (18%)
	SEROQUEL XR 300 mg	197	26 (13%)
Triglycerides ≥ 200 mg/dL	Placebo	223	18 (8%)
	SEROQUEL XR 150 mg	232	36 (16%)
	SEROQUEL XR 300 mg	226	39 (17%)
LDL-Cholesterol ≥ 160 mg/dL	Placebo	219	21 (10%)
	SEROQUEL XR 150 mg	242	29 (12%)
	SEROQUEL XR 300 mg	215	22 (10%)
HDL-Cholesterol ≤ 40 mg/dL	Placebo	230	19 (8%)
	SEROQUEL XR 150 mg	238	14 (6%)
	SEROQUEL XR 300 mg	232	20 (9%)

* 6 weeks duration

Table 9: Percentage of Patients with Weight Gain ≥ 7% of Body Weight (Children and Adolescents)

Vital Sign	Indication	Treatment Arm	N	Patients n (%)
Weight gain ≥ 7% of Body Weight	Schizophrenia*	SEROQUEL	111	23 (21%)
		Placebo	44	3 (7%)
	Bipolar Mania†	SEROQUEL	157	18 (12%)
		Placebo	68	0 (0%)

* 6 weeks duration
† 3 weeks duration

The mean change in body weight in the schizophrenia trial was 2.0 kg in the SEROQUEL group and -0.4 kg in the placebo group and in the bipolar mania trial it was 1.7 kg in the SEROQUEL group and 0.4 kg in the placebo group.

In an open-label study that enrolled patients from the above two pediatric trials, 63% of patients (241/380) completed 26 weeks of therapy with SEROQUEL. After 26 weeks of treatment, the mean increase in body weight was 4.4 kg. Forty-five percent of the patients gained ≥ 7% of their body weight, not adjusted for normal growth. In order to adjust for normal growth over 26 weeks, an increase of at least 0.5 standard deviation from baseline in BMI was used as a measure of a clinically significant change; 18.3% of patients on SEROQUEL met this criterion after 26 weeks of treatment.

When treating pediatric patients with SEROQUEL for any indication, weight gain should be assessed against that expected for normal growth.

5.7 Tardive Dyskinesia

A syndrome of potentially irreversible, involuntary, dyskinetic movements may develop in patients treated with antipsychotic drugs including quetiapine. Although the prevalence of the syndrome appears to be highest among the elderly, especially elderly women, it is impossible to rely upon prevalence estimates to predict, at the inception of antipsychotic treatment, which patients are likely to develop the syndrome. Whether antipsychotic drug products differ in their potential to cause tardive dyskinesia is unknown.

The risk of developing tardive dyskinesia and the likelihood that it will become irreversible are believed to increase as the duration of treatment and the total cumulative dose of antipsychotic drugs administered to the patient increase. However, the syndrome can develop, although much less commonly, after relatively brief treatment periods at low doses or may even arise after discontinuation of treatment.

There is no known treatment for established cases of tardive dyskinesia, although the syndrome may remit, partially or completely, if antipsychotic treatment is with-

Table 6: Percentage of Children and Adolescents with Shifts in Total Cholesterol, Triglycerides LDL-Cholesterol and HDLCholesterol from Baseline to Clinically Significant Levels by Indication

Laboratory Analyte	Indication	Treatment Arm	N	Patients n (%)
Total Cholesterol ≥ 200 mg/dL	Schizophrenia*	SEROQUEL	107	13 (12%)
		Placebo	56	1 (2%)
	Bipolar Mania†	SEROQUEL	159	16 (10%)
		Placebo	66	2 (3%)
Triglycerides ≥150 mg/dL	Schizophrenia*	SEROQUEL	103	17 (17%)
		Placebo	51	4 (8%)
	Bipolar Mania†	SEROQUEL	149	32 (22%)
		Placebo	60	8 (13%)
LDL-Cholesterol ≥ 130 mg/dL	Schizophrenia*	SEROQUEL	112	4 (4%)
		Placebo	60	1 (2%)
	Bipolar Mania†	SEROQUEL	169	13 (8%)
		Placebo	74	4 (5%)
HDL-Cholesterol ≤ 40 mg/dL	Schizophrenia*	SEROQUEL	104	16 (15%)
		Placebo	54	10 (19%)
	Bipolar Mania†	SEROQUEL	154	16 (10%)
		Placebo	61	4 (7%)

* 13-17 years, 6 weeks duration
† 10-17 years, 3 weeks duration

Table 7: Percentage of Patients with Weight Gain ≥ 7% of Body Weight (Adults) by Indication

Vital sign	Indication	Treatment Arm	N	Patients n (%)
Weight Gain≥ 7% of Body Weight	Schizophrenia*	SEROQUEL XR	907	90 (10%)
		Placebo	299	16 (5%)
	Bipolar Mania †	SEROQUEL XR	138	7 (5%)
		Placebo	150	0 (0%)
	Bipolar Depression‡	SEROQUEL XR	110	9 (8%)
		Placebo	125	1 (1%)
	Major Depressive Disorder (Adjunctive Therapy)§	SEROQUEL XR	616	32 (5%)
		Placebo	302	5 (2%)

* 6 weeks duration
† 3 weeks duration
‡ 8 weeks duration
§ 6 weeks duration

drawn. Antipsychotic treatment, itself, however, may suppress (or partially suppress) the signs and symptoms of the syndrome and thereby may possibly mask the underlying process. The effect that symptomatic suppression has upon the longterm course of the syndrome is unknown.

Given these considerations, SEROQUEL XR should be prescribed in a manner that is most likely to minimize the occurrence of tardive dyskinesia. Chronic antipsychotic treatment should generally be reserved for patients who appear to suffer from a chronic illness that (1) is known to respond to antipsychotic drugs, and (2) for whom alternative, equally effective, but potentially less harmful treatments are not available or appropriate. In patients who do require chronic treatment, the smallest dose and the shortest duration of treatment producing a satisfactory clinical response should be sought. The need for continued treatment should be reassessed periodically.

If signs and symptoms of tardive dyskinesia appear in a patient on SEROQUEL XR, drug discontinuation should be considered. However, some patients may require treatment with quetiapine despite the presence of the syndrome.

5.8 Orthostatic Hypotension

Quetiapine may induce orthostatic hypotension associated with dizziness, tachycardia and, in some patients, syncope, especially during the dose-titration period, probably reflecting its α1-adrenergic antagonist properties. Syncope was reported in 0.3% (5/1866) of the patients treated with SEROQUEL XR across all indications, compared with 0.2% (2/928) on placebo. Syncope was reported in 1% (28/3265) of the patients treated with SEROQUEL, compared with 0.2% (2/954) on placebo. Orthostatic hypotension, dizziness, and syncope may lead to falls.

Quetiapine should be used with particular caution in patients with known cardiovascular disease (history of myocardial infarction or ischemic heart disease, heart failure or conduction abnormalities), cerebrovascular disease or conditions which would predispose patients to hypotension (dehydration, hypovolemia and treatment with antihypertensive medications) [see *Adverse Reactions* (6.2)]. If hypotension occurs during titration to the target dose, a return to the previous dose in the titration schedule is appropriate.

5.9 Increases in Blood Pressure (Children and Adolescents)

Safety and effectiveness of SEROQUEL XR have not been established in pediatric patients and SEROQUEL XR is not approved for patients under the age of 18 years. In placebo-controlled trials in children and adolescents with schizophrenia (6-week duration) or bipolar mania (3-week duration), the incidence of increases at any time in systolic blood pressure (≥ 20 mmHg) was 15.2% (51/335) for SEROQUEL and 5.5% (9/163) for placebo; the incidence of increases at any time in diastolic blood pressure (≥ 10 mmHg) was 40.6% (136/335) for SEROQUEL and 24.5% (40/163) for placebo. In the 26-week open-label clinical trial, one child with a reported history of hypertension experienced a hypertensive crisis. Blood pressure in children and adolescents should be measured at the beginning of, and periodically during treatment.

5.10 Leukopenia, Neutropenia and Agranulocytosis

In clinical trial and postmarketing experience, events of leukopenia/neutropenia have been reported temporally related to atypical antipsychotic agents, including quetiapine fumarate. Agranulocytosis (including fatal cases) has also been reported.

Possible risk factors for leukopenia/neutropenia include pre-existing low white cell count (WBC) and history of drug induced leukopenia/neutropenia. Patients with a pre-existing low WBC or a history of drug induced leukopenia/neutropenia should have their complete blood count (CBC) monitored frequently during the first few months of therapy and should discontinue SEROQUEL XR at the first sign of a decline in WBC in absence of other causative factors. Patients with neutropenia should be carefully monitored for fever or other symptoms or signs of infection and treated promptly if such symptoms or signs occur. Patients with severe neutropenia (absolute neutrophil count <1000/mm³) should discontinue SEROQUEL XR and have their WBC followed until recovery [see *Adverse Reactions* (6.2)].

5.11 Cataracts

The development of cataracts was observed in association with quetiapine treatment in chronic dog studies [see *Animal Toxicology* (13.2)]. Lens changes have also been observed in adults, children, and adolescents during long-term quetiapine treatment, but a causal relationship to quetiapine use has not been established. Nevertheless, the possibility of lenticular changes cannot be excluded at this time. Therefore, examination of the lens by methods adequate to detect cataract formation, such as slit lamp exam or other appropriately sensitive methods, is recommended at initiation of treatment or shortly thereafter, and at 6-month intervals during chronic treatment.

5.12 Seizures

During short-term clinical trials with SEROQUEL XR, seizures occurred in 0.05% (1/1866) of patients treated with SEROQUEL XR across all indications compared to 0.3% (3/928) on placebo. During clinical trials with SEROQUEL, seizures occurred in 0.5% (20/3490) of patients treated with SEROQUEL compared to 0.2% (2/954) on placebo. As with other antipsychotics, quetiapine fumarate should be used cautiously in patients with a history of seizures or with conditions that potentially lower the seizure threshold, e.g., Alzheimer's dementia. Conditions that lower the seizure threshold may be more prevalent in a population of 65 years or older.

5.13 Hypothyroidism

Adults: In SEROQUEL XR clinical trials across all indications 1.8% (24/1336) of patients on SEROQUEL XR vs. 0.6% (3/530) on placebo experienced decreased free thyroxine and 1.6% (21/1346) on SEROQUEL XR vs. 1.9% (18/534) on placebo experienced increased thyroid stimulating hormone (TSH); however, no patients experienced a combination of clinically significant decreased free thyroxine and increased TSH. Clinical trials with SEROQUEL demonstrated a dose-related decrease in total and free thyroxine (T4) of approximately 20% at the higher end of the therapeutic dose range and was maximal in the first two to four weeks of treatment and maintained without adaptation or progression during more chronic therapy. Generally, these changes were of no clinical significance and TSH was unchanged in most patients and levels of thyroid binding globulin (TBG) were unchanged. In nearly all cases, cessation of quetiapine treatment was associated with a reversal of the effects on total and free T4, irrespective of the duration of treatment. About 0.7% (26/3489) of SEROQUEL patients did experience TSH increases in monotherapy studies. Six of these patients with TSH increases needed replacement thyroid treatment.

Children and Adolescents: Safety and effectiveness of SEROQUEL XR have not been established in pediatric patients and SEROQUEL XR is not approved for patients under the age of 18 years. In acute placebo-controlled trials in children and adolescent patients with schizophrenia (6-week duration) or bipolar mania (3-week duration), the incidence of shifts to potentially clinically important thyroid function values at any time for SEROQUEL treated patients and placebo-treated patients for elevated TSH was 2.9% (8/280) vs. 0.7% (1/138), respectively and for decreased total thyroxine was 2.8% (8/289) vs. 0% (0/145), respectively. Of the SEROQUEL treated patients with elevated TSH levels, 1 had simultaneous low free T4 level at end of treatment.

5.14 Hyperprolactinemia

Adults: During clinical trials with quetiapine across all indications, the incidence of shifts in prolactin levels to a clinically significant value occurred in 3.6% (158/4416) of patients treated with quetiapine compared to 2.6% (51/1968) on placebo.

Children and Adolescents: Safety and effectiveness of SEROQUEL XR have not been established in pediatric patients and SEROQUEL XR is not approved for patients under the age of 18 years. In acute placebo-controlled trials in children and adolescent patients with bipolar mania (3-week duration) or schizophrenia (6-week duration), the incidence of shifts in prolactin levels to a clinically significant value (>20 µg/L males; > 26 µg/L females at any time) was 13.4% (18/134) for SEROQUEL compared to 4% (3/75) for placebo in males and 8.7% (9/104) for SEROQUEL compared to 0% (0/39) for placebo in females.

Like other drugs that antagonize dopamine D2 receptors, SEROQUEL XR elevates prolactin levels in some patients and the elevation may persist during chronic administration. Hyperprolactinemia, regardless of etiology, may suppress hypothalamic GnRH, resulting in reduced pituitary gonadotrophin secretion. This, in turn, may inhibit reproductive function by impairing gonadal steroidogenesis in both female and male patients. Galactorrhea, amenorrhea, gynecomastia, and impotence have been reported in patients receiving prolactin-elevating compounds. Longstanding hyperprolactinemia when associated with hypogonadism may lead to decreased bone density in both female and male subjects.

Tissue culture experiments indicate that approximately one-third of human breast cancers are prolactin dependent in vitro, a factor of potential importance if the prescription of these drugs is considered in a patient with previously detected breast cancer. As is common with compounds which increase prolactin release, mammary gland, and pancreatic islet cell neoplasia (mammary adenocarcinomas, pituitary and pancreatic adenomas) was observed in carcinogenicity studies conducted in mice and rats. Neither clinical studies nor epidemiologic studies conducted to date have shown an association between chronic administration of this class of drugs and tumorigenesis in humans, but the available evidence is too limited to be conclusive [see *Carcinogenesis, Mutagenesis, Impairment of Fertility* (13.1)].

5.15 Transaminase Elevations

Asymptomatic, transient and reversible elevations in serum transaminases (primarily ALT) have been reported. The proportions of patients with transaminase elevations of >3 times the upper limits of the normal reference range in a pool of placebo-controlled trials ranged between 1% and 2% for SEROQUEL XR compared to 2% for placebo. In schizophrenia trials in adults, the proportions of patients with transaminase elevations of >3 times the upper limits of the normal reference range in a pool of 3- to 6-week placebo-controlled trials were approximately 6% (29/483) for SEROQUEL compared to 1% (3/194) for placebo. These hepatic enzyme elevations usually occurred within the first 3 weeks of drug treatment and promptly returned to pre-study levels with ongoing treatment with quetiapine.

5.16 Potential for Cognitive and Motor Impairment

Somnolence was a commonly reported adverse event reported in patients treated with quetiapine especially during the 3-day period of initial dose titration. In schizophrenia trials, somnolence was reported in 24.7% (235/951) of patients on SEROQUEL XR compared to 10.3% (33/319) of placebo patients. In a bipolar depression clinical trial, somnolence was reported in 51.8% (71/137) of patients on SEROQUEL XR compared to 12.9% (18/140) of placebo patients. In a clinical trial for bipolar mania, somnolence was reported in 50.3% (76/151) of patients on SEROQUEL XR compared to 11.9% (19/160) of placebo patients. Since quetiapine has the potential to impair judgment, thinking, or motor skills, patients should be cautioned about performing activities requiring mental alertness, such as operating a motor vehicle (including automobiles) or operating hazardous machinery until they are reasonably certain that quetiapine therapy does not affect them adversely. Somnolence may lead to falls.

In short-term adjunctive therapy trials for MDD, somnolence was reported in 40% (252/627) of patients on SEROQUEL XR respectively compared to 9% (27/309) of placebo patients. Somnolence was dose-related in these trials (37% (117/315) and 43% (135/312) for the 150 mg and 300 mg groups, respectively).

5.17 Priapism

One case of priapism in a patient receiving quetiapine was reported prior to market introduction. While a causal relationship to use of quetiapine has not been established, other drugs with α-adrenergic blocking effects have been reported to induce priapism, and it is possible that quetiapine may share this capacity. Severe priapism may require surgical intervention.

5.18 Body Temperature Regulation

Disruption of the body's ability to reduce core body temperature has been attributed to antipsychotic agents. Appropriate care is advised when prescribing SEROQUEL XR for patients who will be experiencing conditions which may contribute to an elevation in core body temperature, eg, exercising strenuously, exposure to extreme heat, receiving concomitant medication with anticholinergic activity, or being subject to dehydration.

5.19 Dysphagia

Esophageal dysmotility and aspiration have been associated with antipsychotic drug use. Aspiration pneumonia is a common cause of morbidity and mortality in elderly patients, in particular those with advanced Alzheimer's dementia. SEROQUEL XR and other antipsychotic drugs should be used cautiously in patients at risk for aspiration pneumonia.

5.20 Suicide

The possibility of a suicide attempt is inherent in schizophrenia, bipolar disorder and depression; close supervision of high risk patients should accompany drug therapy. Prescriptions for SEROQUEL XR should be written for the smallest quantity of tablets consistent with good patient management in order to reduce the risk of overdose.

In three, 6-week clinical studies in patients with schizophrenia (N=951) the incidence of treatment emergent suicidal ideation or suicide attempt was 0.6% (n=6) in SEROQUEL XR treated patients and 0.9% (n=3) in placebo-treated patients.

In an 8-week clinical study in patients with bipolar depression (N=137 for SEROQUEL XR and 140 for placebo) the incidence of treatment emergent suicidal ideation or suicide attempt was 0.7% (n=1) for SEROQUEL XR treated patients and 1.4% (n=2) for placebo.

In a 3-week clinical study in patients with bipolar mania (N=311, 151 for SEROQUEL XR and 160 for placebo) the incidence of treatment emergent suicidal ideation or suicide attempt was 1.3% (n=2) for SEROQUEL XR compared to 3.8% (n=6) for placebo.

In two, 6-week MDD adjunctive therapy trials (n=936, 627 on SEROQUEL XR and 309 on placebo) the incidence of treatment emergent suicidal ideation or suicide attempt was 0.5% (n=3) in SEROQUEL XR treated patients and 0.6% (n=2) in placebo.

5.21 Use in Patients with Concomitant Illness

Clinical experience with SEROQUEL XR in patients with certain concomitant systemic illnesses [see *Pharmacokinetics* (12.3)] is limited.

SEROQUEL XR has not been evaluated or used to any appreciable extent in patients with a recent history of myocardial infarction or unstable heart disease. Patients with these diagnoses were excluded from premarketing clinical studies. Because of the risk of orthostatic hypotension with SEROQUEL XR, caution should be observed in cardiac patients [see *Warnings and Precautions* (5.8)].

In clinical trials quetiapine was not associated with a persistent increase in absolute QT intervals. However, in post marketing experience there were cases reported of QT prolongation in patients who overdosed on quetiapine [see *Overdosage* (10.1), in patients with concomitant illness, and in patients taking medicines known to cause electrolyte imbalance or increase QT interval [see *Drug Interactions* (7)]. Caution should be exercised when quetiapine is prescribed in patients with cardiovascular disease or family history of QT prolongation. Also, caution should be exercised when quetiapine is prescribed with medicines known to cause electrolyte imbalance or increase QT interval or with concomitant neuroleptics, especially for patients with increased risk of QT prolongation, i.e., the elderly, patients with congenital long QT syndrome, congestive heart failure, heart hypertrophy, hypokalemia, or hypomagnesemia.

5.22 Withdrawal

Acute withdrawal symptoms, such as insomnia, nausea and vomiting have been described after abrupt cessation of atypical antipsychotic drugs, including quetiapine fumarate. In short-term placebo-controlled, monotherapy clinical trials with SEROQUEL XR that included a discontinuation phase which evaluated discontinuation symptoms, the aggregated incidence of patients experiencing one or more discontinuation symptoms after abrupt cessation was 12.1% (241/1993) for SEROQUEL XR and 6.7% (71/1065) for placebo. The incidence of the individual adverse events (i.e., insomnia, nausea, headache, diarrhea, vomiting, dizziness and irritability) did not exceed 5.3% in any treatment group and usually resolved after 1 week post-discontinuation. Gradual withdrawal is advised.

6 ADVERSE REACTIONS

6.1 Clinical Studies Experience

Because clinical studies are conducted under widely varying conditions, adverse reaction rates observed in the clinical studies of a drug cannot be directly compared to rates in the clinical studies of another drug and may not reflect the rates observed in practice.

The information below is derived from a clinical trial database for SEROQUEL XR consisting of approximately 3400 patients exposed to SEROQUEL XR for the treatment of Schizophrenia, Bipolar Disorder, and Major Depressive Disorder in placebo-controlled trials. This experience corresponds to approximately 1020.1 patient-years. Adverse reactions were assessed by collecting adverse reactions, results of physical examinations, vital signs, body weights, laboratory analyses and ECG results.

Adverse reactions during exposure were obtained by general inquiry and recorded by clinical investigators using terminology of their own choosing. Consequently, it is not possible to provide a meaningful estimate of the proportion of individuals experiencing adverse reactions without first grouping similar types of reactions into a smaller number of standardized event categories. In the tables and tabulations that follow, standard MedDRA terminology has been used to classify reported adverse reactions.

The stated frequencies of adverse reactions represent the proportion of individuals who experienced, at least once, a treatment-emergent adverse reaction of the type listed. An event was considered treatment-emergent if it occurred for the first time or worsened while receiving therapy following baseline evaluation.

Adverse Reactions Associated with Discontinuation of Treatment in Short-Term, Placebo-Controlled Trials

Schizophrenia: There was no difference in the incidence and type of adverse reactions associated with discontinuation (6.4% (61/951) for SEROQUEL XR vs. 7.5% (24/319) for placebo) in a pool of controlled Schizophrenia trials. There were no adverse reactions leading to discontinuation that occurred at an incidence of ≥ 2% for SEROQUEL XR in Schizophrenia trials.

Bipolar Disorder:

Mania: In a single clinical trial in patients with bipolar mania, 4.6% (7/151) of patients on SEROQUEL XR discontinued due to an adverse reaction compared to 8.1% (13/160) on placebo. There were no adverse reactions leading to discontinuation that occurred at an incidence of ≥ 2% for SEROQUEL XR in Bipolar Mania trials.

Depression: In a single clinical trial in patients with bipolar depression, 14% (19/137) of patients on SEROQUEL XR discontinued due to adverse reaction compared to 4% (5/

140) on placebo. Somnolence[#] was the only adverse reaction leading to discontinuation that occurred at an incidence of ≥ 2% in SEROQUEL XR in Bipolar Depression trials.
[#] The adverse reaction term "somnolence" includes both "somnolence" and "sedation."

MDD, Adjunctive Therapy: In adjunctive therapy clinical trials inpatients with MDD, 12.1% (76/627) of patients on SEROQUEL XR discontinued due to adverse reaction compared to 1.9% (6/309) on placebo. Somnolence* was the only adverse reaction leading to discontinuation that occurred at an incidence of ≥ 2% in SEROQUEL XR in MDD trials.

Commonly Observed Adverse Reactions in Short-Term, Placebo-Controlled Trials:

In short-term placebo-controlled studies for schizophrenia the most commonly observed adverse reactions associated with the use of SEROQUEL XR (incidence of 5% or greater) and observed at a rate on SEROQUEL XR at least twice that of placebo were somnolence (25%), dry mouth (12%), dizziness (10%), and dyspepsia (5%).

Adverse Reactions Occurring at an Incidence of 1% or More Among SEROQUEL XR Treated Patients in Short-Term, Placebo-Controlled Trials

Table 10 enumerates the incidence, rounded to the nearest percent, of treatment-emergent adverse reactions that occurred during acute therapy of schizophrenia (up to 6 weeks) in 1% or more in patients treated with SEROQUEL XR (doses ranging from 300 to 800 mg/ day) where the incidence in patients treated with SEROQUEL XR was greater than the incidence in placebo-treated patients.

Table 10: Treatment-Emergent Adverse Reaction Incidence in 6-Week Placebo-Controlled Clinical Trials for the Treatment of Schizophrenia[1]

Table 10: Treatment-Emergent Adverse Reaction Incidence in 6-Week Placebo-Controlled Clinical Trials for the Treatment of Schizophrenia*

Body System/ Preferred Term	PLACEBO (n=319)	SEROQUEL XR (n=951)
Cardiac Disorders		
Tachycardia	1%	3%
Eye Disorders		
Vision blurred	1%	2%
Gastrointestinal Disorders		
Dry Mouth	1%	12%
Constipation	5%	6%
Dyspepsia	2%	5%
Toothache	0%	2%
General Disorders and Administration Site Conditions		
Fatigue	2%	3%
Irritability	0%	1%
Pyrexia	0%	1%
Investigations		
Heart Rate Increased	1%	4%
Metabolism and Nutrition Disorders		
Increased Appetite	0%	2%
Musculoskeletal and Connective Tissue Disorders		
Muscle Spasms	1%	2%
Nervous System Disorders		
Somnolence[†]	10%	25%
Dizziness	4%	10%
Tremor	1%	2%
Akathisia	1%	2%
Extrapyramidal Symptoms[‡]	5%	8%
Psychiatric Disorders		
Anxiety	1%	2%
Schizophrenia	1%	2%
Restlessness	1%	2%
Vascular Disorders		
Orthostatic Hypotension	5%	7%
Hypotension	1%	3%

* Reactions for which the SEROQUEL XR incidence was 1% or more and equal to or less than placebo are not listed in the table, but included the following: headache, insomnia, and nausea, vomiting, diarrhea, stomach discomfort, weight increased, diastolic blood pressure decreased, systolic blood pressure decreased, arthralgia, back pain, pain in extremity, extrapyramidal disorder, agitation, psychotic disorder, sleep disorder, nasal congestion, hypertension.
† Somnolence combines adverse reaction terms somnolence and sedation.
‡ Extrapyramidal symptoms that were reported for SEROQUEL XR or placebo include the terms: akathisia, cogwheel rigidity, drooling, dyskinesia dystonia, extrapyramidal disorder, hypertonia, movement disorder, muscle rigidity, oculogyration, parkinsonism, parkinsonian gait, psychomotor hyperactivity, tardive dyskinesia, restlessness and tremor.

In a 3-week, placebo-controlled study in bipolar mania the most commonly observed adverse reactions associated with the use of SEROQUEL XR (incidence of 5% or greater) and observed at a rate on SEROQUEL XR at least twice that of placebo were somnolence (50%), dry mouth (34%), dizziness (10%), constipation (10%), weight gain (7%), dysarthria (5%), and nasal congestion (5%).

Table 11 enumerates the incidence, rounded to the nearest percent, of treatment-emergent adverse reactions that occurred during acute therapy of bipolar mania (up to 3 weeks) in 1% or more of patients treated with SEROQUEL XR (doses ranging from 400 to 800 mg/day) where the incidence in patients treated with SEROQUEL XR was greater than the incidence in placebo-treated patients.

Table 11: Treatment-Emergent Adverse Reactions in a 3-Week Placebo-Controlled Clinical Trial for the Treatment of Bipolar Mania*

Body System/ Preferred Term	PLACEBO (n=160)	SEROQUEL XR (n=151)
Cardiac Disorders		
Tachycardia	1%	2%
Eye Disorders		
Vision blurred	1%	2%
Gastrointestinal Disorders		
Dry Mouth	7%	34%
Constipation	3%	10%
Dyspepsia	4%	7%
Toothache	1%	3%
General Disorders and Administration Site Conditions		
Fatigue	4%	7%
Sluggishness	1%	2%
Pain	0%	1%
Investigations		
Weight Gain	1%	7%
Heart Rate Increased	0%	3%
Injury, Poisoning And Procedural Complications		
Contusion	0%	1%
Metabolism and Nutrition Disorder		
Increased Appetite	2%	4%
Nervous System Disorders		
Extrapyramidal Symptoms[†]	4%	7%
Somnolence[‡]	12%	50%
Dizziness	4%	10%
Dysarthia	0%	5%
Lethargy	1%	2%
Postural Dizziness	0%	1%
Musculoskeletal And Connective Tissue Disorders		
Back Pain	2%	3%
Arthralgia	0%	1%
Psychiatric Disorders		
Abnormal Dreams	0%	3%
Bipolar I Disorder	0%	1%
Respiratory, Thoracic and Mediastinal Disorders		
Nasal Congestion	1%	5%
Dry Throat	0%	1%
Vascular Disorders		
Orthostatic Hypotension	0%	3%

* Reactions for which the SEROQUEL XR incidence was 1% or more and equal to or less than placebo are not listed in the table, but included the following: headache, peripheral edema, diarrhea, nausea, vomiting, decreased appetite, muscle spasms, musculoskeletal stiffness, myalgia, tremor, akathisia, insomnia, agitation, nightmare, restlessness, erectile dysfunction, pharyngolaryngeal pain, cough, and hypotension.
† Extrapyramidal symptoms that were reported for SEROQUEL XR or placebo include the terms: akathisia, cogwheel rigidity, dystonia, extrapyramidal disorder, restlessness and tremor.
‡ Somnolence combines adverse reaction terms somnolence and sedation.

In the 8-week placebo-controlled bipolar depression study, the most commonly observed adverse reactions associated with the use of SEROQUEL XR (incidence of 5% or greater) and observed at a rate on SEROQUEL XR at least twice that of placebo were somnolence (52%), dry mouth (37%), increased appetite (12%), weight gain (7%), dyspepsia (7%), and fatigue (6%).

Table 12: enumerates the incidence, rounded to the nearest percent, of treatment-emergent adverse reactions that occurred during acute therapy of bipolar depression (up to 8 weeks) in 1% or more of patients treated with SEROQUEL XR 300 mg/day where the incidence in patients treated with SEROQUEL XR was greater than the incidence in placebo-treated patients.

Table 12: Treatment-Emergent Adverse Reactions in an 8-Week Placebo-Controlled Clinical Trial for the Treatment of Bipolar Depression*

Body System/ Preferred Term	Placebo (n=140)	SEROQUEL XR (n=137)
Ear And Labyrinth Disorders		
Ear Pain	1%	2%
Gastrointestinal Disorders		
Dry Mouth	7%	37%
Constipation	6%	8%
Dyspepsia	1%	7%
Toothache	0%	3%
Abdominal Distension	0%	1%
General Disorders and Administration Site Conditions		
Fatigue	2%	6%
Irritability	3%	4%
Immune System Disorders		
Seasonal Allergy	1%	2%
Infections And Infestations		
Viral Gastroenteritis	1%	4%
Urinary Tract Infection	0%	2%
Sinusitis	1%	2%
Investigations		
Weight Gain	1%	7%
Heart Rate Increased	0%	2%
Metabolism and Nutrition Disorder		
Increased Appetite	6%	12%
Decreased Appetite	1%	2%
Musculoskeletal And Connective Tissue Disorders		
Arthralgia	1%	4%
Back Pain	1%	3%
Muscle Spasms	1%	3%
Myalgia	1%	2%
Neck Pain	0%	2%
Nervous System Disorders		
Somnolence[†]	13%	52%
Extrapyramidal Symptoms[‡]	1%	4%
Dizziness	11%	13%
Paraesthesia	2%	3%
Disturbance in Attention	1%	2%
Dysarthria	0%	2%
Akathisia	0%	2%
Hypersomnia	0%	2%
Mental Impairment	0%	2%
Migraine	1%	2%
Restless Legs Syndrome	1%	2%
Sinus Headache	1%	2%
Psychiatric Disorders		
Abnormal Dreams	0%	3%
Anxiety	1%	2%
Confusional State	0%	2%
Disorientation	0%	2%
Libido Decreased	1%	2%
Renal And Urinary Disorders		
Pollakiuria	1%	2%
Respiratory, Thoracic And Mediastinal Disorders		
Sinus Congestion	1%	2%
Skin And Subcutaneous Tissue Disorders		
Hyperhidrosis	1%	2%
Vascular Disorders		
Orthostatic Hypotension	1%	2%

* Reactions for which the SEROQUEL XR incidence was 1% or more and equal to or less than placebo are not listed in the table, but included the following: headache insomnia, nausea, diarrhea, vomiting, nasopharyngitis, upper respiratory tract infection, influenza, pain in extremity, cough and nasal congestion.
† Somnolence combines adverse reaction terms somnolence and sedation.
‡ Extrapyramidal symptoms that were reported for SEROQUEL XR or placebo include the terms: akathisia, dystonia, extrapyramidal disorder, hypertonia, and tremor.

In the 6-week placebo-controlled fixed dose adjunctive therapy clinical trials, for MDD, the most commonly observed adverse reactions associated with the use of SEROQUEL XR (incidence of 5% or greater and observed at a rate on SEROQUEL XR and at least twice that of placebo) were somnolence (150 mg: 37%; 300 mg: 43%), dry mouth (150 mg: 27%; 300 mg: 40%), fatigue (150 mg: 14%; 300 mg: 11%) and constipation (150 mg only: 11%).

Table 13 enumerates the incidence, rounded to the nearest percent, of treatment-emergent adverse reactions that occurred during short-term adjunctive therapy of MDD (up to 6 weeks) in 1% or more of patients treated with SEROQUEL XR (at doses of either 150 mg or 300 mg/day) where the incidence in patients treated with SEROQUEL XR was greater than the incidence in placebo-treated patients.

Table 13: Treatment-Emergent Adverse Reaction Incidence in Placebo-Controlled Adjunctive Therapy Clinical Trials for the Treatment of MDD by Fixed Dose*

Body System/ Preferred Term	Placebo (n=309)	SEROQUEL XR 150 mg (n=315)	SEROQUEL XR 300 mg (n=312)
Ear And Labyrinth Disorders			
Vertigo	1%	2%	2%
Eye Disorders			
Vision Blurred	1%	2%	1%
Gastrointestinal Disorders			
Dry Mouth	8%	27%	40%
Constipation	4%	6%	11%
Nausea	7%	7%	8%
Dyspepsia	2%	2%	3%
Abdominal Distension	0%	0%	1%
Vomiting	1%	3%	1%
General Disorders and Administration Site Conditions			
Fatigue	4%	14%	11%
Irritability	3%	4%	2%
Chills	0%	1%	1%
Infections And Infestations			
Upper Respiratory Tract Infection	2%	3%	2%
Influenza	0%	2%	1%
Injury, Poisoning And Procedural Complications			
Fall	1%	2%	0%
Investigations			
Weight Increased	0%	3%	5%
Metabolism And Nutrition Disorders			
Increased Appetite	3%	3%	5%
Musculoskeletal And Connective Tissue Disorders			
Back pain	1%	3%	3%
Muscle Spasms	1%	2%	1%
Nervous System Disorders			
Somnolence[†]	9%	37%	43%
Dizziness	7%	11%	12%
Extrapyramidal Symptoms[‡]	4%	4%	6%
Hypersomnia	0%	1%	2%
Dysarthia	0%	1%	1%
Dysgeusia	0%	1%	1%
Lethargy	1%	2%	1%
Akathisia	1%	2%	2%
Psychiatric Disorders			
Abnormal Dreams	1%	2%	2%
Anxiety	1%	2%	2%
Restlessness	1%	1%	2%
Libido Decreased	0%	0%	1%
Depression	1%	2%	1%

* Reactions for which the SEROQUEL XR incidence was 1% or more but equal to or less than placebo are not listed in the table, but included the following: headache, insomnia, nausea, disturbance in attention, dysarthria, paraesthesia, tremor, diarrhea, upper abdominal pain, nightmare, nasopharyngitis, sinusitis, decreased appetite, myalgia, arthralgia, pain in extremity, hyperhidrosis, night sweats and nasal congestion.
† Somnolence combines adverse event terms somnolence and sedation.
‡ Extrapyramidal symptoms that were reported for SEROQUEL XR or placebo include the terms: akathisia, cogwheel rigidity, drooling, dyskinesia, extrapyramidal disorder, hypertonia, hypokinesia, psychomotor hyperactivity, restlessness, and tremor.

Adverse Reactions Occurring at an Incidence of 5% or More Among SEROQUEL XR Treated Patients in Long-Term, Placebo-Controlled Trials
In a longer-term placebo-controlled trial, adult patients with schizophrenia who remained clinically stable on SEROQUEL XR during open-label treatment for at least 4 months were randomized to placebo (n=103) or to continue on their current SEROQUEL XR (n=94) for up to 12 months of observation for possible relapse, the adverse reactions reported were generally consistent with those reported in the short-term, placebo-controlled trials. Insomnia (8.5%) and headache (7.4%) were the only adverse events reported by 5% or more patients.
Adverse Reactions that occurred in <5% of patients and were considered drug-related (incidence greater than placebo and consistent with known pharmacology of drug class) in order of decreasing frequency:
heart rate increased, hypotension, weight increased, tremor, akathisia, increased appetite, blurred vision, postural dizziness, pyrexia, dysarthria, dystonia, drooling, syncope, tardive dyskinesia, dysphagia, leukopenia, and rash.

Adverse Reactions in clinical trials with quetiapine and not listed elsewhere in the label:

nightmares, peripheral edema, rhinitis, eosinophilia, hypersensitivity, elevations in gamma-GT levels, and elevations in serum creatine phosphokinase (not associated with NMS).

Extrapyramidal Symptoms (EPS):

Dystonia

Class Effect: Symptoms of dystonia, prolonged abnormal contractions of muscle groups, may occur in susceptible individuals during the first few days of treatment. Dystonic symptoms include: spasm of the neck muscles, sometimes progressing to tightness of the throat, swallowing difficulty, difficulty breathing, and/or protrusion of the tongue. While these symptoms can occur at low doses, they occur more frequently and with greater severity with high potency and at higher doses of first generation antipsychotic drugs. An elevated risk of acute dystonia is observed in males and younger age groups.

Four methods were used to measure EPS: (1) Simpson-Angus total score (mean change from baseline) which evaluates parkinsonism and akathisia, (2) Barnes Akathisia Rating Scale (BARS) Global Assessment Score, (3) incidence of spontaneous complaints of EPS (akathisia, akinesia, cogwheel rigidity, extrapyramidal syndrome, hypertonia, hypokinesia, neck rigidity, and tremor), and (4) use of anticholinergic medications to treat emergent EPS.

Adults: In placebo-controlled clinical trials with quetiapine, utilizing doses up to 800 mg per day, the incidence of any adverse reactions potentially related to EPS ranged from 8% to 11% for quetiapine and 4% to 11% for placebo.

In three-arm placebo-controlled clinical trials for the treatment of schizophrenia, utilizing doses between 300 mg and 800 mg of SEROQUEL XR, the incidence of any adverse reactions potentially related to EPS was 8% for SEROQUEL XR and 8% for SEROQUEL (without evidence of being dose related), and 5% in the placebo group. In these studies, the incidence of the individual adverse reactions (akathisia, extrapyramidal disorder, tremor, dyskinesia, dystonia, restlessness, and muscle rigidity) was generally low and did not exceed 3% for any treatment group.

At the end of treatment, the mean change from baseline in SAS total score and BARS Global Assessment score was similar across the treatment groups. The use of concomitant anticholinergic medications was infrequent and similar across the treatment groups. The incidence of extrapyramidal symptoms was consistent with that seen with the profile of SEROQUEL in schizophrenia patients.

[See table 14 at top right]

In a placebo-controlled clinical trial for the treatment of bipolar mania, utilizing the dose range of 400-800 mg/day of SEROQUEL XR, the incidence of any adverse reactions potentially related to EPS was 6.6% for SEROQUEL XR and 3.8% in the placebo group. In this study, the incidence of the individual adverse reactions (akathisia, extrapyramidal disorder, tremor, dystonia, restlessness, and cogwheel rigidity) did not exceed 2.0% for any adverse reaction.

Table 15: Adverse Experiences Associated with Extrapyramidal Symptoms in a Placebo-controlled Clinical Trial for Bipolar Mania

Preferred term*	Placebo (N=160)		SEROQUEL XR (N=151)	
	n	%	n	%
Dystonic event†	0	0.0	1	0.7
Parkinsonism‡	3	1.9	4	2.7
Akathisia§	1	0.6	2	1.3
Other extrapyramidal event¶	2	1.3	3	2.0

* There were no adverse experiences with the preferred term of dyskinetic event.
† Patients with the following terms were counted in this category: nuchal rigidity, hypertonia, dystonia, muscle rigidity, oculogyration
‡ Patients with the following terms were counted in this category: cogwheel rigidity, tremor, drooling, hypokinesia
§ Patients with the following terms were counted in this category: akathisia, psychomotor agitation
¶ Patients with the following terms were counted in this category: restlessness; extrapyramidal disorder, movement disorder

In a placebo-controlled clinical trial for the treatment of bipolar depression utilizing 300 mg of SEROQUEL XR, the incidence of any adverse reactions potentially related to EPS was 4.4% for SEROQUEL XR and 0.7% in the placebo group. In this study, the incidence of the individual adverse reactions (akathisia, extrapyramidal disorder, tremor, dystonia, hypertonia) did not exceed 1.5% for any individual adverse reaction.

Table 14: Adverse Experiences Associated with Extrapyramidal Symptoms in Placebo-controlled Clinical Trials for Schizophrenia

Preferred Term	Placebo (N-319)		SEROQUEL XR 300 mg/day (N=91)		SEROQUEL XR 400 mg/day (N=227)		SEROQUEL XR 600 mg/day (N=310)		SEROQUEL XR 800 mg/day (N=323)		All Doses (N=951)	
	n	%	n	%	n	%	n	%	n	%	n	%
Dystonic event*	0	0.0	3	3.3	0	0.0	4	1.3	1	0.3	8	0.8
Parkinsonism†	4	1.3	1	1.1	3	1.3	11	3.6	7	2.2	22	2.3
Akathisia‡	4	1.3	0	0.0	3	1.3	7	2.3	7	2.2	17	1.8
Dyskinetic event§	2	0.6	2	2.2	1	0.4	1	0.3	1	0.3	5	0.5
Other extrapyramidal event¶	7	2.2	3	3.3	4	1.8	7	2.3	12	3.7	26	2.7

* Patients with the following terms were counted in this category: nuchal rigidity, hypertonia, dystonia, muscle rigidity, oculogyration
† Patients with the following terms were counted in this category: cogwheel rigidity, tremor, drooling, hypokinesia
‡ Patients with the following terms were counted in this category: akathisia, psychomotor agitation
§ Patients with the following terms were counted in this category: tardive dyskinesia, dyskinesia, choreoathetosis
¶ Patients with the following terms were counted in this category: restlessness; extrapyramidal disorder, movement disorder

Table 17: Adverse Reactions Potentially Associated with EPS in MDD Trials by Dose, Adjunctive Therapy Clinical Trials (6 weeks duration)

Preferred term	Placebo (N=309)		SEROQUEL XR 150 mg/day (N=315)		SEROQUEL XR 300 mg/day (N=312)		All Doses (N=627)	
	n	%	n	%	n	%	n	%
Dystonic event*	0	0.0	1	0.3	0	0.0	1	0.2
Parkinsonism†	5	1.6	3	1.0	4	1.3	7	1.1
Akathisia‡	3	1.0	5	1.6	8	2.6	13	2.1
Dyskinetic event§	0	0.0	0	0.0	1	0.3	1	0.2
Other extrapyramidal event¶	5	1.6	5	1.6	7	2.2	12	1.9

* Patients with the following terms were counted in this category: nuchal rigidity, hypertonia, dystonia, muscle rigidity, oculogyration
† Patients with the following terms were counted in this category: cogwheel rigidity, tremor, drooling, hypokinesia
‡ Patients with the following terms were counted in this category: akathisia, psychomotor agitation
§ Patients with the following terms were counted in this category: tardive dyskinesia, dyskinesia, choreoathetosis
¶ Patients with the following terms were counted in this category: restlessness; extrapyramidal disorder, movement disorder

Table 16: Adverse Experiences Associated with Extrapyramidal Symptoms in a Placebo-controlled Clinical Trial for Bipolar Depression

Preferred Term*	Placebo (N=140)		SEROQUEL XR (N=137)	
	n	%	n	%
Dystonic event†	0	0.0	2	1.5
Parkinsonism‡	1	0.7	1	0.7
Akathisia§	0	0.0	2	1.5
Other extrapyramidal event¶	0	0.0	1	0.7

* There were no adverse experiences with the preferred term of dyskinetic event.
† Patients with the following terms were counted in this category: nuchal rigidity, hypertonia, dystonia, muscle rigidity, oculogyration
‡ Patients with the following terms were counted in this category: cogwheel rigidity, tremor, drooling, hypokinesia
§ Patients with the following terms were counted in this category: akathisia, psychomotor agitation
¶ Patients with the following terms were counted in this category: restlessness; extrapyramidal disorder, movement disorder

In two placebo-controlled short-term adjunctive therapy clinical trials for the treatment of MDD utilizing between 150 mg and 300 mg of SEROQUEL XR, the incidence of any adverse reactions potentially related to EPS was 5.1% for SEROQUEL XR and 4.2% for the placebo group.

Table 17 shows the percentage of patients experiencing adverse reactions potentially associated with EPS in adjunct clinical trials for MDD by dose:

[See table 17 above]

Children and Adolescents: Safety and effectiveness of SEROQUEL XR have not been established in pediatric patients and SEROQUEL XR is not approved for patients under the age of 18 years. In a short-term placebo-controlled monotherapy trial in adolescent patients with schizophrenia (6-week duration), the aggregated incidence of extrapyramidal symptoms was 12.9% for SEROQUEL and 5.3% for placebo, though the incidence of the individual adverse events (eg, akathisia, tremor, extrapyramidal disorder, hypokinesia, restlessness, psychomotor hyperactivity, muscle rigidity, dyskinesia) did not exceed 4.1% in any treatment group. In a short-term placebo-controlled monotherapy trial in children and adolescent patients with bipolar mania (3-

week duration), the aggregated incidence of extrapyramidal symptoms was 3.6% for SEROQUEL and 1.1% for placebo. Table 18 below presents a listing of patients with adverse experiences potentially associated with EPS in the short-term placebo-controlled monotherapy trial in adolescent patients with schizophrenia (6-week duration).

[See table 18 at top of next page]

Table 19 below presents a listing of patients with Adverse Experiences potentially associated with EPS in a short-term placebo-controlled monotherapy trial in children and adolescent patients with bipolar mania (3-week duration)

[See table 19 on next page]

Children and Adolescents: Safety and effectiveness of SEROQUEL XR have not been established in pediatric patients and SEROQUEL XR is not approved for patients under the age of 18 years. In acute placebo-controlled trials in children and adolescent patients with schizophrenia (6-week duration) or bipolar mania (3-week duration), the incidence of increased appetite was 7.6% for SEROQUEL compared to 2.4% for placebo. In a 26-week open-label study that enrolled patients from the above two pediatric trials, the incidence of increased appetite was 10% for SEROQUEL.

6.2 Vital Signs and Laboratory Values

Hyperglycemia, hyperlipidemia, weight gain and orthostatic hypotension have been reported with quetiapine. Increases in blood pressure have also been reported with quetiapine in children and adolescents [see Warnings and Precautions (5.4, 5.5, 5.6, 5.8 and 5.9)].

Laboratory Changes:

Neutrophil Counts

In three-arm SEROQUEL XR placebo-controlled monotherapy clinical trials, among patients with a baseline neutrophil count $\geq 1.5 \times 10^9$/L, the incidence of at least one occurrence of neutrophil count $<1.5 \times 10^9$/L was 1.5% in patients treated with SEROQUEL XR and 1.5% for SEROQUEL, compared to 0.8% in placebo-treated patients. In placebo-controlled monotherapy clinical trials involving 3368 patients on quetiapine fumarate and 1515 on placebo, the incidence of at least one occurrence of neutrophil count $<1.0 \times 10^9$/L among patients with a normal baseline neutrophil count and at least one available follow up laboratory measurement was 0.3% (10/2967) in patients treated with quetiapine, compared to 0.1% (2/1349) in patients treated with placebo. Patients with a pre-existing low WBC or a history of drug induced leukopenia/neutropenia should have their complete blood count (CBC) monitored frequently during the first few months of therapy and should discontinue

SEROQUEL XR at the first sign of a decline in WBC in absence of other causative factors [*see Warnings and Precautions* (5.10)].

Decreased Hemoglobin

In short-term placebo-controlled trials, decreases in hemoglobin to ≤ 13 g/dL males, ≤ 12 g/dL females on at least one occasion occurred in 8.3% (594/7155) of quetiapine-treated patients compared to 6.2% (219/3536) of patients treated with placebo. In a database of controlled and uncontrolled clinical trials, decreases in hemoglobin to ≤ 13 g/dL males, ≤ 12 g/dL females on at least one occasion occurred in 11% (2277/20729) of quetiapine-treated patients.

ECG Changes:

2.5% of SEROQUEL XR patients, and 2.3% of placebo patients, had tachycardia (>120 bpm) at any time during the trials. SEROQUEL XR was associated with a mean increase in heart rate, assessed by ECG, of 6.3 beats per minute compared to a mean increase of 0.4 beats per minute for placebo. This is consistent with the rates for SEROQUEL. The incidence of adverse reactions of tachycardia was 1.9% for SEROQUEL XR compared to 0.5% for placebo. SEROQUEL use was associated with a mean increase in heart rate, assessed by ECG, of 7 beats per minute compared to a mean increase of 1 beat per minute among placebo patients. The slight tendency for tachycardia may be related to quetiapine's potential for inducing orthostatic changes [*see Warnings and Precautions* (5.8)].

Children and Adolescents: Safety and effectiveness of SEROQUEL XR have not been established in pediatric patients. In the acute (6-week) schizophrenia trial in adolescents, potentially clinically significant increases in heart rate (> 110 bpm) occurred in 5.2% of patients receiving SEROQUEL 400 mg and 8.5% of patients receiving SEROQUEL 800 mg compared to 0% of patients receiving placebo. Mean increases in heart rate were 3.8 bpm and 11.2 bpm for SEROQUEL 400 mg and 800 mg groups, respectively, compared to a decrease of 3.3 bpm in the placebo group [*see Warnings and Precautions* (5.8)].

In the acute (3-week) bipolar mania trial in children and adolescents, potentially clinically significant increases in heart rate (> 110 bpm) occurred in 1.1% of patients receiving SEROQUEL 400 mg and 2.4% of patients receiving SEROQUEL 600 mg compared to 0% of patients receiving placebo. Mean increases in heart rate were 12.8 bpm and 13.4 bpm for SEROQUEL 400 mg and 600 mg groups, respectively, compared to a decrease of 1.7 bpm in the placebo group [*see Warnings and Precautions* (5.8)].

6.3 Post Marketing Experience

The following adverse reactions were identified during post approval use of SEROQUEL. Because these reactions are reported voluntarily from a population of uncertain size, it is not always possible to reliably estimate their frequency or establish a causal relationship to drug exposure.

Adverse reactions reported since market introduction which were temporally related to SEROQUEL therapy include anaphylactic reaction and galactorrhea.

Other adverse reactions reported since market introduction, which were temporally related to SEROQUEL therapy, but not necessarily causally related, include the following: agranulocytosis, cardiomyopathy, hyponatremia, myocarditis, rhabdomyolysis, syndrome of inappropriate antidiuretic hormone secretion (SIADH), Stevens-Johnson syndrome (SJS), and decreased platelets.

In post-marketing clinical trials, elevations in total cholesterol (predominantly LDL cholesterol) have been reported.

Table 18: Adverse experiences potentially associated with EPS in the short-term placebo-controlled monotherapy trial in adolescent patients with schizophrenia (6-week duration).

Preferred term	Placebo (N=75)		SEROQUEL 400 mg/day (N=73)		SEROQUEL 800 mg/day (N=74)		All SEROQUEL (N=147)	
	n	%	n	%	n	%	n	%
Dystonic event*	0	0.0	2	2.7	0	0.0	2	1.4
Parkinsonism†	2	2.7	4	5.5	4	5.4	8	5.4
Akathisia‡	3	4.0	3	4.1	4	5.4	7	4.8
Dyskinetic event§	0	0.0	2	2.7	0	0.0	2	1.4
Other extrapyramidal event¶	0	0.0	2	2.7	2	2.7	4	2.7

* Patients with the following terms were counted in this category: nuchal rigidity, hypertonia, dystonia, muscle rigidity
† Patients with the following terms were counted in this category: cogwheel rigidity, tremor
‡ Patients with the following terms were counted in this category: akathisia
§ Patients with the following terms were counted in this category: tardive dyskinesia, dyskinesia, choreoathetosis
¶ Patients with the following terms were counted in this category: restlessness; extrapyramidal disorder

Table 19: Adverse experiences potentially associated with EPS in a short-term placebo-controlled monotherapy trial in children and adolescent patients with bipolar mania (3-week duration)
Table 19

Preferred term*	Placebo (N=90)		SEROQUEL 400 mg/day (N=95)		SEROQUEL 800 mg/day (N=98)		All SEROQUEL (N=193)	
	n	%	n	%	n	%	n	%
Parkinsonism†	1	1.1	2	2.1	1	1.0	3	1.6
Akathisia‡	0	0.0	1	1.0	1	1.0	2	1.0
Other extrapyramidal event§	0	0.0	1	1.1	1	1.0	2	1.0

* There were no adverse experiences with the preferred term of dystonic or dyskinetic events.
† Patients with the following terms were counted in this category: cogwheel rigidity, tremor
‡ Patients with the following terms were counted in this category: akathisia
§ Patients with the following terms were counted in this category: restlessness; extrapyramidal disorder

7 DRUG INTERACTIONS

The risks of using SEROQUEL XR in combination with other drugs have not been extensively evaluated in systematic studies. Given the primary CNS effects of SEROQUEL XR, caution should be used when it is taken in combination with other centrally acting drugs. Quetiapine potentiated the cognitive and motor effects of alcohol in a clinical trial in subjects with selected psychotic disorders, and alcoholic beverages should be limited while taking quetiapine.

Because of its potential for inducing hypotension, SEROQUEL XR may enhance the effects of certain antihypertensive agents.

SEROQUEL XR may antagonize the effects of levodopa and dopamine agonists.

Caution should be exercised when quetiapine is used concomitantly with drugs known to cause electrolyte imbalance or to increase QT interval [*see Warnings and Precautions* (5.21)].

There have been reports of false positive results in urine enzyme immunoassays for methadone and tricyclic antidepressants in patients who have taken quetiapine. If false positive results are suspected, confirmation by an appropriate chromatographic technique is recommended.

7.1 The Effect of Other Drugs on Quetiapine

Phenytoin

Coadministration of quetiapine (250 mg three times/day) and phenytoin (100 mg three times/day) increased the mean oral clearance of quetiapine by 5-fold. Increased doses of SEROQUEL XR may be required to maintain control of symptoms of schizophrenia in patients receiving quetiapine and phenytoin, or other hepatic enzyme inducers (eg, carbamazepine, barbiturates, rifampin, glucocorticoids). Caution should be taken if phenytoin is withdrawn and replaced with a non-inducer (eg, valproate) [*see Dosage and Administration* (2)].

Divalproex

Coadministration of quetiapine (150 mg twice daily) and divalproex (500 mg twice daily) increased the mean maximum plasma concentration of quetiapine at steady-state by 17% without affecting the extent of absorption or mean oral clearance.

Thioridazine

Thioridazine (200 mg twice daily) increased the oral clearance of quetiapine (300 mg twice daily) by 65%.

Cimetidine

Administration of multiple daily doses of cimetidine (400 mg three times daily for 4 days) resulted in a 20% decrease in the mean oral clearance of quetiapine (150 mg three times daily). Dosage adjustment for quetiapine is not required when it is given with cimetidine.

P450 3A Inhibitors

Coadministration of ketoconazole (200 mg once daily for 4 days), a potent inhibitor of cytochrome P450 3A, reduced oral clearance of quetiapine by 84%, resulting in a 335% increase in maximum plasma concentration of quetiapine. Caution (reduced dosage) is indicated when SEROQUEL XR is administered with ketoconazole and other inhibitors of cytochrome P450 3A (eg, itraconazole, fluconazole, erythromycin, protease inhibitors).

Fluoxetine, Imipramine, Haloperidol, and Risperidone

Coadministration of fluoxetine (60 mg once daily), imipramine (75 mg twice daily), haloperidol (7.5 mg twice daily), or risperidone (3 mg twice daily) with quetiapine (300 mg twice daily) did not alter the steady-state pharmacokinetics of quetiapine.

7.2 Effect of Quetiapine on Other Drugs

Lorazepam

The mean oral clearance of lorazepam (2 mg, single dose) was reduced by 20% in the presence of quetiapine administered as 250 mg three times daily dosing.

Divalproex

The mean maximum concentration and extent of absorption of total and free valproic acid at steady-state were decreased by 10 to 12% when divalproex (500 mg twice daily) was administered with quetiapine (150 mg twice daily). The mean oral clearance of total valproic acid (administered as divalproex 500 mg twice daily) was increased by 11% in the presence of quetiapine (150 mg twice daily). The changes were not significant.

Lithium

Concomitant administration of quetiapine (250 mg three times daily) with lithium had no effect on any of the steady-state pharmacokinetic parameters of lithium.

Antipyrine

Administration of multiple daily doses up to 750 mg/day (on a three times daily schedule) of quetiapine to subjects with selected psychotic disorders had no clinically relevant effect on the clearance of antipyrine or urinary recovery of antipyrine metabolites. These results indicate that quetiapine does not significantly induce hepatic enzymes responsible for cytochrome P450 mediated metabolism of antipyrine.

8 USE IN SPECIFIC POPULATIONS

8.1 Pregnancy

Pregnancy Category C:

There are no adequate and well-controlled studies of SEROQUEL XR use in pregnant women. In limited published literature, there were no major malformations associated with quetiapine exposure during pregnancy. In animal studies, embryo-fetal toxicity occurred. Quetiapine should be used during pregnancy only if the potential benefit justifies the potential risk to the fetus.

There are limited published data on the use of quetiapine for treatment of schizophrenia and other psychiatric disorders during pregnancy. In a prospective observational study, 21 women exposed to quetiapine and other psychoactive medications during pregnancy delivered infants with no major malformations. Among 42 other infants born to pregnant women who used quetiapine during pregnancy, there were no major malformations reported (one study of 36 women, 6 case reports). Due to the limited number of exposed pregnancies, these postmarketing data do not reliably estimate the frequency or absence of adverse outcomes.

When pregnant rats and rabbits were exposed to quetiapine during organogenesis, there was no increase in the incidence of major malformations in fetuses at doses up to 2.4 times the maximum recommended human dose for schizophrenia (MRHD, 800 mg/day on a mg/m^2 basis); however, there was evidence of embryo-fetal toxicity. In rats, delays in skeletal ossification occurred at 0.6 and 2.4 times the MRHD and in rabbits at 1.2 and 2.4 times the MRHD. At 2.4 times the MRHD, there was an increased incidence of carpal/ tarsal flexure (minor soft tissue anomaly) in rabbit fetuses and decreased fetal weights in both species. Maternal toxicity (decreased body weights and/or death) occurred at 2.4 times the MRHD in rats and at 0.6-2.4 times the MRHD (all doses) in rabbits.

In a peri/postnatal reproductive study in rats, no drug-related effects were observed when pregnant dams were treated with quetiapine at doses 0.01, 0.12, and 0.24 times the MRHD. However, in a preliminary peri/postnatal study, there were increases in fetal and pup death, and decreases in mean litter weight at 3.0 times the MRHD.

8.2 Labor and Delivery

The effect of SEROQUEL XR on labor and delivery in humans is unknown.

8.3 Nursing Mothers

SEROQUEL XR was excreted into human milk. Caution should be exercised when SEROQUEL XR is administered to a nursing woman.

In published case reports, the level of quetiapine in breast milk ranged from undetectable to 170 μg/L. The estimated infant dose ranged from 0.09% to 0.43% of the weight-adjusted maternal dose. Based on a limited number (N=8) of mother/infant pairs, calculated infant daily doses range from less than 0.01 mg/kg (at a maternal daily dose up to 100 mg quetiapine) to 0.1 mg/kg (at a maternal daily dose of 400 mg).

8.4 Pediatric Use

Safety and effectiveness of SEROQUEL XR have not been established in pediatric patients and SEROQUEL XR is not approved for patients under the age of 18 years [*see Warnings and Precautions* (5) *and Adverse Reactions* (6)].

In general, the adverse reactions observed in children and adolescents during the clinical trials with SEROQUEL were similar to those in the adult population with few exceptions. Increases in systolic and diastolic blood pressure occurred in children and adolescents and did not occur in adults. Orthostatic hypotension occurred more frequently in adults (4-7%) compared to children and adolescents (< 1%).

8.5 Geriatric Use

Sixty-eight patients in clinical studies with SEROQUEL XR were 65 years of age or over. In general, there was no indication of any different tolerability of SEROQUEL XR in the elderly compared to younger adults. Nevertheless, the presence of factors that might decrease pharmacokinetic clearance, increase the pharmacodynamic response to SEROQUEL XR, or cause poorer tolerance or orthostasis, should lead to consideration of a lower starting dose, slower titration, and careful monitoring during the initial dosing period in the elderly. The mean plasma clearance of quetiapine was reduced by 30% to 50% in elderly patients when compared to younger patients [*see Dosage and Administration* (2.4) *and Pharmacokinetics* (12.3)].

8.6 Renal Impairment

Clinical experience with SEROQUEL XR in patients with renal impairment [*see Clinical Pharmacology* (12.3)] is limited.

8.7 Hepatic Impairment

Since quetiapine is extensively metabolized by the liver, higher plasma levels are expected in the hepatically impaired population, and dosage adjustment may be needed [*see Dosage and Administration* (2.3) *and Clinical Pharmacology* (12.3)].

9 DRUG ABUSE AND DEPENDENCE

9.1 Controlled Substance

SEROQUEL XR is not a controlled substance.

9.2 Abuse

SEROQUEL XR has not been systematically studied in animals or humans for its potential for abuse, tolerance or physical dependence. While the clinical trials did not reveal any tendency for any drug-seeking behavior, these observations were not systematic and it is not possible to predict on the basis of this limited experience the extent to which a CNS-active drug will be misused, diverted, and/or abused once marketed. Consequently, patients should be evaluated carefully for a history of drug abuse, and such patients should be observed closely for signs of misuse or abuse of SEROQUEL XR (eg, development of tolerance, increases in dose, drug-seeking behavior).

10 OVERDOSAGE

10.1 Human Experience

In clinical trials, survival has been reported in acute overdoses of up to 30 grams of quetiapine. Most patients who overdosed experienced no adverse events or recovered fully from the reported events. Death has been reported in a clinical trial following an overdose of 13.6 grams of quetiapine alone. In general, reported signs and symptoms were those resulting from an exaggeration of the drug's known pharmacological effects, ie, drowsiness and sedation, tachycardia and hypotension. Patients with pre-existing severe cardiovascular disease may be at an increased risk of the effects of overdose [*see Warnings and Precautions* (5.8)]. One case, involving an estimated overdose of 9600 mg, was associated with hypokalemia and first degree heart block. In postmarketing experience, there were cases reported of QT prolongation with overdose. There were also very rare reports of overdose of SEROQUEL alone resulting in death or coma.

10.2 Management of Overdosage

In case of acute overdosage, establish and maintain an airway and ensure adequate oxygenation and ventilation. Gastric lavage (after intubation, if patient is unconscious) and administration of activated charcoal together with a laxative should be considered. The possibility of obtundation, seizure or dystonic reaction of the head and neck following overdose may create a risk of aspiration with induced emesis. Cardiovascular monitoring should commence immediately and should include continuous electrocardiographic monitoring to detect possible arrhythmias. If antiarrhythmic therapy is administered, disopyramide, procainamide and quinidine carry a theoretical hazard of additive QT-prolonging effects when administered in patients with acute overdosage of SEROQUEL XR. Similarly it is reasonable to expect that the α-adrenergic-blocking properties of bretylium might be additive to those of quetiapine, resulting in problematic hypotension.

There is no specific antidote to SEROQUEL XR. Therefore, appropriate supportive measures should be instituted. The possibility of multiple drug involvement should be considered. Hypotension and circulatory collapse should be treated with appropriate measures such as intravenous fluids and/or sympathomimetic agents (epinephrine and dopamine should not be used, since β stimulation may worsen hypotension in the setting of quetiapine-induced α blockade). In cases of severe extrapyramidal symptoms, anticholinergic medication should be administered. Close medical supervision and monitoring should continue until the patient recovers.

11 DESCRIPTION

SEROQUEL XR (quetiapine fumarate) is a psychotropic agent belonging to a chemical class, the dibenzothiazepine derivatives. The chemical designation is 2-[2-(4-dibenzo [*b,f*] [1,4] thiazepin-11-yl-1-piperazinyl)ethoxy]-ethanol fumarate (2:1) (salt). It is present in tablets as the fumarate salt. All doses and tablet strengths are expressed as milligrams of base, not as fumarate salt. Its molecular formula is $C_{42}H_{50}N_6O_4S_2 \bullet C_4H_4O_4$ and it has a molecular weight of 883.11 (fumarate salt). The structural formula is:

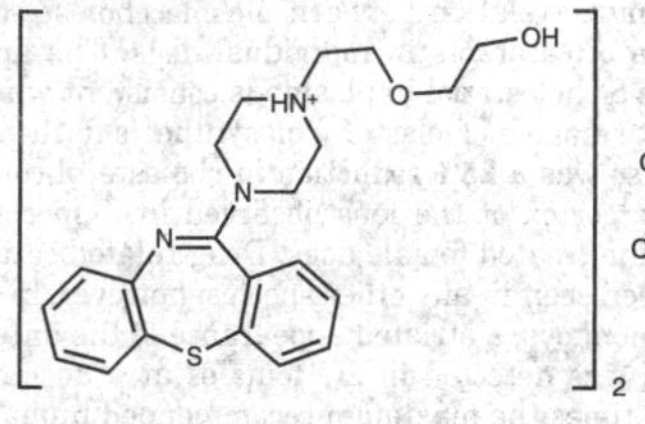

Quetiapine fumarate is a white to off-white crystalline powder which is moderately soluble in water.

SEROQUEL XR is supplied for oral administration as 50 mg (peach), 150 mg (white), 200 mg (yellow), 300 mg (pale yellow), and 400 mg (white). All tablets are capsule shaped and film coated.

Inactive ingredients for SEROQUEL XR are lactose monohydrate, microcrystalline cellulose, sodium citrate, hypromellose, and magnesium stearate. The film coating for all SEROQUEL XR tablets contain hypromellose, polyethylene glycol 400 and titanium dioxide. In addition, yellow iron oxide (50, 200 and 300 mg tablets) and red iron oxide (50 mg tablets) are included in the film coating of specific strengths.

Each 50 mg tablet contains 58 mg of quetiapine fumarate equivalent to 50 mg quetiapine. Each 150 mg tablet contains 173 mg of quetiapine fumarate equivalent to 150 mg quetiapine. Each 200 mg tablet contains 230 mg of quetiapine fumarate equivalent to 200 mg quetiapine. Each 300 mg tablet contains 345 mg of quetiapine fumarate equivalent to 300 mg quetiapine. Each 400 mg tablet contains 461 mg of quetiapine fumarate equivalent to 400 mg quetiapine.

12 CLINICAL PHARMACOLOGY

12.1 Mechanism of Action

The mechanism of action of SEROQUEL XR, as with other drugs having efficacy in the treatment of schizophrenia, bipolar disorder and major depressive disorder (MDD), is unknown. However, it has been proposed that the efficacy of SEROQUEL XR in schizophrenia is mediated through a combination of dopamine type 2 (D2) and serotonin type 2A (5HT2A) antagonism. The active metabolite, N-desalkyl quetiapine (norquetiapine), has similar activity at D2, but greater activity at 5HT2A receptors, than the parent drug (quetiapine). Quetiapine's efficacy in bipolar depression and MDD may partly be explained by the high affinity and potent inhibitory effects that norquetiapine exhibits for the norepinephrine transporter.

Antagonism at receptors other than dopamine and serotonin with similar or greater affinities may explain some of the other effects of quetiapine and norquetiapine: antagonism at histamine H_1 receptors may explain the somnolence, antagonism at adrenergic α_1b receptors may explain the orthostatic hypotension, and antagonism at muscarinic M_1 receptors may explain the anticholinergic effects.

12.2 Pharmacodynamics

Quetiapine and norquetiapine have affinity for multiple neurotransmitter receptors including dopamine D_1 and D_2, serotonin $5HT_{1A}$ and $5HT_{2A}$, histamine H_1, muscarinic M_1, and adrenergic α_1b and α_2 receptors. Quetiapine differs from norquetiapine in having no appreciable affinity for muscarinic M_1 receptors whereas norquetiapine has high affinity. Quetiapine and norquetiapine lack appreciable affinity for benzodiazepine receptors.

Receptor Affinities (K_i, nM) for Quetiapine and Norquetiapine

Receptor	Quetiapine	Norquetiapine
Dopamine D_1	428	99.8
Dopamine D_2	626	489
Serotonin $5HT_{1A}$	1040	191
Serotonin $5HT_{2A}$	38	2.9
Norepinephrine transporter	>10000	34.8
Histamine H_1	4.41	1.15
Adrenergic α_1b	14.6	46.4
Adrenergic α_2	617	1290
Muscarinic M_1	1086	38.3
Benzodiazepine	>10000	> 10000

12.3 Pharmacokinetics

Following multiple dosing of quetiapine up to a total daily dose of 800 mg, administered in divided doses, the plasma concentration of quetiapine and norquetiapine, the major active metabolite of quetiapine, were proportional to the total daily dose. Accumulation is predictable upon multiple dosing. Steady-state mean C_{max} and AUC of norquetiapine are about 21-27% and 46-56%, respectively of that observed for quetiapine. Elimination of quetiapine is mainly via hepatic metabolism. The mean-terminal half-life is approximately 7 hours for quetiapine and approximately 12 hours for norquetiapine within the clinical dose range. Steady-state concentrations are expected to be achieved within two days of dosing. SEROQUEL XR is unlikely to interfere with the metabolism of drugs metabolized by cytochrome P450 enzymes.

Absorption

Quetiapine fumarate reaches peak plasma concentrations approximately 6 hours following administration. SEROQUEL XR dosed once daily at steady-state has comparable bioavailability to an equivalent total daily dose of SEROQUEL administered in divided doses, twice daily. A high-fat meal (approximately 800 to 1000 calories) was found to produce statistically significant increases in the SEROQUEL XR C_{max} and AUC of 44% to 52% and 20% to 22%, respectively, for the 50 mg and 300 mg tablets. In comparison, a light meal (approximately 300 calories) had no significant effect on the C_{max} or AUC of quetiapine. It is recommended that SEROQUEL XR be taken without food or with a light meal [*see Dosage and Administration* (2)].

Distribution

Quetiapine is widely distributed throughout the body with an apparent volume of distribution of 10±4 L/kg. It is 83% bound to plasma proteins at therapeutic concentrations. *In vitro*, quetiapine did not affect the binding of warfarin or diazepam to human serum albumin. In turn, neither warfarin nor diazepam altered the binding of quetiapine.

Metabolism and Elimination

Following a single oral dose of ^{14}C-quetiapine, less than 1% of the administered dose was excreted as unchanged drug, indicating that quetiapine is highly metabolized. Approximately 73% and 20% of the dose was recovered in the urine and feces, respectively. The average dose fraction of free quetiapine and its major active metabolite is <5% excreted in the urine.

Quetiapine is extensively metabolized by the liver. The major metabolic pathways are sulfoxidation to the sulfoxide metabolite and oxidation to the parent acid metabolite; both metabolites are pharmacologically inactive. *In vitro* studies using human liver microsomes revealed that the cytochrome P450 3A4 isoenzyme is involved in the metabolism of quetiapine to its major, but inactive, sulfoxide metabolite and in the metabolism of its active metabolite norquetiapine.

Age

Oral clearance of quetiapine was reduced by 40% in elderly patients (> 65 years, n = 9) compared to young patients (n = 12), and dosing adjustment may be necessary [*see Dosage and Administration* (2.3)].

Gender

There is no gender effect on the pharmacokinetics of quetiapine.

Race

There is no race effect on the pharmacokinetics of quetiapine.

Smoking

Smoking has no effect on the oral clearance of quetiapine.

Renal Insufficiency

Patients with severe renal impairment (CL_{cr}=10-30 mL/min/1.73m^2, n=8) had a 25% lower mean oral clearance than normal subjects (CL_{cr}>80 mL/min/1.73m^2, n=8), but plasma quetiapine concentrations in the subjects with renal insufficiency were within the range of concentrations seen in normal subjects receiving the same dose. Dosage adjustment is therefore not needed in these patients.

Hepatic Insufficiency
Hepatically impaired patients (n=8) had a 30% lower mean oral clearance of quetiapine than normal subjects. In 2 of the 8 hepatically impaired patients, AUC and C_{max} were 3 times higher than those observed typically in healthy subjects. Since quetiapine is extensively metabolized by the liver, higher plasma levels are expected in the hepatically impaired population, and dosage adjustment may be needed [*see Dosage and Administration* (2.4)].

Drug-Drug Interactions
In vitro enzyme inhibition data suggest that quetiapine and 9 of its metabolites would have little inhibitory effect on *in vivo* metabolism mediated by cytochromes P450 1A2, 2C9, 2C19, 2D6 and 3A4.
Quetiapine oral clearance is increased by the prototype cytochrome P450 3A4 inducer, phenytoin, and decreased by the prototype cytochrome P450 3A4 inhibitor, ketoconazole. Dose adjustment of quetiapine will be necessary if it is co-administered with phenytoin or ketoconazole [*see Dosage and Administration* (2.4) *and Drug Interactions* (7.1)].
Quetiapine oral clearance is not inhibited by the non-specific enzyme inhibitor, cimetidine.
Quetiapine at doses of 750 mg/day did not affect the single dose pharmacokinetics of antipyrine, lithium or lorazepam [*see Drug Interactions* (7.2)].

13 NONCLINICAL TOXICOLOGY

13.1 Carcinogenesis, Mutagenesis, Impairment of Fertility

Carcinogenesis
Carcinogenicity studies were conducted in C57BL mice and Wistar rats. Quetiapine was administered in the diet to mice at doses of 20, 75, 250, and 750 mg/kg and to rats by gavage at doses of 25, 75, and 250 mg/kg for two years. These doses are equivalent to 0.1, 0.5, 1.5, and 4.5 times the maximum human dose for schizophrenia and bipolar mania (800 mg/day) on a mg/m^2 basis (mice) or 0.3, 0.9, and 3.0 times the maximum human dose on a mg/m^2 basis (rats). There were statistically significant increases in thyroid gland follicular adenomas in male mice at doses of 250 and 750 mg/kg or 1.5 and 4.5 times the maximum human dose on a mg/m^2 basis and in male rats at a dose of 250 mg/kg or 3.0 times the maximum human dose on a mg/m^2 basis. Mammary gland adenocarcinomas were statistically significantly increased in female rats at all doses tested (25, 75, and 250 mg/kg or 0.3, 0.9, and 3.0 times the maximum recommended human dose on a mg/m^2 basis).
Thyroid follicular cell adenomas may have resulted from chronic stimulation of the thyroid gland by thyroid stimulating hormone (TSH) resulting from enhanced metabolism and clearance of thyroxine by rodent liver. Changes in TSH, thyroxine, and thyroxine clearance consistent with this mechanism were observed in subchronic toxicity studies in rat and mouse and in a 1-year toxicity study in rat; however, the results of these studies were not definitive. The relevance of the increases in thyroid follicular cell adenomas to human risk, through whatever mechanism, is unknown.
Antipsychotic drugs have been shown to chronically elevate prolactin levels in rodents. Serum measurements in a 1-year toxicity study showed that quetiapine increased median serum prolactin levels a maximum of 32- and 13-fold in male and female rats, respectively. Increases in mammary neoplasms have been found in rodents after chronic administration of other antipsychotic drugs and are considered to be prolactin-mediated. The relevance of this increased incidence of prolactin-mediated mammary gland tumors in rats to human risk is unknown [*see Warnings and Precautions* (5.14)].

Mutagenesis
The mutagenic potential of quetiapine was tested in six *in vitro* bacterial gene mutation assays and in an *in vitro* mammalian gene mutation assay in Chinese Hamster Ovary cells. However, sufficiently high concentrations of quetiapine may not have been used for all tester strains. Quetiapine did produce a reproducible increase in mutations in one Salmonella typhimurium tester strain in the presence of metabolic activation. No evidence of clastogenic potential was obtained in an *in vitro* chromosomal aberration assay in cultured human lymphocytes or in the *in vivo* micronucleus assay in rats.

Impairment of Fertility
Quetiapine decreased mating and fertility in male Sprague-Dawley rats at oral doses of 50 and 150 mg/kg or 0.6 and 1.8 times the maximum human dose on a mg/m^2 basis. Drug-related effects included increases in interval to mate and in the number of matings required for successful impregnation. These effects continued to be observed at 150 mg/kg even after a two-week period without treatment. The no-effect dose for impaired mating and fertility in male rats was 25 mg/kg, or 0.3 times the maximum human dose on a mg/m^2 basis. Quetiapine adversely affected mating and fertility in female Sprague-Dawley rats at an oral dose of 50 mg/kg, or 0.6 times the maximum human dose on a mg/m^2 basis. Drug-related effects included decreases in matings and in matings resulting in pregnancy, and an increase in the interval to mate. An increase in irregular estrus cycles was observed at doses of 10 and 50 mg/kg, or 0.1 and 0.6 times the maximum human dose on a mg/m^2 basis. The no-effect dose in female rats was 1 mg/kg, or 0.01 times the maximum human dose on a mg/m^2 basis.

13.2 Animal Toxicology and/or Pharmacology

Quetiapine caused a dose-related increase in pigment deposition in thyroid gland in rat toxicity studies which were 4 weeks in duration or longer and in a mouse 2-year carcinogenicity study. Doses were 10-250 mg/kg in rats, 75-750 mg/kg in mice; these doses are 0.1-3.0, and 0.1-4.5 times the maximum recommended human dose (on a mg/m^2 basis), respectively. Pigment deposition was shown to be irreversible in rats. The identity of the pigment could not be determined, but was found to be co-localized with quetiapine in thyroid gland follicular epithelial cells. The functional effects and the relevance of this finding to human risk are unknown.
In dogs receiving quetiapine for 6 or 12 months, but not for 1 month, focal triangular cataracts occurred at the junction of posterior sutures in the outer cortex of the lens at a dose of 100 mg/kg, or 4 times the maximum recommended human dose on a mg/m^2 basis. This finding may be due to inhibition of cholesterol biosynthesis by quetiapine. Quetiapine caused a dose-related reduction in plasma cholesterol levels in repeat-dose dog and monkey studies; however, there was no correlation between plasma cholesterol and the presence of cataracts in individual dogs. The appearance of delta 8 cholestanol in plasma is consistent with inhibition of a late stage in cholesterol biosynthesis in these species. There also was a 25% reduction in cholesterol content of the outer cortex of the lens observed in a special study in quetiapine treated female dogs. Drug-related cataracts have not been seen in any other species; however, in a 1-year study in monkeys, a striated appearance of the anterior lens surface was detected in 2/7 females at a dose of 225 mg/kg or 5.5 times the maximum recommended human dose on a mg/m^2 basis.

14 CLINICAL STUDIES

14.1 Schizophrenia

The efficacy of SEROQUEL XR in the treatment of schizophrenia was demonstrated in 1 short-term, 6-week, fixed-dose, placebo-controlled trial of inpatients and outpatients with schizophrenia (n=573) who met DSM IV criteria for schizophrenia. SEROQUEL XR (once daily) was administered as 300 mg on Day 1, and the dose was increased to either 400 mg or 600 mg by Day 2, or 800 mg by Day 3. The primary endpoint was the change from baseline of the Positive and Negative Syndrome Scale (PANSS) total score at the end of treatment (Day 42). SEROQUEL XR doses of 400 mg, 600 mg and 800 mg once daily were superior to placebo in the PANSS total score at Day 42.
In a longer-term trial, clinically stable adult outpatients (n=171) meeting DSM-IV criteria for schizophrenia who remained stable following 16 weeks of open-label treatment with flexible doses of SEROQUEL XR (400 mg/day-800 mg/day) were randomized to placebo or to continue on their current SEROQUEL XR (400 mg/day-800 mg/day) for observation for possible relapse during the double-blind continuation (maintenance) phase. Stabilization during the open-label phase was defined as receiving a stable dose of SEROQUEL XR and having a CGI-S≤4 and a PANSS score ≤60 from beginning to end of this open-label phase (with no increase of ≥10 points in PANSS total score). Relapse during the double-blind phase was defined in terms of a ≥30% increase in the PANSS Total score, or CGI-Improvement score of ≥6, or hospitalization due to worsening of schizophrenia, or need for any other antipsychotic medication. Patients on SEROQUEL XR experienced a statistically significant longer time to relapse than did patients on placebo.

14.2 Bipolar Disorder

Bipolar Mania
The efficacy of SEROQUEL XR in the acute treatment of manic episodes was established in one 3-week, placebo-controlled trial in patients who met DSM-IV criteria for bipolar I disorder with manic or mixed episodes with or without psychotic features (N=316). Patients were hospitalized for a minimum of 4 days at randomization. Patients randomized to SEROQUEL XR received 300 mg on Day 1 and 600 mg on Day 2. Afterwards, the dose could be adjusted between 400 mg and 800 mg per day.
The primary rating instrument used for assessing manic symptoms in these trials was the Young Mania Rating Scale (YMRS), an 11-item clinician-rated scale traditionally used to assess the degree of manic symptoms in a range from 0 (no manic features) to 60 (maximum score). SEROQUEL XR was superior to placebo in the reduction of the YMRS total score at week 3.
The efficacy of SEROQUEL in the treatment of acute manic episodes was also established in 3 placebo-controlled trials in patients who met DSM-IV criteria for bipolar I disorder with manic episodes. These trials included patients with or without psychotic features and excluded patients with rapid cycling and mixed episodes. Of these trials, 2 were monotherapy (12 weeks) and 1 was adjunct therapy (3 weeks) to either lithium or divalproex. Key outcomes in these trials were change from baseline in the YMRS score at 3 and 12 weeks for monotherapy and at 3 weeks for adjunct therapy. Adjunct therapy is defined as the simultaneous initiation or subsequent administration of SEROQUEL with lithium or divalproex.
The results of the trials follow:

Monotherapy
In two 12-week trials (n=300, n=299) comparing SEROQUEL to placebo, SEROQUEL was superior to placebo in the reduction of the YMRS total score at weeks 3 and 12. The majority of patients in these trials taking SEROQUEL were dosed in a range between 400 mg/day and 800 mg/day.

Adjunct Therapy
In a 3-week placebo-controlled trial, 170 patients with bipolar mania (YMRS ≥ 20) were randomized to receive SEROQUEL or placebo as adjunct treatment to lithium or divalproex. Patients may or may not have received an adequate treatment course of lithium or divalproex prior to randomization. SEROQUEL was superior to placebo when added to lithium or divalproex alone in the reduction of YMRS total score. The majority of patients in this trial taking SEROQUEL were dosed in a range between 400 mg/day and 800 mg/day.

Depressive Episodes Associated with Bipolar Disorder
The efficacy of SEROQUEL XR for the acute treatment of depressive episodes associated with bipolar disorder in patients who met DSM-IV criteria for bipolar disorder was established in one 8-week, randomized, double-blind, placebo-controlled study (N=280 outpatients). This study included patients with bipolar I and II disorder, and those with and without a rapid cycling course. Patients randomized to SEROQUEL XR were administered 50 mg on Day 1, 100 mg on Day 2, 200 mg on Day 3, and 300 mg on Day 4 and after. The primary rating instrument used to assess depressive symptoms was the Montgomery-Asberg Depression Rating Scale (MADRS), a 10-item clinician-rated scale with scores ranging from 0 (no depressive features) to 60 (maximum score). The primary endpoint was the change from baseline in MADRS score at week 8. SEROQUEL XR was superior to placebo in reduction of MADRS score at week 8.
The efficacy of SEROQUEL for the treatment of depressive episodes associated with bipolar disorder was established in 2 identical 8-week, randomized, double-blind, placebo-controlled studies (N=1045). These studies included patients with either bipolar I or II disorder and those with or without a rapid cycling course. Patients randomized to SEROQUEL were administered fixed doses of either 300 mg or 600 mg once daily.
The primary rating instrument used to assess depressive symptoms in these studies was the MADRS. The primary endpoint in both studies was the change from baseline in MADRS score at week 8. In both studies, SEROQUEL was superior to placebo in reduction of MADRS score at week 8. In these studies, no additional benefit was seen with the 600 mg dose. For the 300 mg dose group, statistically significant improvements over placebo were seen in overall quality of life and satisfaction related to various areas of functioning, as measured using the Q-LES-Q(SF).

Maintenance Treatment as an Adjunct to Lithium or Divalproex
The efficacy of SEROQUEL in the maintenance treatment of bipolar I disorder was established in 2 placebo-controlled trials in patients (n=1326) who met DSM-IV criteria for bipolar I disorder. The trials included patients whose most recent episode was manic, depressed, or mixed, with or without psychotic features. In the open-label phase, patients were required to be stable on SEROQUEL plus lithium or divalproex for at least 12 weeks in order to be randomized. On average, patients were stabilized for 15 weeks. In the randomization phase, patients continued treatment with lithium or divalproex and were randomized to receive either SEROQUEL (administered twice daily totaling 400 mg/day to 800 mg/day or placebo). Approximately 50% of the patients had discontinued from the SEROQUEL group by day 280 and 50% of the placebo group had discontinued by day 117 of double-blind treatment. The primary endpoint in these studies was time to recurrence of a mood event (manic, mixed or depressed episode). A mood event was defined as medication initiation or hospitalization for a mood episode; YMRS score ≥ 20 or MADRS score ≥ 20 at 2 consecutive assessments; or study discontinuation due to a mood event.
In both studies, SEROQUEL was superior to placebo in increasing the time to recurrence of any mood event. The treatment effect was present for increasing time to recurrence of both manic and depressed episodes. The effect of SEROQUEL was independent of any specific subgroup (assigned mood stabilizer, sex, age, race, most recent bipolar episode, or rapid cycling course).

14.3 Major Depressive Disorder, Adjunctive Therapy to Antidepressants

The efficacy of SEROQUEL XR as adjunctive therapy to antidepressants in the treatment of MDD was demonstrated in two 6-week placebo-controlled, fixed-dose trials (n=936). SEROQUEL XR 150 mg/day or 300 mg/day was given as adjunctive therapy to existing antidepressant therapy in patients who had previously shown an inadequate response to at least one antidepressant. SEROQUEL XR was administered as 50 mg/day on Days 1 and 2, and increased to 150 mg/day on Day 3 for both dose groups. On Day 5, the dose was increased to 300 mg/day in the 300 mg/day fixed-dose group. Inadequate response was defined as having continued depressive symptoms for the current episode (HAM-D total score of ≥ 20) despite using an antidepressant for 6 weeks at or above the minimally effective labelled dose. The mean HAM-D total score at entry was 24, and 17% of patients scored 28 or greater. Patients were on various antidepressants prior to study entry including SSRI's (paroxetine, fluoxetine, sertraline, escitalopram, or citalopram), SNRI's, (duloxetine and venlafaxine,) TCA (amitryptiline) and other (bupropion).

The primary endpoint in these trials was change from baseline to week 6 in the Montgomery-Asberg Depression Rating Scale (MADRS), a 10-item clinician-rated scale used to assess the degree of depressive symptomatology (apparent sadness, reported sadness, inner tension, reduced sleep, reduced appetite, concentration difficulties, lassitude, inability to feel, pessimistic thoughts, and suicidal thoughts) with total scores ranging from 0 (no depressive features) to 60 (maximum score).

SEROQUEL XR 300 mg once daily as adjunctive treatment to other antidepressant therapy was superior to antidepressant alone in reduction of MADRS total score in both trials. SEROQUEL XR 150 mg once daily as adjunctive treatment was superior to antidepressant therapy alone in reduction of MADRS total score in one trial.

16 HOW SUPPLIED/STORAGE AND HANDLING

- 50 mg Tablets (NDC 0310-0280) peach, film coated, capsule-shaped, biconvex, intagliated tablet with "XR 50" on one side and plain on the other are supplied in bottles of 60 tablets and hospital unit dose packages of 100 tablets.
- 150 mg Tablets (NDC 0310-0281) white, film-coated, capsule-shaped, biconvex, intagliated tablet with 'XR 150' on one side and plain on the other are supplied in bottles of 60 tablets and hospital unit dose packages of 100 tablets.
- 200 mg Tablets (NDC 0310-0282) yellow, film coated, capsule-shaped, biconvex, intagliated tablet with "XR 200" on one side and plain on the other are supplied in bottles of 60 tablets and hospital unit dose packages of 100 tablets.
- 300 mg Tablets (NDC 0310-0283) pale yellow, film coated, capsule-shaped, biconvex, intagliated tablet with "XR 300" on one side and plain on the other are supplied in bottles of 60 tablets and hospital unit dose packages of 100 tablets.
- 400 mg Tablets (NDC 0310-0284) white, film coated, capsule-shaped, biconvex, intagliated tablet with "XR 400" on one side and plain on the other are supplied in bottles of 60 tablets and hospital unit dose packages of 100 tablets.

Store SEROQUEL XR at 25°C (77°F); excursions permitted to 15-30°C (59-86°F) [See USP].

17 PATIENT COUNSELING INFORMATION

17.1 Information for Patients

[see Medication Guide]

Prescribers or other health professionals should inform patients, their families, and their caregivers about the benefits and risks associated with treatment with SEROQUEL XR and should counsel them in its appropriate use. A patient Medication Guide about "Antidepressant Medicines, Depression and other Serious Mental Illness, and Suicidal Thoughts or Actions" is available for SEROQUEL XR. The prescriber or health professional should instruct patients, their families, and their caregivers to read the Medication Guide and should assist them in understanding its contents. Patients should be given the opportunity to discuss the contents of the Medication Guide and to obtain answers to any questions they may have. The complete text of the Medication Guide is reprinted at the end of this document. Patients should be advised of the following issues and asked to alert their prescriber if these occur while taking SEROQUEL XR.

Increased Mortality in Elderly Patients with Dementia-Related Psychosis

Patients and caregivers should be advised that elderly patients with dementia-related psychoses treated with atypical antipsychotic drugs are at increased risk of death compared with placebo. Quetiapine is not approved for elderly patients with dementia-related psychosis [see Warnings and Precautions (5.1)].

Clinical Worsening and Suicide Risk

Patients, their families, and their caregivers should be encouraged to be alert to the emergence of anxiety, agitation, panic attacks, insomnia, irritability, hostility, aggressiveness, impulsivity, akathisia (psychomotor restlessness), hypomania, mania, other unusual changes in behavior, worsening of depression, and suicidal ideation, especially early during antidepressant treatment and when the dose is adjusted up or down. Families and caregivers of patients should be advised to look for the emergence of such symptoms on a day-to-day basis, since changes may be abrupt. Such symptoms should be reported to the patient's prescriber or health professional, especially if they are severe, abrupt in onset, or were not part of the patient's presenting symptoms. Symptoms such as these may be associated with an increased risk for suicidal thinking and behavior and indicate a need for very close monitoring and possibly changes in the medication [see Warnings and Precautions (5.2)].

Neuroleptic Malignant Syndrome (NMS)

Patients should be advised to report to their physician any signs or symptoms that may be related to NMS. These may include muscle stiffness and high fever [see Warnings and Precautions (5.3)].

Hyperglycemia and Diabetes Mellitus

Patients should be aware of the symptoms of hyperglycemia (high blood sugar) and diabetes mellitus. Patients who are diagnosed with diabetes, those with risk factors for diabetes, or those that develop these symptoms during treatment should have their blood glucose monitored at the beginning of and periodically during treatment [see Warnings and Precautions (5.4)].

Hyperlipidemia

Patients should be advised that elevations in total cholesterol, LDL-cholesterol and triglycerides and decreases in HDL-cholesterol may occur. Patients should have their lipid profile monitored at the beginning of and periodically during treatment [see Warnings and Precautions (5.5)].

Weight Gain

Patients should be advised that they may experience weight gain. Patients should have their weight monitored regularly [see Warnings and Precautions (5.6)].

Orthostatic Hypotension

Patients should be advised of the risk of orthostatic hypotension (symptoms include feeling dizzy or lightheaded upon standing, which may lead to falls) especially during the period of initial dose titration, and also at times of re-initiating treatment or increases in dose [see Warnings and Precautions (5.8)].

Increased Blood Pressure in Children and Adolescents

Blood pressure should be measured at the beginning of, and periodically during, treatment [see Warnings and Precautions (5.9)].

Leukopenia/Neutropenia

Patients with a pre-existing low WBC or a history of drug induced leukopenia/neutropenia should be advised that they should have their CBC monitored while taking SEROQUEL XR [see Warnings and Precautions (5.10)].

Interference with Cognitive and Motor Performance

Patients should be advised of the risk of somnolence or sedation (which may lead to falls), especially during the period of initial dose titration. Patients should be cautioned about performing any activity requiring mental alertness, such as operating a motor vehicle (including automobiles) or operating machinery, until they are reasonably certain quetiapine therapy does not affect them adversely. Patients should limit consumption of alcohol during treatment with quetiapine [see Warnings and Precautions (5.16)].

Heat Exposure and Dehydration

Patients should be advised regarding appropriate care in avoiding overheating and dehydration [see Warnings and Precautions (5.18)].

Concomitant Medication

As with other medications, patients should be advised to notify their physicians if they are taking, or plan to take, any prescription or over-the-counter drugs [see Warnings and Precautions (5.21)].

Pregnancy and Nursing

Patients should be advised to notify their physician if they become pregnant or intend to become pregnant during therapy. Patients should be advised not to breast feed if they are taking quetiapine [see Use in Specific Populations (8.1 and 8.3)].

17.2 MEDICATION GUIDE

Medication Guide

SEROQUEL XR (SER-oh-kwell)

quetiapine fumarate

Read this Medication Guide before you start taking SEROQUEL XR and each time you get a refill. There may be new information. This Medication Guide does not take the place of talking to your healthcare provider about your medical condition or treatment.

What is the most important information I should know about SEROQUEL XR?

Serious side effects may happen when you take SEROQUEL XR, including:

- **Risk of death in the elderly with dementia:** Medicines like SEROQUEL XR can raise the risk of death in elderly people who have lost touch with reality due to confusion and memory loss (dementia). SEROQUEL XR is not approved for treating psychosis in the elderly with dementia.
- **Risk of suicidal thoughts or actions:** Antidepressant medicines, depression and other serious mental illnesses, and suicidal thoughts or actions:

1. **Antidepressant medicines may increase suicidal thoughts or actions in some children, teenagers, and young adults within the first few months of treatment.**
2. **Depression and other serious mental illnesses are the most important causes of suicidal thoughts and actions. Some people may have a particularly high risk of having suicidal thoughts or actions. These include people who have (or have a family history of) depression, bipolar illness (also called manic-depressive illness), or suicidal thoughts or actions.**
3. **How can I watch for and try to prevent suicidal thoughts and actions in myself or a family member?**

- Pay close attention to any changes, especially sudden changes, in mood, behaviors, thoughts, or feelings. This is very important when an antidepressant medicine is started or when the dose is changed.
- Call the healthcare provider right away to report new or sudden changes in mood, behavior, thoughts, or feelings.
- Keep all follow-up visits with the healthcare provider as scheduled. Call the healthcare provider between visits as needed, especially if you have concerns about symptoms.

Call a healthcare provider right away if you or your family member has any of the following symptoms, especially if they are new, worse, or worry you:

- thoughts about suicide or dying
- attempts to commit suicide
- new or worse depression
- new or worse anxiety
- feeling very agitated or restless
- panic attacks
- trouble sleeping (insomnia)
- new or worse irritability
- acting aggressive, being angry, or violent
- acting on dangerous impulses
- an extreme increase in activity and talking (mania)
- other unusual changes in behavior or mood

What else do I need to know about antidepressant medicines?

- Never stop an antidepressant medicine without first talking to a healthcare provider. Stopping an antidepressant medicine suddenly can cause other symptoms.
- Antidepressants are medicines used to treat depression and other illnesses. It is important to discuss all the risks of treating depression and also the risks of not treating it. Patients and their families or other caregivers should discuss all treatment choices with the healthcare provider, not just the use of antidepressants.
- Antidepressant medicines have other side effects. Talk to the healthcare provider about the side effects of the medicine prescribed for you or your family member.
- Antidepressant medicines can interact with other medicines. Know all of the medicines that you or your family member take. Keep a list of all medicines to show the healthcare provider. Do not start new medicines without first checking with your healthcare provider.
- Not all antidepressant medicines prescribed for children are FDA approved for use in children. Talk to your child's healthcare provider for more information.

What is SEROQUEL XR?

- SEROQUEL XR is a prescription medicine used to treat schizophrenia in adults.
- SEROQUEL XR is a prescription medicine used to treat bipolar disorder in adults, including:
  - manic episodes associated with bipolar disorder alone or with lithium or divalproex.
  - depressive episodes associated with bipolar disorder.
  - long-term treatment of bipolar I disorder with lithium or divalproex.
- SEROQUEL XR is a prescription medicine used to treat major depressive disorder as add-on treatment with antidepressant medicines when your doctor determines that one antidepressant alone is not enough to treat your depression.

SEROQUEL XR is not approved for patients under 18 years of age.

What should I tell my healthcare provider before taking SEROQUEL XR?

Before taking SEROQUEL XR, tell your healthcare provider if you have or have had:

- diabetes or high blood sugar in you or your family: your healthcare provider should check your blood sugar before you start SEROQUEL XR and also during therapy.
- high levels of total cholesterol, triglycerides or LDL-cholesterol or low levels of HDL-cholesterol
- low or high blood pressure
- low white blood cell count
- cataracts
- seizures
- abnormal thyroid tests
- high prolactin levels
- heart problems
- liver problems
- any other medical condition
- pregnancy or plans to become pregnant. It is not known if SEROQUEL XR will harm your unborn baby.
- breast-feeding or plans to breast-feed. It is not known if SEROQUEL XR will pass into your breast milk. You and your healthcare provider should decide if you will take SEROQUEL XR or breast-feed. You should not do both.

Tell the healthcare provider about all the medicines that you take or recently have taken including prescription medicines, non-prescription medicines, herbal supplements and vitamins.

SEROQUEL XR and other medicines may affect each other causing serious side effects. SEROQUEL XR may affect the way other medicines work, and other medicines may affect how SEROQUEL XR works.

Especially tell your healthcare provider if you take or plan to take medicines for:
- depression
- high blood pressure
- Parkinson's disease
- trouble sleeping

Also tell your healthcare provider if you take or plan to take any of these medicines:
- phenytoin, divalproex or carbamazepine (for epilepsy)
- barbiturates (to help you sleep)
- rifampin (for tuberculosis)
- glucocorticoids (steroids for inflammation)
- thioridazine (an antipsychotic)
- ketoconazole, fluconazole or itraconazole (for fungal infections)
- erythromycin (an antibiotic)
- protease inhibitors (for HIV)

This is not a complete list of medicines that can affect or be affected by SEROQUEL XR. Your doctor can tell you if it is safe to take SEROQUEL XR with your other medicines. Do not start or stop any medicines while taking SEROQUEL XR without talking to your healthcare provider first. Know the medicines you take. Keep a list of your medicines to show your healthcare provider and pharmacist when you get a new medicine.

Tell your healthcare provider if you are having a urine drug screen because SEROQUEL XR may affect your test results. Tell those giving the test that you are taking SEROQUEL XR.

How should I take SEROQUEL XR?
- Take SEROQUEL XR exactly as your healthcare provider tells you to take it. Do not change the dose yourself.
- Take SEROQUEL XR by mouth, with a light meal or without food.
- SEROQUEL XR should be swallowed whole and not split, chewed or crushed.
- If you feel you need to stop SEROQUEL XR, talk to your healthcare provider first.

If you suddenly stop taking SEROQUEL XR, you may experience side effects such as trouble sleeping or trouble staying asleep (insomnia), nausea, and vomiting.
- If you miss a dose, take it as soon as you remember. If it is close to the next dose, skip the missed dose. Just take the next dose at your regular time. Do not take 2 doses at the same time unless your healthcare provider tells you to. If you are not sure about your dosing, call your healthcare provider.
- If you take too much SEROQUEL XR, call your healthcare provider or poison control center at 1-800-222-1222 right away or go to the nearest hospital emergency room.

What should I avoid while taking SEROQUEL XR?
Do not drive, operate machinery, or do other dangerous activities until you know how SEROQUEL XR affects you. SEROQUEL XR may make you drowsy.
- Avoid getting over-heated or dehydrated.
  - Do not over-exercise.
  - In hot weather, stay inside in a cool place if possible.
  - Stay out of the sun. Do not wear too much or heavy clothing.
  - Drink plenty of water.
- Do not drink alcohol while taking SEROQUEL XR. It may make some side effects of SEROQUEL XR worse.

What are possible side effects of SEROQUEL XR?
Serious side effects have been reported with SEROQUEL XR including:

Also see "What is the most important information I should know about SEROQUEL XR?" at the beginning of this Medication Guide
- **Neuroleptic malignant syndrome (NMS):** Tell your healthcare provider right away if you have some or all of the following symptoms: high fever, stiff muscles, confusion, sweating, changes in pulse, heart rate, and blood pressure. These may be symptoms of a rare and serious condition that can lead to death. Stop SEROQUEL XR and call your healthcare provider right away.
- **High blood sugar (hyperglycemia):** Increases in blood sugar can happen in some people who take SEROQUEL XR. Extremely high blood sugar can lead to coma or death. If you have diabetes or risk factors for diabetes (such as being overweight or a family history of diabetes) your healthcare provider should check your blood sugar before you start SEROQUEL XR and during therapy. Call your healthcare provider if you have any of these symptoms of high blood sugar while taking SEROQUEL XR:
  - feel very thirsty
  - need to urinate more than usual
  - feel very hungry
  - feel weak or tired
  - feel sick to your stomach
  - feel confused, or your breath smells fruity.
- **High cholesterol and triglyceride levels in the blood (fat in the blood)** Increases in total cholesterol, triglycerides and LDL (bad) cholesterol and decreases in HDL (good) cholesterol have been reported in clinical trials with SEROQUEL XR. You may not have any symptoms, so your healthcare provider should do blood tests to check your cholesterol and triglyceride levels before you start taking SEROQUEL XR and during therapy.
- **Increase in weight (weight gain):** Weight gain has been seen in patients who take SEROQUEL XR so you and your healthcare provider should check your weight regularly.
- **Tardive dyskinesia:** Tell your healthcare provider about any movements you cannot control in your face, tongue, or other body parts. These may be signs of a serious condition. Tardive dyskinesia may not go away, even if you stop taking SEROQUEL XR. Tardive dyskinesia may also start after you stop taking SEROQUEL XR.
- **Orthostatic hypotension (decreased blood pressure):** lightheadedness or fainting caused by a sudden change in heart rate and blood pressure when rising too quickly from a sitting or lying position.
- **Increases in blood pressure:** reported in children and teenagers. Your healthcare provider should check blood pressure in children and adolescents before starting SEROQUEL XR and during therapy. SEROQUEL XR is not approved for patients under 18 years of age.
- **Low white blood cell count**
- **Cataracts**
- **Seizures**
- **Abnormal thyroid tests:** Your healthcare provider may do blood tests to check your thyroid hormone level.
- **Increases in prolactin levels:** Your healthcare provider may do blood tests to check your prolactin levels.
- **Increases in liver enzymes:** Your healthcare provider may do blood tests to check your liver enzyme levels.
- **Long lasting and painful erection**
- **Difficulty swallowing**
Common possible side effects with SEROQUEL XR include:
- drowsiness
- dry mouth
- constipation
- dizziness
- increased appetite
- upset stomach
- weight gain
- fatigue
- disturbance in speech and language
- stuffy nose

These are not all the possible side effects of SEROQUEL XR. For more information, ask your healthcare provider or pharmacist.
Call your healthcare provider for medical advice about side effects. You may report side effects to FDA at 1-800-FDA-1088.

How should I store SEROQUEL XR?
- Store SEROQUEL XR at room temperature, between 59°F to 86°F (15°C to 30°C).
- Keep SEROQUEL XR and all medicines out of the reach of children.

General information about SEROQUEL XR
Do not take SEROQUEL XR unless your healthcare provider has prescribed it for you for your condition. Do not share SEROQUEL XR with other people, even if they have the same condition. It may harm them.
This Medication Guide provides a summary of important information about SEROQUEL XR. For more information about SEROQUEL XR, talk with your healthcare provider

or pharmacist or call 1-800-236-9933. You can ask your healthcare provider for information about SEROQUEL XR that is written for health professionals.

What are the ingredients in SEROQUEL XR?
Active ingredient: quetiapine fumarate
Inactive ingredients: lactose monohydrate, microcrystalline cellulose, sodium citrate, hypromellose, and magnesium stearate. The film coating for all SEROQUEL XR tablets contain hypromellose, polyethylene glycol 400 and titanium dioxide. In addition, yellow iron oxide (50, 200 and 300 mg tablets) and red iron oxide (50 mg tablets) are included in the film coating of specific strengths.
The symptoms of Schizophrenia include:
- Having lost touch with reality (psychosis),
- Seeing things that are not there or hearing voices (hallucinations),
- Believing things that are not true (delusions) and
- Being suspicious (paranoia).
The symptoms of Bipolar Disorder include:
- General symptoms of bipolar disorder include: extreme mood swings, along with other specific symptoms and behaviors. These mood swings, or "episodes," include manic (highs) and depressive (lows)
- Common symptoms of a manic episode include feeling extremely happy, being very irritable, restless, talking too fast and too much, and having more energy and needing less sleep than usual
- Common symptoms of a depressive episode include feelings of sadness or emptiness, increased tearfulness, a loss of interest in activities you once enjoyed, loss of energy, difficulty concentrating or making decisions, feelings of worthlessness or guilt, changes in sleep or appetite and
- Thoughts of death or suicide.
The symptoms of Major Depressive Disorder (MDD) include:
- Feeling of sadness, emptiness and increased tearfulness,
- Loss of interest in activities that you once enjoyed and loss of energy,
- Problems focusing and making decisions
- Feeling of worthlessness or guilt
- Changes in sleep or eating patterns
- Thoughts of death or suicide
- MDD symptoms last most of the day, nearly every day for at least two weeks, and interfere with daily life at home and at work.

This Medication Guide has been approved by the U.S. Food and Drug Administration.
SEROQUEL XR is a trademark of the AstraZeneca group of companies
©AstraZeneca 2010
Distributed by:
AstraZeneca Pharmaceuticals LP
Wilmington, DE 19850
SIC 35537–03
Rev. 05/2010
Shown in Product Identification Guide, page 306

VIMOVO™   ℞
[vi-moh'-voh]
(naproxen and esomeprazole magnesium)
delayed-release tablets

HIGHLIGHTS OF PRESCRIBING INFORMATION
These highlights do not include all the information needed to use VIMOVO. See full prescribing information for VIMOVO.
VIMOVO™ (naproxen and esomeprazole magnesium)
DELAYED RELEASE TABLETS
Initial U.S. Approval: 2010

> **WARNING: CARDIOVASCULAR AND GASTROINTESTINAL RISKS**
> *See full prescribing information for complete boxed warning*
> **Cardiovascular Risk**
> • **Naproxen, a component of VIMOVO, may cause an increased risk of serious cardiovascular thrombotic events, myocardial infarction, and stroke, which can be fatal. This risk may increase with duration of use. Patients with cardiovascular disease or risk factors for cardiovascular disease may be at greater risk. (5.1)**
> • **VIMOVO is contraindicated for the treatment of perioperative pain in the setting of coronary artery bypass graft (CABG) surgery. (4, 5.1)**
> **Gastrointestinal Risk**
> • **NSAIDs, including naproxen, a component of VIMOVO, cause an increased risk of serious gastrointestinal adverse events including bleeding, ulceration, and perforation of the stomach or intestines, which can be fatal. These events can occur at any time during use**

and without warning symptoms. Elderly patients are at greater risk for serious gastrointestinal (GI) events. (5.4)

INDICATIONS AND USAGE

Relief of signs and symptoms of osteoarthritis, rheumatoid arthritis, and ankylosing spondylitis and to decrease the risk of developing gastric ulcers in patients at risk of developing NSAID associated gastric ulcers (1)

DOSAGE AND ADMINISTRATION

One tablet twice daily. Use the lowest effective dose. Not recommended in moderate/severe renal insufficiency or in severe hepatic insufficiency. Consider dose reduction in mild/moderate hepatic insufficiency (2)

DOSAGE FORMS AND STRENGTHS

Delayed release tablets: 375 mg/20 mg or 500 mg/20 mg of naproxen and esomeprazole magnesium (3)

CONTRAINDICATIONS

• Known hypersensitivity to any component of VIMOVO or substituted benzimidazoles (4)
• History of asthma, urticaria, or other allergic-type reactions after taking aspirin or other NSAIDs (4, 5.8, 5.9, 5.13)
• Use during the peri-operative period in the setting of coronary artery bypass graft (CABG) surgery (4, 5.1)
• Late pregnancy (4, 5.10, 8.1)

WARNINGS AND PRECAUTIONS

• Serious and potentially fatal cardiovascular (CV) thrombotic events, myocardial infarction, and stroke. Patients with known CV disease/risk factors may be at greater risk (5.1)
• Serious gastrointestinal (GI) adverse events, which can be fatal. The risk is greater in patients with a prior history of ulcer disease or GI bleeding, and in patients at high risk for GI events, especially the elderly. VIMOVO should be used with caution in these patients (5.4, 8.5)
• Treatment should be withdrawn when active and clinically significant bleeding from any source occurs (5.5)
• Elevated liver enzymes and, rarely, severe hepatic reactions. Discontinue use immediately if abnormal liver enzymes persist or worsen (5.11, 8.6, 12.3)
• New onset or worsening of preexisting hypertension. Blood pressure should be monitored closely during treatment with VIMOVO (5.2, 7.1, 7.4)
• Congestive heart failure and edema. VIMOVO should be used with caution in patients with fluid retention or heart failure (5.3)
• Renal papillary necrosis and other renal injury with long-term use. Use VIMOVO with caution in the elderly, those with impaired renal function, hypovolemia, salt depletion, heart failure, liver dysfunction, and those taking diuretics, or ACE-inhibitors. Not recommended for patients with moderate or severe renal impairment (2, 5.6, 5.7, 7.1, 7.4, 8.7)
• Anaphylactoid reactions. Do not use VIMOVO in patients with the aspirin triad (5.8)
• Serious skin adverse reactions such as exfoliative dermatitis, Stevens-Johnson syndrome, and toxic epidermal necrolysis, which can be fatal and can occur without warning. Discontinue VIMOVO at first appearance of skin rash or any other sign of hypersensitivity (5.9)
• Long-term PPI therapy is associated with an increased risk for osteoporosis-related fractures of the hip, wrist or spine (5.16)
• Symptomatic response to esomeprazole does not preclude the presence of gastric malignancy (5.4)
• Atrophic gastritis has been noted on biopsy with long-term omeprazole therapy (5.4)

ADVERSE REACTIONS

Most common adverse reactions in clinical trials (>5%): erosive gastritis, dyspepsia, gastritis, diarrhea, gastric ulcer, upper abdominal pain, nausea (6.1)
To report SUSPECTED ADVERSE REACTIONS, contact AstraZeneca at 1-800-236-9933 or FDA at 1-800-FDA-1088 or www.fda.gov/medwatch.

DRUG INTERACTIONS

• Concomitant use of NSAIDs may reduce the antihypertensive effect of ACE Inhibitors, diuretics, and beta-blockers (7.1, 7.4, 7.9)
• Concomitant use of NSAIDs increases lithium plasma levels (7.5)
• Concomitant use of VIMOVO with methotrexate may increase the toxicity of methotrexate (7.6)
• Concomitant use of VIMOVO and warfarin may result in increased risk of bleeding complications. Monitor for increases in INR and prothrombin time (7.7)
• Esomeprazole inhibits gastric acid secretion and may interfere with the absorption of drugs where gastric pH is an important determinant of bioavailability (eg, ketoconazole, iron salts and digoxin) (7.11)

USE IN SPECIFIC POPULATIONS

• Pregnancy Category C: VIMOVO should not be used in late pregnancy (4, 5.10, 8.1)
• Hepatic Insufficiency: VIMOVO is not recommended in patients with severe hepatic insufficiency (2, 4, 5.11, 8.6, 12.3)

• Renal Insufficiency: VIMOVO is not recommended in patients with moderate or severe renal insufficiency (2, 5.6, 5.7, 8.7, 12.3)
See 17 for PATIENT COUNSELING INFORMATION and Medication Guide

Revised: 05/2010

FULL PRESCRIBING INFORMATION: CONTENTS*

* Sections or subsections omitted from the full prescribing information are not listed

FULL PRESCRIBING INFORMATION

CARDIOVASCULAR RISK

• Non-Steroidal Anti-inflammatory Drugs (NSAIDs), a component of VIMOVO, may cause an increased risk of serious cardiovascular thrombotic events, myocardial infarction, and stroke, which can be fatal. This risk may increase with duration of use. Patients with cardiovascular disease or risk factors for cardiovascular disease may be at greater risk [see Warnings and Precautions (5.1)].
• VIMOVO is contraindicated for the treatment of perioperative pain in the setting of coronary artery bypass graft (CABG) surgery [see Contraindications (4), and Warnings and Precautions (5.1)].

Gastrointestinal Risk

• NSAIDs, including naproxen, a component of VIMOVO, cause an increased risk of serious gastrointestinal adverse events including bleeding, ulceration, and perforation of the stomach or intestines, which can be fatal. These events can occur at any time during use and without warning symptoms. Elderly patients are at greater risk for serious gastrointestinal events [see Warnings and Precautions (5.4)].

1   INDICATIONS AND USAGE

VIMOVO is a combination product that contains naproxen and esomeprazole. It is indicated for the relief of signs and symptoms of osteoarthritis, rheumatoid arthritis and ankylosing spondylitis and to decrease the risk of developing gastric ulcers in patients at risk of developing NSAID associated gastric ulcers. VIMOVO is not recommended for initial treatment of acute pain because the absorption of naproxen is delayed compared to absorption from other naproxen-containing products. Controlled studies do not extend beyond 6 months.

2   DOSAGE AND ADMINISTRATION

Carefully consider the potential benefits and risks of VIMOVO and other treatment options before deciding to use VIMOVO. Use the lowest effective dose for the shortest duration consistent with individual patient treatment goals. VIMOVO does not allow for administration of a lower daily dose of esomeprazole. If a dose of esomeprazole lower than a total daily dose of 40 mg is more appropriate, a different treatment should be considered.
Rheumatoid Arthritis, Osteoarthritis and Ankylosing Spondylitis
The dosage is one tablet twice daily of VIMOVO 375 mg naproxen and 20 mg of esomeprazole or 500 mg naproxen and 20 mg of esomeprazole.
The tablets are to be swallowed whole with liquid. Do not split, chew, crush or dissolve the tablet. VIMOVO is to be taken at least 30 minutes before meals.

Geriatric Patients
Studies indicate that although total plasma concentration of naproxen is unchanged, the unbound plasma fraction of naproxen is increased in the elderly. Use caution when high doses are required and some adjustment of dosage may be required in elderly patients. As with other drugs used in the elderly use the lowest effective dose [see Use in Specific Populations (8.5) and Clinical Pharmacology (12.3)].
Patients With Moderate to Severe Renal Impairment
Naproxen-containing products are not recommended for use in patients with moderate to severe or severe renal impairment (creatinine clearance <30 mL/min) [see Warnings and Precautions (5.6, 5.7) and Use in Specific Populations (8.7)].
Hepatic Insufficiency
Monitor patients with mild to moderate hepatic impairment closely and consider a possible dose reduction based on the naproxen component of VIMOVO.
VIMOVO is not recommended in patients with severe hepatic impairment because esomeprazole doses should not exceed 20 mg daily in these patients [see Warnings and Precautions (5.11), Use in Specific Populations (8.6) and Clinical Pharmacology (12.3)].
Pediatric Patients
The safety and efficacy of VIMOVO in children younger than 18 years has not been established. VIMOVO is therefore not recommended for use in children.

3   DOSAGE FORMS AND STRENGTHS

Oval, yellow, delayed release tablets for oral administration containing either:
• 375 mg enteric coated naproxen and 20 mg esomeprazole (as magnesium trihydrate) tablets printed with 375/20 in black, or
• 500 mg enteric coated naproxen and 20 mg esomeprazole (as magnesium trihydrate) tablets printed with 500/20 in black.

4   CONTRAINDICATIONS

VIMOVO is contraindicated in patients with known hypersensitivity to naproxen, esomeprazole magnesium, substituted benzimidazoles, or to any of the excipients.
VIMOVO is contraindicated in patients who have experienced asthma, urticaria, or allergic-type reactions after taking aspirin or other NSAIDs. Severe, rarely fatal, anaphylactic-like reactions to NSAIDs have been reported in such patients [see Warnings and Precautions (5.8, 5.13)]. Hypersensitivity reactions, eg, angioedema and anaphylactic reaction/shock, have been reported with esomeprazole use.
VIMOVO is contraindicated for the treatment of perioperative pain in the setting of coronary artery bypass graft (CABG) surgery [see Warnings and Precautions (5.1)].
VIMOVO is contraindicated in patients in the late stages of pregnancy [see Warnings and Precautions (5.10) and Use in Specific Populations (8.1)].

5 WARNINGS AND PRECAUTIONS

5.1 Cardiovascular Thrombotic Events

Clinical trials of several COX-2 selective and nonselective NSAIDs of up to three years duration have shown an increased risk of serious cardiovascular (CV) thrombotic events, myocardial infarction, and stroke, which can be fatal. All NSAIDs, both COX-2 selective and nonselective, may have a similar risk. Patients with known CV disease or risk factors for CV disease may be at greater risk. To minimize the potential risk for an adverse CV event in patients treated with an NSAID, the lowest effective dose should be used for the shortest duration possible. Physicians and patients should remain alert for the development of such events, even in the absence of previous CV symptoms. Patients should be informed about the signs and/or symptoms of serious CV events and the steps to take if they occur. There is no consistent evidence that concurrent use of aspirin mitigates the increased risk of serious CV thrombotic events associated with NSAID use.

Two large, controlled, clinical trials of a COX-2 selective NSAID for the treatment of pain in the first 10–14 days following CABG surgery found an increased incidence of myocardial infarction and stroke [see *Contraindications (4)*].

5.2 Hypertension

NSAIDs, including naproxen, a component of VIMOVO, can lead to onset of new hypertension or worsening of pre-existing hypertension, either of which may contribute to the increased incidence of CV events. Patients taking thiazides or loop diuretics may have impaired response to these therapies when taking NSAIDs. NSAIDs should be used with caution in patients with hypertension. Blood pressure (BP) should be monitored closely during the initiation of NSAID treatment and throughout the course of therapy [see *Drug Interactions (7.1, 7.4)*].

5.3 Congestive Heart Failure and Edema

Fluid retention, edema, and peripheral edema have been observed in some patients taking NSAIDs and should be used with caution in patients with fluid retention or heart failure.

5.4 Gastrointestinal Effects — Risk of Ulceration, Bleeding, and Perforation

NSAIDs, including naproxen, a component of VIMOVO, can cause serious gastrointestinal (GI) adverse events including inflammation, bleeding, ulceration, and perforation of the stomach, small intestine, or large intestine, which can be fatal. While VIMOVO has been shown to significantly decrease the occurrence of gastric ulcers compared to naproxen alone, ulceration and associated complications can still occur.

These serious adverse events can occur at any time, with or without warning symptoms, in patients treated with NSAIDs. Only one in five patients who develop a serious upper GI adverse event on NSAID therapy is symptomatic. Upper GI ulcers, gross bleeding, or perforation caused by NSAIDs occur in approximately 1% of patients treated for 3–6 months, and in about 2–4% of patients treated for one year. These trends continue with longer duration of use, increasing the likelihood of developing a serious GI event at some time during the course of therapy. However, even short-term therapy is not without risk. The utility of periodic laboratory monitoring has not been demonstrated, nor has it been adequately assessed.

VIMOVO should be prescribed with caution in those with a prior history of ulcer disease or gastrointestinal bleeding. Patients with a prior history of peptic ulcer disease and/or gastrointestinal bleeding who use NSAIDs have a greater than 10-fold increased risk of developing a GI bleed compared to patients with neither of these risk factors. Other factors that increase the risk for GI bleeding in patients treated with NSAIDs include concomitant use of oral corticosteroids or anticoagulants or antiplatelets (including low-dose aspirin), longer duration of NSAID therapy, smoking, use of alcohol, older age, and poor general health status. Most spontaneous reports of fatal GI events are in elderly or debilitated patients, and therefore special care should be taken in treating this population.

To minimize the potential risk for an adverse GI event in patients treated with an NSAID or NSAID-containing product, the lowest effective dose should be used for the shortest possible duration. Patients and physicians should remain alert for signs and symptoms of GI ulceration and bleeding during NSAID therapy and promptly initiate additional evaluation and treatment if a serious GI adverse event is suspected. This should include discontinuation of the NSAID until a serious GI adverse event is ruled out. For high risk patients, alternate therapies that do not involve NSAIDs should be considered.

Epidemiological studies of the case-control and cohort design have demonstrated an association between use of psychotropic drugs that interfere with serotonin reuptake and the occurrence of upper gastrointestinal bleeding. In two studies, concurrent use of an NSAID, COX-2 inhibitor, or aspirin potentiated the risk of bleeding [see *Drug Interac-*

tions (7.2, 7.8)]. Although these studies focused on upper gastrointestinal bleeding, bleeding at other sites cannot be ruled out.

NSAIDs should be given with care to patients with a history of inflammatory bowel disease (ulcerative colitis, Crohn's disease) as their condition may be exacerbated.

Gastrointestinal symptomatic response to therapy with VIMOVO does not preclude the presence of gastric malignancy.

Atrophic gastritis has been noted occasionally in gastric corpus biopsies from patients treated long-term with omeprazole, of which esomeprazole is an enantiomer and a component of VIMOVO.

5.5 Active Bleeding

When active and clinically significant bleeding from any source occurs in patients receiving VIMOVO, the treatment should be withdrawn.

5.6 Renal Effects

Long-term administration of NSAIDs has resulted in renal papillary necrosis and other renal injury. Renal toxicity has also been seen in patients in whom renal prostaglandins have a compensatory role in the maintenance of renal perfusion. In these patients, administration of an NSAID may cause a dose-dependent reduction in prostaglandin formation and, secondarily, in renal blood flow, which may precipitate overt renal decompensation. Patients at greatest risk of this reaction are those with impaired renal function, hypovolemia, heart failure, liver dysfunction, salt depletion, those taking diuretics and ACE inhibitors, and the elderly. Discontinuation of NSAID therapy is usually followed by recovery to the pretreatment state.

5.7 Advanced Renal Disease

No information is available from controlled clinical studies regarding the use of VIMOVO in patients with advanced renal disease. Therefore, treatment with VIMOVO is not recommended in these patients with advanced renal disease. If VIMOVO therapy must be initiated, close monitoring of the patient's renal function is advisable [see *Dosage and Administration (2), Use in Specific Populations (8.7)* and *Clinical Pharmacology (12.3)*].

5.8 Anaphylactoid Reactions

Anaphylactoid reactions may occur in patients without known prior exposure to either component of VIMOVO. NSAIDs should not be given to patients with the aspirin triad. This symptom complex typically occurs in asthmatic patients who experience rhinitis with or without nasal polyps, or who exhibit severe, potentially fatal bronchospasm after taking aspirin or other NSAIDs [see *Contraindications (4)*]. Emergency help should be sought in cases where an anaphylactoid reaction occurs. Anaphylactoid reactions, like anaphylaxis, may have a fatal outcome.

5.9 Skin Reactions

NSAIDs can cause serious skin adverse events such as exfoliative dermatitis, Stevens-Johnson syndrome, and toxic epidermal necrolysis, which can be fatal. These serious events may occur without warning. Patients should be informed about the signs and symptoms of serious skin manifestations and use of the drug should be discontinued at the first appearance of skin rash or any other sign of hypersensitivity.

5.10 Pregnancy

Pregnancy Category C

In late pregnancy, as with other NSAIDs, naproxen, a component of VIMOVO, should be avoided because it may cause premature closure of the ductus arteriosus [see *Contraindications (4)*, and *Use in Specific Populations (8.1)*].

5.11 Hepatic Effects

Borderline elevations of one or more liver tests may occur in up to 15% of patients taking NSAIDs including naproxen, a component of VIMOVO. Hepatic abnormalities may be the result of hypersensitivity rather than direct toxicity. These laboratory abnormalities may progress, may remain essentially unchanged, or may be transient with continued therapy. The SGPT (ALT) test is probably the most sensitive indicator of liver dysfunction. Notable elevations of ALT or AST (approximately three or more times the upper limit of normal) have been reported in approximately 1% of patients in clinical trials with NSAIDs. In addition, rare cases of severe hepatic reactions, including jaundice and fatal fulminant hepatitis, liver necrosis and hepatic failure, some of them with fatal outcomes, have been reported.

A patient with symptoms and/or signs suggesting liver dysfunction, or in whom an abnormal liver test has occurred, should be evaluated for evidence of the development of more severe hepatic reaction while on therapy with VIMOVO.

If clinical signs and symptoms consistent with liver disease develop, or if systemic manifestations occur (eg, eosinophilia, rash, etc.), VIMOVO should be discontinued.

Chronic alcoholic liver disease and probably other diseases with decreased or abnormal plasma proteins (albumin) reduce the total plasma concentration of naproxen, but the plasma concentration of unbound naproxen is increased. Caution is advised when high doses are required and some adjustment of dosage may be required in these patients. It is prudent to use the lowest effective dose for the shortest possible duration of adequate treatment.

VIMOVO is not recommended in patients with severe hepatic impairment because esomeprazole doses should not exceed 20 mg daily in these patients [see *Dosage and Administration (2)*, and *Use in Specific Populations (8.6)*].

5.12 Hematological Effects

Anemia is sometimes seen in patients receiving NSAIDs. This may be due to fluid retention, occult or gross GI blood loss, or an incompletely described effect upon erythropoiesis. Patients on long-term treatment with NSAIDs should have their hemoglobin or hematocrit checked if they exhibit any signs or symptoms of anemia.

NSAIDs inhibit platelet aggregation and have been shown to prolong bleeding time in some patients. Unlike aspirin, their effect on platelet function is quantitatively less, of shorter duration, and reversible. Patients receiving VIMOVO who may be adversely affected by alterations in platelet function, such as those with coagulation disorders or patients receiving anticoagulants or antiplatelets, should be carefully monitored.

5.13 Pre-existing Asthma

Patients with asthma may have aspirin-sensitive asthma. The use of aspirin in patients with aspirin-sensitive asthma has been associated with severe bronchospasm, which can be fatal. Since cross reactivity, including bronchospasm, between aspirin and other NSAIDs has been reported in such aspirin-sensitive patients, VIMOVO should not be administered to patients with this form of aspirin sensitivity and should be used with caution in patients with pre-existing asthma.

5.14 Concomitant NSAID

Use VIMOVO contains naproxen as one of its active ingredients. It should not be used with other naproxen-containing products since they all circulate in the plasma as the naproxen anion.

The concomitant use of VIMOVO with any dose of a non-aspirin NSAID should be avoided due to the potential for increased risk of adverse reactions.

5.15 Corticosteroid Treatment

VIMOVO cannot be expected to substitute for corticosteroids or to treat corticosteroid insufficiency. Abrupt discontinuation of corticosteroids may lead to disease exacerbation. Patients on prolonged corticosteroid therapy should have their therapy tapered slowly if a decision is made to discontinue corticosteroids and the patient should be observed closely for any evidence of adverse effects, including adrenal insufficiency and exacerbation of symptoms of arthritis.

5.16 Bone Fracture

Several studies and literature reports indicate that proton pump inhibitor (PPI) therapy is associated with an increased risk for osteoporosis-related fractures of the hip, wrist, or spine. Those patients with the highest risk received high-dose or long-term PPI therapy (a year or longer). Patients should use the lowest effective dose and shortest duration of PPI therapy appropriate to the condition being treated. Patients at risk for osteoporosis-related fractures should be managed according to the established treatment guidelines. Adequate vitamin D and calcium intake is recommended.

5.17 Masking of Inflammation and Fever

The pharmacological activity of VIMOVO in reducing fever and inflammation may diminish the utility of these diagnostic signs in detecting complications of presumed noninfectious, noninflammatory painful conditions.

5.18 Laboratory Tests

Because serious GI tract ulcerations and bleeding can occur without warning symptoms, physicians should monitor for signs or symptoms of GI bleeding. Patients on long-term treatment with NSAIDs should have their CBC and a chemistry profile checked periodically. If clinical signs and symptoms consistent with liver or renal disease develop, systemic manifestations occur (eg, eosinophilia, rash, etc.) or if abnormal liver tests persist or worsen, VIMOVO should be discontinued.

Patients with initial hemoglobin values of 10 g or less who are to receive long-term therapy should have hemoglobin values determined periodically.

6 ADVERSE REACTIONS

6.1 Clinical Studies Experience

Because clinical trials are conducted under widely varying conditions, adverse reaction rates observed in the clinical trials of a drug cannot be directly compared to rates in the clinical trials of another drug and may not reflect the rates observed in practice.

The adverse reactions reported below are specific to the clinical trials with VIMOVO. See also the full prescribing information for naproxen and esomeprazole magnesium products.

The safety of VIMOVO was evaluated in clinical studies involving 2317 patients (aged 27 to 90 years) and ranging from 3-12 months. Patients received either 500 mg/20 mg of VIMOVO twice daily (n=1157), 500 mg of enteric-coated naproxen twice daily (n=426), or placebo (n=246). The average number of VIMOVO doses taken over 12 months was 696±44.

The table below lists all adverse reactions, regardless of causality, occurring in >2% of patients receiving VIMOVO from two clinical studies (Study 1 and Study 2). Both of these studies were randomized, multi-center, double-blind, parallel studies. The majority of patients were female (67%), white (86%). The majority of patients were 50-69 years of age (83%). Approximately one quarter were on low-dose aspirin.

Table 1: Adverse Reactions occurring in patients >2% Study 1 and Study 2 (endoscopic studies)

Preferred term (sorted by SOC)	VIMOVO 500 mg/ 20 mg twice daily (n=428) %	EC-Naproxen 500 mg twice daily (n=426) %
Gastrointestinal Disorders		
Gastritis Erosive	19	38
Dyspepsia	18	27
Gastritis	17	14
Diarrhea	6	5
Gastric Ulcer	6	24
Abdominal Pain Upper	6	9
Nausea	5	5
Hiatus Hernia	4	6
Abdominal Distension	4	4
Flatulence	4	3
Esophagitis	4	8
Constipation	3	3
Abdominal pain	2	2
Erosive Duodenitis	2	12
Abdominal pain lower	2	3
Duodenitis	1	7
Gastritis hemorrhagic	1	2
Gastroesophageal reflux disease	<1	4
Duodenal ulcer	<1	5
Erosive esophagitis	<1	6
Infections and infestations		
Upper respiratory tract infection	5	4
Bronchitis	2	2
Urinary tract infection	2	1
Sinusitis	2	2
Nasopharyngitis	<1	2
Musculoskeletal and connective tissue disorders		
Arthralgia	1	2
Nervous system disorders		
Headache	3	1
Dysgeusia	2	1
Respiratory, thoracic and mediastinal disorders		
Cough	2	3

In Study 1 and Study 2, patients taking VIMOVO had fewer premature discontinuations due to adverse reactions compared to patients taking enteric-coated naproxen alone

(7.9% vs. 12.5% respectively). The most common reasons for discontinuations due to adverse events in the VIMOVO treatment group were upper abdominal pain (1.2%, n=5), duodenal ulcer (0.7%, n=3) and erosive gastritis (0.7%, n=3). Among patients receiving enteric-coated naproxen, the most common reasons for discontinuations due to adverse events were duodenal ulcer 5.4% (n=23), dyspepsia 2.8% (n=12) and upper abdominal pain 1.2% (n=5). The proportion of patients discontinuing treatment due to any upper gastrointestinal adverse events (including duodenal ulcers) in patients treated with VIMOVO was 4% compared to 12% for patients taking enteric-coated naproxen.

The table below lists all adverse reactions, regardless of causality, occurring in >2% of patients from 2 clinical studies conducted in patients with osteoarthritis of the knee (Study 3 and Study 4).

Table 2: Adverse Reactions occurring in patients >2% (Study 3 and Study 4)

Preferred term (sorted by SOC)	VIMOVO 500 mg/ 20 mg twice daily (n=490) %	Placebo (n=246) %
Gastrointestinal Disorders		
Dyspepsia	8	12
Diarrhea	6	4
Abdominal Pain Upper	4	3
Constipation	4	1
Nausea	4	4
Nervous System Disorders		
Dizziness	3	2
Headache	3	5
General disorders and administration site conditions		
Peripheral edema	3	1
Respiratory, thoracic and mediastinal disorders		
Cough	1	3
Infections and infestations		
Sinusitis	1	2

The percentage of subjects who withdrew from the VIMOVO treatment group in these studies due to treatment-emergent adverse events was 7%. There were no preferred terms in which more than 1% of subjects withdrew from any treatment group.

The long-term safety of VIMOVO was evaluated in an open-label clinical trial of 239 patients, of which 135 patients received 500 mg/20 mg of VIMOVO for 12 months. There were no differences in frequency or types of adverse reactions seen in the long-term safety study compared to shorter-term treatment in the randomized controlled studies.

6.2 Postmarketing experience
6.2.1 Naproxen
The following adverse reactions have been identified during post-approval use of naproxen. Because these reactions are reported voluntarily from a population of uncertain size, it is not always possible to reliably estimate their frequency or establish a causal relationship to drug exposure. These reports are listed below by body system:
Body as a Whole: anaphylactoid reactions, angioneurotic edema, menstrual disorders, pyrexia (chills and fever)
Cardiovascular: congestive heart failure, vasculitis, hypertension, pulmonary edema
Gastrointestinal: gastrointestinal bleeding and/or perforation, hematemesis, pancreatitis, vomiting, colitis, exacerbation of inflammatory bowel disease (ulcerative colitis, Crohn's disease), nonpeptic gastrointestinal ulceration, ulcerative stomatitis, esophagitis, peptic ulceration
Hepatobiliary: jaundice, abnormal liver function tests, hepatitis (some cases have been fatal)
Hemic and Lymphatic: eosinophilia, leucopenia, melena, thrombocytopenia, agranulocytosis, granulocytopenia, hemolytic anemia, aplastic anemia
Metabolic and Nutritional: hyperglycemia, hypoglycemia

Nervous System: inability to concentrate, depression, dream abnormalities, insomnia, malaise, myalgia, muscle weakness, aseptic meningitis, cognitive dysfunction, convulsions
Respiratory: eosinophilic pneumonitis, asthma
Dermatologic: alopecia, urticaria, skin rashes, toxic epidermal necrolysis, erythema multiforme, erythema nodosum, fixed drug eruption, lichen planus, pustular reaction, systemic lupus erythematoses, bullous reactions, including Stevens-Johnson syndrome, photosensitive dermatitis, photosensitivity reactions, including rare cases resembling porphyria cutanea tarda (pseudoporphyria) or epidermolysis bullosa. If skin fragility, blistering or other symptoms suggestive of pseudoporphyria occur, treatment should be discontinued and the patient monitored.
Special Senses: hearing impairment, corneal opacity, papillitis, retrobulbar optic neuritis, papilledema
Urogenital: glomerular nephritis, hematuria, hyperkalemia, interstitial nephritis, nephrotic syndrome, renal disease, renal failure, renal papillary necrosis, raised serum creatinine
Reproduction (female): infertility
6.2.2 Esomeprazole
The following adverse reactions have been identified during post-approval use of esomeprazole. Because these reactions are reported voluntarily from a population of uncertain size, it is not always possible to reliably estimate their frequency or establish a causal relationship to drug exposure. These reports are listed below by body system:
Blood and Lymphatic: agranulocytosis, pancytopenia;
Eye: blurred vision;
Gastrointestinal: pancreatitis; stomatitis;
Hepatobiliary: hepatic failure, hepatitis with or without jaundice;
Immune System: anaphylactic reaction/shock;
Infections and Infestations: GI candidiasis;
Metabolism and Nutritional Disorders: hypomagnesemia
Musculoskeletal and Connective Tissue: muscular weakness, myalgia;
Nervous System: hepatic encephalopathy, taste disturbance;
Psychiatric: aggression, agitation, depression, hallucination;
Renal and Urinary: interstitial nephritis;
Reproductive System and Breast: gynecomastia;
Respiratory, Thoracic, and Mediastinal: bronchospasm;
Skin and Subcutaneous Tissue: alopecia, erythema multiforme, hyperhidrosis, photosensitivity, Stevens-Johnson syndrome, toxic epidermal necrolysis (some fatal).

7 DRUG INTERACTIONS
Several studies conducted with VIMOVO have shown no interaction between the two components, naproxen and esomeprazole.
7.1 ACE-inhibitors
Reports suggest that NSAIDs may diminish the antihypertensive effect of ACE-inhibitors. This interaction should be given consideration in patients taking VIMOVO concomitantly with ACE-inhibitors.
7.2 Aspirin
VIMOVO can be administered with low-dose aspirin (≤325 mg/day) therapy. The concurrent use of aspirin and VIMOVO may increase the risk of serious adverse events [see *Warnings and Precautions (5.1, 5.4), Adverse Reactions (6),* and *Clinical Studies (14)*]. When naproxen is administered with doses of aspirin (>1 gram/day), its protein binding is reduced. The clinical significance of this interaction is not known. However, as with other NSAIDs, concomitant administration of naproxen and aspirin is not generally recommended because of the potential of increased adverse effects.
7.3 Cholestyramine
As with other NSAIDs, concomitant administration of cholestyramine can delay the absorption of naproxen.
7.4 Diuretics
Clinical studies, as well as postmarketing observations, have shown that NSAIDs can reduce the natriuretic effect of furosemide and thiazides in some patients. This response has been attributed to inhibition of renal prostaglandin synthesis. During concomitant therapy with NSAIDs, the patient should be observed closely both for signs of renal failure, as well as to monitor to assure diuretic efficacy [see *Warnings and Precautions (5.6, 5.7)*].
7.5 Lithium
NSAIDs have produced an elevation of plasma lithium levels and a reduction in renal lithium clearance. The mean minimum lithium concentration increased 15% and the renal clearance was decreased by approximately 20%. These effects have been attributed to inhibition of renal prostaglandin synthesis by the NSAID. Thus, when NSAIDs and lithium are administered concurrently, subjects should be observed carefully for signs of lithium toxicity.

7.6 Methotrexate

NSAIDs have been reported to competitively inhibit methotrexate accumulation in rabbit kidney slices. NSAIDs have been reported to reduce the tubular secretion of methotrexate in an animal model. This may indicate that they could enhance the toxicity of methotrexate. Caution should be used when NSAIDs are administered concomitantly with methotrexate.

7.7 Anticoagulants

Naproxen decreases platelet aggregation and may prolong bleeding time.

The effects of warfarin and NSAIDs on GI bleeding are synergistic, such that users of both drugs together have a risk of serious GI bleeding higher than users of either drug alone. No significant interactions have been observed in clinical studies with naproxen and coumarin-type anticoagulants. However, caution is advised since interactions have been seen with other nonsteroidal agents of this class. The free fraction of warfarin may increase substantially in some subjects and naproxen interferes with platelet function.

Post-marketing reports of changes in prothrombin measures have been reported among patients on concomitant warfarin and esomeprazole therapy. Increases in INR and prothrombin time may lead to abnormal bleeding and even death. Patients treated with proton pump inhibitors and warfarin concomitantly may need to be monitored for increases in INR and prothrombin time.

7.8 Selective Serotonin Reuptake Inhibitors (SSRIs)

There is an increased risk of gastrointestinal bleeding when selective serotonin reuptake inhibitors (SSRIs) are combined with NSAIDs including COX-2 selective inhibitors. Caution should be used when NSAIDs are administered concomitantly with SSRIs [see *Warnings and Precautions (5.4)*].

7.9 Other Information Concerning Drug Interactions

Naproxen is highly bound to plasma albumin; it thus has a theoretical potential for interaction with other albumin-bound drugs such as sulphonylureas, hydantoins, and other NSAIDs. Patients simultaneously receiving VIMOVO and a hydantoin, sulphonamide or sulphonylurea should be observed for adjustment of dose if required.

Naproxen and other NSAIDs can reduce the antihypertensive effect of propranolol and other beta-blockers.

Probenecid given concurrently increases naproxen anion plasma levels and extends its plasma half-life significantly.

7.10 Drug/Laboratory Test Interaction

Naproxen may decrease platelet aggregation and prolong bleeding time. This effect should be kept in mind when bleeding times are determined.

The administration of naproxen may result in increased urinary values for 17-ketogenic steroids because of an interaction between the drug and/or its metabolites with m-di-nitrobenzene used in this assay. Although 17-hydroxy-corticosteroid measurements (Porter-Silber test) do not appear to be artifactually altered, it is suggested that therapy with naproxen be temporarily discontinued 72 hours before adrenal function tests are performed if the Porter-Silber test is to be used.

Naproxen may interfere with some urinary assays of 5-hydroxy indoleacetic acid (5HIAA).

7.11 Interactions related to absorption

Esomeprazole inhibits gastric acid secretion. Therefore, esomeprazole may interfere with the absorption of drugs where gastric pH is an important determinant of bioavailability (eg, ketoconazole, iron salts and digoxin).

7.12 Antiretroviral agents

Concomitant use of atazanavir and nelfinavir with proton pump inhibitors such as esomeprazole is not recommended. Co-administration of atazanavir with proton pump inhibitors is expected to substantially decrease atazanavir plasma concentrations and thereby reduce its therapeutic effect. Omeprazole, the racemate of esomeprazole, has been reported to interact with some antiretroviral drugs. The clinical importance and the mechanisms behind these interactions are not always known. Increased gastric pH during omeprazole treatment may change the absorption of the antiretroviral drug. Other possible interaction mechanisms are via CYP2C19. For some antiretroviral drugs, such as atazanavir and nelfinavir, decreased serum levels have been reported when given together with omeprazole. Following multiple doses of nelfinavir (1250 mg, twice daily) and omeprazole (40 mg once a day), AUC was decreased by 36% and 92%, C_{max} by 37% and 89% and C_{min} by 39% and 75% respectively for nelfinavir and main oxidative metabolite, hydroxy-t-butylamide (M8). Following multiple doses of atazanavir (400 mg, once a day) and omeprazole (40 mg, once a day, 2 hr before atazanavir), AUC was decreased by 94%, C_{max} by 96%, and C_{min} by 95%. Concomitant administration with omeprazole and drugs such as atazanavir and nelfinavir is therefore not recommended. For other antiretroviral drugs, such as saquinavir, elevated serum levels have been reported with an increase in AUC by 82% in C_{max} by 75% and in C_{min} by 106% following multiple dosing of saquinavir/ritonavir (1000/100 mg) twice a day for 15 days with omeprazole 40 mg once a day co-administered on days 11 to 15. Therefore, clinical and laboratory monitoring for saquinavir toxicity is recommended during concurrent use with esomeprazole. Dose reduction of saquinavir should be considered from the safety perspective for individual patients. There are also some antiretroviral drugs of which unchanged serum levels have been reported when given with omeprazole.

7.13 Effects on hepatic metabolism/cytochrome P-450 pathways

Esomeprazole is extensively metabolized in the liver by CYP2C19 and CYP3A4.

In vitro and *in vivo* studies have shown that esomeprazole is not likely to inhibit CYPs 1A2, 2A6, 2C9, 2D6, 2E1 and 3A4. No clinically relevant interactions with drugs metabolized by these CYP enzymes would be expected. Drug interaction studies have shown that esomeprazole does not have any clinically significant interactions with phenytoin, warfarin, quinidine, clarithromycin or amoxicillin.

However, post-marketing reports of changes in prothrombin measures have been received among patients on concomitant warfarin and esomeprazole therapy. Increases in INR and prothrombin time may lead to abnormal bleeding and even death. Patients treated with proton pump inhibitors and warfarin concomitantly may need to be monitored for increases in INR and prothrombin time.

Esomeprazole may potentially interfere with CYP2C19, the major esomeprazole metabolizing enzyme. Co-administration of esomeprazole 30 mg and diazepam, a CYP2C19 substrate, resulted in a 45% decrease in clearance of diazepam.

Concomitant administration of esomeprazole and a combined inhibitor of CYP2C19 and CYP3A4, such as voriconazole, may result in more than doubling of the esomeprazole exposure. Dose adjustment of esomeprazole is not normally required. Omeprazole acts as an inhibitor of CYP2C19. Omeprazole, given in doses of 40 mg daily for one week to 20 healthy subjects in cross-over study, increased C_{max} and AUC of cilostazol by 18% and 26% respectively. C_{max} and AUC of one of its active metabolites, 3,4-dihydrocilostazol, which has 4-7 times the activity of cilostazol, were increased by 29% and 69% respectively. Co-administration of cilostazol with esomeprazole is expected to increase concentrations of cilostazol and its above mentioned active metabolite. Therefore a dose reduction of cilostazol from 100 mg twice daily to 50 mg twice daily should be considered.

7.14 Other pharmacokinetic-based interactions

Co-administration of oral contraceptives, diazepam, phenytoin, or quinidine does not seem to change the pharmacokinetic profile of esomeprazole.

8 USE IN SPECIFIC POPULATIONS

8.1 Pregnancy

Teratogenic Effects: Pregnancy Category C prior to 30 weeks gestation; Category D starting 30 weeks gestation. Starting at 30 weeks gestation, VIMOVO, and other NSAIDs, should be avoided by pregnant women as premature closure of the ductus arteriosus in the fetus may occur. VIMOVO can cause fetal harm when administered to a pregnant woman starting at 30 weeks gestation. If this drug is used during this time period in pregnancy, the patient should be apprised of the potential hazard to a fetus. There are no adequate and well-controlled studies in pregnant women. Prior to 30 weeks gestation, VIMOVO should be used during pregnancy only if the potential benefit justifies the potential risk to the fetus.

Reproductive studies with naproxen have been performed in rats at 20 mg/kg/day (125 mg/m²/day, 0.23 times the human systemic exposure), rabbits at 20 mg/kg/day (220 mg/m²/day, 0.27 times the human systemic exposure), and mice at 170 mg/kg/day (510 mg/m²/day, 0.28 times the human systemic exposure) with no evidence of impaired fertility or harm to the fetus due to the drug [see *Animal Toxicology and/or Pharmacology (13.2)*]. However, animal reproduction studies are not always predictive of human response.

Reproductive studies in rats and rabbits with esomeprazole and multiple cohort studies in pregnant women with omeprazole use during the first trimester do not show an increased risk of congenital anomalies or adverse pregnancy outcomes. There are no adequate and well controlled studies of esomeprazole use in pregnancy. Because animal reproduction studies are not always predictive of human response, this drug should be used during pregnancy only if clearly needed.

Esomeprazole is the S-isomer of omeprazole. In four population-based cohort studies that included 1226 women exposed during the first trimester of pregnancy to omeprazole there was no increased risk of congenital anomalies. Reproductive studies with esomeprazole have been performed in rats at doses up to 57 times the human dose and in rabbits at doses up to 35 times the human dose and have revealed no evidence of impaired fertility or harm to the fetus [see *Animal Toxicology and/or Pharmacology (13.2)*].

Reproductive studies conducted with omeprazole on rats at oral doses up to 56 times the human dose and in rabbits at doses up to 56 times the human dose did not show any evidence of teratogenicity. In pregnant rabbits, omeprazole at doses about 5.5 to 56 times the human dose produced dose-related increases in embryo-lethality, fetal resorptions, and pregnancy loss. In rats treated with omeprazole at doses about 5.6 to 56 times the human dose, dose-related embryo/fetal toxicity and postnatal developmental toxicity occurred in offspring.

8.2 Labor and Delivery

In rat studies with NSAIDs, as with other drugs known to inhibit prostaglandin synthesis, an increased incidence of dystocia, delayed parturition, and decreased pup survival occurred. Naproxen-containing products are not recommended in labor and delivery because, through its prostaglandin synthesis inhibitory effect, naproxen may adversely affect fetal circulation and inhibit uterine contractions, thus increasing the risk of uterine hemorrhage. The effects of VIMOVO on labor and delivery in pregnant women are unknown.

8.3 Nursing Mothers

VIMOVO should not be used in nursing mothers due to the naproxen component.

Naproxen

The naproxen anion has been found in the milk of lactating women at a concentration equivalent to approximately 1% of maximum naproxen concentration in plasma. Because of the possible adverse effects of prostaglandin-inhibiting drugs on neonates, use in nursing mothers should be avoided.

Esomeprazole

The excretion of esomeprazole in milk has not been studied. It is not known whether this drug is excreted in human milk. However, omeprazole concentrations have been measured in breast milk of one woman taking omeprazole 20 mg per day. Because many drugs are excreted in human milk and because of the potential for tumorigenicity shown for esomeprazole in rat carcinogenicity studies, a decision should be made whether to discontinue nursing or to discontinue the drug, taking into account the importance of the drug to the mother.

8.4 Pediatric Use

The safety and efficacy of VIMOVO has not been established in children younger than 18 years.

8.5 Geriatric Use

Of the total number of patients who received VIMOVO (n=1157) in clinical trials, 387 were ≥65 years of age, of which 85 patients were 75 years and over. No meaningful differences in efficacy or safety were observed between these subjects and younger subjects [see *Adverse Reactions (6)*]. Studies indicate that although total plasma concentration of naproxen is unchanged, the unbound plasma fraction of naproxen is increased in the elderly. Caution is advised when high doses are required and some adjustment of dosage may be required in elderly patients. As with other drugs used in the elderly, it is prudent to use the lowest effective dose [see *Dosage and Administration (2)* and *Clinical Pharmacology (12.3)*].

Experience indicates that geriatric patients may be particularly sensitive to certain adverse effects of NSAIDs. Elderly or debilitated patients seem to tolerate peptic ulceration or bleeding less well when these events do occur. Most spontaneous reports of fatal GI events are in the geriatric population [see *Warnings and Precautions (5.4)*].

Naproxen is known to be substantially excreted by the kidney, and the risk of toxic reactions to this drug may be greater in patients with impaired renal function. Because elderly patients are more likely to have decreased renal function, care should be taken in dose selection, and it may be useful to monitor renal function. Geriatric patients may be at a greater risk for the development of a form of renal toxicity precipitated by reduced prostaglandin formation during administration of NSAIDs [see *Warnings and Precautions (5.6, 5.7)*].

8.6 Hepatic Insufficiency

VIMOVO is not recommended for use in patients with severe hepatic impairment because esomeprazole doses should not exceed 20 mg daily in these patients [see *Dosage and Administration (2)*, and *Warnings and Precautions (5.11)*].

8.7 Renal Insufficiency

Naproxen-containing products, including VIMOVO, are not recommended for use in patients with advanced renal disease [see *Dosage and Administration (2)*, and *Warnings and Precautions (5.6, 5.7)*].

10 OVERDOSAGE

There is no clinical data on overdosage with VIMOVO.

Overdosage of naproxen:

Significant naproxen overdosage may be characterized by lethargy, dizziness, drowsiness, epigastric pain, abdominal discomfort, heartburn, indigestion, nausea, transient alterations in liver function, hypoprothrombinemia, renal 24 dysfunction, metabolic acidosis, apnea, disorientation or vomiting. Gastrointestinal bleeding can occur. Hypertension, acute renal failure, respiratory depression, and coma may occur, but are rare. Anaphylactoid reactions have been reported with therapeutic ingestion of NSAIDs, and may occur following an overdose. A few patients have experienced convulsions, but it is not clear whether or not these were drug-related. It is not known what dose of the drug would be life threatening. The oral LD_{50} of the drug is 543 mg/kg in rats, 1234 mg/kg in mice, 4110 mg/kg in hamsters, and greater than 1000 mg/kg in dogs.

Patients should be managed by symptomatic and supportive care following an NSAID overdose. There are no specific antidotes. Hemodialysis does not decrease the plasma concentration of naproxen because of the high degree of its protein binding. Activated charcoal (60 to 100 g in adults, 1 to 2 g/kg in children) and/or osmotic cathartic may be indicated in patients seen within 4 hours of ingestion with symptoms or following a large overdose. Forced diuresis, alkalinization of urine or hemoperfusion may not be useful due to high protein binding.

Overdosage of esomeprazole:

A single oral dose of esomeprazole at 510 mg/kg (about 103 times the human dose on a body surface area basis) was lethal to rats. The major signs of acute toxicity were reduced motor activity, changes in respiratory frequency, tremor, ataxia, and intermittent clonic convulsions.

The symptoms described in connection with deliberate esomeprazole overdose (limited experience of doses in excess of 240 mg/ day) are transient. Single doses of 80 mg of esomeprazole were uneventful. Reports of overdosage with omeprazole in humans may also be relevant. Doses ranged up to 2,400 mg (120 times the usual recommended clinical dose). Manifestations were variable, but included confusion, drowsiness, blurred vision, tachycardia, nausea, diaphoresis, flushing, headache, dry mouth, and other adverse reactions similar to those seen in normal clinical experience (see omeprazole package insert - *Adverse Reactions*). No specific antidote for esomeprazole is known. Since esomeprazole is extensively protein bound, it is not expected to be removed by dialysis. In the event of overdosage, treatment should be symptomatic and supportive.

If overexposure occurs, call the Poison Control Center at 1-800-222-1222.

11   DESCRIPTION

The active ingredients of VIMOVO are naproxen which is a NSAID and esomeprazole magnesium which is a Proton Pump Inhibitor (PPI).

VIMOVO is available as an oval, yellow, multi-layer, delayed release tablet combining an enteric coated naproxen core and an immediate release esomeprazole magnesium layer surrounding the core. Each strength contains either 375 mg of naproxen and 20 mg of esomeprazole (present as 22.3 mg esomeprazole magnesium trihydrate) or 500 mg of naproxen and 20 mg of esomeprazole (present as 22.3 mg esomeprazole magnesium trihydrate) for oral administration. The inactive ingredients are carnauba wax, colloidal silicon dioxide, croscarmellose sodium, iron oxide yellow, glyceryl monostearate, hypromellose, iron oxide black, magnesium stearate, methacrylic acid copolymer dispersion, methylparaben, polysorbate 80, polydextrose, polyethylene glycol, povidone, propylene glycol, propylparaben, titanium dioxide, and triethyl citrate.

The chemical name for naproxen is (S)-6-methoxy-α-methyl-2-naphthaleneacetic acid. Naproxen has the following structure:

Naproxen has a molecular weight of 230.26 and a molecular formula of $C_{14}H_{14}O_3$.

Naproxen is an odorless, white to off-white crystalline substance. It is lipid soluble, practically insoluble in water at low pH and freely soluble in water at high pH. The octanol/water partition coefficient of naproxen at pH 7.4 is 1.6 to 1.8.

The chemical name for esomeprazole is bis(5-methoxy-2-[(S)-[(4-methoxy-3,5-dimethyl-2-pyridinyl)methyl]sulfinyl]-1H-benzimidazole-1-yl) magnesium trihydrate. Esomeprazole is the S-isomer of omeprazole, which is a mixture of the S- and R-isomers. Its molecular formula is $(C_{17}H_{18}N_3O_3S)_2Mg \times 3 H_2O$ with molecular weight of 767.2 as the trihydrate and 713.1 on an anhydrous basis. The structural formula is:

[See chemical structure at top of next column]

The magnesium salt is a white to slightly colored crystalline powder. It contains 3 moles of water of solvation and is slightly soluble in water.

The stability of esomeprazole magnesium is a function of pH; it rapidly degrades in acidic media, but it has accept-

Table 3: Effect on Intragastric pH on Day 9 (N=25)

	Naproxen 500 mg combined with esomeprazole		
	10 mg	20 mg	30 mg
% Time Gastric pH >4* †	41.1 (3.0)	71.5 (3.0)	76.8 (3.0)
Coefficient of variation	55%	18%	16%

*Gastric pH was measured over a 24-hour period
†LS Mean (SE)

able stability under alkaline conditions. At pH 6.8 (buffer), the half-life of the magnesium salt is about 19 hours at 25°C and about 8 hours at 37°C.

12   CLINICAL PHARMACOLOGY

12.1   Mechanism of Action

VIMOVO consists of an immediate-release esomeprazole magnesium layer and an enteric-coated naproxen core. As a result, esomeprazole is released first in the stomach, prior to the dissolution of naproxen in the small intestine. The enteric coating prevents naproxen release at pH levels below 5.5.

Naproxen is a NSAID with analgesic and antipyretic properties. The mechanism of action of the naproxen anion, like that of other NSAIDs, is not completely understood but may be related to prostaglandin synthetase inhibition.

Esomeprazole is a proton pump inhibitor that suppresses gastric acid secretion by specific inhibition of the H^+/K^+-ATPase in the gastric parietal cell. Esomeprazole is protonated and converted in the acidic compartment of the parietal cell forming the active inhibitor, the achiral sulphenamide. By acting specifically on the proton pump, esomeprazole blocks the final step in acid production, thus reducing gastric acidity. This effect is dose-related up to a daily dose of 20 to 40 mg and leads to inhibition of gastric acid secretion.

12.2   Pharmacodynamics

Antisecretory Activity

The effect of VIMOVO on intragastric pH was determined in 25 healthy volunteers in one study. Three VIMOVO combinations (naproxen 500 mg combined with either esomeprazole 10, 20, or 30 mg) were administered twice daily over 9 days. The results are shown in the following table:

[See table 3 above]

Serum Gastrin Effects

The effect of esomeprazole on serum gastrin concentrations was evaluated in approximately 2,700 patients in clinical trials up to 8 weeks and in over 1,300 patients for up to 6-12 months. The mean fasting gastrin level increased in a dose-related manner. This increase reached a plateau within two to three months of therapy and returned to baseline levels within four weeks after discontinuation of therapy.

Enterochromaffin-like (ECL) Cell Effects

In over 1,000 patients treated with esomeprazole (10, 20 or 40 mg/day) up to 6-12 months, the prevalence of ECL cell hyperplasia increased with time and dose. No patient developed ECL cell carcinoids, dysplasia, or neoplasia in the gastric mucosa.

Endocrine Effects

Esomeprazole had no effect on thyroid function when given in oral doses of 20 or 40 mg for 4 weeks. Other effects of esomeprazole on the endocrine system were assessed using omeprazole studies. Omeprazole given in oral doses of 30 or 40 mg for 2 to 4 weeks had no effect on carbohydrate metabolism, circulating levels of parathyroid hormone, cortisol, estradiol, testosterone, prolactin, cholecystokinin or secretin.

Effects on Gastrointestinal Microbial Ecology

Decreased gastric acidity due to any means including proton pump inhibitors, increases gastric counts of bacteria normally present in the gastrointestinal tract. Treatment with proton pump inhibitors may lead to slightly increased risk of gastrointestinal infections such as *Salmonella* and *Campylobacter* and possibly *Clostridium difficile* in hospitalized patients.

12.3   Pharmacokinetics

Absorption

Naproxen

At steady state following administration of VIMOVO twice daily, peak plasma concentrations of naproxen are reached on average 3 hours following both the morning and the evening dose.

Bioequivalence between VIMOVO and enteric coated naproxen, based on both area under the plasma concentration-time curve (AUC) and maximum plasma concentration (C_{max}) of naproxen, has been demonstrated for

both the 375 mg and 500 mg doses. Naproxen is absorbed from the gastrointestinal tract with an *in vivo* bioavailability of 95%.

Steady-state levels of naproxen are reached in 4 to 5 days.

Esomeprazole

Following administration of VIMOVO twice daily, esomeprazole is rapidly absorbed with peak plasma concentration reached within on average, 0.43 to 1.2 hours, following the morning and evening dose on both the first day of administration and at steady state. The peak plasma concentrations of esomeprazole are higher at steady state compared to on first day of dosing of VIMOVO.

Figure 1 represents the pharmacokinetics of naproxen and esomeprazole following administration of VIMOVO 500 mg/20 mg.

Figure 1: Mean plasma concentrations of naproxen and esomeprazole following single dose administration of VIMOVO (500mg/20 mg)

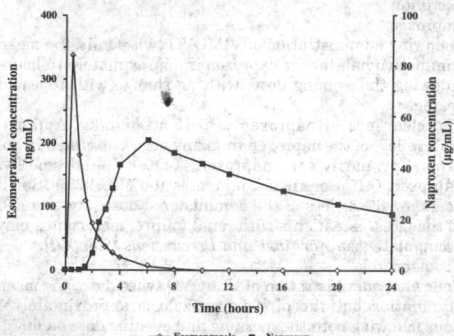

Food effect

Administration of VIMOVO together with high-fat food in healthy volunteers does not affect the extent of absorption of naproxen but significantly prolongs t_{max} by 10 hours and decreases peak plasma concentration (C_{max}) by about 12%. Administration of VIMOVO together with high-fat food in healthy volunteers delays t_{max} of esomeprazole by 1 hour and significantly reduces the extent of absorption, resulting in 52% and 75% reductions of area under the plasma concentration versus time curve (AUC) and peak plasma concentration (C_{max}), respectively.

Administration of VIMOVO 30 minutes before high-fat food intake in healthy volunteers does not affect the extent of absorption of naproxen but delays the absorption by about 4 hours and decreases peak plasma concentration (C_{max}) by about 17%, but has no significant effect on the rate or extent of esomeprazole absorption compared to administration under fasted conditions [see *Dosage and Administration (2)*]. Administration of VIMOVO 60 minutes before high-fat food intake in healthy volunteers has no effect on the rate and extent of naproxen absorption; however, increases the esomeprazole AUC by 25% and C_{max} by 50% compared to administration under fasted conditions. This increase in esomeprazole C_{max} does not raise a safety issue since the approved dosing regimen of esomeprazole at 40 mg QD would result in higher C_{max} [see *Dosage and Administration (2)*].

Therefore, VIMOVO should be taken at least 30 minutes before the meal.

Distribution

Naproxen

Naproxen has a volume of distribution of 0.16 L/kg. At therapeutic levels naproxen is greater than 99% albumin-bound. At doses of naproxen greater than 500 mg/day there is less than proportional increase in plasma levels due to an increase in clearance caused by saturation of plasma protein binding at higher doses (average trough C_{ss} 36.5, 49.2 and 56.4 mg/L with 500, 1000 and 1500 mg daily doses of naproxen, respectively). The naproxen anion has been found in the milk of lactating women at a concentration equivalent to approximately 1% of maximum naproxen concentration in plasma [see *Use in Specific Populations (8.3)*].

Esomeprazole

The apparent volume of distribution at steady state in healthy subjects is approximately 16L. Esomeprazole is 97% plasma protein bound.

Metabolism

Naproxen

Naproxen is extensively metabolized in the liver by the cytochrome P450 system (CYP), CYP2C9 and CYP1A2, to 6-0-desmethyl naproxen. Neither the parent drug nor the metabolites induce metabolizing enzymes. Both naproxen and 6-0-desmethyl naproxen are further metabolized to their respective acylglucuronide conjugated metabolites. Consistent with the half-life of naproxen, the area under the plasma concentration time curve increases with repeated dosing of VIMOVO twice daily.

Esomeprazole

Esomeprazole is extensively metabolized in the liver by the CYP enzyme system. The major part of the metabolism of esomeprazole is dependent on the polymorphic CYP2C19, responsible for the formation of the hydroxyl- and desmethyl metabolites of esomeprazole. The remaining part is dependent on another specific isoform CYP3A4, responsible for the formation of esomeprazole sulphone, the main metabolite in plasma. The major metabolites of esomeprazole have no effect on gastric acid secretion.

The area under the plasma esomeprazole concentration-time curve increases with repeated administration of VIMOVO. This increase is dose-dependent and results in a non-linear dose-AUC relationship after repeated administration. An increased absorption of esomeprazole with repeated administration of VIMOVO probably also contributes to the time-and dose-dependency.

Excretion

Naproxen

Following administration of VIMOVO twice daily, the mean elimination half-life for naproxen is approximately 15 hours following the evening dose, with no change with repeated dosing.

The clearance of naproxen is 0.13 mL/min/kg. Approximately 95% of the naproxen from any dose is excreted in the urine, primarily as naproxen (<1%), 6-0-desmethyl naproxen (<1%) or their conjugates (66% to 92%). Small amounts, 3% or less of the administered dose, are excreted in the feces. In patients with renal failure, metabolites may accumulate [see *Warnings and Precautions (5.6, 5.7)*].

Esomeprazole

Following administration of VIMOVO twice daily, the mean elimination half-life of esomeprazole is approximately 1 hour following both the morning and evening dose on day 1, with a slightly longer elimination half-life at steady state (1.2-1.5 hours).

Almost 80% of an oral dose of esomeprazole is excreted as metabolites in the urine, the remainder in the feces. Less than 1% of the parent drug is found in the urine.

Special Populations

Geriatric Patients

There is no specific data on the pharmacokinetics of VIMOVO in patients over age 65.

Studies indicate that although total plasma concentration of naproxen is unchanged, the unbound plasma fraction of naproxen is increased in the elderly, although the unbound fraction is <1% of the total naproxen concentration. Unbound trough naproxen concentrations in elderly subjects have been reported to range from 0.12% to 0.19% of total naproxen concentration, compared with 0.05% to 0.075% in younger subjects. The clinical significance of this finding is unclear, although it is possible that the increase in free naproxen concentration could be associated with an increase in the rate of adverse events per a given dosage in some elderly patients [see *Adverse Reactions (6)* and *Use in Specific Populations (8.5)*].

The AUC and C_{max} values of esomeprazole were slightly higher (25% and 18%, respectively) in the elderly as compared to younger subjects at steady state. Dosage adjustment for the esomeprazole component based on age is not necessary.

Race

Pharmacokinetic differences due to race have not been studied for naproxen.

Approximately 3% of Caucasians and 15 to 20% of Asians lack a functional CYP2C19 enzyme and are called poor metabolizers. In these individuals the metabolism of esomeprazole is probably mainly catalyzed by CYP3A4. After repeated once-daily administration of 40 mg esomeprazole, the mean area under the plasma concentration-time curve was approximately 100% higher in poor metabolizers than in subjects having a functional CYP2C19 enzyme (extensive metabolizers).

Hepatic Insufficiency

The pharmacokinetics of VIMOVO or naproxen have not been determined in subjects with hepatic impairment.

Chronic alcoholic liver disease and probably also other forms of cirrhosis reduce the total plasma concentration of naproxen, but the plasma concentration of unbound naproxen is increased. The implication of this finding for the naproxen component of VIMOVO dosing is unknown but it is prudent to use the lowest effective dose.

The AUCs of esomeprazole in patients with severe hepatic insufficiency (Child Pugh Class C) have been shown to be 2-3 times higher than in patients with normal liver function. For this reason, it has been recommended that esomeprazole doses not exceed 20 mg daily in patients with severe hepatic impairment. However, there is no dose adjustment necessary for patients with Child Pugh Class A and B for the esomeprazole component of VIMOVO. There is no VIMOVO dosage form that contains less than 20 mg esomeprazole for twice daily dosing.

Renal Insufficiency

The pharmacokinetics of VIMOVO or naproxen have not been determined in subjects with renal impairment.

Given that naproxen, its metabolites and conjugates are primarily excreted by the kidney, the potential exists for naproxen metabolites to accumulate in the presence of renal insufficiency. Elimination of naproxen is decreased in patients with severe renal impairment. Naproxen-containing products, including VIMOVO, is not recommended for use in patients with moderate to severe and severe renal impairment (creatinine clearance <30 ml/min) [see *Dosage and Administration (2)*, *Warnings and Precautions (5.6, 5.7)*, and *Use in Specific Populations (8.7)*].

No studies have been performed with esomeprazole in patients with decreased renal function. Since the kidney is responsible for the excretion of the metabolites of esomeprazole but not for the elimination of the parent compound, the metabolism of esomeprazole is not expected to be changed in patients with impaired renal function.

Gender

The AUC and C_{max} values of esomeprazole were slightly higher (13%) in females than in males at steady state. Dosage adjustment for the esomeprazole component based on gender is not necessary.

13 NONCLINICAL TOXICOLOGY

13.1 Carcinogenesis, Mutagenesis, Impairment of Fertility

Naproxen

A 2-year study was performed in rats to evaluate the carcinogenic potential of naproxen at rat doses of 8, 16, and 24 mg/kg/day (50, 100, and 150 mg/m^2). The maximum dose used was 0.28 times the highest recommended human dose. No evidence of tumorigenicity was found.

Esomeprazole

The carcinogenic potential of esomeprazole was assessed using omeprazole studies. In two 24-month oral carcinogenicity studies in rats, omeprazole at daily doses of 1.7, 3.4, 13.8, 44 and 140.8 mg/kg/day (about 0.7 to 57 times the human dose of 20 mg/day expressed on a body surface area basis) produced gastric ECL cell carcinoids in a dose-related manner in both male and female rats; the incidence of this effect was markedly higher in female rats, which had higher blood levels of omeprazole. Gastric carcinoids seldom occur in the untreated rat. In addition, ECL cell hyperplasia was present in all treated groups of both sexes. In one of these studies, female rats were treated with 13.8 mg omeprazole/kg/day (about 5.6 times the human dose on a body surface area basis) for 1 year, then followed for an additional year without the drug. No carcinoids were seen in these rats. An increased incidence of treatment-related ECL cell hyperplasia was observed at the end of 1 year (94% treated vs 10% controls). By the second year the difference between treated and control rats was much smaller (46% vs 26%) but still showed more hyperplasia in the treated group. Gastric adenocarcinoma was seen in one rat (2%). No similar tumor was seen in male or female rats treated for 2 years. For this strain of rat no similar tumor has been noted historically, but a finding involving only one tumor is difficult to interpret. A 78-week mouse carcinogenicity study of omeprazole did not show increased tumor occurrence, but the study was not conclusive.

Esomeprazole was negative in the Ames mutation test, in the *in vivo* rat bone marrow cell chromosome aberration test, and the *in vivo* mouse micronucleus test. Esomeprazole, however, was positive in the *in vitro* human lymphocyte chromosome aberration test. Omeprazole was positive in the *in vitro* human lymphocyte chromosome aberration test, the *in vivo* mouse bone marrow cell chromosome aberration test, and the *in vivo* mouse micronucleus test.

The potential effects of esomeprazole on fertility and reproductive performance were assessed using omeprazole studies. Omeprazole at oral doses up to 138 mg/kg/day in rats (about 56 times the human dose on a body surface area basis) was found to have no effect on reproductive performance of parental animals.

13.2 Animal Toxicology and/or Pharmacology

Naproxen

Reproductive studies have been performed in rats at 20 mg/kg/day (125 mg/m^2/day, 0.23 times the maximum recommended human dose), rabbits at 20 mg/kg/day (220 mg/m^2/day, 0.27 times the maximum recommended human dose), and mice at 170 mg/kg/day (510 mg/m^2/day, 0.28 times the maximum recommended human dose) with no evidence of impaired fertility or harm to the fetus due to the drug. However, animal reproduction studies are not always predictive of human response.

Esomeprazole

Reproductive studies have been performed in rats at oral doses up to 280 mg/kg/day (about 57 times the human dose on a body surface area basis) and in rabbits at oral doses up to 86 mg/kg/day (about 35 times the human dose on a body surface area basis) and have revealed no evidence of impaired fertility or harm to the fetus due to esomeprazole.

Reproductive studies conducted with omeprazole in rats at oral doses up to 138 mg/kg/day (about 56 times the human dose on a body surface area basis) and in rabbits at doses up to 69 mg/kg/day (about 56 times the human dose on a body surface area basis) did not disclose any evidence for a teratogenic potential of omeprazole. In rabbits, omeprazole in a dose range of 6.9 to 69.1 mg/kg/day (about 5.5 to 56 times the human dose on a body surface area basis) produced dose-related increases in embryo-lethality, fetal resorptions, and pregnancy disruptions. In rats, dose-related embryo/fetal toxicity and postnatal developmental toxicity were observed in offspring resulting from parents treated with omeprazole at 13.8 to 138.0 mg/kg/day (about 5.6 to 56 times the human doses on a body surface area basis).

14 CLINICAL STUDIES

Two randomized, multi-center, double-blind trials (Study 1 and Study 2) compared the incidence of gastric ulcer formation in 428 patients taking VIMOVO and 426 patients taking enteric-coated naproxen. Subjects were at least 18 years of age with a medical condition expected to require daily NSAID therapy for at least 6 months, and, if less than 50 years old, with a documented history of gastric or duodenal ulcer within the past 5 years. The majority of patients were female (67%), white (86%). The majority of patients were 50-69 years of age (83%). Approximately one quarter were on low-dose aspirin.

Studies 1 and 2 showed that VIMOVO given as 500 mg/20 mg twice daily statistically significantly reduced the 6-month cumulative incidence of gastric ulcers compared to enteric-coated naproxen 500 mg twice daily (see Table 4).

Approximately a quarter of the patients in Studies 1 and 2 were taking concurrent low-dose aspirin (≤ 325 mg daily). The results for this subgroup analysis in patients who used aspirin were consistent with the overall findings of the study.

The results at one month, three months, and six months are presented in Table 4.

[See table 4 at bottom left]

In these trials, patients receiving VIMOVO had a mean duration of therapy of 152 days compared to 124 days in patients receiving enteric-coated naproxen alone. A higher proportion of patients taking EC-naproxen (12%) discontinued the study due to upper GI adverse events (including duodenal ulcers) compared to VIMOVO (4%) in both trials [see *Adverse Reactions (6)*].

The efficacy of VIMOVO in treating the signs and symptoms of osteoarthritis was established in two 12-week randomized, double-blind, placebo-controlled trials in patients with osteoarthritis (OA) of the knee. In these two trials, patients were allowed to remain on low-dose aspirin for cardioprophylaxis. VIMOVO was given as 500 mg/20 mg twice daily. In each trial, patients receiving VIMOVO had significantly better results compared to patients receiving placebo as measured by change from baseline of the WOMAC pain subscale and the WOMAC physical function subscale and a Patient Global Assessment Score.

Table 4–Cumulative Observed Incidence of Gastric Ulcers at 1, 3 and 6 Months

	Study 1		Study 2	
	VIMOVO N=218 number (%)	EC-naproxen N=216 number (%)	VIMOVO N=210 number (%)	EC-naproxen N=210 number (%)
0-1 Month	3 (1.4)	28 (13.0)	4 (1.9)	21 (10.0)
0-3 Months	4 (1.8)	42 (19.4)	10 (4.8)	37 (17.6)
0-6 Months*	9 (4.1)	50 (23.1)	15 (7.1)	51 (24.3)

*For both Studies, p < 0.001 for treatment comparisons of cumulative GU incidence at six months.

Based on studies with enteric-coated naproxen, improvement in patients treated for rheumatoid arthritis was demonstrated by a reduction in joint swelling, a reduction in duration of morning stiffness, a reduction in disease activity as assessed by both the investigator and patient, and by increased mobility as demonstrated by a reduction in walking time. In patients with osteoarthritis, the therapeutic action of naproxen has been shown by a reduction in joint pain or tenderness, an increase in range of motion in knee joints, increased mobility as demonstrated by a reduction in walking time, and improvement in capacity to perform activities of daily living impaired by the disease. In patients with ankylosing spondylitis, naproxen has been shown to decrease night pain, morning stiffness and pain at rest.

16 HOW SUPPLIED/STORAGE AND HANDLING

VIMOVO 375 mg/20 mg tablets are oval, yellow film-coated tablets printed with 375/20 in black ink, supplied as:
NDC 0186-0510-60 Bottles of 60 tablets
VIMOVO 500 mg/20 mg tablets are oval, yellow film-coated tablets printed with 500/20 in black ink, supplied as:
NDC 0186-0520-60 Bottles of 60 tablets
NDC 0186-0520-39 Unit Dose Blisters, package of 100 tablets
Storage: Store at 25°C (77°F); excursions permitted to 15-30°C (59-86°F) [see USP Controlled Room Temperature]. Store in the original container and keep the bottle tightly closed to protect from moisture. Dispense in a tight container if package is subdivided.

17 PATIENT COUNSELING INFORMATION

Patients should be informed of the following before initiating therapy with VIMOVO and periodically during the course of ongoing therapy. Patients should also be encouraged to read the NSAID Medication Guide that accompanies each prescription dispensed.

1. VIMOVO, like other NSAID-containing products, may cause serious cardiovascular side effects, such as myocardial infarction or stroke, which may result in hospitalization and even death. Although serious cardiovascular events can occur without warning symptoms, patients should be alert for the signs and symptoms of chest pain, shortness of breath, weakness, slurring of speech, and should ask for medical advice when observing any indicative sign or symptoms. Patients should be apprised of the importance of this follow-up [see *Warnings and Precautions (5.1)*].

2. VIMOVO has been developed with esomeprazole to decrease incidence of ulceration from naproxen. NSAIDs, including naproxen, can cause GI discomfort and, rarely, serious GI side effects, such as ulcers and bleeding, which may result in hospitalization and even death. Although serious GI tract ulcerations and bleeding can occur without warning symptoms, patients should be alert for the signs and symptoms of ulcerations and bleeding, and should ask for medical advice when observing any indicative sign or symptoms including epigastric pain, dyspepsia, melena, and hematemesis. Patients should be apprised of the importance of this follow-up [see *Warnings and Precautions (5.4)*].

3. VIMOVO, like other NSAID-containing products, can cause serious skin side effects such as exfoliative dermatitis, Stevens-Johnson syndrome, and toxic epidermal necrolysis, which may result in hospitalizations and even death. Although serious skin reactions may occur without warning, patients should be alert for the signs and symptoms of skin rash and blisters, fever, or other signs of hypersensitivity such as itching, and should ask for medical advice when observing any indicative signs or symptoms. Patients should be advised to stop the drug immediately if they develop any type of rash and contact their physicians as soon as possible [see *Warnings and Precautions (5.9)*].

4. Patients should promptly report signs or symptoms of unexplained weight gain or edema to their physicians.

5. Patients should be informed of the warning signs and symptoms of hepatotoxicity (eg, nausea, fatigue, lethargy, pruritus, jaundice, right upper quadrant tenderness, and "flu-like" symptoms). If these occur, patients should be instructed to stop therapy and seek immediate medical therapy [see *Contraindications (4)* and *Warnings and Precautions (5.11)*].

6. Patients should be informed of the signs of an anaphylactoid reaction (eg, difficulty breathing, swelling of the face or throat). If these occur, patients should be instructed to seek immediate emergency help [see *Warnings and Precautions (5.8)*].

7. In late pregnancy, as with other NSAIDs, VIMOVO should be avoided because it may cause premature closure of the ductus arteriosus [see *Contraindications (4)*, *Warnings and Precautions (5.10)* and *Use in Specific Populations (8.1)*].

8. Caution should be exercised by patients whose activities require alertness if they experience drowsiness, dizziness, vertigo or depression during therapy with VIMOVO.

9. Patients should be instructed to tell their physicians if they have a history of asthma or aspirin-sensitive asthma

Serious side effects include:
heart attack
stroke
high blood pressure
heart failure from body swelling (fluid retention)
kidney problems including kidney failure
bleeding and ulcers in the stomach and intestine
low red blood cells (anemia)
life-threatening skin reactions
life-threatening allergic reactions
liver problems including liver failure
asthma attacks in people who have asthma

because the use of NSAIDs in patients with aspirin-sensitive asthma has been associated with severe bronchospasm, which can be fatal. Patients with this form of aspirin sensitivity should be instructed not to take VIMOVO. Patients with preexisting asthma should be instructed to seek immediate medical attention if their asthma worsens after taking VIMOVO [see *Warnings and Precautions (5.8, 5.13)*].
10. Antacids may be used while taking VIMOVO.
11. VIMOVO tablets should be swallowed whole with liquid. Tablets should not be split, chewed, crushed or dissolved. VIMOVO tablets should be taken at least 30 minutes before meals [see *Dosage and Administration (2)*].
VIMOVO is a trademark of the AstraZeneca group of companies.
Manufactured by:
Patheon Pharmaceuticals Inc.
Cincinnati, OH 45237
For: AstraZeneca LP, Wilmington, DE 19850
Part 35520–00
April 2010
©AstraZeneca 2010

MEDICATION GUIDE

VIMOVO (vi-moh'-voh)
(naproxen and esomeprazole magnesium)
Delayed Release Tablets
Read this Medication Guide before you start taking VIMOVO and each time you get a refill. There may be new information. This information does not take the place of talking with your health care provider about your medical condition or your treatment.
What is the most important information I should know about VIMOVO?
VIMOVO, which contains naproxen [a nonsteroidal anti-inflammatory drug (NSAID)] and esomeprazole magnesium, may increase the chance of a heart attack or stroke that can lead to death. This chance increases:
• with longer use of NSAID medicines
• in people who have heart disease
NSAID-containing medicines, such as VIMOVO, should never be used right before or after a heart surgery called a coronary artery bypass graft (CABG).
NSAID-containing medicines, such as VIMOVO, can cause ulcers and bleeding in the stomach and intestines at any time during treatment. Ulcers and bleeding:
• can happen without warning symptoms
• may cause death
The chance of a person getting an ulcer or bleeding increases with:
• taking medicines called steroid hormones (corticosteroids) and blood thinners (anticoagulants)
• longer use
• smoking
• drinking alcohol
• older age
• having poor health
NSAID medicines should only be used:
• exactly as prescribed
• at the lowest dose possible for your treatment
• for the shortest time needed
What are Non-Steroidal Anti-Inflammatory Drugs (NSAIDs)?
NSAID medicines are used to treat pain and redness, swelling, and heat (inflammation) from medical conditions such as:
• different types of arthritis
• menstrual cramps and other types of short-term pain
Who should not take a Non-Steroidal Anti-Inflammatory Drug (NSAID)?
Do not take an NSAID medicine:
• if you had an asthma attack, hives, or other allergic reaction with aspirin or any other NSAID medicine
• for pain right before or after heart bypass surgery
Tell your health care provider:
• about all of your medical conditions
• about all of the medicines you take. NSAIDs and some other medicines can interact with each other and cause serious side effects. **Keep a list of your medicines to show to your health care provider and pharmacist**

Other side effects include:
stomach pain
constipation
diarrhea
gas
heartburn
nausea
vomiting
dizziness

• if you are pregnant. **NSAID medicines should not be used by pregnant women late in their pregnancy.**
• if you are breastfeeding. Talk to your health care provider
What are the possible side effects of Non-Steroidal Anti-Inflammatory Drugs (NSAIDs)?
[See table above]
Get emergency help right away if you have any of the following symptoms:
• shortness of breath or trouble breathing
• chest pain
• weakness in one part or side of your body
• slurred speech
• swelling of the face or throat
Stop your NSAID medicine and call your health care provider right away if you have any of the following symptoms:
• nausea
• more tired or weaker than usual
• itching
• your skin or eyes look yellow
• stomach pain
• flu-like symptoms
• vomit blood
• there is blood in your bowel movement or it is black and sticky like tar
• skin rash or blisters with fever
• unusual weight gain
• swelling of the arms and legs, hands and feet
These are not all of the possible side effects with NSAID medicines. Talk to your health care provider or pharmacist for more information about NSAID medicines. Call your health care provider for medical advice about side effects. You may report side effects to FDA at 1-800-FDA-1088.
Other information about Non-Steroidal Anti-Inflammatory Drugs (NSAIDs)
• Aspirin is an NSAID medicine but it does not increase the chance of a heart attack. Aspirin can cause bleeding in the brain, stomach, and intestines. Aspirin can also cause ulcers in the stomach and intestines
• Some of these NSAID medicines are sold in lower doses without a prescription (over-the-counter). Talk to your health care provider before using over-the-counter NSAIDs for more than 10 days

NSAID medicines that need a prescription

Generic Name	TRADENAME
Celecoxib	Celebrex
Diclofenac	Cataflam, Voltaren, Arthrotec (combined with misoprostol) Voltaren
Diflunisal	Dolobid
Etodolac	Lodine, Lodine XL
Fenoprofen	Nalfon, Nalfon 200
Flurbiprofen	Ansaid
Ibuprofen	Motrin, Tab-Profen, Vicoprofen* (combined with hydrocodone) Combunox (combined with oxycodone)
Indomethacin	Indocin, Indocin SR, Indo-Lemmon, Indomethagan
Ketoprofen	Oruvail
Ketorolac	Toradol
Mefenamic Acid	Ponstel
Meloxicam	Mobic
Nabumetone	Relafen
Naproxen	Naprosyn, Anaprox, Anaprox DS, EC-Naproxyn, Naprelan, VIMOVO
Oxaprozin	Daypro
Piroxicam	Feldene
Sulindac	Clinoril
Tolmetin	Tolectin, Tolectin DS, Tolectin 600

*Vicoprofen contains the same dose of ibuprofen as over-the-counter (OTC) NSAIDs, and is usually used for less than 10 days to treat pain. The OTC NSAID label warns that long-term continuous use may increase the risk of heart attack or stroke.

What is VIMOVO?

VIMOVO contains 2 medicines: naproxen, a non-steroidal anti-inflammatory drug (NSAID) and esomeprazole magnesium, a proton pump inhibitor (PPI).

VIMOVO is a prescription medicine used to:
- relieve signs and symptoms of osteoarthritis, rheumatoid arthritis, and ankylosing spondylitis
- decrease the risk of developing stomach (gastric) ulcers in people who are at risk of developing gastric ulcers with NSAIDs

It is not known if VIMOVO is safe or effective in children under the age of 18.

Who should not take VIMOVO?

Do not take VIMOVO:
- If you had an asthma attack, hives, or other allergic reaction after taking aspirin or other NSAID medicine
- If you are allergic to any of the ingredients in VIMOVO See the end of this leaflet for a complete list of ingredients in VIMOVO
- If you are allergic to any other Proton Pump Inhibitor (PPI) medicine
- For pain right before or after heart bypass surgery
- If you are in the late stages of pregnancy (third trimester)

What should I tell my doctor before taking VIMOVO?

Before you take VIMOVO, tell your health care provider about all your medical conditions, including if you:
- have liver or kidney problems
- have ulcerative colitis or Crohn's disease (inflammatory bowel disease or IBD)
- have any other medical conditions
- are pregnant or plan to become pregnant. See "What is the most important information I should know about VIMOVO?"
- are breast-feeding or plan to breast-feed. VIMOVO can pass into your milk and may harm your baby. You should not breast-feed while taking VIMOVO. Talk to your health care provider about the best way to feed your baby if you take VIMOVO

Tell your health care provider about all the medicines you take, including prescription and non-prescription medicines, vitamins, and herbal supplements. Since VIMOVO contains naproxen, talk to your health care provider before taking any other NSAID-containing products.

Using VIMOVO with other medicines can cause serious side effects. VIMOVO may affect the way other medicines work, and other medicines may affect how VIMOVO works.

Know the medicines you take. Keep a list of them to show your health care provider or pharmacist when you get a new medicine.

How should I take VIMOVO?

- Take VIMOVO exactly as your health care provider tells you to take it
- Your health care provider may tell you to take Vitamin D and Calcium supplements during treatment with VIMOVO
- Your health care provider will tell you how many VIMOVO to take and when to take them
- Do not change your dose or stop VIMOVO without first talking to your health care provider
- Take VIMOVO at least 30 minutes before a meal
- Swallow VIMOVO tablets whole with liquid. Do not split, chew, crush or dissolve the VIMOVO tablet. Tell your doctor if you cannot swallow the tablet whole. You may need a different medicine
- You may use antacids while taking VIMOVO
- If you forget to take a dose of VIMOVO, take it as soon as you remember. If it is almost time for your next dose, do not take the missed dose. Take the next dose on time. Do not take 2 doses at one time to make up for a missed dose.
- If you take too much VIMOVO, tell your health care provider or go to the closest hospital emergency room right away. Symptoms that you have taken too much VIMOVO may include:
  - feeling weak and tired
  - dizziness
  - feeling sleepy
  - upper stomach-area pain or discomfort
  - heartburn, indigestion, or nausea
  - a change in breathing or you stop breathing
  - vomiting
  - bleeding
  - movements of a body part that you cannot control
  - coordination problems and decreased movement

If you take more VIMOVO than your doctor recommends, call your Poison Control Center at 1-800-222-1222.
- Your doctor may do certain tests from time to time to check you for side effect of VIMOVO.

What are the possible side effects of VIMOVO?

VIMOVO may cause serious side effects.

See "What is the most important information I should know about VIMOVO?"
- High blood pressure.

- **Heart problems** such as congestive heart failure. Tell your health care provider about any swelling of your body, hands or feet, sudden weight gain or trouble breathing
- **Active bleeding.** Tell your doctor if you have signs of active bleeding including:
  - passing black sticky bowel movements (stools)
  - having bloody diarrhea
  - vomiting or coughing up blood or dark particles that look like coffee grounds
- **Serious allergic reactions.** Tell your health care provider or get medical help right away if you develop sudden wheezing, swelling of your lips, tongue, throat or body, rash, fainting or problems breathing or swallowing (severe allergic reaction)
- **Serious skin reactions.** Tell your health care provider or get medical help right away if you develop:
  - reddening of your skin with blisters or peeling
  - blisters and bleeding of your lips, eye lids, mouth, nose, and genitals
- **Liver problems.** Tell your health care provider if you develop yellowing of the skin or the whites of your eyes, dark urine or feel tired
- **Bone Fracture.** Talk to your health care provider about your risk for fractures if you take VIMOVO for a long period of time

The most common side effects of VIMOVO include
- inflammation of the lining of the stomach, with or without loss of the protective layer of the stomach (erosive gastritis)
- indigestion
- diarrhea
- stomach ulcers
- upper stomach-area (abdominal) pain
- nausea

Tell your health care provider if you have any side effect that bothers you or that does not go away.

These are not all the possible side effects of VIMOVO. For more information, ask your health care provider or pharmacist.

Call your doctor for medical advice about side effects. You may report side effects to FDA at 1-800-FDA-1088.

How should I store VIMOVO?

- Store VIMOVO at 59°F to 86°F (15°C to 30°C)
- Keep VIMOVO in the original container and keep the bottle tightly closed
- Keep VIMOVO dry

Keep VIMOVO and all medicines out of the reach of children.

General Information about VIMOVO

Medicines are sometimes prescribed for purposes other than those listed in this Medication Guide. Do not use VIMOVO for a condition for which it was not prescribed. Do not give VIMOVO to other people, even if they have the same symptoms you have. It may harm them.

This Medication Guide summarizes the most important information about VIMOVO. If you would like more information, ask your health care provider. You can ask your health care provider or pharmacist for information that is written for health care professionals. For more information, call 1-800-236-9933 or go to www.VIMOVO.com

What are the ingredients in VIMOVO?

Active ingredients: naproxen and esomeprazole magnesium

Inactive ingredients: carnauba wax, colloidal silicon dioxide, croscarmellose sodium, iron oxide yellow, glyceryl monostearate, hypromellose, iron oxide black, magnesium stearate, methacrylic acid copolymer dispersion, methylparaben, polysorbate 80, polydextrose, polyethylene glycol, povidone, propylene glycol, propylparaben, titanium dioxide, and triethyl citrate.

Manufactured by:
Patheon Pharmaceuticals Inc.
Cincinnati, OH 45237
For: AstraZeneca LP, Wilmington, DE 19850
Issued April 2010
This Medication Guide has been approved by the U.S. Food and Drug Administration. VIMOVO is a trademark of the AstraZeneca group of companies. Other trademarks are the property of their respective companies.

Shown in Product Identification Guide, page 306

ZOMIG NASAL SPRAY   ℞

[zō'mig]
(zolmitriptan)
spray, metered for nasal use

HIGHLIGHTS OF PRESCRIBING INFORMATION

These highlights do not include all the information needed to use ZOMIG NASAL SPRAY safely and effectively. See full prescribing information for ZOMIG NASAL SPRAY.

ZOMIG NASAL SPRAY (zolmitriptan) spray, metered for nasal use

Initial U.S. Approval: 1997

——RECENT MAJOR CHANGES——
Warning and Precautions, serotonin syndrome (5.5) 10/2008
Drug Interactions, serotonin syndrome (7.5) 10/2008
Use in Specific Populations, pediatric use (8.4) 10/2008

——INDICATIONS AND USAGE——
ZOMIG Nasal Spray is a 5HT$_{1B/1D}$ receptor agonist (triptan) indicated for:
- Acute treatment of migraine with or without aura in adults (1)

Important limitations:
- Use only after a clear diagnosis of migraine has been established (1.2)
- Not intended for the prophylactic therapy of migraine (1.2)
- Not indicated for the treatment of cluster headache (1.2)

——DOSAGE AND ADMINISTRATION——
Single 5 mg dose; may repeat after 2 hours if needed; not to exceed 10 mg in any 24-hour period; benefit of a second dose not established (2)

——DOSAGE FORMS AND STRENGTHS——
Nasal Spray: 5 mg (3)

——CONTRAINDICATIONS——
- Ischemic heart disease, coronary artery vasospasm, or other significant underlying cardiovascular disease (4.1)
- Cerebrovascular syndromes (e.g. history of stroke or TIA) (4.2)
- Peripheral Vascular Disease (including ischemic bowel disease) (4.3)
- Uncontrolled Hypertension (4.4)
- Do not use ZOMIG within 24 hours of another 5-HT$_1$ agonist, ergotamine-containing or ergot-type medication (4.5)
- Hemiplegic or basilar migraine (4.6)
- Do not use ZOMIG within 2 weeks of an MAO-A inhibitor (4.7)
- Hypersensitivity to ZOMIG (4.8)

——WARNINGS AND PRECAUTIONS——
- Serious adverse cardiac events, including acute myocardial infarction, and life-threatening disturbances of cardiac rhythm (5.1)
- It is strongly recommended that ZOMIG not be given to patients in whom unrecognized coronary artery disease (CAD) is predicted by the presence of risk factors. In very rare cases, serious cardiovascular events have been reported in association with ZOMIG in the absence of known cardiovascular disease. If ZOMIG is considered, patients should first have a cardiovascular evaluation. If the evaluation is satisfactory, first dose should take place in a physician's office setting (5.1)
- Sensations of pain, tightness, pressure and heaviness in the chest, throat, neck and jaw: generally not associated with myocardial ischemia, but patients with signs or symptoms suggestive of angina should be evaluated for the presence of CAD (5.2)
- Cerebrovascular events, some fatal (5.3)
- Gastrointestinal ischemic events and peripheral vasospastic reactions (e.g. Raynaud's syndrome) (5.4)
- Patients with symptomatic Wolff-Parkinson-White syndrome or arrhythmias associated with other cardiac accessory conduction pathways should not receive ZOMIG (5.1)
- Potentially life-threatening serotonin syndrome, particularly in combination with SSRIs or SNRIs. Monitor patients carefully if concomitant treatment is clinically warranted (5.5, 7.6)
- Increase in blood pressure, very rarely associated with significant clinical events (4.4, 5.6)

——ADVERSE REACTIONS——
- In controlled studies the most common adverse reactions (≥ 2% and > placebo) were: unusual taste, paresthesia, hyperesthesia, nausea, pain location specified, pain throat, somnolence, asthenia, disorder/discomfort of nasal cavity, dry mouth, tightness throat (6.1)

To report SUSPECTED ADVERSE REACTIONS, contact AstraZeneca at 1-800-236-9933 or FDA at 1-800-FDA-1088 or www.fda.gov/medwatch

——DRUG INTERACTIONS——
- Ergot-type or ergotamine-containing medications other 5HT$_1$ agonists, and ZOMIG: do not use within 24 hours of each other (4.5, 7.1, 7.3)
- Do not use ZOMIG within 2 weeks of an MAO-A inhibitor (4.7, 7.2)
- Cimetidine: half-life and AUC of zolmitriptan doubled (7.4)
- SSRI or SNRI: life-threatening serotonin syndrome reported during combined use with triptans (5.5, 7.5)

——USE IN SPECIFIC POPULATIONS——
- Pregnancy: Based on animal data, may cause fetal harm. Use ZOMIG during pregnancy only if the potential benefit justifies the potential risk to the fetus (8.1)
- Nursing Mothers: Use with caution while nursing, as it is not known if ZOMIG is excreted in human milk. Zolmitriptan has been detected in rat milk at levels equal to or greater than those in maternal plasma (8.3)
- Pediatric Use: Efficacy not established in a study in patients 12-17 years. Adverse reactions similar in nature and frequency to adults. Not studied in patients under 12 years (8.4)

• **Geriatric Use:** Safety and effectiveness in patients over 65 not established (8.5, 12.3).

• **Hepatic Impairment:** Decreased clearance of zolmitriptan and significant elevation in blood pressure observed. Use doses < 2.5 mg of an oral formulation, with blood pressure monitoring (2.2, 8.6, 12.3).

See 17 for PATIENT COUNSELING INFORMATION

Revised: 10/2008

FULL PRESCRIBING INFORMATION: CONTENTS*

*Sections or subsections omitted from the full prescribing information are not listed.

FULL PRESCRIBING INFORMATION

1   INDICATIONS AND USAGE

1.1   Acute Treatment of Migraine Attacks

ZOMIG Nasal Spray is indicated for the acute treatment of migraine with or without aura in adults.

1.2   Important Limitations

ZOMIG should only be used where a clear diagnosis of migraine has been established. If a patient has no response for the first migraine attack treated with ZOMIG, the diagnosis of migraine should be reconsidered before ZOMIG is administered to treat any subsequent attacks.

ZOMIG is not intended for the prophylactic therapy of migraine or for use in the management of hemiplegic or basilar migraine [see Contraindications (4.6)].

Safety and effectiveness of ZOMIG have not been established for cluster headache, which is present in an older, predominantly male population.

2   DOSAGE AND ADMINISTRATION

2.1   Acute Treatment of Migraine Attacks

Administer one dose of ZOMIG Nasal Spray 5 mg for the treatment of acute migraine. If the headache returns, the dose may be repeated after 2 hours. The effectiveness of a second dose has not been established in placebo controlled trials. The maximum daily dose should not exceed 10 mg in any 24-hour period.

In controlled clinical trials, single doses of 5 mg of zolmitriptan nasal spray were administered into one nostril and were effective for the treatment of acute migraines in adults.

Individuals may vary in response to ZOMIG Nasal Spray. The pharmacokinetics of a 5 mg nasal spray dose is similar to the 5 mg oral formulations. Doses lower than 5 mg can only be achieved through the use of an oral formulation. The choice of dose, and route of administration should therefore be made on an individual basis.

The safety of treating an average of more than four headaches in a 30-day period has not been established.

2.2   Hepatic Impairment

Patients with moderate to severe hepatic impairment have decreased clearance of zolmitriptan and significant elevation in blood pressure was observed in some patients. Use of doses less than 2.5 mg of an alternate formulation with blood pressure monitoring is recommended [see Clinical Pharmacology (12.3) and Warnings and Precautions (5.6)].

3   DOSAGE FORMS & STRENGTHS

Nasal Spray 5 mg

4   CONTRAINDICATIONS

4.1   Ischemic or Vasospastic Coronary Artery Disease

ZOMIG should not be given to patients with ischemic heart disease (angina pectoris, history of myocardial infarction, or documented silent ischemia) or to patients who have symptoms or findings consistent with ischemic heart disease, coronary artery vasospasm, including Prinzmetal's variant angina, or other significant underlying cardiovascular disease [see Warnings and Precautions (5.1)].

4.2   Cerebrovascular Syndromes

ZOMIG should not be given to patients with cerebrovascular syndromes including (but not limited to) stroke of any type as well as transient ischemic attacks. [see Warnings and Precautions (5.3)].

4.3   Peripheral Vascular Disease

ZOMIG should not be given to patients with peripheral vascular disease including (but not limited to) ischemic bowel disease [see Warnings and Precautions (5.4)].

4.4   Uncontrolled Hypertension

Because ZOMIG may increase blood pressure, it should not be given to patients with uncontrolled hypertension [see Warnings and Precautions (5.6)].

4.5   Use within 24 hours of treatment with another 5-HT₁ agonist, or ergotamine containing medication, or ergot type medication

ZOMIG and any ergotamine-containing or ergot-type medication (such as dihydroergotamine or methysergide) should not be used within 24 hours of each other, nor should ZOMIG and another 5-HT₁ agonist be used within 24 hours of each other [See Drug Interactions (7.1 and 7.3)].

4.6   Hemiplegic or Basilar Migraine

ZOMIG should not be administered to patients with hemiplegic or basilar migraine.

4.7   Administration of MAO-A inhibitors within 2 weeks

Concurrent administration of MAO-A inhibitors or use of zolmitriptan within 2 weeks of discontinuation of MAO-A inhibitor therapy is contraindicated [see Clinical Pharmacology (12.4) and Drug Interactions (7.2)].

4.8   Hypersensitivity to zolmitriptan

ZOMIG is contraindicated in patients who are hypersensitive to zolmitriptan or any of its inactive ingredients.

5   WARNINGS AND PRECAUTIONS

5.1   Risk of Myocardial Ischemia and/or Infarction and Other Adverse Cardiac Events:

Cardiac Events and Fatalities with 5-HT₁ Agonists Serious adverse cardiac events, including acute myocardial infarction, have been reported within a few hours following administration of zolmitriptan. Life-threatening disturbances of cardiac rhythm, and death have been reported within a few hours following the administration of other 5-HT₁ agonists. Considering the extent of use of 5 HT₁ agonists in patients with migraine, the incidence of these events is extremely low.

ZOMIG can cause coronary artery vasospasm; at least one of these events occurred in a patient with no cardiac disease history and with documented absence of coronary artery disease. Because of the close proximity of the events to ZOMIG use, a causal relationship cannot be excluded. In the cases where there has been known underlying coronary artery disease, the relationship is uncertain. Patients who experience signs or symptoms suggestive of angina following dosing should be evaluated for the presence of CAD or a predisposition to Prinzmetal's variant angina before receiving additional doses of medication, and should be monitored electrocardiographically if dosing is resumed and similar symptoms recur.

Patients with symptomatic Wolff-Parkinson-White syndrome or arrhythmias associated with other cardiac accessory conduction pathway disorders should not receive ZOMIG.

Premarketing experience with zolmitriptan

Among the more than 2,500 patients with migraine who participated in premarketing controlled clinical trials of ZOMIG Tablets, no deaths or serious cardiac events were reported. In a premarketing controlled clinical trial of ZOMIG Nasal Spray, more than 1,300 patients participated and there were no deaths or serious cardiac events to report.

Postmarketing experience with zolmitriptan

Serious cardiovascular events have been reported in association with the use of ZOMIG Tablets, and in very rare cases, these events have occurred in the absence of known cardiovascular disease. The uncontrolled nature of postmarketing surveillance, however, makes it impossible to determine definitively the proportion of the reported cases that were actually caused by zolmitriptan or to reliably assess causation in individual cases.

Patients with documented coronary artery disease

Because of the potential of this class of compound (5-HT₁ agonists) to cause coronary vasospasm, ZOMIG should not be given to patients with documented ischemic or vasospastic coronary artery disease [see Contraindications (4.1)].

Patients with risk factors for CAD

It is strongly recommended that zolmitriptan not be given to patients in whom unrecognized coronary artery disease (CAD) is predicted by the presence of risk factors (eg, hypertension, hypercholesterolemia, smoker, obesity, diabetes, strong family history of CAD, female with surgical or physiological menopause, or male over 40 years of age) unless a cardiovascular evaluation provides satisfactory clinical evidence that the patient is reasonably free of coronary artery and ischemic myocardial disease or other significant underlying cardiovascular disease. The sensitivity of cardiac diagnostic procedures to detect cardiovascular disease or predisposition to coronary artery vasospasm is modest, at best. If, during the cardiovascular evaluation, the patient's medical history, electrocardiographic or other investigations reveal findings indicative of, or consistent with, coronary artery vasospasm or myocardial ischemia, zolmitriptan should not be administered [see Contraindications (4.1)].

For patients with risk factors predictive of CAD, who are determined to have a satisfactory cardiovascular evaluation, it is strongly recommended that administration of the first dose of zolmitriptan take place in the setting of a physician's office or similar medically staffed and equipped facility unless the patient has previously received zolmitriptan. Because cardiac ischemia can occur in the absence of clinical symptoms, consideration should be given to obtaining on the first occasion of use an electrocardiogram (ECG) during the interval immediately following ZOMIG, in these patients with risk factors.

It is recommended that patients who are intermittent long-term users of ZOMIG and who have or acquire risk factors predictive of CAD, as described above, undergo periodic interval cardiovascular evaluation as they continue to use ZOMIG.

The systematic approach described above is intended to reduce the likelihood that patients with unrecognized cardiovascular disease will be inadvertently exposed to zolmitriptan.

5.2   Sensations of pain, tightness, pressure in the chest and or throat, neck and jaw

As with other 5-HT₁ agonists, sensations of tightness, pain, pressure, and heaviness in the precordium, throat, neck, and jaw have been reported after treatment with ZOMIG Tablets. Because 5-HT₁ agonists may cause coronary vasospasm, patients who experience signs or symptoms suggestive of angina following dosing should be evaluated for the presence of CAD or a predisposition to Prinzmetal's variant angina before receiving additional doses of medication, and should be monitored electrocardiographically if dosing is resumed and similar symptoms occur. Patients shown to have CAD and those with Prinzmetal's variant angina should not receive 5-HT₁ agonists [see CONTRAINDICATIONS (4.1)].

5.3   Cerebrovascular Events

Cerebral hemorrhage, subarachnoid hemorrhage, stroke, and other cerebrovascular events have been reported in patients treated with 5-HT$_1$ agonists, and some have resulted in fatalities. In a number of cases, it appears possible that the cerebrovascular events were primary, the agonist having been administered in the incorrect belief that the symptoms experienced were a consequence of migraine, when they were not. As with other acute migraine therapies, before treating headaches in patients not previously diagnosed as migraineurs, and in migraineurs who present with atypical symptoms, care should be taken to exclude other potentially serious neurological conditions. It should be noted that patients with migraine may be at increased risk of certain cerebrovascular events (eg, stroke, hemorrhage, transient ischemic attack) *[see Contraindications (4.2)]*.

5.4   Other Vasospasm-Related Events, including Peripheral Vascular Ischemia and Colonic Ischemia
5-HT$_1$ agonists, including ZOMIG, may cause vasospastic reactions other than coronary artery vasospasm, such as peripheral and gastrointestinal vascular ischemia with abdominal pain and bloody diarrhea.
Very rare reports of transient and permanent blindness and significant partial vision loss have been reported with the use of 5-HT$_1$ agonists. Visual disorders may also be part of a migraine attack.
Patients who experience other symptoms or signs suggestive of decreased arterial flow following the use of any 5-HT agonist, such as ischemic bowel syndrome or Raynaud's syndrome, are candidates for further evaluation *[see Contraindications (4.3)]*.

5.5   Serotonin Syndrome
The development of a potentially life-threatening serotonin syndrome may occur with triptans, including ZOMIG treatment, particularly during combined use with selective serotonin reuptake inhibitors (SSRIs) or serotonin norepinephrine reuptake inhibitors (SNRIs). If concomitant treatment with ZOMIG and an SSRI (e.g., fluoxetine, paroxetine, sertraline, fluvoxamine, citalopram, escitalopram) or SNRI (e.g., venlafaxine, duloxetine) is clinically warranted, careful observation of the patient is advised, particularly during treatment initiation and dose increases. Serotonin syndrome symptoms may include mental status changes (e.g., agitation, hallucinations, coma), autonomic instability (e.g., tachycardia, labile blood pressure, hyperthermia), neuromuscular aberrations (e.g., hyperreflexia, incoordination) and/or gastrointestinal symptoms (e.g., nausea, vomiting, diarrhea) *[See Drug Interactions (7.5)]*.

5.6   Increase in Blood Pressure
As with other 5-HT$_1$ agonists, significant elevations in systemic blood pressure have been reported on rare occasions with ZOMIG Tablet use, in patients with and without a history of hypertension; very rarely these increases in blood pressure have been associated with significant clinical events. Zolmitriptan is contraindicated in patients with uncontrolled hypertension. In volunteers, an increase of 1 and 5 mm Hg in the systolic and diastolic blood pressure, respectively, was seen at 5 mg. In the headache trials, vital signs were measured only in the small inpatient study and no effect on blood pressure was seen. In a study of patients with moderate to severe liver disease, 7 of 27 experienced 20 to 80 mm Hg elevations in systolic and/or diastolic blood pressure after a dose of 10 mg of zolmitriptan *[see Contraindications (4.4)]*.
An 18% increase in mean pulmonary artery pressure was seen following dosing with another 5–HT$_1$ agonist in a study evaluating subjects undergoing cardiac catheterization.

5.7   Binding to Melanin-Containing Tissues:
When pigmented rats were given a single oral dose of 10 mg/kg of radiolabeled zolmitriptan, the radioactivity in the eye after 7 days, the latest time point examined, was still 75% of the value measured after 4 hours. This suggests that zolmitriptan and/or its metabolites may bind to the melanin of the eye. Because there could be accumulation in melanin rich tissues over time, this raises the possibility that zolmitriptan could cause toxicity in these tissues after extended use. However, no effects on the retina related to treatment with zolmitriptan were noted in any of the toxicity studies including those conducted by the nasal route. Although no systematic monitoring of ophthalmologic function was undertaken in clinical trials, and no specific recommendations for ophthalmologic monitoring are offered, prescribers should be aware of the possibility of long-term ophthalmologic effects.

5.8   Laboratory Tests:
No monitoring of specific laboratory tests is recommended.

5.9   Drug/Laboratory Test Interactions
Zolmitriptan is not known to interfere with commonly employed clinical laboratory tests.

6   ADVERSE REACTIONS
6.1   Clinical Studies Experience
Because clinical studies are conducted under widely varying conditions, adverse reaction rates observed in the clinical studies of a drug cannot be directly compared to rates in the clinical studies of another drug and may not reflect the rates observed in practice.

Serious cardiac reactions, including myocardial infarction, have occurred following the use of ZOMIG Tablets. These reactions are extremely rare and most have been reported in patients with risk factors predictive of CAD. Reactions reported, in association with triptans, have included coronary artery vasospasm, transient myocardial ischemia, myocardial infarction, ventricular tachycardia, and ventricular fibrillation *[See Contraindications, (4.1) and Warnings and Precautions (5.1)]*.

Incidence in Controlled Clinical Trials:
Among 464 adult patients treating single attacks with zolmitriptan nasal spray in a blinded placebo controlled trial, there was a low withdrawal rate related to adverse reactions: 5 mg (1.3%), and placebo (0.4%). None of the withdrawals were due to a serious reaction. One patient was withdrawn due to abnormal ECG changes from baseline that was incidentally found 23 days after the last dose of ZOMIG Nasal Spray. The most common adverse reactions in clinical trials for ZOMIG Nasal Spray were: unusual taste, paresthesia, hyperesthesia, and dizziness.
Table 1 lists the adverse reactions that occurred in ≥ 2% of the 236 patients in the 5 mg dose group of the controlled clinical trial.

Table 1: Adverse reactions with an incidence of ≥ 2% of patients in the zolmitriptan 5 mg nasal spray treatment group by body system and greater than placebo.

Body System and Adverse Reaction	Placebo (N=228)	5.0 mg (N=236)
Atypical Sensations		
Hyperesthesia	0%	5%
Paraesthesia	6%	10%
Ear/Nose/Throat		
Disorder/Discomfort of nasal cavity	2%	3%
Pain and Pressure Sensations		
Pain Location Specified	1%	4%
Pain Throat	1%	4%
Tightness Throat	1%	2%
Digestive		
Dry Mouth	0%	2%
Nausea	1%	4%
Neurological		
Somnolence	2%	4%
Unusual Taste	3%	21%
Other		
Asthenia	1%	3%

Adverse clinical reactions occurring in ≥ 1% and < 2% of patients in all attacks of the controlled clinical trial were pain abdominal, pressure throat, vomiting, headache, tightness chest, dysphagia, insomnia, palpitation and reaction aggravation.
The incidence of adverse reactions in controlled clinical trials was not affected by gender, weight, or age of the patients (18-39 vs. 40-65 years of age), or presence of aura. There were insufficient data to assess the impact of race on the incidence of adverse reactions.

Local Adverse Reactions:
Among 922 patients using the zolmitriptan nasal spray to treat 2311 attacks in the controlled clinical study who were exposed, across all doses (0.5 to 5 mg), approximately 3% noted local irritation or soreness at the site of administration. Adverse reactions of any kind, perceived in the nasopharynx (which may include systemic effects of triptans) were severe in about 1% of patients and approximately 60% resolved in 1 hour. Nasopharyngeal examinations, in a subset of patients participating in two long term trials of up to one year duration, failed to demonstrate any clinically significant changes with repeated use of ZOMIG Nasal Spray. All nasopharyngeal adverse reactions with an incidence of ≥ 2% of patients in any zolmitriptan nasal spray dose groups are included in ADVERSE REACTIONS Table 1.

Other Adverse Reactions:
In the paragraphs that follow, the frequencies of less commonly reported adverse clinical reactions are presented. Because the reports include reactions observed in open and

uncontrolled studies, the role of ZOMIG in their causation cannot be reliably determined. Furthermore, variability associated with adverse reaction reporting, the terminology used to describe adverse reactions, etc., limit the value of the quantitative frequency estimates provided. Reaction frequencies are calculated as the number of patients who used ZOMIG Nasal Spray and reported a reaction divided by the total number of patients exposed to ZOMIG Nasal Spray (n=3059). All reported reactions are included except those already listed in the previous table, those too general to be informative, and those not reasonably associated with the use of the drug. Reactions are further classified within body system categories and enumerated in order of decreasing frequency using the following definitions: infrequent adverse reactions are those occurring in 1/100 to 1/1,000 patients and rare adverse reactions are those occurring in fewer than 1/1,000 patients.

Body:
Infrequent: allergic reaction, back pain, chills, cyst, flu syndrome, infection, jaw pain, pressure other, jaw tightening, edema of the face, abnormal laboratory test, neck pain, neoplasm, and neck tightness, chest heaviness, chest pain, and chest pressure
Rare: cellulitis, fever, jaw pressure, and neck heaviness

Cardiovascular:
Infrequent: arrhythmias, hypertension, syncope, thrombophlebitis, and tachycardia
Rare: angina pectoris, bradycardia, atrial fibrillation, myocardial infarct, vasodilation, and vascular disorder

Digestive:
Infrequent: diarrhea, dyspepsia, tongue edema, gastrointestinal disorder, increased saliva, and thirst
Rare: increased appetite, colitis, constipation, eructation, gastritis, gastrointestinal carcinoma, gingivitis, hepatic neoplasia, intestinal obstruction, jaundice, sialadenitis, and stomatitis

Endocrine System:
Rare: hyperthyroidism and thyroid edema

Hemic:
Infrequent: cyanosis
Rare: ecchymosis, lymphadenopathy and leukopenia

Metabolic Nutritional:
Rare: increased weight, dehydration, and peripheral edema

Musculoskeletal:
Infrequent: arthralgia, joint disorder, and myalgia
Rare: bone pain, osteoporosis, tenosynovitis and twitching

Nervous System:
Infrequent: agitation, amnesia, anxiety, ataxia, abnormal coordination, confusion, depersonalization, depression, hypertonia, insomnia, nervousness, speech disorder, abnormal thinking, tremor, vertigo, and circumoral paresthesia
Rare: apathy, convulsions, abnormal dreams, euphoria, hypertonia, irritability, tardive dyskinesia, manic reaction, neuropathy, and psychosis

Respiratory:
Infrequent: bronchitis, increased cough, dyspnea, epistaxis, laryngeal edema, pharyngitis, rhinitis, sinusitis, throat discomfort, and voice alteration
Rare: hiccup, hyperventilation, laryngitis, pneumonia, increased sputum, and yawning

Skin:
Infrequent: pruritus, rash, skin disorder, and sweating
Rare: eczema, erythema, erythema multiforme, hair disorder, and neoplasm

Special Senses:
Infrequent: amblyopia, disorder of lacrimation, ear pain, eye pain, parosmia and tinnitus
Rare: conjunctivitis, dry eye, photophobia, and visual field defect

Urogenital:
Infrequent: polyuria and menorrhagia
Rare: breast carcinoma, dysmenorrhea, metrorrhagia, breast neoplasm, unintended pregnancy, suspicious PAP smear, uterine disorder, enlarged uterine fibroids, fibrocytic breast, vaginitis, urogenital neoplasm, cystitis, urinary tract infection, kidney pain, pyelonephritis, urinary frequency, urine impaired, and urinary tract disorder
The adverse experience profile seen with ZOMIG Nasal Spray is similar to that seen with ZOMIG tablets and ZOMIG-ZMT tablets except for the occurrence of local adverse reactions from the nasal spray (see ZOMIG Tablet Prescribing Information).

6.2   Postmarketing Experience with ZOMIG Tablets
The following adverse reactions were identified during post approval use of ZOMIG. Because these reactions are reported voluntarily from a population of uncertain size, it is not always possible to reliably estimate their frequency or establish a causal relationship to drug exposure.
The following section enumerates potentially important adverse reactions that have occurred in clinical practice and which have been reported spontaneously to various surveillance systems. The reactions enumerated represent reports arising from both domestic and non-domestic use of oral

zolmitriptan. The reactions enumerated include all except those already listed in the ADVERSE REACTIONS section above or those too general to be informative. Because the reports cite reactions reported spontaneously from worldwide postmarketing experience, frequency of reactions and the role of zolmitriptan in their causation cannot be reliably determined.

Cardiovascular:

Coronary artery vasospasm, transient myocardial ischemia, angina pectoris, and myocardial infarction.

Digestive:

Very rare gastrointestinal ischemic reactions including splenic infarction, ischemic colitis and gastrointestinal infarction or necrosis have been reported; these may present as bloody diarrhea or abdominal pain. *[See Warnings and Precautions (5.4)].*

General:

As with other 5-HT $_{1B/1D}$ agonists, there have been very rare reports of anaphylaxis or anaphylactoid reactions in patients receiving ZOMIG. There have been rare reports of hypersensitivity reactions, including angioedema.

Serotonin syndrome has also been reported during the postmarketing period *[see Warnings and Precautions (5.5)].*

Neurological:

As with other acute migraine treatments including other 5–HT_1 agonists, there have been rare reports of headache.

7 DRUG INTERACTIONS

7.1 Ergot-containing drugs

Ergot-containing drugs have been reported to cause prolonged vasospastic reactions. Because there is a theoretical basis that these effects may be additive, use of ergotamine containing or ergot-type medications (like dihydroergotamine or methysergide) and zolmitriptan within 24 hours of each other should be avoided *[see Contraindications (4.5)].*

7.2 MAO-A Inhibitors

MAO-A inhibitors increase the systemic exposure of zolmitriptan. Therefore, the use of zolmitriptan in patients receiving MAO-A inhibitors is contraindicated *[see Clinical Pharmacology (12.4) and Contraindications (4.7)].*

7.3 5-$HT_{1B/1D}$ agonists (e.g. triptans)

Concomitant use of other 5-$HT_{1B/1D}$ agonists within 24 hours of ZOMIG treatment is not recommended *[see Contraindications (4.5)].*

7.4 Cimetidine

Following administration of cimetidine, the half-life and AUC of zolmitriptan and its active metabolites were approximately doubled *[see Clinical Pharmacology (12.4)].*

7.5 Selective Serotonin Reuptake Inhibitors/Serotonin Norepinephrine Reuptake Inhibitors and Serotonin Syndrome

Cases of life-threatening serotonin syndrome have been reported during combined use of selective serotonin reuptake inhibitors (SSRIs) or serotonin norepinephrine reuptake inhibitors (SNRIs) and triptans *[See Warnings and Precautions (5.5)].*

8 USE IN SPECIFIC POPULATIONS

8.1 Pregnancy

Pregnancy Category C. There are no adequate and well controlled studies in pregnant women; therefore, zolmitriptan should be used during pregnancy only if the potential benefit justifies the potential risk to the fetus. In reproductive toxicity studies in rats and rabbits, oral administration of zolmitriptan to pregnant animals resulted in embryolethality and fetal abnormalities (malformations and variations) at clinically relevant exposures.

When zolmitriptan was administered to pregnant rats during the period of organogenesis at oral doses of 100, 400, and 1200 mg/kg/day (plasma exposures (AUCs) ≈280, 1100, and 5000 times the human AUC at the maximum recommended human dose (MRHD) of 10 mg/day), there was a dose-related increase in embryolethality. A no-effect dose for embryolethality was not established. When zolmitriptan was administered to pregnant rabbits during the period of organogenesis at oral doses of 3, 10, and 30 mg/kg/day (plasma AUCs ≈1, 11, and 42 times the human AUC at the MRHD), there were increases in embryolethality and in fetal malformations and variations. The no-effect dose for adverse effects on embryo-fetal development was associated with a plasma AUC similar to that in humans at the MRHD. When female rats were given zolmitriptan during gestation, parturition, and lactation at oral doses of 25, 100, and 400 mg/kg/day (plasma AUCs ≈70, 280, and 1100 times that in human at the MRHD), an increased incidence of hydronephrosis was found in the offspring. The no-effect dose was associated with a plasma AUC ≈280 times that in humans at the MRHD.

8.3 Nursing Mothers

It is not known whether zolmitriptan is excreted in human milk. Because many drugs are excreted in human milk, caution should be exercised when zolmitriptan is administered to a nursing woman. Lactating rats dosed with zolmitriptan had levels in milk equivalent to maternal plasma levels at 1 hour and 4 times higher than plasma levels at 4 hours.

8.4 Pediatric Use

Safety and effectiveness of ZOMIG in pediatric patients have not been established; therefore, ZOMIG is not recommended for use in patients under 18 years of age.

A single, multicenter, double-blind, randomized placebo-controlled, study was conducted to evaluate the efficacy of zolmitriptan 5 mg nasal spray in the acute treatment of migraine headache in 171 evaluable adolescent subjects 12 to 17 years of age. Efficacy was not established in that study. Adverse reactions observed in this study were similar in nature and frequency to those reported in ZOMIG Nasal Spray adult clinical trials. The most commonly reported adverse reactions (≥ 2% and > placebo) were dysgeusia (7%), nasal discomfort (3%), dizziness (2%), nasal congestion (2%), nausea (2%), and throat irritation (2%).

ZOMIG Nasal Spray has not been studied in pediatric patients under 12 years of age.

In the postmarketing experience with triptans, including ZOMIG, there is a limited number of reports that describe pediatric patients who have experienced clinically serious adverse events; those that were reported are similar in nature to those reported rarely in adults.

8.5 Geriatric Use

Although the pharmacokinetic disposition of the drug in the elderly is similar to that seen in younger adults, there is no information about the safety and effectiveness of zolmitriptan in this population because patients over age 65 were excluded from the controlled clinical trials *[see Clinical Pharmacology (12.3)].*

8.6 Hepatic Impairment

The effect of hepatic disease on the pharmacokinetics of zolmitriptan nasal spray has not been evaluated. After oral administration, zolmitriptan exposure was increased in patients with severe hepatic impairment, and significant elevation in blood pressure was observed in some patients. Because of the similarity in exposure, zolmitriptan tablets and nasal spray should have similar dosage adjustments and should be administered with caution in subjects with liver disease, generally using doses less than 2.5 mg. Doses lower than 5 mg can only be achieved through the use of an oral formulation. *[see Dosage and Administration (2.2) and Clinical Pharmacology (12.3)].*

9 DRUG ABUSE AND DEPENDENCE

The abuse potential of ZOMIG has not been assessed in clinical trials.

10 OVERDOSAGE

There is no experience with acute overdose. Clinical study subjects receiving single 50 mg oral doses of zolmitriptan commonly experienced sedation.

The elimination half-life of ZOMIG is 3 hours *[see Clinical Pharmacology (12.1)]* and therefore monitoring of patients after overdose with ZOMIG should continue for at least 15 hours or while symptoms or signs persist.

There is no specific antidote to zolmitriptan. In cases of severe intoxication, intensive care procedures are recommended, including establishing and maintaining a patent airway, ensuring adequate oxygenation and ventilation, and monitoring and support of the cardiovascular system.

It is unknown what effect hemodialysis or peritoneal dialysis has on the plasma concentrations of zolmitriptan.

11 DESCRIPTION

ZOMIG® (zolmitriptan) Nasal Spray contains zolmitriptan, which is a selective 5 hydroxytryptamine $_{1B/1D}$ (5 $HT_{1B/1D}$) receptor agonist. Zolmitriptan is chemically designated as (S)-4-[[3-[2-(dimethylamino)ethyl]-1H-indol-5-yl]methyl]-2-oxazolidinone and has the following chemical structure:

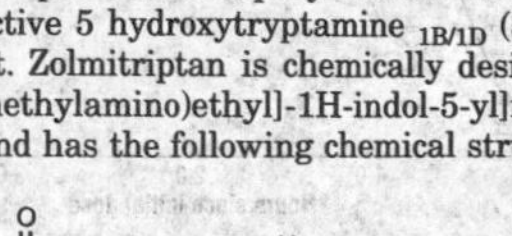

The empirical formula is $C_{16}H_{21}N_3O_2$, representing a molecular weight of 287.36. Zolmitriptan is a white to almost white powder that is readily soluble in water. ZOMIG Nasal Spray is supplied as a clear to pale yellow solution of zolmitriptan, buffered to a pH 5.0. Each ZOMIG Nasal Spray contains 5 mg of zolmitriptan in a 100-µL unit dose aqueous buffered solution containing citric acid, anhydrous, USP, disodium phosphate dodecahydrate USP and purified water USP.

ZOMIG Nasal Spray is hypertonic. The osmolarity of ZOMIG Nasal Spray 5 mg is 420 to 470 mOsmol.

12 CLINICAL PHARMACOLOGY

12.1 Mechanism of Action

Zolmitriptan binds with high affinity to human recombinant 5 HT_{1D} and 5 HT_{1B} receptors. Zolmitriptan exhibits modest affinity for 5-HT_{1A} receptors, but has no significant affinity (as measured by radioligand binding assays) or pharmacological activity at 5 HT2, 5-HT3, 5 HT4, α_1, α_2 or β_1 adrenergic; H_1, H_2, histaminic; muscarinic; D_1, or D_2 receptors. The N-desmethyl metabolite also has high affinity for 5 $HT_{1B/1D}$ and modest affinity for 5 HT_{1A} receptors.

Current theories proposed to explain the etiology of migraine headache suggest that symptoms are due to local cranial vasodilatation and/or to the release of sensory neuropeptides (vasoactive intestinal peptide, substance P and calcitonin gene-related peptide) through nerve endings in the trigeminal system. The therapeutic activity of zolmitriptan for the treatment of migraine headache can most likely be attributed to the agonist effects at the 5 $HT_{1B/1D}$ receptors on intracranial blood vessels (including the arterio-venous anastomoses) and sensory nerves of the trigeminal system which result in cranial vessel constriction and inhibition of pro inflammatory neuropeptide release.

12.3 Pharmacokinetics

Absorption:

Zolmitriptan nasal spray is rapidly absorbed via the nasopharynx as detected in a Photon Emission Tomography (PET) study using ^{11}C zolmitriptan. Zolmitriptan was detected in plasma by 5 minutes and peak plasma concentration generally was achieved by 3 hours. The time at which maximum plasma concentrations were observed was similar after single (1 day) or multiple (4 day) nasal dosing. Plasma concentrations of zolmitriptan are sustained for 4 to 6 hours after dosing. Zolmitriptan displays linear kinetics after multiple doses of 2.5 mg, 5 mg, or 10 mg. The mean relative bioavailability of the nasal spray formulation is 102%, compared with the oral tablet.

Zolmitriptan and its active metabolite display dose proportionality after single or multiple dosing. Dose proportional increases in zolmitriptan and N-desmethyl metabolite C_{max} and AUC were observed for 2.5 and 5 mg nasal spray doses. The pharmacokinetics for elimination of zolmitriptan and its active N-desmethyl metabolite are similar for all nasal spray dosages. The N-desmethyl metabolite is detected in plasma by 15 minutes and peak plasma concentration is generally achieved by 3 hours after administration.

Food has no significant effect on the bioavailability of zolmitriptan.

Distribution:

Plasma protein binding of zolmitriptan is 25% over the concentration range of 10–1000 ng/mL. The mean (±SD) apparent volume of distribution for zolmitriptan nasal spray formulation is 8.4±3.3 L/kg.

Metabolism:

Zolmitriptan is converted to an active N-desmethyl metabolite such that the metabolite concentrations are about two-thirds that of zolmitriptan. Because the $5HT_{1B/1D}$ potency of the metabolite is 2 to 6 times that of the parent compound, the metabolite may contribute a substantial portion of the overall effect after zolmitriptan administration.

Excretion:

The mean elimination half-life for zolmitriptan and its active N-desmethyl metabolite following nasal spray administration are approximately 3 hours, which is similar to the half-life values seen after oral tablet administration. The half-life values were similar for zolmitriptan and the N-desmethyl metabolite after single (1 day) and multiple (4 day) nasal dosing.

Mean total plasma clearance is 25.9 mL/min/kg, of which one-sixth is renal clearance. The renal clearance is greater than the glomerular filtration rate suggesting renal tubular secretion.

Special Populations:

Age:

The pharmacokinetics of oral zolmitriptan in healthy elderly non-migraineur volunteers (age 65–76 yrs) was similar to those in younger non-migraineur volunteers (age 18–39 yrs).

Gender:

Mean plasma concentrations of orally administered zolmitriptan were up to 1.5-fold higher in females than males.

Renal Impairment:

The effect of renal impairment on the pharmacokinetics of zolmitriptan nasal spray has not been evaluated. After orally dosing zolmitriptan, renal clearance was reduced by 25% in patients with severe renal impairment (Clcr ≥ 5 ≤ 25 mL/min) compared with the normal group (Clcr ≥ 70 mL/min); no significant change in renal clearance was observed in the moderately renally impaired group (Clcr ≥ 26 ≤ 50 mL/min).

Hepatic Impairment:

The effect of hepatic disease on the pharmacokinetics of zolmitriptan nasal spray has not been evaluated. In severely hepatically impaired patients, the mean C_{max}, T_{max}, and AUC0-∞ of zolmitriptan dosed orally were increased 1.5, 2, and 3-fold, respectively, compared with normals. Seven out of 27 patients experienced 20 to 80 mm Hg elevations in systolic and/or diastolic blood pressure after a

10 mg dose. Because of the similarity in exposure, zolmitriptan tablets and nasal spray should have similar dosage adjustments and should be administered with caution in subjects with liver disease, generally using doses less than 2.5 mg. Doses lower than 5 mg can only be achieved through the use of an oral formulation *[see Dosing and Administration (2.2) and Use in Special Populations (8.6)].*

Hypertensive Patients:
No differences in the pharmacokinetics of oral zolmitriptan or its effects on blood pressure were seen in mild to moderate hypertensive volunteers compared with normotensive controls.

Race:
Retrospective analysis of pharmacokinetic data between Japanese and Caucasians revealed no significant differences for orally dosed zolmitriptan.

12.4 Drug Interactions
All drug interaction studies were performed in healthy volunteers using a single 10 mg dose of zolmitriptan and a single dose of the other drug except where otherwise noted. Eight drug interaction studies have been performed with zolmitriptan tablets and one study (xylometazoline) was performed with nasal spray.

Xylometazoline:
An *in vivo* drug interaction study with ZOMIG Nasal Spray indicated that 1 spray (100μL dose) of xylometazoline (0.1% w/v), a decongestant, administered 30 minutes prior to a 5 mg nasal dose of zolmitriptan did not alter the pharmacokinetics of zolmitriptan.

Fluoxetine:
The pharmacokinetics of zolmitriptan, as well as its effect on blood pressure, were unaffected by 4 weeks of pretreatment with oral fluoxetine (20 mg/day).

MAO Inhibitors:
Following one week of administration of 150 mg bid moclobemide, a specific MAO-A inhibitor, there was an increase of about 25% in both C_{max} and AUC for zolmitriptan and a 3-fold increase in the C_{max} and AUC of the active N-desmethyl metabolite of zolmitriptan *[see Contraindications (4) and Warnings and Precautions (5)].*
Selegiline, a selective MAO-B inhibitor, at a dose of 10 mg/day for 1 week, had no effect on the pharmacokinetics of zolmitriptan and its metabolite.

Propranolol:
C_{max} and AUC of zolmitriptan increased 1.5-fold after one week of dosing with propranolol (160 mg/day). C_{max} and AUC of the N-desmethyl metabolite were reduced by 30% and 15%, respectively. There were no interactive effects on blood pressure or pulse rate following administration of propranolol with zolmitriptan.

Acetaminophen:
A single 1 g dose of acetaminophen does not alter the pharmacokinetics of zolmitriptan and its N-desmethyl metabolite. However, zolmitriptan delayed the T_{max} of acetaminophen by one hour.

Metoclopramide:
A single 10 mg dose of metoclopramide had no effect on the pharmacokinetics of zolmitriptan or its metabolites.

Oral Contraceptives:
Retrospective analysis of pharmacokinetic data across studies indicated that mean plasma concentrations of zolmitriptan were generally higher in females taking oral contraceptives compared with those not taking oral contraceptives. Mean C_{max} and AUC of zolmitriptan were found to be higher by 30% and 50%, respectively, and T_{max} was delayed by one-half hour in females taking oral contraceptives. The effect of zolmitriptan on the pharmacokinetics of oral contraceptives has not been studied.

Cimetidine:
Following the administration of cimetidine, the half-life and AUC of a 5 mg dose of zolmitriptan and its active metabolite were approximately doubled *[see Drug Interactions (7.4)].*

13 NONCLINICAL TOXICOLOGY
13.1 Carcinogenesis, Mutagenesis, Impairment of Fertility
Carcinogenesis:
Zolmitriptan was administered to mice and rats at doses up to 400 mg/kg/day. Mice were dosed for 85 weeks (males) and 92 weeks (females); rats were dosed for 101 weeks (males) and 86 weeks (females). There was no evidence of drug-induced tumors in mice at plasma exposures (AUC) up to approximately 700 times that in humans at the maximum recommended human dose (MRHD) of 10 mg/day. In rats, there was an increase in the incidence of thyroid follicular cell hyperplasia and thyroid follicular cell adenomas seen in male rats receiving 400 mg/kg/day. The no-effect dose for tumors in rats (100 mg/kg/day) was associated with a plasma AUC ≈700 times that in humans at the MRHD.

13.2 Mutagenesis
Zolmitriptan was positive in an *in vitro* bacterial reverse mutation (Ames) assay and in an *in vitro* chromosomal aberration assay in human lymphocytes. Zolmitriptan was

negative in an *in vitro* mammalian gene cell mutation (CHO/HGPRT) assay and in oral *in vivo* micronucleus assays in mouse and rat.

13.3 Impairment of Fertility
Studies of male and female rats administered zolmitriptan prior to and during mating and up to implantation showed no impairment of fertility at oral doses up to 400 mg/kg/day. The plasma exposure (AUC) at this dose was approximately 3000 times that in humans at the maximum recommended human dose of 10 mg/day.

14 CLINICAL STUDIES
The efficacy of ZOMIG Nasal Spray 5 mg in the acute treatment of migraine headache with or without aura was demonstrated in a randomized, outpatient, double blind, placebo-controlled trial.
Patients were instructed to treat a moderate to severe headache. Headache response, defined as a reduction in headache severity from moderate or severe pain to mild or no pain, was assessed 15, 30, 45 minutes and 1, 2, and 4 hours after dosing. Pain free response rates and associated symptoms such as nausea, photophobia, and phonophobia were also assessed. A dose of escape medication was allowed 4 to 24 hours after the initial treatment for persistent and recurrent headache.
Of the 1372 patients treated in the study, 83% were female and 99% were Caucasian, with a mean age of 40.6 years (range 18 to 65 years).
The two hour headache response rates in patients treated with ZOMIG Nasal Spray were statistically significant among patients receiving ZOMIG Nasal Spray compared with placebo. There was a greater percentage of patients with a headache response at 2 hours in the higher dose groups. The headache response efficacy endpoints of the controlled clinical study, analyzed from the first attack data, are shown in Table 2.

Table 2: First Attack Data: Percentage of Patients with Headache Response to ZOMIG Nasal Spray (Mild or No Headache) 2 Hours Following Treatment (N = number of randomized patients treating a migraine attack). The 2 hour headache response was the primary end-point.

N	PLACEBO (226)	ZOMIG 5 mg (235)
2 hours	31%	69%*

* p<0.0001 in comparison with placebo

The estimated probability of achieving an initial headache response by 4 hours following treatment with ZOMIG Nasal Spray is depicted in Figure 1.

Figure 1: Estimated probability of achieving an initial headache response within 4 hours of initial treatment

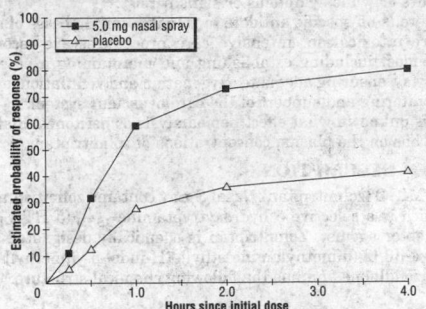

Note: Figure 1 shows the Kaplan-Meier plot of the probability over time of obtaining headache response (moderate or severe headache improving to mild or no pain) following treatment with zolmitriptan nasal spray. The averages displayed are based on a placebo controlled, outpatient trial providing evidence of efficacy. Patients not achieving headache response or taking additional treatment prior to 4 hours were censored to 4 hours.
For patients with migraine associated photophobia, phonophobia, and nausea at baseline, there was a decreased incidence of these symptoms following administration of ZOMIG Nasal Spray as compared with placebo.
Four to 24 hours following the initial dose of study treatment, patients were allowed to use additional treatment for pain relief in the form of a second dose of study treatment or other medication. The estimated probability of patients taking a second dose or other medication for migraine over the 24 hours following the initial dose of study treatment is summarized in Figure 2.
[See figure at top of next column]
The efficacy of ZOMIG was unaffected by presence of aura; presence of headache upon awakening, relationship to menses; gender, age or weight of the patient; or presence of pretreatment nausea.

Figure 2: Estimated probability of patients taking an escape medication within the 24 hours following the initial dose of study treatment

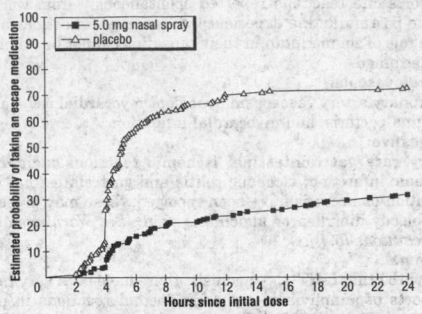

*This Kaplan-Meier plot is based on data obtained from the placebo controlled clinical trial. Patients not using additional treatments were censored at 24 hours. The plot includes both patients who had headache response at 2 hours and those who had no response to the initial dose. It should be noted that the protocol did not allow remediation within 4 hours post dose.

The efficacy of ZOMIG Nasal Spray 5 mg was further supported by an interim analysis of another similarly designed trial. The 2 hour headache response rates for the first 210 subjects in that study for ZOMIG 5 mg and placebo were 70% and 47%, respectively (N=108 and 102, respectively, p=0.0006).

16 HOW SUPPLIED/STORAGE AND HANDLING
The ZOMIG Nasal Spray device is a blue colored plastic device with a gray protection cap, labeled to indicate the nominal dose. Each ZOMIG Nasal Spray device administers a single dose of ZOMIG.
ZOMIG Nasal Spray is supplied as a clear to pale yellow solution of zolmitriptan, buffered to a pH 5.0. Each ZOMIG Nasal Spray device contains 5 mg of zolmitriptan in a 100-μL unit dose aqueous buffered solution containing citric acid, anhydrous, USP, disodium phosphate dodecahydrate USP and purified water USP.
5 mg ZOMIG® Nasal Spray is supplied in boxes of 6 single use nasal spray units. (NDC 310-0208-60).
Each ZOMIG® Nasal Spray single dose unit spray supplies 5 mg of zolmitriptan. The ZOMIG® Nasal Spray unit must be discarded after use.
Store at controlled room temperature, 20-25°C (68-77°F) [see USP].

17 PATIENT COUNSELING INFORMATION
See FDA-Approved Patient Labeling (17.5)
17.1 Risk of Myocardial Ischemia and/or Infarction, Other Adverse Cardiac Events, Other Vasospasm-related Event, and Cerebrovascular Events
Patients should be informed that ZOMIG may cause serious cardiovascular side effects such as myocardial infarction or stroke, which may result in hospitalization and even death. Although serious cardiovascular events can occur without warning symptoms, patients should be alert for the signs and symptoms of chest pain, shortness of breath, weakness, slurring of speech, and should ask for medical advice when observing any indicative sign or symptoms. Patients should be apprised of the importance of this follow-up *[see Warnings and Precautions (5.1, 5.3, 5.4)].*
17.2 Serotonin Syndrome
Patients should be cautioned about the risk of serotonin syndrome with the use of ZOMIG or other triptans, particularly during combined use with selective serotonin reuptake inhibitors (SSRIs) or serotonin norepinephrine reuptake inhibitors (SNRIs) *[See Warnings and Precautions (5.5)].*
17.3 Device Use
The ZOMIG Nasal Spray device is packaged in a carton and is a blue colored plastic device with a gray protection cap, labeled to indicate the nominal dose. Patients should be cautioned to not remove the gray protection cap until prior to dosing. The ZOMIG Nasal Spray device is placed in a nostril and actuated to deliver a single dose. **Patients should be cautioned to avoid spraying the contents of the device in their eyes.**
17.4 Pregnancy
ZOMIG should not be used during pregnancy unless the potential benefit justifies the potential risk to the fetus.
17.5 Approved Patient Labeling
Please read this information before you start taking ZOMIG Nasal Spray and each time you renew your prescription just in case anything has changed. Remember, this summary does not take the place of discussions with your doctor. You and your doctor should discuss ZOMIG Nasal Spray when you start taking your medication and at regular checkups.

What is ZOMIG Nasal Spray?

ZOMIG Nasal Spray is a prescription medication used to treat migraine headaches in adults. ZOMIG Nasal Spray is not for other types of headaches. The safety and efficacy of ZOMIG in patients under 18 have not been established.

What is a Migraine Headache?

Migraine is an intense, throbbing headache. You may have pain on one or both sides of your head. You may have nausea and vomiting, and be sensitive to light and noise. The pain and symptoms of a migraine headache can be worse than a common headache. Some women get migraines around the time of their menstrual period. Some people have visual symptoms before the headache, such as flashing lights or wavy lines, called an aura.

How does ZOMIG Nasal Spray work?

Treatment with ZOMIG Nasal Spray reduces swelling of blood vessels surrounding the brain. This swelling is associated with the headache pain of a migraine attack. ZOMIG Nasal Spray blocks the release of substances from nerve endings that cause more pain and other symptoms like nausea, and sensitivity to light and sound. It is thought that these actions contribute to relief of your symptoms by ZOMIG Nasal Spray.

Who should not take ZOMIG Nasal Spray?

Do not take ZOMIG Nasal Spray if you:
- Have heart disease or a history of heart disease
- Have uncontrolled high blood pressure
- Have hemiplegic or basilar migraine (if you are not sure about this, ask your doctor)
- Have or had a stroke or problems with your blood circulation
- Have serious liver problems
- Have taken any of the following medicines in the last 24 hours: other "triptans" like almotriptan (AXERT®), eletriptan (RELPAX®), frovatriptan (FROVA®), naratriptan (AMERGE®), rizatriptan (MAXALT®), sumatriptan (IMITREX®); sumatriptan/naproxen (TREXIMET); ergotamines like BELLERGAL-S®, CAFERGOT®, ERGOMAR®, WIGRAINE®; dihydroergotamine like D.H.E. 45® or MIGRANAL®; or methysergide (SANSERT®). These medications have side effects similar to ZOMIG Nasal Spray.
- Have taken monoamine oxidase (MAO) inhibitors such as phenelzine sulfate (NARDIL®) or tranylcypromine sulfate (PARNATE®) for depression or other conditions, or if it has been less than 2 weeks since you stopped taking a MAO inhibitor.
- Are allergic to ZOMIG Nasal Spray or any of its ingredients. The active ingredient is zolmitriptan. The inactive ingredients are listed at the end of this leaflet.

Tell your doctor about all the medicines you take or plan to take, including prescription and nonprescription medicines, supplements, and herbal remedies.

Tell your doctor if you are taking selective serotonin reuptake inhibitors (SSRIs) or serotonin norepinephrine reuptake inhibitors (SNRIs), two types of drugs for depression or other disorders. Common SSRIs are CELEXA® (citalopram HBr), LEXAPRO® (escitalopram oxalate), PAXIL® (paroxetine), PROZAC® (fluoxetine), SYMBYAX® (olanzapine/fluoxetine), ZOLOFT® (sertraline), SARAFEM® (fluoxetine) and LUVOX® (fluvoxamine). Common SNRIs are CYMBALTA® (duloxetine) and EFFEXOR® (venlafaxine). Your doctor will decide if you can take ZOMIG Nasal Spray with your other medicines.

Tell your doctor if you know that you have any of the following: risk factors for heart disease like high cholesterol, diabetes, smoking, obesity (overweight), menopause, or a family history of heart disease or stroke.

Tell your doctor if you are pregnant, planning to become pregnant, breast feeding, planning to breast feed, or not using effective birth control.

How should I take ZOMIG NASAL Spray?

The ZOMIG Nasal Spray device is a blue colored plastic sprayer device with a gray protection cap, labeled to indicate the dose. For adults, the usual dose is a single nasal spray taken into one nostril. If your headache comes back after your first dose, you may take a second dose anytime after 2 hours of taking the first dose. For any attack where the first dose didn't work, do not take a second dose without talking with your doctor. Do not take more than a total of 10 mg of ZOMIG (tablets or spray combined) in any 24-hour period. If you take too much medicine, contact your doctor, hospital emergency department, or poison control center right away.

The ZOMIG Nasal Spray device consists of the following parts:

A. **The Tip:** This is the part that you put into your nostril. The medicine comes out of a tiny hole in the top.

B. **The Protective Cap:** This covers the tip to protect it. Do not remove the protective cap until just before you are ready to take your ZOMIG Nasal Spray.

C. **The Finger-grip:** This is the part that you hold when you use the sprayer.

D. **The Plunger:** This is the part that you press when you put the tip into your nostril. This sprayer works only once. Steps for using ZOMIG Nasal Spray (Please read all steps before using for the first time):

1. Blow your nose gently before use. Remove the protective cap (B) (Figure 1). Hold the nasal sprayer device gently with your fingers and thumb as shown in the picture to the right (Figure 2). There is only one dose in the nasal sprayer. Do not try to prime the nasal sprayer or you will lose the dose. Do not press the plunger until you have put the tip into your nostril or you will lose the dose.

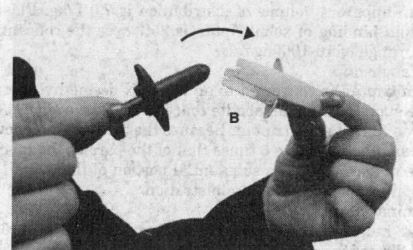

Figure 1

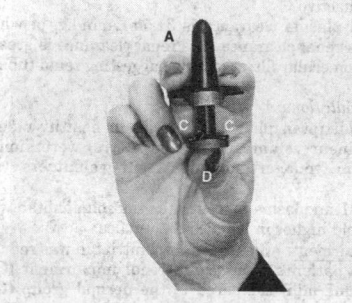

Figure 2

2. Block one nostril by pressing firmly on the side of your nose (Figure 3). Either nostril can be used. Put the tip (A) of the sprayer device into the other nostril as far as feels comfortable and tilt your head slightly as shown in the picture to the right (Figure 4).

Do not press the plunger yet.

Do not spray the contents of the device in your eyes.

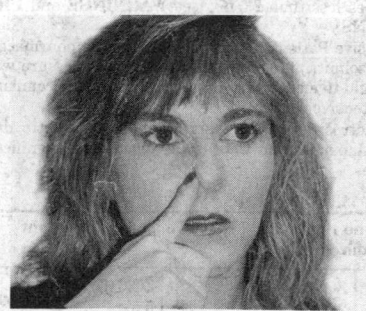

Figure 3

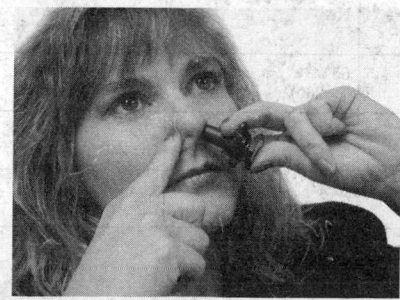

Figure 4

3. Breathe in gently through your nose and at the same time press the plunger (D) firmly with your thumb. The plunger may feel stiff and you may hear a click. Keep your head slightly tilted back and remove the tip from your nose. Breathe gently through your mouth for 5–10 seconds. You may feel liquid in your nose or the back of your throat. This is normal and will soon pass.

What are the possible side effects of ZOMIG Nasal Spray?

ZOMIG Nasal Spray is generally well tolerated. As with any medicine, people taking ZOMIG Nasal Spray may have side effects. The side effects are usually mild and do not last long.

The most common side effects of ZOMIG Nasal Spray are:
- unusual taste, dry mouth
- tingling sensation, skin sensitivity, especially around the nose
- pain, pressure, and tightness sensations (eg, in the nose, throat, or chest)
- drowsiness, weakness, dizziness
- nausea

In very rare cases, patients taking triptans may experience serious side effects, such as heart attacks, high blood pressure, stroke, or serious allergic reactions. Extremely rarely, patients have died. **Call your doctor right away if you have any of the following problems after taking ZOMIG Nasal Spray:**
- **severe tightness, pain, pressure or heaviness in your chest, throat, neck, or jaw**
- **shortness of breath or wheezing**
- **sudden or severe stomach pain**
- **hives; tongue, mouth, or throat swelling**
- **problems seeing**
- **unusual weakness or numbness**

Some people may have a reaction called serotonin syndrome, which can be life-threatening, when they use ZOMIG. In particular, this reaction may occur when they use ZOMIG together with certain types of antidepressants known as SSRIs or SNRIs. Symptoms may include mental changes (hallucinations, agitation, coma), fast heartbeat, changes in blood pressure, high body temperature or sweating, tight muscles, trouble walking, nausea, vomiting, and diarrhea. Call your doctor immediately if you have any of these symptoms after taking ZOMIG.

This is not a complete list of side effects. Talk to your doctor if you develop any symptoms that concern you.

What to do in case of an overdose?

Call your doctor or poison control center or go to the ER.

General advice about ZOMIG Nasal Spray

Medicines are sometimes prescribed for conditions that are not mentioned in patient information leaflets. Do not use ZOMIG Nasal Spray for a condition for which it was not prescribed. Do not give ZOMIG Nasal Spray to other people, even if they have the same symptoms as you. People may be harmed if they take medicines that have not been prescribed for them.

This leaflet summarizes the most important information about ZOMIG Nasal Spray. If you would like more information about ZOMIG Nasal Spray, talk to your doctor. You can ask your doctor or pharmacist for information on ZOMIG Nasal Spray that is written for health professionals. You can also call 1–800–236–9933 or visit our web site at www.ZOMIG.com.

What are the Ingredients in ZOMIG Nasal Spray? Active ingredient: zolmitriptan

Inactive ingredients: anhydrous citric acid, dibasic sodium phosphate, and purified water

Store your medication at controlled room temperature, 20–25°C (68–77°F), and away from children. Discard after use or when it expires.

ZOMIG is a registered trademark of the AstraZeneca group of companies.

Other brands mentioned are trademarks of their respective owners and are not trademarks of the AstraZeneca group of companies. The makers of these brands are not affiliated with AstraZeneca or its products.

©AstraZeneca 2008

Manufactured for:
AstraZeneca Pharmaceuticals LP
Wilmington, Delaware 19850
By: AstraZeneca UK Limited, Macclesfield, Cheshire UK
Made in the United Kingdom

31455-00
Revised: 10/2008   AstraZeneca
308498   8/10

ZOMIG®   ℞
[zō-mĭg]
(zolmitriptan)
TABLETS
ZOMIG-ZMT®
(zolmitriptan)
ORALLY DISINTEGRATING TABLETS
Rx only

DESCRIPTION

ZOMIG® (zolmitriptan) Tablets and ZOMIG-ZMT® (zolmitriptan) Orally Disintegrating Tablets contain zolmitriptan, which is a selective 5-hydroxytryptamine $_{1B/1D}$ (5-HT$_{1B/1D}$) receptor agonist. Zolmitriptan is chemically designated as (S)-4-[[3-[2-(dimethylamino)ethyl]-1H-indol-5-yl]methyl]-2-oxazolidinone and has the following chemical structure:

The empirical formula is $C_{16}H_{21}N_3O_2$, representing a molecular weight of 287.36. Zolmitriptan is a white to almost white powder that is readily soluble in water. ZOMIG Tablets are available as 2.5 mg (yellow) and 5 mg (pink) film coated tablets for oral administration. The film coated tablets contain anhydrous lactose NF, microcrystalline cellulose NF, sodium starch glycolate NF, magnesium stearate NF, hydroxypropyl methylcellulose USP, titanium dioxide USP, polyethylene glycol 400 NF, yellow iron oxide NF (2.5 mg tablet), red iron oxide NF (5 mg tablet), and polyethylene glycol 8000 NF.

ZOMIG-ZMT® Orally Disintegrating Tablets are available as 2.5 mg and 5.0 mg white uncoated tablets for oral administration. The orally disintegrating tablets contain mannitol USP, microcrystalline cellulose NF, crospovidone NF, aspartame NF, sodium bicarbonate USP, citric acid anhydrous USP, colloidal silicon dioxide NF, magnesium stearate NF and orange flavor SN 027512.

CLINICAL PHARMACOLOGY

Mechanism of Action

Zolmitriptan binds with high affinity to human recombinant 5-HT$_{1B}$ and 5-HT$_{1D}$ receptors. Zolmitriptan exhibits modest affinity for 5-HT$_{1A}$ receptors, but has no significant affinity (as measured by radioligand binding assays) or pharmacological activity at 5-HT$_2$, 5-HT$_3$, 5-HT$_4$, alpha$_1$-, alpha$_2$-, or beta$_1$-adrenergic; H$_1$, H$_2$, histaminic; muscarinic; dopamine$_1$, or dopamine$_2$ receptors. The N-desmethyl metabolite also has high affinity for 5-HT$_{1B/1D}$ and modest affinity for 5-HT$_{1A}$ receptors.

Current theories proposed to explain the etiology of migraine headache suggest that symptoms are due to local cranial vasodilatation and/or to the release of sensory neuropeptides (vasoactive intestinal peptide, substance P and calcitonin gene-related peptide) through nerve endings in the trigeminal system. The therapeutic activity of zolmitriptan for the treatment of migraine headache can most likely be attributed to the agonist effects at the 5-HT$_{1B/1D}$ receptors on intracranial blood vessels (including the arterio-venous anastomoses) and sensory nerves of the trigeminal system which result in cranial vessel constriction and inhibition of pro-inflammatory neuropeptide release.

Clinical Pharmacokinetics and Bioavailability

Absorption:
Zolmitriptan is well absorbed after oral administration for both the conventional tablets and the orally disintegrating tablets. Zolmitriptan displays linear kinetics over the dose range of 2.5 to 50 mg.

The AUC and C$_{max}$ of zolmitriptan are similar following administration of ZOMIG Tablets and ZOMIG-ZMT Orally Disintegrating Tablets, but the T$_{max}$ is somewhat later with ZOMIG-ZMT, with a median T$_{max}$ of 3 hours for the orally disintegrating tablet compared with 1.5 hours for the conventional tablet. The AUC, C$_{max}$, and T$_{max}$ for the active N-desmethyl metabolite are similar for the two formulations.

During a moderate to severe migraine attack, mean AUC$_{0-4}$ and C$_{max}$ for zolmitriptan, dosed as a conventional tablet, were decreased by 40% and 25%, respectively, and mean T$_{max}$ was delayed by one-half hour compared to the same patients during a migraine free period.

Food has no significant effect on the bioavailability of zolmitriptan. No accumulation occurred on multiple dosing.

Distribution:
Mean absolute bioavailability is approximately 40%. The mean apparent volume of distribution is 7.0 L/kg. Plasma protein binding of zolmitriptan is 25% over the concentration range of 10-1000ng/mL.

Metabolism:
Zolmitriptan is converted to an active N-desmethyl metabolite such that the metabolite concentrations are about two-thirds that of zolmitriptan. Because the 5HT$_{1B/1D}$ potency of the metabolite is 2 to 6 times that of the parent, the metabolite may contribute a substantial portion of the overall effect after zolmitriptan administration.

Elimination:
Total radioactivity recovered in urine and feces was 65% and 30% of the administered dose, respectively. About 8% of the dose was recovered in the urine as unchanged zolmitriptan. Indole acetic acid metabolite accounted for 31% of the dose, followed by N-oxide (7%) and N-desmethyl (4%) metabolites. The indole acetic acid and N-oxide metabolites are inactive.

Mean total plasma clearance is 31.5mL/min/kg, of which one-sixth is renal clearance. The renal clearance is greater than the glomerular filtration rate suggesting renal tubular secretion.

Special Populations:
Age: Zolmitriptan pharmacokinetics in healthy elderly non-migraineur volunteers (age 65-76 yrs) were similar to those in younger non-migraineur volunteers (age 18-39 yrs).

Gender: Mean plasma concentrations of zolmitriptan were up to 1.5-fold higher in females than males.

Renal Impairment: Clearance of zolmitriptan was reduced by 25% in patients with severe renal impairment (Clcr ≥ 5 ≤ 25 mL/min) compared to the normal group (Clcr ≥ 70 mL/min); no significant change in clearance was observed in the moderately renally impaired group (Clcr ≥ 26 ≤ 50 mL/min).

Hepatic Impairment: In severely hepatically impaired patients, the mean C$_{max}$, T$_{max}$, and AUC$_{0-\infty}$ of zolmitriptan were increased 1.5, 2 (2 vs 4 hr), and 3-fold, respectively, compared to normals. Seven out of 27 patients experienced 20 to 80 mm Hg elevations in systolic and/or diastolic blood pressure after a 10 mg dose. Zolmitriptan should be administered with caution in subjects with liver disease, generally using doses less than 2.5 mg (see WARNINGS and PRECAUTIONS).

Hypertensive Patients: No differences in the pharmacokinetics of zolmitriptan or its effects on blood pressure were seen in mild to moderate hypertensive volunteers compared to normotensive controls.

Race: Retrospective analysis of pharmacokinetic data between Japanese and Caucasians revealed no significant differences.

Drug Interactions:
All drug interaction studies were performed in healthy volunteers using a single 10 mg dose of zolmitriptan and a single dose of the other drug except where otherwise noted.

Fluoxetine: The pharmacokinetics of zolmitriptan, as well as its effect on blood pressure, were unaffected by 4 weeks of pretreatment with oral fluoxetine (20 mg/day).

MAO Inhibitors: Following one week of administration of 150 mg bid moclobemide, a specific MAO-A inhibitor, there was an increase of about 25% in both C$_{max}$ and AUC for zolmitriptan and a 3-fold increase in the C$_{max}$ and AUC of the active N-desmethyl metabolite of zolmitriptan (see CONTRAINDICATIONS and PRECAUTIONS).

Selegiline, a selective MAO-B inhibitor, at a dose of 10 mg/day for 1 week, had no effect on the pharmacokinetics of zolmitriptan and its metabolite.

Propranolol: C$_{max}$ and AUC of zolmitriptan increased 1.5-fold after one week of dosing with propranolol (160 mg/day). C$_{max}$ and AUC of the N-desmethyl metabolite were reduced by 30% and 15%, respectively. There were no interactive effects on blood pressure or pulse rate following administration of propranolol with zolmitriptan.

Acetaminophen: A single 1 g dose of acetaminophen does not alter the pharmacokinetics of zolmitriptan and its N-desmethyl metabolite. However, zolmitriptan delayed the T$_{max}$ of acetaminophen by one hour.

Metoclopramide: A single 10 mg dose of metoclopramide had no effect on the pharmacokinetics of zolmitriptan or its metabolites.

Oral Contraceptives: Retrospective analysis of pharmacokinetic data across studies indicated that mean plasma concentrations of zolmitriptan were generally higher in females taking oral contraceptives compared to those not taking oral contraceptives. Mean C$_{max}$ and AUC of zolmitriptan were found to be higher by 30% and 50%, respectively, and T$_{max}$ was delayed by one-half hour in females taking oral contraceptives. The effect of zolmitriptan on the pharmacokinetics of oral contraceptives has not been studied.

Cimetidine: Following the administration of cimetidine, the half-life and AUC of a 5 mg dose of zolmitriptan and its active metabolite were approximately doubled (see PRECAUTIONS).

Clinical Studies:
The efficacy of ZOMIG Tablets in the acute treatment of migraine headaches was demonstrated in five randomized, double-blind, placebo controlled studies, of which 2 utilized the 1 mg dose, 2 utilized the 2.5 mg dose and 4 utilized the 5 mg dose; all studies used the marketed formulation. In study 1, patients treated their headaches in a clinic setting. In the other studies, patients treated their headaches as outpatients. In study 4, patients who had previously used sumatriptan were excluded, whereas in the other studies no such exclusion was applied. Patients enrolled in these 5 studies were predominantly female (82%) and Caucasian (97%) with a mean age of 40 years (range 12-65). Patients were instructed to treat a moderate to severe headache. Headache response, defined as a reduction in headache severity from moderate or severe pain to mild or no pain, was assessed at 1, 2, and, in most studies, 4 hours after dosing. Associated symptoms such as nausea, photophobia, and phonophobia were also assessed. Maintenance of response was assessed for up to 24 hours postdose. A second dose of ZOMIG Tablets or other medication was allowed 2 to 24 hours after the initial treatment for persistent and recurrent headache. The frequency and time to use of these additional treatments were also recorded. In all studies, the effect of zolmitriptan was compared to placebo in the treatment of a single migraine attack.

In all five studies, the percentage of patients achieving headache response 2 hours after treatment was significantly greater among patients receiving ZOMIG Tablets at all doses (except for the 1 mg dose in the smallest study) compared to those who received placebo. In the two studies that evaluated the 1 mg dose, there was a statistically significant greater percentage of patients with headache response at 2 hours in the higher dose groups (2.5 and/or 5 mg) compared to the 1 mg dose group. There were no statistically significant differences between the 2.5 and 5 mg dose groups (or of doses up to 20 mg) for the primary end point of headache response at 2 hours in any study. The results of these controlled clinical studies are summarized in Table 1.

Comparisons of drug performance based upon results obtained in different clinical trials are never reliable. Because studies are conducted at different times, with different samples of patients, by different investigators, employing different criteria and/or different interpretations of the same criteria, under different conditions (dose, dosing regimen, etc.), quantitative estimates of treatment response and the timing of response may be expected to vary considerably from study to study.

[See table 1 at left]

Table 1: Percentage of Patients with Headache Response (Mild or no Headache) 2 Hours Following Treatment (n=number of patients randomized).

	Placebo	ZOMIG 1.0 mg	ZOMIG 2.5 mg	ZOMIG 5 mg
Study 1*	16% (n=19)	27% (n=22)	NA†	60%‡§ (n=20)
Study 2	19% (n=88)	NA†	NA†	66%‡ (n=179)
Study 3	34% (n=121)	50%‡ (n=140)	65%‡§ (n=260)	67%‡§ (n=245)
Study 4¶	44% (n=55)	NA†	NA†	59%‡ (n=491)
Study 5	36% (n=92)	NA† NA†	62%‡ (n=178)	NA†

* This was the only study in which patients treated the headache in a clinic setting.
† NA - not applicable
‡ p<0.05 in comparison with placebo.
§ p<0.05 in comparison with 1 mg.
¶ This was the only study where patients were excluded who had previously used sumatriptan.

The estimated probability of achieving an initial headache response by 4 hours following treatment is depicted in Figure 1.

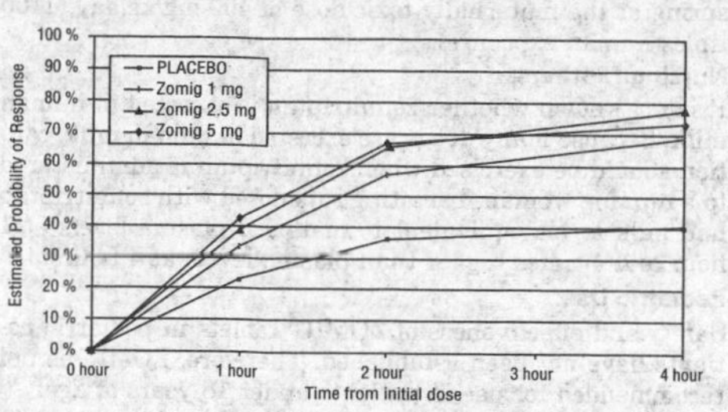

Figure 1: Estimated probability of achieving initial headache response within 4 hours*

*Figure 1 shows the Kaplan-Meier plot of the probability over time of obtaining headache response (no or mild pain) following treatment with zolmitriptan. The averages displayed are based on pooled data from 3 placebo controlled, outpatient trials providing evidence of efficacy (Trials 2, 3 and 5). Patients not achieving headache response or taking additional treatment prior to 4 hours were censored at 4 hours.

For patients with migraine associated photophobia, phonophobia, and nausea at baseline, there was a decreased incidence of these symptoms following administration of ZOMIG as compared to placebo.

Two to 24 hours following the initial dose of study treatment, patients were allowed to use additional treatment for pain relief in the form of a second dose of study treatment or other medication. The estimated probability of patients taking a second dose or other medication for migraine over the 24 hours following the initial dose of study treatment is summarized in Figure 2.

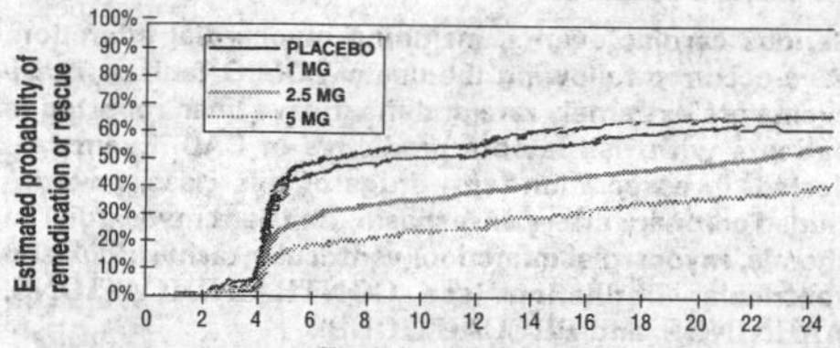

Figure 2: The Estimated Probability Of Patients Taking A Second Dose Or Other Medication For Migraines Over The 24 Hours Following The Initial Dose Of Study Treatment*

*This Kaplan-Meier plot is based on data obtained in 3 placebo controlled clinical trials (Study 2, 3 and 5). Patients not using additional treatments were censored at 24 hours. The plot includes both patients who had headache response at 2 hours and those who had no response to the initial dose. It should be noted that the protocols did not allow remedication within 2 hours postdose.

The efficacy of ZOMIG was unaffected by presence of aura; duration of headache prior to treatment; relationship to menses; gender, age, or weight of the patient; pretreatment nausea, or concomitant use of common migraine prophylactic drugs.

ZOMIG-ZMT Orally Disintegrating Tablets

The efficacy of ZOMIG-ZMT 2.5 mg was demonstrated in a randomized, placebo-controlled trial that was similar in design to the trials of ZOMIG Tablets. Patients were instructed to treat a moderate to severe headache. Of the 471 patients treated in the study, 87% were female and 97% were Caucasian, with a mean age of 41 years (range 18-62). At 2 hours post-dosing response rates in patients treated with ZOMIG-ZMT 2.5 mg were 63% compared to 22% in the placebo group. The difference was statistically significant. The estimated probability of achieving an initial headache response by 2 hours following treatment with ZOMIG-ZMT Tablets is depicted in Figure 3.

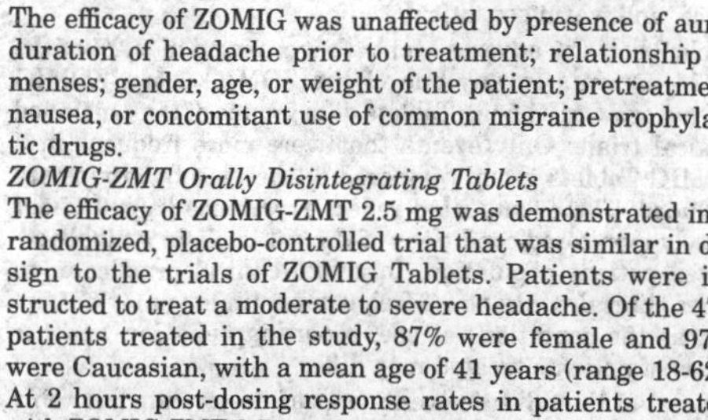

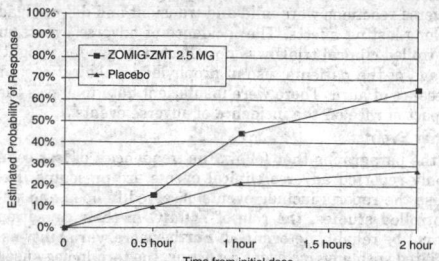

Figure 3: Estimated Probability of Achieving Initial Headache Response by 2 Hours

Figure 3 shows the Kaplan-Meier plot of the probability over time of obtaining headache response (no or mild pain) following treatment with ZOMIG-ZMT Tablets or placebo. Patients taking additional treatment or not achieving headache response prior to 2 hours were censored at 2 hours.

For patients with migraine-associated photophobia, phonophobia and nausea at baseline, there was a decreased incidence of these symptoms following administration of ZOMIG-ZMT as compared to placebo.

Two to 24 hours following the initial dose of study treatment, patients were allowed to use additional treatment in the form of a second dose of study treatment or other medication. The estimated probability of patients taking a second dose or other medication for migraine over the 24 hours following the initial dose of study treatment is summarized in Figure 4.

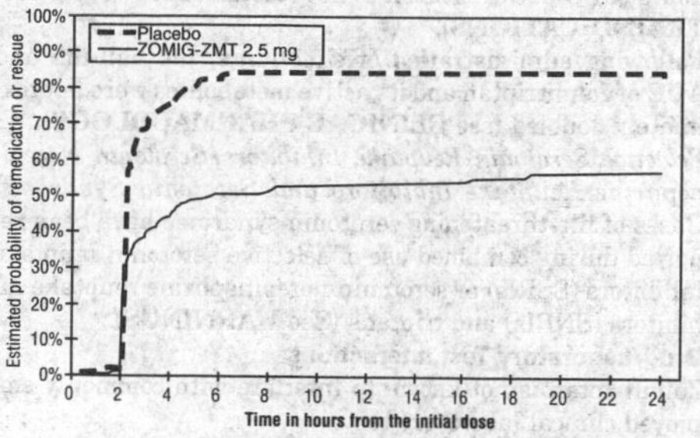

Figure 4: The Estimated Probability of Patients Taking a Second Dose or Other Medication for Migraines Over the 24 Hours Following The Initial Dose of Study Treatment

In this Kaplan-Meier plot, patients not using additional treatments were censored at 24 hours. The plot includes both patients who had headache response at 2 hours and those who had no response to the initial dose. Remedication was allowed 2 hours post-dose, and unlike the conventional tablet, remedication prior to 4 hours was not discouraged.

INDICATIONS AND USAGE

ZOMIG is indicated for the acute treatment of migraine with or without aura in adults.

ZOMIG should only be used where a clear diagnosis of migraine has been established.

ZOMIG is not intended for the prophylactic therapy of migraine or for use in the management of hemiplegic or basilar migraine (see **CONTRAINDICATIONS**). Safety and effectiveness of ZOMIG have not been established for cluster headache, which is present in an older, predominantly male population.

CONTRAINDICATIONS

ZOMIG should not be given to patients with ischemic heart disease (angina pectoris, history of myocardial infarction, or documented silent ischemia) or to patients who have symptoms or findings consistent with ischemic heart disease, coronary artery vasospasm, including Prinzmetal's variant angina, or other significant underlying cardiovascular disease (see WARNINGS and PRECAUTIONS).

ZOMIG should not be given to patients with cerebrovascular syndromes including (but not limited to) stroke of any type as well as transient ischemic attacks (see WARNINGS).

ZOMIG should not be given to patients with peripheral vascular disease including (but not limited to) ischemic bowel disease (see WARNINGS and PRECAUTIONS).

Because ZOMIG may increase blood pressure, it should not be given to patients with uncontrolled hypertension (see WARNINGS).

ZOMIG should not be used within 24 hours of treatment with another 5-HT$_1$ agonist, or an ergotamine-containing or ergot-type medication like dihydroergotamine or methysergide.

ZOMIG should not be administered to patients with hemiplegic or basilar migraine.

Concurrent administration of MAO-A inhibitors or use of zolmitriptan within 2 weeks of discontinuation of MAO-A inhibitor therapy is contraindicated (see CLINICAL PHARMACOLOGY: Drug Interactions and PRECAUTIONS: Drug Interactions).

ZOMIG is contraindicated in patients who are hypersensitive to zolmitriptan or any of its inactive ingredients.

WARNINGS

Risk of Myocardial Ischemia and/or Infarction and Other Adverse Cardiac Events: ZOMIG should not be given to patients with documented ischemic or vasospastic coronary artery disease (see CONTRAINDICATIONS). It is strongly recommended that zolmitriptan not be given to patients in whom unrecognized coronary artery disease (CAD) is predicted by the presence of risk factors (e.g., hypertension, hypercholesterolemia, smoker, obesity, diabetes, strong family history of CAD, female with surgical or physiological menopause, or male over 40 years of age) unless a cardiovascular evaluation provides satisfactory clinical evidence that the patient is reasonably free of coronary artery and ischemic myocardial disease or other significant underlying cardiovascular disease. The sensitivity of cardiac diagnostic procedures to detect cardiovascular disease or predisposition to coronary artery vasospasm is modest, at best. If, during the cardiovascular evaluation, the patient's medical history, electrocardiographic or other investigations reveal findings indicative of, or consistent with, coronary artery vasospasm or myocardial ischemia, zolmitriptan should not be administered (see CONTRAINDICATIONS). For patients with risk factors predictive of CAD, who are determined to have a satisfactory cardiovascular evaluation, it is strongly recommended that administration of the first dose of zolmitriptan take place in the setting of a physician's office or similar medically staffed and equipped facility unless the patient has previously received zolmitriptan. Because cardiac ischemia can occur in the absence of clinical symptoms, consideration should be given to obtaining on the first occasion of use an electrocardiogram (ECG) during the interval immediately following ZOMIG, in these patients with risk factors.

It is recommended that patients who are intermittent long-term users of ZOMIG and who have or acquire risk factors predictive of CAD, as described above, undergo periodic interval cardiovascular evaluation as they continue to use ZOMIG.

The systematic approach described above is intended to reduce the likelihood that patients with unrecognized cardiovascular disease will be inadvertently exposed to zolmitriptan.

Cardiac Events and Fatalities:

Serious adverse cardiac events, including acute myocardial infarction, have been reported within a few hours following administration of zolmitriptan. Life-threatening disturbances of cardiac rhythm, and death have been reported within a few hours following the administration of other 5-HT$_1$ agonists. Considering the extent of use of 5-HT$_1$ agonists in patients with migraine, the incidence of these events is extremely low.

ZOMIG can cause coronary vasospasm; at least one of these events occurred in a patient with no cardiac disease history and with documented absence of coronary artery disease. Because of the close proximity of the events to ZOMIG use, a causal relationship cannot be excluded. In the cases where there has been known underlying coronary artery disease, the relationship is uncertain.

Patients with symptomatic Wolff-Parkinson-White syndrome or arrhythmias associated with other cardiac accessory conduction pathway disorders should not receive ZOMIG.

Premarketing experience with zolmitriptan:

Among the more than 2,500 patients with migraine who participated in premarketing controlled clinical trials of ZOMIG Tablets, no deaths or serious cardiac events were reported.

Postmarketing experience with zolmitriptan:

Serious cardiovascular events have been reported in association with the use of ZOMIG Tablets, and in very rare cases, these events have occurred in the absence of known cardiovascular disease. The uncontrolled nature of postmarketing surveillance, however, makes it impossible to determine definitively the proportion of the reported cases that were actually caused by zolmitriptan or to reliably assess causation in individual cases.

Cerebrovascular Events and Fatalities with 5-HT$_1$ agonists:

Cerebral hemorrhage, subarachnoid hemorrhage, stroke, and other cerebrovascular events have been reported in patients treated with 5-HT$_1$ agonists; and some have resulted in fatalities. In a number of cases, it appears possible that the cerebrovascular events were primary, the agonist having been administered in the incorrect belief that the symptoms experienced were a consequence of migraine, when they were not. It should be noted that patients with migraine may be at increased risk of certain cerebrovascular events (e.g., stroke, hemorrhage, transient ischemic attack). (See **CONTRAINDICATIONS.**)

Serotonin Syndrome:

The development of a potentially life-threatening serotonin syndrome may occur with triptans, including ZOMIG treatment, particularly during combined use with selective serotonin reuptake inhibitors (SSRIs) or serotonin norepinephrine reuptake inhibitors (SNRIs). If concomitant treatment with ZOMIG and an SSRI (e.g. fluoxetine, paroxetine, sertraline, fluvoxamine, citalopram, escitalopram) or SNRI (e.g., venlafaxine, duloxetine) is clinically warranted, careful observation of the patient is advised, particularly during treatment initiation and dose increases. Serotonin syndrome symptoms may include mental status changes (e.g., agitation, hallucinations, coma), autonomic instability (e.g., tachycardia, labile blood pressure, hyperthermia), neuromuscular aberrations (e.g. hyperreflexia, incoordination) and/or gastrointestinal symptoms (e.g. nausea, vomiting, diarrhea). (See **PRECAUTIONS, Drug Interactions**).

Other Vasospasm-Related Events:

5-HT$_1$ agonists may cause vasospastic reactions other than coronary artery vasospasm such as peripheral and gastro-

intestinal vascular ischemia. As with other serotonin $5HT_1$ agonists, very rare gastrointestinal ischemic events including ischemic colitis and gastrointestinal infarction or necrosis have been reported with ZOMIG Tablets; these may present as bloody diarrhea or abdominal pain. (See **CONTRAINDICATIONS**.)

Very rare reports of transient and permanent blindness and significant partial vision loss have been reported with the use of $5-HT_1$ agonists. Visual disorders may also be part of a migraine attack.

Increase in Blood Pressure:
As with other $5-HT_1$ agonists, significant elevations in systemic blood pressure have been reported on rare occasions with ZOMIG Tablet use, in patients with and without a history of hypertension; very rarely these increases in blood pressure have been associated with significant clinical events. Zolmitriptan is contraindicated in patients with uncontrolled hypertension. In volunteers, an increase of 1 and 5 mm Hg in the systolic and diastolic blood pressure, respectively, was seen at 5 mg. In the headache trials, vital signs were measured only in the small inpatient study and no effect on blood pressure was seen. In a study of patients with moderate to severe liver disease, 7 of 27 experienced 20 to 80 mm Hg elevations in systolic and/or diastolic blood pressure after a dose of 10 mg of zolmitriptan (see **CONTRAINDICATIONS**).

An 18% increase in mean pulmonary artery pressure was seen following dosing with another $5-HT_1$ agonist in a study evaluating subjects undergoing cardiac catheterization.

PRECAUTIONS
General:
As with other $5-HT_{1B/1D}$ agonists, sensations of tightness, pain, pressure, and heaviness have been reported after treatment with ZOMIG Tablets in the precordium, throat, neck, and jaw. Because zolmitriptan may cause coronary artery vasospasm, patients who experience signs or symptoms suggestive of angina following dosing should be evaluated for the presence of CAD or a predisposition to Prinzmetal's variant angina before receiving additional doses of medication, and should be monitored electrocardiographically if dosing is resumed and similar symptoms recur. Similarly, patients who experience other symptoms or signs suggestive of decreased arterial flow, such as ischemic bowel syndrome or Raynaud's syndrome following the use of any $5-HT_1$ agonist are candidates for further evaluation. (see **CONTRAINDICATIONS** and **WARNINGS**.)

Zolmitriptan should also be administered with caution to patients with diseases that may alter the absorption, metabolism, or excretion of drugs, such as impaired hepatic function (see **CLINICAL PHARMACOLOGY**).

For a given attack, if a patient does not respond to the first dose of zolmitriptan, the diagnosis of migraine headache should be reconsidered before administration of a second dose.

Binding to Melanin-Containing Tissues:
When pigmented rats were given a single oral dose of 10 mg/kg of radiolabeled zolmitriptan, the radioactivity in the eye after 7 days, the latest time point examined, was still 75% of the value measured after 4 hours. This suggests that zolmitriptan and/or its metabolites may bind to the melanin of the eye. Because there could be accumulation in melanin rich tissues over time, this raises the possibility that zolmitriptan could cause toxicity in these tissues after extended use. However, no effects on the retina related to treatment with zolmitriptan were noted in any of the toxicity studies. Although no systematic monitoring of ophthalmologic function was undertaken in clinical trials, and no specific recommendations for ophthalmologic monitoring are offered, prescribers should be aware of the possibility of long-term ophthalmologic effects.

Phenylketonurics:
Phenylketonuric patients should be informed that ZOMIG-ZMT contain phenylalanine (a component of aspartame). Each 2.5 mg orally disintegrating tablet contains 2.81 mg phenylalanine. Each 5 mg orally disintegrating tablet contains 5.62 mg phenylalanine.

Information for Patients
See **PATIENT INFORMATION** at the end of this labeling for the text of the separate leaflet provided for patients.
ZOMIG-ZMT Orally Disintegrating Tablets
The orally disintegrating tablet is packaged in a blister. Patients should be instructed not to remove the tablet from the blister until just prior to dosing. The blister pack should then be peeled open, and the orally disintegrating tablet placed on the tongue, where it will dissolve and be swallowed with the saliva.

Patients should be cautioned about the risk of serotonin syndrome with the use of ZOMIG or other triptans, especially during combined use with selective serotonin reuptake inhibitors (SSRIs) or serotonin norepinephrine reuptake inhibitors (SNRIs).

Laboratory Tests:
No monitoring of specific laboratory tests is recommended.
Drug Interactions
Ergot-containing drugs have been reported to cause prolonged vasospastic reactions. Because there is a theoretical basis that these effects may be additive, use of ergotamine-containing or ergot-type medications (like dihydroergotamine or methysergide) and zolmitriptan within 24 hours of each other should be avoided (see **CONTRAINDICATIONS**).

MAO-A inhibitors increase the systemic exposure of zolmitriptan. Therefore, the use of zolmitriptan in patients receiving MAO-A inhibitors is contraindicated (see **CLINICAL PHARMACOLOGY** and **CONTRAINDICATIONS**). Concomitant use of other $5-HT_{1B/1D}$ agonists within 24 hours of ZOMIG treatment is not recommended. (see **CONTRAINDICATIONS**).

Following administration of cimetidine, the half-life and AUC of zolmitriptan and its active metabolites were approximately doubled (see **CLINICAL PHARMACOLOGY**).

Selective Serotonin Reuptake Inhibitors / Serotonin Norepinephrine Reuptake Inhibitors and Serotonin Syndrome: Cases of life-threatening serotonin syndrome have been reported during combined use of selective serotonin reuptake inhibitors (SSRIs) or serotonin norepinephrine reuptake inhibitors (SNRIs) and triptans (See **WARNINGS**).

Drug/Laboratory Test Interactions:
Zolmitriptan is not known to interfere with commonly employed clinical laboratory tests.

Carcinogenesis, Mutagenesis, Impairment of Fertility:
Carcinogenesis:
Carcinogenicity studies by oral gavage were carried out in mice and rats at doses up to 400 mg/kg/day. Mice were dosed for 85 weeks (males) and 92 weeks (females). The exposure (plasma AUC of parent drug) at the highest dose level was approximately 800 times that seen in humans after a single 10 mg dose (the maximum recommended total daily dose). There was no effect of zolmitriptan on tumor incidence. Control, low dose, and middle dose rats were dosed for 104-105 weeks; the high dose group was sacrificed after 101 weeks (males) and 86 weeks (females) due to excess mortality. Aside from an increase in the incidence of thyroid follicular cell hyperplasia and thyroid follicular cell adenomas seen in male rats receiving 400 mg/kg/day, an exposure approximately 3000 times that seen in humans after dosing with 10 mg, no tumors were noted.

Mutagenesis:
Zolmitriptan was mutagenic in an Ames test, in 2 of 5 strains of *S. typhimurium* tested, in the presence of, but not in the absence of, metabolic activation. It was not mutagenic in an *in vitro* mammalian gene cell mutation (CHO/HGPRT) assay. Zolmitriptan was clastogenic in an *in vitro* human lymphocyte assay both in the absence of and the presence of metabolic activation; it was not clastogenic in an *in vivo* mouse micronucleus assay. It was also not genotoxic in an unscheduled DNA synthesis study.

Impairment of Fertility:
Studies of male and female rats administered zolmitriptan prior to and during mating and up to implantation have shown no impairment of fertility at doses up to 400 mg/kg/day. Exposure at this dose was approximately 3000 times exposure at the maximum recommended human dose of 10 mg/day.

Pregnancy:
Pregnancy Category C:
There are no adequate and well controlled studies in pregnant women; therefore, zolmitriptan should be used during pregnancy only if the potential benefit justifies the potential risk to the fetus.

In reproductive toxicity studies in rats and rabbits, oral administration of zolmitriptan to pregnant animals was associated with embryolethality and fetal abnormalities. When pregnant rats were administered oral zolmitriptan during the period of organogenesis at doses of 100, 400, and 1200 mg/kg/day, there was a dose-related increase in embryolethality which became statistically significant at the high dose. The maternal plasma exposures at these doses were approximately 280, 1100, and 5000 times the exposure in humans receiving the maximum recommended total daily dose of 10 mg. The high dose was maternally toxic, as evidenced by a decreased maternal body weight gain during gestation. In a similar study in rabbits, embryolethality was increased at the maternally toxic doses of 10 and 30 mg/kg/day (maternal plasma exposures equivalent to 11 and 42 times exposure in humans receiving the maximum recommended total daily dose of 10 mg), and increased incidences of fetal malformations (fused sternebrae, rib anomalies) and variations (major blood vessel variations, irregular ossification pattern of ribs) were observed at 30 mg/kg/day. Three mg/kg/day was a no effect dose (equivalent to human

exposure at a dose of 10 mg). When female rats were given zolmitriptan during gestation, parturition, and lactation, an increased incidence of hydronephrosis was found in the offspring at the maternally toxic dose of 400 mg/kg/day (1100 times human exposure).

Nursing Mothers:
It is not known whether zolmitriptan is excreted in human milk. Because many drugs are excreted in human milk, caution should be exercised when zolmitriptan is administered to a nursing woman. Lactating rats dosed with zolmitriptan had milk levels equivalent to maternal plasma levels at 1 hour and 4 times higher than plasma levels at 4 hours.

Pediatric Use:
Safety and effectiveness of ZOMIG Tablets in pediatric patients have not been established. Therefore, ZOMIG is not recommended for use in patients under 18 years of age.

One randomized, placebo-controlled clinical trial evaluating zolmitriptan tablets (2.5, 5 and 10 mg) in pediatric patients aged 12-17 years evaluated a total of 696 adolescent migraineurs. This study did not establish the efficacy of zolmitriptan compared to placebo in the treatment of migraine in adolescents. Adverse events observed were similar in nature and frequency to those reported in clinical trials in adults.

Postmarketing experience with ZOMIG and other triptans includes a limited number of reports that describe pediatric patients who have experienced clinically serious adverse events that are similar in nature to those reported rarely in adults.

Geriatric Use:
Although the pharmacokinetic disposition of the drug in the elderly is similar to that seen in younger adults, there is no information about the safety and effectiveness of zolmitriptan in this population because patients over age 65 were excluded from the controlled clinical trials. (see **CLINICAL PHARMACOLOGY: Special Populations**)

ADVERSE REACTIONS

Serious cardiac events, including myocardial infarction, have occurred following the use of ZOMIG Tablets. These events are extremely rare and most have been reported in patients with risk factors predictive of CAD. Events reported, in association with drugs of this class, have included coronary artery vasospasm, transient myocardial ischemia, myocardial infarction, ventricular tachycardia, and ventricular fibrillation (see CONTRAINDICATIONS, WARNINGS, and PRECAUTIONS).

Incidence in Controlled Clinical Trials:
Among 2,633 patients treated with ZOMIG Tablets in the active and placebo controlled trials, no patients withdrew for reasons related to adverse events, but as patients treated a single headache in these trials, the opportunity for discontinuation was limited. In a long-term, open label study where patients were allowed to treat multiple migraine attacks for up to 1 year, 8% (167 out of 2,058) withdrew from the trial because of adverse experience. The most common events were paresthesia, asthenia, nausea, dizziness, pain, chest or neck tightness or heaviness, somnolence, and warm sensation.

Table 2 lists the adverse events that occurred in ≥ 2% of the 2,074 patients in any one of the ZOMIG 1 mg, ZOMIG 2.5 mg or ZOMIG 5 mg Tablets dose groups of the controlled clinical trials. Only events that were more frequent in a ZOMIG Tablets group compared to the placebo groups are included. The events cited reflect experience gained under closely monitored conditions of clinical trials in a highly selected patient population. In actual clinical practice or in other clinical trials, these frequency estimates may not apply, as the conditions of use, reporting behavior, and the kinds of patients treated may differ.

Several of the adverse events appear dose related, notably paresthesia, sensation of heaviness or tightness in chest, neck, jaw, and throat, dizziness, somnolence, and possibly asthenia and nausea.

[See table 2 at top of next page]

ZOMIG is generally well tolerated. Across all doses, most adverse reactions were mild and transient and did not lead to long-lasting effects. The incidence of adverse events in controlled clinical trials was not affected by gender, weight, or age of the patients; use of prophylactic medications; or presence of aura. There were insufficient data to assess the impact of race on the incidence of adverse events.

Other Events:
In the paragraphs that follow, the frequencies of less commonly reported adverse clinical events are presented. Because the reports include events observed in open and uncontrolled studies, the role of ZOMIG in their causation cannot be reliably determined. Furthermore, variability associated with adverse event reporting, the terminology used to describe adverse events, etc., limit the value of the quantitative frequency estimates provided. Event frequencies are calculated as the number of patients who used ZOMIG

Tablets (n=4,027) and reported an event divided by the total number of patients exposed to ZOMIG Tablets. All reported events are included except those already listed in the previous table, those too general to be informative, and those not reasonably associated with the use of the drug. Events are further classified within body system categories and enumerated in order of decreasing frequency using the following definitions: infrequent adverse events are those occurring in 1/100 to 1/1,000 patients and rare adverse events are those occurring in fewer than 1/1,000 patients.

Atypical sensations: Infrequent was hyperesthesia.

General: Infrequent were allergy reaction, chills, facial edema, fever, malaise, and photosensitivity.

Cardiovascular: Infrequent were arrhythmias, hypertension, and syncope. Rare were bradycardia, extrasystoles, postural hypotension, QT prolongation, tachycardia, and thrombophlebitis.

Digestive: Infrequent were increased appetite, tongue edema, esophagitis, gastroenteritis, liver function abnormality, and thirst. Rare were anorexia, constipation, gastritis, hematemesis, pancreatitis, melena, and ulcer.

Hemic: Infrequent was ecchymosis. Rare were cyanosis, thrombocytopenia, eosinophilia, and leukopenia.

Metabolic: Infrequent was edema. Rare were hyperglycemia and alkaline phosphatase increased.

Musculoskeletal: Infrequent were back pain, leg cramps, and tenosynovitis. Rare were arthritis, asthenia, tetany, and twitching.

Neurological: Infrequent were agitation, anxiety, depression, emotional lability, and insomnia. Rare were akathisia, amnesia, apathy, ataxia, dystonia, euphoria, hallucinations, cerebral ischemia, hyperkinesia, hypotonia, hypertonia, and irritability.

Respiratory: Infrequent were bronchitis, bronchospasm, epistaxis, hiccup, laryngitis, and yawn. Rare were apnea and voice alteration.

Skin: Infrequent were pruritus, rash, and urticaria.

Special Senses: Infrequent were dry eye, eye pain, hyperacusis, ear pain, parosmia, and tinnitus. Rare were diplopia and lacrimation.

Urogenital: Infrequent were hematuria, cystitis, polyuria, urinary frequency, urinary urgency. Rare were miscarriage and dysmenorrhea.

The adverse experiences profile seen with ZOMIG-ZMT Tablets was similar to that seen with ZOMIG Tablets.

Postmarketing Experience with ZOMIG Tablets:
The following section enumerates potentially important adverse events that have occurred in clinical practice and which have been reported spontaneously to various surveillance systems. The events enumerated represent reports arising from both domestic and non-domestic use of oral zolmitriptan. The events enumerated include all except those already listed in the **ADVERSE REACTIONS** section above or those too general to be informative. Because the reports cite events reported spontaneously from worldwide postmarketing experience, frequency of events and the role of zolmitriptan in their causation cannot be reliably determined.

Cardiovascular:
Coronary artery vasospasm; transient myocardial ischemia, angina pectoris, and myocardial infarction.

Digestive:
Very rare gastrointestinal ischemic events including splenic infarction, ischemic colitis and gastrointestinal infarction or necrosis have been reported; these may present as bloody diarrhea or abdominal pain. (See **WARNINGS**.)

Neurological:
As with other acute migraine treatments including other 5HT₁ agonists, there have been rare reports of headache.

General:
As with other 5-HT_{1B/1D} agonists, there have been very rare reports of anaphylaxis or anaphylactoid reactions in patients receiving ZOMIG. There have been rare reports of hypersensitivity reactions, including angioedema.
Serotonin syndrome has also been reported during the postmarketing period (see **WARNINGS** and **PRECAUTIONS**).

DRUG ABUSE AND DEPENDENCE
The abuse potential of ZOMIG has not been assessed in clinical trials.

OVERDOSAGE
There is no experience with clinical overdose. Volunteers receiving single 50 mg oral doses of zolmitriptan commonly experienced sedation.

The elimination half-life of ZOMIG is 3 hours (see **CLINICAL PHARMACOLOGY**), and therefore monitoring of patients after overdose with ZOMIG should continue for at least 15 hours or while symptoms or signs persist.

There is no specific antidote to zolmitriptan. In cases of severe intoxication, intensive care procedures are recommended, including establishing and maintaining a patent

Table 2: Adverse Experience Incidence in Five Placebo-Controlled Migraine Clinical Trials: Events Reported By ≥ 2% Patients Treated With ZOMIG Tablets

Adverse Event Type	Placebo (n=401)	ZOMIG 1 mg (n=163)	ZOMIG 2.5 mg (n=498)	ZOMIG 5 mg (n=1012)
ATYPICAL SENSATIONS	**6%**	**12%**	**12%**	**18%**
Hypesthesia	1%	1%	1%	2%
Paresthesia (all types)	2%	5%	7%	9%
Sensation warm/cold	4%	6%	5%	7%
PAIN AND PRESSURE SENSATIONS	**7%**	**13%**	**14%**	**22%**
Chest - pain/tightness/pressure and/or heaviness	1%	2%	3%	4%
Neck/throat/jaw - pain/tightness/pressure	3%	4%	7%	10%
Heaviness other than chest or neck	1%	1%	2%	5%
Pain – location specified	1%	2%	2%	3%
Other – Pressure/tightness/heaviness	0%	2%	2%	2%
DIGESTIVE	**8%**	**11%**	**16%**	**14%**
Dry mouth	2%	5%	3%	3%
Dyspepsia	1%	3%	2%	1%
Dysphagia	0%	0%	0%	2%
Nausea	4%	4%	9%	6%
NEUROLOGICAL	**10%**	**11%**	**17%**	**21%**
Dizziness	4%	6%	8%	10%
Somnolence	3%	5%	6%	8%
Vertigo	0%	0%	0%	2%
OTHER				
Asthenia	3%	5%	3%	9%
Palpitations	1%	0%	<1%	2%
Myalgia	<1%	1%	1%	2%
Myasthenia	<1%	0%	1%	2%
Sweating	1%	0%	2%	3%

airway, ensuring adequate oxygenation and ventilation, and monitoring and support of the cardiovascular system.
It is unknown what effect hemodialysis or peritoneal dialysis has on the plasma concentrations of zolmitriptan.

DOSAGE AND ADMINISTRATION
ZOMIG Tablets
In controlled clinical trials, single doses of 1, 2.5 and 5 mg of ZOMIG Tablets were effective for the acute treatment of migraines in adults. A greater proportion of patients had headache response following a 2.5 or 5 mg dose than following a 1 mg dose (see Table 1). In the only direct comparison of 2.5 and 5 mg, there was little added benefit from the larger dose but side effects are generally increased at 5 mg (see Table 2). Patients should, therefore, be started on 2.5 mg or lower. A dose lower than 2.5 mg can be achieved by manually breaking the scored 2.5 mg tablet in half.
If the headache returns, the dose may be repeated after 2 hours, not to exceed 10 mg within a 24-hour period. Controlled trials have not adequately established the effectiveness of a second dose if the initial dose is ineffective.
The safety of treating an average of more than three headaches in a 30-day period has not been established.
ZOMIG-ZMT Orally Disintegrating Tablets
In a controlled clinical trial, a single dose of 2.5 mg of ZOMIG-ZMT Tablets was effective for the acute treatment of migraines in adults.
If the headache returns, the dose may be repeated after 2 hours, not to exceed 10 mg within a 24-hour period. Controlled trials have not adequately established the effectiveness of a second dose if the initial dose is ineffective.
The safety of treating an average of more than three headaches in a 30-day period has not been established.
Administration with liquid is not necessary. The orally disintegrating tablet is packaged in a blister. Patients

should be instructed not to remove the tablet from the blister until just prior to dosing. The blister pack should then be peeled open, and the orally disintegrating tablet placed on the tongue, where it will dissolve and be swallowed with the saliva. It is not recommended to break the orally disintegrating tablet.
Hepatic Impairment:
Patients with moderate to severe hepatic impairment have decreased clearance of zolmitriptan and significant elevation in blood pressure was observed in some patients. Use of a low dose with blood pressure monitoring is recommended (see **CLINICAL PHARMACOLOGY** AND **WARNINGS**).

HOW SUPPLIED
2.5 mg Tablets—Yellow, biconvex, round film-coated, scored tablets containing 2.5 mg of zolmitriptan identified with "ZOMIG" and "2.5" debossed on one side are supplied in cartons containing a blister pack of 6 tablets (NDC 0310-0210-20).
2.5 mg Orally Disintegrating Tablets—White, flat faced, uncoated, bevelled tablet containing 2.5 mg of zolmitriptan identified with a debossed "Z" on one side are supplied in cartons containing a blister pack of 6 tablets (NDC 0310-0209-20).
5 mg Tablets—Pink, biconvex, film-coated tablets containing 5 mg of zolmitriptan identified with "ZOMIG" and "5" debossed on one side are supplied in cartons containing a blister pack of 3 tablets (NDC 0310-0211-25).
5 mg Orally Disintegrating Tablets—White, flat faced, round, uncoated, bevelled tablet containing 5.0 mg of zolmitriptan identified with a debossed "Z" and "5" on one side and plain on the other are supplied in cartons containing a blister pack of 3 tablets (NDC 0310-0213-21).
Store both ZOMIG Tablets and ZOMIG-ZMT Tablets at controlled room temperature, 20-25°C (68-77°F) [see USP].
Protect from light and moisture.

PATIENT INFORMATION

The following wording is contained in a separate leaflet provided for patients.

ZOMIG® (zolmitriptan) Tablets

ZOMIG-ZMT® (zolmitriptan) Orally Disintegrating Tablets

Patient Information about ZOMIG (Zo-mig) for Migraines

Generic Name: zolmitriptan (zol-mi-trip-tan)

Information for the Consumer on ZOMIG (zolmitriptan) Tablets:

Please read this leaflet carefully before you take ZOMIG Tablets. This provides a summary of the information available on your medicine. Please do not throw away this leaflet until you have finished your medicine. You may need to read this leaflet again. This leaflet does not contain all the information on ZOMIG Tablets. For further information or advice, ask your doctor or pharmacist.

Information About Your Medicine:

The name of your medicine is ZOMIG Tablets. It can be obtained only by prescription from your doctor. The decision to use ZOMIG Tablets is one that you and your doctor should make jointly, taking into account your individual preferences and medical circumstances. If you have risk factors for heart disease (such as high blood pressure, high cholesterol, obesity, diabetes, smoking, strong family history of heart disease, or you are postmenopausal or a male over the age of 40), you should tell your doctor, who should evaluate you for heart disease in order to determine if ZOMIG Tablets are appropriate for you. This medicine was prescribed for you to treat your particular condition and should not be used by others or for any other condition.

1. **The Purpose of Your Medicine:** ZOMIG Tablets are intended to relieve your migraine, but not to prevent or reduce the number of attacks you experience. Use ZOMIG Tablets only to treat an actual migraine attack.
2. **Important Questions to Consider Before Taking ZOMIG Tablets:** If the answer to any of the following questions is **YES** or if you do not know the answer, then you must discuss it with your doctor before you use ZOMIG Tablets.
   - Do you have any chest pain, heart disease, shortness of breath, or irregular heartbeats? Have you had a heart attack?
   - Do you have risk factors for heart disease (such as high blood pressure, high cholesterol, obesity, diabetes, smoking, strong family history of heart disease, or you are postmenopausal or a male over the age of 40)?
   - Have you had a stroke or problems with your blood circulation?
   - Do you have high blood pressure?
   - Are you pregnant? Do you think you might be pregnant? Are you trying to become pregnant? Are you not using adequate contraception? Are you breast feeding an infant?
   - If you are taking ZOMIG-ZMT®, are you sensitive to phenylalanine (a component of the artificial sweetener aspartame)?
   - Have you ever had to stop taking this or any other medication because of an allergy or other problems?
   - Are you taking any other migraine medications, including 5-HT_1 agonists (triptans) or migraine medications containing ergotamine, dihydroergotamine, or methysergide?
   - Are you taking selective serotonin reuptake inhibitors (SSRIs) or serotonin norepinephrine reuptake inhibitors (SNRIs), two types of drugs for depression or other disorders? Common SSRIs are CELEXA® (citalopram HBr), LEXAPRO® (escitalopram oxalate), PAXIL® (paroxetine), PROZAC® (fluoxetine), SYMBYAX® (olanzapine/fluoxetine), ZOLOFT® (sertraline), SARAFEM® (fluoxetine), and LUVOX® (fluvoxamine). Common SNRIs are CYMBALTA® (duloxetine) and EFFEXOR® (venlafaxine).
   - Are you taking cimetidine for gastrointestinal symptoms?
   - Have you had, or do you have, any disease of the liver or kidney?
   - Have you had, or do you have, epilepsy or seizures?
   - Is this headache different from your usual migraine attacks?

   Remember, if you answered **YES** to any of the above questions, then you must discuss it with your doctor.
3. **The Use of ZOMIG Tablets During Pregnancy:** Do not use ZOMIG Tablets if you are pregnant, think you might be pregnant, are trying to become pregnant, or are not using adequate contraception, unless you have discussed this with your doctor.
4. **How to Use ZOMIG Tablets and ZOMIG-ZMT Orally Disintegrating Tablets:** Adults should be started on a 2.5 mg dose or lower administered by mouth. A dose lower than 2.5 mg can be achieved by manually breaking the conventional film-coated, scored 2.5 mg tablet in half. It is not recommended to break the ZOMIG-ZMT Tablet. If your headache comes back after your initial dose, a second dose may be administered anytime after 2 hours of taking the dose. For any attack where you have no response to the first dose, do not take a second dose without first consulting with your doctor. Do not take more than a total of 10 mg of ZOMIG in any 24-hour period. Discard any unused tablets or its portion that have been removed from the blister packaging. Do not take ZOMIG with any other drug in the same class (triptans) within 24 hours or within 24 hours of taking ergotamine-type medications such as ergotamine, dihydroergotamine or methysergide to treat your migraine.
   Additionally for ZOMIG-ZMT Tablets, the blister pack should be peeled open and the orally disintegrating tablet placed on the tongue, where it will dissolve and be swallowed with the saliva.
5. **Side Effects to Watch for:**
   - Some patients experience pain or tightness in the chest or throat, including muscle aches and pains, when using ZOMIG. If this happens to you, then discuss it with your doctor before using any more ZOMIG. If the chest pain is severe or does not go away, call your doctor immediately. As with other drugs in this class (triptans), there have been very rare reports of heart attack occurring in patients with and without risk factors for heart and blood vessel disease.
   - Some people experience: alterations of heart rate; temporary increase in blood pressure; sudden and severe stomach pain. Call your doctor immediately if you have any of these symptoms after taking ZOMIG.
   - Shortness of breath; wheeziness; heart throbbing; swelling of eyelids, face, or lips; or a skin rash, skin lumps, or hives happens rarely. If it happens to you, then tell your doctor immediately. Do not take any more ZOMIG unless your doctor tells you to do so.
   - Some people may have feelings of dry mouth, tingling, heat, heaviness, or pressure after treatment with ZOMIG. A few people may feel drowsy, dizzy, tired, or sick. Tell your doctor immediately if you have symptoms that you do not understand.
   - Some people may have a reaction called serotonin syndrome, which can be life-threatening, when they use ZOMIG. In particular, this reaction may occur when they use ZOMIG together with certain types of antidepressants known as SSRIs or SNRIs. Symptoms may include confusion, hallucinations, fast heart beat, feeling faint, fever, sweating, muscle spasm, difficulty walking, and/or diarrhea. Call your doctor immediately if you have any of these symptoms after taking ZOMIG.
6. **What To Do If An Overdose Is Taken:** If you have taken more medication than you have been told, contact either your doctor, hospital emergency department, or nearest poison control center immediately.
7. **Storing Your Medicine:** Keep your medicine in a safe place where children cannot reach it. It may be harmful to children. Store your medication away from light and moisture, and at a controlled room temperature. If your medication has expired (the expiration date is printed on the treatment pack), throw it away as instructed. If your doctor decides to stop your treatment, do not keep any leftover medicine unless your doctor tells you to. Throw away your medicine as instructed. Be sure that discarded tablets are out of the reach of children.

ZOMIG and ZOMIG-ZMT are registered trademarks of the AstraZeneca group of companies.

Other brands mentioned are trademarks of their respective owners and are not trademarks of the AstraZeneca group of companies. The makers of these brands are not affiliated with AstraZeneca or its products.

ZOMIG® (zolmitriptan) Tablets
Manufactured for:
AstraZeneca Pharmaceuticals LP
Wilmington, Delaware 19850
By: IPR Pharmaceuticals, Inc.
Carolina, Puerto Rico 00984-1967

ZOMIG-ZMT® (zolmitriptan) Orally Disintegrating Tablets
Manufactured for:
AstraZeneca Pharmaceuticals LP
Wilmington, Delaware 19850
By: CIMA Labs, Inc.
Eden Prairie, Minnesota 55344
Rev 10/08 SIC 30086–XX
308551 8/10

Axcan Pharma U.S., Inc.

22 INVERNESS CENTER PARKWAY
BIRMINGHAM, AL 35242

Direct Inquiries to:
Customer Service
(800) 472-2634
Fax: (205) 991-8426

CANASA® ℞

[*kă-nă-să*]
mesalamine suppository

DESCRIPTION

The active ingredient in CANASA® 1000 mg suppositories is mesalamine, also known as mesalazine or 5-aminosalicylic acid (5-ASA). Chemically, mesalamine is 5-amino-2-hydroxybenzoic acid, and is classified as an anti-inflammatory drug.

The empirical formula is $C_7H_7NO_3$, representing a molecular weight of 153.14. The structural formula is:

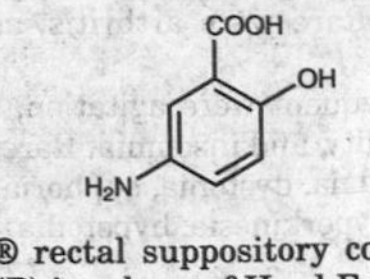

Each CANASA® rectal suppository contains 1000 mg of mesalamine (USP) in a base of Hard Fat, NF.

CLINICAL PHARMACOLOGY

Sulfasalazine has been used in the treatment of ulcerative colitis for over 55 years. It is split by bacterial action in the colon into sulfapyridine (SP) and mesalamine (5-ASA). It is thought that the mesalamine component only is therapeutically active in ulcerative colitis.

Mechanism of Action

The mechanism of action of mesalamine (and sulfasalazine) is not fully understood, but appears to be topical rather than systemic. Although the pathology of inflammatory bowel disease is uncertain, both prostaglandins and leukotrienes have been implicated as mediators of mucosal injury and inflammation. Recently, however, the role of mesalamine as a free radical scavenger or inhibitor of tumor necrosis factor (TNF) has also been postulated.

Pharmacokinetics

Absorption:

Mesalamine (5-ASA) administered as a rectal suppository is variably absorbed. In patients with ulcerative colitis treated with mesalamine 500 mg rectal suppositories, administered once every eight hours for six days, the mean mesalamine peak plasma concentration (C_{max}) was 353 ng/mL (CV=55%) following the initial dose and 361 ng/mL (CV=67%) at steady state. The mean minimum steady state plasma concentration (C_{min}) was 89 ng/mL (CV=89%). Absorbed mesalamine does not accumulate in the plasma.

Distribution:

Mesalamine administered as rectal suppositories distributes in rectal tissue to some extent. In patients with ulcerative proctitis treated with CANASA® (mesalamine, USP) 1000 mg rectal suppositories, rectal tissue concentrations for 5-ASA and N-acetyl-5-ASA have not been rigorously quantified.

Metabolism:

Mesalamine is extensively metabolized, mainly to N-acetyl-5-ASA. The site of metabolism has not been elucidated. In patients with ulcerative colitis treated with one 500 mg mesalamine rectal suppository every eight hours for six days, peak concentration (C_{max}) of N-acetyl-5-ASA ranged from 467 ng/mL to 1399 ng/mL following the initial dose and from 193 ng/mL to 1304 ng/mL at steady state.

Elimination:

Mesalamine is eliminated from plasma mainly by urinary excretion, predominantly as N-acetyl-5-ASA. In patients with ulcerative proctitis treated with one mesalamine 500 mg rectal suppository every eight hours for six days, ≤ 12% of the dose was eliminated in urine as unchanged 5-ASA and 8-77% as N-acetyl-5-ASA following the initial dose. At steady state, ≤ 11% of the dose was eliminated as unchanged 5-ASA and 3-35% as N-acetyl-5-ASA. The mean elimination half-life was five hours (CV=73%) for 5-ASA and six hours (CV=63%) for N-acetyl-5-ASA following the initial dose. At steady state, the mean elimination half-life was seven hours for both 5-ASA and N-acetyl-5-ASA (CV=102% for 5-ASA and 82% for N-acetyl-5-ASA).

Drug-Drug Interactions:

The potential for interactions between mesalamine, administered as 1000 mg rectal suppositories, and other drugs has not been studied.

Special Populations (Patients with Renal or Hepatic Impairment):
The effect of renal or hepatic impairment on elimination of mesalamine in ulcerative proctitis patients treated with mesalamine 1000 mg suppositories has not been studied.

Preclinical Toxicology
Preclinical studies of mesalamine were conducted in rats, mice, rabbits and dogs, and kidney was the main target organ of toxicity. In rats, adverse renal effects were observed at a single oral dose of 600 mg/kg (about 3.2 times the recommended human intra-rectal dose, based on body surface area) and at IV doses of >214 mg/kg (about 1.2 times the recommended human intra-rectal dose, based on body surface area). In a 13-week oral gavage toxicity study in rats, papillary necrosis and/or multifocal tubular injury were observed in males receiving 160 mg/kg (about 0.86 times the recommended human intra-rectal dose, based on body surface area) and in both males and females at 640 mg/kg (about 3.5 times the recommended human intra-rectal dose, based on body surface area). In a combined 52-week toxicity and 127-week carcinogenicity study in rats, degeneration of the kidneys and hyalinization of basement membranes and Bowman's capsule were observed at oral doses of 100 mg/kg/day (about 0.54 times the recommended human intra-rectal dose, based on body surface area) and above. In a 14-day rectal toxicity study of mesalamine suppositories in rabbits, intra-rectal doses up to 800 mg/kg (about 8.6 times the recommended human intra-rectal dose, based on body surface area) was not associated with any adverse effects. In a six-month oral toxicity study in dogs, doses of 80 mg/kg (about 1.4 times the recommended human intra-rectal dose, based on body surface area) and higher caused renal pathology similar to that described for the rat. In a rectal toxicity study of mesalamine suppositories in dogs, a dose of 166.6 mg/kg (about 3.0 times the recommended human intra-rectal dose, based on body surface area) produced chronic nephritis and pyelitis. In the 12-month eye toxicity study in dogs, Keratoconjunctivitis sicca (KCS) occurred at oral doses of 40 mg/kg (about 0.72 times the recommended human intra-rectal dose, based on body surface area) and above.

CLINICAL STUDIES
Two double-blind placebo-controlled multicenter studies were conducted in North America in patients with mild to moderate active ulcerative proctitis. The primary measures of efficacy were the same in all trials (clinical disease activity index, sigmoidoscopic and histologic evaluations). The main difference between the studies was dosage regimen: 500 mg three times daily (1.5 g/d) in Study 1; and 500 mg twice daily (1.0 g/d) in Study 2. A total of 173 patients were studied (Study 1, N=79; Study 2, N=94). Eighty-nine (89) patients received mesalamine suppositories, and eighty-four (84) patients received placebo suppositories. Patients were evaluated clinically and sigmoidoscopically after three and six weeks of suppository treatment. In Study No. 1 patients were 17 to 73 years of age (mean = 39 yrs), 57% were female, and 97% were white. Patients had an average extent of proctitis (upper disease boundary) of 10.8 cm. Eighty-four percent (84%) of the study patients had multiple prior episodes of proctitis. In Study No. 2, patients were 21 to 72 years of age (mean = 39 yrs), 62% were female, and 96% were white. Patients had an average extent of proctitis (upper disease boundary) of 10.3 cm. Seventy-eight percent (78%) of the study patients had multiple prior episodes of proctitis.

Compared to placebo, mesalamine suppository treatment was statistically (p<0.01) superior to placebo in all trials with respect to improvement in stool frequency, rectal bleeding, mucosal appearance, disease severity, and overall disease activity after three and six weeks of treatment. Daily diary records indicated significant improvement in rectal bleeding in the first week of therapy while tenesmus and diarrhea improved significantly within two weeks. Investigators rated patients receiving mesalamine much improved compared to patients receiving placebo (p<0.001).

The effectiveness of mesalamine suppositories was statistically significant irrespective of sex, extent of proctitis, duration of current episode or duration of disease.

A multicenter, open-label, randomized, parallel group study in ninety-nine (99) patients diagnosed with mild to moderate ulcerative proctitis compared the clinical efficacy of the CANASA® 1000 mg suppository to that of the CANASA® 500 mg suppository. The primary measures of efficacy included clinical disease activity index, sigmoidoscopic and histologic evaluations. Patients were randomized to one of two treatment groups, with a dosage regimen of one 500 mg mesalamine suppository BID, morning and HS, or one 1000 mg mesalamine suppository HS for 6 weeks. Patients were evaluated clinically and sigmoidoscopically after three and six weeks of suppository treatment. Of the eighty-one (81) patients in the Per Protocol population, forty-six (46) patients received mesalamine 500 mg suppositories BID, and thirty-five (35) patients received mesalamine 1000 mg suppositories HS.

The efficacy of the 1000 mg HS treatment was not statistically or clinically different after 6 weeks from the 500 mg BID treatment, and both were effective in the treatment of ulcerative proctitis. Both treatments resulted in a significant decrease between Baseline and 6 weeks in the Disease Activity Index (DAI), a composite index reflecting rectal bleeding, stool frequency, mucosal appearance at endoscopy, and a global assessment of disease. In the 500 mg BID group, the mean DAI value decreased from 6.6 to 1.6, and in the 1000 mg HS group, the mean DAI value decreased from 6.2 to 1.3 over 6 weeks of treatment, representing a decrease of greater than 75% in both groups. Seventy-eight percent (78%; 36/46) of patients in the 500 mg BID group and 86% (30/35) of the patients in the 1000 mg HS group achieved a substantial improvement in symptoms (defined as a DAI score of less than 3) after 6 weeks of treatment. These patients regained normal daily stools, lost their rectal bleeding, and lost signs of inflammation at endoscopic visualization. The time to onset of response to the study drug was within 3 weeks of initiation of therapy in each treatment group, but further improvement was observed between 3 and 6 weeks of treatment.

INDICATIONS AND USAGE
CANASA® 1000 mg Suppositories are indicated for the treatment of active ulcerative proctitis.

CONTRAINDICATIONS
CANASA® 1000 mg Suppositories are contraindicated in patients who have demonstrated hypersensitivity to mesalamine (5-aminosalicylic acid) or to the suppository vehicle [saturated vegetable fatty acid esters (Hard Fat, NF)], or to salicylates (including aspirin).

PRECAUTIONS
Mesalamine has been implicated in the production of an acute intolerance syndrome characterized by cramping, acute abdominal pain and bloody diarrhea, sometimes fever, headache and a rash; in such cases prompt withdrawal is required. The patient's history of sulfasalazine intolerance, if any, should be re-evaluated. If a rechallenge is performed later in order to validate the hypersensitivity, it should be carried out under close supervision and only if clearly needed, giving consideration to reduced dosage. In the literature, one patient previously sensitive to sulfasalazine was rechallenged with 400 mg oral mesalamine; within eight hours she experienced headache, fever, intensive abdominal colic, profuse diarrhea and was readmitted as an emergency. She responded poorly to steroid therapy and two weeks later a pancolectomy was required. The possibility of increased absorption of mesalamine and concomitant renal tubular damage as noted in the preclinical studies must be kept in mind. Patients on CANASA® 1000 mg, especially those on concurrent oral products which contain or release mesalamine and those with pre-existing renal disease, should be carefully monitored with urinalysis, BUN and creatinine testing.

In a clinical trial most patients who were hypersensitive to sulfasalazine were able to take mesalamine enemas without evidence of any allergic reaction. Nevertheless, caution should be exercised when mesalamine is initially used in patients known to be allergic to sulfasalazine. These patients should be instructed to discontinue therapy if signs of rash or fever become apparent.

A small proportion of patients have developed pancolitis while using mesalamine. However, extension of upper disease boundary and/or flare-ups occurred less often in the mesalamine-treated group than in the placebo-treated group.

Rare instances of pericarditis have been reported with mesalamine containing products including sulfasalazine. Cases of pericarditis have also been reported as manifestations of inflammatory bowel disease. In the cases reported there have been positive rechallenges with mesalamine or mesalamine containing products. In one of these cases, however, a second rechallenge with sulfasalazine was negative throughout a 2 month follow-up. Chest pain or dyspnea in patients treated with mesalamine should be investigated with this information in mind. Discontinuation of CANASA® suppositories may be warranted in some cases, but rechallenge with mesalamine can be performed under careful clinical observation should the continued therapeutic need for mesalamine be present.

There have been two reports in the literature of additional serious adverse events: one patient who developed leukopenia and thrombocytopenia after seven months of treatment with one 500 mg suppository nightly, and one patient with rash and fever which was a similar reaction to sulfasalazine.

Information for Patients:
See patient information printed at the end of this insert.

Carcinogenesis, Mutagenesis, Impairment of Fertility
Mesalamine caused no increase in the incidence of neoplastic lesions over controls in a two-year study of Wistar rats

fed up to 320 mg/kg/day of mesalamine admixed with diet (about 1.7 times the recommended human intra-rectal dose, based on body surface area).

Mesalamine was not mutagenic in the Ames test, the mouse lymphoma cell (TK$^{+/-}$) forward mutation test, or the mouse micronucleus test.

No effects on fertility or reproductive performance of the male and female rats were observed at oral mesalamine doses up to 320 mg/kg/day (about 1.7 times the recommended human intra-rectal dose, based on body surface area). The oligospermia and infertility in men associated with sulfasalazine have not been reported with mesalamine.

Pregnancy
Teratogenic Effects, Pregnancy Category B
Teratology studies have been performed in rats at oral doses up to 320 mg/kg/day (about 1.7 times the recommended human intra-rectal dose, based on body surface area) and in rabbits at oral doses up to 495 mg/kg/day (about 5.4 times the recommended human intra-rectal dose, based on body surface area) and have revealed no evidence of impaired fertility or harm to the fetus due to mesalamine. There are, however, no adequate and well controlled studies in pregnant women. Because animal reproduction studies are not always predictive of human response, this drug should be used in pregnancy only if clearly needed.

Nursing Mothers
It is not known whether mesalamine or its metabolite(s) are excreted in human milk. Because many drugs are excreted in human milk, caution should be exercised when CANASA® 1000 mg suppositories are administered to a nursing woman.

Pediatric Use
Safety and effectiveness in pediatric patients have not been established.

Geriatric Use
Clinical studies of CANASA® did not include sufficient numbers of subjects aged 65 and over to determine whether they respond differently from younger subjects. Other reported clinical experience has not identified differences in responses between the elderly and younger patients. In general, dose selection for an elderly patient should be cautious, reflecting the greater frequency of decreased hepatic, renal, or cardiac function, and of concomitant disease or other drug therapy.

Mesalamine is known to be substantially excreted by the kidney, and the risk of toxic reactions to this drug may be greater in patients with impaired renal function. Because elderly patients are more likely to have decreased renal function, it may be useful to monitor renal function.

ADVERSE REACTIONS
Clinical Adverse Experience
The most frequent adverse reactions observed in the double-blind, placebo-controlled trials are summarized in the Table below.

ADVERSE REACTIONS OCCURRING IN MORE THAN 1% OF MESALAMINE SUPPOSITORY TREATED PATIENTS (COMPARISON TO PLACEBO)

Symptom	Mesalamine (n=177)		Placebo (n=84)	
	N	%	N	%
Dizziness	5	3.0	2	2.4
Rectal Pain	3	1.8	0	0.0
Fever	2	1.2	0	0.0
Rash	2	1.2	0	0.0
Acne	2	1.2	0	0.0
Colitis	2	1.2	0	0.0

In the multicenter, open-label, randomized, parallel group study comparing the CANASA® 1000 mg suppository (HS) to that of the CANASA® 500 mg suppository (BID), there were no differences between the two treatment groups in the adverse event profile. The most frequent AEs were headache (14.4%), flatulence (5.2%), abdominal pain (5.2%), diarrhea (3.1%), and nausea (3.1%). Three (3) patients had to discontinue medication because of a treatment emergent AE; one of these AEs (headache) was deemed possibly related to study medication.

In addition to the events observed in the clinical trials, the following adverse events have been associated with mesalamine containing products: nephrotoxicity, pancreatitis, fibrosing alveolitis and elevated liver enzymes. Cases of pancreatitis and fibrosing alveolitis have been reported as manifestations of inflammatory bowel disease as well.

Hair Loss

Mild hair loss characterized by "more hair in the comb" but no withdrawal from clinical trials has been observed in seven of 815 mesalamine patients but none of the placebo-treated patients. In the literature there are at least six additional patients with mild hair loss who received either mesalamine or sulfasalazine. Retreatment is not always associated with repeated hair loss.

OVERDOSAGE

There have been no documented reports of serious toxicity in man resulting from massive overdosing with mesalamine. Under ordinary circumstances, mesalamine absorption from the colon is limited.

DOSAGE AND ADMINISTRATION

The usual dosage of CANASA® (mesalamine, USP) 1000 mg suppositories is one rectal suppository 1 time daily at bedtime.

The suppository should be retained for one to three hours or longer, if possible, to achieve the maximum benefit. While the effect of CANASA® suppositories may be seen within three to twenty-one days, the usual course of therapy would be from three to six weeks depending on symptoms and sigmoidoscopic findings. Studies have suggested that CANASA® suppositories will delay relapse after the six-week short-term treatment.

Patient Instructions:
NOTE: CANASA® suppositories will cause staining of direct contact surfaces, including but not limited to fabrics, flooring, painted surfaces, marble, granite, vinyl, and enamel.

1. Detach one suppository from strip of suppositories.
2. Hold suppository upright and carefully remove the plastic wrapper.
3. Avoid excessive handling of suppository, which is designed to melt at body temperature.
4. Insert suppository completely into rectum with gentle pressure, pointed end first.
5. A small amount of lubricating gel may be used on the tip of the suppository to assist insertion.

HOW SUPPLIED

CANASA® (Mesalamine, USP) 1000 mg Suppositories: CANASA® 1000 mg Suppositories for rectal administration are available as bullet shaped, light tan suppositories containing 1000 mg mesalamine supplied in boxes of 30 and 42 individually plastic wrapped suppositories (NDC 58914-501-56 and 58914-501-42).

Store below 25°C (77°F), may be refrigerated. Keep away from direct heat, light or humidity.

Rx only

Axcan Pharma US, Inc.
Birmingham, AL 35242
Date: October 15, 2008

Patient Information

CANASA® Rectal Suppositories
(Mesalamine, USP) 1000 mg

Read this information carefully before you begin treatment. Also, read the information you get whenever you get more medicine. There may be new information. This information does not take the place of talking with your doctor about your medical condition or your treatment. If you have any questions about this medicine, ask your doctor or pharmacist.

What is CANASA®?

CANASA® (can-AH-sah) is a medicine used to treat ulcerative proctitis (ulcerative rectal colitis). CANASA® works inside your rectum (lower intestine) to help reduce bleeding, mucous and bloody diarrhea caused by inflammation (swelling and soreness) of the rectal area. You use CANASA® by inserting it into your rectum.

Who should not use CANASA®?

Do not use CANASA® if you are allergic to the active ingredient mesalamine (also found in drugs such as Rowasa, Asacol, Pentasa, Azulfidine, and Dipentum), if you are allergic to the inactive ingredients, or if you have had any unusual reaction to the ingredients.

Tell your doctor if you:

• Have kidney problems. Using CANASA® may make them worse.
• Have had inflamed pancreas (pancreatitis).
• Are pregnant. You and your doctor will decide if you should use CANASA®.
• Have ever had pericarditis (inflamed sac around your heart).
• Are allergic to sulfasalazine. You may need to watch for signs of an allergic reaction to CANASA®.
• Are allergic to aspirin.
• Are allergic to other things, such as foods, preservatives, or dyes.

How should I use CANASA®?

Follow your doctor's instructions about how often to use CANASA® and how long to use it. For the 1000 mg

suppository, the usual dose is one suppository at bedtime for 3-6 weeks. We do not know if CANASA® will work for children or is safe for them.

Follow these steps to use CANASA®:
1. For best results, empty your rectum (have a bowel movement) just before using CANASA®.
2. Detach one CANASA® suppository from the strip of suppositories.
3. Hold the suppository upright and carefully peel open the plastic at the pre-cut line to take out the suppository.
4. Insert the suppository with the pointed end first completely into your rectum, using gentle pressure.
5. For best results, keep the suppository in your rectum for 3 hours or longer, if possible.

If you have trouble inserting CANASA®, you may put a little bit of lubricating gel on the suppository.

Do not handle the suppository too much, since it may begin to melt from the heat from your hands and body.

If you miss a dose of CANASA®, use it as soon as possible, unless it is almost time for next dose. Do not use two CANASA® suppositories at the same time to make up for a missed dose.

Keep using CANASA® as long as your doctor tells you to use it, even if you feel better.

CANASA® can cause stains on things it touches. Therefore keep it away from clothing and other fabrics, flooring, painted surfaces, marble, granite, plastics, and enamel. Be careful since CANASA® may stain clothing.

What should I avoid while taking CANASA®?

Do not breast feed while using CANASA®. We do not know if CANASA® can pass through the milk and harm the baby. Tell your doctor if you become pregnant while using CANASA®.

What are the possible side effects of CANASA®?

• The most common side effects of CANASA® are: headache, gas or flatulence, and diarrhea. These events also occurred when patients were given an inactive suppository.
• Less common, but possibly serious side effects include a reaction to the medicine (acute intolerance syndrome) that includes cramps, sharp abdominal (stomach area) pain, bloody diarrhea, and sometimes fever, headache and rash. Stop use and tell your doctor right away if you get any of these symptoms.
• In rare cases, the sac around the heart may become inflamed (pericarditis). Tell your doctor right away if you develop chest pain or shortness of breath, which are signs of this problem.
• In rare cases, patients using CANASA® develop worsening colitis (pancolitis).
• A very few patients using CANASA® may have mild hair loss.
• Other side effects not listed above may also occur in some patients.

If you notice any other side effects, check with your doctor or pharmacist.

How should I store CANASA®?

Store CANASA® below 25°C (77°F), may be refrigerated. Keep it away from direct heat, light, or humidity. Keep it out of the reach of children.

General advice about prescription medicines

Medicines are sometimes prescribed for conditions that are not mentioned in patient information leaflets. Do not use CANASA® for a condition for which it was not prescribed. Do not give CANASA® to other people, even if they have the same symptoms you have.

This leaflet summarizes the most important information about CANASA®. If you would like more information, talk with your doctor. You can ask your pharmacist or doctor for information about CANASA® that is written for health professionals.

Revised: 10/2008   Axcan Pharma US, Inc.

Shown in Product Identification Guide, page 306

CARAFATE®   ℞
[kär ʹafăt]
(sucralfate)
Suspension

DESCRIPTION

CARAFATE Suspension contains sucralfate and sucralfate is an α-D-glucopyranoside, β-D-fructofuranosyl-, octakis-(hydrogen sulfate), aluminum complex.
[See chemical structure at top of next column]

CARAFATE Suspension for oral administration contains 1 g of sucralfate per 10 mL.

CARAFATE Suspension also contains: colloidal silicon dioxide NF, FD&C Red #40, flavor, glycerin USP, methylcellulose USP, methylparaben NF, microcrystalline cellulose NF, purified water USP, simethicone USP, and sorbitol solution USP. Therapeutic category: antiulcer.

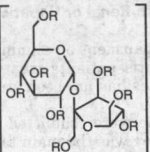

$[Al(OH)_3]_x \times [H_2O]_y$
(x = 8 to 10 and y = 22 to 31)

R = SO₃Al(OH)₂

$R = SO_3Al(OH)_2$

CLINICAL PHARMACOLOGY

Sucralfate is only minimally absorbed from the gastrointestinal tract. The small amounts of the sulfated disaccharide that are absorbed are excreted primarily in the urine.

Although the mechanism of sucralfate's ability to accelerate healing of duodenal ulcers remains to be fully defined, it is known that it exerts its effect through a local, rather than systemic, action.

The following observations also appear pertinent:

1. Studies in human subjects and with animal models of ulcer disease have shown that sucralfate forms an ulcer-adherent complex with proteinaceous exudate at the ulcer site.
2. In vitro, a sucralfate-albumin film provides a barrier to diffusion of hydrogen ions.
3. In human subjects, sucralfate given in doses recommended for ulcer therapy inhibits pepsin activity in gastric juice by 32%.
4. In vitro, sucralfate adsorbs bile salts.

These observations suggest that sucralfate's antiulcer activity is the result of formation of an ulcer-adherent complex that covers the ulcer site and protects it against further attack by acid, pepsin, and bile salts. There are approximately 14 to 16 mEq of acid-neutralizing capacity per 1-g dose of sucralfate.

CLINICAL TRIALS

In a multicenter, double-blind, placebo-controlled study of CARAFATE Suspension, a dosage regiment of 1 g (10 mL) four times daily was demonstrated to be superior to placebo in ulcer healing.

Results From Clinical Trials Healing Rates for Acute Duodenal Ulcer

Treatment	n	Week 2 Healing Rates	Week 4 Healing Rates	Week 8 Healing Rates
CARAFATE Suspension	145	23(16%)*	66(46%)†	95(66%)‡
Placebo	147	10(7%)	39(27%)	58(39%)

* $P=0.016$
† $P=0.001$
‡ $P=0.0001$

Equivalence of sucralfate suspension to sucralfate tablets has not been demonstrated.

INDICATIONS AND USAGE

CARAFATE (sucralfate) Suspension is indicated in the short-term (up to 8 weeks) treatment of active duodenal ulcer.

CONTRAINDICATIONS

There are no known contraindications to the use of sucralfate.

PRECAUTIONS

Duodenal ulcer is a chronic, recurrent disease. While short-term treatment with sucralfate can result in complete healing of the ulcer, a successful course of treatment with sucralfate should not be expected to alter the posthealing frequency or severity of duodenal ulceration.

Special Populations: Chronic Renal Failure and Dialysis Patients

When sucralfate is administered orally, small amounts of aluminum are absorbed from the gastrointestinal tract. Concomitant use of sucralfate with other products that contain aluminum, such as aluminum-containing antacids, may increase the total body burden of aluminum. Patients with normal renal function receiving the recommended doses of sucralfate and aluminum-containing products adequately excrete aluminum in the urine. Patients with chronic renal failure or those receiving dialysis have impaired excretion of absorbed aluminum. In addition, aluminum does not cross dialysis membranes because it is bound to albumin and transferrin plasma proteins. Aluminum accumulation and toxicity (aluminum osteodystrophy, osteomalacia, encephalopathy) have been described in patients with renal impairment. Sucralfate should be used with caution in patients with chronic renal failure.

Drug Interactions

Some studies have shown that simultaneous sucralfate administration in healthy volunteers reduced the extent of absorption (bioavailability) of single doses of the following cimetidine, digoxin, fluoroquinolone antibiotics, ketoconazole, l-thyroxine, phenytoin, quinidine, ranitidine, tetracycline, and theophylline. Subtherapeutic prothrombin times with concomitant warfarin and sucralfate therapy have been reported in spontaneous and published case reports. However, two clinical studies have demonstrated no change in either serum warfarin concentration or prothrombin time with the addition of sucralfate to chronic warfarin therapy.

The mechanism of these interactions appears to be nonsystemic in nature, presumably resulting from sucralfate binding to the concomitant agent in the gastrointestinal tract. In all cases studied to date (cimetidine, ciprofloxacin, digoxin, norfloxacin, ofloxacin, and ranitidine), dosing the concomitant medication 2 hours before sucralfate eliminated the interaction. Because of the potential of CARAFATE to alter the absorption of some drugs, CARAFATE should be administered separately from other drugs when alterations in bioavailability are felt to be critical. In these cases, patients should be monitored appropriately.

Carcinogenesis, Mutagenesis, Impairment of Fertility

Chronic oral toxicity studies of 24 months' duration were conducted in mice and rats at doses up to 1 g/kg (12 times the human dose).

There was no evidence of drug-related tumorigenicity. A reproduction study in rats at doses up to 38 times the human dose did not reveal any indication of fertility impairment. Mutagenicity studies were not conducted.

Pregnancy

Teratogenic effects. Pregnancy Category B.

Teratogenicity studies have been performed in mice, rats, and rabbits at doses up to 50 times the human dose and have revealed no evidence of harm to the fetus due to sucralfate. There are, however, no adequate and well-controlled studies in pregnant women. Because animal reproduction studies are not always predictive of human response, this drug should be used during pregnancy only if clearly needed.

Nursing Mothers

It is not known whether this drug is excreted in human milk. Because many drugs are excreted in human milk, caution should be exercised when sucralfate is administered to a nursing woman.

Pediatric Use

Safety and effectiveness in pediatric patients have not been established.

Geriatric Use

Clinical studies of CARAFATE Suspension did not include sufficient numbers of subjects aged 65 and over to determine whether they respond differently from younger subjects. Other reported clinical experience has not identified differences in responses between the elderly and younger patients. In general, dose selection for an elderly patient should be cautious, usually starting at the low end of the dosing range, reflecting the greater frequency of decreased hepatic, renal, or cardiac function, and of concomitant disease or other drug therapy. (See **DOSAGE AND ADMINISTRATION**)

This drug is known to be substantially excreted by the kidney, and the risk of toxic reactions to this drug may be greater in patients with impaired renal function. (See **PRECAUTIONS Special Populations: Chronic Renal Failure and Dialysis Patients**) Because elderly patients are more likely to have decreased renal function, care should be taken in dose selection, and it may be useful to monitor renal function.

ADVERSE REACTIONS

Adverse reactions to sucralfate tablets in clinical trials were minor and only rarely led to discontinuation of the drug. In studies involving over 2700 patients treated with sucralfate, adverse effects were reported in 129 (4.7%). Constipation was the most frequent complaint (2%). Other adverse effects reported in less than 0.5% of the patients are listed below by body system:

Gastrointestinal: diarrhea, dry mouth, flatulence, gastric discomfort, indigestion, nausea, vomiting

Dermatological: pruritus, rash

Nervous System: dizziness, insomnia, sleepiness, vertigo

Other: back pain, headache

Postmarketing reports of hypersensitivity reactions, including urticaria (hives), angioedema, respiratory difficulty, rhinitis, laryngospasm, and facial swelling have been reported in patients receiving sucralfate tablets. Similar events were reported with sucralfate suspension. However, a causal relationship has not been established.

Bezoars have been reported in patients treated with sucralfate. The majority of patients had underlying medical conditions that may predispose to bezoar formation (such as delayed gastric emptying) or were receiving concomitant enteral tube feedings.

Inadvertent injection of insoluble sucralfate and its insoluble excipients has led to fatal complications, including pulmonary and cerebral emboli. Sucralfate is **not** intended for intravenous administration.

OVERDOSAGE

Due to limited experience in humans with overdosage of sucralfate, no specific treatment recommendations can be given. Acute oral studies in animals, however, using doses up to 12 g/kg body weight, could not find a lethal dose. Sucralfate is only minimally absorbed from the gastrointestinal tract. Risks associated with acute overdosage should, therefore, be minimal. In rare reports describing sucralfate overdose, most patients remained asymptomatic. Those few reports where adverse events were described included symptoms of dyspepsia, abdominal pain, nausea, and vomiting.

DOSAGE AND ADMINISTRATION

Active Duodenal Ulcer. The recommended adult oral dosage for duodenal ulcer is 1 g (10 mL/2 teaspoonfuls) four times per day. CARAFATE should be administered on an empty stomach.

Antacids may be prescribed as needed for relief of pain but should not be taken within one-half hour before or after sucralfate.

While healing with sucralfate may occur during the first week or two, treatment should be continued for 4 to 8 weeks unless healing has been demonstrated by x-ray or endoscopic examination.

Elderly. In general, dose selection for an elderly patient should be cautious, usually starting at the low end of the dosing range, reflecting the greater frequency of decreased hepatic, renal, or cardiac function, and of concomitant disease or other drug therapy. (See **PRECAUTIONS Geriatric Use**) Call your doctor for medical advice about side effects. You may report side effects to FDA at 1-800-FDA-1088.

HOW SUPPLIED

CARAFATE (sucralfate) Suspension 1 g/10 mL is a pink suspension supplied in bottles of 14 fl oz (NDC 58914-170-14).

SHAKE WELL BEFORE USING. AVOID FREEZING

Store at controlled room temperature 20-25°C (68-77°F)[see USP]

Rx Only

Prescribing Information as of April 2007

Axcan Pharma US, Inc.
22 Inverness Center Parkway
Birmingham, AL 35242
www.axcan.com

PHOTOFRIN®   ℞

[fō´tō-frĭn]

(porfimer sodium)

injection, powder, for solution for intravenous use

HIGHLIGHTS OF PRESCRIBING INFORMATION

These highlights do not include all the information needed to use PHOTOFRIN safely and effectively. See full prescribing information for PHOTOFRIN.

PHOTOFRIN (porfimer sodium) injection, powder, for solution for intravenous use
Initial U.S. Approval: 1995

—————RECENT MAJOR CHANGES—————

Contraindications (4) 06/2008
Warnings and Precautions (5.3, 5.4, 5.9) 06/2008
Adverse Reactions (6.1, 6.2) 06/2008
Clinical Studies (14.3) 06/2008

—————INDICATIONS AND USAGE—————

PHOTOFRIN is a photoactivated drug indicated for:

Esophageal Cancer (1.1)
• Palliation of patients with completely obstructing esophageal cancer, or of patients with partially obstructing esophageal cancer who, in the opinion of their physician, cannot be satisfactorily treated with Nd:YAG laser therapy

Endobronchial Cancer (1.2)
• Treatment of microinvasive endobronchial non-small-cell lung cancer (NSCLC) in patients for whom surgery and radiotherapy are not indicated
• Reduction of obstruction and palliation of symptoms in patients with completely or partially obstructing endobronchial NSCLC

High-Grade Dysplasia in Barrett's Esophagus (1.3)
• Ablation of high-grade dysplasia (HGD) in Barrett's esophagus (BE) patients who do not undergo esophagectomy

—————DOSAGE AND ADMINISTRATION—————

PHOTOFRIN (2.1)
• PHOTOFRIN administration: 2 mg/kg intravenous

Photoactivation (2.2)
Esophageal Cancer
• Laser light dose of 300 J/cm of fiber optic diffuser length 40-50 hours following injection with PHOTOFRIN; repeated, if needed, 96-120 hours after initial injection
Endobronchial Cancer
• Laser light dose of 200 J/cm of fiber optic diffuser length 40-50 hours following injection with PHOTOFRIN; repeated, if needed, after gentle debridement of residual tumor 96-120 hours after initial injection
High-Grade Dysplasia in Barrett's Esophagus
• Laser light dose of 130 J/cm of fiber optic diffuser length 40-50 hours following injection with PHOTOFRIN; repeated, if needed, with a light dose of 50 J/cm of fiber optic diffuser length 96-120 hours after initial injection

—————DOSAGE FORMS AND STRENGTHS—————
75 mg vial (3)

—————CONTRAINDICATIONS—————
• Porphyria (4)
• Existing tracheoesophageal or bronchoesophageal fistula (4, 5.1)
• Tumors eroding into a major blood vessel (4, 5.2)
• Emergency treatment of patients with severe acute respiratory distress caused by an obstructing endobronchial lesion because 40 to 50 hours are required between injection of PHOTOFRIN and laser light treatment (4)
• Esophageal or gastric varices or esophageal ulcers >1 cm in diameter (4)

—————WARNINGS AND PRECAUTIONS—————
• Tracheoesophageal or bronchoesophageal fistula can occur if esophageal tumor is eroding into trachea or bronchial tree (5.1)
• High risk of bleeding in patients with esophageal varices (5.1)
• High risk for fatal massive hemoptysis with endobronchial tumors that are: large, centrally located; cavitating; extensive, extrinsic to the bronchus (5.2)
• After treatment of HGD in BE, monitor endoscopic biopsy every three months, until four consecutive negative evaluations for HGD have been recorded (5.3)
• Use with extreme caution for endobronchial tumors in locations where treatment-induced inflammation could obstruct the main airway leading to life-threatening respiratory distress (5.2, 5.8)
• Photosensitivity can be expected; ocular sensitivity is possible (5.4, 5.5)
• Allow 2-4 weeks between PDT and subsequent radiotherapy (5.6)
• Substernal chest pain may occur after treatment and may require analgesics (5.7)
• Esophageal stenosis occur frequently after treatment of HGD in BE (5.9)
• Patients with hepatic or renal impairment may need longer precautionary measures for photosensitivity (5.10)

—————ADVERSE REACTIONS—————
Most common adverse reactions reported during clinical trials (>10% of patients) are (6.2):
• Esophageal Cancer: Anemia, pleural effusion, pyrexia, constipation, nausea, chest pain, pain, abdominal pain, dyspnoea, photosensitivity reaction, pneumonia, vomiting, insomnia, back pain, pharyngitis
• Obstructing Endobronchial Cancer: Dyspnoea, photosensitivity reaction, hemoptysis, pyrexia, cough, pneumonia
• Superficial Endobronchial Tumors: Exudate, photosensitivity reaction, bronchial obstruction, edema, bronchostenosis
• High-Grade Dysplasia in Barrett's Esophagus: Photosensitivity reaction, esophageal stenosis, vomiting, chest pain, nausea, pyrexia, constipation, dysphagia, abdominal pain, pleural effusion, dehydration

To report SUSPECTED ADVERSE REACTIONS, contact AXCAN Pharma US, Inc. at 1-800-472-2634 or drugsafety@axcan.com or FDA at 1-800-FDA-1088 or www.fda.gov/medwatch

—————DRUG INTERACTIONS—————
• Other photosensitizing agents: May increase the risk of photosensitivity reaction (7.1)
• Concomitant therapy: May decrease the efficacy of PDT (7.2)

See 17 for PATIENT COUNSELING INFORMATION
Revised: 08/2008

FULL PRESCRIBING INFORMATION: CONTENTS*

* Sections or subsections omitted from the full prescribing information are not listed

---

FULL PRESCRIBING INFORMATION

1   INDICATIONS AND USAGE

1.1   Esophageal Cancer

PHOTOFRIN® is indicated for the palliation of patients with completely obstructing esophageal cancer, or of patients with partially obstructing esophageal cancer who, in the opinion of their physician, cannot be satisfactorily treated with Nd:YAG laser therapy.

1.2   Endobronchial Cancer

PHOTOFRIN is indicated for the treatment of microinvasive endobronchial non-small-cell lung cancer (NSCLC) in patients for whom surgery and radiotherapy are not indicated.

PHOTOFRIN is indicated for the reduction of obstruction and palliation of symptoms in patients with completely or partially obstructing endobronchial NSCLC.

1.3   High-Grade Dysplasia in Barrett's Esophagus

PHOTOFRIN is indicated for the ablation of high-grade dysplasia in Barrett's esophagus patients who do not undergo esophagectomy.

2   DOSAGE AND ADMINISTRATION

Photodynamic therapy (PDT) with PHOTOFRIN is a two-stage process requiring administration of both drug and light. The first stage of PDT is the intravenous injection of PHOTOFRIN at 2 mg/kg. Illumination with laser light 40-50 hours following injection with PHOTOFRIN constitutes the second stage of therapy. A second laser light application may be given 96-120 hours after injection [see Dosage and Administration (2.2)]. In clinical studies on endobronchial cancer, debridement via endoscopy was required 2-3 days after the initial light application. Standard endoscopic techniques are used for light administration and debride-

ment. Practitioners should be fully familiar with the patient's condition and trained in the safe and efficacious treatment of esophageal or endobronchial cancer, or high-grade dysplasia (HGD) in Barrett's esophagus (BE) using PDT with PHOTOFRIN and associated light delivery devices. PDT with PHOTOFRIN should be applied only in those facilities properly equipped for the procedure.

The laser system must be approved for delivery of a stable power output at a wavelength of 630 ± 3 nm. Light is delivered to the tumor by cylindrical OPTIGUIDE™ fiber optic diffusers passed through the operating channel of an endoscope/bronchoscope. Instructions for use of the fiber optic and the selected laser system should be read carefully before use. OPTIGUIDE™ cylindrical diffusers are available in several lengths. The choice of diffuser tip length depends on the length of the tumor or Barrett's mucosa to be treated. Diffuser length should be sized to avoid exposure of nonmalignant tissue to light and to prevent overlapping of previously treated malignant tissue. Refer to the OPTIGUIDE™ instructions for use for complete instructions concerning the fiber optic diffuser.

2.1   PHOTOFRIN

PHOTOFRIN should be administered as a single slow intravenous injection over 3 to 5 minutes at 2 mg/kg of body weight. Reconstitute each vial of PHOTOFRIN with 31.8 mL of either 5% Dextrose Injection (USP) or 0.9% Sodium Chloride Injection (USP), resulting in a final concentration of 2.5 mg/mL. Shake well until dissolved. Do not mix PHOTOFRIN with other drugs in the same solution. PHOTOFRIN, reconstituted with 5% Dextrose Injection (USP) or with 0.9% Sodium Chloride Injection (USP), has a pH in the range of 7 to 8. PHOTOFRIN has been formulated with an overage to deliver the 75 mg labeled quantity. **The reconstituted product should be protected from bright light and used immediately.** Reconstituted PHOTOFRIN is an opaque solution, in which detection of particulate matter by visual inspection is extremely difficult. Reconstituted PHOTOFRIN, however, like all parenteral drug products, should be inspected visually for particulate matter and discoloration prior to administration whenever solution and container permit.

Precautions should be taken to prevent extravasation at the injection site. If extravasation occurs, care must be taken to protect the area from light. There is no known benefit from injecting the extravasation site with another substance.

2.2   Photoactivation

Esophageal Cancer
Initiate 630 nm wavelength laser light delivery to the patient 40–50 hours following injection with PHOTOFRIN. A second laser light treatment may be given as early as 96 hours or as late as 120 hours after the initial injection with PHOTOFRIN. No further injection of PHOTOFRIN should be given for such retreatment with laser light. Before providing a second laser light treatment, the residual tumor may be debrided. The debridement is optional since the residua will be removed naturally by peristaltic action of the esophagus. Vigorous debridement may cause tumor bleeding.

Photoactivation of PHOTOFRIN is controlled by the total light dose delivered. In the treatment of esophageal cancer, a light dose of 300 Joules/cm (J/cm) of diffuser length should be delivered. The total power output at the fiber tip is set to deliver the appropriate light dose using exposure times of 12 minutes and 30 seconds.

For the treatment of esophageal cancer, patients may receive a second course of PDT a minimum of 30 days after the initial therapy; up to three courses of PDT (each separated by a minimum of 30 days) can be given. Before each course of treatment, patients with esophageal cancer should be evaluated for the presence of a tracheoesophageal or bronchoesophageal fistula [see Contraindications (4)]. All patients should be evaluated for the possibility that the tumor may be eroding into a major blood vessel [see Contraindications (4)].

Endobronchial Cancer
Initiate 630 nm wavelength laser light delivery to the patient 40–50 hours following injection with PHOTOFRIN. A second laser light treatment may be given as early as 96 hours or as late as 120 hours after the initial injection with PHOTOFRIN. No further injection of PHOTOFRIN should be given for such retreatment with laser light. Before providing a second laser light treatment, the residual tumor should be debrided. Vigorous debridement may cause tumor bleeding. For endobronchial tumors, debridement of necrotic tissue should be discontinued when the volume of bleeding increases, as this may indicate that debridement has gone beyond the zone of the PDT effect.

Photoactivation of PHOTOFRIN is controlled by the total light dose delivered. In the treatment of endobronchial cancer, a light dose of 200 J/cm of diffuser length should be delivered. The total power output at the fiber tip is set to deliver the appropriate light dose using exposure times of 8 minutes and 20 seconds. For noncircumferential endobronchial tumors that are soft enough to penetrate, interstitial fiber placement is preferred to intraluminal activation, since this method produces better efficacy and results in less exposure of the normal bronchial mucosa to light. It is important to perform a debridement 2 to 3 days after each light administration to minimize the potential for obstruction caused by necrotic debris [see Warnings and Precautions (5.8)].

For the treatment of endobronchial cancer, patients may receive a second course of PDT a minimum of 30 days after the initial therapy; up to three courses of PDT (each separated by a minimum of 30 days) can be given. In patients with endobronchial lesions who have recently undergone radiotherapy, sufficient time (approximately 4 weeks) should be allowed between the therapies to ensure that the acute inflammation produced by radiotherapy has subsided prior to PDT [see Warnings and Precautions (5.6)]. All patients should be evaluated for the possibility that the tumor may be eroding into a major blood vessel [see Contraindications (4)].

High-Grade Dysplasia (HGD) in Barrett's Esophagus (BE)
Prior to initiating treatment with PHOTOFRIN PDT, the diagnosis of HGD in BE should be confirmed by an expert GI pathologist.

Approximately 40-50 hours after PHOTOFRIN administration light should be delivered by a X-Cell Photodynamic Therapy (PDT) Balloon with Fiber Optic Diffuser. The choice of fiber optic/balloon diffuser combination will depend on the length of Barrett's mucosa to be treated (**Table 1**).

TABLE 1. Fiber Optic Diffuser/Balloon Combination*

Treated Barrett's Mucosa Length (cm)	Fiber Optic Diffuser Length (cm)	Balloon Window Length (cm)
6-7	9	7
4-5	7	5
1-3	5	3

*Whenever possible, the BE segment selected for treatment should include normal tissue margins of a few millimeters at the proximal and distal ends.

Photoactivation is controlled by the total light dose delivered. The objective is to expose and treat all areas of HGD and the entire length of BE. The light dose administered will be 130 J/cm of diffuser length using a centering balloon. Based on the randomized clinical study, acceptable light intensity for the balloon/diffuser combinations range from 200-270 mW/cm of diffuser length.

To calculate the light dose, the following specific light dosimetry equation applies for all fiber optic diffusers:

Light Dose (J/cm) = Power Output From Diffuser (W) × Treatment Time (s)/Diffuser Length (cm)

Table 2 provides the settings that will be used to deliver the dose within the shortest time (light intensity of 270 mW/cm). A second option (light intensity of 200 mW/cm) has also been included where necessary to accommodate lasers with a total capacity that does not exceed 2.5 W.

[See table 2 at left]

Short fiber diffusers (≤2.5 cm) are to be used to pretreat nodules with 50 J/cm of diffuser length prior to regular balloon treatment in the first laser light session or for the treatment of "skip" areas (i.e., an area that does not show sufficient mucosal response) after the first light session. For this treatment, the fiber optic diffuser is used without a centering balloon, and a light intensity of 400 mW/cm should be used. For nodule pretreatment and treatment of skipped areas, care should be taken to minimize exposure to normal tissue as it is also sensitized. **Table 3** lists appropriate fiber optic power outputs and treatment times using a light intensity of 400 mW/cm.

TABLE 2. Fiber Optic Power Outputs and Treatment Times Required to Deliver 130 J/cm of Diffuser Length Using the Centering Balloon

Balloon Window Length (cm)	Fiber Optic Diffuser Length (cm)	Light Intensity (mW/cm)	Required Power Output from Diffuser* (mW)	Treatment Time (sec)	Treatment Time (min:sec)
3	5	270	1350	480	8:00
5	7	270	1900	480	8:00
7	9	270	2440	480	8:00
		200	1800	480	10:50

*As measured by immersing the diffuser into the cuvet in the power meter and slowly increasing the laser power.
Note: No more than 1.5 times the required diffuser power output should be needed from the laser. If more than this is required, the system should be checked.

TABLE 3. Short Fiber Optic Diffusers to be Used Without a Centering Balloon to Deliver 50 J/cm of Diffuser Length at a Light Intensity of 400 mW/cm

Fiber Optic Diffuser Length (cm)	Required Power Output From Diffuser* (mW)	Treatment Time (sec)	Treatment Time (min:sec)
1.0	400	125	2:05
1.5	600	125	2:05
2.0	800	125	2:05
2.5	1000	125	2:05

*As measured by immersing the diffuser into the cuvet in the power meter and slowly increasing the laser power.
Note: No more than 1.5 times the required diffuser power output should be needed from the laser. If more than this is required, the system should be checked.

TABLE 4. High-Grade Dysplasia in Barrett's Esophagus

Procedure	Study Day	Light Delivery Devices	Treatment Intent
PHOTOFRIN Injection	Day 1	NA	Uptake of photosensitizer
Laser Light Application	Day 3*	3, 5 or 7 cm balloon (130 J/cm)	Photoactivation
Laser Light Application *(Optional)*	Day 5	Short (≤2.5 cm) fiber optic diffuser (50 J/cm)	Treatment of "skip" areas only

*Discrete nodules will receive an initial light application of 50 J/cm (using a short fiber optic diffuser without balloon) before the balloon light application.
NA: Not Applicable

A maximum of 7 cm of esophageal mucosa is treated at the first light session using an appropriate size of centering balloon and fiber optic diffuser (**Table 1**). Whenever possible, the segment selected for the first light application should contain all the areas of HGD. Also, whenever possible, the BE segment selected for the first light application should include normal tissue margin of a few millimeters at the proximal and distal ends.
Nodules are to be pretreated at a light dose of 50 J/cm of diffuser length with a short (≤2.5 cm) fiber optic diffuser placed directly against the nodule followed by standard balloon application as described above.
Repeat Light Application
A second laser light application may be given to a previously treated segment that shows a "skip" area, using a short, ≤2.5 cm, fiber optic diffuser without centering balloon at the light dose of 50 J/cm of the diffuser length. Patients with BE >7 cm, should have the remaining untreated length of Barrett's epithelium treated with a second PDT course at least 90 days later.
The treatment regimen is summarized in **Table 4**.
[See table 4 at top right]
For the ablation of HGD in BE, patients may receive an additional course of PDT at a minimum of 90 days after the initial therapy; up to three courses of PDT (each injection separated by a minimum of 90 days) can be given to a previously treated segment which still shows HGD, low-grade dysplasia, or Barrett's metaplasia, or to a new segment if the initial Barrett's segment was >7 cm in length. Both residual and additional segments may be treated in the same light session(s) provided that the total length of the segments treated with the balloon/diffuser combination is not greater than 7 cm. In the case of a previously treated esophageal segment, if it has not sufficiently healed and/or histological assessment of biopsies is not clear, the subsequent course of PDT may be delayed for an additional 1-2 months.

3 DOSAGE FORMS AND STRENGTHS

75 mg vial

4 CONTRAINDICATIONS

- PHOTOFRIN is contraindicated in patients with porphyria.
- Photodynamic therapy (PDT) is contraindicated in patients with an existing tracheoesophageal or bronchoesophageal fistula.
- PDT is contraindicated in patients with tumors eroding into a major blood vessel.
- PDT is not suitable for emergency treatment of patients with severe acute respiratory distress caused by an obstructing endobronchial lesion because 40 to 50 hours are required between injection with PHOTOFRIN and laser light treatment.
- PDT is not suitable for patients with esophageal or gastric varices, or patients with esophageal ulcers >1 cm in diameter.

5 WARNINGS AND PRECAUTIONS

5.1 Esophageal Cancer

If the esophageal tumor is eroding into the trachea or bronchial tree, the likelihood of tracheoesophageal or bronchoesophageal fistula resulting from treatment is sufficiently high that photodynamic therapy (PDT) is not recommended.
Patients with esophageal varices should be treated with extreme caution. Light should not be given directly to the variceal area because of the high risk of bleeding.

5.2 Endobronchial Cancer

Patients should be assessed for the possibility that a tumor may be eroding into a pulmonary blood vessel *[see Contraindications (4)]*. Patients at high risk for fatal massive hemoptysis (FMH) include those with large, centrally located tumors, those with cavitating tumors or those with extensive tumor extrinsic to the bronchus.
If the endobronchial tumor invades deeply into the bronchial wall, the possibility exists for fistula formation upon resolution of tumor.
PDT should be used with extreme caution for endobronchial tumors in locations where treatment-induced inflammation could obstruct the main airway, e.g., long or circumferential tumors of the trachea, tumors of the carina that involve both mainstem bronchi circumferentially, or circumferential tumors in the mainstem bronchus in patients with prior pneumonectomy.

5.3 High-Grade Dysplasia (HGD) in Barrett's Esophagus (BE)

The long-term effect of PDT on HGD in BE is unknown. There is always a risk of cancer or abnormal epithelium that is invisible to the endoscopist beneath the new squamous cell epithelium; these facts emphasize the risk of overlooking cancer in such patients and the need for rigorous continuing surveillance despite the endoscopic appearance of complete squamous cell reepithelialization. It is recommended that endoscopic biopsy surveillance be conducted every three months, until four consecutive negative evaluations for HGD have been recorded; further follow-up may be scheduled every 6 to 12 months, as per judgment of physicians. The follow-up period of the randomized study at the time of analysis was a minimum of two years (ranging from 2 to 5.6 years).

5.4 Photosensitivity

All patients who receive PHOTOFRIN will be photosensitive and must observe precautions to avoid exposure of skin and eyes to direct sunlight or bright indoor light (from examination lamps, including dental lamps, operating room lamps, unshaded light bulbs at close proximity, etc.) for at least 30 days. Some patients may remain photosensitive for up to 90 days or more. The photosensitivity is due to residual drug, which will be present in all parts of the skin. Exposure of the skin to ambient indoor light is, however, beneficial because the remaining drug will be inactivated gradually and safely through a photobleaching reaction. Therefore, patients should not stay in a darkened room during this period and should be encouraged to expose their skin to ambient indoor light. The level of photosensitivity will vary for different areas of the body, depending on the extent of previous exposure to light. Before exposing any area of skin to direct sunlight or bright indoor light, the patient should test it for residual photosensitivity. A small area of skin should be exposed to sunlight for 10 minutes. If no photosensitivity reaction (erythema, edema, blistering) occurs within 24 hours, the patient can gradually resume normal outdoor activities, initially continuing to exercise caution and gradually allowing increased exposure. If some photosensitivity reaction occurs with the limited skin test, the patient should continue precautions for another 2 weeks before retesting. The tissue around the eyes may be more sensitive, and therefore, it is not recommended that the face be used for testing. If patients travel to a different geographical area with greater sunshine, they should retest their level of photosensitivity. Conventional ultraviolet (UV) sunscreens will only protect against UV light-related photosensitivity and will be of no value in protecting against induced photosensitivity reactions caused by visible light.

5.5 Ocular Sensitivity

Ocular discomfort, commonly described as sensitivity to sun, bright lights, or car headlights, has been reported in patients who received PHOTOFRIN. For 30 days, when outdoors, patients should wear dark sunglasses which have an average white light transmittance of <4%.

5.6 Use Before or After Radiotherapy

If PDT is to be used before or after radiotherapy, sufficient time should be allotted between the two therapies to ensure that the inflammatory response produced by the first treatment has subsided before commencing the second treatment. The inflammatory response from PDT will depend on tumor size and extent of surrounding normal tissue that receives light. It is recommended that 2 to 4 weeks be allowed after PDT before commencing radiotherapy. Similarly, if PDT is to be given after radiotherapy, the acute inflammatory reaction from radiotherapy usually subsides within 4 weeks after completing radiotherapy, after which PDT may be given.

5.7 Chest Pain

As a result of PDT treatment, patients may complain of substernal chest pain because of inflammatory responses within the area of treatment. Such pain may be of sufficient intensity to warrant the short-term prescription of opiate analgesics.

5.8 Respiratory Distress

Patients with endobronchial lesions must be closely monitored between the laser light therapy and the mandatory debridement bronchoscopy for any evidence of respiratory distress. Inflammation, mucositis, and necrotic debris may cause obstruction of the airway. If respiratory distress occurs, the physician should be prepared to carry out immediate bronchoscopy to remove secretions and debris to open the airway.

5.9 Esophageal Strictures

Esophageal strictures as a result of PDT of HGD in BE are common adverse reactions. An esophageal stricture was defined as a fixed lumen narrowing with solid food dysphagia and requiring dilation.
Regardless of the indication, esophageal strictures were reported in 122 of the 318 (38%) patients enrolled in the three clinical studies. Overall, esophageal strictures occurred within six months following PDT and were manageable through dilations. Multiple dilations of esophageal strictures may be required, as shown in **Table 5**. Special care should be taken during dilation to avoid perforation of the esophagus.
A high proportion of patients who developed an esophageal stricture received a nodule pretreatment prior to developing the event (49%) and/or had a mucosal segment treated twice (82%). Therefore, nodule pretreatment and re-treating the same mucosal segment more than once may influence the risk of developing an esophageal stricture.

5.10 Hepatic and Renal Impairment

Hepatic or Renal impairment will likely prolong the elimination of porfimer sodium leading to higher rates of toxicity. Patients with severe renal impairment or mild to severe hepatic impairment should be clearly informed that the period requiring the precautionary measures for photosensitivity may be longer than 90 days.

TABLE 5. Esophageal Dilations in Patients with Treatment-Related Strictures

Number of Dilations	Number of Patients with Strictures N=114	Percentage of Patients with Strictures
1–2 Dilations	32	28%
3–5 Dilations	32	28%
6–10 Dilations	24	21%
>10 Dilations	26	23%

6 ADVERSE REACTIONS

6.1 Overall Adverse Reaction Profile

Systemically induced effects of photodynamic therapy (PDT) with PHOTOFRIN consist of photosensitivity and mild constipation. All patients who receive PHOTOFRIN will be photosensitive and must observe precautions to avoid sunlight and bright indoor light *[see Warnings and Precautions (5.4)]*. Photosensitivity reactions occurred in approximately 20% of cancer patients and in 69% of high-grade dysplasia (HGD) in Barrett's esophagus (BE) patients treated with PHOTOFRIN. Typically these reactions were mostly mild to moderate erythema but they also included swelling, pruritus, burning sensation, feeling hot, or blisters. In a single study of 24 healthy subjects, some evidence of photosensitivity reactions occurred in all subjects. Other less common skin manifestations were also reported in areas where photosensitivity reactions had occurred, such as increased hair growth, skin discoloration, skin nodule, skin wrinkling and increased skin fragility. These manifestations may be attributable to a pseudoporphyria state (temporary drug-induced cutaneous porphyria).
Most toxicities of this therapy are local effects seen in the region of illumination and occasionally in surrounding tissues. The local adverse reactions are characteristic of an inflammatory response induced by the photodynamic effect.

A few cases of fluid imbalance have been reported in patients treated with PHOTOFRIN PDT for overtly disseminated intraperitoneal malignancies. Fluid imbalance is an expected PDT-related event.

A case of cataracts has been reported in a 51 year-old obese man treated with PHOTOFRIN PDT for HGD in BE. The patient suffered from a PDT response with development of a deep esophageal ulcer. Within two months post PDT, the patient noted difficulty with his distant vision. A thorough eye examination revealed a change in the refractive error that later progressed to cataracts in both eyes. Both of his parents had a history of cataracts in their 70s. Whether PHOTOFRIN directly caused or accelerated a familial underlying condition is unknown.

6.2 Adverse Reactions in Clinical Trials

Because clinical trials are conducted under widely varying conditions, adverse reaction rates observed in the clinical trials of a drug cannot be directly compared to rates in the clinical trials of another drug and may not reflect the rates observed in practice.

Esophageal Carcinoma

The following adverse reactions were reported over the entire follow-up period in at least 5% of patients treated with PHOTOFRIN PDT, who had completely or partially obstructing esophageal cancer. Table 6 presents data from 88 patients who received the currently marketed formulation. The relationship of many of these adverse reactions to PDT with PHOTOFRIN is uncertain.

TABLE 6. Adverse Reactions Reported in 5% or More of Patients* with Obstructing Esophageal Cancer

SYSTEM ORGAN CLASS/ Adverse Reaction	N=88 n(%)
Patients with at Least One Adverse Reaction	84 (95)
BLOOD and LYMPHATIC SYSTEM DISORDERS	
Anemia	28 (32)
CARDIAC DISORDERS	
Atrial fibrillation	9 (10)
Cardiac failure	6 (7)
Tachycardia	5 (6)
GASTROINTESTINAL DISORDERS	
Constipation	21 (24)
Nausea	21 (24)
Abdominal pain	18 (20)
Vomiting	15 (17)
Dysphagia	9 (10)
Esophageal edema	7 (8)
Hematemesis	7 (8)
Dyspepsia	5 (6)
Esophageal stenosis	5 (6)
Diarrhea	4 (5)
Esophagitis	4 (5)
Eructation	4 (5)
Melena	4 (5)
GENERAL DISORDERS & ADMINISTRATION SITE CONDITIONS	
Pyrexia	27 (31)
Chest pain	19 (22)
Pain	19 (22)
Edema peripheral	6 (7)
Asthenia	5 (6)
Chest pain (substernal)	4 (5)
Edema generalized	4 (5)
INFECTIONS AND INFESTATIONS	
Candidiasis	8 (9)
Urinary tract infection	6 (7)
INJURY, POISONING and PROCEDURAL COMPLICATIONS	
Post procedural complication	4 (5)
INVESTIGATIONS	
Weight decreased	8 (9)
METABOLISM and NUTRITION DISORDERS	
Anorexia	7 (8)
Dehydration	6 (7)
MUSCULOSKELETAL and CONNECTIVE TISSUE DISORDERS	
Back pain	10 (11)
NEOPLASMS BENIGN, MALIGNANT and UNSPECIFIED	
Tumor hemorrhage	7 (8)
PSYCHIATRIC DISORDERS	
Insomnia	12 (14)
Confusional state	7 (8)
Anxiety	6 (7)
RESPIRATORY, THORACIC and MEDIASTINAL DISORDERS	
Pleural effusion	28 (32)
Dyspnoea	18 (20)
Pneumonia	16 (18)
Pharyngitis	10 (11)
Respiratory insufficiency	9 (10)
Cough	6 (7)
Tracheoesophageal fistula	5 (6)
SKIN and SUBCUTANEOUS TISSUE DISORDERS	
Photosensitivity reaction	17 (19)
VASCULAR DISORDERS	
Hypotension	6 (7)
Hypertension	5 (6)

*Based on adverse reactions reported at any time during the entire period of follow-up.

Location of the tumor was a prognostic factor for three adverse reactions: upper-third of the esophagus (esophageal edema), middle-third (atrial fibrillation), and lower-third, the most vascular region (anemia). Also, patients with large tumors (>10 cm) were more likely to experience anemia. Two of 17 patients with complete esophageal obstruction from tumor experienced esophageal perforations, which were considered to be possibly treatment-associated; these perforations occurred during subsequent endoscopies.

Serious and other notable adverse reactions observed in less than 5% of PDT-treated patients with obstructing esophageal cancer in the clinical studies include the following; their relationship to therapy is uncertain. In the gastrointestinal system, esophageal perforation, gastric ulcer, ileus, jaundice, and peritonitis have occurred. Sepsis has been reported occasionally. Cardiovascular reactions have included angina pectoris, bradycardia, myocardial infarction, sick sinus syndrome, and supraventricular tachycardia. Respiratory reactions of bronchitis, bronchospasm, laryngotracheal edema, pneumonitis, pulmonary hemorrhage, pulmonary edema, respiratory failure, and stridor have occurred. The temporal relationship of some gastrointestinal, cardiovascular and respiratory reactions to the administration of light was suggestive of mediastinal inflammation in some patients. Vision-related reactions of abnormal vision, diplopia, eye pain and photophobia have been reported.

Obstructing Endobronchial Cancer

Table 7 presents adverse reactions that were reported over the entire follow-up period in at least 5% of patients with obstructing endobronchial cancer treated with PHOTOFRIN PDT or Nd:YAG. These data are based on the 86 patients who received the currently marketed formula-

TABLE 7. Adverse Reactions Reported in 5% or More of Patients with Obstructing Endobronchial Cancer

SYSTEM ORGAN CLASS/ Adverse Reaction	Within 30 Days of Treatment PDT N=86 n (%)	Within 30 Days of Treatment Nd:YAG N=86 n (%)	Entire Follow-up Period* PDT N=86 n (%)	Entire Follow-up Period* Nd:YAG N=86 n (%)
Patients with at Least One Adverse Reaction	43 (50)	33 (38)	62 (72)	48 (56)
GASTROINTESTINAL DISORDERS				
Dyspepsia	1 (1)	4 (5)	2 (2)	5 (6)
Constipation	4 (5)	1 (1)	4 (5)	2 (2)
GENERAL DISORDERS and ADMINISTRATION SITE CONDITIONS				
Pyrexia	7 (8)	7 (8)	14 (16)	8 (9)
Chest pain	6 (7)	6 (7)	7 (8)	8 (9)
Pain	1 (1)	4 (5)	4 (5)	8 (9)
Edema peripheral	3 (3)	3 (3)	4 (5)	3 (3)
MUSCULOSKELETAL and CONNECTIVE TISSUE DISORDERS				
Back pain	3 (3)	1 (1)	3 (3)	5 (6)
NERVOUS SYSTEM DISORDERS				
Dysphonia	3 (3)	2 (2)	4 (5)	2 (2)
PSYCHIATRIC DISORDERS				
Insomnia	4 (5)	2 (2)	4 (5)	3 (4)
Anxiety	3 (3)	0 (0)	5 (6)	0 (0)
RESPIRATORY, THORACIC and MEDIASTINAL DISORDERS				
Dyspnoea	15 (17)	7 (8)	26 (30)	13 (15)
Cough	5 (6)	8 (9)	13 (15)	11 (13)
Hemoptysis	6 (7)	5 (6)	14 (16)	7 (8)
Pneumonia	5 (6)	4 (5)	10 (12)	5 (6)
Bronchitis	9 (10)	2 (2)	9 (10)	2 (2)
Productive cough	4 (5)	5 (6)	7 (8)	6 (7)
Respiratory insufficiency	0 (0)	0 (0)	5 (6)	1 (1)
Pleural effusion	0 (0)	0 (0)	4 (5)	1 (1)
Pneumothorax	0 (0)	0 (0)	0 (0)	4 (5)
SKIN and SUBCUTANEOUS TISSUE DISORDERS				
Photosensitivity reaction	16 (19)	0 (0)	18 (21)	0 (0)

*Follow-up was 33% longer for the PDT group than for the Nd:YAG group, introducing a bias against PDT when adverse reactions are compared for the entire follow-up period.

tion. Since it seems likely that most adverse reactions caused by these acute acting therapies would occur within 30 days of treatment, Table 7 presents those reactions occurring within 30 days of a treatment procedure, as well as those occurring over the entire follow-up period. It should be noted that follow-up was 33% longer for the PDT group than for the Nd:YAG group, thereby introducing a bias against PDT when adverse reaction rates are compared for the entire follow-up period. The extent of follow-up in the 30-day period following treatment was comparable between groups (only 9% more for PDT).

Transient inflammatory reactions in PDT-treated patients occur in about 10% of patients and manifest as pyrexia, bronchitis, chest pain, and dyspnoea. The incidences of bronchitis and dyspnoea were higher with PDT than with Nd:YAG. Most cases of bronchitis occurred within 1 week of treatment and all but one were mild or moderate in intensity. The reactions usually resolved within 10 days with antibiotic therapy. Treatment-related worsening of dyspnoea is generally transient and self-limiting. Debridement of the treated area is mandatory to remove exudate and necrotic tissue. Life-threatening respiratory insufficiency likely due to therapy occurred in 3% of PDT-treated patients and 2% of Nd:YAG-treated patients [see Warnings and Precautions (5.8)].

There was a trend toward a higher rate of fatal massive hemoptysis (FMH) occurring on the PDT arm (10%) versus the Nd:YAG arm (5%), however, the rate of FMH occurring within 30 days of treatment was the same for PDT and Nd:YAG (4% total events, 3% treatment-associated events). Patients who have received radiation therapy have a higher incidence of FMH after treatment with PDT and after other forms of local therapy than patients who have not received radiation therapy, but analyses suggest that this increased risk may be due to associated prognostic factors such as having a centrally located tumor. The incidence of FMH in patients previously treated with radiotherapy was 21% (6/29) in the PDT group and 10% (3/29) in the Nd:YAG group. In patients with no prior radiotherapy, the overall incidence of FMH was less than 1%. Characteristics of patients at high risk for FMH are described in Contraindications (4) and Warnings and Precautions (5.2).

Other serious or notable adverse reactions were observed in less than 5% of PDT-treated patients with endobronchial cancer; their relationship to therapy is uncertain. In the respiratory system, pulmonary thrombosis, pulmonary embo-

lism, and lung abscess have occurred. Cardiac failure, sepsis, and possible cerebrovascular accident have also been reported in one patient each.
[See table 7 at top of previous page]
Superficial Endobronchial Tumors
The following adverse reactions were reported over the entire follow-up period in at least 5% of patients with superficial tumors (microinvasive or carcinoma *in situ*) who received the currently marketed formulation.

TABLE 8. Adverse Reactions Reported in 5% or More of Patients* with Superficial Endobronchial Tumors

Adverse Reaction	N=90	n(%)
Patients with at Least One Adverse Reaction	44	(49)
RESPIRATORY, THORACIC and MEDIASTINAL DISORDERS		
Exudate	20	(22)
Bronchial mucus plug or bronchial obstruction	19	(21)
Edema	16	(18)
Bronchostenosis	10	(11)
Bronchial ulceration	8	(9)
Cough	8	(9)
Dyspnoea	6	(7)
SKIN and SUBCUTANEOUS TISSUE DISORDERS		
Photosensitivity reaction	20	(22)

*Based on adverse reactions reported at any time during the entire period of follow-up.

In patients with superficial endobronchial tumors, 44 of 90 patients (49%) experienced an adverse reaction, two-thirds of which were related to the respiratory system. The most common reaction to therapy was a mucositis reaction in one-fifth of the patients, which manifested as edema, exudate, and obstruction. The obstruction (mucus plug) is easily removed with suction or forceps. Mucositis can be minimized by avoiding exposure of normal tissue to excessive light *[see Warnings and Precautions (5.8)]*. Three patients experienced life-threatening dyspnoea: one was given a double dose of light, one was treated concurrently in both mainstem bronchi and the other had had prior pneumonectomy and was treated in the sole remaining main airway *[see Warnings and Precautions (5.2)]*. Stent placement was required in 3% of the patients due to endobronchial stricture. Fatal massive hemoptysis occurred within 30 days of treatment in one patient with superficial tumors (1%).
High-Grade Dysplasia (HGD) in Barrett's Esophagus (BE)
Table 9 presents adverse reactions that were reported over the follow-up period in at least 5% of patients with HGD in BE in either controlled or uncontrolled clinical trials.
In the PHOTOFRIN PDT + OM group severe adverse reactions included chest pain of non-cardiac origin, dysphagia, nausea, vomiting, regurgitation, and heartburn. The severity of these symptoms decreased within 4 to 6 weeks following treatment.
The majority of the photosensitivity reactions occurred within 90 days following PHOTOFRIN injection and was of mild (68%) or moderate (24%) intensity. Fourteen (10%) patients reported severe reactions, all of which resolved. The typical reaction was described as skin disorder, sunburn or rash, and affected mostly the face, hands, and neck. Associated symptoms and signs were swelling, pruritis, erythema, blisters, burning sensation, and feeling of heat.
The majority of esophageal stenosis including strictures reported in the PHOTOFRIN PDT + OM group were of mild (57%) or moderate (35%) intensity, while approximately 8% were of severe intensity. The majority of esophageal strictures were reported during Course 2 of treatment. All esophageal strictures were considered to be due to treatment. Most esophageal strictures were manageable through dilations *[see Warnings and Precautions (5.9)]*.
[See table 9 at top right]
Laboratory Abnormalities
In patients with esophageal cancer, PDT with PHOTOFRIN may result in anemia due to tumor bleeding. No significant effects were observed for other parameters in patients with endobronchial carcinoma or with HGD in BE.

7 DRUG INTERACTIONS
7.1 Other Photosensitizing Agents
There have been no formal interaction studies of PHOTOFRIN and any other drugs. However, it is possible that concomitant use of other photosensitizing agents (e.g., tetracyclines, sulfonamides, phenothiazines, sulfonylurea hypoglycemic agents, thiazide diuretics, griseofulvin, and fluoroquinolones) could increase the risk of photosensitivity reaction.
7.2 Concomitant Therapy
Photodynamic therapy (PDT) with PHOTOFRIN causes direct intracellular damage by initiating radical chain reac-

Table 9. Adverse Reactions Reported in ≥5% of Patients Treated with PHOTOFRIN PDT in the Clinical Trials on High-Grade Dysplasia in Barrett's Esophagus

SYSTEM ORGAN CLASS/Adverse Reaction	HGD* PHOPDT +OM	HGD†OM Only	Other‡ PHOPDT +OM	Total PHOPDT +OM
	N=219 n(%)	N=69 n(%)	N=99 n(%)	N=318 n(%)
Patients with at Least One Adverse Reaction	206 (94)	9 (13)	97 (98)	303 (95)
GASTROINTESTINAL DISORDERS	163 (74)	6 (9)	83 (84)	246 (77)
Nausea	57 (26)	1 (1)	61 (62)	118 (37)
Vomiting	63 (29)	1 (1)	34 (34)	97 (31)
Esophageal Stricture§	81 (37)	0	33 (33)	114 (36)
Esophageal Narrowing¶	71 (32)	4 (6)	24 (24)	95 (30)
Dysphagia	49 (22)	0	26 (26)	75 (24)
Constipation	25 (11)	1 (1)	7 (7)	32 (10)
Abdominal pain (Upper, lower, NOS)	11 (5)	1 (1)	6 (6)	17 (5)
Esophageal pain	13 (6)	0	9 (9)	22 (7)
Dyspepsia	10 (5)	0	4 (4)	14 (4)
Hiccups	16 (7)	0	1 (1)	17 (5)
Odynophagia	13 (6)	0	4 (4)	17 (5)
GENERAL and ADMINISTRATION SITE CONDITIONS	110 (50)	0	62 (63)	172 (54)
Chest pain	63 (29)	0	37 (37)	100 (31)
Pyrexia	41 (19)	0	13 (13)	54 (17)
Chest discomfort	13 (6)	0	19 (19)	32 (10)
Pain	11 (5)	0	7 (7)	18 (6)
INJURY, POISONING and PROCEDURAL COMPLICATIONS	24 (11)	0	19 (19)	43 (14)
Post procedural pain	14 (6)	0	14 (14)	28 (9)
INVESTIGATIONS	24 (11)	0	11 (11)	35 (11)
Weight decreased	15 (7)	0	2 (2)	17 (5)
METABOLISM and NUTRITION DISORDERS	28 (13)	0	16 (16)	44 (14)
Dehydration	24 (11)	0	8 (8)	32 (10)
RESPIRATORY, THORACIC and MEDIASTINAL DISORDERS	35 (16)	0	18 (18)	53 (17)
Pleural effusion	22 (10)	0	15 (15)	37 (12)
SKIN and SUBCUTANEOUS TISSUE DISORDERS	115 (53)	1 (1)	28 (28)	143 (45)
Photosensitivity reaction	102 (47)	0	16 (16)	118 (37)

* Includes all HGD patients in the Safety population from PHO BAR 02 (N=133), TCSC 93-07 (N=44), and TCSC 96-01 (N=42).
† Includes all HGD patients in the Safety population from PHO BAR 02 (N=69).
‡ Includes patients with Barrett's metaplasia, indefinite dysplasia, LGD, and adenocarcinoma at baseline in the Safety population from TCSC 93-07 (N=55) and TCSC 96-01 (N=44).
§ Esophageal stricture was defined as a dilated esophageal stenosis.
¶ Esophageal narrowing was defined as an undilated esophageal stenosis.
PHO: PHOTOFRIN
NOTE: Adverse reactions classified using MedDRA 5.0 dictionary with the exception of esophageal stricture and esophageal narrowing.

tions that damage intracellular membranes and mitochondria. Tissue damage also results from ischemia secondary to vasoconstriction, platelet activation and aggregation and clotting. Research in animals and in cell culture has suggested that many drugs could influence the effects of PDT, possible examples of which are described below. There are no human data that support or rebut these possibilities.
Compounds that quench active oxygen species or scavenge radicals, such as dimethyl sulfoxide, β-carotene, ethanol, formate and mannitol would be expected to decrease PDT activity. Preclinical data also suggest that tissue ischemia, allopurinol, calcium channel blockers and some prostaglandin synthesis inhibitors could interfere with PHOTOFRIN PDT. Drugs that decrease clotting, vasoconstriction or platelet aggregation, e.g., thromboxane A_2 inhibitors, could decrease the efficacy of PDT. Glucocorticoid hormones given before or concomitant with PDT may decrease the efficacy of the treatment.

8 USE IN SPECIFIC POPULATIONS
8.1 Pregnancy
Pregnancy Category C. There are no adequate and well-controlled studies of PHOTOFRIN in pregnant women. Porfimer sodium had an embryocidal effect in rats and rabbits at maternal doses 0.64 times the recommended human dose on a mg/m² basis. PHOTOFRIN should be used during pregnancy only if the potential benefit justifies the potential risk to the fetus.
Porfimer sodium given to rat dams during fetal organogenesis intravenously at 0.64 times the clinical dose on a mg/m² basis for 10 days caused no major malformations or developmental changes. This dose caused maternal and fetal toxicity resulting in increased resorptions, decreased litter size, delayed ossification, and reduced fetal weight. Porfimer sodium caused no major malformations when given to rabbits intravenously during organogenesis at 0.65 times the clinical dose on a mg/m² basis for 13 days. This dose caused maternal toxicity resulting in increased resorptions, decreased litter size, and reduced fetal body weight.

Porfimer sodium given to rats during late pregnancy through lactation intravenously at 0.32 times the clinical dose on a mg/m² basis for at least 42 days caused a reversible decrease in growth of offspring. Parturition was unaffected.
8.3 Nursing Mothers
It is not known whether PHOTOFRIN is excreted in human milk. Because many drugs are excreted in human milk and because of the potential for serious adverse reactions in nursing infants from PHOTOFRIN, a decision should be made whether not to treat or to discontinue breastfeeding, taking into account the importance of the drug to the mother.
8.4 Pediatric Use
Safety and effectiveness in children have not been established.
8.5 Geriatric Use
Approximately 70% of the patients treated with PDT using PHOTOFRIN in clinical trials were over 60 years of age. There was no apparent difference in effectiveness or safety in these patients compared to younger people. Dose modification based upon age is not required.

10 OVERDOSAGE
10.1 PHOTOFRIN Overdose
There is no information on overdosage situations involving PHOTOFRIN. Higher than recommended drug doses of two 2 mg/kg doses given two days apart (10 patients) and three 2 mg/kg doses given within two weeks (one patient), were tolerated without notable adverse reactions. Effects of overdosage on the duration of photosensitivity are unknown. Laser treatment should not be given if an overdose of PHOTOFRIN is administered. In the event of an overdose, patients should protect their eyes and skin from direct sunlight or bright indoor lights for 30 days. At this time, patients should test for residual photosensitivity *[see Warnings and Precautions (5.4)]*. PHOTOFRIN is not dialyzable.
10.2 Overdose of Laser Light Following PHOTOFRIN Injection
Light doses of two to three times the recommended dose have been administered to a few patients with superficial

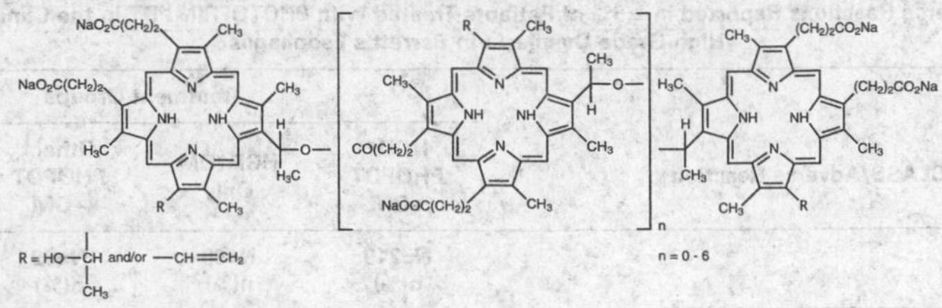

Figure 1 Structure of Porfimer Sodium

endobronchial tumors. One patient experienced life-threatening dyspnoea and the others had no notable complications. Increased symptoms and damage to normal tissue might be expected following an overdose of light. There is no information on overdose of laser light following PHOTOFRIN injection in patients with esophageal cancer or in patients with high-grade dysplasia in Barrett's esophagus.

11 DESCRIPTION

PHOTOFRIN (porfimer sodium) for Injection is a photosensitizing agent used in the photodynamic therapy (PDT) of tumors and of high-grade dysplasia (HGD) in Barrett's esophagus (BE). Following reconstitution of the freeze-dried product with 5% Dextrose Injection (USP) or 0.9% Sodium Chloride Injection (USP), it is injected intravenously. This is followed 40-50 hours later by illumination of the tumor or the esophageal segment with HGD in BE with laser light (630 nm wavelength). PHOTOFRIN is not a single chemical entity; it is a mixture of oligomers formed by ether and ester linkages of up to eight porphyrin units. It is a dark red to reddish brown cake or powder. Each vial of PHOTOFRIN contains 75 mg of porfimer sodium as a sterile freeze-dried cake or powder. Hydrochloric Acid and/or Sodium Hydroxide may be added during manufacture to adjust the pH to within 7.2-7.9. There are no preservatives or other additives. The structural formula below is representative of the components present in PHOTOFRIN.

[See chemical structure above]

12 CLINICAL PHARMACOLOGY

12.1 Mechanism of Action

Cellular damage caused by photodynamic therapy (PDT) with PHOTOFRIN is a consequence of the propagation of radical reactions. Radical initiation may occur after porfimer sodium absorbs light to form a porphyrin excited state. Spin transfer from porfimer sodium to molecular oxygen may then generate singlet oxygen. Subsequent radical reactions can form superoxide and hydroxyl radicals. Tumor death also occurs through ischemic necrosis secondary to vascular occlusion that appears to be partly mediated by thromboxane A_2 release. As opposed to a thermal effect, the laser treatment with porfimer sodium induces a photochemical effect. The necrotic reaction and associated inflammatory responses may evolve over several days.

12.2 Pharmacodynamics

The cytotoxic and antitumor actions of PHOTOFRIN are light and oxygen dependent. PDT with PHOTOFRIN is a two-stage process. The first stage is the intravenous injection of PHOTOFRIN. Clearance from a variety of tissues occurs over 40-72 hours, but tumors, skin, and organs of the reticuloendothelial system (including liver and spleen) retain PHOTOFRIN for a longer period. Illumination with 630 nm wavelength laser light constitutes the second stage of therapy. Tumor selectivity in treatment occurs through a combination of selective retention of PHOTOFRIN and selective delivery of light.

12.3 Pharmacokinetics

Following a 2 mg/kg dose of PHOTOFRIN to 4 male cancer patients, the average peak plasma concentration was 15 ± 3 mcg/mL, the elimination half-life was 250 ± 285 hours, the steady-state volume of distribution was 0.49 ± 0.28 L/kg, and the total plasma clearance was 0.051 ± 0.035 mL/min/kg. The mean plasma concentration at 48 hours was 2.6 ± 0.4 mcg/mL. The influence of impaired hepatic function on PHOTOFRIN disposition has not been evaluated.

PHOTOFRIN was approximately 90% protein bound in human serum, studied *in vitro*. The binding was independent of concentration over the concentration range of 20-100 mcg/mL.

The pharmacokinetics of PHOTOFRIN was also studied in 24 healthy subjects (12 men and 12 women) who received a single dose of 2 mg/kg PHOTOFRIN given via the intravenous route. The serum decay was bi-exponential, with a slow distribution phase and a very long elimination phase. The elimination half-life was 415 ± 104 hours (17 ± 4.3 days). The C_{max} was determined to be 40 ± 11.6 mcg/mL and AUC_{inf} was 2400 ± 552 mcg•hour/mL. Women had a lower C_{max} and a higher AUC. The clinical significance of these differences is unknown. The T_{max} was approximately 1.5 hours in women and 0.17 hours in men. At the time of intended photoactivation 40-50 hours after injection, the pharmacokinetic profiles of PHOTOFRIN in men and women were similar.

13 NONCLINICAL TOXICOLOGY

13.1 Carcinogenesis, Mutagenesis, Impairment of Fertility

No long-term studies have been conducted to evaluate the carcinogenic potential of porfimer sodium. In the presence of light, *in vitro*, porfimer sodium PDT did not cause mutations in the Ames test, nor did it cause chromosome aberrations or mutations (HGPRT locus) in Chinese hamster ovary (CHO) cells. Porfimer sodium PDT caused <2-fold, but significant, increases in sister chromatid exchange in CHO cells irradiated with visible light and a 3-fold increase in Chinese hamster lung fibroblasts irradiated with near UV light. Porfimer sodium PDT caused an increase in thymidine kinase mutants and DNA-protein cross-links in mouse L5178Y cells, but not mouse LYR83 cells. Porfimer sodium PDT caused a light-dose dependant increase in DNA-strand breaks in malignant human cervical carcinoma cells, but not in normal cells. In the absence of light, porfimer sodium was negative in a Chinese hamster ovarian cells (CHO/HGPRT) mutation test. *In vivo*, porfimer sodium did not cause chromosomal aberrations in the mouse micronucleus test. Porfimer sodium given to male and female rats intravenously, at 4 mg/kg/d (0.32 times the clinical dose on a mg/m^2 basis) before conception and through Day 7 of pregnancy caused no impairment of fertility. In this study, long-term dosing with porfimer sodium caused discoloration of testes and ovaries and hypertrophy of the testes. Porfimer sodium also caused decreased body weight in the parent rats.

14 CLINICAL STUDIES

Clinical studies of photodynamic therapy (PDT) with PHOTOFRIN were conducted in patients with obstructing esophageal and endobronchial non-small-cell lung cancers, in patients with early-stage radiologically occult endobronchial cancer, and in patients with high-grade dysplasia (HGD) in Barrett's esophagus (BE). In all clinical studies, the method of PDT administration was essentially identical. A course of therapy consisted of one injection of PHOTOFRIN (2 mg/kg administered as a slow intravenous injection over 3–5 minutes) followed by up to two non-thermal applications of 630 nm laser light. Light doses of 300 J/cm of diffuser length were used in esophageal cancer. Light doses of 200 J/cm of diffuser length were used in endobronchial cancer for both palliation of obstructing cancer and treatment of superficial lesions. For the ablation of HGD in BE, the light dose administered was 130 J/cm of diffuser length using a centering balloon for the first application and 50 J/cm of diffuser length without a centering balloon for the second application *[see Dosage and Administration (2.2)]*. In all cases, the first application of light occurred 40–50 hours after PHOTOFRIN injection.

For treatment of esophageal cancer debridement of residua via endoscopy is optional 96–120 hours after injection, after which any residual tumor could be retreated with a second laser light application at the same light dose used for the initial treatment. Additional courses of PDT with PHOTOFRIN were allowed after one month, up to a maximum of three courses.

For treatment of endobronchial cancer, debridement of residua was performed via bronchoscopy 96–120 hours after injection, after which any residual tumor could be retreated with a second laser light application at the same light dose used for the initial treatment. Additional courses of PDT with PHOTOFRIN were allowed after one month, up to a maximum of three courses.

For ablation of HGD in BE, a second laser light application of 50 J/cm of diffuser length without a centering balloon could be given 96-120 hours after the PHOTOFRIN injection for untreated areas ("skip" areas). Additional courses of PDT with PHOTOFRIN were allowed after three months, up to a maximum of three courses.

14.1 Esophageal Cancer

PDT with PHOTOFRIN was utilized in a multicenter, single-arm study in 17 patients with completely obstructing esophageal carcinoma. Assessments were made at 1 week and 1 month after the last treatment procedure. As shown in **Table 10**, after a single course of therapy, 94% of patients obtained an objective tumor response and 76% of patients experienced some palliation of their dysphagia. On average, before treatment these patients had difficulty swallowing liquids, even saliva. After one course of therapy, there was a statistically significant improvement in mean dysphagia grade (1.5 units, p <0.05) and 13 of 17 patients could swallow liquids without difficulty 1 week and/or 1 month after treatment. Based on all courses, three patients achieved a complete tumor response (CR). In two of these patients, the CR was documented only at Week 1 as they had no further assessments. The third patient achieved a CR after a second course of therapy, which was supported by negative histopathology and maintained for the entire follow-up of 6 months.

Of the 17 treated patients, 11 (65%) received clinically important benefit from PDT. Clinically important benefit was defined hierarchically as a complete tumor response (3 patients), achievement of normal swallowing (2 patients went from Grade 5 dysphagia to Grade 1), or achievement of a marked improvement of two or more grades of dysphagia with minimal adverse reactions (6 patients). The median duration of benefit in these patients was 69 days. Duration of benefit was calculated only for the period with documented evidence of improvement. All of these patients were still in response at their last assessment and, therefore, the estimate of 69 days is conservative. The median survival for these 11 patients was 115 days.

14.2 Endobronchial Cancer

Two randomized multicenter Phase III studies were conducted to compare the safety and efficacy of PHOTOFRIN PDT versus Nd:YAG laser therapy for reduction of obstruction and palliation of symptomatic patients with partially or completely obstructing endobronchial non-small-cell lung cancer. Assessments were made at 1 week and at monthly intervals after treatment. **Table 11** shows the results from all randomized patients in the two studies combined. Objective tumor response rates (CR + PR), which demonstrate reduction of obstruction, were 59% for PDT and 58% for Nd:YAG at Week 1. The response rate at 1 month or later was 60% for PDT and 41% for Nd:YAG.

Patient symptoms were evaluated using a 5- or 6-grade pulmonary symptom severity rating scale for dyspnoea, cough, and hemoptysis. Patients with moderate to severe symptoms are those most in need of palliation. Improvements of 2 or more grades are considered to be clinically significant. **Table 12** shows the percentages of patients with moderate to severe symptoms at baseline who demonstrated a 2-grade improvement at any time during the interval evaluated.

TABLE 10. Course 1 Efficacy Results in Patients with Completely Obstructing Esophageal Cancer

EFFICACY PARAMETER	PDT N=17
OBJECTIVE TUMOR RESPONSE* (% of patients)	
Week 1	82%
Month 1	35%†
Any assessment‡	94%
IMPROVEMENT§ IN DYSPHAGIA (% of patients)	
Week 1	71%
Month 1	47%
Any assessment‡	76%
MEAN DYSPHAGIA GRADE¶ AT BASELINE (units)	4.6
MEAN IMPROVEMENT¶ IN DYSPHAGIA GRADE (units)	
Week 1	1.4
Month 1	1.5
MEAN NUMBER OF LASER APPLICATIONS (units)	1.4

* CR+PR, CR = complete response (absence of endoscopically visible tumor), PR = partial response (appearance of a visible lumen).

† Eight of the 17 treated patients did not have assessments at Month 1.

‡ Week 1 or Month 1.

§ Patients with at least a one-grade improvement in dysphagia grade.

¶ Dysphagia Scale: Grade 1 = normal swallowing, Grade 2 = difficulty swallowing some hard solids; can swallow semisolids, Grade 3 = unable to swallow any solids; can swallow liquids, Grade 4 = difficulty swallowing liquids, Grade 5 = unable to swallow saliva.

TABLE 11. Efficacy Results from Studies in Late-stage Obstructing Endobronchial Cancer—All Randomized Patients*

EFFICACY PARAMETER	PDT N=102 (% of Patients)	Nd:YAG N=109 (% of Patients)
OBJECTIVE TUMOR RESPONSE[†]		
Week 1	59%	58%
Month 1 or later	60%	41%*
ATELECTASIS IMPROVEMENT[‡]	n=60	n=71
Week 1	35%	18%
Month 1 or later	35%	20%

* Statistical comparisons were precluded by the amount of missing data at Month 1 or later (e.g. for tumor response, PDT 28% missing, Nd:YAG 38%).
† CR+PR, CR = complete response (absence of bronchoscopically visible tumor), PR = partial response (increase of ≥50% in the smallest luminal diameter or any appearance of a lumen for completely obstructing tumors).
‡ In patients with atelectasis at baseline.

TABLE 12. Efficacy Results from Studies in Late-stage Obstructing Endobronchial Cancer – Clinically Significant Improvements in Patients with Moderate to Severe Symptoms at Baseline*

CLINICALLY SIGNIFICANT SYMPTOM IMPROVEMENT[†]	PDT N=102 (% of Patients)	Nd:YAG N=109 (% of Patients)
ANY SYMPTOM	n=89	n=89
Week 1	25%	29%
Month 1 or later	40%	27%*
DYSPNOEA	n=60	n=68
Week 1	15%	18%
Month 1 or later	23%	13%
COUGH	n=63	n=65
Week 1	6%	9%
Month 1 or later	24%	8%
HEMOPTYSIS	n=24	n=31
Week 1	58%	29%
Month 1 or later	79%	35%

* Statistical comparisons were precluded by the amount of missing data at Month 1 or later.
† Dyspnoea was graded on a 6-point severity rating scale; cough and hemoptysis on a 5-point scale. Clinically significant improvement was defined as a change of at least two grades from baseline.

In a separate retrospective analysis, patients were individually evaluated to identify those patients whose benefit to risk ratio was most favorable, i.e., those who obtained clinically important benefit with minimal adverse reactions. Clinically important benefit was defined as one of the following:
1. A substantial improvement in pulmonary symptoms at Month 1 or later (dyspnea ≥2 grades, hemoptysis ≥3 grades, cough ≥3 grades or increase in FEV$_1$ ≥40%);
2. A moderate improvement in symptoms at Month 2 or later (dyspnea 1 grade, cough 2 grades, hemoptysis 2 grades or increase in FEV$_1$ ≥20%); or
3. A durable objective tumor response (CR or PR maintained to Month 2 or longer).

Thirty-six (36) of the 99 PDT-treated patients (36%) and 23 of the 99 Nd:YAG-treated patients (23%) received clinically important benefit with only minimal or moderate toxicities of short duration. Thirty-four of 99 PDT-treated patients demonstrated improvements in 2 or more efficacy endpoints (dyspnoea, cough, hemoptysis, sputum, atelectasis, pulmonary function tests of FEV$_1$ or FVC, Karnofsky Performance Score or tumor response) and 29 patients had improvements in 3 or more.

The median duration of documented benefit in the 36 patients was 63 days. In these patients with late-stage obstructing lung cancer, median survival was 174 days in PDT-treated patients and 161 days in Nd: YAG-treated patients.

The efficacy of PHOTOFRIN PDT was also evaluated in the treatment of microinvasive endobronchial tumors in 62 inoperable patients in three noncomparative studies. Microinvasive lung cancer is defined histologically as disease, which invades beyond the basement membrane but not through or into the cartilage. For 11 of the 62 patients, it was clearly documented that surgery and radiotherapy were not indicated. These 11 patients were all inoperable for medical or technical reasons. Radiotherapy was not indicated due to

TABLE 13. Overall Efficacy Results in Patients with Superficial Endobronchial Tumors

EFFICACY PARAMETER	PDT n =11	PDT n=62
COMPLETE TUMOR RESPONSE, BIOPSY-PROVEN AT 3 MONTHS		
Number of Patients (%)	3 (27)	31 (50)*
TIME TO TUMOR RECURRENCE IN PATIENTS WITH COMPLETE RESPONSE		
Number of Patients (%) with Recurrences	1 (33)	11 (35)
Median Time to Tumor Recurrence		>2.7 years
[95% Confidence Interval]		[1.6,—†]
SURVIVAL		
Number of Patients (%) who Died of Any Cause	4 (36)	32 (52)
Median Survival		2.9 years
[95% Confidence Interval]		[2.1, 5.7]
DISEASE-SPECIFIC SURVIVAL		
Number of Patients (%) who Died of Lung Cancer	3 (27)	22 (35)
Median Disease-Specific Survival		4.1 years
[95% Confidence Interval]		[2.5,—†]

* Not included are an additional 18 patients (6 patients not eligible for surgery or radiotherapy) who had complete tumor responses which were documented earlier than 3 months after treatment.
† The upper limit of the confidence interval could not be estimated due to an insufficient number of patients whose tumors recurred (Time to Tumor Recurrence) or who died (Survival).

prior high-dose radiotherapy (7 patients), poor pulmonary function (2 patients), multifocal multilobar disease (1 patient), and poor medical condition (1 patient). As shown in **Table 13**, the complete tumor response rate, biopsy-proven at least 3 months after treatment, was 50%, median time to tumor recurrence was more than 2.7 years, median survival was 2.9 years and disease-specific survival was 4.1 years. [See table 13 above]

14.3 High-Grade Dysplasia in Barrett's Esophagus

The safety and efficacy of PDT with PHOTOFRIN in ablation of HGD in patients with BE was assessed in one controlled randomized clinical study and two supportive studies.

Controlled Randomized Study

A multicenter, pathology blinded, randomized, controlled study was conducted in North America and Europe to assess the efficacy of PDT with PHOTOFRIN for Injection plus omeprazole (PHOTOFRIN PDT + OM) in producing complete ablation of HGD in patients with BE compared to control patients receiving omeprazole alone (OM Only). A total of 485 patients with the diagnosis of HGD were screened for the study; 208 (43%) were randomized to treatment, 237 (49%) were excluded because the diagnosis of HGD was not confirmed and 40 (8%) did not meet other screening criteria or declined to participate in the study. The high patient exclusion rate re-enforces the recommendation by the American College of Gastroenterology that the diagnosis of HGD in BE should be confirmed by an expert GI pathologist. Patients were centrally randomized in a 2:1 proportion to receive PHOTOFRIN PDT + OM (138 patients) or OM Only (70 patients). All patients underwent rigorous systematic quarterly endoscopic biopsy surveillance. Four-quadrant jumbo biopsies at every 2 cm of the entire Barrett's mucosa were obtained at each follow-up visit (every three months or six months if four consecutive quarterly follow-up endoscopic biopsy results were negative for HGD). All histological assessments were carried out at a central pathology laboratory and read by pathologists blinded to the treatment administered.

A total of 208 patients who had biopsy-proven HGD in BE were enrolled in the initial 2-year phase of the study. Of those, 199 patients were considered evaluable: 130 of 138 (94%) patients randomized to the PHOTOFRIN PDT + OM group and 69 of 70 (99%) randomized to the OM Only group had no esophageal invasive cancer, suspicion of esophageal invasive cancer, lymph node involvement, or metastases, and had received at least one PHOTOFRIN PDT course or one week of OM treatment, respectively. A disproportionate percentage of patients were discontinued from the OM Only group during the initial 2-year phase leaving 81 (59%) patients in the PHOTOFRIN PDT + OM group and 21 (30%) patients in the OM Only group at the end of the 2-year phase. Consequently, a total of 102 patients who completed the initial 2-year phase were eligible for continuation into the long-term phase until completion of 5 years; of those, 48 (59%) patients from the PHOTOFRIN PDT + OM group and 13 (62%) patients from the OM Only group consented to pursue the long-term phase until completion of 5 years. The mean age was 66 years (38 to 89 years) in the PHOTOFRIN PDT + OM group, and 67 (36 to 88 years) in the OM Only group. The patients in both treatment groups were predominantly male (85%), Caucasian (99%), and former smokers (64%). These characteristics are typical of patients with HGD in BE. Patients randomized to the PHOTOFRIN PDT + OM treatment received up to three courses of treatment

separated by at least 90 days. Each course consisted of intravenous administration of 2.0 mg/kg of PHOTOFRIN followed 40-50 hours later by a 630 nm laser light dose of 130 J/cm of diffuser length delivered using a centering balloon. A second laser light dose of 50 J/cm of diffuser length could be administered without a centering balloon 96-120 hours after the injection of PHOTOFRIN for treatment of "skip" areas. Since centering balloons are up to 7 cm in length, patients with more extensive HGD were treated with two or three courses. Both the PHOTOFRIN PDT treatment group and the control group received 20 mg of omeprazole BID to decrease reflux esophagitis. The mean duration of the follow-up period was 34 months (0-67 months) for the PHOTOFRIN PDT + OM group and 25 months (0-65 months) for the OM Only group.

The primary efficacy endpoint was the Complete Response rate (CR3 or better) at any one of the endoscopic assessment time points. The CR3 or better response was defined as the complete ablation of HGD and referred to as a composite of the following three response levels.
1. CR1—Complete replacement of all Barrett's metaplasia and dysplasia with normal squamous cell epithelium;
2. CR2—Ablation of all histological grades of dysplasia, including patients with indefinite grade of dysplasia, but some areas of Barrett's epithelium still remain; and
3. CR3—Ablation of all areas of HGD but with some areas of low-grade dysplasia with or without areas which are indefinite for dysplasia, or areas of Barrett's metaplastic epithelium.

Additional efficacy endpoints included:
1. Quality of Complete Response, which consisted of CR1 and CR2 or better.
2. Duration of CR;
3. Time to Progression to Cancer.

Table 14 presents the overall clinical response for both treatment groups in the intent-to-treat (ITT) population whose response was CR3 or better at any one of the evaluation time points. Overall, PHOTOFRIN PDT + OM was effective in eliminating HGD in patients with BE. The proportion of responders was significantly higher in the PHOTOFRIN PDT + OM group than in the OM Only group (77% vs. 39%, respectively; p<0.0001).

The quality of response in the PHOTOFRIN PDT + OM group was significantly better than that measured in the OM Only group at all response levels (p<0.0001). Seventy-two (52%) patients in the PHOTOFRIN PDT + OM group achieved a CR1 response as compared to only five (7%) patients in the OM Only group. Eighty-one (59%) patients in the PHOTOFRIN PDT + OM group achieved a CR2 or better response as compared to ten (14%) patients in the OM Only group.

[See table 14 at top of next page]

At the end of the long-term phase, the median response duration was 44.6 months (95% CI: 15.0-not reached, months) in the PHOTOFRIN PDT + OM group compared to 3.2 months (95% CI: 3.0-3.4, months) in the OM Only group.

At the end of the initial 2 year phase, the time to progression to cancer was significantly longer in the PHOTOFRIN PDT + OM group compared to the OM Only group (HR=0.36 (95% CI: 0.19-0.69), a hazard ratio less than 1 favors the PHOTOFRIN PDT + OM group). The proportion of patients' progression to cancer was lower in the PHOTOFRIN PDT + OM group than in the OM Only group: 13% (18 of 138 patients) vs. 28% (20 of 70 patients).

Complete response was influenced by the following factors: treatment with PHOTOFRIN PDT + OM (vs. OM Only), sin-

Table 14. Complete Response Rates After a Minimum Follow-Up of 24 Months in the ITT Population

Responders		Treatment Groups		
		PHOTOFRIN PDT + OM	OM Only	p-value*
Numbers of patients	N	138	70	
CR3 or better[†]	n	106	27	
	Proportion (%)	0.768 (76.8)	0.386 (; 8.6)	<0.0001
	95% CI	(0.689, 0.836)	(0.272, 0.510)	

* Fisher's Exact test.
† CR3 or better: Ablation of all areas HGD.
NOTE: Six patients in the PHOTOFRIN® PDT + OM group and three patients in the OM Only group without post-baseline biopsy data are considered as non-responders.

gle focus of HGD (vs. multiple foci), and prior omeprazole intake of at least 3 months (yes vs. no). Complete response was not influenced by the duration of HGD, length of BE, nodular conditions, gender, age, smoking history, and study center's size.

Supportive Studies
Two uncontrolled, supportive studies were conducted that were physician-sponsored, single center Phase II trials. Both studies included patients that had low-grade dysplasia (LGD), HGD and early adenocarcinoma. All HGD in BE patients were treated with PHOTOFRIN PDT and omeprazole.

The first study enrolled 99 patients (44 with HGD); the purpose of this study was to determine the required light dose to produce effective results. The second study enrolled 86 patients (42 with HGD), who were randomized to receive either PHOTOFRIN PDT with prednisone or PHOTOFRIN PDT without prednisone to determine whether steroid treatment would reduce the incidence and severity of esophageal strictures.

A CR3 or better response was demonstrated in 93% of 44 patients with HGD in the first study and in 95% of 42 patients with HGD in the second study after a minimum follow-up of 12 months. A CR2 or better response was achieved in 82% of patients in the first study and in 91% of patients in the second study. A CR1 response occurred in 57% of patients in the first study and in 60% of the second study. Progression to cancer during the above follow-up period occurred in 18% of patients in the first study and in 7% of patients in the second study. No reduction in the incidence or severity of esophageal strictures was found in the prednisone group in the second study.

16   HOW SUPPLIED/STORAGE AND HANDLING
PHOTOFRIN (porfimer sodium) for Injection is supplied as a freeze-dried cake or powder as follows:
NDC 58914-155-75, 75 mg vial
Storage
PHOTOFRIN freeze-dried cake or powder should be stored at Controlled Room Temperature 20-25°C (68-77°F) [see USP].
Spills and Disposal
Spills of PHOTOFRIN should be wiped up with a damp cloth. Skin and eye contact should be avoided due to the potential for photosensitivity reactions upon exposure to light; use of rubber gloves and eye protection is recommended. All contaminated materials should be disposed of in a polyethylene bag in a manner consistent with local regulations.
Accidental Exposure
PHOTOFRIN is neither a primary ocular irritant nor a primary dermal irritant. However, because of its potential to induce photosensitivity, PHOTOFRIN might be an eye and/or skin irritant in the presence of bright light. It is important to avoid contact with the eyes and skin during preparation and/or administration. As with therapeutic overdosage, any overexposed person must be protected from bright light.

17   PATIENT COUNSELING INFORMATION
17.1   Photosensitivity
Patients should be warned to avoid exposure of skin and eyes to direct sunlight or bright indoor light for at least 30 days following injection with PHOTOFRIN.
Patients should be informed that photosensitivity might last for more than 90 days if patients suffer from liver impairment.
Patients should be instructed to wear protective clothing and dark sunglasses when outdoors, which have an average white light transmittance of < 4%.
Patients should be encouraged to expose their skin to ambient indoor light to facilitate elimination of PHOTOFRIN from their skin.

17.2   Common Adverse Reactions
Patients should be informed that treatment with photodynamic therapy might lead to adverse reactions which include ocular sensitivity, chest pain, respiratory distress or

esophageal strictures. In such cases, patients should call their physicians.
Revised: 08/2008   AXCAN Pharma US, Inc.
Shown in Product Identification Guide, page 306

PYLERA™ CAPSULES   ℞
[pī-le-ra]
(bismuth subcitrate potassium, metronidazole, and tetracycline hydrochloride)
140 mg/125 mg/125 mg

To reduce the development of drug-resistant bacteria and maintain the effectiveness of PYLERA™ and other antibacterial drugs, PYLERA™ should be used only to treat or prevent infections that are proven or strongly suspected to be caused by bacteria.

> **WARNING**
> Metronidazole has been shown to be carcinogenic in mice and rats. (See **PRECAUTIONS**) Unnecessary use of the drug should be avoided. Its use should be reserved for the conditions described in the **INDICATIONS AND USAGE** section below.

DESCRIPTION
PYLERA™ capsules are a combination antimicrobial product containing bismuth subcitrate potassium, metronidazole, and tetracycline hydrochloride for oral administration. Each size 0 elongated hard gelatin capsule contains:
- bismuth subcitrate potassium, 140 mg
- metronidazole, 125 mg
- smaller capsule (size 3) containing tetracycline hydrochloride, 125 mg

Bismuth subcitrate potassium is a white or almost white powder. It is a soluble, complex bismuth salt of citric acid. The schematized empirical molecular formula of bismuth subcitrate potassium is $Bi(Citrate)_2K_5 \cdot 3\ H_2O$. The equivalent theoretical molecular formula is $BiC_{12}H_{14}K_5O_{17}$. The molecular mass of the theoretical molecular formula of a single unit of bismuth subcitrate potassium is 834.71.
Metronidazole is a white to pale yellow crystalline powder. Metronidazole is 2-methyl-5-nitroimidazole-1-ethanol, with a molecular formula of $C_6H_9N_3O_3$ and the following structural formula:

Molecular weight: 171.2

Tetracycline hydrochloride is a yellow, odorless, crystalline powder. Tetracycline is stable in air, but exposure to strong sunlight causes it to darken. Tetracycline hydrochloride is (4S,4aS,5aS,6S,12aS)-4-(dimethylamino)-1,4,4a,5,5a,6,11,12a-octahydro-3,6,10,12,12a-penta-hydroxy-6-methyl-1,11-dioxo-2-naphthacenecarboxamide hydrochloride, with a molecular formula of $C_{22}H_{24}N_2O_8 \cdot HCl$ and the following structural formula:

Molecular weight: 480.90

Each PYLERA™ capsule contains the following inactive ingredients: Magnesium Stearate NF, Lactose Monohydrate NF, Talc USP, Gelatin USP, and Titanium Dioxide NF. Printed with red ink.

CLINICAL PHARMACOLOGY
Pharmacokinetics
The pharmacokinetics of the individual components of PYLERA™, bismuth subcitrate potassium, metronidazole and tetracycline, are summarized below. In addition, two studies on PYLERA™ were conducted by Axcan to determine the effect of co-administration on the pharmacokinetics of the components.
Bismuth Subcitrate Potassium (Bismuth)
Orally absorbed bismuth is distributed throughout the entire body. Bismuth is highly bound to plasma proteins (>90%). The elimination half-life of bismuth is approximately 5 days in both blood and urine. Elimination of bismuth is primarily through urinary and biliary routes. The rate of renal elimination appears to reach steady state 2 weeks after treatment discontinuation with similar rates of elimination at 6 weeks after discontinuation. The average urinary elimination of bismuth is 2.6% per day in the first two weeks after discontinuation (urine drug concentrations 24 to 250 µg/mL) suggesting tissue accumulation and slow elimination.
Metronidazole
Following oral administration, metronidazole is well absorbed, with peak plasma concentrations occurring between 1 and 2 hours after administration. Plasma concentrations of metronidazole are proportional to the administered dose, with oral administration of 500 mg producing a peak plasma concentration of 12 µg/mL.
Metronidazole appears in the plasma mainly as unchanged compound with lesser quantities of the 2-hydroxymethyl metabolite also present. Less than 20% of the circulating metronidazole is bound to plasma proteins. Metronidazole also appears in cerebrospinal fluid, saliva, and breast milk in concentrations similar to those found in plasma.
The average elimination half-life of metronidazole in normal volunteers is 8 hours. The major route of elimination of metronidazole and its metabolites is via the urine (60% to 80% of the dose), with fecal excretion accounting for 6% to 15% of the dose. The metabolites that appear in the urine result primarily from side-chain oxidation [1-(β-hydroxyethyl)2-hydroxymethyl-5-nitroimidazole and 2-methyl-5-nitroimidazole-1-yl-acetic acid] and glucuronide conjugation, with unchanged metronidazole accounting for approximately 20% of the total. Renal clearance of metronidazole is approximately 10 mL/min/1.73 m^2.
Decreased renal function does not alter the single dose pharmacokinetics of metronidazole. In patients with decreased liver function, plasma clearance of metronidazole is decreased.
Tetracycline Hydrochloride
Tetracycline is absorbed (60%-90%) in the stomach and upper small intestine. The presence of food, milk or cations may significantly decrease the extent of absorption. In the plasma, tetracycline is bound to plasma proteins in varying degrees. It is concentrated by the liver in the bile and excreted in the urine and feces at high concentrations in a biologically active form.
Tetracycline is distributed into most body tissues and fluids. It is distributed into the bile and undergoes varying degrees of enterohepatic recirculation. Tetracycline tends to localize in tumors, necrotic or ischemic tissue, liver and spleen and form tetracycline-calcium orthophosphate complexes at sites of new bone formation or tooth development. Tetracycline readily crosses the placenta and is excreted in high amounts in breast milk.
PYLERA™ Capsules
The clinical significance of systemic, as compared to local, drug concentrations for antimicrobial activity against *Helicobacter pylori*, has not been established. A comparative bioavailability study of metronidazole (375 mg), tetracycline (375 mg) and bismuth subcitrate potassium (420 mg, equivalent to 120 mg Bi_2O_3) administered as PYLERA™ or as 3 separate capsule formulations administered simultaneously was conducted in healthy male volunteers. The pharmacokinetic parameters for the individual drugs when administered as separate capsule formulations or as PYLERA™ are similar, as shown in Table 1.
[See table 1 at top of next page]
The pharmacokinetic parameters for metronidazole, tetracycline and bismuth were also determined when PYLERA™ was administered under fasting and fed conditions, as shown in Table 2. Food reduced the systemic absorption of all three PYLERA™ components, with AUC values for metronidazole, tetracycline and bismuth being reduced by 6%, 34% and 60%, respectively. Reduction in the absorption of all three PYLERA™ components in the presence of food is not considered to be clinically significant. PYLERA™ should be given after meals and at bedtime, in combination with omeprazole twice a day. (See **DOSAGE AND ADMINISTRATION**)
[See table 2 on next page]
Omeprazole Capsules
The effect of omeprazole on bismuth absorption was assessed in 34 healthy volunteers given PYLERA™ (qid) with

---

or without omeprazole (20 mg bid) for 6 days. In the presence of omeprazole, the extent of absorption of bismuth from PYLERA™ was significantly increased, compared to when no omeprazole was given (Table 3). Concentration-dependent neurotoxicity is associated with long-term use of bismuth and not likely to occur with short-term administration or at steady state concentrations below 50 ng/mL. One subject transiently achieved a maximum bismuth concentration (C_{max}) higher than 50 ng/mL (73 ng/mL) following multiple dosing of PYLERA™ with omeprazole. The patient did not exhibit symptoms of neurotoxicity during the study. There is no clinical evidence to suggest that short-term exposure to C_{max} concentrations above 50 ng/mL is associated with neurotoxicity.

[See table 3 at right]

Microbiology

The ingredients in PYLERA™ capsules are active as antibacterial agents. Tetracycline hydrochloride interacts with the 30S subunit of the bacterial ribosome and inhibits protein synthesis. Metronidazole is metabolized through reductive pathways into reactive intermediates that have cytotoxic action. The antibacterial action of bismuth salts is not well understood.

PYLERA™ plus omeprazole therapy has been shown to be active against most strains of *Helicobacter pylori in vitro*, and in clinical infections as described in the **CLINICAL STUDIES** and **INDICATIONS AND USAGE** sections.

Susceptibility Testing for *Helicobacter pylori*

Susceptibility testing of *Helicobacter pylori* isolates was performed for metronidazole using agar dilution methodology according to CLSI[1] guidelines and minimum inhibitory concentrations (MICs) were determined.

Susceptibility testing of *Helicobacter pylori* for metronidazole has not been standardized. No interpretive criteria have been established for testing metronidazole against *H. pylori*.

The clinical significance of metronidazole MIC values against *H. pylori* is unknown. In the North American study, pre-treatment metronidazole MIC values showed no correlation with clinical outcome in patients treated with PYLERA™ and omeprazole therapy.

INDICATIONS AND USAGE

PYLERA™ capsules (bismuth subcitrate potassium, metronidazole, and tetracycline hydrochloride), in combination with omeprazole are indicated for the treatment of patients with *Helicobacter pylori* infection and duodenal ulcer disease (active or history of within the past 5 years) to eradicate *H. pylori*. The eradication of *Helicobacter pylori* has been shown to reduce the risk of duodenal ulcer recurrence.

(See **CLINICAL STUDIES** and **DOSAGE AND ADMINISTRATION**)

To reduce the development of drug-resistant bacteria and maintain the effectiveness of PYLERA™ and other antibacterial drugs, PYLERA™ should be used only to treat or prevent infections that are proven or strongly suspected to be caused by susceptible bacteria. When culture and susceptibility information are available, they should be considered in selecting or modifying antibacterial therapy. In the absence of such data, local epidemiology and susceptibility patterns may contribute to the empiric selection of therapy.

CLINICAL STUDIES

Eradication of *Helicobacter pylori* in Patients with Active Duodenal Ulcer or History of Duodenal Ulcer Disease

An open-label, parallel group, active-controlled, multicenter study in *Helicobacter pylori* positive patients with current duodenal ulcer or a history of duodenal ulcer disease was conducted in the United States and Canada.

Patients were randomized to one of the following 10-day treatment regimens:

- Three (3) PYLERA™ capsules four times daily, after meals and at bedtime plus 20 mg omeprazole twice a day after breakfast and supper (**OBMT**).
- Clarithromycin 500 mg plus 1000 mg amoxicillin plus 20 mg omeprazole twice a day before breakfast and supper (**OAC**).

H. pylori eradication rates, defined as two negative ^{13}C-urea breath tests performed at 4 and 8 weeks post-therapy are shown in Table 4 for OBMT and OAC. The eradication rates for both groups were found to be similar using either the Modified Intent-to-Treat (MITT) or Per Protocol (PP) populations.

[See table 4 at top of next page]

CONTRAINDICATIONS

PYLERA™ therapy is contraindicated in pregnant or nursing women, pediatric patients, in patients with renal or hepatic impairment, and in those with known hypersensitivity to bismuth subcitrate potassium, metronidazole or other nitroimidazole derivatives, or tetracyclines. (See **WARNINGS** and **PRECAUTIONS**)

WARNINGS

Bismuth-containing Products

There have been rare reports of neurotoxicity associated with excessive doses of various bismuth-containing products. Effects have been reversible with discontinuation of therapy.

Table 1. Mean (%CV) Pharmacokinetic Parameters for Metronidazole, Tetracycline, and Bismuth Subcitrate Potassium in Healthy Volunteers (N=18)

		C_{max} (ng/mL) (%C.V.**)	AUC_T (ng · h/mL) (%C.V.**)	AUC_∞ (ng · h/mL) (%C.V.**)
Metronidazole	Metronidazole Capsule	9044.7 (20)	80289 (15)	81849 (16)
	PYLERA™*	8666.3 (22)	83018 (17)	84413 (17)
Tetracycline	Tetracycline Capsules	748.0 (40)	9544 (55)	9864 (53)
	PYLERA™*	773.8 (47)	9674 (50)	9987 (49)
Bismuth	Bismuth Capsule	21.3 (123)	46.5 (129)	65.4 (113)
	PYLERA™*	16.7 (202)	42.5 (191)	56.5 (178)

*PYLERA™ given as a single dose of 3 capsules
**C.V. – Coefficient Variation

Table 2. Mean PYLERA™ Pharmacokinetic Parameters in Fasted and Fed States (N=18)*

	FED			FASTED		
	metronidazole	tetracycline	bismuth	metronidazole	tetracycline	bismuth
C_{max} (ng/mL) (%C.V.)	6835.0	515.8	1.7	8666.3	773.8	16.7
	(13)	(36)	(61)	(22)	(47)	(202)
T_{max} (hours)** (range)	3.0 (1.3 - 4.0)	4.0 (2.5 - 5.0)	3.5 (0.8 - 6.0)	0.75 (0.5 - 3.5)	3.3 (1.3 - 5.0)	0.6 (0.5 - 1.7)
AUC_∞ (ng · h/mL) (%C.V.)	79225.6 (18)	5840.1 (312)	18.4 (116)	84413.6 (17)	9986.7 (49)	56.5 (178)

*PYLERA™ given as a single dose of 3 capsules
**T_{max} is expressed as median (range)

Table 3. Mean Bismuth Pharmacokinetic Parameters following PYLERA™ Administration* With and Without Omeprazole (N=34)

Parameter	Without omeprazole		With omeprazole	
	Mean	%C.V.**	Mean	%C.V.**
C_{max} (ng/mL)	8.1	84	25.5	69
AUC_T (ng · h/mL)	48.5	28	140.9	42

*PYLERA™ given as 3 capsules qid for 6 days with or without 20 mg omeprazole bid
**C.V. – Coefficient Variation

Metronidazole

Central Nervous System Effects

Convulsive seizures and peripheral neuropathy, the latter characterized mainly by numbness or paresthesia of an extremity, have been reported in patients treated with metronidazole. The prevalence and severity of the neuropathy are directly related to the cumulative dose and duration of therapy, being most prevalent in patients taking high doses for prolonged treatment periods. The appearance of abnormal neurologic signs demands the prompt discontinuation of metronidazole therapy. Metronidazole should be administered with caution to patients with central nervous system diseases.

Tetracycline

THE USE OF DRUGS OF THE TETRACYCLINE CLASS DURING TOOTH DEVELOPMENT (LAST HALF OF PREGNANCY, INFANCY, AND CHILDHOOD TO THE AGE OF 8 YEARS) MAY CAUSE PERMANENT DISCOLORATION OF THE TEETH (YELLOW-GRAY-BROWN). This adverse reaction is more common during long-term use of the drugs but has been observed following repeated short-term courses. Enamel hypoplasia has also been reported. TETRACYCLINE HYDROCHLORIDE IS A COMPONENT OF PYLERA™ CAPSULES. THEREFORE, PYLERA™ CAPSULES SHOULD NOT BE USED IN THESE PATIENT POPULATIONS. (See **CONTRAINDICATIONS**)

Tetracycline hydrochloride should not be used during pregnancy (see **WARNINGS** above about use during tooth development). Results of animal studies indicate that tetracycline crosses the placenta, is found in fetal tissues, and can have toxic effects on the developing fetus (often related to retardation of skeletal development). Evidence of embryotoxicity has also been noted in animals treated early in pregnancy. If this drug is used during pregnancy or if the patient becomes pregnant while taking this drug, the patient should be apprised of the potential hazard to the fetus. Photosensitivity, manifested by an exaggerated sunburn reaction, has been observed in some individuals taking tetracycline. Patients apt to be exposed to direct sunlight or ultraviolet light should be advised that this reaction can occur with tetracycline drugs. Treatment should be discontinued at the first evidence of skin erythema.

The antianabolic action of the tetracyclines may cause an increase in blood urea nitrogen (BUN). While this is not a problem in those with normal renal function, in patients with significantly impaired renal function, higher serum levels of tetracycline may lead to azotemia, hyperphosphatemia, and acidosis.

PRECAUTIONS

General

Prescribing PYLERA™ in the absence of a proven or strongly suspected bacterial infection or a prophylactic indication is unlikely to provide benefit to the patient and increases the risk of the development of drug-resistant bacteria.

Bismuth-containing Products

Bismuth subcitrate potassium and other bismuth-containing products may cause a temporary and harmless darkening of the tongue and/or black stool. Stool darkening must not be confused with melena.

Metronidazole

Patients with severe hepatic disease metabolize metronidazole slowly, with resultant accumulation of metronidazole and its metabolites in plasma. (See **CONTRAINDICATIONS**) Metronidazole is a nitroimidazole and should be used with caution in patients with evidence of, or history of, blood dyscrasia. A mild leukopenia has been observed; however, no persistent hematologic abnormalities attributable to metronidazole have been observed.

Known or previously unrecognized candidiasis may present more prominent symptoms during therapy with metronidazole and requires treatment with an antifungal agent.

Tetracycline

As with other antibiotics, use of tetracycline hydrochloride may result in overgrowth of nonsusceptible organisms, including fungi. If superinfection occurs, tetracycline should be discontinued and appropriate therapy should be instituted.

Pseudotumor cerebri (benign intracranial hypertension) in adults has been associated with the use of tetracycline. The usual clinical manifestations are headache and blurred vision. While this condition and related symptoms usually resolve soon after discontinuation of the tetracycline, the possibility for permanent sequelae exists.

Information for Patients

- Each dose of PYLERA™ includes 3 capsules. Each dose of all 3 capsules should be taken 4 times a day, after meals and at bedtime for 10 days. Patients should be instructed to swallow the PYLERA™ capsules whole with a full glass of water (8 ounces). One omeprazole 20 mg capsule should be taken twice a day with PYLERA™ after the morning and evening meal for 10 days.

Daily Dosing Schedule for PYLERA™ and Omeprazole:

Time of dose	Number of capsules of PYLERA™	Number of capsules of Omeprazole 20 mg
After morning meal	3	1
After lunch	3	0
After evening meal	3	1
At bedtime	3	0

- Administration of adequate amounts of fluid, particularly with the bedtime dose of PYLERA™, is recommended to reduce the risk of esophageal irritation and ulceration, which can be associated with tetracycline hydrochloride.
- Concurrent use of tetracyclines may render oral contraceptives less effective. Patients should be advised to use a different or additional form of contraception. Breakthrough bleeding has been reported. Women who become pregnant while taking PYLERA™, which contains tetracycline hydrochloride, should be advised to notify their prescriber immediately. (See **CONTRAINDICATIONS** and **WARNINGS**)
- Patients taking PYLERA™, which contains tetracycline hydrochloride, should be cautioned to avoid exposure to sun or sun lamps. (See **WARNINGS**)
- Alcoholic beverages should be avoided while taking PYLERA™, which contains metronidazole, and for at least one day afterward. (See **Drug Interactions**)
- Bismuth subcitrate potassium, contained in PYLERA™, may cause temporary and harmless darkening of the tongue and/or black stool. Stool darkening should not be confused with melena (blood in the stool).
- Missed doses can be made up by continuing the normal dosing schedule until the medication is gone. Patients should not take double doses. If more than 4 doses are missed, the prescriber should be contacted.

Call your doctor for medical advice about side effects. You may report side effects to FDA at 1-800-FDA-1088.

Drug Interactions

Interactions with Metronidazole

Lithium

In patients stabilized on relatively high doses of lithium, short-term metronidazole therapy has been associated with elevation of serum lithium and, in a few cases, signs of lithium toxicity. Serum lithium and serum creatinine should be obtained several days after beginning metronidazole to detect any increase that may precede clinical symptoms of lithium intoxication.

Alcohol

Alcoholic beverages should not be consumed during metronidazole therapy and for at least 1 day afterward because abdominal cramps, nausea, vomiting, headaches, and flushing may occur. Since some pharmaceutical products may contain alcohol, caution should be exercised in patients taking these medications. Psychotic reactions have been reported in alcoholic patients who are using metronidazole and disulfiram concurrently. Metronidazole should not be given to patients who have taken disulfiram within the last 2 weeks.

Anticoagulants

Metronidazole has been reported to potentiate the anticoagulant effect of warfarin and other oral coumarin anticoagulants, resulting in a prolongation of prothrombin time. Therefore, frequent monitoring therapy with appropriate adjustment of the anticoagulant dosage is warranted with initiation of PYLERA™.

Cimetidine, Phenytoin, or Phenobarbital

The simultaneous administration of drugs that decrease microsomal liver enzyme activity, such as cimetidine, may prolong the half-life and decrease plasma clearance of metronidazole. The simultaneous administration of drugs that induce microsomal liver enzymes, such as phenytoin or phenobarbital, may accelerate the elimination of metronidazole, resulting in reduced plasma levels. Impaired clearance of phenytoin has also been reported in this situation.

Interactions with Tetracycline

Methoxyflurane and Tetracycline

The concurrent use of tetracycline and methoxyflurane has been reported to result in fatal renal toxicity.

Oral Contraceptives and Tetracycline

Concurrent use of tetracycline may render oral contraceptives less effective. Patients should be advised to use a different or additional form of contraception. Breakthrough bleeding has been reported. Women who become pregnant while on PYLERA™ should be advised to notify their prescriber immediately.

Anticoagulants

Tetracycline has been shown to depress plasma prothrombin activity. Therefore, frequent monitoring of anticoagulant therapy with appropriate adjustment of the anticoagulant dosage is warranted with initiation of PYLERA™.

Penicillin

Since bacteriostatic drugs, such as the tetracycline class of antibiotics, may interfere with the bactericidal action of penicillin, it is not advisable to administer these drugs concomitantly.

Antacids, Multivitamins, or Dairy Products

Absorption of tetracyclines is impaired by antacids containing aluminum, calcium, or magnesium; preparations containing iron, zinc, or sodium bicarbonate; or milk or dairy products. The clinical significance of reduced tetracycline systemic exposure is unknown as the relative contribution of systemic versus local antimicrobial activity against *Helicobacter pylori* has not been established. PYLERA™ should be given after meals and at bedtime, in combination with omeprazole twice a day. (See **DOSAGE AND ADMINISTRATION**)

Bismuth

There is an anticipated reduction in tetracycline systemic absorption due to an interaction with bismuth. The clinical significance of reduced tetracycline systemic exposure is unknown as the relative contribution of systemic versus local antimicrobial activity against *Helicobacter pylori* has not been established.

Table 4. *Helicobacter pylori* Eradication at 8 Weeks after 10 Day Treatment Regimen Percent (%) of Patients Cured [95% Confidence Interval] (Number of Patients)

	Treatment Group		Difference
	OBMT*	OAC** c	
Per Protocol[a]	92.5% [87.8, 97.2] (n=120)	85.7% [76.9, 91.8] (n=126)	6.8 [-0.9, 14.5]
Modified Intent-to-Treat[b]	87.7% [82.2, 93.2] (n=138)	83.2% [77.0, 89.5] (n=137)	4.5 [-3.9, 12.8]

* **OBMT**: Omeprazole + PYLERA™ (bismuth subcitrate potassium / metronidazole / tetracycline HCl)

** **OAC**: Omeprazole + Amoxicillin + Clarithromycin

[a] Patients were included in the analysis if they had *H. pylori* infection documented at baseline, defined as a positive ^{13}C-UBT plus histology or culture, had at least one endoscopically verified duodenal ulcer ≥ 0.3 cm at baseline or had a documented history of duodenal ulcer disease, and were not protocol violators. Additionally, if patients dropped out of the study due to an adverse event related to the study drug, they were included in the evaluable analysis as failures of therapy.

[b] Patients were included in the analysis if they had documented *H. pylori* infection at baseline as defined above, and had at least one documented duodenal ulcer at baseline or had a documented history of duodenal ulcer disease, and took at least one dose of study medication. All dropouts were included as failures of therapy.

[c] Results for OAC treatment represent all isolates regardless of clarithromycin susceptibility. Eradication rates for clarithromycin susceptible organisms, as defined by an MIC ≤ 0.25 μg/mL, were 94.6% and 92.1% for the PP and MITT analysis, respectively. Eradication rates for clarithromycin non-susceptible organisms, as defined by an MIC ≥ 0.5 μg/mL, were 23.1% and 21.4% for the PP and MITT analysis, respectively.[1]

Drug/Laboratory Test Interactions

Bismuth absorbs x-rays and may interfere with x-ray diagnostic procedures of the gastrointestinal tract.

Bismuth subcitrate potassium may cause a temporary and harmless darkening of the stool. However, this does not interfere with standard tests for occult blood.

Metronidazole may interfere with certain types of determinations of serum chemistry values, such as aspartate aminotransferase (AST, SGOT), alanine aminotransferase (ALT, SGPT), lactate dehydrogenase (LDH), triglycerides, and hexokinase glucose. Values of zero may be observed. All of the assays in which interference has been reported involve enzymatic coupling of the assay to oxidation-reduction of nicotinamide (NAD+ <=> NADH). Interference is due to the similarity in absorbance peaks of NADH (340 nm) and metronidazole (322 nm) at pH 7.

Carcinogenesis, Mutagenesis, Impairment of Fertility

No long-term studies have been performed to evaluate the effect of the combined use of bismuth subcitrate potassium, metronidazole, and tetracycline on carcinogenesis, mutagenesis, or impairment of fertility.

Bismuth Subcitrate Potassium

No carcinogenicity or reproductive toxicity studies have been conducted with bismuth subcitrate potassium. Bismuth subcitrate potassium did not show mutagenic potential in the NTP *Salmonella* plate assay.

Metronidazole

Metronidazole has shown evidence of carcinogenic activity in a number of studies involving chronic, oral administration in mice and rats. Prominent among the effects in the mouse was an increased incidence of pulmonary tumorigenesis. This has been observed in all six reported studies in that species, including one study in which the animals were dosed on an intermittent schedule (administration during every fourth week only). At the highest dose levels, (approximately 500 mg/kg/day, which is approximately 1.4 times the indicated human dose for a 50 kg adult based on body surface area), there was a statistically significant increase in the incidence of malignant liver tumors in male mice. Also, the published results of one of the mouse studies indicate an increase in the incidence of malignant lymphomas as well as pulmonary neoplasms associated with lifetime feeding of the drug. All these effects are statistically significant. Long-term, oral-dosing studies in the rat showed statistically significant increases in the incidence of various neoplasms, particularly in mammary and hepatic tumors, among female rats administered metronidazole over those noted in the concurrent female control groups. Two lifetime tumorigenicity studies in hamsters have been performed and reported to be negative.

Although metronidazole has shown mutagenic activity in a number of *in vitro* assay systems, studies in mammals (*in vivo*) have failed to demonstrate a potential for genetic damage.

Metronidazole, at doses up to 400 mg/kg/day (approximately 2 times the indicated human dose based on mg/m^2) for 28 days, failed to produce any adverse effects on fertility and testicular function in male rats. Fertility studies have been performed in mice at doses up to six times the maximum recommended human dose based on mg/m^2 and have revealed no evidence of impaired fertility.

IMPORTANT NOTICE: Updated drug information is sent bi-monthly via the PDR® Update Insert. For *monthly* email updates, register at PDR.net.

Tetracycline hydrochloride

There has been no evidence of carcinogenicity for tetracycline hydrochloride in studies conducted with rats and mice. Some related antibiotics (oxytetracycline, minocycline) have shown evidence of oncogenic activity in rats.

There was evidence of mutagenicity by tetracycline hydrochloride in two *in vitro* mammalian cell assay systems (L51784y mouse lymphoma and Chinese hamster lung cells).

Tetracycline hydrochloride had no effect on fertility when administered in the diet to male and female rats at a daily intake of 25 times the human dose.

Pregnancy

Teratogenic Effects. Pregnancy Category D

Category D is based on the pregnancy category for tetracycline hydrochloride. (See **CONTRAINDICATIONS** and **WARNINGS/Tetracycline** subsections)

Metronidazole crosses the placental barrier and its effects on the human fetal organogenesis are not known. No fetotoxicity was observed when metronidazole was administered orally to pregnant mice at 20 mg/kg/day, approximately 5 percent of the indicated human dose (1500 mg/day) based on body surface area; however, in a single small study where the drug was administered intraperitoneally, some intrauterine deaths were observed. The relationship of these findings to the drug is unknown. There are no adequate and well-controlled studies in pregnant women.

Non-teratogenic Effects

Pregnant women with renal disease may be more prone to develop tetracycline-associated liver failure. (See **WARNINGS**)

Labor and Delivery

The effect of this therapy on labor and delivery is unknown.

Nursing Mothers

Metronidazole and tetracycline are both secreted into human milk. Metronidazole is secreted in human milk in concentrations similar to those found in plasma. Because of the potential for tumorigenicity shown for metronidazole in mouse and rat studies, and because of the potential for serious adverse reactions in nursing infants from tetracyclines, a decision should be made whether to discontinue nursing or to discontinue therapy, taking into account the importance of the therapy to the mother. (See **CONTRAINDICATIONS**)

Pediatric Use

Tetracycline use in children may cause permanent discoloration of the teeth. Enamel hypoplasia has also been reported. PYLERA™ should not be used in children less than 8 years of age. Safety and effectiveness of PYLERA™ in pediatric patients infected with *Helicobacter pylori* have not been established. (See **CONTRAINDICATIONS** and **WARNINGS**)

Geriatric Use

Of the 324 patients who received PYLERA™ in clinical studies, 40 were ≥ 65 years old. Clinical studies of PYLERA™ did not include sufficient numbers of subjects aged 65 and over to determine whether they respond differently from younger subjects. Other reported clinical experience has not identified differences in responses between the elderly and younger patients. In general, the greater frequency of decreased hepatic, renal, or cardiac function, and of concomitant disease or other drug therapy in elderly patients should be considered when prescribing PYLERA™. As stated in the **CONTRAINDICATIONS** section, PYLERA™ is contraindicated in patients with renal or hepatic impairment.

ADVERSE REACTIONS

The safety of PYLERA™ plus omeprazole for 10 days to eradicate *Helicobacter pylori* was evaluated in 324 patients (aged 18 to 75 years) in two clinical trials world-wide. One trial was conducted in the US and Canada (North American Trial). The other trial was conducted in Europe, Australia, Canada and the US (International Trial).

In the North American trial, patients with a duodenal ulcer or history of an ulcer were randomized to PYLERA™ plus omeprazole (OBMT) or omeprazole, amoxicillin, and clarithromycin (OAC). The International trial differed from the North American trial in that there was no comparator group and all patients received OBMT. Also, patients enrolled in the International trial all had gastrointestinal symptoms (i.e., non-ulcer dyspepsia). It was not necessary for these patients to have a history or current duodenal ulcer.

Two hundred and ninety-nine (299) patients (147 OBMT and 152 OAC) were exposed to at least one dose of the study drugs in the North American trial. Of these patients, 86/147 (58.5%) in the OBMT group and 90/152 (59.2%) in the OAC group reported adverse events. In the OBMT group there were 212 events reported and 236 events reported in the OAC group. An adverse event was defined as any event not

present prior to exposure to study medication or any event present at study entry that worsens in either intensity or frequency following exposure to study medication.

The most frequent adverse events (incidence >1%) by treatment group from the North American trial in order of decreasing incidence for the OBMT group are shown below in Table 5. For both treatments, gastrointestinal adverse events (e.g., diarrhea, dyspepsia, abdominal pain, and nausea) are the most commonly reported.

Because clinical trials are conducted under widely varying conditions, adverse reaction rates observed in the clinical trials of a drug cannot be directly compared to rates in the clinical trials or another drug and may not reflect the rates observed in practice.

Table 5. Adverse Events of Incidence > 1% in Controlled Clinical Trial By Treatment Group, By Decreasing Frequency [n (%)]

Preferred Term	OBMT* (n = 147)	OAC** (n = 152)
Stool Abnormality	23 (15.6)	7 (4.6)
Diarrhea	13 (8.8)	23 (15.1)
Dyspepsia	13 (8.8)	17 (11.2)
Abdominal Pain	13 (8.8)	15 (9.9)
Nausea	12 (8.2)	16 (10.5)
Headache	12 (8.2)	11 (7.2)
Flu Syndrome	8 (5.4)	5 (3.3)
Taste Perversion	7 (4.8)	18 (11.8)
Asthenia	6 (4.1)	4 (2.6)
Vaginitis	6 (4.1)	4 (2.6)
Dizziness	5 (3.4)	4 (2.6)
Lab Test Abnormality	4 (2.7)	4 (2.6)
Pain	3 (2.0)	7 (4.6)
Infection	3 (2.0)	5 (3.3)
Pharyngitis	3 (2.0)	4 (2.6)
Pain Back	3 (2.0)	2 (1.3)
SGPT Increased	3 (2.0)	0
Urinary abnormality	3 (2.0)	0
Infection	2 (1.4)	6 (3.9)
Rhinitis	2 (1.4)	4 (2.6)
Dry Mouth	2 (1.4)	1 (0.7)
Vomit	2 (1.4)	1 (0.7)
Anxiety	2 (1.4)	0
Gastritis	2 (1.4)	0
Gastroenteritis	2 (1.4)	0
Pain, Chest	2 (1.4)	0
Palpitation	2 (1.4)	0
Rash Maculo-Papular	2 (1.4)	0
SGOT Increase	2 (1.4)	0
Flatulence	1 (0.7)	6 (3.9)
Cough	1 (0.7)	3 (2.0)
Rash	1 (0.7)	3 (2.0)
Sinusitis	1 (0.7)	2 (1.3)
Pruritus	0	4 (2.6)
Glossitis	0	2 (1.3)

* OBMT = Omeprazole+PYLERA™ (bismuth subcitrate potassium/metronidazole/tetracycline HCl);
**OAC = Omeprazole+Amoxicillin+Clarithromycin

The following selected adverse reactions from the labeling for bismuth subsalicylate, a similar bismuth-containing product to bismuth subcitrate potassium, are provided for information.

Gastrointestinal: black stools

Mouth: temporary and harmless darkening of the tongue

The following selected adverse reactions from the labeling for metronidazole are provided for information.

Mouth: A sharp, unpleasant metallic taste is not unusual. Furry tongue, glossitis, stomatitis have occurred; these may be associated with a sudden overgrowth of *Candida* which may occur during therapy.

Blood: Reversible neutropenia (leukopenia); rarely, reversible thrombocytopenia.

Cardiovascular: Flattening of the T-wave may be seen in electrocardiographic tracings.

CNS: Two serious adverse reactions reported in patients treated with metronidazole have been convulsive seizures and peripheral neuropathy, the latter characterized mainly by numbness or paresthesia of an extremity. Since persistent peripheral neuropathy has been reported in some patients receiving prolonged administration of metronidazole, patients should be specifically warned about these reactions and should be told to stop the drug and report immediately to their physicians if any neurologic symptoms occur.

Hypersensitivity: urticaria, erythematous rash, flushing, nasal congestion, dryness of mouth (or vagina or vulva), and fever.

Other: If patients receiving metronidazole drink alcoholic beverages, they may experience abdominal distress, nausea, vomiting, flushing, or headache. A modification of the taste of alcoholic beverages has also been reported. Rare cases of pancreatitis, which abated on withdrawal of the drug, have been reported.

The following selected adverse reactions from the labeling for tetracycline hydrochloride are provided for information.

Gastrointestinal: Rare instances of esophagitis and esophageal ulceration have been reported in patients taking the tetracycline-class antibiotics in capsule and tablet form. Most of the patients who experienced esophageal irritation took the medication immediately before going to bed. (See **DOSAGE AND ADMINISTRATION**)

Liver: Hepatotoxicity and liver failure have been observed in patients receiving large doses of tetracycline and in tetracycline-treated patients with renal impairment. Increases in liver enzymes and hepatic toxicity have been reported rarely.

Teeth: Permanent discoloration of teeth may be caused during tooth development. Enamel hypoplasia has also been reported. (See **WARNINGS**)

Blood: hemolytic anemia, thrombocytopenia, thrombocytopenic purpura, neutropenia, and eosinophilia

CNS: Pseudotumor cerebri (benign intracranial hypertension) in adults and bulging fontanels in infants. (See **PRECAUTIONS/Tetracycline**) Dizziness, tinnitus, and visual disturbances have been reported. Myasthenic syndrome has been reported rarely.

Renal: Rise in BUN has been reported and is apparently dose related. (See **WARNINGS**)

Skin: Maculopapular and erythematous rashes have been reported. Exfoliative dermatitis has been rarely reported. Photosensitivity has been reported rarely. (See **WARNINGS**)

OVERDOSAGE

In case of an overdose, patients should contact a physician, poison control center, or emergency room. There is neither a pharmacological basis nor data suggesting an increased toxicity of the combination compared to individual components.

DOSAGE AND ADMINISTRATION

Each dose of PYLERA™ includes 3 capsules. Each dose of all 3 capsules should be taken 4 times a day, after meals and at bedtime for 10 days. Patients should be instructed to swallow the PYLERA™ capsules whole with a full glass of water (8 ounces). One omeprazole 20 mg capsule should be taken twice a day with PYLERA™ after the morning and evening meal for 10 days.

Table 6: Daily Dosing Schedule for PYLERA™ and Omeprazole

Time of dose	Number of capsules of PYLERA™	Number of capsules of Omeprazole 20 mg
After morning meal	3	1
After lunch	3	0

After evening meal	3	1
At bedtime	3	0

Ingestion of adequate amounts of fluid, particularly with the bedtime dose, is recommended to reduce the risk of esophageal irritation and ulceration by tetracycline hydrochloride.

HOW SUPPLIED

PYLERA™ is supplied as a white opaque capsule containing 140 mg bismuth subcitrate potassium, 125 mg metronidazole, and 125 mg tetracycline hydrochloride, with Axcan Pharma logo printed on body and BMT printed on cap. PYLERA™ is supplied in bottles of 120 capsules.
NDC Number 58914-600-21, Bottle of 120.
Store at controlled room temperature [68° to 77°F or 20° to 25°C].

REFERENCES

1. Clinical and Laboratory Standards Institute. *Methods for Dilution Antimicrobial Susceptibility Tests for Bacteria That Grow Aerobically*; Approved Standard — Seventh Edition. Clinical and Laboratory Standards Institute document M7-A7, Vol. 26, No. 2, CLSI, Wayne, PA, January 2006.
CAUTION: Federal law prohibits dispensing without a prescription.
Pylera(tm) is a trademark owned by Axcan Pharma Inc.
Axcan Pharma™ and the Axcan Pharma™ logo are trademarks of Axcan Pharma Inc., the parent company of AXCAN PHARMA US, INC.
PYLERA™ Capsules are manufactured by Draxis Health Inc. for AXCAN PHARMA US, INC., Birmingham, AL 35242

Bausch & Lomb Incorporated

**ONE BAUSCH & LOMB PLACE
ROCHESTER NY 14604**

**7 GIRALDA FARMS
MADISON, NJ 07940**

Direct Inquiries to:
Main Office
(585) 338-6000
Consumer Affairs
1-800-553-5340

BESIVANCE™   ℞
**(besifloxacin ophthalmic
suspension, 0.6%)**

HIGHLIGHTS OF PRESCRIBING INFORMATION

These highlights do not include all the information needed to use Besivance safely and effectively. See full prescribing information for Besivance.
Besivance™ (besifloxacin ophthalmic suspension) 0.6%
Sterile topical ophthalmic drops
Initial U.S. Approval: 2009

INDICATIONS AND USAGE

Besivance™ (besifloxacin ophthalmic suspension) 0.6%, is a quinolone antimicrobial indicated for the treatment of bacterial conjunctivitis caused by susceptible isolates of the following bacteria:
CDC coryneform group G
Corynebacterium pseudodiphtheriticum*, Corynebacterium striatum*, Haemophilus influenzae, Moraxella lacunata*, Staphylococcus aureus, Staphylococcus epidermidis, Staphylococcus hominis*, Staphylococcus lugdunensis*, Streptococcus mitis group, *Streptococcus oralis, Streptococcus pneumoniae, Streptococcus salivarius**
**Efficacy for this organism was studied in fewer than 10 infections. (1)

DOSAGE AND ADMINISTRATION

Instill one drop in the affected eye(s) 3 times a day, four to twelve hours apart for 7 days. (2)

DOSAGE FORMS AND STRENGTHS

7.5 mL size bottle filled with 5 mL of besifloxacin ophthalmic suspension, 0.6% (3)

CONTRAINDICATIONS

None

WARNINGS AND PRECAUTIONS

Topical Ophthalmic Use Only. (5.1)
Growth of Resistant Organisms with Prolonged Use. (5.2)
Avoidance of Contact Lenses. Patients should not wear contact lenses if they have signs or symptoms of bacterial conjunctivitis or during the course of therapy with Besivance™ (5.3)

ADVERSE REACTIONS

The most common adverse event reported in 2% of patients treated with Besivance™ was conjunctival redness. (6)
To report SUSPECTED ADVERSE REACTIONS, contact Bausch & Lomb Incorporated at 1-800-323-0000 or FDA at 1-800-FDA-1088 or www.fda.gov/medwatch.
See 17 for PATIENT COUNSELING INFORMATION
                Revised 4/2009

FULL PRESCRIBING INFORMATION: CONTENTS*

1. **INDICATIONS AND USAGE**
2. **DOSAGE AND ADMINISTRATION**
3. **DOSAGE FORMS AND STRENGTHS**
4. **CONTRAINDICATIONS**
5. **WARNINGS AND PRECAUTIONS**
   5.1 Topical Ophthalmic Use Only
   5.2 Growth of Resistant Organisms with Prolonged Use
   5.3 Avoidance of Contact Lenses
6. **ADVERSE REACTIONS**
8. **USE IN SPECIFIC POPULATIONS**
   8.1 Pregnancy
   8.3 Nursing Mothers
   8.4 Pediatric Use
   8.5 Geriatric Use
11. **DESCRIPTION**
12. **CLINICAL PHARMACOLOGY**
   12.1 Mechanism Of Action
   12.3 Pharmacokinetics
   12.4 Microbiology
13. **NONCLINICAL TOXICOLOGY**
   13.1 Carcinogenesis, Mutagenesis, Impairment Of Fertility
14. **CLINICAL STUDIES**
16. **HOW SUPPLIED/STORAGE AND HANDLING**
17. **PATIENT COUNSELING INFORMATION**
*Sections or subsections omitted from the full prescribing information are not listed

FULL PRESCRIBING INFORMATION

1. INDICATIONS AND USAGE

Besivance™ (besifloxacin ophthalmic suspension) 0.6%, is indicated for the treatment of bacterial conjunctivitis caused by susceptible isolates of the following bacteria:
CDC coryneform group G
Corynebacterium pseudodiphtheriticum*
Corynebacterium striatum*
Haemophilus influenzae
Moraxella lacunata*
Staphylococcus aureus
Staphylococcus epidermidis
Staphylococcus hominis*
Staphylococcus lugdunensis*
Streptococcus mitis group
Streptococcus oralis
Streptococcus pneumoniae
Streptococcus salivarius*
**Efficacy for this organism was studied in fewer than 10 infections.

2. DOSAGE AND ADMINISTRATION

Invert closed bottle and shake once before use.
Instill one drop in the affected eye(s) 3 times a day, four to twelve hours apart for 7 days.

3. DOSAGE FORMS AND STRENGTHS

7.5 mL bottle filled with 5 mL of besifloxacin ophthalmic suspension, 0.6%.

4. CONTRAINDICATIONS

None

5. WARNINGS AND PRECAUTIONS

5.1 Topical Ophthalmic Use Only
NOT FOR INJECTION INTO THE EYE.
Besivance™ is for topical ophthalmic use only, and should not be injected subconjunctivally, nor should it be introduced directly into the anterior chamber of the eye.
5.2 Growth of Resistant Organisms with Prolonged Use
As with other anti-infectives, prolonged use of Besivance™ (besifloxacin ophthalmic suspension) 0.6% may result in overgrowth of non-susceptible organisms, including fungi. If super-infection occurs, discontinue use and institute alternative therapy. Whenever clinical judgment dictates, the patient should be examined with the aid of magnification, such as slit-lamp biomicroscopy, and, where appropriate, fluorescein staining.
5.3 Avoidance of Contact Lenses
Patients should not wear contact lenses if they have signs or symptoms of bacterial conjunctivitis or during the course of therapy with Besivance™.

6. ADVERSE REACTIONS

Because clinical trials are conducted under widely varying conditions, adverse reaction rates observed in one clinical trial of a drug cannot be directly compared with the rates in the clinical trials of the same or another drug and may not reflect the rates observed in practice. The data described below reflect exposure to Besivance™ in approximately 1,000 patients between 1 and 98 years old with clinical signs and symptoms of bacterial conjunctivitis. The most frequently reported ocular adverse event was conjunctival redness, reported in approximately 2% of patients.
Other adverse events reported in patients receiving Besivance™ occurring in approximately 1-2% of patients included: blurred vision, eye pain, eye irritation, eye pruritus and headache.

8. USE IN SPECIFIC POPULATIONS

8.1 Pregnancy
Pregnancy Category C. Oral doses of besifloxacin up to 1000 mg/kg/day were not associated with visceral or skeletal malformations in rat pups in a study of embryo-fetal development, although this dose was associated with maternal toxicity (reduced body weight gain and food consumption) and maternal mortality. Increased postimplantation loss, decreased fetal body weights, and decreased fetal ossification were also observed. At this dose, the mean C_{max} in the rat dams was approximately 20 mcg/mL, >45,000 times the mean plasma concentrations measured in humans. The No Observed Adverse Effect Level (NOAEL) for this embryo-fetal development study was 100 mg/kg/day (C_{max}, 5 mcg/mL, >11,000 times the mean plasma concentrations measured in humans).
In a prenatal and postnatal development study in rats, the NOAELs for both fetal and maternal toxicity were also 100 mg/kg/day. At 1000 mg/kg/day, the pups weighed significantly less than controls and had a reduced neonatal survival rate. Attainment of developmental landmarks and sexual maturation were delayed, although surviving pups from this dose group that were reared to maturity did not demonstrate deficits in behavior, including activity, learning and memory, and their reproductive capacity appeared normal. Since there are no adequate and well-controlled studies in pregnant women, Besivance™ should be used during pregnancy only if the potential benefit justifies the potential risk to the fetus.
8.3 Nursing Mothers
Besifloxacin has not been measured in human milk, although it can be presumed to be excreted in human milk. Caution should be exercised when Besivance™ is administered to a nursing mother.
8.4 Pediatric Use
The safety and effectiveness of Besivance™ in infants below one year of age have not been established. The efficacy of Besivance™ in treating bacterial conjunctivitis in pediatric patients one year or older has been demonstrated in controlled clinical trials [see 14 CLINICAL STUDIES]. There is no evidence that the ophthalmic administration of quinolones has any effect on weight bearing joints, even though systemic administration of some quinolones has been shown to cause arthropathy in immature animals.
8.5 Geriatric Use
No overall differences in safety and effectiveness have been observed between elderly and younger patients.

11. DESCRIPTION

Besivance™ (besifloxacin ophthalmic suspension) 0.6%, is a sterile ophthalmic suspension of besifloxacin formulated with DuraSite®* (polycarbophil, edetate disodium dihydrate and sodium chloride). Each mL of Besivance™ contains 6.63 mg besifloxacin hydrochloride equivalent to 6 mg besifloxacin base. It is an 8-chloro fluoroquinolone anti-infective for topical ophthalmic use.

$C_{19}H_{21}ClFN_3O_3 \cdot HCl$
Mol Wt 430.30

Chemical Name: (+)-7-[(3R)-3-aminohexahydro-1H-azepin-1-yl]-8-chloro-1-cyclopropyl-6-fluoro-4-oxo-1,4-dihydroquinoline-3-carboxylic acid hydrochloride.
Besifloxacin hydrochloride is a white to pale yellowish-white powder.

Each mL Contains:
Active: besifloxacin 0.6% (6 mg/mL);
Preservative: benzalkonium chloride 0.01%
Inactives: polycarbophil, mannitol, poloxamer 407, sodium chloride, edetate disodium dihydrate, sodium hydroxide and water for injection.
Besivance™ is an isotonic suspension with an osmolality of approximately 290 mOsm/kg.

12. CLINICAL PHARMACOLOGY
12.1 Mechanism Of Action
Besifloxacin is a fluoroquinolone antibacterial [see 12.4 Clinical Pharmacology, Microbiology].
12.3 Pharmacokinetics
Plasma concentrations of besifloxacin were measured in adult patients with suspected bacterial conjunctivitis who received Besivance™ bilaterally three times a day (16 doses total). Following the first and last dose, the maximum plasma besifloxacin concentration in each patient was less than 1.3 ng/mL. The mean besifloxacin C_{max} was 0.37 ng/mL on day 1 and 0.43 ng/mL on day 6. The average elimination half-life of besifloxacin in plasma following multiple dosing was estimated to be 7 hours.
12.4 Microbiology
Besifloxacin is an 8-chloro fluoroquinolone with a N-1 cyclopropyl group. The compound has activity against Gram-positive and Gram-negative bacteria due to the inhibition of both bacterial DNA gyrase and topoisomerase IV. DNA gyrase is an essential enzyme required for replication, transcription and repair of bacterial DNA. Topoisomerase IV is an essential enzyme required for partitioning of the chromosomal DNA during bacterial cell division. Besifloxacin is bactericidal with minimum bactericidal concentrations (MBCs) generally within one dilution of the minimum inhibitory concentrations (MICs).
The mechanism of action of fluoroquinolones, including besifloxacin, is different from that of aminoglycoside, macrolide, and β-lactam antibiotics. Therefore, besifloxacin may be active against pathogens that are resistant to these antibiotics and these antibiotics may be active against pathogens that are resistant to besifloxacin. In vitro studies demonstrated cross-resistance between besifloxacin and some fluoroquinolones.
In vitro resistance to besifloxacin develops via multiple-step mutations and occurs at a general frequency of $< 3.3 \times 10^{-10}$ for Staphylococcus aureus and $< 7 \times 10^{-10}$ for Streptococcus pneumoniae.
Besifloxacin has been shown to be active against most isolates of the following bacteria both in vitro and in conjunctival infections treated in clinical trials as described in the INDICATIONS AND USAGE section:
CDC coryneform group G
Corynebacterium pseudodiphtheriticum*
Corynebacterium striatum*
Haemophilus influenzae
Moraxella lacunata*
Staphylococcus aureus
Staphylococcus epidermidis
Staphylococcus hominis*
Staphylococcus lugdunensis*
Streptococcus mitis group
Streptococcus oralis
Streptococcus pneumoniae
Streptococcus salivarius*
*Efficacy for this organism was studied in fewer than 10 infections.

13. NONCLINICAL TOXICOLOGY
13.1 Carcinogenesis, Mutagenesis, Impairment Of Fertility
Long-term studies in animals to determine the carcinogenic potential of besifloxacin have not been performed.
No in vitro mutagenic activity of besifloxacin was observed in an Ames test (up to 3.33 mcg/plate) on bacterial tester strains Salmonella typhimurium TA98, TA100, TA1535, TA1537 and Escherichia coli WP2uvrA. However, it was mutagenic in S. typhimurium strain TA102 and E. coli strain WP2(pKM101). Positive responses in these strains have been observed with other quinolones and are likely related to topoisomerase inhibition.
Besifloxacin induced chromosomal aberrations in CHO cells in vitro and it was positive in an in vivo mouse micronucleus assay at oral doses ≥ 1500 mg/kg. Besifloxacin did not induce unscheduled DNA synthesis in hepatocytes cultured from rats given the test compound up to 2,000 mg/kg by the oral route. In a fertility and early embryonic development study in rats, besifloxacin did not impair the fertility of male or female rats at oral doses of up to 500 mg/kg/day. This is over 10,000 times higher than the recommended total daily human ophthalmic dose.

14. CLINICAL STUDIES
In a randomized, double-masked, vehicle controlled, multicenter clinical trial, in which patients 1-98 years of age were dosed 3 times a day for 5 days, Besivance™ was superior to its vehicle in patients with bacterial conjunctivitis. Clinical resolution was achieved in 45% (90/198) for the Besivance™ treated group versus 33% (63/191) for the vehicle treated group (difference 12%, 95% CI 3%-22%). Microbiological outcomes demonstrated a statistically significant eradication rate for causative pathogens of 91% (181/198) for the Besivance™ treated group versus 60% (114/191) for the vehicle treated group (difference 31%, 95% CI 23%-40%). Microbiologic eradication does not always correlate with clinical outcome in anti-infective trials.

16. HOW SUPPLIED/STORAGE AND HANDLING
Besivance™ (besifloxacin ophthalmic suspension) 0.6%, is supplied as a sterile ophthalmic suspension in a white low density polyethylene (LDPE) bottle with a controlled dropper tip and tan polypropylene cap. Tamper evidence is provided with a shrink band around the cap and neck area of the package.
5 mL in 7.5 mL bottle
NDC 24208-446-05
Storage: Store at 15°-25°C (59°-77°F). Protect from Light. Invert closed bottle and shake once before use.
Rx Only

17. PATIENT COUNSELING INFORMATION
Patients should be advised to avoid contaminating the applicator tip with material from the eye, fingers or other source.
Although Besivance™ is not intended to be administered systemically, quinolones administered systemically have been associated with hypersensitivity reactions, even following a single dose. Patients should be advised to discontinue use immediately and contact their physician at the first sign of a rash or allergic reaction.
Patients should be told that although it is common to feel better early in the course of the therapy, the medication should be taken exactly as directed. Skipping doses or not completing the full course of therapy may (1) decrease the effectiveness of the immediate treatment and (2) increase the likelihood that bacteria will develop resistance and will not be treatable by Besivance™ or other antibacterial drugs in the future.
Patients should be advised not to wear contact lenses if they have signs or symptoms of bacterial conjunctivitis or during the course of therapy with Besivance™.
Patients should be advised to thoroughly wash hands prior to using Besivance™.
Patients should be instructed to invert closed bottle (upside down) and shake once before each use. Remove cap with bottle still in the inverted position. Tilt head back, and with bottle inverted, gently squeeze bottle to instill one drop into the affected eye(s).

MANUFACTURER INFORMATION
Manufactured by: Bausch & Lomb Incorporated
Tampa, Florida 33637
©Bausch & Lomb Incorporated
U.S. Patent No. 6,685,958
U.S. Patent No. 6,699,492
U.S. Patent No. 5,447,926
Besivance™ is a trademark of Bausch & Lomb Incorporated
*DuraSite is a trademark of InSite Vision Incorporated
April 2009
9142602 (flat)
9142702 (folded)

Baxter Healthcare Corporation
BIOSCIENCE
ONE BAXTER WAY
WESTLAKE VILLAGE, CA 91362

For Medical Information Contact:
Baxter Healthcare Corporation
Baxter Medical Information
(866) 424-6724

ADVATE ℞
[ăd-vāt]
[antihemophilic factor (recombinant), plasma/albumin-free method]

HIGHLIGHTS OF PRESCRIBING INFORMATION
These highlights do not include all the information needed to use ADVATE safely and effectively. See full prescribing information for ADVATE.
ADVATE
[Antihemophilic Factor (Recombinant), Plasma/Albumin-Free Method]
For Intravenous Use, Lyophilized Powder for Reconstitution
Initial U.S. Approval: 2003

---RECENT MAJOR CHANGES---
Dosage and Administration   03/2010

---INDICATIONS AND USAGE---
ADVATE is an Antihemophilic Factor (Recombinant) indicated for:
• Control and prevention of bleeding episodes in adults and children (0-16 years) with Hemophilia A (1.1)
• Peri-operative management in adults and children (0-16 years) with hemophilia A (1.2)
• ADVATE is not indicated for the treatment of von Willebrand's disease. (1.2)

---DOSAGE AND ADMINISTRATION---
• For intravenous use after reconstitution only (2)
• Each vial of ADVATE contains the labeled amount of recombinant Factor VIII in international units (IU) (2)
• The required dosage is determined using the following formulas:
Desired increment in Factor VIII concentration (IU/dL or % of normal)=[Total Dose (IU)/body weight (kg) × 2 [IU/dL]/[IU/kg]
OR Required Dose (IU) = body weight (kg) × Desired Factor VIII Rise (IU/dL or % of normal) × 0.5 (IU/kg per IU/dL).
• Frequency of intravenous injection of the reconstituted product is determined by the type of bleeding episode and the recommendation of the treating physician (2.1, 2.2)

---DOSAGE FORMS AND STRENGTHS---
ADVATE is available as a lyophilized powder in single use vials containing 250, 500, 1000, 1500, 2000, 3000 IU (3)

---CONTRAINDICATIONS---
Known anaphylaxis to mouse or hamster protein or other constituents of the product. (4)

---WARNINGS AND PRECAUTIONS---
• Anaphylaxis and severe hypersensitivity reactions are possible. Should symptoms occur, treatment with ADVATE should be discontinued, and appropriate treatment should be administered (5.1)
• Patients may develop hypersensitivity to mouse or hamster protein, which is present in trace amounts in the product (5.1)
• Development of activity-neutralizing antibodies has been detected in patients receiving Factor VIII-containing products. If expected plasma Factor VIII activity levels are not attained, or if bleeding is not controlled with an appropriate dose, an assay that measures Factor VIII inhibitor concentration should be performed. (5.2)

---ADVERSE REACTIONS---
The most serious adverse drug reactions are hypersensitivity reactions and Factor VIII inhibitors. (6.1)
The most common adverse drug reactions observed in ≥ 2% of patients are: Factor VIII inhibitors (observed predominantly in previously untreated patients (PUPs) and headache. (6.1)
To report SUSPECTED ADVERSE REACTIONS, contact Baxter Healthcare Corporation at 1-866-888-2472 or FDA at 1-800-FDA-1088 or www.fda.gov/medwatch

---USE IN SPECIFIC POPULATIONS---
Pregnancy: No human or animal Pregnancy: No human or animal data. Use only if clearly needed. (8.1)
Pediatric Use: Consider larger or more frequent doses to account for the observed differences in adjusted recovery and terminal half-life. Dose adjustment may be needed (8.4).
See 17 for PATIENT COUNSELING INFORMATION and FDA approved patient labeling
Revised: 03/2010

Table 1.
Guide to ADVATE Dosing for Treatment of Bleeding Episodes in Adults and Children

Degree of Hemorrhage or Type of Bleeding Episodes	Required Peak Postinfusion Factor VIII Activity in the Blood (as % of Normal or IU/dL)	Dosage and Frequency Necessary to Maintain the Therapeutic Plasma Level
Minor Early hemarthrosis, muscle bleeding episode, or mild oral bleeding episode.	20-40	10-20 IU/kg[a] Repeat infusions every 12 to 24 hours (8 to 24 hours for patients under the age of 6) for one to three days until the bleeding episode is resolved (as indicated by relief of pain) or healing is achieved.
Moderate Moderate bleeding into muscles, bleeding into the oral cavity, definite hemarthroses, and known trauma.	30-60	15-30 IU per kg[a] Repeat infusions every 12 to 24 hours (8 to 24 hours for patients under the age of 6) for three days or more until the bleeding episode is resolved (as indicated by relief of pain) or healing is achieved.
Major Significant gastrointestinal bleeding, intracranial, intra-abdominal or intrathoracic bleeding, central nervous system bleeding, bleeding in the retropharyngeal or retroperitoneal spaces or iliopsoas sheath, fractures, head trauma.	60-100	Initial dose 30-50 IU per kg[a] Repeat dose 30-50 IU per kg every 8 to 24 hours (6 to 12 hours for patients under the age of 6) until resolution of the bleeding episode has occurred.

[a] Dose (IU/kg) = Desired factor VIII Rise (IU/dL or % of normal) × 0.5 (IU/kg per IU/dL)

Table 2.
Guide to ADVATE Dosing for Peri-operative Management in Adults and Children

Type of Surgery	Required Peak Post-infusion Factor VIII Activity in the Blood (as % of Normal or IU/dL)	Frequency of Infusion
Minor Including tooth extraction	60-100	A single bolus infusion (30-50 IU/kg[a]) beginning within one hour of the operation. Optional additional dosing every 12 to 24 hours as needed to control bleeding. For dental procedures, adjunctive therapy may be considered.
Major Examples include intracranial, intra-abdominal, or intrathoracic surgery, joint replacement surgery	80-120 (pre- and post-operative)	Preoperative bolus infusion: 40–60 IU/kg[a]. Verify 100% activity has been achieved prior to surgery. Maintenance bolus infusion (40-60 IU/kg[a]) repeat infusions every 8 to 24 hours (6 to 24 hours for patients under the age of 6), depending on the desired level of factor VIII and state of wound healing.

[a] Dose (IU/kg) = Desired factor VIII Rise (IU/dL or % of normal) × 0.5 (IU/kg per IU/dL)

12.1 Mechanism of Action
12.2 Pharmacodynamics
12.3 Pharmacokinetics
13 NONCLINICAL TOXICOLOGY
  13.1 Carcinogenesis, Mutagenesis, Impairment of Fertility
14 CLINICAL STUDIES
  14.1 Original Safety and Efficacy Study
  14.2 Continuation Study
  14.3 Perioperative Management Study
15 REFERENCES
16 HOW SUPPLIED/STORAGE AND HANDLING
  16.1 How Supplied
  16.2 Storage and Handling
17 PATIENT COUNSELING INFORMATION AND FDA-APPROVED PATIENT LABELING
* *Sections or subsections omitted from the full prescribing information are not listed*

FULL PRESCRIBING INFORMATION
ADVATE [Antihemophilic Factor (Recombinant), Plasma/Albumin-Free Method]

1. INDICATIONS AND USAGE
1.1 Control and Prevention of Bleeding Episodes
ADVATE is an Antihemophilic Factor (Recombinant) indicated for control and prevention of bleeding episodes in adults and children (0-16 years) with Hemophilia A.
1.2 Perioperative Management
ADVATE is indicated in the peri-operative management in adults and children (0-16 years) with Hemophilia A.

ADVATE is not indicated for the treatment of von Willebrand's disease.

2. DOSAGE AND ADMINISTRATION
For Intravenous Use After Reconstitution Only
• Treatment with ADVATE should be initiated under the supervision of a physician experienced in the treatment of hemophilia A.
• Each vial of ADVATE has the recombinant Factor VIII potency in international units stated on the label. The expected in vivo peak increase in factor VIII level expressed as IU/dL of plasma or percent normal can be estimated by multiplying the dose administered per kg body weight (IU/kg) by 2.
• The dosage and duration depend on the severity of Factor VIII deficiency, the location and extent of the bleeding, and the patient's clinical condition. Careful control of replacement therapy is especially important in cases of major surgery or life-threatening bleeding episodes. [Control and Prevention of Bleeding Episodes (2.1) and Perioperative Management (2.2)]
The expected in vivo peak increase in Factor VIII level expressed as IU/dL (or % of normal) can be estimated using the following formulas:
IU/dL (or % of normal)=[Total Dose (IU)/body weight (kg)] × 2 [IU/dL]/[IU/kg]
OR
Dose (IU) = body weight (kg) × Desired Factor VIII Rise (IU/dL or % of normal) × 0.5 (IU/kg per IU/dL)
Examples (assuming patient's baseline Factor VIII level is < 1% of normal):

1. A dose of 1750 IU ADVATE administered to a 70 kg patient should be expected to result in a peak postinfusion Factor VIII increase of 1750 IU × {[2 IU/dL]/[IU/kg]}/ [70 kg] = 50 IU/dL (50% of normal).
2. A peak level of 70% is required in a 40 kg child. In this situation, the appropriate dose would be 40 kg × 70 IU/dL/{[2 IU/dL]/[IU/kg]} = 1400 IU.
The dose and frequency of administration should be based on the individual clinical response. Patients may vary in their pharmacokinetic (e.g. half-life, in vivo recovery) and clinical responses to ADVATE. Although you can estimate the dose by the calculations above, it is highly recommended that, whenever possible, appropriate laboratory tests including serial Factor VIII activity assays be performed [see WARNINGS and PRECAUTIONS: Monitoring Laboratory Tests (5.4) and Pharmacokinetics (12.3)].
2.1 Control and Prevention of Bleeding Episodes
A guide for dosing in the treatment of bleeding episodes is provided in Table 1. The careful control of treatment dose is especially important in cases of life-threatening episodes. [See table 1 at left]
2.2 Peri-operative Management
A guide for dosing in perioperative management is provided in Table 2. The careful control of dose and duration of treatment is especially important in cases of major surgery or life-threatening bleeding episodes. [See table 2 at left]
2.3 Instruction for Use
ADVATE is administered by intravenous (IV) injection after reconstitution. Patients should follow the specific reconstitution and administration procedures provided by their physicians.
For instructions, patients should follow the recommendations in the FDA-approved patient labeling. [see FDA Approved Patient Labeling (17)]
Reconstitution, product administration, and handling of the administration set and needles must be done with caution. Percutaneous puncture with a needle contaminated with blood can transmit infectious viruses including HIV (AIDS) and hepatitis. Obtain immediate medical attention if injury occurs. Place needles in a sharps container after single use. Discard all equipment, including any reconstituted ADVATE in an appropriate container.
2.4 Preparation and Reconstitution
The procedures below are provided as general guidelines for the reconstitution and administration of ADVATE. Always work on a clean surface and wash hands before performing the following procedures.
1. Bring the ADVATE (dry factor concentrate) and Sterile Water for Injection, USP (diluent) to room temperature.
2. Remove caps from the factor concentrate and diluent vials.
3. Cleanse stoppers with germicidal solution, and allow to dry prior to use. Place the vials on a flat surface.
4. Open the BAXJECT II device package by peeling away the lid, without touching the inside (Figure A). **Do not remove the device from the package.**
5. Turn the package over. Press straight down to fully insert the clear plastic spike through the diluent vial stopper (Figure B).
6. Grip the BAXJECT II package at its edge and pull the package off the device (Figure C). **Do not remove the blue cap from the BAXJECT II device.** Do not touch the exposed white plastic spike.
7. Turn the system over, so that the diluent vial is on top. Quickly insert the white plastic spike fully into the ADVATE vial stopper by pushing straight down (Figure D). The vacuum will draw the diluent into the ADVATE vial.
8. Swirl gently until ADVATE is completely dissolved.
Do not refrigerate after reconstitution.
2.5 Administration:
ADVATE is intended for intravenous use after reconstitution only.
• Inspect parenteral drug products for particulate matter and discoloration prior to administration, whenever solution and container permit. The solution should be clear and colorless in appearance. If not, do not use the solution and notify Baxter immediately.
• Administer ADVATE at room temperature not more than 3 hours after reconstitution.
• Plastic syringes must be used with this product, since proteins such as ADVATE tend to stick to the surface of glass syringes.
1. Use aseptic technique.
2. Remove the blue cap from the BAXJECT II device. Connect the syringe to the BAXJECT II device (Figure E). DO NOT INJECT AIR.
3. Turn the system upside down (factor concentrate vial now on top). Draw the factor concentrate into the syringe by pulling the plunger back slowly (Figure F).
4. Disconnect the syringe; attach a suitable needle and inject intravenously as instructed under **Administration by Bolus Infusion**.
5. If a patient is to receive more than one vial of ADVATE, the contents of multiple vials may be drawn into the same syringe. **Please note that the BAXJECT II device is intended for use with a single vial of ADVATE and Sterile**

Water for Injection only, therefore reconstituting and withdrawing a second vial into the syringe requires a second BAXJECT II device.

ADMINISTRATION BY BOLUS INFUSION

Administer a dose of ADVATE over a period of ≤ 5 minutes (maximum infusion rate, 10 mL/min). Determine the pulse rate before and during administration of ADVATE. Should a significant increase in pulse rate occur, reducing the rate of administration or temporarily halting the injection usually allows the symptoms to disappear promptly.

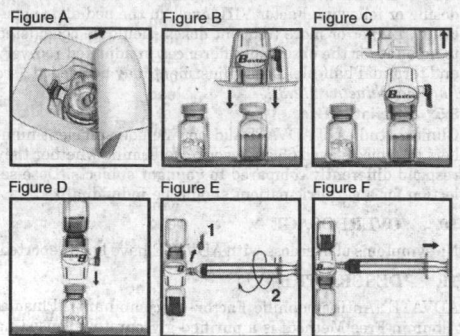

Figure A   Figure B   Figure C
Figure D   Figure E   Figure F

3. DOSAGE FORMS AND STRENGTHS

ADVATE is available as a lyophilized powder in single use glass vials containing nominally 250, 500, 1000, 1500, 2000 or 3000 International Units (IU).

Each vial of ADVATE is labeled with the recombinant antihemophilic factor (rAHF) activity expressed in IU per vial. This potency assignment employs a Factor VIII concentrate standard that is referenced to a WHO International Standard for Factor VIII concentrates, and is evaluated by appropriate methodology to ensure accuracy of the results.

4. CONTRAINDICATIONS

Known anaphylaxis to mouse or hamster protein or other constituents of the product.

5. WARNINGS AND PRECAUTIONS

5.1   Anaphylaxis and Hypersensitivity Reactions

ADVATE. Symptoms have manifested as dizziness, paresthesias, rash, flushing, face swelling, urticaria, dyspnea, and pruritis. *[see Patient Counseling Information (17)]*

ADVATE contains trace amounts of mouse immunoglobulin G (MuIgG; maximum of 0.1 ng/IU ADVATE) and hamster proteins (maximum of 1.5 ng/IU ADVATE). Patients treated with this product may develop hypersensitivity to these non-human mammalian proteins.

Discontinue ADVATE if hypersensitivity symptoms occur and administer appropriate emergency treatment.

5.2   Neutralizing Antibodies

Patients treated with AHF products should be carefully monitored for the development of Factor VIII inhibitors by appropriate clinical observations and laboratory tests. Inhibitors have been reported following administration of ADVATE predominantly in previously untreated patients (PUPs) and previously minimally treated patients (MTPs). If expected plasma Factor VIII activity levels are not attained, or if bleeding is not controlled with an expected dose, an assay that measures Factor VIII inhibitor concentration should be performed *[see Monitoring Laboratory Tests (5.3)]*.

5.3   Monitoring Laboratory Tests

- Monitor plasma Factor VIII activity levels by the one-stage clotting assay to confirm the adequate Factor VIII levels have been achieved and maintained, when clinically indicated *[see Dosage and Administration (2)]*.
- Monitor for development of Factor VIII inhibitors. Perform the Bethesda assay to determine if Factor VIII inhibitor is present. If expected Factor VIII activity plasma levels are not attained, or if bleeding is not controlled with the expected dose of ADVATE. Use Bethesda Units (BU) to titer inhibitors.
  - If the inhibitor is less than 10 BU per mL, the administration of additional Antihemophilic Factor concentrate may neutralize the inhibitor, and may permit an appropriate hemostatic response.
  - Adequate hemostasis may not be achieved if inhibitor titers are above 10 BU per mL. The inhibitor titer may rise following ADVATE infusion as a result of an anamnestic response to Factor VIII. The treatment or prevention of bleeding in such patients requires the use of alternative therapeutic approaches and agents.

The clinical response to ADVATE may vary. If bleeding is not controlled with the recommended dose, the plasma level of Factor VIII should be determined and a sufficient dose of ADVATE should be administered to achieve a satisfactory clinical response. If the patient's plasma Factor VIII level fails to increase as expected or if bleeding is not controlled

Table 3.
Adverse Events Reported by > 5% Treated of Study Subjects[a]

MedDRA[b] System Organ Class	MedDRA Preferred Term	Number of Events	Number of Subjects	Percent[c] of Subjects
Ear and labyrinth disorders	Ear pain	17	14	6.0
Gastrointestinal disorders	Constipation	16	12	5.1
	Diarrhoea	48	34	14.5
	Nausea	25	19	8.1
	Vomiting	53	38	16.2
General disorders and administration site conditions	Influenza like illness	17	13	5.6
	Pain	21	18	7.7
	Pyrexia	173	76	32.5
Infections and infestations	Ear infection	40	25	10.7
	Influenza	22	18	7.7
	Nasopharyngitis	121	62	26.5
	Otitis media	12	12	5.1
	Sinusitis	21	14	6.0
	Upper respiratory tract infection	49	31	13.2
Injury, poisoning and procedural complications	Accident	41	20	8.5
	Fall	22	17	7.3
	Joint sprain	16	14	6.0
	Limb injury	141	44	18.8
	Procedural pain	16	12	5.1
Musculoskeletal and connective tissue disorders	Arthralgia	79	40	17.1
	Joint swelling	15	13	5.6
	Pain in extremity	22	15	6.4
Nervous system disorders	Headache	205	64	27.4
Respiratory, thoracic and mediastinal disorders	Cough	150	68	29.1
	Nasal congestion	64	33	14.1
	Pharyngolaryngeal pain	50	32	13.7
	Rhinorrhoea	40	25	10.7
Skin and subcutaneous tissue disorders	Rash	23	19	8.1

[a] Includes data from 234 treated subjects from 5 completed studies in PTPs, and 1 ongoing study in PUPs as of 27 March 2006.
[b] MedDRA version 8.1 was used.
[c] This percent is calculated relative to 234, the total number of treated subjects.

after the expected dose, the presence of an inhibitor (neutralizing antibodies) should be suspected and appropriate testing performed.

6. ADVERSE REACTIONS

The most serious adverse drug reactions (ADRs) seen with ADVATE are hypersensitivity reactions and the development of high-titer inhibitors necessitating alternative treatments to Factor VIII.

The most common ADRs observed in clinical trials (frequency > 2% of subjects) were: Factor VIII inhibitor formation (observed predominantly in PUPs) and headache (6.1).

6.1   Clinical Trial Experience

Because clinical trials are conducted under widely varying conditions, adverse reaction rates observed in the clinical trials of a drug cannot be directly compared to rates in clinical trials of another drug and may not reflect the rates observed in clinical practice.

ADVATE has been evaluated in five completed studies in previously treated patients (PTPs) and one ongoing study in PUPs with severe to moderately severe Hemophilia A (Factor VIII ≤ 2% of normal). A total of 234 subjects have been treated with ADVATE as of March 2006. Total exposure to ADVATE was 44,926 infusions. The median duration of participation per subject was 370.5 (range: 1 to 1,256) days and the median exposure to ADVATE per subject was 128.0 (range: 1 to 598) days.

There were 2,507 adverse events (AEs) reported in 215 subjects. The most common AEs (product-related and unrelated, according to the investigator's opinion) occurring in at least 5% of subjects who received at least 1 ADVATE study infusion are shown in Table 3. None of the subjects withdrew from the studies due to adverse events. There were no deaths. Nineteen treated subjects reported no AEs during their participation.

[See table 3 above]

The majority of the events in Table 3 appear to have been related to trauma, intercurrent mild respiratory or gastrointestinal disease or well-described complications of hemophilia.

Fifty-six ADRs were reported in 27 subjects. None were reported in neonates, 16 were reported in infants, 7 were reported in children, 8 were reported in adolescents, and 25 were reported in adults. Nearly all ADRs (53/56) were isolated events or occurred once in one subject with numerous subsequent infusions without reoccurrence. The most common ADRs with a frequency greater than or equal to 2% are shown in Table 4.

Table 4.
Summary of Most Common Adverse Drug Reactions (ADRs)[a] with a Frequency ≥ 2%

MedDRA System Organ Class	MedDRA Preferred Term	Number of Patients	ADR Rate (% Patients)[b]
Investigations	Anti-factor VIII antibody positive	5[c]	2.14%
Nervous System Disorders	Headache	5	2.14%

[a] ADR = Adverse Drug Reaction = adverse events considered by the investigator to be at least possibly related to administration of the product.
[b] The ADVATE clinical program included 234 treated subjects from 5 completed studies in PTPs, and 1 ongoing study in PUPs as of 27 March 2006.
[c] All 5 ADRs occurred in (PUPs) from an ongoing clinical study, and all were for the development of factor VIII inhibitors with a titer ≥ 0.6 BU that were to be reported as a serious AE.

ADVATE [Antihemophilic Factor (Recombinant), Plasma/Albumin-Free Method]
IMMUNOGENICITY
The development of Factor VIII inhibitors with the use of ADVATE was evaluated in clinical studies with pediatric PTPs (<6 years of age with >50 Factor VIII exposures) and PTPs (≥10 years of age with >150 Factor VIII exposures). Of 198 subjects who were treated for at least 10 exposure days or on study for a minimum of 120 days, 1 adult developed a low-titer inhibitor (2.0 [BU] in the Bethesda assay) after 26 exposure days. Eight weeks later, the inhibitor was no longer detectable, and in vivo recovery was normal at 1 and 3 hours after infusion of another marketed recombinant Factor VIII concentrate. This single event results in a Factor VIII inhibitor frequency in PTPs of 0.51% (95% CI of 0.03 and 2.91% for the risk of any Factor VIII inhibitor development). No factor VIII inhibitors were detected in the 53 treated pediatric PTPs.
In clinical studies that enrolled previously untreated subjects (defined as having had up to 3 exposures to a Factor VIII product at the time of enrollment, 5 (20%) of 25 subjects who received ADVATE developed inhibitors to Factor VIII. Four patients developed high titer (> 5 BU) and one patient developed low-titer inhibitors. Inhibitors were detected at a median of 11 exposure days (range 7 to 13 exposure days) to investigational product.
Immunogenicity was also evaluated by measuring the development of antibodies to heterologous proteins. 182 treated subjects were assessed for anti-chinese hamster ovary (CHO) cell protein antibodies. Of these patients, 3 showed an upward trend in antibody titer over time and 4 showed repeated but transient elevations of antibodies. 182 treated subjects were assessed for muIgG1 protein antibodies. Of these 10 showed an upward trend in anti-mu IgG antibody titer over time and 2 showed repeated but transient elevations of antibodies. Four subjects who demonstrated antibody elevations reported isolated events of urti-

caria, pruritus, rash, and slightly elevated eosinophil counts. All of these subjects had numerous repeat exposures to the study product without recurrence of the events and a causal relationship between the antibody findings and these clinical events has not been established.
Of the 181 subjects who were treated and assessed for the presence of anti-human von Willebrand Factor (VWF) antibodies, none displayed laboratory evidence indicative of a positive serologic response.
6.2 Post Marketing Experience
The following adverse reactions have been identified during post approval use of ADVATE. Because these reactions are reported voluntarily from a population of uncertain size, it is not always possible to reliably estimate their frequency or establish a causal relationship to drug exposure.
Among patients treated with ADVATE, cases of serious allergic/hypersensitivity reactions including anaphylaxis have been reported and Factor VIII inhibitor formation (observed predominantly in PUPs). Table 5 represents the most frequently reported post-marketing adverse reactions as MedDRA Preferred Terms.

Table 5.
Post-Marketing Experience

Organ System [MedDRA Primary SOC]	Preferred Term
Immune system disorders	Anaphylactic reaction[a] Hypersensitivity[a]
Blood and lymphatic system disorders	Factor VIII inhibition
General disorders and administration site conditions	Injection site reaction Chills Fatigue/Malaise Chest discomfort/pain Vomiting Less-than-expected therapeutic effect Headache

[a] These reactions have been manifested by dizziness, paresthesias, rash, flushing, face swelling, urticaria, and/or pruritus.

7. DRUG INTERACTIONS
There are no known drug interactions reported with ADVATE. Drug interaction studies have not been performed.

8. USE IN SPECIFIC POPULATIONS
8.1 Pregnancy
Pregnancy Category C. Animal reproduction studies have not been conducted with ADVATE. It is not known whether ADVATE can cause fetal harm when administered to a pregnant woman, or whether it can affect reproductive capacity. ADVATE should be given to a pregnant woman only if clearly needed.
8.2 Labor and Delivery
There are no adequate and well-controlled human studies that have investigated the effects of ADVATE during labor and delivery. ADVATE should be used only if clinically needed.

8.3 Nursing Mothers
It is not known whether this drug is excreted in human milk. Because many drugs are excreted in human milk, caution should be exercised when ADVATE is administered to a nursing woman. ADVATE should be given to nursing mothers only if clinically needed.
8.4 Pediatric Use
In comparison to adults, children present with higher Factor VIII clearance values and thus lower half-life and recovery of Factor VIII. This may be explained by differences in body composition and should be taken into account when dosing or following Factor VIII levels in the pediatric population. Larger or more frequent doses should be considered to account for the observed differences in adjusted recovery and terminal half-life. Dose adjustment may be needed. [see Pharmacokinetics (12.3)].
8.5 Geriatric Use
Clinical studies of ADVATE did not include sufficient numbers of subjects aged 65 and over to determine whether they respond differently compared to younger subjects. Dose selection for a geriatric patient should be individualized.

10. OVERDOSAGE
No symptoms of overdose with ADVATE have been reported.

11. DESCRIPTION
ADVATE [Antihemophilic Factor (Recombinant), Plasma/Albumin-Free Method] is a purified glycoprotein consisting of 2,332 amino acids that is synthesized by a genetically engineered CHO cell line. In culture, the CHO cell line expresses rAHF into the cell culture medium. The rAHF is purified from the culture medium using a series of chromatography columns. The purification process includes an immunoaffinity chromatography step in which a monoclonal antibody directed against Factor VIII is employed to selectively isolate the rAHF from the medium. The cell culture and purification processes used in the manufacture of ADVATE employ no additives of human or animal origin. The production process includes a dedicated, viral inactivation solvent-detergent treatment step. The rAHF synthesized by the CHO cells has the same biological effects on clotting as Antihemophilic Factor (Human) [AHF (Human)]. Structurally the recombinant protein has a similar combination of heterogeneous heavy and light chains as found in AHF (Human).
ADVATE is formulated as a sterile, non-pyrogenic, white to off white powder for intravenous injection. ADVATE is available in single-dose vials that contain nominally 250, 500, 1000, 1500, 2000 and 3000 International Units (IU) per vial. When reconstituted with the appropriate volume of diluent, the product contains the following stabilizers in maximal amounts: 38 mg/mL mannitol, 10 mg/mL trehalose, 108 mEq/L sodium, 12 mM histidine, 12 mM Tris, 1.9 mM calcium, 0.15 mg/mL polysorbate-80, and 0.10 mg/mL glutathione. VWF is co-expressed with Factor VIII, and helps to stabilize it in culture. The final product contains no more than 2 ng VWF/IU rAHF, which will not have any clinically relevant effect in patients with von Willebrand's disease. The product contains no preservative.
Each vial of ADVATE is labeled with the rAHF activity expressed in IU per vial. Biological potency is determined by an in vitro assay, which employs a Factor VIII concentrate standard that is referenced to a World Health Organization (WHO) International Standard for Factor VIII concentrates. One IU, as defined by the World Health Organization standard for blood coagulation FVIII, human, is approximately equal to the level of FVIII activity found in 1 mL of fresh pooled human plasma. The specific activity of ADVATE is 4000 to 10000 IU per milligram of protein.

12. CLINICAL PHARMACOLOGY
12.1 Mechanism of Action
ADVATE temporarily replaces the missing clotting Factor VIII that is needed for effective hemostasis.
12.2 Pharmacodynamics
The activated partial thromboplastin time (aPTT) is prolonged in patients with hemophilia. Determination of aPTT is a conventional in vitro assay for biological activity of Factor VIII. Treatment with ADVATE normalizes the aPTT over the effective dosing period.
12.3 Pharmacokinetics
A randomized, crossover pharmacokinetic study of ADVATE produced at Orth, Austria (test) and RECOMBINATE [Antihemophilic Factor (Recombinant)] (reference) was conducted in 56 non-bleeding subjects. The subjects received either of the products as an IV infusion (50 ± 5 IU/kg body weight) and there was a washout period of 72 hours to 4 weeks between the two infusions. The pharmacokinetic parameters were calculated from Factor VIII activity measurements in blood samples obtained up to 48 hours following each infusion. Pharmacokinetic parameters for adults for each study preparation in the per-protocol analysis are presented in Table 6.
[See table 6 at left]

Table 6.
Pharmacokinetic Parameters for ADVATE and RECOMBINATE
(Per-Protocol Analysis, Adult Subjects age > 16 years)

Parameter	RECOMBINATE (n = 20)[a] Mean ± SD	ADVATE (n = 20)[a] Mean ± SD
AUC_{0-48h} (IU•h/dL)[b]	1638 ± 357	1644 ± 338
In vivo recovery (IU/dL/IU/kg)[c]	2.74 ± 0.56	2.57 ± 0.53
Half-life (h)	11.16 ± 2.50	12.03 ± 4.15
C_{max} (IU/dL)	136 ± 29	128 ± 28
MRT (h)	14.68 ± 3.82	15.81 ± 5.91
V_{ss} (dL/kg)	0.43 ± 0.10	0.44 ± 0.10
CL (dL/kg/h)	0.03 ± 0.01	0.03 ± 0.01

[a] 56 subjects were enrolled in the clinical study. The per protocol analysis included 30 patients (20 adults and 10 children). The PK parameters in the table are calculated for adult subjects only.
[b] Area under the plasma factor VIII concentration × time curve from 0 to 48 hours post-infusion
[c] Calculated as (C_{max} – baseline factor VIII) divided by the dose in IU/kg, where C_{max} is the maximal post-infusion factor VIII measurement

The 90% confidence intervals for the ratios of the mean $AUC_{(0-48h)}$ and in vivo recovery values for the test and control products were within the pre-established limits of 0.80 and 1.25. In addition, in vivo recoveries at the onset of treatment and after 75 exposure days were compared for 62 subjects. Results of this analysis indicated no significant change in the in vivo recovery at the onset of treatment and after ≥ 75 exposure days.

See the description of the clinical study results for a discussion of the effect of long-term exposure on the pharmacokinetic properties of ADVATE [CLINICAL STUDIES, Section (14.2)].

In an interim analysis of data from 10 of 25 planned subjects in the Phase 2/3 surgery study, the target Factor VIII level was met or exceeded in all cases following a single loading dose ranging from 48.0 to 69.8 IU/kg.

Pharmacokinetic parameters calculated from interim pharmacokinetic data for 51 subjects ≤ 16 years of age (per-protocol analysis) are available for 0 neonates, 3 infants, 21 children, and 27 adolescents as shown in Table 7. The clearance of ADVATE in infants, children, older children, and adolescents was 26%, 23%, 42%, and 23% higher than adults (0.031 dL/hr/kg). The half-life of ADVATE in infants, children, older children, and adolescents was 27%, 15%, 10%, and 3% lower than adults (12.08 hours). Clinical significance of these differences is not known.

[See table 7 at right]

13. NONCLINICAL TOXICOLOGY

Single doses several fold higher than the recommended clinical dose (related to body weight) did not demonstrate any acute or toxic effect for ADVATE in laboratory animals (mouse, rat, rabbit, and dog). Multiple dose studies were not performed with ADVATE, but were performed with the related product, RECOMBINATE and with formulation buffers of ADVATE.

13.1 Carcinogenesis, Mutagenesis, Impairment of Fertility

No studies have been conducted with the active ingredient in ADVATE to assess its mutagenic or carcinogenic potential. The CHO cell line employed in the production of ADVATE is derived from that used in the biosynthesis of RECOMBINATE [Antihemophilic Factor (Recombinant)]. ADVATE has been shown to be comparable to RECOMBINATE with respect to its biochemical and physicochemical properties, as well as its non-clinical in vivo pharmacology.

RECOMBINATE was tested for mutagenicity at doses considerably exceeding plasma concentrations in vitro, and at doses up to ten times the expected maximal clinical dose *in vivo*. At that concentration, it did not cause reverse mutations, chromosomal aberrations, or an increase in micronuclei formation in bone marrow polychromatic erythrocytes. Studies in animals have not been performed to evaluate carcinogenic potential.

14. CLINICAL STUDIES

The pharmacokinetic properties of ADVATE were investigated at the beginning of treatment in a multicenter study of previously treated subjects, and at the end of treatment in a subset of subjects (N=13) who had completed at least 75 exposure days of treatment with ADVATE. Post-infusion levels and clearance of Factor VIII during the perioperative period were examined in an interim analysis of subjects enrolled in an ongoing surgery study. The pharmacokinetics of ADVATE were investigated in an interim analysis of a study of pediatric previously treated subjects < 6 years of age. [see Pediatric Use (8.4) and Clinical Pharmacology (12)].

14.1 Original Safety and Efficacy Study

The study design, key inclusion and exclusion criteria, treatment, number of subjects and age range for the original study (069901) can be found in Table 8.

[See table 8 at right]

In the safety and efficacy study, a global assessment of efficacy was rendered by the subject (for home treatment) or study site investigator (for treatment under medical supervision) using an ordinal scale of excellent, good, fair, or none, based on the quality of hemostasis achieved with ADVATE produced in the Orth facility for the treatment of each new bleeding episode. A total of 510 bleeding episodes were reported, with a mean (± SD) of 6.1 ± 8.2 bleeding episodes per subject. Of the 510 new bleeding episodes treated with ADVATE, 439 (86%) were rated excellent or good in their response to treatment, 61 (12%) were rated fair, 1 (0.2%) was rated as having no response, and for 9 (2%), the response to treatment was unknown. A total of 411 (81%) new bleeding episodes were managed with a single infusion, 62 (12%) required 2 infusions, 15 (3%) required 3 infusions, and 22 (4%) required 4 or more infusions of ADVATE for satisfactory resolution. A total of 162 (32%) new bleeding episodes occurred spontaneously, 228 (45%) were the result of antecedent trauma, and for 120 (24%) bleeding episodes, the etiology was unknown.

Table 7. Pharmacokinetic Parameters (Mean ± SD) of ADVATE by Age Group (N = 51; Intent to Treat Analysis)

Parameters	Infants (n = 3) (1 month to < 2 years)	Children (n = 8) (2 to < 5 years)	Children (n = 13) (5 to < 12 years)	Adolescents (n = 27) (12 to < 16 years)
AUC (IU*hr/dL)	1385 ± 476	1545 ± 616	1282 ± 509	1447 ± 528
C_{max} (IU/dL)	98.0 ± 10.5	104.6 ± 34.5	111.8 ± 25.7	113.3 ± 21.7
CL (dL/hr/kg)	0.039 ± 0.015	0.038 ± 0.016	0.044 ± 0.012	0.038 ± 0.012
Half-life (hrs)	8.86 ± 1.78	10.27 ± 1.94	10.89 ± 1.60	11.70 ± 3.72
V_d (dL/kg)[a]	0.43 ± 0.08	0.46 ± 0.12	0.54 ± 0.07	0.53 ± 0.08
Recovery[b] IU/dL/IU/kg	1.96 ± 0.21	2.05 ± 0.62	2.21 ± 0.44	2.26 ± 0.42

[a] Volume of distribution
[b] Incremental recovery at C_{max}

Table 8. Study Design, Key Inclusion and Exclusion Criteria, Treatment, Number of Subjects and Age Range for ADVATE Original Study 069901

Type of Study; Study Design	• (Parts 1&3) Randomized, Crossover (nonblinded) with RECOMBINATE rAHF and rAHF-PFM • (Part 2) Open-label with rAHF-PFM, non-controlled, • Multi-center • Prospective • Safety, immunogenicity, efficacy, and pharmacokinetics in previously treated subjects ≥10y with severe or moderately severe hemophilia A
Key Inclusion Criteria	• Severe or moderately severe hemophilia A; baseline FVIII ≤2% • Age ≥10y • Weight >35kg • ≥150 exposure days with FVIII • HIV seronegative or if seropositive, then CD4 >400/mm[3]
Key Exclusion Criteria	• Detectable FVIII inhibitor at enrollment • History of FVIII inhibitor (>1BU) • Portal vein hypertension (INR >1.4), presence of splenomegaly, spider angiomata, and/or history of esophageal hemorrhage or documented esophageal varices • Hypersensitivity to RECOMBINATE rAHF • Scheduled to receive immunomodulating drug • Participation in another clinical study within 30d of enrollment
Treatment(s)	**Parts 1 & 3 Pharmacokinetic** Single Infusion: 50 ±5 IU/kg **Part 2 Prophylaxis:** 25-40 IU/kg, 3-4 times/wk
Number of Subjects	**Final: 111**
Age Range, Race	**Final: ≥ 10 years** Caucasian: 103 Black: 7 Asian: 1

The rate of new bleeding episodes during the protocol-mandated 75 exposure day prophylactic regimen (≥ 25 IU/kg body weight 3-4 times per week) was calculated as a function of the etiology of bleeding episodes for 107 evaluable subjects (n = 274 new bleeding episodes). These rates are presented in Table 9.

Table 9. Rate of New Bleeding Episodes During Prophylaxis

Bleeding Episode Etiology	Mean (± SD) New Bleeding Episodes/Subject/Month
Spontaneous	0.34 ± 0.49
Post-traumatic	0.39 ± 0.46
Unknown[a]	0.33 ± 0.34
Overall	0.52 ± 0.71

[a] Etiology was indeterminate

14.2 Continuation Study

The study design, key inclusion and exclusion criteria, treatment, number of subjects and age range for the original study (060102) can be found in Table 10.

[See table 10 at top of next page]

Additional safety and efficacy data were based on subjects who continued with treatment following participation in the safety and efficacy study. An interim analysis of efficacy from the continuation study was conducted for 27 of 82 enrolled subjects who self-administered ADVATE produced in Neuchâtel on a routine prophylactic regimen during a minimum period of 50 exposure days to ADVATE. New bleeding episodes were treated with ADVATE and the outcome of treatment was rated as excellent, good, fair, or none, based on the quality of hemostasis achieved. A total of 51 new bleeding episodes occurred in 13 of the 27 subjects being treated with ADVATE. By etiology, 53% of these bleeding events resulted from trauma and 27% occurred spontaneously; the other 20% had an undetermined etiology. The response to treatment with ADVATE for the majority (63%) of all new bleeding episodes was rated as excellent or good. 86% of the bleeding episodes resolved with only 1 infusion and an additional 6% were resolved by a second infusion. In vivo recoveries at the onset of treatment and after 75 exposure days were compared for 62 subjects. There were no significant differences between the in vivo recoveries at the onset of treatment and the in vivo recoveries after ≥ 75 exposure days.

ADVATE [Antihemophilic Factor (Recombinant), Plasma/Albumin-Free Method]

14.3 Perioperative Management Study

The study design, key inclusion and exclusion criteria, treatment, number of subjects and age range for the original study (069902) can be found in Table 11.

[See table 11 on next page]

An interim analysis of the hemostatic efficacy of ADVATE during the perioperative management of subjects undergoing surgical procedures was conducted for 10 of 25 planned subjects. Ten subjects underwent 10 surgical procedures while receiving ADVATE. Eight subjects received the test product by intermittent bolus infusion and 2 subjects received a combination of continuous and intermittent bolus infusion. Nine of the 10 subjects completed the study. Six of

the surgical procedures were classified as major, and 4 were minor. Of the 6 major surgeries, 5 were for orthopedic complications of hemophilia. A brief description of each surgical procedure, along with study duration and study medication exposure, are presented in Table 12.
[See table 12 at top of next page]
For each of the 10 subjects, intra- and post-operative quality of hemostasis achieved with ADVATE was assessed by the operating surgeon and study site investigator, respectively, using an ordinal scale of excellent, good, fair, or none. The same rating scale was used to evaluate control of hemorrhage from a surgical drain placed at the incision site in one subject. The quality of hemostasis achieved with ADVATE was rated as excellent or good for all assessments.

15. REFERENCES

1. Aledort L: Inhibitors in hemophilia patients: Current status and management. *Am J Hematol* 1994 47:208-217.
2. Kessler CM: An introduction to Factor VIII inhibitors: The detection and quantitation. *Am J Med* 1991 91 (Suppl 5A):1S-5S.
3. White II GC, Courter S, Bray GL, et al: A multicenter study of recombinant factor VIII (Recombinate) in previously treated patients with hemophilia A. *Thromb Haemost* 1997 77:660-667.
4. Abshire TC, Brackmann H-H, Scharrer I, et al: Sucrose formulated recombinant human antihemophilic factor VIII is safe and efficacious for treatment of hemophilia A in home therapy. *Thromb Haemost* 2000 83:811-816.
5. Lee CA, Owens D, Bray G, et al: Pharmacokinetics of recombinant factor VIII (Recombinate) using one-stage clotting and chromogenic factor VIII assay. *Thromb Haemost* 1999 82:1644-1647.
6. Manco-Johnson MJ, Abshire TC, Shapiro AD et al. Prophylaxis versus episodic treatment to prevent joint disease in boys with severe hemophilia. *N Engl J Med*. 2007; 357:603-5.
7. Ljung R, Aronis-Vournas S, Kurnik-Auberger K, et al. Treatment of children with haemophilia in Europe: a survey of 20 centres in 16 countries. *Haemophilia*. 2000; 6:619-24.
8. Löfqvist T, Nilsson IM, Berntorp E, Pettersson H. Haemophilia prophylaxis in young patients—a long-term follow-up. *J Intern Med*. 1997; 241:395-400.

16. HOW SUPPLIED/STORAGE AND HANDLING

16.1 How Supplied
ADVATE [Antihemophilic Factor (Recombinant), Plasma/Albumin-Free Method] is available in single-dose vials that contain the following nominal product strengths:
[See second table on next page]
Actual Factor VIII activity in IU is stated on the label of each ADVATE carton and vial.

16.2 Storage and Handling
ADVATE is packaged with 5 mL of Sterile Water for Injection, USP, a BAXJECT II Needleless Transfer Device, one full prescribing physician insert, and one patient insert.
ADVATE should be refrigerated (2°-8°C [36°-46°F]) in powder form.
ADVATE may be stored at room temperature (up to 30°C [86°F]) for a period of up to 6 months not to exceed the expiration date.
The date that ADVATE is removed from refrigeration should be noted on the carton.
Do not use beyond the expiration date printed on the vial or six months after date noted on the carton, whichever is earlier. After storage at room temperature, the product must not be returned to the refrigerator. Avoid freezing to prevent damage to the diluent vial.

17. PATIENT COUNSELING INFORMATION

See Patient Product Information (PPI) and Instructions for Use
- Advise patients to report any adverse reactions or problems following ADVATE administration to their physician or healthcare provider.
- Allergic-type hypersensitivity reactions have been reported with ADVATE. Warn patients of the early signs of hypersensitivity reactions, including hives, pruritus, generalized urticaria, angioedema, hypotension, shock, anaphylaxis and acute respiratory distress. Advise patients to discontinue use of the product if these symptoms occur and seek immediate emergency treatment with resuscitative measures such as the administration of epinephrine and oxygen.
- Inhibitor formation may occur with the treatment of a patient with hemophilia A. Advise patients to contact their physician or treatment center for further treatment and/or assessment, if they experience a lack of clinical response to Factor VIII replacement therapy, as this may be a manifestation of an inhibitor.
- Advise patients to consult with their physicians or healthcare provider prior to travel.

- While traveling advise patients to bring an adequate supply of ADVATE, based on their current regimen of treatment.
To enroll in the confidential, industry-wide Patient Notification System, call 1 888 UPDATE U (1-888-873-2838).
Baxter, Advate, Baxject and Recombinate are trademarks of Baxter International Inc. Baxter, Advate and Baxject are registered in the U.S. Patent and Trademark Office.

Patented under U.S. Patent Numbers. 5,733,873; 5,854,021; 5,919,766; 5,955,448; 6,313,102; 6,586,573; 6,649,386; 7,087,723; and, 7,247,707. Made according to the method of U.S. Patent Nos. 5,470,954; 6,100,061; 6,475,725; 6,555,391; 6,936,441; 7,094,574; 7,253,262; and, 7,381,796.
Baxter Healthcare Corporation
Westlake Village, CA 91362 USA
U.S. License No. 140

Table 10.
Study Design, Key Inclusion and Exclusion Criteria, Treatment, Number of Subjects and Age Range for ADVATE Original Study 060102

Type of Study; Study Design	• Open label with rAHF-PFM • Non-controlled • Multi-center • Prospective • Safety, immunogenicity, efficacy, and pharmacokinetics in only subjects who completed Baxter clinical study 069901	
Key Inclusion Criteria	• Completed Baxter clinical study 069901 • HIV seronegative or if seropositive, then CD4 >400/mm^3	
Key Exclusion Criteria	• Received FVIII products other than rAHF-PFM • Developed FVIII inhibitor • Scheduled to receive immunomodulating drug	
Treatment(s)	**Part 1 Pharmacokinetic** Single Infusion: 50 ± 5 IU/kg **Part 2 Therapeutic Regimen** determined by investigator: 1. Standard prophylaxis: 25-40 IU/kg, 3-4 times/wk, 2. Modified prophylaxis: investigator-determined dose and frequency, 3. On demand: investigator-determined dose and frequency	
Number of Subjects	Interim: 33 13 for PK; 27 for safety and efficacy	Final: 82
Age Range, Race	Interim: 19: 10-18y 14: > 18y Caucasian: 32 Black: 1	Final: ≥ 10y Caucasian: 77 Black: 4 Asian: 1

Table 11.
Study Design, Key Inclusion and Exclusion Criteria, Treatment, Number of Subjects and Age Range for ADVATE Original Study 069902

Type of Study; Study Design	• Open label with rAHF-PFM • Non-controlled • Multi-center • Prospective • Safety and efficacy in subjects with severe or moderately severe hemophilia A who require surgical, dental or other invasive procedure • Minimum of 20% of the total study cohort must have major surgical procedures	
Key Inclusion Criteria	• Severe or moderately-severe hemophilia A; baseline FVIII ≤2% • Need for surgical, dental, or other invasive procedure • Age ≥5y • ≥150 exposure days with FVIII • Life expectancy >28d from surgery	
Key Exclusion Criteria	• Detectable FVIII inhibitor at enrollment • History of FVIII inhibitor (>1BU) • Hypersensitivity to RECOMBINATE rAHF • Evidence of abnormal hemostasis (other than hemophilia A) • Participation in another clinical study within 30d of enrollment	
Treatment(s)	**Perioperative Management** **1. Preoperative** Dental loading dose: FVIII level 60-100% of normal; Major/Minor loading dose: FVIII level 80-120% of normal **2. Intra- and Post-Operative** *BI: as clinically indicated; *CI: initial rate for subjects >12y: 4 IU•kg-1•h-1; initial rate subjects 5-12y: 5 IU•kg-1•h-1 for; then investigator-determined **3. Home Replacement Therapy** Prescribed by investigator for up to 6wks for major orthopedic procedures and up to 2wks for all other procedures	
Number of Subjects	Interim: 10 Procedures: Major: 6 Minor: 4 Orthopedic: 5 Dental: 0	Final: 59 Procedures: 65 Major: 22 Minor: 35 Orthopedic: 40 Dental: 8
Age Range, Race	Interim: 14-64y Caucasian: 9 Black: 1	Final: 7-65y Caucasian: 55 Black: 3 Asian: 1

*"BI"is bolus infusion and "CI" as intermittent infusion

Table 12.
Surgical Procedures, Study Duration, and Study Medication Exposure

Surgery Type	Days of Study	ADVATE Exposure Days	Cumulative ADVATE Exposure (IU)
Total hip replacement	16	15	61,600
Knee joint replacement	22	18	76,060
Knee arthrodesis	24	22	66,080
Transposition of the left ulnar nerve	5	3	14,560
Insertion of Mediport	28	8[a]	46,893
Dental extraction	18	6	16,599
Left elbow synovectomy	43	32	102,180
Teeth extraction	2	2	10,350
Right knee arthroscopy, chondroplasty and synovectomy	13	10[a]	32,334
Wisdom teeth extraction	14	5	15,357

[a] ADVATE was administered by continuous infusion for the first 48 hours post-operatively, followed by bolus infusions for the remainder of study treatment.

Nominal Strength	Factor VIII Potency Range	NDC Number
250 IU per vial	200–400 IU/vial	NDC 0944-2941-10
500 IU per vial	401–800 IU/vial	NDC 0944-2942-10
1000 IU per vial	801–1200 IU/vial	NDC 0944-2943-10
1500 IU per vial	1201–1800 IU/vial	NDC 0944-2944-10
2000 IU per vial	1801–2400 IU/vial	NDC 0944-2945-10
3000 IU per vial	2401–3600 IU/vial	NDC 0944-2946-10

cough	headache	joint swelling	sore throat
fever	itching	unusual taste	dizziness
hematoma	abdominal pain	hot flashes	swelling of legs
diarrhea	chills	nausea	sweating

Printed in USA
Issued March 2010
LE-07-14499

FDA-Approved Patient Labeling—Patient Product Information (PPI)

ADVATE (ad-vate) [Antihemophilic Factor (Recombinant), Plasma/Albumin-Free Method]

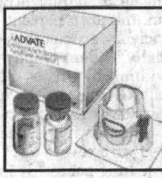

This leaflet summarizes important information about ADVATE. Please read it carefully before using this medicine. This information does not take the place of talking with your healthcare provider, and it does not include all of the important information about ADVATE. If you have any questions after reading this, ask your healthcare provider.

What is the most important information I need to know about ADVATE?

Do not attempt to do an infusion to yourself unless you have been taught how by your doctor or hemophilia center.

You must carefully follow your doctor's or other healthcare provider's instructions regarding the dose and schedule for infusing ADVATE so that your treatment will work best for you.

What is ADVATE?

ADVATE is a medicine used to replace clotting factor (Factor VIII or antihemophilic factor) that is missing in people with hemophilia A (also called "classic" hemophilia). Hemophilia A is an inherited bleeding disorder that prevents blood from clotting normally.

ADVATE is used to prevent and control bleeding in people with hemophilia A.

Your healthcare provider may give you ADVATE when you have surgery.

ADVATE is not used to treat von Willebrand's Disease.

Who should not use ADVATE?

You should not use ADVATE if you
• are allergic to mice or hamsters.
• are allergic to any ingredients in ADVATE.

Tell your healthcare provider if you are pregnant or breast-feeding because ADVATE may not be right for you.

How should I use ADVATE?

ADVATE is given directly into the blood stream.

You may infuse ADVATE at a hemophilia treatment center, at your healthcare provider's office or in your home. You should be trained on how to do infusions by your hemophilia treatment center or healthcare provider. Many people with hemophilia A learn to infuse their ADVATE by themselves or with the help of a family member.

Your healthcare provider will tell you how much ADVATE to use based on your weight, the severity of your hemophilia A, and where you are bleeding.

You may have to have blood tests done after getting ADVATE to be sure that your blood level of Factor VIII is high enough to clot your blood.

Call your healthcare provider right away if your bleeding does not stop after taking ADVATE.

What should I tell my healthcare provider before I use ADVATE?

You should tell your healthcare provider if you
• have or have had any medical problems.
• take any medicines, including prescription and non-prescription medicines, such as over the counter medicines, supplements or herbal remedies.
• have any allergies, including allergies to mice or hamsters.
• are breastfeeding. It is not known if ADVATE passes into your milk and if it can harm your baby.
• are pregnant or planning to become pregnant. It is not known if ADVATE may harm your unborn baby.
• have been told that you have inhibitors to Factor VIII (because ADVATE may not work for you).

What are the possible side effects of ADVATE?

You could have an allergic reaction to ADVATE.

Call your healthcare provider right away and stop treatment if you get a rash or hives, itching, tightness of the throat, chest pain or tightness, difficulty breathing, light-headed, dizziness, nausea or fainting.

Side effects that have been reported with ADVATE include: [See third table above]

Tell your doctor about any side effects that bother you or do not go away

These are not all the possible side effects with ADVATE. You can ask your healthcare provider for information that is for written for healthcare professionals.

What are the ADVATE dosage strengths?

ADVATE comes in six different dosage strengths. The actual strength will be imprinted on the label and on the box. The six different strengths are coded, as follows:

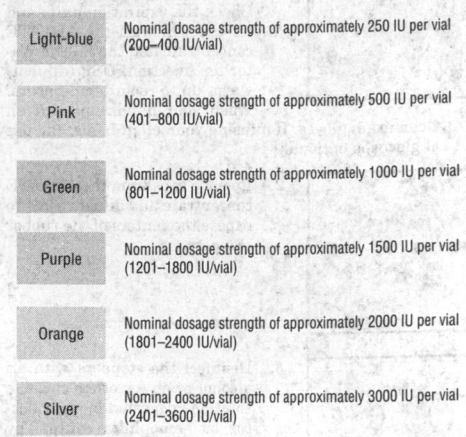

Light-blue	Nominal dosage strength of approximately 250 IU per vial (200–400 IU/vial)
Pink	Nominal dosage strength of approximately 500 IU per vial (401–800 IU/vial)
Green	Nominal dosage strength of approximately 1000 IU per vial (801–1200 IU/vial)
Purple	Nominal dosage strength of approximately 1500 IU per vial (1201–1800 IU/vial)
Orange	Nominal dosage strength of approximately 2000 IU per vial (1801–2400 IU/vial)
Silver	Nominal dosage strength of approximately 3000 IU per vial (2401–3600 IU/vial)

Always check the potency printed on the label to make sure you are using the strength prescribed by your doctor. Always check the expiration date printed on the box. You should not use the product after the expiration date printed on the box.

How do I store ADVATE?

Do not freeze ADVATE.

ADVATE vials containing powdered product (without sterile diluent added) should be stored in a refrigerator (2° to 8°C [36° to 46°F]) or at room temperature (up to 30°C [86°F]) for up to 6 months.

If you choose to store ADVATE at room temperature:
• note the date that the product is removed from refrigeration on the box.
• do not use after six months from this date or the expiration date listed on the vial, whichever is earlier.

Store vials in their original box and protect them from extreme exposure to light.

Reconstituted product (after mixing dry product with wet diluent) must be used within 3 hours and cannot be stored or refrigerated. Any ADVATE left in the vial at the end of your infusion should be discarded.

What else should I know about ADVATE and hemophilia A?

Your body may form inhibitors to Factor VIII. An inhibitor is part of the body's normal defense system. If you form inhibitors, it may stop ADVATE from working properly. Consult with your healthcare provider to make sure you are carefully monitored with blood tests for the development of inhibitors to Factor VIII.

Medicines are sometimes prescribed for purposes other than those listed here. Do not use ADVATE for a condition for which it is not prescribed. Do not share ADVATE with other people, even if they have the same symptoms that you have.

Resources at Baxter available to the patients:

For more product information on ADVATE, please visit www.advate.com or call 1-888-4ADVATE (1-888-423-8283).

For information on patient assistance programs that are available to you, including the Baxter CARE Program, please contact the Baxter Insurance Assistance Helpline at 1-888-BAXTER9 (1-888-229-8379).

For information on additional Baxter patient resources, please visit www.advate.com.

Issued: March 2010

Instructions For Use

ADVATE [Antihemophilic Factor (Recombinant), Plasma/Albumin-Free Method] (For intravenous use only)

Do not attempt to do an infusion to yourself unless you have been taught how by your doctor or hemophilia center.

See below for step-by-step instructions for reconstituting ADVATE at the end of this leaflet.

You should always follow the specific instructions given by your healthcare provider. The steps listed below are general guidelines for using ADVATE. If you are unsure of the procedures, please call your healthcare provider before using. Call your healthcare provider right away if bleeding is not controlled after using ADVATE.

Your healthcare provider will prescribe the dose that you should take.

Your healthcare provider may need to take blood tests from time to time.

Talk to your healthcare provider before traveling. You should plan to bring enough ADVATE for your treatment during this time.

Dispose of all materials, including any leftover reconstituted ADVATE product, in an appropriate container.

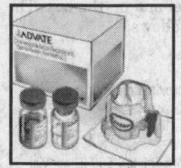

1. Prepare a clean flat surface and gather all the materials you will need for the infusion. Check the expiration date, and let the vial with the ADVATE concentrate and the Sterile Water for Injection, USP (diluent) warm up to room temperature. Wash your hands and put on clean exam gloves. If infusing yourself at home, the use of gloves is optional.

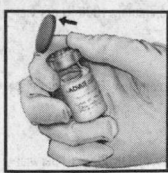

2. Remove caps from the ADVATE concentrate and diluent vials to expose the centers of the rubber stoppers.

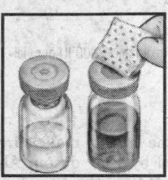

3. Disinfect the stoppers with an alcohol swab (or other suitable solution suggested by your doctor or hemophilia center) by rubbing the stoppers firmly for several seconds, and allow them to dry prior to use. Place the vials on a flat surface.

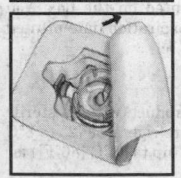

4. Open the BAXJECT II device package by peeling away the lid, without touching the inside of the package. **Do not remove the BAXJECT II device from the package.**

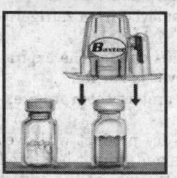

5. Turn the package with the BAXJECT II device upside down, and place it over the top of the diluent vial. Fully insert the clear plastic spike of the device into the center of the diluent vial's stopper by pushing straight down. Grip the package at its edge and lift it off the device. Be careful not to touch the white plastic spike. **Do not remove the blue cap from the BAXJECT II device.** The diluent vial now has the BAXJECT II device connected to it and is ready to be connected to the ADVATE vial.

6. To connect the diluent vial to the ADVATE vial, turn the diluent vial over and place it on top of the vial containing ADVATE concentrate. Fully insert the white plastic spike into the ADVATE vial's stopper by pushing straight down. Diluent will flow into the ADVATE vial. This should be done right away to keep the liquid free of germs.

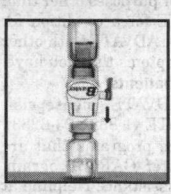

7. Swirl the connected vials gently and continuously until the ADVATE is completely dissolved. **Do not shake.** The ADVATE solution should look clear and colorless. If not, do not use it and notify Baxter immediately.

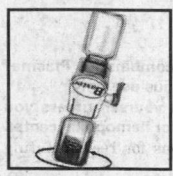

8. Take off the blue cap from the BAXJECT II device and connect the syringe. **BE CAREFUL TO NOT INJECT AIR.**

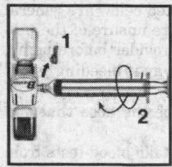

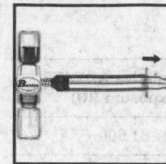

9. Turn over the connected vials so that the ADVATE vial is on top. Draw the ADVATE solution into the syringe by pulling back the plunger slowly. Disconnect the syringe from the vials. Attach the infusion needle to the syringe using a winged (butterfly) infusion set, if available.

Point the needle up and remove any air bubbles by gently tapping the syringe with your finger and slowly and carefully pushing air out of the syringe and needle.

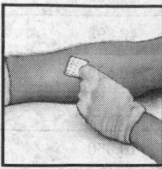

10. If you are using more than one vial of ADVATE, the contents of more than one vial may be drawn into the same syringe. However, you will need a separate diluent and BAXJECT II device to mix each additional vial of ADVATE.

Apply a tourniquet, and get the injection site ready by wiping the skin well with an alcohol swab (or other suitable solution suggested by your doctor or hemophilia center).

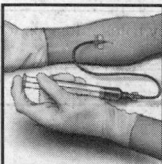

11. Insert the needle into the vein, and remove the tourniquet. Slowly infuse the ADVATE. **Do not infuse any faster than 10 mL per minute.**

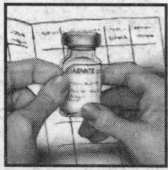

12. Take the needle out of the vein and use sterile gauze to put pressure on the infusion site for several minutes. **Do not recap the needle.** Place it with the used syringe in a hard-walled Sharps container for proper disposal.

Remove the peel-off label from the ADVATE vial and place it in your logbook. Clean any spilled blood with a freshly prepared mixture of 1 part bleach and 9 parts water, soap and water, or any household disinfecting solution.

13. Dispose of the used vials and BAXJECT II system in your hard-walled Sharps container, without taking them apart. Do not dispose of these supplies in ordinary household trash.

Important: Contact your doctor or local Hemophilia Treatment Center if you experience any problems.

Baxter, Advate, Baxject and CARE are trademarks of Baxter International Inc. registered in the U.S. Patent and Trademark Office.

Patented under U.S. Patent Numbers. 5,733,873; 5,854,021; 5,919,766; 5,955,448; 6,313,102; 6,586,573; 6,649,386; 7,087,723; and, 7,247,707. Made according to the method of U.S. Patent Nos. 5,470,954; 6,100,061; 6,475,725; 6,555,391; 6,936,441; 7,094,574; 7,253,262; and, 7,381,796.

Baxter Healthcare Corporation
Westlake Village, CA 91362 USA
U.S. License No. 140
Printed in USA
Issued March 2010
LE-07-14499

ARALAST NP   ℞

[A-ra-last]
[Alpha$_1$-Proteinase Inhibitor (Human)]
Solvent Detergent Treated
Nanofiltered

DESCRIPTION

ARALAST NP is a sterile, stable, lyophilized preparation of purified human alpha$_1$-proteinase inhibitor (α_1-PI), also known as alpha$_1$-antitrypsin.[1] ARALAST NP is a similar product to ARALAST, containing the same active components of plasma α_1-PI with identical formulations.

ARALAST NP is prepared from large pools of human plasma by using the cold ethanol fractionation process, followed by purification steps including polyethylene glycol and zinc chloride precipitations and ion exchange chromatography. All U.S. licensed α_1-PI plasma derived products contain chemical modifications which arise during manufacturing and occur in varying levels from product to product.[11] ARALAST NP contains approximately 2% α_1-PI with truncated C-terminal lysine (removal of Lys394), whereas ARALAST contains approximately 67% α_1-PI with the

---

C-terminal lysine truncation.[12] No known data suggest influence of these structural modifications on the functional activity and immunogenicity of α_1-PI.[13]

To reduce the risk of viral transmission, the manufacturing process includes treatment with a solvent detergent (S/D) mixture [tri-n-butyl phosphate and polysorbate 80] to inactivate enveloped viral agents such as human immunodeficiency virus (HIV), hepatitis B (HBV), and hepatitis C (HCV). In addition, a nanofiltration step is incorporated into the manufacturing process to reduce the risk of transmission of enveloped and non-enveloped viral agents. Based on in vitro studies, the process used to produce ARALAST NP has been shown to inactivate and/or partition various viruses as shown in Table 1 below.[2]

[See table 1 at top of next page]

The unreconstituted, lyophilized cake should be white or off-white to slightly yellow-green or yellow in color. When reconstituted as directed, the concentration of functionally active α_1-PI is ≥ 16 mg/mL and the specific activity is ≥ 0.55 mg active α_1-PI/mg total protein. The composition of the reconstituted product is as follows:

Component	Quantity/mL
Elastase Inhibitory Activity	≥ 400 mg Active α_1-PI/0.5 g vial* ≥ 800 mg Active α_1-PI/1.0 g vial**
Albumin	≤ 5 mg/mL
Polyethylene Glycol	≤ 112 µg/mL
Polysorbate 80	≤ 50 µg/mL
Sodium	≤ 230 mEq/L
Tri-n-butyl Phosphate	≤ 1.0 µg/mL
Zinc	≤ 3 ppm

* Reconstitution volume: 25 mL/0.5 g vial
** Reconstitution volume: 50 mL/1.0 g vial

Each vial of ARALAST NP is labeled with the amount of functionally active α_1-PI expressed in mg/vial. The formulation contains no preservative. The pH of the solution ranges from 7.2 to 7.8. Product must only be administered intravenously.

CLINICAL PHARMACOLOGY

ARALAST NP functions in the lungs to inhibit serine proteases such as neutrophil elastase (NE), which is capable of degrading protein components of the alveolar walls and which is chronically present in the lung. In the normal lung, α_1-PI is thought to provide more than 90% of the anti-NE protection in the lower respiratory tract.[3,4]

α_1-PI deficiency is an autosomal, co-dominant, hereditary disorder characterized by low serum and lung levels of α_1-PI.[1,3,5,6] Severe forms of the deficiency are frequently associated with slowly progressive, moderate-to-severe panacinar emphysema that most often manifests in the third to fourth decades of life, resulting in a significantly lower life expectancy.[1,3,4,6,7] However, an unknown percentage of individuals with severe α_1-PI deficiency are not diagnosed with or may never develop clinically evident emphysema during their lifetimes. Individuals with α_1-PI deficiency have little protection against NE released by a chronic, low-level of neutrophils in their lower respiratory tract, resulting in a protease:protease inhibitor imbalance in the lung.[3,8] The emphysema associated with severe α_1-PI deficiency is typically worse in the lower lung zones.[5] It is believed to develop because there are insufficient amounts of α_1-PI in the lower respiratory tract to inhibit NE. This imbalance allows relatively unopposed destruction of the connective tissue framework of the lung parenchyma.[8]

There are a large number of phenotypic variants of this disorder.[1,3,4] Individuals with the PiZZ variant typically have serum α_1-PI levels less than 35% of the average normal level.[1,5] Individuals with the Pi(null)(null) variant have undetectable α_1-PI protein in their serum.[1,3] Individuals with these low serum α_1-PI levels, i.e., less than 11 µM, have an increased risk of developing emphysema over their lifetimes. In addition, PiSZ individuals, whose serum α_1-PI levels range from approximately 9 to 23 µM[14], are considered to have moderately increased risk for developing emphysema, regardless of whether their serum α_1-PI levels are above or below 11 µM. Two Registry studies have shown 54% and 72% of α_1-PI deficient individuals had emphysema and pulmonary symptoms such as cough, phlegm, wheeze, breathlessness, and chest colds, respectively.[9,10] The risk of accelerated development and progression of emphysema in individuals with severe α_1-PI deficiency is higher in smokers than in ex-smokers or non-smokers.[3]

Not all individuals with severe genetic variants of α_1-PI deficiency have emphysema. **Augmentation therapy with Alpha$_1$-Proteinase Inhibitor (Human) is indicated only in patients with congenital α_1-PI deficiency who have clinically evident emphysema.**

Augmenting the levels of functional α_1-proteinase inhibitor by intravenous infusion is an approach to therapy for patients with α_1-PI deficiency. However, the efficacy of augmentation therapy in affecting the progression of emphysema has not been demonstrated in randomized, controlled clinical trials. The intended theoretical goal is to provide protection to the lower respiratory tract by correcting the imbalance between neutrophil elastase and protease inhibitors. Whether augmentation therapy with ARALAST NP actually protects the lower respiratory tract from progressive emphysematous changes has not been evaluated. Although the maintenance of blood serum levels of α_1-PI (antigenically measured) above 11 µM has been historically postulated to provide therapeutically relevant anti-neutrophil elastase protection, this has not been proven. Individuals with severe α_1-PI deficiency have been shown to have increased neutrophil and neutrophil elastase concentrations in lung epithelial lining fluid compared to normal PiMM individuals, and some PiSZ individuals with α_1-PI above 11 µM have emphysema attributed to α_1-PI deficiency. These observations underscore the uncertainty regarding the appropriate therapeutic target serum level of α_1-PI during augmentation therapy. The clinical benefit of the increased blood levels of Alpha$_1$-Proteinase Inhibitor at the recommended dose has not been established.

The clinical efficacy of ARALAST NP in influencing the course of pulmonary emphysema or the frequency, duration, or severity of pulmonary exacerbations has not been demonstrated in randomized, controlled clinical trials.

Pharmacokinetics

The pharmacokinetics of ARALAST NP were compared with ARALAST in a multicenter, single-dose, randomized, double-blind, crossover clinical study (Study 460501). Twenty-five subjects with congenital α_1-PI deficiency received a single intravenous (IV) infusion of 60 mg/kg ARALAST NP or ARALAST. The 25 subjects in this study were between 20 and 75 years old, with a median age of 59. Plasma α_1-PI concentrations were measured using an enzyme linked immunosorbent assay (ELISA). Figure 1 shows that the mean ± standard deviation (SD) plasma α_1-PI concentration-time profiles after a single IV infusion of ARALAST NP and ARALAST at 60 mg/kg were comparable. Table 2 summarizes the pharmacokinetic parameters of ARALAST NP and ARALAST. The 90% confidence intervals for C_{max} and AUC_{0-inf}/dose were well within the pre-defined acceptance limits of 80 to 125%.

Figure 1. Mean (± SD) Plasma α_1-PI Concentration-Time Profiles After a Single Intravenous Infusion of ARALAST NP and ARALAST (60 mg/kg) in Subjects with Congenital α_1-PI Deficiency

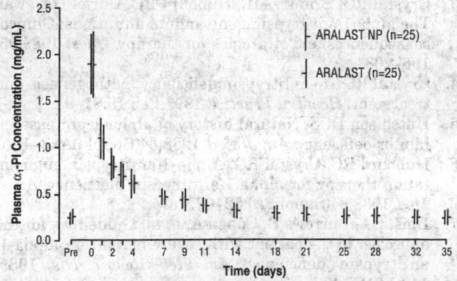

[See table 2 at right]

A clinical study (ATC 97-01) was conducted to compare ARALAST to a commercially available preparation of α_1-PI (Prolastin®, manufactured by Bayer Corporation). All subjects were to have been diagnosed as having congenital α_1-PI deficiency and emphysema but no α_1-PI augmentation therapy within the preceding six months.

Twenty-eight subjects were randomized to receive either ARALAST or Prolastin®, 60 mg/kg intravenously per week, for 10 consecutive weeks. Two subjects withdrew from the study prematurely: 1 subject receiving ARALAST withdrew consent after 6 infusions; 1 subject receiving Prolastin® withdrew after 1 infusion due to pneumonia following unscheduled bronchoscopy to remove a foreign body. Trough levels of α_1-PI (antigenic determination) and anti-NE capacity (functional determination) were measured prior to treatment at Weeks 8 through 11. Following their first 10 weekly infusions, the subjects who were receiving Prolastin® were switched to ARALAST while those who already were receiving ARALAST continued to receive it. Maintenance of mean serum α_1-PI trough levels was assessed prior to treatments at Weeks 12 through 24. Bronchoalveolar lavages (BALs) were performed on subjects at baseline and prior to treatment at Week 7. The epithelial lining fluid (ELF) from each BAL meeting acceptance criteria was analyzed for the α_1-PI level and anti-NE capacity.

With weekly augmentation therapy with ARALAST or Prolastin®, a gradual increase in peak and trough serum

α_1-PI levels was noted, with stabilization after several weeks. The metabolic half-life of ARALAST was 5.9 days. Serum anti-NE capacity trough levels rose substantially in all subjects by Week 2, and by Week 3, serum anti-NE capacity trough levels exceeded 11 µM in the majority of subjects. With few exceptions, levels remained above this recommended threshold level in individual subjects for the duration of the period Weeks 3 through 24 on study. Although only five of fourteen subjects (35.7%) receiving ARALAST had BALs meeting acceptance criteria for analysis at both baseline and Week 7, a statistically significant increase in the antigenic level of α_1-PI in the ELF was observed. No statistically significant increase in the anti-NE capacity in the ELF was detected.

Viral serology of all subjects was determined periodically throughout the study, including testing for antibodies to hepatitis A (HAV) and C (HCV), presence of circulating HBsAg, and presence of antibodies to HIV-1, HIV-2, and Parvovirus B-19. Subjects who were seronegative to parvovirus B-19 at enrollment were retested by PCR at Week 2. There were no seroconversions in subjects treated with ARALAST through Week 24. None of the subjects became HBsAg positive during the study, although five of 13 (38%) evaluable subjects treated with ARALAST and eight of 13 (62%) treated with Prolastin® had not been vaccinated to hepatitis B. No patient developed antibodies against α_1-PI. It was concluded that at a dose of 60 mg/kg administered intravenously once weekly, ARALAST and Prolastin® had similar effects in maintaining target serum α_1-PI trough levels and increasing antigenic levels of α_1-PI in epithelial lining fluid (ELF) with maintenance augmentation therapy.

INDICATIONS AND USAGE

Congenital Alpha$_1$-Proteinase Inhibitor Deficiency

ARALAST NP is indicated for chronic augmentation therapy in patients having congenital deficiency of α_1-PI with clinically evident emphysema. Clinical and biochemical studies have demonstrated that with such therapy, ARALAST is effective in maintaining target serum α_1-PI trough levels and increasing α_1-PI levels in epithelial lining fluid (ELF). ARALAST NP pharmacokinetics are comparable with the pharmacokinetics of ARALAST after single-dose administration in 25 subjects with congenital deficiency of α_1-PI. Clinical data demonstrating the long-term effects of chronic augmentation or replacement therapy of individuals with ARALAST NP or ARALAST are not available.

The effect of augmentation therapy with ARALAST NP on pulmonary exacerbations and on the progression of emphysema in alpha$_1$-antitrypsin deficiency has not been demonstrated in randomized, controlled clinical trials.

ARALAST NP is not indicated as therapy for lung disease patients in whom congenital α_1-PI deficiency has not been established.

CONTRAINDICATIONS

ARALAST NP is contraindicated in IgA deficient patients with antibodies against IgA, due to the risk of severe hypersensitivity.

WARNINGS

Because ARALAST NP is derived from pooled human plasma, it may carry a risk of transmitting infectious agents, e.g., viruses and theoretically, the Creutzfeldt-Jakob disease (CJD) agent. Stringent procedures designed to reduce the risk of adventitious agent transmission have been employed in the manufacture of this product, from the screening of plasma donors and the collection and testing of plasma through the application of viral elimination/reduction steps such as ethanol fractionation, PEG precipitation, solvent detergent treatment, and nanofiltration. Despite these measures, such products can still potentially transmit disease; therefore, the risk of infectious agents cannot be totally eliminated. ALL infections thought to by a physician possibly to have been transmitted by this product should be reported to the manufacturer at 1-800-423-2090 (US). The physician should weigh the risks and benefits of the use of this product and should discuss these with the patient. ARALAST NP may contain trace amounts of IgA. Patients with known antibodies to IgA, which can be present in patients with selective or severe IgA deficiency, have a greater risk of developing potentially severe hypersensitivity and anaphylactic reactions. ARALAST NP is contraindicated in patients with antibodies against IgA due to risk of severe hypersensitivity.

The rate of administration specified in DOSAGE AND ADMINISTRATION should be closely followed, at least until the physician has had sufficient experience with a given patient. Vital signs should be monitored continuously and the patient should be carefully observed throughout the infusion. **IF ANAPHYLACTIC OR SEVERE ANAPHYLACTOID REACTIONS OCCUR, THE INFUSION SHOULD BE DISCONTINUED IMMEDIATELY.** Epinephrine and other appropriate supportive therapy should be available for the treatment of any acute anaphylactic or anaphylactoid reaction.

PRECAUTIONS

General

ARALAST NP should be administered at room temperature within three (3) hours after reconstitution. Partially used vials should be discarded and not saved for future use. The solution contains no preservative.

ARALAST NP should be administered alone, without mixing with other agents or diluting solutions.

Pregnancy Category C

Animal reproduction studies have not been conducted with ARALAST NP. It is also not known whether ARALAST NP can cause fetal harm when administered to pregnant women or can affect reproductive capacity.

Table 1: Virus Log Reduction in ARALAST NP Manufacturing Process

Processing Step	Virus Log Reduction Factors				
	HIV-1	BVDV	PRV	HAV	MMV
Cold ethanol fractionation	4.6	1.4	2.1	1.4	≤ 1.0*
Solvent Detergent-treatment	> 5.8	> 6.0	> 5.5	N/A	N/A
15 N nanofiltration	> 5.3	> 6.0	> 5.6	> 5.1	4.9
Overall reduction factor	**> 15.7**	**> 13.4**	**> 13.2**	**> 6.5**	**4.9**

*Reduction factors ≤ 1.0 are not used for calculation of the overall reduction factor
N/A – Not applicable; study did not test for virus indicated
HIV-1: Human immunodeficiency virus-1, BVDV (Bovine Viral Diarrhea Virus, model for Hepatitis C Virus and other lipid-enveloped RNA viruses), PRV (Pseudorabies Virus, model for lipid-enveloped DNA viruses, to which Hepatitis B also belongs): HAV: Hepatitis A Virus, MMV (Mice Minute Virus, model for small non-lipid-enveloped DNA viruses)

Table 2: Mean (± SD) Pharmacokinetic Parameters of ARALAST NP and ARALAST Following a Single IV infusion of 60 mg/kg (n=25)

Parameters	Units	ARALAST NP	ARALAST
C_{max}	mg/mL	1.6 ± 0.3	1.7 ± 0.3
AUC_{0-inf}/dose	days*kg/mL	0.0868 ± 0.0253	0.0920 ± 0.0238
Half-life	days	4.7 ± 2.7	4.8 ± 2.0
Clearance	mL/day	940 ± 275	862 ± 206
V_{ss}	mL	5632 ± 2006	5618 ± 1618

C_{max} = Maximum increase in plasma α_1-PI concentration following infusion; AUC_{0-inf}/dose = Area under the curve from time 0 to infinity divided by dose; Half-life = terminal phase half-life determined using non-compartmental method; V_{ss} = Volume of distribution at steady state.

Nursing Mothers
It is not known whether alpha$_1$-proteinase inhibitor is excreted in human milk. Because many drugs are excreted in human milk, caution should be exercised when ARALAST NP is administered to a nursing woman.

Pediatric Use
Safety and effectiveness in pediatric patients have not been established.

Geriatric Use
Clinical studies of ARALAST NP did not include sufficient numbers of subjects aged 65 and over to determine whether they respond differently from younger subjects. As for all patients, dosing for geriatric patients should be appropriate to their overall situation. Safety and effectiveness in patients over age 65 years of age have not been established.

Information for Patients
Inform patients that administration of ARALAST NP has been demonstrated to raise the plasma level of α_1-PI, but that the effect of this augmentation on the frequency of pulmonary exacerbations and on the rate of progression of emphysema has not been established by clinical trials.

ADVERSE REACTIONS

The safety of ARALAST NP was evaluated with ARALAST after a single-dose IV infusion in a multicenter, randomized, double-blind, crossover clinical PK comparability study (Study 460501). The number of subjects with one or more adverse events, regardless of causality, was 23 of 25 (92%) when receiving ARALAST NP and 19 of 25 (76%) when receiving ARALAST. Treatment-related adverse events were reported in 8 of 25 subjects (32%) for ARALAST NP and 7 of 25 subjects (28%) for ARALAST. Of a total of 61 adverse events reported for ARALAST NP, 43 (70%) were mild, 16 (26%) moderate, and 2 (3%) severe. Seventeen of 61 (28%) adverse events were deemed possibly or probably related to ARALAST NP of which 14 (82%) were mild and 3 (18%) were moderate. Of a total of 60 adverse events reported for ARALAST, 45 (75%) were mild, 12 (20%) moderate, and 3 (5%) severe. Eleven of 60 (18%) adverse events were deemed possibly or probably related to ARALAST of which 8 (73%) were mild and 3 (27%) were moderate. No serious adverse events or deaths were reported in the study. No clinically significant changes in the peri-infusion vital signs (blood pressure, heart rate, or respiratory rate) were reported. The most common adverse events deemed related to ARALAST NP included: headache (4 of 61 [7%] events) and musculoskeletal discomfort (4 of 61 [7%] events). These adverse events, as well as most of the other adverse events, were also reported in subjects treated with ARALAST.

In Clinical Study ATC 97-01, ARALAST was evaluated for up to 96 weeks in 27 subjects with a congenital deficiency of α_1-PI and clinically evident emphysema. The number of subjects with an adverse event, regardless of causality, was 22 of 27 (81.5%). The number of subjects with an adverse event deemed possibly, probably, or definitely related to study drug was 7 of 27 (25.9%).

The frequency of infusions associated with an adverse event, regardless of causality, was 108 of 1127 (9.6%) infusions administered per protocol. The most common symptoms were pharyngitis (1.6%), headache (0.7%), and increased cough (0.6%). Symptoms of bronchitis, sinusitis, pain, rash, back pain, viral infection, peripheral edema, bloating, dizziness, somnolence, asthma, and rhinitis were each associated with ≥ 0.2% but < 0.6% of infusions. All symptoms were mild to moderate in severity.

The overall frequency of adverse events deemed to be possibly, probably, or definitely related to study drug was 15 of 1127 (1.3%) infusions. The most common symptoms included headache (0.3%) and somnolence (0.3%). Symptoms of chills and fever, vasodilation, dizziness, pruritus, rash, abnormal vision, chest pain, increased cough, and dyspnea were each associated with one (0.1%) infusion. Five (5) of 27 (18.5%) subjects experienced eight (8) serious adverse reactions during the study. None of these serious adverse events were considered to be causally related to the administration of ARALAST.

Twenty-six (26) of 27 (96.3%) subjects experienced a total of 94 upper and lower respiratory-tract infections during the 96-week study (median: 3.0; range: 1 to 8; mean ± SD: 3.6 ± 2.3 infections). Twenty-eight (29.8%) of the respiratory infections occurred in 19 (70.4%) subjects during the first 24 weeks of the 96-week study suggesting that the risk of infection did not change with time on ARALAST. In a post-hoc analysis, subjects experienced a range of 0 to 8 exacerbations of COPD over the 96-week study with a median of less than one exacerbation per year (median: 0.61; mean ± SD: 0.83 ± 0.87 exacerbations per year).

Treatment-emergent elevations (> two times the upper limit of normal) in aminotransferases (ALT or AST), up to 3.7 times the upper limit of normal, were noted in 3 of 27 (11.1%) subjects. Elevations were transient lasting three months or less. No subject developed any evidence of viral hepatitis or hepatitis seroconversion while being treated with ARALAST, including 13 evaluable subjects who were not vaccinated against hepatitis B.

No clinically relevant alterations in blood pressure, heart rate, respiratory rate, or body temperature occurred during infusion of ARALAST. Mean hematology and laboratory parameters were little changed over the duration of the study, with individual variations not clinically meaningful.

During the initial 10 weeks of the study, subjects were randomized to receive either ARALAST or a commercially available preparation of α_1-PI (Prolastin®). The overall frequency, severity and symptomatology of adverse reactions were similar in both the ARALAST and Prolastin® groups. There were two serious adverse events in the Prolastin® group, both of which were considered to be possibly related to Prolastin®. These included chest pain, dyspnea and bilateral pulmonary infiltrates in one individual that withdrew from the study prematurely following an unscheduled bronchoscopy to remove a foreign body and the other, a positive seroconversion to Parvovirus B-19. There were no serious adverse events or seroconversions reported for the ARALAST group during the 96 week study period. No subject developed an antibody to α_1-PI.

DOSAGE AND ADMINISTRATION

Dose ranging studies using efficacy endpoints have not been performed.

Chronic Augmentation Therapy
FOR INTRAVENOUS USE ONLY. The recommended dosage of ARALAST NP is 60 mg/kg body weight administered once weekly by intravenous infusion. Each vial of ARALAST NP has the functional activity, as determined by inhibition of porcine pancreatic elastase, stated on the label. Administration of ARALAST NP within three hours after reconstitution is recommended to avoid the potential ill effect of any inadvertent microbial contamination occurring during reconstitution. Discard any unused contents.

Infusion Rate
ARALAST NP should be administered at a rate not exceeding 0.08 mL/kg body weight/minute. If adverse events occur, the rate should be reduced or the infusion interrupted until the symptoms subside. The infusion may then be resumed at a rate tolerated by the subject.

RECONSTITUTION

Use Aseptic Technique

1. ARALAST NP and diluent should be at room temperature before reconstitution.
2. Remove caps from the diluent and product vials.
3. Swab the exposed stopper surfaces with alcohol.
4. Open the package of the BAXJECT II Hi-Flow device by peeling away the lid without touching the inside contents (Fig. A). Do not remove the transfer system from the package. Do not touch the clear spike.

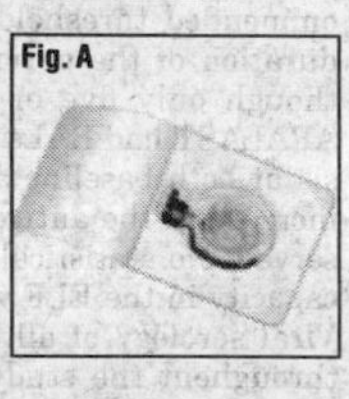
Fig. A

5. Turn the package over and insert the clear plastic spike through the diluent vial by pressing straight down (Fig. B).

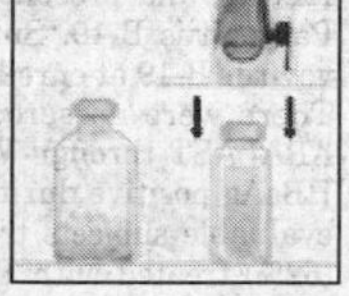
Fig. B

6. Grip the BAXJECT II Hi-Flow package at the edges and pull the package off the device (Fig. C). Do not remove the blue protective cap from the BAXJECT II Hi-Flow device. Do not touch the purple spike.

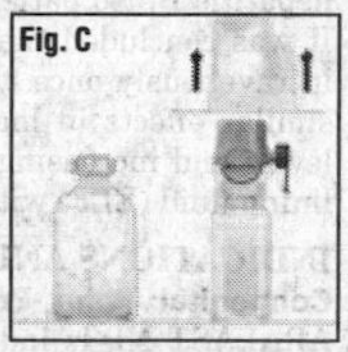
Fig. C

7. Turn the system over so that the diluent vial is on top. Press the purple spike of the BAXJECT II Hi-Flow device into the ARALAST NP vial. The vacuum will draw the diluent into the ARALAST NP vial (Fig. D).

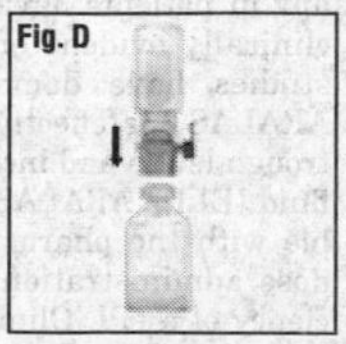
Fig. D

8. Let the vial stand until most of the contents is in solution, then GENTLY swirl until the powder is completely dissolved. Reconstitution requires no more than five minutes for a 0.5 gram vial and no more than 10 minutes for a 1.0 gram vial.
9. DO NOT SHAKE THE CONTENTS OF THE VIAL. DO NOT INVERT THE VIAL UNTIL READY TO WITHDRAW CONTENTS.
10. Use within three hours of reconstitution.

For Intravenous Injection/Infusion

1. After reconstituting the product as described under **Reconstitution**, inspect parenteral drug products visually for particulate matter and discoloration prior to administration. The reconstituted product should be a colorless or slightly yellowish to yellowish-green solution and be essentially free of visible particles.
2. Remove the blue protective cap from the BAXJECT II Hi-Flow device. Connect the syringe to the BAXJECT II Hi-Flow device (DO NOT DRAW AIR INTO THE SYRINGE) (Fig. E).

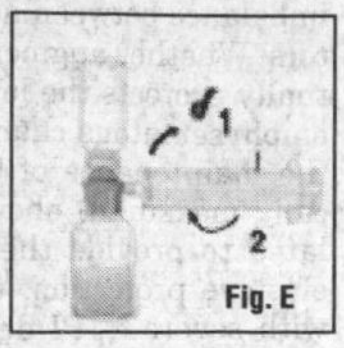

Fig. E

3. Invert the system (with the ARALAST NP concentrate vial on top). Draw the dissolved product into the syringe by pulling the plunger back SLOWLY (Fig. F).

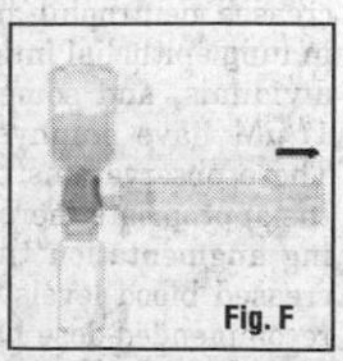
Fig. F

4. Disconnect the syringe. Reconstituted product from several vials may be pooled into an empty, sterile IV solution container by using aseptic technique.

HOW SUPPLIED

ARALAST NP is supplied as a sterile, non-pyrogenic, lyophilized powder in single-dose vials. The following product packages are available:

Fill Size	NDC
0.5 g	0944-2812-01
1.0 g	0944-2822-02

ARALAST NP is packaged with a suitable volume of Sterile Water for Injection, USP diluent (25 mL/0.5 g vial; 50 mL/1.0 g vial), one BAXJECT II Hi-Flow Needleless Transfer Device and one package insert.

STORAGE
ARALAST NP should be stored at temperatures not to exceed 25°C (77°F). Do not freeze. Do not use after the expiration date printed on the label.

Rx only

REFERENCES

1. Brantly M, Nukiwa T, Crystal RG. Molecular basis of alpha-1-antitrypsin deficiency. *Am J Med* 1988 (Suppl 6A);84:13–31.
2. Data on file at Baxter Healthcare Corporation.
3. Crystal RG, Brantly ML, Hubbard RC, Curiel DT, et al. The alpha1-antitrypsin gene and its mutations: Clinical consequences and strategies for therapy. *Chest* 1989;95: 196–208.
4. Crystal RG. α_1-Antitrypsin deficiency: pathogenesis and treatment. *Hospital Practice* 1991;Feb.15:81–94.
5. Hutchison DCS. Natural history of alpha-1-protease inhibitor deficiency. *Am J Med* 1988;84(Suppl 6A):3–12.
6. Hubbard RC, Crystal RG. Alpha-1-antitrypsin augmentation therapy for alpha-1-antitrypsin deficiency. *Am J Med* 1988;84(Suppl 6A):52–62.
7. Buist SA, Burrows B, Cohen A, et al. Guidelines for the approach to the patient with severe hereditary alpha-1-antitrypsin deficiency. *Am Rev Respir Dis* 1989; 140:1494–1497.
8. Gadek JE, Fells GA, Zimmerman RL, et al. Anti-elastases of the human alveolar structures: Implications for the protease-antiprotease theory of emphysema. *J Clin Invest* 1981;68:889-898.
9. Stoller JK, Brantly M, Fleming LE, et al. Formation and current results of a patient-organized registry for α_1-antitrypsin deficiency. *Chest* 2000; 118(3):843-848.
10. McElvaney NG, Stoller JK, Buist AS, et al. Baseline characteristics of enrollees in the National Heart, Lung and Blood Institute Registry of α_1-antitrypsin deficiency. *Chest* 1997;111:394-403.
11. FDA/CBER "Heterogeneity of Alpha-1-Proteinase Inhibitor Products" 27 Mar 2006 <http://www.fda.gov/cber/infosheets/alph1pi.htm>
12. Kolarich D, et al. Biochemical, molecular characterization, and glycoproteomic analyses of α_1-proteinase inhibitor products used for replacement therapy. *Transfusion* 2006;46:1959-1977.
13. Transcript of Blood Products Advisory Committee (BPAC) 85th Meeting; 3-4 Nov 2005.
14. Turino GM, Barker AF, Brantly ML, *et al:* Clinical features of individuals with Pi*SZ phenotype of α_1-antitrypsin deficiency. *Am J Respir Crit Care Med* 154: 1718-25, 1996.

BAXTER, ARALAST NP and BAXJECT are trademarks of Baxter International Inc.

Made by the method of U.S. Patent No. 5,616,693 and 5,981,715

DATE OF REVISION: August 2010
Baxter Healthcare Corporation
Westlake Village, CA 91362
U.S. License No. 140

BUMINATE 25%
[bu-min-ate]
Albumin (Human), USP, 25% Solution

℞

DESCRIPTION

BUMINATE 25%, in 20, 50 and 100 mL glass bottles is a sterile, nonpyrogenic preparation of albumin in a single dosage form for intravenous administration. Each 100 mL contains 25 g of albumin and was prepared from human venous plasma using the Cohn cold ethanol fractionation process. Source material for fractionation may be obtained from another U.S. licensed manufacturer. It has been adjusted to physiological pH with sodium bicarbonate and/or sodium hydroxide and stabilized with N-acetyltryptophan (0.02 M) and sodium caprylate (0.02 M). The sodium content is 145 ± 15 mEq/L. This solution contains no preservative and none of the coagulation factors found in fresh whole blood or plasma. BUMINATE 25% is a transparent or slightly opalescent solution which may have a greenish tint or may vary from a pale straw to an amber color.

The likelihood of the presence of viable hepatitis viruses has been minimized by testing the plasma at three stages for the presence of hepatitis viruses, by fractionation steps with demonstrated virus removal capacity and by heating the product for 10 hours at 60°C. This procedure has been shown to be an effective method of inactivating hepatitis virus in albumin solutions even when those solutions were prepared from plasma known to be infective.[1-3]

CLINICAL PHARMACOLOGY

Albumin is responsible for 70-80% of the colloid osmotic pressure of normal plasma, thus making it useful in regulating the volume of circulating blood.[4-6] Albumin is also a transport protein and binds naturally occurring, therapeutic and toxic materials in the circulation.[5,6]

BUMINATE 25% is osmotically equivalent to approximately five times its volume of human plasma. When injected intravenously, 25% albumin will draw about 3.5 times its volume of additional fluid into the circulation within 15 minutes, except when the patient is markedly dehydrated. This extra fluid reduces hemoconcentration and blood viscosity. The degree and duration of volume expansion depends upon the initial blood volume. With patients treated for diminished blood volume, the effect of infused albumin may persist for many hours; however, in patients with normal volume, the duration will be shorter.[7-9]

Total body albumin is estimated to be 350 g for a 70 kg man and is distributed throughout the extracellular compartments; more than 60% is located in the extravascular fluid compartment. The half-life of albumin is 15 to 20 days with a turnover of approximately 15 g per day.[5]

The minimum plasma albumin level necessary to prevent or reverse peripheral edema is unknown. Some investigators recommend that plasma albumin levels be maintained at approximately 2.5 g/dL. This concentration provides a plasma oncotic pressure value of 20 mm Hg.[4]

BUMINATE 25% is manufactured from human plasma by the modified Cohn-Oncley cold ethanol fractionation process, which includes a series of cold-ethanol precipitation, centrifugation and/or filtration steps followed by pasteurization of the final product at 60 ± 0.5°C for 10–11 hours. This process accomplishes both purification of albumin and the reduction of viruses.

In vitro studies demonstrate that the manufacturing process for BUMINATE 25% provides for significant viral reduction. These viral reduction studies, summarized in Table 1, demonstrate viral clearance during the manufacturing process for BUMINATE 25% using human immunodeficiency virus, type 1 (HIV-1) both as a target virus and as model virus for HIV-2 and other lipid-enveloped RNA viruses; bovine viral diarrhea virus (BVDV), a model for lipid-enveloped RNA viruses, such as hepatitis C virus (HCV); West Nile Virus (WNV), a target virus and model for other similar lipid-enveloped RNA viruses; pseudorabies virus (PRV), a model for other lipid-enveloped DNA viruses such as hepatitis B virus (HBV); mice minute virus (MMV), models for non-enveloped DNA viruses such as human parvovirus B19[10]; hepatitis A virus (HAV), a target virus and a model for other non-enveloped RNA viruses.

These studies indicate that specific steps in the manufacture of BUMINATE 25% are capable of eliminating/inactivating a wide range of relevant and model viruses. Since the mechanism of virus elimination/inactivation by fractionation and by heating is different, the overall manufacturing process of BUMINATE 25% is robust in reducing viral load.
[See table 1]

TABLE 1
Summary of Viral Reduction Factor for Each Virus and Processing Step

Process Step	Viral Reduction Factor (log_{10})					
	Lipid Enveloped				Non-Lipid Enveloped	
	HIV-1	Flaviviridae		PRV	HAV	Parvoviridae
		BVDV	WNV			MMV
Processing of Fraction I+II+III/II+III supernatant to Fraction IV₄ Cuno 70C filtrate*	> 4.9	> 4.8	> 5.7	> 5.5	> 4.5	3.0
Pasteurization	> 7.8	> 6.5	n.d.	> 7.4	3.2	1.6**
Mean Cumulative Reduction Factor, log_{10}	**> 12.7**	**> 11.3**	**> 5.7**	**> 12.9**	**> 7.7**	**4.6**

n.d. = not determined

* Other Albumin fractionation process steps (processing of cryo-poor plasma to Fractionation I+II+III/II+III supernatant and processing of Fraction V suspension to Cuno 90LP filtrate) showed significant virus reduction capacity in *in-vitro* viral clearance studies. These process steps also contribute to the overall viral clearance robustness of the manufacturing process. However, since the mechanism of virus removal is similar to that of this particular process step, the viral inactivation data from other steps were not used in the calculation of the Mean Cumulative Reduction Factor.

** Recent scientific data suggests that the actual human parvovirus B19 (B19V), is far more effectively inactivated by pasteurization than indicated by model virus data.[10]

INDICATIONS AND USAGE

1. Hypovolemia

Hypovolemia is a possible indication for use of BUMINATE 25%. Its effectiveness in reversing hypovolemia depends largely upon its ability to draw interstitial fluid into the circulation. It is most effective with patients who are well hydrated. When the hypovolemia is long standing and hypoalbuminemia exists accompanied by adequate hydration or edema, 25% albumin is preferable to 5% protein solutions.[4,6] However, in the absence of adequate or excessive hydration, 5% protein solutions should be used or 25% albumin should be diluted with crystalloid solutions.

Although crystalloid solutions and colloid-containing plasma substitutes can be used in emergency treatment of shock, Albumin (Human) has a prolonged intravascular half-life.[11] When blood volume deficit is the result of hemorrhage, compatible red blood cells or whole blood should be administered as quickly as possible.

2. Hypoalbuminemia

A. General

Hypoalbuminemia is another possible indication for use of BUMINATE 25%. Hypoalbuminemia can result from one or more of the following:[5]

(1) Inadequate production (malnutrition, burns, major injury, infections, etc.)

(2) Excessive catabolism (burns, major injury, pancreatitis, etc.)

(3) Loss from the body (hemorrhage, excessive renal excretion, burn exudates, etc.)

(4) Redistribution within the body (major surgery, various inflammatory conditions, etc.)

When albumin deficit is the result of excessive protein loss, the effect of administration of albumin will be temporary unless the underlying disorder is reversed. In most cases, increased nutritional replacement of amino acids and/or protein with concurrent treatment of the underlying disorder will restore normal plasma albumin levels more effectively than albumin solutions. Occasionally hypoalbuminemia accompanying severe injuries, infections or pancreatitis cannot be quickly reversed and nutritional supplements may fail to restore serum albumin levels. In these cases, BUMINATE 25% might be a useful therapeutic adjunct.

B. Burns

An optimum regimen for the use of albumin, electrolytes and fluid in the early treatment of burns has not been established, however, in conjunction with appropriate crystalloid therapy, BUMINATE 25% may be indicated for treatment of oncotic deficits after the initial 24-hour period following extensive burns and to replace the protein loss which accompanies any severe burn.[4,6]

C. Adult Respiratory Distress Syndrome (ARDS)

A characteristic of ARDS is a hypoproteinemic state, which may be causally related to the interstitial pulmonary edema. Although uncertainty exists concerning the precise indication of albumin infusion in these patients, if there is a pulmonary overload accompanied by hypoalbuminemia, 25% albumin solution may have a therapeutic effect when used with a diuretic.[4]

D. Nephrosis

BUMINATE 25% may be a useful aid in treating edema in patients with severe nephrosis who are receiving steroids and/or diuretics.

3. Cardiopulmonary Bypass Surgery

BUMINATE 25% has been recommended prior to or during cardiopulmonary bypass surgery, although no clear data exist indicating its advantage over crystalloid solutions.[4,6,12]

4. Hemolytic Disease of the Newborn (HDN)

BUMINATE 25% may be administered in an attempt to bind and detoxify unconjugated bilirubin in infants with severe HDN.

There is no valid reason for use of albumin as an intravenous nutrient.

CONTRAINDICATIONS

A history of allergic reactions to albumin and any of the excipients is a specific contraindication to the use of this product.

BUMINATE 25% is also contraindicated in severely anemic patients and in patients with cardiac failure.

BUMINATE 25% must not be diluted with Sterile Water for Injection as this may cause hemolysis in recipients. There exists a risk of potentially fatal hemolysis and acute renal failure from the use of Sterile Water for Injection as a diluent for Albumin (Human). Acceptable diluents include 0.9% Sodium Chloride or 5% Dextrose in Water.

BUMINATE 25% must not be administered to patients with chronic renal insufficiencies due to the potential for accumulations of aluminum. Accumulations of aluminum in patients with chronic renal insufficiencies have led to toxic manifestations such as hypercalcemia, vitamin D-refractory osteodystrophy, anemia, and severe progressive encephalopathy.[13-15, 19]

WARNINGS

BUMINATE 25% is made from human plasma. Products made from human plasma may contain infectious agents, such as viruses, that can cause disease. This also applies to unknown or emerging viruses and pathogens.

The risk that such products will transmit an infectious agent has been reduced by screening plasma donors for prior exposure to certain viruses, by testing for the presence of certain current virus infections, and by inactivating and/or removing certain viruses (See Description). The measures taken are considered effective for enveloped viruses such as HIV, HBV, and HCV, and for the non-enveloped viruses HAV and Parvovirus B19. Despite these measures, such products can still potentially transmit disease. Based on effective donor screening and product manufacturing processes, albumin carries an extremely remote risk for transmission of viral diseases. A theoretical risk for transmission of Creutzfeldt-Jakob disease (CJD) also is considered extremely remote. No cases of transmission of viral diseases or CJD have ever been identified for albumin. All infections thought by a physician possibly to have been transmitted by this product, should be reported by the physician, or other healthcare provider to Baxter Healthcare Corporation at 1-800-423-2862. The physician should discuss the risks and benefits of this product with the patient. Suspicion of allergic or anaphylactic type reactions requires immediate discontinuation of the injection. In case of shock, standard medical treatment for shock should be implemented.

PRECAUTIONS

Certain components used in the packaging of this product contain natural rubber latex.

Hemodynamics

Do not administer BUMINATE 25% without very close monitoring of hemodynamics; look for evidence of cardiac or respiratory failure, renal failure, or increasing intra-cranial pressure.

Hypervolemia/Hemodilution

BUMINATE 25% should be used with caution in conditions where hypervolemia and its consequences or hemodilution could represent a special risk for the patient. Examples may include but are not limited to: decompensated cardiac insufficiency, hypertension, esophageal varices, pulmonary edema, hemorrhagic diathesis, severe anemia, renal and post-renal failure.

BUMINATE 25% must be administered intravenously. The rate of administration should be adjusted according to the solution concentration and the patient's hemodynamic measurements and should not exceed 1mL/min to patients with normal blood volume. More rapid administration might cause circulatory overload and pulmonary edema.[16] At the first clinical signs of cardiovascular overload (headache, dyspnea, jugular vein congestion), or increased blood pressure, raised central venous pressure and pulmonary edema, the infusion is to be stopped immediately.

Blood Pressure

A rise in blood pressure after 25% albumin infusion necessitates careful observation of the injured or post-operative patient in order to detect and treat severed blood vessels that may not have bled at a lower blood pressure.

Pregnancy–Category C, and Lactation

There are no adequate data from the use of BUMINATE 25% in pregnant or lactating women.

Animal reproduction studies have not been conducted with BUMINATE 25%. It is not known whether BUMINATE 25% can cause fetal harm when administered to a pregnant woman or can affect reproductive capacity. Physicians should carefully consider the potential risks and benefits for each specific patient before prescribing BUMINATE 25%. BUMINATE 25% should be given to a pregnant woman only if clearly needed.

Pediatric Use

The safety of albumin solutions has been demonstrated in children provided the dose is appropriate for body weight. However, the safety of BUMINATE 25% has not been evaluated in pediatric patients.

Large Volumes

If comparatively large volumes are to be replaced, controls of coagulation and hematocrit are necessary. Care must be taken to ensure adequate substitution of other blood constituents (coagulation factors, electrolytes, platelets, and erythrocytes). Appropriate hemodynamic monitoring should be undertaken.

Electrolyte Status

When BUMINATE 25% is given, the electrolyte status of the patient should be monitored and appropriate steps taken to restore or maintain the electrolyte balance.

DRUG INTERACTIONS

No interaction studies have been performed with BUMINATE 25%.

ADVERSE REACTIONS

Adverse Reactions from Clinical Trials

There are no data available on adverse reactions from clinical trials conducted with BUMINATE 25%.

Post-Marketing Adverse Reactions

The following adverse reactions have been reported in the post-marketing experience. These reactions are listed by MedDRA System Organ Class (SOC), then by Preferred Term in order of severity.

IMMUNE SYSTEM DISORDERS: Anaphylactic shock, Anaphylactic reactions, Hypersensitivity/Allergic reactions
NERVOUS SYSTEM DISORDERS: Headache
CARDIAC DISORDERS: Tachycardia
VASCULAR DISORDERS: Hypotension, Flushing
RESPIRATORY, THORACIC, AND MEDIASTINAL DISORDERS: Dyspnea
GASTROINTESTINAL DISORDERS: Vomiting, Nausea, Dysguesia
SKIN AND SUBCUTANEOUS TISSUE DISORDERS: Urticaria, Rash, Pruritis
GENERAL DISORDERS AND ADMINISTRATION SITE CONDITIONS: Pyrexia, Chills

Overdose

Hypervolemia may occur if the dosage and rate of infusion are too high. (See Precautions: Hypervolemia/ Hemodilution)

DOSAGE AND ADMINISTRATION

BUMINATE 25% must be administered intravenously. **Do not use if turbid. Do not begin administration more than 4 hours after the container has been entered. Discard unused portion.**

BUMINATE 25% solutions must not be diluted with Sterile Water for Injection as this may cause hemolysis in recipients (see CONTRAINDICATIONS).

Albumin solutions should not be mixed with other medicinal products including blood and blood components, but can be used concomitantly with other parenterals such as whole blood, plasma, saline, glucose or sodium lactate when deemed medically necessary. The addition of four volumes of normal saline or 5% glucose to 1 volume of BUMINATE 25% gives a solution, which is approximately isotonic and isosmotic with citrated plasma.

Albumin solutions should not be mixed with protein hydrolysates or solutions containing alcohol since these combinations may cause the proteins to precipitate.

Do not add supplementary medication.

Hypervolemia may occur if the dosage and rate of infusion are not adjusted, giving consideration to the solution concentration and the patient's clinical status. Hemodynamic parameters should be monitored in patients receiving BUMINATE 25% and should be used to check for the risk of hypervolemia and cardiovascular overload. (See PRECAUTIONS: Hypervolemia/ Hemodilution).

It is strongly recommended that every time that BUMINATE 25% is administered to a patient, the name and batch number of the product be recorded in order to maintain a link between the patient and the batch of the product.

Recommended Dosages

1. Hypovolemic Shock

The dosage of BUMINATE 25% must be individualized. As a guideline, the initial treatment should be in the range of 100 to 200 mL for adults and 2.5 to 5 mL per kilogram body weight for children. This may be repeated after 15 to 30 minutes, if the response is not adequate. For patients with significant plasma volume deficits, albumin replacement is best administered in the form of 5% Albumin (Human).

Upon administration of additional albumin or if hemorrhage has occurred, hemodilution and a relative anemia will follow. This condition should be controlled by the supplemental administration of compatible red blood cells or compatible whole blood.

2. Burns

The optimal therapeutic regimen for administration of crystalloid and colloid solutions after extensive burns has not been established. When BUMINATE 25% is administered after the first 24 hours following burns, the dose should be determined according to the patient's condition and response to treatment.

3. Hypoalbuminemia

Hypoalbuminemia is usually accompanied by a hidden extravascular albumin deficiency of equal magnitude. This total body albumin deficit must be considered when determining the amount of albumin necessary to reverse the hypoalbuminemia. When using patient's serum albumin concentration to estimate the deficit, the body albumin compartment should be calculated to be 80 to 100 mL per kg of body weight.[5,6] Daily dose should not exceed 2 g of albumin per kilogram of body weight.

4. Hemolytic Disease of the Newborn

BUMINATE 25% may be administered prior to or during exchange transfusion in a dose of 1 g per kilogram body weight.[17]

Preparation for Administration

Do not use unless solution is clear of particulate matter and seal is intact. BUMINATE 25% is a transparent or slightly opalescent solution, which may have a greenish tint or may vary from a pale straw to an amber color. Parenteral drug products should be inspected visually for particulate matter and discoloration prior to administration, whenever solution and container permit.

1. Remove cap from bottle to expose center portion of rubber stopper.
2. Clean stopper with germicidal solution.

Administration

Follow directions for use printed on the administration set container. Make certain that the administration set contains an adequate filter (15-micron or smaller).

HOW SUPPLIED

BUMINATE 25% is supplied in 20 mL (NDC 0944-0490-01), 50 mL (NDC 0944-0490-02) and 100 mL (NDC 0944-0490-03) bottles.

STORAGE

Store BUMINATE 25% at room temperature, not to exceed 30°C (86°F). Avoid freezing to prevent damage to the bottle. Stability testing for BUMINATE 25% showed that aluminum concentration increased over time reaching levels that could exceed 1000 ppb over the shelf life of the product. (See CONTRAINDICATIONS).[18, 19]

REFERENCES

1. Cai K, Gierman T, *et al*: Ensuring the Biologic Safety of Plasma-Derived Therapeutic Proteins. Department of Preclinical Research and Pathogen Safety, Bayer HealthCare LLC, North Carolina, USA. **Biodrugs 19(2)**: 79-96 2005.
2. Gerety RJ, Aronson DL: Plasma derivatives and viral hepatitis. **Transfusion 22**:347-351, 1982.
3. Burnouf T, Padilla A, Current strategies to prevent transmission of prions by human plasma derivatives. **Transfusion Clinique et Biologique 13**:320-328, 2006.
4. Tullis JL: Albumin, 1. Background and use, and 2. Guidelines for clinical use. **JAMA 237**:355-360, 460-463, 1977.
5. Peters T Jr: Serum albumin, in **The Plasma Proteins, 2nd ed, Vol 1.** Putnam FW (ed). New York, Academic Press, 1975, pp 133-181.
6. Finlayson JS: Albumin products. **Semin Thromb Hemostas. 6**:85-120, 1980.
7. Haynes G, Navickis R, Wilkes M, Albumin administration – what is the evidence of clinical benefit? Asystematic review of randomized controlled trials. **European Journal of Anesthesiology 20**:771-793 2003.
8. Mendez, C, McClain C, Marsano L *et al*, Albumin Therapy in Clinical Practice. **Nutrition in Clinical Practice 20** No. 3:314-320, June 2005.
9. Quinlan G, Martin G, Evans T, Albumin: Biochemical Properties and Therapeutic Potential. **HEMATOLOGY** Vol 14, No. 6 1211-1219 2005.
10. J. Blümel *et al*., Inactivation of Parvovirus B19 During Pasteurization of Human Serum Albumin. **Transfusion 42**:1011-1018, 2002.
11. Shoemaker WC, Schluchter M, Hopkins JA, *et al:* Comparison of the relative effectiveness of colloids and crystalloids in emergency resuscitation. **Am J Surg 142:** 73-83, 1981.
12. Lowenstein E, Hallowell P, Bland JHL: Use of colloid and crystalloid solutions in open heart surgery: Physiological basis and clinical results in, **Proceedings of the Workshop on Albumin**. Sgouris JT, Rene A (eds). DHEW Publication No. (NIH) 76-925, Washington, DC, US Government Printing Office, 1976, pp 195-210.
13. Milliner DS, Shenaberger JH, Shuman P, *et al:* Inadvertent aluminum administration during plasma exchange due to aluminum contamination of albumin-replacement solutions. **N Engl J Med 312**: 165-7,1985
14. Ott SM, Maloney NA, Klein GL, *et al:* Aluminum is associated with low bone formation in patients receiving chronic parenteral nutrition. **Ann Intern Med 98:** 910-4,1983
15. Wills MR, Savory J: Aluminum poisoning: dialysis encephalopathy, osteomalacia, and anaemia. **Lancet 2:** 29-34,1983
16. Grocott, Michael P.W., Mythen, Michael G., and Gan, Tong J. Perioperative Fluid Management and Clinical Outcomes in Adults. **Anesth Analg.** 2005;100:1100.
17. Tsao YC, Yu VYH: Albumin in management of neonatal hyperbilirubinaemia. **Arch Dis Childhood 47**:250-256, 1972.
18. Data on file; Baxter Healthcare Corporation.
19. Data on file; Baxter Healthcare Corporation.

Baxter Healthcare Corporation
Westlake Village, CA 91362 USA
U.S. License No. 140
Printed in the USA

To enroll in the confidential industry-wide Patient Notification System, call 1-888-UPDATE U (1-888-873-2838).

Baxter and Buminate are trademarks of Baxter International Inc.

Revised September 2009

FEIBA NF ℞

[*fī-bäh*]

[Anti-Inhibitor Coagulant Complex]
Nanofiltered and Vapor Heated
Lyophilized powder for solution
Intravenous

WARNING

Thrombotic and thromboembolic events have been reported during post-marketing surveillance following infusion of FEIBA VH or FEIBA NF, particularly following the administration of high doses and/or in patients with thrombotic risk factors (See WARNINGS, PRECAUTIONS and ADVERSE REACTIONS).

DESCRIPTION

FEIBA NF (Anti-Inhibitor Coagulant Complex), nanofiltered and vapor heated, is a freeze-dried sterile human plasma fraction with Factor VIII inhibitor bypassing activity. *In vitro*, FEIBA NF shortens the activated partial thromboplastin time (APTT) of plasma containing Factor VIII inhibitor. Factor VIII inhibitor bypassing activity is expressed in arbitrary units. One unit of activity is defined as that amount of FEIBA NF that shortens the APTT of a high titer Factor VIII inhibitor reference plasma to 50% of the blank value.

FEIBA NF contains Factors II, IX, and X, mainly non-activated, and Factor VII mainly in the activated form. The product contains approximately equal unitages of Factor VIII inhibitor bypassing activity and Prothrombin Complex Factors. In addition, 1–6 units of Factor VIII coagulant antigen (FVIII C:Ag) per mL are present. The preparation contains only traces of factors of the kinin generating system. It contains no heparin.

Reconstituted FEIBA NF contains 4 mg of trisodium citrate and 8 mg of sodium chloride per mL.

FEIBA NF is manufactured from large plasma pools of human plasma. Screening against potentially infectious agents begins with the donor selection process and continues throughout plasma collection and plasma preparation. Each individual plasma donation used in the manufacture of FEIBA NF is collected only at FDA approved blood establishments and is tested by FDA licensed serological tests for Hepatitis B Surface Antigen (HBsAg), and for antibodies to Human Immunodeficiency Virus (HIV-1/HIV-2) and Hepatitis C Virus (HCV) in accordance with the U.S. regulatory requirements. As an additional safety measure, mini-pools of the plasma are tested for the presence of HIV-1 and HCV by FDA licensed Nucleic Acid Testing (NAT) and found negative. In addition, two dedicated and independent virus removal/inactivation steps have been integrated into the manufacturing process, namely 35 nm nanofiltration and a vapor heat treatment process. In addition, the DEAE-Sephadex adsorption contributes to the virus safety profile of FEIBA NF. Despite these measures, such products can still potentially transmit disease (see WARNINGS).

In vitro spiking studies have been used to validate the capability of the manufacturing process to remove and inactivate viruses. To establish the minimum applicable virus clearance capacity of the manufacturing process, these virus clearance studies were performed under extreme conditions (e.g. at minimum incubation times and temperatures below specifications for vapor-heat treatment). Virus clearance studies for FEIBA NF performed in accordance with good laboratory practices have demonstrated, that the manufacturing process of FEIBA NF ensures a high margin of safety with respect to adventitious viruses (Table 1).

[See table 1 at top right]

Table 1: Mean $\log_{10}$ Reduction Factors (RFS) For Each Virus and Manufacturing Step

Virus Type	Enveloped RNA			Enveloped DNA	Non-enveloped RNA	Non-enveloped DNA	
Virus Family	Retroviridae	Flaviviridae		Herpesviridae	Picornaviridae	Parvoviridae	
Virus*	HIV-1	BVDV	WNV	PRV	HAV	B19V**	MMV
DEAE Sephadex Adsorption	3.2	1.8	n.d.	2.5	1.5	1.7	1.2
35 nm Nanofiltration	> 5.3	2.1	4.7	> 5.7	2.6	0.2†	1.0
Vapor-Heat Treatment	> 5.9	> 5.6	> 8.1	> 6.7	> 5.2	3.5	0.9†
Overall log reduction factor (ORF)	> 14.4	> 9.5	> 12.8	> 14.9	> 9.3	5.2	2.2

* Abbreviations: HIV-1, Human Immunodeficiency Virus Type 1; BVDV, Bovine Viral Diarrhea Virus (model for Hepatitis C Virus and other lipid enveloped RNA viruses); WNV, West Nile Virus; PRV, Pseudorabies Virus (model for lipid enveloped DNA viruses, including Hepatitis B Virus); HAV, Hepatitis A Virus; MMV, Mice Minute Virus (model for non-lipid enveloped DNA viruses, including B19 virus [B19V]).

** Reduction factor for Parvovirus B19 claimed for the Vapor Heat Treatment is based on results derived from experimental infectivity and titration assays.

† Reduction factors < 1 log are not used for calculation of the overall reduction factor; n.d. (not done).

CLINICAL STUDIES

FEIBA NF is identical in formulation to FEIBA VH. Biochemical and preclinical studies have confirmed the comparability of FEIBA NF and FEIBA VH.

The safety and efficacy of FEIBA has been demonstrated by two prospective clinical trials.[1, 2] The first, conducted by Sixma and collaborators, was a randomized double-blind study comparing the effect of FEIBA and PROTHROMPLEX IMMUNO (a non-activated prothrombin complex concentrate) in 15 patients with hemophilia A and inhibitors to Factor VIII. A total of 150 bleeding episodes (primarily joint and musculoskeletal plus a few mucocutaneous) were treated. A single dose of 88 Units per kg of body weight was used uniformly for treatments with FEIBA. The study showed that, based on subjective patient evaluation, FEIBA was fully effective in 41.0% and partly effective in 24.6% of episodes (i.e. combined effectiveness of 65.6%), while PROTHROMPLEX IMMUNO was rated fully effective in 25.0% and partly effective in 21.4% of episodes (i.e. combined effectiveness of 46.4%).

The second study with FEIBA was a multicenter study conducted by Hilgartner *et al.*[2] This study was conducted in 44 hemophilia A subjects with inhibitors, 3 hemophilia B subjects with inhibitors, and 2 acquired FVIII inhibitor subjects. It was designed to evaluate the efficacy of FEIBA in the treatment of joint, mucous membrane, musculocutaneous and emergency bleeding episodes such as central nervous system hemorrhages and surgical bleedings. In 49 patients with inhibitor titers of greater than 5 Bethesda Units (from nine co-operating hemophilia centers), 489 single doses were given for the treatment of 165 bleeding episodes. The usual dosage was 50 Units per kg of body weight, repeated at 12-hour intervals (6-hour intervals in mucous membrane bleedings), if necessary. Bleeding was controlled in 153 episodes (93%). In 130 (78%) of the episodes, hemostasis was achieved with one or more infusions within 36 hours. Of these, 36% were controlled with one infusion within 12 hours. An additional 14% of episodes responded after more than 36 hours.

Of the 489 single doses, only 18 (3.7%) caused minor transient reactions in recipients. Out of 49 patients, 10 (20%) showed a rise in their inhibitor titers. In 5 of these patients (10%), the rise was tenfold or more. However, of these 10 patients, 3 had received Factor VIII or Factor IX concentrates within 2 weeks prior to treatment with FEIBA. These anamnestic rises have not been observed to interfere with the efficacy of FEIBA.

INDICATIONS AND USAGE

FEIBA NF (Anti-Inhibitor Coagulant Complex) is indicated for the control of spontaneous bleeding episodes or to cover surgical interventions in hemophilia A and hemophilia B patients with inhibitors.

Clinical experience suggests that patients with a Factor VIII inhibitor titer of less than 5 B.U. may be successfully treated with Antihemophilic Factor. Patients with titers ranging between 5 and 10 B.U. may either be treated with Antihemophilic Factor or FEIBA NF. Cases with Factor VIII inhibitor titers greater than 10 B.U. have generally been refractory to treatment with Antihemophilic Factor.

Guidelines to First and Second Choice Treatment

Patient's Inhibitor	Clinical Situation		
Titer	Minor Bleeding	Major Bleeding	Surgery (Emergency)
less than 5 B.U.	AHF*	AHF	AHF
5 to 10 B.U.	AHF	AHF	AHF
	FEIBA NF	FEIBA NF	FEIBA NF
more than 10 B.U.	FEIBA NF	FEIBA NF	FEIBA NF

*AHF = Antihemophilic Factor

Inadequate response to treatment may result from an abnormal platelet count or impaired platelet function[3-5] that were present before treatment with FEIBA NF, nanofiltered and vapor-heated.

CONTRAINDICATIONS

The use of FEIBA NF is contraindicated:

- in patients who are known to have a normal coagulation mechanism.
- for the treatment of bleeding episodes resulting from coagulation factor deficiencies in the absence of inhibitors to coagulation factor VIII or coagulation factor IX.
- in patients with significant signs of disseminated intravascular coagulation (DIC).

WARNINGS

Anaphylactoid Reactions

Allergic reactions, including severe anaphylactoid reactions, have been reported following the infusion of FEIBA. If signs and symptoms of severe allergic reactions occur, immediately discontinue administration of FEIBA NF and provide appropriate supportive care. Epinephrine and other appropriate medications to treat allergic reactions should be available whenever FEIBA NF is administered.

Thrombotic and Thromboembolic Events

Thrombotic and thromboembolic events [including disseminated intravascular coagulation (DIC), venous thrombosis, pulmonary embolism, myocardial infarction, and stroke] have been reported following infusion of FEIBA VH or FEIBA NF, particularly following the administration of high doses and/or in patients with thrombotic risk factors (see ADVERSE REACTIONS). The possible presence of such risk factors should always be considered in patients with congenital and acquired hemophilia. Thromboembolic events are well recognized potential complications of FEIBA infusion. Many of these events occurred with doses above 200 units/kg/day or in patients with other risk factors for thromboembolic events. A single dose of 100 units/kg body weight and a daily dose of 200 units/kg body weight should not be exceeded unless the severity of bleeding warrants and justifies the use of higher doses. Patients receiving more than 100 units/kg of body weight of FEIBA NF must be monitored for the development of DIC and/or symptoms of acute coronary ischemia. High doses of FEIBA NF should be given only as long as absolutely necessary to stop bleeding.

Patients with disseminated intravascular coagulation (DIC), advanced atherosclerotic disease, crush injury, septicemia, or concomitant treatment with recombinant factor VIIa have an increased risk of developing thrombotic events due to circulating tissue factor (TF) or predisposing coagulopathy.

FEIBA VH or FEIBA NF should be used with particular caution and only if there are no therapeutic alternatives in patients:

- at risk of DIC, arterial or venous thrombosis.
- with existing thrombotic conditions (e.g., acute myocardial infarction, or venous thrombosis).

FEIBA NF should not be given to patients with significant signs of disseminated intravascular coagulation (DIC) or fibrinolysis. Infusion of FEIBA NF should not exceed single dosage of 100 units per kg of body weight and daily doses of 200 units per kg body weight. Thrombotic events have been identified through post-marketing surveillance following FEIBA use for each of the approved indications. The incidence of thrombotic events cannot be determined from post-marketing data.

Transmission of Infectious Agents

FEIBA NF (Anti-Inhibitor Coagulant Complex), nanofiltered and vapor heated, is made from human plasma. Products made from plasma may contain infectious agents, such as viruses, that can cause disease. Tthe risk that such products will transmit an infectious agent has been reduced by effective donor screening, testing for the presence of certain current virus infections, by inactivating and/or removing certain viruses. Despite these measures, such products can still potentially transmit disease. Because this product is made from human blood, it may carry a risk of transmitting infectious agents, e.g. viruses, and theoretically the Creutzfeldt-Jakob disease (CJD) agent. Individuals who receive infusions of blood or plasma products may develop signs and/or symptoms of some viral infections, particularly non-A, non-B hepatitis. ALL infections thought by a physician possibly to have been transmitted by this product should be reported by the physician or other health care provider to Baxter Healthcare Corporation, at 1-800-423-2862 (in the U.S.). The physician should discuss the risks and benefits of this product with the patient.

Anamnestic Responses

Anamnestic responses with rise in Factor VIII inhibitor titer have been observed in 20% of the cases (see CLINICAL STUDIES).

PRECAUTIONS

General

Caution should be used when administering FEIBA VH or FEIBA NF to patients with an increased risk of thromboembolic complications. These include, but are not limited to, patients with a history of coronary heart disease, liver disease, disseminated intravascular coagulation, postoperative immobilization, elderly patients and neonates. In each of these situations, the potential benefit of treatment with FEIBA VH or FEIBA NF should be weighed against the risk of these complications.

Patients who receive FEIBA VH or FEIBA NF should be monitored for development of signs or symptoms of DIC, acute coronary ischemia, and signs and symptoms of other thrombotic and thromboembolic events. If clinical signs of intravascular coagulation occur, which include changes in blood pressure, changes in pulse rate, respiratory distress, chest pain and/or cough, the infusion should be stopped promptly and appropriate diagnostic and therapeutic measures are to be initiated.

Laboratory indications of DIC are decreased fibrinogen, decreased platelet count, and/or presence of fibrin-fibrinogen degradation products (FDP). Other indications of DIC include significantly prolonged thrombin time, prothrombin time, or partial thromboplastin time.

It has been reported that FEIBA NF and antifibrinolytics have been given simultaneously without complications. No adequate and well-controlled studies of the combined or sequential use of FEIBA NF and recombinate Factor VIIa or antifibrinolytics have been conducted. The possibility of thrombotic events should be considered when systemic antifibrinolytics such as tranexamic acid and aminocaproic acid are used during treatment with FEIBA NF. It is recommended not to use antifibrinolytics until 12 hours after the administration of FEIBA NF.

Information for Patients

Some viruses, such as parvovirus B19 or hepatitis A, are particularly difficult to remove or inactivate at this time. Parvovirus B19 most seriously affects pregnant women or immune-compromised individuals. Symptoms of parvovirus B19 infection include fever, drowsiness, chills, and runny nose followed about two weeks later by a rash, and joint pain. Evidence of hepatitis A may include several days to weeks of poor appetite, tiredness, and low-grade fever followed by nausea, vomiting, and pain in the belly. Dark urine and a yellowed complexion are also common symptoms. Patients should be encouraged to consult their physician if such symptoms appear.

Non-Hemophilic Patients

Non-hemophilic patients with acquired inhibitors against Factors VIII, IX or XII may have both a bleeding tendency and an increased risk of thrombosis at the same time.

Laboratory Tests and Clinical Efficacy

Tests used to help evaluate hemostasis, such as APTT, WBCT, and TEG, do not correlate with clinical improvement. For this reason, attempts at normalizing these values by increasing the dose of FEIBA NF may not be successful and are strongly discouraged because of the potential hazard of producing DIC by overdose.

Pregnancy Category C

Animal reproduction studies have not been conducted with FEIBA NF. It is also not known whether FEIBA NF can cause fetal harm when administered to a pregnant woman or can affect reproductive capacity. FEIBA NF should be given to a pregnant woman only if clearly needed.

Pediatric Use

No data are available regarding the use of FEIBA NF in newborns.

ADVERSE REACTIONS

The following adverse reactions have been identified during post approval use of FEIBA: Myocardial infarction, disseminated intravascular coagulopathy, injection site pain, anaphylactic reaction, hypersensitivity, urticaria, blood pressure decreased, hypoaesthesia, hypoaesthesia facial, embolism.

Because these reactions are reported voluntarily from a population of uncertain size, it is not always possible to reliably estimate their frequency or establish a causal relationship to drug exposure.

OVERDOSAGE

Overdosage of FEIBA NF may increase the risk of thromboembolism, DIC or myocardial infarction (See WARNINGS).

DOSAGE AND ADMINISTRATION

(See under *Intravenous Injection/Infusion*).

Clinical trials[1, 2] demonstrated that the response to treatment with FEIBA may differ from patient to patient with no correlation to the patient's inhibitor titer. Response may also vary between different types of hemorrhage (e.g. joint hemorrhage vs. CNS hemorrhage). As a general guideline, a dosage range of 50 to 100 Units of FEIBA NF, per kg of body weight is recommended. However, care should be taken to distinguish between the following four indications, all of which have undergone careful clinical evaluation:

Joint Hemorrhage

In joint hemorrhage, a dose of 50 units per kg of body weight is recommended at 12-hour intervals, which may be increased to doses of 100 units per kg of body weight at 12-hour intervals.

Treatment should be continued until clear signs of clinical improvement appear, such as relief of pain, reduction of swelling or mobilization of the joint.

Mucous Membrane Bleeding

A dose of 50 units per kg of body weight is recommended to be given at 6-hour intervals under careful monitoring (visible bleeding site, repeated measurements of the patient's hematocrit). If hemorrhage does not stop, the dose may be increased to 100 units per kg of body weight at 6-hour intervals. Two such administrations or 200 units per kg of body weight a day should not be exceeded.

Soft Tissue Hemorrhage

For serious soft tissue bleeding, such as retroperitoneal bleeding, doses of 100 units per kg of body weight at 12-hour intervals are recommended. A daily dosage of 200 units per kg of body weight should not be exceeded.

Other Severe Hemorrhages

Severe hemorrhages, such as CNS bleedings have been effectively treated with doses of 100 units per kg of body weight at 12-hour intervals. Sometimes, FEIBA NF may be indicated at 6-hour intervals until clear clinical improvement is achieved.

Reconstitution

1. Allow the unopened vials of FEIBA NF (concentrate) and Sterile Water for Injection (diluent) to reach room temperature (not above 37°C, 98°F).
2. Remove caps from the concentrate and diluent vials to expose central portions of the rubber stoppers.
3. Disinfect the rubber stoppers of both vials using a germicidal solution. Place the vials on an even surface and allow them to dry.
4. Open the package of BAXJECT device by peeling away the lid without touching the inside (Fig. A).

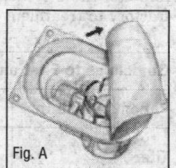

Fig. A

5. **Do not remove the device from the package.** Turn the package over and insert the plastic spike through diluent stopper (Fig. B).

Fig. B

6. Grip the package at its edge and pull the package off the device (Fig. B).

7. Turn the system over, so that the vial is on top. Quickly insert the plastic spike into the FEIBA NF stopper (Fig. C). The vacuum will draw the diluent into the FEIBA NF vial. **Please make sure that the connection of the two vials should be done expeditiously to close the open fluid pathway created by the first insertion of the spike to the diluent vial!**

Fig. C

8. Swirl gently until FEIBA NF is completely dissolved.

Do not refrigerate after reconstitution!

After complete reconstitution of FEIBA NF its injection or infusion should be commenced as promptly as practicable, but must be completed within three hours following reconstitution. The solution must be given by intravenous injection or intravenous drip infusion.

Rate of Administration:

The maximum injection or infusion rate must not exceed 2 units per kg of body weight per minute. For a patient with a body weight of 75 kg, this corresponds to an infusion rate of 2.5–7.5 mL per minute depending on the number of units per vial (see label on vial).

Intravenous Injection or Infusion:

Inspect for particulate matter and discoloration after reconstituting the concentrate as described under *Reconstitution* prior to administration. The appearance of the solution should be colorless to slightly yellowish and essentially free of visible particles. Plastic Luer lock syringes are recommended for use with this product since protein such as FEIBA NF tends to stick to the surface of all-glass syringes.

1. Turn the BAXJECT device handle down towards the FEIBA NF concentrate vial and remove the cap attached to the syringe connection of the BAXJECT device (Fig. D).

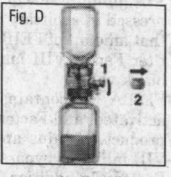

Fig. D

2. Draw air into the syringe, connect the syringe to the BAXJECT device, inject air into the concentrate vial (Fig. E).

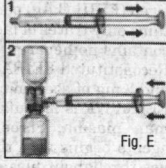

Fig. E

3. While keeping the syringe plunger in place, turn the system upside down (concentrate vial now on top). Draw the concentrate into the syringe by pulling the plunger back slowly (Fig. F).

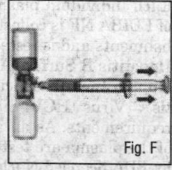

Fig. F

4. Turn the BAXJECT handle to its original position (facing side way).
5. Disconnect the syringe, attach a suitable needle and inject or infuse intravenously as instructed under **Rate of Administration**.

HOW SUPPLIED

FEIBA NF is available in single-dose vials in the following nominal dosage strengths:

Blue   500 Units per vial (NDC 64193-223-02)
Green   1000 Units per vial (NDC 64193-224-02)
Purple   2500 Units per vial (NDC 64193-225-02)

The number of Units of Factor VIII inhibitor bypassing activity is stated on the label of each vial.

FEIBA NF is packaged with a suitable volume (20 mL or 50 mL) of Sterile Water for Injection, U.S.P., one BAXJECT Needleless Transfer Device, and one Package Insert.

Certain components of the packaging material contain Dry Natural Rubber Latex.

STORAGE

Store at refrigerated temperature (2° to 8°C, 35° to 46°F). Within the indicated shelf life, the product may be stored at room temperature (not exceeding 25°C, 77°F) for up to 6 months. After storage at room temperature, the product must not be returned to the refrigerator.

Please note: If you transfer the product from the refrigerator to room temperature, it expires at the end of the 6-month period or at the end of shelf life, whatever comes earlier.

Record the date on the package prior to shifting the product at room temperature.

Avoid freezing, which may damage the diluent vial.

REFERENCES

1. Sjamsoedin L. J. M., Heijnen L., Mauser-Bunschoten E. P., van Geijlswijk J. L., van Houwelingen H., van Asten P., Sixma J. J.: The Effect of Activated Prothrombin-Complex Concentrate (FEIBA) on Joint and Muscle Bleeding in Patients with Hemophilia A and Antibodies to Factor VIII. *The New Engl. J. of Med.* 305: 717, 1981.
2. Hilgartner M. W., Knatterud G. AND THE FEIBA STUDY GROUP: The Use of Factor-Eight-Inhibitor-By-Passing-Activity (FEIBA IMMUNO) Product for Treatment of Bleeding Episodes in Hemophiliacs with Inhibitors. *Blood* 61: 36, 1983.
3. Vermylen J., Schetz J., Semeraro N., Mertens F., Verstraete M.: Evidence that 'Activated' Prothrombin Concentrates Enhance Platelet Coagulant Activity. *Brit. J. Haematol.* 38: 235, 1978.
4. Semeraro N., Vermylen J.: Evidence that Washed Human Platelets Possess Factor-X Activator Activity. *Brit. J. Haematol.* 36: 107, 1977.
5. Wensley R. T.: General Summary of the Use of FEIBA in Haemophiliacs with Inhibitors to FVIII. Presentation at the Second Workshop on Factor VIII Inhibitor Patients, Vienna, 1979.

To enroll in the confidential, Industry-wide Patient Notification System, call 1-888-UPDATE U (1-888-873-2838).

Baxter, FEIBA and PROTHROMPLEX are trademarks of Baxter AG, Vienna, Austria. Baxter, FEIBA and BAXJECT are trademarks of Baxter International Inc., registered in the U.S. Patent and Trademark Office.

Baxter Healthcare Corporation
Westlake Village, CA 91362 USA
U.S. License No. 140
Revised: July 2010
0714149

FLEXBUMIN 25% ℞
[fleks-bew-min]
Albumin (Human), USP, 25% Solution in GALAXY Single Dose Container

DESCRIPTION

FLEXBUMIN 25% in 50 and 100 mL Galaxy plastic container is a sterile, nonpyrogenic preparation of albumin in a single dosage form for intravenous administration. Each 100 mL contains 25 g of albumin and was prepared from human venous plasma using the Cohn cold ethanol fractionation process. Source material for fractionation may be obtained from another U.S. licensed manufacturer. It has been adjusted to physiological pH with sodium bicarbonate and/or sodium hydroxide and stabilized with N-acetyltryptophan (0.02M) and sodium caprylate (0.02M). The sodium content is 145 ± 15 mEq/L. This solution contains no preservative and none of the coagulation factors found in fresh whole blood or plasma. FLEXBUMIN 25% is a transparent or slightly opalescent solution which may have a greenish tint or may vary from a pale straw to an amber color.

The likelihood of the presence of viable hepatitis viruses has been minimized by testing the plasma at three stages for the presence of hepatitis viruses, by fractionation steps with demonstrated virus removal capacity and by heating the product for 10 hours at 60°C. This procedure has been shown to be an effective method of inactivating hepatitis virus in albumin solutions even when those solutions were prepared from plasma known to be infective.[1-3]

The GALAXY plastic container is fabricated from a specially designed multilayered plastic (PL 2501). Solutions are in contact with the polyethylene layer of the container and can leach out certain chemical components of the plastic in very small amounts within the expiration period. The suitability and safety of the plastic have been confirmed in tests in animals according to the USP biological tests for plastic containers, as well as by tissue culture toxicity studies.

CLINICAL PHARMACOLOGY

Albumin is responsible for 70-80% of the colloid osmotic pressure of normal plasma, thus making it useful in regulating the volume of circulating blood.[4-6] Albumin is also a transport protein and binds naturally occurring, therapeutic and toxic materials in the circulation.[5,6]

FLEXBUMIN 25% is osmotically equivalent to approximately five times its volume of human plasma. When injected intravenously, 25% albumin will draw about 3.5 times its volume of additional fluid into the circulation within 15 minutes, except when the patient is markedly dehydrated. This extra fluid reduces hemoconcentration and blood viscosity. The degree and duration of volume expansion depends upon the initial blood volume. With patients treated for diminished blood volume, the effect of infused albumin may persist for many hours; however, in patients with normal volume, the duration will be shorter.[7-9]

Total body albumin is estimated to be 350 g for a 70 kg man and is distributed throughout the extracellular compartments; more than 60% is located in the extravascular fluid compartment. The half-life of albumin is 15 to 20 days with a turnover of approximately 15 g per day.[5]

The minimum plasma albumin level necessary to prevent or reverse peripheral edema is unknown. Some investigators recommend that plasma albumin levels be maintained at approximately 2.5 g/dL. This concentration provides a plasma oncotic value of 20 mm Hg.[4]

FLEXBUMIN 25% is manufactured from human plasma by the modified Cohn-Oncley cold ethanol fractionation process, which includes a series of cold-ethanol precipitation, centrifugation and/or filtration steps followed by pasteurization of the final product at 60 ± 0.5°C for 10-11 hours. This process accomplishes both purification of albumin and reduction of viruses.

In vitro studies demonstrate that the manufacturing process for FLEXBUMIN 25% provides for significant viral reduction. These viral reduction studies, summarized in Table 1, demonstrate viral clearance during the manufacturing process for FLEXBUMIN 25% using human immunodeficiency virus, type 1 (HIV-1) both as a target virus and as model virus for HIV-2 and other lipid-enveloped RNA viruses; bovine viral diarrhea-virus (BVDV), a model for lipid-enveloped RNA viruses, such as hepatitis C virus (HCV); West Nile Virus (WNV), a target virus and model for other similar lipid- enveloped RNA viruses; pseudorabies virus (PRV), a model for other lipid-enveloped DNA viruses such as hepatitis B virus (HBV); mice minute virus (MMV), models for non-enveloped DNA viruses such as human parvovirus B19[10]; hepatitis A virus (HAV), a target virus and a model for other non-enveloped RNA viruses.

These studies indicate that specific steps in the manufacture of FLEXBUMIN 25% are capable of eliminating/inactivating a wide range of relevant and model viruses. Since the mechanism of virus elimination/inactivation by fractionation and by heating is different, the overall manufacturing process of FLEXBUMIN 25% is robust in reducing viral load.

[See table 1 above]

TABLE 1
Summary of Viral Reduction Factor for Each Virus and Processing Step

Process Step	Viral Reduction Factor (log_{10})					
	Lipid Enveloped				Non-Lipid Enveloped	
	HIV-1	*Flaviviridae* BVDV	*Flaviviridae* WNV	PRV	HAV	*Parvoviridae* MMV
Processing of Fraction I+II+III/II+III supernatant to Fraction IV_4 Cuno 70C filtrate*	> 4.9	> 4.8	> 5.7	> 5.5	> 4.5	3.0
Pasteurization	> 7.8	> 6.5	n.d.	> 7.4	3.2	1.6**
Mean Cumulative Reduction Factor, log_{10}	**> 12.7**	**> 11.3**	**> 5.7**	**> 12.9**	**> 7.7**	**4.6**

n.d. = not determined
* Other Albumin fractionation process steps (processing of cryo-poor plasma to Fraction I+II+III/II+III supernatant and processing of Fraction V suspension to Cuno 90LP filtrate) showed significant virus reduction capacity in *in-vitro* viral clearance studies. These process steps also contribute to the overall viral clearance robustness of the manufacturing process. However, since the mechanism of virus removal is similar to that of this particular process step, the viral inactivation data from other steps were not used in the calculation of the Mean Cumulative Reduction Factor.
** Recent scientific data suggest that the actual human parvovirus B19 (B19V), is far more effectively inactivated by pasteurization than indicated by model virus data.[10]

INDICATIONS AND USAGE

1. Hypovolemia

Hypovolemia is a possible indication for FLEXBUMIN 25%. Its effectiveness in reversing hypovolemia depends largely upon its ability to draw interstitial fluid into the circulation. It is most effective with patients who are well hydrated. When hypovolemia is long standing and hypoalbuminemia exists accompanied by adequate hydration or edema, 25% albumin is preferable to 5% protein solutions.[4,6] However, in the absence of adequate or excessive hydration, 5% protein solutions should be used or 25% albumin should be diluted with crystalloid.

Although crystalloid solutions and colloid-containing plasma substitutes can be used in emergency treatment of shock, Albumin (Human) has a prolonged intravascular half-life.[11] When blood volume deficit is the result of hemorrhage, compatible red blood cells or whole blood should be administered as quickly as possible.

2. Hypoalbuminemia

A. General

Hypoalbuminemia is another possible indication for use of FLEXBUMIN 25%.

Hypoalbuminemia can result from one or more of the following:[5]

(1) Inadequate production (malnutrition, burns, major injury, infections, etc.)
(2) Excessive catabolism (burns, major injury, pancreatitis, etc.)
(3) Loss from the body (hemorrhage, excessive renal excretion, burn exudates, etc.)
(4) Redistribution within the body (major surgery, various inflammatory conditions, etc.)

When albumin deficit is the result of excessive protein loss, the effect of administration of albumin will be temporary unless the underlying disorder is reversed. In most cases, increased nutritional replacement of amino acids and/or protein with concurrent treatment of the underlying disorder will restore normal plasma albumin levels more effectively than albumin solutions. Occasionally hypoalbuminemia accompanying severe injuries, infections or pancreatitis cannot be quickly reversed and nutritional supplements may fail to restore serum albumin levels. In these cases, FLEXBUMIN 25% might be a useful therapeutic adjunct.

B. Burns

An optimum regimen for the use of albumin, electrolytes and fluid in the early treatment of burns has not been established, however, in conjunction with appropriate crystalloid therapy, FLEXBUMIN 25% may be indicated for treatment of oncotic deficits after the initial 24 hour period following extensive burns and to replace the protein loss which accompanies any severe burn.[4,6]

C. Adult Respiratory Distress Syndrome (ARDS)

A characteristic of ARDS is a hypoproteinemic state, which may be causally related to the interstitial pulmonary edema. Although uncertainty exists concerning the precise indication of albumin infusion in these patients, if there is a pulmonary overload accompanied by hypoalbuminemia, 25% albumin solution may have a therapeutic effect when used with a diuretic.[4]

D. Nephrosis

FLEXBUMIN 25% may be a useful aid in treating edema in patients with severe nephrosis who are receiving steroids and/or diuretics.

3. Cardiopulmonary Bypass Surgery

FLEXBUMIN 25% has been recommended prior to or during cardiopulmonary bypass surgery, although no clear data exist indicating its advantage over crystalloid solutions.[4,6,12]

4. Hemolytic Disease of the Newborn (HDN)

FLEXBUMIN 25% may be administered in an attempt to bind and detoxify unconjugated bilirubin in infants with severe HDN.

There is no valid reason for use of albumin as an intravenous nutrient.

CONTRAINDICATIONS

A history of allergic reactions to albumin and any of the excipients is a specific contraindication to the use of this product. FLEXBUMIN 25% is also contraindicated in severely anemic patients and in patients with cardiac failure.

FLEXBUMIN 25% must not be diluted with Sterile Water for Injection as this may cause hemolysis in recipients. There exists a risk of potentially fatal hemolysis and acute renal failure from the use of Sterile Water for Injection as a diluent for Albumin (Human). Acceptable diluents include 0.9% Sodium Chloride or 5% Dextrose in Water.

WARNINGS

FLEXBUMIN 25% is made from human plasma. Products made from human plasma may contain infectious agents, such as viruses, that can cause disease. This also applies to unknown or emerging viruses and pathogens. The risk that such products will transmit an infectious agent has been reduced by screening plasma donors for prior exposure to certain viruses, by testing for the presence of certain current virus infections, and by inactivating and/or removing certain viruses (See Description). The measures taken are considered effective for enveloped viruses such as HIV, HBV, and HCV, and for the non-enveloped viruses HAV and Parvovirus B19. Despite these measures, such products can still potentially transmit disease. Based on effective donor screening and product manufacturing processes, albumin carries an extremely remote risk for transmission of viral diseases. A theoretical risk for transmission of Creutzfeldt-Jakob disease (CJD) also is considered extremely remote. No cases of transmission of viral diseases or CJD have ever been identified for albumin. ALL infections thought by a physician possibly to have been transmitted by this product, should be reported by the physician, or other health-care provider to Baxter Healthcare Corporation at 1-800-423-2862. The physician should discuss the risks and benefits of this product with the patient.

Suspicion of allergic or anaphylactic type reactions requires immediate discontinuation of the injection. In case of shock, standard medical treatment for shock should be implemented.

PRECAUTIONS

Hemodynamics

Do not administer FLEXBUMIN 25% without very close monitoring of hemodynamics; look for evidence of cardiac or respiratory failure, renal failure, or increasing intra-cranial pressure.

Hypervolemia/Hemodilution

FLEXBUMIN 25% should be used with caution in conditions where hypervolemia and its consequences or hemodilution could represent a special risk for the patient. Examples may include but are not limited to: decompensated cardiac insufficiency, hypertension, esophageal varices, pulmonary edema, hemorrhagic diathesis, severe anemia, renal and post-renal failure.

FLEXBUMIN 25% must be administered intravenously. The rate of administration should be adjusted according to the solution concentration and the patient's hemodynamic measurements and should not exceed 1 mL/min to patients with normal blood volume. More rapid administration might cause circulatory overload and pulmonary edema.[13]

At the first clinical signs of cardiovascular overload (headache, dyspnea, jugular vein congestion), or increased blood pressure, raised central venous pressure and pulmonary edema, the infusion is to be stopped immediately.

Blood Pressure

A rise in blood pressure after 25% albumin infusion necessitates careful observation of the injured or post-operative patient in order to detect and treat severed blood vessels that may not have bled at a lower blood pressure.

Pregnancy–Category C, and Lactation

There are no adequate data from the use of FLEXBUMIN 25% in pregnant or lactating women. Animal reproduction studies have not been conducted with FLEXBUMIN 25%. It is not known whether FLEXBUMIN 25% can cause fetal harm when administered to a pregnant woman or can affect reproductive capacity. Physicians should carefully consider the potential risks and benefits for each specific patient before prescribing FLEXBUMIN 25%. FLEXBUMIN 25% should be given to a pregnant woman only if clearly needed.

Pediatric Use

The safety of albumin solutions has been demonstrated in children provided the dose is appropriate for body weight, however, the safety of FLEXBUMIN 25% has not been evaluated in pediatric patients.

Large Volumes

If comparatively large volumes are to be replaced, controls of coagulation and hematocrit are necessary. Care must be taken to ensure adequate substitution of other blood constituents (coagulation factors, electrolytes, platelets, and erythrocytes). Appropriate hemodynamic monitoring should be undertaken.

Electrolyte Status

When FLEXBUMIN 25% is given, the electrolyte status of the patient should be monitored and appropriate steps taken to restore or maintain the electrolyte balance.

DRUG INTERACTIONS

No interaction studies have been performed with FLEXBUMIN 25%.

ADVERSE REACTIONS

Adverse Reactions from Clinical Trials

There are no data available on adverse reactions from clinical trials conducted with FLEXBUMIN 25%.

Post-Marketing Adverse Reactions

The following adverse reactions have been reported in the post-marketing experience. These reactions are listed by MedDRA System Organ Class (SOC), then by Preferred Term in order of severity.

IMMUNE SYSTEM DISORDERS: Anaphylactic shock, Anaphylactic reactions, Hypersensitivity/Allergic reactions

NERVOUS SYSTEM DISORDERS: Headache

CARDIAC DISORDERS: Tachycardia

VASCULAR DISORDERS: Hypotension, Flushing

RESPIRATORY, THORACIC, AND MEDIASTINAL DISORDERS: Dyspnea

GASTROINTESTINAL DISORDERS: Vomiting, Nausea, Dysguesia

SKIN AND SUBCUTANEOUS TISSUE DISORDERS: Urticaria, Rash, Pruritis

GENERAL DISORDERS AND ADMINISTRATION SITE CONDITIONS: Pyrexia, Chills

Overdose

Hypervolemia may occur if the dosage and rate of infusion are too high. (See Precautions: Hypervolemia/Hemodilution)

DOSAGE AND ADMINISTRATION

FLEXBUMIN 25% must be administered intravenously. Do not use if turbid. Do not begin administration more than 4 hours after the container has been entered. Discard unused portion.

FLEXBUMIN 25% solutions must not be diluted with Sterile Water for Injection as this may cause hemolysis in recipients (see CONTRAINDICATIONS).

Albumin solutions should not be mixed with other medicinal products including blood and blood components, but can be used concomitantly with other parenterals such as whole blood, plasma, saline, glucose or sodium lactate when deemed medically necessary. The addition of four volumes of normal saline or 5% glucose to 1 volume of FLEXBUMIN 25% gives a solution, which is approximately isotonic and isosmotic with citrated plasma.

Albumin solutions should not be mixed with protein hydrolysates or solutions containing alcohol since these combinations may cause the proteins to precipitate.

Do not add supplementary medication.

Hypervolemia may occur if the dosage and rate of infusion are not adjusted, giving consideration to the solution concentration and the patient's clinical status. Hemodynamic parameters should be monitored in patients receiving FLEXBUMIN 25% and should be used to check for the risk of hypervolemia and cardiovascular overload. (See PRECAUTIONS).

It is strongly recommended that every time that FLEXBUMIN 25% is administered to a patient, the name and batch number of the product be recorded in order to maintain a link between the patient and the batch of the product.

Recommended Dosages

1. Hypovolemic Shock

The dosage of FLEXBUMIN 25% must be individualized. As a guideline, the initial treatment should be in the range of 100 to 200 mL for adults and 2.5 to 5 mL per kilogram body weight for children. This may be repeated after 15 to 30 minutes, if the response is not adequate. For patients with significant plasma volume deficits, albumin replacement is best administered in the form of 5% Albumin (Human).

Upon administration of additional albumin or if hemorrhage has occurred, hemodilution and a relative anemia will follow. This condition should be controlled by the supplemental administration of compatible red blood cells or compatible whole blood.

2. Burns

The optimal therapeutic regimen for administration of crystalloid and colloid solutions after extensive burns has not been established. When FLEXBUMIN 25% is administered after the first 24 hours following burns, the dose should be determined according to the patient's condition and response to treatment.

3. Hypoalbuminemia

Hypoalbuminemia is usually accompanied by a hidden extravascular albumin deficiency of equal magnitude. This total body albumin deficit must be considered when determining the amount of albumin necessary to reverse the hypoalbuminemia. When using patient's serum albumin concentration to estimate the deficit, the body albumin compartment should be calculated to be 80 to 100 mL per kg of body weight.[5,6] Daily dose should not exceed 2 g of albumin per kilogram of body weight.

4. Hemolytic Disease of the Newborn

FLEXBUMIN 25% may be administered prior to or during exchange transfusion in a dose of 1 g per kilogram body weight.[14]

Preparation for Administration

Check the GALAXY container for minute leaks prior to use by squeezing the bag firmly. If leaks are found, discard solution as sterility may be impaired. Do not add supplementary medication. Do not use unless solution is clear of particulate matter and seal is intact. FLEXBUMIN 25% is a transparent or slightly opalescent solution, which may have a greenish tint or may vary from a pale straw to an amber color. Parenteral drug products should be inspected visually for particulate matter and discoloration prior to administration, whenever solution and container permit.

CAUTION: Do not use plastic containers in series connections. Such use could result in air embolism due to residual air being drawn from the primary container before the administration of the fluid from the secondary container is complete.

Administration

1. Suspend container from eyelet support.
2. Remove plastic protector from outlet port at bottom of container.
3. Attach administration set. Refer to complete directions accompanying set. Make certain that the administration set contains an adequate filter (15-micron or smaller).

HOW SUPPLIED

FLEXBUMIN 25% is supplied in 50 mL (NDC 0944-0493-01) and 100 mL (NDC 0944-0493-02) in single dose GALAXY plastic container (PL 2501).

STORAGE

Store FLEXBUMIN 25% at room temperature, not to exceed 30°C (86°F). Protect from freezing.

REFERENCES

1. Cai K, Gierman T, et al: Ensuring the Biologic Safety of Plasma-Derived Therapeutic Proteins. Department of Preclinical Research and Pathogen Safety, Bayer HealthCare LLC, North Carolina, USA. **Biodrugs 19(2)**: 79-96 2005.
2. Gerety RJ, Aronson DL: Plasma derivatives and viral hepatitis. **Transfusion 22**:347-351, 1982.
3. Burnouf T, Padilla A, Current strategies to prevent transmission of prions by human plasma derivatives. **Transfusion Clinique et Biologique 13**:320-328, 2006.
4. Tullis JL: Albumin, 1. Background and use, and 2. Guidelines for clinical use. **JAMA 237**:355-360, 460-463, 1977.
5. Peters T Jr: Serum albumin, in **The Plasma Proteins, 2nd ed, Vol 1.** Putnam FW (ed). New York, Academic Press, 1975, pp 133-181.
6. Finlayson JS: Albumin products. **Semin Thromb Hemostas. 6**:85-120, 1980.
7. Haynes G, Navickis R, Wilkes M, Albumin administration – what is the evidence of clinical benefit? Asystematic review of randomized controlled trials. **European Journal of Anesthesiology 20**:771-793 2003.
8. Mendez, C, McClain C, Marsano L et al, Albumin Therapy in Clinical Practice. **Nutrition in Clinical Practice 20** No. 3:314-320, June 2005.
9. Quinlan G, Martin G, Evans T, Albumin: Biochemical Properties and Therapeutic Potential. **HEMATOLOGY** Vol 14, No. 6 1211-1219 2005.
10. J. Blümel et al., Inactivation of Parvovirus B19 During Pasteurization of Human Serum Albumin. **Transfusion 42**:1011-1018, 2002.
11. Shoemaker WC, Schluchter M, Hopkins JA, *et al:* Comparison of the relative effectiveness of colloids and crystalloids in emergency resuscitation. **Am J Surg 142**: 73-83, 1981.
12. Lowenstein E, Hallowell P, Bland JHL: Use of colloid and crystalloid solutions in open heart surgery: Physiological basis and clinical results in, **Proceedings of the Workshop on Albumin.** Sgouris JT, Rene A (eds). DHEW Publication No. (NIH) 76-925, Washington, DC, US Government Printing Office, 1976, pp 195-210.
13. Grocott, Michael P.W., Mythen, Michael G., and Gan, Tong J. Perioperative Fluid Management and Clinical Outcomes in Adults. **Anesth Analg.** 2005;100:1100.
14. Tsao YC, Yu VYH: Albumin in management of neonatal hyperbilirubinaemia. **Arch Dis Childhood 47**:250-256, 1972.

Baxter Healthcare Corporation
Westlake Village, CA 91362 USA
U.S. License No. 140
Printed in the USA

To enroll in the confidential industry-wide Patient Notification System, call 1-888-UPDATE U (1-888-873-2838).

Baxter, Flexbumin and Galaxy are trademarks of Baxter International Inc.

Revised September 2009

GAMMAGARD LIQUID ℞

[gă-mă-gärd]

[immune globulin intravenous (human)] 10%

DESCRIPTION

GAMMAGARD LIQUID Immune Globulin Intravenous (Human), 10% is a ready-for-use sterile, liquid preparation of highly purified and concentrated immunoglobulin G (IgG) antibodies. The distribution of the IgG subclasses is similar to that of normal plasma.[1,2] The Fc and Fab functions are maintained in GAMMAGARD LIQUID. Pre-kallikrein activator activity is not detectable. GAMMAGARD LIQUID contains 100 mg/mL protein. At least 98% of the protein is gammaglobulin, the average immunoglobulin A (IgA) concentration is 37µg/mL, and immunoglobulin M is present in trace amounts. GAMMAGARD LIQUID contains a broad spectrum of IgG antibodies against bacterial and viral agents. Glycine (0.25M) serves as a stabilizing and buffering agent, and there are no added sugars, sodium or preservatives. The pH is 4.6 to 5.1. The osmolality is 240-300 mOsmol/kg, which is similar to physiological osmolality (285 to 295 mOsmol/kg).[3]

GAMMAGARD LIQUID is manufactured from large pools of human plasma. Screening against potentially infectious agents begins with the donor selection process and continues throughout plasma collection and plasma preparation. Each individual plasma donation used in the manufacture of GAMMAGARD LIQUID is collected only at FDA approved blood establishments and is tested by FDA licensed serological tests for Hepatitis B Surface Antigen (HBsAg), and for antibodies to Human Immunodeficiency Virus (HIV-1/HIV-2) and Hepatitis C Virus (HCV) in accordance with U.S. regulatory requirements. As an additional safety measure, mini-pools of the plasma are tested for the presence of HIV-1 and HCV by FDA licensed Nucleic Acid Testing (NAT) and found negative. IgGs are purified from plasma pools using a modified Cohn-Oncley cold ethanol fractionation process, as well as cation and anion exchange chromatography.

To further improve the margin of safety, three dedicated, independent and effective virus inactivation/removal steps have been integrated into the manufacturing and formulation processes, namely solvent/detergent (S/D) treatment,[4,5] 35 nm nanofiltration,[6,7] and a low pH incubation at elevated temperature.[8,9] The S/D process includes treatment with an organic mixture of tri-n-butyl phosphate, octoxynol 9 and polysorbate 80 at 18°C to 25°C for a minimum of 60 minutes.

In vitro virus spiking studies have been used to validate the capability of the manufacturing process to inactivate and remove viruses. To establish the minimum applicable virus clearance capacity of the manufacturing process, these virus clearance studies were performed under extreme conditions (e.g., at minimum S/D concentrations, incubation time and temperature for the S/D treatment). Virus clearance studies for GAMMAGARD LIQUID performed in accordance with good laboratory practices (Table 1) have demonstrated that:

- S/D treatment inactivates the lipid-enveloped viruses investigated to below detection limits within minutes.
- 35 nm nanofiltration removes lipid-enveloped viruses to below detection limits and reduces the non-lipid enveloped viruses HAV and B19V. As determined by a polymerase chain reaction assay, nanofiltration reduced B19V by a mean $\log_{10}$ reduction factor of 4.8 genome equivalents.
- Treatment with low pH at elevated temperature of 30°C to 32°C inactivates lipid-enveloped virus and encephalomyocarditis virus (EMCV, model for HAV) to below detection limits, and reduces mice minute virus (MMV, model for B19V).

[See table 1 at top right]

CLINICAL PHARMACOLOGY
Clinical Efficacy
Use of GAMMAGARD LIQUID in patients with Primary Immunodeficiency is supported by the Phase 3 clinical study of subjects who were treated with 300 to 600 mg/kg every 21 to 28 days for 12 months. The 61 subjects in this study were between 6 to 72 years of age, 54% female and 46% male, and 93% Caucasian, 5% African-American, and 2% Asian. Three subjects were excluded from the per-protocol analysis due to non-study product related reasons. The primary efficacy endpoint was the annualized rate of specified acute serious bacterial infections, i.e., the mean number of specified acute serious bacterial infections per subject per year (see Table 2).

Table 2: Summary of Validated Acute Serious Bacterial Infections for the Per-Protocol Analysis

	Number of Events
Validated Infections[a]	
Bacteremia/Sepsis	0
Bacterial Meningitis	0
Osteomyelitis/Septic Arthritis	0
Bacterial Pneumonia	0
Visceral Abscess	0
Total	0
Hospitalizations Secondary to Infection	0
Mean Number of Validated Infections per Subject per Year	0
p-value[b]	p < 0.0001
95% Confidence Interval[b]	(0.000, 0.064)

[a] Serious acute bacterial infections were defined by FDA and met specific diagnostic requirements.
[b] The rate of validated infections was compared with a rate of 1 per subject per year, in accordance with recommendations by the FDA Blood Products Advisory Committee.[10]

The secondary efficacy endpoints in this study were the annualized rate of other specified validated bacterial infections (see Table 3), and the number of hospitalizations secondary to all validated infectious complications (see Table 2 and Table 3).

Table 1: Three Dedicated Independent Virus Inactivation/Removal Steps Mean $\log_{10}$ Reduction Factors[a] (RFs) For Each Virus and Manufacturing Step

Virus type Family	Enveloped RNA		Enveloped DNA	Non-enveloped RNA		Non-enveloped DNA
	Retroviridae	Flaviviridae	Herpesviridae	Picornaviridae		Parvoviridae
Virus	HIV-1	BVDV	WNV	PRV	HAV	EMCV	MMV
SD treatment	>4.5	>6.2	n.a.	>4.8	n.d.	n.d.	n.d.
35 nm nanofiltration	>4.5	>5.1	>6.2	>5.6	5.7	1.4	2.0
Low pH treatment	>5.8	>5.5	>6.0	>6.5	n.d.[b]	>6.3	3.1
Overall log reduction factor (ORF)	>14.8	>16.8	>12.2	>16.9	5.7[b]	>7.7	5.1

Abbreviations: HIV-1, Human Immunodeficiency Virus Type 1; BVDV, Bovine Viral Diarrhea Virus (model for Hepatitis C Virus and other lipid enveloped RNA viruses); WNV, West Nile Virus; PRV, Pseudorabies Virus (model for lipid enveloped DNA viruses, including Hepatitis B Virus); EMCV, Encephalomyocarditis Virus (model for non-lipid enveloped RNA viruses, including Hepatitis A virus [HAV]); MMV, Mice Minute Virus (model for non-lipid enveloped DNA viruses, including B19 virus [B19V]); n.d. (not done), n.a. (not applicable).
[a] For the calculation of these RF data from virus clearance study reports, applicable manufacturing conditions were used. $\log_{10}$ RFs on the order of 4 or more are considered effective for virus clearance in accordance with the Committee for Medicinal Products for Human Use (CHMP, formerly CPMP) guidelines.
[b] No RF obtained due to immediate neutralization of HAV by the anti-HAV antibodies present in the product.

Table 3: Summary of Validated Other Bacterial Infections

	Number of Events
Validated Infections[a]	
Urinary Tract Infection	1
Gastroenteritis	1
Lower Respiratory Tract Infection: Tracheobronchitis, Bronchiolitis Without Evidence of Pneumonia	0
Lower Respiratory Tract Infection: Other Infections (e.g., Lung Abscess, Empyema)	0
Otitis Media	2
Total	4
Hospitalizations Secondary to Infection	0
Mean Number of Validated Infections per Subject per Year	0.07
95% Confidence Interval	(0.018, 0.168)

[a] Other bacterial infections that met specific diagnostic requirements.

In this study, there were no validated acute serious bacterial infections in any of the treated subjects. The annualized rate of acute serious bacterial infections was significantly less than ($p < 0.0001$) the rate of one infection per year, in accordance with recommendations by the FDA Blood Products Advisory Committee.[10] Four of the 61 subjects reported a total of 4 other specified validated bacterial infections. None were serious or severe, none resulted in hospitalization, and all resolved completely.

The rate of all clinically-defined but non-validated infections was 3.4 infections per patient per year. These consisted primarily of recurrent episodes of commonly observed infections in this patient population - sinusitis, bronchitis, nasopharyngitis, urinary tract infections, and upper respiratory infections.

Pharmacokinetics
The overall pharmacokinetic characteristics of Immune Globulin Intravenous (Human) [IGIV] products are well-described in the literature.[11,12] Following infusion, IGIV products show a biphasic decay curve. The initial (α) phase is characterized by an immediate post-infusion peak in serum IgG and is followed by rapid decay due to equilibration between the plasma and extravascular fluid compartments. The second (β) phase is characterized by a slower and constant rate of decay.

The commonly cited "normal" half life of 18 to 25 days is based on studies in which tiny quantities of radiolabeled IgG are injected into healthy individuals.[13,14] When radiolabeled IgG was injected into patients with hypogammaglobulinemia or agammaglobulinemia, highly variable half-lives ranging from 12 to 40 days were observed.[13,14] In other radiolabeled studies, high serum concentrations of IgG, and hypermetabolism associated with fever and infection, have been seen to coincide with a shortened half-life of IgG.[14,15,16,17]

In contrast, however, pharmacokinetic studies in immunodeficient patients are based on the decline of IgG concentrations following infusions of large quantities of gammaglobulin. In such trials, investigators have reported uniformly prolonged half-lives of 26 to 35 days.[16,18,19,20,21,22]

Pharmacokinetic parameters for GAMMAGARD LIQUID were determined from total IgG levels following the fourth infusion. A total of 61 subjects were enrolled and treated. Of these, 57 had sufficient pharmacokinetic data to be included in the dataset. Pharmacokinetic parameters are presented in Table 4.

Table 4: Summary of Pharmacokinetic Parameters in 57 Subjects

Parameter	Median	95% Confidence Interval
Elimination Half-Life ($T\,\frac{1}{2}$ days)	35	(31, 42)
AUC_{0-21d} (mg·days/dL)	29139	(27494, 30490)
C_{max} (Peak, mg/dL)	2050	(1980, 2200)
C_{min} (Trough, mg/dL)	1030	(939, 1110)
Incremental recovery (mg/dL)/(mg/kg)	2.3	(2.2, 2.6)

Abbreviations: AUC = area under the curve; C_{max} = maximum concentration; C_{min} = minimum concentration

Median IgG trough levels were maintained between 960-1120 mg/dL. These dosing regimens maintained serum trough IgG levels considerably above 450 mg/dL, which is consistent with levels considered to be effective in the treatment of patients with Primary Immunodeficiency.[23,24] The elimination half-life of GAMMAGARD LIQUID of 35 days was similar to the half-lives reported for other IGIV products.[13,14,15,17,25,26]

INDICATIONS AND USAGE
Primary Immunodeficiency
GAMMAGARD LIQUID is indicated for the treatment of primary immunodeficiency disorders associated with defects in humoral immunity. These include but are not limited to congenital X-linked agammaglobulinemia, common variable immunodeficiency, Wiskott-Aldrich syndrome, and severe combined immunodeficiencies.[15,22]

CONTRAINDICATIONS
GAMMAGARD LIQUID is contraindicated in patients with known anaphylactic or severe hypersensitivity responses to Immune Globulin (Human).

Patients with severe selective IgA deficiency (IgA < 0.05 g/L) may develop anti-IgA antibodies that can result in a severe anaphylactic reaction. Anaphylaxis can occur using GAMMAGARD LIQUID even though it contains low amounts of IgA (average concentration of 37μg/mL). These patients should be treated only if their IgA deficiency is associated with an immune deficiency for which therapy with intravenous immune globulin is clearly indicated. Such patients should only receive intravenous immune globulin with utmost caution and in a setting where supportive care is available for treating life-threatening reactions.

WARNINGS

Immune Globulin Intravenous (Human) products have been reported to be associated with renal dysfunction, acute renal failure, osmotic nephrosis, and death.[27] Patients predisposed to acute renal failure include patients with any degree of pre-existing renal insufficiency, diabetes mellitus, age greater than 65, volume depletion, sepsis, paraproteinemia, or patients receiving known nephrotoxic drugs. Especially in such patients, IGIV products should be administered at the minimum concentration available and the minimum rate of infusion practicable. While these reports of renal dysfunction and acute renal failure have been associated with the use of many of the licensed IGIV products, those containing sucrose as a stabilizer accounted for a disproportionate share of the total number.
Glycine, an amino acid, is used as a stabilizer. GAMMAGARD LIQUID does not contain sucrose.
See PRECAUTIONS and DOSAGE AND ADMINISTRATION sections for important information intended to reduce the risk of acute renal failure.

Immune Globulin Intravenous (Human), 10% is made from human plasma. Products made from human plasma may contain infectious agents, such as viruses, that can cause disease. The risk that such products will transmit an infectious agent has been reduced by screening plasma donors for prior exposure to certain viruses, by testing for the presence of certain current virus infections, and by inactivating and/or removing certain viruses (see DESCRIPTION). Despite these measures, such products can still potentially transmit disease. Because this product is made from human blood, it may carry a risk of transmitting infectious agents, e.g., viruses and theoretically, the Creutzfeldt-Jakob disease (CJD) agent. ALL infections thought by a physician possibly to have been transmitted by this product should be reported by the physician or other healthcare provider to Baxter Healthcare Corporation, at 1-800-423-2862 (in the U.S.). The physician should discuss the risks and benefits of this product with the patient.
GAMMAGARD LIQUID should only be administered intravenously. Other routes of administration have not been evaluated.
Immediate anaphylactic and hypersensitivity reactions are a remote possibility. Epinephrine and antihistamines should be available for treatment of any acute anaphylactoid reactions.

PRECAUTIONS

General

Some viruses, such as B19V (formerly known as Parvovirus B19) or Hepatitis A, are particularly difficult to remove or inactivate. B19V most seriously affects pregnant women, or immune-compromised individuals. Symptoms of B19V infection include fever, drowsiness, chills and runny nose followed about two weeks later by a rash and joint pain. Evidence of Hepatitis A may include several days to weeks of poor appetite, tiredness, and low-grade fever followed by nausea, vomiting and abdominal pain. Dark urine and a yellowed complexion are also common symptoms. Patients should be encouraged to consult their physician if such symptoms appear.
Components used in the packaging of this product are latex-free.

Renal Function

Periodic monitoring of renal function tests and urine output is particularly important in patients judged to have a potential increased risk for developing acute renal failure. Assure that patients are not volume depleted prior to the initiation of infusion of GAMMAGARD LIQUID. Renal function, including measurement of blood urea nitrogen (BUN)/serum creatinine, should be assessed prior to the initial infusion of IGIV products and again at appropriate intervals thereafter. If renal function deteriorates, discontinuation of the product should be considered.
For patients judged to be at risk of developing renal dysfunction, it may be prudent to reduce the rate of infusion to less than 3.3 mg IgG/kg/min (< 2 mL/kg/hr).

Hemolysis

IGIV products can contain blood group antibodies which may act as hemolysins and induce *in vivo* coating of red blood cells with immunoglobulin, causing a positive direct antiglobulin reaction and, rarely, hemolysis.[28,29,30] Hemolytic anemia can develop subsequent to IGIV therapy due to enhanced red blood cells (RBC) sequestration (see ADVERSE REACTIONS).[31] IGIV recipients should be monitored for clinical signs and symptoms of hemolysis (see PRECAUTIONS: Laboratory Tests).

Transfusion-Related Acute Lung Injury (TRALI)

There have been reports of noncardiogenic pulmonary edema (Transfusion-Related Acute Lung Injury [TRALI]) in patients administered IGIV.[32] TRALI is characterized by severe respiratory distress, pulmonary edema, hypoxemia, normal left ventricular function, and fever, and typically occurs within 1 to 6 hours after transfusion. Patients with TRALI may be managed using oxygen therapy with adequate ventilatory support.
IGIV recipients should be monitored for pulmonary adverse reactions. If TRALI is suspected, appropriate tests should be performed for the presence of anti-neutrophil antibodies in both the product and patient serum (see PRECAUTIONS: Laboratory Tests).

Thrombotic Events

Thrombotic events have been reported in association with IGIV (see ADVERSE REACTIONS).[33,34,35,36,37,38,39,40,41] Patients at risk may include those with a history of atherosclerosis, multiple cardiovascular risk factors, advanced age, impaired cardiac output, and/or known or suspected hyperviscosity, hypercoagulable disorders and prolonged periods of immobilization. The potential risks and benefits of IGIV should be weighed against those of alternative therapies for all patients for whom IGIV administration is being considered. Baseline assessment of blood viscosity should be considered in patients at risk for hyperviscosity, including those with cryoglobulins, fasting chylomicronemia/markedly high triacylglycerols (triglycerides), or monoclonal gammopathies (see PRECAUTIONS: Laboratory Tests).

Aseptic Meningitis Syndrome

An aseptic meningitis syndrome (AMS) has been reported to occur infrequently in association with IGIV treatment. Discontinuation of IGIV treatment has resulted in remission of AMS within several days without sequelae. The syndrome usually begins within several hours to two days following IGIV treatment. It is characterized by symptoms and signs including severe headache, nuchal rigidity, drowsiness, fever, photophobia, painful eye movements, and nausea and vomiting. Cerebrospinal fluid (CSF) studies are frequently positive with pleocytosis up to several thousand cells per cubic mm, predominantly from the granulocytic series, and elevated protein levels up to several hundred mg/dL. Patients exhibiting such symptoms and signs should receive a thorough neurological examination, including CSF studies, to rule out other causes of meningitis. AMS may occur more frequently in association with high dose (2 g/kg) IGIV treatment.

Laboratory Tests

If signs and/or symptoms of hemolysis are present after IGIV infusion, appropriate confirmatory laboratory testing should be done [see PRECAUTIONS].
If TRALI is suspected, appropriate tests should be performed for the presence of anti-neutrophil antibodies in both the product and patient serum [see PRECAUTIONS].
Because of the potentially increased risk of thrombosis, baseline assessment of blood viscosity should be considered in patients at risk for hyperviscosity, including those with cryoglobulins, fasting chylomicronemia/markedly high triacylglycerols (triglycerides), or monoclonal gammopathies [see PRECAUTIONS].

Information For Patients

Patients should be instructed to immediately report symptoms of decreased urine output, sudden weight gain, fluid retention/edema, and/or shortness of breath (which may suggest kidney damage) to their physicians.

Drug Interactions

See DOSAGE AND ADMINISTRATION section.

Pregnancy Category C

Animal reproduction studies have not been conducted with GAMMAGARD LIQUID. It is also not known whether GAMMAGARD LIQUID can cause fetal harm when administered to a pregnant woman or can affect reproduction capacity. GAMMAGARD LIQUID should be given to a pregnant woman only if clearly indicated. Maternally administered IGIV products have been shown to cross the placenta, increasingly after 30 weeks gestation.[42,43,44]

Use in Pediatrics

The safety and efficacy of GAMMAGARD LIQUID has not been evaluated in neonates or infants.

ADVERSE REACTIONS

General

Various mild and moderate reactions, such as headache, fever, fatigue, chills, flushing, dizziness, urticaria, wheezing or chest tightness, nausea, vomiting, rigors, back pain, chest pain, muscle cramps, and changes in blood pressure may occur with infusions of Immune Globulin Intravenous (Human). In general, reported adverse reactions to GAMMAGARD LIQUID in patients with Primary Immunodeficiency are similar in kind and frequency to those observed with other IGIV products. Slowing or stopping the infusion usually allows the symptoms to disappear promptly. Although hypersensitivity reactions have not been reported in the clinical studies with GAMMAGARD LIQUID immediate anaphylactic and hypersensitivity reactions are a remote possibility. Epinephrine and antihistamines should be available for treatment of any acute anaphylactic reactions (see WARNINGS).

Clinical Study

Adverse experiences were examined among a total of 61 enrolled subjects with Primary Immunodeficiency who received at least one infusion of GAMMAGARD LIQUID during the Phase 3 multicenter clinical study. For this study, temporally associated adverse events are defined by the FDA as those occurring during or within 72 hours of completion of an infusion. Adverse drug reactions (ADR's) are those adverse events that were deemed by the investigators as causally related to the infusion of GAMMAGARD LIQUID.
Of all adverse experiences, 15 events in 8 subjects were serious. Two serious events, two episodes of aseptic meningitis in one patient, were deemed to be possibly related to the infusion of GAMMAGARD LIQUID.
Among the 896 non-serious adverse experiences, 258 were judged by the investigator to be possibly or probably related to the infusion of GAMMAGARD LIQUID. Of these, 136 were mild, 106 were moderate, and 16 were severe. All of the severe non-serious adverse experiences were transient, did not lead to hospitalization, and resolved without complication. One subject withdrew from the study due to a non-serious adverse experience (papular rash).
Of the 345 temporally related adverse experiences, those occurring in > 5% of subjects are shown in Table 5. Of these events, only headache occurred in association with more than 5% of infusions. All events were expected based on past experiences with intravenous gammaglobulin products.
[See table 5 at left]
The majority (227/258) of the non-serious adverse experiences deemed related to study product were considered expected based on previous experience with IGIV products and 31 were considered unexpected. In virtually every case, these unexpected events were either consistent with the subject's specific type of immunodeficiency or with the subject's medical history prior to entering the study. A total of 14 hospitalizations occurred during the study but none were related to infection.
Hematology and clinical chemistry parameters were monitored in all subjects prior to each infusion throughout the 12-month period of study. Mean values for all laboratory parameters remained consistent throughout the study period. Three of the hematology values in one subject were outside of the normal range and reported as non-serious adverse experiences that resolved completely. These were a red cell count of $3.9 \times 10^6/\mu L$, hematocrit of 31%, and white cell count of $3.88 \times 10^3/\mu L$. All spontaneously returned to baseline. One subject had an elevated BUN (45 mg/dL) and creatinine (1.4 mg/dL) on one occasion that were reported as non-serious adverse experiences and resolved completely. These values improved to 30 mg/dL and 0.8 mg/dL, respec-

Table 5: Adverse Events*, Regardless of Causality, that Occurred within 72 Hours of Infusion

Event	By Infusion		By Subject	
	Number	Percentage	Number	Percentage
Headache	57	6.90	22	36.1
Fever	19	2.30	13	21.3
Fatigue	18	2.18	10	16.4
Vomiting	10	1.21	9	14.8
Chills	14	1.69	8	13.1
Infusion site events	8	0.97	8	13.1
Nausea	9	1.09	6	9.8
Dizziness	7	0.85	6	9.8
Pain in Extremity	7	0.85	5	8.2
Diarrhea	7	0.85	5	8.2
Cough	5	0.61	5	8.2
Pruritus	5	0.61	4	6.5
Pharyngeal Pain	5	0.61	4	6.5

*Excluding Infections

tively, by the next infusion. Six of the patients had a single, transient elevation in serum transaminases. Two additional patients had persistent elevations in transaminases, ALT and AST, which were present at the initiation of the study, prior to the infusion of GAMMAGARD LIQUID. There was no other evidence of liver abnormalities. None of the hematology or chemistry laboratory abnormalities that occurred during the course of the study required clinical intervention and none had clinical consequences.

During the Phase 3 clinical study, viral safety was assessed by serological screening for HBsAg and antibodies to HCV and HIV-1 and HIV-2 prior to, during, and at the end of the study and by Polymerase Chain Reaction (PCR) tests for HBV, HCV, and HIV-1 genomic sequences prior to and at the end of the study. None of the 61 treated subjects were positive prior to study entry and none converted from negative to positive during the 12-month period of study.

Postmarketing:
The following is a list of adverse reactions that have been identified and reported during the post-approval use of IGIV products:

Respiratory
cyanosis, hypoxemia, pulmonary edema, dyspnea, bronchospasm

Cardiovascular
thromboembolism, hypotension

Neurological
seizures, tremor

Hematologic
hemolysis, positive direct antiglobulin (Coombs) test

General/Body as a Whole
pyrexia, rigors

Musculoskeletal
back pain

Gastrointestinal
hepatic dysfunction, abdominal pain

Rare and Uncommon Adverse Events:

Respiratory
apnea, Acute Respiratory Distress Syndrome (ARDS), Transfusion-Related Acute Lung Injury (TRALI)

Integumentary
bullous dermatitis, epidermolysis, erythema multiforme, Stevens-Johnson syndrome

Cardiovascular
cardiac arrest, vascular collapse

Neurological
coma, loss of consciousness

Hematologic
pancytopenia, leukopenia

Because postmarketing reporting of these reactions is voluntary and the at-risk populations are of uncertain size, it is not always possible to reliably estimate the frequency of the reaction to establish a causal relationship to exposure to the product. Such is also the case with literature reports authored independently[45] (see PRECAUTIONS).

DOSAGE AND ADMINISTRATION
GAMMAGARD LIQUID should be at room temperature during administration.

Parenteral drug products should be inspected visually for particulate matter and discoloration prior to administration. Do not use if particulate matter and/or discoloration is observed. Only clear or slightly opalescent and colorless or pale yellow solutions are to be administered. GAMMAGARD LIQUID should only be administered intravenously. Other routes of administration have not been evaluated. The use of an in-line filter is optional.

For patients with Primary Immunodeficiency, monthly doses of approximately 300 to 600 mg/kg infused at 3 to 4 week intervals are commonly used.[23,24] As there are significant differences in the half-life of IgG among patients with Primary Immunodeficiency, the frequency and amount of immunoglobulin therapy may vary from patient to patient. The proper amount can be determined by monitoring clinical response. The minimum serum concentration of IgG necessary for protection varies among patients and has not been established by controlled clinical studies.

Rate of Administration
During the first infusion of the Phase 3 clinical study, GAMMAGARD LIQUID was infused at an initial rate of 0.5 mL/kg/hr (0.8 mg/kg/min). The rate was gradually increased every 30 minutes to a rate of 5.0 mL/kg/hr (8.9 mg/kg/min) if it was well tolerated. However, some patients completed the infusion before the maximum rate could be obtained. During subsequent infusions the initial rate and the rate of escalation were based on their previous infusion history; however, the maximum rate attained during the first infusion was used throughout the remainder of the study. The mean rate attained by all patients was 4.3 mL/kg/hr. Fifty-eight subjects (95%) achieved a maximum rate of 4.0 mL/kg/hr or greater and of these, 16 subjects (26%) attained a rate of 5.0 mL/kg/hr.

In general, it is recommended that patients beginning therapy with IGIV or switching from one IGIV product to another be started at the lower rates and then advanced to the maximal rate if they have tolerated several infusions at intermediate rates of infusion. It is important to individualize rates for each patient.

As noted in the WARNINGS section, **patients who have underlying renal disease or who are judged to be at risk of developing thrombotic events should not be infused rapidly with any IGIV product**. Although there are no prospective studies demonstrating that any concentration or rate of infusion is completely safe, it is believed that risk is decreased at lower rates of infusion.[46] Therefore, as a guideline, it is recommended that these patients who are judged to be at risk of renal dysfunction or thrombotic complications be gradually titrated up to a more conservative maximal rate of less than 3.3 mgIgG/kg/min (< 2mL/kg/hr).

A rate of administration that is too rapid may cause flushing and changes in pulse rate and blood pressure. Slowing or stopping the infusion usually results in the prompt disappearance of signs. The infusion may then be resumed at a rate that is comfortable for the patient.

Drug Interactions
Antibodies in IGIV products may interfere with patient responses to live vaccines, such as those for measles, mumps and rubella.[47,48,49] The immunizing physician should be informed of recent therapy with IGIV products so that appropriate precautions can be taken.

Admixtures of GAMMAGARD LIQUID with other drugs and intravenous solutions have not been evaluated. It is recommended that GAMMAGARD LIQUID be administered separately from other drugs or medications that the patient may be receiving. The product should not be mixed with IGIV products from other manufacturers.

Normal saline should not be used as a diluent. If dilution is preferred, GAMMAGARD LIQUID may be diluted with 5% dextrose in water (D5W).[50] No other drug interactions or compatibilities have been evaluated.

HOW SUPPLIED
GAMMAGARD LIQUID is supplied in single use bottles as follows:

NDC Number	Volume	Grams
0944-2700-02	10 mL	1.0
0944-2700-03	25 mL	2.5
0944-2700-04	50 mL	5.0
0944-2700-05	100 mL	10.0
0944-2700-06	200 mL	20.0

STORAGE
Refrigeration: 36 months storage at refrigerated temperature 2° to 8°C (36°-46°F). Do not freeze.
Room Temperature: 12 months storage at room temperature 25°C (77°F), within the first 24 months of the date of manufacture. See below for detailed storage information.

The total storage time of GAMMAGARD LIQUID depends on the point of time the vial is transferred to room temperature. Examples for total storage times are illustrated in Figure 1. The new expiration date must be recorded on the package when the product is transferred to room temperature.

Figure 1: Storage Guidelines
Months from Date of Manufacture

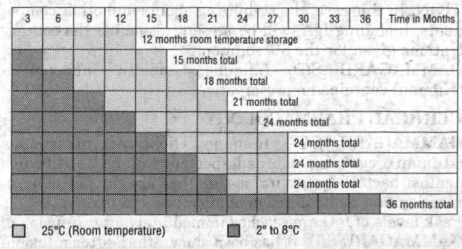

☐ 25°C (Room temperature)   ■ 2° to 8°C

Storage Details:
- Example 1: If the product is taken out of the refrigerator after 3 months from date of manufacture, it can be stored for 12 months at room temperature. Total storage time is 15 months.
- Example 2: If the product is taken out of the refrigerator after 21 months from the date of manufacture, it can be stored for 3 additional months at room temperature. Total storage time is 24 months.
- After 24 months from date of manufacture, product cannot be stored at room temperature.

To enroll in the confidential, industry-wide Patient Notification System, call 1-888-UPDATE U (1-888-873-2838)
BAXTER and GAMMAGARD LIQUID are trademarks of Baxter International Inc.
Baxter Healthcare Corporation
Westlake Village, CA 91362 USA
U.S. License No. 140
[LE-07-03746; LE-07-03747; LE-07-03748]
Revised October 2009

REFERENCES
1. Skvaril F. Qualitative and quantitative aspects of IgG subclasses in i.v. immunoglobulin preparations. In: Nydegger UE, ed. Immunotherapy. London: Academic Press; 1981:118-122.
2. French M. Serum IgG subclasses in normal adults. Monogr Allergy. 1986;19:100-107.
3. Lacy CF, Armstrong LL, Goldman MP, Lance LL. Appendix: Abbreviations and Measurements. Drug Information Handbook. Lexi-Comp; 1999:1254.
4. Horowitz B, Prince AM, Hamman J, Watklevicz C. Viral safety of solvent/detergent-treated blood products. Blood Coagul Fibrinolysis. 1994;5 Suppl 3:S21-S28.
5. Kreil TR, Berting A, Kistner O, Kindermann J. West Nile virus and the safety of plasma derivatives: verification of high safety margins, and the validity of predictions based on model virus data. Transfusion. 2003;43:1023-1028.
6. Hamamoto Y, Harada S, Kobayashi S, et al. A novel method for removal of human immunodeficiency virus: filtration with porous polymeric membranes. Vox Sang. 1989;56:230-236.
7. Yuasa T, Ishikawa G, Manabe S, Sekiguchi S, Takeuchi K, Miyamura T. The particle size of hepatitis C virus estimated by filtration through microporous regenerated cellulose fibre. J Gen Virol. 1991;72 (Pt 8):2021-2024.
8. Kempf C, Jentsch P, Poirier B, et al. Virus inactivation during production of intravenous immunoglobulin. Transfusion. 1991;31:423-427.
9. Louie RE, Galloway CJ, Dumas ML, Wong MF, Mitra G. Inactivation of hepatitis C virus in low pH intravenous immunoglobulin. Biologicals. 1994;22:13-19.
10. Golding B. IGIV Clinical Endpoints. Presented at: Blood Products Advisory Committee, 65th Meeting. 17 March 2000. Silver Spring, MD.
11. Schiff RI. Intravenous immunoglobulins for treatment of antibody deficiencies. In: Good RA, Lindenlaub E, eds. The Nature, Cellular, and Biochemical Basis and Management of Immunodeficiencies. Symposium Vernried, West Germany. 21-25 September. Stuttgart: F. K. Schattauer Verlag; 1986:523-541.
12. Morell A. Pharmacokinetics of intravenous immunoglobulin preparations. In: Lee ML, Strand V, eds. Intravenous Immunoglobulins in Clinical Practice. New York: M. Dekker, Inc.; 1997:1-18.
13. Morell A, Skvaril F. Structure and Biological Properties of Immunoglobulins and γ-Globulin Preparations. II. Properties of γ-Globulin Preparations, Schweizerishche Medizinische Wochenschrift 1980; 110:80-85.
14. Waldmann TA, Strober W. Metabolism of immunoglobulins. Prog Allergy. 1969;13:1-110.
15. Stiehm ER. Standard and special human immune serum globulins as therapeutic agents. Pediatrics. 1979;63:301-319.
16. Lee ML, Mankarious S, Ochs H, Fischer S, Wedgwood RJ. The pharmacokinetics of total IgG, IgG subclasses, and type specific antibodies in immunodeficient patients. Immunol Invest. 1991;20:193-198.
17. Buckley RH. Immunoglobulin replacement therapy: indications and contraindications for use and variable IgG levels achieved. In: Alving BM, Finlayson JS, eds. Immunoglobulins: characteristics and use of intravenous preparations. Washington, D.C.: US Department of Health and Human Services; 1979:3-8.
18. Mankarious S, Lee M, Fischer S, et al. The half-lives of IgG subclasses and specific antibodies in patients with primary immunodeficiency who are receiving intravenously administered immunoglobulin. J Lab Clin Med. 1988;112:634-640.
19. Pirofsky B. Safety and toxicity of a new serum immunoglobulin G intravenous preparation, IGIV pH 4.25. Rev Infect Dis. 1986;8 Suppl 4:S457-63.
20. Pirofsky B. Clinical use of a new pH 4.25 intravenous immunoglobulin preparation (Gamimune-N). J Infect. 1987;15 Suppl 1:29-37.

21. Schiff RI. Half-life and clearance of pH 6.8 and pH 4.25 immunoglobulin G intravenous preparations in patients with primary disorders of humoral immunity. Rev Infect Dis. 1986;8 Suppl 4:S449-56.

22. Schiff RI, Rudd C. Alterations in the half-life and clearance of IgG during therapy with intravenous gammaglobulin in 16 patients with severe primary humoral immunodeficiency. J Clin Immunol. 1986;6:256-264.

23. Eijkhout HW, Der Meer JW, Kallenberg CG, et al. The effect of two different dosages of intravenous immunoglobulin on the incidence of recurrent infections in patients with primary hypogammaglobulinemia. A randomized, double-blind, multicenter crossover trial. Ann Intern Med. 2001;135:165-174.

24. Roifman CM, Gelfand EW. Replacement therapy with high dose intravenous gamma-globulin improves chronic sinopulmonary disease in patients with hypogammaglobulinemia. Pediatr Infect Dis J. 1988;7:S92-S96.

25. Ballow M, Berger M, Bonilla FA, et al. Pharmacokinetics and tolerability of a new intravenous immunoglobulin preparation, IGIV-C, 10% (Gamunex, 10%). Vox Sang. 2003;84:202-210.

26. Ochs HD, Pinciaro PJ, The Octagam Study Group. Octagam(R) 5%, an intravenous IgG product, is efficacious and well tolerated in subjects with primary immunodeficiency diseases. J Clin Immunol. 2004;24:309-314.

27. Cayco AV, Perazella MA, Hayslett JP. Renal insufficiency after intravenous immune globulin therapy: a report of two cases and an analysis of the literature. J Am Soc Nephrol. 1997;8:1788-1794.

28. Copelan EA, Strohm PL, Kennedy MS, Tutschka PJ. Hemolysis following intravenous immune globulin therapy. Transfusion. 1986;26:410-412.

29. Wilson JR, Bhoopalam H, Fisher M. Hemolytic anemia associated with intravenous immunoglobulin. Muscle Nerve. 1997;20:1142-1145.

30. Thomas MJ, Misbah SA, Chapel HM, Jones M, Elrington G, Newsom-Davis J. Hemolysis after high-dose intravenous Ig. Blood. 1993;82:3789.

31. Kessary-Shoham H, Levy Y, Shoenfeld Y, Lorber M, Gershon H. In vivo administration of intravenous immunoglobulin (IVIg) can lead to enhanced erythrocyte sequestration. J Autoimmun. 1999;13:129-135.

32. Rizk A, Gorson KC, Kenney L, Weinstein R. Transfusion-related acute lung injury after the infusion of IVIG. Transfusion. 2001;41:264-268.

33. Brannagan TH, III, Nagle KJ, Lange DJ, Rowland LP. Complications of intravenous immune globulin treatment in neurologic disease. Neurology. 1996;47:674-677.

34. Dalakas MC. High-dose intravenous immunoglobulin and serum viscosity: risk of precipitating thromboembolic events. Neurology. 1994;44:223-226.

35. ElKayam O, Paran D, Milo R, et al. Acute myocardial infarction associated with high dose intravenous immunoglobulin infusion for autoimmune disorders. A study of four cases. Ann Rheum Dis. 2000;59:77-80.

36. Gomperts ED, Darr F. Rapid infusion of intravenous immunoglobulin in patients with neuromuscular diseases. Neurology. 2002;58:1444.

37. Haplea SS, Farrar JT, Gibson GA, Laskin M, Pizzi LT, Ashbury AK. Thromboembolic events associated with intravenous immunoglobulin therapy [abstract]. Neurology. 1997;48:A54.

38. Harkness K, Howell SJ, Davies-Jones GA. Encephalopathy associated with intravenous immunoglobulin treatment for Guillain-Barre syndrome. J Neurol Neurosurg Psychiatry. 1996;60:586.

39. Kwan T, Keith P. Stroke following intravenous immunoglobulin infusion in a 28-year-old male with common variable immune deficiency: a case report and literature review. Can J Allergy Clin Immunol. 1999;4:250-253.

40. Wolberg AS, Kon RH, Monroe DM, Hoffman M. Coagulation factor XI is a contaminant in intravenous immunoglobulin preparations. Am J Hematol. 2000;65:30-34.

41. Woodruff RK, Grigg AP, Firkin FC, Smith IL. Fatal thrombotic events during treatment of autoimmune thrombocytopenia with intravenous immunoglobulin in elderly patients. Lancet. 1986;2:217-218.

42. Hammarstrom L, Smith CI. Placental transfer of intravenous immunoglobulin. Lancet. 1986;1:681.

43. Morell A, Sidiropoulos D, Herrmann U, et al. IgG subclasses and antibodies to group B streptococci, pneumococci, and tetanus toxoid in preterm neonates after intravenous infusion of immunoglobulin to the mothers. Pediatr Res. 1986;20:933-936.

44. Sidiropoulos D, Herrmann U, Jr., Morell A, von Muralt G, Barandun S. Transplacental passage of intravenous immunoglobulin in the last trimester of pregnancy. J Pediatr. 1986;109:505-508.

45. Pierce LR, Jain N. Risks associated with the use of intravenous immunoglobulin. Transfusion Med Rev. 2003;17:241-251.

46. Tan E, Hajinazarian M, Bay W, Neff J, Mendell JR. Acute renal failure resulting from intravenous immunoglobulin therapy. Arch Neurol. 1993;50:137-139.

47. Morbidity and Mortality Weekly Report. Measles, Mumps, and Rubella; Vaccine use and strategies for elimination of measles, rubella, and congenital rubella syndrome and control of mumps. Recommendations for the Advisory Committee on Immunization Practices (ACIP). 98 A.D.;47.

48. Peter G. Summary of major changes in the 1994 Red Book: American Academy of Pediatrics. Report of the Committee on Infectious Disease. Pediatrics. 1994;93:1000-1002.

49. Siber GR, Werner BG, Halsey NA, et al. Interference of immune globulin with measles and rubella immunization. J Pediatr. 1993;122:204-211.

50. Data on file, Baxter Healthcare Corporation.

GAMMAGARD S/D ℞

[ga-ma-gard]
[immune globulin intravenous (human)]
Solvent Detergent Treated
IgA less than 2.2 µg/mL in a 5% Solution

DESCRIPTION

GAMMAGARD S/D, Immune Globulin Intravenous (Human) [IGIV] is a solvent/detergent treated, sterile, freeze-dried preparation of highly purified immunoglobulin G (IgG) derived from large pools of human plasma. The product is manufactured by the Cohn-Oncley cold ethanol fractionation process followed by ultrafiltration and ion exchange chromatography. Source material for fractionation may be obtained from another U.S. licensed manufacturer. The manufacturing process includes treatment with an organic solvent/detergent mixture,[1,2] composed of tri-n-butyl phosphate, octoxynol 9 and polysorbate 80.[3] The GAMMAGARD S/D manufacturing process provides a significant viral reduction in in vitro studies.[3] These studies, summarized in Table 1, demonstrate virus clearance during GAMMAGARD S/D manufacturing using infectious human immunodeficiency virus, Types 1 and 2 (HIV-1, HIV-2); bovine viral diarrhea virus (BVD), a model virus for hepatitis C virus; sindbis virus (SIN), a model virus for lipid-enveloped viruses; pseudorabies virus (PRV), a model virus for lipid-enveloped DNA viruses such as herpes; vesicular stomatitis virus (VSV), a model virus for lipid-enveloped RNA viruses; hepatitis A virus (HAV) and encephalomyocarditis virus (EMC), a model virus for non-lipid-enveloped RNA viruses; and porcine parvovirus (PPV), a model virus for non-lipid-enveloped DNA viruses.[3] These reductions are achieved through a combination of process chemistry, partitioning and/or inactivation during cold ethanol fractionation and the solvent/detergent treatment.[3]

[See table 1 at top of next page]

When reconstituted with the total volume of diluent (Sterile Water for Injection, USP) supplied, this preparation contains approximately 50 mg of protein per mL (5%), of which at least 90% is gamma globulin. The product, reconstituted to 5%, contains a physiological concentration of sodium chloride (approximately 8.5 mg/mL) and has a pH of 6.8 ± 0.4. Stabilizing agents and additional components are present in the following maximum amounts for a 5% solution: 3 mg/mL Albumin (Human), 22.5 mg/mL glycine, 20 mg/mL glucose, 2 mg/mL polyethylene glycol (PEG), 1 µg/mL tri-n-butyl phosphate, 1 µg/mL octoxynol 9, and 100 µg/mL polysorbate 80. The manufacturing process for GAMMAGARD S/D isolates IgG without additional chemical or enzymatic modification, and the Fc portion is maintained intact. GAMMAGARD S/D contains all of the IgG antibody activities which are present in the donor population. On the average, the distribution of IgG subclasses present in this product is similar to that in normal plasma.[3] GAMMAGARD S/D contains trace amounts of IgA (≤ 2.2 µg/mL in a 5% solution). IgM is also present in trace amounts. If it is necessary to prepare a 10% (100 mg/mL) solution for infusion, half the volume of diluent should be added, as described in **DOSAGE AND ADMINISTRATION**. In this case, the stabilizing agents and other components, including IgA, will be present at double the concentrations given for the 5% solution.

GAMMAGARD S/D, Immune Globulin Intravenous (Human) contains no preservative.

CLINICAL PHARMACOLOGY

GAMMAGARD S/D, Immune Globulin Intravenous (Human), contains a broad spectrum of IgG antibodies against bacterial and viral agents that are capable of opsonization and neutralization of microbes and toxins.

Peak levels of IgG are reached immediately after infusion of GAMMAGARD S/D. It has been shown that, after infusion, exogenous IgG is distributed relatively rapidly between plasma and extravascular fluid until approximately half is partitioned in the extravascular space. Therefore, a rapid

initial drop in serum IgG levels is to be expected.[4] As a class, IgG survives longer in vivo than other serum proteins.[4,5] Studies show that the half-life of GAMMAGARD S/D is approximately 37.7 ± 15 days.[3] Previous studies reported IgG half-life values of 21 to 25 days[4,5] using radiolabeled IgG or 17.7 to 37.6 days measuring IgG levels during administration of IGIV to immunodeficient patients.[6] The half-life of IgG can vary considerably from person to person, however. In particular, high concentrations of IgG and hypermetabolism associated with fever and infection have been seen to coincide with a shortened half-life of IgG.[4-7]

Clinical Study

Clinical studies were conducted with lots of GAMMAGARD S/D containing IgA < 2.2 µg/mL. No clinical studies have been specifically conducted using only lots with IgA content of < 1 µg/mL.

INDICATIONS AND USAGE

GAMMAGARD S/D is not indicated in patients with selective IgA deficiency where the IgA deficiency is the only abnormality of concern (see **WARNINGS**).

Primary Immunodeficiency Diseases

GAMMAGARD S/D is indicated for the treatment of primary immunodeficient states, such as: congenital agammaglobulinemia, common variable immunodeficiency, Wiskott-Aldrich syndrome, and severe combined immunodeficiencies.[6,7] This indication was supported by a clinical trial of 17 patients with primary immunodeficiency who received a total of 341 infusions. GAMMAGARD S/D is especially useful when high levels or rapid elevation of circulating IgG are desired or when intramuscular injections are contraindicated (e.g., small muscle mass).

B-cell Chronic Lymphocytic Leukemia (CLL)

GAMMAGARD S/D is indicated for prevention of bacterial infections in patients with hypogammaglobulinemia and/or recurrent bacterial infections associated with B-cell Chronic Lymphocytic Leukemia (CLL). In a study of 81 patients, 41 of whom were treated with GAMMAGARD, Immune Globulin Intravenous (Human), bacterial infections were significantly reduced in the treatment group.[8,9] In this study, the placebo group had approximately twice as many bacterial infections as the IGIV group. The median time to first bacterial infection for the IGIV group was greater than 365 days. By contrast, the time to first bacterial infection in the placebo group was 192 days. The number of viral and fungal infections, which were for the most part minor, was not statistically different between the two groups.

Idiopathic Thrombocytopenic Purpura (ITP)

When a rapid rise in platelet count is needed to prevent and/or to control bleeding in a patient with Idiopathic Thrombocytopenic Purpura, the administration of GAMMAGARD S/D should be considered.

The efficacy of GAMMAGARD has been demonstrated in a clinical study involving 16 patients. Of these 16 patients, 13 had chronic ITP (11 adults, 2 children), and 3 patients had acute ITP (one adult, 2 children). All 16 patients (100%) demonstrated a clinically significant rise in platelet count to a level greater than 40,000/mm[3] following the administration of GAMMAGARD. Ten of the 16 patients (62.5%) exhibited a significant rise to greater than 80,000 platelets/mm[3]. Of these 10 patients, 7 had chronic ITP (5 adults, 2 children), and 3 patients had acute ITP (one adult, 2 children). The rise in platelet count to greater than 40,000/mm[3] occurred after a single 1 g/kg infusion of GAMMAGARD in 8 patients with chronic ITP (6 adults, 2 children), and in 2 patients with acute ITP (one adult, one child). A similar response was observed after two 1 g/kg infusions in 3 adult patients with chronic ITP, and one child with acute ITP. The remaining 2 adult patients with chronic ITP received more than two 1 g/kg infusions before achieving a platelet count greater than 40,000/mm[3]. The rise in platelet count was generally rapid, occurring within 5 days. However, this rise was transient and not considered curative. Platelet count rises lasted 2 to 3 weeks, with a range of 12 days to 6 months. It should be noted that childhood ITP may resolve spontaneously without treatment.

Kawasaki Syndrome

GAMMAGARD S/D is indicated for the prevention of coronary artery aneurysms associated with Kawasaki syndrome. The percentage incidence of coronary artery aneurysm in patients with Kawasaki syndrome receiving GAMMAGARD either at a single dose of 1 g/kg (n=22) or at a dose of 400 mg/kg for four consecutive days (n=22), beginning within seven days of onset of fever, was 3/44 (6.8%). This was significantly different (p=0.008) from a comparable group of patients that received aspirin only in previous trials and of whom 42/185 (22.7%) experienced coronary artery aneurysms.[10,11,12] All patients in the GAMMAGARD trial received concomitant aspirin therapy and none experienced hypersensitivity-type reactions (urticaria, bronchospasm or generalized anaphylaxis).[13]

Several studies have documented the efficacy of intravenous gammaglobulin in reducing the incidence of coronary artery abnormalities resulting from Kawasaki syndrome.[10-12, 14-17]

CONTRAINDICATIONS

GAMMAGARD S/D is contraindicated in patients with selective IgA deficiency where the IgA deficiency is the only abnormality of concern (see **INDICATIONS AND USAGE** and **WARNINGS**). Patients may experience severe hypersensitivity reactions or anaphylaxis in the setting of detectable IgA levels following infusion of GAMMAGARD S/D. The occurrence of severe hypersensitivity reactions or anaphylaxis under such conditions should prompt consideration of an alternative therapy.

WARNINGS

Warning

Immune Globulin Intravenous (Human) products have been reported to be associated with renal dysfunction, acute renal failure, osmotic nephrosis, and death.[18] Patients predisposed to acute renal failure include patients with any degree of pre-existing renal insufficiency, diabetes mellitus, age greater than 65, volume depletion, sepsis, paraproteinemia, or patients receiving known nephrotoxic drugs. Especially in such patients, IGIV products should be administered at the minimum concentration available and the minimum rate of infusion practicable. While these reports of renal dysfunction and acute renal failure have been associated with the use of many of the licensed IGIV products, those containing sucrose as a stabilizer accounted for a disproportionate share of the total number.*

See PRECAUTIONS and DOSAGE AND ADMINISTRATION sections for important information intended to reduce the risk of acute renal failure.

***GAMMAGARD S/D does not contain sucrose.**

GAMMAGARD S/D, Immune Globulin Intravenous (Human), is made from human plasma. Products made from human plasma may contain infectious agents, such as viruses, that can cause disease. The risk that such products will transmit an infectious agent has been reduced by screening plasma donors for prior exposure to certain viruses, by testing for the presence of certain current virus infections, and by inactivating and/or removing certain viruses. (See DESCRIPTION). Despite these measures, such products can still potentially transmit disease. Because this product is made from human blood, it may carry a risk of transmitting infectious agents, e.g., viruses and theoretically, the Creutzfeldt-Jakob disease (CJD) agent. ALL infections thought by a physician possibly to have been transmitted by this product should be reported by the physician or other healthcare provider to Baxter Healthcare Corporation at 1-800-423-2862 (in the U.S.). The physician should discuss the risks and benefits of this product with the patient.

GAMMAGARD S/D, Immune Globulin Intravenous (Human), should only be administered intravenously. Other routes of administration have not been evaluated.

Immediate anaphylactic and hypersensitivity reactions are a remote possibility. Epinephrine and antihistamines should be available for treatment of any acute anaphylactoid reactions.

GAMMAGARD S/D contains trace amounts of IgA ($\le$ 2.2 µg/mL in a 5% solution). GAMMAGARD S/D is not indicated in patients with selective IgA deficiency where the IgA deficiency is the only abnormality of concern. It should be given with caution to patients with antibodies to IgA or IgA deficiencies, that are a component of an underlying primary immunodeficiency disease for which IGIV therapy is indicated.[7,19] IGIV preparations depleted of IgA (0.4 to 2.9 µg/mL) were shown to be better tolerated by a limited number of patients[19,46,47] who reacted to IGIV preparations with higher IgA concentrations. However, the concentration of IgA that will not provoke a reaction is not known, and therefore **all IGIV preparations carry the risk of inducing an anaphylactic reaction to IgA**. In such instances, a risk of anaphylaxis may exist despite the fact that GAMMAGARD S/D contains trace amounts of IgA.

PRECAUTIONS

General

Some viruses, such as parvovirus B19V (formerly known as parvovirus B19) or hepatitis A, are particularly difficult to remove or inactivate at this time. Parvovirus B19V most seriously affects pregnant women, or immune-compromised individuals. Symptoms of parvovirus B19V infection include fever, drowsiness, chills, and runny nose followed about two weeks later by a rash and joint pain. Evidence of hepatitis A may include several days to weeks of poor appetite, tiredness, and low-grade fever followed by nausea, vomiting, and abdominal pain. Dark urine and a yellowed complexion are also common symptoms. Patients should be encouraged to consult their physician if such symptoms appear.

An aseptic meningitis syndrome (AMS) has been reported to occur infrequently in association with Immune Globulin Intravenous (Human) [IGIV] treatment. Discontinuation of IGIV treatment has resulted in remission of AMS within

Table 1
In Vitro Virus Clearance During GAMMAGARD S/D Manufacturing

Process Step Evaluated	Virus Clearance (log$_{10}$)								
	Lipid-Enveloped Viruses						Non-Lipid-Enveloped Viruses		
	BVD	HIV-1	HIV-2	PRV	SIN	VSV	EMC	HAV	PPV
Step 1: Processing of Cryo-Poor Plasma to Fraction I+II+III Precipitate	0.6*	5.7	NT	1.0*	NT	NT	NT	0.5*	0.2*
Step 2: Processing of Resuspended Suspension A Precipitate to Suspension B Filter Press Filtrate	1.3	4.9	NT	3.7	NT	NT	3.7	4.1	3.5
Step 3: Processing of Suspension B Filter Press to Suspension B Cuno 70 Filtrate	0.7*	4.0	NT	4.5	NT	NT	3.0	3.9	3.9
Step 4: Solvent/Detergent Treatment	>4.9	>3.7	5.7	>4.1	5.1	6.0	NA	NA	NA
Cumulative Reduction of Virus (log$_{10}$)	6.2	18.3	5.7	12.3	5.1	6.0	6.7	8.0	7.4

* These values are not included in the computation of the cumulative reduction of virus since the virus clearance is within the variability limit of the assay ($\le$1.0).
NA Not Applicable. Solvent/detergent treatment does not affect non-lipid-enveloped viruses.
NT Not Tested.

several days without sequelae. The syndrome usually begins within several hours to two days following IGIV treatment. It is characterized by symptoms and signs including severe headache, nuchal rigidity, drowsiness, fever, photophobia, painful eye movements, and nausea and vomiting. Cerebrospinal fluid (CSF) studies are frequently positive with pleocytosis up to several thousand cells per mm^3, predominantly from the granulocytic series, and elevated protein levels up to several hundred mg/dL. Patients exhibiting such symptoms and signs should receive a thorough neurological examination, including CSF studies, to rule out other causes of meningitis. AMS may occur more frequently in association with high dose (2 g/kg) IGIV treatment.

Periodic monitoring of renal function tests and urine output is particularly important in patients judged to have a potential increased risk for developing acute renal failure. Assure that patients are not volume depleted prior to the initiation of the infusion of IGIV. Renal function, including measurement of blood urea nitrogen (BUN)/serum creatinine, should be assessed prior to the initial infusion of GAMMAGARD S/D and again at appropriate intervals thereafter. If renal function deteriorates, discontinuation of the product should be considered.

For patients judged to be at risk for developing renal dysfunction, it may be prudent to reduce the rate of infusion to less than 4 mL/kg/Hr (< 3.3 mg IG/kg/min) for a 5% solution or at a rate less than 2 mL/kg/Hr (< 3.3 mg IG/kg/min) for a 10% solution.

Certain components used in the packaging of this product contain natural rubber latex.

Hemolysis

Immune Globulin Intravenous (Human) [IGIV] products can contain blood group antibodies which may act as hemolysins and induce *in vivo* coating of red blood cells with immunoglobulin, causing a positive direct antiglobulin reaction and, rarely, hemolysis.[20-23] Hemolytic anemia can develop subsequent to IGIV therapy due to enhanced RBC sequestration[23] (see **ADVERSE REACTIONS**). IGIV recipients should be monitored for clinical signs and symptoms of hemolysis (see **PRECAUTIONS: Laboratory Tests**).

Transfusion-Related Acute Lung Injury (TRALI)

There have been reports of noncardiogenic pulmonary edema (Transfusion-Related Acute Lung Injury [TRALI]) in patients administered IGIV.[24] TRALI is characterized by severe respiratory distress, pulmonary edema, hypoxemia, normal left ventricular function, and fever and typically occurs within 1 to 6 hours after transfusion. Patients with TRALI may be managed using oxygen therapy with adequate ventilatory support.

IGIV recipients should be monitored for pulmonary adverse reactions. If TRALI is suspected, appropriate tests should be performed for the presence of anti-neutrophil antibodies in both the product and patient serum (see **PRECAUTIONS: Laboratory Tests**).

Thrombotic Events

Thrombotic events have been reported in association with IGIV[25-33] (see **ADVERSE REACTIONS**). Patients at risk may include those with a history of atherosclerosis, multiple cardiovascular risk factors, advanced age, impaired cardiac output, and/or known or suspected hyperviscosity, hypercoagulable disorders and prolonged periods of immobilization. The potential risks and benefits of IGIV should be weighed against those of alternative therapies for all patients for whom IGIV administration is being considered. Baseline assessment of blood viscosity should be considered in patients at risk for hyperviscosity, including those with cryoglobulins, fasting chylomicronemia/markedly high triacylglycerols (triglycerides), or monoclonal gammopathies (see **PRECAUTIONS: Laboratory Tests**). Analysis of adverse event reports[13,34] has indicated that a rapid rate of infusion may be a risk factor for vascular occlusive events.

Laboratory Tests

If signs and/or symptoms of hemolysis are present after IGIV infusion, appropriate confirmatory laboratory testing should be done (see **PRECAUTIONS**).

If TRALI is suspected, appropriate tests should be performed for the presence of anti-neutrophil antibodies in both the product and patient serum (see **PRECAUTIONS**).

Because of the potentially increased risk of thrombosis, baseline assessment of blood viscosity should be considered in patients at risk for hyperviscosity, including those with cryoglobulins, fasting chylomicronemia/markedly high triacylglycerols (triglycerides), or monoclonal gammopathies (see **PRECAUTIONS**).

Information For Patients

Patients should be instructed to immediately report symptoms of decreased urine output, sudden weight gain, fluid retention/edema, and/or shortness of breath (which may suggest kidney damage) to their physician.

Drug Interactions

See **DOSAGE AND ADMINISTRATION**.

Pregnancy Category C

Animal reproduction studies have not been conducted with GAMMAGARD S/D. It is also not known whether GAMMAGARD S/D can cause fetal harm when administered to a pregnant woman or can affect reproduction capacity. GAMMAGARD S/D should be given to a pregnant woman only if clearly needed.

ADVERSE REACTIONS

Increases in creatinine and blood urea nitrogen (BUN) have been observed as soon as one to two days following infusion. Progression to oliguria and anuria requiring dialysis has been observed, although some patients have improved spontaneously following cessation of treatment.[35]

Types of severe renal adverse reactions that have been seen following IGIV therapy include:
• acute renal failure
• acute tubular necrosis[36]

- proximal tubular nephropathy
- osmotic nephrosis[18] (see also 37-39)

In general, reported adverse reactions to GAMMAGARD, in patients with either congenital or acquired immunodeficiencies are similar in kind and frequency. Various minor reactions, such as mild to moderate hypotension, headache, fatigue, chills, backache, leg cramps, lightheadedness, fever, urticaria, flushing, slight elevation of blood pressure, nausea and vomiting may occasionally occur. Slowing or stopping the infusion usually allows the symptoms to disappear promptly.

Immediate anaphylactic and hypersensitivity reactions are a remote possibility. Epinephrine and antihistamines should be available for treatment of any acute anaphylactoid reaction (see **WARNINGS**).

Primary Immunodeficiency Diseases

Twenty-one adverse reactions occurred in 341 infusions (6%), when using GAMMAGARD (5% solution), in a clinical trial of 17 patients with primary immunodeficiency.[40] Of the 17 patients, 12 (71%) were adults, and 5 (29%) were children (16 years or younger).

In a cross-over study comparing GAMMAGARD and GAMMAGARD S/D (5% solutions) conducted in a small number (n=10) of primary immunodeficient patients, no unusual or unexpected adverse reactions were observed in the GAMMAGARD S/D group. The adverse reactions experienced in the GAMMAGARD S/D group were similar in frequency and nature to those observed in the control group consisting of patients receiving GAMMAGARD.

GAMMAGARD, reconstituted to a concentration of 10%, was administered intravenously at rates varying from 2 to 11 mL/kg/Hr. Systemic reactions occurred in 23 (10.5%) of 219 infusions. This compares with an adverse reaction incidence of 6% (only systemic reactions reported) for primary immunodeficient patients previously treated with a 5% solution at infusion rates varying between 2 and 8 mL/kg/Hr, as described above (see reference 40). Local pain or irritation was experienced during 35 (16%) of 219 infusions. Application of a warm compress to the infusion site alleviated local symptoms. These local reactions tended to be associated with hand vein infusions and their incidence may be reduced by infusions via the antecubital vein.

B-cell Chronic Lymphocytic Leukemia (CLL)

In the study of patients with B-cell Chronic Lymphocytic Leukemia, the incidence of adverse reactions associated with GAMMAGARD infusions was approximately 1.3% while that associated with placebo (normal saline) infusions was 0.6%.[9]

Idiopathic Thrombocytopenic Purpura (ITP)

During the clinical study of GAMMAGARD for the treatment of Idiopathic Thrombocytopenic Purpura, the only adverse reaction reported was headache which occurred in 12 of 16 patients (75%). Of these 12 patients, 11 had chronic ITP (9 adults, 2 children), and one child had acute ITP. Oral antihistamines and analgesics alleviated the symptoms and were used as pretreatment for those patients requiring additional IGIV therapy. The remaining 4 patients did not report any side effects and did not require pretreatment.

Kawasaki Syndrome

In a study of patients (n=51) with Kawasaki syndrome, no hypersensitivity-type reactions (urticaria, bronchospasm or generalized anaphylaxis) were reported in patients receiving either a single 1 g/kg dose of IGIV, GAMMAGARD, or 400 mg/kg of IGIV, GAMMAGARD, for four consecutive days.[13] Mild adverse reactions, including chills, flushing, cramping, headache, hypotension, nausea, rash and wheezing, were reported with both dose regimens. These adverse reactions occurred in 7/51 (13.7%) patients and in association with 7/129 (5.4%) infusions. Of the 25 patients who received a single 1 g/kg dose, 4 patients experienced adverse reactions for an incidence of 16%. Of the 26 patients who received 400 mg/kg/day over 4 days, 3 experienced a single adverse reaction for an incidence of 11.5%.[3]

Postmarketing:

The following is a list of adverse reactions that have been identified and reported during the post-approval use of IGIV products:

Respiratory

cyanosis, hypoxemia, pulmonary edema, dyspnea, bronchospasm

Cardiovascular

thromboembolism, hypotension

Neurological

seizures, tremor

Hematologic

hemolysis, positive direct antiglobulin (Coombs) test

General/Body as a Whole

pyrexia, rigors

Musculoskeletal

back pain

Gastrointestinal

hepatic dysfunction, abdominal pain

Rare and Uncommon Adverse Events:

Respiratory

apnea, Acute Respiratory Distress Syndrome (ARDS), Transfusion Associated Lung Injury (TRALI)

Integumentary

bullous dermatitis, epidermolysis, erythema multiforme, Stevens-Johnson syndrome

Cardiovascular

cardiac arrest, vascular collapse

Neurological

coma, loss of consciousness

Hematologic

pancytopenia, leukopenia

Because postmarketing reporting of these reactions is voluntary and the at-risk populations are of uncertain size, it is not always possible to reliably estimate the frequency of the reaction or establish a causal relationship to exposure to the product. Such is also the case with literature reports authored independently[41] (see **PRECAUTIONS**).

DOSAGE AND ADMINISTRATION

Primary Immunodeficiency Diseases

For patients with primary immunodeficiencies, monthly doses of approximately 300-600 mg/kg infused at 3 to 4 week intervals are commonly used.[42,43] As there are significant differences in the half-life of IgG among patients with primary immunodeficiency, the frequency and amount of immunoglobulin therapy may vary from patient to patient. The proper amount can be determined by monitoring clinical response. The minimum serum concentration of IgG necessary for protection varies among patients and has not been established by controlled clinical trials.

B-cell Chronic Lymphocytic Leukemia (CLL)

For patients with hypogammaglobulinemia and/or recurrent bacterial infections due to B-cell Chronic Lymphocytic Leukemia, a dose of 400 mg/kg every 3 to 4 weeks is recommended.

Kawasaki Syndrome

For patients with Kawasaki syndrome, either a single 1 g/kg dose or a dose of 400 mg/kg for four consecutive days beginning within seven days of the onset of fever, administered concomitantly with appropriate aspirin therapy (80-100 mg/kg/day in four divided doses) is recommended.[44]

Idiopathic Thrombocytopenic Purpura (ITP)

For patients with acute or chronic Idiopathic Thrombocytopenic Purpura, a dose of 1 g/kg is recommended. The need for additional doses can be determined by clinical response and platelet count. Up to three separate doses may be given on alternate days if required.

No prospective data are presently available to identify a maximum safe dose, concentration, and rate of infusion in patients determined to be at increased risk of acute renal failure. In the absence of prospective data, the recommended doses should not be exceeded and the concentration and infusion rate selected should be the minimum level practicable. Reduction in dose, concentration, and/or rate of administration in patients at risk of acute renal failure has been proposed in the literature in order to reduce the risk of acute renal failure.[45]

Reconstitution: Use Aseptic Technique

When reconstitution is performed aseptically **outside** of a sterile laminar air flow hood, administration should begin as soon as possible, but not more than 2 hours after reconstitution.

When reconstitution is performed aseptically **inside** of a sterile laminar air flow hood, the reconstituted product may be either maintained in the original glass container or pooled into VIAFLEX bags and stored under constant refrigeration (2-8°C), for up to 24 hours. (The date and time of reconstitution/pooling should be recorded). If these conditions are not met, sterility of the reconstituted product cannot be maintained. Partially used vials should be discarded.

A. 5% Solution

Note: **If refrigerated, allow GAMMAGARD S/D to reach room temperature before administration.**

1. Remove bottle caps and clean stoppers with germicidal solution.
2. Remove spike cap from one end of the transfer device. Do not touch spike.

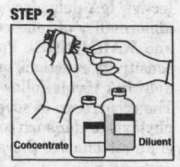

3a. Place diluent bottle on a flat surface. Use exposed end of transfer device to spike diluent bottle through center of the stopper.

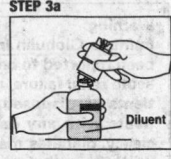

CAUTION: Failure to insert spike into center of the stopper may result in dislodging of the stopper.

3b. Ensure that the collar collapses fully into the device by pushing down on the transfer device firmly.

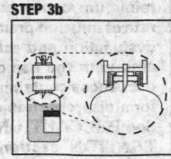

While holding onto transfer device, remove remaining spike cover. Do not touch spike.

4. Hold diluent bottle with attached transfer device at an angle to the concentrate bottle to prevent spilling the diluent.

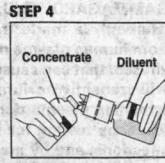

Note: Do not hold diluent bottle upside down, for this can lead to diluent spillage.

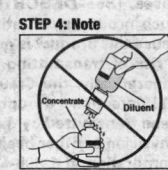

5a. Spike concentrate bottle through center of the stopper while **quickly inverting the diluent vial** to minimize spilling out diluent.

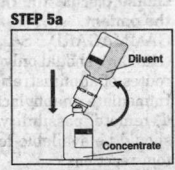

CAUTION: Failure to insert the spike into the center of the stopper may result in dislodging of the stopper and loss of vacuum.

5b. Ensure that the collar collapses fully into the device by pushing down on the diluent bottle firmly.

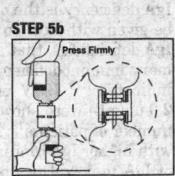

6. After transfer of diluent is complete, remove transfer device and empty diluent bottle. Immediately swirl the concentrate bottle gently to thoroughly mix contents.

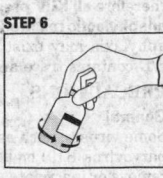

CAUTION: Do not shake. Avoid foaming.
Discard transfer device after single use per local guidelines.

B. 10% Solution

1. Follow step 1 as previously described in **A**.
2. To prepare a 10% solution, it is necessary to remove half of the volume of diluent. Table 2 indicates the volume of diluent that should be **removed from the vial** before attaching the transfer device to produce a 10% concentration. Using aseptic technique, withdraw the unnecessary volume of diluent using a sterile hypodermic syringe and needle. Discard the filled syringe into a suitable puncture proof container (Sharps Container).

3. Using the residual diluent in the diluent vial, follow steps 2-6 as previously described in A.

Table 2
Required Diluent Volume to Be Removed

Concentration	5 g bottle	10 g bottle
5%	Do not remove any diluent for reconstitution of 5% Solution	
10%	48 mL	96 mL

Rate of Administration

It is recommended that initially a 5% solution be infused at a rate of 0.5 mL/kg/Hr. If infusion at this rate and concentration causes the patient no distress, the administration rate may be gradually increased to a maximum rate of 4 mL/kg/Hr for patients with no history of adverse reactions to IGIV and no significant risk factors for renal dysfunction or thrombotic complications. Patients who tolerate the 5% concentration at 4 mL/kg/Hr can be infused with the 10% concentration starting at 0.5 mL/kg/Hr. If no adverse effects occur, the rate can be increased gradually up to a maximum of 8 mL/kg/Hr.

In general, it is recommended that patients beginning therapy with IGIV or switching from one IGIV product to another be started at the lower rates of infusion and should be advanced to the maximal rate only after they have tolerated several infusions at intermediate rates of infusion. It is important to individualize rates for each patient. As noted in the **WARNINGS** section, **patients who have underlying renal disease or who are judged to be at risk of developing thrombotic events should not be infused rapidly with any IGIV product.**

Although there are no prospective studies demonstrating that any concentration or rate of infusion is completely safe, it is believed that risk may be decreased at lower rates of infusion.[45] Therefore, as a guideline, it is recommended that these patients who are judged to be at risk of renal dysfunction or thrombotic complications be gradually titrated up to a more conservative maximal rate of less than 3.3 mg/kg/min (< 2 mL/kg/hr of a 10% or < 4 mL/kg/hr of a 5% solution).

It is recommended that antecubital veins be used especially for 10% solutions, if possible. This may reduce the likelihood of the patient experiencing discomfort at the infusion site (see **ADVERSE REACTIONS**).

A rate of administration which is too rapid may cause flushing and changes in pulse rate and blood pressure. Slowing or stopping the infusion usually allows the symptoms to disappear promptly.

Drug Interactions

Admixtures of GAMMAGARD S/D, Immune Globulin Intravenous (Human), with other drugs and intravenous solutions have not been evaluated. It is recommended that GAMMAGARD S/D be administered separately from other drugs or medications which the patient may be receiving. The product should not be mixed with Immune Globulin Intravenous (Human) from other manufacturers.

Antibodies in immune globulin preparations may interfere with patient responses to live vaccines, such as those for measles, mumps, and rubella. The immunizing physician should be informed of recent therapy with Immune Globulin Intravenous (Human) so that appropriate precautions can be taken.

Administration

GAMMAGARD S/D should be administered as soon after reconstitution as possible, or as described in **DOSAGE AND ADMINISTRATION**.

The reconstituted material should be at room temperature during administration.

Parenteral drug products should be inspected visually for particulate matter and discoloration prior to administration, whenever solution and container permit.

Reconstituted material should be a clear to slightly opalescent and colorless to pale yellow solution. Do not use if particulate matter and/or discoloration is observed.

Follow directions for use which accompany the administration set provided. If another administration set is used, ensure that the set contains a similar filter.

HOW SUPPLIED

GAMMAGARD S/D is supplied in 2.5 g (NDC number 0944-2620-02), 5 g (NDC number 0944-2620-03), or 10 g (NDC number 0944-2620-04) single use bottles. Each bottle of GAMMAGARD S/D is furnished with a suitable volume of Sterile Water for Injection, USP, a transfer device and an administration set which contains an integral airway and a 15 micron filter.

STORAGE

GAMMAGARD S/D is to be stored at a temperature not to exceed 25°C (77°F). Freezing should be avoided to prevent the diluent bottle from breaking.

REFERENCES

1. Prince AM, Horowitz B, Brotman B. Sterilisation of hepatitis and HTLV-III viruses by exposure to tri-n-butyl phosphate and sodium cholate. Lancet. 1986;1: 706-710.
2. Horowitz B, Wiebe ME, Lippin A, et al. Inactivation of viruses in labile blood derivatives: I. Disruption of lipid enveloped viruses by tri-n-butyl phosphate detergent combinations. Transfusion. 1985;25:516-522.
3. Unpublished data in the files of Baxter Healthcare Corporation.
4. Waldmann TA, Storber W. Metabolism of immunoglobulins. Prog Allergy. 1969;13:1-110.
5. Morell A, Riesen W. Structure, function and catabolism of immunoglobulins. In: Nydegger UE, ed. Immunotherapy. London: Academic Press; 1981;17-26.
6. Mankarious S, Lee M, Fischer S, Pyun KH, Ochs HD, Oxelius VA, Wedgwood RJ. The half-lives of IgG subclasses and specific antibodies in patients with primary immunodeficiency who are receiving intravenously administered immunoglobulin. J Lab Clin Med. 1988; 112: 634-40.
7. Buckley RH. Immunoglobulin replacement therapy: Indications and contraindications for use and variable IgG levels achieved In: Alving BM, Finlayson JS eds. Immunoglobulins: characteristics and use of intravenous preparations. Washington, D.C.: US Department of Health and Human Services; 1979;3-8.
8. Bunch C, Chapel HM, Rai K, et al. Intravenous Immune Globulin reduces bacterial infections in Chronic Lymphocytic Leukemia: A controlled randomized clinical trial. Blood. 1987; 70 Suppl 1:753.
9. Cooperative Group for the Study of Immunoglobulin in Chronic Lymphocytic Leukemia: Intravenous immunoglobulin for the prevention of infection in Chronic Lymphocytic Leukemia: A randomized, controlled clinical trial. N Eng J Med. 1988;319:902-907.
10. Newburger J, Takahashi M, Burns JG, et al. The Treatment of Kawasaki Syndrome with Intravenous Gamma Globulin. New England Journal of Medicine. 1986;315: 341-347.
11. Furusho K, Sato K, Soeda T, et al. High Dose Intravenous Gammaglobulin for Kawasaki Disease [letter]. Lancet. 1983;2:1359.
12. Nagashima M, Matsushima M, Matsucka H, Ogawa A, Okumura N. High Dose Gammaglobulin Therapy for Kawasaki Disease. Journal of Pediatrics. 1987; 110: 710-712.
13. Data in the files of Baxter Healthcare Corporation.
14. Furusho K, Hroyuki N, Shinomiya K, et al. High Dose Intravenous Gammaglobulin for Kawasaki Disease. Lancet. 1984;2:1055-1058.
15. Engle MA, Fatica NS, Bussel JB, O'Laughlin JE, Snyder MS, Lesser ML. Clinical Trial of Single-Dose Intravenous Gammaglobulin in Acute Kawasaki Disease. AJDC. 1989;143:1300-1304.
16. Isawa M, Sugiyama K, Kawase A, et al. Prevention of Coronary Artery Involvement in Kawasaki Disease by Early Intravenous High Dose Gammaglobulin. In: Doyle EF, Engle MA, Gersony WM, Rashkind EJ, Talner NS, eds. Pediatric Cardiology. New York. Springer-Verlag. 1986;1083-1085.
17. Okuri M, Harada K, Yamaguchi H, et al. Intravenous Gammaglobulin Therapy in Kawasaki Disease: Trial of Low-Dose Gammaglobulin. In: Shulman ST, ed. Kawasaki Disease. New York. Alan R. Liss, 1987;433-439.
18. Cayco AV, Perazella MA, Hayslett JP. Renal insufficiency after intravenous immune globulin therapy: a report of two cases and an analysis of the literature. J Am Soc Nephrol. 1997;8:1788-1794.
19. Burks AW, Sampson HA, Buckley RH. Anaphylactic reactions after gammaglobulin administration in patients with hypogammaglobulinemia: Detection of IgE antibodies to IgA. N Eng J Med. 1986;314:560-564.
20. Wilson JR, Bhoopalam N, Fisher M. Hemoytic anemia associated with intravenous immunoglobulin. Muscle Nerve. 1997;20:1142-1145.
21. Copelan EA, Strohm PL, Kennedy MS, Tutschka PJ. Hemolysis following intravenous immune globulin therapy. Transfusion. 1986;26:410-412.
22. Thomas MJ, Misbah SA, Chapel HM, Jones M, Elrington G, Newsom-Davis J. Hemolysis after high-dose intravenous Ig. Blood. 1993;82:3789.
23. Kessary-Shoham H, Levy Y, Shoenfeld Y, Lorber M, Gershon H. In vivo administration of intravenous immunoglobulin (IVIg) can lead to enhanced erythrocyte sequestration. J Autoimmune. 1999;13:129-135.
24. Rizk A, Gorson KC, Kenney L, Weinstein R. Transfusion-related acute lung injury after the infusion of IVIG. Transfusion. 2001;41:264-268.
25. Dalakas MC. High-dose intravenous immunoglobulin and serum viscosity: risk of precipitating thromboembolic events. Neurology. 1994;44:223-226.
26. Harkness K, Howell SJL, Davies-Jones GAB. Encephalopathy associated with intravenous immunoglobulin treatment for Guillain-Barre syndrome. Journal of Neurology Neurosurgery, Psychiatry. 1996;60:586-598.
27. Woodruff RK, Grigg AP, Firkin FC, Smith IL. Fatal thrombotic events during treatment of autoimmune thrombocytopenia with intravenous immunoglobulin in elderly patients. Lancet. 1986;2:217-218.
28. Wolberg AS, Kon RH, Monroe DM, Hoffman M. Coagulation factor XI is a contaminant in intravenous immunoglobulin preparations. Am J Hematol. 2000;65:30-34.
29. Brannagan TH, Nagle KJ, Lange DJ, Rowland LP: Complications of intravenous immune globulin treatment in neurologic disease. Neurology. 1996;47:674-677.
30. Haplea SS, Farrar JT, Gibson GA, Laskin M, Pizzi LT, Ashbury AK. Thromboembolic Events Associated with Intravenous Immunoglobulin Therapy. Neurology. 1997;48:A54.
31. Kwan T, and Keith P. Stroke Following Intravenous Immunoglobulin Infusion in a 28-Year-Old Male with Common Variable Immune Deficiency: A Case Report and Literature Review. Canadian Journal of Allergy & Clinical Immunology. 1999;4:250-253.
32. Elkayam O, Paran D, Milo R, Davidovitz Y, Almoznino-Sarafian D, Zelster D, Yaron M, Caspi D. Acute Myocardial Infarction Associated with High Dose Intravenous Immunoglobulin Infusion for Autoimmune Disorders. A study of four cases. Ann Rheum Dis. 2000;59:77-80.
33. Gomperts ED, Darr F. Letter to the Editor. Reference article – Rapid infusion of intravenous immune globulin in patients with neuromuscular disorders. Neurology. 2002. In Press.
34. Grillo JA, Gorson KC, Ropper AH, Lewis J, Weinstein R. Rapid infusion of intravenous immune globulin in patients with neuromuscular disorders. Neurology. 2001;57:1699-1701.
35. Winward DB, Brophy MT. Acute renal failure after administration of intravenous immunoglobulin: review of the literature and case report. Pharmacotherapy. 1995;15:765-772.
36. Phillips AO. Renal failure and intravenous immunoglobulin. Clin Nephrol. 1992;36:83-86.
37. Anderson W, Bethea W. Renal lesions following administration of hypertonic solutions of sucrose. JAMA. 1940;114:1983-1987.
38. Lindberg H, Wald A. Renal changes following the administration of hypertonic solutions. Arch Intern Med. 1939; 63:907-918.
39. Rigdon RH, Cardwell ES. Renal lesions following the intravenous injection of hypertonic solution of sucrose: a clinical and experimental study. Arch Intern Med. 1942;69:670-690.
40. Ochs HD, Lee ML, Fischer SH, et al. Efficacy of a New Intravenous Immunoglobulin Preparation in Primary Immunodeficient Patients. Clinical Therapeutics. 1987;9:512-522.
41. Pierce LR, Jain N. Risks associated with the use of intravenous immunoglobulin. Trans Med Rev. 2003; 17:241-251.
42. Eijkhout HW, Der Meer JW, Kallenbert CG, et al. The effect of two different dosages of intravenous immunoglobulin on the incidence of recurrent infections in patients with primary hypogammaglobulinemia. A randomized, double-blind, multicenter crossover trial. Ann Intern Med. 2001;135:165-174.
43. Roifman CM, Gelfand EW. Replacement therapy with high dose intravenous gammaglobulin improves chronic sinopulmonary disease in patients with hypogammaglobulinemia. Pediatr Infect Dis J. 1988;7:S92-S96.
44. Barron KS, Murphy DJ, Siverman ED, Ruttenberg HD, Wright GB, Franklin W, Goldberg SJ, Higashino SM, Cox DG, Lee M. Treatment of Kawasaki syndrome: a comparison of two dosage regimens of intravenously administered immune globulin. J Pediatr. 1990;117: 638-644.
45. Tan E, Hajinazarian M, Bay W, Neff J, Mendell JR. Acute renal failure resulting from intravenous immunoglobulin therapy. Arch Neurol. 1993;50:137-139.
46. Cunningham-Rundles C, Zhou Z, Mankarious S, Courter S. Long-term use of IgA-Depleted Intravenous Immunoglobulin in Immunodeficient Subjects with Anti-IgA Antibodies. J Clin Immunol 1993; 13:272-8.
47. Björkander J, Hammarström L, Smith CIE, Buckley RH, Cunningham-Rundles C, Hanson LÅ. Immunoglobulin Prophylaxis in Patients with Antibody Deficiency Syndromes and Anti-IgA Antibodies. J Clin Immunol 1987; 7:8-15.

BIBLIOGRAPHY
Bussel JB, Kimberly RP, Inman RD, et al. Intravenous gammaglobulin treatment of chronic idiopathic thrombocytopenic purpura. Blood. 1983;62:480-486.
To enroll in the confidential, industry-wide Patient Notification System, call 1-888-UPDATE U (1-888-873-2838)
Baxter, Gammagard and Viaflex are trademarks of Baxter International Inc., registered in the U.S. Patent and Trademark Office.
Baxter Healthcare Corporation
Westlake Village, CA 91362 USA
U.S. License No. 140
Revised December 2009

HEMOFIL M SINGLE DOSE BOTTLES ℞

[*hē-mō-fĭl*]
Antihemophilic Factor (Human), Method M, Monoclonal Purified

DESCRIPTION

HEMOFIL M, Antihemophilic Factor (Human) (AHF), Method M, Monoclonal Purified, is a sterile, nonpyrogenic, dried preparation of antihemophilic factor (Factor VIII, Factor VIII:C, AHF) in concentrated form with a specific activity range of 2 to 22 AHF International Units/mg of total protein. HEMOFIL M AHF contains a maximum of 12.5 mg/mL Albumin, and per AHF International Unit, 0.07 mg polyethylene glycol (3350), 0.39 mg histidine as stabilizing agents, not more than 0.1 mg glycine, 0.1 ng mouse protein, 18 ng organic solvent (tri-n-butyl phosphate) and 50 ng detergent (octoxynol 9). In the absence of the added Albumin (Human), the specific activity is approximately 2,000 AHF International Units/mg of protein. See **Clinical Pharmacology**.

HEMOFIL M AHF is prepared by the Method M process from pooled human plasma by immunoaffinity chromatography utilizing a murine monoclonal antibody to Factor VIII:C, followed by an ion exchange chromatography step for further purification. Source material may be provided by other US licensed manufacturers. HEMOFIL M AHF also includes an organic solvent (tri-n-butyl phosphate) and detergent (octoxynol 9) virus inactivation step designed to reduce the risk of transmission of hepatitis and other viral diseases. However, no procedure has been shown to be totally effective in removing viral infectivity from coagulation factor products.

Each bottle of HEMOFIL M AHF is labeled with the AHF activity expressed in International Units per bottle, which is referenced to the WHO International Standard.

HEMOFIL M AHF is to be administered only intravenously.

CLINICAL PHARMACOLOGY

Antihemophilic factor (AHF) is a protein found in normal plasma which is necessary for clot formation.

The administration of HEMOFIL M AHF provides an increase in plasma levels of AHF and can temporarily correct the coagulation defect of patients with hemophilia A (classical hemophilia). The administration of HEMOFIL M AHF will also correct deficiencies caused by circulating inhibitors when the inhibitor level does not exceed 10 Bethesda Units per mL.

The half-life of HEMOFIL M, Antihemophilic Factor (Human) (AHF), Method M, Monoclonal Purified, administered to Factor VIII deficient patients has been shown to be 14.8 ± 3.0 hours.

Use of an organic solvent (tri-n-butyl phosphate; TNBP) in the manufacture of Antihemophilic Factor (Human) has little or no effect on AHF activity, while lipid-enveloped viruses, such as hepatitis B and human immunodeficiency virus (HIV) are inactivated.[1] Prince, *et al*, report inactivation of at least 10,000 Chimpanzee Infectious Doses (CID-50) of hepatitis B virus, 10,000 CID-50 of hepatitis non A, non B virus, and 30,000 Tissue Culture Infectious Doses of HIV with TNBP/detergent treatment during manufacture of an Antihemophilic Factor (Human) concentrate.[2]

In vitro studies demonstrate that the HEMOFIL M AHF, manufacturing process provides for significant viral reduction. These studies, summarized in Table 1, demonstrate virus clearance during the HEMOFIL M AHF manufacturing process using human immunodeficiency virus, Type 1 (HIV-1); bovine viral diarrhea virus (BVDV), a generic model for lipid-enveloped RNA viruses, such as hepatitis C virus (HCV); pseudorabies virus (PRV), a model for lipid-enveloped DNA viruses, such as hepatitis B virus (HBV); canine parvovirus (CPV), a model for non-lipid enveloped DNA viruses, such as human parvovirus B19 (B19V); and hepatitis A virus (HAV). These reductions are achieved through a combination of process chemistry, partitioning and/or inactivation during solvent/detergent treatment, and immunoaffinity chromatography.

[See table 1 below]

HEMOFIL M AHF was administered to 11 patients previously untreated with Antihemophilic Factor (Human). They have shown no signs of hepatitis or HIV infection following three to nine months of evaluation.

A study of 25 patients treated with HEMOFIL M AHF, and monitored for three to six months has demonstrated no evidence of antibody response to mouse protein. More than 1,000 infusions of HEMOFIL M AHF have been administered during the clinical trials with no significant reactions. Reported events included a single episode each of chest tightness, fuzziness and dizziness, and one patient reported an unusual taste after each infusion.

INDICATIONS AND USAGE

The use of HEMOFIL M, Antihemophilic Factor (Human) (AHF), Method M, Monoclonal Purified, is indicated in hemophilia A (classical hemophilia) for the prevention and control of hemorrhagic episodes.

HEMOFIL M AHF can be of significant therapeutic value in patients with acquired Factor VIII inhibitors not exceeding 10 Bethesda Units per mL.[3] However, in such uses, the dosage should be controlled by frequent laboratory determinations of circulating AHF.

HEMOFIL M AHF is not indicated in von Willebrand's disease.

CONTRAINDICATIONS

Known hypersensitivity to mouse protein is a contraindication to the use of HEMOFIL M AHF.

WARNINGS

HEMOFIL M, Antihemophilic Factor (Human) (AHF), Method M, Monoclonal Purified, is made from human plasma. Products made from human plasma may contain infectious agents, such as viruses, that can cause disease. The risk that such products will transmit an infectious agent has been reduced by screening plasma donors for prior exposure to certain viruses, by testing for the presence of certain current virus infections, and by inactivating and/or removing certain viruses. Despite these measures, such products can still potentially transmit disease. Because this product is made from human blood, it may carry a risk of transmitting infectious agents, e.g., viruses and theoretically, the Creutzfeldt-Jakob disease (CJD) agent. ALL infections thought by a physician possibly to have been transmitted by this product should be reported by the physician or other healthcare provider to Baxter Healthcare Corporation at 1-800-423-2862 (in the U.S.). The physician should discuss the risks and benefits of this product with the patient.

Individuals who receive infusions of blood or plasma products may develop signs and/or symptoms of some viral infections, particularly non A, non B hepatitis. As indicated under **Clinical Pharmacology**, however, a group of such patients treated with HEMOFIL M AHF did not demonstrate signs or symptoms of non A, non B hepatitis over observation periods ranging from three to nine months.

PRECAUTIONS

General
Certain components used in the packaging of this product contain natural rubber latex.

Identification of the clotting defect as a Factor VIII deficiency is essential before the administration of HEMOFIL M, Antihemophilic Factor (Human) (AHF), Method M, Monoclonal Purified, is initiated.

No benefit may be expected from this product in treating other deficiencies.

The processing of HEMOFIL M, Antihemophilic Factor (Human) (AHF), Method M, Monoclonal Purified, significantly reduces the presence of blood group specific antibodies in the final product.

Formation of Antibodies to Mouse Protein
Although no hypersensitivity reactions have been observed, because HEMOFIL M AHF contains trace amounts of mouse protein (less than 0.1 ng/AHF activity units), the possibility exists that patients treated with this product may develop hypersensitivity to the mouse proteins.

The pulse rate should be determined before and during administration of HEMOFIL M AHF. Should a significant increase occur, reducing the rate of administration or temporarily halting the injection usually allows the symptoms to disappear promptly.

Information for Patients
Some viruses, such as parvovirus B19 or hepatitis A, are particularly difficult to remove or inactivate at this time. Parvovirus B19 most seriously affects pregnant women, or immune-compromised individuals. Symptoms of parvovirus B19 infection include fever, drowsiness, chills, and runny nose followed about two weeks later by a rash, and joint pain. Evidence of hepatitis A may include several days to weeks of poor appetite, tiredness, and low-grade fever followed by nausea, vomiting, and pain in the belly. Dark urine and a yellowed complexion are also common symptoms. Patients should be encouraged to consult their physician if such symptoms appear.

Patients should be informed of the early signs of hypersensitivity reactions including hives, generalized urticaria, tightness of the chest, wheezing, hypotension, and anaphylaxis, and should be advised to discontinue use of the product and contact their physician if these symptoms occur.

Laboratory Tests
Although dosage can be estimated by the calculations which follow, it is strongly recommended that whenever possible, appropriate laboratory tests be performed on the patient's plasma at suitable intervals to assure that adequate AHF levels have been reached and are maintained.

If the AHF content of the patient's plasma fails to reach expected levels or if bleeding is not controlled after apparently adequate dosage, the presence of inhibitor should be suspected. By appropriate laboratory procedures, the presence of inhibitor can be demonstrated and quantified in terms of AHF units neutralized by each mL of plasma or by the total estimated plasma volume.

If the inhibitor is at low levels (i.e., $<$10 Bethesda Units/mL), after administration of sufficient AHF units to neutralize the inhibitor, additional AHF units will elicit the predicted response.

Pregnancy
Pregnancy Category C. Animal reproduction studies have not been conducted with HEMOFIL M, Antihemophilic Factor (Human) (AHF), Method M, Monoclonal Purified. It is not known whether HEMOFIL M AHF can cause fetal harm when administered to a pregnant woman or can affect reproduction capacity. HEMOFIL M AHF should be given to a pregnant woman only if clearly needed.

ADVERSE REACTIONS

Allergic reactions may be encountered from the use of Antihemophilic Factor (Human) preparations. See **Information for Patients**.

The protein in greatest concentration in HEMOFIL M AHF is Albumin (Human). Reactions associated with albumin are extremely rare, although nausea, fever, chills or urticaria have been reported.

DOSAGE AND ADMINISTRATION

Each bottle of HEMOFIL M AHF is labeled with the AHF activity expressed in IU per bottle. This potency assignment is referenced to the World Health Organization International Standard.

The high purity of HEMOFIL M AHF has been thought to influence the difficulty of producing an accurate potency measurement. Experiments have shown that to achieve accurate activity levels, such a potency assay should be conducted using plastic test tubes and pipets as well as substrate containing normal levels of von Willebrand's Factor.

The expected *in vivo* peak AHF level, expressed as IU/dL of plasma or % (percent) of normal, can be calculated by multiplying the dose administered per kg body weight (IU/kg) by two. This calculation is based on the clinical finding by Abildgaard, *et al*,[4] which is supported by data from the collaborative study of *in vivo* recovery and survival with 15 different lots of HEMOFIL M AHF on 56 hemophiliacs that

Table 1
***In Vitro* Virus Clearance During the Manufacture of HEMOFIL M AHF**

Process Step Evaluated	Virus Clearance, log_{10}				
	Lipid-enveloped			Non-Lipid enveloped	
	HIV-1	BVDV	PRV	CPV	HAV
Solvent/Detergent Treatment	> 4.8	> 6.8	> 6.9	*	*
Immunoaffinity Chromatography	N.A.**	N.A.**	N.A.**	≥ 3.9	≥ 4.5
Cumulative Total, log_{10}	**> 4.8**	**> 6.8**	**> 6.9**	**≥ 3.9**	**≥ 4.5**

* Solvent/Detergent treatment inactivates only lipid-enveloped viruses. CPV and HAV are non-lipid enveloped viruses.
** Not Applicable for lipid-enveloped viruses due to the presence of solvent/detergent in the starting material.

HEMORRHAGE

Degree of hemorrhage	Required peak post-infusion AHF activity in the blood (as % of normal or IU/dL plasma)	Frequency of infusion
Early hemarthrosis or muscle bleed or oral bleed	20-40	Begin infusion every 12 to 24 hours for one-three days until the bleeding episode as indicated by pain is resolved or healing is achieved.
More extensive hemarthrosis, muscle bleed, or hematoma	30-60	Repeat infusion every 12 to 24 hours for usually three days or more until pain and disability are resolved.
Life threatening bleeds such as head injury, throat bleed, severe abdominal pain	60-100	Repeat infusion every 8 to 24 hours until threat is resolved.

SURGERY

Type of operation		
Minor surgery, including tooth extraction	60-80	A single infusion plus oral antifibrinolytic therapy within one hour is sufficient in approximately 70% of cases.
Major surgery	80-100 (pre- and post-operative)	Repeat infusion every 8 to 24 hours depending on state of healing.

demonstrated a mean peak recovery point above the mean pre-infusion baseline of about 2.0 IU/dL per infused IU/kg body weight.[5]

Example:

(1) A dose of 1750 IU AHF administered to a 70 kg patient, i.e., 25 IU/kg (1750/70), should be expected to cause a peak post-infusion AHF increase of $25 \times 2 = 50$ IU/dL (50% of normal).

(2) A peak level of 70% is required in a 40 kg child. In this situation the dose would be $70/2 \times 40 = 1400$ IU.

Recommended Dosage Schedule

Physician supervision of the dosage is required. The following dosage schedule may be used as a guide.

[See table above]

The careful control of the substitution therapy is especially important in cases of major surgery or life threatening hemorrhages.

Although dosage can be estimated by the calculations above, it is strongly recommended that whenever possible, appropriate laboratory tests including serial AHF assays be performed on the patient's plasma at suitable intervals to assure that adequate AHF levels have been reached and are maintained.

Other dosage regimens have been proposed such as that of Schimpf, et al, which describes continuous maintenance therapy.[6]

Reconstitution: Use Aseptic Technique

1. Bring HEMOFIL M AHF (dry concentrate) and Sterile Water for Injection, USP, (diluent) to room temperature.
2. Remove caps from concentrate and diluent bottles to expose central portion of rubber stoppers.
3. Cleanse stoppers with germicidal solution.
4. Remove protective covering from one end of double-ended needle and insert exposed needle through diluent stopper.
5. Remove protective covering from other end of double-ended needle. Invert diluent bottle over upright HEMOFIL M AHF bottle, then rapidly insert free end of the needle through the HEMOFIL M AHF bottle stopper at its center. The vacuum in the HEMOFIL M AHF bottle will draw in the diluent.
6. Disconnect the two bottles by removing needle from diluent bottle stopper, then remove needle from HEMOFIL M AHF bottle. Swirl gently until all material is dissolved. Be sure that HEMOFIL M AHF is completely dissolved, otherwise active material will be removed by the filter.

Note: Do not refrigerate after reconstitution.

Administration: Use Aseptic Technique

Administer at room temperature.

HEMOFIL M, Antihemophilic Factor (Human) (AHF), Method M, Monoclonal Purified, should be administered not more than three hours after reconstitution.

Intravenous Syringe Injection

Parenteral drug products should be inspected for particulate matter and discoloration prior to administration, whenever solution and container permit.

Plastic syringes are recommended for use with this product. The ground glass surface of all-glass syringes tend to stick with solutions of this type.

1. Attach filter needle to a disposable syringe and draw back plunger to admit air into syringe.
2. Insert needle into reconstituted HEMOFIL M AHF.
3. Inject air into bottle and then withdraw the reconstituted material into the syringe.

4. Remove and discard the filter needle from the syringe; attach a suitable needle and inject intravenously as instructed under **Rate of Administration**.
5. If a patient is to receive more than one bottle of HEMOFIL M AHF, the contents of two bottles may be drawn into the same syringe by drawing up each bottle through a separate unused filter needle. This practice lessens the loss of HEMOFIL M AHF. Please note, filter needles are intended to filter the contents of a single bottle of HEMOFIL M AHF only.

Rate of Administration

Preparations of HEMOFIL M AHF can be administered at a rate of up to 10 mL per minute with no significant reactions. The pulse rate should be determined before and during administration of HEMOFIL M AHF. Should a significant increase occur, reducing the rate of administration or temporarily halting the injection usually allows the symptoms to disappear promptly.

HOW SUPPLIED

HEMOFIL M AHF is available as single dose bottles that contain nominally 250 (NDC 0944-2930-01), 500 (NDC 0944-2931-01), 1000 (NDC 0944-2932-01), and 1700 (NDC 0944-2933-01) IU per bottle. Each bottle is labeled with the potency in International Units, and is packaged together with 10 mL of Sterile Water for Injection, USP, a double-ended needle, and a filter needle.

STORAGE

HEMOFIL M AHF can be stored at 2°-8°C (36°-46°F) or at room temperature, not to exceed 30°C (86°F), until expiration date noted on the package.

Avoid freezing to prevent damage to the diluent bottle.

REFERENCES

1. Horowitz B, Wiebe ME, Lippin A, et al: Inactivation of viruses in labile blood derivatives: 1. Disruption of lipid enveloped viruses by tri(n-butyl)phosphate detergent combinations. **Transfusion** 25:516-522,1985.
2. Prince AM, Horowitz B, Brotman B: Sterilisation of hepatitis and HTLV-III viruses by exposure to tri(n-butyl)phosphate and sodium cholate. **Lancet 1**: 706-710,1986.
3. Kessler CM: An Introduction to Factor VIII Inhibitors: The Detection and Quantitation. **Am J Med 91 (Suppl 5A)**:1S-5S,1991.
4. Abildgaard CF, Simone JV, Corrigan JJ, et al: Treatment of hemophilia with glycine-precipitated Factor VIII. **New Eng J Med** 275:471-475,1966.
5. Addiego, Jr. JE, Gomperts E, Liu S, et al: Treatment of hemophilia A with a highly purified Factor VIII concentrate prepared by Anti-FVIIIc immunoaffinity chromatography. **Thrombosis and Haemostasis** 67:19-27,1992.
6. Schimpf K, Rothmann P, Zimmermann K: Factor VIII dosis in prophylaxis of hemophilia A; A further controlled study, in **Proc XIth Cong W.F.H.** Kyoto, Japan, Academic Press, 1976, pp 363-366.

To enroll in the confidential, industry-wide Patient Notification System, call 1-888-UPDATE-U (1-888-873-2838).

Baxter and HEMOFIL are trademarks of Baxter International Inc., and are registered in the U.S. Patent and Trademark Office.

Baxter Healthcare Corporation
Westlake Village, CA 91362 USA

U.S. License No. 140
Printed in USA
0710517   Revised January 2009

RECOMBINATE   ℞
[rē-kŏm-bĭnăt]
[Antihemophilic Factor(Recombinant)]
Lyophilized Powder for Reconstitution for Injection

Reconstitute with 10 mL of Sterile Water for Injection using BAXJECT II
Prescribing Information

DESCRIPTION

RECOMBINATE [Antihemophilic Factor (Recombinant)] is a glycoprotein synthesized by a genetically engineered Chinese Hamster Ovary (CHO) cell line. In culture, the CHO cell line secretes recombinant Factor VIII (rFVIII) into the cell culture medium. The rFVIII is purified from the culture medium utilizing a series of chromatography columns. A key step in the purification process is an immunoaffinity chromatography methodology in which a purification matrix, prepared by immobilization of a monoclonal antibody directed to Factor VIII, is utilized to selectively isolate the rFVIII in the medium. The synthesized rFVIII produced by the CHO cells has the same biological effects as human Factor VIII. Structurally the protein has a similar combination of heterogenous heavy and light chains as found in human Factor VIII.

RECOMBINATE is formulated as a sterile, nonpyrogenic, off-white to faint yellow, lyophilized powder preparation of concentrated recombinant Factor VIII for intravenous injection. RECOMBINATE is available in single-dose vials, which contain nominally 250, 500, 1000, 1500, and 2000 International Units per vial. When reconstituted with the appropriate volume of diluent, the product contains the following stabilizers in maximum amounts: For 10 mL reconstitution volume: 12.5 mg/mL Albumin (Human), 0.20 mg/mL calcium, 1.5 mg/mL polyethylene glycol (3350), 180 mEq/L sodium, 55 mM histidine, 1.5 µg/Factor VIII International Unit (IU) polysorbate-80. Recombinant Von Willebrand Factor (rVWF) is coexpressed with the rFVIII and helps to stabilize it. The final product contains not more than 2 ng rVWF/IU rFVIII, which will not have any clinically relevant effect in patients with von Willebrand's disease. The product contains no preservative.

Manufacturing of RECOMBINATE is shared by Baxter Healthcare Corporation and Wyeth BioPharma. The recombinant Antihemophilic Factor Concentrate (For Further Manufacturing Use) is produced by Baxter Healthcare Corporation and Wyeth BioPharma (For Further Manufacturing Use) and subsequently formulated and packaged at Baxter Healthcare Corporation.

Each vial of RECOMBINATE is labeled with the Factor VIII activity expressed in IU per vial. Biological potency is determined by an in vitro assay which is referenced to the World Health Organization (WHO) International Standard for Factor VIII:C Concentrate.

CLINICAL PHARMACOLOGY

Factor VIII is the specific clotting factor deficient in patients with hemophilia A (classical hemophilia). Hemophilia A is a genetic bleeding disorder characterized by hemorrhages, which may occur spontaneously or after minor trauma. The administration of RECOMBINATE provides an increase in plasma levels of Factor VIII and can temporarily correct the coagulation defect in these patients. Pharmacokinetic studies on sixty-nine (69) patients revealed the circulating mean half-life for RECOMBINATE to be 14.6 ± 4.9 hours (n=67), which was not statistically significantly different from plasma-derived HEMOFIL M, [Antihemophilic Factor (Human), Method M, Monoclonal Purified]. The mean half-life of HEMOFIL M was 14.7 ± 5.1 hours (n=61). The actual baseline recovery observed with RECOMBINATE was 123.9 $\pm$ 47.7 IU/dL (n=23), which is significantly higher than the actual HEMOFIL M baseline recovery of 101.7 ± 31.6 IU/dL (n=61). However, the calculated ratio of actual to expected recovery with RECOMBINATE ($121.2 \pm 48.9\%$) is not different on average from HEMOFIL M ($123.4 \pm 16.4\%$).

The clinical study of RECOMBINATE in previously treated patients (individuals with hemophilia A who had been treated with plasma-derived Factor VIII) was based on observations made on a study group of 69 patients. These individuals received cumulative amounts of Factor VIII ranging from 20,914 to 1,383,063 IU over the 48-month study. Patients were given a total of 17,700 infusions totaling 28,090,769 IU RECOMBINATE.

These patients were successfully treated for bleeding episodes on a demand basis and also for the prevention of bleeds (prophylaxis). Spontaneous bleeding episodes successfully managed include hemarthroses, soft tissue and muscle bleeds. Management of hemostasis was also evaluated in surgeries. A total of 24 procedures on 13 patients were performed during this study. These included minor

System Organ Class (SOC)	Preferred MedDRA Term	Number of Subjects	Percent of Evaluable Subjects*
Gastrointestinal disorders	Nausea	1	0.48
General disorders and administration site conditions	Chills	3	1.43
	Fatigue	1	0.48
	Pyrexia	1	0.48
Infections and infestations	Ear infections	1	0.48
Investigations	Acoustic stimulation tests abnormal	1	0.48
Musculoskeletal and connective tissue disorders	Pain in extremity	1	0.48
Nervous system disorders	Dizziness	1	0.48
	Tremors	1	0.48
Respiratory, thoracic and mediastinal disorders	Pharyngolaryngeal pain	1	0.48
Skin and subcutaneous tissue disorders	Hyperhidrosis	1	0.48
	Pruritus	1	0.48
	Rash	2	0.95
	Rash maculopapular	1	0.48
Vascular disorders	Epistaxis	1[†]	0.48
	Flushing	2	0.95
	Hematoma	1	0.48
	Hypotension	1	0.48
	Pallor	1	0.48
	Peripheral coldness	1	0.48

* Number of evaluable subjects experiencing the event/total number of evaluable subjects [% relative to 210, the total number of unique subjects who received at least 1 infusion of RECOMBINATE].

† One subject experienced 11 events for epistaxis.

(e.g. tooth extraction) and major (e.g. bilateral osteotomies, thoracotomy and liver transplant) procedures. Hemostasis was maintained perioperatively and postoperatively with individualized Factor VIII replacement.

A study of RECOMBINATE in previously untreated patients was also performed as part of an ongoing study. The study group was comprised of seventy-nine (79)[1] patients, of whom seventy-six (76) had received at least one infusion of RECOMBINATE. To date, this cohort has been given 12,209 infusions totaling over 11,277,043 IU of RECOMBINATE. Hemostasis was appropriately managed in spontaneous bleeding episodes, intracranial hemorrhage and surgical procedures.

INDICATIONS AND USAGE

The use of RECOMBINATE [Antihemophilic Factor (Recombinant)] is indicated in hemophilia A (classical hemophilia) for the prevention and control of hemorrhagic episodes.[2] RECOMBINATE is also indicated in the perioperative management of patients with hemophilia A (classical hemophilia).

RECOMBINATE can be of therapeutic value in patients with acquired Factor VIII inhibitors not exceeding 10 Bethesda Units per mL.[3] In clinical studies with RECOMBINATE, patients with inhibitors who were entered into the previously treated patient trial and those previously untreated children who had developed inhibitor activity on study showed clinical hemostatic response when the titer of inhibitor was less than 10 Bethesda Units per mL. However, in such uses, the dosage of RECOMBINATE should be controlled by frequent laboratory determinations of circulating Factor VIII levels as well as the clinical status of the patient.

RECOMBINATE is not indicated in von Willebrand's disease.

CONTRAINDICATIONS

RECOMBINATE is contraindicated in patients who have manifested life-threatening immediate hypersensitivity reactions, including anaphylaxis, to the product or its components, including bovine, mouse or hamster proteins.

WARNINGS

General

The clinical response to RECOMBINATE may vary. If bleeding is not controlled with the recommended dose, the plasma level of factor VIII should be determined and a sufficient dose of RECOMBINATE should be administered to achieve a satisfactory clinical response. If the patient's plasma factor VIII level fails to increase as expected or if bleeding is not controlled after the expected dose, the presence of an inhibitor (neutralizing antibodies) should be suspected and appropriate testing performed. (see PRE-CAUTIONS - Monitoring Laboratory Tests).

Anaphylaxis and Severe Hypersensitivity Reactions

Allergic type hypersensitivity reactions, including anaphylaxis, have been reported with RECOMBINATE and have been manifested as dizziness, pruritus, rash, urticaria, flushing, angioedema/face swelling, laryngeal edema, dyspnea, pallor, pyrexia, nausea, paresthesia, hypotension, and loss of consciousness. Discontinue RECOMBINATE if symptoms occur and seek immediate emergency treatment. RECOMBINATE contains trace amounts of bovine proteins, mouse immunoglobulin G (MuIgG), and hamster (CHO) proteins. Patients treated with this product may develop hypersensitivity to these non-human mammalian proteins.

Neutralizing Antibodies

Patients treated with antihemophilic factor (AHF) products should be carefully monitored for the development of factor VIII inhibitors by appropriate clinical observations and laboratory tests. Inhibitors have been reported following administration of RECOMBINATE predominantly in previously untreated and minimally treated patients. The risk of developing inhibitors is highest during the first 20 exposure days. If expected plasma factor VIII activity levels are not attained, or if bleeding is not controlled with an expected dose, an assay that measures factor VIII inhibitor concentration should be performed (see PRECAUTIONS - Monitoring Laboratory Tests).

PRECAUTIONS

General

Certain components used in the packaging of this product contain natural rubber latex.

Identification of the clotting defect as a Factor VIII deficiency is essential before the administration of RECOMBINATE [Antihemophilic Factor (Recombinant)] is initiated. No benefit may be expected from this product in treating other deficiencies.

Formation of Antibodies to Mouse, Hamster or Bovine Protein

As RECOMBINATE contains trace amounts of mouse protein (maximum of 0.1 ng/IU RECOMBINATE), hamster protein (maximum of 1.5 ng CHO protein/IU RECOMBINATE), and bovine protein (maximum of 1 ng BSA/IU RECOMBINATE), the remote possibility exists that patients treated with this product may develop hypersensitivity to these non-human mammalian proteins.

Information for Patients

The patient and physician should discuss the risks and benefits of this product.

Allergic type hypersensitivity reactions have been observed with RECOMBINATE. Patients should be informed of the early signs of hypersensitivity reactions including hives, generalized urticaria, tightness of the chest, wheezing, hypotension, symptoms of laryngeal edema, and anaphylaxis. Patients should be advised to discontinue use of the product and contact their physician if these symptoms occur.

Monitoring Laboratory Tests

• Monitor plasma factor VIII activity levels by the one-stage clotting assay to confirm the adequate factor VIII levels have been achieved and maintained, when clinically indicated. (see DOSAGE and ADMINISTRATION).

• Monitor for development of factor VIII inhibitors. Perform assay to determine if factor VIII inhibitor is present if expected factor VIII activity plasma levels are not attained, or if bleeding is not controlled with the expected dose of RECOMBINATE. Use Bethesda Units (BU) to titer inhibitors.

  ○ If the inhibitor is less than 10 BU per mL, the administration of additional RECOMBINATE concentrate may neutralize the inhibitor, and may permit an appropriate hemostatic response.

  ○ Adequate hemostasis may not be achieved if inhibitor titers are above 10 BU per mL. The inhibitor titer may rise following RECOMBINATE infusion as a result of an anamnestic response to factor VIII. The treatment or prevention of bleeding in such patients requires the use of alternative therapeutic approaches and agents.

Carcinogenesis, Mutagenesis, Impairment of Fertility

RECOMBINATE was tested for mutagenicity at doses considerably exceeding plasma concentrations of Factor VIII in vitro and at doses up to ten times the expected maximum clinical dose in vivo, and did not cause reverse mutations, chromosomal aberrations, or an increase in micronuclei in bone marrow polychromatic erythrocytes. Long-term studies in animals have not been performed to evaluate carcinogenic potential.

Pediatric Use

RECOMBINATE is appropriate for use in children of all ages, including the newborn. Safety and efficacy studies have been performed in both previously treated (n=23) and previously untreated (n=75) children. (See CLINICAL PHARMACOLOGY and PRECAUTIONS).

Pregnancy

Pregnancy Category C. Animal reproduction studies have not been conducted with RECOMBINATE. The safety of RECOMBINATE for use in pregnant women has not been established. It is not known whether RECOMBINATE can cause fetal harm when administered to a pregnant woman or can affect reproductive capacity. Physicians should carefully consider the potential risks and benefits for each specific patient before prescribing RECOMBINATE. RECOMBINATE should be given to a pregnant woman only if clearly needed.

Nursing Mothers

It is not known whether this drug is excreted into human milk. Because many drugs are excreted into human milk, caution should be exercised if RECOMBINATE is administered to nursing mothers. RECOMBINATE should be given to nursing mothers only if clinically needed.

ADVERSE REACTIONS

Adverse Reactions from Clinical Trials

During controlled clinical studies with RECOMBINATE enrolling 210 subjects, the most commonly reported adverse drug reactions were chills, flushing, rash and epistaxis.

[See table at top left]

During the Previously Treated Patients (PTP) study, none of the 71 subjects developed de novo evidence of Factor VIII inhibitor. However, during the phase II/III portion of the study, 1 subject with a history of inhibitors exhibited inhibitor activity at 6 months (0.8 Bethesda Units [BU]), which resolved by 9 months. One other subject in this study had detectable Factor VIII inhibitor at baseline (1.26 BU) and exhibited an anamnestic response at 6 months (10.3 BU). During a prospective pharmaco-surveillance study of subjects who received batches of RECOMBINATE containing modestly increased Chinese Hamster Ovary (CHO) cell protein levels, none of the 34 treated subjects developed a Factor VIII inhibitor.

During the Previously Untreated Patients (PUP) study, 22 of the 73 evaluable subjects developed inhibitors to Factor VIII. Of these, 13 subjects displayed no detectable Factor VIII inhibitors at study exit.

Post-Marketing Adverse Reactions

In addition to the adverse reactions noted in clinical trials, the following adverse reactions have been reported in the post-marketing experience. These adverse reactions are listed by MedDRA (version 12.1) System Organ Class (SOC), then by MedDRA coding system Preferred Term in order of severity.

BLOOD AND LYMPHATIC SYSTEM DISORDERS: Factor VIII inhibition

CARDIAC DISORDERS: Tachycardia, Cyanosis

GASTROINTESTINAL DISORDERS: Vomiting, Abdominal pain

GENERAL DISORDERS AND ADMINISTRATION SITE CONDITIONS: Malaise, Injection site reactions, Chest pain, Chest discomfort

IMMUNE SYSTEM DISORDERS: Anaphylactic reaction, Hypersensitivity

NERVOUS SYSTEM DISORDERS: Loss of consciousness, Headache, Paresthesia

RESPIRATORY, THORACIC AND MEDIASTINAL DISORDERS: Dyspnea, Cough, Laryngeal edema
SKIN AND SUBCUTANEOUS TISSUE DISORDERS: Angioedema, Urticaria, Erythema

DOSAGE AND ADMINISTRATION

Each vial of RECOMBINATE is labeled with the Factor VIII activity expressed in IU per vial. This potency assignment is referenced to the World Health Organization International Standard for Factor VIII:C Concentrate and is evaluated by appropriate methodology to ensure accuracy of the results. The expected *in vivo* peak increase in Factor VIII level expressed as IU/dL of plasma or % (percent) of normal can be estimated by multiplying the dose administered per kg body weight (IU/kg) by two. This calculation is based on the clinical findings of Abildgaard *et al*[4] and is supported by the data generated by 419 clinical pharmacokinetic studies with RECOMBINATE in 67 patients over time. This pharmacokinetic data demonstrated a peak recovery point above the pre-infusion baseline of approximately 2.0 IU/dL per IU/kg body weight.

Examples (Assuming patient's baseline Factor VIII level is at <1%):

(1) A dose of 1750 IU RECOMBINATE administered to a 70 kg patient, *i.e.* 25 IU/kg (1750 IU/70 kg), should be expected to cause a peak post-infusion Factor VIII increase of 25 IU/kg × 2 (IU/dL)/(IU/kg) = 50 IU/dL (50% of normal).

(2) A peak level of 70% is required in a 40 kg child. In this situation, the dose would be 70 IU/dL/[2(IU/dL)/(IU/kg)] × 40 kg = 1400 IU.

Recommended Dosage Schedule

Physician supervision of the dosage is required. The following dosage schedule may be used as a guide.

[See first table at right]

If bleeding is not controlled with the recommended dose, the plasma level of Factor VIII should be determined and a sufficient dose of RECOMBINATE should be administered to achieve a satisfactory clinical response.

The careful control of the substitution therapy is especially important in cases of major surgery or life threatening hemorrhages. In presence of low titer inhibitor, doses larger than those recommended may be necessary as per standard care.

Although dosage can be estimated by the calculations above, it is strongly recommended that whenever possible, appropriate laboratory tests including serial Factor VIII assays be performed on the patient's plasma at suitable intervals to assure that adequate Factor VIII levels have been reached and are maintained.

Patients should be evaluated for the development of Factor VIII inhibitors, if the expected plasma Factor VIII activity levels are not attained, or if bleeding is not controlled with an appropriate dose.

Reconstitution: Use Aseptic Technique

1. Bring RECOMBINATE (dry factor concentrate) and Sterile Water for Injection, USP, (diluent) to room temperature.
2. Remove caps from concentrate and diluent vials.
3. Cleanse stoppers with germicidal solution and allow to dry prior to use. Place vials on a flat surface.
4. Open the BAXJECT II device package by peeling away the lid, without touching the inside. **Do not remove the device from the package.**
5. Turn the package over. Press straight down to fully insert the clear plastic spike through the diluent vial stopper.
6. Grip the BAXJECT II package at its edge and pull the package off the device. **Do not remove the blue cap from the BAXJECT II device.** Do not touch the exposed white plastic spike.
7. Turn the system over, so that the diluent vial is on top. Quickly insert the white plastic spike fully into the RECOMBINATE vial stopper by pushing straight down. The vacuum will draw the diluent into the RECOMBINATE vial.
8. Swirl gently until RECOMBINATE is completely dissolved. After reconstitution, the solution should be colorless to faint yellow, and substantially free from foreign particles.

NOTE: Do not refrigerate after reconstitution. (See **Administration**)

Administration: Use Aseptic Technique

RECOMBINATE is administered by intravenous (IV) injection after reconstitution.

Administer at room temperature.

RECOMBINATE should be administered not more than 3 hours after reconstitution.

Intravenous Syringe Injection

Parenteral drug products should be inspected for particulate matter and discoloration prior to administration, whenever solution and container permit. The solution should be colorless to faint yellow in appearance. If not, do not use the solution and notify Baxter immediately.

	Hemorrhage	
Degree of hemorrhage	**Required peak post-infusion Factor VIII activity in the blood (as % of normal or IU/dL plasma)**	**Frequency of Infusion**
Early hemarthrosis or muscle bleed or oral bleed	20-40	Begin infusion every 12 to 24 hours for one-three days until the bleeding episode is resolved (as indicated by pain) or healing is achieved.
More extensive hemarthrosis, muscle bleed, or hematoma	30-60	Repeat infusion every 12 to 24 hours for (usually) three days or more until pain and disability are resolved.
Life-threatening bleeds such as head injury, throat bleed, severe abdominal pain	60-100	Repeat infusions every 8 to 24 hours until threat is resolved.
	Surgery	
Type of operation		
Minor surgery, including tooth extraction	60-80	A single infusion plus oral antifibrinolytic therapy within one hour is sufficient in approximately 70% of cases.
Major surgery	80-100 (pre- and post-operative)	Repeat infusion every 8 to 24 hours, depending on state of healing.

Color Code	Dosage Strength	RECOMBINATE Supplied with 10 mL sWFI
Light blue bar	220-400 IU per vial	NDC 0944-2831-10
Pink bar	401-800 IU per vial	NDC 0944-2832-10
Green bar	801-1240 IU per vial	NDC 0944-2833-10
Purple bar	1241-1800 IU per vial	NDC 0944-2834-10
Orange bar	1801-2400 IU per vial	NDC 0944-2835-10

Plastic syringes are recommended for use with this product since proteins such as RECOMBINATE tend to stick to the surface of glass syringes.

1. Remove the blue cap from the BAXJECT II device. Connect the syringe to the BAXJECT II device. DO NOT INJECT AIR.
2. Turn over the connected vials so that the RECOMBINATE vial is on top. Draw the factor concentrate into the syringe by pulling the plunger back slowly.
3. Disconnect the syringe; attach a suitable needle and inject intravenously as instructed under **Rate of Administration**.
4. If a patient is to receive more than one vial of RECOMBINATE, the contents of multiple vials may be drawn into the same syringe. **Please note that the BAXJECT II device is intended for use with a single vial of RECOMBINATE and Sterile Water for Injection only, therefore reconstituting and withdrawing a second vial into the syringe requires a second BAXJECT II device.**

Rate of Administration

The rate of administration should be a rate that ensures the comfort of the patient. Preparations of RECOMBINATE can be administered at a rate of up to 10 mL per minute with no significant reactions when reconstituted with 10 mL of sWFI.

The pulse rate should be determined before and during administration of RECOMBINATE. Should a significant increase in pulse rate occur, reducing the rate of administration or temporarily halting the injection usually allows the symptoms to disappear promptly.

HOW SUPPLIED

RECOMBINATE is available in five different strengths in single-dose vials. The strength is designated on the outer box and on the vial label using the following color codes:
[See second table above]

RECOMBINATE is packaged with 10 mL of Sterile Water for Injection, USP, a BAXJECT II Needleless Transfer Device, one physician insert and one patient insert.

STORAGE

RECOMBINATE can be refrigerated [2°-8°C (36°-46°F)] or stored at room temperature, not to exceed 30°C (86°F). Avoid freezing to prevent damage to the diluent vial. Do not use beyond the expiration date printed on the box.

CLINICAL STUDIES

Over the investigational period of the original safety and efficacy study of RECOMBINATE, none of the 69 subjects without an inhibitor at entry into the study developed an inhibitor. In the previously untreated patient group there were 73 eligible subjects with Factor VIII levels less than or equal to 2% who received at least one RECOMBINATE treatment (median days 100, range 3-821) and who were

tested for an inhibitor after treatment with RECOMBINATE. Of this group, 23 individuals (32%) developed a detectable inhibitor (median days on treatment at time of detection 10, range 3-69) and of these, 8 subjects (11%) showed a titer greater than 10 B.U.

REFERENCES

1. Bray GL, Gomperts ED, Courter S, Gruppo R, *et al*: A Multicenter Study of Recombinant Factor VIII (Recombinate): Safety, Efficacy, and Inhibitor Risk in Previously Untreated Patients with Hemophilia A. **Blood 83**: 2428-2435, 1944

2. White GC, McMillan CW, Kingdon HS, *et al*: Use of recombinant antihemophilic factor in the treatment of two patients with classic hemophilia. **New Eng J Med 320**: 166-170, 1989

3. Kessler CM: An Introduction to Factor VIII Inhibitors: The Detection and Quantitation. **Am J Med 91 (Suppl 5A)**:1S-5S, 1991

4. Abildgaard CF, Simone JV, Corrigan JJ, *et al*: Treatment of hemophilia with glycine-precipitated Factor VIII. **New Eng J Med 275**:471-475, 1966

To enroll in the confidential, industry-wide Patient Notification System, call 1-888-UPDATE U (1-888-873-2838).

Baxter, RECOMBINATE, HEMOFIL, and BAXJECT are trademarks of Baxter International Inc.

Manufactured by:

Baxter Healthcare Corporation

Westlake Village, CA 91362 USA

U.S. License No. 140   Printed in USA Issued: March 2010
714470

RECOMBINATE
[Antihemophilic Factor (Recombinant)]
PATIENT INFORMATION

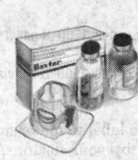

This leaflet summarizes important information about RECOMBINATE. Please read it carefully before using this medicine. This information does not take the place of talking with your healthcare provider, and it does not include all of the important information about RECOMBINATE. If you have any questions after reading this, ask your healthcare provider.

Do not attempt to self-infuse unless you have been taught how by your doctor or hemophilia center.

What is RECOMBINATE [Antihemophilic Factor (Recombinant)]?

RECOMBINATE is a medicine used to replace a clotting factor (Factor VIII or antihemophilic factor) that is missing in people with hemophilia A (also called "classic" hemophilia). Hemophilia A is an inherited bleeding disorder that prevents blood from clotting normally.

RECOMBINATE is used to prevent and control bleeding in people with hemophilia A.

RECOMBINATE is not used to treat von Willebrand's Disease.

Who should not use RECOMBINATE [Antihemophilic Factor (Recombinant)]?

You should not use RECOMBINATE if you
- are allergic to mouse, hamster or bovine proteins.
- are allergic to any ingredients in RECOMBINATE (such as calcium, histidine, human albumin, polyethylene glycol, polysorbate-80 and sodium).

Tell your healthcare provider if you are pregnant or breastfeeding because RECOMBINATE may not be right for you.

How should I use RECOMBINATE [Antihemophilic Factor (Recombinant)]?

RECOMBINATE is given directly into the blood stream.

You may infuse RECOMBINATE at a hemophilia treatment center, at your healthcare provider's office or in your home. You should be trained on how to do infusions by your hemophilia treatment center or healthcare provider. Many people with hemophilia A learn to infuse their RECOMBINATE by themselves or with the help of a family member.

You must carefully follow your doctor's or other healthcare provider's instructions regarding the dose and schedule for infusing RECOMBINATE so that your treatment will work best for you.

Your healthcare provider will tell you how much RECOMBINATE to use based on your weight, the severity of your hemophilia A, and where you are bleeding.

You may have to have blood tests done after getting RECOMBINATE to be sure that your blood level of Factor VIII is high enough to clot your blood.

Call your healthcare provider right away if your bleeding does not stop after taking RECOMBINATE.

What should I tell my healthcare provider before I use RECOMBINATE [Antihemophilic Factor (Recombinant)]?

You should tell your healthcare provider if you
- have or have had any medical problems.
- take any medicines, including non-prescription medicines, dietary supplements and herbal remedies.
- have any allergies, including allergies to mouse, hamster or bovine proteins.
- are nursing.
- are pregnant or planning to become pregnant.
- have been told that you have inhibitors to Factor VIII (because Factor VIII may not work for you).

What are the possible side effects of RECOMBINATE [Antihemophilic Factor (Recombinant)]?

You could have an allergic reaction to RECOMBINATE.

Call your healthcare provider right away and stop treatment if you get:

- Rash or hives
- itching
- tightness of the throat
- chest pain or tightness
- difficulty breathing
- light-headed, dizziness
- fainting

The most common side effects are chills, flushing, rash, and nose bleeds. These are not all possible side effects with RECOMBINATE. You can ask your healthcare provider for information that is written for healthcare professionals. Tell your doctor about any side effect that bothers you or that does not go away.

What are the RECOMBINATE [Antihemophilic Factor (Recombinant)] dosage strengths?

RECOMBINATE comes in five different dosage strengths. The actual strength will be imprinted on the label and on the box. The five different strengths are coded as follows:

Light-Blue	Nominal dosage strength of approximately 250 IU per vial (220 - 400 IU/vial).
Pink	Nominal dosage strength of approximately 500 IU per vial (401 - 800 IU/vial).
Green	Nominal dosage strength of approximately 1000 IU per vial (801 - 1240 IU/vial).
Purple	Nominal dosage strength of approximately 1500 IU per vial (1241 - 1800 IU/vial).
Orange	Nominal dosage strength of approximately 2000 IU per vial (1801 - 2400 IU/vial).

Always check the potency printed on the label to make sure you are using the strength prescribed by your doctor. Always check the expiration date printed on the box. You should not use the product after the expiration date printed on the box.

How do I store RECOMBINATE [Antihemophilic Factor (Recombinant)]?

RECOMBINATE vials containing powdered product (without sterile diluent added) should be stored in a refrigerator (2° to 8°C [36° to 46°F]) or at room temperature (up to 30°C [86°F]).

If you choose to store RECOMBINATE at room temperature:
- it should remain at room temperature until infused.
- do not put room temperature product back in the refrigerator.

Store vials in their original box and protect them from extreme exposure to light.

Do not freeze.

Reconstituted product (after mixing dry product with wet diluent) must be used within 3 hours and cannot be stored or refrigerated. Any RECOMBINATE left in the vial at the end of your infusion should be discarded.

What else should I know about RECOMBINATE [Antihemophilic Factor (Recombinant)] and hemophilia A?

Your body may form inhibitors to Factor VIII. An inhibitor is part of the body's normal defense system. If you form inhibitors, it may stop RECOMBINATE from working properly. Call your healthcare provider right away if your bleeding does not stop after taking RECOMBINATE. Consult with your healthcare provider to make sure you are carefully monitored with blood tests for the development of inhibitors to Factor VIII.

Resources at Baxter available to the patients:

Contact Baxter to receive more product information:
Baxter Customer Service 1-800-423-2090

RECOMBINATE
[Antihemophilic Factor (Recombinant)]
(For intravenous use only)
INSTRUCTIONS FOR USE

1. **Do not attempt to do an infusion to yourself unless you have been taught how by your doctor or hemophilia center.** In a quiet place, prepare a clean flat surface and gather all the materials you will need for the infusion. Check the expiration date, and let the vial with the RECOMBINATE concentrate and the Sterile Water for Injection, USP (diluent) warm up to room temperature. Wash your hands and put on clean exam gloves. If infusing yourself at home, the use of gloves is optional.

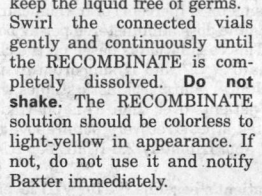

2. Remove caps from the RECOMBINATE concentrate and diluent vials to expose the centers of the rubber stoppers.

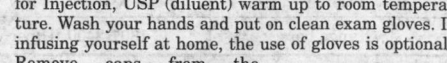

3. Disinfect the stoppers with an alcohol swab (or other suitable solution suggested by your doctor or hemophilia center) by rubbing the stoppers firmly for several seconds, and allow to dry prior to use. Place the vials on a flat surface.

4. Open the BAXJECT II device package by peeling away the lid, without touching the inside of the package. **Do not remove the BAXJECT II device from the package.**

5. Turn the package with the BAXJECT II device upside down, and place it over the top of the diluent vial. Fully insert the clear plastic spike of the device into the center of the diluent vial's stopper by pushing straight down. Grip the package at its edge and lift it off the device. Be careful not to touch the white plastic spike. **Do not remove the blue cap from BAXJECT II device.** The diluent vial now has the BAXJECT II device connected to it and is ready to be connected to the RECOMBINATE vial.

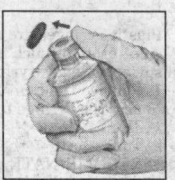

6. To connect the diluent vial to the RECOMBINATE vial, turn the diluent vial over and place it on top of the vial containing RECOMBINATE concentrate. Fully insert the white plastic spike into the RECOMBINATE vial's stopper by pushing straight down. Diluent will flow into the RECOMBINATE vial. This should be done right away to keep the liquid free of germs.

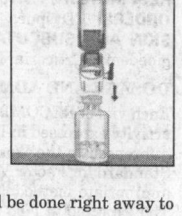
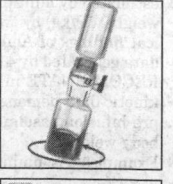

7. Swirl the connected vials gently and continuously until the RECOMBINATE is completely dissolved. **Do not shake.** The RECOMBINATE solution should be colorless to light-yellow in appearance. If not, do not use it and notify Baxter immediately.

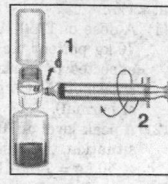

8. Take off the blue cap from the BAXJECT II device and connect the syringe. **BE CAREFUL TO NOT INJECT AIR.**

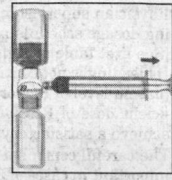

9. Turn over the connected vials so that the RECOMBINATE vial is on top. Draw the RECOMBINATE solution into the syringe by pulling back the plunger slowly. Disconnect the syringe from the vials. Attach the infusion needle to the syringe using a winged (butterfly) infusion set, if available. Point the needle up and remove any air bubbles by gently tapping the syringe with your finger and slowly and carefully pushing air out of the syringe and needle. If you are using more than one vial of RECOMBINATE, the contents of more than one vial may be drawn into the same syringe. However, you will need a separate diluent and BAXJECT II device to mix each additional vial of RECOMBINATE.

10. Apply a tourniquet, and get the injection site ready by wiping the skin well with an alcohol swab (or other suitable solution suggested by your doctor or hemophilia center).

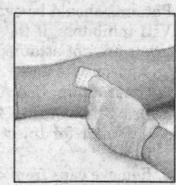

11. Insert the needle into the vein, and remove the tourniquet. Slowly infuse the RECOMBINATE. **Do not infuse any faster than 10 mL per minute for RECOMBINATE dissolved with 10 mL of sWFI.**

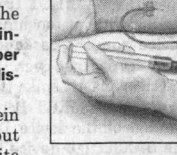

12. Take the needle out of the vein and use sterile gauze to put pressure on the infusion site for several minutes. **Do not recap the needle. Place it with the used syringe in a hard-walled Sharps container for proper disposal.**

13. Remove the peel-off label from the RECOMBINATE vial and place it in your logbook. Clean any spilled blood with a freshly prepared mixture of 1 part bleach and 9 parts water, soap and water, or any household disinfecting solution.

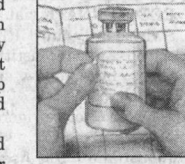

14. Dispose of the used vials and BAXJECT II system in your hard-walled Sharps container, without taking them apart. Do not dispose of these supplies in ordinary household trash.

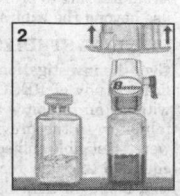

Important: Contact your doctor or local Hemophilia Treatment Center if you experience any problems.
BAXTER, RECOMBINATE, HEMOFIL, AND BAXJECT are trademarks of Baxter International Inc.
Manufactured by:
Baxter Healthcare Corporation
Westlake Village, CA 91362 USA

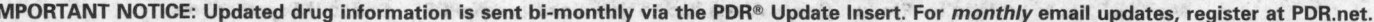

U.S. License No. 140
Printed in USA
Issued: March 2010
714470

Baxter Healthcare Corporation
Anesthesia & Critical Care

**95 SPRING STREET
NEW PROVIDENCE, NJ 07974**

Direct Product Inquiries to:
Professional Services Department
(800) ANA DRUG
(800) 262-3784
Sales and Ordering:
To place an order, call or fax:
(800) 667-0959
Fax 877-702-3580

SUPRANE   ℞
[sū´prān]
(desflurane, USP)
Volatile Liquid for Inhalation
℞ only

DESCRIPTION

SUPRANE (desflurane, USP), a nonflammable liquid administered via vaporizer, is a general inhalation anesthetic. It is (±)1,2,2,2-tetrafluoroethyl difluoromethyl ether:

$$\begin{array}{ccccc} & F & H & F & \\ | & | & | & | & | \\ F-C & - & C-O- & C-H \\ | & | & | & | & | \\ & F & F & F & \end{array}$$

Some physical constants are:

Molecular weight	168.04
Specific gravity (at 20°C/4°C)	1.465
Vapor pressure in mm Hg	669 mm Hg @ 20°C
	731 mm Hg @ 22°C
	757 mm Hg @ 22.8°C
	(boiling point;1atm)
	764 mm Hg @ 23°C
	798 mm Hg @ 24°C
	869 mm Hg @ 26°C

Partition coefficients at 37°C:

Blood/Gas	0.424
Olive Oil/Gas	18.7
Brain/Gas	0.54

Mean Component/Gas Partition Coefficients:

Polypropylene (Y piece)	6.7
Polyethylene (circuit tube)	16.2
Latex rubber (bag)	19.3
Latex rubber (bellows)	10.4
Polyvinylchloride (endotracheal tube)	34.7

Desflurane is nonflammable as defined by the requirements of International Electrotechnical Commission 601-2-13.
Desflurane is a colorless, volatile liquid below 22.8°C. Data indicate that desflurane is stable when stored under normal room lighting conditions according to instructions.
Desflurane is chemically stable. The only known degradation reaction is through prolonged direct contact with soda lime producing low levels of fluoroform (CHF_3). The amount of CHF_3 obtained is similar to that produced with MAC-equivalent doses of isoflurane. No discernible degradation occurs in the presence of strong acids.
Desflurane does not corrode stainless steel, brass, aluminum, anodized aluminum, nickel plated brass, copper, or beryllium.

CLINICAL PHARMACOLOGY

SUPRANE (desflurane, USP) is a volatile liquid inhalation anesthetic minimally biotransformed in the liver in humans. Less than 0.02% of the SUPRANE absorbed can be recovered as urinary metabolites (compared to 0.2% for isoflurane).
Minimum alveolar concentration (MAC) of desflurane in oxygen for a 25 year-old adult is 7.3%. The MAC of SUPRANE (desflurane, USP) decreases with increasing age and with addition of depressants such as opioids or benzodiazepines (see **DOSAGE AND ADMINISTRATION** for details).
Pharmacokinetics
Due to the volatile nature of desflurane in plasma samples, the washin-washout profile of desflurane was used as a surrogate of plasma pharmacokinetics. Eight healthy male volunteers first breathed 70% N_2O/30% O_2 for 30 minutes and

EMERGENCE AND RECOVERY AFTER OUTPATIENT LAPAROSCOPY 178 FEMALES, AGES 20-47
TIMES IN MINUTES: MEAN ± SD (RANGE)

Induction:	Propofol	Propofol	Desflurane/N_2O	Desflurane/O_2
Maintenance:	Propofol/N_2O	Desflurane/N_2O	Desflurane/N_2O	Desflurane/O_2
Number of Pts:	N = 48	N = 44	N = 43	N = 43
Median age	30	26	29	30
	(20-43)	(21-47)	(21-42)	(20-40)
Anesthetic	49 ± 53	45 ± 35	44 ± 29	41 ± 26
Time	(8-336)	(11-178)	(14-149)	(19-126)
Time to open	7 ± 3	5 ± 2*	5 ± 2*	4 ± 2*
eyes	(2-19)	(2-10)	(2-12)	(1-11)
Time to state	9 ± 4	8 ± 3	7 ± 3*	7 ± 3*
name	(4-22)	(3-18)	(3-16)	(2-15)
Time to stand	80 ± 34	86 ± 55	81 ± 38	77 ± 38
	(40-200)	(30-320)	(35-190)	(35-200)
Time to walk	110 ± 6	122 ± 85	108 ± 59	108 ± 66
	(47-285)	(37-375)	(48-220)	(49-250)
Time to fit for	152 ± 75	157 ± 80	150 ± 66	155 ± 73
discharge	(66-375)	(73-385)	(68-310)	(69-325)

*Differences were statistically significant (p < 0.05) by Dunnett's procedure comparing all treatments to the propofol-propofol/N_2O (induction and maintenance) group. Results for comparisons greater than one hour after anesthesia show no differences between groups and considerable variability within groups.

EMERGENCE AND RECOVERY TIMES IN OUTPATIENT SURGERY 46 MALES, 42 FEMALES, AGES 19-70
TIMES IN MINUTES: MEAN ± SD (RANGE)

Induction:	Thiopental	Thiopental	Thiopental	Desflurane/O_2
Maintenance:	Isoflurane/N_2O	Desflurane/N_2O	Desflurane/O_2	Desflurane/O_2
Number of Pts:	N = 23	N = 21	N = 23	N = 21
Median age	43	40	43	41
	(20-70)	(22-67)	(19-70)	(21-64)
Anesthetic	49 ± 23	50 ± 19	50 ± 27	51 ± 23
Time	(11-94)	(16-80)	(16-113)	(19-117)
Time to open	13 ± 7	9 ± 3*	12 ± 8	8 ± 2*
eyes	(5-33)	(4-16)	(4-39)	(4-13)
Time to state	17 ± 10	11 ± 4*	15 ± 10	9 ± 3*
name	(6-44)	(6-19)	(6-46)	(5-14)
Time to walk	195 ± 67	176 ± 60	168 ± 34	181 ± 42
	(124-365)	(101-315)	(119-258)	(92-252)
Time to fit for	205 ± 53	202 ± 41	197 ± 35	194 ± 37
discharge	(153-365)	(144-315)	(155-280)	(134-288)

*Differences were statistically significant (p < 0.05) by Dunnett's procedure comparing all treatments to the thiopental-isoflurane/N_2O (induction and maintenance) group. Results for comparisons greater than one hour after anesthesia show no differences between groups and considerable variability within groups.

then a mixture of SUPRANE (desflurane, USP) 2.0%, isoflurane 0.4%, and halothane 0.2% for another 30 minutes. During this time, inspired and end-tidal concentrations (F_I and F_A) were measured. The F_A/F_I (washin) value at 30 minutes for desflurane was 0.91, compared to 1.00 for N_2O, 0.74 for isoflurane, and 0.58 for halothane (See **Figure 1**). The washin rates for halothane and isoflurane were similar to literature values. The washin was faster for desflurane than for isoflurane and halothane at all time points. The F_A/F_{AO} (washout) value at 5 minutes was 0.12 for desflurane, 0.22 for isoflurane, and 0.25 for halothane (See **Figure 2**). The washout for SUPRANE was more rapid than that for isoflurane and halothane at all elimination time points. By 5 days, the F_A/F_{AO} for desflurane is 1/20th of that for halothane or isoflurane.

Figure 2. Desflurane Washout
Mean ± SD
8 Normal Male Volunteers

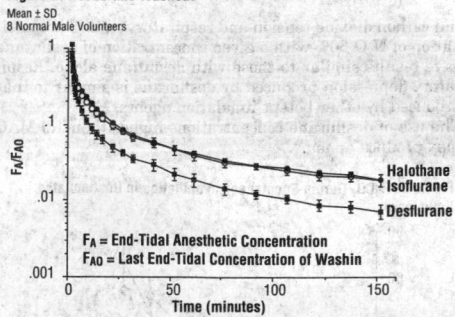

F_A = End-Tidal Anesthetic Concentration
F_{AO} = Last End-Tidal Concentration of Washin

Figure 1. Desflurane Washin
Mean ± SD
8 Normal Male Volunteers

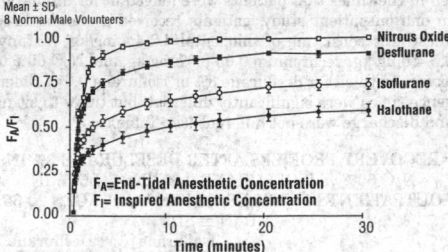

F_A=End-Tidal Anesthetic Concentration
F_I= Inspired Anesthetic Concentration

[See figure at top of next column]
Pharmacodynamics
Changes in the clinical effects of SUPRANE (desflurane, USP) rapidly follow changes in the inspired concentration. The duration of anesthesia and selected recovery measures for SUPRANE are given in the following tables:
In 178 female outpatients undergoing laparoscopy, premedicated with fentanyl (1.5-2.0 μg/kg), anesthesia was initiated with propofol 2.5 mg/kg, desflurane/N_2O 60% in O_2 or desflurane/O_2 alone. Anesthesia was maintained with either propofol 1.5-9.0 mg/kg/hr, desflurane 2.6-8.4% in N_2O 60% in O_2, or desflurane 3.1-8.9% in O_2.
[See first table above]

In 88 unpremedicated outpatients, anesthesia was initiated with thiopental 3-9 mg/kg or desflurane in O_2. Anesthesia was maintained with isoflurane 0.7-1.4% in N_2O 60%, desflurane 1.8-7.7% in N_2O 60%, or desflurane 4.4-11.9% in O_2.
[See second table above]
Recovery from anesthesia was assessed at 30, 60, and 90 minutes following 0.5 MAC desflurane (3%) or isoflurane (0.6%) in N_2O 60% using subjective and objective tests. At 30 minutes after anesthesia, only 43% of the isoflurane group were able to perform the psychometric tests compared to 76% in the desflurane group (p < 0.05).
[See first table at top of next page]
SUPRANE (desflurane, USP) was studied in twelve volunteers receiving no other drugs. Hemodynamic effects during controlled ventilation (PaCO₂ 38mm Hg) were:
[See second table on next page]
When the same volunteers breathed spontaneously during desflurane anesthesia, systemic vascular resistance and mean arterial blood pressure decreased; cardiac index, heart rate, stroke volume, and central venous pressure (CVP) increased compared to values when the volunteers were conscious. Cardiac index, stroke volume, and CVP were greater during spontaneous ventilation than during controlled ventilation.
During spontaneous ventilation in the same volunteers, increasing the concentration of SUPRANE (desflurane, USP) from 3% to 12% decreased tidal volume and increased arte-

RECOVERY TESTS: PERCENT OF PREOPERATIVE BASELINE VALUES 16 MALES, 22 FEMALES, AGES 20-65
PERCENT: MEAN ± SD

| | 60 minutes After Anesthesia | | 90 minutes After Anesthesia | |
Maintenance:	Desflurane/N$_2$O	Isoflurane/N$_2$O	Desflurane/N$_2$O	Isoflurane/N$_2$O
ConfusionΔ	66 ± 6	47 ± 8	75 ± 7*	56 ± 8
FatigueΔ	70 ± 9*	33 ± 6	89 ± 12*	47 ± 8
DrowsinessΔ	66 ± 5*	36 ± 8	76 ± 7*	49 ± 9
ClumsinessΔ	65 ± 5	49 ± 8	80 ± 7*	57 ± 9
Comfort Δ	59 ± 7*	30 ± 6	60 ± 8*	31 ± 7
DSST+ score	74 ± 4*	50 ± 9	75 ± 4*	55 ± 7
Trieger Tests++	67 ± 5	74 ± 6	90 ± 6	83 ± 7

Δ Visual analog scale (values from 0-100; 100 = baseline)
+ DSST = Digit Symbol Substitution Test
++ Trieger Test = Dot Connecting Test
* Differences were statistically significant (p < 0.05) using a two-sample t-test

HEMODYNAMIC EFFECTS OF DESFLURANE DURING CONTROLLED VENTILATION 12 MALE VOLUNTEERS,
AGES 16-26 MEAN ± SD (RANGE)

Total MAC Equivalent	End-Tidal % Des/O$_2$	End-Tidal % Des/N$_2$O	Heart Rate (beats/min)		Mean Arterial Pressure (mm Hg)		Cardiac Index (L/min/m^2)	
			O$_2$	N$_2$O	O$_2$	N$_2$O	O$_2$	N$_2$O
0	0%/21%	0%/0%	69 ± 4 (63-76)	70 ± 6 (62-85)	85 ± 9 (74-102)	85 ± 9 (74-102)	3.7 ± 0.4 (3.0-4.2)	3.7 ± 0.4 (3.0-4.2)
0.8	6%/94%	3%/60%	73 ± 5 (67-80)	77 ± 8 (67-97)	61 ± 5* (55-70)	69 ± 5* (62-80)	3.2 ± 0.5 (2.6-4.0)	3.3 ± 0.5 (2.6-4.1)
1.2	9%/91%	6%/60%	80 ± 5* (72-84)	77 ± 7 (67-90)	59 ± 8* (44-71)	63 ± 8* (47-74)	3.4 ± 0.5 (2.6-4.1)	3.1 ± 0.4* (2.6-3.8)
1.7	12%/88%	9%/60%	94 ± 14* (78-109)	79 ± 9 (61-91)	51 ± 12* (31-66)	59 ± 6* (46-68)	3.5 ± 0.9 (1.7-4.7)	3.0 ± 0.4* (2.4-3.6)

*Differences were statistically significant (p < 0.05) compared to awake values, Newman-Keul's method of multiple comparison.

CARDIOVASCULAR PATIENTS BY AGENT AND TYPE OF SURGERY 418 MALES, 140 FEMALES, AGES 27-87
(MEDIAN 64)

Type of Surgery	13 Centers		1 Center		1 Center	
	Isoflurane	Desflurane	Sufentanil	Desflurane	Fentanyl	Desflurane
CABG	58	57	100	100	25	25
Abd Aorta	29	25	-	-	-	-
Periph Vasc	24	24	-	-	-	-
Carotid Art	45	46	-	-	-	-
Total	156	152	100	100	25	25

rial carbon dioxide tension and respiratory rate. The combination of N$_2$O 60% with a given concentration of desflurane gave results similar to those with desflurane alone. Respiratory depression produced by desflurane is similar to that produced by other potent inhalation agents.
The use of desflurane concentrations higher than 1.5 MAC may produce apnea.

Figure 3. PaCO$_2$ During Spontaneous Ventilation in Unstimulated Volunteers

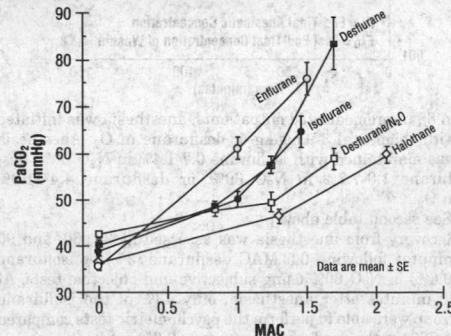

Data are mean ± SE

NOTE: Data for enflurane, halothane and isoflurane are from earlier studies

CLINICAL TRIALS

SUPRANE (desflurane, USP) was evaluated in 1,843 patients including ambulatory (N=1,061), cardiovascular (N=277), geriatric (N=103), neurosurgical (N=40), and pediatric (N=235) patients. Clinical experience with these patients and with 1,087 control patients in these studies not receiving desflurane are described below. Although desflurane can be used in adults for the inhalation induction of anesthesia via mask, it produces a high incidence of respiratory irritation (coughing, breathholding, apnea, increased secretions, laryngospasm). For incidence, see **ADVERSE REACTIONS.** Oxyhemoglobin saturation below 90% occurred in 6% of patients (from pooled data, N = 370 adults).

Ambulatory Surgery
SUPRANE (desflurane, USP) plus N$_2$O was compared to isoflurane plus N$_2$O in multicenter studies (21 sites) of 792 ASA physical status I, II, or III patients aged 18-76 years (median 32).
INDUCTION
Anesthetic induction begun with thiopental and continued with desflurane was associated with a 7% incidence of oxyhemoglobin saturation of 90% or less (from pooled data, N = 307) compared with 5% in patients in whom anesthesia was induced with thiopental and isoflurane (from pooled data, N = 152).
MAINTENANCE & RECOVERY
SUPRANE (desflurane, USP) with or without N$_2$O or other anesthetics was generally well tolerated. There were no differences between desflurane and the other anesthetics studied in the times that patients were judged fit for discharge. In one outpatient study, patients received a standardized anesthetic consisting of thiopental 4.2-4.4 mg/kg, fentanyl 3.5-4.0 µg/kg, vecuronium 0.05-0.07 mg/kg, and N$_2$O 60% in oxygen with either desflurane 3% or isoflurane 0.6%. Emergence times were significantly different; but times to sit up and discharge were not different (see Table).

RECOVERY PROFILES AFTER DESFLURANE 3% IN
N$_2$O 60% vs ISOFLURANE 0.6% IN N$_2$O 60% IN
OUTPATIENTS 16 MALES, 22 FEMALES, AGES 20-65
MEAN ± SD

	Isoflurane	Desflurane
Number	21	17
Anesthetic time (min)	127 ± 80	98 ± 55
Recovery time to:		
Follow commands (min)	11.1 ± 7.9	6.5 ± 2.3*
Sit up (min)	113 ± 27	95 ± 56
Fit for discharge (min)	231 ± 40	207 ± 54

*Difference was statistically significant from the isoflurane group (p < 0.05), unadjusted for multiple comparisons.

Cardiovascular Surgery
Desflurane was compared to isoflurane, sufentanil or fentanyl for the anesthetic management of coronary artery bypass graft (CABG), abdominal aortic aneurysm, peripheral vascular and carotid endarterectomy surgery in 7 studies at 15 centers involving a total of 558 patients. In all patients except the desflurane vs sufentanil study, the volatile anesthetics were supplemented with intravenous opioids, usually fentanyl. Blood pressure and heart rate were controlled by changes in concentration of the volatile anesthetics or opioids and cardiovascular drugs if necessary. Oxygen (100%) was the carrier gas in 253 of 277 desflurane cases (24 of 277 received N$_2$O/O$_2$).
[See third table at left]
No differences were found in cardiovascular outcome (death, myocardial infarction, ventricular tachycardia or fibrillation, heart failure) among desflurane and the other anesthetics.
INDUCTION
Desflurane should not be used as the sole agent for anesthetic induction in patients with coronary artery disease or any patients where increases in heart rate or blood pressure are undesirable. In the desflurane vs sufentanil study, anesthetic induction with desflurane without opioids was associated with new transient ischemia in 14 patients vs 0 in the sufentanil group. In the desflurane group, mean heart rate, arterial pressure, and pulmonary blood pressure increased and stroke volume decreased in contrast to no change in the sufentanil group. Cardiovascular drugs were used frequently in both groups: especially esmolol in the desflurane group (56% vs 0%) and phenylephrine in the sufentanil group (43% vs 27%). When 10 µg/kg of fentanyl was used to supplement induction of anesthesia at one other center, continuous 2-lead ECG analysis showed a low incidence of myocardial ischemia and no difference between desflurane and isoflurane. If desflurane is to be used in patients with coronary artery disease, it should be used in combination with other medications for induction of anesthesia, preferably intravenous opioids and hypnotics.
MAINTENANCE & RECOVERY
In studies where desflurane or isoflurane anesthesia was supplemented with fentanyl, there were no differences in hemodynamic variables or the incidence of myocardial ischemia in the patients anesthetized with desflurane compared to those anesthetized with isoflurane.
During the precardiopulmonary bypass period, in the desflurane vs sufentanil study where the desflurane patients received no intravenous opioid, more desflurane patients required cardiovascular adjuvants to control hemodynamics than the sufentanil patients. During this period, the incidence of ischemia detected by ECG or echocardiography was not statistically different between desflurane (18 of 99) and sufentanil (9 of 98) groups. However, the duration and severity of ECG-detected myocardial ischemia was significantly less in the desflurane group. The incidence of myocardial ischemia after cardiopulmonary bypass and in the ICU did not differ between groups.
Geriatric Surgery
SUPRANE (desflurane, USP) plus N$_2$O was compared to isoflurane plus N$_2$O in a multicenter study (6 sites) of 203 ASA physical status II or III elderly patients, aged 57-91 years (median 71).
INDUCTION
Most patients were premedicated with fentanyl (mean 2 µg/kg), preoxygenated, and received thiopental (mean 4.3 mg/kg IV) or thiamylal (mean 4 mg/kg IV) followed by succinylcholine (mean 1.4 mg/kg IV) for intubation.
MAINTENANCE & RECOVERY
Heart rate and arterial blood pressure remained within 20% of preinduction baseline values during administration of SUPRANE (desflurane, USP) 0.5-7.7% (average 3.6%) with 50-60% N$_2$O. Induction, maintenance, and recovery cardiovascular measurements did not differ from those during isoflurane/N$_2$O administration nor did the postoperative incidence of nausea and vomiting differ. The most common cardiovascular adverse event was hypotension occurring in 8% of the SUPRANE patients and 6% of the isoflurane patients.
Neurosurgery
SUPRANE (desflurane, USP) was studied in 38 patients aged 26-76 years (median 48 years), ASA physical status II or III undergoing neurosurgical procedures for intracranial lesions.
INDUCTION
Induction consisted of standard neuroanesthetic techniques including hyperventilation and thiopental.
MAINTENANCE
No change in cerebrospinal fluid pressure (CSFP) was observed in 8 patients who had intracranial tumors when the dose of desflurane was 0.5 MAC in N$_2$O 50%. In another study of 9 patients with intracranial tumors, 0.8 MAC desflurane/air/O$_2$ did not increase CSFP above postinduction baseline values. In a different study of 10 patients receiving 1.1 MAC desflurane/air/O$_2$, CSFP increased 7 mm Hg (range 3-13 mm Hg increase, with final values of 11-26 mm Hg) above the predrug values.
All volatile anesthetics may increase intracranial pressure in patients with intracranial space occupying lesions. In such patients, desflurane should be administered at 0.8 MAC or less, and in conjunction with a barbiturate induction and hyperventilation (hypocapnia) in the period be-

fore cranial decompression. Appropriate attention must be paid to maintain cerebral perfusion pressure. The use of a lower dose of desflurane and the administration of a barbiturate and mannitol would be predicted to lessen the effect of desflurane on CSFP.

Under hypocapnic conditions ($PaCO_2$ 27 mm Hg) desflurane 1 and 1.5 MAC did not increase cerebral blood flow (CBF) in 9 patients undergoing craniotomies. CBF reactivity to increasing $PaCO_2$ from 27 to 35 mm Hg was also maintained at 1.25 MAC desflurane/air/O_2.

Pediatric Surgery

SUPRANE (desflurane, USP) is not recommended for induction of anesthesia in pediatric patients because of the high incidence of moderate to severe upper airway adverse reactions, including laryngospasm, coughing, breathholding, and secretions, seen in studies of induction of anesthesia in pediatric patients (see **WARNINGS** and **PRECAUTIONS–Pediatric Use**).

SUPRANE is not approved for maintenance of anesthesia in non-intubated pediatric patients due to an increased incidence of respiratory adverse reactions, including coughing, laryngospasm and secretions, seen in one study of maintenance of anesthesia in non-intubated pediatric patients (see **WARNINGS** and **PRECAUTIONS–Pediatric Use**).

MAINTENANCE & RECOVERY IN INTUBATED PEDIATRIC PATIENTS

SUPRANE (desflurane, USP) is approved for maintenance of anesthesia in infants and children after induction of anesthesia with agents other than SUPRANE, and tracheal intubation.

SUPRANE, with or without N_2O, and halothane, with or without N_2O were studied in three clinical trials of pediatric patients aged 2 weeks to 12 years (median 2 years) and ASA physical status I or II. The concentration of SUPRANE (desflurane, USP) required for maintenance of general anesthesia is age-dependent (see **INDIVIDUALIZATION OF DOSE**).

Changes in blood pressure during maintenance of and recovery from anesthesia with desflurane/N_2O/O_2 are similar to those observed with halothane/N_2O/O_2. Heart rate during maintenance of anesthesia is approximately 10 beats per minute faster with desflurane than with halothane. Patients were judged fit for discharge from post-anesthesia care units within one hour with both desflurane and halothane. There were no differences in the incidence of nausea and vomiting between patients receiving desflurane or halothane.

INDIVIDUALIZATION OF DOSE

(Also see **DOSAGE AND ADMINISTRATION**)

Preanesthetic Medication

Issues such as whether or not to premedicate and the choice of premedicant(s) must be individualized. In clinical studies, patients scheduled to be anesthetized with desflurane frequently received IV preanesthetic medication, such as opioid and/or benzodiazepine.

INDUCTION

In adults, some premedicated with opioid, a frequent starting concentration was 3% desflurane, increased in 0.5-1.0% increments every 2 to 3 breaths. End-tidal concentrations of 4-11% SUPRANE (desflurane, USP) with and without N_2O, produced anesthesia within 2 to 4 minutes. When desflurane was tested as the primary anesthetic induction agent, the incidence of upper airway irritation (apnea, breathholding, laryngospasm, coughing and secretions) was high (see **ADVERSE REACTIONS**). During induction in adults, the overall incidence of oxyhemoglobin desaturation ($SpO_2 < 90\%$) was 6%.

After induction in adults with an intravenous drug such as thiopental or propofol, desflurane can be started at approximately 0.5-1 MAC, whether the carrier gas is O_2 or N_2O/O_2.

MAINTENANCE

Surgical levels of anesthesia in adults may be maintained with concentrations of 2.5-8.5% SUPRANE (desflurane, USP) with or without the concomitant use of nitrous oxide. In children, surgical levels of anesthesia may be maintained with concentrations of 5.2-10% SUPRANE with or without the concomitant use of nitrous oxide.

During the maintenance of anesthesia, increasing concentrations of SUPRANE (desflurane, USP) produce dose-dependent decreases in blood pressure. Excessive decreases in blood pressure may be due to depth of anesthesia and in such instances may be corrected by decreasing the inspired concentration of SUPRANE.

Concentrations of desflurane exceeding 1 MAC may increase heart rate. Thus with this drug, an increased heart rate may not serve reliably as a sign of inadequate anesthesia. SUPRANE (desflurane, USP) decreases the doses of neuromuscular blocking agents required (see **PRECAUTIONS, Drug Interactions**).

INDICATIONS AND USAGE

SUPRANE (desflurane, USP) is indicated as an inhalation agent for induction and/or maintenance of anesthesia for inpatient and outpatient surgery in adults (see **PRECAUTIONS**).

DOSAGE OF MUSCLE RELAXANT CAUSING 95% DEPRESSION IN NEUROMUSCULAR BLOCKADE

Desflurane Concentration	Mean ED_{95} (µg/kg) Pancuronium	Atracurium	Succinylcholine
0.65 MAC 60% N_2O/O_2	26	123	-
1.25 MAC 60% N_2O/O_2	18	91	-
1.25 MAC O_2	22	120	362

SUPRANE (desflurane, USP) is not recommended for induction of anesthesia in pediatric patients because of a high incidence of moderate to severe upper airway adverse events (see **WARNINGS**). After induction of anesthesia with agents other than SUPRANE, and tracheal intubation, SUPRANE is indicated for maintenance of anesthesia in infants and children.

CONTRAINDICATIONS

SUPRANE (desflurane, USP) should not be used in patients with a known or suspected genetic susceptibility to malignant hyperthermia.

Known sensitivity to SUPRANE (desflurane, USP) or to other halogenated agents.

WARNINGS

Perioperative Hyperkalemia

Use of inhaled anesthetic agents has been associated with rare increases in serum potassium levels that have resulted in cardiac arrhythmias and death in pediatric patients during the postoperative period. Patients with latent as well as overt neuromuscular disease, particularly Duchenne muscular dystrophy, appear to be most vulnerable. Concomitant use of succinylcholine has been associated with most, but not all, of these cases. These patients also experienced significant elevations in serum creatinine kinase levels and, in some cases, changes in urine consistent with myoglobinuria. Despite the similarity in presentation to malignant hyperthermia, none of these patients exhibited signs or symptoms of muscle rigidity or hypermetabolic state. Early and aggressive intervention to treat the hyperkalemia and resistant arrhythmias is recommended, as is subsequent evaluation for latent neuromuscular disease.

Malignant Hyperthermia

In susceptible individuals, potent inhalation anesthetic agents may trigger a skeletal muscle hypermetabolic state leading to high oxygen demand and the clinical syndrome known as malignant hyperthermia. In genetically susceptible pigs, desflurane induced malignant hyperthermia. The clinical syndrome is signalled by hypercapnia, and may include muscle rigidity, tachycardia, tachypnea, cyanosis, arrhythmias, and/or unstable blood pressure. Some of these nonspecific signs may also appear during light anesthesia: acute hypoxia, hypercapnia, and hypovolemia.

Treatment of malignant hyperthermia includes discontinuation of triggering agents, administration of intravenous dantrolene sodium, and application of supportive therapy. (Consult prescribing information for dantrolene sodium intravenous for additional information on patient management.) Renal failure may appear later, and urine flow should be monitored and sustained if possible.

Respiratory Adverse Reactions in Pediatric Patients

SUPRANE (desflurane, USP) is not recommended for induction of general anesthesia via mask in children due to a high incidence of moderate to severe respiratory adverse reactions seen in clinical studies (see **PRECAUTIONS–Pediatric Use**).

SUPRANE is not approved for maintenance of anesthesia in non-intubated children due to an increased incidence of respiratory adverse reactions, including coughing, laryngospasm and secretions (see **PRECAUTIONS–Pediatric Use**).

Administration of Suprane

SUPRANE (desflurane, USP) should be administered only by persons trained in the administration of general anesthesia, using a vaporizer specifically designed and designated for use with desflurane. Facilities for maintenance of a patent airway, artificial ventilation, oxygen enrichment, and circulatory resuscitation must be immediately available. Hypotension and respiratory depression increase as anesthesia is deepened.

PRECAUTIONS

During the maintenance of anesthesia, increasing concentrations of SUPRANE (desflurane, USP) produce dose-dependent decreases in blood pressure. Excessive decreases in blood pressure may be related to depth of anesthesia and in such instances may be corrected by decreasing the inspired concentration of SUPRANE.

Concentrations of desflurane exceeding 1 MAC may increase heart rate. Thus an increased heart rate may not be a sign of inadequate anesthesia.

In patients with intracranial space occupying lesions, SUPRANE (desflurane, USP) should be administered at 0.8 MAC or less, in conjunction with a barbiturate induction and hyperventilation (hypocapnia). Appropriate measures should be taken to maintain cerebral perfusion pressure (see **CLINICAL TRIALS, Neurosurgery**).

In patients with coronary artery disease, maintenance of normal hemodynamics is important to the avoidance of myocardial ischemia. Desflurane should not be used as the sole agent for anesthetic induction in patients with coronary artery disease or patients where increases in heart rate or blood pressure are undesirable. It should be used with other medications, preferably intravenous opioids and hypnotics (see **CLINICAL TRIALS, Cardiovascular Surgery**).

Inspired concentrations of SUPRANE (desflurane, USP) greater than 12% have been safely administered to patients, particularly during induction of anesthesia. Such concentrations will proportionately dilute the concentration of oxygen; therefore, maintenance of an adequate concentration of oxygen may require a reduction of nitrous oxide or air if these gases are used concurrently.

The recovery from general anesthesia should be assessed carefully before patients are discharged from the post anesthesia care unit (PACU).

SUPRANE (desflurane, USP), like some other inhalational anesthetics, can react with desiccated carbon dioxide (CO_2) absorbents to produce carbon monoxide which may result in elevated levels of carboxyhemoglobin in some patients. Case reports suggest that barium hydroxide lime and soda lime become desiccated when fresh gases are passed through the CO_2 absorber cannister at high flow rates over many hours or days. When a clinician suspects that CO_2 absorbent may be desiccated, it should be replaced before the administration of SUPRANE (desflurane, USP).

As with other halogenated anesthetic agents, SUPRANE (desflurane, USP) may cause sensitivity hepatitis in patients who have been sensitized by previous exposure to halogenated anesthetics (see **CONTRAINDICATIONS**).

Drug Interactions

No clinically significant adverse interactions with commonly used preanesthetic drugs, or drugs used during anesthesia (muscle relaxants, intravenous agents, and local anesthetic agents) were reported in clinical trials. The effect of desflurane on the disposition of other drugs has not been determined.

Like isoflurane, desflurane does not predispose to premature ventricular arrhythmias in the presence of exogenously infused epinephrine in swine.

BENZODIAZEPINES AND OPIOIDS (MAC REDUCTION)

Benzodiazepines (midazolam 25-50 µg/kg) decrease the MAC of desflurane by 16% as do the opioids (fentanyl 3-6 µg/kg) by 50% (see **DOSAGE AND ADMINISTRATION**).

NEUROMUSCULAR BLOCKING AGENTS

Anesthetic concentrations of desflurane at equilibrium (administered for 15 or more minutes before testing) reduced the ED_{95} of succinylcholine by approximately 30% and that of atracurium and pancuronium by approximately 50% compared to N_2O/opioid anesthesia. The effect of desflurane on duration of nondepolarizing neuromuscular blockade has not been studied.

[See table above]

Dosage reduction of neuromuscular blocking agents during induction of anesthesia may result in delayed onset of conditions suitable for endotracheal intubation or inadequate muscle relaxation, because potentiation of neuromuscular blocking agents requires equilibration of muscle with the delivered partial pressure of desflurane.

Among nondepolarizing drugs, only pancuronium and atracurium interactions have been studied. In the absence of specific guidelines:

1. For endotracheal intubation, do not reduce the dose of nondepolarizing muscle relaxants or succinylcholine.
2. During maintenance of anesthesia, the dose of nondepolarizing muscle relaxants is likely to be reduced compared to that during N_2O/opioid anesthesia. Administration of supplemental doses of muscle relaxants should be guided by the response to nerve stimulation.

Renal or Hepatic Insufficiency

Nine patients receiving SUPRANE (desflurane, USP) (N=9) were compared to 9 patients receiving isoflurane, all with chronic renal insufficiency (serum creatinine 1.5-6.9 mg/dL). No differences in hematological or biochemical tests, including renal function evaluation, were seen between the two groups. Similarly, no differences were found in a comparison of patients receiving either SUPRANE (desflurane, USP) (N=28) or isoflurane (N=30) undergoing renal transplant.

Eight patients receiving SUPRANE (desflurane, USP) were compared to six patients receiving isoflurane, all with chronic hepatic disease (viral hepatitis, alcoholic hepatitis, or cirrhosis). No differences in hematological or biochemical tests, including hepatic enzymes and hepatic function evaluation, were seen.

MAINTENANCE IN NONINTUBATED PEDIATRIC PATIENTS (FACE MASK OR LMA USED; N=300)
All Respiratory Events* (>1% of All Pediatric Patients)

	All Ages (N=300)	2-6 yr (N=150)	7-11 yr (N=81)	12-16 yr (N=69)
Any respiratory events	39%	42%	33%	39%
Airway obstruction	4%	5%	4%	3%
Breath-holding	3%	2%	3%	4%
Coughing	26%	33%	19%	22%
Laryngospasm	13%	16%	7%	13%
Secretion	12%	13%	10%	12%
Non-specific desaturation	2%	2%	1%	1%

*Minor, moderate and severe respiratory events

Frequency of Events Occurring in Greater Than 1% of Clinical Trial Patients
(in Reports Deemed "Probably Causally Related")

Induction (use as a mask inhalation agent)

ADULT PATIENTS (N=370):   Coughing 34%, breathholding 30%, apnea 15%, increased secretions*, laryngospasm*, oxyhemoglobin desaturation (SpO₂ < 90%)*, pharyngitis*.

Maintenance or Recovery

ADULT AND INTUBATED PEDIATRIC PATIENTS (N=687):

Body as a Whole	Headache
Cardiovascular	Bradycardia, hypertension, nodal arrhythmia, tachycardia
Digestive	Nausea 27%, vomiting 16%
Nervous System	Increased salivation
Respiratory	Apnea*, breathholding, cough increased*, laryngospasm*, pharyngitis
Special Senses	Conjunctivitis (conjunctival hyperemia)

*Incidence of events: 3%-10%

Frequency of Events Occurring in Less Than 1% of Patients
(in Reports Deemed "Probably Causally Related")

Reported in 3 or more patients, regardless of severity

Adverse reactions reported only from postmarketing experience or in the literature, not seen in clinical trials, are considered rare and are italicized.

Cardiovascular	Arrhythmia, bigeminy, abnormal electrocardiogram, myocardial ischemia, vasodilation
Digestive	*Hepatitis*
Nervous System	Agitation, dizziness
Respiratory	Asthma, dyspnea, hypoxia

Frequency of Events Occurring in Less Than 1% of Clinical Trial Patients
(in Reports Deemed "Causal Relationship Unknown")

Reported in 3 or more patients, regardless of severity

Body as a Whole	Fever
Cardiovascular	Hemorrhage, myocardial infarct
Metabolic and Nutrition	Increased creatinine phosphokinase
Musculoskeletal System	Myalgia
Skin and Appendages	Pruritus

Carcinogenesis, Mutagenesis, Impairment of Fertility

Animal carcinogenicity studies have not been performed with SUPRANE (desflurane, USP). *In vitro* and *in vivo* genotoxicity studies did not demonstrate mutagenicity or chromosomal damage by SUPRANE. Tests for genotoxicity included the Ames mutation assay, the metaphase analysis of human lymphocytes, and the mouse micronucleus assay. Fertility was not affected after 1 MAC-Hour per day exposure (cumulative 63 and 14 MAC-Hours for males and females, respectively). At higher doses, parental toxicity (mortalities and reduced weight gain) was observed which could affect fertility.

Pregnancy

TERATOGENIC EFFECTS

No teratogenic effect was observed at approximately 10 and 13 cumulative MAC-Hour exposures at 1 MAC-Hour per day during organogenesis in rats or rabbits. At higher doses increased incidences of post-implantation loss and maternal toxicity were observed. However, at 10 MAC-Hours cumulative exposure in rats, about 6% decrease in the weight of male pups was observed at preterm caesarean delivery.

PREGNANCY CATEGORY B

There are no adequate and well-controlled studies in pregnant women. SUPRANE (desflurane, USP) should be used during pregnancy only if the potential benefit justifies the potential risk to the fetus.

Rats exposed to desflurane at 1 MAC-Hour per day from gestation day 15 to lactation day 21, did not show signs of dystocia. Body weight of pups delivered by these dams at birth and during lactation were comparable to that of control pups. No treatment related behavioral changes were reported in these pups during lactation.

Labor and Delivery

The safety of desflurane during labor or delivery has not been demonstrated.

Nursing Mothers

The concentrations of desflurane in milk are probably of no clinical importance 24 hours after anesthesia. Because of rapid washout, desflurane concentrations in milk are predicted to be below those found with other volatile potent anesthetics.

Pediatric Use

SUPRANE (desflurane, USP) is approved for maintenance of anesthesia in infants and children after induction of anesthesia with agents other than SUPRANE, and tracheal intubation.

SUPRANE is not recommended for induction of general anesthesia via mask in children because of the high incidence of moderate to severe respiratory adverse reactions, including laryngospasm (50%), coughing (72%), breathholding (68%), increase in secretions (21%) and oxyhemoglobin desaturation (SpO₂ <90%) (26%) seen in clinical studies.

SUPRANE is not approved for maintenance of anesthesia in non-intubated children due to an increased incidence of respiratory adverse reactions (see below).

In a clinical safety trial conducted in children aged 2 to 16 years (mean 7.4 years), following induction with another agent, SUPRANE and isoflurane (in N₂O/O₂) were compared when delivered via face mask or laryngeal mask airway (LMA) for maintenance of anesthesia, after induction with intravenous propofol or inhaled sevoflurane, in order to assess the relative incidence of respiratory adverse events.

[See first table above]

SUPRANE was associated with higher rates (compared with isoflurane) of coughing, laryngospasm and secretions with an overall rate of respiratory events of 39%. Of the pediatric patients exposed to desflurane, 5% experienced severe laryngospasm (associated with significant desaturation; *i.e.* SpO₂ of <90% for >15 seconds, or requiring succinylcholine), across all ages, 2-16 years old. Individual age group incidences of severe laryngospasm were 9% for 2-6 years old, 1% for 7-11 years old, and 1% for 12-16 years old. Removal of LMA under deep anesthesia (MAC range 0.6-2.3 with a mean of 1.12 MAC) was associated with a further increase in frequency of respiratory adverse events as compared to awake LMA removal or LMA removal under deep anesthesia with the comparator. The frequency and severity of non-respiratory adverse events were comparable between the two groups.

The incidence of respiratory events under these conditions was highest in children aged 2-6 years. Therefore, similar studies in children under the age of 2 years were not initiated.

Geriatric Use

The average MAC for SUPRANE (desflurane, USP) in a 70 year old patient is two-thirds the MAC for a 20 year old patient (see **DOSAGE AND ADMINISTRATION**).

Neurosurgical Use

SUPRANE (desflurane, USP) may produce a dose-dependent increase in cerebrospinal fluid pressure (CSFP) when administered to patients with intracranial space occupying lesions. Desflurane should be administered at 0.8 MAC or less, and in conjunction with a barbiturate induction and hyperventilation (hypocapnia) until cerebral decompression in patients with known or suspected increases in CSFP. Appropriate attention must be paid to maintain cerebral perfusion pressure (see **CLINICAL TRIALS, Neurosurgery**).

ADVERSE REACTIONS

Adverse event information is derived from controlled clinical trials, the majority of which were conducted in the United States. The studies were conducted using a variety of premedications, other anesthetics, and surgical procedures of varying length. Most adverse events reported were mild and transient, and may reflect the surgical procedures, patient characteristics (including disease) and/or medications administered.

Of the 2,143 patients exposed to SUPRANE (desflurane, USP) in clinical trials, 370 adults and 152 children were induced with desflurane alone and 987 patients were maintained principally with desflurane. The frequencies given reflect the percent of patients with the event. Each patient was counted once for each type of adverse event. They are presented in alphabetical order according to body system.

[See second table at left]

[See third table at left]

[See fourth table at left]

See **WARNINGS** for information regarding pediatric use and malignant hyperthermia.

Post Marketing Reports

The following adverse reactions have been identified during post-approval use of SUPRANE (desflurane, USP). Because these reactions are reported voluntarily from a population of uncertain size, it is not possible to reliably estimate their frequency or establish a causal relationship to drug exposure.

BLOOD AND LYMPHATIC SYSTEM DISORDERS: Coagulopathy

METABOLISM AND NUTRITION DISORDERS: Hyperkalemia, Hypokalemia, Metabolic acidosis

NERVOUS SYSTEM DISORDERS: Convulsion

EYE DISORDERS: Ocular icterus

CARDIAC DISORDERS: Cardiac arrest, Torsade de pointes, Ventricular failure, Ventricular hypokinesia

VASCULAR DISORDERS: Malignant hypertension, Hemorrhage, Hypotension, Shock

RESPIRATORY, THORACIC AND MEDIASTINAL DISORDERS: Respiratory arrest, Respiratory failure, Respiratory distress, Bronchospasm, Hemoptysis

GASTROINTESTINAL DISORDERS: Pancreatitis acute, Abdominal pain

HEPATOBILIARY DISORDERS: Hepatic failure, Hepatic necrosis, Cytolytic hepatitis, Cholestasis, Jaundice, Hepatic function abnormal, Liver disorder

SKIN AND SUBCUTANEOUS TISSUE DISORDER: Urticaria, Erythema

MUSCULOSKELETAL, CONNECTIVE TISSUE, AND BONE DISORDERS: Rhabdomyolysis

GENERAL DISORDERS AND ADMINISTRATION SITE CONDITIONS: Hyperthermia malignant, Asthenia, Malaise

INVESTIGATIONS: Tranaminases increased, Alanine aminotransferase increased, Aspartate aminotransferase increased, Coagulation test abnormal, Ammonia increased

INJURY, POISONING, AND PROCEDURAL COMPLICATIONS*: Tachyarrhythmia, Palpitations, Eye burns, Blindness transient, Encephalopathy, Ulcerative keratitis, Ocular hyperemia, Visual acuity reduced, Eye irritation, Eye pain, Dizziness, Migraine, Fatigue, Accidental exposure, Skin burning sensation, Drug administration error

*All of reactions categorized within this SOC were accidental exposures to non-patients.

Laboratory Findings

Transient elevations in glucose and white blood cell count may occur as with use of other anesthetic agents.

DRUG ABUSE AND DEPENDENCE

The potential drug abuse liability, and dependence associated with SUPRANE (desflurane, USP) have not been studied.

OVERDOSAGE

In the event of overdosage, or suspected overdosage, take the following actions: discontinue administration of SUPRANE (desflurane, USP), maintain a patent airway, initiate assisted or controlled ventilation with oxygen, and maintain adequate cardiovascular function.

DOSAGE AND ADMINISTRATION

Deliver SUPRANE (desflurane, USP) from a vaporizer specifically designed and designated for use with desflurane. The administration of general anesthesia must be individualized based on the patient's response (see **INDIVIDUALIZATION OF DOSE**). The following two tables provide mean relative potency based upon age and drug interaction studies in predominately ASA physical status I or II patients.

EFFECT OF AGE ON MAC OF DESFLURANE
MEAN ± SD (percent atmospheres)

Age	N	O₂ 100%	N	N₂O 60%
2 weeks	6	9.2 ± 0.0	-	-
10 weeks	5	9.4 ± 0.4	-	-
9 months	4	10.0 ± 0.7	5	7.5 ± 0.8
2 years	3	9.1 ± 0.6	-	-
3 years	-	-	5	6.4 ± 0.4
4 years	4	8.6 ± 0.6	-	-
7 years	5	8.1 ± 0.6	-	-
25 years	4	7.3 ± 0.0	4	4.0 ± 0.3
45 years	4	6.0 ± 0.3	6	2.8 ± 0.6
70 years	6	5.2 ± 0.6	6	1.7 ± 0.4

N = number of crossover pairs (using up-and-down method of quantal response)

Opioids or benzodiazepines decrease the amounts of SUPRANE (desflurane, USP) required to produce anesthesia. The following table is based on studies of drug interaction (MAC reduction).

SUPRANE (desflurane, USP) MAC WITH FENTANYL OR MIDAZOLAM
MEAN ± SD (percent reduction)

Dose	18-30 years	31-65 years
No fentanyl	6.4 ± 0.0	6.3 ± 0.4
3 µg/kg fentanyl	3.5 ± 1.9 (46%)	3.1 ± 0.6 (51%)
6 µg/kg fentanyl	3.0 ± 1.2 (53%)	2.3 ± 1.0 (64%)
No midazolam	6.9 ± 0.1	5.9 ± 0.6
25 µg/kg midazolam	-	4.9 ± 0.9 (16%)
50 µg/kg midazolam	-	4.9 ± 0.5 (17%)

SUPRANE (desflurane, USP) decreases the doses of neuromuscular blocking agents required (see **PRECAUTIONS, Drug Interactions**).

During the maintenance of anesthesia with inflow rates of 2 L/min or more, the alveolar concentration of desflurane will usually be within 10% of the inspired concentration. (F_A/F_I, see **Figure 1** in **Pharmacokinetics** section.)

HOW SUPPLIED

SUPRANE (desflurane, USP), NDC 10019-641-24, is packaged in amber-colored bottles containing 240 mL desflurane.

Safety and Handling

OCCUPATIONAL CAUTION

There is no specific work exposure limit established for SUPRANE (desflurane, USP). However, the National Institute for Occupational Safety and Health Administration (NIOSH) recommends that no worker should be exposed at ceiling concentrations greater than 2 ppm of any halogenated anesthetic agent over a sampling period not to exceed one hour.

The predicted effects of acute overexposure by inhalation of SUPRANE (desflurane, USP) include headache, dizziness or (in extreme cases) unconsciousness.

There are no documented adverse effects of chronic exposure to halogenated anesthetic vapors (Waste Anesthetic Gases or WAGs) in the workplace. Although results of some epidemiological studies suggest a link between exposure to halogenated anesthetics and increased health problems (particularly spontaneous abortion), the relationship is not conclusive. Since exposure to WAGs is one possible factor in the findings for these studies, operating room personnel, and pregnant women in particular, should minimize exposure. Precautions include adequate general ventilation in the operating room, the use of a well-designed and well-maintained scavenging system, work practices to minimize leaks and spills while the anesthetic agent is in use, and routine equipment maintenance to minimize leaks.

Storage

Store at room temperature, 15°-30°C (59°-86°F). SUPRANE (desflurane, USP) has been demonstrated to be stable for the period defined by the expiration dating on the label. The bottle cap should be replaced after each use of SUPRANE. Baxter and Suprane are trademarks of Baxter International Inc.

Manufactured for
Baxter Healthcare Corporation
Deerfield, IL 60015 USA
For Product Inquiry 1 800 ANA DRUG (1-800-262-3784)
MLT-00070/10.0   400-447-16

Bayer HealthCare Pharmaceuticals Inc.
**6 WEST BELT
WAYNE, NJ 07470**

Direct Inquiries to:
Phone: 1-888-84-BAYER
(1-888-842-2937)
http//www.bayerhealthcare.com

For Medical Information contact:
Vice President, Medical Communications
1-888-84-Bayer (1-888-842-2937)

ANGELIQ® TABLETS   ℞
[an"ju-lēk']
(Drospirenone and Estradiol)
0.5 mg/1 mg
Rx Only
PRESCRIBING INFORMATION

> **WARNING**
> Estrogens with or without progestins should not be used for the prevention of cardiovascular disease or dementia. (See **WARNINGS, Cardiovascular disorders** and **Dementia.**)
> The Women's Health Initiative (WHI) study reported increased risks of myocardial infarction, stroke, invasive breast cancer, pulmonary emboli, and deep vein thrombosis in postmenopausal women (50 to 79 years of age) during 5 years of treatment with oral conjugated equine estrogens (CE 0.625mg) combined with medroxyprogesterone acetate (MPA 2.5mg) relative to placebo (see **CLINICAL PHARMACOLOGY, Clinical Studies** and **WARNINGS, Cardiovascular disorders** and **Malignant neoplasms, Breast cancer.**)
> The Women's Health Initiative Memory Study (WHIMS), a substudy of WHI, reported increased risk of developing probable dementia in postmenopausal women 65 years of age or older during 5.2 years of treatment with conjugated estrogens alone and during 4 years of treatment with oral conjugated estrogens plus medroxyprogesterone acetate, relative to placebo. It is unknown whether this finding applies to younger postmenopausal women. (See **CLINICAL PHARMACOLOGY, Clinical Studies, WARNINGS, Dementia** and **PRECAUTIONS, Geriatric Use.**)
> Other doses of oral conjugated estrogens with medroxyprogesterone acetate, and other combinations and dosage forms of estrogens and progestins were not studied in the WHI clinical trials, and, in the absence of comparable data, these risks should be assumed to be similar. Because of these risks, estrogens with or without progestins should be prescribed at the lowest effective doses and for the shortest duration consistent with treatment goals and risks for the individual woman.

DESCRIPTION

ANGELIQ TABLETS provide a hormone regimen consisting of film coated tablets each containing 0.5 mg of drospirenone and 1 mg of estradiol. The inactive ingredients are lactose monohydrate NF, corn starch NF, modified starch NF, povidone 25000 USP, magnesium stearate NF, hydroxylpropylmethyl cellulose USP, macrogol 6000 NF, talc USP, titanium dioxide USP, and ferric oxide pigment NF.

Drospirenone, (6R,7R,8R,9S,10R,13S,14S,15S,16S,17S)-1,3´,4´,6,6a,7,8,9,10,11,12,13,14,15,15a,16-hexadecahydro-10,13-dimethylspiro-[17H-dicyclopropa[6,7:15,16]cyclopenta[a]phenanthrene-17,2´(5H)-furan]-3,5´(2H)-dione (CAS) is

a synthetic progestational compound and has a molecular weight of 366.5 and a molecular formula of $C_{24}H_{30}O_3$. Estradiol USP, (Estra–1,3,5(10)–triene–3,17–diol,17β), has a molecular weight of 272.39 and the molecular formula is $C_{18}H_{24}O_2$. The structural formulas are as follows:

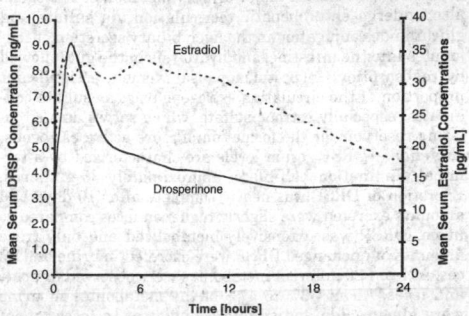

Drospirenone   Estradiol   1/2 H₂O

CLINICAL PHARMACOLOGY

Endogenous estrogens are largely responsible for the development and maintenance of the female reproductive system and secondary sexual characteristics. Although circulating estrogens exist in a dynamic equilibrium of metabolic interconversions, estradiol (E2) is the principal intracellular human estrogen and is substantially more potent than its metabolites, estrone and estriol, at the receptor level.

The primary source of estrogen in normally cycling adult women is the ovarian follicle, which secretes 70 to 500 mcg of estradiol daily, depending on the phase of the menstrual cycle. After menopause, most endogenous estrogen is produced by conversion of androstenedione, secreted by the adrenal cortex, to estrone by peripheral tissues. Thus, estrone and the sulfate-conjugated form, estrone sulfate, are the most abundant circulating estrogens in postmenopausal women.

Estrogens act through binding to nuclear receptors in estrogen-responsive tissues. To date, two estrogen receptors have been identified. These will vary in proportion from tissue to tissue.

Circulating estrogens modulate the pituitary secretion of the gonadotropins, luteinizing hormone (LH), and follicle-stimulating hormone (FSH), through a negative feedback mechanism.

Drospirenone (DRSP) is a synthetic progestin and spironolactone analog with antimineralocorticoid activity. In animals and in vitro, drospirenone has antiandrogenic activity, but no glucocorticoid, antiglucocorticoid, estrogenic, or androgenic activity. Progestins counter estrogenic effects by decreasing the number of nuclear estradiol receptors and suppressing epithelial DNA synthesis in endometrial tissue.

Pharmacokinetics

Absorption: Serum concentrations of DRSP reach peak levels approximately 1 hour after administration of **ANGELIQ** and mean absolute bioavailability of DRSP ranges from 76-85%. Following oral administration, peak serum estradiol concentrations are typically reached 6-8 hours after dosing with **ANGELIQ**. The oral relative bioavailability of estradiol and DRSP following administration of **ANGELIQ** is 107% and 102%, respectively when compared to a combination oral suspension.

The pharmacokinetics of DRSP are dose proportional within the dose range of 0.5-4 mg. Following daily dosing of **ANGELIQ**, steady state DRSP concentrations were observed after 10 days. Mean accumulation ratios for estradiol and DRSP were 1.9 and 2.4, respectively. Mean concentrations at 2 hours for DRSP ranged between 5.9 and 6.7 ng/mL after treatment with **ANGELIQ** for 365 days. Mean steady state serum DRSP and E2 concentrations are shown in Figure 1, and a summary of primary pharmacokinetic parameters following the administration of 1mg E2/1mg DRSP for 28 days is presented in Table 1.

Figure 1: Mean steady state serum drospirenone and estradiol concentrations following daily oral administration of 1 mg E2/0.5 mg DRSP[1]

[1]DRSP levels are simulated based on data obtained after oral administration of 1 mg DRSP/1 mg Estradiol

Table 1: Mean Steady State Pharmacokinetic Parameters of Tablets Containing Drospirenone (1 mg)* and Estradiol (1 mg)

Drospirenone (Mean ± SD)**

Dose	No. of Subjects	C_{max} (ng/mL)	t_{max} (h) Median (range)	AUC (0-24h) (ng·h/mL)	$t_{1/2}$ (h)
1mg E2/1mg DRSP	14	18.3±5.55	1.0 (1.0-2.0)	208±83	42.3±21.3

Estradiol (Mean ± SD)

Dose	No. of Subjects	C_{max} (pg/mL)	t_{max} (h) Median (range)	AUC (0-24h) (pg·h/mL)	$t_{1/2}$ (h)
1mg E2/1mg DRSP	14	43.8±10.0	2.5 (0.5-12.0)	665±178	NA

Estrone (Mean ± SD)

Dose	No. of Subjects	C_{max} (pg/mL)	t_{max} (h) Median (range)	AUC (0-24h) (pg·h/mL)	$t_{1/2}$ (h)
1mg E2/1mg DRSP	14	245±50.6	4.0 (3.0-6.0)	3814±1159	23±6.2

* Angeliq contains 0.5 mg DRSP
** arithmetic mean
NA = Not available, C_{max} = Maximum serum concentration, AUC = area under the curve, t_{max} = time of maximum serum concentration, $t_{1/2}$ = half-life, SD = standard deviation.

[See table 1 above]

Effect of Food: The effect of food on the absorption and bioavailability of DRSP and E2 have not been investigated following the administration of **ANGELIQ**. However, clinical studies with different formulations containing DRSP and E2 have shown that the bioavailability of both drugs is not affected by concomitant food intake.

Distribution: The mean volume of distribution of DRSP is 4.2 L/kg. DRSP does not bind to sex hormone binding globulin (SHBG) or corticosteroid binding globulin (CBG) but binds about 97% to other serum proteins. The distribution of exogenous estrogens is similar to that of endogenous estrogens. Estrogens are widely distributed in the body and are generally found in higher concentrations in the sex hormone target organs. Estradiol circulates in the blood bound to SHBG (37%) and to albumin (61%), while only approximately 1%-2% is unbound.

Metabolism: Mean clearance of DRSP is 1.2 mL/min/kg. DRSP is extensively metabolized after oral administration. The 2 main metabolites of DRSP found in human plasma were identified to be the acid form of DRSP generated by opening of the lactone ring and the 4,5-dihydrodrospirenone-3-sulfate, both of which are formed without the involvement of the cytochrome P450 system. These metabolites were shown not to be pharmacologically active. In *in vitro* studies with human liver microsomes, DRSP was metabolized only to a minor extent mainly by Cytochrome P450 3A4 (CYP3A4).

Exogenous estrogens are metabolized in the same manner as endogenous estrogens. Circulating estrogens exist in a dynamic equilibrium of metabolic interconversions. These transformations take place mainly in the liver. Estradiol is converted reversibly to estrone, and both can be converted to estriol, which is the major urinary metabolite. Estrogens also undergo enterohepatic recirculation via sulfate and glucuronide conjugation in the liver, biliary secretion of conjugates into the intestine, and hydrolysis in the gut followed by reabsorption. In postmenopausal women, a significant proportion of the circulating estrogens exist as sulfate conjugates, especially estrone sulfate, which serves as a circulating reservoir for the formation of more active estrogens.

Excretion: DRSP serum levels are characterized by a terminal elimination half-life of approximately 36-42 hours. Excretion of DRSP was nearly complete after 10 days and amounts excreted were slightly higher in feces compared to urine. DRSP was extensively metabolized and only trace amounts of unchanged DRSP were excreted in urine and feces. At least 20 different metabolites were observed in urine and feces. About 38% to 47% of the metabolites in urine were glucuronide and sulfate conjugates. In feces, about 17% to 20% of the metabolites were excreted as glucuronides and sulfates. Estradiol, estrone, and estriol are ex-creted in the urine along with glucuronide and sulfate conjugates.

Special Populations:
Geriatric: No pharmacokinetic studies were conducted in the geriatric population.
Pediatric: No pharmacokinetic study for **ANGELIQ** has been conducted in a pediatric population.
Gender: **ANGELIQ** is indicated for use in women only.
Race: No studies were done to determine the effect of race on the pharmacokinetics of **ANGELIQ**.
Patients with Hepatic Impairment: **ANGELIQ** is contraindicated in patients with hepatic dysfunction (**also see BOLDED WARNING**). The mean exposure to DRSP in women with moderate liver impairment is approximately three times the exposure in women with normal liver function.
Patients with Renal Impairment: **ANGELIQ** is contraindicated in patients with renal insufficiency (**also see BOLDED WARNING**).
The effect of renal insufficiency on the pharmacokinetics of DRSP (3 mg daily for 14 days) and the effects of DRSP on serum potassium levels were investigated in female subjects (n = 28, age 30-65) with normal renal function (11 patients), and mild (10 patients) and moderate (7 patients) renal impairment. All subjects were on a low potassium diet. During the study 7 subjects continued the use of potassium-sparing drugs for the treatment of the underlying illness. On the 14th day (steady-state) of DRSP treatment, the serum DRSP levels were on average 37% higher in the group with moderate renal impairment (CLcr 30-50 mL/min) compared to those in the group with normal renal function. Serum DRSP levels in the group with mild renal impairment (creatinine clearance CLcr, 50-80 mL/min) were comparable to those in the group with normal renal function (CLcr, >80 mL/min). DRSP treatment was well tolerated by all groups. DRSP treatment did not show any clinically significant effect on serum potassium concentration. Although hyperkalemia was not observed in the study, in 5 of the 7 subjects who continued use of potassium sparing drugs during the study, individual mean serum potassium levels increased by up to 0.33 mEq/L. Therefore, potential exists for hyperkalemia to occur in subjects with renal impairment whose serum potassium is in the upper reference range, and who are concomitantly using potassium sparing drugs.
Drug Interactions:
Effects of Drospirenone on Other Drugs
Metabolic Interactions
Metabolism of DRSP and potential effects of DRSP on hepatic cytochrome P450 (CYP) enzymes have been investigated in *in vitro* and *in vivo* studies (see Metabolism). In *in vitro* studies, DRSP did not affect turnover of model substrates of CYP1A2 and CYP2D6, but had an inhibitory in-fluence on the turnover of model substrates of CYP1A1, CYP2C9, CYP2C19 and CYP3A4 with CYP2C19 being the most sensitive enzyme. The potential effect of DRSP on CYP2C19 activity was investigated in a clinical pharmacokinetic study using omeprazole as a marker substrate. In the study with 24 postmenopausal women [including 12 women with homozygous (wild type) CYP2C19 genotype and 12 women with heterozygous CYP2C19 genotype] the daily oral administration of 3mg DRSP for 14 days did not affect the systemic clearance of the CYP2C19 substrate omeprazole (40 mg) and the CYP2C19 product 5-hydroxy-omeprazole. Furthermore, no significant effect of DRSP on the systemic clearance of the CYP3A4 product omeprazole sulfone was found. These results demonstrated that DRSP did not inhibit CYP2C19 and CYP3A4 *in vivo*.

Two further clinical drug-drug interaction studies using simvastatin and midazolam as marker substrates for CYP3A4, were each performed in 24 healthy, postmenopausal women. The results of these studies demonstrated that pharmacokinetics of the CYP3A4 substrates were not influenced by steady-state DRSP concentrations achieved after administration of 3 mg DRSP/day.

Based on the available results of *in vivo* and *in vitro* studies, it can be concluded that, at clinical dose level, DRSP is unlikely to interact significantly with cytochrome P450 enzymes.

In vitro and *in vivo* studies have shown that estrogens are metabolized partially by cytochrome P450 3A4 (CYP3A4). Therefore, inducers or inhibitors of CYP3A4 may affect estrogen drug metabolism. Inducers of CYP3A4 such as St. John's Wort preparations (Hypericum perforatum), phenobarbital, carbamazepine, and rifampin may reduce plasma concentrations of estrogens, possibly resulting in a decrease in therapeutic effects and/or changes in the uterine bleeding profile. Inhibitors of CYP3A4 such as erythromycin, clarithromycin, ketoconazole, itraconazole, ritonavir and grapefruit juice may increase plasma concentrations of estrogens and may result in side effects.

Co-Administration with Drugs that Have the Potential to Increase Serum Potassium
There is a potential for an increase in serum potassium in women taking drospirenone with other drugs that may affect electrolytes, such as angiotensin converting enzyme (ACE) inhibitors, angiotensin receptor blockers, or non-steroidal anti-inflammatory drugs (NSAIDs).
Electrolytes were studied in 230 postmenopausal women with hypertension and/or diabetes mellitus requiring an ACE inhibitor or angiotensin receptor blocker (ARB). Of these, 26 patients had a creatinine clearance >50 mL/min to <80 mL/min. Patients were given 1 mg estradiol (E2) and 3 mg drospirenone (DRSP) (n=112) or placebo (n=118) over 28 days. Non-diabetic patients also received ibuprofen 1200 mg/day for 5 days during the study. There was a single case of serum potassium >6.0 mEq/L and a single case of serum sodium <130 mEq/L on treatment, both occurring following five days of ibuprofen therapy in two women taking E2/DRSP. Serum potassium levels ≥5.5 mEq/L were observed in 8 (7.3%) E2/DRSP-treated subjects (3 diabetic and 5 non-diabetic) and in 3 (2.6%) placebo-treated subjects (2 diabetic and 1 non-diabetic). After 28 days of exposure, the mean change from baseline in serum potassium was 0.11 mEq/L for the E2/DRSP group and 0.08 mEq/L for the placebo group. None of the subjects with serum potassium levels ≥5.5 mEq/L had cardiovascular adverse events. A drug-drug interaction study of DRSP 3 mg/estradiol (E2) 1 mg versus placebo was performed in 24 mildly hypertensive postmenopausal women taking enalapril maleate 10 mg twice daily. Potassium levels were obtained every other day for a total of 2 weeks in all subjects. Mean serum potassium levels in the DRSP/E2 treatment group relative to baseline were 0.22 mEq/L higher than those in the placebo group. Serum potassium concentrations also were measured at multiple timepoints over 24 hours at baseline and on Day 14. On Day 14, the ratios for serum potassium C_{max} and AUC in the DRSP/E2 group to those in the placebo group were 0.955 (90% CI: 0.914, 0.999) and 1.010 (90% CI: 0.944, 1.080), respectively. No patient in either treatment group developed hyperkalemia (serum potassium concentrations >5.5 mEq/L).
Of note, occasional or chronic use of NSAID medication was not restricted in any of the **ANGELIQ** clinical trials.
Clinical Studies
Support for the indications: Support for treatment of vasomotor symptoms and vaginal and vulvar atrophy was shown through bioequivalence of the E2 component of the combination product with a currently marketed E2 product (Estrace®). The multiple-dose bioequivalence study evaluated the bioequivalence of E2 from a tablet containing DRSP (2 mg) and E2 (1 mg) relative to Estrace (1 mg) tablet. DRSP/E2 tablets met the criteria for bioequivalence to Estrace.
Effects on Endometrium: In a one year clinical trial of 1,142 postmenopausal subjects treated with E2 alone or E2 + 0.5, 1, 2, or 3 mg DRSP, endometrial biopsies were per-

formed on 966 (84.6%) subjects during the treatment period. Eight subjects in the E2 monotherapy group developed endometrial hyperplasia (4 simple hyperplasia with no cytological atypia, 3 complex hyperplasia with no cytological atypia, and 1 complex hyperplasia with cytological atypia), and one subject in the 1 mg E2 + 2 mg DRSP group developed simple hyperplasia with no cytological atypia. Table 2 shows that there were no diagnoses of endometrial hyperplasia in the **ANGELIQ** group.

Table 2: Incidence of Endometrial Hyperplasia after up to 12 Months of Treatment

	E2 1 mg	ANGELIQ
Total No. Subjects	226	227
Total No. of On-Treatment Biopsies	197 (87.2%)	191 (84.1%)
Hyperplasia	8 (4%)	0 (0%)

Effects on Uterine Bleeding or Spotting:
In a cumulative analysis performed over 12 months in a double blind trial, the proportions of women with amenorrhea increased and at one year, 73.5% of subjects on **ANGELIQ** had amenorrhea. Results are shown in Figure 2.

Figure 2: Cumulative proportion of subjects with amenorrhea at a given cycle through cycle 13, LOCF

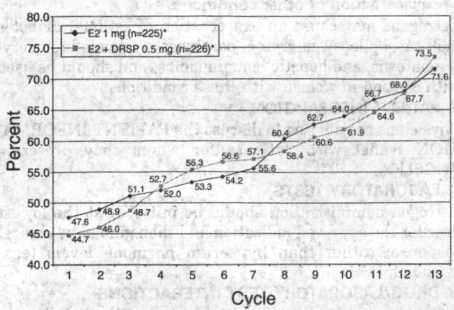

* One patient from each treatment group did not have bleeding diary information

Women's Health Initiative Studies: The Women's Health Initiative (WHI) enrolled a total of 27,000 predominantly healthy postmenopausal women to assess the risks and benefits of either the use of 0.625 mg conjugated equine estrogens (CE) per day alone or the use of 0.625 mg conjugated equine estrogens plus 2.5 mg medroxyprogesterone acetate (MPA) per day compared to placebo in the prevention of certain chronic diseases. The primary endpoint was the incidence of coronary heart disease (CHD) (nonfatal myocardial infarction and CHD death), with invasive breast cancer as the primary adverse outcome studied. A "global index" included the earliest occurrence of CHD, invasive breast cancer, stroke, pulmonary embolism (PE), endometrial cancer, colorectal cancer, hip fracture, or death due to other cause. The study did not evaluate the effects of CE or CE/MPA on menopausal symptoms.
The CE/MPA sub-study was stopped early because, according to the predefined stopping rule, the increased risk of breast cancer and cardiovascular events exceeded the specified benefits included in the "global index". Results of the CE/MPA sub-study, which included 16,608 women (average age of 63 years, range 50 to 79; 83.9% White, 6.5% Black, 5.5% Hispanic), after an average follow-up of 5.2 years are presented in Table 3 below:
[See table 3 above]
For those outcomes included in the "global index," absolute excess risks per 10,000 person-years in the group treated with CE/MPA were 7 more CHD events, 8 more strokes, 8 more PEs, and 8 more invasive breast cancers, while absolute risk reductions per 10,000 person-years were 6 fewer colorectal cancers and 5 fewer hip fractures.
The absolute excess risk of events included in the "global index" was 19 per 10,000 person-years. There was no difference between the groups in terms of all-cause mortality. (See **BOXED WARNINGS, WARNINGS,** and **PRECAUTIONS**.)
Women's Health Initiative Memory Study: The Women's Health Initiative Memory Study (WHIMS), a substudy of WHI, enrolled 4,532 predominantly healthy postmenopausal women 65 years of age and older (47% were age 65 to 69 years, 35% were 70 to 74 years, and 18% were 75 years of age and older) to evaluate the effects of CE/MPA (0.625 mg conjugated estrogens plus 2.5 mg medroxyprogesterone acetate) on the incidence of probable dementia (primary outcome) compared with placebo.

Table 3: Relative and Absolute Risk Seen in the CE/MPA Substudy of WHI[a]

Event[c]	Relative Risk CE/MPA vs placebo at 5.2 Years (95% CI*)	Placebo n = 8102	CE/MPA n = 8506
		Absolute Risk per 10,000 Person-years	
CHD events	1.29 (1.02-1.63)	30	37
Non-fatal MI	*1.32 (1.02-1.72)*	*23*	*30*
CHD death	*1.18 (0.70-1.97)*	*6*	*7*
Invasive breast cancer[b]	1.26 (1.00-1.59)	30	38
Stroke	1.41 (1.07-1.85)	21	29
Pulmonary embolism	2.13 (1.39-3.25)	8	16
Colorectal cancer	0.63 (0.43-0.92)	16	10
Endometrial cancer	0.83 (0.47-1.47)	6	5
Hip fracture	0.66 (0.45-0.98)	15	10
Death due to causes other than the events above	0.92 (0.74-1.14)	40	37
Global Index[c]	1.15 (1.03-1.28)	151	170
Deep vein thrombosis[d]	2.07 (1.49-2.87)	13	26
Vertebral fractures[d]	0.66 (0.44-0.98)	15	9
Other osteoporotic fractures[d]	0.77 (0.69-0.86)	170	131

[a] adapted from JAMA, 2002; 288:321-333
[b] includes metastatic and non-metastatic breast cancer with the exception of in situ breast cancer
[c] a subset of the events was combined in a "global index", defined as the earliest occurrence of CHD events, invasive breast cancer, stroke, pulmonary embolism, endometrial cancer, colorectal cancer, hip fracture, or death due to other causes
[d] not included in Global Index
*nominal confidence intervals unadjusted for multiple looks and multiple comparisons

After an average follow-up of 4 years, 40 women in the estrogen/progestin (45 per 10,000 women-years) and 21 in the placebo group (22 per 10,000 women-years) were diagnosed with probable dementia. The relative risk of probable dementia in the hormone therapy group was 2.05 (95% CI, 1.21 to 3.48) compared to placebo. Differences between groups became apparent in the first year of treatment. It is unknown whether these findings apply to younger postmenopausal women. (See **BOXED WARNING** and **WARNINGS, Dementia.**)

INDICATIONS AND USAGE
ANGELIQ is indicated in women who have a uterus for the:
1. Treatment of moderate to severe vasomotor symptoms associated with the menopause.
2. Treatment of moderate to severe symptoms of vulvar and vaginal atrophy associated with the menopause. When prescribing solely for the treatment of symptoms of vulvar and vaginal atrophy, topical vaginal products should be considered.

CONTRAINDICATIONS
Progestogens/estrogens should not be used in individuals with any of the following conditions:
1. Undiagnosed abnormal genital bleeding.
2. Known, suspected, or history of cancer of the breast.
3. Known or suspected estrogen-dependent neoplasia.
4. Active deep vein thrombosis, pulmonary embolism or history of these conditions.
5. Active or recent (e.g., within the past year) arterial thromboembolic disease (e.g., stroke, myocardial infarction).
6. Renal insufficiency.
7. Liver dysfunction or disease.
8. Adrenal insufficiency.
9. **ANGELIQ** should not be used in patients with known hypersensitivity to its ingredients.
10. Known or suspected pregnancy. There is no indication for **ANGELIQ** in pregnancy. There appears to be little or no increased risk of birth defects in children born to women who have used estrogens and progestins from oral contraceptives inadvertently during early pregnancy. (See **PRECAUTIONS**).

WARNINGS
ANGELIQ contains 0.5 mg of the progestin drospirenone that has antialdosterone activity, including the potential for hyperkalemia in high-risk patients.
ANGELIQ should not be used in patients with conditions that predispose to hyperkalemia (i.e. renal insufficiency, hepatic dysfunction, and adrenal insufficiency).
Use caution when prescribing ANGELIQ to women who regularly take other medications that can increase potassium, such as NSAIDs, potassium-sparing diuretics, potassium supplements, ACE inhibitors, angiotensin-II receptor antagonists, and heparin. Consider checking serum potassium levels during the first treatment cycle in high-risk patients.
See **BOXED WARNINGS.**
1. Cardiovascular disorders
Estrogen and estrogen/progestin therapy has been associated with an increased risk of cardiovascular events such as myocardial infarction and stroke, as well as venous thrombosis and pulmonary embolism (venous thromboembolism or VTE). Should any of these occur or be suspected, estrogens should be discontinued immediately.
Risk factors for cardiovascular disease (e.g., hypertension, diabetes mellitus, tobacco use, hypercholesterolemia, and obesity) and/or venous thromboembolism (e.g., personal history or family history of VTE, obesity, and systemic lupus erythematosus) should be managed appropriately.
a. Coronary heart disease and stroke
In the Women's Health Initiative study (WHI), an increase in the number of myocardial infarctions and strokes has been observed in women receiving oral CE compared to placebo. (See **CLINICAL PHARMACOLOGY, Clinical Studies sections.**)
In the CE/MPA substudy of WHI an increased risk of coronary heart disease (CHD) events (defined as non-fatal myocardial infarction and CHD death) was observed in women receiving CE/MPA compared to women receiving placebo (37 vs 30 per 10,000 person years). The increase in risk was observed in year one and persisted.
In the same substudy of WHI, an increased risk of stroke was observed in women receiving CE/MPA compared to women receiving placebo (29 vs 21 per 10,000 person-years). The increase in risk was observed after the first year and persisted.
In postmenopausal women with documented heart disease (n = 2,763, average age 66.7 years) a controlled clinical trial of secondary prevention of cardiovascular disease (Heart and Estrogen/Progestin Replacement Study; HERS) treatment with CE/MPA-0.625mg/2.5mg per day demonstrated no cardiovascular benefit. During an average follow-up of 4.1 years, treatment with CE/MPA did not reduce the overall rate of CHD events in postmenopausal women with established coronary heart disease. There were more CHD events in the CE/MPA-treated group than in the placebo group in year 1, but not during the subsequent years.
Two thousand three hundred and twenty one women from the original HERS trial agreed to participate in an open label extension of HERS, HERS II. Average follow-up in HERS II was an additional 2.7 years, for a total of 6.8 years overall. Rates of CHD events were comparable among women in the CE/MPA group and the placebo group in HERS, HERS II, and overall.

Large doses of estrogen (5 mg conjugated estrogens per day), comparable to those used to treat cancer of the prostate and breast, have been shown in a large prospective clinical trial in men to increase the risks of nonfatal myocardial infarction, pulmonary embolism, and thrombophlebitis.

b. Venous thromboembolism (VTE)

In the Women's Health Initiative study (WHI), an increase in VTE has been observed in women receiving CE compared to placebo. (See **CLINICAL PHARMACOLOGY** and **Clinical Studies** sections.)

In the CE/MPA substudy of WHI, a 2-fold greater rate of VTE, including deep venous thrombosis and pulmonary embolism, was observed in women receiving CE/MPA compared to women receiving placebo. The rate of VTE was 34 per 10,000 woman-years in the CE/MPA group compared to 16 per 10,000 woman-years in the placebo group. The increase in VTE risk was observed during the first year and persisted.

If feasible, estrogens should be discontinued at least 4 to 6 weeks before surgery of the type associated with an increased risk of thromboembolism, or during periods of prolonged immobilization.

2. Malignant neoplasms

a. Endometrial cancer

The use of unopposed estrogens in women with intact uteri has been associated with an increased risk of endometrial cancer. The reported endometrial cancer risk among unopposed estrogen users is about 2- to 12-fold greater than in non-users, and appears dependent on duration of treatment and on estrogen dose. Most studies show no significant increased risk associated with use of estrogens for less than one year. The greatest risk appears associated with prolonged use, with increased risks of 15- to 24-fold for five to ten years or more and this risk has been shown to persist for at least 8 to 15 years after estrogen therapy is discontinued. Clinical surveillance of all women taking estrogen/progestin combinations is important. Adequate diagnostic measures, including endometrial sampling when indicated, should be undertaken to rule out malignancy in all cases of undiagnosed persistent or recurring abnormal vaginal bleeding. There is no evidence that the use of natural estrogens results in a different endometrial risk profile than synthetic estrogens of equivalent estrogen dose. Adding a progestin to estrogen therapy has been shown to reduce the risk of endometrial hyperplasia, which may be a precursor to endometrial cancer.

b. Breast cancer

The use of estrogens and progestins by postmenopausal women has been reported to increase the risk of breast cancer. The most important randomized clinical trial providing information about this issue is the Women's Health Initiative (WHI) substudy of CE/MPA (see **CLINICAL PHARMACOLOGY, Clinical Studies**). The results from observational studies are generally consistent with those of the WHI clinical trial and report no significant variation in the risk of breast cancer among different estrogens or progestins, doses, or routes of administration.

The CE/MPA substudy of WHI reported an increased risk of breast cancer in women who took CE/MPA for a mean follow-up of 5.6 years. Observational studies have also reported an increased risk for estrogen/progestin combination therapy, and a smaller increased risk for estrogen alone therapy, after several years of use. In the WHI trial and from observational studies, the excess risk increased with duration of use. From observational studies, the risk appeared to return to baseline in about five years after stopping treatment. In addition, observational studies suggest that the risk of breast cancer was greater, and became apparent earlier, with estrogen/progestin combination therapy as compared to estrogen alone therapy.

In the CE/MPA substudy, 26% of the women reported prior use of estrogen alone and/or estrogen/progestin combination hormone therapy. After a mean follow-up of 5.6 years during the clinical trial, the overall relative risk of invasive breast cancer was 1.24 (95% confidence interval 1.01-1.54), and the overall absolute risk was 41 vs. 33 cases per 10,000 women-years, for CE/MPA compared with placebo. Among women who reported prior use of hormone therapy, the relative risk of invasive breast cancer was 1.86, and the absolute risk was 46 vs. 25 cases per 10,000 women-years, for CE/MPA compared with placebo. Among women who reported no prior use of hormone therapy, the relative risk of invasive breast cancer was 1.09, and the absolute risk was 40 vs. 36 cases per 10,000 women-years for CE/MPA compared with placebo. In the same substudy, invasive breast cancers were larger and diagnosed at a more advanced stage in the CE/MPA group compared with the placebo group. Metastatic disease was rare with no apparent difference between the two groups. Other prognostic factors such as histologic subtype, grade and hormone receptor status did not differ between the groups.

The use of estrogen plus progestin has been reported to result in an increase in abnormal mammograms requiring further evaluation. All women should receive yearly breast examinations by a healthcare provider and perform monthly breast self-examinations. In addition, mammography examinations should be scheduled based on patient age, and risk factors, and prior mammogram results.

3. Dementia

In the estrogen alone Women's Health Initiative Memory Study (WHIMS), a substudy of WHI, 2,947 hysterectomized women aged 65 to 79 years were randomized to CE or placebo. In the estrogen plus progestin WHIMS substudy, 4,532 postmenopausal women aged 65 to 79 years were randomized to CE/MPA or placebo.

In the estrogen alone substudy, after an average follow-up of 5.2 years, 28 women in the estrogen alone group and 19 women in the placebo group were diagnosed with probable dementia. The relative risk of probable dementia for estrogen alone versus placebo was 1.49 (95% CI 0.83-2.66). The absolute risk of probable dementia for estrogen alone versus placebo was 37 versus 25 cases per 10,000 women-years. It is unknown whether these findings apply to younger postmenopausal women. (See **CLINICAL PHARMACOLOGY, Clinical Studies** and **PRECAUTIONS, Geriatric Use**.)

After an average follow-up of 4 years, 40 women being treated with CE/MPA (1.8%, n = 2,229) and 21 women in the placebo group (0.9%, n = 2,303) received diagnoses of probable dementia. The relative risk for CE/MPA versus placebo was 2.05 (95% confidence interval 1.21–3.48), and was similar for women with and without histories of menopausal hormone use before WHIMS. The absolute risk of probable dementia for CE/MPA versus placebo was 45 versus 22 cases per 10,000 women-years, and the absolute excess risk for CE/MPA was 23 cases per 10,000 women-years. It is unknown whether these findings apply to younger postmenopausal women. (See **CLINICAL PHARMACOLOGY, Clinical Studies** and **PRECAUTIONS, Geriatric Use**.)

4. Gallbladder disease

A 2- to 4-fold increase in the risk of gallbladder disease requiring surgery in postmenopausal women receiving estrogens has been reported.

5. Hypercalcemia

Estrogen administration may lead to severe hypercalcemia in patients with breast cancer and bone metastases. If hypercalcemia occurs, use of the drug should be stopped and appropriate measures taken to reduce the serum calcium level.

6. Visual abnormalities

Retinal vascular thrombosis has been reported in patients receiving estrogens. Discontinue medication pending examination if there is sudden partial or complete loss of vision, or a sudden onset of proptosis, diplopia, or migraine. If examination reveals papilledema or retinal vascular lesions, estrogens should be permanently discontinued.

PRECAUTIONS

A. GENERAL

1. Addition of a progestin when a woman has not had a hysterectomy

Studies of the addition of a progestin for 10 or more days of a cycle of estrogen administration or daily with estrogen in a continuous regimen, have reported a lowered incidence of endometrial hyperplasia than would be induced by estrogen treatment alone. Endometrial hyperplasia may be a precursor to endometrial cancer.

There are, however, possible risks that may be associated with the use of progestins with estrogens compared to estrogen-alone regimens. These include a possible increased risk of breast cancer.

2. Elevated blood pressure

In a small number of case reports, substantial increases in blood pressure have been attributed to idiosyncratic reactions to estrogens. In a large, randomized, placebo-controlled clinical trial, a generalized effect of estrogen therapy on blood pressure was not seen. Blood pressure should be monitored at regular intervals with estrogen use.

3. Hypertriglyceridemia

In patients with pre-existing hypertriglyceridemia, estrogen therapy may be associated with elevations of plasma triglycerides leading to pancreatitis and other complications.

4. Impaired liver function and past history of cholestatic jaundice

Estrogens may be poorly metabolized in patients with impaired liver function. For patients with a history of cholestatic jaundice associated with past estrogen use or with pregnancy, caution should be exercised and in the case of recurrence, medication should be discontinued.

The clearance of drospirenone was decreased in patients with moderate hepatic impairment.

5. Hypothyroidism

Estrogen administration leads to increased thyroid-binding globulin (TBG) levels. Patients with normal thyroid function can compensate for the increased TBG by making more thyroid hormone, thus maintaining free T4 and T3 serum concentrations in the normal range. Patients dependent on thyroid hormone replacement therapy who are also receiving estrogens may require increased doses of their thyroid replacement therapy. These patients should have their thyroid function monitored in order to maintain their free thyroid hormone levels in an acceptable range.

6. Fluid retention

Because estrogen and estrogen/progestin therapy may cause some degree of fluid retention, patients with conditions that might be influenced by this factor, such as a cardiac or renal dysfunction, warrant careful observation when estrogens are prescribed.

7. Hypocalcemia

Estrogens should be used with caution in individuals with severe hypocalcemia.

8. Hyponatremia

As an aldosterone antagonist, drospirenone may increase the possibility of hyponatremia in high-risk patients.

9. Ovarian cancer

The CE/MPA substudy of WHI reported that estrogen plus progestin increased the risk of ovarian cancer. After an average follow-up of 5.6 years, the relative risk for ovarian cancer for CE/MPA versus placebo was 1.58 (95% confidence interval 0.77–3.24) but was not statistically significant. The absolute risk for CE/MPA versus placebo was 4.2 versus 2.7 cases per 10,000 women-years. In some epidemiologic studies, the use of estrogen alone, in particular for ten or more years, has been associated with an increased risk of ovarian cancer. Other epidemiologic studies have not found these associations.

10. Exacerbation of endometriosis

Endometriosis may be exacerbated with administration of estrogens.

11. Exacerbation of other conditions

Estrogens may cause an exacerbation of asthma, diabetes mellitus, epilepsy, migraine, porphyria, systemic lupus erythematosus, and hepatic hemangiomas, and should be used with caution in women with these conditions.

B. PATIENT INFORMATION

Physicians are advised to discuss the PATIENT INFORMATION leaflet with patients for whom they prescribe ANGELIQ.

C. LABORATORY TESTS

Estrogen administration should be initiated at the lowest dose for the approved indication and then guided by clinical response, rather than by serum hormone levels (e.g., estradiol, FSH).

D. DRUG/LABORATORY TEST INTERACTIONS

1. Accelerated prothrombin time, partial thromboplastin time, and platelet aggregation time; increased platelet count; increased factors II, VII antigen, VIII antigen, VIII coagulant activity; IX, X, XII, VII-X complex, II-VII-X complex, and beta-thromboglobulin; decreased levels of antifactor Xa and antithrombin III, decreased antithrombin III activity; increased levels of fibrinogen and fibrinogen activity; increased plasminogen antigen and activity.

2. Increased thyroid-binding globulin (TBG) levels leading to increased circulating total thyroid hormone, as measured by protein-bound iodine (PBI), T4 levels (by column or by radioimmunoassay) or T3 levels by radioimmunoassay. T3 resin uptake is decreased, reflecting the elevated TBG. Free T4 and free T3 concentrations are unaltered. Patients on thyroid replacement therapy may require higher doses of thyroid hormone.

3. Other binding proteins may be elevated in serum (i.e., corticosteroid binding globulin (CBG), sex hormone-binding globulin (SHBG)) leading to increased circulating corticosteroids and sex steroids, respectively. Free hormone concentrations may be decreased. Other plasma proteins may be increased (angiotensinogen/renin substrate, alpha-1-antitrypsin, ceruloplasmin).

4. Increased plasma HDL and HDL-2 subfraction concentrations, reduced LDL cholesterol concentration, increased triglyceride levels.

5. Impaired glucose tolerance.

6. Reduced response to metyrapone test.

E. CARCINOGENESIS, MUTAGENESIS, AND IMPAIRMENT OF FERTILITY

Long-term continuous administration of estrogen, with and without progestin, in women with and without a uterus, has shown an increased risk of endometrial cancer, breast cancer, and ovarian cancer. (See **BOXED WARNINGS, WARNINGS** and **PRECAUTIONS**.)

Long-term continuous administration of natural and synthetic estrogens in certain animal species increases the frequency of carcinomas of the breast, uterus, cervix, vagina, testis, and liver. (See **BOXED WARNINGS, CONTRAINDICATIONS**, and **WARNINGS** sections.)

In a 24 month oral carcinogenicity study in mice dosed with 10 mg/kg/day drospirenone alone or 1 + 0.01, 3 + 0.03 and 10 + 0.1 mg/kg/day of drospirenone and ethinyl estradiol, 0.24 to 10.3 times the exposure (AUC of drospirenone) of women taking a 1 mg dose, there was an increase in carcinomas of the harderian gland in the group that received the high dose of drospirenone alone. In a similar study in rats given 10 mg/kg/day drospirenone alone or 0.3 + 0.003, 3 + 0.03 and 10 + 0.1 mg/kg/day drospirenone and ethinyl estradiol, 2.3 to 51.2 times the exposure of women taking a 1 mg dose, there was an increased incidence of benign and total (benign and malignant) adrenal gland pheochromocytomas in the group receiving the high dose of drospirenone. Drospirenone was not mutagenic in a number of *in vitro* (Ames, Chinese Hamster Lung gene mutation and chromosomal damage in human lymphocytes) and *in vivo* (mouse micronucleus) genotoxicity tests. Drospirenone increased unscheduled DNA synthesis in rat hepatocytes and formed adducts with rodent liver DNA but not with human liver DNA. (See **WARNINGS** section.)

F. PREGNANCY
ANGELIQ should not be used during pregnancy. (See **CONTRAINDICATIONS**.)

G. NURSING MOTHERS
Estrogen administration to nursing mothers has been shown to decrease the quantity and quality of the milk. Detectable amounts of estrogens have been identified in the milk of mothers receiving this drug. Caution should be exercised when **ANGELIQ** is administered to a nursing woman.

After administration of an oral contraceptive containing drospirenone about 0.02% of the drospirenone dose was excreted into the breast milk of postpartum women within 24 hours. This results in a maximal daily dose of about 3 mcg drospirenone in an infant.

H. PEDIATRIC USE
ANGELIQ is not indicated in children.

I. GERIATRIC USE
There have not been sufficient numbers of geriatric patients involved in clinical studies utilizing **ANGELIQ** to determine whether those over 65 years of age differ from younger subjects in their response to **ANGELIQ**.

In the Women's Health Initiative Memory Study, including 4,532 women 65 years of age and older, followed for an average of 4 years, 82% (n = 3,729) were 65 to 74 while 18% (n = 803) were 75 and over. Most women (80%) had no prior hormone therapy use. Women treated with conjugated estrogens plus medroxyprogesterone acetate were reported to have a two-fold increase in the risk of developing probable dementia. Alzheimer's disease was the most common classification of probable dementia in both the conjugated estrogens plus medroxyprogesterone acetate group and the placebo group. Ninety percent of the cases of probable dementia occurred in the 54% of women who were older than 70. (See **WARNINGS, Dementia**.)

ADVERSE REACTIONS
See BOXED WARNINGS, WARNINGS, AND PRECAUTIONS.

Because clinical trials are conducted under widely varying conditions, adverse reaction rates observed in the clinical trials of a drug cannot be directly compared to rates in the clinical trials of another drug and may not reflect the rates observed in practice. The adverse reaction information from clinical trials does, however, provide a basis for identifying the adverse events that appear to be related to drug use and for approximating rates.

The following are adverse events reported with **ANGELIQ** occurring in >5% of subjects:

Table 4: Adverse Events Regardless of Drug Relationship Reported at a Frequency of >5% in a 1-year Double-blind Clinical Trial

ADVERSE EVENT	E2 1 MG (N=226) n (%)	ANGELIQ (N=227) n (%)
BODY AS A WHOLE		
Abdominal pain	29 (12.8)	25 (11)
Pain in extremity	15 (6.6)	19 (8.4)
Back pain	11 (4.9)	16 (7)
Flu syndrome	15 (6.6)	16 (7)
Accidental injury	15 (6.6)	13 (5.7)
Abdomen enlarged	17 (7.5)	16 (7)
Surgery	6 (2.7)	12 (5.3)
METABOLIC & NUTRITIONAL DISORDERS		
Peripheral edema	12 (5.3)	4 (1.8)
NERVOUS SYSTEM		
Headache	26 (11.5)	22 (9.7)

RESPIRATORY SYSTEM		
Upper respiratory infection	40 (17.7)	43 (18.9)
Sinusitis	8 (3.5)	12 (5.3)
SKIN AND APPENDAGES		
Breast pain	34 (15.0)	43 (18.9)
UROGENITAL		
Vaginal hemorrhage	43 (19.0)	21 (9.3)
Endometrial disorder	22 (9.7)	4 (1.8)
Leukorrhea	14 (6.2)	3 (1.3)

The following additional adverse reactions have been reported with estrogen and or estrogen/progestin therapy:

1. Genitourinary system
Changes in vaginal bleeding pattern and abnormal withdrawal bleeding or flow; breakthrough bleeding, spotting, dysmenorrhea, increase in size of uterine leiomyomata, vaginitis, including vaginal candidiasis, change in amount of cervical secretion, changes in cervical ectropion, ovarian cancer, endometrial hyperplasia, endometrial cancer.

2. Breasts
Tenderness, enlargement, pain, nipple discharge, galactorrhea, fibrocystic breast changes, breast cancer.

3. Cardiovascular
Deep and superficial venous thrombosis, pulmonary embolism, thrombophlebitis, myocardial infarction, stroke, increase in blood pressure.

4. Gastrointestinal
Nausea, vomiting, abdominal cramps, bloating, cholestatic jaundice, increased incidence of gall bladder disease, pancreatitis, enlargement of hepatic hemangiomas.

5. Skin
Chloasma or melasma, which may persist when drug is discontinued, erythema multiforme, erythema nodosum, hemorrhagic eruption, loss of scalp hair, hirsutism, pruritus, rash.

6. Eyes
Retinal vascular thrombosis, intolerance to contact lenses.

7. Central nervous system
Headache, migraine, dizziness, mental depression, chorea, nervousness, mood disturbances, irritability, exacerbation of epilepsy, dementia.

8. Miscellaneous
Increase or decrease in weight, reduced carbohydrate tolerance, aggravation of porphyria, edema, arthralgias, leg cramps, changes in libido, anaphylactoid/anaphylactic reactions including urticaria and angioedema, hypocalcemia, exacerbation of asthma, increased triglycerides.

OVERDOSAGE
In cases of **ANGELIQ** overdose, monitor serum concentrations of potassium and sodium since drospirenone has antimineralocorticoid properties.

Serious ill effects have not been reported following acute ingestion of large doses of progestin/estrogen-containing oral contraceptives by young children. Overdosage may cause nausea and withdrawal bleeding may occur in females.

DOSAGE AND ADMINISTRATION
The dosage of **ANGELIQ** is one tablet daily. Women who are already using a product containing estrogen should stop taking that product before starting **ANGELIQ**.

Use of estrogen, alone or in combination with a progestin, should be limited to the lowest effective dose available and for the shortest duration consistent with treatment goals and risks for the individual woman. Patients should be re-evaluated periodically as clinically appropriate (e.g., 3-month to 6-month intervals) to determine if treatment is still necessary (see **BOXED WARNINGS** and **WARNINGS** sections). For women who have a uterus, adequate diagnostic measures, such as endometrial sampling, when indicated, should be undertaken to rule out malignancy in cases of undiagnosed persistent or recurring abnormal vaginal bleeding.

The lowest effective dose of **ANGELIQ** has not been determined.

HOW SUPPLIED
ANGELIQ TABLETS (drospirenone and estradiol) 0.5 mg/ 1 mg are available as round, biconvex pink film-coated tablets embossed with "CK" inside a hexagon, and supplied in the following packaging:

3 blisters of 28 tablets   NDC 50419-483-03
Storage Conditions
Store at 25°C (77°F); excursions permitted to 15-30°C (59-86°F) [See USP Controlled Room Temperature].
REFERENCES FURNISHED UPON REQUEST

PATIENT INFORMATION
September 2005
ANGELIQ® TABLETS
(drospirenone and estradiol)
(an"ju-lēk')

Read this **PATIENT INFORMATION** before you start taking **ANGELIQ** and read what you get each time you refill **ANGELIQ**. There may be new information. This information does not take the place of talking to your health care provider about your medical condition or your treatment.

> **WHAT IS THE MOST IMPORTANT INFORMATION I SHOULD KNOW ABOUT ANGELIQ (a combination of estrogen and a progestin)?**
> Do not use estrogens with or without progestins to prevent heart disease, heart attacks, or strokes.
> Using estrogens with or without progestins may increase your chances of getting heart attack, strokes, breast cancer, and blood clots. Using estrogens with or without progestins may increase your risk of dementia. You and your healthcare provider should talk regularly about whether you still need treatment with **ANGELIQ**.

What is ANGELIQ?
ANGELIQ is a medicine that contains two kinds of hormones, estrogen and progestin.

What is ANGELIQ used for?
ANGELIQ is used after menopause to:

• **reduce moderate to severe hot flashes.** Estrogens are hormones made by a woman's ovaries. The ovaries normally stop making estrogens when a woman is between 45 to 55 years old. This drop in body estrogen levels causes the "change of life" or menopause (the end of monthly menstrual periods). Sometimes, both ovaries are removed during an operation before natural menopause takes place. The sudden drop in estrogen levels causes "surgical menopause."
When the estrogen levels begin dropping, some women develop very uncomfortable symptoms, such as feelings of warmth in the face, neck, and chest, or sudden strong feelings of heat and sweating ("hot flashes" or "hot flushes"). In some women, the symptoms are mild, and they will not need estrogens. In other women, symptoms can be more severe. You and your health care provider should talk regularly about whether you need treatment with **ANGELIQ**.

• **treat moderate to severe dryness, itching, and burning in or around the vagina.** You and your healthcare provider should talk regularly about whether you still need treatment with **ANGELIQ** to control these problems. If you use **ANGELIQ** only to treat dryness, itching, and burning in and around your vagina, talk with your healthcare provider about whether a topical vaginal product would be better for you.

Who should not use ANGELIQ?
Do not use **ANGELIQ** if you have had your uterus removed (hysterectomy).

ANGELIQ contains a progestin to decrease the chances of getting cancer of the uterus. If you do not have a uterus, you do not need a progestin and you should not use **ANGELIQ**.

Do not start taking ANGELIQ if you:
• have unusual vaginal bleeding.
• currently have or have had certain cancers. Estrogens may increase the chances of getting certain types of cancers, including cancer of the breast or uterus. If you have or had cancer, talk with your health care provider about whether you should take **ANGELIQ**.
• had a stroke or heart attack in the past year.
• currently have or have had blood clots.
• have kidney disease, liver disease, or disease of your adrenal glands.
• are allergic to **ANGELIQ** or any of its ingredients. See the end of this leaflet for a list of ingredients in **ANGELIQ**.
• think you may be pregnant.

Tell your health care provider:
• if you are breastfeeding. The hormone in **ANGELIQ** can pass into your milk.
• about all of your medical problems. Your health care provider may need to check you more carefully if you have certain conditions, such as asthma (wheezing), epilepsy (seizures), migraine, endometriosis, lupus, hypertension (high blood pressure) or problems with your heart, liver, thyroid, kidneys, or have high calcium levels in your blood.
• about all the medicines you take, including prescription and nonprescription medicines, vitamins, and herbal supplements. Some medicines may affect how **ANGELIQ** works. **ANGELIQ** may also affect how your other medicines work.
• if you are going to have surgery or will be on bed rest. You may need to stop taking estrogens.

How should I take ANGELIQ?
1. Take one tablet every day.
2. Estrogens should be used only as long as needed. The lowest effective dose of **ANGELIQ** has not been determined. You and your healthcare provider should talk regularly (for example, every 3 to 6 months) about whether you still need treatment with **ANGELIQ**.

What are the possible side effects of ANGELIQ?
ANGELIQ is different from other hormonal medicines for menopausal symptoms because it contains drospirenone, and drospirenone may increase the potassium or lower the sodium in your blood.

You should not take **ANGELIQ** if you have kidney, liver or adrenal disease because these conditions may also increase the potassium in your blood. Some other medicines also increase potassium. If you regularly take another medicine that increases potassium levels, talk with your healthcare provider about whether **ANGELIQ** is right for you. In some situations, your healthcare provider may recommend testing your blood for potassium.

Less common but serious side effects include the following and should be discussed with your healthcare provider to assess your personal risks:
- Breast cancer
- Cancer of the uterus
- Stroke
- Heart attack
- Blood clots
- Dementia
- Gallbladder disease
- Ovarian cancer

These are some of the warning signs of serious side effects:
- Breast lumps
- Unusual vaginal bleeding
- Dizziness and faintness
- Changes in speech
- Severe headaches
- Chest pain
- Shortness of breath
- Pains in your legs
- Changes in vision
- Vomiting

Call your health care provider right away if you get any of these warning signs, or any other unusual symptom that concerns you.

Common side effects include:
- Headache
- Breast pain
- Irregular vaginal bleeding or spotting
- Stomach/abdominal cramps, bloating
- Nausea and vomiting
- Hair loss

Other side effects include:
- High blood pressure
- Liver problems
- High blood sugar
- Fluid retention
- Enlargement of benign tumors of the uterus ("fibroids")
- Vaginal yeast infection

These are not all the possible side effects of **ANGELIQ**. For more information, ask your health care provider or pharmacist.

What can I do to lower my chances of a serious side effect with ANGELIQ?
Talk with your health care provider regularly about whether you should continue taking **ANGELIQ**.

See your health care provider right away if you get vaginal bleeding while taking **ANGELIQ**.

Have a breast exam and mammogram (breast X-ray) every year unless your health care provider tells you something else. If members of your family have had breast cancer or if you have ever had breast lumps or an abnormal mammogram, you may need to have breast exams more often.

If you have high blood pressure, high cholesterol (fat in the blood), diabetes, are overweight, or if you use tobacco, you may have higher chances for getting heart disease. Ask your health care provider for ways to lower your chances for getting heart disease.

General information about safe and effective use of ANGELIQ.
Medicines are sometimes prescribed for conditions that are not mentioned in patient information leaflets. Do not use **ANGELIQ** for conditions for which it was not prescribed. Do not give **ANGELIQ** to other people, even if they have the same symptoms you have. It may harm them.

Keep ANGELIQ out of the reach of children
This leaflet summarizes the most important information about **ANGELIQ**. If you would like more information, talk with your healthcare provider or pharmacist. You can ask for information about **ANGELIQ** that is written for health professionals. You can get more information by calling our toll free number (1-888-237-5394) or visit www.angeliq-us.com

What are the ingredients in ANGELIQ?
The active ingredients in **ANGELIQ** are drospirenone (a progestin) and estradiol. **ANGELIQ** also contains lactose monohydrate NF, corn starch NF, modified starch NF, povidone USP, magnesium stearate NF, hydroxylpropylmethyl cellulose USP, macrogol NF, talc USP, titanium dioxide USP, and ferric oxide pigment NF.

Do not store above 86°F (30°C).

Manufactured for:
Bayer HealthCare Pharmaceuticals Inc.
Wayne, NJ 07470
Manufactured in Germany
©2008 Bayer HealthCare Pharmaceuticals Inc., All rights reserved.
6702400 US   81587257   March 2008

Shown in Product Identification Guide, page 307

CLIMARA® PATCH
[klĭ-mărä]
(estradiol transdermal system)
Rx only

PRESCRIBING INFORMATION

> **ESTROGENS INCREASE THE RISK OF ENDOMETRIAL CANCER**
> Close clinical surveillance of all women taking estrogens is important. Adequate diagnostic measures, including endometrial sampling when indicated, should be undertaken to rule out malignancy in all cases of undiagnosed persistent or recurring abnormal vaginal bleeding.
> There is no evidence that the use of "natural" estrogens results in a different endometrial risk profile than synthetic estrogens at equivalent estrogen doses. (See **WARNINGS, Malignant neoplasms, Endometrial cancer**.)
> **CARDIOVASCULAR AND OTHER RISKS**
> Estrogens with and without progestins should not be used for the prevention of cardiovascular disease or dementia. (See **WARNINGS, Cardiovascular disorders and Dementia**.)
> The Women's Health Initiative (WHI) study reported increased risks of myocardial infarction, stroke, invasive breast cancer, pulmonary emboli, and deep vein thrombosis in postmenopausal women (50 to 79 years of age) during 5 years of treatment with oral conjugated estrogens (CE 0.625 mg) combined with medroxyprogesterone acetate (MPA 2.5 mg) relative to placebo. (See **CLINICAL PHARMACOLOGY, Clinical Studies** and **WARNINGS, Cardiovascular disorders and Malignant neoplasms**, *Breast cancer*).
> The Women's Health Initiative Memory Study (WHIMS), a substudy of WHI, reported increased risk of developing probable dementia in postmenopausal women 65 years of age or older during 4 years of treatment with oral conjugated estrogens plus medroxyprogesterone acetate relative to placebo. It is unknown whether this finding applies to younger postmenopausal women. (See **CLINICAL PHARMACOLOGY, Clinical Studies** and **WARNINGS, Dementia** and **PRECAUTIONS, Geriatric Use**.)
> Other doses of oral conjugated estrogens with medroxyprogesterone acetate, and other combinations and dosage forms of estrogens and progestins were not studied in the WHI clinical trials and, in the absence of comparable data, these risks should be assumed to be similar. Because of these risks, estrogens with or without progestins should be prescribed at the lowest effective doses and for the shortest duration consistent with treatment goals and risks for the individual woman.

DESCRIPTION
Climara®, estradiol transdermal system, is designed to release estradiol continuously upon application to intact skin. Six (6.5, 9.375, 12.5, 15, 18.75 or 25 cm²) systems are available to provide nominal *in vivo* delivery of 0.025, 0.0375, 0.05, 0.06, 0.075 or 0.1 mg respectively of estradiol per day. The period of use is 7 days. Each system has a contact surface area of either 6.5, 9.375, 12.5, 15, 18.75 or 25 cm², and contains 2, 2.85, 3.8, 4.55, 5.7 or 7.6 mg of estradiol USP respectively. The composition of the systems per unit area is identical. Estradiol USP is a white, crystalline powder, chemically described as estra-1,3,5(10)-triene-3, 17ß-diol. It has an empirical formula of $C_{18}H_{24}O_2$ and molecular weight of 272.39. The structural formula is: [See chemical structure at top of next column]
The Climara system comprises three layers. Proceeding from the visible surface toward the surface attached to the skin, these layers are (1) a translucent polyethylene film, and (2) an acrylate adhesive matrix containing estradiol USP. A protective liner (3) of siliconized or fluoropolymer-

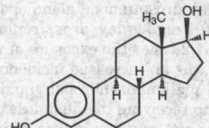

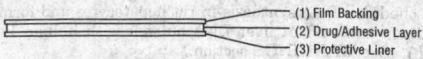

(1) Film Backing
(2) Drug/Adhesive Layer
(3) Protective Liner

coated polyester film is attached to the adhesive surface and must be removed before the system can be used.

The active component of the system is estradiol. The remaining components of the system (acrylate copolymer adhesive, fatty acid esters, and polyethylene backing) are pharmacologically inactive.

CLINICAL PHARMACOLOGY
Endogenous estrogens are largely responsible for the development and maintenance of the female reproductive system and secondary sexual characteristics. Although circulating estrogens exist in a dynamic equilibrium of metabolic interconversions, estradiol is the principal intracellular human estrogen and is substantially more potent than its metabolites, estrone and estriol at the receptor level.

The primary source of estrogen in normally cycling adult women is the ovarian follicle, which secretes 70 to 500 mcg of estradiol daily, depending on the phase of the menstrual cycle. After menopause, most endogenous estrogen is produced by conversion of androstenedione, secreted by the adrenal cortex, to estrone by peripheral tissues. Thus, estrone and the sulfate conjugated form, estrone sulfate, are the most abundant circulating estrogens in postmenopausal women.

Estrogens act through binding to nuclear receptors in estrogen-responsive tissues. To date, two estrogen receptors have been identified. These vary in proportion from tissue to tissue.

Circulating estrogens modulate the pituitary secretion of the gonadotropins, luteinizing hormone (LH) and follicle stimulating hormone (FSH), through a negative feedback mechanism. Estrogens act to reduce the elevated levels of these hormones seen in postmenopausal women.

PHARMACOKINETICS
Transdermal administration of Climara produces mean serum concentrations of estradiol comparable to those produced by premenopausal women in the early follicular phase of the ovulatory cycle. The pharmacokinetics of estradiol following application of the Climara system were investigated in 197 healthy postmenopausal women in six studies. In five of the studies Climara system was applied to the abdomen and in a sixth study application to the buttocks and abdomen were compared.

Absorption: The Climara transdermal delivery system continuously releases estradiol which is transported across intact skin leading to sustained circulating levels of estradiol during a 7-day treatment period. The systemic availability of estradiol after transdermal administration is about 20 times higher than that after oral administration. This difference is due to the absence of first pass metabolism when estradiol is given by the transdermal route.

In a bioavailability study, the Climara 6.5 cm² was studied with the Climara 12.5 cm² as reference. The mean estradiol levels in serum from the two sizes are shown in **Figure 1**.

Figure 1
Mean Serum 17ß-Estradiol Concentrations vs. Time Profile following Application of a 6.5 cm² Transdermal Patch and Application of a 12.5 cm² Climara patch

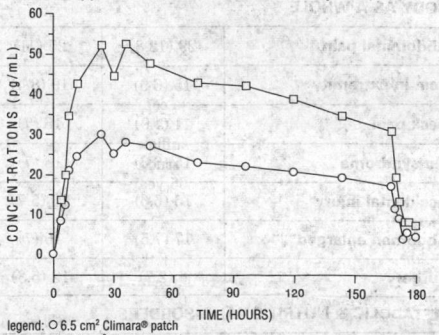

legend: ○ 6.5 cm² Climara® patch
☐ 12.5 cm² Climara® patch

Dose proportionality was demonstrated for the Climara 6.5 cm² transdermal system as compared to the Climara 12.5 cm² transdermal system in a 2-week crossover study with a 1-week washout period between the two transdermal systems in 24 postmenopausal women.

Dose proportionality was also demonstrated for the Climara system (12.5 cm^2 and 25 cm^2) in a 1-week study conducted in 54 postmenopausal women. The mean steady state levels (C_{avg}) of the estradiol during the application of Climara 25 cm^2 and 12.5 cm^2 on the abdomen were about 80 and 40 pg/mL, respectively.

In a 3 week multiple application study in 24 postmenopausal women, the 25 cm^2 Climara system produced average peak estradiol concentrations (C_{max}) of approximately 100 pg/mL. Trough values at the end of each wear interval (C_{min}) were approximately 35 pg/mL. Nearly identical serum curves were seen each week, indicating little or no accumulation of estradiol in the body. Serum estrone peak and trough levels were 60 and 40 pg/mL, respectively.

In a single dose, randomized, crossover study conducted to compare the effect of site of application, 38 postmenopausal women wore a single Climara 25 cm^2 system for 1 week on the abdomen and buttocks. The estradiol serum concentration profiles are shown in **Figure 2**. C_{max} and C_{avg} values were, respectively, 25% and 17% higher with the buttock application than with the abdomen application.

Figure 2
Observed Mean (± S.E.) Estradiol Serum Concentrations for a One Week Application of the Climara system (25 cm²) to the abdomen and buttocks of 38 postmenopausal women

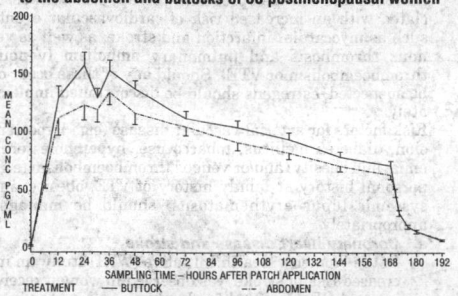

Table 1 provides a summary of estradiol pharmacokinetic parameters determined during evaluation of Climara. [See table 1 above]

The relative standard deviation of each pharmacokinetic parameter after application to the abdomen averaged 50%, which is indicative of the considerable intersubject variability associated with transdermal drug delivery. The relative standard deviation of each pharmacokinetic parameter after application to the buttock was lower than that after application to the abdomen (e.g., for C_{max} 39% vs 62%, and for C_{avg} 35% vs 48%).

Distribution
The distribution of exogenous estrogens is similar to that of endogenous estrogens.

Estrogens are widely distributed in the body and are generally found in higher concentrations in the sex hormone target organs. Estrogens circulate in the blood largely bound to sex hormone binding globulin (SIIBG) and albumin.

Metabolism
Exogenous estrogens are metabolized in the same manner as endogenous estrogens. Circulating estrogens exist in a dynamic equilibrium of metabolic interconversions. These transformations take place mainly in the liver. Estradiol is converted reversibly to estrone, and both can be converted to estriol, which is the major urinary metabolite. Estrogens also undergo enterohepatic recirculation via sulfate and glucuronide conjugation in the liver, biliary secretion of conjugates into the intestine, and hydrolysis in the gut followed by reabsorption. In postmenopausal women, a significant proportion of the circulating estrogens exist as sulfate conjugates, especially estrone sulfate, which serves as a circulating reservoir for the formation of more active estrogens.

Excretion
Estradiol, estrone, and estriol are excreted in the urine along with glucuronide and sulfate conjugates.

Special Populations:
Geriatric: There have not been sufficient numbers of geriatric patients involved in clinical studies utilizing Climara to determine whether those over 65 years of age differ from younger subjects in their response to Climara.

Pediatric: No pharmacokinetic study for Climara has been conducted in a pediatric population.

Gender: Climara is indicated for use in women only.

Race: No studies were done to determine the effect of race on the pharmacokinetics of Climara.

Patients with Renal Impairment: Total estradiol serum levels are higher in postmenopausal women with end stage renal disease (ESRD) receiving maintenance hemodialysis than in normal subjects at baseline and following oral doses of estradiol. Therefore, conventional transdermal estradiol doses used in individuals with normal renal function may be excessive for postmenopausal women with ESRD receiving maintenance hemodialysis.

Patients with Hepatic Impairment: Estrogens may be poorly metabolized in patients with impaired liver function and should be administered with caution.

Drug Interactions
In vitro and *in vivo* studies have shown that estrogens are metabolized partially by cytochrome P450 3A4 (CYP3A4). Therefore, inducers or inhibitors of CYP3A4 may affect estrogen drug metabolism. Inducers of CYP3A4 such as St. John's Wort preparations (Hypericum perforatum), phenobarbital, carbamazepine, and rifampin may reduce plasma concentrations of estrogens, possibly resulting in a decrease in therapeutic effects and/or changes in the uterine bleeding profile. Inhibitors of CYP3A4 such as erythromycin, clarithromycin, ketoconazole, itraconazole, ritonavir and grapefruit juice may increase plasma concentrations of estrogens and may result in side effects.

Adhesion
An open-label study of adhesion potentials of placebo transdermal systems that correspond to the 6.5 cm^2 and 12.5 cm^2 sizes of Climara was conducted in 112 healthy women of 45-75 years of age. Each woman applied both transdermal systems weekly, on the upper outer abdomen, for 3 consecutive weeks. It should be noted that lower abdomen and upper quadrant of the buttock are the approved sites of application for Climara.

The adhesion assessment was done visually on Days 2, 4, 5, 6, 7 of each week of transdermal system wear. A total of 1654 adhesion observations were conducted for 333 transdermal systems of each size.

Of these observations, approximately 90% showed essentially no lift for both the 6.5 cm^2 and 12.5 cm^2 transdermal systems. Of the total number of transdermal systems applied, approximately 5% showed complete detachment for each size. Adhesion potentials of the 18.75 cm^2 and 25cm^2 sizes of transdermal systems (0.075 mg/day and 0.1 mg/day) have not been studied.

Clinical Studies
Effects on vasomotor symptoms
A study of 214 women 25 to 74 years old met the qualification criteria and were randomly assigned to one of the three treatment groups: 72 to the 0.05 mg estradiol patch, 70 to the 0.1 mg estradiol patch, and 72 to placebo. Potential subjects were postmenopausal women in good general health who experienced vasomotor symptoms. Natural menopause patients had not menstruated for at least 12 months and surgical menopause patients had undergone bilateral oophorectomy at least 4 weeks before evaluation for study entry. In order to enter the 11-week treatment phase of the study, potential subjects must have experienced a minimum of five moderate to severe hot flushes per week, or a minimum of 15 hot flushes of any severity per week, for 2 consecutive weeks. Women wore the patches in a cyclical fashion (three weeks on and one week off).

During treatment, all subjects used diaries to record the number and severity of hot flushes. Subjects were monitored by clinic visits at the end of weeks 1, 3, 7, and 11 and by telephone at the end of weeks 4, 5, 8, and 9.

Adequate data for the analysis of efficacy was available from 191 subjects. The results are presented as the mean ± SD number of flushes in each of the 3 treatment weeks of each 4-week cycle. In the 0.05 mg estradiol group, the mean weekly hot flush rate across all treatment cycles decreased from 46 ± 6.5 at baseline to 20 ± 3 (-67.0%). The 0.1 mg estradiol group had a decline in the mean weekly hot flush rate from 52 ± 4.4 at baseline to 16 ± 2.4 (-72%). In the placebo group, the mean weekly hot flush rate declined from 53 ± 4.5 at baseline to 46 ± 6.5 (-18.1%). Compared with placebo, the 0.05 mg and 0.1 mg estradiol groups showed a statistically significantly larger mean decrease in hot flushes across all treatment cycles (P<0.05). When the response to treatment was analyzed for each of the three cycles of therapy, similar statistically significant differences were observed between both estradiol treatment groups and the placebo group during all treatment cycles.

In a double-blind, placebo-controlled, randomized study of 187 women receiving Climara 0.025 mg/day or placebo continuously for up to three 28-day cycles, the Climara 0.025 mg/day dosage was shown to be statistically better than placebo at weeks 4 and 12 for relief of both the frequency and severity of moderate-to-severe vasomotor symptoms.

Table 1
Pharmacokinetic Summary
(Mean Estradiol Values)

Climara® Delivery Rate	Surface Area (cm²)	Application Site	No. of Subjects	Dosing	C_{max} (pg/mL)	C_{min} (pg/mL)	C_{avg} (pg/mL)
0.025	6.5	Abdomen	24	Single	32	17	22
0.05	12.5	Abdomen	102	Single	71	29	41
0.1	25	Abdomen	139	Single	147	60	87
0.1	25	Buttock	38	Single	174	71	106

Table 2
Mean Change from Baseline in the Number of Moderate-to-Severe Vasomotor Symptoms (ITT)

Treatment Group	Statistics	Week 4	Week 8	Week 12
E_2 TDS	N	82	84	68
	Mean	-6.45	-7.69	-7.56
	SD	4.65	4.76	4.64
Placebo	N	83	71	65
	Mean	-5.11	-5.98	-5.98
	SD	7.43	8.63	9.69
	p-Value	<0.002		<0.003

A second active-control trial of 193 randomized subjects was supportive of the placebo-controlled trial.

Effects on bone mineral density
A two-year clinical trial enrolled a total of 175 healthy, hysterectomized, postmenopausal, non-osteoporotic (i.e., lumbar spine bone mineral density >0.9 gm/cm²) women at 10 study centers in the United States. 129 subjects were allocated to receive active treatment with 4 different doses of estradiol patches (6.5, 12.5, 15, 25 cm²) and 46 subjects were allocated to receive placebo patches. 77% of the randomized subjects (100 on active drug and 34 on placebo) contributed data to the analysis of percent change of A-P spine bone mineral density (BMD), the primary efficacy variable (see **Figure 3**). A statistically significant overall treatment effect at each timepoint was noted, implying bone preservation for all active treatment groups at all timepoints, as opposed to bone loss for placebo at all timepoints.

Figure 3
Mean Percent Change from Baseline in Lumbar Spine (A-P View) Bone Mineral Density By Treatment and Time last observation carried forward

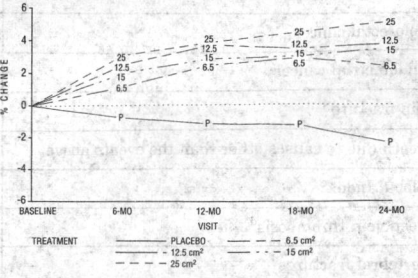

Percent change in BMD of the total hip (see **Figure 4**) was also statistically significantly different from placebo for all active treatment groups. The results of the measurements of biochemical markers supported the finding of efficacy for all doses of transdermal estradiol. Serum osteocalcin levels decreased, indicative of a decrease in bone formation, at all timepoints for all active treatment doses, statistically significantly different from placebo (which generally rose). Urinary deoxypyridinoline and pyridinoline changes also suggested a decrease in bone turnover for all active treatment groups.

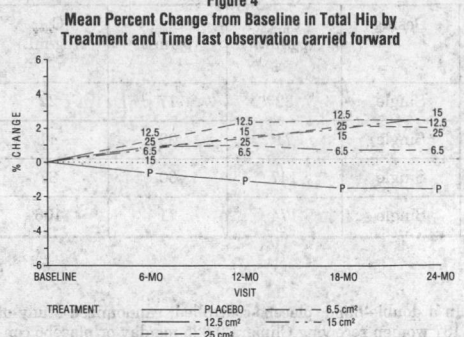

Figure 4
Mean Percent Change from Baseline in Total Hip by Treatment and Time last observation carried forward

Footnote: This figure is based on 74% of the randomized subjects (95 on active drug and 34 on placebo).

Women's Health Initiative Studies

The Women's Health Initiative (WHI) enrolled a total of 27,000 predominantly healthy postmenopausal women to assess the risks and benefits of either the use of oral 0.625 mg conjugated estrogens (CE) per day alone or the use of 0.625 mg conjugated estrogens plus 2.5 mg medroxyprogesterone acetate (MPA) per day compared to placebo in the prevention of certain chronic diseases. The primary endpoint was the incidence of coronary heart disease (CHD) (nonfatal myocardial infarction and CHD death), with invasive breast cancer as the primary adverse outcome studied. A "global index" included the earliest occurrence of CHD, invasive breast cancer, stroke, pulmonary embolism (PB), endometrial cancer, colorectal cancer, hip fixture, or death due to other cause. The study did not evaluate the effects of CE or CE/MPA on menopausal symptoms.

The CE/MPA substudy was stopped early because, according to the predefined stopping rule, the increased risk of breast cancer and cardiovascular events exceeded the specified benefits included in the "global index." Results of the CE/MPA substudy, which included 16,608 women (average age of 63 years, range 50 to 79; 83.9% White, 6.5% Black, 5.5% Hispanic), after an average follow-up of 5.2 years are presented in Table 3 below:

[See table 3 below]

For those outcomes included in the "global index," the absolute excess risks per 10,000 women-years in the group treated with CE/MPA were 7 more CHD events, 8 more

strokes, 8 more PEs, and 8 more invasive breast cancers, while absolute risk reductions per 10,000 women-years were 6 fewer colorectal cancers and 5 fewer hip fractures. The absolute excess risk of events included in the "global index" was 19 per 10,000 women-years. There was no difference between the groups in terms of all-cause mortality. (See **BOXED WARNINGS, WARNINGS,** and **PRECAUTIONS.**)

Women's Health Initiative Memory Study

The Women's Health Initiative Memory Study (WHIMS), a substudy of WHI, enrolled 4,532 predominantly postmenopausal women 65 years of age and older (47% were age 65 to 69 years, 35% were 70 to 74 years, and 18% were 75 years of age and older) to evaluate the effects of CE/MPA (0.625 mg conjugated estrogens plus 2.5 mg medroxyprogesterone acetate) on the incidence of probable dementia (primary outcome) compared with placebo.

After an average follow-up of 4 years, 40 women in the estrogen/progestin group (45 per 10,000 women-years) and 21 in the placebo group (22 per 10,000 women-years) were diagnosed with probable dementia. The relative risk of probable dementia in the hormone therapy group was 2.05 (95% CI, 1.21 to 3.48) compared to placebo. Differences between groups became apparent in the first year of treatment. It is unknown whether these findings apply to younger postmenopausal women. (See **BOXED WARNINGS** and **WARNINGS, Dementia** and **PRECAUTIONS, Geriatric Use.**)

INDICATIONS AND USAGE

Climara is indicated in the:
1. Treatment of moderate to severe vasomotor symptoms associated with the menopause.
2. Treatment of moderate to severe symptoms of vulvar and vaginal atrophy associated with the menopause. When prescribing solely for the treatment of symptoms of vulvar and vaginal atrophy, topical vaginal products should be considered.
3. Treatment of hypoestrogenism due to hypogonadism, castration or primary ovarian failure.
4. Prevention of postmenopausal osteoporosis. When prescribing solely for the prevention of postmenopausal osteoporosis, therapy should only be considered for women at significant risk of osteoporosis and non-estrogen medications should be carefully considered.

The mainstays for decreasing the risk of postmenopausal osteoporosis are weight bearing exercise, adequate calcium and vitamin D intake, and when indicated, pharmacologic therapy. Postmenopausal women require an average of 1500 mg/day of elemental calcium. Therefore, when not contraindicated, calcium supplementation may be helpful for women with suboptimal dietary intake.

Vitamin D supplementation of 400-800 IU/day may also be required to ensure adequate daily intake in postmenopausal women.

CONTRAINDICATIONS

Climara should not be used in women with any of the following conditions:
1. Undiagnosed abnormal genital bleeding.
2. Known, suspected, or history of cancer of the breast.
3. Known or suspected estrogen-dependent neoplasia.
4. Active deep vein thrombosis, pulmonary embolism or a history of these conditions.
5. Active or recent (e.g. within the past year) arterial thromboembolic disease (e.g., stroke, myocardial infarction).
6. Liver dysfunction or disease.
7. Climara should not be used in patients with known hypersensitivity to its ingredients.
8. Known or suspected pregnancy. There is no indication for Climara in pregnancy. There appears to be little or no increased risk of birth defects in children born to women who have used estrogens and progestins from oral contraceptives inadvertently during early pregnancy (see **PRECAUTIONS**).

WARNINGS

See BOXED WARNINGS.

1. Cardiovascular disorders.

Estrogen and estrogen/progestin therapy has been associated with an increased risk of cardiovascular events such as myocardial infarction and stroke, as well as venous thrombosis and pulmonary embolism (venous thromboembolism or VTE). Should any of these occur or be suspected, estrogens should be discontinued immediately.

Risk factors for arterial vascular disease (e.g., hypertension, diabetes mellitus, tobacco use, hypercholesterolemia, and obesity) and/or venous thromboembolism (e.g., personal history or family history of VTE, obesity, and systemic lupus erythematosus) should be managed appropriately.

a. Coronary heart disease and stroke

In the Women's Health Initiative (WHI) study, an increased risk of stroke was observed in women receiving oral CE compared to placebo.

In the CE/MPA substudy of WHI an increased risk of coronary heart disease (CHD) events (defined as nonfatal myocardial infarction and CHD death) was observed in women receiving CE/MPA compared to women receiving placebo (37 vs 30 per 10,000 women years). The increase in risk was observed in year one and persisted. (See **CLINICAL PHARMACOLOGY, Clinical Studies.**)

In the same substudy of WHI, an increased risk of stroke was observed in women receiving CE/MPA compared to women receiving placebo (29 vs 21 per 10,000 women-years). The increase in risk was observed after the first year and persisted.

In postmenopausal women with documented heart disease (n = 2,763, average age 66.7 years) a controlled clinical trial of secondary prevention of cardiovascular disease (Heart and Estrogen/Progestin Replacement Study; HERS) treatment with CE/MPA (0.625mg/2.5mg per day) demonstrated no cardiovascular benefit. During an average follow-up of 4.1 years, treatment with CE/MPA did not reduce the overall rate of CHD events in postmenopausal women with established coronary heart disease. There were more CHD events in the CE/MPA-treated group than in the placebo group in year 1, but not during the subsequent years. Two thousand three hundred and twenty one women from the original HERS trial agreed to participate in an open label extension of HERS, HERS II. Average follow-up in HERS II was an additional 2.7 years, for a total of 6.8 years overall. Rates of CHD events were comparable among women in the CE/MPA group and the placebo group in HERS, HERS II, and overall.

b. Venous thromboembolism (VTE)

In the Women's Health Initiative (WHI) study, an increased risk of deep vein thrombosis was observed in women receiving CE compared to placebo.

In the CE/MPA substudy of WHI, a 2-fold greater rate of VTE, including deep venous thrombosis and pulmonary embolism, was observed in women receiving CE/MPA compared to women receiving placebo. The rate of VTE was 34 per 10,000 women-years in the CE/MPA group compared to 16 per 10,000 women-years in the placebo group. The increase in VTE risk was observed during the first year and persisted. (See **CLINICAL PHARMACOLOGY, Clinical Studies.**)

If feasible, estrogens should be discontinued at least 4 to 6 weeks before surgery of the type associated with an increased risk of thromboembolism, or during periods of prolonged immobilization.

2. Malignant neoplasms

a. Endometrial cancer

The use of unopposed estrogens in women with intact uteri has been associated with an increased risk of endometrial cancer. The reported endometrial cancer risk among unopposed estrogen users is about 2- to

Table 3
Relative and Absolute Risk Seen in the CE/MPA Substudy of WHI[a]

Event[c]	Relative Risk CE/MPA vs placebo at 5.2 Years (95% CI*)	Placebo n = 8102	CE/MPA n = 8506
		Absolute Risk per 10,000 Person-years	
CHD events	1.29 (1.02-1.63)	30	37
Non-fatal MI	*1.32 (1.02-1.72)*	*23*	*30*
CHD death	*1.18 (0.70-1.97)*	*6*	*7*
Invasive breast cancer[b]	1.26 (1.00-1.59)	30	38
Stroke	1.41 (1.07-1.85)	21	29
Pulmonary embolism	2.13 (1.39-3.25)	8	16
Colorectal cancer	0.63 (0.43-0.92)	16	10
Endometrial cancer	0.83 (0.47-1.47)	6	5
Hip fracture	0.66 (0.45-0.98)	15	10
Death due to causes other than the events above	0.92 (0.74-1.14)	40	37
Global Index[c]	1.15 (1.03-1.28)	151	170
Deep vein thrombosis[d]	2.07 (1.49-2.87)	13	26
Vertebral fractures[d]	0.66 (0.44-0.98)	15	9
Other osteoporotic fractures[d]	0.77 (0.69-0.86)	170	131

[a] adapted from JAMA, 2002; 288:321-333
[b] includes metastatic and non-metastatic breast cancer with the exception of in situ breast cancer
[c] a subset of the events was combined in a "global index", defined as the earliest occurrence of CHD events, invasive breast cancer, stroke, pulmonary embolism, endometrial cancer, colorectal cancer, hip fracture, or death due to other causes
[d] not included in Global Index
* nominal confidence intervals unadjusted for multiple looks and multiple comparisons

12-fold greater than in non-users, and appears dependent on duration of treatment and on estrogen dose. Most studies show no significant increased risk associated with use of estrogens for less than one year. The greatest risk appears associated with prolonged use, with increased risks of 15- to 24-fold for five to ten years or more and this risk has been shown to persist for at least 8 to 15 years after estrogen therapy is discontinued.

Clinical surveillance of all women taking estrogen/progestin combinations is important. Adequate diagnostic measures, including endometrial sampling when indicated, should be undertaken to rule out malignancy in all cases of undiagnosed persistent or recurring abnormal vaginal bleeding. There is no evidence that the use of natural estrogens results in a different endometrial risk profile than synthetic estrogens of equivalent estrogen dose. Adding a progestin to estrogen therapy has been shown to reduce the risk of endometrial hyperplasia, which may be a precursor to endometrial cancer.

b. *Breast cancer*

The use of estrogens and progestins by postmenopausal women has been reported to increase the risk of breast cancer. The most important randomized clinical trial providing information about this issue is the Women's Health Initiative (WHI) substudy of CE/MPA (see **CLINICAL PHARMACOLOGY, Clinical Studies**). The results from observational studies are generally consistent with those of the WHI clinical trial and report no significant variation in the risk of breast cancer among different estrogens or progestins, doses, or routes of administration.

The CE/MPA substudy of WHI reported an increased risk of breast cancer in women who took CE/MPA for a mean follow-up of 5.6 years. Observational studies have also reported an increased risk for estrogen/progestin combination therapy, and a smaller increased risk for estrogen alone therapy, after several years of use. In the WHI trial and from observational studies, the excess risk increased with duration of use. From observational studies, the risk appeared to return to baseline in about five years after stopping treatment. In addition, observational studies suggest that the risk of breast cancer was greater, and became apparent earlier, with estrogen/progestin combination therapy as compared to estrogen alone therapy.

In the CE/MPA substudy, 26% of the women reported prior use of estrogen alone and/or estrogen/progestin combination hormone therapy. After a mean follow-up of 5.6 years during the clinical trial, the overall relative risk of invasive breast cancer was 1.24 (95% confidence interval 1.01-1.54), and the overall absolute risk was 41 vs. 33 cases per 10,000 women-years, for CE/MPA compared with placebo. Among women who reported prior use of hormone therapy, the relative risk of invasive breast cancer was 1.86, and the absolute risk was 46 vs. 25 cases per 10,000 women-years, for CE/MPA compared with placebo. Among women who reported no prior use of hormone therapy, the relative risk of invasive breast cancer was 1.09, and the absolute risk was 40 vs. 36 cases per 10,000 women-years for CE/MPA compared with placebo. In the same substudy, invasive breast cancers were larger and diagnosed at a more advanced stage in the CE/MPA group compared with the placebo group. Metastatic disease was rare with no apparent difference between the two groups. Other prognostic factors such as histologic subtype, grade and hormone receptor status did not differ between the groups.

The use of estrogen plus progestin has been reported to result in an increase in abnormal mammograms requiring further evaluation. All women should receive yearly breast examinations by a healthcare provider and perform monthly breast self-examinations. In addition, mammography examinations should be scheduled based on patient age, risk factors, and prior mammogram results.

3. Dementia

In the Women's Health Initiative Memory Study (WHIMS), 4,532 generally healthy postmenopausal women 65 years of age and older were studied, of whom 35% were 70 to 74 years of age and 18% were 75 or older. After an average follow-up of 4 years, 40 women being treated with CE/MPA (1.8%, n=2,229) and 21 women in the placebo group (0.9%, n=2,303) received diagnoses of probable dementia. The relative risk for CE/MPA versus placebo was 2.05 (95% confidence interval 1.21–3.48), and was similar for women with and without histories of menopausal hormone use before WHIMS. The absolute risk of probable dementia for CE/MPA versus placebo was 45 versus 22 cases per 10,000 women-years, and the absolute excess risk for CE/MPA was 23 cases per 10,000 women-years. It is unknown whether these findings apply to younger postmenopausal women. (See **CLINICAL PHARMACOLOGY, Clinical Studies** and **PRECAUTIONS, Geriatric Use.**)

4. Gallbladder disease

A 2- to 4-fold increase in the risk of gallbladder disease requiring surgery in postmenopausal women receiving estrogens has been reported.

5. Hypercalcemia

Estrogen administration may lead to severe hypercalcemia in patients with breast cancer and bone metastases. If hypercalcemia occurs, use of the drug should be stopped and appropriate measures taken to reduce the serum calcium level.

6. Visual abnormalities

Retinal vascular thrombosis has been reported in patients receiving estrogens. Discontinue medication pending examination if there is sudden partial or complete loss of vision, or a sudden onset of proptosis, diplopia, or migraine. If examination reveals papilledema or retinal vascular lesions, estrogens should be permanently discontinued.

PRECAUTIONS

A. General

1. *Addition of a progestin when a woman has not had a hysterectomy.*

Studies of the addition of a progestin for 10 or more days of a cycle of estrogen administration, or daily with estrogen in a continuous regimen, have reported a lowered incidence of endometrial hyperplasia than would be induced by estrogen treatment alone. Endometrial hyperplasia may be a precursor to endometrial cancer. There are, however, possible risks that may be associated with the use of progestins with estrogens compared to estrogen-alone treatment. These include a possible increased risk of breast cancer.

2. *Elevated blood pressure*

In a small number of case reports, substantial increases in blood pressure have been attributed to idiosyncratic reactions to estrogens. In a large, randomized, placebo-controlled clinical trial, a generalized effect of estrogens on blood pressure was not seen. Blood pressure should be monitored at regular intervals with estrogen use.

3. *Hypertriglyceridemia*

In patients with pre-existing hypertriglyceridemia, estrogen therapy may be associated with elevations of plasma triglycerides leading to pancreatitis and other complications.

4. Impaired liver function *and past history of cholestatic jaundice*

Estrogens may be poorly metabolized in patients with impaired liver function. For patients with a history of cholestatic jaundice associated with past estrogen use or with pregnancy, caution should be exercised and in the case of recurrence, medication should be discontinued.

5. *Hypothyroidism*

Estrogen administration leads to increased thyroid-binding globulin (TBG) levels. Patients with normal thyroid function can compensate for the increased TBG by making more thyroid hormone, thus maintaining free T_4 and T_3 serum concentrations in the normal range. Patients dependent on thyroid hormone replacement therapy who are also receiving estrogens may require increased doses of their thyroid replacement therapy. These patients should have their thyroid function monitored in order to maintain their free thyroid hormone levels in an acceptable range.

6. *Fluid retention*

Because estrogens may cause some degree of fluid retention, patients with conditions that might be influenced by this factor, such as a cardiac or renal dysfunction, warrant careful observation when estrogens are prescribed.

7. *Hypocalcemia*

Estrogens should be used with caution in individuals with severe hypocalcemia.

8. *Ovarian cancer*

The CE/MPA sub-study of WHI reported that estrogen plus progestin increased the risk of ovarian cancer. After an average follow-up of 5.6 years, the relative risk for ovarian cancer for CE/MPA versus placebo was 1.58 (95% confidence interval 0.77-3.24) but was not statistically significant. The absolute risk for CE/MPA versus placebo was 4.2 versus 2.7 cases per 10,000 women-years. In some epidemiological studies, the use of estrogen alone, in particular for ten or more years, has been associated with an increased risk of ovarian cancer. Other epidemiologic studies have not found these associations.

9. *Exacerbation of endometriosis*

Endometriosis may be exacerbated with administration of estrogens. A few cases of malignant transformation of residual endometrial implants have been reported in women treated post-hysterectomy with estrogen alone therapy. For patients known to have residual endometriosis post-hysterectomy, the addition of progestin should be considered.

10. *Exacerbation of other conditions*

Estrogens may cause an exacerbation of asthma, diabetes mellitus, epilepsy, migraine or porphyria, systemic lupus erythematosus, and hepatic hemangiomas and should be used with caution in women with these conditions.

B. PATIENT INFORMATION

Physicians are advised to discuss the PATIENT INFORMATION leaflet with patients for whom they prescribe Climara.

C. LABORATORY TESTS

Estrogen administration should be initiated at the lowest dose approved for the indication and then guided by clinical response rather than by serum hormone levels (e.g. estradiol, FSH).

D. DRUG/LABORATORY TEST INTERACTIONS

1. Accelerated prothrombin time, partial thromboplastin time, and platelet aggregation time; increased platelet count; increased factors II, VII antigen, VIII antigen, VIII coagulant activity, IX, X, XII, VII-X complex, II-VII-X complex, and beta-thromboglobulin; decreased levels of antifactor Xa and antithrombin III, decreased antithrombin III activity; increased levels of fibrinogen and fibrinogen activity; increased plasminogen antigen and activity.
2. Increased thyroid-binding globulin (TBG) levels leading to increased circulating total thyroid hormone levels as measured by protein-bound iodine (PBI), T_4 levels (by column or by radioimmunoassay) or T_3 levels by radioimmunoassay. T_3 resin uptake is decreased, reflecting the elevated TBG. Free T_4 and free T_3 concentrations are unaltered. Patients on thyroid replacement therapy may require higher doses of thyroid hormone.
3. Other binding proteins may be elevated in serum (i.e., corticosteroid binding globulin (CBG), sex hormone-binding globulin (SHBG)) leading to increased total circulating corticosteroids and sex steroids, respectively. Free hormone concentrations may be decreased. Other plasma proteins may be increased (angiotensinogen/renin substrate, alpha-l-antitrypsin, ceruloplasmin).
4. Increased plasma HDL and HDL_2 cholesterol subfraction concentrations, reduced LDL cholesterol concentration, and in oral formulations increased triglyceride levels.
5. Impaired glucose tolerance.
6. Reduced response to metyrapone test.

E. CARCINOGENESIS, MUTAGENESIS, AND IMPAIRMENT OF FERTILITY

Long-term continuous administration of estrogen, with and without progestin, in women with and without a uterus, has shown an increased risk of endometrial cancer, breast cancer, and ovarian cancer. (See **BOXED WARNINGS, WARNINGS** and **PRECAUTIONS.**)

Long-term continuous administration of natural and synthetic estrogens in certain animal species increases the frequency of carcinomas of the breast, uterus, cervix, vagina, testis, and liver.

F. PREGNANCY

Climara should not be used during pregnancy. (See **CONTRAINDICATIONS.**)

G. NURSING MOTHERS

Estrogen administration to nursing mothers has been shown to decrease the quantity and quality of the milk. Detectable amounts of estrogens have been identified in the milk of mothers receiving this drug. Caution should be exercised when Climara is administered to a nursing woman.

H. PEDIATRIC USE

Estrogen replacement therapy has been used for the induction of puberty in adolescents with some forms of pubertal delay. Safety and effectiveness in pediatric patients have not otherwise been established. Large and repeated doses of estrogen over an extended time period have been shown to accelerate epiphyseal closure, which could result in short adult stature if treatment is initiated before the completion of physiologic puberty in normally developing children. If estrogen is administered to patients whose bone growth is not complete, periodic monitoring of bone maturation and effects on epiphyseal centers is recommended during estrogen administration. Estrogen treatment of prepubertal girls also induces premature breast development and vaginal cornification, and may induce vaginal bleeding. In boys, estrogen treatment may modify the normal pu-

Summary of Most Frequently Reported Adverse Experiences/Medical Events (≥5%) by Treatment Groups

AE per Body System	Climara®			Placebo (N=72)
	0.025 mg/day (N=219)	0.05 mg/day (N=201)	0.1 mg/day (N=194)	
Body as a Whole	21%	39%	37%	29%
Headache	5%	18%	13%	10%
Pain	1%	8%	11%	7%
Back Pain	4%	8%	9%	6%
Edema	0.5%	13%	10%	6%
Gastro-Intestinal	9%	21%	29%	18%
Abdominal Pain	0%	11%	16%	8%
Nausea	1%	5%	6%	3%
Flatulence	1%	3%	7%	1%
Musculo-Skeletal	7%	9%	11%	4%
Arthralgia	1%	5%	5%	3%
Psychiatric	13%	10%	11%	1%
Depression	1%	5%	8%	0%
Reproductive	12%	18%	41%	11%
Breast Pain	5%	8%	29%	4%
Leukorrhea	1%	6%	7%	1%
Respiratory	15%	26%	29%	14%
URTI	6%	17%	17%	8%
Pharyngitis	0.5%	3%	7%	3%
Sinusitis	4%	4%	5%	3%
Rhinitis	2%	4%	6%	1%
Skin and Appendages	19%	12%	12%	15%
Pruritus	0.5%	6%	3%	6%

bertal process and induce gynecomastia. (See **INDICATIONS** and **DOSAGE AND ADMINISTRATION**.)

I. GERIATRIC USE

There have not been sufficient numbers of geriatric patients involved in clinical studies utilizing Climara to determine whether those over 65 years of age differ from younger subjects in their response to Climara.

In the Women's Health Initiative Memory Study, including 4,532 women 65 years of age and older, followed for an average of 4 years, 82% (n=3,729) were 65 to 74 while 18% (n=803) were 75 and over. Most women (80%) had no prior hormone therapy use. Women treated with conjugated estrogens plus medroxyprogesterone acetate were reported to have a two-fold increase in the risk of developing probable dementia. Alzheimer's disease was the most common classification of probable dementia in both the conjugated estrogens plus medroxyprogesterone acetate group and the placebo group. Ninety percent of the cases of probable dementia occurred in the 54% of women that were older than 70. (See **BOXED WARNING** and **WARNINGS, Dementia**.)

ADVERSE REACTIONS

See **BOXED WARNINGS, WARNINGS** and **PRECAUTIONS**.

Because clinical trials are conducted under widely varying conditions, adverse reaction rates observed in the clinical trials of a drug cannot be directly compared to rates in the clinical trials of another drug and may not reflect the rates observed in practice. The adverse reaction information from clinical trials does, however, provide a basis for identifying the adverse events that appear to be related to drug use and for approximating rates.

[See table above]

Postmarketing Experience: The following adverse reactions have been identified during post approval use of Climara: a few cases in which there were a combination of the symptoms of generalized hives or rash with swelling of the throat or eyelid edema. Because these reactions are reported voluntarily from a population of uncertain size, it is not always possible to reliably estimate their frequency or establish a causal relationship to drug exposure.

The following additional adverse reactions have been reported with estrogen and/or progestin therapy.

1. Genitourinary system
Changes in vaginal bleeding pattern and abnormal withdrawal bleeding or flow; breakthrough bleeding; spotting; dysmenorrhea; increase in size of uterine leiomyomata; vaginitis, including vaginal candidiasis; change in amount of cervical secretion; changes in cervical ectropion; ovarian cancer; endometrial hyperplasia; endometrial cancer.

2. Breasts
Tenderness, enlargement, pain, nipple discharge, galactorrhea; fibrocystic breast changes; breast cancer.

3. Cardiovascular
Deep and superficial venous thrombosis; pulmonary embolism; thrombophlebitis; myocardial infarction; stroke; increase in blood pressure.

4. Gastrointestinal
Nausea, vomiting; abdominal cramps, bloating; cholestatic jaundice; increased incidence of gall bladder disease; pancreatitis; enlargement of hepatic hemangiomas.

5. Skin
Chloasma or melasma, which may persist when drug is discontinued; erythema multiforme; erythema nodosum; hemorrhagic eruption; loss of scalp hair; hirsutism; pruritus, rash.

6. Eyes
Retinal vascular thrombosis, intolerance to contact lenses.

7. Central nervous system
Headache; migraine; dizziness; mental depression; chorea; nervousness; mood disturbances; irritability; exacerbation of epilepsy, dementia.

8. Miscellaneous
Increase or decrease in weight; reduced carbohydrate tolerance; aggravation of porphyria; edema; arthalgias; leg cramps; changes in libido; anaphylactoid/anaphylactic reactions; hypocalcemia; exacerbation of asthma; increased triglycerides.

OVERDOSAGE

Serious ill effects have not been reported following acute ingestion of large doses of estrogen-containing oral contraceptives by young children. Overdosage of estrogen may cause nausea and vomiting, and withdrawal bleeding may occur in females.

DOSAGE AND ADMINISTRATION

When estrogen is prescribed for a postmenopausal woman with a uterus, progestin should also be initiated to reduce the risk of endometrial cancer. A woman without a uterus does not need progestin. Use of estrogen, alone or in combination with a progestin, should be with the lowest effective dose and for the shortest duration consistent with treatment goals and risks for the individual woman. Patients should be reevaluated periodically as clinically appropriate (e.g., 3-month to 6-month intervals) to determine if treatment is still necessary (See **BOXED WARNINGS** and **WARNINGS**.) For women who have a uterus, adequate diagnostic measures, such as endometrial sampling, when indicated, should be undertaken to rule out malignancy in cases of undiagnosed persistent or recurring abnormal vaginal bleeding.

Patients should be started at the lowest dose. Six (6.5, 9.375, 12.5, 15, 18.75 and 25 cm²) Climara systems are available. For the treatment of vasomotor symptoms, treatment should be initiated with the 6.5 cm² (0.025 mg/day) Climara system applied to the skin once weekly. The dose should be adjusted as necessary to control symptoms. Clinical responses (relief of symptoms) at the lowest effective dose should be the guide for establishing administration of the Climara system, especially in women with an intact uterus. Attempts to taper or discontinue the medication should be made at 3- to 6-month intervals. In women who are not currently taking oral estrogens, treatment with the Climara system can be initiated at once. In women who are currently taking oral estrogen, treatment with the Climara system can be initiated 1-week after withdrawal of oral therapy or sooner if symptoms reappear in less than 1-week. For the prevention of postmenopausal osteoporosis, the minimum dose that has been shown to be effective is the 6.5 cm² (0.025 mg/day) Climara system. Response to therapy can be assessed by biochemical markers and measurement of bone mineral density.

Application of the System
The adhesive side of the Climara system should be placed on a clean, dry area of the lower abdomen or the upper quadrant of the buttock. **The Climara system should not be applied to or near the breasts.** The sites of application must be rotated, with an interval of at least 1-week allowed between applications to a particular site. The area selected should not be oily, damaged, or irritated. The waistline should be avoided, since tight clothing may rub or remove the system. Application to areas where sitting would dislodge the system should also be avoided. The system should be applied immediately after opening the pouch and removing the protective liner. The system should be pressed firmly in place with the fingers for about 10 seconds, making sure there is good contact, especially around the edges. If the system lifts, apply pressure to maintain adhesion. In the event that a system should fall off, a new system should be applied for the remainder of the 7-day dosing interval. Only one system should be worn at any one time during the 7-day dosing interval. Swimming, bathing, or using a sauna while using the Climara system has not been studied, and these activities may decrease the adhesion of the system and the delivery of estradiol.

Removal of the System
Removal of the system should be done carefully and slowly to avoid irritation of the skin. Should any adhesive remain on the skin after removal of the system, allow the area to dry for 15 minutes. Then gently rubbing the area with an oil-based cream or lotion should remove the adhesive residue.

Used patches still contain some active hormones. Each patch should be carefully folded in half so that it sticks to itself before throwing it away.

HOW SUPPLIED

Climara (estradiol transdermal system), 0.025 mg/day — each 6.5 cm² system contains 2 mg of estradiol USP Individual Carton of 4 systems .... NDC 50419-454-04
Climara (estradiol transdermal system), 0.0375 mg/day — each 9.375 cm² system contains 2.85 mg of estradiol USP Individual Carton of 4 systems .... NDC 50419-456-04
Climara (estradiol transdermal system), 0.05 mg/day — each 12.5 cm² system contains 3.8 mg of estradiol USP Individual Carton of 4 systems .... NDC 50419-451-04
Climara (estradiol transdermal system), 0.06 mg/day — each 15 cm² system contains 4.55 mg of estradiol USP Individual Carton of 4 systems .... NDC 50419-459-04
Climara (estradiol transdermal system), 0.075 mg/day — each 18.75 cm² system contains 5.7 mg of estradiol USP Individual Carton of 4 systems .... NDC 50419-453-04
Climara (estradiol transdermal system), 0.1 mg/day — each 25 cm² system contains 7.6 mg of estradiol USP Individual Carton of 4 systems .... NDC 50419-452-04
Do not store above 86°F (30°C). Do not store unpouched. Apply immediately upon removal from the protective pouch.

PATIENT INFORMATION Updated June 2005

Climara
(estradiol transdermal system)
Read this PATIENT INFORMATION before you start using Climara and read what you get each time you refill Climara. There may be new information. This information does not take the place of talking to your healthcare provider about your medical condition or your treatment.

What is the most important information I should know about Climara (an estrogen hormone)?
• Estrogens increase the chances of getting cancer of the uterus.
Report any unusual vaginal bleeding right away while you are taking estrogens. Vaginal bleeding after menopause may be a warning sign of cancer of the uterus (womb). Your healthcare provider should check any unusual vaginal bleeding to find out the cause.
• Do not use estrogens with or without progestins to prevent heart disease, heart attacks, strokes, or dementia.

Using estrogens with or without progestins may increase your chances of getting heart attack, strokes, breast cancer, and blood clots. Using estrogens with progestins may increase your risk of dementia. You and your healthcare provider should talk regularly about whether you still need treatment with Climara.

What is Climara?
Climara is a medicine that contains estrogen hormones.
What is Climara used for?
Climara is used after menopause to:
• **reduce moderate to severe hot flashes.** Estrogens are hormones made by a woman's ovaries. The ovaries normally stop making estrogens when a woman is between 45 to 55 years old. This drop in body estrogen levels causes the "change of life" or menopause (the end of monthly menstrual periods). Sometimes, both ovaries are removed during an operation before natural menopause takes place. The sudden drop in estrogen levels causes "surgical menopause."
When the estrogen levels begin dropping, some women develop very uncomfortable symptoms, such as feelings of warmth in the face, neck, and chest, or sudden strong feelings of heat and sweating ("hot flashes" or "hot flushes"). In some women, the symptoms are mild, and they will not need estrogens. In other women, symptoms can be more severe. You and your healthcare provider should talk regularly about whether you still need treatment with Climara.
• **treat moderate to severe dryness, itching, and burning in or around the vagina.** You and your healthcare provider should talk regularly about whether you still need treatment with Climara to control these problems. If you use Climara only to treat your dryness, itching, and burning in and around your vagina, talk with your healthcare provider about whether a topical vaginal product would be better for you.
• **treat certain conditions in which a young woman's ovaries do not produce enough estrogen naturally.**
• **help reduce your chances of getting osteoporosis (thin weak bones).** Osteoporosis from menopause is a thinning of the bones that makes them weaker and easier to break. If you use Climara only to prevent osteoporosis from menopause, talk with your healthcare provider about whether a different treatment or medicine without estrogens might be better for you. You and your healthcare provider should talk regularly about whether you should continue with Climara.
Weight-bearing exercise, like walking or running, and taking calcium and vitamin D supplements may also lower your chances of getting postmenopausal osteoporosis. It is important to talk about exercise and supplements with your healthcare provider before starting them.
Who should not use Climara?
Do not start using Climara if you:
• **have unusual vaginal bleeding.**
• **currently have or have had certain cancers.** Estrogens may increase the chances of getting certain types of cancers, including cancer of the breast or uterus. If you have or had cancer, talk with your healthcare provider about whether you should take Climara.
• **had a stroke or heart attack in the past year.**
• **currently have or have had blood clots.**
• **currently have or have had liver problems.**
• **are allergic to Climara or any of its ingredients.** See the end of this leaflet for a list of ingredients in Climara.
• **think you may be pregnant.**
Tell your healthcare provider:
• **if you are breastfeeding.** The hormone in Climara can pass into your milk.
• **about all of your medical problems.** Your healthcare provider may need to check you more carefully if you have certain conditions, such as asthma (wheezing), epilepsy (seizures), migraine, endometriosis, lupus, problems with your heart, liver, thyroid, kidneys, or have high calcium levels in your blood.
• **about all the medicines you take.** This includes prescription and nonprescription medicines, vitamins, and herbal supplements. Some medicines may affect how Climara works. Climara may also affect how your other medicines work.
• **if you are going to have surgery or will be on bed rest.** You may need to stop taking estrogens.
How should I use Climara?
Climara is a patch that you wear on your skin. The estrogen in the Climara patch passes through your skin. You must change your Climara patch every 7 days (once a week). See the end of this leaflet for complete instructions on how to use Climara.
1. Start at the lowest dose and talk to your health care provider about how well that dose is working for you.
2. Estrogens should be used at the lowest dose possible for your treatment only as long as needed. You and your

healthcare provider should talk regularly (for example, every 3 to 6 months) about the dose you are taking and whether you still need treatment with Climara.
What are the possible side effects of estrogens?
Less common but serious side effects include:
• Breast cancer
• Cancer of the uterus
• Stroke
• Heart attack
• Blood clots
• Dementia
• Gallbladder disease
• Ovarian cancer
These are some of the warning signs of serious side effects:
• Breast lumps
• Unusual vaginal bleeding
• Dizziness and faintness
• Changes in speech
• Severe headaches
• Chest pain
• Shortness of breath
• Pains in your legs
• Changes in vision
• Vomiting
Call your healthcare provider right away if you get any of these warning signs, or any other unusual symptom that concerns you.
Common side effects include:
• Headache
• Breast pain
• Irregular vaginal bleeding or spotting
• Stomach/abdominal cramps, bloating
• Nausea and vomiting
• Hair loss
Other side effects include:
• High blood pressure
• Liver problems
• High blood sugar
• Fluid retention
• Enlargement of benign tumors of the uterus ("fibroids")
• Vaginal yeast infection
These are not all the possible side effects of Climara. For more information, ask your healthcare provider or pharmacist.
What can I do to lower my chances of a serious side effect with Climara?
Talk with your healthcare provider regularly about whether you should continue using Climara:
• If you have a uterus, talk to your healthcare provider about whether the addition of a progestin is right for you.
• See your healthcare provider right away if you get vaginal bleeding while using Climara.
• Have a breast exam and mammogram (breast X-ray) every year unless your healthcare provider tells you something else. If members of your family have had breast cancer or if you have ever had breast lumps or an abnormal mammogram, you may need to have breast exams more often.
• If you have high blood pressure, high cholesterol (fat in the blood), diabetes, are overweight, or if you use tobacco, you may have higher chances for getting heart disease. Ask your healthcare provider for ways to lower your chances for getting heart disease.
General information about safe and effective use of Climara.
Medicines are sometimes prescribed for conditions that are not mentioned in patient information leaflets. Do not take Climara for conditions for which it was not prescribed. Do not give Climara to other people, even if they have the same symptoms you have. **Do not take Climara if you are not sure.**
Keep Climara out of the reach of children.
This leaflet provides a summary of the most important information about Climara. If you would like more information, talk with your healthcare provider or pharmacist. You can ask for information about Climara that is written for health professionals. You can get more information by calling the toll free number (1-888-84BAYER).
What are the ingredients in Climara?
The active ingredient of Climara is estradiol. Climara also contains acrylate copolymer adhesive, fatty acid esters, and polyethylene backing.
Instructions for Use
How and Where to Apply the Climara Patch
Each Climara patch is individually sealed in a protective pouch. To open the pouch, hold it vertically with the Climara name facing you. Tear off the top of the pouch using the top tear notch. Tear off the side of the pouch using the side tear notch. Pull the pouch open. The Climara patch is the see-through plastic film attached to the clear thicker plastic backing. There is a silver foil-sticker attached to the inside of the pouch. **Do not remove it from the pouch.** The sticker contains a moisture protectant (desiccant). **Lift out the Climara patch.** Notice that the patch is attached to a

thicker, hard-plastic backing and that the patch itself is oval and see-through.

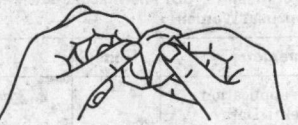

Apply the sticky side of the Climara patch to a clean, dry area of the lower stomach below your belly button or the top of the buttocks (see diagram below). **Do not apply the Climara patch to your breasts.** The sites of application on the lower stomach and buttocks must be rotated, allowing at least 1 week between applications to the same site. The site selected should not be oily, damaged, or irritated. Avoid the waistline, since tight clothing may rub and remove the patch. Also, do not put the patch on areas where sitting would rub it off or loosen it. Apply the patch right after opening the pouch and removing the protective liner. Press the patch firmly in place with your fingers for about 10 seconds. Make sure that it sticks all over, especially around the edges.

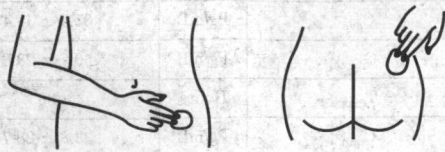

The Climara patch should be worn continuously for one week. You may wish to try different sites when putting on a new patch, to find ones that are most comfortable for you and where clothing will not rub on the patch or loosen it.
When to Apply the Climara System?
The Climara patch should be changed once weekly. Remove the used patch. Carefully fold it in half so that it sticks to itself because used patches still contain active hormones and discard it. Any adhesive that might remain on your skin can be easily rubbed off. Then place the new Climara patch on a different skin site. (The same skin site should not be used again for at least 1 week after removal of the patch.) Contact with water when you are bathing, swimming, or showering may affect the patch. If the patch falls off, the same patch may be reapplied to another area of the lower abdomen. Make sure that there is good contact, especially around the edges. If the patch will not stick completely to your skin, put a new patch on a different area of the lower abdomen. Do not apply two patches at the same time.
Estrogens should be used only as long as needed. You and your health care provider should talk regularly (for example, every 3 to 6 months) about whether you still need treatment with Climara.
© 2007, Bayer HealthCare Pharmaceuticals Inc. All rights reserved.
Manufactured for:
Bayer HealthCare Pharmaceuticals Inc.
Wayne, NJ 07470
Manufactured by:
3M Drug Delivery Systems
Northridge, CA 93124
6705601　　3M 679001　　December 2007
Shown in Product Identification Guide, page 307

CLIMARA PRO®　　　　　　　　　　　　　　℞
[kli-ma ra]
(Estradiol/Levonorgestrel TransdermalSystem)
Rx only
PRESCRIBING INFORMATION

WARNINGS
Estrogens and progestins should not be used for the prevention of cardiovascular disease or dementia. (See **WARNINGS, Cardiovascular disorders** and **Dementia**.)
The Women's Health Initiative (WHI) study reported increased risks of myocardial infarction, stroke, invasive breast cancer, pulmonary emboli, and deep vein thrombosis in postmenopausal women (50 to 79 years of age) during 5 years of treatment with oral conjugated estrogens (CE 0.625 mg) combined with medroxyprogesterone acetate (MPA 2.5 mg) relative to placebo. (See **CLINICAL STUDIES** and **WARNINGS, Cardiovascular disorders** and **Malignant neoplasms**, *Breast cancer*.)
The WHI study reported increased risks of stroke and deep vein thrombosis in postmenopausal women (50 to 79 years of age) during 6.8 years of treatment with oral conjugated estrogens (CE 0.625 mg) relative to placebo.

Table 1: Summary of Mean Pharmacokinetic Parameters

Summary of Mean (± SD) Pharmacokinetic Parameters Following a Single Application of Climara Pro in 24 Healthy Postmenopausal Women

Parameter	Units	Estradiol	Estrone	Levonorgestrel
Single application Week 1 Data				
C_{ave}	Pg/mL	37.7 ± 10.4	41 ± 15	136 ± 52.7
C_{max}	Pg/mL	54.3 ± 18.9	43.9 ± 14.9	138 ± 51.8
T_{max}	Hours	42	84	90
C_{min}	Pg/mL	27.2 ± 7.66	32.6 ± 14.3	110 ± 41.7
AUC	Pg.h/mL	6340 ± 1740	6890 ± 2520	22900 ± 8860

Summary of Mean (± SD) Pharmacokinetic Parameters (Week 4) Following Four Consecutive Weekly Applications of Climara Pro in 44 Healthy Postmenopausal Women

Parameter	Units	Estradiol	Estrone	Levonorgestrel
Multiple application Week 4 Data				
C_{ave}	Pg/mL	35.7 ± 11.4	45.5 ± 62.6	166 ± 97.8
C_{max}	Pg/mL	50.7 ± 28.6	81.6 ± 252	194 ± 111
T_{max}	Hours	36	48	48
C_{min}	Pg/mL	33.8 ± 28.7	72.5 ± 253	153 ± 69.6
AUC	Pg.h/mL	6002 ± 1919	7642 ± 10518	27948 ± 16426

All mean parameters are arithmetic means except T_{max} which is expressed as the median.

(See **CLINICAL STUDIES** and **WARNINGS, Cardiovascular disorders.**)
The Women's Health Initiative Memory Study (WHIMS), a substudy of WHI, reported increased risk of developing probable dementia in postmenopausal women 65 years of age or older during 4 years of treatment with CE 0.625 mg combined with MPA 2.5 mg and during 5.2 years of treatment with CE 0.625 mg alone, relative to placebo. It is unknown whether this finding applies to younger postmenopausal women. (See **CLINICAL STUDIES, WARNINGS, Dementia** and **PRECAUTIONS, Geriatric Use.**)
Other doses of oral conjugated estrogens with medroxyprogesterone acetate, and other combinations and dosage forms of estrogens and progestins were not studied in the WHI clinical trials and, in the absence of comparable data, these risks should be assumed to be similar. Because of these risks, estrogens with or without progestins should be prescribed at the lowest effective doses and for the shortest duration consistent with treatment goals and risks for the individual woman.

DESCRIPTION

Climara Pro® (Estradiol/Levonorgestrel Transdermal System) is an adhesive-based matrix transdermal patch designed to release both estradiol and levonorgestrel, a progestational agent, continuously upon application to intact skin.
The 22 cm² Climara Pro system contains 4.4 mg estradiol and 1.39 mg levonorgestrel and provides a nominal delivery rate (mg per day) of 0.045 estradiol and 0.015 levonorgestrel.
Estradiol USP has a molecular weight of 272.39 and the molecular formula is $C_{18}H_{24}O_2$.
Levonorgestrel USP has a molecular weight of 312.4 and a molecular formula of $C_{21}H_{28}O_2$.
The structural formulas for estradiol and levonorgestrel are:

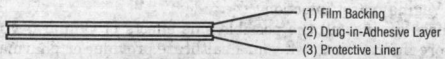

Estradiol (E₂)   Levonorgestrel (LNG)

The Climara Pro system comprises 3 layers. Proceeding from the visible surface towards the surface attached to the skin, these layers are (1) a translucent polyethylene backing film, (2) an acrylate adhesive matrix containing estradiol and levonorgestrel, and (3) a protective liner of either siliconized or fluoropolymer coated polyester film. The protective liner is attached to the adhesive surface and must be removed before the system can be used.

(1) Film Backing
(2) Drug-in-Adhesive Layer
(3) Protective Liner

The active components of the system are estradiol and levonorgestrel. The remaining components of the system (acrylate copolymer adhesive and polyvinylpyrrolidone/vinyl acetate copolymer) are pharmacologically inactive.

CLINICAL PHARMACOLOGY

Endogenous estrogens are largely responsible for the development and maintenance of the female reproductive system and secondary sexual characteristics. Although circulating estrogens exist in a dynamic equilibrium of metabolic interconversions, estradiol is the principal intracellular human estrogen and is substantially more potent than its metabolites, estrone and estriol at the receptor level.
The primary source of estrogen in normally cycling adult women is the ovarian follicle, which secretes 70 to 500 mcg of estradiol daily, depending on the phase of the menstrual cycle. After menopause, most endogenous estrogen is produced by conversion of androstenedione, secreted by the adrenal cortex, to estrone by peripheral tissues. Thus, estrone and the sulfate conjugated form, estrone sulfate, are the most abundant circulating estrogens in postmenopausal women.
Estrogens act through binding to nuclear receptors in estrogen-responsive tissues. To date, two estrogen receptors have been identified. These vary in proportion from tissue to tissue.
Circulating estrogens modulate the pituitary secretion of the gonadotropins, luteinizing hormone (LH) and follicle stimulating hormone (FSH), through a negative feedback mechanism. Estrogens act to reduce the elevated levels of these hormones seen in postmenopausal women.
Levonorgestrel inhibits gonadotropin production resulting in retardation of follicular growth and inhibition of ovulation.
Studies to assess the potency of progestins using estrogen-primed postmenopausal endometrial biochemistry and morphologic features have shown that levonorgestrel counteracts the proliferative effects of estrogens on the endometrium.

A. Absorption

Administration of Climara Pro to postmenopausal women produces mean maximum estradiol concentrations in serum in about 2 to 2.5 days. Estradiol concentrations equivalent to the normal ranges observed at the early follicular phase in premenopausal women are achieved within 12-24 hours after the first application.
In one study, steady state estradiol concentrations in serum were measured during week 4 in 44 healthy, postmenopausal women during four consecutive Climara Pro

applications of two formulations (0.045 mg estradiol/0.03 mg levonorgestrel and 0.045 mg estradiol/0.015 mg levonorgestrel) to the abdomen (each dose was applied for four 7-day periods). Both formulations were bioequivalent in terms of estradiol and estrone C_{max} and AUC parameters. A summary of Climara Pro single and multiple applications estradiol, estrone and levonorgestrel pharmacokinetic parameters is shown in Table 1.
[See table 1 at left]
At steady state, Climara Pro maintains during the application period an average serum estradiol concentration of 35.7 pg/mL as depicted in Figure 1.

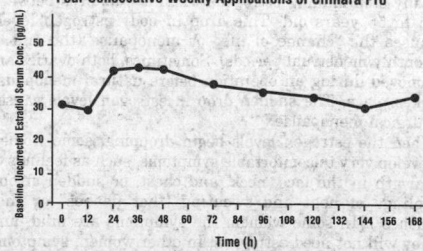

Figure 1: Mean Estradiol Concentration Profile (Week 4) Following Four Consecutive Weekly Applications of Climara Pro

Following the application of the Climara Pro transdermal system, levonorgestrel concentrations are maximum in about 2.5 days. At steady state, Climara Pro maintains during the application period an average serum levonorgestrel concentration of 166 pg/mL as depicted in Figure 2. The mean levonorgestrel pharmacokinetic parameters of Climara Pro are summarized in Table 1.

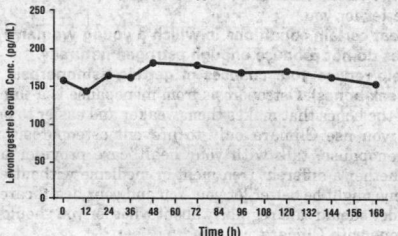

Figure 2: Mean Levonorgestrel Concentration Profile (Week 4) Following Four Consecutive Weekly Applications of Climara Pro

B. Distribution

The distribution of exogenous estrogens is similar to that of endogenous estrogens. Estrogens are widely distributed in the body and are generally found in higher concentrations in the sex hormone target organs. Estrogens circulate in the blood largely bound to sex hormone binding globulin (SHBG) and albumin.
Levonorgestrel in serum is bound to both SHBG and albumin. Following four consecutive weekly applications of Climara Pro mean (± SD) SHBG concentrations declined from a predose value of 47.5 (25.8) to 41.2 (22.4) nmol/L at week 4.

C. Metabolism

Exogenous estrogens are metabolized in the same manner as endogenous estrogens. Circulating estrogens exist in a dynamic equilibrium of metabolic interconversions. These transformations take place mainly in the liver. Estradiol is converted reversibly to estrone, and both can be converted to estriol, which is the major urinary metabolite. Estrogens also undergo enterohepatic recirculation via sulfate and glucuronide conjugation in the liver, biliary secretion of conjugates into the intestine, and hydrolysis in the intestine followed by reabsorption. In postmenopausal women, a significant proportion of the circulating estrogens exist as sulfate conjugates, especially estrone sulfate, which serves as a circulating reservoir for the formation of more active estrogens.
The most important metabolic pathway for levonorgestrel occurs in the reduction of the Δ4- and the 3-oxo-group as well as hydroxylations at positions 2α, 1β, and 16β, followed by conjugation. Most of the metabolites that circulate in the blood are sulfates of 3α, 5β-tetrahydro-levonorgestrel, while excretion occurs predominantly in the form of glucuronides. Some of the parent levonorgestrel also circulates as the 17β-sulfate. *In-vitro* studies on the biotransformation of levonorgestrel in human skin did not indicate any significant metabolism of levonorgestrel during skin penetration.

D. Excretion

Estradiol, estrone, and estriol are excreted in the urine along with glucuronide and sulfate conjugates. Following patch removal, serum estradiol concentrations decline rapidly with a mean (± SD) terminal half-life of 3 ± 0.67 hours. Levonorgestrel and its metabolites are primarily excreted in the urine. Mean (± SD) terminal half-life for levonorgestrel was determined to be 28 ± 6.4 hours.

Table 2

Summary of Mean Daily Number of Moderate to Severe Hot Flushes-ITT

		Baseline*	Week 4	Week 8	Week 12
Placebo	n	88	82	73	69
	Mean (SD)	10.8 (5.803)	6.13 (4.311)	5.35 (4.095)	5.59 (4.93)
	Mean Change from baseline (SD)	NA	-4.23 (4.374)	-4.8 (4.448)	-4.55 (5.407)
0.045/.03	n Mean (SD)	92 10.13 (3.945)	88 2.69 (4.455)	80 1.22 (2.804)	73 1.06 (3.187)
	Mean Change from baseline (SD)	NA	-7.4 (4.715)	-8.68 (4.146)	-8.82 (4.336)
p-Value[a]		NA	<0.001 [*]	NA	<0.001 [*]

ITT= Intent to Treat population; n= Number of subjects in a treatment group in a cycle; SD= standard deviation
Number of subjects varied from cycle to cycle due to missing data
[a] p-Value for comparison to placebo, adjusted by the method of Bonferroni; [*] p <0.025
*A subject was included at baseline only if the subject had a post-baseline mean score. The post-baseline mean score required 3 days in one week.

Table 3

Summary of Mean Severity of Moderate to Severe Hot Flushes-ITT

		Baseline*	Week 4 (day 7)	Week 8 (day 7)	Week 12 (day 7)
Placebo	n	89	76	68	57
	Mean (SD)	2.42 (0.282)	1.99 (0.875)	1.93 (0.955)	1.8 (1.034)
	Mean Change from baseline (SD)	NA	-0.4 (0.865)	-0.48 (0.922)	-0.57 (1.044)
0.045/.03	n	92	83	72	55
	Mean (SD)	2.48 (0.295)	1.1 (1.191)	0.82 (1.226)	0.44 (0.96)
	Mean Change from baseline (SD)	NA	-1.4 (1.164)	-1.67 (1.245)	-2.06 (1.005)
p-Value[a]		NA	<0.001 [*]	NA	<0.001 [*]

ITT= Intent to Treat population; n= Number of subjects in a treatment group in a cycle; SD= standard deviation
Severity scores are: 1 = Mild, 2 = Moderate, 3 = Severe. Mean severity of hot flushes by day is [(2× number of moderate hot flushes) + (3× number of severe hot flushes)]/total number of moderate to severe hot flushes on that day. If no moderate to severe hot flush was indicated, the mean severity was 0.
Number of subjects varied from cycle to cycle due to missing data
[a] p-Value for comparison to placebo, adjusted by the method of Bonferroni; [*] p <0.025
*A subject was included at baseline only if the subject had at least 1 post-baseline value.

E. Special Populations
Climara Pro has been studied only in healthy postmenopausal women.

F. Drug Interactions
In vitro and *in vivo* studies have shown that estrogens are metabolized partially by cytochrome P450 3A4 (CYP3A4). Therefore, inducers or inhibitors of CYP3A4 may affect estrogen drug metabolism. Inducers of CYP3A4, such as St. John's Wort preparations (Hypericum perforatum), phenobarbital, carbamazepine, and rifampin, may reduce plasma concentrations of estrogens, possibly resulting in a decrease in therapeutic effects and/or changes in the uterine bleeding profile. Inhibitors of CYP3A4 such as erythromycin, clarithromycin, ketoconazole, itraconazole, ritonavir and grapefruit juice may increase plasma concentrations of estrogens and may result in side effects.
Hydroxylation of levonorgestrel is a conversion step which is mediated by cytochrome P450 enzymes. Based on in-vitro and in-vivo studies, it can be assumed that CYP3A, CYP2E and CYP2C are involved in the metabolism of levonorgestrel. Likewise, inducers or inhibitors of these enzymes may either, respectively, decrease the therapeutic effects or result in side effects.

G. Adhesion
A study of the adhesion potential of Climara Pro was conducted in 104 healthy women of 45-75 years of age. Each woman applied a placebo patch, containing only the Climara Pro adhesive without active ingredient, to the upper outer abdominal areas weekly for three weeks. The adhesion assessment was done visually on Days 2, 4, 5, 6 and 7 of each of the three weeks using a four-point scale. The mean scores ranked in the highest category possible on the 0 to 4 scale demonstrating clinically acceptable adhesion performance.

CLINICAL STUDIES
Effects on vasomotor symptoms
The efficacy of 0.045 mg estradiol/0.03 mg levonorgestrel administered weekly versus placebo in the relief of moderate to severe vasomotor symptoms in postmenopausal women was studied in one 12-week clinical trial (n=183, average age 52.1 ± 4.93, 82% Caucasian). The 0.045 mg estradiol/0.03 mg levonorgestrel dosage strength was shown to be statistically better than placebo at weeks 4 and 12 for relief of both the number and severity of moderate to severe hot flushes. See Tables 2 and 3. Climara Pro and the 0.045 mg estradiol/0.03 mg levonorgestrel dosage strength are bioequivalent in terms of estradiol delivery. (See CLINICAL PHARMACOLOGY, Absorption.)

[See table 2 above]

[See table 3 above]

Effects on the endometrium
In a 1-year clinical trial of 412 postmenopausal women (with intact uteri) treated with a continuous regimen of Climara Pro or with a continuous estradiol-only transdermal system, results of evaluable endometrial biopsies show that no hyperplasia was seen with Climara Pro. Table 4 below summarizes these results (Intent-to-Treat populations).

Table 4

Incidence of Endometrial Hyperplasia during Continuous Combined treatment with Climara Pro, Intent-to-Treat Population

	Climara Pro E_2 0.045 mg/ LNG 0.015 mg	Estradiol E_2 0.045 mg
	n = 210	n = 202
No. of Patients with Biopsies at ≥6 months[1]	124	139
No. of Patients with Biopsies at 1 year[2]	102	110
No. (%) of Patients with Hyperplasia[3]	0 (0%)[4]	19 (17.3%)
95% Confidence Interval	0-3.55%	9.75-24.79%

n = number of intent-to-treat subjects
[1] Defined as at least 180 days of treatment
[2] Defined as ≥ 323 days of treatment
[3] Includes hyperplasia occurring at any time after initiation of treatment as a proportion of patients with biopsies at 1 year
[4] p < 0.0167 P-value for comparison to unopposed estradiol dose using the Fisher Exact test. P-values were adjusted by the method of Bonferroni.

Effects on uterine bleeding or spotting
The effects of Climara Pro on uterine bleeding or spotting, as recorded using an interactive voice response system, were evaluated in one 12-month clinical trial. Results are shown in Figure 3.

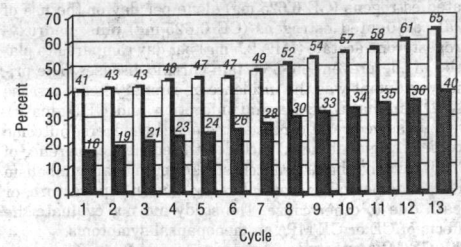

Figure 3: Cumulative proportion of subjects at each cycle with no bleeding/spotting through the end of cycle 13 Last Observation Carried Forward

Percent based upon the number of subjects with data
Last non-missing cycle carried forward through cycle 13
Bleeding associated with endometrial biopsies not included

Effects on bone mineral density
The effects on bone mineral density (BMD) were studied in a randomized, double-blind, placebo-controlled clinical trial of transdermal systems (patches) containing only estradiol (E2). The patients were postmenopausal women with hysterectomies, 40-83 years of age (mean=51.4 years), and 77.3% Caucasian. Patients received calcium supplements if they appeared deficient on a questionnaire. Vitamin D supplements were not given.
A total of 154 patients were randomized in a 2:2:3 ratio to weekly application of 22 cm² patches containing 2.2 mg E2, 4.4 mg E2, or placebo, for 728 days of continuous treatment (26 28-day cycles). Only the results for the estradiol dose in Climara Pro (4.4 mg E2) and for placebo are presented. Statistically significant increases in the primary efficacy variable, BMD of the lumbar spine (A-P view, L2- L4), were seen for 4.4 mg E2 compared to placebo (see Table 5 and Figure 4). BMD was also measured at the hip (total, non-dominant side) and radius (midshaft, non-dominant side) with statistically significant treatment effects only observed for the hip (see Table 5).

Table 5

Mean Bone Mineral Density (Standard Deviation)*

	4.4 mg E2	Placebo
Total Lumbar Spine	n=36	n=46
Baseline (g/cm²)	1.1 (0.2)	1.1 (0.2)
% Change from baseline		
LOCF	+1.7% (4.4)	-2.9% (3.8)
P-value compared to placebo	<0.0001	
Total Hip	n=36	n=48
Baseline (g/cm²)	0.97 (0.1)	0.94 (0.1)
% Change from baseline		
LOCF	+1.3% (4.2)	-0.9% (5.2)
P-value compared to placebo	0.05	

*Intent-to-treat population with on-treatment efficacy data

E2 = estradiol; LOCF = Last Observation Carried Forward

Figure 4: Percent Change From Baseline in Bone Mineral Density (g/cm²) of Lumbar Spine (A-P View, L2 – L4) by Treatment Group and Cycle (Mean ± SE)*

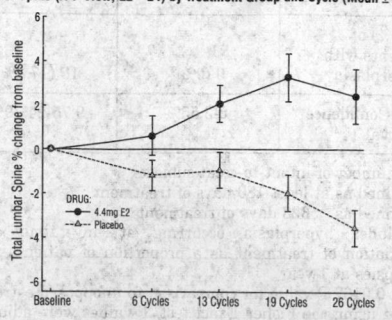

* Data in the figure is for 21 patients on 4.4 mg E2 and 27 placebo patients who completed the study; approximately 44% of randomized patients.

The lumbar spine BMD data were analyzed according to baseline estradiol levels. Estimated treatment effects for 4.4 mg E2 were approximately twice as large in the subgroup with baseline estradiol levels < 5 pg/mL as in the subgroup with baseline estradiol levels ≥ 5 pg/mL.

Women's Health Initiative Studies

The Women's Health Initiative (WHI) enrolled a total of 27,000 predominantly healthy postmenopausal women to assess the risks and benefits of either the use of oral conjugated estrogens (CE 0.625 mg) alone per day or the use of oral conjugated estrogens (CE 0.625 mg) plus medroxyprogesterone acetate (MPA 2.5 mg) per day compared to placebo in the prevention of certain chronic diseases. The primary endpoint was the incidence of coronary heart disease (CHD) (nonfatal myocardial infarction and CHD death), with invasive breast cancer as the primary adverse outcome studied. A "global index" included the earliest occurrence of CHD, invasive breast cancer, stroke, pulmonary embolism (PE), endometrial cancer, colorectal cancer, hip fracture, or death due to other cause. The study did not evaluate the effects of CE or CE/MPA on menopausal symptoms.

The CE/MPA substudy was stopped early because, according to the predefined stopping rule, the increased risk of breast cancer and cardiovascular events exceeded the specified benefits included in the "global index." Results of the CE/MPA substudy, which included 16,608 women (average age of 63 years, range 50 to 79; 83.9% White, 6.5% Black, 5.5% Hispanic), after an average follow-up of 5.2 years is presented in Table 6:

[See table 6 above]

For those outcomes included in the WHI "global index", the absolute excess risks per 10,000 women-years in the group treated with CE/MPA were 7 more CHD events, 8 more strokes, 8 more PEs, and 8 more invasive breast cancers, while absolute risk reductions per 10,000 women-years were 6 fewer colorectal cancers and 5 fewer hip fractures. The absolute excess risk of events included in the "global index" was 19 per 10,000 women-years. There was no difference between the groups in terms of all-cause mortality. (See **BOXED WARNINGS, WARNINGS,** and **PRECAUTIONS.**)

The estrogen-alone substudy was stopped early because an increased risk of stroke was observed. Results of the estrogen-alone substudy, which included 10,739 women (average age of 63 years, range 50 to 79; 75.3 percent white, 15 percent black, 6.1 percent Hispanic), after an average follow-up of 6.8 years are presented in Table 7.

[See table 7 at top of next page]

For those outcomes included in the WHI "global index" that reached statistical significance, the absolute excess risk per

Table 6

RELATIVE AND ABSOLUTE RISK SEEN IN THE CE/MPA SUBSTUDY OF WHI[a]

Event[c]	Relative Risk CE/MPA vs placebo at 5.2 Years (95% CI*)	CE/MPA n = 8506	Placebo n = 8102
		Absolute Risk per 10,000 Women-years	
CHD events	1.29 (1.02-1.63)	37	30
Non-fatal MI	*1.32 (1.02-1.72)*	*30*	*23*
CHD death	*1.18 (0.7-1.97)*	*7*	*6*
Invasive breast cancer[b]	1.26 (1-1.59)	38	30
Stroke	1.41 (1.07-1.85)	29	21
Pulmonary embolism	2.13 (1.39-3.25)	16	8
Colorectal cancer	0.63 (0.43-0.92)	10	16
Endometrial cancer	0.83 (0.47-1.47)	5	6
Hip fracture	0.66 (0.45-0.98)	10	15
Death due to causes other than the events above	0.92 (0.74-1.14)	37	40
Global Index[c]	1.15 (1.03-1.28)	170	151
Deep vein thrombosis[d]	2.07 (1.49-2.87)	26	13
Vertebral fractures[d]	0.66 (0.44-0.98)	9	15
Other osteoporotic fractures[d]	0.77 (0.69-0.86)	131	170

[a] Adapted from JAMA, 2002; 288:321-333

[b] Includes metastatic and non-metastatic breast cancer with the exception of in situ breast cancer

[c] A subset of the events was combined in a "global index", defined as the earliest occurrence of CHD events, invasive breast cancer, stroke, pulmonary embolism, endometrial cancer, colorectal cancer, hip fracture, or death due to other causes

[d] Not included in global index

*Nominal confidence intervals unadjusted for multiple looks and multiple comparisons

10,000 women-years in the group treated with CE 0.625 mg alone was 12 more strokes, while the absolute risk reduction per 10,000 women-years was 6 fewer hip fractures. The absolute excess risk of events included in the "global index" was a nonsignificant 2 events per 10,000 women-years. There was no difference between the groups in terms of all-cause mortality. (See **BOXED WARNINGS, WARNINGS,** and **PRECAUTIONS.**)

Women's Health Initiative Memory Study

The estrogen plus progestin Women's Health Initiative Memory Study (WHIMS), a substudy of WHI, enrolled 4,532 predominantly healthy postmenopausal women 65 years of age and older (47 percent were age 65 to 69 years, 35 percent were 70 to 74 years, and 18 percent were 75 years of age and older) to evaluate the effects of conjugated estrogens (CE 0.625 mg) plus medroxyprogesterone acetate (MPA 2.5 mg) on the incidence of probable dementia (primary outcome) compared with placebo.

After an average follow-up of 4 years, 40 women in the estrogen/progestin group (45 per 10,000 women-years) and 21 in the placebo group (22 per 10,000 women-years) were diagnosed with probable dementia. The relative risk of probable dementia in the hormone therapy group was 2.05 (95% CI, 1.21 to 3.48) compared to placebo. Differences between groups became apparent in the first year of treatment. It is unknown whether these findings apply to younger postmenopausal women. (See **BOXED WARNINGS, WARNINGS, Dementia,** and **PRECAUTIONS, Geriatric Use.**)

The estrogen-alone WHIMS substudy enrolled 2,947 predominantly healthy postmenopausal women 65 years of age and older (45 percent were age 65 to 69 years, 36 percent were 70 to 74 years, and 19 percent were 75 years of age and older) to evaluate the effects of CE.625 mg on the incidence of probable dementia (primary outcome) compared with placebo.

After an average follow-up of 5.2 years, 28 women in the estrogen alone group (37 per 10,000 women-years) and 19 in the placebo group (25 per 10,000 women-years) were diagnosed with probable dementia. The relative risk of probable dementia in the estrogen alone group was 1.49 (95% CI, 0.83 to 2.66) compared to placebo. It is unknown whether these findings apply to younger postmenopausal women. (See **BOXED WARNINGS, WARNINGS, Dementia** and **PRECAUTIONS, Geriatric Use.**)

INDICATIONS AND USAGE

In women with an intact uterus, Climara Pro is indicated in the:

1. Treatment of moderate to severe vasomotor symptoms associated with menopause.
2. Prevention of postmenopausal osteoporosis. When prescribing solely for the prevention of postmenopausal osteoporosis, therapy should only be considered for women at significant risk of osteoporosis and non-estrogen medications should be carefully considered.

The mainstays for decreasing the risk of postmenopausal osteoporosis are weight bearing exercise, adequate calcium and vitamin D intake, and when indicated, pharmacologic therapy. Postmenopausal women require an average of 1500mg/day of elemental calcium. Therefore, when not contraindicated, calcium supplementation may be helpful for women with suboptimal dietary intake. Vitamin D supplementation of 400-800 IU/day may also be required to ensure adequate daily intake in postmenopausal women.

Risk factors for osteoporosis include low bone mineral density, low estrogen levels, family history of osteoporosis, previous fracture, small frame (low BMI), light skin color, smoking, and alcohol intake. Response to therapy can be predicted by pre-treatment serum estradiol, and can be assessed during treatment by measuring biochemical markers of bone formation/resorption, and/or bone mineral density.

CONTRAINDICATIONS

Climara Pro should not be used in women with any of the following conditions:

1. Undiagnosed abnormal genital bleeding.
2. Known, suspected, or history of cancer of the breast.
3. Known or suspected estrogen-dependent neoplasia.
4. Active deep vein thrombosis, pulmonary embolism or a history of these conditions.
5. Active or recent (e.g. within the past year) arterial thromboembolic disease (e.g., stroke, myocardial infarction).
6. Liver dysfunction or disease.
7. Known hypersensitivity to its ingredients of Climara Pro.
8. Known or suspected pregnancy. There is no indication for Climara Pro in pregnancy. There appears to be little or no increased risk of birth defects in children born to women who have used estrogens and progestins from oral contraceptives inadvertently during early pregnancy. (See **PRECAUTIONS.**)

WARNINGS

See **BOXED WARNINGS.**

1. Cardiovascular disorders.

Estrogen and estrogen/progestin therapy have been associated with an increased risk of cardiovascular events such as myocardial infarction and stroke, as well as venous thrombosis and pulmonary embolism (venous thromboembolism or VTE). Should any of these occur or be suspected, estrogens should be discontinued immediately.

Risk factors for arterial vascular disease (e.g., hypertension, diabetes mellitus, tobacco use, hypercholesterolemia, and obesity) and/or venous thromboembolism (e.g., personal history or family history of VTE, obesity, and systemic lupus erythematosus) should be managed appropriately.

a. *Coronary heart disease and stroke*

In the CE/MPA substudy of WHI an increased risk of CHD events (defined as nonfatal myocardial infarction and CHD death) was observed in women receiving CE/MPA compared to women receiving placebo (37 versus 30 per 10,000 women-years). The increase in risk was observed in year 1 and persisted. In the same substudy of WHI, an increased risk of stroke was observed in women receiving CE/MPA compared to women receiving placebo (29 versus 21 per 10,000 women-years). The increase in risk was observed after the first year and persisted. (See **CLINICAL STUDIES.**)

In the WHI estrogen-alone substudy, an increased risk of stroke was observed in women receiving CE compared to placebo (44 versus 32 per 10,000 women-years). The increase in risk was observed in year 1 and persisted.

In postmenopausal women with documented heart disease (n = 2,763, average age 66.7 years), a controlled clinical trial of secondary prevention of cardiovascular disease (Heart and Estrogen/Progestin Replacement Study; HERS) treatment with CE/MPA (0.625 mg/2.5 mg per day) demonstrated no cardiovascular benefit. During an average follow-up of 4.1 years, treatment with CE/MPA did not reduce the overall rate of CHD events in postmenopausal women with established coronary heart disease. There were more CHD events in the CE/MPA-treated group than in the placebo group in year 1, but not during the subsequent years. Participation in an open label extension of the original HERS trial (HERS II) was agreed to by 2,321 women. Average follow-up in HERS II was an additional 2.7 years, for a total of 6.8 years overall. Rates of CHD events were comparable among women in the CE/MPA group and the placebo group in HERS, HERS II, and overall.

b. *Venous thromboembolism (VTE)*

In the CE/MPA substudy of the WHI study, a 2-fold greater rate of VTE, including deep venous thrombosis and pulmonary embolism, was observed in women receiving CE/MPA compared to women receiving placebo. The rate of VTE was 34 per 10,000 women-years in the CE/MPA group compared to 16 per 10,000 women-years in the placebo group. The increase in VTE risk was observed during the first year and persisted. (See **CLINICAL STUDIES.**)

In the WHI estrogen-alone substudy, an increased risk of deep vein thrombosis was observed in women receiving CE compared to placebo (21 versus 15 per 10,000 women-years). The increase in deep vein thrombosis risk was observed during the first year. (See **CLINICAL STUDIES.**)

If feasible, estrogens should be discontinued at least 4 to 6 weeks before surgery of the type associated with an increased risk of thromboembolism, or during periods of prolonged immobilization.

2. Malignant neoplasms

a. *Endometrial cancer*

The use of unopposed estrogens in women with intact uteri has been associated with an increased risk of endometrial cancer. The reported endometrial cancer risk among unopposed estrogen users is about 2 to 12 times greater than in nonusers, and appears dependent on duration of treatment and on estrogen dose. Most studies show no significant increased risk associated with use of estrogens for less than one year. The greatest risk appears associated with prolonged use, with increased risks of 15- to 24-fold for 5 to 10 years or more. This risk has been shown to persist for at least 8 to 15 years after estrogen therapy is discontinued. Clinical surveillance of all women taking estrogen/progestin combinations is important. Adequate diagnostic measures, including endometrial sampling when indicated, should be undertaken to rule out malignancy in all cases of undiagnosed persistent or recurring abnormal vaginal bleeding. There is no evidence that the use of natural estrogens results in a different endometrial risk profile than synthetic estrogens of equivalent estrogen dose. Adding a progestin to estrogen therapy has been shown to reduce the risk of endometrial hyperplasia, which may be a precursor to endometrial cancer.

b. *Breast cancer*

The use of estrogens and progestins by postmenopausal women has been reported to increase the risk of breast cancer. The most important randomized clinical trial providing

Table 7

RELATIVE AND ABSOLUTE RISK SEEN IN THE ESTROGEN-ALONE SUBSTUDY OF WHI[a]

Event[c]	Relative Risk* CE vs. Placebo at 6.8 Years (95% CI)	CE n = 5,310	Placebo n = 5,429
		Absolute Risk per 10,000 Women-years	
CHD events	0.91 (0.75-1.12)	49	54
Non-fatal MI	*0.89 (0.7-1.12)*	*37*	*41*
CHD death	*0.94 (0.65-1.36)*	*15*	*16*
Invasive breast cancer	0.77 (0.59-1.01)	26	33
Stroke	1.39 (1.1-1.77)	44	32
Pulmonary embolism	1.34 (0.87-2.06)	13	10
Colorectal cancer	1.08 (0.75-1.55)	17	16
Hip fracture	0.61 (0.41-0.91)	11	17
Death due to causes other than the events above	1.08 (0.88-1.32)	53	50
Global Index[b]	1.01 (0.91-1.12)	192	190
Deep vein thrombosis[c]	1.47 (1.04-2.08)	21	15
Vertebral fractures[c]	0.62 (0.42-0.93)	11	17
Total fractures[c]	0.7 (0.63-0.79)	139	195

[a] Adapted from JAMA, 2004; 291:1701-1712
[b] A subset of the events was combined in a "global index", defined as the earliest occurrence of CHD events, invasive breast cancer, stroke, pulmonary embolism, endometrial cancer, colorectal cancer, hip fracture, or death due to other causes
[c] Not included in global index
* Nominal confidence intervals unadjusted for multiple looks and multiple comparisons

information about this issue is the CE/MPA substudy of the WHI study (see **CLINICAL STUDIES**). The results from observational studies are generally consistent with those of the WHI clinical trial and report no significant variation in the risk of breast cancer among different estrogens or progestins, doses, or routes of administration.

The CE/MPA substudy of WHI reported an increased risk of breast cancer in women who took CE/MPA for a mean follow-up of 5.6 years. Observational studies have also reported an increased risk for estrogen/progestin combination therapy, and a smaller increased risk for estrogen-alone therapy, after several years of use. In the WHI trial and from observational studies, the excess risk increased with duration of use. From observational studies, the risk appeared to return to baseline in about 5 years after stopping treatment. In addition, observational studies suggest that the risk of breast cancer was greater, and became apparent earlier, with estrogen/progestin combination therapy as compared to estrogen-alone therapy.

In the CE/MPA substudy, 26 percent of the women reported prior use of estrogen-alone and/or estrogen/progestin combination hormone therapy. After a mean follow-up of 5.6 years during the clinical trial, the overall relative risk of invasive breast cancer was 1.24 (95% confidence interval 1.01-1.54), and the overall absolute risk was 41 versus 33 cases per 10,000 women-years, for CE/MPA compared with placebo. Among women who reported prior use of hormone therapy, the relative risk of invasive breast cancer was 1.86, and the absolute risk was 46 versus 25 cases per 10,000 women-years, for CE/MPA compared with placebo. Among women who reported no prior use of hormone therapy, the relative risk of invasive breast cancer was 1.09, and the absolute risk was 40 versus 36 cases per 10,000 women-years for CE/MPA compared with placebo. In the same substudy, invasive breast cancers were larger and diagnosed at a more advanced stage in the CE/MPA group compared with the placebo group. Metastatic disease was rare with no apparent difference between the two groups. Other prognostic factors such as histologic subtype, grade and hormone receptor status did not differ between the groups.

The use of estrogen plus progestin has been reported to result in an increase in abnormal mammograms requiring further evaluation. All women should receive yearly breast examinations by a healthcare provider and perform monthly breast self-examinations. In addition, mammography examinations should be scheduled based on patient age, risk factors, and prior mammogram results.

3. Dementia

In the estrogen plus progestin WHIMS, a population of 4,532 postmenopausal women aged 65 to 79 years was randomized to CE/MPA or placebo. In the estrogen-alone WHIMS, a population of 2,947 hysterectomized women aged 65 to 79 years was randomized to CE or placebo.

In the estrogen plus progestin substudy, after an average follow up of 4 years, 40 women being treated with CE/MPA (1.8 percent, n=2,229) and 21 women in the placebo group (0.9 percent, n=2,303) received diagnoses of probable dementia. The relative risk for CE/MPA versus placebo was 2.05 (95% confidence interval 1.21–3.48), and was similar for women with and without histories of menopausal hormone use before WHIMS. The absolute risk of probable dementia for CE/MPA versus placebo was 45 versus 22 cases per 10,000 women-years, and the absolute excess risk for CE/MPA was 23 cases per 10,000 women-years. It is unknown whether these findings apply to younger postmenopausal women. (See **CLINICAL STUDIES** and **PRECAUTIONS, Geriatric Use.**)

In the estrogen-alone substudy, after an average follow-up of 5.2 years, 28 women in the estrogen-alone group and 19 women in the placebo group were diagnosed with probable dementia. The relative risk of probable dementia for estrogen alone versus placebo was 1.49 (95 percent CI, 0.83-2.66). The absolute risk of probable dementia for estrogen alone versus placebo was 37 versus 25 cases per 10,000 women-years. It is unknown whether these findings apply to younger postmenopausal women. (See **CLINICAL STUDIES** and **PRECAUTIONS, Geriatric Use.**)

4. Gallbladder disease

A 2- to 4-fold increase in the risk of gallbladder disease requiring surgery in postmenopausal women receiving estrogens has been reported.

5. Hypercalcemia

Estrogen administration may lead to severe hypercalcemia in patients with breast cancer and bone metastases. If hypercalcemia occurs, use of the drug should be stopped and appropriate measures taken to reduce the serum calcium level.

6. Visual abnormalities

Retinal vascular thrombosis has been reported in patients receiving estrogens. Discontinue medication pending examination if there is sudden partial or complete loss of vision, or a sudden onset of proptosis, diplopia, or migraine. If examination reveals papilledema or retinal vascular lesions, estrogens should be permanently discontinued.

PRECAUTIONS

A. General

1. Addition of a progestin when a woman has not had a hysterectomy

Studies of the addition of a progestin for 10 or more days of a cycle of estrogen administration, or daily with estrogen in a continuous regimen, have reported a lowered incidence of endometrial hyperplasia than would be induced by estrogen treatment alone. Endometrial hyperplasia may be a precursor to endometrial cancer.

There are, however, possible risks that may be associated with the use of progestins with estrogens compared to estrogen-alone regimens. These include a possible increased risk of breast cancer.

2. Elevated blood pressure

In a small number of case reports, substantial increases in blood pressure have been attributed to idiosyncratic reactions to estrogens. In a large, randomized, placebo-controlled clinical trial, a generalized effect of estrogens on blood pressure was not seen. Blood pressure should be monitored at regular intervals with estrogen use.

3. Hypertriglyceridemia

In patients with pre-existing hypertriglyceridemia, oral estrogen therapy may be associated with elevations of plasma triglycerides leading to pancreatitis and other complications.

4. Impaired liver function and past history of cholestatic jaundice

Estrogens may be poorly metabolized in patients with impaired liver function. For patients with a history of cholestatic jaundice associated with past estrogen use or with pregnancy, caution should be exercised and in the case of recurrence, medication should be discontinued.

5. Hypothyroidism

Estrogen administration leads to increased thyroid-binding globulin (TBG) levels. Patients with normal thyroid function can compensate for the increased TBG by making more thyroid hormone, thus maintaining free T4 and T3 serum concentrations in the normal range. Patients dependent on thyroid hormone replacement therapy who are also receiving estrogens may require increased doses of their thyroid replacement therapy. These patients should have their thyroid function monitored in order to maintain their free thyroid hormone levels in an acceptable range.

6. Fluid retention

Estrogen and estrogen/progestin therapy may cause some degree of fluid retention. Because of this, patients with conditions that might be influenced by this factor, such as a cardiac or renal dysfunction, warrant careful observation when estrogens are prescribed.

7. Hypocalcemia

Estrogens should be used with caution in individuals with severe hypocalcemia.

8. Ovarian cancer

The CE/MPA sub-study of WHI reported that estrogen plus progestin increased the risk of ovarian cancer. After an average follow-up of 5.6 years, the relative risk for ovarian cancer for CE/MPA versus placebo was 1.58 (95% confidence interval 0.77-3.24) but was not statistically significant. The absolute risk for CE/MPA versus placebo was 4.2 versus 2.7 cases per 10,000 women-years. In some epidemiological studies, the use of estrogen alone, in particular for ten or more years, has been associated with an increased risk of ovarian cancer. Other epidemiologic studies have not found these associations.

9. Exacerbation of endometriosis

Endometriosis may be exacerbated with administration of estrogens.

10. Exacerbation of other conditions

Estrogens may cause an exacerbation of asthma, diabetes mellitus, epilepsy, migraine or porphyria, systemic lupus erythematosus, and hepatic hemangiomas and should be used with caution in women with these conditions.

B. Information for Patients

Physicians are advised to discuss the Patient Information leaflet with patients for whom they prescribe Climara Pro.

C. Laboratory Tests

Estrogen administration should be initiated at the lowest dose for the approved indication and then guided by clinical response, rather than by serum hormone levels (e.g., estradiol, FSH).

D. Drug/laboratory Test Interactions

1. Accelerated prothrombin time, partial thromboplastin time, and platelet aggregation time; increased platelet count; increased factors II, VII antigen, VIII antigen, VIII coagulant activity, IX, X, XII, VII-X complex, II-VII-X complex, and beta-thromboglobulin; decreased levels of antifactor Xa and antithrombin III, decreased antithrombin III activity; increased levels of fibrinogen and fibrinogen activity; increased plasminogen antigen and activity.
2. Increased thyroid-binding globulin (TBG) levels leading to increased circulating total thyroid hormone levels as measured by protein-bound iodine (PBI), T_4 levels (by column or by radioimmunoassay) or T_3 levels by radioimmunoassay. T_3 resin uptake is decreased, reflecting the elevated TBG. Free T_4 and free T_3 concentrations are unaltered. Patients on thyroid replacement therapy may require higher doses of thyroid hormone.
3. Other binding proteins may be elevated in serum (i.e., corticosteroid binding globulin (CBG), sex hormone-binding globulin (SHBG) leading to increased total circulating corticosteroids and sex steroids, respectively. Free hormone concentrations may be decreased. Other plasma proteins may be increased (angiotensinogen/renin substrate, alpha-l-antitrypsin, ceruloplasmin).

4. Increased plasma HDL and HDL_2 cholesterol subfraction concentrations, reduced LDL cholesterol concentration, and in oral formulations increased triglycerides levels.
5. Impaired glucose tolerance.
6. Reduced response to metyrapone test.

E. Carcinogenesis, Mutagenesis, Impairment of Fertility

Long-term continuous administration of estrogen, with and without progestin, in women with and without a uterus, has shown an increased risk of endometrial cancer, breast cancer, and ovarian cancer. (See BOXED WARNINGS, WARNINGS and PRECAUTIONS.)

Long-term continuous administration of natural and synthetic estrogens in certain animal species increases the frequency of carcinomas of the breast, uterus, cervix, vagina, testis, and liver.

F. Pregnancy

Climara Pro should not be used during pregnancy. (See CONTRAINDICATIONS.)

G. Nursing Mothers

Estrogen administration to nursing mothers has been shown to decrease the quantity and quality of the milk. Detectable amounts of estrogens and progestins have been identified in the milk of mothers receiving this drug. Caution should be exercised when Climara Pro is administered to a nursing woman.

H. Pediatric Use

Climara Pro is not indicated in children.

I. Geriatric Use

There have not been sufficient numbers of geriatric patients involved in studies utilizing Climara Pro to determine whether those over 65 years of age differ from younger subjects in their response to Climara Pro.

Of the total number of subjects in the estrogen plus progestin substudy of the WHI study, 44 percent (n = 7,320) were 65 years and older, while 6.6 percent (n = 1,095) were 75 years and older. There was a higher relative risk (CE/MPA versus placebo) of stroke and invasive breast cancer in women 75 and older compared to women less than 75 years of age.

In the estrogen plus progestin substudy of WHIMS, a population of 4,532 postmenopausal women, aged 65 to 70 years, was randomized to conjugated estrogens

---

Table 8

All Treatment Emergent Events Regardless of Relationship Reported at a Frequency of > 3% with Climara Pro in the 1 year Endometrial Hyperplasia Study

	Climara Pro 0.045 / 0.015 N = 212	E_2 N = 204
Body as a whole		
Abdominal pain	9 (4.2)	11 (5.4)
Accidental Injury	7 (3.3)	6 (2.9)
Back pain	13 (6.1)	12 (5.9)
Flu syndrome	10 (4.7)	13 (6.4)
Infection	7 (3.3)	10 (4.9)
Pain	11 (5.2)	13 (6.4)
Cardiovascular		
Hypertension	7 (3.3)	9 (4.4)
Digestive		
Flatulence	8 (3.8)	11 (5.4)
Metabolic and Nutritional Disorders		
Edema	8 (3.8)	5 (2.5)
Weight gain	6 (2.8)	10 (4.9)
Musculoskeletal		
Arthralgia	9 (4.2)	10 (4.9)
Nervous		
Depression	12 (5.7)	7 (3.4)
Headache	11 (5.2)	14 (6.9)
Respiratory		
Bronchitis	9 (4.2)	7 (3.4)
Sinusitis	8 (3.8)	12 (5.9)
Upper Respiratory Infection	28 (13.2)	26 (12.7)
Skin and Appendages		
Application site reaction	86 (40.6)	69 (33.8)
Breast pain	40 (18.9)	20 (9.8)
Rash	5 (2.4)	10 (4.9)
Urogenital		
Urinary Tract Infection	7 (3.3)	8 (3.9)
Vaginal Bleeding	78 (36.8)	44 (21.6)
Vaginitis	4 (1.9)	6 (2.9)

N = total number of subjects in a treatment group; n = number of subjects with event

(CE 0.625 mg) plus medroxyprogesterone acetate (MPA 2.5 mg) or placebo. In the estrogen plus progestin group, after an average follow-up of 4 years, the relative risk (CE/MPA versus placebo) of probable dementia was 2.05 (95 percent CI, 1.21-3.48).

Of the total number of subjects in the estrogen-alone substudy of the WHI study, 46 percent (n = 4,943) were 65 years and older, while 7.1 percent (n = 767) were 75 years and older. There was a higher relative risk (CE versus placebo) of stroke in women less than 75 years of age compared to women 75 years and older.

In the estrogen-alone substudy of the WHIMS, a population of 2,947 hysterectomized women, aged 65 to 79 years, was randomized to estrogen alone (CE 0.625 mg) or placebo. In the estrogen-alone group, after an average follow-up of 5.2 years, the relative risk (CE versus placebo) of probable dementia was 1.49 (95 percent CI, 0.83-2.66).

Pooling the events in women receiving CE or CE/MPA in comparison to those in women on placebo, the overall relative risk of probable dementia was 1.76 (95 percent CI, 1.19-2.6). Since both substudies were conducted in women aged 65 to 79 years, it is unknown whether these findings apply to younger postmenopausal women. (See **BOXED WARNINGS** and **WARNINGS, Dementia.**)

ADVERSE REACTIONS

See **BOXED WARNINGS, WARNINGS and PRECAUTIONS.**

Because clinical trials are conducted under widely varying conditions, adverse reaction rates observed in the clinical trials of a drug cannot be directly compared to rates in the clinical trials of another drug and may not reflect the rates observed in practice. The adverse reaction information from clinical trials does, however, provide a basis for identifying the adverse events that appear to be related to drug use and for approximating rates.

[See table 8 at top of previous page]

Irritation potential of Climara Pro was assessed in a 3-week irritation study. The study compared the irritation of a Climara Pro placebo patch (22 cm^2) to a Climara® placebo (25 cm^2). Visual assessments of irritation were made on Day 7 of each wear period, approximately 30 minutes after patch removal using a 7-point scale (0 = no evidence of irritation; 1 = minimal erythema, barely perceptible; 2 = definite erythema, readily visible, or minimal edema, or minimal papular response; 3-7 = erythema and papules, edema, vesicles, strong extensive reaction).

The mean irritation scores were 0.13 (week 1), 0.12 (week 2), and 0.06 (week 3) for the Climara Pro placebo.

The mean scores for the Climara placebo were 0.2 (week 1), 0.26 (week 2), 0.12 (week 3). There were no irritation scores greater than 2 at any timepoint in any subject.

In controlled clinical trials, withdrawals due to application site reactions occurred in 6 (2.1%) of subjects in the 12-week symptom study and in 71 (8.5%) of subjects in the 1-year endometrial protection study.

The following additional adverse reactions have been reported with estrogen and/or estrogen/progestin therapy:

1. Genitourinary system

Changes in vaginal bleeding pattern and abnormal withdrawal bleeding or flow; breakthrough bleeding; spotting; dysmenorrhea; increase in size of uterine leiomyomata; vaginitis, including vaginal candidiasis; change in amount of cervical secretion; changes in cervical ectropion; ovarian cancer; endometrial hyperplasia; endometrial cancer.

2. Breasts

Tenderness, enlargement, pain, nipple discharge, galactorrhea; fibrocystic breast changes; breast cancer.

3. Cardiovascular

Deep and superficial venous thrombosis; pulmonary embolism; thrombophlebitis; myocardial infarction; stroke; increase in blood pressure.

4. Gastrointestinal

Nausea, vomiting; abdominal cramps, bloating; cholestatic jaundice; increased incidence of gallbladder disease; pancreatitis; enlargement of hepatic hemangiomas.

5. Skin

Chloasma or melasma, which may persist when drug is discontinued; erythema multiforme; erythema nodosum; hemorrhagic eruption; loss of scalp hair; hirsutism; pruritus, rash.

6. Eyes

Retinal vascular thrombosis, intolerance to contact lenses.

7. Central nervous system

Headache; migraine; dizziness; mental depression; chorea; nervousness; mood disturbances; irritability; exacerbation of epilepsy, dementia.

8. Miscellaneous

Increase or decrease in weight; reduced carbohydrate tolerance; aggravation of porphyria; edema; arthalgias; leg cramps; changes in libido; urticaria, angioedema, anaphylactoid/anaphylactic reactions; hypocalcemia; exacerbation of asthma; increased triglycerides.

OVERDOSAGE

Serious ill effects have not been reported following acute ingestion of large doses of estrogen/progestin-containing oral contraceptives by young children. Overdosage of estrogen may cause nausea and vomiting, and withdrawal bleeding may occur in females.

DOSAGE AND ADMINISTRATION

When estrogen is prescribed for a postmenopausal woman with a uterus, a progestin should also be initiated to reduce the risk of endometrial cancer. A woman without a uterus does not need progestin. Use of estrogen, alone or in combination with a progestin, should be with the lowest effective dose and for the shortest duration consistent with treatment goals and risks for the individual woman. Patients should be re-evaluated periodically as clinically appropriate (e.g., 3-month to 6-month intervals) to determine if treatment is still necessary. (see **BOXED WARNINGS** and **WARNINGS.**) For women who have a uterus, adequate diagnostic measures, such as endometrial sampling, when indicated, should be undertaken to rule out malignancy in cases of undiagnosed persistent or recurring abnormal vaginal bleeding.

One Climara Pro transdermal system is available for use. Climara Pro delivers 0.045 mg of estradiol per day and 0.015 mg of levonorgestrel per day. The lowest effective dose of Climara Pro has not been determined.

Initiation of Therapy:

Women not currently using continuous estrogen or combination estrogen/progestin therapy may start therapy with Climara Pro at any time. However, women currently using continuous estrogen or combination estrogen/progestin therapy should complete the current cycle of therapy, before initiating Climara Pro therapy. Women often experience withdrawal bleeding at the completion of the cycle. The first day of this bleeding would be an appropriate time to begin Climara Pro therapy.

Therapeutic Regimen:

A Climara Pro 0.045 mg/0.015 mg (22 sq cm) matrix transdermal system is worn continuously on the lower abdomen. A new system should be applied weekly during a 28-day cycle.

Application of the System: Site Selection: Climara Pro should be placed on a smooth (fold free), clean, dry area of the skin on the lower abdomen. **Climara Pro should not be applied to or near the breasts.** The area selected should not be oily (which can impair adherence of the system), damaged, or irritated. The waistline should be avoided, since tight clothing may rub the system off or modify drug delivery. The sites of application must be rotated, with an interval of at least one week allowed between applications to the same site.

Application of the system: After opening the pouch, remove one side of the protective liner, taking care not to touch the adhesive part of the transdermal delivery system with the fingers. Immediately apply the transdermal delivery system to a smooth (fold free) area of skin on the lower abdomen. Remove the second side of the protective liner and press the system firmly in place with the hand for at least 10 seconds, making sure there is good contact, especially around the edges.

Care should be taken that the system does not become dislodged during bathing and other activities. If a system should fall off, the same system may be reapplied to another area of the lower abdomen. If necessary, a new transdermal system may be applied, in which case, the original treatment schedule should be continued. Only one system should be worn at any one time during one week dosing interval.

Once in place, the transdermal system should not be exposed to the sun for prolonged periods of time.

Removal of the System: Removal of the system should be done carefully and slowly to avoid irritation of the skin. Should any adhesive remain on the skin after removal of the system, allow the area to dry for 15 minutes. Then gently rubbing the area with an oil-based cream or lotion should remove the adhesive residue.

Used patches still contain some active hormones. Each patch should be carefully folded in half so that it sticks to itself before throwing it away.

HOW SUPPLIED

Climara Pro (Estradiol/Levonorgestrel Transdermal System) 0.045 mg/day estradiol and 0.015 mg/day levonorgestrel – each 22 cm^2 system contains 4.4 mg of estradiol and 1.39 mg of levonorgestrel.

Individual Carton of 4 systems .... NDC 50419-491-04

Storage Conditions:

Store at 20-25°C (68-77°F); excursions permitted to 15-30°C (59-86°F) [See USP controlled Room Temperature].

Do not store unpouched.

PATIENT INFORMATION

Updated November 16, 2005

Climara Pro®

(Estradiol/Levonorgestrel Transdermal System)

Read this Patient Information leaflet before you start taking Climara Pro and read what you get each time you refill Climara Pro. There may be new information. This information does not take the place of talking to your healthcare provider about your medical condition or your treatment.

WHAT IS THE MOST IMPORTANT INFORMATION I SHOULD KNOW ABOUT CLIMARA PRO (COMBINATION OF ESTROGEN AND PROGESTIN HORMONES)?

- Do not use estrogens with or without progestins to prevent heart disease, heart attacks, or strokes.

Using estrogens and progestins may increase your chances of getting heart attacks, strokes, breast cancer, and blood clots.

- Do not use estrogens with or without progestins to prevent dementia

Using estrogens with progestins may increase your risk of dementia.

You and your healthcare provider should talk regularly about whether you still need treatment with Climara Pro.

What is Climara Pro?

Climara Pro is a medicine that contains two kinds of hormones, estrogen and a progestin.

What is Climara Pro used for?

Climara Pro is used after menopause to:

- **reduce moderate to severe hot flashes.** Estrogens are hormones made by a woman's ovaries. The ovaries normally stop making estrogens when a woman is between 45 to 55 years old. This drop in body estrogen levels causes the "change of life" or menopause (the end of monthly menstrual periods). Sometimes, both ovaries are removed during an operation before natural menopause takes place. The sudden drop in estrogen levels causes "surgical menopause."

  When the estrogen levels begin dropping, some women develop very uncomfortable symptoms, such as feelings of warmth in the face, neck, and chest, or sudden strong feelings of heat and sweating ("hot flashes" or "hot flushes"). In some women, the symptoms are mild, and they will not need estrogens. In other women, symptoms can be more severe. You and your health care provider should talk regularly about whether you still need treatment with Climara Pro.
- **help reduce your chances of getting osteoporosis (thin weak bones).** Osteoporosis from menopause is a thinning of the bones that makes them weaker and easier to break. If you use Climara Pro only to prevent osteoporosis from menopause, talk with your healthcare provider about whether a different treatment or medicine without estrogens might be better for you. You and your healthcare provider should talk regularly about whether you should continue with Climara Pro.

  Weight-bearing exercise, like walking or running, and taking calcium and vitamin D supplements may also lower your chances of getting postmenopausal osteoporosis. It is important to talk about exercise and supplements with your healthcare provider before starting them.

Who should not use Climara Pro?

Do not use Climara Pro if you have had your uterus removed (hysterectomy).

Climara Pro contains a progestin to decrease the chances of getting cancer of the uterus. If you do not have a uterus, you do not need a progestin and you should not use Climara Pro.

Do not start using Climara Pro if you:

- **have unusual vaginal bleeding**
- **currently have or have had certain cancers.** Estrogens may increase the chances of getting certain types of cancers, including cancer of the breast or uterus. If you have or had cancer, talk with your healthcare provider about whether you should use Climara Pro.
- **had a stroke or heart attack in the past year**
- **currently have or have had blood clots**
- **currently have or have had liver problems**
- **are allergic to Climara Pro or any of its ingredients.** See the end of this leaflet for a list of ingredients in Climara Pro.
- **think you may be pregnant**

Tell your health care provider:

- **if you are breastfeeding.** The hormones in Climara Pro can pass into your milk.
- **about all of your medical problems.** Your healthcare provider may need to check you more carefully if you have certain conditions, such as asthma (wheezing), epilepsy (seizures), migraine, endometriosis, lupus, problems with your heart, liver, thyroid, kidneys, or have high calcium levels in your blood.
- **about all the medicines you take,** including prescription and nonprescription medicines, vitamins, and herbal supplements. Some medicines may affect how Climara Pro works. Climara Pro may also affect how your other medicines work.
- **if you are going to have surgery or will be on bed rest.** You may need to stop using estrogens.

How should I use Climara Pro?

Climara Pro is a patch that you wear on your skin. The Climara Pro patch releases two hormones, estradiol and levonorgestrel. See the end of this leaflet for complete instructions on how to use Climara Pro.

1. Start at the lowest dose and talk to your healthcare provider about how well that dose is working for you.
2. Estrogens should be used at the lowest dose possible for your treatment only as long as needed. You and your healthcare provider should talk regularly (for example, every 3 to 6 months) about the dose you are using and whether you still need treatment with Climara Pro.

What are the possible side effects of estrogens?

Less common but serious side effects include:
- Breast cancer
- Cancer of the uterus
- Stroke
- Heart attack
- Blood clots
- Dementia
- Gallbladder disease
- Ovarian cancer

These are some of the warning signs of serious side effects:
- Breast lumps
- Unusual vaginal bleeding
- Dizziness and faintness
- Changes in speech
- Severe headaches
- Chest pain
- Shortness of breath
- Pains in your legs
- Changes in vision
- Vomiting

Call your healthcare provider right away if you get any of these warning signs, or any other unusual symptom that concerns you.

Common side effects include:
- Headache
- Breast pain
- Irregular vaginal bleeding or spotting
- Stomach/abdominal cramps, bloating
- Nausea and vomiting
- Hair loss

Other side effects include:
- High blood pressure
- Liver problems
- High blood sugar
- Fluid retention
- Enlargement of benign tumors of the uterus ("fibroids")
- Vaginal yeast infection

These are not all the possible side effects of Climara Pro. For more information, ask your healthcare provider or pharmacist.

What can I do to lower my chances of a serious side effect with Climara Pro?

- Talk with your healthcare provider regularly about whether you should continue using Climara Pro.
- See your healthcare provider right away if you get vaginal bleeding while using Climara Pro.
- Have a breast exam and mammogram (breast X-ray) every year unless your healthcare provider tells you something else. If members of your family have had breast cancer or if you have ever had breast lumps or an abnormal mammogram, you may need to have breast exams more often.
- If you have high blood pressure, high cholesterol (fat in the blood), diabetes, are overweight, or if you use tobacco, you may have higher chances for getting heart disease. Ask your healthcare provider for ways to lower your chances for getting heart disease.

Have an annual gynecologic exam

General information about safe and effective use of Climara Pro

Medicines are sometimes prescribed for conditions that are not mentioned in patient information leaflets. Do not use Climara Pro for conditions for which it was not prescribed. Do not give Climara Pro to other people, even if they have the same symptoms you have. It may harm them.

Keep Climara Pro out of the reach of children.

This leaflet provides a summary of the most important information about Climara Pro. If you would like more information, talk with your healthcare provider or pharmacist. You can ask for information about Climara Pro that is written for health professionals. You can get more information by calling the toll free number (1-888-84BAYER).

What are the ingredients in Climara Pro?

The active ingredients in Climara Pro are estradiol and levonorgestrel. Climara Pro also contains acrylate copolymer adhesive and polyvinylpyrrolidone/vinyl acetate copolymer.

Do not store above 86°F (30°C).
Do not store unpouched.

Instructions for Use

How and Where do I apply the Climara Pro Patch

- Talk to your healthcare provider or pharmacist if you have questions about applying the Climara Pro patch.
- Each Climara Pro patch is individually sealed in a protective pouch. To open the pouch, hold it up with the Climara Pro name facing you. Tear left to right using the top tear notch. Tear from bottom to top using the side tear notch. Pull the pouch open. **Carefully remove the Climara Pro patch.** You will notice that the patch is attached to a thicker, hard-plastic liner and that the patch itself is oval.

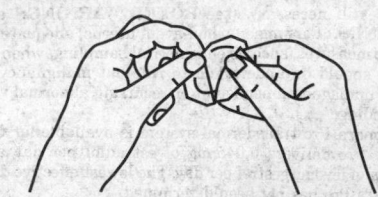

- Apply the adhesive side of the Climara Pro patch to a clean, dry area of the lower abdomen. **Do not apply the Climara Pro patch to your breasts.** The sites of application must be rotated, with an interval of at least 1 week allowed between applications to a particular site. The area selected should not be oily, damaged, or irritated. Avoid the waistline, since tight clothing may rub and remove the patch. Application to areas where sitting would dislodge the patch should also be avoided. Apply the patch immediately after opening the pouch and removing the protective liner. Press the patch firmly in place with the fingers for about 10 seconds, making sure there is good contact, especially around the edges.

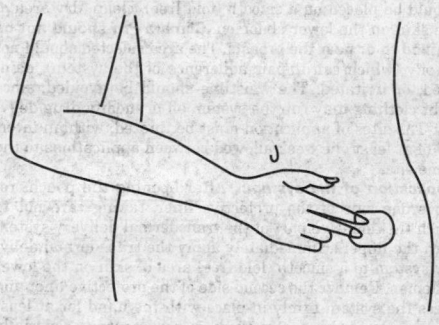

- The Climara Pro patch should be worn continuously for one week. You may wish to experiment with different locations when applying a new patch, to find ones that are most comfortable for you and where clothing will not rub on the patch.
- The Climara Pro patch should be changed once weekly. Remove the used patch. Carefully fold it in half so that it sticks to itself because used patches still contain active hormones and discard it. Any adhesive that might remain on your skin can be easily rubbed off. Then place the new Climara Pro patch on a different skin site. (The same skin site should not be used again for at least 1 week after removal of the patch.)
- Contact with water when you are bathing, swimming, or showering may affect the patch. If the patch falls off, the same patch may be reapplied to another area of the lower abdomen. Make sure that there is good contact, especially around the edges. If the patch will not stick completely to your skin, put a new patch on a different area of the lower abdomen. Do not apply two patches at the same time.
- Once in place, the transdermal system should not be exposed to the sun for prolonged periods of time.

© 2007, Bayer HealthCare Pharmaceuticals Inc. All rights reserved.
Made In USA
Manufactured for:
Bayer HealthCare
Pharmaceuticals
Bayer HealthCare Pharmaceuticals Inc.
Wayne, NJ 07470
Manufactured by:
3M Drug Delivery Systems
Northridge, CA 91324
6705400   3M 678600   May 2007
Shown in Product Identification Guide, page 307

MENOSTAR®   ℞

[men-o-star]
(estradiol transdermal system)
Rx only
Prescribing Information

> **ESTROGENS INCREASE THE RISK OF ENDOMETRIAL CANCER**
> Close clinical surveillance of all women taking estrogens is important. Adequate diagnostic measures, including endometrial sampling when indicated, should be undertaken to rule out malignancy in all cases of undiagnosed persistent or recurring abnormal vaginal bleeding. There is no evidence that the use of "natural" estrogens results in a different endometrial risk profile than synthetic estrogens at equivalent estrogen doses.(See **WARNINGS, Malignant neoplasms,** *Endometrial cancer.*)
> **CARDIOVASCULAR AND OTHER RISKS**
> Estrogens with and without progestins should not be used for the prevention of cardiovascular disease or dementia. (See **WARNINGS, Cardiovascular disorders** and **Dementia**.)
> The Women's Health Initiative (WHI) study reported increased risks of stroke and deep vein thrombosis in postmenopausal women (50 to 79 years of age) during 6.8 years of treatment with oral conjugated estrogens (CE 0.625 mg) alone per day, relative to placebo. (See **CLINICAL STUDIES** and **WARNINGS, Cardiovascular disorders.**)
> The WHI-study reported increased risks of myocardial infarction, stroke, invasive breast cancer, pulmonary emboli, and deep vein thrombosis in postmenopausal women (50 to 79 years of age) during 5 years of treatment with oral conjugated estrogens (CE 0.625 mg) combined with medroxyprogesterone acetate (MPA 2.5mg) per day, relative to placebo (see **CLINICAL STUDIES,** and **WARNINGS, Cardiovascular disorders** and **Malignant neoplasms,** *Breast Cancer.*)
> The Women's Health Initiative Memory Study (WHIMS), a substudy of the WHI study, reported increased risk of developing probable dementia in postmenopausal women 65 years of age or older during 5.2 years of treatment with CE 0.625 mg alone and during 4 years of treatment with CE 0.625 mg combined with MPA 2.5 mg, relative to placebo. It is unknown whether this finding applies to younger postmenopausal women. (See **CLINICAL STUDIES, WARNINGS, Dementia,** and **PRECAUTIONS, geriatric use.**)
> Other doses of oral conjugated estrogens with medroxyprogesterone acetate, and other combinations and dosage forms of estrogens and progestins were not studied in the WHI clinical trials and, in the absence of comparable data, these risks should be assumed to be similar. Because of these risks, estrogens with or without progestins should be prescribed at the lowest effective doses and for the shortest duration consistent with treatment goals and risks for the individual woman.

DESCRIPTION

Menostar®, estradiol transdermal system, is designed to provide nominal *in vivo* delivery of 14 mcg 17β-estradiol per day continuously upon application to intact skin. The period of use is 7 days. The transdermal system has a contact surface area of 3.25 cm², and contains 1 mg of estradiol USP. Estradiol USP (17β-estradiol) is a white, crystalline powder, chemically described as estra-1,3,5(10)-triene-3, 17β-diol. It has an empirical formula of $C_{18}H_{24}O_2$ and molecular weight of 272.39. The structural formula is:

The Menostar transdermal system comprises three layers. Proceeding from the visible surface toward the surface attached to the skin, these layers are (1) a translucent polyethylene film, and (2) an acrylate adhesive matrix containing estradiol USP. A protective liner (3) of siliconized or fluoropolymer-coated polyester film is attached to the adhesive surface and must be removed before the transdermal system can be used.

(1) Film Backing
(2) Drug/Adhesive Layer
(3) Protective Liner

The active component of the transdermal system is 17β-estradiol. The remaining components of the transdermal system (acrylate copolymer adhesive, fatty acid esters, and polyethylene backing) are pharmacologically inactive.

CLINICAL PHARMACOLOGY

The Menostar transdermal system provides systemic estrogen therapy by releasing 17β-estradiol, the major estrogenic hormone secreted by the human ovary.

Endogenous estrogens are largely responsible for the development and maintenance of the female reproductive system and secondary sexual characteristics. Although circulating estrogens exist in a dynamic equilibrium of metabolic interconversions, estradiol is the principal intracellular human estrogen and is substantially more potent than its metabolites, estrone and estriol, at the receptor level.

The primary source of estrogen in normally cycling adult women is the ovarian follicle, which secretes 70 to 500 mcg of estradiol daily, depending on the phase of the menstrual cycle. After menopause, most endogenous estrogen is produced by conversion of androstenedione, secreted by the adrenal cortex, to estrone by peripheral tissues. Thus, estrone and the sulfate conjugated form, estrone sulfate, are the most abundant circulating estrogens in postmenopausal women.

Estrogens act through binding to nuclear receptors in estrogen-responsive tissues. To date, two estrogen receptors have been identified. These vary in proportion from tissue to tissue.

Circulating estrogens modulate the pituitary secretion of the gonadotropins, luteinizing hormone (LH) and follicle stimulating hormone (FSH), through a negative feedback mechanism. Estrogens act to reduce the elevated levels of these hormones seen in postmenopausal women.

The decline of ovarian estrogen production that accompanies menopause or oophorectomy results in the acceleration of bone loss and bone resorption. Bone resorption is increased more than bone formation especially in the early years of menopause where bone loss is the greatest. In some women, these changes will eventually lead to decreased bone mass, osteoporosis and increased risk for fractures, particularly that of the spine, hip, and wrist. Vertebral fractures are the most common type of osteoporotic fracture in postmenopausal women.

Postmenopausal women with low serum estradiol concentrations and high serum concentrations of sex hormone-binding globulin (SHBG) have an increased risk of hip and vertebral fractures. Postmenopausal estrogen therapy decreases bone resorption, helping to reestablish balance between resorption and formation. This effect appears to be effective for as long as treatment is continued.

Pharmacokinetics

The bioavailability of estradiol following application of a Menostar transdermal system, relative to that of a transdermal system delivering 25 mcg/day, was investigated in 18 healthy postmenopausal women mean age 66 years (range 60-80 years). The mean serum estradiol concentrations upon administration of the two patches to the lower abdomen are shown in Figure 1. Transdermal administration of Menostar produced geometric mean serum concentration (Cavg) of estradiol of 13.7 pg/mL. No patches failed to adhere during the one week application period of both transdermal systems. Following application of the Menostar transdermal system to the abdomen, it is estimated to provide an average nominal *in-vivo* daily delivery of 14 mcg estradiol/day.

A. Absorption

The Menostar transdermal delivery system continuously releases estradiol which is transported across intact skin leading to sustained circulating levels of estradiol during a 7-day treatment period. The systemic availability of estradiol after transdermal administration is about 20 times higher than that after oral administration. This difference is due to the absence of first pass metabolism when estradiol is given by the transdermal route.

Table 1. Summary of Estradiol Pharmacokinetic Parameters (Abdomen Application)

Product	Estradiol Daily Delivery Rate, mcg/day	AUC (0-tlast) pg.h/mL	Cmax pg/mL	Cavg pg/mL	Tmax h	Cmin pg/mL
Menostar	14	2296	20.6	13.7	42	12.6
Climara® 6.5 cm²	25	4151	37.2	24.7	42	20.4

Table 2. Mean Percent BMD Change from Baseline in Lumbar Spine and Total Hip (Full Analysis Set)

	Lumbar spine				Total hip		
Time points	Menostar N = 208	Placebo N = 209	p-value	Time points	Menostar N = 208	Placebo N = 209	p-value
12-month Endpoint	n = 189 +2.29	n = 186 +0.51	< 0.001	12-month Endpoint	n = 189 +0.9	n = 184 -0.22	< 0.001
24-month Endpoint	n = 189 +2.99	n = 186 +0.54	< 0.001	24-month Endpoint	n = 189 +0.84	n = 185 -0.71	< 0.001

N = total number of patients; n = number of patients with data available for each variable

Table 1 provides a summary of estradiol pharmacokinetic parameters determined during evaluation of Menostar using baseline uncorrected serum concentrations.

[See table 1 above]

Pharmacokinetic parameters are expressed in geometric means except for the tmax which represents the median estimate and the Cmin which is expressed as the arithmetic mean.

The estimated estradiol daily delivery rate for Climara 6.5 cm² is quoted from the Climara labeling.

B. Distribution

The distribution of exogenous estrogens is similar to that of endogenous estrogens. Estrogens are widely distributed in the body and are generally found in higher concentrations in the sex hormone target organs. Estrogens circulate in the blood largely bound to sex hormone binding globulin (SHBG) and albumin. In the clinical study with 208 patients on Menostar, SHBG concentration (mean ± SD) remained essentially unchanged over the 2 year period (baseline 45.1 ± 20.1 nmol/L, 24 month visit 46.4 ± 20.9 nmol/L).

C. Metabolism

Exogenous estrogens are metabolized in the same manner as endogenous estrogens. Circulating estrogens exist in a dynamic equilibrium of metabolic interconversions. These transformations take place mainly in the liver. Estradiol is converted reversibly to estrone, and both can be converted to estriol, which is the major urinary metabolite. Estrogens also undergo enterohepatic recirculation via sulfate and glucuronide conjugation in the liver, biliary secretion of conjugates into the intestine, and hydrolysis in the intestine followed by reabsorption. In postmenopausal women, a significant proportion of the circulating estrogens exist as sulfate conjugates, especially estrone sulfate, which serves as a circulating reservoir for the formation of more active estrogens.

D. Excretion

Estradiol, estrone, and estriol are excreted in the urine along with glucuronide and sulfate conjugates.

E. Special Populations:

Geriatric: The efficacy and safety of Menostar has been studied in women between 60 and 80 years of age, with approximately half over 65 years old.

Pediatric: No pharmacokinetic study for Menostar has been conducted in a pediatric population.

Gender: Menostar is indicated for use in postmenopausal women only.

Race: No studies were done to determine the effect of race on the pharmacokinetics of Menostar.

Patients with Renal Impairment: Total estradiol serum levels are higher in post-menopausal women with end stage renal disease (ESRD) receiving maintenance hemodialysis than in normal subjects at baseline and following oral doses of estradiol. Therefore, conventional transdermal estradiol doses used in individuals with normal renal function may be excessive for postmenopausal women with ESRD receiving maintenance hemodialysis.

Patients with Hepatic Impairment: Estrogens may be poorly metabolized in patients with impaired liver function and should be administered with caution.

F. Drug Interactions

In vitro and *in vivo* studies have shown that estrogens are metabolized partially by cytochrome P450 3A4 (CYP3A4). Therefore, inducers or inhibitors of CYP3A4 may affect estrogen drug metabolism. Inducers of CYP3A4 such as St. John's Wort preparations (Hypericum perforatum), phenobarbital, carbamazepine, and rifampin may reduce plasma concentrations of estrogens, possibly resulting in a decrease in therapeutic effects and/or changes in the uterine bleeding profile. Inhibitors of CYP3A4 such as erythromycin, clarithromycin, ketoconazole, itraconazole, ritonavir and grapefruit juice may increase plasma concentrations of estrogens and may result in side effects.

G. Adhesion

In a Menostar pharmacokinetic study with 18 postmenopausal women, no patches failed to adhere during the one week application period.

CLINICAL STUDIES

The efficacy of Menostar in the prevention of postmenopausal osteoporosis was investigated in a 2-year double blind, placebo-controlled, multicenter study in the United States. A total of 417 postmenopausal women, 60 to 80 years old, with an intact uterus were enrolled in the study. All patients received supplemental calcium and vitamin D.

Menostar produced larger increases in bone mass than placebo as reflected by dual-energy x-ray absorptiometric (DEXA) measurements of hip and lumbar spine BMD. The changes in BMD from baseline were statistically significantly (p <0.001) greater during treatment with Menostar than during treatment with placebo for hip and spine after 1 and 2 years.

At lumbar spine Menostar increased BMD by 2.3% after 1 year and 3% after 2 years compared with a 0.5% increase after 1 and 2 years of treatment with placebo. At the hip Menostar increased BMD by 0.9% after one year and 0.84% after two years compared with a mean decrease of 0.22% after 1 year and 0.71% after 2 years of placebo treatment (see Table 2 above).

The BMD data of the study were analyzed according to baseline estradiol levels of the patients. Overall, estimated treatment effects on lumbar spine and total hip BMD after 2 years were approximately twice as large in the subgroup with baseline estradiol levels < 5 pg/mL than in the subgroup with baseline estradiol levels ≥ 5 pg/mL [Table 3].

[See table 3 at top of next page]

Menostar therapy also resulted in consistent, statistically significant suppression of bone turnover, as reflected by changes in serum and urine markers of bone formation (osteocalcin and bone-specific alkaline phosphatase) and bone resorption (carboxyterminal telopeptide of type 1 collagen (ICTP) and the urinary deoxypyridinoline/creatinine ratio).

Women's Health Initiative Studies

The WHI-enrolled a total of 27,000 predominantly healthy postmenopausal women to assess the risks and benefits of either the use of oral conjugated estrogens (CE 0.625 mg) alone per day or the use of oral conjugated estrogens (CE 0.625 mg) plus medroxyprogesterone acetate (MPA 2.5 mg) per day compared to placebo in the prevention of certain chronic diseases. The primary end-point was the incidence of coronary heart disease (CHD) (nonfatal myocardial infarction and CHD death), with invasive breast cancer as the primary adverse outcome studied. A "global index" included the earliest occurrence of CHD, invasive breast cancer, stroke, pulmonary embolism (PE), endometrial cancer, colorectal cancer, hip fracture, or death due to other cause. The study did not evaluate the effects of CE or CE/MPA on menopausal symptoms.

The estrogen-alone substudy was stopped early because an increased risk of stroke was observed. Results of the

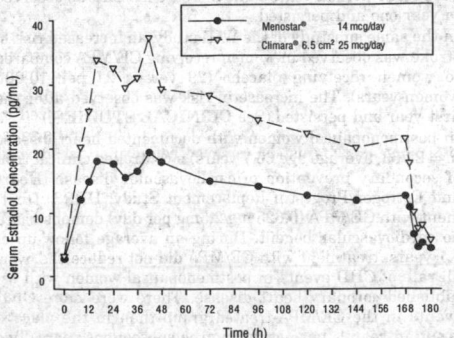

Figure 1
Mean Uncorrected Serum 17β-Estradiol Concentrations vs. Time Profile Following Application of Menostar and Climara® 6.5 cm² Transdermal System

Table 3. Mean percent change in lumbar spine and total hip BMD at 24 months by subgroups of baseline estradiol level (< 5 pg/mL, ≥ 5 pg/mL)

Baseline estradiol levels	Lumbar spine			Total hip		
	Menostar	Placebo	Treatment difference	Menostar	Placebo	Treatment difference
< 5 pg/mL	n = 101 +3.5	n = 97 +0.29	3.21 (p < 0.001)	n = 101 +1.04	n = 96 -1.09	2.13 (p < 0.001)
≥5 pg/mL	n = 88 +2.4	n = 89 +0.81	1.59 (p = 0.002)	n = 88 +0.61	n = 89 -0.31	0.92 (p = 0.045)

n = number of patients with data available for each variable

Table 4. RELATIVE AND ABSOLUTE RISK SEEN IN THE ESTROGEN ALONE SUBSTUDY OF WHI[a]

Event[c]	Relative Risk* CE vs Placebo at 6.8 Years (95% CI)	CE n = 5310	Placebo n = 5429
		Absolute Risk per 10,000 Women-years	
CHD events	0.91 (0.75-1.12)	49	54
Non-fatal MI	*0.89 (0.7-1.12)*	*37*	*41*
CHD death	*0.94 (0.65-1.36)*	*15*	*16*
Invasive breast cancer	0.77 (0.59-1.01)	26	33
Stroke	1.39 (1.1-1.77)	44	32
Pulmonary embolism	1.34 (0.87-2.06)	13	10
Colorectal cancer	1.08 (0.75-1.55)	17	16
Hip fracture	0.61 (0.41-0.91)	11	17
Death due to causes other than the events above	1.08 (0.88-1.32)	53	50
Global Index[b]	1.01 (0.91-1.12)	192	190
Deep vein thrombosis[c]	1.47 (1.04-2.08)	21	15
Vertebral fractures[c]	0.62 (0.42-0.93)	11	17
Total fractures[c]	0.7 (0.63-0.79)	139	195

[a] adapted from JAMA, 2004; 291:1701-1712
[b] a subset of the events was combined in a "global index", defined as the earliest occurrence of CHD events, invasive breast cancer, stroke, pulmonary embolism, endometrial cancer, colorectal cancer, hip fracture, or death due to other causes
[c] Not included in Global Index
* Nominal confidence intervals unadjusted for multiple looks and multiple comparisons

estrogen-alone substudy, which included 10,739 women (average age 63 years, range 50 to 79: 75.3 percent white, 15 percent black, 6.1 percent Hispanic), after an average follow-up of 6.8 years are presented in Table 4.
[See table 4 above]
For those outcomes included in the WHI "global index" that reached statistical significance, the absolute excess risks per 10,000 women-years in the group treated with CE alone was 12 more strokes, while the absolute risk reduction per 10,000 women-years was 6 fewer hip fractures. The absolute excess risk of events included in the "global index" was a nonsignificant 2 events per 10,000 women-years. There was no difference between the groups in terms of all-cause mortality. (See **Boxed WARNINGS, WARNINGS,** and **PRECAUTIONS.**)
The CE/MPA substudy was stopped early because, according to the predefined stopping rule, the increased risk of breast cancer and cardiovascular events exceeded the specified benefits included in the "global index." Results of the CE/MPA substudy, which included 16,608 women (average age of 63 years, range 50 to 79; 83.9% White, 6.5% Black, 5.5% Hispanic), after an average follow-up of 5.2 years are presented in Table 5 below:
[See table 5 at top of next page]
For those outcomes included in the "global index," the absolute excess risks per 10,000 women-years in the group treated with CE/MPA were 7 more CHD events, 8 more strokes, 8 more PEs, and 8 more invasive breast cancers, while absolute risk reductions per 10,000 women-years were 6 fewer colorectal cancers and 5 fewer hip fractures. The absolute excess risk of events included in the "global index" was 19 per 10,000 women-years. There was no differ-

ence between the groups in terms of all-cause mortality. (See **BOXED WARNINGS, WARNINGS,** and **PRECAUTIONS.**)
Women's Health Initiative Memory Study
The estrogen-alone WHIMS, a substudy of the WHI study, enrolled 2,947 predominantly healthy postmenopausal women 65 years of age and older (45 percent were aged 65 to 69 years, 36 percent were 70 to 74 years and 19 percent were 75 years of age and older) to evaluate the effects of conjugated estrogens (CE 0.625 mg) on the incidence of probable dementia (primary outcome) compared with placebo.
After an average follow-up of 5.2 years, 28 women in the estrogen-alone group (37 per 10,000 women-years) and 19 in the placebo group (25 per 10,000 women-years) were diagnosed with probable dementia. The relative risk of probable dementia in the estrogen-alone group was 1.49 (95 percent confidence interval (CI), 0.83-2.66) compared to placebo. It is unknown whether these findings apply to postmenopausal women. (See **BOXED WARNINGS, WARNINGS, Dementia,** and **PRECAUTIONS, Geriatric Use.**)
The estrogen plus progestin WHIMS substudy of WHI enrolled 4,532 predominantly postmenopausal women 65 years of age and older (47% were age 65 to 69 years, 35% were 70 to 74 years, and 18% were 75 years of age and older) to evaluate the effects of CE/MPA (0.625 mg conjugated estrogens plus 2.5 mg medroxyprogesterone acetate) on the incidence of probable dementia (primary outcome) compared with placebo.
After an average follow-up of 4 years, 40 women in the estrogen/progestin group (45 per 10,000 women-years) and 21 in the placebo group (22 per 10,000 women-years) were

diagnosed with probable dementia. The relative risk of probable dementia in the hormone therapy group was 2.05 (95% CI, 1.21 to 3.48) compared to placebo. Differences between groups became apparent in the first year of treatment. It is unknown whether these findings apply to younger postmenopausal women. (See **BOXED WARNINGS, WARNINGS, Dementia,** and **PRECAUTIONS, Geriatric Use.**)

INDICATIONS AND USAGE
Menostar is indicated for the prevention of postmenopausal osteoporosis. When prescribing solely for the prevention of postmenopausal osteoporosis, therapy should be considered only for women at significant risk of osteoporosis and non-estrogen medications should be carefully considered.
The mainstays for decreasing the risk of postmenopausal osteoporosis are weight bearing exercise, adequate calcium and vitamin D intake, and when indicated, pharmacologic therapy. Postmenopausal women require an average of 1500mg/day of elemental calcium. Therefore, when not contraindicated, calcium supplementation may be helpful for women with suboptimal dietary intake. Vitamin D supplementation of 400-800 IU/day may also be required to ensure adequate daily intake in postmenopausal women.
Risk factors for osteoporosis include low bone mineral density, low estrogen levels, family history of osteoporosis, previous fracture, small frame (low BMI), light skin color, smoking, and alcohol intake. Response to therapy can be predicted by pre-treatment serum estradiol (see Table 3), and can be assessed during treatment by measuring biochemical markers of bone formation/resorption, and/or bone mineral density.

CONTRAINDICATIONS
Menostar should not be used in women with any of the following conditions:
1. Undiagnosed abnormal genital bleeding.
2. Known, suspected, or history of cancer of the breast.
3. Known or suspected estrogen-dependent neoplasia.
4. Active deep vein thrombosis, pulmonary embolism or a history of these conditions.
5. Active or recent (e.g. within the past year) arterial thromboembolic disease (e.g., stroke, myocardial infarction).
6. Liver dysfunction or disease.
7. Menostar should not be used in patients with known hypersensitivity to its ingredients.
8. Known or suspected pregnancy. There is no indication for Menostar in pregnancy. There appears to be little or no increased risk of birth defects in children born to women who have used estrogens and progestins from oral contraceptives inadvertently during early pregnancy (See **PRECAUTIONS.**)

WARNINGS
See **BOXED WARNINGS.**
1. Cardiovascular disorders.
Estrogen and estrogen/progestin therapy have been associated with an increased risk of cardiovascular events such as myocardial infarction and stroke, as well as venous thrombosis and pulmonary embolism (venous thromboembolism or VTE). Should any of these occur or be suspected, estrogens should be discontinued immediately.
Risk factors for arterial vascular disease (e.g., hypertension, diabetes mellitus, tobacco use, hypercholesterolemia, and obesity) and/or venous thromboembolism (e.g., personal history or family history of VTE, obesity, and systemic lupus erythematosus) should be managed appropriately.
a. Coronary heart disease and stroke
In the WHI estrogen-alone substudy, an increased risk of stroke was observed in women receiving CE compared to placebo (44 versus 32 per 10,000 women-years). (See **CLINICAL STUDIES.**)
In the CE/MPA substudy of the WHI study, an increased risk of CHD events (defined as non-fatal myocardial infarction and CHD death) was observed in women receiving CE/MPA compared to women receiving placebo (37 versus 30 per 10,000 women-years). The increase in risk was observed in year one and persisted.
In the same substudy of the WHI study, an increased risk of stroke was observed in women receiving CE/MPA compared to women receiving placebo (29 versus 21 per 10,000 women-years). The increase in risk was observed after the first year and persisted.(See **CLINICAL STUDIES.**)
In postmenopausal women with documented heart disease (n = 2,763, average age 66.7 years) a controlled clinical trial of secondary prevention of cardiovascular disease (Heart and Estrogen/Progestin Replacement Study; HERS) treatment with CE/MPA (0.625 mg/2.5mg per day) demonstrated no cardiovascular benefit. During an average follow-up of 4.1 years, treatment with CE/MPA did not reduce the overall rate of CHD events in postmenopausal women with established coronary heart disease. There were more CHD events in the CE/MPA-treated group than in the placebo group in year 1, but not during the subsequent years. Two

thousand three hundred and twenty one women from the original HERS trial agreed to participate in an open label extension of HERS, HERS II. Average follow-up in HERS II was an additional 2.7 years, for a total of 6.8 years overall. Rates of CHD events were comparable among women in the CE/MPA group and the placebo group in HERS, HERS II, and overall.

Large doses of estrogen (5 mg conjugated estrogens per day), comparable to those used to treat cancer of the prostate and breast, have been shown in a large prospective clinical trial in men to increase the risks of nonfatal myocardial infarction, pulmonary embolism, and thrombophlebitis.

b. Venous thromboembolism (VTE)

In the WHI estrogen-alone substudy, an increased risk of deep vein thrombosis was observed in women receiving CE compared to placebo (21 versus 15 per 10,000 women-years). The increase in deep vein thrombosis risk was observed during the first year. (See **CLINICAL STUDIES**.)

In the CE/MPA substudy of WHI, a 2-fold greater rate of VTE, including deep venous thrombosis and pulmonary embolism, was observed in women receiving CE/MPA compared to women receiving placebo. The rate of VTE was 34 per 10,000 women-years in the CE/MPA group compared to 16 per 10,000 women-years in the placebo group. The increase in VTE risk was observed during the first year and persisted. (See **CLINICAL STUDIES**.)

If feasible, estrogens should be discontinued at least 4 to 6 weeks before surgery of the type associated with an increased risk of thromboembolism, or during periods of prolonged immobilization.

2. Malignant neoplasms

a. Endometrial cancer

The use of unopposed estrogens in women with intact uteri has been associated with an increased risk of endometrial cancer. The reported endometrial cancer risk among unopposed estrogen users is about 2- to 12-fold greater than in non-users, and appears dependent on duration of treatment and on estrogen dose. Most studies show no significant increased risk associated with use of estrogens for less than one year. The greatest risk appears associated with prolonged use, with increased risks of 15- to 24-fold for five to ten years or more and this risk has been shown to persist for at least 8 to 15 years after estrogen therapy is discontinued. Clinical surveillance of all women taking estrogen/progestin combinations is important. Adequate diagnostic measures, including endometrial sampling when indicated, should be undertaken to rule out malignancy in all cases of undiagnosed persistent or recurring abnormal vaginal bleeding. There is no evidence that the use of natural estrogens results in a different endometrial risk profile than synthetic estrogens of equivalent estrogen dose. Adding a progestin to estrogen therapy has been shown to reduce the risk of endometrial hyperplasia, which may be a precursor to endometrial cancer.

b. Breast cancer

The use of estrogens and progestins by postmenopausal women has been reported to increase the risk of breast cancer. The most important randomized clinical trial providing information about this issue is the Women's Health Initiative (WHI) substudy of CE/MPA (see **CLINICAL STUDIES**). The results from observational studies are generally consistent with those of the WHI clinical trial and report no significant variation in the risk of breast cancer among different estrogens or progestins, doses, or routes of administration.

The CE/MPA substudy of WHI reported an increased risk of breast cancer in women who took CE/MPA for a mean follow-up of 5.6 years. Observational studies have also reported an increased risk for estrogen/progestin combination therapy, and a smaller increased risk for estrogen alone therapy, after several years of use. In the WHI trial and from observational studies, the excess risk increased with duration of use. From observational studies, the risk appeared to return to baseline in about five years after stopping treatment. In addition, observational studies suggest that the risk of breast cancer was greater, and became apparent earlier, with estrogen/progestin combination therapy as compared to estrogen alone therapy.

In the CE/MPA substudy, 26% of the women reported prior use of estrogen alone and/or estrogen/progestin combination hormone therapy. After a mean follow-up of 5.6 years during the clinical trial, the overall relative risk of invasive breast cancer was 1.24 (95% confidence interval 1.01-1.54), and the overall absolute risk was 41 versus 33 cases per 10,000 women-years, for CE/MPA compared with placebo. Among women who reported prior use of hormone therapy, the relative risk of invasive breast cancer was 1.86, and the absolute risk was 46 versus 25 cases per 10,000 women-years, for CE/MPA compared with placebo. Among women who reported no prior use of hormone therapy, the relative risk of invasive breast cancer was 1.09, and the absolute risk was 40 versus 36 cases per 10,000 women-years for CE/MPA compared with placebo. In the same substudy, invasive breast cancers were larger and diagnosed at a more ad-

Table 5. RELATIVE AND ABSOLUTE RISK SEEN IN THE CE/MPA SUBSTUDY OF WHI[a]			
Event[c]	Relative Risk CE/MPA vs placebo at 5.2 Years (95% CI*)	CE/MPA n = 8506	Placebo n = 8102
		Absolute Risk per 10,000 Person-years	
CHD events	1.29 (1.02-1.63)	37	30
Non-fatal MI	*1.32 (1.02-1.72)*	*30*	*23*
CHD death	*1.18 (0.7-1.97)*	*7*	*6*
Invasive breast cancer[b]	1.26 (1-1.59)	38	30
Stroke	1.41 (1.07-1.85)	29	21
Pulmonary embolism	2.13 (1.39-3.25)	16	8
Colorectal cancer	0.63 (0.43-0.92)	10	16
Endometrial cancer	0.83 (0.47-1.47)	5	6
Hip fracture	0.66 (0.45-0.98)	10	15
Death due to causes other than the events above	0.92 (0.74-1.14)	37	40
Global Index[c]	1.15 (1.03-1.28)	170	151
Deep vein thrombosis[d]	2.07 (1.49-2.87)	26	13
Vertebral fractures[d]	0.66 (0.44-0.98)	9	15
Other osteoporotic fractures[d]	0.77 (0.69-0.86)	131	170

[a] adapted from JAMA, 2002; 288:321-333
[b] includes metastatic and non-metastatic breast cancer with the exception of in situ breast cancer
[c] a subset of the events was combined in a "global index", defined as the earliest occurrence of CHD events, invasive breast cancer, stroke, pulmonary embolism, endometrial cancer, colorectal cancer, hip fracture, or death due to other causes
[d] not included in Global Index
* nominal confidence intervals unadjusted for multiple looks and multiple comparisons

vanced stage in the CE/MPA group compared with the placebo group. Metastatic disease was rare with no apparent difference between the two groups. Other prognostic factors such as histologic subtype, grade and hormone receptor status did not differ between the groups.

The use of estrogen plus progestin has been reported to result in an increase in abnormal mammograms requiring further evaluation. All women should receive yearly breast examinations by a healthcare provider and perform monthly breast self-examinations. In addition, mammography examinations should be scheduled based on patient age, risk factors, and prior mammogram results.

3. Dementia

In the estrogen-alone WHIMS, a population of 2,947 hysterectomized women 65 to 79 years was randomized to CE or placebo. In the estrogen plus progestin WHIMS, a population of 4,532 postmenopausal women 65 to 79 years was randomized to CE/MPA or placebo.

In the estrogen-alone substudy, after an average follow-up of 5.2 years, 28 women in the estrogen-alone group and 19 women in the placebo group were diagnosed with probable dementia. The relative risk of probable dementia for estrogen-alone versus placebo was 1.49 (95 percent CI, 0.83-2.66). The absolute risk of probable dementia for estrogen-alone versus placebo was 37 versus 25 cases per 10,000 women-years. It is unknown whether these findings apply to younger post-menopausal women. (See **CLINICAL STUDIES** and **PRECAUTIONS, Geriatric Use**.)

After an average follow-up of 4 years, 40 women among women being treated with CE/MPA (1.8 percent, n=2,229) and 21 women in the placebo group (0.9 percent, n=2,303) received diagnoses of probable dementia. The relative risk for CE/MPA versus placebo was 2.05 (95 percent CI, 1.21-3.48), and was similar for women with and without histories of menopausal hormone use before WHIMS. The absolute risk of probable dementia for CE/MPA versus placebo was 45 versus 22 cases per 10,000 women-years, and the absolute excess risk for CE/MPA was 23 cases per 10,000 women-years. It is unknown whether these findings apply to younger postmenopausal women. (See **CLINICAL STUDIES** and **PRECAUTIONS, Geriatric Use**.)

It is unknown whether these findings apply to estrogen alone therapy.

4. Gallbladder disease

A 2- to 4-fold increase in the risk of gallbladder disease requiring surgery in postmenopausal women receiving estrogens has been reported.

5. Hypercalcemia

Estrogen administration may lead to severe hypercalcemia in patients with breast cancer and bone metastases. If hy-

percalcemia occurs, use of the drug should be stopped and appropriate measures taken to reduce the serum calcium level.

6. Visual abnormalities

Retinal vascular thrombosis has been reported in patients receiving estrogens. Discontinue medication pending examination if there is sudden partial or complete loss of vision, or a sudden onset of proptosis, diplopia, or migraine. If examination reveals papilledema or retinal vascular lesions, estrogens should be discontinued.

PRECAUTIONS

A. General

1. Addition of a progestin when a woman has not had a hysterectomy

Studies of the addition of a progestin for 10 or more days of a cycle of estrogen administration, or daily with estrogen in a continuous regimen, have reported a lowered incidence of endometrial hyperplasia than would be induced by estrogen treatment alone. Endometrial hyperplasia may be a precursor to endometrial cancer.

There are, however, possible risks that may be associated with the use of progestins with estrogens compared to estrogen-alone regimens. These include a possible increased risk of breast cancer.

2. Elevated blood pressure

In a small number of case reports, substantial increases in blood pressure have been attributed to idiosyncratic reactions to estrogens. In a large, randomized, placebo-controlled clinical trial, a generalized effect of estrogen therapy on blood pressure was not seen. Blood pressure should be monitored at regular intervals with estrogen use.

3. Hypertriglyceridema

In patients with preexisting hypertriglyceridemia, estrogen therapy may be associated with elevations of plasma triglycerides leading to pancreatitis and other complications.

4. Impaired liver function and past history of cholestatic jaundice

Estrogens may be poorly metabolized in patients with impaired liver function. For patients with a history of cholestatic jaundice associated with past estrogen use or with pregnancy, caution should be exercised and in the case of recurrence, medication should be discontinued.

5. Hypothyroidism

Estrogen administration leads to increased thyroid-binding globulin (TBG) levels. Patients with normal thyroid function can compensate for the increased TBG by making more thyroid hormone, thus maintaining free T_4 and T_3 serum concentrations in the normal range. Patients dependent on thyroid hormone replacement therapy who are also receiving estrogens may require increased doses of their thyroid

Summary of Most Frequently Reported Treatment Emergent Adverse Experiences/Medical Events (≥5%) By Treatment Groups

AE per Body System	Menostar 14 mcg/day (N=208)	Placebo (N=209)
Body as a Whole	95 (46%)	100 (48%)
Abdominal Pain	17 (8%)	17 (8%)
Accidental Injury	29 (14%)	23 (11%)
Infection	11 (5%)	10 (5%)
Pain	26 (13%)	26 (12%)
Cardiovascular	20 (10%)	19 (9%)
Digestive System	52 (25%)	44 (21%)
Constipation	11 (5%)	6 (3%)
Dyspepsia	11 (5%)	9 (4%)
Metabolic and Nutritional Disorders	25 (12%)	22 (11%)
Musculoskeletal System	54 (26%)	51 (24%)
Arthralgia	24 (12%)	13 (6%)
Arthritis	11 (5%)	15 (7%)
Myalgia	10 (5%)	6 (3%)
Nervous System	30 (14%)	23 (11%)
Dizziness	11 (5%)	6 (3%)
Respiratory System	62 (30%)	67 (32%)
Bronchitis	12 (6%)	9 (4%)
Upper Respiratory Infection	33 (16%)	35 (17%)
Skin and Appendages	50 (24%)	54 (26%)
Application Site Reaction	18 (9%)	18 (9%)
Breast Pain	10 (5%)	8 (4%)
Urogenital System	66 (32%)	40 (19%)
Cervical Polyps	13 (6%)	4 (2%)
Leukorrhea	22 (11%)	3 (1%)

replacement therapy. These patients should have their thyroid function monitored in order to maintain their free thyroid hormone levels in an acceptable range.

6. Fluid retention

Because estrogens may cause some degree of fluid retention, patients with conditions that might be influenced by this factor, such as a cardiac or renal dysfunction, warrant careful observation when estrogens are prescribed.

7. Hypocalcemia

Estrogens should be used with caution in individuals with severe hypocalcemia.

8. Ovarian cancer

The CE/MPA sub-study of WHI reported that estrogen plus progestin increased the risk of ovarian cancer. After an average follow-up of 5.6 years, the relative risk for ovarian cancer for CE/MPA versus placebo was 1.58 (95 percent CI, 0.77-3.24) but was not statistically significant. The absolute risk for CE/MPA versus placebo was 4.2 versus 2.7 cases per 10,000 women-years. In some epidemiological studies, the use of estrogen alone, in particular for ten or more years, has been associated with an increased risk of ovarian cancer. Other epidemiologic studies have not found these associations.

9. Exacerbation of endometriosis

Endometriosis may be exacerbated with administration of estrogens. A few cases of malignant transformation of residual endometrial implants have been reported in women treated post-hysterectomy with estrogen alone therapy. For patients known to have residual endometriosis post-hysterectomy, the addition of progestin should be considered.

10. Exacerbation of other conditions

Estrogens may cause an exacerbation of asthma, diabetes mellitus, epilepsy, migraine or porphyria, systemic lupus erythematosus, and hepatic hemangiomas and should be used with caution in women with these conditions.

B. Patient Information

Physicians are advised to discuss the Patient Information leaflet with patients for whom they prescribe Menostar.

C. Laboratory Tests

Estrogen administration should be initiated at the lowest dose approved for the indication and then guided by clinical response rather than by serum hormone levels (e.g. estradiol, FSH).

D. Drug/Laboratory Test Interactions

1. Accelerated prothrombin time, partial thromboplastin time, and platelet aggregation time; increased platelet count; increased factors II, VII antigen, VIII antigen, VIII coagulant activity; IX, X, XII, VII-X complex, II-VII-X complex, and beta-thromboglobulin; decreased levels of antifactor Xa and antithrombin III, decreased antithrombin III activity; increased levels of fibrinogen and fibrinogen activity; increased plasminogen antigen and activity.

2. Increased thyroid-binding globulin (TBG) levels leading to increased circulating total thyroid hormone levels as measured by protein-bound iodine (PBI), T_4 levels (by column or by radioimmunoassay) or T_3 levels by radioimmunoassay. T_3 resin uptake is decreased, reflecting the elevated TBG. Free T_4 and free T_3 concentrations are unaltered. Patients on thyroid replacement therapy may require higher doses of thyroid hormone.

3. Other binding proteins may be elevated in serum (i.e., corticosteroid binding globulin (CBG), sex hormone-binding globulin (SHBG) leading to increased total circulating corticosteroids and sex steroids, respectively. Free hormone concentrations may be decreased. Other plasma proteins may be increased (angiotensinogen/renin substrate, alpha-l-antitrypsin, ceruloplasmin).

4. Increased plasma HDL and HDL_2 subfraction concentrations, reduced LDL cholesterol concentration, and in oral formulations increased triglyceride levels.

5. Impaired glucose tolerance.

6. Reduced response to metyrapone test.

E. Carcinogenesis, Mutagenesis, Impairment of Fertility

Long-term continuous administration of estrogen, with and without progestin, in women with and without a uterus, has shown an increased risk of endometrial cancer, breast cancer, and ovarian cancer. (See **BOXED WARNINGS, WARNINGS** and **PRECAUTIONS**.)

Long-term continuous administration of natural and synthetic estrogens in certain animal species increases the frequency of carcinomas of the breast, uterus, cervix, vagina, testis, and liver.

F. Pregnancy

Menostar should not be used during pregnancy. (See **CONTRAINDICATIONS**.)

G. Nursing Mothers

Estrogen administration to nursing mothers has been shown to decrease the quantity and quality of the milk. Detectable amounts of estrogens have been identified in the milk of mothers receiving this drug. Caution should be exercised when Menostar is administered to a nursing woman.

H. Pediatric Use

The safety and efficacy of Menostar in pediatric patients has not been established.

I. Geriatric Use

A total of 417 postmenopausal women 61-79 years old, with an intact uterus, participated in the osteoporosis trial. More than 50% of women receiving study drug, were considered geriatric (65 years or older). Efficacy in older (≥65 years) and younger (<65 years) postmenopausal women in the osteoporosis treatment trial was comparable both at 12 and 24 months. Safety in older (≥65 years) and younger (<65 years) postmenopausal women in the osteoporosis treatment trial was also comparable throughout the study.

Of the total number of subjects in the estrogen-alone substudy of the WHI study, 46 percent (n = 4,943) were 65 years and older, while 7.1 percent (n = 767) were 75 years and older. There was a higher relative risk (CE versus placebo) of stroke in women less than 75 years of age compared to women 75 years and older.

In the estrogen-alone substudy of the WHIMS, a population of 2,947 hysterectomized women, aged 65 to 79 years, was randomized to estrogen-alone (CE 0.625 mg) or placebo. In the estrogen-alone group, after an average follow-up of 5.2 years, the relative risk (CE versus placebo) of probable dementia was 1.49 percent (95 percent CI, 0.83-2.66)

Of the total number of subjects in the estrogen plus progestin substudy of the WHI study, 44 percent (n = 7,320) were 65 years and older, while 6.6 percent (n = 1,095) were 75 years and older. There was a higher relative risk (CE/MPA versus placebo) of stroke and invasive breast cancer in women 75 and older compared to women less than 75 years of age.

In the estrogen plus progestin substudy of WHIMS, a population of 4,532 post-menopausal women, aged 65 to 70 years, was randomized to conjugated estrogens (CE 0.625 mg) plus medroxyprogesterone acetate (MPA 2.5 mg) or placebo. In the estrogen plus progestin group, after an average follow-up of 4 years, the relative risk (CE/MPA versus placebo) of probable dementia was 2.05 (95 percent CI, 1.21-3.48).

Pooling the events in women receiving CE or CE/MPA in comparision to those in women on placebo, the overall relative risk of probable dementia was 1.76 (95 percent CI, 1.19-2.60). Since both substudies were conducted in women 65 to 79 years, it is unknown whether these findings apply to younger post-menopausal women. (See **BOXED WARNINGS** and **WARNINGS, Dementia**.)

ADVERSE REACTIONS

See **BOXED WARNINGS, WARNINGS** and **PRECAUTIONS**.

Because clinical trials are conducted under widely varying conditions, adverse reaction rates observed in the clinical trials of a drug cannot be directly compared to rates in the clinical trials of another drug and may not reflect the rates observed in practice. The adverse reaction information from clinical trials does, however, provide a basis for identifying the adverse events that appear to be related to drug use and for approximating rates.

[See table above]

The following additional adverse reactions have been reported with estrogens and/or progestin therapy.

1. Genitourinary system

Changes in vaginal bleeding pattern and abnormal withdrawal bleeding or flow; breakthrough bleeding; spotting; dysmenorrhea; increase in size of uterine leiomyomata; vaginitis, including vaginal candidiasis; change in amount of cervical secretion; changes in cervical ectropion; ovarian cancer; endometrial hyperplasia; endometrial cancer.

2. Breasts

Tenderness, enlargement, pain, nipple discharge, galactorrhea; fibrocystic breast changes; breast cancer.

3. Cardiovascular

Deep and superficial venous thrombosis; pulmonary embolism; thrombophlebitis; myocardial infarction; stroke; increase in blood pressure.

4. Gastrointestinal

Nausea, vomiting; abdominal cramps, bloating; cholestatic jaundice; increased incidence of gallbladder disease; pancreatitis; enlargement of hepatic hemangiomas.

5. Skin

Chloasma or melasma, which may persist when drug is discontinued; erythema multiforme; erythema nodosum; hemorrhagic eruption; loss of scalp hair; hirsutism; pruritus; rash.

6. Eyes

Retinal vascular thrombosis; intolerance to contact lenses.

7. Central nervous system

Headache; migraine; dizziness; mental depression; chorea; nervousness; mood disturbances; irritability; exacerbation of epilepsy; dementia.

8. Miscellaneous

Increase or decrease in weight; reduced carbohydrate tolerance; aggravation of porphyria; edema; arthalgias; leg cramps; changes in libido; anaphylactoid/anaphylactic reactions including urticaria and angioedema; hypocalcemia; exacerbation of asthma; increased triglycerides.

OVERDOSAGE

Overdosage of estrogen may cause nausea, and withdrawal bleeding may occur in females. Serious ill effects have not been reported following acute ingestion of large doses of estrogen-containing drug products by young children.

DOSAGE AND ADMINISTRATION

Menostar should only be prescribed to postmenopausal women who are at significant risk of osteoporosis. Non-estrogen medications should be carefully considered. Risk factors for osteoporosis include low bone mineral density, low estrogen levels, family history of osteoporosis, previous fracture, small frame (low BMI), light skin color, smoking, and alcohol intake. Response to therapy can be predicted by pre-treatment serum estradiol (see Table 3), and can be assessed during treatment by measuring biochemical markers of bone formation/resorption, and/or bone mineral density.

When estrogen is prescribed for a postmenopausal woman with a uterus, a progestin should also be used, to reduce the risk of endometrial cancer. A woman without a uterus does not need progestin. For women who have a uterus, adequate diagnostic measures, such as endometrial sampling, when indicated, should be undertaken to rule out malignancy in cases of undiagnosed persistent or recurring abnormal vaginal bleeding.

It is recommended that women who have a uterus and are treated with Menostar receive a progestin for 14 days every 6 to 12 months and undergo an endometrial biopsy at yearly intervals or as clinically indicated. (See **BOXED WARNINGS** and **WARNINGS**).

Application of the System

The adhesive side of the Menostar transdermal system should be placed on a clean, dry area of the lower abdomen. **Menostar should not be applied to or near the breasts**. The sites of application must be rotated, with an interval of at least 1-week allowed between applications to a particular site. The area selected should not be oily, damaged, or irritated. The waistline should be avoided, since tight clothing may rub and remove the transdermal system. Application to areas where sitting would dislodge the transdermal system should also be avoided. The transdermal system should be applied immediately after opening the pouch and removing the protective liner. The transdermal system should be pressed firmly in place with the fingers for about 10 seconds, making sure there is good contact, especially around the edges. If the transdermal system lifts, apply pressure to maintain adhesion. In the event that a transdermal system should fall off, a new transdermal system should be applied for the remainder of the 7-day dosing interval. Only one system should be worn at any one time during the 7-day dosing interval. Swimming, bathing, or using a sauna while using Menostar has not been studied, and these activities may decrease the adhesion of the transdermal system and the delivery of estradiol.

Removal of the Transdermal System:

Removal of the system should be done carefully and slowly to avoid irritation of the skin. Should any adhesive remain on the skin after removal of the system, allow the area to dry for 15 minutes. Then gently rubbing the area with an oil-based cream or lotion should remove the adhesive residue.

Used patches still contain some active hormones. Each patch should be carefully folded in half so that it sticks to itself before throwing it away.

HOW SUPPLIED

Menostar (estradiol transdermal system), 14 mcg/day—each 3.25 cm^2 system contains 1 mg of estradiol USP

Individual Carton of 4 systems .... NDC 50419-455-04

Do not store above 86°F (30°C). Do not store unpouched. Apply immediately upon removal from the protective pouch.

PATIENT INFORMATION

Updated December 2005

Menostar® (Men-ō-star)

(estradiol transdermal system)

Read this before you start using Menostar and read what you get each time you refill Menostar. There may be new information. This information does not take the place of talking to your health care provider about your medical condition or your treatment.

What is the most important information I should know about Menostar (an osteoporosis preventative containing an estrogen hormone)?

- Estrogens increase the chances of getting cancer of the uterus.

Report any unusual vaginal bleeding right away while you are taking estrogens. Vaginal bleeding after menopause may be a warning sign of cancer of the uterus (womb). Your health care provider should check any unusual vaginal bleeding to find out the cause.

- Do not use estrogens with or without progestins to prevent heart disease, heart attacks, or strokes.

Using estrogens with or without progestins may increase your chances of getting heart attacks, strokes, breast cancer, or blood clots.

- Using estrogens with or without progestins may increase your risk of dementia.

You and your healthcare provider should talk regularly about whether you still need treatment with Menostar.

What is Menostar?

Menostar is a medicine that contains an estrogen hormone.

What is Menostar used for?

Menostar is used after menopause to:

- **reduce your chances of getting osteoporosis (thin weak bones).**
  Osteoporosis from menopause is a thinning of the bones that makes them weaker and easier to break. Very low doses of estrogen can help keep your bones from becoming weaker. You and your healthcare provider should talk regularly about whether you should continue with Menostar. Weight-bearing exercise, like walking or running, and taking calcium and vitamin D supplements may also lower your chances of getting postmenopausal osteoporosis. It is important to talk about exercise and supplements with your healthcare provider before starting them.

Who should not use Menostar?

Do not start using Menostar if you:

- **have unusual vaginal bleeding**
- **currently have or have had certain cancers.** Estrogens may increase the chances of getting certain types of cancers, including cancer of the breast or uterus. If you have or had cancer, talk with your health care provider about whether you should use Menostar.
- **had a stroke or heart attack in the past year.**
- **currently have or have had blood clots.**
- **currently have or have had liver problems.**
- **are allergic to Menostar or any of its ingredients.** See the end of this leaflet for a list of ingredients in Menostar. If you are allergic to other estrogen patches, you will likely be allergic to Menostar.
- **think you may be pregnant**

Tell your health care provider:

- **if you are breastfeeding.** The hormone in Menostar can pass into your milk.
- **about all of your medical problems.** Your health care provider may need to check you more carefully if you have certain conditions, such as asthma (wheezing), epilepsy (seizures), migraine, endometriosis, lupus, or problems with your heart, liver, thyroid, kidneys, or have high calcium levels in your blood.
- **about all the medicines you take,** including prescription and nonprescription medicines, vitamins, and herbal supplements. Do not use any estrogen pill, patch or injection with Menostar. Some medicines may affect how Menostar works. Menostar may also affect how your other medicines work.
- **if you are going to have surgery or will be on bed rest.** You may need to stop taking estrogens.

How should I use Menostar?

- Menostar is a patch that you wear on your skin. The estrogen in the Menostar patch passes through your skin. You must change your Menostar patch every 7 days (once a week). See the end of this leaflet for complete instructions for using Menostar.
- Estrogens should be used at the lowest dose possible for your treatment, only as long as needed. You and your healthcare provider should talk regularly about whether you still need treatment with Menostar.

What are the possible side effects of estrogens?

Less common but serious side effects include:

- Breast cancer
- Cancer of the uterus
- Stroke
- Heart attack
- Blood clots
- Dementia
- Gallbladder disease
- Ovarian cancer

These are some of the warning signs of serious side effects:

- Breast lumps
- Unusual vaginal bleeding
- Dizziness and faintness
- Changes in speech
- Severe headaches
- Chest pain
- Shortness of breath
- Pains in your legs
- Changes in vision
- Vomiting

Call your health care provider right away if you get any of these warning signs, or any other unusual symptom that concerns you.

Common side effects include:

- Headache
- Breast pain
- Irregular vaginal bleeding or spotting
- Stomach/abdominal cramps, bloating
- Nausea and vomiting
- Hair loss

Other side effects include:

- High blood pressure
- Liver problems
- High blood sugar
- Fluid retention
- Enlargement of benign tumors of the uterus ("fibroids")
- Vaginal yeast infection

These are not all the possible side effects of Menostar. For more information, ask your healthcare provider or pharmacist.

What can I do to lower my chances of a serious side effect with Menostar?

- Talk with your healthcare provider regularly about whether you should continue using Menostar. If you have a uterus, talk to your healthcare provider about whether the addition of a progestin is right for you. In general, the addition of a progestin is recommended for women with a uterus to reduce the chance of getting cancer of the uterus.
- See your healthcare provider right away if you get vaginal bleeding while using Menostar.
- Have a breast exam and mammogram (breast X-ray) every year unless your healthcare provider tells you something else. If members of your family have had breast cancer or if you have ever had breast lumps or an abnormal mammogram, you may need to have breast exams more often.
- If you have high blood pressure, high cholesterol (fat in the blood), diabetes, are overweight, or if you use tobacco, you may have higher chances for getting heart disease. Ask your healthcare provider for ways to lower your chances for getting heart disease.

General information about safe and effective use of Menostar.

Medicines are sometimes prescribed for conditions that are not mentioned in patient information leaflets. Do not use Menostar for conditions for which it was not prescribed. Do not give Menostar to other people, even if they have the same symptoms you have. It may harm them.

Keep Menostar out of the reach of children.

This leaflet provides a summary of the most important information about Menostar. If you would like more information, talk with your healthcare provider or pharmacist. You can ask for information about Menostar that is written for health professionals. You can get more information by calling the toll free number (1-888-237-5394) or visit www.menostar-us.com.

What are the ingredients in Menostar?

The active ingredient of Menostar is estradiol. Menostar also contains acrylate copolymer adhesive, fatty acid esters, and polyethylene backing. Menostar does not contain latex.

Instructions for Use

How and where do I apply the Menostar patch?

- Talk to your healthcare provider or pharmacist if you have questions about applying the Menostar patch.
- 1 Menostar patch is applied and worn for 7 days (1 week). The Menostar patch is changed once a week.
- Each Menostar patch is individually sealed in a protective pouch. To open the pouch, hold it upright with the Menostar name facing you. Tear off the top of the pouch using the top tear notch. Tear off the side of the pouch using the side tear notch. Pull the pouch open. The Menostar patch is the see-through plastic film attached to the clear thicker plastic backing. There is a silver foil-sticker attached to the inside of the pouch. Do not remove it from the pouch. The sticker contains a moisture protectant. Lift out the Menostar patch. Notice that the patch is attached to a thicker, hard-plastic backing and that the patch itself is oval and see-through.

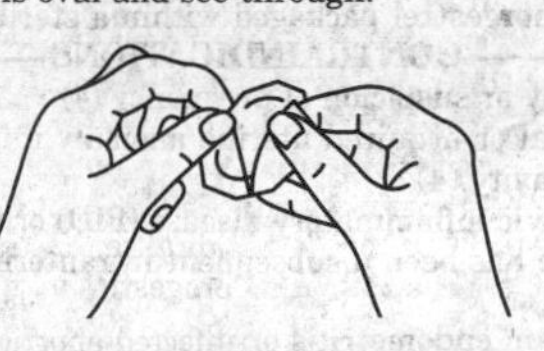

- Apply the sticky side of the Menostar patch to a clean, dry area of the lower stomach area below your belly button (see diagram below). **Do not apply the Menostar patch to your breasts**. The site selected should not be oily, damaged, or irritated. Avoid the waistline area, since tight clothing may rub and remove the patch. Also, do not put the patch on areas where sitting would rub it off or loosen it. Apply the patch right after opening the pouch and removing the protective liner. Press the patch firmly in place with your fingers for about 10 seconds. Make sure that it sticks all over, especially around the edges.

[See figure at top of next page]

- The Menostar patch should be left in place for 7 days (one week). Change the Menostar patch every 7 days (once a week). Remove the used patch. Carefully fold it in half so that it sticks to itself and safely throwaway, away from children and pets. Place a new Menostar patch on a different clean, dry area of the lower stomach area below your belly button. The same skin site should not be used again for at least 1 week after removal of the patch.

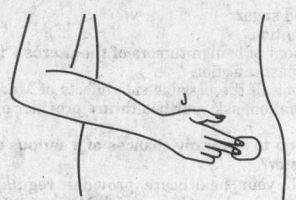

- If the Menostar patch falls off, the same patch may be re-applied to another area of your lower stomach. Make sure that Menostar patch sticks well to your skin, especially around the edges. If the patch will not stick completely to your skin, remove it and safely throwaway. Apply a new patch on a different area of the lower stomach. Do not wear 2 Menostar patches at the same time.
- Bathing, swimming, or showering may affect and loosen the Menostar patch.

Manufactured by 3M Drug Delivery Systems
Northridge, CA 91324
Manufactured for:
Bayer HealthCare
Pharmaceuticals
Bayer HealthCare Pharmaceuticals, Inc.
Wayne, NJ 07470
6705200   3M 677800   March 2007

MIRENA® ℞
[mĭ-rĕ-nä]
(levonorgestrel-releasing intrauterinesystem)

HIGHLIGHTS OF PRESCRIBING INFORMATION
These highlights do not include all the information needed to use Mirena® safely and effectively. See full prescribing information for Mirena.
Mirena (levonorgestrel-releasing intrauterine system)
Initial U.S. Approval: 2000

——————RECENT MAJOR CHANGES——————
Indications and Usage (1)   10/2009

——————INDICATIONS AND USAGE——————
Mirena is a sterile, levonorgestrel-releasing intrauterine system indicated for:
- Intrauterine contraception for up to 5 years (1)
- Treatment of heavy menstrual bleeding for women who choose to use intrauterine contraception as their method of contraception. (1)

It is recommended for women who have had at least one child.

——————DOSAGE AND ADMINISTRATION——————
- Initial release rate of levonorgestrel is 20 mcg per day; this rate is reduced by about 50% after 5 years; Mirena should be replaced after 5 years. (2)
- To be inserted by a trained healthcare provider using strict aseptic technique. Healthcare providers are advised to become thoroughly familiar with the insertion instructions before attempting insertion. (2.1, 2.2, 2.3, 2.4)
- Patient should be re-examined and evaluated 4 to 12 weeks after insertion; then, yearly or more often if indicated. (2.3)

——————DOSAGE FORMS AND STRENGTHS——————
One sterile intrauterine system consisting of a T-shaped polyethylene frame with a steroid reservoir containing 52 mg levonorgestrel packaged within a sterile inserter (3)

——————CONTRAINDICATIONS——————
- Pregnancy or suspicion of pregnancy (4)
- Congenital or acquired uterine anomaly if it distorts the uterine cavity (4)
- Acute pelvic inflammatory disease (PID) or history of unless there has been a subsequent intrauterine pregnancy (4)
- Postpartum endometritis or infected abortion in the past 3 months (4)
- Known or suspected uterine or cervical neoplasia or abnormal Pap smear (4)
- Genital bleeding of unknown etiology (4)
- Untreated acute cervicitis or vaginitis or other lower genital tract infections (4)
- Acute liver disease or liver tumor (benign or malignant) (4)
- Increased susceptibility to pelvic infection (4)
- A previously inserted IUD that has not been removed (4)
- Hypersensitivity to any component of Mirena (4)
- Known or suspected carcinoma of the breast (4)

——————WARNINGS AND PRECAUTIONS——————
- If pregnancy should occur with Mirena in place, remove Mirena. (5.2) There is increased risk of ectopic pregnancy including loss of fertility, pregnancy loss, septic abortion (including septicemia, shock and death) and premature labor and delivery. (5.1, 5.2)
- Group A streptococcal infection has been reported; strict aseptic technique is essential during insertion. (5.3)

- Before using Mirena, consider the risks of PID. (5.4)
- Bleeding patterns become altered, may remain irregular and amenorrhea may ensue. (5.5)
- Perforation may occur during insertion. Risk is increased in women with fixed retroverted uteri, during lactation, and postpartum. (5.6)
- Embedment in the myometrium and partial or complete expulsion may occur. (5.8)
- Persistent enlarged ovarian follicles should be evaluated. (5.9)

——————ADVERSE REACTIONS——————
The most common adverse reactions reported in clinical trials (> 10% users) are uterine/vaginal bleeding alterations (51.9%), amenorrhea (23.9%), intermenstrual bleeding and spotting (23.4%), abdominal /pelvic pain (12.8%) and ovarian cysts (12%). (6)
To report SUSPECTED ADVERSE REACTIONS, contact Bayer HealthCare Pharmaceuticals Inc. at 1-888-842-2937 or FDA at 1-800-FDA-1088 or www.fda.gov/medwatch

——————DRUG INTERACTIONS——————
- Drugs or herbal products that induce certain enzymes, such as CYP3A4, may decrease the serum concentration of progestins. (7)

——————USE IN SPECIFIC POPULATIONS——————
- Small amounts of progestins pass into breast milk resulting in detectable steroid levels in infant serum. (8.3)
- Use of this product before menarche is not indicated. (8.4)
- Use in women over 65 has not been studied and is not approved. (8.5)

See 17 for PATIENT COUNSELING INFORMATION and FDA-Approved Patient Labeling
                                            Revised: 10/2009

FULL PRESCRIBING INFORMATION: CONTENTS*
*Sections or subsections omitted from the full prescribing information are not listed

FULL PRESCRIBING INFORMATION

1 INDICATIONS AND USAGE
- Mirena® is indicated for intrauterine contraception for up to 5 years.

- Mirena is also indicated for the treatment of heavy menstrual bleeding in women who choose to use intrauterine contraception as their method of contraception.
Mirena is recommended for women who have had at least one child. The system should be replaced after 5 years if continued use is desired.

2 DOSAGE AND ADMINISTRATION
Mirena contains 52 mg of levonorgestrel. Initially, levonorgestrel is released at a rate of approximately 20 mcg/day. This rate decreases progressively to half that value after 5 years.
Mirena is packaged sterile within an inserter. Information regarding insertion instructions, patient counseling and record keeping, patient follow-up, removal of Mirena and continuation of contraception after removal is provided below.

2.1. Insertion Instructions
- **NOTE:** Mirena should be inserted by a trained healthcare provider. Healthcare providers are advised to become thoroughly familiar with the insertion instructions before attempting insertion of Mirena.
- Mirena is inserted with the provided inserter **(Figure 1a)** into the uterine cavity within seven days of the onset of menstruation or immediately after a first trimester abortion by carefully following the insertion instructions. It can be replaced by a new Mirena at any time during the menstrual cycle.

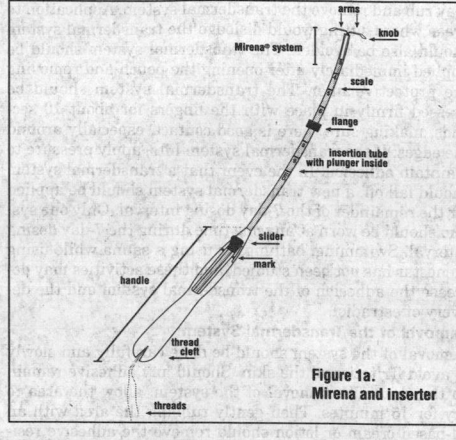

**Figure 1a.
Mirena and inserter**

Preparation for insertion
- Ensure that the patient understands the contents of the Patient Information Booklet and obtain consent. A consent form that includes the lot number is on the last page of the Patient Information Booklet.
- Confirm that there are no contraindications to the use of Mirena.
- Perform a urine pregnancy test, if indicated.
- With the patient comfortably in lithotomy position, gently insert a speculum to visualize the cervix and rule out genital contraindications to the use of Mirena.
- Do a bimanual exam to establish the size and position of the uterus, to detect other genital contraindications, and to exclude pregnancy.
- Thoroughly cleanse the cervix and vagina with a suitable antiseptic solution. Perform a paracervical block, if needed.
- Prepare to sound the uterine cavity. Grasp the upper lip of the cervix with a tenaculum forceps and apply gentle traction to align the cervical canal with the uterine cavity. If the uterus is retroverted, it may be more appropriate to grasp the lower lip of the cervix. Note that the tenaculum forceps should remain in position throughout the insertion procedure to maintain gentle traction on the cervix.
- Gently insert a uterine sound to check the patency of the cervix, measure the depth of the uterine cavity, confirm its direction and exclude the presence of any uterine anomaly. If you encounter cervical stenosis, use dilatation, not force, to overcome resistance.
- The uterus should sound to a depth of 6 to 10 cm. Insertion of Mirena into a uterine cavity less than 6 cm by sounding may increase the incidence of expulsion, bleeding, pain, perforation, and possibly pregnancy.
- After ascertaining that the patient is appropriate for Mirena, open the carton containing Mirena.

Insertion Procedure
Ensure use of sterile technique throughout the entire procedure.
Step 1–Opening of the sterile package
- Open the sterile package completely **(Figure 1b)**.
- Place sterile gloves on your hands.
- Pick up the handle of the inserter containing Mirena and carefully release the threads so that they hang freely.

Place your thumb or forefinger on the slider. Make sure that the slider is in the furthest position away from you, for example, at the top of the handle towards the insertion tube (**Figure 1b**).
NOTE: Keep your thumb or forefinger on the slider until insertion is complete.
• With the centimeter scale of the insertion tube facing up, check that the arms of Mirena are in a horizontal position. If they are not, align them on a flat, sterile surface, for example, the sterile package (**Figures 1b and 1c**).

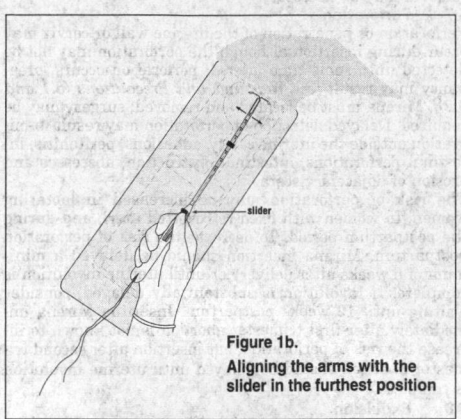

Figure 1b.
Aligning the arms with the slider in the furthest position

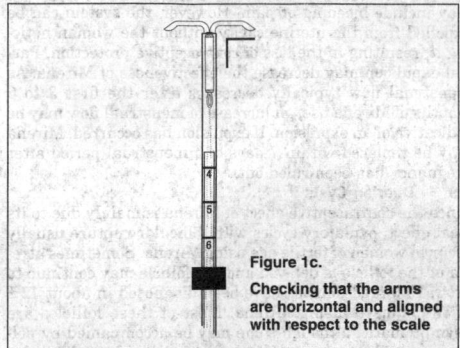

Figure 1c.
Checking that the arms are horizontal and aligned with respect to the scale

Step 2—Load Mirena into the insertion tube
• Holding the slider in the furthest position, pull on both threads to load Mirena into the insertion tube (**Figure 2a**).
• Note that the knobs at the ends of the arms now meet to close the open end of the insertion tube (**Figure 2b**).

If the knobs do not meet properly
If the knobs do not meet properly, release the arms by pulling the slider back to the mark (raised horizontal line on the handle) (**Figure 6a**). Re-load Mirena by aligning the open arms on a sterile surface (**Figure 1b**). Return the slider to its furthermost position and pull on both threads. Check for proper loading (**Figure 2b**).

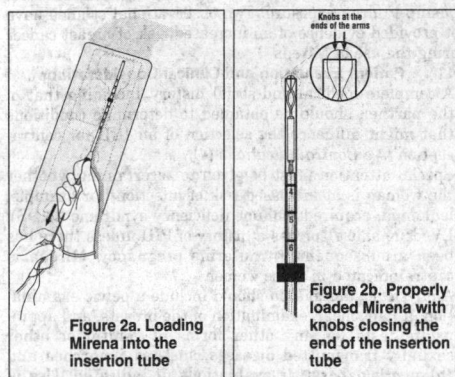

Figure 2a. Loading Mirena into the insertion tube

Figure 2b. Properly loaded Mirena with knobs closing the end of the insertion tube

Step 3—Secure the threads
Secure the threads in the cleft at the bottom end of the handle to keep Mirena in the loaded position (**Figure 3**).
[See first figure at top of next column]
Step 4—Setting the flange
Set the upper edge of the flange to the depth measured during the uterine sounding (**Figure 4**).
[See second figure at top of next column]

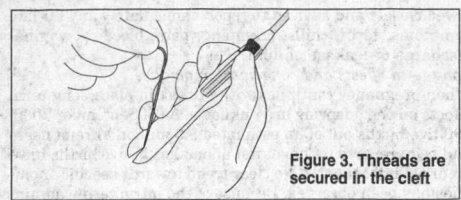

Figure 3. Threads are secured in the cleft

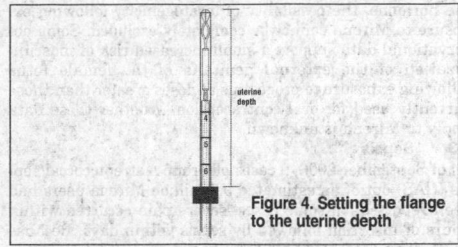

Figure 4. Setting the flange to the uterine depth

Step 5—Mirena is now ready to be inserted
• Continue to hold the slider with the thumb or forefinger firmly in the furthermost position. Grasp the tenaculum forceps with your other hand and apply gentle traction to align the cervical canal with the uterine cavity.
• While maintaining traction on the cervix, gently advance the insertion tube through the cervical canal and into the uterine cavity **until the flange is 1.5 to 2 cm from the external cervical os.**
• **CAUTION: do not advance flange to the cervix at this step.** Maintaining the flange 1.5 to 2 cm from the cervical os allows sufficient space for the arms to open (when released) within the uterine cavity (**Figures 5 and 6b**).
NOTE! Do not force the inserter. If necessary, dilate the cervical canal.

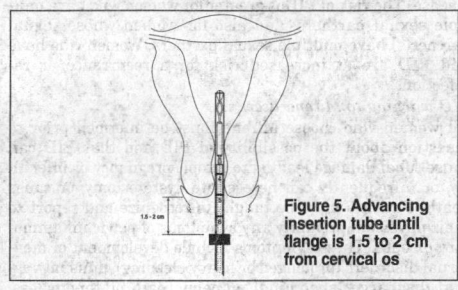

Figure 5. Advancing insertion tube until flange is 1.5 to 2 cm from cervical os

Step 6—Release the arms
• While holding the inserter steady, release the arms of Mirena by pulling the slider back until the top of the slider reaches the mark (raised horizontal line on the handle) (**Figure 6a**).
• Wait approximately 10 seconds to allow the horizontal arms of Mirena to open and regain its T-shape (**Figure 6b**).

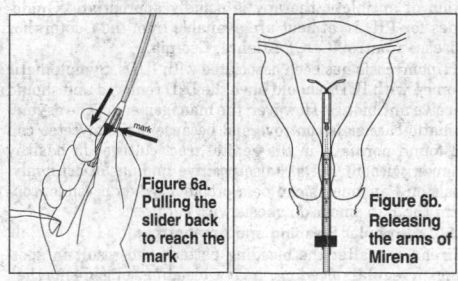

Figure 6a. Pulling the slider back to reach the mark

Figure 6b. Releasing the arms of Mirena

Step 7—Advance to fundal position
Gently advance the inserter into the uterine cavity until the flange meets the cervix and you feel fundal resistance. Mirena should now be in the desired fundal position (**Figure 7**).
[See first figure at top of next column]
Step 8—Release Mirena and withdraw the inserter
• While holding the inserter steady, pull the slider all the way down to release Mirena from the insertion tube (**Figure 8**). The threads will release automatically from the cleft.
• Check that the threads are hanging freely and gently withdraw the inserter from the uterus. Be careful not to pull on the threads as this will displace Mirena.
[See second figure at top of next column]

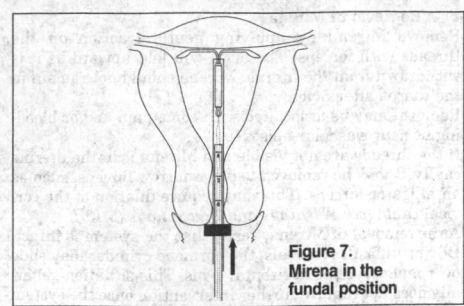

Figure 7. Mirena in the fundal position

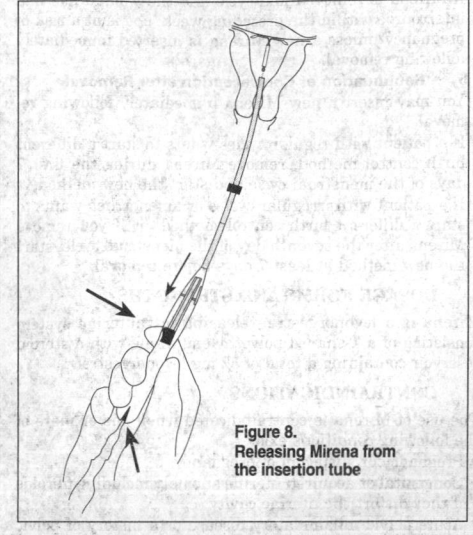

Figure 8. Releasing Mirena from the insertion tube

Step 9—Cut the threads
• Cut the threads perpendicular to the thread length, for example, with sterile curved scissors, leaving about 3 cm visible outside the cervix (**Figure 9**).
NOTE: Cutting threads at an angle may leave sharp ends.

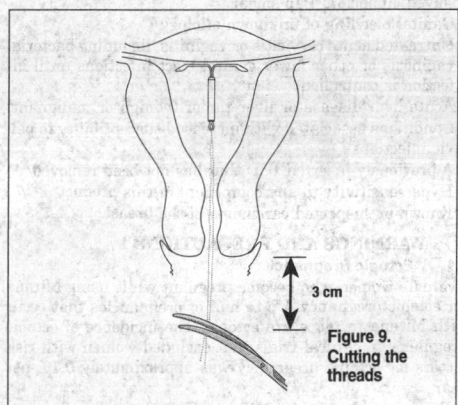

Figure 9. Cutting the threads

Mirena insertion is now complete.
Important information to consider during or after insertion
• If you suspect that Mirena is not in the correct position, check placement (for example, with transvaginal ultrasound). Remove Mirena if it is not positioned completely within the uterus. A removed Mirena must not be reinserted.
• If there is clinical concern and/or exceptional pain or bleeding during or after insertion, appropriate and timely measures and assessments, for example ultrasound, should be performed to exclude perforation.
2.2　Patient Counseling and Record Keeping
• Keep a copy of the consent form and lot number for your records.
• Counsel the patient on what to expect following Mirena insertion. Give the patient the Follow-up Reminder Card that is provided with the product. Discuss expected bleeding patterns during the first months of Mirena use. *[See Patient Counseling Information (17.1).]*
• Prescribe analgesics, if indicated.
2.3　Patient Follow-up
• Patients should be reexamined and evaluated 4 to 12 weeks after insertion and once a year thereafter, or more frequently if clinically indicated.

2.4 Removal of Mirena

- Remove Mirena by applying gentle traction on the threads with forceps. The arms will fold upward as it is withdrawn from the uterus. Mirena should not remain in the uterus after 5 years.
- Removal may be associated with some pain and/or bleeding or neurovascular episodes.
- If the threads are not visible and Mirena is in the uterine cavity, it may be removed using a narrow forceps, such as an alligator forceps. This may require dilation of the cervical canal [see Warnings and Precautions (5.13)].
- After removal of Mirena, verify that the system is intact.
- During difficult removals, the hormone cylinder may slide over and cover the horizontal arms. This situation generally does not require further intervention once the system is verified to be intact.
- If Mirena is removed mid-cycle and the woman has had intercourse within the preceding week, she is at a risk of pregnancy unless a new Mirena is inserted immediately following removal.

2.5 Continuation of Contraception after Removal

- You may insert a new Mirena immediately following removal.
- If a patient with regular cycles wants to start a different birth control method, remove Mirena during the first 7 days of the menstrual cycle and start the new method.
- If a patient with irregular cycles or amenorrhea wants to start a different birth control method, or if you remove Mirena after the seventh day of the menstrual cycle, start the new method at least 7 days before removal.

3 DOSAGE FORMS AND STRENGTHS

Mirena is a levonorgestrel-releasing intrauterine system consisting of a T-shaped polyethylene frame with a steroid reservoir containing a total of 52 mg levonorgestrel.

4 CONTRAINDICATIONS

The use of Mirena is contraindicated when one or more of the following conditions exist:

- Pregnancy or suspicion of pregnancy
- Congenital or acquired uterine anomaly including fibroids if they distort the uterine cavity
- Acute pelvic inflammatory disease or a history of pelvic inflammatory disease unless there has been a subsequent intrauterine pregnancy
- Postpartum endometritis or infected abortion in the past 3 months
- Known or suspected uterine or cervical neoplasia or unresolved, abnormal Pap smear
- Genital bleeding of unknown etiology
- Untreated acute cervicitis or vaginitis, including bacterial vaginosis or other lower genital tract infections until infection is controlled
- Acute liver disease or liver tumor (benign or malignant)
- Conditions associated with increased susceptibility to pelvic infections
- A previously inserted IUD that has not been removed
- Hypersensitivity to any component of this product
- Known or suspected carcinoma of the breast.

5 WARNINGS AND PRECAUTIONS

5.1 Ectopic Pregnancy

Evaluate women who become pregnant while using Mirena for ectopic pregnancy. Up to half of pregnancies that occur with Mirena in place are ectopic. The incidence of ectopic pregnancy in clinical trials that excluded women with risk factors for ectopic pregnancy was approximately 0.1% per year.

Tell women who choose Mirena about the risks of ectopic pregnancy, including the loss of fertility. Teach them to recognize and report to their physician promptly any symptoms of ectopic pregnancy. Women with a previous history of ectopic pregnancy, tubal surgery or pelvic infection carry a higher risk of ectopic pregnancy.

The risk of ectopic pregnancy in women who have a history of ectopic pregnancy and use Mirena is unknown. Clinical trials of Mirena excluded women with a history of ectopic pregnancy.

5.2 Intrauterine Pregnancy

If pregnancy should occur with Mirena in place, Mirena should be removed. Removal or manipulation of Mirena may result in pregnancy loss. In the event of an intrauterine pregnancy with Mirena, consider the following:

Septic abortion

In patients becoming pregnant with an IUD in place, septic abortion—with septicemia, septic shock, and death—may occur.

Continuation of pregnancy

If a woman becomes pregnant with Mirena in place and if Mirena cannot be removed or the woman chooses not to have it removed, she should be warned that failure to remove Mirena increases the risk of miscarriage, sepsis, premature labor and premature delivery. She should be fol-

lowed closely and advised to report immediately any flu-like symptoms, fever, chills, cramping, pain, bleeding, vaginal discharge or leakage of fluid.

Long-term effects and congenital anomalies

When pregnancy continues with Mirena in place, long-term effects on the offspring are unknown. As of September 2006, 390 live births out of an estimated 9.9 million Mirena users had been reported. Congenital anomalies in live births have occurred infrequently. No clear trend towards specific anomalies has been observed. Because of the intrauterine administration of levonorgestrel and local exposure of the fetus to the hormone, the possibility of teratogenicity following exposure to Mirena cannot be completely excluded. Some observational data support a small increased risk of masculinization of the external genitalia of the female fetus following exposure to progestins at doses greater than those currently used for oral contraception. Whether these data apply to Mirena is unknown.

5.3 Sepsis

As of September 2006, 9 cases of Group A streptococcal sepsis (GAS) out of an estimated 9.9 million Mirena users had been reported. In some cases, severe pain occurred within hours of insertion followed by sepsis within days. Because death from GAS is more likely if treatment is delayed, it is important to be aware of these rare but serious infections. Aseptic technique during insertion of Mirena is essential. GAS sepsis may also occur postpartum, after surgery, and from wounds.

5.4 Pelvic Inflammatory Disease (PID)

Mirena is contraindicated in the presence of known or suspected PID or in women with a history of PID unless there has been a subsequent intrauterine pregnancy. Use of IUDs has been associated with an increased risk of PID. The highest risk of PID occurs shortly after insertion (usually within the first 20 days thereafter) [see Warnings and Precautions (5.12)]. A decision to use Mirena must include consideration of the risks of PID.

Women at increased risk for PID

PID is often associated with a sexually transmitted disease, and Mirena does not protect against sexually transmitted disease. The risk of PID is greater for women who have multiple sexual partners, and also for women whose sexual partner(s) have multiple sexual partners. Women who have had PID are at increased risk for a recurrence or reinfection.

PID warning to Mirena users

All women who choose Mirena must be informed prior to insertion about the possibility of PID and that PID can cause tubal damage leading to ectopic pregnancy or infertility, or infrequently can necessitate hysterectomy, or cause death. Patients must be taught to recognize and report to their physician promptly any symptoms of pelvic inflammatory disease. These symptoms include development of menstrual disorders (prolonged or heavy bleeding), unusual vaginal discharge, abdominal or pelvic pain or tenderness, dyspareunia, chills, and fever.

Asymptomatic PID

PID may be asymptomatic but still result in tubal damage and its sequelae.

Treatment of PID

Following a diagnosis of PID, or suspected PID, bacteriologic specimens should be obtained and antibiotic therapy should be initiated promptly. Removal of Mirena after initiation of antibiotic therapy is usually appropriate. Guidelines for PID treatment are available from the Centers for Disease Control (CDC), Atlanta, Georgia.

Actinomycosis has been associated with IUDs. Symptomatic women with IUDs should have the IUD removed and should receive antibiotics. However, the management of the asymptomatic carrier is controversial because actinomycetes can be found normally in the genital tract cultures in healthy women without IUDs. False positive findings of actinomycosis on Pap smears can be a problem. When possible, confirm the Pap smear diagnosis with cultures.

5.5 Irregular Bleeding and Amenorrhea

Mirena can alter the bleeding pattern and result in spotting, irregular bleeding, heavy bleeding, oligomenorrhea and amenorrhea. During the first three to six months of Mirena use, the number of bleeding and spotting days may be increased and bleeding patterns may be irregular. Thereafter the number of bleeding and spotting days usually decreases but bleeding may remain irregular. If bleeding irregularities develop during prolonged treatment, appropriate diagnostic measures should be taken to rule out endometrial pathology.

Amenorrhea develops in approximately 20% of Mirena users by one year. The possibility of pregnancy should be considered if menstruation does not occur within six weeks of the onset of previous menstruation. Once pregnancy has been excluded, repeated pregnancy tests are generally not necessary in amenorrheic women unless indicated, for example, by other signs of pregnancy or by pelvic pain [see Clinical Studies (14.1)].

In most women with heavy menstrual bleeding, the number of bleeding and spotting days may also increase during the initial months of therapy but usually decrease with continued use; the volume of blood loss per cycle progressively becomes reduced [see Clinical Studies (14.2)].

5.6 Embedment

Embedment of Mirena in the myometrium may occur. Embedment may decrease contraceptive effectiveness and result in pregnancy [see Warnings and Precautions (5.1 and 5.2)]. An embedded Mirena should be removed. Embedment can result in difficult removal and, in some cases surgical removal may be necessary.

5.7 Perforation

Perforation or penetration of the uterine wall or cervix may occur during insertion although the perforation may not be detected until some time later. If perforation occurs, pregnancy may result [see Warnings and Precautions (5.1 and 5.2)]. Mirena must be located and removed; surgery may be required. Delayed detection of perforation may result in migration outside the uterine cavity, adhesions, peritonitis, intestinal perforations, intestinal obstruction, abscesses and erosion of adjacent viscera.

The risk of perforation may be increased in lactating women, in women with fixed retroverted uteri, and during the postpartum period. To decrease the risk of perforation postpartum, Mirena insertion should be delayed a minimum of 6 weeks after delivery or until uterine involution is complete. If involution is substantially delayed, consider waiting until 12 weeks postpartum. Inserting Mirena immediately after first trimester abortion is not known to increase the risk of perforation, but insertion after second trimester abortion should be delayed until uterine involution is complete.

5.8 Expulsion

Partial or complete expulsion of Mirena may occur [see Warnings and Precautions (5.13)].

Symptoms of the partial or complete expulsion of any IUD may include bleeding or pain. However, the system can be expelled from the uterine cavity without the woman noticing it, resulting in the loss of contraceptive protection. Partial expulsion may decrease the effectiveness of Mirena. As menstrual flow typically decreases after the first 3 to 6 months of Mirena use, an increase of menstrual flow may be indicative of an expulsion. If expulsion has occurred, Mirena may be replaced within 7 days of a menstrual period after pregnancy has been ruled out.

5.9 Ovarian Cysts

Since the contraceptive effect of Mirena is mainly due to its local effect, ovulatory cycles with follicular rupture usually occur in women of fertile age using Mirena. Sometimes atresia of the follicle is delayed and the follicle may continue to grow. Enlarged follicles have been diagnosed in about 12% of the subjects using Mirena. Most of these follicles are asymptomatic, although some may be accompanied by pelvic pain or dyspareunia. In most cases the enlarged follicles disappear spontaneously during two to three months observation. Persistent enlarged follicles should be evaluated. Surgical intervention is not usually required.

5.10 Breast Cancer

Women who currently have or have had breast cancer, or have a suspicion of breast cancer, should not use hormonal contraception because breast cancer is a hormone-sensitive tumor.

Spontaneous reports of breast cancer have been received during postmarketing experience with Mirena. Because spontaneous reports are voluntary and from a population of uncertain size, it is not possible to use postmarketing data to reliably estimate the frequency or establish causal relationship to drug exposure. Two observational studies have not provided evidence of an increased risk of breast cancer during the use of Mirena.

5.11 Patient Evaluation and Clinical Considerations

- A complete medical and social history, including that of the partner, should be obtained to determine conditions that might influence the selection of an IUD for contraception [see Contraindications (4)].
- Special attention must be given to ascertaining whether the woman is at increased risk of infection (for example, leukemia, acquired immune deficiency syndrome (AIDS), I.V. drug abuse), or has a history of PID unless there has been a subsequent intrauterine pregnancy. Mirena is contraindicated in these women.
- A physical examination should include a pelvic examination, a Pap smear, examination of the breasts, and appropriate tests for any other forms of genital or other sexually transmitted diseases, such as gonorrhea and chlamydia laboratory evaluations, if indicated. Use of Mirena in patients with vaginitis or cervicitis should be postponed until proper treatment has eradicated the infection and until it has been shown that the cervicitis is not due to gonorrhea or chlamydia [see Contraindications (4)].
- Irregular bleeding may mask symptoms and signs of endometrial polyps or cancer. Because irregular bleeding/spotting is common during the first months of Mirena use, exclude endometrial pathology prior to the insertion of

Mirena in women with persistent or uncharacteristic bleeding. If unexplained bleeding irregularities develop during the prolonged use of Mirena, appropriate diagnostic measures should be taken *[see Warnings and Precautions (5.5)]*.

- **The healthcare provider should determine that the patient is not pregnant.** The possibility of insertion of Mirena in the presence of an existing undetermined pregnancy is reduced if insertion is performed within 7 days of the onset of a menstrual period. Mirena can be replaced by a new system at any time in the cycle. Mirena can be inserted immediately after first trimester abortion.
- Mirena should not be inserted until 6 weeks postpartum or until involution of the uterus is complete in order to reduce the incidence of perforation and expulsion. If involution is substantially delayed, consider waiting until 12 weeks postpartum *[see Warnings and Precautions (5.7)]*.
- Patients with certain types of valvular or congenital heart disease and surgically constructed systemic-pulmonary shunts are at increased risk of infective endocarditis. Use of Mirena in these patients may represent a potential source of septic emboli. Patients with known congenital heart disease who may be at increased risk should be treated with appropriate antibiotics at the time of insertion and removal.
- Patients requiring chronic corticosteroid therapy or insulin for diabetes should be monitored with special care for infection.

Mirena should be used with caution in patients who have:

- Coagulopathy or are receiving anticoagulants
- Migraine, focal migraine with asymmetrical visual loss or other symptoms indicating transient cerebral ischemia
- Exceptionally severe headache
- Marked increase of blood pressure
- Severe arterial disease such as stroke or myocardial infarction.

5.12 Insertion Precautions

- Observe strict asepsis during insertion. The presence of organisms capable of establishing PID cannot be determined by appearance, and IUD insertion may be associated with introduction of vaginal bacteria into the uterus. Administration of antibiotics may be considered, but the utility of this treatment is unknown.
- Carefully sound the uterus prior to Mirena insertion to determine the degree of patency of the endocervical canal and the internal os, and the direction and depth of the uterine cavity. In occasional cases, severe cervical stenosis may be encountered. Do not use excessive force to overcome this resistance.
- Fundal positioning of Mirena is important to prevent expulsion and maximize efficacy. Therefore, follow the instructions for the insertion carefully.
- If the patient develops decreased pulse, perspiration, or pallor, have her remain supine until these signs resolve. Insertion may be associated with some pain and/or bleeding. Syncope, bradycardia, or other neurovascular episodes may occur during insertion of Mirena, especially in patients with a predisposition to these conditions or cervical stenosis.

5.13 Continuation and Removal

- Reexamine and evaluate patients 4 to 12 weeks after insertion and once a year thereafter, or more frequently if clinically indicated.
- If the threads are not visible, they may have retracted into the uterus or broken, or Mirena may have broken, perforated the uterus, or been expelled *[see Warnings and Precautions (5.7 and 5.8)]*. If the length of the threads has changed from the length at time of insertion, the system may have become displaced. Pregnancy must be excluded and the location of Mirena verified, for example, by sonography, X-ray, or by gentle exploration of the uterine cavity with a probe. If Mirena is displaced, remove it. A new Mirena may be inserted at that time or during the next menses if it is certain that conception has not occurred. If Mirena is in place with no evidence of perforation, no intervention is indicated.
- Promptly examine users with complaints of pain, odorous discharge, unexplained bleeding *[see Warnings and Precautions (5.5)]*, fever, genital lesions or sores.
- Consider the possibility of ectopic pregnancy in the case of lower abdominal pain especially in association with missed periods or if an amenorrheic woman starts bleeding *[see Warnings and Precautions (5.1)]*.

In the event a pregnancy is confirmed during Mirena use:

- Determine whether pregnancy is ectopic and, if so, take appropriate measures.
- Inform patient of the risks of leaving Mirena in place or removing it during pregnancy and of the lack of data on long-term effects on the offspring of women who have had Mirena in place during conception or gestation *[see Warnings and Precautions (5.2)]*.
- If possible, Mirena should be removed after the patient has been warned of the risks of removal. If removal is difficult, the patient should be counseled and offered pregnancy termination.
- If Mirena is left in place, the patient's course should be followed closely.

In the event of a sexually transmitted disease during Mirena use:

Should the patient's relationship cease to be mutually monogamous, or should her partner become HIV positive, or acquire a sexually transmitted disease, she should be instructed to report this change to her clinician immediately. The use of a barrier method as a partial protection against acquiring sexually transmitted diseases should be strongly recommended.

Removal of Mirena should be considered.

Mirena should be removed for the following medical reasons:

- New onset menorrhagia and/or metrorrhagia producing anemia
- Sexually transmitted disease
- Pelvic infection; endometritis
- Symptomatic genital actinomycosis
- Intractable pelvic pain
- Severe dyspareunia
- Pregnancy
- Endometrial or cervical malignancy
- Uterine or cervical perforation.

Removal of the system should also be considered if any of the following conditions arise for the first time:

- Migraine, focal migraine with asymmetrical visual loss or other symptoms indicating transient cerebral ischemia
- Exceptionally severe headache
- Jaundice
- Marked increase of blood pressure
- Severe arterial disease such as stroke or myocardial infarction.

Removal may be associated with some pain and/or bleeding or neurovascular episodes.

5.14 Glucose Tolerance

Levonorgestrel may affect glucose tolerance, and the blood glucose concentration should be monitored in diabetic users of Mirena.

6 ADVERSE REACTIONS

The following most serious adverse reactions associated with the use of Mirena are discussed in greater detail in the *Warnings and Precautions section (5)*:

- Ectopic Pregnancy *[see Warnings and Precautions (5.1)]*
- Intrauterine Pregnancy *[see Warnings and Precautions (5.2)]*
- Group A streptococcal sepsis (GAS) *[see Warnings and Precautions (5.3)]*
- Pelvic Inflammatory Disease *[see Warnings and Precautions (5.4)]*
- Embedment *[see Warnings and Precautions (5.6)]*
- Perforation *[see Warnings and Precautions (5.7)]*
- Breast Cancer *[see Warnings and Precautions (5.10)]*

6.1 Clinical Trial Experience

Because clinical trials are conducted under widely varying conditions, adverse reaction rates observed in the clinical studies of a drug cannot be directly compared to rates in the clinical trials of another drug and may not reflect the rates observed in practice.

The data provided reflect the experience with the use of Mirena in the adequate and well-controlled studies for contraception (n=2,339) and heavy menstrual bleeding (n=80). For the contraception indication, Mirena was compared to a copper IUD (n=1,855), to another formulation of levonorgestrel intrauterine system (n=390) and to a combined oral contraceptive (n=94) in women 18 to 35 years old. The data cover more than 92,000 woman-months of exposure. For the treatment of heavy menstrual bleeding indication (n=80), the subjects included women aged 26 to 50 with confirmed heavy bleeding and exposed for a median of 183 treatment days of Mirena (range 7 to 295 days). The frequencies of reported adverse drug reactions represent crude incidences.

The adverse reactions seen across the 2 indications overlapped, and are reported using the frequencies from the contraception studies.

The most common adverse reactions (≥5% users) are uterine/vaginal bleeding alterations (51.9%), amenorrhea (23.9%), intermenstrual bleeding and spotting (23.4%), abdominal/pelvic pain (12.8%), ovarian cysts (12%), headache/migraine (7.7%), acne (7.2%), depressed/altered mood (6.4%), menorrhagia (6.3%), breast tenderness/pain (4.9%), vaginal discharge (4.9%) and IUD expulsion (4.9%).

Other relevant adverse reactions occurring in <5% of subjects include nausea, nervousness, vulvovaginitis, dysmenorrhea, back pain, weight increase, decreased libido, cervicitis/Papanicolaou smear normal/class II, hypertension, dyspareunia, anemia, alopecia, skin disorders including eczema, pruritus, rash and urticaria, abdominal distention, hirsutism and edema.

6.2 Postmarketing Experience

The following adverse reactions have been identified during post approval use of Mirena: device breakage and angioedema. Because these reactions are reported voluntarily from a population of uncertain size, it is not always possible to reliably estimate their frequency or establish a causal relationship to drug exposure.

7 DRUG INTERACTIONS

Drugs or herbal products that induce enzymes, including CYP3A4, that metabolize progestins may decrease the serum concentrations of progestins.

Some drugs or herbal products that may decrease the serum concentration of levonorgestrel include:

- barbiturates
- bosentan
- carbamazepine
- felbamate
- griseofulvin
- oxcarbazepine
- phenytoin
- rifampin
- St. John's wort
- topiramate.

Significant changes (increase or decrease) in the serum concentrations of the progestin have been noted in some cases of co-administration with HIV protease inhibitors or with non-nucleoside reverse transcriptase inhibitors. Consult the labeling of all concurrently used drugs to obtain further information about interactions with Mirena or the potential for enzyme alterations.

8 USE IN SPECIFIC POPULATIONS

8.1 Pregnancy

Many studies have found no harmful effects on fetal development associated with long-term use of contraceptive doses of oral progestins. The few studies of infant growth and development that have been conducted with progestin-only pills have not demonstrated significant adverse effects. *[Also see Contraindications (4), Warnings and Precautions (5.1 and 5.2).]*

8.3 Nursing Mothers

In general, no adverse effects have been found on breastfeeding performance or on the health, growth, or development of the infant. However, isolated postmarketing cases of decreased milk production have been reported. Small amounts of progestins pass into the breast milk of nursing mothers, resulting in detectable steroid levels in infant serum. *[Also, see Warnings and Precautions (5.7).]*

8.4 Pediatric Use

Safety and efficacy of Mirena have been established in women of reproductive age. Use of this product before menarche is not indicated.

8.5 Geriatric Use

Mirena has not been studied in women over age 65 and is not currently approved for use in this population.

8.6 Hepatic Impairment

No studies were conducted to evaluate the effect of hepatic disease on the disposition of levonorgestrel released from Mirena *[see Contraindications (4)]*.

8.7 Renal Impairment

No studies were conducted to evaluate the effect of renal disease on the disposition of levonorgestrel released from Mirena.

11 DESCRIPTION

Mirena is intended to provide an initial release rate of 20 mcg/day of levonorgestrel

Levonorgestrel USP, (-)-13-Ethyl-17-hydroxy-18,19-dinor-17α-pregn-4-en-20-yn-3-one, the active ingredient in Mirena, has a molecular weight of 312.4, a molecular formula of $C_{21}H_{28}O_2$, and the following structural formula:

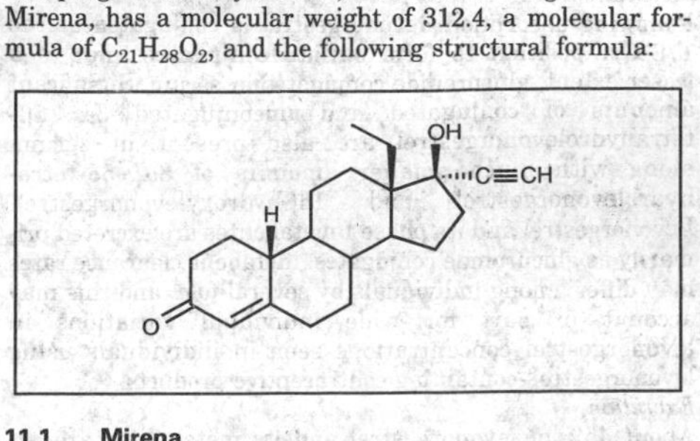

11.1 Mirena

Mirena (levonorgestrel-releasing intrauterine system) consists of a T-shaped polyethylene frame (T-body) with a steroid reservoir (hormone elastomer core) around the vertical stem. The reservoir consists of a white or almost white cylinder, made of a mixture of levonorgestrel and silicone (polydimethylsiloxane), containing a total of 52 mg levonorgestrel. The reservoir is covered by a semi-opaque silicone (polydimethylsiloxane) membrane. The T-body is 32 mm in both the horizontal and vertical directions. The polyethylene of the T-body is compounded with barium sulfate, which makes it radiopaque. A monofilament brown polyethylene removal thread is attached to a loop at the end of the vertical stem of the T-body.

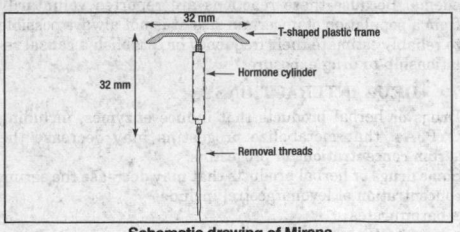

Schematic drawing of Mirena

11.2 Inserter

Mirena is packaged sterile within an inserter. The inserter, which is used for insertion of Mirena into the uterine cavity, consists of a symmetric two-sided body and slider that are integrated with flange, lock, pre-bent insertion tube and plunger. Once Mirena is in place, the inserter is discarded.

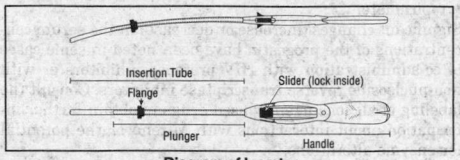

Diagram of Inserter

12 CLINICAL PHARMACOLOGY

12.1 Mechanism of Action

The local mechanism by which continuously released levonorgestrel enhances contraceptive effectiveness of Mirena has not been conclusively demonstrated. Studies of Mirena prototypes have suggested several mechanisms that prevent pregnancy: thickening of cervical mucus preventing passage of sperm into the uterus, inhibition of sperm capacitation or survival, and alteration of the endometrium.

12.2 Pharmacodynamics

Mirena has mainly local progestogenic effects in the uterine cavity. The high local levels of levonorgestrel[1] lead to morphological changes including stromal pseudodecidualization, glandular atrophy, a leukocytic infiltration and a decrease in glandular and stromal mitoses.
Ovulation is inhibited in some women using Mirena. In a 1-year study approximately 45% of menstrual cycles were ovulatory and in another study after 4 years 75% of cycles were ovulatory.

12.3 Pharmacokinetics

Absorption
Low doses of levonorgestrel are administered into the uterine cavity with the Mirena intrauterine delivery system. Initially, levonorgestrel is released at a rate of approximately 20 mcg/day. This rate decreases progressively to half that value after 5 years. A stable serum concentration, without peaks and troughs, of levonorgestrel of 150–200 pg/mL occurs after the first few weeks following insertion of Mirena. Levonorgestrel concentrations after long-term use of 12, 24, and 60 months were 180±66 pg/mL, 192±140 pg/mL, and 159±59 pg/mL, respectively.

Distribution
The apparent volume of distribution of levonorgestrel is reported to be approximately 1.8 L/kg. It is about 97.5 to 99% protein-bound, principally to sex hormone binding globulin (SHBG) and, to a lesser extent, serum albumin.

Metabolism
Following absorption, levonorgestrel is conjugated at the 17β-OH position to form sulfate conjugates and, to a lesser extent, glucuronide conjugates in serum. Significant amounts of conjugated and unconjugated 3α, 5β-tetrahydrolevonorgestrel are also present in serum, along with much smaller amounts of 3α, 5α-tetrahydrolevonorgestrel and 16βhydroxylevonorgestrel. Levonorgestrel and its phase I metabolites are excreted primarily as glucuronide conjugates. Metabolic clearance rates may differ among individuals by several-fold, and this may account in part for wide individual variations in levonorgestrel concentrations seen in individuals using levonorgestrel–containing contraceptive products.

Excretion
About 45% of levonorgestrel and its metabolites are excreted in the urine and about 32% are excreted in feces, mostly as glucuronide conjugates. The elimination half-life of levonorgestrel after daily oral doses is approximately 17 hours.

Specific Populations
Pediatric: Safety and efficacy of Mirena have been established in women of reproductive age. Use of this product before menarche is not indicated.
Geriatric: Mirena has not been studied in women over age 65 and is not currently approved for use in this population.

Race: No studies have evaluated the effect of race on pharmacokinetics of Mirena.
Hepatic Impairment: No studies were conducted to evaluate the effect of hepatic disease on the disposition of Mirena.
Renal Impairment: No formal studies were conducted to evaluate the effect of renal disease on the disposition of Mirena.

Drug-Drug Interactions
No drug-drug interaction studies were conducted with Mirena *[see Drug Interactions (7)]*.

13 NONCLINICAL TOXICOLOGY

13.1 Carcinogenesis, Mutagenesis, Impairment of Fertility

Carcinogenicity
Long-term studies in animals to assess the carcinogenic potential of levonorgestrel releasing intrauterine system have not been performed. There is no evidence of increased risk of cancer with short-term use of progestins. There was no increase in tumorigenicity following parenteral administration of levonorgestrel to rats for 2 years at approximately 5 mcg/day, or following oral administration to dogs for 7 years at up to 0.125 mg/kg/day, or to rhesus monkeys for 10 years at up to 250 mcg/kg/day. In another 7 year dog study, oral administration of levonorgestrel at 0.5 mg/kg/day did increase the number of mammary adenomas in treated dogs compared to controls. There were no malignancies. The nonclinical doses above are respectively 16, 200, 240 and 810 times the release rate of levonorgestrel by Mirena (20 mcg/day), based on body surface area *[see Warnings and Precautions (5.10)]*.

Mutagenicity
Levonorgestrel was not found to be genotoxic in the Ames assay, *in vitro* mammalian culture assays utilizing mouse lymphoma cells and Chinese hamster ovary cells, and in an *in vivo* micronucleus assay in mice.

Impairment of Fertility
There are no irreversible effects on fertility following cessation of exposures to levonorgestrel or progestins in general.

14 CLINICAL STUDIES

14.1 Clinical Trials on Intrauterine Contraception

Mirena has been studied for safety and efficacy in two large clinical trials in Finland and Sweden. In study sites having verifiable data and informed consent, 1,169 women 18 to 35 years of age at enrollment used Mirena for up to 5 years, for a total of 45,000 women-months of exposure. Subjects had previously been pregnant, had no history of ectopic pregnancy, had no history of pelvic inflammatory disease over the preceding 12 months, were predominantly Caucasian, and over 70% of the participants had previously used IUDs (intrauterine devices). The reported 12-month pregnancy rates were less than or equal to 0.2 per 100 women (0.2%) and the cumulative 5-year pregnancy rate was approximately 0.7 per 100 women (0.7%).
About 80% of women wishing to become pregnant conceived within 12 months after removal of Mirena.

14.2 Clinical Trial on Heavy Menstrual Bleeding

The efficacy of Mirena in the treatment of heavy menstrual bleeding was studied in a randomized, open-label, active-control, parallel-group trial comparing Mirena (n=79) to an approved therapy, medroxyprogesterone acetate (MPA) (n=81), over 6 cycles. The subjects included reproductive-aged women in good health, with no contraindications to the drug products and with confirmed heavy menstrual bleeding (≥ 80 mL menstrual blood loss [MBL]) determined using the alkaline hematin method. Excluded were women with organic or systemic conditions that may cause heavy uterine bleeding (except small fibroids, with total volume not > 5 mL). Treatment with Mirena showed a statistically significantly greater reduction in MBL *(see Figure 10)* and a statistically significantly greater number of subjects with successful treatment *(see Figure 11)*. Successful treatment was defined as proportion of subjects with (1) end-of-study MBL < 80 mL and (2) a ≥ 50% decrease in MBL from baseline to end-of-study.

Figure 10. Median Menstrual Blood Loss (MBL) by Time and Treatment

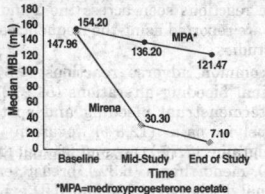

[See figure 11 at top of next column]

15 REFERENCES

[1] Nilsson CG, Haukkamaa M, Vierola H, Luukkainen T. Tissue Concentrations of Levonorgestrel in Women Using a Levonorgestrel-releasing IUD. Clinical Endocrinol 1982;17: 529-536.

Figure 11. Proportion of Subjects with Successful Treatment

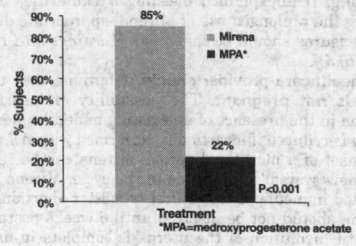

16 HOW SUPPLIED/STORAGE AND HANDLING

Mirena (levonorgestrel-releasing intrauterine system), containing a total of 52 mg levonorgestrel, is available in a carton of one sterile unit NDC# 50419-421-01. Each Mirena is packaged together with an inserter in a thermoformed blister package with a peelable lid.
Mirena is supplied sterile. Mirena is sterilized with ethylene oxide. Do not resterilize. For single use only. Do not use if the inner package is damaged or open. Insert before the end of the month shown on the label.
Store at 25°C (77°F); with excursions permitted between 15–30°C (59–86°F) *[see USP Controlled Room Temperature]*.

17 PATIENT COUNSELING INFORMATION

17.1 Information for Patients

• Patients should be counseled that this product does not protect against HIV infection (AIDS) and other sexually transmitted diseases (STDs).
• Prior to insertion, give the patient the Patient Information Booklet. She should be given the opportunity to read the information and discuss fully any questions she may have concerning Mirena as well as other methods of contraception and therapies for heavy menstrual bleeding. Also, advise the patient that the prescribing information is available to her upon request.
• Inform the patient that irregular or prolonged bleeding and spotting, and/or cramps may occur during the first few weeks after insertion. If her symptoms continue or are severe she should report them to her healthcare provider.
• Instruct the patient to contact her healthcare provider if she experiences any of the following:
  ◦ A stroke or heart attack
  ◦ Develops very severe or migraine headaches
  ◦ Unexplained fever
  ◦ Yellowing of the skin or whites of the eyes, as these may be signs of serious liver problems
  ◦ She thinks she is pregnant
  ◦ Pelvic pain or pain during sex
  ◦ She or her partner becomes HIV positive
  ◦ She might be exposed to sexually transmitted diseases (STDs)
  ◦ Unusual vaginal discharge or genital sores
  ◦ Severe vaginal bleeding or bleeding that lasts a long time, or if she misses a menstrual period
  ◦ Cannot feel Mirena's threads.
Instruct the patient on how to check after her menstrual period to make certain that the threads still protrude from the cervix and caution her not to pull on the threads and displace Mirena. Inform her that there is no contraceptive protection if Mirena is displaced or expelled.
FDA-Approved Patient Information
PATIENT INFORMATION
Mirena® (Mur-ā-nah)
(levonorgestrel-releasing intrauterine system)
Mirena does not protect against HIV infection (AIDS) and other sexually transmitted diseases (STDs).
Read this Patient Information carefully before you decide if Mirena is right for you. This information does not take the place of talking with your gynecologist or other healthcare provider who specializes in women's health. If you have any questions about Mirena, ask your healthcare provider. You should also learn about other birth control methods to choose the one that is best for you.
What is Mirena?
• Mirena is a hormone-releasing system placed in your uterus to prevent pregnancy for up to 5 years.
• Mirena can also lessen menstrual blood loss in women who have heavy menstrual flow and who also want to use a birth control method that is placed in the uterus to prevent pregnancy.
• Mirena is recommended for women who have had at least one child.
Mirena is T-shaped. It is made of flexible plastic and contains a progestin hormone called levonorgestrel that is often used in birth control pills. Mirena does not contain estrogen. Mirena releases the hormone into the uterus. Only small amounts of the hormone enter your blood.

Two threads are attached to the stem of Mirena. The threads are the only part of Mirena you can feel when Mirena is in your uterus.

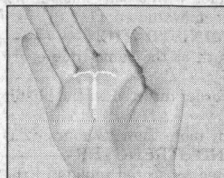 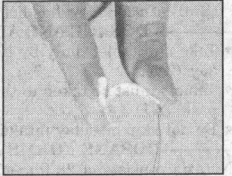

Mirena is small...　　　　and flexible

What if I need birth control for more than 5 years?
Mirena must be removed after 5 years. Your healthcare provider can insert a new Mirena during the same office visit if you choose to continue using Mirena.

What if I change my mind about birth control and want to become pregnant in less than 5 years?
Your healthcare provider can remove Mirena at any time. You may become pregnant as soon as Mirena is removed. About 8 out of 10 women who want to become pregnant will become pregnant some time in the first year after Mirena is removed.

How does Mirena work?
It is not known exactly how Mirena works. Mirena may work in several ways. It may thicken your cervical mucus, thin the lining of your uterus, inhibit sperm movement and reduce sperm survival. Mirena may stop release of your egg from your ovary, but this is not the way it works in most cases. Most likely, these actions work together to prevent pregnancy. Mirena can cause your menstrual bleeding to be less by thinning the lining of the uterus.

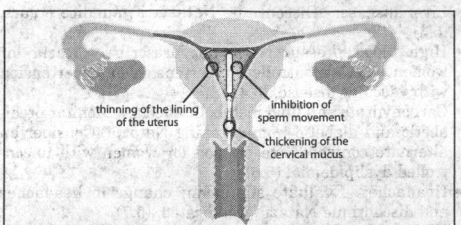

thinning of the lining of the uterus
inhibition of sperm movement
thickening of the cervical mucus

How well does Mirena work for contraception?
The following chart shows the chance of getting pregnant for women who use different methods of birth control. Each box on the chart contains a list of birth control methods that are similar in effectiveness. The most effective methods are in the box at the top of the chart. Mirena, an intrauterine device, is in the box at the top of the chart. The box on the bottom of the chart shows the chance of getting pregnant for women who do not use birth control and are trying to get pregnant.

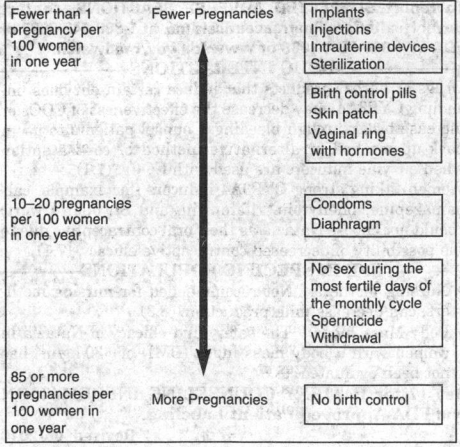

Fewer than 1 pregnancy per 100 women in one year	Fewer Pregnancies	Implants Injections Intrauterine devices Sterilization
		Birth control pills Skin patch Vaginal ring with hormones
10–20 pregnancies per 100 women in one year		Condoms Diaphragm
		No sex during the most fertile days of the monthly cycle Spermicide Withdrawal
85 or more pregnancies per 100 women in one year	More Pregnancies	No birth control

How well does Mirena work for heavy menstrual bleeding?
In the clinical trial performed in women with heavy menstrual bleeding and treated with Mirena, almost 9 out of 10 were treated successfully and their blood loss was reduced by more than half.

Who might use Mirena?
You might choose Mirena if you:
• Want birth control that provides a low chance of getting pregnant (less than 1 in 100)
• Want birth control that is reversible
• Want a birth control method that does not require taking it daily
• Have had at least one child

• Want treatment for heavy periods and want to use a birth control method that is placed in the uterus to prevent pregnancy.

Who should not use Mirena?
Do not use Mirena if you:
• Might be pregnant
• Have had a serious pelvic infection called pelvic inflammatory disease (PID) unless you have had a normal pregnancy after the infection went away
• Have an untreated pelvic infection now
• Have had a serious pelvic infection in the past 3 months after a pregnancy
• Can get infections easily. For example, if you have:
  ○ More than one sexual partner or your partner has more than one partner
  ○ Problems with your immune system
  ○ Intravenous drug abuse.
• Have or suspect you might have cancer of the uterus or cervix
• Have bleeding from the vagina that has not been explained
• Have liver disease or liver tumor
• Have breast cancer now or in the past or suspect you have breast cancer
• Have an intrauterine device in your uterus already
• Have a condition of the uterus that changes the shape of the uterine cavity, such as large fibroid tumors
• Are allergic to levonorgestrel, silicone, or polyethylene.

Before having Mirena placed, tell your healthcare provider if you:
• Have had a heart attack
• Have had a stroke
• Were born with heart disease or have problems with your heart valves
• Have problems with blood clotting or take medicine to reduce clotting
• Have high blood pressure
• Recently had a baby or if you are breast feeding
• Have diabetes (high blood sugar)
• Use corticosteroid medications on a long-term basis
• Have severe migraine headaches.

How is Mirena placed?
First, your healthcare provider will examine your pelvis to find the exact position of your uterus. Your healthcare provider will then clean your vagina and cervix with an antiseptic solution, and slide a thin plastic tube containing Mirena into your uterus. Your healthcare provider will then remove the plastic tube, and leave Mirena in your uterus. Your healthcare provider will cut the threads to the right length. Placement takes only a few minutes during an office visit.

You may experience pain, bleeding or dizziness during and after placement. If these symptoms do not pass 30 minutes after placement, Mirena may not have been placed correctly. Your healthcare provider will examine you to see if Mirena needs to be removed or replaced.

Should I check that Mirena is in the proper position?
Yes, you should check that Mirena is in proper position by feeling the removal threads. You should do this after each menstrual period. First, wash your hands with soap and water. Feel for the threads at the top of your vagina with your clean fingers. The threads are the only part of Mirena you should feel when Mirena is in your uterus. Be careful not to pull on the threads. If you feel more than just the threads, Mirena is not in the right position and may not prevent pregnancy. Call your healthcare provider to have it removed. If you cannot feel the threads at all, ask your healthcare provider to check that Mirena is still in the right place. In either case, use a non-hormonal birth control method (such as condoms or spermicide) until otherwise advised by your healthcare provider.

How soon after placement of Mirena should I return to my healthcare provider?
Call your healthcare provider if you have any questions or concerns (see "When should I call my healthcare provider"). Otherwise, you should return to your healthcare provider for a follow-up visit 4 to 12 weeks after Mirena is placed to make sure that Mirena is in the right position.

Can I use tampons with Mirena?
Tampons may be used with Mirena.

What if I become pregnant while using Mirena?
Call your healthcare provider right away if you think you are pregnant. If you get pregnant while using Mirena, you may have an ectopic pregnancy. This means that the pregnancy is not in the uterus. Unusual vaginal bleeding or abdominal pain may be a sign of ectopic pregnancy.

Ectopic pregnancy is a medical emergency that often requires surgery.

Ectopic pregnancy can cause internal bleeding, infertility, and even death.

There are also risks if you get pregnant while using Mirena and the pregnancy is in the uterus. Severe infection, miscarriage, premature delivery, and even death can occur with pregnancies that continue with an intrauterine device

(IUD). Because of this, your healthcare provider may try to remove Mirena, even though removing it may cause a miscarriage. If Mirena cannot be removed, talk with your healthcare provider about the benefits and risks of continuing the pregnancy.

If you continue your pregnancy, see your healthcare provider regularly. Call your healthcare provider right away if you get flu-like symptoms, fever, chills, cramping, pain, bleeding, vaginal discharge, or fluid leaking from your vagina. These may be signs of infection.

It is not known if Mirena can cause long-term effects on the fetus if it stays in place during a pregnancy.

How will Mirena change my periods?
For the first 3 to 6 months, your monthly period may become irregular and the number of bleeding days may increase at first. You may also have frequent spotting or light bleeding. A few women have heavy bleeding during this time. After your body adjusts, the number of bleeding days is likely to lessen, and you may even find that your periods stop altogether. In some women with heavy bleeding, the total blood loss per cycle progressively decreases with continued use. The number of spotting and bleeding days may initially increase but then typically decreases in the months that follow.

Is it safe to breast-feed while using Mirena?
You may use Mirena when you are breastfeeding if more than six weeks have passed since you had your baby. If you are breastfeeding, Mirena is not likely to affect the quality or amount of your breast milk or the health of your nursing baby. However, isolated cases of decreased milk production have been reported among women using progestin-only birth control pills.

Will Mirena interfere with sexual intercourse?
You and your partner should not feel Mirena during intercourse. Mirena is placed in the uterus, not in the vagina. Sometimes male partners feel the threads.

What are the possible side effects of using Mirena?
Mirena can cause serious side effects including:
• *Pelvic inflammatory disease (PID)*. Some IUD users get a serious pelvic infection called pelvic inflammatory disease. PID is usually sexually transmitted. You have a higher chance of getting PID if you or your partner have sex with other partners. PID can cause serious problems such as infertility, ectopic pregnancy or pelvic pain that does not go away. PID is usually treated with antibiotics. More serious cases of PID may require surgery. A hysterectomy (removal of the uterus) is sometimes needed. In rare cases, infections that start as PID can even cause death.
• Tell your healthcare provider right away if you have any of these signs of PID: long-lasting or heavy bleeding, unusual vaginal discharge, low abdominal (stomach area) pain, painful sex, chills, or fever.
• *Life-threatening infection*. Life-threatening infection can occur within the first few days after Mirena is placed. Call your healthcare provider if you develop severe pain within a few hours after Mirena is placed.
• *Embedment*. Mirena may become attached to the uterine wall. This is called embedment. If embedment happens, Mirena may no longer prevent pregnancy and you may need surgery to have it removed.
• *Perforation*. Mirena may go through the uterus. This is called perforation. If your uterus is perforated, Mirena may no longer prevent pregnancy. It may move outside the uterus and can cause internal scarring, infection, or damage to other organs, and you may need surgery to have Mirena removed.

Common side effects of Mirena include:
• Pain, bleeding or dizziness during and after placement. If these symptoms do not stop 30 minutes after placement, Mirena may not have been placed correctly. Your healthcare provider will examine you to see if Mirena needs to be removed or replaced.
• *Expulsion*. Mirena may come out by itself. This is called expulsion. You may become pregnant if Mirena comes out. If you notice that Mirena has come out, use a backup birth control method like condoms and call your healthcare provider.
• *Missed menstrual periods*. About 2 out of 10 women stop having periods after 1 year of Mirena use. If you do not have a period for 6 weeks during Mirena use, call your healthcare provider. When Mirena is removed, your menstrual periods will come back.
• *Changes in bleeding*. You may have bleeding and spotting between menstrual periods, especially during the first 3 to 6 months. Sometimes the bleeding is heavier than usual at first. However, the bleeding usually becomes lighter than usual and may be irregular. Call your healthcare provider if the bleeding remains heavier than usual or if the bleeding becomes heavy after it has been light for a while.
• *Cyst on the ovary*. About 12 out of 100 women using Mirena develop a cyst on the ovary. These cysts usually

disappear on their own in a month or two. However, cysts can cause pain and sometimes cysts will need surgery.

This is not a complete list of possible side effects with Mirena. For more information, ask your healthcare provider.

Call your doctor for medical advice about side effects. You may report side effects to the manufacturer at 1-888-842-2937, or FDA at 1-800-FDA-1088 or www.fda.gov/medwatch.

After Mirena has been placed, when should I call my healthcare provider?

Call your healthcare provider if you have any concerns about Mirena. Be sure to call if you:

• Think you are pregnant.
• Have pelvic pain or pain during sex.
• Have unusual vaginal discharge or genital sores.
• Have unexplained fever.
• Might be exposed to sexually transmitted diseases (STDs).
• Cannot feel Mirena's threads.
• Develop very severe or migraine headaches.
• Have yellowing of the skin or whites of the eyes. These may be signs of liver problems.
• Have a stroke or heart attack.
• Or your partner becomes HIV positive.
• Have severe vaginal bleeding or bleeding that lasts a long time.

General advice about prescription medicines

Medicines are sometimes prescribed for conditions that are not mentioned in patient information leaflets. This leaflet summarizes the most important information about Mirena. If you would like more information, talk with your healthcare provider. You can ask your healthcare provider for information about Mirena that is written for health providers.

© 2009, Bayer HealthCare Pharmaceuticals Inc. All rights reserved.

Manufactured for:
Bayer HealthCare Pharmaceuticals Inc.
Wayne, NJ 07470

This patient information booklet was updated October 2009.

Fill out the following checklist. Your answers will help you and your healthcare provider decide if Mirena is a good choice for you.

Do you have any of these conditions?

	Yes	No	Don't know—will discuss with my healthcare provider
Abnormalities of the uterus	☐	☐	☐
Acquired immune deficiency syndrome (AIDS)	☐	☐	☐
Anemia or blood clotting problems	☐	☐	☐
Bleeding between periods	☐	☐	☐
Cancer of the uterus or cervix	☐	☐	☐
History of other types of cancer	☐	☐	☐
Steroid therapy (for example, prednisone)	☐	☐	☐
Possible pregnancy	☐	☐	☐
Diabetes	☐	☐	☐
Ectopic pregnancy in the past	☐	☐	☐
Fainting attacks	☐	☐	☐
Genital sores	☐	☐	☐
Heart disease	☐	☐	☐
Heart murmur	☐	☐	☐
Heavy menstrual flow	☐	☐	☐
Hepatitis or other liver disease	☐	☐	☐
Infection of the uterus or cervix	☐	☐	☐
IUD in place now or in the past	☐	☐	☐
IV drug abuse now or in the past	☐	☐	☐
Leukemia	☐	☐	☐
More than one sexual partner	☐	☐	☐
A sexual partner who has more than one sexual partner	☐	☐	☐
Pelvic infection	☐	☐	☐
Abortion or miscarriage in the past 2 months	☐	☐	☐
Pregnancy in the past 2 months	☐	☐	☐
Severe menstrual cramps	☐	☐	☐
Severe Headache	☐	☐	☐
Sexually transmitted disease (STD), such as gonorrhea or chlamydia	☐	☐	☐
Stroke	☐	☐	☐
Abnormal Pap smear	☐	☐	☐
Unexplained genital bleeding	☐	☐	☐
Uterine or pelvic surgery	☐	☐	☐
Vaginal discharge or infection	☐	☐	☐
HIV infection	☐	☐	☐
Breastfeeding	☐	☐	☐
High blood pressure	☐	☐	☐

Manufactured for:
Bayer HealthCare Pharmaceuticals Inc.
Wayne, NJ 07470
Manufactured in Finland
Bayer HealthCare Pharmaceuticals Mirena Hotline - 1-866-647-3646
© 2009, Bayer HealthCare Pharmaceuticals Inc.
All rights reserved.
October 2009
Bayer HealthCare Pharmaceuticals Inc.
6705104 82174630
Shown in Product Identification Guide, page 307

NATAZIA
[na-ta-zi-a]
(estradiol valerate and estradiol valerate/dienogest)
Tablets for Oral Use   ℞

HIGHLIGHTS OF PRESCRIBING INFORMATION

These highlights do not include all the information needed to use Natazia safely and effectively. See full prescribing information for Natazia.

Natazia (estradiol valerate and estradiol valerate/ dienogest) tablets for oral use
Initial U.S. Approval: 2010

WARNING: CIGARETTE SMOKING AND SERIOUS CARDIOVASCULAR EVENTS

See full prescribing information for complete boxed warning.

• Women who are over 35 years old and smoke should not use Natazia.
• Cigarette smoking increases the risk of serious cardiovascular events from combination oral contraceptive (COC) use.

——————INDICATIONS AND USAGE——————
• Natazia is an estrogen/progestin COC indicated for use by women to prevent pregnancy. (1)
• The efficacy of Natazia in women with a body mass index (BMI) of >30 kg/m² has not been evaluated. (1, 8.8)

————DOSAGE AND ADMINISTRATION————
• Take one tablet daily by mouth at the same time every day. (2.1)
• Tablets must be taken in the order directed on the blister pack. (2.1)
• Do not skip or delay intake by more than 12 hours. (2.1)

————DOSAGE FORMS AND STRENGTHS————
Natazia consists of 28 film-coated, unscored tablets in the following order:
• 2 dark yellow tablets each containing 3 mg estradiol valerate
• 5 medium red tablets each containing 2 mg estradiol valerate and 2 mg dienogest
• 17 light yellow tablets each containing 2 mg estradiol valerate and 3 mg dienogest
• 2 dark red tablets each containing 1 mg estradiol valerate
• 2 white tablets (inert) (3)

——————CONTRAINDICATIONS——————
• A high risk of arterial or venous thrombotic diseases (4)
• Undiagnosed abnormal genital bleeding (4)
• Breast cancer or other estrogen- or progestin-sensitive cancer (4)
• Liver tumors or liver disease (4)
• Pregnancy (4)

————WARNINGS AND PRECAUTIONS————
• Vascular risks: Stop Natazia if a thrombotic event occurs. Stop Natazia at least 4 weeks before and through 2 weeks after major surgery. Start Natazia no earlier than 4 weeks after delivery, in women who are not breastfeeding. (5.1)
• Liver disease: Discontinue Natazia if jaundice occurs. (5.3)
• High blood pressure: Do not prescribe Natazia for women with uncontrolled hypertension or hypertension with vascular disease. (5.4)
• Carbohydrate and lipid metabolic effects: Monitor prediabetic and diabetic women taking Natazia. Consider an alternate contraceptive method for women with uncontrolled dyslipidemia. (5.6)
• Headache: Evaluate significant change in headaches and discontinue Natazia if indicated. (5.7)
• Uterine bleeding: Evaluate irregular bleeding or amenorrhea. (5.8)
• CYP3A4 induction: Women taking strong CYP3A4 inducers (for example, carbamazepine, phenytoin, rifampicin, and St. John's wort) should not choose Natazia as their oral contraceptive due to the possibility of decreased contraceptive efficacy. (5.13)

——————ADVERSE REACTIONS——————
The most common adverse reactions (≥2%) in clinical trials for Natazia are headaches, irregular uterine bleeding, breast tenderness, nausea/vomiting, acne and increased weight. (6)

To report SUSPECTED ADVERSE REACTIONS, contact Bayer HealthCare Pharmaceuticals Inc. at 1-888-842-2937 or FDA at 1-800-FDA-1088 or www.fda.gov/medwatch.

——————DRUG INTERACTIONS——————
Drugs or herbal products that induce certain enzymes, including CYP3A4, may decrease the effectiveness of COCs or increase breakthrough bleeding. Counsel patients to use a back-up method or alternative method of contraception when enzyme inducers are used with COCs. (7.1)
Women taking strong CYP3A4 inducers (for example, carbamazepine, phenytoin, rifampicin, and St. John's wort) should not choose Natazia as their oral contraceptive due to the possibility of decreased contraceptive efficacy. (7.1)

————USE IN SPECIFIC POPULATIONS————
• Nursing mothers: Not recommended for nursing mothers; can decrease milk production. (8.3)
• Body Mass Index: The safety and efficacy of Natazia in women with a body mass index (BMI) of >30 kg/m² has not been evaluated. (8.8)

See 17 for PATIENT COUNSELING INFORMATION and FDA-Approved Patient Labeling.

Revised: 05/2010

*Sections or subsections omitted from the full prescribing information are not listed

---

FULL PRESCRIBING INFORMATION

> **WARNING: CIGARETTE SMOKING AND SERIOUS CARDIOVASCULAR EVENTS**
> **Cigarette smoking increases the risk of serious cardiovascular events from combination oral contraceptive (COC) use. This risk increases with age, particularly in women over 35 years of age, and with the number of cigarettes smoked. For this reason, COCs should not be used by women who are over 35 years of age and smoke. [See Contraindications (4).]**

1 INDICATIONS AND USAGE

Natazia™ is indicated for use by women to prevent pregnancy.
The efficacy of Natazia in women with a body mass index (BMI) of > 30 kg/m² has not been evaluated.

2 DOSAGE AND ADMINISTRATION

2.1 How to take Natazia

To achieve maximum contraceptive effectiveness, Natazia must be taken exactly as directed. Take one tablet by mouth the same time every day. Tablets must be taken in the order directed on the blister pack. Tablets should not be skipped or intake delayed by more than 12 hours. For patient instructions for missed pills, see FDA-Approved Patient Labeling.

2.2 How to start Natazia

Instruct the patient to begin taking Natazia on Day 1 of her menstrual cycle (that is, the first day of her menstrual bleeding) [see FDA-Approved Patient Labeling]. Instruct the patient to use a non-hormonal contraceptive as back-up during the first 9 days.
For postpartum women who do not breastfeed or after a second trimester abortion, Natazia may be started no earlier than 4 weeks postpartum. Recommend use of a non-hormonal back-up method for the first 9 days. When combined oral contraceptives (COCs) are used during the postpartum period, the increased risk of thromboembolic disease associated with the postpartum period must be considered. The possibility of ovulation and conception before starting COCs should also be considered.
If the patient is switching from a combination hormonal method such as:

- Another pill
- Vaginal ring
- Patch

- Instruct her to take the first dark yellow pill on the first day of her withdrawal bleed. She should not continue taking the pills from her previous birth control pack. If she does not have a withdrawal bleed, rule out pregnancy before starting Natazia.
- If she previously used a vaginal ring or transdermal patch, she should start using Natazia on the day the ring or patch is removed.
- Instruct the patient to use a non-hormonal back-up method such as a condom or spermicide for the first 9 days.

If the patient is switching from a progestin-only method such as a:

- Progestin-only pill
- Implant
- Intrauterine system
- Injection

- Instruct her to take the first dark yellow pill on the day she would have taken her next progestin-only pill or on the day of removal of her implant or intrauterine system or on the day when she would have had her next injection.
- Instruct the patient to use a non-hormonal back-up method such as a condom or spermicide for the first 9 days.

2.3 Advice in case of Gastrointestinal Disturbances

In case of severe vomiting or diarrhea, absorption may not be complete and additional contraceptive measures should be taken. If vomiting or diarrhea occurs within 3-4 hours after taking a colored tablet, this can be regarded as a missed tablet. [See FDA-Approved Patient Labeling.]

3 DOSAGE FORMS AND STRENGTHS

Natazia (estradiol valerate and estradiol valerate/dienogest) tablets are available in blister packs.
Each blister pack (28 film-coated tablets) contains in the following order:

- 2 dark yellow tablets each containing 3 mg estradiol valerate
- 5 medium red tablets each containing 2 mg estradiol valerate and 2 mg dienogest
- 17 light yellow tablets each containing 2 mg estradiol valerate and 3 mg dienogest
- 2 dark red tablets each containing 1 mg estradiol valerate
- 2 white tablets (inert)

4 CONTRAINDICATIONS

Do not prescribe Natazia to women who are known to have the following:

- A high risk of arterial or venous thrombotic diseases. Examples include women who are known to:
  - Smoke, if over age 35 [see Boxed Warning and Warnings and Precautions (5.1)]
  - Have deep vein thrombosis or pulmonary embolism, now or in the past [see Warnings and Precautions (5.1)]
  - Have cerebrovascular disease [see Warnings and Precautions (5.1)]
  - Have coronary artery disease [see Warnings and Precautions (5.1)]
  - Have thrombogenic valvular or thrombogenic rhythm diseases of the heart (for example, subacute bacterial endocarditis with valvular disease, or atrial fibrillation) [see Warnings and Precautions (5.1)]
  - Have inherited or acquired hypercoagulopathies [see Warnings and Precautions (5.1)]
  - Have uncontrolled hypertension [see Warnings and Precautions (5.4)]
  - Have diabetes with vascular disease [see Warnings and Precautions (5.6)]
  - Have headaches with focal neurological symptoms or have migraine headaches with or without aura if over age 35 [see Warnings and Precautions (5.7)]
- Undiagnosed abnormal genital bleeding [see Warnings and Precautions (5.8)]
- Breast cancer or other estrogen- or progestin-sensitive cancer, now or in the past [see Warnings and Precautions (5.2)]
- Liver tumors, benign or malignant, or liver disease [see Warnings and Precautions (5.3), Use in Specific Populations (8.7) and Clinical Pharmacology (12.3)].
- Pregnancy, because there is no reason to use COCs during pregnancy [see Warnings and Precautions (5.9) and Use in Specific Populations (8.1)].

5 WARNINGS AND PRECAUTIONS

5.1 Thrombotic and Other Vascular Events

Stop COCs if an arterial or deep venous thrombotic (VTE) event occurs. Although the use of COCs increases the risk of venous thromboembolism, pregnancy increases the risk of venous thromboembolism as much or more than the use of COCs. The risk of venous thromboembolism in women using COCs is 3 to 9 per 10,000 woman-years. The excess risk is highest during the first year of use of a COC. Use of COCs also increases the risk of arterial thromboses such as strokes and myocardial infarctions, especially in women with other risk factors for these events. The risk of thromboembolic disease due to oral contraceptives gradually disappears after COC use is discontinued.
If feasible, stop COCs at least 4 weeks before and through 2 weeks after major surgery or other surgeries known to have an elevated risk of thromboembolism.
Start COCs no earlier than 4 weeks after delivery, in women who are not breastfeeding. The risk of postpartum thromboembolism decreases after the third postpartum week, whereas the risk of ovulation increases after the third postpartum week.
COCs have been shown to increase both the relative and attributable risks of cerebrovascular events (thrombotic and hemorrhagic strokes), although, in general, the risk is greatest among older (>35 years of age), hypertensive women who also smoke. COCs also increase the risk for stroke in women with other underlying risk factors.
Oral contraceptives must be used with caution in women with cardiovascular disease risk factors. Stop COCs if there is unexplained loss of vision, proptosis, diplopia, papilledema, or retinal vascular lesions. Evaluate for retinal vein thrombosis immediately. [See Adverse Reactions (6).]

5.2 Carcinoma of the Breasts and Reproductive Organs

Women who currently have or have had breast cancer should not use COCs because breast cancer is a hormonally-sensitive tumor.
There is substantial evidence that COCs do not increase the incidence of breast cancer. Although some past studies have suggested that COCs might increase the incidence of breast cancer, more recent studies have not confirmed such findings.
Some studies suggest that COCs are associated with an increase in the risk of cervical cancer or intraepithelial neoplasia. However, there is controversy about the extent to which these findings may be due to differences in sexual behavior and other factors.
Endometrial biopsies performed in a subset of subjects in a Phase 3 Natazia clinical trial did not reveal any unexpected or concerning findings for subjects taking COCs. [See Adverse Reactions (6.1).]

5.3 Liver Disease

Discontinue COCs if jaundice develops. Steroid hormones may be poorly metabolized in patients with impaired liver function. Acute or chronic disturbances of liver function may necessitate the discontinuation of COC use until markers of liver function return to normal and COC causation has been excluded.
Hepatic adenomas are associated with COC use. An estimate of the attributable risk is 3.3 cases/100,000 COC users. Rupture of hepatic adenomas may cause death through intra-abdominal hemorrhage.
Studies have shown an increased risk of developing hepatocellular carcinoma in long-term (> 8 years) COC users. However, the attributable risk of liver cancers in COC users is less than one case per million users. Oral contraceptive-related cholestasis may occur in women with a history of pregnancy-related cholestasis. Women with a history of COC-related cholestasis may have the condition recur with subsequent COC use.

5.4 High Blood Pressure

For women with well-controlled hypertension, monitor blood pressure and stop COCs if blood pressure rises significantly. Women with uncontrolled hypertension or hypertension with vascular disease should not use COCs. An increase in blood pressure has been reported in women taking COCs, and this increase is more likely in older women and with extended duration of use. The incidence of hypertension increases with increasing concentration of progestin.

5.5 Gallbladder Disease

Studies suggest a small increased relative risk of developing gallbladder disease among COC users.

5.6 Carbohydrate and Lipid Metabolic Effects

Carefully monitor prediabetic and diabetic women who are taking COCs. COCs may decrease glucose tolerance in a dose-related fashion.
Consider alternative contraception for women with uncontrolled dyslipidemia. A small proportion of women will have adverse lipid changes while on COCs.
Women with hypertriglyceridemia, or a family history thereof, may be at an increased risk of pancreatitis when using COCs.

5.7 Headache

If a woman taking COCs develops new headaches that are recurrent, persistent, or severe, evaluate the cause and discontinue COCs if indicated.
An increase in frequency or severity of migraine during COC use (which may be prodromal of a cerebrovascular event) may be a reason for immediate discontinuation of the COC. [See Adverse Reactions (6).]

5.8 Bleeding Irregularities

Breakthrough bleeding and spotting sometimes occur in patients on COCs, especially during the first three months of use. If bleeding persists or occurs after previously regular cycles, check for causes such as pregnancy or malignancy. If pathology and pregnancy are excluded, bleeding irregularities may resolve over time or with a change to a different COC.

Women who are not pregnant and use Natazia, may experience amenorrhea. Based on patient diaries, amenorrhea occurs in approximately 16% of cycles in women using Natazia. Pregnancy should be ruled out in the event of amenorrhea occurring in two or more consecutive cycles. Some women may encounter amenorrhea or oligomenorrhea after stopping COCs, especially when such a condition was pre-existent.

Based on patient diaries from three clinical trials evaluating the safety and efficacy of Natazia, 10-23% of women experienced intracyclic bleeding per cycle. A total of 38 subjects out of 2,266 (1.7%) discontinued due to metrorrhagia or irregular menstruation.

5.9 COC Use Before or During Early Pregnancy

Extensive epidemiological studies have revealed no increased risk of birth defects in women who have used oral contraceptives prior to pregnancy. Studies also do not suggest a teratogenic effect, particularly in so far as cardiac anomalies and limb-reduction defects are concerned, when taken inadvertently during early pregnancy. Oral contraceptive use should be discontinued if pregnancy is confirmed.

The administration of oral contraceptives to induce withdrawal bleeding should not be used as a test for pregnancy *[see Use in Specific Populations (8.1)]*.

5.10 Emotional Disorders

Women with a history of depression should be carefully observed and the COC discontinued if depression recurs to a serious degree.

5.11 Interference with Laboratory Tests

The use of COCs may change the results of some laboratory tests, such as coagulation factors, lipids, glucose tolerance, and binding proteins. Women on thyroid hormone replacement therapy may need increased doses of thyroid hormone because serum concentrations of thyroid-binding globulin increase with use of COCs.

5.12 Monitoring

A woman who is taking COCs should have a yearly visit with her healthcare provider for a blood pressure check and for other indicated healthcare.

5.13 Drug Interactions

Women who take medications that are strong CYP3A4 inducers (for example, carbamazepine, phenytoin, rifampicin, and St. John's wort) should not choose Natazia as their oral contraceptive while using these inducers and for at least 28 days after discontinuation of these inducers due to the possibility of decreased contraceptive efficacy. *[See Drug Interactions (7.1) and Clinical Pharmacology (12.3).]*

5.14 Other Conditions

In women with hereditary angioedema, exogenous estrogens may induce or exacerbate symptoms of angioedema. Chloasma may occasionally occur, especially in women with a history of chloasma gravidarum. Women with a tendency to chloasma should avoid exposure to the sun or ultraviolet radiation while taking COCs.

6 ADVERSE REACTIONS

The following serious adverse reactions with the use of COCs are discussed elsewhere in the labeling:

- Serious cardiovascular events and smoking *[see Boxed Warning and Warnings and Precautions (5.1)]*
- Vascular events *[see Warnings and Precautions (5.1)]*
- Liver disease *[see Warnings and Precautions (5.3)]*

Adverse reactions commonly reported by COC users are:

- Irregular uterine bleeding
- Nausea
- Breast tenderness
- Headache

6.1 Clinical Trials Experience

Because clinical trials are conducted under widely varying conditions, adverse reaction rates observed in the clinical trials of a drug cannot be directly compared to rates in the clinical trials of another drug and may not reflect the rates observed in practice.

Contraception Studies

Two multicenter phase 3 clinical trials evaluated the safety and efficacy of Natazia for pregnancy prevention. Both were non-comparative, open-labeled, single-arm studies with a treatment duration up to 28 cycles. A total of 1,867 women aged 18–50 were enrolled and took at least one dose of Natazia. *[See Clinical Studies (14.1).]*

Adverse Reactions Leading to Study Discontinuation: 11.5% of the women discontinued from the clinical trials due to an adverse reaction; the most frequent adverse reactions leading to discontinuation were metrorrhagia and irregular menstruation (1.9%), acne (1.2%), headache and migraine (1.0%), and weight increase (0.7%).

Common Treatment-Emergent Adverse Reactions (≥ 2%): headache (including migraines) (13.2%), metrorrhagia and irregular menstruation (8.0%), breast pain, discomfort or tenderness (6.6%), nausea or vomiting (6.5%), acne (3.9%) and increased weight (2.8%).

Serious Adverse Reactions: deep vein thrombosis, myocardial infarction, focal nodular hyperplasia of the liver, uterine leiomyoma, and ruptured ovarian cyst.

7 DRUG INTERACTIONS

7.1 Effects of Other Drugs on Combined Hormonal Contraceptives

Interactions between oral contraceptives and other drugs may lead to breakthrough bleeding and/or contraceptive failure. The following interactions have been reported in the literature for COCs in general or were studied in clinical trials with Natazia.

CYP3A4 Inducers: Drugs or herbal products that induce certain enzymes, including CYP3A4, may decrease the effectiveness of COCs or increase breakthrough bleeding. Some drugs or herbal products that may decrease the effectiveness of hormonal contraceptives include barbiturates, bosentan, felbamate, griseofulvin, oxcarbazepine, and topiramate. Counsel women to use an alternative method of contraception or a back-up method when moderate or weak enzyme inducers are used with COCs, and to continue back-up contraception for 28 days after discontinuing the enzyme inducer to ensure contraceptive reliability.

Dienogest is a substrate of cytochrome P450 (CYP) 3A4. Women who take medications that are strong CYP3A4 inducers (for example, carbamazepine, phenytoin, rifampicin, and St. John's wort) should not choose Natazia as their oral contraceptive while using these inducers and for at least 28 days after discontinuation of these inducers due to the possibility of decreased contraceptive efficacy.

The effect of the CYP3A4 inducer rifampicin was studied in healthy postmenopausal women. Co-administration of rifampicin with estradiol valerate/dienogest tablets led to a 52% and 83% decrease in the mean C_{max} and AUC(0–24hr), respectively, for dienogest and a 25% and 44% decrease in C_{max} and AUC(0–24hr), respectively, for estradiol at steady state.

Strong CYP3A4 Inhibitors: Strong CYP3A4 inhibitors such as ketoconazole increased hormone serum concentrations. In a study investigating the effect of ketoconazole on dienogest and estradiol pharmacokinetics, co-administration with the strong CYP3A4 inhibitor ketoconazole resulted in a 186% increase of AUC (0–24hr) at steady state for dienogest and a 57% increase for estradiol. There was also a 94% and 65% increase of C_{max} at steady state for dienogest and estradiol when co-administered with ketoconazole.

Moderate CYP3A4 Inhibitors: The AUC (0–24hr) of dienogest and estradiol at steady state were increased by 62% and 33%, respectively, when co-administered with a moderate CYP3A4 inhibitor, erythromycin. There was also a 33% and 51% increase of Cmax at steady state for dienogest and estradiol, respectively, when co-administered with erythromycin.

Other known CYP.3A4 inhibitors like azole antifungals, cimetidine, verapamil, macrolides, diltiazem, antidepressants, and grapefruit juice may increase plasma levels of dienogest.

HIV Protease Inhibitors: Significant changes (increase or decrease) in the plasma levels of estrogen and progestin have been noted in some cases of co-administration of HIV protease inhibitors.

Antibiotics: There have been reports of pregnancy while taking hormonal contraceptives and antibiotics, but clinical pharmacokinetic studies have not shown consistent effects of antibiotics on plasma concentrations of synthetic steroids.

Consult the labeling of all concurrently-used drugs to obtain further information about interactions with hormonal contraceptives or the potential for enzyme alterations.

7.2 Effects of Combined Hormonal Contraceptives on Other Drugs

COCs containing ethinyl estradiol (or mestranol), may inhibit the metabolism of other compounds. COCs have been shown to significantly decrease plasma concentrations of lamotrigine, likely due to induction of lamotrigine glucuronidation. This may reduce seizure control; therefore, dosage adjustments of lamotrigine may be necessary. Consult the labeling of the concurrently-used drug to obtain further information about interactions with COCs or the potential for enzyme alterations.

In vitro studies with human CYP enzymes did not indicate an inhibitory potential of dienogest at clinically relevant concentrations.

8 USE IN SPECIFIC POPULATIONS

8.1 Pregnancy

Pregnancy category X. *[See Contraindications (4) and Warnings and Precautions (5.9).]*

8.3 Nursing Mothers

When possible, advise the nursing mother to use other forms of contraception until she has weaned her child. Estrogen-containing OCs can reduce milk production in breastfeeding mothers. This is less likely to occur once breastfeeding is well-established; however, it can occur at any time in some women. Small amounts of oral contraceptive steroids and/or metabolites are present in breast milk.

8.4 Pediatric Use

Safety and efficacy of Natazia have been established in women of reproductive age. Efficacy is expected to be the same for postpubertal adolescents under the age of 18 as for users 18 years and older. Use of this product before menarche is not indicated. *[See Clinical Pharmacology (12.3).]*

8.5 Geriatric Use

Natazia has not been studied in postmenopausal women and is not indicated in this population. *[See Clinical Pharmacology (12.3).]*

8.6 Renal Impairment

The pharmacokinetics of Natazia has not been studied in subjects with renal impairment, but an effect requiring dose adjustment is unlikely to be present *[See Clinical Pharmacology (12.3)]*.

8.7 Hepatic Impairment

The pharmacokinetics of Natazia has not been studied in subjects with hepatic impairment. Steroid hormones may be poorly metabolized in patients with impaired liver function. Acute or chronic disturbances of liver function may necessitate the discontinuation of COC use until markers of liver function return to normal. *[See Contraindications (4), Warnings and Precautions (5.3) and Clinical Pharmacology (12.3)]*

8.8 Body Mass Index

The safety and efficacy of Natazia in women with a BMI of > 30 kg/m^2 has not been evaluated. *[See Clinical Pharmacology (12.3).]*

10 OVERDOSAGE

There have been no reports of serious ill effects from overdose of oral contraceptives, including ingestion by children. Overdosage may cause nausea, and withdrawal bleeding may occur in females.

11 DESCRIPTION

Natazia (estradiol valerate and estradiol valerate/dienogest) tablets provide an oral contraceptive regimen consisting of 26 active film-coated tablets that contain the active ingredients specified for each tablet below, followed by two inert tablets:

- 2 dark yellow tablets each containing 3 mg estradiol valerate
- 5 medium red tablets each containing 2 mg estradiol valerate and 2 mg dienogest
- 17 light yellow tablets each containing 2 mg estradiol valerate and 3 mg dienogest
- 2 dark red tablets each containing 1 mg estradiol valerate
- 2 white tablets (inert)

Natazia also contains the excipients lactose monohydrate, maize starch, maize starch pre-gelatinized, povidone 25, magnesium stearate, hypromellose, macrogol 6000, talc, titanium dioxide, and ferric oxide pigment, yellow, or ferric oxide pigment, red.

The empirical formula of estradiol valerate is C_{23} H_{32} O_3 and the chemical structure is:

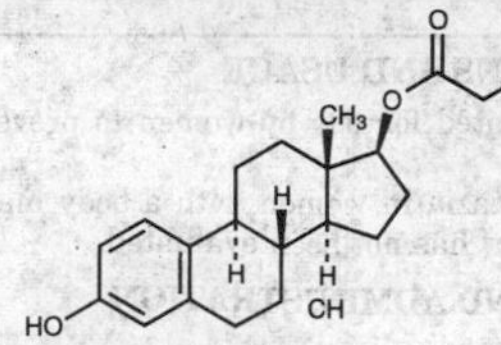

Estradiol Valerate

The chemical name of estradiol valerate is Estra-1,3,5(10)-triene-3,17-diol(17β)-,17-pentanoate.

The empirical formula of dienogest is C_{20} H_{25} NO_2 and the chemical structure is:

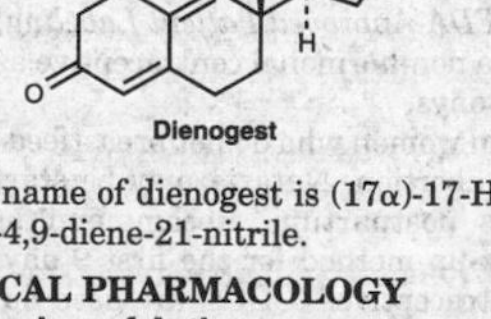

Dienogest

The chemical name of dienogest is (17α)-17-Hydroxy-3-oxo-19-norpregna-4,9-diene-21-nitrile.

12 CLINICAL PHARMACOLOGY

12.1 Mechanism of Action

COCs lower the risk of becoming pregnant primarily by suppressing ovulation. Other possible mechanisms may include cervical mucus changes that inhibit sperm penetration and endometrial changes that reduce the likelihood of implantation.

12.2 Pharmacodynamics

The contraceptive effect of COCs is based on the interaction of various factors, the most important of which are the inhibition of ovulation and the changes in the cervical secretion. The estrogen in Natazia is estradiol valerate, a synthetic prodrug of 17β-estradiol.

The progestin in Natazia is dienogest (DNG). DNG displays properties of 19-nortestosterone derivatives as well as properties associated with progesterone derivatives. *[See Nonclinical Toxicology (13.2).]*

Cardiac Electrophysiology

The effect of Natazia on QT prolongation was evaluated in a randomized, double-blind, positive (moxifloxacin 400 mg) and negative (placebo) controlled crossover study in healthy subjects. A total of 53 subjects were administered Natazia (containing 3 mg dienogest and 2 mg estradiol valerate), dienogest 10 mg, and placebo as once daily doses for 4 days, and moxifloxacin 400 mg as a single oral dose. The upper bound of the 90% confidence interval for the largest placebo-adjusted, baseline-corrected QTc based on Fridericia's correction method (QTcF) was below 10 msec, the threshold for regulatory concern.

12.3 Pharmacokinetics

Absorption

After oral administration of estradiol valerate, cleavage to 17β-estradiol and valeric acid takes place during absorption by the intestinal mucosa or in the course of the first liver passage. This gives rise to estradiol and its metabolites, estrone and other metabolites. Maximum serum estradiol concentrations of 73.3 pg/mL are reached at a median of approximately 6 hours (range: 1.5–12 hours) and the area under the estradiol concentration curve [AUC(0–24hr)] was 1301 pg•hr/mL after single ingestion of a tablet containing 3 mg estradiol valerate under fasted condition on Day 1 of the 28-day sequential regimen.

Bioavailability of dienogest is about 91%. Maximum serum dienogest concentrations of 91.7 ng/mL are reached at a median of approximately 1 hour (range: 0.5–1.5 hour) and the area under the dienogest concentration curve [AUC(0–24hr)] was 964 ng/mL after single oral administration of Natazia tablet containing 2 mg estradiol valerate/ 3 mg dienogest under fasted condition. The pharmacokinetics of dienogest are dose-proportional within the dose range of 1–8 mg. Steady state is reached after 4 days of the same dosage of 2 mg dienogest. The mean accumulation ratio for AUC (0–24hr) is approximately 1.24.

The mean plasma pharmacokinetic parameters at steady state following repeated oral doses of a 2 mg estradiol valerate/3 mg dienogest combination tablet in fertile women under fasted condition are reported in Table 1.

[See table 1 above]

Table 1: Arithmetic Mean (SD) Serum Pharmacokinetic Parameters at Steady-state (on Day 24) following Repeated Oral Doses of 2 mg EV/3 mg DNG on Days 8–24 of the 28 day Regimen in Fertile Women under Fasted Condition (N=15)

Parameter	Dienogest	Estradiol	Estrone
C_{max}	85.2 (19.7) ng/ml	70.5 (25.9) pg/ml	483 (198) pg/ml
T_{max} (hr)[a]	1.5 (1–2)	3 (1.5–12)	4 (3–12)
AUC(0–24hr)	828 (187) ng•hr/ml	1323 (480) pg•hr/ml	7562 (3403) pg•hr/ml
$t_{1/2}$ (hr)	12.3 (1.4)	NA	NA

[a] Median (range) for T_{max}
C_{max} = Maximum serum concentration
T_{max} = Time to reach maximum concentration
AUC(0–24hr) = Area under the concentration-time curve from 0 hr data point up to 48 hr post-administration
NA: Data not available

Food Effect

Concomitant food intake in women resulted in a 28% decrease for dienogest C_{max} and 23% increase of estradiol C_{max} while the exposure (AUC) of both dienogest and estradiol did not change.

Distribution

In serum, 38% of estradiol is bound to sex hormone-binding globulin (SHBG), 60% to albumin and 2–3% circulates in free form. An apparent volume of distribution of approximately 1.2 L/kg was determined after intravenous (IV) administration.

A relatively high fraction (10%) of circulating dienogest is present in the free form, with approximately 90% being bound non-specifically to albumin. Dienogest does not bind to SHBG and corticosteroid-binding globulin (CBG). The volume of distribution at steady state ($V_{d,ss}$) of dienogest is 46 L after the IV administration of 85 mcg ^{3}H-dienogest.

Metabolism

After oral administration of estradiol valerate, approximately 3% of the dose is directly bioavailable as estradiol. Estradiol undergoes an extensive first-pass effect and a considerable part of the dose administered is already metabolized in the gastrointestinal mucosa. The CYP 3A family is known to play the most important role in human estradiol metabolism. Together with the pre-systemic metabolism in the liver, about 95% of the orally administered dose becomes metabolized before entering the systemic circulation. The main metabolites are estrone and its sulfate or glucuronide conjugates.

Dienogest is extensively metabolized by the known pathways of steroid metabolism (hydroxylation, conjugation), with the formation of endocrinologically mostly inactive metabolites. CYP3A4 was identified as a predominant enzyme catalyzing the metabolism of dienogest.

Excretion

Estradiol and its metabolites are mainly excreted in urine, with about 10% being excreted in the feces. The terminal half-life of estradiol is approximately 14 hours.

Dienogest is mainly excreted renally in the form of metabolites and unchanged dienogest is the dominating fraction in plasma. The terminal half-life of dienogest is approximately 11 hours.

Specific Populations

Pediatric Use: Safety and efficacy of Natazia has been established in women of reproductive age. Efficacy is expected to be the same for postpubertal adolescents under the age of 18 as for users 18 years and older. Use of this product before menarche is not indicated. *[See Use in Specific Populations (8.4)]*

Geriatric Use: Natazia has not been studied in postmenopausal women and is not indicated in this population. *[See Use in Specific Populations (8.5)]*

Renal Impairment: The pharmacokinetics of Natazia has not been studied in subjects with renal impairment. *[See Use in Specific Populations (8.6)]*

Hepatic Impairment: The pharmacokinetics of Natazia has not been studied in subjects with hepatic impairment. Steroid hormones may be poorly metabolized in patients with impaired liver function. Acute or chronic disturbances of liver function may necessitate the discontinuation of COC use until markers of liver function return to normal. *[See Contraindications (4), Warnings and Precautions (5.3) and Use in Specific Populations (8.7)]*

Body Mass Index: The efficacy of Natazia in women with a BMI of > 30 kg/m^2 has not been evaluated. *[See Use in Specific Populations (8.8)]*

Drug Interactions

CYP3A4 Inducers: Drugs or herbal products that induce certain enzymes, including CYP3A4, may decrease the effectiveness of COCs or increase breakthrough bleeding. Some drugs or herbal products that may decrease the effectiveness of hormonal contraceptives include barbiturates, bosentan, felbamate, griseofulvin, oxcarbazepine, and topiramate. Counsel women to use an alternative method of contraception or a back-up method when moderate or weak enzyme inducers are used with COCs, and to continue back-up contraception for 28 days after discontinuing the enzyme inducer to ensure contraceptive reliability.

Dienogest is a substrate of CYP3A4. Women who take medications that are strong CYP3A4 inducers (for example, carbamazepine, phenytoin, rifampicin, and St. John's wort) should not choose Natazia as their oral contraceptive while using these inducers and for at least 28 days after discontinuation of these inducers due to the possibility of decreased contraceptive efficacy.

The effect of the CYP3A4 inducer rifampicin was studied in an open-label, non-randomized, single center study in 16 healthy postmenopausal women. All volunteers received a treatment regimen of 2 mg estradiol valerate and 3 mg dienogest combination tablets, dosed once daily over 17 days, and of rifampicin, which was administered once daily in an oral dose of 600 mg on Days 12 to 16. 24–hr pharmacokinetics of estradiol and dienogest on Days 11 and 17 were compared. Co-administration of rifampicin with estradiol valerate/dienogest tablets led to a 52 % and 83% decrease in the mean C_{max} and AUC(0–24hr), respectively, for dienogest and a 25% and 44% decrease in C_{max} and AUC(0–24hr), respectively, for estradiol at steady state. *[See Drug Interactions (7.1)]*

Strong CYP3A4 Inhibitors: Strong CYP3A4 inhibitors such as ketoconazole increase hormone serum levels. The effect of a strong CYP3A4 inhibitor, ketoconazole, on dienogest and estradiol pharmacokinetics was studied in an open-label, two parallel-groups, one-sequence, one-way crossover study in healthy postmenopausal Caucasian women. One tablet of 2 mg estradiol valerate and 3 mg dienogest was administered orally once a day for 14 days. Twelve volunteers received an oral dose of 400 mg ketoconazole (that is, 2 tablets containing 200 mg ketoconazole) once daily for 7 days (Days 8–14). Twenty-four hour pharmacokinetics of estradiol and dienogest on Days 7 and 14 were compared. Co-administration with the strong inhibitor ketoconazole resulted in a 186% and 57% increase of AUC (0–24hr) at steady state for dienogest and estradiol. There was also a 94% and 65% increase of C_{max} at steady state for dienogest and estradiol when co-administered with ketoconazole. *[See Drug Interactions (7.1).]*

Moderate CYP3A4 Inhibitors: Moderate CYP3A4 inhibitors such as erythromycin increase hormone serum levels. The effect of a moderate CYP3A4 inhibitor, erythromycin on dienogest and estradiol pharmacokinetics was studied in an open-label, two parallel-groups, one-sequence, one-way crossover study in healthy postmenopausal Caucasian women. One tablet of 2 mg estradiol valerate and 3 mg dienogest was administered orally once a day for 14 days. Twelve volunteers received an oral dose of 500 mg erythromycin three times a day for 7 days (Days 8–14). Twenty-four hour pharmacokinetics of estradiol and dienogest on Days 7 and 14 were compared. When co-administered with the moderate inhibitor erythromycin, the AUC (0–24hr) of dienogest and estradiol at steady state were increased by 62% and 33%, respectively. There was also a 33% and 51% increase of C_{max} at steady state for dienogest and estradiol when co-administered with erythromycin. *[See Drug Interactions (7.1).]*

Other known CYP3A4 inhibitors such as azole antifungals, cimetidine, verapamil, macrolides, diltiazem, antidepressants, and grapefruit juice may increase plasma levels of dienogest and estradiol. *[See Drug Interactions (7.1).]*

HIV Protease Inhibitors: Significant changes (increase or decrease) in the plasma levels of the estrogen and progestin have been noted in some cases of co-administration of HIV protease inhibitors.

Antibiotics: There have been reports of pregnancy while taking hormonal contraceptives and antibiotics, but clinical pharmacokinetic studies have not shown consistent effects of antibiotics on plasma concentrations of synthetic steroids.

Consult the labeling of all concurrently-used drugs to obtain further information about interactions with hormonal contraceptives or the potential for enzyme alterations.

Effects of Combined Hormonal Contraceptives on Other Drugs: COCs containing ethinyl estradiol (or mestranol), may inhibit the metabolism of other compounds. COCs have been shown to significantly decrease plasma concentrations of lamotrigine, likely due to induction of lamotrigine glucuronidation. This may reduce seizure control; therefore, dosage adjustments of lamotrigine may be necessary. Consult the labeling of the concurrently-used drug to obtain further information about interactions with COCs or the potential for enzyme alterations.

In vitro studies with human CYP enzymes did not indicate an inhibitory potential of dienogest at clinically relevant concentrations.

13 NONCLINICAL TOXICOLOGY

13.1 Carcinogenesis, Mutagenesis, Impairment of Fertility

In a 24 month carcinogenicity study in mice dosed orally with dienogest by gavage with doses of 5, 15 and 50 mg/kg/ day (males) and 10, 30 and 100 mg/kg/day (females), the systemic exposures in the females were 1.1, 3.5, and 10.6 times the exposure (AUC of dienogest) of women taking a 3 mg dose. A statistically significantly higher incidence of stromal polyps of the uterus was observed in females given 100 mg/kg. In a similar study in rats given 1, 3, and 10 mg/kg for 104 weeks, 0.2, 1.4, and 6.1 times the exposure of women taking a 3 mg dose, there were no statistically significant drug-related neoplasms.

Dienogest was not mutagenic in *in vitro* reverse mutation tests in bacteria, in chromosome aberration tests in human peripheral lymphocytes, mouse lymphoma cells, and Chinese hamster lung cells, and tests of unscheduled DNA synthesis (UDS) in rat and human liver cells. Dienogest was also negative in an *in vivo* mouse micronucleus test, a rat liver initiation-promotion model, and an *in vitro/in vivo* UDS test in female rats.

13.2 Animal Toxicology and/or Pharmacology

Nonclinical studies in animals and *in vitro*, have shown that besides progestogenic activities, DNG is devoid of estrogenic, androgenic, glucocorticoid and mineralocorticoid activities.

Table 2: Summary of the Pearl Indexes and the Cumulative Contraceptive Failure Rates

Study	Age Group	Relative Treatment Exposure Cycles[1]	Number of Pregnancies within 13 Cycles and 7 Days after Last Treatment	Pearl Index	Upper Limit of 95% CI	Contraceptive Failure Rate at the End of First Year
North America	18–35	3,969	5	1.64	3.82	0.016
Europe	18–35	11,275	9	1.04	1.97	0.010

[1] Total treatment exposure time without back-up contraception

14   CLINICAL STUDIES

14.1   Oral Contraceptive Clinical Trials

The study conducted in North America (U.S. and Canada) was a multicenter, open-label, single-arm, unintended pregnancy study. There were 490 healthy subjects between 18 and 35 years of age (mean age: 25.1 years) who were treated for up to 28 cycles of 28 days each. The racial demographic of enrolled women was: Caucasian (76%), Hispanic (13%), African-American (7%), Asian (3%), and Other (1%). The weight range for treated women was 40 to 100 kg (mean weight: 62.5 kg) and the BMI range was 14 to 30 kg/m² (mean BMI: 23.3 kg/m²). Of treated women, 15% discontinued the study treatment due to an adverse event, 13% were lost to follow up, 10% withdrew their consent, 8% discontinued due to other reason, 1% discontinued due to protocol deviation, and 1% discontinued due to pregnancy.

The study conducted in Europe (Germany, Austria and Spain) was a multicenter, open-label, single-arm contraceptive reliability study. There were 1,377 healthy subjects between 18 and 50 years of age (mean age: 30.3 years) who were treated for 20 cycles of 28 days each. The racial demographic of enrolled women was predominantly Caucasian (99.2%). The weight range for treated women was 38 to 98 kg (mean weight: 63.8 kg) and the BMI range was 15 to 31.8 kg/m² (mean BMI: 22.8 kg/m²). Of treated women, 10% discontinued the study treatment due to an adverse event, 5% discontinued due to other reason, 2% were lost to follow up, 2% discontinued due to protocol deviation, 2% withdrew their consent, and 1% discontinued due to pregnancy.

The Pearl Index (PI) was the primary efficacy endpoint used to assess contraceptive reliability and was assessed in each of the two studies, assuming all subjects were at risk of pregnancy in all medication cycles unless back-up contraception was documented. The PI is based on pregnancies that occurred after the onset of treatment and within 7 days after the last pill intake. Cycles in which conception did not occur, but which included the use of back-up contraception, were not included in the calculation of the PI. The PI also includes patients who did not take the drug correctly. The estimated PI for the North American study is 1.64 and the estimated PI for the European study is 1.04. The Kaplan-Meier method was also used to calculate the contraceptive failure rate.

The summary of the Pearl Indexes and cumulative contraceptive failure rates are provided in Table 2:

[See table 2 above]

16   HOW SUPPLIED/STORAGE AND HANDLING

16.1   How Supplied

Natazia (estradiol valerate and estradiol valerate/dienogest) tablets are available in packages of three blister packs (NDC 50419-409-03).

The active and inert film-coated tablets are rounded with biconvex faces, one side is embossed with a regular hexagon shape with the letters DD or DJ or DH or DN or DT.

Each blister pack (28 film-coated tablets) contains in the following order:

- 2 round biconvex dark yellow film-coated tablets with embossed "DD" in a regular hexagon on one side each containing 3 mg estradiol valerate
- 5 round biconvex medium red film-coated tablets with embossed "DJ" in a regular hexagon on one side each containing 2 mg estradiol valerate and 2 mg dienogest
- 17 round biconvex light yellow film-coated tablets with embossed "DH" in a regular hexagon on one side each containing 2 mg estradiol valerate and 3 mg dienogest
- 2 round biconvex dark red film-coated tablets with embossed "DN" in a regular hexagon on one side each containing 1 mg estradiol valerate
- 2 white round biconvex white film-coated tablets with embossed "DT" in a regular hexagon on one side (inert)

Keep out of reach of children.

16.2   Storage Conditions

Store at 25° C (77° F); excursions permitted to 15–30°C (59–86°F) [see USP Controlled Room Temperature].

17   PATIENT COUNSELING INFORMATION

See FDA-Approved Patient Labeling.

17.1   Information for Patients

- Counsel patients that cigarette smoking increases the risk of serious cardiovascular events from COC use, and that women who are over 35 years old and smoke should not use COCs.
- Counsel patients that this product does not protect against HIV infection (AIDS) and other sexually transmitted diseases.
- Counsel patients on Warnings and Precautions associated with COCs.
- Counsel patients to take one tablet daily by mouth at the same time every day in the exact order noted on the blister. Instruct patients what to do in the event pills are missed. See *What Should I Do if I Miss any Pills* section or *FDA-Approved Patient Labeling*.
- Counsel women who are taking strong CYP3A4 inducers (for example, carbamazepine, phenytoin, rifampicin, and St. John's wort) not to choose Natazia as their oral contraceptive due to the possibility of decreased contraceptive efficacy.
- Counsel patients to use a back-up or alternative method of contraception when weak or moderate enzyme inducers are used with Natazia.
- Counsel patients who are breastfeeding or who desire to breastfeed that COCs may reduce breast milk production. This is less likely to occur if breastfeeding is well established.
- Counsel any patient who starts COCs postpartum, and who has not yet had a period, to use an additional method of contraception until she has taken Natazia for 9 consecutive days.
- Counsel patients that amenorrhea may occur. Pregnancy should be ruled out in the event of amenorrhea in two or more consecutive cycles.

FDA-Approved Patient Labeling
Guide for Using Natazia

WARNING TO WOMEN WHO SMOKE

Do not use Natazia if you smoke cigarettes and are over 35 years old. Smoking increases your risk of serious cardiovascular side effects (heart and blood vessel problems) from birth control pills, including death from heart attack, blood clots or stroke. This risk increases with age and the number of cigarettes you smoke.

Birth control pills help to lower the chances of becoming pregnant when taken as directed. They do not protect against HIV infection (AIDS) and other sexually transmitted diseases.

What Is Natazia?

Natazia is a birth control pill. It contains two female hormones, an estrogen called estradiol valerate and a progestin called dienogest. Estradiol valerate is a synthetic estrogen that is converted to estradiol in your body.

How Well Does Natazia Work?

Your chance of getting pregnant depends on how well you follow the directions for taking your birth control pills. The more carefully you follow the directions, the less chance you have of getting pregnant.

Based on the results of two clinical studies, 1 to 2 women out of 100 women, may get pregnant during the first year they use Natazia.

The following chart shows the chance of getting pregnant for women who use different methods of birth control. Each box on the chart contains a list of birth control methods that are similar in effectiveness. The most effective methods are at the top of the chart. The box on the bottom of the chart shows the chance of getting pregnant for women who do not use birth control and are trying to get pregnant.

[See figure at top of next column]

How Do I Take Natazia?

- Take one pill every day at the same time. Take the pills in the order directed on the blister pack.
- Do not skip pills or delay taking your pill by more than 12 hours. If you miss pills (including starting the pack late), you could get pregnant. The more pills you miss, the more likely you are to get pregnant.
- If you have trouble remembering to take Natazia, talk to your healthcare provider about how to make pill-taking easier, or about using another method of birth control.

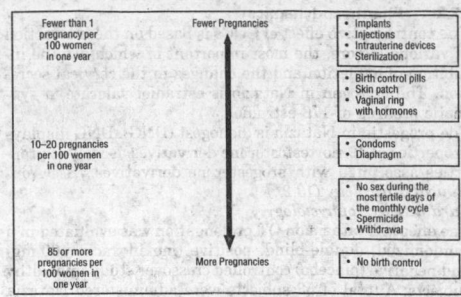

- You may have spotting or light bleeding when you first take Natazia. Spotting or light bleeding is normal at first.
- You may feel sick to your stomach (nauseous), especially during the first few months that you take Natazia. If you feel sick to your stomach, do not stop taking the pill. The problem will usually go away. If your nausea doesn't go away, call your healthcare provider.
- If you vomit or have diarrhea within 4 hours of taking your pill, follow the instructions for "What Should I Do if I Miss any Pills."
- Missing pills can also cause spotting or light bleeding, even when you take the missed pills later. On the days you take 2 pills to make up for missed pills, you could also feel a little sick to your stomach.

Before you start taking Natazia

- Decide what time of day you want to take your pill. It is important to take it at the same time every day and in the order as directed on the blister pack.

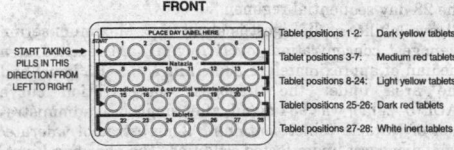

- Look at your Natazia blister pack. The blister pack has four rows of 7 pills each, for a total of 28 pills. Find:
  - where on the pack to start taking your pills
  - in what order to take the pills
- Each NATAZIA blister pack has 28 pills.
  - 2 dark yellow pills with hormones, for Days 1 and 2
  - 5 medium red pills with hormones for Days 3–7
  - 17 light yellow pills with hormones for Days 8–24
  - 2 dark red pills with hormones for Days 25 and 26
  - 2 white pills without hormones for Days 27 and 28
- After taking the last white pill (day 28) of the blister pack, start taking the first dark yellow pill from a new blister pack the very next day whether or not you are having your period.
- Be sure to have ready at all times another kind of birth control (such as condoms or spermicides) to use as a back-up in case you miss pills.
- It is not uncommon to miss a period. However, if you miss 2 periods in a row or feel like you may be pregnant, call your healthcare provider. If you are pregnant, you should stop taking Natazia.

When to Start Natazia

If you start taking Natazia and you did not use a hormonal birth control method before:

- Take the first dark yellow pill on the first day (Day 1) of your natural menstrual cycle. The first day of your menstrual cycle is the first day you start spotting or bleeding.
- Use non-hormonal back-up contraception such as a condom or spermicide for the first 9 days that you take Natazia.

If you start taking Natazia and you are switching from a combination hormonal method such as:

- another pill
- vaginal ring
- patch
- Take the first dark yellow pill on the first day of your period. Do not continue taking the pills from your previous birth control pack. If you do not have a period, contact your healthcare provider before you start Natazia.
- If you previously used a vaginal ring or transdermal patch, you should start using Natazia on the day the ring or patch is removed.
- Use a non-hormonal back-up method such as a condom or spermicide for the first 9 days you take Natazia.

If you start taking Natazia and you are switching from a progestin-only method such as a:

- progestin-only pill
- implant
- intrauterine system
- injection
- Take the first dark yellow pill on the day you would have taken your next progestin-only pill or on the day of re-

moval of your implant or intrauterine system or on the day when you would have had your next injection.
• Use a non-hormonal back-up method such as a condom or spermicide for the first 9 days you take Natazia.

What Should I Do if I Miss any Pills?
If you forgot to start a new blister pack, **you may already be pregnant.** Use back-up contraception (such as condoms and spermicides) anytime you have sex. Call your healthcare provider if you are unsure whether you are pregnant.
• Do not take more than 2 pills in one day. On the days you take 2 pills to make up for missed pills, you may feel a little sick to your stomach (nauseous).
• If you start vomiting or have diarrhea within 4 hours of taking your pill, take another pill of the same color from your extra blister pack.

If you are less than 12 hours late taking your pill
• Take your pill as soon as you remember
• Take the next pill at the usual time
• You do not need to use back-up contraception

If you miss ONE PILL for more than 12 hours
Days 1–17
• Take your missed pill immediately
• Take your next pill at the usual time (you may have to take two pills that day)
• Use back-up contraception for the next 9 days
• Continue taking one pill each day at the same time for the rest of your cycle
Days 18–24
• Do not take any pills from your current blister pack and throw the pack away
• Take Day 1 pill from a new blister pack
• Use back-up contraception for the next 9 days
• Continue taking one pill from the new blister pack at the same time each day
Days 25–28
• Take your missed pill immediately
• Take your next pill at the usual time (you may have to take two pills that day)
• No back-up contraception is needed
• Continue taking one pill each day at the same time for the rest of your cycle

If you miss TWO PILLS in a row
Days 1–17 (if you miss the pills for Days 17 and 18, follow the instructions for Days 17–25 instead)
• Do not take the missed pills. Instead, take the pill for the day on which you first noticed you had missed pills.
• Use back-up contraception for the next 9 days
• Continue taking one pill each day at the same time for the rest of your cycle
Days 17–25 (if you miss the pills for Days 25 and 26, follow the instructions for Days 25–28 instead)
• Do not take any pills from your current blister pack and throw the pack away
• Take Day 3 pill from a new blister pack
• Use back-up contraception for the next 9 days
• Continue taking one pill from the new blister pack at the same time each day
Days 25–28
• Do not take any pills from your current blister pack and throw the pack away
• Start a new pack on the same day or start a new pack on the day you usually start a new pack
• No back-up contraception is needed
• Continue taking one pill from the new pack at the same time each day, for the rest of your cycle

---

You may already be pregnant or COULD BECOME PREGNANT if you had sex on the days after the pills were missed. The more pills missed and the closer they are to the end of the cycle, the higher the risk of a pregnancy. You should call your doctor or healthcare provider if you are unsure whether you are already pregnant.

If you are still not sure of what to do about the pills you have missed:
• Call your healthcare provider
• Use back-up contraception (such as condoms and spermicides) anytime you have sex and keep taking 1 pill each day

Who Should Not Take Natazia?
Your healthcare provider will not give you Natazia if you have:
• Ever had breast cancer or any cancer that is sensitive to female hormones
• Liver disease, including liver tumors
• Ever had blood clots in your arms, legs, or lungs
• Ever had a stroke
• Ever had a heart attack
• Certain heart valve problems or heart rhythm abnormalities that can cause blood clots to form in the heart

• An inherited problem with your blood that makes it clot more than normal
• High blood pressure that medicine can't control
• Diabetes with kidney, eye, or blood vessel damage
• Certain kinds of severe migraine headaches with aura, numbness, weakness or changes in vision
Also, do not take birth control pills if you:
• Smoke and are over 35 years old
• Are pregnant
Birth control pills may not be a good choice for you if you have ever had jaundice (yellowing of the skin or eyes) caused by pregnancy (also called cholestasis of pregnancy).

What Else Should I Know about Taking Natazia?
Birth control pills do not protect you against any sexually transmitted disease, including HIV, the virus that causes AIDS.
Do not skip any pills, even if you do not have sex often.
If you miss a period, you could be pregnant. However, some women miss periods or have light periods on birth control pills, even when they are not pregnant. Contact your healthcare provider for advice if you:
• Think you are pregnant
• Miss one period and have not taken your birth control pills according to directions
• Miss two periods in a row
Birth control pills should not be taken during pregnancy. However, birth control pills taken by accident during pregnancy are not known to cause birth defects.
If you are breastfeeding, consider another birth control method until you are ready to stop breastfeeding. Birth control pills that contain estrogen, like Natazia, may decrease the amount of milk you make. A small amount of the pill's hormones pass into breast milk.
Tell your healthcare provider about all medicines and herbal products that you take. You should not choose Natazia as your birth control pill if you take carbemazepine, phenytoin, rifampicin or St. John's wort, because these medicines may make Natazia ineffective. Some other medicines and herbal products may make birth control pills less effective, including:
• Barbiturates
• Bosentan
• Felbamate
• Griseofulvin
• Oxcarbazepine
• Topiramate
Consider using another birth control method when you take medicines that may make birth control pills less effective. Birth control pills may interact with lamotrigine, an anticonvulsant used for epilepsy. This may increase the risk of seizures, so your healthcare provider may need to adjust the dose of lamotrigine.
If you have vomiting or diarrhea, your birth control pills may not work as well. Use another birth control method, like condoms and a spermicide, until you check with your healthcare provider.

What are the Most Serious Risks of Taking Birth Control Pills?
Like pregnancy, birth control pills increase the risk of serious blood clots, especially in women who have other risk factors, such as smoking, obesity, or age greater than 35. It is possible to die from a problem caused by a blood clot, such as a heart attack or a stroke. Some examples of serious blood clots are blood clots in the:
• Legs (thrombophlebitis)
• Lungs (pulmonary embolus)
• Eyes (loss of eyesight)
• Heart (heart attack)
• Brain (stroke)
A few women who take birth control pills may get:
• High blood pressure
• Gallbladder problems
• Rare cancerous or noncancerous liver tumors
All of these events are uncommon in healthy women.
Call your healthcare provider right away if you have:
• Persistent leg pain
• Sudden shortness of breath
• Sudden blindness, partial or complete
• Severe pain in your chest
• Sudden, severe headache unlike your usual headaches
• Weakness or numbness in an arm or leg, or trouble speaking
• Yellowing of the skin or eyeballs
What are the Common Side Effects of Birth Control Pills?
The most common side effects of birth control pills are:
• Spotting or bleeding between menstrual periods
• Nausea
• Breast tenderness
• Headache
These side effects are usually mild and usually disappear with time.
Less common side effects are:
• Acne
• Less sexual desire

• Bloating or fluid retention
• Blotchy darkening of the skin, especially on the face
• High blood sugar, especially in women who already have diabetes
• High fat levels in the blood
• Depression, especially if you have had depression in the past.
Call your healthcare provider immediately if you have any thoughts of harming yourself.
• Problems tolerating contact lenses
• Weight changes
This is not a complete list of possible side effects. Talk to your healthcare provider if you develop any side effects that concern you. You may report side effects to the FDA at 1-800-FDA-1088.
No serious problems have been reported from a birth control pill overdose, even when accidentally taken by children.
Do Birth Control Pills Cause Cancer?
Birth control pills do not seem to cause breast cancer. However, if you have breast cancer now, or have had it in the past, do not use birth control pills because some breast cancers are sensitive to hormones.
Women who use birth control pills may have a slightly higher chance of getting cervical cancer. However, this may be due to other reasons such as having more sexual partners.
What Should I Know about My Period when Taking Natazia?
Irregular vaginal bleeding or spotting may occur while you are taking Natazia. Irregular bleeding may vary from slight staining between menstrual periods to breakthrough bleeding, which is a flow much like a regular period. Irregular bleeding occurs most often during the first few months of oral contraceptive use, but may also occur after you have been taking the pill for some time. Such bleeding may be temporary and usually does not indicate any serious problems. It is important to continue taking your pills on schedule. If the bleeding occurs in more than one cycle, is unusually heavy, or lasts for more than a few days, call your healthcare provider.
Also, your menstrual period while using oral contraceptives may be shorter and lighter than usual. Some women may not have a menstrual period but this should not be cause for alarm as long has you have taken the pills according to direction.
What If I Miss My Scheduled Period when Taking Natazia?
It is not uncommon to miss your period. However, if you miss more than two periods in a row or miss one period when you have not taken your birth control pills according to directions, call your healthcare provider. Also notify your healthcare provider if you have symptoms of pregnancy such as morning sickness or unusual breast tenderness. It is important that your healthcare provider checks you to find out if you are pregnant. Stop taking Natazia if you are pregnant.
What If I Want to Become Pregnant?
You may stop taking the pill whenever you wish. Consider a visit with your healthcare provider for a pre-pregnancy checkup before you stop taking the pill.
General Advice about Natazia
Your healthcare provider prescribed Natazia for you. Please do not share Natazia with anyone else. Keep Natazia out of the reach of children.
If you have concerns or questions, ask your healthcare provider. You may also ask your healthcare provider for a more detailed label written for medical professionals.
Manufactured by:
Bayer HealthCare Pharmaceuticals Inc.
Wayne, NJ 07470
Manufactured in Germany
© 2010, Bayer HealthCare Pharmaceuticals Inc., All Rights Reserved.
Bayer HealthCare Pharmaceuticals Inc.
6704300   Revised: 05/2010
                                                        US 82775308
Shown in Product Identification Guide, page 307

YASMIN 28 TABLETS   ℞
[yaz-min]
(drospirenone and ethinyl estradiol)
PHYSICIAN LABELING
Rx only

PATIENTS SHOULD BE COUNSELED THAT THIS PRODUCT DOES NOT PROTECT AGAINST HIV INFECTION (AIDS) AND OTHER SEXUALLY TRANSMITTED DISEASES.
DESCRIPTION
YASMIN® provides an oral contraceptive regimen consisting of 21 active film coated tablets each containing 3 mg of drospirenone and 0.03 mg of ethinyl estradiol and 7 inert film coated tablets. The inactive ingredients are lactose monohydrate NF, corn starch NF, modified starch NF, povidone 25000 USP, magnesium stearate NF, hydroxylpropyl-

methyl cellulose USP, macrogol 6000 NF, talc USP, titanium dioxide USP, ferric oxide pigment, yellow NF. The inert film coated tablets contain lactose monohydrate NF, corn starch NF, povidone 25000 USP, magnesium stearate NF, hydroxylpropylmethyl cellulose USP, talc USP, titanium dioxide USP.

Drospirenone (6R,7R,8R,9S,10R,13S,14S,15S,16S,17S)-1,3′,4′,6,6a,7,8,9,10,11,12,13, 14,15,15a,16-hexadecahydro-10,13-dimethylspiro-[17H-dicyclopropa-6,7:15,16] cyclopenta [a]phenanthrene-17,2′(5H)-furan]-3,5′(2H)-dione) is a synthetic progestational compound and has a molecular weight of 366.5 and a molecular formula of $C_{24}H_{30}O_3$. Ethinyl estradiol (19-nor-17α-pregna 1,3,5(10)-triene-20-yne-3,17-diol) is a synthetic estrogenic compound and has a molecular weight of 296.4 and a molecular formula of $C_{20}H_{24}O_2$. The structural formulas are as follows:

Drospirenone   Ethinyl estradiol

CLINICAL PHARMACOLOGY
PHARMACODYNAMICS

Combination oral contraceptives (COCs) act by suppression of gonadotropins. Although the primary mechanism of this action is inhibition of ovulation, other alterations include changes in the cervical mucus (which increases the difficulty of sperm entry into the uterus) and the endometrium (which reduces the likelihood of implantation).

Drospirenone is a spironolactone analogue with antimineralocorticoid activity. Preclinical studies in animals and in vitro have shown that drospirenone has no androgenic, estrogenic, glucocorticoid, and antiglucocorticoid activity. Preclinical studies in animals have also shown that drospirenone has antiandrogenic activity.

PHARMACOKINETICS
Absorption

The absolute bioavailability of drospirenone (DRSP) from a single entity tablet is about 76%. The absolute bioavailability of ethinyl estradiol (EE) is approximately 40% as a result of presystemic conjugation and first-pass metabolism. The absolute bioavailability of YASMIN which is a combination tablet of drospirenone and ethinyl estradiol has not been evaluated. Serum concentrations of DRSP and EE reached peak levels within 1–3 hours after administration of YASMIN. After single dose administration of YASMIN, the relative bioavailability, compared to a suspension, was 107% and 117% for DRSP and EE, respectively.

The pharmacokinetics of DRSP are dose proportional following single doses ranging from 1–10 mg. Following daily dosing of YASMIN, steady state DRSP concentrations were observed after 10 days. There was about 2 to 3 fold accumulation in serum C_{max} and AUC(0–24h) values of DRSP following multiple dose administration of YASMIN (see TABLE I).

For EE, steady-state conditions are reported during the second half of a treatment cycle. Following daily administration of YASMIN serum C_{max} and AUC(0–24h) values of EE accumulate by a factor of about 1.5 to 2.

[See table I below]

Effect of Food

The rate of absorption of DRSP and EE following single administration of two YASMIN tablets was slower under fed conditions with the serum Cmax being reduced about 40% for both components. The extent of absorption of DRSP, however, remained unchanged. In contrast the extent of absorption of EE was reduced by about 20% under fed conditions.

Distribution

DRSP and EE serum levels decline in two phases. The apparent volume of distribution of DRSP is approximately 4 L/kg and that of EE is reported to be approximately 4–5 L/kg.

DRSP does not bind to sex hormone binding globulin (SHBG) or corticosteroid binding globulin (CBG) but binds about 97% to other serum proteins. Multiple dosing over 3 cycles resulted in no change in the free fraction (as measured at trough levels). EE is reported to be highly but non-specifically bound to serum albumin (approximately 98.5%) and induces an increase in the serum concentrations of both SHBG and CBG. EE induced effects on SHBG and CBG were not affected by variation of the DRSP dosage in the range of 2 to 3 mg.

Metabolism

The two main metabolites of DRSP found in human plasma were identified to be the acid form of DRSP generated by opening of the lactone ring and the 4,5-dihydrodrospirenone- 3-sulfate. These metabolites were shown not to be pharmacologically active. In in vitro studies with human liver microsomes, DRSP was metabolized only to a minor extent mainly by cytochrome P450 3A4 (CYP3A4).

EE has been reported to be subject to presystemic conjugation in both small bowel mucosa and the liver. Metabolism occurs primarily by aromatic hydroxylation but a wide variety of hydroxylated and methylated metabolites are formed. These are present as free metabolites and as conjugates with glucuronide and sulfate. CYP3A4 in the liver are responsible for the 2-hydroxylation which is the major oxidative reaction. The 2-hydroxy metabolite is further transformed by methylation and glucuronidation prior to urinary and fecal excretion.

Excretion

DRSP serum levels are characterized by a terminal disposition phase half-life of approximately 30 hours after both single and multiple dose regimens. Excretion of DRSP was nearly complete after ten days and amounts excreted were slightly higher in feces compared to urine. DRSP was extensively metabolized and only trace amounts of unchanged DRSP were excreted in urine and feces. At least 20 different metabolites were observed in urine and feces. About 38–47% of the metabolites in urine were glucuronide and sulfate conjugates. In feces, about 17–20% of the metabolites were excreted as glucuronides and sulfates.

For EE the terminal disposition phase half-life has been reported to be approximately 24 hours. EE is not excreted unchanged. EE is excreted in the urine and feces as glucuronide and sulfate conjugates and undergoes enterohepatic circulation.

Special Populations
Race

The effect of race on the disposition of YASMIN has not been evaluated.

Hepatic Dysfunction

YASMIN is contraindicated in patients with hepatic dysfunction (also see BOLDED WARNINGS). The mean exposure to DRSP in women with moderate liver impairment is approximately three times the exposure in women with normal liver function.

Renal Insufficiency

YASMIN is contraindicated in patients with renal insufficiency (also see WARNINGS).

The effect of renal insufficiency on the pharmacokinetics of DRSP (3 mg daily for 14 days) and the effect of DRSP on serum potassium levels were investigated in female subjects (n=28, age 30–65) with normal renal function and mild and moderate renal impairment. All subjects were on a low potassium diet. During the study 7 subjects continued the use of potassium sparing drugs for the treatment of the underlying illness. On the 14th day (steadystate) of DRSP treatment, the serum DRSP levels in the group with mild renal impairment (creatinine clearance CLcr, 50–80 mL/min) were comparable to those in the group with normal renal function (CLcr, >80 mL/min). The serum DRSP levels were on average 37% higher in the group with moderate renal impairment (CLcr, 30–50 mL/min) compared to those in the group with normal renal function. DRSP treatment was well tolerated by all groups. DRSP treatment did not show any clinically significant effect on serum potassium concentration. Although hyperkalemia was not observed in the study, in five of the seven subjects who continued use of potassium sparing drugs during the study, mean serum potassium levels increased by up to 0.33 mEq/L. Therefore, potential exists for hyperkalemia to occur in subjects with renal impairment whose serum potassium is in the upper reference range, and who are concomitantly using potassium sparing drugs.

INDICATIONS AND USAGE

YASMIN is indicated for the prevention of pregnancy in women who elect to use an oral contraceptive.

Oral contraceptives are highly effective. TABLE II lists the typical accidental pregnancy rates for users of combination oral contraceptives and other methods of contraception. The efficacy of these contraceptive methods, except sterilization, depends upon the reliability with which they are used. Correct and consistent use of methods can result in lower failure rates.

[See table II at top of next page]

In clinical efficacy studies of YASMIN of up to 2 years duration, 2,629 subjects completed 33,160 cycles of use without any other contraception. The mean age of the subjects was 25.5 ± 4.7 years. The age range was 16 to 37 years. The racial demographic was: 83% Caucasian, 1% Hispanic, 1% Black, <1% Asian, <1% other, <1% missing data, 14% not inquired and <1% unspecified. Pregnancy rates in the clinical trials were less than one per 100 woman-years of use.

CONTRAINDICATIONS

YASMIN should not be used in women who have the following:

- Renal insufficiency
- Hepatic dysfunction
- Adrenal insufficiency
- Thrombophlebitis or thromboembolic disorders
- A past history of deep-vein thrombophlebitis or thromboembolic disorders
- Cerebral-vascular or coronary-artery disease
- Valvular heart disease with thrombogenic complications
- Severe hypertension
- Diabetes with vascular involvement
- Headaches with focal neurological symptoms
- Known or suspected carcinoma of the breast
- Carcinoma of the endometrium or other known or suspected estrogen-dependent neoplasia
- Undiagnosed abnormal genital bleeding
- Cholestatic jaundice of pregnancy or jaundice with prior pill use
- Liver tumor (benign or malignant) or active liver disease
- Known or suspected pregnancy
- Heavy smoking (≥15 cigarettes per day) and over age 35

TABLE I TABLE OF MEAN PHARMACOKINETIC PARAMETERS OF YASMIN (Drospirenone 3 mg and Ethinyl Estradiol 0.03 mg)

Drospirenone Mean (%CV) Values

Cycle/Day	No. of Subjects	C_{max} (ng/mL)	T_{max} (h)	AUC(0-24h) (ng·h/mL)	$t_{1/2}$ (h)
1/1	12	36.9 (13)	1.7 (47)	288 (25)	NA[a]
1/21	12	87.5 (59)	1.7 (20)	827 (23)	30.9 (44)
6/21	12	84.2 (19)	1.8 (19)	930 (19)	32.5 (38)
9/21	12	81.3 (19)	1.6 (38)	957 (23)	31.4 (39)
13/21	12	78.7 (18)	1.6 (26)	968 (24)	31.1 (36)

Ethinyl Estradiol Mean (%CV) Values

Cycle/Day	No. of Subjects	C_{max} (pg/mL)	T_{max} (h)	AUC(0-24h) (pg·h/mL)	$t_{1/2}$ (h)
1/1	11	53.5 (43)	1.9 (45)	280.3 (87)	NA[a]
1/21	11	92.1 (35)	1.5 (40)	461.3 (94)	NA[a]
6/21	11	99.1 (45)	1.5 (47)	346.4 (74)	NA[a]
9/21	11	87 (43)	1.5 (42)	485.3 (92)	NA[a]
13/21	10	90.5 (45)	1.6 (38)	469.5 (83)	NA[a]

a) NA = Not available

WARNINGS

> Cigarette smoking increases the risk of serious cardio-vascular side effects from oral contraceptive use. This risk increases with age and with heavy smoking (15 or more cigarettes per day) and is quite marked in women over 35 years of age. Women who use oral contraceptives should be strongly advised not to smoke.

YASMIN contains 3 mg of the progestin drospirenone that has antimineralocorticoid activity, including the potential for hyperkalemia in high-risk patients, comparable to a 25 mg dose of spironolactone. YASMIN should not be used in patients with conditions that predispose to hyperkalemia (i.e. renal insufficiency, hepatic dysfunction and adrenal insufficiency). Women receiving daily, long-term treatment for chronic conditions or diseases with medications that may increase serum potassium, should have their serum potassium level checked during the first treatment cycle. Drugs that may increase serum potassium include ACE inhibitors, angiotensin–II receptor antagonists, potassium-sparing diuretics, heparin, aldosterone antagonists, and NSAIDs.

The use of oral contraceptives is associated with increased risks of several serious conditions including myocardial infarction, thromboembolism, stroke, hepatic neoplasia, gallbladder disease, and hypertension, although the risk of serious morbidity or mortality is very small in healthy women without underlying risk factors. The risk of morbidity and mortality increases significantly in the presence of other underlying risk factors such as hypertension, hyperlipidemias, obesity and diabetes.

Practitioners prescribing oral contraceptives should be familiar with the following information relating to these risks. The information contained in this package insert is based principally on studies carried out in patients who used oral contraceptives with higher formulations of estrogens and progestogens than those in common use today. The effect of long-term use of the oral contraceptives with lower formulations of both estrogens and progestogens remains to be determined.

Throughout this labeling, epidemiologic studies reported are of two types. retrospective or case control studies and prospective or cohort studies. Case control studies provide a measure of the relative risk of a disease, namely, a ratio of the incidence of a disease among oral contraceptive users to that among nonusers. The relative risk does not provide information on the actual clinical occurrence of a disease. Cohort studies provide a measure of attributable risk, which is the difference in the incidence of disease between oral contraceptive users and nonusers. The attributable risk does provide information about the actual occurrence of a disease in the population. For further information, the reader is referred to a text on epidemiologic methods.

1. THROMBOEMBOLIC DISORDERS AND OTHER VASCULAR PROBLEMS

a. Myocardial infarction

An increased risk of myocardial infarction has been attributed to oral contraceptive use. This risk is primarily in smokers or women with other underlying risk factors for coronary-artery disease such as hypertension, hypercholesterolemia, morbid obesity, and diabetes. The relative risk of heart attack for current oral contraceptive users has been estimated to be two to six. The risk is very low under the age of 30.

Smoking in combination with oral contraceptive use has been shown to contribute substantially to the incidence of myocardial infarctions in women in their mid-thirties or older with smoking accounting for the majority of excess cases. Mortality rates associated with circulatory disease have been shown to increase substantially in smokers over the age of 35 and nonsmokers over the age of 40 (Table III) among women who use oral contraceptives.

[See table III at right]

Oral contraceptives may compound the effects of well-known risk factors, such as hypertension, diabetes, hyperlipidemias, age and obesity. In particular, some progestogens are known to decrease HDL cholesterol and cause glucose intolerance, while estrogens may create a state of hyperinsulinism. Oral contraceptives have been shown to increase blood pressure among users (see **section 9** in **WARNINGS**). Similar effects on risk factors have been associated with an increased risk of heart disease. Oral contraceptives must be used with caution in women with cardiovascular disease risk factors.

b. Thromboembolism

An increased risk of thromboembolic and thrombotic disease associated with the use of oral contraceptives is well established. Case control studies have found the relative risk of users compared to nonusers to be 3 for the first episode of superficial venous thrombosis, 4 to 11 for deep vein thrombosis or pulmonary embolism, and 1.5 to 6 for women with predisposing conditions for venous thromboembolic

TABLE II Percentage of women experiencing an unintended pregnancy during the first year of typical use and first year of perfect use of contraception and the percentage continuing use at the end of the first year: United States.

Method (1)	% of Women Experiencing an Accidental Pregnancy Within the First Year of Use		% of Women Continuing Use At One Year[a] (4)
	Typical Use[b] (2)	Perfect Use[c] (3)	
Chance[d]	85	85	
Spermicides[e]	26	6	40
Periodic abstinence	25		63
Calendar		9	
Ovulation method		3	
Sympto-thermal[f]		2	
Post-ovulation		1	
Withdrawal	19	4	
Cap[g]			
Parous women	40	26	42
Nulliparous women	20	9	56
Sponge			
Parous women	40	20	42
Nulliparous women	20	9	56
Diaphragm[g]	20	6	56
Condom[h]			
Female (Reality)	21	5	56
Male	14	3	61
Pill	5		71
progestin only		0.5	
combined		0.1	
IUD			
Progesterone T:	2	1.5	81
Copper T 380A	0.8	0.6	78
Lng 20	0.1	0.1	81
Depo Provera	0.3	0.3	70
Norplant and Norplant-2	0.05	0.05	88
Female Sterilization	0.5	0.5	100
Male Sterilization	0.15	0.1	100

Emergency Contraceptive Pills: Treatment initiated within 72 hours after unprotected intercourse reduces the risk of pregnancy by at least 75%[i]

Lactational Amenorrhea Method: LAM is highly effective, *temporary* method of contraception[j]

Source: Trussell J, Contraceptive efficacy. In Hatcher RA, Trussell J, Stewart F, Cates W, Stewart GK, Kowal D, Guest F, Contraceptive Technology: Seventeenth Revised Edition. New York NY: Irvington Publishers, 1998.

a) Among couples attempting to avoid pregnancy, the percentage who continue to use a method for one year.

b) Among *typical* couples who initiate use of a method (not necessarily for the first time), the percentage who experience an accidental pregnancy during the first year if they do not stop use for any other reason.

c) Among couples who initiate use of a method (not necessarily for the first time) and who use it *perfectly* (both consistently and correctly), the percentage who experience an accidental pregnancy during the first year if they do not stop use for any reason.

d) The percents becoming pregnant in columns (2) and (3) are based on data from populations where contraception is not used and from women who cease using contraception in order to become pregnant. Among such populations, about 89% become pregnant within one year. This estimate was lowered slightly (to 85%) to represent the percentage who would become pregnant within one year among women now relying on reversible methods of contraception if they abandoned contraception altogether.

e) Foams, creams, gels, vaginal suppositories, and vaginal film.

f) Cervical mucus (ovulation) method supplemented by calendar in the pre-ovulatory and basal body temperature in the post-ovulatory phases.

g) With spermicidal cream or jelly.

h) Without spermicides.

i) The treatment schedule is one dose within 72 hours after unprotected intercourse, and a second dose 12 hours after the first dose. The Food and Drug Administration has declared the following brands of oral contraceptives to be safe and effective for emergency contraception: Ovral (1 dose is 2 white pills), Alesse (1 dose is 5 pink pills), Nordette or Levlen (1 dose is 2 light-orange pills), Lo/Ovral (1 dose is 4 white pills), Triphasil or Tri-Levlen (1 dose is 4 yellow pills).

j) However, to maintain effective protection against pregnancy, another method of contraception must be used as soon as menstruation resumes, the frequency or duration of breastfeeds is reduced, bottle feeds are introduced, or the baby reaches six months of age.

TABLE III. (Adapted from P.M. Layde and V. Beral)
CIRCULATORY DISEASE MORTALITY RATES PER 100,000 WOMAN-YEARS BY AGE SMOKING STATUS AND ORAL CONTRACEPTIVE USE

AGE	EVER-USERS NON-SMOKERS	EVER-USERS SMOKERS	CONTROL NON-SMOKERS	CONTROL SMOKERS
15–24	0	10.5	0	0
25–34	4.4	14.2	2.7	4.2
35–44	21.5	63.4	6.4	15.2
45+	52.4	206.7	11.4	27.9

disease. Cohort studies have shown the relative risk to be somewhat lower, about 3 for new cases and about 4.5 for new cases requiring hospitalization. The risk of thromboembolic disease due to oral contraceptives is not related to length of use and disappears after pill use is stopped.

A two- to four-fold increase in the relative risk of postoperative thromboembolic complications has been reported with the use of oral contraceptives. The relative risk of venous thrombosis in women who have predisposing conditions is twice that of women without such medical conditions. If feasible, oral contraceptives should be discontinued from at least four weeks prior to and for two weeks after elective surgery of a type associated with an increase in risk of thromboembolism and during and following prolonged immobilization. Since the immediate postpartum period is also associated with an increased risk of thromboembolism,

TABLE IV
ANNUAL NUMBER OF BIRTH-RELATED OR METHOD-RELATED DEATHS ASSOCIATED WITH CONTROL OF FERTILITY PER 100,000 NONSTERILE WOMEN, BY FERTILITY-CONTROL METHOD ACCORDING TO AGE

Method of Control and Outcome	15–19	20–24	25–29	30–34	35–39	40–44
No fertility control methods[a]	7	7.4	9.1	14.8	25.7	28.2
Oral contraceptives nonsmoker[b]	0.3	0.5	0.9	1.9	13.8	31.6
Oral contraceptives smoker[b]	2.2	3.4	6.6	13.5	51.1	117.2
IUD[b]	0.8	0.8	1	1	1.4	1.4
Condom[a]	1.1	1.6	0.7	0.2	0.3	0.4
Diaphragm/spermicide[a]	1.9	1.2	1.2	1.3	2.2	2.8
Periodic abstinence[a]	2.5	1.6	1.6	1.7	2.9	3.6

a) Deaths are birth-related
b) Deaths are method-related
Adapted from H.W. Ory, Family Planning Perspectives, 15:57-63, 1983.

oral contraceptives should be started no earlier than four to six weeks after delivery.

Several studies have investigated the relative risks of thromboembolism in women using **YASMIN** compared to those in women using COCs containing other progestins. Two prospective cohort studies, both evaluating the risk of venous and arterial thromboembolism and death, were initiated at the time of **YASMIN** approval.[1, 2] The first (EURAS) showed the risk of thromboembolism (particularly venous thromboembolism) and death in **YASMIN** users to be comparable to that of other oral contraceptive preparations, including those containing levonorgestrel (a so-called second generation COC). The second prospective cohort study (Ingenix) also showed a comparable risk of thromboembolism in **YASMIN** users compared to users of other COCs, including those containing levonorgestrel. In the second study, COC comparator groups were selected based on their having similar characteristics to those being prescribed **YASMIN**.

Two additional epidemiological studies, one case-control study (van Hylckama Vlieg et al.[3]) and one retrospective cohort study (Lidegaard et al.[4]) suggested that the risk of venous thromboembolism occurring in **YASMIN** users was higher than that for users of levonorgestrel-containing COCs and lower than that for users of desogestrel/gestodenecontaining COCs (so-called third generation COCs). In the case-control study, however, the number of **YASMIN** cases was very small (1.2% of all cases) making the risk estimates unreliable. The relative risk for **YASMIN** users in the retrospective cohort study was greater than that for users of other COC products when considering women who used the products for less than one year. However, these one-year estimates may not be reliable because the analysis may include women of varying risk levels. Among women who used the product for 1 to 4 years, the relative risk was similar for users of **YASMIN** to that for users of other COC products.

c. Cerebrovascular diseases
Oral contraceptives have been shown to increase both the relative and attributable risks of cerebrovascular events (thrombotic and hemorrhagic strokes), although, in general, the risk is greatest among older (>35 years), hypertensive women who also smoke. Hypertension was found to be a risk factor, for both users and nonusers, for both types of strokes, while smoking interacted to increase the risk for hemorrhagic strokes.

In a large study, the relative risk of thrombotic strokes has been shown to range from 3 for normotensive users to 14 for users with severe hypertension. The relative risk of hemorrhagic stroke is reported to be 1.2 for nonsmokers who used oral contraceptives, 2.6 for smokers who did not use oral contraceptives, 7.6 for smokers who used oral contraceptives, 1.8 for normotensive users and 25.7 for users with severe hypertension. The attributable risk is also greater in older women.

d. Dose-related risk of vascular disease from oral contraceptives
A positive association has been observed between the amount of estrogen and progestogen in oral contraceptives and the risk of vascular disease. A decline in serum high-density lipoproteins (HDL) has been reported with many progestational agents. A decline in serum high-density lipoproteins has been associated with an increased incidence of ischemic heart disease. Because estrogens increase HDL cholesterol, the net effect of an oral contraceptive depends

on a balance achieved between doses of estrogen and progestogen and the nature and absolute amount of progestogen used in the contraceptive. The amount of both hormones should be considered in the choice of an oral contraceptive.

Minimizing exposure to estrogen and progestogen is in keeping with good principles of therapeutics. For any particular estrogen/progestogen combination, the dosage regimen prescribed should be one which contains the least amount of estrogen and progestogen that is compatible with a low failure rate and the needs of the individual patient. New acceptors of oral contraceptive agents should be started on preparations containing the lowest estrogen content which provides satisfactory results in the individual.

e. Persistence of risk of vascular disease
There are two studies which have shown persistence of risk of vascular disease for ever-users of oral contraceptives. In a study in the United States, the risk of developing myocardial infarction after discontinuing oral contraceptives persists for at least 9 years for women aged 40 to 49 years who had used oral contraceptives for five or more years, but this increased risk was not demonstrated in other age groups. In another study in Great Britain, the risk of developing cerebrovascular disease persisted for at least 6 years after discontinuation of oral contraceptives, although excess risk was very small. However, both studies were performed with oral contraceptive formulations containing 50 micrograms or higher of estrogens.

2. ESTIMATES OF MORTALITY FROM CONTRACEPTIVE USE
One study gathered data from a variety of sources which have estimated the mortality rate associated with different methods of contraception at different ages (Table IV). These estimates include the combined risk of death associated with contraceptive methods plus the risk attributable to pregnancy in the event of method failure. Each method of contraception has its specific benefits and risks. The study concluded that with the exception of oral contraceptive users 35 and older who smoke and 40 and older who do not smoke, mortality associated with all methods of birth control is below that associated with childbirth.

The observation of a possible increase in risk of mortality with age for oral contraceptive users is based on data gathered in the 1970's – but not reported until 1983. However, current clinical practice involves the use of lower estrogen dose formulations combined with careful restriction of oral contraceptive use to women who do not have the various risk factors listed in this labeling.

Because of these changes in practice and, also, because of some limited new data which suggest that the risk of cardiovascular disease with the use of oral contraceptives may now be less than previously observed, the Fertility and Maternal Health Drugs Advisory Committee was asked to review the topic in 1989. The Committee concluded that although cardiovascular disease risks may be increased with oral contraceptive use after age 40 in healthy nonsmoking women (even with the newer low-dose formulations), there are greater potential health risks associated with pregnancy in older women and with the alternative surgical and medical procedures which may be necessary if such women do not have access to effective and acceptable means of contraception.

Therefore, the Committee recommended that the benefits of oral contraceptive use by healthy nonsmoking women over

40 may outweigh the possible risks. Of course, women of all ages who take oral contraceptives, should take the lowest possible dose formulation that is effective.
[See table IV at left]

3. CARCINOMA OF THE REPRODUCTIVE ORGANS AND BREASTS
Numerous epidemiological studies have been performed on the incidence of breast, endometrial, ovarian and cervical cancer in women using oral contraceptives.

The risk of having breast cancer diagnosed may be slightly increased among current and recent users of COCs. However, this excess risk appears to decrease over time after COC discontinuation and by 10 years after cessation the increased risk disappears. The risk does not appear to increase with duration of use and no consistent relationships have been found with dose or type of steroid. Most studies show a similar pattern of risk with COC use regardless of a woman's reproductive history or her family breast cancer history. Some studies have found a small increase in risk for women who first use COCs before age 20.

Breast cancers diagnosed in current or previous OC users tend to be less clinically advanced than in nonusers.

Women who currently have or have had breast cancer should not use oral contraceptives because breast cancer is a hormonally-sensitive tumor.

Some studies suggest that oral contraceptive use has been associated with an increase in the risk of cervical intraepithelial neoplasia in some populations of women. However, there continues to be controversy about the extent to which such findings may be due to differences in sexual behavior and other factors.

In spite of many studies of the relationship between oral contraceptive use and breast and cervical cancers, a cause-and-effect relationship has not been established.

4. HEPATIC NEOPLASIA
Benign hepatic adenomas are associated with oral contraceptive use, although the incidence of benign tumors is rare in the United States. Indirect calculations have estimated the attributable risk to be in the range of 3.3 cases/100,000 for users, a risk that increases after four or more years of use. Rupture of rare, benign, hepatic adenomas may cause death through intra-abdominal hemorrhage.

Studies from Britain have shown an increased risk of developing hepatocellular carcinoma in long-term (>8 years) oral contraceptive users. However, these cancers are extremely rare in the U.S. and the attributable risk (the excess incidence) of liver cancers in oral contraceptive users approaches less than one per million users.

5. OCULAR LESIONS
There have been clinical case reports of retinal thrombosis associated with the use of oral contraceptives. Oral contraceptives should be discontinued if there is unexplained partial or complete loss of vision; onset of proptosis or diplopia; papilledema; or retinal vascular lesions. Appropriate diagnostic and therapeutic measures should be undertaken immediately.

6. ORAL CONTRACEPTIVE USE BEFORE OR DURING EARLY PREGNANCY
Extensive epidemiological studies have revealed no increased risk of birth defects in women who have used oral contraceptives prior to pregnancy. Studies also do not suggest a teratogenic effect, particularly in so far as cardiac anomalies and limb-reduction defects are concerned, when taken inadvertently during early pregnancy.

The administration of oral contraceptives to induce withdrawal bleeding should not be used as a test for pregnancy. Oral contraceptives should not be used during pregnancy to treat threatened or habitual abortion.

It is recommended that for any patient who has missed two consecutive periods, pregnancy should be ruled out. If the patient has not adhered to the prescribed dosing schedule, the possibility of pregnancy should be considered at the time of the first missed period. Oral contraceptive use should be discontinued if pregnancy is confirmed.

7. GALLBLADDER DISEASE
Earlier studies have reported an increased lifetime relative risk of gallbladder surgery in users of oral contraceptives and estrogens. More recent studies, however, have shown that the relative risk of developing gallbladder disease among oral contraceptive users may be minimal. The recent findings of minimal risk may be related to the use of oral contraceptive formulations containing lower hormonal doses of estrogens and progestogens.

8. CARBOHYDRATE AND LIPID METABOLIC EFFECTS
Oral contraceptives have been shown to cause glucose intolerance in a significant percentage of users. Oral contraceptives containing greater than 75 micrograms of estrogens cause hyperinsulinism, while lower doses of estrogen cause less glucose intolerance. Progestogens increase insulin secretion and create insulin resistance, this effect varying with different progestational agents. However, in the non-diabetic woman, oral contraceptives appear to have no effect on fasting blood glucose. Because of these demonstrated effects, prediabetic and diabetic women should be carefully observed while taking oral contraceptives.

A small proportion of women will have persistent hypertriglyceridemia while on the pill. As discussed earlier (see

WARNINGS, **1a** and **1d**), changes in serum triglycerides and lipoprotein levels have been reported in oral contraceptive users.

9. ELEVATED BLOOD PRESSURE

An increase in blood pressure has been reported in women taking oral contraceptives and this increase is more likely in older oral contraceptive users and with continued use. Data from the Royal College of General Practitioners and subsequent randomized trials have shown that the incidence of hypertension increases with increasing concentrations of progestogens.

Women with a history of hypertension or hypertension-related diseases, or renal disease should be encouraged to use another method of contraception. If women with hypertension elect to use oral contraceptives, they should be monitored closely, and if significant elevation of blood pressure occurs, oral contraceptives should be discontinued. For most women, elevated blood pressure will return to normal after stopping oral contraceptives and there is no difference in the occurrence of hypertension among ever- and never-users.

10. HEADACHE

The onset or exacerbation of migraine or development of headache with a new pattern which is recurrent, persistent or severe requires discontinuation of oral contraceptives and evaluation of the cause.

11. BLEEDING IRREGULARITIES

Breakthrough bleeding and spotting are sometimes encountered in patients on oral contraceptives, especially during the first three months of use. Nonhormonal causes should be considered and adequate diagnostic measures taken to rule out malignancy or pregnancy in the event of breakthrough bleeding, as in the case of any abnormal vaginal bleeding. If pathology has been excluded, time or a change to another formulation may solve the problem. In the event of amenorrhea, pregnancy should be ruled out.

Some women may encounter post-pill amenorrhea or oligomenorrhea, especially when such a condition was pre-existent.

PRECAUTIONS

1. GENERAL

Patients should be counseled that this product does not protect against HIV infection (AIDS) and other sexually transmitted diseases.

2. PHYSICAL EXAMINATION AND FOLLOW-UP

It is good medical practice for all women to have annual history and physical examinations, including women using oral contraceptives. The physical examination, however, may be deferred until after initiation of oral contraceptives if requested by the woman and judged appropriate by the clinician. The physical examination should include special reference to blood pressure, breasts, abdomen and pelvic organs, including cervical cytology and relevant laboratory tests. In case of undiagnosed, persistent or recurrent abnormal vaginal bleeding, appropriate measures should be conducted to rule out malignancy. Women with a strong family history of breast cancer or who have breast nodules should be monitored with particular care.

3. LIPID DISORDERS

Women who are being treated for hyperlipidemias should be followed closely if they elect to use oral contraceptives. Some progestogens may elevate LDL levels and may render the control of hyperlipidemias more difficult.

4. LIVER FUNCTION

If jaundice develops in any woman receiving oral contraceptives, the medication should be discontinued. Steroid hormones may be poorly metabolized in patients with impaired liver function.

5. FLUID RETENTION

Oral contraceptives may cause some degree of fluid retention. They should be prescribed with caution, and only with careful monitoring, in patients with conditions which might be aggravated by fluid retention.

6. EMOTIONAL DISORDERS

Women with a history of depression should be carefully observed and the drug discontinued if depression recurs to a serious degree.

7. CONTACT LENSES

Contact-lens wearers who develop visual changes or changes in lens tolerance should be assessed by an ophthalmologist.

8. DRUG INTERACTIONS

Effects of Other Drugs on Combined Hormonal Contraceptives

Rifampin

Metabolism of ethinyl estradiol and some progestins (e.g., norethindrone) is increased by rifampin. A reduction in contraceptive effectiveness and an increase in menstrual irregularities have been associated with concomitant use of rifampin.

Anticonvulsants

Anticonvulsants such as phenobarbital, phenytoin, and carbamazepine have been shown to increase the metabolism of ethinyl estradiol and/or some progestins, which could result in a reduction of contraceptive effectiveness.

Antibiotics

Pregnancy while taking combined hormonal contraceptives has been reported when the combined hormonal contraceptives were administered with antimicrobials such as ampicillin, tetracycline, and griseofulvin. However, clinical pharmacokinetic studies have not demonstrated any consistent effects of antibiotics (other than rifampin) on plasma concentrations of synthetic steroids.

Atorvastatin

Coadministration of atorvastatin and an oral contraceptive increased AUC values for norethindrone and ethinyl estradiol by approximately 30% and 20%, respectively.

St. John's Wort

Herbal products containing St. John's Wort (hypericum perforatum) may induce hepatic enzymes (cytochrome P450) and p-glycoprotein transporter and may reduce the effectiveness of oral contraceptives and emergency contraceptive pills. This may also result in breakthrough bleeding.

Other

Ascorbic acid and acetaminophen may increase plasma concentrations of some synthetic estrogens, possibly by inhibition of conjugation. A reduction in contraceptive effectiveness and an increased incidence of menstrual irregularities has been suggested with phenylbutazone.

Effects of Drospirenone on Other Drugs

Metabolic Interactions

Metabolism of DRSP and potential effects of DRSP on hepatic cytochrome P450 (CYP) enzymes have been investigated in *in vitro* and *in vivo* studies (see **Metabolism**). In *in vitro* studies DRSP did not affect turnover of model substrates of CYP1A2 and CYP2D6, but had an inhibitory influence on the turnover of model substrates of CYP1A1, CYP2C9, CYP2C19 and CYP3A4 with CYP2C19 being the most sensitive enzyme.

The potential effect of DRSP on CYP2C19 activity was investigated in a clinical pharmacokinetic study using omeprazole as a marker substrate. In the study with 24 postmenopausal women [including 12 women with homozygous (wild type) CYP2C19 genotype and 12 women with heterozygous CYP2C19 genotype] the daily oral administration of 3 mg DRSP for 14 days did not affect the oral clearance of omeprazole (40 mg, single oral dose). Based on the available results of *in vivo* and *in vitro* studies it can be concluded that, at clinical dose level, DRSP shows little propensity to interact to a significant extent with cytochrome P450 enzymes.

Interactions With Drugs That Have The Potential To Increase Serum Potassium

There is a potential for an increase in serum potassium in women taking **YASMIN** with other drugs (see **BOLDED WARNINGS**). Of note, occasional or chronic use of NSAID medication was not restricted in any of the **YASMIN** clinical trials.

A drug-drug interaction study of DRSP 3 mg/estradiol (E2) 1 mg versus placebo was performed in 24 mildly hypertensive postmenopausal women taking enalapril maleate 10 mg twice daily. Potassium levels were obtained every other day for a total of 2 weeks in all subjects. Mean serum potassium levels in the DRSP/E2 treatment group relative to baseline were 0.22 mEq/L higher than those in the placebo group. Serum potassium concentrations also were measured at multiple timepoints over 24 hours at baseline and on Day 14. On Day 14, the ratios for serum potassium C_{max} and AUC in the DRSP/E2 group to those in the placebo group were 0.955 (90% CI: 0.914, 0.999) and 1.01 (90% CI: 0.944, 1.08), respectively. No patient in either treatment group developed hyperkalemia (serum potassium concentrations > 5.5 mEq/L).

Effects of Combined Hormonal Contraceptives on Other Drugs

Combined oral contraceptives containing ethinyl estradiol may inhibit the metabolism of other compounds. Increased plasma concentrations of cyclosporine, prednisolone, and theophylline have been reported with concomitant administration of oral contraceptives. In addition, oral contraceptives may induce the conjugation of other compounds. Decreased plasma concentrations of acetaminophen and increased clearance on temazepam, salicylic acid, morphine, and clofibric acid have been noted when these drugs were administered with oral contraceptives.

9. INTERACTIONS WITH LABORATORY TESTS

Certain endocrine- and liver-function tests and blood components may be affected by oral contraceptives:

a. Increased prothrombin and factors VII, VIII, IX and X; decreased antithrombin 3; increased norepinephrine-induced platelet aggregability.

b. Increased thyroid-binding globulin (TBG) leading to increased circulating total thyroid hormone, as measured by protein-bound iodine (PBI), T4 by column or by radio-immunoassay. Free T3 resin uptake is decreased, reflecting the elevated TBG, free T4 concentration is unaltered.

c. Other binding proteins may be elevated in serum.

d. Sex-hormone-binding globulins are increased and result in elevated levels of total circulating sex steroids and corticoids; however, free or biologically active levels remain unchanged.

e. Triglycerides may be increased.

f. Glucose tolerance may be decreased.

g. Serum folate levels may be depressed by oral contraceptive therapy. This may be of clinical significance if a woman becomes pregnant shortly after discontinuing oral contraceptives.

10. CARCINOGENESIS, MUTAGENESIS, IMPAIRMENT OF FERTILITY

In a 24 month oral carcinogenicity study in mice dosed with 10 mg/kg/day drospirenone alone or 1 + 0.01, 3 + 0.03 and 10 + 0.1 mg/kg/day of drospirenone and ethinyl estradiol, 0.1 to 2 times the exposure (AUC of drospirenone) of women taking a contraceptive dose, there was an increase in carcinomas of the harderian gland in the group that received the high dose of drospirenone alone. In a similar study in rats given 10 mg/kg/day drospirenone alone or 0.3 + 0.003, 3 + 0.03 and 10 + 0.1 mg/kg/day drospirenone and ethinyl estradiol, 0.8 to 10 times the exposure of women taking a contraceptive dose, there was an increased incidence of benign and total (benign and malignant) adrenal gland pheochromocytomas in the group receiving the high dose of drospirenone. Drospirenone was not mutagenic in a number of *in vitro* (Ames, Chinese Hamster Lung gene mutation and chromosomal damage in human lymphocytes) and *in vivo* (mouse micronucleus) genotoxicity tests. Drospirenone increased unscheduled DNA synthesis in rat hepatocytes and formed adducts with rodent liver DNA but not with human liver DNA. See **WARNINGS**.

11. PREGNANCY

Pregnancy category X. See **CONTRAINDICATIONS** and **WARNINGS**.

Estrogens and progestins should not be used during pregnancy. Fourteen pregnancies that occurred with **YASMIN** exposure *in utero* (none with more than a single cycle of exposure) have been identified. One infant was born with esophageal atresia. A causal association with **YASMIN** is unknown.

A teratology study in pregnant rats given drospirenone orally at doses of 5, 15 and 45 mg/kg/day, 6 to 50 times the human exposure based on AUC of drospirenone, resulted in an increased number of fetuses with delayed ossification of bones of the feet in the two higher doses. A similar study in rabbits dosed orally with 1, 30 and 100 mg/kg/day drospirenone, 2 to 27 times the human exposure, resulted in an increase in fetal loss and retardation of fetal development (delayed ossification of small bones, multiple fusions of ribs) at the high dose only. When drospirenone was administered with ethinyl estradiol (100:1) during late pregnancy (the period of genital development) at doses of 5, 15 and 45 mg/kg, there was a dose dependent increase in feminization of male rat fetuses. In a study in 36 cynomolgous monkeys, no teratogenic or feminization effects were observed with orally administered drospirenone and ethinyl estradiol (100:1) at doses up to 10 mg/kg/day drospirenone, 30 times the human exposure.

12. NURSING MOTHERS

Small amounts of oral contraceptive steroids have been identified in the milk of nursing mothers, and a few adverse effects on the child have been reported, including jaundice and breast enlargement. In addition, oral contraceptives given in the postpartum period may interfere with lactation by decreasing the quantity and quality of breast milk. If possible, the nursing mother should be advised not to use oral contraceptives but to use other forms of contraception until she has completely weaned her child.

After oral administration of **YASMIN** about 0.02% of the drospirenone dose was excreted into the breast milk of postpartum women within 24 hours. This results in a maximal daily dose of about 3 mcg drospirenone in an infant.

13. PEDIATRIC USAGE

Safety and efficacy of **YASMIN** have been established in women of reproductive age. Safety and efficacy are expected to be the same for postpubertal adolescents under the age of 16 and for users 16 years and older. Use of this product before menarche is not indicated.

INFORMATION FOR THE PATIENT

See Patient Labeling printed below.

ADVERSE REACTIONS

An increased risk of the following serious adverse reactions has been associated with the use of oral contraceptives (see **WARNINGS**).

- Thrombophlebitis
- Arterial thromboembolism
- Pulmonary embolism
- Myocardial infarction

- Cerebral hemorrhage
- Cerebral thrombosis
- Hypertension
- Gallbladder disease
- Hepatic adenomas or benign liver tumors

There is evidence of an association between the following conditions and the use of oral contraceptives, although additional confirmatory studies are needed:

- Mesenteric thrombosis
- Retinal thrombosis

The following adverse reactions have been reported in patients receiving oral contraceptives and are believed to be drug-related:

- Nausea
- Vomiting
- Gastrointestinal symptoms (such as abdominal cramps and bloating)
- Breakthrough bleeding
- Spotting
- Change in menstrual flow
- Amenorrhea
- Temporary infertility after discontinuation of treatment
- Edema
- Melasma which may persist
- Breast changes: tenderness, enlargement, secretion
- Change in weight (increase or decrease)
- Change in cervical erosion and secretion
- Diminution in lactation when given immediately postpartum
- Cholestatic jaundice
- Migraine
- Rash (allergic)
- Mental depression
- Reduced tolerance to carbohydrates
- Vaginal candidiasis
- Change in corneal curvature (steepening)
- Intolerance to contact lenses

The following adverse reactions have been reported in users of oral contraceptives and a causal association has been neither confirmed nor refuted:

- Acne
- Budd-Chiari syndrome
- Cataracts
- Changes in appetite
- Changes in libido
- Colitis
- Cystitis-like syndrome
- Dizziness
- Erythema multiforme
- Erythema nodosum
- Headache
- Hemolytic uremic syndrome
- Hemorrhagic eruption
- Hirsutism
- Impaired renal function
- Loss of scalp hair
- Nervousness
- Porphyria
- Pre-menstrual syndrome
- Vaginitis

The following are the most common adverse events reported with use of **YASMIN** during the clinical trials, occurring in > 1% of subjects and which may or may not be drug-related: Headache, Menstrual Disorder, Breast Pain, Abdominal Pain, Nausea, Leukorrhea, Flu Syndrome, Acne, Vaginal Moniliasis, Depression, Diarrhea, Asthenia, Dysmenorrhea, Back Pain, Infection, Pharyngitis, Intermenstrual Bleeding, Migraine, Vomiting, Dizziness, Nervousness, Vaginitis, Sinusitis, Cystitis, Bronchitis, Gastroenteritis, Allergic Reaction, Urinary Tract Infection, Pruritus, Emotional Lability, Surgery, Rash, Upper Respiratory Infection.

OVERDOSAGE

Serious ill effects have not been reported following acute ingestion of large doses of other oral contraceptives by young children. Overdosage may cause nausea, and withdrawal bleeding may occur in females. Drospirenone, however, is a spironolactone analogue which has antimineralocorticoid properties. Serum concentration of potassium and sodium, and evidence of metabolic acidosis, should be monitored in cases of overdose.

NON-CONTRACEPTIVE HEALTH BENEFITS

The following non-contraceptive health benefits related to the use of oral contraceptives are supported by epidemiological studies which largely utilized oral contraceptive formulations containing doses exceeding 0.035 mg of ethinyl estradiol or 0.05 mg mestranol.
Effects on menses

- increased menstrual cycle regularity
- decreased blood loss and decreased incidence of iron-deficiency anemia
- decreased incidence of dysmenorrhea

Effects related to inhibition of ovulation

- decreased incidence of functional ovarian cysts
- decreased incidence of ectopic pregnancies

Effects from long-term use

- decreased incidence of fibroadenomas and fibrocystic disease of the breast
- decreased incidence of acute pelvic inflammatory disease
- decreased incidence of endometrial cancer
- decreased incidence of ovarian cancer

DOSAGE AND ADMINISTRATION

YASMIN

To achieve maximum contraceptive effectiveness, **YASMIN** (drospirenone and ethinyl estradiol) must be taken exactly as directed at intervals not exceeding 24 hours.

YASMIN consists of 21 tablets of a monophasic combined hormonal preparation plus 7 inert tablets. The dosage of **YASMIN** is one yellow tablet daily for 21 consecutive days followed by 7 white inert tablets per menstrual cycle. A patient should begin to take **YASMIN** either on the first day of her menstrual period (Day 1 Start) or on the first Sunday after the onset of her menstrual period (Sunday Start).

Day 1 Start. During the first cycle of **YASMIN** use, the patient should be instructed to take one yellow **YASMIN** daily, beginning on day one (1) of her menstrual cycle. (The first day of menstruation is day one.) She should take one yellow **YASMIN** daily for 21 consecutive days, followed by one white inert tablet daily on menstrual cycle days 22 through 28. It is recommended that **YASMIN** be taken at the same time each day, preferably after the evening meal or at bedtime. If **YASMIN** is first taken later than the first day of the menstrual cycle, **YASMIN** should not be considered effective as a contraceptive until after the first 7 consecutive days of product administration. The possibility of ovulation and conception prior to initiation of medication should be considered.

Sunday Start. During the first cycle of **YASMIN** use, the patient should be instructed to take one yellow **YASMIN** daily, beginning on the first Sunday after the onset of her menstrual period. She should take one yellow **YASMIN** daily for 21 consecutive days, followed by one white inert tablet daily on menstrual cycle days 22 through 28. It is recommended that **YASMIN** be taken at the same time each day, preferably after the evening meal or at bedtime. **YASMIN** should not be considered effective as a contraceptive until after the first 7 consecutive days of product administration. The possibility of ovulation and conception prior to initiation of medication should be considered.

The patient should begin her next and all subsequent 28-day regimens of **YASMIN** on the same day of the week that she began her first regimen, following the same schedule. She should begin taking her yellow tablets on the next day after ingestion of the last white tablet, regardless of whether or not a menstrual period has occurred or is still in progress. Anytime a subsequent cycle of **YASMIN** is started later than the day following administration of the last white tablet, the patient should use another method of contraception until she has taken a yellow **YASMIN** daily for seven consecutive days.

When switching from another oral contraceptive, **YASMIN** should be started on the same day that a new pack of the previous oral contraceptive would have been started.

Withdrawal bleeding usually occurs within 3 days following the last yellow tablet. If spotting or breakthrough bleeding occurs while taking **YASMIN**, the patient should be instructed to continue taking her **YASMIN** as instructed and by the regimen described above. She should be instructed that this type of bleeding is usually transient and without significance; however, if the bleeding is persistent or prolonged, the patient should be advised to consult her physician.

Although the occurrence of pregnancy is unlikely if **YASMIN** is taken according to directions, if withdrawal bleeding does not occur, the possibility of pregnancy must be considered. If the patient has not adhered to the prescribed dosing schedule (missed one or more active tablets or started taking them on a day later than she should have), the possibility of pregnancy should be considered at the time of the first missed period and appropriate diagnostic measures taken. If the patient has adhered to the prescribed regimen and misses two consecutive periods, pregnancy should be ruled out. Hormonal contraception should be discontinued if pregnancy is confirmed.

The risk of pregnancy increases with each active yellow tablet missed. For additional patient instructions regarding missed pills, see the "WHAT TO DO IF YOU MISS PILLS" section in the DETAILED PATIENT LABELING which follows. If breakthrough bleeding occurs following missed tablets, it will usually be transient and of no consequence. If the patient misses one or more white tablets, she should still be protected against pregnancy provided she begins taking yellow tablets again on the proper day.

In the nonlactating mother, **YASMIN** may be initiated 4 weeks postpartum, for contraception. When the tablets are administered in the postpartum period, the increased risk of thromboembolic disease associated with the postpartum period must be considered. (See **CONTRAINDICATIONS, WARNINGS,** and **PRECAUTIONS** concerning thromboembolic disease.)

HOW SUPPLIED

YASMIN 28 Tablets (drospirenone and ethinyl estradiol) are available in packages of 3 BLISTER packs (NDC 50419-402-03).

Each pack contains 21 active yellow round, unscored, film coated tablets each containing 3 mg drospirenone and 0.03 mg ethinyl estradiol, and 7 inert white round, unscored, film coated tablets.

Store at 25° C (77°F); excursions permitted to 15–30°C (59–86°F). [See USP Controlled Room Temperature.]

REFERENCES

1. Dinger JC, Heinemann LAJ, et al: The safety of a drospirenone-containing oral contraceptive: final results from the European active surveillance study on oral contraceptives based on 142,475 women-years of observation. *Contraception* 2007;75:344-354.
2. Seeger JD, Loughlin J, Eng PM, et al: Risk of thromboembolism in women taking ethinylestradiol/drospirenone and other oral contraceptives. *Obstetrics & Gynecology* 2007;110(3):587-593.
3. van Hylckama Vlieg A, Helmerhorst FM, Vandenbroucke JP, et al: The venous thrombotic risk of oral contraceptives, effects of oestrogen dose and progestogen type: results of the MEGA case-control study. *BMJ* 2009;339:b2921.
4. Lidegaard O, Lokkegaard E, Svendsen AL, et al: Hormonal contraception and risk of venous thromboembolism: national follow-up study. *BMJ* 2009; 339:b2890.

Manufactured for:
Bayer HealthCare Pharmaceuticals Inc.
Manufactured in: Germany

BRIEF SUMMARY PATIENT PACKAGE INSERT

YASMIN® 28 Tablets
(drospirenone and ethinyl estradiol)
28 tablets containing the following:
21 yellow – "active" tablets
7 white – "inert" tablets

This product (like all oral contraceptives) is intended to prevent pregnancy. It does not protect against HIV infection (AIDS) and other sexually transmitted diseases.

YASMIN is different from other birth-control pills because it contains the progestin drospirenone. Drospirenone may increase potassium. Therefore, you should not take YASMIN if you have kidney, liver or adrenal disease because this could cause serious heart and health problems. Other drugs may also increase potassium. If you are currently on daily, long-term treatment for a chronic condition with any of the medications below, you should consult your healthcare provider about whether YASMIN is right for you, and during the first month that you take YASMIN, you should have a blood test to check your potassium level.

- **NSAIDs (ibuprofen [Motrin®, Advil®], naproxen [Naprosyn®, Aleve® and others] when taken long-term and for treatment of arthritis or other problems)**
- **Potassium-sparing diuretics (spironolactone and others)**
- **Potassium supplementation**
- **ACE inhibitors (Capoten®, Vasotec®, Zestril® and others)**
- **Angiotensin-II receptor antagonists (Cozaar®, Diovan®, Avapro® and others)**
- **Heparin**

Oral contraceptives, also known as "birth-control pills" or "the pill," are taken to prevent pregnancy, and when taken correctly, have a failure rate of less than 1% per year when used without missing any pills. The typical failure rate of large numbers of pill users is less than 5% per year when women who miss pills are included. However, forgetting to take pills considerably increases the chances of pregnancy. For the majority of women, oral contraceptives can be taken safely. But there are some women who are at high risk of developing certain serious diseases that can be life-threatening or may cause temporary or permanent disability or death. The risks associated with taking oral contraceptives increase significantly if you:

- smoke
- have high blood pressure, diabetes, high cholesterol
- have or have had clotting disorders, heart attack, stroke, angina pectoris, cancer of the breast or sex organs, jaundice, or malignant or benign liver tumors.

You should not take the pill if you suspect you are pregnant or have unexplained vaginal bleeding.

Cigarette smoking increases the risk of serious adverse effects on the heart and blood vessels from oral contraceptive use. This risk increases with age and with heavy smoking (15 or more cigarettes per day) and is quite marked in women over 35 years of age. Women who use oral contraceptives should not smoke.

Most side effects of the pill are not serious. The most common such effects are nausea, vomiting, bleeding between menstrual periods, weight gain, breast tenderness, and difficulty wearing contact lenses. These side effects, especially nausea and vomiting may subside within the first three months of use.

The serious side effects of the pill occur very infrequently, especially if you are in good health and are young. However, you should know that the following medical conditions have been associated with or made worse by the pill:

1. Blood clots in the legs (thrombophlebitis), lungs (pulmonary embolism), blockage or rupture of a blood vessel in the brain (stroke), blockage of blood vessels in the heart (heart attack and angina pectoris) or other organs of the body. As mentioned above, smoking increases the risk of heart attacks and strokes and subsequent serious medical consequences.

2. Liver tumors, which may rupture and cause severe bleeding. A possible but not definite association has been found with the pill and liver cancer. However, liver cancers are extremely rare. The chance of developing liver cancer from using the pill is thus even rarer.

3. High blood pressure, although blood pressure usually returns to normal when the pill is stopped.

4. Cancer of the breast. Various studies give conflicting reports on the relationship between breast cancer and oral contraceptive use. Oral contraceptive use may slightly increase your chance of having breast cancer diagnosed, particularly after using hormonal contraceptives at a younger age. After you stop using hormonal contraceptives, the chances of getting breast cancer begin to go back down. You should have regular breast examinations by a healthcare provider and examine your own breasts monthly. Tell your healthcare provider if you have a family history of breast cancer or if you have had breast nodules or an abnormal mammogram. Women who currently have or have had breast cancer should not use oral contraceptives because breast cancer is a hormone-sensitive tumor.

The symptoms associated with these serious side effects are discussed in the detailed leaflet given to you with your supply of pills. Notify your doctor or healthcare provider if you notice any unusual physical disturbances while taking the pill. In addition, drugs such as rifampin, as well as some anticonvulsants, some antibiotics and some herbal products such as St. John's Wort, may decrease oral contraceptive effectiveness.

Taking the pill provides some important non-contraceptive benefits. These include less painful menstruation, less menstrual blood loss and anemia, fewer pelvic infections, and fewer cancers of the ovary and the lining of the uterus.

Be sure to discuss any medical condition you may have with your healthcare provider. Your healthcare provider will take a medical and family history before prescribing oral contraceptives and will examine you. The physical examination may be delayed to another time if you request it and the healthcare provider believes that it is appropriate to postpone it. You should be reexamined at least once a year while taking oral contraceptives. The detailed patient information booklet gives you further information which you should read and discuss with your healthcare provider.

This product (like all oral contraceptives) is intended to prevent pregnancy. It does not protect against transmission of HIV (AIDS) and other sexually transmitted diseases such as chlamydia, genital herpes, genital warts, gonorrhea, hepatitis B, and syphilis.

INSTRUCTIONS TO PATIENTS

HOW TO TAKE THE PILL

IMPORTANT POINTS TO REMEMBER

***BEFORE* YOU START TAKING YOUR PILLS**

1. BE SURE TO READ THESE DIRECTIONS:
   Before you start taking your pills. Anytime you are not sure what to do.
2. THE RIGHT WAY TO TAKE THE PILL IS TO TAKE ONE PILL EVERY DAY AT THE SAME TIME.
   If you miss pills you could get pregnant. This includes starting the pack late. The more pills you miss, the more likely you are to get pregnant.
3. MANY WOMEN HAVE SPOTTING OR LIGHT BLEEDING, OR MAY FEEL SICK TO THEIR STOMACH DURING THE FIRST 1–3 PACKS OF PILLS.
   If you do have spotting or light bleeding or feel sick to your stomach, do not stop taking the pill. The problem will usually go away. If it does not go away, check with your doctor or healthcare provider.
4. MISSING PILLS CAN ALSO CAUSE SPOTTING OR LIGHT BLEEDING, even when you make up these missed pills.
   On the days you take two pills, to make up for missed pills, you could also feel a little sick to your stomach.
5. IF YOU HAVE VOMITING OR DIARRHEA, or IF YOU TAKE SOME MEDICINES, including some antibiotics and some herbal products such as St. John's Wort, your pills may not work as well.
   Use a back-up method (such as condoms or spermicides) until you check with your doctor or healthcare provider.
6. IF YOU HAVE TROUBLE REMEMBERING TO TAKE THE PILL, talk to your doctor or healthcare provider about how to make pill-taking easier or about using another method of birth control.
7. IF YOU HAVE ANY QUESTIONS OR ARE UNSURE ABOUT THE INFORMATION IN THIS LEAFLET, call your doctor or healthcare provider.

***BEFORE* YOU START TAKING YOUR PILLS**

1. DECIDE WHAT TIME OF DAY YOU WANT TO TAKE YOUR PILL.
   It is important to take it at about the same time every day.
2. LOOK AT YOUR PILL PACK - IT HAS 28 PILLS:
   The YASMIN pill pack has 21 yellow "active" pills (with hormones) to be taken for three weeks, followed by 7 white "reminder" pills (without hormones) to be taken for one week.
3. ALSO FIND:
   1) where on the pack to start taking pills,
   2) in what order to take the pills (follow the arrows)
   3) the week numbers as shown in the diagram below

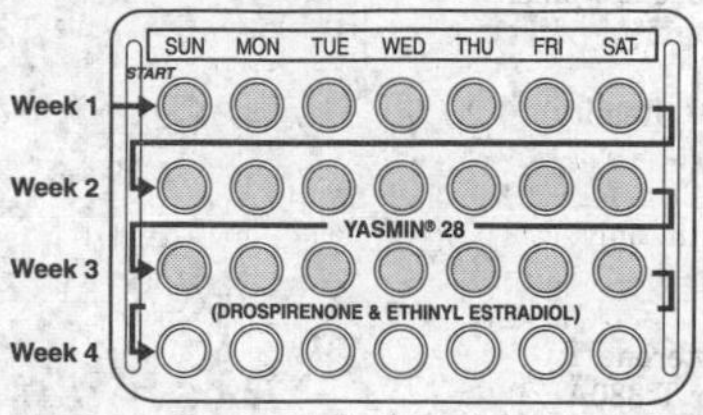

4. BE SURE YOU HAVE READY AT ALL TIMES:
   ANOTHER KIND OF BIRTH CONTROL such as condoms or spermicides) to use as a back-up in case you miss pills.
   AN EXTRA, FULL PILL PACK.

WHEN TO START THE FIRST PACK OF PILLS

You have a choice for which day to start taking your first pack of pills. Decide with your doctor or healthcare provider which is the best day for you. Pick a time of day which will be easy to remember.

DAY 1 START:

1. Take the first yellow "active" pill of the first pack during the *first 24 hours of your period.*
2. You will not need to use a back-up method of birth control, since you are starting the pill at the beginning of your period.

SUNDAY START:

1. Take the first yellow "active" pill of the first pack on the *Sunday after your period starts*, even if you are still bleeding. If your period begins on Sunday, start the pack that same day.
2. *Use another method of birth control* (such as condoms or spermicides) as a back-up method if you have sex any time from the Sunday you start your first pack until the next Sunday (7 days).

WHAT TO DO DURING THE MONTH

1. **TAKE ONE PILL AT THE SAME TIME EVERY DAY UNTIL THE PACK IS EMPTY**
   Do not skip pills even if you are spotting or bleeding between monthly periods or feel sick to your stomach (nausea).
   Do not skip pills even if you do not have sex very often.
2. **WHEN YOU FINISH A PACK OR SWITCH YOUR BRAND OF PILLS:**
   Start the next pack on the day after your last white "reminder" pill. Do not wait any days between packs.

WHAT TO DO IF YOU MISS PILLS

If you **MISS 1** yellow "active" pill:

1. Take it as soon as you remember. Take the next pill at your regular time. This means you may take two pills in one day.
2. You do not need to use a back-up birth control method if you have sex.

If you **MISS 2** yellow "active" pills in a row in **WEEK 1 OR WEEK 2** of your pack:

1. Take two pills on the day you remember and two pills the next day.
2. Then take one pill a day until you finish the pack.
3. You MAY BECOME PREGNANT if you have sex in the 7 *days* after you miss pills. You MUST use another birth control method (such as condoms or spermicides) as a back-up for those 7 days.

If you **MISS 2** yellow "active" pills in a row in the **3RD WEEK:**

1. ***If you are a Day 1 Starter:***
   THROW OUT the rest of the pill pack and start a new pack that same day.
   If you are a Sunday Starter:
   Keep taking one pill every day until Sunday. On Sunday, THROW OUT the rest of the pack and start a new pack of pills that same day.
2. You may not have your period this month but this is expected. However, if you miss your period two months in a row, call your doctor or healthcare provider because you might be pregnant.
3. You MAY BECOME PREGNANT if you have sex in the 7 *days* after you miss pills. You MUST use another birth control method (such as condoms or spermicides) as a back-up for those 7 days.

If you **MISS 3 OR MORE** yellow "active" pills in a row (during the first 3 weeks):

1. **If you are a Day 1 Starter:**
   THROW OUT the rest of the pill pack and start a new pack that same day.
   If you are a Sunday Starter:
   Keep taking 1 pill every day until Sunday. On Sunday, THROW OUT the rest of the pack and start a new pack of pills that same day.
2. You may not have your period this month but this is expected. However, if you miss your period two months in a row, call your doctor or healthcare provider because you might be pregnant.
3. You MAY BECOME PREGNANT if you have sex in the 7 days after you miss pills. You MUST use another birth control method (such as condoms or spermicides) as a back-up for those 7 days.

If you forget any of the 7 white "reminder" pills in Week 4:

THROW AWAY the pills you missed.

Keep taking one pill each day until the pack is empty.

You do not need a back-up method.

FINALLY, IF YOU ARE STILL NOT SURE WHAT TO DO ABOUT THE PILLS YOU HAVE MISSED:

Use a BACK-UP METHOD (such as condoms or spermicides) anytime you have sex.

KEEP TAKING ONE ACTIVE PILL EACH DAY until you can reach your doctor or healthcare provider.

For additional information see Detailed Patient Labeling

DETAILED PATIENT PACKAGE INSERT

This product (like all oral contraceptives) is intended to prevent pregnancy. It does not protect against HIV infection (AIDS) and other sexually transmitted diseases.

YASMIN is different from other birth-control pills because it contains the progestin drospirenone. Drospirenone may increase potassium. Therefore, you should not take YASMIN if you have kidney, liver or adrenal disease because this could cause serious heart and health problems. Other drugs may also increase potassium. If you are currently on daily, long-term treatment for a chronic condition with any of the medications below, you should consult your healthcare provider about whether YASMIN is right for you, and during the first month that you take YASMIN, you should have a blood test to check your potassium level.

- NSAIDs (ibuprofen [Motrin®, Advil®], naproxen [Naprosyn®, Aleve®and others] when taken long-term and for treatment of arthritis or other problems)
- Potassium-sparing diuretics (spironolactone and others)
- Potassium supplementation
- ACE inhibitors (Capoten®, Vasotec®, Zestril® and others)
- Angiotensin-II receptor antagonists (Cozaar®, Diovan®, Avapro® and others)
- Heparin

INTRODUCTION

Any woman who considers using oral contraceptives (the birth-control pill or "the pill") should understand the benefits and risks of using this form of birth control. This leaflet will give you much of the information you will need to make this decision and will also help you determine if you are at risk of developing any of the serious side effects of the pill. It will tell you how to use the pill properly so that it will be as effective as possible. However, this leaflet is not a replacement for a careful discussion between you and your healthcare provider. You should discuss the information provided in this leaflet with him or her, both when you first start taking the pill and during your revisits. You should also follow your healthcare provider's advice with regard to regular check-ups while you are on the pill.

EFFECTIVENESS OF ORAL CONTRACEPTIVES

Oral contraceptives or "birth-control pills" or "the pill" are used to prevent pregnancy and are more effective than other nonsurgical methods of birth control. When they are taken correctly, the chance of becoming pregnant is less than 1% (one pregnancy per 100 women per year of use) when used perfectly, without missing any pills. Typical failure rates, including women who don't always follow the instructions exactly, are about 5% per year. The chance of becoming pregnant increases with each missed pill during a menstrual cycle.

In comparison, typical failure rates for other nonsurgical methods of birth control during the first year of use are as follows:

[See table at right]

WHO SHOULD NOT TAKE ORAL CONTRACEPTIVES

Cigarette smoking increases the risk of serious adverse effects on the heart and blood vessels from oral contraceptive use. This risk increases with age and with heavy smoking (15 or more cigarettes per day) and is quite marked in women over 35 years of age. Women who use YASMIN should not smoke.

Some women should not use the pill. For example, you should not take YASMIN if you are pregnant or think you may be pregnant. You should also not use YASMIN if you have had any of the following conditions:

- A history of heart attack or stroke
- Blood clots in the legs (thrombophlebitis), lungs (pulmonary embolism), brain (stroke) or eyes
- A history of blood clots in the deep veins of your legs
- Chest pain (angina pectoris)
- Known or suspected breast cancer or cancer of the lining of the uterus, cervix or vagina
- Unexplained vaginal bleeding (until a diagnosis is reached by your doctor)
- Yellowing of the whites of the eyes or of the skin (jaundice) during pregnancy or during previous use of the pill
- Liver tumor (benign or cancerous)
- Known or suspected pregnancy

In addition, you should not use YASMIN if you have any of the following conditions:

- Kidney Disease
- Liver Disease
- Adrenal Disease

Tell your healthcare provider if you have ever had any of the above conditions (Your healthcare provider can recommend another method of birth control). If you are currently on daily, long-term treatment for a chronic condition with any of the following medications, you should consult your healthcare provider before taking YASMIN:

- NSAIDs (ibuprofen, naproxen and others)
- Potassium-sparing diuretics (spironolactone and others)
- Potassium supplementation
- ACE inhibitors (captopril, enalapril, lisinopril and others)
- Angiotensin-II receptor antagonists (Cozaar®, Diovan®, Avapro® and others)
- Heparin

OTHER CONSIDERATIONS BEFORE TAKING ORAL CONTRACEPTIVES

Tell your healthcare provider if you or any family member has ever had:

- Breast nodules, fibrocystic disease of the breast, an abnormal breast X-ray or mammogram
- Diabetes
- Elevated cholesterol or triglycerides
- High blood pressure
- Migraine or other headaches or epilepsy
- Mental depression
- Gallbladder, heart or kidney disease
- History of scanty or irregular menstrual periods

Women with any of these conditions should be checked often by their healthcare provider if they choose to use oral contraceptives.

Also, be sure to inform your doctor or healthcare provider if you smoke or take any medications.

RISKS OF TAKING ORAL CONTRACEPTIVES

1. RISK OF DEVELOPING BLOOD CLOTS

Blood clots and blockage of blood vessels are the most serious side effects of taking oral contraceptives and can be fatal. In particular, a clot in the legs can cause thrombophlebitis and a clot that travels to the lungs can cause sudden blocking of the vessel carrying blood to the lungs. Rarely, clots occur in the blood vessels of the eye and may cause blindness, double vision, or impaired vision.

If you take oral contraceptives and need elective surgery, need to stay in bed for a prolonged illness or have recently delivered a baby, you may be at risk of developing blood clots. You should consult your doctor about stopping oral contraceptives three to four weeks before surgery and not taking oral contraceptives for two weeks after surgery or during bed rest. You should also not take oral contraceptives soon after delivery of a baby or a mid-trimester pregnancy loss or termination. It is advisable to wait for at least four weeks after delivery if you are not breast-feeding. If you are breast-feeding, you should wait until you have weaned your child before using the pill. (See also the section on breast-feeding in GENERAL PRECAUTIONS.)

2. HEART ATTACKS AND STROKES

Oral contraceptives may increase the tendency to develop strokes (stoppage or rupture of blood vessels in the brain) and angina pectoris and heart attacks (blockage of blood vessels in the heart). Any of these conditions can cause death or serious disability.

Smoking greatly increases the possibility of suffering heart attacks and strokes. Furthermore, smoking and the use of oral contraceptives greatly increase the chances of developing and dying of heart disease.

Percentage of women experiencing an unintended pregnancy during the first year of typical use and first year of perfect use of contraception and the percentage continuing use at the end of the first year: United States.

Method (1)	% of Women Experiencing an Accidental Pregnancy Within the First Year of Use		% of Women Continuing Use At One Year[a] (4)
	Typical Use[b] (2)	Perfect Use[c] (3)	
Chance[d]	85	85	
Spermicides[e]	26	6	40
Periodic abstinence	25		63
Calendar		9	
Ovulation method		3	
Sympto-thermal[f]		2	
Post-ovulation		1	
Withdrawal	19	4	
Cap[g]			
Parous women	40	26	42
Nulliparous women	20	9	56
Sponge			
Parous women	40	20	42
Nulliparous women	20	9	56
Diaphragm[g]	20	6	56
Condom[h]			
Female (Reality)	21	5	56
Male	14	3	61
Pill	5		71
progestin only		0.5	
combined		0.1	
IUD			
Progesterone T:	2	1.5	81
Copper T 380A	0.8	0.6	78
Lng 20	0.1	0.1	81
Depo Provera	0.3	0.3	70
Norplant and Norplant-2	0.05	0.05	88
Female Sterilization	0.5	0.5	100
Male Sterilization	0.15	0.1	100

Emergency Contraceptive Pills: Treatment initiated within 72 hours after unprotected intercourse reduces the risk of pregnancy by at least 75%[i]

Lactational Amenorrhea Method: LAM is highly effective, *temporary* method of contraception[j]

Source: Trussell J, Contraceptive efficacy. In Hatcher RA, Trussell J, Stewart F, Cates W, Stewart GK, Kowal D, Guest F, Contraceptive Technology: Seventeenth Revised Edition. New York NY: Irvington Publishers, 1998.

a) Among couples attempting to avoid pregnancy, the percentage who continue to use a method for one year.

b) Among *typical* couples who initiate use of a method (not necessarily for the first time), the percentage who experience an accidental pregnancy during the first year if they do not stop use for any other reason.

c) Among couples who initiate use of a method (not necessarily for the first time) and who use it *perfectly* (both consistently and correctly), the percentage who experience an accidental pregnancy during the first year if they do not stop use for any reason.

d) The percents becoming pregnant in columns (2) and (3) are based on data from populations where contraception is not used and from women who cease using contraception in order to become pregnant. Among such populations, about 89% become pregnant within one year. This estimate was lowered slightly (to 85%) to represent the percentage who would become pregnant within one year among women now relying on reversible methods of contraception if they abandoned contraception altogether.

e) Foams, creams, gels, vaginal suppositories, and vaginal film.

f) Cervical mucus (ovulation) method supplemented by calendar in the pre-ovulatory and basal body temperature in the post-ovulatory phases.

g) With spermicidal cream or jelly.

h) Without spermicides.

i) The treatment schedule is one dose within 72 hours after unprotected intercourse, and a second dose 12 hours after the first dose. The Food and Drug Administration has declared the following brands of oral contraceptives to be safe and effective for emergency contraception: Ovral (1 dose is 2 white pills), Alesse (1 dose is 5 pink pills), Nordette or Levlen (1 dose is 2 light-orange pills), Lo/Ovral (1 dose is 4 white pills), Triphasil or Tri-Levlen (1 dose is 4 yellow pills).

j) However, to maintain effective protection against pregnancy, another method of contraception must be used as soon as menstruation resumes, the frequency or duration of breastfeeds is reduced, bottle feeds are introduced, or the baby reaches six months of age.

3. GALLBLADDER DISEASE

Oral contraceptive users probably have a greater risk than nonusers of having gallbladder disease, although this risk may be related to pills containing high doses of estrogens.

4. LIVER TUMORS

In rare cases, oral contraceptives can cause benign but dangerous liver tumors. These benign liver tumors can rupture and cause fatal internal bleeding. In addition, a possible but not definite association has been found with the pill and liver cancers in two studies, in which a few women who developed these very rare cancers were found to have used oral contraceptives for long periods. However, liver cancers are extremely rare. The chance of developing liver cancer from using the pill is thus even rarer.

5. CANCER OF THE REPRODUCTIVE ORGANS AND BREASTS

Various studies give conflicting reports on the relationship between breast cancer and oral contraceptive use. Oral contraceptive use may slightly increase your chance of having breast cancer diagnosed, particularly after using hormonal contraceptives at a younger age. After you stop using hormonal contraceptives, the chances of getting breast cancer begin to go back down. You should have regular breast examinations by a healthcare provider and examine your own breasts monthly. Tell your healthcare provider if you have a family history of breast cancer or if you have had breast nodules or an abnormal mammogram. Women who currently have or have had breast cancer should not use oral contraceptives because breast cancer is a hormone-sensitive tumor.

Some studies have found an increase in the incidence of cancer of the cervix in women who use oral contraceptives. However, this finding may be related to factors other than the use of oral contraceptives.

ESTIMATED RISK OF DEATH FROM A BIRTH CONTROL METHOD OR PREGNANCY

All methods of birth control and pregnancy are associated with a risk of developing certain diseases which may lead to disability or death. An estimate of the number of deaths associated with different methods of birth control and pregnancy has been calculated and is shown in the following table.

[See table at top of next page]

In the above table, the risk of death from any birth-control method is less than the risk of childbirth, except for oral contraceptive users over the age of 35 who smoke and pill users over the age of 40 even if they do not smoke. It can be seen in the table that for women aged 15 to 39, the risk of death was highest with pregnancy (7–26 deaths per 100,000 women, depending on age). Among pill users who do not smoke, the risk of death was always lower than that associated with pregnancy for any age group, except for those women over the age of 40, when the risk increases to 32 deaths per 100,000 women, compared to 28 associated with pregnancy at that age. However, for pill users who smoke and are over the age of 35, the estimated number of deaths exceeds those for other methods of birth control. If a woman is over the age of 40 and smokes, her estimated risk of death is four times higher (117/100,000 women) than the estimated risk associated with pregnancy (28/100,000 women) in that age group.

The suggestion that women over 40 who do not smoke should not take oral contraceptives is based on information from older high-dose pills and on less-selective use of pills than is practiced today. An Advisory Committee of the FDA discussed this issue in 1989 and recommended that the benefits of oral contraceptive use by healthy, non-smoking women over 40 years of age may outweigh the possible risks. However, all women, especially older women, are cautioned to use the lowest-dose pill that is effective.

WARNING SIGNALS

If any of these adverse effects occur while you are taking oral contraceptives, call your doctor immediately:

- Sharp chest pain, coughing of blood, or sudden shortness of breath (indicating a possible clot in the lung)
- Pain in the calf (indicating a possible clot in the leg)
- Crushing chest pain or heaviness in the chest (indicating a possible heart attack)
- Sudden severe headache or vomiting, dizziness or fainting, disturbances of vision or speech, weakness, or numbness in an arm or leg (indicating a possible stroke)
- Sudden partial or complete loss of vision (indicating a possible clot in the eye)
- Breast lumps (indicating possible breast cancer or fibrocystic disease of the breast; ask your doctor or healthcare provider to show you how to examine your breasts)
- Severe pain or tenderness in the stomach area (indicating a possibly ruptured liver tumor)
- Difficulty in sleeping, weakness, lack of energy, fatigue, or change in mood (possibly indicating severe depression)
- Jaundice or a yellowing of the skin or eyeballs, accompanied frequently by fever, fatigue, loss of appetite, dark-colored urine, or light-colored bowel movements (indicating possible liver problems)

SIDE EFFECTS OF ORAL CONTRACEPTIVES

1. VAGINAL BLEEDING

Irregular vaginal bleeding or spotting may occur while you are taking the pills. Irregular bleeding may vary from slight staining between menstrual periods to breakthrough bleeding, which is a flow much like a regular period. Irregular bleeding occurs most often during the first few months of oral contraceptive use, but may also occur after you have been taking the pill for some time. Such bleeding may be temporary and usually does not indicate any serious problems. It is important to continue taking your pills on schedule. If the bleeding occurs in more than one cycle or lasts for more than a few days, talk to your doctor or healthcare provider.

2. CONTACT LENSES

If you wear contact lenses and notice a change in vision or an inability to wear your lenses, contact your doctor or healthcare provider.

3. FLUID RETENTION

Oral contraceptives may cause edema (fluid retention) with swelling of the fingers or ankles and may raise your blood pressure. If you experience fluid retention, contact your doctor or healthcare provider.

4. MELASMA

A spotty darkening of the skin is possible, particularly of the face.

5. OTHER SIDE EFFECTS

Other side effects may include nausea, vomiting, change in appetite, headache, nervousness, depression, dizziness, loss of scalp hair, rash, and vaginal infections.

If any of these side effects occur, call your doctor or healthcare provider.

GENERAL PRECAUTIONS

1. Missed periods and use of oral contraceptives before or during early pregnancy.

There may be times when you may not menstruate regularly after you have completed taking a cycle of pills. If you have taken your pills regularly and miss one menstrual period, continue taking your pills for the next cycle but be sure to inform your healthcare provider before doing so. If you have not taken the pills daily as instructed and missed a menstrual period, or if you missed two consecutive menstrual periods, you may be pregnant. Check with your healthcare provider immediately to determine whether you are pregnant. Stop taking oral contraceptives if pregnancy is confirmed.

There is no conclusive evidence that oral contraceptive use is associated with an increase in birth defects when taken inadvertently during early pregnancy. Previously, a few studies had reported that oral contraceptives might be associated with birth defects, but these studies have not been

ANNUAL NUMBER OF BIRTH-RELATED OR METHOD-RELATED DEATHS ASSOCIATED WITH CONTROL OF FERTILITY PER 100,000 NONSTERILE WOMEN, BY FERTILITY-CONTROL METHOD ACCORDING TO AGE

Method of Control and Outcome	15–19	20–24	25–29	30–34	35–39	40–44
No fertility control methods[a]	7	7.4	9.1	14.8	25.7	28.2
Oral contraceptives nonsmoker[b]	0.3	0.5	0.9	1.9	13.8	31.6
Oral contraceptives smoker[b]	2.2	3.4	6.6	13.5	51.1	117.2
IUD[b]	0.8	0.8	1	1	1.4	1.4
Condom[a]	1.1	1.6	0.7	0.2	0.3	0.4
Diaphragm/spermicide[a]	1.9	1.2	1.2	1.3	2.2	2.8
Periodic abstinence[a]	2.5	1.6	1.6	1.7	2.9	3.6

a) Deaths are birth-related
b) Deaths are method-related
Adapted from H.W. Ory, Family Planning Perspectives, 15:57-63, 1983.

confirmed. Nevertheless, oral contraceptives should not be used during pregnancy. You should check with your doctor about risks to your unborn child of any medication taken during pregnancy.

2. While Breast-Feeding

If you are breast-feeding, consult your doctor before starting oral contraceptives. Some of the drug will be passed on to the child in the milk. A few adverse effects on the child have been reported, including yellowing of the skin (jaundice) and breast enlargement. In addition, oral contraceptives may decrease the amount and quality of your milk. If possible, do not use oral contraceptives while breast-feeding. You should use another method of contraception since breast-feeding provides only partial protection from becoming pregnant, and this partial protection decreases significantly as you breast-feed for longer periods of time. You should consider starting oral contraceptives only after you have weaned your child completely.

3. Laboratory Tests

If you are scheduled for any laboratory tests, tell your doctor you are taking birth-control pills. Certain blood tests may be affected by birth-control pills.

4. Drug Interactions

Certain drugs may interact with birth-control pills to make them less effective in preventing pregnancy or cause an increase in breakthrough bleeding. Such drugs include rifampin, drugs used for epilepsy such as barbiturates (for example, phenobarbital) and phenytoin (Dilantin is one brand of this drug), phenylbutazone (Butazolidin is one brand) and possibly certain antibiotics. Herbal products containing St. John's Wort (hypericum perforatum) may reduce the effectiveness of oral contraceptives. This may also result in breakthrough bleeding. You may need to use an additional method of contraception during any cycle in which you take drugs that can make oral contraceptives less effective (also see BOLDED TEXT AT BEGINNING).

5. Sexually Transmitted Diseases

This product (like all oral contraceptives) is intended to prevent pregnancy. It does not protect against transmission of HIV (AIDS) and other sexually transmitted diseases such as chlamydia, genital herpes, genital warts, gonorrhea, hepatitis B, and syphilis.

HOW TO TAKE THE PILL

IMPORTANT POINTS TO REMEMBER

BEFORE YOU START TAKING YOUR PILLS

1. BE SURE TO READ THESE DIRECTIONS:
   Before you start taking your pills.
   Any time you are not sure what to do.
2. THE RIGHT WAY TO TAKE THE PILL IS TO TAKE ONE PILL EVERY DAY AT THE SAME TIME.
   If you miss pills you could get pregnant. This includes starting the pack late. The more pills you miss, the more likely you are to get pregnant.
3. MANY WOMEN HAVE SPOTTING OR LIGHT BLEEDING, OR MAY FEEL SICK TO THEIR STOMACH DURING THE FIRST 1–3 PACKS OF PILLS.
   If you do have spotting or light bleeding or feel sick to your stomach, do not stop taking the pill. The problem will usually go away. If it does not go away, check with your doctor or healthcare provider.
4. MISSING PILLS CAN ALSO CAUSE SPOTTING OR LIGHT BLEEDING,
   even when you make up these missed pills.
   On the days you take two pills, to make up for missed pills, you could also feel a little sick to your stomach.

5. IF YOU HAVE VOMITING OR DIARRHEA, for any reason, or IF YOU TAKE SOME MEDICINES, including some antibiotics and some herbal products such as St. John's Wort, your pills may not work as well.
   Use a back-up method (such as condoms or spermicides) until you check with your doctor or healthcare provider.
6. IF YOU HAVE TROUBLE REMEMBERING TO TAKE THE PILL, talk to your doctor or healthcare provider about how to make pill-taking easier or about using another method of birth control.
7. IF YOU HAVE ANY QUESTIONS OR ARE UNSURE ABOUT THE INFORMATION IN THIS LEAFLET, call your doctor or healthcare provider.

BEFORE YOU START TAKING YOUR PILLS

1. DECIDE WHAT TIME OF DAY YOU WANT TO TAKE YOUR PILL.
   It is important to take it at about the same time every day.
2. LOOK AT YOUR PILL PACK - IT HAS 28 PILLS: The YASMIN pill pack has 21 yellow "active" pills (with hormones) to be taken for three weeks, followed by 7 white "reminder" pills (without hormones) to be taken for one week.
3. ALSO FIND:
   1) where on the pack to start taking pills,
   2) in what order to take the pills (follow the arrows)
   3) the week numbers as shown in the diagram below

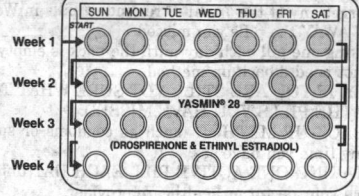

4. BE SURE YOU HAVE READY AT ALL TIMES: ANOTHER KIND OF BIRTH CONTROL (such as condoms or spermicides) to use as a back-up in case you miss pills.
   AN EXTRA, FULL PILL PACK.

WHEN TO START THE FIRST PACK OF PILLS

You have a choice for which day to start taking your first pack of pills. Decide with your doctor or healthcare provider which is the best day for you. Pick a time of day which will be easy to remember.

DAY 1 START:

1. Take the first yellow "active" pill of the first pack during the first 24 hours of your period.
2. You will not need to use a back-up method of birth control, since you are starting the pill at the beginning of your period.

SUNDAY START:

1. Take the first yellow "active" pill of the first pack on the Sunday after your period starts, even if you are still bleeding. If your period begins on Sunday, start the pack that same day.
2. Use another method of birth control (such as condoms or spermicides) as a back-up method if you have sex any time from the Sunday you start your first pack until the next Sunday (7 days).

WHAT TO DO DURING THE MONTH

1. TAKE ONE PILL AT THE SAME TIME EVERY DAY UNTIL THE PACK IS EMPTY Do not skip pills even if you are spotting or bleeding between monthly periods or feel sick to your stomach (nausea).

2. Do not skip pills even if you do not have sex very often.
3. **WHEN YOU FINISH A PACK OR SWITCH YOUR BRAND OF PILLS:** Start the next pack on the day after your last white "reminder" pill. Do not wait any days between packs.

WHAT TO DO IF YOU MISS PILLS

If you **MISS 1** yellow "active" pill:

1. Take it as soon as you remember. Take the next pill at your regular time. This means you may take two pills in one day.
2. You do not need to use a back-up birth control method if you have sex.

If you **MISS 2** yellow "active" pills in a row in **WEEK 1 OR WEEK 2** of your pack:

1. Take two pills on the day you remember and two pills the next day.
2. Then take one pill a day until you finish the pack.
3. You MAY BECOME PREGNANT if you have sex in the 7 *days* after you miss pills. You MUST use another birth control method (such as condoms or spermicides) as a back-up for those 7 days.

If you **MISS 2** yellow "active" pills in a row in the **3RD WEEK:**

1. **If you are a Day 1 Starter:**
   THROW OUT the rest of the pill pack and start a new pack that same day.
   If you are a Sunday Starter:
   Keep taking one pill every day until Sunday. On Sunday, THROW OUT the rest of the pack and start a new pack of pills that same day.
2. You may not have your period this month but this is expected. However, if you miss your period two months in a row, call your doctor or healthcare provider because you might be pregnant.
3. You MAY BECOME PREGNANT if you have sex in the 7 days after you miss pills. You MUST use another birth control method (such as condoms or spermicides) as a back-up for those 7 days.

If you **MISS 3 OR MORE** yellow "active" pills in a row (during the first 3 weeks):

1. **If you are a Day 1 Starter:**
   THROW OUT the rest of the pill pack and start a new pack that same day.
   If you are a Sunday Starter:
   Keep taking 1 pill every day until Sunday. On Sunday, THROW OUT the rest of the pack and start a new pack of pills that same day.
2. You may not have your period this month but this is expected. However, if you miss your period two months in a row, call your doctor or healthcare provider because you might be pregnant.

You MAY BECOME PREGNANT if you have sex in the 7 days after you miss pills. You MUST use another birth control method (such as condoms or spermicides) as a back-up for those 7 days.

If you forget any of the 7 white "reminder" pills in Week 4: THROW AWAY the pills you missed.
Keep taking one pill each day until the pack is empty.
You do not need a back-up method.

FINALLY, IF YOU ARE STILL NOT SURE WHAT TO DO ABOUT THE PILLS YOU HAVE MISSED:
Use a BACK-UP METHOD (such as condoms or spermicides) any time you have sex.
KEEP TAKING ONE ACTIVE PILL EACH DAY until you can reach your doctor or healthcare provider.

PREGNANCY DUE TO PILL FAILURE

The incidence of pill failure resulting in pregnancy is approximately less than 1% (one pregnancy per 100 women per year of use) if taken every day as directed, but more typical failure rates are about 5%. If failure does occur with **YASMIN** use, the risk to the fetus is unknown.

PREGNANCY AFTER STOPPING THE PILL

There may be some delay in becoming pregnant after you stop using oral contraceptives, especially if you had irregular menstrual cycles before you used oral contraceptives. It may be advisable to postpone conception until you begin menstruating regularly once you have stopped taking the pill and desire pregnancy.
There does not appear to be any increase in birth defects in newborn babies when pregnancy occurs soon after stopping the pill.

OVERDOSAGE

Serious ill effects have not been reported following ingestion of large doses of other oral contraceptives by young children. Overdosage of **YASMIN** may cause nausea and withdrawal bleeding in females and may increase blood levels of potassium or decrease blood levels of sodium, which could be dangerous. In case of overdosage, contact your healthcare provider.

OTHER INFORMATION

Your healthcare provider will take a medical and family history before prescribing oral contraceptives and will examine you. The physical examination may be delayed to another time if you request it and the healthcare provider believes

---

that it is appropriate to postpone it. You should be re-examined at least once a year. Be sure to inform your healthcare provider if there is a family history of any of the conditions listed previously in this leaflet. Be sure to keep all appointments with your healthcare provider, because this is a time to determine if there are early signs of side effects of oral contraceptive use.

Do not use the drug for any condition other than the one for which it was prescribed. This drug has been prescribed specifically for you; do not give it to others who may want birth-control pills.

HEALTH BENEFITS FROM ORAL CONTRACEPTIVES

In addition to preventing pregnancy, use of oral contraceptives may provide certain benefits. They are:

- Menstrual cycles may become more regular
- Blood flow during menstruation may be lighter and less iron may be lost. Therefore, anemia due to iron deficiency is less likely to occur.
- Pain or other symptoms during menstruation may be encountered less frequently
- Ovarian cysts may occur less frequently
- Ectopic (tubal) pregnancy may occur less frequently
- Noncancerous cysts or lumps in the breast may occur less frequently
- Acute pelvic inflammatory disease may occur less frequently
- Oral contraceptive use may provide some protection against developing two forms of cancer: cancer of the ovaries and cancer of the lining of the uterus

If you want more information about birth-control pills, ask your doctor or pharmacist. They have a more technical leaflet called the Prescribing Information which you may wish to read.

Manufactured for:
Bayer HealthCare Pharmaceuticals Inc.
Wayne, NJ 07470
Manufactured in Germany
© 2010, Bayer HealthCare Pharmaceuticals Inc. All Rights Reserved.
6701401 US   April 2010
Shown in Product Identification Guide, page 307

YAZ®   ℞

[yăz]
(drospirenone and ethinyl estradiol) Tablets
PHYSICIAN LABELING
Rx only

PATIENTS SHOULD BE COUNSELED THAT THIS PRODUCT DOES NOT PROTECT AGAINST HIV INFECTION (AIDS) AND OTHER SEXUALLY TRANSMITTED DISEASES

DESCRIPTION

YAZ® provides an oral contraceptive regimen consisting of 24 active film coated tablets each containing 3 mg of drospirenone and 0.02 mg of ethinyl estradiol stabilized by betadex as a clathrate (molecular inclusion complex) and 4 inert film coated tablets. Other ingredients are lactose monohydrate NF, corn starch NF, magnesium stearate NF, hypromellose USP, talc USP, titanium dioxide USP, ferric oxide pigment, red NF. The inert film coated tablets contain lactose monohydrate NF, corn starch NF, povidone 25000 USP, magnesium stearate NF, hypromellose USP, talc USP, titanium dioxide USP.

Drospirenone (6R,7R,8R,9S,10R,13S,14S,15S,16S,17S)-1,3',4',6,6a,7,8,9,10,11,12,13,14,15,15a,16-hexadecahydro-10,13-dimethylspiro-[17H-dicyclopropa-[6,7:15,16] cyclopenta[a]phenanthrene-17,2'(5H)-furan]-3,5'(2H)-dione) is a synthetic progestational compound and has a molecular weight of 366.5 and a molecular formula of $C_{24}H_{30}O_3$. Ethinyl estradiol (19-nor-17α-pregna 1,3,5(10)-triene-20-yne-3, 17-diol) is a synthetic estrogenic compound and has a molecular weight of 296.4 and a molecular formula of $C_{20}H_{24}O_2$. The structural formulas are as follows:

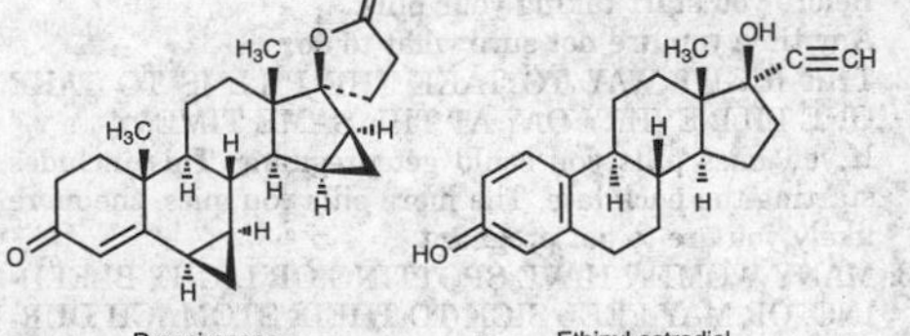

Drospirenone   Ethinyl estradiol

CLINICAL PHARMACOLOGY
PHARMACODYNAMICS
Oral Contraception

Combination oral contraceptives (COCs) act by suppression of gonadotropins. Although the primary mechanism of this action is inhibition of ovulation, other alterations include changes in the cervical mucus (which increases the difficulty of sperm entry into the uterus) and the endometrium (which reduces the likelihood of implantation).

Drospirenone is a spironolactone analogue with antimineralocorticoid activity. Preclinical studies in animals and *in vitro* have shown that drospirenone has no androgenic, estrogenic, glucocorticoid, or antiglucocorticoid activity. Preclinical studies in animals have also shown that drospirenone has antiandrogenic activity.

Acne

Acne vulgaris is a skin condition with a multifactorial etiology including androgen stimulation of sebum production. While the combination of ethinyl estradiol and drospirenone increases sex hormone binding globulin (SHBG) and decreases free testosterone, the relationship between these changes and a decrease in the severity of facial acne in otherwise healthy women with this skin condition has not been established. The impact of the antiandrogenic activity of drospirenone on acne is not known.

PHARMACOKINETICS
Absorption

The absolute bioavailability of drospirenone (DRSP) from a single entity tablet is about 76%. The absolute bioavailability of ethinyl estradiol (EE) is approximately 40% as a result of presystemic conjugation and first-pass metabolism. The absolute bioavailability of YAZ, which is a combination tablet of drospirenone and ethinyl estradiol stabilized by betadex as a clathrate (molecular inclusion complex), has not been evaluated. The bioavailability of EE is similar when dosed via a betadex clathrate formulation compared to when it is dosed as a free steroid. Serum concentrations of DRSP and EE reached peak levels within 1-2 hours after administration of YAZ.

The pharmacokinetics of DRSP are dose proportional following single doses ranging from 1-10 mg. Following daily dosing of YAZ, steady state DRSP concentrations were observed after 8 days. There was about 2 to 3 fold accumulation in serum Cmax and AUC (0-24h) values of DRSP following multiple dose administration of YAZ (see Table I).

For EE, steady-state conditions are reported during the second half of a treatment cycle. Following daily administration of YAZ serum Cmax and AUC (0-24h) values of EE accumulate by a factor of about 1.5 to 2 (see Table I).

[See table I at top of next page]

Effect of Food

The rate of absorption of DRSP and EE following single administration of a formulation similar to YAZ was slower under fed (high fat meal) conditions with the serum Cmax being reduced about 40% for both components. The extent of absorption of DRSP, however, remained unchanged. In contrast, the extent of absorption of EE was reduced by about 20% under fed conditions.

Distribution

DRSP and EE serum levels decline in two phases. The apparent volume of distribution of DRSP is approximately 4 L/kg and that of EE is reported to be approximately 4-5 L/kg.

DRSP does not bind to sex hormone binding globulin (SHBG) or corticosteroid binding globulin (CBG) but binds about 97% to other serum proteins. Multiple dosing over 3 cycles resulted in no change in the free fraction (as measured at trough levels). EE is reported to be highly but non-specifically bound to serum albumin (approximately 98.5 %) and induces an increase in the serum concentrations of both SHBG and CBG. EE induced effects on SHBG and CBG were not affected by variation of the DRSP dosage in the range of 2 to 3 mg.

Metabolism

The two main metabolites of DRSP found in human plasma were identified to be the acid form of DRSP generated by opening of the lactone ring and the 4,5-dihydrodrospirenone-3-sulfate. These metabolites were shown not to be pharmacologically active. In *in vitro* studies with human liver microsomes, DRSP was metabolized only to a minor extent mainly by Cytochrome P450 3A4 (CYP3A4).

EE has been reported to be subject to presystemic conjugation in both small bowel mucosa and the liver. Metabolism occurs primarily by aromatic hydroxylation but a wide variety of hydroxylated and methylated metabolites are formed. These are present as free metabolites and as conjugates with glucuronide and sulfate. CYP3A4 in the liver is responsible for the 2-hydroxylation which is the major oxidative reaction. The 2-hydroxy metabolite is further transformed by methylation and glucuronidation prior to urinary and fecal excretion.

Excretion

DRSP serum levels are characterized by a terminal disposition phase half-life of approximately 30 hours after both single and multiple dose regimens. Excretion of DRSP was nearly complete after ten days and amounts excreted were slightly higher in feces compared to urine. DRSP was extensively metabolized and only trace amounts of unchanged DRSP were excreted in urine and feces. At least 20 different metabolites were observed in urine and feces. About 38-47%

TABLE I: TABLE OF PHARMACOKINETIC PARAMETERS OF YAZ
(Drospirenone 3 mg and Ethinyl Estradiol 0.02 mg)

Drospirenone

Cycle/Day	No. of Subjects	Cmax[1] (ng/mL)	Tmax[2] (h)	AUC(0-24h)[1] (ng·h/mL)	$t_{1/2}$[1] (h)
1/1	23	38.4 (25)	1.5 (1-2)	268 (19)	NA
1/21	23	70.3 (15)	1.5 (1-2)	763 (17)	30.8 (22)

Ethinyl Estradiol

Cycle/Day	No. of Subjects	Cmax[1] (pg/mL)	Tmax[2] (h)	AUC(0-24h)[1] (pg·h/mL)	$t_{1/2}$[1] (h)
1/1	23	32.8 (45)	1.5 (1-2)	108 (52)	NA
1/21	23	45.1 (35)	1.5 (1-2)	220 (57)	NA

NA = Not available [1]: geometric mean (geometric coefficient of variation) [2]: median (range)

of the metabolites in urine were glucuronide and sulfate conjugates. In feces, about 17-20% of the metabolites were excreted as glucuronides and sulfates.

For EE the terminal disposition phase half-life has been reported to be approximately 24 hours. EE is not excreted unchanged. EE is excreted in the urine and feces as glucuronide and sulfate conjugates and undergoes enterohepatic circulation.

Special Populations
Ethnic groups
No clinically significant difference was observed between the pharmacokinetics of DRSP or EE in Japanese versus Caucasian women (age 20-35) when YAZ was administered daily for 21 days. Other ethnic groups have not been studied.

Hepatic Dysfunction
YAZ is contraindicated in patients with hepatic dysfunction **(see CONTRAINDICATIONS and BOLDED WARNING).** The mean exposure to DRSP in women with moderate liver impairment is approximately three times higher than the exposure in women with normal liver function. YAZ has not been studied in women with severe hepatic impairment.

Renal Insufficiency
YAZ is contraindicated in patients with renal insufficiency **(see CONTRAINDICATIONS and BOLDED WARNING).** The effect of renal insufficiency on the pharmacokinetics of DRSP (3 mg daily for 14 days) and the effect of DRSP on serum potassium levels were investigated in female subjects (n = 28, age 30-65) with normal renal function and mild and moderate renal impairment. All subjects were on a low potassium diet. During the study 7 subjects continued the use of potassium sparing drugs for the treatment of the underlying illness. On the 14th day (steady-state) of DRSP treatment, serum DRSP levels in the group with mild renal impairment (creatinine clearance CLcr, 50-80 mL/min) were comparable to those in the group with normal renal function (CLcr, >80 mL/min). The serum DRSP levels were on average 37 % higher in the group with moderate renal impairment (CLcr, 30-50 mL/min) compared to those in the group with normal renal function. DRSP treatment was well tolerated by all groups. DRSP treatment did not show any clinically significant effect on serum potassium concentration. Although hyperkalemia was not observed in the study, in five of the seven subjects who continued use of potassium sparing drugs during the study, mean serum potassium levels increased by up to 0.33 mEq/L. Therefore, potential exists for hyperkalemia to occur in subjects with renal impairment whose serum potassium is in the upper reference range, and who are concomitantly using potassium sparing drugs.

INDICATIONS AND USAGE

YAZ is indicated for the prevention of pregnancy in women who elect to use an oral contraceptive.

Oral contraceptives are highly effective. Table II lists the typical unintended pregnancy rates for users of combination oral contraceptives and other methods of contraception. The efficacy of these contraceptive methods, except sterilization and contraceptive implants and IUDs, depends upon the reliability with which they are used. Correct and consistent use of methods can result in lower failure rates.

YAZ is also indicated for the treatment of symptoms of premenstrual dysphoric disorder (PMDD) in women who choose to use an oral contraceptive as their method of contraception. The effectiveness of YAZ for PMDD when used for more than three menstrual cycles has not been evaluated.

The essential features of PMDD according to the Diagnostic and Statistical Manual-4th edition (DSM-IV) include markedly depressed mood, anxiety or tension, affective lability, and persistent anger or irritability. Other features include decreased interest in usual activities, difficulty concentrating, lack of energy, change in appetite or sleep, and feeling out of control. Physical symptoms associated with PMDD include breast tenderness, headache, joint and muscle pain, bloating and weight gain. In this disorder, these symptoms occur regularly during the luteal phase and remit within a few days following onset of menses; the disturbance markedly interferes with work or school, or with usual social activities and relationships with others. Diagnosis is made by healthcare providers according to DSM-IV criteria, with symptomatology assessed prospectively over at least two menstrual cycles. In making the diagnosis, care should be taken to rule out other cyclical mood disorders.

YAZ has not been evaluated for the treatment of premenstrual syndrome (PMS).

YAZ is indicated for the treatment of moderate acne vulgaris in women at least 14 years of age, who have no known contraindications to oral contraceptive therapy and have achieved menarche. YAZ should be used for the treatment of acne only if the patient desires an oral contraceptive for birth control.

TABLE II: Percentage of women experiencing an unintended pregnancy during the first year of typical use and first year of perfect use of contraception and the percentage continuing use at the end of the first year: United States.

Method (1)	% of Women Experiencing an Unintended Pregnancy Within the First Year of Use — Typical Use[1] (2)	% of Women Experiencing an Unintended Pregnancy Within the First Year of Use — Perfect Use[2] (3)	% of Women Continuing Use at One Year[3] (4)
Chance[4]	85	85	40
Spermicides[5]	26	6	63
Periodic abstinence	25		
Calendar		9	
Ovulation method		3	
Sympto-thermal[6]		2	
Post-ovulation		1	
Withdrawal	19	4	
Cap[7]			
Parous women	40	26	42
Nulliparous women	20	9	56
Sponge			
Parous women	40	20	42
Nulliparous women	20	9	56
Diaphragm[7]	20	6	56
Condom[8]			
Female (Reality)	21	5	56
Male	14	3	61
Pill	5		71
progestin only		0.5	
combined		0.1	
IUD			
Progesterone T	2	1.5	81
Copper T 380A	0.8	0.6	78
Lng 20	0.1	0.1	81
Depo Provera	0.3	0.3	70
Norplant and Norplant-2	0.05	0.05	88
Female sterilization	0.5	0.5	100
Male sterilization	0.15	0.1	100

Emergency Contraceptive Pills: Treatment initiated within 72 hours after unprotected intercourse reduces the risk of pregnancy by at least 75%.[9]
Lactational Amenorrhea Method: LAM is highly effective, *temporary* method of contraception.[10]
Source: Trussell J, Contraceptive efficacy. In Hatcher RA, Trussell J, Stewart F, Cates W, Stewart GK, Guest F, Kowal D, *Contraceptive Technology: Seventeenth Revised Edition.* New York NY: Irvington Publishers, 1998.

1 Among typical couples who initiate use of a method (not necessarily for the first time), the percentage who experience an accidental pregnancy during the first year if they do not stop use for any other reason.
2 Among couples who initiate use of a method (not necessarily for the first time) and who use it perfectly (both consistently and correctly). The percentage who experience an accidental pregnancy during the first year if they do not stop use for any reason.
3 Among couples attempting to avoid pregnancy, the percentage who continue to use a method for one year.
4 The percents becoming pregnant in columns (2) and (3) are based on data from populations where contraception is not used and from women who cease using contraception in order to become pregnant. Among such populations, about 89% become pregnant within one year. This estimate was lowered slightly (to 85%) to represent the percentage who would become pregnant within one year among women now relying on reversible methods of contraception if they abandoned contraception altogether.
5 Foams, creams, gels, vaginal suppositories, and vaginal film.
6 Cervical mucus (ovulation) method supplemented by calendar in the pre-ovulatory and basal body temperature in the post-ovulatory phases.
7 With spermicidal cream or jelly.
8 Without spermicides.
9 The treatment schedule is one dose within 72 hours after unprotected intercourse, and a second dose 12 hours after the first dose. The Food and Drug Administration has declared the following brands of oral contraceptives to be safe and effective for emergency contraception: Ovral (1 dose is 2 white pills), Alesse (1 dose is 5 pink pills), Nordette or Levlen (1 dose is 2 light-orange pills), Lo/Ovral (1 dose is 4 white pills), Triphasil or Tri-Levlen (1 dose is 4 yellow pills).
10 However, to maintain effective protection against pregnancy, another method of contraception must be used as soon as menstruation resumes, the frequency or duration of breastfeeds is reduced, bottle feeds are introduced, or the baby reaches six months of age.

Oral Contraceptive Clinical Trial
In the primary contraceptive efficacy study of YAZ (3 mg DRSP/0.02 mg EE) of up to 1 year duration, 1,027 subjects were enrolled and completed 11,480 28-day cycles of use. The age range was 17 to 36 years. The racial demographic was: 87.8% Caucasian, 4.6% Hispanic, 4.3% Black, 1.2% Asian, and 2.1% other. Women with a BMI greater than 35 were excluded from the trial. The pregnancy rate (Pearl Index) was 1.41 per 100 woman-years of use based on 12 pregnancies that occurred after the onset of treatment and within 14 days after the last dose of YAZ in women 35 years of age or younger during cycles in which no other form of contraception was used.

Premenstrual Dysphoric Disorder Clinical Trials
Two multicenter, double-blind, randomized, placebo-controlled studies were conducted to evaluate the effectiveness of YAZ in treating the symptoms of PMDD. Women aged 18-42 who met DSM-IV criteria for PMDD, confirmed by prospective daily ratings of their symptoms, were enrolled. Both studies measured the treatment effect of YAZ using the Daily Record of Severity of Problems scale, a patient-rated instrument that assesses the symptoms that constitute the DSM-IV diagnostic criteria. The primary study was a parallel group design that included 384 evaluable reproductive-aged women with PMDD who were randomly assigned to receive YAZ or placebo treatment for 3 menstrual cycles. The supportive study, a crossover design, was terminated prematurely prior to achieving recruitment goals due to enrollment difficulties. A total of 64 women of reproductive age with PMDD were treated initially with YAZ or placebo for up to 3 cycles followed by a washout cycle and then crossed over to the alternate medication for 3 cycles.

Efficacy was assessed in both studies by the change from baseline during treatment using a scoring system based on the first 21 items of the Daily Record of Severity of Problems. Each of the 21 items was rated on a scale from 1 (not

Table III: Efficacy Results for Acne Trials*

	Study 1		Study 2	
	YAZ N=228	Placebo N=230	YAZ N=218	Placebo N=213
ISGA Success Rate	35 (15%)	10 (4%)	46 (21%)	19 (9%)
Inflammatory Lesions				
Mean Baseline Count	33	33	32	32
Mean Absolute (%) Reduction	15 (48%)	11 (32%)	16 (51%)	11 (34%)
Non-inflammatory Lesions				
Mean Baseline Count	47	47	44	44
Mean Absolute (%) Reduction	18 (39%)	10 (18%)	17 (42%)	11 (26%)
Total lesions				
Mean Baseline Count	80	80	76	76
Mean Absolute (%) reduction	33 (42%)	21 (25%)	33 (46%)	22 (31%)

*Evaluated at day 15 of cycle 6, last observation carried forward for the Intent to treat population

TABLE IV: CIRCULATORY DISEASE MORTALITY RATES PER 100,000 WOMAN-YEARS BY AGE, SMOKING STATUS AND ORAL CONTRACEPTIVE USE

AGE	EVER-USERS NON-SMOKERS	EVER-USERS SMOKERS	CONTROLS NON-SMOKERS	CONTROL SMOKERS
15-24	0	10.5	0	0
25-34	4.4	14.2	2.7	4.2
35-44	21.5	63.4	6.4	15.2
45+	52.4	206.7	11.4	27.9

(Adapted from P.M. Layde and V. Beral)

at all) to 6 (extreme); thus a maximum score of 126 was possible. In both trials, women who received YAZ had statistically significantly greater improvement in their Daily Record of Severity of Problems scores. In the primary study, the average decrease (improvement) from baseline was 37.5 points in women taking YAZ, compared to 30 points in women taking placebo.

Acne Clinical Trials
In two multicenter, double blind, randomized, placebo-controlled studies, 889 subjects, ages 14 to 45 years, with moderate acne received YAZ or placebo for six 28 day cycles. The primary efficacy endpoints were the percent change in inflammatory lesions, non-inflammatory lesions, total lesions, and the percentage of subjects with a "clear" or "almost clear" rating on the Investigator's Static Global Assessment (ISGA) scale on day 15 of cycle 6, as presented in Table III:
[See table III above]

CONTRAINDICATIONS
YAZ should not be used in women who have the following:
- Renal insufficiency
- Hepatic dysfunction
- Adrenal Insufficiency
- Thrombophlebitis or thromboembolic disorders
- A past history of deep-vein thrombophlebitis or thromboembolic disorders
- Cerebral-vascular or coronary-artery disease (current or history)
- Valvular heart disease with thrombogenic complications
- Severe hypertension
- Diabetes with vascular involvement
- Headaches with focal neurological symptoms
- Major surgery with prolonged immobilization
- Known or suspected carcinoma of the breast
- Carcinoma of the endometrium or other known or suspected estrogen-dependent neoplasia
- Undiagnosed abnormal genital bleeding
- Cholestatic jaundice of pregnancy or jaundice with prior Pill use
- Known or suspected pregnancy
- Liver tumor (benign or malignant) or active liver disease
- Heavy smoking (≥15 cigarettes per day) and over age 35
- Hypersensitivity to any component of this product

WARNINGS

Cigarette smoking increases the risk of serious cardiovascular side effects from oral contraceptive use. This risk increases with age and with heavy smoking (15 or more cigarettes per day) and is quite marked in women over 35 years of age. Women who use oral contraceptives should be strongly advised not to smoke.

YAZ contains 3 mg of the progestin drospirenone that has antimineralocorticoid activity, including the potential for hyperkalemia in high-risk patients, comparable to a 25 mg dose of spironolactone. YAZ should not be used in patients with conditions that predispose to hyperkalemia (i.e. renal insufficiency, hepatic dysfunction and adrenal insufficiency). Women receiving daily, long-term treatment for chronic conditions or diseases with medications that may increase serum potassium should have their serum potassium level checked during the first treatment cycle. Medications that may increase serum potassium include ACE inhibitors, angiotensin – II receptor antagonists, potassium-sparing diuretics, potassium supplementation, heparin, aldosterone antagonists, and NSAIDS.

The use of oral contraceptives is associated with increased risks of several serious conditions including venous and arterial thrombotic and thromboembolic events (such as myocardial infarction, thromboembolism, stroke), hepatic neoplasia, gallbladder disease, and hypertension. The risk of serious morbidity or mortality is very small in healthy women without underlying risk factors. The risk of morbidity and mortality increases significantly in the presence of other underlying risk factors such as hypertension, hyperlipidemias, obesity and diabetes.

Practitioners prescribing oral contraceptives should be familiar with the following information relating to these risks. The information contained in this package insert is based principally on studies carried out in patients who used oral contraceptives with higher formulations of estrogens and progestogens than those in common use today. The effect of long-term use of the oral contraceptives with lower formulations of both estrogens and progestogens remains to be determined.

Throughout this labeling, epidemiologic studies reported are of two types: retrospective or case control studies and prospective or cohort studies. Case control studies provide a measure of the relative risk of a disease, namely, a ratio of the incidence of a disease among oral contraceptive users to that among nonusers. The relative risk does not provide information on the actual clinical occurrence of a disease. Cohort studies provide a measure of attributable risk, which is the difference in the incidence of disease between oral contraceptive users and nonusers. The attributable risk does provide information about the actual occurrence of a disease in the population. For further information, the reader is referred to a text on epidemiologic methods.

1. THROMBOEMBOLIC DISORDERS AND OTHER VASCULAR PROBLEMS
a. Myocardial infarction
An increased risk of myocardial infarction has been attributed to oral contraceptive use. This risk is primarily in smokers or women with other underlying risk factors for coronary-artery disease such as hypertension, hypercholesterolemia, morbid obesity, and diabetes. The relative risk of heart attack for current oral contraceptive users has been estimated to be two to six. The risk is very low under the age of 30.

Smoking in combination with oral contraceptive use has been shown to contribute substantially to the incidence of myocardial infarctions in women in their mid-thirties or older with smoking accounting for the majority of excess cases. Mortality rates associated with circulatory disease have been shown to increase substantially in smokers over the age of 35 and nonsmokers over the age of 40 (Table IV) among women who use oral contraceptives.
[See table IV at left]
Oral contraceptives may compound the effects of well-known risk factors, such as hypertension, diabetes, hyperlipidemias, age and obesity. In particular, some progestogens are known to decrease HDL cholesterol and cause glucose intolerance, while estrogens may create a state of hyperinsulinism. Oral contraceptives have been shown to increase blood pressure among users (see section 9 in WARNINGS). Similar effects on risk factors have been associated with an increased risk of heart disease. Oral contraceptives must be used with caution in women with cardiovascular disease risk factors.
b. Thromboembolism
An increased risk of thromboembolic and thrombotic disease associated with the use of oral contraceptives is well established. Case control studies have found the relative risk of users compared to nonusers to be 3 for the first episode of superficial venous thrombosis, 4 to 11 for deep vein thrombosis or pulmonary embolism, and 1.5 to 6 for women with predisposing conditions for venous thromboembolic disease. Cohort studies have shown the relative risk to be somewhat lower, about 3 for new cases and about 4.5 for new cases requiring hospitalization. The risk of thromboembolic disease due to oral contraceptives is not related to length of use and disappears after Pill use is stopped.
A two- to four-fold increase in the relative risk of postoperative thromboembolic complications has been reported with the use of oral contraceptives. The relative risk of venous thrombosis in women who have predisposing conditions is twice that of women without such medical conditions. If feasible, oral contraceptives should be discontinued from at least four weeks prior to and for two weeks after elective surgery of a type associated with an increase in risk of thromboembolism and during and following prolonged immobilization. Since the immediate postpartum period is also associated with an increased risk of thromboembolism, combined oral contraceptives should be started no earlier than four to six weeks after delivery and at that time only in women who elect not to breast feed.
Several studies have investigated the relative risks of thromboembolism in women using a different drospirenone-containing COC (Yasmin, which contains 0.03 mg of ethinyl estradiol and 3 mg of drospirenone) compared to those in women using COCs containing other progestins. Two prospective cohort studies, both evaluating the risk of venous and arterial thromboembolism and death, were initiated at the time of Yasmin approval.[1, 2] The first (EURAS) showed the risk of thromboembolism (particularly venous thromboembolism) and death in Yasmin users to be comparable to that of other oral contraceptive preparations, including those containing levonorgestrel (a so-called second generation COC). The second prospective cohort study (Ingenix) also showed a comparable risk of thromboembolism in Yasmin users compared to users of other COCs, including those containing levonorgestrel. In the second study, COC comparator groups were selected based on their having similar characteristics to those being prescribed Yasmin.
Two additional epidemiological studies, one case-control study (van Hylckama Vlieg et al.[3]) and one retrospective cohort study (Lidegaard et al.[4]) suggested that the risk of venous thromboembolism occurring in Yasmin users was higher than that for users of levonorgestrel-containing COCs and lower than that for users of desogestrel/gestodene-containing COCs (so-called third generation COCs). In the case-control study, however, the number of Yasmin cases was very small (1.2% of all cases) making the risk estimates unreliable. The relative risk for Yasmin users in the retrospective cohort study was greater than that for users of other COC products when considering women who used the products for less than one year. However, these one-year estimates may not be reliable because the analysis may include women of varying risk levels. Among women who used the product for 1 to 4 years, the relative risk was similar for users of Yasmin to that for users of other COC products.
c. Cerebrovascular diseases
Oral contraceptives have been shown to increase both the relative and attributable risks of cerebrovascular events (thrombotic and hemorrhagic strokes), although, in general, the risk is greatest among older (>35 years), hypertensive women who also smoke. Hypertension was found to be a

risk factor, for both users and nonusers, for both types of strokes, while smoking interacted to increase the risk for hemorrhagic strokes.

In a large study, the relative risk of thrombotic strokes has been shown to range from 3 for normotensive users to 14 for users with severe hypertension. The relative risk of hemorrhagic stroke is reported to be 1.2 for nonsmokers who used oral contraceptives, 2.6 for smokers who did not use oral contraceptives, 7.6 for smokers who used oral contraceptives, 1.8 for normotensive users and 25.7 for users with severe hypertension. The attributable risk is also greater in older women. Oral contraceptives also increase the risk for stroke in women with other underlying risk factors such as certain inherited or acquired thrombophilias, hyperlipidemias, and obesity. Women with migraine (particularly migraine with aura) who take combination oral contraceptives may be at an increased risk of stroke.

d. Dose-related risk of vascular disease from oral contraceptives

A positive association has been observed between the amount of estrogen and progestogen in oral contraceptives and the risk of vascular disease. A decline in serum high-density lipoproteins (HDL) has been reported with many progestational agents. A decline in serum high-density lipoproteins has been associated with an increased incidence of ischemic heart disease. Because estrogens increase HDL cholesterol, the net effect of an oral contraceptive depends on a balance achieved between doses of estrogen and progestogen and the nature and absolute amount of progestogen used in the contraceptive. The amount of both hormones should be considered in the choice of an oral contraceptive.

Minimizing exposure to estrogen and progestogen is in keeping with good principles of therapeutics. For any particular estrogen/progestogen combination, the dosage regimen prescribed should be one which contains the least amount of estrogen and progestogen that is compatible with a low failure rate and the needs of the individual patient. New acceptors of oral contraceptive agents should be started on preparations containing the lowest estrogen content that is judged appropriate for the individual patient.

e. Persistence of risk of vascular disease

There are two studies which have shown persistence of risk of vascular disease for ever-users of oral contraceptives. In a study in the United States, the risk of developing myocardial infarction after discontinuing oral contraceptives persists for at least 9 years for women aged 40 to 49 years who had used oral contraceptives for five or more years, but this increased risk was not demonstrated in other age groups. In another study in Great Britain, the risk of developing cerebrovascular disease persisted for at least 6 years after discontinuation of oral contraceptives, although excess risk was very small. However, both studies were performed with oral contraceptive formulations containing 50 micrograms or higher of estrogens.

2. ESTIMATES OF MORTALITY FROM CONTRACEPTIVE USE

One study gathered data from a variety of sources which have estimated the mortality rate associated with different methods of contraception at different ages (Table V). These estimates include the combined risk of death associated with contraceptive methods plus the risk attributable to pregnancy in the event of method failure. Each method of contraception has its specific benefits and risks. The study concluded that with the exception of oral contraceptive users 35 and older who smoke and 40 and older who do not smoke, mortality associated with all methods of birth control is below that associated with childbirth.

The observation of a possible increase in risk of mortality with age for oral contraceptive users is based on data gathered in the 1970's—but not reported until 1983. However, current clinical practice involves the use of lower estrogen dose formulations combined with careful restriction of oral contraceptive use to women who do not have the various risk factors listed in this labeling.

Because of these changes in practice and, also, because of some limited new data which suggest that the risk of cardiovascular disease with the use of oral contraceptives may now be less than previously observed, the Fertility and Maternal Health Drugs Advisory Committee was asked to review the topic in 1989. The Committee concluded that although cardiovascular disease risks may be increased with oral contraceptive use after age 40 in healthy nonsmoking women (even with the newer low-dose formulations), there are greater potential health risks associated with pregnancy in older women and with the alternative surgical and medical procedures which may be necessary if such women do not have access to effective and acceptable means of contraception.

Therefore, the Committee recommended that the benefits of oral contraceptive use by healthy nonsmoking women over 40 may outweigh the possible risks. Of course, women of all ages who take oral contraceptives, should take the lowest possible dose formulation that is effective.

[See table V above]

Table V: ANNUAL NUMBER OF BIRTH-RELATED OR METHOD-RELATED DEATHS ASSOCIATED WITH CONTROL OF FERTILITY PER 100,000 NONSTERILE WOMEN, BY FERTILITY-CONTROL METHOD ACCORDING TO AGE

Method of Control and Outcome	15-19 years	20-24 years	25-29 years	30-34 years	35-39 years	40-44 years
No fertility control methods\1\	7	7.4	9.1	14.8	25.7	28.2
Oral contraceptives non-smoker\2\	0.3	0.5	0.9	1.9	13.8	31.6
Oral contraceptives smoker\2\	2.2	3.4	6.6	13.5	51.1	117.2
IUD\2\	0.8	0.8	1	1	1.4	1.4
Condom\1\	1.1	1.6	0.7	0.2	0.3	0.4
Diaphragm/spermicide\1\	1.9	1.2	1.2	1.3	2.2	2.8
Periodic abstinence\1\	2.5	1.6	1.6	1.7	2.9	3.6

\1\ Deaths are birth-related
\2\ Deaths are method-related
Adapted from H.W. Ory, Family Planning Perspectives, 15:57-63, 1983.

3. CARCINOMA OF THE REPRODUCTIVE ORGANS AND BREASTS

Numerous epidemiological studies have been performed on the incidence of breast, endometrial, ovarian and cervical cancer in women using oral contraceptives.

Although the risk of having breast cancer diagnosed may be slightly increased among current and recent users of combined oral contraceptives (RR=1.24), this excess risk decreases over time after combination oral contraceptive discontinuation and by 10 years after cessation the increased risk disappears. The risk does not increase with duration of use and no consistent relationships have been found with dose or type of steroid. The patterns of risk are also similar regardless of a woman's reproductive history or her family breast cancer history. The subgroup for whom risk has been found to be significantly elevated is women who first used oral contraceptives before age 20, but because breast cancer is so rare at these young ages, the number of cases attributable to this early oral contraceptive use is extremely small.

Breast cancers diagnosed in current or previous OC users tend to be less clinically advanced than in never users.

Women who currently have or have had breast cancer should not use oral contraceptives because breast cancer is a hormonally-sensitive tumor.

Some studies suggest that oral contraceptive use has been associated with an increase in the risk of cervical intraepithelial neoplasia in some populations of women. However, there continues to be controversy about the extent to which such findings may be due to differences in sexual behavior and other factors.

In spite of many studies of the relationship between oral contraceptive use and breast and cervical cancers, a cause-and-effect relationship has not been established.

4. HEPATIC NEOPLASIA

Benign hepatic adenomas are associated with oral contraceptive use, although the incidence of benign tumors is rare in the United States. Indirect calculations have estimated the attributable risk to be in the range of 3.3 cases/100,000 for users, a risk that increases after four or more years of use. Rupture of rare, benign, hepatic adenomas may cause death through intra-abdominal hemorrhage.

Studies from Britain have shown an increased risk of developing hepatocellular carcinoma in long-term (>8 years) oral contraceptive users. However, these cancers are extremely rare in the U.S. and the attributable risk (the excess incidence) of liver cancers in oral contraceptive users approaches less than one per million users.

5. OCULAR LESIONS

There have been clinical case reports of retinal thrombosis associated with the use of oral contraceptives, which may lead to partial or complete loss of vision. Oral contraceptives should be discontinued if there is unexplained partial or complete loss of vision; onset of proptosis or diplopia; papilledema; or retinal vascular lesions. Appropriate diagnostic and therapeutic measures should be undertaken immediately.

6. ORAL CONTRACEPTIVE USE BEFORE OR DURING EARLY PREGNANCY

Extensive epidemiological studies have revealed no increased risk of birth defects in women who have used oral contraceptives prior to pregnancy. Studies also do not suggest a teratogenic effect, particularly in so far as cardiac anomalies and limb-reduction defects are concerned, when taken inadvertently during early pregnancy.

The administration of oral contraceptives to induce withdrawal bleeding should not be used as a test for pregnancy. Oral contraceptives should not be used during pregnancy to treat threatened or habitual abortion. (see **CONTRAINDICATIONS**)

It is recommended that for any patient who has missed two consecutive periods, pregnancy should be ruled out. If the patient has not adhered to the prescribed dosing schedule, the possibility of pregnancy should be considered at the time of the first missed period. Oral contraceptive use should be discontinued if pregnancy is confirmed.

7. GALLBLADDER DISEASE

Earlier studies have reported an increased lifetime relative risk of gallbladder surgery in users of oral contraceptives and estrogens. More recent studies, however, have shown that the relative risk of developing gallbladder disease among oral contraceptive users may be minimal. The recent findings of minimal risk may be related to the use of oral contraceptive formulations containing lower hormonal doses of estrogens and progestogens.

8. CARBOHYDRATE AND LIPID METABOLIC EFFECTS

Oral contraceptives have been shown to cause glucose intolerance in a significant percentage of users. Oral contraceptives containing greater than 75 micrograms of estrogens cause hyperinsulinism, while lower doses of estrogen cause less glucose intolerance. Progestogens increase insulin secretion and create insulin resistance, this effect varying with different progestational agents. However, in the nondiabetic woman, oral contraceptives appear to have no effect on fasting blood glucose. Because of these demonstrated effects, prediabetic and diabetic women should be carefully observed while taking oral contraceptives.

A small proportion of women will have persistent hypertriglyceridemia while on the Pill. As discussed earlier (see **WARNINGS** 1a. and 1d.), changes in serum triglycerides and lipoprotein levels have been reported in oral contraceptive users.

9. ELEVATED BLOOD PRESSURE

Women with severe hypertension should not be started on hormonal contraceptives (see **CONTRAINDICATIONS**).

An increase in blood pressure has been reported in women taking oral contraceptives and this increase is more likely in older oral contraceptive users and with continued use. Data from the Royal College of General Practitioners and subsequent randomized trials have shown that the incidence of hypertension increases with increasing concentrations of progestogens.

Women with a history of hypertension or hypertension-related diseases, or renal disease should be encouraged to use another method of contraception. If women with hypertension elect to use oral contraceptives, they should be monitored closely, and if significant elevation of blood pressure occurs, oral contraceptives should be discontinued. For most women, elevated blood pressure will return to normal after stopping oral contraceptives and there is no difference in the occurrence of hypertension among ever- and never-users.

10. HEADACHE

The onset or exacerbation of migraine or development of headache with a new pattern which is recurrent, persistent or severe requires discontinuation of oral contraceptives and evaluation of the cause.

11. BLEEDING IRREGULARITIES

Breakthrough bleeding and spotting are sometimes encountered in patients on oral contraceptives, especially during the first three months of use. Nonhormonal causes should be considered and adequate diagnostic measures taken to rule out malignancy or pregnancy in the event of breakthrough bleeding, as in the case of any abnormal vaginal bleeding. If pathology has been excluded, time or a change to another formulation may solve the problem. In the event of amenorrhea, pregnancy should be ruled out.

Some women may encounter post-pill amenorrhea or oligomenorrhea, especially when such a condition was preexistent.

PRECAUTIONS

1. GENERAL

Patients should be counseled that this product does not protect against HIV infection (AIDS) and other sexually transmitted diseases.

2. PHYSICAL EXAMINATION AND FOLLOW-UP
A periodic personal and family medical history and complete physical examination are appropriate for all women, including women using oral contraceptives. The physical examination, however, may be deferred until after initiation of oral contraceptives if requested by the woman and judged appropriate by the clinician. The physical examination should include special reference to blood pressure, breasts, abdomen and pelvic organs, including cervical cytology and relevant laboratory tests. In case of undiagnosed, persistent or recurrent abnormal vaginal bleeding, appropriate measures should be conducted to rule out malignancy. Women with a strong family history of breast cancer or who have breast nodules should be monitored with particular care.
3. LIPID DISORDERS
Women who are being treated for hyperlipidemias should be followed closely if they elect to use oral contraceptives. Some progestogens may elevate LDL levels and may render the control of hyperlipidemias more difficult. (See **WARNINGS** 1.d.)
In patients with familial defects of lipoprotein metabolism receiving estrogen-containing preparations, there have been case reports of significant elevations of plasma triglycerides leading to pancreatitis.
4. LIVER FUNCTION
If jaundice develops in any woman receiving oral contraceptives, the medication should be discontinued. Steroid hormones may be poorly metabolized in patients with impaired liver function.
5. FLUID RETENTION
Oral contraceptives may cause some degree of fluid retention. They should be prescribed with caution, and only with careful monitoring, in patients with conditions which might be aggravated by fluid retention.
6. EMOTIONAL DISORDERS
Women with a history of depression should be carefully observed and the drug discontinued if depression recurs to a serious degree.
Patients becoming significantly depressed while taking oral contraceptives should stop the medication and use an alternate method of contraception in an attempt to determine whether the symptom is drug related.
7. CONTACT LENSES
Contact-lens wearers who develop visual changes or changes in lens tolerance should be assessed by an ophthalmologist.
8. DRUG INTERACTIONS
Effects of Other Drugs on Combined Hormonal Contraceptives
Rifampin: Metabolism of ethinyl estradiol and some progestins (e.g., norethindrone) is increased by rifampin. A reduction in contraceptive effectiveness and an increase in menstrual irregularities have been associated with concomitant use of rifampin.
Minocycline: Minocycline-related changes in estradiol, progesterone, FSH and LH plasma levels, breakthrough bleeding, or contraceptive failure cannot be ruled out.
Anticonvulsants: Anticonvulsants such as phenobarbital, phenytoin, and carbamazepine have been shown to increase the metabolism of ethinyl estradiol and/or some progestins, which could result in a reduction of contraceptive effectiveness.
Antibiotics: Pregnancy while taking combined hormonal contraceptives has been reported when the combined hormonal contraceptives were administered with antimicrobials such as ampicillin, tetracycline, and griseofulvin. However, clinical pharmacokinetic studies have not demonstrated any consistent effects of antibiotics (other than rifampin—see above) on plasma concentrations of synthetic steroids. See also separate discussion on minocycline (above).
Atorvastatin: Coadministration of atorvastatin and an oral contraceptive increased AUC values for norethindrone and ethinyl estradiol by approximately 30% and 20%, respectively.
St. John's Wort: Herbal products containing St. John's Wort (hypericum perforatum) may induce hepatic enzymes (cytochrome P450) and p-glycoprotein transporter and may reduce the effectiveness of oral contraceptives and emergency contraceptive pills. This may also result in breakthrough bleeding.
Other: Ascorbic acid and acetaminophen may increase plasma concentrations of some synthetic estrogens, possibly by inhibition of conjugation.
Effects of Drospirenone on Other Drugs
Metabolic Interactions
Metabolism of DRSP and potential effects of DRSP on hepatic cytochrome P450 (CYP) enzymes have been investigated in *in vitro* and *in vivo* studies (see Metabolism). In *in vitro* studies DRSP did not affect turnover of model substrates of CYP1A2 and CYP2D6, but had an inhibitory influence on the turnover of model substrates of CYP1A1, CYP2C9, CYP2C19 and CYP3A4 with CYP2C19 being the most sensitive enzyme. The potential effect of DRSP on CYP2C19 activity was investigated in a clinical pharmacokinetic study using omeprazole as a marker substrate. In the study with 24 postmenopausal women [including 12 women with homozygous (wild type) CYP2C19 genotype and 12 women with heterozygous CYP2C19 genotype] the daily oral administration of 3 mg DRSP for 14 days did not affect the oral clearance of omeprazole (40 mg, single oral dose) and the CYP2C19 product 5-hydroxy omeprazole. Furthermore, no significant effect of DRSP on the systemic clearance of the CYP3A4 product omeprazole sulfone was found. These results demonstrate that DRSP did not inhibit CYP2C19 and CYP3A4 *in vivo*.
Two additional clinical drug-drug interaction studies using simvastatin and midazolam as marker substrates for CYP3A4 were each performed in 24 healthy postmenopausal women. The results of these studies demonstrated that pharmacokinetics of the CYP3A4 substrates were not influenced by steady state DRSP concentrations achieved after administration of 3 mg DRSP/day.
Interactions with Drugs that Have the Potential to Increase Serum Potassium
There is a potential for an increase in serum potassium in women taking YAZ with other drugs (see **BOLDED WARNING**). Of note, occasional or chronic use of NSAID medication was not restricted in any of the clinical trials with YAZ.
A drug-drug interaction study of DRSP 3 mg/estradiol (E2) 1 mg versus placebo was performed in 24 mildly hypertensive postmenopausal women taking enalapril maleate 10 mg twice daily. Potassium levels were obtained every other day for a total of 2 weeks in all subjects. Mean serum potassium levels in the DRSP/E2 treatment group relative to baseline were 0.22 mEq/L higher than those in the placebo group. Serum potassium concentrations also were measured at multiple timepoints over 24 hours at baseline and on Day 14. On Day 14, the ratios for serum potassium Cmax and AUC in the DRSP/E2 group to those in the placebo group were 0.955 (90% CI: 0.914, 0.999) and 1.01 (90% CI: 0.944, 1.08), respectively. No patient in either treatment group developed hyperkalemia (serum potassium concentrations >5.5 mEq/L).
Effects of Combined Hormonal Contraceptives on Other Drugs
Combined oral contraceptives containing ethinyl estradiol may inhibit the metabolism of other compounds. Increased plasma concentrations of cyclosporine, prednisolone, and theophylline have been reported with concomitant administration of oral contraceptives. In addition, oral contraceptives may induce the conjugation of other compounds. Decreased plasma concentrations of acetaminophen and increased clearance on temazepam, salicylic acid, morphine, and clofibric acid have been noted when these drugs were administered with oral contraceptives.
9. INTERACTIONS WITH LABORATORY TESTS
Certain endocrine- and liver-function tests and blood components may be affected by oral contraceptives:
a. Increased prothrombin and factors VII, VIII, IX and X; decreased antithrombin 3; increased norepinephrine-induced platelet aggregability.
b. Increased thyroid-binding globulin (TBG) leading to increased circulating total thyroid hormone, as measured by protein-bound iodine (PBI), T4 by column or by radioimmunoassay. Free T3 resin uptake is decreased, reflecting the elevated TBG, free T4 concentration is unaltered.
c. Other binding proteins may be elevated in serum.
d. Sex-hormone-binding globulins are increased and result in elevated levels of total circulating sex steroids and corticoids; however, free or biologically active levels remain unchanged.
e. Triglycerides may be increased.
f. Glucose tolerance may be decreased.
g. Serum folate levels may be depressed by oral contraceptive therapy. This may be of clinical significance if a woman becomes pregnant shortly after discontinuing oral contraceptives.
10. CARCINOGENESIS, MUTAGENESIS, IMPAIRMENT OF FERTILITY
In a 24 month oral carcinogenicity study in mice dosed with 10 mg/kg/day drospirenone alone or 1 + 0.01, 3 + 0.03 and 10 + 0.1 mg/kg/day of drospirenone and ethinyl estradiol, 0.1 to 2 times the exposure (AUC of drospirenone) of women taking a contraceptive dose, there was an increase in carcinomas of the harderian gland in the group that received the high dose of drospirenone alone. In a similar study in rats given 10 mg/kg/day drospirenone alone or 0.3 + 0.003, 3 + 0.03 and 10 + 0.1 mg/kg/day drospirenone and ethinyl estradiol, 0.8 to 10 times the exposure of women taking a contraceptive dose, there was an increased incidence of benign and total (benign and malignant) adrenal gland pheochromocytomas in the group receiving the high dose of drospirenone. Drospirenone was not mutagenic in a number of *in vitro* (Ames, Chinese Hamster Lung gene mutation and chromosomal damage in human lymphocytes) and *in vivo* (mouse micronucleus) genotoxicity tests. Drospirenone increased unscheduled DNA synthesis in rat hepatocytes and formed adducts with rodent liver DNA but not with human liver DNA. (See **WARNINGS**.)
11. PREGNANCY
Pregnancy category X. (See **CONTRAINDICATIONS** and **WARNINGS**)
Estrogens and progestins should not be used during pregnancy. Fourteen pregnancies that occurred during exposure with 3 mg DRSP/0.03 mg EE tablets *in utero* (none with more than a single cycle of exposure) have been identified. One infant was born with esophageal atresia. A causal association with the 3 mg DRSP/0.03 mg EE tablet is unknown.
Twelve pregnancies that occurred with YAZ exposure *in utero* (none with more than a single cycle of exposure) have been identified. There were no known cases of congenital anomalies.
A teratology study in pregnant rats given drospirenone orally at doses of 5, 15 and 45 mg/kg/day, 6 to 50 times the human exposure based on AUC of drospirenone, resulted in an increased number of fetuses with delayed ossification of bones of the feet in the two higher doses. A similar study in rabbits dosed orally with 1, 30 and 100 mg/kg/day drospirenone, 2 to 27 times the human exposure, resulted in an increase in fetal loss and retardation of fetal development (delayed ossification of small bones, multiple fusions of ribs) at the high dose only. When drospirenone was administered with ethinyl estradiol (100:1) during late pregnancy (the period of genital development) at doses of 5, 15 and 45 mg/kg, there was a dose dependent increase in feminization of male rat fetuses. In a study in 36 cynomolgous monkeys, no teratogenic or feminization effects were observed with orally administered drospirenone and ethinyl estradiol (100:1) at doses up to 10 mg/kg/day drospirenone, 30 times the human exposure.
12. NURSING MOTHERS
Small amounts of oral contraceptive steroids have been identified in the milk of nursing mothers, and a few adverse effects on the child have been reported, including jaundice and breast enlargement. In addition, oral contraceptives given in the postpartum period may interfere with lactation by decreasing the quantity and quality of breast milk. If possible, the nursing mother should be advised not to use oral contraceptives but to use other forms of contraception until she has completely weaned her child.
After oral administration of 3 mg DRSP/0.03 mg EE tablets about 0.02% of the drospirenone dose was excreted into the breast milk of postpartum women within 24 hours. This results in a maximal daily dose of about 3 mcg drospirenone in an infant.
13. PEDIATRIC USAGE
Safety and efficacy of YAZ has been established in women of reproductive age. Safety and efficacy are expected to be the same for postpubertal adolescents under the age of 16 and for users 16 years and older. Use of this product before menarche is not indicated.
INFORMATION FOR THE PATIENT
See "Patient Labeling" printed below.

ADVERSE REACTIONS

An increased risk of the following serious adverse reactions has been associated with the use of oral contraceptives (see **WARNINGS**).
- Thrombophlebitis
- Arterial thromboembolism
- Pulmonary embolism
- Myocardial infarction
- Cerebral hemorrhage
- Cerebral thrombosis
- Hypertension
- Gallbladder disease
- Hepatic adenomas or benign liver tumors

There is evidence of an association between the following conditions and the use of oral contraceptives:
- Mesenteric thrombosis
- Retinal thrombosis

The following adverse reactions have been reported in patients receiving oral contraceptives and are believed to be drug-related:
- Nausea
- Vomiting
- Gastrointestinal symptoms (such as abdominal cramps and bloating)
- Breakthrough bleeding
- Spotting
- Change in menstrual flow
- Amenorrhea
- Temporary infertility after discontinuation of treatment
- Edema
- Melasma which may persist
- Breast changes: tenderness, enlargement, secretion
- Change in weight or appetite (increase or decrease)
- Change in cervical ectropion and secretion

- Possible diminution in lactation when given immediately postpartum
- Cholestatic jaundice
- Migraine
- Rash (allergic)
- Mood changes, including depression
- Reduced tolerance to carbohydrates
- Vaginitis, including candidiasis
- Change in corneal curvature (steepening)
- Intolerance to contact lenses
- Decrease in serum folate levels
- Exacerbation of systemic lupus erythematosus
- Exacerbation of porphyria
- Exacerbation of chorea
- Aggravation of varicose veins
- Anaphylactic/anaphylactoid reactions, including urticaria, angioedema, and severe reactions with respiratory and circulatory symptoms

The following adverse reactions have been reported in users of oral contraceptives and a causal association has been neither confirmed nor refuted:

- Acne
- Budd-Chiari syndrome
- Cataracts
- Changes in libido
- Colitis
- Cystitis-like syndrome
- Dizziness
- Dysmenorrhea
- Erythema multiforme
- Erythema nodosum
- Headache
- Hemolytic uremic syndrome
- Hemorrhagic eruption
- Hirsutism
- Impaired renal function
- Loss of scalp hair
- Nervousness
- Optic neuritis, which may lead to partial or complete loss of vision
- Pancreatitis
- Premenstrual syndrome

The most frequent (> 1%) treatment-emergent adverse events, listed in descending order, reported with the use of YAZ in the contraception clinical trials, which may or not be drug related, included: upper respiratory infection, headache, breast pain, vaginal moniliasis, leukorrhea, diarrhea, nausea, vomiting, vaginitis, abdominal pain, flu syndrome, dysmenorrhea, moniliasis, allergic reaction, urinary tract infection, accidental injury, cystitis, tooth disorder, sore throat, infection, fever, surgery, sinusitis, back pain, emotional lability, migraine, suspicious Papanicolaou smear, dyspepsia, rhinitis, acne, gastroenteritis, bronchitis, pharyngitis, skin disorder, intermenstrual bleeding, decreased libido, weight gain, pain, depression, increased cough, dizziness, menstrual disorder, pain in extremity, pelvic pain, and asthenia.

The most frequent (> 1%) treatment-emergent adverse events, listed in descending order, reported with the use of YAZ in the PMDD clinical trials, which may or not be drug related, included: intermenstrual bleeding, headache, nausea, breast pain, upper respiratory infection, asthenia, abdominal pain, decreased libido, emotional lability, suspicious Papanicolaou smear, nervousness, menorrhagia, pain in extremity, depression, menstrual disorder, migraine, sinusitis, weight gain, vaginal moniliasis, vaginitis, hyperlipidemia, back pain, diarrhea, increased appetite, enlarged abdomen, accidental injury, acne, dysmenorrhea, and urinary tract infection.

The most frequent (> 1%) treatment-emergent adverse events, listed in descending order, reported with the use of YAZ in the acne clinical trials, which may or not be drug related, included: upper respiratory infection, metrorrhagia, headache, suspicious Papanicolaou smear, nausea, sinusitis, vaginal moniliasis, flu syndrome, menorrhagia, depression, emotional lability, abdominal pain, gastroenteritis, urinary tract infection, tooth disorder, infection, vomiting, pharyngitis, breast pain, dysmenorrhea, menstrual disorder, accidental injury, asthenia, sore throat, weight gain, arthralgia, bronchitis, rhinitis, amenorrhea, and urine abnormality.

OVERDOSAGE

Serious ill effects have not been reported following acute ingestion of large doses of other oral contraceptives by young children. Overdosage may cause nausea, and withdrawal bleeding may occur in females. Drospirenone, however, is a spironolactone analogue which has antimineralocorticoid properties. Serum concentration of potassium and sodium, and evidence of metabolic acidosis, should be monitored in cases of overdose.

NON-CONTRACEPTIVE HEALTH BENEFITS

The following non-contraceptive health benefits related to the use of oral contraceptives are supported by epidemiological studies which largely utilized oral contraceptive formulations containing doses exceeding 0.035 mg of ethinyl estradiol or 0.05 mg mestranol.

Effects on menses:

- increased menstrual cycle regularity
- decreased blood loss and decreased incidence of iron-deficiency anemia
- decreased incidence of dysmenorrhea

Effects related to inhibition of ovulation:

- decreased incidence of functional ovarian cysts
- decreased incidence of ectopic pregnancies

Effects from long-term use:

- decreased incidence of fibroadenomas and fibrocystic disease of the breast
- decreased incidence of acute pelvic inflammatory disease
- decreased incidence of endometrial cancer
- decreased incidence of ovarian cancer

DOSAGE AND ADMINISTRATION

ORAL CONTRACEPTION and PMDD

To achieve maximum contraceptive and PMDD effectiveness, YAZ (drospirenone and ethinyl estradiol) must be taken exactly as directed at intervals not exceeding 24 hours.

YAZ consists of 24 light pink active tablets of a monophasic combined hormonal preparation plus 4 inert white tablets. The dosage of YAZ is one light pink tablet daily for 24 consecutive days followed by 4 white inert tablets per menstrual cycle. A patient should begin to take YAZ either on the first day of her menstrual period (Day 1 Start) or on the first Sunday after the onset of her menstrual period (Sunday Start).

Day 1 Start. During the first cycle of YAZ use, the patient should be instructed to take one light pink YAZ daily, beginning on Day one (1) of her menstrual cycle. (The first day of menstruation is Day one.) She should take one light pink YAZ daily for 24 consecutive days, followed by one white inert tablet daily on menstrual cycle days 25 through 28. It is recommended that YAZ be taken at the same time each day, preferably after the evening meal or at bedtime. YAZ can be taken without regard to meals. If YAZ is first taken later than the first day of the menstrual cycle, YAZ should not be considered effective as a contraceptive until after the first 7 consecutive days of product administration. The possibility of ovulation and conception prior to initiation of medication should be considered.

Sunday Start. During the first cycle of YAZ use, the patient should be instructed to take one light pink YAZ daily, beginning on the first Sunday after the onset of her menstrual period. She should take one light pink YAZ daily for 24 consecutive days, followed by one white inert tablet daily on menstrual cycle days 25 through 28. It is recommended that YAZ be taken at the same time each day, preferably after the evening meal or at bedtime. YAZ can be taken without regard to meals. YAZ should not be considered effective as a contraceptive until after the first 7 consecutive days of product administration. The possibility of ovulation and conception prior to initiation of medication should be considered.

The patient should begin her next and all subsequent 28-day regimens of YAZ on the same day of the week that she began her first regimen, following the same schedule. She should begin taking her light pink tablets on the next day after ingestion of the last white tablet, regardless of whether or not a menstrual period has occurred or is still in progress. Anytime a subsequent cycle of YAZ is started later than the day following administration of the last white tablet, the patient should use another method of contraception until she has taken a light pink YAZ daily for seven consecutive days.

When switching from another oral contraceptive, YAZ should be started on the same day that a new pack of the previous oral contraceptive would have been started.

Withdrawal bleeding usually occurs within 3 days following the last light pink tablet. If spotting or breakthrough bleeding occurs while taking YAZ, the patient should be instructed to continue taking her YAZ as instructed and by the regimen described above. She should be instructed that this type of bleeding is usually transient and without significance; however, if the bleeding is persistent or prolonged, the patient should be advised to consult her physician.

Although the occurrence of pregnancy is low if YAZ is taken according to directions, if withdrawal bleeding does not occur, the possibility of pregnancy must be considered. If the patient has not adhered to the prescribed dosing schedule (missed one or more active tablets or started taking them on a day later than she should have), the possibility of pregnancy should be considered at the time of the first missed period and appropriate diagnostic measures taken. If the patient has adhered to the prescribed regimen and misses two consecutive periods, pregnancy should be ruled out. Hormonal contraceptives should be discontinued if pregnancy is confirmed.

The risk of pregnancy increases with each active light pink tablet missed. For additional patient instructions regarding missed pills, see the **"WHAT TO DO IF YOU MISS PILLS"** section in the **DETAILED PATIENT LABELING** which follows. If breakthrough bleeding occurs following missed tablets, it will usually be transient and of no consequence. If the patient misses one or more white tablets, she should still be protected against pregnancy provided she begins taking light pink tablets again on the proper day.

In the nonlactating mother, YAZ may be initiated 4-6 weeks postpartum, for contraception. When the tablets are administered in the postpartum period, the increased risk of thromboembolic disease associated with the postpartum period must be considered. (See **CONTRAINDICATIONS, WARNINGS,** and **PRECAUTIONS** concerning thromboembolic disease.)

ACNE

The timing and initiation of dosing with YAZ in women with acne should follow the guideline for use of YAZ as an oral contraceptive. The 28-day dosage regimen for YAZ for treating facial acne consists of one active tablet daily for 24 consecutive days followed by one inert tablet daily for 4 days. After 28 tablets are taken, a new course is started the next day.

HOW SUPPLIED

YAZ (drospirenone and ethinyl estradiol) Tablets are available in packages of 3 BLISTER packs (NDC 50419-405-03). Each pack contains 24 active light pink round, unscored, film-coated tablets debossed with a "DS" in a regular hexagon on one side, each containing 3 mg drospirenone and 0.02 mg ethinyl estradiol, and 4 inert white round, unscored, film-coated tablets debossed with a "DP" in a regular hexagon on one side.

Store at 25° C (77° F); excursions permitted to 15–30° C (59–86° F) [See USP Controlled Room Temperature].

REFERENCES

1. Dinger JC, Heinemann LAJ, et al: The safety of a drospirenone-containing oral contraceptive: final results from the European active surveillance study on oral contraceptives based on 142,475 women-years of observation. *Contraception* 2007;75:344-354.
2. Seeger JD, Loughlin J, Eng PM, et al: Risk of thromboembolism in women taking ethinylestradiol/drospirenone and other oral contraceptives. *Obstetrics & Gynecology* 2007;110(3):587-593.
3. van Hylckama Vlieg A, Helmerhorst FM, Vandenbroucke JP, et al: The venous thrombotic risk of oral contraceptives, effects of oestrogen dose and progestogen type: results of the MEGA case-control study. *BMJ* 2009;339: b2921.
4. Lidegaard O, Lokkegaard E, Svendsen AL, et al: Hormonal contraception and risk of venous thromboembolism: national follow-up study. *BMJ* 2009; 339:b2890.

Manufactured for: Bayer HealthCare Pharmaceuticals Inc.
Manufactured in: Germany

BRIEF SUMMARY PATIENT PACKAGE INSERT

YAZ
(drospirenone and ethinyl estradiol) Tablets
containing the following:
24 light pink–"active" tablets
4 white–"inert" tablets

This product (like all oral contraceptives) is intended to prevent pregnancy. It does not protect against HIV infection (AIDS) and other sexually transmitted diseases.

YAZ is different from other birth control pills because it contains the progestin drospirenone. Drospirenone may increase potassium. Therefore, you should not take YAZ if you have kidney, liver or adrenal disease because this could cause serious heart and health problems. Other drugs may also increase potassium. If you are currently on daily, long-term treatment for a chronic condition with any of the medications below, you should consult your healthcare provider about whether YAZ is right for you, and during the first month that you take YAZ, you should have a blood test to check your potassium level.

- **NSAIDs (ibuprofen [Motrin, Advil], naprosyn [Aleve and others] when taken long-term and daily for treatment of arthritis or other problems)**
- **Potassium-sparing diuretics (spironolactone and others)**
- **Potassium supplementation**
- **ACE inhibitors (Capoten, Vasotec, Zestril and others)**
- **Angiotensin-II receptor antagonists (Cozaar, Diovan, Avapro and others)**
- **Heparin**
- **Aldosterone antagonists**

YAZ is an oral contraceptive, also known as a "birth control pill" or "the Pill." Oral contraceptives are taken to prevent pregnancy, and, when taken correctly without missing any pills, have a failure rate of approximately 1% per year (1 pregnancy per 100 women per year of use). The typical failure rate in pill users is approximately 5% per year (5 pregnancies per 100 women per year of use) when women who miss pills are included. Forgetting to take pills considerably increases the chances of pregnancy.

YAZ may also be taken to treat premenstrual dysphoric disorder (PMDD) if you choose to use the Pill for birth control. Unless you have already decided to use the Pill for birth control, you should not start YAZ to treat your PMDD because there are other medical therapies for PMDD that do not have the same risks as the Pill. PMDD is a mood disorder related to the menstrual cycle. PMDD significantly interferes with work or school, or with usual social activities and relationships with others. Symptoms include markedly depressed mood, anxiety or tension, mood swings, and persistent anger or irritability. Other features include decreased interest in usual activities, difficulty concentrating, lack of energy, change in appetite or sleep, and feeling out of control. Physical symptoms associated with PMDD may include breast tenderness, headache, joint and muscle pain, bloating and weight gain. These symptoms occur regularly before menstruation starts and go away within a few days following the start of the period. Diagnosis of PMDD should be made by healthcare providers.

You should only use YAZ for treatment of PMDD if you:

- Have already decided to use oral contraceptives for birth control, and
- Have been diagnosed with PMDD by your healthcare provider.

YAZ has not been shown to be effective for the treatment of premenstrual syndrome (PMS), a less serious cluster of symptoms occurring before menstruation. If you or your healthcare provider believes you have PMS, you should only take YAZ if you want to prevent pregnancy; and not for the treatment of PMS.

YAZ may also be taken to treat moderate acne in women who are able to and wish to use the Pill for birth control.

Any woman who needs contraception (birth control) and chooses to use an oral contraceptive should understand the benefits and risks of using the Pill. This leaflet will give you much of the information you will need to help you decide if you should use the Pill for contraception and will also help you determine if you are at risk of developing any of the serious side effects of the Pill. It will tell you how to use the Pill properly so that it will be as effective as possible. However, this leaflet is not a replacement for a careful discussion between you and your healthcare professional. You should discuss the information provided in this leaflet with him or her, both when you first start taking the Pill and during your revisits. You should also follow your healthcare professional's advice with regard to regular check-up while you are on the Pill.

For the majority of women, oral contraceptives can be taken safely. But there are some women who are at high risk of developing certain serious diseases that can be life-threatening or may cause temporary or permanent disability or death. The risks associated with taking oral contraceptives increase significantly if you:

- smoke
- have high blood pressure, diabetes, high cholesterol, or are obese
- have or have had clotting disorders, heart attack, stroke, angina pectoris (severe chest pains), cancer of the breast or sex organs, jaundice, or malignant or benign liver tumors.

You should not take the Pill if you suspect you are pregnant or have unexplained vaginal bleeding.

Although cardiovascular disease risks may be increased with oral contraceptive use after age 40 in healthy, non-smoking women (even with the newer low-dose formulations), there are also greater potential health risks associated with pregnancy in older women.

Cigarette smoking increases the risk of serious adverse effects on the heart and blood vessels from oral contraceptive use. This risk increases with age and with heavy smoking (15 or more cigarettes per day) and is quite marked in women over 35 years of age. Women who use oral contraceptives should not smoke.

Most side effects of the Pill are not serious. The most common such effects are nausea, vomiting, bleeding between menstrual periods, weight gain, breast tenderness, and difficulty wearing contact lenses. These side effects, especially nausea and vomiting may subside within the first three months of use.

The serious side effects of the Pill occur very infrequently, especially if you are in good health and are young. However, you should know that the following medical conditions have been associated with or made worse by the Pill:

1. Blood clots in the legs (thrombophlebitis), lungs (pulmonary embolism), blockage or rupture of a blood vessel in the brain (stroke), blockage of blood vessels in the heart (heart attack and angina pectoris) or other organs of the body. As mentioned above, smoking increases the risk of heart attacks and strokes and subsequent serious medical consequences. Women with migraine headaches also may be at increased risk of stroke when taking the Pill.
2. Liver tumors, which may rupture and cause severe bleeding. A possible but not definite association has been found with the Pill and liver cancer. However, liver cancers are extremely rare. The chance of developing liver cancer from using the Pill is thus even rarer.
3. High blood pressure, although blood pressure usually returns to normal when the Pill is stopped.
4. Cancer of the breast. Various studies give conflicting reports on the relationship between breast cancer and oral contraceptive use. Oral contraceptive use may slightly increase your chance of having breast cancer diagnosed, particularly after using hormonal contraceptives at a younger age. After you stop using hormonal contraceptives, the chances of getting breast cancer begin to go back down. You should have regular breast examinations by a healthcare provider and examine your own breasts monthly. Tell your healthcare provider if you have a family history of breast cancer or if you have had breast nodules or an abnormal mammogram. Women who currently have or have had breast cancer should not use oral contraceptives because breast cancer is a hormone-sensitive tumor.

Some studies have found an increase in the incidence of cancer or precancerous lesions of the cervix in women who use the Pill. However, this finding may be related to factors other than the use of the Pill.

The symptoms associated with these serious side effects are discussed in the detailed leaflet given to you with your supply of pills. Notify your doctor or healthcare provider if you notice any unusual physical disturbances while taking the Pill. In addition, drugs such as rifampin, as well as some anticonvulsants, some antibiotics and some herbal products such as St. John's Wort, may decrease oral contraceptive effectiveness.

Taking the Pill may provide some important non-contraceptive benefits. These include less painful menstruation, less menstrual blood loss and anemia, fewer pelvic infections, and fewer cancers of the ovary and the lining of the uterus.

Be sure to discuss any medical condition you may have with your healthcare provider. Your healthcare provider will take a medical and family history before prescribing oral contraceptives and will examine you. The physical examination may be delayed to another time if you request it and the healthcare provider believes that it is appropriate to postpone it. You should be reexamined at least once a year while taking oral contraceptives. The detailed patient information booklet gives you further information which you should read and discuss with your healthcare provider.

This product (like all oral contraceptives) is intended to prevent pregnancy. Oral contraceptives do not protect against HIV infection (AIDS) and other sexually transmitted diseases such as chlamydia, genital herpes, genital warts, gonorrhea, hepatitis B, and syphilis.

INSTRUCTIONS TO PATIENTS

HOW TO TAKE THE PILL

IMPORTANT POINTS TO REMEMBER

BEFORE YOU START TAKING YOUR PILLS:

1. BE SURE TO READ THESE DIRECTIONS:
   Before you start taking your pills.
   Anytime you are not sure what to do.
2. THE RIGHT WAY TO TAKE THE PILL IS TO TAKE ONE PILL EVERY DAY AT THE SAME TIME. YAZ CAN BE TAKEN WITHOUT REGARD TO MEALS.
   If you miss pills you could get pregnant. This includes starting the pack late. The more pills you miss, the more likely you are to get pregnant. See **"WHAT TO DO IF YOU MISS PILLS"** below.
3. MANY WOMEN HAVE SPOTTING OR LIGHT BLEEDING, OR MAY FEEL SICK TO THEIR STOMACH DURING THE FIRST 1-3 PACKS OF PILLS.
   If you do have spotting or light bleeding or feel sick to your stomach, do not stop taking the Pill. The problem will usually go away. If it does not go away, check with your healthcare provider.
4. MISSING PILLS CAN ALSO CAUSE SPOTTING OR LIGHT BLEEDING, even when you make up these missed pills.
   On the days you take two pills, to make up for missed pills, you could also feel a little sick to your stomach.
5. IF YOU HAVE VOMITING (within 3 to 4 hours after you take your pill), you should follow the instructions for **"WHAT TO DO IF YOU MISS PILLS"**. IF YOU HAVE DIARRHEA, or IF YOU TAKE CERTAIN MEDICINES, including some antibiotics and some herbal products such as St. John's Wort, your pills may not work as well.
   Use a back-up method (such as condoms or spermicides) until you check with your healthcare provider.
6. IF YOU HAVE TROUBLE REMEMBERING TO TAKE THE PILL, talk to your healthcare provider about how to make pill-taking easier or about using another method of birth control.
7. IF YOU HAVE ANY QUESTIONS OR ARE UNSURE ABOUT THE INFORMATION IN THIS LEAFLET, call your healthcare provider.

***BEFORE* YOU START TAKING YOUR PILLS**

1. DECIDE WHAT TIME OF DAY YOU WANT TO TAKE YOUR PILL.
   It is important to take YAZ at about the same time every day. YAZ can be taken without regard to meals.
2. LOOK AT YOUR PILL PACK:–IT HAS 28 PILLS:
   The YAZ-*pill pack* has 24 light pink "active" pills (with hormones) to be taken for 24 days, followed by 4 white "reminder" pills (without hormones) to be taken for four days.
3. ALSO FIND:
   1) Where on the pack to start taking pills,
   2) In what order to take the pills (follow the arrows)
   3) The week numbers as shown in the diagram below
4. BE SURE YOU HAVE READY AT ALL TIMES:
   ANOTHER KIND OF BIRTH CONTROL (such as condoms or spermicides) to use as a back-up in case you miss pills.
   AN EXTRA, FULL PILL PACK.

WHEN TO START THE FIRST PACK OF PILLS

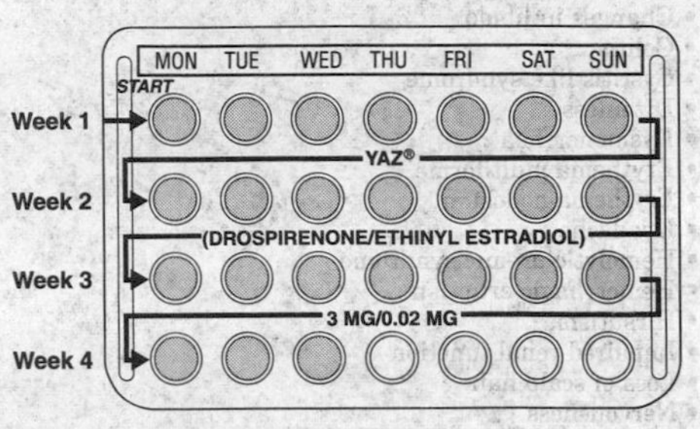

You have a choice for which day to start taking your first pack of pills. Decide with your healthcare provider which is the best day for you. Pick a time of day which will be easy to remember.

DAY 1 START:

1. Take the first light pink "active" pill of the first pack during the *first 24 hours of your period.*
2. You will not need to use a back-up method of birth control, since you are starting the Pill at the beginning of your period.

SUNDAY START:

1. Take the first light pink "active" pill of the first pack on the *Sunday after your period starts*, even if you are still bleeding. If your period begins on Sunday, start the pack that same day.
2. *Use another method of birth control* (such as condoms or spermicides) as a back-up method if you have sex anytime from the Sunday you start your first pack until the next Sunday (7 days).

WHEN YOU SWITCH FROM A DIFFERENT BIRTH CONTROL PILL

When switching from another birth control pill, YAZ should be started on the same day that a new pack of the previous birth control pills would have been started.

WHAT TO DO DURING THE MONTH

1. **TAKE ONE PILL AT THE SAME TIME EVERY DAY UNTIL THE PACK IS EMPTY**
   Do not skip pills even if you are spotting or bleeding between monthly periods or feel sick to your stomach (nausea).
   Do not skip pills even if you do not have sex very often.
2. **WHEN YOU FINISH A PACK OF PILLS:**
   Start the next pack on the day after your last white "reminder" pill. Do not wait any days between packs.

WHAT TO DO IF YOU MISS PILLS

If you **MISS 1** light pink "active" pill in Week 1 of your pack:

1. Take it as soon as you remember. Take the next pill at your regular time. This means you may take two pills in one day.
2. You do not need to use a back-up birth control method if you have sex.

If you **MISS 2** light pink "active" pills in a row in **WEEK 1** or **WEEK 2** of your pack:

1. Take two pills on the day you remember and two pills the next day.
2. Then take one pill a day until you finish the pack.
3. You COULD BECOME PREGNANT if you have sex in the 7 *days* after you restart your pills. You MUST use another birth control method (such as condoms or spermicides) as a back-up for those 7 days.

If you **MISS 2** light pink "active" pills in a row in **WEEK 3** or **Week 4** of your pack:

1. **If you are a Day 1 Starter:**
   THROW OUT the rest of the pill pack and start a new pack that same day.

If you are a Sunday Starter:
Keep taking one pill every day until Sunday. On Sunday, THROW OUT the rest of the pack and start a new pack of pills that same day.

2. You COULD BECOME PREGNANT if you have sex in the 7 *days* after you restart your pills. You MUST use another birth control method (such as condoms or spermicides) as a back-up for those 7 days.
3. You may not have your period this month but this is expected. However, if you miss your period two months in a row, call your healthcare provider because you might be pregnant.

If you **MISS 3 OR MORE** light pink "active" pills in a row during **ANY Week:**

1. ***If you are a Day 1 Starter:***
THROW OUT the rest of the pill pack and start a new pack that same day.
If you are a Sunday Starter:
Keep taking 1 pill every day until Sunday. On Sunday, THROW OUT the rest of the pack and start a new pack of pills that same day.
2. You COULD BECOME PREGNANT if you have sex in the 7 *days* after you restart pills. You MUST use another birth control method (such as condoms or spermicides) as a back-up for those 7 days.
3. You may not have your period this month but this is expected. However, if you miss your period two months in a row, call your healthcare provider because you might be pregnant.

If you **MISS ANY** of the **4** white "reminder" pills in **Week 4:**
THROW AWAY the pills you missed.
Keep taking one pill each day until the pack is empty.
You do not need a back-up method of birth control.

FINALLY, IF YOU ARE STILL NOT SURE WHAT TO DO ABOUT THE PILLS YOU HAVE MISSED:
Use a BACK-UP METHOD (such as condoms or spermicides) anytime you have sex.
KEEP TAKING ONE ACTIVE LIGHT PINK PILL EACH DAY until you can contact your healthcare provider.
For additional information see "Detailed Patient Labeling"

DETAILED PATIENT PACKAGE INSERT

This product (like all oral contraceptives) is intended to prevent pregnancy. Oral contraceptives do not protect against HIV infection (AIDS) and other sexually transmitted diseases.

YAZ is different from other birth control pills because it contains the progestin drospirenone. Drospirenone may increase potassium. Therefore, you should not take YAZ if you have kidney, liver or adrenal disease because this could cause serious heart and health problems. Other drugs may also increase potassium. If you are currently on daily, long-term treatment for a chronic condition with any of the medications below, you should consult your healthcare provider about whether YAZ is right for you, and during the first month that you take YAZ, you should have a blood test to check your potassium level.

- **NSAIDs (ibuprofen [Motrin, Advil], naprosyn [Aleve and others] when taken long-term and daily for treatment of arthritis or other problems)**
- **Potassium-sparing diuretics (spironolactone and others)**
- **Potassium supplementation**
- **ACE inhibitors (Capoten, Vasotec, Zestril and others)**
- **Angiotensin-II receptor antagonists (Cozaar, Diovan, Avapro and others)**
- **Heparin**
- **Aldosterone antagonists**

YAZ is an oral contraceptive, also known as a "birth control pill" or "the Pill." Oral contraceptives are taken to prevent pregnancy, and, when taken correctly without missing any pills, have a failure rate of approximately 1% per year (1 pregnancy per 100 women per year of use). The typical failure rate in pill users is approximately 5% per year (5 pregnancies per 100 women per year of use) when women who miss pills are included. Forgetting to take pills considerably increases the chances of pregnancy.

YAZ may also be taken to treat premenstrual dysphoric disorder (PMDD) if you choose to use the Pill for birth control. Unless you have already decided to use the Pill for birth control, you should not start YAZ to treat your PMDD because there are other medical therapies for PMDD that do not have the same risks as the Pill. PMDD is a mood disorder related to the menstrual cycle. PMDD significantly interferes with work or school, or with usual social activities and relationships with others. Symptoms include markedly depressed mood, anxiety or tension, mood swings, and persistent anger or irritability. Other features include decreased interest in usual activities, difficulty concentrating, lack of energy, change in appetite or sleep, and feeling out of control. Physical symptoms associated with PMDD may include breast tenderness, headache, joint and muscle pain, bloating and weight gain. These symptoms occur regularly before menstruation starts and go away within a few days following the start of the period. Diagnosis of PMDD should be made by healthcare providers.

You should only use YAZ for treatment of PMDD if you:

- Have already decided to use oral contraceptives for birth control, and
- Have been diagnosed with PMDD by your healthcare provider.

YAZ has not been shown to be effective for the treatment of premenstrual syndrome (PMS), a less serious cluster of symptoms occurring before menstruation. If you or your healthcare provider believes you have PMS, you should only take YAZ if you want to prevent pregnancy; and not for the treatment of PMS.

YAZ may also be taken to treat moderate acne in women who are able to and wish to use the Pill for birth control.

INTRODUCTION

Any woman who needs contraception (birth control) and chooses to use an oral contraceptive should understand the benefits and risks of using the Pill. This leaflet will give you much of the information you will need to help you decide if you should use the Pill for contraception and will also help you determine if you are at risk of developing any of the serious side effects of the Pill. It will tell you how to use the Pill properly so that it will be as effective as possible. However, this leaflet is not a replacement for a careful discussion between you and your healthcare professional. You should discuss the information provided in this leaflet with him or her, both when you first start taking the Pill and during your revisits. You should also follow your healthcare professional's advice with regard to regular check-ups while you are on the Pill.

EFFECTIVENESS OF YAZ FOR PREVENTION OF PREGNANCY

Oral contraceptives or "birth control pills" or "the Pill" are used to prevent pregnancy and are more effective than most other nonsurgical methods of birth control. When they are taken correctly, the chance of becoming pregnant is less than 1% (one pregnancy per 100 women per year of use) when used perfectly, without missing any pills. Typical failure rates, including women who don't always follow the instructions exactly, are about 5% per year. The chance of becoming pregnant increases with each missed pill during a menstrual cycle.

In comparison, typical failure rates for other nonsurgical methods of birth control during the first year of use are as follows:

Percentage of women experiencing an unintended pregnancy during the first year of typical use and first year of perfect use of contraception and the percentage continuing use at the end of the first year: United States.

	% of Women Experiencing an Unintended Pregnancy Within the First Year of Use		% of Women Continuing Use at One Year[3]
Method (1)	Typical Use[1] (2)	Perfect Use[2] (3)	(4)
Chance[4]	85	85	
Spermicides[5]	26	6	40
Periodic abstinence	25		63
Calendar		9	
Ovulation method		3	
Sympto-thermal[6]		2	
Post-ovulation		1	
Withdrawal	19	4	
Cap[7]			
Parous women	40	26	42
Nulliparous women	20	9	56
Sponge			
Parous women	40	20	42
Nulliparous women	20	9	56
Diaphragm[7]	20	6	56
Condom[8]			
Female (Reality)	21	5	56
Male	14	3	61
Pill	5		71
progestin only		0.5	
combined		0.1	
IUD:			
Progesterone T	2	1.5	81
Copper T 380A	0.8	0.6	78
Lng 20	0.1	0.1	81
Depo Provera	0.3	0.3	70
Norplant and Norplant-2	0.05	0.05	88
Female sterilization	0.5	0.5	100
Male sterilization	0.15	0.1	100

Emergency Contraceptive Pills: Treatment initiated within 72 hours after unprotected intercourse reduces the risk of pregnancy by at least 75%.[9]
Lactational Amenorrhea Method: LAM is highly effective, *temporary* method of contraception.[10]
Source: Trussell J, Contraceptive efficacy. In Hatcher RA, Trussell J, Stewart F, Cates W, Stewart GK, Guest F, Kowal D, *Contraceptive Technology: Seventeenth Revised Edition*. New York NY: Irvington Publishers, 1998.

1 Among typical couples who initiate use of a method (not necessarily for the first time), the percentage who experience an accidental pregnancy during the first year if they do not stop use for any other reason.
2 Among couples who initiate use of a method (not necessarily for the first time) and who use it perfectly (both consistently and correctly). The percentage who experience an accidental pregnancy during the first year if they do not stop use for any reason.
3 Among couples attempting to avoid pregnancy, the percentage who continue to use a method for one year.
4 The percents becoming pregnant in columns (2) and (3) are based on data from populations where contraception is not used and from women who cease using contraception in order to become pregnant. Among such populations, about 89% become pregnant within one year. This estimate was lowered slightly (to 85%) to represent the percentage who would become pregnant within one year among women now relying on reversible methods of contraception if they abandoned contraception altogether.
5 Foams, creams, gels, vaginal suppositories, and vaginal film.
6 Cervical mucus (ovulation) method supplemented by calendar in the pre-ovulatory and basal body temperature in the post-ovulatory phases.
7 With spermicidal cream or jelly.
8 Without spermicides.
9 The treatment schedule is one dose within 72 hours after unprotected intercourse, and a second dose 12 hours after the first dose. The Food and Drug Administration has declared the following brands of oral contraceptives to be safe and effective for emergency contraception: Ovral (1 dose is 2 white pills), Alesse (1 dose is 5 pink pills), Nordette or Levlen (1 dose is 2 light-orange pills), Lo/Ovral (1 dose is 4 white pills), Triphasil or Tri-Levlen (1 dose is 4 yellow pills).
10 However, to maintain effective protection against pregnancy, another method of contraception must be used as soon as menstruation resumes, the frequency or duration of breastfeeds is reduced, bottle feeds are introduced, or the baby reaches six months of age.

YAZ may also be taken to treat moderate acne if **all** of the following are true:

- Your doctor says it is safe for you to use the Pill.
- You are at least 14 years old.
- You have started having menstrual periods.
- You want to use the Pill for birth control.

WHO SHOULD NOT TAKE YAZ or ORAL CONTRACEPTIVES

Cigarette smoking increases the risk of serious adverse effects on the heart and blood vessels from oral contraceptive use. This risk increases with age and with heavy smoking (15 or more cigarettes per day) and is quite marked in women over 35 years of age. Women who use oral contraceptives should not smoke.

Some women should not use YAZ. For example, you should not take YAZ if you are pregnant or think you may be pregnant. You should also not use YAZ if you have had any of the following conditions:

- A history of heart attack or stroke
- A history of blood clots in the legs (deep vein thrombosis), lungs (pulmonary embolism), or eyes (retinal thrombosis)
- Chest pain (angina pectoris)
- Known or suspected breast cancer or cancer of the lining of the uterus, cervix or vagina
- Unexplained vaginal bleeding (until a diagnosis is reached by your doctor)
- Yellowing of the whites of the eyes or of the skin (jaundice) during pregnancy or during previous use of the Pill or other hormonal contraceptives
- Liver tumor (benign or cancerous)
- Known or suspected pregnancy
- Heart valve or heart rhythm disorders that may be associated with formation of blood clots
- Diabetes with complications of the kidneys, eyes, nerves, or blood vessels
- Severe high blood pressure

ANNUAL NUMBER OF BIRTH-RELATED OR METHOD-RELATED DEATHS ASSOCIATED WITH CONTROL OF FERTILITY PER 100,000 NONSTERILE WOMEN, BY FERTILITY-CONTROL METHOD ACCORDING TO AGE

Method of Control and Outcome	15-19 years	20-24 years	25-29 years	30-34 years	35-39 years	40-44 years
No fertility control methods\1\	7	7.4	9.1	14.8	25.7	28.2
Oral contraceptives non-smoker\2\	0.3	0.5	0.9	1.9	13.8	31.6
Oral contraceptives smoker\2\	2.2	3.4	6.6	13.5	51.1	117.2
IUD\2\	0.8	0.8	1	1	1.4	1.4
Condom\1\	1.1	1.6	0.7	0.2	0.3	0.4
Diaphragm/spermicide\1\	1.9	1.2	1.2	1.3	2.2	2.8
Periodic abstinence\1\	2.5	1.6	1.6	1.7	2.9	3.6

\1\ Deaths are birth-related
\2\ Deaths are method-related
Adapted from H.W. Ory, *Family Planning Perspectives*, 15:57-63, 1983.

- A need for surgery with prolonged bedrest
- Headaches with neurological symptoms
- Allergy or hypersensitivity to any of the components of YAZ

In addition, you should not use YAZ if you have any of the following conditions:
- Kidney Disease
- Liver Disease
- Adrenal Disease

Tell your healthcare provider if you have ever had any of the above conditions (Your healthcare provider can recommend another method of birth control). If you are currently on daily, long-term treatment for a chronic condition with any of the following medications, you should consult your healthcare provider before taking YAZ:
- NSAIDs (ibuprofen, naprosyn and others)
- Potassium-sparing diuretics (spironolactone and others)
- Potassium supplementation
- ACE inhibitors (captopril, enalapril, lisinopril and others)
- Angiotensin-II receptor antagonists (Cozaar, Diovan, Avapro and others)
- Heparin
- Aldosterone antagonists

OTHER CONSIDERATIONS BEFORE TAKING ORAL CONTRACEPTIVES
Tell your healthcare provider if you have or ever had:
- Breast nodules, fibrocystic disease of the breast, an abnormal breast X-ray or mammogram
- Diabetes
- Elevated cholesterol or triglycerides
- High blood pressure
- A blood test indicating a higher risk of having blood clots
- Migraine or other headaches or epilepsy
- Mental depression
- Gallbladder, heart or kidney disease
- History of scanty or irregular menstrual periods

Women with any of these conditions should be checked often by their healthcare provider if they choose to use oral contraceptives.

Also, be sure to inform your doctor or healthcare provider if you smoke, are on any medications, recently had a baby or miscarriage, or are breast feeding.

RISKS OF TAKING ORAL CONTRACEPTIVES
1. RISK OF DEVELOPING BLOOD CLOTS
Blood clots and blockage of blood vessels are the most serious side effects of taking oral contraceptives and can be fatal. In particular, a clot in the legs (deep vein thrombosis) can cause pain and swelling, and a clot that travels to the lungs can cause sudden blocking of the vessel carrying blood to the lungs. Rarely, clots occur in the blood vessels of the eye and may cause blindness, double vision, or impaired vision.

If you take oral contraceptives and need elective surgery, need to stay in bed for a prolonged illness or have recently delivered a baby, you may be at risk of developing blood clots. You should consult your doctor about stopping oral contraceptives three to four weeks before surgery and not taking oral contraceptives for two weeks after surgery or during bed rest. You should also not take oral contraceptives soon after delivery of a baby or a mid-trimester pregnancy loss or termination. It is advisable to wait for at least four to six weeks after delivery if you are not breastfeeding. If you are breast-feeding, you should wait until you have weaned your child before using the Pill. (See also the section on breast-feeding in **GENERAL PRECAUTIONS**.)

2. HEART ATTACKS AND STROKES
Oral contraceptives may increase the tendency to develop strokes (stoppage or rupture of blood vessels in the brain) and angina pectoris and heart attacks (blockage of blood vessels in the heart). Any of these conditions can cause death or serious disability.

Smoking greatly increases the possibility of suffering heart attacks and strokes. Furthermore, smoking and the use of oral contraceptives greatly increase the chances of developing and dying of heart disease.

3. GALLBLADDER DISEASE
Oral contraceptive users probably have a greater risk than nonusers of having gallbladder disease, although this risk may be related to pills containing high doses of estrogens.

4. LIVER TUMORS
In rare cases, oral contraceptives can cause benign but dangerous liver tumors. These benign liver tumors can rupture and cause fatal internal bleeding. In addition, a possible but not definite association has been found with the pill and liver cancers in two studies, in which a few women who developed these very rare cancers were found to have used oral contraceptives for long periods. However, liver cancers are extremely rare. The chance of developing liver cancer from using the Pill is thus even rarer.

5. CANCER OF THE REPRODUCTIVE ORGANS AND BREASTS
Various studies give conflicting reports on the relationship between breast cancer and oral contraceptive use. Oral contraceptive use may slightly increase your chance of having breast cancer diagnosed, particularly after using hormonal contraceptives at a younger age. After you stop using hormonal contraceptives, the chances of getting breast cancer begin to go back down. You should have regular breast examinations by a healthcare provider and examine your own breasts monthly. Tell your healthcare provider if you have a family history of breast cancer or if you have had breast nodules or an abnormal mammogram. Women who currently have or have had breast cancer should not use oral contraceptives because breast cancer is a hormone-sensitive tumor.

Some studies have found an increase in the incidence of cancer of the cervix in women who use oral contraceptives. However, this finding may be related to factors other than the use of oral contraceptives.

ESTIMATED RISK OF DEATH FROM A BIRTH CONTROL METHOD OR PREGNANCY
All methods of birth control and pregnancy are associated with a risk of developing certain diseases which may lead to disability or death. An estimate of the number of deaths associated with different methods of birth control and pregnancy has been calculated and is shown in the following table.
[See table above]
In the above table, the risk of death from any birth control method is less than the risk of childbirth, except for oral contraceptive users over the age of 35 who smoke and Pill users over the age of 40 even if they do not smoke. It can be seen in the table that for women aged 15 to 39, the risk of death was highest with pregnancy (7-26 deaths per 100,000 women, depending on age). Among Pill users who do not smoke, the risk of death was always lower than that associated with pregnancy for any age group, except for those women over the age of 40, when the risk increases to 32 deaths per 100,000 women, compared to 28 associated with pregnancy at that age. However, for Pill users who smoke and are over the age of 35, the estimated number of deaths exceeds those for other methods of birth control. If a woman is over the age of 40 and smokes, her estimated risk of death is four times higher (117/100,000 women) than the estimated risk associated with pregnancy (28/100,000 women) in that age group.

The suggestion that women over 40 who do not smoke should not take oral contraceptives is based on information from older high-dose pills and on less-selective use of pills than is practiced today. An Advisory Committee of the FDA discussed this issue in 1989 and recommended that the benefits of oral contraceptive use by healthy, non-smoking women over 40 years of age may outweigh the possible risks. However, all women, especially older women, are cautioned to use the lowest-dose pill that is effective.

WARNING SIGNALS
If any of these adverse effects occur while you are taking oral contraceptives, call your doctor immediately:
- Sharp chest pain, coughing of blood, or sudden shortness of breath (indicating a possible clot in the lung)
- Pain in the calf (indicating a possible clot in the leg)
- Crushing chest pain or heaviness in the chest (indicating a possible heart attack)
- Sudden severe headache or vomiting, dizziness or fainting, disturbances of vision or speech, weakness, or numbness in an arm or leg (indicating a possible stroke)
- Sudden partial or complete loss of vision (indicating a possible clot in the eye)
- Breast lumps (indicating possible breast cancer or fibrocystic disease of the breast; ask your doctor or healthcare provider to show you how to examine your breasts)
- Severe pain or tenderness in the stomach area (indicating a possibly ruptured liver tumor)
- Difficulty in sleeping, weakness, lack of energy, fatigue, or change in mood (possibly indicating severe depression)
- Jaundice or a light yellowing of the skin or eyeballs, accompanied frequently by fever, fatigue, loss of appetite, dark-colored urine, or light-colored bowel movements (indicating possible liver problems)

SIDE EFFECTS OF ORAL CONTRACEPTIVES
1. VAGINAL BLEEDING
Irregular vaginal bleeding or spotting may occur while you are taking the pills. Irregular bleeding may vary from slight staining between menstrual periods to breakthrough bleeding, which is a flow much like a regular period. Irregular bleeding occurs most often during the first few months of oral contraceptive use, but may also occur after you have been taking the Pill for some time. Such bleeding may be temporary and usually does not indicate any serious problems. It is important to continue taking your pills on schedule. If the bleeding occurs in more than one cycle or lasts for more than a few days, talk to your doctor or healthcare provider.

2. CONTACT LENSES
If you wear contact lenses and notice a change in vision or an inability to wear your lenses, contact your doctor or healthcare provider.

3. FLUID RETENTION
Oral contraceptives may cause edema (fluid retention) with swelling of the fingers or ankles and may raise your blood pressure. If you experience fluid retention, contact your doctor or healthcare provider.

4. MELASMA
A spotty darkening of the skin is possible, particularly of the face.

5. OTHER SIDE EFFECTS
Other side effects may include nausea, vomiting, change in appetite, headache, nervousness, depression, dizziness, loss of scalp hair, rash, and vaginal infections.

If any of these side effects bother you, call your doctor or healthcare provider.

GENERAL PRECAUTIONS
1. Missed periods and use of oral contraceptives before or during early pregnancy.
There may be times when you may not menstruate regularly after you have completed taking a cycle of pills. If you have taken your pills regularly and miss one menstrual period, continue taking your pills for the next cycle but be sure to inform your healthcare provider. If you have not taken the pills daily as instructed and missed a menstrual period, or if you missed two consecutive menstrual periods, you may be pregnant. Check with your healthcare provider immediately to determine whether you are pregnant. Stop taking oral contraceptives if pregnancy is confirmed. There is no conclusive evidence that oral contraceptive use is associated with an increase in birth defects when taken inadvertently during early pregnancy. Previously, a few studies had reported that oral contraceptives might be associated with birth defects, but these studies have not been confirmed. Nevertheless, oral contraceptives should not be used during pregnancy. You should check with your doctor about risks to your unborn child of any medication taken during pregnancy.

2. While Breast-Feeding

If you are breast-feeding, consult your doctor before starting oral contraceptives. Some of the drug will be passed on to the child in the milk. A few adverse effects on the child have been reported, including light yellowing of the skin (jaundice) and breast enlargement. In addition, oral contraceptives may decrease the amount and quality of your milk. If possible, do not use oral contraceptives while breast-feeding. You should use another method of contraception since breast-feeding provides only partial protection from becoming pregnant, and this partial protection decreases significantly as you breast-feed for longer periods of time. You should consider starting oral contraceptives only after you have weaned your child completely.

3. Laboratory Tests

If you are scheduled for any laboratory tests, tell your doctor you are taking birth control pills. Certain blood tests may be affected by birth control pills.

4. Drug Interactions

Certain drugs may interact with birth control pills to make them less effective in preventing pregnancy or cause an increase in breakthrough bleeding. Such drugs include rifampin, drugs used for epilepsy such as barbiturates (for example, phenobarbital) and phenytoin (Dilantin is one brand of this drug), phenylbutazone (Butazolidin is one brand) and possibly certain antibiotics. Herbal products containing St. John's Wort (hypericum perforatum) may reduce the effectiveness of oral contraceptives. This may also result in breakthrough bleeding. You may need to use an additional method of contraception during any cycle in which you take drugs that can make oral contraceptives less effective (See **BOLDED TEXT AT BEGINNING**).

5. Sexually Transmitted Diseases

This product (like all oral contraceptives) is intended to prevent pregnancy. It does not protect against transmission of HIV (AIDS) and other sexually transmitted diseases such as chlamydia, genital herpes, genital warts, gonorrhea, hepatitis B, and syphilis.

INSTRUCTIONS TO PATIENTS

HOW TO TAKE THE PILL

IMPORTANT POINTS TO REMEMBER

BEFORE YOU START TAKING YOUR PILLS:

1. BE SURE TO READ THESE DIRECTIONS:
   Before you start taking your pills.
   Anytime you are not sure what to do.

2. THE RIGHT WAY TO TAKE THE PILL IS TO TAKE ONE PILL EVERY DAY AT THE SAME TIME. YAZ CAN BE TAKEN WITHOUT REGARD TO MEALS.
   If you miss pills you could get pregnant. This includes starting the pack late. The more pills you miss, the more likely you are to get pregnant. See **"WHAT TO DO IF YOU MISS PILLS"** below.

3. MANY WOMEN HAVE SPOTTING OR LIGHT BLEEDING, OR MAY FEEL SICK TO THEIR STOMACH DURING THE FIRST 1-3 PACKS OF PILLS.
   If you do have spotting or light bleeding or feel sick to your stomach, do not stop taking the Pill. The problem will usually go away. If it does not go away, check with your healthcare provider.

4. MISSING PILLS CAN ALSO CAUSE SPOTTING OR LIGHT BLEEDING, even when you make up these missed pills.
   On the days you take two pills, to make up for missed pills, you could also feel a little sick to your stomach.

5. IF YOU HAVE VOMITING (within 3 to 4 hours after you take your pill), you should follow the instructions for **"WHAT TO DO IF YOU MISS PILLS"**. IF YOU HAVE DIARRHEA OR IF YOU TAKE CERTAIN MEDICINES, including some antibiotics and some herbal products such as St. John's Wort, your pills may not work as well.
   Use a back-up method (such as condoms or spermicides) until you check with your healthcare provider.

6. IF YOU HAVE TROUBLE REMEMBERING TO TAKE THE PILL, talk to your healthcare provider about how to make pill-taking easier or about using another method of birth control.

7. IF YOU HAVE ANY QUESTIONS OR ARE UNSURE ABOUT THE INFORMATION IN THIS LEAFLET, call your healthcare provider.

BEFORE YOU START TAKING YOUR PILLS

1. DECIDE WHAT TIME OF DAY YOU WANT TO TAKE YOUR PILL.
   It is important to take YAZ at about the same time every day. YAZ can be taken without regard to meals.

2. LOOK AT YOUR PILL PACK: – IT HAS 28 PILLS
   The YAZ-pill pack has 24 light pink "active" pills (with hormones) to be taken for 24 days, followed by 4 white "reminder" pills (without hormones) to be taken for four days.

3. ALSO FIND:
   1) Where on the pack to start taking pills,
   2) In what order to take the pills (follow the arrows)
   3) The week numbers as shown in the diagram below

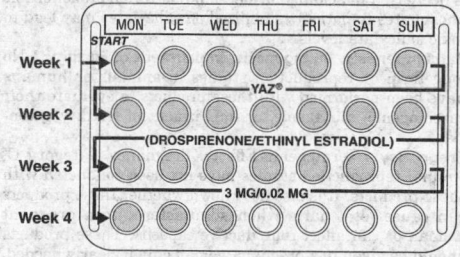

4. BE SURE YOU HAVE READY AT ALL TIMES:
   ANOTHER KIND OF BIRTH CONTROL (such as condoms or spermicides) to use as a back-up in case you miss pills.
   AN EXTRA, FULL PILL PACK.

WHEN TO START THE *FIRST* PACK OF PILLS

You have a choice for which day to start taking your first pack of pills. Decide with your healthcare provider which is the best day for you. Pick a time of day which will be easy to remember.

DAY 1 START:

1. Take the first light pink "active" pill of the first pack during the *first 24 hours of your period.*
2. You will not need to use a back-up method of birth control, since you are starting the Pill at the beginning of your period.

SUNDAY START:

1. Take the first light pink "active" pill of the first pack on the *Sunday after your period starts,* even if you are still bleeding. If your period begins on Sunday, start the pack that same day.
2. *Use another method of birth control* (such as condoms or spermicides) as a back-up method if you have sex anytime from the Sunday you start your first pack until the next Sunday (7 days).

WHEN YOU SWITCH FROM A DIFFERENT BIRTH CONTROL PILL

When switching from another birth control pill, YAZ should be started on the same day that a new pack of the previous birth control pill would have been started.

WHAT TO DO DURING THE MONTH

1. TAKE ONE PILL AT THE SAME TIME EVERY DAY UNTIL THE PACK IS EMPTY.

Do not skip pills even if you are spotting or bleeding between monthly periods or feel sick to your stomach (nausea).

Do not skip pills even if you do not have sex very often.

2. WHEN YOU FINISH A PACK OF PILLS:

Start the next pack on the day after your last white "reminder" pill. Do not wait any days between packs.

WHAT TO DO IF YOU MISS PILLS

If you **MISS 1** light pink "active" pill:

1. Take it as soon as you remember. Take the next pill at your regular time. This means you may take two pills in one day.
2. You do not need to use a back-up birth control method if you have sex.

If you **MISS 2** light pink "active" pills in a row in **WEEK 1 OR WEEK 2** of your pack:

1. Take two pills on the day you remember and two pills the next day.
2. Then take one pill a day until you finish the pack.
3. You COULD BECOME PREGNANT if you have sex in the 7 *days* after you restart your pills. You MUST use another birth control method (such as condoms or spermicides) as a back-up for those 7 days.

If you **MISS 2** light pink "active" pills in a row in **WEEK 3** or **Week 4** of your pack:

1. If you are a Day 1 Starter:
   THROW OUT the rest of the pill pack and start a new pack that same day.
   If you are a Sunday Starter:
   Keep taking one pill every day until Sunday. On Sunday, THROW OUT the rest of the pack and start a new pack of pills that same day.
2. You COULD BECOME PREGNANT if you have sex in the 7 *days* after you restart your pills. You MUST use another birth control method (such as condoms or spermicides) as a back up for those 7 days.
3. You may not have your period this month but this is expected. However, if you miss your period two months in a row, call your doctor or clinic because you might be pregnant.

If you **MISS 3 OR MORE** light pink "active" pills in a row during **ANY Week:**

1. **If you are a Day 1 Starter:**
   THROW OUT the rest of the pill pack and start a new pack that same day.
   If you are a Sunday Starter:
   Keep taking 1 pill every day until Sunday. On Sunday, THROW OUT the rest of the pack and start a new pack of pills that same day.
2. You COULD BECOME PREGNANT if you have sex in the 7 *days* after you restart your pills. You MUST use another birth control method (such as condoms or spermicides) as a back-up for those 7 days.
3. You may not have your period this month but this is expected. However, if you miss your period two months in a row, call your doctor or clinic because you might be pregnant.

If you **MISS ANY** of the **4 white** "reminder" pills in **Week 4:** THROW AWAY the pills you missed.

Keep taking one pill each day until the pack is empty.

You do not need a back-up method.

FINALLY, IF YOU ARE STILL NOT SURE WHAT TO DO ABOUT THE PILLS YOU HAVE MISSED:

Use a BACK-UP METHOD (such as condoms or spermicides) anytime you have sex.

KEEP TAKING ONE ACTIVE LIGHT PINK PILL EACH DAY until you contact your healthcare provider.

PREGNANCY AFTER STOPPING THE PILL

There may be some delay in becoming pregnant after you stop using oral contraceptives, especially if you had irregular menstrual cycles before you used oral contraceptives. It may be advisable to postpone conception until you begin menstruating regularly once you have stopped taking the Pill and desire pregnancy.

There does not appear to be any increase in birth defects in newborn babies when pregnancy occurs soon after stopping the Pill.

OVERDOSAGE

Serious ill effects have not been reported following ingestion of large doses of oral contraceptives by young children. Overdosage of YAZ may cause nausea and withdrawal bleeding in females and may increase blood levels of potassium or decrease blood levels of sodium, which could be dangerous. In case of overdosage, contact your healthcare provider.

OTHER INFORMATION

Your healthcare provider will take a medical and family history before prescribing oral contraceptives and will examine you. The physical examination may be delayed to another time if you request it and the healthcare provider believes that it is appropriate to postpone it. You should be re-examined at least once a year. Be sure to inform your healthcare provider if there is a family history of any of the conditions listed previously in this leaflet. Be sure to keep all appointments with your healthcare provider, because this is a time to determine if there are early signs of side effects of oral contraceptive use.

Do not use the drug for any condition other than the one for which it was prescribed. This drug has been prescribed specifically for you; do not give it to others who may want birth control pills.

HEALTH BENEFITS FROM ORAL CONTRACEPTIVES

In addition to preventing pregnancy, use of oral contraceptives may provide certain benefits. They are:

• Menstrual cycles may become more regular.
• Blood flow during menstruation may be lighter and less iron may be lost. Therefore, anemia due to iron deficiency is less likely to occur.
• Pain or other symptoms during menstruation may be encountered less frequently.
• Ovarian cysts may occur less frequently.
• Ectopic (tubal) pregnancy may occur less frequently.
• Noncancerous cysts or lumps in the breast may occur less frequently.
• Acute pelvic inflammatory disease may occur less frequently.
• Oral contraceptive use may provide some protection against developing two forms of cancer: cancer of the ovaries and cancer of the lining of the uterus.

If you want more information about birth control pills, ask your doctor or pharmacist. They have a more technical leaflet called the Prescribing Information which you may wish to read.

Manufactured by:

Bayer HealthCare

Pharmaceuticals

Bayer HealthCare Pharmaceuticals Inc.

Wayne, NJ 07470

Manufactured in Germany

© 2010, Bayer HealthCare Pharmaceuticals Inc. All Rights Reserved.

6700401 US   April 2010

Shown in Product Identification Guide, page 307

Beach Pharmaceuticals
Division of Beach Products, Inc.
5220 SOUTH MANHATTAN AVENUE
TAMPA, FL 33611

Direct Inquiries to:
Richard Stephen Jenkins
(813) 839-6565
FAX (813) 837-2511

K-PHOS® M.F.   ℞
[K - phos]
K-PHOS® No. 2
Urinary Acidifiers

DESCRIPTION
K-PHOS® M.F.: Each tablet contains potassium acid phosphate 155 mg and sodium acid phosphate, anhydrous 350 mg. Each tablet yields approximately 125.6 mg of phosphorus, 44.5 mg of potassium or 1.1 mEq and 67 mg of sodium or 2.9 mEq. **K-PHOS® No. 2:** Each tablet contains potassium acid phosphate 305 mg and sodium acid phosphate, anhydrous 700 mg. Each tablet yields approximately 250 mg of phosphorus, 88 mg of potassium or 2.3 mEq and 134 mg of sodium or 5.8 mEq.

CLINICAL PHARMACOLOGY
Phosphorus has a number of important functions in the biochemistry of the body. The bulk of the body's phosphorus is located in the bones, where it plays a key role in osteoblastic and osteoclastic activities. Enzymatically catalyzed phosphate-transfer reactions are numerous and vital in the metabolism of carbohydrate, lipid and protein, and a proper concentration of the anion is of primary importance in assuring an orderly biochemical sequence. In addition, phosphorus plays an important role in modifying steady-state tissue concentration of calcium. Phosphate ions are important buffers of the intracellular fluid, and also play a primary role in the renal excretion of hydrogen ion.
In general, in adults, about two thirds of the ingested phosphate is absorbed from the bowel, most of which is rapidly excreted into the urine.

INDICATIONS AND USAGE
These products are highly effective urinary acidifiers for use in patients with elevated urinary pH. These products help keep calcium soluble and reduce odor and rash caused by ammoniacal urine. Also, by acidifying the urine, they increase the antibacterial activity of methenamine mandelate and methenamine hippurate.

CONTRAINDICATIONS
These products are contraindicated in patients with infected phosphate stones, in patients with severely impaired renal function (less than 30% of normal), and in the presence of hyperphosphatemia.

PRECAUTIONS
General: These products contain potassium and sodium and should be used with caution if regulation of these elements is desired. Occasionally, some individuals may experience a mild laxative effect during the first few days of phosphate therapy. If laxation persists to an unpleasant degree, reduce the daily dosage until this effect subsides or, if necessary, discontinue the use of the product. Use of these medications should be carefully considered when the following medical problems exist: Cardiac disease (particularly in digitalized patients), Addison's disease, acute dehydration, extensive tissue breakdown, myotonia congenita, cardiac failure, cirrhosis of the liver or severe hepatic disease, peripheral and pulmonary edema, hypernatremia, hypertension, toxemia of pregnancy, hypoparathyroidism, and acute pancreatitis. Rickets may benefit from phosphate therapy, but caution should be observed. High serum phosphate levels increase the risk of extraskeletal calcification.
Information for Patients: Patients with kidney stones may pass old stones when phosphate therapy is started and should be warned of this possibility. Patients should be advised to avoid the use of antacids containing aluminum, magnesium, or calcium which may prevent the absorption of phosphate.
Laboratory Tests: Careful monitoring of renal function and serum calcium, phosphorus, potassium, and sodium may be required at periodic intervals. Other tests may be warranted in some patients, depending on conditions.
Drug Interactions: Use of antacids containing magnesium, aluminum or calcium in conjunction with phosphate preparations may bind the phosphate and prevent its absorption. Concurrent use of antihypertensives, especially diazoxide, guanethidine, hydralazine, methyldopa or rauwolfia alkaloid; or corticosteroids, especially mineralocorticoids or corticotropin, with sodium phosphate may result in hyper-

natremia. Potassium-containing medications, or potassium-sparing diuretics may cause hyperkalemia when used with potassium phosphate. Patients should have serum potassium level determinations at periodic intervals. Plasma levels of salicylates may be increased since salicylate excretion is decreased in acidified urine. Administration of monobasic phosphates to patients stabilized on salicylates may lead to toxic salicylate levels.
Carcinogenesis, Mutagenesis, Impairment of Fertility: No long term or reproduction studies in animals or humans have been performed with these products to evaluate their carcinogenic, mutagenic, or impairment of fertility potential.
Pregnancy: Teratogenic Effects. Pregnancy Category C. Animal reproduction studies have not been conducted with these products. It is also not known whether these products can cause fetal harm when administered to a pregnant woman or can affect reproductive capacity. These products should be given to a pregnant woman only if clearly needed.
Nursing Mothers: It is not known whether these drugs are excreted in human milk. Because many drugs are excreted in human milk, caution should be exercised when these products are administered to a nursing woman.

ADVERSE REACTIONS
Gastrointestinal upset (diarrhea, nausea, stomach pain and vomiting) may occur with phosphate therapy. Also, bone and joint pain (possible phosphate-induced osteomalacia) could occur. The following adverse effects may be observed (primarily from sodium or potassium): headaches; dizziness; mental confusion; seizures; weakness or heaviness of legs; unusual tiredness or weakness; muscle cramps; numbness, tingling, pain, or weakness of hands or feet; numbness or tingling around lips; fast or irregular heartbeat; shortness of breath or troubled breathing; swelling of feet or lower legs; unusual weight gain; low urine output; unusual thirst.

DOSAGE AND ADMINISTRATION
K-PHOS® M.F.: Two tablets four times daily with a full glass of water.
K-PHOS® No. 2: One tablet four times daily with a full glass of water. When the urine is difficult to acidify, administer one tablet every two hours not to exceed eight tablets in a 24 hour period.

HOW SUPPLIED
K-PHOS® M.F.: White, scored tablet with the name **BEACH** and the number **1135** imprinted on each tablet. Bottles of 100 (NDC 0486-1135-01) and bottles of 500 (NDC 0486-1135-05) tablets. **K-PHOS® No. 2:** Brown, capsule-shaped tablet with the name **BEACH** and the number **1134** imprinted on each tablet. Bottles of 100 (NDC 0486-1134-01) and bottles of 500 (NDC 0486-1134-05) tablets.
Dispense in tight, light-resistant containers with child-resistant closures.
STORAGE: Keep tightly closed. Store at controlled room temperature, 20°-25°C (68°-77°F).
Rx ONLY
Beach
Pharmaceuticals
Div. of
Beach Products, Inc.,
Tampa, FL 33611

R10/98

Shown in Product Identification Guide, page 307

K-PHOS® NEUTRAL   ℞
Supplies 250 mg of phosphorus per tablet.
Rx Only

DESCRIPTION
Each tablet contains 852 mg dibasic sodium phosphate anhydrous, 155 mg monobasic potassium phosphate, and 130 mg monobasic sodium phosphate monohydrate. Each tablet yields approximately 250 mg of phosphorus, 298 mg of sodium (13.0 mEq) and 45 mg of potassium (1.1 mEq).
INACTIVE INGREDIENTS
Hydroxypropyl methylcellulose, magnesium stearate, polyethylene glycol, povidone, sodium starch glycolate and titanium dioxide. May contain: glycerol triacetate, lactose monohydrate, maltodextrin, microcrystalline cellulose, polysorbate 80, sodium citrate, stearic acid, sugar and triacetin.
CLINICAL PHARMACOLOGY
Phosphorus has a number of important functions in the biochemistry of the body. The bulk of the body's phosphorus is located in the bones, where it plays a key role in osteoblastic and osteoclastic activities. Enzymatically catalyzed phosphate-transfer reactions are numerous and vital in the metabolism of carbohydrate, lipid and protein, and a proper concentration of the anion is of primary importance in assuring an orderly biochemical sequence. In addition, phosphorus plays an important role in modifying steady-state

tissue concentrations of calcium. Phosphate ions are important buffers of the intracellular fluid, and also play a primary role in the renal excretion of hydrogen ion.
Oral administration of inorganic phosphates increases serum phosphate levels. Phosphates lower urinary calcium levels in idiopathic hypercalciuria.
In general, in adults, about two thirds of the ingested phosphate is absorbed from the bowel, most of which is rapidly excreted into the urine.

INDICATIONS AND USAGE
K-PHOS® NEUTRAL increases urinary phosphate and pyrophosphate. As a phosphorus supplement, each tablet supplies 25% of the U.S. Recommended Daily Allowance (U.S. RDA) of phosphorus for adults and children over 4 years of age.

CONTRAINDICATIONS
This product is contraindicated in patients with infected phosphate stones, in patients with severely impaired renal function (less than 30% of normal) and in the presence of hyperphosphatemia.

PRECAUTIONS
General: This product contains potassium and sodium and should be used with caution if regulation of these elements is desired. Occasionally, some individuals may experience a mild laxative effect during the first few days of phosphate therapy. If laxation persists to an unpleasant degree, reduce the daily dosage until this effect subsides or, if necessary, discontinue the use of this product.
Caution should be exercised when prescribing this product in the following conditions: Cardiac disease (particularly in digitalized patients); severe adrenal insufficiency (Addison's disease); acute dehydration; severe renal insufficiency; renal function impairment or chronic renal disease; extensive tissue breakdown (such as severe burns); myotonia congenita; cardiac failure; cirrhosis of the liver or severe hepatic disease; peripheral or pulmonary edema; hypernatremia; hypertension; toxemia of pregnancy; hypoparathyroidism; and acute pancreatitis. Rickets may benefit from phosphate therapy, but caution should be exercised. High serum phosphate levels may increase the incidence of extra-skeletal calcification.
Information for Patients: Patients with kidney stones may pass old stones when phosphate therapy is started and should be warned of this possibility. Patients should be advised to avoid the use of antacids containing aluminum, magnesium, or calcium which may prevent the absorption of phosphate.
Laboratory Tests: Careful monitoring of renal function and serum calcium, phosphorus, potassium, and sodium may be required at periodic intervals during phosphate therapy. Other tests may be warranted in some patients, depending on conditions.
Drug Interactions: The use of antacids containing magnesium, aluminum, or calcium in conjunction with phosphate preparations may bind the phosphate and prevent its absorption. Concurrent use of antihypertensives, especially diazoxide, guanethidine, hydralazine, methyldopa, or rauwolfia alkaloid; or corticosteroids, especially mineralocorticoids or corticotropin, with sodium phosphate may result in hypernatremia. Calcium-containing preparations and/or Vitamin D may antagonize the effects of phosphates in the treatment of hypercalcemia. Potassium-containing medications or potassium-sparing diuretics may cause hyperkalemia. Patients should have serum potassium level determinations at periodic intervals.
Carcinogenesis, Mutagenesis, Impairment of Fertility: No long term or reproduction studies in animals or humans have been performed with **K-PHOS® NEUTRAL** to evaluate its carcinogenic, mutagenic, or impairment of fertility potential.
Pregnancy: Teratogenic Effects: Pregnancy Category C. Animal reproduction studies have not been conducted with **K-PHOS® NEUTRAL**. It is also not known whether this product can cause fetal harm when administered to a pregnant woman or can affect reproductive capacity. This product should be given to a pregnant woman only if clearly needed.
Nursing Mothers: It is not known whether this drug is excreted in human milk. Because many drugs are excreted in human milk, caution should be exercised when this product is administered to a nursing woman.
Pediatric Use: See **DOSAGE AND ADMINISTRATION.**

ADVERSE REACTIONS
Gastrointestinal upset (diarrhea, nausea, stomach pain, and vomiting) may occur with phosphate therapy. Also, bone and joint pain (possible phosphate-induced osteomalacia) could occur. The following adverse effects may be observed (primarily from sodium or potassium): headaches; dizziness; mental confusion; seizures; weakness or heaviness of legs; unusual tiredness or weakness; muscle cramps; numbness, tingling, pain, or weakness of hands or feet; numbness or

tingling around lips; fast or irregular heartbeat; shortness of breath or troubled breathing; swelling of feet or lower legs; unusual weight gain; low urine output; unusual thirst.

DOSAGE AND ADMINISTRATION

K-PHOS® NEUTRAL tablets should be taken with a full glass of water, with meals and at bedtime. Adults: One or two tablets four times daily; Pediatric Patients over 4 years of age: One tablet four times daily. For Pediatric Patients under 4 years of age, use only as directed by a physician.

HOW SUPPLIED

White, film-coated, capsule-shaped tablet with the name **BEACH** and number **1125** imprinted on each tablet. Bottles of 100 (NDC 0486-1125-01) and 500 (NDC 0486-1125-05) tablets.

Shown in Product Identification Guide, page 307

K–PHOS® ORIGINAL (Sodium Free) ℞

(Potassium Acid Phosphate)
Urinary Acidifier
Supplies 114 mg of phosphorus per tablet.
Rx Only

DESCRIPTION

Each tablet contains potassium acid phosphate 500 mg. Each tablet yields approximately 114 mg of phosphorus and 144 mg of potassium or 3.7 mEq.

INACTIVE INGREDIENTS

Magnesium stearate, microcrystalline cellulose, silicon dioxide, and starch. May also contain stearic acid.

ACTIONS

K-PHOS® ORIGINAL (Sodium Free) is a highly effective urinary acidifier.

INDICATIONS AND USAGE

For use in patients with elevated urinary pH. Helps keep calcium soluble and reduces odor and rash caused by ammoniacal urine. Also, by acidifying the urine, it increases the antibacterial activity of methenamine mandelate and methenamine hippurate.

CONTRAINDICATIONS

This product is contraindicated in patients with infected phosphate stones; in patients with severely impaired renal function (less than 30% of normal) and in the presence of hyperphosphatemia and hyperkalemia.

PRECAUTIONS

General: This product contains potassium and should be used with caution if regulation of this element is desired. Occasionally, some individuals may experience a mild laxative effect during the first few days of phosphate therapy. If laxation persists to an unpleasant degree, reduce the daily dosage until this effect subsides or, if necessary, discontinue the use of this product.

Caution should be exercised when prescribing this product in the following conditions: Cardiac disease (particularly in digitalized patients); severe adrenal insufficiency (Addison's disease); acute dehydration; severe renal insufficiency or chronic renal disease; extensive tissue breakdown (such as severe burns); myotonia congenita; hypoparathyroidism; and acute pancreatitis. Rickets may benefit from phosphate therapy, but caution should be exercised. High serum phosphate levels may increase the incidence of extraskeletal calcification.

Information for Patients: Patients with kidney stones may pass old stones when phosphate therapy is started and should be warned of this possibility. Patients should be advised to avoid the use of antacids containing aluminum, calcium, or magnesium which may prevent the absorption of phosphate. To assure against gastrointestinal injury associated with oral ingestion of concentrated potassium salt preparations, patients should be instructed to dissolve tablets completely in an appropriate amount of water before taking.

Laboratory Tests: Careful monitoring of renal function and serum electrolytes (calcium, phosphorus, potassium) may be required at periodic intervals during potassium phosphate therapy. Other tests may be warranted in some patients, depending on conditions.

Drug Interactions: The use of antacids containing magnesium, calcium, or aluminum in conjunction with phosphate preparations may bind the phosphate and prevent its absorption. Potassium-containing medications or potassium-sparing diuretics may cause hyperkalemia when used concurrently with potassium salts. Patients should have serum potassium level determinations at periodic intervals. Concurrent use of salicylates may lead to increased serum salicylate levels since excretion of salicylates is reduced in acidified urine. Serum salicylate levels should be closely monitored to avoid toxicity.

Carcinogenesis, Mutagenesis, Impairment of Fertility: There have been no studies in animals or humans to evaluate the carcinogenesis, mutagenesis, or impairment of fertility for this product.

Pregnancy: Pregnancy Category C. Animal reproduction studies have not been conducted with this product. It is also not known whether this product can cause fetal harm when administered to a pregnant woman or can affect reproductive capacity. This product should be given to a pregnant woman only if clearly needed.

Nursing Mothers: It is not known whether this drug is excreted in human milk. Because many drugs are excreted in human milk, caution should be exercised when this product is administered to a nursing woman.

ADVERSE REACTIONS

Gastrointestinal upset (diarrhea, nausea, stomach pain, and vomiting) may occur with the use of potassium phosphate. Also, bone and joint pain (possible phosphate-induced osteomalacia) could occur. The following adverse effects may be observed with potassium administration: irregular heartbeat; dizziness; mental confusion; weakness or heaviness of legs; unusual tiredness; muscle cramps; numbness, tingling, pain, or weakness in hands or feet; numbness or tingling around lips; shortness of breath or troubled breathing.

DOSAGE AND ADMINISTRATION

Two tablets dissolved in 6–8 oz. of water 4 times daily with meals and at bedtime. For best results, let the tablets soak in water for 2 to 5 minutes, or more if necessary, and stir. If any tablet particles remain undissolved, they may be crushed and stirred vigorously to speed dissolution.

HOW SUPPLIED

White scored tablet with the name **BEACH** and the number **1111** imprinted on each tablet. Bottles of 100 (NDC 0486-1111-01) and bottles of 500 (NDC 0486-1111-05) tablets.

Shown in Product Identification Guide, page 307

UROQID-Acid® No. 2 Tablets ℞

Rx Only

DESCRIPTION

Each **UROQID-Acid® No. 2** tablet contains methenamine mandelate 500 mg and sodium acid phosphate, monohydrate 500 mg.

INACTIVE INGREDIENTS

D&C Yellow #10, Aluminum Lake, FD&C Yellow #6 Aluminum Lake, hydroxypropyl methylcellulose, magnesium stearate, methylcellulose, microcrystalline cellulose, povidone, sodium starch glycolate, starch, talc and titanium dioxide. May contain: calcium phosphate, FD&C Blue #2 Lake, glycerine, glycerol triacetate, polysorbate 80, polydextrose, polyethylene glycol, silicon dioxide, sugar, syloid and triacetin.

CLINICAL PHARMACOLOGY

Methenamine mandelate is rapidly absorbed and excreted in the urine. Formaldehyde is released by acid hydrolysis from methenamine with bactericidal levels rapidly reached at pH 5.0–5.5. Proportionally less formaldehyde is released as urinary pH approaches 6.0 and insufficient quantities are released above this level for therapeutic response. In acid urine, mandelic acid exerts its antibacterial action and also contributes to the acidification of the urine. Mandelic acid is excreted by both glomerular filtration and tubular excretion. In acid urine, there is equally effective antibacterial activity against both gram-positive and gram-negative organisms, since the antibacterial action of mandelic acid and formaldehyde is nonspecific. With Proteus vulgaris and urea splitting strains of Pseudomonas and Aerobacter, results may be discouraging and particular attention is required in monitoring urinary pH and overall management.

INDICATIONS AND USAGE

For the suppression or elimination of bacteriuria associated with chronic and recurrent infections of the urinary tract, including pyelitis, pyelonephritis, cystitis, and infected residual urine accompanying neurogenic bladder. When used as recommended, **UROQID-Acid® No. 2** is particularly suitable for long-term therapy because of its relative safety and because resistance to the nonspecific bactericidal action of formaldehyde does not develop. Pathogens resistant to other antibacterial agents may respond because of the nonspecific effect of formaldehyde formed in an acid urine.

Prophylactic Use Rationale: Urine is a good culture medium for many urinary pathogens. Inoculation by a few organisms (relapse or reinfection) may lead to bacteriuria in susceptible individuals. Thus, the rationale of management in recurring urinary tract infection (bacteriuria) is to change the urine from a growth-supporting to a growth-inhibiting medium. There is a growing body of evidence that long-term administration of methenamine can prevent recurrence of bacteriuria in patients with chronic pyelonephritis.

Therapeutic Use Rationale: Helps to sterilize the urine and, in some situations in which underlying pathologic conditions prevent sterilization by any means, can help to suppress bacteriuria. As part of the overall management of the urinary tract infection, a thorough diagnostic evaluation should accompany the use of this product.

CONTRAINDICATIONS

UROQID-Acid® No.2 is contraindicated in patients with renal insufficiency, severe hepatic disease, severe dehydration, hyperphosphatemia, and in patients who have exhibited hypersensitivity to any components of this product.

PRECAUTIONS

General

This product should not be used as the sole therapeutic agent in acute parenchymal infections causing systemic symptoms such as chills and fever.

UROQID-Acid® No. 2 contains approximately 83 mg of sodium per tablet and should be used with caution in patients on a sodium-restricted diet.

Sodium phosphates should be used with caution in the following conditions: cardiac failure; peripheral or pulmonary edema; hypernatremia; hypertension; toxemia of pregnancy; hypoparathyroidism; and acute pancreatitis. High serum phosphate levels increase the incidence of extraskeletal calcification.

Large doses of methenamine (8 grams daily for 3 to 4 weeks) have caused bladder irritation, painful and frequent micturition, albuminuria and gross hematuria. Dysuria may occur, although usually at higher than recommended doses, and can be controlled by reducing the dosage. This product contains a urinary acidifier and can cause metabolic acidosis.

Care should be taken to maintain an acidic urinary pH (below 5.5), especially when treating infections due to urea-splitting organisms such as Proteus and strains of Pseudomonas.

Drugs and/or foods which produce an alkaline urine should be restricted. Frequent urine pH tests are essential. If acidification of the urine is contraindicated or unattainable, use of this product should be discontinued.

Information For Patients: To assure an acidic pH, patients should be instructed to restrict or avoid most fruits, milk and milk products, and antacids containing sodium carbonate or bicarbonate.

Laboratory Tests: As with all urinary tract infections, the efficacy of therapy should be monitored by repeated urine cultures. During long-term therapy, careful monitoring of renal function, serum phosphorus and sodium may be required at periodic intervals.

Drug Interactions: Formaldehyde and sulfamethizole form an insoluble precipitate in acid urine and increase the risk of crystalluria; therefore, these products should not be used concurrently. Thiazide diuretics, carbonic anhydrase inhibitors, antacids, or urinary alkalinizing agents should not be used concurrently since they may cause the urine to become alkaline and reduce the effectiveness of methenamine by inhibiting its conversion to formaldehyde. Concurrent use of antihypertensives, especially diazoxide, guanethidine, hydralazine, methyldopa, or rauwolfia alkaloids; or corticosteroids, especially mineralocorticoids or corticotropin, with sodium phosphates may result in hypernatremia. Concurrent use of salicylates may lead to increased serum salicylate levels since excretion of salicylates is reduced in acidified urine. Serum salicylate levels should be closely monitored to avoid toxicity.

Laboratory Test Interactions: Formaldehyde interferes with fluorometric procedures for determination of urinary catecholamines and vanilmandelic acid (VMA) causing erroneously high results. Formaldehyde also causes falsely decreased urine estriol levels by reacting with estriol when acid hydrolysis techniques are used; estriol determinations which use enzymatic hydrolysis are unaffected by formaldehyde. Formaldehyde causes falsely elevated 17-hydroxycorticosteroid levels when the Porter-Silber method is used and falsely decreased 5-hydroxyindoleacetic acid (5HIAA) levels by inhibiting color development when nitrosonaphthol methods are used.

Carcinogenesis, Mutagenesis, Impairment Of Fertility: Long-term animal studies to evaluate the carcinogenic, mutagenic, or impairment of fertility potential of this product have not been performed.

Pregnancy: Teratogenic Effects. Pregnancy Category C. Animal reproduction studies have not been conducted with **UROQID-Acid® No.2**. It is also not known whether this product can cause fetal harm when administered to a pregnant woman or can affect reproductive capacity. Since methenamine is known to cross the placental barrier, this product should be given to a pregnant woman only if clearly needed.

Nursing Mothers: Methenamine is excreted in breast milk. Caution should be exercised when this product is administered to a nursing woman.

ADVERSE REACTIONS

Gastrointestinal disturbances (nausea, stomach upset), generalized skin rash, dysuria, painful or difficult urination may occur occasionally with the use of methenamine preparations. Microscopic and rarely, gross hematuria have also been reported.

Gastrointestinal upset (diarrhea, nausea, stomach pain, and vomiting) may occur with the use of sodium phosphates. Also, bone or joint pain (possible phosphate induced osteomalacia) could occur. The following adverse effects may be observed (primarily from sodium): headaches; dizziness; mental confusion; seizures; weakness or heaviness of legs; unusual tiredness or weakness; muscle cramps; numbness, tingling, pain, or weakness of hands or feet; numbness or tingling around lips; fast or irregular heartbeat; shortness of breath or troubled breathing; swelling of feet or lower legs; unusual weight gain; low urine output, unusual thirst.

DOSAGE AND ADMINISTRATION

UROQID-Acid® No. 2: *Adults:* Initially, 2 tablets 4 times daily with a full glass of water. For maintenance, 2 to 4 tablets daily, in divided doses with a full glass of water.

HOW SUPPLIED

UROQID-Acid® No. 2 is a yellow, film-coated, capsule-shaped tablet with the name **BEACH** and the number **1114** imprinted on each tablet. Packaged in bottles of 100 tablets (NDC 0486-1114-01).

Shown in Product Identification Guide, page 307

Bertek Pharmaceuticals, Inc.

for further product information see Mylan Pharmaceuticals Inc.

Boehringer Ingelheim

**900 RIDGEBURY ROAD
P.O. BOX 368
RIDGEFIELD, CT 06877-0368**

Direct inquiries to:
(800) 243-0127
TTY (800) 246-6196

For medical information or to report an adverse drug experience contact:
(800) 542-6257
TTY (800) 459-9906
(option 4)
http://us.boehringer-ingelheim.com

AGGRENOX®   ℞
[AG-reh-nox]
**(aspirin/extended-release dipyridamole)
Capsules**

**HIGHLIGHTS OF PRESCRIBING INFORMATION
These highlights do not include all the information needed to use Aggrenox Capsules safely and effectively. See full prescribing information for Aggrenox Capsules.
AGGRENOX® (aspirin/extended-release dipyridamole)
Capsules
Initial U.S. Approval: 1999**

————————INDICATIONS AND USAGE————————
• AGGRENOX is a combination antiplatelet agent indicated to reduce the risk of stroke in patients who have had transient ischemia of the brain or completed ischemic stroke due to thrombosis (1)

————DOSAGE AND ADMINISTRATION————
• One capsule twice daily (morning and evening) with or without food (2)
• In case of intolerable headaches during initial treatment, switch to one capsule at bedtime and low-dose aspirin in the morning; resume BID dosing within one week (2)
• Do not chew capsule (2)
• **Not interchangeable with the individual components of aspirin and dipyridamole tablets (2)**
• Dispense in this unit-of-use container (16)

————DOSAGE FORMS AND STRENGTHS————
• Capsule: 25 mg aspirin/200 mg extended-release dipyridamole (3)

————————CONTRAINDICATIONS————————
• Hypersensitivity to any product ingredients (4.1)
• Patients with known allergy to NSAIDs (4.2)
• Patients with the syndrome of asthma, rhinitis, and nasal polyps (4.2)

————WARNINGS AND PRECAUTIONS————
• The risk of GI bleeding is increased, especially in patients who are heavy alcohol users, have a history of peptic ulcer, or have coagulation abnormalities due to liver disease or vitamin K deficiency (5.1)

• As with other antiplatelets, there is a risk of intracranial hemorrhage (5.1)
• Avoid use in patients with severe hepatic or renal insufficiency (5.2, 5.3)
• Can cause fetal harm when administered to a pregnant woman, especially in the third trimester (5.4)

————————ADVERSE REACTIONS————————
• The most frequently reported adverse reactions (>10% and greater than placebo) were headache, dyspepsia, abdominal pain, nausea, and diarrhea (6)

To report SUSPECTED ADVERSE REACTIONS, contact Boehringer Ingelheim Pharmaceuticals, Inc. at (800) 542-6257 or (800) 459-9906 TTY or FDA at 1-800-FDA-1088 or www.fda.gov/medwatch.

————————DRUG INTERACTIONS————————
• Co-administration with anti-coagulants or NSAIDS can increase risk of bleeding (7.4, 7.10)
• Decreased renal function can occur with co-administration with NSAIDS (7.10)

————USE IN SPECIFIC POPULATIONS————
• Pregnancy Category D (8.1)

See 17 for PATIENT COUNSELING INFORMATION and FDA-approved patient labeling

Revised: 10/2009

FULL PRESCRIBING INFORMATION*
1   INDICATIONS AND USAGE
2   DOSAGE AND ADMINISTRATION
       2.1   Alternative Regimen in Case of Intolerable Headaches
3   DOSAGE FORMS AND STRENGTHS
4   CONTRAINDICATIONS
       4.1   Hypersensitivity
       4.2   Allergy
       4.3   Reye Syndrome
5   WARNINGS AND PRECAUTIONS
       5.1   Risk of Bleeding
       5.2   Renal Failure
       5.3   Hepatic Insufficiency
       5.4   Pregnancy
       5.5   Coronary Artery Disease
       5.6   Hypotension
       5.7   General
6   ADVERSE REACTIONS
       6.1   Clinical Trials Experience
       6.2   Post-Marketing Experience
7   DRUG INTERACTIONS
       7.1   Adenosine
       7.2   Angiotensin Converting Enzyme (ACE) Inhibitors
       7.3   Acetazolamide
       7.4   Anticoagulant Therapy (heparin and warfarin)
       7.5   Anticonvulsants
       7.6   Beta Blockers
       7.7   Cholinesterase Inhibitors
       7.8   Diuretics
       7.9   Methotrexate
       7.10   Nonsteroidal Anti-Inflammatory Drugs (NSAIDs)
       7.11   Oral Hypoglycemics
       7.12   Uricosuric Agents (probenecid and sulfinpyrazone)
8   USE IN SPECIFIC POPULATIONS
       8.1   Pregnancy
       8.2   Labor and Delivery
       8.3   Nursing Mothers
       8.4   Pediatric Use
       8.5   Geriatric Use
       8.6   Patients with Severe Hepatic or Severe Renal Dysfunction
10   OVERDOSAGE
11   DESCRIPTION
12   CLINICAL PHARMACOLOGY
       12.1   Mechanism of Action
       12.2   Pharmacodynamics
       12.3   Pharmacokinetics
13   NONCLINICAL TOXICOLOGY
       13.1   Carcinogenesis, Mutagenesis, Impairment of Fertility
14   CLINICAL STUDIES
16   HOW SUPPLIED/STORAGE AND HANDLING
17   PATIENT COUNSELING INFORMATION
       17.1   Risk of Bleeding
       17.2   Pregnancy
       17.3   Headaches
       17.4   Dosage and Administration
       17.5   Storage

* Sections or subsections omitted from the full prescribing information are not listed

---

FULL PRESCRIBING INFORMATION

1   INDICATIONS AND USAGE

AGGRENOX is indicated to reduce the risk of stroke in patients who have had transient ischemia of the brain or completed ischemic stroke due to thrombosis.

2   DOSAGE AND ADMINISTRATION

AGGRENOX is not interchangeable with the individual components of aspirin and dipyridamole tablets.
The recommended dose of AGGRENOX is one capsule given orally twice daily, one in the morning and one in the evening. Swallow capsules whole without chewing. AGGRENOX can be administered with or without food.

2.1   Alternative Regimen in Case of Intolerable Headaches
In the event of intolerable headaches during initial treatment, switch to one capsule at bedtime and low-dose aspirin in the morning. Because there are no outcome data with this regimen and headaches become less of a problem as treatment continues, patients should return to the usual regimen as soon as possible, usually within one week.

3   DOSAGE FORMS AND STRENGTHS

25 mg/200 mg capsules with a red cap and an ivory-colored body, containing yellow extended-release pellets incorporating dipyridamole and a round white tablet incorporating immediate-release aspirin. The capsule body is imprinted in red with the Boehringer Ingelheim logo and with "01A".

4   CONTRAINDICATIONS

4.1   Hypersensitivity
AGGRENOX is contraindicated in patients with known hypersensitivity to any of the product components.

4.2   Allergy
Aspirin is contraindicated in patients with known allergy to nonsteroidal anti-inflammatory drug products and in patients with the syndrome of asthma, rhinitis, and nasal polyps. Aspirin may cause severe urticaria, angioedema or bronchospasm.

4.3   Reye Syndrome
Do not use aspirin in children or teenagers with viral infections because of the risk of Reye syndrome.

5   WARNINGS AND PRECAUTIONS

5.1   Risk of Bleeding
Intracranial Hemorrhage
In ESPS2 the incidence of intracranial hemorrhage was 0.6% in the AGGRENOX group, 0.5% in the extended-release dipyridamole (ER-DP) group, 0.4% in the aspirin (ASA) group and 0.4% in the placebo groups.
Coagulation Abnormalities
Even low doses of aspirin can inhibit platelet function leading to an increase in bleeding time. This can adversely affect patients with inherited or acquired (liver disease or vitamin K deficiency) bleeding disorders [see Drug Interactions (7.4)].
Gastrointestinal (GI) Side Effects
GI side effects include stomach pain, heartburn, nausea, vomiting, and gross GI bleeding. Although minor upper GI symptoms, such as dyspepsia, are common and can occur anytime during therapy, physicians should remain alert for signs of ulceration and bleeding, even in the absence of previous GI symptoms. Inform patients about the signs and symptoms of GI side effects and what steps to take if they occur.
In ESPS2 the incidence of gastrointestinal bleeding was 4.1% in the AGGRENOX group, 2.2% in the extended-release dipyridamole group, 3.2% in the aspirin group, and 2.1% in the placebo groups.
Peptic Ulcer Disease
Avoid using aspirin in patients with a history of active peptic ulcer disease, which can cause gastric mucosal irritation and bleeding.
Alcohol Warning
Because AGGRENOX contains aspirin, counsel patients who consume three or more alcoholic drinks every day about the bleeding risks involved with chronic, heavy alcohol use while taking aspirin.

5.2   Renal Failure
Avoid aspirin in patients with severe renal failure (glomerular filtration rate less than 10 mL/minute) [see Use in Specific Populations (8.6) and Clinical Pharmacology (12.3)].

5.3   Hepatic Insufficiency
Elevations of hepatic enzymes and hepatic failure have been reported in association with dipyridamole administration [see Use in Specific Populations (8.6) and Clinical Pharmacology (12.3)].

5.4   Pregnancy
Because AGGRENOX contains aspirin, AGGRENOX can cause fetal harm when administered to a pregnant woman. Maternal aspirin use during later stages of pregnancy may cause low birth weight, increased incidence for intracranial hemorrhage in premature infants, stillbirths and neonatal death. Because of the above and because of the known effects of nonsteroidal anti-inflammatory drugs (NSAIDs) on

the fetal cardiovascular system (closure of the ductus arteriosus), avoid AGGRENOX in the third trimester of pregnancy [see *Use in Specific Populations (8.1)*].

Aspirin has been shown to be teratogenic in rats (spina bifida, exencephaly, microphthalmia and coelosomia) and rabbits (congested fetuses, agenesis of skull and upper jaw, generalized edema with malformation of the head, and diaphanous skin) at oral doses of 330 mg/kg/day and 110 mg/kg/day, respectively. These doses, which also resulted in a high resorption rate in rats (63% of implantations versus 5% in controls), are, on a mg/m² basis, about 66 and 44 times, respectively, the dose of aspirin contained in the maximum recommended daily human dose of AGGRENOX. Reproduction studies with dipyridamole have been performed in mice, rabbits and rats at oral doses of up to 125 mg/kg, 40 mg/kg and 1000 mg/kg, respectively (about 1½, 2 and 25 times the maximum recommended daily human oral dose, respectively, on a mg/m² basis) and have revealed no evidence of harm to the fetus due to dipyridamole. When 330 mg aspirin/kg/day was combined with 75 mg dipyridamole/kg/day in the rat, the resorption rate approached 100%, indicating potentiation of aspirin-related fetal toxicity. There are no adequate and well-controlled studies of the use of AGGRENOX in pregnant women. If AGGRENOX is used during pregnancy, or if the patient becomes pregnant while taking AGGRENOX, inform the patient of the potential hazard to the fetus.

5.5 Coronary Artery Disease

Dipyridamole has a vasodilatory effect. Chest pain may be precipitated or aggravated in patients with underlying coronary artery disease who are receiving dipyridamole.

For stroke or TIA patients for whom aspirin is indicated to prevent recurrent myocardial infarction (MI) or angina pectoris, the aspirin in this product may not provide adequate treatment for the cardiac indications.

5.6 Hypotension

Dipyridamole produces peripheral vasodilation, which can exacerbate pre-existing hypotension.

5.7 General

AGGRENOX capsules are not interchangeable with the individual components of aspirin and dipyridamole tablets.

6 ADVERSE REACTIONS

The following adverse reactions are discussed elsewhere in the labeling:

- Hypersensitivity [see *Contraindications (4.1)*].
- Allergy [see *Contraindications (4.2)*].
- Risk of Bleeding [see *Warnings and Precautions (5.1)*].

6.1 Clinical Trials Experience

Because clinical trials are conducted under widely varying conditions, adverse reaction rates observed in the clinical trials of a drug cannot be directly compared to rates in the clinical trials of another drug and may not reflect the rates observed in practice.

The efficacy and safety of AGGRENOX was established in the European Stroke Prevention Study-2 (ESPS2). ESPS2 was a double-blind, placebo controlled study that evaluated 6602 patients over the age of 18 years who had a previous ischemic stroke or transient ischemic attack within ninety days prior to entry. Patients were randomized to either AGGRENOX, aspirin, ER-DP, or placebo [see *Clinical Studies (14)*]; primary endpoints included stroke (fatal or nonfatal) and death from all causes.

This 24-month, multicenter, double-blind, randomized study (ESPS2) was conducted to compare the efficacy and safety of AGGRENOX with placebo, extended-release dipyridamole alone and aspirin alone. The study was conducted in a total of 6602 male and female patients who had experienced a previous ischemic stroke or transient ischemia of the brain within three months prior to randomization.

Table 1 presents the incidence of adverse events that occurred in 1% or more of patients treated with AGGRENOX where the incidence was also greater than in those patients treated with placebo. There is no clear benefit of the dipyridamole/aspirin combination over aspirin with respect to safety.

[See table 1 at right and on next page]

Discontinuation due to adverse events in ESPS2 was 25% for AGGRENOX, 25% for extended-release dipyridamole, 19% for aspirin, and 21% for placebo (refer to Table 2)

[See table 2 on next page]

Headache was most notable in the first month of treatment.

Other Adverse Events

Adverse reactions that occurred in less than 1% of patients treated with AGGRENOX in the ESPS2 study and that were medically judged to be possibly related to either dipyridamole or aspirin are listed below.

Body as a Whole: Allergic reaction, fever
Cardiovascular: Hypotension
Central Nervous System: Coma, dizziness, paresthesia, cerebral hemorrhage, intracranial hemorrhage, subarachnoid hemorrhage

Table 1 Incidence of Adverse Events in ESPS2*

Body System/Preferred Term	Individual Treatment Group			
	AGGRENOX	ER-DP Alone	ASA Alone	Placebo
Total Number of Patients	1650	1654	1649	1649
Total Number (%) of Patients With at Least One On-Treatment Adverse Event	1319 (80%)	1305 (79%)	1323 (80%)	1304 (79%)
Central and Peripheral Nervous System Disorders				
Headache	647 (39%)	634 (38%)	558 (34%)	543 (33%)
Convulsions	28 (2%)	15 (1%)	28 (2%)	26 (2%)
Gastrointestinal System Disorders				
Dyspepsia	303 (18%)	288 (17%)	299 (18%)	275 (17%)
Abdominal Pain	289 (18%)	255 (15%)	262 (16%)	239 (14%)
Nausea	264 (16%)	254 (15%)	210 (13%)	232 (14%)
Diarrhea	210 (13%)	257 (16%)	112 (7%)	161 (10%)
Vomiting	138 (8%)	129 (8%)	101 (6%)	118 (7%)
Hemorrhage Rectum	26 (2%)	22 (1%)	16 (1%)	13 (1%)
Melena	31 (2%)	10 (1%)	20 (1%)	13 (1%)
Hemorrhoids	16 (1%)	13 (1%)	10 (1%)	10 (1%)
GI Hemorrhage	20 (1%)	5 (0%)	15 (1%)	7 (0%)
Body as a Whole - General Disorders				
Pain	105 (6%)	88 (5%)	103 (6%)	99 (6%)
Fatigue	95 (6%)	93 (6%)	97 (6%)	90 (5%)
Back Pain	76 (5%)	77 (5%)	74 (4%)	65 (4%)
Accidental Injury	42 (3%)	24 (1%)	51 (3%)	37 (2%)
Malaise	27 (2%)	23 (1%)	26 (2%)	22 (1%)
Asthenia	29 (2%)	19 (1%)	17 (1%)	18 (1%)
Syncope	17 (1%)	13 (1%)	16 (1%)	8 (0%)
Psychiatric Disorders				
Amnesia	39 (2%)	40 (2%)	57 (3%)	34 (2%)
Confusion	18 (1%)	9 (1%)	22 (1%)	15 (1%)
Anorexia	19 (1%)	17 (1%)	10 (1%)	15 (1%)
Somnolence	20 (1%)	13 (1%)	18 (1%)	9 (1%)
Musculoskeletal System Disorders				
Arthralgia	91 (6%)	75 (5%)	91 (6%)	76 (5%)
Arthritis	34 (2%)	25 (2%)	17 (1%)	19 (1%)
Arthrosis	18 (1%)	22 (1%)	13 (1%)	14 (1%)
Myalgia	20 (1%)	16 (1%)	11 (1%)	11 (1%)
Respiratory System Disorders				
Coughing	25 (2%)	18 (1%)	32 (2%)	21 (1%)
Upper Respiratory Tract Infection	16 (1%)	9 (1%)	16 (1%)	14 (1%)

(Table continued on next page)

Gastrointestinal: Gastritis, ulceration and perforation
Hearing and Vestibular Disorders: Tinnitus, and deafness. Patients with high frequency hearing loss may have difficulty perceiving tinnitus. In these patients, tinnitus cannot be used as a clinical indicator of salicylism
Heart Rate and Rhythm Disorders: Tachycardia, palpitation, arrhythmia, supraventricular tachycardia
Liver and Biliary System Disorders: Cholelithiasis, jaundice, hepatic function abnormal
Metabolic and Nutritional Disorders: Hyperglycemia, thirst
Platelet, Bleeding and Clotting Disorders: Hematoma, gingival bleeding

Psychiatric Disorders: Agitation
Reproductive: Uterine hemorrhage
Respiratory: Hyperpnea, asthma, bronchospasm, hemoptysis, pulmonary edema
Special Senses Other Disorders: Taste loss
Skin and Appendages Disorders: Pruritus, urticaria
Urogenital: Renal insufficiency and failure, hematuria
Vascular (Extracardiac) Disorders: Flushing
Laboratory Changes
Over the course of the 24-month study (ESPS2), patients treated with AGGRENOX showed a decline (mean change from baseline) in hemoglobin of 0.25 g/dL, hematocrit of 0.75%, and erythrocyte count of 0.13×10⁶/mm³.

6.2 Post-Marketing Experience

The following is a list of additional adverse reactions that have been reported either in the literature or are from post-marketing spontaneous reports for either dipyridamole or aspirin. Because these reactions are reported voluntarily from a population of uncertain size, it is not always possible to estimate reliably their frequency or establish a causal relationship to drug exposure. Decisions to include these reactions in labeling are typically based on one or more of the following factors: (1) seriousness of the reaction, (2) frequency of reporting, or (3) strength of causal connection to AGGRENOX.

Body as a Whole: Hypothermia, chest pain
Cardiovascular: Angina pectoris
Central Nervous System: Cerebral edema
Fluid and Electrolyte: Hyperkalemia, metabolic acidosis, respiratory alkalosis, hypokalemia
Gastrointestinal: Pancreatitis, Reye syndrome, hematemesis
Hearing and Vestibular Disorders: Hearing loss
Immune System Disorders: Hypersensitivity, acute anaphylaxis, laryngeal edema
Liver and Biliary System Disorders: Hepatitis, hepatic failure
Musculoskeletal: Rhabdomyolysis
Metabolic and Nutritional Disorders: Hypoglycemia, dehydration
Platelet, Bleeding and Clotting Disorders: Prolongation of the prothrombin time, disseminated intravascular coagulation, coagulopathy, thrombocytopenia
Reproductive: Prolonged pregnancy and labor, stillbirths, lower birth weight infants, antepartum and postpartum bleeding
Respiratory: Tachypnea, dyspnea
Skin and Appendages Disorders: Rash, alopecia, angioedema, Stevens-Johnson syndrome, skin hemorrhages such as bruising, ecchymosis, and hematoma
Urogenital: Interstitial nephritis, papillary necrosis, proteinuria
Vascular (Extracardiac Disorders): Allergic vasculitis
Other adverse events: anorexia, aplastic anemia, migraine, pancytopenia, thrombocytosis.

7 DRUG INTERACTIONS

No pharmacokinetic drug-drug interaction studies were conducted with AGGRENOX capsules. The following information was obtained from the literature.

7.1 Adenosine
Dipyridamole has been reported to increase the plasma levels and cardiovascular effects of adenosine. Adjustment of adenosine dosage may be necessary.

7.2 Angiotensin Converting Enzyme (ACE) Inhibitors
Due to the indirect effect of aspirin on the renin-angiotensin conversion pathway, the hyponatremic and hypotensive effects of ACE inhibitors may be diminished by concomitant administration of aspirin.

7.3 Acetazolamide
Concurrent use of aspirin and acetazolamide can lead to high serum concentrations of acetazolamide (and toxicity) due to competition at the renal tubule for secretion.

7.4 Anticoagulant Therapy (heparin and warfarin)
Patients on anticoagulation therapy are at increased risk for bleeding because of drug-drug interactions and effects on platelets. Aspirin can displace warfarin from protein binding sites, leading to prolongation of both the prothrombin time and the bleeding time. Aspirin can increase the anticoagulant activity of heparin, increasing bleeding risk.

7.5 Anticonvulsants
Salicylic acid can displace protein-bound phenytoin and valproic acid, leading to a decrease in the total concentration of phenytoin and an increase in serum valproic acid levels.

7.6 Beta Blockers
The hypotensive effects of beta blockers may be diminished by the concomitant administration of aspirin due to inhibition of renal prostaglandins, leading to decreased renal blood flow and salt and fluid retention.

7.7 Cholinesterase Inhibitors
Dipyridamole may counteract the anticholinesterase effect of cholinesterase inhibitors, thereby potentially aggravating myasthenia gravis.

7.8 Diuretics
The effectiveness of diuretics in patients with underlying renal or cardiovascular disease may be diminished by the concomitant administration of aspirin due to inhibition of renal prostaglandins, leading to decreased renal blood flow and salt and fluid retention.

7.9 Methotrexate
Salicylate can inhibit renal clearance of methotrexate, leading to bone marrow toxicity, especially in the elderly or renal impaired.

7.10 Nonsteroidal Anti-Inflammatory Drugs (NSAIDs)
The concurrent use of aspirin with other NSAIDs may increase bleeding or lead to decreased renal function.

Table 1 *(cont.)* **Incidence of Adverse Events in ESPS2***

Body System/Preferred Term	Individual Treatment Group			
	AGGRENOX	ER-DP Alone	ASA Alone	Placebo
Cardiovascular Disorders, General				
Cardiac Failure	26 (2%)	17 (1%)	30 (2%)	25 (2%)
Platelet, Bleeding & Clotting Disorders				
Hemorrhage NOS	52 (3%)	24 (1%)	46 (3%)	24 (2%)
Epistaxis	39 (2%)	16 (1%)	45 (3%)	25 (1%)
Purpura	23 (1%)	8 (0%)	9 (1%)	7 (0%)
Neoplasm				
Neoplasm NOS	28 (2%)	16 (1%)	23 (1%)	20 (1%)
Red Blood Cell Disorders				
Anemia	27 (2%)	16 (1%)	19 (1%)	9 (1%)

* Reported by ≥1% of patients during AGGRENOX treatment where the incidence was greater than in those treated with placebo.
Note: ER-DP = extended-release dipyridamole 200 mg; ASA = aspirin 25 mg. The dosage regimen for all treatment groups is BID
NOS = not otherwise specified.

Table 2 **Incidence of Adverse Events that Led to the Discontinuation of Treatment: Adverse Events with an Incidence of ≥1% in the AGGRENOX Group**

	Treatment Groups			
	AGGRENOX	ER-DP	ASA	Placebo
Total Number of Patients	1650	1654	1649	1649
Patients with at least one Adverse Event that led to treatment discontinuation	417 (25%)	419 (25%)	318 (19%)	352 (21%)
Headache	165 (10%)	166 (10%)	57 (3%)	69 (4%)
Dizziness	85 (5%)	97 (6%)	69 (4%)	68 (4%)
Nausea	91 (6%)	95 (6%)	51 (3%)	53 (3%)
Abdominal Pain	74 (4%)	64 (4%)	56 (3%)	52 (3%)
Dyspepsia	59 (4%)	61 (4%)	49 (3%)	46 (3%)
Vomiting	53 (3%)	52 (3%)	28 (2%)	24 (1%)
Diarrhea	35 (2%)	41 (2%)	9 (<1%)	16 (<1%)
Stroke	39 (2%)	48 (3%)	57 (3%)	73 (4%)
Transient Ischemic Attack	35 (2%)	40 (2%)	26 (2%)	48 (3%)
Angina Pectoris	23 (1%)	20 (1%)	16 (<1%)	26 (2%)

Note: ER-DP = extended-release dipyridamole 200 mg; ASA = aspirin 25 mg. The dosage regimen for all treatment groups is BID

7.11 Oral Hypoglycemics
Moderate doses of aspirin may increase the effectiveness of oral hypoglycemic drugs, leading to hypoglycemia.

7.12 Uricosuric Agents (probenecid and sulfinpyrazone)
Salicylates antagonize the uricosuric action of uricosuric agents.

8 USE IN SPECIFIC POPULATIONS

8.1 Pregnancy
Teratogenic Effects, Pregnancy Category D. [*see Warnings and Precautions (5.4)*].

8.2 Labor and Delivery
Aspirin can result in excessive blood loss at delivery as well as prolonged gestation and prolonged labor. Because of these effects on the mother and because of adverse fetal effects seen with aspirin during the later stages of pregnancy [*see Warnings and Precautions (5.4)*], avoid AGGRENOX in the third trimester of pregnancy and during labor and delivery.

8.3 Nursing Mothers
Both dipyridamole and aspirin are excreted in human milk. Exercise caution when AGGRENOX capsules are administered to a nursing woman.

8.4 Pediatric Use
Safety and effectiveness of AGGRENOX in pediatric patients have not been studied. Due to the aspirin component, use of this product in the pediatric population is not recommended [*see Contraindications (4.3)*].

8.5 Geriatric Use
Of the total number of subjects in ESPS2, 61 percent were 65 and over, while 27 percent were 75 and over. No overall differences in safety or effectiveness were observed between these subjects and younger subjects, and other reported clinical experience has not identified differences in responses between the elderly and younger patients, but greater sensitivity of some older individuals cannot be ruled out [*see Clinical Pharmacology (12.3)*].

8.6 Patients with Severe Hepatic or Severe Renal Dysfunction
AGGRENOX has not been studied in patients with hepatic or renal impairment. Avoid using aspirin containing products, such as Aggrenox in patients with severe hepatic or severe renal (glomerular filtration rate < 10 mL/min) dysfunction [*see Warnings and Precautions (5.2, 5.3) and Clinical Pharmacology (12.3)*].

10 OVERDOSAGE

Because of the dose ratio of dipyridamole to aspirin, overdosage of AGGRENOX is likely to be dominated by signs and symptoms of dipyridamole overdose. In case of real or suspected overdose, seek medical attention or contact a Poison Control Center immediately. Careful medical management is essential.
Based upon the known hemodynamic effects of dipyridamole, symptoms such as warm feeling, flushes,

sweating, restlessness, feeling of weakness and dizziness may occur. A drop in blood pressure and tachycardia might also be observed.

Salicylate toxicity may result from acute ingestion (overdose) or chronic intoxication. Severity of aspirin intoxication is determined by measuring the blood salicylate level. The early signs of salicylic overdose (salicylism), including tinnitus (ringing in the ears), occur at plasma concentrations approaching 200 µg/mL. In severe cases, hyperthermia and hypovolemia are the major immediate threats to life. Plasma concentrations of aspirin above 300 µg/mL are clearly toxic. Severe toxic effects are associated with levels above 400 µg/mL. A single lethal dose of aspirin in adults is not known with certainty but death may be expected at 30 g.

Treatment of overdose consists primarily of supporting vital functions, increasing drug elimination, and correcting acid-base disturbances. Consider gastric emptying and/or lavage as soon as possible after ingestion, even if the patient has vomited spontaneously. After lavage and/or emesis, administration of activated charcoal as a slurry may be beneficial if less than 3 hours have passed since ingestion. Charcoal absorption should not be employed prior to emesis and lavage. Follow acid base status closely with serial blood gas and serum pH measurements. Maintain fluid and electrolyte balance. Administer replacement fluid intravenously and augment with correction of acidosis. Treatment may require the use of a vasopressor. Infusion of glucose may be required to control hypoglycemia.

Administration of xanthine derivatives (e.g., aminophylline) may reverse the hemodynamic effects of dipyridamole overdose. Plasma electrolytes and pH should be monitored serially to promote alkaline diuresis of salicylate if renal function is normal. In patients with renal insufficiency or in cases of life-threatening intoxication, dialysis is usually required to treat salicylic overdose, however since dipyridamole is highly protein bound, dialysis is not likely to remove dipyridamole. Exchange transfusion may be indicated in infants and young children.

11 DESCRIPTION

AGGRENOX is a combination antiplatelet agent intended for oral administration. Each hard gelatin capsule contains 200 mg dipyridamole in an extended-release form and 25 mg aspirin, as an immediate-release sugar-coated tablet. In addition, each capsule contains the following inactive ingredients: acacia, aluminum stearate, colloidal silicon dioxide, corn starch, dimethicone, hypromellose, hypromellose phthalate, lactose monohydrate, methacrylic acid copolymer, microcrystalline cellulose, povidone, stearic acid, sucrose, talc, tartaric acid, titanium dioxide and triacetin.

Each capsule shell contains gelatin, red iron oxide and yellow iron oxide, titanium dioxide and water.

Dipyridamole

Dipyridamole is an antiplatelet agent chemically described as 2,2′,2″,2‴-[(4,8-Dipiperidinopyrimido[5,4-*d*]pyrimidine-2,6-diyl)dinitrilo]-tetraethanol. It has the following structural formula:

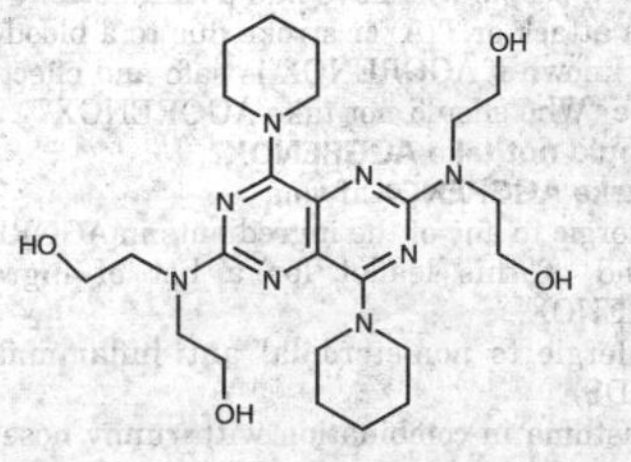

$C_{24}H_{40}N_8O_4$ Mol. Wt. 504.63

Dipyridamole is an odorless yellow crystalline substance, having a bitter taste. It is soluble in dilute acids, methanol and chloroform, and is practically insoluble in water.

Aspirin

The antiplatelet agent aspirin (acetylsalicylic acid) is chemically known as benzoic acid, 2-(acetyloxy)-, and has the following structural formula:

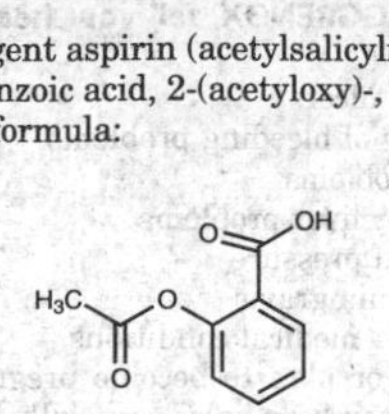

$C_9H_8O_4$ Mol. Wt. 180.16

Aspirin is an odorless white needle-like crystalline or powdery substance. When exposed to moisture, aspirin hydrolyzes into salicylic and acetic acids, and gives off a vinegary odor. It is highly lipid soluble and slightly soluble in water.

12 CLINICAL PHARMACOLOGY

12.1 Mechanism of Action

The antithrombotic action of AGGRENOX is the result of the additive antiplatelet effects of dipyridamole and aspirin.

Dipyridamole

Dipyridamole inhibits the uptake of adenosine into platelets, endothelial cells and erythrocytes *in vitro* and *in vivo*; the inhibition occurs in a dose-dependent manner at therapeutic concentrations (0.5-1.9 µg/mL). This inhibition results in an increase in local concentrations of adenosine which acts on the platelet A_2-receptor thereby stimulating platelet adenylate cyclase and increasing platelet cyclic-3′,5′-adenosine monophosphate (cAMP) levels. Via this mechanism, platelet aggregation is inhibited in response to various stimuli such as platelet activating factor (PAF), collagen and adenosine diphosphate (ADP).

Dipyridamole inhibits phosphodiesterase (PDE) in various tissues. While the inhibition of cAMP-PDE is weak, therapeutic levels of dipyridamole inhibit cyclic-3′,5′-guanosine monophosphate-PDE (cGMP-PDE), thereby augmenting the increase in cGMP produced by EDRF (endothelium-derived relaxing factor, now identified as nitric oxide).

Aspirin

Aspirin inhibits platelet aggregation by irreversible inhibition of platelet cyclooxygenase and thus inhibits the generation of thromboxane A_2, a powerful inducer of platelet aggregation and vasoconstriction.

12.2 Pharmacodynamics

The effect of either agent on the other's inhibition of platelet reactivity has not been evaluated.

12.3 Pharmacokinetics

There are no significant interactions between aspirin and dipyridamole. The kinetics of the components are unchanged by their co-administration as AGGRENOX.

Dipyridamole

Absorption

Peak plasma levels of dipyridamole are achieved 2 hours (range 1-6 hours) after administration of a daily dose of 400 mg AGGRENOX (given as 200 mg BID). The peak plasma concentration at steady-state is 1.98 µg/mL (1.01-3.99 µg/mL) and the steady-state trough concentration is 0.53 µg/mL (0.18–1.01 µg/mL).

Effect of Food

When AGGRENOX capsules were taken with a high fat meal, dipyridamole peak plasma levels (C_{max}) and total absorption (AUC) were decreased at steady-state by 20-30% compared to fasting. Due to the similar degree of inhibition of adenosine uptake at these plasma concentrations, this food effect is not considered clinically relevant.

Distribution

Dipyridamole is highly lipophilic (log P=3.71, pH=7); however, it has been shown that the drug does not cross the blood-brain barrier to any significant extent in animals. The steady-state volume of distribution of dipyridamole is about 92 L. Approximately 99% of dipyridamole is bound to plasma proteins, predominantly to alpha 1-acid glycoprotein and albumin.

Metabolism and Elimination

Dipyridamole is metabolized in the liver, primarily by conjugation with glucuronic acid, of which monoglucuronide which has low pharmacodynamic activity is the primary metabolite. In plasma, about 80% of the total amount is present as parent compound and 20% as monoglucuronide. Most of the glucuronide metabolite (about 95%) is excreted via bile into the feces, with some evidence of enterohepatic circulation. Renal excretion of parent compound is negligible and urinary excretion of the glucuronide metabolite is low (about 5%). With intravenous (i.v.) treatment of dipyridamole, a triphasic profile is obtained: a rapid alpha phase, with a half-life of about 3.4 minutes, a beta phase, with a half-life of about 39 minutes, (which, together with the alpha phase accounts for about 70% of the total area under the curve, AUC) and a prolonged elimination phase λ_z with a half-life of about 15.5 hours. Due to the extended absorption phase of the dipyridamole component, only the terminal phase is apparent from oral treatment with AGGRENOX which, in Trial 9.123 was 13.6 hours.

Special Populations

Geriatric Patients: In ESPS2 [*see Clinical Studies (14)*], plasma concentrations (determined as AUC) of dipyridamole in healthy elderly subjects (>65 years) were about 40% higher than in subjects younger than 55 years receiving treatment with AGGRENOX.

Hepatic Dysfunction: No study has been conducted with AGGRENOX in patients with hepatic dysfunction.

In a study conducted with an intravenous formulation of dipyridamole, patients with mild to severe hepatic insufficiency showed no change in plasma concentrations of dipyridamole but showed an increase in the pharmacologically inactive monoglucuronide metabolite. Dipyridamole can be dosed without restriction as long as there is no evidence of hepatic failure.

Renal Dysfunction: No study has been conducted with AGGRENOX in patients with renal dysfunction.

In ESPS2 patients [*see Clinical Studies (14)*], with creatinine clearances ranging from about 15 mL/min to >100 mL/min, no changes were observed in the pharmacokinetics of dipyridamole or its glucuronide metabolite if data were corrected for differences in age.

Aspirin

Absorption

Peak plasma levels of aspirin are achieved 0.63 hours (0.5–1 hour) after administration of a 50 mg aspirin daily dose from AGGRENOX (given as 25 mg BID). The peak plasma concentration at steady-state is 319 ng/mL (175–463 ng/mL). Aspirin undergoes moderate hydrolysis to salicylic acid in the liver and the gastrointestinal wall, with 50%–75% of an administered dose reaching the systemic circulation as intact aspirin.

Effect of Food

When AGGRENOX capsules were taken with a high fat meal, there was no difference for aspirin in AUC at steady-state, and the approximately 50% decrease in C_{max} was not considered clinically relevant based on a similar degree of cyclooxygenase inhibition comparing the fed and fasted state.

Distribution

Aspirin is poorly bound to plasma proteins and its apparent volume of distribution is low (10 L). Its metabolite, salicylic acid, is highly bound to plasma proteins, but its binding is concentration-dependent (nonlinear). At low concentrations (<100 µg/mL), approximately 90% of salicylic acid is bound to albumin. Salicylic acid is widely distributed to all tissues and fluids in the body, including the central nervous system, breast milk, and fetal tissues. Early signs of salicylate overdose (salicylism), including tinnitus (ringing in the ears), occur at plasma concentrations approximating 200 µg/mL [*see Adverse Reactions (6) and Overdosage (10)*].

Metabolism and Elimination

Aspirin is rapidly hydrolyzed in plasma to salicylic acid, with a half-life of 20 minutes. Plasma levels of aspirin are essentially undetectable 2-2.5 hours after dosing and peak salicylic acid concentrations occur 1 hour (range: 0.5-2 hours) after administration of aspirin. Salicylic acid is primarily conjugated in the liver to form salicyluric acid, a phenolic glucuronide, an acyl glucuronide, and a number of minor metabolites. Salicylate metabolism is saturable and total body clearance decreases at higher serum concentrations due to the limited ability of the liver to form both salicyluric acid and phenolic glucuronide. Following toxic doses (10-20 g), the plasma half-life may be increased to over 20 hours.

The elimination of acetylsalicylic acid follows first-order kinetics with AGGRENOX and has a half-life of 0.33 hours. The half-life of salicylic acid is 1.71 hours. Both values correspond well with data from the literature at lower doses which state a resultant half-life of approximately 2-3 hours. At higher doses, the elimination of salicylic acid follows zero-order kinetics (i.e., the rate of elimination is constant in relation to plasma concentration), with an apparent half-life of 6 hours or higher. Renal excretion of unchanged drug depends upon urinary pH. As urinary pH rises above 6.5, the renal clearance of free salicylate increases from <5% to >80%. Alkalinization of the urine is a key concept in the management of salicylate overdose [*see Overdosage (10)*]. Following therapeutic doses, about 10% is excreted as salicylic acid and 75% as salicyluric acid, as the phenolic and acyl glucuronides, in urine.

Special Populations

Hepatic Dysfunction: Avoid aspirin in patients with severe hepatic insufficiency.

Renal Dysfunction: Avoid aspirin in patients with severe renal failure (glomerular filtration rate less than 10 mL/min).

13 NONCLINICAL TOXICOLOGY

13.1 Carcinogenesis, Mutagenesis, Impairment of Fertility

In studies in which dipyridamole was administered in the feed to mice (up to 111 weeks in males and females) and rats (up to 128 weeks in males and up to 142 weeks in females), there was no evidence of drug-related carcinogenesis. The highest dose administered in these studies (75 mg/kg/day) was, on a mg/m^2 basis, about equivalent to the maximum recommended daily human oral dose (MRHD) in mice and about twice the MRHD in rats.

Combinations of dipyridamole and aspirin (1:5 ratio) tested negative in the Ames test, *in vivo* chromosome aberration tests (in mice and hamsters), oral micronucleus tests (in mice and hamsters) and oral dominant lethal test (in mice). Aspirin, alone, induced chromosome aberrations in cultured human fibroblasts. Mutagenicity tests of dipyridamole alone with bacterial and mammalian cell systems were negative.

Combinations of dipyridamole and aspirin have not been evaluated for effects on fertility and reproductive performance. There was no evidence of impaired fertility when dipyridamole was administered to male and female rats at

Table 4   Summary of First Stroke (Fatal or Nonfatal): ESPS2: Intent-to-Treat Population

	Total Number of Patients n	Number of Patients With Stroke Within 2 Years n (%)	Kaplan-Meier Estimate of Survival at 2 Years (95% C.I.)	Gehan-Wilcoxon Test P-value	Risk Reduction at 2 Years	Odds Ratio (95% C.I.)
Individual Treatment Group						
AGGRENOX	1650	157 (9.5%)	89.9% (88.4%, 91.4%)	-	-	-
ER-DP	1654	211 (12.8%)	86.7% (85.0%, 88.4%)	-	-	-
ASA	1649	206 (12.5%)	87.1% (85.4%, 88.7%)	-	-	-
Placebo	1649	250 (15.2%)	84.1% (82.2%, 85.9%)	-	-	-
Pairwise Treatment Group Comparisons						
AGGRENOX vs. ER-DP	-	-	-	0.002**	24.4%	0.72 (0.58, 0.90)
AGGRENOX vs. ASA	-	-	-	0.008**	22.1%	0.74 (0.59, 0.92)
AGGRENOX vs. Placebo	-	-	-	<0.001**	36.8%	0.59 (0.48, 0.73)
ER-DP vs. Placebo	-	-	-	0.036*	16.5%	0.82 (0.67, 1.00)
ASA vs. Placebo	-	-	-	0.009**	18.9%	0.80 (0.66, 0.97)

*0.010 < p-value ≤0.050; **p-value ≤0.010.
Note: ER-DP = extended-release dipyridamole 200 mg; ASA = aspirin 25 mg. The dosage regimen for all treatment groups is BID

oral doses up to 500 mg/kg/day (about 12 times the MRHD on a mg/m² basis). A significant reduction in number of corpora lutea with consequent reduction in implantations and live fetuses was, however, observed at 1250 mg/kg (more than 30 times the MRHD on a mg/m² basis). Aspirin inhibits ovulation in rats.

14   CLINICAL STUDIES

ESPS2 (European Stroke Prevention Study 2) was a double-blind, placebo-controlled, 24-month study in which 6602 patients over the age of 18 years had an ischemic stroke (76%) or transient ischemic attack (TIA, 24%) within three months prior to entry. Patients were enrolled in 13 European countries between February 1989 and May 1995 and were randomized to one of four treatment groups: AGGRENOX (aspirin/extended-release dipyridamole) 25 mg/200 mg; extended-release dipyridamole (ER-DP) 200 mg alone; aspirin (ASA) 25 mg alone; or placebo. The mean age in this population was 66.7 years with 58% of them being males. Patients received one capsule twice daily (morning and evening). Efficacy assessments included analyses of stroke (fatal or nonfatal) and death (from all causes) as confirmed by a blinded morbidity and mortality assessment group. There were no differences with regard to efficacy based on age or gender; patients who were older had a trend towards more events.

Stroke Endpoint
AGGRENOX reduced the risk of stroke by 22.1% compared to aspirin 50 mg/day alone (p = 0.008) and reduced the risk of stroke by 24.4% compared to extended-release dipyridamole 400 mg/day alone (p = 0.002) (Table 4). AGGRENOX reduced the risk of stroke by 36.8% compared to placebo (p <0.001).
[See table 4 above]

ESP2: Cumulative Stroke Rate (Fatal or Nonfatal)
Over 24 months of Follow-UP

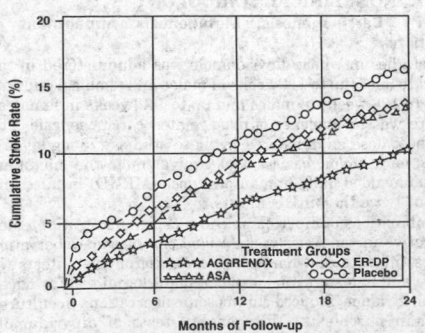

Note: ER-DP = extended-release dipyridamole 200 mg; ASA = aspirin 25 mg. The dosage regimen for all treatment groups is b.i.d.

Combined Stroke or Death Endpoint
In ESPS2, AGGRENOX reduced the risk of stroke or death by 12.1% compared to aspirin alone and by 10.3% compared

to extended-release dipyridamole alone. These results were not statistically significant. AGGRENOX reduced the risk of stroke or death by 24.2% compared to placebo.
Death Endpoint
The incidence rate of all cause mortality was 11.3% for AGGRENOX, 11.0% for aspirin alone, 11.4% for extended-release dipyridamole alone and 12.3% for placebo alone. The differences between the AGGRENOX, aspirin alone and extended-release dipyridamole alone treatment groups were not statistically significant. These incidence rates for AGGRENOX and aspirin alone are consistent with previous aspirin studies in stroke and TIA patients.

16   HOW SUPPLIED/STORAGE AND HANDLING

AGGRENOX capsules are available as a hard gelatin capsule, with a red cap and an ivory-colored body, 24.0 mm in length, containing yellow extended-release pellets incorporating dipyridamole and a round white tablet incorporating immediate-release aspirin. The capsule body is imprinted in red with the Boehringer Ingelheim logo and with "01A".
AGGRENOX capsules are supplied in unit-of-use bottles of 60 capsules (NDC 0597-0001-60).
Store at 25°C (77°F); excursions permitted to 15°-30°C (59°-86°F) [see USP Controlled Room Temperature]. Protect from excessive moisture.

17   PATIENT COUNSELING INFORMATION

See FDA-approved Patient Labeling
17.1   Risk of Bleeding
Inform patients that as with other antiplatelet agents, there is a general risk of bleeding including intracranial and gastrointestinal bleeding. Inform patients about the signs and symptoms of bleeding, including occult bleeding. Tell patients to notify their physician if they are prescribed any drug which may increase risk of bleeding.
Counsel patients who consume three or more alcoholic drinks daily about the bleeding risks involved with chronic, heavy alcohol use while taking aspirin.
17.2   Pregnancy
Inform patients that aspirin is known to be harmful to fetuses and ask the patient to notify them if they are or become pregnant.
17.3   Headaches
Some patients may experience headaches upon treatment initiation; these are usually transient. In case of intolerable headaches, tell the patient to contact their physician.
17.4   Dosage and Administration
Tell patients that AGGRENOX capsules should be swallowed whole, and not chewed or crushed. If you miss a dose, continue with your next dose on your regular schedule. Do not take a double dose.
17.5   Storage
Inform patients to protect AGGRENOX from moisture.
Distributed by:
Boehringer Ingelheim Pharmaceuticals, Inc.
Ridgefield, CT 06877 USA

Licensed from:
Boehringer Ingelheim International GmbH
©Copyright 2009 Boehringer Ingelheim International GmbH
ALL RIGHTS RESERVED
Patent No. 6,015,577
Rev: October 2009
OT1000FJ0709
42633/US/8
PATIENT INFORMATION
Aggrenox® (AG-reh-nox)
(aspirin/extended-release dipyridamole)
Capsules
Read this Patient Information before you start taking AGGRENOX and each time you get a refill. There may be new information. This information does not take the place of talking to your healthcare provider about your medical condition or your treatment.
What is AGGRENOX?
AGGRENOX is a prescription medicine that contains aspirin and a medicine that is slowly released in your body, called dipyridamole. AGGRENOX is used to lower the risk of stroke in people who have had a "mini-stroke" (transient ischemia attack or TIA) or stroke due to a blood clot.
It is not known if AGGRENOX is safe and effective in children. See "Who should not take AGGRENOX?"
Who should not take AGGRENOX?
Do not take AGGRENOX if you:
• are allergic to any of the ingredients in AGGRENOX. See the end of this leaflet for a list of ingredients in AGGRENOX.
• are allergic to non-steroidal anti-inflammatory drugs (NSAIDS)
• have asthma in combination with runny nose and nasal polyps
Do not give AGGRENOX to a child or teenager with a viral illness. Reye's syndrome, a life-threatening condition, can happen when aspirin (an ingredient in AGGRENOX) is used in children and teenagers who have certain viral illnesses.
What should I tell my doctor before using AGGRENOX? Before taking AGGRENOX, tell your healthcare provider if you:
• have stomach ulcers
• have a history of bleeding problems
• have heart problems
• have kidney or liver problems
• have low blood pressure
• have myasthenia gravis
• have any other medical conditions
• are pregnant or plan to become pregnant. AGGRENOX can harm your unborn baby, especially if you take it in the last (third) trimester of pregnancy. You should not take AGGRENOX during pregnancy without first talking to your healthcare provider. Tell your healthcare provider right away if you become pregnant while taking AGGRENOX.
• are breast-feeding or plan to breast-feed. AGGRENOX can pass into your milk and may harm your baby. Talk to

your healthcare provider about the best way to feed your baby if you take AGGRENOX.

Tell your doctor about all the medicines you take including, prescription and non-prescription medicines, vitamins and herbal supplements. AGGRENOX and other medicines may affect each other causing side effects. AGGRENOX may affect the way other medicines work, and other medicines may affect how AGGRENOX works.

Especially tell your healthcare provider if you take:

- **a medicine for high blood pressure, irregular heart beat, or heart failure**
- **acetazolamide [Diamox®]**
- **the blood thinner medicine warfarin sodium [Coumadin®, Jantoven®] or a heparin medicine**
- **a seizure medicine**
- **a medicine for Alzheimer's disease**
- **a water pill**
- **methotrexate sodium [Trexall®]**
- **aspirin or a non-steroidal anti-inflammatory drug (NSAIDS). You should not take NSAIDs during treatment with AGGRENOX.** Using these medicines with AGGRENOX can increase your risk of bleeding.
- **a medicine for diabetes**
- **probenecid [Probalan®, Col-Probenecid®]**

Ask your healthcare provider or pharmacist if you are not sure if your medicine is one that is listed above.

Know the medicines you take. Keep a list of them and show your healthcare provider and pharmacist when you get a new medicine.

How should I take AGGRENOX?

- Take AGGRENOX exactly as prescribed. Your healthcare provider will tell you how many AGGRENOX to take and when to take them.
- Headaches are not uncommon when you first start taking AGGRENOX, but often lessen as treatment continues. Tell your healthcare provider if you have a severe headache. Your healthcare provider may change the instructions for taking AGGRENOX.
- Swallow AGGRENOX whole. Do not crush or chew the capsules.
- You can take AGGRENOX with or without food.
- *If you miss a dose, take your next dose at the usual time. Do not take two doses at one time.*
- If you take more AGGRENOX (overdose) than prescribed, call your healthcare provider or Poison Control Center, or get emergency help right away.

Symptoms of an overdose of AGGRENOX include:
- a warm feeling or flushing
- sweating
- restlessness
- weakness or dizziness
- a fast heart rate
- ringing in the ears

What should I avoid while using AGGRENOX?
- heavy alcohol use. People who drink three or more alcoholic drinks every day have a higher risk of bleeding during treatment with AGGRENOX, because it contains aspirin.

What are the possible side effects of AGGRENOX?
AGGRENOX may cause serious side effects, including:
- **increased risk of bleeding.** You may bleed more easily during AGGRENOX treatment, and it may take longer than usual for bleeding to stop. This can include:
  - **bleeding into your brain (intracranial hemorrhage).** This can be a medical emergency. Get medical help right away if you have any of these symptoms while taking AGGRENOX:
    - severe headache with drowsiness
    - confusion or memory change
    - pass out (become unconscious)
  - **bleeding in your stomach or intestine.**
    - stomach pain
    - heartburn or nausea
    - vomiting blood or vomit looks like "coffee grounds"
    - red or bloody stools
    - black stools that look like tar
- **new or worsening chest pain in some people with heart disease.** Tell your healthcare provider if you have new chest pain or have any change in your chest pain during treatment with AGGRENOX.
- **liver problems,** including increased liver function tests and liver failure. Tell your healthcare provider if you have any of these symptoms of a liver problem while taking AGGRENOX:
  - loss of appetite
  - pale colored stool
  - stomach area (abdomen) pain
  - yellowing of your skin or whites of your eyes
  - dark urine
  - itching

Call your healthcare provider right away if you have any of the symptoms listed above.

The most common side effects of AGGRENOX include:
- headache

- upset stomach
- diarrhea

These are not all the possible side effects of AGGRENOX. Tell your healthcare provider or pharmacist if you have any side effect that bothers you or that does not go away. Call your healthcare provider for medical advice about side effects. You may report side effects to FDA at 1-800-FDA-1088.

How should I store AGGRENOX?
- Store AGGRENOX at 59°F to 86°F (15°C to 30°C).
- Keep AGGRENOX capsules dry.
- Safely throw away medicine that is out of date or no longer needed.

Keep AGGRENOX and all medicines out of the reach of children.

General information about AGGRENOX
Medicines are sometimes prescribed for purposes other than those listed in the Patient Information. Do not use AGGRENOX for a condition for which it was not prescribed. Do not give AGGRENOX to other people, even if they have the same symptoms that you have. It may harm them.

This Patient Information summarizes the most important information about AGGRENOX. If you would like more information, talk with your healthcare provider. You can ask your pharmacist or healthcare provider for information about AGGRENOX that is written for health professionals. For more information, call Boehringer Ingelheim Pharmaceuticals, Inc. at 1-800-542-6257 or (TTY) 1-800-459-9906.

What are the ingredients in AGGRENOX?
Active Ingredients: dipyridamole in an extended-release form and aspirin
Inactive Ingredients: acacia, aluminum stearate, colloidal silicon dioxide, corn starch, dimethicone, hypromellose, hypromellose phthalate, lactose monohydrate, methacrylic acid copolymer, microcrystalline cellulose, povidone, stearic acid, sucrose, talc, tartaric acid, titanium dioxide and triacetin. Each capsule shell contains gelatin, red iron oxide and yellow iron oxide, titanium dioxide, and water.

Distributed by:
Boehringer Ingelheim Pharmaceuticals, Inc.
Ridgefield, CT 06877 USA
Licensed from:
Boehringer Ingelheim International GmbH
©Copyright 2009 Boehringer Ingelheim International GmbH
ALL RIGHTS RESERVED
Patent No. 6,015,577
Rev: October 2009
OT1000FJ0709
42633/US/8

Shown in Product Identification Guide, page 307

SPIRIVA® HANDIHALER®   ℞
[speh REE vah]
(tiotropium bromide inhalation powder)
Capsules for Respiratory Inhalation
DO NOT Swallow SPIRIVA Capsules
FOR ORAL INHALATION ONLY with the HandiHaler Device

HIGHLIGHTS OF PRESCRIBING INFORMATION

These highlights do not include all the information needed to use SPIRIVA HandiHaler safely and effectively. See full prescribing information for SPIRIVA HandiHaler.

SPIRIVA® HandiHaler® (tiotropium bromide inhalation powder)
Capsules for Respiratory Inhalation
DO NOT Swallow SPIRIVA Capsules
FOR ORAL INHALATION ONLY with the HandiHaler Device
Initial U.S. Approval: 2004

————RECENT MAJOR CHANGES————

Indications and Usage (1)	12/2009
Dosage and Administration (2)	12/2009
Contraindications (4)	12/2009
Warnings and Precautions, Immediate Hypersensitivity Reactions (5.2)	12/2009
Worsening of Narrow-Angle Glaucoma (5.4)	12/2009
Worsening of Urinary Retention (5.5)	12/2009
Renal Impairment (5.6)	12/2009

————INDICATIONS AND USAGE————
SPIRIVA HandiHaler is an anticholinergic indicated for the long-term, once-daily, maintenance treatment of bronchospasm associated with chronic obstructive pulmonary disease (COPD), and for reducing COPD exacerbations (1)

————DOSAGE AND ADMINISTRATION————
DO NOT swallow SPIRIVA capsules (2)
For Use with the HandiHaler Device ONLY (2)
For Oral Inhalation ONLY (2)
- Two inhalations of the powder contents of a single SPIRIVA capsule (18 mcg) once daily (2)

————DOSAGE FORMS AND STRENGTHS————
SPIRIVA capsules for oral inhalation: 18 mcg tiotropium powder, for use with HandiHaler device (3)
————CONTRAINDICATIONS————
- Hypersensitivity to ipratropium or tiotropium (4)
————WARNINGS AND PRECAUTIONS————
- Not for acute use: Not for use as a rescue medication (5.1)
- Immediate hypersensitivity reactions: Discontinue SPIRIVA HandiHaler at once and consider alternatives if immediate hypersensitivity reactions, including angioedema, occur. Use with caution in patients with severe hypersensitivity to milk proteins. (5.2)
- Paradoxical bronchospasm: Discontinue SPIRIVA HandiHaler and consider other treatments if paradoxical bronchospasm occurs (5.3)
- Worsening of narrow-angle glaucoma may occur. Use with caution in patients with narrow-angle glaucoma and instruct patients to consult a physician immediately if this occurs. (5.4)
- Worsening of urinary retention may occur. Use with caution in patients with prostatic hyperplasia or bladder-neck obstruction and instruct patients to consult a physician immediately if this occurs. (5.5)
————ADVERSE REACTIONS————
- The most common adverse reactions (>5% incidence in the 1-year placebo-controlled trials) were upper respiratory tract infection, dry mouth, sinusitis, pharyngitis, non-specific chest pain, urinary tract infection, dyspepsia, and rhinitis (6.1)

To report SUSPECTED ADVERSE REACTIONS, contact Boehringer Ingelheim Pharmaceuticals, Inc. at (800) 542-6257 or (800) 459-9906 TTY, or FDA at 1-800-FDA-1088 or www.fda.gov/medwatch.
————DRUG INTERACTIONS————
Not recommended for use with other anticholinergics since this has not been studied (7.2)
————USE IN SPECIFIC POPULATIONS————
Patients with moderate to severe renal impairment should be monitored closely for potential anticholinergic side effects (2, 8.6)

See 17 for PATIENT COUNSELING INFORMATION and FDA-approved patient labeling.

Revised: 12/2009

FULL PRESCRIBING INFORMATION

1 INDICATIONS AND USAGE

SPIRIVA HandiHaler (tiotropium bromide inhalation powder) is indicated for the long-term, once-daily, maintenance treatment of bronchospasm associated with chronic obstructive pulmonary disease (COPD), including chronic bronchitis and emphysema. SPIRIVA HandiHaler is indicated to reduce exacerbations in COPD patients.

2 DOSAGE AND ADMINISTRATION

DO NOT SWALLOW SPIRIVA CAPSULES
FOR USE WITH HANDIHALER DEVICE ONLY
FOR ORAL INHALATION ONLY
SPIRIVA capsules must not be swallowed as the intended effects on the lungs will not be obtained. The contents of the SPIRIVA capsules are only for oral inhalation and should only be used with the HandiHaler device [see Overdosage (10)].

The recommended dose of SPIRIVA HandiHaler is two inhalations of the powder contents of one SPIRIVA capsule, once-daily, with the HandiHaler device [see Patient Counseling Information (17.6)].

For administration of SPIRIVA HandiHaler, a SPIRIVA capsule is placed into the center chamber of the HandiHaler device. The SPIRIVA capsule is pierced by pressing and releasing the green piercing button on the side of the HandiHaler device. The tiotropium formulation is dispersed into the air stream when the patient inhales through the mouthpiece [see Patient Counseling Information (17.6)].

No dosage adjustment is required for geriatric, hepatically-impaired, or renally-impaired patients. However, patients with moderate to severe renal impairment given SPIRIVA HandiHaler should be monitored closely for anticholinergic effects [see Warnings and Precautions (5.6), Use in Specific Populations (8.5, 8.6, 8.7), and Clinical Pharmacology (12.3)].

3 DOSAGE FORMS AND STRENGTHS

SPIRIVA HandiHaler consists of SPIRIVA capsules and a HandiHaler device. SPIRIVA capsules contain 18 mcg dry powder formulation of tiotropium in a light green, hard gelatin capsule with TI 01 printed on one side and Boehringer Ingelheim company logo on the other side. Supplied with a HandiHaler device.

4 CONTRAINDICATIONS

SPIRIVA HandiHaler is contraindicated in patients with a hypersensitivity to ipratropium or tiotropium. In clinical trials and postmarketing experience with SPIRIVA HandiHaler, immediate hypersensitivity reactions, including angioedema (including swelling of the lips, tongue, or throat), itching, or rash have been reported.

5 WARNINGS AND PRECAUTIONS

5.1 Not for Acute Use

SPIRIVA HandiHaler is intended as a once-daily maintenance treatment for COPD and is not indicated for the initial treatment of acute episodes of bronchospasm (i.e., rescue therapy).

5.2 Immediate Hypersensitivity Reactions

Immediate hypersensitivity reactions, including angioedema (including swelling of the lips, tongue, or throat), itching, or rash may occur after administration of SPIRIVA HandiHaler. If such a reaction occurs, therapy with SPIRIVA HandiHaler should be stopped at once and alternative treatments should be considered. Given the similar structural formula of atropine to tiotropium, patients with a history of hypersensitivity reactions to atropine should be closely monitored for similar hypersensitivity reactions to SPIRIVA HandiHaler. In addition, SPIRIVA HandiHaler should be used with caution in patients with severe hypersensitivity to milk proteins.

5.3 Paradoxical Bronchospasm

Inhaled medicines, including SPIRIVA HandiHaler, may cause paradoxical bronchospasm. If this occurs, treatment with SPIRIVA HandiHaler should be stopped and other treatments considered.

5.4 Worsening of Narrow-Angle Glaucoma

SPIRIVA HandiHaler should be used with caution in patients with narrow-angle glaucoma. Prescribers and patients should be alert for signs and symptoms of acute narrow-angle glaucoma (e.g., eye pain or discomfort, blurred vision, visual halos or colored images in association with red eyes from conjunctival congestion and corneal edema). Instruct patients to consult a physician immediately should any of these signs or symptoms develop.

5.5 Worsening of Urinary Retention

SPIRIVA HandiHaler should be used with caution in patients with urinary retention. Prescribers and patients should be alert for signs and symptoms of prostatic hyperplasia or bladder-neck obstruction (e.g., difficulty passing urine, painful urination). Instruct patients to consult a physician immediately should any of these signs or symptoms develop.

5.6 Renal Impairment

As a predominantly renally excreted drug, patients with moderate to severe renal impairment (creatinine clearance of ≤50 mL/min) treated with SPIRIVA HandiHaler should be monitored for anticholinergic side effects [see Clinical Pharmacology (12.3)].

6 ADVERSE REACTIONS

The following adverse reactions are described, or described in greater detail, in other sections:

- Immediate hypersensitivity reactions [see Warnings and Precautions (5.2)]
- Paradoxical bronchospasm [see Warnings and Precautions (5.3)]
- Worsening of narrow-angle glaucoma [see Warnings and Precautions (5.4)]
- Worsening of urinary retention [see Warnings and Precautions (5.5)]

6.1 Clinical Trials Experience

Because clinical trials are conducted under widely varying conditions, adverse reaction rates observed in the clinical trials of a drug cannot be directly compared to rates in the clinical trials of another drug and may not reflect the rates observed in practice.

6-Month to 1-Year Trials
The data described below reflect exposure to SPIRIVA HandiHaler in 2663 patients. SPIRIVA HandiHaler was studied in two 1-year placebo-controlled trials, two 1-year active-controlled trials, and two 6-month placebo-controlled trials in patients with COPD. In these trials, 1308 patients were treated with SPIRIVA HandiHaler at the recommended dose of 18 mcg once a day. The population had an age ranging from 39 to 87 years with 65% to 85% males, 95% Caucasian, and had COPD with a mean prebronchodilator forced expiratory volume in one second (FEV$_1$) percent predicted of 39% to 43%.

Patients with narrow-angle glaucoma, or symptomatic prostatic hypertrophy or bladder outlet obstruction were excluded from these trials. An additional 6-month trial conducted in a Veteran's Affairs setting is not included in this safety database because only serious adverse events were collected.

The most commonly reported adverse drug reaction was dry mouth. Dry mouth was usually mild and often resolved during continued treatment. Other reactions reported in individual patients and consistent with possible anticholinergic effects included constipation, tachycardia, blurred vision, glaucoma (new onset or worsening), dysuria, and urinary retention.

Four multicenter, 1-year, placebo-controlled and active-controlled trials evaluated SPIRIVA HandiHaler in patients with COPD. Table 1 shows all adverse reactions that occurred with a frequency of ≥3% in the SPIRIVA HandiHaler group in the 1-year placebo-controlled trials where the rates in the SPIRIVA HandiHaler group exceeded placebo by ≥1%. The frequency of corresponding reactions in the ipratropium-controlled trials is included for comparison. [See table 1 at left]

Arthritis, coughing, and influenza-like symptoms occurred at a rate of ≥3% in the SPIRIVA HandiHaler treatment group, but were <1% in excess of the placebo group.

Other reactions that occurred in the SPIRIVA HandiHaler group at a frequency of 1% to 3% in the placebo-controlled trials where the rates exceeded that in the placebo group include: *Body as a Whole:* allergic reaction, leg pain; *Central and Peripheral Nervous System:* dysphonia, paresthesia; *Gastrointestinal System Disorders:* gastrointestinal disorder not otherwise specified (NOS), gastroesophageal reflux, stomatitis (including ulcerative stomatitis); *Metabolic and Nutritional Disorders:* hypercholesterolemia, hyperglycemia; *Musculoskeletal System Disorders:* skeletal pain; *Cardiac Events:* angina pectoris (including aggravated angina pectoris); *Psychiatric Disorder:* depression; *Infections:* herpes zoster; *Respiratory System Disorder (Upper):* laryngitis; *Vision Disorder:* cataract. In addition, among the adverse reactions observed in the clinical trials with an incidence of <1% were atrial fibrillation, supraventricular tachycardia, angioedema, and urinary retention.

In the 1-year trials, the incidence of dry mouth, constipation, and urinary tract infection increased with age [see Use in Specific Populations (8.5)].

Two multicenter, 6-month, controlled studies evaluated SPIRIVA HandiHaler in patients with COPD. The adverse reactions and the incidence rates were similar to those seen in the 1-year controlled trials.

4-Year Trial
The data described below reflect exposure to SPIRIVA HandiHaler in 5592 COPD patients in a 4-year placebo-controlled trial. In this trial, 2986 patients were treated with SPIRIVA HandiHaler at the recommended dose of 18 mcg once a day. The population had an age range from 40

Table 1 Adverse Reactions (% Patients) in One-Year COPD Clinical Trials

Body System (Event)	Placebo-Controlled Trials		Ipratropium-Controlled Trials	
	SPIRIVA (n = 550)	Placebo (n = 371)	SPIRIVA (n = 356)	Ipratropium (n = 179)
Body as a Whole				
Chest Pain (non-specific)	7	5	5	2
Edema, Dependent	5	4	3	5
Gastrointestinal System Disorders				
Dry Mouth	16	3	12	6
Dyspepsia	6	5	1	1
Abdominal Pain	5	3	6	6
Constipation	4	2	1	1
Vomiting	4	2	1	2
Musculoskeletal System				
Myalgia	4	3	4	3
Resistance Mechanism Disorders				
Infection	4	3	1	3
Moniliasis	4	2	3	2
Respiratory System (Upper)				
Upper Respiratory Tract Infection	41	37	43	35
Sinusitis	11	9	3	2
Pharyngitis	9	7	7	3
Rhinitis	6	5	3	2
Epistaxis	4	2	1	1
Skin and Appendage Disorders				
Rash	4	2	2	2
Urinary System				
Urinary Tract Infection	7	5	4	2

to 88 years, was 75% male, 90% Caucasian, and had COPD with a mean pre-bronchodilator FEV_1 percent predicted of 40%. Patients with narrow-angle glaucoma, or symptomatic prostatic hypertrophy or bladder outlet obstruction were excluded from these trials. When the adverse reactions were analyzed with a frequency of ≥3% in the SPIRIVA HandiHaler group where the rates in the SPIRIVA HandiHaler group exceeded placebo by ≥1%, adverse reactions included (SPIRIVA HandiHaler, placebo): pharyngitis (12.5%, 10.8%), sinusitis (6.5%, 5.3%), headache (5.7%, 4.5%), constipation (5.1%, 3.7%), dry mouth (5.1%, 2.7%), depression (4.4%, 3.3%), insomnia (4.4%, 3.0%), and arthralgia (4.2%, 3.1%).

Additional Adverse Reactions

Other adverse reactions not previously listed that were reported more frequently in COPD patients treated with SPIRIVA HandiHaler than placebo include: dehydration, skin ulcer, stomatitis, gingivitis, oropharyngeal candidiasis, dry skin, skin infection, and joint swelling.

6.2 Postmarketing Experience

Adverse reactions have been identified during worldwide post-approval use of SPIRIVA HandiHaler. Because these reactions are reported voluntarily from a population of uncertain size, it is not always possible to reliably estimate their frequency or establish a causal relationship to drug exposure. These adverse reactions are: application site irritation (glossitis, mouth ulceration, and pharyngolaryngeal pain), dizziness, dysphagia, hoarseness, intestinal obstruction including ileus paralytic, intraocular pressure increased, oral candidiasis, palpitations, pruritus, tachycardia, throat irritation, and urticaria.

7 DRUG INTERACTIONS

7.1 Sympathomimetics, Methylxanthines, Steroids

SPIRIVA HandiHaler has been used concomitantly with short-acting and long-acting sympathomimetic (beta-agonists) bronchodilators, methylxanthines, and oral and inhaled steroids without increases in adverse drug reactions.

7.2 Anticholinergics

The co-administration of SPIRIVA HandiHaler with other anticholinergic-containing drugs (e.g., ipratropium) has not been studied and is therefore not recommended.

7.3 Cimetidine, Ranitidine

No clinically significant interaction occurred between tiotropium and cimetidine or ranitidine [*see Clinical Pharmacology (12.3)*].

8 USE IN SPECIFIC POPULATIONS

8.1 Pregnancy

Teratogenic Effects, Pregnancy Category C.

There are no adequate and well-controlled studies in pregnant women. SPIRIVA HandiHaler should be used during pregnancy only if the potential benefit justifies the potential risk to the fetus.

No evidence of structural alterations was observed in rats and rabbits at inhalation tiotropium doses of up to approximately 660 and 6 times the recommended human daily inhalation dose (RHDID) on a mg/m^2 basis, respectively. However, in rats, tiotropium caused fetal resorption, litter loss, decreases in the number of live pups at birth and the mean pup weights, and a delay in pup sexual maturation at inhalation tiotropium doses of approximately 35 times the RHDID on a mg/m^2 basis. In rabbits, tiotropium caused an increase in post-implantation loss at an inhalation dose of approximately 360 times the RHDID on a mg/m^2 basis. Such effects were not observed at inhalation doses of approximately 4 and 80 times the RHDID on a mg/m^2 basis, respectively. These dose multiples may be over-estimated due to difficulties in measuring deposited doses in animal inhalation studies.

8.2 Labor and Delivery

The safety and effectiveness of SPIRIVA HandiHaler has not been studied during labor and delivery.

8.3 Nursing Mothers

Clinical data from nursing women exposed to tiotropium are not available. Based on lactating rodent studies, tiotropium is excreted into breast milk. It is not known whether tiotropium is excreted in human milk, but because many drugs are excreted in human milk and given these findings in rats, caution should be exercised if SPIRIVA HandiHaler is administered to a nursing woman.

8.4 Pediatric Use

SPIRIVA HandiHaler is approved for use in the maintenance treatment of bronchospasm associated with COPD and for the reduction of COPD exacerbations. COPD does not normally occur in children. The safety and effectiveness of SPIRIVA HandiHaler in pediatric patients have not been established.

8.5 Geriatric Use

Of the total number of patients who received SPIRIVA HandiHaler in the 1-year clinical trials, 426 were <65 years, 375 were 65 to 74 years, and 105 were ≥75 years of age. Within each age subgroup, there were no differences between the proportion of patients with adverse events in the SPIRIVA HandiHaler and the comparator groups for most events. Dry mouth increased with age in the SPIRIVA HandiHaler group (differences from placebo were 9.0%, 17.1%, and 16.2% in the aforementioned age subgroups). A higher frequency of constipation and urinary tract infections with increasing age was observed in the SPIRIVA HandiHaler group in the placebo-controlled studies. The differences from placebo for constipation were 0%, 1.8%, and 7.8% for each of the age groups. The differences from placebo for urinary tract infections were –0.6%, 4.6%, and 4.5%. No overall differences in effectiveness were observed among these groups. Based on available data, no adjustment of SPIRIVA HandiHaler dosage in geriatric patients is warranted [*see Clinical Pharmacology (12.3)*].

8.6 Renal Impairment

Patients with moderate to severe renal impairment (creatinine clearance of ≤50 mL/min) treated with SPIRIVA HandiHaler should be monitored closely for anticholinergic side effects [*see Dosage and Administration (2), Warnings and Precautions (5.4), and Clinical Pharmacology (12.3)*].

8.7 Hepatic Impairment

The effects of hepatic impairment on the pharmacokinetics of tiotropium were not studied.

10 OVERDOSAGE

High doses of tiotropium may lead to anticholinergic signs and symptoms. However, there were no systemic anticholinergic adverse effects following a single inhaled dose of up to 282 mcg tiotropium in 6 healthy volunteers. In a study of 12 healthy volunteers, bilateral conjunctivitis and dry mouth were seen following repeated once-daily inhalation of 141 mcg of tiotropium.

Accidental Ingestion

Acute intoxication by inadvertent oral ingestion of SPIRIVA capsules is unlikely since it is not well-absorbed systemically.

A case of overdose has been reported from postmarketing experience. A female patient was reported to have inhaled 30 capsules over a 2.5 day period, and developed altered mental status, tremors, abdominal pain, and severe constipation. The patient was hospitalized, SPIRIVA HandiHaler was discontinued, and the constipation was treated with an enema. The patient recovered and was discharged on the same day.

No mortality was observed at inhalation tiotropium doses up to 32.4 mg/kg in mice, 267.7 mg/kg in rats, and 0.6 mg/kg in dogs. These doses correspond to 7300, 120,000, and 850 times the recommended human daily inhalation dose on a mg/m^2 basis, respectively. These dose multiples may be over-estimated due to difficulties in measuring deposited doses in animal inhalation studies.

11 DESCRIPTION

SPIRIVA HandiHaler consists of a capsule dosage form containing a dry powder formulation of tiotropium intended for oral inhalation only with the HandiHaler device.

Each light green, hard gelatin SPIRIVA capsule contains 18 mcg tiotropium (equivalent to 22.5 mcg tiotropium bromide monohydrate) blended with lactose monohydrate (which may contain milk proteins) as the carrier.

The dry powder formulation within the SPIRIVA capsule is intended for oral inhalation only.

The active component of SPIRIVA HandiHaler is tiotropium. The drug substance, tiotropium bromide monohydrate, is an anticholinergic with specificity for muscarinic receptors. It is chemically described as (1α, 2ß, 4ß, 5α, 7ß)-7-[(Hydroxydi-2-thienylacetyl)oxy]-9,9-dimethyl-3-oxa-9-azoniatricyclo[$3.3.1.0^{2,4}$]nonane bromide monohydrate. It is a synthetic, non-chiral, quaternary ammonium compound. Tiotropium bromide is a white or yellowish white powder. It is sparingly soluble in water and soluble in methanol.

The structural formula is:

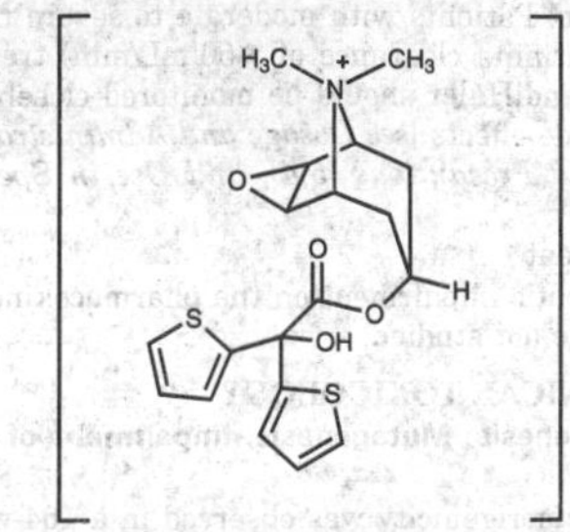

Tiotropium bromide (monohydrate) has a molecular mass of 490.4 and a molecular formula of $C_{19}H_{22}NO_4S_2Br \cdot H_2O$.

The HandiHaler device is an inhalation device used to inhale the dry powder contained in the SPIRIVA capsule. The dry powder is delivered from the HandiHaler device at flow rates as low as 20 L/min. Under standardized *in vitro* testing, the HandiHaler device delivers a mean of 10.4 mcg tiotropium when tested at a flow rate of 39 L/min for 3.1 seconds (2 L total). In a study of 26 adult patients with COPD and severely compromised lung function [mean FEV_1 1.02 L (range 0.45 to 2.24 L); 37.6% of predicted (range 16% to 65%)], the median peak inspiratory flow (PIF) through the HandiHaler device was 30.0 L/min (range 20.4 to 45.6 L/min). The amount of drug delivered to the lungs will vary depending on patient factors such as inspiratory flow and peak inspiratory flow through the HandiHaler device, which may vary from patient to patient, and may vary with the exposure time of the SPIRIVA capsule outside the blister pack.

12 CLINICAL PHARMACOLOGY

12.1 Mechanism of Action

Tiotropium is a long-acting, antimuscarinic agent, which is often referred to as an anticholinergic. It has similar affinity to the subtypes of muscarinic receptors, M_1 to M_5. In the airways, it exhibits pharmacological effects through inhibition of M_3-receptors at the smooth muscle leading to bronchodilation. The competitive and reversible nature of antagonism was shown with human and animal origin receptors and isolated organ preparations. In preclinical *in vitro* as well as *in vivo* studies, prevention of methacholine-induced bronchoconstriction effects was dose-dependent and lasted longer than 24 hours. The bronchodilation following inhalation of tiotropium is predominantly a site-specific effect.

12.2 Pharmacodynamics

Cardiovascular Effects

In a multicenter, randomized, double-blind trial that enrolled 198 patients with COPD, the number of subjects with changes from baseline-corrected QT interval of 30 to 60 msec was higher in the SPIRIVA HandiHaler group as compared with placebo. This difference was apparent using both the Bazett (QTcB) [20 (20%) patients vs 12 (12%) patients] and Fredericia (QTcF) [16 (16%) patients vs 1 (1%) patient] corrections of QT for heart rate. No patients in either group had either QTcB or QTcF of >500 msec. Other clinical studies with SPIRIVA HandiHaler did not detect an effect of the drug on QTc intervals.

The effect of SPIRIVA HandiHaler on QT interval was also evaluated in a randomized, placebo- and positive-controlled crossover study in 53 healthy volunteers. Subjects received SPIRIVA HandiHaler 18 mcg, 54 mcg (3 times the recommended dose), or placebo for 12 days. ECG assessments were performed at baseline and throughout the dosing interval following the first and last dose of study medication. Relative to placebo, the maximum mean change from baseline in study-specific QTc interval was 3.2 msec and 0.8 msec for SPIRIVA HandiHaler 18 mcg and 54 mcg, respectively. No subject showed a new onset of QTc >500 msec or QTc changes from baseline of ≥60 msec.

12.3 Pharmacokinetics

Tiotropium is administered by dry powder inhalation. In common with other inhaled drugs, the majority of the delivered dose is deposited in the gastrointestinal tract and, to a lesser extent, in the lung, the intended organ. Many of the pharmacokinetic data described below were obtained with higher doses than recommended for therapy.

Absorption

Following dry powder inhalation by young healthy volunteers, the absolute bioavailability of 19.5% suggests that the fraction reaching the lung is highly bioavailable. It is expected from the chemical structure of the compound (quaternary ammonium compound) that tiotropium is poorly absorbed from the gastrointestinal tract. The effect of food on tiotropium's bioavailability has not been studied. Oral solutions of tiotropium have an absolute bioavailability of 2% to 3%. Maximum tiotropium plasma concentrations were observed 5 minutes after inhalation.

Distribution

Tiotropium shows a volume of distribution of 32 L/kg indicating that the drug binds extensively to tissues. The human plasma protein binding for tiotropium is 72%. At steady state, peak tiotropium plasma levels in COPD patients were 17 to 19 pg/mL when measured 5 minutes after dry powder inhalation of an 18 mcg dose and decreased in a multi-compartmental manner. Steady-state trough plasma concentrations were 3 to 4 pg/mL. Local concentrations in the lung are not known, but the mode of administration suggests substantially higher concentrations in the lung. Studies in rats have shown that tiotropium does not readily penetrate the blood-brain barrier.

Metabolism

The extent of metabolism appears to be small. This is evident from a urinary excretion of 74% of unchanged substance after an intravenous dose to young healthy volunteers. Tiotropium, an ester, is nonenzymatically cleaved to the alcohol *N*-methylscopine and dithienylglycolic acid, neither of which bind to muscarinic receptors.

Figure 1 Mean FEV$_1$ Over Time (prior to and after administration of study drug) on Days 1 and 169 for Trial A (a Six-Month Placebo-Controlled Study)*

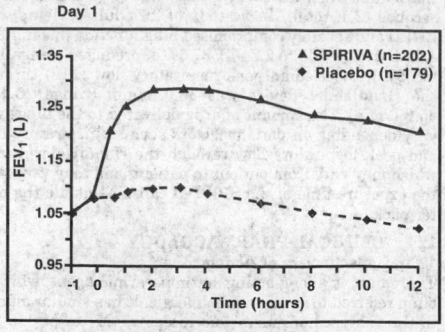 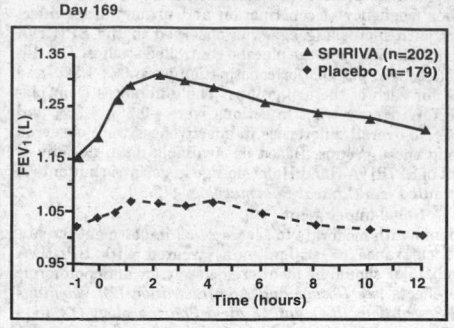

*Means adjusted for center, treatment, and baseline effect. On Day 169, a total of 183 and 149 patients in the SPIRIVA HandiHaler and placebo groups, respectively, completed the trial. The data for the remaining patients were imputed using the last observation or least favorable observation carried forward.

Figure 2 Mean FEV$_1$ Over Time (0 to 6 hours post-dose) on Days 1 and 92, Respectively for One of the Two Ipratropium-Controlled Studies*

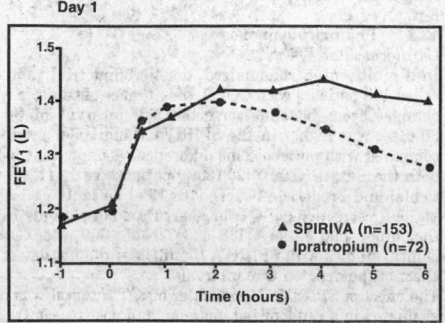 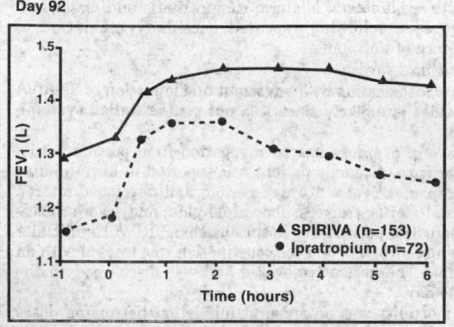

*Means adjusted for center, treatment, and baseline effect. On Day 92 (primary endpoint), a total of 151 and 69 patients in the SPIRIVA HandiHaler and ipratropium groups, respectively, completed through 3 months of observation. The data for the remaining patients were imputed using the last observation or least favorable observation carried forward.

In vitro experiments with human liver microsomes and human hepatocytes suggest that a fraction of the administered dose (74% of an intravenous dose is excreted unchanged in the urine, leaving 25% for metabolism) is metabolized by cytochrome P450-dependent oxidation and subsequent glutathione conjugation to a variety of Phase II metabolites. This enzymatic pathway can be inhibited by CYP450 2D6 and 3A4 inhibitors, such as quinidine, ketoconazole, and gestodene. Thus, CYP450 2D6 and 3A4 are involved in the metabolic pathway that is responsible for the elimination of a small part of the administered dose. *In vitro* studies using human liver microsomes showed that tiotropium in supratherapeutic concentrations did not inhibit CYP450 1A1, 1A2, 2B6, 2C9, 2C19, 2D6, 2E1, or 3A4.

Elimination

The terminal elimination half-life of tiotropium was between 5 and 6 days following inhalation. Total clearance was 880 mL/min after an intravenous dose in young healthy volunteers with an inter-individual variability of 22%. Intravenously administered tiotropium was mainly excreted unchanged in urine (74%). After dry powder inhalation, urinary excretion was 14% of the dose, the remainder being mainly non-absorbed drug in the gut which was eliminated via the feces. The renal clearance of tiotropium exceeds the creatinine clearance, indicating active secretion into the urine. After chronic once-daily inhalation by COPD patients, pharmacokinetic steady state was reached after 2 to 3 weeks with no accumulation thereafter.

Drug Interactions

An interaction study with tiotropium (14.4 mcg intravenous infusion over 15 minutes) and cimetidine 400 mg three times daily or ranitidine 300 mg once daily was conducted. Concomitant administration of cimetidine with tiotropium resulted in a 20% increase in the AUC$_{0-4h}$, a 28% decrease in the renal clearance of tiotropium and no significant change in the C$_{max}$ and amount excreted in urine over 96 hours. Co-administration of tiotropium with ranitidine did not affect the pharmacokinetics of tiotropium.

Specific Populations

Geriatric Patients

As expected for drugs predominantly excreted renally, advanced age was associated with a decrease of tiotropium renal clearance (326 mL/min in COPD patients <58 years to 163 mL/min in COPD patients >70 years), which may be explained by decreased renal function. Tiotropium excretion in urine after inhalation decreased from 14% (young healthy volunteers) to about 7% (COPD patients). Plasma concentrations were numerically increased with advancing age within COPD patients (43% increase in AUC$_{0-4}$ after dry powder inhalation), which was not significant when considered in relation to inter- and intra-individual variability [*see Dosage and Administration (2) and Use in Specific Populations (8.5)*].

Renal Impairment

Since tiotropium is predominantly renally excreted, renal impairment was associated with increased plasma drug concentrations and reduced drug clearance after both intravenous infusion and dry powder inhalation. Mild renal impairment (creatinine clearance of 50 to 80 mL/min), which is often seen in elderly patients, increased tiotropium plasma concentrations (39% increase in AUC$_{0-4}$ after intravenous infusion). In COPD patients with moderate to severe renal impairment (creatinine clearance of <50 mL/min), the intravenous administration of tiotropium resulted in doubling of the plasma concentrations (82% increase in AUC$_{0-4}$), which was confirmed by plasma concentrations after dry powder inhalation. Patients with moderate to severe renal impairment (creatinine clearance of ≤50 mL/min) treated with SPIRIVA HandiHaler should be monitored closely for anticholinergic side effects [*see Dosage and Administration (2), Warnings and Precautions (5.4), and Use in Specific Populations (8.6)*].

Hepatic Impairment

The effects of hepatic impairment on the pharmacokinetics of tiotropium were not studied.

13 NONCLINICAL TOXICOLOGY

13.1 Carcinogenesis, Mutagenesis, Impairment of Fertility

No evidence of tumorigenicity was observed in a 104-week inhalation study in rats at tiotropium doses up to 0.059 mg/kg/day, in an 83-week inhalation study in female mice at doses up to 0.145 mg/kg/day, and in a 101-week inhalation study in male mice at doses up to 0.002 mg/kg/day. These doses correspond to approximately 25, 35, and 0.5 times the recommended human daily inhalation dose (RHDID) on a mg/m^2 basis, respectively. These dose multiples may be over-estimated due to difficulties in measuring deposited doses in animal inhalation studies.

Tiotropium bromide demonstrated no evidence of mutagenicity or clastogenicity in the following assays: the bacterial gene mutation assay, the V79 Chinese hamster cell mutagenesis assay, the chromosomal aberration assays in human lymphocytes *in vitro* and mouse micronucleus formation *in vivo*, and the unscheduled DNA synthesis in primary rat hepatocytes *in vitro* assay.

In rats, decreases in the number of corpora lutea and the percentage of implants were noted at inhalation tiotropium doses of 0.078 mg/kg/day or greater (approximately 35 times the RHDID on a mg/m^2 basis). No such effects were observed at 0.009 mg/kg/day (approximately 4 times than the RHDID on a mg/m^2 basis). The fertility index, however, was not affected at inhalation doses up to 1.689 mg/kg/day (approximately 760 times the RHDID on a mg/m^2 basis). These dose multiples may be over-estimated due to difficulties in measuring deposited doses in animal inhalation studies.

13.2 Animal Toxicology and Pharmacology

Reproductive Toxicology Studies

No evidence of fetal structural alteration was observed in rats and rabbits at inhalation tiotropium doses of up to 1.471 and 0.007 mg/kg/day, respectively. These doses correspond to approximately 660 and 6 times the RHDID on a mg/m^2 basis, respectively. However, in rats, fetal resorption, litter loss, decreases in the number of live pups at birth and the mean pup weights, and a delay in pup sexual maturation were observed at inhalation tiotropium doses of ≥0.078 mg/kg (approximately 35 times the RHDID on a mg/m^2 basis). In rabbits, an increase in post-implantation loss was observed at an inhalation dose of 0.4 mg/kg/day (approximately 360 times the RHDID on a mg/m^2 basis). Such effects were not observed at inhalation doses of 0.009 and up to 0.088 mg/kg/day in rats and rabbits, respectively. These doses correspond to approximately 4 and 80 times the RHDID on a mg/m^2 basis, respectively. These dose multiples may be over-estimated due to difficulties in measuring deposited doses in animal inhalation studies.

14 CLINICAL STUDIES

The SPIRIVA HandiHaler (tiotropium bromide inhalation powder) clinical development program consisted of six Phase 3 studies in 2663 patients with COPD (1308 receiving SPIRIVA HandiHaler): two 1-year, placebo–controlled studies, two 6-month, placebo-controlled studies and two 1-year, ipratropium-controlled studies. These studies enrolled patients who had a clinical diagnosis of COPD, were 40 years of age or older, had a history of smoking greater than 10 pack-years, had a forced expiratory volume in one second (FEV$_1$) less than or equal to 60% or 65% of predicted, and a ratio of FEV$_1$/FVC of less than or equal to 0.7.

In these studies, SPIRIVA HandiHaler, administered once-daily in the morning, provided improvement in lung function (FEV$_1$), with peak effect occurring within 3 hours following the first dose.

Two additional trials evaluated exacerbations: a 6-month, randomized, double-blind, placebo-controlled, multicenter clinical trial of 1829 COPD patients in a US Veterans Affairs setting and a 4-year, randomized, double-blind, placebo-controlled, multicenter, clinical trial of 5992 COPD patients. Long-term effects on lung function and other outcomes were also evaluated in the 4-year multicenter trial.

6-Month to 1-Year Effects on Lung Function

In the 1-year, placebo-controlled trials, the mean improvement in FEV$_1$ at 30 minutes was 0.13 liters (13%) with a peak improvement of 0.24 liters (24%) relative to baseline after the first dose (Day 1). Further improvements in FEV$_1$ and forced vital capacity (FVC) were observed with pharmacodynamic steady state reached by Day 8 with once-daily treatment. The mean peak improvement in FEV$_1$, relative to baseline, was 0.28 to 0.31 liters (28% to 31%), after 1 week (Day 8) of once-daily treatment. Improvement of lung function was maintained for 24 hours after a single dose and consistently maintained over the 1-year treatment period with no evidence of tolerance.

In the two 6-month, placebo-controlled trials, serial spirometric evaluations were performed throughout daytime hours in Trial A (12 hours) and limited to 3 hours in Trial B. The serial FEV$_1$ values over 12 hours (Trial A) are displayed in Figure 1. These trials further support the improvement in pulmonary function (FEV$_1$) with SPIRIVA HandiHaler, which persisted over the spirometric observational period. Effectiveness was maintained for 24 hours after administration over the 6-month treatment period.

[See figure 1 above]

Results of each of the 1-year ipratropium-controlled trials were similar to the results of the 1-year placebo-controlled trials. The results of one of these trials are shown in Figure 2.

[See figure 2 above]

A randomized, placebo-controlled clinical study in 105 patients with COPD demonstrated that bronchodilation was maintained throughout the 24-hour dosing interval in comparison to placebo, regardless of whether SPIRIVA HandiHaler was administered in the morning or in the evening.

Throughout each week of the one-year treatment period in the two placebo-controlled trials, patients taking SPIRIVA HandiHaler had a reduced requirement for the use of rescue short-acting beta$_2$-agonists. Reduction in the use of rescue short-acting beta$_2$-agonists, as compared to placebo, was demonstrated in one of the two 6-month studies.

4-Year Effects on Lung Function

A 4-year, randomized, double-blind, placebo-controlled, multicenter clinical trial involving 5992 COPD patients was conducted to evaluate the long-term effects of SPIRIVA HandiHaler on disease progression (rate of decline in FEV$_1$). Patients were permitted to use all respiratory medications (including short-acting and long-acting beta-agonists, inhaled and systemic steroids, and theophyllines) other than inhaled anticholinergics. The patients were 40 to 88 years of age, 75% male, and 90% Caucasian with a diagnosis of COPD and a mean pre-bronchodilator FEV$_1$ of 39% predicted (range = 9% to 76%) at study entry. There was no difference between the groups in either of the co-primary efficacy endpoints, yearly rate of decline in pre- and post-bronchodilator FEV$_1$, as demonstrated by similar slopes of FEV$_1$ decline over time (Figure 3).

SPIRIVA HandiHaler maintained improvements in trough (pre-dose) FEV$_1$ (adjusted means over time: 87 to 103 mL) throughout the 4 years of the study (Figure 3).

Figure 3 Trough (pre-dose) FEV$_1$ Mean Values at Each Time Point

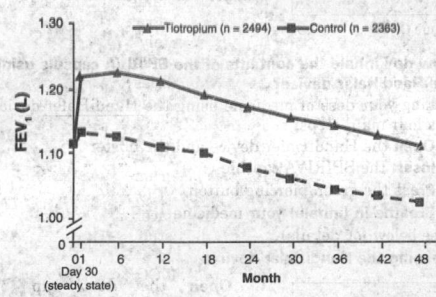

Repeated measure ANOVA was used to estimate means. Means are adjusted for baseline measurements. Baseline trough FEV$_1$ (observed mean) = 1.12. Patients with ≥3 acceptable pulmonary function tests after Day 30 and non-missing baseline value were included in the analysis.

Exacerbations

The effect of SPIRIVA HandiHaler on COPD exacerbations was evaluated in two clinical trials: a 4-year clinical trial described above and a 6-month clinical trial of 1829 COPD patients in a Veterans Affairs setting. In the 6-month trial, COPD exacerbations were defined as a complex of respiratory symptoms (increase or new onset) of more than one of the following: cough, sputum, wheezing, dyspnea, or chest tightness with a duration of at least 3 days requiring treatment with antibiotics, systemic steroids, or hospitalization. The population had an age ranging from 40 to 90 years with 99% males, 91% Caucasian, and had COPD with a mean pre-bronchodilator FEV$_1$ percent predicted of 36% (range = 8% to 93%). Patients were permitted to use respiratory medications (including short-acting and long-acting beta-agonists, inhaled and systemic steroids, and theophyllines) other than inhaled anticholinergics. In the 6-month trial, the co-primary endpoints were the proportion of patients with COPD exacerbation and the proportion of patients with hospitalization due to COPD exacerbation. SPIRIVA HandiHaler significantly reduced the proportion of COPD patients who experienced exacerbations compared to placebo (27.9% vs 32.3%, respectively; Odds Ratio (OR) (tiotropium/placebo) = 0.81; 95% CI = 0.66, 0.99; p = 0.037). The proportion of patients with hospitalization due to COPD exacerbations in patients who used SPIRIVA HandiHaler compared to placebo was 7.0% vs 9.5%, respectively; OR = 0.72; 95% CI = 0.51, 1.01; p = 0.056.

Exacerbations were evaluated as a secondary outcome in the 4-year multicenter trial. In this trial, COPD exacerbations were defined as an increase or new onset of more than one of the following respiratory symptoms (cough, sputum, sputum purulence, wheezing, dyspnea) with a duration of three or more days requiring treatment with antibiotics and/or systemic (oral, intramuscular, or intravenous) ster-

oids. SPIRIVA HandiHaler significantly reduced the risk of an exacerbation by 14% (Hazard Ratio (HR) = 0.86; 95% CI = 0.81, 0.91; p<0.001) and reduced the risk of exacerbation-related hospitalization by 14% (HR = 0.86; 95% CI = 0.78, 0.95; p<0.002) compared to placebo. The median time to first exacerbation was delayed from 12.5 months (95% CI = 11.5, 13.8) in the placebo group to 16.7 months (95% CI = 14.9, 17.9) in the SPIRIVA HandiHaler group.

16   HOW SUPPLIED/STORAGE AND HANDLING

SPIRIVA HandiHaler consists of SPIRIVA capsules and the HandiHaler device. SPIRIVA capsules contain 18 mcg of tiotropium and are light green, with the Boehringer Ingelheim company logo on the SPIRIVA capsule cap and TI 01 on the SPIRIVA capsule body, or vice versa.

The HandiHaler device is gray colored with a green piercing button. It is imprinted with SPIRIVA HandiHaler (tiotropium bromide inhalation powder), the Boehringer Ingelheim company logo, and the Pfizer company logo. It is also imprinted to indicate that SPIRIVA capsules should not be stored in the HandiHaler device and that the HandiHaler device is only to be used with SPIRIVA capsules.

SPIRIVA capsules are packaged in an aluminum/aluminum blister card and joined along a perforated-cut line. SPIRIVA capsules should always be stored in the blister and only removed immediately before use. The drug should be used immediately after the packaging over an individual SPIRIVA capsule is opened.

The following packages are available:

- carton containing 5 SPIRIVA capsules (1 unit-dose blister card) and 1 HandiHaler inhalation device (NDC 0597-0075-75)
- carton containing 30 SPIRIVA capsules (3 unit-dose blister cards) and 1 HandiHaler inhalation device (NDC 0597-0075-41)
- carton containing 90 SPIRIVA capsules (9 unit-dose blister cards) and 1 HandiHaler inhalation device (NDC 0597-0075-47)

Storage

Store at 25°C (77°F); excursions permitted to 15°–30°C (59°–86°F) [see USP Controlled Room Temperature].

The SPIRIVA capsules should not be exposed to extreme temperature or moisture. Do not store SPIRIVA capsules in the HandiHaler device.

17   PATIENT COUNSELING INFORMATION

See FDA-approved Patient Labeling (17.6)

17.1   Instructions for Administering SPIRIVA HandiHaler

It is important for patients to understand how to correctly administer SPIRIVA capsules using the HandiHaler device [*see Patient Counseling Information (17.6)*]. Patients should be instructed that SPIRIVA capsules should only be administered via the HandiHaler device and the HandiHaler device should not be used for administering other medications. **The contents of SPIRIVA capsules are for oral inhalation only and must not be swallowed.**

SPIRIVA capsules should always be stored in sealed blisters. Only one SPIRIVA capsule should be removed immediately before use or its effectiveness may be reduced. Additional SPIRIVA capsules that are exposed to air (i.e., not intended for immediate use) should be discarded.

17.2   Paradoxical Bronchospasm

Patients should be informed that SPIRIVA HandiHaler can produce paradoxical bronchospasm. If paradoxical bronchospasm occurs, patients should discontinue SPIRIVA HandiHaler.

17.3   Urinary Retention

Difficulty passing urine and dysuria may be symptoms of new or worsening prostatic hyperplasia or bladder outlet obstruction. Patients should be instructed to consult a physician immediately should any of these signs or symptoms develop.

17.4   Visual Effects

Eye pain or discomfort, blurred vision, visual halos or colored images in association with red eyes from conjunctival congestion and corneal edema may be signs of acute narrow-angle glaucoma. Patients should be told to consult a physician immediately should any of these signs and symptoms develop. Miotic eye drops alone are not considered to be effective treatment.

Patients should be told that care must be taken not to allow the powder to enter into the eyes as this may cause blurring of vision and pupil dilation.

17.5   Acute Exacerbation

Patients should understand that SPIRIVA HandiHaler is a once-daily maintenance bronchodilator and should not be used for immediate relief of breathing problems (i.e., as a rescue medication).

17.6   FDA-approved Patient Labeling

Patient Information and Patient's Instructions for Use are supplied as tear-off leaflets following the full prescribing information and should be dispensed with each new prescription and refill.

Distributed by:
Boehringer Ingelheim Pharmaceuticals, Inc.
Ridgefield, CT 06877 USA
Marketed by:
Boehringer Ingelheim Pharmaceuticals, Inc.
Ridgefield, CT 06877 USA
and
Pfizer Inc
New York, NY 10017 USA
Licensed from:
Boehringer Ingelheim International GmbH
Address medical inquiries to: (800) 542-6257 or (800) 459-9906 TTY.

SPIRIVA® and HandiHaler® are registered trademarks and are used under license from Boehringer Ingelheim International GmbH.

©Copyright 2009 Boehringer Ingelheim International GmbH

ALL RIGHTS RESERVED

SPIRIVA® (tiotropium bromide inhalation powder) is covered by U.S. Patent Nos. RE38,912, RE39,820, 5,478,578, 6,777,423, 6,908,928, 7,070,800, and 7,309,707 with other patents pending. The HandiHaler® inhalation device is covered by U.S. Design Patent No. D355,029 with other patents pending.

Rev: December 2009
IT1600WL1609
10004551/07
65626-08

PATIENT INFORMATION

**SPIRIVA® (speh REE vah) HandiHaler®
(tiotropium bromide inhalation powder)**

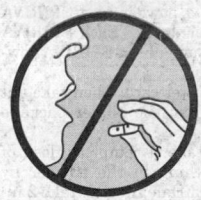
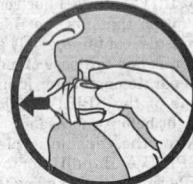

Do NOT swallow SPIRIVA capsules.

After putting the SPIRIVA capsule into the HandiHaler device, breathe in your medicine through your mouth.

Important Information: Do not swallow SPIRIVA capsules. SPIRIVA capsules should only be used with the HandiHaler device. SPIRIVA HandiHaler should only be inhaled by mouth (oral inhalation).

Read the information that comes with your SPIRIVA HandiHaler before you start using it and each time you refill your prescription. There may be new information. This leaflet does not take the place of talking with your doctor about your medical condition or your treatment.

What is SPIRIVA HandiHaler?

SPIRIVA HandiHaler is a prescription medicine that you use one time every day (a maintenance medicine) to control symptoms of chronic obstructive pulmonary disease (COPD). SPIRIVA HandiHaler helps make your lungs work better for 24 hours. SPIRIVA HandiHaler relaxes your airways and helps keep them open. You may start to feel like it is easier to breathe on the first day, but it may take longer for you to feel the full effects of the medicine. SPIRIVA HandiHaler works best and may help make it easier to breathe when you use it every day.

SPIRIVA HandiHaler also reduces the likelihood of flare-ups and worsening of COPD symptoms (COPD exacerbations). A COPD exacerbation is defined as an increase or new onset of more than one COPD symptom such as cough, mucus, shortness of breath, and wheezing that requires medicine beyond your rescue medicine.

SPIRIVA HandiHaler is **not** a rescue medicine and should not be used for treating sudden breathing problems. Your doctor may give you other medicine to use for sudden breathing problems.

SPIRIVA HandiHaler has not been studied in children.

Who should not take SPIRIVA HandiHaler?

Do not use SPIRIVA HandiHaler if you:

- are allergic to tiotropium. See the end of this leaflet for a complete list of ingredients.
- have had an allergic reaction to ipratropium (Atrovent®). Allergic reactions may include itching, rash, or swelling of the lips, tongue, or throat (trouble swallowing).

What should I tell my doctor before using SPIRIVA HandiHaler?

Before taking SPIRIVA HandiHaler, tell your doctor about all your medical conditions, including if you:
- have kidney problems.
- have glaucoma. SPIRIVA HandiHaler may make your glaucoma worse.
- have an enlarged prostate, problems passing urine, or a blockage in your bladder. SPIRIVA HandiHaler may make these problems worse.
- are pregnant or plan to become pregnant. It is not known if SPIRIVA HandiHaler could harm your unborn baby.
- are breast-feeding or plan to breast-feed. It is not known if SPIRIVA HandiHaler passes into breast milk. You and your doctor will decide if SPIRIVA HandiHaler is right for you while you breast-feed.
- have a severe allergy to milk proteins. Ask your doctor if you are not sure.

Tell your doctor about all the medicines you take, including prescription and non-prescription medicines and eye drops, vitamins, and herbal supplements. Some of your other medicines or supplements may affect the way SPIRIVA HandiHaler works. SPIRIVA HandiHaler is an anticholinergic medicine. You should not take other anticholinergic medicines while using SPIRIVA HandiHaler, including ipratropium. Ask your doctor or pharmacist if you are not sure if one of your medicines is an anticholinergic.

Know the medicines you take. Keep a list of your medicines with you to show your doctor and pharmacist when you get a new medicine.

How should I take SPIRIVA HandiHaler?

- Use SPIRIVA HandiHaler exactly as prescribed. Use SPIRIVA HandiHaler one time every day.
- Read the "Patient's Instructions for Use" at the end of this leaflet before you use SPIRIVA HandiHaler. Talk with your doctor if you do not understand the instructions.
- **Do not swallow SPIRIVA capsules.**
- **Only use SPIRIVA capsules with the HandiHaler device.**
- **Do not use the HandiHaler device to take any other medicine**
- SPIRIVA HandiHaler comes as a powder in a SPIRIVA capsule that fits the HandiHaler device. Each SPIRIVA capsule, containing only a small amount of SPIRIVA powder, is one full dose of medicine.
- Separate one blister from the blister card. Then take out one of the SPIRIVA capsules from the blister package right before you use it.
- After the capsule is pierced, take a complete dose of SPIRIVA HandiHaler by breathing in the powder by mouth two times, using the HandiHaler device (take 2 inhalations from one SPIRIVA capsule). See the "Patient's Instructions for Use" at the end of this leaflet.
- Throw away any SPIRIVA capsule that is not used right away after it is taken out of the blister package. Do not leave the SPIRIVA capsules open to air; they may not work as well.
- If you miss a dose, take it as soon as you remember. Do not use SPIRIVA HandiHaler more than one time every 24 hours.
- If you use more than your prescribed dose of SPIRIVA HandiHaler, call your doctor or a poison control center.

What should I avoid while using SPIRIVA HandiHaler?

Do not let the powder from the SPIRIVA capsule get into your eyes. Your vision may get blurry and the pupil in your eye may get larger (dilate). If this happens, call your doctor.

What are the possible side effects of SPIRIVA HandiHaler?

SPIRIVA HandiHaler can cause serious side effects. If you get any of the following side effects, stop taking SPIRIVA HandiHaler and get medical help right away.

- **Allergic reaction.** Symptoms may include: itching, rash, swelling of the lips, tongue, or throat (trouble swallowing).
- **Sudden narrowing and blockage of the airways into the lungs (bronchospasm).** Your breathing suddenly gets worse.
- **New or worsened increased pressure in the eyes (acute narrow-angle glaucoma).** Symptoms of acute narrow-angle glaucoma may include: eye pain, blurred vision, seeing halos (visual halos) or colored images along with red eyes.
- **New or worsened urinary retention.** Symptoms of blockage in your bladder and/or enlarged prostate may include: difficulty passing urine, painful urination.

Other side effects with SPIRIVA HandiHaler include:
- upper respiratory tract infection
- dry mouth
- sinus infection
- sore throat
- non-specific chest pain
- urinary tract infection
- indigestion
- runny nose
- constipation

- increased heart rate
- blurred vision

These are not all the possible side effects with SPIRIVA HandiHaler. Tell your doctor if you have any side effect that bothers you or that does not go away.

Call your doctor for medical advice about side effects. You may report side effects to FDA at 1-800-FDA-1088.

How do I store SPIRIVA HandiHaler?

- **Do not store SPIRIVA capsules in the HandiHaler device.**
- Store SPIRIVA capsules in the sealed blister package at room temperature between 68°F–77°F (20°–25°C).
- Keep SPIRIVA capsules away from heat and cold (do not freeze).
- Store SPIRIVA capsules in a dry place. Throw away any unused SPIRIVA capsules that have been open to air.

Ask your doctor or pharmacist if you have any questions about storing your SPIRIVA capsules.

Keep SPIRIVA HandiHaler, SPIRIVA capsules, and all medicines out of the reach of children.

General information about SPIRIVA HandiHaler

Medicines are sometimes prescribed for purposes other than those listed in Patient Information leaflets. Do not use SPIRIVA HandiHaler for a purpose for which it has not been prescribed. Do not give SPIRIVA HandiHaler to other people even if they have the same symptoms that you have. It may harm them.

For more information about SPIRIVA HandiHaler, talk with your doctor. You can ask your doctor or pharmacist for information about SPIRIVA HandiHaler that is written for health professionals.

For more information about SPIRIVA HandiHaler, you may call Boehringer Ingelheim Pharmaceuticals, Inc. at 1-800-542-6257 or (TTY) 1-800-459-9906.

What are the ingredients in SPIRIVA HandiHaler?

Active ingredient: tiotropium
Inactive ingredient: lactose monohydrate

What is COPD (Chronic Obstructive Pulmonary Disease)?

COPD is a serious lung disease that includes chronic bronchitis, emphysema, or both. Most COPD is caused by smoking. When you have COPD, your airways become narrow. So, air moves out of your lungs more slowly. This makes it hard to breathe.

Distributed by:
Boehringer Ingelheim Pharmaceuticals, Inc.
Ridgefield, CT 06877 USA

Marketed by:
Boehringer Ingelheim Pharmaceuticals, Inc.
Ridgefield, CT 06877 USA
and
Pfizer Inc
New York, NY 10017 USA

Licensed from:
Boehringer Ingelheim International GmbH
SPIRIVA® and HandiHaler® are registered trademarks and are used under license from Boehringer Ingelheim International GmbH.
©Copyright 2009 Boehringer Ingelheim International GmbH
ALL RIGHTS RESERVED
Rev: December 2009
IT1600WL1609
10004551/07
65626-08

PATIENT'S INSTRUCTIONS FOR USE
SPIRIVA® HandiHaler®
(tiotropium bromide inhalation powder)

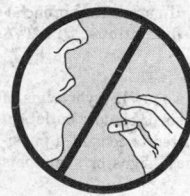
Do NOT swallow SPIRIVA capsules.

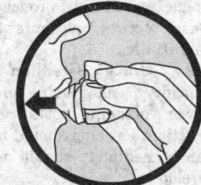
Step 1: Put the SPIRIVA capsule into the HandiHaler device.
Step 2: Inhale the medicine through your mouth.

Important Information: Do not swallow SPIRIVA capsules. SPIRIVA capsules should only be used with the HandiHaler device. SPIRIVA HandiHaler should only be inhaled through your mouth (oral inhalation).

First read the Patient Information that comes with SPIRIVA HandiHaler for important information about using SPIRIVA HandiHaler.

Read these Patient's Instructions for Use before you start to use SPIRIVA HandiHaler and each time you refill your prescription. There may be new information.

For more information, ask your doctor or pharmacist.

SPIRIVA HandiHaler comes with SPIRIVA capsules and a HandiHaler device. The HandiHaler device is an inhalation device that is for use only with SPIRIVA capsules. Do not use the HandiHaler device to take any other medicine.

Becoming familiar with SPIRIVA HandiHaler:

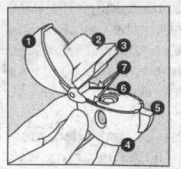
Figure A

Remove the HandiHaler device from the pouch and become familiar with its components. (Figure A)
1. dust cap
2. mouthpiece
3. mouthpiece ridge
4. base
5. green piercing button
6. center chamber
7. air intake vents

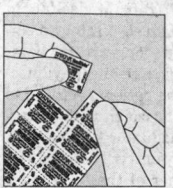
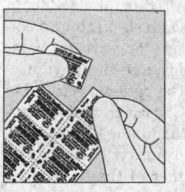
Figure B

Each SPIRIVA capsule is packaged in a blister. Each blister can be separated from the blister card by tearing along the perforation. (Figure B)

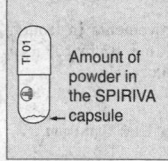
Amount of powder in the SPIRIVA capsule
Figure C

Do not open the SPIRIVA capsule before you insert it into the HandiHaler device. If you open the SPIRIVA capsule, it may not work. Each SPIRIVA capsule contains only a small amount of powder. (Figure C) This is one full dose. The product was designed this way.

How do I inhale the contents of the SPIRIVA capsule using the HandiHaler device?

Taking your dose of medicine using the HandiHaler device has four main steps:
1. **Open** the HandiHaler device and the blister
2. **Insert** the SPIRIVA capsule
3. **Press** the green piercing button
4. **Breathe in (inhale)** your medicine
(See below for details)

Opening the HandiHaler device:

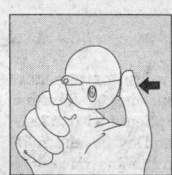
Figure 1

1. Open the dust cap by pressing the green piercing button. (Figure 1)

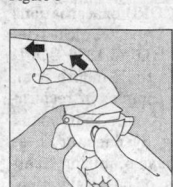
Figure 2

Pull the dust cap upwards to expose the mouthpiece. (Figure 2)

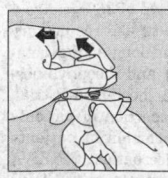
Figure 3

Open the mouthpiece by pulling the mouthpiece ridge upwards away from the base. (Figure 3)

Removing a SPIRIVA capsule:

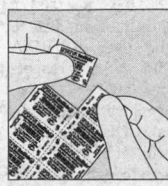
Figure 4

Before removing a SPIRIVA capsule from the blister, separate one of the blisters from the blister card by tearing along the perforation. (Figure 4)

Do not swallow SPIRIVA capsules. Always store SPIRIVA capsules in the sealed blisters. Remove only one SPIRIVA capsule from the blister right before use. Do not store SPIRIVA capsules in the HandiHaler device. Inhale the contents of the SPIRIVA capsule using the HandiHaler device right away af-

ter the blister packaging of an individual SPIRIVA capsule is opened, or else it may not work as well.

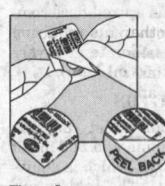
Figure 5

Right before you are ready to use your SPIRIVA HandiHaler:
Bend back and forth one of the corners of the blister that has an arrow and then with your finger separate the aluminum foil layers. Carefully peel back the printed foil until you can see the whole SPIRIVA capsule. (Figure 5)

Turn the blister upside down and tip the SPIRIVA capsule out, tapping the back of the blister, if needed.

Do not cut the foil or use sharp instruments to take out the SPIRIVA capsule from the blister.
If more SPIRIVA capsules are opened to air, they should not be used and should be thrown away.

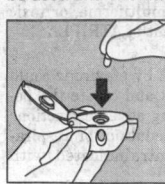
Figure 6

2. Insert (put) the SPIRIVA capsule in the center chamber of the HandiHaler device. It does not matter which end of the SPIRIVA capsule you put in the chamber. (Figure 6)

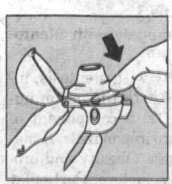
Figure 7

Close the mouthpiece **until you hear a click,** but leave the dust cap open. (Figure 7)
Be sure that you have the mouthpiece sitting firmly against the gray base.

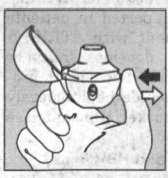
Figure 8

Taking your dose using the HandiHaler device: Hold the HandiHaler device with the mouthpiece upright. It is important that you hold the HandiHaler device in an upright position (Figure 8) when pressing the green piercing button.
3. Press the green piercing button until it is flat (flush) against the base, and release. This is how you make holes in the SPIRIVA capsule so that you get the medicine when you breathe in.
Do not press the green button more than one time.

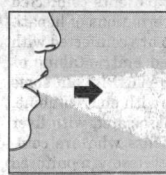
Figure 9

Breathe out completely. (Figure 9)
Important: Do not breathe (exhale) into the mouthpiece of the HandiHaler device at any time.

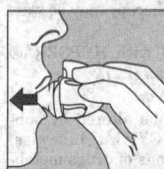
Figure 10

4. Breathe in (inhale)
• Hold the HandiHaler device by the gray base. Do not block the air intake vents.
• Raise the HandiHaler device to your mouth and close your lips tightly around the mouthpiece.
• **Keep your head in an upright position. The HandiHaler device should be in a horizontal position.** (Figure 10)

• Breathe in **slowly and deeply** so that you **hear or feel the SPIRIVA capsule vibrate.**
• Breathe in until your lungs are full.
• Hold your breath as long as is comfortable and at the same time take the HandiHaler device out of your mouth. Breathe normally again.

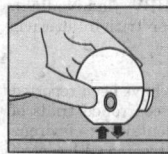
Figure 11

To make sure you get the full dose, you must breathe out completely, and inhale again as in Step 4 above. (Figure 10). Do not press the green piercing button again. If you do not hear or feel the SPIRIVA capsule vibrate, **do not press the green piercing button again.** Instead, hold the HandiHaler device in an upright position and tap the HandiHaler device gently on a table. (Figure 11)

Check to see that the mouthpiece is completely closed. Then, breathe in again – slowly and deeply.
If you still do not hear or feel the SPIRIVA capsule vibrate after repeating the above steps, throw away the SPIRIVA capsule. Open the base by lifting the green piercing button and check the center chamber for pieces of the SPIRIVA capsule (SPIRIVA capsule fragments). SPIRIVA capsule fragments in the center chamber can cause a SPIRIVA capsule not to vibrate. Turn the HandiHaler device upside down and gently tap to remove the SPIRIVA capsule fragments. Call your doctor for instructions.

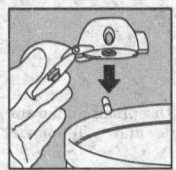
Figure 12

After you finish taking your daily dose of SPIRIVA HandiHaler, open the mouthpiece again. Tip out the used SPIRIVA capsule and throw it away. (Figure 12)

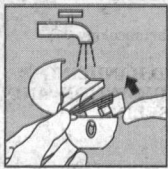
Figure 13

Close the mouthpiece and dust cap for storage of your HandiHaler device. (Figure 13)
Do not store used or unused SPIRIVA capsules in the HandiHaler device.

When and how should I clean my HandiHaler device?
Clean the HandiHaler device one time each month or as needed. (Figure 14)
• Open the dust cap and mouthpiece.
• Open the base by lifting the green piercing button.
• Look at the center chamber for SPIRIVA capsule fragments or powder residue.
• Rinse the HandiHaler device with warm water. Check that any powder buildup or SPIRIVA capsule fragments are removed.
• Do not use cleaning agents or detergents.
• Do not place the HandiHaler device in the dishwasher for cleaning.
• Dry the HandiHaler device well by tipping the excess water out on a paper towel. Air-dry afterwards, leaving the dust cap, mouthpiece, and base open.
• Do not use a hair dryer to dry the HandiHaler device.
• **It takes 24 hours to air dry, so clean the HandiHaler device right after you use it so that it will be ready for your next dose.**
• Do not use the HandiHaler device when it is wet. If needed, you may clean the outside of the mouthpiece with a clean damp cloth.

Distributed by:
Boehringer Ingelheim Pharmaceuticals, Inc.
Ridgefield, CT 06877 USA
Marketed by:
Boehringer Ingelheim Pharmaceuticals, Inc.
Ridgefield, CT 06877 USA
and
Pfizer Inc
New York, NY 10017 USA
Licensed from:
Boehringer Ingelheim International GmbH
SPIRIVA® and HandiHaler® are registered trademarks and are used under license from Boehringer Ingelheim International GmbH
©Copyright 2009 Boehringer Ingelheim International GmbH
ALL RIGHTS RESERVED
Rev: December 2009
IT1600WL1609
10004551/07
65626-08

Shown in Product Identification Guide, page 307

Bristol-Myers Squibb & Gilead Sciences, LLC
333 LAKESIDE DRIVE
FOSTER CITY, CA 94404

For Medical Information Contact:
1-888-547-4267
Medicalinformation@BMS-Gilead.com
To Report Adverse Events, Contact:
1-800-445-3235 press option 3
For Business Operations Contact:
1-800-445-3235 press option 8

ATRIPLA®
[*uh TRIP luh*]   ℞
(Efavirenz/emtricitabine/tenofovir disoproxilfumarate) tablets

HIGHLIGHTS OF PRESCRIBING INFORMATION
These highlights do not include all the information needed to use ATRIPLA safely and effectively. See full prescribing information for ATRIPLA.
ATRIPLA® (efavirenz/emtricitabine/tenofovir disoproxil fumarate) tablets
Initial U.S. Approval: 2006

> **WARNINGS: LACTIC ACIDOSIS/SEVERE HEPATO-MEGALY WITH STEATOSIS and POST TREATMENT EXACERBATION OF HEPATITIS B**
> *See full prescribing information for complete boxed warning.*
> • Lactic acidosis and severe hepatomegaly with steatosis, including fatal cases, have been reported with the use of nucleoside analogs, including tenofovir disoproxil fumarate, a component of ATRIPLA. (5.1)
> • ATRIPLA is not approved for the treatment of chronic hepatitis B virus (HBV) infection. Severe acute exacerbations of hepatitis B have been reported in patients coinfected with HBV and HIV-1 who have discontinued EMTRIVA or VIREAD, two of the components of ATRIPLA. Hepatic function should be monitored closely in these patients. If appropriate, initiation of anti-hepatitis B therapy may be warranted. (5.2)

——————————**RECENT MAJOR CHANGES**——————————

Boxed Warning	1/2010
Warnings and Precautions	
Patients Coinfected with HIV-1 and HBV (5.2)	1/2010
New Onset or Worsening Renal Impairment (5.7)	1/2010
Reproductive Risk Potential (5.8)	5/2010
Decrease in Bone Mineral Density (5.11)	1/2010
Hepatotoxicity (5.10)	5/2010

——————————**INDICATIONS AND USAGE**——————————
ATRIPLA, a combination of 2 nucleoside analog HIV-1 reverse transcriptase inhibitors and 1 non-nucleoside HIV-1 reverse transcriptase inhibitor, is indicated for use alone as a complete regimen or in combination with other antiretroviral agents for the treatment of HIV-1 infection in adults. (1)

——————————**DOSAGE AND ADMINISTRATION**——————————
• Recommended dose: One tablet once daily taken orally on an empty stomach, preferably at bedtime. (2)
• Dose in renal impairment: Should not be administered in patients with creatinine clearance <50 mL/min. (2)

——————————**DOSAGE FORMS AND STRENGTHS**——————————
Tablet containing 600 mg of efavirenz, 200 mg of emtricitabine and 300 mg of tenofovir disoproxil fumarate. (3)

——————————**CONTRAINDICATIONS**——————————
• Previously demonstrated hypersensitivity (e.g., Stevens-Johnson syndrome, erythema multiforme, or toxic skin eruptions) to efavirenz, a component of ATRIPLA. (4.1)
• For some drugs, competition for CYP3A by efavirenz could result in inhibition of their metabolism and create the potential for serious and/or life-threatening adverse reactions (e.g., cardiac arrhythmias, prolonged sedation, or respiratory depression). (4.2)

---WARNINGS AND PRECAUTIONS---

- Serious psychiatric symptoms: Immediate medical evaluation is recommended. (5.5, 6.1)
- Nervous system symptoms (NSS): NSS are frequent, usually begin 1–2 days after initiating therapy and resolve in 2–4 weeks. Dosing at bedtime may improve tolerability. NSS are not predictive of onset of psychiatric symptoms. (2, 5.6)
- New onset or worsening renal impairment: Can include acute renal failure and Fanconi syndrome. Assess creatinine clearance (CrCl) before initiating treatment with ATRIPLA. Monitor CrCl and serum phosphorus in patients at risk. Avoid administering ATRIPLA with concurrent or recent use of nephrotoxic drugs. (5.7)
- Pregnancy: Fetal harm can occur when administered to a pregnant woman during the first trimester. Women should be apprised of the potential harm to the fetus. (5.8)
- Rash: Discontinue if severe rash develops. (5.9, 6.1)
- Hepatotoxicity: Monitor liver function tests before and during treatment in patients with underlying hepatic disease, including hepatitis B or C coinfection, marked transaminase elevations, or who are taking medications associated with liver toxicity. Among reported cases of hepatic failure, a few occurred in patients with no pre-existing hepatic disease. (5.10, 6.3, 8.6)
- Decreases in bone mineral density (BMD): Consider monitoring BMD in patients with a history of pathological fracture or who are at risk for osteopenia. (5.11)
- Convulsions: Use caution in patients with a history of seizures. (5.12)
- Immune reconstitution syndrome: May necessitate further evaluation and treatment. (5.13)
- Redistribution/accumulation of body fat: Observed in patients receiving antiretroviral therapy. (5.14)
- Coadministration with other products: Do not use with drugs containing efavirenz, emtricitabine or tenofovir disoproxil fumarate including SUSTIVA, TRUVADA, EMTRIVA, VIREAD; or with drugs containing lamivudine. Do not administer in combination with HEPSERA. (5.4)

---ADVERSE REACTIONS---

Most common adverse reactions (incidence ≥10%) observed in an active-controlled clinical study of efavirenz, emtricitabine, and tenofovir DF are diarrhea, nausea, fatigue, headache, dizziness, depression, insomnia, abnormal dreams, and rash. (6)

To report SUSPECTED ADVERSE REACTIONS, contact Gilead Sciences, Inc. at 1-800-GILEAD-5 or FDA at 1-800-FDA-1088 or www.fda.gov/medwatch

---DRUG INTERACTIONS---

- Efavirenz: Coadministration of efavirenz can alter the concentrations of other drugs and other drugs may alter the concentrations of efavirenz. The potential for drug-drug interactions must be considered before and during therapy. (4.2, 7.1, 12.3)
- Didanosine: Tenofovir disoproxil fumarate increases didanosine concentrations. Use with caution and monitor for evidence of didanosine toxicity (e.g., pancreatitis, neuropathy) when coadministered. Consider dose reductions or discontinuations of didanosine if warranted. (7.2)
- Atazanavir: Coadministration of ATRIPLA and atazanavir or atazanavir/ritonavir is not recommended. (7.3)
- Lopinavir/ritonavir: Coadministration increases tenofovir concentrations. Monitor for evidence of tenofovir toxicity. (7.3)

---USE IN SPECIFIC POPULATIONS---

- Pregnancy: Women should avoid pregnancy while receiving ATRIPLA and for 12 weeks after discontinuation. (5.8)
- Nursing mothers: Women infected with HIV should be instructed not to breast feed. (8.3)
- Hepatic impairment: Use caution in patients with hepatic impairment. (5.10, 8.6)
- Pediatrics: Safety and efficacy not established in patients less than 18 years of age. (2, 8.4)

See 17 for PATIENT COUNSELING INFORMATION and FDA-approved patient labeling

Revised: 05/2010

FULL PRESCRIBING INFORMATION: CONTENTS*
WARNINGS: LACTIC ACIDOSIS/SEVERE HEPATOMEGALY WITH STEATOSIS AND POST TREATMENT EXACERBATION OF HEPATITIS B

* Sections or subsections omitted from the full prescribing information are not listed

---

FULL PRESCRIBING INFORMATION

> **WARNINGS: LACTIC ACIDOSIS/SEVERE HEPATO-MEGALY WITH STEATOSIS AND POST TREATMENT EXACERBATION OF HEPATITIS B**
>
> **Lactic acidosis and severe hepatomegaly with steatosis, including fatal cases, have been reported with the use of nucleoside analogs, including tenofovir disoproxil fumarate, a component of ATRIPLA, in combination with other antiretrovirals *[See Warnings and Precautions (5.1)]*.**
>
> **ATRIPLA is not approved for the treatment of chronic hepatitis B virus (HBV) infection and the safety and efficacy of ATRIPLA have not been established in patients coinfected with HBV and HIV-1. Severe acute exacerbations of hepatitis B have been reported in patients who have discontinued EMTRIVA or VIREAD, which are components of ATRIPLA. Hepatic function should be monitored closely with both clinical and laboratory follow-up for at least several months in patients who are coinfected with HIV-1 and HBV and discontinue ATRIPLA. If appropriate, initiation of anti-hepatitis B therapy may be warranted *[See Warnings and Precautions (5.2)]*.**

1   INDICATIONS AND USAGE

ATRIPLA® is indicated for use alone as a complete regimen or in combination with other antiretroviral agents for the treatment of HIV-1 infection in adults.

2   DOSAGE AND ADMINISTRATION

Adults: The dose of ATRIPLA is one tablet once daily taken orally on an empty stomach. Dosing at bedtime may improve the tolerability of nervous system symptoms.

Pediatrics: ATRIPLA is not recommended for use in patients <18 years of age.

Renal Impairment: Because ATRIPLA is a fixed-dose combination, it should not be prescribed for patients requiring dosage adjustment such as those with moderate or severe renal impairment (creatinine clearance <50 mL/min).

3   DOSAGE FORMS AND STRENGTHS

ATRIPLA is available as tablets. Each tablet contains 600 mg of efavirenz, 200 mg of emtricitabine and 300 mg of tenofovir disoproxil fumarate (tenofovir DF, which is equivalent to 245 mg of tenofovir disoproxil). The tablets are pink, capsule-shaped, film-coated, debossed with "123" on one side and plain-faced on the other side.

4   CONTRAINDICATIONS

4.1   Hypersensitivity

ATRIPLA is contraindicated in patients with previously demonstrated clinically significant hypersensitivity (e.g., Stevens-Johnson syndrome, erythema multiforme, or toxic skin eruptions) to efavirenz, a component of ATRIPLA.

4.2   Contraindicated Drugs

For some drugs, competition for CYP3A by efavirenz could result in inhibition of their metabolism and create the potential for serious and/or life-threatening adverse reactions (e.g., cardiac arrhythmias, prolonged sedation, or respiratory depression). Drugs that are contraindicated with ATRIPLA are listed in Table 1.

[See table 1 at top of next page]

5   WARNINGS AND PRECAUTIONS

5.1   Lactic Acidosis/Severe Hepatomegaly with Steatosis

Lactic acidosis and severe hepatomegaly with steatosis, including fatal cases, have been reported with the use of nucleoside analogs including tenofovir DF, a component of ATRIPLA, in combination with other antiretrovirals. A majority of these cases have been in women. Obesity and prolonged nucleoside exposure may be risk factors. Particular caution should be exercised when administering nucleoside analogs to any patient with known risk factors for liver disease; however, cases have also been reported in patients with no known risk factors. Treatment with ATRIPLA should be suspended in any patient who develops clinical or laboratory findings suggestive of lactic acidosis or pronounced hepatotoxicity (which may include hepatomegaly and steatosis even in the absence of marked transaminase elevations).

5.2   Patients Coinfected with HIV-1 and HBV

It is recommended that all patients with HIV-1 be tested for the presence of chronic HBV before initiating antiretroviral therapy. ATRIPLA is not approved for the treatment of chronic HBV infection, and the safety and efficacy of ATRIPLA have not been established in patients coinfected with HBV and HIV-1. Severe acute exacerbations of hepatitis B have been reported in patients who are coinfected with HBV and HIV-1 and have discontinued emtricitabine or tenofovir DF, two of the components of ATRIPLA. In some patients infected with HBV and treated with emtricitabine, the exacerbations of hepatitis B were associated with liver decompensation and liver failure. Patients who are coinfected with HIV-1 and HBV should be closely monitored with both clinical and laboratory follow up for at least several months after stopping treatment with ATRIPLA. If appropriate, initiation of anti-hepatitis B therapy may be warranted.

ATRIPLA should not be administered with HEPSERA® (adefovir dipivoxil) *[See Drug Interactions (7.2)]*.

5.3   Drug Interactions

Efavirenz plasma concentrations may be altered by substrates, inhibitors, or inducers of CYP3A. Likewise, efavirenz may alter plasma concentrations of drugs metabolized by CYP3A *[See Contraindications (4.2), Drug Interactions (7.1)]*.

5.4   Coadministration with Related Products

Related drugs not for coadministration with ATRIPLA include EMTRIVA (emtricitabine), VIREAD (tenofovir DF), TRUVADA (emtricitabine/tenofovir DF), and SUSTIVA (efavirenz), which contain the same active components as ATRIPLA. Due to similarities between emtricitabine and lamivudine, ATRIPLA should not be coadministered with drugs containing lamivudine, including Combivir (lamivudine/zidovudine), Epivir, or Epivir-HBV (lamivudine), Epzicom (abacavir sulfate/lamivudine), or Trizivir (abacavir sulfate/lamivudine/zidovudine).

5.5   Psychiatric Symptoms

Serious psychiatric adverse experiences have been reported in patients treated with efavirenz. In controlled trials of 1008 subjects treated with regimens containing efavirenz for a mean of 2.1 years and 635 subjects treated with control regimens for a mean of 1.5 years, the frequency (regardless of causality) of specific serious psychiatric events among subjects who received efavirenz or control regimens, respectively, were: severe depression (2.4%, 0.9%), suicidal ideation (0.7%, 0.3%), nonfatal suicide attempts (0.5%, 0%), aggressive behavior (0.4%, 0.5%), paranoid reactions (0.4%, 0.3%), and manic reactions (0.2%, 0.3%). When psychiatric symptoms similar to those noted above were combined and evaluated as a group in a multifactorial analysis of data from Study AI266006 (006), treatment with efavirenz was associated with an increase in the occurrence of these selected psychiatric symptoms. Other factors associated with an increase in the occurrence of these psychiatric symptoms were history of injection drug use, psychiatric history, and receipt of psychiatric medication at study entry; similar associations were observed in both the efavirenz and control treatment groups. In Study 006, onset of new serious psychiatric symptoms occurred throughout the study for both efavirenz-treated and control-treated subjects. One percent of efavirenz-treated subjects discontinued or interrupted treatment because of one or more of these selected psychiatric symptoms. There have also been occasional postmarketing reports of death by suicide, delusions, and psychosis-like behavior, although a causal relationship to the use of efavirenz cannot be determined from these reports. Patients with serious psychiatric adverse experiences should seek immediate medical evaluation to assess the possibility that the symptoms may be related to the use of efavirenz, and if so, to determine whether the risks of continued therapy outweigh the benefits *[See Adverse Reactions (6)]*.

5.6 Nervous System Symptoms

Fifty-three percent (531/1008) of subjects receiving efavirenz in controlled trials reported central nervous system symptoms (any grade, regardless of causality) compared to 25% (156/635) of subjects receiving control regimens. These symptoms included dizziness (28.1% of the 1008 subjects), insomnia (16.3%), impaired concentration (8.3%), somnolence (7.0%), abnormal dreams (6.2%), and hallucinations (1.2%). Other reported symptoms were euphoria, confusion, agitation, amnesia, stupor, abnormal thinking, and depersonalization. The majority of these symptoms were mild-moderate (50.7%); symptoms were severe in 2.0% of subjects. Overall, 2.1% of subjects discontinued therapy as a result. These symptoms usually begin during the first or second day of therapy and generally resolve after the first 2–4 weeks of therapy. After 4 weeks of therapy, the prevalence of nervous system symptoms of at least moderate severity ranged from 5% to 9% in subjects treated with regimens containing efavirenz and from 3% to 5% in subjects treated with a control regimen. Patients should be informed that these common symptoms were likely to improve with continued therapy and were not predictive of subsequent onset of the less frequent psychiatric symptoms *[See Warnings and Precautions (5.5)]*. Dosing at bedtime may improve the tolerability of these nervous system symptoms *[See Dosage and Administration (2)]*.

Analysis of long-term data from Study 006, (median follow-up 180 weeks, 102 weeks, and 76 weeks for subjects treated with efavirenz + zidovudine + lamivudine, efavirenz + indinavir, and indinavir + zidovudine + lamivudine, respectively) showed that, beyond 24 weeks of therapy, the incidences of new-onset nervous system symptoms among efavirenz-treated subjects were generally similar to those in the indinavir-containing control arm.

Patients receiving ATRIPLA should be alerted to the potential for additive central nervous system effects when ATRIPLA is used concomitantly with alcohol or psychoactive drugs.

Patients who experience central nervous system symptoms such as dizziness, impaired concentration, and/or drowsiness should avoid potentially hazardous tasks such as driving or operating machinery.

5.7 New Onset or Worsening Renal Impairment

Emtricitabine and tenofovir are principally eliminated by the kidney; however, efavirenz is not. Since ATRIPLA is a combination product and the dose of the individual components cannot be altered, patients with creatinine clearance <50 mL/min should not receive ATRIPLA.

Renal impairment, including cases of acute renal failure and Fanconi syndrome (renal tubular injury with severe hypophosphatemia), has been reported with the use of tenofovir DF *[See Adverse Reactions (6.3)]*.

It is recommended that creatinine clearance be calculated in all patients prior to initiating therapy and as clinically appropriate during therapy with ATRIPLA. Routine monitoring of calculated creatinine clearance and serum phosphorus should be performed in patients at risk for renal impairment, including patients who have previously experienced renal events while receiving HEPSERA.

ATRIPLA should be avoided with concurrent or recent use of a nephrotoxic agent.

5.8 Reproductive Risk Potential

Pregnancy Category D: Efavirenz may cause fetal harm when administered during the first trimester to a pregnant woman. Pregnancy should be avoided in women receiving ATRIPLA. Barrier contraception must always be used in combination with other methods of contraception (e.g., oral or other hormonal contraceptives). Because of the long half-life of efavirenz, use of adequate contraceptive measures for 12 weeks after discontinuation of ATRIPLA is recommended. Women of childbearing potential should undergo pregnancy testing before initiation of ATRIPLA. If this drug is used during the first trimester of pregnancy, or if the patient becomes pregnant while taking this drug, the patient should be apprised of the potential harm to the fetus.

There are no adequate and well-controlled studies of ATRIPLA in pregnant women. ATRIPLA should be used during pregnancy only if the potential benefit justifies the potential risk to the fetus, such as in pregnant women without other therapeutic options.

Antiretroviral Pregnancy Registry: To monitor fetal outcomes of pregnant women, an Antiretroviral Pregnancy Registry has been established. Physicians are encouraged to register patients who become pregnant by calling (800) 258-4263.

Efavirenz: As of July 2009, the Antiretroviral Pregnancy Registry has received prospective reports of 661 pregnancies exposed to efavirenz-containing regimens, nearly all of which were first-trimester exposures (606 pregnancies). Birth defects occurred in 14 of 501 live births (first-trimester exposure) and 2 of 55 live births (second/third-trimester exposure). One of these prospectively reported defects with first-trimester exposure was a neural tube defect. A single case of anophthalmia with first-trimester exposure to efavirenz has also been prospectively reported; however, this case included severe oblique facial clefts and amniotic banding, a known association with anophthalmia. There have been six retrospective reports of findings consistent with neural tube defects, including meningomyelocele. All mothers were exposed to efavirenz-containing regimens in the first trimester. Although a causal relationship of these events to the use of efavirenz has not been established, similar defects have been observed in preclinical studies of efavirenz.

Malformations have been observed in 3 of 20 fetuses/infants from efavirenz-treated cynomolgus monkeys (versus 0 of 20 concomitant controls) in a developmental toxicity study. The pregnant monkeys were dosed throughout pregnancy (postcoital days 20–150) with efavirenz 60 mg/kg daily, a dose which resulted in plasma drug concentrations similar to those in humans given 600 mg/day of efavirenz. Anencephaly and unilateral anophthalmia were observed in one fetus, microphthalmia was observed in another fetus, and cleft palate was observed in a third fetus. Efavirenz crosses the placenta in cynomolgus monkeys and produces fetal blood concentrations similar to maternal blood concentrations. Efavirenz has been shown to cross the placenta in rats and rabbits and produces fetal blood concentrations of efavirenz similar to maternal concentrations. An increase in fetal resorptions was observed in rats at efavirenz doses that produced peak plasma concentrations and AUC values in female rats equivalent to or lower than those achieved in humans given 600 mg once daily of efavirenz. Efavirenz produced no reproductive toxicities when given to pregnant rabbits at doses that produced peak plasma concentrations similar to and AUC values approximately half of those achieved in humans given 600 mg once daily of efavirenz.

5.9 Rash

In controlled clinical trials, 26% (266/1008) of subjects treated with 600 mg efavirenz experienced new-onset skin rash compared with 17% (111/635) of subjects treated in control groups. Rash associated with blistering, moist desquamation, or ulceration occurred in 0.9% (9/1008) of subjects treated with efavirenz. The incidence of Grade 4 rash (e.g., erythema multiforme, Stevens-Johnson syndrome) in subjects treated with efavirenz in all studies and expanded access was 0.1%. Rashes are usually mild-to-moderate maculopapular skin eruptions that occur within the first 2 weeks of initiating therapy with efavirenz (median time to onset of rash in adults was 11 days) and, in most subjects continuing therapy with efavirenz, rash resolves within 1 month (median duration, 16 days). The discontinuation rate for rash in clinical trials was 1.7% (17/1008). ATRIPLA can be reinitiated in patients interrupting therapy because of rash. ATRIPLA should be discontinued in patients developing severe rash associated with blistering, desquamation, mucosal involvement, or fever. Appropriate antihistamines and/or corticosteroids may improve the tolerability and hasten the resolution of rash.

Experience with efavirenz in subjects who discontinued other antiretroviral agents of the NNRTI class is limited. Nineteen subjects who discontinued nevirapine because of rash have been treated with efavirenz. Nine of these subjects developed mild-to-moderate rash while receiving therapy with efavirenz, and two of these subjects discontinued because of rash.

5.10 Hepatotoxicity

Monitoring of liver enzymes before and during treatment is recommended for patients with underlying hepatic disease, including hepatitis B or C infection; patients with marked transaminase elevations; and patients treated with other medications associated with liver toxicity *[See also Warnings and Precautions (5.2)]*. A few of the postmarketing reports of hepatic failure occurred in patients with no pre-existing hepatic disease or other identifiable risk factors *[See Adverse Reactions (6.3)]*. Liver enzyme monitoring should also be considered for patients without pre-existing hepatic dysfunction or other risk factors. In patients with persistent elevations of serum transaminases to greater than five times the upper limit of the normal range, the benefit of continued therapy with ATRIPLA needs to be weighed against the unknown risks of significant liver toxicity *[See Adverse Reactions (6.2)]*.

5.11 Decreases in Bone Mineral Density

Bone mineral density (BMD) monitoring should be considered for HIV-1 infected subjects who have a history of pathologic bone fracture or are at risk for osteopenia. Although the effect of supplementation with calcium and vitamin D was not studied, such supplementation may be beneficial for all patients. If bone abnormalities are suspected then appropriate consultation should be obtained.

Table 1 Drugs That Are Contraindicated or Not Recommended for Use With ATRIPLA

Drug Class: Drug Name	Clinical Comment
Antifungal: voriconazole	Efavirenz significantly decreases voriconazole plasma concentrations, and coadministration may decrease the therapeutic effectiveness of voriconazole. Also, voriconazole significantly increases efavirenz plasma concentrations, which may increase the risk of efavirenz-associated side effects. Because ATRIPLA is a fixed-dose combination product, the dose of efavirenz cannot be altered. *[See Clinical Pharmacology (12.3) Tables 5 and 6]*
Ergot derivatives (dihydroergotamine, ergonovine, ergotamine, methylergonovine)	Potential for serious and/or life-threatening reactions such as acute ergot toxicity characterized by peripheral vasospasm and ischemia of the extremities and other tissues.
Benzodiazepines: midazolam, triazolam	Potential for serious and/or life-threatening reactions such as prolonged or increased sedation or respiratory depression.
Calcium channel blocker: bepridil	Potential for serious and/or life-threatening reactions such as cardiac arrhythmias.
GI motility agent: cisapride	Potential for serious and/or life-threatening reactions such as cardiac arrhythmias.
Neuroleptic: pimozide	Potential for serious and/or life-threatening reactions such as cardiac arrhythmias.
St. John's wort (*Hypericum perforatum*)	May lead to loss of virologic response and possible resistance to efavirenz or to the class of non-nucleoside reverse transcriptase inhibitors (NNRTIs).

In a 144-week study of treatment-naive subjects receiving tenofovir DF, decreases in BMD were seen at the lumbar spine and hip in both arms of the study. At Week 144, there was a significantly greater mean percentage decrease from baseline in BMD at the lumbar spine in subjects receiving tenofovir DF + lamivudine + efavirenz compared with subjects receiving stavudine + lamivudine + efavirenz. Changes in BMD at the hip were similar between the two treatment groups. In both groups, the majority of the reduction in BMD occurred in the first 24–48 weeks of the study and this reduction was sustained through 144 weeks. Twenty-eight percent of tenofovir DF-treated subjects vs. 21% of the comparator subjects lost at least 5% of BMD at the spine or 7% of BMD at the hip. Clinically relevant fractures (excluding fingers and toes) were reported in 4 subjects in the tenofovir DF group and 6 subjects in the comparator group. Tenofovir DF was associated with significant increases in biochemical markers of bone metabolism (serum bone-specific alkaline phosphatase, serum osteocalcin, serum C-telopeptide, and urinary N-telopeptide), suggesting increased bone turnover. Serum parathyroid hormone levels and 1,25 Vitamin D levels were also higher in subjects receiving tenofovir DF. The effects of tenofovir DF-associated changes in BMD and biochemical markers on long-term bone health and future fracture risk are unknown. For additional information, consult the tenofovir DF prescribing information.

Cases of osteomalacia (associated with proximal renal tubulopathy and which may contribute to fractures) have been reported in association with the use of tenofovir DF [See Adverse Reactions (6.3)].

5.12 Convulsions
Convulsions have been observed in patients receiving efavirenz, generally in the presence of known medical history of seizures. Caution must be taken in any patient with a history of seizures.

Patients who are receiving concomitant anticonvulsant medications primarily metabolized by the liver, such as phenytoin and phenobarbital, may require periodic monitoring of plasma levels [See Drug Interactions (7.3)].

5.13 Immune Reconstitution Syndrome
Immune reconstitution syndrome has been reported in patients treated with combination antiretroviral therapy, including the components of ATRIPLA. During the initial phase of combination antiretroviral treatment, patients whose immune system responds may develop an inflammatory response to indolent or residual opportunistic infections [such as Mycobacterium avium infection, cytomegalovirus, Pneumocystis jirovecii pneumonia (PCP), or tuberculosis], which may necessitate further evaluation and treatment.

5.14 Fat Redistribution
Redistribution/accumulation of body fat including central obesity, dorsocervical fat enlargement (buffalo hump), peripheral wasting, facial wasting, breast enlargement, and "cushingoid appearance" have been observed in patients receiving antiretroviral therapy. The mechanism and long-term consequences of these events are currently unknown. A causal relationship has not been established.

6 ADVERSE REACTIONS
Efavirenz, Emtricitabine and Tenofovir Disoproxil Fumarate: The following adverse reactions are discussed in other sections of the labeling:
- Lactic Acidosis/Severe Hepatomegaly with Steatosis [See Boxed Warning, Warnings and Precautions (5.1)].
- Severe Acute Exacerbations of Hepatitis B [See Boxed Warning, Warnings and Precautions (5.2)].
- Psychiatric Symptoms [See Warnings and Precautions (5.5)].
- Nervous System Symptoms [See Warnings and Precautions (5.6)].
- New Onset or Worsening Renal Impairment [See Warnings and Precautions (5.7)].
- Rash [See Warnings and Precautions (5.9)].
- Hepatotoxicity [See Warnings and Precautions (5.10)].
- Decreases in Bone Mineral Density [See Warnings and Precautions (5.11)].
- Immune Reconstitution Syndrome [See Warnings and Precautions (5.13)].
- Drug Interactions [See Contraindications (4.2), Warnings and Precautions (5.3) and Drug Interactions (7)].

For additional safety information about SUSTIVA (efavirenz), EMTRIVA (emtricitabine), or VIREAD (tenofovir DF) in combination with other antiretroviral agents, consult the prescribing information for these products.

6.1 Adverse Reactions from Clinical Trials Experience
Because clinical trials are conducted under widely varying conditions, adverse reaction rates observed in the clinical trials of a drug cannot be directly compared to rates in the clinical trials of another drug and may not reflect the rates observed in practice.

Study 934
Study 934 was an open-label active-controlled study in which 511 antiretroviral-naive subjects received either

emtricitabine + tenofovir DF administered in combination with efavirenz (N=257) or zidovudine/lamivudine administered in combination with efavirenz (N=254).

The most common adverse reactions (incidence ≥ 10%, any severity) occurring in Study 934 include diarrhea, nausea, fatigue, headache, dizziness, depression, insomnia, abnormal dreams, and rash. Adverse reactions observed in Study 934 were generally consistent with those seen in previous studies of the individual components (Table 2).

Table 2 Selected Treatment-Emergent Adverse Reactions* (Grades 2–4) Reported in ≥5% in Either Treatment Group in Study 934 (0–144 Weeks)

	FTC + TDF + EFV[†]	AZT/3TC + EFV
	N=257	N=254
Gastrointestinal Disorder		
Diarrhea	9%	5%
Nausea	9%	7%
Vomiting	2%	5%
General Disorders and Administration Site Condition		
Fatigue	9%	8%
Infections and Infestations		
Sinusitis	8%	4%
Upper respiratory tract infections	8%	5%
Nasopharyngitis	5%	3%
Nervous System Disorders		
Headache	6%	5%
Dizziness	8%	7%
Psychiatric Disorders		
Anxiety	5%	4%
Depression	9%	7%
Insomnia	5%	7%
Skin and Subcutaneous Tissue Disorders		
Rash Event[‡]	7%	9%

* Frequencies of adverse reactions are based on all treatment-emergent adverse events, regardless of relationship to study drug.
† From Weeks 96 to 144 of the study, subjects received emtricitabine/tenofovir DF administered in combination with efavirenz in place of emtricitabine + tenofovir DF with efavirenz.
‡ Rash event includes rash, exfoliative rash, rash generalized, rash macular, rash maculo-papular, rash pruritic, and rash vesicular.

Study 073
In Study 073, subjects with stable, virologic suppression on antiretroviral therapy and no history of virologic failure were randomized to receive ATRIPLA or to stay on their baseline regimen. The adverse reactions observed in Study 073 were generally consistent with those seen in Study 934 and those seen with the individual components of ATRIPLA when each was administered in combination with other antiretroviral agents.

Efavirenz, Emtricitabine, or Tenofovir Disoproxil Fumarate
In addition to the adverse reactions in Study 934 and Study 073 the following adverse reactions were observed in clinical trials of efavirenz, emtricitabine, or tenofovir DF in combination with other antiretroviral agents.

Efavirenz: The most significant adverse reactions observed in subjects treated with efavirenz are nervous system symptoms [See Warnings and Precautions (5.6)], psychiatric symptoms [See Warnings and Precautions (5.5)], and rash [See Warnings and Precautions (5.9)].

Selected adverse reactions of moderate-severe intensity observed in ≥2% of efavirenz-treated subjects in two controlled clinical trials included pain, impaired concentration, abnormal dreams, somnolence, anorexia, dyspepsia, abdominal pain, nervousness, and pruritus.

Pancreatitis has also been reported, although a causal relationship with efavirenz has not been established. Asymptomatic increases in serum amylase levels were observed in a significantly higher number of subjects treated with efavirenz 600 mg than in control subjects.

Emtricitabine and Tenofovir Disoproxil Fumarate: Adverse reactions that occurred in at least 5% of treatment-experienced or treatment-naive subjects receiving emtricitabine or tenofovir DF with other antiretroviral agents in clinical trials include arthralgia, increased cough, dyspepsia, fever, myalgia, pain, abdominal pain, back pain,

paresthesia, peripheral neuropathy (including peripheral neuritis and neuropathy), pneumonia, rhinitis and rash event (including rash, pruritus, maculopapular rash, urticaria, vesiculobullous rash, pustular rash and allergic reaction).

Skin discoloration has been reported with higher frequency among emtricitabine-treated subjects; it was manifested by hyperpigmentation on the palms and/or soles and was generally mild and asymptomatic. The mechanism and clinical significance are unknown.

6.2 Laboratory Abnormalities
Efavirenz, Emtricitabine and Tenofovir Disoproxil Fumarate: Laboratory abnormalities observed in Study 934 were generally consistent with those seen in previous studies (Table 3).

Table 3 Significant Laboratory Abnormalities Reported in ≥1% of Subjects in Either Treatment Group in Study 934 (0–144 Weeks)

	FTC + TDF + EFV*	AZT/3TC + EFV
	(N=257)	(N=254)
Any ≥ Grade 3 Laboratory Abnormality	30%	26%
Fasting Cholesterol (>240 mg/dL)	22%	24%
Creatine Kinase (M: >990 U/L) (F: >845 U/L)	9%	7%
Serum Amylase (>175 U/L)	8%	4%
Alkaline Phosphatase (>550 U/L)	1%	0%
AST (M: >180 U/L) (F: >170 U/L)	3%	3%
ALT (M: >215 U/L) (F: >170 U/L)	2%	3%
Hemoglobin (<8.0 mg/dL)	0%	4%
Hyperglycemia (>250 mg/dL)	2%	1%
Hematuria (>75 RBC/HPF)	3%	2%
Glycosuria (≥3+)	<1%	1%
Neutrophils (<750/mm³)	3%	5%
Fasting Triglycerides (>750 mg/dL)	4%	2%

* From Weeks 96 to 144 of the study, subjects received emtricitabine/tenofovir DF administered in combination with efavirenz in place of emtricitabine + tenofovir DF with efavirenz.

Laboratory abnormalities observed in Study 073 were generally consistent with those in Study 934.

In addition to the laboratory abnormalities described for Study 934 (Table 3), Grade 3/4 elevations of bilirubin (>2.5 × ULN), pancreatic amylase (>2.0 × ULN), serum glucose (<40 or >250 mg/dL), and serum lipase (>2.0 × ULN) occurred in up to 3% of subjects treated with emtricitabine or tenofovir DF with other antiretroviral agents in clinical trials.

Hepatic Events: In Study 934, 19 subjects treated with efavirenz, emtricitabine, and tenofovir DF and 20 subjects treated with efavirenz and fixed-dose zidovudine/lamivudine were hepatitis B surface antigen or hepatitis C antibody positive. Among these coinfected subjects, one subject (1/19) in the efavirenz, emtricitabine and tenofovir DF arm had elevations in transaminases to greater than five times ULN through 144 weeks. In the fixed-dose zidovudine/lamivudine arm, two subjects (2/20) had elevations in transaminases to greater than five times ULN through 144 weeks. No HBV and/or HCV coinfected subject discontinued from the study due to hepatobiliary disorders [See Warnings and Precautions (5.10)].

6.3 Postmarketing Experience
The following adverse reactions have been identified during postapproval use of efavirenz, emtricitabine, or tenofovir DF. Because postmarketing reactions are reported voluntarily from a population of uncertain size, it is not always possible to reliably estimate their frequency or establish a causal relationship to drug exposure.

Efavirenz:
Cardiac Disorders
Palpitations
Ear and Labyrinth Disorders
Tinnitus
Endocrine Disorders
Gynecomastia
Eye Disorders
Abnormal vision
Gastrointestinal Disorders
Constipation, malabsorption
General Disorders and Administration Site Conditions
Asthenia
Hepatobiliary Disorders
Hepatic enzyme increase, hepatic failure, hepatitis. A few of the postmarketing reports of hepatic failure, including cases in patients with no pre-existing hepatic disease or other identifiable risk factors, were characterized by a fulminant course, progressing in some cases to transplantation or death.
Immune System Disorders
Allergic reactions
Metabolism and Nutrition Disorders
Redistribution/accumulation of body fat *[See Warnings and Precautions (5.14)]*, hypercholesterolemia, hypertriglyceridemia
Musculoskeletal and Connective Tissue Disorders
Arthralgia, myalgia, myopathy
Nervous System Disorders
Abnormal coordination, ataxia, cerebellar coordination and balance disturbances, convulsions, hypoesthesia, paresthesia, neuropathy, tremor
Psychiatric Disorders
Aggressive reactions, agitation, delusions, emotional lability, mania, neurosis, paranoia, psychosis, suicide
Respiratory, Thoracic and Mediastinal Disorders
Dyspnea
Skin and Subcutaneous Tissue Disorders
Flushing, erythema multiforme, photoallergic dermatitis, Stevens-Johnson syndrome
Emtricitabine: No postmarketing adverse reactions have been identified for inclusion in this section.
Tenofovir Disoproxil Fumarate:
Immune System Disorders
Allergic reaction, including angioedema
Metabolism and Nutrition Disorders
Lactic acidosis, hypokalemia, hypophosphatemia
Respiratory, Thoracic, and Mediastinal Disorders
Dyspnea
Gastrointestinal Disorders
Pancreatitis, increased amylase, abdominal pain
Hepatobiliary Disorders
Hepatic steatosis, hepatitis, increased liver enzymes (most commonly AST, ALT, gamma GT)
Skin and Subcutaneous Tissue Disorders
Rash
Musculoskeletal and Connective Tissue Disorders
Rhabdomyolysis, osteomalacia (manifested as bone pain and which may contribute to fractures), muscular weakness, myopathy
Renal and Urinary Disorders
Acute renal failure, renal failure, acute tubular necrosis, Fanconi syndrome, proximal renal tubulopathy, interstitial nephritis (including acute cases), nephrogenic diabetes insipidus, renal insufficiency, increased creatinine, proteinuria, polyuria
General Disorders and Administration Site Conditions
Asthenia
The following adverse reactions, listed under the body system headings above, may occur as a consequence of proximal renal tubulopathy: rhabdomyolysis, osteomalacia, hypokalemia, muscular weakness, myopathy, hypophosphatemia.

7   DRUG INTERACTIONS
This section describes clinically relevant drug interactions with ATRIPLA. Drug interaction studies are described elsewhere in the labeling *[See Clinical Pharmacology (12.3)]*.

7.1   Efavirenz
Efavirenz has been shown in vivo to induce CYP3A. Other compounds that are substrates of CYP3A may have decreased plasma concentrations when coadministered with efavirenz. In vitro studies have demonstrated that efavirenz inhibits CYP2C9, 2C19, and 3A4 isozymes in the range of observed efavirenz plasma concentrations. Coadministration of efavirenz with drugs primarily metabolized by these isozymes may result in altered plasma concentrations of the coadministered drug. Therefore, appropriate dose adjustments may be necessary for these drugs.
Drugs that induce CYP3A activity (e.g., phenobarbital, rifampin, rifabutin) would be expected to increase the clearance of efavirenz resulting in lowered plasma concentrations.

Table 4 Established and Other Potentially Significant* Drug Interactions: Alteration in Dose or Regimen May Be Recommended Based on Drug Interaction Studies or Predicted Interaction

Concomitant Drug Class: Drug Name	Effect	Clinical Comment
Antiretroviral agents		
Protease inhibitor: atazanavir	↓ atazanavir concentration ↑ tenofovir concentration	Coadministration of atazanavir with ATRIPLA is not recommended. Coadministration of atazanavir with either efavirenz or tenofovir DF decreases plasma concentrations of atazanavir. The combined effect of efavirenz plus tenofovir DF on atazanavir plasma concentrations is not known. Also, atazanavir has been shown to increase tenofovir concentrations. There are insufficient data to support dosing recommendations for atazanavir or atazanavir/ritonavir in combination with ATRIPLA.
Protease inhibitor: fosamprenavir calcium	↓ amprenavir concentration	Fosamprenavir (unboosted): Appropriate doses of fosamprenavir and ATRIPLA with respect to safety and efficacy have not been established. Fosamprenavir/ritonavir: An additional 100 mg/day (300 mg total) of ritonavir is recommended when ATRIPLA is administered with fosamprenavir/ritonavir once daily. No change in the ritonavir dose is required when ATRIPLA is administered with fosamprenavir plus ritonavir twice daily.
Protease inhibitor: indinavir	↓ indinavir concentration	The optimal dose of indinavir, when given in combination with efavirenz, is not known. Increasing the indinavir dose to 1000 mg every 8 hours does not compensate for the increased indinavir metabolism due to efavirenz.
Protease inhibitor: lopinavir/ritonavir	↓ lopinavir concentration ↑ tenofovir concentration	A dose increase of lopinavir/ritonavir to 600/150 mg (3 tablets) twice daily may be considered when used in combination with efavirenz in treatment-experienced patients where decreased susceptibility to lopinavir is clinically suspected (by treatment history or laboratory evidence). **Patients should be monitored for tenofovir-associated adverse reactions. ATRIPLA should be discontinued in patients who develop tenofovir-associated adverse reactions.**
Protease inhibitor: ritonavir	↑ ritonavir concentration ↑ efavirenz concentration	When ritonavir 500 mg every 12 hours was coadministered with efavirenz 600 mg once daily, the combination was associated with a higher frequency of adverse clinical experiences (e.g., dizziness, nausea, paresthesia) and laboratory abnormalities (elevated liver enzymes). Monitoring of liver enzymes is recommended when ATRIPLA is used in combination with ritonavir.
Protease inhibitor: saquinavir	↓ saquinavir concentration	Should not be used as sole protease inhibitor in combination with ATRIPLA.
CCR5 co-receptor antagonist: Maraviroc	↓ maraviroc concentration	Efavirenz decreases plasma concentrations of maraviroc. Refer to the full prescribing information for maraviroc for guidance on coadministration with ATRIPLA.
NRTI: didanosine	↑ didanosine concentration	Higher didanosine concentrations could potentiate didanosine-associated adverse reactions, including pancreatitis and neuropathy. **In adults weighing >60 kg, the didanosine dose should be reduced to 250 mg if coadministered with ATRIPLA. Data are not available to recommend a dose adjustment of didanosine for patients weighing <60 kg. Coadministration of ATRIPLA and didanosine should be undertaken with caution and patients receiving this combination should be monitored closely for didanosine-associated adverse reactions. For additional information, please consult the Videx/Videx EC (didanosine) prescribing information.**

(Table continued on next page)

7.2   Emtricitabine and Tenofovir Disoproxil Fumarate
Since emtricitabine and tenofovir are primarily eliminated by the kidneys, coadministration of ATRIPLA with drugs that reduce renal function or compete for active tubular secretion may increase serum concentrations of emtricitabine, tenofovir, and/or other renally eliminated drugs. Some examples include, but are not limited to, acyclovir, adefovir dipivoxil, cidofovir, ganciclovir, valacyclovir, and valganciclovir.
Coadministration of tenofovir DF and didanosine should be undertaken with caution and patients receiving this combination should be monitored closely for didanosine-associated adverse reactions. Didanosine should be discontinued in patients who develop didanosine-associated

adverse reactions [for didanosine dosing adjustment recommendations, see *Table 4*]. Suppression of CD4+ cell counts has been observed in patients receiving tenofovir DF with didanosine 400 mg daily.
Lopinavir/ritonavir has been shown to increase tenofovir concentrations. The mechanism of this interaction is unknown. Patients receiving lopinavir/ritonavir with ATRIPLA should be monitored for tenofovir-associated adverse reactions. ATRIPLA should be discontinued in patients who develop tenofovir-associated adverse reactions [See *Table 4*].
Coadministration of atazanavir with ATRIPLA is not recommended since coadministration of atazanavir with either

efavirenz or tenofovir DF has been shown to decrease plasma concentrations of atazanavir. Also, atazanavir has been shown to increase tenofovir concentrations. There are insufficient data to support dosing recommendations for atazanavir or atazanavir/ritonavir in combination with ATRIPLA [See Table 4].

7.3 Efavirenz, Emtricitabine and Tenofovir Disoproxil Fumarate

Other important drug interaction information for ATRIPLA is summarized in Table 1 and Table 4. The drug interactions described are based on studies conducted with efavirenz, emtricitabine or tenofovir DF as individual agents or are potential drug interactions; no drug interaction studies have been conducted using ATRIPLA [for pharmacokinetics data see *Clinical Pharmacology (12.3)*, Tables 5–9]. The tables include potentially significant interactions, but are not all inclusive.

[See table 4 on pages 895 through 897]

7.4 Efavirenz Assay Interference

Cannabinoid Test Interaction: Efavirenz does not bind to cannabinoid receptors. False-positive urine cannabinoid test results have been observed in non-HIV-infected volunteers receiving efavirenz when the Microgenics Cedia DAU Multi-Level THC assay was used for screening. Negative results were obtained when more specific confirmatory testing was performed with gas chromatography/mass spectrometry. For more information, please consult the SUSTIVA prescribing information.

8 USE IN SPECIFIC POPULATIONS

8.1 Pregnancy

Pregnancy Category D [See Warnings and Precautions (5.8)]

8.3 Nursing Mothers

The Centers for Disease Control and Prevention recommend that HIV-1 infected mothers not breast-feed their infants to avoid risking postnatal transmission of HIV-1. Studies in rats have demonstrated that both efavirenz and tenofovir are secreted in milk. It is not known whether efavirenz, emtricitabine, or tenofovir is excreted in human milk. Because of both the potential for HIV-1 transmission and the potential for serious adverse reactions in nursing infants, **mothers should be instructed not to breast-feed if they are receiving ATRIPLA.**

8.4 Pediatric Use

ATRIPLA is not recommended for patients less than 18 years of age because it is a fixed-dose combination tablet containing a component, tenofovir DF, for which safety and efficacy have not been established in this age group.

8.5 Geriatric Use

Clinical studies of efavirenz, emtricitabine, or tenofovir DF did not include sufficient numbers of subjects aged 65 and over to determine whether they respond differently from younger subjects. In general, dose selection for the elderly patients should be cautious, keeping in mind the greater frequency of decreased hepatic, renal, or cardiac function, and of concomitant disease or other drug therapy.

8.6 Hepatic Impairment

The pharmacokinetics of efavirenz have not been adequately studied in subjects with hepatic impairment. Because of the extensive cytochrome P450-mediated metabolism of efavirenz and limited clinical experience in patients with hepatic impairment, caution should be exercised in administering ATRIPLA to these patients [See Warnings and Precautions (5.10)].

8.7 Renal Impairment

Because ATRIPLA is a fixed-dose combination, it should not be prescribed for patients requiring dosage adjustment such as those with moderate or severe renal impairment (creatinine clearance <50 mL/min) [See Warnings and Precautions (5.7)].

10 OVERDOSAGE

If overdose occurs, the patient should be monitored for evidence of toxicity, including monitoring of vital signs and observation of the patient's clinical status; standard supportive treatment should then be applied as necessary. Administration of activated charcoal may be used to aid removal of unabsorbed efavirenz. Hemodialysis can remove both emtricitabine and tenofovir DF (refer to detailed information below), but is unlikely to significantly remove efavirenz from the blood.

Efavirenz: Some patients accidentally taking 600 mg twice daily have reported increased nervous system symptoms. One patient experienced involuntary muscle contractions.

Emtricitabine: Limited clinical experience is available at doses higher than the therapeutic dose of emtricitabine. In one clinical pharmacology study single doses of emtricitabine 1200 mg were administered to 11 subjects. No severe adverse reactions were reported. Hemodialysis treatment removes approximately 30% of the emtricitabine dose over a 3-hour dialysis period starting within 1.5 hours of emtricitabine dosing (blood flow rate of 400 mL/min and a dialysate flow rate of 600 mL/min). It is not known whether emtricitabine can be removed by peritoneal dialysis.

Tenofovir Disoproxil Fumarate: Limited clinical experience at doses higher than the therapeutic dose of tenofovir DF 300 mg is available. In one study, 600 mg tenofovir DF was administered to 8 subjects orally for 28 days, and no severe adverse reactions were reported. The effects of higher doses are not known. Tenofovir is efficiently removed by hemodialysis with an extraction coefficient of approximately 54%. Following a single 300 mg dose of tenofovir DF, a 4-hour hemodialysis session

Table 4 (cont.) Established and Other Potentially Significant* Drug Interactions: Alteration in Dose or Regimen May Be Recommended Based on Drug Interaction Studies or Predicted Interaction

Concomitant Drug Class: Drug Name	Effect	Clinical Comment
Other agents		
Anticoagulant: warfarin	↑ or ↓ warfarin concentration	Plasma concentrations and effects potentially increased or decreased by efavirenz.
Anticonvulsants: carbamazepine phenytoin phenobarbital	↓ carbamazepine concentration ↓ efavirenz concentration ↓ anticonvulsant concentration ↓ efavirenz concentration	There are insufficient data to make a dose recommendation for ATRIPLA. Alternative anticonvulsant treatment should be used. Potential for reduction in anticonvulsant and/or efavirenz plasma levels; periodic monitoring of anticonvulsant plasma levels should be conducted.
Antidepressant: sertraline	↓ sertraline concentration	Increases in sertraline dose should be guided by clinical response.
Antifungals: itraconazole	↓ itraconazole concentration ↓ hydroxy-itraconazole concentration	Since no dose recommendation for itraconazole can be made, alternative antifungal treatment should be considered.
ketoconazole	↓ ketoconazole concentration	Drug interaction studies with ATRIPLA and ketoconazole have not been conducted. Efavirenz has the potential to decrease plasma concentrations of ketoconazole.
posaconazole	↓ posaconazole concentration	Avoid concomitant use unless the benefit outweighs the risks.
Anti-infective: clarithromycin	↓ clarithromycin concentration ↑ 14-OH metabolite concentration	Clinical significance unknown. In uninfected volunteers, 46% developed rash while receiving efavirenz and clarithromycin. No dose adjustment of ATRIPLA is recommended when given with clarithromycin. Alternatives to clarithromycin, such as azithromycin, should be considered. Other macrolide antibiotics, such as erythromycin, have not been studied in combination with ATRIPLA.
Antimycobacterial: rifabutin	↓ rifabutin concentration	Increase daily dose of rifabutin by 50%. Consider doubling the rifabutin dose in regimens where rifabutin is given 2 or 3 times a week.
Antimycobacterial: rifampin	↓ efavirenz concentration	Clinical significance of reduced efavirenz concentration is unknown. Dosing recommendations for concomitant use of ATRIPLA and rifampin have not been established.
Calcium channel blockers: diltiazem	↓ diltiazem concentration ↓ desacetyl diltiazem concentration ↓ N-monodes-methyl diltiazem concentration	Diltiazem dose adjustments should be guided by clinical response (refer to the full prescribing information for diltiazem). No dose adjustment of ATRIPLA is necessary when administered with diltiazem.
Others (eg, felodipine, nicardipine, nifedipine, verapamil)	↓ calcium channel blocker	No data are available on the potential interactions of efavirenz with other calcium channel blockers that are substrates of CYP3A. The potential exists for reduction in plasma concentrations of the calcium channel blocker. Dose adjustments should be guided by clinical response (refer to the full prescribing information for the calcium channel blocker).
HMG-CoA reductase inhibitors: atorvastatin pravastatin simvastatin	↓ atorvastatin concentration ↓ pravastatin concentration ↓ simvastatin concentration	Plasma concentrations of atorvastatin, pravastatin, and simvastatin decreased with efavirenz. Consult the full prescribing information for the HMG-CoA reductase inhibitor for guidance on individualizing the dose.
Hormonal contraceptives: Oral: Ethinyl estradiol/Norgestimate	↓ active metabolites of norgestimate	A reliable method of barrier contraception must be used in addition to hormonal contraceptives. Efavirenz had no effect on ethinyl estradiol concentrations, but progestin levels (norelgestromin and levonorgestrel) were markedly decreased. No effect of ethinyl estradiol/norgestimate on efavirenz plasma concentrations was observed.
Implant: Etonogestrel	↓ etonogestrel	A reliable method of barrier contraception must be used in addition to hormonal contraceptives. The interaction between etonogestrel and efavirenz has not been studied. Decreased exposure of etonogestrel may be expected. There have been postmarketing reports of contraceptive failure with etonogestrel in efavirenz-exposed patients.

(Table continued on next page)

removed approximately 10% of the administered tenofovir dose.

11 DESCRIPTION

ATRIPLA is a fixed-dose combination tablet containing efavirenz, emtricitabine, and tenofovir disoproxil fumarate (tenofovir DF). SUSTIVA is the brand name for efavirenz, a non-nucleoside reverse transcriptase inhibitor. EMTRIVA is the brand name for emtricitabine, a synthetic nucleoside analog of cytidine. VIREAD is the brand name for tenofovir DF, which is converted in vivo to tenofovir, an acyclic nucleoside phosphonate (nucleotide) analog of adenosine 5'-monophosphate. VIREAD and EMTRIVA are the components of TRUVADA.

ATRIPLA tablets are for oral administration. Each tablet contains 600 mg of efavirenz, 200 mg of emtricitabine, and 300 mg of tenofovir DF (which is equivalent to 245 mg of tenofovir disoproxil) as active ingredients. The tablets include the following inactive ingredients: croscarmellose sodium, hydroxypropyl cellulose, magnesium stearate, microcrystalline cellulose, and sodium lauryl sulfate. The tablets are film-coated with a coating material containing black iron oxide, polyethylene glycol, polyvinyl alcohol, red iron oxide, talc, and titanium dioxide.

Efavirenz: Efavirenz is chemically described as (S)-6-chloro-4-(cyclopropylethynyl)-1,4-dihydro-4-(trifluoromethyl)-2H-3,1-benzoxazin-2-one. Its molecular formula is $C_{14}H_9ClF_3NO_2$ and its structural formula is:

Efavirenz is a white to slightly pink crystalline powder with a molecular mass of 315.68. It is practically insoluble in water (<10 μg/mL).

Emtricitabine: The chemical name of emtricitabine is 5-fluoro-1-(2R,5S)-[2-(hydroxymethyl)-1,3-oxathiolan-5-yl]cytosine. Emtricitabine is the (-) enantiomer of a thio analog of cytidine, which differs from other cytidine analogs in that it has a fluorine in the 5-position.

It has a molecular formula of $C_8H_{10}FN_3O_3S$ and a molecular weight of 247.24. It has the following structural formula:

Emtricitabine is a white to off-white crystalline powder with a solubility of approximately 112 mg/mL in water at 25 °C.

Tenofovir Disoproxil Fumarate: Tenofovir DF is a fumaric acid salt of the *bis*-isopropoxycarbonyloxymethyl ester derivative of tenofovir. The chemical name of tenofovir disoproxil fumarate is 9-[(R)-2-[[bis[[(isopropoxycarbonyl)oxy]-methoxy]phosphinyl]methoxy]propyl]adenine fumarate (1:1). It has a molecular formula of $C_{19}H_{30}N_5O_{10}P$ • $C_4H_4O_4$ and a molecular weight of 635.52. It has the following structural formula:

Tenofovir DF is a white to off-white crystalline powder with a solubility of 13.4 mg/mL in water at 25 °C.

12 CLINICAL PHARMACOLOGY

For additional information on Mechanism of Action, Antiviral Activity, Resistance and Cross Resistance, please consult the SUSTIVA, EMTRIVA and VIREAD prescribing information.

12.1 Mechanism of Action

ATRIPLA is a fixed-dose combination of antiviral drugs efavirenz, emtricitabine and tenofovir disoproxil fumarate. [See Clinical Pharmacology (12.4)].

12.3 Pharmacokinetics

ATRIPLA: One ATRIPLA tablet is bioequivalent to one SUSTIVA tablet (600 mg) plus one EMTRIVA capsule (200 mg) plus one VIREAD tablet (300 mg) following single-dose administration to fasting healthy subjects (N=45).

Efavirenz: In HIV-1 infected subjects time-to-peak plasma concentrations were approximately 3–5 hours and steady-

Table 4 *(cont.)* Established and Other Potentially Significant* Drug Interactions: Alteration in Dose or Regimen May Be Recommended Based on Drug Interaction Studies or Predicted Interaction

Concomitant Drug Class: Drug Name	Effect	Clinical Comment
Other agents (continued)		
Immunosuppressants: Cyclosporine, tacrolimus, sirolimus, and others metabolized by CYP3A	↓ immuno-suppressant	Decreased exposure of the immunosuppressant may be expected due to CYP3A induction by efavirenz. These immunosuppressants are not anticipated to affect exposure of efavirenz. Dose adjustments of the immunosuppressant may be required. Close monitoring of immunosuppressant concentrations for at least 2 weeks (until stable concentrations are reached) is recommended when starting or stopping treatment with ATRIPLA.
Narcotic analgesic: methadone	↓ methadone concentration	Coadministration of efavirenz in HIV-1 infected individuals with a history of injection drug use resulted in decreased plasma levels of methadone and signs of opiate withdrawal. Methadone dose was increased by a mean of 22% to alleviate withdrawal symptoms. Patients should be monitored for signs of withdrawal and their methadone dose increased as required to alleviate withdrawal symptoms.

*This table is not all inclusive.

state plasma concentrations were reached in 6–10 days. In 35 HIV-1 infected subjects receiving efavirenz 600 mg once daily, steady-state C_{max} was 12.9 ± 3.7 μM (mean ± SD), C_{min} was 5.6 ± 3.2 μM, and AUC was 184 ± 73 μM•hr. Efavirenz is highly bound (approximately 99.5–99.75%) to human plasma proteins, predominantly albumin. Following administration of ^{14}C-labeled efavirenz, 14–34% of the dose was recovered in the urine (mostly as metabolites) and 16–61% was recovered in feces (mostly as parent drug). In vitro studies suggest CYP3A and CYP2B6 are the major isozymes responsible for efavirenz metabolism. Efavirenz has been shown to induce CYP enzymes, resulting in induction of its own metabolism. Efavirenz has a terminal half-life of 52–76 hours after single doses and 40–55 hours after multiple doses.

Emtricitabine: Following oral administration, emtricitabine is rapidly absorbed with peak plasma concentrations occurring at 1–2 hours post-dose. Following multiple dose oral administration of emtricitabine to 20 HIV-1 infected subjects, the steady-state plasma emtricitabine C_{max} was 1.8 ± 0.7 μg/mL (mean ± SD) and the AUC over a 24-hour dosing interval was 10.0 ± 3.1 μg•hr/mL. The mean steady state plasma trough concentration at 24 hours post-dose was 0.09 μg/mL. The mean absolute bioavailability of emtricitabine was 93%. In vitro binding of emtricitabine to human plasma proteins is <4% and is independent of concentration over the range of 0.02–200 μg/mL. Following administration of radiolabeled emtricitabine, approximately 86% is recovered in the urine and 13% is recovered as metabolites. The metabolites of emtricitabine include 3'-sulfoxide diastereomers and their glucuronic acid conjugate. Emtricitabine is eliminated by a combination of glomerular filtration and active tubular secretion with a renal clearance in adults with normal renal function of 213 ± 89 mL/min (mean ± SD). Following a single oral dose, the plasma emtricitabine half-life is approximately 10 hours.

Tenofovir Disoproxil Fumarate: Following oral administration of a single 300 mg dose of tenofovir DF to HIV-1 infected subjects in the fasted state, maximum serum concentrations (C_{max}) were achieved in 1.0 ± 0.4 hrs (mean ± SD) and C_{max} and AUC values were 296 ± 90 ng/mL and 2287 ± 685 ng•hr/mL, respectively. The oral bioavailability of tenofovir from tenofovir DF in fasted subjects is approximately 25%. In vitro binding of tenofovir to human plasma proteins is <0.7% and is independent of concentration over the range of 0.01–25 μg/mL. Approximately 70–80% of the intravenous dose of tenofovir is recovered as unchanged drug in the urine. Tenofovir is eliminated by a combination of glomerular filtration and active tubular secretion with a renal clearance in adults with normal renal function of 243 ± 33 mL/min (mean ± SD). Following a single oral dose, the terminal elimination half-life of tenofovir is approximately 17 hours.

Effects of Food on Oral Absorption

ATRIPLA has not been evaluated in the presence of food. Administration of efavirenz tablets with a high fat meal increased the mean AUC and C_{max} of efavirenz by 28% and 79%, respectively, compared to administration in the fasted state. Compared to fasted administration, dosing of tenofovir DF and emtricitabine in combination with either a high fat meal or a light meal increased the mean AUC and C_{max} of tenofovir by 35% and 15%, respectively, without affecting emtricitabine exposures [See Dosage and Administration (2) and Patient Counseling Information (17.3)].

Special Populations

Race

Efavirenz: The pharmacokinetics of efavirenz in HIV-1 infected subjects appear to be similar among the racial groups studied.

Emtricitabine: No pharmacokinetic differences due to race have been identified following the administration of emtricitabine.

Tenofovir Disoproxil Fumarate: There were insufficient numbers from racial and ethnic groups other than Caucasian to adequately determine potential pharmacokinetic differences among these populations following the administration of tenofovir DF.

Gender

Efavirenz, Emtricitabine, and Tenofovir Disoproxil Fumarate: Efavirenz, emtricitabine, and tenofovir pharmacokinetics are similar in male and female subjects.

Pediatric and Geriatric Patients

Pharmacokinetic studies of tenofovir DF have not been performed in pediatric subjects (<18 years). Efavirenz has not been studied in pediatric subjects below 3 years of age or who weigh less than 13 kg. Emtricitabine has been studied in pediatric subjects from 3 months to 17 years of age. ATRIPLA is not recommended for pediatric administration. Pharmacokinetics of efavirenz, emtricitabine and tenofovir have not been fully evaluated in the elderly (>65 years) [See Use in Specific Populations (8)].

Patients with Impaired Renal Function

Efavirenz: The pharmacokinetics of efavirenz have not been studied in subjects with renal insufficiency; however, less than 1% of efavirenz is excreted unchanged in the urine, so the impact of renal impairment on efavirenz elimination should be minimal.

Emtricitabine and Tenofovir Disoproxil Fumarate: The pharmacokinetics of emtricitabine and tenofovir DF are altered in subjects with renal impairment. In subjects with creatinine clearance <50 mL/min, C_{max} and $AUC_{0-\infty}$ of emtricitabine and tenofovir were increased [See Warnings and Precautions (5.7)].

Patients with Hepatic Impairment

Efavirenz: The pharmacokinetics of efavirenz have not been adequately studied in subjects with hepatic impairment [See Warnings and Precautions (5.10) and Use in Specific Populations (8.6)].

Emtricitabine: The pharmacokinetics of emtricitabine have not been studied in subjects with hepatic impairment; however, emtricitabine is not significantly metabolized by liver enzymes, so the impact of liver impairment should be limited.

Tenofovir Disoproxil Fumarate: The pharmacokinetics of tenofovir following a 300 mg dose of tenofovir DF have been studied in non-HIV infected subjects with moderate to severe hepatic impairment. There were no substantial alterations in tenofovir pharmacokinetics in subjects with hepatic impairment compared with unimpaired subjects.

Assessment of Drug Interactions

The drug interaction studies described were conducted with efavirenz, emtricitabine, or tenofovir DF as individual agents; no drug interaction studies have been conducted using ATRIPLA.

Efavirenz: The steady-state pharmacokinetics of efavirenz and tenofovir were unaffected when efavirenz and tenofovir DF were administered together versus each agent dosed alone. Specific drug interaction studies have not been performed with efavirenz and NRTIs other than tenofovir, lamivudine, and zidovudine. Clinically significant interactions would not be expected based on NRTIs elimination pathways.

Efavirenz has been shown in vivo to cause hepatic enzyme induction, thus increasing the biotransformation of some drugs metabolized by CYP3A. In vitro studies have shown that efavirenz inhibited CYP isozymes 2C9, 2C19, and 3A4 with K_i values (8.5–17 μM) in the range of observed efavirenz plasma concentrations. In in vitro studies, efavirenz did not inhibit CYP2E1 and inhibited CYP2D6 and CYP1A2 (K_i values 82–160 μM) only at concentrations well above those achieved clinically. Coadministration of efavirenz with drugs primarily metabolized by 2C9, 2C19, and 3A4 isozymes may result in altered plasma concentrations of the coadministered drug. Drugs which induce CYP3A activity would be expected to increase the clearance of efavirenz resulting in lowered plasma concentrations. Drug interaction studies were performed with efavirenz and other drugs likely to be coadministered or drugs commonly used as probes for pharmacokinetic interaction. There was no clinically significant interaction observed between efavirenz and zidovudine, lamivudine, azithromycin, fluconazole, lorazepam, cetirizine, or paroxetine. Single doses of famotidine or an aluminum and magnesium antacid with simethicone had no effects on efavirenz exposures. The effects of coadministration of efavirenz on C_{max}, AUC, and C_{min} are summarized in Table 5 (effect of other drugs on efavirenz) and Table 6 (effect of efavirenz on other drugs). For information regarding clinical recommendations see *Drug Interactions (7)*.
[See table 5 below]
[See table 6 on pages 899 and 900]

Emtricitabine and Tenofovir Disoproxil Fumarate: The steady-state pharmacokinetics of emtricitabine and tenofovir were unaffected when emtricitabine and tenofovir DF were administered together versus each agent dosed alone.

In vitro and clinical pharmacokinetic drug-drug interaction studies have shown that the potential for CYP mediated interactions involving emtricitabine and tenofovir with other medicinal products is low.

Emtricitabine and tenofovir are primarily excreted by the kidneys by a combination of glomerular filtration and active tubular secretion. No drug-drug interactions due to competition for renal excretion have been observed; however, coadministration of emtricitabine and tenofovir DF with drugs that are eliminated by active tubular secretion may increase concentrations of emtricitabine, tenofovir, and/or the coadministered drug.

Drugs that decrease renal function may increase concentrations of emtricitabine and/or tenofovir.

No clinically significant drug interactions have been observed between emtricitabine and famciclovir, indinavir, stavudine, tenofovir DF and zidovudine. Similarly, no clinically significant drug interactions have been observed between tenofovir DF and abacavir, efavirenz, emtricitabine, entecavir, indinavir, lamivudine, lopinavir/ritonavir, methadone, nelfinavir, oral contraceptives, ribavirin, saquinavir/ritonavir or tacrolimus in studies conducted in healthy volunteers.

Following multiple dosing to HIV-negative subjects receiving either chronic methadone maintenance therapy, oral contraceptives, or single doses of ribavirin, steady-state tenofovir pharmacokinetics were similar to those observed in previous studies, indicating a lack of clinically significant drug interactions between these agents and tenofovir DF. The effects of coadministered drugs on the C_{max}, AUC, and C_{min} of tenofovir are shown in Table 7. The effects of coadministration of tenofovir DF on C_{max}, AUC, and C_{min} of coadministered drugs are shown in Table 8 and Table 9.
[See table 7 at top of page 901]
[See table 8 on page 901]

Coadministration of tenofovir DF with didanosine results in changes in the pharmacokinetics of didanosine that may be of clinical significance. Table 9 summarizes the effects of tenofovir DF on the pharmacokinetics of didanosine. Concomitant dosing of tenofovir DF with didanosine buffered tablets or enteric-coated capsules significantly increases the C_{max} and AUC of didanosine. When didanosine 250 mg enteric-coated capsules were administered with tenofovir DF, systemic exposures of didanosine were similar to those seen with the 400 mg enteric-coated capsules alone under fasted conditions. The mechanism of this interaction is unknown [for didanosine dosing adjustment recommendations see *Drug Interactions (7.3)*, Table 4].
[See table 9 at top of page 902]

12.4 Microbiology
Mechanism of Action
Efavirenz: Efavirenz is a non-nucleoside reverse transcriptase (RT) inhibitor of HIV-1. Efavirenz activity is mediated predominantly by noncompetitive inhibition of HIV-1 reverse transcriptase (RT). HIV-2 RT and human cellular DNA polymerases α, β, γ, and δ are not inhibited by efavirenz.

Emtricitabine: Emtricitabine, a synthetic nucleoside analog of cytidine, is phosphorylated by cellular enzymes to form emtricitabine 5'-triphosphate. Emtricitabine 5'-triphosphate inhibits the activity of the HIV-1 RT by competing with the natural substrate deoxycytidine 5'-triphosphate and by being incorporated into nascent viral DNA which results in chain termination. Emtricitabine 5'-triphosphate is a weak inhibitor of mammalian DNA polymerase α, β, ε, and mitochondrial DNA polymerase γ.

Tenofovir Disoproxil Fumarate: Tenofovir DF is an acyclic nucleoside phosphonate diester analog of adenosine monophosphate. Tenofovir DF requires initial diester hydrolysis for conversion to tenofovir and subsequent phosphorylations by cellular enzymes to form tenofovir diphosphate. Tenofovir diphosphate inhibits the activity of HIV-1 RT by competing with the natural substrate deoxyadenosine 5'-triphosphate and, after incorporation into DNA, by DNA chain termination. Tenofovir diphosphate is a weak inhibitor of mammalian DNA polymerases α, β, and mitochondrial DNA polymerase γ.

Antiviral Activity
Efavirenz, Emtricitabine, and Tenofovir Disoproxil Fumarate: In combination studies evaluating the antiviral activity in cell culture of emtricitabine and efavirenz together, efavirenz and tenofovir together, and emtricitabine and tenofovir together, additive to synergistic antiviral effects were observed.

Efavirenz: The concentration of efavirenz inhibiting replication of wild-type laboratory adapted strains and clinical isolates in cell culture by 90–95% ($EC_{90–95}$) ranged from 1.7–25 nM in lymphoblastoid cell lines, peripheral blood mononuclear cells, and macrophage/monocyte cultures.

Table 5 Drug Interactions: Changes in Pharmacokinetic Parameters for Efavirenz in the Presence of the Coadministered Drug

Coadministered Drug	Dose of Coadministered Drug (mg)	Efavirenz Dose (mg)	N	Mean % Change of Efavirenz Pharmacokinetic Parameters* (90% CI)		
				C_{max}	AUC	C_{min}
Indinavir	800 mg q8h × 14 days	200 mg qd × 14 days	11	↔	↔	↔
Lopinavir/ritonavir	400/100 mg q12h × 9 days	600 mg qd × 9 days	11, 12[†]	↔	↓ 16 (↓ 38 to ↑ 15)	↓ 16 (↓ 42 to ↑ 20)
Nelfinavir	750 mg q8h × 7 days	600 mg qd × 7 days	10	↓ 12 (↓ 32 to ↑ 13)[‡]	↓ 12 (↓ 35 to ↑ 18)[‡]	↓ 21 (↓ 53 to ↑ 33)
Ritonavir	500 mg q12h × 8 days	600 mg qd × 10 days	9	↑ 14 (↑ 4 to ↑ 26)	↑ 21 (↑ 10 to ↑ 34)	↑ 25 (↑ 7 to ↑ 46)[‡]
Saquinavir SGC[§]	1200 mg q8h × 10 days	600 mg qd × 10 days	13	↓ 13 (↓ 5 to ↓ 20)	↓ 12 (↓ 4 to ↓ 19)	↓ 14 (↓ 2 to ↓ 24)[‡]
Clarithromycin	500 mg q12h × 7 days	400 mg qd × 7 days	12	↑ 11 (↑ 3 to ↑ 19)	↔	↔
Itraconazole	200 mg q12h × 14 days	600 mg qd × 28 days	16	↔	↔	↔
Rifabutin	300 mg qd × 14 days	600 mg qd × 14 days	11	↔	↔	↓ 12 (↓ 24 to ↑ 1)
Rifampin	600 mg × 7 days	600 mg qd × 7 days	12	↓ 20 (↓ 11 to ↓ 28)	↓ 26 (↓ 15 to ↓ 36)	↓ 32 (↓ 15 to ↓ 46)
Atorvastatin	10 mg qd × 4 days	600 mg qd × 15 days	14	↔	↔	↔
Pravastatin	40 mg qd × 4 days	600 mg qd × 15 days	11	↔	↔	↔
Simvastatin	40 mg qd × 4 days	600 mg qd × 15 days	14	↓ 12 (↓ 28 to ↑ 8)	↔	↓ 12 (↓ 25 to ↑ 3)
Carbamazepine	200 mg qd × 3 days, 200 mg bid × 3 days, then 400 mg qd × 15 days	600 mg qd × 35 days	14	↓ 21 (↓ 15 to ↓ 26)	↓ 36 (↓ 32 to ↓ 40)	↓ 47 (↓ 41 to ↓ 53)
Diltiazem	240 mg × 14 days	600 mg qd × 28 days	12	↑ 16 (↑ 6 to ↑ 26)	↑ 11 (↑ 5 to ↑ 18)	↑ 13 (↑ 1 to ↑ 26)
Sertraline	50 mg qd × 14 days	600 mg qd × 14 days	13	↑ 11 (↑ 6 to ↑ 16)	↔	↔
	400 mg po q12h × 1 day then 200 mg po q12h × 8 days	400 mg qd × 9 days	NA	↑ 38[¶]	↑ 44[¶]	NA
Voriconazole	300 mg po q12h days 2–7	300 mg qd × 7 days	NA	↓ 14[#] (↓ 7 to ↓ 21)	↔[#]	NA
	400 mg po q12h days 2–7	300 mg qd × 7 days	NA	↔[#]	↑ 17[#] (↑ 6 to ↑ 29)	NA

NA = not available
* Increase = ↑; Decrease = ↓; No Effect = ↔
† Parallel-group design; N for efavirenz + lopinavir/ritonavir, N for efavirenz alone.
‡ 95% CI
§ Soft Gelatin Capsule.
¶ 90% CI not available
# Relative to steady-state administration of efavirenz (600 mg once daily for 9 days).

Table 6 Drug Interactions: Changes in Pharmacokinetic Parameters for Coadministered Drug in the Presence of Efavirenz

Coadministered Drug	Dose of Coadministered Drug (mg)	Efavirenz Dose (mg)	N	C_{max}	AUC	C_{min}
				Mean % Change of Coadministered Drug Pharmacokinetic Parameters* (90% CI)		
Atazanavir	400 mg qd with a light meal d 1–20	600 mg qd with a light meal d 7–20	27	↓ 59 (↓ 49 to ↓ 67)	↓ 74 (↓ 68 to ↓ 78)	↓ 93 (↓ 90 to ↓ 95)
	400 mg qd d 1–6, then 300 mg qd d 7–20 with ritonavir 100 mg qd and a light meal	600 mg qd 2 h after atazanavir and ritonavir d 7–20	13	↑ 14[†] (↓ 17 to ↑ 58)	↑ 39[†] (↑ 2 to ↑ 88)	↑ 48[†] (↑ 24 to ↑ 76)
	300 mg qd/ritonavir 100 mg qd d 1–10 (pm), then 400 mg qd/ritonavir 100 mg qd d 11–24 (pm) (simultaneous with efavirenz)	600 mg qd with a light snack d 11–24 (pm)	14	↑ 17 (↑ 8 to ↑ 27)	↔	↓ 42 (↓ 31 to ↓ 51)
Indinavir	1000 mg q8h × 10 days	600 mg qd × 10 days	20			
	After morning dose			↔[‡]	↓ 33[‡] (↓ 26 to ↓ 39)	↓ 39[‡] (↓ 24 to ↓ 51)
	After afternoon dose			↔[‡]	↓ 37[‡] (↓ 26 to ↓ 46)	↓ 52[‡] (↓ 47 to ↓ 57)
	After evening dose			↓ 29[‡] (↓ 11 to ↓ 43)	↓ 46[‡] (↓ 37 to ↓ 54)	↓ 57[‡] (↓ 50 to ↓ 63)
Lopinavir/ritonavir	400/100 mg q12h × 9 days	600 mg qd × 9 days	11, 7[§]	↔[¶]	↓ 19[¶] (↓ 36 to ↑ 3)	↓ 39[¶] (↓ 3 to ↓ 62)
Nelfinavir	750 mg q8h × 7 days	600 mg qd × 7 days	10	↑ 21 (↑ 10 to ↑ 33)	↑ 20 (↑ 8 to ↑ 34)	↔
Metabolite AG-1402				↓ 40 (↓ 30 to ↓ 48)	↓ 37 (↓ 25 to ↓ 48)	↓ 43 (↓ 21 to ↓ 59)
Ritonavir	500 mg q12h × 8 days	600 mg qd × 10 days	11			
	After AM dose			↑ 24 (↑ 12 to ↑ 38)	↑ 18 (↑ 6 to ↑ 33)	↑ 42 (↑ 9 to ↑ 86)[#]
	After PM dose			↔	↔	↑ 24 (↑ 3 to ↑ 50)[#]
Saquinavir SGC[b]	1200 mg q8h × 10 days	600 mg qd × 10 days	12	↓ 50 (↓ 28 to ↓ 66)	↓ 62 (↓ 45 to ↓ 74)	↓ 56 (↓ 16 to ↓ 77)[#]
Maraviroc	100 mg bid	600 mg qd	12	↓ 51 (↓ 37 to ↓ 62)	↓ 45 (↓ 38 to ↓ 51)	↓ 45 (↓ 28 to ↓ 57)
Clarithromycin	500 mg q12h × 7 days	400 mg qd × 7 days	11	↓ 26 (↓ 15 to ↓ 35)	↓ 39 (↓ 30 to ↓ 46)	↓ 53 (↓ 42 to ↓ 63)
14-OH metabolite				↑ 49 (↑ 32 to ↑ 69)	↑ 34 (↑ 18 to ↑ 53)	↑ 26 (↑ 9 to ↑ 45)
Itraconazole	200 mg q12h × 28 days	600 mg qd × 14 days	18	↓ 37 (↓ 20 to ↓ 51)	↓ 39 (↓ 21 to ↓ 53)	↓ 44 (↓ 27 to ↓ 58)
Hydroxy-itraconazole				↓ 35 (↓ 12 to ↓ 52)	↓ 37 (↓ 14 to ↓ 55)	↓ 43 (↓ 18 to ↓ 60)
Posaconazole	400 mg (oral suspension) bid × 10 and 20 days	400 mg qd × 10 and 20 days	11	↓ 45 (↓ 34 to ↓ 53)	↓ 50 (↓ 40 to ↓ 57)	NA
Rifabutin	300 mg qd × 14 days	600 mg qd × 14 days	9	↓ 32 (↓ 15 to ↓ 46)	↓ 38 (↓ 28 to ↓ 47)	↓ 45 (↓ 31 to ↓ 56)
Atorvastatin	10 mg qd × 4 days	600 mg qd × 15 days	14	↓ 14 (↓ 1 to ↓ 26)	↓ 43 (↓ 34 to ↓ 50)	↓ 69 (↓ 49 to ↓ 81)
Total active (including metabolites)				↓ 15 (↓ 2 to↓ 26)	↓ 32 (↓ 21 to↓ 41)	↓ 48 (↓ 23 to ↓ 64)

(Table continued on next page)

Efavirenz demonstrated additive antiviral activity against HIV-1 in cell culture when combined with non-nucleoside reverse transcriptase inhibitors (NNRTIs) (delavirdine and nevirapine), nucleoside reverse transcriptase inhibitors (NRTIs) (abacavir, didanosine, lamivudine, stavudine, zalcitabine, and zidovudine), protease inhibitors (PIs) (amprenavir, indinavir, lopinavir, nelfinavir, ritonavir, and saquinavir), and the fusion inhibitor enfuvirtide. Efavirenz demonstrated additive to antagonistic antiviral activity in cell culture with atazanavir. Efavirenz demonstrated antiviral activity against clade B and most non-clade B isolates (subtypes A, AE, AG, C, D, F, G, J, and N), but had reduced antiviral activity against group O viruses. Efavirenz is not active against HIV-2.

Emtricitabine: The antiviral activity in cell culture of emtricitabine against laboratory and clinical isolates of HIV-1 was assessed in lymphoblastoid cell lines, the MAGI-CCR5 cell line, and peripheral blood mononuclear cells. The 50% effective concentration (EC_{50}) values for emtricitabine were in the range of 0.0013–0.64 μM (0.0003–0.158 μg/mL). In drug combination studies of emtricitabine with NRTIs (abacavir, lamivudine, stavudine, zalcitabine, and zidovudine), NNRTIs (delavirdine, efavirenz, and nevirapine), and PIs (amprenavir, nelfinavir, ritonavir, and saquinavir), ad-

ditive to synergistic effects were observed. Emtricitabine displayed antiviral activity in cell culture against HIV-1 clades A, B, C, D, E, F, and G (EC_{50} values ranged from 0.007–0.075 μM) and showed strain specific activity against HIV-2 (EC_{50} values ranged from 0.007–1.5 μM).

Tenofovir Disoproxil Fumarate: The antiviral activity in cell culture of tenofovir against laboratory and clinical isolates of HIV-1 was assessed in lymphoblastoid cell lines, primary monocyte/macrophage cells and peripheral blood lymphocytes. The EC_{50} values for tenofovir were in the range of 0.04–8.5 μM. In drug combination studies of tenofovir with NRTIs (abacavir, didanosine, lamivudine, stavudine, zalcit-

Table 6 *(cont.)* Drug Interactions: Changes in Pharmacokinetic Parameters for Coadministered Drug in the Presence of Efavirenz

Coadministered Drug	Dose of Coadministered Drug (mg)	Efavirenz Dose (mg)	N	Mean % Change of Coadministered Drug Pharmacokinetic Parameters* (90% CI)		
				C_{max}	AUC	C_{min}
Pravastatin	40 mg qd × 4 days	600 mg qd × 15 days	13	↓ 32 (↓ 59 to ↑ 12)	↓ 44 (↓ 26 to ↓ 57)	↓ 19 (↓ 0 to ↓ 35)
Simvastatin	40 mg qd × 4 days	600 mg qd × 15 days	14	↓ 72 (↓ 63 to ↓ 79)	↓ 68 (↓ 62 to ↓ 73)	↓ 45 (↓ 20 to ↓ 62)
Total active (including metabolites)				↓ 68 (↓ 55 to ↓ 78)	↓ 60 (↓ 52 to ↓ 68)	NA^ß
Carbamazepine	200 mg qd × 3 days, 200 mg bid × 3 days, then 400 mg qd × 29 days	600 mg qd × 14 days	12	↓ 20 (↓ 15 to ↓ 24)	↓ 27 (↓ 20 to ↓ 33)	↓ 35 (↓ 24 to ↓ 44)
Epoxide metabolite				↔	↔	↓ 13 (↓ 30 to ↑ 7)
Diltiazem	240 mg × 21 days	600 mg qd × 14 days	13	↓ 60 (↓ 50 to ↓ 68)	↓ 69 (↓ 55 to ↓ 79)	↓ 63 (↓ 44 to ↓ 75)
Desacetyl diltiazem				↓ 64 (↓ 57 to ↓ 69)	↓ 75 (↓ 59 to ↓ 84)	↓ 62 (↓ 44 to ↓ 75)
N-monodesmethyl diltiazem				↓ 28 (↓ 7 to ↓ 44)	↓ 37 (↓ 17 to ↓ 52)	↓ 37 (↓ 17 to ↓ 52)
Ethinyl estradiol/ Norgestimate	0.035 mg/0.25 mg × 14 days	600 mg qd × 14 days				
Ethinyl estradiol			21	↔	↔	↔
Norelgestromin			21	↓ 46 (↓ 39 to ↓ 52)	↓ 64 (↓ 62 to ↓ 67)	↓ 82 (↓ 79 to ↓ 85)
Levonorgestrel			6	↓ 80 (↓ 77 to ↓ 83)	↓ 83 (↓ 79 to ↓ 87)	↓ 86 (↓ 80 to ↓ 90)
Methadone	Stable maintenance 35–100 mg daily	600 mg qd 14–21 days	11	↓ 45 (↓ 25 to ↓ 59)	↓ 52 (↓ 33 to ↓ 66)	NA
Sertraline	50 mg qd × 14 days	600 mg qd × 14 days	13	↓ 29 (↓ 15 to ↓ 40)	↓ 39 (↓ 27 to ↓ 50)	↓ 46 (↓ 31 to ↓ 58)
	400 mg po q12h × 1 day then 200 mg po q12h × 8 days	400 mg qd × 9 days	NA	↓ 61^à	↓ 77^à	NA
Voriconazole	300 mg po q12h days 2–7	300 mg qd × 7 days	NA	↓ 36^è (↓ 21 to ↓ 49)	↓ 55^è (↓ 45 to ↓ 62)	NA
	400 mg po q12h days 2–7	300 mg qd × 7 days	NA	↑ 23^è (↓ 1 to ↑ 53)	↓ 7^è (↓ 23 to ↑ 13)	NA

NA = not available
* Increase = ↑; Decrease = ↓; No Effect = ↔
† Compared with atazanavir 400 mg qd alone.
‡ Comparator dose of indinavir was 800 mg q8h × 10 days.
§ Parallel-group design; N for efavirenz + lopinavir/ritonavir, N for lopinavir/ritonavir alone.
¶ Values are for lopinavir. The pharmacokinetics of ritonavir 100 mg q12h are unaffected by concurrent efavirenz.
# 95% CI
Þ Soft Gelatin Capsule
ß Not available because of insufficient data.
à 90% CI not available
è Relative to steady-state administration of voriconazole (400 mg for 1 day, then 200 mg po q12h for 2 days).

abine, and zidovudine), NNRTIs (delavirdine, efavirenz, and nevirapine), and PIs (amprenavir, indinavir, nelfinavir, ritonavir, and saquinavir), additive to synergistic effects were observed. Tenofovir displayed antiviral activity in cell culture against HIV-1 clades A, B, C, D, E, F, G and O (EC_{50} values ranged from 0.5–2.2 µM) and showed strain specific activity against HIV-2 (EC_{50} values ranged from 1.6 µM to 5.5 µM).

Resistance
Efavirenz, Emtricitabine, and Tenofovir Disoproxil Fumarate: HIV-1 isolates with reduced susceptibility to the combination of emtricitabine and tenofovir have been selected in cell culture and in clinical studies. Genotypic analysis of these isolates identified the M184V/I and/or K65R amino acid substitutions in the viral RT.
In a clinical study of treatment-naive subjects *[Study 934, see Clinical Studies (14)]* resistance analysis was performed on HIV-1 isolates from all confirmed virologic failure subjects with >400 copies/mL of HIV-1 RNA at Week 144 or early discontinuations. Genotypic resistance to efavirenz, predominantly the K103N substitution, was the most common form of resistance that developed. Resistance to efavirenz occurred in 13/19 analyzed subjects in the emtricitabine + tenofovir DF group and in 21/29 analyzed subjects in the zidovudine/lamivudine fixed-dose combina-

tion group. The M184V amino acid substitution, associated with resistance to emtricitabine and lamivudine, was observed in 2/19 analyzed subject isolates in the emtricitabine + tenofovir DF group and in 10/29 analyzed subject isolates in the zidovudine/lamivudine group. Through 144 weeks of Study 934, no subjects developed a detectable K65R substitution in their HIV-1 as analyzed through standard genotypic analysis.
In a clinical study of treatment-naive subjects, isolates from 8/47 (17%) analyzed subjects receiving tenofovir DF developed the K65R substitution through 144 weeks of therapy; 7 of these occurred in the first 48 weeks of treatment and one at Week 96. In treatment experienced subjects, 14/304 (5%) of tenofovir DF treated subjects with virologic failure through Week 96 showed >1.4 fold (median 2.7) reduced susceptibility to tenofovir. Genotypic analysis of the resistant isolates showed a substitution in the HIV-1 RT gene resulting in the K65R amino acid substitution.
Efavirenz: Clinical isolates with reduced susceptibility in cell culture to efavirenz have been obtained. The most frequently observed amino acid substitution in clinical studies with efavirenz is K103N (54%). One or more RT substitutions at amino acid positions 98, 100, 101, 103, 106, 108, 188, 190, 225, 227, and 230 were observed in subjects failing treatment with efavirenz in combination with other antire-

trovirals. Other resistance substitutions observed to emerge commonly included L100I (7%), K101E/Q/R (14%), V108I (11%), G190S/T/A (7%), P225H (18%), and M230I/L (11%). HIV-1 isolates with reduced susceptibility to efavirenz (>380-fold increase in EC_{90} value) emerged rapidly under selection in cell culture. Genotypic characterization of these viruses identified substitutions resulting in single amino acid substitutions L100I or V179D, double substitutions L100I/V108I, and triple substitutions L100I/V179D/Y181C in RT.
Emtricitabine: Emtricitabine-resistant isolates of HIV-1 have been selected in cell culture and in clinical studies. Genotypic analysis of these isolates showed that the reduced susceptibility to emtricitabine was associated with a substitution in the HIV-1 RT gene at codon 184 which resulted in an amino acid substitution of methionine by valine or isoleucine (M184V/I).
Tenofovir Disoproxil Fumarate: HIV-1 isolates with reduced susceptibility to tenofovir have been selected in cell culture. These viruses expressed a K65R substitution in RT and showed a 2–4 fold reduction in susceptibility to tenofovir.
Cross Resistance
Efavirenz, Emtricitabine, and Tenofovir Disoproxil Fumarate: Cross-resistance has been recognized among

NNRTIs. Cross resistance has also been recognized among certain NRTIs. The M184V/I and/or K65R substitutions selected in cell culture by the combination of emtricitabine and tenofovir are also observed in some HIV-1 isolates from subjects failing treatment with tenofovir in combination with either lamivudine or emtricitabine, and either abacavir or didanosine. Therefore, cross-resistance among these drugs may occur in patients whose virus harbors either or both of these amino acid substitutions.

Efavirenz: Clinical isolates previously characterized as efavirenz-resistant were also phenotypically resistant in cell culture to delavirdine and nevirapine compared to baseline. Delavirdine- and/or nevirapine-resistant clinical viral isolates with NNRTI resistance-associated substitutions (A98G, L100I, K101E/P, K103N/S, V106A, Y181X, Y188X, G190X, P225H, F227L, or M230L) showed reduced susceptibility to efavirenz in cell culture. Greater than 90% of NRTI-resistant isolates tested in cell culture retained susceptibility to efavirenz.

Emtricitabine: Emtricitabine-resistant isolates (M184V/I) were cross-resistant to lamivudine and zalcitabine but retained susceptibility in cell culture to didanosine, stavudine, tenofovir, zidovudine, and NNRTIs (delavirdine, efavirenz, and nevirapine). HIV-1 isolates containing the K65R substitution, selected in vivo by abacavir, didanosine, tenofovir, and zalcitabine, demonstrated reduced susceptibility to inhibition by emtricitabine. Viruses harboring substitutions conferring reduced susceptibility to stavudine and zidovudine (M41L, D67N, K70R, L210W, T215Y/F, and K219Q/E) or didanosine (L74V) remained sensitive to emtricitabine.

Tenofovir Disoproxil Fumarate: The K65R substitution selected by tenofovir is also selected in some HIV-1 infected patients treated with abacavir, didanosine, or zalcitabine. HIV-1 isolates with the K65R substitution also showed reduced susceptibility to emtricitabine and lamivudine. Therefore, cross-resistance among these drugs may occur in patients whose virus harbors the K65R substitution. HIV-1 isolates from patients (N=20) whose HIV-1 expressed a mean of 3 zidovudine-associated RT amino acid substitutions (M41L, D67N, K70R, L210W, T215Y/F, or K219Q/E/N) showed a 3.1-fold decrease in the susceptibility to tenofovir. Subjects whose virus expressed an L74V substitution without zidovudine resistance associated substitutions (N=8) had reduced response to VIREAD. Limited data are available for patients whose virus expressed a Y115F substitution (N=3), Q151M substitution (N=2), or T69 insertion (N=4), all of whom had a reduced response.

13 NONCLINICAL TOXICOLOGY

13.1 Carcinogenesis, Mutagenesis, Impairment of Fertility

Efavirenz: Long-term carcinogenicity studies in mice and rats were carried out with efavirenz. Mice were dosed with 0, 25, 75, 150, or 300 mg/kg/day for 2 years. Incidences of hepatocellular adenomas and carcinomas and pulmonary alveolar/bronchiolar adenomas were increased above background in females. No increases in tumor incidence above background were seen in males. In studies in which rats were administered efavirenz at doses of 0, 25, 50, or 100 mg/kg/day for 2 years, no increases in tumor incidence above background were observed. The systemic exposure (based on AUCs) in mice was approximately 1.7-fold that in humans receiving the 600-mg/day dose. The exposure in rats was lower than that in humans. The mechanism of the carcinogenic potential is unknown. However, in genetic toxicology assays, efavirenz showed no evidence of mutagenic or clastogenic activity in a battery of in vitro and in vivo studies. These included bacterial mutation assays in *S. typhimurium* and *E. coli*, mammalian mutation assays in Chinese hamster ovary cells, chromosome aberration assays in human peripheral blood lymphocytes or Chinese hamster ovary cells, and an in vivo mouse bone marrow micronucleus assay. Given the lack of genotoxic activity of efavirenz, the relevance to humans of neoplasms in efavirenz-treated mice is not known.

Efavirenz did not impair mating or fertility of male or female rats, and did not affect sperm of treated male rats. The reproductive performance of offspring born to female rats given efavirenz was not affected. As a result of the rapid clearance of efavirenz in rats, systemic drug exposures achieved in these studies were equivalent to or below those achieved in humans given therapeutic doses of efavirenz.

Emtricitabine: In long-term carcinogenicity studies of emtricitabine, no drug-related increases in tumor incidence were found in mice at doses up to 750 mg/kg/day (26 times the human systemic exposure at the therapeutic dose of 200 mg/day) or in rats at doses up to 600 mg/day (31 times the human systemic exposure at the therapeutic dose).

Emtricitabine was not genotoxic in the reverse mutation bacterial test (Ames test), mouse lymphoma or mouse micronucleus assays.

Emtricitabine did not affect fertility in male rats at approximately 140-fold or in male and female mice at approxi-

mately 60-fold higher exposures (AUC) than in humans given the recommended 200 mg daily dose. Fertility was normal in the offspring of mice exposed daily from before birth (in utero) through sexual maturity at daily exposures (AUC) of approximately 60-fold higher than human exposures at the recommended 200 mg daily dose.

Tenofovir Disoproxil Fumarate: Long-term oral carcinogenicity studies of tenofovir DF in mice and rats were carried out at exposures up to approximately 16 times (mice) and 5 times (rats) those observed in humans at the therapeutic dose for HIV-1 infection. At the high dose in female mice, liver adenomas were increased at exposures 16 times that in humans. In rats, the study was negative for carcinogenic findings at exposures up to 5 times that observed in humans at the therapeutic dose.

Tenofovir DF was mutagenic in the in vitro mouse lymphoma assay and negative in an in vitro bacterial mutagenicity test (Ames test). In an in vivo mouse micronucleus assay, tenofovir DF was negative when administered to male mice.

There were no effects on fertility, mating performance or early embryonic development when tenofovir DF was administered to male rats at a dose equivalent to 10 times the human dose based on body surface area comparisons for 28 days prior to mating and to female rats for 15 days prior to mating through day seven of gestation. There was, however, an alteration of the estrous cycle in female rats.

13.2 Animal Toxicology and/or Pharmacology

Efavirenz: Nonsustained convulsions were observed in 6 of 20 monkeys receiving efavirenz at doses yielding plasma AUC values 4- to 13-fold greater than those in humans given the recommended dose.

Tenofovir Disoproxil Fumarate: Tenofovir and tenofovir DF administered in toxicology studies to rats, dogs and monkeys at exposures (based on AUCs) greater than or

equal to 6-fold those observed in humans caused bone toxicity. In monkeys the bone toxicity was diagnosed as osteomalacia. Osteomalacia observed in monkeys appeared to be reversible upon dose reduction or discontinuation of tenofovir. In rats and dogs, the bone toxicity manifested as reduced bone mineral density. The mechanism(s) underlying bone toxicity is unknown.

Evidence of renal toxicity was noted in 4 animal species administered tenofovir and tenofovir DF. Increases in serum creatinine, BUN, glycosuria, proteinuria, phosphaturia and/or calciuria and decreases in serum phosphate were observed to varying degrees in these animals. These toxicities were noted at exposures (based on AUCs) 2–20 times higher than those observed in humans. The relationship of the renal abnormalities, particularly the phosphaturia, to the bone toxicity is not known.

14 CLINICAL STUDIES

Clinical Study 934 supports the use of ATRIPLA tablets in antiretroviral treatment-naive HIV-1 infected patients. Additional data in support of the use of ATRIPLA in treatment-naive patients can be found in the prescribing information for VIREAD.

Clinical Study 073 provides clinical experience in subjects with stable, virologic suppression and no history of virologic failure who switched from their current regimen to ATRIPLA.

In antiretroviral treatment-experienced patients, the use of ATRIPLA tablets may be considered for patients with HIV-1 strains that are expected to be susceptible to the components of ATRIPLA as assessed by treatment history or by genotypic or phenotypic testing [See Clinical Pharmacology (12.4)].

Study 934: Data through 144 weeks are reported for Study 934, a randomized, open-label, active-controlled multicenter study comparing emtricitabine + tenofovir DF administered

Table 7 Drug Interactions: Changes in Pharmacokinetic Parameters for Tenofovir in the Presence of the Coadministered Drug*,†

Coadministered Drug	Dose of Coadministered Drug (mg)	N	Mean % Change of Tenofovir Pharmacokinetic Parameters‡ (90% CI)		
			C_{max}	AUC	C_{min}
Atazanavir§	400 once daily × 14 days	33	↑ 14 (↑ 8 to ↑ 20)	↑ 24 (↑ 21 to ↑ 28)	↑ 22 (↑ 15 to ↑ 30)
Didanosine (enteric-coated)	400 once	25	↔	↔	↔
Didanosine (buffered)	250 or 400 once daily × 7 days	14	↔	↔	↔
Lopinavir/ritonavir	400/100 twice daily × 14 days	24	↔	↑ 32 (↑ 25 to ↑ 38)	↑ 51 (↑ 37 to ↑ 66)

* All interaction studies conducted in healthy volunteers.
† Subjects received tenofovir DF 300 mg once daily.
‡ Increase = ↑; Decrease = ↓; No Effect = ↔
§ Reyataz Prescribing Information

Table 8 Drug Interactions: Changes in Pharmacokinetic Parameters for Coadministered Drug in the Presence of Tenofovir Disoproxil Fumarate*,†

Coadministered Drug	Dose of Coadministered Drug (mg)	N	Mean % Change of Coadministered Drug Pharmacokinetic Parameters‡ (90% CI)		
			C_{max}	AUC	C_{min}
Atazanavir§	400 once daily × 14 days	34	↓ 21 (↓ 27 to ↓ 14)	↓ 25 (↓ 30 to ↓ 19)	↓ 40 (↓ 48 to ↓ 32)
	Atazanavir/ritonavir 300/100 once daily × 42 days	10	↓ 28 (↓ 50 to ↑ 5)	↓ 25¶ (↓ 42 to ↓ 3)	↓ 23¶ (↓ 46 to ↑ 10)
Lopinavir	Lopinavir/ritonavir 400/100 twice daily × 14 days	24	↔	↔	↔
Ritonavir	Lopinavir/ritonavir 400/100 twice daily × 14 days	24	↔	↔	↔

* All interaction studies conducted in healthy volunteers.
† Subjects received tenofovir DF 300 mg once daily.
‡ Increase = ↑; Decrease = ↓; No Effect = ↔
§ Reyataz Prescribing Information
¶ In HIV-infected patients, addition of tenofovir DF to atazanavir 300 mg plus ritonavir 100 mg, resulted in AUC and C_{min} values of atazanavir that were 2.3- and 4-fold higher than the respective values observed for atazanavir 400 mg when given alone.

Table 9 Drug Interactions: Changes in Pharmacokinetic Parameters for Didanosine in the Presence of Tenofovir Disoproxil Fumarate[*,†]

Didanosine Dose (mg)/Method of Administration[‡]	Tenofovir DF Method of Administration[†,‡]	N	Mean % Change (90% CI) vs. Didanosine 400 mg Alone, Fasted[§]	
			C_{max}	AUC
Buffered tablets				
400 once daily[¶] × 7 days	Fasted 1 hour after didanosine	14	↑ 28 (↑ 11 to ↑ 48)	↑ 44 (↑ 31 to ↑ 59)
Enteric coated capsules				
400 once, fasted	With food, 2 hr after didanosine	26	↑ 48 (↑ 25 to ↑ 76)	↑ 48 (↑ 31 to ↑ 67)
400 once, with food	Simultaneously with didanosine	26	↑ 64 (↑ 41 to ↑ 89)	↑ 60 (↑ 44 to ↑ 79)
250 once, fasted	With food, 2 hr after didanosine	28	↓ 10 (↓ 22 to ↑ 3)	↔
250 once, fasted	Simultaneously with didanosine	28	↔	↑ 14 (0 to ↑ 31)
250 once, with food	Simultaneously with didanosine	28	↓ 29 (↓ 39 to ↓ 18)	↓ 11 (↓ 23 to ↑ 2)

* All interaction studies conducted in healthy volunteers.
† Subjects received tenofovir DF 300 mg once daily.
‡ Administration with food was with a light meal (~373 kcal, 20% fat).
§ Increase = ↑; Decrease = ↓; No Effect = ↔
¶ Includes 4 subjects weighing <60 kg receiving ddI 250 mg.

Table 10 Outcomes of Randomized Treatment at Weeks 48 and 144 (Study 934)

Outcomes	At Week 48		At Week 144	
	FTC + TDF +EFV (N=244)	AZT/3TC +EFV (N=243)	FTC + TDF +EFV (N=227)*	AZT/3TC +EFV (N=229)*
Responder[†]	84%	73%	71%	58%
Virologic failure[‡]	2%	4%	3%	6%
Rebound	1%	3%	2%	5%
Never suppressed	0%	0%	0%	0%
Change in antiretroviral regimen	1%	1%	1%	1%
Death	<1%	1%	1%	1%
Discontinued due to adverse event	4%	9%	5%	12%
Discontinued for other reasons[§]	10%	14%	20%	22%

* Subjects who were responders at Week 48 or Week 96 (HIV-1 RNA <400 copies/mL) but did not consent to continue study after Week 48 or Week 96 were excluded from analysis.
† Subjects achieved and maintained confirmed HIV-1 RNA <400 copies/mL through Weeks 48 and 144.
‡ Includes confirmed viral rebound and failure to achieve confirmed HIV-1 RNA <400 copies/mL through Weeks 48 and 144.
§ Includes lost to follow-up, patient withdrawal, noncompliance, protocol violation and other reasons.

in combination with efavirenz versus zidovudine/lamivudine fixed-dose combination administered in combination with efavirenz in 511 antiretroviral-naive subjects. From weeks 96 to 144 of the study, subjects received emtricitabine/tenofovir DF fixed-dose combination with efavirenz in place of emtricitabine + tenofovir DF with efavirenz. Subjects had a mean age of 38 years (range 18–80), 86% were male, 59% were Caucasian and 23% were Black. The mean baseline CD4[+] cell count was 245 cells/mm³ (range 2–1191) and median baseline plasma HIV-1 RNA was 5.01 log_{10} copies/mL (range 3.56–6.54). Subjects were stratified by baseline CD4[+] cell count (< or ≥ 200 cells/mm³) and 41% had CD4[+] cell counts <200 cells/mm³. Fifty-one percent (51%) of subjects had baseline viral loads >100,000 copies/mL. Treatment outcomes through 48 and 144 weeks for those subjects who did not have efavirenz resistance at baseline (n=487) are presented in Table 10. [See table 10 above]
Through Week 48, 84% and 73% of subjects in the emtricitabine + tenofovir DF group and the zidovudine/lamivudine group, respectively, achieved and maintained HIV-1 RNA <400 copies/mL (71% and 58% through Week 144). The difference in the proportion of subjects who achieved and maintained HIV-1 RNA <400 copies/mL through 48 weeks largely results from the higher number of discontinuations due to adverse events and other reasons in

the zidovudine/lamivudine group in this open-label study. In addition, 80% and 70% of subjects in the emtricitabine + tenofovir DF group and the zidovudine/lamivudine group, respectively, achieved and maintained HIV-1 RNA <50 copies/mL through Week 48 (64% and 56% through Week 144). The mean increase from baseline in CD4[+] cell count was 190 cells/mm³ in the emtricitabine + tenofovir DF group and 158 cells/mm³ in the zidovudine/lamivudine group at Week 48 (312 and 271 cells/mm³ at Week 144).
Through 48 weeks, 7 subjects in the emtricitabine + tenofovir DF group and 5 subjects in the zidovudine/lamivudine group experienced a new CDC Class C event (10 and 6 subjects through 144 weeks).
Study 073: Study 073 was a 48-week open-label, randomized clinical trial in subjects with stable, virologic suppression on combination antiretroviral therapy consisting of at least two nucleoside reverse transcriptase inhibitors (NRTIs) administered in combination with a protease inhibitor (with or without ritonavir) or a non-nucleoside reverse transcriptase inhibitor (NNRTI). To be enrolled, subjects were to have HIV-1 RNA <200 copies/mL for at least 12 weeks on their current regimen prior to study entry with no known HIV-1 substitutions conferring resistance to the components of ATRIPLA and no history of virologic failure. The study compared the efficacy of switching to ATRIPLA or staying on the baseline antiretroviral regimen (SBR). Subjects were

randomized in a 2:1 ratio to switch to ATRIPLA (N=203) or stay on SBR (N=97). Subjects had a mean age of 43 years (range 22 to 73 years), 88% were male, 68% were white, 29% were black or African-American, and 3% were of other races. At baseline, median CD4[+] cell count was 516 cells/mm³ and 96% had HIV-1 RNA <50 copies/mL. The median time since onset of antiretroviral therapy was 3 years and 88% of subjects were receiving their first antiretroviral regimen at study enrollment.
At Week 48, 89% and 87% of subjects who switched to ATRIPLA maintained HIV-1 RNA <200 copies/mL and <50 copies/mL, respectively, compared to 88% and 85% who remained on SBR; this difference was not statistically significant. No changes in CD4+ cell counts from baseline to Week 48 were observed in either treatment arm.

16   HOW SUPPLIED/STORAGE AND HANDLING
ATRIPLA tablets are pink, capsule-shaped, film-coated, debossed with "123" on one side and plain-faced on the other side. Each bottle contains 30 tablets (NDC 15584-0101-1) and silica gel desiccant, and is closed with a child-resistant closure.
Store at 25 °C (77 °F); excursions permitted to 15–30 °C (59–86 °F) [See USP Controlled Room Temperature].
• Keep container tightly closed.
• Dispense only in original container.
• Do not use if seal over bottle opening is broken or missing.

17   PATIENT COUNSELING INFORMATION AND FDA-APPROVED PATIENT LABELING
17.1   Drug Interactions
A statement to patients and healthcare providers is included on the product's bottle labels: *ALERT: Find out about medicines that should NOT be taken with ATRIPLA.* ATRIPLA may interact with some drugs; therefore, patients should be advised to report to their doctor the use of any other prescription, nonprescription medication, or herbal products, particularly St. John's wort.
17.2   Information for Patients
Patients should be advised that:
• ATRIPLA is not a cure for HIV-1 infection and that they may continue to experience illnesses associated with HIV-1 infection, including opportunistic infections. Patients should remain under the care of a physician when using ATRIPLA.
• The use of ATRIPLA has not been shown to reduce the risk of transmission of HIV-1 to others through sexual contact or blood contamination. Patients should be advised to continue to practice safer sex and to use latex or polyurethane condoms to lower the chance of sexual contact with any body fluids such as semen, vaginal secretions or blood. Patients should be advised never to re-use or share needles.
• The long term effects of ATRIPLA are unknown.
• Redistribution or accumulation of body fat may occur in patients receiving antiretroviral therapy and that the cause and long-term health effects of these conditions are not known.
• ATRIPLA should not be coadministered with SUSTIVA, EMTRIVA, VIREAD, or TRUVADA, or drugs containing lamivudine, including Combivir, Epivir, Epivir-HBV, Epzicom, or Trizivir.
• ATRIPLA should not be administered with HEPSERA [See Warnings and Precautions (5.2)].
17.3   Lactic Acidosis/Severe Hepatomegaly with Steatosis
Patients should be informed that lactic acidosis and severe hepatomegaly with steatosis, including fatal cases, have been reported. Treatment will be suspended in any patients who develop clinical symptoms suggestive of lactic acidosis or pronounced hepatotoxicity (including nausea, vomiting, unusual or unexpected stomach discomfort, and weakness) [See Warnings and Precautions (5.1)].
17.4   Patients Coinfected with HIV-1 and HBV
Patients with HIV-1 should be tested for hepatitis B virus (HBV) before initiating antiretroviral therapy.
Patients should be advised that severe acute exacerbations of hepatitis B have been reported in patients who are coinfected with HBV and HIV-1 and have discontinued EMTRIVA (emtricitabine) or VIREAD (tenofovir DF), which are components of ATRIPLA.
17.5   New Onset or Worsening Renal Impairment
Renal impairment, including cases of acute renal failure and Fanconi syndrome, has been reported. ATRIPLA should be avoided with concurrent or recent use of a nephrotoxic agent [See Warnings and Precautions (5.7)].
17.6   Decreases in Bone Mineral Density
Patients should be informed that decreases in bone mineral density have been observed with the use of tenofovir DF. Bone mineral density monitoring may be performed in patients who have a history of pathologic bone fracture or are at risk for osteopenia [See Warnings and Precautions (5.11)].
17.7   Dosing Instructions
Patients should be advised to take ATRIPLA orally on an empty stomach and that it is important to take ATRIPLA on a regular dosing schedule to avoid missing doses.

17.8 Nervous System Symptoms

Patients should be informed that central nervous system symptoms (NSS) including dizziness, insomnia, impaired concentration, drowsiness, and abnormal dreams are commonly reported during the first weeks of therapy with efavirenz. Dosing at bedtime may improve the tolerability of these symptoms, which are likely to improve with continued therapy. Patients should be alerted to the potential for additive effects when ATRIPLA is used concomitantly with alcohol or psychoactive drugs. Patients should be instructed that if they experience NSS they should avoid potentially hazardous tasks such as driving or operating machinery [See Warnings and Precautions (5.6), and Dosage and Administration (2)].

17.9 Psychiatric Symptoms

Patients should be informed that serious psychiatric symptoms including severe depression, suicide attempts, aggressive behavior, delusions, paranoia, and psychosis-like symptoms have been reported in patients receiving efavirenz. If they experience severe psychiatric adverse experiences they should seek immediate medical evaluation. Patients should be advised to inform their physician of any history of mental illness or substance abuse [See Warnings and Precautions (5.5)].

17.10 Rash

Patients should be informed that a common side effect is rash. Rashes usually go away without any change in treatment. However, since rash may be serious, patients should be advised to contact their physician promptly if rash occurs.

17.11 Reproductive Risk Potential

Women receiving ATRIPLA should be instructed to avoid pregnancy [See Warnings and Precautions (5.8)]. A reliable form of barrier contraception must always be used in combination with other methods of contraception, including oral or other hormonal contraception. Because of the long half-life of efavirenz, use of adequate contraceptive measures for 12 weeks after discontinuation of ATRIPLA is recommended. Women should be advised to notify their physician if they become pregnant or plan to become pregnant while taking ATRIPLA. If this drug is used during the first trimester of pregnancy, or if the patient becomes pregnant while taking this drug, she should be apprised of the potential harm to the fetus.

FDA-APPROVED PATIENT LABELING

Patient Information

ATRIPLA® (uh TRIP luh) Tablets

ALERT: Find out about medicines that should NOT be taken with ATRIPLA.

Please also read the section "MEDICINES YOU SHOULD NOT TAKE WITH ATRIPLA."

Generic name: efavirenz, emtricitabine and tenofovir disoproxil fumarate

(eh FAH vih renz, em tri SIT uh bean and te NOE' fo veer dye soe PROX il FYOU mar ate)

Read the Patient Information that comes with ATRIPLA before you start taking it and each time you get a refill since there may be new information. This information does not take the place of talking to your healthcare provider about your medical condition or treatment. You should stay under a healthcare provider's care when taking ATRIPLA. **Do not change or stop your medicine without first talking with your healthcare provider.** Talk to your healthcare provider or pharmacist if you have any questions about ATRIPLA.

What is the most important information I should know about ATRIPLA?

- **Some people who have taken medicine like ATRIPLA (which contains nucleoside analogs) have developed a serious condition called lactic acidosis** (build up of an acid in the blood). Lactic acidosis can be a medical emergency and may need to be treated in the hospital. **Call your healthcare provider right away if you get the following signs or symptoms of lactic acidosis:**
  - You feel very weak or tired.
  - You have unusual (not normal) muscle pain.
  - You have trouble breathing.
  - You have stomach pain with nausea and vomiting.
  - You feel cold, especially in your arms and legs.
  - You feel dizzy or lightheaded.
  - You have a fast or irregular heartbeat.
- **Some people who have taken medicines like ATRIPLA have developed serious liver problems called hepatotoxicity, with liver enlargement (hepatomegaly) and fat in the liver (steatosis). Call your healthcare provider right away if you get the following signs or symptoms of liver problems:**
  - Your skin or the white part of your eyes turns yellow (jaundice).
  - Your urine turns dark.
  - Your bowel movements (stools) turn light in color.
  - You don't feel like eating food for several days or longer.
  - You feel sick to your stomach (nausea).
  - You have lower stomach area (abdominal) pain.

- **You may be more likely to get lactic acidosis or liver problems** if you are female, very overweight (obese), or have been taking nucleoside analog-containing medicines, like ATRIPLA, for a long time.
- **If you also have hepatitis B virus (HBV) infection and you stop taking ATRIPLA, you may get a "flare-up" of your hepatitis.** A "flare-up" is when the disease suddenly returns in a worse way than before. Patients with HBV who stop taking ATRIPLA need close medical follow-up for several months, including medical exams and blood tests to check for hepatitis that could be getting worse. ATRIPLA is not approved for the treatment of HBV, so you must discuss your HBV therapy with your healthcare provider.

What is ATRIPLA?

ATRIPLA contains 3 medicines, SUSTIVA® (efavirenz), EMTRIVA® (emtricitabine) and VIREAD® (tenofovir disoproxil fumarate also called tenofovir DF) combined in one pill. EMTRIVA and VIREAD are HIV-1 (human immunodeficiency virus) nucleoside analog reverse transcriptase inhibitors (NRTIs) and SUSTIVA is an HIV-1 non-nucleoside analog reverse transcriptase inhibitor (NNRTI). VIREAD and EMTRIVA are the components of TRUVADA®. ATRIPLA can be used alone as a complete regimen, or in combination with other anti-HIV-1 medicines to treat people with HIV-1 infection. ATRIPLA is for adults age 18 and over. ATRIPLA has not been studied in children under age 18 or adults over age 65.

HIV infection destroys CD4+ T cells, which are important to the immune system. The immune system helps fight infection. After a large number of T cells are destroyed, acquired immune deficiency syndrome (AIDS) develops.

ATRIPLA helps block HIV-1 reverse transcriptase, a viral chemical in your body (enzyme) that is needed for HIV-1 to multiply. ATRIPLA lowers the amount of HIV-1 in the blood (viral load). ATRIPLA may also help to increase the number of T cells (CD4+ cells), allowing your immune system to improve. Lowering the amount of HIV-1 in the blood lowers the chance of death or infections that happen when your immune system is weak (opportunistic infections).

Does ATRIPLA cure HIV-1 or AIDS?

ATRIPLA **does not cure HIV-1 infection or AIDS.** The long-term effects of ATRIPLA are not known at this time. People taking ATRIPLA may still get opportunistic infections or other conditions that happen with HIV-1 infection. Opportunistic infections are infections that develop because the immune system is weak. Some of these conditions are pneumonia, herpes virus infections, and *Mycobacterium avium complex* (MAC) infection. **It is very important that you see your healthcare provider regularly while taking ATRIPLA.**

Does ATRIPLA reduce the risk of passing HIV-1 to others?

ATRIPLA **has not been shown to lower your chance of passing HIV-1 to other people through sexual contact, sharing needles, or being exposed to your blood.**

- **Do not share needles or other injection equipment.**
- **Do not share personal items that can have blood or body fluids on them, like toothbrushes or razor blades.**
- **Do not have any kind of sex without protection.** Always practice safer sex by using a latex or polyurethane condom or other barrier to reduce the chance of sexual contact with semen, vaginal secretions, or blood.

Who should not take ATRIPLA?

Together with your healthcare provider, you need to decide whether ATRIPLA is right for you.

Do not take ATRIPLA if you are allergic to ATRIPLA or any of its ingredients. The active ingredients of ATRIPLA are efavirenz, emtricitabine, and tenofovir DF. See the end of this leaflet for a complete list of ingredients.

What should I tell my healthcare provider before taking ATRIPLA?

Tell your healthcare provider if you:

- **Are pregnant or planning to become pregnant** (see "What should I avoid while taking ATRIPLA?").
- **Are breastfeeding** (see "What should I avoid while taking ATRIPLA?").
- **Have kidney problems or are undergoing kidney dialysis treatment.**
- **Have bone problems.**
- **Have liver problems, including hepatitis B virus infection.** Your healthcare provider may want to do tests to check your liver while you take ATRIPLA.
- **Have ever had mental illness or are using drugs or alcohol.**
- **Have ever had seizures or are taking medicine for seizures.**

What important information should I know about taking other medicines with ATRIPLA?

ATRIPLA may change the effect of other medicines, including the ones for HIV-1, and may cause serious side effects. Your healthcare provider may change your other medicines or change their doses. Other medicines, including herbal products, may affect ATRIPLA. For this reason, **it is very**

important to let all your healthcare providers and pharmacists know what medications, herbal supplements, or vitamins you are taking.

MEDICINES YOU SHOULD NOT TAKE WITH ATRIPLA

- The following medicines may cause serious and life-threatening side effects when taken with ATRIPLA. You should not take any of these medicines while taking ATRIPLA: Vascor (bepridil), Propulsid (cisapride), Versed (midazolam), Orap (pimozide), Halcion (triazolam), ergot medications (for example, Wigraine and Cafergot).
- ATRIPLA also should not be used with Combivir (lamivudine/zidovudine), EMTRIVA, Epivir, Epivir-HBV (lamivudine), Epzicom (abacavir sulfate/lamivudine), Trizivir (abacavir sulfate/lamivudine/zidovudine), SUSTIVA, TRUVADA, or VIREAD.
- Vfend (voriconazole) should not be taken with ATRIPLA since it may lose its effect or may increase the chance of having side effects from ATRIPLA.
- **Do not take St. John's wort (*Hypericum perforatum*), or products containing St. John's wort with ATRIPLA.** St. John's wort is an herbal product sold as a dietary supplement. Talk with your healthcare provider if you are taking or are planning to take St. John's wort. Taking St. John's wort may decrease ATRIPLA levels and lead to increased viral load and possible resistance to ATRIPLA or cross-resistance to other anti-HIV-1 drugs.
- ATRIPLA should not be used with HEPSERA® (adefovir dipivoxil).

It is also important to tell your healthcare provider if you are taking any of the following:

- Fortovase, Invirase (saquinavir), Biaxin (clarithromycin), Noxafil (posaconazole), or Sporanox (itraconazole); **these medicines may need to be replaced with another medicine when taken with ATRIPLA.**
- Calcium channel blockers such as Cardizem or Tiazac (diltiazem), Covera HS or Isoptin (verapamil) and others; Crixivan (indinavir), Selzentry (maraviroc); the immunosuppressant medicines cyclosporine (Gengraf, Neoral, Sandimmune, and others), Prograf (tacrolimus), or Rapamune (sirolimus); Methadone; Mycobutin (rifabutin); Rifampin; cholesterol-lowering medicines such as Lipitor (atorvastatin), Pravachol (pravastatin sodium), and Zocor (simvastatin); or Zoloft (sertraline); **these medicines may need to have their dose changed when taken with ATRIPLA.**
- Videx, Videx EC (didanosine); tenofovir DF (a component of ATRIPLA) may increase the amount of didanosine in your blood, which could result in more side effects. **You may need to be monitored more carefully** if you are taking ATRIPLA and didanosine together. Also, the dose of didanosine may need to be changed.
- Reyataz (atazanavir sulfate) or Kaletra (lopinavir/ritonavir); these medicines may increase the amount of tenofovir DF (a component of ATRIPLA) in your blood, which could result in more side effects. Reyataz is not recommended with ATRIPLA. **You may need to be monitored more carefully** if you are taking ATRIPLA and Kaletra together. Also, the dose of Kaletra may need to be changed.
- Medicine for seizures [for example, Dilantin (phenytoin), Tegretol (carbamazepine), or phenobarbital]; your healthcare provider may want to switch you to another medicine or check drug levels in your blood from time to time.

These are not all the medicines that may cause problems if you take ATRIPLA. Be sure to tell your healthcare provider about all medicines that you take.

Keep a complete list of all the prescription and nonprescription medicines as well as any herbal remedies that you are taking, how much you take, and how often you take them. Make a new list when medicines or herbal remedies are added or stopped, or if the dose changes. Give copies of this list to all of your healthcare providers and pharmacists every time you visit your healthcare provider or fill a prescription. This will give your healthcare provider a complete picture of the medicines you use. Then he or she can decide the best approach for your situation.

How should I take ATRIPLA?

- Take the exact amount of ATRIPLA your healthcare provider prescribes. Never change the dose on your own. Do not stop this medicine unless your healthcare provider tells you to stop.
- You should take ATRIPLA on an empty stomach.
- Swallow ATRIPLA with water.
- Taking ATRIPLA at bedtime may make some side effects less bothersome.
- Do not miss a dose of ATRIPLA. If you forget to take ATRIPLA, take the missed dose right away, unless it is almost time for your next dose. Do not double the next dose. Carry on with your regular dosing schedule. If you need help in planning the best times to take your medicine, ask your healthcare provider or pharmacist.
- If you believe you took more than the prescribed amount of ATRIPLA, contact your local poison control center or emergency room right away.

- Tell your healthcare provider if you start any new medicine or change how you take old ones. Your doses may need adjustment.
- When your ATRIPLA supply starts to run low, get more from your healthcare provider or pharmacy. This is very important because the amount of virus in your blood may increase if the medicine is stopped for even a short time. The virus may develop resistance to ATRIPLA and become harder to treat.
- Your healthcare provider may want to do blood tests to check for certain side effects while you take ATRIPLA.

What should I avoid while taking ATRIPLA?
- **Women should not become pregnant while taking ATRIPLA and for 12 weeks after stopping it.** Serious birth defects have been seen in the babies of animals and women treated with efavirenz (a component of ATRIPLA) during pregnancy. It is not known whether efavirenz caused these defects. **Tell your healthcare provider right away if you are pregnant.** Also talk with your healthcare provider if you want to become pregnant.
- Women should not rely only on hormone-based birth control, such as pills, injections, or implants, because ATRIPLA may make these contraceptives ineffective. Women must use a reliable form of barrier contraception, such as a condom or diaphragm, even if they also use other methods of birth control. Efavirenz, a component of ATRIPLA, may remain in your blood for a time after therapy is stopped. Therefore, you should continue to use contraceptive measures for 12 weeks after you stop taking ATRIPLA.
- **Do not breast-feed if you are taking ATRIPLA.** The Centers for Disease Control and Prevention recommend that mothers with HIV not breast-feed because they can pass the HIV through their milk to the baby. Also, ATRIPLA may pass through breast milk and cause serious harm to the baby. Talk with your healthcare provider if you are breast-feeding. You should stop breast-feeding or may need to use a different medicine.
- Taking ATRIPLA with alcohol or other medicines causing similar side effects as ATRIPLA, such as drowsiness, may increase those side effects.
- Do not take any other medicines, including prescription and nonprescription medicines and herbal products, without checking with your healthcare provider.
- **Avoid doing things that can spread HIV-1 infection** since ATRIPLA does not stop you from passing the HIV-1 infection to others.

What are the possible side effects of ATRIPLA?
ATRIPLA may cause the following serious side effects:
- **Lactic acidosis** (buildup of an acid in the blood). Lactic acidosis can be a medical emergency and may need to be treated in the hospital. **Call your healthcare provider right away if you get signs of lactic acidosis.** (See "What is the most important information I should know about ATRIPLA?")
- **Serious liver problems (hepatotoxicity),** with liver enlargement (hepatomegaly) and fat in the liver (steatosis). Call your healthcare provider right away if you get any signs of liver problems. (See "What is the most important information I should know about ATRIPLA?")
- **"Flare-ups" of hepatitis B virus (HBV) infection,** in which the disease suddenly returns in a worse way than before, can occur if you have HBV and you stop taking ATRIPLA. Your healthcare provider will monitor your condition for several months after stopping ATRIPLA if you have both HIV-1 and HBV infection and may recommend treatment for your HBV. ATRIPLA is not approved for the treatment of hepatitis B virus infection. If you have advanced liver disease and stop treatment with ATRIPLA, the "flare-up" of hepatitis B may cause your liver function to decline.
- **Serious psychiatric problems.** A small number of patients may experience severe depression, strange thoughts, or angry behavior while taking ATRIPLA. Some patients have thoughts of suicide and a few have actually committed suicide. These problems may occur more often in patients who have had mental illness. Contact your healthcare provider right away if you think you are having these psychiatric symptoms, so your healthcare provider can decide if you should continue to take ATRIPLA.
- **Kidney problems** (including decline or failure of kidney function). If you have had kidney problems in the past or take other medicines that can cause kidney problems, your healthcare provider should do regular blood tests to check your kidneys. Symptoms that may be related to kidney problems include a high volume of urine, thirst, muscle pain, and muscle weakness.
- **Other serious liver problems.** Some patients have experienced serious liver problems including liver failure resulting in transplantation or death. Most of these serious side effects occurred in patients with a chronic liver disease such as hepatitis infection, but there have also been a few reports in patients without any existing liver disease.
- **Changes in bone mineral density (thinning bones).** Laboratory tests show changes in the bones of patients treated

with tenofovir DF, a component of ATRIPLA. Some HIV patients treated with tenofovir DF developed thinning of the bones (osteopenia) which could lead to fractures. If you have had bone problems in the past, your healthcare provider may need to do tests to check your bone mineral density or may prescribe medicines to help your bone mineral density. Additionally, bone pain and softening of the bone (which may contribute to fractures) may occur as a consequence of kidney problems.

Common side effects:
Patients may have dizziness, headache, trouble sleeping, drowsiness, trouble concentrating, and/or unusual dreams during treatment with ATRIPLA. These side effects may be reduced if you take ATRIPLA at bedtime on an empty stomach. They also tend to go away after you have taken the medicine for a few weeks. If you have these common side effects, such as dizziness, it does not mean that you will also have serious psychiatric problems, such as severe depression, strange thoughts, or angry behavior. Tell your healthcare provider right away if any of these side effects continue or if they bother you. It is possible that these symptoms may be more severe if ATRIPLA is used with alcohol or mood altering (street) drugs.
If you are dizzy, have trouble concentrating, or are drowsy, avoid activities that may be dangerous, such as driving or operating machinery.
Rash may be common. Rashes usually go away without any change in treatment. In a small number of patients, rash may be serious. If you develop a rash, call your healthcare provider right away.
Other common side effects include tiredness, upset stomach, vomiting, gas, and diarrhea.

Other possible side effects with ATRIPLA:
- Changes in body fat. Changes in body fat develop in some patients taking anti HIV-1 medicine. These changes may include an increased amount of fat in the upper back and neck ("buffalo hump"), in the breasts, and around the trunk. Loss of fat from the legs, arms, and face may also happen. The cause and long-term health effects of these fat changes are not known.
- Skin discoloration (small spots or freckles) may also happen with ATRIPLA.
- In some patients with advanced HIV infection (AIDS), signs and symptoms of inflammation from previous infections may occur soon after anti-HIV treatment is started. It is believed that these symptoms are due to an improvement in the body's immune response, enabling the body to fight infections that may have been present with no obvious symptoms. If you notice any symptoms of infection, please inform your doctor immediately.
- Additional side effects are inflammation of the pancreas, allergic reaction (including swelling of the face, lips, tongue, or throat), shortness of breath, pain, stomach pain, weakness and indigestion.

Tell your healthcare provider or pharmacist if you notice any side effects while taking ATRIPLA.
Contact your healthcare provider before stopping ATRIPLA because of side effects or for any other reason.
This is not a complete list of side effects possible with ATRIPLA. Ask your healthcare provider or pharmacist for a more complete list of side effects of ATRIPLA and all the medicines you will take.

How do I store ATRIPLA?
- **Keep ATRIPLA and all other medicines out of reach of children.**
- Store ATRIPLA at room temperature 77 °F (25 °C).
- Keep ATRIPLA in its original container and keep the container tightly closed.
- Do not keep medicine that is out of date or that you no longer need. If you throw any medicines away make sure that children will not find them.

General information about ATRIPLA:
Medicines are sometimes prescribed for conditions that are not mentioned in patient information leaflets. Do not use ATRIPLA for a condition for which it was not prescribed. Do not give ATRIPLA to other people, even if they have the same symptoms you have. It may harm them.
This leaflet summarizes the most important information about ATRIPLA. If you would like more information, talk with your healthcare provider. You can ask your healthcare provider or pharmacist for information about ATRIPLA that is written for health professionals.
Do not use ATRIPLA if the seal over bottle opening is broken or missing.

What are the ingredients of ATRIPLA?
Active Ingredients: efavirenz, emtricitabine, and tenofovir disoproxil fumarate
Inactive Ingredients: croscarmellose sodium, hydroxypropyl cellulose, microcrystalline cellulose, magnesium stearate, sodium lauryl sulfate. The film coating contains black iron oxide, polyethylene glycol, polyvinyl alcohol, red iron oxide, talc, and titanium dioxide.

℞ Only
May 2010

ATRIPLA is a trademark of Bristol-Myers Squibb & Gilead Sciences, LLC. EMTRIVA, TRUVADA, HEPSERA and VIREAD are trademarks of Gilead Sciences, Inc. SUSTIVA is a trademark of Bristol-Myers Squibb Pharma Company. Reyataz and Videx are trademarks of Bristol-Myers Squibb Company. Pravachol is a trademark of ER Squibb & Sons, LLC. Other brands listed are the trademarks of their respective owners.
21-937-GS-007 May 2010

Celltech Pharmaceuticals, Inc.
for product information, please see UCB Inc.

Centocor Ortho Biotech Inc.
**800 RIDGEVIEW DRIVE
HORSHAM, PA 19044
USA**
www.centocororthobiotech.com

Direct General Inquiries to:
Ph: (610) 651-6000
Fax: (610) 651-6100
Medical Emergency Contact:
Ph: (800) 457-6399
For Medical Information/Adverse Experience Reporting Contact:
Medical Information
Ph: (800) 457-6399

REMICADE®   ℞
[rem-eh-kaid]
(infliximab)
Lyophilized Concentrate for Intravenous (IV) Injection

HIGHLIGHTS OF PRESCRIBING INFORMATION
These highlights do not include all the information needed to use REMICADE® safely and effectively. See full prescribing information for REMICADE.
REMICADE (infliximab)
Lyophilized Concentrate for Intravenous (IV) Injection
Initial U.S. Approval: 1998

> **WARNINGS:**
> *See full prescribing information for complete boxed warning*
> **SERIOUS INFECTIONS**
> - **Increased risk of serious infections leading to hospitalization or death, including tuberculosis (TB), bacterial sepsis, invasive fungal infections (such as histoplasmosis) and infections due to other opportunistic pathogens.**
> - **REMICADE should be discontinued if a patient develops a serious infection or sepsis during treatment.**
> - **Perform test for latent TB; if positive, start treatment for TB prior to starting REMICADE.**
> - **Monitor all patients for active TB during treatment, even if initial latent TB test is negative. (5.1)**
> **MALIGNANCY**
> - **Lymphoma and other malignancies, some fatal, have been reported in children and adolescent patients treated with TNF blockers, including REMICADE. (5.2)**
> - **Postmarketing cases of hepatosplenic T-cell lymphoma (HSTCL), a rare type of T-cell lymphoma, have been reported in patients treated with TNF blockers including REMICADE. All cases were reported in patients with Crohn's disease and ulcerative colitis, the majority of whom were adolescent or young adult males. This rare, aggressive T-cell lymphoma is fatal. All of these patients had received treatment with azathioprine or 6-mercaptopurine concomitantly with REMICADE at or prior to diagnosis. (5.2)**

──────RECENT MAJOR CHANGES──────

Boxed Warnings: MALIGNANCY (Lymphoma)	11/2009
Boxed Warnings: MALIGNANCY (HSTCL)	4/2009
Dosage and Administration (2.7)	4/2010
Warnings and Precautions: Malignancy, (Lymphoma) (5.2)	11/2009
Warnings and Precautions: Malignancy, (HSTCL) (5.2)	4/2009

──────INDICATIONS AND USAGE──────
REMICADE is a tumor necrosis factor (TNF) blocker indicated for:
Crohn's Disease (1.1):
- reducing signs and symptoms and inducing and maintaining clinical remission in adult and pediatric patients with

moderately to severely active disease who have had an inadequate response to conventional therapy.

• reducing the number of draining enterocutaneous and rectovaginal fistulas and maintaining fistula closure in adult patients with fistulizing disease.

Ulcerative Colitis (1.2):

• reducing signs and symptoms, inducing and maintaining clinical remission and mucosal healing, and eliminating corticosteroid use in patients with moderately to severely active disease who have had an inadequate response to conventional therapy.

Rheumatoid Arthritis (1.3) in combination with methotrexate:

• reducing signs and symptoms, inhibiting the progression of structural damage, and improving physical function in patients with moderately to severely active disease.

Ankylosing Spondylitis (1.4):

• reducing signs and symptoms in patients with active disease.

Psoriatic Arthritis (1.5):

• reducing signs and symptoms of active arthritis, inhibiting the progression of structural damage, and improving physical function.

Plaque Psoriasis (1.6):

• treatment of adult patients with chronic severe (i.e., extensive and /or disabling) plaque psoriasis who are candidates for systemic therapy and when other systemic therapies are medically less appropriate.

──────────DOSAGE AND ADMINISTRATION──────────

REMICADE is administered by intravenous infusion.

Crohn's Disease (2.1)

• 5 mg/kg at 0, 2 and 6 weeks, then every 8 weeks. Some adult patients who initially respond to treatment may benefit from increasing the dose to 10 mg/kg if they later lose their response.

Ulcerative Colitis (2.2)

• 5 mg/kg at 0, 2 and 6 weeks, then every 8 weeks.

Rheumatoid Arthritis (2.3)

• In conjunction with methotrexate, 3 mg/kg at 0, 2 and 6 weeks, then every 8 weeks. Some patients may benefit from increasing the dose up to 10 mg/kg or treating as often as every 4 weeks.

Ankylosing Spondylitis (2.4)

• 5 mg/kg at 0, 2 and 6 weeks, then every 6 weeks.

Psoriatic Arthritis (2.5)

• 5 mg/kg at 0, 2 and 6 weeks, then every 8 weeks.

Plaque Psoriasis (2.6)

• 5 mg/kg at 0, 2 and 6 weeks, then every 8 weeks.

──────────DOSAGE FORMS AND STRENGTHS──────────

100 mg of lyophilized infliximab in a 20 mL vial to be reconstituted in 10 mL of sterile water for injection. (3)

──────────CONTRAINDICATIONS──────────

• REMICADE doses >5 mg/kg in moderate to severe heart failure. (4)

• Previous severe hypersensitivity reaction to REMICADE or known hypersensitivity to inactive components of REMICADE or to any murine proteins. (4)

──────────WARNINGS AND PRECAUTIONS──────────

• Serious infections–do not give REMICADE during an active infection. If an infection develops, monitor carefully and stop REMICADE if infection becomes serious. (5.1)

• Malignancies–seen more often than in controls. Lymphoma seen more often than in the general population; carefully assess the risks and benefits of treatment and monitor for malignancies in children and adolescents. (5.2)

• Hepatosplenic T-cell Lymphoma–carefully assess the risk benefit especially if the patient has Crohn's disease or ulcerative colitis, is male, and is receiving azathioprine or 6-mercaptopurine treatment (5.2)

• Hepatitis B virus reactivation–monitor HBV carriers during and several months after therapy. If reactivation occurs, stop REMICADE and begin anti-viral therapy. (5.3)

• Hepatotoxicity–rare severe hepatic reactions, some fatal or necessitating liver transplantation. Stop REMICADE in cases of jaundice and/or marked liver enzyme elevations. (5.4)

• Heart failure–closely monitor patients with heart failure and stop REMICADE if new or worsening symptoms occur. (4, 5.5)

• Cytopenias–advise patients to seek immediate medical attention if signs and symptoms develop, and consider stopping REMICADE. (5.6)

• Hypersensitivity–serious infusion reactions including anaphylaxis or serum sickness-like reactions may occur. (5.7)

• Demyelinating disease–consider stopping REMICADE if exacerbation or new onset occurs. (5.8)

• Lupus-like syndrome–stop REMICADE if syndrome develops. (5.10)

──────────ADVERSE REACTIONS──────────

Most common adverse reactions (>10%)–infections (e.g. upper respiratory, sinusitis, and pharyngitis), infusion-related reactions, headache, and abdominal pain. (6.1)

To report SUSPECTED ADVERSE REACTIONS, contact Centocor at 1-800-457-6399 or FDA at 1-800-FDA-1088 or *www.fda.gov/medwatch.*

──────────DRUG INTERACTIONS──────────

• Anakinra–increased risk of serious infections (7.1)

• Live vaccines–should not be given with REMICADE. Bring pediatric Crohn's patients up to date with all vaccinations prior to initiating REMICADE. (5.11)

──────────USE IN SPECIFIC POPULATIONS──────────

• Pediatric Use–Although indicated for use in pediatric Crohn's disease, REMICADE has not been studied in children with Crohn's disease <6 years of age. (8.3)

See 17 for PATIENT COUNSELING INFORMATION and Medication Guide

Revised: 04/2010

FULL PRESCRIBING INFORMATION

WARNINGS
SERIOUS INFECTIONS

Patients treated with REMICADE® are at increased risk for developing serious infections that may lead to hospitalization or death *[see Warnings and Precautions (5.1) and Adverse Reactions (6.1)]*. Most patients who developed these infections were taking concomitant immunosuppressants such as methotrexate or corticosteroids.

REMICADE should be discontinued if a patient develops a serious infection or sepsis.

Reported infections include:

• Active tuberculosis, including reactivation of latent tuberculosis. Patients with tuberculosis have frequently presented with disseminated or extrapulmonary disease. Patients should be tested for latent tuberculosis before REMICADE use and during therapy.[1,2] Treatment for latent infection should be initiated prior to REMICADE use.

• Invasive fungal infections, including histoplasmosis, coccidioidomycosis, candidiasis, aspergillosis, blastomycosis, and pneumocystosis. Patients with histoplasmosis or other invasive fungal infections may present with disseminated, rather than localized, disease. Antigen and antibody testing for histoplasmosis may be negative in some patients with active infection. Empiric anti-fungal therapy should be considered in patients at risk for invasive fungal infections who develop severe systemic illness.

• Bacterial, viral and other infections due to opportunistic pathogens.

The risks and benefits of treatment with REMICADE should be carefully considered prior to initiating therapy in patients with chronic or recurrent infection.

Patients should be closely monitored for the development of signs and symptoms of infection during and after treatment with REMICADE, including the possible development of tuberculosis in patients who tested negative for latent tuberculosis infection prior to initiating therapy.

MALIGNANCY

Lymphoma and other malignancies, some fatal, have been reported in children and adolescent patients treated with TNF blockers, including REMICADE *[see Warnings and Precautions (5.2)]*.

Postmarketing cases of hepatosplenic T-cell lymphoma (HSTCL), a rare type of T-cell lymphoma, have been reported in patients treated with TNF blockers including REMICADE. These cases have had a very aggressive disease course and have been fatal. All reported REMICADE cases have occurred in patients with Crohn's disease or ulcerative colitis and the majority were in adolescent and young adult males. All of these patients had received treatment with azathioprine or 6-mercaptopurine concomitantly with REMICADE at or prior to diagnosis.

1 INDICATIONS AND USAGE

1.1 Crohn's Disease

REMICADE is indicated for reducing signs and symptoms and inducing and maintaining clinical remission in adult and pediatric patients with moderately to severely active Crohn's disease who have had an inadequate response to conventional therapy *[see Use in Specific Populations (8.4)]*. REMICADE is indicated for reducing the number of draining enterocutaneous and rectovaginal fistulas and maintaining fistula closure in adult patients with fistulizing Crohn's disease.

1.2 Ulcerative Colitis

REMICADE is indicated for reducing signs and symptoms, inducing and maintaining clinical remission and mucosal healing, and eliminating corticosteroid use in patients with moderately to severely active ulcerative colitis who have had an inadequate response to conventional therapy.

1.3 Rheumatoid Arthritis

REMICADE, in combination with methotrexate, is indicated for reducing signs and symptoms, inhibiting the progression of structural damage, and improving physical function in patients with moderately to severely active rheumatoid arthritis.

1.4 Ankylosing Spondylitis

REMICADE is indicated for reducing signs and symptoms in patients with active ankylosing spondylitis.

1.5 Psoriatic Arthritis

REMICADE is indicated for reducing signs and symptoms of active arthritis, inhibiting the progression of structural damage, and improving physical function in patients with psoriatic arthritis.

1.6 Plaque Psoriasis

REMICADE is indicated for the treatment of adult patients with chronic severe (i.e., extensive and/or disabling) plaque psoriasis who are candidates for systemic therapy and when other systemic therapies are medically less appropriate. REMICADE should only be administered to patients who will be closely monitored and have regular follow-up visits with a physician [see Boxed WARNINGS, Warnings and Precautions (5)].

2 DOSAGE AND ADMINISTRATION

2.1 Crohn's Disease or Fistulizing Crohn's Disease

The recommended dose of REMICADE is 5 mg/kg given as an intravenous induction regimen at 0, 2 and 6 weeks followed by a maintenance regimen of 5 mg/kg every 8 weeks thereafter for the treatment of adults with moderately to severely active Crohn's disease or fistulizing Crohn's disease. For adult patients who respond and then lose their response, consideration may be given to treatment with 10 mg/kg. Patients who do not respond by Week 14 are unlikely to respond with continued dosing and consideration should be given to discontinue REMICADE in these patients.

The recommended dose of REMICADE for children with moderately to severely active Crohn's disease is 5 mg/kg given as an intravenous induction regimen at 0, 2 and 6 weeks followed by a maintenance regimen of 5 mg/kg every 8 weeks.

2.2 Ulcerative Colitis

The recommended dose of REMICADE is 5 mg/kg given as an intravenous induction regimen at 0, 2 and 6 weeks followed by a maintenance regimen of 5 mg/kg every 8 weeks thereafter for the treatment of moderately to severely active ulcerative colitis.

2.3 Rheumatoid Arthritis

The recommended dose of REMICADE is 3 mg/kg given as an intravenous induction regimen at 0, 2, and 6 weeks followed by a maintenance regimen of 3 mg/kg every 8 weeks thereafter for the treatment of moderately to severely active rheumatoid arthritis. REMICADE should be given in combination with methotrexate. For patients who have an incomplete response, consideration may be given to adjusting the dose up to 10 mg/kg or treating as often as every 4 weeks bearing in mind that risk of serious infections is increased at higher doses [see Adverse Reactions (6.1)].

2.4 Ankylosing Spondylitis

The recommended dose of REMICADE is 5 mg/kg given as an intravenous induction regimen at 0, 2 and 6 weeks followed by a maintenance regimen of 5 mg/kg every 6 weeks thereafter for the treatment of active ankylosing spondylitis.

2.5 Psoriatic Arthritis

The recommended dose of REMICADE is 5 mg/kg given as an intravenous induction regimen at 0, 2, and 6 weeks followed by maintenance regimen of 5 mg/kg every 8 weeks thereafter for the treatment of psoriatic arthritis. REMICADE can be used with or without methotrexate.

2.6 Plaque Psoriasis

The recommended dose of REMICADE is 5 mg/kg given as an intravenous induction regimen at 0, 2, and 6 weeks followed by maintenance regimen of 5 mg/kg every 8 weeks thereafter for the treatment of chronic severe (i.e., extensive and/or disabling) plaque psoriasis.

2.7 Monitoring to Assess Safety

Prior to initiating REMICADE and periodically during therapy, patients should be evaluated for active tuberculosis and tested for latent infection [see Warnings and Precautions (5.1)].

2.8 Administration Instructions Regarding Infusion Reactions

Adverse effects during administration of REMICADE have included flu-like symptoms, headache, dyspnea, hypotension, transient fever, chills, gastrointestinal symptoms, and skin rashes. Anaphylaxis might occur at any time during REMICADE infusion. Approximately 20% of REMICADE-treated patients in all clinical trials experienced an infusion reaction compared with 10% of placebo-treated patients [see Adverse Reactions (6.1)]. Prior to infusion with REMICADE, premedication may be administered at the physician's discretion. Premedication could include antihistamines (anti-H1 +/- anti-H2), acetaminophen and/or corticosteroids.

During infusion, mild to moderate infusion reactions may improve following slowing or suspension of the infusion, and upon resolution of the reaction, reinitiation at a lower infusion rate and/or therapeutic administration of antihistamines, acetaminophen, and/ or corticosteroids. For patients that do not tolerate the infusion following these interventions, REMICADE should be discontinued.

During or following infusion, patients who have severe infusion-related hypersensitivity reactions should be discontinued from further REMICADE treatment. The management of severe infusion reactions should be dictated by the signs and symptoms of the reaction. Appropriate personnel and medication should be available to treat anaphylaxis if it occurs.

2.9 General Considerations and Instructions for Preparation and Administration

REMICADE is intended for use under the guidance and supervision of a physician. The reconstituted infusion solution should be prepared by a trained medical professional using aseptic technique by the following procedure:

1. Calculate the dose, total volume of reconstituted REMICADE solution required and the number of REMICADE vials needed. Each REMICADE vial contains 100 mg of the infliximab antibody.
2. Reconstitute each REMICADE vial with 10 mL of Sterile Water for Injection, USP, using a syringe equipped with a 21-gauge or smaller needle as follows: Remove the fliptop from the vial and wipe the top with an alcohol swab. Insert the syringe needle into the vial through the center of the rubber stopper and direct the stream of Sterile Water for Injection, USP, to the glass wall of the vial. Gently swirl the solution by rotating the vial to dissolve the lyophilized powder. Avoid prolonged or vigorous agitation. DO NOT SHAKE. Foaming of the solution on reconstitution is not unusual. Allow the reconstituted solution to stand for 5 minutes. The solution should be colorless to light yellow and opalescent, and the solution may develop a few translucent particles as infliximab is a protein. Do not use if the lyophilized cake has not fully dissolved or if opaque particles, discoloration, or other foreign particles are present.
3. Dilute the total volume of the reconstituted REMICADE solution dose to 250 mL with sterile 0.9% Sodium Chloride Injection, USP, by withdrawing a volume equal to the volume of reconstituted REMICADE from the 0.9% Sodium Chloride Injection, USP, 250 mL bottle or bag. Slowly add the total volume of reconstituted REMICADE solution to the 250 mL infusion bottle or bag. Gently mix. The resulting infusion concentration should range between 0.4 mg/mL and 4 mg/mL.
4. The infusion solution must be administered over a period of not less than 2 hours and must use an infusion set with an in-line, sterile, non-pyrogenic, low-protein-binding filter (pore size of 1.2 µm or less). The vials do not contain antibacterial preservatives. Therefore, any unused portion of the infusion solution should not be stored for reuse.
5. No physical biochemical compatibility studies have been conducted to evaluate the co-administration of REMICADE with other agents. REMICADE should not be infused concomitantly in the same intravenous line with other agents.
6. Parenteral drug products should be inspected visually before and after reconstitution for particulate matter and discoloration prior to administration, whenever solution and container permit. If visibly opaque particles, discoloration or other foreign particulates are observed, the solution should not be used.

3 DOSAGE FORMS AND STRENGTHS

100 mg vial: 100 mg lyophilized infliximab in a 20 mL vial.

4 CONTRAINDICATIONS

REMICADE at doses >5 mg/kg should not be administered to patients with moderate to severe heart failure. In a randomized study evaluating REMICADE in patients with moderate to severe heart failure (New York Heart Association [NYHA] Functional Class III/IV), REMICADE treatment at 10 mg/kg was associated with an increased incidence of death and hospitalization due to worsening heart failure [see Warnings and Precautions (5.5) and Adverse Reactions (6.1)].

REMICADE should not be re-administered to patients who have experienced a severe hypersensitivity reaction to REMICADE. Additionally, REMICADE should not be administered to patients with known hypersensitivity to inactive components of the product or to any murine proteins.

5 WARNINGS AND PRECAUTIONS
(see Boxed WARNINGS)

5.1 Serious Infections

Serious and sometimes fatal infections due to bacterial, mycobacterial, invasive fungal, viral, or other opportunistic pathogens have been reported in patients receiving TNF-blocking agents. Among opportunistic infections, tuberculosis, histoplasmosis, aspergillosis, candidiasis, coccidioidomycosis, listeriosis, and pneumocystosis were the most commonly reported. Patients have frequently presented with disseminated rather than localized disease, and are often taking concomitant immunosuppressants such as methotrexate or corticosteroids with REMICADE.

Treatment with REMICADE should not be initiated in patients with an active infection, including clinically important localized infections. The risks and benefits of treatment should be considered prior to initiating therapy in patients:

• with chronic or recurrent infection;
• who have been exposed to tuberculosis;
• who have resided or traveled in areas of endemic tuberculosis or endemic mycoses, such as histoplasmosis, coccidioidomycosis, or blastomycosis; or
• with underlying conditions that may predispose them to infection.

Cases of reactivation of tuberculosis or new tuberculosis infections have been observed in patients receiving REMICADE, including patients who have previously received treatment for latent or active tuberculosis. Patients should be evaluated for tuberculosis risk factors and tested for latent infection prior to initiating REMICADE and periodically during therapy.

Treatment of latent tuberculosis infection prior to therapy with TNF blocking agents has been shown to reduce the risk of tuberculosis reactivation during therapy. Induration of 5 mm or greater with tuberculin skin testing should be considered a positive test result when assessing if treatment for latent tuberculosis is needed prior to initiating REMICADE, even for patients previously vaccinated with Bacille Calmette-Guerin (BCG).

Anti-tuberculosis therapy should also be considered prior to initiation of REMICADE in patients with a past history of latent or active tuberculosis in whom an adequate course of treatment cannot be confirmed, and for patients with a negative test for latent tuberculosis but having risk factors for tuberculosis infection. Consultation with a physician with expertise in the treatment of tuberculosis is recommended to aid in the decision whether initiating anti-tuberculosis therapy is appropriate for an individual patient.

Tuberculosis should be strongly considered in patients who develop a new infection during REMICADE treatment, especially in patients who have previously or recently traveled to countries with a high prevalence of tuberculosis, or who have had close contact with a person with active tuberculosis.

Patients should be closely monitored for the development of signs and symptoms of infection during and after treatment with REMICADE, including the development of tuberculosis in patients who tested negative for latent tuberculosis infection prior to initiating therapy. Tests for latent tuberculosis infection may also be falsely negative while on therapy with REMICADE.

REMICADE should be discontinued if a patient develops a serious infection or sepsis. A patient who develops a new infection during treatment with REMICADE should be closely monitored, undergo a prompt and complete diagnostic workup appropriate for an immunocompromised patient, and appropriate antimicrobial therapy should be initiated. For patients who reside or travel in regions where mycoses are endemic, invasive fungal infection should be suspected if they develop a serious systemic illness. Appropriate empiric antifungal therapy should be considered while a diagnostic workup is being performed. Antigen and antibody testing for histoplasmosis may be negative in some patients with active infection. When feasible, the decision to administer empiric antifungal therapy in these patients should be made in consultation with a physician with expertise in the diagnosis and treatment of invasive fungal infections and should take into account both the risk for severe fungal infection and the risks of antifungal therapy.

5.2 Malignancies

Malignancies, some fatal, have been reported among children, adolescents and young adults who received treatment with TNF-blocking agents (initiation of therapy ≤ 18 years of age), including REMICADE. Approximately half of these cases were lymphomas, including Hodgkin's and non-Hodgkin's lymphoma. The other cases represented a variety of malignancies, including rare malignancies that are usually associated with immunosuppression and malignancies that are not usually observed in children and adolescents. The malignancies occurred after a median of 30 months (range 1 to 84 months) after the first dose of TNF blocker therapy. Most of the patients were receiving concomitant immunosuppressants. These cases were reported postmarketing and are derived from a variety of sources, including registries and spontaneous postmarketing reports.

Postmarketing cases of hepatosplenic T-cell lymphoma (HSTCL), a rare type of T-cell lymphoma, have been reported in patients treated with TNF blockers including REMICADE. These cases have had a very aggressive disease course and have been fatal. All reported REMICADE cases have occurred in patients with Crohn's disease or ulcerative colitis and the majority were in adolescent and young adult males. All of these patients had received treatment with the immunosuppressants azathioprine or 6-mercaptopurine concomitantly with REMICADE at or prior to diagnosis. It is uncertain whether the occurrence of HSTCL is related to REMICADE or REMICADE in combination with these other immunosuppressants.

In the controlled portions of clinical trials of some TNF-blocking agents including REMICADE, more malignancies (excluding lymphoma and nonmelanoma skin cancer [NMSC]) have been observed in patients receiving those

TNF-blockers compared with control patients. During the controlled portions of REMICADE trials in patients with moderately to severely active rheumatoid arthritis, Crohn's disease, psoriatic arthritis, ankylosing spondylitis, ulcerative colitis, and plaque psoriasis, 14 patients were diagnosed with malignancies (excluding lymphoma and NMSC) among 4019 REMICADE-treated patients vs. 1 among 1597 control patients (at a rate of 0.52/100 patient-years among REMICADE-treated patients vs. a rate of 0.11/100 patient-years among control patients), with median duration of follow-up 0.5 years for REMICADE-treated patients and 0.4 years for control patients. Of these, the most common malignancies were breast, colorectal, and melanoma. The rate of malignancies among REMICADE-treated patients was similar to that expected in the general population whereas the rate in control patients was lower than expected.

In the controlled portions of clinical trials of all the TNF-blocking agents, more cases of lymphoma have been observed among patients receiving a TNF blocker compared with control patients. In the controlled and open-label portions of REMICADE clinical trials, 5 patients developed lymphomas among 5707 patients treated with REMICADE (median duration of follow-up 1.0 years) vs. 0 lymphomas in 1600 control patients (median duration of follow-up 0.4 years). In rheumatoid arthritis patients, 2 lymphomas were observed for a rate of 0.08 cases per 100 patient-years of follow-up, which is approximately three-fold higher than expected in the general population. In the combined clinical trial population for rheumatoid arthritis, Crohn's disease, psoriatic arthritis, ankylosing spondylitis, ulcerative colitis, and plaque psoriasis, 5 lymphomas were observed for a rate of 0.10 cases per 100 patient-years of follow-up, which is approximately four-fold higher than expected in the general population. Patients with Crohn's disease, rheumatoid arthritis or plaque psoriasis, particularly patients with highly active disease and/or chronic exposure to immunosuppressant therapies, may be at a higher risk (up to several fold) than the general population for the development of lymphoma, even in the absence of TNF-blocking therapy. Cases of acute and chronic leukemia have been reported with post-marketing TNF-blocker use in rheumatoid arthritis and other indications. Even in the absence of TNF blocker therapy, patients with rheumatoid arthritis may be at a higher risk (approximately 2-fold) than the general population for the development of leukemia.

In a clinical trial exploring the use of REMICADE in patients with moderate to severe chronic obstructive pulmonary disease (COPD), more malignancies, the majority of lung or head and neck origin, were reported in REMICADE-treated patients compared with control patients. All patients had a history of heavy smoking *[see Adverse Reactions (6.1)]*. Prescribers should exercise caution when considering the use of REMICADE in patients with moderate to severe COPD.

Psoriasis patients should be monitored for nonmelanoma skin cancers (NMSCs), particularly those patients who have had prior prolonged phototherapy treatment. In the maintenance portion of clinical trials for REMICADE, NMSCs were more common in patients with previous phototherapy *[see Adverse Reactions (6.1)]*.

The potential role of TNF-blocking therapy in the development of malignancies is not known *[see Adverse Reactions (6.1)]*. Rates in clinical trials for REMICADE cannot be compared to rates in clinical trials of other TNF-blockers and may not predict rates observed in a broader patient population. Caution should be exercised in considering REMICADE treatment in patients with a history of malignancy or in continuing treatment in patients who develop malignancy while receiving REMICADE.

5.3 Hepatitis B Virus Reactivation

Use of TNF blockers, including REMICADE has been associated with reactivation of hepatitis B virus (HBV) in patients who are chronic carriers of this virus. In some instances, HBV reactivation occurring in conjunction with TNF blocker therapy has been fatal. The majority of these reports have occurred in patients concomitantly receiving other medications that suppress the immune system, which may also contribute to HBV reactivation. Patients at risk for HBV infection should be evaluated for prior evidence of HBV infection before initiating TNF blocker therapy. Prescribers should exercise caution in prescribing TNF blockers, including REMICADE, for patients identified as carriers of HBV. Adequate data are not available on the safety or efficacy of treating patients who are carriers of HBV with anti-viral therapy in conjunction with TNF blocker therapy to prevent HBV reactivation. Patients who are carriers of HBV and require treatment with TNF blockers should be closely monitored for clinical and laboratory signs of active HBV infection throughout therapy and for several months following termination of therapy. In patients who develop HBV reactivation, TNF blockers should be stopped and antiviral therapy with appropriate supportive treatment should be initiated. The safety of resuming TNF blocker therapy after HBV reactivation is controlled is not known.

Therefore, prescribers should exercise caution when considering resumption of TNF blocker therapy in this situation and monitor patients closely.

5.4 Hepatotoxicity

Severe hepatic reactions, including acute liver failure, jaundice, hepatitis and cholestasis have been reported rarely in postmarketing data in patients receiving REMICADE. Autoimmune hepatitis has been diagnosed in some of these cases. Severe hepatic reactions occurred between 2 weeks to more than 1 year after initiation of REMICADE; elevations in hepatic aminotransferase levels were not noted prior to discovery of the liver injury in many of these cases. Some of these cases were fatal or necessitated liver transplantation. Patients with symptoms or signs of liver dysfunction should be evaluated for evidence of liver injury. If jaundice and/or marked liver enzyme elevations (e.g., ≥5 times the upper limit of normal) develop, REMICADE should be discontinued, and a thorough investigation of the abnormality should be undertaken. In clinical trials, mild or moderate elevations of ALT and AST have been observed in patients receiving REMICADE without progression to severe hepatic injury *[see Adverse Reactions (6.1)]*.

5.5 Patients with Heart Failure

REMICADE has been associated with adverse outcomes in patients with heart failure, and should be used in patients with heart failure only after consideration of other treatment options. The results of a randomized study evaluating the use of REMICADE in patients with heart failure (NYHA Functional Class III/IV) suggested higher mortality in patients who received 10 mg/kg REMICADE, and higher rates of cardiovascular adverse events at doses of 5 mg/kg and 10 mg/kg. There have been post-marketing reports of worsening heart failure, with and without identifiable precipitating factors, in patients taking REMICADE. There have also been rare post-marketing reports of new onset heart failure, including heart failure in patients without known pre-existing cardiovascular disease. Some of these patients have been under 50 years of age. If a decision is made to administer REMICADE to patients with heart failure, they should be closely monitored during therapy, and REMICADE should be discontinued if new or worsening symptoms of heart failure appear *[see Contraindications (4) and Adverse Reactions (6.1)]*.

5.6 Hematologic Events

Cases of leukopenia, neutropenia, thrombocytopenia, and pancytopenia, some with a fatal outcome, have been reported in patients receiving REMICADE. The causal relationship to REMICADE therapy remains unclear. Although no high-risk group(s) has been identified, caution should be exercised in patients being treated with REMICADE who have ongoing or a history of significant hematologic abnormalities. All patients should be advised to seek immediate medical attention if they develop signs and symptoms suggestive of blood dyscrasias or infection (e.g., persistent fever) while on REMICADE. Discontinuation of REMICADE therapy should be considered in patients who develop significant hematologic abnormalities.

5.7 Hypersensitivity

REMICADE has been associated with hypersensitivity reactions that vary in their time of onset and required hospitalization in some cases. Most hypersensitivity reactions, which include urticaria, dyspnea, and/or hypotension, have occurred during or within 2 hours of REMICADE infusion. However, in some cases, serum sickness-like reactions have been observed in patients after initial REMICADE therapy (i.e., as early as after the second dose), and when REMICADE therapy was reinstituted following an extended period without REMICADE treatment. Symptoms associated with these reactions include fever, rash, headache, sore throat, myalgias, polyarthralgias, hand and facial edema and/or dysphagia. These reactions were associated with marked increase in antibodies to infliximab, loss of detectable serum concentrations of infliximab, and possible loss of drug efficacy.

REMICADE should be discontinued for severe hypersensitivity reactions. Medications for the treatment of hypersensitivity reactions (e.g., acetaminophen, antihistamines, corticosteroids and/or epinephrine) should be available for immediate use in the event of a reaction *[see Adverse Reactions (6.1)]*.

5.8 Neurologic Events

REMICADE and other agents that inhibit TNF have been associated in rare cases with optic neuritis, seizure and new onset or exacerbation of clinical symptoms and/or radiographic evidence of central nervous system demyelinating disorders, including multiple sclerosis, and CNS manifestation of systemic vasculitis, and peripheral demyelinating disorders, including Guillain-Barré syndrome. Prescribers should exercise caution in considering the use of REMICADE in patients with pre-existing or recent onset of demyelinating or seizure disorders. Discontinuation of REMICADE should be considered in patients who develop significant central nervous system adverse reactions.

5.9 Use with Anakinra

Serious infections were seen in clinical studies with concurrent use of anakinra and another TNFα-blocking agent, etanercept, with no added clinical benefit compared to etanercept alone. Because of the nature of the adverse events seen with combination of etanercept and anakinra therapy, similar toxicities may also result from the combination of anakinra and other TNFα-blocking agents. Therefore, the combination of REMICADE and anakinra is not recommended.

5.10 Autoimmunity

Treatment with REMICADE may result in the formation of autoantibodies and, rarely, in the development of a lupus-like syndrome. If a patient develops symptoms suggestive of a lupus-like syndrome following treatment with REMICADE, treatment should be discontinued *[see Adverse Reactions (6.1)]*.

5.11 Vaccinations

No data are available on the response to vaccination with live vaccines or on the secondary transmission of infection by live vaccines in patients receiving anti-TNF therapy. It is recommended that live vaccines not be given concurrently. It is recommended that all pediatric Crohn's disease patients be brought up to date with all vaccinations prior to initiating REMICADE therapy. The interval between vaccination and initiation of REMICADE therapy should be in accordance with current vaccination guidelines.

6 ADVERSE REACTIONS

6.1 Clinical Studies Experience

The data described herein reflect exposure to REMICADE in 4779 adult patients (1304 patients with rheumatoid arthritis, 1106 patients with Crohn's disease, 202 with ankylosing spondylitis, 293 with psoriatic arthritis, 484 with ulcerative colitis, 1373 with plaque psoriasis, and 17 patients with other conditions), including 2625 patients exposed beyond 30 weeks and 374 exposed beyond 1 year. *[For information on adverse reactions in pediatric patients see Adverse Reactions (6.1).]* One of the most-common reasons for discontinuation of treatment was infusion-related reactions (e.g. dyspnea, flushing, headache and rash). Adverse events have been reported in a higher proportion of rheumatoid arthritis patients receiving the 10 mg/kg dose than the 3 mg/kg dose, however, no differences were observed in the frequency of adverse events between the 5 mg/kg dose and 10 mg/kg dose in patients with Crohn's disease.

Infusion-related Reactions

An infusion reaction was defined in clinical trials as any adverse event occurring during an infusion or within 1 to 2 hours after an infusion. Approximately 20% of REMICADE-treated patients in all clinical studies experienced an infusion reaction compared to approximately 10% of placebo-treated patients. Among all REMICADE infusions, 3% were accompanied by nonspecific symptoms such as fever or chills, 1% were accompanied by cardiopulmonary reactions (primarily chest pain, hypotension, hypertension or dyspnea), and <1% were accompanied by pruritus, urticaria, or the combined symptoms of pruritus/urticaria and cardiopulmonary reactions. Serious infusion reactions occurred in <1% of patients and included anaphylaxis, convulsions, erythematous rash and hypotension. Approximately 3% of patients discontinued REMICADE because of infusion reactions, and all patients recovered with treatment and/or discontinuation of the infusion. REMICADE infusions beyond the initial infusion were not associated with a higher incidence of reactions. The infusion reaction rates remained stable in psoriasis through 1 year in psoriasis Study I. In psoriasis Study II, the rates were variable over time and somewhat higher following the final infusion than after the initial infusion. Across the 3 psoriasis studies, the percent of total infusions resulting in infusion reactions (i.e. an adverse event occurring within 1 to 2 hours) was 7% in the 3 mg/kg group, 4% in the 5 mg/kg group, and 1% in the placebo group.

Patients who became positive for antibodies to infliximab were more likely (approximately two- to three-fold) to have an infusion reaction than were those who were negative. Use of concomitant immunosuppressant agents appeared to reduce the frequency of both antibodies to infliximab and infusion reactions *[see Adverse Reactions (6.1) and Drug Interactions (7.3)]*.

In post-marketing experience, cases of anaphylactic-like reactions, including laryngeal/pharyngeal edema and severe bronchospasm, and seizure have been associated with REMICADE administration.

Delayed Reactions/Reactions Following Re-administration

Plaque Psoriasis

In psoriasis studies, approximately 1% of REMICADE-treated patients experienced a possible delayed hypersensitivity reaction, generally reported as serum sickness or a combination of arthralgia and/or myalgia with fever and/or rash. These reactions generally occurred within 2 weeks after repeat infusion.

Crohn's disease

In a study where 37 of 41 patients with Crohn's disease were retreated with infliximab following a 2- to 4-year period without infliximab treatment, 10 patients experienced adverse events manifesting 3 to 12 days following infusion of which 6 were considered serious. Signs and symptoms included myalgia and/or arthralgia with fever and/or rash, with some patients also experiencing pruritus, facial, hand or lip edema, dysphagia, urticaria, sore throat, and headache. Patients experiencing these adverse events had not experienced infusion-related adverse events associated with their initial infliximab therapy. These adverse events occurred in 39% (9/23) of patients who had received liquid formulation which is no longer in use and 7% (1/14) of patients who received lyophilized formulation. The clinical data are not adequate to determine if occurrence of these reactions is due to differences in formulation. Patients' signs and symptoms improved substantially or resolved with treatment in all cases. There are insufficient data on the incidence of these events after drug-free intervals of 1 to 2 years. These events have been observed only infrequently in clinical studies and post-marketing surveillance with retreatment intervals up to 1 year.

Infections

In REMICADE clinical studies, treated infections were reported in 36% of REMICADE-treated patients (average of 51 weeks of follow-up) and in 25% of placebo-treated patients (average of 37 weeks of follow-up). The infections most frequently reported were respiratory tract infections (including sinusitis, pharyngitis, and bronchitis) and urinary tract infections. Among REMICADE-treated patients, serious infections included pneumonia, cellulitis, abscess, skin ulceration, sepsis, and bacterial infection. In clinical trials, 7 opportunistic infections were reported; 2 cases each of coccidioidomycosis (1 case was fatal) and histoplasmosis (1 case was fatal), and 1 case each of pneumocystosis, nocardiosis and cytomegalovirus. Tuberculosis was reported in 14 patients, 4 of whom died due to miliary tuberculosis. Other cases of tuberculosis, including disseminated tuberculosis, also have been reported post-marketing. Most of these cases of tuberculosis occurred within the first 2 months after initiation of therapy with REMICADE and may reflect recrudescence of latent disease [see *Warnings and Precautions (5.1)*]. In the 1-year placebo-controlled studies RA I and RA II, 5.3% of patients receiving REMICADE every 8 weeks with MTX developed serious infections as compared to 3.4% of placebo patients receiving MTX. Of 924 patients receiving REMICADE, 1.7% developed pneumonia and 0.4% developed TB, when compared to 0.3% and 0.0% in the placebo arm respectively. In a shorter (22-week) placebo-controlled study of 1082 RA patients randomized to receive placebo, 3 mg/kg or 10 mg/kg REMICADE infusions at 0, 2, and 6 weeks, followed by every 8 weeks with MTX, serious infections were more frequent in the 10 mg/kg REMICADE group (5.3%) than the 3 mg/kg or placebo groups (1.7% in both). During the 54-week Crohn's II Study, 15% of patients with fistulizing Crohn's disease developed a new fistula-related abscess.

In REMICADE clinical studies in patients with ulcerative colitis, infections treated with antimicrobials were reported in 27% of REMICADE-treated patients (average of 41 weeks of follow-up) and in 18% of placebo-treated patients (average 32 weeks of follow-up). The types of infections, including serious infections, reported in patients with ulcerative colitis were similar to those reported in other clinical studies. In post-marketing experience in the various indications, infections have been observed with various pathogens including viral, bacterial, fungal, and protozoal organisms. Infec-

tions have been noted in all organ systems and have been reported in patients receiving REMICADE alone or in combination with immunosuppressive agents.

The onset of serious infections may be preceded by constitutional symptoms such as fever, chills, weight loss, and fatigue. The majority of serious infections, however, may also be preceded by signs or symptoms localized to the site of the infection.

Autoantibodies/Lupus-like Syndrome

Approximately half of REMICADE-treated patients in clinical trials who were antinuclear antibody (ANA) negative at baseline developed a positive ANA during the trial compared with approximately one-fifth of placebo-treated patients. Anti-dsDNA antibodies were newly detected in approximately one-fifth of REMICADE-treated patients compared with 0% of placebo-treated patients. Reports of lupus and lupus-like syndromes, however, remain uncommon.

Malignancies

In controlled trials, more REMICADE-treated patients developed malignancies than placebo-treated patients [see *Warnings and Precautions (5.2)*].

In a randomized controlled clinical trial exploring the use of REMICADE in patients with moderate to severe COPD who were either current smokers or ex-smokers, 157 patients were treated with REMICADE at doses similar to those used in rheumatoid arthritis and Crohn's disease. Of these REMICADE-treated patients, 9 developed a malignancy, including 1 lymphoma, for a rate of 7.67 cases per 100 patient-years of follow-up (median duration of follow-up 0.8 years; 95% CI 3.51–14.56). There was 1 reported malignancy among 77 control patients for a rate of 1.63 cases per 100 patient-years of follow-up (median duration of follow-up 0.8 years; 95% CI 0.04–9.10). The majority of the malignancies developed in the lung or head and neck.

Malignancies, including non-Hodgkin's lymphoma and Hodgkin's disease, have also been reported in patients receiving REMICADE during post-approval use.

Patients with Heart Failure

In a randomized study evaluating REMICADE in moderate to severe heart failure (NYHA Class III/IV; left ventricular ejection fraction ≤35%), 150 patients were randomized to receive treatment with 3 infusions of REMICADE 10 mg/kg, 5 mg/kg, or placebo, at 0, 2, and 6 weeks. Higher incidences of mortality and hospitalization due to worsening heart failure were observed in patients receiving the 10 mg/kg REMICADE dose. At 1 year, 8 patients in the 10 mg/kg REMICADE group had died compared with 4 deaths each in the 5 mg/kg REMICADE and the placebo groups. There were trends toward increased dyspnea, hypotension, angina, and dizziness in both the 10 mg/kg and 5 mg/kg REMICADE treatment groups, versus placebo. REMICADE has not been studied in patients with mild heart failure (NYHA Class I/II) [see *Contraindications (4)* and *Warnings and Precautions (5.5)*].

Immunogenicity

Treatment with REMICADE can be associated with the development of antibodies to infliximab. The incidence of antibodies to infliximab in patients given a 3-dose induction regimen followed by maintenance dosing was approximately 10% as assessed through 1 to 2 years of REMICADE treatment. A higher incidence of antibodies to infliximab was observed in Crohn's disease patients receiving REMICADE after drug-free intervals >16 weeks. In a study of psoriatic arthritis in which 191 patients received 5 mg/kg with or without MTX, antibodies to infliximab occurred in 15% of patients. The majority of antibody-positive patients had low titers. Patients who were antibody-positive were

more likely to have higher rates of clearance, reduced efficacy and to experience an infusion reaction [see *Adverse Reactions (6.1)*] than were patients who were antibody negative. Antibody development was lower among rheumatoid arthritis and Crohn's disease patients receiving immunosuppressant therapies such as 6-MP/AZA or MTX.

In the psoriasis Study II, which included both the 5 mg/kg and 3 mg/kg doses, antibodies were observed in 36% of patients treated with 5 mg/kg every 8 weeks for 1 year, and in 51% of patients treated with 3 mg/kg every 8 weeks for 1 year. In the psoriasis Study III, which also included both the 5 mg/kg and 3 mg/kg doses, antibodies were observed in 20% of patients treated with 5 mg/kg induction (weeks 0, 2 and 6), and in 27% of patients treated with 3 mg/kg induction. Despite the increase in antibody formation, the infusion reaction rates in Studies I and II in patients treated with 5 mg/kg induction followed by every 8 week maintenance for 1 year and in Study III in patients treated with 5 mg/kg induction (14.1%–23.0%) and serious infusion reaction rates (<1%) were similar to those observed in other study populations. The clinical significance of apparent increased immunogenicity on efficacy and infusion reactions in psoriasis patients as compared to patients with other diseases treated with REMICADE over the long term is not known.

The data reflect the percentage of patients whose test results were positive for antibodies to infliximab in an ELISA assay, and they are highly dependent on the sensitivity and specificity of the assay. Additionally, the observed incidence of antibody positivity in an assay may be influenced by several factors including sample handling, timing of sample collection, concomitant medication, and underlying disease. For these reasons, comparison of the incidence of antibodies to infliximab with the incidence of antibodies to other products may be misleading.

Hepatotoxicity

Severe liver injury, including acute liver failure and autoimmune hepatitis, has been reported rarely in patients receiving REMICADE [see *Warnings and Precautions (5.4)*]. Reactivation of hepatitis B virus has occurred in patients receiving TNF-blocking agents, including REMICADE, who are chronic carriers of this virus [see *Warnings and Precautions (5.3)*].

In clinical trials in rheumatoid arthritis, Crohn's disease, ulcerative colitis, ankylosing spondylitis, plaque psoriasis, and psoriatic arthritis, elevations of aminotransferases were observed (ALT more common than AST) in a greater proportion of patients receiving REMICADE than in controls (Table 1), both when REMICADE was given as monotherapy and when it was used in combination with other immunosuppressive agents. In general, patients who developed ALT and AST elevations were asymptomatic, and the abnormalities decreased or resolved with either continuation or discontinuation of REMICADE, or modification of concomitant medications.

[See table 1 below]

Adverse Reactions in Pediatric Crohn's Disease

There were some differences in the adverse reactions observed in the pediatric patients receiving REMICADE compared to those observed in adults with Crohn's disease. These differences are discussed in the following paragraphs. The following adverse events were reported more commonly in 103 randomized pediatric Crohn's disease patients administered 5 mg/kg REMICADE through 54 weeks than in 385 adult Crohn's disease patients receiving a similar treatment regimen: anemia (11%), blood in stool (10%), leukopenia (9%), flushing (9%), viral infection (8%), neutropenia (7%), bone fracture (7%), bacterial infection (6%), and respiratory tract allergic reaction (6%).

Infections were reported in 56% of randomized pediatric patients in Study Peds Crohn's and in 50% of adult patients in Study Crohn's I. In Study Peds Crohn's, infections were reported more frequently for patients who received every 8-week as opposed to every 12-week infusions (74% and 38%, respectively), while serious infections were reported for 3 patients in the every 8-week and 4 patients in the every 12-week maintenance treatment group. The most commonly reported infections were upper respiratory tract infection and pharyngitis, and the most commonly reported serious infection was abscess. Pneumonia was reported for 3 patients, (2 in the every 8-week and 1 in the every 12-week maintenance treatment groups). Herpes zoster was reported for 2 patients in the every 8-week maintenance treatment group.

In Study Peds Crohn's, 18% of randomized patients experienced 1 or more infusion reactions, with no notable difference between treatment groups. Of the 112 patients in Study Peds Crohn's, there were no serious infusion reactions, and 2 patients had non-serious anaphylactoid reactions.

Antibodies to REMICADE developed in 3% of pediatric patients in Study Peds Crohn's.

Table 1 Proportion of patients with elevated ALT in clinical trials

	Proportion of patients with elevated ALT					
	>1 to <3 × ULN		≥3 × ULN		≥5 × ULN	
	Placebo	REMICADE	Placebo	REMICADE	Placebo	REMICADE
Rheumatoid arthritis*	24%	34%	3%	4%	<1%	<1%
Crohn's disease†	34%	39%	4%	5%	0%	2%
Ulcerative colitis‡	12%	17%	1%	2%	<1%	<1%
Ankylosing spondylitis§	15%	51%	0%	10%	0%	4%
Psoriatic arthritis¶	16%	50%	0%	7%	0%	2%
Plaque psoriasis#	24%	49%	<1%	8%	0%	3%

*Placebo patients received methotrexate while REMICADE patients received both REMICADE and methotrexate. Median follow-up was 58 weeks.
†Placebo patients in the 2 Phase 3 trials in Crohn's disease received an initial dose of 5 mg/kg REMICADE at study start and were on placebo in the maintenance phase. Patients who were randomized to the placebo maintenance group and then later crossed over to REMICADE are included in the REMICADE group in ALT analysis. Median follow-up was 54 weeks.
‡Median follow-up was 30 weeks. Specifically, the median duration of follow-up was 30 weeks for placebo and 31 weeks for REMICADE.
§Median follow-up was 24 weeks for placebo group and 102 weeks for REMICADE group.
¶Median follow-up was 39 weeks for REMICADE group and 18 weeks for placebo group.
#ALT values are obtained in 2 Phase 3 psoriasis studies with median follow-up of 50 weeks for REMICADE and 16 weeks for placebo.

Elevations of ALT up to 3 times the upper limit of normal (ULN) were seen in 18% of pediatric patients in Crohn's disease clinical trials; 4% had ALT elevations ≥3 × ULN, and 1% had elevations ≥5 × ULN. (Median follow-up was 53 weeks.)

Adverse Reactions in Psoriasis Studies
During the placebo-controlled portion across the 3 clinical trials up to week 16, the proportion of patients who experienced at least 1 SAE (defined as resulting in death, life threatening, requires hospitalization, or persistent or significant disability/incapacity) was 1.7% in the 3 mg/kg REMICADE group, 3.2% in the placebo group, and 3.9% in the 5 mg/kg REMICADE group.

Among patients in the 2 Phase 3 studies, 12.4% of patients receiving REMICADE 5 mg/kg every 8 weeks through 1 year of maintenance treatment experienced at least 1 SAE in Study I. In Study II, 4.1% and 4.7% of patients receiving REMICADE 3 mg/kg and 5 mg/kg every 8 weeks, respectively, through 1 year of maintenance treatment experienced at least 1 SAE.

One death due to bacterial sepsis occurred 25 days after the second infusion of 5 mg/kg REMICADE. Serious infections included sepsis, and abscesses. In Study I, 2.7% of patients receiving REMICADE 5 mg/kg every 8 weeks through 1 year of maintenance treatment experienced at least 1 serious infection. In Study II, 1.0% and 1.3% of patients receiving REMICADE 3 mg/kg and 5 mg/kg, respectively, through 1 year of treatment experienced at least 1 serious infection. The most common serious infection (requiring hospitalization) was abscess (skin, throat, and peri-rectal) reported by 5 (0.7%) patients in the 5 mg/kg REMICADE group. Two active cases of tuberculosis were reported: 6 weeks and 34 weeks after starting REMICADE.

In the placebo-controlled portion of the psoriasis studies, 7 of 1123 patients who received REMICADE at any dose were diagnosed with at least one NMSC compared to 0 of 334 patients who received placebo.

In the psoriasis studies, 1% (15/1373) of patients experienced serum sickness or a combination of arthralgia and/or myalgia with fever, and/or rash, usually early in the treatment course. Of these patients, 6 required hospitalization due to fever, severe myalgia, arthralgia, swollen joints, and immobility.

Other Adverse Reactions
Safety data are available from 4779 REMICADE-treated adult patients, including 1304 with rheumatoid arthritis, 1106 with Crohn's disease, 484 with ulcerative colitis, 202 with ankylosing spondylitis, 293 with psoriatic arthritis, 1373 with plaque psoriasis and 17 with other conditions. *[For information on other adverse reactions in pediatric patients, see Adverse Reactions (6.1)].* Adverse events reported in ≥5% of all patients with rheumatoid arthritis receiving 4 or more infusions are in Table 2. The types and frequencies of adverse reactions observed were similar in REMICADE-treated rheumatoid arthritis, ankylosing spondylitis, psoriatic arthritis, plaque psoriasis and Crohn's disease patients except for abdominal pain, which occurred in 26% of REMICADE-treated patients with Crohn's disease. In the Crohn's disease studies, there were insufficient numbers and duration of follow-up for patients who never received REMICADE to provide meaningful comparisons.

Table 2 Adverse reactions occurring in 5% or more of patients receiving 4 or more infusions for rheumatoid arthritis

	Placebo	REMICADE
	(n=350)	(n=1129)
Average weeks of follow-up	59	66
Gastrointestinal		
Nausea	20%	21%
Abdominal pain	8%	12%
Diarrhea	12%	12%
Dyspepsia	7%	10%
Respiratory		
Upper respiratory tract infection	25%	32%
Sinusitis	8%	14%
Pharyngitis	8%	12%
Coughing	8%	12%
Bronchitis	9%	10%
Skin and appendages disorders		
Rash	5%	10%
Pruritus	2%	7%
Body as a whole-general disorders		
Fatigue	7%	9%
Pain	7%	8%
Resistance mechanism disorders		
Fever	4%	7%
Moniliasis	3%	5%
Central and peripheral nervous system disorders		
Headache	14%	18%
Musculoskeletal system disorders		
Arthralgia	7%	8%
Urinary system disorders		
Urinary tract infection	6%	8%
Cardiovascular disorders, general		
Hypertension	5%	7%

Because clinical trials are conducted under widely varying conditions, adverse reaction rates observed in clinical trials of a drug cannot be directly compared to rates in clinical trials of another drug and may not predict the rates observed in broader patient populations in clinical practice. The most common serious adverse reactions observed in clinical trials were infections *[see Adverse Reactions (6.1)].* Other serious, medically relevant adverse reactions ≥0.2% or clinically significant adverse reactions by body system were as follows:

- *Body as a whole:* allergic reaction, edema
- *Blood:* pancytopenia
- *Cardiovascular:* hypotension
- *Gastrointestinal:* constipation, intestinal obstruction
- *Central and Peripheral Nervous:* dizziness
- *Heart Rate and Rhythm:* bradycardia
- *Liver and Biliary:* hepatitis
- *Metabolic and Nutritional:* dehydration
- *Platelet, Bleeding and Clotting:* thrombocytopenia
- *Neoplasms:* lymphoma
- *Red Blood Cell:* anemia, hemolytic anemia
- *Resistance Mechanism:* cellulitis, sepsis, serum sickness
- *Respiratory:* lower respiratory tract infection (including pneumonia), pleurisy, pulmonary edema
- *Skin and Appendages:* increased sweating
- *Vascular (Extracardiac):* thrombophlebitis
- *White Cell and Reticuloendothelial:* leukopenia, lymphadenopathy

6.2 Post-marketing Experience
The following adverse reactions, some with fatal outcome, have been reported during post-approval use of REMICADE: neutropenia *[see Warnings and Precautions (5.6)],* interstitial lung disease (including pulmonary fibrosis/interstitial pneumonitis and very rare rapidly progressive disease), idiopathic thrombocytopenic purpura, thrombotic thrombocytopenic purpura, pericardial effusion, systemic and cutaneous vasculitis, erythema multiforme, Stevens-Johnson Syndrome, toxic epidermal necrolysis, peripheral demyelinating disorders (such as Guillain-Barré syndrome, chronic inflammatory demyelinating polyneuropathy, and multifocal motor neuropathy), new onset and worsening psoriasis (all subtypes including pustular, primarily palmoplantar), transverse myelitis, and neuropathies (additional neurologic events have also been observed) *[see Warnings and Precautions (5.8)]* and acute liver failure, jaundice, hepatitis, and cholestasis *[see Warnings and Precautions (5.4)].* Because these events are reported voluntarily from a population of uncertain size, it is not always possible to reliably estimate their frequency or establish a causal relationship to REMICADE exposure.

The following serious adverse reactions have been reported in the post-marketing experience in children: infections (some fatal) including opportunistic infections and tuberculosis, infusion reactions, and hypersensitivity reactions.

Serious adverse reactions in the post-marketing experience with REMICADE in the pediatric population have also included malignancies, including hepatosplenic T-cell lymphomas *[see Boxed WARNINGS and Warnings and Precautions (5.2)],* transient hepatic enzyme abnormalities, lupus-like syndromes, and the development of autoantibodies.

7 DRUG INTERACTIONS

7.1 Anakinra
Serious infections were seen in clinical studies with concurrent use of anakinra and another TNFα-blocking agent, etanercept, with no added clinical benefit compared to etanercept alone. Because of the nature of the adverse events seen with combination of etanercept and anakinra therapy, similar toxicities may also result from the combination of anakinra and other TNFα-blocking agents. Therefore, the combination of REMICADE and anakinra is not recommended *[see Warnings and Precautions (5.1)].*

7.2 Methotrexate (MTX) and Other Concomitant Medications
Specific drug interaction studies, including interactions with MTX, have not been conducted. The majority of patients in rheumatoid arthritis or Crohn's disease clinical studies received one or more concomitant medications. In rheumatoid arthritis, concomitant medications besides MTX were nonsteroidal anti-inflammatory agents (NSAIDs), folic acid, corticosteroids and/or narcotics. Concomitant Crohn's disease medications were antibiotics, antivirals, corticosteroids, 6-MP/AZA and aminosalicylates. In psoriatic arthritis clinical trials, concomitant medications included MTX in approximately half of the patients as well as NSAIDs, folic acid and corticosteroids. Concomitant MTX use may decrease the incidence of anti-infliximab antibody production and increase infliximab concentrations.

7.3 Immunosuppressants
Patients with Crohn's disease who received immunosuppressants tended to experience fewer infusion reactions compared to patients on no immunosuppressants *[see Adverse Reactions (6.1)].* Serum infliximab concentrations appeared to be unaffected by baseline use of medications for the treatment of Crohn's disease including corticosteroids, antibiotics (metronidazole or ciprofloxacin) and aminosalicylates.

8 USE IN SPECIFIC POPULATIONS

8.1 Pregnancy
Pregnancy Category B. It is not known whether REMICADE can cause fetal harm when administered to a pregnant woman or can affect reproduction capacity. REMICADE should be given to a pregnant woman only if clearly needed. Because infliximab does not cross-react with TNFα in species other than humans and chimpanzees, animal reproduction studies have not been conducted with REMICADE. No evidence of maternal toxicity, embryotoxicity or teratogenicity was observed in a developmental toxicity study conducted in mice using an analogous antibody that selectively inhibits the functional activity of mouse TNFα. Doses of 10 to 15 mg/kg in pharmacodynamic animal models with the anti-TNF analogous antibody produced maximal pharmacologic effectiveness. Doses up to 40 mg/kg were shown to produce no adverse effects in animal reproduction studies.

8.3 Nursing Mothers
It is not known whether REMICADE is excreted in human milk or absorbed systemically after ingestion. Because many drugs and immunoglobulins are excreted in human milk, and because of the potential for adverse reactions in nursing infants from REMICADE, women should not breast-feed their infants while taking REMICADE. A decision should be made whether to discontinue nursing or to discontinue the drug, taking into account the importance of the drug to the mother.

8.4 Pediatric Use
REMICADE is indicated for reducing signs and symptoms and inducing and maintaining clinical remission in pediatric patients with moderately to severely active Crohn's disease who have had an inadequate response to conventional therapy *[see Boxed WARNINGS, Warnings and Precautions (5), Indications and Usage (1.1), Dosage and Administration (2.1), Clinical Studies (14.1) and Adverse Reactions (6.1)].* Remicade has been studied only in combination with conventional immunosuppressive therapy in children with Crohn's disease. REMICADE has not been studied in children with Crohn's disease <6 years of age. The longer term (greater than 1 year) safety and effectiveness of REMICADE in pediatric Crohn's disease patients have not been established in clinical trials.

Safety and effectiveness of REMICADE in pediatric patients with ulcerative colitis and plaque psoriasis have not been established.

The safety and efficacy of REMICADE in patients with juvenile rheumatoid arthritis (JRA) were evaluated in a multicenter, randomized, placebo-controlled, double-blind study for 14 weeks, followed by a double-blind, all-active treatment extension, for a maximum of 44 weeks. Patients with active JRA between the ages of 4 and 17 years who had been treated with MTX for at least 3 months were enrolled. Concurrent use of folic acid, oral corticosteroids (≤0.2 mg/kg/day of prednisone or equivalent), NSAIDs, and/or disease modifying antirheumatic drugs (DMARDs) was permitted. Doses of 3 mg/kg REMICADE or placebo were administered intravenously at Weeks 0, 2 and 6. Patients randomized to placebo crossed-over to receive 6 mg/kg REMICADE at Weeks 14, 16, and 20, and then every 8 weeks through Week 44. Patients who completed the study continued to receive open-label treatment with REMICADE for up to 2 years in a companion extension study.

The study failed to establish the efficacy of REMICADE in the treatment of JRA. Key observations in the study included a high placebo response rate and a higher rate of immunogenicity than what has been observed in adults. Additionally, a higher rate of clearance of infliximab was observed than had been observed in adults *[see Clinical Pharmacology (12.3)].*

A total of 60 patients with JRA were treated with doses of 3 mg/kg and 57 patients were treated with doses of 6 mg/kg. The proportion of patients with infusion reactions who received 3 mg/kg REMICADE was 35% (21/60) over 52 weeks compared with 18% (10/57) in patients who received 6 mg/kg over 38 weeks. The most common infusion reactions reported were vomiting, fever, headache, and hypotension. In the 3 mg/kg REMICADE group, 4 patients had a serious infusion reaction and 3 patients reported a possible anaphylactic reaction (2 of which were among the serious infusion reactions). In the 6 mg/kg REMICADE group, 2 patients had a serious infusion reaction, 1 of whom had a possible anaphylactic reaction. Two of the 6 patients who experienced serious infusion reactions received REMICADE by rapid infusion (duration of less than 2 hours). Antibodies to infliximab developed in 38% (20/53) of patients who received 3 mg/kg REMICADE compared with 12% (6/49) of patients who received 6 mg/kg.

A total of 68% (41/60) of patients who received 3 mg/kg REMICADE in combination with MTX experienced an infection over 52 weeks compared with 65% (37/57) of patients who received 6 mg/kg REMICADE in combination with MTX over 38 weeks. The most commonly reported infections were upper respiratory tract infection and pharyngitis, and the most commonly reported serious infection was pneumonia. Other notable infections included primary varicella infection in 1 patient and herpes zoster in 1 patient.

8.5 Geriatric Use

In rheumatoid arthritis and plaque psoriasis clinical trials, no overall differences were observed in effectiveness or safety in 181 patients with rheumatoid arthritis and 75 patients with plaque psoriasis, aged 65 or older who received REMICADE, compared to younger patients - although the incidence of serious adverse events in patients aged 65 or older was higher in both REMICADE and control groups compared to younger patients. In Crohn's disease, ulcerative colitis, ankylosing spondylitis and psoriatic arthritis studies, there were insufficient numbers of patients aged 65 and over to determine whether they respond differently from patients aged 18 to 65. Because there is a higher incidence of infections in the elderly population in general, caution should be used in treating the elderly *[see Adverse Reactions (6.1)]*.

10 OVERDOSAGE

Single doses up to 20 mg/kg have been administered without any direct toxic effect. In case of overdosage, it is recommended that the patient be monitored for any signs or symptoms of adverse reactions or effects and appropriate symptomatic treatment instituted immediately.

11 DESCRIPTION

Infliximab, the active ingredient in REMICADE, is a chimeric IgG1κ monoclonal antibody (composed of human constant and murine variable regions) specific for human tumor necrosis factor-alpha (TNFα). It has a molecular weight of approximately 149.1 kilodaltons. Infliximab is produced by a recombinant cell line cultured by continuous perfusion and is purified by a series of steps that includes measures to inactivate and remove viruses.

REMICADE is supplied as a sterile, white, lyophilized powder for intravenous infusion. Following reconstitution with 10 mL of Sterile Water for Injection, USP, the resulting pH is approximately 7.2. Each single-use vial contains 100 mg infliximab, 500 mg sucrose, 0.5 mg polysorbate 80, 2.2 mg monobasic sodium phosphate, monohydrate, and 6.1 mg dibasic sodium phosphate, dihydrate. No preservatives are present.

12 CLINICAL PHARMACOLOGY

12.1 Mechanism of Action

Infliximab neutralizes the biological activity of TNFα by binding with high affinity to the soluble and transmembrane forms of TNFα and inhibits binding of TNFα with its receptors. Infliximab does not neutralize TNFβ (lymphotoxin-α), a related cytokine that utilizes the same receptors as TNFα. Biological activities attributed to TNFα include: induction of pro-inflammatory cytokines such as interleukins (IL) 1 and 6, enhancement of leukocyte migration by increasing endothelial layer permeability and expression of adhesion molecules by endothelial cells and leukocytes, activation of neutrophil and eosinophil functional activity, induction of acute phase reactants and other liver proteins, as well as tissue degrading enzymes produced by synoviocytes and/or chondrocytes. Cells expressing transmembrane TNFα bound by infliximab can be lysed *in vitro* or *in vivo*.

Infliximab inhibits the functional activity of TNFα in a wide variety of *in vitro* bioassays utilizing human fibroblasts, endothelial cells, neutrophils, B and T- lymphocytes and epithelial cells. The relationship of these biological response markers to the mechanism(s) by which REMICADE exerts its clinical effects is unknown. Anti-TNFα antibodies reduce disease activity in the cotton-top tamarin colitis model, and decrease synovitis and joint erosions in a murine model of collagen-induced arthritis. Infliximab prevents disease in transgenic mice that develop polyarthritis as a result of constitutive expression of human TNFα, and when administered after disease onset, allows eroded joints to heal.

12.2 Pharmacodynamics

Elevated concentrations of TNFα have been found in involved tissues and fluids of patients with rheumatoid arthritis, Crohn's disease, ulcerative colitis, ankylosing spondylitis, psoriatic arthritis and plaque psoriasis. In rheumatoid arthritis, treatment with REMICADE reduced infiltration of inflammatory cells into inflamed areas of the joint as well as expression of molecules mediating cellular adhesion [E-selectin, intercellular adhesion molecule-1 (ICAM-1) and vascular cell adhesion molecule-1 (VCAM-1)], chemoattraction [IL-8 and monocyte chemotactic protein (MCP-1)] and tissue degradation [matrix metalloproteinase (MMP) 1 and 3]. In Crohn's disease, treatment with REMICADE reduced infiltration of inflammatory cells and TNFα production in inflamed areas of the intestine, and reduced the proportion of mononuclear cells from the lamina propria able to express TNFα and interferon. After treatment with REMICADE, patients with rheumatoid arthritis or Crohn's disease exhibited decreased levels of serum IL-6 and C-reactive protein (CRP) compared to baseline. Peripheral blood lymphocytes from REMICADE-treated patients showed no significant decrease in number or in proliferative responses to *in vitro* mitogenic stimulation when compared to cells from untreated patients. In psoriatic arthritis, treatment with REMICADE resulted in a reduction in the number of T-cells and blood vessels in the synovium and psoriatic skin lesions as well as a reduction of macrophages in the synovium. In plaque psoriasis, REMICADE treatment may reduce the epidermal thickness and infiltration of inflammatory cells. The relationship between these pharmacodynamic activities and the mechanism(s) by which REMICADE exerts its clinical effects is unknown.

12.3 Pharmacokinetics

In adults, single intravenous (IV) infusions of 3 mg/kg to 20 mg/kg showed a linear relationship between the dose administered and the maximum serum concentration. The volume of distribution at steady state was independent of dose and indicated that infliximab was distributed primarily within the vascular compartment. Pharmacokinetic results for single doses of 3 mg/kg to 10 mg/kg in rheumatoid arthritis, 5 mg/kg in Crohn's disease, and 3 mg/kg to 5 mg/kg in plaque psoriasis indicate that the median terminal half-life of infliximab is 7.7 to 9.5 days.

Following an initial dose of REMICADE, repeated infusions at 2 and 6 weeks resulted in predictable concentration-time profiles following each treatment. No systemic accumulation of infliximab occurred upon continued repeated treatment with 3 mg/kg or 10 mg/kg at 4- or 8-week intervals. Development of antibodies to infliximab increased infliximab clearance. At 8 weeks after a maintenance dose of 3 to 10 mg/kg of REMICADE, median infliximab serum concentrations ranged from approximately 0.5 to 6 mcg/mL; however, infliximab concentrations were not detectable (<0.1 mcg/mL) in patients who became positive for antibodies to infliximab. No major differences in clearance or volume of distribution were observed in patient subgroups defined by age, weight, or gender. It is not known if there are differences in clearance or volume of distribution in patients with marked impairment of hepatic or renal function.

Infliximab peak and trough concentrations were similar in pediatric (aged 6 to 17 years old) and adult patients with Crohn's disease following the administration of the recommended regimen *[see Dosage and Administration (2.1)]*.

Table 3 Clinical remission and steroid withdrawal

	Single 5-mg/kg Dose*	Three-Dose Induction†	
	Placebo Maintenance	REMICADE Maintenance q 8 wks	
		5 mg/kg	10 mg/kg
Week 30	25/102	41/104	48/105
Clinical remission	25%	39%	46%
P-value‡		0.022	0.001
Week 54			
Patients in remission able to	6/54	14/56	18/53
discontinue corticosteroid use§	11%	25%	34%
P-value‡		0.059	0.005

*REMICADE at Week 0
†REMICADE 5 mg/kg administered at Weeks 0, 2 and 6
‡*P*-values represent pairwise comparisons to placebo
§Of those receiving corticosteroids at baseline

Population pharmacokinetic analysis showed that in children with juvenile rheumatoid arthritis (JRA) with a body weight of up to 35 kg receiving 6 mg/kg REMICADE and children with JRA with body weight greater than 35 kg up to adult body weight receiving 3mg/kg REMICADE, the steady state area under the concentration curve (AUCss) was similar to that observed in adults receiving 3 mg/kg of REMICADE.

13 NONCLINICAL TOXICOLOGY

13.1 Carcinogenesis, Mutagenesis, Impairment of Fertility

The significance of the results of nonclinical studies for human risk is unknown. A repeat dose toxicity study was conducted with mice given cV1q anti-mouse TNFα to evaluate tumorigenicity. CV1q is an analogous antibody that inhibits the function of TNFα in mice. Animals were assigned to 1 of 3 dose groups: control, 10 mg/kg or 40 mg/kg cV1q given weekly for 6 months. The weekly doses of 10 mg/kg and 40 mg/kg are 2 and 8 times, respectively, the human dose of 5 mg/kg for Crohn's disease. Results indicated that cV1q did not cause tumorigenicity in mice. No clastogenic or mutagenic effects of infliximab were observed in the *in vivo* mouse micronucleus test or the *Salmonella-Escherichia coli* (Ames) assay, respectively. Chromosomal aberrations were not observed in an assay performed using human lymphocytes. It is not known whether infliximab can impair fertility in humans. No impairment of fertility was observed in a fertility and general reproduction toxicity study with the analogous mouse antibody used in the 6-month chronic toxicity study.

14 CLINICAL STUDIES

14.1 Crohn's Disease

Active Crohn's Disease

The safety and efficacy of single and multiple doses of REMICADE were assessed in 2 randomized, double-blind, placebo-controlled clinical studies in 653 patients with moderate to severely active Crohn's disease [Crohn's Disease Activity Index (CDAI) ≥220 and ≤400] with an inadequate response to prior conventional therapies. Concomitant stable doses of aminosalicylates, corticosteroids and/or immunomodulatory agents were permitted and 92% of patients continued to receive at least one of these medications.

In the single-dose trial of 108 patients, 16% (4/25) of placebo patients achieved a clinical response (decrease in CDAI ≥70 points) at Week 4 vs. 81% (22/27) of patients receiving 5 mg/kg REMICADE (p<0.001, two-sided, Fisher's Exact test). Additionally, 4% (1/25) of placebo patients and 48% (13/27) of patients receiving 5 mg/kg REMICADE achieved clinical remission (CDAI<150) at Week 4.

In a multidose trial (ACCENT I [Study Crohn's I]), 545 patients received 5 mg/kg at Week 0 and were then randomized to one of three treatment groups; the placebo maintenance group received placebo at Weeks 2 and 6, and then every 8 weeks; the 5 mg/kg maintenance group received 5 mg/kg at Weeks 2 and 6, and then every 8 weeks; and the 10 mg/kg maintenance group received 5 mg/kg at Weeks 2 and 6, and then 10 mg/kg every 8 weeks. Patients in response at Week 2 were randomized and analyzed separately from those not in response at Week 2. Corticosteroid taper was permitted after Week 6.

At Week 2, 57% (311/545) of patients were in clinical response. At Week 30, a significantly greater proportion of these patients in the 5 mg/kg and 10 mg/kg maintenance groups achieved clinical remission compared to patients in the placebo maintenance group (Table 3).

Additionally, a significantly greater proportion of patients in the 5 mg/kg and 10 mg/kg REMICADE maintenance groups were in clinical remission and were able to discontinue corticosteroid use compared to patients in the placebo maintenance group at Week 54 (Table 3).

[See table 3 at left]

Patients in the REMICADE maintenance groups (5 mg/kg and 10 mg/kg) had a longer time to loss of response than patients in the placebo maintenance group (Figure 1). At Weeks 30 and 54, significant improvement from baseline was seen among the 5 mg/kg and 10 mg/kg REMICADE-treated groups compared to the placebo group in the disease-specific inflammatory bowel disease questionnaire (IBDQ), particularly the bowel and systemic components, and in the physical component summary score of the general health-related quality of life questionnaire SF-36.

[See figure at top of next page]

In a subset of 78 patients who had mucosal ulceration at baseline and who participated in an endoscopic substudy, 13 of 43 patients in the REMICADE maintenance group had endoscopic evidence of mucosal healing compared to 1 of 28 patients in the placebo group at Week 10. Of the REMICADE-treated patients showing mucosal healing at Week 10, 9 of 12 patients also showed mucosal healing at Week 54.

Patients who achieved a response and subsequently lost response were eligible to receive REMICADE on an episodic basis at a dose that was 5 mg/kg higher than the dose to

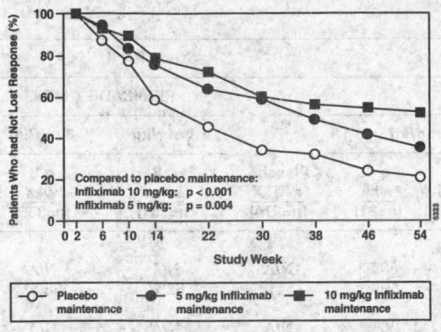

Figure 1 Kaplan-Meier estimate of the proportion of patients who had not lost response through Week 54

which they were randomized. The majority of such patients responded to the higher dose. Among patients who were not in response at Week 2, 59% (92/157) of REMICADE maintenance patients responded by Week 14 compared to 51% (39/77) of placebo maintenance patients. Among patients who did not respond by Week 14, additional therapy did not result in significantly more responses [see Dosage and Administration (2)].

Fistulizing Crohn's Disease
The safety and efficacy of REMICADE were assessed in 2 randomized, double-blind, placebo-controlled studies in patients with fistulizing Crohn's disease with fistula(s) that were of at least 3 months duration. Concurrent use of stable doses of corticosteroids, 5-aminosalicylates, antibiotics, MTX, 6-mercaptopurine (6-MP) and/or azathioprine (AZA) was permitted.

In the first trial, 94 patients received 3 doses of either placebo or REMICADE at Weeks 0, 2 and 6. Fistula response (≥50% reduction in number of enterocutaneous fistulas draining upon gentle compression on at least 2 consecutive visits without an increase in medication or surgery for Crohn's disease) was seen in 68% (21/31) of patients in the 5 mg/kg REMICADE group (P=0.002) and 56% (18/32) of patients in the 10 mg/kg REMICADE group (P=0.021) vs. 26% (8/31) of patients in the placebo arm. The median time to onset of response and median duration of response in REMICADE-treated patients was 2 and 12 weeks, respectively. Closure of all fistulas was achieved in 52% of REMICADE-treated patients compared with 13% of placebo-treated patients (P<0.001).

In the second trial (ACCENT II [Study Crohn's II]), patients who were enrolled had to have at least 1 draining enterocutaneous (perianal, abdominal) fistula. All patients received 5 mg/kg REMICADE at Weeks 0, 2 and 6. Patients were randomized to placebo or 5 mg/kg REMICADE maintenance at Week 14. Patients received maintenance doses at Week 14 and then every 8 weeks through Week 46. Patients who were in fistula response (fistula response was defined the same as in the first trial) at both Weeks 10 and 14 were randomized separately from those not in response. The primary endpoint was time from randomization to loss of response among those patients who were in fistula response. Among the randomized patients (273 of the 296 initially enrolled), 87% had perianal fistulas and 14% had abdominal fistulas. Eight percent also had rectovaginal fistulas. Greater than 90% of the patients had received previous immunosuppressive and antibiotic therapy.

At Week 14, 65% (177/273) of patients were in fistula response. Patients randomized to REMICADE maintenance had a longer time to loss of fistula response compared to the placebo maintenance group (Figure 2). At Week 54, 38% (33/87) of REMICADE-treated patients had no draining fistulas compared with 22% (20/90) of placebo-treated patients (P=0.02). Compared to placebo maintenance, patients on REMICADE maintenance had a trend toward fewer hospitalizations.

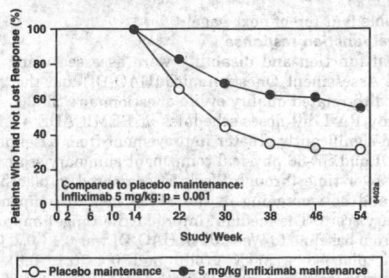

Figure 2 Life table estimates of the proportion of patients who had not lost fistula response through Week 54

Patients who achieved a fistula response and subsequently lost response were eligible to receive REMICADE maintenance therapy at a dose that was 5 mg/kg higher than the dose to which they were randomized. Of the placebo maintenance patients, 66% (25/38) responded to 5 mg/kg REMICADE, and 57% (12/21) of REMICADE maintenance patients responded to 10 mg/kg.

Patients who had not achieved a response by Week 14 were unlikely to respond to additional doses of REMICADE.

Similar proportions of patients in either group developed new fistulas (17% overall) and similar numbers developed abscesses (15% overall).

Active Crohn's Disease in Pediatric Patients
The safety and efficacy of REMICADE were assessed in a randomized, open-label study (Study Peds Crohn's) in 112 pediatric patients aged 6 to 17 years old with moderately to severely active Crohn's disease and an inadequate response to conventional therapies. The median age was 13 years and the median Pediatric Crohn's Disease Activity Index (PCDAI) was 40 (on a scale of 0 to 100). All patients were required to be on a stable dose of 6-MP, AZA, or MTX; 35% were also receiving corticosteroids at baseline.

All patients received induction dosing of 5 mg/kg REMICADE at Weeks 0, 2, and 6. At Week 10, 103 patients were randomized to a maintenance regimen of 5 mg/kg REMICADE given either every 8 weeks or every 12 weeks. At Week 10, 88% of patients were in clinical response (defined as a decrease from baseline in the PCDAI score of ≥15 points and total PCDAI score of ≤30 points), and 59% were in clinical remission (defined as PCDAI score of ≤10 points). The proportion of pediatric patients achieving clinical response at Week 10 compared favorably with the proportion of adults achieving a clinical response in Study Crohn's I. The study definition of clinical response in Study Peds Crohn's was based on the PCDAI score, whereas the CDAI score was used in the adult Study Crohn's I.

At both Week 30 and Week 54, the proportion of patients in clinical response was greater in the every 8-week treatment group than in the every 12-week treatment group (73% vs. 47% at Week 30, and 64% vs. 33% at Week 54). At both Week 30 and Week 54, the proportion of patients in clinical remission was also greater in the every 8-week treatment group than in the every 12-week treatment group (60% vs. 35% at Week 30, and 56% vs. 24% at Week 54), (Table 4).

For patients in Study Peds Crohn's receiving corticosteroids at baseline, the proportion of patients able to discontinue

corticosteroids while in remission at Week 30 was 46% for the every 8 week maintenance group and 33% for the every 12 week maintenance group. At Week 54, the proportion of patients able to discontinue corticosteroids while in remission was 46% for the every 8-week maintenance group and 17% for the every 12-week maintenance group.

Table 4 Response and remission in study peds Crohn's

	5 mg/kg REMICADE	
	Every 8 Week	Every 12 Week
	Treatment Group	Treatment Group
Patients randomized	52	51
Clinical Response*		
Week 30	73%[†]	47%
Week 54	64%[†]	33%
Clinical Remission[‡]		
Week 30	60%[§]	35%
Week 54	56%[†]	24%

* Defined as a decrease from baseline in the PCDAI score of ≥15 points and total score of ≤30 points.
[†]P<0.01
[‡]Defined as a PCDAI score of ≤10 points.
[§]P-value <0.05

14.2   Ulcerative Colitis
The safety and efficacy of REMICADE were assessed in 2 randomized, double-blind, placebo-controlled clinical studies in 728 patients with moderately to severely active ulcerative colitis (UC) (Mayo score[5] 6 to 12 [of possible range 0 to12], Endoscopy subscore ≥2) with an inadequate response to conventional oral therapies (Studies UC I and UC II). Concomitant treatment with stable doses of aminosalicylates, corticosteroids and/or immunomodulatory agents was permitted. Corticosteroid taper was permitted after Week 8. Patients were randomized at week 0 to receive either placebo, 5 mg/kg REMICADE or 10 mg/kg REMICADE at Weeks 0, 2, 6, and every 8 weeks thereafter through Week 46 in Study UC I, and at Weeks 0, 2, 6, and every 8 weeks thereafter through Week 22 in Study UC II. In Study UC II, patients were allowed to continue blinded therapy to Week 46 at the investigator's discretion.

Table 5 Response, remission, and mucosal healing in ulcerative colitis studies

	Study UC I			Study UC II		
	Placebo	5 mg/kg REMICADE	10 mg/kg REMICADE	Placebo	5 mg/kg REMICADE	10 mg/kg REMICADE
Patients randomized	121	121	122	123	121	120
Clinical Response*,[†]						
Week 8	37%	69%[‡]	62%[‡]	29%	65%[‡]	69%[‡]
Week 30	30%	52%[‡]	51%[§]	26%	47%[‡]	60%[‡]
Week 54	20%	45%[‡]	44%[‡]	NA	NA	NA
Sustained Response[†]						
(Clinical response at both Week 8 and 30)	23%	49%[‡]	46%[‡]	15%	41%[‡]	53%[‡]
(Clinical response at Weeks 8, 30, and 54)	14%	39%[‡]	37%[‡]	NA	NA	NA
Clinical Remission¶,[†]						
Week 8	15%	39%[‡]	32%[§]	6%	34%[‡]	28%[‡]
Week 30	16%	34%[§]	37%[‡]	11%	26%[§]	36%[‡]
Week 54	17%	35%[‡]	34%[§]	NA	NA	NA
Sustained Remission[†]						
(Clinical remission at both Week 8 and 30)	8%	23%[§]	26%[‡]	2%	15%[‡]	23%[‡]
(Clinical remission at Weeks 8, 30 and 54)	7%	20%[§]	20%[§]	NA	NA	NA
Mucosal Healing#,[†]						
Week 8	34%	62%[‡]	59%[‡]	31%	60%[‡]	62%[‡]
Week 30	25%	50%[‡]	49%[‡]	30%	46%[§]	57%[‡]
Week 54	18%	45%[‡]	47%[‡]	NA	NA	NA

*Defined as a decrease from baseline in the Mayo score by ≥30% and ≥3 points, accompanied by a decrease in the rectal bleeding subscore of ≥1 or a rectal bleeding subscore of 0 or 1. (The Mayo score consists of the sum of four subscores: stool frequency, rectal bleeding, physician's global assessment and endoscopy findings.)
[†]Patients who had a prohibited change in medication, had an ostomy or colectomy, or discontinued study infusions due to lack of efficacy are considered to not be in clinical response, clinical remission or mucosal healing from the time of the event onward.
[‡]P<0.001
[§]P<0.01
¶Defined as a Mayo score ≤2 points, no individual subscore >1.
#Defined as a 0 or 1 on the endoscopy subscore of the Mayo score.

Patients in Study UC I had failed to respond or were intolerant to oral corticosteroids, 6-MP, or AZA. Patients in Study UC II had failed to respond or were intolerant to the above treatments and/or aminosalicylates. Similar proportions of patients in Studies UC I and UC II were receiving corticosteroids (61% and 51%, respectively), 6-MP/AZA (49% and 43%) and aminosalicylates (70% and 75%) at baseline. More patients in Study UC II than UC I were taking solely aminosalicylates for UC (26% vs. 11%, respectively). Clinical response was defined as a decrease from baseline in the Mayo score by ≥30% and ≥3 points, accompanied by a decrease in the rectal bleeding subscore of ≥1 or a rectal bleeding subscore of 0 or 1.

Clinical Response, Clinical Remission, and Mucosal Healing

In both Study UC I and Study UC II, greater percentages of patients in both REMICADE groups achieved clinical response, clinical remission and mucosal healing than in the placebo group. Each of these effects was maintained through the end of each trial (Week 54 in Study UC I, and Week 30 in Study UC II). In addition, a greater proportion of patients in REMICADE groups demonstrated sustained response and sustained remission than in the placebo groups (Table 5).

Of patients on corticosteroids at baseline, greater proportions of patients in the REMICADE treatment groups were in clinical remission and able to discontinue corticosteroids at Week 30 compared with the patients in the placebo treatment groups (22% in REMICADE treatment groups vs. 10% in placebo group in Study UC I; 23% in REMICADE treatment groups vs. 3% in placebo group in Study UC II). In Study UC I, this effect was maintained through Week 54 (21% in REMICADE treatment groups vs. 9% in placebo group). The REMICADE-associated response was generally similar in the 5 mg/kg and 10 mg/kg dose groups.
[See table 5 at top of previous page]

The improvement with REMICADE was consistent across all Mayo subscores through Week 54 (Study UC I shown in Table 6; Study UC II through Week 30 was similar).

Table 6 Proportion of patients in Study UC I with Mayo subscores indicating inactive or mild disease through Week 54

	Study UC I		
	Placebo	REMICADE	
		5 mg/kg	10 mg/kg
	(n=121)	(n=121)	(n=122)
Stool frequency			
Baseline	17%	17%	10%
Week 8	35%	60%	58%
Week 30	35%	51%	53%
Week 54	31%	52%	51%
Rectal bleeding			
Baseline	54%	40%	48%
Week 8	74%	86%	80%
Week 30	65%	74%	71%
Week 54	62%	69%	67%
Physician's global assessment			
Baseline	4%	6%	3%
Week 8	44%	74%	64%
Week 30	36%	57%	55%
Week 54	26%	53%	53%
Endoscopy findings			
Baseline	0%	0%	0%
Week 8	34%	62%	59%
Week 30	26%	51%	52%
Week 54	21%	50%	51%

14.3 Rheumatoid Arthritis

The safety and efficacy of REMICADE were assessed in 2 multicenter, randomized, double-blind, pivotal trials: ATTRACT (Study RA I) and ASPIRE (Study RA II). Concurrent use of stable doses of folic acid, oral corticosteroids (≤10 mg/day) and/or non-steroidal anti-inflammatory drugs (NSAIDs) was permitted.

Study RA I was a placebo-controlled study of 428 patients with active rheumatoid arthritis despite treatment with MTX. Patients enrolled had a median age of 54 years, median disease duration of 8.4 years, median swollen and tender joint count of 20 and 31 respectively, and were on a median dose of 15 mg/wk of MTX. Patients received either placebo + MTX or one of 4 doses/schedules of REMICADE + MTX: 3 mg/kg or 10 mg/kg of REMICADE by IV infusion at Weeks 0, 2 and 6 followed by additional infusions every 4 or 8 weeks in combination with MTX.

Study RA II was a placebo-controlled study of 3 active treatment arms in 1004 MTX naive patients of 3 or fewer years' duration active rheumatoid arthritis. Patients enrolled had a median age of 51 years with a median disease duration of

Table 7 ACR response (percent of patients)

	Study RA I						Study RA II		
		REMICADE + MTX						REMICADE + MTX	
		3 mg/kg		10 mg/kg				3 mg/kg	6 mg/kg
Response	Placebo + MTX (n=88)	q 8 wks (n=86)	q 4 wks (n=86)	q 8 wks (n=87)	q 4 wks (n=81)	Placebo + MTX (n=274)	q 8 wks (n=351)	q 8 wks (n=355)
ACR 20								
Week 30	20%	50%*	50%*	52%*	58%*	N/A	N/A	N/A
Week 54	17%	42%*	48%*	59%*	59%*	54%	62%†	66%*
ACR 50								
Week 30	5%	27%*	29%*	31%*	26%*	N/A	N/A	N/A
Week 54	9%	21%†	34%*	40%*	38%*	32%	46%*	50%*
ACR 70								
Week 30	0%	8%‡	11%‡	18%*	11%*	N/A	N/A	N/A
Week 54	2%	11%†	18%*	26%*	19%*	21%	33%‡	37%*
Major clinical response§	0%	7%†	8%‡	15%*	6%†	8%	12%	17%*

*P ≤ 0.001
†P < 0.05
‡P < 0.01
§A major clinical response was defined as a 70% ACR response for 6 consecutive months (consecutive visits spanning at least 26 weeks) through week 102 for Study RA I and week 54 for Study RA II.

Table 8 Components of ACR 20 at baseline and 54 weeks (Study RA I)

| | Placebo + MTX | | REMICADE + MTX* | |
| | (n=88) | | (n=340) | |
Parameter (medians)	Baseline	Week 54	Baseline	Week 54
No. of Tender Joints	24	16	32	8
No. of Swollen Joints	19	13	20	7
Pain†	6.7	6.1	6.8	3.3
Physician's Global Assessment†	6.5	5.2	6.2	2.1
Patient's Global Assessment†	6.2	6.2	6.3	3.2
Disability Index (HAQ-DI)‡	1.8	1.5	1.8	1.3
CRP (mg/dL)	3.0	2.3	2.4	0.6

*All doses/schedules of REMICADE + MTX
†Visual Analog Scale (0=best, 10=worst)
‡Health Assessment Questionnaire, measurement of 8 categories: dressing and grooming, arising, eating, walking, hygiene, reach, grip, and activities (0=best, 3=worst)

0.6 years, median swollen and tender joint count of 19 and 31, respectively, and >80% of patients had baseline joint erosions. At randomization, all patients received MTX (optimized to 20 mg/wk by Week 8) and either placebo, 3 mg/kg or 6 mg/kg REMICADE at Weeks 0, 2, and 6 and every 8 weeks thereafter.

Data on use of REMICADE without concurrent MTX are limited [see Adverse Reactions (6.1)].

Clinical response

In Study RA I, all doses/schedules of REMICADE + MTX resulted in improvement in signs and symptoms as measured by the American College of Rheumatology response criteria (ACR 20) with a higher percentage of patients achieving an ACR 20, 50 and 70 compared to placebo + MTX (Table 7). This improvement was observed at Week 2 and maintained through Week 102. Greater effects on each component of the ACR 20 were observed in all patients treated with REMICADE + MTX compared to placebo + MTX (Table 8). More patients treated with REMICADE reached a major clinical response than placebo-treated patients (Table 7).

In Study RA II, after 54 weeks of treatment, both doses of REMICADE + MTX resulted in statistically significantly greater response in signs and symptoms compared to MTX alone as measured by the proportion of patients achieving ACR 20, 50 and 70 responses (Table 7). More patients treated with REMICADE reached a major clinical response than placebo-treated patients (Table 7).
[See table 7 above]
[See table 8 above]

Radiographic response

Structural damage in both hands and feet was assessed radiographically at Week 54 by the change from baseline in the van der Heijde-modified Sharp (vdH-S) score, a composite score of structural damage that measures the number and size of joint erosions and the degree of joint space narrowing in hands/wrists and feet.[3]

In Study RA I, approximately 80% of patients had paired X-ray data at 54 weeks and approximately 70% at 102 weeks. The inhibition of progression of structural damage was observed at 54 weeks (Table 9) and maintained through 102 weeks.

In Study RA II, >90% of patients had at least 2 evaluable X-rays. Inhibition of progression of structural damage was observed at Weeks 30 and 54 (Table 9) in the REMICADE + MTX groups compared to MTX alone. Patients treated with REMICADE + MTX demonstrated less progression of structural damage compared to MTX alone, whether baseline acute-phase reactants (ESR and CRP) were normal or elevated: patients with elevated baseline acute-phase reactants treated with MTX alone demonstrated a mean progression in vdH-S score of 4.2 units compared to patients treated with REMICADE + MTX who demonstrated 0.5 units of progression; patients with normal baseline acute phase reactants treated with MTX alone demonstrated a mean progression in vdH-S score of 1.8 units compared to REMICADE + MTX who demonstrated 0.2 units of progression. Of patients receiving REMICADE + MTX, 59% had no progression (vdH-S score ≤ 0 unit) of structural damage compared to 45% of patients receiving MTX alone. In a subset of patients who began the study without erosions, REMICADE + MTX maintained an erosion-free state at 1 year in a greater proportion of patients than MTX alone, 79% (77/98) vs. 58% (23/40), respectively (P<0.01). Fewer patients in the REMICADE + MTX groups (47%) developed erosions in uninvolved joints compared to MTX alone (59%).
[See table 9 at top of next page]

Physical function response

Physical function and disability were assessed using the Health Assessment Questionnaire (HAQ-DI) and the general health-related quality of life questionnaire SF-36.

In Study RA I, all doses/schedules of REMICADE + MTX showed significantly greater improvement from baseline in HAQ-DI and SF-36 physical component summary score averaged over time through Week 54 compared to placebo + MTX, and no worsening in the SF-36 mental component summary score. The median (interquartile range) improvement from baseline to Week 54 in HAQ-DI was 0.1 (-0.1, 0.5) for the placebo + MTX group and 0.4 (0.1, 0.9) for REMICADE + MTX (p<0.001). Both HAQ-DI and SF-36 effects were maintained through Week 102. Approximately 80% of patients in all doses/schedules of REMICADE + MTX remained in the trial through 102 weeks.

In Study RA II, both REMICADE treatment groups showed greater improvement in HAQ-DI from baseline averaged over time through Week 54 compared to MTX alone; 0.7 for REMICADE + MTX vs. 0.6 for MTX alone (P≤0.001). No worsening in the SF-36 mental component summary score was observed.

14.4 Ankylosing Spondylitis

The safety and efficacy of REMICADE were assessed in a randomized, multicenter, double-blind, placebo-controlled study in 279 patients with active ankylosing spondylitis. Patients were between 18 and 74 years of age, and had ankylosing spondylitis as defined by the modified New York criteria for Ankylosing Spondylitis.[4] Patients were to have had active disease as evidenced by both a Bath Ankylosing Spondylitis Disease Activity Index (BASDAI) score >4 (possible range 0–10) and spinal pain >4 (on a Visual Analog Scale [VAS] of 0–10). Patients with complete ankylosis of the spine were excluded from study participation, and the use of Disease Modifying Anti-Rheumatic Drugs (DMARDs) and systemic corticosteroids were prohibited. Doses of REMICADE 5 mg/kg or placebo were administered intravenously at Weeks 0, 2, 6, 12 and 18.

At 24 weeks, improvement in the signs and symptoms of ankylosing spondylitis, as measured by the proportion of patients achieving a 20% improvement in ASAS response criteria (ASAS 20), was seen in 60% of patients in the REMICADE-treated group vs. 18% of patients in the placebo group (p<0.001). Improvement was observed at Week 2 and maintained through Week 24 (Figure 3 and Table 10).

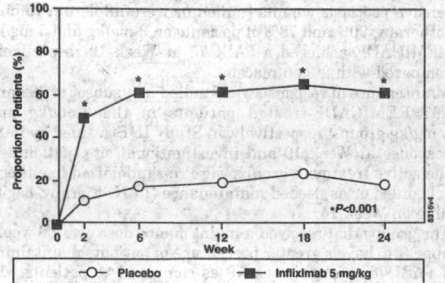

Figure 3 Proportion of patients achieving ASAS 20 response

At 24 weeks, the proportions of patients achieving a 50% and a 70% improvement in the signs and symptoms of ankylosing spondylitis, as measured by ASAS response criteria (ASAS 50 and ASAS 70, respectively), were 44% and 28%, respectively, for patients receiving REMICADE, compared to 9% and 4%, respectively, for patients receiving placebo (P<0.001, REMICADE vs. placebo). A low level of disease activity (defined as a value <20 [on a scale of 0–100 mm] in each of the 4 ASAS response parameters) was achieved in 22% of REMICADE-treated patients vs. 1% in placebo-treated patients (P<0.001).

[See table 10 at right]

The median improvement from baseline in the general health-related quality-of-life questionnaire SF-36 physical component summary score at Week 24 was 10.2 for the REMICADE group vs. 0.8 for the placebo group (P<0.001). There was no change in the SF-36 mental component summary score in either the REMICADE group or the placebo group.

Results of this study were similar to those seen in a multicenter double-blind, placebo-controlled study of 70 patients with ankylosing spondylitis.

14.5 Psoriatic Arthritis

Safety and efficacy of REMICADE were assessed in a multicenter, double-blind, placebo-controlled study in 200 adult patients with active psoriatic arthritis despite DMARD or NSAID therapy (≥5 swollen joints and ≥5 tender joints) with 1 or more of the following subtypes: arthritis involving DIP joints (n=49), arthritis mutilans (n=3), asymmetric peripheral arthritis (n=40), polyarticular arthritis (n=100), and spondylitis with peripheral arthritis (n=8). Patients also had plaque psoriasis with a qualifying target lesion ≥2 cm in diameter. Forty-six percent of patients continued on stable doses of methotrexate (≤25 mg/week). During the 24-week double-blind phase, patients received either 5 mg/kg REMICADE or placebo at Weeks 0, 2, 6, 14, and 22 (100 patients in each group). At Week 16, placebo patients with <10% improvement from baseline in both swollen and tender joint counts were switched to REMICADE induction (early escape). At Week 24, all placebo-treated patients crossed over to REMICADE induction. Dosing continued for all patients through Week 46.

Clinical response

Treatment with REMICADE resulted in improvement in signs and symptoms, as assessed by the ACR criteria, with 58% of REMICADE-treated patients achieving ACR 20 at Week 14, compared with 11% of placebo-treated patients (P< 0.001). The response was similar regardless of concomitant use of methotrexate. Improvement was observed as early as Week 2. At 6 months, the ACR 20/50/70 responses were achieved by 54%, 41%, and 27%, respectively, of patients receiving REMICADE compared to 16%, 4%, and 2%, respectively, of patients receiving placebo. Similar responses were seen in patients with each of the subtypes of psoriatic arthritis, although few patients were enrolled with the arthritis mutilans and spondylitis with peripheral arthritis subtypes.

Compared to placebo, treatment with REMICADE resulted in improvements in the components of the ACR response criteria, as well as in dactylitis and enthesopathy (Table 11). The clinical response was maintained through Week 54. Similar ACR responses were observed in an earlier randomized, placebo-controlled study of 104 psoriatic arthritis patients, and the responses were maintained through 98 weeks in an open-label extension phase.

[See table 11 at top of next page]

Improvement in Psoriasis Area and Severity Index (PASI) in psoriatic arthritis patients with baseline body surface area (BSA) ≥3% (n=87 placebo, n=83 REMICADE) was achieved at Week 14, regardless of concomitant methotrexate use, with 64% of REMICADE- treated patients achieving at least 75% improvement from baseline vs. 2% of placebo-treated patients; improvement was observed in some patients as early as Week 2. At 6 months, the PASI 75 and PASI 90 responses were achieved by 60% and 39%, respectively, of patients receiving REMICADE compared to 1% and 0%, respectively, of patients receiving placebo. The PASI response was generally maintained through Week 54. [See also Clinical Studies (14.6)].

Radiographic response

Structural damage in both hands and feet was assessed radiographically by the change from baseline in the van der Heijde-Sharp (vdH-S) score, modified by the addition of hand DIP joints. The total modified vdH-S score is a composite score of structural damage that measures the number and size of joint erosions and the degree of joint space narrowing (JSN) in the hands and feet. At Week 24, REMICADE-treated patients had less radiographic progression than placebo-treated patients (mean change of -0.70 vs.

Table 9 Radiographic change from baseline to Week 54

	Study RA I			Study RA II		
		REMICADE + MTX			REMICADE + MTX	
	Placebo + MTX (n=64)	3 mg/kg q 8 wks (n=71)	10 mg/kg q 8 wks (n=77)	Placebo + MTX (n=282)	3 mg/kg q 8 wks (n=359)	6 mg/kg q 8 wks (n=363)
Total Score						
Baseline						
Mean	79	78	65	11.3	11.6	11.2
Median	55	57	56	5.1	5.2	5.3
Change from baseline						
Mean	6.9	1.3*	0.2*	3.7	0.4*	0.5*
Median	4.0	0.5	0.5	0.4	0.0	0.0
Erosion Score						
Baseline						
Mean	44	44	33	8.3	8.8	8.3
Median	25	29	22	3.0	3.8	3.8
Change from baseline						
Mean	4.1	0.2*	0.2*	3.0	0.3*	0.1*
Median	2.0	0.0	0.5	0.3	0.0	0.0
JSN Score						
Baseline						
Mean	36	34	31	3.0	2.9	2.9
Median	26	29	24	1.0	1.0	1.0
Change from baseline						
Mean	2.9	1.1*	0.0*	0.6	0.1*	0.2
Median	1.5	0.0	0.0	0.0	0.0	0.0

*P<0.001 for each outcome against placebo.

Table 10 Components of ankylosing spondylitis disease activity

	Placebo (n=78)		REMICADE 5 mg/kg (n=201)		
	Baseline	24 Weeks	Baseline	24 Weeks	*P-value*
ASAS 20 response					
Criteria (Mean)					
Patient global assessment*	6.6	6.0	6.8	3.8	<0.001
Spinal pain*	7.3	6.5	7.6	4.0	<0.001
BASFI†	5.8	5.6	5.7	3.6	<0.001
Inflammation‡	6.9	5.8	6.9	3.4	<0.001
Acute Phase Reactants					
Median CRP§ (mg/dL)	1.7	1.5	1.5	0.4	<0.001
Spinal Mobility (cm, Mean)					
Modified Schober's test¶	4.0	5.0	4.3	4.4	0.75
Chest expansion¶	3.6	3.7	3.3	3.9	0.04
Tragus to wall¶	17.3	17.4	16.9	15.7	0.02
Lateral spinal flexion¶	10.6	11.0	11.4	12.9	0.03

*Measured on a VAS with 0="none" and 10="severe"
†Bath Ankylosing Spondylitis Functional Index (BASFI), average of 10 questions
‡Inflammation, average of last 2 questions on the 6-question BASDAI
§CRP normal range 0-1.0 mg/dL
¶Spinal mobility normal values: modified Schober's test: >4 cm; chest expansion:>6 cm; tragus to wall: <15 cm; lateral spinal flexion: >10 cm

Table 11 Components of ACR 20 and percentage of patients with 1 or more joints with dactylitis and percentage of patients with enthesopathy at baseline and Week 24

Patients Randomized	Placebo (n=100)		REMICADE 5mg/kg* (n=100)	
	Baseline	Week 24	Baseline	Week 24
Parameter (medians)				
No. of Tender Joints†	24	20	20	6
No. of Swollen Joints‡	12	9	12	3
Pain§	6.4	5.6	5.9	2.6
Physician's Global Assessment§	6.0	4.5	5.6	1.5
Patient's Global Assessment§	6.1	5.0	5.9	2.5
Disability Index (HAQ-DI)¶	1.1	1.1	1.1	0.5
CRP (mg/dL)#	1.2	0.9	1.0	0.4
% Patients with 1 or more digits with dactylitis	41	33	40	15
% Patients with enthesopathy	35	36	42	22

*P<0.001 for percent change from baseline in all components of ACR 20 at Week 24, P<0.05 for % of patients with dactylitis, and P=0.004 for % of patients with enthesopathy at Week 24
†Scale 0-68
‡Scale 0-66
§Visual Analog Scale (0=best, 10=worst)
¶Health Assessment Questionnaire, measurement of 8 categories: dressing and grooming, arising, eating, walking, hygiene, reach, grip, and activities (0=best, 3=worst)
#Normal range 0-0.6 mg/dL

Table 12 Psoriasis studies I, II, and III, Week 10 percentage of patients who achieved PASI 75 and percentage who achieved treatment "success" with physician's global assessment

	Placebo	REMICADE	
		3 mg/kg	5 mg/kg
Psoriasis Study I - patients randomized*	77	—	301
PASI 75	2 (3%)	—	242 (80%)†
sPGA	3 (4%)	—	242 (80%)†
Psoriasis Study II - patients randomized*	208	313	314
PASI 75	4 (2%)	220 (70%)†	237 (75%)†
rPGA	2 (1%)	217 (69%)†	234 (75%)†
Psoriasis Study III - patients randomized‡	51	99	99
PASI 75	3 (6%)	71 (72%)†	87 (88%)†
sPGA	5 (10%)	71 (72%)†	89 (90%)†

*Patients with missing data at Week 10 were considered as nonresponders.
†P<0.001 compared with placebo
‡Patients with missing data at Week 10 were imputed by last observation.

0.82, P<0.001). REMICADE-treated patients also had less progression in their erosion scores (-0.56 vs 0.51) and JSN scores (-0.14 vs 0.31). The patients in the REMICADE group demonstrated continued inhibition of structural damage at Week 54. Most patients showed little or no change in the vdH-S score during this 12-month study (median change of 0 in both patients who initially received REMICADE or placebo). More patients in the placebo group (12%) had readily apparent radiographic progression compared with the REMICADE group (3%).

Physical function
Physical function status was assessed using the HAQ Disability Index (HAQ-DI) and the SF-36 Health Survey. REMICADE-treated patients demonstrated significant improvement in physical function as assessed by HAQ-DI (median percent improvement in HAQ-DI score from baseline to Week 14 and 24 of 43% for REMICADE-treated patients vs 0% for placebo-treated patients).
During the placebo-controlled portion of the trial (24 weeks), 54% of REMICADE-treated patients achieved a clinically meaningful improvement in HAQ-DI (≥0.3 unit decrease) compared with 22% of placebo-treated patients. REMICADE-treated patients also demonstrated greater improvement in the SF-36 physical and mental component summary scores than placebo-treated patients. The responses were maintained for up to 2 years in an open-label extension study.

14.6 Plaque Psoriasis
The safety and efficacy of REMICADE were assessed in 3 randomized, double-blind, placebo-controlled studies in patients 18 years of age and older with chronic, stable plaque psoriasis involving ≥10% BSA, a minimum PASI score of 12, and who were candidates for systemic therapy or phototherapy. Patients with guttate, pustular, or erythrodermic psoriasis were excluded from these studies. No concomitant anti-psoriatic therapies were allowed during the study, with the exception of low-potency topical corticosteroids on the face and groin after Week 10 of study initiation.
Study I (EXPRESS) evaluated 378 patients who received placebo or REMICADE at a dose of 5 mg/kg at Weeks 0, 2, and 6 (induction therapy), followed by maintenance therapy every 8 weeks. At Week 24, the placebo group crossed over to REMICADE induction therapy (5 mg/kg), followed by maintenance therapy every 8 weeks. Patients originally randomized to REMICADE continued to receive REMICADE 5 mg/kg every 8 weeks through Week 46. Across all treatment groups, the median baseline PASI score was 21 and the baseline Static Physician Global Assessment (sPGA) score ranged from moderate (52% of patients) to severe (36%) to severe (2%). In addition, 75% of patients had a BSA >20%. Seventy-one percent of patients previously received systemic therapy, and 82% received phototherapy.
Study II (EXPRESS II) evaluated 835 patients who received placebo or REMICADE at doses of 3 mg/kg or 5 mg/kg at Weeks 0, 2, and 6 (induction therapy). At Week 14, within each REMICADE dose group, patients were randomized to either scheduled (every 8 weeks) or as needed (PRN) maintenance treatment through Week 46. At Week 16, the placebo group crossed over to REMICADE induction therapy (5 mg/kg), followed by maintenance therapy every 8 weeks. Across all treatment groups, the median baseline PASI score was 18, and 63% of patients had a BSA >20%. Fifty-five percent of patients previously received systemic therapy, and 64% received a phototherapy.
Study III (SPIRIT) evaluated 249 patients who had previously received either psoralen plus ultraviolet A treatment (PUVA) or other systemic therapy for their psoriasis. These patients were randomized to receive either placebo or REMICADE at doses of 3 mg/kg or 5 mg/kg at Weeks 0, 2, and 6. At Week 26, patients with a sPGA score of moderate or worse (greater than or equal to 3 on a scale of 0 to 5) received an additional dose of the randomized treatment. Across all treatment groups, the median baseline PASI score was 19, and the baseline sPGA score ranged from moderate (62% of patients) to marked (22%) to severe (3%). In addition, 75% of patients had a BSA >20%. Of the enrolled patients, 114 (46%) received the Week 26 additional dose.
In Studies I, II and III, the primary endpoint was the proportion of patients who achieved a reduction in score of at least 75% from baseline at Week 10 by the PASI (PASI 75).
In Study I and Study III, another evaluated outcome included the proportion of patients who achieved a score of

"cleared" or "minimal" by the sPGA. The sPGA is a 6-category scale ranging from "5 = severe" to "0 = cleared" indicating the physician's overall assessment of the psoriasis severity focusing on induration, erythema, and scaling. Treatment success, defined as "cleared" or "minimal," consisted of none or minimal elevation in plaque, up to faint red coloration in erythema, and none or minimal fine scale over <5% of the plaque.
Study II also evaluated the proportion of patients who achieved a score of "clear" or "excellent" by the relative Physician's Global Assessment (rPGA). The rPGA is a 6-category scale ranging from "6 = worse" to "1 = clear" that was assessed relative to baseline. Overall lesions were graded with consideration to the percent of body involvement as well as overall induration, scaling, and erythema. Treatment success, defined as "clear" or "excellent," consisted of some residual pinkness or pigmentation to marked improvement (nearly normal skin texture; some erythema may be present). The results of these studies are presented in Table 12.
[See table 12 at left]
In Study I, in the subgroup of patients with more extensive psoriasis who had previously received phototherapy, 85% of patients on 5 mg/kg REMICADE achieved a PASI 75 at Week 10 compared with 4% of patients on placebo.
In Study II, in the subgroup of patients with more extensive psoriasis who had previously received phototherapy, 72% and 77% of patients on 3 mg/kg and 5 mg/kg REMICADE achieved a PASI 75 at Week 10 respectively compared with 1% on placebo. In Study II, among patients with more extensive psoriasis who had failed or were intolerant to phototherapy, 70% and 78% of patients on 3 mg/kg and 5 mg/kg REMICADE achieved a PASI 75 at Week 10 respectively, compared with 2% on placebo.
Maintenance of response was studied in a subset of 292 and 297 REMICADE-treated patients in the 3 mg/kg and 5 mg/kg groups; respectively, in Study II. Stratified by PASI response at Week 10 and investigational site, patients in the active treatment groups were re-randomized to either a scheduled or as needed maintenance (PRN) therapy, beginning on Week 14.
The groups that received a maintenance dose every 8 weeks appear to have a greater percentage of patients maintaining a PASI 75 through week 50 as compared to patients who received the as-needed or PRN doses, and the best response was maintained in the 5 mg/kg every 8-week dose. These results are shown in Figure 4. At Week 46, when REMICADE serum concentrations were at trough level, in the every 8-week dose group, 54% of patients in the 5 mg/kg group compared to 36% in the 3 mg/kg group achieved PASI 75. The lower percentage of PASI 75 responders in the 3 mg/kg every 8-week dose group compared to the 5 mg/kg group was associated with a lower percentage of patients with detectable trough serum infliximab levels. This may be related in part to higher antibody rates [see Adverse Reactions (6.1)]. In addition, in a subset of patients who had achieved a response at Week 10, maintenance of response appears to be greater in patients who received REMICADE every 8 weeks at the 5 mg/kg dose. Regardless of whether the maintenance doses are PRN or every 8 weeks, there is a decline in response in a subpopulation of patients in each group over time. The results of Study I through Week 50 in the 5 mg/kg every 8 weeks maintenance dose group were similar to the results from Study II.

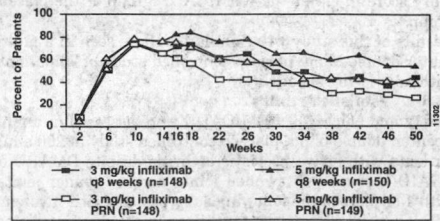

Figure 4 Proportion of patients achieving ≥75% improvement in PASI from baseline through Week 50; patients randomized at Week 14

Efficacy and safety of REMICADE treatment beyond 50 weeks have not been evaluated in patients with plaque psoriasis.

15 REFERENCES
1. American Thoracic Society, Centers for Disease Control and Prevention. Targeted tuberculin testing and treatment of latent tuberculosis infection. Am J Respir Crit Care Med 2000;161:S221–S247.
2. See latest Centers for Disease Control guidelines and recommendations for tuberculosis testing in immunocompromised patients.
3. van der Heijde DM, van Leeuwen MA, van Riel PL, et al. Biannual radiographic assessments of hands and feet in a three-year prospective follow-up of patients with early rheumatoid arthritis. Arthritis Rheum. 1992;35(1):26–34.

4. van der Linden S, Valkenburg HA, Cats A. Evaluation of diagnostic criteria for ankylosing spondylitis. A proposal for modification of the New York criteria. *Arthritis Rheum*. 1984;27(4):361–368.

5. Schroeder KW, Tremaine WJ, Ilstrup DM. Coated oral 5-aminosalicylic acid therapy for mildly to moderately active ulcerative colitis. A randomized study. *N Engl J Med*. 1987;317(26):1625–1629.

16 HOW SUPPLIED/STORAGE AND HANDLING

Each REMICADE 20 mL vial is individually packaged in a carton. REMICADE is supplied in an accumulator carton containing 10 vials.

• NDC 57894-030-01   100 mg vial

Each single dose vial contains 100 mg of infliximab for final reconstitution volume of 10 mL.

Storage and Stability

REMICADE must be refrigerated at 2°C to 8°C (36°F to 46°F). Do not use REMICADE beyond the expiration date (Exp) located on the carton and the vial. This product contains no preservative.

17 PATIENT COUNSELING INFORMATION

17.1 Patient Counseling

Patients or their caregivers should be advised of the potential benefits and risks of REMICADE. Physicians should instruct their patients to read the Medication Guide before starting REMICADE therapy and to reread it each time they receive an infusion. It is important that the patient's overall health be assessed at each treatment visit and that any questions resulting from the patient's or their caregiver's reading of the Medication Guide be discussed.

• Immunosuppression

Inform patients that REMICADE may lower the ability of their immune system to fight infections. Instruct patients of the importance of contacting their doctors if they develop any symptoms of an infection, including tuberculosis and reactivation of hepatitis B virus infections. Patients should be counseled about the risk of lymphoma and other malignancies while receiving REMICADE.

• Other Medical Conditions

Advise patients to report any signs of new or worsening medical conditions such as heart disease, neurological disease, or autoimmune disorders. Advise patients to report any symptoms of a cytopenia such as bruising, bleeding or persistent fever.

Product developed and manufactured by:
Centocor Ortho Biotech Inc.
200 Great Valley Parkway
Malvern, PA 19355
Revised April 2010
License # 1821
©Centocor Ortho Biotech Inc. 2010

17.2 Medication Guide

MEDICATION GUIDE

REMICADE® (Rem-eh-kaid)
(infliximab)

Read the Medication Guide that comes with REMICADE before you receive the first treatment, and before each time you get a treatment of REMICADE. This Medication Guide does not take the place of talking with your doctor about your medical condition or treatment.

What is the most important information I should know about REMICADE?

REMICADE may cause serious side effects, including:

1. Risk of infection

REMICADE is a medicine that affects your immune system. REMICADE can lower the ability of your immune system to fight infections. Serious infections have happened in patients receiving REMICADE. These infections include tuberculosis (TB) and infections caused by viruses, fungi or bacteria that have spread throughout the body. Some patients have died from these infections.

• Your doctor should test you for TB before starting REMICADE.

• Your doctor should monitor you closely for signs and symptoms of TB during treatment with REMICADE.

Before starting REMICADE, tell your doctor if you:

• think you have an infection. You should not start taking REMICADE if you have any kind of infection.

• are being treated for an infection

• have signs of an infection, such as a fever, cough, flu-like symptoms

• have any open cuts or sores on your body

• get a lot of infections or have infections that keep coming back

• have diabetes or an immune system problem. People with these conditions have a higher chance for infections.

• Have TB, or have been in close contact with someone with TB

• live or have lived in certain parts of the country (such as the Ohio and Mississippi River valleys) where there is an increased risk for getting certain kinds of fungal infections (histoplasmosis, coccidioidomycosis, or blastomycosis). These infections may develop or become more severe

if you take REMICADE. If you do not know if you have lived in an area where histoplasmosis, coccidioidomycosis, or blastomycosis is common, ask your doctor.

• have or have had hepatitis B

• use the medicine Kineret (anakinra)

After starting REMICADE, if you have an infection, any sign of an infection including a fever, cough, flu-like symptoms, or have open cuts or sores on your body, call your doctor right away. REMICADE can make you more likely to get infections or make any infection that you have worse.

2. Risk of Cancer

• There have been cases of unusual cancers in children and teenage patients using TNF-blocking agents.

• For children and adults taking TNF-blocker medicines, including REMICADE, the chances of getting lymphoma or other cancers may increase.

• People who have been treated for rheumatoid arthritis, Crohn's disease, ankylosing spondylitis, psoriatic arthritis and plaque psoriasis for a long time may be more likely to develop lymphoma. This is especially true for people with very active disease.

• Some patients with Crohn's disease or ulcerative colitis who have received REMICADE have developed a rare type of cancer called Hepatosplenic T-cell Lymphoma. Most of these patients were teenage or young adult males. This type of cancer results in death. All of these patients had also received drugs known as azathioprine or 6-mercaptopurine together with REMICADE.

• Patients with COPD (a specific type of lung disease) may have an increased risk for getting cancer while being treated with REMICADE.

• Tell your doctor if you have ever had any type of cancer. Discuss with your doctor any need to adjust medicines you may be taking.

See the section **"What are the possible side effects of REMICADE?"** below for more information.

What is REMICADE?

REMICADE is a prescription medicine that is approved for patients with:

• Rheumatoid Arthritis–adults with moderately to severely active rheumatoid arthritis, along with the medicine methotrexate

• Crohn's Disease–children over the age of 6 and adults with Crohn's disease who have not responded well enough to other medicines

• Ankylosing Spondylitis

• Psoriatic Arthritis

• Plaque Psoriasis–adult patients with plaque psoriasis that is chronic (doesn't go away) severe, extensive, and/or disabling

• Ulcerative Colitis–adults with moderately to severely active ulcerative colitis who have not responded well enough to other medicines.

REMICADE blocks the action of a protein in your body called tumor necrosis factor-alpha (TNF-alpha). TNF-alpha is made by your body's immune system. People with certain diseases have too much TNF-alpha that can cause the immune system to attack normal healthy parts of the body. REMICADE can block the damage caused by too much TNF-alpha.

Who should not receive REMICADE?

You should not receive REMICADE if you have:

• heart failure, unless your doctor has examined you and decided that you are able to take REMICADE. Talk to your doctor about your heart failure.

• had an allergic reaction to REMICADE, or any of the other ingredients in REMICADE. See the end of this Medication Guide for a complete list of ingredients in REMICADE.

What should I tell my doctor before starting treatment with REMICADE?

Your doctor will assess your health before each treatment. Tell your doctor about all of your medical conditions, including if you:

• have an infection (see **"What is the most important information I should know about REMICADE?"**).

• have other liver problems including liver failure.

• have heart failure or other heart conditions. If you have heart failure, it may get worse while you take REMICADE.

• have or have had any type of cancer.

• have had phototherapy (treatment with ultraviolet light or sunlight along with a medicine to make your skin sensitive to light) for psoriasis. You may have a higher chance of getting skin cancer while receiving REMICADE.

• have COPD (Chronic Obstructive Pulmonary Disease), a specific type of lung disease. Patients with COPD may have an increased risk of getting cancer while taking REMICADE.

• have or have had a condition that affects your nervous system such as

  • multiple sclerosis, or Guillain-Barré syndrome, or

• if you experience any numbness or tingling, or

• if you have had a seizure.

• have recently received or are scheduled to receive a vaccine. **Adults and children should not receive a live vaccine while taking REMICADE.** Children with Crohn's disease should have all of their vaccines brought up to date before starting treatment with REMICADE.

• are pregnant or planning to become pregnant. It is not known if REMICADE harms your unborn baby. REMICADE should be given to a pregnant woman only if clearly needed. Talk to your doctor about stopping REMICADE if you are pregnant or planning to become pregnant.

• are breast-feeding or planning to breast-feed. It is not known whether REMICADE passes into your breast milk. Talk to your doctor about the best way to feed your baby while taking REMICADE. You should not breast-feed while taking REMICADE.

How should I receive REMICADE?

• You will be given REMICADE through a needle placed in a vein (IV or intravenous infusion) in your arm.

• Your doctor may decide to give you medicine before starting the REMICADE infusion to prevent or lessen side effects.

• Only a healthcare professional should prepare the medicine and administer it to you.

• REMICADE will be given to you over a period of about 2 hours.

• If you have side effects from REMICADE, the infusion may need to be adjusted or stopped. In addition, your healthcare professional may decide to treat your symptoms.

• A healthcare professional will monitor you during the REMICADE infusion and for a period of time afterward for side effects. Your doctor may do certain tests while you are taking REMICADE to monitor you for side effects and to see how well you respond to the treatment.

• Your doctor will determine the right dose of REMICADE for you and how often you should receive it. Make sure to discuss with your doctor when you will receive infusions and to come in for all your infusions and follow-up appointments.

What should I avoid while receiving REMICADE?

Do not take REMICADE and the medication KINERET (anakinra) together.

Tell your doctor about all the medicines you take, including prescription and non-prescription medicines, vitamins, and herbal supplements.

Know the medicines you take. Keep a list of your medicines and show them to your doctor and pharmacist when you get a new medicine.

What are the possible side effects of REMICADE?

Remicade can cause serious side effects, including:

See **"What is the most important information I should know about REMICADE?"**.

Serious Infections

• Some patients have had serious infections while receiving REMICADE. These serious infections include TB and infections caused by viruses, fungi, or bacteria that have spread throughout the body. Some patients die from these infections. If you get an infection while receiving treatment with REMICADE your doctor will treat your infection and may need to stop your REMICADE treatment.

• Tell your doctor right away if you have any of the following signs of an infection while taking or after taking REMICADE:

  • a fever

  • feel very tired

  • have a cough

  • have flu-like symptoms

  • warm, red, or painful skin

• Your doctor will examine you for TB and perform a test to see if you have TB. If your doctor feels that you are at risk for TB, you may be treated with medicine for TB before you begin treatment with REMICADE and during treatment with REMICADE.

• Even if your TB test is negative, your doctor should carefully monitor you for TB infections while you are taking REMICADE. Patients who had a **negative** TB skin test before receiving REMICADE have developed active TB.

• If you are a chronic carrier of the hepatitis B virus, the virus can become active while you are being treated with REMICADE. In some cases, patients have died as a result of hepatitis B virus being reactivated. Your doctor may do a blood test before you start treatment with REMICADE and occasionally while you are being treated. Tell your doctor if you have any of the following symptoms:

  • feel unwell

  • poor appetite

  • tiredness (fatigue)

  • fever, skin rash and/or joint pain

Heart Failure
If you have a heart problem called congestive heart failure, your doctor should check you closely while you are taking REMICADE. Your congestive heart failure may get worse while you are taking REMICADE. Be sure to tell your doctor of any new or worse symptoms including:
- shortness of breath
- swelling of ankles or feet
- sudden weight gain

Treatment with REMICADE may need to be stopped if you get new or worse congestive heart failure.

Liver Injury
In rare cases, some patients taking REMICADE have developed serious liver problems. Tell your doctor if you have
- jaundice (skin and eyes turning yellow)
- dark brown-colored urine
- pain on the right side of your stomach area (right-sided abdominal pain)
- fever
- extreme tiredness (severe fatigue)

Blood Problems
In some patients taking REMICADE, the body may not make enough of the blood cells that help fight infections or help stop bleeding.
Tell your doctor if you
- have a fever that does not go away
- bruise or bleed very easily
- look very pale

Nervous System Disorders
In rare cases, patients taking REMICADE have developed problems with their nervous system. Tell your doctor if you have
- changes in your vision
- weakness in your arms and/or legs
- numbness or tingling in any part of your body
- seizures

Allergic Reactions
Some patients have had allergic reactions to REMICADE. Some of these reactions were severe. These reactions can happen while you are getting your REMICADE treatment or shortly afterward. Your doctor may need to stop or pause your treatment with REMICADE and may give you medicines to treat the allergic reaction. Signs of an allergic reaction can include:
- hives (red, raised, itchy patches of skin)
- difficulty breathing
- chest pain
- high or low blood pressure
- fever
- chills

Some patients treated with REMICADE have had delayed allergic reactions. The delayed reactions occurred 3 to 12 days after receiving treatment with REMICADE. Tell your doctor right away if you have any of these signs of delayed allergic reaction to REMICADE:
- fever
- rash
- headache
- sore throat
- muscle or joint pain
- swelling of the face and hands
- difficulty swallowing

Lupus-like Syndrome
Some patients have developed symptoms that are like the symptoms of Lupus. If you develop any of the following symptoms, your doctor may decide to stop your treatment with REMICADE.
- chest discomfort or pain that does not go away
- shortness of breath
- joint pain
- rash on the cheeks or arms that gets worse in the sun

Psoriasis
Some people using REMICADE had new psoriasis or worsening of psoriasis they already had. Tell your doctor if you develop red scaly patches or raised bumps on the skin that are filled with pus. Your doctor may decide to stop your treatment with REMICADE.

The most common side effects of REMICADE are
- respiratory infections, such as sinus infections and sore throat
- headache
- rash
- coughing
- stomach pain

Children who took REMICADE in studies for Crohn's disease showed some differences in side effects compared with adults who took REMICADE for Crohn's disease. The side effects that happened more in children were: anemia (low red blood cells), blood in stool, leukopenia (low white blood cells), flushing (redness or blushing), viral infections, neutropenia (low neutrophils, the white blood cells that fight infection), bone fracture, bacterial infection and allergic reactions of the breathing tract.

Tell your doctor about any side effect that bothers you or does not go away.
These are not all of the side effects with REMICADE. Ask your doctor or pharmacist for more information.

General information about REMICADE
Medicines are sometimes prescribed for purposes that are not mentioned in Medication Guides or patient information sheets. Do not use REMICADE for a condition for which it was not prescribed.
This information sheet summarizes the most important information about REMICADE. You can ask your doctor or pharmacist for information about REMICADE that is written for health professionals.
Call your doctor for medical advice about side effects. You may report side effects to FDA at 1-800-FDA-1088.
For more information go to www.remicade.com, or call 1-800-457-6399.

What are the ingredients in REMICADE?
The active ingredient is Infliximab.
The inactive ingredients in REMICADE include: sucrose, polysorbate 80, monobasic sodium phosphate monohydrate, and dibasic sodium phosphate dihydrate. No preservatives are present.
Product developed and manufactured by:
Centocor Ortho Biotech Inc.
200 Great Valley Parkway
Malvern, PA 19355
License # 1821
Revised November 2009
©Centocor Ortho Biotech Inc. 2009
This Medication Guide has been approved by the U.S. Food and Drug Administration
Shown in Product Identification Guide, page 307

SIMPONI™ ℞
[*SIM-po-nee*]
(golimumab)
Injection, solution for subcutaneous use

HIGHLIGHTS OF PRESCRIBING INFORMATION
These highlights do not include all the information needed to use SIMPONI (golimumab) safely and effectively. See full prescribing information for SIMPONI.
SIMPONI (golimumab)
Injection, solution for subcutaneous use
Initial U.S. Approval: 2009

WARNINGS:
SERIOUS INFECTIONS
See full prescribing information for complete boxed warning
- Serious infections leading to hospitalization or death including tuberculosis (TB), bacterial sepsis, invasive fungal, and other opportunistic infections have occurred in patients receiving SIMPONI (5.1).
- SIMPONI should be discontinued if a patient develops a serious infection or sepsis (5.1).
- Perform test for latent TB; if positive, start treatment for TB prior to starting SIMPONI (5.1).
- Monitor all patients for active TB during treatment, even if initial latent TB test is negative (5.1)

MALIGNANCY
- Lymphoma and other malignancies, some fatal, have been reported in children and adolescent patients treated with TNF blockers, of which SIMPONI is a member (5.2)

RECENT MAJOR CHANGES

Boxed Warning, MALIGNANCY	11/2009
Warnings and Precautions, Malignancies (5.2)	11/2009

INDICATIONS AND USAGE
SIMPONI is a tumor necrosis factor (TNF) blocker indicated for the treatment of:
- Moderately to severely active Rheumatoid Arthritis (RA) in adults, in combination with methotrexate (1.1)
- Active Psoriatic Arthritis (PsA) in adults, alone or in combination with methotrexate (1.2)
- Active Ankylosing Spondylitis in adults (AS) (1.3)

DOSAGE AND ADMINISTRATION
Rheumatoid Arthritis, Psoriatic Arthritis, and Ankylosing Spondylitis (2.1)
- 50 mg administered by subcutaneous injection once a month.

DOSAGE FORMS AND STRENGTHS
- 50 mg/0.5 mL in a single dose prefilled SmartJect autoinjector (3)
- 50 mg/0.5 mL in a single dose prefilled syringe (3)

CONTRAINDICATIONS
- None (4)

WARNINGS AND PRECAUTIONS
- Serious Infections—Do not start SIMPONI during an active infection. If an infection develops, monitor carefully, and stop SIMPONI if infection becomes serious (5.1).
- Invasive fungal infections—For patients who develop a systemic illness on SIMPONI, consider empiric antifungal therapy for those who reside or travel to regions where mycoses are endemic (5.1).
- Hepatitis B reactivation—Monitor HBV carriers during and several months after therapy. If reactivation occurs, stop SIMPONI and begin anti-viral therapy (5.1).
- Malignancies—The incidence of lymphoma was seen more often than in the general U.S. population. Cases of other malignancies have been observed among patients receiving TNF-blockers (5.2).
- Heart failure—Worsening, or new onset, may occur. Stop SIMPONI if new or worsening symptoms occur (5.3).
- Demyelinating disease, exacerbation or new onset, may occur (5.4).

ADVERSE REACTIONS
Most common adverse reactions (incidence > 5%): upper respiratory tract infection, nasopharyngitis (6.1).
To report SUSPECTED ADVERSE REACTIONS, contact Centocor Ortho Biotech Inc. at 1-800-457-6399 or FDA at 1-800-FDA-1088 or *www.fda.gov/medwatch*.

DRUG INTERACTIONS
- Abatacept—increased risk of serious infection (5.1, 5.5, 7.2).
- Anakinra—increased risk of serious infection (5.1, 5.6, 7.2).
- Live vaccines—should not be given with SIMPONI (5.8, 7.3).

See 17 for PATIENT COUNSELING INFORMATION and Medication Guide

Revised: 11/2009

FULL PRESCRIBING INFORMATION: CONTENTS*
WARNINGS: SERIOUS INFECTIONS
MALIGNANCY

* Sections or subsections omitted from the full prescribing information are not listed

FULL PRESCRIBING INFORMATION

> **WARNINGS**
> **SERIOUS INFECTIONS**
> Patients treated with SIMPONI™ are at increased risk for developing serious infections that may lead to hospitalization or death [see Warnings and Precautions (5.1)]. Most patients who developed these infections were taking concomitant immunosuppressants such as methotrexate or corticosteroids.
> SIMPONI should be discontinued if a patient develops a serious infection.
> Reported infections include:
> • Active tuberculosis, including reactivation of latent tuberculosis. Patients with tuberculosis have frequently presented with disseminated or extrapulmonary disease. Patients should be tested for latent tuberculosis before SIMPONI use and during therapy. Treatment for latent infection should be initiated prior to SIMPONI use.
> • Invasive fungal infections, including histoplasmosis, coccidioidomycosis, and pneumocystosis. Patients with histoplasmosis or other invasive fungal infections may present with disseminated, rather than localized, disease. Antigen and antibody testing for histoplasmosis may be negative in some patients with active infection. Empiric anti-fungal therapy should be considered in patients at risk for invasive fungal infections who develop severe systemic illness.
> • Bacterial, viral, and other infections due to opportunistic pathogens.
> The risks and benefits of treatment with SIMPONI should be carefully considered prior to initiating therapy in patients with chronic or recurrent infection.
> Patients should be closely monitored for the development of signs and symptoms of infection during and after treatment with SIMPONI, including the possible development of tuberculosis in patients who tested negative for latent tuberculosis infection prior to initiating therapy [see Warning and Precautions (5.1)].
> **MALIGNANCY**
> • Lymphoma and other malignancies, some fatal, have been reported in children and adolescent patients treated with TNF blockers, of which SIMPONI is a member [see Warning and Precautions (5.2)].

1.0   INDICATIONS AND USAGE

1.1   Rheumatoid Arthritis
SIMPONI, in combination with methotrexate, is indicated for the treatment of adult patients with moderately to severely active rheumatoid arthritis.

1.2   Psoriatic Arthritis
SIMPONI, alone or in combination with methotrexate, is indicated for the treatment of adult patients with active psoriatic arthritis.

1.3   Ankylosing Spondylitis
SIMPONI is indicated for the treatment of adult patients with active ankylosing spondylitis.

2.0   DOSAGE AND ADMINISTRATION

2.1   Rheumatoid Arthritis, Psoriatic Arthritis, Ankylosing Spondylitis
The SIMPONI dose regimen is 50 mg administered by subcutaneous (SC) injection once a month.
For patients with rheumatoid arthritis (RA), SIMPONI should be given in combination with methotrexate and for patients with psoriatic arthritis (PsA) or ankylosing spondylitis (AS), SIMPONI may be given with or without methotrexate or other non-biologic DMARDs. For patients with RA, PsA, or AS, corticosteroids, non-biologic DMARDs, and/or NSAIDs may be continued during treatment with SIMPONI.

2.2   Monitoring to Assess Safety
Prior to initiating SIMPONI and periodically during therapy, patients should be evaluated for active tuberculosis and tested for latent infection [see Warnings and Precautions (5.1)].

2.3   General Considerations for Administration
SIMPONI is intended for use under the guidance and supervision of a physician. After proper training in subcutaneous injection technique, a patient may self inject with SIMPONI if a physician determines that it is appropriate. Patients should be instructed to follow the directions provided in the Medication Guide [see Medication Guide (17.3)]. To ensure proper use, allow the prefilled syringe or autoinjector to sit at room temperature outside the carton for 30 minutes prior to subcutaneous injection. Do not warm SIMPONI in any other way.
Prior to administration, visually inspect the solution for particles and discoloration through the viewing window. SIMPONI should be clear to slightly opalescent and color-less to light yellow. The solution should not be used if discolored, or cloudy, or if foreign particles are present. Any leftover product remaining in the prefilled syringe or prefilled autoinjector should not be used. NOTE: The needle cover on the prefilled syringe as well as the prefilled syringe in the autoinjector contains dry natural rubber (a derivative of latex), which should not be handled by persons sensitive to latex.
Injection sites should be rotated and injections should never be given into areas where the skin is tender, bruised, red, or hard.

3.0   DOSAGE FORMS AND STRENGTHS

SmartJect™ Autoinjector
Each single dose SmartJect autoinjector contains a prefilled glass syringe (27 gauge ½ inch) providing 50 mg of SIMPONI per 0.5 mL of solution.

Prefilled Syringe
Each single dose prefilled glass syringe (27 gauge ½ inch) contains 50 mg of SIMPONI per 0.5 mL of solution.

4.0   CONTRAINDICATIONS

None.

5.0   WARNINGS AND PRECAUTIONS

(see Boxed WARNINGS)

5.1   Serious Infections
Serious and sometimes fatal infections due to bacterial, mycobacterial, invasive fungal, viral, protozoal, or other opportunistic pathogens have been reported in patients receiving TNF-blockers including SIMPONI. Among opportunistic infections, tuberculosis, histoplasmosis, aspergillosis, candidiasis, coccidioidomycosis, listeriosis, and pneumocystosis were the most commonly reported with TNF-blockers. Patients have frequently presented with disseminated rather than localized disease, and were often taking concomitant immunosuppressants such as methotrexate or corticosteroids. The concomitant use of a TNF-blocker and abatacept or anakinra was associated with a higher risk of serious infections; therefore, the concomitant use of SIMPONI and these biologic products is not recommended [see Warning and Precautions (5.5, 5.6) and Drug Interactions (7.2)].
Treatment with SIMPONI should not be initiated in patients with an active infection, including clinically important localized infections. The risks and benefits of treatment should be considered prior to initiating SIMPONI in patients:
• with chronic or recurrent infection;
• who have been exposed to tuberculosis;
• with a history of an opportunistic infection;
• who have resided or traveled in areas of endemic tuberculosis or endemic mycoses, such as histoplasmosis, coccidioidomycosis, or blastomycosis; or
• with underlying conditions that may predispose them to infection.
Patients should be closely monitored for the development of signs and symptoms of infection during and after treatment with SIMPONI. SIMPONI should be discontinued if a patient develops a serious infection, an opportunistic infection, or sepsis. A patient who develops a new infection during treatment with SIMPONI should undergo a prompt and complete diagnostic workup appropriate for an immunocompromised patient, appropriate antimicrobial therapy should be initiated, and the patient should be closely monitored.
In controlled Phase 3 trials through Week 16 in patients with RA, PsA, and AS, serious infections were observed in 1.4% of SIMPONI-treated patients and 1.3% of control-treated patients. In the controlled Phase 3 trials through Week 16 in patients with RA, PsA, and AS, the incidence of serious infections per 100 patient-years of follow-up was 5.4 (95% CI: 4.0, 7.2) for the SIMPONI group and 5.3 (95% CI: 3.1, 8.7) for the placebo group. Serious infections observed in SIMPONI-treated patients included sepsis, pneumonia, cellulitis, abscess, tuberculosis, invasive fungal infections, and hepatitis B infection.

Tuberculosis
Cases of reactivation of tuberculosis or new tuberculosis infections have been observed in patients receiving TNF-blockers, including patients who have previously received treatment for latent or active tuberculosis. Patients should be evaluated for tuberculosis risk factors and tested for latent infection prior to initiating SIMPONI and periodically during therapy.
Treatment of latent tuberculosis infection prior to therapy with TNF-blockers has been shown to reduce the risk of tuberculosis reactivation during therapy. Induration of 5 mm or greater with tuberculin skin testing should be considered a positive test result when assessing if treatment for latent tuberculosis is needed prior to initiating SIMPONI, even for patients previously vaccinated with Bacille Calmette-Guerin (BCG).
Anti-tuberculosis therapy should also be considered prior to initiation of SIMPONI in patients with a past history of latent or active tuberculosis in whom an adequate course of treatment cannot be confirmed, and for patients with a negative test for latent tuberculosis but having risk factors for tuberculosis infection. Consultation with a physician with expertise in the treatment of tuberculosis is recommended to aid in the decision whether initiating anti-tuberculosis therapy is appropriate for an individual patient.
Patients should be closely monitored for the development of signs and symptoms of tuberculosis including patients who tested negative for latent tuberculosis infection prior to initiating therapy.
Tuberculosis should be strongly considered in patients who develop a new infection during SIMPONI treatment, especially in patients who have previously or recently traveled to countries with a high prevalence of tuberculosis, or who have had close contact with a person with active tuberculosis.
In the controlled and uncontrolled portions of the Phase 2 RA and Phase 3 RA, PsA, and AS trials, the incidence of active TB was 0.23 and 0 per 100 patient-years in 2347 SIMPONI-treated patients and 674 placebo-treated patients, respectively. Cases of TB included pulmonary and extra pulmonary TB. The overwhelming majority of the TB cases occurred in countries with a high incidence rate of TB.

Invasive Fungal Infections
For SIMPONI-treated patients who reside or travel in regions where mycoses are endemic, invasive fungal infection should be suspected if they develop a serious systemic illness. Appropriate empiric antifungal therapy should be considered while a diagnostic workup is being performed. Antigen and antibody testing for histoplasmosis may be negative in some patients with active infection. When feasible, the decision to administer empiric antifungal therapy in these patients should be made in consultation with a physician with expertise in the diagnosis and treatment of invasive fungal infections and should take into account both the risk for severe fungal infection and the risks of antifungal therapy.

Hepatitis B Virus Reactivation
The use of TNF-blockers including SIMPONI has been associated with reactivation of hepatitis B virus (HBV) in patients who are chronic hepatitis B carriers (i.e., surface antigen positive). In some instances, HBV reactivation occurring in conjunction with TNF-blocker therapy has been fatal. The majority of these reports have occurred in patients who received concomitant immunosuppressants.
Patients at risk for HBV infection should be evaluated for prior evidence of HBV infection before initiating TNF-blocker therapy. The risks and benefits of treatment should be considered prior to prescribing TNF-blockers, including SIMPONI, to patients who are carriers of HBV. Adequate data are not available on whether anti-viral therapy can reduce the risk of HBV reactivation in HBV carriers who are treated with TNF-blockers. Patients who are carriers of HBV and require treatment with TNF-blockers should be closely monitored for clinical and laboratory signs of active HBV infection throughout therapy and for several months following termination of therapy.
In patients who develop HBV reactivation, TNF-blockers should be stopped and antiviral therapy with appropriate supportive treatment should be initiated. The safety of resuming TNF-blockers after HBV reactivation has been controlled is not known. Therefore, prescribers should exercise caution when considering resumption of TNF-blockers in this situation and monitor patients closely.

5.2   Malignancies
Malignancies, some fatal, have been reported among children, adolescents, and young adults who received treatment with TNF-blocking agents (initiation of therapy ≤ 18 years of age), of which SIMPONI is a member. Approximately half the cases were lymphomas, including Hodgkin's and non-Hodgkin's lymphoma. The other cases represented a variety of malignancies, including rare malignancies that are usually associated with immunosuppression, and malignancies that are not usually observed in children and adolescents. The malignancies occurred after a median of 30 months (range 1 to 84 months) after the first dose of TNF blocker therapy. Most of the patients were receiving concomitant immunosuppressants. These cases were reported postmarketing and are derived from a variety of sources, including registries and spontaneous postmarketing reports.
The risks and benefits of TNF-blocker treatment including SIMPONI should be considered prior to initiating therapy in patients with a known malignancy other than a successfully treated non-melanoma skin cancer (NMSC) or when considering continuing a TNF-blocker in patients who develop a malignancy.
In the controlled portions of clinical trials of TNF-blockers including SIMPONI, more cases of lymphoma have been observed among patients receiving anti-TNF treatment compared with patients in the control groups. During the controlled portions of the Phase 2 trials in RA, and the Phase 3 trials in RA, PsA and AS, the incidence of lymphoma per 100 patient-years of follow-up was 0.21 (95% CI: 0.03, 0.77) in the combined SIMPONI group compared with an incidence of 0 (95% CI: 0., 0.96) in the placebo group. In the controlled

and uncontrolled portions of these clinical trials in 2347 SIMPONI-treated patients with a median follow-up of 1.4 years, the incidence of lymphoma was 3.8-fold higher than expected in the general U.S. population according to the SEER database (adjusted for age, gender, and race).[1] Patients with RA and other chronic inflammatory diseases, particularly patients with highly active disease and/or chronic exposure to immunosuppressant therapies, may be at higher risk (up to several fold) than the general population for the development of lymphoma, even in the absence of TNF-blocking therapy. Cases of acute and chronic leukemia have been reported with postmarketing TNF-blocker use in rheumatoid arthritis and other indications. Even in the absence of TNF blocker therapy, patients with rheumatoid arthritis may be at a higher risk (approximately 2-fold) than the general population for the development of leukemia.

During the controlled portions of the Phase 2 trial in RA, and the Phase 3 trials in RA, PsA and AS, the incidence of malignancies other than lymphoma per 100 patient-years of follow-up was not elevated in the combined SIMPONI group compared with the placebo group. In the controlled and uncontrolled portions of these trials, the incidence of malignancies, other than lymphoma, in SIMPONI-treated patients was similar to that expected in the general U.S. population according to the SEER database (adjusted for age, gender, and race).[1]

In controlled trials of other TNF-blockers in patients at higher risk for malignancies (e.g., patients with COPD, patients with Wegener's granulomatosis treated with concomitant cyclophosphamide) a greater portion of malignancies occurred in the TNF-blocker group compared to the controlled group. In an exploratory 1-year clinical trial evaluating the use of 50, 100 and 200 mg of SIMPONI in 309 patients with severe persistent asthma, 6 patients developed malignancies other than NMSC in the SIMPONI groups compared to none in the control group. Three of the 6 patients were in the 200 mg SIMPONI group.

5.3 Congestive Heart Failure

Cases of worsening congestive heart failure (CHF) and new onset CHF have been reported with TNF-blockers. In several exploratory trials of other TNF-blockers in the treatment of CHF, there were greater proportions of TNF-blocker treated patients who had CHF exacerbations requiring hospitalization or increased mortality. SIMPONI has not been studied in patients with a history of CHF and SIMPONI should be used with caution in patients with CHF. If a decision is made to administer SIMPONI to patients with CHF, these patients should be closely monitored during therapy, and SIMPONI should be discontinued if new or worsening symptoms of CHF appear.

5.4 Demyelinating Disorders

Use of TNF-blockers has been associated with cases of new onset or exacerbation of central nervous system (CNS) demyelinating disorders, including multiple sclerosis (MS). While no trials have been performed evaluating SIMPONI in the treatment of patients with MS, another TNF-blocker was associated with increased disease activity in patients with MS. Therefore, prescribers should exercise caution in considering the use of TNF-blockers including SIMPONI in patients with CNS demyelinating disorders including MS.

5.5 Use with Abatacept

In controlled trials, the concurrent administration of another TNF-blocker and abatacept was associated with a greater proportion of serious infections than the use of a TNF-blocker alone; and the combination therapy, compared to the use of a TNF-blocker alone, has not demonstrated improved clinical benefit in the treatment of RA. Therefore, the combination of TNF-blockers including SIMPONI and abatacept is not recommended [*see Drug Interactions (7.2)*].

5.6 Use with Anakinra

Concurrent administration of anakinra (an interleukin-1 antagonist) and another TNF-blocker, was associated with a greater portion of serious infections and neutropenia and no additional benefits compared with the TNF-blocker alone. Therefore, the combination of anakinra with TNF-blockers, including SIMPONI, is not recommended [*see Drug Interactions 7.2*].

5.7 Hematologic Cytopenias

There have been post-marketing reports of pancytopenia, leukopenia, neutropenia, aplastic anemia, and thrombocytopenia in patients receiving TNF-blockers. Although, there were no cases of severe cytopenias seen in the SIMPONI clinical trials, caution should be exercised when using TNF-blockers, including SIMPONI, in patients who have significant cytopenias.

5.8 Vaccinations

Patients treated with SIMPONI may receive vaccinations, except for live vaccines. No data are available on the response to live vaccination or the risk of infection, or transmission of infection after the administration of live vaccines to patients receiving SIMPONI. In the Phase 3 PsA study, after pneumococcal vaccination, a similar proportion of SIMPONI-treated and placebo-treated patients were able to mount an adequate immune response of at least a 2-fold increase in antibody titers to pneumococcal polysaccharide vaccine. In both SIMPONI-treated and placebo-treated patients, the proportions of patients with response to pneumococcal vaccine were lower among patients receiving MTX compared with patients not receiving MTX. The data suggest that SIMPONI does not suppress the humoral immune response to the pneumococcal vaccine.

6.0 ADVERSE REACTIONS

Because clinical trials are conducted under widely varying conditions, adverse reaction rates observed in the clinical trials of a drug cannot be directly compared to rates in the clinical trials of another drug and may not reflect the rates observed in clinical practice.

6.1 Clinical Studies Experience

The safety data described below are based on 5 pooled, randomized, double-blind, controlled Phase 3 trials in patients with RA, PsA, and AS (Studies RA-1, RA-2, RA-3, PsA, and AS) [*see Clinical Studies (14.1, 14.2 and 14.3)*]. These 5 trials included 639 control-treated patients and 1659 SIMPONI-treated patients including 1089 with RA, 292 with PsA, and 278 with AS. The proportion of patients who discontinued treatment due to adverse reactions in the controlled Phase 3 trials through Week 16 in RA, PsA and AS was 2% for SIMPONI-treated patients and 3% for placebo-treated patients. The most common adverse reactions leading to discontinuation of SIMPONI in the controlled Phase 3 trials through Week 16 were sepsis (0.2%), alanine aminotransferase increased (0.2%), and aspartate aminotransferase increased (0.2%).

The most serious adverse reactions were:

- Serious Infections [*see Warnings and Precautions (5.1)*]
- Malignancies [*see Warnings and Precautions (5.2)*]

Upper respiratory tract infection and nasopharyngitis were the most common adverse reactions reported in the combined Phase 3 RA, PsA and AS trials through Week 16, occurring in 7% and 6% of SIMPONI-treated patients as compared with 6% and 5% of control-treated patients, respectively.

Infections

In controlled Phase 3 trials through Week 16 in RA, PsA, and AS, infections were observed in 28% of SIMPONI-treated patients compared to 25% of control-treated patients [for Serious Infections, *see Warnings and Precautions (5.1)*].

Liver Enzyme Elevations

There have been reports of severe hepatic reactions including acute liver failure in patients receiving TNF-blockers. In controlled Phase 3 trials of SIMPONI in patients with RA, PsA, and AS through Week 16, ALT elevations $\geq 5 \times$ ULN occurred in 0.2% of control-treated patients and 0.7% of SIMPONI-treated patients and ALT elevations $\geq 3 \times$ ULN occurred in 2% of control-treated patients and 2% of SIMPONI-treated patients. Since many of the patients in the Phase 3 trials were also taking medications that cause liver enzyme elevations (e.g., NSAIDS, MTX), the relationship between golimumab and liver elevation is not clear.

Autoimmune Disorders and Autoantibodies

The use of TNF-blockers has been associated with the formation of autoantibodies and, rarely, with the development of a lupus-like syndrome. In the controlled Phase 3 trials in patients with RA, PsA, and AS through Week 14, there was no association of SIMPONI treatment and the development of newly positive anti-dsDNA antibodies.

Injection Site Reactions

In controlled Phase 3 trials through Week 16 in RA, PsA and AS, 6% of SIMPONI-treated patients had injection site reactions compared with 2% of control-treated patients. The majority of the injection site reactions were mild and the most frequent manifestation was injection site erythema. In controlled Phase 2 and 3 trials in RA, PsA, and AS, no patients treated with SIMPONI developed anaphylactic reactions.

Psoriasis: New-Onset and Exacerbations

Cases of new onset psoriasis, including pustular psoriasis and palmoplantar psoriasis, have been reported with the use of TNF-blockers, including SIMPONI. Cases of exacerbation of pre-existing psoriasis have also been reported with the use of TNF-blockers. Many of these patients were taking concomitant immunosuppressants (e.g., MTX, corticosteroids). Some of these patients required hospitalization. Most patients had improvement of their psoriasis following discontinuation of their TNF-blocker. Some patients have had recurrences of the psoriasis when they were re-challenged with a different TNF-blocker. Discontinuation of SIMPONI should be considered for severe cases and those that do not improve or that worsen despite topical treatments.

Immunogenicity

Antibodies to SIMPONI were detected in 57 (4%) of SIMPONI-treated patients across the Phase 3 RA, PsA and AS trials through Week 24. Similar rates were observed in each of the three indications. Patients who received SIMPONI with concomitant MTX had a lower proportion of antibodies to SIMPONI than patients who received SIMPONI without MTX (approximately 2% versus 7%, respectively). Of the patients with a positive antibody response to SIMPONI in the Phase 2 and 3 trials, most were determined to have neutralizing antibodies to golimumab as measured by a cell-based functional assay. The small number of patients positive for antibodies to SIMPONI limits the ability to draw definitive conclusions regarding the relationship between antibodies to golimumab and clinical efficacy or safety measures.

The data above reflect the percentage of patients whose test results were considered positive for antibodies to SIMPONI in an ELISA assay, and are highly dependent on the sensitivity and specificity of the assay. Additionally, the observed incidence of antibody positivity in an assay may be influenced by several factors including sample handling, timing of sample collection, concomitant medications, and underlying disease. For these reasons, comparison of the incidence of antibodies to SIMPONI with the incidence of antibodies to other products may be misleading.

Other Adverse Reactions

Table 1 summarizes the adverse drug reactions that occurred at a rate of at least 1% in the combined SIMPONI groups during the controlled period of the 5 pooled Phase 3 trials through Week 16 in patients with RA, PsA, and AS.

Table 1. Adverse Drug Reactions Reported by ≥ 1% of Patients in the Phase 3 Trials of RA, PsA, and AS through Week 16*

	Placebo ± DMARDs	SIMPONI ± DMARDs
Patients treated	639	1659
Adverse Reaction (Preferred Term)		
Upper respiratory tract infection	37 (6%)	120 (7%)
Nasopharyngitis	31 (5%)	91 (6%)
Alanine aminotransferase increased	18 (3%)	58 (4%)
Injection site erythema	6 (1%)	56 (3%)
Hypertension	9 (1%)	48 (3%)
Aspartate aminotransferase increased	10 (2%)	44 (3%)
Bronchitis	9 (1%)	31 (2%)
Dizziness	7 (1%)	32 (2%)
Sinusitis	7 (1%)	27 (2%)
Influenza	7 (1%)	25 (2%)
Pharyngitis	8 (1%)	22 (1%)
Rhinitis	4 (< 1%)	20 (1%)
Pyrexia	4 (< 1%)	20 (1%)
Oral herpes	2 (< 1%)	16 (1%)
Paraesthesia	2 (< 1%)	16 (1%)

*Patients may have taken concomitant MTX, sulfasalazine, hydroxychloroquine, low dose corticosteroids (≤ 10 mg of prednisone/day or equivalent), and/or NSAIDs during the trials).

7.0 DRUG INTERACTIONS

7.1 Methotrexate

For the treatment of RA, SIMPONI should be used with methotrexate (MTX) [*see Clinical Studies (14.1)*]. Since the presence or absence of concomitant MTX did not appear to influence the efficacy or safety of SIMPONI in the treatment of PsA or AS, SIMPONI can be used with or without MTX in the treatment of PsA and AS [*see Clinical Studies (14.1) and Clinical Pharmacology (12.3)*].

7.2 Biologic Products for RA, PsA, and/or AS

An increased risk of serious infections has been seen in clinical RA studies of other TNF-blockers used in combination with anakinra or abatacept, with no added benefit; therefore, use of SIMPONI with abatacept or anakinra is not recommended [*see Warnings and Precautions (5.5 and 5.6)*]. A higher rate of serious infections has also been observed in RA patients treated with rituximab who received subsequent treatment with a TNF-blocker. There is insufficient information to provide recommendations regarding the concomitant use of SIMPONI and other biologic products approved to treat RA, PsA, or AS.

7.3 Live Vaccines

Live vaccines should not be given concurrently with SIMPONI [*see Warnings and Precautions (5.8)*].

7.4 Cytochrome P450 Substrates

The formation of CYP450 enzymes may be suppressed by increased levels of cytokines (e.g., TNFα) during chronic inflammation. Therefore, it is expected that for a molecule that antagonizes cytokine activity, such as golimumab, the formation of CYP450 enzymes could be normalized. Upon initiation or discontinuation of SIMPONI in patients being treated with CYP450 substrates with a narrow therapeutic index, monitoring of the effect (e.g., warfarin) or drug concentration (e.g., cyclosporine or theophylline) is recommended and the individual dose of the drug product may be adjusted as needed.

8.0 USE IN SPECIFIC POPULATIONS

8.1 Pregnancy

Pregnancy Category B—There are no adequate and well-controlled studies of SIMPONI in pregnant women. Because animal reproduction and developmental studies are not always predictive of human response, it is not known whether SIMPONI can cause fetal harm when administered to a pregnant woman or can affect reproduction capacity. SIMPONI should be used during pregnancy only if clearly needed.

An embryofetal developmental toxicology study was performed in which pregnant cynomolgus monkeys were treated subcutaneously with golimumab during the first trimester with doses up to 50 mg/kg twice weekly (360 times greater than the maximum recommended human dose-MHRD) and has revealed no evidence of harm to maternal animals or fetuses. Umbilical cord blood samples collected at the end of the second trimester showed that fetuses were exposed to golimumab during gestation. In this study, *in utero* exposure to golimumab produced no developmental defects to the fetus.

A pre- and post-natal developmental study was performed in which pregnant cynomolgus monkeys were treated with golimumab during the second and third trimesters, and during lactation at doses up to 50 mg/kg twice weekly (860 times and 310 times greater than the maximal steady state human blood levels for maternal animals and neonates, respectively) and has revealed no evidence of harm to maternal animals or neonates. Golimumab was present in the neonatal serum from the time of birth and for up to six months postpartum. Exposure to golimumab during gestation and during the postnatal period caused no developmental defects in the infants.

8.3 Nursing Mothers

It is not known whether SIMPONI is excreted in human milk or absorbed systemically after ingestion. Because many drugs and immunoglobulins are excreted in human milk, and because of the potential for adverse reactions in nursing infants from SIMPONI, a decision should be made whether to discontinue nursing or to discontinue the drug, taking into account the importance of the drug to the mother.

In the pre- and post-natal development study in cynomolgus monkeys in which golimumab was administered subcutaneously during pregnancy and lactation, golimumab was detected in the breast milk at concentrations that were approximately 400-fold lower than the maternal serum concentrations.

8.4 Pediatric Use

Safety and effectiveness of SIMPONI in pediatric patients less than 18 years of age have not been established.

8.5 Geriatric Use

In the Phase 3 trials in RA, PsA, and AS, there were no overall differences in SAEs, serious infections, and AEs in SIMPONI-treated patients ages 65 or older (N = 155) compared with younger SIMPONI-treated patients. Because there is a higher incidence of infections in the geriatric population in general, caution should be used in treating geriatric patients with SIMPONI.

10.0 OVERDOSAGE

In a clinical study, 5 patients received protocol-directed single infusions of 10 mg/kg of intravenous SIMPONI without serious adverse reactions or other significant reactions. The highest weight patient was 100 kg, and therefore received a single intravenous infusion of 1000 mg of SIMPONI. There were no SIMPONI overdoses in the clinical studies.

11.0 DESCRIPTION

SIMPONI (golimumab) is a human IgG1κ monoclonal antibody specific for human tumor necrosis factor alpha (TNFα) that exhibits multiple glycoforms with molecular masses of approximately 150 to 151 kilodaltons. SIMPONI was created using genetically engineered mice immunized with human TNF, resulting in an antibody with human-derived antibody variable and constant regions. SIMPONI is produced by a recombinant cell line cultured by continuous perfusion and is purified by a series of steps that includes measures to inactivate and remove viruses.

The SIMPONI drug product is a sterile solution of the golimumab antibody supplied as either a single dose prefilled syringe (with a passive needle safety guard) or a single dose prefilled autoinjector. The Type 1 glass syringe has a coated stopper. The fixed stainless steel needle (5 bevel, 27G, half-inch) is covered with a needle shield to prevent leakage of the solution through the needle and to protect the needle during handling prior to administration. The needle shield is made of a dry natural rubber containing latex.

SIMPONI does not contain preservatives. The solution is clear to slightly opalescent, colorless to light yellow with a pH of approximately 5.5. SIMPONI is provided in one strength: 50 mg of the golimumab antibody in 0.5 mL of solution. Each 0.5 mL of SIMPONI contains 50 mg of the golimumab antibody, 0.44 mg of L-histidine and L-histidine monohydrochloride monohydrate, 20.5 mg of sorbitol, 0.08 mg of polysorbate 80, and Water for Injection.

12.0 CLINICAL PHARMACOLOGY

12.1 Mechanism of Action

Golimumab is a human monoclonal antibody that binds to both the soluble and transmembrane bioactive forms of human TNFα. This interaction prevents the binding of TNFα to its receptors, thereby inhibiting the biological activity of TNFα (a cytokine protein). There was no evidence of the golimumab antibody binding to other TNF superfamily ligands; in particular, the golimumab antibody did not bind or neutralize human lymphotoxin. Golimumab did not lyse human monocytes expressing transmembrane TNF in the presence of complement or effector cells.

Elevated TNFα levels in the blood, synovium, and joints have been implicated in the pathophysiology of several chronic inflammatory diseases such as rheumatoid arthritis, psoriatic arthritis, and ankylosing spondylitis. TNFα is an important mediator of the articular inflammation that is characteristic of these diseases. Golimumab modulated the *in vitro* biological effects mediated by TNF in several bioassays, including the expression of adhesion proteins responsible for leukocyte infiltration (E-selectin, ICAM-1 and VCAM-1) and the secretion of proinflammatory cytokines (IL-6, IL-8, G-CSF and GM-CSF).

12.2 Pharmacodynamics

In clinical studies, decreases in C-reactive protein (CRP), interleukin (IL)-6, matrix metalloproteinase 3 (MMP-3), intercellular adhesion molecule (ICAM)-1 and vascular endothelial growth factor (VEGF) were observed following SIMPONI administration in patients with RA, PsA, and AS.

12.3 Pharmacokinetics

Following subcutaneous (SC) administration of SIMPONI to healthy subjects and patients with active RA, the median time to reach maximum serum concentrations (T_{max}) ranged from 2 to 6 days. A SC injection of 50 mg SIMPONI to healthy subjects produced a mean maximum serum concentration (C_{max}) of approximately 2.5 μg/mL. SIMPONI exhibited dose-proportional pharmacokinetics (PK) in patients with active RA over the dose range of 0.1 to 10.0 mg/kg following a single intravenous (IV) dose. Following a single IV administration over the same dose range in patients with active RA, mean systemic clearance of SIMPONI was estimated to be 4.9 to 6.7 mL/day/kg, and mean volume of distribution ranged from 58 to 126 mL/kg. The volume of distribution for SIMPONI indicates that SIMPONI is distributed primarily in the circulatory system with limited extravascular distribution. Median terminal half-life values were estimated to be approximately 2 weeks in healthy subjects and patients with active RA, PsA or AS. By cross-study comparisons of mean AUC_{inf} values following an IV or SC administration of SIMPONI, the absolute bioavailability of SC SIMPONI was estimated to be approximately 53%.

When 50 mg SIMPONI was administered SC to patients with RA, PsA or AS every 4 weeks, serum concentrations appeared to reach steady state by Week 12. With concomitant use of methotrexate (MTX), treatment with 50 mg SIMPONI SC every 4 weeks resulted in a mean steady-state trough serum concentration of approximately 0.4–0.6 μg/mL in patients with active RA, approximately 0.5 μg/mL in patients with active PsA, and approximately 0.8 μg/mL in patients with active AS. Patients with RA, PsA and AS treated with SIMPONI 50 mg and MTX had approximately 52%, 36% and 21% higher mean steady-state trough concentrations of golimumab, respectively compared with those treated with SIMPONI 50 mg without MTX. The presence of MTX also decreased anti-golimumab antibody incidence from 7% to 2% [*see Adverse Reactions (6.1)*]. For RA, SIMPONI should be used with MTX. In the PsA and AS trials, the presence or absence of concomitant MTX did not appear to influence clinical efficacy and safety parameters [*see Drug Interactions (7.1) and Clinical Studies (14.1)*].

Population PK analyses indicated that concomitant use of NSAIDs, oral corticosteroids, or sulfasalazine did not influence the apparent clearance of SIMPONI.

Population PK analyses showed there was a trend toward higher apparent clearance of SIMPONI with increasing weight. However, across the PsA and AS populations, no meaningful differences in clinical efficacy were observed among the subgroups by weight quartile. The RA trial in MTX-experienced and TNF-blocker-naïve patients (Study RA-2) did show evidence of a reduction in clinical efficacy with increasing body weight, but this effect was observed for both tested doses of SIMPONI (50 mg and 100 mg). Therefore, there is no need to adjust the dosage of SIMPONI based on a patient's weight.

Population PK analyses suggested no PK differences between male and female patients after body weight adjustment in the RA and PsA trials. In the AS trial, female patients showed 13% higher apparent clearance than male patients after body weight adjustment. Subgroup analysis based on gender showed that both female and male patients achieved clinically significant response at the proposed clinical dose. Dosage adjustment based on gender is not needed. Population PK analyses indicated that PK parameters of SIMPONI were not influenced by age in adult patients. Patients with age $\geq$ 65 years had apparent clearance of SIMPONI similar to patients with age $<$ 65 years. No ethnicity-related PK differences were observed between Caucasians and Asians, and there were too few patients of other races to assess for PK differences.

Patients who developed anti-SIMPONI antibodies generally had lower steady-state serum trough concentrations of SIMPONI.

No formal study of the effect of renal or hepatic impairment on the PK of golimumab was conducted.

13.0 NONCLINICAL TOXICOLOGY

13.1 Carcinogenesis, Mutagenesis, Impairment of Fertility

Long-term animal studies of golimumab have not been conducted to evaluate its carcinogenic potential. Mutagenicity studies have not been conducted with golimumab. A fertility study conducted in mice using an analogous anti-mouse TNFα antibody showed no impairment of fertility.

14.0 CLINICAL STUDIES

14.1 Rheumatoid Arthritis

The efficacy and safety of SIMPONI were evaluated in 3 multicenter, randomized, double-blind, controlled trials (Studies RA-1, RA-2, and RA-3) in 1542 patients $\geq$ 18 years of age with moderately to severely active RA, diagnosed according to the American College of Rheumatology (ACR) criteria, for at least 3 months prior to administration of study agent. Patients were required to have at least 4 swollen and 4 tender joints. SIMPONI was administered subcutaneously at doses of 50 mg or 100 mg every 4 weeks. Double-blinded controlled efficacy data were collected and analyzed through Week 24. Patients were allowed to continue stable doses of concomitant low dose corticosteroids (equivalent to $\leq$ 10 mg of prednisone a day) and/or NSAIDs and patients may have received oral MTX during the trials.

Study RA-1 evaluated 461 patients who were previously treated (at least 8 to 12 weeks prior to administration of study agent) with one or more doses of a biologic TNF-blocker without a serious adverse reaction. Patients may have discontinued the biologic TNF-blocker for a variety of reasons. Patients were randomized to receive placebo (n = 155), SIMPONI 50 mg (n = 153), or SIMPONI 100 mg (n = 153). Patients were allowed to continue stable doses of concomitant MTX, sulfasalazine (SSZ), and/or hydroxychloroquine (HCQ) during the trial. The use of other DMARDs including cytotoxic agents or other biologics was prohibited.

Study RA-2 evaluated 444 patients who had active RA despite a stable dose of at least 15 mg/week of MTX and who had not been previously treated with a biologic TNF-blocker. Patients were randomized to receive background MTX (n = 133), SIMPONI 50 mg + background MTX (n = 89), SIMPONI 100 mg + background MTX (n = 89), or SIMPONI 100 mg monotherapy (n = 133). The use of other DMARDs including SSZ, HCQ, cytotoxic agents, or other biologics was prohibited.

Study RA-3 evaluated 637 patients with active RA who were MTX-naïve and had not previously been treated with a biologic TNF-blocker. Patients were randomized to receive MTX (n = 160), SIMPONI 50 mg + MTX (n = 159), SIMPONI 100 mg + MTX (n = 159), or SIMPONI 100 mg monotherapy (n = 159). For patients receiving MTX, MTX was administered at a dose of 10 mg/week beginning at Week 0 and increased to 20 mg/week by Week 8. The use of other DMARDs including SSZ, HCQ, cytotoxic agents, or other biologics was prohibited.

The primary endpoint in Study RA-1 and Study RA-2 was the percentage of patients achieving an ACR 20 response at Week 14 and the primary endpoint in Study RA-3 was the percentage of patients achieving an ACR 50 response at Week 24.

In Studies RA-1, RA-2, and RA-3, the median duration of RA disease was 9.4, 5.7, and 1.2 years; and 99%, 75%, and 54% of the patients used at least one DMARD in the past, respectively. Approximately 77% and 57% of patients received concomitant NSAIDs and low dose corticosteroids, respectively, in the 3 pooled RA trials.

Clinical Response

In the 3 RA trials, a greater percentage of patients treated with the combination of SIMPONI and MTX achieved ACR responses at Week 14 (Studies RA-1 and RA-2) and Week 24 (Studies RA-1, RA-2, and RA-3) versus patients treated with the MTX alone. There was no clear evidence of improved ACR response with the higher SIMPONI dose group (100 mg) compared to the lower SIMPONI dose group (50 mg). In Studies RA-2 and RA-3, the SIMPONI monotherapy groups were not statistically different from the MTX monotherapy groups in ACR responses. Table 2 shows

Table 2. Studies RA-1, RA-2, and RA-3 Proportion of Patients with an ACR Response*

| | Study RA-1 Active RA previously treated with one or more doses of TNF-blockers | | Study RA-2 Active RA, despite MTX | | Study RA-3 Active RA, MTX Naïve | |
	Placebo ± DMARDs[†]	SIMPONI 50 mg ± DMARDs[†]	Background MTX	SIMPONI 50 mg + Background MTX	MTX	SIMPONI 50 mg + MTX
N[‡]	155	153	133	89	160	159
ACR 20						
Week 14	18%	35%	33%	55%	NA	NA
Week 24	17%	34%	28%	60%	49%	62%
ACR 50						
Week 14	6%	16%	10%	35%	NA	NA
Week 24	5%	18%	14%	37%	29%	40%
ACR 70						
Week 14	2%	10%	4%	13%	NA	NA
Week 24	3%	12%	5%	20%	16%	24%[§]

NA Not applicable, as data was not collected at Week 14 in Study RA-3.
*Approximately 78% and 58% of the patients received concomitant low dose corticosteroids (equivalent to ≤ 10 mg of prednisone a day) and NSAIDs, respectively, during the 3 pooled RA trials.
†DMARDs in Study RA-1 included MTX, HCQ, and/or SSZ (about 68%, 8%, and 5% of patients received MTX, HCQ, and SSZ, respectively).
‡N reflects randomized patients.
§Not significantly different from MTX monotherapy.

the proportion of patients with the ACR response for the SIMPONI 50 mg and control groups in Studies RA-1, RA-2, and RA-3. In the subset of patients who received SIMPONI in combination with MTX in Study RA-1, the proportion of patients achieving ACR 20, 50 and 70 responses at week 14 were 40%, 18%, and 13%, respectively, in the SIMPONI 50 mg + MTX group (N = 103) compared with 17%, 6%, and 2%, respectively, in the placebo + MTX group (N = 107). Table 3 shows the percent improvement in the components of the ACR response criteria for the SIMPONI 50 mg + MTX and MTX groups in Study RA-2. The percent of patients achieving ACR 20 responses by visit for Study RA-2 is shown in Figure 1. ACR 20 responses were observed in 38% of patients in the SIMPONI 50 mg + MTX group at the first assessment (Week 4) after the initial SIMPONI administration.
[See table 2 above]

Table 3. Study RA-2—Median Percent Improvement from Baseline in the Individual ACR Components at Weeks 14*

	Background MTX	SIMPONI 50 mg + Background MTX
N[†]	133	89
Number of swollen joints (0–66)		
Baseline	12	13
Week 14	38%	62%
Number of tender joints (0–68)		
Baseline	21	26
Week 14	30%	60%
Patient's assessment of pain (0–10)		
Baseline	5.7	6.1
Week 14	18%	55%
Patient's global assessment of disease activity (0–10)		
Baseline	5.3	6.0
Week 14	15%	45%
Physician's global assessment of disease activity (0–10)		
Baseline	5.7	6.1

Week 14	35%	55%
HAQ score (0–3)		
Baseline	1.25	1.38
Week 14	10%	29%
CRP (mg/dL)		
Baseline	0.8	1.0
Week 14	2%	44%

Note: Baseline values are medians.
*In Study RA-2, about 70% and 85% of patients received concomitant low dose corticosteroids (equivalent to ≤ 10 mg of prednisone a day) and/or NSAIDs during the trials, respectively.
†N reflects randomized patients; actual number of patients evaluable for each endpoint may vary.

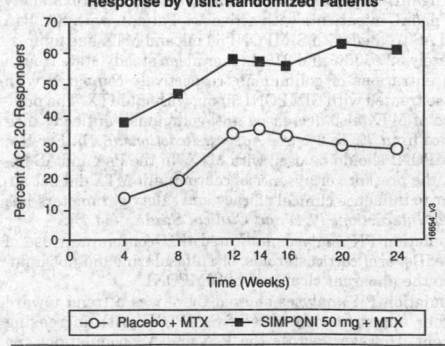

Figure 1. Study RA-2 – Percent of Patients Achieving ACR 20 Response by Visit: Randomized Patients*

○— Placebo + MTX   ■— SIMPONI 50 mg + MTX

*The same patients may not have responded at each timepoint.

Physical Function Response in Patients with RA
In Studies RA-1 and RA-2, the SIMPONI 50 mg groups demonstrated a greater improvement compared to the control groups in the change in mean Health Assessment Questionnaire Disability Index (HAQ-DI) score from baseline to Week 24: 0.25 vs. 0.05 in RA-1, 0.47 vs. 0.13 in RA-2, respectively. Also in Studies RA-1 and RA-2, the SIMPONI 50 mg groups compared to the control groups had a greater propor-

tion of HAQ responders (change from baseline > 0.22) at Week 24: 44% vs. 28%, 65% vs. 35%, respectively.

14.2   Psoriatic Arthritis
The safety and efficacy of SIMPONI were evaluated in a multi-center, randomized, double-blind, placebo-controlled trial in 405 adult patients with moderately to severely active PsA (≥ 3 swollen joints and ≥ 3 tender joints) despite NSAID or DMARD therapy (Study PsA). Patients in this study had a diagnosis of PsA for at least 6 months with a qualifying psoriatic skin lesion of at least 2 cm in diameter. Previous treatment with a biologic TNF-blocker was not allowed. Patients were randomly assigned to placebo (n = 113), SIMPONI 50 mg (n = 146), or SIMPONI 100 mg (n = 146) given subcutaneously every 4 weeks. Patients were allowed to receive stable doses of concomitant MTX (≤ 25 mg/week), low dose oral corticosteroids (equivalent to ≤ 10 mg of prednisone a day), and/or NSAIDs during the trial. The use of other DMARDs including SSZ, HCQ, cytotoxic agents, or other biologics was prohibited. The primary endpoint was the percentage of patients achieving ACR 20 response at Week 14. Placebo-controlled efficacy data were collected and analyzed through Week 24.
Patients with each subtype of PsA were enrolled, including polyarticular arthritis with no rheumatoid nodules (43%), asymmetric peripheral arthritis (30%), distal interphalangeal (DIP) joint arthritis (15%), spondylitis with peripheral arthritis (11%), and arthritis mutilans (1%). The median duration of PsA disease was 5.1 years, 78% of patients received at least one DMARD in the past, and approximately 48% of patients received MTX, and 16% received low dose oral steroids.

Clinical Response in Patients with PsA
SIMPONI ± MTX, compared with placebo ± MTX, resulted in significant improvement in signs and symptoms as demonstrated by the proportion of patients with an ACR 20 response at Week 14 in Study PsA (see Table 4). There was no clear evidence of improved ACR response with the higher SIMPONI dose group (100 mg) compared to the lower SIMPONI dose group (50 mg). ACR responses observed in the SIMPONI-treated groups were similar in patients receiving and not receiving concomitant MTX. Similar ACR 20 responses at Week 14 were observed in patients with different PsA subtypes. However, the number of patients with arthritis mutilans was too small to allow meaningful assessment. SIMPONI 50 mg treatment also resulted in significantly greater improvement compared with placebo for each ACR component in Study PsA (Table 5). Treatment with SIMPONI resulted in improvement in enthesitis and skin manifestations in patients with PsA. However, the safety and efficacy of SIMPONI in the treatment of patients with plaque psoriasis has not been established.
The percent of patients achieving ACR 20 responses by visit for Study PsA is shown in Figure 2. ACR 20 responses were observed in 31% of patients in the SIMPONI 50 mg + MTX group at the first assessment (Week 4) after the initial SIMPONI administration.

Table 4. Study PsA - Proportion of Patients with ACR Responses

	Placebo ± MTX*	SIMPONI 50 mg ± MTX*
N[†]	113	146
ACR 20		
Week 14	**9%**	**51%**
Week 24	12%	52%
ACR 50		
Week 14	2%	30%
Week 24	4%	32%
ACR 70		
Week 14	1%	12%
Week 24	1%	19%

Bold text indicates primary endpoint
*In Study PsA, about 48%, 16%, and 72% of the patients received stable doses of MTX (≤ 25 mg/day), low dose corticosteroids (equivalent to ≤ 10 mg of prednisone a day), and NSAIDs, respectively.
†N reflects randomized patients.

Table 5. Study PsA - Percent Improvement in ACR Components at Week 14

	Placebo ± MTX*	SIMPONI 50 mg ± MTX*
N†	113	146
Number of swollen joints (0–66)		
Baseline	10.0	11.0
Week 14	8%	60%
Number of tender joints (0–68)		
Baseline	18.0	19.0
Week 14	0%	54%
Patient's assessment of pain (0–10)		
Baseline	5.4	5.8
Week 14	-1%	48%
Patient's global assessment of disease activity (0–10)		
Baseline	5.2	5.2
Week 14	2%	49%
Physician's global assessment of disease activity (0–10)		
Baseline	5.2	5.4
Week 14	7%	59%
HAQ score (0–10)		
Baseline	1.0	1.0
Week 14	0%	28%
CRP (mg/dL) (0–10)		
Baseline	0.6	0.6
Week 14	0%	40%

Note: Baseline are median values
*In Study PsA, about 48%, 16%, and 78% of the patients received stable doses of MTX (≤ 25 mg/day), low dose corticosteroids (equivalent to ≤ 10 mg of prednisone a day), and NSAIDs, respectively.
†N reflects randomized patients; actual number of patients evaluable for each endpoint may vary by timepoint

Figure 2. Study PsA – Percent of ACR 20 PsA Responders by Visit: Randomized Patients*

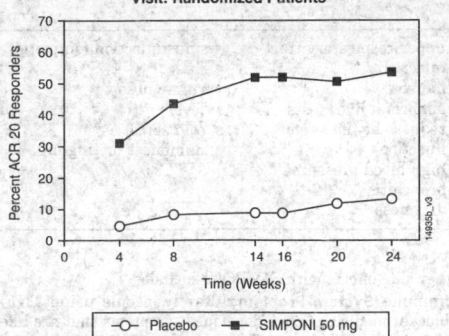

*The same patients may not have responded at each timepoint.

Physical Function Response in Patients with PsA
In Study PsA, SIMPONI 50 mg demonstrated a greater improvement compared to placebo in the change in mean Health Assessment Questionnaire Disability Index (HAQ-DI) score from baseline to Week 24 (0.33 and -0.01, respectively). In addition, the SIMPONI 50 mg group compared to the placebo group had a greater proportion of HAQ responders (≥ 0.3 change from baseline) at Week 24: 43% vs. 22%, respectively.

14.3 Ankylosing Spondylitis
The safety and efficacy of SIMPONI were evaluated in a multi-center, randomized, double-blind, placebo-controlled trial in 356 adult patients with active ankylosing spondylitis according to modified New York criteria for at least 3 months (Study AS). Patients had symptoms of active disease [defined as a Bath AS Disease Activity Index (BASDAI) ≥ 4 and VAS for total back pain of ≥ 4, on scales of 0 to 10 cm] despite current or previous NSAID therapy. Patients were excluded if they were previously treated with a biologic TNF-blocker or if they had complete ankylosis of the spine. Patients were randomly assigned to placebo (n = 78), SIMPONI 50 mg (n = 138), or SIMPONI 100 mg (n = 140) administered subcutaneously every 4 weeks. Patients were allowed to continue stable doses of concomitant MTX, sulfasalazine (SSZ), hydroxychloroquine (HCQ), low dose corticosteroids (equivalent to < 10 mg of prednisone a day), and/or NSAIDs during the trial. The use of other DMARDs including cytotoxic agents or other biologics was prohibited. The primary endpoint was the percentage of patients achieving an ASsessment in Ankylosing Spondylitis (ASAS) 20 response at Week 14. Placebo-controlled efficacy data were collected and analyzed through Week 24.
In Study AS, the median duration of AS disease was 5.6 years, median duration of inflammatory back pain was 12 years, 83% were HLA-B27 positive, 24% had prior joint surgery or procedure, and 55% received at least one DMARD in the past. During the trial, the use of concomitant DMARDs and/or NSAIDs was as follows: MTX (20%), SSZ (26%), HCQ (1%), low dose oral steroids (16%), and NSAIDs (90%).

Clinical Response in Patients with AS
In Study AS, SIMPONI ± DMARDs treatment, compared with placebo ± DMARDs, resulted in a significant improvement in signs and symptoms as demonstrated by the proportion of patients with an ASAS 20 response at Week 14 (see Table 6). There was no clear evidence of improved ASAS response with the higher SIMPONI dose group (100 mg) compared to the lower SIMPONI dose group (50 mg). Table 7 shows the percent improvement in the components of the ASAS response criteria for the SIMPONI 50 mg ± DMARDs and placebo ± DMARDs groups in Study AS.
The percent of patients achieving ASAS 20 responses by visit for Study AS is shown in Figure 3. ASAS 20 responses were observed in 48% of patients in the SIMPONI 50 mg + MTX group at the first assessment (Week 4) after the initial SIMPONI administration.

Table 6. Study AS – Proportion of ASAS Responders at Weeks 14 and 24

	Placebo ± DMARDs*	SIMPONI 50 mg ± DMARDs*
N†	78	138
Responders, % of patients		
ASAS 20		
Week 14	**22%**	**59%**
Week 24	23%	56%
ASAS 40		
Week 14	15%	45%
Week 24	15%	44%

Bold text indicates primary endpoint
*During the trial, the concomitant use of stable doses of DMARDS was as follows: MTX (21%), SSZ (25%), and HCQ (1%). About 16% and 89% of patients received stable doses of low dose oral steroids and NSAIDs during the trial, respectively.
†N reflects randomized patients.

Table 7. Study AS — Median Percent Improvement in ASAS Components at Week 14

	Placebo ± DMARDs*	SIMPONI 50 mg ± DMARDs*
N†	78	138
ASAS components		
Patient global assessment (0–10)		
Baseline	7.2	7.0
Week 14	13%	47%
Total back pain (0–10)		
Baseline	7.6	7.5
Week 14	9%	50%
BASFI (0–10)‡		
Baseline	4.9	5.0
Week 14	-3%	37%
Inflammation (0–10)§		
Baseline	7.1	7.1
Week 14	6%	59%

*During the trial, the concomitant use of stable doses of DMARDS was as follows: MTX (21%), SSZ (25%), and HCQ (1%). About 16% and 89% of patients received stable doses of low dose oral steroids and NSAIDs during the trial, respectively.
†N reflects randomized patients
‡BASFI is Bath Ankylosing Spondylitis Functional Index
§Inflammation is the mean of two patient-reported stiffness self-assessments in the Bath AS Disease Activity Index (BASDAI)

Figure 3. Study AS – Percent of AS Patients Achieving ASAS 20 Response by Visit: Randomized Patients*

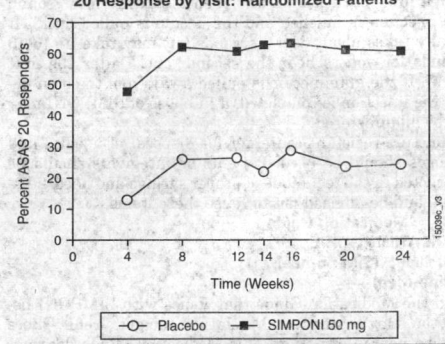

*The same patients may not have responded at each timepoint.

15.0 REFERENCES
1. SEER [database online]. US Population Data – 1969–2004. Bethesda, MD: National Cancer Institute. Release date: January 3, 2007. Available at: http://seer.cancer.gov/popdata/.

16.0 HOW SUPPLIED/STORAGE AND HANDLING
Each SIMPONI prefilled autoinjector or prefilled syringe is packaged in a light-blocking, cardboard outer carton. SIMPONI is available in packs of 1 prefilled syringe NDC 57894-070-01 or 1 prefilled SmartJect autoinjector NDC 57894-070-02.

Prefilled SmartJect Autoinjector
Each single dose SmartJect autoinjector contains a prefilled glass syringe (27 gauge ½ inch) providing 50 mg of SIMPONI per 0.5 mL of solution.

Prefilled Syringe
Each single dose prefilled glass syringe (27 gauge ½ inch) contains 50 mg of SIMPONI per 0.5 mL of solution.

Storage and Stability
SIMPONI must be refrigerated at 2°C to 8°C (36°F to 46°F) and protected from light. Keep the product in the original carton to protect from light until the time of use. Do not freeze. Do not shake. Do not use SIMPONI beyond the expiration date (EXP) on the carton or the expiration date on the prefilled syringe (observed through the viewing window) or the prefilled SmartJect autoinjector.

17.0 PATIENT COUNSELING INFORMATION
See Medication Guide (17.3)
17.1 Patient Counseling
Patients should be advised of the potential benefits and risks of SIMPONI. Physicians should instruct their patients to read the Medication Guide before starting SIMPONI therapy and to read it each time the prescription is renewed.
Infections
Inform patients that SIMPONI may lower the ability of their immune system to fight infections. Instruct the pa-

tient of the importance of contacting their doctor if they develop any symptoms of infection, including tuberculosis, invasive fungal infections, and hepatitis B reactivation.

Malignancies

Patients should be counseled about the risk of lymphoma and other malignancies while receiving SIMPONI.

Allergic Reactions

Advise latex-sensitive patients that the needle cover on the prefilled syringe as well as the prefilled syringe in the prefilled SmartJect autoinjector contains dry natural rubber (a derivative of latex).

Other Medical Conditions

Advise patients to report any signs of new or worsening medical conditions such as congestive heart failure, demyelinating disorders, autoimmune diseases, liver disease, cytopenias, or psoriasis.

17.2   Instruction on Injection Technique

The first self-injection should be performed under the supervision of a qualified healthcare professional. If a patient or caregiver is to administer SIMPONI, he/she should be instructed in injection techniques and their ability to inject subcutaneously should be assessed to ensure the proper administration of SIMPONI [see Medication Guide (17.3)].

Prior to use, remove the prefilled syringe or the prefilled SmartJect autoinjector from the refrigerator and allow SIMPONI to sit at room temperature outside of the carton for 30 minutes and out of the reach of children.

Do not warm SIMPONI in any other way. For example, do not warm SIMPONI in a microwave or in hot water.

Do not remove the prefilled syringe needle cover or SmartJect autoinjector cap while allowing SIMPONI to reach room temperature. Remove these immediately before injection.

Do not pull the autoinjector away from the skin until you hear a first "click" sound and then a second "click" sound (the injection is finished and the needle is pulled back). It usually takes about 3 to 6 seconds but may take up to 15 seconds for you to hear the second "click" after the first "click". If the autoinjector is pulled away from the skin before the injection is completed, a full dose of SIMPONI may not be administered.

A puncture-resistant container for disposal of needles and syringes should be used. Patients or caregivers should be instructed in the technique of proper syringe and needle disposal, and be advised not to reuse these items.

17.3   Medication Guide

MEDICATION GUIDE

SIMPONI™ (SIM-po-nee)

(golimumab)

Read the Medication Guide that comes with SIMPONI before you start taking it and each time you get a refill. There may be new information. This Medication Guide does not take the place of talking with your doctor about your medical condition or treatment. It is important to remain under your doctor's care while using SIMPONI.

What is the most important information I should know about SIMPONI?

SIMPONI is a medicine that affects your immune system. SIMPONI can lower the ability of your immune system to fight infections. Some people have serious infections while taking SIMPONI, including tuberculosis (TB), and infections caused by bacteria, fungi, or viruses that spread throughout their body. Some people have died from these serious infections.

• Your doctor should test you for TB before starting SIMPONI.

• Your doctor should monitor you closely for signs and symptoms of TB during treatment with SIMPONI.

You should not start taking SIMPONI if you have any kind of infection unless your doctor says it is okay.

Before starting SIMPONI, tell your doctor if you:

• think you have an infection or have symptoms of an infection such as:

• fever, sweat, or chills	• warm, red, or painful skin or sores on your body
• muscle aches	• diarrhea or stomach pain
• cough	• burning when you urinate
• shortness of breath	or urinate more often than
• blood in phlegm	normal
• weight loss	• feel very tired

• are being treated for an infection

• get a lot of infections or have infections that keep coming back

• have diabetes, HIV, or a weak immune system. People with these conditions have a higher chance for infections.

• have TB, or have been in close contact with someone with TB

• live, have lived, or traveled to certain parts of the country (such as the Ohio and Mississippi River valleys and the Southwest) where there is an increased chance for getting

certain kinds of fungal infections (histoplasmosis, coccidioidomycosis, blastomycosis). These infections may happen or become more severe if you use SIMPONI. Ask your doctor, if you do not know if you have lived in an area where these infections are common.

• have or have had hepatitis B

• use the medicine Orencia (abatacept), Kineret (anakinra), or Rituxan (rituximab)

After starting SIMPONI, call your doctor right away if you have any symptoms of an infection. SIMPONI can make you more likely to get infections or make worse any infection that you have.

Cancer

• There have been cases of unusual cancers in children and teenage patients taking TNF-blocking agents.

• For children and adults taking TNF-blocker medicines, including SIMPONI, the chances of getting lymphoma or other cancers may increase.

• People with inflammatory diseases including rheumatoid arthritis, psoriatic arthritis, or ankylosing spondylitis, especially those with very active disease, may be more likely to get lymphoma.

What is SIMPONI?

SIMPONI is a prescription medicine called a Tumor Necrosis Factor (TNF) blocker. SIMPONI is used in adults:

• with the medicine methotrexate to treat moderately to severely active rheumatoid arthritis (RA)

• to treat active psoriatic arthritis (PsA) alone or with methotrexate

• to treat active ankylosing spondylitis (AS)

You may continue to use other medicines that help treat your condition while taking SIMPONI, such as nonsteroidal anti-inflammatory drugs (NSAIDs) and prescription steroids, as recommended by your doctor.

What should I tell my doctor before starting treatment with SIMPONI?

SIMPONI may not be right for you. Before starting SIMPONI, tell your doctor about all your medical conditions, including if you:

• have an infection (see "What is the most important information I should know about SIMPONI?").

• have or have had lymphoma or any other type of cancer.

• have or had heart failure.

• have or have had a condition that affects your nervous system, such as multiple sclerosis.

• have recently received or are scheduled to receive a vaccine. People taking SIMPONI should not receive live vaccines. People taking SIMPONI can receive non-live vaccines.

• are allergic to rubber or latex. The needle cover on the prefilled syringe and SmartJect autoinjector contains dry natural rubber.

• are pregnant or planning to become pregnant. It is not known if SIMPONI will harm your unborn baby.

• are breastfeeding. You and your doctor should decide if you will take SIMPONI or breastfeed. You should not do both without talking to your doctor first.

Tell your doctor about all the medicines you take, including prescription and non-prescription medicines, vitamins, and herbal supplements. Especially, tell your doctor if you use:

• ORENCIA (abatacept), KINERET (anakinra), or RITUXAN (rituximab). You should not take SIMPONI while you are also taking ORENCIA or KINERET. Your doctor may not want to give you SIMPONI if you have received RITUXAN recently.

• Another TNF-blocker medicine. You should not take SIMPONI while you are also taking REMICADE (infliximab), HUMIRA (adalimumab), ENBREL (etanercept), or CIMZIA (certolizumab pegol).

Ask your doctor if you are not sure if your medicine is one listed above.

Keep a list of all your medications with you to show your doctor and pharmacist each time you get a new medicine.

How should I use SIMPONI?

• SIMPONI is given as an injection under the skin (subcutaneous injection or SC).

• SIMPONI should be injected one time each month.

• If your doctor decides that you or a caregiver may be able to give your injections of SIMPONI at home, you should receive training on the right way to prepare and inject SIMPONI. Do not try to inject SIMPONI yourself until you have been shown the right way to give the injections by your doctor or nurse.

• Use SIMPONI exactly as prescribed by your doctor.

• SIMPONI comes in a prefilled syringe or SmartJect™ autoinjector. Your doctor will prescribe the type that is best for you.

• See the detailed *Patient Instructions for Use* at the end of this Medication Guide for instructions about the right

way to prepare and give your SIMPONI injections at home.

• Do not miss any doses of SIMPONI. If you forget to use SIMPONI, inject your dose as soon as you remember. Then, take your next dose at your regular scheduled time. In case you are not sure when to inject SIMPONI, call your doctor or pharmacist.

What are the possible side effects with SIMPONI?

SIMPONI can cause serious side effects, including:

See **"What is the most important information I should know about SIMPONI?"**

Serious Infections

Hepatitis B infection in people who carry the virus in their blood.

• If you are a carrier of the hepatitis B virus (a virus that affects the liver), the virus can become active while you use SIMPONI. Your doctor may do blood tests before you start treatment with SIMPONI and while you are using SIMPONI. Tell your doctor if you have any of the following symptoms of a possible hepatitis B infection:

• feel very tired	• clay-colored bowel
• skin or eyes look yellow	movements
• little or no appetite	• fevers
• vomiting	• chills
• muscle aches	• stomach discomfort
• dark urine	• skin rash

Heart failure, including new heart failure or worsening of heart failure that you already have. New or worse heart failure can happen in people who use TNF-blocker medicines like SIMPONI.

• If you have heart failure, your condition should be watched closely while you take SIMPONI.

• Call your doctor right away if you get new or worsening symptoms of heart failure while taking SIMPONI (such as shortness of breath or swelling of your lower legs or feet).

Nervous System Problems

Rarely, people using TNF-blocker medicine have nervous system problems such as multiple sclerosis.

• Tell your doctor right away if you get any of these symptoms:

  • vision changes

  • weakness in your arms or legs

  • numbness or tingling in any part of your body

Liver Problems

Liver problems can happen in people who use TNF-blocker medicines, including SIMPONI. These problems can lead to liver failure and death. Call your doctor right away if you have any of these symptoms:

• feel very tired

• skin or eyes look yellow

• poor appetite or vomiting

• pain on the right side of your stomach (abdomen)

Blood Problems

Low blood counts have been seen with other TNF-blockers. Your body may not make enough blood cells that help fight infections or help stop bleeding. Symptoms include fever, bruising or bleeding easily, or looking pale. Your doctor will check your blood counts before and during treatment with SIMPONI.

Common side effects with SIMPONI include:

• upper respiratory tract infection	• sinus infection (sinusitis)
• nausea	• flu
• abnormal liver tests	• runny nose
• redness at the site of injection	• fever
• high blood pressure	• cold sores
• bronchitis	• numbness or tingling
• dizziness	

Other side effects with SIMPONI include:

• **Immune System Problems.** Rarely, people using TNF-blocker medicines have developed symptoms that are like the symptoms of Lupus. Tell your doctor if you have any of these symptoms:

• a rash on your cheeks or other parts of the body

• sensitivity to the sun

• new joint or muscle pains

• becoming very tired

• chest pain or shortness of breath

• swelling of the feet, ankles, and/or legs

- **Psoriasis.** Some people using SIMPONI had new psoriasis or worsening of psoriasis they already had. Tell your doctor if you develop red scaly patches or raised bumps that are filled with pus. Your doctor may decide to stop your treatment with SIMPONI.
- **Allergic Reactions.** Allergic reactions can happen in people who use TNF-blocker medicines. Call your doctor right away if you have any of these symptoms of an allergic reaction:
  - hives
  - swollen face
  - breathing trouble
  - chest pain

These are not all of the side effects with SIMPONI. Tell your doctor about any side effect that bothers you or does not go away. Call your doctor for medical advice about side effects. You may report side effects to the FDA at 1-800-FDA-1088.

How do I store SIMPONI?
- Refrigerate SIMPONI at 36°F to 46°F (2°C to 8°C).
- Do not freeze SIMPONI.
- Keep SIMPONI in the carton to protect it from light when not being used.
- Do not shake SIMPONI.

Keep SIMPONI and all medicines out of the reach of children.

General Information about SIMPONI
- Medicines are sometimes prescribed for purposes other than those listed in the Medication Guide. Do not use SIMPONI for a condition for which it was not prescribed.
- Do not give SIMPONI to other people, even if they have the same condition that you have. It may harm them.
- This Medication Guide summarizes the most important information about SIMPONI. If you would like more information, talk to your doctor. You can ask your doctor or pharmacist for information about SIMPONI that is written for health professionals. For more information go to www.simponi.com or call 1-800-457-6399.

What are the ingredients in SIMPONI?
Active ingredient: golimumab.
Inactive ingredients: L-histidine, L-histidine monohydrochloride monohydrate, sorbitol, polysorbate 80, and water for injection. SIMPONI does not contain preservatives.

Patient Instructions for Use
SIMPONI™ (SIM-po-nee)
(golimumab)
SmartJect™ autoinjector
If your doctor decides that you or a caregiver may be able to give your injections of SIMPONI at home, you should receive training on the right way to prepare and inject SIMPONI. **Do not** try to inject SIMPONI yourself until you have been shown the right way to give the injections by your doctor or nurse.
It is important to read, understand, and follow these instructions so that you inject SIMPONI the right way. Call your doctor if you or your caregiver has any questions about the right way to inject SIMPONI.
Important information about your SmartJect autoinjector:
- When the button on the SmartJect autoinjector is pressed to give the dose of SIMPONI you will hear a loud 'click' sound. It is very important that you practice injecting SIMPONI with your doctor or nurse so that you are not startled by this click when you start giving the injections to yourself at home.
- If you pull the SmartJect autoinjector away from the skin before the injection is completed, you may not get your full dose of medicine and may lose some of the medicine.

Do not:
- shake the SmartJect autoinjector at any time
- remove the SmartJect autoinjector cap until you get to that step

Step 1:   Gather and inspect the supplies for your injection
You will need these supplies for an injection of SIMPONI. See Figure 1.
- 1 alcohol swab
- 1 cotton ball or gauze
- 1 SIMPONI prefilled SmartJect autoinjector
- sharps container for autoinjector disposal

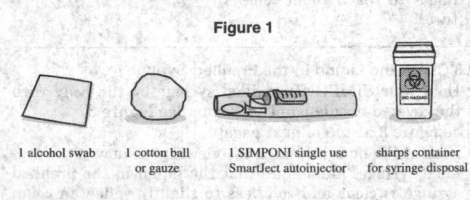

Figure 1

1 alcohol swab   1 cotton ball or gauze   1 SIMPONI single use SmartJect autoinjector   sharps container for syringe disposal

The figure below shows what the SmartJect autoinjector looks like. See Figure 2.

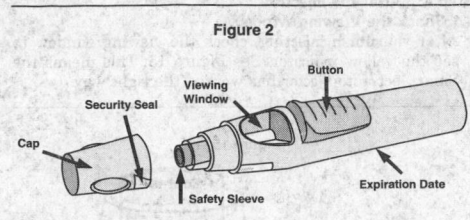

Figure 2

Security Seal — Cap — Viewing Window — Button — Safety Sleeve — Expiration Date

1.1 Check Expiration Date
- Check the expiration date ("EXP") on the SmartJect autoinjector.
- You can also check the expiration date printed on the carton.
- If the expiration date has passed, do not use the SmartJect autoinjector. Call your doctor or pharmacist, or call 1-800-457-6399 for help.

1.2 Check Security Seal
- Check the security seal around the cap of the SmartJect autoinjector. If the security seal is broken, do not use the SmartJect autoinjector.

1.3 Wait 30 minutes

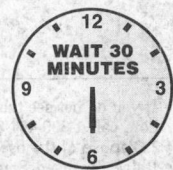

- To ensure proper injection, allow the autoinjector to sit at room temperature outside the carton for 30 minutes and out of the reach of children.

WAIT 30 MINUTES

Do not warm the SmartJect autoinjector in any other way (For example, **do not** warm it in a microwave or in hot water).
Do not remove the SmartJect autoinjector cap while allowing it to reach room temperature.

1.4 Check the Liquid in the SmartJect autoinjector
- Look through the viewing window of the SmartJect autoinjector. See Figure 3. Make sure that the liquid in the prefilled syringe is clear and colorless to slightly yellow in color. You may see a small amount of tiny particles that are white, or that you can see through. Do not inject the liquid if it is cloudy or discolored, or has large particles in it.
- You may also notice an air bubble. This is normal. See Figure 3.

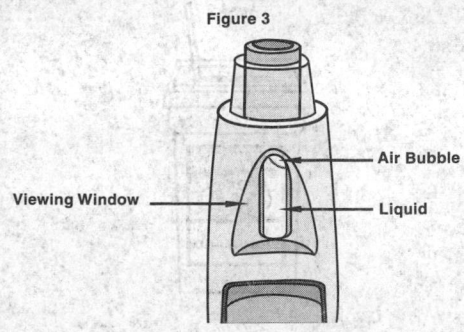

Figure 3

Viewing Window — Air Bubble — Liquid

Step 2:   Choose and prepare the injection site

2.1 Choose the Injection Site
- The recommended injection site is the front of your middle thighs. See Figure 4.

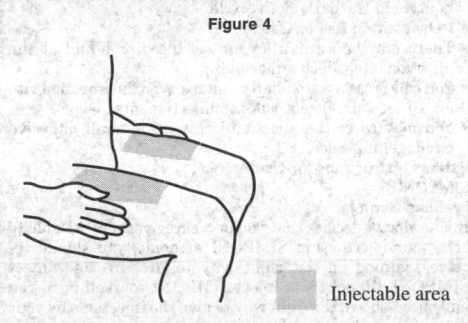

Figure 4

Injectable area

- You can also use the lower part of the abdomen below the navel (belly button), except for the two-inch area directly around the navel. See Figure 5.
- If a caregiver is giving you the injection, the outer area of the upper arms may also be used. See Figure 5.

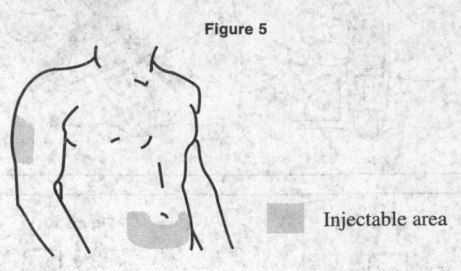

Figure 5

Injectable area

- **Do not** inject into areas where the skin is tender, bruised, red, scaly, or hard. Avoid areas with scars or stretch marks.

2.2 Prepare the Injection Site
- Wash your hands well with soap and warm water.
- Wipe the injection site with an alcohol swab.
- **Do not** touch this area again before giving the injection. Allow the skin to dry before injecting.
- **Do not** fan or blow on the clean area.

Step 3: Injecting SIMPONI using the single dose SmartJect autoinjector

3.1 Remove the Cap
- Do not remove the cap until you are ready to inject SIMPONI. Inject SIMPONI within 5 minutes after the cap has been removed.
- When you are ready to inject, twist the cap slightly to break the security seal. See Figure 6.

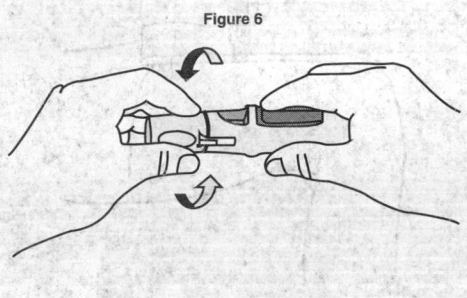

Figure 6

- Pull the cap off and throw it in the trash right away. See Figure 7.

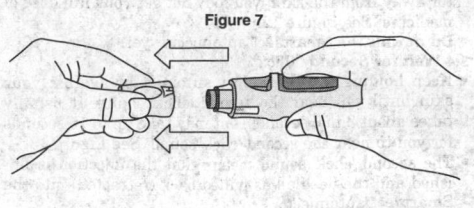

Figure 7

- **Do not** put the cap back on because it may damage the needle inside the SmartJect autoinjector.
- **Do not** use your SmartJect autoinjector if it is dropped without the cap in place.

3.2 Push the SmartJect autoinjector against the skin
- Hold the SmartJect autoinjector comfortably in your hand.
- Do not press the button. Push the open end of the SmartJect autoinjector firmly against the skin at **90-degree angle**. See Figure 8.
[See figure 8 at top of next page]
- **Use your** free hand to pinch and hold the skin at the injection site. This may make injecting easier.

3.3 Press button to inject
- Continue to hold the SmartJect autoinjector firmly against the skin, and press the button with your fingers (see Figure 9) or thumb (see Figure 10). You will not be able to push in the button unless the SmartJect autoinjector is pushed firmly against your skin.

Figure 8

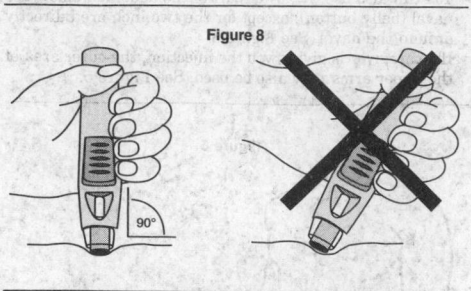

Figure 9

Figure 10

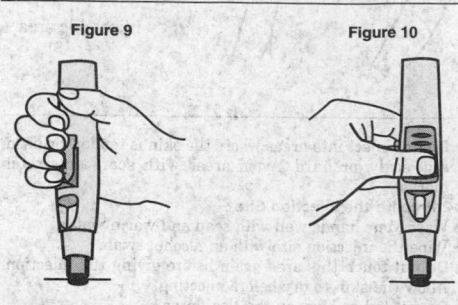

• After the button is pressed, it will stay pressed in so you do not need to keep pressure on it. See Figure 11.

Figure 11

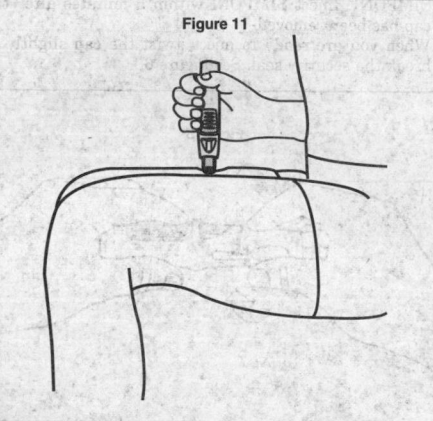

• You will hear a loud 'click' sound. This means that the injection has started. Do not pull the SmartJect autoinjector away from your skin. If you pull the SmartJect autoinjector away from the skin, you may not get your full dose of medicine. See Figure 12.
• **Do not** lift the SmartJect autoinjector yet.

3.4 Wait for Second "Click"
• Keep holding the SmartJect autoinjector against your skin until you hear the second 'click' sound. It usually takes about 3 to 6 seconds, but may take up to 15 seconds for you to hear the second 'click' sound. See Figure 13.
• The second 'click' sound means that the injection is finished and the needle has pulled back (retracted) into the SmartJect autoinjector.
• Lift the SmartJect autoinjector from the injection site. See Figure 14.
• If you have hearing problems, count for 15 seconds from the time you pressed the button and then lift the SmartJect autoinjector from the injection site.

Figure 12   **Figure 13**   **Figure 14**

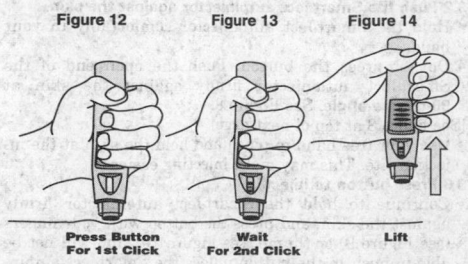

Press Button   Wait   Lift
For 1st Click   For 2nd Click

Step 4:   After the injection
4.1 Check the Viewing Window
• After you finish injecting, check the viewing window to see the yellow indicator. See Figure 15. This means the SmartJect autoinjector has worked the right way.

Figure 15

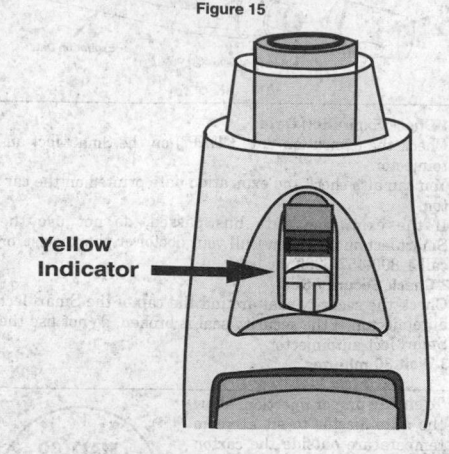

Yellow Indicator →

• If you do not see the yellow indicator in the viewing window, call 1-800-457-6399 for help.
4.2 Dispose of the used SmartJect autoinjector
• Place the used SmartJect autoinjector into a closable puncture-resistant container. You may use a sharps container (such as a red biohazard container), a hard plastic container (such as a detergent bottle), or a metal container (such as an empty coffee can). See Figure 16.

Figure 16

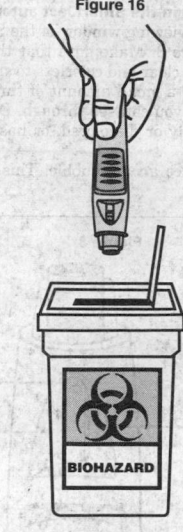

BIOHAZARD

• Ask your doctor for instructions on the right way to throw away (dispose of) the container. There may be local or state laws about how you should throw away used needles and syringes.
• Do not throw away your used SmartJect autoinjector in household trash. Do not recycle.
4.3 Use Cotton Ball or Gauze
• There may be a small amount of blood or liquid at the injection site, which is normal.
• You can press a cotton ball or gauze over the injection site for 10 seconds. Do not rub the injection site.
• You may cover the injection site with a small adhesive bandage, if needed.
Patient Instructions for Use
SIMPONI™
Prefilled Syringe
If your doctor decides that you or a caregiver may be able to give your injections of SIMPONI at home, you should receive training on the right way to prepare and inject SIMPONI. **Do not** try to inject SIMPONI yourself until you have been shown the right way to give the injections by your doctor or nurse.

It is important to read, understand, and follow these instructions so that you inject SIMPONI the right way. Call your doctor if you or your caregiver has any questions about the right way to inject SIMPONI.
Important information about your prefilled syringe:
• Always hold the prefilled syringe by the body of the syringe.
Do not:
• pull back on the plunger at any time.
• shake the SIMPONI prefilled syringe. This may damage the medicine.
• remove the needle cover from the prefilled syringe until you get to that step.
• touch the needle guard activation clips to prevent covering the needle with the needle guard too soon (See Figure 2).
• use SIMPONI if it has been frozen or if it has been kept at a room temperature that is too warm. See the Medication Guide section: "How should I store SIMPONI?"
• use your SIMPONI prefilled syringe if it looks damaged.
Step 1:   Gather the supplies for your injection
You will need these supplies for an injection of SIMPONI. See Figure 1.
• 1 alcohol swab
• 1 cotton ball or gauze
• 1 SIMPONI prefilled syringe
• sharps container for syringe disposal

Figure 1

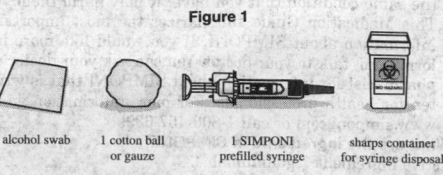

1 alcohol swab   1 cotton ball   1 SIMPONI   sharps container
                  or gauze   prefilled syringe   for syringe disposal

The diagram below shows what the prefilled syringe looks like. See Figure 2.

Figure 2

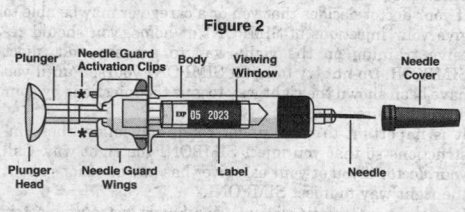

Plunger   Needle Guard   Body   Viewing   Needle
          Activation Clips   Window   Cover

Plunger   Needle Guard   Label   Needle
Head   Wings

Step 2:   Get ready to use your prefilled syringe
2.1 Check the Expiration Date
• Look for the expiration date printed on the back panel of the SIMPONI carton.
• **If the expiration date has passed, do not use the prefilled syringe. Call your doctor** or pharmacist or call 1-800-457-6399 for help.
2.2 Wait 30 minutes

• To ensure proper injection, allow the prefilled syringe to sit at room temperature outside of the carton for 30 minutes and out of the reach of children.
• **Do not** warm the prefilled syringe in any other way (For example, **Do not** warm it in a microwave or in hot water).
• **Do not** remove the prefilled syringe needle cover while allowing it to reach room temperature.

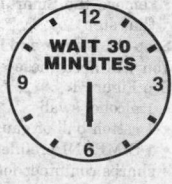

WAIT 30 MINUTES

2.3 Check the Liquid in the Prefilled Syringe
• Hold your SIMPONI prefilled syringe by the body with the covered needle pointing down. See Figure 3.
[See figure 3 at top of next page]
• Look at the liquid through the viewing window of the prefilled syringe. Make sure that the liquid in the prefilled syringe is clear and colorless to slightly yellow in color. You may see a small amount of tiny particles that are white, or that you can see through. Do not inject the liquid if it is cloudy or discolored, or has large particles in it.
• You may also see an air bubble. This is normal.

Figure 3

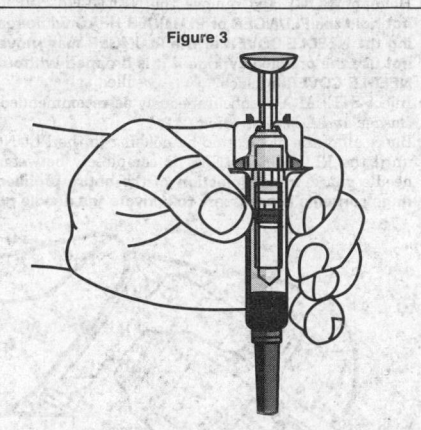

Step 3: Choose and prepare the injection site

3.1 Choose the Injection Site

• The recommended injection site is the front of your middle thighs. See Figure 4.

Figure 4

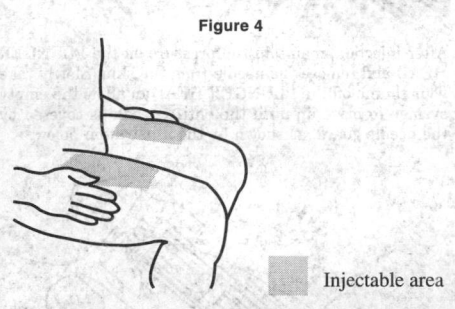

Injectable area

• You can also use the lower part of the abdomen below the navel (belly button), except for the two-inch area directly around the navel. See Figure 5.
• If a caregiver is giving you the injection, the outer area of the upper arms may also be used. See Figure 5.

Figure 5

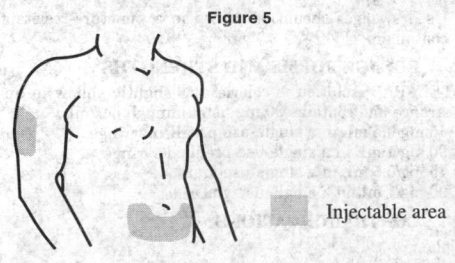

Injectable area

Do not inject into areas where the skin is tender, bruised, red, scaly, or hard. Avoid areas with scars or stretch marks.

3.2 Prepare the Injection Site

• Wash your hands well with soap and warm water.
• Wipe the injection site with an alcohol swab.
• **Do not** touch this area again before giving the injection. Let your skin dry before injecting.
• **Do not** fan or blow on the clean area.

Step 4: Inject SIMPONI

Do not remove the needle cover until you are ready to inject SIMPONI. Inject SIMPONI within 5 minutes after you remove the needle cover.

4.1 Remove the Needle Cover

• **Do not** touch the plunger while removing the needle cover.
• Hold the body of the prefilled syringe with one hand, and pull the needle cover straight off. See Figure 6.

[See figure 6 at top of next column]

• Put the needle cover in the trash.
• You may see an air bubble in the prefilled syringe. This is normal.

Figure 6

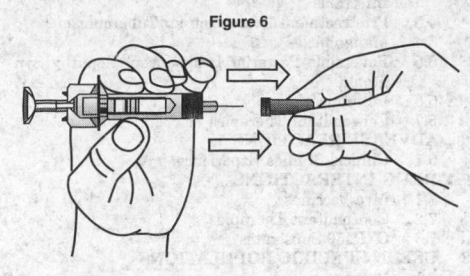

• You may also see a drop of liquid at the end of the needle. This is normal.
• **Do not** touch the needle or let it touch any surface.
• **Do not** use the prefilled syringe if it is dropped without the needle cover in place.

4.2 Position the prefilled syringe and inject SIMPONI

• Hold the body of the prefilled syringe in one hand between the thumb and index fingers. See Figure 7.

Figure 7

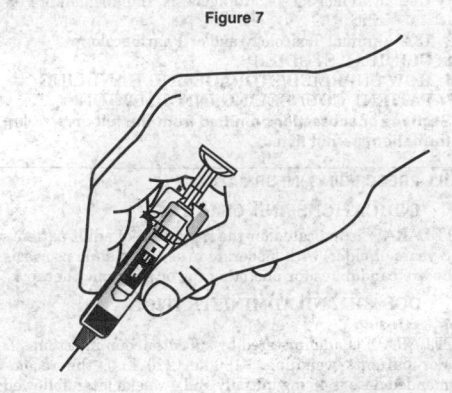

• **Do not** pull back on the plunger at any time.
• Use the other hand to gently pinch the area of skin that you previously cleaned. Hold firmly.
• Use a quick, dart-like motion to insert the needle into the pinched skin at about a **45-degree angle**. See Figure 8.

Figure 8

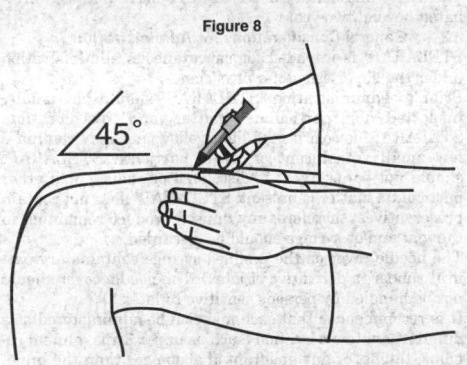

45°

• Inject all of the medicine by using your thumb to push in the plunger until the plunger head is completely between the needle guard wings. See Figure 9.

Figure 9

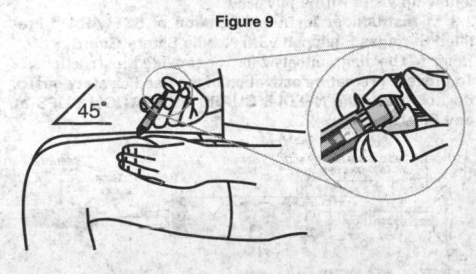

45°

• When the plunger is pushed as far as it will go, keep pressure on the plunger head. Take the needle out of the skin and let go of the skin.
• Slowly take your thumb off the plunger head. This will let the empty syringe move up until the entire needle is covered by the needle guard. See Figure 10.

Figure 10

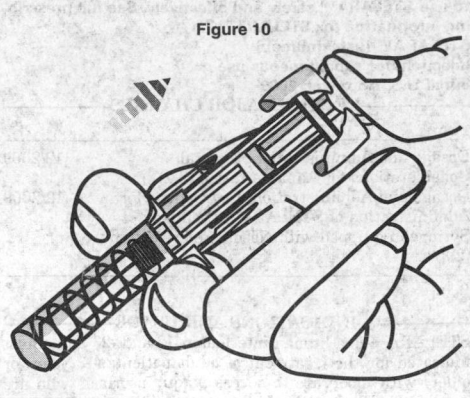

Step 5: After the injection

5.1 Dispose of the used prefilled syringe

• Place the used prefilled syringe in a closable puncture-resistant container. You may use a sharps container (such as a red biohazard container), a hard plastic container (such as a detergent bottle), or a metal container (such as an empty coffee can). For the safety and health of you and others, needles and used syringes **must never** be re-used. See Figure 11.

Figure 11

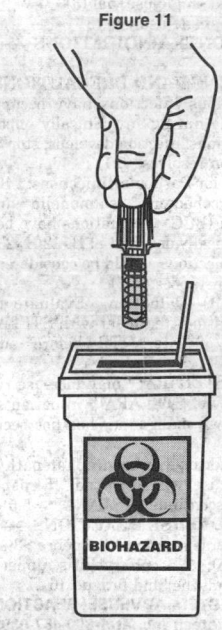

BIOHAZARD

• Ask your doctor for instructions on the right way to throw away (dispose of) the container. There may be local or state laws about how you should throw away used needles and syringes.
• Do not throw away your used prefilled syringe in household trash. Do not recycle.

5.2 Use Cotton Ball or Gauze

• There may be a small amount of blood or liquid at the injection site, which is normal.
• You can press a cotton ball or gauze over the injection site and hold for 10 seconds. Do not rub the injection site.
• You may cover the injection site with a small adhesive bandage, if needed.

Manufactured by:
Centocor Ortho Biotech Inc.
Horsham, PA 19044
US License No. 1821
Revised: 11/2009
This Medication Guide has been approved by the U.S. Food and Drug Administration.

Shown in Product Identification Guide, page 307

STELARA™   ℞
[stel ar' a]
(ustekinumab)
Injection, for subcutaneous use

HIGHLIGHTS OF PRESCRIBING INFORMATION
These highlights do not include all the information needed to use STELARA™ safely and effectively. See full prescribing information for STELARA™.
STELARA™ (ustekinumab)
Injection, for subcutaneous use
Initial U.S. Approval: 2009

————RECENT MAJOR CHANGES————

Dosage and Administration, General Considerations for Administration (2.2)	12/2009
Dosage and Administration, Instructions for Administration of STELARA™ Prefilled Syringes Equipped with Needle Safety Guard (2.3)	12/2009

————INDICATIONS AND USAGE————
STELARA™ is a human interleukin-12 and -23 antagonist indicated for the treatment of adult patients (18 years or older) with moderate to severe plaque psoriasis who are candidates for phototherapy or systemic therapy. (1)

————DOSAGE AND ADMINISTRATION————
STELARA™ is administered by subcutaneous injection. (2)
• For patients weighing ≤100 kg (220 lbs), the recommended dose is 45 mg initially and 4 weeks later, followed by 45 mg every 12 weeks. (2.1)
• For patients weighing >100 kg (220 lbs), the recommended dose is 90 mg initially and 4 weeks later, followed by 90 mg every 12 weeks. (2.1)

————DOSAGE FORMS AND STRENGTHS————
• 45 mg/0.5 mL in a single-use prefilled syringe (3)
• 90 mg/1 mL in a single-use prefilled syringe (3)
• 45 mg/0.5 mL in a single-use vial (3)
• 90 mg/1 mL in a single-use vial (3)

————CONTRAINDICATIONS————
None (4)

————WARNINGS AND PRECAUTIONS————
• Infections: Serious infections have occurred. Do not start STELARA™ during any clinically important active infection. If a serious infection develops, stop STELARA™ until the infection resolves. (5.1)
• Theoretical Risk for Particular Infections: Serious infections from mycobacteria, salmonella and Bacillus Calmette-Guerin (BCG) vaccinations have been reported in patients genetically deficient in IL-12/IL-23. Diagnostic tests for these infections should be considered as dictated by clinical circumstances. (5.2)
• Tuberculosis (TB) evaluation: Evaluate patients for TB prior to initiating treatment with STELARA™. Initiate treatment of latent TB before administering STELARA™. (5.3)
• Malignancies: STELARA™ may increase risk of malignancy. The safety of STELARA™ in patients with a history of or a known malignancy has not been evaluated. (5.4)
• Reversible Posterior Leukoencephalopathy Syndrome (RPLS): One case was reported. If suspected, treat promptly and discontinue STELARA™. (5.5)

————ADVERSE REACTIONS————
Most common adverse reactions (incidence >3% and greater than with placebo): Nasopharyngitis, upper respiratory tract infection, headache, and fatigue. (6.1)
To report SUSPECTED ADVERSE REACTIONS, contact Centocor Ortho Biotech Inc. at 1-800-457-6399 or FDA at 1-800-FDA-1088 or www.fda.gov/medwatch.

————DRUG INTERACTIONS————
• Live vaccines: Live vaccines should not be given with STELARA™. (7.1)
• Concomitant therapy: The safety of concomitant use of STELARA™ with immunosuppressants or phototherapy has not been evaluated. (7.2)

See 17 for PATIENT COUNSELING INFORMATION and Medication Guide

Revised: 12/2009

FULL PRESCRIBING INFORMATION: CONTENTS*

FULL PRESCRIBING INFORMATION

1   INDICATIONS AND USAGE
STELARA™ is indicated for the treatment of adult patients (18 years or older) with moderate to severe plaque psoriasis who are candidates for phototherapy or systemic therapy.

2   DOSAGE AND ADMINISTRATION
2.1   Dosing
STELARA™ is administered by subcutaneous injection.
• For patients weighing ≤100 kg (220 lbs), the recommended dose is 45 mg initially and 4 weeks later, followed by 45 mg every 12 weeks.
• For patients weighing >100 kg (220 lbs), the recommended dose is 90 mg initially and 4 weeks later, followed by 90 mg every 12 weeks.
In subjects weighing >100 kg, 45 mg was also shown to be efficacious. However, 90 mg resulted in greater efficacy in these subjects [see Clinical Studies (14)].
The safety and efficacy of STELARA™ have not been evaluated beyond two years.

2.2   General Considerations for Administration
STELARA™ is intended for subcutaneous administration under the supervision of a physician.
Prior to administration, STELARA™ should be visually inspected for particulate matter and discoloration. STELARA™ is colorless to light yellow and may contain a few small translucent or white particles. STELARA™ should not be used if it is discolored or cloudy, or if other particulate matter is present. STELARA™ does not contain preservatives; therefore, any unused product remaining in the vial and/or syringe should be discarded.
The needle cover on the prefilled syringe contains dry natural rubber (a derivative of latex). The needle cover should not be handled by persons sensitive to latex.
It is recommended that each injection be administered at a different anatomic location (such as upper arms, gluteal regions, thighs, or any quadrant of abdomen) than the previous injection, and not into areas where the skin is tender, bruised, erythematous, or indurated. When using the single-use vial, a 27 gauge, ½ inch needle is recommended. STELARA™ should only be administered by a healthcare provider. STELARA™ should only be administered to patients who will be closely monitored and have regular follow-up visits with a physician.

2.3   Instructions for Administration of STELARA™ Prefilled Syringes Equipped with Needle Safety Guard
Refer to the diagram below for the provided instructions.
To prevent premature activation of the needle safety guard, do not touch the NEEDLE GUARD ACTIVATION CLIPS at any time during use.

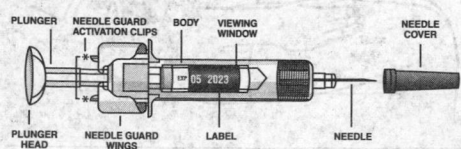

PLUNGER   NEEDLE GUARD ACTIVATION CLIPS   BODY   VIEWING WINDOW   NEEDLE COVER
PLUNGER HEAD   NEEDLE GUARD WINGS   LABEL   NEEDLE

• Hold the BODY and remove the NEEDLE COVER. Do not hold the PLUNGER or PLUNGER HEAD while removing the NEEDLE COVER or the PLUNGER may move. Do not use the prefilled syringe if it is dropped without the NEEDLE COVER in place.
• Inject STELARA™ subcutaneously as recommended [see Dosage and Administration (2.2)].
• Inject all of the medication by pushing in the PLUNGER until the PLUNGER HEAD is completely between the needle guard wings. Injection of the entire prefilled syringe contents is necessary to activate the needle guard.

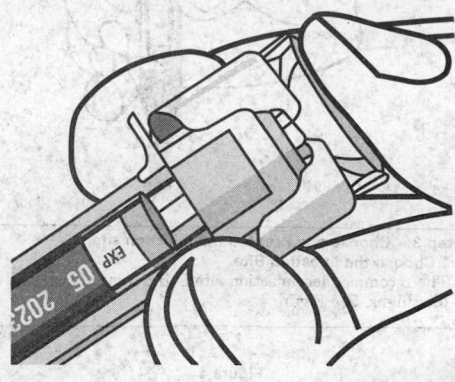

• After injection, maintain the pressure on the PLUNGER HEAD and remove the needle from the skin. Slowly take your thumb off the PLUNGER HEAD to allow the empty syringe to move up until the entire needle is covered by the needle guard, as shown by the illustration below:

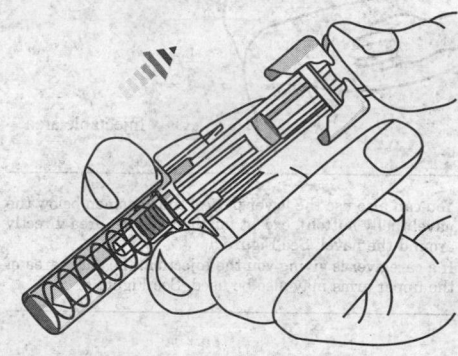

• Used syringes should be placed in a puncture-resistant container.

3   DOSAGE FORMS AND STRENGTHS
STELARA™ solution is colorless to slightly yellow in appearance and contains 90 mg ustekinumab per mL.
• 45 mg/0.5 mL in a single-use prefilled syringe
• 90 mg/1 mL in a single-use prefilled syringe
• 45 mg/0.5 mL in a single-use vial
• 90 mg/1 mL in a single-use vial

4   CONTRAINDICATIONS
None.

5   WARNINGS AND PRECAUTIONS
5.1   Infections
STELARA™ may increase the risk of infections and reactivation of latent infections. Serious bacterial, fungal, and viral infections were observed in subjects receiving STELARA™ [see Adverse Reactions (6.1)].
STELARA™ should not be given to patients with any clinically important active infection. STELARA™ should not be administered until the infection resolves or is adequately treated. Instruct patients to seek medical advice if signs or symptoms suggestive of an infection occur. Exercise caution when considering the use of STELARA™ in patients with a chronic infection or a history of recurrent infection.
Serious infections requiring hospitalization occurred in the psoriasis development program. These serious infections included cellulitis, diverticulitis, osteomyelitis, viral infections, gastroenteritis, pneumonia, and urinary tract infections.

5.2   Theoretical Risk for Vulnerability to Particular Infections
Individuals genetically deficient in IL-12/IL-23 are particularly vulnerable to disseminated infections from mycobacteria (including nontuberculous, environmental mycobacteria), salmonella (including nontyphi strains), and Bacillus Calmette-Guerin (BCG) vaccinations. Serious infections and fatal outcomes have been reported in such patients.

It is not known whether patients with pharmacologic blockade of IL-12/IL-23 from treatment with STELARA™ will be susceptible to these types of infections. Appropriate diagnostic testing should be considered, e.g., tissue culture, stool culture, as dictated by clinical circumstances.

5.3 Pre-treatment Evaluation for Tuberculosis
Evaluate patients for tuberculosis infection prior to initiating treatment with STELARA™.

Do not administer STELARA™ to patients with active tuberculosis. Initate treatment of latent tuberculosis prior to administering STELARA™. Consider anti-tuberculosis therapy prior to initiation of STELARA™ in patients with a past history of latent or active tuberculosis in whom an adequate course of treatment cannot be confirmed. Patients receiving STELARA™ should be monitored closely for signs and symptoms of active tuberculosis during and after treatment.

5.4 Malignancies
STELARA™ is an immunosuppressant and may increase the risk of malignancy. Malignancies were reported among subjects who received STELARA™ in clinical studies [see Adverse Reactions (6.1)]. In rodent models, inhibition of IL-12/IL-23p40 increased the risk of malignancy [see Nonclinical Toxicology (13)].

The safety of STELARA™ has not been evaluated in patients who have a history of malignancy or who have a known malignancy.

5.5 Reversible Posterior Leukoencephalopathy Syndrome
One case of reversible posterior leukoencephalopathy syndrome (RPLS) was observed during the clinical development program which included 3523 STELARA™-treated subjects. The subject, who had received 12 doses of STELARA™ over approximately two years, presented with headache, seizures and confusion. No additional STELARA™ injections were administered and the subject fully recovered with appropriate treatment.

RPLS is a neurological disorder, which is not caused by demyelination or a known infectious agent. RPLS can present with headache, seizures, confusion and visual disturbances. Conditions with which it has been associated include preeclampsia, eclampsia, acute hypertension, cytotoxic agents and immunosuppressive therapy. Fatal outcomes have been reported.

If RPLS is suspected, STELARA™ should be discontinued and appropriate treatment administered.

5.6 Immunizations
Prior to initiating therapy with STELARA™, patients should receive all immunizations appropriate for age as recommended by current immunization guidelines. Patients being treated with STELARA™ should not receive live vaccines. BCG vaccines should not be given during treatment with STELARA™ or for one year prior to initiating treatment or one year following discontinuation of treatment. Caution is advised when administering live vaccines to household contacts of patients receiving STELARA™ because of the potential risk for shedding from the household contact and transmission to patient.

Non-live vaccinations received during a course of STELARA™ may not elicit an immune response sufficient to prevent disease.

5.7 Concomitant Therapies
The safety of STELARA™ in combination with other immunosuppressive agents or phototherapy has not been evaluated. Ultraviolet-induced skin cancers developed earlier and more frequently in mice genetically manipulated to be deficient in both IL-12 and IL-23 or IL-12 alone [see Nonclinical Toxicology (13)].

6 ADVERSE REACTIONS
The following serious adverse reactions are discussed elsewhere in the label:
• Infections [see Warnings and Precautions (5.1)]
• Malignancies [see Warnings and Precautions (5.4)]
• Reversible Posterior Leukoencephalopathy Syndrome [see Warnings and Precautions (5.5)]

6.1 Clinical Studies Experience
The safety data reflect exposure to STELARA™ in 2266 psoriasis subjects, including 1970 exposed for at least 6 months, 1285 exposed for at least one year, and 373 exposed for at least 18 months.

Because clinical trials are conducted under widely varying conditions, adverse reaction rates observed in the clinical trials of a drug cannot be directly compared to rates in the clinical trials of another drug and may not reflect the rates observed in practice.

Table 1 summarizes the adverse reactions that occurred at a rate of at least 1% and at a higher rate in the STELARA™ groups than the placebo group during the placebo-controlled period of STUDY 1 and STUDY 2.

Table 1. Adverse reactions reported by ≥1% of subjects through Week 12 in STUDY 1 and STUDY 2

		STELARA™	
	Placebo	45 mg	90 mg
Subjects treated	665	664	666
Nasopharyngitis	51 (8%)	56 (8%)	49 (7%)
Upper respiratory tract infection	30 (5%)	36 (5%)	28 (4%)
Headache	23 (3%)	33 (5%)	32 (5%)
Fatigue	14 (2%)	18 (3%)	17 (3%)
Diarrhea	12 (2%)	13 (2%)	13 (2%)
Back pain	8 (1%)	9 (1%)	14 (2%)
Dizziness	8 (1%)	8 (1%)	14 (2%)
Pharyngolaryngeal pain	7 (1%)	9 (1%)	12 (2%)
Pruritus	9 (1%)	10 (2%)	9 (1%)
Injection site erythema	3 (<1%)	6 (1%)	13 (2%)
Myalgia	4 (1%)	7 (1%)	8 (1%)
Depression	3 (<1%)	8 (1%)	4 (1%)

Adverse drug reactions that occurred at rates less than 1% included: cellulitis and certain injection site reactions (pain, swelling, pruritus, induration, hemorrhage, bruising, and irritation). One case of RPLS occurred during clinical trials [see Warnings and Precautions (5.5)].

Infections
In the placebo-controlled period of clinical studies of psoriasis subjects (average follow-up of 12.6 weeks for placebo-treated subjects and 13.4 weeks for STELARA™-treated subjects), 27% of STELARA™-treated subjects reported infections (1.39 per subject-year of follow-up) compared with 24% of placebo-treated subjects (1.21 per subject-year of follow-up). Serious infections occurred in 0.3% of STELARA™-treated subjects (0.01 per subject-year of follow-up) and in 0.4% of placebo-treated subjects (0.02 per subject-year of follow-up) [see Warnings and Precautions (5.1)].
In the controlled and non-controlled portions of psoriasis clinical trials, 61% of STELARA™-treated subjects reported infections (1.24 per subject-year of follow-up). Serious infections were reported in 0.9% of subjects (0.01 per subject-year of follow-up).

Malignancies
In the controlled and non-controlled portions of psoriasis clinical trials, 0.4% of STELARA™-treated subjects reported malignancies excluding non-melanoma skin cancers (0.36 per 100 subject-years of follow-up). Non-melanoma skin cancer was reported in 0.8% of STELARA™-treated subjects (0.80 per 100 subject-years of follow-up) [see Warnings and Precautions (5.4)].
Serious malignancies included breast, colon, head and neck, kidney, prostate, and thyroid cancers.

Immunogenicity
The presence of ustekinumab in the serum can interfere with the detection of anti-ustekinumab antibodies resulting in inconclusive results due to assay interference. In STUDIES 1 and 2, antibody testing was done at time points when ustekinumab may have been present in the serum. Table 2 summarizes the antibody results from STUDIES 1 and 2. In STUDY 1 the last ustekinumab injection was between Weeks 28 and 48 and the last test for anti-ustekinumab antibodies was at Week 52. In STUDY 2 the last ustekinumab injection was at Week 16 and the last test for anti-ustekinumab antibodies was at Week 24.

Table 2

Antibody Results	STUDY 1 (N=743)	STUDY 2 (N=1198)
Positive	38 (5%)	33 (3%)
Negative	351 (47%)	90 (8%)
Inconclusive	354 (48%)	1075 (90%)

The data reflect the percentage of subjects whose test results were positive for antibodies to ustekinumab in a bridging immunoassay, and are highly dependent on the sensitivity and specificity of the assay. Additionally, the observed incidence of antibody positivity in an assay may be influenced by several factors, including sample handling, timing of sample collection, concomitant medications and underlying disease. For these reasons, comparison of the incidence of antibodies to ustekinumab with the incidence of antibodies to other products may be misleading.

7 DRUG INTERACTIONS
Drug interaction studies have not been conducted with STELARA™.

7.1 Live Vaccines
Live vaccines should not be given concurrently with STELARA™ [see Warnings and Precautions (5.6)].

7.2 Concomitant Therapies
The safety of STELARA™ in combination with immunosuppressive agents or phototherapy has not been evaluated [see Warnings and Precautions (5.7)].

7.3 CYP450 Substrates
The formation of CYP450 enzymes can be altered by increased levels of certain cytokines (e.g., IL-1, IL-6, IL-10, TNFα, IFN) during chronic inflammation. Thus, ustekinumab could normalize the formation of CYP450 enzymes. A role for IL-12 or IL-23 in the regulation of CYP450 enzymes has not been reported. However, upon initiation of ustekinumab in patients who are receiving concomitant CYP450 substrates, particularly those with a narrow therapeutic index, monitoring for therapeutic effect (e.g., for warfarin) or drug concentration (e.g., for cyclosporine) should be considered and the individual dose of the drug adjusted as needed [see Clinical Pharmacology (12.3)].

8 USE IN SPECIFIC POPULATIONS

8.1 Pregnancy
Pregnancy Category B
There are no studies of STELARA™ in pregnant women. STELARA™ should be used during pregnancy only if the potential benefit justifies the potential risk to the fetus. No teratogenic effects were observed in the developmental and reproductive toxicology studies performed in cynomolgus monkeys at doses up to 45 mg/kg ustekinumab, which is 45 times (based on mg/kg) the highest intended clinical dose in psoriasis patients (approximately 1 mg/kg based on administration of a 90 mg dose to a 90 kg psoriasis patient).
Ustekinumab was tested in two embryo-fetal development toxicity studies. Pregnant cynomolgus monkeys were administered ustekinumab at doses up to 45 mg/kg during the period of organogenesis either twice weekly via subcutaneous injections or weekly by intravenous injections. No significant adverse developmental effects were noted in either study.

In an embryo-fetal development and pre- and post-natal development toxicity study, three groups of 20 pregnant cynomolgus monkeys were administered subcutaneous doses of 0, 22.5, or 45 mg/kg ustekinumab twice weekly from the beginning of organogenesis in cynomolgus monkeys to Day 33 after delivery. There were no treatment-related effects on mortality, clinical signs, body weight, food consumption, hematology, or serum biochemistry in dams. Fetal losses occurred in six control monkeys, six 22.5 mg/kg-treated monkeys, and five 45 mg/kg-treated monkeys. Neonatal deaths occurred in one 22.5 mg/kg-treated monkey and in one 45 mg/kg-treated monkey. No ustekinumab-related abnormalities were observed in the neonates from birth through six months of age in clinical signs, body weight, hematology, or serum biochemistry. There were no treatment-related effects on functional development until weaning, functional development after weaning, morphological development, immunological development, and gross and histopathological examinations of offsprings by the age of 6 months.

8.3 Nursing Mothers
Caution should be exercised when STELARA™ is administered to a nursing woman. The unknown risks to the infant from gastrointestinal or systemic exposure to ustekinumab should be weighed against the known benefits of breastfeeding. Ustekinumab is excreted in the milk of lactating monkeys administered ustekinumab. IgG is excreted in human milk, so it is expected that STELARA™ will be present in human milk. It is not known if ustekinumab is absorbed systemically after ingestion; however, published data suggest that antibodies in breast milk do not enter the neonatal and infant circulation in substantial amounts.

8.4 Pediatric Use
Safety and effectiveness of STELARA™ in pediatric patients have not been evaluated.

8.5 Geriatric Use
Of the 2266 psoriasis subjects exposed to STELARA™, a total of 131 were 65 years or older, and 14 subjects were 75 years or older. Although no differences in safety or efficacy were observed between older and younger subjects, the number of subjects aged 65 and over is not sufficient to determine whether they respond differently from younger subjects.

10 OVERDOSAGE
Single doses up to 4.5 mg/kg intravenously have been administered in clinical studies without dose-limiting toxicity. In case of overdosage, it is recommended that the patient be monitored for any signs or symptoms of adverse reactions or effects and appropriate symptomatic treatment be instituted immediately.

11 DESCRIPTION
STELARA™ is a human IgG1κ monoclonal antibody against the p40 subunit of the IL-12 and IL-23 cytokines.

Table 3. Clinical Outcomes STUDY 1 and STUDY 2

Week 12	STUDY 1			STUDY 2		
		STELARA™			STELARA™	
	Placebo	45 mg	90 mg	Placebo	45 mg	90 mg
Subjects randomized	255	255	256	410	409	411
PASI 75 response	8 (3%)	171 (67%)	170 (66%)	15 (4%)	273 (67%)	311 (76%)
PGA of Cleared or Minimal	10 (4%)	151 (59%)	156 (61%)	18 (4%)	277 (68%)	300 (73%)

Table 4. Clinical Outcomes by Weight STUDY 1 and STUDY 2

	STUDY 1			STUDY 2		
		STELARA™			STELARA™	
	Placebo	45 mg	90 mg	Placebo	45 mg	90 mg
Subjects randomized	255	255	256	410	409	411
Week 12						
PASI 75 response						
≤ 100 kg	4%	74%	65%	4%	73%	78%
	6/166	124/168	107/164	12/290	218/297	225/289
>100 kg	2%	54%	68%	3%	49%	71%
	2/89	47/87	63/92	3/120	55/112	86/121
PGA of Cleared or Minimal						
≤ 100 kg	4%	64%	63%	5%	74%	75%
	7/166	108/168	103/164	14/290	220/297	216/289
>100 kg	3%	49%	58%	3%	51%	69%
	3/89	43/87	53/92	4/120	57/112	84/121

Using DNA recombinant technology, STELARA™ is produced in a well characterized recombinant cell line and is purified using standard bio-processing technology. The manufacturing process contains steps for the clearance of viruses. STELARA™ is comprised of 1326 amino acids and has an estimated molecular mass that ranges from 148,079 to 149,690 Daltons.

STELARA™ is available as: 45 mg of ustekinumab in 0.5 mL and 90 mg of ustekinumab in 1 mL. STELARA™ is supplied as a sterile solution in a single-use prefilled syringe with a 27 gauge fixed ½ inch needle, or a single-use 2 mL Type I glass vial with a coated stopper. The syringe is fitted with a passive needle guard and a needle cover that is manufactured using a dry natural rubber (a derivative of latex).

Each 45 mg ustekinumab prefilled syringe also contains: L-histidine and L-histidine monohydrochloride monohydrate (0.5 mg), Polysorbate 80 (0.02 mg), and sucrose (38 mg) to fill to a final volume of 0.5 mL.

Each 90 mg ustekinumab prefilled syringe also contains: L-histidine and L-histidine monohydrochloride monohydrate (1 mg), Polysorbate 80 (0.04 mg), and sucrose (76 mg) to fill to a final volume of 1 mL.

Each 45 mg ustekinumab vial also contains: L-histidine and L-histidine monohydrochloride monohydrate (0.5 mg), Polysorbate 80 (0.02 mg), and sucrose (38 mg) to fill to a final volume of 0.5 mL.

Each 90 mg ustekinumab vial also contains: L-histidine and L-histidine monohydrochloride monohydrate (1 mg), Polysorbate 80 (0.04 mg), and sucrose (76 mg) to fill to a final volume of 1 mL.

The STELARA™ solution is colorless to slightly yellow in appearance and has a pH of 5.7–6.3. STELARA™ does not contain preservatives.

12 CLINICAL PHARMACOLOGY

12.1 Mechanism of Action

Ustekinumab is a human IgG1κ monoclonal antibody that binds with high affinity and specificity to the p40 protein subunit used by both the interleukin (IL)-12 and IL-23 cytokines. IL-12 and IL-23 are naturally occurring cytokines that are involved in inflammatory and immune responses, such as natural killer cell activation and CD4+ T-cell differentiation and activation. In *in vitro* models, ustekinumab was shown to disrupt IL-12 and IL-23 mediated signaling and cytokine cascades by disrupting the interaction of these cytokines with a shared cell-surface receptor chain, IL-12 β1.

12.2 Pharmacodynamics

In a small exploratory study, a decrease was observed in the expression of mRNA of its molecular targets IL-12 and IL-23 in lesional skin biopsies measured at baseline and up to two weeks post-treatment in psoriatic subjects.

12.3 Pharmacokinetics

Absorption

In psoriasis subjects, the median time to reach the maximum serum concentration (T_{max}) was 13.5 days and 7 days, respectively, after a single subcutaneous administration of 45 mg (N=22) and 90 mg (N=24) of ustekinumab. In healthy subjects (N=30), the median T_{max} value (8.5 days) following a single subcutaneous administration of 90 mg of ustekinumab was comparable to that observed in psoriasis subjects. Following multiple subcutaneous doses of STELARA™, the steady-state serum concentrations of ustekinumab were achieved by Week 28. The mean (±SD) steady-state trough serum concentration ranged from 0.31 ± 0.33 mcg/mL (45 mg) to 0.64 ± 0.64 mcg/mL (90 mg). There was no apparent accumulation in serum ustekinumab concentration over time when given subcutaneously every 12 weeks.

Distribution

Following subcutaneous administration of 45 mg (N=18) and 90 mg (N=21) of ustekinumab to psoriasis subjects, the mean (±SD) apparent volume of distribution during the terminal phase (Vz/F) was 161 ± 65 mL/kg and 179 ± 85 mL/kg, respectively. The mean (± SD) volume of distribution during the terminal phase (Vz) following a single intravenous administration to subjects with psoriasis ranged from 56.1 ± 6.5 to 82.1 ± 23.6 mL/kg.

Metabolism

The metabolic pathway of ustekinumab has not been characterized. As a human IgG1κ monoclonal antibody ustekinumab is expected to be degraded into small peptides and amino acids via catabolic pathways in the same manner as endogenous IgG.

Elimination

The mean (± SD) systemic clearance (CL) following a single intravenous administration of ustekinumab to psoriasis subjects ranged from 1.90 ± 0.28 to 2.22 ± 0.63 mL/day/kg. The mean (±SD) half-life ranged from 14.9 ± 4.6 to 45.6 ± 80.2 days across all psoriasis studies following intravenous and subcutaneous administration.

Weight

When given the same dose, subjects weighing >100 kg had lower median serum ustekinumab concentrations compared with those subjects weighing ≤100 kg.

Hepatic and Renal Impairment

No pharmacokinetic data are available in patients with hepatic or renal impairment.

Elderly

A population pharmacokinetic analysis (N=106/1937 subjects greater than or equal to 65 years old) was performed to evaluate the effect of age on the pharmacokinetics of ustekinumab. There were no apparent changes in pharmacokinetic parameters (clearance and volume of distribution) in subjects older than 65 years old.

Drug-Drug Interactions

Upon initiation of ustekinumab in patients who are receiving concomitant CYP450 substrates, particularly those with narrow therapeutic index, monitoring for therapeutic effect (e.g., for warfarin) or drug concentration (e.g., for cyclosporine) should be considered and the individual dose of the drug adjusted as needed *[see Drug Interactions (7.3)]*.

13 NONCLINICAL TOXICOLOGY

13.1 Carcinogenesis, Mutagenesis, Impairment of Fertility

Animal studies have not been conducted to evaluate the carcinogenic or mutagenic potential of STELARA™. Published literature showed that administration of murine IL-12 caused an anti-tumor effect in mice that contained transplanted tumors and IL-12/IL-23p40 knockout mice or mice treated with anti-IL-12/IL-23p40 antibody had decreased host defense to tumors. Mice genetically manipulated to be deficient in both IL-12 and IL-23 or IL-12 alone developed UV-induced skin cancers earlier and more frequently compared to wild-type mice. The relevance of these experimental findings in mouse models for malignancy risk in humans is unknown.

A male fertility study was conducted with only 6 male monkeys per group administered subcutaneous doses of 0, 22.5, or 45 mg/kg ustekinumab twice weekly prior to mating and during the mating period for 13 weeks, followed by a 13-week treatment-free period. Although fertility and pregnancy outcomes were not evaluated in mated females, there were no treatment-related effects on parental toxicity or male fertility parameters.

A female fertility study was conducted in mice using an analogous IL-12/IL-23p40 antibody by subcutaneous administration at doses up to 50 mg/kg, twice weekly, beginning 15 days before cohabitation and continuing through GD 7. There were no treatment-related effects on maternal toxicity or female fertility parameters.

13.2 Animal Toxicology and/or Pharmacology

In a 26-week toxicology study, one out of 10 monkeys subcutaneously administered 45 mg/kg ustekinumab twice weekly for 26 weeks had a bacterial infection.

14 CLINICAL STUDIES

Two multicenter, randomized, double-blind, placebo-controlled studies (STUDY 1 and STUDY 2) enrolled a total of 1996 subjects 18 years of age and older with plaque psoriasis who had a minimum body surface area involvement of 10%, and Psoriasis Area and Severity Index (PASI) score ≥12, and who were candidates for phototherapy or systemic therapy. Subjects with guttate, erythrodermic, or pustular psoriasis were excluded from the studies.

STUDY 1 enrolled 766 subjects and STUDY 2 enrolled 1230 subjects. The studies had the same design through Week 28. In both studies, subjects were randomized in equal proportion to placebo, 45 mg or 90 mg of STELARA™. Subjects randomized to STELARA™ received 45 mg or 90 mg doses, regardless of weight, at Weeks 0, 4, and 16. Subjects randomized to receive placebo at Weeks 0 and 4 crossed over to receive STELARA™ (either 45 mg or 90 mg) at Weeks 12 and 16.

In both studies, the endpoints were the proportion of subjects who achieved at least a 75% reduction in PASI score (PASI 75) from baseline to Week 12 and treatment success (cleared or minimal) on the Physician's Global Assessment (PGA). The PGA is a 6-category scale ranging from 0 (cleared) to 5 (severe) that indicates the physician's overall assessment of psoriasis focusing on plaque thickness/induration, erythema, and scaling.

In both studies, subjects in all treatment groups had a median baseline PASI score ranging from approximately 17 to 18. Baseline PGA score was marked or severe in 44% of subjects in STUDY 1 and 40% of subjects in STUDY 2. Approximately two-thirds of all subjects had received prior phototherapy, 69% had received either prior conventional systemic or biologic therapy for the treatment of psoriasis, with 56% receiving prior conventional systemic therapy and 43% receiving prior biologic therapy. A total of 28% of study subjects had a history of psoriatic arthritis.

Clinical Response

The results of STUDY 1 and STUDY 2 are presented in Table 3 below.

[See table 3 above]

Examination of age, gender, and race subgroups did not identify differences in response to STELARA™ among these subgroups.

In subjects who weighed <100 kg, response rates were similar with both the 45 mg and 90 mg doses; however, in subjects who weighed >100 kg, higher response rates were seen with 90 mg dosing compared with 45 mg dosing (Table 4 below).

[See table 4 above]

Subjects in STUDY 1 were evaluated through Week 52. At Week 40, those who were PASI 75 responders at both Weeks 28 and 40 were re-randomized to either continued dosing of STELARA™ (STELARA™ at Week 40) or to withdrawal of therapy (placebo at Week 40). At Week 52, 89% (144/162) of subjects re-randomized to STELARA™ treatment were PASI 75 responders compared with 63% (100/159) of subjects re-randomized to placebo (treatment withdrawal after Week 28 dose).

16 HOW SUPPLIED/STORAGE AND HANDLING

STELARA™ does not contain preservatives. STELARA™ is available in prefilled syringes or single-use vials containing 45 mg or 90 mg of ustekinumab. Each prefilled syringe is equipped with a needle safety guard.

The NDC number for the 45 mg prefilled syringe is 57894-060-03.

The NDC number for the 90 mg prefilled syringe is 57894-061-03.

The NDC number for the 45 mg vial is 57894-060-02.

The NDC number for the 90 mg vial is 57894-061-02.

Storage and Stability
Store STELARA™ upright and refrigerated at 2°C to 8°C (36°F to 46°F). Keep the product in the original carton to protect from light until the time of use. Do not freeze. Do not shake. STELARA™ does not contain a preservative; discard any unused portion.

17 PATIENT COUNSELING INFORMATION

Instruct patients to read the Medication Guide before starting STELARA™ therapy and to reread the Medication Guide each time the prescription is renewed.
Infections
Inform patients that STELARA™ may lower the ability of their immune system to fight infections. Instruct patients of the importance of communicating any history of infections to the doctor, and contacting their doctor if they develop any symptoms of infection.
Malignancies
Patients should be counseled about the risk of malignancies while receiving STELARA™.

Prefilled Syringe Manufactured by: Centocor Ortho Biotech Inc., Horsham, PA 19044, License No. 1821 at Baxter Pharmaceutical Solutions, Bloomington, IN 47403
Vial Manufactured by: Centocor Ortho Biotech Inc., Horsham, PA 19044, License No. 1821 at Cilag AG, Schaffhausen, Switzerland
© Centocor Ortho Biotech Inc. 2009

MEDICATION GUIDE
STELARA™ (stel ar′ a)
(ustekinumab)
Injection

Read this Medication Guide before you start taking STELARA™ and each time before you get an injection. There may be new information. This Medication Guide does not take the place of talking with your doctor about your medical condition or treatment with STELARA™.

What is the most important information I should know about STELARA™?
STELARA™ is a medicine that affects your immune system. STELARA™ can increase your chances of having serious side effects, including:
Serious Infections: STELARA™ may lower the ability of your immune system to fight infections and may increase your risk of infections. Some people have serious infections while taking STELARA™, including tuberculosis (TB), and infections caused by bacteria, fungi, or viruses. Some people have to be hospitalized for treatment of their infection.
• Your doctor should check you for TB before starting STELARA™.
• If your doctor feels that you are at risk for TB, you may be treated with medicine for TB before you begin treatment with STELARA™ and during treatment with STELARA™.
• Your doctor should watch you closely for signs and symptoms of TB during treatment with STELARA™.
You should not start taking STELARA™ if you have any kind of infection unless your doctor says it is okay.
Before starting STELARA™, tell your doctor if you think you have an infection or have symptoms of an infection such as:
• fever, sweats, or chills
• muscle aches
• cough
• shortness of breath
• blood in your phlegm
• weight loss
• warm, red, or painful skin or sores on your body
• diarrhea or stomach pain
• burning when you urinate or urinate more often than normal
• feel very tired
• are being treated for an infection
• get a lot of infections or have infections that keep coming back
• have TB, or have been in close contact with someone who has TB.
After starting STELARA™, call your doctor right away if you have any symptoms of an infection (see above).
STELARA™ can make you more likely to get infections or make an infection that you have worse.
People who have a genetic problem where the body does not make any of the proteins interleukin 12 (IL-12) and interleukin 23 (IL-23) are at a higher risk for certain serious infections. These infections can spread throughout the body and cause death. It is not known if people who take STELARA™ will get any of these infections, because of the effects of STELARA™ on these proteins in your body.
Cancers:
STELARA™ may decrease the activity of your immune system and increase your risk for certain types of cancers. Tell your doctor if you have ever had any type of cancer.

Reversible Posterior Leukoencephalopathy Syndrome (RPLS):
RPLS is a rare condition that affects the brain and can cause death. The cause of RPLS is not known. If RPLS is found early and treated, most people recover. Tell your doctor right away if you have any new or worsening medical problems including:
• headache
• seizures
• confusion
• vision problems
What is STELARA™?
STELARA™ is a prescription medicine used to treat adults 18 years and older with moderate or severe psoriasis that involves large areas or many areas of their body, who may benefit from taking injections or pills (systemic therapy) or phototherapy (treatment using ultraviolet light alone or with pills).
STELARA™ may improve your psoriasis but may also lower the ability of your immune system to fight infections. This may also increase your risk for certain types of cancer. It is not known if STELARA™ is safe and effective in children.
It is not known if taking STELARA™ for more than 2 years is safe and effective.
What should I tell my doctor before receiving STELARA™?
Before receiving STELARA™, tell your doctor if you:
• have any of the conditions or symptoms listed in the section "What is the most important information I should know about STELARA™?"
• have recently received or are scheduled to receive an immunization (vaccine). People who take STELARA™ should not receive live vaccines. Tell your doctor if anyone in your house needs a vaccine. The viruses used in some types of vaccines can spread to people with a weakened immune system, and can cause serious problems. **You should not receive the BCG vaccine during the one year before taking STELARA™ or one year after you stop taking STELARA™.**
• receive phototherapy for your psoriasis.
• have any other medical conditions.
• are pregnant or planning to become pregnant. It is not known if STELARA™ will harm your unborn baby. You and your doctor should decide if you will take STELARA™.
• are breast-feeding or plan to breast-feed. It is thought that STELARA™ passes into your breast milk. You should not breast-feed while taking STELARA™ without first talking with your doctor.
Tell your doctor about all the medicines you take, including prescription and non-prescription medicines, vitamins, and herbal supplements. Especially tell your doctor if you take:
• other medicines that affect your immune system.
• certain medicines that can affect how your liver breaks down other medicines.
Ask your doctor or pharmacist if you are not sure if your medicine is one that is listed above.
Know the medicines you take. Keep a list of them to show your doctor and pharmacist when you get a new medicine.
How will I receive STELARA™?
• STELARA™ is given by injection under the skin (subcutaneous injection).
• STELARA™ should only be given by a healthcare provider as directed by your doctor.
• Your doctor will decide the right dose of STELARA™ for you and how often you should receive it.
• Be sure to keep all of your scheduled follow-up appointments.
What should I avoid while receiving STELARA™?
You should not receive a live vaccine while taking STELARA™. See "What should I tell my doctor before taking STELARA™?"
What are the possible side effects of STELARA™?
STELARA™ can increase your chances of having serious side effects. See "What is the most important information I should know about STELARA™?"
Common side effects of STELARA™ include:
• upper respiratory infections
• headache
• tiredness
These are not all of the possible side effects of STELARA™. Tell your doctor about any side effect that bothers you or that does not go away. For more information, ask your doctor or pharmacist.
Call your doctor for medical advice about side effects. You may report side effects to FDA at 1-800-FDA-1088 or to Centocor Ortho Biotech Inc. at 1-800-457-6399.
General information about STELARA™.
Medicines are sometimes prescribed for purposes other than those listed in a Medication Guide.
This Medication Guide summarizes the most important information about STELARA™. If you would like more infor-

mation, talk with your doctor. You can ask your doctor or pharmacist for information about STELARA™ that was written for healthcare professionals.
What are the ingredients in STELARA™?
Active ingredient: ustekinumab
Inactive ingredients: L-histidine, L-histidine monohydrochloride monohydrate, polysorbate 80, and sucrose.
Prefilled Syringe Manufactured by: Centocor Ortho Biotech Inc., Horsham, PA 19044, License No. 1821 at Baxter Pharmaceutical Solutions, Bloomington, IN 47403
Vial Manufactured by: Centocor Ortho Biotech Inc., Horsham, PA 19044, License No. 1821 at Cilag AG, Schaffhausen, Switzerland
Revised December 2009
This Medication Guide has been approved by the U.S. Food and Drug Administration.
U.S. License No. 1821
© Centocor Ortho Biotech Inc. 2009
Shown in Product Identification Guide, page 307

Centocor Ortho Biotech Products, L.P.
800 RIDGEVIEW DRIVE
HORSHAM, PA 19044
www.centocororthobiotech.com

For Medical Information and Adverse Event Reporting:
(800) 457-6399

For General Inquiries:
(610) 651-6000

For Customer Service (Sales, Ordering & Returns):
(800) 325-7504, Prompt #1

DOXIL®   ℞
[däk′sil]
(doxorubicin HCl liposome injection)
for intravenous infusion

HIGHLIGHTS OF PRESCRIBING INFORMATION
These highlights do not include all the information needed to use DOXIL safely and effectively. See full prescribing information for DOXIL.
DOXIL® (doxorubicin HCl liposome injection) for intravenous infusion
Initial U.S. Approval: 1995

> **WARNING: INFUSION REACTIONS, MYELOSUP-
> PRESSION, CARDIOTOXICITY, LIVER IMPAIRMENT,
> SUBSTITUTION**
> *See full prescribing information for complete boxed warning.*
> • Myocardial damage may lead to congestive heart failure and may occur as the total cumulative dose of doxorubicin HCl approaches 550 mg/m². Cardiac toxicity may also occur at lower cumulative doses with mediastinal irradiation or concurrent cardiotoxic agents (5.1).
> • Acute infusion-related reactions, sometimes reversible upon terminating or slowing infusion, occurred in up to 10% of patients. Serious and sometimes fatal allergic/anaphylactoid-like infusion reactions have been reported. Medications/emergency equipment to treat such reactions should be available for immediate use (5.2).
> • Severe myelosuppression may occur (5.3)
> • Reduce dosage in patients with impaired hepatic function (2.6).
> • Accidental substitution of DOXIL resulted in severe side effects. Do not substitute on mg per mg basis with doxorubicin HCl (2.1).

────────RECENT MAJOR CHANGES────────
Indications and Usage, AIDS-related
Kaposi's Sarcoma (1.2)   6/2008
────────INDICATIONS AND USAGE────────
DOXIL is an anthracycline topoisomerase inhibitor indicated for:
• **Ovarian cancer (1.1)**
After failure of platinum-based chemotherapy.
• **AIDS-related Kaposi's Sarcoma (1.2)**
After failure of prior systemic chemotherapy or intolerance to such therapy.
• **Multiple Myeloma (1.3)**
In combination with bortezomib in patients who have not previously received bortezomib and have received at least one prior therapy.

DOSAGE AND ADMINISTRATION

Administer DOXIL at an initial rate of 1 mg/min to minimize the risk of infusion reactions. If no infusion related reactions occur, increase rate of infusion to complete administration over 1 hour. Do not administer as bolus injection or undiluted solution (2.1).

- **Ovarian cancer:** 50 mg/m^2 IV every 4 weeks for 4 courses minimum (2.2)
- **AIDS-related Kaposi's Sarcoma:** 20 mg/m^2 IV every 3 weeks (2.3)
- **Multiple Myeloma:** 30 mg/m^2 IV on day 4 following bortezomib which is administered at 1.3 mg/m^2 bolus on days 1, 4, 8 and 11, every 3 weeks (2.4)

DOSAGE FORMS AND STRENGTHS

Single dose vial: 20 mg/10 mL and 50 mg/30 mL (3)

CONTRAINDICATIONS

- Hypersensitivity reactions to a conventional formulation of doxorubicin HCl or the components of DOXIL (4, 5.2)
- Nursing mothers (4, 8.3)

WARNINGS AND PRECAUTIONS

- Hand-Foot Syndrome may occur. Dose modification or discontinuation may be required (5.4)
- Radiation recall reaction may occur (5.5)

ADVERSE REACTIONS

Most common adverse reactions (>20%) are asthenia, fatigue, fever, anorexia, nausea, vomiting, stomatitis, diarrhea, constipation, hand and foot syndrome, rash, neutropenia, thrombocytopenia and anemia (6).

To report SUSPECTED ADVERSE REACTIONS contact Ortho Biotech Products, LP at (888) 227-5624 or FDA at 1-800-FDA-1088 or www.fda.gov/medwatch.

DRUG INTERACTIONS

- DOXIL may interact with drugs known to interact with conventional formulations of Doxorubicin HCl. (7)

USE IN SPECIFIC POPULATIONS

- DOXIL can cause fetal harm when used during pregnancy. (5.6, 8.1)

See 17 for PATIENT COUNSELING INFORMATION.

Revised: 06/2008

FULL PRESCRIBING INFORMATION

WARNING: INFUSION REACTIONS, MYELOSUPPRESSION, CARDIOTOXICITY, LIVER IMPAIRMENT, ACCIDENTAL SUBSTITUTION

1. The use of DOXIL (doxorubicin HCl liposome injection) may lead to cardiac toxicity. Myocardial damage may lead to congestive heart failure and may occur as the total cumulative dose of doxorubicin HCl approaches 550 mg/m^2. In a clinical study in patients with advanced breast cancer, 250 patients received DOXIL at a starting dose of 50 mg/m^2 every 4 weeks. At all cumulative anthracycline doses between 450-500 mg/m^2 or between 500-550 mg/m^2, the risk of cardiac toxicity for patients treated with DOXIL was 11%. Prior use of other anthracyclines or anthracenediones should be included in calculations of total cumulative dosage. Cardiac toxicity may also occur at lower cumulative doses in patients with prior mediastinal irradiation or who are receiving concurrent cyclophosphamide therapy [see Warnings and Precautions (5.1)].

2. Acute infusion-related reactions including, but not limited to, flushing, shortness of breath, facial swelling, headache, chills, back pain, tightness in the chest or throat, and/or hypotension have occurred in up to 10% of patients treated with DOXIL. In most patients, these reactions resolve over the course of several hours to a day once the infusion is terminated. In some patients, the reaction has resolved with slowing of the infusion rate. Serious and sometimes life-threatening or fatal allergic/anaphylactoid-like infusion reactions have been reported. Medications to treat such reactions, as well as emergency equipment, should be available for immediate use. DOXIL should be administered at an initial rate of 1 mg/min to minimize the risk of infusion reactions [see Warnings and Precautions (5.2)].

3. Severe myelosuppression may occur [see Warnings and Precautions (5.3)].

4. Dosage should be reduced in patients with impaired hepatic function [see Dosage and Administration (2.6) and Use in Specific Populations (8.6)].

5. Accidental substitution of DOXIL for doxorubicin HCl has resulted in severe side effects. DOXIL should not be substituted for doxorubicin HCl on a mg per mg basis [see Dosage and Administration (2.1)].

---

1   INDICATIONS AND USAGE

1.1   Ovarian Cancer
DOXIL (doxorubicin HCl liposome injection) is indicated for the treatment of patients with ovarian cancer whose disease has progressed or recurred after platinum-based chemotherapy.

1.2   AIDS-Related Kaposi's Sarcoma
DOXIL is indicated for the treatment of AIDS-related Kaposi's sarcoma in patients after failure of prior systemic chemotherapy or intolerance to such therapy.

1.3   Multiple Myeloma
DOXIL in combination with bortezomib is indicated for the treatment of patients with multiple myeloma who have not previously received bortezomib and have received at least one prior therapy.

2   DOSAGE AND ADMINISTRATION

2.1   Usage and Administration Precautions
Liposomal encapsulation can substantially affect a drug's functional properties relative to those of the unencapsulated drug. Therefore DO NOT SUBSTITUTE one drug for the other.

Do not administer as a bolus injection or an undiluted solution. Rapid infusion may increase the risk of infusion-related reactions [see Warnings and Precautions (5.2)]. DOXIL must not be given by the intramuscular or subcutaneous route.

Until specific compatibility data are available, it is not recommended that DOXIL be mixed with other drugs.

DOXIL should be considered an irritant and precautions should be taken to avoid extravasation. With intravenous administration of DOXIL, extravasation may occur with or without an accompanying stinging or burning sensation, even if blood returns well on aspiration of the infusion needle. If any signs or symptoms of extravasation have occurred, the infusion should be immediately terminated and restarted in another vein. The application of ice over the site of extravasation for approximately 30 minutes may be helpful in alleviating the local reaction.

2.2   Patients With Ovarian Cancer
DOXIL (doxorubicin HCl liposome injection) should be administered intravenously at a dose of 50 mg/m^2 (doxorubicin HCl equivalent) at an initial rate of 1 mg/min to minimize the risk of infusion reactions. If no infusion-related adverse reactions are observed, the rate of infusion can be increased to complete administration of the drug over one hour. The patient should be dosed once every 4 weeks, for as long as the patient does not progress, shows no evidence of cardiotoxicity [see Warnings and Precautions (5.1)], and continues to tolerate treatment. A minimum of 4 courses is recommended because median time to response in clinical trials was 4 months. To manage adverse reactions such as hand-foot syndrome (HFS), stomatitis, or hematologic toxicity the doses may be delayed or reduced [see Dosage and Administration (2.5)]. Pretreatment with or concomitant use of antiemetics should be considered.

2.3   Patients With AIDS-Related Kaposi's Sarcoma
DOXIL (doxorubicin HCl liposome injection) should be administered intravenously at a dose of 20 mg/m^2 (doxorubicin HCl equivalent). An initial rate of 1 mg/min should be used to minimize the risk of infusion-related reactions. If no infusion-related adverse reactions are observed, the infusion rate should be increased to complete the administration of the drug over one hour. The dose should be repeated once every three weeks, for as long as patients respond satisfactorily and tolerate treatment.

2.4   Patients With Multiple Myeloma
Bortezomib is administered at a dose of 1.3 mg/m^2 as intravenous bolus on days 1, 4, 8 and 11, every three weeks. DOXIL 30 mg/m^2 should be administered as a 1-hr intravenous infusion on day 4 following bortezomib. With the first DOXIL dose, an initial rate of 1 mg/min should be used to minimize the risk of infusion-related reactions. If no infusion-related adverse reactions are observed, the infusion rate should be increased to complete the administration of the drug over one hour. Patients may be treated for up to 8 cycles until disease progression or the occurrence of unacceptable toxicity.

2.5   Dose Modification Guidelines
DOXIL exhibits nonlinear pharmacokinetics at 50 mg/m^2; therefore, dose adjustments may result in a nonproportional greater change in plasma concentration and exposure to the drug [see Clinical Pharmacology (12.3)]. Patients should be carefully monitored for toxicity. Adverse reactions, such as HFS, hematologic toxicities, and stomatitis may be managed by dose delays and adjustments. Following the first appearance of a Grade 2 or higher adverse reactions, the dosing should be adjusted or delayed as described in the following tables. Once the dose has been reduced, it should not be increased at a later time.
Recommended Dose Modification Guidelines

Table 1: Hand-Foot Syndrome (HFS)

Toxicity Grade	Dose Adjustment
1 (mild erythema, swelling, or desquamation not interfering with daily activities)	Redose unless patient has experienced previous Grade 3 or 4 HFS. If so, delay up to 2 weeks and decrease dose by 25%. Return to original dose interval.
2 (erythema, desquamation, or swelling interfering with, but not precluding normal physical activities; small blisters or ulcerations less than 2 cm in diameter)	Delay dosing up to 2 weeks or until resolved to Grade 0-1. If after 2 weeks there is no resolution, DOXIL should be discontinued. If resolved to Grade 0-1 within 2 weeks, and there are no prior Grade 3-4 HFS, continue treatment at previous dose and return to original dose interval. If patient experienced previous Grade 3-4 toxicity, continue treatment with a 25% dose reduction and return to original dose interval.
3 (blistering, ulceration, or swelling interfering with walking or normal daily activities; cannot wear regular clothing)	Delay dosing up to 2 weeks or until resolved to Grade 0-1. Decrease dose by 25% and return to original dose interval. If after 2 weeks there is no resolution, DOXIL should be discontinued.
4 (diffuse or local process causing infectious complications, or a bed ridden state or hospitalization)	Delay dosing up to 2 weeks or until resolved to Grade 0-1. Decrease dose by 25% and return to original dose interval. If after 2 weeks there is no resolution, DOXIL should be discontinued.

[See table 2 at right]

Table 3: Stomatitis

Toxicity Grade	Dose Adjustment
1 (painless ulcers, erythema, or mild soreness)	**Redose unless patient has experienced previous Grade 3 or 4 toxicity.** If so, delay up to 2 weeks and decrease dose by 25%. Return to original dose interval.
2 (painful erythema, edema, or ulcers, but can eat)	**Delay dosing up to 2 weeks or until resolved to Grade 0-1.** If after 2 weeks there is no resolution, DOXIL should be discontinued. If resolved to Grade 0-1 within 2 weeks and there was no prior Grade 3-4 stomatitis, continue treatment at previous dose and return to original dose interval. If patient experienced previous Grade 3-4 toxicity, continue treatment with a 25% dose reduction and return to original dose interval.
3 (painful erythema, edema, or ulcers, and cannot eat)	**Delay dosing up to 2 weeks or until resolved to Grade 0-1.** Decrease dose by 25% and return to original dose interval. If after 2 weeks there is no resolution, DOXIL should be discontinued.
4 (requires parenteral or enteral support)	**Delay dosing up to 2 weeks or until resolved to Grade 0-1.** Decrease dose by 25% and return to DOXIL original dose interval. If after 2 weeks there is no resolution, DOXIL should be discontinued.

Multiple Myeloma

For patients treated with DOXIL in combination with bortezomib who experience hand-foot syndrome or stomatitis, the DOXIL dose should be modified as described in Tables 1 and 3 above. Table 4 describes dosage adjustments for DOXIL and bortezomib combination therapy. For bortezomib dosing and dosage adjustments, see manufacturer's prescribing information.

[See table 4 above]

2.6 Patients With Impaired Hepatic Function

Limited clinical experience exists in treating patients with hepatic impairment with DOXIL. Based on experience with doxorubicin HCl, it is recommended that the DOXIL dosage be reduced if the bilirubin is elevated as follows: serum bilirubin 1.2 to 3.0 mg/dL – give ½ normal dose; serum bilirubin > 3 mg/dL – give ¼ normal dose.

No information, including dosage adjustments, is available for patients with multiple myeloma with hepatic impairment.

2.7 Preparation for Intravenous Administration

Each 10-mL vial contains 20 mg doxorubicin HCl at a concentration of 2 mg/mL.

Each 30-mL vial contains 50 mg doxorubicin HCl at a concentration of 2 mg/mL.

DOXIL doses up to 90 mg must be diluted in 250 mL of 5% Dextrose Injection, USP prior to administration. Doses exceeding 90 mg should be diluted in 500 mL of 5% Dextrose Injection, USP prior to administration. Aseptic technique must be strictly observed since no preservative or bacteriostatic agent is present in DOXIL. Diluted DOXIL should be refrigerated at 2°C to 8°C (36°F to 46°F) and administered within 24 hours.

Do not use with in-line filters.

Do not mix with other drugs.

Do not use with any diluent other than 5% Dextrose Injection.

Do not use any bacteriostatic agent, such as benzyl alcohol.

DOXIL is not a clear solution but a translucent, red liposomal dispersion.

Parenteral drug products should be inspected visually for particulate matter and discoloration prior to administration, whenever solution and container permit. Do not use if a precipitate or foreign matter is present.

Rapid flushing of the infusion line should be avoided.

2.8 Procedure for Proper Handling and Disposal

Caution should be exercised in the handling and preparation of DOXIL.

The use of gloves is required.

If DOXIL comes into contact with skin or mucosa, immediately wash thoroughly with soap and water.

DOXIL should be considered an irritant and precautions should be taken to avoid extravasation. With intravenous administration of DOXIL, extravasation may occur with or without an accompanying stinging or burning sensation,

Table 2: Hematological Toxicity

Grade	ANC	Platelets	Modification
1	1,500–1,900	75,000–150,000	Resume treatment with no dose reduction
2	1,000–<1,500	50,000–<75,000	Wait until ANC ≥1,500 and platelets ≥75,000; redose with no dose reduction
3	500–999	25,000–<50,000	Wait until ANC ≥1,500 and platelets ≥75,000; redose with no dose reduction
4	<500	<25,000	Wait until ANC ≥1,500 and platelets ≥75,000; redose at 25% dose reduction or continue full dose with cytokine support

Table 4: Dosage adjustments for DOXIL + bortezomib combination therapy

Patient status	DOXIL	bortezomib
Fever ≥ 38°C and ANC <1,000/mm³	Do not dose this cycle if before Day 4; if after Day 4, reduce next dose by 25%.	Reduce next dose by 25%
On any day of drug administration after Day 1 of each cycle: Platelet count <25,000/mm³ Hemoglobin <8g/dL ANC <500/mm³	Do not dose this cycle if before Day 4; if after Day 4 reduce next dose by 25% in the following cycles if bortezomib is reduced for hematologic toxicity.	Do not dose; if 2 or more doses are not given in a cycle, reduce dose by 25% in following cycles.
Grade 3 or 4 non-hematologic drug related toxicity	Do not dose until recovered to Grade <2 and reduce dose by 25% for all subsequent doses.	Do not dose until recovered to Grade <2 and reduce dose by 25% for all subsequent doses.
Neuropathic pain or peripheral neuropathy	No dosage adjustments.	See bortezomib manufacturer's prescribing information for dosage adjustments in patients with neuropathic pain.

even if blood returns well on aspiration of the infusion needle. If any signs or symptoms of extravasation have occurred, the infusion should be immediately terminated and restarted in another vein. **DOXIL must not be given by the intramuscular or subcutaneous route.**

DOXIL should be handled and disposed of in a manner consistent with other anticancer drugs. Several guidelines on this subject exist [see References (15)].

3 DOSAGE FORMS AND STRENGTHS

- 20 mg/10 mL single use vial
- 50 mg/30 mL single use vial

4 CONTRAINDICATIONS

DOXIL (doxorubicin HCl liposome injection) is contraindicated in patients who have a history of hypersensitivity reactions to a conventional formulation of doxorubicin HCl or the components of DOXIL [see Warnings and Precautions (5.2)].

DOXIL is contraindicated in nursing mothers [see Use in Specific Populations (8.3)].

5 WARNINGS AND PRECAUTIONS

5.1 Cardiac Toxicity

Special attention must be given to the risk of myocardial damage from cumulative doses of doxorubicin HCl. Acute left ventricular failure may occur with doxorubicin, particularly in patients who have received a total cumulative dosage of doxorubicin exceeding the currently recommended limit of 550 mg/m². Lower (400 mg/m²) doses appear to cause heart failure in patients who have received radiotherapy to the mediastinal area or concomitant therapy with other potentially cardiotoxic agents such as cyclophosphamide.

Prior use of other anthracyclines or anthracenodiones should be included in calculations of total cumulative dosage. Congestive heart failure or cardiomyopathy may be encountered after discontinuation of anthracycline therapy. Patients with a history of cardiovascular disease should be administered DOXIL only when the potential benefit of treatment outweighs the risk.

Cardiac function should be carefully monitored in patients treated with DOXIL. The most definitive test for anthracycline myocardial injury is endomyocardial biopsy. Other methods, such as echocardiography or multigated radionuclide scans, have been used to monitor cardiac function during anthracycline therapy. Any of these methods should be employed to monitor potential cardiac toxicity in patients treated with DOXIL. If these test results indicate possible cardiac injury associated with DOXIL therapy, the benefit of continued therapy must be carefully weighed against the risk of myocardial injury.

In a clinical study in patients with advanced breast cancer, 250 patients received DOXIL at starting dose of 50 mg/m² every 4 weeks. At all cumulative anthracycline doses between 450-500 mg/m², or between 500-550 mg/m², the risk of cardiac toxicity for patients treated with DOXIL was 11%.

In this study, cardiotoxicity was defined as a decrease of >20% from baseline if the resting left ventricular ejection fraction (LVEF) remained in the normal range, or a de-

crease of >10% if the resting LVEF became abnormal (less than the institutional lower limit of normal). The data on left ventricular ejection fraction (LVEF) defined cardiotoxicity and congestive heart failure (CHF) are in the table below.

Table 5: Number of Patients With Advanced Breast Cancer

	DOXIL (n=250)
Patients who Developed Cardiotoxicity (LVEF Defined)	10
Cardiotoxicity (With Signs & Symptoms of CHF)	0
Cardiotoxicity (no Signs & Symptoms of CHF)	10
Patients With Signs and Symptoms of CHF Only	2

In the randomized multiple myeloma study, the incidence of heart failure events (ventricular dysfunction, cardiac failure, right ventricular failure, congestive cardiac failure, chronic cardiac failure, acute pulmonary edema and pulmonary edema) was similar in the DOXIL+bortezomib group and the bortezomib monotherapy group, 3% in each group. LVEF decrease was defined as an absolute decrease of ≥15% over baseline or a ≥5% decrease below the institutional lower limit of normal. Based on this definition, 25 patients in the bortezomib arm (8%) and 42 patients in the DOXIL+bortezomib arm (13%) experienced a reduction in LVEF.

5.2 Infusion Reactions

Acute infusion-related reactions were reported in 7.1% of patients treated with DOXIL in the randomized ovarian cancer study. These reactions were characterized by one or more of the following symptoms: flushing, shortness of breath, facial swelling, headache, chills, chest pain, back pain, tightness in the chest and throat, fever, tachycardia, pruritus, rash, cyanosis, syncope, bronchospasm, asthma, apnea, and hypotension. In most patients, these reactions resolve over the course of several hours to a day once the infusion is terminated. In some patients, the reaction resolved when the rate of infusion was slowed. In this study, two patients treated with DOXIL (0.8%) discontinued due to infusion-related reactions. In clinical studies, six patients with AIDS-related Kaposi's sarcoma (0.9%) and 13 (1.7%) solid tumor patients discontinued DOXIL therapy because of infusion-related reactions.

Serious and sometimes life-threatening or fatal allergic/anaphylactoid-like infusion reactions have been reported. Medications to treat such reactions, as well as emergency equipment, should be available for immediate use.

The majority of infusion-related events occurred during the first infusion. Similar reactions have not been reported with conventional doxorubicin and they presumably represent a reaction to the DOXIL liposomes or one of its surface components.

The initial rate of infusion should be 1 mg/min to help minimize the risk of infusion reactions [see Dosage and Administration (2)].

5.3 Myelosuppression

Because of the potential for bone marrow suppression, careful hematologic monitoring is required during use of DOXIL, including white blood cell, neutrophil, platelet counts, and Hgb/Hct. With the recommended dosage schedule, leukopenia is usually transient. Hematologic toxicity may require dose reduction or delay or suspension of DOXIL therapy. Persistent severe myelosuppression may result in superinfection, neutropenic fever, or hemorrhage. Development of sepsis in the setting of neutropenia has resulted in discontinuation of treatment and, in rare cases, death. DOXIL may potentiate the toxicity of other anticancer therapies. In particular, hematologic toxicity may be more severe when DOXIL is administered in combination with other agents that cause bone marrow suppression.

In patients with relapsed ovarian cancer, myelosuppression was generally moderate and reversible. In the three single-arm studies, anemia was the most common hematologic adverse reaction (52.6%), followed by leukopenia (WBC <4,000 mm^3; 42.2%), thrombocytopenia (24.2%), and neutropenia (ANC <1,000; 19.0%). In the randomized study, anemia was the most common hematologic adverse reaction (40.2%), followed by leukopenia (WBC <4,000 mm^3; 36.8%), neutropenia (ANC <1,000; 35.1%), and thrombocytopenia (13.0%) [see Adverse Reactions (6.2)].

In patients with relapsed ovarian cancer, 4.6% received G-CSF (or GM-CSF) to support their blood counts [see Dosage and Administrations (2.5)].

For patients with AIDS-related Kaposi's sarcoma who often present with baseline myelosuppression due to such factors as their HIV disease or concomitant medications, myelosuppression appears to be the dose-limiting adverse reaction at the recommended dose of 20 mg/m^2 [see Adverse Reactions (6.2)]. Leukopenia is the most common adverse reaction experienced in this population; anemia and thrombocytopenia can also be expected. Sepsis occurred in 5% of patients; for 0.7% of patients the event was considered possibly or probably related to DOXIL. Eleven patients (1.6%) discontinued study because of bone marrow suppression or neutropenia. Table 10 presents data on myelosuppression in patients with multiple myeloma receiving DOXIL and bortezomib in combination [see Adverse Reactions (6.2)].

5.4 Hand-Foot Syndrome (HFS)

In the randomized ovarian cancer study, 50.6% of patients treated with DOXIL at 50 mg/m^2 every 4 weeks experienced HFS (developed palmar-plantar skin eruptions characterized by swelling, pain, erythema and, for some patients, desquamation of the skin on the hands and the feet), with 23.8% of the patients reporting HFS Grade 3 or 4 events. Ten subjects (4.2%) discontinued treatment due to HFS or other skin toxicity. HFS toxicity grades are described above [see definitions of HFS grades in Dosage and Administration (2.5)].

Among 705 patients with AIDS-related Kaposi's sarcoma treated with DOXIL at 20 mg/m^2 every 2 weeks, 24 (3.4%) developed HFS, with 3 (0.9%) discontinuing.

In the randomized multiple myeloma study, 19% of patients treated with DOXIL at 30 mg/m^2 every three weeks experienced HFS.

HFS was generally observed after 2 or 3 cycles of treatment but may occur earlier. In most patients the reaction is mild and resolves in one to two weeks so that prolonged delay of therapy need not occur. However, dose modification may be required to manage HFS [see Dosage and Administration (2.5)]. The reaction can be severe and debilitating in some patients and may require discontinuation of treatment.

5.5 Radiation Recall Reaction

Recall reaction has occurred with DOXIL administration after radiotherapy.

5.6 Fetal Mortality

Pregnancy Category D

DOXIL can cause fetal harm when administered to a pregnant woman. There are no adequate and well-controlled studies in pregnant women. If DOXIL is to be used during pregnancy, or if the patient becomes pregnant during therapy, the patient should be apprised of the potential hazard to the fetus. If pregnancy occurs in the first few months following treatment with DOXIL, the prolonged half-life of the drug must be considered. Women of childbearing potential should be advised to avoid pregnancy during treatment with Doxil. [see Use in Specific Populations (8.1)].

5.7 Toxicity Potentiation

The doxorubicin in DOXIL may potentiate the toxicity of other anticancer therapies. Exacerbation of cyclophosphamide-induced hemorrhagic cystitis and enhancement of the hepatotoxicity of 6-mercaptopurine have been reported with the conventional formulation of doxorubicin HCl. Radiation-induced toxicity to the myocardium, mucosae, skin, and liver have been reported to be increased by the administration of doxorubicin HCl.

5.8 Monitoring: Laboratory Tests

Complete blood counts, including platelet counts, should be obtained frequently and at a minimum prior to each dose of DOXIL [see Warnings and Precautions (5.3)].

6 ADVERSE REACTIONS

6.1 Overall Adverse Reactions Profile

The following adverse reactions are discussed in more detail in other sections of the labeling.

• Cardiac Toxicity [see Warnings and Precautions (5.1)]
• Infusion reactions [see Warnings and Precautions (5.2)]
• Myelosuppression [see Warnings and Precautions (5.3)]
• Hand-Foot syndrome [see Warnings and Precautions (5.4)]

The most common adverse reactions observed with DOXIL are asthenia, fatigue, fever, nausea, stomatitis, vomiting, diarrhea, constipation, anorexia, hand-foot syndrome, rash and neutropenia, thrombocytopenia and anemia.

The most common serious adverse reactions observed with DOXIL are described in Section 6.2.

The safety data described below reflect exposure to DOXIL in 1310 patients including: 239 patients with ovarian cancer, 753 patients with AIDS-related Kaposi's sarcoma and 318 patients with multiple myeloma [see Adverse Reactions in Clinical Trials (6.2)].

6.2 Adverse Reactions in Clinical Trials

Because clinical trials are conducted under widely varying conditions, the adverse reaction rates observed cannot be directly compared to rates on other clinical trials and may not reflect the rates observed in clinical practice.

The following tables present adverse reactions from clinical trials of DOXIL in ovarian cancer and AIDS-Related Kaposi's sarcoma.

Patients With Ovarian Cancer

The safety data described below are from 239 patients with ovarian cancer treated with DOXIL (doxorubicin HCl liposome injection) at 50 mg/m^2 once every 4 weeks for a minimum of 4 courses in a randomized, multicenter, open-label study. In this study, patients received DOXIL for a median number of 98.0 days (range 1-785 days). The population studied was 27-87 years of age, 91% Caucasian, 6% Black and 3% Hispanic and other.

Table 6 presents the hematologic adverse reactions from the randomized study of DOXIL compared to topotecan.

Table 6: Ovarian Cancer Randomized Study Hematology Data Reported in Patients With Ovarian Cancer

	DOXIL Patients (n = 239)	Topotecan Patients (n = 235)
Neutropenia		
500-<1000/mm^3	19 (7.9%)	33 (14.0%)
<500/mm^3	10 (4.2%)	146 (62.1%)
Anemia		
6.5-< 8 g/dL	13 (5.4%)	59 (25.1%)
<6.5 g/dL	1 (0.4%)	10 (4.3%)
Thrombocytopenia		
10,000-<50,000/mm^3	3 (1.3%)	40 (17.0%)
<10,000/mm^3	0 (0.0%)	40 (17.0%)

Table 7 presents a comparative profile of the non-hematologic adverse reactions from the randomized study of DOXIL compared to topotecan.

Table 7: Ovarian Cancer Randomized Study

Non-Hematologic Adverse Reaction 10% or Greater	DOXIL (%) treated (n = 239)		Topotecan (%) treated (n = 235)	
	All grades	Grades 3-4	All grades	Grades 3-4
Body as a Whole				
Asthenia	40.2	7.1	51.5	8.1
Fever	21.3	0.8	30.6	5.5
Mucous Membrane Disorder	14.2	3.8	3.4	0
Back Pain	11.7	1.7	10.2	0.9
Infection	11.7	2.1	6.4	0.9
Headache	10.5	0.8	14.9	0
Digestive				
Nausea	46.0	5.4	63.0	8.1
Stomatitis	41.4	8.3	15.3	0.4
Vomiting	32.6	7.9	43.8	9.8
Diarrhea	20.9	2.5	34.9	4.2
Anorexia	20.1	2.5	21.7	1.3
Dyspepsia	12.1	0.8	14.0	0
Nervous				
Dizziness	4.2	0	10.2	0

Respiratory				
Pharyngitis	15.9	0	17.9	0.4
Dyspnea	15.1	4.1	23.4	4.3
Cough increased	9.6	0	11.5	0
Skin and Appendages				
Hand-foot syndrome	50.6	23.8	0.9	0
Rash	28.5	4.2	12.3	0.4
Alopecia	19.2	N/A	52.3	N/A

The following additional adverse reactions (not in table) were observed in patients with ovarian cancer with doses administered every four weeks.

Incidence 1% to 10%

Cardiovascular: vasodilation, tachycardia, deep thrombophlebitis, hypotension, cardiac arrest.

Digestive: oral moniliasis, mouth ulceration, esophagitis, dysphagia, rectal bleeding, ileus.

Hemic and Lymphatic: ecchymosis.

Metabolic and Nutritional: dehydration, weight loss, hyperbilirubinemia, hypokalemia, hypercalcemia, hyponatremia.

Nervous: somnolence, dizziness, depression.

Respiratory: rhinitis, pneumonia, sinusitis, epistaxis.

Skin and Appendages: pruritus, skin discoloration, vesiculobullous rash, maculopapular rash, exfoliative dermatitis, herpes zoster, dry skin, herpes simplex, fungal dermatitis, furunculosis, acne.

Special Senses: conjunctivitis, taste perversion, dry eyes.

Urinary: urinary tract infection, hematuria, vaginal moniliasis.

Patients With AIDS-Related Kaposi's Sarcoma

The safety data below is based on the experience reported in 753 patients with AIDS-related Kaposi's sarcoma enrolled in four studies. The median age of the population was 38.7 years (range 24-70 years), which was 99% male, 1% female, 88% Caucasian, 6% Hispanic, 4% Black, and 2% Asian/other/unknown. The majority of patients were treated with 20 mg/m^2 of DOXIL every two to three weeks. The median time on study was 127 days and ranged from 1 to 811 days. The median cumulative dose was 120 mg/m^2 and ranged from 3.3 to 798.6 mg/m^2. Twenty-six patients (3.0%) received cumulative doses of greater than 450 mg/m^2.

Of these 753 patients, 61.2% were considered poor risk for KS tumor burden, 91.5% poor for immune system, and 46.9% for systemic illness; 36.2% were poor risk for all three categories. Patients median CD4 count was 21.0 cells/mm^3, with 50.8% of patients having less than 50 cells/mm^3. The mean absolute neutrophil count at study entry was approximately 3,000 cells/mm^3.

Patients received a variety of potentially myelotoxic drugs in combination with DOXIL. Of the 693 patients with concomitant medication information, 58.7% were on one or more antiretroviral medications; 34.9% patients were on zidovudine (AZT), 20.8% on didanosine (ddI), 16.5% on zalcitabine (ddC), and 9.5% on stavudine (D4T). A total of 85.1% patients were on PCP prophylaxis, most (54.4%) on sulfamethoxazole/trimethoprim. Eighty-five percent of patients were receiving antifungal medications, primarily fluconazole (75.8%). Seventy-two percent of patients were receiving antivirals, 56.3% acyclovir, 29% ganciclovir, and 16% foscarnet. In addition, 47.8% patients received colony-stimulating factors (sargramostim/filgrastim) sometime during their course of treatment.

Adverse reactions led to discontinuation of treatment in 5% of patients with AIDS related Kaposi's sarcoma. Those that did so included bone marrow suppression, cardiac adverse reactions, infusion-related reactions, toxoplasmosis, HFS, pneumonia, cough/dyspnea, fatigue, optic neuritis, progression of a non-KS tumor, allergy to penicillin, and unspecified reasons.

Table 8: Hematology Data Reported in Patients With AIDS-Related Kaposi's Sarcoma

	Patients With Refractory or Intolerant AIDS-Related Kaposi's Sarcoma (n = 74)		Total Patients With AIDS-Related Kaposi's Sarcoma (n = 720)	
Neutropenia				
<1000/mm^3	34	(45.9%)	352	(48.9%)
<500/mm^3	8	(10.8%)	96	(13.3%)
Anemia				
<10 g/dL	43	(58.1%)	399	(55.4%)
<8 g/dL	12	(16.2%)	131	(18.2%)
Thrombocytopenia				
<150,000/mm^3	45	(60.8%)	439	(60.9%)
<25,000/mm^3	1	(1.4%)	30	(4.2%)

Table 9: Probably and Possibly Drug-Related Non-Hematologic Adverse Reactions Reported in ≥5% of Patients With AIDS-Related Kaposi's Sarcoma

Adverse Reactions	Patients With Refractory or Intolerant AIDS-Related Kaposi's Sarcoma (n = 77)		Total Patients With AIDS-Related Kaposi's Sarcoma (n = 705)	
Nausea	14	(18.2%)	119	(16.9%)
Asthenia	5	(6.5%)	70	(9.9%)
Fever	6	(7.8%)	64	(9.1%)
Alopecia	7	(9.1%)	63	(8.9%)
Alkaline Phosphatase Increase	1	(1.3%)	55	(7.8%)
Vomiting	6	(7.8%)	55	(7.8%)
Diarrhea	4	(5.2%)	55	(7.8%)
Stomatitis	4	(5.2%)	48	(6.8%)
Oral Moniliasis	1	(1.3%)	39	(5.5%)

The following additional (not in table) adverse reactions were observed in patients with AIDS-related Kaposi's sarcoma.
Incidence 1% to 5%
Body as a Whole: headache, back pain, infection, allergic reaction, chills.
Cardiovascular: chest pain, hypotension, tachycardia.
Cutaneous: herpes simplex, rash, itching.
Digestive: mouth ulceration, anorexia, dysphagia.
Metabolic and Nutritional: SGPT increase, weight loss, hyperbilirubinemia.
Other: dyspnea, pneumonia, dizziness, somnolence.
Incidence Less Than 1%
Body As A Whole: sepsis, moniliasis, cryptococcosis.
Cardiovascular: thrombophlebitis, cardiomyopathy, palpitation, bundle branch block, congestive heart failure, heart arrest, thrombosis, ventricular arrhythmia.
Digestive: hepatitis.
Metabolic and Nutritional Disorders: dehydration
Respiratory: cough increase, pharyngitis.
Skin and Appendages: maculopapular rash, herpes zoster.
Special Senses: taste perversion, conjunctivitis.
Patients With Multiple Myeloma
The safety data below are from 318 patients treated with DOXIL (30 mg/m² as a 1-hr i.v. infusion) administered on day 4 following bortezomib (1.3 mg/m² i.v. bolus on days 1, 4, 8 and 11) every three weeks, in a randomized, open-label, multicenter study. In this study, patients in the DOXIL + bortezomib combination group were treated for a median number of 138 days (range 21-410 days). The population was 28-85 years of age, 58% male, 42% female, 90% Caucasian, 6% Black, and 4% Asian and other. Table 10 lists adverse reactions reported in 10% or more of patients treated with DOXIL in combination with bortezomib for multiple myeloma.
[See table 10 above]

6.3 Post Marketing Experience
The following additional adverse reactions have been identified during post approval use of DOXIL. Because these reactions are reported voluntarily from a population of uncertain size, it is not always possible to reliably estimate their frequency or establish a causal relationship to drug exposure.
Musculoskeletal and Connective Tissue Disorders: rare cases of muscle spasms.
Respiratory, Thoracic and Mediastinal Disorders: rare cases of pulmonary embolism (in some cases fatal).
Hematologic disorders: Secondary acute myelogenous leukemia with and without fatal outcome has been reported in patients whose treatment included DOXIL.
Skin and subcutaneous tissue disorders: rare cases of erythema multiforme, Stevens-Johnson syndrome and toxic epidermal necrolysis have been reported.

7 DRUG INTERACTIONS
No formal drug interaction studies have been conducted with DOXIL. DOXIL may interact with drugs known to interact with the conventional formulation of doxorubicin HCl.

8 USE IN SPECIFIC POPULATIONS
8.1 Pregnancy
Pregnancy Category D *[see Warnings and Precautions (5.6)].*
DOXIL is embryotoxic at doses of 1 mg/kg/day in rats and is embryotoxic and abortifacient at 0.5 mg/kg/day in rabbits (both doses are about one-eighth the 50 mg/m² human dose on a mg/m² basis). Embryotoxicity was characterized by increased embryo-fetal deaths and reduced live litter sizes.

Table 10: Frequency of treatment emergent adverse reactions reported in ≥10% patients treated for multiple myeloma with DOXIL in combination with bortezomib, by Severity, Body System, and MedDRA Terminology.

Adverse Reaction	DOXIL + bortezomib (n=318)			Bortezomib (n=318)		
	Any (%)	Grade 3	Grade 4	Any (%)	Grade 3	Grade 4
Blood and lymphatic system disorders						
Neutropenia	36	22	10	22	11	5
Thrombocytopenia	33	11	13	28	9	8
Anemia	25	7	2	21	8	2
General disorders and administration site conditions						
Fatigue	36	6	1	28	3	0
Pyrexia	31	1	0	22	1	0
Asthenia	22	6	0	18	4	0
Gastrointestinal disorders						
Nausea	48	3	0	40	1	0
Diarrhea	46	7	0	39	5	0
Vomiting	32	4	0	22	1	0
Constipation	31	1	0	31	1	0
Mucositis/Stomatitis	20	2	0	5	<1	0
Abdominal pain	11	1	0	8	1	0
Infections and infestations						
Herpes zoster	11	2	0	9	2	0
Herpes simplex	10	0	0	6	1	0
Investigations						
Weight decreased	12	0	0	4	0	0
Metabolism and Nutritional disorders						
Anorexia	19	2	0	14	<1	0
Nervous system disorders						
Peripheral Neuropathy*	42	7	<1	45	10	1
Neuralgia	17	3	0	20	4	1
Paresthesia/dysesthesia	13	<1	0	10	0	0
Respiratory, thoracic and mediastinal disorders						
Cough	18	0	0	12	0	0
Skin and subcutaneous tissue disorders						
Rash**	22	1	0	18	1	0
Hand-foot syndrome	19	6	0	<1	0	0

* Peripheral neuropathy includes the following adverse reactions: peripheral sensory neuropathy, neuropathy peripheral, polyneuropathy, peripheral motor neuropathy, and neuropathy NOS.
**Rash includes the following adverse reactions: rash, rash erythematous, rash macular, rash maculo-papular, rash pruritic, exfoliative rash, and rash generalized.

8.3 Nursing Mothers
It is not known whether this drug is excreted in human milk. Because many drugs, including anthracyclines, are excreted in human milk and because of the potential for serious adverse reactions in nursing infants from DOXIL, mothers should discontinue nursing prior to taking this drug.

8.4 Pediatric Use
The safety and effectiveness of DOXIL in pediatric patients have not been established.

8.5 Geriatric Use
Of the patients treated with DOXIL in the randomized ovarian cancer study, 34.7% (n=83) were 65 years of age or older while 7.9% (n=19) were 75 years of age or older. Of the 318 patients treated with DOXIL in combination with bortezomib for multiple myeloma, 37% were 65 years of age or older and 8% were 75 years of age or older. No overall differences in safety or efficacy were observed between these patients and younger patients.

8.6 Hepatic Impairment
The pharmacokinetics of DOXIL has not been adequately evaluated in patients with hepatic impairment. Doxorubicin is eliminated in large part by the liver. Thus, DOXIL dosage should be reduced in patients with impaired hepatic function *[see Dosage and Administration (2.6)].*
Prior to DOXIL administration, evaluation of hepatic function is recommended using conventional clinical laboratory tests such as SGOT, SGPT, alkaline phosphatase, and bilirubin *[see Dosage and Administration (2.6)].*

10 OVERDOSAGE
Acute overdosage with doxorubicin HCl causes increases in mucositis, leucopenia, and thrombocytopenia.
Treatment of acute overdosage consists of treatment of the severely myelosuppressed patient with hospitalization, antibiotics, platelet and granulocyte transfusions, and symptomatic treatment of mucositis.

11 DESCRIPTION
DOXIL (doxorubicin HCl liposome injection) is doxorubicin hydrochloride (HCl) encapsulated in STEALTH® liposomes for intravenous administration.
Doxorubicin is an anthracycline topoisomerase inhibitor isolated from *Streptomyces peucetius* var. *caesius.*
Doxorubicin HCl, which is the established name for (8S, 10S)-10-[(3-amino-2,3,6-trideoxy-α-L-lyxo-hexopyranosyl) oxy]-8-glycoloyl-7,8,9,10-tetrahydro-6,8,11-trihydroxy-1-methoxy-5,12-naphthacenedione hydrochloride, has the following structure:

The molecular formula of the drug is $C_{27}H_{29}NO_{11}\cdot HCl$; its molecular weight is 579.99.
DOXIL is provided as a sterile, translucent, red liposomal dispersion in 10-mL or 30-mL glass, single use vials. Each vial contains 20 mg or 50 mg doxorubicin HCl at a concentration of 2 mg/mL and a pH of 6.5. The STEALTH® liposome carriers are composed of N-(carbonyl-methoxypolyethylene glycol 2000)-1,2-distearoyl-sn-glycero-3 phosphoethanolamine sodium salt (MPEG-DSPE), 3.19 mg/mL; fully hydrogenated soy phosphatidylcholine (HSPC), 9.58 mg/mL; and cholesterol, 3.19 mg/mL. Each mL also contains ammonium sulfate, approximately 2 mg; histidine as a buffer; hydrochloric acid and/or sodium hydroxide for pH control; and sucrose to maintain isotonicity. Greater than 90% of the drug is encapsulated in the STEALTH® liposomes.
MPEG-DSPE has the following structural formula:

n = ca. 45

HSPC has the following structural formula:

m, n = 14 or 16

12 CLINICAL PHARMACOLOGY
12.1 Mechanism of Action
The active ingredient of DOXIL is doxorubicin HCl. The mechanism of action of doxorubicin HCl is thought to be re-

Table 11: Pharmacokinetic Parameters of DOXIL in Patients With AIDS-Related Kaposi's Sarcoma

Parameter (units)	Dose	
	10 mg/m^2	20 mg/m^2
Peak Plasma Concentration (µg/mL)	4.12 ± 0.215	8.34 ± 0.49
Plasma Clearance (L/h/m²)	0.056 ± 0.01	0.041 ± 0.004
Steady State Volume of Distribution (L/m²)	2.83 ± 0.145	2.72 ± 0.120
AUC (µg/mL•h)	277 ± 32.9	590 ± 58.7
First Phase (λ_1) Half-Life (h)	4.7 ± 1.1	5.2 ± 1.4
Second Phase (λ_1) Half-Life (h)	52.3 ± 5.6	55.0 ± 4.8

N = 23
Mean ± Standard Error

Table 12: Patient Demographics for Patients With Refractory Ovarian Cancer From Single Arm Ovarian Cancer Studies

	Study 1 (U.S.) (n = 27)	Study 2 (U.S.) (n = 82)	Study 3 (non-U.S.) (n = 36)
Age at Diagnosis (Years)			
Median	64	61.5	51.5
Range	46–75	34–85	22–80
Drug-Free Interval (Months)			
Median	1.8	1.7	2.6
Range	0.5–15.6	0.6–7.0	0.7–15.2
Sum of Lesions at Baseline (cm)²			
Median	25	18.3	32.4
Range	1.2–230.0	1.3–285.0	0.3–114.0
FIGO Staging			
I	1 (3.7%)	3 (3.7%)	4 (11.1%)
II	3 (11.1%)	3 (3.7%)	1 (2.8%)
III	15 (55.6%)	60 (73.2%)	24 (66.7%)
IV	8 (29.6%)	16 (19.5%)	6 (16.7%)
Not Specified	—	—	1 (2.8%)
CA-125 at Baseline			
Median	123.5	199.0	1004.5
Range	20–14,012	7–46,594	20–12,089
Number of Prior Chemotherapy Regimens			
1	7 (25.9%)	13 (15.9%)	9 (25.0%)
2	11 (40.7%)	44 (53.7%)	19 (52.8%)
3	6 (22.2%)	25 (30.5%)	8 (22.8%)
4	3 (11.1%)	—	—

Table 13: Response Rates in Patients With Refractory Ovarian Cancer From Single Arm Ovarian Cancer Studies

	Study 1 (U.S.)	Study 2 (U.S.)	Study 3 (non-U.S.)
Response Rate	22.2% (6/27)	17.1% (14/82)	0% (0/36)
95% Confidence Interval	8.6%-42.3%	9.7%-27.0%	0.0%-9.7%

lated to its ability to bind DNA and inhibit nucleic acid synthesis. Cell structure studies have demonstrated rapid cell penetration and perinuclear chromatin binding, rapid inhibition of mitotic activity and nucleic acid synthesis, and induction of mutagenesis and chromosomal aberrations.

DOXIL is doxorubicin HCl encapsulated in long-circulating STEALTH® liposomes. Liposomes are microscopic vesicles composed of a phospholipid bilayer that are capable of encapsulating active drugs. The STEALTH® liposomes of DOXIL are formulated with surface-bound methoxypolyethylene glycol (MPEG), a process often referred to as pegylation, to protect liposomes from detection by the mononuclear phagocyte system (MPS) and to increase blood circulation time.

Representation of a STEALTH® liposome:

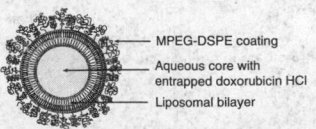

MPEG-DSPE coating
Aqueous core with entrapped doxorubicin HCl
Liposomal bilayer

STEALTH® liposomes have a half-life of approximately 55 hours in humans. They are stable in blood, and direct measurement of liposomal doxorubicin shows that at least 90% of the drug (the assay used cannot quantify less than 5-10% free doxorubicin) remains liposome-encapsulated during circulation.

It is hypothesized that because of their small size (ca. 100 nm) and persistence in the circulation, the pegylated DOXIL liposomes are able to penetrate the altered and often compromised vasculature of tumors. This hypothesis is supported by studies using colloidal gold-containing STEALTH® liposomes, which can be visualized microscopi-

cally. Evidence of penetration of STEALTH® liposomes from blood vessels and their entry and accumulation in tumors has been seen in mice with C-26 colon carcinoma tumors and in transgenic mice with Kaposi's sarcoma-like lesions. Once the STEALTH® liposomes distribute to the tissue compartment, the encapsulated doxorubicin HCl becomes available. The exact mechanism of release is not understood.

12.3 Pharmacokinetics

The plasma pharmacokinetics of DOXIL were evaluated in 42 patients with AIDS-related Kaposi's sarcoma (KS) who received single doses of 10 or 20 mg/m² administered by a 30-minute infusion. Twenty-three of these patients received single doses of both 10 and 20 mg/m² with a 3-week washout period between doses. The pharmacokinetic parameter values of DOXIL, given for total doxorubicin (mostly liposomally bound), are presented in Table 11.

[See table 11 above]

DOXIL displayed linear pharmacokinetics over the range of 10 to 20 mg/m². Disposition occurred in two phases after DOXIL administration, with a relatively short first phase (≈ 5 hours) and a prolonged second phase (≈ 55 hours) that accounted for the majority of the area under the curve (AUC).

The pharmacokinetics of DOXIL at a 50 mg/m² dose is reported to be nonlinear. At this dose, the elimination half-life of DOXIL is expected to be longer and the clearance lower compared to a 20 mg/m² dose. The exposure (AUC) is thus expected to be more than proportional at a 50 mg/m² dose when compared with the lower doses.

Distribution:
In contrast to the pharmacokinetics of doxorubicin, which displays a large volume of distribution, ranging from 700 to 1100 L/m², the small steady state volume of distribution of DOXIL shows that DOXIL is confined mostly to the vascular

fluid volume. Plasma protein binding of DOXIL has not been determined; the plasma protein binding of doxorubicin is approximately 70%.

Metabolism:
Doxorubicinol, the major metabolite of doxorubicin, was detected at very low levels (range: of 0.8 to 26.2 ng/mL) in the plasma of patients who received 10 or 20 mg/m² DOXIL.

Excretion:
The plasma clearance of DOXIL was slow, with a mean clearance value of 0.041 L/h/m² at a dose of 20 mg/m². This is in contrast to doxorubicin, which displays a plasma clearance value ranging from 24 to 35 L/h/m².

Because of its slower clearance, the AUC of DOXIL, primarily representing the circulation of liposome-encapsulated doxorubicin, is approximately two to three orders of magnitude larger than the AUC for a similar dose of conventional doxorubicin HCl as reported in the literature.

Special Populations:
The pharmacokinetics of DOXIL have not been separately evaluated in women, in members of different ethnic groups, or in individuals with renal or hepatic insufficiency.

Drug-Drug Interactions:
Drug-drug interactions between DOXIL and other drugs, including antiviral agents, have not been adequately evaluated in patients with ovarian cancer, AIDS-related Kaposi's sarcoma or multiple myeloma.

Tissue Distribution in Patients with Kaposi's Sarcoma:
Kaposi's sarcoma lesions and normal skin biopsies were obtained at 48 and 96 hours post infusion of 20 mg/m² DOXIL in 11 patients. The concentration of DOXIL in KS lesions was a median of 19 (range, 3-53) times higher than in normal skin at 48 hours post treatment; however, this was not corrected for likely differences in blood content between KS lesions and normal skin. The corrected ratio may lie between 1 and 22 times. Thus, higher concentrations of DOXIL are delivered to KS lesions than to normal skin.

13 NON-CLINICAL TOXICOLOGY

13.1 Carcinogenesis, Mutagenesis, and Impairment of Fertility

Although no studies have been conducted with DOXIL, doxorubicin HCl and related compounds have been shown to have mutagenic and carcinogenic properties when tested in experimental models.

STEALTH® liposomes without drug were negative when tested in Ames, mouse lymphoma and chromosomal aberration assays in vitro, and mammalian micronucleus assay in vivo.

The possible adverse effects on fertility in males and females in humans or experimental animals have not been adequately evaluated. However, DOXIL resulted in mild to moderate ovarian and testicular atrophy in mice after a single dose of 36 mg/kg (about twice the 50 mg/m² human dose on a mg/m² basis). Decreased testicular weights and hypospermia were present in rats after repeat doses ≥ 0.25 mg/kg/day (about one thirtieth the 50 mg/m² human dose on a mg/m² basis), and diffuse degeneration of the seminiferous tubules and a marked decrease in spermatogenesis were observed in dogs after repeat doses of 1 mg/kg/day (about one half the 50 mg/m² human dose on a mg/m² basis).

14 CLINICAL STUDIES

14.1 Ovarian Cancer

DOXIL (doxorubicin HCl liposome injection) was studied in three open-label, single-arm, clinical studies of 176 patients with metastatic ovarian cancer. One hundred forty-five (145) of these patients were refractory to both paclitaxel- and platinum-based chemotherapy regimens. Refractory ovarian cancer is defined as disease progression while on treatment, or relapse within 6 months of completing treatment. Patients in these studies received DOXIL at 50 mg/m² infused over one hour every 3 or 4 weeks for 3-6 cycles or longer in the absence of dose-limiting toxicity or progression of disease.

The baseline demographics and clinical characteristics of the patients with refractory ovarian cancer are provided in **Table 12** below.

[See table 12 above]

The primary efficacy parameter was response rate for the population of patients refractory to both paclitaxel- and a platinum-containing regimen. Assessment of response was based on Southwest Oncology Group (SWOG) criteria, and required confirmation four weeks after the initial observation. Secondary efficacy parameters were time to response, duration of response, and time to progression.

The response rates for the individual single arm studies are given in **Table 13** below.

[See table 13 above]

When the data from the single arm studies are combined, the response rate for all patients refractory to paclitaxel and platinum agents was 13.8% (20/145) (95% CI 8.1% to 19.3%). The median time to progression was 15.9 weeks, the median time to response was 17.6 weeks, and the duration of response was 39.4 weeks.

DOXIL (doxorubicin HCl liposome injection) was also studied in a randomized, multicenter, open-label, study in 474 patients with epithelial ovarian cancer after platinum-based chemotherapy. Patients in this study received an initial dose of either DOXIL 50 mg/m² infused over one hour every 4 weeks or topotecan 1.5 mg/m² infused daily for 5 consecutive days every 3 weeks. Patients were stratified according to platinum sensitivity and the presence of bulky disease (presence of tumor mass greater than 5 cm in size). Platinum sensitivity is defined by response to initial platinum-based therapy and a progression-free interval of greater than 6 months off treatment. The primary efficacy endpoint for this study was time to progression (TTP). Other efficacy endpoints included overall survival and objective response rate.

The baseline patient demographic and clinical characteristics are provided in **Table 14** below.

Table 14: Ovarian Cancer Randomized Study Baseline Demographic and Clinical Characteristics

	DOXIL (n = 239)	Topotecan (n = 235)
Age at Diagnosis (Years)		
Median	60.0	60.0
Range	27-87	25-85
Drug-Free Interval (Months)		
Median	7.0	6.7
Range	0.9-82.1	0.5-109.6
FIGO Staging		
I	11 (4.6%)	15 (6.4%)
II	13 (5.4%)	8 (3.4%)
III	175 (73.2%)	164 (69.8%)
IV	40 (16.7%)	48 (20.4%)
Platinum Sensitivity		
Sensitive	109 (45.6%)	110 (46.8%)
Refractory	130 (54.4%)	125 (53.2%)
Bulky Disease		
Present	108 (45.2%)	105 (44.7%)
Absent	131 (54.8%)	130 (55.3%)

Study results are provided in **Table 15**. There was no statistically significant difference in TTP between the two treatment arms.

Table 15: Results of Efficacy Analyses[a]

	Protocol Defined ITT Population	
	DOXIL (n = 239)	Topotecan (n = 235)
TTP (Protocol Specified Primary Endpoint)		
Median (Months)[b]	4.1	4.2
p-value[c]	0.617	
Hazard Ratio[d]	0.955	
95% CI for Hazard Ratio	(0.762, 1.196)	
Overall Survival		
Median (Months)[b]	14.4	13.7
p-value*	0.05	
Hazard Ratio[d]	0.822	
95% CI for Hazard Ratio	(0.676, 1.000)	
Response Rate		
Overall Response n (%)	47 (19.7)	40 (17.0)
Complete Response n (%)	9 (3.8)	11 (4.7)
Partial Response n (%)	38 (15.9)	29 (12.3)
Median Duration of Response (Months)[b]	6.9	5.9

[a] Analysis based on investigator's strata for protocol defined ITT population.
[b] Kaplan-Meier estimates.
[c] p-value is based on the stratified log-rank test.
[d] Hazard ratio is based on Cox proportional-hazard model with the treatment as single independent variable. A hazard ratio less than 1 indicates an advantage for DOXIL.
*p-value not adjusted for multiple comparisons.

14.2 AIDS-Related Kaposi's Sarcoma
DOXIL was studied in an open-label, single-arm, multicenter study utilizing DOXIL at 20 mg/m² by intravenous infusion every three weeks, generally until progression or intolerance occurred. In an interim analysis, the treatment history of 383 patients was reviewed, and a cohort of 77 patients was retrospectively identified as having disease progression on prior systemic combination chemotherapy (at least 2 cycles of a regimen containing at least two of three treatments: bleomycin, vincristine or vinblastine, or doxorubicin) or as being intolerant to such therapy. Forty-nine of the 77 patients (64%) had received prior doxorubicin HCl.

These 77 patients were predominantly Caucasian, homosexual males with a median CD4 count of 10 cells/mm³. Their

age ranged from 24 to 54 years, with a mean age of 38 years. Using the ACTG staging criteria, 78% of the patients were at poor risk for tumor burden, 96% at poor risk for immune system, and 58% at poor risk for systemic illness at baseline. Their mean Karnofsky status score was 74%. All 77 patients had cutaneous or subcutaneous lesions, 40% also had oral lesions, 26% pulmonary lesions, and 14% of patients had lesions of the stomach/intestine.

The majority of these patients had disease progression on prior systemic combination chemotherapy.

Investigator Assessment
Investigator response was based on modified ACTG criteria. Partial response was defined as no new lesions, sites of disease, or worsening edema; flattening of ≥ 50% of previously raised lesions or area of indicator lesions decreasing by ≥ 50%; and response lasting at least 21 days with no prior progression.

Indicator Lesion Assessment
A retrospectively defined analysis was conducted based on assessment of the response of up to five prospectively identified representative indicator lesions. A partial response was defined as flattening of ≥50% of previously raised indicator lesions, or >50% decrease in the area of indicator lesions and lasting at least 21 days with no prior progression. Only patients with adequate documentation of baseline status and follow-up assessments were considered evaluable for response. Patients who received concomitant KS treatment during study, who completed local radiotherapy to sites encompassing one or more of the indicator lesions within two months of study entry, who had less than four indicator lesions, or who had less than three raised indicator lesions at baseline (the latter applies solely to indicator lesion assessment) were considered nonevaluable for response. Of the 77 patients who had disease progression on prior systemic combination chemotherapy or who were intolerant to such therapy, 34 were evaluable for investigator assessment and 42 were evaluable for indicator lesion assessment.

Table 16: Response in Patients with Refractory[a] AIDS-related Kaposi's Sarcoma

Investigator Assessment	All Evaluable Patients (n = 34)	Evaluable Patients Who Received Prior Doxorubicin (n = 20)
Response[b]		
Partial (PR)	27%	30%
Stable	29%	40%
Progression	44%	30%

Duration of PR (Days)		
Median	73	89
Range	42+-210+	42+-210+
Time to PR (Days)		
Median	43	53
Range	15-133	15-109

Indicator Lesion Assessment	All Evaluable Patients (n = 42)	Evaluable Patients Who Received Prior Doxorubicin (n = 23)
Response[b]		
Partial (PR)	48%	52%
Stable	26%	30%
Progression	26%	17%
Duration of PR (Days)		
Median	71	79
Range	22+-210+	35-210+
Time to PR (Days)		
Median	22	48
Range	15-109	15-109

[a] Patients with disease that progressed on prior combination chemotherapy or who were intolerant to such therapy.
[b] There were no complete responses in this population.

Retrospective efficacy analyses were performed on two studies that had subsets of patients who received single agent DOXIL and who were on stable antiretroviral therapy for at least 60 days prior to enrollment and at least until a response was demonstrated. In one cooperative group trial that was closed early due to slow accrual, 7 of 17 patients (40%) on stable antiretroviral therapy had a durable response. The median duration was not reached but was longer than 11.6 months. In another trial, 4 of 11 patients (40%) on stable antiretroviral therapy demonstrated durable responses.

14.3 Multiple Myeloma
The safety and efficacy of DOXIL in combination with bortezomib in the treatment of multiple myeloma were evaluated in a randomized, open label, international multicenter study. This study included 646 patients who have not previously received bortezomib and whose disease progressed during or after at least one prior therapy. Patients were randomized (1:1 ratio) to receive either DOXIL (30 mg/m² as a 1-hr i.v. infusion) administered on day 4 following bortezomib (1.3 mg/m² i.v. bolus on days 1, 4, 8 and 11) or bortezomib alone (1.3 mg/m² i.v. bolus on days 1, 4, 8 and 11). Treatment was administered every 3 weeks. Patients were treated for up to 8 cycles until disease progression or the occurrence of unacceptable toxicity. Patients who maintained a response were allowed to receive further treatment. The median number of cycles in each treatment arm was 5 (range 1-18). The baseline demographics and clinical characteristics of the patients with multiple myeloma are provided in **Table 17** below.
[See table 17 above]

Table 17: Summary of Baseline Patient and Disease Characteristics

Patient Characteristics	DOXIL + bortezomib n=324	bortezomib n=322
Median age in years (range)	61 (28, 85)	62 (34, 88)
% Male/female	58 / 42	54 / 46
% Caucasian/Black/other	90 / 6 / 4	94 / 4 / 2
Disease Characteristics		
% with IgG/IgA/Light chain	57 / 27 / 12	62 / 24 / 11
% β₂-microglobulin group		
≤2.5 mg/L	14	14
>2.5 mg/L and ≤5.5 mg/L	56	55
>5.5 mg/L	30	31
Serum M-protein (g/dL):		
Median (Range)	2.5 (0-10.0)	2.7 (0-10.0)
Urine M-protein (mg/24 hours):		
Median (Range)	107 (0-24883)	66 (0-39657)
Median Months Since Diagnosis	35.2	37.5
% Prior Therapy		
One	34	34
More than one	66	66
Prior Systemic Therapies for Multiple Myeloma		
Corticosteroid (%)	99	>99
Anthracyclines	68	67
Alkylating agent (%)	92	90
Thalidomide/lenalidomide (%)	40	43
Stem cell transplantation (%)	57	54

The primary endpoint in this study was time to progression (TTP). TTP was defined as the time from randomization to the first occurrence of progressive disease or death due to progressive disease. The combination arm demonstrated significant improvement in TTP. As the prespecified primary objective was achieved at the interim analysis, patients in the bortezomib monotherapy group were then allowed to receive the DOXIL + bortezomib combination. Survival continued to be followed after the interim analysis and survival data are not mature at this time. Efficacy results are as shown in **Table 18** and **Figure 1**.

Table 18: Efficacy of DOXIL in combination with bortezomib in the treatment of patients with multiple myeloma

Endpoint	DOXIL + bortezomib n=324	Bortezomib n=322
Time to Progression[a]		
Progression or death due to progression (n)	99	150
Censored (n)	225	172
Median in days (months)	282 (9.3)	197 (6.5)
95% CI	250;338	170;217
Hazard ratio[b]	0.55	
(95% CI)	(0.43, 0.71)	
p-value[c]	<0.0001	
Response (n)[d]	303	310
% Complete Response (CR)	5	3
% Partial Response (PR)	43	40
% CR + PR	48	43
p-value[e]	0.251	
Median Duration of Response (months)	10.2	7.0
(95% CI)	(10.2;12.9)	(5.9;8.3)

[a] Kaplan Meier estimate.
[b] Hazard ratio based on stratified Cox proportional hazards regression. A hazard ratio <1 indicates an advantage for DOXIL+bortezomib.
[c] Stratified log-rank test.
[d] RR as per EBMT criteria.
[e] Cochran-Mantel-Haenszel test adjusted for the stratification factors.

Time to progression outcomes were consistent with the overall result across most subgroups defined by patient demographic and baseline characteristics. There were too few Blacks or Asian patients to adequately assess differences in effects for the race subgroup.

Figure 1- Time to Progression Kaplan-Meier Curve

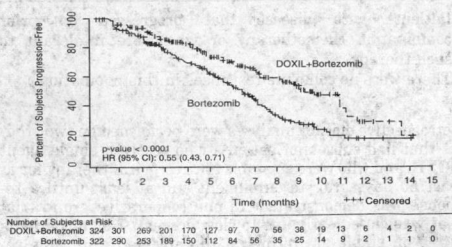

Number of Subjects at Risk														
DOXIL+Bortezomib	324	301	269	201	170	127	97	70	56	38	19	13	6	4	2	0
Bortezomib	322	290	253	189	150	112	84	56	35	25	14	9	2	1	1	0

15 REFERENCES

1. NIOSH Alert: Preventing occupational exposures to antineoplastic and other hazardous drugs in healthcare settings. 2004. U.S. Department of Health and Human Services, Public Health Service, Centers for Disease Control and Prevention, National Institute for Occupational Safety and Health, DHHS (NIOSH) Publication No. 2004-165.
2. OSHA Technical Manual, TED 1-0.15A, Section VI: Chapter 2. Controlling Occupational Exposure to Hazardous Drugs. OSHA, 1999. http://www.osha.gov/dts/osta/otm/otm_vi/otm_vi_2.html
3. NIH [2002]. 1999 recommendations for the safe handling of cytotoxic drugs. U.S. Department of Health and Human Services, Public Health Service, National Institutes of Health, NIH Publication No. 92-2621.
4. American Society of Health-System Pharmacists. (2006) ASHP Guidelines on Handling Hazardous Drugs.
5. Polovich, M., White, J. M., & Kelleher, L.O. (eds.) 2005. Chemotherapy and biotherapy guidelines and recommendations for practice (2nd. ed.) Pittsburgh, PA: Oncology Nursing Society.

16 HOW SUPPLIED/STORAGE AND HANDLING

DOXIL (doxorubicin HCl liposome injection) is supplied as a sterile, translucent, red liposomal dispersion in 10-mL or 30-mL glass, single use vials.
Each 10-mL vial contains 20 mg doxorubicin HCl at a concentration of 2 mg/mL.
Each 30-mL vial contains 50 mg doxorubicin HCl at a concentration of 2 mg/mL.
Refrigerate unopened vials of DOXIL at 2°-8°C (36°-46°F). Avoid freezing. Prolonged freezing may adversely affect liposomal drug products; however, short-term freezing (less than 1 month) does not appear to have a deleterious effect on DOXIL.
The following packages of six individually cartoned vials are available:

Table 19

mg in vial	fill volume	vial size	NDC #s
20 mg vial	10-mL	10-mL	17314-9600-1
50 mg vial	25-mL	30-mL	17314-9600-2

17 PATIENT COUNSELING INFORMATION

Patients and patient's caregivers should be informed of the expected adverse effects of DOXIL, particularly hand-foot syndrome, stomatitis, and neutropenia and related complications of neutropenic fever, infection, and sepsis.
Hand-Foot Syndrome (HFS): Patients who experience tingling or burning, redness, flaking, bothersome swelling, small blisters, or small sores on the palms of their hands or soles of their feet (symptoms of Hand-Foot Syndrome) should notify their physician.
Stomatitis: Patients who experience painful redness, swelling, or sores in the mouth (symptoms of stomatitis) should notify their physician.
Fever and Neutropenia: Patients who develop a fever of 100.5°F or higher should notify their physician.
Nausea, vomiting, tiredness, weakness, rash, or mild hair loss: Patients who develop any of these symptoms should notify their physician.
Following its administration, DOXIL may impart a reddish-orange color to the urine and other body fluids. This nontoxic reaction is due to the color of the product and will dissipate as the drug is eliminated from the body.
0016716-5
Manufactured by:
Ben Venue Laboratories, Inc.
Bedford, OH 44146
Distributed by:
Ortho Biotech Products, LP
Raritan, NJ 08869-0670
ORTHO BIOTECH
alza™
An ALZA STEALTH®
Technology Product
STEALTH® and DOXIL® are registered trademarks of ALZA Corporation.
Shown in Product Identification Guide, page 307

LEUSTATIN®   ℞
[lew'stăt-in]
(cladribine)
Injection
For Intravenous Infusion Only

> **WARNING**
> LEUSTATIN (cladribine) Injection should be administered under the supervision of a qualified physician experienced in the use of antineoplastic therapy. Suppression of bone marrow function should be anticipated. This is usually reversible and appears to be dose dependent. Serious neurological toxicity (including irreversible paraparesis and quadraparesis) has been reported in patients who received LEUSTATIN Injection by continuous infusion at high doses (4 to 9 times the recommended dose for Hairy Cell Leukemia). Neurologic toxicity appears to demonstrate a dose relationship; however, severe neurological toxicity has been reported rarely following treatment with standard cladribine dosing regimens.
> Acute nephrotoxicity has been observed with high doses of LEUSTATIN (4 to 9 times the recommended dose for Hairy Cell Leukemia), especially when given concomitantly with other nephrotoxic agents/therapies.

DESCRIPTION

LEUSTATIN (cladribine) Injection (also commonly known as 2-chloro-2'-deoxy-β-D-adenosine) is a synthetic antineoplastic agent for continuous intravenous infusion. It is a clear, colorless, sterile, preservative-free, isotonic solution. LEUSTATIN Injection is available in single-use vials containing 10 mg (1 mg/mL) of cladribine, a chlorinated purine nucleoside analog. Each milliliter of LEUSTATIN Injection contains 1 mg of the active ingredient and 9 mg (0.15 mEq) of sodium chloride as an inactive ingredient. The solution has a pH range of 5.5 to 8.0. Phosphoric acid and/or dibasic sodium phosphate may have been added to adjust the pH to 6.3±0.3.
The chemical name for cladribine is 2-chloro-6-amino-9-(2-deoxy-β-D-erythropento-furanosyl) purine and the structure is represented below:

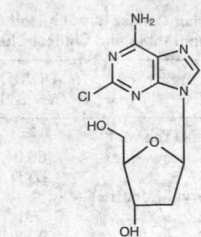

cladribine

MW 285.7

CLINICAL PHARMACOLOGY

Cellular Resistance and Sensitivity:
The selective toxicity of 2-chloro-2'-deoxy-β-D-adenosine towards certain normal and malignant lymphocyte and monocyte populations is based on the relative activities of deoxycytidine kinase and deoxynucleotidase. Cladribine passively crosses the cell membrane. In cells with a high ratio of deoxycytidine kinase to deoxynucleotidase, it is phosphorylated by deoxycytidine kinase to 2-chloro-2'-deoxy-β-D-adenosine monophosphate (2-CdAMP). Since 2-chloro-2'-deoxy-β-D-adenosine is resistant to deamination by adenosine deaminase and there is little deoxynucleotide deaminase in lymphocytes and monocytes, 2-CdAMP accumulates intracellularly and is subsequently converted into the active triphosphate deoxynucleotide, 2-chloro-2'-deoxy-β-D-adenosine triphosphate (2-CdATP). It is postulated that cells with high deoxycytidine kinase and low deoxynucleotidase activities will be selectively killed by 2-chloro-2'-deoxy-β-D-adenosine as toxic deoxynucleotides accumulate intracellularly.
Cells containing high concentrations of deoxynucleotides are unable to properly repair single-strand DNA breaks. The broken ends of DNA activate the enzyme poly (ADP-ribose) polymerase resulting in NAD and ATP depletion and disruption of cellular metabolism. There is evidence, also, that 2-CdATP is incorporated into the DNA of dividing cells, resulting in impairment of DNA synthesis. Thus, 2-chloro-2'-deoxy-β-D-adenosine can be distinguished from other chemotherapeutic agents affecting purine metabolism in that it is cytotoxic to both actively dividing and quiescent lymphocytes and monocytes, inhibiting both DNA synthesis and repair.

Pharmacokinetics
In a clinical investigation, 17 patients with Hairy Cell Leukemia and normal renal function were treated for 7 days with the recommended treatment regimen of LEUSTATIN Injection (0.09 mg/kg/day) by continuous intravenous infusion. The mean steady-state serum concentration was estimated to be 5.7 ng/mL with an estimated systemic clearance of 663.5 mL/h/kg when LEUSTATIN was given by continuous infusion over 7 days. In Hairy Cell Leukemia patients, there does not appear to be a relationship between serum concentrations and ultimate clinical outcome.
In another study, 8 patients with hematologic malignancies received a two (2) hour infusion of LEUSTATIN Injection (0.12 mg/kg). The mean end-of-infusion plasma LEUSTATIN concentration was 48±19 ng/mL. For 5 of these patients, the disappearance of LEUSTATIN could be described by either a biphasic or triphasic decline. For these patients with normal renal function, the mean terminal half-life was 5.4 hours. Mean values for clearance and steady-state volume of distribution were 978±422 mL/h/kg and 4.5±2.8 L/kg, respectively.
Cladribine plasma concentration after intravenous administration declines multi-exponentially with an average half-life of 6.7±2.5 hours. In general, the apparent volume of distribution of cladribine is approximately 9 L/kg, indicating an extensive distribution in body tissues.
Cladribine penetrates into cerebrospinal fluid. One report indicates that concentrations are approximately 25% of those in plasma.
LEUSTATIN is bound approximately 20% to plasma proteins.
Except for some understanding of the mechanism of cellular toxicity, no other information is available on the metabolism

of LEUSTATIN in humans. An average of 18% of the administered dose has been reported to be excreted in urine of patients with solid tumors during a 5-day continuous intravenous infusion of 3.5-8.1 mg/m²/day of LEUSTATIN. The effect of renal and hepatic impairment on the elimination of cladribine has not been investigated in humans.

CLINICAL STUDIES

Two single-center open label studies of LEUSTATIN (cladribine) have been conducted in patients with Hairy Cell Leukemia with evidence of active disease requiring therapy. In the study conducted at the Scripps Clinic and Research Foundation (Study A), 89 patients were treated with a single course of LEUSTATIN Injection given by continuous intravenous infusion for 7 days at a dose of 0.09 mg/kg/day. In the study conducted at the M.D. Anderson Cancer Center (Study B), 35 patients were treated with a 7-day continuous intravenous infusion of LEUSTATIN Injection at a comparable dose of 3.6 mg/m²/day. A complete response (CR) required clearing of the peripheral blood and bone marrow of hairy cells and recovery of the hemoglobin to 12 g/dL, platelet count to 100×10^9/L, and absolute neutrophil count to 1500×10^6/L. A good partial response (GPR) required the same hematologic parameters as a complete response, and that fewer than 5% hairy cells remain in the bone marrow. A partial response (PR) required that hairy cells in the bone marrow be decreased by at least 50% from baseline and the same response for hematologic parameters as for complete response. A pathologic relapse was defined as an increase in bone marrow hairy cells to 25% of pretreatment levels. A clinical relapse was defined as the recurrence of cytopenias, specifically, decreases in hemoglobin $\geq$ 2 g/dL, ANC $\geq$ 25% or platelet counts $\geq$ 50,000. Patients who met the criteria for a complete response but subsequently were found to have evidence of bone marrow hairy cells (< 25% of pretreatment levels) were reclassified as partial responses and were not considered to be complete responses with relapse.

Among patients evaluable for efficacy (N=106), using the hematologic and bone marrow response criteria described above, the complete response rates in patients treated with LEUSTATIN Injection were 65% and 68% for Study A and Study B, respectively, yielding a combined complete response rate of 66%. Overall response rates (i.e., Complete plus Good Partial plus Partial Responses) were 89% and 86% in Study A and Study B, respectively, for a combined overall response rate of 88% in evaluable patients treated with LEUSTATIN Injection.

Using an intent-to-treat analysis (N=123) and further requiring no evidence of splenomegaly as a criterion for CR (i.e., no palpable spleen on physical examination and $\leq$ 13 cm on CT scan), the complete response rates for Study A and Study B were 54% and 53%, respectively, giving a combined CR rate of 54%. The overall response rates (CR + GPR + PR) were 90% and 85%, for Studies A and B, respectively, yielding a combined overall response rate of 89%.

RESPONSE RATES TO LEUSTATIN TREATMENT IN PATIENTS WITH HAIRY CELL LEUKEMIA

	CR	Overall
Evaluable Patients N=106	66%	88%
Intent-to-treat Population N=123	54%	89%

In these studies, 60% of the patients had not received prior chemotherapy for Hairy Cell Leukemia or had undergone splenectomy as the only prior treatment and were receiving LEUSTATIN as a first-line treatment. The remaining 40% of the patients received LEUSTATIN as a second-line treatment, having been treated previously with other agents, including α-interferon and/or deoxycoformycin. The overall response rate for patients without prior chemotherapy was 92%, compared with 84% for previously treated patients. LEUSTATIN is active in previously treated patients; however, retrospective analysis suggests that the overall response rate is decreased in patients previously treated with splenectomy or deoxycoformycin and in patients refractory to α-interferon.

OVERALL RESPONSE RATES (CR + GPR + PR) TO LEUSTATIN TREATMENT IN PATIENTS WITH HAIRY CELL LEUKEMIA

	OVERALL RESPONSE (N = 123)	NR + RELAPSE
No Prior Chemotherapy	68/74 92%	6 + 4 14%
Any Prior Chemotherapy	41/49 84%	8 + 3 22%
Previous Splenectomy	32/41* 78%	9 + 1 24%
Previous Interferon	40/48 83%	8 + 3 23%
Interferon Refractory	6/11* 55%	5 + 2 64%
Previous Deoxycoformycin	3/6* 50%	3 + 1 66%

NR = No Response
*P < 0.05

After a reversible decline, normalization of peripheral blood counts (Hemoglobin >12.0 g/dL, Platelets >100 × 10⁹/L, Absolute Neutrophil Count (ANC) >1500 × 10⁶/L) was achieved by 92% of evaluable patients. The median time to normalization of peripheral counts was 9 weeks from the start of treatment (Range: 2 to 72). The median time to normalization of Platelet Count was 2 weeks, the median time to normalization of ANC was 5 weeks and the median time to normalization of Hemoglobin was 8 weeks. With normalization of Platelet Count and Hemoglobin, requirements for platelet and RBC transfusions were abolished after Months 1 and 2, respectively, in those patients with complete response. Platelet recovery may be delayed in a minority of patients with severe baseline thrombocytopenia. Corresponding to normalization of ANC, a trend toward a reduced incidence of infection was seen after the third month, when compared to the months immediately preceding LEUSTATIN therapy (see also WARNINGS, PRECAUTIONS and ADVERSE REACTIONS).

LEUSTATIN TREATMENT IN PATIENTS WITH HAIRY CELL LEUKEMIA TIME TO NORMALIZATION OF PERIPHERAL BLOOD COUNTS

Parameter	Median Time to Normalization of Count*
Platelet Count	2 weeks
Absolute Neutrophil Count	5 weeks
Hemoglobin	8 weeks
ANC, Hemoglobin and Platelet Count	9 weeks

*Day 1 = First day of infusion

For patients achieving a complete response, the median time to response (i.e., absence of hairy cells in bone marrow and peripheral blood together with normalization of peripheral blood parameters), measured from treatment start, was approximately 4 months. Since bone marrow aspiration and biopsy were frequently not performed at the time of peripheral blood normalization, the median time to complete response may actually be shorter than that which was recorded. At the time of data cut-off, the median duration of complete response was greater than 8 months and ranged to 25+ months. Among 93 responding patients, seven had shown evidence of disease progression at the time of the data cut-off. In four of these patients, disease was limited to the bone marrow without peripheral blood abnormalities (pathologic progression), while in three patients there were also peripheral blood abnormalities (clinical progression). Seven patients who did not respond to a first course of LEUSTATIN received a second course of therapy. In the five patients who had adequate follow-up, additional courses did not appear to improve their overall response.

INDICATIONS FOR USE

LEUSTATIN Injection is indicated for the treatment of active Hairy Cell Leukemia as defined by clinically significant anemia, neutropenia, thrombocytopenia or disease-related symptoms.

CONTRAINDICATIONS

LEUSTATIN Injection is contraindicated in those patients who are hypersensitive to this drug or any of its components.

WARNINGS

Severe bone marrow suppression, including neutropenia, anemia and thrombocytopenia, has been commonly observed in patients treated with LEUSTATIN, especially at high doses. At initiation of treatment, most patients in the clinical studies had hematologic impairment as a manifestation of active Hairy Cell Leukemia. Following treatment with LEUSTATIN, further hematologic impairment occurred before recovery of peripheral blood counts began. During the first two weeks after treatment initiation, mean Platelet Count, ANC, and Hemoglobin concentration declined and subsequently increased with normalization of mean counts by Day 12, Week 5 and Week 8, respectively. The myelosuppressive effects of LEUSTATIN were most notable during the first month following treatment. Forty-four percent (44%) of patients received transfusions with RBCs and 14% received transfusions with platelets during Month 1. Careful hematologic monitoring, especially during the first 4 to 8 weeks after treatment with LEUSTATIN Injection, is recommended (see PRECAUTIONS).

Fever (T $\geq$ 100°F) was associated with the use of LEUSTATIN in approximately two-thirds of patients (131/196) in the first month of therapy. Virtually all of these patients were treated empirically with parenteral antibiotics. Overall, 47% (93/196) of all patients had fever in the setting of neutropenia (ANC $\leq$ 1000), including 62 patients (32%) with severe neutropenia (i.e., ANC $\leq$ 500).

In a Phase I investigational study using LEUSTATIN in high doses (4 to 9 times the recommended dose for Hairy Cell Leukemia) as part of a bone marrow transplant conditioning regimen, which also included high dose cyclophosphamide and total body irradiation, acute nephrotoxicity and delayed onset neurotoxicity were observed. Thirty-one (31) poor-risk patients with drug-resistant acute leukemia in relapse (29 cases) or non-Hodgkins Lymphoma (2 cases) received LEUSTATIN for 7 to 14 days prior to bone marrow transplantation. During infusion, 8 patients experienced gastrointestinal symptoms. While the bone marrow was initially cleared of all hematopoietic elements, including tumor cells, leukemia eventually recurred in all treated patients. Within 7 to 13 days after starting treatment with LEUSTATIN, 6 patients (19%) developed manifestations of renal dysfunction (e.g., acidosis, anuria, elevated serum creatinine, etc.) and 5 required dialysis. Several of these patients were also being treated with other medications having known nephrotoxic potential. Renal dysfunction was reversible in 2 of these patients. In the 4 patients whose renal function had not recovered at the time of death, autopsies were performed; in 2 of these, evidence of tubular damage was noted. Eleven (11) patients (35%) experienced delayed onset neurologic toxicity. In the majority, this was characterized by progressive irreversible motor weakness (paraparesis/quadriparesis) of the upper and/or lower extremities, first noted 35 to 84 days after starting high dose therapy with LEUSTATIN. Non-invasive testing (electromyography and nerve conduction studies) was consistent with demyelinating disease. Severe neurologic toxicity has also been noted with high doses of another drug in this class.

Axonal peripheral polyneuropathy was observed in a dose escalation study at the highest dose levels (approximately 4 times the recommended dose for Hairy Cell Leukemia) in patients not receiving cyclophosphamide or total body irradiation. Severe neurological toxicity has been reported rarely following treatment with standard cladribine dosing regimens.

In patients with Hairy Cell Leukemia treated with the recommended treatment regimen (0.09 mg/kg/day for 7 consecutive days), there have been no reports of nephrologic toxicities.

Of the 196 Hairy Cell Leukemia patients entered in the two trials, there were 8 deaths following treatment. Of these, 6 were of infectious etiology, including 3 pneumonias, and 2 occurred in the first month following LEUSTATIN therapy. Of the 8 deaths, 6 occurred in previously treated patients who were refractory to α interferon.

Benzyl alcohol is a constituent of the recommended diluent for the 7-day infusion solution. Benzyl alcohol has been reported to be associated with a fatal "Gasping Syndrome" in premature infants (see DOSAGE AND ADMINISTRATION).

Pregnancy Category D:

LEUSTATIN Injection should not be given during pregnancy.

Cladribine is teratogenic in mice and rabbits and consequently has the potential to cause fetal harm when administered to a pregnant woman. A significant increase in fetal variations was observed in mice receiving 1.5 mg/kg/day (4.5 mg/m²) and increased resorptions, reduced litter size and increased fetal malformations were observed when mice received 3.0 mg/kg/day (9 mg/m²). Fetal death and malformations were observed in rabbits that received 3.0 mg/kg/day (33.0 mg/m²). No fetal effects were seen in mice at 0.5 mg/kg/day (1.5 mg/m²) or in rabbits at 1.0 mg/kg/day (11.0 mg/m²).

Although there is no evidence of teratogenicity in humans due to LEUSTATIN, other drugs which inhibit DNA synthesis (e.g., methotrexate and aminopterin) have been reported to be teratogenic in humans. LEUSTATIN has been shown to be embryotoxic in mice when given at doses equivalent to the recommended dose.

There are no adequate and well controlled studies in pregnant women. If LEUSTATIN is used during pregnancy, or if the patient becomes pregnant while taking this drug, the patient should be apprised of the potential hazard to the fetus. Women of childbearing age should be advised to avoid becoming pregnant.

PRECAUTIONS

General:

LEUSTATIN Injection is a potent antineoplastic agent with potentially significant toxic side effects. It should be administered only under the supervision of a physician experienced with the use of cancer chemotherapeutic agents. Patients undergoing therapy should be closely observed for signs of hematologic and non-hematologic toxicity. Periodic assessment of peripheral blood counts, particularly during the first 4 to 8 weeks post-treatment, is recommended to detect the development of anemia, neutropenia and thrombocytopenia and for early detection of any potential sequelae (e.g., infection or bleeding). As with other potent chemotherapeutic agents, monitoring of renal and hepatic function is also recommended, especially in patients with underlying kidney or liver dysfunction (see **WARNINGS** and **ADVERSE REACTIONS**).

Fever was a frequently observed side effect during the first month on study. Since the majority of fevers occurred in neutropenic patients, patients should be closely monitored during the first month of treatment and empiric antibiotics should be initiated as clinically indicated. Although 69% of patients developed fevers, less than 1/3 of febrile events were associated with documented infection. Given the known myelosuppressive effects of LEUSTATIN, practitioners should carefully evaluate the risks and benefits of administering this drug to patients with active infections (see **WARNINGS** and **ADVERSE REACTIONS**).

There are inadequate data on dosing of patients with renal or hepatic insufficiency. Development of acute renal insufficiency in some patients receiving high doses of LEUSTATIN has been described. Until more information is available, caution is advised when administering the drug to patients with known or suspected renal or hepatic insufficiency (see **WARNINGS**).

Rare cases of tumor lysis syndrome have been reported in patients treated with cladribine with other hematologic malignancies having a high tumor burden.

LEUSTATIN Injection must be diluted in designated intravenous solutions prior to administration (see **DOSAGE AND ADMINISTRATION**).

Laboratory Tests:

During and following treatment, the patient's hematologic profile should be monitored regularly to determine the degree of hematopoietic suppression. In the clinical studies, following reversible declines in all cell counts, the mean Platelet Count reached 100×10^9/L by Day 12, the mean Absolute Neutrophil Count reached 1500×10^6/L by Week 5 and the mean Hemoglobin reached 12 g/dL by Week 8. After peripheral counts have normalized, bone marrow aspiration and biopsy should be performed to confirm response to treatment with LEUSTATIN. Febrile events should be investigated with appropriate laboratory and radiologic studies. Periodic assessment of renal function and hepatic function should be performed as clinically indicated.

Drug Interactions:

There are no known drug interactions with LEUSTATIN Injection. Caution should be exercised if LEUSTATIN Injection is administered before, after, or in conjunction with other drugs known to cause immunosuppression or myelosuppression. (see **WARNINGS**).

Carcinogenesis:

No animal carcinogenicity studies have been conducted with cladribine. However, its carcinogenic potential cannot be excluded based on demonstrated genotoxicity of cladribine.

Mutagenesis:

As expected for compounds in this class, the actions of cladribine yield DNA damage. In mammalian cells in culture, cladribine caused the accumulation of DNA strand breaks. Cladribine was also incorporated into DNA of human lymphoblastic leukemia cells. Cladribine was not mutagenic *in vitro* (Ames and Chinese hamster ovary cell gene mutation tests) and did not induce unscheduled DNA synthesis in primary rat hepatocyte cultures. However, cladribine was clastogenic both *in vitro* (chromosome aberrations in Chinese hamster ovary cells) and *in vivo* (mouse bone marrow micronucleus test).

Impairment of Fertility:

When administered intravenously to Cynomolgus monkeys, cladribine has been shown to cause suppression of rapidly generating cells, including testicular cells. The effect on human fertility is unknown.

Pregnancy:

Pregnancy Category D: (see **WARNINGS**).

Nursing Mothers:

It is not known whether this drug is excreted in human milk. Because many drugs are excreted in human milk and because of the potential for serious adverse reactions in nursing infants from cladribine, a decision should be made whether to discontinue nursing or discontinue the drug, taking into account the importance of the drug for the mother.

Pediatric Use:

Safety and effectiveness in pediatric patients have not been established. In a Phase I study involving patients 1-21 years old with relapsed acute leukemia, LEUSTATIN was given by continuous intravenous infusion in doses ranging from 3 to 10.7 mg/m^2/day for 5 days (one-half to twice the dose recommended in Hairy Cell Leukemia). In this study, the dose-limiting toxicity was severe myelosuppression with profound neutropenia and thrombocytopenia. At the highest dose (10.7 mg/m^2/day), 3 of 7 patients developed irreversible myelosuppression and fatal systemic bacterial or fungal infections. No unique toxicities were noted in this study[1] (see **WARNINGS** and **ADVERSE REACTIONS**).

Geriatric Use:

Clinical studies of LEUSTATIN did not include sufficient numbers of subjects aged 65 and over to determine whether they respond differently from younger subjects. Other reported clinical experience has not identified differences in responses between the elderly and younger patients. In general, dose selection for an elderly patient should be cautious, reflecting the greater frequency of decreased hepatic, renal, or cardiac function, and of concomitant disease or other drug therapy in elderly patients.

ADVERSE REACTIONS

Safety data are based on 196 patients with Hairy Cell Leukemia: the original cohort of 124 patients plus an additional 72 patients enrolled at the same two centers after the original enrollment cutoff. In Month 1 of the Hairy Cell Leukemia clinical trials, severe neutropenia was noted in 70% of patients, fever in 69%, and infection was documented in 28%. Other adverse experiences reported frequently during the first 14 days after initiating treatment included: fatigue (45%), nausea (28%), rash (27%), headache (22%) and injection site reactions (19%). Most non-hematologic adverse experiences were mild to moderate in severity.

Myelosuppression was frequently observed during the first month after starting treatment. Neutropenia (ANC $< 500 \times 10^6$/L) was noted in 70% of patients, compared with 26% in whom it was present initially. Severe anemia (Hemoglobin < 8.5 g/dL) developed in 37% of patients, compared with 10% initially and thrombocytopenia (Platelets $< 20 \times 10^9$/L) developed in 12% of patients, compared to 4% in whom it was noted initially.

During the first month, 54 of 196 patients (28%) exhibited documented evidence of infection. Serious infections (e.g., septicemia, pneumonia) were reported in 6% of all patients; the remainder were mild or moderate. Several deaths were attributable to infection and/or complications related to the underlying disease. During the second month, the overall rate of documented infection was 6%; these infections were mild to moderate and no severe systemic infections were seen. After the third month, the monthly incidence of infection was either less than or equal to that of the months immediately preceding LEUSTATIN therapy.

During the first month, 11% of patients experienced severe fever (i.e., ≥104°F). Documented infections were noted in fewer than one-third of febrile episodes. Of the 196 patients studied, 19 were noted to have a documented infection in the month prior to treatment. In the month following treatment, there were 54 episodes of documented infection: 23 (42%) were bacterial, 11 (20%) were viral and 11 (20%) were fungal. Seven (7) of 8 documented episodes of herpes zoster occurred during the month following treatment. Fourteen (14) of 16 episodes of documented fungal infections occurred in the first two months following treatment. Virtually all of these patients were treated empirically with antibiotics. (see **WARNINGS** and **PRECAUTIONS**).

Analysis of lymphocyte subsets indicates that treatment with cladribine is associated with prolonged depression of the CD4 counts. Prior to treatment, the mean CD4 count was 766/μL. The mean CD4 count nadir, which occurred 4 to 6 months following treatment, was 272/μL. Fifteen (15) months after treatment, mean CD4 counts remained below 500/μL. CD8 counts behaved similarly, though increasing counts were observed after 9 months. The clinical significance of the prolonged CD4 lymphopenia is unclear.

Another event of unknown clinical significance includes the observation of prolonged bone marrow hypocellularity. Bone marrow cellularity of < 35% was noted after 4 months in 42 of 124 patients (34%) treated in the two pivotal trials. This hypocellularity was noted as late as day 1010. It is not known whether the hypocellularity is the result of disease related marrow fibrosis or if it is the result of cladribine toxicity. There was no apparent clinical effect on the peripheral blood counts.

The vast majority of rashes were mild and occurred in patients who were receiving or had recently been treated with other medications (e.g., allopurinol or antibiotics) known to cause rash.

Most episodes of nausea were mild, not accompanied by vomiting, and did not require treatment with antiemetics. In patients requiring antiemetics, nausea was easily controlled, most frequently with chlorpromazine.

Adverse reactions reported during the first 2 weeks following treatment initiation (regardless of relationship to drug) by > 5% of patients included:

Body as a Whole: fever (69%), fatigue (45%), chills (9%), asthenia (9%), diaphoresis (9%), malaise (7%), trunk pain (6%)
Gastrointestinal: nausea (28%), decreased appetite (17%), vomiting (13%), diarrhea (10%), constipation (9%), abdominal pain (6%)
Hemic/Lymphatic: purpura (10%), petechiae (8%), epistaxis (5%)
Nervous System: headache (22%), dizziness (9%), insomnia (7%)
Cardiovascular System: edema (6%), tachycardia (6%)
Respiratory System: abnormal breath sounds (11%), cough (10%), abnormal chest sounds (9%), shortness of breath (7%)
Skin/Subcutaneous Tissue: rash (27%), injection site reactions (19%), pruritis (6%), pain (6%), erythema (6%)
Musculoskeletal System: myalgia (7%), arthralgia (5%)

Adverse experiences related to intravenous administration included: injection site reactions (9%) (i.e., redness, swelling, pain), thrombosis (2%), phlebitis (2%) and a broken catheter (1%). These appear to be related to the infusion procedure and/or indwelling catheter, rather than the medication or the vehicle. From Day 15 to the last follow-up visit, the only events reported by > 5% of patients were: fatigue (11%), rash (10%), headache (7%), cough (7%), and malaise (5%).

For a description of adverse reactions associated with use of high doses in non-Hairy Cell Leukemia patients, see **WARNINGS**.

The following additional adverse events have been reported since the drug became commercially available. These adverse events have been reported primarily in patients who received multiple courses of LEUSTATIN Injection:

Hematologic: bone marrow suppression with prolonged pancytopenia, including some reports of aplastic anemia; hemolytic anemia, which was reported in patients with lymphoid malignancies, occurring within the first few weeks following treatment. Rare cases of myelodysplastic syndrome have been reported.

Hepatic: reversible, generally mild increases in bilirubin and transaminases.

Nervous System: Neurological toxicity; however, severe neurotoxicity has been reported rarely following treatment with standard cladribine dosing regimens.

Respiratory System: pulmonary interstitial infiltrates; in most cases, an infectious etiology was identified.

Skin/Subcutaneous: urticaria, hypereosinophilia. In isolated cases Stevens-Johnson and toxic epidermal necrolysis have been reported in patients who were receiving or had recently been treated with other medications (e.g., allopurinol or antibiotics) known to cause these syndromes.

Opportunistic infections have occurred in the acute phase of treatment due to the immunosuppression mediated by LEUSTATIN Injection.

OVERDOSAGE

High doses of LEUSTATIN have been associated with: irreversible neurologic toxicity (paraparesis/quadriparesis), acute nephrotoxicity, and severe bone marrow suppression resulting in neutropenia, anemia and thrombocytopenia (see **WARNINGS**). There is no known specific antidote to overdosage. Treatment of overdosage consists of discontinuation of LEUSTATIN, careful observation and appropriate supportive measures. It is not known whether the drug can be removed from the circulation by dialysis or hemofiltration.

DOSAGE AND ADMINISTRATION

Usual Dose:

The recommended dose and schedule of LEUSTATIN Injection for active Hairy Cell Leukemia is as a single course given by continuous infusion for 7 consecutive days at a dose of 0.09 mg/kg/day. Deviations from this dosage regimen are not advised. If the patient does not respond to the initial course of LEUSTATIN Injection for Hairy Cell Leukemia, it is unlikely that they will benefit from additional courses. Physicians should consider delaying or discontinuing the drug if neurotoxicity or renal toxicity occurs (see **WARNINGS**).

Specific risk factors predisposing to increased toxicity from LEUSTATIN have not been defined. In view of the known toxicities of agents of this class, it would be prudent to proceed carefully in patients with known or suspected renal insufficiency or severe bone marrow impairment of any etiology. Patients should be monitored closely for hematologic and non-hematologic toxicity (see **WARNINGS** and **PRECAUTIONS**).

Preparation and Administration of Intravenous Solutions:

LEUSTATIN Injection must be diluted with the designated diluent prior to administration. Since the drug product does not contain any anti-microbial preservative or bacteriostatic agent, **aseptic technique and proper environmental precautions must be observed in preparation of LEUSTATIN Injection solutions.**

To prepare a single daily dose:

Add the calculated dose (0.09 mg/kg or 0.09 mL/kg) of LEUSTATIN Injection to an infusion bag containing 500 mL of 0.9% Sodium Chloride Injection, USP. Infuse continuously over 24 hours. Repeat daily for a total of 7 consecutive days. **The use of 5% dextrose as a diluent is not recommended because of increased degradation of cladribine.** Admixtures of LEUSTATIN Injection are chemically and physically stable for at least 24 hours at room temperature under normal room fluorescent light in Baxter Viaflex®† PVC infusion containers. **Since limited compatibility data are available, adherence to the recommended diluents and infusion systems is advised.**

	Dose of LEUSTATIN Injection	Recommended Diluent	Quantity of Diluent
24-hour infusion method	1 (day) × 0.09 mg/kg	0.9% Sodium Chloride Injection, USP	500 mL

To prepare a 7-day infusion:

The 7-day infusion solution should only be prepared with Bacteriostatic 0.9% Sodium Chloride Injection, USP (0.9% benzyl alcohol preserved). In order to minimize the risk of microbial contamination, both LEUSTATIN Injection and the diluent should be passed through a sterile 0.22µ disposable hydrophilic syringe filter as each solution is being introduced into the infusion reservoir. First add the calculated dose of LEUSTATIN Injection (7 days × 0.09 mg/kg or mL/kg) to the infusion reservoir through the sterile filter. Then add a calculated amount of Bacteriostatic 0.9% Sodium Chloride Injection, USP (0.9% benzyl alcohol preserved) also through the filter to bring the total volume of the solution to 100 mL. After completing solution preparation, clamp off the line, disconnect and discard the filter. Aseptically aspirate air bubbles from the reservoir as necessary using the syringe and a dry second sterile filter or a sterile vent filter assembly. Reclamp the line and discard the syringe and filter assembly. Infuse continuously over 7 days. Solutions prepared with Bacteriostatic Sodium Chloride Injection for individuals weighing more than 85 kg may have reduced preservative effectiveness due to greater dilution of the benzyl alcohol preservative. Admixtures for the 7-day infusion have demonstrated acceptable chemical and physical stability for at least 7 days in the SIMS Deltec MEDICATION CASSETTE™ Reservoir‡.

	Dose of LEUSTATIN Injection	Recommended Diluent	Quantity of Diluent
7-day infusion method (use sterile 0.22µ filter when preparing infusion solution)	7 (days) × 0.09 mg/kg	Bacteriostatic 0.9% Sodium Chloride Injection, USP (0.9% benzyl alcohol)	q.s. to 100 mL

Since limited compatibility data are available, adherence to the recommended diluents and infusion systems is advised. Solutions containing LEUSTATIN Injection should not be mixed with other intravenous drugs or additives or infused simultaneously via a common intravenous line, since compatibility testing has not been performed. Preparations containing benzyl alcohol should not be used in neonates (see **WARNINGS**).

Care must be taken to assure the sterility of prepared solutions. Once diluted, solutions of LEUSTATIN Injection should be administered promptly or stored in the refrigerator (2° to 8° C) for no more than 8 hours prior to start of administration. Vials of LEUSTATIN Injection are for single-use only. Any unused portion should be discarded in an appropriate manner (see Handling and Disposal).

Parenteral drug products should be inspected visually for particulate matter and discoloration prior to administration, whenever solution and container permit. A precipitate may occur during the exposure of LEUSTATIN Injection to low temperatures; it may be resolubilized by allowing the solution to warm naturally to room temperature and by shaking vigorously. **DO NOT HEAT OR MICROWAVE.**

Chemical Stability of Vials:

When stored in refrigerated conditions between 2° to 8°C (36° to 46°F) protected from light, unopened vials of LEUSTATIN Injection are stable until the expiration date indicated on the package. Freezing does not adversely affect the solution. If freezing occurs, thaw naturally to room temperature. DO NOT heat or microwave. Once thawed, the

vial of LEUSTATIN Injection is stable until expiry if refrigerated. DO NOT refreeze. Once diluted, solutions containing LEUSTATIN Injection should be administered promptly or stored in the refrigerator (2° to 8°C) for no more than 8 hours prior to administration.

Handling and Disposal:

The potential hazards associated with cytotoxic agents are well established and proper precautions should be taken when handling, preparing, and administering LEUSTATIN Injection. The use of disposable gloves and protective garments is recommended. If LEUSTATIN Injection contacts the skin or mucous membranes, wash the involved surface immediately with copious amounts of water. Several guidelines on this subject have been published.[2-8] There is no general agreement that all of the procedures recommended in the guidelines are necessary or appropriate. Refer to your Institution's guidelines and all applicable state/local regulations for disposal of cytotoxic waste.

HOW SUPPLIED

LEUSTATIN Injection is supplied as a sterile, preservative-free, isotonic solution containing 10 mg (1 mg/mL) of cladribine as 10 mL filled into a single-use clear flint glass 20 mL vial. LEUSTATIN Injection is supplied in 10 mL (1 mg/mL) single-use vials (NDC 59676-201-01) available in a treatment set (case) of seven vials.

Store refrigerated 2° to 8°C (36° to 46°F). Protect from light during storage.

REFERENCES:

1. Santana VM, Mirro J, Harwood FC, et al: A phase I clinical trial of 2-Chloro-deoxyadenosine in pediatric patients with acute leukemia. J. Clin. Onc., 9: 416 (1991).
2. Recommendations for the Safe Handling of Parenteral Antineoplastic Drugs. NIH Publication No. 83-2621. For sale by the Superintendent of Documents, U. S. Government Printing Office, Washington, D. C. 20402.
3. AMA Council Report. Guidelines for Handling Parenteral Antineoplastics, JAMA, March 15 (1985).
4. National Study Commission on Cytotoxic Exposure–Recommendations for Handling Cytotoxic Agents. Available from Louis P. Jeffrey, Sc.D., Chairman, National Study Commission on Cytotoxic Exposure, Massachusetts College of Pharmacy and Allied Health Sciences, 179 Longwood Avenue, Boston, Massachusetts 02115.
5. Clinical Oncological Society of Australia: Guidelines and Recommendations for Safe Handling of Antineoplastic Agents, Med. J. Australia 1:425 (1983).
6. Jones RB, et al. Safe Handling of Chemotherapeutic Agents: A Report from the Mount Sinai Medical Center. Ca—A Cancer Journal for Clinicians Sept/Oct. 258-263 (1983).
7. American Society of Hospital Pharmacists Technical Assistance Bulletin on Handling Cytotoxic Drugs in Hospitals. Am. J. Hosp. Pharm., 42:131 (1985).
8. OSHA Work-Practice Guidelines for Personnel Dealing with Cytotoxic (antineoplastic) Drugs. Am. J. Hosp. Pharm., 43:1193 (1986).
† Viaflex® containers, manufactured by Baxter Healthcare Corporation - Code No. 2B8013 (tested in 1991)
‡ MEDICATION CASSETTE™ Reservoir, manufactured by SIMS Deltec, Inc. - Reorder No. 602100A (tested in 1991)

Ortho Biotech Products, L.P.   10259601
Raritan, NJ 08869   Revised August 2007

ORTHOCLONE OKT®3 Sterile Solution   ℞
[or'tho-klon]
(muromonab-CD3)
For Intravenous Use Only

WARNING:

Only physicians experienced in immunosuppressive therapy and management of solid organ transplant patients should use ORTHOCLONE OKT3 (muromonab-CD3). Patients treated with ORTHOCLONE OKT3 must be managed in a facility equipped and staffed for cardiopulmonary resuscitation and where the patient can be closely monitored for an appropriate period based on his or her health status.

Anaphylactic and anaphylactoid reactions may occur following administration of any dose or course of ORTHOCLONE OKT3. In addition, serious, occasionally life-threatening or lethal, systemic, cardiovascular, and central nervous system reactions have been reported following administration of ORTHOCLONE OKT3. These have included: pulmonary edema, especially in patients with volume overload; shock, cardiovascular collapse, cardiac or respiratory arrest, seizures, coma, cerebral edema, cerebral herniation, blindness, and paralysis. Fluid status should be carefully monitored prior to and during ORTHOCLONE OKT3 administration. Pretreatment with methylprednisolone is recommended to minimize symptoms of Cy-

tokine Release Syndrome. (See: WARNINGS: Cytokine Release Syndrome, Central Nervous System Events, Anaphylactic Reactions; DOSAGE AND ADMINISTRATION.)

DESCRIPTION

ORTHOCLONE OKT3 (muromonab-CD3) Sterile Solution is a murine monoclonal antibody to the CD3 antigen of human T cells which functions as an immunosuppressant. It is for intravenous use only. The antibody is a biochemically purified IgG$_{2a}$ immunoglobulin with a heavy chain of approximately 50,000 daltons and a light chain of approximately 25,000 daltons. It is directed to a glycoprotein with a molecular weight of 20,000 in the human T cell surface which is essential for T cell functions. Because it is a monoclonal antibody preparation, ORTHOCLONE OKT3 Sterile Solution is a homogeneous, reproducible antibody product with consistent, measurable reactivity to human T cells. Each 5 mL ampule of ORTHOCLONE OKT3 Sterile Solution contains 5 mg (1 mg/mL) of muromonab-CD3 in a clear colorless solution which may contain a few fine translucent protein particles. Each ampule contains a buffered solution (pH 7.0 ± 0.5) of monobasic sodium phosphate (2.25 mg), dibasic sodium phosphate (9.0 mg), sodium chloride (43 mg), and polysorbate 80 (1.0 mg) in water for injection. The proper name, muromonab-CD3, is derived from the descriptive term murine monoclonal antibody. The CD3 designation identifies the specificity of the antibody as the Cell Differentiation (CD) cluster 3 defined by the First International Workshop on Human Leukocyte Differentiation Antigens.

CLINICAL PHARMACOLOGY

ORTHOCLONE OKT3 reverses graft rejection, probably by blocking the function of T cells which play a major role in acute allograft rejection. ORTHOCLONE OKT3 reacts with and blocks the function of a 20,000 dalton molecule (CD3) in the membrane of human T cells that has been associated in vitro with the antigen recognition structure of T cells and is essential for signal transduction. In in vitro cytolytic assays, ORTHOCLONE OKT3 blocks both the generation and function of effector cells. Binding of ORTHOCLONE OKT3 to T lymphocytes results in early activation of T cells, which leads to cytokine release, followed by blocking T cell functions. After termination of ORTHOCLONE OKT3 therapy, T cell function usually returns to normal within one week. In vivo, ORTHOCLONE OKT3 reacts with most peripheral blood T cells and T cells in body tissues, but has not been found to react with other hematopoietic elements or other tissues of the body.

A rapid and concomitant decrease in the number of circulating CD3 positive cells, including those that are CD2, CD4, or CD8 positive has been observed in patients studied within minutes after the administration of ORTHOCLONE OKT3. This decrease in the number of CD3 positive T cells results from the specific interaction between ORTHOCLONE OKT3 and the CD3 antigen on the surface of all T lymphocytes. T cell activation results in the release of numerous cytokines/lymphokines, which are felt to be responsible for many of the acute clinical manifestations seen following ORTHOCLONE OKT3 administration. (See: WARNINGS: Cytokine Release Syndrome, Central Nervous System Events.)

While CD3 positive cells are not detectable between days two and seven, increasing numbers of circulating CD2, CD4, and CD8 positive cells have been observed. The presence of these CD2, CD4, and CD8 positive cells has not been shown to affect reversal of rejection. After termination of ORTHOCLONE OKT3 therapy, CD3 positive cells reappear rapidly and reach pre-treatment levels within a week. In some patients however, increasing numbers of CD3 positive cells have been observed prior to termination of ORTHOCLONE OKT3 therapy. This reappearance of CD3 positive cells has been attributed to the development of neutralizing antibodies to ORTHOCLONE OKT3, which in turn block its ability to bind to the CD3 antigen on T lymphocytes. (See: PRECAUTIONS: Sensitization.)

Pediatric patients are known to have higher CD3 lymphocyte counts than adults. Pediatric patients receiving ORTHOCLONE OKT®3 therapy often require progressively higher doses of ORTHOCLONE OKT3 to achieve depletion of CD3 positive cells (<25 cells/mm^3) and ensure therapeutic ORTHOCLONE OKT3 serum concentrations (>800 ng/mL). (See: DOSAGE AND ADMINISTRATION; PRECAUTIONS: Laboratory Tests.)

Serum levels of ORTHOCLONE OKT3 are measurable using an enzyme-linked immunosorbent assay (ELISA). During the initial clinical trials in renal allograft rejection, in patients treated with 5 mg per day for 14 days, mean serum trough levels of the drug rose over the first three days and then averaged 900 ng/mL on days 3 to 14. Serum concentrations measured daily during treatment with ORTHOCLONE OKT3 in renal, hepatic, and cardiac allograft recipients revealed that pediatric patients less than 10 years of age have higher levels than patients 10-50 years of age. Subsequent clinical experience has demonstrated that serum levels greater than or equal to 800 ng/mL of ORTHOCLONE OKT3 blocks the function of cytotoxic T cells *in vitro* and *in vivo*. Reduced T cell clearance or low plasma ORTHOCLONE OKT3 levels provide a basis for adjusting ORTHOCLONE OKT3 dosage or for discontinuing therapy. (See: WARNINGS: Anaphylactic Reactions; PRECAUTIONS: Laboratory Tests; ADVERSE EVENTS: Hypersensitivity Reactions; DOSAGE AND ADMINISTRATION.) Following administration of ORTHOCLONE OKT3 *in vivo*, leukocytes have been observed in cerebrospinal and peritoneal fluids. The mechanism for this effect is not completely understood, but probably is related to cytokines altering membrane permeability, rather than an active inflammatory process. (See: WARNINGS: Cytokine Release Syndrome, Central Nervous System Events.)

CLINICAL STUDIES

Acute Renal Rejection:

In a controlled randomized clinical trial, ORTHOCLONE OKT3 was compared with conventional high-dose steroid therapy in reversing acute renal allograft rejection. In this trial, 122 evaluable patients undergoing acute rejection of cadaveric renal transplants were treated either with ORTHOCLONE OKT3 daily for a mean of 14 days, with concomitant lowering of the dosage of azathioprine and maintenance steroids (62 patients), or with conventional high-dose steroids (60 patients). ORTHOCLONE OKT3 reversed 94% of the rejections compared to a 75% reversal rate obtained with conventional high-dose steroid treatment (p=0.006). The one year Kaplan-Meier (actuarial) estimates of graft survival rates for these patients who had acute rejection were 62% and 45% for ORTHOCLONE OKT3 and steroid-treated patients, respectively (p=0.04). At two years the rates were 56% and 42%, respectively (p=0.06).

One- and two-year patient survivals were not significantly different between the two groups, being 85% and 75% for ORTHOCLONE OKT3 treated patients and 90% and 85% for steroid-treated patients.

In additional open clinical trials, the observed rate of reversal of acute renal allograft rejection was 92% (n=126) for ORTHOCLONE OKT3 therapy. ORTHOCLONE OKT3 was also effective in reversing acute renal allograft rejections in 65% (n=225) of cases where steroids and lymphocyte immune globulin preparations were contraindicated or were not successful.

The effectiveness of ORTHOCLONE OKT3 for prophylaxis of renal allograft rejection has not been established.

Acute Cardiac or Hepatic Allograft Rejection:

ORTHOCLONE OKT3 was studied for use in reversing acute cardiac and hepatic allograft rejection in patients who are unresponsive to high-doses of steroids. The rate of reversal in acute cardiac allograft rejection was 90% (n=61) and was 83% for hepatic allograft rejection (n=124) in patients unresponsive to treatment with steroids.

Controlled randomized trials have not been conducted to evaluate the effectiveness of ORTHOCLONE OKT3 compared to conventional therapy as first line treatment for acute cardiac and hepatic allograft rejection.

INDICATIONS AND USAGE

ORTHOCLONE OKT3 is indicated for the treatment of acute allograft rejection in renal transplant patients.

ORTHOCLONE OKT3 is indicated for the treatment of steroid-resistant acute allograft rejection in cardiac and hepatic transplant patients.

The dosage of other immunosuppressive agents used in conjunction with ORTHOCLONE OKT3 should be reduced to the lowest level compatible with an effective therapeutic response. (See: WARNINGS and ADVERSE EVENTS: Infections, Neoplasia; DOSAGE AND ADMINISTRATION.)

CONTRAINDICATIONS

ORTHOCLONE OKT3 should not be given to patients who:
- are hypersensitive to this or any other product of murine origin;
- have anti-mouse antibody titers ≥1:1000;
- are in (uncompensated) heart failure or in fluid overload, as evidenced by chest X-ray or a greater than 3 percent weight gain within the week prior to planned ORTHOCLONE OKT3 administration;
- have uncontrolled hypertension;
- have a history of seizures, or are predisposed to seizures;
- are determined or suspected to be pregnant, or who are breast-feeding. (See: PRECAUTIONS: Pregnancy Nursing Mothers.)

WARNINGS

SEE BOXED WARNING

Cytokine Release Syndrome

Most patients develop an acute clinical syndrome [i.e., Cytokine Release Syndrome (CRS)] that has been attributed to the release of cytokines by activated lymphocytes or monocytes and is temporally associated with the administration of the first few doses of ORTHOCLONE OKT®3 (particularly, the first two to three doses). This clinical syndrome has ranged from a more frequently reported mild, self-limited, "flu-like" illness to a less frequently reported severe, life-threatening shock-like reaction, which may include serious cardiovascular and central nervous system manifestations. The syndrome typically begins approximately 30 to 60 minutes after administration of a dose of ORTHOCLONE OKT3 (but may occur later) and may persist for several hours. The frequency and severity of this symptom complex is usually greatest with the first dose. With each successive dose of ORTHOCLONE OKT3, both the frequency and severity of the Cytokine Release Syndrome tends to diminish. Increasing the amount of ORTHOCLONE OKT3 or resuming treatment after a hiatus may result in a reappearance of the CRS.

Common clinical manifestations of CRS may include: high fever (often spiking, up to 107°F), chills/rigors, headache, tremor, nausea/vomiting, diarrhea, abdominal pain, malaise, muscle/joint aches and pains, and generalized weakness. Less frequently reported adverse experiences include: minor dermatologic reactions (e.g., rash, pruritus, etc.) and a spectrum of often serious, occasionally fatal, cardiorespiratory and central nervous system adverse experiences. Cardiorespiratory findings may include: dyspnea, shortness of breath, bronchospasm/wheezing, tachypnea, respiratory arrest/failure/distress, cardiovascular collapse, cardiac arrest, angina/myocardial infarction, chest pain/tightness, tachycardia (including ventricular), hypertension, hemodynamic instability, hypotension including profound shock, heart failure, pulmonary edema (cardiogenic and noncardiogenic), adult respiratory distress syndrome, hypoxemia, apnea, and arrhythmias. (See: BOXED WARNING; PRECAUTIONS; ADVERSE EVENTS.)

In the initial studies of renal allograft rejection, potentially fatal, severe pulmonary edema occurred in 5% of the initial 107 patients. Fluid overload was present before treatment in all of these cases. It occurred in none of the subsequent 311 patients treated with first-dose volume/weight restrictions. In subsequent trials and in post-marketing experience, severe pulmonary edema has occurred in patients who appeared to be euvolemic. The pathogenesis of pulmonary edema may involve all or some of the following: volume overload; increased pulmonary vascular permeability; and/or reduced left ventricular compliance/contractility. During the first 1 to 3 days of ORTHOCLONE OKT3 therapy, some patients have experienced an acute and transient decline in the glomerular filtration rate (GFR) and diminished urine output with a resulting increase in the level of serum creatinine. Massive release of cytokines appears to lead to reversible renal functional impairment and/or delayed renal allograft function. Similarly, transient elevations in hepatic transaminases have been reported following administration of the first few doses of ORTHOCLONE OKT3.

Patients at risk for more serious complications of CRS may include those with the following conditions: unstable angina; recent myocardial infarction or symptomatic ischemic heart disease; heart failure of any etiology; pulmonary edema of any etiology; any form of chronic obstructive pulmonary disease; intravascular volume overload or depletion of any etiology (e.g., excessive dialysis, recent intensive diuresis, blood loss, etc.); cerebrovascular disease; patients with advanced symptomatic vascular disease or neuropathy; a history of seizures; and septic shock. Efforts should be made to correct or stabilize background conditions prior to the initiation of therapy. (See: PRECAUTIONS.)

Prior to administration of ORTHOCLONE OKT3, the patient's volume (fluid) status and a chest X-ray should be assessed to rule out volume overload, uncontrolled hypertension, or uncompensated heart failure. Patients should not weigh >3% above their minimum weight during the week prior to injection.

The Cytokine Release Syndrome is associated with increased serum levels of cytokines (e.g., TNF-α, IL-2, IL-6, IFN-γ) that peak between 1 and 4 hours following administration of ORTHOCLONE OKT3. The serum levels of cytokines and the manifestations of CRS may be reduced by pretreatment with 8 mg/kg of methylprednisolone (i.e., high-dose steroids), given 1 to 4 hours prior to administration of the first dose of ORTHOCLONE OKT3, and by closely following recommendations for dosage and treatment duration. (See: DOSAGE AND ADMINISTRATION.) It is not known if corticosteroid pretreatment decreases organ damage and sequelae associated with CRS. For example, increased intracranial pressure and cerebral herniation have occurred despite pretreatment with currently recommended doses and schedules of methylprednisolone.

If any of the more serious presentations of the Cytokine Release Syndrome occur, intensive treatment including oxygen, intravenous fluids, corticosteroids, pressor amines, antihistamines, intubation, etc., may be required.

Central Nervous System Events

Seizures, encephalopathy, cerebral edema, aseptic meningitis, and headache have been reported, even following the first dose, during therapy with ORTHOCLONE OKT®3. Seizures, some accompanied by loss of consciousness or cardiorespiratory arrest, or death, have occurred independently or in conjunction with any of the neurologic syndromes described below.

A few cases of fatal cerebral herniations subsequent to cerebral edema have been reported. All patients, particularly pediatric patients, must be carefully evaluated for fluid retention and hypertension before the initiation of ORTHOCLONE OKT3 therapy. Close monitoring for neurologic symptoms must be performed during the first twenty-four (24) hours following each of the first few doses of ORTHOCLONE OKT3 injection.

Patients should be closely monitored for convulsions and manifestations of encephalopathy, including: impaired cognition, confusion, obtundation, altered mental status, disorientation, auditory/visual hallucinations, psychosis (delirium, paranoia), mood changes (e.g., mania, agitation, combativeness, etc.), diffuse hypotonus, hyperreflexia, myoclonus, tremor, asterixis, involuntary movements, major motor seizures, lethargy/stupor/coma, and diffuse weakness. Approximately one-third of patients with a diagnosis of encephalopathy may have had coexisting aseptic meningitis syndrome.

Signs and symptoms of the aseptic meningitis syndrome described in association with the use of ORTHOCLONE OKT3 have included: fever, headache, meningismus (stiff neck), and photophobia. Diagnosis is confirmed by cerebrospinal fluid (CSF) analysis demonstrating leukocytosis with pleocytosis, elevated protein and normal or decreased glucose, with negative viral, bacterial, and fungal cultures. The possibility of infection should be evaluated in any immunosuppressed transplant patient with clinical findings suggesting meningitis. Approximately one-third of the patients with a diagnosis of aseptic meningitis had coexisting signs and symptoms of encephalopathy. Most patients with the aseptic meningitis syndrome had a benign course and recovered without any permanent sequelae during therapy or subsequent to its completion or discontinuation. However, because meningitis is a frequent infection encountered in pediatric allograft recipients, and the immunosuppression associated with transplantation increases the risk of opportunistic infection, pediatric patients with signs or symptoms suggestive of meningeal irritation while receiving ORTHOCLONE OKT3 should have lumbar punctures performed to rule out an infectious etiology. (See: PRECAUTIONS: Pediatric Use.)

Signs or symptoms of encephalopathy, meningitis, seizures, and cerebral edema, with or without headache, typically have been reversible. Headache, aseptic meningitis, seizures, and less severe forms of encephalopathy resolved in most patients despite continued treatment with ORTHOCLONE OKT3. However, some events resulted in permanent neurologic impairment.

The following additional central nervous system events have each been reported: irreversible blindness, impaired vision, quadri- or paraparesis/plegia, cerebrovascular accident (hemiparesis/plegia), aphasia, transient ischemic attack, subarachnoid hemorrhage, palsy of the VI cranial nerve, hearing decrease, and deafness.

Patients who may be at greater risk for CNS adverse experiences include those: with known or suspected CNS disorders (e.g., history of seizure disorder, etc.); with cerebrovascular disease (small or large vessel); with conditions having associated neurologic problems (e.g., head trauma, uremia, infection, fluid and electrolyte disturbance, etc.); with underlying vascular diseases; or who are receiving a medication concomitantly that may, by itself, affect the central nervous system. (See: WARNINGS, PRECAUTIONS and ADVERSE EVENTS: Cytokine Release Syndrome.)

Anaphylactic Reactions

Serious and occasionally fatal, immediate (usually within 10 minutes) hypersensitivity (anaphylactic) reactions have been reported in patients treated with ORTHOCLONE OKT3. **Manifestations of anaphylaxis may appear similar to manifestations of the Cytokine Release Syndrome (described above). It may be impossible to determine the mechanism responsible for any systemic reaction(s).** Reactions attributed to hypersensitivity have been reported less frequently than those attributed to cytokine release. Acute hypersensitivity reactions may be characterized by: cardiovascular collapse, cardiorespiratory arrest, loss of consciousness, hypotension/shock, tachycardia, tingling, angioedema (including laryngeal, pharyngeal, or facial edema), airway obstruction, bronchospasm, dyspnea, urticaria, and pruritus.

Serious allergic events, including anaphylactic or anaphylactoid reactions, have been reported in patients re-exposed to ORTHOCLONE OKT3 subsequent to their initial course of therapy. Pretreatment with antihistamines and/or steroids may not reliably prevent anaphylaxis in this setting. Possible allergic hazards of retreatment should be weighed against expected therapeutic benefits and alternatives. If a patient is retreated with

ORTHOCLONE OKT3, it is particularly important that epinephrine and other emergency life-support equipment should be immediately available.

If hypersensitivity is suspected, discontinue the drug immediately; do not resume therapy or re-expose the patient to ORTHOCLONE OKT3. Serious acute hypersensitivity reactions may require emergency treatment with 0.3 mL to 0.5 mL aqueous epinephrine (1:1000 dilution) subcutaneously and other resuscitative measures including oxygen, intravenous fluids, antihistamines, corticosteroids, pressor amines, and airway management, as clinically indicated. (See: PRECAUTIONS: Cytokine Release Syndrome vs. anaphylactic Reactions; ADVERSE EVENTS: Hypersensitivity Reactions.)

Consequences of Immunosuppression

Serious and sometimes fatal infections and neoplasias have been reported in association with all immunosuppressive therapies, including those regimens containing ORTHOCLONE OKT®3.

Infections: ORTHOCLONE OKT3 is usually added to immunosuppressive therapeutic regimens, thereby augmenting the degree of immunosuppression. This increase in the total amount of immunosuppression may alter the spectrum of infections observed and increase the risk, the severity, and the morbidity of infectious complications. During the first month post-transplant, patients are at greatest risk for the following infections: (1) those present prior to transplant, perhaps exacerbated by post-transplant immunosuppression; (2) infection conveyed by the donor organ; and (3) the usual post-operative urinary tract, intravenous line related, wound, or pulmonary infections due to bacterial pathogens. (See: ADVERSE EVENTS: Infections.)

Approximately one to six months post-transplant, patients are at risk for viral infections [e.g., cytomegalovirus (CMV), Epstein-Barr virus (EBV), herpes simplex virus (HSV), etc.] which produce serious systemic disease and which also increase the overall state of immunosuppression.

Reactivation (1 to 4 months post-transplant) of EBV and CMV has been reported. When administration of an antilymphocyte antibody, including ORTHOCLONE OKT3, is followed by an immunosuppressive regimen including cyclosporine, there is an increased risk of reactivating CMV and impaired ability to limit its proliferation, resulting in symptomatic and disseminated disease. EBV infection, either primary or reactivated, may play an important role in the development of post-transplant lymphoproliferative disorders. (See: WARNINGS and ADVERSE EVENTS: Neoplasia.)

In the pediatric transplant population, viral infections often include pathogens uncommon in adults, such as varicella zoster virus (VZV), adenovirus, and respiratory syncytial virus (RSV). A large proportion of pediatric patients have not been infected with the herpes viruses prior to transplantation and, therefore, are susceptible to developing primary infections from the grafted organ and/or blood products.

Geriatric patients may have a reduced capability to overcome infections during intense immunosuppression. There is no information on the use of OKT3 in geriatric patients. In an age-stratification analysis, no overall difference in the safety of OKT3 was noted between older (51 to 64 years) and younger (≤30 years) patients. Caution should be used when prescribing immunosuppressive agents to elderly patients. Anti-infective prophylaxis may reduce the morbidity associated with certain potential pathogens and should be considered for pediatric and other high-risk patients. Judicious use of immunosuppressive drugs, including type, dosage, and duration, may limit the risk and seriousness of some opportunistic infections. It is also possible to reduce the risk of serious CMV or EBV infection by avoiding transplantation of a CMV-seropositive (donor) and/or EBV-seropositive (donor) organ into a seronegative patient.

Neoplasia: As a result of depressed cell-mediated immunity from immunosuppressive agents, organ transplant patients have an increased risk of developing malignancies. This risk is evidenced almost exclusively by the occurrence of lymphoproliferative disorders, squamous cell carcinomas of the skin and lip, and sarcomas. In immunosuppressed patients, T cell cytotoxicity is impaired allowing for transformation and proliferation of EBV-infected B lymphocytes. Transformed B lymphocytes are thought to initiate oncogenesis, which ultimately culminates in the development of most post-transplant lymphoproliferative disorders. Patients, especially pediatric patients, with primary EBV infection may be at a higher risk for the development of EBV-associated lymphoproliferative disorders. Data support an association between the development of lymphoproliferative disorders at the time of active EBV infection and ORTHOCLONE OKT3 administration in pediatric liver allograft recipients. (See: ADVERSE EVENTS, Infections, Neoplasia.)

Following the initiation of ORTHOCLONE OKT3 therapy, patients should be continuously monitored for evidence of lymphoproliferative disorders through physical examination and histological evaluation of any suspect lymphoid tissue. Close surveillance is advised, since early detection with subsequent reduction of total immunosuppression may result in regression of some of these lymphoproliferative disorders. Since the potential for the development of lymphoproliferative disorders is related to the duration and extent (intensity) of total immunosuppression, physicians are advised: to adhere to the recommended dosage and duration of ORTHOCLONE OKT3 therapy; to limit the number of courses of ORTHOCLONE OKT3 and other anti- T lymphocyte antibody preparations administered within a short period of time; and, if appropriate, to reduce the dosage(s) of immunosuppressive drugs used concomitantly to the lowest level compatible with an effective therapeutic response. (See: DOSAGE AND ADMINISTRATION.)

A recent study examined the incidence of non-Hodgkin's lymphoma (NHL) among 45,000 kidney transplant recipients and over 7,500 heart transplant recipients. This study suggested that all transplant patients, regardless of the immunosuppressive regimen employed, are at increased risk of NHL over the general population. The relative risk was highest among those receiving the most aggressive regimens.

The long-term risk of neoplastic events in patients being treated with ORTHOCLONE OKT3 has not been determined.

PRECAUTIONS

General

When using combinations of immunosuppressive agents, the dose of each agent, including ORTHOCLONE OKT®3, should be reduced to the lowest level compatible with an effective therapeutic response so as to reduce the potential for and severity of infections and malignant transformations.

Fever: If the temperature of the patient exceeds 37.8°C (100°F), it should be lowered by antipyretics before administration of each dose of ORTHOCLONE OKT3. The possibility of infection should be evaluated.

Severe Cytokine Release Syndrome Versus Anaphylactic Reactions: It may not be possible to distinguish between an acute hypersensitivity reaction (e.g., anaphylaxis, angioedema, etc.) and the Cytokine Release Syndrome. Potentially serious signs and symptoms having an immediate onset (usually within 10 minutes) following administration of ORTHOCLONE OKT3 are probably due to acute hypersensitivity. If hypersensitivity is suspected, discontinue the drug immediately; do not resume therapy or re-expose the patient to ORTHOCLONE OKT3. Clinical manifestations beginning approximately 30 to 60 minutes (or later) following administration of ORTHOCLONE OKT3 are more likely cytokine-mediated. (See: WARNINGS: Cytokine Release Syndrome, Anaphylactic Reactions.)

Central Nervous System Events: Since some seizures (and other serious central nervous system events) following ORTHOCLONE OKT3 administration have been life-threatening, anti-seizure precautions (e.g., an airway ready for use, if needed) should be taken. (See: WARNINGS and ADVERSE EVENTS: Central Nervous System Events.)

Infection/Viral-Induced Lymphoproliferative Disorders: If infection or a viral induced lymphoproliferative disorder occurs, culture or biopsy as soon as possible, promptly institute appropriate anti-infective therapy, and (if possible) reduce/discontinue immunosuppressive therapy. (See: WARNINGS, ADVERSE EVENTS.)

Low Protein-Binding Filter: Use a low protein-binding 0.2 or 0.22 micrometer (μm) filter to prepare the injections. (See: ADMINISTRATION INSTRUCTIONS.)

Sensitization: ORTHOCLONE OKT3 is a mouse (immunoglobulin) protein that can induce human anti-mouse antibody production (i.e., sensitization) in some patients following exposure; a titer ≥1:1000 is a contraindication for use. (See: WARNINGS, ADVERSE EVENTS.)

In the initial clinical trials using low doses of prednisone and azathioprine during ORTHOCLONE OKT3 therapy for renal allograft rejection, antibodies to ORTHOCLONE OKT3 were observed with an incidence of 21% (n=43) for IgM, 86% (n=43) for IgG and 29% (n=35) for IgE. The mean time of appearance of IgG antibodies was 20 ± 2 days (mean $\pm$ SD). Early IgG antibodies appeared towards the end of the second week of treatment in 3% (n=86) of the patients. Subsequent clinical experience has shown that the dose, duration, and type of immunosuppressive medications used in combination with ORTHOCLONE OKT3 may affect both the incidence and magnitude of the host antibody response. Furthermore, immunosuppressive agents used concomitantly with ORTHOCLONE OKT3 (i.e., steroids, azathioprine, prednisone, or cyclosporine) have altered the time course of anti-mouse antibody development and the specificity of the antibodies formed (i.e., idiotypic, isotypic, allotypic).

Thrombosis: As with other immunosuppressive therapies, arterial, venous, and capillary thromboses of allografts and other vascular beds (e.g., heart, lungs, brain, bowel, etc.) have been reported in patients treated with ORTHOCLONE OKT3. In addition, microangiopathic changes (e.g., platelet microthrombi) in the renal allograft associated in some patients with microangiopathic hemolytic anemia have been reported. This was observed in 5 of 93 (5%) patients receiving doses above the recommended dose. The relationship to dose remains uncertain; however, the relative risk appears to be greater with doses above the recommended dose. Patients with a history of thrombosis or underlying vascular disease should be given ORTHOCLONE OKT3 only when the potential benefits clearly outweigh the increased risks of therapy.

Information for Patients:

Patients should be advised:
- of the signs and symptoms associated with the Cytokine Release Syndrome and the potentially serious nature of this syndrome (e.g., systemic, cardiovascular, central nervous system events).
- to seek medical attention for skin rash, urticaria, rapid heart beat, respiratory distress, dysphagia, or any swelling suggesting an allergic reaction or angioedema.
- that ORTHOCLONE OKT3 may impair mental alertness and coordination and may effect the ability to operate an automobile or machinery.
- of other risks associated with the use of ORTHOCLONE OKT3. (See: BOXED WARNING; WARNINGS; PRECAUTIONS; ADVERSE EVENTS.)

Laboratory Tests: The following tests should be monitored prior to and during ORTHOCLONE OKT®3 therapy:
- Renal: BUN, serum creatinine, etc.;
- Hepatic: transaminases, alkaline phosphatase, bilirubin;
- Hematopoietic: WBCs and differential, platelet count, etc.;
- Chest X-ray within 24 hours before initiating ORTHOCLONE OKT3 treatment to rule out heart failure or fluid overload.
- Blood Tests: Periodic assessment of organ system functions (renal, hepatic, and hematopoietic) should be performed.

During therapy with ORTHOCLONE OKT3: In adults, periodic monitoring to ensure plasma ORTHOCLONE OKT3 levels (≥800 ng/mL) or T cell clearance (CD3 positive T cells <25 cells/mm^3) is recommended. In pediatric patients, both plasma ORTHOCLONE OKT3 levels (≥800 ng/mL) and T cell clearance (CD3 positive T cells <25 cells/mm^3) should be monitored daily. (See: CLINICAL PHARMACOLOGY.)

Carcinogenesis: Long-term studies have not been performed in laboratory animals to evaluate the carcinogenic potential of ORTHOCLONE OKT3; however, neoplasia has been reported in patients receiving this product. (See: WARNINGS and ADVERSE EVENTS: Neoplasia.)

Pregnancy Category C: Animal reproductive studies have not been conducted with ORTHOCLONE OKT3. It is also not known whether ORTHOCLONE OKT3 can cause fetal harm when administered to a pregnant woman or can affect reproduction capacity. However, ORTHOCLONE OKT3 is an IgG antibody and may cross the human placenta. The effect on the fetus of the release of cytokines and/or immunosuppression after treatment with ORTHOCLONE OKT3 is not known. ORTHOCLONE OKT3 should be given to a pregnant woman only if clearly needed. If this drug is used during pregnancy, or the patient becomes pregnant while taking this drug, the patient should be apprised of the potential hazard to the fetus. (See: CONTRAINDICATIONS, WARNINGS, and ADVERSE EVENTS.)

Nursing Mothers: It is not known whether ORTHOCLONE OKT3 is excreted in human milk. Because many drugs are excreted in human milk and because of the potential for serious adverse events/oncogenesis shown for ORTHOCLONE OKT3 in human studies, a decision should be made to discontinue nursing or to discontinue the drug, taking into account the importance of the drug to the mother. (See: CONTRAINDICATIONS.)

Pediatric Use: Safety and effectiveness have been established in infants (1 mo. up to 2 yr.); children (2 yr. up to 12 yr.); and adolescents (12 yr. up to 16 yr.). Use of ORTHOCLONE OKT3 in these age groups is supported by clinical studies that included adults and pediatric patients. In those studies, the safety and efficacy of ORTHOCLONE OKT3 in pediatric patients receiving renal or hepatic transplants was similar to that in the overall cohort. There were insufficient data to compare the safety and efficacy of ORTHOCLONE OKT3 in pediatric patients in a study of patients receiving cardiac transplants. Additional pharmacokinetic, pharmacodynamic, and clinical studies in infants, children, and adolescents have been reported in published literature.

Pediatric patients are known to have higher CD3 lymphocyte counts than adults; therefore, progressively higher doses of ORTHOCLONE OKT3 are often required to achieve therapeutic levels of lymphocyte clearance. (See: DOSAGE AND ADMINISTRATION.)

Specific Safety Concerns in Pediatric Patients
Deaths Due to Cerebral Herniation:
The postmarketing data base indicates that pediatric patients may be at increased risk of developing cerebral

edema with or without herniation compared to adults. In the period between 1986 and 1996, twenty-five cases (6 in pediatric patients) of cerebral edema were identified with subsequent cerebral herniation and death in five cases (4 in pediatric patients). Herniation in the pediatric patients and one 19 year old subject occurred within a few hours to one day after the first dose (2.5 or 5 mg) of ORTHOCLONE OKT3 administered in the investigational setting for prophylaxis of renal allograft rejection. All pediatric patients and especially those receiving a renal allograft must be carefully evaluated for fluid retention and hypertension before the initiation of ORTHOCLONE OKT3 therapy. (See: WARNINGS: Cytokine Release Syndrome; DOSAGE AND ADMINISTRATION: General.) Patients should be closely monitored for neurologic symptoms during the first twenty four (24) hours following each of the first few doses of ORTHOCLONE OKT3 injection.

Other Serious Central Nervous System Adverse Events:
Other significant neurologic complications reported in pediatric transplant recipients receiving ORTHOCLONE OKT3 include status epilepticus, cerebral edema, diffuse encephalopathy, cerebritis, seizures, cortical dysfunction, and intracranial hemorrhage. Permanent neurologic impairments (e.g., blindness, deafness, paralysis) have been reported rarely. Because meningitis is a frequent infection encountered in pediatric allograft recipients, and the immunosuppression associated with transplantation increases the risk of opportunistic infection, patients with meningeal irritation following treatment with ORTHOCLONE OKT3 therapy should be evaluated with lumbar puncture as early as possible to rule out an infectious etiology.

Viral Infection:
The overall incidence of infections appeared to be similar in pediatric patients compared to the overall population studied. In the pediatric population, viral infections often include pathogens uncommon in adults, such as varicella zoster virus (VZV), adenovirus, enterovirus, parainfluenza virus, and respiratory syncytial virus (RSV). In addition, many viral diseases often manifest differently in pediatric patients than they do in adults. Because a large proportion of pediatric patients have not been infected by herpes viruses (e.g., EBV, HSV, CMV) prior to transplantation they may be more susceptible to acquiring primary infections from the grafted organ and/or blood products when immunosuppressed. Antiviral prophylactic therapy may be particularly useful in high risk pediatric patients. (See: ADVERSE EVENTS: Infections.)

Neoplasia:
Patients with primary EBV infection may be at higher risk for the development of EBV-associated lymphoproliferative disorders. There are data to support an association between the development of lymphoproliferative disorders at the time of active EBV infection and ORTHOCLONE OKT®3 administration in pediatric liver allograft recipients. Antiviral prophylactic therapy may be particularly useful in these high risk pediatric patients.

Gastrointestinal Fluid Losses:
Parenteral hydration may be required for gastrointestinal fluid loss secondary to diarrhea and/or vomiting resulting from the "Cytokine Release Syndrome."

Thrombosis:
Pediatric patients may be at an increased risk of thrombosis. Pediatric patients weighing less than 15 kg are at high-risk for hepatic artery thrombosis. Thrombosis has been reported in pediatric transplant recipients treated with ORTHOCLONE OKT3. A number of factors, including surgical technique, the presence of a hypercoaguable state, and the absence of prior dialysis experience may be relevant to the pathophysiology of the increased risk of thrombosis. (See: BOXED WARNING; WARNINGS; PRECAUTIONS; ADVERSE EVENTS; DOSAGE AND ADMINISTRATION.)

Geriatric Use:
There is no information on the use of OKT3 in geriatric patients. Caution should be used when prescribing immunosuppressive agents to elderly patients.

ADVERSE EVENTS

Cytokine Release Syndrome
In controlled clinical trials for treatment of acute renal allograft rejection, patients treated with ORTHOCLONE OKT3 plus concomitant low-dose immunosuppressive therapy (primarily azathioprine and corticosteroids) were observed to have an increased incidence of adverse experiences during the first two days of treatment, as compared with the group of patients receiving azathioprine and high-dose steroid therapy. During this period the majority of patients experienced pyrexia (90%), of which 19% were 40.0°C (104°F) or above, and chills (59%). In addition, other adverse experiences occurring in 8% or more of the patients during the first two days of ORTHOCLONE OKT3 therapy included: dyspnea (21%), nausea (19%), vomiting (19%), chest pain (14%), diarrhea (14%), tremor (13%), wheezing (13%), headache (11%), tachycardia (10%), rigor (8%), and hypertension (8%). A similar spectrum of clinical manifestations has been observed in open clinical studies and in post-marketing experience involving patients treated with ORTHOCLONE OKT3 for rejection following renal, cardiac, and hepatic transplantation.
Additional serious and occasionally fatal cardiorespiratory manifestations have been reported following any of the first few doses. (See: WARNINGS: Cytokine Release Syndrome; ADVERSE EVENTS: Cardiovascular, Respiratory.)
In the acute renal allograft rejection trials, potentially fatal pulmonary edema had been reported following the first two doses in less than 2% of the patients treated with ORTHOCLONE OKT3. Pulmonary edema was usually associated with fluid overload. However, post-marketing experience revealed that pulmonary edema has occurred in patients who appeared to be euvolemic, presumably as a consequence of cytokine-mediated increased vascular permeability ("leaky capillaries") and/or reduced myocardial contractility/compliance (i.e., left ventricular dysfunction). (See: WARNINGS: Cytokine Release Syndrome; DOSAGE AND ADMINISTRATION.)

Infections
In the controlled randomized renal allograft rejection trial conducted before cyclosporine was marketed, the most common infections during the first 45 days of ORTHOCLONE OKT3 therapy were due to herpes simplex virus (27%) and cytomegalovirus (19%). Other severe and life-threatening infections were *Staphylococcus epidermidis* (5%), *Pneumocystis carinii* (3%), *Legionella* (2%), *Cryptococcus* (2%), *Serratia* (2%) and gram-negative bacteria (2%). The incidence of infections was similar in patients treated with ORTHOCLONE OKT3 and in patients treated with high-dose steroids.
In a clinical trial of acute hepatic allograft rejection, refractory to conventional treatment, the most common infections reported in patients treated with ORTHOCLONE OKT3 during the first 45 days of the study were cytomegalovirus (16% of patients, of which 43% of infections were severe), fungal infections (15% of patients, of which 30% were severe), and herpes simplex virus (8% of patients, of which 10% were severe). Other severe and life-threatening infections were gram-positive infections (9% of patients), gram-negative infections (8% of patients), viral infections (2% of patients), and *Legionella* (1% of patients). In another trial studying the use of ORTHOCLONE OKT®3 in patients with hepatic allografts, the incidence of fungal infections was 34% and infections with the herpes simplex virus was 31%.
In a clinical trial studying the use of ORTHOCLONE OKT3 in patients with acute cardiac rejection refractory to conventional treatment, the most common infections in the ORTHOCLONE OKT3 group reported during the first 45 days of the study were herpes simplex virus (5% of patients, of which 20% were severe), fungal infections (4% of patients, of which 75% were severe), and cytomegalovirus (3% of patients, of which 33% were severe). No other severe or life-threatening infections were reported during this period.
In a retrospective analysis of pediatric patients treated for acute hepatic rejection, the most common infections reported in patients treated with ORTHOCLONE OKT3 therapy were due to bacterial infections (47%), fungal infections (21%), cytomegalovirus (19%), herpes simplex virus (15%), adenovirus (8%), and Epstein-Barr virus (8%). The overall rates of viral, fungal, and bacterial infections were similar in patients treated with ORTHOCLONE OKT3 (n=53) and in patients whose rejection was treated with steroids alone (n=27). In another study of 149 pediatric liver allograft patients where 59 episodes of steroid-resistant rejection were treated with ORTHOCLONE OKT3, the incidence of invasive cytomegalovirus infection was higher in patients receiving ORTHOCLONE OKT3 than in those receiving steroids alone.
Clinically significant infections (e.g., pneumonia, sepsis, etc.) due to the following pathogens have been reported:
Bacterial: Clostridiumspecies (including perfringens), Corynebacterium, Enterococcus, *Enterobacter aerogenes, Escherichia coli Klebsiella* species, *Lactobacillus, Legionella, Listeria monocytogenes, Mycobacteria* species, *Nocardia asteroides, Proteus* species, *Providencia* species, *Pseudomonas aeruginosa, Serratia* species, *Staphylococcus* species, *Streptococcus* species, *Yersinia enterocolitica,* and other gram-negative bacteria.
Fungal: Aspergillus, Candida, Cryptococcus, Dermatophytes.*
Protozoa: Pneumocystis carinii, Toxoplasma gondii.
Viral: cytomegalovirus* (CMV), Epstein-Barr virus* (EBV), herpes simplex virus* (HSV), hepatitis viruses, varicella zoster virus (VZV), adenovirus, enterovirus, respiratory syncytial virus (RSV), parainfluenza virus.
As a consequence of being a potent immunosuppressive, the incidence and severity of infections with designated(*) pathogens, especially the herpes family of viruses, may be increased. (See: WARNINGS: Infections.)

Neoplasia
In patients treated with ORTHOCLONE OKT3, post-transplant lymphoproliferative disorders have ranged from lymphadenopathy or benign polyclonal B cell hyperplasias to malignant and often fatal monoclonal B cell lymphomas. In post-marketing experience, approximately one-third of the lymphoproliferations reported were benign and two-thirds were malignant. Lymphoma types included: B cell, large cell, polyclonal, non-Hodgkin's, lymphocytic, T cell, Burkitt's. The majority were not histologically classified. Malignant lymphomas appear to develop early after transplantation, the majority within the first four months post-treatment. Many of these have been rapidly progressive. Some were fulminant, involving the allografted organ and were widely disseminated at the time of diagnosis. Carcinomas of the skin included: basal cell, squamous cell, sarcoma, melanoma, and keratoacanthoma. Other neoplasms infrequently reported include: multiple myeloma, leukemia, carcinoma of the breast, adenocarcinoma, cholangiocarcinoma, and recurrences of pre-existing hepatoma and renal cell carcinoma. (See: WARNINGS: Neoplasia.)

Hypersensitivity Reactions
Reported adverse reactions resulting from the formation of antibodies to ORTHOCLONE OKT3 have included antigen-antibody (immune complex) mediated syndromes and IgE-mediated reactions. Hypersensitivity reactions have ranged from a mild, self-limited rash or pruritus to severe, life-threatening anaphylactic reactions/shock or angioedema (including: swelling of lips, eyelids, laryngeal spasm and airway obstruction with hypoxia). (See: WARNINGS: Anaphylactic Reactions.)
Other hypersensitivity reactions have included: ineffectiveness of treatment, serum sickness, arthritis, allergic interstitial nephritis, immune complex deposition resulting in glomerulonephritis, vasculitis (including temporal and retinal), and eosinophilia.

Adverse Reactions by Body System
Adverse events reported in greater than or equal to 1% of clinical trial patients treated with ORTHOCLONE OKT3 (n=393) are shown in Table 1:

Table 1: Adverse Events Reported in Clinical Trials (≥1% incidence, n=393)

Body System	Incidence (%)
Autonomic Nervous System Disorders	
Diaphoresis	7
Vasodilation	7
Body as a Whole, General Disorders	
Anorexia	4
Asthenia	10
Chills	43
Fatigue	9
Lethargy	6
Malaise	5
Pain, trunk	6
Pyrexia	77
Cardiovascular Disorders, General	
Arrhythmia	4
Bradycardia	4
Hypertension	19
Hypotension	25
Pain, chest	9
Tachycardia	26
Vascular Occlusion	2
Central & Peripheral Nervous System Disorders	
Convulsions	1
Dizziness	6
Headache	28
Meningitis	1
Tremor	14
Gastrointestinal System Disorders	
Diarrhea	37
Nausea	32
Pain, abdominal	6
Pain, GI	7
Vomiting	25
Hematopoietic Disorders	
Anemia	2
Leukocytosis	1
Thrombocytopenia	2
Metabolic and Nutritional Disorders	
Edema	12
Musculoskeletal System Disorders	
Arthralgia	7
Myalgia	1
Psychiatric Disorders	
Confusion	6
Depression	3
Nervousness	5
Somnolence	2
Renal Disorders	
Renal Dysfunction	3
Respiratory System Disorders	
Abnormal Chest Sound	10

Dyspnea	16
Hyperventilation	7
Hypoxia	1
Pneumonia	1
Pulmonary Edema	2
Respiratory Congestion	4
Wheezing	6
Skin and Appendages Disorders	
Pruritus	7
Rash	14
Rash Erythematous	2
Special Senses	
Photophobia	1
Tinnitus	1
White Cell and Reticuloendothelial System Disorders	
Leukopenia	7

Selected Adverse Events Reported In Clinical Trials (< 1% incidence, n=393):

Cardiovascular Disorders, General: Angina, Cardiac Arrest, Fluctuation in Blood Pressure, Heart Failure, Myocardial Infarction, Shock, Thrombosis.

Central and Peripheral Nervous System Disorders: Coma, Encephalopathy, Epilepsy, Hypotonia.

Gastrointestinal Disorders: Gastrointestinal Hemorrhage.

Hemapoietic Disorders: Coagulation Disorder, Lymphadenopathy, Lymphopenia.

Hepatobiliary: Hepatitis, SGOT Increased, SGPT Increased.

Psychiatric Disorders: Hallucinations, Mood Changes, Paranoia, Psychosis.

Renal Disorders: Anuria, Oliguria.

Respiratory System Disorders: Apnea, Pneumonitis.

Special Senses: Conjunctivitis, Hearing Decrease.

Worldwide Postmarketing Experience - Body Systems/Events Listed Alphabetically:

Body as a Whole, General Disorders: Fever (including spiking temperatures as high as 107°F), Flu-like Syndrome.

Cardiovascular Disorders: Cardiovascular Collapse, Hemodynamic Instability, Left Ventricular Dysfunction.

Central and Peripheral Nervous System Disorders: Agitation, Aphasia, Asterixis, Cerebritis, Cerebral Edema, Cerebral Herniation, Cerebrovascular Accident, CNS Infection, CNS Malignancy, Cranial Nerve VI Palsy, Encephalitis, Hyperreflexia, Involuntary Movements, Intracranial Hemorrhage, Impaired Cognition, Myoclonus, Obnubilation, Paresis/plegia including quadriparesis/plegia, Status Epilepticus, Stupor, Transient Ischemic Attack, Vertigo.

In a post-marketing survey involving 214 renal transplant patients, the incidence of aseptic meningitis syndrome was 6%. Fever (89%), headache (44%), neck stiffness (14%), and photophobia (10%) were the most commonly reported symptoms; a combination of these four symptoms occurred in 5% of patients.

Between 1987 and 1992, 75 post-marketing reports have described seizures, averaging about 12 per year, and including 23 fatalities. More than two-thirds of these reports (53) were of domestic spontaneous origin, and their age and sex distributions were broad. Post-licensure reports generally provide insufficient data to allow accurate estimation of risk or of incidence.

Gastrointestinal Disorders: Bowel Infarction.

Hematopoietic Disorders: Aplastic anemia, Arterial, Venous and Capillary Thrombosis of allografts and other vascular beds e.g., heart, lung, brain and bowel etc., Disseminated Intravascular Coagulation, Microangiopathic Changes (e.g., platelet microthrombi), Microangiopathic Hemolytic Anemia, Neutropenia, Pancytopenia.

Hepatobiliary: Hepatitis or Hepato/splenomegaly, usually secondary to viral infection or lymphoma.

Musculoskeletal Disorders: Arthritis, Stiffness/Aches/Pains.

Renal Disorders: Azotemia, Abnormal Urinary Cytology including exfoliation of damaged lymphocytes, collecting duct cells and cellular casts, Delayed Graft Function, Renal Insufficiency/Renal Failure, usually transient and reversible and occasionally in association with Cytokine Release Syndrome.

Respiratory System Disorders: Adult Respiratory Distress Syndrome, Respiratory Arrest, Respiratory Failure.

Skin and Appendages: Erythema, Flushing, Stevens-Johnson Syndrome, Urticaria.

Special Senses: Blindness, Blurred Vision, Deafness, Diplopia, Otitis Media, Nasal and Ear Stuffiness, Papilledema.

OVERDOSAGE

Symptoms of overdosage with ORTHOCLONE OKT®3 may include hyperthermia, severe chills, myalgia, vomiting, diarrhea, edema, oliguria, pulmonary edema, and acute renal failure. A high incidence (5%) of microangiopathic hemolytic anemia/HUS syndrome in patients receiving 10 mg per day of ORTHOCLONE OKT3 was also reported. In the event of acute overdosage with ORTHOCLONE OKT3, the patient should be carefully observed and given symptomatic and supportive treatment.

DOSAGE AND ADMINISTRATION
Adults
The recommended dose of ORTHOCLONE OKT3 for the treatment of acute renal, steroid-resistant cardiac, or steroid-resistant hepatic allograft rejection is 5 mg per day in a single (bolus) intravenous injection in less than one minute for 10 to 14 days. For acute renal rejection, treatment should begin upon diagnosis. For steroid-resistant cardiac or hepatic allograft rejection, treatment should begin when the treating physician deems a rejection has not been reversed by an adequate course of corticosteroid therapy. (See: CLINICAL PHARMACOLOGY; PRECAUTIONS: Sensitization, Laboratory Tests.)

Pediatric Patients
The initial recommended dose is 2.5 mg per day in pediatric patients weighing less than or equal to 30 kg and 5 mg per day in pediatric patients weighing greater than 30 kg in a single (bolus) intravenous injection in less than one minute for 10 to 14 days. Daily increases in ORTHOCLONE OKT3 doses (i.e., 2.5 mg increments) may be required to achieve depletion of CD3 positive cells (<25 cells/mm^3) and ensure therapeutic ORTHOCLONE OKT3 serum concentrations (>800 ng/mL). Pediatric patients may require augmentation of the ORTHOCLONE OKT3 dose. For acute renal rejection, treatment should begin upon diagnosis. For steroid-resistant cardiac or hepatic allograft rejection, treatment should begin when the treating physician deems a rejection has not been reversed by an adequate course of corticosteroid therapy. (See: CLINICAL PHARMACOLOGY; PRECAUTIONS: Laboratory Tests; Pediatric Use.)

General
For the first few doses, patients should be monitored in a facility equipped and staffed for cardiopulmonary resuscitation (CPR). Patients receiving subsequent doses of ORTHOCLONE OKT3, should also be monitored in a facility equipped and staffed for CPR. Vital signs should be monitored frequently. Patients receiving ORTHOCLONE OKT3 should also be carefully monitored for signs and symptoms of Cytokine Release Syndrome, particularly after the first few doses but also after a treatment hiatus with resumption of therapy. The patient's temperature should be lowered to <37.8°C (100°F) before the administration of any dose of ORTHOCLONE OKT3.

Prior to administration of ORTHOCLONE OKT3, the patient's volume status should be assessed carefully. It is imperative, especially prior to the first few doses, that there be no clinical evidence of volume overload, uncontrolled hypertension, or uncompensated heart failure. Patients should have a clear chest X-ray and should not weigh more than 3% above their minimum weight during the week prior to injection.

To decrease the incidence and severity of Cytokine Release Syndrome, associated with the first dose of ORTHOCLONE OKT3, it is strongly recommended that methylprednisolone sodium succinate 8.0 mg/kg be administered intravenously 1 to 4 hours prior to the initial dose of ORTHOCLONE OKT3. Acetaminophen and antihistamines given concomitantly with ORTHOCLONE OKT3 may also help to reduce some early reactions. (See: WARNINGS and ADVERSE EVENTS: Cytokine Release Syndrome.)

When using concomitant immunosuppressive drugs, the dose of each should be reduced to the lowest level compatible with an effective therapeutic response in order to reduce the potential for malignancy and infections. Maintenance immunosuppression should be resumed approximately three days prior to the cessation of ORTHOCLONE OKT®3 therapy. (See: WARNINGS and ADVERSE EVENTS: Infection, Neoplasia.)

Reduced T cell clearance or low plasma ORTHOCLONE OKT3 levels provide a basis for adjusting ORTHOCLONE OKT3 dosage or for discontinuing therapy. (See: WARNINGS: Anaphylactic Reactions; PRECAUTIONS: Laboratory Tests; ADVERSE EVENTS: Hypersensitivity Reactions.)

ADMINISTRATION INSTRUCTIONS
1. Before administration, ORTHOCLONE OKT3 should be inspected for particulate matter and discoloration. Because ORTHOCLONE OKT3 is a protein solution, it may develop fine translucent particles (shown not to affect potency).
2. No bacteriostatic agent is present in this product. Adherence to aseptic technique is advised. Once the ampule is opened, use immediately and discard the unused portion.
3. Prepare ORTHOCLONE OKT3 for injection by drawing solution into a syringe through a low protein-binding 0.2 or 0.22 micrometer (µm) filter. Detach filter and attach a new needle for a single intravenous (bolus) injection.
4. Because no data is available on compatibility of ORTHOCLONE OKT3 with other intravenous substances or additives, other medications/substances should not be added or infused simultaneously through the same intravenous line. If the same intravenous line is used for sequential infusion of several different drugs, the line should be flushed with saline before and after injection of ORTHOCLONE OKT3.
5. Administer ORTHOCLONE OKT3 as a single intravenous (bolus) injection in less than one minute. Do **not** administer by intravenous infusion or in conjunction with other drug solutions.

HOW SUPPLIED

ORTHOCLONE OKT3 is supplied as a sterile solution in packages of 5 ampules (NDC 59676-101-01). Each 5 mL ampule contains 5 mg of muromonab-CD3.

Storage: Store in a refrigerator at 2° to 8°C (36° to 46°F). DO NOT FREEZE OR SHAKE.

REFERENCES
1. Adair JC, Woodley SL, O'Connell JB, et al. Aseptic Meningitis following Cardiac Transplantation: Clinical Characteristics and Relationship to Immunosuppressive Regimen. Neurology 41:249-252, 1991.
2. Chatenoud L, Legendre C, Ferran C, et al. Corticosteroid Inhibition of the OKT3 - Induced Cytokine-Related Syndrome - Dosage and Kinetics Prerequisites. Transplantation 51:334-338, 1991.
3. Cockfield SM, Preiksaitis J, Harvey E, Jones C, Herbert D, Keown P, and Halloran PF, et al. Is Sequential Use of ALG and OKT3 in Renal Transplants Associated with an Increased Incidence of Fulminant Post Transplant Lymphoproliferative Disorders? Transplant. Proc. 23:1106-1107, 1991.
4. Ettenger RB, Marik J, Rosenthal JT, et al. OKT3 for Rejection Reversal in Pediatric Renal Transplantation. Clin. Transplantation 2:180-184, 1988.
5. Gaston RS, Deierhoi MH, Patterson T, et al. OKT3 First-Dose Reaction: Association with T Cell Subsets and Cytokine Release. Kid. International 39:141-148, 1991.
6. Goldman M, Abramowicz D, DePauw L, et al. OKT3-Induced Cytokine Released Attenuation by High-Dose Methylprednisolone. Lancet 2:802-803, 1989.
7. Ortho Multicenter Transplant Study Group. A Randomized Clinical Trial of OKT3 Monoclonal Antibody for Acute Rejection of Cadaveric Renal Transplants. N. Engl. J. Med. 313:337-342, 1985.
8. Penn I. The Changing Patterns of Posttransplant Malignancies. Transplant. Proc. 23:1101-1103,1991.
9. Rubin RH and Tolkoff-Rubin NE. The Impact of Infection on the Outcome of Transplantation. Transplant. Proc. 23:2068-2074, 1991.
10. Schroeder TJ, Ryckman FC, Hurtubise PE, et al. Immunological Monitoring During and Following OKT3 Therapy in Children. Clin. Transplantation 5:191-196, 1991.
11. Goldstein G, Fuccello AJ, Norman DJ, et al. OKT3 Monoclonal Antibody Plasma Levels During Therapy and the Subsequent Development of Host Antibodies to OKT3. Transplantation 42:507-511, 1986.
12. Schroeder TJ, Michael AT, First MR, et al. Variations in Serum OKT3 Concentration Based Upon Age, Sex, Transplanted Organ, Treatment Regimen, and Anti-OKT3 Status. Therapeutic Drug Monitoring 16:361-367, 1994.
13. First MR, Schroeder TJ, Hurtubise PE, et al. Immune Monitoring During Retreatment with OKT3. Transplan. Proc. 21:1753-1754, 1989.

ORTHO BIOTECH PRODUCTS, L.P.
ORTHO BIOTECH
Raritan, New Jersey 08869
U.S.A.
© OBPLP 2001
631-10-191-5
Revised November 2004

PROCRIT®   ℞

[pro' – krit]
(Epoetin alfa)
FOR INJECTION

WARNINGS: INCREASED MORTALITY, SERIOUS CARDIOVASCULAR EVENTS, THROMBOEMBOLIC EVENTS, STROKE and INCREASED RISK OF TUMOR PROGRESSION OR RECURRENCE
Chronic Renal Failure
- In clinical studies, patients experienced greater risks for death, serious cardiovascular events, and stroke when administered erythropoiesis-stimulating agents (ESAs) to target hemoglobin levels of 13 g/dL and above.
- Individualize dosing to achieve and maintain hemoglobin levels within the range of 10 to 12 g/dL.
Cancer
- ESAs shortened overall survival and/or increased the risk of tumor progression or recurrence in some clin-

ical studies in patients with breast, non-small cell lung, head and neck, lymphoid, and cervical cancers (see WARNINGS: Table 1).

- To decrease these risks, as well as the risk of serious cardio- and thrombovascular events, use the lowest dose needed to avoid red blood cell transfusion.
- Because of these risks, prescribers and hospitals must enroll in and comply with the ESA APPRISE Oncology Program to prescribe and/or dispense PROCRIT® to patients with cancer. To enroll in the ESA APPRISE Oncology Program, visit www.esa-apprise.com or call 1-866-284-8089 for further assistance.
- Use ESAs only for treatment of anemia due to concomitant myelosuppressive chemotherapy.
- ESAs are not indicated for patients receiving myelosuppressive therapy when the anticipated outcome is cure.
- Discontinue following the completion of a chemotherapy course.

Perisurgery: PROCRIT® increased the rate of deep venous thromboses in patients not receiving prophylactic anticoagulation. Consider deep venous thrombosis prophylaxis.

(See WARNINGS: Increased Mortality, Serious Cardiovascular Events, Thromboembolic Events, and Stroke, WARNINGS: Increased Mortality and/or Increased Risk of Tumor Progression or Recurrence, INDICATIONS AND USAGE, and DOSAGE AND ADMINISTRATION.)

DESCRIPTION

Erythropoietin is a glycoprotein which stimulates red blood cell production. It is produced in the kidney and stimulates the division and differentiation of committed erythroid progenitors in the bone marrow. PROCRIT® (Epoetin alfa), a 165 amino acid glycoprotein manufactured by recombinant DNA technology, has the same biological effects as endogenous erythropoietin.[1] It has a molecular weight of 30,400 daltons and is produced by mammalian cells into which the human erythropoietin gene has been introduced. The product contains the identical amino acid sequence of isolated natural erythropoietin.

PROCRIT® is formulated as a sterile, colorless liquid in an isotonic sodium chloride/sodium citrate buffered solution or a sodium chloride/sodium phosphate buffered solution for intravenous (IV) or subcutaneous (SC) administration.

Single-dose, Preservative-free Vial

Each 1 mL of solution contains 2000, 3000, 4000 or 10,000 Units of Epoetin alfa, 2.5 mg Albumin (Human), 5.8 mg sodium citrate, 5.8 mg sodium chloride, and 0.06 mg citric acid in Water for Injection, USP (pH 6.9 ± 0.3). This formulation contains no preservative.

Single-dose, Preservative-free Vial

1 mL (40,000 Units/mL). Each 1 mL of solution contains 40,000 Units of Epoetin alfa, 2.5 mg Albumin (Human), 1.2 mg sodium phosphate monobasic monohydrate, 1.8 mg sodium phosphate dibasic anhydrate, 0.7 mg sodium citrate, 5.8 mg sodium chloride, and 6.8 mcg citric acid in Water for Injection, USP (pH 6.9 ± 0.3). This formulation contains no preservative.

Multidose, Preserved Vial

2 mL (20,000 Units, 10,000 Units/mL). Each 1 mL of solution contains 10,000 Units of Epoetin alfa, 2.5 mg Albumin (Human), 1.3 mg sodium citrate, 8.2 mg sodium chloride, 0.11 mg citric acid, and 1% benzyl alcohol as preservative in Water for Injection, USP (pH 6.1 ± 0.3).

Multidose, Preserved Vial

1 mL (20,000 Units/mL). Each 1 mL of solution contains 20,000 Units of Epoetin alfa, 2.5 mg Albumin (Human), 1.3 mg sodium citrate, 8.2 mg sodium chloride, 0.11 mg citric acid, and 1% benzyl alcohol as preservative in Water for Injection, USP (pH 6.1 ± 0.3).

CLINICAL PHARMACOLOGY

Chronic Renal Failure Patients

Endogenous production of erythropoietin is normally regulated by the level of tissue oxygenation. Hypoxia and anemia generally increase the production of erythropoietin, which in turn stimulates erythropoiesis.[2] In normal subjects, plasma erythropoietin levels range from 0.01 to 0.03 Units/mL and increase up to 100- to 1000-fold during hypoxia or anemia.[2] In contrast, in patients with chronic renal failure (CRF), production of erythropoietin is impaired, and this erythropoietin deficiency is the primary cause of their anemia.[3,4]

Chronic renal failure is the clinical situation in which there is a progressive and usually irreversible decline in kidney function. Such patients may manifest the sequelae of renal dysfunction, including anemia, but do not necessarily require regular dialysis. Patients with end-stage renal disease (ESRD) are those patients with CRF who require regular dialysis or kidney transplantation for survival.

PROCRIT® has been shown to stimulate erythropoiesis in anemic patients with CRF, including both patients on dialysis and those who do not require regular dialysis.[4-12] The first evidence of a response to the three times weekly (TIW) administration of PROCRIT® is an increase in the reticulocyte count within 10 days, followed by increases in the red cell count, hemoglobin, and hematocrit, usually within 2 to 6 weeks.[4,5] Because of the length of time required for erythropoiesis — several days for erythroid progenitors to mature and be released into the circulation — a clinically significant increase in hematocrit is usually not observed in less than 2 weeks and may require up to 6 weeks in some patients. Once the hematocrit reaches the suggested target range (30% to 36%), that level can be sustained by PROCRIT® therapy in the absence of iron deficiency and concurrent illnesses.

The rate of hematocrit increase varies between patients and is dependent upon the dose of PROCRIT®, within a therapeutic range of approximately 50 to 300 Units/kg TIW.[4] A greater biologic response is not observed at doses exceeding 300 Units/kg TIW.[6] Other factors affecting the rate and extent of response include availability of iron stores, the baseline hematocrit, and the presence of concurrent medical problems.

Zidovudine-treated HIV-infected Patients

Responsiveness to PROCRIT® in HIV-infected patients is dependent upon the endogenous serum erythropoietin level prior to treatment. Patients with endogenous serum erythropoietin levels ≤ 500 mUnits/mL, and who are receiving a dose of zidovudine ≤ 4200 mg/week, may respond to PROCRIT® therapy. Patients with endogenous serum erythropoietin levels > 500 mUnits/mL do not appear to respond to PROCRIT® therapy. In a series of four clinical trials involving 255 patients, 60% to 80% of HIV-infected patients treated with zidovudine had endogenous serum erythropoietin levels ≤ 500 mUnits/mL.

Response to PROCRIT® in zidovudine-treated HIV-infected patients is manifested by reduced transfusion requirements and increased hematocrit.

Cancer Patients on Chemotherapy

A series of clinical trials enrolled 131 anemic cancer patients who received PROCRIT® TIW and who were receiving cyclic cisplatin- or non cisplatin-containing chemotherapy. Endogenous baseline serum erythropoietin levels varied among patients in these trials with approximately 75% (n = 83/110) having endogenous serum erythropoietin levels ≤ 132 mUnits/mL, and approximately 4% (n = 4/110) of patients having endogenous serum erythropoietin levels > 500 mUnits/mL. In general, patients with lower baseline serum erythropoietin levels responded more vigorously to PROCRIT® than patients with higher baseline erythropoietin levels. Although no specific serum erythropoietin level can be stipulated above which patients would be unlikely to respond to PROCRIT® therapy, treatment of patients with grossly elevated serum erythropoietin levels (eg, > 200 mUnits/mL) is not recommended.

Pharmacokinetics

In adult and pediatric patients with CRF, the elimination half-life of plasma erythropoietin after intravenously administered PROCRIT® ranges from 4 to 13 hours.[13-15] The half-life is approximately 20% longer in CRF patients than that in healthy subjects. After SC administration, peak plasma levels are achieved within 5 to 24 hours. The half-life is similar between adult patients with serum creatinine level greater than 3 and not on dialysis and those maintained on dialysis. The pharmacokinetic data indicate no apparent difference in PROCRIT® half-life among adult patients above or below 65 years of age.

The pharmacokinetic profile of PROCRIT® in children and adolescents appears to be similar to that of adults. Limited data are available in neonates.[16] A study of 7 preterm very low birth weight neonates and 10 healthy adults given IV erythropoietin suggested that distribution volume was approximately 1.5 to 2 times higher in the preterm neonates than in the healthy adults, and clearance was approximately 3 times higher in the preterm neonates than in the healthy adults.[39]

The pharmacokinetics of PROCRIT® have not been studied in HIV-infected patients.

A pharmacokinetic study comparing 150 Units/kg SC TIW to 40,000 Units SC weekly dosing regimen was conducted for 4 weeks in healthy subjects (n = 12) and for 6 weeks in anemic cancer patients (n = 32) receiving cyclic chemotherapy. There was no accumulation of serum erythropoietin after the 2 dosing regimens during the study period. The 40,000 Units weekly regimen had a higher C_{max} (3- to 7-fold), longer T_{max} (2- to 3-fold), higher AUC_{0-168h} (2- to 3-fold) of erythropoietin and lower clearance (50%) than the 150 Units/kg TIW regimen. In anemic cancer patients, the average $t_{1/2}$ was similar (40 hours with range of 16 to 67 hours) after both dosing regimens. After the 150 Units/kg TIW dosing, the values of T_{max} and clearance are similar (13.3 ± 12.4 vs. 14.2 ± 6.7 hours, and 20.2 ± 15.9 vs. 23.6 ± 9.5 mL/h/kg) between Week 1 when patients were receiving chemotherapy (n = 14) and Week 3 when patients were not receiving chemotherapy (n = 4). Differences were observed after the 40,000 Units weekly dosing with longer T_{max} (38 ± 18 hours) and lower clearance (9.2 ± 4.7 mL/h/kg) during Week 1 when patients were receiving chemotherapy (n = 18) compared with those (22 ± 4.5 hours, 13.9 ± 7.6 mL/h/kg) during Week 3 when patients were not receiving chemotherapy (n = 7).

The bioequivalence between the 10,000 Units/mL citrate-buffered Epoetin alfa formulation and the 40,000 Units/mL phosphate-buffered Epoetin alfa formulation has been demonstrated after SC administration of single 750 Units/kg doses to healthy subjects.

INDICATIONS AND USAGE

Treatment of Anemia of Chronic Renal Failure Patients

PROCRIT® is indicated for the treatment of anemia associated with CRF, including patients on dialysis and patients not on dialysis. PROCRIT® is indicated to elevate or maintain the red blood cell level (as manifested by the hematocrit or hemoglobin determinations) and to decrease the need for transfusions in these patients.

Non-dialysis patients with symptomatic anemia considered for therapy should have a hemoglobin less than 10 g/dL. PROCRIT® is not intended for patients who require immediate correction of severe anemia. PROCRIT® may obviate the need for maintenance transfusions but is not a substitute for emergency transfusion.

Prior to initiation of therapy, the patient's iron stores should be evaluated. Transferrin saturation should be at least 20% and ferritin at least 100 ng/mL. Blood pressure should be adequately controlled prior to initiation of PROCRIT® therapy, and must be closely monitored and controlled during therapy.

Treatment of Anemia in Zidovudine-treated HIV-infected Patients

PROCRIT® is indicated for the treatment of anemia related to therapy with zidovudine in HIV-infected patients. PROCRIT® is indicated to elevate or maintain the red blood cell level (as manifested by the hematocrit or hemoglobin determinations) and to decrease the need for transfusions in these patients. PROCRIT® is not indicated for the treatment of anemia in HIV-infected patients due to other factors such as iron or folate deficiencies, hemolysis, or gastrointestinal bleeding, which should be managed appropriately. PROCRIT® use has not been demonstrated in controlled clinical trials to improve symptoms of anemia, quality of life, fatigue, or patient well-being.

PROCRIT®, at a dose of 100 Units/kg TIW, is effective in decreasing the transfusion requirement and increasing the red blood cell level of anemic, HIV-infected patients treated with zidovudine, when the endogenous serum erythropoietin level is ≤ 500 mUnits/mL and when patients are receiving a dose of zidovudine ≤ 4200 mg/week.

Treatment of Anemia in Cancer Patients on Chemotherapy

PROCRIT® is indicated for the treatment of anemia due to the effect of concomitantly administered chemotherapy based on studies that have shown a reduction in the need for RBC transfusions in patients with metastatic, non-myeloid malignancies receiving chemotherapy for a minimum of 2 months. Studies to determine whether PROCRIT® increases mortality or decreases progression-free/recurrence-free survival are ongoing.

- PROCRIT® is not indicated for use in patients receiving hormonal agents, therapeutic biologic products, or radiotherapy unless receiving concomitant myelosuppressive chemotherapy.
- PROCRIT® is not indicated for patients receiving myelosuppressive therapy when the anticipated outcome is cure due to the absence of studies that adequately characterize the impact of PROCRIT® on progression-free and overall survival (see WARNINGS: Increased Mortality and/or Increased Risk of Tumor Progression or Recurrence).
- PROCRIT® is not indicated for the treatment of anemia in cancer patients due to other factors such as iron or folate deficiencies, hemolysis, or gastrointestinal bleeding (see PRECAUTIONS: Lack or Loss of Response).
- PROCRIT® use has not been demonstrated in controlled clinical trials to improve symptoms of anemia, quality of life, fatigue, or patient well-being.

Reduction of Allogeneic Blood Transfusion in Surgery Patients

PROCRIT® is indicated for the treatment of anemic patients (hemoglobin > 10 to ≤ 13 g/dL) who are at high risk for perioperative blood loss from elective, noncardiac, nonvascular surgery to reduce the need for allogeneic blood transfusions.[17-19] PROCRIT® is not indicated for anemic patients who are willing to donate autologous blood (see BOXED WARNINGS and DOSAGE AND ADMINISTRATION).

CLINICAL EXPERIENCE: RESPONSE TO PROCRIT®

Chronic Renal Failure Patients

When dosed with PROCRIT®, patients responded with an increase in hematocrit.[5] After 3 months on study, more than 95% of patients were transfusion-independent.

In the presence of adequate iron stores (see IRON EVALUATION), the time to reach the target hematocrit is a function of the baseline hematocrit and the rate of hematocrit rise.

The rate of increase in hematocrit is dependent upon the dose of PROCRIT® administered and individual patient variation. In clinical trials at starting doses of 50 to 150 Units/kg TIW, adult patients responded with an average rate of hematocrit rise of:

Starting Dose (TIW IV)	Hematocrit Increase Points/Day	Points/2 Weeks
50 Units/kg	0.11	1.5
100 Units/kg	0.18	2.5
150 Units/kg	0.25	3.5

In a 26 week, double-blind, placebo-controlled trial, 118 anemic dialysis patients with an average hemoglobin of approximately 7 g/dL were randomized to either PROCRIT® or placebo. By the end of the study, average hemoglobin increased to approximately 11 g/dL in the PROCRIT®-treated patients and remained unchanged in patients receiving placebo. PROCRIT®-treated patients experienced improvements in exercise tolerance and patient-reported physical functioning at month 2 that was maintained throughout the study.

Adult Patients on Dialysis: Thirteen clinical studies were conducted, involving IV administration to a total of 1010 anemic patients on dialysis for 986 patient-years of PROCRIT® therapy. In the three largest of these clinical trials, the median maintenance dose necessary to maintain the hematocrit between 30% to 36% was approximately 75 Units/kg TIW. In the US multicenter phase 3 study, approximately 65% of the patients required doses of 100 Units/kg TIW, or less, to maintain their hematocrit at approximately 35%. Almost 10% of patients required a dose of 25 Units/kg, or less, and approximately 10% required a dose of more than 200 Units/kg TIW to maintain their hematocrit at this level.

A multicenter unit dose study was also conducted in 119 patients receiving peritoneal dialysis who self-administered PROCRIT® subcutaneously for approximately 109 patient-years of experience. Patients responded to PROCRIT® administered SC in a manner similar to patients receiving IV administration.[20]

Pediatric Patients on Dialysis: One hundred twenty-eight children from 2 months to 19 years of age with CRF requiring dialysis were enrolled in 4 clinical studies of PROCRIT®. The largest study was a placebo-controlled, randomized trial in 113 children with anemia (hematocrit ≤ 27%) undergoing peritoneal dialysis or hemodialysis. The initial dose of PROCRIT® was 50 Units/kg IV or SC TIW. The dose of study drug was titrated to achieve either a hematocrit of 30% to 36% or an absolute increase in hematocrit of 6 percentage points over baseline.

At the end of the initial 12 weeks, a statistically significant rise in mean hematocrit (9.4% vs 0.9%) was observed only in the PROCRIT® arm. The proportion of children achieving a hematocrit of 30%, or an increase in hematocrit of 6 percentage points over baseline, at any time during the first 12 weeks was higher in the PROCRIT® arm (96% vs 58%). Within 12 weeks of initiating PROCRIT® therapy, 92.3% of the pediatric patients were transfusion-independent as compared to 65.4% who received placebo. Among patients who received 36 weeks of PROCRIT®, hemodialysis patients required a higher median maintenance dose (167 Units/kg/week [n = 28] vs 76 Units/kg/week [n = 36]) and took longer to achieve a hematocrit of 30% to 36% (median time to response 69 days vs 32 days) than patients undergoing peritoneal dialysis.

Patients With CRF Not Requiring Dialysis

Four clinical trials were conducted in patients with CRF not on dialysis involving 181 patients treated with PROCRIT® for approximately 67 patient-years of experience. These patients responded to PROCRIT® therapy in a manner similar to that observed in patients on dialysis. Patients with CRF not on dialysis demonstrated a dose-dependent and sustained increase in hematocrit when PROCRIT® was administered by either an IV or SC route, with similar rates of rise of hematocrit when PROCRIT® was administered by either route. Moreover, PROCRIT® doses of 75 to 150 Units/kg per week have been shown to maintain hematocrits of 36% to 38% for up to 6 months.[21–22]

Zidovudine-treated HIV-infected Patients

Efficacy in HIV-infected patients with anemia related to therapy with zidovudine was demonstrated based on reduction in the requirement for RBC transfusions.

PROCRIT® has been studied in four placebo-controlled trials enrolling 297 anemic (hematocrit < 30%) HIV-infected (AIDS) patients receiving concomitant therapy with zidovudine (all patients were treated with Epoetin alfa manufactured by Amgen Inc). In the subgroup of patients (89/125 PROCRIT® and 88/130 placebo) with prestudy endogenous serum erythropoietin levels ≤ 500 mUnits/mL, PROCRIT® reduced the mean cumulative number of units of blood transfused per patient by approximately 40% as compared to the placebo group.[24] Among those patients who required transfusions at baseline, 43% of patients treated with PROCRIT® versus 18% of placebo-treated patients were transfusion-independent during the second and third months of therapy. PROCRIT® therapy also resulted in significant increases in hematocrit in comparison to placebo. When examining the results according to the weekly dose of zidovudine received during month 3 of therapy, there was a statistically significant ($p < 0.003$) reduction in transfusion requirements in patients treated with PROCRIT® (n = 51) compared to placebo treated patients (n = 54) whose mean weekly zidovudine dose was ≤ 4200 mg/week.[23]

Approximately 17% of the patients with endogenous serum erythropoietin levels ≤ 500 mUnits/mL receiving PROCRIT® in doses from 100 to 200 Units/kg TIW achieved a hematocrit of 38% without administration of transfusions or significant reduction in zidovudine dose. In the subgroup of patients whose prestudy endogenous serum erythropoietin levels were > 500 mUnits/mL, PROCRIT® therapy did not reduce transfusion requirements or increase hematocrit, compared to the corresponding responses in placebo-treated patients.

In a 6 month open-label PROCRIT® study, patients responded with decreased transfusion requirements and sustained increases in hematocrit and hemoglobin with doses of PROCRIT® up to 300 Units/kg TIW.[23–25]

Responsiveness to PROCRIT® therapy may be blunted by intercurrent infectious/inflammatory episodes and by an increase in zidovudine dosage. Consequently, the dose of PROCRIT® must be titrated based on these factors to maintain the desired erythropoietic response.

Cancer Patients on Chemotherapy

Adult Patients

Efficacy in patients with anemia due to concomitant chemotherapy was demonstrated based on reduction in the requirement for RBC transfusions.

Three-Times Weekly (TIW) Dosing

PROCRIT® administered TIW has been studied in a series of six placebo-controlled, double-blind trials that enrolled 131 anemic cancer patients receiving PROCRIT® or matching placebo. Across all studies, 72 patients were treated with concomitant non cisplatin-containing chemotherapy regimens and 59 patients were treated with concomitant cisplatin-containing chemotherapy regimens. Patients were randomized to PROCRIT® 150 Units/kg or placebo subcutaneously TIW for 12 weeks in each study.

The results of the pooled data from these six studies are shown in the table below. Because of the length of time required for erythropoiesis and red cell maturation, the efficacy of PROCRIT® (reduction in proportion of patients requiring transfusions) is not manifested until 2 to 6 weeks after initiation of PROCRIT®.

[See table above]

Proportion of Patients Transfused During Chemotherapy (Efficacy Population*)

Chemotherapy Regimen	On Study†		During Months 2 and 3‡	
	PROCRIT®	Placebo	PROCRIT®	Placebo
Regimens without cisplatin	44% (15/34)	44% (16/36)	21% (6/29)	33% (11/33)
Regimens containing cisplatin	50% (14/28)	63% (19/30)	23% (5/22)§	56% (14/25)
Combined	47% (29/62)	53% (35/66)	22% (11/51)§	43% (25/58)

* Limited to patients remaining on study at least 15 days (1 patient excluded from PROCRIT®, 2 patients excluded from placebo).
† Includes all transfusions from day 1 through the end of study.
‡ Limited to patients remaining on study beyond week 6 and includes only transfusions during weeks 5–12.
§ Unadjusted 2-sided $p < 0.05$

Intensity of chemotherapy in the above trials was not directly assessed, however the degree and timing of neutropenia was comparable across all trials. Available evidence suggests that patients with lymphoid and solid cancers respond similarly to PROCRIT® therapy, and that patients with or without tumor infiltration of the bone marrow respond similarly to PROCRIT® therapy.

Weekly (QW) Dosing

PROCRIT® was also studied in a placebo-controlled, double-blind trial utilizing weekly dosing in a total of 344 anemic cancer patients. In this trial, 61 (35 placebo arm and 26 in the PROCRIT® arm) patients were treated with concomitant cisplatin containing regimens and 283 patients received concomitant chemotherapy regimens that did not contain cisplatinum. Patients were randomized to PROCRIT® 40,000 Units weekly (n = 174) or placebo (n = 170) SC for a planned treatment period of 16 weeks. If hemoglobin had not increased by > 1 g/dL after 4 weeks of therapy or the patient received RBC transfusion during the first 4 weeks of therapy, study drug was increased to 60,000 Units weekly. Forty-three percent of patients in the Epoetin alfa group required an increase in PROCRIT® dose to 60,000 Units weekly.[23]

Results demonstrated that PROCRIT® therapy reduced the proportion of patients transfused in day 29 through week 16 of the study as compared to placebo. Twenty-five patients (14%) in the PROCRIT® group received transfusions compared to 48 patients (28%) in the placebo group ($p = 0.0010$) between day 29 and week 16 or the last day on study.

Comparable intensity of chemotherapy for patients enrolled in the two study arms was suggested by similarities in mean dose and frequency of administration for the 10 most commonly administered chemotherapy agents, and similarity in the incidence of changes in chemotherapy during the trial in the two arms.

Pediatric Patients

The safety and effectiveness of PROCRIT® were evaluated in a randomized, double-blind, placebo-controlled, multicenter study in anemic patients ages 5 to 18 receiving chemotherapy for the treatment of various childhood malignancies. Two hundred twenty-two patients were randomized (1:1) to PROCRIT® or placebo. PROCRIT® was administered at 600 Units/kg (maximum 40,000 Units) intravenously once per week for 16 weeks. If hemoglobin had not increased by 1g/dL after the first 4–5 weeks of therapy, PROCRIT® was increased to 900 Units/kg (maximum 60,000 Units). Among the PROCRIT®-treated patients 60% required dose escalation to 900 Units/kg/week.

The effect of PROCRIT® on transfusion requirements is shown in the table below:

Percentage of Patients Transfused:

On Study*		After 28 Days Post-Randomization	
PROCRIT® (n=111)	Placebo (n=111)	PROCRIT® (n=111)	Placebo (n=111)
65% (72)	77% (86)	51% (57)†	69% (77)

* Includes all transfusions from day 1 through the end of study
† Adjusted 2 sided $p < 0.05$

There was no evidence of an improvement in health-related quality of life, including no evidence of an effect on fatigue, energy or strength, in patients receiving PROCRIT® as compared to those receiving placebo.

Surgery Patients

PROCRIT® has been studied in a placebo-controlled, double-blind trial enrolling 316 patients scheduled for major, elective orthopedic hip or knee surgery who were expected to require ≥ 2 units of blood and who were not able or willing to participate in an autologous blood donation program. Based on previous studies which demonstrated that pretreatment hemoglobin is a predictor of risk of receiving transfusion,[19,26] patients were stratified into one of three groups based on their pretreatment hemoglobin [≤ 10 (n = 2), > 10 to ≤ 13 (n = 96), and > 13 to ≤ 15 g/dL (n = 218)] and then randomly assigned to receive 300 Units/kg PROCRIT®, 100 Units/kg PROCRIT® or placebo by SC injection for 10 days before surgery, on the day of surgery, and for 4 days after surgery.[17] All patients received oral iron and a low-dose post-operative warfarin regimen.[17]

Treatment with PROCRIT® 300 Units/kg significantly ($p = 0.024$) reduced the risk of allogeneic transfusion in patients with a pretreatment hemoglobin of > 10 to ≤ 13; 5/31 (16%) of PROCRIT® 300 Units/kg, 6/26 (23%) of PROCRIT®

100 Units/kg, and 13/29 (45%) of placebo-treated patients were transfused.[17] There was no significant difference in the number of patients transfused between PROCRIT® (9% 300 Units/kg, 6% 100 Units/kg) and placebo (13%) in the > 13 to ≤ 15 g/dL hemoglobin stratum. There were too few patients in the ≤ 10 g/dL group to determine if PROCRIT® is useful in this hemoglobin strata. In the > 10 to ≤ 13 g/dL pretreatment stratum, the mean number of units transfused per PROCRIT®-treated patient (0.45 units blood for 300 Units/kg, 0.42 units blood for 100 Units/kg) was less than the mean transfused per placebo-treated patient (1.14 units) (overall p = 0.028). In addition, mean hemoglobin, hematocrit, and reticulocyte counts increased significantly during the presurgery period in patients treated with PROCRIT®.[17]

PROCRIT® was also studied in an open-label, parallel-group trial enrolling 145 subjects with a pretreatment hemoglobin level of ≥ 10 to ≤ 13 g/dL who were scheduled for major orthopedic hip or knee surgery and who were not participating in an autologous program.[18] Subjects were randomly assigned to receive one of two SC dosing regimens of PROCRIT® (600 Units/kg once weekly for 3 weeks prior to surgery and on the day of surgery, or 300 Units/kg once daily for 10 days prior to surgery, on the day of surgery and for 4 days after surgery). All subjects received oral iron and appropriate pharmacologic anticoagulation therapy.

From pretreatment to presurgery, the mean increase in hemoglobin in the 600 Units/kg weekly group (1.44 g/dL) was greater than observed in the 300 Units/kg daily group.[18] The mean increase in absolute reticulocyte count was smaller in the weekly group (0.11 × 10⁶/mm³) compared to the daily group (0.17 × 10⁶/mm³). Mean hemoglobin levels were similar for the two treatment groups throughout the postsurgical period.

The erythropoietic response observed in both treatment groups resulted in similar transfusion rates [11/69 (16%) in the 600 Units/kg weekly group and 14/71 (20%) in the 300 Units/kg daily group].[18] The mean number of units transfused per subject was approximately 0.3 units in both treatment groups.

CONTRAINDICATIONS

PROCRIT® is contraindicated in patients with:
1. Uncontrolled hypertension.
2. Known hypersensitivity to mammalian cell-derived products.
3. Known hypersensitivity to Albumin (Human).

WARNINGS
Pediatrics
Risk in Premature Infants
The multidose preserved formulation contains benzyl alcohol. Benzyl alcohol has been reported to be associated with an increased incidence of neurological and other complications in premature infants which are sometimes fatal.
Adults
Increased Mortality, Serious Cardiovascular Events, Thromboembolic Events, and Stroke
Patients with chronic renal failure experienced greater risks for death, serious cardiovascular events, and stroke when administered erythropoiesis-stimulating agents (ESAs) to target hemoglobin levels of 13 g/dL and above in clinical studies. Patients with chronic renal failure and an insufficient hemoglobin response to ESA therapy may be at even greater risk for cardiovascular events and mortality than other patients. PROCRIT® and other ESAs increased the risks for death and serious cardiovascular events in controlled clinical trials of patients with cancer. These events included myocardial infarction, stroke, congestive heart failure, and hemodialysis vascular access thrombosis. A rate of hemoglobin rise of > 1 g/dL over 2 weeks may contribute to these risks.

In a randomized prospective trial, 1432 anemic chronic renal failure patients who were not undergoing dialysis were assigned to Epoetin alfa (rHuEPO) treatment targeting a maintenance hemoglobin concentration of 13.5 g/dL or 11.3 g/dL. A major cardiovascular event (death, myocardial infarction, stroke, or hospitalization for congestive heart failure) occurred among 125 (18%) of the 715 patients in the higher hemoglobin group compared to 97 (14%) among the 717 patients in the lower hemoglobin group (HR 1.3, 95% CI: 1.0, 1.7, p = 0.03).[40]

In a randomized, double-blind, placebo-controlled study of 4038 patients, there was an increased risk of stroke when darbepoetin alfa was administered to patients with anemia, type 2 diabetes, and CRF who were not on dialysis. Patients were randomized to darbepoetin alfa treatment targeted to a hemoglobin level of 13 g/dL or to placebo. Placebo patients received darbepoetin alfa only if their hemoglobin levels were less than 9 g/dL. A total of 101 patients receiving darbepoetin alfa experienced stroke compared to 53 patients receiving placebo (5% vs. 2.6%; HR 1.92, 95% CI: 1.38, 2.68; p < 0.001).

Increased risk for serious cardiovascular events was also reported from a randomized, prospective trial of 1265 hemo-

dialysis patients with clinically evident cardiac disease (ischemic heart disease or congestive heart failure). In this trial, patients were assigned to PROCRIT® treatment targeted to a maintenance hematocrit of either 42 ± 3% or 30 ± 3%.[37] Increased mortality was observed in 634 patients randomized to a target hematocrit of 42% [221 deaths (35% mortality)] compared to 631 patients targeted to remain at a hematocrit of 30% [185 deaths (29% mortality)]. The reason for the increased mortality observed in this study is unknown, however, the incidence of non-fatal myocardial infarctions (3.1% vs. 2.3%), vascular access thromboses (39% vs. 29%), and all other thrombotic events (22% vs. 18%) were also higher in the group randomized to achieve a hematocrit of 42%. An increased incidence of thrombotic events has also been observed in patients with cancer treated with erythropoietic agents.

In a randomized controlled study (referred to as Cancer Study 1 - the 'BEST' study) with another ESA in 939 women with metastatic breast cancer receiving chemotherapy, patients received either weekly Epoetin alfa or placebo for up to a year. This study was designed to show that survival was superior when an ESA was administered to prevent anemia (maintain hemoglobin levels between 12 and 14 g/dL or hematocrit between 36% and 42%). The study was terminated prematurely when interim results demonstrated that a higher mortality at 4 months (8.7% vs. 3.4%) and a higher rate of fatal thrombotic events (1.1% vs. 0.2%) in the first 4 months of the study were observed among patients treated with Epoetin alfa. Based on Kaplan-Meier estimates, at the time of study termination, the 12-month survival was lower in the Epoetin alfa group than in the placebo group (70% vs. 76%; HR 1.37, 95% CI: 1.07, 1.75; p = 0.012).[43]

A systematic review of 57 randomized controlled trials (including Cancer Studies 1 and 5 - the 'BEST' and 'ENHANCE' studies) evaluating 9353 patients with cancer compared ESAs plus red blood cell transfusion with red blood cell transfusion alone for prophylaxis or treatment of anemia in cancer patients with or without concurrent antineoplastic therapy. An increased relative risk of thromboembolic events (RR 1.67, 95% CI: 1.35, 2.06; 35 trials and 6769 patients) was observed in ESA-treated patients. An overall survival hazard ratio of 1.08 (95% CI: 0.99, 1.18; 42 trials and 8167 patients) was observed in ESA-treated patients.[41]

An increased incidence of deep vein thrombosis (DVT) in patients receiving Epoetin alfa undergoing surgical orthopedic procedures has been observed (see ADVERSE REACTIONS, Surgery Patients: Thrombotic/Vascular Events). In a randomized controlled study (referred to as the 'SPINE' study), 681 adult patients, not receiving prophylactic anticoagulation and undergoing spinal surgery, received either 4 doses of 600 U/kg Epoetin alfa (7, 14, and 21 days before surgery, and the day of surgery) and standard of care (SOC) treatment, or SOC treatment alone. Preliminary analysis showed a higher incidence of DVT, determined by either Color Flow Duplex Imaging or by clinical symptoms, in the Epoetin alfa group [16 patients (4.7%)] compared to the SOC group [7 patients (2.1%)]. In addition, 12 patients in the Epoetin alfa group and 7 patients in the SOC group had other thrombotic vascular events. Deep venous thrombosis prophylaxis should be strongly considered when ESAs are used for the reduction of allogeneic RBC transfusions in surgical patients (see BOXED WARNINGS and DOSAGE AND ADMINISTRATION).

Increased mortality was also observed in a randomized placebo-controlled study of PROCRIT® in adult patients who were undergoing coronary artery bypass surgery (7 deaths in 126 patients randomized to PROCRIT® versus no deaths among 56 patients receiving placebo). Four of these deaths occurred during the period of study drug administration and all four deaths were associated with thrombotic events.[42] ESAs are not approved for reduction of allogeneic red blood cell transfusions in patients scheduled for cardiac surgery.

Increased Mortality and/or Increased Risk of Tumor Progression or Recurrence
Erythropoiesis-stimulating agents resulted in decreased locoregional control/progression-free survival and/or overall survival (see Table 1). These findings were observed in studies of patients with advanced head and neck cancer receiving radiation therapy (Cancer Studies 5 and 6), in patients receiving chemotherapy for metastatic breast cancer (Cancer Study 1) or lymphoid malignancy (Cancer Study 2), and in patients with non-small cell lung cancer or various malignancies who were not receiving chemotherapy or radiotherapy (Cancer Studies 7 and 8).

[See table 1 at left]

Decreased overall survival
Cancer Study 1 (the 'BEST' study) was previously described (see WARNINGS: Increased Mortality, Serious Cardiovascular Events, Thromboembolic Events, and Stroke). Mortality at 4 months (8.7% vs. 3.4%) was significantly higher in the Epoetin alfa arm. The most common investigator-attributed cause of death within the first 4 months was dis-

Table 1: Randomized, Controlled Trials with Decreased Survival and/or Decreased Locoregional Control

Study / Tumor / (n)	Hemoglobin Target	Achieved Hemoglobin (Median Q1,Q3)	Primary Endpoint	Adverse Outcome for ESA-containing Arm
Chemotherapy				
Cancer Study 1 Metastatic breast cancer (n=939)	12–14 g/dL	12.9 g/dL 12.2, 13.3 g/dL	12-month overall survival	Decreased 12-month survival
Cancer Study 2 Lymphoid malignancy (n=344)	13–15 g/dL (M) 13–14 g/dL (F)	11.0 g/dL 9.8, 12.1 g/dL	Proportion of patients achieving a hemoglobin response	Decreased overall survival
Cancer Study 3 Early breast cancer (n=733)	12.5–13 g/dL	13.1 g/dL 12.5, 13.7 g/dL	Relapse-free and overall survival	Decreased 3 yr. relapse-free and overall survival
Cancer Study 4 Cervical Cancer (n=114)	12–14 g/dL	12.7 g/dL 12.1, 13.3 g/dL	Progression-free and overall survival and locoregional control	Decreased 3 yr. progression-free and overall survival and locoregional control
Radiotherapy Alone				
Cancer Study 5 Head and neck cancer (n=351)	≥15 g/dL (M) ≥14 g/dL (F)	Not available	Locoregional progression-free survival	Decreased 5-year locoregional progression-free survival Decreased overall survival
Cancer Study 6 Head and neck cancer (n=522)	14–15.5 g/dL	Not available	Locoregional disease control	Decreased locoregional disease control
No Chemotherapy or Radiotherapy				
Cancer Study 7 Non-small cell lung cancer (n=70)	12–14 g/dL	Not available	Quality of life	Decreased overall survival
Cancer Study 8 Non-myeloid malignancy (n=989)	12–13 g/dL	10.6 g/dL 9.4, 11.8 g/dL	RBC transfusions	Decreased overall survival

ease progression; 28 of 41 deaths in the Epoetin alfa arm and 13 of 16 deaths in the placebo arm were attributed to disease progression. Investigator assessed time to tumor progression was not different between the two groups. Survival at 12 months was significantly lower in the Epoetin alfa arm (70% vs. 76%, HR 1.37, 95% CI: 1.07, 1.75; p = 0.012).[43]

Cancer Study 2 was a Phase 3, double-blind, randomized (darbepoetin alfa vs. placebo) study conducted in 344 anemic patients with lymphoid malignancy receiving chemotherapy. With a median follow-up of 29 months, overall mortality rates were significantly higher among patients randomized to darbepoetin alfa as compared to placebo (HR 1.36, 95% CI: 1.02, 1.82).

Cancer Study 7 was a Phase 3, multicenter, randomized (Epoetin alfa vs. placebo), double-blind study, in which patients with advanced non-small cell lung cancer receiving only palliative radiotherapy or no active therapy were treated with Epoetin alfa to achieve and maintain hemoglobin levels between 12 and 14 g/dL. Following an interim analysis of 70 of 300 patients planned, a significant difference in survival in favor of the patients on the placebo arm of the trial was observed (median survival 63 vs. 129 days; HR 1.84; p = 0.04).

Cancer Study 8 was a Phase 3, double-blind, randomized (darbepoetin alfa vs. placebo), 16-week study in 989 anemic patients with active malignant disease, neither receiving nor planning to receive chemotherapy or radiation therapy. There was no evidence of a statistically significant reduction in proportion of patients receiving RBC transfusions. The median survival was shorter in the darbepoetin alfa treatment group (8 months) compared with the placebo group (10.8 months); HR 1.30, 95% CI: 1.07, 1.57.

Decreased progression-free survival and overall survival

Cancer Study 3 (the 'PREPARE' study) was a randomized controlled study in which darbepoetin alfa was administered to prevent anemia conducted in 733 women receiving neo-adjuvant breast cancer treatment. After a median follow-up of approximately 3 years, the survival rate (86% vs. 90%, HR 1.42, 95% CI: 0.93, 2.18) and relapse-free survival rate (72% vs. 78%, HR 1.33, 95% CI: 0.99, 1.79) were lower in the darbepoetin alfa-treated arm compared to the control arm.

Cancer Study 4 (protocol GOG 191) was a randomized controlled study that enrolled 114 of a planned 460 cervical cancer patients receiving chemotherapy and radiotherapy. Patients were randomized to receive Epoetin alfa to maintain hemoglobin between 12 and 14 g/dL or to transfusion support as needed. The study was terminated prematurely due to an increase in thromboembolic events in Epoetin alfa-treated patients compared to control (19% vs. 9%). Both local recurrence (21% vs. 20%) and distant recurrence (12% vs. 7%) were more frequent in Epoetin alfa-treated patients compared to control. Progression-free survival at 3 years was lower in the Epoetin alfa-treated group compared to control (59% vs. 62%, HR 1.06, 95% CI: 0.58, 1.91). Overall survival at 3 years was lower in the Epoetin alfa-treated group compared to control (61% vs. 71%, HR 1.28, 95% CI: 0.68, 2.42).

Cancer Study 5 (the 'ENHANCE' study) was a randomized controlled study in 351 head and neck cancer patients where Epoetin beta or placebo was administered to achieve target hemoglobin of 14 and 15 g/dL for women and men, respectively. Locoregional progression-free survival was significantly shorter in patients receiving Epoetin beta (HR 1.62, 95% CI: 1.22, 2.14; p = 0.0008) with a median of 406 days Epoetin beta vs. 745 days placebo. Overall survival was significantly shorter in patients receiving Epoetin beta (HR 1.39, 95% CI: 1.05, 1.84; p = 0.02).[38]

Decreased locoregional control

Cancer Study 6 (DAHANCA 10) was conducted in 522 patients with primary squamous cell carcinoma of the head and neck receiving radiation therapy randomized to darbepoetin alfa with radiotherapy or radiotherapy alone. An interim analysis on 484 patients demonstrated that locoregional control at 5 years was significantly shorter in patients receiving darbepoetin alfa (RR 1.44, 95% CI: 1.06, 1.96; p = 0.02). Overall survival was shorter in patients receiving darbepoetin alfa (RR 1.28, 95% CI: 0.98, 1.68; p = 0.08).

ESA APPRISE Oncology Program

Prescribers and hospitals must enroll in and comply with the ESA APPRISE Oncology Program to prescribe and/or dispense PROCRIT® to patients with cancer. To enroll, visit www.esa-apprise.com or call 1-866-284-8089 for further assistance. Additionally, prescribers and patients must provide written acknowledgement of a discussion of the risks associated with PROCRIT®.

Pure Red Cell Aplasia

Cases of pure red cell aplasia (PRCA) and of severe anemia, with or without other cytopenias, associated with neutralizing antibodies to erythropoietin have been reported in patients treated with PROCRIT®. This has been reported predominantly in patients with CRF receiving ESAs by subcutaneous administration. PRCA has also been reported in patients receiving ESAs while undergoing treatment for hepatitis C with interferon and ribavirin. Any patient who develops a sudden loss of response to PROCRIT®, accompanied by severe anemia and low reticulocyte count, should be evaluated for the etiology of loss of effect, including the presence of neutralizing antibodies to erythropoietin (see PRECAUTIONS: Lack or Loss of Response). If anti-erythropoietin antibody-associated anemia is suspected, withhold PROCRIT® and other ESAs. Contact CENTOCOR ORTHO BIOTECH at 1 888 2ASK OBI (1-888-227-5624) to perform assays for binding and neutralizing antibodies. PROCRIT® should be permanently discontinued in patients with antibody-mediated anemia. Patients should not be switched to other ESAs as antibodies may cross-react (see ADVERSE REACTIONS: Immunogenicity).

Albumin (Human)

PROCRIT® contains albumin, a derivative of human blood. Based on effective donor screening and product manufacturing processes, it carries an extremely remote risk for transmission of viral diseases. A theoretical risk for transmission of Creutzfeldt-Jakob disease (CJD) also is considered extremely remote. No cases of transmission of viral diseases or CJD have ever been identified for albumin.

Chronic Renal Failure Patients

Hypertension: Patients with uncontrolled hypertension should not be treated with PROCRIT®; blood pressure should be controlled adequately before initiation of therapy. Although there do not appear to be any direct pressor effects of PROCRIT®, blood pressure may rise during PROCRIT® therapy. During the early phase of treatment when the hematocrit is increasing, approximately 25% of patients on dialysis may require initiation of, or increases in, antihypertensive therapy. Hypertensive encephalopathy and seizures have been observed in patients with CRF treated with PROCRIT®.

Special care should be taken to closely monitor and aggressively control blood pressure in patients treated with PROCRIT®. Patients should be advised as to the importance of compliance with antihypertensive therapy and dietary restrictions. If blood pressure is difficult to control by initiation of appropriate measures, the hemoglobin may be reduced by decreasing or withholding the dose of PROCRIT®. A clinically significant decrease in hemoglobin may not be observed for several weeks.

It is recommended that the dose of PROCRIT® be decreased if the hemoglobin increase exceeds 1 g/dL in any 2-week period, because of the possible association of excessive rate of rise of hemoglobin with an exacerbation of hypertension. In CRF patients on hemodialysis with clinically evident ischemic heart disease or congestive heart failure, the dose of PROCRIT® should be carefully adjusted to achieve and maintain hemoglobin levels between 10–12 g/dL (see WARNINGS: Increased Mortality, Serious Cardiovascular Events, Thromboembolic Events, and Stroke, and DOSAGE AND ADMINISTRATION: Chronic Renal Failure Patients).

Seizures: Seizures have occurred in patients with CRF participating in PROCRIT® clinical trials.

In adult patients on dialysis, there was a higher incidence of seizures during the first 90 days of therapy (occurring in approximately 2.5% of patients) as compared with later timepoints.

Given the potential for an increased risk of seizures during the first 90 days of therapy, blood pressure and the presence of premonitory neurologic symptoms should be monitored closely. Patients should be cautioned to avoid potentially hazardous activities such as driving or operating heavy machinery during this period.

While the relationship between seizures and the rate of rise of hemoglobin is uncertain, it is recommended that the dose of PROCRIT® be decreased if the hemoglobin increase exceeds 1 g/dL in any 2-week period.

Thrombotic Events: During hemodialysis, patients treated with PROCRIT® may require increased anticoagulation with heparin to prevent clotting of the artificial kidney (see ADVERSE REACTIONS for more information about thrombotic events).

Other thrombotic events (eg, myocardial infarction, cerebrovascular accident, transient ischemic attack) have occurred in clinical trials at an annualized rate of less than 0.04 events per patient year of PROCRIT® therapy. These trials were conducted in adult patients with CRF (whether on dialysis or not) in whom the target hematocrit was 32% to 40%. However, the risk of thrombotic events, including vascular access thrombosis, was significantly increased in adult patients with ischemic heart disease or congestive heart failure receiving PROCRIT® therapy with the goal of reaching a normal hematocrit (42%) as compared to a target hematocrit of 30%. Patients with pre-existing cardiovascular disease should be monitored closely.

Zidovudine-treated HIV-infected Patients

In contrast to CRF patients, PROCRIT® therapy has not been linked to exacerbation of hypertension, seizures, and thrombotic events in HIV-infected patients. However, the clinical data do not rule out an increased risk for serious cardiovascular events.

PRECAUTIONS

The parenteral administration of any biologic product should be attended by appropriate precautions in case allergic or other untoward reactions occur (see CONTRAINDICATIONS). In clinical trials, while transient rashes were occasionally observed concurrently with PROCRIT® therapy, no serious allergic or anaphylactic reactions were reported (see ADVERSE REACTIONS for more information regarding allergic reactions).

The safety and efficacy of PROCRIT® therapy have not been established in patients with a known history of a seizure disorder or underlying hematologic disease (eg, sickle cell anemia, myelodysplastic syndromes, or hypercoagulable disorders).

In some female patients, menses have resumed following PROCRIT® therapy; the possibility of pregnancy should be discussed and the need for contraception evaluated.

Hematology

Exacerbation of porphyria has been observed rarely in patients with CRF treated with PROCRIT®. However, PROCRIT® has not caused increased urinary excretion of porphyrin metabolites in normal volunteers, even in the presence of a rapid erythropoietic response. Nevertheless, PROCRIT® should be used with caution in patients with known porphyria.

In preclinical studies in dogs and rats, but not in monkeys, PROCRIT® therapy was associated with subclinical bone marrow fibrosis. Bone marrow fibrosis is a known complication of CRF in humans and may be related to secondary hyperparathyroidism or unknown factors. The incidence of bone marrow fibrosis was not increased in a study of adult patients on dialysis who were treated with PROCRIT® for 12 to 19 months, compared to the incidence of bone marrow fibrosis in a matched group of patients who had not been treated with PROCRIT®.

Hemoglobin in CRF patients should be measured twice a week; zidovudine-treated HIV-infected and cancer patients should have hemoglobin measured once a week until hemoglobin has been stabilized, and measured periodically thereafter.

Lack or Loss of Response

If the patient fails to respond or to maintain a response to doses within the recommended dosing range, the following etiologies should be considered and evaluated:

1. Iron deficiency: Virtually all patients will eventually require supplemental iron therapy (see IRON EVALUATION).
2. Underlying infectious, inflammatory, or malignant processes.
3. Occult blood loss.
4. Underlying hematologic diseases (ie, thalassemia, refractory anemia, or other myelodysplastic disorders).
5. Vitamin deficiencies: Folic acid or vitamin B$_{12}$.
6. Hemolysis.
7. Aluminum intoxication.
8. Osteitis fibrosa cystica.
9. Pure Red Cell Aplasia (PRCA) or anti-erythropoietin antibody-associated anemia: In the absence of another etiology, the patient should be evaluated for evidence of PRCA and sera should be tested for the presence of antibodies to erythropoietin (see WARNINGS: Pure Red Cell Aplasia).

See DOSAGE AND ADMINISTRATION: Chronic Renal Failure Patients for management of patients with an insufficient hemoglobin response to PROCRIT® therapy.

Iron Evaluation

During PROCRIT® therapy, absolute or functional iron deficiency may develop. Functional iron deficiency, with normal ferritin levels but low transferrin saturation, is presumably due to the inability to mobilize iron stores rapidly enough to support increased erythropoiesis. Transferrin saturation should be at least 20% and ferritin should be at least 100 ng/mL.

Prior to and during PROCRIT® therapy, the patient's iron status, including transferrin saturation (serum iron divided by iron binding capacity) and serum ferritin, should be evaluated. Virtually all patients will eventually require supplemental iron to increase or maintain transferrin saturation to levels which will adequately support erythropoiesis stimulated by PROCRIT®. All surgery patients being treated with PROCRIT® should receive adequate iron supplementation throughout the course of therapy in order to support erythropoiesis and avoid depletion of iron stores.

Drug Interaction

No evidence of interaction of PROCRIT® with other drugs was observed in the course of clinical trials.

Carcinogenesis, Mutagenesis, and Impairment of Fertility

Carcinogenic potential of PROCRIT® has not been evaluated. PROCRIT® does not induce bacterial gene mutation (Ames Test), chromosomal aberrations in mammalian cells, micronuclei in mice, or gene mutation at the HGPRT locus. In female rats treated IV with PROCRIT®, there was a trend for slightly increased fetal wastage at doses of 100 and 500 Units/kg.

Pregnancy Category C

PROCRIT® has been shown to have adverse effects in rats when given in doses 5 times the human dose. There are no adequate and well-controlled studies in pregnant women. PROCRIT® should be used during pregnancy only if potential benefit justifies the potential risk to the fetus.

In studies in female rats, there were decreases in body weight gain, delays in appearance of abdominal hair, delayed eyelid opening, delayed ossification, and decreases in the number of caudal vertebrae in the F1 fetuses of the 500 Units/kg group. In female rats treated IV, there was a trend for slightly increased fetal wastage at doses of 100 and 500 Units/kg. PROCRIT® has not shown any adverse effect at doses as high as 500 Units/kg in pregnant rabbits (from day 6 to 18 of gestation).

Nursing Mothers

Postnatal observations of the live offspring (F1 generation) of female rats treated with PROCRIT® during gestation and lactation revealed no effect of PROCRIT® at doses of up to 500 Units/kg. There were, however, decreases in body weight gain, delays in appearance of abdominal hair, eyelid opening, and decreases in the number of caudal vertebrae in the F1 fetuses of the 500 Units/kg group. There were no PROCRIT®-related effects on the F2 generation fetuses.

It is not known whether PROCRIT® is excreted in human milk. Because many drugs are excreted in human milk, caution should be exercised when PROCRIT® is administered to a nursing woman.

Pediatric Use

See WARNINGS: Pediatrics.

Pediatric Patients on Dialysis: PROCRIT® is indicated in infants (1 month to 2 years), children (2 years to 12 years), and adolescents (12 years to 16 years) for the treatment of anemia associated with CRF requiring dialysis. Safety and effectiveness in pediatric patients less than 1 month old have not been established (see CLINICAL EXPERIENCE: CHRONIC RENAL FAILURE, PEDIATRIC PATIENTS ON DIALYSIS). The safety data from these studies show that there is no increased risk to pediatric CRF patients on dialysis when compared to the safety profile of PROCRIT® in adult CRF patients (see ADVERSE REACTIONS and WARNINGS). Published literature[27-30] provides supportive evidence of the safety and effectiveness of PROCRIT® in pediatric CRF patients on dialysis.

Pediatric Patients Not Requiring Dialysis: Published literature[30,31] has reported the use of PROCRIT® in 133 pediatric patients with anemia associated with CRF not requiring dialysis, ages 3 months to 20 years, treated with 50 to 250 Units/kg SC or IV, QW to TIW. Dose-dependent increases in hemoglobin and hematocrit were observed with reductions in transfusion requirements.

Pediatric HIV-infected Patients: Published literature[32,33] has reported the use of PROCRIT® in 20 zidovudine-treated anemic HIV-infected pediatric patients ages 8 months to 17 years, treated with 50 to 400 Units/kg SC or IV, 2 to 3 times per week. Increases in hemoglobin levels and in reticulocyte counts, and decreases in or elimination of blood transfusions were observed.

Pediatric Cancer Patients on Chemotherapy: The safety and effectiveness of PROCRIT® were evaluated in a randomized, double-blind, placebo-controlled, multicenter study (see CLINICAL EXPERIENCE, Weekly (QW) Dosing, Pediatric Patients).

Geriatric Use

Among 1051 patients enrolled in the 5 clinical trials of PROCRIT® for reduction of allogeneic blood transfusions in patients undergoing elective surgery 745 received PROCRIT® and 306 received placebo. Of the 745 patients who received PROCRIT®, 432 (58%) were aged 65 and over, while 175 (23%) were 75 and over. No overall differences in safety or effectiveness were observed between geriatric and younger patients. The dose requirements for PROCRIT® in geriatric and younger patients within the 4 trials using the TIW schedule were similar. Insufficient numbers of patients were enrolled in the study using the weekly dosing regimen to determine whether the dosing requirements differ for this schedule.

Of the 882 patients enrolled in the 3 studies of chronic renal failure patients on dialysis, 757 received PROCRIT® and 125 received placebo. Of the 757 patients who received PROCRIT®, 361 (47%) were aged 65 and over, while 100 (13%) were 75 and over. No differences in safety or effectiveness were observed between geriatric and younger patients. Dose selection and adjustment for an elderly patient should be individualized to achieve and maintain the target hematocrit (See DOSAGE AND ADMINISTRATION).

Insufficient numbers of patients age 65 or older were enrolled in clinical studies of PROCRIT® for the treatment of anemia associated with pre-dialysis chronic renal failure,

cancer chemotherapy, and Zidovudine-treatment of HIV infection to determine whether they respond differently from younger subjects.

Information for Patients

Patients should be informed of the increased risks of mortality, serious cardiovascular events, thromboembolic events, and increased risk of tumor progression or recurrence (see WARNINGS). In those situations in which the physician determines that a patient or their caregiver can safely and effectively administer PROCRIT® at home, instruction as to the proper dosage and administration should be provided. Patients should be instructed to read the PROCRIT® Medication Guide and Patient Instructions for Use and should be informed that the Medication Guide is not a disclosure of all possible side effects. Patients should be informed of the possible side effects of PROCRIT® and of the signs and symptoms of allergic drug reaction and advised of appropriate actions. If home use is prescribed for a patient, the patient should be thoroughly instructed in the importance of proper disposal and cautioned against the reuse of needles, syringes, or drug product. A puncture-resistant container should be available for the disposal of used syringes and needles, and guidance provided on disposal of the full container.

Chronic Renal Failure Patients

Patients with CRF Not Requiring Dialysis

Blood pressure and hemoglobin should be monitored no less frequently than for patients maintained on dialysis. Renal function and fluid and electrolyte balance should be closely monitored.

Hematology

Sufficient time should be allowed to determine a patient's responsiveness to a dosage of PROCRIT® before adjusting the dose. Because of the time required for erythropoiesis and the red cell half-life, an interval of 2 to 6 weeks may occur between the time of a dose adjustment (initiation, increase, decrease, or discontinuation) and a significant change in hemoglobin.

For patients who respond to PROCRIT® with a rapid increase in hemoglobin (eg, more than 1 g/dL in any 2-week period), the dose of PROCRIT® should be reduced because of the possible association of excessive rate of rise of hemoglobin with an exacerbation of hypertension.

The elevated bleeding time characteristic of CRF decreases toward normal after correction of anemia in adult patients treated with PROCRIT®. Reduction of bleeding time also occurs after correction of anemia by transfusion.

Laboratory Monitoring

The hemoglobin should be determined twice a week until it has stabilized in the suggested hemoglobin range and the maintenance dose has been established. After any dose adjustment, the hemoglobin should also be determined twice weekly for at least 2 to 6 weeks until it has been determined that the hemoglobin has stabilized in response to the dose change. The hemoglobin should then be monitored at regular intervals.

A complete blood count with differential and platelet count should be performed regularly. During clinical trials, modest increases were seen in platelets and white blood cell counts. While these changes were statistically significant, they were not clinically significant and the values remained within normal ranges.

In patients with CRF, serum chemistry values (including blood urea nitrogen [BUN], uric acid, creatinine, phosphorus, and potassium) should be monitored regularly. During clinical trials in adult patients on dialysis, modest increases were seen in BUN, creatinine, phosphorus, and potassium. In some adult patients with CRF not on dialysis treated with PROCRIT®, modest increases in serum uric acid and phosphorus were observed. While changes were statistically significant, the values remained within the ranges normally seen in patients with CRF.

Diet

The importance of compliance with dietary and dialysis prescriptions should be reinforced. In particular, hyperkalemia is not uncommon in patients with CRF. In US studies in patients on dialysis, hyperkalemia has occurred at an annualized rate of approximately 0.11 episodes per patient-year of PROCRIT® therapy, often in association with poor compliance to medication, diet, and/or dialysis.

Dialysis Management

Therapy with PROCRIT® results in an increase in hematocrit and a decrease in plasma volume which could affect dialysis efficiency. In studies to date, the resulting increase in hematocrit did not appear to adversely affect dialyzer function[8,9] or the efficiency of high flux hemodialysis.[10] During hemodialysis, patients treated with PROCRIT® may require increased anticoagulation with heparin to prevent clotting of the artificial kidney.

Patients who are marginally dialyzed may require adjustments in their dialysis prescription. As with all patients on dialysis, the serum chemistry values (including BUN, creatinine, phosphorus, and potassium) in patients treated

with PROCRIT® should be monitored regularly to assure the adequacy of the dialysis prescription.

Renal Function

In adult patients with CRF not on dialysis, renal function and fluid and electrolyte balance should be closely monitored. In patients with CRF not on dialysis, placebo-controlled studies of progression of renal dysfunction over periods of greater than 1 year have not been completed. In shorter term trials in adult patients with CRF not on dialysis, changes in creatinine and creatinine clearance were not significantly different in patients treated with PROCRIT® compared with placebo-treated patients. Analysis of the slope of 1/serum creatinine versus time plots in these patients indicates no significant change in the slope after the initiation of PROCRIT® therapy.

Zidovudine-treated HIV-infected Patients

Hypertension

Exacerbation of hypertension has not been observed in zidovudine-treated HIV-infected patients treated with PROCRIT®. However, PROCRIT® should be withheld in these patients if pre-existing hypertension is uncontrolled, and should not be started until blood pressure is controlled. In double-blind studies, a single seizure has been experienced by a patient treated with PROCRIT®.[23]

Cancer Patients on Chemotherapy

Hypertension

Hypertension, associated with a significant increase in hemoglobin, has been noted rarely in patients treated with PROCRIT®. Nevertheless, blood pressure in patients treated with PROCRIT® should be monitored carefully, particularly in patients with an underlying history of hypertension or cardiovascular disease.

Seizures

In double-blind, placebo-controlled trials, 3.2% (n = 2/63) of patients treated with PROCRIT® TIW and 2.9% (n = 2/68) of placebo-treated patients had seizures. Seizures in 1.6% (n = 1/63) of patients treated with PROCRIT® TIW occurred in the context of a significant increase in blood pressure and hematocrit from baseline values. However, both patients treated with PROCRIT® also had underlying CNS pathology which may have been related to seizure activity.

In a placebo-controlled, double-blind trial utilizing weekly dosing with PROCRIT®, 1.2% (n = 2/168) of safety-evaluable patients treated with PROCRIT® and 1% (n = 1/165) of placebo-treated patients had seizures. Seizures in the patients treated with weekly PROCRIT® occurred in the context of a significant increase in hemoglobin from baseline values however significant increases in blood pressure were not seen. These patients may have had other CNS pathology.

Thrombotic Events

In double-blind, placebo-controlled trials, 3.2% (n = 2/63) of patients treated with PROCRIT® TIW and 11.8% (n = 8/68) of placebo-treated patients had thrombotic events (eg, pulmonary embolism, cerebrovascular accident), (see WARNINGS: Increased Mortality, Serious Cardiovascular Events, Thromboembolic Events, and Stroke).

In a placebo-controlled, double-blind trial utilizing weekly dosing with PROCRIT®, 6.0% (n = 10/168) of safety-evaluable patients treated with PROCRIT® and 3.6% (n = 6/165) (p = 0.444) of placebo-treated patients had clinically significant thrombotic events (deep vein thrombosis requiring anticoagulant therapy, embolic event including pulmonary embolism, myocardial infarction, cerebral ischemia, left ventricular failure and thrombotic microangiopathy). A definitive relationship between the rate of hemoglobin increase and the occurrence of clinically significant thrombotic events could not be evaluated due to the limited schedule of hemoglobin measurements in this study.

The safety and efficacy of PROCRIT® were evaluated in a randomized, double-blind, placebo-controlled, multicenter study that enrolled 222 anemic patients ages 5 to 18 receiving treatment for a variety of childhood malignancies. Due to the study design (small sample size and the heterogeneity of the underlying malignancies and of anti-neoplastic treatments employed), a determination of the effect of PROCRIT® on the incidence of thrombotic events could not be performed. In the PROCRIT® arm, the overall incidence of thrombotic events was 10.8% and the incidence of serious or life-threatening events was 7.2%.

Surgery Patients

Hypertension

Blood pressure may rise in the perioperative period in patients being treated with PROCRIT®. Therefore, blood pressure should be monitored carefully.

ADVERSE REACTIONS

Immunogenicity

As with all therapeutic proteins, there is the potential for immunogenicity. Neutralizing antibodies to erythropoietin, in association with PRCA or severe anemia (with or without other cytopenias), have been reported in patients receiving PROCRIT® (see WARNINGS: Pure Red Cell Aplasia) during post-marketing experience.

There has been no systematic assessment of immune responses, i.e., the incidence of either binding or neutralizing antibodies to PROCRIT®, in controlled clinical trials. Where reported, the incidence of antibody formation is highly dependent on the sensitivity and specificity of the assay. Additionally, the observed incidence of antibody (including neutralizing antibody) positivity in an assay may be influenced by several factors including assay methodology, sample handling, timing of sample collection, concomitant medications, and underlying disease. For these reasons, comparison of the incidence of antibodies across products within this class (erythropoietic proteins) may be misleading.

Chronic Renal Failure Patients
In double-blind, placebo-controlled studies involving over 300 patients with CRF, the events reported in greater than 5% of patients treated with PROCRIT® during the blinded phase were:

Percent of Patients Reporting Event

Event	Patients Treated With PROCRIT® (n = 200)	Placebo-treated Patients (n = 135)
Hypertension	24%	19%
Headache	16%	12%
Arthralgias	11%	6%
Nausea	11%	9%
Edema	9%	10%
Fatigue	9%	14%
Diarrhea	9%	6%
Vomiting	8%	5%
Chest Pain	7%	9%
Skin Reaction (Administration Site)	7%	12%
Asthenia	7%	12%
Dizziness	7%	13%
Clotted Access	7%	2%

Significant adverse events of concern in patients with CRF treated in double-blind, placebo-controlled trials occurred in the following percent of patients during the blinded phase of the studies:

Seizure	1.1%	1.1%
CVA/TIA	0.4%	0.6%
MI	0.4%	1.1%
Death	0%	1.7%

In the US PROCRIT® studies in adult patients on dialysis (over 567 patients), the incidence (number of events per patient-year) of the most frequently reported adverse events were: hypertension (0.75), headache (0.40), tachycardia (0.31), nausea/vomiting (0.26), clotted vascular access (0.25), shortness of breath (0.14), hyperkalemia (0.11), and diarrhea (0.11). Other reported events occurred at a rate of less than 0.10 events per patient per year.

Events reported to have occurred within several hours of administration of PROCRIT® were rare, mild, and transient, and included injection site stinging in dialysis patients and flu-like symptoms such as arthralgias and myalgias.

In all studies analyzed to date, PROCRIT® administration was generally well-tolerated, irrespective of the route of administration.

Pediatric CRF Patients
In pediatric patients with CRF on dialysis, the pattern of most adverse events was similar to that found in adults. Additional adverse events reported during the double-blind phase in >10% of pediatric patients in either treatment group were: abdominal pain, dialysis access complications including access infections and peritonitis in those receiving peritoneal dialysis, fever, upper respiratory infection, cough, pharyngitis, and constipation. The rates are similar between the treatment groups for each event.

Hypertension
Increases in blood pressure have been reported in clinical trials, often during the first 90 days of therapy. On occasion,

hypertensive encephalopathy and seizures have been observed in patients with CRF treated with PROCRIT®. When data from all patients in the US phase 3 multicenter trial were analyzed, there was an apparent trend of more reports of hypertensive adverse events in patients on dialysis with a faster rate of rise of hematocrit (greater than 4 hematocrit points in any 2-week period). However, in a double-blind, placebo-controlled trial, hypertensive adverse events were not reported at an increased rate in the group treated with PROCRIT® (150 Units/kg TIW) relative to the placebo group.

Seizures
There have been 47 seizures in 1010 patients on dialysis treated with PROCRIT® in clinical trials, with an exposure of 986 patient-years for a rate of approximately 0.048 events per patient-year. However, there appeared to be a higher rate of seizures during the first 90 days of therapy (occurring in approximately 2.5% of patients) when compared to subsequent 90-day periods. The baseline incidence of seizures in the untreated dialysis population is difficult to determine; it appears to be in the range of 5% to 10% per patient-year.[34-36]

Thrombotic Events
In clinical trials where the maintenance hematocrit was 35 ± 3% on PROCRIT®, clotting of the vascular access (A-V shunt) has occurred at an annualized rate of about 0.25 events per patient-year, and other thrombotic events (eg, myocardial infarction, cerebral vascular accident, transient ischemic attack, and pulmonary embolism) occurred at a rate of 0.04 events per patient-year. In a separate study of 1111 untreated dialysis patients, clotting of the vascular access occurred at a rate of 0.50 events per patient-year. However, in CRF patients on hemodialysis who also had clinically evident ischemic heart disease or congestive heart failure, the risk of A-V shunt thrombosis was higher (39% vs 29%, p < 0.001), and myocardial infarctions, vascular ischemic events, and venous thrombosis were increased, in patients targeted to a hematocrit of 42 ± 3% compared to those maintained at 30 ± 3% (see WARNINGS).

In patients treated with commercial PROCRIT®, there have been rare reports of serious or unusual thromboembolic events including migratory thrombophlebitis, microvascular thrombosis, pulmonary embolus, and thrombosis of the retinal artery, and temporal and renal veins. A causal relationship has not been established.

Allergic Reactions
There have been no reports of serious allergic reactions or anaphylaxis associated with PROCRIT® administration during clinical trials. Skin rashes and urticaria have been observed rarely and when reported have generally been mild and transient in nature.

There have been rare reports of potentially serious allergic reactions including urticaria with associated respiratory symptoms or circumoral edema, or urticaria alone. Most reactions occurred in situations where a causal relationship could not be established. Symptoms recurred with rechallenge in a few instances, suggesting that allergic reactivity may occasionally be associated with PROCRIT® therapy. If an anaphylactoid reaction occurs, PROCRIT® should be immediately discontinued and appropriate therapy initiated.

Zidovudine-treated HIV-infected Patients
In double-blind, placebo-controlled studies of 3 months duration involving approximately 300 zidovudine-treated HIV-infected patients, adverse events with an incidence of ≥ 10% in either patients treated with PROCRIT® or placebo-treated patients were:

Percent of Patients Reporting Event

Event	Patients Treated With PROCRIT® (n = 144)	Placebo-treated Patients (n = 153)
Pyrexia	38%	29%
Fatigue	25%	31%
Headache	19%	14%
Cough	18%	14%
Diarrhea	16%	18%
Rash	16%	8%
Congestion, Respiratory	15%	10%
Nausea	15%	12%
Shortness of Breath	14%	13%
Asthenia	11%	14%
Skin Reaction Medication Site	10%	7%
Dizziness	9%	10%

In the 297 patients studied, PROCRIT® was not associated with significant increases in opportunistic infections or mor-

tality.[23] In 71 patients from this group treated with PROCRIT® at 150 Units/kg TIW, serum p24 antigen levels did not appear to increase.[25] Preliminary data showed no enhancement of HIV replication in infected cell lines in vitro.[23]

Peripheral white blood cell and platelet counts are unchanged following PROCRIT® therapy.

Allergic Reactions
Two zidovudine-treated HIV-infected patients had urticarial reactions within 48 hours of their first exposure to study medication. One patient was treated with PROCRIT® and one was treated with placebo (PROCRIT® vehicle alone). Both patients had positive immediate skin tests against their study medication with a negative saline control. The basis for this apparent pre-existing hypersensitivity to components of the PROCRIT® formulation is unknown, but may be related to HIV-induced immunosuppression or prior exposure to blood products.

Seizures
In double-blind and open-label trials of PROCRIT® in zidovudine-treated HIV-infected patients, 10 patients have experienced seizures.[23] In general, these seizures appear to be related to underlying pathology such as meningitis or cerebral neoplasms, not PROCRIT® therapy.

Cancer Patients on Chemotherapy
In double-blind, placebo-controlled studies of up to 3 months duration involving 131 cancer patients, adverse events with an incidence > 10% in either patients treated with PROCRIT® or placebo-treated patients were as indicated below:

Percent of Patients Reporting Event

Event	Patients Treated With PROCRIT® (n = 63)	Placebo-treated Patients (n = 68)
Pyrexia	29%	19%
Diarrhea	21%*	7%
Nausea	17%*	32%
Vomiting	17%	15%
Edema	17%*	1%
Asthenia	13%	16%
Fatigue	13%	15%
Shortness of Breath	13%	9%
Paresthesia	11%	6%
Upper Respiratory Infection	11%	4%
Dizziness	5%	12%
Trunk Pain	3%*	16%

*Statistically significant

Although some statistically significant differences between patients being treated with PROCRIT® and placebo-treated patients were noted, the overall safety profile of PROCRIT® appeared to be consistent with the disease process of advanced cancer. During double-blind and subsequent open-label therapy in which patients (n = 72 for total exposure to PROCRIT®) were treated for up to 32 weeks with doses as high as 927 Units/kg, the adverse experience profile of PROCRIT® was consistent with the progression of advanced cancer.

Three hundred thirty-three (333) cancer patients enrolled in a placebo-controlled double-blind trial utilizing Weekly dosing with PROCRIT® for up to 4 months were evaluable for adverse events. The incidence of adverse events was similar in both the treatment and placebo arms.

Surgery Patients
Adverse events with an incidence of ≥ 10% are shown in the following table:
[See first table at top of next page]

Thrombotic/Vascular Events
In three double-blind, placebo-controlled orthopedic surgery studies, the rate of deep venous thrombosis (DVT) was similar among Epoetin alfa and placebo-treated patients in the recommended population of patients with a pretreatment hemoglobin of > 10 g/dL to ≤ 13 g/dL.[17,19,26] However, in 2 of 3 orthopedic surgery studies the overall rate (all pretreatment hemoglobin groups combined) of DVTs detected by postoperative ultrasonography and/or surveillance venography was higher in the group treated with Epoetin alfa than in the placebo-treated group (11% vs. 6%). This finding was attributable to the difference in DVT rates observed in the subgroup of patients with pretreatment hemoglobin > 13 g/dL.

In the orthopedic surgery study of patients with pretreatment hemoglobin of > 10 g/dL to ≤ 13 g/dL which compared two dosing regimens (600 Units/kg weekly × 4 and 300 Units/kg daily × 15), 4 subjects in the 600 Units/kg weekly PROCRIT® group (5%) and no subjects in the 300 Units/kg daily group had a thrombotic vascular event during the study period.[18]

Event	Percent of Patients Reporting Event				
	Patients Treated With PROCRIT® 300 U/kg (n = 112)*	Patients Treated With PROCRIT® 100 U/kg (n = 101)*	Placebo-treated Patients (n = 103)*	Patients Treated With PROCRIT® 600 U/kg (n = 73)†	Patients Treated With PROCRIT® 300 U/kg (n = 72)†
Pyrexia	51%	50%	60%	47%	42%
Nausea	48%	43%	45%	45%	58%
Constipation	43%	42%	43%	51%	53%
Skin Reaction, Medication Site	25%	19%	22%	26%	29%
Vomiting	22%	12%	14%	21%	29%
Skin Pain	18%	18%	17%	5%	4%
Pruritus	16%	16%	14%	14%	22%
Insomnia	13%	16%	13%	21%	18%
Headache	13%	11%	9%	10%	19%
Dizziness	12%	9%	12%	11%	21%
Urinary Tract Infection	12%	3%	11%	11%	8%
Hypertension	10%	11%	10%	5%	10%
Diarrhea	10%	7%	12%	10%	6%
Deep Venous Thrombosis	10%	3%	5%	0%‡	0%‡
Dyspepsia	9%	11%	6%	7%	8%
Anxiety	7%	2%	11%	11%	4%
Edema	6%	11%	8%	11%	7%

* Study including patients undergoing orthopedic surgery treated with PROCRIT® or placebo for 15 days
† Study including patients undergoing orthopedic surgery treated with PROCRIT® 600 Units/kg weekly × 4 or 300 Units/kg daily × 15
‡ Determined by clinical symptoms

Starting Dose:	
Adults	50 to 100 Units/kg TIW; IV or SC
Pediatric Patients	50 Units/kg TIW; IV or SC
Increase Dose by 25% If:	1. Hemoglobin is < 10 g/dL and has not increased by 1 g/dL after 4 weeks of therapy or
	2. Hemoglobin decreases below 10 g/dL
Reduce Dose by 25% When:	1. Hemoglobin approaches 12 g/dL or,
	2. Hemoglobin increases > 1 g/dL in any 2-week period

In a study examining the use of Epoetin alfa in 182 patients scheduled for coronary artery bypass graft surgery, 23% of patients treated with Epoetin alfa and 29% treated with placebo experienced thrombotic/vascular events. There were 4 deaths among the Epoetin alfa-treated patients that were associated with a thrombotic/vascular event (see WARNINGS).

OVERDOSAGE

The expected manifestations of PROCRIT® overdosage include signs and symptoms associated with an excessive and/or rapid increase in hemoglobin concentration, including any of the cardiovascular events described in WARNINGS and listed in ADVERSE REACTIONS. Patients receiving an overdosage of PROCRIT® should be monitored closely for cardiovascular events and hematologic abnormalities. Polycythemia should be managed acutely with phlebotomy, as clinically indicated. Following resolution of the effects due to PROCRIT® overdosage, reintroduction of PROCRIT® therapy should be accompanied by close monitoring for evidence of rapid increases in hemoglobin concentration (>1 gm/dL per 14 days). In patients with an excessive hematopoietic response, reduce the PROCRIT® dose in accordance with the recommendations described in DOSAGE AND ADMINISTRATION.

DOSAGE AND ADMINISTRATION

IMPORTANT: See BOXED WARNINGS and WARNINGS: Increased Mortality, Serious Cardiovascular Events, Thromboembolic Events, and Stroke.

Chronic Renal Failure Patients

The recommended range for the starting dose of PROCRIT® is 50 to 100 Units/kg TIW for adult patients. The recommended starting dose for pediatric CRF patients on dialysis is 50 Units/kg TIW. Individualize dosing to achieve and maintain hemoglobin levels between 10–12 g/dL. The dose of PROCRIT® should be reduced as the hemoglobin approaches 12 g/dL or increases by more than 1 g/dL in any 2-week period. If hemoglobin excursions outside the recommended range occur, the PROCRIT® dose should be adjusted as described below.

PROCRIT® may be given either as an IV or SC injection. *In patients on hemodialysis, the IV route is recommended* (see WARNINGS: Pure Red Cell Aplasia). While the administration of PROCRIT® is independent of the dialysis procedure, PROCRIT® may be administered into the venous line at the end of the dialysis procedure to obviate the need for additional venous access. In adult patients with CRF not on dialysis, PROCRIT® may be given either as an IV or SC injection.

Patients who have been judged competent by their physicians to self-administer PROCRIT® without medical or other supervision may give themselves either an IV or SC injection. The table below provides general therapeutic guidelines for patients with CRF:

Individually titrate to achieve and maintain hemoglobin levels between 10 to 12 g/dL.

[See second table above]

During therapy, hematological parameters should be monitored regularly. Doses must be individualized to ensure that hemoglobin is maintained at an appropriate level for each patient.

For patients whose hemoglobin does not attain a level within the range of 10 to 12 g/dL despite the use of appropriate PROCRIT® dose titrations over a 12-week period:

• do not administer higher PROCRIT® doses and use the lowest dose that will maintain a hemoglobin level sufficient to avoid the need for recurrent RBC transfusions,
• evaluate and treat for other causes of anemia (see PRECAUTIONS: Lack or Loss of Response), and
• thereafter, hemoglobin should continue to be monitored and if responsiveness improves, PROCRIT® dose adjustments should be made as described above; discontinue PROCRIT® if responsiveness does not improve and the patient needs recurrent RBC transfusions.

Pretherapy Iron Evaluation

Prior to and during PROCRIT® therapy, the patient's iron stores, including transferrin saturation (serum iron divided by iron binding capacity) and serum ferritin, should be evaluated. Transferrin saturation should be at least 20%, and ferritin should be at least 100 ng/mL. Virtually all patients will eventually require supplemental iron to increase or maintain transferrin saturation to levels that will adequately support erythropoiesis stimulated by PROCRIT®.

Dose Adjustment

The dose should be adjusted for each patient to achieve and maintain hemoglobin levels between 10 to 12 g/dL.

Increases in dose should not be made more frequently than once a month. If the hemoglobin is increasing and approaching 12 g/dL, the dose should be reduced by approximately 25%. If the hemoglobin continues to increase, dose should be temporarily withheld until the hemoglobin begins to decrease, at which point therapy should be reinitiated at a dose approximately 25% below the previous dose. If the hemoglobin increases by more than 1 g/dL in a 2-week period, the dose should be decreased by approximately 25%.

If the increase in the hemoglobin is less than 1 g/dL over 4 weeks and iron stores are adequate (see PRECAUTIONS: Laboratory Monitoring), the dose of PROCRIT® may be increased by approximately 25% of the previous dose. Further increases may be made at 4-week intervals until the specified hemoglobin is obtained.

Maintenance Dose

The maintenance dose must be individualized for each patient on dialysis. In the US phase 3 multicenter trial in patients on hemodialysis, the median maintenance dose was 75 Units/kg TIW, with a range from 12.5 to 525 Units/kg TIW. Almost 10% of the patients required a dose of 25 Units/kg, or less, and approximately 10% of the patients required more than 200 Units/kg TIW to maintain their hematocrit in the suggested target range. In pediatric hemodialysis and peritoneal dialysis patients, the median maintenance dose was 167 Units/kg/week (49 to 447 Units/kg per week) and 76 Units/kg per week (24 to 323 Units/kg/week) administered in divided doses (TIW or BIW), respectively to achieve the target range of 30% to 36%.

If the transferrin saturation is greater than 20%, the dose of PROCRIT® may be increased. Such dose increases should not be made more frequently than once a month, unless clinically indicated, as the response time of the hemoglobin to a dose increase can be 2 to 6 weeks. Hemoglobin should be measured twice weekly for 2 to 6 weeks following dose increases. In adult patients with CRF not on dialysis, the dose should also be individualized to maintain hemoglobin levels between 10 to 12 g/dL. PROCRIT® doses of 75 to 150 Units/kg/week have been shown to maintain hematocrits of 36% to 38% for up to 6 months.

Lack or Loss of Response

If a patient fails to respond or maintain a response, an evaluation for causative factors should be undertaken (see WARNINGS: Pure Red Cell Aplasia, PRECAUTIONS: Lack or Loss of Response, and PRECAUTIONS: Iron Evaluation). If the transferrin saturation is less than 20%, supplemental iron should be administered.

Zidovudine-treated HIV-infected Patients

Prior to beginning PROCRIT®, it is recommended that the endogenous serum erythropoietin level be determined (prior to transfusion). Available evidence suggests that patients receiving zidovudine with endogenous serum erythropoietin levels > 500 mUnits/mL are unlikely to respond to therapy with PROCRIT®.

In zidovudine-treated HIV-infected patients the dosage of PROCRIT® should be titrated for each patient to achieve and maintain the lowest hemoglobin level sufficient to avoid the need for blood transfusion and not to exceed the upper safety limit of 12 g/dL.

Starting Dose

For adult patients with serum erythropoietin levels ≤ 500 mUnits/mL who are receiving a dose of zidovudine ≤ 4200 mg/week, the recommended starting dose of PROCRIT® is 100 Units/kg as an IV or SC injection TIW for 8 weeks. For pediatric patients, see PRECAUTIONS: PEDIATRIC USE.

Increase Dose

During the dose adjustment phase of therapy, the hemoglobin should be monitored weekly. If the response is not satisfactory in terms of reducing transfusion requirements or increasing hemoglobin after 8 weeks of therapy, the dose of PROCRIT® can be increased by 50 to 100 Units/kg TIW. Response should be evaluated every 4 to 8 weeks thereafter and the dose adjusted accordingly by 50 to 100 Units/kg increments TIW. If patients have not responded satisfactorily to a PROCRIT® dose of 300 Units/kg TIW, it is unlikely that they will respond to higher doses of PROCRIT®.

Maintenance Dose

After attainment of the desired response (ie, reduced transfusion requirements or increased hemoglobin), the dose of PROCRIT® should be titrated to maintain the response based on factors such as variations in zidovudine dose and the presence of intercurrent infectious or inflammatory episodes. If the hemoglobin exceeds the upper safety limit of 12 g/dL, the dose should be discontinued until the hemoglobin drops below 11 g/dL. The dose should be reduced by 25% when treatment is resumed and then titrated to maintain the desired hemoglobin.

Cancer Patients on Chemotherapy

Only prescribers enrolled in the ESA APPRISE Oncology Program may prescribe and/or dispense PROCRIT® (see WARNINGS: ESA APPRISE Oncology Program).

Although no specific serum erythropoietin level has been established which predicts which patients would be unlikely to respond to PROCRIT® therapy, treatment of patients with grossly elevated serum erythropoietin levels (eg, > 200 mUnits/mL) is not recommended. Therapy should not be initiated at hemoglobin levels ≥ 10 g/dL. The hemoglobin should be monitored on a weekly basis in patients receiving PROCRIT® therapy until hemoglobin becomes stable. The dose of PROCRIT® should be titrated for each patient to achieve and maintain the lowest hemoglobin level sufficient to avoid the need for blood transfusion (see recommended Dose Modifications, below).

Recommended Dose

The initial recommended dose of PROCRIT® in adults is 150 Units/kg SC TIW or 40,000 Units SC Weekly. The initial recommended dose of PROCRIT® in pediatric patients is

600 Units/kg IV weekly. Discontinue PROCRIT® following the completion of a chemotherapy course (see BOXED WARNINGS: Cancer).

Dose Modification
[See table at right]

Surgery Patients

Prior to initiating treatment with PROCRIT® a hemoglobin should be obtained to establish that it is > 10 to ≤ 13 g/dL.[17] The recommended dose of PROCRIT® is 300 Units/kg/day subcutaneously for 10 days before surgery, on the day of surgery, and for 4 days after surgery.

An alternate dose schedule is 600 Units/kg PROCRIT® subcutaneously in once weekly doses (21, 14, and 7 days before surgery) plus a fourth dose on the day of surgery.[18]

All patients should receive adequate iron supplementation. Iron supplementation should be initiated no later than the beginning of treatment with PROCRIT® and should continue throughout the course of therapy. Deep venous thrombosis prophylaxis should be strongly considered (see BOXED WARNINGS).

PREPARATION AND ADMINISTRATION OF PROCRIT®

1. Do not shake. It is not necessary to shake PROCRIT®. Prolonged vigorous shaking may denature any glycoprotein, rendering it biologically inactive.

2. Protect the solution from light. Parenteral drug products should be inspected visually for particulate matter and discoloration prior to administration. Do not use any vials exhibiting particulate matter or discoloration.

3. Using aseptic techniques, attach a sterile needle to a sterile syringe. Remove the flip top from the vial containing PROCRIT®, and wipe the septum with a disinfectant. Insert the needle into the vial, and withdraw into the syringe an appropriate volume of solution.

4. **Single-dose:** 1 mL vial contains no preservative. Use one dose per vial; do not re-enter the vial. Discard unused portions.
   Multidose: 1 mL and 2 mL vials contain preservative. Store at 2° to 8° C after initial entry and between doses. Discard 21 days after initial entry.

5. Do not dilute or administer in conjunction with other drug solutions. However, at the time of SC administration, preservative-free PROCRIT® from single-use vials may be admixed in a syringe with bacteriostatic 0.9% sodium chloride injection, USP, with benzyl alcohol 0.9% (bacteriostatic saline) at a 1:1 ratio using aseptic technique. The benzyl alcohol in the bacteriostatic saline acts as a local anesthetic which may ameliorate SC injection site discomfort. Admixing is not necessary when using the multidose vials of PROCRIT® containing benzyl alcohol.

HOW SUPPLIED

PROCRIT®, containing Epoetin alfa, is available in the following packages:

1 mL **Single-Dose, Preservative-free** Solution
Cartons containing six (6) **single-dose** vials:
2000 Units/mL (NDC 59676-302-01)
3000 Units/mL (NDC 59676-303-01)
4000 Units/mL (NDC 59676-304-01)
10,000 Units/mL (NDC 59676-310-01)
Cartons containing four (4) **single-dose** vials:
40,000 Units/mL (NDC 59676-340-01)
Trays containing twenty-five (25) **single-dose** vials:
2000 Units/mL (NDC 59676-302-02)
3000 Units/mL (NDC 59676-303-02)
4000 Units/mL (NDC 59676-304-02)
10,000 Units/mL (NDC 59676-310-02)
2 mL **Multidose, Preserved** Solution
Cartons containing four (4) **multidose** vials:
10,000 Units/mL (NDC 59676-312-04)
Cartons containing six (6) **multidose** vials:
10,000 Units/mL (NDC 59676-312-01)
1 mL **Multidose, Preserved** Solution
Cartons containing four (4) **multidose** vials:
20,000 Units/mL (NDC 59676-320-04)
Cartons containing six (6) **multidose** vials:
20,000 Units/mL (NDC 59676-320-01)

STORAGE

Store at 2° to 8° C (36 ° to 46° F). Do not freeze or shake. Protect from light.

TIW Dosing

Starting Dose:	
Adults	150 Units/kg SC TIW
Reduce Dose by 25% when:	Hemoglobin reaches a level needed to avoid transfusion or increases > 1 g/dL in any 2-week period
Withhold Dose if:	Hemoglobin exceeds a level needed to avoid transfusion. Restart at 25% below the previous dose when the hemoglobin approaches a level where transfusions may be required.
Increase Dose to 300 Units/kg TIW if:	Response is not satisfactory (no reduction in transfusion requirements or rise in hemoglobin) after 4 weeks to achieve and maintain the lowest hemoglobin level sufficient to avoid the need for RBC transfusion.
Discontinue:	If after 8 weeks of therapy there is no response as measured by hemoglobin levels or if transfusions are still required.

Weekly Dosing

Starting Dose:	
Adults	40,000 Units SC
Pediatrics	600 Units/kg IV (maximum 40,000 Units)
Reduce Dose by 25% when:	Hemoglobin reaches a level needed to avoid transfusion or increases > 1 g/dL in any 2-weeks.
Withhold Dose if:	Hemoglobin exceeds a level needed to avoid transfusion and restart at 25% below the previous dose when the hemoglobin approaches a level where transfusions may be required.
Increase Dose if: For Adults: 60,000 Units SC Weekly For Pediatrics: 900 Units/kg IV (maximum 60,000 Units) if:	Response is not satisfactory (no increase in hemoglobin by ≥ 1g/dL after 4 weeks of therapy, in the absence of a RBC transfusion) to achieve and maintain the lowest hemoglobin level sufficient to avoid the need for RBC transfusion.
Discontinue:	If after 8 weeks of therapy there is no response as measured by hemoglobin levels or if transfusions are still required.

REFERENCES

1. Egrie JC, Strickland TW, Lane J, et al. Characterization and Biological Effects of Recombinant Human Erythropoietin. *Immunobiol.* 1986;72:213–224.

2. Graber SE, Krantz SB. Erythropoietin and the Control of Red Cell Production. *Ann Rev Med.* 1978;29:51–66.

3. Eschbach JW, Adamson JW. Anemia of End-Stage Renal Disease (ESRD). *Kidney Intl.* 1985;28:1–5.

4. Eschbach JW, Egrie JC, Downing MR, et al. Correction of the Anemia of End-Stage Renal Disease with Recombinant Human Erythropoietin. *NEJM.* 1987;316:73–78.

5. Eschbach JW, Abdulhadi MH, Browne JK, et al. Recombinant Human Erythropoietin in Anemic Patients with End-Stage Renal Disease. *Ann Intern Med.* 1989; 111:992–1000.

6. Eschbach JW, Egrie JC, Downing MR, et al. The Use of Recombinant Human Erythropoietin (r-HuEPO): Effect in End-Stage Renal Disease (ESRD). In: Friedman, Beyer, DeSanto, Giordano, eds. *Prevention of Chronic Uremia.* Philadelphia, PA: Field and Wood Inc. 1989: 148–155.

7. Egrie JC, Eschbach JW, McGuire T, Adamson JW. Pharmacokinetics of Recombinant Human Erythropoietin (r-HuEPO) Administered to Hemodialysis (HD) Patients. *Kidney Intl.* 1988;33:262.

8. Paganini E, Garcia J, Ellis P, et al. Clinical Sequelae of Correction of Anemia with Recombinant Human Erythropoietin (r-HuEPO); Urea Kinetics, Dialyzer Function and Reuse. *Am J Kid Dis.* 1988;11:16.

9. Delano BG, Lundin AP, Golansky R, et al. Dialyzer Urea and Creatinine Clearances Not Significantly Changed in r-HuEPO Treated Maintenance Hemodialysis (MD) Patients. *Kidney Intl.* 1988;33:219.

10. Stivelman J, Van Wyck D, Ogden D. Use of Recombinant Erythropoietin (r-HuEPO) with High Flux Dialysis (HFD) Does Not Worsen Azotemia or Shorten Access Survival. *Kidney Intl.* 1988;33:239.

11. Lim VS, DeGowin RL, Zavala D, et al. Recombinant Human Erythropoietin Treatment in Pre-Dialysis Patients: A Double-Blind Placebo Controlled Trial. *Ann Int Med.* 1989;110:108–114.

12. Stone WJ, Graber SE, Krantz SB, et al. Treatment of the Anemia of Pre-Dialysis Patients with Recombinant Human Erythropoietin: A Randomized, Placebo-Controlled Trial. *Am J Med Sci.* 1988;296:171–179.

13. Braun A, Ding R, Seidel C, Fies T, Kurtz A, Scharer K. Pharmacokinetics of recombinant human erythropoietin applied subcutaneously to children with chronic renal failure. *Pediatr Nephrol.* 1993;7:61–64.

14. Geva P, Sherwood JB. Pharmacokinetics of recombinant human erythropoietin (rHuEPO) in pediatric patients on chronic cycling peritoneal dialysis (CCPD). *Blood.* 1991;78 (Suppl 1):91a.

15. Jabs K, Grant JR, Harmon W, et al. Pharmacokinetics of Epoetin alfa (rHuEPO) in pediatric hemodialysis (HD) patients. *J Am Soc Nephrol.* 1991;2:380.

16. Kling PJ, Widness JA, Guillery EN, Veng-Pedersen P, Peters C, DeAlarcon PA. Pharmacokinetics and pharmacodynamics of erythropoietin during therapy in an infant with renal failure. *J Pediatr.* 1992;121:822–825.

17. deAndrade JR and Jove M. Baseline Hemoglobin as a Predictor of Risk of Transfusion and Response to Epoetin alfa in Orthopedic Surgery Patients. *Am. J. of Orthoped.* 1996;25 (8):533–542.

18. Goldberg MA and McCutchen JW. A Safety and Efficacy Comparison Study of Two Dosing Regimens of Epoetin alfa in Patients Undergoing Major Orthopedic Surgery. *Am. J. of Orthoped.* 1996;25 (8):544–552.

19. Faris PM and Ritter MA. The Effects of Recombinant Human Erythropoietin on Perioperative Transfusion Requirements in Patients Having a Major Orthopedic Operation. *J. Bone and Joint Surgery.* 1996;78-A:62–72.

20. Amgen Inc., data on file.

21. Eschbach JW, Kelly MR, Haley NR, et al. Treatment of the Anemia of Progressive Renal Failure with Recombinant Human Erythropoietin. *NEJM.* 1989;321:158–163.

22. The US Recombinant Human Erythropoietin Predialysis Study Group. Double-Blind, Placebo-Controlled Study of the Therapeutic Use of Recombinant Human Erythropoietin for Anemia Associated with Chronic Renal Failure in Predialysis Patients. *Am J Kid Dis.* 1991;18:50–59.

23. Ortho Biologics, Inc., data on file.

24. Danna RP, Rudnick SA, Abels RI. Erythropoietin Therapy for the Anemia Associated with AIDS and AIDS Therapy and Cancer. In: MB Garnick, ed. *Erythropoietin in Clinical Applications — An International Perspective.* New York, NY: Marcel Dekker; 1990:301–324.

25. Fischl M, Galpin JE, Levine JD, et al. Recombinant Human Erythropoietin for Patients with AIDS Treated with Zidovudine. *NEJM.* 1990;322:1488–1493.

26. Laupacis A. Effectiveness of Perioperative Recombinant Human Erythropoietin in Elective Hip Replacement. *Lancet.* 1993;341:1228–1232.

27. Campos A, Garin EH. Therapy of renal anemia in children and adolescents with recombinant human erythropoietin (rHuEPO). *Clin Pediatr (Phila).* 1992;31:94–99.

28. Montini G, Zacchello G, Baraldi E, et al. Benefits and risks of anemia correction with recombinant human erythropoietin in children maintained by hemodialysis. *J Pediatr.* 1990;117:556–560.

29. Offner G, Hoyer PF, Latta K, Winkler L, Brodehl J, Scigalla P. One year's experience with recombinant erythropoietin in children undergoing continuous ambulatory or cycling peritoneal dialysis. *Pediatr Nephrol.* 1990;4:498–500.

30. Muller-Wiefel DE, Scigalla P. Specific problems of renal anemia in childhood. *Contrib Nephrol.* 1988;66:71–84.

31. Scharer K, Klare B, Dressel P, Gretz N. Treatment of renal anemia by subcutaneous erythropoietin in children with preterminal chronic renal failure. *Acta Paediatr.* 1993;82:953–958.

32. Mueller BU, Jacobsen RN, Jarosinski P, et al. Erythropoietin for zidovudine-associated anemia in children with HIV infection. *Pediatr AIDS and HIV Infect: Fetus to Adolesc.* 1994;5:169–173.

33. Zuccotti GV, Plebani A, Biasucci G, et al. Granulocyte-colony stimulating factor and erythropoietin therapy in children with human immunodeficiency virus infection. *J Int Med Res.* 1996;24:115–121.

34. Raskin NH, Fishman RA. Neurologic Disorders in Renal Failure (First of Two Parts). *NEJM.* 1976;294:143–148.

35. Raskin NH and Fishman RA. Neurologic Disorders in Renal Failure (Second of Two Parts). *NEJM.* 1976;294: 204–210.

36. Messing RO, Simon RP. Seizures as a Manifestation of Systemic Disease. *Neurologic Clinics.* 1986;4:563–584.

37. Besarab A, Bolton WK, Browne JK, et al. The effects of normal as compared with low hematocrit values in patients with cardiac disease who are receiving hemodialysis and epoetin. *NEJM.* 1998;339:584–90.

38. Henke, M, Laszig, R, Rübe, C., et al. Erythropoietin to treat head and neck cancer patients with anaemia un-

dergoing radiotherapy: randomized, double-blind, placebo-controlled trial. *The Lancet.* 2003; 362: 1255–1260.
39. Widness JA, Veng-Pedersen P, Peters C, Pereira LM, Schmidt RL, Lowe SL. Erythropoietin Pharmacokinetics in Premature Infants: Developmental, Nonlinearity, and Treatment Effects. *J Appl Physiol.* 1996;80 (1): 140–148.
40. Singh AK, Szczech L, Tang KL, et al. Correction of Anemia with Epoetin Alfa in Chronic Kidney Disease, *N Engl j Med.* 2006; 355:2085–98.
41. Bohlius J, Wilson J, Seidenfeld J, et at. Recombinant Human Erythropoietins and Cancer Patients: Updated Meta-Analysis of 57 Studies Including 9353 Patients. *J Natl Cancer Inst.* 2006; 98:708–14.
42. D'Ambra MN, Gray RJ, Hillman R, et al. Effect of Recombinant Human Erythropoietin on Transfusion Risk in Coronary Bypass Patients. *Ann Thorac Surg.* 1997; 64: 1686–93.
43. Leyland-Jones B, Semiglazov V, Pawlicki M, et al. Maintaining Normal Hemoglobin Levels With Epoetin Alfa in Mainly Nonanemic Patients With Metastatic Breast Cancer Receiving First-Line Chemotherapy: A Survival Study. *JCO.* 2005; 23(25): 1–13.

This product's label may have been revised after this insert was used in production. For further product information and the current package insert, please visit www.PROCRIT.com or call our Medical Information Group toll-free at 1 888 2ASK OBI (1-888-227-5624).

Manufactured by:
Amgen Inc.
One Amgen Center Drive
Thousand Oaks, CA 91320-1799
Manufactured for:
Centocor Ortho Biotech Products, L.P.
Raritan, New Jersey 08869-0670
Revised: 02/2010 10112805

Printed in U. S. A.

MEDICATION GUIDE

PROCRIT® (PRO'-KRIT)
(epoetin alfa)

Read this Medication Guide before you start PROCRIT, each time you refill your prescription, and if you are told by your healthcare provider that there is new information about PROCRIT. This Medication Guide does not take the place of talking to your healthcare provider about your medical condition or your treatment. Talk with your healthcare provider regularly about the use of PROCRIT and ask if there is new information about PROCRIT.

What is the most important information I should know about PROCRIT?

Using PROCRIT can lead to death or other serious side effects.

Patients with cancer:

Your healthcare provider has received special training through the ESA APPRISE Oncology Program in order to prescribe PROCRIT. Before you can begin to receive PROCRIT, you must sign the ESA APPRISE Oncology Patient and Healthcare Professional (HCP) Acknowledgement Form to document that your healthcare provider discussed the risks of PROCRIT with you. When you sign this form, you are stating that you are aware of the risks associated with use of PROCRIT.

These risks include that your tumor may grow faster and you may die sooner when PROCRIT is used experimentally to try to raise your hemoglobin beyond the amount needed to avoid red blood cell transfusion or if you are not getting strong doses of chemotherapy. It is not known whether these risks exist when PROCRIT is given according to the FDA-approved directions for use.

You should discuss with your doctor:
- Why PROCRIT treatment is being prescribed.
- What are the chances you will get red blood cell transfusions if you do not take PROCRIT.
- What are the chances you will get red blood cell transfusions even if you take PROCRIT.
- How taking PROCRIT may affect the success of your cancer treatment.

If you decide to take PROCRIT, your healthcare provider should prescribe the smallest dose of PROCRIT to lower the chance of getting red blood cell transfusions.
- After you have finished your chemotherapy course, PROCRIT treatment should be stopped.
- PROCRIT does not improve the symptoms of anemia (lower than normal number of red blood cells), quality of life, fatigue, or well-being for patients with cancer.

All patients, including patients with cancer or chronic kidney failure:
- You may get serious heart problems such as heart attack, stroke, heart failure, and may die sooner if you are treated with PROCRIT to a hemoglobin level above 12 g/dL.
- You may get blood clots at any time while taking PROCRIT. If you are receiving PROCRIT and you are going to have surgery, talk to your healthcare provider about whether or not you need to take a blood thinner to lessen the chance of blood clots during or following surgery. Clots can form in blood vessels (veins), especially in your leg (deep venous thrombosis or DVT). Pieces of a blood clot may travel to the lungs and block the blood circulation in the lungs (pulmonary embolus).

Call your healthcare provider or get medical help right away if you have any of these symptoms of blood clots:
- Chest pain
- Trouble breathing or shortness of breath
- Pain in your legs, with or without swelling
- A cool or pale arm or leg
- Sudden confusion, trouble speaking, or trouble understanding others' speech
- Sudden numbness or weakness in your face, arm, or leg, especially on one side of your body
- Sudden trouble seeing
- Sudden trouble walking, dizziness, loss of balance or coordination
- Loss of consciousness (fainting)
- Hemodialysis vascular access stops working. If you are a patient with chronic kidney failure and have a hemodialysis vascular access, blood clots may form in this access.

Also see **"What are the possible side effects of PROCRIT?"** below.

What is PROCRIT?

PROCRIT is a man-made form of the protein human erythropoietin that is given to patients to lessen the need for red blood cell transfusions. PROCRIT stimulates your bone marrow to make more red blood cells. Having more red blood cells raises your hemoglobin level. If your hemoglobin level stays too high or if your hemoglobin goes up too quickly, this may lead to serious health problems which may result in death. These serious health problems may happen even if you take PROCRIT and do not have an increase in your hemoglobin level.

PROCRIT may be used to treat a lower than normal number of red blood cells (anemia) if it is caused by:
- Chronic kidney failure (you may or may not be on dialysis)
- Chemotherapy that is used for at least two months to treat some types of cancer
- A medicine called zidovudine (AZT) used to treat HIV infection

PROCRIT may also be used if you are scheduled for certain surgeries with a lot of blood loss to reduce the chance you will need red blood cell transfusions.

PROCRIT should not be used for treatment of anemia:
- In place of emergency treatment (red blood cell transfusions)
- If you have cancer and you are not receiving chemotherapy that may cause anemia
- If your cancer has a high chance of being cured

PROCRIT should not be used if you are scheduled for certain surgeries and you are able and willing to donate blood prior to surgery.

Who should not take PROCRIT?

Do not take PROCRIT if you:
- Have cancer and have not been counseled by your healthcare provider regarding the risks of PROCRIT and signed the ESA APPRISE Oncology Program Patient and Healthcare Professional (HCP) Acknowledgement Form before you begin to receive PROCRIT.
- Have high blood pressure that is not controlled (uncontrolled hypertension).
- Have been told by your healthcare provider that you have or have ever had a type of anemia called Pure Red Cell Aplasia (PRCA) that starts after treatment with PROCRIT or other erythropoietin medicines.
- Have allergies to any of the ingredients in PROCRIT. See the end of this Medication Guide for a complete list of ingredients in PROCRIT.

Do not give PROCRIT from multidose vials to premature babies.

What should I tell my healthcare provider before taking PROCRIT?

PROCRIT may not be right for you. **Tell your healthcare provider about all your health conditions,** including if you:
- Have heart disease.
- Have high blood pressure.
- Have had a seizure (convulsion) or stroke.
- Are pregnant or planning to become pregnant. It is not known if PROCRIT may harm your unborn baby. Talk with your healthcare provider about possible pregnancy and birth control choices that are right for you.
- Are breast-feeding or planning to breast-feed. It is not known if PROCRIT passes into breast milk.

Tell your healthcare provider about all the medicines you take, including prescription and nonprescription medicines, vitamins, and herbal supplements.

Know the medicines you take. Keep a list of your medicines with you and show it to your healthcare provider when you get a new medicine.

How should I take PROCRIT?

Patients with cancer:

Before you begin to receive PROCRIT, your healthcare provider will:
- Ask you to review this PROCRIT Medication Guide
- Explain the risks of PROCRIT and answer all your questions about PROCRIT
- Have you sign the ESA APPRISE Oncology Program Patient and Healthcare Professional (HCP) Acknowledgement Form

All patients:
- Continue to follow your healthcare provider's instructions for diet, dialysis, and medicines, including medicines for high blood pressure, while taking PROCRIT.
- Have your blood pressure checked as instructed by your healthcare provider.
- If you or your caregiver has been trained to give PROCRIT shots (injections) at home:
  - Be sure that you read, understand, and follow the "Patient Instructions for Use" that come with PROCRIT.
  - Take PROCRIT exactly as your healthcare provider tells you to. Do not change the dose of PROCRIT unless told to do so by your healthcare provider.
  - Your healthcare provider will show you how much PROCRIT to use, how to inject it, how often it should be injected, and how to safely throw away the used vial, syringes, and needles.
  - If you miss a dose of PROCRIT, call your healthcare provider right away and ask what to do.
  - If you take more than the prescribed amount of PROCRIT, call your healthcare provider right away.

What are the possible side effects of PROCRIT?

PROCRIT may cause serious side effects. See **"What is the most important information I should know about PROCRIT?"**

Other side effects of PROCRIT, which may also be serious, include:
- **High blood pressure in patients with chronic kidney failure.** Your blood pressure may go up or be difficult to control with blood pressure medicines while taking PROCRIT. This can happen even if you have never had high blood pressure before. Your healthcare provider should check your blood pressure often. If your blood pressure does go up, your healthcare provider may prescribe new or more blood pressure medicine.
- **Seizures.** If you have any seizures while taking PROCRIT, get medical help right away and tell your healthcare provider.
- **Antibodies to PROCRIT.** Your body may make antibodies to PROCRIT. These antibodies can block or lessen your body's ability to make red blood cells and cause you to have severe anemia. Call your healthcare provider if you have unusual tiredness, lack of energy, dizziness, or fainting. You may need to stop taking PROCRIT.
- **Serious allergic reactions.** Serious allergic reactions can cause a rash over your whole body, shortness of breath, wheezing, dizziness and fainting because of a drop in blood pressure, swelling around your mouth or eyes, fast pulse, or sweating. If you have a serious allergic reaction, stop using PROCRIT and call your healthcare provider or get medical help right away.
- **Dangers of giving PROCRIT to premature babies.** PROCRIT from multi-dose vials contain benzyl alcohol. Do not give PROCRIT from multidose vials to premature babies because it can cause death and brain damage.

Common side effects of PROCRIT include:
- Rash
- Swelling in your legs and arms
- Injection site reaction, including irritation and pain

These are not all of the possible side effects of PROCRIT. Your healthcare provider can give you a more complete list. Tell your healthcare provider about any side effects that bother you or that do not go away.

Call your doctor for medical advice about side effects. You may report side effects to FDA at 1-800-FDA-1088.

How should I store PROCRIT?
- Store PROCRIT in the refrigerator between 36°F to 46°F (2°C to 8°C).
- **Do not freeze.** Do not use a vial of PROCRIT that has been frozen.
- Keep away from direct light.
- Do not shake PROCRIT.
- Throw away multidose vials of PROCRIT after 21 days from the first day that you put a needle into the vial.
- Single use vials of PROCRIT should be used only one time. Throw the vial away after use even if there is medicine left in the vial.

Keep PROCRIT and all medicines out of the reach of children.

General information about PROCRIT

Medicines are sometimes prescribed for purposes other than those listed in a Medication Guide. Use PROCRIT only for the condition for which it has been prescribed. Do not give PROCRIT to other people even if they have the same symptoms that you have. It may harm them.

This Medication Guide summarizes the most important information about PROCRIT. If you would like more information about PROCRIT, talk to your healthcare provider. You can ask your healthcare provider or pharmacist for information about PROCRIT that is written for healthcare professionals. For more information, go to the following website: www.PROCRIT.com or call 1 888 2ASK OBI (1-888-227-5624).

What are the ingredients in PROCRIT?

Active Ingredient: epoetin alfa

Inactive Ingredients: All formulations include albumin (human), sodium citrate, sodium chloride, and citric acid in Water for Injection. Multidose vials contain benzyl alcohol. Certain formulations also contain sodium phosphate monobasic monohydrate and sodium phosphate dibasic anhydrate.

Manufactured by:
Amgen Manufacturing, Limited, a subsidiary of Amgen Inc.
One Amgen Center Drive
Thousand Oaks, CA 91320-1799

Manufactured for:
Centocor Ortho Biotech Products, L.P.
Raritan, New Jersey 08869-0670
© COBPLP 2000
Printed in U. S. A.
Revised: 02/2010
This Medication Guide has been approved by the U.S. Food and Drug Administration.

Patient Instructions for Use

PROCRIT® (PRO´-KRIT)
(epoetin alfa)

Use these instructions if you or your caregiver has been trained to give PROCRIT injections at home. Do not give yourself the injection unless you have received training from your healthcare provider. If you are not sure about giving the injection or you have questions, ask your healthcare provider for help.

Before reading these instructions for use, read the Medication Guide that comes with PROCRIT for the most important information you need to know.

When you receive your PROCRIT vial and syringes make sure that:

- The name PROCRIT appears on the carton and vial label.
- The expiration date on the vial label has not passed. Do not use a vial of PROCRIT after the expiration date on the label.
- The dose strength of the PROCRIT vial (number of Units per mL on the vial label) is the same as your healthcare provider prescribed.
- You understand what the dose strength of PROCRIT means. PROCRIT vials come in several dose strengths. For example, the dose strength may be described as 10,000 Units/mL on the vial label. This strength means that 10,000 Units of medicine are contained in each 1 mL (milliliter) of liquid. Your healthcare provider may also refer to a mL as a "cc." One mL is the same as one "cc."
- The PROCRIT liquid in the vial is clear and colorless. Do not use PROCRIT if the liquid in the vial looks discolored or cloudy, or if the liquid has lumps, flakes, or particles.
- The PROCRIT vial has a color cap on the top of the vial. Do not use a vial of PROCRIT if the color cap on the top of the vial has been removed or is missing.
- Use only the type of disposable syringe and needle that your healthcare provider has prescribed.
- Do not shake PROCRIT. If shaking has occurred, the solution in the vial may look foamy and should not be used.
- Do not freeze PROCRIT. Do not use a vial of PROCRIT that has been frozen.
- Keep PROCRIT away from light.

How should I prepare for an injection of PROCRIT?

- Always keep an extra syringe and needle on hand.
- Follow your healthcare provider's instructions on how to measure your dose of PROCRIT. This dose will be measured in Units per mL or cc (1 mL is the same as 1 cc). Use a syringe that is marked in tenths of mL (for example, 0.2 mL or 0.2 cc). Using the wrong syringe can lead to a mistake in your dose and you could inject too much or too little PROCRIT.

Only use disposable syringes and needles. Use the syringes and needles only one time and then throw them away as instructed by your healthcare provider.

What do I need to know about the different types of PROCRIT vials?

PROCRIT comes in two different types of vials.
- Single-Use Vials
- Multidose-Use Vials

Single-Use Vials

If you have been prescribed PROCRIT vials for single use:
- Single-Use vials of PROCRIT come in several different strengths (Units per mL). For example, the vial label may say the strength is 2,000 Units/mL, which means the vial contains 2,000 Units of medicine in 1 mL. Injecting 1 mL of this strength means you will receive 2,000 Units of PROCRIT.
- Double-check to be sure you are using a vial that contains the correct strength of PROCRIT.
- The Single-Use Vials cannot be used more than one time and any unused medicine in the vial should be thrown away as directed by your healthcare provider.

Multidose-Use Vials

If you have been prescribed PROCRIT vials for use multiple times:
- Multidose vials of PROCRIT may be used to inject more than one dose of PROCRIT, as prescribed by your healthcare provider.
- Multidose vials of PROCRIT come in 1 mL and 2 mL vials.
  ○ 1 mL vials contain 20,000 Units of PROCRIT in 1 mL of liquid (this means each vial contains a total of 20,000 Units of PROCRIT).
  ○ 2 mL vials contain 10,000 Units of PROCRIT in each 1 mL of liquid, and since the vials contain a total of 2 mL of liquid, each vial contains a total of 20,000 Units of PROCRIT.
- After removing a dose from the vial, store the vial in the refrigerator (but not the freezer). Do not store the vial for more than 21 days.
- If the vial is stored for more than 21 days, or when a vial no longer contains a full dose of medicine, throw the vial away as directed by your healthcare provider.

Important: Follow these instructions exactly to help avoid infections.

Preparing the dose:
1. Remove the vial of PROCRIT from the refrigerator. During this time, protect the solution from light.
2. Do not use a Single-Use vial of PROCRIT more than one time.
3. Do not shake PROCRIT.
4. Gather the other supplies you will need for your injection (vial, syringe, alcohol wipes, cotton ball, and a puncture-proof container for throwing away the syringe and needle). See Figure 1.

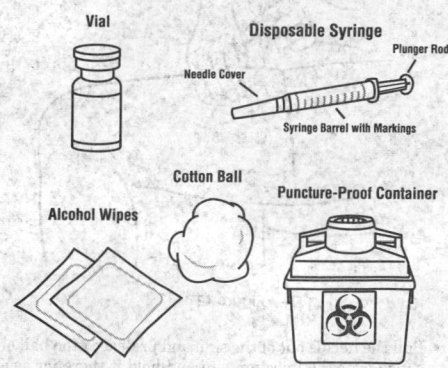

Vial
Disposable Syringe
Needle Cover
Plunger Rod
Syringe Barrel with Markings
Cotton Ball
Alcohol Wipes
Puncture-Proof Container

Figure 1

5. Check the date on the PROCRIT vial to be sure that the drug has not expired.
6. Wash your hands well with soap and water before preparing the medicine. See Figure 2.

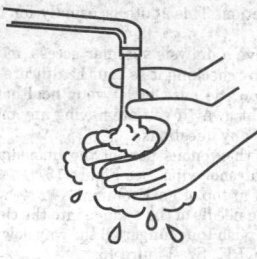

Figure 2

7. Flip off the protective color cap on the top of the vial. Do not remove the grey rubber stopper. Wipe the top of the grey rubber stopper with an alcohol wipe. See Figures 3 and 4.

[See figures 3 and 4 at top of next column]

8. Check the package containing the syringe. If the package has been opened or damaged, do not use that sy-

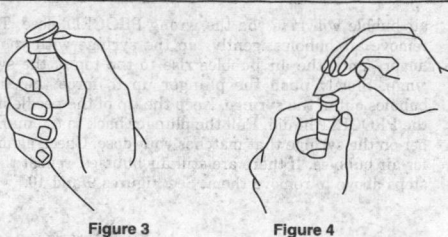

Figure 3   Figure 4

ringe. Throw away the syringe in the puncture-proof disposable container. If the syringe package is undamaged, open the package and remove the syringe.

9. Using a syringe and needle that has been recommended by your healthcare provider, carefully remove the needle cover. See Figure 5. Then draw air into the syringe by pulling back on the plunger. The amount of air drawn into the syringe should be equal to the amount (mL or cc) of the PROCRIT dose prescribed by your healthcare provider. See Figure 6.

Pull Straight Off

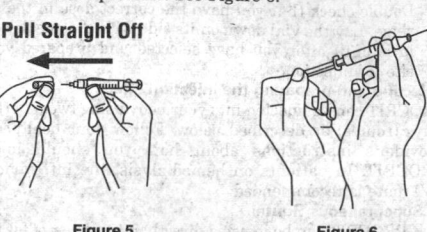

Figure 5   Figure 6

10. With the vial on a flat work surface, insert the needle straight down through the grey rubber stopper of the PROCRIT vial. See Figure 7.
11. Push the plunger of the syringe down to inject the air from the syringe into the vial of PROCRIT. The air injected into the vial will allow PROCRIT to be easily withdrawn into the syringe. See Figure 7.

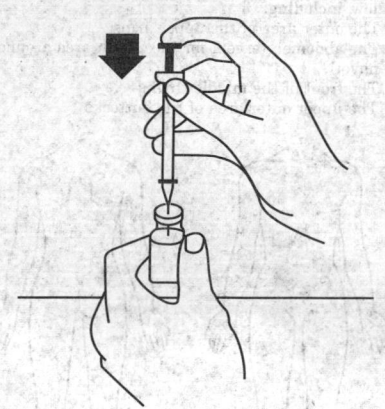

Figure 7

12. Keep the needle inside the vial. Turn the vial and syringe upside down. Be sure the tip of the needle is in the PROCRIT liquid. Keep the vial upside down. Slowly pull back on the plunger to fill the syringe with PROCRIT liquid to the number (mL or cc) that matches the dose your healthcare provider prescribed. See Figure 8.

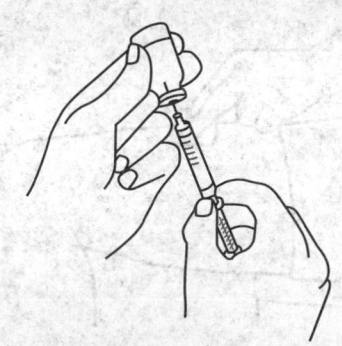

Figure 8

13. Keep the needle in the vial. Check for air bubbles in the syringe. A small amount of air is harmless. Too large an

air bubble will give you the wrong PROCRIT dose. To remove air bubbles, gently tap the syringe with your fingers until the air bubbles rise to the top of the syringe. Slowly push the plunger up to force the air bubbles out of the syringe. Keep the tip of the needle in the PROCRIT liquid. Pull the plunger back to the number on the syringe that matches your dose. Check again for air bubbles. If there are still air bubbles, repeat the steps above to remove them. See Figures 9 and 10.

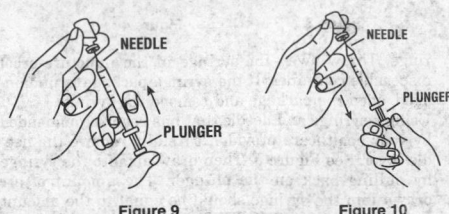

Figure 9   **Figure 10**

14. Double-check that you have the correct dose in the syringe. Lay the vial down on its side with the needle still in it until after you have selected and prepared your site for injection.

Selecting and preparing the injection site:
PROCRIT can be injected into your body using two different ways (routes) as described below. Follow your healthcare provider's instructions about how you should inject PROCRIT. In patients on hemodialysis, the intravenous (IV) route is recommended.

1. Subcutaneous Route:
- PROCRIT can be injected directly into a layer of fat under your skin. This is called a subcutaneous injection. When giving subcutaneous injections, follow your healthcare provider's instructions about changing the site for each injection. You may wish to write down the site where you have injected.
- Do not inject PROCRIT into an area that is tender, red, bruised, hard, or has scars or stretch marks. Recommended sites for injection are presented in Figure 11 below, including:
  - The outer area of the upper arms
  - The abdomen (except for the 2-inch area around the navel)
  - The front of the middle thighs
  - The upper outer area of the buttocks

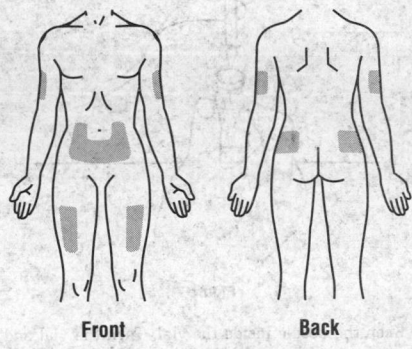

Front   **Back**

Figure 11

- Clean the skin with an alcohol wipe where the injection is to be made. Be careful not to touch the skin that has been wiped clean. See Figure 12.

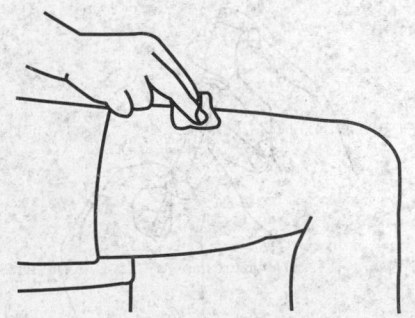

Figure 12

- Double-check that the correct amount of PROCRIT is in the syringe.

- Remove the prepared syringe and needle from the vial of PROCRIT and hold it in the hand that you will use to inject the medicine.
- Use the other hand to pinch a fold of skin at the cleaned injection site. Do not touch the cleaned area of skin. See Figure 13.

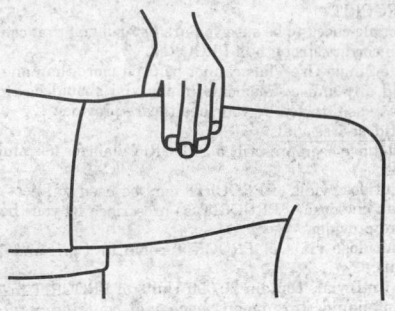

Figure 13

- Hold the syringe like you would hold a pencil. Use a quick "dart-like" motion to insert the needle either straight up and down (90-degree angle) or at a slight angle (45 degrees) into the skin. Let go of the skin and pull the plunger back slightly. If blood comes into the syringe, do not inject PROCRIT since the needle may have entered a blood vessel; instead, withdraw the syringe, discard it in the puncture-proof container. Prepare a new syringe of PROCRIT using the instructions above. Clean a new area of skin. In this new area of clean skin, again insert a new needle (as you did before), and again pull the plunger back slightly. If blood does not enter the syringe, inject the PROCRIT by pushing the plunger all the way down. See Figure 14.

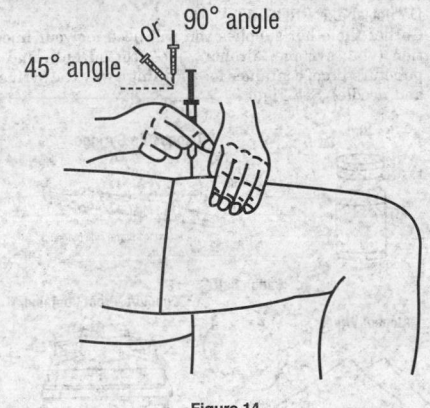

Figure 14

- Pull the needle out of the skin and press a cotton ball or gauze over the injection site and hold it there for several seconds. Do not recap the needle.
- Dispose of the used syringe and needle as described below. Do not reuse syringes and needles.

2. Intravenous Route:
- PROCRIT can be injected in your vein through a special access port put in by your healthcare provider. This type of PROCRIT injection is called an intravenous (IV) injection. This route is usually for hemodialysis patients.
- If you have a dialysis vascular access, make sure it is working by checking it as your healthcare provider has shown you. Be sure to let your healthcare provider know right away if you are having any problems, or if you have any questions.
- Wipe off the venous port of the hemodialysis tubing with an alcohol wipe. See Figure 15.

[See figure 15 at top of next column]

- Insert the needle of the syringe into the cleaned venous port and push the plunger all the way down to inject all the PROCRIT. See Figure 16.

[See figure 16 at top of next column]

- Remove the syringe from the venous port. Do not recap the needle.
- Dispose of the used syringe and needle as described below.

How should I dispose of syringes and needles?
- Do not reuse disposable syringes and needles. Throw away syringes and needles as instructed by your healthcare provider by following these steps:

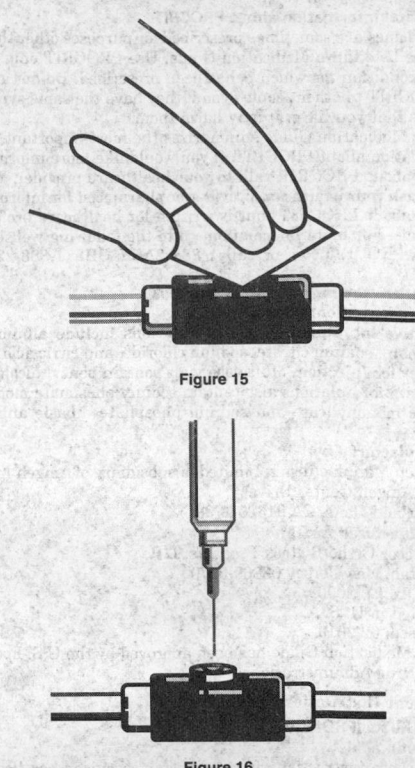

Figure 15

Figure 16

- Do not throw the needle, syringe, or disposable container in the household trash or recycle.
- Do not put the needle cover back on the needle.
- Place all used needles and syringes in a puncture-proof disposable container with a lid. Do not use glass or clear plastic containers, or any container that will be recycled or returned to a store.
- Keep the container out of the reach of children.
- When the container is full, tape around the cap or lid to make sure the cap or lid does not come off. Throw away the puncture-proof disposable container as instructed by your healthcare provider. There may be special state and local laws for disposing of used needles and syringes. **Do not throw the disposable container in the household trash. Do not recycle.**

Manufactured by:
Amgen Inc.
One Amgen Center Drive
Thousand Oaks, CA 91320-1799
Manufactured for:
Centocor Ortho Biotech Products, L.P.
Raritan, New Jersey 08869-0670
Revised: 10/2009
10112805
© COBPLP 2000
Printed in U. S. A.
Shown in Product Identification Guide, page 307

Cephalon, Inc.
41 MOORES ROAD
PO BOX 4011
FRAZER, PA 19355

For Medical Information and Adverse Drug Experience/ Product Complaint Reporting Contact:
(800) 896-5855
Fax 866-996-5211

AMRIX®   Rx
[ăm-rĭks]
(Cyclobenzaprine Hydrochloride Extended-Release Capsules)

DESCRIPTION
AMRIX® (Cyclobenzaprine Hydrochloride Extended-Release Capsules) is a skeletal muscle relaxant which relieves muscle spasm of local origin without interfering with muscle function. The active ingredient in AMRIX extended-release capsules is cyclobenzaprine hydrochloride, USP.

Cyclobenzaprine hydrochloride (HCl) is a white, crystalline tricyclic amine salt with the empirical formula $C_{20}H_{21}N \bullet HCl$ and a molecular weight of 311.9. It has a melting point of 217°C, and a pK_a of 8.47 at 25°C. It is freely soluble in water and alcohol, sparingly soluble in isopropanol, and insoluble in hydrocarbon solvents. If aqueous solutions are made alkaline, the free base separates. Cyclobenzaprine HCl is designated chemically as 3-(5H-dibenzo[a,d] cyclohepten-5-ylidene)-N,N-dimethyl-1-propanamine hydrochloride, and has the following structural formula:

HCCH$_2$CH$_2$N(CH$_3$)$_2$ • HCl

AMRIX extended-release capsules for oral administration are supplied in 15 and 30 mg strengths. AMRIX capsules contain the following inactive ingredients: diethyl phthalate NF, ethylcellulose NF (Ethocel Standard 10 Premium), gelatin, Opadry® Clear YS-1-7006, sugar spheres NF (20-25 mesh), and titanium dioxide. AMRIX 15 mg capsules also contain D&C yellow #10, FD&C green #3, and FD&C red #40. AMRIX 30 mg capsules also contain FD&C blue #1, FD&C blue #2, FD&C red #40, and FD&C yellow #6.

CLINICAL PHARMACOLOGY

Cyclobenzaprine relieves skeletal muscle spasm of local origin without interfering with muscle function. Cyclobenzaprine has not been shown to be effective in muscle spasm due to central nervous system disease. In animal models, cyclobenzaprine reduced or abolished skeletal muscle hyperactivity. Animal studies indicate that cyclobenzaprine does not act at the neuromuscular junction or directly on skeletal muscle. Such studies show that cyclobenzaprine acts primarily within the central nervous system at the brain stem as opposed to the spinal cord level, although an overlapping action on the latter may contribute to its overall skeletal muscle relaxant activity. Evidence suggests that the net effect of cyclobenzaprine is a reduction of tonic somatic motor activity, influencing both gamma (γ) and alpha (α) motor systems. Pharmacological studies in animals demonstrated a similarity between the effects of cyclobenzaprine and the structurally related tricyclic antidepressants, including reserpine antagonism, norepinephrine potentiation, potent peripheral and central anticholinergic effects, and sedation. Cyclobenzaprine caused slight to moderate increase in heart rate in animals.

Pharmacokinetics
Absorption
In a single-dose study comprised of healthy adult males (n=15), the dose adjusted ratios of the arithmetic means of AUC_{0-168} and $AUC_{0-\infty}$ indicated that exposure of the AMRIX 30 mg was about 16% and 10% higher than that of AMRIX 15 mg, respectively. The dose-adjusted ratios of the arithmetic means of C_{max} indicated that the peak plasma concentration of AMRIX 30 mg was about 20% higher than that of AMRIX 15 mg. The half-lives and time to peak plasma cyclobenzaprine concentration were similar for both AMRIX 15 mg and 30 mg. These data are summarized below.

Table 1: Summary of Pharmacokinetic Parameters in Healthy Adult Subjects

Parameter Mean ± SD	AMRIX 15 mg (N=15)	AMRIX 30 mg (N=14)
AUC_{0-168} (ng•hr/mL)	318.3 ± 114.7	736.6 ± 259.4
$AUC_{0-\infty}$ (ng•hr/mL)	354.1 ± 119.8	779.9 ± 277.6
C_{max} (ng/mL)	8.3 ± 2.2	19.9 ± 5.9
T_{max} (hrs)	8.1 ± 2.9	7.1 ± 1.6
$t_{1/2}$ (hrs)	33.4 ± 10.3	32.0 ± 10.1

SD = standard deviation

A food effect study conducted in healthy adult subjects (n=15) utilizing a single dose of AMRIX 30 mg demonstrated a statistically significant increase in bioavailability when AMRIX 30 mg was given with food relative to the fasted state. There was a 35% increase in peak plasma cyclobenzaprine concentration (C_{max}) and a 20% increase in exposure (AUC_{0-168} and $AUC_{0-\infty}$) in the presence of food. No effect, however, was noted in T_{lag}, T_{max}, or the shape of the mean plasma cyclobenzaprine concentration versus time profile. Cyclobenzaprine in plasma was first detectable in both the fed and fasted states at 1.5 hours.

In a multiple-dose study utilizing AMRIX 30 mg administered once daily for 7 days in a group of healthy adult volunteers (n=35) a 2.5-fold accumulation of plasma cyclobenzaprine levels was noted at steady-state.

Metabolism and Elimination
Cyclobenzaprine is extensively metabolized and is excreted primarily as glucuronides via the kidney. Cytochromes P-450 3A4, 1A2, and, to a lesser extent, 2D6, mediate N-demethylation, one of the oxidative pathways for cyclobenzaprine. Cyclobenzaprine has an elimination half-life of 32 hours (range 8-37 hours; n=18); plasma clearance is 0.7 L/min following single dose administration of AMRIX.

Special Populations
Elderly
Although there were no notable differences in C_{max} or T_{max}, cyclobenzaprine plasma AUC is increased by 40% and the plasma half-life of cyclobenzaprine is prolonged in elderly subjects greater than 65 years of age (50 hours) after dosing with AMRIX compared to younger subjects (32 hours). Pharmacokinetic characteristics of cyclobenzaprine following multiple-dose administration of AMRIX in the elderly were not evaluated.

Table 2: Summary of Pharmacokinetic Parameters of AMRIX 30 mg Extended-Release Capsules, By Age Group

Parameter Mean ± SD	AMRIX 30 mg QD	
	18 to 45 years (N=18)	65 to 75 years (N=17)
AUC_{0-168} (ng•hr/mL)	715.1 ± 264.2	945.9 ± 255.2
$AUC_{0-\infty}$ (ng•hr/mL)	751.2 ± 271.5	1055.2 ± 301.9
C_{max} (ng/mL)*	19.2 ± 5.6	19.2 ± 5.1
T_{max} (hrs)*	6.8 ± 1.9	8.5 ± 2.3
$t_{1/2}$ (hrs)	32.4 ± 8.1	49.0 ± 8.3

* Measured over the entire 24 hour period
SD = standard deviation

Hepatic Impairment
In a pharmacokinetic study of immediate-release cyclobenzaprine in 16 subjects with hepatic impairment (15 mild, 1 moderate per Child-Pugh score), both AUC and C_{max} were approximately double the values seen in the healthy control group. The pharmacokinetics of cyclobenzaprine in subjects with severe hepatic impairment is not known.

CLINICAL STUDIES
Efficacy was assessed in two double-blind, parallel-group, placebo-controlled studies of identical design of AMRIX 15 mg and 30 mg taken once daily in patients with muscle spasms associated with acute painful musculoskeletal conditions.

There were significant differences in the primary efficacy analysis, the patient's rating of medication helpfulness, between the AMRIX 15 mg group and the placebo group at Days 4 and 14 in one study and between the AMRIX 30 mg group and the placebo group at Day 4 in the second study. [See table 3 above]
[See table 4 above]

In addition, one of the two studies demonstrated significant differences between the AMRIX 30 mg group and the placebo group in terms of patient-rated relief from local pain due to muscle spasm at Day 4 and Day 8, in subject-rated restriction of movement at Day 4 and Day 8, and in patient-rated global impression of change at Day 4, Day 8, and Day 14.

There were no significant treatment differences between the AMRIX treatment groups and the placebo group in physician's global assessment, in subject-rated restriction in activities of daily living, or quality of night-time sleep.

INDICATIONS AND USAGE
AMRIX is indicated as an adjunct to rest and physical therapy for relief of muscle spasm associated with acute, painful musculoskeletal conditions. Improvement is manifested by relief of muscle spasm and its associated signs and symptoms, namely, pain, tenderness, and limitation of motion.

AMRIX should be used only for short periods (up to two or three weeks) because adequate evidence of effectiveness for more prolonged use is not available and because muscle spasm associated with acute, painful musculoskeletal conditions is generally of short duration and specific therapy for longer periods is seldom warranted.

AMRIX has not been found effective in the treatment of spasticity associated with cerebral or spinal cord disease or in children with cerebral palsy.

CONTRAINDICATIONS
- Hypersensitivity to any component of this product.
- Concomitant use of monoamine oxidase (MAO) inhibitors or within 14 days after their discontinuation.
- Hyperpyretic crisis seizures and deaths have occurred in patients receiving cyclobenzaprine (or structurally similar tricyclic antidepressants) concomitantly with MAO inhibitor drugs.
- During the acute recovery phase of myocardial infarction, and in patients with arrhythmias, heart block conduction disturbances, or congestive heart failure.
- Hyperthyroidism.

Table 3: Subject's Rating of Medication Helpfulness - Study 1105

	Day 4		Day 14	
	Number of Subjects (%)		Number of Subjects (%)	
	Placebo (N = 64)	AMRIX 30 mg (N = 64)	Placebo (N = 64)	AMRIX 30 mg (N = 64)
Excellent	1 (1.6%)	3 (4.7%)	12 (18.8%)	15 (23.4%)
Very Good	5 (7.8%)	13 (20.3%)	9 (14.1%)	19 (29.7%)
Good	15 (23.4%)	22 (34.4%)	10 (15.6%)	15 (23.4%)
Fair	24 (37.5%)	20 (31.3%)	16 (25.0%)	10 (15.6%)
Poor	10 (15.6%)	5 (7.8%)	9 (14.1%)	4 (6.3%)
Missing	9 (14.1%)	1 (1.6%)	8 (12.5%)	1 (1.6%)

Table 4: Subject's Rating of Medication Helpfulness - Study 1106

	Day 4		Day 14	
	Number of Subjects (%)		Number of Subjects (%)	
	Placebo (N = 64)	AMRIX 15 mg (N = 63)	Placebo (N = 64)	AMRIX 15 mg (N = 63)
Excellent	1 (1.6%)	2 (3.2%)	10 (15.6%)	13 (20.6%)
Very Good	10 (15.6%)	12 (19.0%)	12 (18.8%)	21 (33.3%)
Good	14 (21.9%)	21 (33.3%)	13 (20.3%)	9 (14.3%)
Fair	16 (25.0%)	17 (27.0%)	14 (21.9%)	10 (15.9%)
Poor	19 (29.7%)	6 (9.5%)	12 (18.8%)	5 (7.9%)
Missing	4 (6.3%)	5 (17.9%)	3 (4.7%)	5 (7.9%)

WARNINGS

AMRIX is closely related to the tricyclic antidepressants, e.g., amitriptyline and imipramine. In short term studies for indications other than muscle spasm associated with acute musculoskeletal conditions, and usually at doses somewhat greater than those recommended for skeletal muscle spasm, some of the more serious central nervous system reactions noted with the tricyclic antidepressants have occurred (see **WARNINGS**, below, and **ADVERSE REACTIONS**).

Tricyclic antidepressants have been reported to produce arrhythmias, sinus tachycardia, prolongation of the conduction time leading to myocardial infarction and stroke. AMRIX may enhance the effects of alcohol, barbiturates, and other CNS depressants.

As a result of a two-fold higher cyclobenzaprine plasma levels in subjects with mild hepatic impairment, as compared to healthy subjects, following administration of immediate-release cyclobenzaprine and because there is limited dosing flexibility with AMRIX, use of AMRIX is not recommended in subjects with mild, moderate or severe hepatic impairment.

As a result of a 40% increase in cyclobenzaprine plasma levels and a 56% increase in plasma half-life following administration of AMRIX in elderly subjects as compared to young adults, use of AMRIX is not recommended in elderly.

PRECAUTIONS

General

Because of its atropine-like action, AMRIX should be used with caution in patients with a history of urinary retention, angle-closure glaucoma, increased intraocular pressure, and in patients taking anticholinergic medication.

Information for Patients

AMRIX, especially when used with alcohol or other CNS depressants, may impair mental and/or physical abilities required for performance of hazardous tasks, such as operating machinery or driving a motor vehicle.

Drug Interactions

AMRIX may have life-threatening interactions with MAO inhibitors. (See **CONTRAINDICATIONS**.) AMRIX may enhance the effects of alcohol, barbiturates, and other CNS depressants. Tricyclic antidepressants may block the antihypertensive action of guanethidine and similarly acting compounds. Tricyclic antidepressants may enhance the seizure risk in patients taking tramadol (ULTRAM® [tramadol HCl tablets, Ortho-McNeil Pharmaceutical] or ULTRACET® [tramadol HCl and acetaminophen tablets, Ortho-McNeil Pharmaceutical]).

Carcinogenesis, Mutagenesis, Impairment of Fertility

In rats treated with cyclobenzaprine for up to 67 weeks at doses of approximately 5 to 40 times the maximum recommended human dose, pale, sometimes enlarged, livers were noted and there was a dose-related hepatocyte vacuolation with lipidosis. In the higher dose groups, this microscopic change was seen after 26 weeks and even earlier in rats that died prior to 26 weeks; at lower doses, the change was not seen until after 26 weeks. Cyclobenzaprine did not affect the onset, incidence, or distribution of neoplasia in an 81-week study in the mouse or in a 105-week study in the rat. At oral doses of up to 10 times the human dose, cyclobenzaprine did not adversely affect the reproductive performance or fertility of male or female rats. Cyclobenzaprine did not demonstrate mutagenic activity in the male mouse at dose levels of up to 20 times the human dose.

A battery of mutagenicity tests using bacterial and mammalian systems for point mutations and cytogenic effects have provided no evidence for a mutagenic potential for cyclobenzaprine. An in vivo mouse bone micronucleus assay, an assessment of chromosomal aberrations (Chinese hamster ovary), and a mammalian microsome reverse mutation assay were negative.

Pregnancy

Pregnancy Category B: Reproduction studies have been performed in rats, mice, and rabbits at doses up to 20 times the human dose and have revealed no evidence of impaired fertility or harm to the fetus due to cyclobenzaprine. There are, however, no adequate and well-controlled studies in pregnant women. Because animal reproduction studies are not always predictive of human response, this drug should be used during pregnancy only if clearly needed.

Nursing Mothers

It is not known whether this drug is excreted in human milk. Because cyclobenzaprine is closely related to the tricyclic antidepressants, some of which are known to be excreted in human milk, caution should be exercised when AMRIX is administered to a nursing woman.

Pediatric Use

Safety and effectiveness of AMRIX has not been studied in pediatric patients.

Use in the Elderly

The plasma concentration and half-life of cyclobenzaprine are substantially increased in the elderly when compared to the general patient population (see **CLINICAL PHARMACOLOGY**, *Pharmacokinetics*, **Special Populations**, *Elderly*). Accordingly, AMRIX should not be used in the elderly.

ADVERSE REACTIONS

The most common adverse reactions in the two 14-day clinical efficacy trials and in the 7-day repeat-dose pharmacokinetic study are presented in Tables 5 and 6, respectively.

Table 5: Incidence of the Most Common Adverse Reactions Occurring in ≥ 3% of Subjects in Any Treatment Group in the Two Phase 3, Double-Blind AMRIX Trials

	AMRIX 15 mg N=127	AMRIX 30 mg N=126	Placebo N=128
Dry mouth	6%	14%	2%
Dizziness	3%	6%	2%
Fatigue	3%	3%	2%
Constipation	1%	3%	0%
Somnolence	1%	2%	0%
Nausea	3%	3%	1%
Dyspepsia	0%	4%	1%

Table 6: Incidence of the Most Common Adverse Reactions Occurring in ≥ 3% of Subjects in Any Treatment Group in the Seven-Day Pharmacokinetic Study of AMRIX

	AMRIX 30 mg N = 36
Somnolence	100%
Dry mouth	58%
Headache NOS	17%
Dizziness	19%
Vision blurred	3%
Nausea	8%
Dysgeusia	6%
Palpitations	6%
Tremor	6%
Dry throat	8%
Acne NOS	6%
Disturbance in attention	6%
Insomnia	0

In a postmarketing surveillance program (7607 patients treated with cyclobenzaprine 10 mg TID), the adverse reactions reported most frequently were drowsiness, dry mouth, and dizziness. The incidence of these common adverse reactions was lower in the surveillance program than in the controlled clinical studies:

Table 7: Most Common Adverse Reactions from Postmarketing Surveillance Program

	Clinical Studies cyclobenzaprine 10 mg TID	Surveillance Program cyclobenzaprine 10 mg TID
Drowsiness	39%	16%
Dry mouth	27%	7%
Dizziness	11%	3%

Among the less frequent adverse reactions, there was no appreciable difference in incidence in controlled clinical studies or in the surveillance program. Adverse reactions which were reported in 1% to 3% of the patients were: fatigue/tiredness, asthenia, nausea, constipation, dyspepsia, unpleasant taste, blurred vision, headache, nervousness, and

confusion. The following adverse reactions have been reported in post-marketing experience or with an incidence of less than 1% of patients in clinical trials with the 10 mg TID tablet:

Body as a Whole: Syncope; malaise.
Cardiovascular: Tachycardia; arrhythmia; vasodilatation; palpitation; hypotension.
Digestive: Vomiting; anorexia; diarrhea; gastrointestinal pain; gastritis; thirst; flatulence; edema of the tongue; abnormal liver function and rare reports of hepatitis, jaundice, and cholestasis.
Hypersensitivity: Anaphylaxis; angioedema; pruritus; facial edema; urticaria; rash.
Musculoskeletal: Local weakness.
Nervous System and Psychiatric: Seizures, ataxia; vertigo; dysarthria; tremors; hypertonia; convulsions; muscle twitching; disorientation; insomnia; depressed mood; abnormal sensations; anxiety; agitation; psychosis, abnormal thinking and dreaming; hallucinations; excitement; paresthesia; diplopia.
Skin: Sweating.
Special Senses: Ageusia; tinnitus.
Urogenital: Urinary frequency and/or retention.
Causal Relationship Unknown
Other reactions, reported rarely for cyclobenzaprine under circumstances where a causal relationship could not be established or reported for other tricyclic drugs, are listed to serve as alerting information to physicians:
Body as a Whole: Chest pain; edema.
Cardiovascular: Hypertension; myocardial infarction; heart block; stroke.
Digestive: Paralytic ileus, tongue discoloration; stomatitis; parotid swelling.
Endocrine: Inappropriate ADH syndrome.
Hematic and Lymphatic: Purpura; bone marrow depression; leukopenia; eosinophilia; thrombocytopenia.
Metabolic, Nutritional and Immune: Elevation and lowering of blood sugar levels; weight gain or loss.
Musculoskeletal: Myalgia.
Nervous System and Psychiatric: Decreased or increased libido; abnormal gait; delusions; aggressive behavior; paranoia; peripheral neuropathy; Bell's palsy; alteration in EEG patterns; extrapyramidal symptoms.
Respiratory: Dyspnea.
Skin: Photosensitization; alopecia.
Urogenital: Impaired urination; dilatation of urinary tract; impotence; testicular swelling; gynecomastia; breast enlargement; galactorrhea.

DRUG ABUSE AND DEPENDENCE

Pharmacologic similarities among the tricyclic drugs require that certain withdrawal symptoms be considered when AMRIX is administered, even though they have not been reported to occur with this drug. Abrupt cessation of treatment after prolonged administration rarely may produce nausea, headache, and malaise. These are not indicative of addiction.

OVERDOSAGE

Although rare, deaths may occur from overdosage with AMRIX. Multiple drug ingestion (including alcohol) is common in deliberate cyclobenzaprine overdose. **As management of overdose is complex and changing, it is recommended that the physician contact a poison control center for current information on treatment**. Signs and symptoms of toxicity may develop rapidly after cyclobenzaprine overdose; therefore, hospital monitoring is required as soon as possible. The acute oral LD_{50} of cyclobenzaprine is approximately 338 and 425 mg/kg in mice and rats, respectively.

Manifestations

The most common effects associated with cyclobenzaprine overdose are drowsiness and tachycardia. Less frequent manifestations include tremor, agitation, coma, ataxia, hypertension, slurred speech, confusion, dizziness, nausea, vomiting, and hallucinations. Rare but potentially critical manifestations of overdose are cardiac arrest, chest pain, cardiac dysrhythmias, severe hypotension, seizures, and neuroleptic malignant syndrome. Changes in the electrocardiogram, particularly in QRS axis or width, are clinically significant indicators of cyclobenzaprine toxicity. Other potential effects of overdosage include any of the symptoms listed under **ADVERSE REACTIONS**.

Management

General
As management of overdose is complex and changing, it is recommended that the physician contact a poison control center for current information on treatment.
In order to protect against the rare but potentially critical manifestations described above, obtain an ECG and immediately initiate cardiac monitoring. Protect the patient's airway, establish an intravenous line, and initiate gastric decontamination. Observation with cardiac monitoring and observation for signs of CNS or respiratory depression, hypotension, cardiac dysrhythmias and/or conduction blocks, and seizures is necessary. If signs of toxicity occur at any time during this period, extended monitoring is re-

quired. Monitoring of plasma drug levels should not guide management of the patient. Dialysis is probably of no value because of low plasma concentrations of the drug.

Gastrointestinal Decontamination

All patients suspected of an overdose with AMRIX should receive gastrointestinal decontamination. This should include large volume gastric lavage followed by activated charcoal. If consciousness is impaired, the airway should be secured prior to lavage and emesis is contraindicated.

Cardiovascular

A maximal limb-lead QRS duration of 0.10 seconds may be the best indication of the severity of the overdose. Serum alkalinization, to a pH of 7.45 to 7.55, using intravenous sodium bicarbonate and hyperventilation (as needed), should be instituted for patients with dysrhythmias and/or QRS widening. A pH >7.60 or a pCO_2 <20 mmHg is undesirable. Dysrhythmias unresponsive to sodium bicarbonate therapy/hyperventilation may respond to lidocaine, bretylium, or phenytoin. Type 1A and 1C antiarrhythmics are generally contraindicated (e.g., quinidine, disopyramide, and procainamide).

CNS

In patients with CNS depression, early intubation is advised because of the potential for abrupt deterioration. Seizures should be controlled with benzodiazepines or, if these are ineffective, other anticonvulsants (e.g., phenobarbital, phenytoin). Physostigmine is not recommended except to treat life-threatening symptoms that have been unresponsive to other therapies, and then only in close consultation with a poison control center.

Psychiatric Follow-up

Since overdosage is often deliberate, patients may attempt suicide by other means during the recovery phase. Psychiatric referral may be appropriate.

Pediatric Management

The principles of management of child and adult overdosage are similar. It is strongly recommended that the physician contact the local poison control center for specific pediatric treatment.

DOSAGE AND ADMINISTRATION

The recommended adult dose for most patients is one (1) AMRIX 15 mg capsule taken once daily. Some patients may require up to 30 mg/day, given as one (1) AMRIX 30 mg capsule taken once daily or as two (2) AMRIX 15 mg capsules taken once daily.

It is recommended that doses be taken at approximately the same time each day.

Use of AMRIX for periods longer than two or three weeks is not recommended (see INDICATIONS AND USAGE).

Dosage Considerations for Special Patient Populations: AMRIX should not be used in the elderly or in patients with impaired hepatic function. (see WARNINGS)

HOW SUPPLIED

AMRIX extended-release capsules are available in 15 and 30 mg strengths, packaged in bottles of 60 capsules. AMRIX 15 mg capsules (NDC 63459-700-60) are orange/orange and are embossed in blue ink with "15 mg" on the body, and Cephalon "C" logo, "Cephalon", and a dashed band on the cap. AMRIX 30 mg capsules (NDC 63459-701-60) are blue/orange and are embossed in white ink with "30 mg" on the body, and Cephalon "C" logo, "Cephalon", and a dashed band on the cap.

Dispense in a tight, light-resistant container as defined in the USP/NF.

Store at 25°C (77°F); excursions permitted to 15 - 30°C (59 - 86°F); [see USP Controlled Room Temperature].

KEEP THIS AND ALL MEDICATION OUT OF THE REACH OF CHILDREN. IN CASE OF ACCIDENTAL OVERDOSE, SEEK PROFESSIONAL ASSISTANCE OR CONTACT A POISON CONTROL CENTER IMMEDIATELY.

Distributed by:
Cephalon, Inc.
Frazer, PA 19355
Manufactured by:
Eurand Inc.
Vandalia, Ohio 45377
AMRIX is a trademark of Cephalon, Inc. or its affiliates.
U.S. Patent No. 7,387,793

© 2004, 2006, 2007, 2008 Cephalon, Inc., or its affiliates. All rights reserved.

PI-40018-01
Revised December 2008

Shown in Product Identification Guide, page 307

FENTORA®

[fen-tor'-ah]
(fentanyl buccal tablet)

CII ℞

Each tablet contains fentanyl citrate equivalent to fentanyl base: 100, 200, 300, 400, 600, 800 mcg

PHYSICIANS AND OTHER HEALTHCARE PROVIDERS MUST BECOME FAMILIAR WITH THE IMPORTANT WARNINGS IN THIS LABEL.

Reports of serious adverse events, including deaths in patients treated with *FENTORA* have been reported. Deaths occurred as a result of improper patient selection (e.g., use in opioid non-tolerant patients) and/or improper dosing. The substitution of *FENTORA* for any other fentanyl product may result in fatal overdose.

***FENTORA* is indicated only for the management of breakthrough pain in patients with cancer who are already receiving and who are tolerant to around-the-clock opioid therapy for their underlying persistent cancer pain.** Patients considered opioid tolerant are those who are taking around-the-clock medicine consisting of at least 60 mg of oral morphine daily, at least 25 mcg of transdermal fentanyl/hour, at least 30 mg of oxycodone daily, at least 8 mg of oral hydromorphone daily or an equianalgesic dose of another opioid daily for a week or longer.

***FENTORA* is not indicated for use in opioid non-tolerant patients including those with only as needed (PRN) prior exposure.**

***FENTORA* is contraindicated in the management of acute or postoperative pain including headache/migraine. Life-threatening respiratory depression could occur at any dose in opioid non-tolerant patients. Deaths have occurred in opioid non-tolerant patients.**

When prescribing, do not convert patients on a mcg per mcg basis from Actiq® to *FENTORA*. Carefully consult the Initial Dosing Recommendations table. (See DOSAGE AND ADMINISTRATION, Table 7.)

When dispensing, do not substitute a *FENTORA* prescription for other fentanyl products. Substantial differences exist in the pharmacokinetic profile of *FENTORA* compared to other fentanyl products that result in clinically important differences in the extent of absorption of fentanyl. As a result of these differences, the substitution of *FENTORA* for any other fentanyl product may result in fatal overdose.

Special care must be used when dosing ***FENTORA***. If the breakthrough pain episode is not relieved after 30 minutes, patients may take ONLY one additional dose using the same strength and must wait at least 4 hours before taking another dose. **(See DOSAGE AND ADMINISTRATION.)**

***FENTORA* contains fentanyl, an opioid agonist and a Schedule II controlled substance, with an abuse liability similar to other opioid analgesics. *FENTORA* can be abused in a manner similar to other opioid agonists, legal or illicit. This should be considered when prescribing or dispensing *FENTORA* in situations where the physician or pharmacist is concerned about an increased risk of misuse, abuse or diversion. Schedule II opioid substances which include morphine, oxycodone, hydromorphone, oxymorphone, and methadone have the highest potential for abuse and risk of fatal overdose due to respiratory depression.**

Patients and their caregivers must be instructed that *FENTORA* contains a medicine in an amount which can be fatal to a child. Patients and their caregivers must be instructed to keep all tablets out of the reach of children. (See Information for Patients and Caregivers for disposal instructions.)

***FENTORA* is intended to be used only in the care of opioid tolerant cancer patients and only by healthcare professionals who are knowledgeable of and skilled in the use of Schedule II opioids to treat cancer pain.**

The concomitant use of ***FENTORA*** with strong and moderate cytochrome P450 3A4 inhibitors may result in an increase in fentanyl plasma concentrations, and may cause potentially fatal respiratory depression.

DESCRIPTION

FENTORA (fentanyl buccal tablet) is a potent opioid analgesic, intended for buccal mucosal administration. *FENTORA* is formulated as a flat-faced, round, beveled-edge white tablet.

FENTORA is designed to be placed and retained within the buccal cavity for a period sufficient to allow disintegration of the tablet and absorption of fentanyl across the oral mucosa.

FENTORA employs the OraVescent® drug delivery technology, which generates a reaction that releases carbon dioxide when the tablet comes in contact with saliva. It is believed that transient pH changes accompanying the reaction may optimize dissolution (at a lower pH) and membrane permeation (at a higher pH) of fentanyl through the buccal mucosa.

Active Ingredient: Fentanyl citrate, USP is N-(1-Phenethyl-4-piperidyl) propionanilide citrate (1:1). Fentanyl is a highly lipophilic compound (octanol-water partition coefficient at pH 7.4 is 816:1) that is freely soluble in organic solvents and sparingly soluble in water (1:40). The molecular weight of the free base is 336.5 (the citrate salt is 528.6). The pKa of the tertiary nitrogens are 7.3 and 8.4. The compound has the following structural formula:

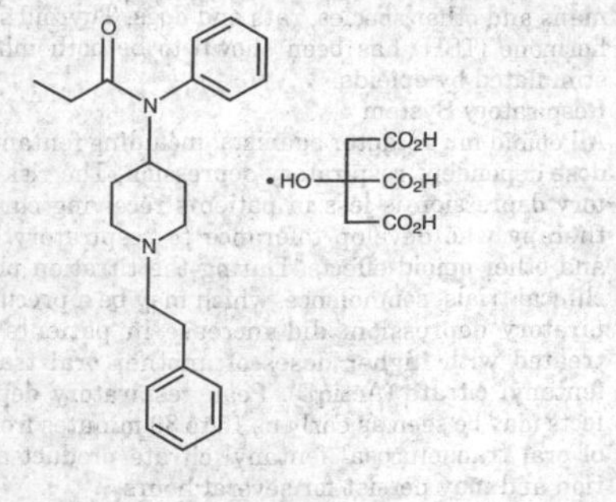

All tablet strengths are expressed as the amount of fentanyl free base, e.g., the 100 microgram strength tablet contains 100 micrograms of fentanyl free base.

Inactive Ingredients: Mannitol, sodium starch glycolate, sodium bicarbonate, sodium carbonate, citric acid, and magnesium stearate.

CLINICAL PHARMACOLOGY

Pharmacology:

Fentanyl is a pure opioid agonist whose principal therapeutic action is analgesia. Other members of the class known as opioid agonists include substances such as morphine, oxycodone, hydromorphone, codeine, and hydrocodone. Pharmacological effects of opioid agonists include anxiolysis, euphoria, feelings of relaxation, respiratory depression, constipation, miosis, cough suppression, and analgesia. Like all pure opioid agonist analgesics, with increasing doses there is increasing analgesia, unlike with mixed agonist/antagonists or non-opioid analgesics, where there is a limit to the analgesic effect with increasing doses. With pure opioid agonist analgesics, there is no defined maximum dose; the ceiling to analgesic effectiveness is imposed only by side effects, the more serious of which may include somnolence and respiratory depression.

Analgesia

The analgesic effects of fentanyl are related to the blood level of the drug, if proper allowance is made for the delay into and out of the CNS (a process with a 3-to-5-minute half-life).

In general, the effective concentration and the concentration at which toxicity occurs increase with increasing tolerance with any and all opioids. The rate of development of tolerance varies widely among individuals. As a result, the dose of *FENTORA* should be individually titrated to achieve the desired effect. (See **DOSAGE AND ADMINISTRATION.**)

Central Nervous System

The precise mechanism of the analgesic action is unknown although fentanyl is known to be a mu opioid receptor agonist. Specific CNS opioid receptors for endogenous compounds with opioid-like activity have been identified throughout the brain and spinal cord and play a role in the analgesic effects of this drug.

Fentanyl produces respiratory depression by direct action on brain stem respiratory centers. The respiratory depression involves both a reduction in the responsiveness of the brain stem to increases in carbon dioxide and to electrical stimulation.

Fentanyl depresses the cough reflex by direct effect on the cough center in the medulla. Antitussive effects may occur with doses lower than those usually required for analgesia.

Fentanyl causes miosis even in total darkness. Pinpoint pupils are a sign of opioid overdose but are not pathognomonic (e.g., pontine lesions of hemorrhagic or ischemic origin may produce similar findings).

Gastrointestinal System

Fentanyl causes a reduction in motility associated with an increase in smooth muscle tone in the antrum of the stomach and in the duodenum. Digestion of food is delayed in the small intestine and propulsive contractions are decreased. Propulsive peristaltic waves in the colon are decreased, while tone may be increased to the point of spasm resulting in constipation. Other opioid-induced effects may include a reduction in gastric, biliary and pancreatic secretions, spasm of the sphincter of Oddi, and transient elevations in serum amylase.

Cardiovascular System

Fentanyl may produce release of histamine with or without associated peripheral vasodilation. Manifestations of histamine release and/or peripheral vasodilation may include pruritus, flushing, red eyes, sweating, and/or orthostatic hypotension.

Endocrine System

Opioid agonists have been shown to have a variety of effects on the secretion of hormones. Opioids inhibit the secretion of ACTH, cortisol, and luteinizing hormone (LH) in humans. They also stimulate prolactin, growth hormone (GH) secretion, and pancreatic secretion of insulin and glucagon in humans and other species, rats and dogs. Thyroid stimulating hormone (TSH) has been shown to be both inhibited and stimulated by opioids.

Respiratory System

All opioid mu-receptor agonists, including fentanyl, produce dose dependent respiratory depression. The risk of respiratory depression is less in patients receiving chronic opioid therapy who develop tolerance to respiratory depression and other opioid effects. During the titration phase of the clinical trials, somnolence, which may be a precursor to respiratory depression, did increase in patients who were treated with higher doses of another oral transmucosal fentanyl citrate (Actiq®). Peak respiratory depressive effects may be seen as early as 15 to 30 minutes from the start of oral transmucosal fentanyl citrate product administration and may persist for several hours.

Serious or fatal respiratory depression can occur even at recommended doses. Fentanyl depresses the cough reflex as a result of its CNS activity. Although not observed with oral transmucosal fentanyl products in clinical trials, fentanyl given rapidly by intravenous injection in large doses may interfere with respiration by causing rigidity in the muscles of respiration. Therefore, physicians and other healthcare providers should be aware of this potential complication.

(See **BOXED WARNING, CONTRAINDICATIONS, WARNINGS, PRECAUTIONS, ADVERSE REACTIONS,** and **OVERDOSAGE** for additional information on hypoventilation.)

Pharmacokinetics

Fentanyl exhibits linear pharmacokinetics. Systemic exposure to fentanyl following administration of *FENTORA* increases linearly in an approximate dose-proportional manner over the 100- to 800-mcg dose range.

Absorption:

Following buccal administration of *FENTORA*, fentanyl is readily absorbed with an absolute bioavailability of 65%. The absorption profile of *FENTORA* is largely the result of an initial absorption from the buccal mucosa, with peak plasma concentrations following venous sampling generally attained within an hour after buccal administration. Approximately 50% of the total dose administered is absorbed transmucosally and becomes systemically available. The remaining half of the total dose is swallowed and undergoes more prolonged absorption from the gastrointestinal tract. In a study that compared the absolute and relative bioavailability of *FENTORA* and Actiq (oral transmucosal fentanyl citrate), the rate and extent of fentanyl absorption were considerably different (approximately 30% greater exposure with *FENTORA*) (Table 1).

Table 1. Pharmacokinetic Parameters* in Adult Subjects Receiving FENTORA or Actiq

Pharmacokinetic Parameter (mean)	*FENTORA* 400 mcg	Actiq 400 mcg (adjusted dose)***
Absolute Bioavailability	65% ± 20%	47% ± 10.5%
Fraction Absorbed Transmucosally	48% ± 31.8%	22% ± 17.3%
T_{max} (minute)**	46.8 (20-240)	90.8 (35-240)
C_{max} (ng/mL)	1.02 ± 0.42	0.63 ± 0.21
AUC_{0-tmax} (ng•hr/mL)	0.40 ± 0.18	0.14 ± 0.05
AUC_{0-inf} (ng•hr/mL)	6.48 ± 2.98	4.79 ± 1.96

* Based on venous blood samples.
** Data for T_{max} presented as median (range).
*** Actiq data was dose adjusted (800 mcg to 400 mcg).

Similarly, in another bioavailability study exposure following administration of *FENTORA* was also greater (approximately 50%) compared to Actiq.

Due to differences in drug delivery, measures of exposure (C_{max}, AUC_{0-tmax}, AUC_{0-inf}) associated with a given dose of fentanyl were substantially greater with *FENTORA* compared to Actiq (see Figure 1). Therefore, caution must be exercised when switching patients from one product to another. (See **DOSAGE AND ADMINISTRATION.**) Figure 1 includes an inset which shows the mean plasma concentration versus time profile to 6 hours. The vertical line denotes the median T_{max} for *FENTORA*.

[See figure 1 at top of next column]

Systemic exposure to fentanyl following administration of *FENTORA* increases linearly in an approximate dose-proportional manner over the 100- to 800-mcg dose range. Mean pharmacokinetic parameters are presented in Table 2. Mean plasma concentration versus time profiles are presented in Figure 2.

[See table 2 above]
[See figure 2 in next column]

Table 2. Pharmacokinetic Parameters* Following Single 100, 200, 400, and 800 mcg Doses of FENTORA in Healthy Subjects

Pharmacokinetic Parameter (mean ± SD)	100 mcg	200 mcg	400 mcg	800 mcg
C_{max} (ng/mL)	0.25 ± 0.14	0.40 ± 0.18	0.97 ± 0.53	1.59 ± 0.90
T_{max}, minute** (range)	45.0 (25.0-181.0)	40.0 (20.0-180.0)	35.0 (20.0-180.0)	40.0 (25.0-180.0)
AUC_{0-inf} (ng•hr/mL)	0.98 ± 0.37	2.11 ± 1.13	4.72 ± 1.95	9.05 ± 3.72
AUC_{0-tmax} (ng•hr/mL)	0.09 ± 0.06	0.13 ± 0.09	0.34 ± 0.23	0.52 ± 0.34
T1/2, hr**	2.63 (1.47-13.57)	4.43 (1.85-20.76)	11.09 (4.63-20.59)	11.70 (4.63-28.63)

* Based on venous sampling.
** Data for T_{max} presented as median (range).

Table 3. Pharmacokinetic Parameters in Patients with Mucositis

Patient status	C_{max} (ng/mL)	t_{max} (min)	AUC_{0-tmax} (ng-hr/mL)	AUC_{0-8} (ng-hr/mL)
Mucositis	1.25 ± 0.78	25.0 (15-45)	0.21 ± 0.16	2.33 ± 0.93
No mucositis	1.24 ± 0.77	22.5 (10-121)	0.25 ± 0.24	1.86 ± 0.86

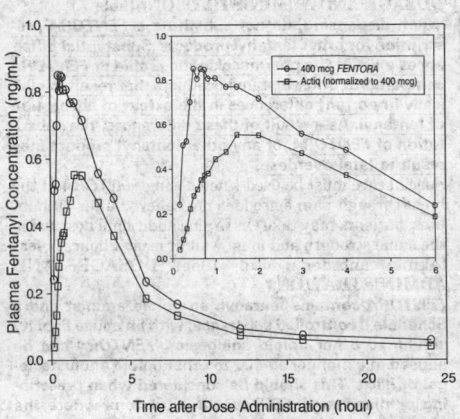

Figure 1. Mean Plasma Concentration Versus Time Profiles Following Single Doses of *FENTORA* and Actiq in Healthy Subjects

Actiq data was dose adjusted (800 mcg to 400 mcg).

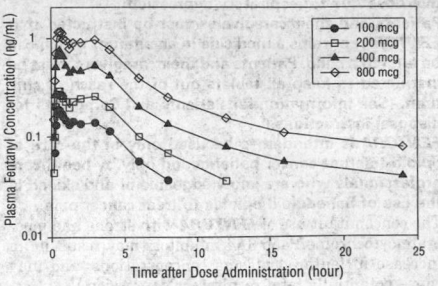

Figure 2. Mean Plasma Concentration Versus Time Profiles Following Single 100, 200, 400, and 800 mcg Doses of FENTORA in Healthy Subjects

Dwell time (defined as the length of time that the tablet takes to fully disintegrate following buccal administration), does not appear to affect early systemic exposure to fentanyl.

The effect of mucositis (Grade 1) on the pharmacokinetic profile of *FENTORA* was studied in a group of patients with (N = 8) and without mucositis (N = 8) who were otherwise matched. A single 200 mcg tablet was administered, followed by sampling at appropriate intervals. Mean summary statistics (standard deviation in parentheses, expected t_{max} where range was used) are presented in Table 3.

[See table 3 above]

Distribution:

Fentanyl is highly lipophilic. The plasma protein binding of fentanyl is 80-85%. The main binding protein is alpha-1-acid glycoprotein, but both albumin and lipoproteins contribute to some extent. The mean oral volume of distribution at steady state (Vss/F) was 25.4 L/kg.

Metabolism:

The metabolic pathways following buccal administration of *FENTORA* have not been characterized in clinical studies. The progressive decline of fentanyl plasma concentrations results from the uptake of fentanyl in the tissues and biotransformation in the liver. Fentanyl is metabolized in the liver and in the intestinal mucosa to norfentanyl by cytochrome P450 3A4 isoform. In animal studies, norfentanyl was not found to be pharmacologically active. (See **PRECAUTIONS: Drug Interactions** for additional information.)

Elimination:

Disposition of fentanyl following buccal administration of *FENTORA* has not been characterized in a mass balance study. Fentanyl is primarily (more than 90%) eliminated by biotransformation to N-dealkylated and hydroxylated inactive metabolites. Less than 7% of the administered dose is excreted unchanged in the urine, and only about 1% is excreted unchanged in the feces. The metabolites are mainly excreted in the urine, while fecal excretion is less important.

The total plasma clearance of fentanyl following intravenous administration is approximately 42 L/h.

Special Populations:

The pharmacokinetics of *FENTORA* has not been studied in Special Populations.

Race

The pharmacokinetic effects of race with the use of *FENTORA* have not been systematically evaluated. In studies conducted in healthy Japanese subjects, systemic exposure was generally higher than that observed in US subjects (mean C_{max} and AUC values were approximately 50% and 20% higher, respectively). The observed differences were largely attributed to the lower mean weight of the Japanese subjects compared to US subjects (57.4 kg versus 73 kg).

Age

The effect of age on the pharmacokinetics of *FENTORA* has not been studied.

Gender

Systemic exposure was higher for women than men (mean C_{max} and AUC values were approximately 28% and 22% higher, respectively). The observed differences between men and women were largely attributable to differences in weight.

Renal or Hepatic Impairment:

The effect of renal or hepatic impairment on the pharmacokinetics of *FENTORA* has not been studied. Although fentanyl kinetics are known to be altered as a result of hepatic and renal disease due to alterations in metabolic clearance and plasma protein binding, the duration of effect for the initial dose of fentanyl is largely determined by the rate of distribution of the drug.

Diminished metabolic clearance may, therefore, become significant, primarily with repeated dosing or at very high single doses. For these reasons, while it is recommended that *FENTORA* is titrated to clinical effect for all patients, special care should be taken in patients with severe hepatic or renal disease. (See **PRECAUTIONS.**)

Drug Interactions

The interaction between ritonavir and fentanyl was investigated in eleven healthy volunteers in a randomized crossover study. Subjects received oral ritonavir or placebo for 3 days. The ritonavir dose was 200 mg tid on Day 1 and 300 mg tid on Day 2 followed by one morning dose of 300 mg on Day 3. On Day 2, fentanyl was given as a single IV dose at 5 mcg/kg two hours after the afternoon dose of oral ritonavir or placebo. Naloxone was administered to counteract the side effects of fentanyl. The results suggested that ritonavir might decrease the clearance of fentanyl by 67%, resulting in a 174% (range 52%-420%) increase in fentanyl AUC_{0-inf}. Coadministration of ritonavir in patients receiving *FENTORA* has not been studied; however, an increase in fentanyl AUC is expected. (See **DOSAGE AND ADMINISTRATION** and **PRECAUTIONS.**)

CLINICAL TRIALS

Breakthrough Pain:

The efficacy of *FENTORA* was demonstrated in a double-blind, placebo-controlled, cross-over study in opioid tolerant patients with cancer and breakthrough pain. Patients considered opioid tolerant were those who were taking at least 60 mg of oral morphine/day, at least 25 mcg of transdermal fentanyl/hour, at least 30 mg of oxycodone daily, at least 8 mg of oral hydromorphone daily or an equianalgesic dose of another opioid for a week or longer.

In this trial, patients were titrated in an open-label manner to a successful dose of *FENTORA*. A successful dose was defined as the dose in which a patient obtained adequate analgesia with tolerable side effects. Patients who identified a successful dose were randomized to a sequence of 10 treatments with 7 being the successful dose of *FENTORA* and 3 being placebo. Patients used one tablet (either *FENTORA* or Placebo) per breakthrough pain episode.

Patients assessed pain intensity on a scale that rated the pain as 0=none to 10=worst possible pain. With each episode of breakthrough pain, pain intensity was assessed first and then treatment was administered. Pain intensity (0-10) was measured at 15, 30, 45 and 60 minutes after the start of administration. The sum of differences in pain intensity scores at 15 and 30 minutes from baseline ($SPID_{30}$) was the primary efficacy measure.

Sixty five percent of patients who entered the study achieved a successful dose during the titration phase. The distribution of successful doses is shown in Table 4. The median dose was 400 mcg.

Table 4. Successful Dose of *FENTORA* Following Initial Titration

FENTORA Dose	(N=80) n(%)
100 mcg	13 (16)
200 mcg	11 (14)
400 mcg	21 (26)
600 mcg	10 (13)
800 mcg	25 (31)

The LS mean (SE) $SPID_{30}$ for *FENTORA*-treated episodes was 3.0 (0.12) while for placebo-treated episodes it was 1.8 (0.18) (p<0.0001).

Figure 3. Mean Pain Intensity Difference (PID) at Each Time Point During the Double-Blind Treatment Period

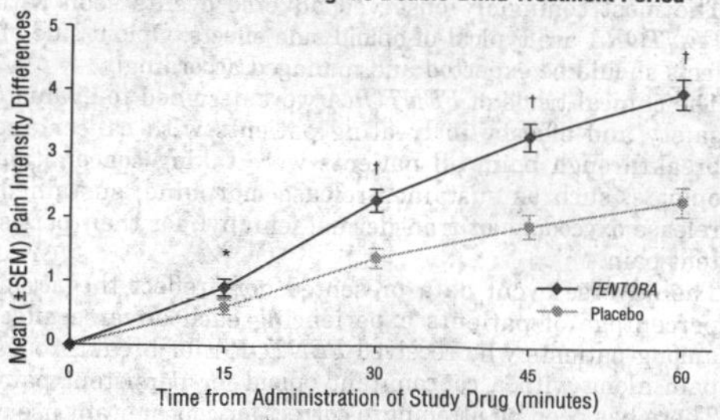

*p<0.01 *FENTORA* versus placebo, in favor of *FENTORA*, by one-sample Wilcoxon signed rank test
†p<0.0001 *FENTORA* versus placebo, in favor of *FENTORA*, by one-sample Wilcoxon signed rank test
PID=pain intensity difference; *FENTORA* fentanyl; SEM=standard error of the mean

INDICATIONS AND USAGE

(See BOXED WARNING and CONTRAINDICATIONS.)

FENTORA is indicated only for the management of breakthrough pain in patients with cancer who are **already receiving and who are tolerant to around-the-clock opioid therapy for their underlying persistent cancer pain.** Patients considered opioid tolerant are those who are taking around-the-clock medicine consisting of at least 60 mg of oral morphine daily, at least 25 mcg of transdermal fentanyl/hour, at least 30 mg of oxycodone daily, at least 8 mg of oral hydromorphone daily or an equianalgesic dose of another opioid daily for a week or longer.

This product **must not** be used in opioid non-tolerant patients because life-threatening hypoventilation and death could occur at any dose in patients not on a chronic regimen of opioids. For this reason, *FENTORA* is contraindicated in the management of acute or postoperative pain.

FENTORA is intended to be used only in the care of opioid tolerant cancer patients and only by healthcare professionals who are knowledgeable of and skilled in the use of Schedule II opioids to treat cancer pain.

CONTRAINDICATIONS

FENTORA is contraindicated in opioid non-tolerant patients. *FENTORA* is contraindicated in the management of acute or postoperative pain including headache/migraine. Life-threatening respiratory depression and death could occur at any dose in opioid non-tolerant patients.

FENTORA is contraindicated in patients with known intolerance or hypersensitivity to any of its components or the drug fentanyl.

WARNINGS

See BOXED WARNING

When prescribing, DO NOT convert a patient from Actiq to *FENTORA* without following the instructions found in the prescribing information as Actiq and *FENTORA* are not equivalent on a microgram per microgram basis. *FENTORA* is NOT a generic version of Actiq.

When dispensing, DO NOT substitute a *FENTORA* prescription for an Actiq prescription under any circumstances. *FENTORA* and Actiq are not equivalent. Substantial differences exist in the pharmacokinetic profile of *FENTORA* compared to other fentanyl products including Actiq that result in clinically important differences in the rate and extent of absorption of fentanyl. **As a result of these differences, the substitution of the same dose of *FENTORA* for the same dose of Actiq or any other fentanyl product may result in a fatal overdose.**

There are no safe conversion directions available for patients on any other fentanyl products. (Note: This includes oral, transdermal, or parenteral formulations of fentanyl.)

Therefore, for opioid tolerant patients, the initial dose of *FENTORA* should be 100 mcg. Each patient should be individually titrated to provide adequate analgesia while minimizing side effects. (See **DOSAGE AND ADMINISTRATION.**)

Use with CNS Depressants

The concomitant use of other CNS depressants, including other opioids, sedatives or hypnotics, general anesthetics, phenothiazines, tranquilizers, skeletal muscle relaxants, sedating antihistamines, potent inhibitors of cytochrome P450 3A4 isoform (e.g., erythromycin, ketoconazole, and certain protease inhibitors), and alcoholic beverages may produce increased depressant effects. Hypoventilation, hypotension, and profound sedation may occur.

FENTORA is not recommended for use in patients who have received MAO inhibitors within 14 days, because severe and unpredictable potentiation by MAO inhibitors has been reported with opioid analgesics.

Pediatric Use:

The safety and efficacy of *FENTORA* have not been established in pediatric patients below the age of 18 years.

Patients and their caregivers must be instructed that *FENTORA* contains a medicine in an amount which can be fatal to a child. Patients and their caregivers must be instructed to keep tablets out of the reach of children. (See **SAFETY AND HANDLING, PRECAUTIONS,** and **MEDICATION GUIDE** for specific patient instructions.)

Drug Abuse, Addiction and Diversion of Opioids

FENTORA contains fentanyl, a mu-opioid agonist and a Schedule II controlled substance with high potential for abuse similar to hydromorphone, methadone, morphine, oxycodone, and oxymorphone. Fentanyl can be abused and is subject to misuse, and criminal diversion.

Concerns about abuse, addiction, and diversion should not prevent the proper management of pain. However, all patients treated with opioids require careful monitoring for signs of abuse and addiction, since use of opioid analgesic products carries the risk of addiction even under appropriate medical use.

Addiction is a primary, chronic, neurobiologic disease, with genetic, psychosocial, and environmental factors influencing its development and manifestations. It is characterized by behaviors that include one or more of the following: impaired control over drug use, compulsive use, continued use despite harm, and craving. Drug addiction is a treatable disease, utilizing a multidisciplinary approach, but relapse is common.

"Drug-seeking" behavior is very common in addicts and drug abusers. *FENTORA* should be prescribed with caution to patients who have a higher risk of substance abuse, including patients with bipolar disorder and/or schizophrenia.

Patients with chronic pain may be at a higher risk for suicide.

Abuse and addiction are separate and distinct from physical dependence and tolerance. Physicians should be aware that addiction may not be accompanied by concurrent tolerance and symptoms of physical dependence in all addicts. In addition, abuse of opioids can occur in the absence of addiction and is characterized by misuse for non-medical purposes, often in combination with other psychoactive substances.

Since *FENTORA* tablets may be diverted for non-medical use, careful record keeping of prescribing information, including quantity, frequency, and renewal requests is strongly advised.

Proper assessment of patients, proper prescribing practices, periodic re-evaluation of therapy, and proper dispensing and storage are appropriate measures that help to limit abuse of opioid drugs.

FENTORA should be handled appropriately to minimize the risk of diversion, including restriction of access and accounting procedures as appropriate to the clinical setting and as required by law.

Healthcare professionals should contact their State Professional Licensing Board, or State Controlled Substances Authority for information on how to prevent and detect abuse or diversion of this product.

Physical Dependence and Withdrawal

The administration of *FENTORA* should be guided by the response of the patient. Physical dependence, per se, is not ordinarily a concern when one is treating a patient with cancer and chronic pain, and fear of tolerance and physical dependence should not deter using doses that adequately relieve the pain.

Opioid analgesics may cause physical dependence. Physical dependence results in withdrawal symptoms in patients who abruptly discontinue the drug. Withdrawal also may be precipitated through the administration of drugs with opioid antagonist activity, e.g., naloxone, nalmefene, or mixed agonist/antagonist analgesics (pentazocine, butorphanol, buprenorphine, nalbuphine).

Physical dependence usually does not occur to a clinically significant degree until after several weeks of continued opioid usage. Tolerance, in which increasingly larger doses are required in order to produce the same degree of analgesia, is initially manifested by a shortened duration of analgesic effect, and subsequently, by decreases in the intensity of analgesia.

Respiratory Depression

Respiratory depression is the chief hazard of opioid agonists, including fentanyl, the active ingredient in *FENTORA*. Respiratory depression is more likely to occur in patients with underlying respiratory disorders and elderly or debilitated patients, usually following large initial doses in opioid non-tolerant patients, or when opioids are given in conjunction with other drugs that depress respiration.

Respiratory depression from opioids is manifested by a reduced urge to breathe and a decreased rate of respiration, often associated with the "sighing" pattern of breathing (deep breaths separated by abnormally long pauses). Carbon dioxide retention from opioid-induced respiratory depression can exacerbate the sedating effects of opioids. This makes overdoses involving drugs with sedative properties and opioids especially dangerous.

PRECAUTIONS

General

Opioid analgesics impair the mental and/or physical ability required for the performance of potentially dangerous tasks (e.g., driving a car or operating machinery). Patients taking *FENTORA* should be warned of these dangers and should be counseled accordingly.

The use of concomitant CNS active drugs requires special patient care and observation. (See **WARNINGS.**)

Chronic Pulmonary Disease

Because potent opioids can cause respiratory depression, *FENTORA* should be titrated with caution in patients with chronic obstructive pulmonary disease or pre-existing medical conditions predisposing them to respiratory depression. In such patients, even normal therapeutic doses of *FENTORA* may further decrease respiratory drive to the point of respiratory failure.

Head Injuries and Increased Intracranial Pressure

FENTORA should only be administered with extreme caution in patients who may be particularly susceptible to the intracranial effects of CO_2 retention such as those with evidence of increased intracranial pressure or impaired consciousness. Opioids may obscure the clinical course of a patient with a head injury and should be used only if clinically warranted.

Application Site Reactions

In clinical trials, 10% of all patients exposed to *FENTORA* reported application site reactions. These reactions ranged from paresthesia to ulceration and bleeding. Application site reactions occurring in ≥1% of patients were pain (4%), ulcer (3%), and irritation (3%). Application site reactions tended to occur early in treatment, were self-limited and only resulted in treatment discontinuation for 2% of patients.

Cardiac Disease

Intravenous fentanyl may produce bradycardia. Therefore, *FENTORA* should be used with caution in patients with bradyarrhythmias.

Hepatic or Renal Disease

Insufficient information exists to make recommendations regarding the use of *FENTORA* in patients with impaired renal or hepatic function. Fentanyl is metabolized primarily via human cytochrome P450 3A4 isoenzyme system and mostly eliminated in urine. If the drug is used in these patients, it should be used with caution because of the hepatic metabolism and renal excretion of fentanyl.

Information for Patients and Caregivers

1. **Patients and their caregivers must be instructed that children, especially small children, exposed to *FENTORA* are at high risk of FATAL RESPIRATORY DEPRESSION.** Patients and their caregivers must be in-

structed to keep *FENTORA* tablets out of the reach of children. (See **SAFETY AND HANDLING, WARNINGS,** and **MEDICATION GUIDE** for specific patient instructions.)

2. Patients and their caregivers must be provided a Medication Guide each time *FENTORA* is dispensed because new information may be available.

3. Patients must be instructed not to take *FENTORA* for acute pain, postoperative pain, pain from injuries, headache, migraine or any other short term pain, even if they have taken other opioid analgesics for these conditions.

4. Patients must be instructed on the meaning of opioid tolerance and that *FENTORA* is only to be used as a supplemental pain medication for patients with pain requiring around-the-clock opioids, who have developed tolerance to the opioid medication, and who need additional opioid treatment of breakthrough pain episodes.

5. Patients must be instructed that, if they are not taking an opioid medication on a scheduled basis (around-the-clock), they should not take *FENTORA*.

6. Patients should be instructed that the titration phase is the only period in which they may take more than ONE tablet to achieve a desired dose (e.g., two 100 mcg tablets for a 200 mcg dose).

7. Patients must be instructed that, if the breakthrough pain episode is not relieved after 30 minutes, they may take **ONLY ONE ADDITIONAL DOSE OF** *FENTORA* **USING THE SAME STRENGTH FOR THAT EPISODE. Thus, patients should take a maximum of two doses of** *FENTORA* for any breakthrough pain episode.

8. Patients must be instructed that they MUST wait at least 4 hours before treating another episode of breakthrough pain with *FENTORA*.

9. Patients must be instructed NOT to share *FENTORA* and that sharing *FENTORA* with anyone else could result in the other individual's death due to overdose.

10. Patients must be aware that *FENTORA* contains fentanyl which is a strong pain medication similar to hydromorphone, methadone, morphine, oxycodone, and oxymorphone.

11. Patients must be instructed that the active ingredient in *FENTORA*, fentanyl, is a drug that some people abuse. *FENTORA* should be taken only by the patient it was prescribed for, and it should be protected from theft or misuse in the work or home environment.

12. Patients should be instructed that *FENTORA* tablets are not to be swallowed whole; this will reduce the effectiveness of the medication. Tablets are to be placed between the cheek and gum above a molar tooth and allowed to dissolve. After 30 minutes if remnants of the tablet still remain, patients may swallow it with a glass of water.

13. Patients must be cautioned to talk to their doctor if breakthrough pain is not alleviated or worsens after taking *FENTORA*.

14. Patients must be instructed to use *FENTORA* exactly as prescribed by their doctor and not to take *FENTORA* more often than prescribed.

15. Patients must be cautioned that *FENTORA* can affect a person's ability to perform activities that require a high level of attention (such as driving or using heavy machinery). Patients taking *FENTORA* should be warned of these dangers and counseled accordingly.

16. Patients must be warned to not combine *FENTORA* with alcohol, sleep aids, or tranquilizers except by the orders of the prescribing physician, because dangerous additive effects may occur, resulting in serious injury or death.

17. Female patients must be informed that if they become pregnant or plan to become pregnant during treatment with *FENTORA*, they should ask their doctor about the effects that *FENTORA* (or any medicine) may have on them and their unborn children.

18. Patients and caregivers must be advised that if they have been receiving treatment with *FENTORA* and the medicine is no longer needed they should flush any re-

maining product down the toilet, and if they then need further assistance, contact Cephalon at 1-800-896-5855.

Disposal of Unopened *FENTORA* Blister Packages When No Longer Needed
Patients and members of their household must be advised to dispose of any unopened blister packages remaining from a prescription as soon as they are no longer needed.
To dispose of unused *FENTORA*, remove *FENTORA* tablets from blister packages and flush down the toilet. Do not flush the *FENTORA* blister packages or cartons down the toilet. (See **SAFETY AND HANDLING.**)
Detailed instructions for the proper storage, administration, disposal, and important instructions for managing an overdose of *FENTORA* are provided in the *FENTORA* Medication Guide. Patients should be encouraged to read this information in its entirety and be given an opportunity to have their questions answered.
In the event that a caregiver requires additional assistance in disposing of excess unusable tablets that remain in the home after a patient has expired, they should be instructed to call the Cephalon toll-free number (1-800-896-5855) or seek assistance from their local DEA office.

Laboratory Tests
The effects of *FENTORA* on laboratory tests have not been evaluated.

Drug Interactions
See **WARNINGS.**
Fentanyl is metabolized mainly via the human cytochrome P450 3A4 isoenzyme system (CYP3A4); therefore potential interactions may occur when *FENTORA* is given concurrently with agents that affect CYP3A4 activity. The concomitant use of *FENTORA* with strong CYP3A4 inhibitors (e.g., ritonavir, ketoconazole, itraconazole, troleandomycin, clarithromycin, nelfinavir, and nefazadone) or moderate CYP3A4 inhibitors (e.g., amprenavir, aprepitant, diltiazem, erythromycin, fluconazole, fosamprenavir, and verapamil) may result in increased fentanyl plasma concentrations, potentially causing serious adverse drug effects including fatal respiratory depression. Patients receiving *FENTORA* concomitantly with moderate or strong CYP 3A4 inhibitors should be carefully monitored for an extended period of time. Dosage increase should be done conservatively. (See **PHARMACOKINETICS, Drug Interactions and DOSAGE AND ADMINISTRATION.**)
Grapefruit and grapefruit juice decrease CYP3A4 activity, increasing blood concentrations of fentanyl, thus should be avoided.
Drugs that induce cytochrome P450 3A4 activity may have the opposite effects.
Concomitant use of *FENTORA* with an MAO inhibitor, or within 14 days of discontinuation, is not recommended.

Carcinogenesis, Mutagenesis, and Impairment of Fertility
Long-term studies in animals have not been performed to evaluate the carcinogenic potential of fentanyl.
Fentanyl citrate was not mutagenic in the *in vitro* Ames reverse mutation assay in *S. tymphimurium* or *E. coli*, or the mouse lymphoma mutagenesis assay. Fentanyl citrate was not clastogenic in the *in vivo* mouse micronucleus assay.
Fentanyl impairs fertility in rats at doses of 30 mcg/kg IV and 160 mcg/kg SC. Conversion to human equivalent doses indicates this is within the range of the human recommended dosing for *FENTORA*.

Pregnancy - Category C
There are no adequate and well-controlled studies in pregnant women. *FENTORA* should be used during pregnancy only if the potential benefit justifies the potential risk to the fetus. No epidemiological studies of congenital anomalies in infants born to women treated with fentanyl during pregnancy have been reported.
Chronic maternal treatment with fentanyl during pregnancy has been associated with transient respiratory depression, behavioral changes, or seizures characteristic of neonatal abstinence syndrome in newborn infants. Symptoms of neonatal respiratory or neurological depression were no more frequent than expected in most studies of infants born to women treated acutely during labor with in-

travenous or epidural fentanyl. Transient neonatal muscular rigidity has been observed in infants whose mothers were treated with intravenous fentanyl.
Fentanyl is embryocidal as evidenced by increased resorptions in pregnant rats at doses of 30 mcg/kg IV or 160 mcg/kg SC. Conversion to human equivalent doses indicates this is within the range of the human recommended dosing for *FENTORA*.
Fentanyl citrate was not teratogenic when administered to pregnant animals. Published studies demonstrated that administration of fentanyl (10, 100, or 500 mcg/kg/day) to pregnant rats from day 7 to 21, of their 21 day gestation, via implanted microosmotic minipumps was not teratogenic (the high dose was approximately 3-times the human dose of 1600 mcg per pain episode on a mg/m² basis). Intravenous administration of fentanyl (10 or 30 mcg/kg) to pregnant female rats from gestation day 6 to 18, was embryo or fetal toxic, and caused a slightly increased mean delivery time in the 30 mcg/kg/day group, but was not teratogenic.

Labor and Delivery
Fentanyl readily passes across the placenta to the fetus; therefore *FENTORA* is not recommended for analgesia during labor and delivery.

Nursing Mothers
Fentanyl is excreted in human milk; therefore *FENTORA* should not be used in nursing women because of the possibility of sedation and/or respiratory depression in their infants. Symptoms of opioid withdrawal may occur in infants at the cessation of nursing by women using *FENTORA*.

Pediatric Use
See **WARNINGS.**

Geriatric Use
Of the 304 patients with cancer in clinical studies of *FENTORA*, 69 (23%) were 65 years of age and older.
Patients over the age of 65 years tended to titrate to slightly lower doses than younger patients.
Patients over the age of 65 years reported a slightly higher frequency for some adverse events specifically vomiting, constipation, and abdominal pain. Therefore, caution should be exercised in individually titrating *FENTORA* in elderly patients to provide adequate efficacy while minimizing risk.

ADVERSE REACTIONS
Pre-Marketing Clinical Trial Experience
The safety of *FENTORA* has been evaluated in 304 opioid tolerant cancer patients with breakthrough pain. The average duration of therapy was 76 days with some patients being treated for over 12 months.
The most commonly observed adverse events seen with *FENTORA* are typical of opioid side effects. Opioid side effects should be expected and managed accordingly.
The clinical trials of *FENTORA* were designed to evaluate safety and efficacy in treating patients with cancer and breakthrough pain; all patients were taking concomitant opioids, such as sustained-release morphine, sustained-release oxycodone or transdermal fentanyl, for their persistent pain.
The adverse event data presented here reflect the actual percentage of patients experiencing each adverse effect among patients who received *FENTORA* for breakthrough pain along with a concomitant opioid for persistent pain. There has been no attempt to correct for concomitant use of other opioids, duration of *FENTORA* therapy or cancer-related symptoms.
Table 5 lists, by maximum dose received, adverse events with an overall frequency of 5% or greater within the total population that occurred during titration. The ability to assign a dose-response relationship to these adverse events is limited by the titration schemes used in these studies.
[See table 5 at left]
Table 6 lists, by successful dose, adverse events with an overall frequency of ≥ 5% within the total population that occurred after a successful dose had been determined.
[See table 6 at top of next page]
In addition, a small number of patients (n=11) with Grade 1 mucositis were included in clinical trials designed to support the safety of *FENTORA*. There was no evidence of excess toxicity in this subset of patients.
The duration of exposure to *FENTORA* varied greatly, and included open-label and double-blind studies. The frequencies listed below represent the ≥1% of patients from three clinical trials (titration and post-titration periods combined) who experienced that event while receiving *FENTORA*. Events are classified by system organ class.
Adverse Events (≥1%)
Blood and Lymphatic System Disorders: Anemia, Neutropenia, Thrombocytopenia, Leukopenia
Cardiac Disorders: Tachycardia
Gastrointestinal Disorders: Nausea, Vomiting, Constipation, Abdominal Pain, Diarrhea, Stomatitis, Dry Mouth, Dyspepsia, Upper Abdominal Pain, Abdominal Distension, Dysphagia, Gingival Pain, Stomach Discomfort, Gastroesophageal Reflux Disease, Glossodynia, Mouth Ulceration

Table 5. Adverse Events Which Occurred During Titration at a Frequency of ≥ 5%

System Organ Class MeDRA preferred term, n (%)	100 mcg (N=45)	200 mcg (N=34)	400 mcg (N=53)	600 mcg (N=56)	800 mcg (N=113)	Total (N=304)*
Gastrointestinal disorders						
Nausea	4 (9)	5 (15)	10 (19)	13 (23)	18 (16)	50 (17)
Vomiting	0	2 (6)	2 (4)	7 (13)	3 (3)	14 (5)
General disorders and administration site conditions						
Fatigue	3 (7)	1 (3)	9 (17)	1 (2)	5 (4)	19 (6)
Nervous system disorders						
Dizziness	5 (11)	2 (6)	12 (23)	18 (32)	21 (19)	58 (19)
Somnolence	2 (4)	2 (6)	6 (12)	7 (13)	3 (3)	20 (7)
Headache	1 (2)	3 (9)	4 (8)	8 (14)	10 (9)	26 (9)

*Three hundred and two (302) patients were included in the safety analysis.

General Disorders and Administration Site Conditions: Fatigue, Edema Peripheral, Asthenia, Pyrexia, Application Site Pain, Application Site Ulcer, Chest Pain, Chills, Application Site Irritation, Edema, Mucosal Inflammation, Pain

Hepatobiliary Disorders: Jaundice

Infections and Infestations: Pneumonia, Oral Candidiasis, Urinary Tract Infection, Cellulitis, Nasopharyngitis, Sinusitis, Upper Respiratory Tract Infection, Influenza, Tooth Abscess

Injury, Poisoning and Procedural Complications: Fall, Spinal Compression Fracture

Investigations: Decreased Weight, Decreased Hemoglobin, Increased Blood Glucose, Decreased Hematocrit, Decreased Platelet Count

Metabolism and Nutrition Disorders: Dehydration, Anorexia, Hypokalemia, Decreased Appetite, Hypoalbuminemia, Hypercalcemia, Hypomagnesemia, Hyponatremia, Reduced Oral Intake

Musculoskeletal and Connective Tissue Disorders: Arthralgia, Back Pain, Pain in Extremity, Myalgia, Chest Wall Pain, Muscle Spasms, Neck Pain, Shoulder Pain

Nervous System Disorders: Dizziness, Headache, Somnolence, Hypoesthesia, Dysgeusia, Lethargy, Peripheral Neuropathy, Paresthesia, Balance Disorder, Migraine, Neuropathy

Psychiatric Disorders: Confusional State, Depression, Insomnia, Anxiety, Disorientation, Euphoric Mood, Hallucination, Nervousness

Renal and Urinary Disorders: Renal Failure

Respiratory, Thoracic and Mediastinal Disorders: Dyspnea, Cough, Pharyngolaryngeal Pain, Exertional Dyspnea, Pleural Effusion, Decreased Breathing Sounds, Wheezing

Skin and Subcutaneous Tissue Disorders: Pruritus, Rash, Hyperhidrosis, Cold Sweat

Vascular Disorders: Hypertension, Hypotension, Pallor, Deep Vein Thrombosis

OVERDOSAGE

Clinical Presentation

The manifestations of *FENTORA* overdosage are expected to be similar in nature to intravenous fentanyl and other opioids, and are an extension of its pharmacological actions with the most serious significant effect being hypoventilation. (See **CLINICAL PHARMACOLOGY**.)

General

Immediate management of opioid overdose includes removal of the *FENTORA* tablet, if still in the mouth, ensuring a patent airway, physical and verbal stimulation of the patient, and assessment of level of consciousness, as well as ventilatory and circulatory status.

Treatment of Overdosage in the Opioid Non-Tolerant Person

Ventilatory support should be provided, intravenous access obtained, and naloxone or other opioid antagonists should be employed as clinically indicated. The duration of respiratory depression following overdose may be longer than the effects of the opioid antagonist's action (e.g., the half-life of naloxone ranges from 30 to 81 minutes) and repeated administration may be necessary. Consult the package insert of the individual opioid antagonist for details about such use.

Treatment of Overdose in Opioid-Tolerant Patients

Ventilatory support should be provided and intravenous access obtained as clinically indicated. Judicious use of naloxone or another opioid antagonist may be warranted in some instances, but it is associated with the risk of precipitating an acute withdrawal syndrome.

General Considerations for Overdose

Management of severe *FENTORA* overdose includes: securing a patent airway, assisting or controlling ventilation, establishing intravenous access, and GI decontamination by lavage and/or activated charcoal, once the patient's airway is secure. In the presence of hypoventilation or apnea, ventilation should be assisted or controlled and oxygen administered as indicated.

Patients with overdose should be carefully observed and appropriately managed until their clinical condition is well controlled.

Although muscle rigidity interfering with respiration has not been seen following the use of *FENTORA*, this is possible with fentanyl and other opioids. If it occurs, it should be managed by the use of assisted or controlled ventilation, by an opioid antagonist, and as a final alternative, by a neuromuscular blocking agent.

DOSAGE AND ADMINISTRATION

Physicians should individualize treatment using a progressive plan of pain management. Healthcare professionals should follow appropriate pain management principles of careful assessment and ongoing monitoring. (See **BOXED WARNING** and Dosing.)

It is important to minimize the number of strengths available to patients at any time to prevent confusion and possible overdose.

Table 6. Adverse Events Which Occurred During Long-Term Treatment at a Frequency of ≥ 5%

System Organ Class MeDRA preferred term, n (%)	100 mcg (N=19)	200 mcg (N=31)	400 mcg (N=44)	600 mcg (N=48)	800 mcg (N=58)	Total (N=200)
Blood and lymphatic system disorders						
Anemia	6 (32)	4 (13)	4 (9)	5 (10)	7 (13)	26 (13)
Neutropenia	0	2 (6)	1 (2)	4 (8)	4 (7)	11 (6)
Gastrointestinal disorders						
Nausea	8 (42)	5 (16)	14 (32)	13 (27)	17 (31)	57 (29)
Vomiting	7 (37)	5 (16)	9 (20)	8 (17)	11 (20)	40 (20)
Constipation	5 (26)	4 (13)	5 (11)	4 (8)	6 (11)	24 (12)
Diarrhea	3 (16)	0	4 (9)	3 (6)	5 (9)	15 (8)
Abdominal pain	2 (11)	1 (3)	4 (9)	7 (15)	4 (7)	18 (9)
General disorders and administration site conditions						
Edema peripheral	6 (32)	5 (16)	4 (9)	5 (10)	3 (5)	23 (12)
Asthenia	3 (16)	5 (16)	2 (5)	3 (6)	8 (15)	21 (11)
Fatigue	3 (16)	3 (10)	9 (20)	9 (19)	8 (15)	32 (16)
Infections and infestations						
Pneumonia	1 (5)	5 (16)	1 (2)	1 (2)	4 (7)	12 (6)
Investigations						
Weight decreased	1 (5)	1 (3)	3 (7)	2 (4)	6 (11)	13 (7)
Metabolism and nutrition disorders						
Dehydration	4 (21)	0	4 (9)	6 (13)	7 (13)	21 (11)
Anorexia	1 (5)	2 (6)	4 (9)	3 (6)	6 (11)	16 (8)
Hypokalemia	0	2 (6)	0	1 (2)	8 (15)	11 (6)
Musculoskeletal and connective tissue disorders						
Back pain	2 (11)	0	2 (5)	3 (6)	2 (4)	9 (5)
Arthralgia	0	1 (3)	3 (7)	4 (8)	3 (5)	11 (6)
Neoplasms benign, malignant and unspecified (including cysts and polyps)						
Cancer pain	3 (16)	1 (3)	3 (7)	2 (4)	1 (2)	10 (5)
Nervous system disorders						
Dizziness	5 (26)	3 (10)	5 (11)	6 (13)	6 (11)	25 (13)
Headache	2 (11)	1 (3)	4 (9)	5 (10)	8 (15)	20 (10)
Somnolence	0	1 (3)	4 (9)	4 (8)	8 (15)	17 (9)
Psychiatric disorders						
Confusional state	3 (16)	1 (3)	2 (5)	3 (6)	5 (9)	14 (7)
Depression	2 (11)	1 (3)	4 (9)	3 (6)	5 (9)	15 (8)
Insomnia	2 (11)	1 (3)	3 (7)	2 (4)	4 (7)	12 (6)
Respiratory, thoracic, and mediastinal disorders						
Cough	1 (5)	1 (3)	2 (5)	4 (8)	5 (9)	13 (7)
Dyspnea	1 (5)	6 (19)	0	7 (15)	4 (7)	18 (9)

Dosing

1. **Initial Dose**

a. For opioid-tolerant patients **not** being converted from Actiq, the initial dose of *FENTORA* is **always** 100 mcg.

b. For patients being converted from Actiq, prescribers must use the Initial Dosing Recommendations table below (Table 7). The doses of *FENTORA* in this table are starting doses and not intended to represent equianalgesic doses to Actiq. Patients must be instructed to stop the use of Actiq and dispose of any remaining units.

Table 7. Initial Dosing Recommendations for Patients on Actiq

Current Actiq Dose (mcg)	Initial *FENTORA* Dose (mcg)
200	100 mcg tablet
400	100 mcg tablet
600	200 mcg tablet
800	200 mcg tablet
1200	2 × 200 mcg tablets
1600	2 × 200 mcg tablets

c. For patients converting from Actiq doses equal to or greater than 600 mcg, titration should be initiated with the 200 mcg *FENTORA* tablet and should proceed using multiples of this tablet strength.

d. In cases where the breakthrough pain episode is not relieved after 30 minutes, patients may take **ONLY ONE** additional dose using the same strength for that episode. Thus patients should take a maximum of two doses of *FENTORA* for any episode of breakthrough pain.

e. Patients MUST wait **at least 4 hours** before treating another episode of breakthrough pain with *FENTORA*.

2. **Titration**

a. From an initial dose, patients should be closely followed by the prescriber and the dosage strength changed until the patient reaches a dose that provides adequate analgesia with tolerable side effects. Patients should record their use of *FENTORA* over several episodes of breakthrough pain and discuss their experience with their physician to determine if a dosage adjustment is warranted.

b. Patients whose initial dose is 100 mcg and who need to titrate to a higher dose, can be instructed to use two 100-mcg tablets (one on each side of the mouth in the buccal cavity) with their next breakthrough pain episode. If this dosage is not successful, the patient may be instructed to place two 100-mcg tablets on each side of the mouth in the buccal cavity (total of four 100-mcg tablets). Titrate using multiples of the 200-mcg *FENTORA* tablet for doses above 400 mcg (600 mcg and 800 mcg). Note: Do not use more than 4 tablets simultaneously.

c. In cases where the breakthrough pain episode is not relieved after 30 minutes, patients may take **ONLY ONE** additional dose of the same strength for that episode. Thus patients should take a maximum of two doses of *FENTORA* for any breakthrough pain episode. During titration, one **dose** of *FENTORA* may include administration of 1 to 4 tablets of the same dosage strength (100 mcg or 200 mcg).

d. Patients MUST wait **at least 4 hours** before treating another episode of breakthrough pain with *FENTORA*. To reduce the risk of overdosing during titration, patients should have only one strength of *FENTORA* tablets available at any one time.

e. Patients should be strongly encouraged to use all of their *FENTORA* tablets of one strength prior to being prescribed the next strength. If this is not practical, unused *FENTORA* should be disposed of safely. (See **DISPOSAL OF FENTORA**.) Dispose of any unopened *FENTORA* tablets remaining from a prescription as soon as they are no longer needed.

3. **Maintenance Dosing**

a. Once titrated to an effective dose, patients should generally use **only ONE** *FENTORA* tablet of the appropriate strength per breakthrough pain episode.

b. On occasion when the breakthrough pain episode is not relieved after 30 minutes, patients may take **ONLY ONE** additional dose using the same strength for that episode.

c. Patients MUST wait **at least 4 hours** before treating another episode of breakthrough pain with *FENTORA*.

d. Dosage adjustment of *FENTORA* may be required in some patients in order to continue to provide adequate relief of breakthrough pain.

Generally, the *FENTORA* dose should be increased only when a single administration of the current dose fails to adequately treat the breakthrough pain episode for several consecutive episodes.

If the patient experiences greater than four breakthrough pain episodes per day, the dose of the maintenance (around-the-clock) opioid used for persistent pain should be re-evaluated.

Patients With Hepatic and/or Renal Impairment

Caution should be exercised for patients with hepatic and/or renal impairment, and the lowest possible dose should be used in these patients. (See **PRECAUTIONS**.)

Patients Receiving CYP3A4 Inhibitors

Particular caution should be exercised for patients receiving CYP3A4 inhibitors, and the lowest possible dose should be used in these patients. (See **PRECAUTIONS**.)

Patients With Mucositis

No dose adjustment appears necessary in patients with Grade 1 mucositis. The safety and efficacy of *FENTORA* when used in patients with mucositis more severe than Grade 1 have not been studied.

Opening the Blister Package

1. Patients should be instructed not to open the blister until ready to administer *FENTORA*.
2. A single blister unit should be separated from the blister card by bending and tearing apart at the perforations.
3. The blister unit should then be bent along the line where indicated.
4. The blister backing should then be peeled back to expose the tablet. **Patients should NOT attempt to push the tablet through the blister as this may cause damage to the tablet.**
5. The tablet should not be stored once it has been removed from the blister package as the tablet integrity may be compromised, and more importantly, because this increases the risk of accidental exposure to the tablet.

Tablet Administration

Once the tablet is removed from the blister unit, the patient should **immediately** place the entire *FENTORA* tablet in the buccal cavity (above a rear molar, between the upper cheek and gum). **Patients should not split the tablet.**

The *FENTORA* tablet should not be sucked, chewed or swallowed, as this will result in lower plasma concentrations than when taken as directed.

The *FENTORA* tablet should be left between the cheek and gum until it has disintegrated, which usually takes approximately 14-25 minutes.

After 30 minutes, if remnants from the *FENTORA* tablet remain, they may be swallowed with a glass of water.

It is recommended that patients alternate sides of the mouth when administering subsequent doses of *FENTORA*.

SAFETY AND HANDLING

FENTORA is supplied in individually sealed, child-resistant blister packages. The amount of fentanyl contained in *FENTORA* can be fatal to a child. **Patients and their caregivers must be instructed to keep *FENTORA* out of the reach of children. (See BOXED WARNING, WARNINGS, PRECAUTIONS, and MEDICATION GUIDE.)**

Store at 20-25°C (68-77°F) with excursions permitted between 15° and 30°C (59° to 86°F) until ready to use. (See USP Controlled Room Temperature.)

FENTORA should be protected from freezing and moisture. Do not use if the blister package has been tampered with.

DISPOSAL OF *FENTORA*

Patients and members of their household must be advised to dispose of any tablets remaining from a prescription as soon as they are no longer needed. Information is available in the **Information for Patients and Caregivers** and in the **Medication Guide**. If additional assistance is required, referral to the Cephalon 800# (1-800-896-5855) should be made.

To dispose of unused *FENTORA*, remove *FENTORA* tablets from blister packages and flush down the toilet. Do not flush *FENTORA* blister packages or cartons down the toilet. If you need additional assistance with disposal of *FENTORA*, call Cephalon, Inc., at 1-800-896-5855.

HOW SUPPLIED

Each carton contains 7 blister cards with 4 white tablets in each card. The blisters are child-resistant, encased in peelable foil, and provide protection from moisture. Each tablet is debossed on one side with [C], and the other side of each dosage strength is uniquely identified by the debossing on the tablet as described in the table below. The dosage strength of each tablet is marked on the tablet, the blister package and the carton. See blister package and carton for product information.

Dosage Strength (fentanyl base)	Debossing	Carton/Blister Package Color	NDC Number
100 mcg	1	Blue	NDC 63459-541-28
200 mcg	2	Orange	NDC 63459-542-28
300 mcg	3	Gray	NDC 63459-543-28
400 mcg	4	Sage green	NDC 63459-544-28
600 mcg	6	Magenta (pink)	NDC 63459-546-28
800 mcg	8	Yellow	NDC 63459-548-28

Note: Carton/blister package colors are a secondary aid in product identification. Please be sure to confirm the printed dosage before dispensing.

Rx only.

DEA order form required. A Schedule CII narcotic.

Manufactured for:
Cephalon, Inc.
Frazer, PA 19355
By:
CIMA LABS, INC.
10000 Valley View Road
Eden Prairie, MN 55344
and
Cephalon, Inc.
4745 Wiley Post Way
Salt Lake City, UT 84116
U. S. Patent Nos. 6,200,604 and 6,974,590
Printed in USA
FENTORA® is a registered trademark of Cephalon, Inc., or its affiliates.
Label code 00010583.04
December 2009
© 2006-2009 Cephalon, Inc., or its affiliates. All rights reserved.

Shown in Product Identification Guide, page 308

GABITRIL® ℞

[găb-ĭ-trĭl]
(tiagabine hydrochloride)
Tablets

DESCRIPTION

GABITRIL® (tiagabine HCl) is an antiepilepsy drug available as 2 mg, 4 mg, 12 mg, and 16 mg tablets for oral administration. Its chemical name is (-)-(R)-1-[4,4-Bis(3-methyl-2-thienyl)-3-butenyl]nipecotic acid hydrochloride, its molecular formula is $C_{20}H_{25}NO_2S_2$ HCl, and its molecular weight is 412.0. Tiagabine HCl is a white to off-white, odorless, crystalline powder. It is insoluble in heptane, sparingly soluble in water, and soluble in aqueous base. The structural formula is:

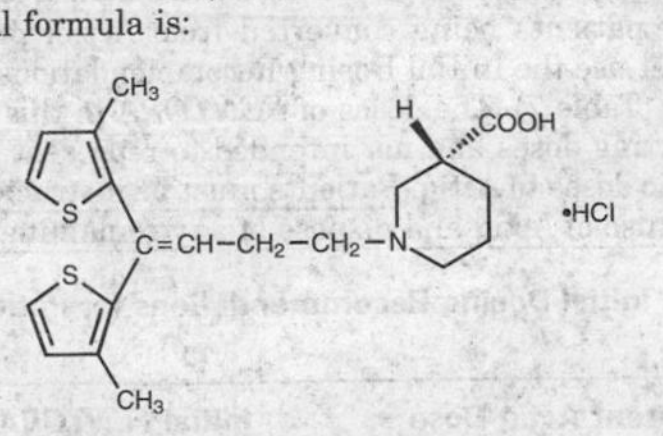

Inactive Ingredients

GABITRIL tablets contain the following inactive ingredients: Ascorbic acid, colloidal silicon dioxide, crospovidone, hydrogenated vegetable oil wax, hydroxypropyl cellulose, hypromellose, lactose, magnesium stearate, microcrystalline cellulose, pregelatinized starch, stearic acid, and titanium dioxide.

In addition, individual tablets contain:

2 mg tablets: FD&C Yellow No. 6.
4 mg tablets: D&C Yellow No. 10.
12 mg tablets: D&C Yellow No. 10 and FD&C Blue No. 1.
16 mg tablets: FD&C Blue No. 2.

CLINICAL PHARMACOLOGY

Mechanism of Action

The precise mechanism by which tiagabine exerts its antiseizure effect is unknown, although it is believed to be related to its ability, documented in *in vitro* experiments, to enhance the activity of gamma aminobutyric acid (GABA), the major inhibitory neurotransmitter in the central nervous system. These experiments have shown that tiagabine binds to recognition sites associated with the GABA uptake carrier. It is thought that, by this action, tiagabine blocks GABA uptake into presynaptic neurons, permitting more GABA to be available for receptor binding on the surfaces of post-synaptic cells. Inhibition of GABA uptake has been shown for synaptosomes, neuronal cell cultures, and glial cell cultures. In rat-derived hippocampal slices, tiagabine has been shown to prolong GABA-mediated inhibitory post-synaptic potentials. Tiagabine increases the amount of GABA available in the extracellular space of the globus pallidus, ventral palladum, and substantia nigra in rats at the ED_{50} and ED_{85} doses for inhibition of pentylenetetrazol (PTZ)-induced tonic seizures. This suggests that tiagabine prevents the propagation of neural impulses that contribute to seizures by a GABA-ergic action.

Tiagabine has shown efficacy in several animal models of seizures. It is effective against the tonic phase of subcutaneous PTZ-induced seizures in mice and rats, seizures induced by the proconvulsant DMCM in mice, audiogenic seizures in genetically epilepsy-prone rats (GEPR), and amygdala-kindled seizures in rats. Tiagabine has little efficacy against maximal electroshock seizures in rats and is only partially effective against subcutaneous PTZ-induced clonic seizures in mice, picrotoxin-induced tonic seizures in the mouse, bicuculline-induced seizures in the rat, and photic seizures in photosensitive baboons. Tiagabine produces a biphasic dose-response curve against PTZ- and DMCM-induced convulsions, with attenuated effectiveness at higher doses.

Based on *in vitro* binding studies, tiagabine does not significantly inhibit the uptake of dopamine, norepinephrine, serotonin, glutamate, or choline and shows little or no binding to dopamine D1 and D2, muscarinic, serotonin $5HT_{1A}$, $5HT_2$, and $5HT_3$, beta-1 and 2 adrenergic, alpha-1 and alpha-2 adrenergic, histamine H2 and H3, adenosine A_1 and A_2, opiate μ and K_1, NMDA glutamate, and $GABA_A$ receptors at 100 μM. It also lacks significant affinity for sodium or calcium channels. Tiagabine binds to histamine H1, serotonin $5HT_{1B}$, benzodiazepine, and chloride channel receptors at concentrations 20 to 400 times those inhibiting the uptake of GABA.

Pharmacokinetics

Tiagabine is well absorbed, with food slowing absorption rate but not altering the extent of absorption. The elimination half-life of tiagabine is 7 to 9 hours in normal volunteers. In epilepsy clinical trials, most patients were receiving hepatic enzyme-inducing agents (e.g., carbamazepine, phenytoin, primidone, and phenobarbital). The pharmacokinetic profile in induced patients is significantly different from the non-induced population (see **PRECAUTIONS, General, Use in Non-Induced Patients**). The systemic clearance of tiagabine in induced patients is approximately 60% greater resulting in considerably lower plasma concentrations and an elimination half-life of 2 to 5 hours. Given this difference in clearance, the systemic exposure after a dose of 32 mg/day in an induced population is expected to be comparable to the systemic exposure after a dose of 12 mg/day in a non-induced population. Similarly, the systemic exposure after a dose of 56 mg/day in an induced population is expected to be comparable to the systemic exposure after a dose of 22 mg/day in a non-induced population.

Absorption and Distribution

Absorption of tiagabine is rapid, with peak plasma concentrations occurring at approximately 45 minutes following an oral dose in the fasting state. Tiagabine is nearly completely absorbed (>95%), with an absolute oral bioavailability of about 90%. A high fat meal decreases the rate (mean T_{max} was prolonged to 2.5 hours, and mean C_{max} was reduced by about 40%) but not the extent (AUC) of tiagabine absorption. In all clinical trials, tiagabine was given with meals. The pharmacokinetics of tiagabine are linear over the single dose range of 2 to 24 mg. Following multiple dosing, steady state is achieved within 2 days.

Tiagabine is 96% bound to human plasma proteins, mainly to serum albumin and α1-acid glycoprotein over the concentration range of 10 ng/mL to 10,000 ng/mL. While the relationship between tiagabine plasma concentrations and clinical response is not currently understood, trough plasma concentrations observed in controlled clinical trials at doses from 30 to 56 mg/day ranged from <1 ng/mL to 234 ng/mL.

Metabolism and Elimination

Although the metabolism of tiagabine has not been fully elucidated, *in vivo* and *in vitro* studies suggest that at least two metabolic pathways for tiagabine have been identified in humans: 1) thiophene ring oxidation leading to the formation of 5-oxo-tiagabine; and 2) glucuronidation. The 5-oxo-tiagabine metabolite does not contribute to the pharmacologic activity of tiagabine.

Based on *in vitro* data, tiagabine is likely to be metabolized primarily by the 3A isoform subfamily of hepatic cytochrome P450 (CYP 3A), although contributions to the metabolism of tiagabine from CYP 1A2, CYP 2D6 or CYP 2C19 have not been excluded.

Approximately 2% of an oral dose of tiagabine is excreted unchanged, with 25% and 63% of the remaining dose excreted into the urine and feces, respectively, primarily as metabolites, at least 2 of which have not been identified. The mean systemic plasma clearance is 109 mL/min (CV = 23%) and the average elimination half-life for tiagabine in healthy subjects ranged from 7 to 9 hours. The elimination half-life decreased by 50 to 65% in hepatic enzyme-induced patients with epilepsy compared to uninduced patients with epilepsy.

A diurnal effect on the pharmacokinetics of tiagabine was observed. Mean steady-state C_{min} values were 40% lower in the evening than in the morning. Tiagabine steady-state AUC values were also found to be 15% lower following the evening tiagabine dose compared to the AUC following the morning dose.

Special Populations

Renal Insufficiency

The pharmacokinetics of total and unbound tiagabine were similar in subjects with normal renal function (creatinine clearance >80 mL/min) and in subjects with mild (creatinine clearance 40 to 80 mL/min), moderate (creatinine clearance 20 to 39 mL/min), or severe (creatinine clearance 5 to 19 mL/min) renal impairment. The pharmacokinetics of total and unbound tiagabine were also unaffected in subjects with renal failure requiring hemodialysis.

Hepatic Insufficiency

In patients with moderate hepatic impairment (Child-Pugh Class B), clearance of unbound tiagabine was reduced by about 60%. Patients with impaired liver function may require reduced initial and maintenance doses of tiagabine and/or longer dosing intervals compared to patients with normal hepatic function (see **PRECAUTIONS**).

Geriatric

The pharmacokinetic profile of tiagabine was similar in healthy elderly and healthy young adults.

Pediatric

Tiagabine has not been investigated in adequate and well-controlled clinical trials in patients below the age of 12. The apparent clearance and volume of distribution of tiagabine per unit body surface area or per kg were fairly similar in 25 children (age: 3 to 10 years) and in adults taking enzyme-inducing antiepilepsy drugs ([AEDs] e.g., carbamazepine or phenytoin). In children who were taking a non-inducing AED (e.g., valproate), the clearance of tiagabine based upon body weight and body surface area was 2 and 1.5-fold higher, respectively, than in non-induced adults with epilepsy.

Gender, Race and Cigarette Smoking

No specific pharmacokinetic studies were conducted to investigate the effect of gender, race and cigarette smoking on the disposition of tiagabine. Retrospective pharmacokinetic analyses, however, suggest that there is no clinically important difference between the clearance of tiagabine in males and females, when adjusted for body weight. Population pharmacokinetic analyses indicated that tiagabine clearance values were not significantly different in Caucasian (N=463), Black (N=23), or Hispanic (N=17) patients with epilepsy, and that tiagabine clearance values were not significantly affected by tobacco use.

Interactions with other Antiepilepsy Drugs

The clearance of tiagabine is affected by the co-administration of hepatic enzyme-inducing antiepilepsy drugs. Tiagabine is eliminated more rapidly in patients who have been taking hepatic enzyme-inducing drugs, e.g., carbamazepine, phenytoin, primidone and phenobarbital than in patients not receiving such treatment (see **PRECAUTIONS, Drug Interactions**).

Interactions with Other Drugs

See **PRECAUTIONS, Drug Interactions.**

CLINICAL STUDIES

The effectiveness of GABITRIL as adjunctive therapy (added to other antiepilepsy drugs) was examined in three multi-center, double-blind, placebo-controlled, parallel-group, clinical trials in 769 patients with refractory partial seizures who were taking at least one hepatic enzyme-inducing antiepilepsy drug (AED), and two placebo-controlled cross-over studies in 90 patients. In the parallel-group trials, patients had a history of at least six complex partial seizures (Study 1 and Study 2, U.S. studies), or six partial seizures of any type (Study 3, European study), occurring alone or in combination with any other seizure type within the 8-week period preceding the first study visit in spite of receiving one or more AEDs at therapeutic concentrations.

In the first two studies, the primary protocol-specified outcome measure was the median reduction from baseline in the 4-week complex partial seizure (CPS) rates during treatment. In the third study, the protocol-specified primary outcome measure was the proportion of patients achieving a 50% or greater reduction from baseline in the 4-week seizure rate of all partial seizures during treatment. The results given below include data for complex partial seizures and all partial seizures for the intent-to-treat population (all patients who received at least one dose of treatment and at least one seizure evaluation) in each study.

Study 1 was a double-blind, placebo-controlled, parallel-group trial comparing GABITRIL 16 mg/day, GABITRIL 32 mg/day, GABITRIL 56 mg/day, and placebo. Study drug was given as a four times a day regimen. After a prospective Baseline Phase of 12 weeks, patients were randomized to one of the four treatment groups described above. The 16-week Treatment Phase consisted of a 4-week Titration Period, followed by a 12-week Fixed-Dose Period, during which concomitant AED doses were held constant. The primary outcome was assessed for the combined 32 and 56 mg/day groups compared to placebo.

Study 2 was a double-blind, placebo-controlled, parallel-group trial consisting of an 8-week Baseline Phase and a

12-week Treatment Phase, the first 4 weeks of which constituted a Titration Period and the last 8 weeks a Fixed-Dose Period. This study compared GABITRIL 16 mg BID and 8 mg QID to placebo. The protocol-specified primary outcome measure was assessed separately for each group treated with GABITRIL.

The following tables display the results of the analyses of these two trials.

[See table 1 above]

[See table 2 above]

Figures 1 to 4 present the proportion of patients (X-axis) whose percent reduction from baseline in the all partial seizure rate was at least as great as that indicated on the Y axis in the three placebo-controlled adjunctive studies (Studies 1, 2, and 3). A positive value on the Y axis indicates an improvement from baseline (i.e., a decrease in seizure rate), while a negative value indicates a worsening from baseline (i.e., an increase in seizure rate). Thus, in a display of this type, the curve for an effective treatment is shifted to the left of the curve for placebo.

Figure 1 indicates that the proportion of patients achieving any particular level of reduction in seizure rate was consistently higher for the combined GABITRIL 32 mg and 56 mg groups compared to the placebo group in Study 1. For example, Figure 1 indicates that approximately 24% of patients treated with GABITRIL experienced a 50% or greater reduction, compared to 4% in the placebo group.

Figure 1, Study 1

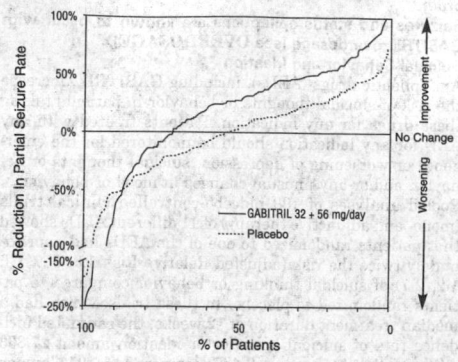

Figure 2 also displays the results for Study 1, which was a dose-response study, by treatment group, without combining GABITRIL dosage groups. Figure 2 indicates a dose-response relationship across the three GABITRIL groups. The proportion of patients achieving any particular level of reduction in all partial seizure rates was consistently higher as the dose of GABITRIL was increased. For example, Figure 2 indicates that approximately 4% of patients in the placebo group experienced a 50% or greater reduction in all partial seizure rate, compared to approximately 10% of the GABITRIL 16 mg/day group, 21% of the GABITRIL 32 mg/day group, and 30% of the GABITRIL 56 mg/day group.

Figure 2, Study 1

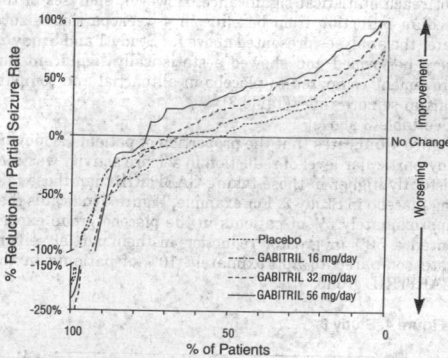

Figure 3 indicates that the proportion of patients achieving any particular level of reduction in partial seizure rate was consistently greater in patients taking GABITRIL than in those taking placebo in Study 2. (Study 2 compared placebo to GABITRIL 32 mg/day; one of the GABITRIL groups received 8 mg QID, while the other GABITRIL group received 16 mg BID). For example, Figure 3 indicates that approximately 7% of patients in the placebo group experienced a 50% or greater reduction in their partial seizure rate, compared to approximately 23% of patients in the GABITRIL 8 mg QID group and 28% of patients in the GABITRIL 16 mg BID group.

Figure 3, Study 2

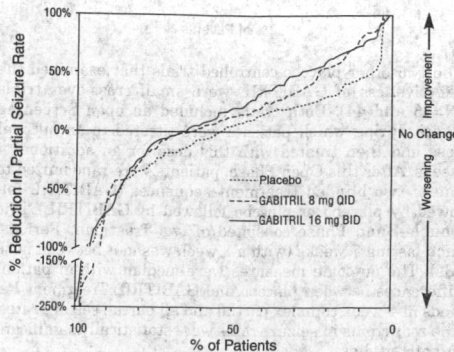

Study 3 was a double-blind, placebo-controlled, parallel-group trial that compared GABITRIL 10 mg TID (N=77) with placebo (N=77). In this trial, patients were followed prospectively during a 12-week Baseline Phase and then randomized to receive study drug during an 18-week Treatment Phase. During the first 6 weeks of treatment (Titration Period), patients were titrated to 30 mg/day, after which they were maintained on this dose during the 12-

Table 1: Median Reduction and Median Percent Reduction from Baseline in 4-Week Seizure Rates in Study 1

		Placebo (N=91)	GABITRIL 16 mg/day (N=61)	GABITRIL 32 mg/day (N=87)	GABITRIL 56 mg/day (N=56)	Combined 32 and 56 mg/day (N=143)
Complex Partial	Median Reduction	0.6	0.8	2.2*	2.9*	2.6*
	Median % Reduction[†]	9%	13%	25%	32%	29%
All Partial	Median Reduction	0.2	1.2	2.7*	3.5*	2.9*
	Median % Reduction[†]	3%	12%	24%	36%	27%

*p < 0.05
[†]Statistical significance was not assessed for median % reduction.

Table 2: Median Reduction and Median Percent Reduction from Baseline in 4-Week Seizure Rates in Study 2

		Placebo (N=107)	GABITRIL 16 mg BID (N=106)	GABITRIL 8 mg QID (N=104)
Complex Partial	Median Reduction	0.3	1.6	1.3*
	Median % Reduction[†]	4%	22%	15%
All Partial	Median Reduction	0.5	1.6	1.3
	Median % Reduction[†]	5%	19%	13%

*p < 0.027, necessary for statistical significance due to multiple comparisons.
[†]Statistical significance was not assessed for median % reduction.

Table 3: Median Reduction and Median Percent Reduction from Baseline in 4-Week Seizure Rates in Study 3

		Placebo (N=77)	GABITRIL 30 mg/day (N=77)
Complex Partial‡	Median Reduction	-0.1	1.3*
	Median % Reduction†	-1%	14%
All Partial	Median Reduction	-0.5	1.1*
	Median % Reduction†	-7%	11%

*p < 0.05
†Statistical significance was not assessed for median % reduction.
‡N=72 and 75 for placebo and GABITRIL, respectively.

Table 4: Risk by Indication for Antiepileptic Drugs in the Pooled Analysis

Indication	Placebo Patients with Events per 1000 Patients	Drug Patients with Events per 1000 Patients	Relative Risk: Incidence of Events in Drug Patients/Incidence in Placebo Patients	Risk Difference: Additional Drug Patients with Events per 1000 Patients
Epilepsy	1.0	3.4	3.5	2.4
Psychiatric	5.7	8.5	1.5	2.9
Other	1.0	1.8	1.9	0.9
Total	2.4	4.3	1.8	1.9

week Fixed-Dose Period. The protocol-specified primary outcome measure (proportion of patients who achieved at least a 50% reduction from baseline in partial seizure rate) did not reach statistical significance. However, analyses of the median reduction from baseline in 4-week partial seizure rate (the analyses presented above for Study 1 and Study 2) were performed and showed a statistically significant improvement compared to placebo in all partial and complex partial seizure rates (Table 3):

[See table 3 above]

Figure 4 indicates that the proportion of patients achieving any particular level of reduction in seizure activity was consistently higher in those taking GABITRIL than those taking placebo in Study 3. For example, Figure 4 indicates that approximately 5% of patients in the placebo group experienced a 50% or greater reduction in their partial seizure rate compared to approximately 10% of patients in the GABITRIL group.

Figure 4, Study 3

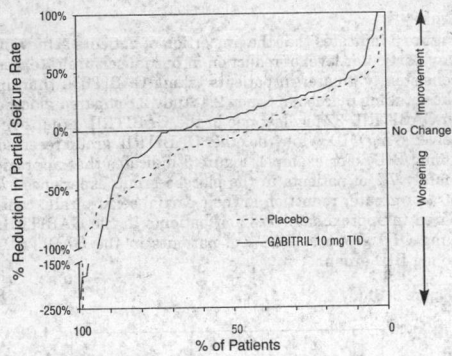

The two other placebo-controlled trials that examined the effectiveness of GABITRIL were small cross-over trials (N=46 and 44). Both trials included an open Screening Phase during which patients were titrated to an optimal dose and then treated with this dose for an additional 4 weeks. After this Open Phase, patients were randomized to one of two blinded treatment sequences (GABITRIL followed by placebo or placebo followed by GABITRIL). The Double-Blind Phase consisted of two Treatment Periods, each lasting 7 weeks (with a 3 week washout between periods). The outcome measures were median with-in patient differences between placebo and GABITRIL Treatment Periods in 4-week complex partial and all partial seizure rates. The reductions in seizure rates were statistically significant in both studies.

INDICATIONS AND USAGE

GABITRIL (tiagabine hydrochloride) is indicated as adjunctive therapy in adults and children 12 years and older in the treatment of partial seizures.

CONTRAINDICATIONS

GABITRIL is contraindicated in patients who have demonstrated hypersensitivity to the drug or its ingredients.

WARNINGS

Seizures in Patients Without Epilepsy: Post-marketing reports have shown that GABITRIL use has been associated with new onset seizures and status epilepticus in patients without epilepsy. Dose may be an important predisposing factor in the development of seizures, although seizures have been reported in patients taking daily doses of GABITRIL as low as 4 mg/day. In most cases, patients were using concomitant medications (antidepressants, antipsychotics, stimulants, narcotics) that are thought to lower the seizure threshold. Some seizures occurred near the time of a dose increase, even after periods of prior stable dosing.

The GABITRIL dosing recommendations in current labeling for treatment of epilepsy were based on use in patients with partial seizures 12 years of age and older, most of whom were taking enzyme-inducing antiepileptic drugs (AEDs; e.g., carbamazepine, phenytoin, primidone and phenobarbital) which lower plasma levels of GABITRIL by inducing its metabolism. Use of GABITRIL without enzyme-inducing antiepileptic drugs results in blood levels about twice those attained in the studies on which current dosing recommendations are based (see DOSAGE AND ADMINISTRATION).

Safety and effectiveness of GABITRIL have not been established for any indication other than as adjunctive therapy for partial seizures in adults and children 12 years and older.

In nonepileptic patients who develop seizures while on GABITRIL treatment, GABITRIL should be discontinued and patients should be evaluated for an underlying seizure disorder.

Seizures and status epilepticus are known to occur with GABITRIL overdosage (see OVERDOSAGE).

Suicidal Behavior and Ideation

Antiepileptic drugs (AEDs), including GABITRIL, increase the risk of suicidal thoughts or behavior in patients taking these drugs for any indication. Patients treated with any AED for any indication should be monitored for the emergence or worsening of depression, suicidal thoughts or behavior, and/or any unusual changes in mood or behavior.

Pooled analyses of 199 placebo-controlled clinical trials (mono- and adjunctive therapy) of 11 different AEDs showed that patients randomized to one of the AEDs had approximately twice the risk (adjusted Relative Risk 1.8, 95% CI: 1.2, 2.7) of suicidal thinking or behavior compared to patients randomized to placebo. In these trials, which had a median treatment duration of 12 weeks, the estimated incidence rate of suicidal behavior or ideation among 27,863 AED-treated patients was 0.43%, compared to 0.24% among 16,029 placebo-treated patients, representing an increase of approximately one case of suicidal thinking or behavior for every 530 patients treated. There were four suicides in drug-treated patients in the trials and none in placebo-treated patients, but the number is too small to allow any conclusion about drug effect on suicide.

The increased risk of suicidal thoughts or behavior with AEDs was observed as early as one week after starting drug treatment with AEDs and persisted for the duration of treatment assessed. Because most trials included in the analysis did not extend beyond 24 weeks, the risk of suicidal thoughts or behavior beyond 24 weeks could not be assessed.

The risk of suicidal thoughts or behavior was generally consistent among drugs in the data analyzed. The finding of increased risk with AEDs of varying mechanisms of action and across a range of indications suggests that the risk applies to all AEDs used for any indication. The risk did not vary substantially by age (5-100 years) in the clinical trials analyzed.

Table 4 shows absolute and relative risk by indication for all evaluated AEDs.

[See table 4 at left]

The relative risk for suicidal thoughts or behavior was higher in clinical trials for epilepsy than in clinical trials for psychiatric or other conditions, but the absolute risk differences were similar for the epilepsy and psychiatric indications.

Anyone considering prescribing GABITRIL or any other AED must balance the risk of suicidal thoughts or behavior with the risk of untreated illness. Epilepsy and many other illnesses for which AEDs are prescribed are themselves associated with morbidity and mortality and an increased risk of suicidal thoughts and behavior. Should suicidal thoughts and behavior emerge during treatment, the prescriber needs to consider whether the emergence of these symptoms in any given patient may be related to the illness being treated.

Patients, their caregivers, and families should be informed that AEDs increase the risk of suicidal thoughts and behavior and should be advised of the need to be alert for the emergence or worsening of the signs and symptoms of depression, any unusual changes in mood or behavior, or the emergence of suicidal thoughts, behavior, or thoughts about self-harm. Behaviors of concern should be reported immediately to healthcare providers.

Withdrawal Seizures

As a rule, antiepilepsy drugs should not be abruptly discontinued because of the possibility of increasing seizure frequency. In a placebo-controlled, double-blind, dose-response study (Study 1 described in CLINICAL STUDIES) designed, in part, to investigate the capacity of GABITRIL to induce withdrawal seizures, study drug was tapered over a 4-week period after 16 weeks of treatment. Patients' seizure frequency during this 4-week withdrawal period was compared to their baseline seizure frequency (before study drug). For each partial seizure type, for all partial seizure types combined, and for secondarily generalized tonic-clonic seizures, more patients experienced increases in their seizure frequencies during the withdrawal period in the three GABITRIL groups than in the placebo group. The increase in seizure frequency was not affected by dose. GABITRIL should be withdrawn gradually to minimize the potential of increased seizure frequency, unless safety concerns require a more rapid withdrawal.

Cognitive/Neuropsychiatric Adverse Events

Adverse events most often associated with the use of GABITRIL were related to the central nervous system. The most significant of these can be classified into 2 general categories: 1) impaired concentration, speech or language problems, and confusion (effects on thought processes); and 2) somnolence and fatigue (effects on level of consciousness). The majority of these events were mild to moderate. In controlled clinical trials, these events led to discontinuation of treatment with GABITRIL in 6% (31 of 494) of patients compared to 2% (5 of 275) of the placebo-treated patients. A total of 1.6% (8 of 494) of the GABITRIL treated patients in the controlled trials were hospitalized secondary to the occurrence of these events compared to 0% of the placebo treated patients. Some of these events were dose related and usually began during initial titration.

Patients with a history of spike and wave discharges on EEG have been reported to have exacerbations of their EEG abnormalities associated with these cognitive/neuropsychiatric events. This raises the possibility that these clinical events may, in some cases, be a manifestation of underlying seizure activity (see PRECAUTIONS, Laboratory Tests, EEG). In the documented cases of spike and wave discharges on EEG with cognitive/neuropsychiatric events, patients usually continued tiagabine, but required dosage adjustment.

Additionally, there have been postmarketing reports of patients who have experienced cognitive/neuropsychiatric symptoms, some accompanied by EEG abnormalities such as generalized spike and wave activity, that have been reported as nonconvulsant status epilepticus. Some reports describe recovery following reduction of dose or discontinuation of GABITRIL.

Status Epilepticus

In the three double-blind, placebo-controlled, parallel-group studies (Studies 1, 2, and 3), the incidence of any type of status epilepticus (simple, complex, or generalized tonic-clonic) in patients receiving GABITRIL was 0.8% (4 of 494 patients) versus 0.7% (2 of 275 patients) receiving placebo. Among the patients treated with GABITRIL across all epilepsy studies (controlled and uncontrolled), 5% had some form of status epilepticus. Of the 5%, 57% of patients experienced complex partial status epilepticus. A critical risk factor for status epilepticus was the presence of a previous history; 33% of patients with a history of status epilepticus had recurrence during GABITRIL treatment. Because adequate information about the incidence of status epilepticus in a similar population of patients with epilepsy who have not received treatment with GABITRIL is not available, it is impossible to state whether or not treatment with GABITRIL is associated with a higher or lower rate of status epilepticus than would be expected to occur in a similar population not treated with GABITRIL.

Sudden Unexpected Death In Epilepsy (SUDEP)

There have been as many as 10 cases of sudden unexpected deaths during the clinical development of tiagabine among 2531 patients with epilepsy (3831 patient-years of exposure).

This represents an estimated incidence of 0.0026 deaths per patient-year. This rate is within the range of estimates for the incidence of sudden and unexpected deaths in patients with epilepsy not receiving GABITRIL (ranging from 0.0005 for the general population with epilepsy, 0.003 to 0.004 for clinical trial populations similar to that in the clinical development program for GABITRIL, to 0.005 for patients with refractory epilepsy. The estimated SUDEP rates in patients receiving GABITRIL are also similar to those observed in patients receiving other antiepilepsy drugs, chemically unrelated to GABITRIL, that underwent clinical testing in similar populations at about the same time. This evidence suggests that the SUDEP rates reflect population rates, not a drug effect.

PRECAUTIONS

General

Use in Non-Induced Patients

Virtually all experience with GABITRIL has been obtained in patients with epilepsy receiving at least one concomitant enzyme-inducing antiepilepsy drug (AED), which lowers the plasma levels of tiagabine. Use in non-induced patients requires lower doses of GABITRIL. These patients may also require a slower titration of GABITRIL compared to that of induced patients (see **DOSAGE AND ADMINISTRATION**). Patients taking a combination of inducing and non-inducing agents (e.g., carbamazepine and valproate) should be considered to be induced. Patients not receiving hepatic enzyme-inducing agents are referred to as non-induced patients.

Generalized Weakness

Moderately severe to incapacitating generalized weakness has been reported following administration of GABITRIL in 28 of 2531 (approximately 1%) patients with epilepsy. The weakness resolved in all cases after a reduction in dose or discontinuation of GABITRIL.

Binding in the Eye and Other Melanin-Containing Tissues

When dogs received a single dose of radiolabeled tiagabine, there was evidence of residual binding in the retina and uvea after 3 weeks (the latest time point measured). Although not directly measured, melanin binding is suggested. The ability of available tests to detect potentially adverse consequences, if any, of the binding of tiagabine to melanin-containing tissue is unknown and there was no systematic monitoring for relevant ophthalmological changes during the clinical development of GABITRIL. However, long term (up to one year) toxicological studies of tiagabine in dogs showed no treatment-related ophthalmoscopic changes and macro- and microscopic examinations of the eye were unremarkable. Accordingly, although there are no specific recommendations for periodic ophthalmologic monitoring, prescribers should be aware of the possibility of long-term ophthalmologic effects.

Use in Hepatically-Impaired Patients

Because the clearance of tiagabine is reduced in patients with liver disease, dosage reduction may be necessary in these patients.

Serious Rash

Four patients treated with tiagabine during the product's premarketing clinical testing developed what were considered to be serious rashes. In two patients, the rash was described as maculopapular; in one it was described as vesiculobullous; and in the 4th case, a diagnosis of Stevens-Johnson Syndrome was made. In none of the 4 cases is it certain that tiagabine was the primary, or even a contributory, cause of the rash. Nevertheless, drug associated rash can, if extensive and serious, cause irreversible morbidity, even death.

Information for Patients

Suicidal Thinking and Behavior

Patients, their caregivers, and families should be counseled that AEDs, including GABITRIL, may increase the risk of suicidal thoughts and behavior and should be advised of the need to be alert for the emergence or worsening of symptoms of depression, any unusual changes in mood or behavior, or the emergence of suicidal thoughts, behavior, or thoughts about self-harm. Behaviors of concern should be reported immediately to healthcare providers.

Patients should be advised that GABITRIL may cause dizziness, somnolence, and other symptoms and signs of CNS depression. Accordingly, patients should be advised neither to drive nor to operate other complex machinery until they have gained sufficient experience on GABITRIL to gauge whether or not it affects their mental and/or motor performance adversely. Because of the possible additive depressive effects, caution should also be used when patients are taking other CNS depressants in combination with GABITRIL.

Because teratogenic effects were seen in the offspring of rats exposed to maternally toxic doses of tiagabine and because experience in humans is limited, patients should be advised to notify their physicians if they become pregnant or intend to become pregnant during therapy.

Because of the possibility that tiagabine may be excreted in breast milk, patients should be advised to notify those providing care to themselves and their children if they intend to breast-feed or are breast-feeding an infant.

Patients should be encouraged to enroll in the North American Antiepileptic Drug (NAAED) Pregnancy Registry if they become pregnant. This registry is collecting information about the safety of antiepileptic drugs during pregnancy. To enroll, patients can call the toll free number 1-888-233-2334 (see **PRECAUTIONS, Pregnancy**).

Laboratory Tests

Therapeutic Monitoring of Plasma Concentrations of Tiagabine

A therapeutic range for tiagabine plasma concentrations has not been established. In controlled trials, trough plasma concentrations observed among patients randomized to doses of tiagabine that were statistically significantly more effective than placebo ranged from <1 ng/mL to 234 ng/mL (median, 10th and 90th percentiles are 23.7 ng/mL, 5.4 ng/mL, and 69.8 ng/mL, respectively). Because of the potential for pharmacokinetic interactions between GABITRIL and drugs that induce or inhibit hepatic metabolizing enzymes, it may be useful to obtain plasma levels of tiagabine before and after changes are made in the therapeutic regimen.

Clinical Chemistry and Hematology

During the development of GABITRIL, no systematic abnormalities on routine laboratory testing were noted. Therefore, no specific guidance is offered regarding routine monitoring; the practitioner retains responsibility for determining how best to monitor the patient in his/her care.

EEG

Patients with a history of spike and wave discharges on EEG have been reported to have exacerbations of their EEG abnormalities associated with cognitive/neuropsychiatric events. This raises the possibility that these clinical events may, in some cases, be a manifestation of underlying seizure activity (see **WARNINGS, Cognitive/Neuropsychiatric Adverse Events**). In the documented cases of spike and wave discharges on EEG with cognitive/neuropsychiatric events, patients usually continued tiagabine, but required dosage adjustment.

Drug Interactions

In evaluating the potential for interactions among co-administered antiepilepsy drugs (AEDs), whether or not an AED induces or does not induce metabolic enzymes is an important consideration. Carbamazepine, phenytoin, primidone, and phenobarbital are generally classified as enzyme inducers; valproate and gabapentin are not. GABITRIL is considered to be a non-enzyme inducing AED (see **PRECAUTIONS, General, Use in Non-Induced Patients**).

The drug interaction data described in this section were obtained from studies involving either healthy subjects or patients with epilepsy.

Effects of GABITRIL on other Antiepilepsy Drugs (AEDs):

Phenytoin: Tiagabine had no effect on the steady-state plasma concentrations of phenytoin in patients with epilepsy.

Carbamazepine: Tiagabine had no effect on the steady-state plasma concentrations of carbamazepine or its epoxide metabolite in patients with epilepsy.

Valproate: Tiagabine causes a slight decrease (about 10%) in steady-state valproate concentrations.

Phenobarbital or Primidone: No formal pharmacokinetic studies have been performed examining the addition of tiagabine to regimens containing phenobarbital or primidone. The addition of tiagabine in a limited number of patients in three well-controlled studies caused no systematic changes in phenobarbital or primidone concentrations when compared to placebo.

Effects of other Antiepilepsy Drugs (AEDs) on GABITRIL:

Carbamazepine: Population pharmacokinetic analyses indicate that tiagabine clearance is 60% greater in patients taking carbamazepine with or without other enzyme-inducing AEDs.

Phenytoin: Population pharmacokinetic analyses indicate that tiagabine clearance is 60% greater in patients taking phenytoin with or without other enzyme-inducing AEDs.

Phenobarbital (Primidone): Population pharmacokinetic analyses indicate that tiagabine clearance is 60% greater in patients taking phenobarbital (primidone) with or without other enzyme-inducing AEDs.

Valproate: The addition of tiagabine to patients taking valproate chronically had no effect on tiagabine pharmacokinetics, but valproate significantly decreased tiagabine binding in vitro from 96.3 to 94.8%, which resulted in an increase of approximately 40% in the free tiagabine concentration. The clinical relevance of this in vitro finding is unknown.

Interaction of GABITRIL with Other Drugs:

Cimetidine: Co-administration of cimetidine (800 mg/day) to patients taking tiagabine chronically had no effect on tiagabine pharmacokinetics.

Theophylline: A single 10 mg dose of tiagabine did not affect the pharmacokinetics of theophylline at steady state.

Warfarin: No significant differences were observed in the steady-state pharmacokinetics of R-warfarin or S-warfarin with the addition of tiagabine given as a single dose. Prothrombin times were not affected by tiagabine.

Digoxin: Concomitant administration of tiagabine did not affect the steady-state pharmacokinetics of digoxin or the mean daily trough serum level of digoxin.

Ethanol or Triazolam: No significant differences were observed in the pharmacokinetics of triazolam (0.125 mg) and tiagabine (10 mg) when given together as a single dose. The pharmacokinetics of ethanol were not affected by multiple-dose administration of tiagabine. Tiagabine has shown no clinically important potentiation of the pharmacodynamic effects of triazolam or alcohol. Because of the possible additive effects of drugs that may depress the nervous system, ethanol or triazolam should be used cautiously in combination with tiagabine.

Oral Contraceptives: Multiple dose administration of tiagabine (8 mg/day monotherapy) did not alter the pharmacokinetics of oral contraceptives in healthy women of child-bearing age.

Antipyrine: Antipyrine pharmacokinetics were not significantly different before and after tiagabine multiple-dose regimens. This indicates that tiagabine does not cause induction or inhibition of the hepatic microsomal enzyme systems responsible for the metabolism of antipyrine.

Interaction of GABITRIL with Highly Protein Bound Drugs:

In vitro data showed that tiagabine is 96% bound to human plasma protein and therefore has the potential to interact with other highly protein bound compounds. Such an interaction can potentially lead to higher free fractions of either tiagabine or the competing drug.

Carcinogenesis, Mutagenesis, Impairment of Fertility

Carcinogenesis: In rats, a study of the potential carcinogenicity associated with tiagabine HCl administration showed that 200 mg/kg/day (plasma exposure [AUC] 36 to 100 times that at the maximum recommended human dosage [MRHD] of 56 mg/day) for 2 years resulted in small, but statistically significant increases in the incidences of hepatocellular adenomas in females and Leydig cell tumors of the testis in males. The significance of these findings relative to the use of GABITRIL in humans is unknown. The no effect dosage for induction of tumors in this study was 100 mg/kg/day (17 to 50 times the exposure at the MRHD). No statistically significant increases in tumor formation were noted in mice at dosages up to 250 mg/kg/day (20 times the MRHD on a mg/m² basis).

Mutagenesis: Tiagabine produced an increase in structural chromosome aberration frequency in human lymphocytes in vitro in the absence of metabolic activation. No increase in chromosomal aberration frequencies was demonstrated in this assay in the presence of metabolic activation. No evidence of genetic toxicity was found in the in vitro bacterial gene mutation assays, the in vitro HGPRT forward mutation assay in Chinese hamster lung cells, the in vivo mouse micronucleus test, or an unscheduled DNA synthesis assay.

Impairment of Fertility: Studies of male and female rats administered dosages of tiagabine HCl prior to and during mating, gestation, and lactation have shown no impairment of fertility at doses up to 100 mg/kg/day. This dose represents approximately 16 times the maximum recommended human dose (MRHD) of 56 mg/day, based on body surface area (mg/m²). Lowered maternal weight gain and decreased viability and growth in the rat pups were found at 100 mg/kg, but not at 20 mg/kg/day (3 times the MRHD on a mg/m² basis).

Pregnancy:

Pregnancy Category C: Tiagabine has been shown to have adverse effects on embryo-fetal development, including teratogenic effects, when administered to pregnant rats and rabbits at doses greater than the human therapeutic dose. An increased incidence of malformed fetuses (various craniofacial, appendicular, and visceral defects) and decreased fetal weights were observed following oral administration of 100 mg/kg/day to pregnant rats during the period of organogenesis. This dose is approximately 16 times the maximum recommended human dose (MRHD) of 56 mg/day, based on body surface area (mg/m^2). Maternal toxicity (transient weight loss/reduced maternal weight gain during gestation) was associated with this dose, but there is no evidence to suggest that the teratogenic effects were secondary to the maternal effects. No adverse maternal or embryofetal effects were seen at a dose of 20 mg/kg/day (3 times the MRHD on a mg/m^2 basis).

Decreased maternal weight gain, increased resorption of embryos and increased incidences of fetal variations, but not malformations, were observed when pregnant rabbits were given 25 mg/kg/day (8 times the MRHD on a mg/m^2 basis) during organogenesis. The no effect level for maternal and embryo-fetal toxicity in rabbits was 5 mg/kg/day (equivalent to the MRHD on a mg/m^2 basis).

When female rats were given tiagabine 100 mg/kg/day during late gestation and throughout parturition and lactation, decreased maternal weight gain during gestation, an increase in stillbirths, and decreased postnatal offspring viability and growth were found. There are no adequate and well-controlled studies in pregnant women. Tiagabine should be used during pregnancy only if clearly needed.

To provide additional information regarding the effects of in utero exposure to GABITRIL, physicians are advised to recommend that pregnant patients taking GABITRIL enroll in the NAAED Pregnancy Registry. This can be done by calling the toll free number 1-888-233-2334, and must be done by patients themselves. Information on the registry can also be found at the website http://www.aedpregnancyregistry.org/.

Use in Nursing Mothers:
Studies in rats have shown that tiagabine HCl and/or its metabolites are excreted in the milk of that species. Levels of excretion of tiagabine and/or its metabolites in human milk have not been determined and effects on the nursing infant are unknown. GABITRIL should be used in women who are nursing only if the benefits clearly outweigh the risks.

Pediatric Use:
Safety and effectiveness in pediatric patients below the age of 12 have not been established. The pharmacokinetics of tiagabine were evaluated in pediatric patients age 3 to 10 years (see CLINICAL PHARMACOLOGY, Special Populations, Pediatric).

Geriatric Use:
Because few patients over the age of 65 (approximately 20) were exposed to GABITRIL during its clinical evaluation,

no specific statements about the safety or effectiveness of GABITRIL in this age group could be made.

ADVERSE REACTIONS

The most commonly observed adverse events in placebo-controlled, parallel-group, add-on epilepsy trials associated with the use of GABITRIL in combination with other antiepilepsy drugs not seen at an equivalent frequency among placebo-treated patients were dizziness/light-headedness, asthenia/lack of energy, somnolence, nausea, nervousness/irritability, tremor, abdominal pain, and thinking abnormal/difficulty with concentration or attention.

Approximately 21% of the 2531 patients who received GABITRIL in clinical trials of epilepsy discontinued treatment because of an adverse event. The adverse events most commonly associated with discontinuation were dizziness (1.7%), somnolence (1.6%), depression (1.3%), confusion (1.1%), and asthenia (1.1%).

In Studies 1 and 2 (U.S. studies), the double-blind, placebo-controlled, parallel-group, add-on studies, the proportion of patients who discontinued treatment because of adverse events was 11% for the group treated with GABITRIL and 6% for the placebo group. The most common adverse events considered the primary reason for discontinuation were confusion (1.2%), somnolence (1.0%), and ataxia (1.0%).

Adverse Event Incidence in Controlled Clinical Trials
Table 5 lists treatment-emergent signs and symptoms that occurred in at least 1% of patients treated with GABITRIL for epilepsy participating in parallel-group, placebo-controlled trials and were numerically more common in the GABITRIL group. In these studies, either GABITRIL or placebo was added to the patient's current antiepilepsy drug therapy. Adverse events were usually mild or moderate in intensity.

The prescriber should be aware that these figures, obtained when GABITRIL was added to concurrent antiepilepsy drug therapy, cannot be used to predict the frequency of adverse events in the course of usual medical practice when patient characteristics and other factors may differ from those prevailing during clinical studies. Similarly, the cited frequencies cannot be directly compared with figures obtained from other clinical investigations involving different treatments, uses, or investigators. An inspection of these frequencies, however, does provide the prescribing physician with one basis to estimate the relative contribution of drug and non-drug factors to the adverse event incidences in the population studied.

Table 5: Treatment-Emergent Adverse Event[1] Incidence in Parallel-Group, Placebo-Controlled, Add-On Trials (events in at least 1% of patients treated with GABITRIL and numerically more frequent than in the placebo group)

Body System/ COSTART	GABITRIL N=494 %	Placebo N=275 %
Body as a Whole		
Abdominal Pain	7	3
Pain (unspecified)	5	3
Cardiovascular		
Vasodilation	2	1
Digestive		
Nausea	11	9
Diarrhea	7	3
Vomiting	7	4
Increased Appetite	2	0
Mouth Ulceration	1	0
Musculoskeletal		
Myasthenia	1	0
Nervous System		
Dizziness	27	15
Asthenia	20	14
Somnolence	18	15
Nervousness	10	3
Tremor	9	3
Difficulty with Concentration/Attention*	6	2
Insomnia	6	4
Ataxia	5	3
Confusion	5	3
Speech Disorder	4	2
Difficulty With Memory*	4	3
Paresthesia	4	2
Depression	3	1
Emotional Lability	3	2
Abnormal Gait	3	2
Hostility	2	1
Nystagmus	2	1
Language Problems*	2	0
Agitation	1	0
Respiratory System		
Pharyngitis	7	4
Cough Increased	4	3
Skin and Appendages		
Rash	5	4
Pruritus	2	0

[1]Patients in these add-on studies were receiving one to three concomitant enzyme-inducing antiepilepsy drugs in addition to GABITRIL or placebo. Patients may have reported multiple adverse experiences; thus, patients may be included in more than one category.
*COSTART term substituted with a more clinically descriptive term.

Other events reported by 1% or more of patients treated with GABITRIL but equally or more frequent in the placebo group were: accidental injury, chest pain, constipation, flu syndrome, rhinitis, anorexia, back pain, dry mouth, flatulence, ecchymosis, twitching, fever, amblyopia, conjunctivitis, urinary tract infection, urinary frequency, infection, dyspepsia, gastroenteritis, nausea and vomiting, myalgia, diplopia, headache, anxiety, acne, sinusitis, and incoordination.

Study 1 was a dose-response study including doses of 32 mg and 56 mg. Table 6 shows adverse events reported at a rate of ≥ 5% in at least one GABITRIL group and more frequent than in the placebo group. Among these events, depression, tremor, nervousness, difficulty with concentration/attention, and perhaps asthenia exhibited a positive relationship to dose.

[See table 6 at left]

The effects of GABITRIL in relation to those of placebo on the incidence of adverse events and the types of adverse events reported were independent of age, weight, and gender. Because only 10% of patients were non-Caucasian in parallel-group, placebo-controlled trials, there is insufficient data to support a statement regarding the distribution of adverse experience reports by race.

Other Adverse Events Observed During All Clinical Trials
GABITRIL has been administered to 2531 patients during all phase 2/3 clinical trials, only some of which were placebo-controlled. During these trials, all adverse events were recorded by the clinical investigators using terminology of their own choosing. To provide a meaningful estimate of the proportion of individuals having adverse events, similar types of events were grouped into a smaller number of standardized categories using modified COSTART dictionary terminology. These categories are used in the listing below. The frequencies presented represent the proportion of the 2531 patients exposed to GABITRIL who experienced

Table 6: Treatment-Emergent Adverse Event Incidence in Study 1[†] (events in at least 5% of patients treated with GABITRIL 32 or 56 mg and numerically more frequent than in the placebo group)

Body System/ COSTART Term	GABITRIL 56 mg (N=57) %	GABITRIL 32 mg (N=88) %	Placebo (N=91) %
Body as a Whole			
Accidental Injury	21	15	20
Infection	19	10	12
Flu Syndrome	9	6	3
Pain	7	2	3
Abdominal Pain	5	7	4
Digestive System			
Diarrhea	2	10	6
Hemic and Lymphatic System			
Ecchymosis	0	6	1
Musculoskeletal System			
Myalgia	5	2	3
Nervous System			
Dizziness	28	31	12
Asthenia	23	18	15
Tremor	21	14	1
Somnolence	19	21	17
Nervousness	14	11	6
Difficulty with Concentration/Attention*	14	7	3
Ataxia	9	6	0
Depression	7	1	0
Insomnia	5	6	3
Abnormal Gait	5	5	3
Hostility	5	5	2
Respiratory System			
Pharyngitis	7	8	6
Special Senses			
Amblyopia	4	9	8
Urogenital System			
Urinary Tract Infection	5	0	2

[†] Patients in this study were receiving one to three concomitant enzyme-inducing antiepilepsy drugs in addition to GABITRIL or placebo. Patients may have reported multiple adverse experiences; thus, patients may be included in more than one category.
* COSTART term substituted with a more clinically descriptive term.

events of the type cited on at least one occasion while receiving GABITRIL. All reported events are included except those already listed above, events seen only three times or fewer (unless potentially important), events very unlikely to be drug-related, and those too general to be informative. Events are included without regard to determination of a causal relationship to tiagabine.

Events are further classified within body system categories and enumerated in order of decreasing frequency using the following definitions: frequent adverse events are defined as those occurring in at least 1/100 patients; infrequent adverse events are those occurring in 1/100 to 1/1000 patients; rare events are those occurring in fewer than 1/1000 patients.

Body as a Whole: *Frequent:* Allergic reaction, chest pain, chills, cyst, neck pain, and malaise. *Infrequent:* Abscess, cellulitis, facial edema, halitosis, hernia, neck rigidity, neoplasm, pelvic pain, photosensitivity reaction, sepsis, sudden death, and suicide attempt.

Cardiovascular System: *Frequent:* Hypertension, palpitation, syncope, and tachycardia. *Infrequent:* Angina pectoris, cerebral ischemia, electrocardiogram abnormal, hemorrhage, hypotension, myocardial infarct, pallor, peripheral vascular disorder, phlebitis, postural hypotension, and thrombophlebitis.

Digestive System: *Frequent:* Gingivitis and stomatitis. *Infrequent:* Abnormal stools, cholecystitis, cholelithiasis, dysphagia, eructation, esophagitis, fecal incontinence, gastritis, gastrointestinal hemorrhage, glossitis, gum hyperplasia, hepatomegaly, increased salivation, liver function tests abnormal, melena, periodontal abscess, rectal hemorrhage, thirst, tooth caries, and ulcerative stomatitis.

Endocrine System: *Infrequent:* Goiter and hypothyroidism.

Hemic and Lymphatic System: *Frequent:* Lymphadenopathy. *Infrequent:* Anemia, erythrocytes abnormal, leukopenia, petechia, and thrombocytopenia.

Metabolic and Nutritional: *Frequent:* Edema, peripheral edema, weight gain, and weight loss. *Infrequent:* Dehydration, hypercholesteremia, hyperglycemia, hyperlipemia, hypoglycemia, hypokalemia, and hyponatremia.

Musculoskeletal System: *Frequent:* Arthralgia. *Infrequent:* Arthritis, arthrosis, bursitis, generalized spasm, and tendinous contracture.

Nervous System: *Frequent:* Depersonalization, dysarthria, euphoria, hallucination, hyperkinesia, hypertonia, hypesthesia, hypokinesia, hypotonia, migraine, myoclonus, paranoid reaction, personality disorder, reflexes decreased, stupor, twitching, and vertigo. *Infrequent:* Abnormal dreams, apathy, choreoathetosis, circumoral paresthesia, CNS neoplasm, coma, delusions, dry mouth, dystonia, encephalopathy, hemiplegia, leg cramps, libido increased, libido decreased, movement disorder, neuritis, neurosis, paralysis, peripheral neuritis, psychosis, reflexes increased, and urinary retention.

Respiratory System: *Frequent:* Bronchitis, dyspnea, epistaxis, and pneumonia. *Infrequent:* Apnea, asthma, hemoptysis, hiccups, hyperventilation, laryngitis, respiratory disorder, and voice alteration.

Skin and Appendages: *Frequent:* Alopecia, dry skin, and sweating. *Infrequent:* Contact dermatitis, eczema, exfoliative dermatitis, furunculosis, herpes simplex, herpes zoster, hirsutism, maculopapular rash, psoriasis, skin benign neoplasm, skin carcinoma, skin discolorations, skin nodules, skin ulcer, subcutaneous nodule, urticaria, and vesiculobullous rash.

Special Senses: *Frequent:* Abnormal vision, ear pain, otitis media, and tinnitus. *Infrequent:* Blepharitis, blindness, deafness, eye pain, hyperacusis, keratoconjunctivitis, otitis externa, parosmia, photophobia, taste loss, taste perversion, and visual field defect.

Urogenital System: *Frequent:* Dysmenorrhea, dysuria, metrorrhagia, urinary incontinence, and vaginitis. *Infrequent:* Abortion, amenorrhea, breast enlargement, breast pain, cystitis, fibrocystic breast, hematuria, impotence, kidney failure, menorrhagia, nocturia, papanicolaou smear suspicious, polyuria, pyelonephritis, salpingitis, urethritis, urinary urgency, and vaginal hemorrhage.

DRUG ABUSE AND DEPENDENCE

The abuse and dependence potential of GABITRIL have not been evaluated in human studies.

OVERDOSAGE

Human Overdose Experience: Human experience of acute overdose with GABITRIL is limited. Eleven patients in clinical trials took single doses of GABITRIL up to 800 mg. All patients fully recovered, usually within one day. The most common symptoms reported after overdose included somnolence, impaired consciousness, agitation, confusion, speech difficulty, hostility, depression, weakness, and myoclonus. One patient who ingested a single dose of 400 mg experienced generalized tonic-clonic status epilepticus, which responded to intravenous phenobarbital.

Table 7: Typical Dosing Titration Regimen for Patients Already Taking Enzyme-Inducing AEDs

	Initiation and Titration Schedule	Total Daily Dose
Week 1	Initiate at 4 mg once daily	4 mg/day
Week 2	Increase total daily dose by 4 mg	8 mg/day (in two divided doses)
Week 3	Increase total daily dose by 4 mg	12 mg/day (in three divided doses)
Week 4	Increase total daily dose by 4 mg	16 mg/day (in two to four divided doses)
Week 5	Increase total daily dose by 4 to 8 mg	20 to 24 mg/day (in two to four divided doses)
Week 6	Increase total daily dose by 4 to 8 mg	24 to 32 mg/day (in two to four divided doses)

Usual Adult Maintenance Dose in Induced Patients: 32 to 56 mg/day in two to four divided doses

From post-marketing experience, there have been no reports of fatal overdoses involving GABITRIL alone (doses up to 720 mg), although a number of patients required intubation and ventilatory support as part of the management of their status epilepticus. Overdoses involving multiple drugs, including GABITRIL, have resulted in fatal outcomes. Symptoms most often accompanying GABITRIL overdose, alone or in combination with other drugs, have included: seizures including status epilepticus in patients with and without underlying seizure disorders, nonconvulsive status epilepticus, coma, ataxia, confusion, somnolence, drowsiness, impaired speech, agitation, lethargy, myoclonus, spike wave stupor, tremors, disorientation, vomiting, hostility, and temporary paralysis. Respiratory depression was seen in a number of patients, including children, in the context of seizures.

Management of Overdose: There is no specific antidote for overdose with GABITRIL. If indicated, elimination of unabsorbed drug should be achieved by emesis or gastric lavage; usual precautions should be observed to maintain the airway. General supportive care of the patient is indicated including monitoring of vital signs and observation of clinical status of the patient. Since tiagabine is mostly metabolized by the liver and is highly protein bound, dialysis is unlikely to be beneficial. A Certified Poison Control Center should be consulted for up to date information on the management of overdose with GABITRIL.

DOSAGE AND ADMINISTRATION

General:

The blood level of tiagabine obtained after a given dose depends on whether the patient also is receiving a drug that induces the metabolism of tiagabine. The presence of an inducer means that the attained blood level will be substantially reduced. Dosing should take the presence of concomitant medications into account.

GABITRIL (tiagabine HCl) is recommended as adjunctive therapy for the treatment of partial seizures in patients 12 years and older.

The following dosing recommendations apply to all patients taking GABITRIL:

- GABITRIL is given orally and should be taken with food.
- Do not use a loading dose of GABITRIL.
- Dose titration: Rapid escalation and/or large dose increments of GABITRIL should not be used.
- Missed dose(s): If the patient forgets to take the prescribed dose of GABITRIL at the scheduled time, the patient should not attempt to make up for the missed dose by increasing the next dose. If a patient has missed multiple doses, patient should refer back to his or her physician for possible re-titration as clinically indicated.
- Dosage adjustment of GABITRIL should be considered whenever a change in patient's enzyme-inducing status occurs as a result of the addition, discontinuation, or dose change of the enzyme-inducing agent.

Induced Adults and Adolescents 12 Years or Older:

The following dosing recommendations apply to patients who are already taking enzyme-inducing antiepilepsy drugs (AEDs) (e.g., carbamazepine, phenytoin, primidone, and phenobarbital). Such patients are considered induced patients when administering GABITRIL.

In adolescents 12 to 18 years old, GABITRIL should be initiated at 4 mg once daily. Modification of concomitant antiepilepsy drugs is not necessary, unless clinically indicated. The total daily dose of GABITRIL may be increased by 4 mg at the beginning of Week 2. Thereafter, the total daily dose may be increased by 4 to 8 mg at weekly intervals until clinical response is achieved or up to 32 mg/day. The total daily dose should be given in divided doses two to four times daily. Doses above 32 mg/day have been tolerated in a small number of adolescent patients for a relatively short duration.

In adults, GABITRIL should be initiated at 4 mg once daily. Modification of concomitant antiepilepsy drugs is not necessary, unless clinically indicated. The total daily dose of GABITRIL may be increased by 4 to 8 mg at weekly intervals until clinical response is achieved or, up to 56 mg/day. The total daily dose should be given in divided doses two to four times daily. Doses above 56 mg/day have not been systematically evaluated in adequate and well-controlled clinical trials.

Experience is limited in patients taking total daily doses above 32 mg/day using twice daily dosing. A typical dosing titration regimen for patients taking enzyme-inducing AEDs (induced patients) is provided in Table 7.

[See table 7 above]

Non-Induced Adults and Adolescents 12 Years or Older:

The following dosing recommendations apply to patients who are taking only non-enzyme-inducing AEDs. Such patients are considered non-induced patients:

Following a given dose of GABITRIL, the estimated plasma concentration in the non-induced patients is more than twice that in patients receiving enzyme-inducing agents. Use in non-induced patients requires lower doses of GABITRIL. These patients may also require a slower titration of GABITRIL compared to that of induced patients (see **CLINICAL PHARMACOLOGY, Pharmacokinetics** and **PRECAUTIONS, General, Use in Non-Induced Patients**).

HOW SUPPLIED

GABITRIL tablets are available in four dosage strengths.

- 2 mg orange-peach, round tablets, debossed with C on one side and 402 on the opposite side, are available in bottles of 30 (**NDC** 63459-402-30).
- 4 mg yellow, round tablets, debossed with C on one side and 404 on the opposite side, are available in bottles of 30 (**NDC** 63459-404-30).
- 12 mg green, ovaloid tablets, debossed with C on one side and 412 on the opposite side, are available in bottles of 30 (**NDC** 63459-412-30).
- 16 mg blue, ovaloid tablets, debossed with C on one side and 416 on the opposite side, are available in bottles of 30 (**NDC** 63459-416-30).

Recommended Storage: Store tablets at controlled room temperature, between 20-25°C (68-77°F). See USP. Protect from light and moisture.

ANIMAL TOXICOLOGY

In repeat dose toxicology studies, dogs receiving daily oral doses of 5 mg/kg/day or greater experienced unexpected CNS effects throughout the study. These effects occurred acutely and included marked sedation and apparent visual impairment which was characterized by a lack of awareness of objects, failure to fix on and follow moving objects, and absence of a blink reaction. Plasma exposures (AUCs) at 5 mg/kg/day were equal to those in humans receiving the maximum recommended daily human dose of 56 mg/day. The effects were reversible upon cessation of treatment and were not associated with any observed structural abnormality. The implications of these findings for humans are unknown.

GAB-012

Revised: September 2009

Manufactured for:

Cephalon, Inc.

Frazer, PA 19355

GABITRIL is a trademark of Cephalon, Inc., or its affiliates.

©1997-2009 Cephalon, Inc., or its affiliates. All rights reserved.

U.S. Patent Nos. 5,010,090; 5,354,760; 5,866,590; 5,958,951

Printed in U.S.A.

Shown in Product Identification Guide, page 308

NUVIGIL® CIV ℞

[nu-vij-el]

(armodafinil)

Tablets

DESCRIPTION

NUVIGIL® (armodafinil) is a wakefulness-promoting agent for oral administration. Armodafinil is the R-enantiomer of modafinil which is a mixture of the R- and S-enantiomers.

The chemical name for armodafinil is 2-[(R)-(diphenylmethyl)sulfinyl]acetamide. The molecular formula is $C_{15}H_{15}NO_2S$ and the molecular weight is 273.35.
The chemical structure is:

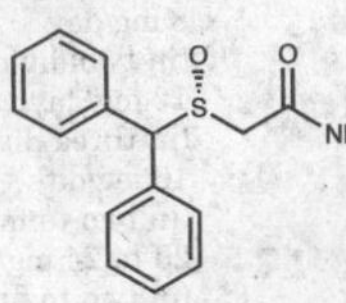

Armodafinil is a white to off-white, crystalline powder that is very slightly soluble in water, sparingly soluble in acetone and soluble in methanol. NUVIGIL tablets contain 50, 150, or 250 mg of armodafinil and the following inactive ingredients: croscarmellose sodium, lactose monohydrate, magnesium stearate, microcrystalline cellulose, povidone, and pregelatinized starch.

CLINICAL PHARMACOLOGY

Mechanism of Action and Pharmacology

The precise mechanism(s) through which armodafinil (R-enantiomer) or modafinil (mixture of R- and S-enantiomers) promote wakefulness is unknown. Both armodafinil and modafinil have shown similar pharmacological properties in nonclinical animal and in vitro studies, to the extent tested.
At pharmacologically relevant concentrations, armodafinil does not bind to or inhibit several receptors and enzymes potentially relevant for sleep/wake regulation, including those for serotonin, dopamine, adenosine, galanin, melatonin, melanocortin, orexin-1, orphanin, PACAP or benzodiazepines, or transporters for GABA, serotonin, norepinephrine, and choline or phosphodiesterase VI, COMT, GABA transaminase, and tyrosine hydroxylase. Modafinil does not inhibit the activity of MAO-B or phosphodiesterases II-IV.
Modafinil-induced wakefulness can be attenuated by the α1-adrenergic receptor antagonist, prazosin; however, modafinil is inactive in other in vitro assay systems known to be responsive to α-adrenergic agonists such as the rat vas deferens preparation.
Armodafinil is not a direct- or indirect-acting dopamine receptor agonist. However, in vitro, both armodafinil and modafinil bind to the dopamine transporter and inhibit dopamine reuptake. For modafinil, this activity has been associated in vivo with increased extracellular dopamine levels in some brain regions of animals. In genetically engineered mice lacking the dopamine transporter (DAT), modafinil lacked wake-promoting activity, suggesting that this activity was DAT-dependent. However, the wake-promoting effects of modafinil, unlike those of amphetamine, were not antagonized by the dopamine receptor antagonist haloperidol in rats. In addition, alpha-methyl-p-tyrosine, a dopamine synthesis inhibitor, blocks the action of amphetamine, but does not block locomotor activity induced by modafinil.
Armodafinil and modafinil have wake-promoting actions similar to sympathomimetic agents including amphetamine and methylphenidate, although their pharmacologic profile is not identical to that of the sympathomimetic amines. In addition to its wake-promoting effects and ability to increase locomotor activity in animals, modafinil produces psychoactive and euphoric effects, alterations in mood, perception, thinking, and feelings typical of other CNS stimulants in humans. Modafinil has reinforcing properties, as evidenced by its self-administration in monkeys previously trained to self-administer cocaine; modafinil was also partially discriminated as stimulant-like.
Based on nonclinical studies, two major metabolites, acid and sulfone, of modafinil or armodafinil, do not appear to contribute to the CNS-activating properties of the parent compounds.

Pharmacokinetics

The active component of NUVIGIL is armodafinil, which is the longer-lived enantiomer of modafinil. NUVIGIL exhibits linear time-independent kinetics following single and multiple oral dose administration. Increase in systemic exposure is proportional over the dose range of 50 to 400 mg. No time-dependent change in kinetics was observed through 12 weeks of dosing. Apparent steady state for NUVIGIL was reached within 7 days of dosing. At steady state, the systemic exposure for NUVIGIL is 1.8 times the exposure observed after a single dose. The concentration-time profiles of the pure R-enantiomer following administration of 50 mg NUVIGIL or 100 mg PROVIGIL® (modafinil) are nearly superimposable.

Absorption

NUVIGIL is readily absorbed after oral administration. The absolute oral bioavailability was not determined due to the aqueous insolubility of armodafinil, which precluded intravenous administration. Peak plasma concentrations are attained at approximately 2 hours in the fasted state. Food effect on the overall bioavailability of NUVIGIL is considered minimal; however, time to reach peak concentration (t_{max}) may be delayed by approximately 2-4 hours in the fed state. Since the delay in t_{max} is also associated with elevated plasma levels later in time, food can potentially affect the onset and time course of pharmacologic action for NUVIGIL.

Distribution

NUVIGIL has an apparent volume of distribution of approximately 42 L. Data specific to armodafinil protein binding are not available. However, modafinil is moderately bound to plasma protein (approximately 60%), mainly to albumin. The potential for interactions of NUVIGIL with highly protein-bound drugs is considered to be minimal.

Metabolism

In vitro and in vivo data show that armodafinil undergoes hydrolytic deamidation, S-oxidation, and aromatic ring hydroxylation, with subsequent glucuronide conjugation of the hydroxylated products. Amide hydrolysis is the single most prominent metabolic pathway, with sulfone formation by cytochrome P450 (CYP) 3A4/5 being next in importance. The other oxidative products are formed too slowly in vitro to enable identification of the enzyme(s) responsible. Only two metabolites reach appreciable concentrations in plasma (i.e., R-modafinil acid and modafinil sulfone).
Data specific to NUVIGIL disposition are not available. However, modafinil is mainly eliminated via metabolism, predominantly in the liver, with less than 10% of the parent compound excreted in the urine. A total of 81% of the administered radioactivity was recovered in 11 days post-dose, predominantly in the urine (80% vs. 1.0% in the feces).

Elimination

After oral administration of NUVIGIL, armodafinil exhibits an apparent monoexponential decline from the peak plasma concentration. The apparent terminal t½ is approximately 15 hours. The oral clearance of NUVIGIL is approximately 33 mL/min.

Drug-Drug Interactions

The existence of multiple pathways for armodafinil metabolism, as well as the fact that a non-CYP-related pathway is the most rapid in metabolizing armodafinil, suggest that there is a low probability of substantive effects on the overall pharmacokinetic profile of NUVIGIL due to CYP inhibition by concomitant medications.
In vitro data demonstrated that armodafinil shows a weak inductive response for CYP1A2 and possibly CYP3A activities in a concentration-related manner and that CYP2C19 activity is reversibly inhibited by armodafinil. Other CYP activities did not appear to be affected by armodafinil. An in vitro study demonstrated that armodafinil is a substrate of P-glycoprotein.
Chronic administration of NUVIGIL at 250 mg reduced the systemic exposure to midazolam by 32% and 17% after single oral (5 mg) and intravenous (2 mg) doses, respectively, suggesting that administration of NUVIGIL moderately induces CYP3A activity. Drugs that are substrates for CYP3A4/5, such as cyclosporine, may require dosage adjustment. (See **PRECAUTIONS, Drug Interactions**).
Chronic administration of NUVIGIL at 250 mg did not affect the pharmacokinetics of caffeine (200 mg), a probe substrate for CYP1A2 activity.
Coadministration of a single 400-mg dose of NUVIGIL with omeprazole (40 mg) increased systemic exposure to omeprazole by approximately 40%, indicating that armodafinil moderately inhibits CYP2C19 activity. Drugs that are substrates for CYP2C19 may require dosage reduction. (See **PRECAUTIONS, Drug Interactions**).

Gender Effect:

Population pharmacokinetic analysis suggests no gender effect on the pharmacokinetics of armodafinil.

Special Populations

Data specific to armodafinil in special populations are not available.

Age Effect:

A slight decrease (~20%) in the oral clearance (CL/F) of modafinil was observed in a single dose study at 200 mg in 12 subjects with a mean age of 63 years (range 53–72 years), but the change was considered not likely to be clinically significant. In a multiple dose study (300 mg/day) in 12 patients with a mean age of 82 years (range 67–87 years), the mean levels of modafinil in plasma were approximately two times those historically obtained in matched younger subjects. Due to potential effects from the multiple concomitant medications with which most of the patients were being treated, the apparent difference in modafinil pharmacokinetics may not be attributable solely to the effects of aging. However, the results suggest that the clearance of modafinil may be reduced in the elderly (See **DOSAGE AND ADMINISTRATION**).

Race Effect:

The influence of race on the pharmacokinetics of modafinil has not been studied.

Renal Impairment:

In a single dose 200 mg modafinil study, severe chronic renal failure (creatinine clearance ≤20 mL/min) did not significantly influence the pharmacokinetics of modafinil, but exposure to modafinil acid was increased 9-fold (See **PRECAUTIONS**).

Hepatic Impairment:

The pharmacokinetics and metabolism of modafinil were examined in patients with cirrhosis of the liver (6 men and 3 women). Three patients had stage B or B+ cirrhosis and 6 patients had stage C or C+ cirrhosis (per the Child-Pugh score criteria). Clinically 8 of 9 patients were icteric and all had ascites. In these patients, the oral clearance of modafinil was decreased by about 60% and the steady state concentration was doubled compared to normal patients. The dose of NUVIGIL should be reduced in patients with severe hepatic impairment (See **PRECAUTIONS** and **DOSAGE AND ADMINISTRATION**).

CLINICAL TRIALS

The effectiveness of NUVIGIL in improving wakefulness has been established in the following sleep disorders: obstructive sleep apnea/hypopnea syndrome (OSAHS), narcolepsy and shift work sleep disorder (SWSD).
For each clinical trial, a p-value of ≤ 0.05 was required for statistical significance.

Obstructive Sleep Apnea/Hypopnea Syndrome (OSAHS)

The effectiveness of NUVIGIL in improving wakefulness in patients with excessive sleepiness associated with OSAHS was established in two 12-week, multi-center, placebo-controlled, parallel-group, double-blind studies of outpatients who met the International Classification of Sleep Disorders (ICSD) criteria for OSAHS (which are also consistent with the American Psychiatric Association DSM-IV criteria). These criteria include either, 1) excessive sleepiness or insomnia, plus frequent episodes of impaired breathing during sleep, and associated features such as loud snoring, morning headaches or dry mouth upon awakening; or 2) excessive sleepiness or insomnia; and polysomnography demonstrating one of the following: more than five obstructive apneas, each greater than 10 seconds in duration, per hour of sleep; and one or more of the following: frequent arousals from sleep associated with the apneas, bradytachycardia, or arterial oxygen desaturation in association with the apneas. In addition, for entry into these studies, all patients were required to have excessive sleepiness as demonstrated by a score ≥ 10 on the Epworth Sleepiness Scale, despite treatment with continuous positive airway pressure (CPAP). Evidence that CPAP was effective in reducing episodes of apnea/hypopnea was required along with documentation of CPAP use.
Patients were required to be compliant with CPAP, defined as CPAP use ≥ 4 hours/night on ≥ 70% of nights. CPAP use continued throughout the study. In both studies, the primary measures of effectiveness were 1) sleep latency, as assessed by the Maintenance of Wakefulness Test (MWT) and 2) the change in the patient's overall disease status, as measured by the Clinical Global Impression of Change (CGI-C) at the final visit. For a successful trial both measures had to show statistically significant improvement.
The MWT measures latency (in minutes) to sleep onset. An extended MWT was performed with test sessions at 2 hour intervals between 9AM and 7PM. The primary analysis was the average of the sleep latencies from the first four test sessions (9AM to 3PM). For each test session, the subject was asked to attempt to remain awake without using extraordinary measures. Each test session was terminated after 30 minutes if no sleep occurred or immediately after sleep onset. The CGI-C is a 7-point scale, centered at *No Change*, and ranging from *Very Much Worse* to *Very Much Improved*. Evaluators were not given any specific guidance about the criteria they were to apply when rating patients.
In the first study, a total of 395 patients with OSAHS were randomized to receive NUVIGIL 150 mg/day, NUVIGIL 250 mg/day or matching placebo. Patients treated with NUVIGIL showed a statistically significant improvement in the ability to remain awake compared to placebo-treated patients as measured by the MWT at final visit. A statistically significant greater number of patients treated with NUVIGIL showed improvement in overall clinical condition as rated by the CGI-C scale at final visit. The average sleep latencies (in minutes) in the MWT at baseline for the trials are shown in Table 1 below, along with the average change from baseline on the MWT at final visit. The percentages of patients who showed any degree of improvement on the CGI-C in the clinical trials are shown in Table 2 below. The two doses of NUVIGIL produced statistically significant effects of similar magnitudes on the MWT, and also on the CGI-C.
In the second study, 263 patients with OSAHS were randomized to either NUVIGIL 150 mg/day or placebo. Patients treated with NUVIGIL showed a statistically significant improvement in the ability to remain awake compared to placebo-treated patients as measured by the MWT [Table 1]. A statistically significant greater number of patients treated with NUVIGIL showed improvement in overall clinical condition as rated by the CGI-C scale [Table 2].

Table 1. Average Baseline Sleep Latency and Change from Baseline at Final Visit (MWT and MSLT in minutes)

Disorder	Measure	NUVIGIL 150 mg*		NUVIGIL 250 mg*		Placebo	
		Baseline	Change from Baseline	Baseline	Change from Baseline	Baseline	Change from Baseline
OSAHS I	MWT	21.5	1.7	23.3	2.2	23.2	-1.7
OSAHS II	MWT	23.7	2.3	-	-	23.3	-1.3
Narcolepsy	MWT	12.1	1.3	9.5	2.6	12.5	-1.9
SWSD	MSLT	2.3	3.1	-	-	2.4	0.4

*Significantly different than placebo for all trials (p<0.05)

Nighttime sleep measured with polysomnography was not affected by the use of NUVIGIL in either study.

Narcolepsy

The effectiveness of NUVIGIL in improving wakefulness in patients with excessive sleepiness (ES) associated with narcolepsy was established in one 12-week, multi-center, placebo-controlled, parallel-group, double-blind study of outpatients who met the ICSD criteria for narcolepsy. A total of 196 patients were randomized to receive NUVIGIL 150 or 250 mg/day, or matching placebo. The ICSD criteria for narcolepsy include either 1) recurrent daytime naps or lapses into sleep that occur almost daily for at least three months, plus sudden bilateral loss of postural muscle tone in association with intense emotion (cataplexy), or 2) a complaint of excessive sleepiness or sudden muscle weakness with associated features: sleep paralysis, hypnagogic hallucinations, automatic behaviors, disrupted major sleep episode; and polysomnography demonstrating one of the following: sleep latency less than 10 minutes or rapid eye movement (REM) sleep latency less than 20 minutes and a Multiple Sleep Latency Test (MSLT) that demonstrates a mean sleep latency of less than 5 minutes and two or more sleep onset REM periods and no medical or mental disorder accounts for the symptoms. For entry into these studies, all patients were required to have objectively documented excessive daytime sleepiness, via MSLT with a sleep latency of 6 minutes or less and the absence of any other clinically significant active medical or psychiatric disorder. The MSLT, an objective polysomnographic assessment of the patient's ability to fall asleep in an unstimulating environment, measured latency (in minutes) to sleep onset averaged over 4 test sessions at 2-hour intervals. For each test session, the subject was told to lie quietly and attempt to sleep. Each test session was terminated after 20 minutes if no sleep occurred or immediately after sleep onset.

The primary measures of effectiveness were: 1) sleep latency as assessed by the Maintenance of Wakefulness Test (MWT) and 2) the change in the patient's overall disease status, as measured by the Clinical Global Impression of Change (CGI-C) at the final visit (See **CLINICAL TRIALS**, *OSAHS* section above for a description of these measures). Each MWT test session was terminated after 20 minutes if no sleep occurred or immediately after sleep onset in this study.

Patients treated with NUVIGIL showed a statistically significantly enhanced ability to remain awake on the MWT at each dose compared to placebo at final visit [Table 1]. A statistically significant greater number of patients treated with NUVIGIL at each dose showed improvement in overall clinical condition as rated by the CGI-C scale at final visit [Table 2].

The two doses of NUVIGIL produced statistically significant effects of similar magnitudes on the CGI-C. Although a statistically significant effect on the MWT was observed for each dose, the magnitude of effect was observed to be greater for the higher dose.

Nighttime sleep measured with polysomnography was not affected by the use of NUVIGIL.

Shift Work Sleep Disorder (SWSD)

The effectiveness of NUVIGIL in improving wakefulness in patients with excessive sleepiness associated with SWSD was demonstrated in a 12-week, multi-center, double-blind, placebo-controlled, parallel-group, clinical trial. A total of 254 patients with chronic SWSD were randomized to receive NUVIGIL 150 mg/day or placebo. All patients met the ICSD criteria for chronic SWSD [which are consistent with the American Psychiatric Association DSM-IV criteria for Circadian Rhythm Sleep Disorder: Shift Work Type]. These criteria include 1) either: a) a primary complaint of excessive sleepiness or insomnia which is temporally associated with a work period (usually night work) that occurs during the habitual sleep phase, or b) polysomnography and the MSLT demonstrate loss of a normal sleep-wake pattern (i.e., disturbed chronobiological rhythmicity); and 2) no other medical or mental disorder accounts for the symptoms, and 3) the symptoms do not meet criteria for any other sleep disorder producing insomnia or excessive sleepiness (e.g., time zone change [jet lag] syndrome).

It should be noted that not all patients with a complaint of sleepiness who are also engaged in shift work meet the criteria for the diagnosis of SWSD. In the clinical trial, only patients who were symptomatic for at least 3 months were enrolled.

Enrolled patients were also required to work a minimum of 5 night shifts per month, have excessive sleepiness at the time of their night shifts (MSLT score ≤ 6 minutes), and have daytime insomnia documented by a daytime polysomnogram (PSG).

The primary measures of effectiveness were 1) sleep latency, as assessed by the Multiple Sleep Latency Test (MSLT) performed during a simulated night shift at the final visit, and 2) the change in the patient's overall disease status, as measured by the Clinical Global Impression of Change (CGI-C) at the final visit. (See **CLINICAL TRIALS**, *Narcolepsy* and *OSAHS* sections above for description of these measures).

Patients treated with NUVIGIL showed a statistically significant prolongation in the time to sleep onset compared to placebo-treated patients, as measured by the nighttime MSLT at final visit [Table 1]. A statistically significant greater number of patients treated with NUVIGIL showed improvement in overall clinical condition as rated by the CGI-C scale at final visit [Table 2].

Daytime sleep measured with polysomnography was not affected by the use of NUVIGIL.

[See table 1 above]

Table 2. Clinical Global Impression of Change (CGI-C) (Percent of Patients Who Improved at Final Visit)

Disorder	NUVIGIL 150 mg*	NUVIGIL 250 mg*	Placebo
OSAHS I	71%	74%	37%
OSAHS II	71%	-	53%
Narcolepsy	69%	73%	33%
SWSD	79%	-	59%

*Significantly different than placebo for all trials (p<0.05)

INDICATIONS AND USAGE

NUVIGIL is indicated to improve wakefulness in patients with excessive sleepiness associated with obstructive sleep apnea/hypopnea syndrome, narcolepsy and shift work sleep disorder.

In OSAHS, NUVIGIL is indicated as an adjunct to standard treatment(s) for the underlying obstruction. If continuous positive airway pressure (CPAP) is the treatment of choice for a patient, a maximal effort to treat with CPAP for an adequate period of time should be made prior to initiating NUVIGIL. If NUVIGIL is used adjunctively with CPAP, the encouragement of and periodic assessment of CPAP compliance is necessary.

In all cases, careful attention to the diagnosis and treatment of the underlying sleep disorder(s) is of utmost importance. Prescribers should be aware that some patients may have more than one sleep disorder contributing to their excessive sleepiness.

The effectiveness of NUVIGIL in long-term use (greater than 12 weeks) has not been systematically evaluated in placebo-controlled trials. The physician who elects to prescribe NUVIGIL for an extended time in patients should periodically re-evaluate long-term usefulness for the individual patient.

CONTRAINDICATIONS

NUVIGIL is contraindicated in patients with known hypersensitivity to modafinil and armodafinil or its inactive ingredients.

WARNINGS

Serious Rash, including Stevens-Johnson Syndrome

Serious rash requiring hospitalization and discontinuation of treatment has been reported in adults in association with the use of armodafinil and in adults and children in association with the use of modafinil, a racemic mixture of S and R modafinil (the latter is armodafinil).

Armodafinil has not been studied in pediatric patients in any setting and is not approved for use in pediatric patients for any indication.

No serious skin rashes have been reported in adult clinical trials (0 per 1,595) of armodafinil. However, cases of serious rash have been reported in adults in postmarketing experience. Because armodafinil is the R isomer of racemic modafinil, a similar risk of serious rash in pediatric patients with armodafinil cannot be ruled out.

In clinical trials of modafinil (the racemate), the incidence of rash resulting in discontinuation was approximately 0.8% (13 per 1,585) in pediatric patients (age <17 years); these rashes included 1 case of possible Stevens-Johnson Syndrome (SJS) and 1 case of apparent multi-organ hypersensitivity reaction. Several of the cases were associated with fever and other abnormalities (e.g., vomiting, leukopenia). The median time to rash that resulted in discontinuation was 13 days. No such cases were observed among 380 pediatric patients who received placebo. No serious skin rashes have been reported in adult clinical trials (0 per 4,264) of modafinil. Rare cases of serious or life-threatening rash, including SJS, Toxic Epidermal Necrolysis (TEN), and Drug Rash with Eosinophilia and Systemic Symptoms (DRESS) have been reported in adults and children in worldwide post-marketing experience. The reporting rate of TEN and SJS associated with modafinil use, which is generally accepted to be an underestimate due to underreporting, exceeds the background incidence rate. Estimates of the background incidence rate for these serious skin reactions in the general population range between 1 to 2 cases per million-person years.

There are no factors that are known to predict the risk of occurrence or the severity of rash associated with armodafinil or modafinil. Nearly all cases of serious rash associated with armodafinil or modafinil occurred within 1 to 5 weeks after treatment initiation. However, isolated cases have been reported after prolonged treatment with modafinil (e.g., 3 months). Accordingly, duration of therapy cannot be relied upon as a means to predict the potential risk heralded by the first appearance of a rash.

Although benign rashes also occur with armodafinil, it is not possible to reliably predict which rashes will prove to be serious. Accordingly, armodafinil should ordinarily be discontinued at the first sign of rash, unless the rash is clearly not drug-related. Discontinuation of treatment may not prevent a rash from becoming life-threatening or permanently disabling or disfiguring.

Angioedema and Anaphylactoid Reactions

One serious case of angioedema and one case of hypersensitivity (with rash, dysphagia, and bronchospasm), were observed among 1,595 patients treated with armodafinil. Patients should be advised to discontinue therapy and immediately report to their physician any signs or symptoms suggesting angioedema or anaphylaxis (e.g., swelling of face, eyes, lips, tongue or larynx; difficulty in swallowing or breathing; hoarseness).

Multi-organ Hypersensitivity Reactions

Multi-organ hypersensitivity reactions, including at least one fatality in postmarketing experience, have occurred in close temporal association (median time to detection 13 days: range 4-33) to the initiation of modafinil. A similar risk of multi-organ hypersensitivity reactions with armodafinil cannot be ruled out.

Although there have been a limited number of reports, multi-organ hypersensitivity reactions may result in hospitalization or be life-threatening. There are no factors that are known to predict the risk of occurrence or the severity of multi-organ hypersensitivity reactions associated with modafinil. Signs and symptoms of this disorder were diverse; however, patients typically, although not exclusively, presented with fever and rash associated with other organ system involvement. Other associated manifestations included myocarditis, hepatitis, liver function test abnormalities, hematological abnormalities (e.g., eosinophilia, leukopenia, thrombocytopenia), pruritus, and asthenia. Because multi-organ hypersensitivity is variable in its expression, other organ system symptoms and signs, not noted here, may occur.

If a multi-organ hypersensitivity reaction is suspected, NUVIGIL should be discontinued. Although there are no case reports to indicate cross-sensitivity with other drugs that produce this syndrome, the experience with drugs associated with multi-organ hypersensitivity would indicate this to be a possibility.

Persistent Sleepiness

Patients with abnormal levels of sleepiness who take NUVIGIL should be advised that their level of wakefulness may not return to normal. Patients with excessive sleepiness, including those taking NUVIGIL, should be frequently reassessed for their degree of sleepiness and, if appropriate, advised to avoid driving or any other potentially dangerous activity. Prescribers should also be aware that patients may not acknowledge sleepiness or drowsiness until directly questioned about drowsiness or sleepiness during specific activities.

Psychiatric Symptoms

Psychiatric adverse experiences have been reported in patients treated with modafinil. Modafinil and armodafinil (NUVIGIL) are very closely related. Therefore, the incidence and type of psychiatric symptoms associated with armodafinil are expected to be similar to the incidence and type of these events with modafinil.

Postmarketing adverse events associated with the use of modafinil have included mania, delusions, hallucinations, suicidal ideation and aggression, some resulting in hospitalization. Many, but not all, patients had a prior psychiatric history. One healthy male volunteer developed ideas of reference, paranoid delusions, and auditory hallucinations in association with multiple daily 600 mg doses of modafinil and sleep deprivation. There was no evidence of psychosis 36 hours after drug discontinuation.

In the controlled trial NUVIGIL database, anxiety, agitation, nervousness, and irritability were reasons for treatment discontinuation more often in patients on NUVIGIL compared to placebo (NUVIGIL 1.2% and placebo 0.3%). In the NUVIGIL controlled studies, depression was also a reason for treatment discontinuation more often in patients on NUVIGIL compared to placebo (NUVIGIL 0.6% and placebo 0.2%). Two cases of suicide ideation were observed in clinical trials. Caution should be exercised when NUVIGIL is given to patients with a history of psychosis, depression, or mania. If psychiatric symptoms develop in association with NUVIGIL administration, consider discontinuing NUVIGIL.

PRECAUTIONS

Diagnosis of Sleep Disorders

NUVIGIL should be used only in patients who have had a complete evaluation of their excessive sleepiness, and in whom a diagnosis of either narcolepsy, OSAHS, and/or SWSD has been made in accordance with ICSD or DSM diagnostic criteria (See **CLINICAL TRIALS**). Such an evaluation usually consists of a complete history and physical examination, and it may be supplemented with testing in a laboratory setting. Some patients may have more than one sleep disorder contributing to their excessive sleepiness (e.g., OSAHS and SWSD coincident in the same patient).

CPAP Use in Patients with OSAHS

In OSAHS, NUVIGIL is indicated as an adjunct to standard treatment(s) for the underlying obstruction. If continuous positive airway pressure (CPAP) is the treatment of choice for a patient, a maximal effort to treat with CPAP for an adequate period of time should be made prior to initiating NUVIGIL. If NUVIGIL is used adjunctively with CPAP, the encouragement of and periodic assessment of CPAP compliance is necessary. There was a slight trend for reduced CPAP use over time (mean reduction of 18 minutes for patients treated with NUVIGIL and a 6 minute reduction for placebo-treated patients from a mean baseline use of 6.9 hours per night) in NUVIGIL trials.

General

Although NUVIGIL has not been shown to produce functional impairment, any drug affecting the CNS may alter judgment, thinking or motor skills. Patients should be cautioned about operating an automobile or other hazardous machinery until they are reasonably certain that NUVIGIL therapy will not adversely affect their ability to engage in such activities.

Cardiovascular System

NUVIGIL has not been evaluated or used to any appreciable extent in patients with a recent history of myocardial infarction or unstable angina, and such patients should be treated with caution.

In clinical studies of PROVIGIL, signs and symptoms including chest pain, palpitations, dyspnea and transient ischemic T-wave changes on ECG were observed in three subjects in association with mitral valve prolapse or left ventricular hypertrophy. It is recommended that NUVIGIL tablets not be used in patients with a history of left ventricular hypertrophy or in patients with mitral valve prolapse who have experienced the mitral valve prolapse syndrome when previously receiving CNS stimulants. Signs of mitral valve prolapse syndrome include but are not limited to ischemic ECG changes, chest pain, or arrhythmia. If new onset of any of these symptoms occurs, consider cardiac evaluation.

Blood pressure monitoring in short-term (≤ 3 months) controlled trials showed only small average increases in mean systolic and diastolic blood pressure in patients receiving NUVIGIL as compared to placebo (1.2 to 4.3 mmHg in the various experimental groups). There was also a slightly greater proportion of patients on NUVIGIL requiring new or increased use of antihypertensive medications (2.9%) compared to patients on placebo (1.8%). Increased monitoring of blood pressure may be appropriate in patients on NUVIGIL.

Patients Using Steroidal Contraceptives

The effectiveness of steroidal contraceptives may be reduced when used with NUVIGIL and for one month after discon-

tinuation of therapy (See **PRECAUTIONS, Drug Interactions**). Alternative or concomitant methods of contraception are recommended for patients treated with NUVIGIL and for one month after discontinuation of NUVIGIL treatment.

Patients Using Cyclosporine

The blood levels of cyclosporine may be reduced when used with NUVIGIL (See **PRECAUTIONS, Drug Interactions**). Monitoring of circulating cyclosporine concentrations and appropriate dosage adjustment for cyclosporine should be considered when these drugs are used concomitantly.

Patients with Severe Hepatic Impairment

In patients with severe hepatic impairment, with or without cirrhosis (See **CLINICAL PHARMACOLOGY**), NUVIGIL should be administered at a reduced dose (See **DOSAGE AND ADMINISTRATION**).

Patients with Severe Renal Impairment

There is inadequate information to determine safety and efficacy of dosing in patients with severe renal impairment (For pharmacokinetics in renal impairment, see **CLINICAL PHARMACOLOGY**).

Elderly Patients

In elderly patients, elimination of armodafinil and its metabolites may be reduced as a consequence of aging. Therefore, consideration should be given to the use of lower doses in this population (See **CLINICAL PHARMACOLOGY** and **DOSAGE AND ADMINISTRATION**).

Information for Patients

Physicians are advised to discuss the following issues with patients for whom they prescribe NUVIGIL.

NUVIGIL is indicated for patients who have abnormal levels of sleepiness. NUVIGIL has been shown to improve, but not eliminate, this abnormal tendency to fall asleep. Therefore, patients should not alter their previous behavior with regard to potentially dangerous activities (e.g., driving, operating machinery) or other activities requiring appropriate levels of wakefulness, until and unless treatment with NUVIGIL has been shown to produce levels of wakefulness that permit such activities. Patients should be advised that NUVIGIL is not a replacement for sleep.

Patients should be informed that it may be critical that they continue to take their previously prescribed treatments (e.g., patients with OSAHS receiving CPAP should continue to do so).

Patients should be informed of the availability of a patient information leaflet, and they should be instructed to read the leaflet prior to taking NUVIGIL. See Patient Information at the end of this labeling for the text of the leaflet provided for patients.

Patients should be advised to contact their physician if they experience rash, depression, anxiety, or signs of psychosis or mania.

Pregnancy

Patients should be advised to notify their physician if they become pregnant or intend to become pregnant during therapy. Patients should be cautioned regarding the potential increased risk of pregnancy when using steroidal contraceptives (including depot or implantable contraceptives) with NUVIGIL and for one month after discontinuation of therapy (See *Carcinogenesis, Mutagenesis, Impairment of Fertility* and **Pregnancy**).

Nursing

Patients should be advised to notify their physician if they are breastfeeding an infant.

Concomitant Medication

Patients should be advised to inform their physician if they are taking, or plan to take, any prescription or over-the-counter drugs, because of the potential for interactions between NUVIGIL and other drugs.

Alcohol

Patients should be advised that the use of NUVIGIL in combination with alcohol has not been studied. Patients should be advised that it is prudent to avoid alcohol while taking NUVIGIL.

Allergic Reactions

Patients should be advised to stop taking NUVIGIL and to notify their physician if they develop a rash, hives, mouth sores, blisters, peeling skin, trouble swallowing or breathing or a related allergic phenomenon.

Drug Interactions

Potential Interactions with Drugs That Inhibit, Induce, or Are Metabolized by Cytochrome P450 Isoenzymes and Other Hepatic Enzymes

Due to the partial involvement of CYP3A enzymes in the metabolic elimination of armodafinil, coadministration of potent inducers of CYP3A4/5 (e.g., carbamazepine, phenobarbital, rifampin) or inhibitors of CYP3A4/5 (e.g., ketoconazole, erythromycin) could alter the plasma levels of armodafinil.

The Potential of NUVIGIL to Alter the Metabolism of Other Drugs by Enzyme Induction or Inhibition

Drugs Metabolized by CYP1A2

In vitro data demonstrated that armodafinil shows a weak inductive response for CYP1A2 and possibly CYP3A activities in a concentration related manner and demon-

strated that CYP2C19 activity is reversibly inhibited by armodafinil. However, the effect on CYP1A2 activity was not observed clinically in an interaction study performed with caffeine (See **Pharmacokinetics**, *Drug-Drug Interactions*).

Drugs Metabolized by CYP3A4/5 (e.g., cyclosporine, ethinyl estradiol, midazolam and triazolam)

Chronic administration of NUVIGIL resulted in moderate induction of CYP3A activity. Hence, the effectiveness of drugs that are substrates for CYP3A enzymes (e.g., cyclosporine, ethinyl estradiol, midazolam and triazolam) may be reduced after initiation of concurrent treatment with NUVIGIL. A 32% reduction in systemic exposure of oral midazolam was seen upon concomitant administration of armodafinil with midazolam. Dose adjustment may be required (See **Pharmacokinetics**, *Drug-Drug Interactions*). Such effects (reduced concentrations) were also seen upon concomitant administration of modafinil with cyclosporine, ethinyl estradiol, and triazolam.

Drugs Metabolized by CYP2C19 (e.g., omeprazole, diazepam, phenytoin, and propranolol)

Administration of NUVIGIL resulted in moderate inhibition of CYP2C19 activity. Hence, dosage reduction may be required for some drugs that are substrates for CYP2C19 (e.g., phenytoin, diazepam, and propranolol, omeprazole and clomipramine) when used concurrently with NUVIGIL. A 40% increase in exposure was seen upon concomitant administration of armodafinil with omeprazole. (See **Pharmacokinetics**, *Drug-Drug Interactions*).

Interactions with CNS Active Drugs

Data specific to armodafinil drug-drug interaction potential with CNS active drugs are not available. However, the following available drug-drug interaction information on modafinil should be applicable to armodafinil (See **DESCRIPTION** and **CLINICAL PHARMACOLOGY**).

Concomitant administration of modafinil with methylphenidate, or dextroamphetamine produced no significant alterations on the pharmacokinetic profile of modafinil or either stimulant, even though the absorption of modafinil was delayed for approximately one hour.

Concomitant modafinil or clomipramine did not alter the PK profile of either drug; however, one incident of increased levels of clomipramine and its active metabolite desmethylclomipramine was reported in a patient with narcolepsy during treatment with modafinil.

Data specific to armodafinil or modafinil drug-drug interaction potential with Monoamine Oxidase (MAO) inhibitors are not available. Therefore, caution should be used when concomitantly administering MAO inhibitors and NUVIGIL.

Interactions with Other Drugs

Data specific to armodafinil drug-drug interaction potential for additional other drugs are not available. However, the following available drug-drug interaction information on modafinil should be applicable to armodafinil.

Warfarin

Concomitant administration of modafinil with warfarin did not produce significant changes in the pharmacokinetic profiles of R- and S-warfarin. However, since only a single dose of warfarin was tested in this study, a pharmacodynamic interaction cannot be ruled out. Therefore, more frequent monitoring of prothrombin times/INR should be considered whenever NUVIGIL is coadministered with warfarin.

Carcinogenesis, Mutagenesis, Impairment of Fertility

Carcinogenesis

Carcinogenicity studies have not been conducted with armodafinil alone.

Carcinogenicity studies were conducted in which modafinil was administered in the diet to mice for 78 weeks and to rats for 104 weeks at doses of 6, 30, and 60 mg/kg/day. The highest dose studied represents 1.5 (mouse) or 3 (rat) times greater than the recommended adult human daily dose of modafinil (200 mg) on a mg/m^2 basis. There was no evidence of tumorigenesis associated with modafinil administration in these studies. However, since the mouse study used an inadequate high dose that was not representative of a maximum tolerated dose, a subsequent carcinogenicity study was conducted in the Tg.AC transgenic mouse. Doses evaluated in the Tg.AC assay were 125, 250, and 500 mg/kg/day, administered dermally. There was no evidence of tumorigenicity associated with modafinil administration; however, this dermal model may not adequately assess the carcinogenic potential of an orally administered drug.

Mutagenesis

Armodafinil was evaluated in an in vitro bacterial reverse mutation assay and in an in vitro mammalian chromosomal aberration assay in human lymphocytes. Armodafinil was negative in these assays, both in the absence and presence of metabolic activation.

Modafinil demonstrated no evidence of mutagenic or clastogenic potential in a series of in vitro (i.e., bacterial reverse mutation assay, mouse lymphoma tk assay, chromosomal aberration assay in human lymphocytes, cell transformation assay in BALB/3T3 mouse embryo cells) assays in the absence or presence of metabolic activation, or in vivo (mouse bone marrow micronucleus) assays. Modafinil was also negative in the unscheduled DNA synthesis assay in rat hepatocytes.

Impairment of Fertility

A fertility and early embryonic development (to implantation) study was not conducted with armodafinil alone.

Oral administration of modafinil (doses of up to 480 mg/kg/day) to male and female rats prior to and throughout mating, and continuing in females through day 7 of gestation produced an increase in the time to mate at the highest dose; no effects were observed on other fertility or reproductive parameters. The no-effect dose of 240 mg/kg/day was associated with a plasma modafinil exposure (AUC) approximately equal to that in humans at the recommended dose of 200 mg.

Pregnancy

Pregnancy Category C.

In studies conducted in rats (armodafinil, modafinil) and rabbits (modafinil), developmental toxicity was observed at clinically relevant exposures.

Oral administration of armodafinil (60, 200, or 600 mg/kg/day) to pregnant rats throughout the period of organogenesis resulted in increased incidences of fetal visceral and skeletal variations at the intermediate dose or greater and decreased fetal body weights at the highest dose. The no-effect dose for rat embryofetal developmental toxicity was associated with a plasma armodafinil exposure (AUC) approximately 0.03 times the AUC in humans at the maximum recommended daily dose of 250 mg.

Modafinil (50, 100, or 200 mg/kg/day) administered orally to pregnant rats throughout the period of organogenesis caused, in the absence of maternal toxicity, an increase in resorptions and an increased incidence of visceral and skeletal variations in the offspring at the highest dose. The higher no-effect dose for rat embryofetal developmental toxicity was associated with a plasma modafinil exposure approximately 0.5 times the AUC in humans at the recommended daily dose (RHD) of 200 mg. However, in a subsequent study of up to 480 mg/kg/day (plasma modafinil exposure approximately 2 times the AUC in humans at the RHD) no adverse effects on embryofetal development were observed.

Modafinil administered orally to pregnant rabbits throughout the period of organogenesis at doses of up to 100 mg/kg/day (plasma modafinil AUC approximately equal to the AUC in humans at the RHD) had no effect on embryofetal development; however, the doses used were too low to adequately assess the effects of modafinil on embryofetal development. In a subsequent developmental toxicity study evaluating doses of 45, 90, and 180 mg/kg/day in pregnant rabbits, the incidences of fetal structural alterations and embryofetal death were increased at the highest dose. The highest no-effect dose for developmental toxicity was associated with a plasma modafinil AUC approximately equal to the AUC in humans at the RHD.

Modafinil administration to rats throughout gestation and lactation at oral doses of up to 200 mg/kg/day resulted in decreased viability in the offspring at doses greater than 20 mg/kg/day (plasma modafinil AUC approximately 0.1 times the AUC in humans at the RHD). No effects on postnatal developmental and neurobehavioral parameters were observed in surviving offspring.

There are no adequate and well-controlled studies of either armodafinil or modafinil in pregnant women. Two cases of intrauterine growth retardation and one case of spontaneous abortion have been reported in association with armodafinil and modafinil. Although the pharmacology of armodafinil is not identical to that of the sympathomimetic amines, it does share some pharmacologic properties with this class. Certain of these drugs have been associated with intrauterine growth retardation and spontaneous abortions. Whether the cases reported with armodafinil are drug-related is unknown.

Armodafinil or modafinil should be used during pregnancy only if the potential benefit justifies the potential risk to the fetus.

Labor and Delivery

The effect of armodafinil on labor and delivery in humans has not been systematically investigated.

Nursing Mothers

It is not known whether armodafinil or its metabolites are excreted in human milk. Because many drugs are excreted in human milk, caution should be exercised when NUVIGIL tablets are administered to a nursing woman.

Pediatric Use

Safety and effectiveness of armodafinil use in individuals below 17 years of age have not been established. Serious rash has been seen in pediatric patients receiving modafinil (See **WARNINGS, Serious Rash, including Stevens-Johnson Syndrome**).

Table 4. Incidence (In Percent) Of Dose-Dependent, Treatment-Emergent Adverse Experiences By Dose and By Treatment In Parallel-Group, Placebo-Controlled Clinical Trials[a] In OSAHS, Narcolepsy and SWSD With NUVIGIL (150 mg and 250 mg)

System Organ Class MedDRA preferred term	NUVIGIL 250 mg (Percent, N=198)	NUVIGIL 150 mg (Percent, N=447)	NUVIGIL Combined (Percent, N=645)	Placebo (Percent, N=445)
Gastrointestinal Disorders				
Nausea	9	6	7	3
Dry Mouth	7	2	4	<1
Nervous System Disorders				
Headache	23	14	17	9
Psychiatric Disorders				
Insomnia	6	4	5	1
Depression	3	1	2	<1
Skin And Subcutaneous Tissue Disorders				
Rash	4	1	2	<1

[a] Four double-blind, placebo-controlled clinical studies in SWSD, OSAHS, and narcolepsy.

Geriatric Use

Safety and effectiveness in individuals above 65 years of age have not been established.

ADVERSE REACTIONS

Armodafinil has been evaluated for safety in over 1100 patients with excessive sleepiness associated with primary disorders of sleep and wakefulness. In clinical trials, NUVIGIL has been found to be generally well tolerated and most adverse experiences were mild to moderate.

In the placebo-controlled clinical studies, the most commonly observed adverse events (≥ 5%) associated with the use of NUVIGIL occurring more frequently than in the placebo-treated patients were headache, nausea, dizziness, and insomnia. The adverse event profile was similar across the studies.

In the placebo-controlled clinical trials, 44 of the 645 patients (7%) who received NUVIGIL discontinued due to an adverse experience compared to 16 of the 445 (4%) of patients that received placebo. The most frequent reason for discontinuation was headache (1%).

Incidence in Controlled Trials

The following table (Table 3) presents the adverse experiences that occurred at a rate of 1% or more and were more frequent in patients treated with NUVIGIL than in placebo group patients in the placebo-controlled clinical trials.

The prescriber should be aware that the figures provided below cannot be used to predict the frequency of adverse experiences in the course of usual medical practice, where patient characteristics and other factors may differ from those occurring during clinical studies. Similarly, the cited frequencies cannot be directly compared with figures obtained from other clinical investigations involving different treatments, uses, or investigators. Review of these frequencies, however, provides prescribers with a basis to estimate the relative contribution of drug and non-drug factors to the incidence of adverse events in the population studied.

Table 3. Incidence > 1% (In Percent) Of Treatment-Emergent Adverse Experiences In Parallel-Group, Placebo-Controlled Clinical Trials[a] In OSAHS, Narcolepsy and SWSD With NUVIGIL (150 mg and 250 mg)

System Organ Class MedDRA preferred term	NUVIGIL (Percent, N = 645)	Placebo (Percent, N = 445)
Cardiac Disorders		
Palpitations	2	1
Gastrointestinal Disorders		
Nausea	7	3
Diarrhea	4	2
Dry Mouth	4	1
Dyspepsia	2	0
Abdominal Pain Upper	2	1
Constipation	1	0
Vomiting	1	0
Loose Stools	1	0
General Disorders And Administration Site Conditions		
Fatigue	2	1
Thirst	1	0
Influenza-Like Illness	1	0
Pain	1	0
Pyrexia	1	0
Immune System Disorders		
Seasonal Allergy	1	0
Investigations		
Gamma-Glutamyltransferase Increased	1	0
Heart Rate Increased	1	0

Metabolism And Nutrition Disorders		
Anorexia	1	0
Decreased Appetite	1	0
Nervous System Disorders		
Headache	17	9
Dizziness	5	2
Disturbance In Attention	1	0
Tremor	1	0
Migraine	1	0
Paraesthia	1	0
Psychiatric Disorders		
Insomnia	5	1
Anxiety	4	1
Depression	2	0
Agitation	1	0
Nervousness	1	0
Depressed Mood	1	0
Renal And Urinary Disorders		
Polyuria	1	0
Respiratory, Thoracic And Mediastinal Disorders		
Dyspnea	1	0
Skin And Subcutaneous Tissue Disorders		
Rash	2	0
Contact Dermatitis	1	0
Hyperhydrosis	1	0

[a] Four double-blind, placebo-controlled clinical studies in SWSD, OSAHS, and narcolepsy; incidence is rounded to the nearest whole percent. Included are only those events for which NUVIGIL incidence is greater than that of placebo.

Dose Dependency of Adverse Events

In the placebo-controlled clinical trials which compared doses of 150 mg/day and 250 mg/day of NUVIGIL and placebo, the only adverse events that appeared to be dose-related were headache, rash, depression, dry mouth, insomnia, and nausea.

[See table 4 above]

Vital Sign Changes

There were small, but consistent, increases in average values for mean systolic and diastolic blood pressure in controlled trials (See **PRECAUTIONS**). There was a small, but consistent, average increase in pulse rate over placebo in controlled trials. This increase varied from 0.9 to 3.5 BPM.

Laboratory Changes

Clinical chemistry, hematology, and urinalysis parameters were monitored in the studies. Mean plasma levels of gamma glutamyltransferase (GGT) and alkaline phosphatase (AP) were found to be higher following administration of NUVIGIL, but not placebo. Few subjects, however, had GGT or AP elevations outside of the normal range. No differences were apparent in alanine aminotransferase, aspartate aminotransferase, total protein, albumin, or total bilirubin, although there were rare cases of isolated elevations of AST and/or ALT. A single case of mild pancytopenia was observed after 35-days of treatment and resolved with drug discontinuation. A small mean decrease from baseline in serum uric acid compared to placebo was seen in clinical trials. The clinical significance of this finding is unknown.

ECG Changes

No pattern of ECG abnormalities could be attributed to NUVIGIL administration in placebo-controlled clinical trials.

DRUG ABUSE AND DEPENDENCE

Controlled Substance Class

Armodafinil (NUVIGIL) is a Schedule IV controlled substance.

Abuse Potential and Dependence

Although the abuse potential of armodafinil has not been specifically studied, its abuse potential is likely to be similar to that of modafinil (PROVIGIL). In humans, modafinil produces psychoactive and euphoric effects, alterations in mood, perception, thinking and feelings typical of other CNS stimulants. In in vitro binding studies, modafinil binds to the dopamine reuptake site and causes an increase in extracellular dopamine, but no increase in dopamine release. Modafinil is reinforcing, as evidenced by its self-administration in monkeys previously trained to self-administer cocaine. In some studies, modafinil was also partially discriminated as stimulant-like. Physicians should follow patients closely, especially those with a history of drug and/or stimulant (e.g., methylphenidate, amphetamine, or cocaine) abuse. Patients should be observed for signs of misuse or abuse (e.g., incrementation of doses or drug-seeking behavior).

The abuse potential of modafinil (200, 400, and 800 mg) was assessed relative to methylphenidate (45 and 90 mg) in an inpatient study in individuals experienced with drugs of abuse. Results from this clinical study demonstrated that modafinil produced psychoactive and euphoric effects and feelings consistent with other scheduled CNS stimulants (methylphenidate).

OVERDOSAGE

Human Experience

There were no overdoses reported in the NUVIGIL clinical studies. Symptoms of NUVIGIL overdose are likely to be similar to those of modafinil. Overdose in modafinil clinical trials included excitation or agitation, insomnia, and slight or moderate elevations in hemodynamic parameters. From post-marketing experience with modafinil, there have been no reports of fatal overdoses involving modafinil alone (doses up to 12 grams). Overdoses involving multiple drugs, including modafinil, have resulted in fatal outcomes. Symptoms most often accompanying modafinil overdose, alone or in combination with other drugs have included; insomnia; central nervous system symptoms such as restlessness, disorientation, confusion, excitation and hallucination; digestive changes such as nausea and diarrhea; and cardiovascular changes such as tachycardia, bradycardia, hypertension and chest pain.

Overdose Management

No specific antidote exists for the toxic effects of a NUVIGIL overdose. Such overdoses should be managed with primarily supportive care, including cardiovascular monitoring. If there are no contraindications, induced emesis or gastric lavage should be considered. There are no data to suggest the utility of dialysis or urinary acidification or alkalinization in enhancing drug elimination. The physician should consider contacting a poison-control center for advice in the treatment of any overdose.

DOSAGE AND ADMINISTRATION

Obstructive Sleep Apnea/Hypopnea Syndrome (OSAHS) and Narcolepsy

The recommended dose of NUVIGIL for patients with OSAHS or narcolepsy is 150 mg or 250 mg given as a single dose in the morning. In patients with OSAHS, doses up to 250 mg/day, given as a single dose, have been well tolerated, but there is no consistent evidence that this dose confers additional benefit beyond that of the 150 mg/day dose (See **CLINICAL PHARMACOLOGY** and **CLINICAL TRIALS**).

Shift Work Sleep Disorder (SWSD)

The recommended dose of NUVIGIL for patients with SWSD is 150 mg given daily approximately 1 hour prior to the start of their work shift.

Dosage adjustment should be considered for concomitant medications that are substrates for CYP3A4/5, such as steroidal contraceptives, triazolam, and cyclosporine (See **PRECAUTIONS, Drug Interactions**).

Drugs that are largely eliminated via CYP2C19 metabolism, such as diazepam, propranolol, and phenytoin may have prolonged elimination upon coadministration with NUVIGIL and may require dosage reduction and monitoring for toxicity (See **PRECAUTIONS, Drug Interactions**).

In patients with severe hepatic impairment, NUVIGIL should be administered at a reduced dose (See **CLINICAL PHARMACOLOGY** and **PRECAUTIONS**).

There is inadequate information to determine safety and efficacy of dosing in patients with severe renal impairment (See **CLINICAL PHARMACOLOGY** and **PRECAUTIONS**).

In elderly patients, elimination of armodafinil and its metabolites may be reduced as a consequence of aging. Therefore, consideration should be given to the use of lower doses in this population (See **CLINICAL PHARMACOLOGY** and **PRECAUTIONS**).

HOW SUPPLIED

NUVIGIL® (armodafinil) Tablets [C-IV]

50 mg: Each round, white to off-white tablet is debossed with [C] on one side and "205" on the other.
NDC 63459-205-60 - Bottles of 60

150 mg: Each oval, white to off-white tablet is debossed with [C] on one side and "215" on the other.
NDC 63459-215-60 - Bottles of 60

250 mg: Each oval, white to off-white tablet is debossed with [C] on one side and "225" on the other.
NDC 63459-225-60 - Bottles of 60

Store at 20°-25° C (68°-77° F).

Manufactured for:
Cephalon, Inc.
Frazer, PA 19355
U.S. Patent Nos. RE37,516; 4,927,855; 7,132,570; 7,297,346
NUVIGIL is a trademark of Cephalon, Inc. or its affiliates.
© 2007-2010 Cephalon, Inc. All rights reserved.
January 2010
NUV-004

PATIENT INFORMATION

NUVIGIL® (nu-vij-el) Tablets [C-IV]

Generic name: armodafinil

Read the Patient Information that comes with NUVIGIL before you start taking it and each time you get a refill. There may be new information. This leaflet does not take the place of talking with your doctor about your condition or treatment.

What is the most important information I should know about NUVIGIL?

1. **NUVIGIL may cause you to have a serious rash or a serious allergic reaction. Stop NUVIGIL and call your doctor right away or get emergency treatment if you have any of the following:**
   - skin rash, hives, sores in your mouth, or your skin blisters and peels
   - swelling of your face, eyes, lips, tongue, or throat
   - trouble swallowing or breathing
   - hoarse voice

2. **NUVIGIL has not been studied in children under the age of 17. NUVIGIL is not approved for children for any condition.**

What is NUVIGIL?

NUVIGIL is a prescription medicine used to improve awakeness in adults who are very sleepy due to one of the following diagnosed sleep problems:
- shift work sleep disorder (SWSD)
- obstructive sleep apnea/hypopnea syndrome (OSAHS). NUVIGIL is used along with other medical treatments for this sleep problem. NUVIGIL is not a replacement for your CPAP machine. It is important that you continue to use your CPAP machine while sleeping.
- narcolepsy

You should be diagnosed with one of these sleep disorders before taking NUVIGIL. Sleepiness can be a symptom of other medical conditions that need to be treated.

- NUVIGIL will not cure the above sleep disorders. NUVIGIL may help the sleepiness caused by these conditions, but it may not stop all your sleepiness.
- NUVIGIL does not take the place of getting enough sleep.
- Follow your doctor's advice about good sleep habits and using other treatments.

NUVIGIL is a federally controlled substance (C-IV) because it can be abused or lead to dependence. Keep NUVIGIL in a safe place to prevent misuse and abuse. Selling or giving away NUVIGIL may harm others, and is against the law. Tell your doctor if you have ever abused or been dependent on alcohol, prescription medicines or street drugs.

Who should not take NUVIGIL?

Do not take NUVIGIL if you:
- are allergic to any of its ingredients. The active ingredient is armodafinil. See the end of this leaflet for a complete list of ingredients.
- have had a rash or allergic reaction to modafinil, the active ingredient in PROVIGIL, because these medicines are very similar.

It is not known if NUVIGIL works in or is safe for use in children under 17 years old.

What should I tell my doctor before starting NUVIGIL?

Tell your doctor about all of your health conditions including, if you:
- have a history of mental health problems
- have heart problems or had a heart attack
- have high blood pressure
- have liver or kidney problems
- have a history of drug or alcohol abuse or addiction
- have ever had a mental problem called psychosis.
- are pregnant or planning to become pregnant. It is not known if NUVIGIL may harm your unborn baby.
- are breastfeeding. It is not known if NUVIGIL passes into your milk or if it can harm your baby.

Tell your doctor about all the medicines you take, including prescription and non-prescription medicines, vitamins, and herbal supplements. NUVIGIL and many other medicines can interact with each other, sometimes causing side effects. NUVIGIL may affect the way other medicines work, and other medicines may affect how NUVIGIL works. Especially, tell your doctor if you use a hormonal birth control method. NUVIGIL can affect hormonal birth control methods. Hormonal birth control methods include pills, shots, implants, patches, vaginal rings, and intrauterine devices (IUDs). Women who use hormonal birth control with NUVIGIL may have a higher chance for getting pregnant while taking NUVIGIL, and for one month after stopping NUVIGIL. Talk to your doctor about birth control methods that are right for you while using NUVIGIL.

Keep a list of all the medicines you take. Your doctor or pharmacist will tell you if it is safe to take NUVIGIL and other medicines together. Do not take other medicines with NUVIGIL unless your doctor has told you it is okay.

How should I take NUVIGIL?

- Take NUVIGIL exactly as prescribed by your doctor. Your doctor will prescribe the dose of NUVIGIL that is right for you. Do not change your dose of NUVIGIL without talking to your doctor. Do not take more NUVIGIL than prescribed.
- Your doctor will tell you the right time of day to take NUVIGIL.
  - Patients with narcolepsy or OSAHS usually take one dose of NUVIGIL every day in the morning.
  - Patients with SWSD usually take NUVIGIL about 1 hour before their work shift. Do not change the time of day you take NUVIGIL unless you have talked to your doctor. If you take NUVIGIL too close to your bedtime, you may find it harder to go to sleep.
- If you take more than your prescribed dose or overdose, call your doctor or poison control center right away.

What should I avoid while taking NUVIGIL?

- Do not drive a car or do other dangerous activities until you know how NUVIGIL affects you. People with sleep disorders should always be careful about doing things that could be dangerous. Do not change your daily habits until your doctor tells you it is okay.
- Avoid drinking alcohol.

What are the possible side effects of NUVIGIL?

NUVIGIL may cause serious side effects. Call your doctor or get emergency help if you get any of the following:
- **a serious rash or serious allergic reaction.** (See, "What is the most important information I should know about NUVIGIL?")
- **mental (psychiatric) symptoms.** Symptoms include depression, anxiety, hallucinations, mania, thoughts of suicide, aggression, or other mental problems.
- **heart problems including chest pain**

The most common side effects of NUVIGIL are headache, nausea, dizziness, and trouble sleeping.

NUVIGIL may cause allergic reactions. If you get a rash, hives or other allergic reaction, stop taking NUVIGIL and call your doctor right away.

If you have either of the problems listed below or any other serious side effects while taking NUVIGIL stop taking NUVIGIL and call your doctor or get emergency help:
- chest pain.
- mental problems.

Some effects of NUVIGIL on the brain are the same as other medicines called "stimulants". These effects may lead to abuse or dependence on NUVIGIL. Before starting NUVIGIL, tell your doctor if you have ever abused drugs, including other stimulant medicines.

Tell your doctor if you get any side effect that bothers you or that does not go away while taking NUVIGIL.

These are not all the side effects of NUVIGIL. For more information, ask your doctor or pharmacist.

How should I store NUVIGIL?

- Store NUVIGIL at room temperature, 68° to 77° F (20° to 25° C).
- Keep NUVIGIL and all medicines out of the reach of children.

General information about NUVIGIL

Medicines are sometimes prescribed for conditions that are not listed in patient information leaflets. Do not use NUVIGIL for a condition for which it was not prescribed. **Do not give NUVIGIL to other people, even if they have the same symptoms you have. It may harm them and it is against the law.**

This leaflet summarizes the most important information about NUVIGIL. If you would like more information, talk with your doctor. You can ask your doctor or pharmacist for information about NUVIGIL that is written for health professionals. For more information, please call 1-800-896-5855, or go to www.NUVIGIL.com.

What are the ingredients in NUVIGIL?

Active Ingredient: armodafinil

Inactive Ingredients: croscarmellose sodium, lactose monohydrate, magnesium stearate, microcrystalline cellulose, povidone, and pregelatinized starch.

Rx Only
November 2010
NUVPIL - 004
Cephalon, Inc. Frazer, PA 19355

This Patient Information Leaflet has been approved by the U.S. Food and Drug Administration.

Shown in Product Identification Guide, page 308

PROVIGIL® Ⓒ ℞
[*pro-vij-el*]
(modafinil)
Tablet

DESCRIPTION

PROVIGIL (modafinil) is a wakefulness-promoting agent for oral administration. Modafinil is a racemic compound. The chemical name for modafinil is 2-[(diphenylmethyl)-sulfinyl]acetamide. The molecular formula is $C_{15}H_{15}NO_2S$ and the molecular weight is 273.35.
The chemical structure is:

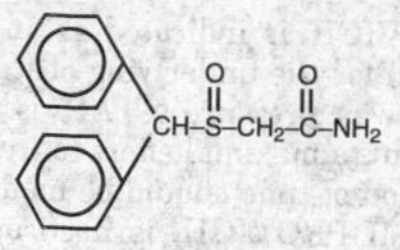

Modafinil is a white to off-white, crystalline powder that is practically insoluble in water and cyclohexane. It is sparingly to slightly soluble in methanol and acetone. PROVIGIL tablets contain 100 mg or 200 mg of modafinil and the following inactive ingredients: lactose, microcrystalline cellulose, pregelatinized starch, croscarmellose sodium, povidone, and magnesium stearate.

CLINICAL PHARMACOLOGY

Mechanism of Action and Pharmacology

The precise mechanism(s) through which modafinil promotes wakefulness is unknown. Modafinil has wake-promoting actions similar to sympathomimetic agents like amphetamine and methylphenidate, although the pharmacologic profile is not identical to that of sympathomimetic amines.
Modafinil has weak to negligible interactions with receptors for norepinephrine, serotonin, dopamine, GABA, adenosine, histamine-3, melatonin, and benzodiazepines. Modafinil also does not inhibit the activities of MAO-B or phosphodiesterases II-V.
Modafinil-induced wakefulness can be attenuated by the α_1-adrenergic receptor antagonist prazosin; however, modafinil is inactive in other in vitro assay systems known to be responsive to α-adrenergic agonists, such as the rat vas deferens preparation.
Modafinil is not a direct- or indirect-acting dopamine receptor agonist. However, in vitro, modafinil binds to the dopamine transporter and inhibits dopamine reuptake. This activity has been associated in vivo with increased extracellular dopamine levels in some brain regions of animals. In genetically engineered mice lacking the dopamine transporter (DAT), modafinil lacked wake-promoting activity, suggesting that this activity was DAT-dependent. However, the wake-promoting effects of modafinil, unlike those of amphetamine, were not antagonized by the dopamine receptor antagonist haloperidol in rats. In addition, alpha-methyl-p-tyrosine, a dopamine synthesis inhibitor, blocks the action of amphetamine, but does not block locomotor activity induced by modafinil.
In the cat, equal wakefulness-promoting doses of methylphenidate and amphetamine increased neuronal activation throughout the brain. Modafinil at an equivalent wakefulness-promoting dose selectively and prominently increased neuronal activation in more discrete regions of the brain. The relationship of this finding in cats to the effects of modafinil in humans is unknown.
In addition to its wake-promoting effects and ability to increase locomotor activity in animals, modafinil produces psychoactive and euphoric effects, alterations in mood, perception, thinking, and feelings typical of other CNS stimulants in humans. Modafinil has reinforcing properties, as evidenced by its self-administration in monkeys previously trained to self-administer cocaine. Modafinil was also partially discriminated as stimulant-like.
The optical enantiomers of modafinil have similar pharmacological actions in animals. Two major metabolites of modafinil, modafinil acid and modafinil sulfone, do not appear to contribute to the CNS-activating properties of modafinil.

Pharmacokinetics

Modafinil is a racemic compound, whose enantiomers have different pharmacokinetics (e.g., the half-life of the *l*-isomer is approximately three times that of the *d*-isomer in adult humans). The enantiomers do not interconvert. At steady state, total exposure to the *l*-isomer is approximately three times that for the *d*-isomer. The trough concentration (C_{minss}) of circulating modafinil after once daily dosing consists of 90% of the *l*-isomer and 10% of the *d*-isomer. The effective elimination half-life of modafinil after multiple doses is about 15 hours. The enantiomers of modafinil exhibit linear kinetics upon multiple dosing of 200-600 mg/day once daily in healthy volunteers. Apparent steady states of total modafinil and *l*-(-)-modafinil are reached after 2-4 days of dosing.

Absorption

Absorption of PROVIGIL tablets is rapid, with peak plasma concentrations occurring at 2-4 hours. The bioavailability of PROVIGIL tablets is approximately equal to that of an aqueous suspension. The absolute oral bioavailability was not determined due to the aqueous insolubility (<1 mg/mL) of modafinil, which precluded intravenous administration. Food has no effect on overall PROVIGIL bioavailability; however, its absorption (t_{max}) may be delayed by approximately one hour if taken with food.

Distribution

Modafinil is well distributed in body tissue with an apparent volume of distribution (~0.9 L/kg) larger than the volume of total body water (0.6 L/kg). In human plasma, in vitro, modafinil is moderately bound to plasma protein (~60%, mainly to albumin). At serum concentrations obtained at steady state after doses of 200 mg/day, modafinil exhibits no displacement of protein binding of warfarin, diazepam or propranolol. Even at much larger concentrations (1000μM; > 25 times the C_{max} of 40μM at steady state at 400 mg/day), modafinil has no effect on warfarin binding. Modafinil acid at concentrations >500μM decreases the extent of warfarin binding, but these concentrations are >35 times those achieved therapeutically.

Metabolism and Elimination

The major route of elimination is metabolism (~90%), primarily by the liver, with subsequent renal elimination of the metabolites. Urine alkalinization has no effect on the elimination of modafinil.
Metabolism occurs through hydrolytic deamidation, S-oxidation, aromatic ring hydroxylation, and glucuronide conjugation. Less than 10% of an administered dose is excreted as the parent compound. In a clinical study using radiolabeled modafinil, a total of 81% of the administered radioactivity was recovered in 11 days post-dose, predominantly in the urine (80% vs. 1.0% in the feces). The largest fraction of the drug in urine was modafinil acid, but at least six other metabolites were present in lower concentrations. Only two metabolites reach appreciable concentrations in plasma, i.e., modafinil acid and modafinil sulfone. In preclinical models, modafinil acid, modafinil sulfone, 2-[(diphenylmethyl)sulfonyl]acetic acid and 4-hydroxy modafinil, were inactive or did not appear to mediate the arousal effects of modafinil.
In adults, decreases in trough levels of modafinil have sometimes been observed after multiple weeks of dosing, suggesting auto-induction, but the magnitude of the decreases and the inconsistency of their occurrence suggest that their clinical significance is minimal. Significant accumulation of modafinil sulfone has been observed after multiple doses due to its long elimination half-life of 40 hours. Induction of metabolizing enzymes, most importantly cytochrome P-450 (CYP) 3A4, has also been observed in vitro after incubation of primary cultures of human hepatocytes with modafinil and in vivo after extended administration of modafinil at 400 mg/day. (For further discussion of the effects of modafinil on CYP enzyme activities, see **PRECAUTIONS, Drug Interactions**.)
Drug-Drug Interactions: Based on in vitro data, modafinil is metabolized partially by the 3A isoform subfamily of hepatic cytochrome P450 (CYP3A4). In addition, modafinil has the potential to inhibit CYP2C19, suppress CYP2C9, and induce CYP3A4, CYP2B6, and CYP1A2. Because modafinil and modafinil sulfone are reversible inhibitors of the drug-metabolizing enzyme CYP2C19, co-administration of modafinil with drugs such as diazepam, phenytoin and propranolol, which are largely eliminated via that pathway, may increase the circulating levels of those compounds. In addition, in individuals deficient in the enzyme CYP2D6 (i.e., 7-10% of the Caucasian population; similar or lower in other populations), the levels of CYP2D6 substrates such as tricyclic antidepressants and selective serotonin reuptake inhibitors, which have ancillary routes of elimination through CYP2C19, may be increased by co-administration of modafinil. Dose adjustments may be necessary for patients being treated with these and similar medications (See **PRECAUTIONS, Drug Interactions**). An in vitro study demonstrated that armodafinil (one of the enantiomers of modafinil) is a substrate of P-glycoprotein.
Coadministration of modafinil with other CNS active drugs such as methylphenidate and dextroamphetamine did not significantly alter the pharmacokinetics of either drug.
Chronic administration of modafinil 400 mg was found to decrease the systemic exposure to two CYP3A4 substrates, ethinyl estradiol and triazolam, after oral administration suggesting that CYP3A4 had been induced. Chronic administration of modafinil can increase the elimination of substrates of CYP3A4. Dose adjustments may be necessary for patients being treated with these and similar medications (See **PRECAUTIONS, Drug Interactions**).
An apparent concentration-related suppression of CYP2C9 activity was observed in human hepatocytes after exposure to modafinil in vitro suggesting that there is a potential for a metabolic interaction between modafinil and the substrates of this enzyme (e.g., S-warfarin, phenytoin). However, in an interaction study in healthy volunteers, chronic modafinil treatment did not show a significant effect on the pharmacokinetics of warfarin when compared to placebo. (See **PRECAUTIONS, Drug Interactions**, *Other Drugs*, Warfarin).
Special Populations
Gender Effect: The pharmacokinetics of modafinil are not affected by gender.
Age Effect: A slight decrease (~20%) in the oral clearance (CL/F) of modafinil was observed in a single dose study at 200 mg in 12 subjects with a mean age of 63 years (range 53 – 72 years), but the change was considered not likely to be clinically significant. In a multiple dose study (300 mg/day) in 12 patients with a mean age of 82 years (range 67 – 87 years), the mean levels of modafinil in plasma were approximately two times those historically obtained in matched younger subjects. Due to potential effects from the multiple concomitant medications with which most of the patients were being treated, the apparent difference in modafinil pharmacokinetics may not be attributable solely to the effects of aging. However, the results suggest that the clearance of modafinil may be reduced in the elderly (See **DOSAGE AND ADMINISTRATION**).
Race Effect: The influence of race on the pharmacokinetics of modafinil has not been studied.
Renal Impairment: In a single dose 200 mg modafinil study, severe chronic renal failure (creatinine clearance ≤ 20 mL/min) did not significantly influence the pharmacokinetics of modafinil, but exposure to modafinil acid (an inactive metabolite) was increased 9-fold (See **PRECAUTIONS**).
Hepatic Impairment: Pharmacokinetics and metabolism were examined in patients with cirrhosis of the liver (6 males and 3 females). Three patients had stage B or B+ cirrhosis (per the Child criteria) and 6 patients had stage C or C+ cirrhosis. Clinically 8 of 9 patients were icteric and all had ascites. In these patients, the oral clearance of modafinil was decreased by about 60% and the steady state concentration was doubled compared to normal patients. The dose of PROVIGIL should be reduced in patients with severe hepatic impairment (See **PRECAUTIONS** and **DOSAGE AND ADMINISTRATION**).

CLINICAL TRIALS

The effectiveness of PROVIGIL in reducing excessive sleepiness has been established in the following sleep disorders: narcolepsy, obstructive sleep apnea/hypopnea syndrome (OSAHS), and shift work sleep disorder (SWSD).

Narcolepsy

The effectiveness of PROVIGIL in reducing the excessive sleepiness (ES) associated with narcolepsy was established in two US 9-week, multicenter, placebo-controlled, two-dose (200 mg per day and 400 mg per day) parallel-group, double-blind studies of outpatients who met the ICD-9 and American Sleep Disorders Association criteria for narcolepsy (which are also consistent with the American Psychiatric Association DSM-IV criteria). These criteria include either 1) recurrent daytime naps or lapses into sleep that occur almost daily for at least three months, plus sudden bilateral loss of postural muscle tone in association with intense emotion (cataplexy) or 2) a complaint of excessive sleepiness or sudden muscle weakness with associated features: sleep paralysis, hypnagogic hallucinations, automatic behaviors, disrupted major sleep episode; and polysomnography demonstrating one of the following: sleep latency less than 10 minutes or rapid eye movement (REM) sleep latency less than 20 minutes. In addition, for entry into these studies, all patients were required to have objectively documented excessive daytime sleepiness, a Multiple Sleep Latency Test (MSLT) with two or more sleep onset REM periods, and the absence of any other clinically significant active medical or psychiatric disorder. The MSLT, an objective daytime polysomnographic assessment of the patient's ability to fall asleep in an unstimulating environment, measures latency (in minutes) to sleep onset averaged over 4 test sessions at 2-hour intervals following nocturnal polysomnography. For each test session, the subject was told to lie quietly and attempt to sleep. Each test session was terminated after 20 minutes if no sleep occurred or 15 minutes after sleep onset.
In both studies, the primary measures of effectiveness were 1) sleep latency, as assessed by the Maintenance of Wakefulness Test (MWT) and 2) the change in the patient's overall disease status, as measured by the Clinical Global Impression of Change (CGI-C). For a successful trial, both measures had to show significant improvement.

Table 1. Average Baseline Sleep Latency and Change from Baseline at Final Visit in Adults (MWT and MSLT in minutes)

Disorder	Measure	PROVIGIL 200 mg*		PROVIGIL 400 mg*		Placebo	
		Baseline	Change from Baseline	Baseline	Change from Baseline	Baseline	Change from Baseline
Narcolepsy I	MWT	5.8	2.3	6.6	2.3	5.8	-0.7
Narcolepsy II	MWT	6.1	2.2	5.9	2.0	6.0	-0.7
OSAHS	MWT	13.1	1.6	13.6	1.5	13.8	-1.1
SWSD	MSLT	2.1	1.7	–	–	2.0	0.3

*Significantly different than placebo for all trials (p<0.01 for all trials but SWSD, which was p<0.05)

Table 2. Clinical Global Impression of Change (CGI-C) (Percent of Adult Patients Who Improved at Final Visit)

Disorder	PROVIGIL 200 mg*	PROVIGIL 400 mg*	Placebo
Narcolepsy I	64%	72%	37%
Narcolepsy II	58%	60%	38%
OSAHS	61%	68%	37%
SWSD	74%	–	36%

*Significantly different than placebo for all trials (p<0.01)

The MWT measures latency (in minutes) to sleep onset averaged over 4 test sessions at 2 hour intervals following nocturnal polysomnography. For each test session, the subject was asked to attempt to remain awake without using extraordinary measures. Each test session was terminated after 20 minutes if no sleep occurred or 10 minutes after sleep onset. The CGI-C is a 7-point scale, centered at *No Change*, and ranging from *Very Much Worse* to *Very Much Improved*. Patients were rated by evaluators who had no access to any data about the patients other than a measure of their baseline severity. Evaluators were not given any specific guidance about the criteria they were to apply when rating patients.

Other assessments of effect included the Multiple Sleep Latency Test (MSLT), Epworth Sleepiness Scale (ESS; a series of questions designed to assess the degree of sleepiness in everyday situations) the Steer Clear Performance Test (SCPT; a computer-based evaluation of a patient's ability to avoid hitting obstacles in a simulated driving situation), standard nocturnal polysomnography, and patient's daily sleep log. Patients were also assessed with the Quality of Life in Narcolepsy (QOLIN) scale, which contains the validated SF-36 health questionnaire.

Both studies demonstrated improvement in objective and subjective measures of excessive daytime sleepiness for both the 200 mg and 400 mg doses compared to placebo. Patients treated with either dose of PROVIGIL showed a statistically significantly enhanced ability to remain awake on the MWT (all p values <0.001) at weeks 3, 6, 9, and final visit compared to placebo and a statistically significantly greater global improvement, as rated on the CGI-C scale (all p values <0.05).

The average sleep latencies (in minutes) on the MWT at baseline for the 2 controlled trials are shown in Table 1 below, along with the average change from baseline on the MWT at final visit.

The percentages of patients who showed any degree of improvement on the CGI-C in the two clinical trials are shown in Table 2 below.

Similar statistically significant treatment-related improvements were seen on other measures of impairment in narcolepsy, including a patient assessed level of daytime sleepiness on the ESS (p<0.001 for each dose in comparison to placebo).

Nighttime sleep measured with polysomnography was not affected by the use of PROVIGIL.

Obstructive Sleep Apnea/Hypopnea Syndrome (OSAHS)
The effectiveness of PROVIGIL in reducing the excessive sleepiness associated with OSAHS was established in two clinical trials. In both studies, patients were enrolled who met the International Classification of Sleep Disorders (ICSD) criteria for OSAHS (which are also consistent with the American Psychiatric Association DSM-IV criteria). These criteria include either, 1) excessive sleepiness or insomnia, plus frequent episodes of impaired breathing during sleep, and associated features such as loud snoring, morning headaches and dry mouth upon awakening; or 2) excessive sleepiness or insomnia and polysomnography demonstrating one of the following: more than five obstructive apneas, each greater than 10 seconds in duration, per hour of sleep and one or more of the following: frequent arousals from sleep associated with the apneas, bradytachycardia, and arterial oxygen desaturation in association with the apneas. In addition, for entry into these studies, all patients were required to have excessive sleepiness as demonstrated by a score ≥10 on the Epworth Sleepiness Scale, despite treatment with continuous positive airway pressure (CPAP). Evidence that CPAP was effective in reducing episodes of apnea/hypopnea was required along with documentation of CPAP use.

In the first study, a 12-week multicenter placebo-controlled trial, a total of 327 patients were randomized to receive PROVIGIL 200 mg/day, PROVIGIL 400 mg/day, or matching placebo. The majority of patients (80%) were fully compliant with CPAP, defined as CPAP use > 4 hours/night on

> 70% nights. The remainder were partially CPAP compliant, defined as CPAP use < 4 hours/night on >30% nights. CPAP use continued throughout the study. The primary measures of effectiveness were 1) sleep latency, as assessed by the Maintenance of Wakefulness Test (MWT) and 2) the change in the patient's overall disease status, as measured by the Clinical Global Impression of Change (CGI-C) at week 12 or the final visit. (See **CLINICAL TRIALS**, *Narcolepsy* section above for a description of these tests.)
Patients treated with PROVIGIL showed a statistically significant improvement in the ability to remain awake compared to placebo-treated patients as measured by the MWT (p<0.001) at endpoint [Table 1]. PROVIGIL-treated patients also showed a statistically significant improvement in clinical condition as rated by the CGI-C scale (p<0.001) [Table 2]. The two doses of PROVIGIL performed similarly.
In the second study, a 4-week multicenter placebo-controlled trial, 157 patients were randomized to either PROVIGIL 400 mg/day or placebo. Documentation of regular CPAP use (at least 4 hours/night on 70% of nights) was required for all patients. The primary outcome measure was the change from baseline on the ESS at week 4 or final visit. The baseline ESS scores for the PROVIGIL and placebo groups were 14.2 and 14.4, respectively. At week 4, the ESS was reduced by 4.6 in the PROVIGIL group and by 2.0 in the placebo group, a difference that was statistically significant (p<0.0001).
Nighttime sleep measured with polysomnography was not affected by the use of PROVIGIL.

Shift Work Sleep Disorder (SWSD)
The effectiveness of PROVIGIL for the excessive sleepiness associated with SWSD was demonstrated in a 12-week placebo-controlled clinical trial. A total of 209 patients with chronic SWSD were randomized to receive PROVIGIL 200 mg/day or placebo. All patients met the International Classification of Sleep Disorders (ICSD-10) criteria for chronic SWSD (which are consistent with the American Psychiatric Association DSM-IV criteria for Circadian Rhythm Sleep Disorder: Shift Work Type). These criteria include 1) either: a) a primary complaint of excessive sleepiness or insomnia which is temporally associated with a work period (usually night work) that occurs during the habitual sleep phase, or b) polysomnography and the MSLT demonstrate loss of a normal sleep-wake pattern (i.e., disturbed chronobiological rhythmicity); and 2) no other medical or mental disorder accounts for the symptoms, and 3) the symptoms do not meet criteria for any other sleep disorder producing insomnia or excessive sleepiness (e.g., time zone change [jet lag] syndrome).
It should be noted that not all patients with a complaint of sleepiness who are also engaged in shift work meet the criteria for the diagnosis of SWSD. In the clinical trial, only patients who were symptomatic for at least 3 months were enrolled.
Enrolled patients were also required to work a minimum of 5 night shifts per month, have excessive sleepiness at the time of their night shifts (MSLT score < 6 minutes), and have daytime insomnia documented by a daytime polysomnogram (PSG).
The primary measures of effectiveness were 1) sleep latency, as assessed by the Multiple Sleep Latency Test (MSLT) performed during a simulated night shift at week 12 or the final visit and 2) the change in the patient's overall disease status, as measured by the Clinical Global Impression of Change (CGI-C) at week 12 or the final visit. Patients treated with PROVIGIL showed a statistically significant prolongation in the time to sleep onset compared to placebo-treated patients, as measured by the nighttime MSLT [Table 1] (p<0.05). Improvement on the CGI-C was also observed to be statistically significant (p<0.001). (See **CLINICAL TRIALS**, *Narcolepsy* section above for a description of these tests.)
Daytime sleep measured with polysomnography was not affected by the use of PROVIGIL.
[See table 1 above]

INDICATIONS AND USAGE
PROVIGIL is indicated to improve wakefulness in adult patients with excessive sleepiness associated with narcolepsy, obstructive sleep apnea/hypopnea syndrome, and shift work sleep disorder.
In OSAHS, PROVIGIL is indicated as an adjunct to standard treatment(s) for the underlying obstruction. If continuous positive airway pressure (CPAP) is the treatment of choice for a patient, a maximal effort to treat with CPAP for an adequate period of time should be made prior to initiating PROVIGIL. If PROVIGIL is used adjunctively with CPAP, the encouragement of and periodic assessment of CPAP compliance is necessary.
In all cases, careful attention to the diagnosis and treatment of the underlying sleep disorder(s) is of utmost importance. Prescribers should be aware that some patients may have more than one sleep disorder contributing to their excessive sleepiness.
The effectiveness of modafinil in long-term use (greater than 9 weeks in Narcolepsy clinical trials and 12 weeks in OSAHS and SWSD clinical trials) has not been systematically evaluated in placebo-controlled trials. The physician who elects to prescribe PROVIGIL for an extended time in patients with Narcolepsy, OSAHS, or SWSD should periodically reevaluate long-term usefulness for the individual patient.

CONTRAINDICATIONS
PROVIGIL is contraindicated in patients with known hypersensitivity to modafinil, armodafinil or its inactive ingredients.

WARNINGS
Serious Rash, including Stevens-Johnson Syndrome
Serious rash requiring hospitalization and discontinuation of treatment has been reported in adults and children in association with the use of modafinil.
Modafinil is not approved for use in pediatric patients for any indication.
In clinical trials of modafinil, the incidence of rash resulting in discontinuation was approximately 0.8% (13 per 1,585) in pediatric patients (age <17 years); these rashes included 1 case of possible Stevens-Johnson Syndrome (SJS) and 1 case of apparent multi-organ hypersensitivity reaction. Several of the cases were associated with fever and other abnormalities (e.g., vomiting, leukopenia). The median time to rash that resulted in discontinuation was 13 days. No such cases were observed among 380 pediatric patients who received placebo. No serious skin rashes have been reported in adult clinical trials (0 per 4,264) of modafinil.
Rare cases of serious or life-threatening rash, including SJS, Toxic Epidermal Necrolysis (TEN), and Drug Rash with Eosinophilia and Systemic Symptoms (DRESS) have been reported in adults and children in worldwide postmarketing experience. The reporting rate of TEN and SJS associated with modafinil use, which is generally accepted to be an underestimate due to underreporting, exceeds the background incidence rate. Estimates of the background incidence rate for these serious skin reactions in the general population range between 1 to 2 cases per million-person years.
There are no factors that are known to predict the risk of occurrence or the severity of rash associated with modafinil. Nearly all cases of serious rash associated with modafinil occurred within 1 to 5 weeks after treatment initiation. However, isolated cases have been reported after prolonged treatment (e.g., 3 months). Accordingly, duration of therapy cannot be relied upon as a means to predict the potential risk heralded by the first appearance of a rash.
Although benign rashes also occur with modafinil, it is not possible to reliably predict which rashes will prove to be serious. Accordingly, modafinil should ordinarily be discontinued at the first sign of rash, unless the rash is clearly not drug-related. Discontinuation of treatment may not prevent a rash from becoming life-threatening or permanently disabling or disfiguring.
Angioedema and Anaphylactoid Reactions
One serious case of angioedema and one case of hypersensitivity (with rash, dysphagia, and bronchospasm), were observed among 1,595 patients treated with armodafinil, the

R enantiomer of modafinil (which is the racemic mixture). No such cases were observed in modafinil clinical trials. However, angioedema has been reported in postmarketing experience with modafinil. Patients should be advised to discontinue therapy and immediately report to their physician any signs or symptoms suggesting angioedema or anaphylaxis (e.g., swelling of face, eyes, lips, tongue or larynx; difficulty in swallowing or breathing; hoarseness).

Multi-organ Hypersensitivity Reactions

Multi-organ hypersensitivity reactions, including at least one fatality in postmarketing experience, have occurred in close temporal association (median time to detection 13 days: range 4-33) to the initiation of modafinil.

Although there have been a limited number of reports, multi-organ hypersensitivity reactions may result in hospitalization or be life-threatening. There are no factors that are known to predict the risk of occurrence or the severity of multi-organ hypersensitivity reactions associated with modafinil. Signs and symptoms of this disorder were diverse; however, patients typically, although not exclusively, presented with fever and rash associated with other organ system involvement. Other associated manifestations included myocarditis, hepatitis, liver function test abnormalities, hematological abnormalities (e.g., eosinophilia, leukopenia, thrombocytopenia), pruritus, and asthenia. Because multi-organ hypersensitivity is variable in its expression, other organ system symptoms and signs, not noted here, may occur.

If a multi-organ hypersensitivity reaction is suspected, PROVIGIL should be discontinued. Although there are no case reports to indicate cross-sensitivity with other drugs that produce this syndrome, the experience with drugs associated with multi-organ hypersensitivity would indicate this to be a possibility.

Persistent Sleepiness

Patients with abnormal levels of sleepiness who take PROVIGIL should be advised that their level of wakefulness may not return to normal. Patients with excessive sleepiness, including those taking PROVIGIL, should be frequently reassessed for their degree of sleepiness and, if appropriate, advised to avoid driving or any other potentially dangerous activity. Prescribers should also be aware that patients may not acknowledge sleepiness or drowsiness until directly questioned about drowsiness or sleepiness during specific activities.

Psychiatric Symptoms

Psychiatric adverse experiences have been reported in patients treated with modafinil. Postmarketing adverse events associated with the use of modafinil have included mania, delusions, hallucinations, suicidal ideation and aggression, some resulting in hospitalization. Many, but not all, patients had a prior psychiatric history. One healthy male volunteer developed ideas of reference, paranoid delusions, and auditory hallucinations in association with multiple daily 600 mg doses of modafinil and sleep deprivation. There was no evidence of psychosis 36 hours after drug discontinuation.

In the adult modafinil controlled trials database, psychiatric symptoms resulting in treatment discontinuation (at a frequency ≥0.3%) and reported more often in patients treated with modafinil compared to those treated with placebo were anxiety (1%), nervousness (1%), insomnia (<1%), confusion (<1%), agitation (<1%), and depression (<1%). Caution should be exercised when PROVIGIL is given to patients with a history of psychosis, depression, or mania. Consideration should be given to the possible emergence or exacerbation of psychiatric symptoms in patients treated with PROVIGIL. If psychiatric symptoms develop in association with PROVIGIL administration, consider discontinuing PROVIGIL.

PRECAUTIONS

Diagnosis of Sleep Disorders

PROVIGIL should be used only in patients who have had a complete evaluation of their excessive sleepiness, and in whom a diagnosis of either narcolepsy, OSAHS, and/or SWSD has been made in accordance with ICSD or DSM diagnostic criteria (See CLINICAL TRIALS). Such an evaluation usually consists of a complete history and physical examination, and it may be supplemented with testing in a laboratory setting. Some patients may have more than one sleep disorder contributing to their excessive sleepiness (e.g., OSAHS and SWSD coincident in the same patient).

General

Although modafinil has not been shown to produce functional impairment, any drug affecting the CNS may alter judgment, thinking or motor skills. Patients should be cautioned about operating an automobile or other hazardous machinery until they are reasonably certain that PROVIGIL therapy will not adversely affect their ability to engage in such activities.

CPAP Use in Patients with OSAHS

In OSAHS, PROVIGIL is indicated as an adjunct to standard treatment(s) for the underlying obstruction. If contin-

uous positive airway pressure (CPAP) is the treatment of choice for a patient, a maximal effort to treat with CPAP for an adequate period of time should be made prior to initiating PROVIGIL. If PROVIGIL is used adjunctively with CPAP, the encouragement of and periodic assessment of CPAP compliance is necessary.

Cardiovascular System

Modafinil has not been evaluated in patients with a recent history of myocardial infarction or unstable angina, and such patients should be treated with caution.

In clinical studies of PROVIGIL, signs and symptoms including chest pain, palpitations, dyspnea and transient ischemic T-wave changes on ECG were observed in three subjects in association with mitral valve prolapse or left ventricular hypertrophy. It is recommended that PROVIGIL tablets not be used in patients with a history of left ventricular hypertrophy or in patients with mitral valve prolapse who have experienced the mitral valve prolapse syndrome when previously receiving CNS stimulants. Such signs may include but are not limited to ischemic ECG changes, chest pain, or arrhythmia. If new onset of any of these symptoms occurs, consider cardiac evaluation.

Blood pressure monitoring in short-term (<3 months) controlled trials showed no clinically significant changes in mean systolic and diastolic blood pressure in patients receiving PROVIGIL as compared to placebo. However, a retrospective analysis of the use of antihypertensive medication in these studies showed that a greater proportion of patients on PROVIGIL required new or increased use of antihypertensive medications (2.4%) compared to patients on placebo (0.7%). The differential use was slightly larger when only studies in OSAHS were included, with 3.4% of patients on PROVIGIL and 1.1% of patients on placebo requiring such alterations in the use of antihypertensive medication. Increased monitoring of blood pressure may be appropriate in patients on PROVIGIL.

Patients Using Steroidal Contraceptives

The effectiveness of steroidal contraceptives may be reduced when used with PROVIGIL tablets and for one month after discontinuation of therapy (See PRECAUTIONS, Drug Interactions). Alternative or concomitant methods of contraception are recommended for patients treated with PROVIGIL tablets, and for one month after discontinuation of PROVIGIL.

Patients Using Cyclosporine

The blood levels of cyclosporine may be reduced when used with PROVIGIL (See PRECAUTIONS, Drug Interactions). Monitoring of circulating cyclosporine concentrations and appropriate dosage adjustment for cyclosporine should be considered when these drugs are used concomitantly.

Patients with Severe Hepatic Impairment

In patients with severe hepatic impairment, with or without cirrhosis (See CLINICAL PHARMACOLOGY), PROVIGIL should be administered at a reduced dose (See DOSAGE AND ADMINISTRATION).

Patients with Severe Renal Impairment

There is inadequate information to determine safety and efficacy of dosing in patients with severe renal impairment. (For pharmacokinetics in renal impairment, see CLINICAL PHARMACOLOGY.)

Elderly Patients

In elderly patients, elimination of modafinil and its metabolites may be reduced as a consequence of aging. Therefore, consideration should be given to the use of lower doses in this population. (See CLINICAL PHARMACOLOGY and DOSAGE AND ADMINISTRATION).

Information for Patients

Physicians are advised to discuss the following issues with patients for whom they prescribe PROVIGIL.

PROVIGIL is indicated for patients who have abnormal levels of sleepiness. PROVIGIL has been shown to improve, but not eliminate this abnormal tendency to fall asleep. Therefore, patients should not alter their previous behavior with regard to potentially dangerous activities (e.g., driving, operating machinery) or other activities requiring appropriate levels of wakefulness, until and unless treatment with PROVIGIL has been shown to produce levels of wakefulness that permit such activities. Patients should be advised that PROVIGIL is not a replacement for sleep.

Patients should be informed that it may be critical that they continue to take their previously prescribed treatments (e.g., patients with OSAHS receiving CPAP should continue to do so).

Patients should be informed of the availability of a patient information leaflet, and they should be instructed to read the leaflet prior to taking PROVIGIL. See Patient Information at the end of this labeling for the text of the leaflet provided for patients.

Patients should be advised to contact their physician if they experience chest pain, rash, depression, anxiety, or signs of psychosis or mania.

Pregnancy

Patients should be advised to notify their physician if they become pregnant or intend to become pregnant during ther-

apy. Patients should be cautioned regarding the potential increased risk of pregnancy when using steroidal contraceptives (including depot or implantable contraceptives) with PROVIGIL and for one month after discontinuation of therapy (See Carcinogenesis, Mutagenesis, Impairment of Fertility and Pregnancy).

Nursing

Patients should be advised to notify their physician if they are breast feeding an infant.

Concomitant Medication

Patients should be advised to inform their physician if they are taking, or plan to take, any prescription or over-the-counter drugs, because of the potential for interactions between PROVIGIL and other drugs.

Alcohol

Patients should be advised that the use of PROVIGIL in combination with alcohol has not been studied. Patients should be advised that it is prudent to avoid alcohol while taking PROVIGIL.

Allergic Reactions

Patients should be advised to stop taking PROVIGIL and to notify their physician if they develop a rash, hives, mouth sores, blisters, peeling skin, trouble swallowing or breathing or a related allergic phenomenon.

Drug Interactions

CNS Active Drugs

Methylphenidate-In a single-dose study in healthy volunteers, simultaneous administration of modafinil (200 mg) with methylphenidate (40 mg) did not cause any significant alterations in the pharmacokinetics of either drug. However, the absorption of PROVIGIL may be delayed by approximately one hour when coadministered with methylphenidate.

In a multiple-dose, steady-state study in healthy volunteers, modafinil was administered once daily at 200 mg/day for 7 days followed by 400 mg/day for 21 days. Administration of methylphenidate (20 mg/day) during days 22-28 of modafinil treatment 8 hours after the daily dose of modafinil did not cause any significant alterations in the pharmacokinetics of modafinil.

Dextroamphetamine-In a single dose study in healthy volunteers, simultaneous administration of modafinil (200 mg) with dextroamphetamine (10 mg) did not cause any significant alterations in the pharmacokinetics of either drug. However, the absorption of PROVIGIL may be delayed by approximately one hour when coadministered with dextroamphetamine.

In a multiple-dose, steady-state study in healthy volunteers, modafinil was administered once daily at 200 mg/day for 7 days followed by 400 mg/day for 21 days. Administration of dextroamphetamine (20 mg/day) during days 22-28 of modafinil treatment 7 hours after the daily dose of modafinil did not cause any significant alterations in the pharmacokinetics of modafinil.

Clomipramine-The coadministration of a single dose of clomipramine (50 mg) on the first of three days of treatment with modafinil (200 mg/day) in healthy volunteers did not show an effect on the pharmacokinetics of either drug. However, one incident of increased levels of clomipramine and its active metabolite desmethylclomipramine has been reported in a patient with narcolepsy during treatment with modafinil.

Triazolam-In the drug interaction study between PROVIGIL and ethinyl estradiol (EE_2), on the same days as those for the plasma sampling for EE_2 pharmacokinetics, a single dose of triazolam (0.125 mg) was also administered. Mean C_{max} and $AUC_{0-\infty}$ of triazolam were decreased by 42% and 59%, respectively, and its elimination half-life was decreased by approximately an hour after the modafinil treatment.

Monoamine Oxidase (MAO) Inhibitors-Interaction studies with monoamine oxidase inhibitors have not been performed. Therefore, caution should be used when concomitantly administering MAO inhibitors and modafinil.

Other Drugs

Warfarin-There were no significant changes in the pharmacokinetic profiles of R- and S-warfarin in healthy subjects given a single dose of racemic warfarin (5 mg) following chronic administration of modafinil (200 mg/day for 7 days followed by 400 mg/day for 27 days) relative to the profiles in subjects given placebo. However, more frequent monitoring of prothrombin times/INR is advisable whenever PROVIGIL is coadministered with warfarin (See CLINICAL PHARMACOLOGY, Pharmacokinetics, Drug-Drug Interactions).

Ethinyl Estradiol-Administration of modafinil to female volunteers once daily at 200 mg/day for 7 days followed by 400 mg/day for 21 days resulted in a mean 11% decrease in C_{max} and 18% decrease in AUC_{0-24} of ethinyl estradiol (EE_2; 0.035 mg; administered orally with norgestimate). There was no apparent change in the elimination rate of ethinyl estradiol.

Cyclosporine-One case of an interaction between modafinil and cyclosporine, a substrate of CYP3A4, has been reported in a 41 year old woman who had undergone an organ transplant. After one month of administration of 200 mg/day of modafinil, cyclosporine blood levels were decreased by 50%. The interaction was postulated to be due to the increased metabolism of cyclosporine, since no other factor expected to affect the disposition of the drug had changed. Dosage adjustment for cyclosporine may be needed.

Potential Interactions with Drugs That Inhibit, Induce, or are Metabolized by Cytochrome P-450 Isoenzymes and Other Hepatic Enzymes

In in vitro studies using primary human hepatocyte cultures, modafinil was shown to slightly induce CYP1A2, CYP2B6 and CYP3A4 in a concentration-dependent manner. Although induction results based on in vitro experiments are not necessarily predictive of response in vivo, caution needs to be exercised when PROVIGIL is coadministered with drugs that depend on these three enzymes for their clearance. Specifically, lower blood levels of such drugs could result (See *Other Drugs*, Cyclosporine above).

The exposure of human hepatocytes to modafinil in vitro produced an apparent concentration-related suppression of expression of CYP2C9 activity suggesting that there is a potential for a metabolic interaction between modafinil and the substrates of this enzyme (e.g., S-warfarin and phenytoin). In a subsequent clinical study in healthy volunteers, chronic modafinil treatment did not show a significant effect on the single-dose pharmacokinetics of warfarin when compared to placebo (See **PRECAUTIONS, Drug Interactions**, Warfarin).

In vitro studies using human liver microsomes showed that modafinil reversibly inhibited CYP2C19 at pharmacologically relevant concentrations of modafinil. CYP2C19 is also reversibly inhibited, with similar potency, by a circulating metabolite, modafinil sulfone. Although the maximum plasma concentrations of modafinil sulfone are much lower than those of parent modafinil, the combined effect of both compounds could produce sustained partial inhibition of the enzyme. Drugs that are largely eliminated via CYP2C19 metabolism, such as diazepam, propranolol, phenytoin (also via CYP2C9) or S-mephenytoin may have prolonged elimination upon coadministration with PROVIGIL and may require dosage reduction and monitoring for toxicity.

Tricyclic antidepressants-CYP2C19 also provides an ancillary pathway for the metabolism of certain tricyclic antidepressants (e.g., clomipramine and desipramine) that are primarily metabolized by CYP2D6. In tricyclic-treated patients deficient in CYP2D6 (i.e., those who are poor metabolizers of debrisoquine; 7-10% of the Caucasian population; similar or lower in other populations), the amount of metabolism by CYP2C19 may be substantially increased. PROVIGIL may cause elevation of the levels of the tricyclics in this subset of patients. Physicians should be aware that a reduction in the dose of tricyclic agents might be needed in these patients.

In addition, due to the partial involvement of CYP3A4 in the metabolic elimination of modafinil, coadministration of potent inducers of CYP3A4 (e.g., carbamazepine, phenobarbital, rifampin) or inhibitors of CYP3A4 (e.g., ketoconazole, itraconazole) could alter the plasma levels of modafinil.

Carcinogenesis, Mutagenesis, Impairment of Fertility

Carcinogenesis

Carcinogenicity studies were conducted in which modafinil was administered in the diet to mice for 78 weeks and to rats for 104 weeks at doses of 6, 30, and 60 mg/kg/day. The highest dose studied is 1.5 (mouse) or 3 (rat) times greater than the recommended adult human daily dose of modafinil (200 mg) on a mg/m^2 basis. There was no evidence of tumorigenesis associated with modafinil administration in these studies. However, since the mouse study used an inadequate high dose that was not representative of a maximum tolerated dose, a subsequent carcinogenicity study was conducted in the Tg.AC transgenic mouse. Doses evaluated in the Tg.AC assay were 125, 250, and 500 mg/kg/day, administered dermally. There was no evidence of tumorigenicity associated with modafinil administration; however, this dermal model may not adequately assess the carcinogenic potential of an orally administered drug.

Mutagenesis

Modafinil demonstrated no evidence of mutagenic or clastogenic potential in a series of in vitro (i.e., bacterial reverse mutation assay, mouse lymphoma tk assay, chromosomal aberration assay in human lymphocytes, cell transformation assay in BALB/3T3 mouse embryo cells) assays in the absence or presence of metabolic activation, or in vivo (mouse bone marrow micronucleus) assays. Modafinil was also negative in the unscheduled DNA synthesis assay in rat hepatocytes.

Impairment of Fertility

Oral administration of modafinil (doses of up to 480 mg/kg/day) to male and female rats prior to and throughout mating, and continuing in females through day 7 of gestation produced an increase in the time to mate at the highest dose; no effects were observed on other fertility or reproductive parameters. The no-effect dose of 240 mg/kg/day was associated with a plasma modafinil exposure (AUC) approximately equal to that in humans at the recommended dose of 200 mg.

Pregnancy

Pregnancy Category C: In studies conducted in rats and rabbits, developmental toxicity was observed at clinically relevant exposures.

Modafinil (50, 100, or 200 mg/kg/day) administered orally to pregnant rats throughout the period of organogenesis caused, in the absence of maternal toxicity, an increase in resorptions and an increased incidence of visceral and skeletal variations in the offspring at the highest dose. The higher no-effect dose for rat embryofetal developmental toxicity was associated with a plasma modafinil exposure approximately 0.5 times the AUC in humans at the recommended daily dose (RHD) of 200 mg. However, in a subsequent study of up to 480 mg/kg/day (plasma modafinil exposure approximately 2 times the AUC in humans at the RHD) no adverse effects on embryofetal development were observed.

Modafinil administered orally to pregnant rabbits throughout the period of organogenesis at doses of 45, 90, and 180 mg/kg/day increased the incidences of fetal structural alterations and embryofetal death at the highest dose. The highest no-effect dose for developmental toxicity was associated with a plasma modafinil AUC approximately equal to the AUC in humans at the RHD.

Oral administration of armodafinil (the R-enantiomer of modafinil; 60, 200, or 600 mg/kg/day) to pregnant rats throughout the period of organogenesis resulted in increased incidences of fetal visceral and skeletal variations at the intermediate dose or greater and decreased fetal body weights at the highest dose. The no-effect dose for rat embryofetal developmental toxicity was associated with a plasma armodafinil exposure (AUC) approximately one-tenth times the AUC for armodafinil in humans treated with modafinil at the RHD.

Modafinil administration to rats throughout gestation and lactation at oral doses of up to 200 mg/kg/day resulted in decreased viability in the offspring at doses greater than 20 mg/kg/day (plasma modafinil AUC approximately 0.1 times the AUC in humans at the RHD). No effects on postnatal developmental and neurobehavioral parameters were observed in surviving offspring.

There are no adequate and well-controlled studies in pregnant women. Two cases of intrauterine growth retardation and one case of spontaneous abortion have been reported in association with armodafinil and modafinil. Although the pharmacology of modafinil and armodafinil is not identical to that of the sympathomimetic amines, they do share some pharmacologic properties with this class. Certain of these drugs have been associated with intrauterine growth retardation and spontaneous abortions. Whether the cases reported are drug-related is unknown.

Modafinil should be used during pregnancy only if the potential benefit justifies the potential risk to the fetus.

Labor and Delivery

The effect of modafinil on labor and delivery in humans has not been systematically investigated.

Nursing Mothers

It is not known whether modafinil or its metabolites are excreted in human milk. Because many drugs are excreted in human milk, caution should be exercised when PROVIGIL tablets are administered to a nursing woman.

Pediatric Use

Safety and effectiveness in pediatric patients, below age 16, have not been established. Serious skin rashes, including erythema multiforme major (EMM) and Stevens-Johnson Syndrome (SJS) have been associated with modafinil use in pediatric patients (see **WARNINGS, Serious Rash, including Stevens-Johnson Syndrome**).

In a controlled 6-week study, 165 pediatric patients (aged 5-17 years) with narcolepsy were treated with modafinil (n=123), or placebo (n=42). There were no statistically significant differences favoring modafinil over placebo in prolonging sleep latency as measured by MSLT, or in perceptions of sleepiness as determined by the clinical global impression-clinician scale (CGI-C).

In the controlled and open-label clinical studies, treatment emergent adverse events of the psychiatric and nervous system included Tourette's syndrome, insomnia, hostility, increased cataplexy, increased hypnagogic hallucinations and suicidal ideation. Transient leukopenia, which resolved without medical intervention, was also observed. In the controlled clinical study, 3 of 38 girls, ages 12 or older, treated with modafinil experienced dysmenorrhea compared to 0 of 10 girls who received placebo.

Geriatric Use

Safety and effectiveness in individuals above 65 years of age have not been established. Experience in a limited number of patients who were greater than 65 years of age in clinical trials showed an incidence of adverse experiences similar to other age groups.

ADVERSE REACTIONS

Modafinil has been evaluated for safety in over 3500 patients, of whom more than 2000 patients with excessive sleepiness associated with primary disorders of sleep and wakefulness were given at least one dose of modafinil. In clinical trials, modafinil has been found to be generally well tolerated and most adverse experiences were mild to moderate.

The most commonly observed adverse events (≥5%) associated with the use of PROVIGIL more frequently than placebo-treated patients in the placebo-controlled clinical studies in primary disorders of sleep and wakefulness were headache, nausea, nervousness, rhinitis, diarrhea, back pain, anxiety, insomnia, dizziness, and dyspepsia. The adverse event profile was similar across these studies.

In the placebo-controlled clinical trials, 74 of the 934 patients (8%) who received PROVIGIL discontinued due to an adverse experience compared to 3% of patients that received placebo. The most frequent reasons for discontinuation that occurred at a higher rate for PROVIGIL than placebo patients were headache (2%), nausea, anxiety, dizziness, insomnia, chest pain and nervousness (each <1%). In a Canadian clinical trial, a 35 year old obese narcoleptic male with a prior history of syncopal episodes experienced a 9-second episode of asystole after 27 days of modafinil treatment (300 mg/day in divided doses).

Incidence in Controlled Trials

The following table (Table 3) presents the adverse experiences that occurred at a rate of 1% or more and were more frequent in adult patients treated with PROVIGIL than in placebo-treated patients in the principal, placebo-controlled clinical trials.

The prescriber should be aware that the figures provided below cannot be used to predict the frequency of adverse experiences in the course of usual medical practice, where patient characteristics and other factors may differ from those occurring during clinical studies. Similarly, the cited frequencies cannot be directly compared with figures obtained from other clinical investigations involving different treatments, uses, or investigators. Review of these frequencies, however, provides prescribers with a basis to estimate the relative contribution of drug and non-drug factors to the incidence of adverse events in the population studied.

[See table 3 at top of next page]

Dose Dependency of Adverse Events

In the adult placebo-controlled clinical trials which compared doses of 200, 300, and 400 mg/day of PROVIGIL and placebo, the only adverse events that were clearly dose related were headache and anxiety.

Vital Sign Changes

While there was no consistent change in mean values of heart rate or systolic and diastolic blood pressure, the requirement for antihypertensive medication was slightly greater in patients on PROVIGIL compared to placebo (See **PRECAUTIONS**).

Weight Changes

There were no clinically significant differences in body weight change in patients treated with PROVIGIL compared to placebo-treated patients in the placebo-controlled clinical trials.

Laboratory Changes

Clinical chemistry, hematology, and urinalysis parameters were monitored in Phase 1, 2, and 3 studies. In these studies, mean plasma levels of gamma glutamyltransferase (GGT) and alkaline phosphatase (AP) were found to be higher following administration of PROVIGIL, but not placebo. Few subjects, however, had GGT or AP elevations outside of the normal range. Shifts to higher, but not clinically significantly abnormal, GGT and AP values appeared to increase with time in the population treated with PROVIGIL in the Phase 3 clinical trials. No differences were apparent in alanine aminotransferase, aspartate aminotransferase, total protein, albumin, or total bilirubin.

ECG Changes

No treatment-emergent pattern of ECG abnormalities was found in placebo-controlled clinical trials following administration of PROVIGIL.

Postmarketing Reports

The following adverse reactions have been identified during post-approval use of PROVIGIL. Because these reactions are reported voluntarily from a population of uncertain size, it is not possible to reliably estimate their frequency or establish a causal relationship to drug exposure. Decisions to include these reactions in labeling are typically based on one or more of the following factors: (1) seriousness of the reaction, (2) frequency of the reporting, or (3) strength of causal connection to PROVIGIL.

Hematologic: agranulocytosis

DRUG ABUSE AND DEPENDENCE

Controlled Substance Class

Modafinil (PROVIGIL) is listed in Schedule IV of the Controlled Substances Act.

Abuse Potential and Dependence

In addition to its wakefulness-promoting effect and increased locomotor activity in animals, in humans, PROVIGIL produces psychoactive and euphoric effects, alterations in mood, perception, thinking and feelings typical of other CNS stimulants. In in vitro binding studies, modafinil binds to the dopamine reuptake site and causes an increase in extracellular dopamine, but no increase in dopamine release. Modafinil is reinforcing, as evidenced by its self-administration in monkeys previously trained to self-administer cocaine. In some studies, modafinil was also partially discriminated as stimulant-like. Physicians should follow patients closely, especially those with a history of drug and/or stimulant (e.g., methylphenidate, amphetamine, or cocaine) abuse. Patients should be observed for signs of misuse or abuse (e.g., incrementation of doses or drug-seeking behavior).

The abuse potential of modafinil (200, 400, and 800 mg) was assessed relative to methylphenidate (45 and 90 mg) in an inpatient study in individuals experienced with drugs of abuse. Results from this clinical study demonstrated that modafinil produced psychoactive and euphoric effects and feelings consistent with other scheduled CNS stimulants (methylphenidate).

Withdrawal

The effects of modafinil withdrawal were monitored following 9 weeks of modafinil use in one US Phase 3 controlled clinical trial. No specific symptoms of withdrawal were observed during 14 days of observation, although sleepiness returned in narcoleptic patients.

OVERDOSAGE

Human Experience

In clinical trials, a total of 151 protocol-specified doses ranging from 1000 to 1600 mg/day (5 to 8 times the recommended daily dose of 200 mg) have been administered to 32 subjects, including 13 subjects who received doses of 1000 or 1200 mg/day for 7 to 21 consecutive days. In addition, several intentional acute overdoses occurred; the two largest being 4500 mg and 4000 mg taken by two subjects participating in foreign depression studies. None of these study subjects experienced any unexpected or life-threatening effects. Adverse experiences that were reported at these doses included excitation or agitation, insomnia, and slight or moderate elevations in hemodynamic parameters. Other observed high-dose effects in clinical studies have included anxiety, irritability, aggressiveness, confusion, nervousness, tremor, palpitations, sleep disturbances, nausea, diarrhea and decreased prothrombin time.

From post-marketing experience, there have been no reports of fatal overdoses involving modafinil alone (doses up to 12 grams). Overdoses involving multiple drugs, including modafinil, have resulted in fatal outcomes. Symptoms most often accompanying modafinil overdose, alone or in combination with other drugs, have included: insomnia; central nervous system symptoms such as restlessness, disorientation, confusion, excitation and hallucination; digestive changes such as nausea and diarrhea; and cardiovascular changes such as tachycardia, bradycardia, hypertension and chest pain.

Cases of accidental ingestion/overdose have been reported in children as young as 11 months of age. The highest reported accidental ingestion on a mg/kg basis occurred in a three-year-old boy who ingested 800-1000 mg (50-63 mg/kg) of modafinil. The child remained stable. The symptoms associated with overdose in children were similar to those observed in adults.

Overdose Management

No specific antidote to the toxic effects of modafinil overdose has been identified to date. Such overdoses should be managed with primarily supportive care, including cardiovascular monitoring. If there are no contraindications, induced emesis or gastric lavage should be considered. There are no data to suggest the utility of dialysis or urinary acidification or alkalinization in enhancing drug elimination. The physician should consider contacting a poison-control center on the treatment of any overdose.

DOSAGE AND ADMINISTRATION

The recommended dose of PROVIGIL is 200 mg given once a day.

For patients with narcolepsy and OSAHS, PROVIGIL should be taken as a single dose in the morning.

For patients with SWSD, PROVIGIL should be taken approximately 1 hour prior to the start of their work shift.

Doses up to 400 mg/day, given as a single dose, have been well tolerated, but there is no consistent evidence that this dose confers additional benefit beyond that of the 200 mg dose (See **CLINICAL PHARMACOLOGY** and **CLINICAL TRIALS**).

General Considerations

Dosage adjustment should be considered for concomitant medications that are substrates for CYP3A4, such as triazolam and cyclosporine (See **PRECAUTIONS, Drug Interactions**).

Drugs that are largely eliminated via CYP2C19 metabolism, such as diazepam, propranolol, phenytoin (also via CYP2C9) or S-mephenytoin may have prolonged elimination upon coadministration with PROVIGIL and may require dosage reduction and monitoring for toxicity.

In patients with severe hepatic impairment, the dose of PROVIGIL should be reduced to one-half of that recommended for patients with normal hepatic function (See **CLINICAL PHARMACOLOGY** and **PRECAUTIONS**).

There is inadequate information to determine safety and efficacy of dosing in patients with severe renal impairment (See **CLINICAL PHARMACOLOGY** and **PRECAUTIONS**).

In elderly patients, elimination of PROVIGIL and its metabolites may be reduced as a consequence of aging. Therefore, consideration should be given to the use of lower doses in this population (See **CLINICAL PHARMACOLOGY** and **PRECAUTIONS**).

Table 3. Incidence Of Treatment-Emergent Adverse Experiences In Parallel-Group, Placebo-Controlled Clinical Trials[1] With PROVIGIL In Adults With Narcolepsy, OSAHS, and SWSD (200mg, 300mg and 400mg)*

Body System	Preferred Term	Modafinil (n = 934)	Placebo (n = 567)
Body as a Whole	Headache	34%	23%
	Back Pain	6%	5%
	Flu Syndrome	4%	3%
	Chest Pain	3%	1%
	Chills	1%	0%
	Neck Rigidity	1%	0%
Cardiovascular	Hypertension	3%	1%
	Tachycardia	2%	1%
	Palpitation	2%	1%
	Vasodilatation	2%	0%
Digestive	Nausea	11%	3%
	Diarrhea	6%	5%
	Dyspepsia	5%	4%
	Dry Mouth	4%	2%
	Anorexia	4%	1%
	Constipation	2%	1%
	Abnormal Liver Function[2]	2%	1%
	Flatulence	1%	0%
	Mouth Ulceration	1%	0%
	Thirst	1%	0%
Hemic/Lymphatic	Eosinophilia	1%	0%
Metabolic/Nutritional	Edema	1%	0%
Nervous	Nervousness	7%	3%
	Insomnia	5%	1%
	Anxiety	5%	1%
	Dizziness	5%	4%
	Depression	2%	1%
	Paresthesia	2%	1%
	Somnolence	2%	0%
	Hypertonia	1%	1%
	Dyskinesia[3]	1%	0%
	Hyperkinesia	1%	0%
	Agitation	1%	0%
	Confusion	1%	0%
	Tremor	1%	0%
	Emotional Lability	1%	0%
	Vertigo	1%	0%
Respiratory	Rhinitis	7%	6%
	Pharyngitis	4%	2%
	Lung Disorder	2%	1%
	Epistaxis	1%	0%
	Asthma	1%	0%
Skin/Appendages	Sweating	1%	0%
	Herpes Simplex	1%	0%
Special Senses	Amblyopia	1%	0%
	Abnormal Vision	1%	0%
	Taste Perversion	1%	0%
	Eye Pain	1%	0%
Urogenital	Urine Abnormality	1%	0%
	Hematuria	1%	0%
	Pyuria	1%	0%

* Six double-blind, placebo-controlled clinical studies in narcolepsy, OSAHS, and SWSD.

[1] Events reported by at least 1% of patients treated with PROVIGIL that were more frequent than in the placebo group are included; incidence is rounded to the nearest 1%. The adverse experience terminology is coded using a standard modified COSTART Dictionary.
Events for which the PROVIGIL incidence was at least 1%, but equal to or less than placebo are not listed in the table. These events included the following: infection, pain, accidental injury, abdominal pain, hypothermia, allergic reaction, asthenia, fever, viral infection, neck pain, migraine, abnormal electrocardiogram, hypotension, tooth disorder, vomiting, periodontal abscess, increased appetite, ecchymosis, hyperglycemia, peripheral edema, weight loss, weight gain, myalgia, leg cramps, arthritis, cataplexy, thinking abnormality, sleep disorder, increased cough, sinusitis, dyspnea, bronchitis, rash, conjunctivitis, ear pain, dysmenorrhea[4], urinary tract infection.

[2] Elevated liver enzymes.

[3] Oro-facial dyskinesias.

[4] Incidence adjusted for gender.

HOW SUPPLIED

PROVIGIL® (modafinil) Tablets

100 mg: Each capsule-shaped, white, uncoated tablet is debossed with "PROVIGIL" on one side and "100 MG" on the other.
NDC 63459-101-01 - Bottles of 100

200 mg: Each capsule-shaped, white, scored, uncoated tablet is debossed with "PROVIGIL" on one side and "200 MG" on the other.
NDC 63459-201-01 - Bottles of 100

Store at 20°-25° C (68°-77° F).

Manufactured for:
Cephalon, Inc.
Frazer, PA 19355
U.S. Patent Nos. RE37,516 / 4,927,855
© Cephalon, Inc., 2008. All rights reserved
March 2008
PROV-011

PATIENT INFORMATION

PROVIGIL® (pro-vij-el) Tablets [C-IV]

Generic name: modafinil

Read the Patient Information that comes with PROVIGIL before you start taking it and each time you get a refill. There may be new information. This leaflet does not take the place of talking with your doctor about your condition or treatment.

What is the most important information I should know about PROVIGIL?

1. **PROVIGIL may cause you to have a serious rash or a serious allergic reaction. Stop PROVIGIL and call your doctor right away or get emergency treatment if you have any of the following:**
   - skin rash, hives, sores in your mouth, or your skin blisters and peels
   - swelling of your face, eyes, lips, tongue, or throat
   - trouble swallowing or breathing
   - hoarse voice
2. **PROVIGIL is not approved for use in children.**

What is PROVIGIL?

PROVIGIL is a prescription medicine used to improve awakeness in adults who are very sleepy due to one of the following diagnosed sleep problems:
- shift work sleep disorder (SWSD)
- obstructive sleep apnea/hypopnea syndrome (OSAHS). PROVIGIL is used along with other medical treatments for this sleep problem. PROVIGIL is not a replacement for your CPAP machine. It is important that you continue to use your CPAP machine while sleeping.
- narcolepsy

You should be diagnosed with one of these sleep disorders before taking PROVIGIL. Sleepiness can be a symptom of other medical conditions that need to be treated.
- PROVIGIL will not cure the above sleep disorders. PROVIGIL may help the sleepiness caused by these conditions, but it may not stop all your sleepiness.
- PROVIGIL does not take the place of getting enough sleep.
- Follow your doctor's advice about good sleep habits and using other treatments.

> PROVIGIL is a federally controlled substance (C-IV) because it can be abused or lead to dependence. Keep PROVIGIL in a safe place to prevent misuse and abuse. Selling or giving away PROVIGIL may harm others, and is against the law. Tell your doctor if you have ever abused or been dependent on alcohol, prescription medicines or street drugs.

Who should not take PROVIGIL?

Do not take PROVIGIL if you:
- are allergic to any of its ingredients. The active ingredient is modafinil. See the end of this leaflet for a complete list of ingredients.
- have had a rash or allergic reaction to armodafinil, the active ingredient in NUVIGIL™, because these medicines are very similar.

PROVIGIL is not approved for use in children.

What should I tell my doctor before starting PROVIGIL?

Tell your doctor about all of your health conditions including, if you:
- have a history of mental health problems
- have heart problems or had a heart attack
- have high blood pressure
- have liver or kidney problems
- have a history of drug or alcohol abuse or addiction
- have ever had a mental problem called psychosis.
- are pregnant or planning to become pregnant. It is not known if PROVIGIL may harm your unborn baby.
- are breastfeeding. It is not known if PROVIGIL passes into your milk or if it can harm your baby.

Tell your doctor about all the medicines you take, including prescription and non-prescription medicines, vitamins, and herbal supplements. PROVIGIL and many other medicines can interact with each other, sometimes causing side effects. PROVIGIL may affect the way other medicines work, and other medicines may affect how PROVIGIL works. Especially, tell your doctor if you use a hormonal birth control method. PROVIGIL can affect hormonal birth control methods. Hormonal birth control methods include pills, shots, implants, patches, vaginal rings, and intrauterine devices (IUDs). Women who use hormonal birth control with PROVIGIL may have a higher chance for getting pregnant while taking PROVIGIL, and for one month after stopping PROVIGIL. Talk to your doctor about birth control methods that are right for you while using PROVIGIL.

Keep a list of all the medicines you take. Your doctor or pharmacist will tell you if it is safe to take PROVIGIL and other medicines together. Do not take other medicines with PROVIGIL unless your doctor has told you it is okay.

How should I take PROVIGIL?
- Take PROVIGIL exactly as prescribed by your doctor. Your doctor will prescribe the dose of PROVIGIL that is right for you. Do not change your dose of PROVIGIL without talking to your doctor. Do not take more PROVIGIL than prescribed.
- Your doctor will tell you the right time of day to take PROVIGIL.
  - Patients with narcolepsy or OSAHS usually take one dose of PROVIGIL every day in the morning.
  - Patients with SWSD usually take PROVIGIL about 1 hour before their work shift. Do not change the time of day you take PROVIGIL unless you have talked to your doctor. If you take PROVIGIL too close to your bedtime, you may find it harder to go to sleep.
  - You can take PROVIGIL with or without food.
- If you take more than your prescribed dose or overdose, call your doctor or poison control center right away.

What should I avoid while taking PROVIGIL?
- Do not drive a car or do other dangerous activities until you know how PROVIGIL affects you. People with sleep disorders should always be careful about doing things that could be dangerous. Do not change your daily habits until your doctor tells you it is okay.
- Avoid drinking alcohol.

What are the possible side effects of PROVIGIL?

PROVIGIL may cause serious side effects. Call your doctor or get emergency help if you get any of the following:
- **a serious rash or serious allergic reaction.** (See, "What is the most important information I should know about PROVIGIL.")
- **mental (psychiatric) symptoms.** Symptoms include depression, anxiety, hallucinations, mania, thoughts of suicide, aggression, or other mental problems.
- **heart problems including chest pain**

The most common side effects of PROVIGIL are headache, nausea, nervousness, stuffy nose, diarrhea, back pain, anxiety, trouble sleeping, dizziness, and upset stomach.

PROVIGIL may cause allergic reactions. If you get a rash, hives or other allergic reaction, stop taking PROVIGIL and call your doctor right away.

If you have either of the problems listed below or any other serious side effects while taking PROVIGIL stop taking PROVIGIL and call your doctor or get emergency help:
- chest pain.
- mental problems.

Some effects of PROVIGIL on the brain are the same as other medicines called "stimulants". These effects may lead to abuse or dependence on PROVIGIL. Before starting PROVIGIL, tell your doctor if you have ever abused drugs, including other stimulant medicines.

Tell your doctor if you get any side effect that bothers you or that does not go away while taking PROVIGIL.

These are not all the side effects of PROVIGIL. For more information, ask your doctor or pharmacist.

How should I store PROVIGIL?
- Store PROVIGIL at room temperature, 68° to 77° F (20° to 25° C).
- Keep PROVIGIL and all medicines out of the reach of children.

General information about PROVIGIL

Medicines are sometimes prescribed for conditions that are not listed in patient information leaflets. Do not use PROVIGIL for a condition for which it was not prescribed. **Do not give PROVIGIL to other people, even if they have the same symptoms you have. It may harm them and it is against the law.**

This leaflet summarizes the most important information about PROVIGIL. If you would like more information, talk with your doctor. You can ask your doctor or pharmacist for information about PROVIGIL that is written for health professionals. For more information, please call 1-800-896-5855, or go to www.PROVIGIL.com.

What are the ingredients in PROVIGIL?

Active Ingredient: modafinil

Inactive Ingredients: croscarmellose sodium, lactose, magnesium stearate, microcrystalline cellulose, povidone, and pregelatinized starch.

Rx Only

March 2008
Manufactured for:
Cephalon, Inc.
Frazer, PA 19355
This Patient Information Leaflet has been approved by the U.S. Food and Drug Administration.

Shown in Product Identification Guide, page 308

TREANDA® ℞

[tree-and-uh]

(bendamustine hydrochloride)

for Injection, for Intravenous infusion

HIGHLIGHTS OF PRESCRIBING INFORMATION

These highlights do not include all the information needed to use TREANDA safely and effectively. See full prescribing information for TREANDA.

TREANDA® (bendamustine hydrochloride) injection, powder, lyophilized, for solution for intravenous use

Initial U.S. Approval: 2008

RECENT MAJOR CHANGES

Warnings and Precautions, Extravasation (5.7) 01/2010

INDICATIONS AND USAGE

TREANDA for Injection is an alkylating drug indicated for treatment of patients with:
- Chronic lymphocytic leukemia (CLL). Efficacy relative to first line therapies other than chlorambucil has not been established. (1.1)
- Indolent B-cell non-Hodgkin's lymphoma (NHL) that has progressed during or within six months of treatment with rituximab or a rituximab-containing regimen. (1.2)

DOSAGE AND ADMINISTRATION

For CLL:
- 100 mg/m² infused intravenously over 30 minutes on Days 1 and 2 of a 28-day cycle, up to 6 cycles (2.1)
- Dose modifications for hematologic toxicity: for Grade 3 or greater toxicity, reduce dose to 50 mg/m² on Days 1 and 2; if Grade 3 or greater toxicity recurs, reduce dose to 25 mg/m² on Days 1 and 2. (2.1)
- Dose modifications for non-hematologic toxicity: for clinically significant Grade 3 or greater toxicity, reduce the dose to 50 mg/m² on Days 1 and 2 of each cycle. (2.1)
- Dose re-escalation may be considered. (2.1)

For NHL:
- 120 mg/m² infused intravenously over 60 minutes on Days 1 and 2 of a 21-day cycle, up to 8 cycles (2.2)
- Dose modifications for hematologic toxicity: for Grade 4 toxicity, reduce the dose to 90 mg/m² on Days 1 and 2 of each cycle; if Grade 4 toxicity recurs, reduce the dose to 60 mg/m² on Days 1 and 2 of each cycle. (2.2)
- Dose modifications for non-hematologic toxicity: for Grade 3 or greater toxicity, reduce the dose to 90 mg/m² on Days 1 and 2 of each cycle; if Grade 3 or greater toxicity recurs, reduce the dose to 60 mg/m² on Days 1 and 2 of each cycle. (2.2)

General Dosing Considerations:
- Delay treatment for Grade 4 hematologic toxicity or clinically significant ≥ Grade 2 non-hematologic toxicity. (2.1, 2.2)
- TREANDA for Injection must be reconstituted and further diluted prior to infusion. (2.3)

DOSAGE FORMS AND STRENGTHS

TREANDA for Injection single-use vial containing either 25 mg or 100 mg of bendamustine HCl as lyophilized powder (3)

CONTRAINDICATIONS

Known hypersensitivity to bendamustine or mannitol. (4)

WARNINGS AND PRECAUTIONS
- Myelosuppression: May warrant treatment delay or dose reduction. Monitor closely and restart treatment based on ANC and platelet count recovery. Complications of myelosuppression may lead to death. (5.1)
- Infections: Monitor for fever and other signs of infection and treat promptly. (5.2)
- Infusion Reactions and Anaphylaxis: Severe anaphylactic reactions have occurred. Monitor clinically and discontinue drug for severe reactions. Ask patients about reactions after the first cycle. Consider pre-treatment for cycles subsequent to milder reactions. (5.3)
- Tumor Lysis Syndrome: May lead to acute renal failure and death. Take precautions in patients at high risk. (5.4)
- Skin Reactions: Discontinue for severe skin reactions. Cases of SJS and TEN, some fatal, have been reported when TREANDA was administered concomitantly with allopurinol and other medications known to cause these syndromes. (5.5)
- Other Malignancies: Pre-malignant and malignant diseases have been reported. (5.6)
- Extravasation: Take precautions to avoid extravasation, including monitoring intravenous infusion site during and after administration. (5.7)
- Use in Pregnancy: Fetal harm can occur when administered to a pregnant woman. Women should be advised to avoid becoming pregnant when receiving TREANDA. (5.8, 8.1)

ADVERSE REACTIONS

Most common non-hematologic adverse reactions for CLL (frequency ≥15%) are pyrexia, nausea, and vomiting. (6.1)

Most common non-hematologic adverse reactions for NHL (frequency ≥15%) are nausea, fatigue, vomiting, diarrhea, pyrexia, constipation, anorexia, cough, headache, weight decreased, dyspnea, rash, and stomatitis. (6.2)

Most common hematologic abnormalities for both indications (frequency ≥15%) are lymphopenia, anemia, leukopenia, thrombocytopenia, and neutropenia. (6.1, 6.2)

To report SUSPECTED ADVERSE REACTIONS, contact Cephalon, Inc. at 1-800-896-5855 or FDA at 1-800-FDA-1088 or www.fda.gov/medwatch

---DRUG INTERACTIONS---

Concomitant CYP1A2 inducers or inhibitors have the potential to affect the exposure of bendamustine. (7)

---USE IN SPECIFIC POPULATIONS---

• Renal impairment: Do not use if CrCL is <40 mL/min. Use with caution in lesser degrees of renal impairment. (8.6)

• Hepatic impairment: Do not use in moderate or severe hepatic impairment. Use with caution in mild hepatic impairment. (8.7)

See 17 for PATIENT COUNSELING INFORMATION
Revised: 07/2010

FULL PRESCRIBING INFORMATION: CONTENTS*

* Sections or subsections omitted from the full prescribing information are not listed

FULL PRESCRIBING INFORMATION

1   INDICATIONS AND USAGE
1.1   Chronic Lymphocytic Leukemia (CLL)
TREANDA® is indicated for the treatment of patients with chronic lymphocytic leukemia. Efficacy relative to first line therapies other than chlorambucil has not been established.
1.2   Non-Hodgkin's Lymphoma (NHL)
TREANDA for Injection is indicated for the treatment of patients with indolent B-cell non-Hodgkin's lymphoma that has progressed during or within six months of treatment with rituximab or a rituximab-containing regimen.

2   DOSAGE AND ADMINISTRATION
2.1   Dosing Instructions for CLL
Recommended Dosage:
The recommended dose is 100 mg/m² administered intravenously over 30 minutes on Days 1 and 2 of a 28-day cycle, up to 6 cycles.
Dose Delays, Dose Modifications and Reinitiation of Therapy for CLL:
TREANDA administration should be delayed in the event of Grade 4 hematologic toxicity or clinically significant

≥ Grade 2 non-hematologic toxicity. Once non-hematologic toxicity has recovered to ≤ Grade 1 and/or the blood counts have improved [Absolute Neutrophil Count (ANC) ≥ 1 × 10⁹/L, platelets ≥ 75 × 10⁹/L], TREANDA can be reinitiated at the discretion of the treating physician. In addition, dose reduction may be warranted. [See Warnings and Precautions (5.1)]

Dose modifications for hematologic toxicity: for Grade 3 or greater toxicity, reduce the dose to 50 mg/m² on Days 1 and 2 of each cycle; if Grade 3 or greater toxicity recurs, reduce the dose to 25 mg/m² on Days 1 and 2 of each cycle

Dose modifications for non-hematologic toxicity: for clinically significant Grade 3 or greater toxicity, reduce the dose to 50 mg/m² on Days 1 and 2 of each cycle.

Dose re-escalation in subsequent cycles may be considered at the discretion of the treating physician.

2.2   Dosing Instructions for NHL
Recommended Dosage:
The recommended dose is 120 mg/m² administered intravenously over 60 minutes on Days 1 and 2 of a 21-day cycle, up to 8 cycles.
Dose Delays, Dose Modifications and Reinitiation of Therapy for NHL:
TREANDA administration should be delayed in the event of a Grade 4 hematologic toxicity or clinically significant ≥ Grade 2 non-hematologic toxicity. Once non-hematologic toxicity has recovered to ≤ Grade 1 and/or the blood counts have improved [Absolute Neutrophil Count (ANC) ≥ 1 × 10⁹/L, platelets ≥ 75 × 10⁹/L], TREANDA can be reinitiated at the discretion of the treating physician. In addition, dose reduction may be warranted. [See Warnings and Precautions (5.1)]

Dose modifications for hematologic toxicity: for Grade 4 toxicity, reduce the dose to 90 mg/m² on Days 1 and 2 of each cycle; if Grade 4 toxicity recurs, reduce the dose to 60 mg/m² on Days 1 and 2 of each cycle.

Dose modifications for non-hematologic toxicity: for Grade 3 or greater toxicity, reduce the dose to 90 mg/m² on Days 1 and 2 of each cycle; if Grade 3 or greater toxicity recurs, reduce the dose to 60 mg/m² on Days 1 and 2 of each cycle.

2.3   Reconstitution/Preparation for Intravenous Administration
• Aseptically reconstitute each TREANDA vial as follows:
  • 25 mg TREANDA vial: Add 5 mL of only **Sterile Water for Injection, USP.**
  • 100 mg TREANDA vial: Add 20 mL of only **Sterile Water for Injection, USP.**
  Shake well to yield a clear, colorless to a pale yellow solution with a bendamustine HCl concentration of 5 mg/mL. The lyophilized powder should completely dissolve in 5 minutes. If particulate matter is observed, the reconstituted product should not be used.
• Aseptically withdraw the volume needed for the required dose (based on 5 mg/mL concentration) and immediately transfer to a 500 mL infusion bag of 0.9% Sodium Chloride Injection, USP (normal saline). As an alternative to 0.9% Sodium Chloride Injection, USP (normal saline), a 500 mL infusion bag of 2.5% Dextrose/0.45% Sodium Chloride Injection, USP, may be considered. The resulting final concentration of bendamustine HCl in the infusion bag should be within 0.2–0.6 mg/mL. The reconstituted solution must be transferred to the infusion bag within 30 minutes of reconstitution. After transferring, thoroughly mix the contents of the infusion bag. The admixture should be a clear and colorless to slightly yellow solution.
  Use Sterile Water for Injection, USP, for reconstitution and then either 0.9% Sodium Chloride Injection, USP, or 2.5% Dextrose/0.45% Sodium Chloride Injection, USP, for dilution, as outlined above. No other diluents have been shown to be compatible.
  Parenteral drug products should be inspected visually for particulate matter and discoloration prior to administration whenever solution and container permit. Any unused solution should be discarded according to institutional procedures for antineoplastics.

2.4   Admixture Stability
TREANDA contains no antimicrobial preservative. The admixture should be prepared as close as possible to the time of patient administration.
Once diluted with either 0.9% Sodium Chloride Injection, USP, or 2.5% Dextrose/0.45% Sodium Chloride Injection, USP, the final admixture is stable for 24 hours when stored refrigerated (2-8°C or 36-47°F) or for 3 hours when stored at room temperature (15-30°C or 59-86°F) and room light. Administration of TREANDA must be completed within this period.

3   DOSAGE FORMS AND STRENGTHS
TREANDA for Injection single-use vial containing either 25 mg or 100 mg of bendamustine HCl as white to off-white lyophilized powder.

4   CONTRAINDICATIONS
TREANDA is contraindicated in patients with a known hypersensitivity (e.g., anaphylactic and anaphylactoid reac-

tions) to bendamustine or mannitol. [See Warnings and Precautions (5.3)]

5   WARNINGS AND PRECAUTIONS
5.1   Myelosuppression
Patients treated with TREANDA are likely to experience myelosuppression. In the two NHL studies, 98% of patients had Grade 3-4 myelosuppression (see Table 4). Three patients (2%) died from myelosuppression-related adverse reactions; one each from neutropenic sepsis, diffuse alveolar hemorrhage with Grade 3 thrombocytopenia, and pneumonia from an opportunistic infection (CMV).
In the event of treatment-related myelosuppression, monitor leukocytes, platelets, hemoglobin (Hgb), and neutrophils closely. In the clinical trials, blood counts were monitored every week initially. Hematologic nadirs were observed predominantly in the third week of therapy. Hematologic nadirs may require dose delays if recovery to the recommended values have not occurred by the first day of the next scheduled cycle. Prior to the initiation of the next cycle of therapy, the ANC should be ≥ 1 × 10⁹/L and the platelet count should be ≥ 75 × 10⁹/L. [See Dosage and Administration (2.1) and (2.2)]
5.2   Infections
Infection, including pneumonia and sepsis, has been reported in patients in clinical trials and in post-marketing reports. Infection has been associated with hospitalization, septic shock and death. Patients with myelosuppression following treatment with TREANDA are more susceptible to infections. Patients with myelosuppression following TREANDA treatment should be advised to contact a physician if they have symptoms or signs of infection.
5.3   Infusion Reactions and Anaphylaxis
Infusion reactions to TREANDA have occurred commonly in clinical trials. Symptoms include fever, chills, pruritus and rash. In rare instances severe anaphylactic and anaphylactoid reactions have occurred, particularly in the second and subsequent cycles of therapy. Monitor clinically and discontinue drug for severe reactions. Patients should be asked about symptoms suggestive of infusion reactions after their first cycle of therapy. Patients who experienced Grade 3 or worse allergic-type reactions were not typically rechallenged. Measures to prevent severe reactions, including antihistamines, antipyretics and corticosteroids should be considered in subsequent cycles in patients who have previously experienced Grade 1 or 2 infusion reactions. Discontinuation should be considered in patients with Grade 3 or 4 infusion reactions.
5.4   Tumor Lysis Syndrome
Tumor lysis syndrome associated with TREANDA treatment has been reported in patients in clinical trials and in post-marketing reports. The onset tends to be within the first treatment cycle of TREANDA and, without intervention, may lead to acute renal failure and death. Preventive measures include maintaining adequate volume status, and close monitoring of blood chemistry, particularly potassium and uric acid levels. Allopurinol has also been used during the beginning of TREANDA therapy. However, there may be an increased risk of severe skin toxicity when TREANDA and allopurinol are administered concomitantly [see Warnings and Precautions (5.5)].
5.5   Skin Reactions
A number of skin reactions have been reported in clinical trials and post-marketing safety reports. These events have included rash, toxic skin reactions and bullous exanthema. Some events occurred when TREANDA was given in combination with other anticancer agents, so the precise relationship to TREANDA is uncertain.
In a study of TREANDA (90 mg/m²) in combination with rituximab, one case of toxic epidermal necrolysis (TEN) occurred. TEN has been reported for rituximab (see rituximab package insert). Cases of Stevens-Johnson syndrome (SJS) and TEN, some fatal, have been reported when TREANDA was administered concomitantly with allopurinol and other medications known to cause these syndromes. The relationship to TREANDA cannot be determined.
Where skin reactions occur, they may be progressive and increase in severity with further treatment. Therefore, patients with skin reactions should be monitored closely. If skin reactions are severe or progressive, TREANDA should be withheld or discontinued.
5.6   Other Malignancies
There are reports of pre-malignant and malignant diseases that have developed in patients who have been treated with TREANDA, including myelodysplastic syndrome, myeloproliferative disorders, acute myeloid leukemia and bronchial carcinoma. The association with TREANDA therapy has not been determined.
5.7   Extravasation
There are postmarketing reports of bendamustine extravasations resulting in hospitalizations from erythema, marked swelling, and pain. Precautions should be taken to avoid extravasation, including monitoring of the intravenous infusion site for redness, swelling, pain, infection, and necrosis during and after administration of TREANDA.

Table 1: Non-Hematologic Adverse Reactions Occurring in Randomized CLL Clinical Study in at Least 5% of Patients

System organ class Preferred term	TREANDA (N=153) All Grades	TREANDA (N=153) Grade 3/4	Chlorambucil (N=143) All Grades	Chlorambucil (N=143) Grade 3/4
Total number of patients with at least 1 adverse reaction	121 (79)	52 (34)	96 (67)	25 (17)
Gastrointestinal disorders	31 (20)	1 (<1)	21 (15)	1 (<1)
Nausea	24 (16)	1 (<1)	9 (6)	0
Vomiting	14 (9)	2 (1)	5 (3)	0
Diarrhea				
General disorders and administration site conditions	36 (24)	6 (4)	8 (6)	2 (1)
Pyrexia	14 (9)	2 (1)	8 (6)	0
Fatigue	13 (8)	0	6 (4)	0
Asthenia	9 (6)	0	1 (<1)	0
Chills				
Immune system disorders	7 (5)	2 (1)	3 (2)	0
Hypersensitivity				
Infections and infestations	10 (7)	0	12 (8)	0
Nasopharyngitis	9 (6)	3 (2)	1 (<1)	1 (<1)
Infection	5 (3)	0	7 (5)	0
Herpes simplex				
Investigations	11 (7)	0	5 (3)	0
Weight decreased				
Metabolism and nutrition disorders	11 (7)	3 (2)	2 (1)	0
Hyperuricemia				
Respiratory, thoracic and mediastinal disorders	6 (4)	1 (<1)	7 (5)	1 (<1)
Cough				
Skin and subcutaneous tissue disorders	12 (8)	4 (3)	7 (5)	3 (2)
Rash	8 (5)	0	2 (1)	0
Pruritus				

Table 2: Incidence of Hematology Laboratory Abnormalities in Patients Who Received TREANDA or Chlorambucil in the Randomized CLL Clinical Study

Laboratory Abnormality	TREANDA N=150 All Grades n (%)	TREANDA N=150 Grade 3/4 n (%)	Chlorambucil N=141 All Grades n (%)	Chlorambucil N=141 Grade 3/4 n (%)
Hemoglobin Decreased	134 (89)	20 (13)	115 (82)	12 (9)
Platelets Decreased	116 (77)	16 (11)	110 (78)	14 (10)
Leukocytes Decreased	92 (61)	42 (28)	26 (18)	4 (3)
Lymphocytes Decreased	102 (68)	70 (47)	27 (19)	6 (4)
Neutrophils Decreased	113 (75)	65 (43)	86 (61)	30 (21)

5.8   Use in Pregnancy

TREANDA can cause fetal harm when administered to a pregnant woman. Single intraperitoneal doses of bendamustine in mice and rats administered during organogenesis caused an increase in resorptions, skeletal and visceral malformations, and decreased fetal body weights. *[See Use in Specific Populations (8.1)]*

6   ADVERSE REACTIONS

The data described below reflect exposure to TREANDA in 349 patients who participated in an actively-controlled trial (N=153) for the treatment of CLL and two single-arm studies (N=176) for the treatment of indolent B-cell NHL. Because clinical trials are conducted under widely varying conditions, adverse reaction rates observed in the clinical trials of a drug cannot be directly compared to rates in the clinical trials of another drug and may not reflect the rates observed in practice.

The following serious adverse reactions have been associated with TREANDA in clinical trials and are discussed in greater detail in other sections of the label.
- Myelosuppression *[See Warnings and Precautions (5.1)]*
- Infections *[See Warnings and Precautions (5.2)]*
- Infusion Reactions and Anaphylaxis *[See Warnings and Precautions (5.3)]*
- Tumor Lysis Syndrome *[See Warnings and Precautions (5.4)]*
- Skin Reactions *[See Warnings and Precautions (5.5)]*
- Other Malignancies *[See Warnings and Precautions (5.6)]*

6.1   Clinical Trials Experience in CLL

The data described below reflect exposure to TREANDA in 153 patients. TREANDA was studied in an active-controlled trial. The population was 45-77 years of age, 63% male, 100% white, and had treatment naïve CLL. All patients started the study at a dose of 100 mg/m² intravenously over 30 minutes on Days 1 and 2 every 28 days.

Adverse reactions were reported according to NCI CTC v.2.0. In the randomized CLL clinical study, non-hematologic adverse reactions (any grade) in the TREANDA group that occurred with a frequency greater than 15% were pyrexia (24%), nausea (20%), and vomiting (16%).

Other adverse reactions seen frequently in one or more studies included asthenia, fatigue, malaise, and weakness; dry mouth; somnolence; cough; constipation; headache; mucosal inflammation and stomatitis.

Worsening hypertension was reported in 4 patients treated with TREANDA in the randomized CLL clinical study and none treated with chlorambucil. Three of these 4 adverse reactions were described as a hypertensive crisis and were managed with oral medications and resolved.

The most frequent adverse reactions leading to study withdrawal for patients receiving TREANDA were hypersensitivity (2%) and pyrexia (1%).

Table 1 contains the treatment emergent adverse reactions, regardless of attribution, that were reported in ≥ 5% of patients in either treatment group in the randomized CLL clinical study.

[See table 1 above]

The Grade 3 and 4 hematology laboratory test values by treatment group in the randomized CLL clinical study are described in Table 2. These findings confirm the myelosuppressive effects seen in patients treated with TREANDA. Red blood cell transfusions were administered to 20% of patients receiving TREANDA compared with 6% of patients receiving chlorambucil.

[See table 2 above]

In the randomized CLL clinical study, 34% of patients had bilirubin elevations, some without associated significant elevations in AST and ALT. Grade 3 or 4 increased bilirubin occurred in 3% of patients. Increases in AST and ALT of Grade 3 or 4 were limited to 1% and 3% of patients, respec-

tively. Patients treated with TREANDA may also have changes in their creatinine levels. If abnormalities are detected, monitoring of these parameters should be continued to ensure that significant deterioration does not occur.

6.2   Clinical Trials Experience in NHL

The data described below reflect exposure to TREANDA in 176 patients with indolent B-cell NHL treated in two single-arm studies. The population was 31-84 years of age, 60% male, and 40% female. The race distribution was 89% White, 7% Black, 3% Hispanic, 1% other, and <1% Asian. These patients received TREANDA at a dose of 120 mg/m² intravenously on Days 1 and 2 for up to 8 21-day cycles.

The adverse reactions occurring in at least 5% of the NHL patients, regardless of severity, are shown in Table 3. The most common non-hematologic adverse reactions (≥30%) were nausea (75%), fatigue (57%), vomiting (40%), diarrhea (37%) and pyrexia (34%). The most common non-hematologic Grade 3 or 4 adverse reactions (≥5%) were fatigue (11%), febrile neutropenia (6%), and pneumonia, hypokalemia and dehydration, each reported in 5% of patients.

[See table 3 at top of next page]

Hematologic toxicities, based on laboratory values and CTC grade, in NHL patients treated in both single arm studies combined are described in Table 4. Clinically important chemistry laboratory values that were new or worsened from baseline and occurred in >1% of patients at Grade 3 or 4, in NHL patients treated in both single arm studies combined were hyperglycemia (3%), elevated creatinine (2%), hyponatremia (2%), and hypocalcemia (2%).

Table 4: Incidence of Hematology Laboratory Abnormalities in Patients Who Received TREANDA in the NHL Studies

Hematology variable	Percent of Patients All Grades	Percent of Patients Grade 3/4
Lymphocytes Decreased	99	94
Leukocytes Decreased	94	56
Hemoglobin Decreased	88	11
Neutrophils Decreased	86	60
Platelets Decreased	86	25

In both studies, serious adverse reactions, regardless of causality, were reported in 37% of patients receiving TREANDA. The most common serious adverse reactions occurring in ≥5% of patients were febrile neutropenia and pneumonia. Other important serious adverse reactions reported in clinical trials and/or post-marketing experience were acute renal failure, cardiac failure, hypersensitivity, skin reactions, pulmonary fibrosis, and myelodysplastic syndrome.

Serious drug-related adverse reactions reported in clinical trials included myelosuppression, infection, pneumonia, tumor lysis syndrome and infusion reactions *[see Warnings and Precautions (5)]*. Adverse reactions occurring less frequently but possibly related to TREANDA treatment were hemolysis, dysgeusia/taste disorder, atypical pneumonia, sepsis, herpes zoster, erythema, dermatitis, and skin necrosis.

6.3   Post-Marketing Experience

The following adverse reactions have been identified during post-approval use of TREANDA. Because these reactions are reported voluntarily from a population of uncertain size, it is not always possible to reliably estimate their frequency or establish a causal relationship to drug exposure: anaphylaxis; and injection or infusion site reactions including phlebitis, pruritus, irritation, pain, and swelling.

Skin reactions including SJS and TEN have occurred when TREANDA was administered concomitantly with allopurinol and other medications known to cause these syndromes. *[See Warnings and Precautions (5.5)]*.

7   DRUG INTERACTIONS

No formal clinical assessments of pharmacokinetic drug-drug interactions between TREANDA and other drugs have been conducted.

Bendamustine's active metabolites, gamma-hydroxy bendamustine (M3) and N-desmethyl-bendamustine (M4), are formed via cytochrome P450 CYP1A2. Inhibitors of CYP1A2 (e.g., fluvoxamine, ciprofloxacin) have potential to increase plasma concentrations of bendamustine and decrease plasma concentrations of active metabolites. Inducers of CYP1A2 (e.g., omeprazole, smoking) have potential to decrease plasma concentrations of bendamustine and increase plasma concentrations of its active metabolites. Caution should be used, or alternative treatments considered if concomitant treatment with CYP1A2 inhibitors or inducers is needed.

The role of active transport systems in bendamustine distribution has not been fully evaluated. *In vitro* data suggest that P-glycoprotein, breast cancer resistance protein (BCRP), and/or other efflux transporters may have a role in bendamustine transport.

Based on *in vitro* data, bendamustine is not likely to inhibit metabolism via human CYP isoenzymes CYP1A2, 2C9/10, 2D6, 2E1, or 3A4/5, or to induce metabolism of substrates of cytochrome P450 enzymes.

8 USE IN SPECIFIC POPULATIONS

8.1 Pregnancy

Pregnancy Category D *[See Warnings and Precautions (5.8)]* TREANDA can cause fetal harm when administered to a pregnant woman. Single intraperitoneal doses of bendamustine from 210 mg/m^2 (70 mg/kg) in mice administered during organogenesis caused an increase in resorptions, skeletal and visceral malformations (exencephaly, cleft palates, accessory rib, and spinal deformities) and decreased fetal body weights. This dose did not appear to be maternally toxic and lower doses were not evaluated. Repeat intraperitoneal dosing in mice on gestation days 7-11 resulted in an increase in resorptions from 75 mg/m^2 (25 mg/kg) and an increase in abnormalities from 112.5 mg/m^2 (37.5 mg/kg) similar to those seen after a single intraperitoneal administration. Single intraperitoneal doses of bendamustine from 120 mg/m^2 (20 mg/kg) in rats administered on gestation days 4, 7, 9, 11, or 13 caused embryo and fetal lethality as indicated by increased resorptions and a decrease in live fetuses. A significant increase in external [effect on tail, head, and herniation of external organs (exomphalos)] and internal (hydronephrosis and hydrocephalus) malformations were seen in dosed rats. There are no adequate and well-controlled studies in pregnant women. If this drug is used during pregnancy, or if the patient becomes pregnant while taking this drug, the patient should be apprised of the potential hazard to the fetus.

8.3 Nursing Mothers

It is not known whether this drug is excreted in human milk. Because many drugs are excreted in human milk and because of the potential for serious adverse reactions in nursing infants and tumorigenicity shown for bendamustine in animal studies, a decision should be made whether to discontinue nursing or to discontinue the drug, taking into account the importance of the drug to the mother.

8.4 Pediatric Use

The safety and effectiveness of TREANDA in pediatric patients have not been established.

8.5 Geriatric Use

In CLL and NHL studies, there were no clinically significant differences in the adverse reaction profile between geriatric (≥ 65 years of age) and younger patients.

Chronic Lymphocytic Leukemia

In the randomized CLL clinical study, 153 patients received TREANDA. The overall response rate for patients younger than 65 years of age was 70% (n=82) for TREANDA and 30% (n = 69) for chlorambucil. The overall response rate for patients 65 years or older was 47% (n=71) for TREANDA and 22% (n = 79) for chlorambucil. In patients younger than 65 years of age, the median progression-free survival was 19 months in the TREANDA group and 8 months in the chlorambucil group. In patients 65 years or older, the median progression-free survival was 12 months in the TREANDA group and 8 months in the chlorambucil group.

Non-Hodgkin's Lymphoma

Efficacy (Overall Response Rate and Duration of Response) was similar in patients < 65 years of age and patients ≥ 65 years. Irrespective of age, all of the 176 patients experienced at least one adverse reaction.

8.6 Renal Impairment

No formal studies assessing the impact of renal impairment on the pharmacokinetics of bendamustine have been conducted. TREANDA should be used with caution in patients with mild or moderate renal impairment. TREANDA should not be used in patients with CrCL < 40 mL/min. *[See Clinical Pharmacology (12.3)]*

8.7 Hepatic Impairment

No formal studies assessing the impact of hepatic impairment on the pharmacokinetics of bendamustine have been conducted. TREANDA should be used with caution in patients with mild hepatic impairment. TREANDA should not be used in patients with moderate (AST or ALT 2.5-10 × ULN and total bilirubin 1.5-3 × ULN) or severe (total bilirubin > 3 × ULN) hepatic impairment. *[See Clinical Pharmacology (12.3)]*

8.8 Effect of Gender

No clinically significant differences between genders were seen in the overall incidences of adverse reactions in either CLL or NHL studies.

Chronic Lymphocytic Leukemia

In the randomized CLL clinical study, the overall response rate (ORR) for men (n=97) and women (n=56) in the TREANDA group was 60% and 57%, respectively. The ORR for men (n=90) and women (n=58) in the chlorambucil group was 24% and 28%, respectively. In this study, the median progression-free survival for men was 19 months in the TREANDA treatment group and 6 months in the chlorambucil treatment group. For women, the median progression-free survival was 13 months in the TREANDA treatment group and 8 months in the chlorambucil treatment group.

Non-Hodgkin's Lymphoma

The pharmacokinetics of bendamustine were similar in male and female patients with indolent NHL. No clinically-relevant differences between genders were seen in efficacy (ORR and DR).

Table 3: Non-Hematologic Adverse Reactions Occurring in at Least 5% of NHL Patients Treated with TREANDA by System Organ Class and Preferred Term (N=176)

System organ class / Preferred term	Number (%) of patients* All Grades	Grade 3/4
Total number of patients with at least 1 adverse reaction	176 (100)	94 (53)
Cardiac Disorders		
Tachycardia	13 (7)	0
Gastrointestinal disorders		
Nausea	132 (75)	7 (4)
Vomiting	71 (40)	5 (3)
Diarrhea	65 (37)	6 (3)
Constipation	51 (29)	1 (<1)
Stomatitis	27 (15)	1 (<1)
Abdominal pain	22 (13)	2 (1)
Dyspepsia	20 (11)	0
Gastroesophageal reflux disease	18 (10)	0
Dry mouth	15 (9)	1 (<1)
Abdominal pain upper	8 (5)	0
Abdominal distension	8 (5)	0
General disorders and administration site conditions		
Fatigue	101 (57)	19 (11)
Pyrexia	59 (34)	3 (2)
Chills	24 (14)	0
Edema peripheral	23 (13)	1 (<1)
Asthenia	19 (11)	4 (2)
Chest pain	11 (6)	1 (<1)
Infusion site pain	11 (6)	0
Pain	10 (6)	0
Catheter site pain	8 (5)	0
Infections and infestations		
Herpes zoster	18 (10)	5 (3)
Upper respiratory tract infection	18 (10)	0
Urinary tract infection	17 (10)	4 (2)
Sinusitis	15 (9)	0
Pneumonia	14 (8)	9 (5)
Febrile neutropenia	11 (6)	11 (6)
Oral candidiasis	11 (6)	2 (1)
Nasopharyngitis	11 (6)	0
Investigations		
Weight decreased	31 (18)	3 (2)
Metabolism and nutrition disorders		
Anorexia	40 (23)	3 (2)
Dehydration	24 (14)	8 (5)
Decreased appetite	22 (13)	1 (<1)
Hypokalemia	15 (9)	9 (5)
Musculoskeletal and connective tissue disorders		
Back pain	25 (14)	5 (3)
Arthralgia	11 (6)	0
Pain in extremity	8 (5)	2 (1)
Bone pain	8 (5)	0
Nervous system disorders		
Headache	36 (21)	0
Dizziness	25 (14)	0
Dysgeusia	13 (7)	0
Psychiatric disorder		
Insomnia	23 (13)	0
Anxiety	14 (8)	1 (<1)
Depression	10 (6)	0
Respiratory, thoracic and mediastinal disorders		
Cough	38 (22)	1 (<1)
Dyspnea	28 (16)	3 (2)
Pharyngolaryngeal pain	14 (8)	1 (<1)
Wheezing	8 (5)	0
Nasal congestion	8 (5)	0
Skin and subcutaneous tissue disorders		
Rash	28 (16)	1 (<1)
Pruritus	11 (6)	0
Dry skin	9 (5)	0
Night sweats	9 (5)	0
Hyperhidrosis	8 (5)	0
Vascular disorders		
Hypotension	10 (6)	2 (1)

*Patients may have reported more than 1 adverse reaction.

NOTE: Patients counted only once in each preferred term category and once in each system organ class category.

10 OVERDOSAGE

The intravenous LD$_{50}$ of bendamustine HCl is 240 mg/m^2 in the mouse and rat. Toxicities included sedation, tremor, ataxia, convulsions and respiratory distress.

Across all clinical experience, the reported maximum single dose received was 280 mg/m^2. Three of four patients treated at this dose showed ECG changes considered dose-limiting at 7 and 21 days post-dosing. These changes included QT prolongation (one patient), sinus tachycardia (one patient), ST and T wave deviations (two patients) and left anterior fascicular block (one patient). Cardiac enzymes and ejection fractions remained normal in all patients.

No specific antidote for TREANDA overdose is known. Management of overdosage should include general supportive measures, including monitoring of hematologic parameters and ECGs.

11   DESCRIPTION

TREANDA contains bendamustine hydrochloride, an alkylating drug, as the active ingredient. The chemical name of bendamustine hydrochloride is 1H-benzimidazole-2-butanoic acid, 5-[bis(2-chloroethyl)amino]-1 methyl-, monohydrochloride. Its empirical molecular formula is $C_{16}H_{21}Cl_2N_3O_2$ · HCl, and the molecular weight is 394.7. Bendamustine hydrochloride contains a mechlorethamine group and a benzimidazole heterocyclic ring with a butyric acid substituent, and has the following structural formula:

$$Cl\text{-}CH_2\text{-}CH_2 \diagdown N \diagup \quad \diagup N \diagdown \quad (CH_2)_3\text{-}COOH \cdot HCl$$
$$Cl\text{-}CH_2\text{-}CH_2 \diagup \qquad \diagdown N \diagup$$
$$\qquad\qquad CH_3$$

TREANDA (bendamustine hydrochloride) for Injection is intended for intravenous infusion only after reconstitution with Sterile Water for Injection, USP, and after further dilution with either 0.9% Sodium Chloride Injection, USP, or 2.5% Dextrose/0.45% Sodium Chloride Injection, USP. It is supplied as a sterile non-pyrogenic white to off-white lyophilized powder in a single-use vial. Each 25-mg vial contains 25 mg of bendamustine hydrochloride and 42.5 mg of mannitol, USP. Each 100-mg vial contains 100 mg of bendamustine hydrochloride and 170 mg of mannitol, USP. The pH of the reconstituted solution is 2.5-3.5.

12   CLINICAL PHARMACOLOGY

12.1   Mechanism of Action

Bendamustine is a bifunctional mechlorethamine derivative containing a purine-like benzimidazole ring. Mechlorethamine and its derivatives form electrophilic alkyl groups. These groups form covalent bonds with electron-rich nucleophilic moieties, resulting in interstrand DNA crosslinks. The bifunctional covalent linkage can lead to cell death via several pathways. Bendamustine is active against both quiescent and dividing cells. The exact mechanism of action of bendamustine remains unknown.

12.3   Pharmacokinetics

Absorption
Following a single IV dose of bendamustine hydrochloride C_{max} typically occurred at the end of infusion. The dose proportionality of bendamustine has not been studied.

Distribution
In vitro, the binding of bendamustine to human serum plasma proteins ranged from 94-96% and was concentration independent from 1-50 µg/mL. Data suggest that bendamustine is not likely to displace or to be displaced by highly protein-bound drugs. The blood to plasma concentration ratios in human blood ranged from 0.84 to 0.86 over a concentration range of 10 to 100 µg/mL indicating that bendamustine distributes freely in human red blood cells. In humans, the mean steady state volume of distribution (V_{ss}) was approximately 25 L.

Metabolism
In vitro data indicate that bendamustine is primarily metabolized via hydrolysis to metabolites with low cytotoxic activity. In vitro, studies indicate that two active minor metabolites, M3 and M4, are primarily formed via CYP1A2. However, concentrations of these metabolites in plasma are 1/10 and 1/100 that of the parent compound, respectively, suggesting that the cytotoxic activity is primarily due to bendamustine.

In vitro studies using human liver microsomes indicate that bendamustine does not inhibit CYP1A2, 2C9/10, 2D6, 2E1, or 3A4/5. Bendamustine did not induce metabolism of CYP1A2, CYP2A6, CYP2B6, CYP2C8, CYP2C9, CYP2C19, CYP2E1, or CYP3A4/5 enzymes in primary cultures of human hepatocytes.

Elimination
No mass balance study has been undertaken in humans. Preclinical radiolabeled bendamustine studies showed that approximately 90% of drug administered was recovered in excreta primarily in the feces.
Bendamustine clearance in humans is approximately 700 mL/minute. After a single dose of 120 mg/m² bendamustine IV over 1-hour the intermediate $t_{1/2}$ of the parent compound is approximately 40 minutes. The mean apparent terminal elimination $t_{1/2}$ of M3 and M4 are approximately 3 hours and 30 minutes respectively. Little or no accumulation in plasma is expected for bendamustine administered on Days 1 and 2 of a 28-day cycle.

Renal Impairment
In a population pharmacokinetic analysis of bendamustine in patients receiving 120 mg/m² there was no meaningful effect of renal impairment (CrCL 40 - 80 mL/min, N=31) on the pharmacokinetics of bendamustine. Bendamustine has not been studied in patients with CrCL < 40 mL/min. These results are however limited, and therefore bendamustine should be used with caution in patients with mild or moderate renal impairment. Bendamustine should not be used in patients with CrCL < 40 mL/min. [See Use in Specific Populations (8.6)]

Hepatic Impairment
In a population pharmacokinetic analysis of bendamustine in patients receiving 120 mg/m² there was no meaningful effect of mild (total bilirubin ≤ ULN, AST ≥ ULN to 2.5 × ULN, and/or ALP ≥ ULN to 5.0 × ULN, N=26) hepatic impairment on the pharmacokinetics of bendamustine. Bendamustine has not been studied in patients with moderate or severe hepatic impairment.
These results are however limited, and therefore bendamustine should be used with caution in patients with mild hepatic impairment. Bendamustine should not be used in patients with moderate (AST or ALT 2.5 - 10 × ULN and total bilirubin 1.5 - 3 × ULN) or severe (total bilirubin > 3 × ULN) hepatic impairment. [See Use in Specific Populations (8.7)]

Effect of Age
Bendamustine exposure (as measured by AUC and C_{max}) has been studied in patients ages 31 through 84 years. The pharmacokinetics of bendamustine (AUC and C_{max}) were not significantly different between patients less than or greater than/equal to 65 years of age. [See Use in Specific Populations (8.4, 8.5)]

Effect of Gender
The pharmacokinetics of bendamustine were similar in male and female patients. [See Use in Specific Populations (8.8)]

Effect of Race
The effect of race on the safety, and/or efficacy of TREANDA has not been established. Based on a cross-study comparison, Japanese subjects (n = 6) had on average exposures that were 40% higher than non-Japanese subjects receiving the same dose. The significance of this difference on the safety and efficacy of TREANDA in Japanese subjects has not been established.

12.4   Pharmacokinetics/Pharmacodynamics

Based on the pharmacokinetics/pharmacodynamics analyses of data from NHL patients, a correlation was observed between nausea and bendamustine C_{max}.

13   NONCLINICAL TOXICOLOGY

13.1   Carcinogenesis, Mutagenesis, Impairment of Fertility

Bendamustine was carcinogenic in mice. After intraperitoneal injections at 37.5 mg/m²/day (12.5 mg/kg/day, the lowest dose tested) and 75 mg/m²/day (25 mg/kg/day) for four days, peritoneal sarcomas in female AB/jena mice were produced. Oral administration at 187.5 mg/m²/day (62.5 mg/kg/day, the only dose tested) for four days induced mammary carcinomas and pulmonary adenomas.
Bendamustine is a mutagen and clastogen. In a reverse bacterial mutation assay (Ames assay), bendamustine was shown to increase revertant frequency in the absence and presence of metabolic activation. Bendamustine was clastogenic in human lymphocytes in vitro, and in rat bone marrow cells in vivo (increase in micronucleated polychromatic erythrocytes) from 37.5 mg/m², the lowest dose tested.
Impaired spermatogenesis, azoospermia, and total germinal aplasia have been reported in male patients treated with alkylating agents, especially in combination with other drugs. In some instances spermatogenesis may return in patients in remission, but this may occur only several years after intensive chemotherapy has been discontinued. Patients should be warned of the potential risk to their reproductive capacities.

14   CLINICAL STUDIES

14.1   Chronic Lymphocytic Leukemia (CLL)

The safety and efficacy of TREANDA were evaluated in an open-label, randomized, controlled multicenter trial comparing TREANDA to chlorambucil. The trial was conducted in 301 previously-untreated patients with Binet Stage B or C (Rai Stages I - IV) CLL requiring treatment. Need-to-treat criteria included hematopoietic insufficiency, B-symptoms, rapidly progressive disease or risk of complications from bulky lymphadenopathy. Patients with autoimmune hemolytic anemia or autoimmune thrombocytopenia, Richter's syndrome, or transformation to prolymphocytic leukemia were excluded from the study.
The patient populations in the TREANDA and chlorambucil treatment groups were balanced with regard to the following baseline characteristics: age (median 63 vs. 66 years), gender (63% vs. 61% male), Binet stage (71% vs. 69% Binet B), lymphadenopathy (79% vs. 82%), enlarged spleen (76% vs. 80%), enlarged liver (48% vs. 46%), hypercellular bone marrow (79% vs. 73%), "B" symptoms (51% vs. 53%), lymphocyte count (mean 65.7×10⁹/L vs. 65.1×10⁹/L), and serum lactate dehydrogenase concentration (mean 370.2 vs. 388.4 U/L). Ninety percent of patients in both treatment groups had immuno-phenotypic confirmation of CLL (CD5, CD23 and either CD19 or CD20 or both).
Patients were randomly assigned to receive either TREANDA at 100 mg/m², administered intravenously over a period of 30 minutes on Days 1 and 2 or chlorambucil at 0.8 mg/kg (Broca's normal weight) administered orally on Days 1 and 15 of each 28-day cycle. Efficacy endpoints of objective response rate and progression-free survival were calculated using a pre-specified algorithm based on NCI working group criteria for CLL[1].
The results of this open-label randomized study demonstrated a higher rate of overall response and a longer progression-free survival for TREANDA compared to chlorambucil (see Table 5). Survival data are not mature.
[See table 5 above]
Kaplan-Meier estimates of progression-free survival comparing TREANDA with chlorambucil are shown in Figure 1.

Table 5: Efficacy Data for CLL

	TREANDA (N=153)	Chlorambucil (N=148)	p-value
Response Rate n(%)			
Overall response rate	90 (59)	38 (26)	<0.0001
(95% CI)	(51.0, 66.6)	(18.6, 32.7)	
Complete response (CR)*	13 (8)	1 (<1)	
Nodular partial response (nPR)**	4 (3)	0	
Partial response (PR)†	73 (48)	37 (25)	
Progression-Free Survival††			
Median, months (95% CI)	18 (11.7, 23.5)	6 (5.6, 8.6)	
Hazard ratio (95% CI)	0.27 (0.17, 0.43)		<0.0001

CI = confidence interval
* CR was defined as peripheral lymphocyte count ≤ 4.0 × 10⁹/L, neutrophils ≥ 1.5 × 10⁹/L, platelets >100 × 10⁹/L, hemoglobin > 110g/L, without transfusions, absence of palpable hepatosplenomegaly, lymph nodes ≤ 1.5 cm, < 30% lymphocytes without nodularity in at least a normocellular bone marrow and absence of "B" symptoms. The clinical and laboratory criteria were required to be maintained for a period of at least 56 days.
** nPR was defined as described for CR with the exception that the bone marrow biopsy shows persistent nodules.
† PR was defined as ≥50% decrease in peripheral lymphocyte count from the pretreatment baseline value, and either ≥50% reduction in lymphadenopathy, or ≥50% reduction in the size of spleen or liver, as well as one of the following hematologic improvements: neutrophils ≥ 1.5 × 10⁹/L or 50% improvement over baseline, platelets >100 × 10⁹/L or 50% improvement over baseline, hemoglobin >110g/L or 50% improvement over baseline without transfusions, for a period of at least 56 days.
†† PFS was defined as time from randomization to progression or death from any cause.

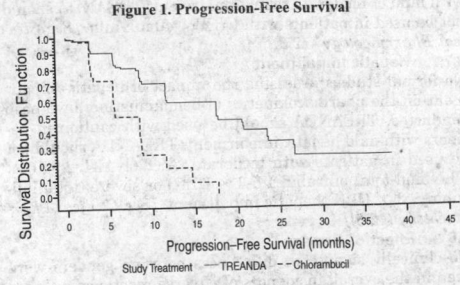

Figure 1. Progression-Free Survival

14.2   Non-Hodgkin's Lymphoma (NHL)

The efficacy of TREANDA was evaluated in a single arm study of 100 patients with indolent B-cell NHL that had progressed during or within six months of treatment with rituximab or a rituximab-containing regimen. Patients were included if they relapsed within 6 months of either the first dose (monotherapy) or last dose (maintenance regimen or combination therapy) of rituximab. All patients received TREANDA intravenously at a dose of 120 mg/m^2, on Days 1 and 2 of a 21-day treatment cycle. Patients were treated for up to 8 cycles.

The median age was 60 years, 65% were male, and 95% had a baseline WHO performance status of 0 or 1. Major tumor subtypes were follicular lymphoma (62%), diffuse small lymphocytic lymphoma (21%), and marginal zone lymphoma (16%). Ninety-nine percent of patients had received previous chemotherapy, 91% of patients had received previous alkylator therapy, and 97% of patients had relapsed within 6 months of either the first dose (monotherapy) or last dose (maintenance regimen or combination therapy) of rituximab.

Efficacy was based on the assessments by a blinded independent review committee (IRC) and included overall response rate (complete response + complete response unconfirmed + partial response) and duration of response (DR) as summarized in Table 6.

Table 6: Efficacy Data for NHL*

	TREANDA (N=100)
Response Rate (%)	
Overall response rate (CR+CRu+PR)	74
(95% CI)	(64.3, 82.3)
Complete response (CR)	13
Complete response unconfirmed (CRu)	4
Partial response (PR)	57
Duration of Response (DR)	
Median, months (95% CI)	9.2 months (7.1, 10.8)

CI = confidence interval

*IRC assessment was based on modified International Working Group response criteria (IWG-RC)[2]. Modifications to IWG-RC specified that a persistently positive bone marrow in patients who met all other criteria for CR would be scored as PR. Bone marrow sample lengths were not required to be ≥20 mm.

15 REFERENCES

1. Cheson et al. National Cancer Institute – sponsored Working Group Guidelines for Chronic Lymphocytic Leukemia. Blood Vol 87 1996:pp 4990.
2. Report of an International Workshop to Standardize Response Criteria for Non-Hodgkin's Lymphomas. *J Clin Oncol*. 1999;17:1244-1253.
3. Preventing occupational exposures to Antineoplastic and Other Hazardous Drugs in Health Care Settings. NIOSH Alert 2004-165.
4. OSHA Technical Manual, TED 1-0.15A, Section VI: Chapter 2. Controlling Occupational Exposure to Hazardous Drugs. OSHA, 1999. http://www.osha.gov/dts/osta/otm/otm_vi/otm_vi_2.html.
5. American Society of Health-System Pharmacists. ASHP Guidelines on Handling Hazardous Drugs. *Am J Health-Syst Pharm.* 2006; 63:1172-1193.
6. Polovich, M., White, J. M., & Kelleher, L.O. (eds.) 2005. Chemotherapy and biotherapy guidelines and recommendations for practice (2nd. ed.) Pittsburgh, PA: Oncology Nursing Society.

16 HOW SUPPLIED/STORAGE AND HANDLING

16.1 Safe Handling and Disposal

As with other potentially toxic anticancer agents, care should be exercised in the handling and preparation of solutions prepared from TREANDA. The use of gloves and safety glasses is recommended to avoid exposure in case of breakage of the vial or other accidental spillage. If a solution of TREANDA contacts the skin, wash the skin immediately and thoroughly with soap and water. If TREANDA contacts the mucous membranes, flush thoroughly with water.

Procedures for the proper handling and disposal of anticancer drugs should be considered. Several guidelines on the subject have been published[3-6]. There is no general agreement that all of the procedures recommended in the guidelines are necessary or appropriate.

16.2 How Supplied

TREANDA (bendamustine hydrochloride) for Injection is supplied in individual cartons as follows:

NDC 63459-390-08	TREANDA (bendamustine hydrochloride) for Injection, 25 mg in 8 mL amber single-use vial
NDC 63459-391-20	TREANDA (bendamustine hydrochloride) for Injection, 100 mg in 20 mL amber single-use vial

16.3 Storage

TREANDA may be stored up to 25°C (77°F) with excursions permitted up to 30°C (86°F) (see USP Controlled Room Temperature). Retain in original package until time of use to protect from light.

17 PATIENT COUNSELING INFORMATION

- Allergic (Hypersensitivity) Reactions

Patients should be informed of the possibility of mild or serious allergic reactions and to immediately report rash, facial swelling, or difficulty breathing during or soon after infusion.

- Myelosuppression

Patients should be informed of the likelihood that TREANDA will cause a decrease in white blood cells, platelets, and red blood cells. They will need frequent monitoring of these parameters. They should be instructed to report shortness of breath, significant fatigue, bleeding, fever, or other signs of infection.

- Pregnancy and Nursing

TREANDA can cause fetal harm. Women should be advised to avoid becoming pregnant throughout treatment and for 3 months after TREANDA therapy has stopped. Men receiving TREANDA should use reliable contraception for the same time period. Advise patients to report pregnancy immediately. Advise patients to avoid nursing while receiving TREANDA.

- Fatigue

Advise patients that TREANDA may cause tiredness and to avoid driving any vehicle or operating any dangerous tools or machinery if they experience this side effect.

- Nausea and Vomiting

Advise patients that TREANDA may cause nausea and/or vomiting. Patients should report nausea and vomiting so that symptomatic treatment may be provided.

- Diarrhea

Advise patients that TREANDA may cause diarrhea. Patients should report diarrhea to the physician so that symptomatic treatment may be provided.

- Rash

Advise patients that a mild rash or itching may occur during treatment with TREANDA. Advise patients to immediately report severe or worsening rash or itching.

TRE-006

Distributed by
Cephalon, Inc.
Frazer, PA 19355

Label Code: 00016287.06

Shown in Product Identification Guide, page 308

TRISENOX® ℞

[trī-sĕ-nŏks]
(arsenic trioxide) injection
For Intravenous Use Only
10 mg/10 mL (1mg/mL) ampule

WARNING

Experienced Physician and Institution: TRISENOX (arsenic trioxide) injection should be administered under the supervision of a physician who is experienced in the management of patients with acute leukemia.

APL Differentiation Syndrome: Some patients with APL treated with TRISENOX have experienced symptoms similar to a syndrome called the retinoic-acid-Acute Promyelocytic Leukemia (RA-APL) or APL differentiation syndrome, characterized by fever, dyspnea, weight gain, pulmonary infiltrates and pleural or pericardial effusions, with or without leukocytosis. This syndrome can be fatal. The management of the syndrome has not been fully studied, but high-dose steroids have been used at the first suspicion of the APL differentiation syndrome and appear to mitigate signs and symptoms. At the first signs that could suggest the syndrome (unexplained fever, dyspnea and/or weight gain, abnormal chest auscultatory findings or radiographic abnormalities), high-dose steroids (dexamethasone 10 mg intravenously BID) should be immediately initiated, irrespective of the leukocyte count, and continued for at least 3 days or longer until signs and symptoms have abated. The majority of patients do not require termination of TRISENOX therapy during treatment of the APL differentiation syndrome.

ECG Abnormalities: Arsenic trioxide can cause QT interval prolongation and complete atrioventricular block. QT prolongation can lead to a torsade de pointes-type ventricular arrhythmia, which can be fatal. The risk of torsade de pointes is related to the extent of QT prolongation, concomitant administration of QT prolonging drugs, a history of torsade de pointes, preexisting QT interval prolongation, congestive heart failure, administration of potassium-wasting diuretics, or other conditions that result in hypokalemia or hypomagnesemia. One patient (also receiving amphotericin B) had torsade de pointes during induction therapy for relapsed APL with arsenic trioxide.

ECG and Electrolyte Monitoring Recommendations: Prior to initiating therapy with TRISENOX, a 12-lead ECG should be performed and serum electrolytes (potassium, calcium, and magnesium) and creatinine should be assessed; preexisting electrolyte abnormalities should be corrected and, if possible, drugs that are known to prolong the QT interval should be discontinued. For QTc greater than 500 msec, corrective measures should be completed and the QTc reassessed with serial ECGs prior to considering using TRISENOX. During therapy with TRISENOX, potassium concentrations should be kept above 4 mEq/L and magnesium concentrations should be kept above 1.8 mg/dL. Patients who reach an absolute QT interval value > 500 msec should be reassessed and immediate action should be taken to correct concomitant risk factors, if any, while the risk/benefit of continuing versus suspending TRISENOX therapy should be considered. If syncope, rapid or irregular heartbeat develops, the patient should be hospitalized for monitoring, serum electrolytes should be assessed, TRISENOX therapy should be temporarily discontinued until the QTc interval regresses to below 460 msec, electrolyte abnormalities are corrected, and the syncope and irregular heartbeat cease. There are no data on the effect of TRISENOX on the QTc interval during the infusion.

DESCRIPTION

TRISENOX is a sterile injectable solution of arsenic trioxide. The molecular formula of the drug substance in the solid state is As_2O_3, with a molecular weight of 197.8 g. TRISENOX is available in 10 mL, single-use ampules containing 10 mg of arsenic trioxide. TRISENOX is formulated as a sterile, nonpyrogenic, clear solution of arsenic trioxide in water for injection using sodium hydroxide and dilute hydrochloric acid to adjust to pH 8. TRISENOX is preservative-free. Arsenic trioxide, the active ingredient, is present at a concentration of 1.0 mg/mL. Inactive ingredients and their respective approximate concentrations are sodium hydroxide (1.2 mg/mL) and hydrochloric acid, which is used to adjust the pH to 7.5-8.5.

CLINICAL PHARMACOLOGY

Mechanism of Action

The mechanism of action of TRISENOX is not completely understood. Arsenic trioxide causes morphological changes and DNA fragmentation characteristic of apoptosis in NB4 human promyelocytic leukemia cells *in vitro*. Arsenic trioxide also causes damage or degradation of the fusion protein PML/RAR-alpha.

Pharmacokinetics

The inorganic, lyophilized form of arsenic trioxide, when placed into solution, immediately forms the hydrolysis product arsenious acid (As^{III}). As^{III} is the pharmacologically active species of arsenic trioxide. Monomethylarsonic acid (MMA^V), and dimethylarsinic acid (DMA^V) are the main pentavalent metabolites formed during metabolism, in addition to arsenic acid (As^V) a product of As^{III} oxidation. The pharmacokinetics of arsenical species ([As^{III}], [As^V], [MMA^V], [DMA^V]) were determined in 6 APL patients following once daily doses of 0.15 mg/kg for 5 days per week. Over the total single dose range of 7 to 32 mg (administered as 0.15 mg/kg), systemic exposure (AUC) appears to be linear. Peak plasma concentrations of arsenious acid (As^{III}), the primary active arsenical species were reached at the end of infusion (2 hours). Plasma concentration of As^{III} declined in a biphasic manner with a mean elimination half-life of 10 to 14 hours and is characterized by an initial rapid distribution phase followed by a slower terminal elimination phase. The daily exposure to As^{III} (mean AUC_{0-24}) was 194 ng•hr/mL (n=5) on Day 1 of Cycle 1 and 332 ng•hr/mL (n=6) on Day 25 of Cycle 1, which represents an approximate 2-fold accumulation. The primary pentavalent metabolites, MMA^V and DMA^V, are slow to appear in plasma (approximately 10-24 hours after first administration of arsenic trioxide), but, due to their longer half-life, accumulate more upon multiple dosing than does As^{III}. The mean estimated terminal elimination half-lives of the metabolites MMA^V and DMA^V are 32 hours and 72 hours, respectively. Approximate accumulation ranged from 1.4- to 8-fold following multiple dosing as compared to single dose administration. As^V is present in plasma only at relatively low levels.

Distribution

The volume of distribution (V_{ss}) for As^{III} is large (mean 562 L, N=10) indicating that As^{III} is widely distributed throughout body tissues. V_{ss} is also dependent on body weight and increases as body weight increases.

Metabolism

Much of the As^{III} is distributed to the tissues where it is methylated to the less cytotoxic metabolites, monomethylarsonic acid (MMA^V) and dimethylarsinic acid (DMA^V) by methyltransferases primarily in the liver. The metabolism of arsenic trioxide also involves oxidation of As^{III} to As^V, which may occur in numerous tissues via enzymatic or non-enzymatic processes. As^V is present in plasma only at relatively low levels following administration of arsenic trioxide.

Excretion

Approximately 15% of the administered TRISENOX dose is excreted in the urine as unchanged As^{III}. The methylated metabolites of As^{III} (MMA^V, DMA^V) are primarily excreted in the urine. The total clearance of As^{III} is 49 L/h and the renal clearance is 9 L/h. Clearance is not dependent on body weight or dose administered over the range of 7-32 mg.

Special Populations

Effect of Age, Gender, and Race

The effect of age, gender, or race on the pharmacokinetics of TRISENOX has not been studied.

Pediatric Patients

Following IV administration of 0.15 mg/kg/day of arsenic trioxide in 10 APL patients (median age = 13.5 years, range 4-20 years), the daily exposure to As^{III} (mean AUC_{0-24h}) was 317 ng•hr/mL on Day 1 of Cycle 1 (see **PRECAUTIONS, Pediatric Use**).

Effect of Renal Impairment

The effect of renal impairment on the pharmacokinetics of As^{III}, As^V, and the pentavalent metabolites MMA^V and DMA^V was evaluated in 20 patients with advanced malignancies. Patients were classified as having normal renal function (creatinine clearance [CrCl] > 80 mL/min, n=6), mild renal impairment (CrCl 50-80 mL/min, n=5), moderate renal impairment (CrCl 30-49 mL/min, n=6), or severe renal impairment (CrCl < 30 mL/min, n=3). Following twice weekly administration of 0.15 mg/kg over a 2-hour infusion, the mean $AUC_{0-\infty}$ for As^{III} was comparable among the normal, mild and moderate renal impairment groups. However, in the severe renal impairment group, the mean $AUC_{0-\infty}$ for As^{III} was approximately 48% higher than that in the normal group.

Systemic exposure to MMA^V and DMA^V tended to be larger in patients with renal impairment; however, the clinical consequences of this increased exposure are not known. As^V plasma levels were generally below the limit of assay quantitation in patients with impaired renal function (see **PRECAUTIONS**). The use of arsenic trioxide in patients on dialysis has not been studied.

Effect of Hepatic Impairment

The effect of pharmacokinetics of As^{III}, As^V, and the pentavalent metabolites MMA^V and DMA^V was evaluated following administration of 0.25-0.50 mg/kg of arsenic trioxide in patients with hepatocellular carcinoma. Patients were classified as having normal hepatic function (n=4), mild hepatic impairment (Child-Pugh class A, n=12), moderate hepatic impairment (Child-Pugh class B, n=3), or severe hepatic impairment (Child-Pugh class C, n=1). No clear trend toward an increase in systemic exposure to As^{III}, As^V, MMA^V or DMA^V was observed with decreasing level of hepatic function as assessed by dose-normalized (per mg dose) AUC in the mild and moderate hepatic impairment groups. However, the one patient with severe hepatic impairment had mean dose-normalized AUC_{0-24} and C_{max} values 40% and 70% higher, respectively, than those patients with normal hepatic function. The mean dose-normalized trough plasma levels for both MMA^V and DMA^V in this severely hepatically impaired patient were 2.2-fold and 4.7-fold higher, respectively, than those in the patients with normal hepatic function (see **PRECAUTIONS**).

Drug Interactions

No formal assessments of pharmacokinetic drug-drug interactions between TRISENOX and other drugs have been conducted. The methyltransferases responsible for metabolizing arsenic trioxide are not members of the cytochrome P450 family of isoenzymes.

In vitro incubation of arsenic trioxide with human liver microsomes showed no inhibitory activity on substrates of the major cytochrome P450 (CYP) enzymes such as 1A2, 2A6, 2B6, 2C8, 2C9, 2C19, 2D6, 2E1, 3A4/5, and 4A9/11. The pharmacokinetics of drugs that are substrates for these CYP enzymes are not expected to be affected by concomitant treatment with arsenic trioxide (see **PRECAUTIONS**).

CLINICAL STUDIES

Clinical Studies Experience

TRISENOX has been investigated in 40 relapsed or refractory APL patients, previously treated with an anthracycline and a retinoid regimen, in an open-label, single-arm, non-comparative study. Patients received 0.15 mg/kg/day intravenously over 1 to 2 hours until the bone marrow was cleared of leukemic cells or up to a maximum of 60 days. The CR (absence of visible leukemic cells in bone marrow and peripheral recovery of platelets and white blood cells with a confirmatory bone marrow ≥ 30 days later) rate in this population of previously treated patients was 28 of 40 (70%). Among the 22 patients who had relapsed less than one year after treatment with ATRA, there were 18 complete responders (82%). Of the 18 patients receiving TRISENOX ≥ one year from ATRA treatment, there were 10 complete responders (55%). The median time to bone marrow remission was 44 days and to onset of CR was 53 days. Three of 5 children, 5 years or older, achieved CR. No children less than 5 years old were treated.

Three to six weeks following bone marrow remission, 31 patients received consolidation therapy with TRISENOX, at the same dose, for 25 additional days over a period up to 5 weeks. In follow-up treatment, 18 patients received further arsenic trioxide as a maintenance course. Fifteen patients had bone marrow transplants. At last follow-up, 27 of 40 patients were alive with a median follow-up time of 484 days (range 280 to 755) and 23 of 40 patients remained in complete response with a median follow-up time of 483 days (range 280 to 755).

Cytogenetic conversion to no detection of the APL chromosome rearrangement was observed in 24 of 28 (86%) patients who met the response criteria defined above, in 5 of 5 (100%) patients who met some but not all of the response criteria, and 3 of 7 (43%) of patients who did not respond. Reverse Transcriptase – Polymerase Chain Reaction conversions to no detection of the APL gene rearrangement were demonstrated in 22 of 28 (79%) of patients who met the response criteria, in 3 of 5 (60%) of patients who met some but not all of the response criteria, and in 2 of 7 (29%) of patients who did not respond.

Responses were seen across all age groups tested, ranging from 6 to 72 years. The ability to achieve a CR was similar for both genders. There were insufficient patients of Black, Hispanic or Asian derivation to estimate relative response rates in these groups, but responses were seen in members of each group.

Another single center study in 12 patients with relapsed or refractory APL, where patients received TRISENOX (arsenic trioxide) injection doses generally similar to the recommended dose, had similar results with 9 of 12 (75%) patients attaining a CR.

INDICATIONS AND USAGE

TRISENOX is indicated for induction of remission and consolidation in patients with acute promyelocytic leukemia (APL) who are refractory to, or have relapsed from, retinoid and anthracycline chemotherapy, and whose APL is characterized by the presence of the t(15;17) translocation or PML/RAR-alpha gene expression.

The response rate of other acute myelogenous leukemia subtypes to TRISENOX has not been examined.

CONTRAINDICATIONS

TRISENOX is contraindicated in patients who are hypersensitive to arsenic.

WARNINGS

(See Boxed WARNING)

TRISENOX should be administered under the supervision of a physician who is experienced in the management of patients with acute leukemia.

APL Differentiation Syndrome

(See Boxed WARNING)

Nine of 40 patients with APL treated with TRISENOX, at a dose of 0.15 mg/kg, experienced the APL differentiation syndrome (see **Boxed WARNING and ADVERSE REACTIONS**).

Hyperleukocytosis

Treatment with TRISENOX has been associated with the development of hyperleukocytosis ($\geq 10 \times 10^3/uL$) in 20 of 40 patients. A relationship did not exist between baseline WBC counts and development of hyperleukocytosis nor baseline WBC counts and peak WBC counts. Hyperleukocytosis was not treated with additional chemotherapy. WBC counts during consolidation were not as high as during induction treatment.

QT Prolongation

(See Boxed WARNING)

QT/QTc prolongation should be expected during treatment with arsenic trioxide and torsade de pointes as well as complete heart block has been reported. Over 460 ECG tracings from 40 patients with refractory or relapsed APL treated with TRISENOX were evaluated for QTc prolongation. Sixteen of 40 patients (40%) had at least one ECG tracing with a QTc interval greater than 500 msec. Prolongation of the QTc was observed between 1 and 5 weeks after TRISENOX infusion, and then returned towards baseline by the end of 8 weeks after TRISENOX infusion. In these ECG evaluations, women did not experience more pronounced QT prolongation than men, and there was no correlation with age.

Complete AV block

Complete AV block has been reported with arsenic trioxide in the published literature including a case of a patient with APL.

Carcinogenesis

Carcinogenicity studies have not been conducted with TRISENOX by intravenous administration. The active ingredient of TRISENOX, arsenic trioxide is a human carcinogen.

Pregnancy

TRISENOX may cause fetal harm when administered to a pregnant woman. Studies in pregnant mice, rats, hamsters, and primates have shown that inorganic arsenicals cross the placental barrier when given orally or by injection. The reproductive toxicity of arsenic trioxide has been studied in a limited manner. An increase in resorptions, neural-tube defects, anophthalmia and microphthalmia were observed in rats administered 10 mg/kg of arsenic trioxide on gestation day 9 (approximately 10 times the recommended human daily dose on a mg/m^2 basis). Similar findings occurred in mice administered a 10 mg/kg dose of a related trivalent arsenic, sodium arsenite, (approximately 5 times the projected human dose on a mg/m^2 basis) on gestation days 6, 7, 8 or 9. Intravenous injection of 2 mg/kg sodium arsenite (approximately equivalent to the projected human daily dose on a mg/m^2 basis) on gestation day 7 (the lowest dose tested) resulted in neural-tube defects in hamsters.

There are no studies in pregnant women using TRISENOX. If this drug is used during pregnancy or if the patient becomes pregnant while taking this drug, the patient should be apprised of the potential harm to the fetus. One patient who became pregnant while receiving arsenic trioxide had a miscarriage. Women of childbearing potential should be advised to avoid becoming pregnant.

PRECAUTIONS

Laboratory Tests

The patient's electrolyte, hematologic and coagulation profiles should be monitored at least twice weekly, and more frequently for clinically unstable patients during the induction phase and at least weekly during the consolidation phase. ECGs should be obtained weekly, and more frequently for clinically unstable patients, during induction and consolidation.

Drug Interactions

No formal assessments of pharmacokinetic drug-drug interactions between TRISENOX and other agents have been conducted. Caution is advised when TRISENOX is coadministered with other medications that can prolong the QT interval (e.g., certain antiarrhythmics or thioridazine) or lead to electrolyte abnormalities (such as diuretics or amphotericin B).

Carcinogenesis, Mutagenesis, Impairment of Fertility

See **WARNINGS** section for information on carcinogenesis. Arsenic trioxide and trivalent arsenite salts have not been demonstrated to be mutagenic to bacteria, yeast or mammalian cells. Arsenite salts are clastogenic *in vitro* (human fibroblast, human lymphocytes, Chinese hamster ovary cells, Chinese hamster V79 lung cells). Trivalent arsenic produced an increase in the incidence of chromosome aberrations and micronuclei in bone marrow cells of mice. The effect of arsenic on fertility has not been adequately studied.

Pregnancy

Pregnancy Category D. See **WARNINGS** section.

Nursing Mothers

Arsenic is excreted in human milk. Because of the potential for serious adverse reactions in nursing infants from TRISENOX, a decision should be made whether to discontinue nursing or to discontinue the drug, taking into account the importance of the drug to the mother.

Pediatric Use

There are limited clinical data on the pediatric use of TRISENOX. Of 5 patients below the age of 18 years (age range: 5 to 16 years) treated with TRISENOX, at the recommended dose of 0.15 mg/kg/day, 3 achieved a complete response.

In an additional study, the toxicity profile observed in 13 pediatric patients with APL between the ages of 4 and 20 receiving TRISENOX at 0.15 mg/kg/day was similar to that observed in adult patients (see **ADVERSE REACTIONS**). Safety and effectiveness in relapsed APL pediatric patients below the age of 4 years have not been studied.

Patients with Renal Impairment

Exposure of arsenic trioxide may be higher in patients with severe renal impairment (See **CLINICAL PHARMACOLOGY, Special Populations**.). Patients with severe renal impairment (creatinine clearance less than 30 mL/min) should be closely monitored for toxicity when these patients are treated with TRISENOX, and a dose reduction may be warranted.

The use of TRISENOX in patients on dialysis has not been studied.

Patients with Hepatic Impairment

Since limited data are available across all hepatic impairment groups, caution is advised in the use of TRISENOX in patients with hepatic impairment (see **CLINICAL PHARMACOLOGY, Special Populations**). Patients with severe hepatic impairment (Child-Pugh class C) should be closely monitored for toxicity when these patients are treated with TRISENOX.

ADVERSE REACTIONS

Safety information was available for 52 patients with relapsed or refractory APL who participated in clinical trials of TRISENOX. Forty patients in the Phase 2 study received the recommended dose of 0.15 mg/kg of which 28 completed both induction and consolidation treatment cycles. An additional 12 patients with relapsed or refractory APL received doses generally similar to the recommended dose. Most patients experienced some drug-related toxicity, most commonly leukocytosis, gastrointestinal (nausea, vomiting, diarrhea, and abdominal pain), fatigue, edema, hyperglycemia, dyspnea, cough, rash or itching, headaches, and dizziness. These adverse effects have not been observed to be permanent or irreversible nor do they usually require interruption of therapy.

Serious adverse events (SAEs), grade 3 or 4 according to version 2 of the NCI Common Toxicity Criteria, were common. Those SAEs attributed to TRISENOX in the Phase 2 study of 40 patients with refractory or relapsed APL included APL differentiation syndrome (n=3), hyperleukocytosis (n=3), QTc interval ≥ 500 msec (n=16, 1 with torsade de pointes), atrial dysrhythmias (n=2), and hyperglycemia (n=2).

The following table describes the adverse events that were observed in patients between the ages of 5-73 years treated for APL with TRISENOX at the recommended dose at a rate of 5% or more. Similar adverse event profiles were seen in the other patient populations who received TRISENOX.

Adverse Events (any grade) Occurring in ≥ 5% of 40 Patients with APL who Received TRISENOX (arsenic trioxide) injection at a dose of 0.15 mg/kg/day

System organ class/Adverse Event	All Adverse Events, Any Grade		Grade 3 & 4 Events	
	n	%	n	%
General disorders and administration site conditions				
Fatigue	25	63	2	5
Pyrexia (fever)	25	63	2	5
Edema - non-specific	16	40		
Rigors	15	38		
Chest pain	10	25	2	5
Injection site pain	8	20		
Pain - non-specific	6	15	1	3
Injection site erythema	5	13		
Injection site edema	4	10		
Weakness	4	10	2	5
Hemorrhage	3	8		
Weight gain	5	13		
Weight loss	3	8		
Drug hypersensitivity	2	5	1	3
Gastrointestinal disorders				
Nausea	30	75		
Anorexia	9	23		
Appetite decreased	6	15		
Diarrhea	21	53		
Vomiting	23	58		
Abdominal pain (lower & upper)	23	58	4	10
Sore throat	14	35		
Constipation	11	28	1	3
Loose stools	4	10		
Dyspepsia	4	10		
Oral blistering	3	8		
Fecal incontinence	3	8		
Gastrointestinal hemorrhage	3	8		
Dry mouth	3	8		
Abdominal tenderness	3	8		
Diarrhea hemorrhagic	3	8		
Abdominal distension	3	8		
Metabolism and nutrition disorders				
Hypokalemia	20	50	5	13
Hypomagnesemia	18	45	5	13
Hyperglycemia	18	45	5	13
ALT increased	8	20	2	5
Hyperkalemia	7	18	2	5
AST increased	5	13	1	3
Hypocalcemia	4	10		
Hypoglycemia	3	8		
Acidosis	2	5		

System organ class/Adverse Event	All Adverse Events, Any Grade		Grade 3 & 4 Events	
Nervous system disorders				
Headache	24	60	1	3
Insomnia	17	43	1	3
Paresthesia	13	33	2	5
Dizziness (excluding vertigo)	9	23		
Tremor	5	13		
Convulsion	3	8	2	5
Somnolence	3	8		
Coma	2	5	2	5
Respiratory				
Cough	26	65		
Dyspnea	21	53	4	10
Epistaxis	10	25		
Hypoxia	9	23	4	10
Pleural effusion	8	20	1	3
Post nasal drip	5	13		
Wheezing	5	13		
Decreased breath sounds	4	10		
Crepitations	4	10		
Rales	4	10		
Hemoptysis	3	8		
Tachypnea	3	8		
Rhonchi	3	8		
Skin & subcutaneous tissue disorders				
Dermatitis	17	43		
Pruritus	13	33	1	3
Ecchymosis	8	20		
Dry Skin	6	15		
Erythema - non-specific	5	13		
Increased sweating	5	13		
Facial edema	3	8		
Night sweats	3	8		
Petechiae	3	8		
Hyperpigmentation	3	8		
Non-specific skin lesions	3	8		
Urticaria	3	8		
Local exfoliation	2	5		
Eyelid edema	2	5		
Cardiac disorders				
Tachycardia	22	55		
ECG QT corrected interval prolonged > 500 msec	16	40		
Palpitations	4	10		
ECG abnormal other than QT interval prolongation	3	8		
Infections and infestations				
Sinusitis	8	20		
Herpes simplex	5	13		
Upper respiratory tract infection	5	13	1	3
Bacterial infection - non-specific	3	8	1	3
Herpes zoster	3	8		
Nasopharyngitis	2	5		
Oral candidiasis	2	5		
Sepsis	2	5	2	5
Musculoskeletal, connective tissue and bone disorders				
Arthralgia	13	33	3	8
Myalgia	10	25	2	5
Bone pain	9	23	4	10
Back pain	7	18	1	3
Neck pain	5	13		
Pain in limb	5	13	2	5
Hematologic disorders				
Leukocytosis	20	50	1	3
Anemia	8	20	2	5
Thrombocytopenia	7	18	5	13
Febrile neutropenia	5	13	3	8
Neutropenia	4	10	4	10
Disseminated intravascular coagulation	3	8	3	8
Lymphadenopathy	3	8		
Vascular disorders				
Hypotension	10	25	2	5
Flushing	4	10		
Hypertension	4	10		
Pallor	4	10		
Psychiatric disorders				
Anxiety	12	30		
Depression	8	20		
Agitation	2	5		
Confusion	2	5		
Ocular disorders				
Eye irritation	4	10		
Blurred vision	4	10		
Dry eye	3	8		
Painful red eye	2	5		
Renal and urinary disorders				
Renal failure	3	8	1	3
Renal impairment	3	8		
Oliguria	2	5		
Incontinence	2	5		

System organ class/Adverse Event	All Adverse Events, Any Grade		Grade 3 & 4 Events	
Reproductive system disorders				
Vaginal hemorrhage	5	13		
Intermenstrual bleeding	3	8		
Ear disorders				
Earache	3	8		
Tinnitus	2	5		

The following additional adverse events were reported as related to TRISENOX treatment in 13 pediatric patients (defined as ages 4 through 20): gastrointestinal (dysphagia, mucosal inflammation/stomatitis, oropharyngeal pain, caecitis), metabolic and nutrition disorders (hyponatremia, hypoalbuminemia, hypophosphatemia, and lipase increased), cardiac failure congestive, respiratory (acute respiratory distress syndrome, lung infiltration, pneumonitis, pulmonary edema, respiratory distress, capillary leak syndrome), neuralgia, and enuresis. Pulmonary edema (n=1) and caecitis (n=1) were considered serious reactions.

Post-Marketing Experience

The following reactions have been reported from clinical trials and/or world-wide post-marketing surveillance. Because they are reported from a population of unknown size, precise estimates of frequency cannot be made.

Cardiac disorders: ventricular extrasystoles in association with QT prolongation, and ventricular tachycardia in association with QT prolongation

Nervous system disorders: peripheral neuropathy

Hematologic disorders: pancytopenia

Respiratory, thoracic, and mediastinal disorders: A differentiation syndrome, like retinoic acid syndrome, has been reported with the use of TRISENOX for the treatment of malignancies other than APL. See **Boxed WARNING**.

OVERDOSAGE

If symptoms suggestive of serious acute arsenic toxicity (e.g., convulsions, muscle weakness and confusion) appear, TRISENOX (arsenic trioxide) injection should be immediately discontinued and chelation therapy should be considered. A conventional protocol for acute arsenic intoxication includes dimercaprol administered at a dose of 3 mg/kg intramuscularly every 4 hours until immediate life-threatening toxicity has subsided. Thereafter, penicillamine at a dose of 250 mg orally, up to a maximum frequency of four times per day (≤ 1 g per day), may be given.

DOSAGE AND ADMINISTRATION

TRISENOX should be diluted with 100 to 250 mL 5% Dextrose Injection, USP or 0.9% Sodium Chloride Injection, USP, using proper aseptic technique, immediately after withdrawal from the ampule. The TRISENOX ampule is single-use and does not contain any preservatives. Unused portions of each ampule should be discarded properly. Do not save any unused portions for later administration. Do not mix TRISENOX with other medications.

TRISENOX should be administered intravenously over 1-2 hours. The infusion duration may be extended up to 4 hours if acute vasomotor reactions are observed. A central venous catheter is not required.

Stability

After dilution, TRISENOX is chemically and physically stable when stored for 24 hours at room temperature and 48 hours when refrigerated.

Dosing Regimen

TRISENOX is recommended to be given according to the following schedule:

Induction Treatment Schedule: TRISENOX should be administered intravenously at a dose of 0.15 mg/kg daily until bone marrow remission. Total induction dose should not exceed 60 doses.

Consolidation Treatment Schedule: Consolidation treatment should begin 3 to 6 weeks after completion of induction therapy. TRISENOX should be administered intravenously at a dose of 0.15 mg/kg daily for 25 doses over a period up to 5 weeks.

HANDLING AND DISPOSAL

Procedures for proper handling and disposal of anticancer drugs should be considered. Several guidelines on this subject have been published.[1-4] There is no general agreement that all of the procedures recommended in the guidelines are necessary or appropriate.

HOW SUPPLIED

TRISENOX (arsenic trioxide) injection is supplied as a sterile, clear, colorless solution in 10 mL glass, single-use ampules.

NDC 63459-600-10 10 mg/10 mL (1 mg/mL) ampule in packages of ten ampules.

Store at 25°C (77°F); excursions permitted to 15-30°C (59-86°F). Do not freeze.

Do not use beyond expiration date printed on the label.

REFERENCES

1. Preventing Occupational Exposures to Antineoplastic and Other Hazardous Drugs in Health Care Settings. NIOSH Alert 2004:165.

2. OSHA Technical Manual. TED 1-0.15A, Section VI: Chapter 2. Controlling Occupational Exposure to Hazardous Drugs. OSHA, 1999. http://www.osha.gov/dts/osta/otm/otm_vi_2.html

3. American Society of Health-System Pharmacists. ASHP guidelines on handling hazardous drugs. *Am J Health-Syst Pharm.* 2006; 63:1172-1193.

4. Polovich, M., White, J.M., & Kelleher, L.O. (eds.) 2005. Chemotherapy and biotherapy guidelines and recommendations for practice (2nd ed.) Pittsburgh, PA: Oncology Nursing Society

Rx only
Manufactured for:
Cephalon, Inc.
Frazer, PA 19355
TRI-007
Revised June 2010
TRISENOX is a trademark of Cephalon, Inc. or its affiliates.
U.S. Patent Nos. 6,723,351; 6,855,339; 6,861,076; 6,884,439; 6,982,096
©2000-2010 Cephalon, Inc. or its affiliates. All rights reserved.
Label Code: 00016790.01
Shown in Product Identification Guide, page 308

Cumberland Pharmaceuticals Inc.

2525 WEST END AVENUE
SUITE 950
NASHVILLE, TN 37203

Ph. 615-255-0068
Fx. 615-255-0094
www.cumberlandpharma.com

ACETADOTE®   ℞
(acetylcysteine)
Injection

HIGHLIGHTS OF PRESCRIBING INFORMATION
These highlights do not include all the information needed to use Acetadote safely and effectively. See full prescribing information for Acetadote.
ACETADOTE (acetylcysteine) Injection
Initial U.S. Approval: 2004

――――RECENT MAJOR CHANGES――――
Adverse Reactions, Postmarketing Safety
Study (6.1)   12/2008

――――― INDICATIONS AND USAGE―――――
Acetadote, administered intravenously within 8 to 10 hours after ingestion of a potentially hepatotoxic quantity of acetaminophen, is indicated to prevent or lessen hepatic injury (1)

―――DOSAGE AND ADMINISTRATION―――
Patients ≥40 kg (2.1):
Loading Dose: 150 mg/kg in 200 mL of diluent administered over 60 min
Dose 2: 50 mg/kg in 500 mL of diluent administered over 4 hr
Dose 3: 100 mg/kg in 1000 mL of diluent administered over 16 hr
Patients >20-<40 kg (2.1):
Loading Dose: 150 mg/kg in 100 mL of diluent administered over 60 min
Dose 2: 50 mg/kg in 250 mL of diluent administered over 4 hr
Dose 3: 100 mg/kg in 500 mL of diluent administered over 16 hr
Patients ≤20 kg (2.1):
Loading Dose: 150 mg/kg in 3 mL/kg of body weight of diluent administered over 60 min
Dose 2: 50 mg/kg in 7 mL/kg of body weight of diluent administered over 4 hr
Dose 3: 100 mg/kg in 14 mL/kg of body weight of diluent administered over 16 hr

――――DOSAGE FORMS AND STRENGTHS――――
Vials: 200 mg/mL, 30 mL (20% solution) (3)
――――――CONTRAINDICATIONS――――――
Patients with previous anaphylactoid reaction to acetylcysteine (4)

――――WARNINGS AND PRECAUTIONS――――
• Monitor as acute flushing and erythema of the skin may occur; usually associated with the loading dose; often resolves spontaneously despite continued infusion (5.1)
• Monitor for serious anaphylactoid reactions; infusion may be interrupted until treatment of anaphylactoid symptoms has been initiated (5.1)
• Should be used with caution in patients with asthma, or where there is a history of bronchospasm (5.2)

• Total volume administered should be adjusted for patients less than 40kg and for those requiring fluid restriction (5.3)

―――――――ADVERSE REACTIONS―――――――
Most common adverse reactions (incidence >2%) are rash, urticaria/facial flushing and pruritus (6.1)
To report SUSPECTED ADVERSE REACTIONS, contact Cumberland Pharmaceuticals Inc. at 1-877-484-2700 or FDA at 1-800-FDA-1088 or www.fda.gov/medwatch.
―――――――DRUG INTERACTIONS―――――――
No drug-drug interaction studies have been conducted. (7)
――――USE IN SPECIFIC POPULATIONS――――
Pregnancy: This drug should be used during pregnancy only if clearly needed (8.1)
Nursing Mothers: Unknown if drug is excreted in human milk (8.3)
Pediatric Use: See dose adjustment for patients < 40 kg (2)
See 17 for PATIENT COUNSELING INFORMATION
                                        Revised: 12/2008

FULL PRESCRIBING INFORMATION: CONTENTS*
1   INDICATIONS AND USAGE
    1.1   Acetaminophen Assays Interpretation and Methodology – Acute Ingestion
    1.2   Acetaminophen Assays Interpretation and Methodology – Repeated Supratherapeutic Ingestion
2   DOSAGE AND ADMINISTRATION
    2.1   Administration Instructions (Three-Bag Method: Loading, Second and Third dose)
    2.2   Renal Impairment
    2.3   Hepatic Impairment
3   DOSAGE FORMS AND STRENGTHS
4   CONTRAINDICATIONS
5   WARNINGS AND PRECAUTIONS
    5.1   Anaphylactoid Reactions
    5.2   Monitoring Patients with Asthma
    5.3   Volume Adjustment: Patients <40 kg and Requiring Fluid Restriction
6   ADVERSE REACTIONS
    6.1   Clinical Studies Experience
7   DRUG INTERACTIONS
8   USE IN SPECIFIC POPULATIONS
    8.1   Pregnancy
    8.3   Nursing mothers
    8.4   Pediatric use
    8.5   Geriatric use
10 OVERDOSAGE
11 DESCRIPTION
12 CLINICAL PHARMACOLOGY
    12.1 Mechanism of action
    12.3 Pharmacokinetics
13 NONCLINICAL TOXICOLOGY
    13.1 Carcinogenesis, Mutagenesis, Impairment of Fertility
    13.3 Reproductive and Developmental Toxicology
14 CLINICAL STUDIES
16 HOW SUPPLIED/STORAGE AND HANDLING
17 PATIENT COUNSELING INFORMATION
* Sections or subsections omitted from the Full Prescribing Information are not listed.

―――――――――――――――――――――――――――――
FULL PRESCRIBING INFORMATION

1   INDICATIONS AND USAGE
Acetadote, administered intravenously within 8 to 10 hours after ingestion of a potentially hepatotoxic quantity of acetaminophen, is indicated to prevent or lessen hepatic injury [see *Dosage and Administration (2) and Acetaminophen Assays – Interpretation and Methodology (1.1, 1.2)*].
On admission for suspected acetaminophen overdose, a serum blood sample should be drawn at least 4 hours after ingestion to determine the acetaminophen level and will serve as a basis for determining the need for treatment with acetylcysteine. If the patient presents after 4 hours post-ingestion, the serum acetaminophen sample should be determined immediately.
Acetadote should be administered within 8 hours from acetaminophen ingestion for maximal protection against hepatic injury for patients whose serum acetaminophen levels fall above the "possible" toxicity line on the Rumack-Matthew nomogram (line connecting 150 mcg/mL at 4 hours with 37.5 mcg/mL at 12 hours); [see *Acetaminophen Assays – Interpretation and Methodology [(1.1, 1.2)]*. If the time of ingestion is unknown, or the serum acetaminophen level is not available, cannot be interpreted, or is not available within the 8 hour time interval from acetaminophen ingestion, Acetadote should be administered immediately if 24 hours or less have elapsed from the reported time of ingestion of an overdose of acetaminophen, regardless of the quantity reported to have been ingested.
The aspartate aminotransferase (AST, SGOT), alanine aminotransferase (ALT, SGPT), bilirubin, prothrombin time, creatinine, blood urea nitrogen (BUN), blood glucose, and elec-

---

trolytes also should be determined in order to monitor hepatic and renal function and electrolyte and fluid balance.
NOTE: The critical ingestion-treatment interval for maximal protection against severe hepatic injury is between 0–8 hours. Efficacy diminishes progressively after 8 hours and treatment initiation between 15 and 24 hours post-ingestion of acetaminophen yields limited efficacy. However, it does not appear to worsen the condition of patients and it should not be withheld, since the reported time of ingestion may not be correct.

1.1   Acetaminophen Assays Interpretation and Methodology – Acute Ingestion
The acute ingestion of acetaminophen in quantities of 150 mg/kg or greater may result in hepatic toxicity. However, the reported history of the quantity of a drug ingested as an overdose is often inaccurate and is not a reliable guide to therapy of the overdose. Therefore, plasma or serum acetaminophen concentrations, determined as early as possible, but no sooner than four hours following an acute overdose, are essential in assessing the potential risk of hepatotoxicity. If an assay for acetaminophen cannot be obtained, it is necessary to assume that the overdose is potentially toxic.

Interpretation of Acetaminophen Assays
1. When results of the plasma acetaminophen assay are available, refer to the nomogram in Figure 1 to determine if plasma concentration is in the potentially toxic range. Values above the line connecting 200 mcg/mL at 4 hours with 50 mcg/mL at 12 hours (probable line) are associated with a probability of hepatic toxicity if an antidote is not administered.
2. If the predetoxification plasma level is above the line connecting 150 mcg/mL at 4 hours with 37.5 mcg/mL at 12 hours (possible line), continue with maintenance doses of acetylcysteine. It is better to err on the safe side and thus this line, defining possible toxicity, is plotted 25% below the line defining probable toxicity.
3. If the predetoxification plasma level is below the line connecting 150 mcg/mL at 4 hours with 37.5 mcg/mL at 12 hours (possible line), there is minimal risk of hepatic toxicity, and acetylcysteine treatment may be discontinued.
Estimating Potential for Hepatotoxicity: The following depiction of the Rumack-Matthew nomogram has been developed to estimate the probability that plasma levels in relation to intervals post-ingestion will result in hepatotoxicity.

Figure 1. Rumack-Matthew Nomogram: Plasma or Serum Acetaminophen Concentration vs. Time Post Acetaminophen Ingestion (Rumack BH, Matthew H. Acetaminophen poisoning and toxicity. Pediatrics. 1975;55:871-876 and Rumack BH, Peterson RC, Kock GG, Amara IA. Acetaminophen overdose. 662 cases with evaluation of oral acetylcysteine treatment. Arch Intern Med. 1981;141:380-385).

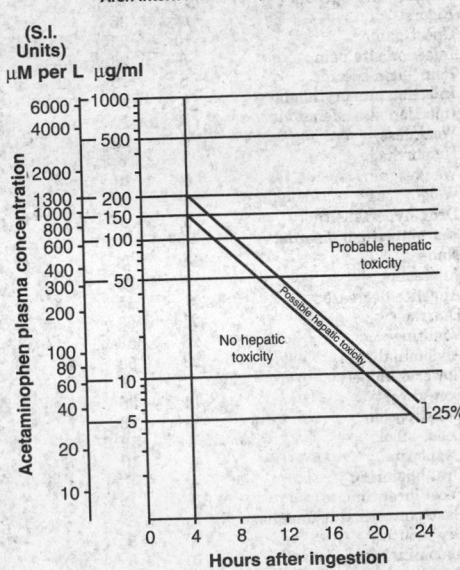

1.2   Acetaminophen Assays Interpretation and Methodology – Repeated Supratherapeutic Ingestion
Repeated Supratherapeutic Ingestion (RSI) is defined as ingestion of acetaminophen at doses higher than those recommended for extended periods of time. The nomogram does not apply to patients with RSI. Treatment is based on the acetaminophen and elevated AST/ALT levels indicative of potential toxicity due to acetaminophen. For specific treatment information regarding the clinical management of repeated supratherapeutic acetaminophen overdose, please contact your regional poison center at 1-800-222-1222, or al-

ternatively, a special health professional assistance line for acetaminophen overdose at 1-800-525-6115.

Figure 2. Acetadote Treatment Flow Chart

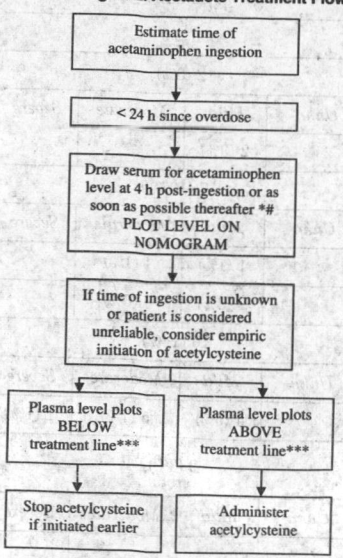

*Acetaminophen levels drawn less than 4 hours post-ingestion may be misleading.

\# With an extended-release preparation, an acetaminophen level drawn less than 8 hours post-ingestion may be misleading. Draw a second level at 4 to 6 hours after the initial level. If either falls above the toxicity line, acetylcysteine treatment should be initiated.

***Acetylcysteine may be withheld until acetaminophen assay results are available as long as initiation of treatment is not delayed beyond 8 hours post-ingestion. If more than 8 hours post-ingestion, start acetylcysteine treatment immediately.

2   DOSAGE AND ADMINISTRATION

The total dose of Acetadote is 300 mg/kg administered over 21 hours. Please refer to the guidelines below for dose preparation based upon patient weight.

2.1   Administration Instructions (Three-Bag Method: Loading, Second and Third Dose)

Patients ≥40 kg (Table 1):

Loading Dose: 150 mg/kg in 200 mL of diluent[1] administered over 60 min

Second Dose: 50 mg/kg in 500 mL of diluent administered over 4 hr

Third Dose: 100 mg/kg in 1000 mL of diluent administered over 16 hr

[See table 1 at top right]

The total volume administered should be adjusted for patients less than 40 kg and for those requiring fluid restriction:

Patients >20 - <40 kg (Table 2):

Loading Dose: 150 mg/kg in 100 mL of diluent[1] administered over 60 min

Second Dose: 50 mg/kg in 250 mL of diluent administered over 4 hr

Third Dose: 100 mg/kg in 500 mL of diluent administered over 16 hr

[See table 2 at right]

Patients ≤20 kg (Table 3):

Loading Dose: 150 mg/kg in 3 mL/kg of body weight of diluent[1] administered over 60 min

Second Dose: 50 mg/kg in 7 mL/kg of body weight of diluent administered over 4 hr

Third Dose: 100 mg/kg in 14 mL/kg of body weight of diluent administered over 16 hr

[See table 3 at right]

Single dose vial, preservative-free, discard unused portion. If vial was previously opened, do not use for I.V. administration.

Stability studies indicate that the diluted solution is stable for 24 hours at controlled room temperature.

Note: The color of Acetadote may turn from essentially colorless to a slight pink or purple once the stopper is punctured. The color change does not affect the quality of the product.

2.2   Renal Impairment

No data are available to determine if a dose adjustment in patients with moderate or severe renal impairment is required.

2.3   Hepatic Impairment

Although there was a threefold increase in acetylcysteine plasma concentrations in patients with hepatic cirrhosis, no data are available to determine if a dose adjustment in these patients is required. The published medical literature does not indicate that the dose of acetylcysteine in patients with hepatic impairment should be reduced.

3   DOSAGE FORMS AND STRENGTHS

Acetadote (acetylcysteine) Injection is available as a 20% solution (200 mg/mL) in 30 mL single dose glass vials. Acetadote is sterile and can be used for I.V. administration.

4   CONTRAINDICATIONS

Acetadote is contraindicated in patients with previous anaphylactoid reactions to acetylcysteine.

5   WARNINGS AND PRECAUTIONS

5.1   Anaphylactoid Reactions

Serious anaphylactoid reactions, including death in a patient with asthma, have been reported in patients administered acetylcysteine intravenously.

Acute flushing and erythema of the skin may occur in patients receiving acetylcysteine intravenously. These reactions usually occur 30 to 60 minutes after initiating the infusion and often resolve spontaneously despite continued infusion of acetylcysteine. Anaphylactoid reactions (defined as the occurrence of an acute hypersensitivity reaction during acetylcysteine administration including rash, hypotension, wheezing, and/or shortness of breath) have been observed in patients receiving I.V. acetylcysteine for acetaminophen overdose and occurred soon after initiation of the infusion [see Adverse Reactions (6.1)]. If a reaction to acetylcysteine involves more than simply flushing and erythema of the skin, it should be treated as an anaphylactoid reaction. This usually entails administering antihistaminic drugs and in severe cases may require administration of epinephrine. In addition, the acetylcysteine infusion may be interrupted until treatment of the anaphylactoid symptoms has been initiated and then carefully restarted. If the anaphylactoid reaction returns upon reinitiation of treatment or increases in severity, intravenous acetylcysteine should be discontinued and alternative patient management should be considered.

5.2   Monitoring Patients with Asthma

Acetadote should be used with caution in patients with asthma, or where there is a history of bronchospasm.

5.3   Volume Adjustment: Patients <40 kg and Requiring Fluid Restriction

The total volume administered should be adjusted for patients less than 40 kg and for those requiring fluid restriction. To avoid fluid overload, the volume of diluent should be reduced as needed [see Dosage and Administration (2)]. If volume is not adjusted fluid overload can occur, potentially resulting in hyponatremia, seizure and death.

For specific treatment information regarding the clinical management of acetaminophen overdose, please contact your regional poison center at 1-800-222-1222, or alternatively, a special health professional assistance line for acetaminophen overdose at 1-800-525-6115.

6   ADVERSE REACTIONS

6.1   Clinical Studies Experience

Because clinical trials are conducted under widely varying conditions, adverse reaction rates observed in the clinical trials of a drug cannot be directly compared to rates in the clinical trials of another drug and may not reflect the rates observed in practice.

In the literature the most frequently reported adverse reactions attributed to I.V. acetylcysteine administration were rash, urticaria and pruritus. The frequency of adverse reactions has been reported to be between 0.2% and 20.8%, and they most commonly occur during the initial loading dose of acetylcysteine.

Loading Dose/Infusion Rate Study

The incidence of drug-related adverse reactions occurring within the first 2 hours following acetylcysteine administration reported in a randomized study in patients with acetaminophen poisoning is presented in Table 4 by preferred term. In this study patients were randomized to a 15-minute or a 60-minute loading dose regimen.

Within the first 2 hours following I.V. acetylcysteine administration, 17% developed an anaphylactoid reaction (18% in

Table 1. Three-Bag Method Dosage Guide by Weight, patients ≥ 40 kg

Body Weight		LOADING Dose 150 mg/kg in 200 mL diluent[1] over 60 min	SECOND Dose 50 mg/kg in 500 mL diluent over 4 hours	THIRD Dose 100 mg/kg in 1000 mL diluent over 16 hours
(kg)	(lb)	Acetadote (mL)	Acetadote (mL)	Acetadote (mL)
100	220	75	25	50
90	198	67.5	22.5	45
80	176	60	20	40
70	154	52.5	17.5	35
60	132	45	15	30
50	110	37.5	12.5	25
40	88	30	10	20

Table 2. Three-Bag Method Dosage Guide by Weight, Patients >20 - < 40 kg

Body Weight		LOADING Dose 150 mg/kg over 60 minutes		SECOND Dose 50 mg/kg over 4 hours		THIRD Dose 100 mg/kg over 16 hours	
(kg)	(lb)	Acetadote (mL)	Diluent[1] (mL)	Acetadote (mL)	Diluent (mL)	Acetadote (mL)	Diluent (mL)
30	66	22.5	100	7.5	250	15	500
25	55	18.75	100	6.25	250	12.5	500

Table 3. Three-Bag Method Dosage Guide by Weight, patients ≤ 20 kg

Body Weight		LOADING Dose 150 mg/kg over 60 minutes		SECOND Dose 50 mg/kg over 4 hours		THIRD Dose 100 mg/kg over 16 hours	
(kg)	(lb)	Acetadote (mL)	Diluent[1] (mL)	Acetadote (mL)	Diluent (mL)	Acetadote (mL)	Diluent (mL)
20	44	15	60	5	140	10	280
15	33	11.25	45	3.75	105	7.5	210
10	22	7.5	30	2.5	70	5	140

[1]Acetadote is hyperosmolar (2600 mOsm/L) and is compatible with 5% Dextrose (D5W), ½ Normal Saline (0.45% Sodium Chloride Injection, ½ NS), and Water for Injection (WFI).

the 15-minute treatment group; 14% in the 60-minute treatment group) in this randomized, open-label, multi-center clinical study conducted in Australia to compare the rates of anaphylactoid reactions between two rates of infusion for the I.V. acetylcysteine loading dose. [see Warnings (Section 5) and Clinical Studies - Loading Dose/Infusion Rate Study (Section 14)].

[See table 4 at right]

Postmarketing Safety Study
A large multi-center study was performed in Canada where data were collected from patients who were treated with I.V. NAC for acetaminophen overdose between 1980 and 2005. This study evaluated 4709 adult cases and 1905 pediatric cases. The incidence of anaphylactoid reactions in adult (overall incidence 7.9%) and pediatric (overall incidence 9.5%) patients is presented in Tables 5 and 6.

Table 5. Distribution of reported reactions in adult patients receiving I.V. NAC

Reaction	Incidence (%) % of Patients (N=4709)
Urticaria/Facial Flushing	6.1%
Pruritus	4.3%
Respiratory Symptoms*	1.9%
Edema	1.6%
Hypotension	0.1%
Anaphylaxis	0.1%

Table 6. Distribution of reported reactions in pediatric patients receiving I.V. NAC

Reaction	Incidence (%) % of Patients (N=1905)
Urticaria/Facial Flushing	7.6%
Pruritus	4.1%
Respiratory Symptoms*	2.2%
Edema	1.2%
Anaphylaxis	0.2%
Hypotension	0.1%

*Respiratory symptoms are defined as presence of any of the following: cough, wheezing, stridor, shortness of breath, chest tightness, respiratory distress, or bronchospasm.

Table 4. Incidence of Drug-Related Adverse Reactions Occurring Within the First 2 Hours Following Study Drug Administration by Preferred Term: Loading Dose/Infusion Rate Study

Treatment Group	15-min				60-min			
Number of Patients	n=109				n=71			
Cardiac disorders	5 (5%)				2 (3%)			
Severity:	Unkn	Mild	Moderate	Severe	Unkn	Mild	Moderate	Severe
Tachycardia NOS		4 (4%)	1 (1%)			2 (3%)		
Gastrointestinal disorders	16 (15%)				7 (10%)			
Severity:	Unkn	Mild	Moderate	Severe	Unkn	Mild	Moderate	Severe
Nausea	1 (1%)		6 (6%)			1 (1%)	1 (1%)	
Vomiting NOS		2 (2%)	11 (10%)			2 (3%)	4 (6%)	
Immune System Disorders	20 (18%)				10 (14%)			
Severity:	Unkn	Mild	Moderate	Severe	Unkn	Mild	Moderate	Severe
Anaphylactoid reaction	2 (2%)	6 (6%)	11 (10%)	1 (1%)		4 (6%)	5 (7%)	1 (1%)
Respiratory, thoracic and mediastinal disorders	2 (2%)				2 (3%)			
Severity:	Unkn	Mild	Moderate	Severe	Unkn	Mild	Moderate	Severe
Pharyngitis			1 (1%)					
Rhinorrhoea		1 (1%)						
Rhonchi						1 (1%)		
Throat tightness						1 (1%)		
Skin & subcutaneous tissue disorders	6 (6%)				5 (7%)			
Severity:	Unkn	Mild	Moderate	Severe	Unkn	Mild	Moderate	Severe
Pruritis		1 (1%)				2 (3%)		
Rash NOS		3 (3%)	2 (2%)			3 (4%)		
Vascular disorders	2 (2%)				3 (4%)			
Severity:	Unkn	Mild	Moderate	Severe	Unkn	Mild	Moderate	Severe
Flushing		1 (1%)	1 (1%)			2 (3%)	1 (1%)	
Unkn=Unknown								

7   DRUG INTERACTIONS
No drug-drug interaction studies have been conducted.

8   USE IN SPECIFIC POPULATIONS
8.1   Pregnancy
Pregnancy Category B
There are no adequate and well-controlled studies of Acetadote in pregnant women. However, limited case reports of pregnant women exposed to acetylcysteine during various trimesters did not report any adverse maternal, fetal or neonatal outcomes.
There are published reports on four pregnant women with acetaminophen toxicity, who were treated with oral or intravenous acetylcysteine at the time of delivery. Acetylcysteine crossed the placenta and was measurable following delivery in serum and cord blood of three viable infants and in cardiac blood of a fourth infant at autopsy (22 weeks gestational age who died 3 hours after birth). No adverse sequelae developed in the three viable infants. All mothers recovered and none of the infants had evidence of acetaminophen poisoning.
Reproductive and developmental toxicity studies performed in rats at oral doses up to 6.7 times the recommended human intravenous dose and in rabbits at doses up to 3.3 times the recommended human intravenous dose revealed no evidence of impaired fertility or embryofetal toxicity [see Reproductive and Developmental Toxicology (13.3)].

8.3   Nursing mothers
It is not known whether Acetadote is present in human milk. Because many drugs are excreted in human milk, caution should be exercised when acetylcysteine is administered to a nursing woman. Based on the pharmacokinetics

of acetylcysteine, it should be nearly completely cleared 30 hours after administration. Nursing women may consider resuming nursing 30 hours after administration.

8.4   Pediatric use
No adverse effects were noted during I.V. infusion with acetylcysteine at a mean rate of 4.2 mg/kg/h for 24 hours to 10 preterm newborns ranging in gestational age from 25 to 31 weeks and in weight from 500 to 1380 grams in one study or in 6 newborns ranging in gestational age from 26 to 30 weeks and in weight from 520 to 1335 grams infused with acetylcysteine at 0.1 to 1.3 mg/kg/h for 6 days. Elimination of acetylcysteine was slower in these infants than in adults; mean elimination half-life was 11 hours. There are no adequate and well-controlled studies in pediatric patients.

8.5   Geriatric use
The clinical studies do not provide a sufficient number of geriatric subjects to determine whether the elderly respond differently.

10   OVERDOSAGE
Single intravenous doses of acetylcysteine at 1000 mg/kg in mice, 2445 mg/kg in rats, 1500 mg/kg in guinea pigs, 1200 mg/kg in rabbits and 500 mg/kg in dogs were lethal. Symptoms of acute toxicity were ataxia, hypoactivity, labored respiration, cyanosis, loss of righting reflex and convulsions.

11   DESCRIPTION
Acetylcysteine injection is an intravenous (I.V.) medication for the treatment of acetaminophen overdose. Acetylcysteine is the nonproprietary name for the N-acetyl derivative of the naturally occurring amino acid, L-cysteine (N-acetyl-L-cysteine, NAC). The compound is a white crystalline powder, which melts in the range of 104° to 110°C and has a very slight odor. The molecular formula of the compound is $C_5H_9NO_3S$, and its molecular weight is 163.2. Acetylcysteine has the following structural formula:

Acetadote is supplied as a sterile solution in vials containing 20% w/v (200 mg/mL) acetylcysteine. The pH of the solution ranges from 6.0 to 7.5. Acetadote contains the following inactive ingredients: 0.5 mg/mL disodium edetate, sodium hydroxide (used for pH adjustment), and Sterile Water for Injection, USP.

12   CLINICAL PHARMACOLOGY
12.1   Mechanism of action
Acetaminophen Overdose:
Acetaminophen is absorbed from the upper gastrointestinal tract with peak plasma levels occurring between 30 and 60 minutes after therapeutic doses and usually within 4 hours following an overdose. It is extensively metabolized in the liver to form principally the sulfate and glucuronide conjugates which are excreted in the urine. A small fraction of an ingested dose is metabolized in the liver by isozyme CYP2E1 of the cytochrome P-450 mixed function oxidase enzyme system to form a reactive, potentially toxic, intermediate metabolite. The toxic metabolite preferentially conjugates with hepatic glutathione to form nontoxic cysteine and mercapturic acid derivatives, which are then excreted by the kidney. Recommended therapeutic doses of acetaminophen are not believed to saturate the glucuronide and sulfate conjugation pathways and therefore are not expected to result in the formation of sufficient reactive metabolite to deplete glutathione stores. However, following ingestion of a large overdose, the glucuronide and sulfate conjugation pathways are saturated resulting in a larger fraction of the drug being metabolized via the cytochrome P-450 pathway and therefore, the amount of acetaminophen

metabolized to the reactive intermediate increases. The increased formation of the reactive metabolite may deplete the hepatic stores of glutathione with subsequent binding of the metabolite to protein molecules within the hepatocyte resulting in cellular necrosis.

Acetylcysteine I.V. Treatment:
Acetylcysteine has been shown to reduce the extent of liver injury following acetaminophen overdose. It is most effective when given early, with benefit seen principally in patients treated within 8-10 hours of the overdose. Acetylcysteine likely protects the liver by maintaining or restoring the glutathione levels, or by acting as an alternate substrate for conjugation with, and thus detoxification of, the reactive metabolite.

12.3 Pharmacokinetics

Distribution:
The steady-state volume of distribution (Vd_{ss}) and the protein binding for acetylcysteine were reported to be 0.47 liter/kg and 83%, respectively.

Metabolism:
Acetylcysteine may form cysteine, disulfides and conjugates in vivo (N, N'-diacetylcysteine, N-acetylcysteine-cysteine, N-acetylcysteine-glutathione, N-acetylcysteine-protein, etc). Based on published data, it was reported that after an oral dose of ^{35}S-acetylcysteine, about 22% of total radioactivity was excreted in urine after 24 hours. No metabolites were identified.

Elimination:
After a single intravenous dose of acetylcysteine, the plasma concentration of total acetylcysteine declined in a poly-exponential decay manner with a mean terminal half-life ($T_{1/2}$) of 5.6 hours. The mean clearance (CL) for acetylcysteine was reported to be 0.11 liter/hr/kg and renal CL constituted about 30% of total CL.

Special Populations:
Gender: Adequate information is not available to assess if there are differences in pharmacokinetics (PK) between males and females.
Pediatric: The mean elimination $T_{1/2}$ of acetylcysteine is longer in newborns (11 hours) than in adults (5.6 hours). Pharmacokinetic information is not available in other age groups.
Pregnant Women: In four pregnant women with acetaminophen toxicity, oral or I.V. acetylcysteine was administered at the time of delivery. Acetylcysteine was detected in the cord blood of 3 viable infants and in cardiac blood of a fourth infant sampled at autopsy [see Pregnancy (8.1)].
Hepatic Impairment: In subjects with severe liver damage, i.e., cirrhosis due to alcohol (with Child-Pugh score of 7-13), or primary and/or secondary biliary cirrhosis (with Child-Pugh score of 5-7), mean $T_{1/2}$ increased by 80% while mean CL decreased by 30% compared to the control group.
Renal Impairment: Pharmacokinetic information is not available in patients with renal impairment.
Geriatric Patients: Adequate information on acetylcysteine PK in geriatric patients is not available.

13 NONCLINICAL TOXICOLOGY

13.1 Carcinogenesis, Mutagenesis, Impairment of Fertility

Long-term studies in animals have not been performed to evaluate the carcinogenic potential of acetylcysteine.
Acetylcysteine was not genotoxic in the Ames test or the in vivo mouse micronucleus test. It was, however, positive in the in vitro mouse lymphoma cell (L5178Y/TK+/-) forward mutation test.
Treatment of male rats with acetylcysteine at an oral dose of 250 mg/kg/day for 15 weeks (0.8 times the recommended human dose of 300 mg/kg) did not affect the fertility or general reproductive performance.

13.3 Reproductive and Developmental Toxicology

Reproduction studies were performed in rats at oral doses up to 2000 mg/kg/day (6.7 times the recommended human dose of 300 mg/kg) and in rabbits at oral doses up to 1000 mg/kg/day (3.3 times the recommended human dose of 300 mg/kg) and revealed no evidence of impaired fertility or harm to the fetus due to acetylcysteine [see Pregnancy (8.1)].

14 CLINICAL STUDIES

Loading Dose/Infusion Rate Study
A randomized, open-label, multi-center clinical study was conducted in Australia to compare the rates of anaphylactoid reactions between two rates of infusion for the I.V. acetylcysteine loading dose. One hundred nine subjects were randomized to a 15 minute infusion rate and seventy-one subjects were randomized to a 60 minute infusion rate. The loading dose was 150 mg/kg followed by a maintenance dose of 50 mg/kg over 4 hours and then 100 mg/kg over 16 hours. Of the 180 patients, 27% were male and 73% were female. Ages ranged from 15 to 83 years, with the mean age being 29.9 years (±13.0).
A subgroup of 58 subjects (33 in the 15-minute treatment group; 25 in the 60-minute treatment group) was treated within 8 hours of acetaminophen ingestion. No hepatotoxicity occurred within this subgroup; however with 95% confi-

dence, the true hepatotoxicity rates could range from 0% to 9% for the 15-minute treatment group and from 0% to 12% for the 60-minute treatment group.

Observational Study
An open-label, observational database contained information on 1749 patients who sought treatment for acetaminophen overdose over a 16-year period. Of the 1749 patients, 65% were female, 34% were male and <1% was transgender. Ages ranged from 2 months to 96 years, with 71.4% of the patients falling in the 16-40 year old age bracket. A total of 399 patients received acetylcysteine treatment. A post-hoc analysis identified 56 patients who (1) were at high or probable risk for hepatotoxicity (APAP >150 mg/L at the four hours line according to the Australian nomogram) and (2) had a liver function test. Of the 53 patients who were treated with I.V. acetylcysteine (300 mg/kg I.V. acetylcysteine administered over 20-21 hours) within 8 hours, two (4%) developed hepatotoxicity (AST or ALT>1000U/L). Twenty-one of 48 (44%) patients treated with acetylcysteine after 15 hours developed hepatotoxicity. The actual number of hepatotoxicity outcomes may be higher than what is reported here. For patients with multiple admissions for acetaminophen overdose, only the first overdose treated with I.V. acetylcysteine was examined. Hepatotoxicity may have occurred in subsequent admissions.
Evaluable data were available from a total of 148 pediatric patients (less than 16 years of age) who were admitted for poisoning following ingestion of acetaminophen, of whom 23 were treated with I.V. acetylcysteine. Of the 23 patients who received I.V. acetylcysteine treatment, 3 patients (13%) had an adverse reaction (anaphylactoid reaction, rash and flushing, transient erythema). There were no deaths of pediatric patients. None of the pediatric patients receiving I.V. acetylcysteine developed hepatotoxicity while two patients not receiving I.V. acetylcysteine developed hepatotoxicity. The number of pediatric patients is too small to provide a statistically significant finding of efficacy, however the results appear to be consistent to those observed for adults.

Postmarketing Safety Study [see 6.1 Clinical Studies Experience]

16 HOW SUPPLIED/STORAGE AND HANDLING

Acetadote (acetylcysteine) Injection is available as a 20% solution (200 mg/mL) in 30 mL single dose glass vials. Acetadote is sterile and can be used for I.V. administration. It is available as follows:

• 30 mL vials, carton of 4 (NDC 66220-107-30)

Do not use previously opened vials for I.V. administration.

Note: The color of Acetadote may turn from essentially colorless to a slight pink or purple once the stopper is punctured. The color change does not affect the quality of the product.

The stopper in the Acetadote vial is formulated with a synthetic base-polymer and does not contain Natural Rubber Latex, Dry Natural Rubber, or blends of Natural Rubber.

Storage
Store unopened vials at controlled room temperature, 20° to 25°C (68° to 77°F) [See USP Controlled Room Temperature].

17 PATIENT COUNSELING INFORMATION

Sensitivity to acetylcysteine: Patients should be advised to report to their physician any history of sensitivity to acetylcysteine [see Contraindications (4)].
Asthma: Patients should be advised to report to their physician any history of asthma [see Warnings and Precautions (5)].
For all questions concerning adverse reactions associated with the use of this product or for inquiries concerning our products, please contact us at 1-877-484-2700.
For specific treatment information regarding the clinical management of acetaminophen overdose, please contact your regional poison center at 1-800-222-1222, or alternatively, a special health professional assistance line for acetaminophen overdose at 1-800-525-6115.
Manufactured for:
Cumberland Pharmaceuticals Inc.
Nashville, TN 37203
Revised: 12/2008   Cumberland Pharmaceuticals Inc.
*Sections or subsetions omitted from the Full Prescribing Information are not listed.

Shown in Product Identification Guide, page 308

CALDOLOR

(ibuprofen)   ℞

Injection, for intravenous use

HIGHLIGHTS OF PRESCRIBING INFORMATION

These highlights do not include all the information needed to use Caldolor safely and effectively. See full prescribing information for Caldolor.

CALDOLOR (ibuprofen) Injection, for intravenous use
Initial U.S. Approval: 1974

WARNING: RISK OF SERIOUS CARDIOVASCULAR AND GASTROINTESTINAL EVENTS
See full prescribing information for complete boxed warning

Cardiovascular Risk
• **Non-steroidal anti-inflammatory drugs (NSAIDs) may increase the risk of serious cardiovascular (CV) thrombotic events, myocardial infarction, and stroke, which can be fatal. Risk may increase with duration of use. (5.1)**
• **Caldolor is contraindicated for the treatment of perioperative pain in the setting of coronary artery bypass graft (CABG) surgery. (4.3, 5.1)**

Gastrointestinal Risk
• **NSAIDs increase the risk of serious gastrointestinal (GI) adverse events including bleeding, ulceration, and perforation of the stomach or intestines, which can be fatal. Events can occur at any time without warning symptoms. Elderly patients are at greater risk. (5.2)**

---INDICATIONS AND USAGE---
Caldolor is an NSAID indicated in adults for the:
• Management of mild to moderate pain (1.1)
• Management of moderate to severe pain as an adjunct to opioid analgesics (1.1)
• Reduction of fever (1.2)

---DOSAGE AND ADMINISTRATION---
• Pain: 400 mg to 800 mg intravenously over 30 minutes every 6 hours as necessary. (2.1)
• Fever: 400 mg intravenously over 30 minutes, followed by 400 mg every 4 to 6 hours or 100-200 mg every 4 hours as necessary. (2.2)
• Patients must be well hydrated before Caldolor administration.
• Caldolor must be diluted before administration. (2.3)

---DOSAGE FORMS AND STRENGTHS---
Vials: 400 mg/4 mL or 800 mg/8 mL (3)

---CONTRAINDICATIONS---
• Known hypersensitivity to ibuprofen or other NSAIDs (4.1)
• Asthma, urticaria, or allergic-type reactions after taking aspirin or other NSAIDs (4.2)
• Use during the peri-operative period in the setting of coronary artery bypass graft (CABG) surgery (4.3, 5.1)

---WARNINGS AND PRECAUTIONS---
• Serious and potentially fatal CV thrombotic events: Use lowest effective dose of Caldolor for shortest possible duration. (5.1)
• Serious and potentially fatal GI reactions: Use lowest effective dose of Caldolor for shortest possible duration. Use with caution in patients with prior history of ulcer disease or GI bleeding. (5.2)
• Hepatic effects: Range from transaminase elevations to liver failure. Discontinue Caldolor immediately if abnormal liver tests persist or worsen. (5.3, 5.15)
• Hypertension: Can occur with NSAID treatment. Monitor blood pressure closely during treatment with Caldolor. (5.4)
• Congestive heart failure and edema: Fluid retention and edema can occur with NSAID treatment. Use Caldolor with caution in patients with fluid retention or heart failure. (5.5)
• Renal effects: Long-term administration of NSAIDs can result in renal papillary necrosis and other renal injury. Use Caldolor with caution in patients at risk (e.g., the elderly, those with renal impairment, heart failure, liver impairment, and those taking diuretics or ACE inhibitors). (5.6)
• Anaphylactoid reactions: May occur in patients with the aspirin triad or in patients without prior exposure to Caldolor. Discontinue Caldolor immediately if an anaphylactoid reaction occurs. (5.7, 5.12)
• Serious skin reactions: Include exfoliative dermatitis, Stevens-Johnson Syndrome, and toxic epidermal necrolysis, which can be fatal. Discontinue Caldolor if rash or other signs of local skin reaction occur. (5.8)

---ADVERSE REACTIONS---
The most common adverse reactions are nausea, flatulence, vomiting, headache, hemorrhage and dizziness (>5%). (6.1)
To report SUSPECTED ADVERSE REACTIONS, contact Cumberland Pharmaceuticals Inc. at 1-877-484-2700 or FDA at 1-800-FDA-1088 or www.fda.gov/medwatch

---DRUG INTERACTIONS---
• ACE inhibitors: NSAIDs may diminish the antihypertensive effect of ACE inhibitors. (7.3)
• Aspirin: Concomitant administration of ibuprofen and aspirin is not generally recommended because of the potential for increased adverse effects. (7.1)

---USE IN SPECIFIC POPULATIONS---
• Pregnancy: Avoid use after 30 weeks gestation because premature closure of the ductus arteriosus in the fetus may occur. (8.1)
• Nursing Mothers: Use with caution as it is not known if ibuprofen is excreted in human milk. (8.3)

- Pediatric Use: Safety and effectiveness not established in patients less than 17 years of age. (8.4)

See 17 for PATIENT COUNSELING INFORMATION
Revised: 06/2009

FULL PRESCRIBING INFORMATION: CONTENTS*

FULL PRESCRIBING INFORMATION

WARNING: RISK OF SERIOUS CARDIOVASCULAR AND GASTROINTESTINAL EVENTS
Cardiovascular Risk

- Non-steroidal anti-inflammatory drugs (NSAIDs) may increase the risk of serious cardiovascular (CV) thrombotic events, myocardial infarction, and stroke, which can be fatal. This risk may increase with duration of use. Patients with cardiovascular disease or risk factors for cardiovascular disease may be at greater risk [see Warnings and Precautions (5.1)].
- Caldolor is contraindicated for the treatment of perioperative pain in the setting of coronary artery bypass graft (CABG) surgery [see Contraindications (4.3) and Warnings and Precautions (5.1)].

Gastrointestinal Risk

- NSAIDs increase the risk of serious gastrointestinal (GI) adverse events including bleeding, ulceration, and perforation of the stomach or intestines, which can be fatal. These events can occur at any time during use and without warning symptoms. Elderly patients are at greater risk for serious gastrointestinal events [see Warnings and Precautions (5.2)].

1 INDICATIONS AND USAGE

1.1 Analgesia (Pain)
Caldolor is indicated in adults for the management of mild to moderate pain and the management of moderate to severe pain as an adjunct to opioid analgesics.

1.2 Antipyretic (Fever)
Caldolor is indicated for the reduction of fever in adults.

2 DOSAGE AND ADMINISTRATION

Use the lowest effective dose for the shortest duration consistent with individual patient treatment goals [see Warnings and Precautions (5)]. After observing the response to initial therapy with Caldolor, the dose and frequency should be adjusted to suit an individual patient's needs. Do not exceed 3200 mg total daily dose.
To reduce the risk of renal adverse reactions, patients must be well hydrated prior to administration of Caldolor.

2.1 Analgesia (Pain)
Administer 400 mg to 800 mg intravenously every 6 hours as necessary. Infusion time must be no less than 30 minutes.

2.2 Antipyretic (Fever)
Administer 400 mg intravenously, followed by 400 mg every 4 to 6 hours or 100-200 mg every 4 hours as necessary. Infusion time must be no less than 30 minutes.

2.3 Preparation and Administration
Caldolor **must be diluted** prior to intravenous infusion. Dilute to a final concentration of 4 mg/mL or less. Appropriate diluents include 0.9% Sodium Chloride Injection USP (normal saline), 5% Dextrose Injection USP (D5W), or Lactated Ringers Solution.

- **800 mg dose:** Dilute 8 mL of Caldolor in no less than 200 mL of diluent.
- **400 mg dose:** Dilute 4 mL of Caldolor in no less than 100 mL of diluent.

Visually inspect parenteral drug products for particulate matter and discoloration prior to administration, whenever solution and container permit. If visibly opaque particles, discoloration or other foreign particulates are observed, the solution should not be used.
Diluted solutions are stable for up to 24 hours at ambient temperature (approximately 20 to 25° C) and room lighting. Infusion time must be no less than 30 minutes.

3 DOSAGE FORMS AND STRENGTHS

Caldolor is available as a 400 mg/4 mL single-dose vial (100 mg/mL) and 800 mg/8 mL single-dose vial (100 mg/mL).

4 CONTRAINDICATIONS

4.1 Hypersensitivity
Caldolor is contraindicated in patients with known hypersensitivity (e.g., anaphylactoid reactions and serious skin reactions) to ibuprofen [see Warnings and Precautions (5.7, 5.8)].

4.2 Asthma and Allergic Reactions
Caldolor is contraindicated in patients who have experienced asthma, urticaria, or allergic-type reactions after taking aspirin or other NSAIDs. Severe, rarely fatal anaphylactic-like reactions to NSAIDs have been reported in such patients [see Warnings and Precautions (5.7, 5.12)].

4.3 Coronary Artery Bypass Graft (CABG)
Caldolor is contraindicated for the treatment of perioperative pain in the setting of coronary artery bypass graft (CABG) surgery [see Warnings and Precautions (5.1)].

5 WARNINGS AND PRECAUTIONS

5.1 Cardiovascular Thrombotic Events
Clinical trials of several COX-2 selective and nonselective NSAIDs of up to three years duration have shown an increased risk of serious cardiovascular (CV) thrombotic events, myocardial infarction and stroke, which can be fatal. All NSAIDs, both COX-2 selective and nonselective, may have a similar risk. Patients with known CV disease or risk factors for CV disease may be at greater risk. To minimize the potential risk for an adverse CV event in patients treated with an NSAID, use the lowest effective dose for the shortest duration possible. Physicians and patients should remain alert for the development of such events, even in the absence of previous CV symptoms. Patients should be informed about the signs and/or symptoms of serious CV events and the steps to take if they occur.
Two large, controlled clinical trials of a COX-2 selective NSAID for the treatment of pain in the first 10-14 days following CABG surgery found an increased incidence of myocardial infarction and stroke [see Contraindications (4.3)].
There is no consistent evidence that concurrent use of aspirin mitigates the increased risk of serious CV thrombotic events associated with NSAID use. The concurrent use of aspirin and an NSAID does increase the risk of serious gastrointestinal (GI) events [see Warnings and Precautions (5.2)].

5.2 Gastrointestinal Effects: Risk of Ulceration, Bleeding, and Perforation
NSAIDs, including ibuprofen, can cause serious GI adverse events including inflammation, bleeding, ulceration, and perforation of the stomach, small intestine, or large intestine, which can be fatal. These serious adverse events can occur at any time, with or without warning symptoms, in patients treated with NSAIDs. Only one in five patients who develop a serious upper GI adverse event on NSAID therapy is symptomatic. Upper GI ulcers, gross bleeding, or perforation caused by NSAIDs occur in approximately 1% of patients treated for 3-6 months and in about 2-4% of patients treated for one year. These trends continue with longer duration of use, increasing the likelihood of developing a serious GI event at some time during the course of therapy. However, even short-term therapy is not without risk.
Prescribe NSAIDs, including Caldolor, with extreme caution in those with a prior history of ulcer disease or GI bleeding. Patients with a prior history of peptic ulcer disease and/or GI bleeding who use NSAIDs have a greater than 10-fold increased risk for developing a GI bleed compared to treated patients with neither of these risk factors. Other factors that increase the risk of GI bleeding in patients treated with NSAIDs include concomitant use of oral corticosteroids or anticoagulants, longer duration of NSAID therapy, smoking, use of alcohol, older age, and poor general health status. Most reports of spontaneous fatal GI events are in elderly or debilitated patients, and therefore special care should be taken in treating this population.
To minimize the potential risk for an adverse GI event in patients treated with an NSAID, use the lowest effective dose for the shortest possible duration. Patients and physicians should remain alert for signs and symptoms of GI ulcerations and bleeding during NSAID therapy and promptly initiate additional evaluation and treatment if a serious GI event is suspected. This should include discontinuation of the NSAID until a serious GI adverse event is ruled out. For high-risk patients, alternate therapies that do not involve NSAIDs should be considered.

5.3 Hepatic Effects
Borderline elevations of one or more liver tests may occur in up to 15% of patients taking NSAIDs, including ibuprofen. These laboratory abnormalities may progress, may remain unchanged, or may be transient with continuing therapy. Notable elevations of ALT or AST (approximately three or more times the upper limit of normal) have been reported in approximately 1% of patients in clinical trials with NSAIDs. In addition, rare cases of severe hepatic reactions have been reported, including jaundice, fulminant hepatitis, liver necrosis and hepatic failure, some with fatal outcomes. A patient with symptoms and/or signs suggesting liver dysfunction, or with abnormal liver test values, should be evaluated for evidence of the development of a more severe hepatic reaction while on therapy with ibuprofen. If clinical signs and symptoms consistent with liver disease develop, or if systemic manifestations occur (e.g., eosinophilia, rash, etc.), ibuprofen should be discontinued.

5.4 Hypertension
NSAIDs, including ibuprofen, can lead to onset of new hypertension or worsening of pre-existing hypertension, either of which may contribute to the increased incidence of CV events. Use NSAIDs, including ibuprofen, with caution in patients with hypertension. Monitor blood pressure closely during the initiation of NSAID treatment and throughout the course of therapy.
Patients taking ACE inhibitors, thiazides, or loop diuretics may have impaired response to these therapies when taking NSAIDs.

5.5 Congestive Heart Failure and Edema
Fluid retention and edema have been observed in some patients taking NSAIDs. Use Caldolor with caution in patients with fluid retention or heart failure.

5.6 Renal Effects
Use caution when initiating treatment with Caldolor in patients with considerable dehydration.
Long-term administration of NSAIDs has resulted in renal papillary necrosis and other renal injury. Renal toxicity has also been seen in patients in whom renal prostaglandins have a compensatory role in the maintenance of renal perfusion. In these patients, administration of an NSAID may cause a dose dependent reduction in prostaglandin formation and, secondarily, in renal blood flow, which may precipitate overt renal decompensation. Patients at greatest risk of this reaction are those with impaired renal function, heart failure, liver dysfunction, those taking diuretics or ACE inhibitors, and the elderly. Discontinuation of NSAID therapy is usually followed by recovery to the pretreatment state.
No information is available from controlled clinical studies regarding the use of Caldolor in patients with advanced re-

nal disease. If Caldolor therapy must be initiated in patients with advanced renal disease, closely monitor the patient's renal function.

5.7 Anaphylactoid Reactions

As with other NSAIDs, anaphylactoid reactions may occur in patients without known prior exposure to ibuprofen. Caldolor is contraindicated in patients with the aspirin triad. This symptom complex typically occurs in asthmatic patients who experience rhinitis with or without nasal polyps, or who exhibit severe, potentially fatal bronchospasm after taking aspirin or other NSAIDs [see Contraindications (4.2)].

5.8 Serious Skin Reactions

NSAIDs, including ibuprofen, can cause serious skin adverse reactions such as exfoliative dermatitis, Stevens-Johnson Syndrome (SJS), and toxic epidermal necrolysis (TEN), which can be fatal. These serious events may occur without warning. Inform patients about the signs and symptoms of serious skin manifestations, and to discontinue Caldolor at the first appearance of skin rash or any other sign of hypersensitivity.

5.9 Pregnancy

Starting at 30 weeks gestation, Caldolor, and other NSAIDs, should be avoided by pregnant women as premature closure of the ductus arteriosus in the fetus may occur [see Use in Specific Populations (8.1)].

5.10 Masking Inflammation and Fever

The pharmacological activity of ibuprofen in reducing fever and inflammation may diminish the utility of these diagnostic signs in detecting complications of presumed noninfectious, painful conditions.

5.11 Hematological Effects

Caldolor must be diluted prior to use. Infusion of the drug product without dilution can cause hemolysis [see Dosage and Administration (2.3)].

Anemia may occur in patients receiving NSAIDs, including ibuprofen. This may be due to fluid retention, occult or gross GI blood loss, or an incompletely described effect on erythropoiesis. In patients on long-term treatment with NSAIDs, including ibuprofen, check hemoglobin or hematocrit if they exhibit any signs or symptoms of anemia or blood loss.

NSAIDs inhibit platelet aggregation and have been shown to prolong bleeding time in some patients. Unlike aspirin, their effects on platelet function are less severe quantitatively, of shorter duration, and reversible. Carefully monitor patients who may be adversely affected by alterations in platelet function, such as those with coagulation disorders or patients receiving anticoagulants.

5.12 Pre-existing Asthma

Patients with asthma may have aspirin-sensitive asthma. The use of aspirin in patients with aspirin-sensitive asthma has been associated with severe bronchospasm, which can be fatal. Since cross-reactivity between aspirin and NSAIDs has been reported in such aspirin-sensitive patients, including bronchospasm, Caldolor is contraindicated in patients with this form of aspirin sensitivity and should be used with caution in all patients with pre-existing asthma.

5.13 Ophthalmological Effects

Blurred or diminished vision, scotomata, and changes in color vision have been reported with oral ibuprofen. Discontinue ibuprofen if a patient develops such complaints, and refer the patient for an ophthalmologic examination that includes central visual fields and color vision testing.

5.14 Aseptic Meningitis

Aseptic meningitis with fever and coma has been observed in patients on oral ibuprofen therapy. Although it is probably more likely to occur in patients with systemic lupus erythematosus and related connective tissue diseases, it has been reported in patients who do not have underlying chronic disease. If signs or symptoms of meningitis develop in a patient on ibuprofen, give consideration to whether or not the signs or symptoms are related to ibuprofen therapy.

5.15 Monitoring

Because serious GI tract ulcerations and bleeding can occur without warning symptoms, physicians should monitor for signs or symptoms of GI bleeding.

Patients on long-term treatment with NSAIDs should have CBC and chemistry profiles checked periodically. If clinical signs and symptoms consistent with liver or renal disease develop, systemic manifestations occur (e.g., eosinophilia, rash), or abnormal liver tests persist or worsen, discontinue Caldolor.

6 ADVERSE REACTIONS

The following serious adverse reactions are discussed elsewhere in the labeling:

- Cardiovascular thrombotic events [see Boxed Warning and Warnings and Precautions (5.1)]
- Gastrointestinal effects [see Boxed Warning and Warnings and Precautions (5.2)]
- Hepatic effects [see Warnings and Precautions (5.3)]
- Hypertension [see Warnings and Precautions (5.4)]
- Congestive heart failure and edema [see Warnings and Precautions (5.5)]
- Renal effects [see Warnings and Precautions (5.6)]
- Anaphylactoid reactions [see Warnings and Precautions (5.7)]
- Serious skin reactions [see Warnings and Precautions (5.8)]

The most common adverse reactions reported in clinical studies are nausea, flatulence, vomiting, and headache.

The most common reason for discontinuation due to adverse events in controlled trials of Caldolor is pruritus (<1%).

6.1 Clinical Studies Experience

Because clinical trials are conducted under widely varying conditions, adverse reaction rates observed in the clinical trials of a drug cannot be compared directly to rates in the clinical trials of another drug and may not reflect the rates observed in practice.

During clinical development, 560 patients were exposed to Caldolor, 438 in pain and 122 with fever. In the pain studies, Caldolor was started intra-operatively and administered at a dose of 400 mg or 800 mg every six hours for up to three days. In the fever studies, Caldolor was administered at doses of 100 mg, 200 mg, or 400 mg every four or six hours for up to 3 days.

The most frequent type of adverse reaction occurring with oral ibuprofen is gastrointestinal.

Table 1: Post-operative Patients with Adverse Reactions Observed in ≥ 3% of Patients in any Caldolor Treatment Group in Pain Studies*

Event	Caldolor 400 mg (N=134)	Caldolor 800 mg (N=304)	Placebo (N=287)
Any Reaction	118 (88%)	260 (86%)	258 (90%)
Nausea	77 (57%)	161 (53%)	179 (62%)
Vomiting	30 (22%)	46 (15%)	50 (17%)
Flatulence	10 (7%)	49 (16%)	44 (15%)
Headache	12 (9%)	35 (12%)	31 (11%)
Hemorrhage	13 (10%)	13 (4%)	16 (6%)
Dizziness	8 (6%)	13 (4%)	5 (2%)
Edema peripheral	1 (<1%)	9 (3%)	4 (1%)
Urinary retention	7 (5%)	10 (3%)	10 (3%)
Anemia	5 (4%)	7 (2%)	6 (2%)
Decreased hemoglobin	4 (3%)	6 (2%)	3 (1%)
Dyspepsia	6 (4%)	4 (1%)	2 (<1%)
Wound hemorrhage	4 (3%)	4 (1%)	4 (1%)
Abdominal discomfort	4 (3%)	2 (<1%)	0
Cough	4 (3%)	2 (<1%)	1 (<1%)
Hypokalemia	5 (4%)	3 (<1%)	8 (3%)

*All patients received concomitant morphine during these studies.

Table 2: Patients with Adverse Reactions Observed in ≥ 3% of Patients in any Caldolor Treatment Group in All-Cause Fever Study

Event	Caldolor 100 mg N=30	Caldolor 200 mg N=30	Caldolor 400 mg N=31	Placebo N=28
Any Reaction	27 (87%)	25 (83%)	23 (74%)	25 (89%)
Anemia	5 (17%)	6 (20%)	11 (36%)	4 (14%)
Eosinophilia	7 (23%)	7 (23%)	8 (26%)	7 (25%)
Hypokalemia	4 (13%)	4 (13%)	6 (19%)	5 (18%)
Hypoproteinemia	3 (10%)	0	4 (13%)	2 (7%)
Neutropenia	2 (7%)	2 (7%)	4 (13%)	2 (7%)
Blood urea increased	0	0	3 (10%)	0
Hypernatremia	2 (7%)	0	3 (10%)	0
Hypertension	0	0	3 (10%)	0
Hypoalbuminemia	3 (10%)	1 (3%)	3 (10%)	1 (4%)
Hypotension	0	2 (7%)	3 (10%)	1 (4%)
Diarrhea	3 (10%)	3 (10%)	2 (7%)	2 (7%)
Pneumonia bacterial	3 (10%)	1 (3%)	2 (7%)	0
Blood LDH increased	3 (10%)	2 (7%)	1 (3%)	1 (4%)
Thrombocythemia	3 (10%)	2 (7%)	1 (3%)	0
Bacteremia	4 (13%)	0	0	0

Table 3: Pharmacokinetic Parameters of Intravenous Ibuprofen

	400 mg* Caldolor Mean (CV%)	800 mg* Caldolor Mean (CV%)
Number of Patients	12	12
AUC (mcg.h/mL)	109.3 (26.4)	192.8 (18.5)
Cmax (mcg/mL)	39.2 (15.5)	72.6 (13.2)
KEL (1/h)	0.32 (17.9)	0.29 (12.8)
$T_{1/2}$ (h)	2.22 (20.1)	2.44 (12.9)

AUC = Area-under-the-curve
Cmax = Peak plasma concentration
CV = Coefficient of Variation
KEL = First-order elimination rate constant
$T_{1/2}$ = Elimination half-life
* = 60 minute infusion time

Pain Studies
The incidence rates of adverse reactions listed in the following table were derived from multi-center, controlled clinical studies in post-operative patients comparing Caldolor to placebo in patients also receiving morphine as needed for post-operative pain.
[See table 1 at top of previous page]
Fever Studies
Fever studies were conducted in febrile hospitalized patients with malaria and febrile hospitalized patients with varying causes of fever. In hospitalized febrile patients with malaria, the adverse reactions observed in at least two Caldolor-treated patients included abdominal pain and nasal congestion.
In hospitalized febrile patients (all causes), adverse reactions observed in more than two patients in any given treatment group are presented in the table below.
[See table 2 on previous page]

7 DRUG INTERACTIONS
7.1 Aspirin
When ibuprofen is administered with aspirin, ibuprofen's protein binding is reduced, although the clearance of free ibuprofen is not altered. The clinical significance of this interaction is not known; however, as with other NSAIDs, concomitant administration of Caldolor and aspirin is not generally recommended because of the potential for increased adverse effects.
7.2 Anticoagulants
The effects of warfarin and NSAIDs on GI bleeding are synergistic, such that the users of both drugs together have a higher risk of serious GI bleeding than users of either drug alone [see Warnings and Precautions (5.2)].
7.3 ACE Inhibitors
NSAIDs may diminish the antihypertensive effect of ACE inhibitors. This interaction should be given consideration in patients taking NSAIDs concomitantly with ACE inhibitors.
7.4 Diuretics
Clinical studies and postmarketing observations have shown that ibuprofen can reduce the natriuretic effects of furosemide and thiazides in some patients. This response has been attributed to inhibition of renal prostaglandin synthesis. During concomitant therapy with NSAIDs, observe patients closely for signs of renal failure, as well as to assure diuretic efficacy [see Warnings and Precautions (5.6)].
7.5 Lithium
NSAIDs have produced elevations of plasma lithium levels and a reduction in renal lithium clearance. The mean minimum lithium concentration increased 15%, and the renal clearance of lithium decreased by 20%. This effect has been attributed to inhibition of renal prostaglandin synthesis by the NSAID. Thus, when NSAIDs and lithium are administered concurrently, observe patients carefully for signs of lithium toxicity.
7.6 Methotrexate
NSAIDs have been reported to competitively inhibit methotrexate accumulation in rabbit kidney slices. This indicates that NSAIDs may enhance the toxicity of methotrexate. Use caution when NSAIDs are administered concomitantly with methotrexate.
7.7 H-2 Antagonists
In studies of human volunteers, co-administration of cimetidine or ranitidine with ibuprofen had no substantive effect on ibuprofen serum concentrations.

8 USE IN SPECIFIC POPULATIONS
8.1 Pregnancy
Teratogenic effects — Pregnancy Category C prior to 30 weeks gestation; Category D starting at 30 weeks gestation. Starting at 30 weeks gestation, Caldolor, and other NSAIDs, should be avoided by pregnant women as premature closure of the ductus arteriosus in the fetus may occur. Caldolor can cause fetal harm when administered to a pregnant woman starting at 30 weeks gestation.
There are no adequate, well-controlled studies in pregnant women. Prior to 30 weeks gestation, Caldolor should be used during pregnancy only if the potential benefit justifies the potential risk to the fetus.
Reproductive studies conducted in rats and rabbits have not demonstrated evidence of developmental abnormalities.
8.2 Labor and Delivery
The effects of Caldolor on labor and delivery in pregnant women are unknown. In rat studies, maternal exposure to NSAIDs, as with other drugs known to inhibit prostaglandin synthesis, increased the incidence of dystocia and delayed parturition, and decreased pup survival.
8.3 Nursing Mothers
It is not known whether this drug is excreted in human milk. Because many drugs are excreted in human milk and because of the potential for serious adverse reactions in nursing infants from Caldolor, a decision should be made whether to discontinue nursing or discontinue the drug, taking into account the importance of the drug to the mother.
8.4 Pediatric Use
Safety and effectiveness of Caldolor for management of pain and reduction of fever has not been established in pediatric patients below the age of 17 years.
8.5 Geriatric Use
Clinical studies of Caldolor did not include sufficient numbers of subjects aged 65 and over to determine whether they respond differently from younger subjects. Dose selection for an elderly patient should be cautious, usually starting at the low end of the dosing range, reflecting the greater frequency of decreased hepatic, renal, or cardiac function, and of concomitant disease or other drug therapy. Elderly patients are at increased risk for serious GI adverse events.

10 OVERDOSAGE
The following signs and symptoms have occurred in individuals following an overdose of oral ibuprofen: abdominal pain, nausea, vomiting, drowsiness, and dizziness. There are no specific measures to treat acute overdosage with Caldolor. There is no known antidote to ibuprofen. In case of an overdosage, discontinue Caldolor therapy and consider contacting a regional poison control center at 1-800-222-1222.

11 DESCRIPTION
Caldolor contains the active ingredient ibuprofen, which is (±)-2-(p-isobutylphenyl) propionic acid. Ibuprofen is a white powder with a melting point of 74-77°C. It has a molecular weight of 206.28. It is very slightly soluble in water (<1 mg/mL) and readily soluble in organic solvents such as ethanol and acetone. The structural formula of ibuprofen is represented below:

$$H_3C-HC-CH_2- -CH(CH_3)-COOH$$

Each 1 mL of solution contains 100 mg of ibuprofen in Water for Injection, USP. The product also contains 78 mg/mL arginine at a molar ratio of 0.92:1 arginine:ibuprofen. The solution pH is about 7.4.
Caldolor is sterile and is intended for intravenous administration only.

12 CLINICAL PHARMACOLOGY
12.1 Mechanism of Action
Ibuprofen's mechanism of action, like that of other NSAIDs, is not completely understood but may be related to prostaglandin synthetase inhibition. Caldolor possesses anti-inflammatory, analgesic, and antipyretic activity.
12.3 Pharmacokinetics
Ibuprofen is a racemic mixture of [-]R- and [+]S-isomers. In vivo and in vitro studies indicate that the [+]S-isomer is responsible for clinical activity. The [-]R-form, while thought to be pharmacologically inactive, is slowly and incompletely (~60%) interconverted into the active [+]S species in adults. The [-]R-isomer serves as a circulating reservoir to maintain levels of active drug. The pharmacokinetic parameters of Caldolor determined in a study with volunteers are presented below.
[See table 3 at left]
Ibuprofen, like most NSAIDs, is highly protein bound (>99% bound at 20 mcg/mL). Protein binding is saturable, and at concentrations >20 mcg/mL binding is nonlinear. Based on oral dosing data, there is an age- or fever-related change in volume of distribution for ibuprofen.

14 CLINICAL STUDIES
14.1 Analgesia (Pain)
The effect of Caldolor on acute pain was evaluated in two multi-center, randomized, double-blind, placebo-controlled studies.
In a study of women who had undergone an elective abdominal hysterectomy, 319 patients were randomized and treated with Caldolor 800 mg or placebo administered every 6 hours (started intra-operatively) and morphine administered on an as needed basis. Efficacy was demonstrated as a statistically significant greater reduction in the mean morphine consumption through 24 hours in patients who received Caldolor as compared to those receiving placebo (47 mg and 56 mg, respectively). The clinical relevance of this finding is supported by a greater reduction in pain intensity over 24 hours for patients treated with Caldolor, even though morphine was available on an as needed basis.
In a study of patients who had undergone an elective abdominal or orthopedic surgery, 406 patients (87 men, 319 women) were randomized to receive Caldolor 400 mg, Caldolor 800 mg, or placebo administered every 6 hours (started intra-operatively), and morphine on an as needed basis. This study failed to demonstrate a statistically significant difference in outcome between patients receiving Caldolor 800 mg or 400 mg and placebo, although there were trends favoring the active treatments.
14.2 Antipyretic (Fever)
The effect of Caldolor on fever was evaluated in two randomized, double-blind studies.
In a multi-center study, 120 hospitalized patients (88 men, 32 women) with temperatures of 101°F or greater were randomized to Caldolor 400 mg, 200 mg, 100 mg or placebo, administered every 4 hours for 24 hours. Each of the three Caldolor doses, 100 mg, 200 mg, and 400 mg, resulted in a statistically greater percentage of patients with a reduced temperature (<101°F) after 4 hours, compared to placebo (65%, 73%, 77% and 32%, respectively). The dose response is shown in the figure below.

Figure 1: Temperature Reduction by Treatment Group, Hospitalized Febrile Patients

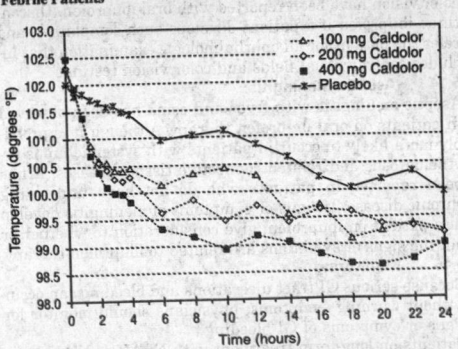

In a single-center study, 60 hospitalized patients (48 men, 12 women) with uncomplicated *P. falciparum* malaria having temperatures ≥100.4°F were randomized to Caldolor 400 mg or placebo, administered every 6 hours for 72 hours of treatment. There was a significant reduction in fever within the first 24 hours of treatment, measured as the area above the temperature 98.6°F vs. time curve for patients treated with Caldolor.

16 HOW SUPPLIED/STORAGE AND HANDLING
Caldolor is available in the following strengths:
400 mg/4 mL (100 mg/mL)
Carton of 25 vials, NDC 66220-247-04
800 mg/8 mL (100 mg/mL)
Carton of 25 vials, NDC 66220-287-08
Store at controlled room temperature 20° to 25°C (68° to 77°F) [see USP].

The stopper in the Caldolor vial does not contain natural rubber latex, dry natural rubber, or blends of natural rubber.

17 PATIENT COUNSELING INFORMATION

Patients should be informed of the following information before initiating therapy with an NSAID.

17.1 Cardiovascular Effects

Ibuprofen, like other NSAIDs, may cause serious CV events such as myocardial infarction or stroke, which may result in hospitalization and even death. Although serious CV events can occur without warning symptoms, advise patients to be alert for the signs and symptoms of chest pain, shortness of breath, weakness, and slurring of speech, and to ask for medical advice when observing any indicative sign or symptoms. Inform patients of the importance of this follow-up [see Warnings and Precautions (5.1)].

17.2 Gastrointestinal Effects

Ibuprofen, like other NSAIDs, can cause GI discomfort and, rarely, serious GI side effects such as ulcers and bleeding, which may result in hospitalization and even death. Although serious GI tract ulcerations and bleeding can occur without warning symptoms, advise patients to be alert for the signs and symptoms of ulcerations and bleeding, and to ask for medical advice when observing any indicative signs or symptoms including epigastric pain, dyspepsia, melena, and hematemesis. Inform patients of the importance of this follow-up [see Warnings and Precautions (5.2)].

17.3 Hepatotoxicity

Inform patients of the warning signs and symptoms of hepatotoxicity (e.g., nausea, fatigue, lethargy, pruritus, jaundice, right upper quadrant tenderness, and "flulike" symptoms). Instruct patients to stop therapy with Caldolor and seek immediate medical therapy if any of these occur [see Warnings and Precautions (5.3)].

17.4 Adverse Skin Reactions

Ibuprofen, like other NSAIDs, can cause serious skin side effects such as exfoliative dermatitis, SJS and TEN, which may result in hospitalization and even death. Although serious skin reactions may occur without warning, advise patients to be alert for the signs and symptoms of skin rash and blisters, fever, or other signs of hypersensitivity such as itching, and to ask for medical advice when observing any indicative sign or symptoms. Advise patients to stop Caldolor immediately if they develop any type of rash, and to contact a physician as soon as possible [see Warnings and Precautions (5.8)].

17.5 Weight Gain and Edema

Advise patients to promptly report to their physicians signs or symptoms of unexplained weight gain or edema during treatment with Caldolor [see Warnings and Precautions (5.5)].

17.6 Anaphylactoid Reactions

Inform patients of the signs of an anaphylactoid reaction (e.g. difficulty in breathing, swelling of the face or throat). If these occur, therapy should be discontinued and medical therapy initiated [see Warnings and Precautions (5.7)].

17.7 Effects During Pregnancy

Starting at 30 weeks gestation, Caldolor and other NSAIDs should be avoided by pregnant women as premature closure of the ductus arteriosus in the fetus may occur [see Use in Specific Populations (8.1)].
Manufactured for:
Cumberland Pharmaceuticals Inc.
Nashville, TN 37203
US Patent Number 6,727,286
Shown in Product Identification Guide, page 308

KRISTALOSE®
[krĭs' tă lōsĕ]
(LACTULOSE)
For Oral Solution

℞

DESCRIPTION

KRISTALOSE® (LACTULOSE) is a synthetic disaccharide in the form of crystals for reconstitution prior to use for oral administration. Each 10 g of lactulose contains less than 0.3 g galactose and lactose as a total sum. The pH range is 3.0 to 7.0.
Lactulose is a colonic acidifier which promotes laxation.
The chemical name for lactulose is 4-O-β-D-Galactopyranosyl-D-fructofuranose. It has the following structural formula:

The molecular formula is $C_{12}H_{22}O_{11}$. The molecular weight is 342.30. It is freely soluble in water.

CLINICAL PHARMACOLOGY

KRISTALOSE® (LACTULOSE) is poorly absorbed from the gastrointestinal tract and no enzyme capable of hydrolysis of this disaccharide is present in human gastrointestinal tissue. As a result, oral doses of lactulose reach the colon virtually unchanged. In the colon, lactulose is broken down primarily to lactic acid, and also to small amounts of formic and acetic acids, by the action of colonic bacteria, which results in an increase in osmotic pressure and slight acidification of the colonic contents. This in turn causes an increase in stool water content and softens the stool.
Since lactulose does not exert its effect until it reaches the colon, and since transit time through the colon may be slow, 24 to 48 hours may be required to produce desired bowel movement.
Lactulose given orally to man and experimental animals resulted in only small amounts reaching the blood. Urinary excretion has been determined to be 3% or less and is essentially complete within 24 hours.

INDICATIONS AND USAGE

KRISTALOSE® (LACTULOSE) For Oral Solution is indicated for the treatment of constipation. In patients with a history of chronic constipation, lactulose therapy increases the number of bowel movements per day and the number of days on which bowel movements occur.

CONTRAINDICATIONS

Since KRISTALOSE® (LACTULOSE) For Oral Solution contains galactose (less than 0.3 g/10 g as a total sum with lactose), it is contraindicated in patients who require a low galactose diet.

WARNINGS

A theoretical hazard may exist for patients being treated with lactulose who may be required to undergo electrocautery procedures during proctoscopy or colonoscopy. Accumulation of H_2 gas in significant concentration in the presence of an electrical spark may result in an explosive reaction. Although this complication has not been reported with lactulose, patients on lactulose therapy undergoing such procedures should have a thorough bowel cleansing with a non-fermentable solution. Insufflation of CO_2 as an additional safeguard may be pursued but is considered to be a redundant measure.

PRECAUTIONS

General
Since KRISTALOSE® (LACTULOSE) For Oral Solution contains galactose and lactose (less than 0.3 g/10 g as a total sum), it should be used with caution in diabetics.
Information for Patients
In the event that an unusual diarrheal condition occurs, contact your physician.
Laboratory Tests
Elderly, debilitated patients who receive lactulose for more than six months should have serum electrolytes (potassium, chloride, carbon dioxide) measured periodically.
Drug Interactions
Results of preliminary studies in humans and rats suggest that nonabsorbable antacids given concurrently with lactulose may inhibit the desired lactulose-induced drop in colonic pH. Therefore, a possible lack of desired effect of treatment should be taken into consideration before such drugs are given concomitantly with lactulose.
Carcinogenesis, Mutagenesis, Impairment of Fertility
There are no known human data on long-term potential for carcinogenicity, mutagenicity, or impairment of fertility. There are no known animal data on long-term potential for mutagenicity.
Administration of lactulose syrup in the diet of mice for 18 months in concentrations of 3 and 10 percent (v/w) did not produce any evidence of carcinogenicity.
In studies in mice, rats, and rabbits, doses of lactulose syrup up to 6 or 12 mL/kg/day produced no deleterious effects in breeding, conception, or parturition.
Pregnancy
Teratogenic Effects
Pregnancy Category B
Reproduction studies have been performed in mice, rats, and rabbits at doses up to 3 or 6 times the usual human oral dose and have revealed no evidence of impaired fertility or harm to the fetus due to lactulose. There are, however, no adequate and well-controlled studies in pregnant women. Because animal reproduction studies are not always predictive of human response, this drug should be used during pregnancy only if clearly needed.
Nursing Mothers
It is not known whether this drug is excreted in human milk. Because many drugs are excreted in human milk, caution should be exercised when lactulose is administered to a nursing woman.
Pediatric Use
Safety and effectiveness in pediatric patients have not been established.

ADVERSE REACTIONS

Precise frequency data are not available.
Initial dosing may produce flatulence and intestinal cramps, which are usually transient. Excessive dosage can lead to diarrhea with potential complications such as loss of fluids, hypokalemia, and hypernatremia.
Nausea and vomiting have been reported.

OVERDOSAGE

Signs and Symptoms
There have been no reports of accidental overdosage. In the event of overdosage, it is expected that diarrhea and abdominal cramps would be the major symptoms. Medication should be terminated.
Oral LD_{50}
The acute oral LD_{50} of the drug is 48.8 mL/kg in mice and greater than 30 mL/kg in rats.
Dialysis
Dialysis data are not available for lactulose. Its molecular similarity to sucrose, however, would suggest that it should be dialyzable.

DOSAGE AND ADMINISTRATION

The usual adult dosage is 10 g to 20 g of lactulose daily. The dose may be increased to 40 g daily if necessary. Twenty-four to 48 hours may be required to produce a normal bowel movement.

DIRECTIONS FOR PREPARATION

Dissolve contents of packet in half a glass (4 ounces) of water.
When Lactulose For Oral Solution is dissolved in water, the resulting solution may be colorless to a slightly pale yellow color.

HOW SUPPLIED

KRISTALOSE® (LACTULOSE) For Oral Solution is available in single dose packets of 10 g (NDC 66220-719-01) and single dose packets of 20 g (NDC 66220-729-01). The packets are supplied as follows:
NDC 66220-719-30 (Carton of thirty 10 g packets)
NDC 66220-729-30 (Carton of thirty 20 g packets)
STORE AT ROOM TEMPERATURE, 15°–30°C (59°–86°F).
To report adverse events associated with this product, please call 1-877-484-2700.
www.kristalose.com
Distributed by
CUMBERLAND PHARMACEUTICALS INC.
Nashville, TN 37203
Manufactured by
Inalco S.p.A.
Milan, Italy

LB1700406
Issued: May 2008
1108.2
Shown in Product Identification Guide, page 308

Dermik Laboratories
For product information, please see
The sanofi-aventis Group

Eisai Inc.
100 TICE BOULEVARD
WOODCLIFF LAKE, NJ 07677

Direct Inquiries to:
Eisai Medical Services
1 (888) 274-2378
(888) 422-4743
(877) 873-4724
FAX: (201) 746-3207
For Reporting Adverse Events:
Medical Emergencies:
24 hours/day, 7 days/week
1 (888) 274-2378
FAX: 201-746-3207

ACIPHEX®
[a-se-feks]
(rabeprazole sodium)
Delayed-Release Tablets

℞

HIGHLIGHTS OF PRESCRIBING INFORMATION
These highlights do not include all the information needed to use ACIPHEX safely and effectively. See full prescribing information for ACIPHEX.
ACIPHEX® (rabeprazole sodium) Delayed Release Tablets
Initial U.S. Approval: 1999

RECENT MAJOR CHANGES

Indications and Usage (1.3)
Dosage and Administration, Pediatric Patients (2.7)
Use in Specific Populations, Pediatric Use (8.4) June/2008

INDICATIONS AND USAGE

ACIPHEX is a proton-pump inhibitor indicated in adults for:
- Healing of Erosive or Ulcerative Gastroesophageal Reflux Disease (GERD) (1.1)
- Maintenance of Healing of Erosive or Ulcerative GERD (1.2)
- Treatment of Symptomatic GERD (1.3)
- Healing of Duodenal Ulcers (1.4)
- *Helicobacter pylori* Eradication to Reduce the Risk of Duodenal Ulcer Recurrence (1.5)
- Treatment of Pathological Hypersecretory Conditions, Including Zollinger-Ellison Syndrome (1.6)

ACIPHEX is a proton-pump inhibitor indicated for adolescent patients 12 years of age and above for:
- Short-term treatment of Symptomatic GERD (1.3)

DOSAGE AND ADMINISTRATION

ACIPHEX tablets should be swallowed whole. The tablets should not be chewed, crushed or split.

Healing of Erosive or Ulcerative Gastroesophageal Reflux Disease (GERD) (2.1)	20 mg once daily
Maintenance of Healing of Erosive or Ulcerative GERD (2.2)	20 mg once daily
Treatment of Symptomatic GERD (2.3)	20 mg once daily
Healing of Duodenal Ulcers (2.4)	20 mg once daily after morning meal
Helicobacter pylori Eradication to Reduce the Risk of Duodenal Ulcer Recurrence (2.5) Three Drug Regimen: ACIPHEX 20 mg Amoxicillin 1000 mg Clarithromycin 500 mg	*All three medications should be taken twice daily with morning and evening meals for 7 days*
Treatment of Pathological Hypersecretory Conditions, Including Zollinger-Ellison Syndrome (2.6)	Starting dose 60 mg once daily then adjust to patient needs
Short-term Treatment of GERD in Adolescent Patients 12 Years of Age and Above (2.7)	20 mg once daily for up to 8 weeks

DOSAGE FORMS AND STRENGTHS
- Tablets: 20 mg (3)

CONTRAINDICATIONS
- History of hypersensitivity to rabeprazole (4.1)

WARNINGS AND PRECAUTIONS
- Symptomatic response to therapy with rabeprazole does not preclude the presence of gastric malignancy. (5.4)
- Patients treated with a proton pump inhibitor and warfarin may need to be monitored for increases in INR and prothrombin time due to risk of abnormal bleeding (5.5)

ADVERSE REACTIONS
- In the adult studies (4 to 8 weeks), there are no adverse reactions that occur at a rate greater than 5% and greater than placebo (6.1)
- In the adolescent patient studies, adverse reactions were similar to those found in adults (6.1)

To report SUSPECTED ADVERSE REACTIONS, contact Eisai Inc. at 1-888-274-2378 (fax 1-201-746-3207) or FDA at 1-800-FDA-1088 or www.fda.gov/medwatch

DRUG INTERACTIONS
- Increased INR and prothrombin times have been reported with concomitant use with warfarin. Patients need to be monitored (7.2)
- Rabeprazole has been shown to inhibit cyclosporine metabolism *in vitro* (7.3)
- ACIPHEX inhibits gastric acid secretion and may interfere with the absorption of drugs where gastric pH is an important determinant of bioavailability (e.g., ketoconazole, iron salts and digoxin) (7.4)
- ACIPHEX may reduce the plasma levels of atazanavir (7.4)

USE IN SPECIFIC POPULATIONS
- The safety and efficacy of ACIPHEX for GERD have not been established for pediatric patients less than 12 years of age.
- The safety and efficacy of ACIPHEX for the other adult indications have not been established for pediatric patients.

See 17 for PATIENT COUNSELING INFORMATION

Revised: January/2009

FULL PRESCRIBING INFORMATION: CONTENTS*

FULL PRESCRIBING INFORMATION

1. INDICATIONS AND USAGE

1.1. Healing of Erosive or Ulcerative GERD
ACIPHEX is indicated for short-term (4 to 8 weeks) treatment in the healing and symptomatic relief of erosive or ulcerative gastroesophageal reflux disease (GERD). For those patients who have not healed after 8 weeks of treatment, an additional 8-week course of ACIPHEX may be considered.

1.2. Maintenance of Healing of Erosive or Ulcerative GERD
ACIPHEX is indicated for maintaining healing and reduction in relapse rates of heartburn symptoms in patients with erosive or ulcerative gastroesophageal reflux disease (GERD Maintenance). Controlled studies do not extend beyond 12 months.

1.3. Treatment of Symptomatic GERD
ACIPHEX is indicated for the treatment of daytime and nighttime heartburn and other symptoms associated with GERD in adults and adolescents 12 years of age and above.

1.4. Healing of Duodenal Ulcers
ACIPHEX is indicated for short-term (up to four weeks) treatment in the healing and symptomatic relief of duodenal ulcers. Most patients heal within four weeks.

1.5. *Helicobacter pylori* Eradication to Reduce the Risk of Duodenal Ulcer Recurrence
ACIPHEX in combination with amoxicillin and clarithromycin as a three drug regimen, is indicated for the treatment of patients with *H. pylori* infection and duodenal ulcer disease (active or history within the past 5 years) to eradicate *H. pylori*. Eradication of *H. pylori* has been shown to reduce the risk of duodenal ulcer recurrence. [See CLINICAL STUDIES (14.5) and DOSAGE AND ADMINISTRATION (2.5)].
In patients who fail therapy, susceptibility testing should be done. If resistance to clarithromycin is demonstrated or susceptibility testing is not possible, alternative antimicrobial therapy should be instituted. [See CLINICAL PHARMACOLOGY, Microbiology (12.2) and the clarithromycin package insert, CLINICAL PHARMACOLOGY, Microbiology.]

1.6. Treatment of Pathological Hypersecretory Conditions, Including Zollinger-Ellison Syndrome
ACIPHEX is indicated for the long-term treatment of pathological hypersecretory conditions, including Zollinger-Ellison syndrome.

2. DOSAGE AND ADMINISTRATION
ACIPHEX tablets should be swallowed whole. The tablets should not be chewed, crushed, or split. ACIPHEX can be taken with or without food.

2.1. Healing of Erosive or Ulcerative GERD
The recommended adult oral dose is one ACIPHEX 20 mg delayed-release tablet to be taken once daily for four to eight weeks. [See INDICATIONS AND USAGE (1.1)]. For those patients who have not healed after 8 weeks of treatment, an additional 8-week course of ACIPHEX may be considered.

2.2. Maintenance of Healing of Erosive or Ulcerative GERD
The recommended adult oral dose is one ACIPHEX 20 mg delayed-release tablet to be taken once daily. [See INDICATIONS AND USAGE (1.2)].

2.3. Treatment of Symptomatic GERD
The recommended adult oral dose is one ACIPHEX 20 mg delayed-release tablet to be taken once daily for 4 weeks. [See INDICATIONS AND USAGE (1.3)]. If symptoms do not resolve completely after 4 weeks, an additional course of treatment may be considered. The recommended adolescent dosing is listed in Section 2.7.

2.4. Healing of Duodenal Ulcers
The recommended adult oral dose is one ACIPHEX 20 mg delayed-release tablet to be taken once daily after the morning meal for a period up to four weeks. [See INDICATIONS AND USAGE (1.4)]. Most patients with duodenal ulcer heal within four weeks. A few patients may require additional therapy to achieve healing.

2.5. *Helicobacter pylori* Eradication to Reduce the Risk of Duodenal Ulcer Recurrence

TABLE 1
THREE DRUG REGIMEN[a]

ACIPHEX	20 mg	Twice Daily for 7 Days
Amoxicillin	1000 mg	Twice Daily for 7 Days
Clarithromycin	500 mg	Twice Daily for 7 Days

All three medications should be taken twice daily with the morning and evening meals.
[a] It is important that patients comply with the full 7-day regimen. [See CLINICAL STUDIES section (14.5)].

2.6. Treatment of Pathological Hypersecretory Conditions, Including Zollinger-Ellison Syndrome
The dosage of ACIPHEX in patients with pathologic hypersecretory conditions varies with the individual patient. The recommended adult oral starting dose is 60 mg once a day. Doses should be adjusted to individual patient needs and should continue for as long as clinically indicated. Some patients may require divided doses. Doses up to

100 mg QD and 60 mg BID have been administered. Some patients with Zollinger-Ellison syndrome have been treated continuously with ACIPHEX for up to one year.

2.7. Short-term Treatment of GERD in Adolescent Patients 12 Years of Age and Above

The recommended oral dose for adolescents 12 years of age and above is 20 mg once daily for up to 8 weeks [See *Pediatric Use* (8.4)].

2.8. Elderly, Renal and Hepatic Impaired Patients

No dosage adjustment is necessary in elderly patients, in patients with renal disease or in patients with mild to moderate hepatic impairment. Administration of rabeprazole to patients with mild to moderate liver impairment resulted in increased exposure and decreased elimination. Due to the lack of clinical data on rabeprazole in patients with severe hepatic impairment, caution should be exercised in those patients.

3. DOSAGE FORMS AND STRENGTHS

20 mg light yellow enteric-coated delayed release tablets. The name and strength, in mg, (ACIPHEX 20) is imprinted on one side.

4. CONTRAINDICATIONS

4.1. Hypersensitivity to rabeprazole

Rabeprazole is contraindicated in patients with known hypersensitivity to rabeprazole, substituted benzimidazoles or to any component of the formulation.

4.2. Use of Clarithromycin and hypersensitivity to macrolide antibiotics

Clarithromycin is contraindicated in patients with known hypersensitivity to any macrolide antibiotic.

4.3. Concomitant use of Clarithromycin with pimozide and cisapride

Concomitant administration of clarithromycin with pimozide and cisapride is contraindicated. There have been postmarketing reports of drug interactions when clarithromycin and/or erythromycin are co-administered with pimozide resulting in cardiac arrhythmias (QT prolongation, ventricular tachycardia, ventricular fibrillation, and torsade de pointes) most likely due to inhibition of hepatic metabolism of pimozide by erythromycin and clarithromycin. Fatalities have been reported. (Please refer to full prescribing information for clarithromycin.)

4.4. Amoxicillin and hypersensitivity to penicillin

Amoxicillin is contraindicated in patients with a known hypersensitivity to any penicillin. (Please refer to full prescribing information for amoxicillin.)

5. WARNINGS AND PRECAUTIONS

5.1. Clarithromycin use in pregnant women

CLARITHROMYCIN SHOULD NOT BE USED IN PREGNANT WOMEN EXCEPT IN CLINICAL CIRCUMSTANCES WHERE NO ALTERNATIVE THERAPY IS APPROPRIATE.

If pregnancy occurs while taking clarithromycin, the patient should be apprised of the potential hazard to the fetus. (See *WARNINGS* in prescribing information for clarithromycin.)

5.2. Anaphylactic reactions associated with antibiotic use

Amoxicillin:

Serious and occasionally fatal hypersensitivity (anaphylactic) reactions have been reported in patients on penicillin therapy. These reactions are more likely to occur in individuals with a history of penicillin hypersensitivity and/or a history of sensitivity to multiple allergens.

There have been well-documented reports of individuals with a history of penicillin hypersensitivity reactions that have experienced severe hypersensitivity reactions when treated with a cephalosporin. Before initiating therapy with any penicillin, careful inquiry should be made concerning previous hypersensitivity reactions to penicillin, cephalosporin, and other allergens. If an allergic reaction occurs, amoxicillin should be discontinued and the appropriate therapy instituted. (See *WARNINGS* in prescribing information for amoxicillin.)

SERIOUS ANAPHYLACTIC REACTIONS REQUIRE IMMEDIATE EMERGENCY TREATMENT WITH EPINEPHRINE. OXYGEN, INTRAVENOUS STEROIDS, AND AIRWAY MANAGEMENT, INCLUDING INTUBATION, SHOULD ALSO BE ADMINISTERED AS INDICATED.

5.3. Pseudomembranous colitis associated with antibiotic use

Pseudomembranous colitis has been reported with nearly all antibacterial agents, including clarithromycin and amoxicillin, and may range in severity from mild to life threatening. Therefore, it is important to consider this diagnosis in patients who present with diarrhea subsequent to the administration of antibacterial agents.

Treatment with antibacterial agents alters the normal flora of the colon and may permit overgrowth of clostridia. Studies indicate that a toxin produced by *Clostridium difficile* is a primary cause of "antibiotic-associated colitis".

After the diagnosis of pseudomembranous colitis has been established, therapeutic measures should be initiated. Mild cases of pseudomembranous colitis usually respond to discontinuation of the drug alone. In moderate to severe cases, consideration should be given to management with fluid and electrolytes, protein supplementation, and treatment with an antibacterial drug clinically effective against *Clostridium difficile colitis.*

5.4. Presence of gastric malignancy

Symptomatic response to therapy with rabeprazole does not preclude the presence of gastric malignancy.

Patients with healed GERD were treated for up to 40 months with rabeprazole and monitored with serial gastric biopsies. Patients without *H. pylori* infection (221 of 326 patients) had no clinically important pathologic changes in the gastric mucosa. Patients with *H. pylori* infection at baseline (105 of 326 patients) had mild or moderate inflammation in the gastric body or mild inflammation in the gastric antrum. Patients with mild grades of infection or inflammation in the gastric body tended to change to moderate, whereas those graded moderate at baseline tended to remain stable. Patients with mild grades of infection or inflammation in the gastric antrum tended to remain stable. At baseline 8% of patients had atrophy of glands in the gastric body and 15% had atrophy in the gastric antrum. At endpoint, 15% of patients had atrophy of glands in the gastric body and 11% had atrophy in the gastric antrum. Approximately 4% of patients had intestinal metaplasia at some point during follow-up, but no consistent changes were seen.

5.5. Concomitant use with warfarin

Steady state interactions of rabeprazole and warfarin have not been adequately evaluated in patients. There have been reports of increased INR and prothrombin time in patients receiving a proton pump inhibitor and warfarin concomitantly. Increases in INR and prothrombin time may lead to abnormal bleeding and even death. Patients treated with a proton pump inhibitor and warfarin concomitantly may need to be monitored for increases in INR and prothrombin time.

6. ADVERSE REACTIONS

Worldwide, over 2900 patients have been treated with rabeprazole in Phase II-III clinical trials involving various dosages and durations of treatment.

Because clinical trials are conducted under varying conditions, adverse reaction rates observed in the clinical trials of a drug cannot be directly compared to rates in the clinical trials of another drug and may not reflect the rates observed in practice.

6.1. Clinical Studies Experience

The data described below reflect exposure to ACIPHEX in 1064 patients exposed for up to 8 weeks. The studies were primarily placebo- and active-controlled trials in patients with Erosive or Ulcerative Gastroesophageal Reflux Disease (GERD), Duodenal Ulcers and Gastric Ulcers. The population had a mean age of 53 years (range 18-89 years) and had a ratio of approximately 60% male/40% female. The racial distribution was 86% Caucasian, 8% African American, 2% Asian and 5% other. Most patients received either 10 mg, 20 mg or 40 mg/day of ACIPHEX.

An analysis of adverse reactions appearing in ≥ 2% of ACIPHEX patients (n=1064) and with a greater frequency than placebo (n=89) in controlled North American and European acute treatment trials, revealed the following adverse reactions: pain (3% vs. 1%), pharyngitis (3% vs. 2%), flatulence (3% vs. 1%), infection (2% vs. 1%), and constipation (2% vs. 1%). The 3 long-term maintenance studies consisted of a total of 740 patients; at least 54% of patients were exposed to rabeprazole for 6 months while at least 33% were exposed for 12 months. Of the 740 patients, 247 (33%) and 241 (33%) patients received 10 mg and 20 mg of ACIPHEX, respectively, while 169 (23%) patients received placebo and 83 (11%) received omeprazole.

The safety profile of rabeprazole in the maintenance studies was consistent with what was observed in the acute studies.

Other adverse reactions that were seen in controlled clinical trials which do not meet the above criteria (≥ 2% of ACIPHEX treated patients and > placebo) and for which there is a possibility of a causal relationship to rabeprazole include the following: headache, abdominal pain, diarrhea, dry mouth, dizziness, peripheral edema, hepatic enzyme increase, hepatitis, hepatic encephalopathy, myalgia, and arthralgia.

In a multicenter, open-label study of adolescent patients aged 12 to 16 years with a clinical diagnosis of symptomatic GERD or endoscopically proven GERD, the adverse event profile was similar to that of adults. The adverse reactions reported without regard to relationship to ACIPHEX that occurred in ≥ 2% of 111 patients were headache (9.9%), diarrhea (4.5%), nausea (4.5%), vomiting (3.6%), and abdominal pain (3.6%). The related reported adverse reactions that occurred in ≥ 2% of patients were headache (5.4%) and nausea (1.8%). There were no adverse reactions reported in these studies that were not previously observed in adults.

Combination Treatment with Amoxicillin and Clarithromycin: In clinical trials using combination therapy with rabeprazole plus amoxicillin and clarithromycin (RAC), no adverse reactions unique to this drug combination were observed. In the U.S. multicenter study, the most frequently reported drug related adverse reactions for patients who received RAC therapy for 7 or 10 days were diarrhea (8% and 7%) and taste perversion (6% and 10%), respectively.

No clinically significant laboratory abnormalities particular to the drug combinations were observed.

For more information on adverse reactions or laboratory changes with amoxicillin or clarithromycin, refer to their respective package prescribing information, **ADVERSE REACTIONS** section.

6.2. Postmarketing Experience

The following adverse reactions have been identified during postapproval use of ACIPHEX. Because these reactions are reported voluntarily from a population of uncertain size, it is not always possible to reliably estimate their frequency or establish a causal relationship to drug exposure: sudden death; coma, hyperammonemia; jaundice; rhabdomyolysis; disorientation and delirium; anaphylaxis; angioedema; bullous and other drug eruptions of the skin; severe dermatologic reactions, including toxic epidermal necrolysis (some fatal), Stevens-Johnson syndrome, and erythema multiforme; interstitial pneumonia; interstitial nephritis; and TSH elevations. In addition, agranulocytosis, hemolytic anemia, leukopenia, pancytopenia, and thrombocytopenia have been reported. Increases in prothrombin time/INR in patients treated with concomitant warfarin have been reported.

7. DRUG INTERACTIONS

7.1. Drugs metabolized by CYP450

Rabeprazole is metabolized by the cytochrome P450 (CYP450) drug metabolizing enzyme system. Studies in healthy subjects have shown that rabeprazole does not have clinically significant interactions with other drugs metabolized by the CYP450 system, such as warfarin and theophylline given as single oral doses, diazepam as a single intravenous dose, and phenytoin given as a single intravenous dose (with supplemental oral dosing). Steady state interactions of rabeprazole and other drugs metabolized by this enzyme system have not been studied in patients.

7.2. Warfarin

There have been reports of increased INR and prothrombin time in patients receiving proton pump inhibitors, including rabeprazole, and warfarin concomitantly. Increases in INR and prothrombin time may lead to abnormal bleeding and even death. [See *WARNINGS AND PRECAUTIONS* (5.5)].

7.3. Cyclosporine

In vitro incubations employing human liver microsomes indicated that rabeprazole inhibited cyclosporine metabolism with an IC_{50} of 62 micromolar, a concentration that is over 50 times higher than the C_{max} in healthy volunteers following 14 days of dosing with 20 mg of rabeprazole. This degree of inhibition is similar to that by omeprazole at equivalent concentrations.

7.4. Compounds dependent on gastric pH for absorption

Rabeprazole produces sustained inhibition of gastric acid secretion. An interaction with compounds which are dependent on gastric pH for absorption may occur due to the magnitude of acid suppression observed with rabeprazole. For example, in normal subjects, co-administration of rabeprazole 20 mg QD resulted in an approximately 30% decrease in the bioavailability of ketoconazole and increases in the AUC and C_{max} for digoxin of 19% and 29%, respectively. Therefore, patients may need to be monitored when such drugs are taken concomitantly with rabeprazole. Co-administration of rabeprazole and antacids produced no clinically relevant changes in plasma rabeprazole concentrations.

Concomitant use of atazanavir and proton pump inhibitors is not recommended. Co-administration of atazanavir with proton pump inhibitors is expected to substantially decrease atazanavir plasma concentrations and thereby reduce its therapeutic effect.

7.5. Drugs metabolized by CYP2C19

In a clinical study in Japan evaluating rabeprazole in patients categorized by CYP2C19 genotype (n=6 per genotype category), gastric acid suppression was higher in poor metabolizers as compared to extensive metabolizers. This could be due to higher rabeprazole plasma levels in poor metabolizers. Whether or not interactions of rabeprazole sodium with other drugs metabolized by CYP2C19 would be different between extensive metabolizers and poor metabolizers has not been studied.

7.6. Combined Administration with Clarithromycin

Combined administration consisting of rabeprazole, amoxicillin, and clarithromycin resulted in increases in plasma concentrations of rabeprazole and 14-hydroxyclarithromycin. [See *CLINICAL PHARMACOLOGY, Combination Therapy with Antimicrobials* (12.3)].

Concomitant administration of clarithromycin with pimozide and cisapride is contraindicated. (See *PRECAUTIONS* in prescribing information for clarithromycin.) (See *PRECAUTIONS* in prescribing information for amoxicillin.)

TABLE 3
AUC ACIDITY (MMOL•HR/L)
ACIPHEX VERSUS PLACEBO ON DAY 7 OF ONCE DAILY DOSING (MEAN±SD)

AUC interval (hrs)	Treatment			
	10 mg RBP (N=24)	20 mg RBP (N=24)	40 mg RBP (N=24)	Placebo (N=24)
08:00–13:00	19.6±21.5*	12.9±23*	7.6±14.7*	91.1±39.7
13:00–19:00	5.6±9.7*	8.3±29.8*	1.3±5.2*	95.5±48.7
19:00–22:00	0.1±0.1*	0.1±0.06*	0.0±0.02*	11.9±12.5
22:00–08:00	129.2±84*	109.6±67.2*	76.9±58.4*	479.9±165
AUC 0-24 hours	155.5±90.6*	130.9±81*	85.8±64.3*	678.5±216

*(p<0.001 versus placebo)

TABLE 4
GASTRIC ACID PARAMETERS
ACIPHEX ONCE DAILY DOSING VERSUS PLACEBO ON DAY 1 AND DAY 8

Parameter	ACIPHEX 20 mg QD		Placebo	
	Day 1	Day 8	Day 1	Day 8
Mean AUC_{0-24} Acidity	340.8*	176.9*	925.5	862.4
Median trough pH (23-hr)[a]	3.77	3.51	1.27	1.38
% Time Gastric pH>3[b]	54.6*	68.7*	19.1	21.7
% Time Gastric pH>4[b]	44.1*	60.3*	7.6	11.0

[a] No inferential statistics conducted for this parameter.

*(p<0.001 versus placebo)

[b] Gastric pH was measured every hour over a 24-hour period.

8. USE IN SPECIFIC POPULATIONS

8.1. Pregnancy
Teratogenic Effects. Pregnancy Category B: Teratology studies have been performed in rats at intravenous doses up to 50 mg/kg/day (plasma AUC of 11.8 µg•hr/mL, about 13 times the human exposure at the recommended dose for GERD) and rabbits at intravenous doses up to 30 mg/kg/day (plasma AUC of 7.3 µg•hr/mL, about 8 times the human exposure at the recommended dose for GERD) and have revealed no evidence of impaired fertility or harm to the fetus due to rabeprazole. There are, however, no adequate and well-controlled studies in pregnant women. Because animal reproduction studies are not always predictive of human response, this drug should be used during pregnancy only if clearly needed.

8.3. Nursing Mothers
Following intravenous administration of ^{14}C-labeled rabeprazole to lactating rats, radioactivity in milk reached levels that were 2- to 7-fold higher than levels in the blood. It is not known if unmetabolized rabeprazole is excreted in human breast milk. Administration of rabeprazole to rats in late gestation and during lactation at doses of 400 mg/kg/day (about 195-times the human dose based on mg/m²) resulted in decreases in body weight gain of the pups. Since many drugs are excreted in milk, and because of the potential for adverse reactions to nursing infants from rabeprazole, a decision should be made to discontinue nursing or discontinue the drug, taking into account the importance of the drug to the mother.

8.4. Pediatric Use
Use of ACIPHEX in adolescent patients 12 years of age and above for short-term treatment of GERD is supported by a) extrapolation of results from adequate and well-controlled studies that supported the approval of ACIPHEX for adults (see CLINICAL STUDIES (14.1, 14.2, 14.3) and INDICATIONS AND USAGE (1.1, 1.2, 1.3)); b) safety and pharmacokinetic studies performed in adolescent patients (see Pharmacokinetics, Pediatric (12.3)). The safety and effectiveness of ACIPHEX for the treatment of GERD patients <12 years of age have not been established. The safety and effectiveness of ACIPHEX for other uses have not been established in pediatric patients.

In a multicenter, randomized, open-label, parallel-group study, 111 adolescent patients 12 to 16 years of age with a clinical diagnosis of symptomatic GERD or suspected or endoscopically proven GERD were randomized and treated with either ACIPHEX 10 mg or ACIPHEX 20 mg once daily for up to 8 weeks for the evaluation of safety and efficacy. The adverse event profile in adolescent patients was similar to that of adults. The related reported adverse reactions that occurred in ≥ 2% of patients were headache (5.4%) and nausea (1.8%). There were no adverse reactions reported in these studies that were not previously observed in adults.

8.5. Geriatric Use
Of the total number of subjects in clinical studies of ACIPHEX, 19% were 65 years and over, while 4% were 75 years and over. No overall differences in safety or effectiveness were observed between these subjects and younger subjects, and other reported clinical experience has not identified differences in responses between the elderly and younger patients, but greater sensitivity of some older individuals cannot be ruled out.

8.6. Gender
Duodenal ulcer and erosive esophagitis healing rates in women are similar to those in men. Adverse reactions and laboratory test abnormalities in women occurred at rates similar to those in men.

10. OVERDOSAGE

Because strategies for the management of overdose are continually evolving, it is advisable to contact a Poison Control Center to determine the latest recommendations for the management of an overdose of any drug. There has been no experience with large overdoses with rabeprazole. Seven reports of accidental overdosage with rabeprazole have been received. The maximum reported overdose was 80 mg. There were no clinical signs or symptoms associated with any reported overdose. Patients with Zollinger-Ellison syndrome have been treated with up to 120 mg rabeprazole QD. No specific antidote for rabeprazole is known. Rabeprazole is extensively protein bound and is not readily dialyzable. In the event of overdosage, treatment should be symptomatic and supportive.

Single oral doses of rabeprazole at 786 mg/kg and 1024 mg/kg were lethal to mice and rats, respectively. The single oral dose of 2000 mg/kg was not lethal to dogs. The major symptoms of acute toxicity were hypoactivity, labored respiration, lateral or prone position and convulsion in mice and rats and watery diarrhea, tremor, convulsion and coma in dogs.

11. DESCRIPTION

The active ingredient in ACIPHEX Delayed-Release Tablets is rabeprazole sodium, a substituted benzimidazole that inhibits gastric acid secretion. Rabeprazole sodium is known chemically as 2-[[[4-(3-methoxypropoxy)-3-methyl-2-pyridinyl]-methyl]sulfinyl]-1H-benzimidazole sodium salt. It has an empirical formula of $C_{18}H_{20}N_3NaO_3S$ and a molecular weight of 381.43. Rabeprazole sodium is a white to slightly yellowish-white solid. It is very soluble in water and methanol, freely soluble in ethanol, chloroform and ethyl acetate and insoluble in ether and n-hexane. The stability of rabeprazole sodium is a function of pH; it is rapidly degraded in acid media, and is more stable under alkaline conditions. The structural formula is:

FIGURE 1

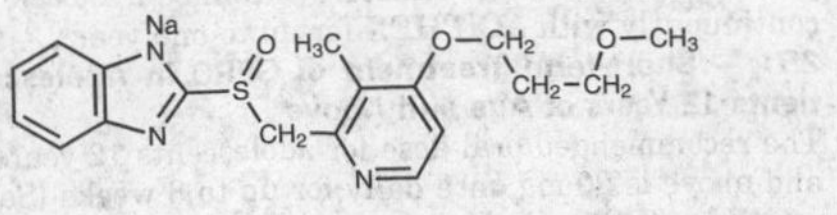

ACIPHEX is available for oral administration as delayed-release, enteric-coated tablets containing 20 mg of rabeprazole sodium.

Inactive ingredients of the 20 mg tablet are carnauba wax, crospovidone, diacetylated monoglycerides, ethylcellulose, hydroxypropyl cellulose, hypromellose phthalate, magnesium stearate, mannitol, propylene glycol, sodium hydroxide, sodium stearyl fumarate, talc, and titanium dioxide. Iron oxide yellow is the coloring agent for the tablet coating. Iron oxide red is the ink pigment.

12. CLINICAL PHARMACOLOGY

12.1. Mechanism of Action
Rabeprazole belongs to a class of antisecretory compounds (substituted benzimidazole proton-pump inhibitors) that do not exhibit anticholinergic or histamine H_2-receptor antagonist properties, but suppress gastric acid secretion by inhibiting the gastric H^+, $K^+ATPase$ at the secretory surface of the gastric parietal cell. Because this enzyme is regarded as the acid (proton) pump within the parietal cell, rabeprazole has been characterized as a gastric proton-pump inhibitor. Rabeprazole blocks the final step of gastric acid secretion. In gastric parietal cells, rabeprazole is protonated, accumulates, and is transformed to an active sulfenamide. When studied in vitro, rabeprazole is chemically activated at pH 1.2 with a half-life of 78 seconds. It inhibits acid transport in porcine gastric vesicles with a half-life of 90 seconds.

12.2. Pharmacodynamics
Antisecretory Activity
The antisecretory effect begins within one hour after oral administration of 20 mg ACIPHEX. The median inhibitory effect of ACIPHEX on 24 hour gastric acidity is 88% of maximal after the first dose. ACIPHEX 20 mg inhibits basal and peptone meal-stimulated acid secretion versus placebo by 86% and 95%, respectively, and increases the percent of a 24-hour period that the gastric pH>3 from 10% to 65% (see table below). This relatively prolonged pharmacodynamic action compared to the short pharmacokinetic half-life (1-2 hours) reflects the sustained inactivation of the H^+, $K^+ATPase$.

TABLE 2
GASTRIC ACID PARAMETERS
ACIPHEX VERSUS PLACEBO AFTER 7 DAYS OF ONCE DAILY DOSING

Parameter	ACIPHEX (20 mg QD)	Placebo
Basal Acid Output (mmol/hr)	0.4*	2.8
Stimulated Acid Output (mmol/hr)	0.6*	13.3
% Time Gastric pH>3	65*	10

*(p<0.01 versus placebo)

Compared to placebo, ACIPHEX, 10 mg, 20 mg, and 40 mg, administered once daily for 7 days significantly decreased intragastric acidity with all doses for each of four meal-related intervals and the 24-hour time period overall. In this study, there were no statistically significant differences between doses; however, there was a significant dose-related decrease in intragastric acidity. The ability of rabeprazole to cause a dose-related decrease in mean intragastric acidity is illustrated below.

[See table 3 at top left]

After administration of 20 mg ACIPHEX once daily for eight days, the mean percent of time that gastric pH>3 or gastric pH>4 after a single dose (Day 1) and multiple doses (Day 8) was significantly greater than placebo (see table below). The decrease in gastric acidity and the increase in gastric pH observed with 20 mg ACIPHEX administered once daily for eight days were compared to the same parameters for placebo, as illustrated below:

[See table 4 at left]

Effects on Esophageal Acid Exposure
In patients with gastroesophageal reflux disease (GERD) and moderate to severe esophageal acid exposure, ACIPHEX 20 mg and 40 mg per day decreased 24-hour esophageal acid exposure. After seven days of treatment, the percentage of time that esophageal pH<4 decreased from baselines of 24.7% for 20 mg and 23.7% for 40 mg, to 5.1% and 2.0%, respectively. Normalization of 24-hour intraesophageal acid exposure was correlated to gastric pH>4 for at least 35% of the 24-hour period; this level was achieved in 90% of subjects receiving ACIPHEX 20 mg and

in 100% of subjects receiving ACIPHEX 40 mg. With ACIPHEX 20 mg and 40 mg per day, significant effects on gastric and esophageal pH were noted after one day of treatment, and more pronounced after seven days of treatment.

Effects on Serum Gastrin

In patients given daily doses of ACIPHEX for up to eight weeks to treat ulcerative or erosive esophagitis and in patients treated for up to 52 weeks to prevent recurrence of disease the median fasting gastrin level increased in a dose-related manner. The group median values stayed within the normal range.

In a group of subjects treated daily with ACIPHEX 20 mg for 4 weeks a doubling of mean serum gastrin concentrations were observed. Approximately 35% of these treated subjects developed serum gastrin concentrations above the upper limit of normal. In a study of CYP2C19 genotyped subjects in Japan, poor metabolizers developed statistically significantly higher serum gastrin concentrations than extensive metabolizers.

Effects on Enterochromaffin-like (ECL) Cells

Increased serum gastrin secondary to antisecretory agents stimulates proliferation of gastric ECL cells which, over time, may result in ECL cell hyperplasia in rats and mice and gastric carcinoids in rats, especially in females [see *Carcinogenesis, Mutagenesis, Impairment of Fertility* (13.1)].

In over 400 patients treated with ACIPHEX (10 or 20 mg/day) for up to one year, the incidence of ECL cell hyperplasia increased with time and dose, which is consistent with the pharmacological action of the proton-pump inhibitor. No patient developed the adenomatoid, dysplastic or neoplastic changes of ECL cells in the gastric mucosa. No patient developed the carcinoid tumors observed in rats.

Endocrine Effects

Studies in humans for up to one year have not revealed clinically significant effects on the endocrine system. In healthy male volunteers treated with ACIPHEX for 13 days, no clinically relevant changes have been detected in the following endocrine parameters examined: 17 β-estradiol, thyroid stimulating hormone, tri-iodothyronine, thyroxine, thyroxine-binding protein, parathyroid hormone, insulin, glucagon, renin, aldosterone, follicle-stimulating hormone, luteotrophic hormone, prolactin, somatotrophic hormone, dehydroepiandrosterone, cortisol-binding globulin, and urinary 6β-hydroxycortisol, serum testosterone and circadian cortisol profile.

Other Effects

In humans treated with ACIPHEX for up to one year, no systemic effects have been observed on the central nervous, lymphoid, hematopoietic, renal, hepatic, cardiovascular, or respiratory systems. No data are available on long-term treatment with ACIPHEX and ocular effects.

Microbiology

The following *in vitro* data are available but the clinical significance is unknown.

Rabeprazole sodium, amoxicillin and clarithromycin as a three drug regimen has been shown to be active against most strains of *Helicobacter pylori in vitro* and in clinical infections as described in the *CLINICAL STUDIES* (14) and *INDICATIONS AND USAGE* (1) sections.

Helicobacter pylori

Susceptibility testing of *H. pylori* isolates was performed for amoxicillin and clarithromycin using agar dilution methodology[1], and minimum inhibitory concentrations (MICs) were determined. The clarithromycin and amoxicillin MIC values should be interpreted according to the following criteria:

TABLE 5
INTERPRETATION OF CLARITHROMYCIN AND AMOXICILLIN MIC VALUES

Clarithromycin MIC (μg/mL)[a]	Interpretation
≤ 0.25	Susceptible (S)
0.5	Intermediate (I)
≥ 1.0	Resistant (R)
Amoxicillin MIC (μg/mL)[a,b]	**Interpretation**
≤ 0.25	Susceptible (S)

[a] These are breakpoints for the agar dilution methodology and they should not be used to interpret results using alternative methods.
[b] There were not enough organisms with MICs > 0.25 μg/mL to determine a resistance breakpoint.

Standardized susceptibility test procedures require the use of laboratory control microorganisms to control the technical aspects of the laboratory procedures. Standard clarithromycin and amoxicillin powders should provide the following MIC values:

TABLE 6
MIC VALUES FOR STANDARD CLARITHROMYCIN AND AMOXICILLIN POWDERS

Microorganism	Antimicrobial Agent	MIC (μg/mL)[a]
H. pylori ATCC 43504	Clarithromycin	0.015–0.12 μg/mL
H. pylori ATCC 43504	Amoxicillin	0.015–0.12 μg/mL

[a] These are quality control ranges for the agar dilution methodology and they should not be used to control test results obtained using alternative methods.

Incidence of Antibiotic-Resistant Organisms Among Clinical Isolates

Pretreatment Resistance: Clarithromycin pretreatment resistance rate (MIC ≥ 1 μg/mL) to *H. pylori* was 9% (51/560) at baseline in all treatment groups combined. A total of > 99% (558/560) of patients had *H. pylori* isolates which were considered to be susceptible (MIC ≤ 0.25 μg/mL) to amoxicillin at baseline. Two patients had baseline *H. pylori* isolates with an amoxicillin MIC of 0.5 μg/mL.

Clarithromycin Susceptibility Test Results and Clinical/Bacteriologic Outcomes: For the U.S. multicenter study, the baseline *H. pylori* clarithromycin susceptibility results and the *H. pylori* eradication results post-treatment are shown in the table below:

TABLE 7
CLARITHROMYCIN SUSCEPTIBILITY TEST RESULTS AND CLINICAL/BACTERIOLOGIC OUTCOMES[a] FOR A THREE DRUG REGIMEN (RABEPRAZOLE 20 MG TWICE DAILY, AMOXICILLIN 1000 MG TWICE DAILY, AND CLARITHROMYCIN 500 MG TWICE DAILY FOR 7 OR 10 DAYS)

Days of RAC Therapy	Clarithromycin Pretreatment Results	Total Number	*H. pylori* Negative (Eradicated)
7	Susceptible[b]	129	103
7	Intermediate[b]	0	0
7	Resistant[b]	16	5
10	Susceptible[b]	133	111
10	Intermediate[b]	0	0
10	Resistant[b]	9	1

H. pylori Positive (Persistent) Post-Treatment Susceptibility Results

Days of RAC Therapy	S[b]	I[b]	R[b]	No MIC
7	2	0	1	23
7	0	0	0	0
7	2	1	4	4
10	3	1	2	16
10	0	0	0	0
10	0	0	5	3

[a] Includes only patients with pretreatment and post-treatment clarithromycin susceptibility test results.
[b] Susceptible (S) MIC ≤ 0.25 μg/mL, Intermediate (I) MIC = 0.5 μg/mL, Resistant (R) MIC ≥ 1 μg/mL

Patients with persistent *H. pylori* infection following rabeprazole, amoxicillin, and clarithromycin therapy will likely have clarithromycin resistant clinical isolates. Therefore, clarithromycin susceptibility testing should be done when possible. If resistance to clarithromycin is demonstrated or susceptibility testing is not possible, alternative antimicrobial therapy should be instituted.

Amoxicillin Susceptibility Test Results and Clinical/Bacteriologic Outcomes: In the U.S. multicenter study, a total of >99% (558/560) of patients had *H. pylori* isolates which were considered to be susceptible (MIC ≤ 0.25 μg/mL) to amoxicillin at baseline. The other 2 patients had baseline *H. pylori* isolates with an amoxicillin MIC of 0.5 μg/mL, and both isolates were clarithromycin-resistant at baseline; in one case the *H. pylori* was eradicated. In the 7- and 10-day treatment groups 75% (107/145) and 79% (112/142), respectively, of the patients who had pretreatment amoxicillin susceptible MICs (≤ 0.25 μg/mL) were eradicated of *H. pylori*. No patients developed amoxicillin-resistant *H. pylori* during therapy.

12.3. Pharmacokinetics

ACIPHEX delayed-release tablets are enteric-coated to allow rabeprazole sodium, which is acid labile, to pass through the stomach relatively intact. After oral administration of 20 mg ACIPHEX, peak plasma concentrations (C_{max}) of rabeprazole occur over a range of 2.0 to 5.0 hours (T_{max}). The rabeprazole C_{max} and AUC are linear over an oral dose range of 10 mg to 40 mg. There is no appreciable accumulation when doses of 10 mg to 40 mg are administered every 24 hours; the pharmacokinetics of rabeprazole is not altered by multiple dosing. The plasma half-life ranges from 1 to 2 hours.

Absorption: Absolute bioavailability for a 20 mg oral tablet of rabeprazole (compared to intravenous administration) is approximately 52%. When rabeprazole is administered with a high fat meal, its T_{max} is variable and may delay its absorption up to 4 hours or longer, however, the C_{max} and the extent of rabeprazole absorption (AUC) are not significantly altered. Thus rabeprazole may be taken without regard to timing of meals.

Distribution: Rabeprazole is 96.3% bound to human plasma proteins.

Metabolism: Rabeprazole is extensively metabolized. A significant portion of rabeprazole is metabolized via systemic nonenzymatic reduction to a thioether compound. Rabeprazole is also metabolized to sulphone and desmethyl compounds via cytochrome P450 in the liver. The thioether and sulphone are the primary metabolites measured in human plasma. These metabolites were not observed to have significant antisecretory activity. *In vitro* studies have demonstrated that rabeprazole is metabolized in the liver primarily by cytochromes P450 3A (CYP3A) to a sulphone metabolite and cytochrome P450 2C19 (CYP2C19) to desmethyl rabeprazole. CYP2C19 exhibits a known genetic polymorphism due to its deficiency in some sub-populations (e.g. 3 to 5% of Caucasians and 17 to 20% of Asians). Rabeprazole metabolism is slow in these sub-populations, therefore, they are referred to as poor metabolizers of the drug.

Elimination: Following a single 20 mg oral dose of ^{14}C-labeled rabeprazole, approximately 90% of the drug was eliminated in the urine, primarily as thioether carboxylic acid; its glucuronide, and mercapturic acid metabolites. The remainder of the dose was recovered in the feces. Total recovery of radioactivity was 99.8%. No unchanged rabeprazole was recovered in the urine or feces.

Geriatric: In 20 healthy elderly subjects administered 20 mg rabeprazole once daily for seven days, AUC values approximately doubled and the C_{max} increased by 60% compared to values in a parallel younger control group. There was no evidence of drug accumulation after once daily administration. [see *USE IN SPECIAL POPULATIONS Geriatric Use* (8.5)].

Pediatric: The pharmacokinetics of rabeprazole was studied in 12 adolescent patients with GERD 12 to 16 years of age, in a multicenter study. Patients received rabeprazole 20 mg once daily for five or seven days. An approximate 40% increase in exposure was noted following 5 to 7 days of dosing compared with the exposure after 1 day dosing. Pharmacokinetic parameters in adolescent patients with GERD 12 to 16 years of age were within the range observed in healthy adult volunteers.

Gender and Race: In analyses adjusted for body mass and height, rabeprazole pharmacokinetics showed no clinically significant differences between male and female subjects. In studies that used different formulations of rabeprazole, $AUC_{0-\infty}$ values for healthy Japanese men were approximately 50-60% greater than values derived from pooled data from healthy men in the United States.

Renal Disease: In 10 patients with stable end-stage renal disease requiring maintenance hemodialysis (creatinine clearance ≤ 5 mL/min/1.73 m^2), no clinically significant differences were observed in the pharmacokinetics of rabeprazole after a single 20 mg oral dose when compared to 10 healthy volunteers. [see *DOSAGE AND ADMINISTRATION* (2.7)].

Hepatic Disease: In a single dose study of 10 patients with chronic mild to moderate compensated cirrhosis of the liver who were administered a 20 mg dose of rabeprazole, AUC_{0-24} was approximately doubled, the elimination half-life was 2- to 3-fold higher, and total body clearance was decreased to less than half compared to values in healthy men. In a multiple dose study of 12 patients with mild to moderate hepatic impairment administered 20 mg rabeprazole once daily for eight days, $AUC_{0-\infty}$ and C_{max} values increased approximately 20% compared to values in healthy age- and gender-matched subjects. These increases were not statistically significant.

No information exists on rabeprazole disposition in patients with severe hepatic impairment. Please refer to the *DOSAGE AND ADMINISTRATION section* (2.7) for information on dosage adjustment in patients with hepatic impairment.

TABLE 8

HEALING OF EROSIVE OR ULCERATIVE GASTROESOPHAGEAL REFLUX DISEASE (GERD) PERCENTAGE OF PATIENTS HEALED

Week	10 mg ACIPHEX QD N=27	20 mg ACIPHEX QD N=25	40 mg ACIPHEX QD N=26	Placebo N=25
4	63%*	56%*	54%*	0%
8	93%*	84%*	85%*	12%

*(p<0.001 versus placebo)

Combined Administration with Antimicrobials: Sixteen healthy volunteers genotyped as extensive metabolizers with respect to CYP2C19 were given 20 mg rabeprazole sodium, 1000 mg amoxicillin, 500 mg clarithromycin, or all 3 drugs in a four-way crossover study. Each of the four regimens was administered twice daily for 6 days. The AUC and C_{max} for clarithromycin and amoxicillin were not different following combined administration compared to values following single administration. However, the rabeprazole AUC and C_{max} increased by 11% and 34%, respectively, following combined administration. The AUC and C_{max} for 14-hydroxyclarithromycin (active metabolite of clarithromycin) also increased by 42% and 46%, respectively. This increase in exposure to rabeprazole and 14-hydroxyclarithromycin is not expected to produce safety concerns.

13. NONCLINICAL PHARMACOLOGY

13.1. Carcinogenesis, Mutagenesis, Impairment of Fertility

In a 88/104-week carcinogenicity study in CD-1 mice, rabeprazole at oral doses up to 100 mg/kg/day did not produce any increased tumor occurrence. The highest tested dose produced a systemic exposure to rabeprazole (AUC) of 1.40 µg•hr/mL which is 1.6 times the human exposure (plasma $AUC_{0-\infty} = 0.88$ µg•hr/mL) at the recommended dose for GERD (20 mg/day). In a 28-week carcinogenicity study in p53[+/-] transgenic mice, rabeprazole at oral doses of 20, 60 and 200 mg/kg/day did not cause an increase in the incidence rates of tumors but produced gastric mucosal hyperplasia at all doses. The systemic exposure to rabeprazole at 200 mg/kg/day is about 17-24 times the human exposure at the recommended dose for GERD. In a 104-week carcinogenicity study in Sprague-Dawley rats, males were treated with oral doses of 5, 15, 30 and 60 mg/kg/day and females with 5, 15, 30, 60 and 120 mg/kg/day. Rabeprazole produced gastric enterochromaffin-like (ECL) cell hyperplasia in male and female rats and ECL cell carcinoid tumors in female rats at all doses including the lowest tested dose. The lowest dose (5 mg/kg/day) produced a systemic exposure to rabeprazole (AUC) of about 0.1 µg•hr/mL which is about 0.1 times the human exposure at the recommended dose for GERD. In male rats, no treatment related tumors were observed at doses up to 60 mg/kg/day producing a rabeprazole plasma exposure (AUC) of about 0.2 µg•hr/mL (0.2 times the human exposure at the recommended dose for GERD). Rabeprazole was positive in the Ames test, the Chinese hamster ovary cell (CHO/HGPRT) forward gene mutation test and the mouse lymphoma cell (L5178Y/TK+/-) forward gene mutation test. Its demethylated-metabolite was also positive in the Ames test. Rabeprazole was negative in the *in vitro* Chinese hamster lung cell chromosome aberration test, the *in vivo* mouse micronucleus test, and the *in vivo* and *ex vivo* rat hepatocyte unscheduled DNA synthesis (UDS) tests.

Rabeprazole at intravenous doses up to 30 mg/kg/day (plasma AUC of 8.8 µg•hr/mL, about 10 times the human exposure at the recommended dose for GERD) was found to have no effect on fertility and reproductive performance of male and female rats.

14. CLINICAL STUDIES

14.1. Healing of Erosive or Ulcerative GERD

In a U.S., multicenter, randomized, double-blind, placebo-controlled study, 103 patients were treated for up to eight weeks with placebo, 10 mg, 20 mg or 40 mg ACIPHEX QD. For this and all studies of GERD healing, only patients with GERD symptoms and at least grade 2 esophagitis (modified Hetzel-Dent grading scale) were eligible for entry. Endoscopic healing was defined as grade 0 or 1. Each rabeprazole dose was significantly superior to placebo in producing endoscopic healing after four and eight weeks of treatment. The percentage of patients demonstrating endoscopic healing was as follows:

[See table 8 above]

In addition, there was a statistically significant difference in favor of the ACIPHEX 10 mg, 20 mg, and 40 mg doses compared to placebo at Weeks 4 and 8 regarding complete resolution of GERD heartburn frequency (p≤ 0.026). All ACIPHEX groups reported significantly greater rates of complete resolution of GERD daytime heartburn severity compared to placebo at Weeks 4 and 8 (p≤ 0.036). Mean reductions from baseline in daily antacid dose were statistically significant for all ACIPHEX groups when compared to placebo at both Weeks 4 and 8 (p≤ 0.007).

In a North American multicenter, randomized, double-blind, active-controlled study of 336 patients, ACIPHEX was statistically superior to ranitidine with respect to the percentage of patients healed at endoscopy after four and eight weeks of treatment (see table below):

TABLE 9

HEALING OF EROSIVE OR ULCERATIVE GASTROESOPHAGEAL REFLUX DISEASE (GERD) PERCENTAGE OF PATIENTS HEALED

Week	ACIPHEX 20 mg QD N=167	Ranitidine 150 mg QID N=169
4	59%*	36%
8	87%*	66%

*(p<0.001 versus ranitidine)

ACIPHEX 20 mg once daily was significantly more effective than ranitidine 150 mg QID in the percentage of patients with complete resolution of heartburn at Weeks 4 and 8 (p<0.001). ACIPHEX 20 mg once daily was also more effective in complete resolution of daytime heartburn (p≤ 0.025), and nighttime heartburn (p≤ 0.012) at both Weeks 4 and 8, with significant differences by the end of the first week of the study.

14.2. Long-term Maintenance of Healing of Erosive or Ulcerative GERD

The long-term maintenance of healing in patients with erosive or ulcerative GERD previously healed with gastric antisecretory therapy was assessed in two U.S., multicenter, randomized, double-blind, placebo-controlled studies of identical design of 52 weeks duration. The two studies randomized 209 and 285 patients, respectively, to receive either 10 mg or 20 mg of ACIPHEX QD or placebo. As demonstrated in the tables below, ACIPHEX was significantly superior to placebo in both studies with respect to the maintenance of healing of GERD and the proportions of patients remaining free of heartburn symptoms at 52 weeks:

TABLE 10

PERCENT OF PATIENTS IN ENDOSCOPIC REMISSION

	ACIPHEX 10 mg	ACIPHEX 20 mg	Placebo
Study 1	N=66	N=67	N=70
Week 4	83%*	96%*	44%
Week 13	79%*	93%*	39%
Week 26	77%*	93%*	31%
Week 39	76%*	91%*	30%
Week 52	73%*	90%*	29%
Study 2	N=93	N=93	N=99
Week 4	89%*	94%*	40%
Week 13	86%*	91%*	33%
Week 26	85%*	89%*	30%
Week 39	84%*	88%*	29%
Week 52	77%*	86%*	29%
COMBINED STUDIES	N=159	N=160	N=169
Week 4	87%*	94%*	42%
Week 13	83%*	92%*	36%
Week 26	82%*	91%*	31%
Week 39	81%*	89%*	30%
Week 52	75%*	87%*	29%

*(p<0.001 versus placebo)

[See table 11 at top of next page]

14.3. Treatment of Symptomatic GERD

Two U.S., multicenter, double-blind, placebo controlled studies were conducted in 316 patients with daytime and nighttime heartburn. Patients reported 5 or more periods of moderate to very severe heartburn during the placebo treatment phase the week prior to randomization. Patients were confirmed by endoscopy to have no esophageal erosions. The percentage of heartburn free daytime and/or nighttime periods was greater with ACIPHEX 20 mg compared to placebo over the 4 weeks of study in Study RAB-USA-2 (47% vs. 23%) and Study RAB-USA-3 (52% vs. 28%). The mean decreases from baseline in average daytime and nighttime heartburn scores were significantly greater for ACIPHEX 20 mg as compared to placebo at week 4. Graphical displays depicting the daily mean daytime and nighttime scores are provided in Figures 2 to 5.

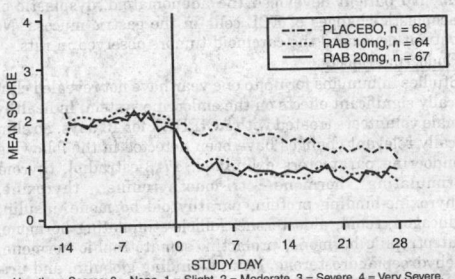

FIGURE 2: MEAN DAYTIME HEARTBURN SCORES RAB-USA-2

PLACEBO, n = 68
RAB 10mg, n = 64
RAB 20mg, n = 67

Heartburn Scores: 0 = None, 1 = Slight, 2 = Moderate, 3 = Severe, 4 = Very Severe.

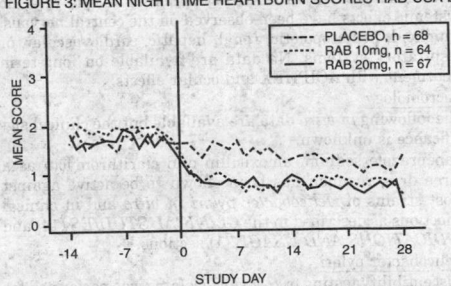

FIGURE 3: MEAN NIGHTTIME HEARTBURN SCORES RAB-USA-2

PLACEBO, n = 68
RAB 10mg, n = 64
RAB 20mg, n = 67

Heartburn Scores: 0 = None, 1 = Slight, 2 = Moderate, 3 = Severe, 4 = Very Severe.

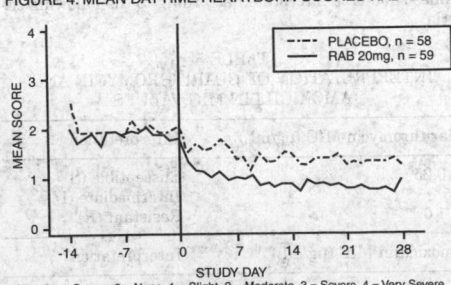

FIGURE 4: MEAN DAYTIME HEARTBURN SCORES RAB-USA-3

PLACEBO, n = 58
RAB 20mg, n = 59

Heartburn Scores: 0 = None, 1 = Slight, 2 = Moderate, 3 = Severe, 4 = Very Severe.

[See figure at top of next column]

In addition, the combined analysis of these two studies showed ACIPHEX 20 mg significantly improved other GERD-associated symptoms (regurgitation, belching and early satiety) by week 4 compared with placebo (all p values < 0.005).

ACIPHEX 20 mg also significantly reduced daily antacid consumption versus placebo over 4 weeks (p<0.001).

14.4. Healing of Duodenal Ulcers

In a U.S., randomized, double-blind, multicenter study assessing the effectiveness of 20 mg and 40 mg of ACIPHEX QD versus placebo for healing endoscopically defined duo-

FIGURE 5: MEAN NIGHTTIME HEARTBURN SCORES RAB-USA-3

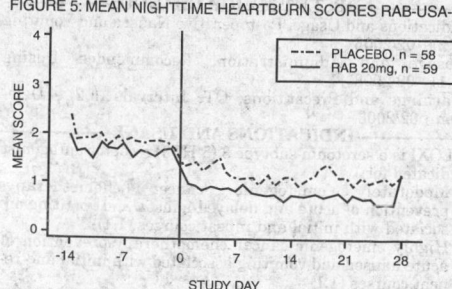

Heartburn Scores: 0 = None, 1 = Slight, 2 = Moderate, 3 = Severe, 4 = Very Severe.

denal ulcers, 100 patients were treated for up to four weeks. ACIPHEX was significantly superior to placebo in producing healing of duodenal ulcers. The percentages of patients with endoscopic healing are presented below:

TABLE 12
HEALING OF DUODENAL ULCERS PERCENTAGE OF PATIENTS HEALED

Week	ACIPHEX 20 mg QD N=34	ACIPHEX 40 mg QD N=33	Placebo N=33
2	44%	42%	21%
4	79%*	91%*	39%

*p≤ 0.001 versus placebo

At Weeks 2 and 4, significantly more patients in the ACIPHEX 20 and 40 mg groups reported complete resolution of ulcer pain frequency (p≤ 0.018), daytime pain severity (p≤ 0.023), and nighttime pain severity (p≤ 0.035) compared with placebo patients. The only exception was the ACIPHEX 40 mg group versus placebo at Week 2 for duodenal ulcer pain frequency (p=0.094). Significant differences in resolution of daytime and nighttime pain were noted in both ACIPHEX groups relative to placebo by the end of the first week of the study. Significant reductions in daily antacid use were also noted in both ACIPHEX groups compared to placebo at Weeks 2 and 4 (p<0.001).

An international randomized, double-blind, active-controlled trial was conducted in 205 patients comparing 20 mg ACIPHEX QD with 20 mg omeprazole QD. The study was designed to provide at least 80% power to exclude a difference of at least 10% between ACIPHEX and omeprazole, assuming four-week healing response rates of 93% for both groups. In patients with endoscopically defined duodenal ulcers treated for up to four weeks, ACIPHEX was comparable to omeprazole in producing healing of duodenal ulcers. The percentages of patients with endoscopic healing at two and four weeks are presented below:
[See table 13 at right]
ACIPHEX and omeprazole were comparable in providing complete resolution of symptoms.

14.5. *Helicobacter pylori* **Eradication in Patients with Peptic Ulcer Disease or Symptomatic Non-Ulcer Disease**
The U.S. multicenter study was a double-blind, parallel-group comparison of rabeprazole, amoxicillin, and clarithromycin for 3, 7, or 10 days vs. omeprazole, amoxicillin and clarithromycin for 10 days. Therapy consisted of rabeprazole 20 mg twice daily, amoxicillin 1000 mg twice daily, and clarithromycin 500 mg twice daily (RAC) or omeprazole 20 mg twice daily, amoxicillin 1000 mg twice daily, and clarithromycin 500 mg twice daily (OAC). Patients with *H. pylori* infection were stratified in a 1:1 ratio for those with peptic ulcer disease (active or a history of ulcer in the past five years) [PUD] and those who were symptomatic but without peptic ulcer disease [NPUD], as determined by upper gastrointestinal endoscopy. The overall *H. pylori* eradication rates, defined as negative ^{13}C-UBT for *H. pylori* ≥ 6 weeks from the end of the treatment are shown in the following table. The eradication rates in the 7-day and 10-day RAC regimens were found to be similar to 10-day OAC regimen using either the Intent-to-Treat (ITT) or Per-Protocol (PP) populations. Eradication rates in the RAC 3-day regimen were inferior to the other regimens.
[See table 14 at right]

14.6. **Pathological Hypersecretory Conditions Including Zollinger-Ellison Syndrome**
Twelve patients with idiopathic gastric hypersecretion or Zollinger-Ellison syndrome have been treated successfully with ACIPHEX at doses from 20 to 120 mg for up to 12 months. ACIPHEX produced satisfactory inhibition of gastric acid secretion in all patients and complete resolution of signs and symptoms of acid-peptic disease where present. ACIPHEX also prevented recurrence of gastric hypersecretion and manifestations of acid-peptic disease in all pa-

tients. The high doses of ACIPHEX used to treat this small cohort of patients with gastric hypersecretion were well tolerated.

15.   REFERENCES
1. National Committee for Clinical Laboratory Standards. *Methods for Dilution Antimicrobial Susceptibility Tests for Bacteria That Grow Aerobically*—Fifth Edition. Approved Standard NCCLS Document M7-A5, Vol. 20, No. 2, NCCLS, Wayne, PA, January 2000.

16.   HOW SUPPLIED/STORAGE AND HANDLING
ACIPHEX 20 mg is supplied as delayed-release light yellow enteric-coated tablets. The name and strength, in mg, (ACIPHEX 20) is imprinted on one side.

TABLE 11
PERCENT OF PATIENTS WITHOUT RELAPSE IN HEARTBURN FREQUENCY AND DAYTIME AND NIGHTTIME HEARTBURN SEVERITY AT WEEK 52

	ACIPHEX 10 mg	ACIPHEX 20 mg	Placebo
Heartburn Frequency			
Study 1	46/55 (84%)*	48/52 (92%)*	17/45 (38%)
Study 2	50/72 (69%)*	57/72 (79%)*	22/79 (28%)
Daytime Heartburn Severity			
Study 1	61/64 (95%)*	60/62 (97%)*	42/61 (69%)
Study 2	73/84 (87%)†	82/87 (94%)*	67/90 (74%)
Nighttime Heartburn Severity			
Study 1	57/61 (93%)*	60/61 (98%)*	37/56 (66%)
Study 2	67/80 (84%)	79/87 (91%)†	64/87 (74%)

*   p≤0.001 versus placebo
†   0.001<p<0.05 versus placebo

TABLE 13
HEALING OF DUODENAL ULCERS PERCENTAGE OF PATIENTS HEALED

Week	ACIPHEX 20 mg QD N=102	Omeprazole 20 mg QD N=103	95% Confidence Interval for the Treatment Difference (ACIPHEX - Omeprazole)
2	69%	61%	(−6%, 22%)
4	98%	93%	(−3%, 15%)

TABLE 14
HELICOBACTER PYLORI ERADICATION AT ≥ 6 WEEKS AFTER THE END OF TREATMENT

	Treatment Group Percent (%) of Patients Cured (Number of Patients)		Difference (RAC–OAC) [95% Confidence Interval]
	7-day RAC*	**10-day OAC**	
Per Protocol[a]	84.3% (N=166)	81.6% (N=179)	2.8 [-5.2, 10.7]
Intent-to-Treat[b]	77.3% (N=194)	73.3% (N=206)	4.0 [-4.4, 12.5]
	10-day RAC*	**10-day OAC**	
Per Protocol[a]	86.0% (N=171)	81.6% (N=179)	4.4 [-3.3, 12.1]
Intent-to-Treat[b]	78.1% (N=196)	73.3% (N=206)	4.8 [-3.6, 13.2]
	3-day RAC	**10-day OAC**	
Per Protocol[a]	29.9% (N=167)	81.6% (N=179)	-51.6 [-60.6, -42.6]
Intent-to-Treat[b]	27.3% (N=187)	73.3% (N=206)	-46.0 [-54.8, -37.2]

[a] Patients were included in the analysis if they had *H. pylori* infection documented at baseline, defined as a positive ^{13}C-UBT plus rapid urease test or culture and were not protocol violators. Patients who dropped out of the study due to an adverse event related to the study drug were included in the evaluable analysis as failures of therapy.
[b] Patients were included in the analysis if they had documented *H. pylori* infection at baseline as defined above and took at least one dose of study medication. All dropouts were included as failures of therapy.
*The 95% confidence intervals for the difference in eradication rates for 7-day RAC minus 10-day RAC are (-9.3, 6.0) in the PP population and (-9.0, 7.5) in the ITT population.

Bottles of 30 (NDC#62856-243-30)
Bottles of 90 (NDC#62856-243-90)
Unit Dose Blisters Package of 100 (10 × 10) (NDC#62856-243-41)
Store at 25°C (77°F); excursions permitted to 15-30°C (59-86°F). [see USP Controlled Room Temperature] Protect from moisture.

17.   PATIENT COUNSELING INFORMATION
17.1.   How to Take ACIPHEX
Patients should be cautioned that ACIPHEX delayed-release tablets should be swallowed whole. The tablets should not be chewed, crushed, or split. ACIPHEX can be taken with or without food.

17.2.   FDA-approved patient labeling

PATIENT INFORMATION
ACIPHEX (a-se-feks)
(rabeprazole sodium)
Delayed-Release Tablets
Read the Patient Information that comes with ACIPHEX before you start taking it and each time you get a refill. There may be new information. This leaflet does not take the place of talking to your healthcare provider about your medical condition or treatment.

What is ACIPHEX?
ACIPHEX is a medicine called a proton pump inhibitor or an "acid pump inhibitor". This means it reduces the amount of acid that is made by your stomach. ACIPHEX is used in adults:

• for the short-term (4 to 8 weeks) treatment in the healing and symptom relief of damaging (erosive) Gastro-esophageal Reflux Disease (GERD).
• to maintain healing of damage (erosions) and relief of heartburn symptoms with GERD. ACIPHEX has not been studied for treatment lasting longer than 12 months (1 year).
• for the treatment of daytime and nighttime heartburn and other symptoms that happen with GERD.
• for short-term treatment (up to 4 weeks) in the healing and relief of stomach-area (duodenal) ulcers. The duodenal area is the area where food passes when it leaves the stomach. The main symptom of a duodenal ulcer is a steady pain in the stomach area.
• with certain antibiotic medicines for the treatment of an infection caused by bacteria called H. pylori. Sometimes H. pylori bacteria can cause duodenal ulcers. The infection needs to be treated to prevent the ulcers from coming back.
• for the long-term treatment of conditions where your stomach makes too much acid. This includes a condition called Zollinger-Ellison syndrome.

ACIPHEX is used in adolescents 12 years of age and above:
• for the short-term (up to 8 weeks) treatment of GERD.
• The safety and effectiveness of ACIPHEX has not been established for children under the age of 12.

Who should not take ACIPHEX?
Do not take ACIPHEX if you:
• are allergic to any of the ingredients in ACIPHEX. See the end of this leaflet for a complete list of ingredients in ACIPHEX.
• are allergic to any other Proton Pump Inhibitor (PPI) medicine.

What should I tell my doctor before I take ACIPHEX?
Tell your doctor about all of your medical conditions, including if you:
• have any liver problems.
• have any allergies.
• are pregnant or planning to become pregnant. It is not known if ACIPHEX can harm your unborn baby.
• are breastfeeding. It is not known if ACIPHEX passes into your breast milk or if it can harm your baby. You should choose to breastfeed or take ACIPHEX, but not both. Talk to your doctor about other ways to feed your baby while taking ACIPHEX.

Tell your doctor about all the medicines you take, including prescription and non-prescription medicines, vitamins and herbal supplements. ACIPHEX and certain medicines can affect each other. This can cause serious side effects. Know the medicines that you take. Keep a list of them with you and show it to your doctor when you get a new medicine. Be sure to tell your doctor if you are taking:
• atazanavir (Reyataz)
• cyclosporine (Sandimmune, Neoral)
• digoxin (Lanoxin)
• ketoconazole (Nizoral)
• warfarin (Coumadin)
• antibiotics

How should I take ACIPHEX?
• Take ACIPHEX exactly as prescribed. Your doctor will prescribe the dose that is right for you and your medical condition. Do not change your dose or stop taking ACIPHEX unless you talk to your doctor. Take ACIPHEX for as long as it is prescribed even if you feel better.
• ACIPHEX is usually taken once a day. Your doctor will tell you the time of day to take ACIPHEX, based on your medical condition.
• ACIPHEX can be taken with or without food. Your healthcare provider will tell you whether to take this medicine with or without food based on your medical condition.
• Swallow each ACIPHEX tablet whole with water. **Do not chew, crush, or split ACIPHEX tablets** because this will damage the tablet and the medicine will not work. Tell your doctor if you cannot swallow tablets whole. You may need a different medicine.
• **If you miss a dose** of ACIPHEX, take it as soon as possible. If it is almost time for your next dose, skip the missed dose and go back to your normal schedule. Do not take 2 doses at the same time.

• If you take too much ACIPHEX, call your doctor or Poison Control Center right away, or go to the emergency department.
• Your doctor may prescribe antibiotic medicines with ACIPHEX to help treat a stomach infection and heal stomach-area (duodenal) ulcers that are caused by bacteria called H. pylori. Make sure you read the patient information that comes with an antibiotic before you start taking it.

What are the possible side effects of ACIPHEX?
ACIPHEX, like other proton pump inhibitors, may cause serious allergic reactions. See the end of this leaflet for a complete list of ingredients in ACIPHEX.
The most common side effects with ACIPHEX may include:
• headache
• pain
• pharyngitis
• flatulence
• infection
• constipation
These are not all the side effects of ACIPHEX. For more information, ask your doctor or pharmacist.
Call your healthcare provider for medical advice about side effects. You may report side effects to FDA at 1-800-FDA-1088.

How should I store ACIPHEX?
• Store ACIPHEX in a dry place at room temperature, 59°F to 86°F (15°C to 30°C).
• **Keep ACIPHEX and all medicines out of the reach of children.**

General Information about ACIPHEX
Medicines are sometimes prescribed for conditions other than those described in patient information leaflets. Do not use ACIPHEX for any condition for which it was not prescribed by your doctor. Do not give ACIPHEX to other people, even if they have the same symptoms as you. It may harm them.
This leaflet summarizes the most important information about ACIPHEX. If you would like more information, talk to your doctor. You can also ask your doctor or pharmacist for information about ACIPHEX that is written for healthcare professionals. For full product information, visit the website at http://www.aciphex.com/ or call the toll-free numbers 1-888-4-ACIPHEX or 1-800 JANSSEN.

What are the ingredients in ACIPHEX?
Active Ingredient: rabeprazole sodium
Inactive ingredients of the 20 mg tablet are carnauba wax, crospovidone, diacetylated monoglycerides, ethylcellulose, hydroxypropyl cellulose, hypromellose phthalate, magnesium stearate, mannitol, propylene glycol, sodium hydroxide, sodium stearyl fumarate, talc, and titanium dioxide. Iron oxide yellow is the coloring agent for the tablet coating. Iron oxide red is the ink pigment.
The following are registered trademarks of their respective manufacturers: Reyataz (Bristol-Myers Squibb Company), Sandimmune and Neoral (Novartis Pharmaceuticals Corporation), Lanoxin (GlaxoSmithKline), Nizoral (Janssen Pharmaceutica Products, LP), and Coumadin (Bristol-Myers Squibb Company).

What is GERD?
Your stomach needs acid to help your body digest food. Stomach acid is made by tiny acid pumps in the cells that line your stomach. If your body makes too much acid or cannot protect itself against a normal amount of acid, medical problems such as GERD can happen.
GERD happens when acid in your stomach backs up into the tube (esophagus) that connects your mouth to your stomach. Stomach acid can damage (erode) the lining of your esophagus. Some symptoms of GERD are heartburn, sour taste in the back of your throat and burping.

For prescription only
Revised January 2009
ACIPHEX is a registered trademark of
Eisai Co., Ltd., Tokyo, Japan.
Manufactured and Marketed by Eisai Inc.,
Woodcliff Lake, NJ 07677
Marketed by PRICARA,
Division of Ortho-McNeil-Janssen Pharmaceuticals, Inc.,
Raritan, NJ 08869
AC0109
Shown in Product Identification Guide, page 308

ALOXI®   ℞
[a-lŏk-sē]
(palonosetron HCl)
Injection for Intravenous Use

HIGHLIGHTS OF PRESCRIBING INFORMATION
These highlights do not include all the information needed to use ALOXI safely and effectively. See full prescribing information for ALOXI.
ALOXI® (palonosetron HCl) Injection for Intravenous Use
Initial U.S. Approval: 2003

———RECENT MAJOR CHANGES———
Indications and Usage, Postoperative Nausea and Vomiting (1.2) 02/2008
Dosage and Administration, Recommended Dosing (2.1) 02/2008
Warnings and Precautions, QTc Intervals (5.2) - Deletion 02/2008

———INDICATIONS AND USAGE———
ALOXI is a serotonin subtype 3 (5-HT3) receptor antagonist indicated for:
• Moderately emetogenic cancer chemotherapy-prevention of acute and delayed nausea and vomiting associated with initial and repeat courses (1.1)
• Highly emetogenic cancer chemotherapy-prevention of acute nausea and vomiting associated with initial and repeat courses (1.1)
• Prevention of postoperative nausea and vomiting (PONV) for up to 24 hours following surgery. Efficacy beyond 24 hours has not been demonstrated (1.2)

———DOSAGE AND ADMINISTRATION———
Chemotherapy-Induced Nausea and Vomiting (2.1)
• Adult Dosage: a single 0.25 mg I.V. dose administered over 30 seconds. Dosing should occur approximately 30 minutes before the start of chemotherapy.
Postoperative Nausea and Vomiting (2.1)
• Adult Dosage: a single 0.075 mg I.V. dose administered over 10 seconds immediately before the induction of anesthesia.

———DOSAGE FORMS AND STRENGTHS———
0.25 mg/5 mL (free base) single-use vial (3)
0.075 mg/1.5 mL (free base) single-use vial (3)

———CONTRAINDICATIONS———
ALOXI is contraindicated in patients known to have hypersensitivity to the drug or any of its components (4)

———WARNINGS AND PRECAUTIONS———
• Hypersensitivity reactions may occur in patients who have exhibited hypersensitivity to other selective 5-HT3 receptor antagonists (5.1)

———ADVERSE REACTIONS———
The most common adverse reactions in chemotherapy-induced nausea and vomiting (incidence ≥ 5%) are and constipation (6.1)
The most common adverse reactions in postoperative nausea and vomiting (incidence ≥ 2%) are QT prolongation, bradycardia, headache, and constipation.
To report SUSPECTED ADVERSE REACTIONS, contact EISAI at 1-888-422-4743 or FDA at 1-800-FDA-1088 or www.fda.gov/medwatch.

———DRUG INTERACTIONS———
The potential for clinically significant drug interactions with palonosetron appears to be low (7)

———USE IN SPECIFIC POPULATIONS———
Safety and effectiveness in patients below the age of 18 years have not been established (8.4)
See 17 for PATIENT COUNSELING INFORMATION
Revised: 09/2008

FULL PRESCRIBING INFORMATION: CONTENTS*
RECENT MAJOR CHANGES

16 HOW SUPPLIED/STORAGE AND HANDLING
17 PATIENT COUNSELING INFORMATION
17.1 Instructions for Patients
17.2 FDA-Approved Patient Labeling
PRINCIPAL DISPLAY PANEL
*** Sections or subsections omitted from the full prescribing information are not listed**

FULL PRESCRIBING INFORMATION

1 INDICATIONS AND USAGE

1.1 Chemotherapy-Induced Nausea and Vomiting

ALOXI is indicated for:
- Moderately emetogenic cancer chemotherapy-prevention of acute and delayed nausea and vomiting associated with initial and repeat courses
- Highly emetogenic cancer chemotherapy-prevention of acute nausea and vomiting associated with initial and repeat courses

1.2 Postoperative Nausea and Vomiting

ALOXI is indicated for:
- Prevention of postoperative nausea and vomiting (PONV) for up to 24 hours following surgery. Efficacy beyond 24 hours has not been demonstrated.

As with other antiemetics, routine prophylaxis is not recommended in patients in whom there is little expectation that nausea and/or vomiting will occur postoperatively. In patients where nausea and vomiting must be avoided during the postoperative period, ALOXI is recommended even where the incidence of postoperative nausea and/or vomiting is low.

2 DOSAGE AND ADMINISTRATION

2.1 Recommended Dosing

Chemotherapy-Induced Nausea and Vomiting

Dosage for Adults-a single 0.25 mg I.V. dose administered over 30 seconds. Dosing should occur 30 minutes before the start of chemotherapy.

Postoperative Nausea and Vomiting

Dosage for Adults-a single 0.075 mg I.V. dose administered over 10 seconds immediately before the induction of anesthesia.

2.2 Instructions for I.V. Administration

ALOXI is supplied ready for intravenous injection. ALOXI should not be mixed with other drugs. Flush the infusion line with normal saline before and after administration of ALOXI.

Parenteral drug products should be inspected visually for particulate matter and discoloration before administration, whenever solution and container permit.

3 DOSAGE FORM AND STRENGTHS

ALOXI is supplied as a single-use sterile, clear, colorless solution in glass vials that provide:
- 0.25 mg (free base) per 5 mL
- 0.075 mg (free base) per 1.5 mL

4 CONTRAINDICATIONS

ALOXI is contraindicated in patients known to have hypersensitivity to the drug or any of its components. *[see Adverse Reactions (6.2)]*

5 WARNINGS AND PRECAUTIONS

5.1 Hypersensitivity

Hypersensitivity reactions may occur in patients who have exhibited hypersensitivity to other 5-HT_3 receptor antagonists.

6 ADVERSE REACTIONS

Because clinical trials are conducted under widely varying conditions, adverse reaction rates observed in the clinical trials of a drug cannot be directly compared to rates in the clinical trials of another drug and may not reflect the rates observed in practice.

6.1 Chemotherapy-Induced Nausea and Vomiting

In clinical trials for the prevention of nausea and vomiting induced by moderately or highly emetogenic chemotherapy, 1374 adult patients received palonosetron. Adverse reactions were similar in frequency and severity with ALOXI and ondansetron or dolasetron. Following is a listing of all adverse reactions reported by ≥ 2% of patients in these trials (Table 1).

Table 1: Adverse Reactions from Chemotherapy-Induced Nausea and Vomiting Studies ≥ 2% in any Treatment Group

Event	ALOXI 0.25 mg (N=633)	Ondansetron 32 mg I.V. (N=410)	Dolasetron 100 mg I.V. (N=194)
Headache	60 (9%)	34 (8%)	32 (16%)
Constipation	29 (5%)	8 (2%)	12 (6%)
Diarrhea	8 (1%)	7 (2%)	4 (2%)
Dizziness	8 (1%)	9 (2%)	4 (2%)
Fatigue	3 (< 1%)	4 (1%)	4 (2%)
Abdominal Pain	1 (< 1%)	2 (< 1%)	3 (2%)
Insomnia	1 (< 1%)	3 (1%)	3 (2%)

In other studies, 2 subjects experienced severe constipation following a single palonosetron dose of 0.75 mg, three times the recommended dose. One patient received a 10 mcg/kg oral dose in a post-operative nausea and vomiting study and one healthy subject received a 0.75 mg I.V. dose in a pharmacokinetic study.

In clinical trials, the following infrequently reported adverse reactions, assessed by investigators as treatment-related or causality unknown, occurred following administration of ALOXI to adult patients receiving concomitant cancer chemotherapy:

Cardiovascular: 1%: non-sustained tachycardia, bradycardia, hypotension, < 1%: hypertension, myocardial ischemia, extrasystoles, sinus tachycardia, sinus arrhythmia, supraventricular extrasystoles and QT prolongation. In many cases, the relationship to ALOXI was unclear.

Dermatological: < 1%: allergic dermatitis, rash.

Hearing and Vision: < 1%: motion sickness, tinnitus, eye irritation and amblyopia.

Gastrointestinal System: 1% diarrhea, < 1% dyspepsia, abdominal pain, dry mouth, hiccups and flatulence.

General: 1% weakness, < 1% fatigue, fever, hot flash, flu-like syndrome.

Liver: < 1%: transient, asymptomatic increases in AST and/or ALT and bilirubin. These changes occurred predominantly in patients receiving highly emetogenic chemotherapy.

Metabolic: 1%: hyperkalemia, < 1%: electrolyte fluctuations, hyperglycemia, metabolic acidosis, glycosuria, appetite decrease, anorexia.

Musculoskeletal: < 1%: arthralgia.

Nervous System: 1%: dizziness, < 1%: somnolence, insomnia, hypersomnia, paresthesia.

Psychiatric: 1%: anxiety, < 1%: euphoric mood.

Urinary System: < 1%: urinary retention.

Vascular: < 1%: vein discoloration, vein distention.

6.2 Postoperative Nausea and Vomiting

The adverse reactions cited in Table 2 were reported in ≥ 2% of adults receiving I.V. Aloxi 0.075 mg immediately before induction of anesthesia in one phase 2 and two phase 3 randomized placebo-controlled trials. Rates of events between palonosetron and placebo groups were indistinguishable. Some events are known to be associated with, or may be exacerbated by concomitant perioperative and intraoperative medications administered in this surgical population. Please refer to Section 12.2, thorough QTc study results, for definitive data demonstrating the lack of palonosetron effect on QT/QTc.

Table 2: Adverse Reactions from Postoperative Nausea and Vomiting Studies ≥ 2% in any Treatment Group

Event	ALOXI 0.075 mg (N=336)	Placebo (N=369)
Electrocardiogram QT prolongation	16 (5%)	11 (3%)
Bradycardia	13 (4%)	16 (4%)
Headache	11 (3%)	14 (4%)
Constipation	8 (2%)	11 (3%)

In these clinical trials, the following infrequently reported adverse reactions, assessed by investigators as treatment-related or causality unknown, occurred following administration of ALOXI to adult patients receiving concomitant perioperative and intraoperative medications including those associated with anesthesia:

Cardiovascular: 1% electrocardiogram QTc prolongation, sinus bradycardia, tachycardia; < 1%: blood pressure decreased, hypotension, hypertension, arrhythmia, ventricular extrasystoles, generalized edema; ECG T wave amplitude decreased, platelet count decreased. The frequency of these adverse effects did not appear to be different from placebo.

Dermatological: 1%: pruritus.

Gastrointestinal System: 1%: flatatulence, < 1%: dry mouth, upper abdominal pain, salivary hypersecretion, dyspepsia, diarrhea, intestinal hypomotility, anorexia.

General: < 1%: chills.

Liver: 1%: increases in AST and/or ALT, < 1%: hepatic enzyme increased.

Metabolic: < 1%: hypokalemia, anorexia.

Nervous System: < 1%: dizziness.

Respiratory: < 1%: hypoventilation, laryngospasm.

Urinary System: 1%: urinary retention.

6.3 Postmarketing Experience

The following adverse reactions have been identified during postapproval use of ALOXI. Because these reactions are reported voluntarily from a population of uncertain size, it is not always possible to reliably estimate their frequency or establish a causal relationship to drug exposure.

Very rare cases (<1/10,000) of hypersensitivity reactions and injection site reactions (burning, induration, discomfort and pain) were reported from postmarketing experience of ALOXI 0.25 mg in the prevention of Chemotherapy Induced Nausea and Vomiting.

7 DRUG INTERACTIONS

Palonosetron is eliminated from the body through both renal excretion and metabolic pathways with latter mediated via multiple CYP enzymes. Further *in vitro* studies indicated that palonosetron is not an inhibitor of CYP1A2, CYP2A6, CYP2B6, CYP2C9, CYP2D6, CYP2E1 and CYP3A4/5 (CYP2C19 was not investigated) nor does it induce the activity of CYP1A2, CYP2D6, or CYP3A4/5. Therefore, the potential for clinically significant drug interactions with palonosetron appears to be low.

Coadministration of 0.25 mg I.V. palonosetron and 20 mg I.V. dexamethasone in healthy subjects no pharmacokinetic drug-interactions between palonosetron and dexamethasone.

In an interaction study in healthy subjects where palonosetron 0.25 mg (I.V. bolus) was administered on day 1 and oral aprepitant for 3 days (125 mg/80 mg/80 mg), the pharmacokinetics of palonosetron were not significantly altered (AUC: no change, C_{max}: 15% increase).

A study in healthy volunteers involving single-dose I.V. palonosetron (0.75 mg) and steady state oral (10 mg four times daily) demonstrated no significant pharmacokinetic interaction.

In controlled clinical trials, ALOXI injection has been safely administered with corticosteroids, analgesics, antiemetics/antinauseants, antispasmodics and anticholinergic agents.

Palonosetron did not inhibit the antitumor activity of the five chemotherapeutic agents tested (cisplatin, cytarabine, doxorubicin and mitomycin C) in murine tumor models.

8 USE IN SPECIFIC POPULATIONS

8.1 Pregnancy

Teratogenic Effects: Category B

Teratology studies have been performed in rats at oral doses up to 60 mg/kg/day (1894 times the recommended human intravenous dose based on body surface area) and rabbits at oral doses up to 60 mg/kg/day (3789 times the recommended human intravenous dose based on body surface area) and have revealed no evidence of impaired fertility or harm to the fetus due to palonosetron. There are, however, no adequate and well-controlled studies in pregnant women. Because animal reproduction studies are not always predictive of human response, palonosetron should be used during pregnancy only if clearly needed.

8.2 Labor and Delivery

Palonosetron has not been administered to patients undergoing labor and delivery, so its effects on the mother or child are unknown.

8.3 Nursing Mothers

It is not known whether palonosetron is excreted in human milk. Because many drugs are excreted in human milk and because of the potential for serious adverse reactions in nursing infants and the potential for tumorigenicity shown for palonosetron in the rat carcinogenicity study, a decision should be made whether to discontinue nursing or to discontinue the drug, taking into account the importance of the drug to the mother.

8.4 Pediatric Use

Safety and effectiveness in patients below the age of 18 years have not been established.

8.5 Geriatric Use

Population pharmacokinetics analysis did not reveal any differences in palonosetron pharmacokinetics between cancer patients ≥ 65 years of age and younger patients (18 to 64 years). Of the 1374 adult cancer patients in clinical studies of palonosetron, 316 (23%) were ≥ 65 years old, while 71 (5%) were ≥ 75 years old. No overall differences in safety or effectiveness were observed between these subjects and the younger subjects, but greater sensitivity in some older individuals cannot be ruled out. No dose adjustment or special monitoring are required for geriatric patients.

Of the 1520 adult patients in Aloxi PONV clinical studies, 73 (5%) were ≥ 65 years old. No overall differences in safety were observed between older and younger subjects in these studies, though the possibility of heightened sensitivity in some older individuals cannot be excluded. No differences in efficacy were observed in geriatric patients for the CINV indication and none are expected for geriatric PONV patients. However, Aloxi efficacy in geriatric patients has not been adequately evaluated.

8.6 Renal Impairment

Mild to moderate renal impairment does not significantly affect palonosetron pharmacokinetic parameters. Total systemic exposure increased by approximately 28% in severe renal impairment relative to healthy subjects. Dosage adjustment is not necessary in patients with any degree of renal impairment.

8.7 Hepatic Impairment

Hepatic impairment does not significantly affect total body clearance of palonosetron compared to the healthy subjects. Dosage adjustment is not necessary in patients with any degree of hepatic impairment.

8.8 Race

Intravenous palonosetron pharmacokinetics was characterized in twenty-four healthy Japanese subjects over the dose range of 3-90 mcg/kg. Total body clearance was 25% higher in Japanese subjects compared to Whites, however, no dose adjustment is required. The pharmacokinetics of palonosetron in Blacks has not been adequately characterized.

10 OVERDOSAGE

There is no known antidote to ALOXI. Overdose should be managed with supportive care.

Fifty adult cancer patients were administered palonosetron at a dose of 90 mcg/kg (equivalent to 6 mg fixed dose) as part of a dose ranging study. This is approximately 25 times the recommended dose of 0.25 mg. This dose group had a similar incidence of adverse events compared to the other dose groups and no dose response effects were observed. Dialysis studies have not been performed, however, due to the large volume of distribution, dialysis is unlikely to be an effective treatment for palonosetron overdose. A single intravenous dose of palonosetron at 30 mg/kg (947 and 474 times the human dose for rats and mice, respectively, based on body surface area) was lethal to rats and mice. The major signs of toxicity were convulsions, gasping, pallor, cyanosis and collapse.

11 DESCRIPTION

ALOXI (palonosetron hydrochloride) is an antiemetic and antinauseant agent. It is a serotonin subtype 3 (5-HT$_3$) receptor antagonist with a strong binding affinity for this receptor. Chemically, palonosetron hydrochloride is: (3aS)-2-[(S)-1-Azabicyclo [2.2.2]oct-3-yl]-2,3,3a,4,5,6-hexahydro-1-oxo-1Hbenz[de]isoquinoline hydrochloride. The empirical formula is $C_{19}H_{24}N_2O \cdot HCl$, with a molecular weight of 332.87. Palonosetron hydrochloride exists as a single isomer and has the following structural formula:

Palonosetron hydrochloride is a white to off-white crystalline powder. It is freely soluble in water, soluble in propylene glycol, and slightly soluble in ethanol and 2-propanol. ALOXI injection is a sterile, clear, colorless, non pyrogenic, isotonic, buffered solution for intravenous administration. ALOXI injection is available as 5 mL single use vial or 1.5 mL single use vial. Each 5 mL vial contains 0.25 mg palonosetron base as 0.28 mg palonosetron hydrochloride, 207.5 mg mannitol, disodium edetate and citrate buffer in water for intravenous administration.

Each 1.5 mL vial contains 0.075 mg palonosetron base as 0.084 mg palonosetron hydrochloride, 83 mg mannitol, disodium edetate and citrate buffer in water for intravenous administration. The pH of the solution in the 5 mL and 1.5 mL vials is 4.5 to 5.5.

12 CLINICAL PHARMACOLOGY

12.1 Mechanism of Action

Palonosetron is a 5-HT$_3$ receptor antagonist with a strong binding affinity for this receptor and little or no affinity for other receptors.

Cancer chemotherapy may be associated with a high incidence of nausea and vomiting, particularly when certain agents, such as cisplatin, are used. 5-HT$_3$ receptors are located on the nerve terminals of the vagus in the periphery and centrally in the chemoreceptor trigger zone of the area postrema. It is thought that chemotherapeutic agents produce nausea and vomiting by releasing serotonin from the enterochromaffin cells of the small intestine and that the released serotonin then activates 5-HT$_3$ receptors located on vagal afferents to initiate the vomiting reflex.

Postoperative nausea and vomiting is influenced by multiple patient, surgical and anesthesia related factors and is triggered by release of 5-HT in a cascade of neuronal events

involving both the central nervous system and the gastrointestinal tract. The 5-HT$_3$ receptor has been demonstrated to selectively participate in the emetic response.

12.2 Pharmacodynamics

The effect of palonosetron on blood pressure, heart rate, and ECG parameters including QTc were comparable to ondansetron and dolasetron in CINV clinical trials. In PONV clinical trials the effect of palonosetron on the QTc interval was no different from placebo. In non-clinical studies palonosetron possesses the ability to block ion channels involved in ventricular de- and re-polarization and to prolong action potential duration.

The effect of palonosetron on QTc interval was evaluated in a double blind, randomized, parallel, placebo and positive (moxifloxacin) controlled trial in adult men and women. The objective was to evaluate the ECG effects of I.V. administered palonosetron at single doses of 0.25, 0.75 or 2.25 mg in 221 healthy subjects. The study demonstrated no significant effect on any ECG interval including QTc duration (cardiac repolarization) at doses up to 2.25 mg.

12.3 Pharmacokinetics

After intravenous dosing of palonosetron in healthy subjects and cancer patients, an initial decline in concentrations is followed by a slow elimination from the body. Mean maximum plasma concentration (C$_{max}$) and area under the concentration-time curve (AUC$_{0-\infty}$) are generally dose-proportional over the dose range of 0.3-90 mcg/kg in healthy subjects and in cancer patients. Following single I.V. dose of palonosetron at 3 mcg/kg (or 0.21 mg/70 kg) to six cancer patients, mean (±SD) maximum plasma concentration was estimated to be 5.6 ± 5.5 ng/mL and mean AUC was 35.8 ± 20.9 ng•hr/mL.

Following I.V. administration of palonosetron 0.25 mg once every other day for 3 doses in 11 cancer the mean increase in plasma palonosetron concentration from Day 1 to Day 5 was 42 ± 34%. Following I.V. administration of palonosetron 0.25 mg once daily for 3 days in 12 healthy subjects, the mean ±SD) increase in plasma palonosetron concentration from Day 1 to Day 3 was 110 ± 45%.

After intravenous dosing of palonosetron in patients undergoing surgery (abdominal surgery or vaginal hysterectomy), the pharmacokinetic characteristics of palonosetron were similar to those observed in cancer patients.

Distribution

Palonosetron has a volume of distribution of approximately 8.3 ± 2.5 L/kg. Approximately 62% of palonosetron is bound to plasma proteins.

Metabolism

Palonosetron is eliminated by multiple routes with approximately 50% metabolized to form two primary metabolites: N-oxide-palonosetron and 6-S-hydroxy-palonosetron. These metabolites each have less than 1% of the 5-HT$_3$ receptor antagonist activity of palonosetron. In vitro metabolism studies have suggested that CYP2D6 and to a lesser extent, CYP3A4 and CYP1A2 are involved in the metabolism of palonosetron.

However, clinical pharmacokinetic parameters are not significantly different between poor and extensive metabolizers of CYP2D6 substrates.

Elimination

After a single intravenous dose of 10 mcg/kg [^{14}C]-palonosetron, approximately 80% of the dose was recovered within 144 hours in the urine with palonosetron representing approximately 40% of the administered dose. In healthy subjects, the total body clearance of palonosetron was 160 ± 35 mL/h/kg and renal clearance was 66.5 ± 18.2 mL/h/kg. Mean terminal elimination half-life is approximately 40 hours.

Special Populations

[See USE IN SPECIFIC POPULATIONS (8.5-8.8)]

13 NONCLINICAL TOXICOLOGY

13.1 Carcinogenesis, Mutagenesis, Impairment of Fertility

In a 104-week carcinogenicity study in CD-1 mice, animals were treated with oral doses of palonosetron at 10, 30 and 60 mg/kg/day. Treatment with palonosetron was not tumorigenic. The highest tested dose produced a systemic exposure to palonosetron (Plasma AUC) of about 150 to 289 times the human exposure (AUC = 29.8 ng•h/mL) at the recommended intravenous dose of 0.25 mg. In a 104-week carcinogenicity study in Sprague-Dawley rats, male and female rats were treated with oral doses of 15, 30 and 60 mg/kg/day and 15, 45 and 90 mg/kg/day, respectively. The highest doses produced a systemic exposure to palonosetron (Plasma AUC) of 137 and 308 times the human exposure at the recommended dose. Treatment with palonosetron produced increased incidences of adrenal benign pheochromocytoma and combined benign and malignant pheochromocytoma, increased incidences of pancreatic Islet cell adenoma and combined adenoma and carcinoma and pituitary adenoma in male rats. In female rats, it produced hepatocellular adenoma and carcinoma and increased the incidences of thyroid C-cell adenoma and combined adenoma and carcinoma.

Palonosetron was not genotoxic in the Ames test, the Chinese hamster ovarian cell (CHO/HGPRT) forward mutation test, the ex vivo hepatocyte unscheduled DNA synthesis (UDS) test or the mouse micronucleus test. It was, however, positive for clastogenic effects in the Chinese hamster ovarian (CHO) cell chromosomal aberration test.

Palonosetron at oral doses up to 60 mg/kg/day (about 1894 times the recommended human intravenous dose based on body surface area) was found to have no effect on fertility and reproductive performance of male and female rats.

14 CLINICAL STUDIES

14.1 Chemotherapy-Induced Nausea and Vomiting

Efficacy of single-dose palonosetron injection in preventing acute and delayed nausea and vomiting induced by both moderately and highly emetogenic chemotherapy was studied in three Phase 3 trials and one Phase 2 trial. In these double-blind studies, complete response rates (no emetic episodes and no rescue medication) and other efficacy parameters were assessed through at least 120 hours after administration of chemotherapy. The safety and efficacy of palonosetron in repeated courses of chemotherapy was also assessed.

Table 3: Prevention of Acute Nausea and Vomiting (0-24 hours): Complete Response Rates

Chemotherapy	Study	Treatment Group	N[a]	% with Complete Response	p-value[b]	97.5% Confidence Interval ALOXI minus Comparator[c]
Moderately Emetogenic	1	ALOXI 0.25 mg	189	81	0.009	[2%, 23%]
		Ondansetron 32 mg I.V.	185	69		
	2	ALOXI 0.25 mg	189	63	NS	
		Dolasetron 100 mg I.V.	191	53		
Highly Emetogenic	3	ALOXI 0.25 mg	223	59	NS	[-2%, 22%]
		Ondasetron 32 mg I.V.	221	57		[-9%, 13%]

a Intent-to-treat cohort

b 2-sided Fisher's exact test. Significance level at α=0.025.

c These studies were designed to show non-inferiority. A lower bound greater than -15% demonstrates non-inferiority between ALOXI and comparator.

Table 4: Prevention of Delayed Nausea and Vomiting (24-120 hours): Complete Response Rates

Chemotherapy	Study	Treatment Group	N[a]	% with Complete Response	p-value[b]	97.5% Confidence Interval ALOXI minus Comparator[c]
Moderately Emetogenic	1	ALOXI 0.25 mg	189	74	<0.001	
		Ondansetron 32 mg I.V.	185	55		[8%, 30%]
	2	ALOXI 0.25 mg	189	54	0.004	
		Dolasetron 100 mg I.V.	191	39		[3%, 27%]

Difference in Complete Response Rates

a Intent-to-treat cohort

b 2-sided Fisher's exact test. Significance level at α=0.025.

c These studies were designed to show non-inferiority. A lower bound greater than -15% demonstrates non-inferiority between ALOXI and comparator.

Table 5: Prevention of Overall Nausea and Vomiting (0-120 hours): Complete Response Rates

Chemotherapy	Study	Treatment Group	N[a]	% with Complete Response	p-value[b]	97.5% Confidence Interval ALOXI minus Comparator[c]
Moderately Emetogenic	1	ALOXI 0.25 mg	189	69	<0.001	
		Ondansetron 32 mg I.V.	185	50		[7%, 31%]
	2	ALOXI 0.25 mg	189	46	0.021	
		Dolasetron 100 mg I.V.	191	34		[0%, 24%]

Difference in Complete Response Rates

a Intent-to-treat cohort

b 2-sided Fisher's exact test. Significance level at α=0.025.

c These studies were designed to show non-inferiority. A lower bound greater than -15% demonstrates non-inferiority between ALOXI and comparator.

Moderately Emetogenic Chemotherapy

Two Phase 3, double-blind trials involving 1132 patients compared single-dose I.V. ALOXI with either single-dose I.V. ondansetron (study 1) or dolasetron (study 2) given 30 minutes prior to moderately emetogenic chemotherapy including carboplatin, cisplatin $\leq$ 50 mg/m^2, cyclophosphamide < 1500 mg/m^2, doxorubicin > 25 mg/m^2, epirubicin, irinotecan, and methotrexate > 250 mg/m^2. Concomitant corticosteroids were not administered prophylactically in study 1 and were only used by 4-6% of patients in study 2. The majority of patients in these studies were women (77%), White (65%) and naive to previous chemotherapy (54%). The mean age was 55 years.

Highly Emetogenic Chemotherapy

A Phase 2, double-blind, dose-ranging study evaluated the efficacy of single-dose I.V. palonosetron from 0.3 to 90 mcg/kg (equivalent to < 0.1 mg to 6 mg fixed dose) in 161 chemotherapy-naive adult cancer patients receiving highly-emetogenic chemotherapy (either cisplatin $\geq$ 70 mg/m^2 or cyclophosphamide > 1100 mg/m^2). Concomitant corticosteroids were not administered prophylactically. Analysis of

data from this trial indicates that 0.25 mg is the lowest effective dose in preventing acute nausea and vomiting induced by highly emetogenic chemotherapy.

A Phase 3, double-blind trial involving 667 patients compared single-dose I.V. ALOXI with single-dose I.V. ondansetron (study 3) given 30 minutes prior to highly emetogenic chemotherapy including cisplatin $\geq$ 60 mg/m^2, cyclophosphamide > 1500 mg/m^2, and dacarbazine. Corticosteroids were co-administered prophylactically before chemotherapy in 67% of patients. Of the 667 patients, 51% were women, 60% White, and 59% naive to previous chemotherapy. The mean age was 52 years.

Efficacy Results

The antiemetic activity of ALOXI was evaluated during the acute phase (0-24 hours) [Table 3], delayed phase (24-120 hours) [Table 4], and overall phase (0-120 hours) [Table 5] post-chemotherapy in Phase 3 trials

[See table at top of previous page]

These studies show that ALOXI was effective in the prevention of acute nausea and vomiting associated with initial and repeat courses of moderately and highly emetogenic

cancer chemotherapy. In study 3, efficacy was greater when prophylactic corticosteroids were administered concomitantly. Clinical superiority over other 5-HT$_3$ receptor antagonists has not been adequately demonstrated in the acute phase.

[See table 4 at left]

These studies show that ALOXI was effective in the prevention of delayed nausea and vomiting associated with initial and repeat courses of moderately emetogenic chemotherapy.

[See table 5 at left]

These studies show that ALOXI was effective in the prevention of nausea and vomiting throughout the 120 hours (5 days) following initial and repeat courses of moderately emetogenic cancer chemotherapy.

14.2 Postoperative Nausea and Vomiting

In one multicenter, randomized, stratified, double-blind, parallel-group, phase 3 clinical study (Study 1), palonosetron was compared with placebo for the prevention of PONV in 546 patients undergoing abdominal and gynecological surgery. All patients received general anesthesia. Study 1 was a pivotal study conducted predominantly in the US in the out-patient setting for patients undergoing elective gynecologic or abdominal laparoscopic surgery and stratified at randomization for the following risk factors: gender, non-smoking status, history of post operative nausea and vomiting and/or motion sickness.

In Study 1 patients were randomized to receive palonosetron 0.025 mg, 0.050 mg or 0.075 mg or placebo, each given intravenously immediately prior to induction of anesthesia. The antiemetic activity of palonosetron was evaluated during the 0 to 72 hour time period after surgery. Of the 138 patients treated with 0.075 mg palonosetron in Study 1 and evaluated for efficacy, 96% were women; 66% had a history of PONV or motion sickness; 85% were non-smokers. As for race, 63% were White, 20% were Black, 15% were Hispanic, and 1% were Asian. The age of patients ranged from 21 to 74 years, with a mean age of 37.9 years. Three patients were greater than 65 years of age.

Co-primary efficacy measures were Complete Response (CR) defined as no emetic episode and no use of rescue medication in the 0-24 and in the 24-72 hours postoperatively. Secondary efficacy endpoints included:

• Complete Response (CR) 0-48 and 0-72 hours

• Complete Control (CC) defined as CR and no more than mild nausea

• Severity of nausea (none, mild, moderate, severe)

The primary hypothesis in Study 1 was that at least one of the three palonosetron doses were superior to placebo.

Results for Complete Response in Study 1 for 0.075 mg ALOXI versus placebo are described in the following table.

Table 6: Prevention of Postoperative Nausea and Vomiting: Complete Response (CR), Study 1, ALOXI 0.075 mg Vs Placebo

Treatment	n/N (%)	ALOXI Vs Placebo	
		Δ	p-value*
Co-primary Endpoints			
Complete Response 0-24 hours			
ALOXI	59/138 (42.8%)	16.8%	0.004
Placebo	35/135 (25.9%)		
Complete Response 24-72 hours			
ALOXI	67/138 (48.6%)	7.8%	0.188
Placebo	55/135 (40.7%)		

* To reach statistical significance for each co-primary endpoint, the required significance limit for the lowest p-value was p<0.017.

Δ Difference (%): ALOXI 0.075 mg minus placebo

ALOXI 0.075 mg reduced the severity of nausea compared to placebo. Analyses of other secondary endpoints indicate that ALOXI 0.075 mg was numerically better than placebo, however, statistical significance was not formally demonstrated.

A phase 2 randomized, double-blind, multicenter, placebo-controlled, dose ranging study was performed to evaluate I.V. palonosetron for the prevention of post-operative nausea and vomiting following abdominal or vaginal hysterectomy. Five I.V. palonosetron doses (0.1, 0.3, 1.0, 3.0 and 30 μg/kg) were evaluated in a total of 381 intent-to-treat patients. The primary efficacy measure was the proportion of patients with CR in the first 24 hours after recovery from surgery. The lowest effective dose was palonosetron 1 μg/kg (approximately 0.075 mg) which had a CR rate of 44% versus 19% for placebo, p=0.004. Palonosetron 1 µg/kg also significantly reduced the severity of nausea versus placebo, p=0.009.

16 HOW SUPPLIED/STORAGE AND HANDLING

NDC # 62856-797-01, ALOXI Injection 0.25 mg/5 mL (free base) single-use vial individually packaged in a carton.
NDC # 62856-798-01, ALOXI Injection 0.075 mg/1.5 mL (free base) single-use vial packaged in a carton containing 5 vials.

Storage

- Store at controlled temperature of 20-25°C (68°F-77°F). Excursions permitted to 15-30°C (59-86°F).
- Protect from freezing.
- Protect from light.

17 PATIENT COUNSELING INFORMATION

See FDA-Approved Patient Labeling (17.2)

17.1 Instructions for Patients

Patients should be advised to report to their physician all of their medical conditions, any pain, redness, or swelling in and around the infusion site [*see Adverse Reactions (6.2)*]. Patients should be instructed to read the patient insert.

17.2 FDA-Approved Patient Labeling

Patient Information

Aloxi (Ah-lock-see)

Read the Patient Information that comes with ALOXI before your treatment with ALOXI and each time you get ALOXI. There may be new information. This information does not take the place of talking with your doctor about your medical condition or your treatment. If you have questions about ALOXI, ask your doctor or pharmacist.

What is ALOXI?

ALOXI is a medicine called an "antiemetic." ALOXI is used in adults to help prevent the nausea and vomiting that happens:

- right away with certain anti-cancer medicines (chemotherapy)
- or later with certain anti-cancer medicines
- right away after recovery from anesthesia after surgery

What is ALOXI used for?

ALOXI is used to prevent nausea and vomiting that may happen:

- soon after taking certain anti-cancer medicines
- later after taking certain anti-cancer medicines
- soon after recovery from anesthesia after surgery

Who should not take ALOXI?

Do not take ALOXI if you are allergic to any of the ingredients in ALOXI. The active ingredient is palonosetron hydrochloride. See the end of this leaflet for a complete list of ingredients in ALOXI. ALOXI has not been studied in children under 18 years of age.

What should I tell my doctor before using ALOXI?

Tell your doctor about all of your medical conditions, including if you:

- are pregnant. It is not known if ALOXI may harm your unborn baby. You and your doctor should decide if ALOXI is right for you.
- are breastfeeding. It is not known if ALOXI passes into your milk and if it can harm your baby. You should choose to either take ALOXI or breastfeed, but not both.

Tell your doctor about all of the medicines you take including prescription and nonprescription medicines, vitamins and herbal supplements.

How should I use ALOXI?

ALOXI is given in your vein by I.V. (intravenous) injection. It is only given to you by a healthcare provider in a hospital or clinic. ALOXI is usually injected into your vein about 30 minutes before you get your anti-cancer medicine (chemotherapy) or immediately before anesthesia for surgery.

What are the possible side effects of ALOXI?

The most common side effects of ALOXI are headache and constipation. Diarrhea and dizziness have also been observed.

These are not all the side effects from ALOXI. For more information ask your doctor or pharmacist.

General information about ALOXI

Medicines are sometimes prescribed for conditions other than those listed in patient information leaflets. ALOXI was prescribed for your medical condition.

This leaflet summarizes the most important information about ALOXI. If you would like more information, talk with your doctor. You can ask your doctor or pharmacist for information about ALOXI that is written for health professionals. You can also visit the ALOXI web site at www.ALOXI.com.

What are the ingredients in ALOXI?

Active ingredient: palonosetron hydrochloride
Inactive ingredients: mannitol, disodium edetate, and citrate buffer in water
Rx Only

Mfd by OSO Biopharmaceuticals, LLC, Albuquerque, NM, USA or Pierre Fabre, Medicament Production, Idron, Aquitaine, France and Helsinn Birex Pharmaceuticals, Dublin, Ireland
HELSINN, Mfd for Helsinn Healthcare SA, Switzerland
Eisai, Inc. Distributed and marketed by Eisai Inc., Woodcliff Lake, NJ 07677 under license of Helsinn Healthcare SA, Switzerland
ALOXI is a registered trademark of Helsinn Healthcare, SA, Lugano, Switzerland
©2009 Eisai, Woodcliff Lake, NJ 07677 U.S.A. 201227
06/09

Shown in Product Identification Guide, page 308

ARICEPT®
[ă'rĭ-sĕpt]
(donepezil hydrochloride)
Tablets

℞

HIGHLIGHTS OF PRESCRIBING INFORMATION

These highlights do not include all the information needed to use ARICEPT safely and effectively. See full prescribing information for ARICEPT Tablets and ARICEPT Orally Disintegrating Tablets (ODT).

ARICEPT® (donepezil hydrochloride) tablets
Initial U.S. Approval: 1996

————RECENT MAJOR CHANGES————
Addition of new dosage strength: ARICEPT 23 mg

————INDICATIONS AND USAGE————

ARICEPT is indicated for the treatment of dementia of the Alzheimer's type. Efficacy has been demonstrated in patients with mild, moderate, and severe Alzheimer's Disease (1).

————DOSAGE AND ADMINISTRATION————

- **Mild to Moderate Alzheimer's disease**—5 mg or 10 mg administered once daily (2.1)
- **Moderate to Severe Alzheimer's disease**—10 mg or 23 mg administered once daily (2.2)

A dose of 10 mg once daily can be administered once patients have been on a daily dose of 5 mg for 4 to 6 weeks. A dose of 23 mg once daily can be administered once patients have been on a dose of 10 mg once daily for at least 3 months (2.3).

————DOSAGE FORMS AND STRENGTHS————

- Tablets: 5 mg, 10 mg and 23 mg (3)
- Orally Disintegrating Tablets (ODT): 5 mg and 10 mg (3)

————CONTRAINDICATIONS————

- Patients with known hypersensitivity to donepezil hydrochloride or to piperidine derivatives (4)

————WARNINGS AND PRECAUTIONS————

- Cholinesterase inhibitors are likely to exaggerate succinylcholine-type muscle relaxation during anesthesia (5.1).
- Cholinesterase inhibitors may have vagotonic effects on the sinoatrial and atrioventricular nodes manifesting as bradycardia or heart block (5.2).
- ARICEPT can cause vomiting. Patients should be observed closely at initiation of treatment and after dose increases (5.3).
- Patients should be monitored closely for symptoms of active or occult gastrointestinal (GI) bleeding, especially those at increased risk for developing ulcers (5.4).
- The use of ARICEPT in a dose of 23 mg once daily is associated with weight loss (5.5).
- Cholinomimetics may cause bladder outflow obstructions (5.6).
- Cholinomimetics are believed to have some potential to cause generalized convulsions (5.7).
- Cholinesterase inhibitors should be prescribed with care to patients with a history of asthma or obstructive pulmonary disease (5.8).

————ADVERSE REACTIONS————

The most common adverse reactions in clinical studies of ARICEPT are nausea, diarrhea, insomnia, vomiting, muscle cramps, fatigue, and anorexia (6.1).

To report SUSPECTED ADVERSE REACTIONS, contact Eisai Inc. at 1-888-274-2378 (fax 1-201-746-3207) or FDA at 1-800-FDA-1088 or www.fda.gov/medwatch.

————DRUG INTERACTIONS————

- Cholinesterase inhibitors have the potential to interfere with the activity of anticholinergic medications (7.3).
- A synergistic effect may be expected with concomitant administration of succinylcholine, similar neuromuscular blocking agents, or cholinergic agonists (7.4).

————USE IN SPECIFIC POPULATIONS————

- Based on animal data, ARICEPT may cause fetal harm (8.1).

See 17 for PATIENT COUNSELING INFORMATION
Revised: 07/2010

FULL PRESCRIBING INFORMATION: CONTENTS*

* Sections or subsections omitted from the full prescribing information are not listed

FULL PRESCRIBING INFORMATION

1. INDICATIONS AND USAGE

ARICEPT is indicated for the treatment of dementia of the Alzheimer's type. Efficacy has been demonstrated in patients with mild, moderate, and severe Alzheimer's disease.

2. DOSAGE AND ADMINISTRATION

ARICEPT should be taken in the evening, just prior to retiring.
ARICEPT can be taken with or without food and should be swallowed whole with water. ARICEPT should not be split or crushed.
The 23 mg tablet should not be crushed or chewed because this may increase its rate of absorption.
Allow ARICEPT ODT tablet to dissolve on the tongue and follow with water.

2.1. Mild to Moderate Alzheimer's Disease

The dosages of ARICEPT shown to be effective in controlled clinical trials are 5 mg and 10 mg administered once per day.
The higher dose of 10 mg did not provide a statistically significantly greater clinical benefit than 5 mg. There is a suggestion, however, based upon order of group mean scores and dose trend analyses of data from these clinical trials, that a daily dose of 10 mg of ARICEPT might provide additional benefit for some patients. Accordingly, whether or not to employ a dose of 10 mg is a matter of prescriber and patient preference.

2.2. Moderate to Severe Alzheimer's Disease

ARICEPT has been shown to be effective in controlled clinical trials at doses of 10 mg and 23 mg administered once daily. Results of a controlled clinical trial in moderate to severe Alzheimer's Disease that compared ARICEPT 23 mg once daily to 10 mg once daily suggest that a 23 mg dose of ARICEPT provided additional benefit.

2.3. Titration

The recommended starting dose of ARICEPT is 5 mg once daily. Evidence from the controlled trials in mild to moderate Alzheimer's disease indicates that the 10 mg dose, with a one week titration, is likely to be associated with a higher incidence of cholinergic adverse events compared to the

5 mg dose. In open-label trials using a 6 week titration, the type and frequency of these same adverse events were similar between the 5 mg and 10 mg dose groups. Therefore, because ARICEPT steady state is achieved about 15 days after it is started and because the incidence of untoward effects may be influenced by the rate of dose escalation, a dose of 10 mg should not be administered until patients have been on a daily dose of 5 mg for 4 to 6 weeks. A dose of 23 mg once daily can be administered once patients have been on a dose of 10 mg once daily for at least 3 months.

3.   DOSAGE FORMS AND STRENGTHS

ARICEPT is supplied as film-coated, round tablets containing 5 mg, 10 mg, or 23 mg of donepezil hydrochloride.

The 5 mg tablets are white. The strength, in mg (5), is debossed on one side and ARICEPT is debossed on the other side.

The 10 mg tablets are yellow. The strength, in mg (10), is debossed on one side and ARICEPT is debossed on the other side.

The 23 mg tablets are reddish. The strength, in mg (23), is debossed on one side, and ARICEPT is debossed on the other side.

ARICEPT ODT is supplied as round tablets containing either 5 mg or 10 mg of donepezil hydrochloride.

The 5 mg orally disintegrating tablets are white. The strength, in mg (5), is embossed on one side and ARICEPT is embossed on the other side.

The 10 mg orally disintegrating tablets are yellow. The strength, in mg (10), is embossed on one side and ARICEPT is embossed on the other side.

4.   CONTRAINDICATIONS

ARICEPT is contraindicated in patients with known hypersensitivity to donepezil hydrochloride or to piperidine derivatives.

5.   WARNINGS AND PRECAUTIONS
5.1.   Anesthesia
ARICEPT, as a cholinesterase inhibitor, is likely to exaggerate succinylcholine-type muscle relaxation during anesthesia.

5.2.   Cardiovascular Conditions
Because of their pharmacological action, cholinesterase inhibitors may have vagotonic effects on the sinoatrial and atrioventricular nodes. This effect may manifest as bradycardia or heart block in patients both with and without known underlying cardiac conduction abnormalities. Syncopal episodes have been reported in association with the use of ARICEPT.

5.3.   Nausea and Vomiting
ARICEPT, as a predictable consequence of its pharmacological properties, has been shown to produce diarrhea, nausea, and vomiting. These effects, when they occur, appear more frequently with the 10 mg/day dose than with the 5 mg/day dose, and more frequently with the 23 mg dose than with the 10 mg dose. Specifically, in a controlled trial that compared a dose of 23 mg/day to 10 mg/day in patients who had been treated with donepezil 10 mg/day for at least three months, the incidence of nausea in the 23 mg group was markedly greater than in the patients who continued on 10 mg/day (11.8% vs. 3.4%, respectively), and the incidence of vomiting in the 23 mg group was markedly greater than in the 10 mg group (9.2% vs. 2.5%, respectively). The percent of patients who discontinued treatment due to vomiting in the 23 mg group was markedly higher than in the 10 mg group (2.9% vs. 0.4%, respectively).

Although in most cases, these effects have been mild and transient, sometimes lasting one to three weeks, and have resolved during continued use of ARICEPT, patients should be observed closely at the initiation of treatment and after dose increases.

5.4.   Peptic Ulcer Disease and GI Bleeding
Through their primary action, cholinesterase inhibitors may be expected to increase gastric acid secretion due to increased cholinergic activity. Therefore, patients should be monitored closely for symptoms of active or occult gastrointestinal bleeding, especially those at increased risk for developing ulcers, e.g., those with a history of ulcer disease or those receiving concurrent nonsteroidal anti-inflammatory drugs (NSAIDs). Clinical studies of ARICEPT in a dose of 5 mg/day to 10 mg/day have shown no increase, relative to placebo, in the incidence of either peptic ulcer disease or gastrointestinal bleeding. Results of a controlled clinical study with 23 mg/day showed an increase, relative to 10 mg/day, in the incidence of peptic ulcer disease (0.4% vs. 0.2%) and gastrointestinal bleeding from any site (1.1% vs. 0.6%).

5.5.   Weight Loss
Weight loss was reported as an adverse event in 4.7% of patients assigned to ARICEPT in a dose of 23 mg/day compared to 2.5% of patients assigned to 10 mg/day. Compared to their baseline weights, 8.4% of patients taking 23 mg/day were found to have a weight decrease of ≥ 7% by the end of the study, while 4.9% of patients taking 10 mg/day were found to have weight loss of ≥ 7% at the end of the study.

5.6.   Genitourinary Conditions
Although not observed in clinical trials of ARICEPT, cholinomimetics may cause bladder outflow obstruction.

5.7.   Neurological Conditions: Seizures
Cholinomimetics are believed to have some potential to cause generalized convulsions. However, seizure activity also may be a manifestation of Alzheimer's disease.

5.8.   Pulmonary Conditions
Because of their cholinomimetic actions, cholinesterase inhibitors should be prescribed with care to patients with a history of asthma or obstructive pulmonary disease.

6.   ADVERSE REACTIONS
6.1.   Clinical Studies Experience
ARICEPT 5 mg/day and 10 mg/day
Mild to Moderate Alzheimer's Disease
Adverse Events Leading to Discontinuation
The rates of discontinuation from controlled clinical trials of ARICEPT due to adverse events for the ARICEPT 5 mg/day treatment groups were comparable to those of placebo treatment groups at approximately 5%. The rate of discontinuation of patients who received 7-day escalations from 5 mg/day to 10 mg/day was higher at 13%.

The most common adverse events leading to discontinuation, defined as those occurring in at least 2% of patients and at twice or more the incidence seen in placebo patients, are shown in Table 1.

Table 1. Most Frequent Adverse Events Leading to Discontinuation from Controlled Clinical Trials by Dose Group

Dose Group	Placebo	5 mg/day ARICEPT	10 mg/day ARICEPT
Patients Randomized	355	350	315
Event/%Discontinuing			
Nausea	1%	1%	3%
Diarrhea	0%	<1%	3%
Vomiting	<1%	<1%	2%

Most Frequent Adverse Events Seen in Association with the Use of ARICEPT
The most common adverse events, defined as those occurring at a frequency of at least 5% in patients receiving 10 mg/day and twice the placebo rate, are largely predicted by ARICEPT's cholinomimetic effects. These include nausea, diarrhea, insomnia, vomiting, muscle cramp, fatigue and anorexia. These adverse events were often of mild intensity and transient, resolving during continued ARICEPT treatment without the need for dose modification.

There is evidence to suggest that the frequency of these common adverse events may be affected by the rate of titration. An open-label study was conducted with 269 patients who received placebo in the 15 and 30-week studies. These patients were titrated to a dose of 10 mg/day over a 6-week period. The rates of common adverse events were lower than those seen in patients titrated to 10 mg/day over one week in the controlled clinical trials and were comparable to those seen in patients on 5 mg/day.

See Table 2 for a comparison of the most common adverse events following one and six week titration regimens.

Table 2. Comparison of Rates of Adverse Events in Mild to Moderate Patients Titrated to 10 mg/day over 1 and 6 Weeks

Adverse Event	No titration Placebo (n=315)	No titration 5 mg/day (n=311)	One week titration 10 mg/day (n=315)	Six week titration 10 mg/day (n=269)
Nausea	6%	5%	19%	6%
Diarrhea	5%	8%	15%	9%
Insomnia	6%	6%	14%	6%
Fatigue	3%	4%	8%	3%
Vomiting	3%	3%	8%	5%
Muscle cramps	2%	6%	8%	3%
Anorexia	2%	3%	7%	3%

Adverse Events Reported in Controlled Trials
The events cited reflect experience gained under closely monitored conditions of clinical trials in a highly selected patient population. In actual clinical practice or in other clinical trials, these frequency estimates may not apply, as the conditions of use, reporting behavior, and the kinds of patients treated may differ. Table 3 lists treatment emergent signs and symptoms that were reported in at least 2% of patients in placebo-controlled clinical trials who received ARICEPT and for which the rate of occurrence was greater for patients treated with ARICEPT than with placebo. In general, adverse events occurred more frequently in female patients and with advancing age.

Table 3. Adverse Events Reported in Controlled Clinical Trials in Mild to Moderate Alzheimer's Disease in at Least 2% of Patients Receiving ARICEPT and at a Higher Frequency than Placebo Treated Patients

Body System/Adverse Event	Placebo (n=355)	ARICEPT (n=747)
Percent of Patients with any Adverse Event	72	74
Body as a Whole		
Headache	9	10
Pain, various locations	8	9
Accident	6	7
Fatigue	3	5
Cardiovascular System		
Syncope	1	2
Digestive System		
Nausea	6	11
Diarrhea	5	10
Vomiting	3	5
Anorexia	2	4
Hemic and Lymphatic System		
Ecchymosis	3	4
Metabolic and Nutritional Systems		
Weight Decrease	1	3
Musculoskeletal System		
Muscle Cramps	2	6
Arthritis	1	2
Nervous System		
Insomnia	6	9
Dizziness	6	8
Depression	<1	3
Abnormal Dreams	0	3
Somnolence	<1	2
Urogenital System		
Frequent Urination	1	2

Other Adverse Events Observed During Clinical Trials
ARICEPT has been administered to over 1700 individuals during clinical trials worldwide. Approximately 1200 of these patients have been treated for at least 3 months and more than 1000 patients have been treated for at least 6 months. Controlled and uncontrolled trials in the United States included approximately 900 patients. In regards to the highest dose of 23 mg/day, this population includes 650 patients treated for 3 months, 475 patients treated for 6 months and 116 patients treated for over 1 year. The range of patient exposure is from 1 to 1214 days.

Treatment emergent signs and symptoms that occurred during three controlled clinical trials and two open-label trials in the United States were recorded as adverse events by the clinical investigators using terminology of their own choosing. To provide an overall estimate of the proportion of individuals having similar types of events, the events were grouped into a smaller number of standardized categories using a modified COSTART dictionary, and event frequencies were calculated across all studies. These categories are used in the listing below. The frequencies represent the proportion of 900 patients from these trials who experienced that event while receiving ARICEPT. All adverse events occurring at least twice are included, except for those already listed in Tables 2 or 3, COSTART terms too general to be informative, or events less likely to be drug related. Events are classified by body system and listed using the following definitions: *Frequent adverse events* - those occurring in at least 1/100 patients; *Infrequent adverse events* - those occurring in 1/100 to 1/1000 patients. These adverse events are not necessarily related to ARICEPT treatment and in most cases were observed at a similar frequency in placebo treated patients in the controlled studies. No important additional adverse events were seen in studies conducted outside the United States.

Body as a Whole: *Frequent:* influenza, chest pain, toothache; *Infrequent:* fever, edema face, periorbital edema, hernia hiatal, abscess, cellulitis, chills, generalized coldness, head fullness, listlessness.

Cardiovascular System: *Frequent:* hypertension, vasodilation, atrial fibrillation, hot flashes, hypotension; *Infrequent:* angina pectoris, postural hypotension, myocardial infarction, AV block (first degree), congestive heart failure, arteritis, bradycardia, peripheral vascular disease, supraventricular tachycardia, deep vein thrombosis.

Digestive System: *Frequent:* fecal incontinence, gastrointestinal bleeding, bloating, epigastric pain; *Infrequent:* eructation, gingivitis, increased appetite, flatulence, periodontal abscess, cholelithiasis, diverticulitis, drooling, dry mouth, fever sore, gastritis, irritable colon, tongue edema, epigastric distress, gastroenteritis, increased transaminases, hemorrhoids, ileus, increased thirst, jaundice, melena, polydipsia, duodenal ulcer, stomach ulcer.

Endocrine System: *Infrequent:* diabetes mellitus, goiter.

Hemic and Lymphatic System: *Infrequent:* anemia, thrombocythemia, thrombocytopenia, eosinophilia, erythrocytopenia.

Metabolic and Nutritional Disorders: *Frequent:* dehydration; *Infrequent:* gout, hypokalemia, increased creatine kinase, hyperglycemia, weight increase, increased lactate dehydrogenase.

Musculoskeletal System: *Frequent:* bone fracture; *Infrequent:* muscle weakness, muscle fasciculation.

Nervous System: *Frequent:* delusions, tremor, irritability, paresthesia, aggression, vertigo, ataxia, increased libido, restlessness, abnormal crying, nervousness, aphasia; *Infrequent:* cerebrovascular accident, intracranial hemorrhage, transient ischemic attack, emotional lability, neuralgia, coldness (localized), muscle spasm, dysphoria, gait abnormality, hypertonia, hypokinesia, neurodermatitis, numbness (localized), paranoia, dysarthria, dysphasia, hostility, decreased libido, melancholia, emotional withdrawal, nystagmus, pacing.

Respiratory System: *Frequent:* dyspnea, sore throat, bronchitis; *Infrequent:* epistaxis, post nasal drip, pneumonia, hyperventilation, pulmonary congestion, wheezing, hypoxia, pharyngitis, pleurisy, pulmonary collapse, sleep apnea, snoring.

Skin and Appendages: *Frequent:* pruritus, diaphoresis, urticaria; *Infrequent:* dermatitis, erythema, skin discoloration, hyperkeratosis, alopecia, fungal dermatitis, herpes zoster, hirsutism, skin striae, night sweats, skin ulcer.

Special Senses: *Frequent:* cataract, eye irritation, vision blurred; *Infrequent:* dry eyes, glaucoma, earache, tinnitus, blepharitis, decreased hearing, retinal hemorrhage, otitis externa, otitis media, bad taste, conjunctival hemorrhage, ear buzzing, motion sickness, spots before eyes.

Urogenital System: *Frequent:* urinary incontinence, nocturia; *Infrequent:* dysuria, hematuria, urinary urgency, metrorrhagia, cystitis, enuresis, prostate hypertrophy, pyelonephritis, inability to empty bladder, breast fibroadenosis, fibrocystic breast, mastitis, pyuria, renal failure, vaginitis.

Severe Alzheimer's Disease
Adverse Events Leading to Discontinuation
The rates of discontinuation from controlled clinical trials of ARICEPT due to adverse events for the ARICEPT patients were approximately 12% compared to 7% for placebo patients. The most common adverse events leading to discontinuation, defined as those occurring in at least 2% of ARICEPT patients and at twice or more the incidence seen in placebo, were anorexia (2% vs. 1% placebo), nausea (2% vs. <1% placebo), diarrhea (2% vs. 0% placebo) and urinary tract infection (2% vs. 1% placebo).

Most Frequent Adverse Events Seen in Association with the Use of ARICEPT
The most common adverse events, defined as those occurring at a frequency of at least 5% in patients receiving ARICEPT and at twice or more the placebo rate, are largely predicted by ARICEPT's cholinomimetic effects. These include diarrhea, anorexia, vomiting, nausea, and ecchymosis.

These adverse events were often of mild intensity and transient, resolving during continued ARICEPT treatment without the need for dose modification.

Adverse Events Reported in Controlled Trials
Table 4 lists adverse events that were reported in at least 2% of patients in placebo-controlled trials who received ARICEPT and for which the rate of occurrence was greater for patients treated with ARICEPT than with placebo.

Table 4. Adverse Events Reported in Controlled Clinical Trials in Severe Alzheimer's Disease in at Least 2% of Patients Receiving ARICEPT and at a Higher Frequency than Placebo Treated Patients

Body System/Adverse Event	Placebo (n=392)	ARICEPT (n=501)
Percent of Patients with any Adverse Event	73	81
Body as a Whole		
Accident	12	13
Infection	9	11
Headache	3	4
Pain	2	3
Back Pain	2	3
Fever	1	2
Chest Pain	<1	2
Cardiovascular System		
Hypertension	2	3
Hemorrhage	1	2
Syncope	1	2
Digestive System		
Diarrhea	4	10
Vomiting	4	8
Anorexia	4	8
Nausea	2	6
Hemic and Lymphatic System		
Ecchymosis	2	5
Metabolic and Nutritional Systems		
Creatine Phosphokinase Increased	1	3
Dehydration	1	2
Hyperlipemia	<1	2
Nervous System		
Insomnia	4	5
Hostility	2	3
Nervousness	2	3
Hallucinations	1	3
Somnolence	1	2
Dizziness	1	2
Depression	1	2
Confusion	1	2
Emotional Lability	1	2
Personality Disorder	1	2
Skin and Appendages		
Eczema	2	3
Urogenital System		
Urinary Incontinence	1	2

Other Adverse Events Observed During Clinical Trials
ARICEPT has been administered to over 600 patients with severe Alzheimer's disease during clinical trials of at least 6 months duration, including three double-blind placebo-controlled trials, two of which had an open label extension. All adverse events occurring at least twice are included, except for those already listed in Table 4, COSTART terms too general to be informative, or events less likely to be drug related. Events are classified by body system and listed using the following COSTART dictionary and listed using the following definitions: *Frequent adverse events* - those occurring in at least 1/100 patients; *Infrequent adverse events* - those occurring in 1/100 to 1/1000 patients. These adverse events are not necessarily related to ARICEPT treatment and in most cases were observed at a similar frequency in placebo treated patients in the controlled studies.

Body as a Whole: *Frequent:* abdominal pain, asthenia, fungal infection, flu syndrome; *Infrequent:* allergic reaction, cellulitis, malaise, sepsis, face edema, hernia.

Cardiovascular System: *Frequent:* hypotension, bradycardia, ECG abnormal, heart failure; *Infrequent:* myocardial infarction, angina pectoris, atrial fibrillation, congestive heart failure, peripheral vascular disorder, supraventricular extrasystoles, ventricular extrasystoles, cardiomegaly.

Digestive System: *Frequent:* constipation, gastroenteritis, fecal incontinence, dyspepsia; *Infrequent:* gamma glutamyl transpeptidase increase, gastritis, dysphagia, periodontitis, stomach ulcer, periodontal abscess, flatulence, liver function tests abnormal, eructation, esophagitis, rectal hemorrhage.

Endocrine System: *Infrequent:* diabetes mellitus.

Hemic and Lymphatic System: *Frequent:* anemia; *Infrequent:* leukocytosis.

Metabolic and Nutritional Disorders: *Frequent:* weight loss, peripheral edema, edema, lactic dehydrogenase increased, alkaline phosphatase increased; *Infrequent:* hypercholesteremia, hypokalemia, hypoglycemia, weight gain, bilirubinemia, BUN increased, B12 deficiency anemia, cachexia, creatinine increased, gout, hyponatremia, hypoproteinemia, iron deficiency anemia, SGOT increased, SGPT increased.

Musculoskeletal System: *Frequent:* arthritis; *Infrequent:* arthrosis, bone fracture, arthralgia, leg cramps, osteoporosis, myalgia.

Nervous System: *Frequent:* agitation, anxiety, tremor, convulsion, wandering, abnormal gait; *Infrequent:* apathy, vertigo, delusions, abnormal dreams, cerebrovascular accident, increased salivation, ataxia, euphoria, vasodilatation, cerebral hemorrhage, cerebral infarction, cerebral ischemia, dementia, extrapyramidal syndrome, grand mal convulsion, hemiplegia, hypertonia, hypokinesia.

Respiratory System: *Frequent:* pharyngitis, pneumonia, cough increased, bronchitis; *Infrequent:* dyspnea, rhinitis, asthma.

Skin and Appendages: *Frequent:* rash, skin ulcer, pruritus; *Infrequent:* psoriasis, skin discoloration, herpes zoster, dry skin, sweating, urticaria, vesiculobullous rash.

Special Senses: *Infrequent:* conjunctivitis, glaucoma, abnormal vision, ear pain, lacrimation disorder.

Urogenital System: *Frequent:* urinary tract infection, cystitis, hematuria, glycosuria; *Infrequent:* vaginitis, dysuria, urinary frequency, albuminuria.

ARICEPT 23 mg/day
Moderate to Severe Alzheimer's Disease
ARICEPT 23 mg/day has been administered to over 1300 individuals globally in clinical trials. Approximately 1050 of these patients have been treated for at least three months and more than 950 patients have been treated for at least six months. The range of patient exposure was from 1 to over 500 days.

Adverse Events Leading to Discontinuation
The rate of discontinuation from a controlled clinical trial of ARICEPT 23 mg/day due to adverse events was higher (18.6%) than for the 10 mg/day treatment group (7.9%). The most common adverse events leading to discontinuation, defined as those occurring in at least 1% of patients and greater than those occurring with 10 mg/day are shown in Table 5.

Table 5. Most Frequent Adverse Events Leading to Discontinuation from a Controlled Clinical Trial by Treatment Group

Dose Group	23 mg/day ARICEPT	10 mg/day ARICEPT
Safety Population	963	471
Event/%Discontinuing		
Vomiting	3	0
Diarrhea	2	0
Nausea	2	0
Dizziness	1	0

The majority of discontinuations due to adverse events in the 23 mg group occurred during the first month of treatment.

Most Frequent Adverse Events Seen in Association with the Use of 23 mg

The most common adverse events, defined as those occurring at a frequency of at least 5%, include nausea, diarrhea, vomiting, and anorexia. These adverse events were often of mild to moderate intensity.

Adverse Events Reported in Controlled Trials

The events cited reflect experience gained under closely monitored conditions of a controlled clinical trial in a highly selected patient population. In actual clinical practice or in other clinical trials, these frequency estimates may not apply, as the conditions of use, reporting behavior, and the kinds of patients treated may differ. Table 6 lists adverse events that were reported in at least 2% of patients who received 23 mg/day of ARICEPT and at a higher frequency than those receiving 10 mg/day of ARICEPT in a controlled clinical trial that compared the two doses. In this study, there were no important differences in the type of adverse events in patients taking ARICEPT with or without memantine.

Table 6. Adverse Events Reported in a Controlled Clinical Trial in Moderate to Severe Alzheimer's Disease in at Least 2% of Patients and Higher in the 23 mg/day Group

Body System/Adverse Event	23 mg/day ARICEPT	10 mg/day ARICEPT
Safety Population	963	471
Percent of Patients with any Adverse Event	74	64
Gastrointestinal disorders		
Nausea	12	3
Vomiting	9	3
Diarrhea	8	5
General disorders and administration site conditions		
Fatigue	2	1
Asthenia	2	1
Injury, poisoning and procedural complications		
Contusion	2	0
Investigations		
Weight decreased	5	3
Metabolism and nutrition disorders		
Anorexia	5	2
Nervous system		
Dizziness	5	3
Headache	4	3
Somnolence	2	1
Psychiatric disorders		
Insomnia	3	2
Renal and urinary disorders		
Urinary incontinence	3	1

6.2. Postmarketing Experience

Voluntary reports of adverse events temporally associated with ARICEPT that have been received since market introduction that are not listed above, and for which there are inadequate data to determine the causal relationship with the drug include the following: abdominal pain, agitation, cholecystitis, confusion, convulsions, hallucinations, heart block (all types), hemolytic anemia, hepatitis, hyponatremia, neuroleptic malignant syndrome, pancreatitis, and rash.

7. DRUG INTERACTIONS

7.1. Effect of ARICEPT on the Metabolism of Other Drugs

No in vivo clinical trials have investigated the effect of ARICEPT on the clearance of drugs metabolized by CYP 3A4 (e.g. cisapride, terfenadine) or by CYP 2D6 (e.g. imipramine). However, in vitro studies show a low rate of binding to these enzymes (mean K_i about 50-130 μM), that, given the therapeutic plasma concentrations of donepezil (164 nM), indicates little likelihood of interference.

Whether ARICEPT has any potential for enzyme induction is not known. Formal pharmacokinetic studies evaluated the potential of ARICEPT for interaction with theophylline, cimetidine, warfarin, digoxin and ketoconazole. No effects of ARICEPT on the pharmacokinetics of these drugs were observed.

7.2. Effect of Other Drugs on the Metabolism of ARICEPT

Ketoconazole and quinidine, inhibitors of CYP450, 3A4 and 2D6, respectively, inhibit donepezil metabolism in vitro. Whether there is a clinical effect of quinidine is not known. In a 7-day crossover study in 18 healthy volunteers, ketoconazole (200 mg q.d.) increased mean donepezil (5 mg q.d.) concentrations (AUC_{0-24} and C_{max}) by 36%. The clinical relevance of this increase in concentration is unknown.

A small effect of CYP2D6 inhibitors was identified in a population pharmacokinetic analysis of plasma donepezil concentrations measured in patients with Alzheimer's disease. Donepezil clearance was reduced by approximately 17% in patients taking 10 or 23 mg in combination with a known CYP2D6 inhibitor. This result is consistent with the conclusion that CYP2D6 is a minor metabolic pathway of donepezil.

Inducers of CYP 2D6 and CYP 3A4 (e.g., phenytoin, carbamazepine, dexamethasone, rifampin, and phenobarbital) could increase the rate of elimination of ARICEPT.

Formal pharmacokinetic studies demonstrated that the metabolism of ARICEPT is not significantly affected by concurrent administration of digoxin or cimetidine.

7.3. Use with Anticholinergics

Because of their mechanism of action, cholinesterase inhibitors have the potential to interfere with the activity of anticholinergic medications.

7.4. Use with Cholinomimetics and Other Cholinesterase Inhibitors

A synergistic effect may be expected when cholinesterase inhibitors are given concurrently with succinylcholine, similar neuromuscular blocking agents or cholinergic agonists such as bethanechol.

8. USE IN SPECIFIC POPULATIONS

8.1. Pregnancy

Pregnancy Category C: There are no adequate or well-controlled studies in pregnant women. ARICEPT should be used during pregnancy only if the potential benefit justifies the potential risk to the fetus.

Oral administration of donepezil to pregnant rats and rabbits during the period of organogenesis did not produce any teratogenic effects at doses up to 16 mg/kg/day (approximately 6 times the maximum recommended human dose [MRHD] of 23 mg/day on a mg/m² basis) and 10 mg/kg/day (approximately 7 times the MRHD on a mg/m² basis), respectively. Oral administration of donepezil (1, 3, 10 mg/kg/day) to rats during late gestation and throughout lactation to weaning produced an increase in stillbirths and reduced offspring survival through postpartum day 4 at the highest dose. The no-effect dose of 3 mg/kg/day is approximately equal to the MRHD on a mg/m² basis.

8.2. Nursing Mothers

It is not known whether donepezil is excreted in human breast milk. Caution should be exercised when ARICEPT is administered to a nursing woman.

8.3. Pediatric Use

The safety and effectiveness of ARICEPT in children have not been established.

8.4. Geriatric Use

Alzheimer's disease is a disorder occurring primarily in individuals over 55 years of age. The mean age of patients enrolled in the clinical studies with ARICEPT was 73 years; 80% of these patients were between 65 and 84 years old, and 49% of patients were at or above the age of 75. The efficacy and safety data presented in the clinical trials section were obtained from these patients. There were no clinically significant differences in most adverse events reported by patient groups ≥ 65 years old and < 65 years old.

8.5. Lower Weight Individuals

In the controlled clinical trial, among patients in the ARICEPT 23 mg treatment group, those patients weighing < 55 kg reported more nausea, vomiting, and decreased weight than patients weighing 55 kg or more. There were more withdrawals due to adverse events as well. This finding may be related to higher plasma exposure associated with lower weight.

10. OVERDOSAGE

Because strategies for the management of overdose are continually evolving, it is advisable to contact a Poison Control Center to determine the latest recommendations for the management of an overdose of any drug.

As in any case of overdose, general supportive measures should be utilized. Overdosage with cholinesterase inhibitors can result in cholinergic crisis characterized by severe nausea, vomiting, salivation, sweating, bradycardia, hypotension, respiratory depression, collapse and convulsions. Increasing muscle weakness is a possibility and may result in death if respiratory muscles are involved. Tertiary anticholinergics such as atropine may be used as an antidote for ARICEPT overdosage. Intravenous atropine sulfate titrated to effect is recommended: an initial dose of 1.0 to 2.0 mg IV with subsequent doses based upon clinical response. Atypical responses in blood pressure and heart rate have been reported with other cholinomimetics when co-administered with quaternary anticholinergics such as glycopyrrolate. It is not known whether ARICEPT and/or its metabolites can be removed by dialysis (hemodialysis, peritoneal dialysis, or hemofiltration).

Dose-related signs of toxicity in animals included reduced spontaneous movement, prone position, staggering gait, lacrimation, clonic convulsions, depressed respiration, salivation, miosis, tremors, fasciculation and lower body surface temperature.

11. DESCRIPTION

ARICEPT (donepezil hydrochloride) is a reversible inhibitor of the enzyme acetylcholinesterase, known chemically as (±)-2, 3-dihydro-5, 6-dimethoxy-2-[[1-(phenylmethyl)-4-piperidinyl]methyl]-1H-inden-1-one hydrochloride. Donepezil hydrochloride is commonly referred to in the pharmacological literature as E2020. It has an empirical formula of $C_{24}H_{29}NO_3HCl$ and a molecular weight of 415.96. Donepezil hydrochloride is a white crystalline powder and is freely soluble in chloroform, soluble in water and in glacial acetic acid, slightly soluble in ethanol and in acetonitrile and practically insoluble in ethyl acetate and in n-hexane.

ARICEPT is available for oral administration in film-coated tablets containing 5, 10, or 23 mg of donepezil hydrochloride.

Inactive ingredients in 5 mg and 10 mg tablets are lactose monohydrate, corn starch, microcrystalline cellulose, hydroxypropyl cellulose, and magnesium stearate. The film coating contains talc, polyethylene glycol, hypromellose and titanium dioxide. Additionally, the 10 mg tablet contains yellow iron oxide (synthetic) as a coloring agent.

Inactive ingredients in 23 mg tablets include ethylcellulose, hydroxypropyl cellulose, lactose monohydrate, magnesium stearate and methacrylic acid copolymer, Type C. The film coating includes ferric oxide, hypromellose 2910, polyethylene glycol 8000, talc and titanium dioxide.

ARICEPT ODT tablets are available for oral administration. Each ARICEPT ODT tablet contains 5 or 10 mg of donepezil hydrochloride. Inactive ingredients are carrageenan, mannitol, colloidal silicon dioxide and polyvinyl alcohol. Additionally, the 10 mg tablet contains ferric oxide (yellow) as a coloring agent.

12. CLINICAL PHARMACOLOGY

12.1. Mechanism of Action

Current theories on the pathogenesis of the cognitive signs and symptoms of Alzheimer's disease attribute some of them to a deficiency of cholinergic neurotransmission.

Donepezil hydrochloride is postulated to exert its therapeutic effect by enhancing cholinergic function. This is accomplished by increasing the concentration of acetylcholine through reversible inhibition of its hydrolysis by acetylcholinesterase. There is no evidence that donepezil alters the course of the underlying dementing process.

12.2. Pharmacokinetics

Pharmacokinetics of donepezil are linear over a dose range of 1-10 mg given once daily. The rate and extent of absorption of ARICEPT tablets are not influenced by food.

Based on population pharmacokinetic analysis of plasma donepezil concentrations measured in patients with Alzheimer's disease, following oral dosing, peak plasma concentration is achieved for ARICEPT 23 mg tablets in approximately 8 hours, compared with 3 hours for ARICEPT 10 mg tablets. Peak plasma concentrations are almost 2-fold higher for ARICEPT 23 mg tablets than ARICEPT 10 mg tablets.

ARICEPT ODT 5 mg and 10 mg are bioequivalent to ARICEPT 5 mg and 10 mg tablets, respectively. A food effect study has not been conducted with ARICEPT ODT; however, the effect of food with ARICEPT ODT is expected to be minimal. ARICEPT ODT can be taken without regard to meals.

The elimination half life of donepezil is about 70 hours, and the mean apparent plasma clearance (Cl/F) is 0.13-0.19 L/hr/kg. Following multiple dose administration, donepezil accumulates in plasma by 4-7 fold, and steady state is reached within 15 days. The steady state volume of distribution is 12-16 L/kg. Donepezil is approximately 96% bound to human plasma proteins, mainly to albumins (about 75%) and alpha$_1$ - acid glycoprotein (about 21%) over the concentration range of 2-1000 ng/mL.

Donepezil is both excreted in the urine intact and extensively metabolized to four major metabolites, two of which are known to be active, and a number of minor metabolites, not all of which have been identified. Donepezil is metabolized by CYP 450 isoenzymes 2D6 and 3A4 and undergoes glucuronidation. Following administration of ^{14}C-labeled donepezil, plasma radioactivity, expressed as a percent of the administered dose, was present primarily as intact donepezil (53%) and as 6-O-desmethyl donepezil (11%), which has been reported to inhibit AChE to the same extent as donepezil *in vitro* and was found in plasma at concentrations equal to about 20% of donepezil. Approximately 57% and 15% of the total radioactivity was recovered in urine and feces, respectively, over a period of 10 days, while 28% remained unrecovered, with about 17% of the donepezil dose recovered in the urine as unchanged drug. Examination of the effect of CYP2D6 genotype in Alzheimer's patients showed differences in clearance values among CYP2D6 genotype subgroups. When compared to the extensive metabolizers, poor metabolizers had a 31.5% slower clearance and ultra-rapid metabolizers had a 24% faster clearance. These results suggest CYP2D6 has a minor role in the metabolism of donepezil.

Hepatic Disease: In a study of 10 patients with stable alcoholic cirrhosis, the clearance of ARICEPT was decreased by 20% relative to 10 healthy age- and sex-matched subjects.

Renal Disease: In a study of 11 patients with moderate to severe renal impairment (Cl_C < 18 mL/min/1.73 m^2) the clearance of ARICEPT did not differ from 11 age- and sex-matched healthy subjects.

Age: No formal pharmacokinetic study was conducted to examine age-related differences in the pharmacokinetics of ARICEPT. Population pharmacokinetic analysis suggested that the clearance of donepezil in patients decreases with increasing age. When compared with 65-year old, subjects, 90-year old subjects have a 17% decrease in clearance, while 40-year old subjects have a 33% increase in clearance. The effect of age on donepezil clearance may not be clinically significant.

Gender and Race: No specific pharmacokinetic study was conducted to investigate the effects of gender and race on the disposition of ARICEPT. However, retrospective pharmacokinetic analysis and population pharmacokinetic analysis of plasma donepezil concentrations measured in patients with Alzheimer's disease indicates that gender and race (Japanese and Caucasians) did not affect the clearance of ARICEPT to an important degree.

Body weight: There was a relationship noted between body weight and clearance. Over the range of body weight from 50 kg to 110 kg, clearance increased from 7.77 L/h to 14.04 L/h, with a value of 10 L/hr for 70 kg individuals.

Drugs Highly Bound to Plasma Proteins: Drug displacement studies have been performed *in vitro* between this highly bound drug (96%) and other drugs such as furosemide, digoxin, and warfarin. ARICEPT at concentrations of 0.3-10 micrograms/mL did not affect the binding of furosemide (5 micrograms/mL), digoxin (2 ng/mL), and warfarin (3 micrograms/mL) to human albumin. Similarly, the binding of ARICEPT to human albumin was not affected by furosemide, digoxin and warfarin.

13. NONCLINICAL TOXICOLOGY

13.1. Carcinogenesis, Mutagenesis, Impairment of Fertility

No evidence of a carcinogenic potential was obtained in an 88-week carcinogenicity study of donepezil hydrochloride conducted in CD-1 mice at doses up to 180 mg/kg/day (approximately 90 times the maximum recommended human dose on a mg/m^2 basis), or in a 104-week carcinogenicity study in Sprague-Dawley rats at doses up to 30 mg/kg/day (approximately 30 times the maximum recommended human dose on a mg/m^2 basis).

Donepezil was not mutagenic in the Ames reverse mutation assay in bacteria, or in a mouse lymphoma forward mutation assay *in vitro*. In the chromosome aberration test in cultures of Chinese hamster lung (CHL) cells, some clastogenic effects were observed. Donepezil was not clastogenic in the *in vivo* mouse micronucleus test and was not genotoxic in an *in vivo* unscheduled DNA synthesis assay in rats.

Donepezil had no effect on fertility in rats at doses up to 10 mg/kg/day (approximately 8 times the maximum recommended human dose on a mg/m^2 basis).

14. CLINICAL STUDIES

The effectiveness of ARICEPT as a treatment for Alzheimer's disease is demonstrated by the results of randomized, double-blind, placebo-controlled clinical investigations

14.1. Mild to Moderate Alzheimer's disease

The effectiveness of ARICEPT as a treatment for mild to moderate Alzheimer's disease is demonstrated by the results of two randomized, double-blind, placebo-controlled clinical investigations in patients with Alzheimer's disease (diagnosed by NINCDS and DSM III-R criteria, Mini-Mental State Examination ≥ 10 and ≤ 26 and Clinical Dementia Rating of 1 or 2). The mean age of patients participating in ARICEPT trials was 73 years with a range of 50 to 94. Approximately 62% of patients were women and 38% were men. The racial distribution was white 95%, black 3% and other races 2%.

Study Outcome Measures: In each study, the effectiveness of treatment with ARICEPT was evaluated using a dual outcome assessment strategy.

The ability of ARICEPT to improve cognitive performance was assessed with the cognitive subscale of the Alzheimer's Disease Assessment Scale (ADAS-cog), a multi-item instrument that has been extensively validated in longitudinal cohorts of Alzheimer's disease patients. The ADAS-cog examines selected aspects of cognitive performance including elements of memory, orientation, attention, reasoning, language and praxis. The ADAS-cog scoring range is from 0 to 70, with higher scores indicating greater cognitive impairment. Elderly normal adults may score as low as 0 or 1, but it is not unusual for non-demented adults to score slightly higher.

The patients recruited as participants in each study had mean scores on the ADAS-cog of approximately 26 points, with a range from 4 to 61. Experience based on longitudinal studies of ambulatory patients with mild to moderate Alzheimer's disease suggest that scores on the ADAS-cog increase (worsen) by 6-12 points per year. However, smaller changes may be seen in patients with very mild or very advanced disease since the ADAS-cog is not uniformly sensitive to change over the course of the disease. The annualized rate of decline in the placebo patients participating in ARICEPT trials was approximately 2 to 4 points per year.

The ability of ARICEPT to produce an overall clinical effect was assessed using a Clinician's Interview-Based Impression of Change that required the use of caregiver information, the CIBIC-plus. The CIBIC-plus is not a single instrument and is not a standardized instrument like the ADAS-cog. Clinical trials for investigational drugs have used a variety of CIBIC formats, each different in terms of depth and structure.

As such, results from a CIBIC-plus reflect clinical experience from the trial or trials in which it was used and cannot be compared directly with the results of CIBIC-plus evaluations from other clinical trials. The CIBIC-plus used in ARICEPT trials was a semi-structured instrument that was intended to examine four major areas of patient function: General, Cognitive, Behavioral and Activities of Daily Living. It represents the assessment of a skilled clinician based upon his/her observations at an interview with the patient, in combination with information supplied by a caregiver familiar with the behavior of the patient over the interval rated. The CIBIC-plus is scored as a seven point categorical rating, ranging from a score of 1, indicating "markedly improved," to a score of 4, indicating "no change" to a score of 7, indicating "markedly worse." The CIBIC-plus has not been systematically compared directly to assessments not using information from caregivers (CIBIC) or other global methods.

Thirty-Week Study

In a study of 30 weeks duration, 473 patients were randomized to receive single daily doses of placebo, 5 mg/day or 10 mg/day of ARICEPT. The 30-week study was divided into a 24-week double-blind active treatment phase followed by a 6-week single-blind placebo washout period. The study was designed to compare 5 mg/day or 10 mg/day fixed doses of ARICEPT to placebo. However, to reduce the likelihood of cholinergic effects, the 10 mg/day treatment was started following an initial 7-day treatment with 5 mg/day doses.

Effects on the ADAS-cog: Figure 1 illustrates the time course for the change from baseline in ADAS-cog scores for all three dose groups over the 30 weeks of the study. After 24 weeks of treatment, the mean differences in the ADAS-cog change scores for ARICEPT treated patients compared to the patients on placebo were 2.8 and 3.1 points for the 5 mg/day and 10 mg/day treatments, respectively. These differences were statistically significant. While the treatment effect size may appear to be slightly greater for the 10 mg/day treatment, there was no statistically significant difference between the two active treatments.

Following 6 weeks of placebo washout, scores on the ADAS-cog for both the ARICEPT treatment groups were indistinguishable from those patients who had received only placebo for 30 weeks. This suggests that the beneficial effects of ARICEPT abate over 6 weeks following discontinuation of treatment and do not represent a change in the underlying disease. There was no evidence of a rebound effect 6 weeks after abrupt discontinuation of therapy.

Figure 1. Time-course of the Change from Baseline in ADAS-cog Score for Patients Completing 24 Weeks of Treatment.

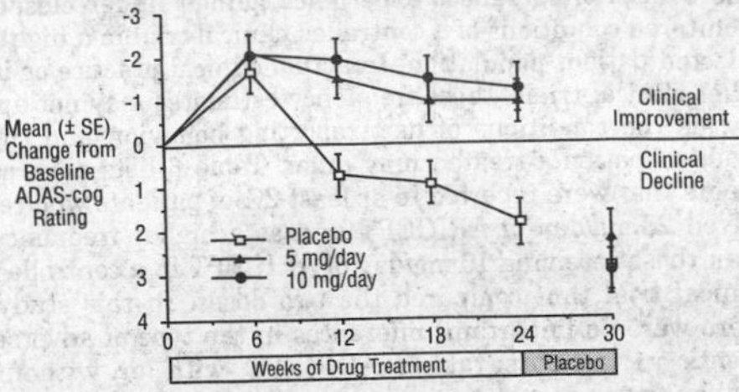

Figure 2 illustrates the cumulative percentages of patients from each of the three treatment groups who had attained the measure of improvement in ADAS-cog score shown on the X axis. Three change scores, (7-point and 4-point reductions from baseline or no change in score) have been identified for illustrative purposes, and the percent of patients in each group achieving that result is shown in the inset table. The curves demonstrate that both patients assigned to placebo and ARICEPT have a wide range of responses, but that the active treatment groups are more likely to show greater improvements. A curve for an effective treatment would be shifted to the left of the curve for placebo, while an ineffective or deleterious treatment would be superimposed upon or shifted to the right of the curve for placebo.

Figure 2. Cumulative Percentage of Patients Completing 24 Weeks of Double-blind Treatment with Specified Changes from Baseline ADAS-cog Scores. The Percentages of Randomized Patients who Completed the Study were: Placebo 80%, 5 mg/day 85% and 10 mg/day 68%.

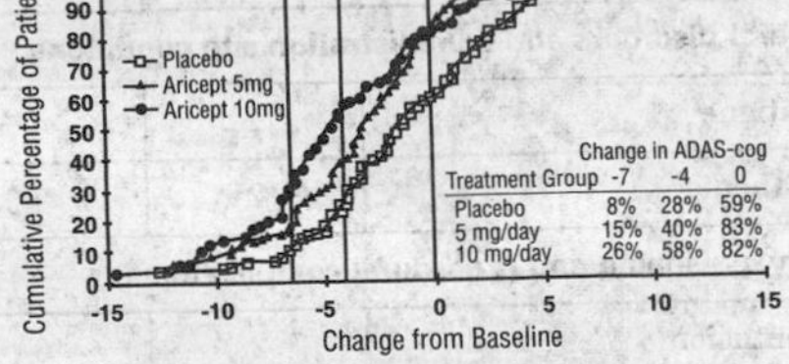

Effects on the CIBIC-plus: Figure 3 is a histogram of the frequency distribution of CIBIC-plus scores attained by patients assigned to each of the three treatment groups who completed 24 weeks of treatment. The mean drug-placebo differences for these groups of patients were 0.35 points and 0.39 points for 5 mg/day and 10 mg/day of ARICEPT, respectively. These differences were statistically significant. There was no statistically significant difference between the two active treatments.

Figure 3. Frequency Distribution of CIBIC plus Scores at Week 24

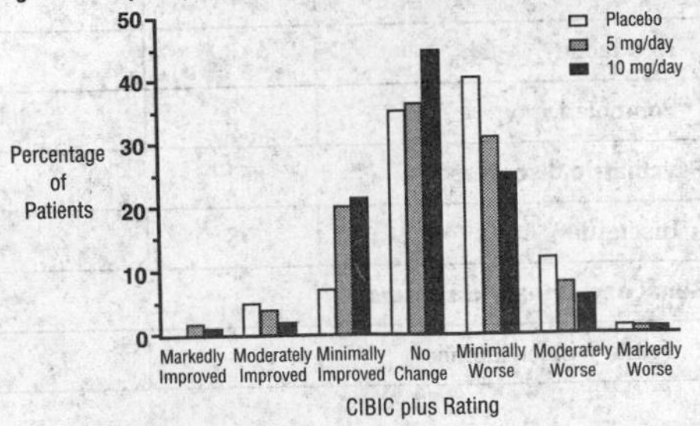

Fifteen-Week Study

In a study of 15 weeks duration, patients were randomized to receive single daily doses of placebo or either 5 mg/day or 10 mg/day of ARICEPT for 12 weeks, followed by a 3-week placebo washout period. As in the 30-week study, to avoid acute cholinergic effects, the 10 mg/day treatment followed an initial 7-day treatment with 5 mg/day doses.

Effects on the ADAS-Cog: Figure 4 illustrates the time course of the change from baseline in ADAS-cog scores for all three dose groups over the 15 weeks of the study. After 12 weeks of treatment, the differences in mean ADAS-cog change scores for the ARICEPT treated patients compared to the patients on placebo were 2.7 and 3.0 points each, for the 5 and 10 mg/day ARICEPT treatment groups, respectively. These differences were statistically significant. The effect size for the 10 mg/day group may appear to be slightly larger than that for 5 mg/day. However, the differences between active treatments were not statistically significant.

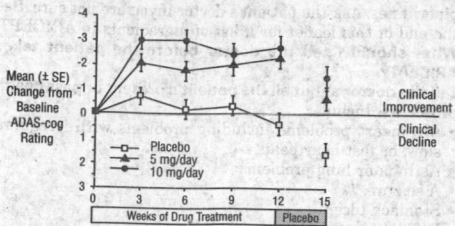

Figure 4. Time-course of the Change from Baseline in ADAS-cog Score for Patients Completing the 15-week Study.

Following 3 weeks of placebo washout, scores on the ADAS-cog for both the ARICEPT treatment groups increased, indicating that discontinuation of ARICEPT resulted in a loss of its treatment effect. The duration of this placebo washout period was not sufficient to characterize the rate of loss of the treatment effect, but, the 30-week study (see above) demonstrated that treatment effects associated with the use of ARICEPT abate within 6 weeks of treatment discontinuation.

Figure 5 illustrates the cumulative percentages of patients from each of the three treatment groups who attained the measure of improvement in ADAS-cog score shown on the X axis. The same three change scores, (7-point and 4-point reductions from baseline or no change in score) as selected for the 30-week study have been used for this illustration. The percentages of patients achieving those results are shown in the inset table.

As observed in the 30-week study, the curves demonstrate that patients assigned to either placebo or to ARICEPT have a wide range of responses, but that the ARICEPT treated patients are more likely to show greater improvements in cognitive performance.

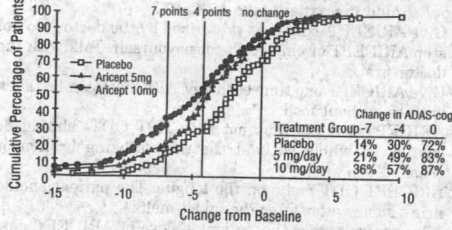

Figure 5. Cumulative Percentage of Patients with Specified Changes from Baseline ADAS-cog Scores. The Percentages of Randomized Patients Within Each Treatment Group Who Completed the Study Were: Placebo 93%, 5 mg/day 90% and 10 mg/day 82%.

Treatment Group	Change in ADAS-cog		
	-7	-4	0
Placebo	14%	30%	72%
5 mg/day	21%	49%	83%
10 mg/day	36%	57%	87%

Effects on the CIBIC-plus: Figure 6 is a histogram of the frequency distribution of CIBIC-plus scores attained by patients assigned to each of the three treatment groups who completed 12 weeks of treatment. The differences in mean scores for ARICEPT treated patients compared to the patients on placebo at Week 12 were 0.36 and 0.38 points for the 5 mg/day and 10 mg/day treatment groups, respectively. These differences were statistically significant.

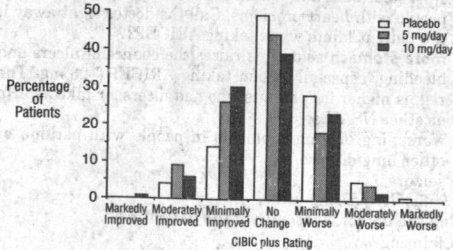

Figure 6. Frequency Distribution of CIBIC plus Scores at Week 12

In both studies, patient age, sex and race were not found to predict the clinical outcome of ARICEPT treatment.

14.2. Moderate to Severe Alzheimer's disease
The effectiveness of ARICEPT in the treatment of patients with moderate to severe Alzheimer's Disease was established in studies employing doses of 10 mg/day and 23 mg/day.

Studies of 10 mg/day
Swedish 6 Month Study
The effectiveness of ARICEPT as a treatment for severe Alzheimer's disease is demonstrated by the results of a randomized, double-blind, placebo-controlled clinical study conducted in Sweden (6 month study) in patients with probable or possible Alzheimer's disease diagnosed by NINCDS-ADRDA and DSM-IV criteria, MMSE: range of 1-10. Two

hundred and forty eight (248) patients with severe Alzheimer's disease were randomized to ARICEPT or placebo. For patients randomized to ARICEPT, treatment was initiated at 5 mg once daily for 28 days and then increased to 10 mg once daily. At the end of the 6 month treatment period, 90.5% of the ARICEPT treated patients were receiving the 10 mg/day dose. The mean age of patients was 84.9 years, with a range of 59 to 99. Approximately 77% of patients were women, and 23% were men. Almost all patients were Caucasian. Probable AD was diagnosed in the majority of the patients (83.6% of ARICEPT treated patients and 84.2% of placebo treated patients).

Study Outcome Measures: The effectiveness of treatment with ARICEPT was determined using a dual outcome assessment strategy that evaluated cognitive function using an instrument designed for more impaired patients and overall function through caregiver- rated assessment. This study showed that patients on ARICEPT experienced significant improvement on both measures compared to placebo. The ability of ARICEPT to improve cognitive performance was assessed with the Severe Impairment Battery (SIB). The SIB, a multi-item instrument, has been validated for the evaluation of cognitive function in patients with moderate to severe dementia. The SIB evaluates selective aspects of cognitive performance, including elements of memory, language, orientation, attention, praxis, visuospatial ability, construction, and social interaction. The SIB scoring range is from 0 to 100, with lower scores indicating greater cognitive impairment.

Daily function was assessed using the Modified Alzheimer's Disease Cooperative Study Activities of Daily Living Inventory for Severe Alzheimer's Disease (ADCS-ADL-severe). The ADCS-ADL-severe is derived from the Alzheimer's Disease Cooperative Study Activities of Daily Living Inventory, which is a comprehensive battery of ADL questions used to measure the functional capabilities of patients. Each ADL item is rated from the highest level of independent performance to complete loss. The ADCS-ADL-severe is a subset of 19 items, including ratings of the patient's ability to eat, dress, bathe, use the telephone, get around (or travel), and perform other activities of daily living; it has been validated for the assessment of patients with moderate to severe dementia. The ADCS-ADL-severe has a scoring range of 0 to 54, with the lower scores indicating greater functional impairment. The investigator performs the inventory by interviewing a caregiver, in this study a nurse staff member, familiar with the functioning of the patient.

Effects on the SIB:
Figure 7 shows the time course for the change from baseline in SIB score for the two treatment groups over the 6 months of the study. At 6 months of treatment, the mean difference in the SIB change scores for ARICEPT treated patients compared to patients on placebo was 5.9 points. ARICEPT treatment was statistically significantly superior to placebo.

Figure 7. Time course of the change from baseline in SIB score for patients completing 6 months of treatment.

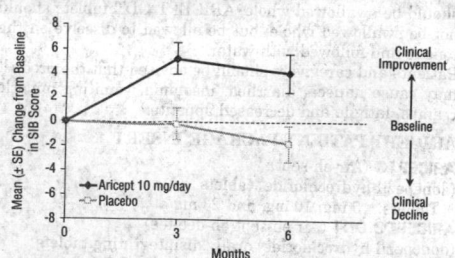

Figure 8 illustrates the cumulative percentages of patients from each of the two treatment groups who attained the measure of improvement in SIB score shown on the X-axis. While patients assigned both to ARICEPT and to placebo have a wide range of responses, the curves show that the ARICEPT group is more likely to show a greater improvement in cognitive performance.

[See figure 8 at top of next column]
[See figure 9 at top of next column]

Effects on the ADCS-ADL-severe: Figure 9 illustrates the time course for the change from baseline in ADCS-ADL-severe scores for patients in the two treatment groups over the 6 months of the study. After 6 months of treatment, the mean difference in the ADCS-ADL-severe change scores for ARICEPT treated patients compared to patients on placebo was 1.8 points. ARICEPT treatment was statistically significantly superior to placebo.

Figure 10 shows the cumulative percentages of patients from each treatment group with specified changes from baseline ADCS-ADL-severe scores. While both patients assigned to ARICEPT and placebo have a wide range of responses, the curves demonstrate that the ARICEPT group is more likely to show a smaller decline or an improvement.

[See figure 10 at top of next column]

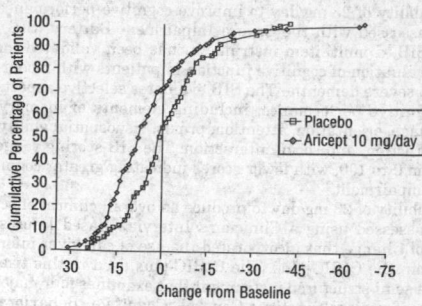

Figure 8. Cumulative percentage of patients completing 6 months of double-blind treatment with particular changes from baseline in SIB scores.

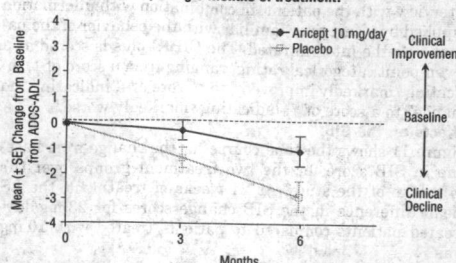

Figure 9. Time course of the change from baseline in ADCS-ADL-severe score for patients completing 6 months of treatment.

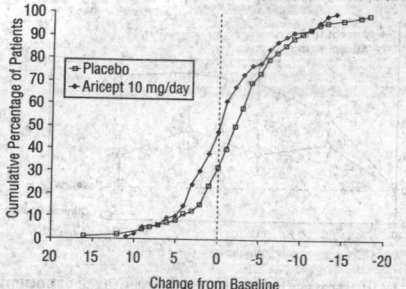

Figure 10. Cumulative percentage of patients completing 6 months of double-blind treatment with particular changes from baseline in ADCS-ADL-severe scores.

Japanese 24-Week Study
In a study of 24 weeks duration conducted in Japan, 325 patients with severe Alzheimer's disease were randomized to doses of 5 mg/day or 10 mg/day of donepezil, administered once daily, or placebo. Patients randomized to treatment with donepezil were to achieve their assigned doses by titration, beginning at 3 mg/day, and extending over a maximum of 6 weeks. Two hundred and forty eight (248) patients completed the study, with similar proportions of patients completing the study in each treatment group. The primary efficacy measures for this study were the SIB and CIBIC-plus.

At 24 weeks of treatment, statistically significant treatment differences were observed between the 10 mg/day dose of donepezil and placebo on both the SIB and CIBIC-plus. The 5 mg/day dose of donepezil showed a statistically significant superiority to placebo on the SIB, but not on the CIBIC-plus.

Study of 23 mg/day
The effectiveness of ARICEPT 23 mg/day as a treatment for moderate to severe Alzheimer's disease has been demonstrated by the results of a randomized, double-blind, controlled clinical investigation in patients with moderate to severe Alzheimer's disease. The controlled clinical study was conducted globally in patients with probable Alzheimer's disease diagnosed by NINCDS-ADRDA and DSM-IV criteria, MMSE: range of 0-20. Patients were required to have been on a stable dose of ARICEPT 10 mg/day for at least 3 months prior to screening. One thousand four hundred and thirty four (1434) patients with moderate to severe Alzheimer's disease were randomized to 23 mg/day or 10 mg/day. The mean age of patients was 73.8 years, with a range of 47 to 90. Approximately 63% of patients were women, and 37% were men. Approximately 36% of the patients were taking memantine throughout the study.

Study Outcome Measures: The effectiveness of treatment with 23 mg/day was determined using a dual outcome assessment strategy that evaluated cognitive function using an instrument designed for more impaired patients and overall function through caregiver- rated assessment. This study showed that patients on 23 mg/day experienced important clinical benefit on both measures compared to 10 mg/day.

The ability of 23 mg/day to improve cognitive performance was assessed with the Severe Impairment Battery (SIB). The SIB, a multi-item instrument, has been validated for the evaluation of cognitive function in patients with moderate to severe dementia. The SIB evaluates selective aspects of cognitive performance, including elements of memory, language, orientation, attention, praxis, visuospatial ability, construction, and social interaction. The SIB scoring range is from 0 to 100, with lower scores indicating greater cognitive impairment.

The ability of 23 mg/day to produce an overall clinical effect was assessed using a Clinician's Interview-Based Impression of Change that incorporated the use of caregiver information, the CIBIC-plus. The CIBIC-plus used in this trial was a semi-structured instrument that examines four major areas of patient function: General, Cognitive, Behavioral and Activities of Daily Living. It represents the assessment of a skilled clinician based upon his/her observations at an interview with the patient, in combination with information supplied by a caregiver familiar with the behavior of the patient over the interval rated. The CIBIC-plus is scored as a seven-point categorical rating, ranging from a score of 1, indicating "markedly improved," to a score of 4, indicating "no change" to a score of 7, indicating "markedly worse."

Effects on the SIB:
Figure 11 shows the time course for the change from baseline in SIB score for the two treatment groups over the 24 weeks of the study. At 24 weeks of treatment, the LS mean difference in the SIB change scores for 23 mg/day-treated patients compared to patients treated with 10 mg/day was

2.2 units (p = 0.0001). The dose of 23 mg/day was statistically significantly superior to the dose of 10 mg/day.

Figure 11. Time-course of the Change from Baseline in SIB Score for Patients Completing 24 Weeks of Treatment.

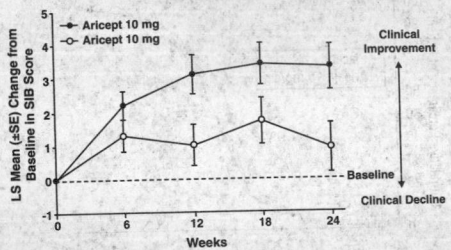

Figure 12 illustrates the cumulative percentages of patients from each of the two treatment groups who attained the measure of improvement in SIB score shown on the X-axis. While patients assigned both to 23 mg/day and to 10 mg/day have a wide range of responses, the curves show that the 23 mg-group is more likely to show a greater improvement in cognitive performance. When such curves are shifted to the left, this indicates a greater percentage of patients responding to treatment on the SIB.

Figure 12. Cumulative Percentage of Patients Completing 24 Weeks of Double-blind Treatment with Specified Changes from Baseline SIB Scores

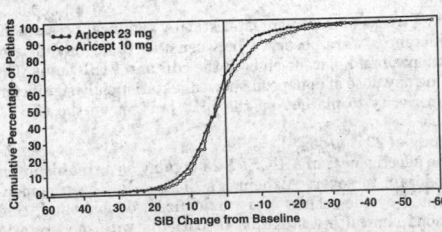

Effects on the CIBIC-plus: Figure 13 is a histogram of the frequency distribution of CIBIC-plus scores attained by patients at the end of 24 weeks of treatment. The mean difference between the 23 mg/day and 10 mg/day treatment groups was 0.06 units. This difference was not statistically significant.
[See figure at top of next column]

16. HOW SUPPLIED/STORAGE AND HANDLING
16.1. ARICEPT Tablets
Supplied as film-coated, round tablets containing 5 mg, 10 mg, or 23 mg of donepezil hydrochloride. The 5 mg tablets are white. The strength, in mg (5), is debossed on one side and ARICEPT is debossed on the other side.
Bottles of 30 (NDC# 62856-245-30)
Bottles of 90 (NDC# 62856-245-90)
Bottles of 1000 (NDC# 62856-245-11)

Figure 13. Frequency Distribution of CIBIC plus Scores at Week 24

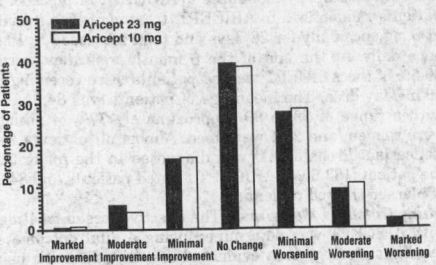

Unit Dose Blister Package 100 (10×10) (NDC# 62856-245-41)
The 10 mg tablets are yellow. The strength, in mg (10), is debossed on one side and ARICEPT is debossed on the other side.
Bottles of 30 (NDC# 62856-246-30)
Bottles of 90 (NDC# 62856-246-90)
Bottles of 1000 (NDC# 62856-246-11)
Unit Dose Blister Package 100 (10×10) (NDC# 62856-246-41)
The 23 mg tablets are reddish in color. The strength, in mg (23), is debossed on one side and ARICEPT is debossed on the other side.
Bottles of 30 (NDC# 62856-247-30)
Bottles of 90 (NDC# 62856-247-90)

16.2. ARICEPT ODT
Supplied as round tablets containing either 5 mg or 10 mg of donepezil hydrochloride.
The 5 mg orally disintegrating tablets are white. The strength, in mg (5), is embossed on one side and ARICEPT is embossed on the other side.
5 mg (White) Unit Dose Blister Package 30 (10×3) (NDC# 62856-831-30)
The 10 mg orally disintegrating tablets are yellow. The strength, in mg (10), is embossed on one side and ARICEPT is embossed on the other side.
10 mg (Yellow) Unit Dose Blister Package 30 (10×3) (NDC# 62856-832-30)
Storage: Store at controlled room temperature, 15°C to 30°C (59°F to 86°F).

17. PATIENT COUNSELING INFORMATION
See FDA-approved Patient Package Insert attached to this label.
To assure safe and effective use of ARICEPT, the information and instructions provided in the attached Patient Package Insert should be discussed with patients and caregivers. Patients and caregivers should be instructed to take ARICEPT only once per day, as prescribed.
Patients and caregivers should be instructed that ARICEPT tablets should not be split or crushed. ARICEPT tablets should be swallowed whole. ARICEPT ODT tablets should not be swallowed whole, but be allowed to dissolve on the tongue and followed with water.
Patients and caregivers should be advised that the product may cause nausea, diarrhea, insomnia, vomiting, muscle cramps, fatigue and decreased appetite.

ARICEPT PATIENT PACKAGE INSERT
ARICEPT® (Air-eh-sept)
(donepezil hydrochloride) tablets
• Tablets: 5 mg, 10 mg, and 23 mg
ARICEPT® ODT (Air-eh-sept oh-dee-tee)
(donepezil hydrochloride) orally disintegrating tablets
• ODT Tablets: 5 mg and 10 mg
Read the Patient Information that comes with ARICEPT before the patient starts taking it and each time you get a refill. There may be new information. This leaflet does not take the place of talking with the doctor about Alzheimer's disease or treatment for it. If you have questions, ask the doctor or pharmacist.
What is ARICEPT?
ARICEPT comes as ARICEPT film-coated tablets in dosage strengths of 5 mg, 10 mg, and 23 mg, and as ARICEPT Orally Disintegrating Tablets (ODT; 5 mg and 10 mg). Except where indicated, all the information about ARICEPT in this leaflet also applies to ARICEPT ODT.
ARICEPT is a prescription medicine to treat mild Alzheimer's disease (up to 10 mg) and moderate to severe Alzheimer's disease (up to 23 mg). ARICEPT can help with mental function and with doing daily tasks. ARICEPT does not work the same in all people. Some people may:
• Seem much better
• Get better in small ways or stay the same
• Get worse over time but slower than expected
• Not change and then get worse as expected
ARICEPT does not cure Alzheimer's disease. All patients with Alzheimer's disease get worse over time, even if they take ARICEPT.

ARICEPT has not been approved as a treatment for any medical condition in children.
Who should not take ARICEPT?
The patient should not take ARICEPT if allergic to any of the ingredients in ARICEPT or to medicines that contain piperidines. Ask the patient's doctor if you are not sure. See the end of this leaflet for a list of ingredients in ARICEPT.
What should I tell the doctor before the patient takes ARICEPT?
Tell the doctor about all the patient's present or past health problems. Include:
• Any heart problems including problems with irregular, slow, or fast heartbeats
• Asthma or lung problems
• A seizure
• Stomach ulcers
• Difficulty passing urine
• Liver or kidney problems
• Trouble swallowing tablets
• Present pregnancy or plans to become pregnant. It is not known if ARICEPT can harm an unborn baby.
• Present breast-feeding. It is not known if ARICEPT passes into breast milk. ARICEPT is not for women who are breast-feeding.
Tell the doctor about all the medicines the patient takes, including prescription and non-prescription medicines, vitamins, and herbal products. ARICEPT and other medicines may affect each other.
Be particularly sure to tell the doctor if the patient takes aspirin or medicines called nonsteroidal anti-inflammatory drugs (NSAIDs). There are many NSAID medicines, both prescription and non-prescription. Ask the doctor or pharmacist if you are not sure if any of the patient's medicines are NSAIDs. Taking NSAIDs and ARICEPT together may make the patient more likely to get stomach ulcers.
ARICEPT taken with certain medicines used for anesthesia may cause side effects. Tell the responsible doctor or dentist that the patient takes ARICEPT before the patient has:
• surgery
• medical procedures
• dental surgery or procedures.
Know the medicines that the patient takes. Keep a list of all the patient's medicines. Show it to the doctor or pharmacist before the patient starts a new medicine.
How should the patient take ARICEPT?
• Give ARICEPT exactly as prescribed by the doctor. Do not stop ARICEPT or change the dose yourself. Talk with the doctor first.
• Give ARICEPT one time each day. ARICEPT can be taken with or without food.
• ARICEPT Tablets (but not ARICEPT ODT) should be swallowed whole without the tablets being broken or crushed.
• ARICEPT ODT melts on the tongue. The patient should drink some water after the tablet melts.
• If you miss giving the patient a dose of ARICEPT, just wait. Give only the next dose at the usual time. Do not give 2 doses at the same time.
• If ARICEPT is missed for 7 days or more, talk with the doctor before starting again.
• If the patient takes too much ARICEPT at one time, call the doctor or poison control center, or go to the emergency room right away.
What are the possible side effects of ARICEPT?
ARICEPT may cause the following serious side effects:
• **slow heartbeat and fainting.** This happens more often in people with heart problems. Call the doctor right away if the patient faints while taking ARICEPT.
• **more stomach acid.** This raises the chance of ulcers and bleeding, especially when taking ARICEPT 23 mg. The risk is higher for patients who had ulcers, or take aspirin or other NSAIDs.
• worsening of lung problems in people with asthma or other lung disease.
• seizures.
• difficulty passing urine.
Call the doctor *right away* if the patient has:
• fainting.
• heartburn or stomach pain that is new or won't go away.
• nausea or vomiting, blood in the vomit, dark vomit that looks like coffee grounds.
• bowel movements or stools that look like black tar.
• new or worse asthma or breathing problems.
• seizures.
• difficulty passing urine.
The most common side effects of ARICEPT are:
• nausea
• diarrhea
• not sleeping well
• vomiting
• muscle cramps
• feeling tired
• not wanting to eat

These side effects may get better after the patient takes ARICEPT for a while. This is not a complete list of side effects with ARICEPT. For more information, ask the doctor or pharmacist.

Call your doctor for medical advice about side effects. You may report side effects to FDA at 1-800-FDA-1088.

How should ARICEPT be stored?

Store ARICEPT at room temperature between 59° to 86°F (15° to 30°C).

Keep ARICEPT and all medicines out of the reach of children.

General information about ARICEPT

Medicines are sometimes prescribed for conditions that are not mentioned in this Patient Information Leaflet. Do not use ARICEPT for a condition for which it was not prescribed. Do not give ARICEPT to people other than the patient, even if they have the same symptoms as the patient, as it may harm them.

This leaflet summarizes the most important information about ARICEPT. If you would like more information talk with the patient's doctor. You can ask your pharmacist or doctor for information about ARICEPT that is written for health professionals. For more information, go to www.ARICEPT.com, or call 1-800-760-6029.

What are the ingredients in ARICEPT?

Active ingredient: donepezil hydrochloride

Inactive ingredients:

- **ARICEPT 5 mg and 10 mg film-coated tablets:** lactose monohydrate, cornstarch, microcrystalline cellulose, hydroxypropyl cellulose, and magnesium stearate. The film coating contains talc, polyethylene glycol, hypromellose, and titanium dioxide. Additionally, the 10 mg tablet contains yellow iron oxide (synthetic) as a coloring agent.
- **ARICEPT 23 mg film-coated tablets:** ethylcellulose, hydroxypropyl cellulose, lactose monohydrate, magnesium stearate and methacrylic acid copolymer, Type C. The reddish color film coating includes ferric oxide, hypromellose 2910, polyethylene glycol 8000, talc and titanium dioxide.
- **ARICEPT ODT 5 mg and 10 mg tablets:** carrageenan, mannitol, colloidal silicon dioxide, and polyvinyl alcohol. The 10 mg tablet contains yellow iron oxide (synthetic) as a coloring agent.

ARICEPT® is a registered trademark of Eisai Co., Ltd.

Manufactured and Marketed by Eisai Inc., Woodcliff Lake, NJ 07677

Marketed by Pfizer Inc, New York, NY 10017

Rx Only

© 2010 Eisai Inc.

Shown in Product Identification Guide, page 308

BANZEL™
[ban-'zel]
(rufinamide)
Tablets

℞

DESCRIPTION

BANZEL (rufinamide) is a triazole derivative structurally unrelated to currently marketed antiepileptic drugs (AEDs). Rufinamide has the chemical name 1-[(2,6-difluorophenyl)methyl]-1H-1,2,3-triazole-4 carboxamide. It has an empirical formula of $C_{10}H_8F_2N_4O$ and a molecular weight of 238.2. The drug substance is a white, crystalline, odorless and slightly bitter tasting neutral powder. Rufinamide is practically insoluble in water, slightly soluble in tetrahydrofuran and in methanol, and very slightly soluble in ethanol and in acetonitrile.

BANZEL is available for oral administration in film-coated tablets, scored on both sides, containing 200 and 400 mg of rufinamide. Inactive ingredients are colloidal silicon dioxide, corn starch crosscarmellose sodium, hypromellose, lactose monohydrate, magnesium stearate, microcrystalline cellulose, and sodium lauryl sulphate. The film coating contains hypromellose, iron oxide red, polyethylene glycol, talc, and titanium dioxide.

CLINICAL PHARMACOLOGY

Mechanism of Action

The precise mechanism(s) by which rufinamide exerts its antiepileptic effect is unknown. The results of in vitro studies suggest that the principal mechanism of action of rufinamide is modulation of the activity of sodium channels and, in particular, prolongation of the inactive state of the channel. Rufinamide (≥ 1 µM) significantly slowed sodium channel recovery from inactivation after a prolonged prepulse in cultured cortical neurons, and limited sustained

repetitive firing of sodium-dependent action potentials (EC_{50} of 3.8 µM).

Pharmacokinetics

Overview

BANZEL is well absorbed after oral administration. However, the rate of absorption is relatively slow and the extent of absorption is decreased as dose is increased. The pharmacokinetics does not change with multiple dosing. Most elimination of rufinamide is via metabolism, with the primary metabolite resulting from enzymatic hydrolysis of the carboxamide moiety to form the carboxylic acid. This metabolic route is not cytochrome P450 dependent. There are no known active metabolites. Plasma half-life of rufinamide is approximately 6–10 hours.

Absorption and Distribution

Following oral administration of BANZEL, peak plasma concentrations occur between 4 and 6 hours (T_{max}) both under fed and fasted conditions. BANZEL tablets display decreasing bioavailability with increasing dose after single and multiple dose administration. Based on urinary excretion, the extent of absorption was at least 85% following oral administration of a single dose of 600 mg rufinamide under fed conditions.

Multiple dose pharmacokinetics can be predicted from single dose data for both rufinamide and its metabolite. Given the dosing frequency of every 12 hours and the half-life of 6 to 10 hours, the observed steady-state peak concentration of about two to three times the peak concentration after a single dose is expected.

Food increased the extent of absorption of rufinamide in healthy volunteers by 34% and increased peak exposure by 56% after a single dose of 400 mg, although the T_{max} was not elevated. Clinical trials were performed under fed conditions and dosing is recommended with food (see DOSAGE AND ADMINISTRATION).

Only a small fraction of rufinamide (34%) is bound to human serum proteins, predominantly to albumin (27%), giving little risk of displacement drug-drug interactions. Rufinamide was evenly distributed between erythrocytes and plasma. The apparent volume of distribution is dependent upon dose and varies with body surface area. The apparent volume of distribution was about 50 L at 3200 mg/day.

Metabolism

Rufinamide is extensively metabolized but has no active metabolites. Following a radiolabeled dose of rufinamide, less than 2% of the dose was recovered unchanged in urine. The primary biotransformation pathway is carboxylesterase(s) mediated hydrolysis of the carboxylamide group to the acid derivative CGP 47292. A few minor additional metabolites were detected in urine, which appeared to be acyl-glucuronides of CGP 47292. There is no involvement of oxidizing cytochrome P450 enzymes or glutathione in the biotransformation process.

Rufinamide is a weak inhibitor of CYP 2E1. It did not show significant inhibition of other CYP enzymes. Rufinamide is a weak inducer of CYP 3A4 enzymes.

Elimination/Excretion

Renal excretion is the predominant route of elimination for drug related material, accounting for 85% of the dose based on a radiolabeled study. Of the metabolites identified in urine, at least 66% of the rufinamide dose was excreted as the acid metabolite CGP 47292, with 2% of the dose excreted as rufinamide.

The plasma elimination half-life is approximately 6–10 hours in healthy subjects and patients with epilepsy.

Special Populations

Gender: Population pharmacokinetic analyses of females show a 6–14% lower apparent clearance of rufinamide compared to males. This effect is not clinically important.

Race: In a population pharmacokinetic analysis of clinical studies, no difference in clearance or volume of distribution of rufinamide was observed between the Black and Caucasian subjects, after controlling for body size. Information on other races could not be obtained because of smaller numbers of these subjects.

Pediatrics: Based on a population analysis in 117 children (age 4–11 years) and 99 adolescents (age 12–17 years), the pharmacokinetics of rufinamide in these patients is similar to the pharmacokinetics in adults.

Elderly: The results of a study evaluating single-dose (400 mg) and multiple dose (800 mg/day for 6 days) pharmacokinetics of rufinamide in 8 healthy elderly subjects (65–80 years old) and 7 younger healthy subjects (18–45 years old) found no significant age-related differences in the pharmacokinetics of rufinamide.

Renal Impairment: Rufinamide pharmacokinetics in 9 patients with severe renal impairment (creatinine clearance <30 mL/min) was similar to that of healthy subjects. Patients undergoing dialysis 3 hours post rufinamide dosing showed a reduction in AUC and C_{max} by 29% and 16% respectively. Adjusting rufinamide dose for the loss of drug upon dialysis should be considered.

Hepatic Impairment: There have been no specific studies investigating the effect of hepatic impairment on the phar-

macokinetics of rufinamide. Therefore, use in patients with severe hepatic impairment is not recommended. Caution should be exercised in treating patients with mild to moderate hepatic impairment.

Drug Interactions

Based on in vitro studies, rufinamide shows little or no inhibition of most cytochrome P450 enzymes at clinically relevant concentrations, with weak inhibition of CYP 2E1. Drugs that are substrates of CYP 2E1 (e.g. chlorzoxazone) may have increased plasma levels in the presence of rufinamide, but this has not been studied.

Based on in vivo drug interaction studies with triazolam and oral contraceptives, rufinamide is a weak inducer of the CYP 3A4 enzyme and can decrease exposure of drugs that are substrates of CYP 3A4 (see Effects of BANZEL on other medications).

Rufinamide is metabolized by carboxylesterases. Drugs that may induce the activity of carboxylesterases may increase the clearance of rufinamide. Broad-spectrum inducers such as carbamazepine and phenobarbital may have minor effects on rufinamide metabolism via this mechanism. Drugs that are inhibitors of carboxylesterases may decrease metabolism of rufinamide.

Antiepileptic Drugs

Effects of BANZEL on other AEDs

Population pharmacokinetic analysis of average concentration at steady state of carbamazepine, lamotrigine, phenobarbital, phenytoin, topiramate, and valproate showed that typical rufinamide C_{avss} levels had little effect on the pharmacokinetics of other AEDs. Any effects, when they occur, have been more marked in the pediatric population.

Table 1 summarizes the drug-drug interactions of BANZEL with other AEDs.

Table 1: Summary of drug-drug interactions of BANZEL with other antiepileptic drugs

AED Co-administered	Influence of Rufinamide on AED concentration[a]	Influence of AED on Rufinamide concentration
Carbamazepine	Decrease by 7 to 13%[b]	Decrease by 19 to 26% Dependent on dose of carbamazepine
Lamotrigine	Decrease by 7 to 13%[b]	No Effect
Phenobarbital	Increase by 8 to 13%[b]	Decrease by 25 to 46%[c, d] Independent of dose or concentration of phenobarbital
Phenytoin	Increase by 7 to 21%[b]	Decrease by 25 to 46%[c, d] Independent of dose or concentration of phenytoin
Topiramate	No Effect	No Effect
Valproate	No Effect	Increase by <16 to 70%[c] Dependent on concentration of valproate
Primidone	Not Investigated	Decrease by 25 to 46%[c, d] Independent of dose or concentration of primidone
Benzodiazepines[e]	Not Investigated	No Effect

a) Predictions are based on BANZEL concentrations at the maximum recommended dose of BANZEL.

b) Maximum changes predicted to be in children and in patients who achieve significantly higher levels of BANZEL, as the effect of rufinamide on these AEDs is concentration-dependent.

c) Larger effects in children at high doses/concentrations of AEDs.

d) Phenobarbital, primidone and phenytoin were treated as a single covariate (phenobarbital-type inducers) to examine the effect of these agents on BANZEL clearance.

e) All compounds of the benzodiazepine class were pooled to examine for 'class effect' on BANZEL clearance.

Phenytoin: The decrease in clearance of phenytoin estimated at typical levels of rufinamide (C_{avss} 15 µg/mL) is predicted to increase plasma levels of phenytoin by 7 to 21%. As phenytoin is known to have non-linear pharmacokinetics (clearance becomes saturated at higher doses), it is possible that exposure will be greater than the model prediction.

Effects of Other AEDs on BANZEL

Potent cytochrome P450 enzyme inducers, such as carbamazepine, phenytoin, primidone, and phenobarbital appear to increase the clearance of BANZEL (see Table 1). Given that the majority of clearance of BANZEL is via a non-CYP-dependent route, the observed decreases in blood levels seen with carbamazepine, phenytoin, phenobarbital, and primidone are unlikely to be entirely attributable to induction of a P450 enzyme. Other factors explaining this interaction are not understood.

Any effects, where they occurred were likely to be more marked in the pediatric population.

Valproate: Based on a population pharmacokinetic analysis, rufinamide clearance was decreased by valproate. In children, valproate administration may lead to elevated levels of rufinamide by up to 70%. Patients stabilized on BANZEL before being prescribed valproate should begin valproate therapy at a low dose, and titrate to a clinically effective dose. Similarly, patients on valproate should begin at a BANZEL dose lower than 400 mg.

Effects of BANZEL on other Medications

Hormonal contraceptives: Co-administration of BANZEL (800 mg BID for 14 days) and Ortho-Novum 1/35® resulted in a mean decrease in the ethinyl estradiol AUC_{0-24} of 22% and C_{max} by 18% and norethindrone AUC_{0-24} by 14% and C_{max} by 18%, respectively. The clinical significance of this decrease is unknown. Female patients of childbearing age should be warned that the concurrent use of BANZEL with hormonal contraceptives may render this method of contraception less effective. Additional non-hormonal forms of contraception are recommended when using BANZEL (see Information for Patients).

Triazolam: Co-administration and pre-treatment with BANZEL (400 mg bid) resulted in a 37% decrease in AUC and a 23% decrease in C_{max} of triazolam, a CYP 3A4 substrate.

Olanzapine: Co-administration and pre-treatment with BANZEL (400mg bid) resulted in no change in AUC and C_{max} of olanzapine, a CYP 1A2 substrate.

CLINICAL STUDIES

The effectiveness of BANZEL as adjunctive treatment for the seizures associated with Lennox-Gastaut syndrome (LGS) was established in a single multicenter, double-blind, placebo-controlled, randomized, parallel-group study (n=138). Male and female patients (between 4 and 30 years of age) were included if they had a diagnosis of inadequately controlled seizures associated with LGS (including both atypical absence seizures and drop attacks) and were being treated with 1 to 3 concomitant stable dose AEDs. Each patient must have had at least 90 seizures in the month prior to study entry. After completing a 4 week Baseline Phase on stable therapy, patients were randomized to have BANZEL or placebo added to their ongoing therapy during the 12 week Double-blind Phase. The Double-blind Phase consisted of 2 periods: the Titration Period (1 to 2 weeks) and the Maintenance Period (10 weeks). During the Titration Period, the dose was increased to a target dosage of approximately 45 mg/kg/day (3200 mg in adults of ≥ 70kg), given on a b.i.d. schedule. Dosage reductions were permitted during titration if problems in tolerability were encountered. Final doses at titration were to remain stable during the maintenance period. Target dosage was achieved in 88% of the BANZEL-treated patients. The majority of these patients reached the target dose within 7 days, with the remaining patients achieving the target dose within 14 days.

The primary efficacy variables were:

- The percent change in total seizure frequency per 28 days;
- The percent change in tonic-atonic (drop attacks) seizure frequency per 28 days;
- Seizure severity from the Parent/Guardian Global Evaluation of the patient's condition. This was a 7-point assessment performed at the end of the Double-blind Phase. A score of +3 indicated that the patient's seizure severity was very much improved, a score of 0 that the seizure severity was unchanged, and a score of -3 that the seizure severity was very much worse.

The results of the three primary endpoints are shown in Table 2 below.

Table 2: Lennox-Gastaut Syndrome Trial Seizure Frequency Primary Efficacy Variable Results

Variable	Placebo	Rufinamide
Median percent change in total seizure frequency per 28 days	-11.7	-32.7 (p=0.0015)
Median percent change in tonic-atonic seizure frequency per 28 days	1.4	-42.5 (p<0.0001)
Improvement in Seizure Severity Rating from Global Evaluation	30.6	53.4 (p=0.0041)

INDICATIONS AND USAGE

BANZEL (rufinamide) is indicated for adjunctive treatment of seizures associated with Lennox-Gastaut syndrome in children 4 years and older and adults.

CONTRAINDICATIONS

BANZEL is contraindicated in patients with Familial Short QT syndrome (see PRECAUTIONS, QT Shortening).

WARNINGS

Suicidal Behavior and Ideation

Antiepileptic drugs increase the risk of suicidal thoughts or behavior in patients taking these drugs for any indication. Patients treated with any antiepileptic drug for any indication should be monitored for the emergence or worsening of depression, suicidal thoughts or behavior, or any unusual changes in mood or behavior.

Pooled analyses of 199 placebo-controlled clinical trials (mono- and adjunctive therapy) of 11 different antiepileptic drugs showed that patients randomized to one of the antiepileptic drugs had approximately twice the risk (adjusted Relative Risk 1.8, 95% CI:1.2, 2.7) of suicidal thinking or behavior compared to patients randomized to placebo. In these trials, which had a median treatment duration of 12 weeks, the estimated incidence rate of suicidal behavior or ideation among 27,863 antiepileptic drug-treated patients was 0.43%, compared to 0.24% among 16,029 placebo-treated patients, representing an increase of approximately one case of suicidal thinking or behavior for every 530 patients treated. There were four suicides in drug-treated patients in the trials and none in placebo-treated patients, but the number of events is too small to allow any conclusion about drug effect on suicide.

The increased risk of suicidal thoughts or behavior was observed as early as one week after starting drug treatment and persisted for at least 24 weeks. Because most trials included in the analysis did not extend beyond 24 weeks, the risk of suicidal thoughts or behavior beyond 24 weeks could not be assessed.

The risk of suicidal thoughts or behavior was generally consistent among drugs in the data analyzed. The finding of increased risk with antiepileptic drugs of varying mechanisms of action and across a range of indications suggests that the risk applies to all antiepileptic drugs used for any indication. The risk did not vary substantially by age in the clinical trials analyzed.

The following table (Table 3) shows absolute and relative risk of suicidal behavior and ideation by indication.

[See table 3 below]

Table 3: Absolute and Relative Risk of Suicidal Behavior and Ideation

Indication	Placebo Patients with Events Per 1000 Patients	Drug Patients with Events Per 1000 Patients	Relative Risk: Incidence of Events in Drug Patients/ Incidence in Placebo Patients	Risk Difference: Additional Drug Patients with Events Per 1000 Patients
Epilepsy	1.0	3.4	3.5	2.4
Psychiatric	5.7	8.5	1.5	2.9
Other	1.0	1.8	1.9	0.9
Total	2.4	4.3	1.8	1.9

The relative risk for suicidal thoughts or behavior was higher in clinical trials for epilepsy than in clinical trials for psychiatric or other conditions, but the absolute risk differences were similar.

Anyone considering prescribing BANZEL or any other antiepileptic drug must balance this risk with the risk of untreated illness. Epilepsy and many other illnesses for which antiepileptics are prescribed are themselves associated with morbidity and mortality and an increased risk of suicidal thoughts and behavior. Should suicidal thoughts and behavior emerge during treatment, the prescriber needs to consider whether the emergence of these symptoms in any given patient may be related to the illness being treated.

Patients, their caregivers, and families should be informed that antiepileptic drugs increase the risk of suicidal thoughts and behavior and should be advised of the need to be alert for the emergence or worsening of the signs and symptoms of depression, any unusual changes in mood or behavior, or the emergence of suicidal thoughts, behavior, or thoughts about self-harm. Behaviors of concern should be reported immediately to healthcare providers.

Central Nervous System Reactions:

Use of BANZEL has been associated with central nervous system-related adverse reactions. The most significant of these can be classified into two general categories:

1) somnolence or fatigue, and 2) coordination abnormalities, dizziness, gait disturbances, and ataxia (see ADVERSE REACTIONS).

PRECAUTIONS

QT Shortening

Formal cardiac ECG studies demonstrated shortening of the QT interval (up to 20 msec) with BANZEL treatment. In a placebo-controlled study of the QT interval, a higher percentage of BANZEL-treated subjects (46% at 2400 mg, 46% at 3200 mg, and 65% at 4800 mg) had a QT shortening of greater than 20 msec at T_{max} compared to placebo (5–10%). Reductions of the QT interval below 300 msec were not observed in the formal QT studies with doses up to 7200 mg/day. Moreover, there was no signal for drug-induced sudden death or ventricular arrhythmias.

The degree of QT shortening induced by BANZEL is without any known clinical risk. Familial Short QT syndrome is associated with an increased risk of sudden death and ventricular arrhythmias, particularly ventricular fibrillation. Such events in this syndrome are believed to occur primarily when the corrected QT interval falls below 300 msec. Nonclinical data also indicate that QT shortening is associated with ventricular fibrillation.

Patients with Familial Short QT syndrome should not be treated with BANZEL (see CONTRAINDICATIONS). Caution should be used when administering BANZEL with other drugs that shorten the QT interval.

Multi-organ Hypersensitivity Reactions

Multi-organ hypersensitivity syndrome, a serious condition sometimes induced by antiepileptic drugs, has occurred in association with BANZEL therapy in clinical trials. One patient experienced rash, urticaria, facial edema, fever, elevated eosinophils, stuporous state, and severe hepatitis, beginning on day 29 of BANZEL therapy and extending over a course of 30 days of continued BANZEL therapy with resolution 11 days after discontinuation. Additional possible cases presented with rash and one or more of the following: fever, elevated liver function studies, hematuria, and lymphadenopathy. These cases occurred in children less than 12 years of age, within four weeks of treatment initiation, and were noted to resolve and/or improve upon BANZEL discontinuation. This syndrome has been reported with other anticonvulsants and typically, although not exclusively, presents with fever and rash associated with other organ system involvement. Because this disorder is variable in its expression, other organ system signs and symptoms not noted here may occur. If this reaction is suspected, BANZEL should be discontinued and alternative treatment started.

All patients who develop a rash while taking BANZEL must be closely supervised.

Withdrawal of AEDs

As with all antiepileptic drugs, BANZEL should be withdrawn gradually to minimize the risk of precipitating seizures, seizure exacerbation, or status epilepticus. If abrupt discontinuation of the drug is medically necessary, the transition to another AED should be made under close medical supervision. In clinical trials, BANZEL discontinuation was achieved by reducing the dose by approximately 25% every two days.

Status Epilepticus

Estimates of the incidence of treatment emergent status epilepticus among patients treated with BANZEL are difficult because standard definitions were not employed. In a controlled Lennox Gastaut syndrome trial, 3 of 74 (4.1 %) BANZEL-treated patients had episodes that could be described as status epilepticus in the BANZEL-treated patients compared with none of the 64 patients in the placebo-treated patients. In all controlled trials that included patients with different epilepsies, 11 of 1240 (0.9%) BANZEL-treated patients had episodes that could be described as status epilepticus compared with none of 635 patients in the placebo-treated patients.

Information for Patients
Prescribers or other health professionals should inform patients, their families, and their caregivers about the benefits and risks associated with treatment with BANZEL and should counsel them in its appropriate use. A patient Medication Guide is available for BANZEL. The prescriber or healthcare professional should instruct patients, their families, and their caregivers to read the Medication Guide and should assist them in understanding its contents. Patients should be given the opportunity to discuss the contents of the Medication Guide and to obtain answers to any questions they may have. The complete text of the Medication Guide is reprinted at the end of this document.
Patients should be advised of the following issues and asked to alert their prescriber if these occur while taking BANZEL.
Suicidal Thinking and Behavior—Patients, their caregivers, and families should be informed that antiepileptic drugs increase the risk of suicidal thoughts and behavior and should be advised of the need to be alert for the emergence or worsening of the signs and symptoms of depression, any unusual changes in mood or behavior, or the emergence of suicidal thoughts, behavior, or thoughts about self-harm. Behaviors of concern should be reported immediately to healthcare providers.
Patients should be instructed to take BANZEL only as prescribed.
BANZEL should be taken with food.
As with all centrally acting medications, alcohol in combination with BANZEL may cause additive central nervous system effects.
Patients should be advised about the potential for somnolence or dizziness and advised not to drive or operate machinery until they have gained sufficient experience on BANZEL to gauge whether it adversely affects their mental and/or motor performance.
Female patients of childbearing age should be warned that the concurrent use of BANZEL with hormonal contraceptives may render this method of contraception less effective (see Drug Interactions). Additional non-hormonal forms of contraception are recommended when using BANZEL.
Patients should be advised to notify their physician if they become pregnant or intend to become pregnant during therapy. Patients should be advised to notify their physician if they are breast-feeding or intend to breast-feed.
Patients should be advised to notify their physician if they experience a rash associated with fever.
Laboratory Tests
Leucopenia (white cell count $< 3 \times 10^9$ L) was more commonly observed in BANZEL-treated patients (43 of 1171, 3.7%) than placebo-treated patients (7 of 579, 1.2%) in all controlled trials.
Drug Interactions
In vitro and in vivo studies have shown that BANZEL is unlikely to be involved in significant pharmacokinetic interactions.
BANZEL can increase plasma concentrations of phenytoin by 21% or more due to non-linear pharmacokinetics.
Valproate can increase BANZEL concentrations up to 70%. Patients stabilized on BANZEL before being prescribed valproate should begin valproate therapy at a low dose, and titrate to a clinically effective dose. Similarly, patients on valproate should begin at a BANZEL dose lower than 400 mg.
Coadministration of BANZEL with ethinyl estradiol and norethindrone can decrease AUC_{0-24} of these hormonal contraceptives by 22% and 14% and C_{max} by 31% and 18%, respectively. Female patients of childbearing age should be warned that the concurrent use of BANZEL with hormonal contraceptives may render this method of contraception less effective. Additional non-hormonal forms of contraception are recommended when using BANZEL (see CLINICAL PHARMACOLOGY and Information for Patients).
Drug/Laboratory Test Interactions
There are no known interactions of BANZEL with commonly used laboratory tests.
Carcinogenicity, Mutagenicity, Impairment of Fertility
Carcinogenicity: Rufinamide was given in the diet to mice at 40, 120, and 400 mg/kg/day and to rats at 20, 60, and 200 mg/kg/day for two years. The doses in mice were associated with plasma AUCs 0.1 to 1 times the human plasma AUC at the maximum recommended human dose (MRHD, 3200 mg/day). Increased incidences of tumors (benign bone tumors (osteomas) and/or hepatocellular adenomas and carcinomas) were observed in mice at all doses. Increased incidences of thyroid follicular adenomas were observed in rats at all but the low dose; the low dose is <0.1 times the MRHD on a mg/m² basis.

Mutagenicity: Rufinamide was not mutagenic in the in vitro bacterial reverse mutation (Ames) assay or the in vitro mammalian cell point mutation assay. Rufinamide was not clastogenic in the in vitro mammalian cell chromosomal aberration assay or the in vivo rat bone marrow micronucleus assay.
Impairment of Fertility: Oral administration of rufinamide (doses of 20, 60, 200, and 600 mg/kg/day) to male and female rats prior to mating and throughout mating, and continuing in females up to day 6 of gestation resulted in impairment of fertility (decreased conception rates and mating and fertility indices; decreased numbers of corpora lutea, implantations, and live embryos; increased preimplantation loss; decreased sperm count and motility) at all doses tested. Therefore, a no-effect dose was not established. The lowest dose tested was associated with a plasma AUC ≈ 0.2 times the human plasma AUC at the MRHD.
PREGNANCY
Pregnancy Category C
Rufinamide produced developmental toxicity when administered orally to pregnant animals at clinically relevant doses.
Rufinamide was administered orally to rats at doses of 20, 100, and 300 mg/kg/day and to rabbits at doses of 30, 200, and 1000 mg/kg/day during the period of organogenesis (implantation to closure of the hard palate); the high doses are associated with plasma AUCs ≈2 times the human plasma AUC at the maximum recommended human dose (MRHD, 3200 mg/day). Decreased fetal weights and increased incidences of fetal skeletal abnormalities were observed in rats at doses associated with maternal toxicity. In rabbits, embryo-fetal death, decreased fetal body weights, and increased incidences of fetal visceral and skeletal abnormalities occurred at all but the low dose. The highest dose tested in rabbits was associated with abortion. The no-effect doses for adverse effects on rat and rabbit embryo-fetal development (20 and 30 mg/kg/day, respectively) were associated with plasma AUCs ≈ 0.2 times that in humans at the MRHD.
In a rat pre- and post-natal development study (dosing from implantation through weaning) conducted at oral doses of 5, 30, and 150 mg/kg/day (associated with plasma AUCs up to ≈1.5 times that in humans at the MRHD), decreased offspring growth and survival were observed at all doses tested. A no-effect dose for adverse effects on pre- and postnatal development was not established. The lowest dose tested was associated with plasma AUC < 0.1 times that in humans at the MRHD.
There are no adequate and well-controlled studies in pregnant women. BANZEL should be used during pregnancy only if the potential benefit justifies the potential risk to the fetus.
Labor and Delivery
The effect of BANZEL on labor and delivery in humans is not known.
Nursing Mothers
Rufinamide is likely to be excreted in breast milk. Because of the potential for serious adverse reactions in nursing infants from BANZEL, a decision should be made whether to discontinue nursing or discontinue the drug taking into account the importance of the drug to the mother.
Pediatric Use
The safety and effectiveness in patients with Lennox-Gastaut syndrome have not been established in children less than 4 years.
Geriatric Use
Clinical studies of BANZEL did not include sufficient numbers of subjects aged 65 and over to determine whether they respond differently from younger subjects. In general, dose selection for an elderly patient should be cautious, usually starting at the low end of the dosing range, reflecting the greater frequency of decreased hepatic, renal, or cardiac function, and of concomitant disease or other drug therapy. A study evaluating the pharmacokinetics of rufinamide in elderly subjects showed that there were no significant differences in the plasma and urine pharmacokinetic parameters of rufinamide between the younger and elderly subjects under both single and multiple dose treatments (see Special Populations: Elderly).

ADVERSE REACTIONS
Placebo-controlled double-blind studies were performed in adults and in pediatric patients, down to age of 4, in other forms of epilepsy, in addition to the trial in Lennox-Gastaut syndrome. Data on CNS Reactions (see WARNINGS) from the Lennox-Gastaut study are presented first. Because there is no reason to suspect that adverse reactions would substantially differ between these patient populations, safety data from all of these controlled studies are then presented. Most of these adverse reactions were mild to moderate and transient in nature.
Common central nervous system reactions in the controlled trial of patients 4 years or older with Lennox-Gastaut syndrome treated with BANZEL as adjunctive therapy (see WARNINGS):
Somnolence was reported in 24.3% of BANZEL-treated patients compared to 12.5% of placebo patients and led to study discontinuation in 2.7% of treated patients compared to 0% of placebo patients. Fatigue was reported in 9.5% of BANZEL-treated patients compared to 7.8% of placebo patients. It led to study discontinuation in 1.4% of treated patients and 0% of placebo patients.
Dizziness was reported in 2.7% of BANZEL-treated patients compared to 0% of placebo patients, and did not lead to study discontinuation.
Ataxia and gait disturbance were reported in 5.4% and 1.4% of BANZEL-treated patients, respectively, and in no placebo patients. Balance disorder and abnormal coordination were each reported in 0% of BANZEL-treated patients and 1.6% of placebo patients. None of these reactions led to study discontinuation.
All Adverse Reactions for All Treated Patients with Epilepsy, Double-blind Adjunctive Therapy Studies: The most commonly observed (≥10%) adverse reactions in BANZEL-treated patients, when used as adjunctive therapy at all doses studied (200 to 3200 mg/day) with a higher frequency than in placebo were: headache, dizziness, fatigue, somnolence, and nausea.
At the target dose of 45 mg/kg/day in children, the most commonly observed (≥5%) adverse reactions in BANZEL-treated patients, given as adjunctive therapy, with a higher frequency than placebo were: somnolence, vomiting, headache, fatigue, dizziness, nausea, and convulsion.
At doses up to 3200 mg/day in adults, the most commonly observed (≥5%) adverse reactions in BANZEL-treated patients, given as adjunctive therapy, at all doses studied, with a higher frequency than placebo were: headache, dizziness, fatigue, nausea, somnolence, diplopia, nasopharyngitis, tremor, nystagmus, vision blurred and vomiting.
Table 4 lists treatment-emergent adverse reactions that occurred in at least 3% of pediatric patients with epilepsy treated with BANZEL in controlled adjunctive studies and were numerically more common in patients treated with BANZEL than placebo.

Table 4: Incidence (%) of Treatment-Emergent Adverse Reactions in all Pediatric Double-Blind Adjunctive Trials by Preferred Term at the Recommended Dose of 45 mg/kg/day (Adverse Reactions occurred in at least 3% of BANZEL-treated patients and occurred more frequently than in Placebo Patients)

Preferred Term	BANZEL (N=187) %	Placebo (N=182) %
Somnolence	17	9
Vomiting	17	7
Headache	16	8
Fatigue	9	8
Dizziness	8	6
Nausea	7	3
Influenza	5	4
Nasopharyngitis	5	3
Decreased Appetite	5	2
Rash	4	2
Ataxia	4	1
Diplopia	4	1
Bronchitis	3	2
Sinusitis	3	2
Psychomotor Hyperactivity	3	1
Abdominal Pain Upper	3	2
Aggression	3	2
Ear Infection	3	1
Disturbance in Attention	3	1
Pruritis	3	0

Table 5 lists treatment-emergent adverse reactions that occurred in at least 3% of adult patients with epilepsy treated with BANZEL (up to 3200mg/day) in adjunctive controlled studies and were numerically more common in patients treated with BANZEL than placebo. In these studies, either BANZEL or placebo was added to current AED therapy.

Table 5: Incidence (%) of Treatment-Emergent Adverse Reactions in all Adult Double-Blind Adjunctive Trials (up to 3200mg/day) by Preferred Term (Adverse Reactions occurred in at least 3% of BANZEL-treated patients and occurred more frequently than in Placebo Patients)

Preferred Term	BANZEL (N=823) %	Placebo (N=376) %
Headache	27	26
Dizziness	19	12
Fatigue	16	10
Nausea	12	9
Somnolence	11	9
Diplopia	9	3
Tremor	6	5
Nystagmus	6	5
Vision Blurred	6	2
Vomiting	5	4
Ataxia	4	0
Abdominal Pain Upper	3	2
Anxiety	3	2
Constipation	3	2
Dyspepsia	3	2
Back Pain	3	1
Gait Disturbance	3	1
Vertigo	3	1

Discontinuation in Controlled Clinical Studies

In controlled double-blind adjunctive clinical studies, 9.0% of patients receiving BANZEL as adjunctive therapy and 4.4% receiving placebo discontinued as a result of an adverse reaction. The adverse reactions most commonly leading to discontinuation of BANZEL (>1%) used as adjunctive therapy were generally similar in adults and children.

In pediatric double-blind adjunctive clinical studies, 8.0% of patients receiving BANZEL as adjunctive therapy and 2.2% receiving placebo discontinued as a result of an adverse reaction. The adverse reactions most commonly leading to discontinuation of BANZEL (>1%) used as adjunctive therapy are presented in Table 6.

Table 6: Adverse Reactions Most Commonly Leading to Discontinuation in Double-Blind Adjunctive Trials (At The Recommended Dose of 45mg/kg/day) in Pediatric Patients

Preferred Term	BANZEL (N=187) %	Placebo (N=182) %
Convulsion	2	1
Rash	2	1
Fatigue	2	0
Vomiting	1	0

In adult double-blind adjunctive clinical studies (up to 3200 mg/day), 9.5% of patients receiving BANZEL as adjunctive therapy and 5.9% receiving placebo discontinued as a result of an adverse reaction. The adverse reactions most commonly leading to discontinuation of BANZEL (>1%) used as adjunctive therapy are presented in Table 7.

Table 7: Adverse Reactions Most Commonly Leading to Discontinuation in Double-Blind Adjunctive Trials (up to 3200 mg/day) in Adult Patients

Preferred Term	BANZEL (N=823) %	Placebo (N=376) %
Dizziness	3	1
Fatigue	2	1
Headache	2	1
Nausea	1	0
Ataxia	1	0

Other Adverse Events Observed During Clinical Trials:

BANZEL has been administered to 1978 individuals during all epilepsy clinical trials (placebo-controlled and open-label). Adverse events occurring during these studies were recorded by the investigators using terminology of their own choosing. To provide a meaningful estimate of the proportion of patients having adverse events, these events were grouped into standardized categories using the MedDRA dictionary. Adverse events occurring at least three times and considered possibly related to treatment are included in the System Organ Class listings below. Terms not included in the listings are those already included in the tables above, those too general to be informative, those related to procedures and terms describing events common in the population. Some events occurring fewer than 3 times are also included based on their medical significance. Because the reports include events observed in open-label, uncontrolled observations, the role of BANZEL in their causation cannot be reliably determined.

Events are classified by body system and listed in order of decreasing frequency as follows: *frequent adverse events*-those occurring in at least 1/100 patients; *infrequent adverse events*- those occurring in 1/100 to 1/1000 patients; *rare*- those occurring in fewer than 1/1000 patients.

Blood and Lymphatic System Disorders: *Frequent:* anemia. *Infrequent:* lymphadenopathy, leukopenia, neutropenia, iron deficiency anemia, thrombocytopenia.

Cardiac Disorders: *Infrequent:* bundle branch block right, atrioventricular block first degree.

Metabolic and Nutritional Disorders: *Frequent:* decreased appetite, increased appetite.

Renal and Urinary Disorders: *Frequent:* pollakiuria. *Infrequent:* urinary incontinence, dysuria, hematuria, nephrolithiasis, polyuria, enuresis, nocturia, incontinence.

DRUG ABUSE AND DEPENDENCE

The abuse and dependence potential of BANZEL has not been evaluated in human studies.

OVERDOSAGE

Because strategies for the management of overdose are continually evolving, it is advisable to contact a Certified Poison Control Center to determine the latest recommendations for the management of an overdose of any drug.

One overdose of 7200 mg/day BANZEL was reported in an adult during the clinical trials. The overdose was associated with no major signs or symptoms, no medical intervention was required, and the patient continued in the study at the target dose.

Treatment or Management of Overdose: There is no specific antidote for overdose with BANZEL. If clinically indicated, elimination of unabsorbed drug should be attempted by induction of emesis or gastric lavage. Usual precautions should be observed to maintain the airway. General supportive care of the patient is indicated including monitoring of vital signs and observation of the clinical status of the patient.

Hemodialysis: Standard hemodialysis procedures may result in limited clearance of rufinamide. Although there is no experience to date in treating overdose with hemodialysis, the procedure may be considered when indicated by the patient's clinical state.

DOSAGE AND ADMINISTRATION

Children four years and older with Lennox-Gastaut syndrome: Treatment should be initiated at a daily dose of approximately 10 mg/kg/day administered in two equally divided doses. The dose should be increased by approximately 10 mg/kg increments every other day to a target dose of 45 mg/kg/day or 3200 mg/day, whichever is less, administered in two equally divided doses. It is not known whether doses lower than the target doses are effective.

Adults with Lennox-Gastaut syndrome: Treatment should be initiated at a daily dose of 400–800 mg/day administered in two equally divided doses. The dose should be increased by 400–800 mg/day every 2 days until a maximum daily dose of 3200 mg/day, administered in two equally divided doses is reached. It is not known whether doses lower than 3200 mg are effective.

BANZEL tablets are scored on both sides and can be cut in half for dosing flexibility. Tablets can be administered whole, as half tablets or crushed.

BANZEL should be given with food.

Patients with Renal Impairment

Renally impaired patients (creatinine clearance less than 30 mL/min) do not require any special dosage change when taking BANZEL.

Patients Undergoing Hemodialysis

Hemodialysis may reduce exposure to a limited (about 30%) extent. Accordingly, adjusting the BANZEL dose during the dialysis process can be considered.

Patients with Hepatic Disease

Use of BANZEL in patients with hepatic impairment has not been studied. Therefore, use in patients with severe hepatic impairment is not recommended. Caution should be exercised in treating patients with mild to moderate hepatic impairment.

HOW SUPPLIED

BANZEL 200 mg tablets (containing 200 mg rufinamide) are pink in color, film-coated, oblong-shape tablets, with a score on both sides, imprinted with "Є 262" on one side. They are available in bottles of 30 (NDC 62856-582-30).

BANZEL 400 mg tablets (containing 400 mg rufinamide) are pink in color, film-coated, oblong-shape tablets, with a score on both sides, imprinted with "Є 263" on one side. They are available in bottles of 120 (NDC 62856-583-52).

Store at 25°C (77°F); excursions permitted to 15°–30°C (59°F–86°F). Protect from moisture. Replace cap securely after opening.

Rx Only

BANZEL™ is a trademark of Novartis Pharma AG, used under license.

Manufactured by Eisai Co., Ltd.

Marketed by Eisai Inc., Woodcliff Lake, NJ 07677

© 2008 Eisai Inc. Printed in U.S.A.

Revised November 2008

Medication Guide

BANZEL™ (ban-'zel)

[rufinamide]

BANZEL and Suicidal Thoughts or Actions

Read this Medication Guide before you start taking BANZEL and each time you get a refill. There may be new information. This information does not take the place of talking to your healthcare provider about your medical condition or treatment. This Medication Guide is only about the risk of suicidal thoughts and actions with BANZEL.

What is the most important information I should know about BANZEL?

1. **BANZEL may cause suicidal thoughts or actions in a very small number of people, about 1 in 500.**

2. **Call a healthcare provider right away if you have any of these symptoms, especially if they are new, worse, or worry you:**
   - thoughts about suicide or dying
   - attempt to commit suicide
   - new or worse depression
   - new or worse anxiety
   - feeling agitated or restless
   - panic attacks
   - trouble sleeping (insomnia)
   - new or worse irritability
   - acting aggressive, being angry, or violent
   - acting on dangerous impulses
   - an extreme increase in activity and talking (mania)
   - other unusual changes in behavior or mood

3. **Do not stop BANZEL without first talking to a healthcare provider.**
   - Stopping BANZEL suddenly can cause serious problems.
   - Suicidal thoughts or actions can be caused by things other than medicines. If you have suicidal thoughts or actions, your healthcare provider may check for other causes.

4. **How can I watch for early symptoms of suicidal thoughts and actions?**
   - Pay attention to any changes, especially sudden changes, in mood, behaviors, thoughts, or feelings.
   - Keep all follow-up visits with your healthcare provider as scheduled.
   - Call your healthcare provider between visits as needed, especially if you are worried about symptoms.

What else should I know about BANZEL?

- BANZEL has other side effects. For more information ask your healthcare provider or pharmacist. Tell your healthcare provider if you have any side effect that bothers you. **Call your doctor for medical advice about side effects. You may report side effects to FDA at 1-800-FDA-1088.**
- BANZEL can interact with other medicines. Tell your healthcare provider about all the medicines you take, in-

cluding prescription and non-prescription medicines, vitamins, and herbal supplements. Using BANZEL with certain other medicines can affect each other causing side effects.

Know the medicines you take. Keep a list of them and show it to your healthcare provider and pharmacist each time you get a new medicine. Do not start a new medicine without first talking with your healthcare provider.

Medicines are sometimes prescribed for purposes other than those listed in a Medication Guide. Do not use BANZEL for a condition for which it was not prescribed. Do not give BANZEL to other people, even if they have the same symptoms that you have. It may harm them.

This Medication Guide summarizes the most important information about BANZEL. If you would like more information, talk with your doctor. You can ask your pharmacist or doctor for information about BANZEL that is written for health professionals.

For more information, go to www.banzel.com or call 1-888-274-2378.

Issued November 2008

This Medication Guide has been approved by the U.S. Food and Drug Administration.

BANZEL™ is a trademark of Novartis Pharma AG, used under license.

Manufactured by Eisai Co., Ltd.
Marketed by Eisai Inc.
Woodcliff Lake, NJ 07677

© 2008 Eisai Inc. Printed in U.S.A.
Shown in Product Identification Guide, page 308

DACOGEN®
[dăk-ō-jĕn]
(decitabine)
for INJECTION

℞

HIGHLIGHTS OF PRESCRIBING INFORMATION
These highlights do not include all the information needed to use Dacogen safely and effectively. See full prescribing information for Dacogen.
DACOGEN® (decitabine) for INJECTION
Initial U.S. Approval: 2006

——————RECENT MAJOR CHANGES——————
Dosage and Administration (2.2)   03/2010

——————INDICATIONS AND USAGE——————
Dacogen is a nucleoside metabolic inhibitor indicated for treatment of patients with myelodysplastic syndromes (MDS) including previously treated and untreated, *de novo* and secondary MDS of all French-American-British subtypes (refractory anemia, refractory anemia with ringed sideroblasts, refractory anemia with excess blasts, refractory anemia with excess blasts in transformation, and chronic myelomonocytic leukemia) and intermediate-1, intermediate-2, and high-risk International Prognostic Scoring System groups. (1)

——————DOSAGE AND ADMINISTRATION——————
There are two regimens for Dacogen administration. With either regimen it is recommended that patients be treated for a minimum of 4 cycles; however, a complete or partial response may take longer than 4 cycles. (2)
• Treatment Regimen - Option 1
Administer Dacogen at a dose of 15 mg/m² by continuous intravenous infusion over 3 hours repeated every 8 hours for 3 days. Repeat cycle every 6 weeks. (2.1)
• Treatment Regimen - Option 2
Administer Dacogen at a dose of 20 mg/m² by continuous intravenous infusion over 1 hour repeated daily for 5 days. Repeat cycle every 4 weeks. (2.2)

——————DOSAGE FORMS AND STRENGTHS——————
Lyophilized powder in a single-dose vial, 50 mg/vial. (3)

——————CONTRAINDICATIONS——————
None

——————WARNINGS AND PRECAUTIONS——————
• Neutropenia and thrombocytopenia: Perform complete blood counts and platelet counts. (5.1)
• Pregnancy: Can cause fetal harm. Advise women of potential risk to the fetus (5.2, 8.1)
• Women of childbearing potential and men with female partners of childbearing potential should use effective contraception and avoid pregnancy (5.3, 5.4)

——————ADVERSE REACTIONS——————
Most common adverse reactions (> 50%) are neutropenia, thrombocytopenia, anemia, and pyrexia. (6.1)

To report SUSPECTED ADVERSE REACTIONS, contact Eisai, Inc. at 1-888-274-2378 or FDA at 1-800-FDA-1088 or www.fda.gov/medwatch.

See 17 for PATIENT COUNSELING INFORMATION
Revised: 03/2010

Table 1 Adverse Events Reported in ≥ 5% of Patients in the Dacogen Group and at a Rate Greater than Supportive Care in Phase 3 MDS Trial

	Dacogen N = 83 (%)	Supportive Care N = 81 (%)
Blood and lymphatic system disorders		
Neutropenia	75 (90)	58 (72)
Thrombocytopenia	74 (89)	64 (79)
Anemia NOS	68 (82)	60 (74)
Febrile neutropenia	24 (29)	5 (6)
Leukopenia NOS	23 (28)	11 (14)
Lymphadenopathy	10 (12)	6 (7)
Thrombocythemia	4 (5)	1 (1)
Cardiac disorders		
Pulmonary edema NOS	5 (6)	0 (0)
Eye disorders		
Vision blurred	5 (6)	0 (0)
Gastrointestinal disorders		
Nausea	35 (42)	13 (16)
Constipation	29 (35)	11 (14)
Diarrhea NOS	28 (34)	13 (16)
Vomiting NOS	21 (25)	7 (9)
Abdominal pain NOS	12 (14)	5 (6)
Oral mucosal petechiae	11 (13)	4 (5)
Stomatitis	10 (12)	5 (6)
Dyspepsia	10 (12)	1 (1)
Ascites	8 (10)	2 (2)
Gingival bleeding	7 (8)	5 (6)
Hemorrhoids	7 (8)	3 (4)
Loose stools	6 (7)	3 (4)
Tongue ulceration	6 (7)	2 (2)
Dysphagia	5 (6)	2 (2)
Oral soft tissue disorder NOS	5 (6)	1 (1)
Lip ulceration	4 (5)	3 (4)
Abdominal distension	4 (5)	1 (1)
Abdominal pain upper	4 (5)	1 (1)
Gastro-esophageal reflux disease	4 (5)	0 (0)
Glossodynia	4 (5)	0 (0)
General disorders and administrative site disorders		
Pyrexia	44 (53)	23 (28)
Edema peripheral	21 (25)	13 (16)
Rigors	18 (22)	14 (17)
Edema NOS	15 (18)	5 (6)
Pain NOS	11 (13)	5 (6)
Lethargy	10 (12)	3 (4)
Tenderness NOS	9 (11)	0 (0)
Fall	7 (8)	3 (4)
Chest discomfort	6 (7)	3 (4)
Intermittent pyrexia	5 (6)	3 (4)
Malaise	4 (5)	1 (1)

(Table continued on next page)

FULL PRESCRIBING INFORMATION

1   INDICATIONS AND USAGE

Dacogen is indicated for treatment of patients with myelodysplastic syndromes (MDS) including previously treated and untreated, *de novo* and secondary MDS of all French-American-British subtypes (refractory anemia, refractory anemia with ringed sideroblasts, refractory anemia with excess blasts, refractory anemia with excess blasts in transformation, and chronic myelomonocytic leukemia) and intermediate-1, intermediate-2, and high-risk International Prognostic Scoring System groups.

2   DOSAGE AND ADMINISTRATION

There are two regimens for Dacogen administration. With either regimen it is recommended that patients be treated for a minimum of 4 cycles; however, a complete or partial response may take longer than 4 cycles.

Complete blood counts and platelet counts should be performed as needed to monitor response and toxicity, but at a minimum, prior to each cycle. Liver chemistries and serum creatinine should be obtained prior to initiation of treatment.

2.1   Treatment Regimen - Option 1

Dacogen is administered at a dose of 15 mg/m^2 by continuous intravenous infusion over 3 hours repeated every 8 hours for 3 days. This cycle should be repeated every 6 weeks. Patients may be premedicated with standard antiemetic therapy.

If hematologic recovery (ANC $\geq$ 1,000/μL and platelets $\geq$ 50,000/μL) from a previous Dacogen treatment cycle requires more than 6 weeks, then the next cycle of Dacogen therapy should be delayed and dosing temporarily reduced by following this algorithm:

- Recovery requiring more than 6, but less than 8 weeks - Dacogen dosing to be delayed for up to 2 weeks and the dose temporarily reduced to 11 mg/m^2 every 8 hours (33 mg/m^2/day, 99 mg/m^2/cycle) upon restarting therapy.
- Recovery requiring more than 8, but less than 10 weeks - Patient should be assessed for disease progression (by bone marrow aspirates); in the absence of progression, the Dacogen dose should be delayed up to 2 more weeks and the dose reduced to 11 mg/m^2 every 8 hours (33 mg/m^2/day, 99 mg/m^2/cycle) upon restarting therapy, then maintained or increased in subsequent cycles as clinically indicated.

Table 1 *(cont.)* Adverse Events Reported in $\geq$ 5% of Patients in the Dacogen Group and at a Rate Greater than Supportive Care in Phase 3 MDS Trial

	Dacogen N = 83 (%)	Supportive Care N = 81 (%)
Crepitations NOS	4 (5)	1 (1)
Catheter site erythema	4 (5)	1 (1)
Catheter site pain	4 (5)	0 (0)
Injection site swelling	4 (5)	0 (0)
Hepatobiliary Disorders		
Hyperbilirubinemia	12 (14)	4 (5)
Infections and Infestations		
Pneumonia NOS	18 (22)	11 (14)
Cellulitis	10 (12)	6 (7)
Candidal infection NOS	8 (10)	1 (1)
Catheter related infection	7 (8)	0 (0)
Urinary tract infection NOS	6 (7)	1 (1)
Staphylococcal infection	6 (7)	0 (0)
Oral candidiasis	5 (6)	2 (2)
Sinusitis NOS	4 (5)	2 (2)
Bacteremia	4 (5)	0 (0)
Injury, poisoning and procedural complications		
Transfusion reaction	6 (7)	3 (4)
Abrasion NOS	4 (5)	1 (1)
Investigations		
Cardiac murmur NOS	13 (16)	9 (11)
Blood alkaline phosphatase NOS increased	9 (11)	7 (9)
Aspartate aminotransferase increased	8 (10)	7 (9)
Blood urea increased	8 (10)	1 (1)
Blood lactate dehydrogenase increased	7 (8)	5 (6)
Blood albumin decreased	6 (7)	0 (0)
Blood bicarbonate increased	5 (6)	1 (1)
Blood chloride decreased	5 (6)	1 (1)
Protein total decreased	4 (5)	3 (4)
Blood bicarbonate decreased	4 (5)	1 (1)
Blood bilirubin decreased	4 (5)	1 (1)
Metabolism and nutrition disorders		
Hyperglycemia NOS	27 (33)	16 (20)
Hypoalbuminemia	20 (24)	14 (17)
Hypomagnesemia	20 (24)	6 (7)
Hypokalemia	18 (22)	10 (12)
Hyponatremia	16 (19)	13 (16)
Appetite decreased NOS	13 (16)	12 (15)
Anorexia	13 (16)	8 (10)
Hyperkalemia	11 (13)	3 (4)
Dehydration	5 (6)	4 (5)
Musculoskeletal and connective tissue disorders		
Arthralgia	17 (20)	8 (10)
Pain in limb	16 (19)	8 (10)
Back pain	14 (17)	5 (6)

(Table continued on next page)

Table 1 *(cont.)* Adverse Events Reported in ≥ 5% of Patients in the Dacogen Group and at a Rate Greater than Supportive Care in Phase 3 MDS Trial

	Dacogen N = 83 (%)	Supportive Care N = 81 (%)
Chest wall pain	6 (7)	1 (1)
Musculoskeletal discomfort	5 (6)	0 (0)
Myalgia	4 (5)	1 (1)
Nervous system disorders		
Headache	23 (28)	11 (14)
Dizziness	15 (18)	10 (12)
Hypoesthesia	9 (11)	1 (1)
Psychiatric disorders		
Insomnia	23 (28)	11 (14)
Confusional state	10 (12)	3 (4)
Anxiety	9 (11)	8 (10)
Renal and urinary disorders		
Dysuria	5 (6)	3 (4)
Urinary frequency	4 (5)	1 (1)
Respiratory, thoracic and Mediastinal disorders		
Cough	33 (40)	25 (31)
Pharyngitis	13 (16)	6 (7)
Crackles lung	12 (14)	1 (1)
Breath sounds decreased	8 (10)	7 (9)
Hypoxia	8 (10)	4 (5)
Rales	7 (8)	2 (2)
Postnasal drip	4 (5)	2 (2)
Skin and subcutaneous tissue disorders		
Ecchymosis	18 (22)	12 (15)
Rash NOS	16 (19)	7 (9)
Erythema	12 (14)	5 (6)
Skin lesion NOS	9 (11)	3 (4)
Pruritus	9 (11)	2 (2)
Alopecia	7 (8)	1 (1)
Urticaria NOS	5 (6)	1 (1)
Swelling face	5 (6)	0 (0)
Vascular disorders		
Petechiae	32 (39)	13 (16)
Pallor	19 (23)	10 (12)
Hypotension NOS	5 (6)	4 (5)
Hematoma NOS	4 (5)	3 (4)

2.2 Treatment Regimen - Option 2

Dacogen is administered at a dose of 20 mg/m² by continuous intravenous infusion over 1 hour repeated daily for 5 days. This cycle should be repeated every 4 weeks. Patients may be premedicated with standard anti-emetic therapy. If myelosuppression is present, subsequent treatment cycles of Dacogen should be delayed until there is hematologic recovery (ANC ≥ 1,000/µL platelets ≥ 50,000/µL).

2.3 Patients with Non-hematologic Toxicity

Following the first cycle of Dacogen treatment, if any of the following non-hematologic toxicities are present, Dacogen treatment should not be restarted until the toxicity is resolved: 1) serum creatinine ≥ 2 mg/dL; 2) SGPT, total bilirubin ≥ 2 times ULN; 3) and active or uncontrolled infection.

2.4 Instructions for Intravenous Administration

Dacogen is a cytotoxic drug and caution should be exercised when handling and preparing Dacogen. Procedures for proper handling and disposal of antineoplastic drugs should be applied. Several guidances on this subject have been published.[1][4].

Dacogen should be aseptically reconstituted with 10 mL of Sterile Water for Injection (USP); upon reconstitution, each mL contains approximately 5.0 mg of decitabine at pH 6.7-7.3. Immediately after reconstitution, the solution should be further diluted with 0.9% Sodium Chloride Injection, 5% Dextrose Injection, or Lactated Ringer's Injection to a final drug concentration of 0.1-1.0 mg/mL. Unless used within 15 minutes of reconstitution, the diluted solution must be prepared using cold (2°C-8°C) infusion fluids and

stored at 2°C-8°C (36°F-46°F) for up to a maximum of 7 hours until administration.

Parenteral drug products should be inspected visually for particulate matter and discoloration prior to administration, whenever solution and container permit. Do not use if there is evidence of particulate matter or discoloration.

3 DOSAGE FORMS AND STRENGTHS

Dacogen (decitabine) for Injection is supplied as a sterile, lyophilized white to almost white powder, in a single-dose vial, packaged in cartons of 1 vial. Each vial contains 50 mg of decitabine.

4 CONTRAINDICATIONS

None

5 WARNINGS AND PRECAUTIONS

5.1 Neutropenia and Thrombocytopenia

Treatment with Dacogen is associated with neutropenia and thrombocytopenia. Complete blood and platelet counts should be performed as needed to monitor response and toxicity, but at a minimum, prior to each dosing cycle. After administration of the recommended dosage for the first cycle, treatment for subsequent cycles should be adjusted [see *Dosage and Administration* (2.1, 2.2)]. Clinicians should consider the need for early institution of growth factors and/or antimicrobial agents for the prevention or treatment of infections in patients with MDS. Myelosuppression and worsening neutropenia may occur more frequently in the first or second treatment cycles, and may not necessarily indicate progression of underlying MDS.

5.2 Use in Pregnancy

Dacogen can cause fetal harm when administered to a pregnant woman. Based on its mechanism of action, Dacogen is expected to result in adverse reproductive effects. In preclinical studies in mice and rats, decitabine was teratogenic, fetotoxic, and embryotoxic. There are no adequate and well-controlled studies of Dacogen in pregnant women. If this drug is used during pregnancy, or if a patient becomes pregnant while receiving this drug, the patient should be apprised of the potential hazard to the fetus. Women of childbearing potential should be advised to avoid becoming pregnant while taking Dacogen [see *Use in Specific Populations* (8.1)]

5.3 Use in Women of Childbearing Potential

Women of childbearing potential should be advised to avoid becoming pregnant while receiving Dacogen and for 1 month following completion of treatment. Women of childbearing potential should be counseled to use effective contraception during this time [see *Use in Specific Populations* (8.1)]. Based on its mechanism of action, Dacogen can cause fetal harm if used during pregnancy.

5.4 Use in Men

Men should be advised not to father a child while receiving treatment with Dacogen, and for 2 months following completion of treatment [see *Nonclinical Toxicology* (13.1)]. Men with female partners of childbearing potential should use effective contraception during this time. Based on its mechanism of action, Dacogen alters DNA synthesis and can cause fetal harm.

6 ADVERSE REACTIONS

6.1 Clinical Studies Experience

Because clinical trials are conducted under widely varying conditions, adverse reaction rates observed in the clinical trials of a drug cannot be directly compared to rates in the clinical trials of another drug and may not reflect the rates observed in practice.

Most Commonly Occurring Adverse Reactions: neutropenia, thrombocytopenia, anemia, fatigue, pyrexia, nausea, cough, petechiae, constipation, diarrhea, and hyperglycemia.

Adverse Reactions Most Frequently (≥ 1%) Resulting in Clinical Intervention in the Phase 3 Trial in the Dacogen Arm:

- Discontinuation: thrombocytopenia, neutropenia, pneumonia, Mycobacterium avium complex infection, cardiorespiratory arrest, increased blood bilirubin, intracranial hemorrhage, abnormal liver function tests.
- Dose Delayed: neutropenia, pulmonary edema, atrial fibrillation, central line infection, febrile neutropenia.
- Dose Reduced: neutropenia, thrombocytopenia, anemia, lethargy, edema, tachycardia, depression, pharyngitis.

Discussion of Adverse Reactions Information

Dacogen was studied in 3 single-arm studies (N = 66, N = 98, N = 99) and 1 controlled supportive care study (N = 83 Dacogen, N = 81 supportive care). The data described below reflect exposure to Dacogen in 83 patients in the MDS trial. In the trial, patients received 15 mg/m² intravenously every 8 hours for 3 days every 6 weeks. The median number of Dacogen cycles was 3 (range 0 to 9).

Table 1 presents all adverse events regardless of causality occurring in at least 5% of patients in the Dacogen group and at a rate greater than supportive care.

[See table 1 on pages 1015, 1016 and above]

Discussion of Clinically Important Adverse Reactions

In the controlled trial using Dacogen dosed at 15 mg/m^2, administered by continuous intravenous infusion over 3 hours repeated every 8 hours for 3 days, the highest incidence of Grade 3 or Grade 4 adverse events in the Dacogen arm were neutropenia (87%), thrombocytopenia (85%), febrile neutropenia (23%) and leukopenia (22%). Bone marrow suppression was the most frequent cause of dose reduction, delay and discontinuation. Six patients had fatal events associated with their underlying disease and myelosuppression (anemia, neutropenia, and thrombocytopenia) that were considered at least possibly related to drug treatment [See *Warnings and Precautions* (5.1)]. Of the 83 Dacogen-treated patients, 8 permanently discontinued therapy for adverse events; compared to 1 of 81 patients in the supportive care arm.

In a single-arm study (N=99) Dacogen was dosed at 20 mg/m^2 intravenous, infused over one hour daily for 5 consecutive days of a 4 week cycle. Table 2 presents all adverse events regardless of causality occurring in at least 5% of patients.

Table 2 Adverse Events Reported in ≥ 5% of Patients in a Single-arm Study*

	Dacogen N = 99 (%)
Blood and lymphatic system disorders	
Anemia	31 (31%)
Febrile neutropenia	20 (20%)
Leukopenia	6 (6%)
Neutropenia	38 (38%)
Pancytopenia	5 (5%)
Thrombocythemia	5 (5%)
Thrombocytopenia	27 (27%)
Cardiac disorders	
Cardiac failure congestive	5 (5%)
Tachycardia	8 (8%)
Ear and labyrinth disorders	
Ear pain	6 (6%)
Gastrointestinal disorders	
Abdominal pain	14 (14%)
Abdominal pain upper	6 (6%)
Constipation	30 (30%)
Diarrhea	28 (28%)
Dyspepsia	10 (10%)
Dysphagia	5 (5%)
Gastro-esophageal reflux disease	5 (5%)
Nausea	40 (40%)
Oral pain	5 (5%)
Stomatitis	11 (11%)
Toothache	6 (6%)
Vomiting	16 (16%)
General disorders and administration site conditions	
Asthenia	15 (15%)
Chest pain	6 (6%)
Chills	16 (16%)
Fatigue	46 (46%)
Mucosal inflammation	9 (9%)
Edema	5 (5%)
Edema peripheral	27 (27%)
Pain	5 (5%)
Pyrexia	36 (36%)
Infections and infestations	
Cellulitis	9 (9%)
Oral candidiasis	6 (6%)
Pneumonia	20 (20%)
Sinusitis	6 (6%)
Staphylococcal bacteremia	8 (8%)
Tooth abscess	5 (5%)
Upper respiratory tract infection	10 (10%)
Urinary tract infection	7 (7%)
Injury, poisoning and procedural complications	
Contusion	9 (9%)
Investigations	
Blood bilirubin increased	6 (6%)
Breath sounds abnormal	5 (5%)
Weight decreased	9 (9%)
Metabolism and nutrition disorders	
Anorexia	23 (23%)
Decreased appetite	8 (8%)
Dehydration	8 (8%)
Hyperglycemia	6 (6%)
Hypokalemia	12 (12%)
Hypomagnesemia	5 (5%)
Musculoskeletal and connective tissue disorders	
Arthralgia	17 (17%)
Back pain	18 (18%)
Bone pain	6 (6%)
Muscle spasms	7 (7%)
Muscular weakness	5 (5%)
Musculoskeletal pain	5 (5%)
Myalgia	9 (9%)
Pain in extremity	18 (18%)
Nervous system disorders	
Dizziness	21 (21%)
Headache	23 (23%)
Psychiatric disorders	
Anxiety	9 (9%)
Confusional state	8 (8%)
Depression	9 (9%)
Insomnia	14 (14%)
Respiratory, thoracic and mediastinal disorders	
Cough	27 (27%)
Dyspnea	29 (29%)
Epistaxis	13 (13%)
Pharyngolaryngeal pain	8 (8%)
Pleural effusion	5 (5%)
Sinus congestion	5 (5%)
Skin and subcutaneous tissue disorders	
Dry skin	8 (8%)
Ecchymosis	9 (9%)
Erythema	5 (5%)
Night sweats	5 (5%)
Petechiae	12 (12%)
Pruritus	9 (9%)
Rash	11 (11%)
Skin lesion	5 (5%)
Vascular disorders	
Hypertension	6 (6%)
Hypotension	11 (11%)

* In this single arm study, investigators reported adverse events based on clinical signs and symptoms rather than predefined laboratory abnormalities. Thus not all laboratory abnormalities were recorded as adverse events.

Discussion of Clinically Important Adverse Reactions

In the single-arm study (N=99) when Dacogen was dosed at 20 mg/m^2 intravenous, infused over one hour daily for 5 consecutive days, the highest incidence of Grade 3 or Grade 4 adverse events were neutropenia (37%), thrombocytopenia (24%) and anemia (22%). Seventy-eight percent of patients had dose delays, the median duration of this delay was 7 days and the largest percentage of delays were due to hematologic toxicities. Hematologic toxicities and infections were the most frequent causes of dose delays and discontinuation. Eight patients had fatal events due to infection and/or bleeding (seven of which occurred in the clinical setting of myelosuppression) that were considered at least possibly related to drug treatment. Nineteen of 99 patients permanently discontinued therapy for adverse events.

No overall difference in safety was detected between patients > 65 years of age and younger patients in these myelodysplasia trials. No significant gender differences in safety or efficacy were detected. Patients with renal or hepatic dysfunction were not studied. Insufficient numbers of non-white patients were available to draw conclusions in these clinical trials.

Serious Adverse Events that occurred in patients receiving Dacogen regardless of causality, not previously reported in **Tables 1 and 2** include:

• Blood and Lymphatic System Disorders: myelosuppression, splenomegaly.
• Cardiac Disorders: myocardial infarction, cardio-respiratory arrest, cardiomyopathy, atrial fibrillation, supraventricular tachycardia.
• Gastrointestinal Disorders: gingival pain, upper gastrointestinal hemorrhage.
• General Disorders and Administrative Site Conditions: chest pain, catheter site hemorrhage.
• Hepatobiliary Disorders: cholecystitis.
• Infections and Infestations: fungal infection, sepsis, bronchopulmonary aspergillosis, peridiverticular abscess, respiratory tract infection, pseudomonal lung infection, Mycobacterium avium complex infection.
• Injury, Poisoning and Procedural Complications: post procedural pain, post procedural hemorrhage.
• Nervous System Disorders: intracranial hemorrhage.
• Psychiatric Disorders: mental status changes.
• Renal and Urinary Disorders: renal failure, urethral hemorrhage.
• Respiratory, Thoracic and Mediastinal Disorders: hemoptysis, lung infiltration, pulmonary embolism, respiratory arrest, pulmonary mass.
• Allergic Reaction: Hypersensitivity (anaphylactic reaction) to Dacogen has been reported in a Phase 2 trial.

6.2   Post-marketing Experience

The following adverse reactions have been identified during post-approval use of Dacogen. Because these reactions are reported voluntarily from a population of uncertain size, it is not always possible to reliably estimate their frequency or establish a causal relationship to drug exposure.

Cases of Sweet's Syndrome (acute febrile neutrophilic dermatosis) have been reported.

7   DRUG INTERACTIONS

Drug interaction studies with decitabine have not been conducted. *In vitro* studies in human liver microsomes suggest that decitabine is unlikely to inhibit or induce cytochrome P450 enzymes. *In vitro* metabolism studies have suggested that decitabine is not a substrate for human liver cytochrome P450 enzymes. As plasma protein binding of

Table 3 Mean (CV% or 95% CI) Pharmacokinetic Parameters of Decitabine

Dose	C_{max} (ng/mL)	$AUC_{0-\infty}$ (ng·h/mL)	$T_{1/2}$(h)	CL (L/h/m²)	$AUC_{Cumulative}$*** (ng·h/mL)
15 mg/m² 3-hr infusion every 8 hours for 3 days (Option 1)*	73.8 (66)	163 (62)	0.62 (49)	125 (53)	1332 (1010-1730)
20 mg/m² 1-hr infusion daily for 5 days (Option 2)**	147 (49)	115 (43)	0.54 (43)	210 (47)	570 (470-700)

* N=14,
** N=11,
*** N=35 Cumulative AUC per cycle

decitabine is negligible (<1%), interactions due to displacement of more highly protein bound drugs from plasma proteins are not expected.

8 USE IN SPECIFIC POPULATIONS

8.1 Pregnancy

Pregnancy Category D [see *Warnings and Precautions* (5.2)] Dacogen can cause fetal harm when administered to a pregnant woman. There are no adequate and well-controlled studies of Dacogen in pregnant women.

The developmental toxicity of decitabine was examined in mice exposed to single IP (intraperitoneal) injections (0, 0.9 and 3.0 mg/m², approximately 2% and 7% of the recommended daily clinical dose, respectively) over gestation days 8, 9, 10 or 11. No maternal toxicity was observed but reduced fetal survival was observed after treatment at 3 mg/m² and decreased fetal weight was observed at both dose levels. The 3 mg/m² dose elicited characteristic fetal defects for each treatment day, including supernumerary ribs (both dose levels), fused vertebrae and ribs, cleft palate, vertebral defects, hind-limb defects and digital defects of fore- and hind-limbs. In rats given a single IP injection of 2.4, 3.6 or 6 mg/m² (approximately 5, 8, or 13% the daily recommended clinical dose, respectively) on gestation days 9-12, no maternal toxicity was observed. No live fetuses were seen at any dose when decitabine was injected on gestation day 9. A significant decrease in fetal survival and reduced fetal weight at doses greater than 3.6 mg/m² was seen when decitabine was given on gestation day 10. Increased incidences of vertebral and rib anomalies were seen at all dose levels, and induction of exophthalmia, exencephaly, and cleft palate were observed at 6.0 mg/m². Increased incidence of foredigit defects was seen in fetuses at doses greater than 3.6 mg/m². Reduced size and ossification of long bones of the fore-limb and hind-limb were noted at 6.0 mg/m². If this drug is used during pregnancy, or if the patient becomes pregnant while taking this drug, the patient should be apprised of the potential hazard to the fetus. Women of child bearing potential should be advised to avoid becoming pregnant while taking Dacogen.

8.3 Nursing Mothers

It is not known whether decitabine or its metabolites are excreted in human milk. Because many drugs are excreted in human milk, and because of the potential for serious adverse reactions from Dacogen in nursing infants, a decision should be made whether to discontinue nursing or to discontinue the drug, taking into account the importance of the drug to the mother.

8.4 Pediatric Use

The safety and effectiveness of Dacogen in pediatric patients have not been established.

8.5 Geriatric Use

Of the total number of patients exposed to Dacogen in the controlled clinical trial, 61 of 83 patients were age 65 and over, while 21 of 83 patients were age 75 and over. No overall differences in safety or effectiveness were observed between these subjects and younger subjects, and other reported clinical experience has not identified differences in responses between the elderly and younger patients, but greater sensitivity of some older individuals cannot be ruled out.

8.6 Renal Impairment

There are no data on the use of Dacogen in patients with renal dysfunction; therefore, Dacogen should be used with caution in these patients.

8.7 Hepatic Impairment

There are no data on the use of Dacogen in patients with hepatic dysfunction; therefore, Dacogen should be used with caution in these patients.

10 OVERDOSAGE

There is no known antidote for overdosage with Dacogen. Higher doses are associated with increased myelosuppression including prolonged neutropenia and thrombocytopenia. Standard supportive measures should be taken in the event of an overdose.

11 DESCRIPTION

Dacogen (decitabine) for Injection contains decitabine (5-aza-2′-deoxycitidine), an analogue of the natural nucleoside 2′-deoxycytidine. Decitabine is a fine, white to almost white powder with the molecular formula of $C_8H_{12}N_4O_4$ and a molecular weight of 228.21. Its chemical name is 4-amino-1-(2-deoxy-β-D-erythro-pentofuranosyl)-1,3,5-triazin-2(1H)-one and it has the following structural formula:

Decitabine is slightly soluble in ethanol/water (50/50), methanol/water (50/50) and methanol; sparingly soluble in water and soluble in dimethylsulfoxide (DMSO).
Dacogen (decitabine) for Injection is a white to almost white sterile lyophilized powder supplied in a clear colorless glass vial. Each 20 mL, single dose, glass vial contains 50 mg decitabine, 68 mg monobasic potassium phosphate (potassium dihydrogen phosphate) and 11.6 mg sodium hydroxide.

12 CLINICAL PHARMACOLOGY

12.1 Mechanism of Action

Decitabine is believed to exert its antineoplastic effects after phosphorylation and direct incorporation into DNA and inhibition of DNA methyltransferase, causing hypomethylation of DNA and cellular differentiation or apoptosis. Decitabine inhibits DNA methylation *in vitro*, which is achieved at concentrations that do not cause major suppression of DNA synthesis. Decitabine-induced hypomethylation in neoplastic cells may restore normal function to genes that are critical for the control of cellular differentiation and proliferation. In rapidly dividing cells, the cytotoxicity of decitabine may also be attributed to the formation of covalent adducts between DNA methyltransferase and decitabine incorporated into DNA. Non-proliferating cells are relatively insensitive to decitabine.

12.2 Pharmacodynamics

Decitabine has been shown to induce hypomethylation both *in vitro* and *in vivo*. However, there have been no studies of decitabine-induced hypomethylation and pharmacokinetic parameters.

12.3 Pharmacokinetics

Pharmacokinetic parameters were evaluated in patients. Eleven patients received 20 mg/m² infused over 1 hour intravenously (treatment Option 2), Fourteen patients received 15 mg/m² infused over 3 hours (treatment Option 1). PK parameters are shown in Table 3. Plasma concentration-time profiles after discontinuation of infusion showed a biexponential decline. The CL of decitabine was higher following treatment Option 2. Upon repeat doses there was no systemic accumulation of decitabine or any changes in PK parameters. Population PK analysis (N=35) showed that the cumulative AUC per cycle for treatment Option 2 was 2.3-fold lower than the cumulative AUC per cycle following treatment Option 1.
[See table 3 above]

The exact route of elimination and metabolic fate of decitabine is not known in humans. One of the pathways of elimination of decitabine appears to be deamination by cytidine deaminase found principally in the liver but also in granulocytes, intestinal epithelium and whole blood.

13 NONCLINICAL TOXICOLOGY

13.1 Carcinogenesis, Mutagenesis and Impairment of Fertility

Carcinogenicity studies with decitabine have not been conducted.

The mutagenic potential of decitabine was tested in several *in vitro* and *in vivo* systems. Decitabine increased mutation frequency in L5178Y mouse lymphoma cells, and mutations were produced in an *Escherichia coli lac-I* transgene in colonic DNA of decitabine-treated mice. Decitabine caused chromosomal rearrangements in larvae of fruit flies.

The effect of decitabine on postnatal development and reproductive capacity was evaluated in mice administered a single 3 mg/m² IP injection (approximately 7% the recommended daily clinical dose) on day 10 of gestation. Body weights of males and females exposed *in utero* to decitabine were significantly reduced relative to controls at all postnatal time points. No consistent effect on fertility was seen when female mice exposed *in utero* were mated to untreated males. Untreated females mated to males exposed *in utero* showed decreased fertility at 3 and 5 months of age (36% and 0% pregnancy rate, respectively). In male mice given IP injections of 0.15, 0.3 or 0.45 mg/m² decitabine (approximately 0.3% to 1% the recommended clinical dose) 3 times a week for 7 weeks, decitabine did not affect survival, body weight gain or hematological measures (hemoglobin and WBC counts). Testes weights were reduced, abnormal histology was observed and significant decreases in sperm number were found at doses ≥ 0.3 mg/m². In females mated to males dosed with ≥ 0.3 mg/m² decitabine, pregnancy rate was reduced and preimplantation loss was significantly increased.

14 CLINICAL STUDIES

14.1 Controlled Trial

A randomized open-label, multicenter, controlled trial evaluated 170 adult patients with myelodysplastic syndromes (MDS) meeting French-American-British (FAB) classification criteria and International Prognostic Scoring System (IPSS) High-Risk, Intermediate-2 and Intermediate-1 prognostic scores. Eighty-nine patients were randomized to Dacogen therapy plus supportive care (only 83 received Dacogen), and 81 to Supportive Care (SC) alone. Patients with Acute Myeloid Leukemia (AML) were not intended to be included. Of the 170 patients included in the study, independent review (adjudicated diagnosis) found that 12 patients (9 in the Dacogen arm and 3 in the SC arm) had the diagnosis of AML at baseline. Baseline demographics and other patient characteristics in the Intent-to-Treat (ITT) population were similar between the 2 groups, as shown in Table 4.

Table 4 Baseline Demographics and Other Patient Characteristics (ITT)

Demographic or Other Patient Characteristic	Dacogen N = 89	Supportive Care N= 81
Age (years)		
Mean (±SD)	69±10	67±10
Median (IQR)	70 (65-76)	70 (62-74)
(Range: min-max)	(31-85)	(30-82)
Gender n (%)		
Male	59 (66)	57 (70)
Female	30 (34)	24 (30)
Race n (%)		
White	83 (93)	76 (94)
Black	4 (4)	2 (2)
Other	2 (2)	3 (4)
Weeks Since MDS Diagnosis		
Mean (±SD)	86±131	77±119
Median (IQR)	29 (10-87)	35 (7-98)
(Range: min-max)	(2-667)	(2-865)
Previous MDS Therapy n (%)		
Yes	27 (30)	19 (23)
No	62 (70)	62 (77)
RBC Transfusion Status n (%)		
Independent	23 (26)	27 (33)
Dependent	66 (74)	54 (67)
Platelet Transfusion Status n (%)		
Independent	69 (78)	62 (77)
Dependent	20 (22)	19 (23)
IPSS Classification n (%)		
Intermediate–1	28 (31)	24 (30)
Intermediate–2	38 (43)	36 (44)
High Risk	23 (26)	21 (26)
FAB Classification n (%)		
RA	12 (13)	12 (15)
RARS	7 (8)	4 (5)
RAEB	47 (53)	43 (53)
RAEB-t	17 (19)	14 (17)
CMML	6 (7)	8 (10)

Patients randomized to the Dacogen arm received Dacogen intravenously infused at a dose of 15 mg/m² over a 3-hour period, every 8 hours, for 3 consecutive days. This cycle was repeated every 6 weeks, depending on the patient's clinical response and toxicity. Supportive care consisted of blood and blood product transfusions, prophylactic antibiotics, and hematopoietic growth factors. The study endpoints were overall response rate (complete response + partial response) and time to AML or death. Responses were classified using the MDS International Working Group (IWG) criteria; patients were required to be RBC and platelet transfusion independent during the time of response. Response criteria are given in **Table 5**:

[See table 5 at right]

The overall response rate (CR+PR) in the ITT population was 17% in Dacogen-treated patients and 0% in the SC group (p<0.001). (**See Table 6**) The overall response rate was 21% (12/56) in Dacogen-treated patients considered evaluable for response (i.e., those patients with pathologically confirmed MDS at baseline who received at least 2 cycles of treatment). The median duration of response (range) for patients who responded to Dacogen was 288 days (116-388) and median time to response (range) was 93 days (55-272). All but one of the Dacogen-treated patients who responded did so by the fourth cycle. Benefit was seen in an additional 13% of Dacogen-treated patients who had hematologic improvement, defined as a response less than PR lasting at least 8 weeks, compared to 7% of SC patients. Dacogen treatment did not significantly delay the median time to AML or death versus supportive care.

[See table 6 at right]

All patients with a CR or PR were RBC and platelet transfusion independent in the absence of growth factors. Responses occurred in patients with an adjudicated baseline diagnosis of AML.

14.2   Single-arm Studies

Three open-label, single-arm, multicenter studies were conducted to evaluate the safety and efficacy of Dacogen in MDS patients with any of the FAB subtypes. In one study conducted in North America, 99 patients with IPSS Intermediate-1, Intermediate-2, or high risk prognostic scores received Dacogen by intravenous infusion at a dose of 20 mg/m² IV over 1-hour daily, on days 1-5 of week 1 every 4 weeks (1 cycle). The results were consistent with the results of the controlled trial and summarized in Table 8.

Table 7 Baseline Demographics and Other Patient Characteristics (ITT)

Demographic or Other Patient Characteristic	Dacogen N = 99
Age (years)	
Mean (±SD)	71±9
Median (Range: min-max)	72 (34-87)
Gender n (%)	
Male	71 (72)
Female	28 (28)
Race n (%)	
White	86 (87)
Black	6 (6)
Asian	4 (4)
Other	3 (3)
Days From MDS Diagnosis to First Dose	
Mean (±SD)	444±626
Median (Range: min-max)	154 (7-3079)
Previous MDS Therapy n (%)	
Yes	27 (27)
No	72 (73)
RBC Transfusion Status n (%)	
Independent	33 (33)
Dependent	66 (67)
Platelet Transfusion Status n (%)	
Independent	84 (85)
Dependent	15 (15)
IPSS Classification n (%)	
Low Risk	1 (1)
Intermediate-1	52 (53)
Intermediate-2	23 (23)
High Risk	23 (23)
FAB Classification n (%)	
RA	20 (20)
RARS	17 (17)
RAEB	45 (45)
RAEB-t	6 (6)
CMML	11 (11)

Table 5 Response Criteria for Phase 3 Trial*

Complete Response (CR) ≥ 8 weeks	Bone Marrow	On repeat aspirates: • < 5% myeloblasts • No dysplastic changes
	Peripheral Blood	In all samples during response: • Hgb > 11g/dL (no transfusions or erythropoietin • ANC ≥ 1500/µL (no growth factor) • Platelets ≥ 100,000/µL (no thrombopoietic agent) • No blasts and no dysplasia
Partial Response (PR) ≥ 8 weeks	Bone Marrow	On repeat aspirates: • ≥ 50% decrease in blasts over pretreatment values OR • Improvement to a less advanced MDS FAB classification
	Peripheral Blood	Same as for CR

* Cheson BD, Bennett JM, et al. Report of an International Working Group to Standardize Response Criteria for MDS. *Blood.* 2000; 96:3671-3674.

Table 6 Analysis of Response (ITT)

Parameter	Dacogen N=89	Supportive Care N=81
Overall Response Rate (CR+PR)⁺	15 (17%)**	0 (0%)
Complete Response (CR)	8 (9%)	0 (0%)
Partial Response (PR)	7 (8%)	0 (0%)
Duration of Response		
Median time to (CR+PR) response - Days (range)	93 (55-272)	NA
Median Duration of (CR+PR) response - Days (range)	288 (116-388)	NA

**p-value <0.001 from two-sided Fisher's Exact Test comparing Dacogen vs. Supportive Care.
⁺In the statistical analysis plan, a p-value of ≤ 0.024 was required to achieve statistical significance.

Table 8 Analysis of Response (ITT)*

Parameter	Dacogen N=99
Overall Response Rate (CR+PR)	16 (16%)
Complete Response (CR)	15 (15%)
Partial Response (PR)	1 (1%)
Duration of Response	
Median time to (CR+PR) response - Days (range)	162 (50-267)
Median Duration of (CR+PR) response - Days (range)	443 (72-722+)

+ indicates censored observation
* Cheson BD, Bennett JM, et al. Report of an International Working Group to Standardize Response Criteria for MDS. *Blood.* 2000; 96:3671-3674.

15   REFERENCES

1. NIOSH Alert: Preventing occupational exposures to antineoplastic and other hazardous drugs in healthcare settings. 2004. U.S. Department of Health and Human Services, Public Health Service, Centers for Disease Control and Prevention, National Institute for Occupational Safety and Health, DHHS (NIOSH) Publication No. 2004-165.
2. OSHA Technical Manual, TED 1-0.15A, Section VI: Chapter 2. Controlling Occupational Exposure to Hazardous Drugs. OSHA, 1999. http://www.osha.gov/dts/osta/otm/otm_vi/otm_vi_2.html
3. American Society of Health-System Pharmacists. ASHP Guidelines on Handling Hazardous Drugs: *Am J Health-Syst Pharm.* 2006;63:1172-1193.
4. Polovich M., White JM, Kelleher LO (eds). Chemotherapy and biotherapy guidelines and recommendations for practice (2nd ed.) 2005. Pittsburgh, PA: Oncology Nursing Society.

16   HOW SUPPLIED/STORAGE AND HANDLING
NDC 62856-600-01, 50 mg single-dose vial individually packaged in a carton.
Storage
Store vials at 25°C (77°F); excursions permitted to 15-30°C (59°-86°F).

17   PATIENT COUNSELING INFORMATION
17.1   Instructions for Patients
Women of childbearing potential should be advised to avoid becoming pregnant while receiving treatment with Dacogen

and for 1 month afterwards, and to use effective contraception during this time, [See Warnings and Precautions (5.3)]. Men should be advised not to father a child while receiving treatment with Dacogen, and for 2 months afterwards. During these times, men with female partners of childbearing potential should use effective contraception [See Warnings and Precautions (5.4) and Nonclinical Toxicology (13.1)].
Patients should be advised to monitor and report any symptoms of neutropenia, thrombocytopenia, or fever to their physician as soon as possible [See Warnings and Precautions (5.1)].
Eisai Inc.
Manufactured by Pharmachemie B.V. Haarlem, The Netherlands
Manufactured for Eisai Inc., Woodcliff Lake, NJ 07677
Dacogen® is a registered trademark of SuperGen, Inc., Dublin, CA, U.S.A. used under license.
Shown in Product Identification Guide, page 308

FRAGMIN®   ℞
[*FRAG - min*]
(dalteparin sodium injection)
for Subcutaneous Use Only

HIGHLIGHTS OF PRESCRIBING INFORMATION
These highlights do not include all the information needed to use FRAGMIN® safely and effectively. See full prescribing information for FRAGMIN.
FRAGMIN (dalteparin sodium injection) for Subcutaneous Use Only
Initial U.S. Approval: 1994

WARNING: SPINAL/EPIDURAL HEMATOMA
Epidural or spinal hematomas may occur in patients who are anticoagulated with low molecular weight heparins (LMWH) or heparinoids and are receiving neuraxial anesthesia or undergoing spinal puncture. These hematomas may result in long-term or permanent paralysis. Consider these risks when scheduling patients for spinal procedures. Factors that can increase the risk of developing epidural or spinal hematomas in these patients include: • Use of indwelling epidural catheters • Concomitant use of other drugs that affect hemostasis, such as non-steroidal anti-inflammatory drugs (NSAIDs), platelet inhibitors, other anticoagulants. • A history of traumatic or repeated epidural or spinal punctures • A history of spinal deformity or spinal surgery Monitor patients frequently for signs and symptoms of neurological impairment. If neurological compromise is noted, urgent treatment is necessary.

Consider the benefits and risks before neuraxial intervention in patients anticoagulated or to be anticoagulated for thromboprophylaxis [see *Warnings and Precautions* (5.1) and *Drug Interactions* (7)].

---RECENT MAJOR CHANGES---

Boxed Warning,	(12/2009)
Indications and Usage (1.3)	(12/2009)

---INDICATIONS AND USAGE---

FRAGMIN is a low molecular weight heparin (LMWH) indicated for

- Prophylaxis of ischemic complications of unstable angina and non-Q-wave myocardial infarction (1.1)
- Prophylaxis of deep vein thrombosis (DVT) in abdominal surgery, hip replacement surgery or medical patients with severely restricted mobility during acute illness (1.2)
- Extended treatment of symptomatic venous thromboembolism (VTE) to reduce the recurrence in patients with cancer. In these patients, the FRAGMIN therapy begins with the initial VTE treatment and continues for six months. (1.3)

Limitations of Use

FRAGMIN is not indicated for the acute treatment of VTE

---DOSAGE AND ADMINISTRATION---

Indication	Dosing Regimen
Unstable angina and non-Q-wave MI	120 IU/kg subcutaneous every 12 hours (with aspirin) (2.1)
DVT prophylaxis in abdominal surgery	2500 IU subcutaneous once daily or 5000 IU subcutaneous once daily or 2500 IU subcutaneous followed by 2500 IU subcutaneous 12 hours later and then 5000 IU subcutaneous once daily (2.1)
DVT prophylaxis in hip replacement surgery	**Postoperative start** - 2500 IU subcutaneous 4 to 8 hours after surgery, then 5000 IU subcutaneous once daily or **Preoperative start - day of surgery** 2500 IU subcutaneous 2 hours before surgery followed by 2500 IU subcutaneous 4 to 8 hours after surgery, then 5000 IU subcutaneous once daily (2.1) **Preoperative start - Evening Before Surgery** 5000 IU subcutaneous followed by 5000 IU subcutaneous 4 to 8 hours after surgery (2.1)
DVT prophylaxis in medical patients	5000 IU subcutaneous once daily (2.1)
Extended treatment of VTE in patients with cancer	Month 1: 200 IU/kg subcutaneous once daily (2.1) Months 2-6: 150 IU/kg subcutaneous once daily (2.1)

Do not use as intramuscular injection. FRAGMIN should not be mixed with other injections or infusions (2)

---DOSAGE FORMS AND STRENGTHS---

- Single-dose prefilled syringe: 2,500 IU/0.2 mL, 5,000 IU/0.2 mL. 7500 IU/0.3 mL, 10,000 IU/0.4 mL, 12,500 IU/0.5 mL, 15,000 IU/0.6 mL, 18,000 IU/0.72 mL (3)
- Single-dose graduated syringe: 10,000 IU/1 mL (3)
- Multiple dose vial: 95,000/3.8 mL, 95,000 IU/9.5 mL (3)

---CONTRAINDICATIONS---

- Active major bleeding (4)
- History of heparin induced thrombocytopenia or heparin induced thrombocytopenia with thrombosis (4)
- Hypersensitivity to dalteparin sodium (4, 6.1)
- In patients undergoing Epidural/Neuraxial anesthesia, do not administer FRAGMIN [see *Boxed Warning* and (4)];
- As a treatment for unstable angina and non-Q-wave MI
- For prolonged VTE prophylaxis
- Hypersensitivity to heparin or pork products (4)

---WARNINGS AND PRECAUTIONS---

- Use caution in conditions with increased risk of hemorrhage (5.1)
- Monitor thrombocytopenia of any degree closely (5.2)
- Multiple-dose formulations contain benzyl alcohol (5.3)
- Periodic blood counts recommended (5.4)

---ADVERSE REACTIONS---

Most common adverse reaction is hematoma at the injection site (6)

To report SUSPECTED ADVERSE REACTIONS, contact Eisai at (1-888-274-2378) or FDA at 1-800-FDA-1088 or *www.fda.gov/medwatch*.

Table 1

Volume of FRAGMIN to be Administered by Patient Weight, Based on 9.5 mL Vial (10,000 IU/mL)

Patient weight (lb)	< 110	110 to 131	132 to 153	154 to 175	176 to 197	≥198
Patient weight (kg)	< 50	50 to 59	60 to 69	70 to 79	80 to 89	≥90
Volume of FRAGMIN (mL)	0.55	0.65	0.75	0.90	1.0	1.0

---DRUG INTERACTIONS---

- Use FRAGMIN with care in patients receiving oral anticoagulants, platelet inhibitors, and thrombolytic agents (7)

---USE IN SPECIFIC POPULATIONS---

- Safety and effectiveness in pediatric patients have not been established. (8.4)

See 17 for PATIENT COUNSELING INFORMATION

Revised: 12/2009

FULL PRESCRIBING INFORMATION: CONTENTS*
WARNING: SPINAL/EPIDURAL HEMATOMAS

FULL PRESCRIBING INFORMATION

WARNING: SPINAL/EPIDURAL HEMATOMAS
Epidural or spinal hematomas may occur in patients who are anticoagulated with low molecular weight heparins (LMWH) or heparinoids and are receiving neuraxial anesthesia or undergoing spinal puncture. These hematomas may result in long-term or permanent paralysis. Consider these risks when scheduling patients for spinal procedures. Factors that can increase the risk of developing epidural or spinal hematomas in these patients include:

- **Use of indwelling epidural catheters**
- **Concomitant use of other drugs that affect hemostasis, such as non-steroidal anti-inflammatory drugs (NSAIDs), platelet inhibitors, other anticoagulants.**
- **A history of traumatic or repeated epidural or spinal punctures**
- **A history of spinal deformity or spinal surgery**

Monitor patients frequently for signs and symptoms of neurological impairment. If neurological compromise is noted, urgent treatment is necessary.

Consider the benefits and risks before neuraxial intervention in patients anticoagulated or to be anticoagulated for thromboprophylaxis [see *Warnings and Precautions* (5.1) and *Drug Interactions* (7)].

1 INDICATIONS AND USAGE

1.1 Prophylaxis of Ischemic Complications in Unstable Angina and Non-Q-Wave Myocardial Infarction

FRAGMIN® Injection is indicated for the prophylaxis of ischemic complications in unstable angina and non-Q-wave myocardial infarction, when concurrently administered with aspirin therapy [see *Clinical Studies* (14.1)].

1.2 Prophylaxis of Deep Vein Thrombosis

FRAGMIN is also indicated for the prophylaxis of deep vein thrombosis (DVT), which may lead to pulmonary embolism (PE):

- In patients undergoing hip replacement surgery [see *Clinical Studies* (14.2)];
- In patients undergoing abdominal surgery who are at risk for thromboembolic complications [see *Clinical Studies* (14.3)];
- In medical patients who are at risk for thromboembolic complications due to severely restricted mobility during acute illness [see *Clinical Studies* (14.4)].

1.3 Extended Treatment of Symptomatic Venous Thromboembolism in Patients with Cancer

FRAGMIN is also indicated for the extended treatment of symptomatic venous thromboembolism (VTE) (proximal DVT and/or PE), to reduce the recurrence of VTE in patients with cancer. In these patients, the FRAGMIN therapy begins with the initial VTE treatment and continues for six months [see *Clinical Studies* (14.5)].

Limitations of Use

FRAGMIN is not indicated for the acute treatment of VTE.

2 DOSAGE AND ADMINISTRATION

FRAGMIN is administered by subcutaneous injection. It must not be administered by intramuscular injection.

FRAGMIN Injection should not be mixed with other injections or infusions unless specific compatibility data are available that support such mixing.

Routine coagulation tests such as Prothrombin Time (PT) and Activated Partial Thromboplastin Time (APTT) are relatively insensitive measures of FRAGMIN activity and, therefore, unsuitable for monitoring the anticoagulant effect of FRAGMIN [see *Warnings and Precautions* (5)].

2.1 Adult Dosage

Prophylaxis of Ischemic Complications in Unstable Angina and Non-Q-Wave Myocardial Infarction: In patients with unstable angina or non-Q-wave myocardial infarction, the recommended dose of FRAGMIN Injection is 120 IU/kg of body weight, but not more than 10,000 IU, subcutaneously every 12 hours with concurrent oral aspirin (75 to 165 mg once daily) therapy. Treatment should be continued until the patient is clinically stabilized. The usual duration of administration is 5 to 8 days. Concurrent aspirin therapy is recommended except when contraindicated.

Table 1 lists the volume of FRAGMIN, based on the 9.5 mL multiple-dose vial (10,000 IU/mL), to be administered for a range of patient weights.

[See table 1 above]

Prophylaxis of Venous Thromboembolism Following Hip Replacement Surgery: Table 2 presents the dosing options for patients undergoing hip replacement surgery. The usual duration of administration is 5 to 10 days after surgery; up to 14 days of treatment with FRAGMIN have been well tolerated in clinical trials.

[See table 2 at top of next page]

Abdominal Surgery: In patients undergoing abdominal surgery with a risk of thromboembolic complications, the recommended dose of FRAGMIN is 2500 IU administered by subcutaneous injection once daily, starting 1 to 2 hours prior to surgery and repeated once daily postoperatively. The usual duration of administration is 5 to 10 days.

In patients undergoing abdominal surgery associated with a high risk of thromboembolic complications, such as malignant disorder, the recommended dose of FRAGMIN is 5000 IU subcutaneously the evening before surgery, then once daily postoperatively. The usual duration of administration is 5 to 10 days. Alternatively, in patients with malignancy, 2500 IU of FRAGMIN can be administered subcutaneously 1 to 2 hours before surgery followed by 2500 IU subcutaneously 12 hours later, and then 5000 IU once daily postoperatively. The usual duration of administration is 5 to 10 days.

Medical Patients During Acute Illness: In medical patients with severely restricted mobility during acute illness, the recommended dose of FRAGMIN is 5000 IU administered by subcutaneous injection once daily. In clinical trials, the usual duration of administration was 12 to 14 days.

Extended Treatment of Symptomatic Venous Thromboembolism in Patients with Cancer: In patients with cancer and symptomatic venous thromboembolism, the recommended dosing of FRAGMIN is as follows: for the first 30 days of treatment administer FRAGMIN 200 IU/kg total body weight subcutaneously once daily. The total daily dose should not exceed 18,000 IU. Table 3 lists the dose of FRAGMIN to be administered once daily during the first month for a range of patient weights

Month 1

Table 3

Dose of FRAGMIN to be Administered Subcutaneously by Patient Weight during the First Month

Body Weight (lbs)	Body Weight (kg)	FRAGMIN Dose (IU) (prefilled syringe) once daily
≤ 124	≤ 56	10,000
125 to 150	57 to 68	12,500
151 to 181	69 to 82	15,000
182 to 216	83 to 98	18,000
≥ 217	≥ 99	18,000

Months 2 to 6
Administer FRAGMIN at a dose of approximately 150 IU/kg, subcutaneously once daily during Months 2 through 6. The total daily dose should not exceed 18,000 IU. Table 4 lists the dose of FRAGMIN to be administered once daily for a range of patient weights during months 2-6.

Table 4

Dose of FRAGMIN to be Administered Subcutaneously by Patient Weight during Months 2-6

Body Weight (lbs)	Body Weight (kg)	FRAGMIN Dose (IU) (prefilled syringe) once daily
≤ 124	≤ 56	7,500
125 to 150	57 to 68	10,000
151 to 181	69 to 82	12,500
182 to 216	83 to 98	15,000
≥ 217	≥ 99	18,000

Safety and efficacy beyond six months have not been evaluated in patients with cancer and acute symptomatic VTE *[see Warnings and Precautions (5) and Adverse Reactions (6.1)]*.

2.2   Dose reductions for thrombocytopenia in patients with cancer and acute symptomatic VTE
In patients receiving FRAGMIN who experience platelet counts between 50,000 and 100,000/mm³, reduce the daily dose of FRAGMIN by 2,500 IU until the platelet count recovers to ≥100,000/mm³. In patients receiving FRAGMIN who experience platelet counts < 50,000/mm³, discontinue FRAGMIN until the platelet count recovers above 50,000/mm³.

Table 2

Dosing Options for Patients Undergoing Hip Replacement Surgery

Timing of First Dose of FRAGMIN	Dose of FRAGMIN to be Given Subcutaneously			
	10 to 14 Hours Before Surgery	Within 2 Hours Before Surgery	4 to 8 Hours After Surgery[1]	Postoperative Period[2]
Postoperative Start	—	—	2500 IU[3]	5000 IU once daily
Preoperative Start - Day of Surgery	—	2500 IU	2500 IU[3]	5000 IU once daily
Preoperative Start - Evening Before Surgery[4]	5000 IU	—	5000 IU	5000 IU once daily

[1] Or later, if hemostasis has not been achieved.
[2] Up to 14 days of treatment was well tolerated in controlled clinical trials, where the usual duration of treatment was 5 to 10 days postoperatively.
[3] Allow a minimum of 6 hours between this dose and the dose to be given on Postoperative Day 1. Adjust the timing of the dose on Postoperative Day 1 accordingly.
[4] Allow approximately 24 hours between doses.

2.3   Dose reductions for renal insufficiency in extended treatment of acute symptomatic venous thromboembolism in patients with cancer
In patients with severely impaired renal function (CrCl < 30 mL/min), monitor anti-Xa levels to determine the appropriate FRAGMIN dose. Target anti-Xa range is 0.5-1.5 IU/mL. When monitoring anti-Xa in these patients, perform sampling 4-6 hrs after FRAGMIN dosing and only after the patient has received 3-4 doses.

2.4   Administration
Subcutaneous injection technique: Patients should be sitting or lying down and FRAGMIN administered by deep subcutaneous injection. FRAGMIN may be injected in a U-shape area around the navel, the upper outer side of the thigh or the upper outer quadrangle of the buttock. The injection site should be varied daily. When the area around the navel or the thigh is used, using the thumb and forefinger, you **must** lift up a fold of skin while giving the injection. The entire length of the needle should be inserted at a 45 to 90 degree angle.
Inspect FRAGMIN prefilled syringes and vials visually for particulate matter and discoloration prior to administration. After first penetration of the rubber stopper, store the multiple-dose vials at room temperature for up to 2 weeks. Discard any unused solution after 2 weeks.

Instructions for using the prefilled single-dose syringes preassembled with needle guard devices

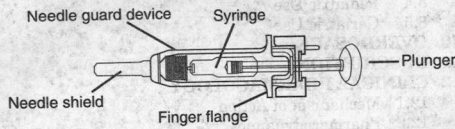

Fixed dose syringes: To ensure delivery of the full dose, do not expel the air bubble from the prefilled syringe before injection. Hold the syringe assembly by the open sides of the device. Remove the needle shield. Insert the needle into the injection area as instructed above. Depress the plunger of the syringe while holding the finger flange **until the entire dose has been given**. The needle guard will **not** be activated unless the **entire** dose has been given. Remove needle from the patient. Let go of the plunger and allow syringe to move up inside the device until the entire needle is guarded. Discard the syringe assembly in approved containers.
Graduated syringes: Hold the syringe assembly by the open sides of the device. Remove the needle shield. With the needle pointing up, prepare the syringe by expelling the air bubble and then continuing to push the plunger to the desired dose or volume, discarding the extra solution in an appropriate manner. Insert the needle into the injection area as instructed above. Depress the plunger of the syringe while holding the finger flange **until the entire dose remaining in the syringe has been given**. The needle guard will **not** be activated unless the **entire** dose has been given. Remove needle from the patient. Let go of the plunger and allow syringe to move up inside the device until the entire needle is guarded. Discard the syringe assembly in approved containers.

3   DOSAGE FORMS AND STRENGTHS
2,500 IU/0.2 mL single-dose prefilled syringe
5,000 IU/0.2 mL single-dose prefilled syringe
7,500 IU/0.3 mL single-dose prefilled syringe
10,000 IU/0.4 mL single-dose prefilled syringe
10,000 IU/1 mL single-dose graduated syringe
12,500 IU/0.5 mL single-dose prefilled syringe
15,000 IU/0.6 mL single-dose prefilled syringe

18,000 IU/0.72 mL single-dose prefilled syringe
95,000 IU/3.8 mL multiple-dose vial
95,000 IU/9.5 mL multiple-dose vial

4   CONTRAINDICATIONS
• Active major bleeding
• History of heparin induced thrombocytopenia or heparin induced thrombocytopenia with thrombosis.
• Hypersensitivity to dalteparin sodium (e.g., pruritis, rash, anaphylactic reactions) [see *Adverse Reactions* (6.1)]
• In patients undergoing Epidural/Neuraxial anesthesia, do not administer FRAGMIN [*See Boxed Warning*];
• As a treatment for unstable angina and non-Q-wave MI
• For prolonged VTE prophylaxis.
• Hypersensitivity to heparin or pork products

5   WARNINGS AND PRECAUTIONS
5.1   Hemorrhage
Spinal or epidural hematomas can occur with the associated use of low molecular weight heparins or heparinoids and neuraxial (spinal/epidural) anesthesia or spinal puncture [*see Boxed Warning and Adverse Reactions (6.2)*].
Use FRAGMIN with extreme caution in patients who have an increased risk of hemorrhage, such as those with severe uncontrolled hypertension, bacterial endocarditis, congenital or acquired bleeding disorders, active ulceration and angiodysplastic gastrointestinal disease, hemorrhagic stroke, or shortly after brain, spinal or ophthalmological surgery. FRAGMIN may enhance the risk of bleeding in patients with thrombocytopenia or platelet defects; severe liver or kidney insufficiency, hypertensive or diabetic retinopathy, and recent gastrointestinal bleeding. Bleeding can occur at any site during therapy with FRAGMIN.
5.2   Thrombocytopenia
Heparin-induced thrombocytopenia can occur with the administration of FRAGMIN. The incidence of this complication is unknown at present. In clinical practice, cases of thrombocytopenia with thrombosis, amputation and death have been observed. [*See Contraindications (4)*] Closely monitor thrombocytopenia of any degree.
In FRAGMIN clinical trials supporting non-cancer indications, platelet counts of < 50,000/mm³ occurred in < 1% of patients. In the clinical trial of patients with cancer and acute symptomatic venous thromboembolism treated for up to 6 months in the FRAGMIN treatment arm, platelet counts of < 100,000/mm³ occurred in 13.6% of patients, including 6.5% who also had platelet counts less than 50,000/mm³. In the same clinical trial, thrombocytopenia was reported as an adverse event in 10.9% of patients in the FRAGMIN arm and 8.1% of patients in the OAC arm. FRAGMIN dose was decreased or interrupted in patients whose platelet counts fell below 100,000/mm³.
5.3   Benzyl Alcohol
Each multiple-dose vial of FRAGMIN contains benzyl alcohol as a preservative. Benzyl alcohol has been reported to be associated with a fatal "Gasping Syndrome" in premature infants. Because benzyl alcohol may cross the placenta, use caution when administering FRAGMIN preserved with benzyl alcohol to pregnant women. If anticoagulation with FRAGMIN is needed during pregnancy, use preservative-free FRAGMIN, where possible [*See Use in Specific Populations (8.1)*].
5.4   Laboratory Tests
Periodic routine complete blood counts, including platelet count, blood chemistry, and stool occult blood tests are recommended during the course of treatment with FRAGMIN. When administered at recommended prophylaxis doses, routine coagulation tests such as Prothrombin Time (PT)

Table 5

Major Bleeding Reactions in Unstable Angina and Non-Q-Wave Myocardial Infarction

Indication	Dosing Regimen		
Unstable Angina and Non-Q-Wave MI	FRAGMIN 120 IU/kg/12 hr subcutaneous[1] n (%)	Heparin[2] intravenous and subcutaneous[2] n (%)	Placebo every 12 hr subcutaneous n (%)
Major Bleeding Reactions[3,4]	15/1497 (1.0)	7/731 (1.0)	4/760 (0.5)

[1] Treatment was administered for 5 to 8 days.
[2] Heparin intravenous infusion for at least 48 hours, APTT 1.5 to 2 times control, then 12,500 U subcutaneously every 12 hours for 5 to 8 days.
[3] Aspirin (75 to 165 mg per day) and beta blocker therapies were administered concurrently.
[4] Bleeding reactions were considered major if: 1) accompanied by a decrease in hemoglobin of ≥2 g/dL in connection with clinical symptoms; 2) a transfusion was required; 3) bleeding led to interruption of treatment or death; or 4) intracranial bleeding.

Table 6

Bleeding Reactions Following Hip Replacement Surgery

Indication	FRAGMIN vs Warfarin Sodium		FRAGMIN vs Heparin	
	Dosing Regimen		Dosing Regimen	
Hip Replacement Surgery	FRAGMIN[2] 5000 IU once daily subcutaneous n (%)	Warfarin Sodium[1] oral n (%)	FRAGMIN[4] 5000 IU once daily subcutaneous n (%)	Heparin 5000 U three times a day subcutaneous n (%)
Major Bleeding Reactions[3]	7/274 (2.6)	1/279 (0.4)	0	3/69 (4.3)
Other Bleeding Reactions[5] Hematuria	8/274 (2.9)	5/279 (1.8)	0	0
Wound Hematoma	6/274 (2.2)	0	0	0
Injection Site Hematoma	3/274 (1.1)	NA	2/69 (2.9)	7/69 (10.1)

[1] Warfarin sodium dosage was adjusted to maintain a prothrombin time index of 1.4 to 1.5, corresponding to an International Normalized Ratio (INR) of approximately 2.5.
[2] Includes three treated patients who did not undergo a surgical procedure.
[3] A bleeding event was considered major if: 1) hemorrhage caused a significant clinical event, 2) it was associated with a hemoglobin decrease of ≥2 g/dL or transfusion of 2 or more units of blood products, 3) it resulted in reoperation due to bleeding, or 4) it involved retroperitoneal or intracranial hemorrhage.
[4] Includes two treated patients who did not undergo a surgical procedure.
[5] Occurred at a rate of at least 2% in the group treated with FRAGMIN 5000 IU once daily.

Table 7

Bleeding Reactions Following Abdominal Surgery

Indication	FRAGMIN vs Placebo		FRAGMIN vs FRAGMIN	
	Dosing Regimen		Dosing Regimen	
Abdominal Surgery	FRAGMIN 2500 IU once daily subcutaneous n (%)	Placebo once daily subcutaneous n (%)	FRAGMIN 2500 IU once daily subcutaneous n (%)	FRAGMIN 5000 IU once daily subcutaneous n (%)
Postoperative Transfusions	14/182 (7.7)	13/182 (7.1)	89/1025 (8.7)	125/1033 (12.1)
Wound Hematoma	2/79 (2.5)	2/77 (2.6)	1/1030 (0.1)	4/1039 (0.4)
Reoperation Due to Bleeding	1/79 (1.3)	1/78 (1.3)	2/1030 (0.2)	13/1038 (1.3)
Injection Site Hematoma	8/172 (4.7)	2/174 (1.1)	36/1026 (3.5)	57/1035 (5.5)
Postoperative Transfusions	26/459 (5.7)	36/454 (7.9)	81/508 (15.9)	63/498 (12.7)
Wound Hematoma	16/467 (3.4)	18/467 (3.9)	12/508 (2.4)	6/498 (1.2)
Reoperation Due to Bleeding	2/392 (0.5)	3/392 (0.8)	4/508 (0.8)	2/498 (0.4)
Injection Site Hematoma	1/466 (0.2)	5/464 (1.1)	36/506 (7.1)	47/493 (9.5)

and Activated Partial Thromboplastin Time (APTT) are relatively insensitive measures of FRAGMIN activity and, therefore, unsuitable for monitoring the anticoagulant effect of FRAGMIN. Anti-Factor Xa may be used to monitor the anticoagulant effect of FRAGMIN, such as in patients with severe renal impairment or if abnormal coagulation parameters or bleeding occurs during FRAGMIN therapy.

6 ADVERSE REACTIONS

6.1 Clinical Trials Experience

Because clinical trials are conducted under widely varying conditions, adverse reaction rates observed in the clinical trials of a drug cannot be directly compared to rates in the clinical trials of another drug and may not accurately reflect the rates observed in practice.

Hemorrhage

The incidence of hemorrhagic complications during treatment with FRAGMIN Injection has been low. The most commonly reported side effect is hematoma at the injection site. The risk for bleeding varies with the indication and may increase with higher doses.

Unstable Angina and Non-Q-Wave Myocardial Infarction

Table 5 summarizes major bleeding reactions that occurred with FRAGMIN, heparin, and placebo in clinical trials of unstable angina and non-Q-wave myocardial infarction. [See table 5 at left]

Hip Replacement Surgery

Table 6 summarizes: 1) all major bleeding reactions and, 2) other bleeding reactions possibly or probably related to treatment with FRAGMIN (preoperative dosing regimen), warfarin sodium, or heparin in two hip replacement surgery clinical trials. [See table 6 at left]

Six of the patients treated with FRAGMIN experienced seven major bleeding reactions. Two of the reactions were wound hematoma (one requiring reoperation), three were bleeding from the operative site, one was intraoperative bleeding due to vessel damage, and one was gastrointestinal bleeding. None of the patients experienced retroperitoneal or intracranial hemorrhage or died of bleeding complications.

In the third hip replacement surgery clinical trial, the incidence of major bleeding reactions was similar in all three treatment groups: 3.6% (18/496) for patients who started FRAGMIN before surgery; 2.5% (12/487) for patients who started FRAGMIN after surgery; and 3.1% (15/489) for patients treated with warfarin sodium.

Abdominal Surgery

Table 7 summarizes bleeding reactions that occurred in clinical trials which studied FRAGMIN 2500 and 5000 IU administered once daily to abdominal surgery patients. [See table 7 at left]

In a trial comparing FRAGMIN 5000 IU once daily to FRAGMIN 2500 IU once daily in patients undergoing surgery for malignancy, the incidence of bleeding reactions was 4.6% and 3.6%, respectively (n.s.). In a trial comparing FRAGMIN 5000 IU once daily to heparin 5000 U twice daily, in the malignancy subgroup the incidence of bleeding reactions was 3.2% and 2.7%, respectively for FRAGMIN and Heparin (n.s.).

Medical Patients with Severely Restricted Mobility During Acute Illness

Table 8 summarizes major bleeding reactions that occurred in a clinical trial of medical patients with severely restricted mobility during acute illness.

Table 8

Bleeding Reactions in Medical Patients with Severely Restricted Mobility During Acute Illness

Indication	Dosing Regimen	
Medical Patients with Severely Restricted Mobility	FRAGMIN 5000 IU once daily subcutaneous n (%)	Placebo once daily subcutaneous n (%)
Major Bleeding Reactions[1] at Day 14	8/1848 (0.4)	0/1833 (0)
Major Bleeding Reactions[1] at Day 21	9/1848 (0.5)	3/1833 (0.2)

[1] A bleeding event was considered major if: 1) it was accompanied by a decrease in hemoglobin of ≥2 g/dL in connection with clinical symptoms; 2) intraocular, spinal/epidural, intracranial, or retroperitoneal bleeding; 3) required transfusion of ≥2 units of blood products; 4) required significant medical or surgical intervention; or 5) led to death.

Three of the major bleeding reactions that occurred by Day 21 were fatal, all due to gastrointestinal hemorrhage (two patients in the group treated with FRAGMIN and one in the group receiving placebo).

Patients with Cancer and Acute Symptomatic Venous Thromboembolism

Table 9 summarizes the number of patients with bleeding reactions that occurred in the clinical trial of patients with cancer and acute symptomatic venous thromboembolism. A bleeding event was considered major if it: 1) was accompanied by a decrease in hemoglobin of ≥ 2 g/dL in connection with clinical symptoms; 2) occurred at a critical site (intraocular, spinal/epidural, intracranial, retroperitoneal, or pericardial bleeding); 3) required transfusion of ≥ 2 units of blood products; or 4) led to death. Minor bleeding was classified as clinically overt bleeding that did not meet criteria for major bleeding.

At the end of the six-month study, a total of 46 (13.6%) patients in the FRAGMIN arm and 62 (18.5%) patients in the OAC arm experienced any bleeding event. One bleeding event (hemoptysis in a patient in the FRAGMIN arm at Day 71) was fatal.

[See table 9 at right]

Thrombocytopenia

[*See Warnings and Precautions (5.2)*]

Elevations of Serum Transaminases

In FRAGMIN clinical trials supporting non-cancer indications, where hepatic transaminases were measured, asymptomatic increases in transaminase levels (SGOT/AST and SGPT/ALT) greater than three times the upper limit of normal of the laboratory reference range were seen in 4.7% and 4.2%, respectively, of patients during treatment with FRAGMIN.

In the FRAGMIN clinical trial of patients with cancer and acute symptomatic venous thromboembolism treated with FRAGMIN for up to 6 months, asymptomatic increases in transaminase levels, AST and ALT, greater than three times the upper limit of normal of the laboratory reference range were reported in 8.9% and 9.5% of patients, respectively. The frequencies of Grades 3 and 4 increases in AST and ALT, as classified by the National Cancer Institute, Common Toxicity Criteria (NCI-CTC) Scoring System, were 3% and 3.8%, respectively. Grades 2, 3 & 4 combined have been reported in 12% and 14% of patients, respectively.

Other

Allergic Reactions: Allergic reactions (i.e., pruritus, rash, fever, injection site reaction, bullous eruption) have occurred. Cases of anaphylactoid reactions have been reported.

Local Reactions: Pain at the injection site, the only non-bleeding event determined to be possibly or probably related to treatment with FRAGMIN and reported at a rate of at least 2% in the group treated with FRAGMIN, was reported in 4.5% of patients treated with FRAGMIN 5000 IU once daily vs 11.8% of patients treated with heparin 5000 U twice daily in the abdominal surgery trials. In the hip replacement trials, pain at injection site was reported in 12% of patients treated with FRAGMIN 5000 IU once daily vs 13% of patients treated with heparin 5000 U three times a day.

6.2   Post-Marketing Experience

The following adverse reactions have been identified during postapproval use of FRAGMIN. Because these reactions are reported voluntarily from a population of uncertain size, it is not always possible to reliably estimate their frequency or establish a causal relationship to drug exposure.

Since first international market introduction in 1985, there have been more than 15 reports of epidural or spinal hematoma formation with concurrent use of dalteparin sodium and spinal/epidural anesthesia or spinal puncture. The majority of patients had postoperative indwelling epidural catheters placed for analgesia or received additional drugs affecting hemostasis. In some cases the hematoma resulted in long-term or permanent paralysis (partial or complete). [*see Boxed Warning*]

Skin necrosis has occurred. There have been cases of alopecia reported that improved on drug discontinuation.

7   DRUG INTERACTIONS

Use FRAGMIN with care in patients receiving oral anticoagulants, platelet inhibitors, and thrombolytic agents because of increased risk of bleeding [*see Warning and Precautions (5)*].

8   USE IN SPECIFIC POPULATIONS

8.1   Pregnancy

Pregnancy Category B

There are no adequate and well-controlled studies of FRAGMIN use in pregnant women. In reproductive and developmental toxicity studies, pregnant rats and rabbits received dalteparin sodium at intravenous doses up to 2400 IU/kg (14,160 IU/m^2) (rats) and 4800 IU/kg (40,800 IU/m^2) (rabbits). These exposures were 2 to 4 times (rats) and 4 times (rabbits) the human dose of 100 IU/kg dalteparin based on the body surface area. No evidence of impaired fertility or harm to the fetuses occurred in these studies. Because animal reproduction studies are not always predictive of human response, this drug should be used during pregnancy only if clearly needed. Cases of "Gasping Syndrome" have occurred in premature infants when large amounts of benzyl alcohol have been administered (99-404 mg/kg/day). The 9.5 mL and the 3.8 mL multiple-dose vials of FRAGMIN contain 14 mg/mL of benzyl alcohol [*see Warnings and Precautions (5.3)*].

8.3   Nursing Mothers

Based on limited published data dalteparin is minimally excreted in human milk. One study of 15 lactating women receiving prophylactic doses of dalteparin, in the immediate postpartum period, detected small amounts of anti-Xa activity (range < 0.005 to 0.037 IU/mL) in breast milk that were

equivalent to a milk/plasma ratio of <0.025-0.224. Oral absorption of LMWH is extremely low, but the clinical implications, if any, of this small amount of anticoagulant activity on a nursing infant are unknown. Caution should be exercised when FRAGMIN is administered to a nursing woman.

8.4   Pediatric Use

Safety and effectiveness in pediatric patients have not been established.

8.5   Geriatric Use

Of the total number of patients in clinical studies of FRAGMIN, 5516 patients were 65 years of age or older and 2237 were 75 or older. No overall differences in effectiveness were observed between these subjects and younger subjects. Some studies suggest that the risk of bleeding increases with age. Postmarketing surveillance and literature reports have not revealed additional differences in the safety of FRAGMIN between elderly and younger patients. Give careful attention to dosing intervals and concomitant medications (especially antiplatelet medications) in geriatric patients, particularly in those with low body weight (< 45 kg) and those predisposed to decreased renal function [*see Warnings and Precautions (5)* and *Clinical Pharmacology (12)*].

10   OVERDOSAGE

An excessive dosage of FRAGMIN Injection may lead to hemorrhagic complications. These may generally be stopped by slow intravenous injection of protamine sulfate (1% solution), at a dose of 1 mg protamine for every 100 anti-Xa IU of FRAGMIN given. If the APTT measured 2 to 4 hours after the first infusion remains prolonged, a second infusion of

0.5 mg protamine sulfate per 100 anti-Xa IU of FRAGMIN may be administered. Even with these additional doses of protamine, the APTT may remain more prolonged than would usually be found following administration of unfractionated heparin. In all cases, the anti-Factor Xa activity is never completely neutralized (maximum about 60 to 75%). Take particular care to avoid overdosage with protamine sulfate. Administration of protamine sulfate can cause severe hypotensive and anaphylactoid reactions. Because fatal reactions, often resembling anaphylaxis, have been reported with protamine sulfate, give protamine sulfate only when resuscitation techniques and treatment for anaphylactic shock are readily available. For additional information, consult the labeling of Protamine Sulfate Injection, USP, products.

11   DESCRIPTION

FRAGMIN Injection (dalteparin sodium injection) is a sterile, low molecular weight heparin. It is available in single-dose, prefilled syringes preassembled with a needle guard device, and multiple-dose vials. With reference to the W.H.O. First International Low Molecular Weight Heparin Reference Standard, each syringe contains either 2500, 5000, 7500, 10,000, 12,500, 15,000 or 18,000 anti-Factor Xa international units (IU), equivalent to 16, 32, 48, 64, 80, 96 or 115.2 mg dalteparin sodium, respectively. Each multiple-dose vial contains either 10,000 or 25,000 anti-Factor Xa IU per 1 mL (equivalent to 64 or 160 mg dalteparin sodium, respectively), for a total of 95,000 anti-Factor Xa IU per vial. Each prefilled syringe also contains Water for Injection and sodium chloride, when required, to maintain physiologic ionic strength. The prefilled syringes are preservative-free.

Table 9

Bleeding Reactions (Major and Any) (As treated population)[1]

Study period	FRAGMIN 200 IU/kg (max. 18,000 IU) subcutaneous once daily × 1 month, then 150 IU/kg (max. 18,000 IU) subcutaneous once daily × 5 months			OAC FRAGMIN 200 IU/kg (max 18,000 IU) subcutaneous once daily × 5-7 days and OAC for 6 months (target INR 2-3)		
	Number at risk	Patients with Major Bleeding n (%)	Patients with Any Bleeding n (%)	Number at risk	Patients with Major Bleeding n (%)	Patients with Any Bleeding n (%)
Total during study	338	19 (5.6)	46 (13.6)	335	12 (3.6)	62 (18.5)
Week 1	338	4 (1.2)	15 (4.4)	335	4 (1.2)	12 (3.6)
Weeks 2-4	332	9 (2.7)	17 (5.1)	321	1 (0.3)	12 (3.7)
Weeks 5-28	297	9 (3.0)	26 (8.8)	267	8 (3.0)	40 (15.0)

[1] Patients with multiple bleeding episodes within any time interval were counted only once in that interval. However, patients with multiple bleeding episodes that occurred at different time intervals were counted once in each interval in which the event occurred.

STRUCTURAL FORMULA

R = H or SO$_3$Na
R$_1$ = COCH$_3$ or SO$_3$Na
R$_2$ = H R$_3$ = COONa
or
R$_2$ = COONa R$_3$ = H

n = 3–20

Table 10

Efficacy of FRAGMIN in the Prophylaxis of Ischemic Complications in Unstable Angina and Non-Q-Wave Myocardial Infarction

Indication	Dosing Regimen	
	FRAGMIN 120 IU/kg/every 12 hr subcutaneous n (%)	Placebo every 12 hr subcutaneous n (%)
All Treated Unstable Angina and Non-Q-Wave MI Patients	746	760
Primary Endpoints - 6 day timepoint Death, MI	13/741 (1.8)[1]	36/757 (4.8)
Secondary Endpoints - 6 day timepoint Death, MI, intravenous heparin, i.v. nitroglycerin, Revascularization	59/739 (8.0)[1]	106/756 (14.0)

[1] p-value = 0.001

Each multiple-dose vial also contains Water for Injection and 14 mg of benzyl alcohol per mL as a preservative. The pH of both formulations is 5.0 to 7.5. [See *Dosage Forms and Strengths* (3) and *How Supplied* (16)]

Dalteparin sodium is produced through controlled nitrous acid depolymerization of sodium heparin from porcine intestinal mucosa followed by a chromatographic purification process. It is composed of strongly acidic sulfated polysaccharide chains (oligosaccharide, containing 2,5-anhydro-D-mannitol residues as end groups) with an average molecular weight of 5000 and about 90% of the material within the range 2000-9000. The molecular weight distribution is:

< 3000 daltons 3.0-15%
3000 to 8000 daltons 65.0-78.0%
> 8000 daltons 14.0-26.0%

[See chemical structure on previous page]

12   CLINICAL PHARMACOLOGY

12.1   Mechanism of Action

Dalteparin is a low molecular weight heparin with antithrombotic properties. It acts by enhancing the inhibition of Factor Xa and thrombin by antithrombin. In humans, dalteparin potentiates preferentially the inhibition of coagulation Factor Xa, while only slightly affecting the activated partial thromboplastin time (APTT).

12.2   Pharmacodynamics

Doses of FRAGMIN Injection of up to 10,000 anti-Factor Xa IU administered subcutaneously as a single dose or two 5000 IU doses 12 hours apart to healthy subjects did not produce a significant change in platelet aggregation, fibrinolysis, or global clotting tests such as prothrombin time (PT), thrombin time (TT) or APTT. Subcutaneous administration of doses of 5000 IU twice daily of FRAGMIN for seven consecutive days to patients undergoing abdominal surgery did not markedly affect APTT, Platelet Factor 4 (PF4), or lipoprotein lipase.

12.3   Pharmacokinetics

Mean peak levels of plasma anti-Factor Xa activity following single subcutaneous doses of 2500, 5000 and 10,000 IU were 0.19 ± 0.04, 0.41 ± 0.07 and 0.82 ± 0.10 IU/mL, respectively, and were attained in about 4 hours in most subjects. Absolute bioavailability in healthy volunteers, measured as the anti-Factor Xa activity, was $87 \pm 6\%$. Increasing the dose from 2500 to 10,000 IU resulted in an overall increase in anti-Factor Xa AUC that was greater than proportional by about one-third.

Peak anti-Factor Xa activity increased more or less linearly with dose over the same dose range. There appeared to be no appreciable accumulation of anti-Factor Xa activity with twice-daily dosing of 100 IU/kg subcutaneously for up to 7 days.

The volume of distribution for dalteparin anti-Factor Xa activity was 40 to 60 mL/kg. The mean plasma clearances of dalteparin anti-Factor Xa activity in normal volunteers following single intravenous bolus doses of 30 and 120 anti-Factor Xa IU/kg were 24.6 ± 5.4 and 15.6 ± 2.4 mL/hr/kg, respectively. The corresponding mean disposition half-lives were 1.47 ± 0.3 and 2.5 ± 0.3 hours.

Following intravenous doses of 40 and 60 IU/kg, mean terminal half-lives were 2.1 ± 0.3 and 2.3 ± 0.4 hours, respectively. Longer apparent terminal half-lives (3 to 5 hours) are observed following subcutaneous dosing, possibly due to delayed absorption. In patients with chronic renal insufficiency requiring hemodialysis, the mean terminal half-life of anti-Factor Xa activity following a single intravenous dose of 5000 IU FRAGMIN was 5.7 ± 2.0 hours, i.e. considerably longer than values observed in healthy volunteers, therefore, greater accumulation can be expected in these patients.

13   NONCLINICAL TOXICOLOGY

13.1   Carcinogenicity, Mutagenesis, Impairment of Fertility

Dalteparin sodium has not been tested for its carcinogenic potential in long-term animal studies. It was not mutagenic in the *in vitro* Ames Test, mouse lymphoma cell forward mutation test and human lymphocyte chromosomal aberration test and in the *in vivo* mouse micronucleus test. Dalteparin sodium at subcutaneous doses up to 1200 IU/kg (7080 IU/m²) did not affect the fertility or reproductive performance of male and female rats.

14   CLINICAL STUDIES

14.1   Prophylaxis of Ischemic Complications in Unstable Angina and Non-Q-Wave Myocardial Infarction

In a double-blind, randomized, placebo-controlled clinical trial, patients who recently experienced unstable angina with EKG changes or non-Q-wave myocardial infarction (MI) were randomized to FRAGMIN Injection 120 IU/kg or placebo every 12 hours subcutaneously. In this trial, unstable angina was defined to include only angina with EKG changes. All patients, except when contraindicated, were treated concurrently with aspirin (75 mg once daily) and beta blockers. Treatment was initiated within 72 hours of the event (the majority of patients received treatment within 24 hours) and continued for 5 to 8 days. A total of

Table 11

Efficacy of FRAGMIN in the Prophylaxis of Deep Vein Thrombosis Following Hip Replacement Surgery

Indication	Dosing Regimen	
	FRAGMIN 5000 IU once daily[1] subcutaneous n (%)	Warfarin Sodium once daily[2] oral n (%)
All Treated Hip Replacement Surgery Patients	271	279
Treatment Failures in Evaluable Patients DVT, Total	28/192 (14.6)[3]	49/190 (25.8)
Proximal DVT	10/192 (5.2)[4]	16/190 (8.4)
PE	2/271 (0.7)	2/279 (0.7)

[1] The daily dose on the day of surgery was divided: 2500 IU was given two hours before surgery and again in the evening of the day of surgery.
[2] Warfarin sodium dosage was adjusted to maintain a prothrombin time index of 1.4 to 1.5, corresponding to an International Normalized Ratio (INR) of approximately 2.5
[3] p-value = 0.006
[4] p-value = 0.185

Table 12

Efficacy of FRAGMIN in the Prophylaxis of Deep Vein Thrombosis Following Abdominal Surgery

Indication	Dosing Regimen	
	FRAGMIN 2500 IU once daily subcutaneous n (%)	Placebo once daily subcutaneous n (%)
All Treated Abdominal Surgery Patients	102	102
Treatment Failures in Evaluable Patients Total Thromboembolic Reactions	4/91 (4.4)[1]	16/91 (17.6)
Proximal DVT	0	5/91 (5.5)
Distal DVT	4/91 (4.4)	11/91 (12.1)
PE	0	2/91 (2.2)[2]

[1] p-value = 0.008
[2] Both patients also had DVT, 1 proximal and 1 distal

Table 13

Efficacy of FRAGMIN in the Prophylaxis of Deep Vein Thrombosis Following Abdominal Surgery

Indication	Dosing Regimen	
	FRAGMIN 2500 IU once daily subcutaneous n (%)	Heparin 5000 U twice daily subcutaneous n (%)
All Treated Abdominal Surgery Patients	195	196
Treatment Failures in Evaluable Patients Total Thromboembolic Reactions	7/178 (3.9)[1]	7/174 (4.0)
Proximal DVT	3/178 (1.7)	4/174 (2.3)
Distal DVT	3/178 (1.7)	3/174 (1.7)
PE	1/178 (0.6)	0

[1] p-value = 0.74

1506 patients were enrolled and treated; 746 received FRAGMIN and 760 received placebo. The mean age of the study population was 68 years (range 40 to 90 years) and the majority of patients were white (99.7%) and male (63.9%). The combined incidence of the endpoint of death or myocardial infarction was lower for FRAGMIN compared with placebo at 6 days after initiation of therapy. These results were observed in an analysis of all-randomized and all-treated patients. The combined incidence of death, MI, need for intravenous heparin or intravenous. nitroglycerin, and revascularization was also lower for FRAGMIN than for placebo (see Table 10).

[See table 10 on previous page]

In a second randomized, controlled trial designed to evaluate long term treatment with FRAGMIN (days 6 to 45), data were also collected comparing 1-week (5 to 8 days) treatment of FRAGMIN 120 IU/kg every 12 hours subcutaneously with heparin at an APTT-adjusted dosage. All patients, except when contraindicated, were treated concur-

rently with aspirin (100 to 165 mg per day). Of the 1499 patients enrolled, 1482 patients were treated; 751 received FRAGMIN and 731 received heparin. The mean age of the study population was 64 years (range 25 to 92 years) and the majority of patients were white (96.0%) and male (64.2%). The incidence of the combined endpoint of death, myocardial infarction, or recurrent angina during this 1-week treatment period (5 to 8 days) was 9.3% for FRAGMIN and 7.6% for heparin (p=0.323).

14.2   Prophylaxis of Deep Vein Thrombosis in Patients Following Hip Replacement Surgery

In an open-label randomized study, FRAGMIN 5000 IU administered once daily subcutaneously was compared with warfarin sodium, administered orally, in patients undergoing hip replacement surgery. Treatment with FRAGMIN was initiated with a 2500 IU dose subcutaneously within 2 hours before surgery, followed by a 2500 IU dose subcutaneously the evening of the day of surgery. Then, a dosing regimen of FRAGMIN 5000 IU subcutaneously once daily

Table 14

Efficacy of FRAGMIN in the Prophylaxis of Deep Vein Thrombosis Following Abdominal Surgery

Indication	Dosing Regimen	
	FRAGMIN 2500 IU once daily subcutaneous n (%)	FRAGMIN 5000 IU once daily subcutaneous n (%)
All Treated Abdominal Surgery Patients[1]	696	679
Treatment Failures in Evaluable Patients Total Thromboembolic Reactions	99/656 (15.1)[2]	60/645 (9.3)
Proximal DVT	18/657 (2.7)	14/646 (2.2)
Distal DVT	80/657 (12.2)	41/646 (6.3)
PE		
Fatal	1/674 (0.1)	1/669 (0.1)
Non-fatal	2	4

[1] Major abdominal surgery with malignancy
[2] p-value = 0.001

Table 15

Efficacy of FRAGMIN in the Prophylaxis of Deep Vein Thrombosis in Medical Patients with Severely Restricted Mobility During Acute Illness

Indication	Dosing Regimen	
	FRAGMIN 5000 IU once daily subcutaneous n (%)	Placebo once daily subcutaneous n (%)
All Treated Medical Patients During Acute Illness	1848	1833
Treatment failure in evaluable patients (Day 21)[1] DVT, PE, or sudden death	42/1518 (2.8)[2]	73/1473 (5.0)
Total thromboembolic reactions (Day 21)	37/1513 (2.5)	70/1470 (4.8)
Total DVT	32/1508 (2.1)	64/1464 (4.4)
Proximal DVT	29/1518 (1.9)	60/1474 (4.1)
Symptomatic VTE	10/1759 (0.6)	17/1740 (1.0)
PE	5/1759 (0.3)	6/1740 (0.3)
Sudden Death	5/1829 (0.3)	3/1807 (0.2)

[1] Defined as DVT (diagnosed by compression ultrasound at Day 21 + 3), confirmed symptomatic DVT, confirmed PE or sudden death.
[2] p-value = 0.0015

was initiated on the first postoperative day. The first dose of warfarin sodium was given the evening before surgery, then continued daily at a dose adjusted for INR 2 to 3. Treatment in both groups was then continued for 5 to 9 days postoperatively. Of the 580 patients enrolled, 553 were treated and 550 underwent surgery. Of those who underwent surgery, 271 received FRAGMIN and 279 received warfarin sodium. The mean age of the study population was 63 years (range 20 to 92 years) and the majority of patients were white (91.1%) and female (52.9%). The incidence of deep vein thrombosis (DVT), as determined by evaluable venography, was significantly lower for the group treated with FRAGMIN compared with patients treated with warfarin sodium (see Table 11).
[See table 11 at top of previous page]
In a second single-center, double-blind study of patients undergoing hip replacement surgery, FRAGMIN 5000 IU once daily subcutaneously starting the evening before surgery, was compared with heparin 5000 U subcutaneously three times a day, starting the morning of surgery. Treatment in both groups was continued for up to 9 days postoperatively. Of the 140 patients enrolled, 139 were treated and 136 underwent surgery. Of those who underwent surgery, 67 received FRAGMIN and 69 received heparin. The mean age of the study population was 69 years (range 42 to 87 years) and the majority of patients were female (58.8%). In the intent-to-treat analysis, the incidence of proximal DVT was significantly lower for patients treated with FRAGMIN compared with patients treated with heparin (6/67 vs 18/69; p=0.012). The incidence of pulmonary embolism detected by lung scan was also significantly lower in the group treated with FRAGMIN (9/67 vs 19/69; p=0.032).

A third multi-center, double-blind, randomized study evaluated a postoperative dosing regimen of FRAGMIN for thromboprophylaxis following total hip replacement surgery. Patients received either FRAGMIN or warfarin sodium, randomized into one of three treatment groups. One group of patients received the first dose of FRAGMIN 2500 IU subcutaneous within 2 hours before surgery, followed by another dose of FRAGMIN 2500 IU subcutaneous at least 4 hours (6.6 ± 2.3 hr) after surgery. Another group received the first dose of FRAGMIN 2500 IU subcutaneous at least 4 hours (6.6 ± 2.4 hr) after surgery. Then, **both** of these groups began a dosing regimen of FRAGMIN 5000 IU once daily subcutaneous on postoperative day 1. The third group of patients received warfarin sodium the evening of the day of surgery, then continued daily at a dose adjusted to maintain INR 2 to 3. Treatment for all groups was continued for 4 to 8 days postoperatively, after which time all patients underwent bilateral venography.
In the total enrolled study population of 1501 patients, 1472 patients were treated; 496 received FRAGMIN (first dose before surgery), 487 received FRAGMIN (first dose after surgery) and 489 received warfarin sodium. The mean age of the study population was 63 years (range 18 to 91 years) and the majority of patients were white (94.4%) and female (51.8%).
Administration of the first dose of FRAGMIN after surgery was as effective in reducing the incidence of thromboembolic reactions as administration of the first dose of FRAGMIN before surgery (44/336 vs 37/338; p=0.448). Both dosing regimens of FRAGMIN were more effective than warfarin sodium in reducing the incidence of thromboembolic reactions following hip replacement surgery.

14.3 Prophylaxis of Deep Vein Thrombosis Following Abdominal Surgery in Patients at Risk for Thromboembolic Complications

Abdominal surgery patients at risk include those who are over 40 years of age, obese, undergoing surgery under general anesthesia lasting longer than 30 minutes, or who have additional risk factors such as malignancy or a history of deep vein thrombosis or pulmonary embolism.
FRAGMIN administered once daily subcutaneously beginning prior to surgery and continued for 5 to 10 days after surgery, reduced the risk of DVT in patients at risk for thromboembolic complications in two double-blind, randomized, controlled clinical trials performed in patients undergoing major abdominal surgery. In the first study, a total of 204 patients were enrolled and treated; 102 received FRAGMIN and 102 received placebo. The mean age of the study population was 64 years (range 40 to 98 years) and the majority of patients were female (54.9%). In the second study, a total of 391 patients were enrolled and treated; 195 received FRAGMIN and 196 received heparin. The mean age of the study population was 59 years (range 30 to 88 years) and the majority of patients were female (51.9%). FRAGMIN 2500 IU was superior to placebo and similar to heparin in reducing the risk of DVT (see Tables 12 and 13).
[See table 12 on previous page]
[See table 13 on previous page]
In a third double-blind, randomized study performed in patients undergoing major abdominal surgery with malignancy, FRAGMIN 5000 IU subcutaneous once daily was compared with FRAGMIN 2500 IU subcutaneous once daily. Treatment was continued for 6 to 8 days. A total of 1375 patients were enrolled and treated; 679 received FRAGMIN 5000 IU and 696 received 2500 IU. The mean age of the combined groups was 71 years (range 40 to 95 years). The majority of patients were female (51.0%). FRAGMIN 5000 IU once daily was more effective than FRAGMIN 2500 IU once daily in reducing the risk of DVT in patients undergoing abdominal surgery with malignancy (see Table 14).
[See table 14 at left]

14.4 Prophylaxis of Deep Vein Thrombosis in Medical Patients at Risk for Thromboembolic Complications Due to Severely Restricted Mobility During Acute Illness

In a double-blind, multi-center, randomized, placebo-controlled clinical trial, general medical patients with severely restricted mobility who were at risk of venous thromboembolism were randomized to receive either FRAGMIN 5000 IU or placebo subcutaneously once daily during Days 1 to 14 of the study. These patients had an acute medical condition requiring a projected hospital stay of at least 4 days, and were confined to bed during waking hours. The study included patients with congestive heart failure (NYHA Class III or IV), acute respiratory failure not requiring ventilatory support, and the following acute conditions with at least one risk factor occurring in > 1% of treated patients: acute infection (excluding septic shock), acute rheumatic disorder, acute lumbar or sciatic pain, vertebral compression, or acute arthritis of the lower extremities. Risk factors include > 75 years of age, cancer, previous DVT/PE, obesity and chronic venous insufficiency. A total of 3681 patients were enrolled and treated: 1848 received FRAGMIN and 1833 received placebo. The mean age of the study population was 69 years (range 26 to 99 years), 92.1% were white and 51.9% were female. The primary efficacy endpoint was evaluated at Day 21 and was defined as at least one of the following within Days 1 to 21 of the study: asymptomatic DVT (diagnosed by compression ultrasound), a confirmed symptomatic DVT, a confirmed pulmonary embolism or sudden death. The follow-up extended through Day 90
When given at a dose of 5000 IU once a day subcutaneously, FRAGMIN significantly reduced the incidence of thromboembolic reactions including verified DVT by Day 21 (see Table 15). The prophylactic effect was sustained through Day 90.
[See table 15 at left]

14.5 Patients with Cancer and Acute Symptomatic Venous Thromboembolism

In a prospective, multi-center, open-label, clinical trial, 676 patients with cancer and newly diagnosed, objectively confirmed acute deep vein thrombosis (DVT) and/or pulmonary embolism (PE) were studied. Patients were randomized to either FRAGMIN 200 IU/kg subcutaneous (max 18,000 IU subcutaneous daily for one month) then 150 IU/kg subcutaneous (max 18,000 IU subcutaneous daily for five months (FRAGMIN arm) or FRAGMIN 200 IU/kg subcutaneous (max 18,000 IU subcutaneous daily for five to seven days and oral anticoagulant for six months (OAC arm). In the OAC arm, oral anticoagulation was adjusted to maintain an INR of 2 to 3. Patients were evaluated for recurrence of symptomatic venous thromboembolism (VTE) every two weeks for six months.
The median age of the patients was 64 years (range: 22 to 89 years); 51.5% of patients were females; 95.3% of patients were Caucasians. Types of tumors were: gastrointestinal

Table 16

Recurrent VTE in Patients with Cancer (Intention to treat population)[1]

Study Period	FRAGMIN arm			OAC arm		
	FRAGMIN 200 IU/kg (max. 18,000 IU) subcutaneous once daily × 1 month, then 150 IU/kg (max. 18,000 IU) subcutaneous once daily × 5 months			FRAGMIN 200 IU/kg (max 18,000 IU) subcutaneous once daily × 5-7 days and OAC for 6 months (target INR 2-3)		
	Number at Risk	Patients with VTE	%	Number at Risk	Patients with VTE	%
Total	338	27	8.0	338	53	15.7
Week 1	338	5	1.5	338	8	2.4
Weeks 2-4	331	6	1.8	327	25	7.6
Weeks 5-28	307	16	5.2	284	20	7.0

[1] Three patients in the FRAGMIN arm and 5 patients in the OAC arm experienced more than 1 VTE over the 6-month study period.

Dosage Form	Strength	Package Size	NDC Number
Single-dose prefilled syringe[1]	2,500 IU/0.2 mL	10 Syringes	62856-250-10
	5,000 IU/0.2 mL	10 Syringes	62856-500-10
	7,500 IU/0.3 mL	10 Syringes	62856-750-10
	10,000 IU/0.4 mL	10 Syringes	62856-100-10
Single-dose graduated syringe[2]	10,000 IU/1 mL	10 Syringes	62856-101-10
Single-dose prefilled syringe[1]	12,500 IU/0.5 mL	10 Syringes	62856-125-10
	15,000 IU/0.6 mL	10 Syringes	62856-150-10
	18,000 IU/0.72 mL	10 Syringes	62856-180-10
Multiple dose vial	95,000 IU/3.8 mL	3.8 mL vial	62856-251-01
Multiple dose vial	95,000 IU/9.5 mL	9.5 mL Vial	62856-102-01

[1] Single-dose prefilled syringe, affixed with a 27-gauge × 1/2 inch needle and preassembled with UltraSafe Passive™ Needle Guard devices.
[2] Single-dose graduated syringe, affixed with a 27-gauge × 1/2 inch needle and preassembled with UltraSafe Passive™ Needle Guard devices. UltraSafe Passive™ Needle Guard is a trademark of Safety Syringes, Inc.

tract (23.7%), genito-urinary (21.5%), breast (16%), lung (13.3%), hematological tumors (10.4%) and other tumors (15.1%).
A total of 27 (8.0%) and 53 (15.7%) patients in the FRAGMIN and OAC arms, respectively, experienced at least one episode of an objectively confirmed, symptomatic DVT and/or PE during the 6-month study period. Most of the difference occurred during the first month of treatment (see Table 16). The benefit was maintained over the 6-month study period.
[See table 16 above]
In the intent-to-treat population that included all randomized patients, the primary comparison of the cumulative probability of the first VTE recurrence over the 6-month study period was statistically significant (p < 0.01) in favor of the FRAGMIN arm, with most of the treatment difference evident in the first month.

16 HOW SUPPLIED/STORAGE AND HANDLING
After first penetration of the rubber stopper, store the multiple-dose vials at room temperature for up to 2 weeks.
[See second table above]
Store at controlled room temperature 20° to 25°C (68° to 77°F) [see USP].

17 PATIENT COUNSELING INFORMATION
If patients have had neuraxial anesthesia or spinal puncture, and particularly, if they are taking concomitant NSAIDs, platelet inhibitors, or other anticoagulants, inform the patients to watch for signs and symptoms of spinal or epidural hematoma, such as tingling, numbness (especially in the lower limbs) and muscular weakness. If any of these symptoms occur the patient should contact his or her physician immediately.
Additionally, the use of aspirin and other NSAIDs may enhance the risk of hemorrhage. Discontinue their use prior to dalteparin therapy whenever possible; if co-administration is essential, the patient's clinical and laboratory status should be closely monitored [see Drug Interactions (7)].
Inform patients:
• of the instructions for injecting FRAGMIN if their therapy is to continue after discharge from the hospitals.

• it may take them longer than usual to stop bleeding.
• they may bruise and/or bleed more easily when they are treated with FRAGMIN.
• they should report any unusual bleeding, bruising, or signs of thrombocytopenia (such as a rash of dark red spots under the skin) to their physician [see Warnings and Precautions (5.1, 5.2)].
• to tell their physicians and dentists they are taking FRAGMIN and/or any other product known to affect bleeding before any surgery is scheduled and before any new drug is taken [see Warnings and Precautions (5.1)].
• to tell their physicians and dentists of all medications they are taking, including those obtained without a prescription, such as aspirin or other NSAIDs [see Drug Interactions (7)].
FRAGMIN is a registered trademark of Pfizer Health AB and is licensed to Eisai Inc.
Manufactured for
Eisai Inc.
Woodcliff Lake, NJ 07677
Manufactured by
Pfizer Inc
New York, NY 10017
Made in Belgium
(multiple-dose vials)
Jointly manufactured by
Pfizer Inc, New York, NY 10017
and Vetter Pharma-Fertigung, GmbH & Co. KG
Ravensburg, Germany
(prefilled syringes)
Insert Code
Revised December 2009
Shown in Product Identification Guide, page 308

GLIADEL® WAFER ℞
[gli-uh-del]
(polifeprosan 20 with carmustine implant)
Rx only

DESCRIPTION
GLIADEL® Wafer (polifeprosan 20 with carmustine implant) is a sterile, off-white to pale yellow wafer approx-

imately 1.45 cm in diameter and 1 mm thick. Each wafer contains 192.3 mg of a biodegradable polyanhydride copolymer and 7.7 mg of carmustine [1,3-bis (2-chloroethyl)-1-nitrosourea, or BCNU]. Carmustine is a nitrosourea oncolytic agent. The copolymer, polifeprosan 20, consists of poly[bis(p-carboxyphenoxy) propane: sebacic acid] in a 20:80 molar ratio and is used to control the local delivery of carmustine. Carmustine is homogeneously distributed in the copolymer matrix.
The structural formula for polifeprosan 20 is:

$$\left[O-C(=O)-C_6H_4-O(CH_2)_3O-C_6H_4-C(=O)-O \right]_m \left[O-C(=O)-CH_2(CH_2)_6CH_2-C(=O) \right]_n$$

Ratio m:n = 20:80; random copolymer

The structural formula for carmustine is:

$$Cl-CH_2-CH_2-N(NO)CNHCH_2-CH_2-Cl \quad (C=O)$$

CLINICAL PHARMACOLOGY
GLIADEL® Wafer is designed to deliver carmustine directly into the surgical cavity created when a brain tumor is resected. On exposure to the aqueous environment of the resection cavity, the anhydride bonds in the copolymer are hydrolyzed, releasing carmustine, carboxyphenoxypropane, and sebacic acid. The carmustine released from GLIADEL® Wafer diffuses into the surrounding brain tissue and produces an antineoplastic effect by alkylating DNA and RNA. Carmustine has been shown to degrade both spontaneously and metabolically. The production of an alkylating moiety, hypothesized to be chloroethyl carbonium ion, leads to the formation of DNA cross-links.
The tumoricidal activity of GLIADEL® Wafer is dependent on release of carmustine to the tumor cavity in concentrations sufficient for effective cytotoxicity.
More than 70% of the copolymer degrades by three weeks. The metabolic disposition and excretion of the monomers differ. Carboxyphenoxypropane is eliminated by the kidney and sebacic acid, an endogenous fatty acid, is metabolized by the liver and expired as CO_2 in animals.
The absorption, distribution, metabolism, and excretion of the copolymer in humans is unknown. Carmustine concentrations delivered by GLIADEL® Wafer in human brain tissue have not been determined. Plasma levels of carmustine after GLIADEL® Wafer implant were not determined. In rabbits implanted with wafers containing 3.85% carmustine, no detectible levels of carmustine were found in the plasma or cerebrospinal fluid.
Following an intravenous infusion of carmustine at doses ranging from 30 to 170 mg/m², the average terminal half-life, clearance, and steady-state volume of distribution were 22 minutes, 56 mL/min/kg, and 3.25 L/kg, respectively. Approximately 60% of the intravenous 200 mg/m² dose of ¹⁴C-carmustine was excreted in the urine over 96 hours and 6% was expired as CO_2.
GLIADEL® Wafers are biodegradable in human brain when implanted into the cavity after tumor resection. The rate of biodegradation is variable from patient to patient. During the biodegradation process, a wafer remnant may be observed on brain imaging scans or at re-operation even though extensive degradation of all components has occurred. Data obtained from review of CT scans obtained 49 days after implantation of GLIADEL® Wafer demonstrated that images consistent with wafers were visible to varying degrees in the scans of 11 of 18 patients. Data obtained at re-operation and autopsies have demonstrated wafer remnants up to 232 days after GLIADEL® Wafer implantation.
Wafer remnants removed at re-operation from two patients with recurrent malignant glioma, one at 64 days and the second at 92 days after implantation, were analyzed for content. The following table presents the results of analyses completed on these remnants.

COMPOSITION OF WAFER REMNANTS REMOVED FROM TWO PATIENTS ON RE-OPERATION

Component	Patient A	Patient B
Days After GLIADEL® Wafer Implantation	64	92
Anhydride Bonds	None detected	None detected
Water Content (% of wafer remnant weight)	95-97%	74-86%

	<0.0004%	0.034%
Carmustine Content (% of initial)	<0.0004%	0.034%
Carboxyphenoxypropane Content (% of initial)	9%	14%
Sebacic Acid Content (% of initial)	4%	3%

The wafer remnants consisted mostly of water and monomeric components with minimal detectable carmustine present.

CLINICAL STUDIES

Primary Surgery

A randomized, double-blind, placebo-controlled clinical trial was conducted in adult patients with newly-diagnosed high-grade malignant glioma undergoing initial craniotomy for tumor resection. This trial determined the safety and efficacy of GLIADEL® Wafer implants plus surgery and radiation therapy compared to placebo implants plus surgery and radiation therapy. Two hundred and forty patients with newly-diagnosed malignant glioma were enrolled. The most common tumor type was Glioblastoma Multiforme (GBM) (n=207), followed by anaplastic oligoastrocytoma (n=11), anaplastic oligodendroglioma (n=11), and anaplastic astrocytoma (n=2). GLIADEL® Wafers were implanted at the time of the surgery in 120 patients and placebo wafers were implanted in 120 patients. The majority of patients received 6-8 wafers. The majority of patients (93/120, 77.5% in the GLIADEL® Wafer group and 98/120, 81.7% in the placebo group) with newly-diagnosed malignant glioma received a standard course of radiotherapy (55 to 60 Gy) typically starting 3 weeks after surgery. There were 17 patients (14.2%) in the GLIADEL® Wafer group and 12 patients (10.0%) in the placebo group who received systemic chemotherapy during the study. All six patients with anaplastic oligodendroglioma received chemotherapy within 30 days of GLIADEL® Wafer implantation. Patients were followed for at least three years or until death. Only one patient was lost to follow-up. Median survival increased from 11.6 months with placebo to 13.8 months with GLIADEL® Wafer (p-value <0.05, log-rank test). The hazard ratio for GLIADEL® Wafer treatment was 0.73 (95% CI: 0.56-0.95).

Kaplan-Meier Overall Survival Curves for Patients Undergoing Initial Surgery for a High-Grade Malignant Glioma

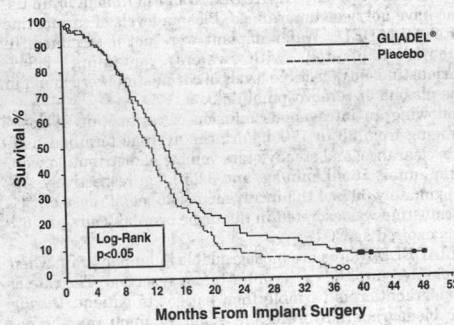

When only patients with Glioblastoma multiforme were included in the analysis, the hazard ratio with GLIADEL® Wafer treatment was 0.78 (95% CI: 0.59-1.03, p=0.08, log-rank test).

Surgery for Recurrent Disease

A randomized, double-blind, placebo-controlled clinical trial was conducted in adult patients with recurrent malignant glioma. This trial determined the safety and efficacy of GLIADEL® Wafer implants plus surgery compared to placebo implants plus surgery.

Ninety-five percent of the patients treated with GLIADEL® Wafer had 7-8 wafers implanted. Chemotherapy was withheld at least four weeks (six weeks for nitrosoureas) prior to and two weeks after surgery in patients undergoing re-operation for malignant glioma. In 222 patients with recurrent malignant glioma who had failed initial surgery and radiation therapy, the six-month survival rate after repeat surgery increased from 47% (53/112) for patients receiving placebo to 60% (66/110) for patients treated with GLIADEL® Wafer. Median survival increased by 33%, from 24 weeks (5.5 months) with placebo to 32 weeks (7.4 months) with GLIADEL® Wafer treatment. In patients with GBM, the six-month survival rate increased from 36% (26/73) with placebo to 56% (40/72) with GLIADEL® Wafer treatment. Median survival of GBM patients increased by 41% from 20 weeks (4.6 months) with placebo to 28 weeks (6.4 months) with GLIADEL® Wafer treatment. In patients with pathologic diagnoses other than GBM at the time of surgery for tumor recurrence, GLIADEL® Wafer produced no survival prolongation.

6-MONTH KAPLAN-MEIER SURVIVAL CURVES FOR PATIENTS UNDERGOING SURGERY FOR RECURRENT GBM

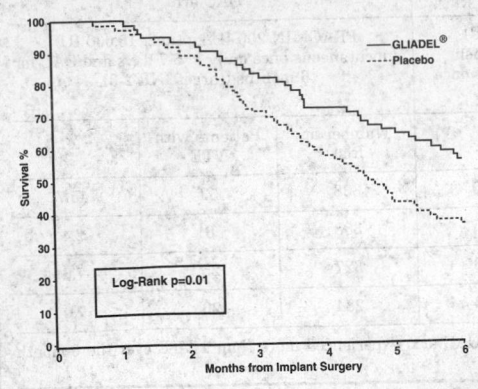

KAPLAN-MEIER OVERALL SURVIVAL CURVES FOR PATIENTS UNDERGOING SURGERY FOR RECURRENT GBM

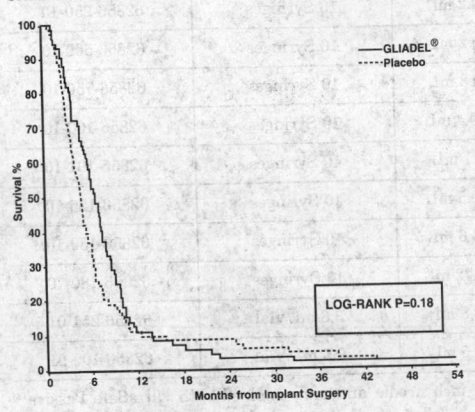

INDICATIONS AND USAGE

GLIADEL® Wafer is indicated in newly-diagnosed high-grade malignant glioma patients as an adjunct to surgery and radiation. GLIADEL® Wafer is indicated in recurrent glioblastoma multiforme patients as an adjunct to surgery.

CONTRAINDICATIONS

GLIADEL® Wafer contains carmustine. GLIADEL® Wafer should not be given to individuals who have demonstrated a previous hypersensitivity to carmustine or any of the components of GLIADEL® Wafer.

WARNINGS

Patients undergoing craniotomy for malignant glioma and implantation of GLIADEL® Wafer should be monitored closely for known complications of craniotomy, including seizures, intracranial infections, abnormal wound healing, and brain edema. Cases of intracerebral mass effect unresponsive to corticosteroids have been described in patients treated with GLIADEL® Wafer, including one case leading to brain herniation.

Pregnancy: There are no studies assessing the reproductive toxicity of GLIADEL® Wafer. Carmustine, the active component of GLIADEL® Wafer, can cause fetal harm when administered to a pregnant woman. Carmustine has been shown to be embryotoxic and teratogenic in rats at i.p. doses of 0.5, 1, 2, 4, or 8 mg/kg/day when given on gestation days 6 through 15. Carmustine caused fetal malformations (anophthalmia, micrognathia, omphalocele) at 1.0 mg/kg/day (about 1/6 the recommended human dose (eight wafers of 7.7 mg carmustine/wafer) on a mg/m^2 basis). Carmustine was embryotoxic in rabbits at i.v. doses of 4.0 mg/kg/day (about 1.2 times the recommended human dose on a mg/m^2 basis). Embryotoxicity was characterized by increased embryo-fetal deaths, reduced numbers of litters, and reduced litter sizes.

There are no studies of GLIADEL® Wafer in pregnant women. If GLIADEL® Wafer is used during pregnancy, or if the patient becomes pregnant after GLIADEL® Wafer implantation, the patient must be warned of the potential hazard to the fetus.

PRECAUTIONS

GENERAL

Communication between the surgical resection cavity and the ventricular system should be avoided to prevent the wafers from migrating into the ventricular system and causing obstructive hydrocephalus. If a communication larger than the diameter of a wafer exists, it should be closed prior to wafer implantation.

Computed tomography and magnetic resonance imaging of the head may demonstrate enhancement in the brain tissue surrounding the resection cavity after implantation of GLIADEL® Wafers. This enhancement may represent edema and inflammation caused by GLIADEL® Wafer or tumor progression.

THERAPEUTIC INTERACTIONS

Interactions of GLIADEL® Wafer with other drugs have not been formally evaluated.

The short-term and long-term toxicity profiles of GLIADEL® Wafer when given in conjunction with chemotherapy have not been fully explored. GLIADEL® Wafer, when given in conjunction with radiotherapy does not appear to have any short-term or chronic toxicities.

CARCINOGENESIS, MUTAGENESIS, IMPAIRMENT OF FERTILITY

No carcinogenicity, mutagenicity or impairment of fertility studies have been conducted with GLIADEL® Wafer. Carcinogenicity, mutagenicity and impairment of fertility studies have been conducted with carmustine, the active component of GLIADEL® Wafer. Carmustine was given three times a week for six months, followed by 12 months observation, to Swiss mice at i.p. doses of 2.5 and 5.0 mg/kg (about 1/5 and 1/3 the recommended human dose (eight wafers of 7.7 mg carmustine/wafer) on a mg/m^2 basis) and to SD rats at i.p. dose of 1.5 mg/kg (about 1/4 the recommended human dose on a mg/m^2 basis). There were increases in tumor incidence in all treated animals, predominantly subcutaneous and lung neoplasms. *Mutagenesis:* Carmustine was mutagenic *in vitro* (Ames assay, human lymphoblast HGPRT assay) and clastogenic both *in vitro* (V79 hamster cell micronucleus assay) and *in vivo* (SCE assay in rodent brain tumors, mouse bone marrow micronucleus assay). *Impairment of Fertility:* Carmustine caused testicular degeneration at i.p. doses of 8 mg/kg/week for eight weeks (about 1.3 times the recommended human dose on a mg/m^2 basis) in male rats.

PREGNANCY

Pregnancy Category D: see WARNINGS.

NURSING MOTHERS

It is not known if either carmustine, carboxyphenoxypropane, or sebacic acid is excreted in human milk. Because many drugs are excreted in human milk and because of the potential for serious adverse reactions from carmustine in nursing infants, it is recommended that patients receiving GLIADEL® Wafer discontinue nursing.

PEDIATRIC USE

The safety and effectiveness of GLIADEL® Wafer in pediatric patients have not been established.

ADVERSE REACTIONS

Adverse reactions for the trials are described in the tables below.

Primary Surgery

The following data are the most frequently occurring adverse events observed in 5% or more of the newly-diagnosed malignant glioma patients during the trial.

COMMON ADVERSE EVENTS OBSERVED IN ≥ 5% OF PATIENTS RECEIVING GLIADEL® WAFER AT INITIAL SURGERY

Body System Adverse event	GLIADEL® Wafer [N=120] n (%)	Placebo [N=120] n (%)
Body as a Whole		
Aggravation reaction*	98 (82)	95 (79)
Headache	33 (28)	44 (37)
Asthenia	26 (22)	18 (15)
Infection	22 (18)	24 (20)
Fever	21 (18)	21 (18)
Pain	16 (13)	18 (15)
Abdominal pain	10 (8)	2 (2)
Back pain	8 (7)	4 (3)
Face edema	7 (6)	6 (5)
Abscess	6 (5)	3 (3)
Accidental injury	6 (5)	8 (7)
Chest pain	6 (5)	0

Allergic reaction	2 (2)	6 (5)
Cardiovascular system		
Deep thrombophlebitis	12 (10)	11 (9)
Pulmonary embolus	10 (8)	10 (8)
Hemorrhage	8 (7)	7 (6)
Digestive system		
Nausea	26 (22)	20 (17)
Vomiting	25 (21)	19 (16)
Constipation	23 (19)	14 (12)
Diarrhea	6 (5)	5 (4)
Liver function tests abnormal	1 (1)	6 (5)
Endocrine system		
Diabetes mellitus	6 (5)	5 (4)
Cushings syndrome	4 (3)	6 (5)
Metabolic and nutritional disorders		
Healing abnormal	19 (16)	14 (12)
Peripheral edema	11 (9)	11 (9)
Musculoskeletal system		
Myasthenia	5 (4)	6 (5)
Nervous system		
Hemiplegia	49 (41)	53 (44)
Convulsion	40 (33)	45 (38)
Confusion	28 (23)	25 (21)
Brain edema	27 (23)	23 (19)
Aphasia	21 (18)	22 (18)
Depression	19 (16)	12 (10)
Somnolence	13 (11)	18 (15)
Speech disorder	13 (11)	10 (8)
Amnesia	11 (9)	12 (10)
Intracranial hypertension	11 (9)	2 (2)
Personality disorder	10 (8)	9 (8)
Anxiety	8 (7)	5 (4)
Facial paralysis	8 (7)	5 (4)
Neuropathy	8 (7)	12 (10)
Ataxia	7 (6)	5 (4)
Hypesthesia	7 (6)	6 (5)
Paresthesia	7 (6)	10 (8)
Thinking abnormal	7 (6)	10 (8)
Abnormal gait	6 (5)	6 (5)
Dizziness	6 (5)	11 (9)
Grand mal convulsion	6 (5)	5 (4)
Hallucinations	6 (5)	4 (3)
Insomnia	6 (5)	7 (6)
Tremor	6 (5)	8 (7)
Coma	5 (4)	6 (5)
Incoordination	3 (3)	8 (7)
Hypokinesia	2 (2)	8 (7)

COMMON ADVERSE EVENTS OBSERVED IN ≥ 4% OF PATIENTS RECEIVING GLIADEL® WAFER AT SURGERY FOR RECURRENT DISEASE

Body System Adverse Event	GLIADEL® Wafer with Carmustine [N=110] n (%)	PLACEBO Wafer without Carmustine [N=112] n (%)
Body as a Whole		
Fever	13 (12)	9 (8)
Pain*	8 (7)	1 (1)
Digestive System		
Nausea and Vomiting	9 (8)	7 (6)
Metabolic and Nutritional Disorders		
Healing Abnormal*	15 (14)	6 (5)
Nervous System		
Convulsion	21 (19)	21 (19)
Hemiplegia	21 (19)	22 (20)
Headache	16 (15)	14 (13)
Somnolence	15 (14)	12 (11)
Confusion	11 (10)	9 (8)
Aphasia	10 (9)	12 (11)
Stupor	7 (6)	7 (6)
Brain Edema	4 (4)	1 (1)
Intracranial Hypertension	4 (4)	7 (6)
Meningitis or Abscess	4 (4)	1 (1)
Skin and Appendages		
Rash	6 (5)	4 (4)
Urogenital System		
Urinary Tract Infection	23 (21)	19 (17)

*p < 0.05 for comparison of GLIADEL® Wafer versus placebo groups

Respiratory system		
Pneumonia	10 (8)	9 (8)
Dyspnea	4 (3)	8 (7)
Skin and appendages		
Rash	14 (12)	13 (11)
Alopecia	12 (10)	14 (12)
Special senses		
Conjunctival edema	8 (7)	8 (7)
Abnormal vision	7 (6)	7 (6)
Visual field defect	6 (5)	8 (7)
Eye disorder	3 (3)	6 (5)
Diplopia	1 (1)	6 (5)
Urogenital system		
Urinary tract infection	10 (8)	13 (11)
Urinary incontinence	9 (8)	9 (8)

*Adverse events coded to the COSTART term "aggravation reaction" were usually events involving tumor/disease progression or general deterioration of condition (e.g. condition/health/Karnofsky/neurological/physical deterioration).

Surgery for Recurrent Disease
The following post-operative adverse events were observed in 4% or more of the patients receiving GLIADEL® Wafer at recurrent surgery. Except for nervous system effects, where there is a possibility that the placebo wafers could have been responsible, only events more common in the GLIADEL® Wafer group are listed. These adverse events were either not present pre-operatively or worsened post-operatively during the follow-up period. The follow-up period was up to 71 months.
[See table above]

Post-marketing experience includes spontaneous reports of cyst formation after GLIADEL® wafer implantation. These occurred at varying time intervals post-implantation. Cyst formation has also been reported in patients following resection of malignant glioma who have not had Gliadel® implanted.

The following four categories of adverse events are possibly related to treatment with GLIADEL® Wafer. The frequency with which they occurred in the randomized trials along with descriptive detail is provided below.

1. Seizures: In the initial surgery trial, the incidence of seizures was 33.3% in patients receiving GLIADEL® Wafer and 37.5% in patients receiving placebo. Grand mal seizures occurred in 5% of GLIADEL® Wafer-treated patients and 4.2% of placebo treated patients. The incidence of seizures within the first 5 days after wafer implantation was 2.5% in the GLIADEL® Wafer group and 4.2% in the placebo group. The time from surgery to the onset of the first post-operative seizure did not differ between the GLIADEL® Wafer and placebo treated patients.
In the surgery for recurrent disease trial, the incidence of post-operative seizures was 19% in both patients receiving GLIADEL® Wafer and placebo. In this study, 12/22 (54%) of patients treated with GLIADEL® Wafer and 2/22 (9%) of placebo patients experienced the first new or worsened seizure within the first five post-operative days. The median time to onset of the first new or worsened post-operative seizure was 3.5 days in patients treated with GLIADEL® Wafer and 61 days in placebo patients.
2. Brain Edema: In the initial surgery trial, brain edema was noted in 22.5% of patients treated with GLIADEL® Wafer and in 19.2% of patients treated with placebo. Devel-

opment of brain edema with mass effect (due to tumor recurrence, intracranial infection, or necrosis) may necessitate re-operation and, in some cases, removal of GLIADEL® Wafer or its remnants.

3. Healing Abnormalities: The following healing abnormalities have been reported in clinical trials of GLIADEL® Wafer: wound dehiscence, delayed wound healing, subdural, subgaleal or wound effusions, and cerebrospinal fluid leak. In the initial surgery trial, healing abnormalities occurred in 15.8% of GLIADEL® Wafer treated patients and in 11.7% of placebo recipients. Cerebrospinal fluid leaks occurred in 5% of GLIADEL® Wafer recipients and 0.8% of those given placebo. During surgery, a water-tight dural closure should be obtained to minimize the risk of cerebrospinal fluid leak. In the surgery for recurrent disease trial, the incidence of healing abnormalities was 14% in GLIADEL® Wafer treated patients and 5% in patients receiving placebo wafers.

4. Intracranial Infection: In the initial surgery trial, the incidence of brain abscess or meningitis was 5% in patients treated with GLIADEL® Wafer and 6% in patients receiving placebo. In the recurrent setting, the incidence of brain abscess or meningitis was 4% in patients treated with GLIADEL® Wafer and 1% in patients receiving placebo. The following adverse events, not listed in the table above, were reported in less than 4% but at least 1% of patients treated with GLIADEL® Wafer in all studies. The events listed were either not present pre-operatively or worsened post-operatively. Whether GLIADEL® Wafer caused these events cannot be determined.

Body as a Whole: peripheral edema (2%); neck pain (2%); accidental injury (1%); back pain (1%); allergic reaction (1%); asthenia (1%); chest pain (1%); sepsis (1%)
Cardiovascular System: hypertension (3%); hypotension (1%)
Digestive System: diarrhea (2%); constipation (2%); dysphagia (1%); gastrointestinal hemorrhage (1%); fecal incontinence (1%)
Hemic and Lymphatic System: thrombocytopenia (1%); leukocytosis (1%)
Metabolic and Nutritional Disorders: hyponatremia (3%); hyperglycemia (3%); hypokalemia (1%)
Musculoskeletal System: infection (1%)
Nervous System: hydrocephalus (3%); depression (3%); abnormal thinking (2%); ataxia (2%); dizziness (2%); insomnia (2%); monoplegia (1%); coma (1%); amnesia (1%); diplopia (1%); paranoid reaction (1%). In addition, cerebral hemorrhage and cerebral infarct were each reported in less than 1% of patients treated with GLIADEL® Wafer.
Respiratory System: infection (2%); aspiration pneumonia (1%)
Skin and Appendages: rash (2%)
Special Senses: visual field defect (2%); eye pain (1%)
Urogenital System: urinary incontinence (2%)

OVERDOSAGE

There is no clinical experience with use of more than eight GLIADEL® Wafers per surgical procedure.

DOSAGE AND ADMINISTRATION

Each GLIADEL® Wafer contains 7.7 mg of carmustine, resulting in a dose of 61.6 mg when eight wafers are implanted. It is recommended that eight wafers be placed in the resection cavity if the size and shape of it allows. Should the size and shape not accommodate eight wafers, the maximum number of wafers as allowed should be placed. Since there is no clinical experience, no more than eight wafers should be used per surgical procedure.

Handling and Disposal[1-7]**:** Wafers should only be handled by personnel wearing surgical gloves because exposure to carmustine can cause severe burning and hyperpigmentation of the skin. Use of double gloves is recommended and the outer gloves should be discarded into a biohazard waste container after use. A surgical instrument dedicated to the handling of the wafers should be used for wafer implantation. If repeat neurosurgical intervention is indicated, any wafer or wafer remnant should be handled as a potentially cytotoxic agent.
GLIADEL® Wafer should be handled with care. The aluminum foil laminate pouches containing GLIADEL® Wafer should be delivered to the operating room and remain unopened until ready to implant the wafers. **The outside surface of the outer foil pouch is not sterile.**

Instructions for Opening Pouch Containing GLIADEL® Wafer
Figure 1: To remove the sterile inner pouch from the outer pouch, locate the folded corner and slowly pull in an outward motion.

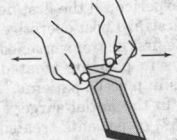

Figure 2: Do NOT pull in a downward motion rolling knuckles over the pouch. This may exert pressure on the wafer and cause it to break.

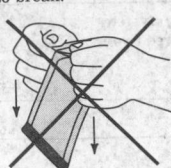

Figure 3: Remove the inner pouch by grabbing hold of the crimped edge and pulling upward.

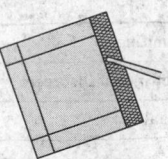

Figure 4: To open the inner pouch, gently hold the crimped edge and cut in an arc-like fashion around the wafer.

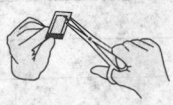

Figure 5: To remove the GLIADEL® Wafer, gently grasp the wafer with the aid of forceps and place it onto a designated sterile field.

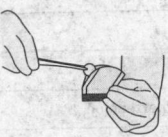

Once the tumor is resected, tumor pathology is confirmed, and hemostasis is obtained, up to eight GLIADEL® Wafers (polifeprosan 20 with carmustine implant) may be placed to cover as much of the resection cavity as possible. Slight overlapping of the wafers is acceptable. Wafers broken in half may be used, but wafers broken in more than two pieces should be discarded in a biohazard container. Oxidized regenerated cellulose (Surgicel®) may be placed over the wafers to secure them against the cavity surface. After placement of the wafers, the resection cavity should be irrigated and the dura closed in a water tight fashion.
Unopened foil pouches may be kept at ambient room temperature for a maximum of six hours at a time.

HOW SUPPLIED

GLIADEL® Wafer is available in a single dose treatment box containing eight individually pouched wafers. Each wafer contains 7.7 mg of carmustine and is packaged in two aluminum foil laminate pouches. The inner pouch is sterile and is designed to maintain product sterility and protect the product from moisture. The outer pouch is a peelable overwrap. **The outside surface of the outer pouch is not sterile.** GLIADEL® Wafer must be stored at or below -20°C (-4°F).

REFERENCES

1. Recommendations for the Safe Handling of Parenteral Antineoplastic Drugs, NIH Publication No. 83-2621. For sale by the Superintendent of Documents, U.S. Government Printing Office, Washington, DC 20402.
2. AMA Council Report, Guidelines for Handling Parenteral Antineoplastics. JAMA, 1985; 253(11):1590-1592.
3. National Study Commission on Cytotoxic Exposure—Recommendations for Handling Cytotoxic Agents. Available from Louis P. Jeffrey, ScD., Chairman, National Study Commission on Cytotoxic Exposure, Massachusetts College of Pharmacy and Allied Health Sciences, 179 Longwood Avenue, Boston, Massachusetts 02115.
4. Clinical Oncological Society of Australia, Guidelines and Recommendations for Safe Handling of Antineoplastic Agents. Med J Australia, 1983; 1:426-428.
5. Jones RB, et al: Safe Handling of Chemotherapeutic Agents: A Report from the Mount Sinai Medical Center. CA—A Cancer Journal for Clinicians, 1983; (Sept/Oct) 258-263.
6. American Society of Hospital Pharmacists Technical Assistance Bulletin on Handling Cytotoxic and Hazardous Drugs. Am J. Hosp Pharm, 1990; 47:1033-1049.
7. OSHA Work-Practice Guidelines for Personnel Dealing with Cytotoxic (Antineoplastic) Drugs. Am J Hosp Pharm, 1986; 43:1193-1204.
NDC: 62856-177-08
CAUTION: FEDERAL LAW PROHIBITS DISPENSING WITHOUT PRESCRIPTION.

Manufactured by
Eisai Inc.
Woodcliff Lake, NJ 07677
Rev. 04/2010
201241
Shown in Product Identification Guide, page 308

LUSEDRA ©℞
[Lu-se-dra]
(fospropofol disodium)
Injection, for intravenous use

HIGHLIGHTS OF PRESCRIBING INFORMATION
These highlights do not include all the information needed to use LUSEDRA safely and effectively. See full prescribing information for LUSEDRA.
LUSEDRA (fospropofol disodium) Injection, for intravenous use, CIV
Initial U.S. Approval: 2008

——INDICATIONS AND USAGE——
LUSEDRA is a sedative-hypnotic agent indicated for monitored anesthesia care (MAC) sedation in adult patients undergoing diagnostic or therapeutic procedures.(1)

——DOSAGE AND ADMINISTRATION——
• Use supplemental oxygen in all patients undergoing sedation with LUSEDRA. (2.1) Continuously monitor with pulse oximetry, electrocardiogram, and frequent blood pressure measurements.(5.1)
• Standard dosing regimen: initial intravenous bolus dose of 6.5 mg/kg followed by supplemental doses of 1.6 mg/kg as needed. No initial dose should exceed 16.5 mL; no supplemental dose should exceed 4 mL. (2.2)
• Modified dosing regimen [for patients who are ≥65 years of age or who have severe systemic disease (ASA P3 or P4)]: 75% of the standard dosing regimen. (2.3)
• Administer supplemental doses only when patients can demonstrate purposeful movement in response to verbal or light tactile stimulation and no more frequently than every 4 minutes. (2.1)
• Adults who weigh >90 kg should be dosed as if they are 90 kg; adults who weigh <60 kg should be dosed as if they are 60 kg. (2.2)
• Intended for single-use administration only.

——DOSAGE FORMS AND STRENGTHS——
Injection, solution containing 1,050 mg fospropofol disodium per 30 mL. (3)

——CONTRAINDICATIONS——
None

——WARNINGS AND PRECAUTIONS——
• A person trained in the administration of general anesthesia and not involved in the conduct of the diagnostic/therapeutic procedure should manage treatment of patients with LUSEDRA. (5.1)
• Respiratory depression (5.2)
• Hypoxemia (5.3)
• Hypotension (5.5)

——ADVERSE REACTIONS——
Most common adverse reactions (> 20%) are paresthesia and pruritus. (6)
To report SUSPECTED ADVERSE REACTIONS, contact Eisai Inc. at 1-888-422-4743 or FDA at 1-800-FDA-1088 or www.fda.gov/medwatch.

——DRUG INTERACTIONS——
As with other sedative-hypnotic agents, LUSEDRA may produce additive cardiorespiratory effects when administered with other cardiorespiratory depressants such as benzodiazepines and narcotic analgesics. (7)

——USE IN SPECIFIC POPULATIONS——
• Patients ≥65 years of age should receive the modified dosing regimen. (2.3, 8.5)
• Patients with severe systemic disease (ASA P3 or P4) should receive the modified dosing regimen. (2.3)
See 17 for PATIENT COUNSELING INFORMATION
Revised: 10/2009

FULL PRESCRIBING INFORMATION: CONTENTS*
1 INDICATIONS AND USAGE
2 DOSAGE AND ADMINISTRATION
   2.1 Dosing Guidelines
   2.2 Standard Dosing Regimen for Sedation
   2.3 Modified Dosing Regimen for Sedation in Patients ≥65 years or Those with Severe Systemic Disease (ASA P3 or P4)
   2.4 Preparation
3 DOSAGE FORM AND STRENGTH
4 CONTRAINDICATIONS
5 WARNINGS AND PRECAUTIONS
   5.1 Monitoring
   5.2 Respiratory Depression
   5.3 Hypoxemia
   5.4 Patient Unresponsiveness to Vigorous Tactile or Painful Stimulation
   5.5 Hypotension

FULL PRESCRIBING INFORMATION

1 INDICATIONS AND USAGE

LUSEDRA™ (fospropofol disodium) injection is an intravenous sedative-hypnotic agent indicated for monitored anesthesia care (MAC) sedation in adult patients undergoing diagnostic or therapeutic procedures.

2 DOSAGE AND ADMINISTRATION

2.1 Dosing Guidelines

- Administer LUSEDRA intravenously as a bolus injection.
- Use supplemental oxygen for all patients undergoing sedation with LUSEDRA.
- Individualize the dosage of LUSEDRA and titrate to the level of sedation required for the procedure.
- In adults aged 18 to <65 years who are healthy or have mild systemic disease as categorized by the American Society of Anesthesiologists (ASA P1 or P2), the standard dosing regimen of LUSEDRA should be followed [see *Standard Dosing Regimen for Sedation (2.2)*].
- In adults who are ≥ 65 years of age or who have severe systemic disease (ASA P3 or P4), the modified dosing regimen should be followed [see *Modified Dosing Regimen for Sedation in Patients ≥ 65 years or Those with Severe Systemic Disease (2.3)*].
- Administer supplemental doses of LUSEDRA based on the patient's level of sedation and the level of sedation required for the procedure. Give supplemental doses only when patients can demonstrate purposeful movement in response to verbal or light tactile stimulation and no more frequently than every 4 minutes. Use only the minimum dosage required to facilitate the procedure.
- Consider the potential for worsened cardiorespiratory depression prior to using LUSEDRA concomitantly with other drugs that have the same potential (e.g., sedative-hypnotics or narcotic analgesics) [see *Warnings and Precautions (5.2, 5.3)*].
- In clinical studies, an opioid premedication (fentanyl citrate 50 mcg intravenously) was administered five minutes prior to the initial dose of LUSEDRA.

2.2 Standard Dosing Regimen for Sedation

In adults aged 18 to <65 years who are healthy or have mild systemic disease (ASA P1 or P2)[1], the standard dosing regimen of LUSEDRA is an initial intravenous bolus of 6.5 mg/kg followed by supplemental doses of 1.6 mg/kg intravenously (25% of initial dosage) as needed to achieve the desired level of sedation as shown in Table 1.

The dosage of LUSEDRA is limited by lower and upper weight bounds of 60 kg and 90 kg. Adults who weigh >90 kg should be dosed as if they weigh 90 kg. **No initial dose should exceed 16.5 mL; no supplemental dose should exceed 4 mL.** Adults who weigh <60 kg should be dosed as if they weigh 60 kg. Dosages lower than those specified for the lower weight limit may be used to achieve lesser levels of sedation. In clinical studies, an opioid premedication (fentanyl citrate 50 mcg IV) was administered five minutes prior to the initial dose of LUSEDRA.

[See table 1 at top right]

Table 1. Standard Dosing Regimen, Adults 18 to <65 Years of Age Who are Healthy or Have Mild Systemic Disease (ASA P1 or P2)

Weight (kg)	Initial Dose		Supplemental Dose No more frequently than every 4 min.	
	mg	mL	mg	mL
≤60	385	11	105	3
61 to 63	402.5	11.5	105	3
64 to 65	420	12	105	3
66 to 68	437.5	12.5	105	3
69 to 71	455	13	105	3
72 to 74	472.5	13.5	122.5	3.5
75 to 76	490	14	122.5	3.5
77 to 79	507.5	14.5	122.5	3.5
80 to 82	525	15	140	4
83 to 84	542.5	15.5	140	4
85 to 87	560	16	140	4
88 to 89	577.5	16.5	140	4
≥90	577.5	16.5	140	4

Note: Doses in this table are rounded to the nearest half-milliliter volume to facilitate practical measurement; hence, they may differ slightly from the dose recommended on the basis of mg/kg.

2.3 Modified Dosing Regimen for Sedation in Patients ≥65 years or Those with Severe Systemic Disease (ASA P3 or P4)

Adults ≥65 years of age or those with severe systemic disease (ASA P3 or P4)[1] should receive initial and supplemental intravenous dosages of 75% of the standard dosing regimen, as presented in Table 2. LUSEDRA is administered intravenously as a bolus injection. In clinical studies, an opioid premedication (fentanyl citrate 50 mcg IV) was administered five minutes prior to the initial dose of LUSEDRA.

[See table 2 at top of next page]

2.4 Preparation

LUSEDRA is provided as a ready to use formulation intended for single-patient use only. Prepare LUSEDRA following strict aseptic techniques. Draw LUSEDRA into sterile syringes immediately after vials are opened. Discard any unused portion at the end of the procedure.

Parenteral drug products should be inspected visually for particulate matter and discoloration prior to administration. Do not use if there is evidence of particulate matter or discoloration.

LUSEDRA has been shown to be compatible with the following fluids:
- 5% Dextrose Injection, USP
- 5% Dextrose and 0.2% Sodium Chloride, USP
- 5% Dextrose and 0.45% Sodium Chloride Injection, USP
- 0.9% Sodium Chloride Injection, USP
- Lactated Ringer's Injection, USP
- Lactated Ringer's and 5% Dextrose Injection, USP
- 0.45% Sodium Chloride Injection, USP
- 5% Dextrose, 0.45% NaCl and 20 mEq KCl, USP

Do not mix LUSEDRA with other drugs or fluids prior to administration. LUSEDRA is not physically compatible with midazolam HCl or meperidine HCl, and compatibility with other agents has not been adequately evaluated.

Administer LUSEDRA through a secure, freely flowing, peripheral intravenous line using commonly available intravenous administration sets. Flush the infusion line with normal saline before and after administration of LUSEDRA.

LUSEDRA is not light sensitive. LUSEDRA does not need to be filtered before use.

3 DOSAGE FORM AND STRENGTH

Single-use vial contents: Solution for intravenous administration containing 35 mg of fospropofol disodium per mL (1,050 mg of fospropofol disodium in 30 mL).

4 CONTRAINDICATIONS

None.

5 WARNINGS AND PRECAUTIONS

5.1 Monitoring

LUSEDRA should be administered only by persons trained in the administration of general anesthesia and not involved in the conduct of the diagnostic or therapeutic procedure. Sedated patients should be continuously monitored, and facilities for maintenance of a patent airway, providing artificial ventilation, administering supplemental oxygen, and instituting cardiovascular resuscitation must be immediately available. Patients should be continuously monitored during sedation and through the recovery process for early signs of hypotension, apnea, airway obstruction, and/or oxygen desaturation.

5.2 Respiratory Depression

LUSEDRA may cause loss of spontaneous respiration. Apnea was reported in 1/455 (< 1%) patients treated with LUSEDRA using the standard or modified dosing regimen [see *Dosage and Administration (2.2, 2.3)*]. In patients treated with greater than the recommended LUSEDRA dose, apnea was reported in 14/556 (3%).

Supplemental oxygen is recommended for all patients receiving LUSEDRA. Dosages of LUSEDRA must be individualized for each patient and titrated to effect [see *Dosage and Administration (2.1) and Clinical Pharmacology (12.2)*]. Use lower doses of LUSEDRA in patients who are ≥65 years of age or who have severe systemic disease [see *Dosage and Administration (2.3)*]. The additive cardiorespiratory effects of narcotic analgesics and sedative-hypnotic agents should be considered when administered concomitantly with LUSEDRA.

Patients should be assessed for their ability to demonstrate purposeful response while sedated with LUSEDRA as patients who are unable to do so may lose protective reflexes. Airway assistance maneuvers may be required in the management of respiratory depression (see Table 4).

5.3 Hypoxemia

LUSEDRA may cause hypoxemia detectable by pulse oximetry. Hypoxemia was reported in 20/455 (4%) patients treated with LUSEDRA using the standard or modified dosing regimen [see *Dosage and Administration (2.2, 2.3)*]. Hypoxemia was reported among patients who retained the ability to respond purposefully to their health care provider following administration of LUSEDRA. Therefore, retention of purposeful responsiveness did not prevent patients from becoming hypoxemic following administration of LUSEDRA. In patients treated with greater than the recommended LUSEDRA dose, hypoxemia was reported in 151/556 (27%).

The risk of hypoxemia is reduced by appropriate positioning of the patient and the use of supplemental oxygen in all patients receiving LUSEDRA. Airway assistance maneuvers may be required in the management of hypoxemia (see Table 4). The additive cardiorespiratory effects of narcotic analgesics and other sedative-hypnotic agents should be considered when administered concomitantly with LUSEDRA.

5.4 Patient Unresponsiveness to Vigorous Tactile or Painful Stimulation

LUSEDRA has not been studied for use in general anesthesia. However, administration of LUSEDRA may inadvertently cause patients to become unresponsive or minimally responsive to vigorous tactile or painful stimulation. The incidence of patients sedated for colonoscopy who became

Table 2. Modified Dosing Regimen, Ages ≥ 65 Years Or Those with Severe Systemic Disease (ASA P3 or P4)

Weight (kg)	Initial Dose		Supplemental Dose No more frequently than every 4 min.	
	mg	mL	mg	mL
≤60	297.5	8.5	70	2
61 to 62	297.5	8.5	70	2
63 to 64	315	9	87.5	2.5
65 to 66	315	9	87.5	2.5
67 to 69	332.5	9.5	87.5	2.5
70 to 73	350	10	87.5	2.5
74 to 77	367.5	10.5	87.5	2.5
78 to 80	385	11	105	3
81 to 84	402.5	11.5	105	3
85 to 87	420	12	105	3
88 to 89	437.5	12.5	105	3
≥90	437.5	12.5	105	3

Note: Doses in this table are rounded to the nearest half-milliliter volume to facilitate practical measurement; hence, they may differ slightly from the dose recommended on the basis of mg/kg.

Table 3. Common Adverse Reactions for Patients Receiving the Standard or Modified Dosing Regimen (Reactions Occurring at a Rate ≥ 2%)

Reaction Term	Colonoscopy (N=183) n (%)	Minor Surgical Procedures (N=123) n (%)	Bronchoscopy (N=149) n (%)
Gastrointestinal disorders			
Nausea	0	5 (4)	2 (1)
Vomiting	0	4 (3)	0
Injury, poisoning, and procedural complications			
Procedural Pain	0	0	3 (2)
Nervous system disorders			
Paresthesia[a]	135 (74)	77 (63)	78 (52)
Headache	1 (1)	3 (2)	1 (1)
Respiratory, thoracic, and mediastinal disorders			
Hypoxemia	3 (2)	1 (1)	16 (11)
Skin and subcutaneous tissue disorders			
Pruritus[b]	30 (16)	34 (28)	24 (16)
Vascular disorders			
Hypotension	4 (2)	4 (3)	10 (7)

[a] Paresthesia includes the following terms: Paresthesia genital male; Burning sensation; Genital burning sensation; Vaginal burning sensation; Skin burning sensation; Genital pain (reported as burning); Perineal pain (reported as burning); Anal discomfort (reported as burning); Chest pain (reported as burning); Ear discomfort (reported as burning); Nasal discomfort (reported as burning); Buttock pain (reported as stinging); Groin pain (reported as stinging); Pain (reported as stinging); Sensory disturbance (reported as non-specific sensation in pubic area).
[b] Pruritus includes the following terms: Genital pruritus female; Genital pruritus male; Pruritus genital; Pruritus ani; Pruritus generalized.

minimally responsive or unresponsive to vigorous tactile or painful stimulation was 7/183 (4%). The duration of minimal or complete unresponsiveness in colonoscopy patients ranged from 2 to 16 minutes. Among patients sedated for bronchoscopy, the incidence of patients who became minimally or completely unresponsive to vigorous tactile or painful stimulation was 24/149 (16%). The duration of minimal to complete unresponsiveness in bronchoscopy patients ranged from 2 to 20 minutes.

5.5 Hypotension
Hypotension following the use of LUSEDRA may occur. Hypotension was reported in 18/455 (4%) patients treated with LUSEDRA using the standard or modified dosing regimen [see *Dosage and Administration* (2.2, 2.3)]. In patients treated with greater than the recommended LUSEDRA dose, hypotension was reported in 31/556 (6%). Patients with compromised myocardial function, reduced vascular tone, or who have reduced intravascular volume may be at an increased risk for hypotension. A secure intravenous access catheter and supplemental volume replacement fluids should be readily available during the procedure. Additional pharmacological management may be necessary.

6 ADVERSE REACTIONS
The following serious adverse reactions are discussed elsewhere in the labeling:
- Respiratory depression [see *Warnings and Precautions* (5.2)]
- Hypoxemia [see *Warnings and Precautions* (5.3)]
- Loss of purposeful responsiveness [see *Warnings and Precautions* (5.4)]
- Hypotension [see *Warnings and Precautions* (5.5)]

The most common adverse reactions (reported in greater than 20%) are paresthesia and pruritus.
The most commonly reported reasons for discontinuation are paresthesia and cough.

6.1 Clinical Trials Experience
Adverse reactions presented in this section are derived from 332 patients in 3 controlled clinical trials in patients undergoing colonoscopy or flexible bronchoscopy and 123 patients in one open-label study in patients undergoing minor procedures. Patients enrolled in the studies who received the standard or modified dosing regimen included males and females, ≥18 years of age and ranging from healthy (359/455 [79%] ASA P1 or P2) to those with severe systemic disease

(96/455 [21%] ASA P3 or P4). Of the 455 patients enrolled, 345 (76%) were ≥18 to <65 years of age and 110 (24%) were ≥65 years of age. Adverse reactions are reported for patients who received the standard or the modified dosing regimen [see *Dosage and Administration* (2)]. The majority of procedures were less than thirty minutes in duration. All patients in these studies received 50 mcg fentanyl citrate intravenously as premedication, and some of the patients received additional 25 mcg fentanyl citrate supplemental doses. Adverse reactions occurring in ≥2% of patients in these studies are presented in Table 3.
Because clinical trials are conducted under widely varying conditions, adverse reaction rates observed in the clinical trials of a drug cannot be directly compared to rates in the clinical trials of another drug and may not accurately reflect the rates observed in practice.
[See table 3 at left]
Paresthesias (including burning, tingling, stinging) and/or pruritus, usually manifested in the perineal region, were the most frequently recorded adverse reactions in clinical trials. Paresthesias and pruritus generally occurred within 5 minutes after administration of the initial dose of LUSEDRA and were generally transient and mild to moderate in intensity. The pharmacologic basis of these sensory phenomena is unknown. No pretreatments, including the use of nonsteroidal anti-inflammatory drugs, opioids, or lidocaine, are known to have an effect on or to reduce the incidence of these sensations.
Sedation-related adverse reactions were experienced at the following rates for subjects receiving the standard or modified LUSEDRA dosing regimen: 20/455 (4%) hypoxemia, 18/455 (4%) hypotension, 1/455 (< 1%) apnea. A greater rate of sedation-related adverse reactions necessitating intervention was observed in patients undergoing bronchoscopy compared with colonoscopy and minor surgical procedures. In the colonoscopy studies, 5/183 (3%) patients were ASA P3. In the minor surgical procedures study, 23/123 (19%) patients were ASA P3 or P4. In the flexible bronchoscopy study, 68/150 (46%) patients were ASA P3 or P4. The type and incidence of airway assistance interventions required for patients who experienced sedation-related adverse reactions are presented in Table 4.
[See table 4 at top of next page]

6.2 Adverse Reactions in Prolonged Exposure in Adults
The safety of LUSEDRA for continuous sedation has not been established and therefore its use is not recommended. LUSEDRA was administered to 38 intubated and mechanically ventilated patients in postoperative and intensive care settings. An occurrence of nonsustained ventricular tachycardia was observed as a serious adverse reaction in one patient in the study. Another patient with acute myeloid leukemia with renal and hepatic insufficiency experienced a further increase in plasma formate concentration from a baseline of 66 mcg/mL to a post-dose level of 212 mcg/mL after a 12-hour infusion. The clinical significance of these findings is unknown.

7 DRUG INTERACTIONS
LUSEDRA may produce additive cardiorespiratory effects when administered with other cardiorespiratory depressants such as sedative-hypnotics and narcotic analgesics.

8 USE IN SPECIFIC POPULATIONS
8.1 Pregnancy
Teratogenic Effects:
Pregnancy Category B.
There are no adequate and well-controlled studies in pregnant women. Because animal reproduction studies are not always predictive of human response, this drug should be used during pregnancy only if clearly needed.
Reproduction studies have been performed in rats and rabbits at doses up to 0.6 and 1.7 times the anticipated human dose for a procedure of 16 minutes based on a comparison of doses expressed as mg/m² and have revealed no evidence of impaired fertility or harm to the fetus due to LUSEDRA.
Pregnant rats were treated with fospropofol disodium (5, 20, or 45 mg/kg/day, IV) from gestation day 7 through 17 (the highest dose is 0.6 times the anticipated human dose for a procedure of 16 minutes based on a comparison of doses expressed as mg/m²). Doses of 20 and 45 mg/kg/day produced significant maternal toxicity. No drug-related adverse effects on embryo-fetal development were noted.
Pregnant rabbits were treated with fospropofol disodium (14, 28, 56 or 70 mg/kg/day, IV) from gestation day 6 through 18 (the highest dose is 1.7 times the anticipated human dose for a procedure of 16 minutes based on a comparison of doses expressed as mg/m²). Significant maternal toxicity was noted at all doses. No drug-related adverse effects on embryo-fetal development were noted.
Nonteratogenic Effects.
Pregnant rats were administered 0, 5, 10, or 20 mg/kg/day fospropofol disodium from gestation day 7 through lactation day 20 to evaluate perinatal and postnatal development (the highest dose is 0.2 times the anticipated human dose for a procedure of 16 minutes based on a comparison of

doses expressed as mg/m²). There were no clear treatment-related effects on growth, development, behavior (passive avoidance and water maze) or fertility and mating capacity of the offspring.

8.2 Labor and Delivery
LUSEDRA is not recommended for use in labor and delivery, including Cesarean section deliveries. It is not known if fospropofol crosses the placenta; however, propofol is known to cross the placenta, and as with other sedative-hypnotic agents, the administration of LUSEDRA may be associated with neonatal respiratory and cardiovascular depression.

8.3 Nursing Mothers
It is not known whether fospropofol is excreted in human milk; however, propofol has been reported to be excreted in human milk, and the effects of oral absorption of fospropofol or propofol are not known. LUSEDRA is not recommended for use in nursing mothers.

8.4 Pediatric Use
Safety and effectiveness in pediatric patients have not been established because LUSEDRA has not been studied in persons <18 years of age. LUSEDRA is not recommended for use in this population.

8.5 Geriatric Use
In studies of LUSEDRA for sedation in brief diagnostic and therapeutic procedures, 17% of patients were ≥65 years of age and 5% of patients were ≥75 years of age. Patients ≥65 years of age should receive the modified dosing regimen [see *Dosage and Administration (2.3)*]. Hypoxemia was reported more frequently among patients aged ≥75 years than among patients aged 65 to <75 years and less frequently among younger patients, aged 18 to < 65 years.

8.6 Patients with Renal Impairment
In studies of LUSEDRA for sedation in brief diagnostic and therapeutic procedures, 21% of patients had a creatinine clearance <80 mL/min, and 4% had a creatinine clearance <50 mL/min. Pharmacokinetics of fospropofol or propofol were not altered in patients with mild to moderate renal insufficiency. No dosing adjustments are required for patients with creatinine clearance ≥30 mL/min. Limited safety and efficacy data are available for LUSEDRA in patients with creatinine clearance < 30 mL/min.

8.7 Patients with Hepatic Impairment
LUSEDRA has not been adequately studied in patients with hepatic impairment. Caution should be exercised when using fospropofol disodium in patients with hepatic impairment.

9 DRUG ABUSE AND DEPENDENCE
9.1 Controlled Substance
LUSEDRA is a Schedule IV controlled substance.
9.2 Abuse
No formal studies of the abuse potential of LUSEDRA have been conducted. Administration of LUSEDRA resulted in euphoria in a small number of subjects who received intravenous or oral dosing.
9.3 Dependence
No formal studies of dependence have been conducted.

10 OVERDOSE
Overdosage with LUSEDRA can cause cardiorespiratory depression. If overdosage occurs, LUSEDRA administration should be discontinued immediately. Respiratory depression may require manual or mechanical ventilation. Cardiovascular depression may require elevation of lower extremities, intravascular volume replacement, and/or pharmacological management.

Formate and phosphate are metabolites of LUSEDRA and may contribute to signs of toxicity following overdosage. Signs of formate toxicity are similar to those of methanol toxicity and are associated with anion-gap metabolic acidosis. Intravenous exposure to a large amount of phosphate could potentially cause hypocalcemia with paresthesia, muscle spasms, and seizures.

11 DESCRIPTION
LUSEDRA is an injection solution intended for intravenous administration as a sedative-hypnotic agent. LUSEDRA is an aqueous, sterile, nonpyrogenic, clear, colorless, iso-osmotic solution containing 35 mg/mL of fospropofol disodium. Fospropofol disodium is a water-soluble prodrug of propofol, chemically described as 2,6-diisopropylphenoxymethyl phosphate, disodium salt. The structural and molecular formulas are shown in Figure 1. [See chemical structure at top of next column]

The inactive components include monothioglycerol (0.25 wt%) and tromethamine (0.12 wt%). LUSEDRA has a pH of 8.2 to 9.0. LUSEDRA does not contain any antimicrobial preservatives and is intended for single-use administration.

12 CLINICAL PHARMACOLOGY
12.1 Mechanism of Action
Fospropofol disodium is a prodrug of propofol. Following intravenous injection, fospropofol is metabolized by alkaline phosphatases. For every millimole of fospropofol disodium

Table 4. Patient Incidence of Airway Management Events

	Healthy Subjects[a] 6 mg/kg N=69 n (%)	Colonoscopy[b] 6.5 mg/kg (or modified dosing regimen) N=183 n (%)	Minor Procedures[b] 6.5 mg/kg (or modified dosing regimen) N=123 n (%)	Flexible Bronchoscopy[b] 6.5 mg/kg (or modified dosing regimen) N=149 n (%)
Increased O_2	0	0	0	21 (14)
Patient Repositioning	0	0	0	2 (1)
Verbal Stimulation	0	2 (1)	1 (1)	5 (3)
Tactile Stimulation	0	0	0	3 (2)
Face Mask (100% O_2)	0	0	0	1 (1)
Jaw Thrust	0	0	0	2 (1)
Chin Lift	0	0	1 (1)	3 (2)
Nasal Trumpet	0	0	0	0
Oral Airway	0	0	0	0
Suction	0	0	0	2 (1)
Manual Ventilation (bag valve mask)	0	0	0	1 (1)
Mechanical Ventilation	0	0	0	

[a] No concomitant medications administered. All subjects were healthy volunteers.
[b] All patients premedicated with 50 mcg fentanyl citrate. Subjects ranged from healthy to those with severe systemic disease that is a constant threat to life (ASA P1 to P4).

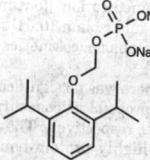

Molecular Formula: $C_{13}H_{19}O_5PNa_2$
Molecular Weight: 332.24
Figure 1. Structural and Molecular Formulas of Fospropofol Disodium

administered, one millimole of propofol is produced (1.86 mg of fospropofol disodium is the molar equivalent of 1 mg propofol).

12.2 Pharmacodynamics
The pharmacology of fospropofol, once metabolized to propofol, is comparable to that of propofol lipid emulsion; however, the liberation of propofol from fospropofol results in differences in the timing of the pharmacodynamic effects. To characterize the pharmacokinetic/pharmacodynamic (PK/PD) profile of propofol derived from LUSEDRA, 12 healthy subjects were administered a 10-mg/kg intravenous bolus dose of LUSEDRA, and the sedative effect was measured as a decrease in Modified Observer's Assessment of Alertness/Sedation (MOAA/S) score (Table 5).[2] The PK and PD results are shown in Figure 2. Peak plasma levels of propofol (2.2 ± 0.4 μg/mL) released from fospropofol were noted by 8 minutes (range 4-13 minutes) and minimum mean MOAA/S score of 1.2 (range 0-3) was noted in 7 minutes (range 1-15 minutes). Subjects completely recovered from sedative effects between 21 to 45 minutes after LUSEDRA administration.

Table 5. Modified Observer's Assessment of Alertness/Sedation Scale[2]

Responsiveness	Score
Responds readily to name spoken in normal tone	5
Lethargic response to name spoken in normal tone	4
Responds only after name is called loudly and/or repeatedly	3
Responds only after mild prodding or shaking	2
Responds only after painful trapezius squeeze	1
Does not respond to painful trapezius squeeze	0

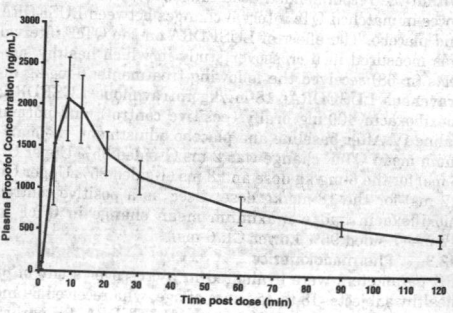

Mean (SD) Propofol

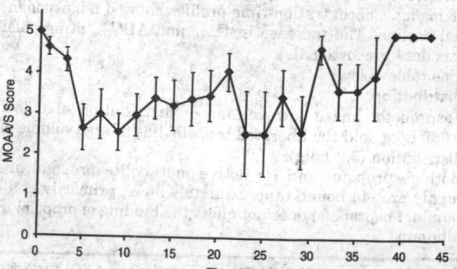

Mean (SE) MOAA/S

Figure 2. Pharmacokinetic and Pharmacodynamic Profiles after a 10-mg/kg Bolus Dose of LUSEDRA

LUSEDRA was evaluated in randomized, blinded, dose-controlled studies for sedation in patients undergoing colonoscopy and flexible bronchoscopy [see *Clinical Studies (14.1)*]. Figure 3 shows MOAA/S scores over time in each of the studies for those patients who received the standard and modified dosing regimens. In the study of patients undergoing colonoscopy, patients who received the standard and modified dosing regimens had a median [range] time to sedation (time from first dose of sedative to the first of 2 consecutive MOAA/S scores of ≤ 4) of 8.0 [2, 28] minutes and a median time to Fully Alert (3 consecutive responses to their name spoken in a normal tone, measured every 2 minutes beginning at or after the end of the procedure) of 5.0 [0,

7] minutes. In the study of patients undergoing flexible bronchoscopy, patients who received the standard and modified LUSEDRA dosing regimens had a median time to sedation of 4 [2, 22] minutes and a median time to Fully Alert of 5.5 [0, 61] minutes.

Patients Undergoing Colonoscopy

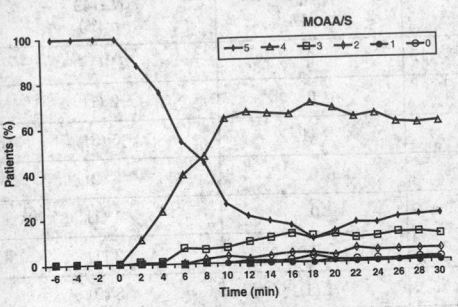

Patients Undergoing Flexible Bronchoscopy

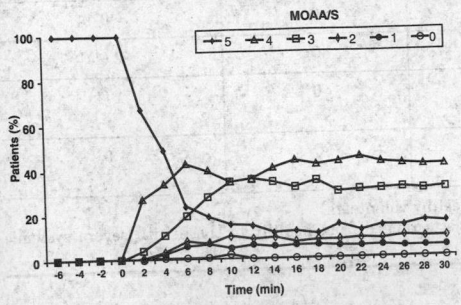

Figure 3. Percentage of Patients at Each MOAA/S Score Over Time

Within the recommended dose range, there were no differences in matched QTc interval changes between LUSEDRA and placebo. The effect of LUSEDRA on the QTcF interval was measured in a crossover study in which healthy subjects (n=68) received the following treatments: 6-mg/kg intravenous LUSEDRA; 18-mg/kg intravenous LUSEDRA; moxifloxacin 400 mg orally (positive control); and normal saline IV. After baseline and placebo adjustment, the maximum mean QTcF change was 2 ms (1-sided 95% Upper CI: 6 ms) for the 6-mg/kg dose and 8 ms (1-sided 95% Upper CI: 12 ms) for the 18-mg/kg dose. Used as a positive control, moxifloxacin had a maximum mean change in QTcF of 12 ms (1-sided 95% Lower CI: 6 ms).

12.3 Pharmacokinetics

PK parameters were evaluated in a crossover study of 68 healthy subjects, 18 to 45 years of age, who received 6- and 18-mg/kg intravenous bolus doses of LUSEDRA. PK parameters are shown in Table 6. The C_{max} and $AUC_{0-\infty}$ values of fospropofol were dose proportional. The intersubject variability in C_{max} and $AUC_{0-\infty}$ was low. Propofol was rapidly liberated reaching plasma C_{max} at a median T_{max} of 12 minutes for LUSEDRA 6 mg/kg and 8 minutes for LUSEDRA 18 mg/kg. Concentration-time profiles showed a biexponential decline. The increase in C_{max} and $AUC_{0-\infty}$ of propofol was dose proportional.

[See table below]

Distribution

Fospropofol has a low volume of distribution of 0.33± 0.069 L/kg, and the liberated propofol has a large volume of distribution (5.8 L/kg).

Both fospropofol and its active metabolite propofol are highly protein bound (approximately 98%), primarily to albumin. Fospropofol does not affect the binding of propofol to albumin.

Metabolism

Fospropofol is completely metabolized by alkaline phosphatases to propofol, formaldehyde, and phosphate. Formaldehyde and phosphate plasma concentrations are comparable to endogenous levels when fospropofol disodium is administered as recommended. Formaldehyde is further metabolized to formate by several enzyme systems, including formaldehyde dehydrogenase, present in various tissues. Propofol liberated from fospropofol is further metabolized to major metabolites propofol glucuronide (34.8%), quinol-4-sulfate (4.6%), quinol-1-glucuronide (11.1%), and quinol-4-glucuronide (5.1%). Oxidation to CO_2 is the primary means of eliminating excess formate.

Fospropofol is not a substrate of CYP450 enzymes.

Elimination

After a single 400 mg intravenous dose of [^{14}C]-fospropofol disodium in humans, approximately 71% of radioactivity was recovered in the urine within 192 hours. Total body clearance (CLp) of fospropofol was 0.280±0.053 L/h/kg, and renal elimination of fospropofol was insignificant (<0.02% of dose). The terminal phase elimination half-life ($t_{1/2}$) of fospropofol was 0.81±0.08 and 0.88±0.08 hours in healthy subjects and patients, respectively. In healthy subjects, the apparent total body clearance of liberated propofol (CLp/F) was 1.95±0.345 L/h/kg and $t_{1/2}$ was 2.06±0.77 hours. In patients, the CLp of fospropofol was 0.31±0.14 L/h/kg and CLp/F for propofol was 2.74±0.80 L/h/kg and is similar to that observed in healthy subjects.

Special Populations

Population pharmacokinetic analysis indicated no influence of race, gender, age, renal impairment or alkaline phosphatase concentrations on the pharmacokinetics of fospropofol. Pharmacokinetics of propofol derived from fospropofol was not influenced by race, gender, or renal impairment.

LUSEDRA has not been adequately studied in patients with hepatic impairment. Caution should be exercised when using fospropofol disodium in patients with hepatic impairment.

Drug Interactions

There was no effect of analgesic premedication [fentanyl (1 mcg/kg); meperidine (0.75 mg/kg); midazolam (0.01 mg/kg); morphine (0.1 mg/kg)] on plasma pharmacokinetics of fospropofol.

In an in vitro protein-binding study, there was no significant interaction between fospropofol and propofol at concentrations up to 200 mcg/mL and 5 mcg/mL, respectively. The interaction of fospropofol with other highly protein-bound drugs given concomitantly has not been studied.

Potential of fospropofol or its major metabolite, propofol, to inhibit or induce major cytochrome P450 enzymes is not known.

13 NONCLINICAL TOXICOLOGY

13.1 Carcinogenesis, Mutagenesis, Impairment of Fertility

Carcinogenesis

Long-term studies in animals have not been performed to evaluate the carcinogenic potential of fospropofol disodium.

Mutagenesis

Fospropofol was not genotoxic in the Ames bacterial reverse mutation assay, with or without metabolic activation, and in the in vivo mouse micronucleus assay. Fospropofol was positive in the L5178Y TK$^{+/-}$ mouse lymphoma forward mutation assay in the presence of metabolic activation. In contrast, fospropofol was negative in this assay in the presence of formaldehyde-metabolizing enzymes suggesting that the positive finding is likely due to an artifact of the culture conditions.

Impairment of Fertility

Male rats were treated with 5, 10, or 20 mg/kg fospropofol for 4 weeks prior to mating. Male fertility was not altered in animals treated with 20 mg/kg (0.3-fold the total human dose for a procedure of 16 minutes based on a mg/m² basis). Female rats were treated with 5, 10, or 20 mg/kg fospropofol for two weeks prior to mating. There were no clear treatment-related effects on female fertility at a dose of 20 mg/kg (0.3-fold the total human dose for a procedure of 16 minutes based on a mg/m² basis).

14 CLINICAL STUDIES

14.1 Use in Sedation for Diagnostic or Therapeutic Procedures

The standard and modified LUSEDRA dosing regimens were evaluated in two controlled studies in patients dosed with LUSEDRA who were over 18 years of age and undergoing diagnostic or therapeutic procedures. All patients received 50 mcg of fentanyl citrate intravenously before study sedative medication. The primary endpoint was the rate of "sedation success," defined as the proportion of patients who did not respond readily to their name spoken in a normal tone of voice (Modified Observer's Assessment of Alertness/Sedation Scale score of 4 or less) on 3 consecutive measurements taken every 2 minutes and who completed the procedure without the use of alternative sedative medication and without the use of manual or mechanical ventilation.[2]

In both studies, an initial bolus dose and up to 3 supplemental doses at 25% of the initial bolus of study sedative medication were administered intravenously to sedate patients so that they did not respond readily to their name spoken in a normal tone and to allow the investigator to start the procedure. During the procedure, supplemental doses at 25% of the initial bolus were allowed to maintain sedation. Patients who were not adequately sedated with study drug received alternative sedative medication per the site's standard of care; however, sites were instructed not to use propofol as it would interfere with PK measurements.

The standard and modified LUSEDRA dosing regimens were evaluated in a randomized, blinded, dose-controlled study for sedation in patients undergoing colonoscopy. All of the patients who received alternative sedative medication (n=19) received midazolam. Patients randomized to receive the LUSEDRA standard or modified dosing regimen had a sedation success rate of 87% and required a mean number of supplemental doses of 2.3 (±1.4 SD). Patients randomized to receive LUSEDRA had a median procedure duration of 11 minutes.

The standard and modified LUSEDRA dosing regimens were also evaluated in a randomized, blinded, dose-controlled study for sedation in patients undergoing flexible bronchoscopy. All of the patients who received alternative sedative medication (n=12) received midazolam. Patients randomized to receive the LUSEDRA standard or modified dosing regimen had a sedation success rate of 89% and required a mean number of supplemental doses of 1.7 (±1.6 SD). Patients randomized to LUSEDRA had a median procedure duration of 10 minutes.

15 REFERENCES

1. Kost, M. *Moderate Sedation/Analgesia: Core Competencies for Practice.* Elsevier Health Sciences, 2004; 62-63.
2. Chernik DA, Gillings D, Laine H, Hendler J, Silver JM, Davidson AB, et al. Validity and reliability of the Observer's Assessment of Alertness/Sedation Scale: study with intravenous midazolam. *J Clin Psychopharmacol.* 1990;10(4):244-251.

16 HOW SUPPLIED/STORAGE AND HANDLING

LUSEDRA, 35 mg/mL (total of 1,050 mg/30 mL) fospropofol disodium, is supplied as a single-use, aqueous, sterile, non-pyrogenic, clear, colorless solution in glass vials ready for intravenous injection. Each vial is filled with 32.1 mL intended to deliver a minimum of 30 mL of fospropofol disodium solution. Store at controlled room temperature 25°C (77°F). Excursions permitted between 15° and 30°C (59° and 86°F).

NDC 62856-350-08.

17 PATIENT COUNSELING INFORMATION

Paresthesias (including burning, tingling, stinging) and/or pruritus, usually manifested in the perineal region are frequently experienced upon injection of the initial dose of LUSEDRA. Inform the patient that these sensations are typically mild to moderate in intensity, last a short time, and require no treatment.

Requirement for a patient escort should be considered. The decision as to when patients who have received LUSEDRA, particularly on an outpatient basis, may again engage in activities requiring complete mental alertness, coordination and/or physical dexterity (e.g., operate hazardous machinery, sign legal documents, or drive a motor vehicle) must be individualized.

Eisai Inc.
100 Tice Boulevard
Woodcliff Lake, NJ 07677
USA

LUSEDRA is a trademark used by Eisai Inc. under license from Eisai R&D Management Co., Ltd.

©2009 Eisai Inc.

All rights reserved. 10/09

Shown in Product Identification Guide, page 308

Table 6. Pharmacokinetic Parameters (mean ± SD) for Fospropofol and Propofol from LUSEDRA Administration

Parameter	Fospropofol			Propofol from LUSEDRA		
	Healthy (6 mg/kg) N=68	Healthy (18 mg/kg) N=68	Patient (6.5 mg/kg) N=667	Healthy (6 mg/kg) N=68	Healthy (18 mg/kg) N=68	Patient (6.5 mg/kg) N=400
C_{max} (mcg/mL)	78.7±15.4	211±48.6	—	1.08±0.33	3.90±0.822	—
T_{max} (min)	4	2	—	12	8	—
$AUC_{0-\infty}$ (mcg•h/mL)	19.2±3.59	50.3±8.4	19.0±7.2	1.70±0.29	5.67±1.28	1.2±0.39
CLp (L/h/kg)	0.28±0.053	0.32±0.058	0.36±0.16	1.95±0.34	1.79±0.39	3.2±0.92
$t_{1/2}$ (h)	0.81±0.08	0.81±0.09	0.88±0.08	2.06±0.77	1.76±0.54	1.13±0.28

HEXALEN®
[hex-uh-len]
(Altretamine)
Capsules
50 mg
℞ Only

℞

WARNINGS

1. **HEXALEN® capsules should only be given under the supervision of a physician experienced in the use of antineoplastic agents.**
2. **Peripheral blood counts should be monitored at least monthly, prior to the initiation of each course of HEXALEN® capsules, and as clinically indicated (see Adverse Reactions).**
3. **Because of the possibility of HEXALEN® capsules-related neurotoxicity, neurologic examination should be performed regularly during HEXALEN® capsules administration (see Adverse Reactions).**

DESCRIPTION

HEXALEN® (altretamine) capsules, is a synthetic cytotoxic antineoplastic s-triazine derivative. HEXALEN® capsules contain 50 mg of altretamine for oral administration. Inert ingredients include lactose, anhydrous and calcium stearate. Altretamine, known chemically as N,N,N′,N′,N″,N″-hexamethyl-1,3,5-triazine-2,4,6-triamine, has the following structural formula:

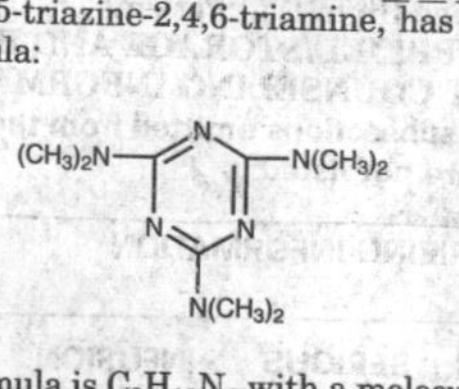

Its empirical formula is $C_9H_{18}N_6$ with a molecular weight of 210.28. Altretamine is a white crystalline powder, melting at 172° ± 1°C. Altretamine is practically insoluble in water but is increasingly soluble at pH 3 and below.

CLINICAL PHARMACOLOGY

The precise mechanism by which HEXALEN® capsules exerts its cytotoxic effect is unknown, although a number of theoretical possibilities have been studied. Structurally, HEXALEN® capsules resembles the alkylating agent triethylenemelamine, yet *in vitro* tests for alkylating activity of HEXALEN® capsules and its metabolites have been negative. HEXALEN® capsules has been demonstrated to be efficacious for certain ovarian tumors resistant to classical alkylating agents. Metabolism of altretamine is a requirement for cytotoxicity. Synthetic monohydroxymethylmelamines, and products of altretamine metabolism, *in vitro* and *in vivo*, can form covalent adducts with tissue macromolecules including DNA, but the relevance of these reactions to antitumor activity is unknown.

HEXALEN® capsules is well-absorbed following oral administration in humans, but undergoes rapid and extensive demethylation in the liver, producing variation in altretamine plasma levels. The principal metabolites are pentamethylmelamine and tetramethylmelamine.

Pharmacokinetic studies were performed in a limited number of patients and should be considered preliminary. After oral administration of HEXALEN® capsules to 11 patients with advanced ovarian cancer in doses of 120-300 mg/m^2, peak plasma levels (as measured by gas-chromatographic assay) were reached between 0.5 and 3 hours, varying from 0.2 to 20.8 mg/l. Half-life of the β-phase of elimination ranged from 4.7 to 10.2 hours. Altretamine and metabolites show binding to plasma proteins. The free fractions of altretamine, pentamethylmelamine and tetramethylmelamine are 6%, 25% and 50%, respectively.

Following oral administration of ^{14}C-ring-labeled altretamine (4 mg/kg), urinary recovery of radioactivity was 61% at 24 hours and 90% at 72 hours. Human urinary metabolites were N-demethylated homologues of altretamine with <1% unmetabolized altretamine excreted at 24 hours. After intraperitoneal administration of ^{14}C-ring-labeled altretamine to mice, tissue distribution was rapid in all organs, reaching a maximum at 30 minutes. The excretory organs (liver and kidney) and the small intestine showed high concentrations of radioactivity, whereas relatively low concentrations were found in other organs, including the brain.

There have been no formal pharmacokinetic studies in patients with compromised hepatic and/or renal function, though HEXALEN® capsules has been administered both concurrently and following nephrotoxic drugs such as cisplatin.

HEXALEN® capsules has been administered in 4 divided doses, with meals and at bedtime, though there is no pharmacokinetic data on this schedule nor information from formal interaction studies about the effect of food on its bioavailability or pharmacokinetics.

In two studies in patients with persistent or recurrent ovarian cancer following first-line treatment with cisplatin and/or alkylating agent-based combinations, HEXALEN® capsules was administered as a single agent for 14 or 21 days of a 28 day cycle. In the 51 patients with measurable or evaluable disease, there were 6 clinical complete responses, 1 pathologic complete response, and 2 partial responses for an overall response rate of 18%. The duration of these responses ranged from 2 months in a patient with a palpable pelvic mass to 36 months in a patient who achieved a pathologic complete response. In some patients, tumor regression was associated with improvement in symptoms and performance status.

INDICATIONS and USAGE

HEXALEN® (altretamine) capsules is indicated for use as a single agent in the palliative treatment of patients with persistent or recurrent ovarian cancer following first-line therapy with a cisplatin and/or alkylating agent-based combination.

CONTRAINDICATIONS

HEXALEN® capsules is contraindicated in patients who have shown hypersensitivity to it. HEXALEN® capsules should not be employed in patients with preexisting severe bone marrow depression or severe neurologic toxicity. HEXALEN® capsules has been administered safely, however, to patients heavily pretreated with cisplatin and/or alkylating agents, including patients with preexisting cisplatin neuropathies. Careful monitoring of neurologic function in these patients is essential.

WARNINGS

See boxed Warnings.

Concurrent administration of HEXALEN® capsules and antidepressants of the monoamine oxidase (MAO) inhibitor class may cause severe orthostatic hypotension. Four patients, all over 60 years of age, were reported to have experienced symptomatic hypotension after 4 to 7 days of concomitant therapy with HEXALEN® capsules and MAO inhibitors.

HEXALEN® capsules causes mild to moderate myelosuppression and neurotoxicity. Blood counts and a neurologic examination should be performed prior to the initiation of each course of therapy and the dose of HEXALEN® capsules adjusted as clinically indicated (see Dosage and Administration).

Pregnancy: Category D

HEXALEN® capsules has been shown to be embryotoxic and teratogenic in rats and rabbits when given at doses 2 and 10 times the human dose. HEXALEN® capsules may cause fetal damage when administered to a pregnant woman. If HEXALEN® capsules is used during pregnancy, or if the patient becomes pregnant while taking the drug, the patient should be apprised of the potential hazard to the fetus. Women of childbearing potential should be advised to avoid becoming pregnant.

PRECAUTIONS

General

Neurologic examination should be performed regularly (see Adverse Reactions).

Laboratory Tests

Peripheral blood counts should be monitored at least monthly, prior to the initiation of each course of HEXALEN® capsules, and as clinically indicated (see Adverse Reactions).

Drug Interactions

Concurrent administration of HEXALEN® capsules and antidepressants of the MAO inhibitor class may cause severe orthostatic hypotension (see Warnings section). Cimetidine, an inhibitor of microsomal drug metabolism, increased altretamine's half-life and toxicity in a rat model.

Data from a randomized trial of HEXALEN® capsules and cisplatin plus or minus pyridoxine in ovarian cancer indicated that pyridoxine significantly reduced neurotoxicity; however, it adversely affected response duration suggesting that pyridoxine should not be administered with HEXALEN® capsules and/or cisplatin (1).

Carcinogenesis, Mutagenesis and Impairment of Fertility

The carcinogenic potential of HEXALEN® capsules has not been studied in animals, but drugs with similar mechanisms of action have been shown to be carcinogenic. HEXALEN® capsules was weakly mutagenic when tested in strain TA100 of *Salmonella typhimurium*. HEXALEN® capsules administered to female rats 14 days prior to breeding through the gestation period had no adverse effect on fertility, but decreased post-natal survival at 120 mg/m^2/day and was embryocidal at 240 mg/m^2/day. Administration of 120 mg/m^2/day HEXALEN® capsules to male rats for 60 days prior to mating resulted in testicular atrophy, reduced fertility and a possible dominant lethal mutagenic effect. Male rats treated with HEXALEN® capsules at 450 mg/m^2/day for 10 days had decreased spermatogenesis, atrophy of testes, seminal vesicles and ventral prostate.

Pregnancy

Pregnancy Category D: see Warnings section.

Nursing Mothers

It is not known whether altretamine is excreted in human milk. Because there is a possibility of toxicity in nursing infants secondary to HEXALEN® capsules treatment of the mother, it is recommended that breast feeding be discontinued if the mother is treated with HEXALEN® capsules.

Pediatric Use

The safety and effectiveness of HEXALEN® capsules in children have not been established.

ADVERSE REACTIONS

Gastrointestinal

With continuous high-dose daily HEXALEN® capsules, nausea and vomiting of gradual onset occur frequently. Although in most instances these symptoms are controllable with anti-emetics, at times the severity requires HEXALEN® capsules dose reduction or, rarely, discontinuation of HEXALEN® capsules therapy. In some instances, a tolerance of these symptoms develops after several weeks of therapy. The incidence and severity of nausea and vomiting are reduced with moderate-dose administration of HEXALEN® capsules. In 2 clinical studies of single-agent HEXALEN® capsules utilizing a moderate, intermittent dose and schedule, only 1 patient (1%) discontinued HEXALEN® capsules due to severe nausea and vomiting.

Neurotoxicity

Peripheral neuropathy and central nervous system symptoms (mood disorders, disorders of consciousness, ataxia, dizziness, vertigo) have been reported. They are more likely to occur in patients receiving continuous high-dose daily HEXALEN® (altretamine) capsules than moderate-dose HEXALEN® capsules administered on an intermittent schedule. Neurologic toxicity has been reported to be reversible when therapy is discontinued. Data from a randomized trial of HEXALEN® capsules and cisplatin plus or minus pyridoxine in ovarian cancer indicated that pyridoxine significantly reduced neurotoxicity; however, it adversely affected response duration suggesting that pyridoxine should not be administered with HEXALEN® capsules and/or cisplatin (1).

Hematologic

HEXALEN® capsules causes mild to moderate dose-related myelosuppression. Leukopenia below 3000 WBC/mm^3 occurred in <15% of patients on a variety of intermittent or continuous dose regimens. Less than 1% had leukopenia below 1000 WBC/mm^3. Thrombocytopenia below 50,000 platelets/mm^3 was seen in <10% of patients. When given in doses of 8-12 mg/kg/day over a 21 day course, nadirs of leukocyte and platelet counts were reached by 3-4 weeks, and normal counts were regained by 6 weeks. With continuous administration at doses of 6-8 mg/kg/day, nadirs are reached in 6-8 weeks (median).

Data in the following table are based on the experience of 76 patients with ovarian cancer previously treated with a cisplatin-based combination regimen who received single-agent HEXALEN® capsules. In one study, HEXALEN® capsules, 260 mg/m^2/day, was administered for 14 days of a 28 day cycle. In another study, HEXALEN® capsules, 6-8 mg/kg/day, was administered for 21 days of a 28 day cycle.

ADVERSE EXPERIENCES IN 76 PREVIOUSLY TREATED OVARIAN CANCER PATIENTS RECEIVING SINGLE-AGENT HEXALEN® CAPSULES

Adverse Experiences	% Patients	
Gastrointestinal		
Nausea and Vomiting	33	
Mild to Moderate		32
Severe		1
Increased Alkaline Phosphatase	9	
Neurologic		
Peripheral Sensory Neuropathy	31	
Mild		22
Moderate to Severe		9
Anorexia and Fatigue	1	
Seizures	1	
Hematologic		
Leukopenia	5	
WBC 2000-2999/mm^3		4
WBC <2000/mm^3		1
Thrombocytopenia	9	
Platelets 75,000-99,000/mm^3		6
Platelets <75,000/mm^3		3
Anemia	33	
Mild		20
Moderate to Severe		13
Renal		
Serum Creatinine 1.6-3.75 mg/dl	7	
BUN	9	
25-40 mg%		5
41-60 mg%		3
>60 mg%		1

dditional adverse reaction information is available from 3 single-agent altretamine studies (total of 1014 patients) conducted under the auspices of the National Cancer Institute. The treated patients had a variety of tumors and many were heavily pretreated with other chemotherapies; most of these trials utilized high, continuous daily doses of altretamine (612 mg/kg/day). In general, adverse reaction experiences were similar in the two trials described above. Additional toxicities, not reported in the above table, included hepatic toxicity, skin rash, pruritus and alopecia, each occurring in <1% of patients.

OVERDOSAGE

No case of acute overdosage in humans has been described. The oral LD50 dose in rats was 1050 mg/kg and 437 mg/kg in mice.

DOSAGE AND ADMINISTRATION

HEXALEN® capsules is administered orally. Doses are calculated on the basis of body surface area.

HEXALEN® capsules may be administered either for 14 or 21 consecutive days in a 28 day cycle at a dose of 260 mg/m^2/day. The total daily dose should be given as 4 divided oral doses after meals and at bedtime. There is no pharmacokinetic information supporting this dosing regimen and the effect of food on HEXALEN® capsules bioavailability or pharmacokinetics has not been evaluated.

HEXALEN® capsules should be temporarily discontinued (for 14 days or longer) and subsequently restarted at 200 mg/m^2/day for any of the following situations:
1) Gastrointestinal intolerance unresponsive to symptomatic measures;
2) White blood count <2000/mm^3 or granulocyte count <1000/mm^3;
3) Platelet count <75,000/mm^3;
4) Progressive neurotoxicity.
If neurologic symptoms fail to stabilize on the reduced dose schedule, HEXALEN® capsules should be discontinued indefinitely.

Procedures for proper handling and disposal of anticancer drugs should be considered. Several guidelines on this subject have been published (2-9). There is no general agreement that all of the procedures recommended in the guidelines are necessary or appropriate.

HOW SUPPLIED

HEXALEN® (altretamine) capsules is available in 50 mg clear, hard gelatin capsules imprinted with the following inscription:
USB 001.
Bottles of 100 capsules
(NDC 62856-001-10)
Store up to 25°C (77°F); excursions permitted to 15° to 30°C (59° to 86°F).

REFERENCES

1. Wiernik PH, et al. Hexamethylmelamine and Low or Moderate Dose Cisplatin With or Without Pyridoxine for Treatment of Advanced Ovarian Carcinoma: A Study of the Eastern Cooperative Oncology Group. *Cancer Invest.* 1992; 10(1): 1-9.
2. ONS Clinical Practice Committee. Cancer Chemotherapy Guidelines and Recommendations for Practice. Pittsburgh, Pa: Oncology Nursing Society; 1999:32-41.
3. U.S. Department of Health and Human Services. Recommendations for the Safe Handling of Parenteral Antineoplastic Drugs. Washington DC: Division of Safety, National Institutes of Health; 1983 Public Health Service publication NIH 83-2621.
4. AMA Council on Scientific Affairs. Guidelines for Handling Parenteral Antineoplastics. *JAMA.* 1985; 253:1590-1591.
5. National Study Commission on Cytotoxic Exposure. Recommendations for Handling Cytotoxic Agents. Boston, MA: Available from Louis P. Jeffrey, Chairman, National Study Commission on Cytotoxic Exposure, Massachusetts College of Pharmacy and Allied Health Sciences, 179 Longwood Avenue, Boston, MA 02115; 1987.
6. Clinical Oncological Society of Australia: Guidelines and Recommendations for Safe Handling of Antineoplastic Agents. *Med J Australia.* 1983;1:426-428.
7. Jones RB, Frank R, Mass T. Safe Handling of Chemotherapeutic Agents: A Report from the Mount Sinai Medical Center. CA *Cancer J Clin.* 1983;33:258-263.
8. American Society of Hospital Pharmacists. ASHP Technical Assistance Bulletin on Handling Cytotoxic and Hazardous Drugs. *Am J Hosp Pharm.* 1990; 47:1033-1049.
9. OSHA Work Practice Guidelines. Controlling Occupational Exposure to Hazardous Drugs. *Am J Health Syst Pharm.* 1996;53:1669-1685.

HEXALEN® (altretamine) capsules is a registered trademark of Eisai Inc.
Manufactured by:
AAI Pharma Inc.
Wilmington, NC 28405
Manufactured for:
Eisai Inc.
Woodcliff Lake, NJ 07677
For Medical Inquiries
call: 1-877-873-4724
Revision Date May 2009

ONTAK® ℞
[ŏn-tăk]
(denileukin diftitox)
Solution for Intravenous use

HIGHLIGHTS OF PRESCRIBING INFORMATION
These highlights do not include all the information needed to use Ontak safely and effectively. See full prescribing information for Ontak.
ONTAK® (denileukin diftitox)
Solution for Intravenous use
Initial U.S. Approval: 1999

> **WARNING: SERIOUS INFUSION REACTIONS, CAPILLARY LEAK SYNDROME AND LOSS OF VISUAL ACUITY.**
> *See full prescribing information for complete boxed warning.*
> The following adverse reactions have been reported:
> • Serious and fatal infusion reactions. Administer Ontak in a facility equipped and staffed for cardiopulmonary resuscitation. (5.1)
> • Capillary leak syndrome resulting in death. (5.2)
> • Loss of visual acuity and color vision. (5.3)

———RECENT MAJOR CHANGES———
———INDICATIONS AND USAGE———
Ontak is a CD25-directed cytotoxin indicated for the treatment of patients with persistent or recurrent cutaneous T-cell lymphoma whose malignant cells express the CD25 component of the IL-2 receptor. (1)
———DOSAGE AND ADMINISTRATION———
• Premedicate with an antihistamine and acetaminophen prior to each Ontak infusion.
• Administer at 9 or 18 mcg/kg/day by intravenous infusion over 30 to 60 minutes for 5 consecutive days every 21 days for 8 cycles. (2.1, 2.2)
———DOSAGE FORMS AND STRENGTHS———
• Single-use vial containing 150 mcg/mL (300 mcg in 2 mL). (3)
———CONTRAINDICATIONS———
None.
———WARNINGS AND PRECAUTIONS———
• **Infusion reactions:** Immediately stop and permanently discontinue Ontak for serious infusion reactions. Monitor patients following infusion. (5.1)
• **Capillary leak syndrome:** Monitor weight, edema, blood pressure and serum albumin levels. (5.2)
• **Loss of Visual Acuity and Color Vision:** Monitor visual acuity and color vision. (5.3)
• **Laboratory Tests:** Monitor serum albumin levels prior to the initiation of each treatment course. Delay administration of Ontak until serum albumin levels are at least 3.0 g/dL. (5.5)
———ADVERSE REACTIONS———
The most common adverse reactions (≥20%) were pyrexia, nausea, fatigue, rigors, vomiting, diarrhea, headache, peripheral edema, cough, dyspnea and pruritus. (6)
To report SUSPECTED ADVERSE REACTIONS, contact Eisai Inc. at 1-888-274-2378 (by fax 1-201-746-3207) or FDA at 1-800-FDA-1088 or www.fda.gov/medwatch.
———USE IN SPECIFIC POPULATIONS———
• **Pregnancy:** No human or animal data. Use only if clearly needed. (8.1)
• **Nursing Mothers:** Discontinue drug or nursing taking into consideration importance of drug to mother. (8.3)
See 17 for PATIENT COUNSELING INFORMATION
Revised: 03/2010

FULL PRESCRIBING INFORMATION: CONTENTS*
WARNING: SERIOUS INFUSION REACTIONS, CAPILLARY LEAK SYNDROME AND LOSS OF VISUAL ACUITY.
1 INDICATIONS AND USAGE
2 DOSAGE AND ADMINISTRATION
   2.1 Dosing Schedule and Administration
   2.2 Preparation and Administration
3 DOSAGE FORMS AND STRENGTHS
4 CONTRAINDICATIONS

5 WARNINGS AND PRECAUTIONS
   5.1 Infusion Reactions
   5.2 Capillary Leak Syndrome
   5.3 Visual Loss
   5.4 CD25 Tumor Expression and Evaluation
   5.5 Laboratory Monitoring/Hypoalbuminemia
6 ADVERSE REACTIONS
   6.1 Clinical Studies Experience
   6.2 Immunogenicity
   6.3 Postmarketing Experience
7 DRUG INTERACTIONS
8 USE IN SPECIFIC POPULATIONS
   8.1 Pregnancy
   8.3 Nursing Mothers
   8.4 Pediatric Use
   8.5 Geriatric Use
10 OVERDOSAGE
11 DESCRIPTION
12 CLINICAL PHARMACOLOGY
   12.1 Mechanism Of Action
   12.3 Pharmacokinetics
13 NONCLINICAL TOXICOLOGY
   13.1 Carcinogenesis, Mutagenesis, Impairment of Fertility
14 CLINICAL STUDIES
   14.1 Study 1: Placebo Controlled Study in CTCL (Stage Ia to III) Patients
   14.2 Study 2: Dose Evaluation Study in CTCL (Stage IIb to IVa) Patients
16 HOW SUPPLIED/STORAGE AND HANDLING
17 PATIENT COUNSELING INFORMATION
* Sections or subsections omitted from the full prescribing information are not listed

FULL PRESCRIBING INFORMATION

> **WARNING: SERIOUS INFUSION REACTIONS, CAPILLARY LEAK SYNDROME AND LOSS OF VISUAL ACUITY.**
> The following adverse reactions have been reported:
> • Serious and fatal infusion reactions. Administer Ontak in a facility equipped and staffed for cardiopulmonary resuscitation. Immediately stop and permanently discontinue Ontak for serious infusion reactions [see *Warnings and Precautions* (5.1)].
> • Capillary leak syndrome resulting in death. Monitor weight, edema, blood pressure and serum albumin levels prior to and during Ontak treatment [see *Warnings and Precautions* (5.2)].
> • Loss of visual acuity and color vision [see *Warnings and Precautions* (5.3)].

1 INDICATIONS AND USAGE
Ontak® is indicated for the treatment of patients with persistent or recurrent cutaneous T-cell lymphoma whose malignant cells express the CD25 component of the IL-2 receptor [see *Warnings and Precautions* (5.4)].

2 DOSAGE AND ADMINISTRATION
2.1 Dosing Schedule and Administration
• Premedicate with an antihistamine and acetaminophen prior to each Ontak infusion.
• Administer at 9 or 18 mcg/kg/day by intravenous infusion over 30-60 minutes for 5 consecutive days every 21 days for 8 cycles.
• Do **not** administer as a bolus injection.
• Withhold administration of Ontak if serum albumin levels are less than 3.0 g/dL.
• Discontinue for adverse infusion reactions.
2.2 Preparation and Administration
• Thaw vials in the refrigerator at 2 to 8°C (36 to 46°F) for not more than 24 hours or at room temperature for 1 to 2 hours.
• Bring Ontak to room temperature, before preparing the dose.
• Mix the solution in the vial by gentle swirling; do not shake.
• Visually inspect for particulate matter and discoloration prior to administration, whenever solution and container permit. Use only if the solution is clear, colorless and without visible particulate matter. After thawing, a haze may be visible which should clear when the solution is at room temperature.
• Do not refreeze Ontak after thawing.
• Prepare and hold diluted Ontak in plastic syringes or soft plastic IV bags. Do not use glass containers.
• Maintain concentration of Ontak at 15 mcg/mL or higher during all steps in the preparation of the solution for IV infusion.
• Withdraw the calculated dose from the vial(s) and inject it into an empty IV infusion bag. Do not add more than 9 mL of sterile saline without preservative to the IV bag for each 1 mL of Ontak.

- Do not mix Ontak with other drugs.
- Do not administer Ontak through an in-line filter.
- Administer prepared solutions of Ontak within 6 hours, using a syringe pump or IV infusion bag.
- Discard unused portions of Ontak immediately.

3 DOSAGE FORMS AND STRENGTHS

Single-use vial containing 150 mcg/mL (300 mcg in 2 mL).

4 CONTRAINDICATIONS

None.

5 WARNINGS AND PRECAUTIONS

5.1 Infusion Reactions

Infusion reactions, defined as symptoms occurring within 24 hours of infusion and resolving within 48 hours of the last infusion in that course, were reported in 70.5% (165/234) of Ontak-treated patients across 3 clinical studies utilizing the approved doses and schedule. Serious infusion reactions were reported in 8.1% (19/234) of Ontak-treated patients. There have been post-marketing reports of infusion reactions resulting in death.

For patients completing at least 4 courses of Ontak treatment in Study 1 [see *Clinical Studies* (14.1)], the incidence of infusion reactions was lower in the 3rd and 4th cycles as compared to the 1st and 2nd cycles of Ontak.

Resuscitative equipment should be available during Ontak administration. Immediately stop and permanently discontinue Ontak for serious infusion reactions.

5.2 Capillary Leak Syndrome

Capillary leak syndrome was defined as the occurrence of at least 2 of the following 3 symptoms (hypotension, edema, serum albumin <3.0 g/dL) at any time during Ontak therapy. These symptoms were not required to occur simultaneously to be characterized as capillary leak syndrome. As defined, capillary leak syndrome was reported in 32.5% (76/234) of Ontak-treated patients. Among these 76 patients with capillary leak syndrome, one-third required hospitalization or medical intervention to prevent hospitalization. There have been post-marketing reports of capillary leak syndrome resulting in death.

The onset of symptoms in patients with capillary leak syndrome may be delayed, occurring up to 2 weeks following infusion. Symptoms may persist or worsen after the cessation of Ontak.

Regularly assess patients for weight gain, new onset or worsening edema, hypotension (including orthostatic changes) and monitor serum albumin levels prior to the initiation of each course of therapy and more often as clinically indicated. Withhold Ontak for serum albumin levels of less than 3.0 g/dL [see *Warnings and Precautions* (5.5)].

5.3 Visual Loss

Loss of visual acuity, usually with loss of color vision, with or without retinal pigment mottling has been reported following administration of Ontak. Recovery was reported in some of the affected patients; however, most patients reported persistent visual impairment.

5.4 CD25 Tumor Expression and Evaluation

Confirm that the patient's malignant cells express CD25 prior to administration of Ontak. A testing service for the assay of CD25 expression in tumor biopsy samples is available. For information on this service call 877-873-4724.

5.5 Laboratory Monitoring/Hypoalbuminemia

Monitor serum albumin levels prior to the initiation of each treatment course. Withhold administration of Ontak if serum albumin levels are less than 3.0 g/dL [see *Dosage and Administration* (2.1) and *Warnings and Precautions* (5.2)].

6 ADVERSE REACTIONS

The following adverse reactions are discussed in greater detail in other sections of the label:
- Infusion Reactions [see *Warnings and Precautions* (5.1)]
- Capillary Leak Syndrome [see *Warnings and Precautions* (5.2)]
- Visual Loss [see *Warnings and Precautions* (5.3)]

6.1 Clinical Studies Experience

Because clinical trials are conducted under widely varying conditions, adverse reaction rates observed in the clinical trials of a drug cannot be directly compared to rates in the clinical trials of another drug and may not reflect the rates observed in practice.

Safety data are available for 3 clinical studies in which 234 patients received Ontak at 9 mcg/kg (n=80) or 18 mcg/kg (n=154) at the recommended schedule. Of these studies, 1 was placebo-controlled and dose-ranging (Study 1, 100 Ontak-treated patients), one was a dose-comparison of 9 and 18 mcg/kg (Study 2, n=71), and the third was a single-arm study using 18 mcg/kg (n=63); all studies were limited to adult patients with CTCL. The median age of patients across the clinical studies was 60 years (range 23-91 years) and 36% (n=85) were 65 years of age or older; 55% were men and 85% were Caucasian.

Across all 3 studies, the most common adverse reactions in Ontak-treated patients (≥20%) were pyrexia, nausea, fatigue, rigors, vomiting, diarrhea, headache, peripheral edema, cough, dyspnea and pruritus. The most common serious adverse reactions were capillary leak syndrome (11.1%), infusion reactions (8.1%), and visual changes including loss of visual acuity (4%). Ontak was discontinued in 28.2% (66/234) of patients due to adverse reactions.

The data described in Table 1 reflect exposure to Ontak in 100 patients administered as a single agent at the recommended dosing schedule in the randomized placebo-controlled trial (Study 1). The median number of Ontak cycles was 7 (range 1-10) for the 9 mcg/kg cohort and 6 (range 1-11) for the 18 mcg/kg cohort. The median age of patients was 59 years (range 23-84 years) and 34% (n=34) were 65 years of age or older; 55% were men and 86% were Caucasian.

Table 1: Incidence of Adverse Reactions Occurring in ≥10% of Ontak-treated patients (18 mcg/kg group) and at a higher rate than Placebo in Study 1

MedDRA version 6.1 Preferred Term	Placebo N=44 n (%)	Ontak 9 mcg/kg N=45 n (%)	Ontak 18 mcg/kg N=55 n (%)
Pyrexia	7 (15.9)	22 (48.9)	35 (63.6)
Nausea	10 (22.7)	21 (46.7)	33 (60.0)
Rigors	9 (20.5)	19 (42.2)	26 (47.3)
Fatigue	14 (31.8)	21 (46.7)	24 (43.6)
Vomiting	3 (6.8)	6 (13.3)	19 (34.5)
Headache	8 (18.2)	13 (28.9)	14 (25.5)
Edema peripheral	10 (22.7)	9 (20.0)	14 (25.5)
Diarrhea	4 (9.1)	10 (22.2)	12 (21.8)
Anorexia	2 (4.5)	4 (8.9)	11 (20.0)
Rash	2 (4.5)	11 (24.4)	11 (20.0)
Myalgia	2 (4.5)	8 (17.8)	11 (20.0)
Cough	3 (6.8)	9 (20.0)	10 (18.2)
Pruritus	4 (9.1)	7 (15.6)	10 (18.2)
Back pain	1 (2.3)	7 (15.6)	10 (18.2)
Asthenia	2 (4.5)	8 (17.8)	10 (18.2)
Hypotension	1 (2.3)	3 (6.7)	9 (16.4)
Upper respiratory tract infection	5 (11.4)	6 (13.3)	7 (12.7)
Dizziness	5 (11.4)	5 (11.1)	7 (12.7)
Arthralgia	5 (11.4)	7 (15.6)	7 (12.7)
Pain	3 (6.8)	5 (11.1)	7 (12.7)
Chest pain	1 (2.3)	2 (4.4)	7 (12.7)
Dysgeusia	1 (2.3)	0 (0)	6 (10.9)
Dyspnea	2 (4.5)	6 (13.3)	6 (10.9)

Hepatobiliary Disorders: Increase in serum alanine aminotransferase (ALT) or aspartate aminotransferase (AST) from baseline occurred in 84% of subjects treated with Ontak (197/234). In the majority of subjects, these enzyme elevations occurred during either the first or the second cycle; enzyme elevation resolved without medical intervention and did not require discontinuation of Ontak.

6.2 Immunogenicity

An immune response to denileukin diftitox was assessed using 2 enzyme-linked immunoassays (ELISA). The first assay measured reactivity directed against intact denileukin diftitox calibrated against anti-diphtheria toxin, and the second assay measured reactivity against the IL-2 portion of the protein. An additional *in vitro* cell-based assay that measured the ability of antibodies in serum to protect a human IL-2R-expressing cell line from toxicity by denileukin diftitox, was used to detect the presence of neutralizing antibodies which inhibited functional activity. The immunogenicity data reflect the percentage of patients whose test results were considered positive for antibodies to the intact fusion protein denileukin diftitox. These results are highly dependent on the sensitivity and the specificity of the assays. Additionally, the observed incidence of the antibody positivity may be influenced by several factors, including sample handling, concomitant medication, and underlying disease. For these reasons, the comparison of the incidence of antibodies to denileukin diftitox with the incidence of antibodies to other products may be misleading.

In Study 1 [see *Clinical Studies* (14.1)], of 95 patients treated with denileukin diftitox, 66% tested positive for antibodies at baseline probably due to a prior exposure to diphtheria toxin or its vaccine. After 1, 2, and 3 courses of treatment, 94%, 99%, and 100% of patients tested positive respectively. Mean titers of anti-denileukin diftitox antibodies were similarly increased in the 9 and 18 mcg/kg/day dose groups after 2 courses of treatment. Meanwhile, pharmacokinetic parameters decreased substantially (C_{max} ~57%, AUC ~80%), and clearance increased 2- to 8-fold.

In Study 2 [see *Clinical Studies* (14.2)], 131 patients were assessed for binding antibodies. Of these, 51 patients (39%) had antibodies at baseline. Seventy-six percent of patients tested positive after 1 course of treatment and 97% after 3 courses of treatment. Neutralizing antibodies were assessed in 60 patients; 45%, 73%, and 97% had evidence of inhibited functional activity in the cellular assay at baseline and after 1 and 3 courses of treatment, respectively.

6.3 Postmarketing Experience

The following adverse reactions have been identified during postapproval use of Ontak. Because these reactions are reported voluntarily from a population of uncertain size, it is not always possible to reliably estimate their frequency or establish a causal relationship to drug exposure.

Thyroid conditions: hyperthyroidism, thyroiditis, thyrotoxicosis, and hypothyroidism.

7 DRUG INTERACTIONS

No formal drug-drug interaction studies have been conducted with Ontak.

8 USE IN SPECIFIC POPULATIONS

8.1 Pregnancy

It is not known whether Ontak can cause fetal harm when administered to a pregnant woman or can affect reproductive capacity. Animal reproduction studies have not been conducted with Ontak. Ontak should be given to a pregnant woman only if clearly needed.

8.3 Nursing Mothers

It is not known whether Ontak is excreted in human milk. Because many drugs are excreted in human milk, and because of the potential for serious adverse reactions in nursing infants from Ontak, a decision should be made whether to discontinue nursing or to discontinue Ontak, taking into account the importance of the drug to the mother.

8.4 Pediatric Use

Safety and effectiveness in pediatric patients have not been established.

8.5 Geriatric Use

Clinical studies of Ontak did not include sufficient numbers of subjects aged 65 and older to determine whether they respond differently from younger subjects.

10 OVERDOSAGE

Doses of approximately twice the recommended dose (31 mcg/kg/day) resulted in moderate-to-severe nausea, vomiting, fever, chills and/or persistent asthenia.

11 DESCRIPTION

Ontak (denileukin diftitox), is a recombinant DNA-derived cytotoxic protein composed of the amino acid sequences for diphtheria toxin fragments A and B (Met_1-Thr_{387})-His and the sequences for human interleukin-2 (IL-2; Ala_1-Thr_{133}). It is produced in an *E. coli* expression system and has a molecular weight of 58 kD. Neomycin is used in the fermentation process but is undetectable in the final product. Ontak is supplied in single use vials as a sterile, frozen solution intended for intravenous (IV) administration. Each 2 mL vial of Ontak contains 300 mcg of recombinant denileukin diftitox in a sterile solution of citric acid (20 mM), EDTA (0.05 mM) and polysorbate 20 (<1%) in Water for Injection, USP. The solution has a pH range of 6.9 to 7.2.

12 CLINICAL PHARMACOLOGY

12.1 Mechanism Of Action

Denileukin diftitox is a fusion protein designed to direct the cytocidal action of diphtheria toxin to cells which express the IL-2 receptor. *Ex vivo* studies report that after binding to the IL-2 receptor on the cell surface, denileukin diftitox is internalized by receptor-mediated endocytosis. The fusion protein is subsequently cleaved, releasing diphtheria toxin enzymatic and translocation domains from the IL-2 fragment, resulting in the inhibition of protein synthesis and ultimately, cell death.

12.3 Pharmacokinetics

Pharmacokinetic parameters associated with denileukin diftitox were determined over a range of doses (3 to 31 mcg/kg/day) in patients with lymphoma. Denileukin diftitox was administered as an IV infusion following the schedule used in the clinical trials. Following the first dose, denileukin iftitox displayed 2-compartment behavior with a distribu-on phase (half-life approximately 2 to 5 minutes) and a erminal phase (half-life approximately 70 to 80 minutes). ystemic exposure was variable but proportional to dose. Iean clearance was approximately 0.6 to 2.0 mL/min/kg nd the mean volume of distribution was similar to that of irculating blood (0.06 to 0.09 L/kg). The mean clearance in-reased approximately 2- to 8-fold from course 1 to course 3 orresponding to a decrease in exposure of approximately '5%. No accumulation was evident between the first and ifth doses. Gender and age have no effect on pharmacoki-ietics of denileukin diftitox.

3 NONCLINICAL TOXICOLOGY

3.1 Carcinogenesis, Mutagenesis, Impairment of Fer-ility

There have been no studies to assess the carcinogenic po-tential of denileukin diftitox. Denileukin diftitox showed no evidence of mutagenicity in the Ames test and the chromo-somal aberration assay. There have been no studies to as-sess the effect of denileukin diftitox on fertility.

14 CLINICAL STUDIES

14.1 Study 1: Placebo Controlled Study in CTCL (Stage Ia to III) Patients

The safety and efficacy of Ontak were evaluated in a ran-domized, double-blind, placebo-controlled, 3-arm trial in pa-tients with Stage Ia to III CD25(+) CTCL. Eligible patients were required to have expression of CD25 on ≥ 20% of bi-opsied malignant cells by immunohistochemistry [see *Warnings and Precautions* (5.4)]. Patients were randomized to re-ceive 0, 9 or 18 mcg/kg/day Ontak via intravenous infusion days 1-5 of each 21-day cycle, for up to 8 cycles. Randomiza-tion was stratified by disease stage (≤IIa vs. ≥IIb). The main efficacy outcome was objective response rate (ORR), using a Weighted Skin Severity Index, in conjunction with assessment of lymph node involvement and percentage of abnormal blood lymphocytes. A total of 144 patients were randomized: 44 patients to placebo, 45 patients to 9 mcg/kg/day Ontak and 55 patients to 18 mcg/kg/day Ontak. Ran-domization for the study was carried out at 1:1:1 for the first 73 patients, 4:1:4 for the next 31 patients, and 1:4:4 for the remaining 40 patients. The median age of patients was 59 years (range 23 to 84 years); 34% were ≥ 65 years. Fifty-five percent were men and 86% were Caucasian. Sixty-seven percent had early stage disease (≤ IIa). Patients had re-ceived a median of 2 anti-CTCL therapies (range 0 to 6) prior to study entry. Results for objective response rate (ORR) and progression-free survival (PFS) are shown in the table below.

Table 2: Efficacy Results in Study 1

Efficacy Endpoint	Ontak 18 mcg/kg/day (N=55)	Ontak 9 mcg/kg/day (N=45)	Placebo (N=44)
ORR %[a] p-value[b]	46% p=0.002	37% p=0.03	15% —
Median Response Duration	220 days	277 days	81 days
PFS[c] Hazard ratio (95% CI) p-value	0.27 (0.14, 0.54) p=0.0002	0.42 (0.20, 0.86) p=0.02	—

[a] Adjusted for disease stage and changes in randomization ratios.
[b] Logistic regression model adjusting for disease stage and changes in randomization ratios over the course of the study; comparisons relative to placebo.
[c] Cox regression analysis stratified by randomization ratio and adjusted for disease stage; comparisons relative to placebo.

14.2 Study 2: Dose Evaluation Study in CTCL (Stage IIb to IVa) Patients

A randomized, double-blind study was conducted to evalu-ate doses of 9 or 18 mcg/kg/day in 71 patients with recur-rent or persistent, Stage Ib to IVa CTCL. Entry to this study required demonstration of CD25 expression on at least 20% of the cells in any relevant tumor tissue sample (skin bi-opsy) or circulating cells. Tumor biopsies were not evaluated for expression of other IL-2 receptor subunit components (CD122/CD132). Ontak was administered as an IV infusion daily for 5 days every 3 weeks. Patients received a median of 6 courses of Ontak therapy (range 1 to 11). The study pop-ulation had received a median of 5 prior therapies (range 1 to 12) with 63% of patients entering the trial with Stage IIb or more advanced stage disease. The median age of patients was 64 years (range 26 to 91 years); 49% were ≥ 65 years. Fifty-two percent were men and 75% were Caucasian.

Overall, 30% (95% CI: 18-41%) of patients treated with Ontak experienced an objective tumor response (50% reduc-tion in tumor burden which was sustained for ≥6 weeks; Table 3). Seven patients (10%) achieved a complete response and 14 patients (20%) achieved a partial response. The over-all median duration of response, measured from first day of response, was 4 months with a median duration for com-plete response of 9 months and for partial response of 4 months.

Table 3: Efficacy Results in Study 2

Clinical Response	9 mcg/kg/day	18 mcg/kg/day
Complete Response 95% Confidence Interval	9% (3/35) (2%, 23%)	11% (4/36) (3%, 26%)
Partial Response 95% Confidence Interval	14% (5/35) (9%, 30%)	25% (9/36) (12%, 42%)
Overall Response 95% Confidence Interval	23% (8/35) (10%, 40%)	36% (13/36) (21%, 54%)

16 HOW SUPPLIED/STORAGE AND HANDLING

Ontak is supplied as 150 mcg/ml, sterile, frozen solution (300 mcg in 2 mL) in a sterile single-use vial.
NDC 62856-603-01, 6 vials in a package.
Store frozen at or below -10°C (14°F).
Manufactured by:
Eisai Medical Research Inc.
Woodcliff Lake, NJ 07677
US License No. 1763
Manufactured at:
Hollister-Stier Labs LLC
Spokane, WA 99207
Distributed by:
Eisai Inc.
Woodcliff Lake, NJ 07677

17 PATIENT COUNSELING INFORMATION

Advise patients to report:

- Fever, chills, breathing problems, chest pain, tachycardia, and urticaria following infusion.
- Rapid weight gain, edema, and orthostatic hypotension following infusion. Instruct patients to weigh themselves daily.
- Visual loss, including loss of color vision.

Shown in Product Identification Guide, page 308

PANRETIN® ℞

[*păn-rĕtĭn*]
(alitretinoin)
gel 0.1%
(For topical use only)
Rx only

DESCRIPTION

Panretin® gel 0.1% contains alitretinoin and is intended for topical application only. The chemical name is 9-*cis*-retinoic acid and the structural formula is as follows:

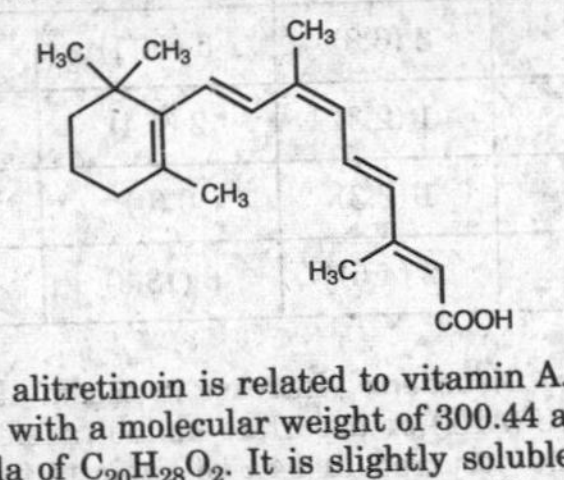

Chemically, alitretinoin is related to vitamin A. It is a yel-low powder with a molecular weight of 300.44 and a molec-ular formula of $C_{20}H_{28}O_2$. It is slightly soluble in ethanol (7.01 mg/g at 25°C) and insoluble in water. Panretin® gel is a clear, yellow gel containing 0.1% (w/w) alitretinoin in a base of dehydrated alcohol USP, polyethylene glycol 400 NF, hydroxypropyl cellulose NF, and butylated hydroxy-toluene NF.

CLINICAL PHARMACOLOGY

Mechanism of Action

Alitretinoin (9-*cis*-retinoic acid) is a naturally-occurring en-dogenous retinoid that binds to and activates all known in-tracellular retinoid receptor subtypes (RARα, RARβ, RARγ, RXRα, RXRβ and RXRγ). Once activated these receptors function as transcription factors that regulate the expres-sion of genes that control the process of cellular differenti-ation and proliferation in both normal and neoplastic cells. Alitretinoin inhibits the growth of Kaposi's sarcoma (KS) cells in vitro.

Pharmacokinetics

No studies have examined plasma 9-*cis*-retinoic acid con-centrations before and after treatment with Panretin® gel. There is, however, indirect evidence that absorption is not extensive. Plasma concentrations of 9-*cis*-retinoic acid were evaluated during clinical studies in patients with cutaneous lesions of AIDS-related KS after repeated multiple-daily dose application of Panretin® gel for up to 60 weeks. The range of 9-*cis*-retinoic acid plasma concentrations in these patients was similar to the range of circulating, naturally-occurring 9-*cis*-retinoic acid plasma concentrations in un-treated healthy volunteers.

Although there are no detectable plasma concentrations of 9-*cis*-retinoic acid metabolites after topical application of Panretin® gel, in vitro studies indicate that the drug is me-tabolized to 4-hydroxy-9-*cis*-retinoic acid and 4-oxo-9-*cis*-retinoic acid by CYP 2C9, 3A4, 1A1, and 1A2 enzymes. In vivo, 4-oxo-9-*cis*-retinoic acid is the major circulating me-tabolite following oral administration of 9-*cis*-retinoic acid. No formal pharmacokinetic drug interaction studies be-tween Panretin® gel and antiretroviral agents have been conducted.

Clinical Studies

Panretin® gel is not a systemic therapy; it therefore cannot treat visceral Kaposi's sarcoma (KS) nor prevent the devel-opment of new KS lesions where it has not been applied. Visceral KS disease was not monitored in these trials, and the appearance of new KS lesions was not considered part of the response assessment in clinical trials.

Panretin® gel was evaluated in two multicenter, prospec-tive, randomized, double-blind, vehicle-controlled studies in patients with cutaneous lesions of AIDS-related KS. In both studies the primary efficacy endpoint was the patients' cu-taneous KS tumor response rate through 12 weeks of study drug treatment which was assessed by evaluating from 3 to 8 KS index lesions according to the modified AIDS Clinical Trials Group (ACTG) response criteria as applied to topical therapy (i.e., evaluation of height and area reductions of the index lesions only; progressive disease in non-index lesions and new lesions were not considered progressive disease; progressive disease was scored only in the treated index le-sions). A global evaluation by physicians was also carried out. It considered all of the patient's treated lesions (index and other) compared to baseline. In this evaluation, pa-tients with at least a 50% improvement in the KS lesions were considered responders. In addition, photographs of le-sions in patients considered responders by the modified ACTG criteria were examined by the FDA for a cosmetically beneficial response, defined as at least a 50% improvement in appearance compared to baseline, considering both the KS lesions and dermal toxicity at the lesion site, in at least 50% of the index lesions and maintained for at least 3 weeks. Patients were also asked about their satisfaction with the treatment.

In Study 1, a total of 268 patients were entered from centers in the U.S. and Canada. Patients were treated topically three to four times a day with either Panretin® gel or a matching vehicle gel for a minimum of 12 weeks, followed by an open-label phase in patients who had not yet pro-gressed on Panretin® gel. Responses during the double-blind phase are shown in Table 1. Responses to Panretin® gel were seen in both previously untreated patients and in patients with prior systemic and/or topical KS treatment. A total of 72 patients responded to Panretin® gel during the randomized or crossover portions of the study. At a median duration of monitoring of 16 weeks, only 15% of the 72 pa-tients had relapsed. Panretin® gel would not be expected to affect development of new lesions in untreated areas and these were seen in about 50% of patients, at similar rates in treated and untreated patients, responders and non-responders. The patients' assessment of their overall satis-faction with the effect on all treated lesions signifi-cantly favored Panretin® gel.

Study 2 was an international study with a planned enroll-ment of 270 patients. Patients were treated topically twice a day with Panretin® gel or a matching vehicle for 12 weeks. The study was stopped early because of positive interim re-sults in the initial 82 patient data set. Results of the study are shown in Table 1. Responses to Panretin® gel were seen both in previously untreated patients and in patients with prior systemic and/or topical KS treatment.

[See table 1 at top of next page]

In the clinical trials, responses were seen as early as two (2) weeks; most patients, however, required four (4) to eight (8) weeks of treatment, and some patients did not experience significant improvement until 14 or more weeks of treat-ment. The cumulative percentage of patients who achieved a response was less than 1% at 2 weeks, 10% at 4 weeks, and 28% at 8 weeks.

In both studies, responses occurred in patients with a wide range of baseline CD4+ lymphocyte counts, including pa-tients with CD4+ lymphocyte counts less than 50 cells/mm^3. Nearly all patients received concomitant combination anti-retroviral therapy.

Photographs of patients revealed a substantial erythematous and edematous response in some cases, leading to a cosmetically mixed outcome even in apparent responders. Nonetheless, in Study 1 it appeared that a cosmetically satisfactory result occurred at about the same rate as the Physician's Global response rate and in both studies such a response was more frequent than in the vehicle control.

INDICATIONS AND USAGE

Panretin® gel is indicated for topical treatment of cutaneous lesions in patients with AIDS-related Kaposi's sarcoma. Panretin® gel is not indicated when systemic anti-KS therapy is required (e.g., more than 10 new KS lesions in the prior month, symptomatic lymphedema, symptomatic pulmonary KS, or symptomatic visceral involvement). There is no experience to date using Panretin® gel with systemic anti-KS treatment.

CONTRAINDICATIONS

Panretin® gel is contraindicated in patients with a known hypersensitivity to retinoids or to any of the ingredients of the product.

WARNINGS

Pregnancy: Panretin® gel could cause fetal harm if significant absorption were to occur in a pregnant woman. 9-cis-retinoic acid has been shown to be teratogenic in rabbits and mice. An increased incidence of fused sternebrae and limb and craniofacial defects occurred in rabbits given oral doses of 0.5 mg/kg/day (about five times the estimated daily human topical dose on a mg/m² basis, assuming complete systemic absorption of 9-cis-retinoic acid, when Panretin® gel is administered as a 60 g tube over 1 month in a 60 kg human) during the period of organogenesis. Limb and craniofacial defects also occurred in mice given a single oral dose of 50 mg/kg on day eleven of gestation (about 127 times the estimated daily human topical dose on a mg/m² basis). Oral 9-cis-retinoic acid was also embryocidal, as indicated by early resorptions and post-implantation loss when it was given during the period of organogenesis to rabbits at doses of 1.5 mg/kg/day (about 15 times the estimated daily human topical dose on a mg/m² basis) and to rats at doses of 5 mg/kg/day (about 25 times the estimated daily human topical dose on a mg/m² basis). Animal reproduction studies with topical 9-cis-retinoic acid have not been conducted. It is not known whether topical Panretin® gel can modulate endogenous 9-cis-retinoic acid levels in a pregnant woman nor whether systemic exposure is increased by application to ulcerated lesions or by duration of treatment. There are no adequate and well-controlled studies in pregnant women. If Panretin® gel is used during pregnancy, or if the patient becomes pregnant while taking it, the patient should be apprised of the potential hazard to the fetus. Women of childbearing potential should be advised to avoid becoming pregnant.

PRECAUTIONS

Panretin® gel is indicated for topical treatment of Kaposi's sarcoma. Patients with cutaneous T-cell lymphoma were less tolerant of topical Panretin® gel; five of seven patients had 6 episodes of treatment-limiting toxicities—grade 3 dermal irritation—with Panretin® gel (0.01% or 0.05%).

Photosensitivity

Retinoids as a class have been associated with photosensitivity. There were no reports of photosensitivity associated with the use of Panretin® gel in the clinical studies. Nonetheless, because in vitro data indicate that 9-cis-retinoic acid may have a weak photosensitizing effect, patients should be advised to minimize exposure of treated areas to sunlight and sunlamps during the use of Panretin® gel.

Drug Interactions

Patients who are applying Panretin® gel should not concurrently use products that contain DEET (N,N-diethyl-m-toluamide), a common component of insect repellent products. Animal toxicology studies showed increased DEET toxicity when DEET was included as part of the formulation.

Although there was no clinical evidence in the vehicle-controlled studies of drug interactions with systemic antiretroviral agents, including protease inhibitors, macrolide antibiotics, and azole antifungals, the effect of Panretin® gel on the steady-state concentrations of these drugs is not known. No drug interaction data are available on concomitant administration of Panretin® gel and systemic anti-KS agents.

Drug/Laboratory Test Interactions

No interference with laboratory tests has been observed.

Carcinogenesis, Mutagenesis, Impairment of Fertility

Long-term studies in animals to assess the carcinogenic potential of 9-cis-retinoic acid have not been conducted. 9-cis-retinoic acid was not mutagenic in vitro (bacterial assays, Chinese hamster ovary cell HGPRT mutation assay) and

was not clastogenic in vitro (chromosome aberration test in human lymphocytes) nor in vivo (mouse micronucleus test).

Pregnancy Category D (see "Warnings" section)

Nursing Mothers

It is not known whether alitretinoin or its metabolites are excreted in human milk. Because many drugs are excreted in human milk and because of the potential for adverse reactions from Panretin® gel in nursing infants, mothers should discontinue nursing prior to using the drug.

Pediatric Use

Safety and effectiveness in pediatric patients have not been established.

Geriatric Use

Inadequate information is available to assess safety and efficacy in patients age 65 years or older.

ADVERSE REACTIONS

The safety of Panretin® gel has been assessed in clinical studies of 385 patients with AIDS-related KS. Adverse events associated with the use of Panretin® gel in patients with AIDS-related KS occurred almost exclusively at the site of application. The dermal toxicity begins as erythema; with continued application of Panretin® gel, erythema may increase and edema may develop. Dermal toxicity may become treatment-limiting, with intense erythema, edema, and vesiculation. Usually, however, adverse events are mild to moderate in severity; they led to withdrawal from the study in only 7% of the patients. Severe local (application site) skin adverse events occurred in about 10% of patients in the U.S. study (versus 0% in the vehicle control). Table 2 lists the adverse events that occurred at the application site with an incidence of at least 5% during the double-blind phase in the Panretin® gel-treated group and in the vehicle control group in either of the two controlled studies. Adverse events were reported at other sites but generally were similar in the two groups.
[See table 2 above]

OVERDOSAGE

There has been no experience with acute overdose of Panretin® gel in humans. Systemic toxicity following acute overdosage with topical application of Panretin® gel is unlikely because of limited systemic plasma levels observed

with normal therapeutic doses. There is no specific antidote for overdosage.

DOSAGE AND ADMINISTRATION

Panretin® gel should initially be applied two (2) times a day to cutaneous KS lesions. The application frequency can be gradually increased to three (3) or four (4) times a day according to individual lesion tolerance. If application site toxicity occurs, the application frequency can be reduced. Should severe irritation occur, application of drug can be temporarily discontinued for a few days until the symptoms subside.

Sufficient gel should be applied to cover the lesion with a generous coating. The gel should be allowed to dry for three to five minutes before covering with clothing. Because unaffected skin may become irritated, application of the gel to normal skin surrounding the lesions should be avoided. In addition, do not apply the gel on or near mucosal surfaces of the body.

A response of KS lesions may be seen as soon as two weeks after initiation of therapy but most patients require longer application. With continued application, further benefit may be attained. Some patients have required over 14 weeks to respond. In clinical trials, Panretin® gel was applied for up to 96 weeks. Panretin® gel should be continued as long as the patient is deriving benefit.

Occlusive dressings should not be used with Panretin® gel.

HOW SUPPLIED

Panretin® gel is available in tubes containing 60 grams, (60 mg active ingredient alitretinoin). NDC 62856-601-22 Store at 25° C (77° F); excursions permitted to 15-30° C (59-86° F) [see USP Controlled Room Temperature].

Manufactured for:
Eisai Inc.
Woodcliff Lake, NJ 07677
by:
Contract Pharmaceuticals Limited Niagara
Buffalo, NY 14213-1091
Panretin is a registered trademark of Eisai Inc.
Revised February 2007
© 2007 Eisai Inc.

TABLE 1: Summary of Tumor Responses

	STUDY 1		STUDY 2	
	Panretin® Gel N=134	Vehicle Gel N=134	Panretin® Gel N=36	Vehicle Gel N=46
Modified ACTG Response (index lesions)	34% PR 1% CR	16% PR p=0.0012	36% PR	7% PR
Physician's Global/Subjective Assessment (all treated lesions)	19% PR	4% PR p=0.00014	47% PR	11% PR
Beneficial Response Photographs (index lesions only)	15%	4% p=0.0026	19%	2%

TABLE 2: Adverse Events with an Incidence of at Least 5% at the Application Site in Either Controlled Study in Patients Receiving Panretin® Gel or Vehicle Control

Adverse Event Term	Study 1		Study 2	
	Panretin® Gel N=134 Pts. %	Vehicle Gel N=134 Pts. %	Panretin® Gel N=36 Pts. %	Vehicle Gel N=46 Pts. %
Rash[1]	77	11	25	4
Pain[2]	34	7	0	4
Pruritus[3]	11	4	8	4
Exfoliative dermatitis[4]	9	2	3	0
Skin disorder[5]	8	1	0	0
Paresthesia[6]	3	0	22	7
Edema[7]	8	3	3	0

Includes Investigator terms:
[1] Erythema, scaling, irritation, redness, rash, dermatitis
[2] Burning, pain
[3] Itching, pruritus
[4] Flaking, peeling, desquamation, exfoliation
[5] Excoriation, cracking, scab, crusting, drainage, eschar, fissure or oozing
[6] Stinging, tingling
[7] Edema, swelling, inflammation

Panretin®

(alitretinoin)

gel 0.1%

Patient's Instructions for Use

(For topical use only)

Your health care provider has prescribed Panretin® gel for the management of the Kaposi's sarcoma (KS) lesions on your skin. The following simple instructions will help you successfully begin and continue your treatment.

WARNINGS

DO NOT apply gel on or near mucosal surfaces of the body such as eyes, nostrils, mouth, lips, vagina, tip of the penis, rectum or anus.

DO NOT use insect repellents containing DEET (N,N-diethyl-m-toluamide) or other products containing DEET while using Panretin® gel.

Keep Out of Reach of Children.

Product contains alcohol and should be kept away from open flame.

DO NOT use Panretin® gel if you are pregnant or breast-feeding. Precautions should be taken to avoid becoming pregnant while using Panretin® gel. If you are pregnant, thinking of becoming pregnant, or breastfeeding, speak with your health care provider for more information.

Topical Panretin® gel does not treat lung or intestinal Kaposi's sarcoma.

Topical Panretin® gel does not prevent the appearance of new KS lesions or the increased growth of KS lesions not treated with Panretin® gel.

Topical Panretin® gel does not treat extremity swelling associated with KS. It is important to understand that KS lesions can appear and affect other parts of your body, including internal organs (e.g., lungs and intestines). You should regularly consult your health care provider about the status of your KS disease, especially if you note changes.

HOW TO APPLY

Apply Panretin® gel to your KS lesions using a clean finger. Place a generous coating of gel over the entire surface of each lesion that you want to treat. It is not necessary to physically rub the gel into the lesion. You should make every effort not to apply gel to the healthy skin around the lesion. The extra effort you take in carefully applying the gel only to the area of the KS lesion will help to lessen any irritation or redness which may occur. Proper application should leave some gel visible on the surface of the lesion when you are finished with the application.

Immediately following application, wipe the finger(s) you have used to apply the gel with a disposable tissue and wash your hands using soap and water.

Allow the gel to dry before covering a treated area with clothing. This will usually take from three (3) to five (5) minutes.

A mild soap is recommended when bathing or showering.

WHEN TO APPLY

Panretin® gel should be applied at an initial frequency of two (2) times daily. Your health care provider may instruct you to apply Panretin® gel at a different frequency (up to four [4] times daily). Applications should be spaced as evenly as possible throughout the day. If you apply Panretin® gel after your shower or bath, you should wait 20 minutes before application.

YOU SHOULD AVOID...

You should avoid applying the gel to areas of healthy skin around a KS lesion. Exposure of healthy skin to Panretin® gel may cause unnecessary irritation or redness.

You should avoid showering, bathing, or swimming until at least three (3) hours after any application, if possible.

You should avoid covering the KS lesions treated with gel with any bandage or material other than loose clothing.

You should avoid prolonged exposure of the treated area to sunlight or other ultraviolet (UV) light (such as tanning lamps).

You should avoid the use of other topical products on your treated KS lesions. Mineral oil may be used between Panretin® gel applications in order to help prevent excessive dryness or itching. However, mineral oil should not be applied for at least two (2) hours before or after the application of Panretin® gel.

You should avoid scratching the treated areas.

WHAT TO EXPECT

Do not be discouraged if you do not see immediate improvement.

Do not stop treatment at the first sign of improvement.

While using Panretin® gel, you may experience some local effects such as redness, discomfort, itching, and skin peeling or flaking at the area of application. Other possible local skin effects include: rawness, surface or deep cracking, scabbing, crusting, drainage, oozing, or infection. Should these or other effects become troublesome to you, consult your health care provider. He or she can provide information on how to manage these effects.

HOW QUICKLY CAN I EXPECT PANRETIN® GEL TO WORK?

Be patient. Panretin® gel takes time to work, up to 14 weeks or more of treatment. In clinical trials, few patients experienced the onset of response as early as two (2) weeks; most patients who responded required at least four (4) to eight (8) weeks of treatment, and some patients did not experience significant improvement until 14 or more weeks of treatment. Continue to use Panretin® gel as instructed by your health care provider.

OTHER INFORMATION

The opening of the Panretin® gel tube is covered by a metal safety seal. If this seal has been punctured or is not visible when you open the package, DO NOT USE and promptly return the product to your pharmacy or place of purchase. To open, use the pointed portion of the cap to puncture the metal safety seal.

Always use the cap to close the tube tightly after each use. Store at room temperature. Keep away from heat.

IF YOU HAVE QUESTIONS...

If you have any questions about your treatment, talk with your health care provider.

Eisai Inc.
Woodcliff Lake, NJ 07677
200602 Revised 03/07

SALAGEN® ℞

[sā-lā-jěn]

(pilocarpine hydrochloride)

Tablets

DESCRIPTION

SALAGEN® Tablets contain pilocarpine hydrochloride, a cholinergic agonist for oral use. Pilocarpine hydrochloride is a hygroscopic, odorless, bitter tasting white crystal or powder which is soluble in water and alcohol and virtually insoluble in most non-polar solvents. Pilocarpine hydrochloride, with a chemical name of (3S-*cis*)-2-(3*H*)-Furanone, 3-ethyldihydro-4-[(1-methyl-1*H*-imidazol-5-yl)methyl] monohydrochloride, has a molecular weight of 244.72.

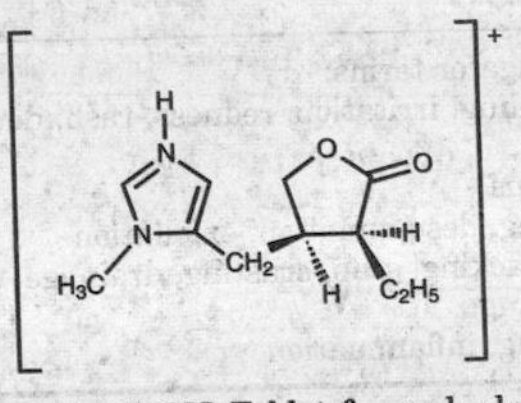

Each 5 mg SALAGEN® Tablet for oral administration contains 5 mg of pilocarpine hydrochloride. Inactive ingredients in the tablet, the tablet's film coating, and polishing are: carnauba wax, hypromellose, microcrystalline cellulose, stearic acid, titanium dioxide and other ingredients.

Each 7.5 mg SALAGEN® Tablet for oral administration contains 7.5 mg of pilocarpine hydrochloride. Inactive ingredients in the tablet, the tablet's film coating, and polishing are: carnauba wax, hypromellose, microcrystalline cellulose, stearic acid, titanium dioxide, FD&C blue#2 aluminum lake, and other ingredients.

CLINICAL PHARMACOLOGY

Pharmacodynamics: Pilocarpine is a cholinergic parasympathomimetic agent exerting a broad spectrum of pharmacologic effects with predominant muscarinic action. Pilocarpine, in appropriate dosage, can increase secretion by the exocrine glands. The sweat, salivary, lacrimal, gastric, pancreatic, and intestinal glands and the mucous cells of the respiratory tract may be stimulated. When applied topically to the eye as a single dose it causes miosis, spasm of accommodation, and may cause a transitory rise in intraocular pressure followed by a more persistent fall. Dose-related smooth muscle stimulation of the intestinal tract may cause increased tone, increased motility, spasm, and tenesmus. Bronchial smooth muscle tone may increase. The tone and motility of urinary tract, gallbladder, and biliary duct smooth muscle may be enhanced. Pilocarpine may have paradoxical effects on the cardiovascular system. The expected effect of a muscarinic agonist is vasodepression, but administration of pilocarpine may produce hypertension after a brief episode of hypotension. Bradycardia and tachycardia have both been reported with use of pilocarpine.

In a study of 12 healthy male volunteers there was a dose-related increase in unstimulated salivary flow following single 5 and 10 mg oral doses of SALAGEN® Tablets. This effect of pilocarpine on salivary flow was time-related with an onset at 20 minutes and a peak effect at 1 hour with a duration of 3 to 5 hours (See **Pharmacokinetics** section).

Head & Neck Cancer Patients: In a 12 week randomized, double-blind, placebo-controlled study in 207 patients (placebo, N=65; 5 mg, N=73; 10 mg, N=69), increases from baseline (means 0.072 and 0.112 mL/min, ranges -0.690 to 0.728 and -0.380 to 1.689) of whole saliva flow for the 5 mg (63%) and 10 mg (90%) tablet, respectively, were seen 1 hour after the first dose of SALAGEN® Tablets. Increases in unstimulated parotid flow were seen following the first dose (means 0.025 and 0.046 mL/min, ranges 0 to 0.414 and -0.070 to 1.002 mL/min for the 5 and 10 mg dose, respectively). In this study, no correlation existed between the amount of increase in salivary flow and the degree of symptomatic relief.

Sjogren's Syndrome Patients: In two 12 week randomized, double-blind, placebo-controlled studies in 629 patients (placebo, N=253; 2.5 mg, N=121; 5 mg, N=255; 5-7.5 mg, N=114), the ability of SALAGEN® Tablets to stimulate saliva production was assessed. In these trials using varying doses of SALAGEN® Tablets (2.5-7.5 mg), the rate of saliva production was plotted against time. An Area Under the Curve (AUC) representing the total amount of saliva produced during the observation interval was calculated. Relative to placebo, an increase in the amount of saliva being produced was observed following the first dose of SALAGEN® Tablets and was maintained throughout the duration (12 weeks) of the trials in an approximate dose response fashion (See **Clinical Studies** section).

Pharmacokinetics: In a multiple-dose pharmacokinetic study in male volunteers following 2 days of 5 or 10 mg of oral pilocarpine hydrochloride tablets given at 8 a.m., noontime, and 6 p.m., the mean elimination half-life was 0.76 hours for the 5 mg dose and 1.35 hours for the 10 mg dose. T_{max} values were 1.25 hours and 0.85 hours. C_{max} values were 15 ng/mL and 41 ng/mL. The AUC trapezoidal values were 33 h(ng/mL) and 108 h(ng/mL), respectively, for the 5 and 10 mg doses following the last 6 hour dose.

Pharmacokinetics in elderly male volunteers (N=11) were comparable to those in younger men. In five healthy elderly female volunteers, the mean C_{max} and AUC were approximately twice that of elderly males and young normal male volunteers.

When taken with a high fat meal by 12 healthy male volunteers, there was a decrease in the rate of absorption of pilocarpine from SALAGEN® Tablets. Mean $T_{max's}$ were 1.47 and 0.87 hours, and mean $C_{max's}$ were 51.8 and 59.2 ng/mL for fed and fasted, respectively.

Limited information is available about the metabolism and elimination of pilocarpine in humans. Inactivation of pilocarpine is thought to occur at neuronal synapses and probably in plasma. Pilocarpine and its minimally active or inactive degradation products, including pilocarpic acid, are excreted in the urine. Pilocarpine does not bind to human or rat plasma proteins over a concentration range of 5 to 25,000 ng/mL. The effect of pilocarpine on plasma protein binding of other drugs has not been evaluated.

In patients with mild to moderate hepatic impairment (N=12), administration of a single 5 mg dose resulted in a 30% decrease in total plasma clearance and a doubling of exposure (as measured by AUC). Peak plasma levels were also increased by about 30% and half-life was increased to 2.1 hrs.

There were no significant differences in the pharmacokinetics of oral pilocarpine in volunteer subjects (N=8) with renal insufficiency (mean creatinine clearances 25.4 mL/min; range 9.8-40.8 mL/min) compared to the pharmacokinetics previously observed in normal volunteers.

Clinical Studies: Head & Neck Cancer Patients: A 12 week randomized, double-blind, placebo-controlled study in 207 patients (142 men, 65 women) was conducted in patients whose mean age was 58.5 years with a range of 19 to 77; the racial distribution was Caucasian 95%, Black 4%, and other 1%. In this population, a statistically significant improvement in mouth dryness occurred in the 5 and 10 mg SALAGEN® Tablet treated patients compared to placebo treated patients. The 5 and 10 mg treated patients could not be distinguished. (See **Pharmacodynamics** section for flow study details.)

Another 12 week, double-blind, randomized, placebo-controlled study was conducted in 162 patients whose mean age was 57.8 years with a range of 27 to 80; the racial distribution was Caucasian 88%, Black 10%, and other 2%. The effects of placebo were compared to 2.5 mg three times a day of SALAGEN® Tablets for 4 weeks followed by adjustment to 5 mg three times a day and 10 mg three times a day. Lowering of the dose was necessary because of adverse events in 3 of 67 patients treated with 5 mg of SALAGEN® Tablets and in 7 of 66 patients treated with 10 mg of SALAGEN® Tablets. After 4 weeks of treatment, 2.5 mg of SALAGEN® Tablets three times a day was comparable to placebo in relieving dryness. In patients treated with 5 mg and 10 mg of SALAGEN® Tablets, the greatest improvement in dryness was noted in patients with no measurable salivary flow at baseline.

In both studies, some patients noted improvement in the global assessment of their dry mouth, speaking without liquids, and a reduced need for supplemental oral comfort agents.

In the two placebo-controlled clinical trials, the most common adverse events related to drug, and increasing in rate as dose increases, were sweating, nausea, rhinitis, diarrhea, chills, flushing, urinary frequency, dizziness, and asthenia. The most common adverse experience causing withdrawal from treatment was sweating (5 mg t.i.d. ≤1%; 10 mg t.i.d. =12%).

Sjogren's Syndrome Patients: Two separate studies were conducted in patients with primary or secondary Sjogren's Syndrome. In both studies, the majority of patients best fit the European criteria for having primary Sjogren's Syndrome. ["Criteria for the Classification of Sjogren's Syndrome" (Vitali C, Bombardieri S, Moutsopoulos HM, et al: Preliminary criteria for the classification of Sjogren's Syndrome. *Arthritis Rheum.* 1993; 36:340-347.)]

A 12-week, randomized, double-blind, parallel-group, placebo-controlled study was conducted in 256 patients (14 men, 242 women) whose mean age was 57 years with a range of 24 to 85 years. The racial distribution was as follows: Caucasian 91%, Black 6%, and other 3%.

The effects of placebo were compared with those of SALAGEN® Tablets 5 mg four times a day (20 mg/day) for 6 weeks. At 6 weeks, the patients' dosage was increased from 5 mg SALAGEN® Tablets q.i.d. to 7.5 mg q.i.d. The data collected during the first 6 weeks of the trial were evaluated for safety and efficacy, and the data of the second 6 weeks of the trial were used to provide additional evidence of safety.

After 6 weeks of treatment, statistically significant global improvement of dry mouth was observed compared to placebo. "Global improvement" is defined as a score of 55 mm or more on a 100 mm visual analogue scale in response to the question, "Please rate your present condition of dry mouth (xerostomia) compared with your condition at the start of this study. Consider the changes to your dry mouth and other symptoms related to your dry mouth that have occurred since you have taken this medication." Patients' assessments of specific dry mouth symptoms such as severity of dry mouth, mouth discomfort, ability to speak without water, ability to sleep without drinking water, ability to swallow food without drinking, and a decreased use of saliva substitutes were found to be consistent with the significant global improvement described.

Another 12 week randomized, double-blind, parallel-group, placebo-controlled study was conducted in 373 patients (16 men, 357 women) whose mean age was 55 years with a range of 21 to 84. The racial distribution was Caucasian 80%, Oriental 14%, Black 2%, and 4% of other origin. The treatment groups were 2.5 mg pilocarpine tablets, 5 mg SALAGEN® Tablets, and placebo. All treatments were administered on a four times a day regimen.

After 12 weeks of treatment, statistically significant global improvement of dry mouth was observed at a dose of 5 mg compared with placebo. The 2.5 mg (10 mg/day) group was not significantly different than placebo. However, a subgroup of patients with rheumatoid arthritis tended to improve in global assessments at both the 2.5 mg q.i.d. (9 patients) and 5 mg q.i.d. (16 patients) dose (10-20 mg/day). The clinical significance of this finding is unknown.

Patients' assessments of specific dry mouth symptoms such as severity of dry mouth, mouth discomfort, ability to sleep without drinking water, and decreased use of saliva substitutes were also found to be consistent with the significant global improvement described when measured after 6 weeks and 12 weeks of SALAGEN® Tablets use.

INDICATIONS AND USAGE

SALAGEN® Tablets are indicated for 1) the treatment of symptoms of dry mouth from salivary gland hypofunction caused by radiotherapy for cancer of the head and neck; and 2) the treatment of symptoms of dry mouth in patients with Sjogren's Syndrome.

CONTRAINDICATIONS

SALAGEN® Tablets are contraindicated in patients with uncontrolled asthma, known hypersensitivity to pilocarpine, and when miosis is undesirable, e.g., in acute iritis and in narrow-angle (angle closure) glaucoma.

WARNINGS

Cardiovascular Disease: Patients with significant cardiovascular disease may be unable to compensate for transient changes in hemodynamics or rhythm induced by pilocarpine. Pulmonary edema has been reported as a complication of pilocarpine toxicity from high ocular doses given for acute angle-closure glaucoma. Pilocarpine should be administered with caution in and under close medical supervision of patients with significant cardiovascular disease.

Ocular: Ocular formulations of pilocarpine have been reported to cause visual blurring which may result in decreased visual acuity, especially at night and in patients with central lens changes, and to cause impairment of depth perception. Caution should be advised while driving at night or performing hazardous activities in reduced lighting.

Pulmonary Disease: Pilocarpine has been reported to increase airway resistance, bronchial smooth muscle tone, and bronchial secretions. Pilocarpine hydrochloride should be administered with caution to and under close medical supervision in patients with controlled asthma, chronic bronchitis, or chronic obstructive pulmonary disease requiring pharmacotherapy.

PRECAUTIONS

General: Pilocarpine toxicity is characterized by an exaggeration of its parasympathomimetic effects. These may include: headache, visual disturbance, lacrimation, sweating, respiratory distress, gastrointestinal spasm, nausea, vomiting, diarrhea, atrioventricular block, tachycardia, bradycardia, hypotension, hypertension, shock, mental confusion, cardiac arrhythmia, and tremors.

The dose-related cardiovascular pharmacologic effects of pilocarpine include hypotension, hypertension, bradycardia, and tachycardia.

Pilocarpine should be administered with caution to patients with known or suspected cholelithiasis or biliary tract disease. Contractions of the gallbladder or biliary smooth muscle could precipitate complications including cholecystitis, cholangitis, and biliary obstruction.

Pilocarpine may increase ureteral smooth muscle tone and could theoretically precipitate renal colic (or "ureteral reflux"), particularly in patients with nephrolithiasis.

Cholinergic agonists may have dose-related central nervous system effects. This should be considered when treating patients with underlying cognitive or psychiatric disturbances.

Hepatic Insufficiency: Based on decreased plasma clearance observed in patients with moderate hepatic impairment, the starting dose in these patients should be 5 mg twice daily, followed by adjustment based on therapeutic response and tolerability. Patients with mild hepatic insufficiency (Child-Pugh score of 5-6) do not require dosage reductions. To date, pharmacokinetic studies in subjects with severe hepatic impairment (Child-Pugh score of 10-15) have not been carried out. The use of pilocarpine in these patients is not recommended.

[See table above]

Child-Pugh Scoring System for Hepatic Impairment

Clinical and Biochemical Measurements	Points Scored for Increasing Abnormality		
	1	2	3
Encephalopathy (grade)*	None	1 and 2	3 and 4
Ascites	Absent	Slight	Moderate
Bilirubin (mg. per 100 ml.)	1-2	2-3	>3
Albumin (g. per 100 ml.)	3-5	2.8–3.5	<2.8
Prothrombin Time (sec. Prolonged)	1-4	4-6	>6
For Primary Biliary Cirrhosis:- Bilirubin (mg. per 100 ml.)	1-4	4-10	>10

*According to grading of Trey C, Burns D, and Saunders S. Treatment of hepatic coma by exchange blood transfusion. *N Engl J Med.* 1966; 274:473-481.

Reference: Pugh RNH, Murray-Lyon IM, Dawson JL, Pietroni MC, Williams R. Transection of the oesophagus for bleeding oesophageal varices. *Brit J Surg.* 1973; 60:646-9.

Information for Patients: Patients should be informed that pilocarpine may cause visual disturbances, especially at night, that could impair their ability to drive safely.

If a patient sweats excessively while taking pilocarpine hydrochloride and cannot drink enough liquid, the patient should consult a physician. Dehydration may develop.

Drug Interactions: Pilocarpine should be administered with caution to patients taking beta-adrenergic antagonists because of the possibility of conduction disturbances. Drugs with parasympathomimetic effects administered concurrently with pilocarpine would be expected to result in additive pharmacologic effects. Pilocarpine might antagonize the anticholinergic effects of drugs used concomitantly. These effects should be considered when anticholinergic properties may be contributing to the therapeutic effect of concomitant medication (e.g., atropine, inhaled ipratropium).

While no formal drug interaction studies have been performed, the following concomitant drugs were used in at least 10% of patients in either or both Sjogren's efficacy studies: acetylsalicylic acid, artificial tears, calcium, conjugated estrogens, hydroxychloroquine sulfate, ibuprofen, levothyroxine sodium, medroxyprogesterone acetate, methotrexate, multivitamins, naproxen, omeprazole, paracetamol, and prednisone.

Carcinogenesis, Mutagenesis, Impairment of Fertility: Lifetime oral carcinogenicity studies were conducted in CD-1 mice and Sprague-Dawley rats. Pilocarpine did not induce tumors in mice at any dosage studied (up to 30 mg/kg/day, which yielded a systemic exposure approximately 50 times larger than the maximum systemic exposure observed clinically). In rats, a dosage of 18 mg/kg/day, which yielded a systemic exposure approximately 100 times larger than the maximum systemic exposure observed clinically, resulted in a statistically significant increase in the incidence of benign pheochromocytomas in both males and females, and a statistically significant increase in the incidence of hepatocellular adenomas in female rats. The tumorigenicity observed in rats was observed only at a large multiple of the maximum labeled clinical dose, and may not be relevant to clinical use.

No evidence that pilocarpine has the potential to cause genetic toxicity was obtained in a series of studies that included: 1) bacterial assays (*Salmonella* and *E. coli*) for reverse gene mutations; 2) an *in vitro* chromosome aberration assay in a Chinese hamster ovary cell line; 3) an *in vivo* chromosome aberration assay (micronucleus test) in mice; and 4) a primary DNA damage assay (unscheduled DNA synthesis) in rat hepatocyte primary cultures.

Oral administration of pilocarpine to male and female rats at a dosage of 18 mg/kg/day, which yielded a systemic exposure approximately 100 times larger than the maximum systemic exposure observed clinically, resulted in impaired reproductive function, including reduced fertility, decreased sperm motility, and morphologic evidence of abnormal sperm. It is unclear whether the reduction in fertility was due to effects on male animals, female animals, or both males and females. In dogs, exposure to pilocarpine at a dosage of 3 mg/kg/day (approximately 3 times the maximum recommended human dose when compared on the basis of body surface area (mg/m^2) estimates) for six months resulted in evidence of impaired spermatogenesis. The data obtained in these studies suggest that pilocarpine may impair the fertility of male and female humans. SALAGEN® Tablets should be administered to individuals who are attempting to conceive a child only if the potential benefit justifies potential impairment of fertility.

Pregnancy: Teratogenic Effects

Pregnancy Category C: Pilocarpine was associated with a reduction in the mean fetal body weight and an increase in the incidence of skeletal variations when given to pregnant rats at a dosage of 90 mg/kg/day (approximately 26 times the maximum recommended dose for a 50 kg human when compared on the basis of body surface area (mg/m^2) estimates). These effects may have been secondary to maternal toxicity. In another study, oral administration of pilocarpine to female rats during gestation and lactation at a dosage of 36 mg/kg/day (approximately 10 times the maximum recommended dose for a 50 kg human when compared on the basis of body surface area (mg/m^2) estimates) resulted in an increased incidence of stillbirths; decreased neonatal survival and reduced mean body weight of pups were observed at dosages of 18 mg/kg/day (approximately 5 times the maximum recommended dose for a 50 kg human when compared on the basis of body surface area (mg/m^2) estimates) and above. There are no adequate and well-controlled studies in pregnant women. SALAGEN® Tablets should be used during pregnancy only if the potential benefit justifies the potential risk to the fetus.

Nursing Mothers: It is not known whether this drug is excreted in human milk. Because many drugs are excreted in human milk and because of the potential for serious adverse reactions in nursing infants from SALAGEN® Tablets, a decision should be made whether to discontinue nursing or to discontinue the drug, taking into account the importance of the drug to the mother.

Pediatric Use: Safety and effectiveness in pediatric patients have not been established.

Geriatric Use: Head & Neck Cancer Patients: In the placebo-controlled clinical trials (See **Clinical Studies** section) the mean age of patients was approximately 58 years (range 19 to 80). Of these patients, 97/369 (61/217 receiving ilocarpine) were over the age of 65 years. In the healthy olunteer studies, 15/150 subjects were over the age of 65 ears. In both study populations, the adverse events reorted by those over 65 years and those 65 years and ounger were comparable. Of the 15 elderly volunteers (5 women, 10 men), the 5 women had higher C_{max}'s and AUC's han the men. (See **Pharmacokinetics** section.)

jogren's Syndrome Patients: In the placebo-controlled linical trials (See **Clinical Studies** section), the mean age of patients was approximately 55 years (range 21 to 85). The adverse events reported by those over 65 years and those 65 years and younger were comparable except for notable trends for urinary frequency, diarrhea, and dizziness (See **ADVERSE REACTIONS** section).

ADVERSE REACTIONS

Head & Neck Cancer Patients: In controlled studies, 217 patients received pilocarpine, of whom 68% were men and 32% were women. Race distribution was 91% Caucasian, 8% Black, and 1% of other origin. Mean age was approximately 58 years. The majority of patients were between 50 and 64 years (51%), 33% were 65 years and older and 16% were younger than 50 years of age.

The most frequent adverse experiences associated with SALAGEN® Tablets were a consequence of the expected pharmacologic effects of pilocarpine.

Adverse Event	Pilocarpine HCl		Placebo
	10 mg t.i.d. (30 mg/day)	5 mg t.i.d. (15 mg/day)	(t.i.d.)
	N=121	N=141	N=152
	68%	29%	9%
Sweating	68%	29%	9%
Nausea	15	6	4
Rhinitis	14	5	7
Diarrhea	7	4	5
Chills	15	3	<1
Flushing	13	8	3
Urinary Frequency	12	9	7
Dizziness	12	5	4
Asthenia	12	6	3

In addition, the following adverse events (≥3% incidence) were reported at dosages of 15-30 mg/day in the controlled clinical trials:

Adverse Event	Pilocarpine HCl	Placebo
	5-10 mg t.i.d. (15-30 mg/day)	(t.i.d.)
	N=212	N=152
	11%	8%
Headache	7	5
Dyspepsia	6	8
Lacrimation	5	4
Edema	4	4
Abdominal Pain	4	2
Amblyopia	4	1
Vomiting	4	8
Pharyngitis	3	8
Hypertension	3	1

The following events were reported with treated head and neck cancer patients at incidences of 1% to 2% at dosages of 7.5 to 30 mg/day: abnormal vision, conjunctivitis, dysphagia, epistaxis, myalgias, pruritus, rash, sinusitis, tachycardia, taste perversion, tremor, voice alteration.

The following events were reported rarely in treated head and neck cancer patients (<1%):

Causal relation is unknown.

Body as a whole: body odor, hypothermia, mucous membrane abnormality

Cardiovascular: bradycardia, ECG abnormality, palpitations, syncope

Digestive: anorexia, increased appetite, esophagitis, gastrointestinal disorder, tongue disorder

Hematologic: leukopenia, lymphadenopathy

Nervous: anxiety, confusion, depression, abnormal dreams, hyperkinesia, hypesthesia, nervousness, parethesias, speech disorder, twitching

Respiratory: increased sputum, stridor, yawning

Skin: seborrhea

Special senses: deafness, eye pain, glaucoma

Urogenital: dysuria, metrorrhagia, urinary impairment

In long-term treatment were two patients with underlying cardiovascular disease of whom one experienced a myocardial infarct and another an episode of syncope. The association with drug is uncertain.

Sjogren's Syndrome Patients: In controlled studies, 376 patients received pilocarpine, of whom 5% were men and 95% were women. Race distribution was 84% Caucasian, 9% Oriental, 3% Black, and 4% of other origin. Mean age was 55 years. The majority of patients were between 40 and 69 years (70%), 16% were 70 years and older and 14% were younger than 40 years of age. Of these patients, 161/629 (89/376 receiving pilocarpine) were over the age of 65 years.

The adverse events reported by those over 65 years and

those 65 years and younger were comparable except for notable trends for urinary frequency, diarrhea, and dizziness. The incidences of urinary frequency and diarrhea in the elderly were about double those of the non-elderly. The incidence of dizziness was about three times as high in the elderly as in the non-elderly. These adverse experiences were not considered to be serious. In the 2 placebo-controlled studies, the most common adverse events related to drug use were sweating, urinary frequency, chills, and vasodilatation (flushing). The most commonly reported reason for patient discontinuation of treatment was sweating. Expected pharmacologic effects of pilocarpine include the following adverse experiences associated with SALAGEN® Tablets:

Adverse Event	Pilocarpine HCl	Placebo
	5 mg q.i.d. (20 mg/day)	(q.i.d.)
	N=255	N=253
Sweating	40%	7%
Urinary Frequency	10	4
Nausea	9	9
Flushing	9	2
Rhinitis	7	8
Diarrhea	6	7
Chills	4	2
Increased Salivation	3	0
Asthenia	2	2

In addition, the following adverse events (≥3% incidence) were reported at dosages of 20 mg/day in the controlled clinical trials:

Adverse Event	Pilocarpine HCl	Placebo
	5 mg q.i.d. (20 mg/day)	(q.i.d.)
	N=255	N=253
	13%	19%
Headache	13%	19%
Flu Syndrome	9	9
Dyspepsia	7	7
Dizziness	6	7
Pain	4	2
Sinusitis	4	5
Abdominal Pain	3	1
Vomiting	3	1
Pharyngitis	2	5
Rash	2	3
Infection	2	6

The following events were reported in Sjogren's patients at incidences of 1% to 2% at dosing of 20 mg/day: accidental injury, allergic reaction, back pain, blurred vision, constipation, increased cough, edema, epistaxis, face edema, fever, flatulence, glossitis, lab test abnormalities, including chemistry, hematology, and urinalysis, myalgia, palpitation, pruritus, somnolence, stomatitis, tachycardia, tinnitus, urinary incontinence, urinary tract infection, and vaginitis.

The following events were reported rarely in treated Sjogren's patients (<1%) at dosing of 10-30 mg/day: Causal relation is unknown.

Body as a whole: chest pain, cyst, death, moniliasis, neck pain, neck rigidity, photosensitivity reaction

Cardiovascular: angina pectoris, arrhythmia, ECG abnormality, hypotension, hypertension, intracranial hemorrhage, migraine, myocardial infarction

Digestive: anorexia, bilirubinemia, cholelithiasis, colitis, dry mouth, eructation, gastritis, gastroenteritis, gastrointestinal disorder, gingivitis, hepatitis, abnormal liver function tests, melena, nausea & vomiting, pancreatitis, parotid gland enlargement, salivary gland enlargement, sputum increased, taste loss, tongue disorder, tooth disorder

Hematologic: hematuria, lymphadenopathy, abnormal platelets, thrombocythemia, thrombocytopenia, thrombosis, abnormal WBC

Metabolic and Nutritional: peripheral edema, hypoglycemia

Musculoskeletal: arthralgia, arthritis, bone disorder, spontaneous bone fracture, pathological fracture, myasthenia, tendon disorder, tenosynovitis

Nervous: aphasia, confusion, depression, abnormal dreams, emotional lability, hyperkinesia, hypesthesia, insomnia, leg cramps, nervousness, parethesias, abnormal thinking, tremor

Respiratory: bronchitis, dyspnea, hiccup, laryngismus, laryngitis, pneumonia, viral infection, voice alteration

Skin: alopecia, contact dermatitis, dry skin, eczema, erythema nodosum, exfoliative dermatitis, herpes simplex, skin ulcer, vesiculobullous rash

Special Senses: cataract, conjunctivitis, dry eyes, ear disorder, ear pain, eye disorder, eye hemorrhage, glaucoma, lacrimation disorder, retinal disorder, taste perversion, abnormal vision

Urogenital: breast pain, dysuria, mastitis, menorrhagia, metrorrhagia, ovarian disorder, pyuria, salpingitis, urethral pain, urinary urgency, vaginal hemorrhage, vaginal moniliasis

The following adverse experiences have been reported rarely with ocular pilocarpine: A-V block, agitation, ciliary congestion, confusion, delusion, depression, dermatitis, middle ear disturbance, eyelid twitching, malignant glaucoma, iris cysts, macular hole, shock, and visual hallucination.

MANAGEMENT OF OVERDOSE

Fatal overdosage with pilocarpine has been reported in the scientific literature at doses presumed to be greater than 100 mg in two hospitalized patients. 100 mg of pilocarpine is considered potentially fatal. Overdosage should be treated with atropine titration (0.5 mg to 1.0 mg given subcutaneously or intravenously) and supportive measures to maintain respiration and circulation. Epinephrine (0.3 mg to 1.0 mg, subcutaneously or intramuscularly) may also be of value in the presence of severe cardiovascular depression or bronchoconstriction. It is not known if pilocarpine is dialyzable.

DOSAGE AND ADMINISTRATION

Regardless of the indication, the starting dose in patients with moderate hepatic impairment should be 5 mg twice daily, followed by adjustment based on therapeutic response and tolerability. Patients with mild hepatic insufficiency do not require dosage reductions. The use of pilocarpine in patients with severe hepatic insufficiency is not recommended. If needed, refer to the *Hepatic Insufficiency* subsection of the **Precautions** section of this label for definitions of mild, moderate and severe hepatic impairment.

Head & Neck Cancer Patients: The recommended initial dose of SALAGEN® Tablets is 5 mg taken three times a day. Dosage should be titrated according to therapeutic response and tolerance. The usual dosage range is up to 15-30 mg per day. (Not to exceed 10 mg per dose.) Although early improvement may be realized, at least 12 weeks of uninterrupted therapy with SALAGEN® Tablets may be necessary to assess whether a beneficial response will be achieved. The incidence of the most common adverse events increases with dose. The lowest dose that is tolerated and effective should be used for maintenance.

Sjogren's Syndrome Patients: The recommended dose of SALAGEN® Tablets is 5 mg taken four times a day. Efficacy was established by 6 weeks of use.

HOW SUPPLIED

SALAGEN® Tablets, 5 mg, are white, film coated, debossed round tablets, coded SAL 5. Each tablet contains 5 mg pilocarpine hydrochloride. They are supplied as follows:
NDC 62856-705-10 bottles of 100
Store up to 25°C (77°F); excursions permitted to 15°-30°C (59°-86°F).

SALAGEN® Tablets, 7.5 mg, are blue, film coated, debossed round tablets, coded SAL 7.5. Each tablet contains 7.5 mg pilocarpine hydrochloride. They are supplied as follows:
NDC 62856-775-10 bottles of 100
Store up to 25°C (77°F); excursions permitted to 15°-30°C (59°-86°F).

Manufactured by:
Patheon Inc.,
Ontario, L5N 7K9
Manufactured for:
Eisai Inc.
Woodcliff Lake, NJ 07677
© 2009 Eisai Inc.   January 2009
SALAGEN® is a registered trademark of Eisai Inc.

201370

TARGRETIN®
[tahr-greh'-tən]
(bexarotene)
capsules, 75 mg
Rx only.

Rx

> Targretin® capsules are a member of the retinoid class of drugs that is associated with birth defects in humans. Targretin® capsules also caused birth defects when administered orally to pregnant rats. Targretin® capsules must not be administered to a pregnant woman. See CONTRAINDICATIONS.

DESCRIPTION

Targretin® (bexarotene) is a member of a subclass of retinoids that selectively activate retinoid X receptors (RXRs). These retinoid receptors have biologic activity distinct from that of retinoic acid receptors (RARs). Each soft gelatin capsule for oral administration contains 75 mg of bexarotene.

The chemical name is 4-[1-(5,6,7,8-tetrahydro-3,5,5,8,8-pentamethyl-2-naphthalenyl)ethenyl] benzoic acid, and the structural formula is as follows:

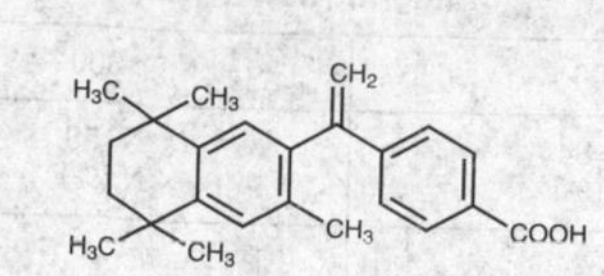

Bexarotene is an off-white to white powder with a molecular weight of 348.48 and a molecular formula of $C_{24}H_{28}O_2$. It is insoluble in water and slightly soluble in vegetable oils and ethanol, USP.

Each Targretin® (bexarotene) capsule also contains the following inactive ingredients: polyethylene glycol 400, NF; polysorbate 20, NF; povidone, USP; and butylated hydroxyanisole, NF. The capsule shell contains gelatin, NF; sorbitol special-glycerin blend; and titanium dioxide, USP.

CLINICAL PHARMACOLOGY

Mechanism of Action

Bexarotene selectively binds and activates retinoid X receptor subtypes (RXRα, RXRβ, RXRγ). RXRs can form heterodimers with various receptor partners such as retinoic acid receptors (RARs), vitamin D receptor, thyroid receptor, and peroxisome proliferator activator receptors (PPARs). Once activated, these receptors function as transcription factors that regulate the expression of genes that control cellular differentiation and proliferation. Bexarotene inhibits the growth *in vitro* of some tumor cell lines of hematopoietic and squamous cell origin. It also induces tumor regression *in vivo* in some animal models. The exact mechanism of action of bexarotene in the treatment of cutaneous T-cell lymphoma (CTCL) is unknown.

Pharmacokinetics

General

After oral administration of Targretin® capsules, bexarotene is absorbed with a T_{max} of about two hours. Terminal half-life of bexarotene is about seven hours. Studies in patients with advanced malignancies show approximate single-dose linearity within the therapeutic range and low accumulation with multiple doses. Plasma bexarotene AUC and C_{max} values resulting from a 75- to 300-mg dose were 35% and 48% higher, respectively, after a fat-containing meal than after a glucose solution (see **PRECAUTIONS: Drug-Food Interaction** and **DOSAGE AND ADMINISTRATION**). Bexarotene is highly bound (>99%) to plasma proteins. The plasma proteins to which bexarotene binds have not been elucidated, and the ability of bexarotene to displace drugs bound to plasma proteins and the ability of drugs to displace bexarotene binding have not been studied (see **PRECAUTIONS: Protein Binding**). The uptake of bexarotene by organs or tissues has not been evaluated.

Metabolism

Four bexarotene metabolites have been identified in plasma: 6- and 7-hydroxy-bexarotene and 6- and 7-oxo-bexarotene. *In vitro* studies suggest that cytochrome P450 3A4 is the major cytochrome P450 responsible for formation of the oxidative metabolites and that the oxidative metabolites may be glucuronidated. The oxidative metabolites are active in *in vitro* assays of retinoid receptor activation, but the relative contribution of the parent and any metabolites to the efficacy and safety of Targretin® capsules is unknown.

Elimination

The renal elimination of bexarotene and its metabolites was examined in patients with Type 2 diabetes mellitus. Neither bexarotene nor its metabolites were excreted in urine in appreciable amounts. Bexarotene is thought to be eliminated primarily through the hepatobiliary system.

Special Populations

Elderly: Bexarotene C_{max} and AUC were similar in advanced cancer patients <60 years old and in patients >60 years old, including a subset of patients >70 years old.

Pediatric: Studies to evaluate bexarotene pharmacokinetics in the pediatric population have not been conducted (see **PRECAUTIONS: Pediatric Use**).

Gender: The pharmacokinetics of bexarotene were similar in male and female patients with advanced cancer.

Ethnic Origin: The effect of ethnic origin on bexarotene pharmacokinetics is unknown.

Renal Insufficiency: No formal studies have been conducted with Targretin® capsules in patients with renal insufficiency. Urinary elimination of bexarotene and its known metabolites is a minor excretory pathway (<1% of administered dose), but because renal insufficiency can result in significant protein binding changes, pharmacokinetics may be altered in patients with renal insufficiency (see **PRECAUTIONS: Renal Insufficiency**).

Hepatic Insufficiency: No specific studies have been conducted with Targretin® capsules in patients with hepatic insufficiency. Because less than 1% of the dose is excreted in the urine unchanged and there is *in vitro* evidence of extensive hepatic contribution to bexarotene elimination, hepatic impairment would be expected to lead to greatly decreased clearance (see **WARNINGS:** Hepatic insufficiency).

Drug-Drug Interactions

No specific studies to evaluate drug interactions with bexarotene have been conducted. Bexarotene oxidative metabolites appear to be formed by cytochrome P450 3A4.

Because bexarotene is metabolized by cytochrome P450 3A4, ketoconazole, itraconazole, erythromycin, gemfibrozil, grapefruit juice, and other inhibitors of cytochrome P450 3A4 would be expected to lead to an increase in plasma bexarotene concentrations. Furthermore, rifampin, phenytoin, phenobarbital, and other inducers of cytochrome P450 3A4 may cause a reduction in plasma bexarotene concentrations.

Concomitant administration of Targretin® capsules and gemfibrozil resulted in substantial increases in plasma concentrations of bexarotene, probably at least partially related to cytochrome P450 3A4 inhibition by gemfibrozil. Under similar conditions, bexarotene concentrations were not affected by concomitant atorvastatin administration. Concomitant administration of gemfibrozil with Targretin® capsules is not recommended (see **PRECAUTIONS: Drug-Drug Interactions**).

Based on interim data, concomitant administration of Targretin® capsules and tamoxifen resulted in approximately a 35% decrease in plasma concentrations of tamoxifen, possibly through an induction of cytochrome P450 3A4. Based on this known interaction, bexarotene may theoretically increase the rate of metabolism and reduce plasma concentrations of other substrates metabolized by cytochrome P450 3A4, including oral or other systemic hormonal contraceptives (see **CONTRAINDICATIONS: Pregnancy: Category X** and **PRECAUTIONS: Drug-Drug Interactions**).

Clinical Studies

Targretin® capsules were evaluated in 152 patients with advanced and early-stage cutaneous T-cell lymphoma (CTCL) in two multicenter, open-label, historically controlled clinical studies conducted in the U.S., Canada, Europe, and Australia.

The advanced disease patients had disease refractory to at least one prior systemic therapy (median of two, range one to six prior systemic therapies) and had been treated with a median of five (range 1 to 11) prior systemic, irradiation, and/or topical therapies. Early disease patients were intolerant to, had disease that was refractory to, or had reached a response plateau of six months on, at least two prior therapies. The patients entered had been treated with a median of 3.5 (range 2 to 12) therapies (systemic, irradiation, and/or topical).

The two clinical studies enrolled a total of 152 patients, 102 of whom had disease refractory to at least one prior systemic therapy, 90 with advanced disease and 12 with early disease. This is the patient population for whom Targretin® capsules are indicated.

Patients were initially treated with a starting dose of 650 mg/m^2/day with a subsequent reduction of starting dose to 500 mg/m^2/day. Neither of these starting doses was tolerated, and the starting dose was then reduced to 300 mg/m^2/day. If, however, a patient on 300 mg/m^2/day of Targretin® capsules showed no response after eight or more weeks of therapy, the dose could be increased to 400 mg/m^2/day.

Tumor response was assessed in both studies by observation of up to five baseline-defined index lesions using a Composite Assessment of Index Lesion Disease Severity (CA). This endpoint was based on a summation of the grades, for all index lesions, of erythema, scaling, plaque elevation, hypopigmentation or hyperpigmentation, and area of involvement. Also considered in response assessment was the presence or absence of cutaneous tumors and extracutaneous disease manifestations.

All tumor responses required confirmation over at least two assessments separated by at least four weeks. A partial response was defined as an improvement of at least 50% in the index lesions without worsening, or development of new cutaneous tumors or non-cutaneous manifestations. A complete clinical response required complete disappearance of all manifestations of disease, but did not require confirmation by biopsy.

At the initial dose of 300 mg/m^2/day, 1/62 (1.6%) of patients had a complete clinical tumor response and 19/62 (30%) of patients had a partial tumor response. The rate of relapse (25% increase in CA or worsening of other aspects of disease) in the 20 patients who had a tumor response was 6/20 (30%) over a median duration of observation of 21 weeks, and the median duration of tumor response had not been reached. Responses were seen as early as four weeks and new responses continued to be seen at later visits.

INDICATIONS AND USAGE

Targretin® (bexarotene) capsules are indicated for the treatment of cutaneous manifestations of cutaneous T-cell lymphoma in patients who are refractory to at least one prior systemic therapy.

CONTRAINDICATIONS

Targretin® capsules are contraindicated in patients with a known hypersensitivity to bexarotene or other components of the product.

Pregnancy: Category X

Targretin® (bexarotene) capsules may cause fetal harm when administered to a pregnant woman. Targretin® capsules must not be given to a pregnant woman or a woman who intends to become pregnant. If a woman becomes pregnant while taking Targretin® capsules, Targretin® capsules must be stopped immediately and the woman given appropriate counseling.

Bexarotene caused malformations when administered orally to pregnant rats during days 7–17 of gestation. Developmental abnormalities included incomplete ossification at 4 mg/kg/day and cleft palate, depressed eye bulge/microphthalmia, and small ears at 16 mg/kg/day. The plasma AUC of bexarotene in rats at 4 mg/kg/day is approximately one third the AUC in humans at the recommended daily dose. At doses greater than 10 mg/kg/day, bexarotene caused developmental mortality. The no-effect dose for fetal effects in rats was 1 mg/kg/day (producing an AUC approximately one sixth of the AUC at the recommended human daily dose).

Women of child-bearing potential should be advised to avoid becoming pregnant when Targretin® capsules are used. The possibility that a woman of child-bearing potential is pregnant at the time therapy is instituted should be considered. A negative pregnancy test (e.g., serum beta-human chorionic gonadotropin, beta-HCG) with a sensitivity of at least 50 mIU/L should be obtained within one week prior to Targretin® capsules therapy, and the pregnancy test must be repeated at monthly intervals while the patient remains on Targretin® capsules. Effective contraception must be used for one month prior to the initiation of therapy, during therapy and for at least one month following discontinuation of therapy; it is recommended that two reliable forms of contraception be used simultaneously unless abstinence is the chosen method. Bexarotene can potentially induce metabolic enzymes and thereby theoretically reduce the plasma concentrations of oral or other systemic hormonal contraceptives (see **CLINICAL PHARMACOLOGY: Drug-Drug Interactions** and **PRECAUTIONS: Drug-Drug Interactions**). Thus, if treatment with Targretin® capsules is intended in a woman with child-bearing potential, it is strongly recommended that one of the two reliable forms of contraception should be non-hormonal. Male patients with sexual partners who are pregnant, possibly pregnant, or who could become pregnant must use condoms during sexual intercourse while taking Targretin® capsules and for at least one month after the last dose of drug. Targretin® capsules therapy should be initiated on the second or third day of a normal menstrual period. No more than a one-month supply of Targretin® capsules should be given to the patient so that the results of pregnancy testing can be assessed and counseling regarding avoidance of pregnancy and birth defects can be reinforced.

WARNINGS

Lipid abnormalities: Targretin® capsules induce major lipid abnormalities in most patients. These must be monitored and treated during long-term therapy. About 70% of patients with CTCL who received an initial dose of ≥300 mg/m^2/day of Targretin® capsules had fasting triglyceride levels greater than 2.5 times the upper limit of normal. About 55% had values over 800 mg/dL with a median of about 1200 mg/dL in those patients. Cholesterol elevations above 300 mg/dL occurred in approximately 60% and 75% of patients with CTCL who received an initial dose of 300 mg/m^2/day or greater than 300 mg/m^2/day, respectively. Decreases in high density lipoprotein (HDL) cholesterol to less than 25 mg/dL were seen in about 55% and 90% of patients receiving an initial dose of 300 mg/m /day or greater than 300 mg/m /day, respectively, of Targretin® capsules. The effects on triglycerides, HDL cholesterol, and total cholesterol were reversible with cessation of therapy, and could generally be mitigated by dose reduction or concomitant antilipemic therapy.

Fasting blood lipid determinations should be performed before Targretin® capsules therapy is initiated and weekly until the lipid response to Targretin® capsules is established, which usually occurs within two to four weeks, and at eight-week intervals thereafter. Fasting triglycerides should be normal or normalized with appropriate intervention prior to initiating Targretin® capsules therapy. Attempts should be made to maintain triglyceride levels below

00 mg/dL to reduce the risk of clinical sequelae (see **WARNINGS: Pancreatitis**). If fasting triglycerides are elevated or become elevated during treatment, antilipemic therapy should be instituted, and if necessary, the dose of Targretin® capsules reduced or suspended. In the 300 mg/m²/day initial dose group, 60% of patients were given lipid-lowering drugs. Atorvastatin was used in 48% (73/152) of patients with CTCL. Because of a potential drug-drug interaction (see **PRECAUTIONS: Drug-Drug Interactions**), gemfibrozil is not recommended for use with Targretin® capsules.

Pancreatitis: Acute pancreatitis has been reported in four patients with CTCL and in six patients with non-CTCL cancers treated with Targretin® capsules; the cases were associated with marked elevations of fasting serum triglycerides, the lowest being 770 mg/dL in one patient. One patient with advanced non-CTCL cancer died of pancreatitis. Patients with CTCL who have risk factors for pancreatitis (e.g., prior pancreatitis, uncontrolled hyperlipidemia, excessive alcohol consumption, uncontrolled diabetes mellitus, biliary tract disease, and medications known to increase triglyceride levels or to be associated with pancreatic toxicity) should generally not be treated with Targretin® capsules (see **WARNINGS: Lipid abnormalities** and **PRECAUTIONS: Laboratory Tests**).

Liver function test abnormalities: For patients with CTCL receiving an initial dose of 300 mg/m²/day of Targretin® capsules, elevations in liver function tests (LFTs) have been observed in 5% (SGOT/AST), 2% (SGPT/ALT), and 0% (bilirubin). In contrast, with an initial dose greater than 300 mg/m²/day of Targretin® capsules, the incidence of LFT elevations was higher at 7% (SGOT/AST), 9% (SGPT/ALT), and 6% (bilirubin). Two patients developed cholestasis, including one patient who died of liver failure. In clinical trials, elevation of LFTs resolved within one month in 80% of patients following a decrease in dose or discontinuation of therapy. Baseline LFTs should be obtained, and LFTs should be carefully monitored after one, two and four weeks of treatment initiation, and if stable, at least every eight weeks thereafter during treatment. Consideration should be given to a suspension or discontinuation of Targretin® capsules if test results reach greater than three times the upper limit of normal values for SGOT/AST, SGPT/ALT, or bilirubin.

Hepatic insufficiency: No specific studies have been conducted with Targretin® capsules in patients with hepatic insufficiency. Because less than 1% of the dose is excreted in the urine unchanged and there is *in vitro* evidence of extensive hepatic contribution to bexarotene elimination, hepatic impairment would be expected to lead to greatly decreased clearance. Targretin® capsules should be used only with great caution in this population.

Thyroid axis alterations: Targretin® capsules induce biochemical evidence of or clinical hypothyroidism in about half of all patients treated, causing a reversible reduction in thyroid hormone (total thyroxine [total T4]) and thyroid-stimulating hormone (TSH) levels. The incidence of decreases in TSH and total T4 were about 60% and 45%, respectively, in patients with CTCL receiving an initial dose of 300 mg/m²/day. Hypothyroidism was reported as an adverse event in 29% of patients. Treatment with thyroid hormone supplements should be considered in patients with laboratory evidence of hypothyroidism. In the 300 mg/m²/day initial dose group, 37% of patients were treated with thyroid hormone replacement. Baseline thyroid function tests should be obtained and patients monitored during treatment.

Leukopenia: A total of 18% of patients with CTCL receiving an initial dose of 300 mg/m²/day of Targretin® capsules had reversible leukopenia in the range of 1000 to <3000 WBC/mm³. Patients receiving an initial dose greater than 300 mg/m²/day of Targretin® capsules had an incidence of leukopenia of 43%. No patient with CTCL treated with Targretin® capsules developed leukopenia of less than 1000 WBC/mm³. The time to onset of leukopenia was generally four to eight weeks. The leukopenia observed in most patients was explained by neutropenia. In the 300 mg/m²/day initial dose group, the incidence of NCI Grade 3 and Grade 4 neutropenia, respectively, was 12% and 4%. The leukopenia and neutropenia experienced during Targretin® capsules therapy resolved after dose reduction or discontinuation of treatment, on average within 30 days in 93% of the patients with CTCL and 82% of patients with non-CTCL cancers. Leukopenia and neutropenia were rarely associated with severe sequelae or serious adverse events. Determination of WBC with differential should be obtained at baseline and periodically during treatment.

Cataracts: Posterior subcapsular cataracts were observed in preclinical toxicity studies in rats and dogs administered bexarotene daily for 6 months. In 15 of 79 patients who had serial slit lamp examinations, new cataracts or worsening of previous cataracts were found. Because of the high prevalence and rate of cataract formation in older patient populations, the relationship of Targretin® capsules and cataracts cannot be determined in the absence of an appropriate control group. Patients treated with Targretin® capsules who experience visual difficulties should have an appropriate ophthalmologic evaluation.

PRECAUTIONS
Pregnancy: Category X
See **CONTRAINDICATIONS.**
General:
Targretin® capsules should be used with caution in patients with a known hypersensitivity to retinoids. Clinical instances of cross-reactivity have not been noted.

Vitamin A Supplementation: In clinical studies, patients were advised to limit vitamin A intake to ≤15,000 IU/day. Because of the relationship of bexarotene to vitamin A, patients should be advised to limit vitamin A supplements to avoid potential additive toxic effects.

Patients with Diabetes Mellitus: Caution should be used when administering Targretin® capsules in patients using insulin, agents enhancing insulin secretion (e.g., sulfonylureas), or insulin-sensitizers (e.g., thiazolidinedione class). Based on the mechanism of action, Targretin® capsules could enhance the action of these agents, resulting in hypoglycemia. Hypoglycemia has not been associated with the use of Targretin® capsules as monotherapy.

Photosensitivity: Retinoids as a class have been associated with photosensitivity. *In vitro* assays indicate that bexarotene is a potential photosensitizing agent. Mild phototoxicity manifested as sunburn and skin sensitivity to sunlight was observed in patients who were exposed to direct sunlight while receiving Targretin® capsules. Patients should be advised to minimize exposure to sunlight and artificial ultraviolet light while receiving Targretin® capsules.

Laboratory Tests
Blood lipid determinations should be performed before Targretin® capsules are given. Fasting triglycerides should be normal or normalized with appropriate intervention prior to therapy. Hyperlipidemia usually occurs within the initial two to four weeks. Therefore, weekly lipid determinations are recommended during this interval. Subsequently, in patients not hyperlipidemic, determinations can be performed less frequently (see **WARNINGS: Lipid abnormalities**).

A white blood cell count with differential should be obtained at baseline and periodically during treatment. Baseline liver function tests should be obtained and should be carefully monitored after one, two and four weeks of treatment initiation, and if stable, periodically thereafter during treatment. Baseline thyroid function tests should be obtained and then monitored during treatment as indicated (see **WARNINGS: Leukopenia, Liver function test abnormalities, and Thyroid axis alterations**).

Drug-Food Interaction
In all clinical trials, patients were instructed to take Targretin® capsules with or immediately following a meal. In one clinical study, plasma bexarotene AUC and C_{max} values were substantially higher following a fat-containing meal versus those following the administration of a glucose solution. Because safety and efficacy data are based upon administration with food, it is recommended that Targretin® capsules be administered with food (see **CLINICAL PHARMACOLOGY: Pharmacokinetics** and **DOSAGE AND ADMINISTRATION**).

Table 1. Adverse Events with Incidence ≥10% in CTCL Trials

Body System Adverse Event[1,2]	Initial Assigned Dose Group (mg/m²/day)	
	300	>300
	N=84 N (%)	N=53 N (%)
METABOLIC AND NUTRITIONAL DISORDERS		
Hyperlipemia	66 (78.6)	42 (79.2)
Hypercholesteremia	27 (32.1)	33 (62.3)
Lactic dehydrogenase increased	6 (7.1)	7 (13.2)
BODY AS A WHOLE		
Headache	25 (29.8)	22 (41.5)
Asthenia	17 (20.2)	24 (45.3)
Infection	11 (13.1)	12 (22.6)
Abdominal pain	9 (10.7)	2 (3.8)
Chills	8 (9.5)	7 (13.2)
Fever	4 (4.8)	9 (17.0)
Flu syndrome	3 (3.6)	7 (13.2)
Back pain	2 (2.4)	6 (11.3)
Infection bacterial	1 (1.2)	7 (13.2)
ENDOCRINE		
Hypothyroidism	24 (28.6)	28 (52.8)
SKIN AND APPENDAGES		
Rash	14 (16.7)	12 (22.6)
Dry skin	9 (10.7)	5 (9.4)
Exfoliative dermatitis	8 (9.5)	15 (28.3)
Alopecia	3 (3.6)	6 (11.3)
HEMIC AND LYMPHATIC SYSTEM		
Leukopenia	14 (16.7)	25 (47.2)
Anemia	5 (6.0)	13 (24.5)
Hypochromic anemia	3 (3.6)	7 (13.2)
DIGESTIVE SYSTEM		
Nausea	13 (15.5)	4 (7.5)
Diarrhea	6 (7.1)	22 (41.5)
Vomiting	3 (3.6)	7 (13.2)
Anorexia	2 (2.4)	12 (22.6)
CARDIOVASCULAR SYSTEM		
Peripheral edema	11 (13.1)	6 (11.3)
NERVOUS SYSTEM		
Insomnia	4 (4.8)	6 (11.3)

[1] Preferred English term coded according to Ligand-modified COSTART 5 Dictionary.
[2] Patients are counted at most once in each AE category.

Drug-Drug Interactions

No formal studies to evaluate drug interactions with bexarotene have been conducted. Bexarotene oxidative metabolites appear to be formed by cytochrome P450 3A4. On the basis of the metabolism of bexarotene by cytochrome P450 3A4, ketoconazole, itraconazole, erythromycin, gemfibrozil, grapefruit juice, and other inhibitors of cytochrome P450 3A4 would be expected to lead to an increase in plasma bexarotene concentrations. Furthermore, rifampin, phenytoin, phenobarbital, and other inducers of cytochrome P450 3A4 may cause a reduction in plasma bexarotene concentrations.

Concomitant administration of Targretin® capsules and gemfibrozil resulted in substantial increases in plasma concentrations of bexarotene, probably at least partially related to cytochrome P450 3A4 inhibition by gemfibrozil. Under similar conditions, bexarotene concentrations were not affected by concomitant atorvastatin administration. Concomitant administration of gemfibrozil with Targretin® capsules is not recommended.

Based on interim data, concomitant administration of Targretin® capsules and tamoxifen resulted in approximately a 35% decrease in plasma concentrations of tamoxifen, possibly through an induction of cytochrome P450 3A4. Based on this known interaction, bexarotene may theoretically increase the rate of metabolism and reduce plasma concentrations of other substrates metabolized by cytochrome P450 3A4, including oral or other systemic hormonal contraceptives (see **CLINICAL PHARMACOLOGY: Drug-Drug Interactions** and **CONTRAINDICATIONS: Pregnancy: Category X**). Thus, if treatment with Targretin® capsules is intended in a woman with childbearing potential, it is strongly recommended that two reliable forms of contraception be used concurrently, one of which should be non-hormonal.

Renal Insufficiency

No formal studies have been conducted with Targretin® capsules in patients with renal insufficiency. Urinary elimination of bexarotene and its known metabolites is a minor excretory pathway for bexarotene (<1% of administered dose), but because renal insufficiency can result in significant protein binding changes, and bexarotene is >99% protein bound, pharmacokinetics may be altered in patients with renal insufficiency.

Protein Binding

Bexarotene is highly bound (>99%) to plasma proteins. The plasma proteins to which bexarotene binds have not been elucidated, and the ability of bexarotene to displace drugs bound to plasma proteins and the ability of drugs to displace bexarotene binding have not been studied.

Drug/Laboratory Test Interactions

CA125 assay values in patients with ovarian cancer may be increased by Targretin® capsule therapy.

Carcinogenesis, Mutagenesis, Impairment of Fertility

Long-term studies in animals to assess the carcinogenic potential of bexarotene have not been conducted. Bexarotene is not mutagenic to bacteria (Ames assay) or mammalian cells (mouse lymphoma assay). Bexarotene was not clastogenic *in vivo* (micronucleus test in mice). No formal fertility studies were conducted with bexarotene. Bexarotene caused testicular degeneration when oral doses of 1.5 mg/kg/day were given to dogs for 91 days (producing an AUC of approximately one fifth the AUC at the recommended human daily dose).

Use in Nursing Mothers

It is not known whether bexarotene is excreted in human milk. Because many drugs are excreted in human milk and because of the potential for serious adverse reactions in nursing infants from bexarotene, a decision should be made whether to discontinue nursing or to discontinue the drug, taking into account the importance of the drug to the mother.

Pediatric Use

Safety and effectiveness in pediatric patients have not been established.

Geriatric Use

Of the total patients with CTCL in clinical studies of Targretin® capsules, 64% were 60 years or older, while 33% were 70 years or older. No overall differences in safety were observed between patients 70 years or older and younger patients, but greater sensitivity of some older individuals to Targretin® capsules cannot be ruled out. Responses to Targretin® capsules were observed across all age group decades, without preference for any individual age group decade.

ADVERSE REACTIONS

The safety of Targretin® capsules has been evaluated in clinical studies of 152 patients with CTCL who received Targretin® capsules for up to 97 weeks and in 352 patients in other studies. The mean duration of therapy for the 152 patients with CTCL was 166 days. The most common adverse events reported with an incidence of at least 10% in patients with CTCL treated at an initial dose of 300 mg/m²/day of Targretin® capsules are shown in Table 1. The events at least possibly related to treatment are lipid abnormalities (elevated triglycerides, elevated total and LDL cholesterol and decreased HDL cholesterol), hypothyroidism, headache, asthenia, rash, leukopenia, anemia, nausea, infection, peripheral edema, abdominal pain, and dry skin. Most adverse events occurred at a higher incidence in patients treated at starting doses of greater than 300 mg/m²/day (see Table 1).

Adverse events leading to dose reduction or study drug discontinuation in at least two patients were hyperlipemia,

Table 2. Incidence of Moderately Severe and Severe Adverse Events Reported in at Least Two Patients (CTCL Trials)

Body System Adverse Event[1,2]	Initial Assigned Dose Group (mg/m²/day)			
	300 (N=84)		>300 (N=53)	
	Mod Sev N (%)	Severe N (%)	Mod Sev N (%)	Severe N (%)
BODY AS A WHOLE				
Asthenia	1 (1.2)	0 (0.0)	11 (20.8)	0 (0.0)
Headache	3 (3.6)	0 (0.0)	5 (9.4)	1 (1.9)
Infection bacterial	1 (1.2)	0 (0.0)	0 (0.0)	2 (3.8)
CARDIOVASCULAR SYS.				
Peripheral edema	2 (2.4)	1 (1.2)	0 (0.0)	0 (0.0)
DIGESTIVE SYSTEM				
Anorexia	0 (0.0)	0 (0.0)	3 (5.7)	0 (0.0)
Diarrhea	1 (1.2)	1 (1.2)	2 (3.8)	1 (1.9)
Pancreatitis	1 (1.2)	0 (0.0)	2 (3.8)	0 (0.0)
Vomiting	0 (0.0)	0 (0.0)	2 (3.8)	0 (0.0)
ENDOCRINE				
Hypothyroidism	1 (1.2)	1 (1.2)	2 (3.8)	0 (0.0)
HEM. & LYMPH. SYS.				
Leukopenia	3 (3.6)	0 (0.0)	6 (11.3)	1 (1.9)
META. AND NUTR. DIS.				
Bilirubinemia	0 (0.0)	1 (1.2)	2 (3.8)	0 (0.0)
Hypercholesteremia	2 (2.4)	0 (0.0)	5 (9.4)	0 (0.0)
Hyperlipemia	16 (19.0)	6 (7.1)	17 (32.1)	5 (9.4)
SGOT/AST increased	0 (0.0)	0 (0.0)	2 (3.8)	0 (0.0)
SGPT/ALT increased	0 (0.0)	0 (0.0)	2 (3.8)	0 (0.0)
RESPIRATORY SYSTEM				
Pneumonia	0 (0.0)	0 (0.0)	2 (3.8)	2 (3.8)
SKIN AND APPENDAGES				
Exfoliative dermatitis	0 (0.0)	1 (1.2)	3 (5.7)	1 (1.9)
Rash	1 (1.2)	2 (2.4)	1 (1.9)	0 (0.0)

[1] Preferred English term coded according to Ligand-modified COSTART 5 Dictionary.
[2] Patients are counted at most once in each AE category. Patients are classified by the highest severity within each row.

Table 3. Treatment-Emergent Abnormal Laboratory Values in CTCL Trials

Analyte	Initial Assigned Dose (mg/m²/day)			
	300 N=83[1]		>300 N=53[1]	
	Grade 3[2] (%)	Grade 4[2] (%)	Grade 3 (%)	Grade 4 (%)
Triglycerides[3]	21.3	6.7	31.8	13.6
Total Cholesterol[3]	18.7	6.7	15.9	29.5
Alkaline Phosphatase	1.2	0.0	0.0	1.9
Hyperglycemia	1.2	0.0	5.7	0.0
Hypocalcemia	1.2	0.0	0.0	0.0
Hyponatremia	1.2	0.0	9.4	0.0
SGPT/ALT	1.2	0.0	1.9	1.9
Hyperkalemia	0.0	0.0	1.9	0.0
Hypernatremia	0.0	1.2	0.0	0.0
SGOT/AST	0.0	0.0	1.9	1.9
Total Bilirubin	0.0	0.0	0.0	1.9
ANC	12.0	3.6	18.9	7.5
ALC	7.2	0.0	15.1	0.0
WBC	3.6	0.0	11.3	0.0
Hemoglobin	0.0	0.0	1.9	0.0

[1] Number of patients with at least one analyte value post-baseline.
[2] Adapted from NCI Common Toxicity Criteria, Grade 3 and 4, Version 2.0. Patients are considered to have had a Grade 3 or 4 value if either of the following occurred: a) Value becomes Grade 3 or 4 during the study; b) Value is abnormal at baseline and worsens to Grade 3 or 4 on study, including all values beyond study drug discontinuation, as defined in data handling conventions.
[3] The denominator used to calculate the incidence rates for fasting Total Cholesterol and Triglycerides were N=75 for the 300 mg/m²/day initial dose group and N=44 for the >300 mg/m²/day initial dose group.

eutropenia/leukopenia, diarrhea, fatigue/lethargy, hypothyroidism, headache, liver function test abnormalities, rash, pancreatitis, nausea, anemia, allergic reaction, muscle spasm, pneumonia, and confusion.

The moderately severe (NCI Grade 3) and severe (NCI Grade 4) adverse events reported in two or more patients with CTCL treated at an initial dose of 300 mg/m²/day of Targretin® capsules (see Table 2) were hypertriglyceridemia, pruritus, headache, peripheral edema, leukopenia, rash, and hypercholesteremia. Most of these moderately severe or severe adverse events occurred at a higher rate in patients treated at starting doses of greater than 300 mg/m²/day than in patients treated at a starting dose of 300 mg/m²/day.

As shown in Table 3, in patients with CTCL receiving an initial dose of 300 mg/m²/day, the incidence of NCI Grade 3 or 4 elevations in triglycerides and total cholesterol was 28% and 25%, respectively. In contrast, in patients with CTCL receiving greater than 300 mg/m²/day, the incidence of NCI Grade 3 or 4 elevated triglycerides and total cholesterol was 45% and 45%, respectively. Other Grade 3 and 4 laboratory abnormalities are shown in Table 3.

In addition to the 152 patients enrolled in the two CTCL studies, 352 patients received Targretin® capsules as monotherapy for various advanced malignancies at doses from 5 mg/m²/day to 1000 mg/m²/day. The common adverse events (incidence greater than 10%) were similar to those seen in patients with CTCL.

In the 504 patients (CTCL and non-CTCL) who received Targretin® capsules as monotherapy, drug-related serious adverse events that were fatal, in one patient each, were acute pancreatitis, subdural hematoma, and liver failure.

In the patients with CTCL receiving an initial dose of 300 mg/m²/day of Targretin® capsules, adverse events reported at an incidence of less than 10% and not included in Tables 1–3 or discussed in other parts of labeling and possibly related to treatment were as follows:

Body as a Whole: chills, cellulitis, chest pain, sepsis, and monilia.

Cardiovascular: hemorrhage, hypertension, angina pectoris, right heart failure, syncope, and tachycardia.

Digestive: constipation, dry mouth, flatulence, colitis, dyspepsia, cheilitis, gastroenteritis, gingivitis, liver failure, and melena.

Hemic and Lymphatic: eosinophilia, thrombocythemia, coagulation time increased, lymphocytosis, and thrombocytopenia.

Metabolic and Nutritional: LDH increased, creatinine increased, hypoproteinemia, hyperglycemia, weight decreased, weight increased, and amylase increased.

Musculoskeletal: arthralgia, myalgia, bone pain, myasthenia, and arthrosis.

Nervous: depression, agitation, ataxia, cerebrovascular accident, confusion, dizziness, hyperesthesia, hypesthesia, and neuropathy.

Respiratory: pharyngitis, rhinitis, dyspnea, pleural effusion, bronchitis, cough increased, lung edema, hemoptysis, and hypoxia.

Skin and Appendages: skin ulcer, acne, alopecia, skin nodule, macular papular rash, pustular rash, serous drainage, and vesicular bullous rash.

Special Senses: dry eyes, conjunctivitis, ear pain, blepharitis, corneal lesion, keratitis, otitis externa, and visual field defect.

Urogenital: albuminuria, hematuria, urinary incontinence, urinary tract infection, urinary urgency, dysuria, kidney function abnormal, and breast pain.

[See table 1 at top of page 1044]
[See table 2 at top of previous page]
[See table 3 on previous page]

OVERDOSAGE

Doses up to 1000 mg/m²/day of Targretin® capsules have been administered in short-term studies in patients with advanced cancer without acute toxic effects. Single doses of 1500 mg/kg and 720 mg/kg were tolerated without significant toxicity in rats and dogs, respectively. These doses are approximately 30 and 50 times, respectively, the recommended human dose on a mg/m² basis.

No clinical experience with an overdose of Targretin® capsules has been reported. Any overdose with Targretin® capsules should be treated with supportive care for the signs and symptoms exhibited by the patient.

DOSAGE AND ADMINISTRATION

The recommended initial dose of Targretin® capsules is 300 mg/m²/day. (See Table 4.) Targretin® capsules should be taken as a single oral daily dose with a meal. See **CONTRAINDICATIONS: Pregnancy: Category X** section for precautions to prevent pregnancy and birth defects in women of child-bearing potential.

Table 4. Targretin® Capsule Initial Dose Calculation According to Body Surface Area

Body Surface Area (m²)	Total Daily Dose (mg/day)	Number of 75 mg Targretin® Capsules
0.88–1.12	300	4
1.13–1.37	375	5
1.38–1.62	450	6
1.63–1.87	525	7
1.88–2.12	600	8
2.13–2.37	675	9
2.38–2.62	750	10

Initial Dose Level (300 mg/m²/day)

Dose Modification Guidelines: The 300 mg/m²/day dose level of Targretin® capsules may be adjusted to 200 mg/m²/day then to 100 mg/m²/day, or temporarily suspended, if necessitated by toxicity. When toxicity is controlled, doses may be carefully readjusted upward. If there is no tumor response after eight weeks of treatment and if the initial dose of 300 mg/m²/day is well tolerated, the dose may be escalated to 400 mg/m²/day with careful monitoring.

Duration of Therapy: In clinical trials in CTCL, Targretin® capsules were administered for up to 97 weeks. Targretin® capsules should be continued as long as the patient is deriving benefit.

HOW SUPPLIED

Targretin® capsules are supplied as 75 mg off-white, oblong soft gelatin capsules, imprinted with "Targretin", in high density polyethylene bottles with child-resistant closures.
Bottles of 100 capsules   NDC 62856-602-10
Store at 2°–25°C (36°–77°F). Avoid exposing to high temperatures and humidity after the bottle is opened. Protect from light.

Manufactured for: Eisai Inc.
                      Woodcliff Lake, NJ 07677
Targretin® is a registered trademark of Eisai Inc.
200606
© 2007 Eisai Inc.
Revised May 2007

Patient's Instructions for Use
Targretin® (bexarotene) capsules, 75 mg

To help you get the full benefits from this medicine, you should read this leaflet carefully and ask your doctor to explain anything you do not understand.

What are the most important things I should know about Targretin® capsules?
• Targretin® capsules can cause major damage to a fetus. Pregnancy must be avoided in patients receiving Targretin® capsules.
• Targretin® capsules can greatly increase blood levels of lipids (triglycerides and cholesterol) and these levels must be monitored and, if elevated, treated.
• Targretin® capsules can cause an underactive thyroid and periodic blood tests will be needed to detect this. Medication to control the condition may be necessary.

Do not take Targretin® capsules if you are pregnant or if you plan to become pregnant.
• Targretin® capsules may harm your fetus (unborn baby). You should contact your doctor immediately if you believe or suspect you are pregnant while you are taking Targretin® capsules and until one month after you stop taking Targretin® capsules.
• If you are capable of becoming pregnant, you must have a pregnancy test, within one week before you start Targretin® capsule therapy and monthly while you are taking Targretin® capsules, confirming you are not pregnant.
• You must use effective contraception (birth control) continuously starting one month before beginning treatment with Targretin® capsules until one month after you stop taking Targretin® capsules. It is strongly recommended that two reliable forms of contraception be used together. At least one of these two forms of contraception should include condoms, diaphragms, cervical caps, IUDs, or spermicides.
• If you are male and your partner is pregnant or capable of becoming pregnant, you should discuss with your doctor the precautions you should take.

What are Targretin® capsules?
Targretin (tar-GRET-in) capsules contain bexarotene (beks-AIR-oh-teen). Targretin® capsules belong to a class of medicines known as retinoids. Each off-white, oblong soft gelatin Targretin® capsule contains 75 mg of bexarotene. Each capsule is imprinted with the name "Targretin" in blue.

What are the uses for Targretin® capsules?
This medicine is used to treat the skin problems arising from a disease called cutaneous T-cell lymphoma, or CTCL. Your doctor must supervise the use of Targretin® capsules.

Do not take Targretin® capsules if you are allergic to this medicine.

If you have any of the following conditions, make sure you have discussed them with your doctor before you start to take this medicine.
• You are pregnant or think you may be pregnant.
• You have or previously had an inflamed pancreas (pancreatitis).
• You are breastfeeding.
• You are taking gemfibrozil (Lopid®)*, a medication to reduce high triglyceride cholesterol (fats) levels in the blood.
• You are taking tamoxifen (Nolvadex®)†

Medical conditions you should tell your doctor about.
• If you are allergic to retinoid medications (for example: Accutane® [isotretinoin], Soriatane® [acitretin], Tegison® [etretinate], Vesanoid® [tretinoin])‡
• If you have or ever had high triglyceride (a fatty substance) levels in your blood.
• If you have diabetes mellitus (sugar diabetes).
• If you have a history of or currently have gall bladder disease.
• If you have or have had any liver disease.
• If you regularly drink more than a small amount of alcohol.
• If you are currently taking any prescription medication especially for fungal infections, bacterial infections, or seizures.
• If you eat a lot of grapefruit or drink a lot of grapefruit juice.

When should you be extra careful while taking Targretin® capsules?
• Because vitamin A in large doses may cause some side effects which are similar to those seen in patients taking Targretin® capsules, do not take more than the recommended daily dietary allowance of vitamin A (4000 to 5000 International Units). If you take vitamins, check the label to see how much vitamin A they contain. If you are not sure, ask your doctor or pharmacist.
• Your skin may become more sensitive to sunlight while taking this medicine. Minimize exposure to sunlight and do not use a sunlamp.

How should Targretin capsules be taken?
• Always take Targretin® capsules the way your doctor tells you.
• Your doctor will tell you how many Targretin® capsules to take each day. You should take your daily dose of Targretin® capsules all at once. It is best to take them once each day with or immediately following a meal. For example, you might always take your daily amount of Targretin® capsules with your evening meal.
• Always swallow each capsule whole; do not chew them or dissolve them in liquid or in your mouth. Depending on your health and condition, your doctor may change your daily dose (the number of capsules you are taking) during your treatment.
• If you miss a dose, take it as soon as possible, with food. However, if it is nearly time for your next dose, skip the missed dose and continue your dose schedule as before. Do not take a double dose.
• If you take too many Targretin® capsules or someone else accidentally takes your medicine, contact your doctor, emergency room or the nearest hospital immediately.

How long before you can expect your CTCL to improve on Targretin® capsule treatment?
• Although some patients saw improvement within the first several weeks of Targretin® capsule treatment, most patients required several months or more of treatment to improve.
• Your doctor should determine how long you should be taking Targretin® capsules, and when treatment may be stopped.

What side effects do Targretin® capsules have?
The most common side effect is an increase in blood lipids (fats in the blood). Periodic blood tests will be needed to determine blood levels of lipids, including triglycerides and cholesterol. Medication may be needed to control high fat levels in the blood.
Another common side effect is underactive thyroid. The symptoms of underactive thyroid may be difficult to detect because they may develop very gradually and may be very mild. For example, you may begin to feel always tired, low on energy, or feeling unusually cold all the time. A thyroid hormone medication is readily available to fully control

these temporary symptoms, so contact your doctor early if you feel you are beginning to experience any of these symptoms. Periodic blood tests will be needed to detect this.

When should you call your doctor about possible complications of Targretin® capsule treatment?

As an infrequent side effect of Targretin® capsule treatment, pancreatitis (inflamed pancreas) may occur. Symptoms of pancreatitis include persistent nausea, vomiting, and abdominal or back pain. If you develop any of these symptoms while taking Targretin® capsules, contact your doctor immediately.

All medications have side effects. You should call your physician regarding any questions or concerns you may have when taking Targretin® capsules.

How should Targretin® capsules be stored?

- The capsules should be stored in a dry place in a closed container, away from light and heat, at room temperature.
- The capsules should not be used after the expiration date printed on the bottle.
- Keep this medicine out of the reach and sight of children.

If Targretin® capsules are broken or leaking, do not touch the capsules or the contents and notify your pharmacist immediately. Should the contents of a broken capsule get on your skin, immediately wash the area with soap and water and notify your physician.

Further Information

- You can get more information on Targretin® capsules from your doctor or pharmacist.

[*] Lopid® (gemfibrozil tablets, USP) is a registered trademark of Parke-Davis, Division of Warner-Lambert Co.

[†] Nolvadex® (tamoxifen citrate) is a registered trademark of AstraZeneca LP.

[‡] Accutane® (isotretinoin) is a registered trademark of Roche Pharmaceuticals, Roche Laboratories Inc.

[‡] Soriatane® (acitretin) is a registered trademark of Roche Pharmaceuticals, Roche Laboratories Inc.

[‡] Tegison® (etretinate) is a registered trademark of Roche Pharmaceuticals, Roche Laboratories, Inc.

[‡] Vesanoid® (tretinoin) is a registered trademark of Roche Pharmaceuticals, Roche Laboratories Inc.

Targretin® (bexarotene) is a registered trademark of Eisai Inc.

Manufactured for:
Eisai Inc.
Woodcliff Lake, NJ 07677
© 2007 Eisai Inc. 200607 (Rev. 0307)

Shown in Product Identification Guide, page 308

TARGRETIN®
[tahr-greh' tən]
(bexarotene)
Gel 1%
Rx only. ℞

DESCRIPTION

Targretin® (bexarotene) gel 1% contains bexarotene and is intended for topical application only. Bexarotene is a member of a subclass of retinoids that selectively activate retinoid X receptors (RXRs). These retinoid receptors have biologic activity distinct from that of retinoic acid receptors (RARs).

The chemical name is 4-[1-(5,6,7,8-tetrahydro-3,5,5,8,8-pentamethyl-2-naphthalenyl)ethenyl] benzoic acid, and the structural formula is as follows:

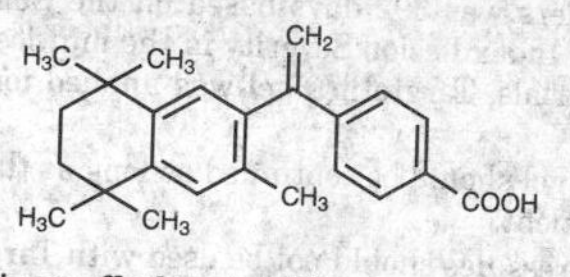

Bexarotene is an off-white to white powder with a molecular weight of 348.48 and a molecular formula of $C_{24}H_{28}O_2$. It is insoluble in water and slightly soluble in vegetable oils and ethanol, USP.

Targretin® gel is a clear gelled solution containing 1.0% (w/w) bexarotene in a base of dehydrated alcohol, USP, polyethylene glycol 400, NF, hydroxypropyl cellulose, NF, and butylated hydroxytoluene, NF.

CLINICAL PHARMACOLOGY

Mechanism of Action

Bexarotene selectively binds and activates retinoid X receptor subtypes (RXRα, RXRβ, RXRγ). RXRs can form heterodimers with various receptor partners such as retinoic acid receptors (RARs), vitamin D receptor, thyroid receptor, and peroxisome proliferator activator receptors (PPARs). Once activated, these receptors function as transcription factors that regulate the expression of genes that control cellular differentiation and proliferation. Bexarotene inhibits the growth *in vitro* of some tumor cell lines of hematopoietic and squamous cell origin. It also induces tumor regression *in vivo* in some animal models. The exact mechanism of action of bexarotene in the treatment of cutaneous T-cell lymphoma (CTCL) is unknown.

Pharmacokinetics

General

Plasma concentrations of bexarotene were determined during clinical studies in patients with CTCL or following repeated single or multiple-daily dose applications of Targretin® gel 1% for up to 132 weeks. Plasma bexarotene concentrations were generally less than 5 ng/mL and did not exceed 55 ng/mL. However, only two patients with very intense dosing regimens (> 40% BSA lesions and QID dosing) were sampled. Plasma bexarotene concentrations and the frequency of detecting quantifiable plasma bexarotene concentrations increased with increasing percent body surface area treated and increasing quantity of Targretin® gel applied. The sporadically observed and generally low plasma bexarotene concentrations indicated that, in patients receiving doses of low to moderate intensity, there is a low potential for significant plasma concentrations following repeated application of Targretin® gel. Bexarotene is highly bound (>99%) to plasma proteins. The plasma proteins to which bexarotene binds have not been elucidated, and the ability of bexarotene to displace drugs bound to plasma proteins and the ability of drugs to displace bexarotene binding have not been studied (see PRECAUTIONS: Protein Binding). The uptake of bexarotene by organs or tissues has not been evaluated.

Metabolism

Four bexarotene metabolites have been identified in plasma following oral administration of bexarotene: 6- and 7-hydroxy-bexarotene and 6- and 7-oxo-bexarotene. *In vitro* studies suggest that cytochrome P450 3A4 is the major cytochrome P450 responsible for formation of the oxidative metabolites and that the oxidative metabolites may be glucuronidated. The oxidative metabolites are active in *in vitro* assays of retinoid receptor activation, but the relative contribution of the parent and any metabolites to the efficacy and safety of Targretin® gel is unknown.

Elimination

The renal elimination of bexarotene and its metabolites was examined in patients with Type 2 diabetes mellitus following oral administration of bexarotene. Neither bexarotene nor its metabolites were excreted in urine in appreciable amounts.

Special Populations

Elderly, Gender, Race: Because of a large number of immeasurable plasma concentrations (< 1 ng/mL), any potential pharmacokinetic differences between Special Populations could not be assessed.

Pediatric: Studies to evaluate bexarotene pharmacokinetics in the pediatric population have not been conducted (see PRECAUTIONS: Pediatric Use).

Renal Insufficiency: No formal studies have been conducted with Targretin® gel in patients with renal insufficiency. Urinary elimination of bexarotene and its known metabolites is a minor excretory pathway (<1% of an orally administered dose), but because renal insufficiency can result in significant protein binding changes, pharmacokinetics may be altered in patients with renal insufficiency (see PRECAUTIONS: Renal Insufficiency).

Hepatic Insufficiency: No specific studies have been conducted with Targretin® gel in patients with hepatic insufficiency. Because less than 1% of the dose of oral bexarotene is excreted in the urine unchanged and there is *in vitro* evidence of extensive hepatic contribution to bexarotene elimination, hepatic impairment would be expected to lead to greatly decreased clearance (see PRECAUTIONS: Hepatic Insufficiency).

Drug-Drug Interactions

No formal studies to evaluate drug interactions with bexarotene or Targretin® gel have been conducted. Bexarotene oxidative metabolites appear to be formed through cytochrome P450 3A4. Drugs that affect levels or activity of cytochrome P450 3A4 may potentially affect the disposition of bexarotene. Concomitant gemfibrozil was associated with increased bexarotene concentrations following oral administration of bexarotene.

Clinical Studies

Targretin® gel was evaluated for the treatment of patients with early stage (Stage IA-IIA) CTCL in one multicenter, open-label, clinical trial as well as in a Phase I-II program (dose-seeking trials with different response criteria than the multicenter trial). These clinical studies enrolled a total of 117 patients.

In the multicenter, open-label clinical trial, Targretin® gel was evaluated for the treatment of patients with early stage CTCL who were refractory to, intolerant to, or reached a response plateau for at least six months on at least two prior therapies. The study was conducted in the U.S., Canada, Europe, and Australia and enrolled a total of 50 patients; 46% of these patients were male, 80% were Caucasian, and the median age was 64 years (range 13 to 85).

Targretin® gel was also evaluated for the treatment of patients with CTCL in a U.S. Phase I-II program involving patients with early stage CTCL. This program enrolled a total of 67 patients; 55% of these patients were male, 85% were Caucasian, and the median age was 61 years (range 30 to 87).

In the multicenter, open-label clinical trial, considering prior systemic, irradiation, and topical treatments, patients had been exposed to a median of three prior therapies (range 2-7). All patients failed at least two treatments; the majority (68%) of patients were either refractory to two or more therapies or were refractory to one therapy and intolerant to at least one therapy.

Patients were treated with Targretin® gel 1% for a planned 16-week period with an option to continue provided that no unacceptable toxicity was occurring.

Tumor response was assessed in the multicenter study by observation of up to five baseline-defined index lesions using a Composite Assessment of Index Lesion Disease Severity (CA). This endpoint was based on a summation of the grades, for all index lesions, of erythema, scaling, plaque elevation, hypopigmentation or hyperpigmentation, and area of involvement. New cutaneous lesions or tumors and extracutaneous disease manifestations were not considered in response or disease progression assessments.

All tumor responses required confirmation over at least two assessments separated by at least four weeks. A partial response was defined as an improvement of at least 50% in the index lesions. A complete clinical response required complete disappearance of the index lesions, but did not require confirmation by biopsy.

Targretin® gel produced an overall response rate of 26% (13/50) with a corresponding exact 95% confidence interval from 14.6% to 40.3% by the Composite Assessment of Index Lesion Severity. For the Stage IA and IB patients, the response rate was 28% (13/47) with a corresponding exact 95% confidence interval from 15.6% to 42.6%. For the Stage II patients the response rate was 0% (0/3). Two percent of patients (1/50) had a clinical complete response. The median time to best response on the Composite Assessment of Index Lesion Severity (n=13) was 85 days (range: 36-154). The rate of relapse in responding patients by the Composite Assessment of Index Lesion Severity was 23% (3/13) over a median observation period of 149 days (range 56-342). Fourteen patients developed new lesions in untreated areas (14/50; 28%). Four patients developed clinically abnormal lymph nodes (≥ 1 cm diam) (4/50; 8%). One patient developed a cutaneous tumor (1/50; 2%).

The Phase I-II program (dose-seeking trials with different response criteria than the multicenter trial) was supportive of the multicenter study results.

INDICATIONS AND USAGE

Targretin® (bexarotene) gel 1% is indicated for the topical treatment of cutaneous lesions in patients with CTCL (Stage IA and IB) who have refractory or persistent disease after other therapies or who have not tolerated other therapies.

CONTRAINDICATIONS

Targretin® gel 1% is contraindicated in patients with a known hypersensitivity to bexarotene or other components of the product.

Pregnancy: Category X

Targretin® gel 1% may cause fetal harm when administered to a pregnant woman.

Targretin® gel must not be given to a pregnant woman or a woman who intends to become pregnant. If a woman becomes pregnant while taking Targretin® gel, Targretin® gel must be stopped immediately and the woman given appropriate counseling.

Bexarotene caused malformations when administered orally to pregnant rats during days 7-17 of gestation. Developmental abnormalities included incomplete ossification at 4 mg/kg/day and cleft palate, depressed eye bulge/microphthalmia, and small ears at 16 mg/kg/day. At doses greater than 10 mg/kg/day, bexarotene caused developmental mortality. The no-effect oral dose in rats was 1 mg/kg/day. Plasma bexarotene concentrations in patients with CTCL applying Targretin® gel 1% were generally less than one hundredth the Cmax associated with dysmorphogenesis in rats, although some patients had Cmax levels that were approximately one eighth the concentration associated with dysmorphogenesis in rats.

Women of child-bearing potential should be advised to avoid becoming pregnant when Targretin® gel is used. The possibility that a woman of child-bearing potential is pregnant at the time therapy is instituted should be considered. A negative pregnancy test (e.g., serum beta-human chorionic gonadotropin, beta-HCG) with a sensitivity of at least 50 mIU/L should be obtained within one week prior to Targretin® gel therapy, and the pregnancy test must be repeated at monthly intervals while the patient remains on Targretin® gel. Effective contraception must be used for one month prior to the initiation of therapy, during therapy and or at least one month following discontinuation of therapy; it is recommended that two reliable forms of contraception be used simultaneously unless abstinence is the chosen method. Male patients with sexual partners who are pregnant, possibly pregnant, or who could become pregnant must use condoms during sexual intercourse while applying Targretin® gel and for at least one month after the last dose of drug. Targretin® gel therapy should be initiated on the second or third day of a normal menstrual period. No more than a one month supply of Targretin® gel should be given to the patient so that the results of pregnancy testing can be assessed and counseling regarding avoidance of pregnancy and birth defects can be reinforced.

PRECAUTIONS
Pregnancy
Category X. See CONTRAINDICATIONS.
General
Targretin® gel should be used with caution in patients with a known hypersensitivity to other retinoids. No clinical instances of cross-reactivity have been noted.
Vitamin A Supplementation: In clinical studies, patients were advised to limit vitamin A intake to ≤ 15,000 IU/day. Because of the relationship of bexarotene to vitamin A, patients should be advised to limit vitamin A supplements to avoid potential additive toxic effects.
Photosensitivity: Retinoids as a class have been associated with photosensitivity. *In vitro* assays indicate that bexarotene is a potential photosensitizing agent. There were no reports of photosensitivity in patients in the clinical studies. Patients should be advised to minimize exposure to sunlight and artificial ultraviolet light during the use of Targretin® gel.
Information for Patients
Please see accompanying "Patient's Instructions for Use"
Drug-Drug Interactions
Patients who are applying Targretin® gel should not concurrently use products that contain DEET (*N,N*-diethyl-*m*-toluamide), a common component of insect repellent products. An animal toxicology study showed increased DEET toxicity when DEET was included as part of the formulation.
No formal studies to evaluate drug interactions with bexarotene have been conducted. Bexarotene oxidative metabolites appear to be formed through cytochrome P450 3A4.
On the basis of the metabolism of bexarotene by cytochrome P450 3A4, concomitant ketoconazole, itraconazole, erythromycin and grapefruit juice could increase bexarotene plasma concentrations. Similarly, based on data that gemfibrozil increases bexarotene concentrations following oral bexarotene administration, concomitant gemfibrozil could increase bexarotene plasma concentrations. However, due to the low systemic exposure to bexarotene after low to moderately intense gel regimens (see Clinical Pharmacology), increases that occur are unlikely to be of sufficient magnitude to result in adverse effects.
No drug interaction data are available on concomitant administration of Targretin® gel and other CTCL therapies.
Renal Insufficiency
No formal studies have been conducted with Targretin® gel in patients with renal insufficiency. Urinary elimination of bexarotene and its known metabolites is a minor excretory pathway for bexarotene (<1% of an orally administered dose), but because renal insufficiency can result in significant protein binding changes, and bexarotene is >99% protein bound, pharmacokinetics may be altered in patients with renal insufficiency.
Hepatic Insufficiency
No specific studies have been conducted with Targretin® gel in patients with hepatic insufficiency. Because less than 1% of the dose of oral bexarotene is excreted in the urine unchanged and there is *in vitro* evidence of extensive hepatic contribution to bexarotene elimination, hepatic impairment would be expected to lead to greatly decreased clearance.
Protein Binding
Bexarotene is highly bound (>99%) to plasma proteins. The plasma proteins to which bexarotene binds have not been elucidated, and the ability of bexarotene to displace drugs bound to plasma proteins and the ability of drugs to displace bexarotene binding have not been studied.
Carcinogenesis, Mutagenesis, Impairment of Fertility
Long-term studies in animals to assess the carcinogenic potential of bexarotene have not been conducted. Bexarotene was not mutagenic to bacteria (Ames assay) or mammalian cells (mouse lymphoma assay). Bexarotene was not clastogenic *in vivo* (micronucleus test in mice). No formal fertility studies were conducted with bexarotene. Bexarotene caused testicular degeneration when oral doses of 1.5 mg/kg/day were given to dogs for 91 days.
Use in Nursing Mothers
It is not known whether bexarotene is excreted in human milk. Because many drugs are excreted in human milk and because of the potential for serious adverse reactions in nursing infants from bexarotene, a decision should be made whether to discontinue nursing or to discontinue the drug, taking into account the importance of the drug to the mother.
Pediatric Use
Safety and effectiveness in pediatric patients have not been established.
Geriatric Use
Of the total patients with CTCL in clinical studies of Targretin® gel, 62% were under 65 years and 38% were 65 years or older. No overall differences in safety were observed between patients 65 years of age or older and younger patients, but greater sensitivity of some older individuals to Targretin® gel cannot be ruled out. Responses to Targretin® gel were observed across all age group decades, without preference for any individual age group decade.

ADVERSE REACTIONS
The safety of Targretin® gel has been assessed in clinical studies of 117 patients with CTCL who received Targretin® gel for up to 172 weeks. In the multicenter open-label study, 50 patients with CTCL received Targretin® gel for up to 98 weeks. The mean duration of therapy for these 50 patients was 199 days. The most common adverse events reported with an incidence at the application site of at least 10% in patients with CTCL were rash, pruritus, skin disorder, and pain.
Adverse events leading to dose reduction or study drug discontinuation in at least two patients were rash, contact dermatitis, and pruritus.
Of the 49 patients (98%) who experienced any adverse event, most experienced events categorized as mild (9 patients, 18%) or moderate (27 patients, 54%). There were 12 patients (24%) who experienced at least one moderately severe adverse event. The most common moderately severe events were rash (7 patients, 14%) and pruritus (3 patients, 6%). Only one patient (2%) experienced a severe adverse event (rash).
In the patients with CTCL receiving Targretin® gel, adverse events reported regardless of relationship to study drug at an incidence of ≥5% are presented in Table 1.
A similar safety profile for Targretin® gel was demonstrated in the Phase I-II program. For the 67 patients enrolled in the Phase I-II program, the mean duration of treatment was 436 days (range 12-1203 days). As in the multicenter study, the most common adverse events regardless of relationship to study drug in the Phase I-II program were rash (78%), pain (40%), and pruritus (40%).

Table 1. Incidence of All Adverse Events* and Application Site Adverse Events with Incidence ≥5% for All Application Frequencies of Targretin® Gel in the Multicenter CTCL Study

COSTART 5 Body System/Preferred Term	All Adverse Events N = 50 n (%)	Application Site Adverse Events N = 50 n (%)
Skin and Appendages		
Contact Dermatitis[1]	7 (14)	4 (8)
Exfoliative Dermatitis	3 (6)	0
Pruritus[2]	18 (36)	9 (18)
Rash[3]	36 (72)	28 (56)
Maculopapular Rash	3 (6)	0
Skin Disorder (NOS)[4]	13 (26)	9 (18)
Sweating	3 (6)	0
Body as a Whole		
Asthenia	3 (6)	0
Headache	7 (14)	0
Infection	9 (18)	0
Pain	15 (30)	9 (18)
Cardiovascular		
Edema	5 (10)	0
Peripheral Edema	3 (6)	0
Hemic and Lymphatic		
Leukopenia	3 (6)	0
Lymphadenopathy	3 (6)	0
WBC Abnormal	3 (6)	0
Metabolic and Nutritional		
Hyperlipemia	5 (10)	0
Nervous		
Paresthesia	3 (6)	3 (6)
Respiratory		
Cough Increased	3 (6)	0
Pharyngitis	3 (6)	0

* Regardless of association with treatment
  Includes Investigator terms such as:
[1] Contact dermatitis, irritant contact dermatitis, irritant dermatitis
[2] Pruritus, itching, itching of lesion
[3] Erythema, scaling, irritation, redness, rash, dermatitis
[4] Skin inflammation, excoriation, sticky or tacky sensation of skin; NOS = Not Otherwise Specified

OVERDOSAGE
Systemic toxicity following acute overdosage with topical application of Targretin® gel is unlikely because of low systemic plasma levels observed with normal therapeutic doses. There is no specific antidote for overdosage.
There has been no experience with acute overdose of Targretin® gel in humans. Any overdose with Targretin® gel should be treated with supportive care for the signs and symptoms exhibited by the patient.

DOSAGE AND ADMINISTRATION
Targretin® gel should be initially applied once every other day for the first week. The application frequency should be increased at weekly intervals to once daily, then twice daily, then three times daily and finally four times daily according to individual lesion tolerance. Generally, patients were able to maintain a dosing frequency of two to four times per day. Most responses were seen at dosing frequencies of two times per day and higher. If application site toxicity occurs, the application frequency can be reduced. Should severe irritation occur, application of drug can be temporarily discontinued for a few days until the symptoms subside. See CONTRAINDICATIONS: Pregnancy: Category X.
Sufficient gel should be applied to cover the lesion with a generous coating. The gel should be allowed to dry before covering with clothing. Because unaffected skin may become irritated, application of the gel to normal skin surrounding the lesions should be avoided. In addition, do not apply the gel near mucosal surfaces of the body.
A response may be seen as soon as four weeks after initiation of therapy but most patients require longer application. With continued application, further benefit may be attained. The longest onset time for the first response among the responders was 392 days based on the Composite Assessment of Index Lesion Severity in the multicenter study. In clinical trials, Targretin® gel was applied for up to 172 weeks.
Targretin® gel should be continued as long as the patient is deriving benefit.
Occlusive dressings should not be used with Targretin® gel.
Targretin® gel is a topical therapy and is not intended for systemic use. Targretin® gel has not been studied in combination with other CTCL therapies.

HOW SUPPLIED
Targretin® gel is supplied in tubes containing 60 g (600 mg active bexarotene).
60 g tube
NDC 62856-604-22
Store at 25°C (77°F); with excursions permitted to 15°-30°C (59°-86°F) [see USP]. Avoid exposing to high temperatures and humidity after the tube is opened. Protect from light.
Manufactured for: Eisai Inc.
Woodcliff Lake, NJ 07677
by: Contract Pharmaceuticals Limited Niagara
Buffalo, NY 14213-1091
© 2009 Eisai Inc.
Revised (07/09)

TARGRETIN® (BEXAROTENE) 1% GEL

PATIENT'S INSTRUCTIONS FOR USE

(For Topical Use Only)

To help you get the full benefits from this medicine, you should read this leaflet carefully and ask your doctor to explain anything you do not understand.

What are the most important things I should know about Targretin® gel?

Do not use Targretin® gel if you are pregnant or if you plan to become pregnant.

- Targretin® gel may harm your fetus (unborn baby). You should contact your doctor immediately if you believe or suspect you are pregnant while you are using Targretin® gel and until one month after you stop using Targretin® gel.
- If you are capable of becoming pregnant, you must have a pregnancy test, within one week before you start Targretin® gel therapy and monthly while you are using Targretin® gel, confirming you are not pregnant.
- You must use effective contraception (birth control) continuously starting one month before beginning treatment with Targretin® gel until one month after you stop using Targretin® gel. It is recommended that two reliable forms of contraception be used together.
- If you are male and your partner is pregnant or capable of becoming pregnant, you should discuss with your doctor the precautions you should take.

What is Targretin® gel?

Targretin (tar-GRET-in) gel contains bexarotene (beks-AIR-oh-teen). Targretin® gel belongs to a class of medicines known as retinoids.

What are the uses for Targretin® gel?

This medicine is used to treat the skin problems arising from a disease called cutaneous T-cell lymphoma, or CTCL. Your health care provider has prescribed Targretin® for the topical treatment of the cutaneous T-cell lymphoma (CTCL), or mycosis fungoides (MF), lesions (sometimes referred to as patches or plaques) on your skin. Your doctor must instruct you on the proper use of Targretin® gel. The following instructions will help you successfully begin and continue your treatment.

Do not use Targretin® gel if you are allergic to this medicine.

Do not use Targretin® gel if you are pregnant or believe you may be pregnant.

If you have any of the following conditions, make sure you have discussed them with your doctor before you start to take this medicine.

- If you are breast feeding.
- If you are allergic to retinoid medications (for example: Accutane® [isotretinoin], Soriatane® [acitretin], Tegison® [etretinate], Vesinoid® [tretinoin]).

When should you be extra careful while using Targretin® gel?

- Because vitamin A in large doses may cause some side effects which are similar to those seen in patients applying Targretin® gel, do not take more than the recommended daily dietary allowance of vitamin A (4000 to 5000 International Units). If you take vitamins, check the label to see how much vitamin A they contain. If you are not sure, ask your doctor or pharmacist.
- Your skin may become more sensitive to sunlight while using this medicine. Minimize exposure to sunlight and do not use a sunlamp.

WARNINGS

For external use only.

DO NOT apply the gel on or near mucosal surfaces of the body such as eyes, nostrils, mouth, lips, vagina, tip of the penis, rectum, or anus.

DO NOT use insect repellents containing DEET (*N,N*-diethyl-*m*-toluamide) or other products containing DEET while using Targretin® gel.

Keep out of reach of children.

Product contains alcohol and should be kept away from open flame.

DO NOT use Targretin® gel if you are pregnant or breast-feeding. Speak to your health care provider if you have any questions or need more information.

HOW TO APPLY

Apply Targretin® gel to your CTCL lesions using a clean washed finger. Place a **generous coating** of gel over the entire surface of each lesion. You should not apply gel to the healthy skin around the lesion. The extra effort you take in carefully applying the gel only to the area of the CTCL lesion will help to lessen any irritation or redness that may occur. Proper application should leave some gel visible on the surface of the lesion when you are finished with the application.

Immediately following application, wipe the finger(s) you have used to apply the gel with a disposable tissue and wash your hands using soap and water.

Allow five (5) to ten (10) minutes for the gel to dry before covering a treated area with clothing.

A mild non-deodorant soap is recommended when bathing or showering. If you apply Targretin® gel after your shower or bath, you should wait 20 minutes before application.

WHEN TO APPLY

Targretin® gel should be applied at an initial frequency of once every other day for the first week. The frequency of application should then be increased as tolerated at weekly intervals to once daily, then twice daily, then three times daily, and finally four times daily. Your health care provider may instruct you to apply Targretin® gel at a different frequency.

YOU SHOULD AVOID...

You should avoid applying Targretin® gel to areas of healthy skin around a CTCL lesion. Exposure of healthy skin to Targretin® gel may cause unnecessary irritation or redness.

You should avoid showering, bathing, or swimming until at least three (3) hours after any application, if possible.

You should avoid covering the CTCL lesions treated with Targretin® gel with any bandage or material other than loose clothing.

You should avoid prolonged exposure of the treated area to sunlight or other ultraviolet (UV) light (such as tanning lamps).

You should avoid the use of other topical products on your treated CTCL lesions.

You should avoid scratching the treated areas.

WHAT SIDE EFFECTS DOES TARGRETIN® GEL HAVE?

While using Targretin® gel, you may experience some local effects such as redness, itching, burning, irritation, and scaling at the area of application. In clinical trials, the majority of these effects were mild or moderate, but some patients did experience more severe rash, itching, irritation, and inflammation. A few patients discontinued treatment due to these types of effects. Should these or other effects become troublesome to you, consult your health care provider. He or she can provide information on how to manage these effects.

All medications have side effects. You should call your physician regarding any questions or concerns you may have when using Targretin® gel.

HOW QUICKLY CAN I EXPECT TARGRETIN® GEL TO WORK?

Be patient. Targretin® gel takes time to work. In clinical trials, some patients began to respond as early as 4 weeks, but most patients did not experience their best response until 48 to 62 weeks of treatment. Do not stop treatment at the first sign of improvement. Continue to use Targretin® gel as instructed by your health care provider.

OTHER INFORMATION

The opening of the Targretin® gel tube is covered by a metal safety seal. If this seal has been punctured or is not visible when you first open the package, DO NOT USE this tube and promptly return the product to your pharmacy or place of purchase.

To open, use the pointed portion of the cap to puncture the metal safety seal.

Always use the cap to close the tube tightly after each use.

Store at room temperature. Keep away from heat or flame.

The gel should not be used after the expiration date printed on the tube.

Keep this medicine out of the reach and sight of children.

IF YOU HAVE QUESTIONS....

If you have questions about your treatment, talk with your health care provider.

Eisai Inc.

Woodcliff Lake, NJ 07677

Shown in Product Identification Guide, page 308

ZONEGRAN® ℞

[*ZO-nuh-gran*]

(zonisamide)

capsules

Rx only

DESCRIPTION

ZONEGRAN® (zonisamide) is an antiseizure drug chemically classified as a sulfonamide and unrelated to other antiseizure agents. The active ingredient is zonisamide, 1,2-benzisoxazole-3-methanesulfonamide. The empirical formula is $C_8H_8N_2O_3S$ with a molecular weight of 212.23. Zonisamide is a white powder, pKa = 10.2, and is moderately soluble in water (0.80 mg/mL) and 0.1 N HCl (0.50 mg/mL).

The chemical structure is:

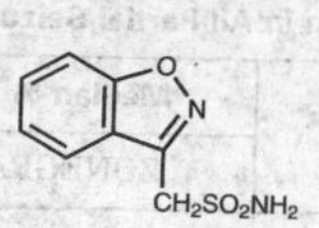

ZONEGRAN is supplied for oral administration as capsul containing 25 mg or 100 mg zonisamide. Each capsule co tains the labeled amount of zonisamide plus the followir inactive ingredients: microcrystalline cellulose, hydrog nated vegetable oil, sodium lauryl sulfate, gelatin, and col rants.

CLINICAL PHARMACOLOGY

Mechanism of Action: The precise mechanism(s) by whic zonisamide exerts its antiseizure effect is unknowr Zonisamide demonstrated anticonvulsant activity in severa experimental models. In animals, zonisamide was effectiv against tonic extension seizures induced by maximal elec troshock but ineffective against clonic seizures induced b subcutaneous pentylenetetrazol. Zonisamide raised th threshold for generalized seizures in the kindled rat mode and reduced the duration of cortical focal seizures inducec by electrical stimulation of the visual cortex in cats. Fur thermore, zonisamide suppressed both interictal spikes anc the secondarily generalized seizures produced by cortical application of tungstic acid gel in rats or by cortical freezing in cats. The relevance of these models to human epilepsy is unknown.

Zonisamide may produce these effects through action at sodium and calcium channels. *In vitro* pharmacological studies suggest that zonisamide blocks sodium channels and reduces voltage-dependent, transient inward currents (T-type Ca^{2+} currents), consequently stabilizing neuronal membranes and suppressing neuronal hypersynchronization. *In vitro* binding studies have demonstrated that zonisamide binds to the GABA/benzodiazepine receptor ionophore complex in an allosteric fashion which does not produce changes in chloride flux. Other *in vitro* studies have demonstrated that zonisamide (10–30 μg/mL) suppresses synaptically-driven electrical activity without affecting postsynaptic GABA or glutamate responses (cultured mouse spinal cord neurons) or neuronal or glial uptake of [^{3}H]-GABA (rat hippocampal slices). Thus, zonisamide does not appear to potentiate the synaptic activity of GABA. *In vivo* microdialysis studies demonstrated that zonisamide facilitates both dopaminergic and serotonergic neurotransmission.

Zonisamide is a carbonic anhydrase inhibitor. The contribution of this pharmacological action to the therapeutic effects of zonisamide is unknown. However, as a carbonic anhydrase inhibitor, zonisamide may cause metabolic acidosis (see **WARNINGS, Metabolic Acidosis** subsection).

Pharmacokinetics: Following a 200–400 mg oral zonisamide dose, peak plasma concentrations (range: 2–5 μg/mL) in normal volunteers occur within 2–6 hours. In the presence of food, the time to maximum concentration is delayed, occurring at 4–6 hours, but food has no effect on the bioavailability of zonisamide. Zonisamide extensively binds to erythrocytes, resulting in an eight-fold higher concentration of zonisamide in red blood cells (RBC) than in plasma. The pharmacokinetics of zonisamide is dose proportional in the range of 200–400 mg, but the C_{max} and AUC increase disproportionately at 800 mg, perhaps due to saturable binding of zonisamide to RBC. Once a stable dose is reached, steady state is achieved within 14 days. The elimination half-life of zonisamide in plasma is about 63 hours. The elimination half-life of zonisamide in RBC is approximately 105 hours.

The apparent volume of distribution (V/F) of zonisamide is about 1.45 L/kg following a 400 mg oral dose. Zonisamide, at concentrations of 1.0–7.0 μg/mL, is approximately 40% bound to human plasma proteins. Protein binding of zonisamide is unaffected in the presence of therapeutic concentrations of phenytoin, phenobarbital or carbamazepine.

Metabolism and Excretion: Following oral administration of ^{14}C-zonisamide to healthy volunteers, only zonisamide was detected in plasma. Zonisamide is excreted primarily in urine as parent drug and as the glucuronide of a metabolite. Following multiple dosing, 62% of the ^{14}C dose was recovered in the urine, with 3% in the feces by day 10. Zonisamide undergoes acetylation to form N-acetyl zonisamide and reduction to form the open ring metabolite, 2–sulfamoylacetyl phenol (SMAP). Of the excreted dose, 35% was recovered as zonisamide, 15% as N-acetyl zonisamide, and 50% as the glucuronide of SMAP. Reduction of zonisamide to SMAP is mediated by cytochrome P450 isozyme 3A4 (CYP3A4). Zonisamide does not induce its own metabolism. Plasma clearance of zonisamide is approximately 0.30–0.35 mL/min/kg in patients not receiving enzyme-inducing antiepilepsy drugs (AEDs). The clearance of zonisamide is increased to 0.5 mL/min/kg in patients concurrently on enzyme-inducing AEDs.

Table 1.
Median % Reduction in All Partial Seizures and % Responders in Primary Efficacy Analyses: Intent-To-Treat Analysis

Study	Median % reduction in partial seizures		% Responders	
	ZONEGRAN	Placebo	ZONEGRAN	Placebo
Study 1:	n=98	n=72	n=98	n=72
Weeks 8–12:	40.5%*	9.0%	41.8%*	22.2%
Study 2:	n=69	n=72	n=69	n=72
Weeks 5–12:	29.6%*	-3.2%	29.0%	15.0%
Study 3:	n=67	n=66	n=67	n=66
Weeks 5–12:	27.2%*	-1.1%	28.0%*	12.0%

*p<0.05 compared to placebo

Table 2.
Median % Reduction in All Partial Seizures and % Responders for Dose Analyses in Study 1: Intent-To-Treat Analysis

Dose Group	Median % reduction in partial seizures		% Responders	
	ZONEGRAN	Placebo	ZONEGRAN	Placebo
100–400 mg/day:	n=112	n=83	n=112	n=83
Weeks 1–12:	32.3%*	5.6%	32.1%*	9.6%
100 mg/day:	n=56	n=80	n=56	n=80
Weeks 1–5:	24.7%*	8.3%	25.0%*	11.3%
200 mg/day:	n=55	n=82	n=55	n=82
Weeks 2–6:	20.4%*	4.0%	25.5%*	9.8%

*p<0.05 compared to placebo

Renal clearance is about 3.5 mL/min. The clearance of an oral dose of zonisamide from RBC is 2 mL/min.

Special Populations:
Renal Insufficiency: Single 300 mg zonisamide doses were administered to three groups of volunteers. Group 1 was a healthy group with a creatinine clearance ranging from 70–152 mL/min. Group 2 and Group 3 had creatinine clearances ranging from 14.5–59 mL/min and 10–20 mL/min, respectively. Zonisamide renal clearance decreased with decreasing renal function (3.42, 2.50, 2.23 mL/min, respectively). Marked renal impairment (creatinine clearance < 20 mL/min) was associated with an increase in zonisamide AUC of 35% (see **DOSAGE AND ADMINIS-TRATION** section).

Hepatic Disease: The pharmacokinetics of zonisamide in patients with impaired liver function has not been studied (see **DOSAGE AND ADMINISTRATION** section).

Age: The pharmacokinetics of a 300 mg single dose of zonisamide was similar in young (mean age 28 years) and elderly subjects (mean age 69 years).

Gender and Race: Information on the effect of gender and race on the pharmacokinetics of zonisamide is not available.

Interactions of Zonisamide with Other Antiepilepsy Drugs (AEDs): Concurrent medication with drugs that either induce or inhibit CYP3A4 may alter serum concentrations of zonisamide. Concomitant administration of phenytoin and carbamazepine increases zonisamide plasma clearance from 0.30–0.35 mL/min/kg to 0.35–0.5 mL/min/kg. The half-life of zonisamide is decreased to 27 hours by phenytoin, to 38 hours by phenobarbital and carbamazepine, and to 46 hours by valproate. Plasma protein binding of phenytoin and carbamazepine was not affected by zonisamide administration (see **PRECAUTIONS, Drug Interactions** subsection).

Clinical Studies: The effectiveness of ZONEGRAN as adjunctive therapy (added to other antiepilepsy drugs) has been established in three multicenter, placebo-controlled, double blind, 3-month clinical trials (two domestic, one European) in 499 patients with refractory partial onset seizures with or without secondary generalization. Each patient had a history of at least four partial onset seizures per month in spite of receiving one or two antiepilepsy drugs at therapeutic concentrations. The 499 patients (209 women, 290 men) ranged in age from 13–68 years with a mean age of about 35 years. In the two US studies, over 80% of patients were Caucasian; 100% of patients in the European study were Caucasian. ZONEGRAN or placebo was added to the existing therapy. The primary measure of effectiveness was median percent reduction from baseline in partial seizure frequency. The secondary measure was proportion of patients achieving a 50% or greater seizure reduction from

baseline (responders). The results described below are for all partial seizures in the intent-to-treat populations.
In the first study (n = 203), all patients had a 1-month baseline observation period, then received placebo or ZONEGRAN in one of two dose escalation regimens; either 1) 100 mg/day for five weeks, 200 mg/day for one week, 300 mg/day for one week, and then 400 mg/day for five weeks; or 2) 100 mg/day for one week, followed by 200 mg/day for five weeks, then 300 mg/day for one week, then 400 mg/day for five weeks. This design allowed a 100 mg vs. placebo comparison over weeks 1–5, and a 200 mg vs. placebo comparison over weeks 2–6; the primary comparison was 400 mg (both escalation groups combined) vs. placebo over weeks 8–12. The total daily dose was given as twice a day dosing. Statistically significant treatment differences favoring ZONEGRAN were seen for doses of 100, 200, and 400 mg/day.
In the second (n = 152) and third (n = 138) studies, patients had a 2–3 month baseline, then were randomly assigned to placebo or ZONEGRAN for three months. ZONEGRAN was introduced by administering 100 mg/day for the first week, 200 mg/day the second week, then 400 mg/day for two weeks, after which the dose (ZONEGRAN or placebo) could be adjusted as necessary to a maximum dose of 20 mg/kg/day or a maximum plasma level of 40 µg/mL. In the second study, the total daily dose was given as twice a day dosing; in the third study, it was given as a single daily dose. The average final maintenance doses received in the studies were 530 and 430 mg/day in the second and third studies, respectively. Both studies demonstrated statistically significant differences favoring ZONEGRAN for doses of 400–600 mg/day, and there was no apparent difference between once daily and twice daily dosing (in different studies). Analysis of the data (first 4 weeks) during titration demonstrated statistically significant differences favoring ZONEGRAN at doses between 100 and 400 mg/day. The primary comparison in both trials was for any dose over Weeks 5–12.
[See table 1 above]
[See table 2 above]
Figure 1 presents the proportion of patients (X-axis) whose percentage reduction from baseline in the all partial seizure rate was at least as great as that indicated on the Y-axis in the second and third placebo-controlled trials. A positive value on the Y-axis indicates an improvement from baseline (i.e., a decrease in seizure rate), while a negative value indicates a worsening from baseline (i.e., an increase in seizure rate). Thus, in a display of this type, the curve for an effective treatment is shifted to the left of the curve for placebo. The proportion of patients achieving any particular

level of reduction in seizure rate was consistently higher for the ZONEGRAN groups compared to the placebo groups. For example, Figure 1 indicates that approximately 27% of patients treated with ZONEGRAN experienced a 75% or greater reduction, compared to approximately 12% in the placebo groups.

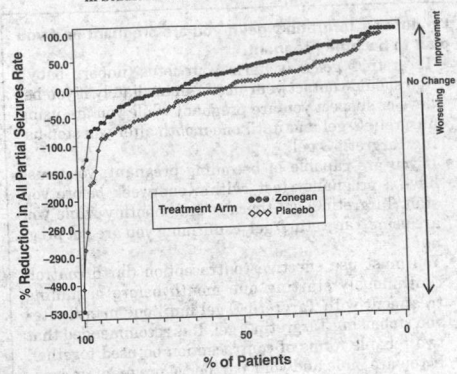

Figure 1 Proportion of Patients Achieving Differing Levels of Seizure Reduction in ZONEGRAN and Placebo Groups in Studies 2 and 3

No differences in efficacy based on age, sex or race, as measured by a change in seizure frequency from baseline, were detected.

INDICATIONS AND USAGE
ZONEGRAN is indicated as adjunctive therapy in the treatment of partial seizures in adults with epilepsy.

CONTRAINDICATIONS
ZONEGRAN is contraindicated in patients who have demonstrated hypersensitivity to sulfonamides or zonisamide.

WARNINGS
Potentially Fatal Reactions to Sulfonamides: Fatalities have occurred, although rarely, as a result of severe reactions to sulfonamides (zonisamide is a sulfonamide) including Stevens-Johnson syndrome, toxic epidermal necrolysis, fulminant hepatic necrosis, agranulocytosis, aplastic anemia, and other blood dyscrasias. Such reactions may occur when a sulfonamide is readministered irrespective of the route of administration. If signs of hypersensitivity or other serious reactions occur, discontinue zonisamide immediately. Specific experience with sulfonamide-type adverse reaction to zonisamide is described below.

Serious Skin Reactions: Consideration should be given to discontinuing ZONEGRAN in patients who develop an otherwise unexplained rash. If the drug is not discontinued, patients should be observed frequently. Seven deaths from severe rash [i.e. Stevens-Johnson syndrome (SJS) and toxic epidermal necrolysis (TEN)] were reported in the first 11 years of marketing in Japan. All of the patients were receiving other drugs in addition to zonisamide. In post-marketing experience from Japan, a total of 49 cases of SJS or TEN have been reported, a reporting rate of 46 per million patient-years of exposure. Although this rate is greater than background, it is probably an underestimate of the true incidence because of under-reporting. There were no confirmed cases of SJS or TEN in the US, European, or Japanese development programs.
In the US and European randomized controlled trials, 6 of 269 (2.2%) zonisamide patients discontinued treatment because of rash compared to none on placebo. Across all trials during the US and European development, rash that led to discontinuation of zonisamide was reported in 1.4% of patients (12.0 events per 1000 patient-years of exposure). During Japanese development, serious rash or rash that led to study drug discontinuation was reported in 2.0% of patients (27.8 events per 1000 patient-years). Rash usually occurred early in treatment, with 85% reported within 16 weeks in the US and European studies and 90% reported within two weeks in the Japanese studies. There was no apparent relationship of dose to the occurrence of rash.

Serious Hematologic Events: Two confirmed cases of aplastic anemia and one confirmed case of agranulocytosis were reported in the first 11 years of marketing in Japan, rates greater than generally accepted background rates. There were no cases of aplastic anemia and two confirmed cases of agranulocytosis in the US, European, or Japanese development programs. There is inadequate information to assess the relationship, if any, between dose and duration of treatment and these events.

Oligohidrosis and Hyperthermia in Pediatric Patients: Oligohidrosis, sometimes resulting in heat stroke and hospitalization, is seen in association with zonisamide in pediatric patients.
During the pre-approval development program in Japan, one case of oligohidrosis was reported in 403 pediatric patients, an incidence of 1 case per 285 patient-years of exposure. While there were no cases reported in the US or European development programs, fewer than 100 pediatric patients participated in these trials.

In the first 11 years of marketing in Japan, 38 cases were reported, an estimated reporting rate of about 1 case per 10,000 patient-years of exposure. In the first year of marketing in the US, 2 cases were reported, an estimated reporting rate of about 12 cases per 10,000 patient-years of exposure. These rates are underestimates of the true incidence because of under-reporting. There has also been one report of heat stroke in an 18-year-old patient in the US. Decreased sweating and an elevation in body temperature above normal characterized these cases. Many cases were reported after exposure to elevated environmental temperatures. Heat stroke, requiring hospitalization, was diagnosed in some cases. There have been no reported deaths. Pediatric patients appear to be at an increased risk for zonisamide-associated oligohidrosis and hyperthermia. Patients, especially pediatric patients, treated with ZONEGRAN should be monitored closely for evidence of decreased sweating and increased body temperature, especially in warm or hot weather. Caution should be used when zonisamide is prescribed with other drugs that predispose patients to heat-related disorders; these drugs include, but are not limited to, carbonic anhydrase inhibitors and drugs with anticholinergic activity.

The practitioner should be aware that the safety and effectiveness of zonisamide in pediatric patients have not been established, and that zonisamide is not approved for use in pediatric patients.

Suicidal Behavior and Ideation: Antiepileptic drugs (AEDs), including ZONEGRAN, increase the risk of suicidal thoughts or behavior in patients taking these drugs for any indication. Patients treated with any AED for any indication should be monitored for the emergence or worsening of depression, suicidal thoughts or behavior, and/or any unusual changes in mood or behavior.

Pooled analyses of 199 placebo-controlled clinical trials (mono- and adjunctive therapy) of 11 different AEDs showed that patients randomized to one of the AEDs had approximately twice the risk (adjusted Relative Risk 1.8, 95% CI:1.2, 2.7) of suicidal thinking or behavior compared to patients randomized to placebo. In these trials, which had a median treatment duration of 12 weeks, the estimated incidence rate of suicidal behavior or ideation among 27,863 AED-treated patients was 0.43%, compared to 0.24% among 16,029 placebo-treated patients, representing an increase of approximately one case of suicidal thinking or behavior for every 530 patients treated. There were four suicides in drug-treated patients in the trials and none in placebo-treated patients, but the number is too small to allow any conclusion about drug effect on suicide.

The increased risk of suicidal thoughts or behavior with AEDs was observed as early as one week after starting drug treatment with AEDs and persisted for the duration of treatment assessed. Because most trials included in the analysis did not extend beyond 24 weeks, the risk of suicidal thoughts or behavior beyond 24 weeks could not be assessed.

The risk of suicidal thoughts or behavior was generally consistent among drugs in the data analyzed. The finding of increased risk with AEDs of varying mechanisms of action and across a range of indications suggests that the risk applies to all AEDs used for any indication. The risk did not vary substantially by age (5–100 years) in the clinical trials analyzed.

Table 3 shows absolute and relative risk by indication for all evaluated AEDs.

[See table 3 above]

Table 3:
Risk by indication for antiepileptic drugs in the pooled analysis

Indication	Placebo Patients with Events Per 1000 Patients	Drug Patients with Events Per 1000 Patients	Relative Risk: Incidence of Events in Drug Patients/Incidence in Placebo Patients	Risk Difference: Additional Drug Patients with Events Per 1000 Patients
Epilepsy	1.0	3.4	3.5	2.4
Psychiatric	5.7	8.5	1.5	2.9
Other	1.0	1.8	1.9	0.9
Total	2.4	4.3	1.8	1.9

The relative risk for suicidal thoughts or behavior was higher in clinical trials for epilepsy than in clinical trials for psychiatric or other conditions, but the absolute risk differences were similar for the epilepsy and psychiatric indications.

Anyone considering prescribing ZONEGRAN or any other AED must balance the risk of suicidal thoughts or behavior with the risk of untreated illness. Epilepsy and many other illnesses for which AEDs are prescribed are themselves associated with morbidity and mortality and an increased risk of suicidal thoughts and behavior. Should suicidal thoughts and behavior emerge during treatment, the prescriber needs to consider whether the emergence of these symptoms in any given patient may be related to the illness being treated.

Patients, their caregivers, and families should be informed that AEDs increase the risk of suicidal thoughts and behavior and should be advised of the need to be alert for the emergence or worsening of the signs and symptoms of depression, any unusual changes in mood or behavior, or the emergence of suicidal thoughts, behavior, or thoughts about self-harm. Behaviors of concern should be reported immediately to healthcare providers (see **WARNINGS, Cognitive/ Neuropsychiatric Adverse Events** subsection below).

Metabolic Acidosis: Zonisamide causes hyperchloremic, non-anion gap, metabolic acidosis (i.e., decreased serum bicarbonate below the normal reference range in the absence of chronic respiratory alkalosis). This metabolic acidosis is caused by renal bicarbonate loss due to the inhibitory effect of zonisamide on carbonic anhydrase. Generally, zonisamide-induced metabolic acidosis occurs early in treatment, but it can develop at any time during treatment. Metabolic acidosis generally appears to be dose-dependent and can occur at doses as low as 25 mg daily.

Conditions or therapies that predispose to acidosis (such as renal disease, severe respiratory disorders, status epilepticus, diarrhea, ketogenic diet, or specific drugs) may be additive to the bicarbonate lowering effects of zonisamide.

Some manifestations of acute or chronic metabolic acidosis include hyperventilation, nonspecific symptoms such as fatigue and anorexia, or more severe sequelae including cardiac arrhythmias or stupor. Chronic, untreated, metabolic acidosis may increase the risk for nephrolithiasis or nephrocalcinosis. Nephrolithiasis has been observed in the clinical development program in 4% of adults treated with ZONEGRAN, has also been detected by renal ultrasound in 8% of pediatric treated patients who had at least one ultrasound prospectively collected, and was reported as an adverse event in 3% (4/133) of pediatric patients (see **PRECAUTIONS, Kidney Stones** subsection).

Chronic, untreated metabolic acidosis may result in osteomalacia (referred to as rickets in pediatric patients) and/or osteoporosis with an increased risk for fracture. Of potential relevance, zonisamide treatment was associated with reductions in serum phosphorus and increases in serum alkaline phosphatase, changes that may be related to metabolic acidosis and osteomalacia (see **PRECAUTIONS, Laboratory Tests** subsection).

Chronic, untreated metabolic acidosis in pediatric patients may reduce growth rates. A reduction in growth rate may eventually decrease the maximal height achieved. The effect of zonisamide on growth and bone-related sequelae has not been systematically investigated.

Measurement of baseline and periodic serum bicarbonate during treatment is recommended. If metabolic acidosis develops and persists, consideration should be given to reducing the dose or discontinuing zonisamide (using dose tapering). If the decision is made to continue patients on zonisamide in the face of persistent acidosis, alkali treatment should be considered.

Serum bicarbonate was not measured in the adjunctive controlled trials of adults with epilepsy. However, serum bicarbonate was studied in three clinical trials for indications which have not been approved: a placebo-controlled trial for migraine prophylaxis in adults, a controlled trial for monotherapy in epilepsy in adults, and an open label trial for adjunctive treatment of epilepsy in pediatric patients (3–16 years). In adults, mean serum bicarbonate reductions ranged from approximately 2 mEq/L at daily doses of 100 mg to nearly 4 mEq/L at daily doses of 300 mg. In pediatric patients, mean serum bicarbonate reductions ranged from approximately 2 mEq/L at daily doses from above 100 mg up to 300 mg, to nearly 4 mEq/L at daily doses from above 400 mg up to 600 mg.

In two controlled studies in adults, the incidence of a persistent treatment-emergent decrease in serum bicarbonate to less than 20 mEq/L (observed at 2 or more consecutive visits or the final visit) was dose-related at relatively low zonisamide doses. In the monotherapy trial of epilepsy, the incidence of a persistent treatment-emergent decrease in serum bicarbonate was 21% for daily zonisamide doses of 25 mg or 100 mg, and was 43% at a daily dose of 300 mg. In a placebo-controlled trial for prophylaxis of migraine, the incidence of a persistent treatment-emergent decrease in serum bicarbonate was 7% for placebo, 29% for 150 mg daily, and 34% for 300 mg daily. The incidence of persistent markedly abnormally low serum bicarbonate (decrease to less than 17 mEq/L and more than 5 mEq/L from a pretreatment value of at least 20 mEq/L in these controlled trials was 2% or less.

In the pediatric study, the incidence of persistent treatment-emergent decreases in serum bicarbonate to levels less than 20 mEq/L was 52% at doses up to 100 mg daily, was 90% for a wide range of doses up to 600 mg daily, and generally appeared to increase with higher doses. The incidence of a persistent markedly abnormally low serum bicarbonate value was 4% at doses up to 100 mg daily, was 18% for a wide range of doses up to 600 mg daily, and generally appeared to increase with higher doses. Some patients experienced moderately severe serum bicarbonate decrements down to a level as low as 10 mEq/L.

The relatively high frequencies of varying severities of metabolic acidosis observed in this study of pediatric patients (compared to the frequency and severity observed in various clinical trial development programs in adults) suggest that pediatric patients may be more likely to develop metabolic acidosis than adults.

Seizures on Withdrawal: As with other AEDs, abrupt withdrawal of ZONEGRAN in patients with epilepsy may precipitate increased seizure frequency or status epilepticus. Dose reduction or discontinuation of zonisamide should be done gradually.

Teratogenicity: Women of child bearing potential who are given zonisamide should be advised to use effective contraception. Zonisamide was teratogenic in mice, rats, and dogs and embryolethal in monkeys when administered during the period of organogenesis. A variety of fetal abnormalities, including cardiovascular defects, and embryo-fetal deaths occurred at maternal plasma levels similar to or lower than therapeutic levels in humans. These findings suggest that the use of ZONEGRAN during pregnancy in humans may present a significant risk to the fetus (see **PRECAUTIONS, Pregnancy** subsection). It cannot be said with any confidence, however, that even mild seizures do not pose some hazards to the developing fetus. Zonisamide should be used during pregnancy only if the potential benefit justifies the potential risk to the fetus.

Cognitive/Neuropsychiatric Adverse Events: Use of ZONEGRAN was frequently associated with central nervous system-related adverse events. The most significant of these can be classified into three general categories: 1) psychiatric symptoms, including depression and psychosis, 2) psychomotor slowing, difficulty with concentration, and speech or language problems, in particular, word-finding difficulties, and 3) somnolence or fatigue.

In placebo-controlled trials, 2.2% of patients discontinued ZONEGRAN or were hospitalized for depression compared to 0.4% of placebo patients. Among all epilepsy patients treated with ZONEGRAN, 1.4% were discontinued and 1.0% were hospitalized because of reported depression or suicide attempts. In placebo-controlled trials, 2.2% of patients discontinued ZONEGRAN or were hospitalized due to psychosis or psychosis-related symptoms compared to none of the placebo patients. Among all epilepsy patients treated with ZONEGRAN, 0.9% were discontinued and 1.4% were hospitalized because of reported psychosis or related symptoms.

Psychomotor slowing and difficulty with concentration occurred in the first month of treatment and were associated with doses above 300 mg/day. Speech and language problems tended to occur after 6–10 weeks of treatment and at doses above 300 mg/day. Although in most cases these events were of mild to moderate severity, they at times led to withdrawal from treatment.

Somnolence and fatigue were frequently reported CNS adverse events during clinical trials with ZONEGRAN. Although in most cases these events were of mild to moderate severity, they led to withdrawal from treatment in 0.2% of the patients enrolled in controlled trials. Somnolence and fatigue tended to occur within the first month of treatment.

mnolence and fatigue occurred most frequently at doses 300–500 mg/day. **Patients should be cautioned about this possibility and special care should be taken by patients if they drive, operate machinery, or perform any hazardous task.**

PRECAUTIONS

General: Somnolence is commonly reported, especially at higher doses of ZONEGRAN (see **WARNINGS: Cognitive/Neuropsychiatric Adverse Events** subsection). Zonisamide is metabolized by the liver and eliminated by the kidneys; caution should therefore be exercised when administering ZONEGRAN to patients with hepatic and renal dysfunction (see **CLINICAL PHARMACOLOGY, Special Populations** subsection).

Kidney Stones: Among 991 patients treated during the development of ZONEGRAN, 40 patients (4.0%) with epilepsy receiving ZONEGRAN developed clinically possible or confirmed kidney stones (e.g. clinical symptomatology, sonography, etc.), a rate of 34 per 1000 patient-years of exposure (40 patients with 1168 years of exposure). Of these, 12 were symptomatic, and 28 were described as possible kidney stones based on sonographic detection. In nine patients, the diagnosis was confirmed by a passage of a stone or by a definitive sonographic finding. The rate of occurrence of kidney stones was 28.7 per 1000 patient-years of exposure in the first six months, 62.6 per 1000 patient-years of exposure between 6 and 12 months, and 24.3 per 1000 patient-years of exposure after 12 months of use. There are no normative sonographic data available for either the general population or patients with epilepsy. Although the clinical significance of the sonographic findings may not be certain, the development of nephrolithiasis may be related to metabolic acidosis (see **WARNINGS, Metabolic Acidosis** subsection). The analyzed stones were composed of calcium or urate salts. In general, increasing fluid intake and urine output can help reduce the risk of stone formation, particularly in those with predisposing risk factors. It is unknown, however, whether these measures will reduce the risk of stone formation in patients treated with ZONEGRAN.

Although not approved in pediatric patients, sonographic findings consistent with nephrolithiasis were also detected in 8% of a subset of ZONEGRAN treated pediatric patients who had at least one renal ultrasound prospectively performed in a clinical development program investigating open-label treatment. The incidence of kidney stone as an adverse event was 3% (see **WARNINGS, Metabolic Acidosis** subsection).

Effect on Renal Function: In several clinical studies, zonisamide was associated with a statistically significant 8% mean increase from baseline of serum creatinine and blood urea nitrogen (BUN) compared to essentially no change in the placebo patients. The increase appeared to persist over time but was not progressive; this has been interpreted as an effect on glomerular filtration rate (GFR). There were no episodes of unexplained acute renal failure in clinical development in the US, Europe, or Japan. The decrease in GFR appeared within the first 4 weeks of treatment. In a 30-day study, the GFR returned to baseline within 2–3 weeks of drug discontinuation. There is no information about reversibility, after drug discontinuation, of the effects on GFR after long-term use. ZONEGRAN should be discontinued in patients who develop acute renal failure or a clinically significant sustained increase in the creatinine/BUN concentration. ZONEGRAN should not be used in patients with renal failure (estimated GFR < 50 mL/min) as there has been insufficient experience concerning drug dosing and toxicity.

Sudden Unexplained Death in Epilepsy: During the development of ZONEGRAN, nine sudden unexplained deaths occurred among 991 patients with epilepsy receiving ZONEGRAN for whom accurate exposure data are available. This represents an incidence of 7.7 deaths per 1000 patient-years. Although this rate exceeds that expected in a healthy population, it is within the range of estimates for the incidence of sudden unexplained deaths in patients with refractory epilepsy not receiving ZONEGRAN (ranging from 0.5 per 1000 patient-years for the general population of patients with epilepsy, to 2–5 per 1000 patient-years for patients with refractory epilepsy; higher incidences range from 9–15 per 1000 patient-years among surgical candidates and surgical failures). Some of the deaths could represent seizure-related deaths in which the seizure was not observed.

Status Epilepticus: Estimates of the incidence of treatment emergent status epilepticus in ZONEGRAN-treated patients are difficult because a standard definition was not employed. Nonetheless, in controlled trials, 1.1% of patients treated with ZONEGRAN had an event labeled as status epilepticus compared to none of the patients treated with placebo. Among patients treated with ZONEGRAN across all epilepsy studies (controlled and uncontrolled), 1.0% of patients had an event reported as status epilepticus.

Creatine Phosphokinase (CPK) Elevation and Pancreatitis: In the post-market setting, the following rare adverse events have been observed (<1:1000):

If patients taking zonisamide develop severe muscle pain and/or weakness, either in the presence or absence of a fever, markers of muscle damage should be assessed, including serum CPK and aldolase levels. If elevated, in the absence of another obvious cause such as trauma, grand mal seizures, etc., tapering and/or discontinuance of zonisamide should be considered and appropriate treatment initiated. Patients taking zonisamide that manifest clinical signs and symptoms of pancreatitis should have pancreatic lipase and amylase levels monitored. If pancreatitis is evident, in the absence of another obvious cause, tapering and/or discontinuation of zonisamide should be considered and appropriate treatment initiated.

Information for Patients: Patients should be informed of the availability of a Medication Guide, and they should be instructed to read the Medication Guide prior to taking ZONEGRAN. Patients should be instructed to take ZONEGRAN only as prescribed.

Patients should be advised as follows: (See Medication Guide)

1. **ZONEGRAN may produce drowsiness, especially at higher doses. Patients should be advised not to drive a car or operate other complex machinery until they have gained experience on ZONEGRAN sufficient to determine whether it affects their performance. Because of the potential of zonisamide to cause CNS depression, as well as other cognitive and/or neuropsychiatric adverse events, zonisamide should be used with caution if used in combination with alcohol or other CNS depressants.**
2. Patients should contact their physician immediately if a skin rash develops or seizures worsen.
3. Patients should contact their physician immediately if they develop signs or symptoms, such as sudden back pain, abdominal pain, and/or blood in the urine, that could indicate a kidney stone. Increasing fluid intake and urine output may reduce the risk of stone formation, particularly in those with predisposing risk factors for stones.
4. Patients should contact their physician immediately if a child has been taking ZONEGRAN and is not sweating as usual with or without a fever.
5. Because zonisamide can cause hematological complications, patients should contact their physician immediately if they develop a fever, sore throat, oral ulcers, or easy bruising.
6. **Suicidal Thinking and Behavior**—Patients, their caregivers, and families should be counseled that AEDs, including ZONEGRAN, may increase the risk of suicidal thoughts and behavior and should be advised of the need to be alert for the emergence or worsening of symptoms of depression, any unusual changes in mood or behavior, or the emergence of suicidal thoughts, behavior, or thoughts about self-harm. Behaviors of concern should be reported immediately to healthcare providers.
7. Patients should contact their physician immediately if they develop fast breathing, fatigue/tiredness, loss of appetite, or irregular heartbeat or palpitations (possible manifestations of metabolic acidosis).
8. As with other AEDs, patients should contact their physician if they intend to become pregnant or are pregnant during ZONEGRAN therapy. Patients should notify their physician if they intend to breast-feed or are breast-feeding an infant.
   Patients should be encouraged to enroll in the North American Antiepileptic Drug (NAAED) Pregnancy Registry if they become pregnant. This registry is collecting information about the safety of antiepileptic drugs during pregnancy. To enroll, patients can call the toll free number 1-888-233-2334 (see **PRECAUTIONS, Pregnancy** subsection).
9. Patients should contact their physician immediately if they develop severe muscle pain and/or weakness.

Laboratory Tests: In several clinical studies, zonisamide was associated with a mean increase in the concentration of serum creatinine and blood urea nitrogen (BUN) of approximately 8% over the baseline measurement. Consideration should be given to monitoring renal function periodically (see **PRECAUTIONS, Effect on Renal Function** subsection).

Zonisamide increases serum chloride and alkaline phosphatase and decreases serum phosphorus, calcium, and albumin.

Drug Interactions: *Effects of ZONEGRAN on the pharmacokinetics of other antiepilepsy drugs (AEDs):* Zonisamide had no appreciable effect on the steady state plasma concentrations of phenytoin, carbamazepine, or valproate during clinical trials. Zonisamide did not inhibit mixed-function liver oxidase enzymes (cytochrome P450), as measured in human liver microsomal preparations, *in vitro*. Zonisamide is not expected to interfere with the metabolism of other drugs that are metabolized by cytochrome P450 isozymes.

Effects of other drugs on ZONEGRAN pharmacokinetics: Drugs that induce liver enzymes increase the metabolism and clearance of zonisamide and decrease its half-life. The half-life of zonisamide following a 400 mg dose in patients concurrently on enzyme-inducing AEDs such as phenytoin, carbamazepine, or phenobarbital was between 27–38 hours; the half-life of zonisamide in patients concurrently on the non-enzyme inducing AED, valproate, was 46 hours. Concurrent medication with drugs that either induce or inhibit CYP3A4 would be expected to alter serum concentrations of zonisamide.

Interaction with cimetidine: Zonisamide single dose pharmacokinetic parameters were not affected by cimetidine (300 mg four times a day for 12 days).

Drug Interactions with CNS depressants: Concomitant administration of ZONEGRAN and alcohol or other CNS depressant drugs has not been evaluated in clinical studies. Because of the potential of zonisamide to cause CNS depression, as well as other cognitive and/or neuropsychiatric adverse events, zonisamide should be used with caution if used in combination with alcohol or other CNS depressants.

Carcinogenicity, Mutagenesis, Impairment of Fertility: No evidence of carcinogenicity was found in mice or rats following dietary administration of zonisamide for two years at doses of up to 80 mg/kg/day. In mice, this dose is approximately equivalent to the maximum recommended human dose (MRHD) of 400 mg/day on a mg/m^2 basis. In rats, this dose is 1–2 times the MRHD on a mg/m^2 basis.

Zonisamide increased mutation frequency in Chinese hamster lung cells in the absence of metabolic activation. Zonisamide was not mutagenic or clastogenic in the Ames test, mouse lymphoma assay, sister chromatid exchange test, and human lymphocyte cytogenetics assay *in vitro*, and the rat bone marrow cytogenetics assay *in vivo*.

Rats treated with zonisamide (20, 60, or 200 mg/kg) before mating and during the initial gestation phase showed signs of reproductive toxicity (decreased corpora lutea, implantations, and live fetuses) at all doses. The low dose in this study is approximately 0.5 times the maximum recommended human dose (MRHD) on a mg/m^2 basis. The effect of zonisamide on human fertility is unknown.

Pregnancy: Pregnancy Category C (see **WARNINGS, Teratogenicity** subsection): Zonisamide may cause serious adverse fetal effects, based on clinical and nonclinical data. Zonisamide was teratogenic in multiple animal species. Zonisamide treatment causes metabolic acidosis in humans. The effect of zonisamide-induced metabolic acidosis has not been studied in pregnancy; however, metabolic acidosis in pregnancy (due to other causes) may be associated with decreased fetal growth, decreased fetal oxygenation, and fetal death, and may affect the fetus' ability to tolerate labor. Pregnant patients should be monitored for metabolic acidosis and treated as in the non-pregnant state. (See **WARNINGS, Metabolic Acidosis** subsection.)

Newborns of mothers treated with zonisamide should be monitored for metabolic acidosis because of transfer of zonisamide to the fetus and possible occurrence of transient metabolic acidosis following birth. Transient metabolic acidosis has been reported in neonates born to mothers treated during pregnancy with a different carbonic anhydrase inhibitor.

Zonisamide was teratogenic in mice, rats, and dogs and embryolethal in monkeys when administered during the period of organogenesis. Fetal abnormalities or embryo-fetal deaths occurred in these species at zonisamide dosage and maternal plasma levels similar to or lower than therapeutic levels in humans, indicating that use of this drug in pregnancy entails a significant risk to the fetus. A variety of external, visceral, and skeletal malformations was produced in animals by prenatal exposure to zonisamide. Cardiovascular defects were prominent in both rats and dogs.

Following administration of zonisamide (10, 30, or 60 mg/kg/day) to pregnant dogs during organogenesis, increased incidences of fetal cardiovascular malformations (ventricular septal defects, cardiomegaly, various valvular and arterial anomalies) were found at doses of 30 mg/kg/day or greater. The low effect dose for malformations produced peak maternal plasma zonisamide levels (25 μg/mL) about 0.5 times the highest plasma levels measured in patients receiving the maximum recommended human dose (MRHD) of 400 mg/day. In dogs, cardiovascular malformations were found in approximately 50% of all fetuses exposed to the high dose, which was associated with maternal plasma levels (44 μg/mL) approximately equal to the highest levels measured in humans receiving the MRHD. Incidences of skeletal malformations were also increased at the high dose, and fetal growth retardation and increased frequencies of skeletal variations were seen at all doses in this study. The low dose produced maternal plasma levels (12 μg/mL) about 0.25 times the highest human levels.

In cynomolgus monkeys, administration of zonisamide (10 or 20 mg/kg/day) to pregnant animals during organogenesis resulted in embryo-fetal deaths at both doses. The possibility that these deaths were due to malformations cannot be ruled out. The lowest embryolethal dose in monkeys was associated with peak maternal plasma zonisamide levels (5 μg/mL) approximately 0.1 times the highest levels measured in patients at the MRHD.

In a mouse embryo-fetal development study, treatment of pregnant animals with zonisamide (125, 250, or 500 mg/kg/day) during the period of organogenesis resulted in increased incidences of fetal malformations (skeletal and/or craniofacial defects) at all doses tested. The low dose in this study is approximately 1.5 times the MRHD on a mg/m² basis. In rats, increased frequencies of malformations (cardiovascular defects) and variations (persistent cords of thymic tissue, decreased skeletal ossification) were observed among the offspring of dams treated with zonisamide (20, 60, or 200 mg/kg/day) throughout organogenesis at all doses. The low effect dose is approximately 0.5 times the MRHD on a mg/m² basis.

Perinatal death was increased among the offspring of rats treated with zonisamide (10, 30, or 60 mg/kg/day) from the latter part of gestation up to weaning at the high dose, or approximately 1.4 times the MRHD on a mg/m² basis. The no effect level of 30 mg/kg/day is approximately 0.7 times the MRHD on a mg/m² basis.

There are no adequate and well-controlled studies in pregnant women. ZONEGRAN should be used during pregnancy only if the potential benefit justifies the potential risk to the fetus.

To provide information regarding the effects of *in utero* exposure to ZONEGRAN, physicians are advised to recommend that pregnant patients taking ZONEGRAN enroll in the NAAED Pregnancy Registry. This can be done by calling the toll free number 1-888-233-2334, and must be done by patients themselves. Information on the registry can also be found at the website http://www.aedpregnancyregistry.org/.

Labor and Delivery: The effect of ZONEGRAN on labor and delivery in humans is not known.

Use in Nursing Mothers: It is not known whether zonisamide is excreted in human milk. Because many drugs are excreted in human milk and because of the potential for serious adverse reactions in nursing infants from zonisamide, a decision should be made whether to discontinue nursing or to discontinue drug, taking into account the importance of the drug to the mother. ZONEGRAN should be used in nursing mothers only if the benefits outweigh the risks.

Pediatric Use: The safety and effectiveness of ZONEGRAN in children under age 16 have not been established. Cases of oligohidrosis and hyperpyrexia have been reported (see **WARNINGS, Oligohidrosis and Hyperthermia in Pediatric Patients** subsection). Zonisamide commonly causes metabolic acidosis in pediatric patients (see **WARNINGS, Metabolic Acidosis** subsection). Chronic untreated metabolic acidosis in pediatric patients may cause nephrolithiasis and/or nephrocalcinosis, osteoporosis and/or osteomalacia (potentially resulting in rickets), and may reduce growth rates. A reduction in growth rate may eventually decrease the maximal height achieved. The effect of zonisamide on growth and bone-related sequelae has not been systematically investigated.

Geriatric Use: Single dose pharmacokinetic parameters are similar in elderly and young healthy volunteers (see **CLINICAL PHARMACOLOGY, Special Populations** subsection). Clinical studies of zonisamide did not include sufficient numbers of subjects aged 65 and over to determine whether they respond differently from younger subjects. Other reported clinical experience has not identified differences in responses between the elderly and younger patients. In general, dose selection for an elderly patient should be cautious, usually starting at the low end of the dosing range, reflecting the greater frequency of decreased hepatic, renal, or cardiac function, and of concomitant disease or other drug therapy.

ADVERSE REACTIONS

The most commonly observed adverse events associated with the use of ZONEGRAN in controlled clinical trials that were not seen at an equivalent frequency among placebo-treated patients were somnolence, anorexia, dizziness, headache, nausea, and agitation/irritability.

In controlled clinical trials, 12% of patients receiving ZONEGRAN as adjunctive therapy discontinued due to an adverse event compared to 6% receiving placebo. Approximately 21% of the 1,336 patients with epilepsy who received ZONEGRAN in clinical studies discontinued treatment because of an adverse event. The adverse events most commonly associated with discontinuation were somnolence, fatigue and/or ataxia (6%), anorexia (3%), difficulty concentrating (2%), difficulty with memory, mental slowing, nausea/vomiting (2%), and weight loss (1%). Many of these adverse events were dose-related (see **WARNINGS** and **PRECAUTIONS**).

Adverse Event Incidence in Controlled Clinical Trials: Table 4 lists treatment-emergent adverse events that occurred in at least 2% of patients treated with ZONEGRAN in controlled clinical trials that were numerically more common in the ZONEGRAN group. In these studies, either ZONEGRAN or placebo was added to the pa-

tient's current AED therapy. Adverse events were usually mild or moderate in intensity.

The prescriber should be aware that these figures, obtained when ZONEGRAN was added to concurrent AED therapy, cannot be used to predict the frequency of adverse events in the course of usual medical practice when patient characteristics and other factors may differ from those prevailing during clinical studies. Similarly, the cited frequencies cannot be directly compared with figures obtained from other clinical investigations involving different treatments, uses, or investigators. An inspection of these frequencies, however, does provide the prescriber with one basis by which to estimate the relative contribution of drug and non-drug factors to the adverse event incidences in the population studied.

TABLE 4.
Incidence (%) of Treatment-Emergent Adverse Events in Placebo-Controlled, Add-On Trials (Events that occurred in at least 2% of ZONEGRAN-treated patients and occurred more frequently in ZONEGRAN-treated than placebo-treated patients)

BODY SYSTEM/ PREFERRED TERM	ZONEGRAN (n=269) %	PLACEBO (n=230) %
BODY AS A WHOLE		
Headache	10	8
Abdominal Pain	6	3
Flu Syndrome	4	3
DIGESTIVE		
Anorexia	13	6
Nausea	9	6
Diarrhea	5	2
Dyspepsia	3	1
Constipation	2	1
Dry Mouth	2	1
HEMATOLOGIC AND LYMPHATIC		
Ecchymosis	2	1
METABOLIC AND NUTRITIONAL		
Weight Loss	3	2
NERVOUS SYSTEM		
Dizziness	13	7
Ataxia	6	1
Nystagmus	4	2
Paresthesia	4	1
NEUROPSYCHIATRIC AND COGNITIVE DYSFUNCTION-ALTERED COGNITIVE FUNCTION		
Confusion	6	3
Difficulty Concentrating	6	2
Difficulty with Memory	6	2
Mental Slowing	4	2
NEUROPSYCHIATRIC AND COGNITIVE DYSFUNCTION-BEHAVIORAL ABNORMALITIES (NON-PSYCHOSIS-RELATED)		
Agitation/Irritability	9	4
Depression	6	3
Insomnia	6	3
Anxiety	3	3
Nervousness	2	1
NEUROPSYCHIATRIC AND COGNITIVE DYSFUNCTION-BEHAVIORAL ABNORMALITIES (PSYCHOSIS-RELATED)		
Schizophrenic/ Schizophreniform Behavior	2	0
NEUROPSYCHIATRIC AND COGNITIVE DYSFUNCTION-CNS DEPRESSION		
Somnolence	17	7
Fatigue	8	6
Tiredness	7	5
NEUROPSYCHIATRIC AND COGNITIVE DYSFUNCTION-SPEECH AND LANGUAGE ABNORMALITIES		
Speech Abnormalities	5	2
Difficulties in Verbal Expression	2	<1
RESPIRATORY		
Rhinitis	2	1
SKIN AND APPENDAGES		
Rash	3	1
SPECIAL SENSES		
Diplopia	6	3
Taste Perversion	2	0

Other Adverse Events Observed During Clinical Trials: ZONEGRAN has been administered to 1,598 individuals during all clinical trials, only some of which were placebo-controlled. During these trials, all events were recorded by the investigators using their own terms. To provide a useful estimate of the proportion of individuals having adverse events, similar events have been grouped into a smaller number of standardized categories using a modified COSTART dictionary. The frequencies represent the proportion of the 1,598 individuals exposed to ZONEGRAN who experienced an event on at least one occasion. All events are included except those already listed in the previous table or discussed in **WARNINGS** or **PRECAUTIONS**, trivial events, those too general to be informative, and those not reasonably associated with ZONEGRAN.

Events are further classified within each category and listed in order of decreasing frequency as follows: frequent occurring in at least 1:100 patient; infrequent occurring in 1:100 to 1:1000 patients; rare occurring in fewer than 1:1000 patients.

Body as a Whole: *Frequent:* Accidental injury, asthenia. *Infrequent:* Chest pain, flank pain, malaise, allergic reaction, face edema, neck rigidity. *Rare:* Lupus erythematosus.
Cardiovascular: *Infrequent:* Palpitation, tachycardia, vascular insufficiency, hypotension, hypertension, thrombophlebitis, syncope, bradycardia. *Rare:* Atrial fibrillation, heart failure, pulmonary embolus, ventricular extrasystoles.
Digestive: *Frequent:* Vomiting. *Infrequent:* Flatulence, gingivitis, gum hyperplasia, gastritis, gastroenteritis, stomatitis, cholelithiasis, glossitis, melena, rectal hemorrhage, ulcerative stomatitis, gastro-duodenal ulcer, dysphagia, gum hemorrhage. *Rare:* Cholangitis, hematemesis, cholecystitis, cholestatic jaundice, colitis, duodenitis, esophagitis, fecal incontinence, mouth ulceration.
Hematologic and Lymphatic: *Infrequent:* Leukopenia, anemia, immunodeficiency, lymphadenopathy. *Rare:* Thrombocytopenia, microcytic anemia, petechia.
Metabolic and Nutritional: *Infrequent:* Peripheral edema, weight gain, edema, thirst, dehydration. *Rare:* Hypoglycemia, hyponatremia, lactic dehydrogenase increased, SGOT increased, SGPT increased.
Musculoskeletal: *Infrequent:* Leg cramps, myalgia, myasthenia, arthralgia, arthritis.
Nervous System: *Frequent:* Tremor, convulsion, abnormal gait, hyperesthesia, incoordination. *Infrequent:* Hypertonia, twitching, abnormal dreams, vertigo, libido decreased, neu-

pathy, hyperkinesia, movement disorder, dysarthria, cerebrovascular accident, hypotonia, peripheral neuritis, paresthesia, reflexes increased. *Rare:* Circumoral paresthesia, dyskinesia, dystonia, encephalopathy, facial paralysis, hypokinesia, hyperesthesia, myoclonus, oculogyric crisis.

Behavioral Abnormalities –Non-Psychosis-Related: *Frequent:* Euphoria.

Respiratory: *Frequent:* Pharyngitis, cough increased. *Infrequent:* Dyspnea. *Rare:* Apnea, hemoptysis.

Skin and Appendages: *Frequent:* Pruritus. *Infrequent:* Maculopapular rash, acne, alopecia, dry skin, sweating, eczema, urticaria, hirsutism, pustular rash, vesiculobullous rash.

Special Senses: *Frequent:* Amblyopia, tinnitus. *Infrequent:* Conjunctivitis, parosmia, deafness, visual field defect, glaucoma. *Rare:* Photophobia, iritis.

Urogenital: *Infrequent:* Urinary frequency, dysuria, urinary incontinence, hematuria, impotence, urinary retention, urinary urgency, amenorrhea, polyuria, nocturia. *Rare:* Albuminuria, enuresis, bladder pain, bladder calculus, gynecomastia, mastitis, menorrhagia.

DRUG ABUSE AND DEPENDENCE

The abuse and dependence potential of ZONEGRAN has not been evaluated in human studies (see **WARNINGS, Cognitive/Neuropsychiatric Adverse Events** subsection). In a series of animal studies, zonisamide did not demonstrate abuse liability and dependence potential. Monkeys did not self-administer zonisamide in a standard reinforcing paradigm. Rats exposed to zonisamide did not exhibit signs of physical dependence of the CNS-depressant type. Rats did not generalize the effects of diazepam to zonisamide in a standard discrimination paradigm after training, suggesting that zonisamide does not have abuse potential of the benzodiazepine-CNS depressant type.

OVERDOSAGE

Human Experience: Experience with ZONEGRAN daily doses over 800 mg/day is limited. During ZONEGRAN clinical development, three patients ingested unknown amounts of ZONEGRAN as suicide attempts, and all three were hospitalized with CNS symptoms. One patient became comatose and developed bradycardia, hypotension, and respiratory depression; the zonisamide plasma level was 100.1 µg/mL measured 31 hours post-ingestion. Zonisamide plasma levels fell with a half-life of 57 hours, and the patient became alert five days later.

Management: No specific antidotes for ZONEGRAN overdosage are available. Following a suspected recent overdose, emesis should be induced or gastric lavage performed with the usual precautions to protect the airway. General supportive care is indicated, including frequent monitoring of vital signs and close observation. Zonisamide has a long half-life (see **CLINICAL PHARMACOLOGY** section). Due to the low protein binding of zonisamide (40%), renal dialysis may be effective. The effectiveness of renal dialysis as a treatment of overdose has not been formally studied. A poison control center should be contacted for information on the management of ZONEGRAN overdosage.

DOSAGE AND ADMINISTRATION

ZONEGRAN (zonisamide) is recommended as adjunctive therapy for the treatment of partial seizures in adults. Safety and efficacy in pediatric patients below the age of 16 have not been established. ZONEGRAN should be administered once or twice daily, using 25 mg or 100 mg capsules. ZONEGRAN is given orally and can be taken with or without food. Capsules should be swallowed whole.

Adults over Age 16: The prescriber should be aware that, because of the long half-life of zonisamide, up to two weeks may be required to achieve steady state levels upon reaching a stable dose or following dosage adjustment. Although the regimen described below is one that has been shown to be tolerated, the prescriber may wish to prolong the duration of treatment at the lower doses in order to fully assess the effects of zonisamide at steady state, noting that many of the side effects of zonisamide are more frequent at doses of 300 mg per day and above. Although there is some evidence of greater response at doses above 100–200 mg/day, the increase appears small and formal dose-response studies have not been conducted.

The initial dose of ZONEGRAN should be 100 mg daily. After two weeks, the dose may be increased to 200 mg/day for at least two weeks. It can be increased to 300 mg/day and 400 mg/day, with the dose stable for at least two weeks to achieve steady state at each level. Evidence from controlled trials suggests that ZONEGRAN doses of 100–600 mg/day are effective, but there is no suggestion of increasing response above 400 mg/day (see **CLINICAL PHARMACOLOGY, Clinical Studies** subsection). There is little experience with doses greater than 600 mg/day.

Patients with Renal or Hepatic Disease: Because zonisamide is metabolized in the liver and excreted by the kidneys, patients with renal or hepatic disease should be treated with caution, and might require slower titration and

more frequent monitoring (see **CLINICAL PHARMACOLOGY** and **PRECAUTIONS**).

HOW SUPPLIED

ZONEGRAN is available as 25 mg and 100 mg two-piece hard gelatin capsules. The capsules are printed in black with "Eisai" and "ZONEGRAN 25" or "ZONEGRAN 100," respectively. ZONEGRAN is available in bottles of 100 with strengths and colors as follows:

Dosage Strength	Capsule Colors	NDC #
25 mg	White opaque body with white opaque cap.	62856-681-10
100 mg	White opaque body with red opaque cap.	62856-680-10

Store at 25°C (77°F), excursions permitted to 15–30°C (59–86°F) [see USP Controlled Room Temperature], in a dry place and protected from light.
US Patent #6,342,515.

ANIMAL TOXICOLOGY

In dogs treated with zonisamide (10, 30, or 75 mg/kg/day) for 1 year, dark brown discoloration of the liver and concentric lamellar bodies in the cytoplasm of hepatocytes were observed in association with clinical chemistry changes indicative of liver damage (elevated alkaline phosphatase, gamma glutamyl transferase, and alanine amino transferase; decreased albumin) and altered drug metabolism at the highest dose, which is approximately 6 times the maximum recommended human dose (MRHD) of 400 mg/day on a mg/m² basis. Gross liver changes not clearly accompanied by biochemical evidence of hepatotoxicity were noted at 30 mg/kg/day, or approximately 2.4 times the MRHD on mg/m² basis. The no effect dose of 10 mg/kg/day is slightly less than the MRHD on mg/m² basis. The significance of these findings for humans is not known.

Manufactured by:
Elan Pharma International Ltd.
Distributed by:
Eisai Inc., Woodcliff Lake, NJ 07677
ZONEGRAN® is a registered trademark of Dainippon Pharmaceutical Co. Ltd. and licensed exclusively to Eisai Inc.
© 2009 Eisai Inc.
Revised May 2009

Medication Guide

ZONEGRAN® (ZO-nuh-gran)
(zonisamide)
capsules

Read this Medication Guide before you start taking ZONEGRAN and each time you get a refill. There may be new information. This information does not take the place of talking to your healthcare provider about your medical condition or treatment.

What is the most important information I should know about ZONEGRAN?

1. ZONEGRAN may cause a serious skin rash that can cause death. These serious skin reactions are more likely to happen when you begin taking ZONEGRAN within the first 4 months of treatment but may occur at later times.

2. ZONEGRAN may cause you to sweat less and to increase your body temperature (fever). You may need to be hospitalized for this. You should watch for decreased sweating and fever, especially when it is hot and especially in children taking ZONEGRAN.
Call your healthcare provider right away if you have:
• a skin rash
• fever
• less sweat than normal

3. **ZONEGRAN can cause blood cell abnormalities such as reduced red and white blood cell counts.** Call your healthcare provider if you develop fever, sore throat, sores in your mouth, or unusual bruising.

4. **Like other antiepileptic drugs, ZONEGRAN may cause suicidal thoughts or actions in a very small number of people, about 1 in 500.**
Call a healthcare provider right away if you have any of these symptoms, especially if they are new, worse, or worry you:
• thoughts about suicide or dying
• attempt to commit suicide
• new or worse depression
• new or worse anxiety
• feeling agitated or restless
• panic attacks
• trouble sleeping (insomnia)
• new or worse irritability
• acting aggressive, being angry, or violent
• acting on dangerous impulses
• an extreme increase in activity and talking (mania)
• other unusual changes in behavior or mood

5. ZONEGRAN can cause metabolic acidosis, which is a condition that happens when there is too much acid in your blood. Metabolic acidosis can cause symptoms such as tiredness, loss of appetite, irregular heartbeat, and impaired consciousness. **Call your healthcare professional right away if you get these symptoms with ZONEGRAN.** Your healthcare professional should do a blood test (measurement of serum bicarbonate) to monitor your bicarbonate level while you are taking ZONEGRAN.

Do not stop ZONEGRAN without first talking to a healthcare provider.
• Stopping ZONEGRAN suddenly can cause serious problems.
• Suicidal thoughts or actions can be caused by things other than medicines. If you have suicidal thoughts or actions, your healthcare provider may check for other causes.

How can I watch for early symptoms of suicidal thoughts and actions?
• Pay attention to any changes, especially sudden changes, in mood, behaviors, thoughts, or feelings.
• Keep all follow-up visits with your healthcare provider as scheduled.
• Call your healthcare provider between visits as needed, especially if you are worried about symptoms.

What is ZONEGRAN?
ZONEGRAN is a prescription medicine that is used with other medicines to treat partial seizures in adults.
It is not known if ZONEGRAN is safe or effective in children under 16 years of age.

Who should not take ZONEGRAN?
Do not take ZONEGRAN if you are allergic to medicines that contain sulfa.

What should I tell my healthcare provider before taking ZONEGRAN?
Before taking ZONEGRAN, tell your healthcare provider about all your medical conditions, including if you:
• have or have had depression, mood problems or suicidal thoughts or behavior
• have kidney problems
• have liver problems
• are pregnant or plan to become pregnant. You and your healthcare provider will have to decide if you should take ZONEGRAN while you are pregnant. If you become pregnant while taking ZONEGRAN, talk to your healthcare provider about registering with the North American Antiepileptic Drug Pregnancy Registry. You can enroll in this registry by calling 1-888-233-2334. The purpose of this registry is to collect information about the safety of antiepileptic drugs during pregnancy.
• are breast-feeding. It is not known if ZONEGRAN passes into breast milk and if it can harm your baby. Talk to your healthcare provider about the best way to feed your baby if you take ZONEGRAN.
Tell your healthcare provider about all the medicines you take including prescription and non-prescription medicines, vitamins or herbal supplements. ZONEGRAN and other medicines may affect each other causing side effects.
Know the medicines you take. Keep a list of them with you to show your healthcare provider and pharmacist each time you get a new medicine.

How should I take ZONEGRAN?
• Take ZONEGRAN exactly as prescribed. Your healthcare provider may change your dose. Your healthcare provider will tell you how much ZONEGRAN to take.
• Take ZONEGRAN with or without food.
• Swallow the capsules whole.
• If you take too much ZONEGRAN, call your local Poison Control Center or go to the nearest emergency room right away.
• Do not stop taking ZONEGRAN without talking to your healthcare provider. Stopping ZONEGRAN suddenly can cause serious problems, including seizures that will not stop (status epilepticus).
• Do not drive a car, work with machines, or do other dangerous activities until you know how ZONEGRAN affects you. ZONEGRAN may make you drowsy.

What are the possible side effects of ZONEGRAN?
ZONEGRAN can cause serious side effects including:
• The side effects mentioned above (see "What is the most important information I should know about ZONEGRAN?")
• **worsening seizures**
• **kidney stones** (sudden back pain, stomach pain, or blood in your urine)
• **problems with mood or thinking** (new or worse depression; sudden changes in mood, behavior, or loss of contact with reality, sometimes associated with hearing voices or seeing things that are not really there; feeling sleepy or tired; trouble concentrating; speech and language problems)
Call your healthcare provider right away if you have any of the symptoms listed above.

The most common side effects of ZONEGRAN include:
- drowsiness
- loss of appetite
- dizziness
- trouble with walking and coordination
- headache
- nausea
- agitation
- irritability

Tell your healthcare provider about any side effect that bothers you or that does not go away. These are not all of the possible side effects of ZONEGRAN. For more information, ask your healthcare provider or pharmacist.

Call your doctor for medical advice about side effects. You may report side effects to the FDA at 1-800-FDA-1088.

How should I store ZONEGRAN?
- Store ZONEGRAN between 59° F to 86° F (15° C to 30° C)
- dry and away from light

Keep ZONEGRAN and all medicines out of the reach of children.

General information about the safe and effective use of ZONEGRAN

Medicines are sometimes prescribed for purposes other than those listed in a Medication Guide. Do not use ZONEGRAN for a condition for which it was not prescribed. Do not give ZONEGRAN to other people, even if they have the same symptoms that you have. It may harm them.

This Medication Guide summarizes the most important information about ZONEGRAN. If you would like more information, talk with your healthcare provider. You can ask your pharmacist or healthcare provider for information about ZONEGRAN that is written for health professionals. For more information, go to www.ZONEGRAN.com or call 1-888-274-2378.

What are the ingredients in ZONEGRAN?

Active ingredient: zonisamide

Inactive ingredients: microcrystalline cellulose, hydrogenated vegetable oil, sodium lauryl sulfate, gelatin, and colorants.

Issued May 2009

This Medication Guide has been approved by the U.S. Food and Drug Administration.

ZONEGRAN® is a registered trademark of Dainippon Pharmaceutical Co. Ltd. and licensed exclusively to Eisai, Inc.
Manufactured by Elan Pharma International Ltd.
Distributed by Eisai Inc.
Woodcliff Lake, NJ 07677

EMD Serono, Inc.
ONE TECHNOLOGY PLACE
ROCKLAND, MA 02370

Direct Inquiries to:
Customer Service, Sales and Ordering
(888) 398-4567
(781) 982-9000
For Medical Information or to report Adverse Drug Experiences contact the U.S. Medical Information or U.S. Product Surveillance Department at
(888) 275-7376
(781) 982-9000
www.emdserono.com
www.howkidsgrow.com
www.easypodus.com
www.mslifelines.com
www.rebif.com
www.fertilitylifelines.com
www.saizenus.com
www.serostim.com
www.zorbtive.com

EMD Serono, Inc. will be pleased to answer inquiries about the following products:

GONAL-F® ℞
[gŏn əl f]
(follitropin alfa for injection)
For subcutaneous injection

DESCRIPTION

Gonal-f® (follitropin alfa for injection) is a human follicle stimulating hormone (FSH) preparation of recombinant DNA origin, which consists of two non-covalently linked, non-identical glycoproteins designated as the α- and β-subunits. The α- and β-subunits have 92 and 111 amino acids, respectively, and their primary and tertiary structure are indistinguishable from those of human follicle stimulating hormone. Recombinant FSH production occurs in genetically modified Chinese Hamster Ovary (CHO) cells cultured in bioreactors. Purification by immuno-chromatography using an antibody specifically binding FSH results in a highly purified preparation with a consistent FSH isoform profile, and a high specific activity. The biological activity of follitropin alfa is determined by measuring the increase in ovary weight in female rats. The *in vivo* biological activity of follitropin alfa has been calibrated against the first International Standard for Recombinant Human Follicle Stimulation Hormone established in 1995 by the Expert Committee on Biological Standards of the World Health Organization. Gonal-f® contains no luteinizing hormone (LH) activity. Based on available data derived from physico-chemical tests and bioassays, follitropin alfa and follitropin beta, another recombinant follicle stimulating hormone product, are indistinguishable.

Gonal-f® is a sterile, lyophilized powder intended for subcutaneous injection after reconstitution.

Each Gonal-f® Multi-Dose vial is filled with 600 IU (44 μg) or 1200 IU (87 μg) follitropin alfa to deliver 450 IU (33 μg) or 1050 IU (77 μg) follitropin alfa, respectively, and contains 30 mg sucrose, 1.11 mg dibasic sodium phosphate dihydrate and 0.45 mg monobasic sodium phosphate monohydrate. O-phosphoric acid and/or sodium hydroxide may be used prior to lyophilization for pH adjustment. Multiple Dose vials are reconstituted with Bacteriostatic Water for Injection (0.9% benzyl alcohol), USP.

Under current storage conditions, Gonal-f® may contain up to 10% of oxidized follitropin alfa.

Therapeutic Class: Infertility

CLINICAL PHARMACOLOGY

Gonal-f® (follitropin alfa for injection) stimulates ovarian follicular growth in women who do not have primary ovarian failure. FSH, the active component of Gonal-f® is the primary hormone responsible for follicular recruitment and development. In order to effect final maturation of the follicle and ovulation in the absence of an endogenous LH surge, human chorionic gonadotropin (hCG) must be given following the administration of Gonal-f® when monitoring of the patient indicates that sufficient follicular development has occurred. There is interpatient variability in response to FSH administration. The physico-chemical, immunological, and biological activities of recombinant FSH (r-hFSH) are comparable to those of pituitary and human menopausal urine-derived FSH. Gonal-f® (follitropin alfa for injection), when administered with hCG, stimulates spermatogenesis in men with hypogonadotropic hypogonadism. FSH, the active component of Gonal-f®, is the primary hormone responsible for spermatogenesis.

Pharmacokinetics

Single dose pharmacokinetics of follitropin alfa were determined following intravenous, subcutaneous and intramuscular administration of 150 IU Gonal-f® to 12 healthy, down-regulated female volunteers. Steady-state pharmacokinetics were also determined in 12 healthy down-regulated female volunteers who were administered a single daily dose of 150 IU for seven days. These pharmacokinetics were confirmed in pituitary down-regulated women undergoing *in vitro* fertilization and embryo transfer (IVF/ET), treated with FSH doses of up to 450 IU per day. Additionally, single dose pharmacokinetics of follitropin alfa were determined following subcutaneous administration of 225 IU Gonal-f® to 12 healthy adult male volunteers in a cross-over design. Steady state pharmacokinetics were also determined in 6 healthy adult male volunteers who were administered a single daily dose of 225 IU Gonal-f® for 7 days. No significant difference in pharmacokinetics is expected in males versus females when administered Gonal-f® subcutaneously. The pharmacokinetic parameters from these studies are included in Table 1.

[See table 1 above]

Absorption

The absorption rate of Gonal-f® following subcutaneous or intramuscular administration was found to be slower than the elimination rate. Hence the pharmacokinetics of Gonal-f® are absorption rate-limited.

Distribution

Human tissue or organ distribution of FSH has not been determined for Gonal-f®.

After intravenous administration to pituitary down-regulated, healthy female volunteers, the serum profile of FSH appears to be described by a two compartment open model with a distribution half-life of about 2-2.5 hours. Steady-state serum levels were reached after 4 to 5 days of daily administration.

Metabolism/Excretion

FSH metabolism following administration of Gonal-f® has not been studied in humans. Total clearance after IV administration in healthy females was 0.6 L/hr; mean residence time was 17-20 hours. FSH renal clearance was 0.07 L/hr after intravenous administration representing approximately 1/8 of total clearance.

Pharmacodynamics

Following daily subcutaneous administration of 150 IU of Gonal-f® for 7 days in healthy female volunteers, serum inhibin and estradiol, and total follicular volume responded as a function of time, with pronounced inter-individual variability. Pharmacodynamic effect lagged behind FSH serum concentration. Of the three pharmacodynamic parameters, serum inhibin levels responded with the least delay and declined rapidly after discontinuation of Gonal-f®. Follicular growth was most delayed and continued even after discontinuation of Gonal-f® administration, and after serum FSH levels had declined. Maximum follicular volume was better correlated with either inhibin or estradiol peak levels than with FSH concentration. Inhibin rise was an early index of follicular development. In healthy male volunteers, despite high interindividual variation and the absence of down-regulation, daily administration of 225 IU Gonal-f® was shown to increase the levels of inhibin to reach a plateau during the whole administration period and then return to baseline.

Population pharmacokinetics and pharmacodynamics

To establish the pharmacokinetics and pharmacodynamics of FSH in a target population, measurements performed during a clinical study of *in vitro* fertilization/embryo transfer were used in conjunction with pharmacokinetic data from studies in healthy female volunteers. The apparent clearance was comparable to that in healthy volunteers. The absorption rate was found to be influenced by the body mass index (BMI), suggesting that the higher the BMI, the lower the rate of absorption. However, FSH serum levels following fixed (during the first five days) and then adjusted doses of Gonal-f® were found to be poor predictors of follicular growth rate. High pre-treatment serum FSH levels may predict lower follicular growth rates.

Special populations: Safety, efficacy, and pharmacokinetics of Gonal-f® in patients with renal or hepatic insufficiency have not been established.

Drug-Drug interactions: No drug-drug interaction studies have been conducted (see PRECAUTIONS).

Table 1: Pharmacokinetic parameters (mean ± SD) of FSH following administration of Gonal-f®

Population	Healthy Female Volunteers			IVF/ET Patients	Healthy Male Volunteers	
Dose (IU)	Single Dose IM (150 IU)	Single Dose SC (150 IU)	Multiple Dose SC (7 × 150 IU)	Multiple Dose SC (5 × 225 IU)*	Single Dose SC (225 IU)	Multiple Dose SC (7 × 225 IU)
AUC (IU-hr/L)	206 ± 66	176 ± 87	187 ± 61#	–	–	–
C_{max} (IU/L)	3 ± 1	3 ± 1	9 ± 3	–	220 ± 109	186 ± 23#
t_{max} (hr)	25 ± 10	16 ± 10	8 ± 6	–	2.5 ± 0.8	8.3 ± 0.9
$t_{1/2}$ terminal (hr)	50 ± 27	24 ± 11	24 ± 8	–	20 ± 14	10.7 ± 6.7
CL/F (L/hr)	–	–	–	32**	41 ± 14	32 ± 4
V/F (L)	–	–	–	0.7 ± 0.2	0.86 ± 0.48	0.90 ± 0.12
F (%)	76 ± 30	66 ± 39	–	10 ± 3	–	–

Abbreviations are: IVF/ET: *in vitro* fertilization/embryo transfer;
C_{max}: peak concentration (above baseline);
t_{max}: time of C_{max};
CL/F: apparent clearance;
V/F: apparent volume of distribution; calculated using a one-compartment model.
$t_{1/2}$: absorption half-life;
F: bioavailability compared to IV
Steady-state $AUC_{144-168}$ (After the 7th daily SC dose)
* First five days of fixed regimen followed by adjustment of the dose depending on response
** increases with body mass index

Clinical Studies:

Women:

The safety and efficacy of Gonal-f® have been examined in four clinical studies, two studies for ovulation induction and two studies for assisted reproductive technologies (ART). In these comparative studies, there were no clinically significant differences between treatment groups in study outcomes.

Ovulation Induction:

The safety and efficacy of Gonal-f® administered subcutaneously vs. urofollitropin administered intramuscularly were assessed in a phase III, open-label, randomized, comparative, multinational, multicenter study in oligo-anovulatory infertile women who failed to ovulate or conceive following adequate clomiphene citrate therapy (Study 5642). The primary efficacy parameter was the ovulation rate. Two hundred and twenty-two patients entered into the first cycle of treatment, of whom 110 received Gonal-f® and 112 received urofollitropin. Ovulation rates were similar between Gonal-f® and urofollitropin treatment groups. The study results for the 222 patients who received treatment in at least one cycle are summarized in Table 2.

Table 2: Cumulative Patient Ovulation and Clinical Pregnancy Rates by Treatment Group in Ovulation Induction

Study 5642	Gonal-f® (n=110)	Urofollitropin (n=112)
Cumulative Ovulation Rate		
Cycle 1	64%	59%
Cycle 2	78%	82%
Cycle 3	84%	91%
Cumulative Clinical Pregnancy* Rate		
Cycle 1	21%	21%
Cycle 2	28%	38%
Cycle 3	35%	46%

* A clinical pregnancy was defined as a pregnancy during which a fetal sac (with or without heart activity) was visualized by ultrasound on day 34-36 after hCG administration.

For the 90 patients who had a clinical pregnancy (39 in Gonal-f® group; 51 in urofollitropin group), the outcome of the pregnancy was:

Table 3: Pregnancy Outcome by Treatment Group in Ovulation Induction

Study 5642	Gonal-f® (n=39)	Urofollitropin (n=51)
Pregnancies not reaching term	20.5%	13.7%
Single births	74.4%	74.5%
Multiple births	5.1%	11.8%

A second randomized, comparative, open-label, multicenter study was conducted in 23 U.S. centers (Study 5727). The primary efficacy parameter was ovulation rate. Ovulation rates were similar between Gonal-f® and urofollitropin treatment groups. Two hundred and thirty-two patients with oligo-anovulatory infertility received treatment with up to three cycles of Gonal-f® administered subcutaneously (118 patients) or urofollitropin administered intramuscularly (114 patients).

The cumulative patient ovulation rate and clinical pregnancy rates by cycle are presented for the 232 patients who received treatment in at least one cycle.

Table 4: Cumulative Patient Ovulation and Clinical Pregnancy Rates by Treatment Group in Ovulation Induction

Study 5727	Gonal-f® (n=118)	Urofollitropin (n=114)
Cumulative Ovulation Rate		
Cycle 1	58%	68%
Cycle 2	72%	86%
Cycle 3	81%	93%
Cumulative Clinical Pregnancy* Rate		
Cycle 1	13%	14%
Cycle 2	25%	25%
Cycle 3	37%	36%

* A clinical pregnancy was defined as a pregnancy during which a fetal sac (with or without heart activity) was visualized by ultrasound on day 34-36 after hCG administration.

For the 85 patients who had a clinical pregnancy (44 in Gonal-f® group; 41 in urofollitropin group), the outcome of the pregnancy is shown in Table 5.

Table 5: Pregnancy Outcome by Treatment Group in Ovulation Induction

Study 5727	Gonal-f® (n=44)	Urofollitropin (n=41)
Pregnancies not reaching term	22.7%	22.0%
Single births	63.6%	65.9%
Multiple births	13.7%	12.2%

2. Assisted Reproductive Technologies (ART):

The safety and efficacy of Gonal-f® administered subcutaneously vs. urofollitropin administered intramuscularly were assessed in a phase III, open-label, randomized, comparative, multinational, multicenter study in ovulatory, infertile women undergoing stimulation of multiple follicles for *In Vitro* Fertilization and Embryo Transfer (IVF/ET) after pituitary down-regulation with a GnRH agonist (Study 5503). The purpose of the study was to demonstrate that Gonal-f®, administered subcutaneously, was clinically not different in terms of safety and efficacy from urofollitropin, administered intramuscularly. The initial and maximal doses of Gonal-f® were 225 and 450 IU, respectively. The primary efficacy parameter was the number of mature pre-ovulatory follicles on the day of hCG administration. One hundred and twenty-three patients were randomized and received either Gonal-f® (60 patients) or urofollitropin (63 patients). The results summarized in Table 6 are mean data with Gonal-f® and urofollitropin administered to ovulatory infertile women undergoing multiple follicular development for IVF/ET.

Table 6: Treatment Outcomes by Treatment Group in ART

Study 5503	Gonal-f® (n=60)	Urofollitropin (n=63)
Mean number of follicles ≥ 14mm diameter on day of hCG	7.8	9.2
Mean number of oocytes recovered per patient	9.3	10.7
Mean Serum E2 (pg/mL) on day of hCG	1576	2193
Mean treatment duration in days (range)	9.9 (5-20)	9.4 (5-14)
Clinical pregnancy* rate per attempt	20%	16%
Clinical pregnancy* rate per embryo transfer	24%	19%

* A clinical pregnancy was defined as a pregnancy during which a fetal sac (with or without heart activity) was visualized by ultrasound on day 34-36 after hCG administration.

For the 22 patients who had a clinical pregnancy (12 in Gonal-f® group; 10 in urofollitropin group), the outcome of the pregnancy is shown in Table 7.

Table 7: Pregnancy Outcome by Treatment Group in ART

Study 5503	Gonal-f® (n=12)	Urofollitropin (n=10)
Pregnancies not reaching term	25.0%	20.0%
Single births	41.7%	50.0%
Multiple births	33.3%	30.0%

A second randomized, comparative, open-label, multicenter study was conducted in 7 U.S. centers (Study 5533). One hundred and fourteen patients with ovulatory infertility undergoing IVF/ET were randomized and received either Gonal-f® by subcutaneous administration (56 patients) or urofollitropin by intramuscular administration (58 patients) following pituitary down-regulation with a GnRH agonist. The primary efficacy parameter was the number of mature pre-ovulatory follicles on the day of hCG administration. Results are summarized in Table 8.

Table 8: Treatment Outcomes by Treatment Group in ART

Study 5533	Gonal-f® (n=56)	urofollitropin (n=58)
Mean number of follicles ≥ 14mm diameter on day of hCG	7.2	8.3
Mean number of oocytes recovered per patient	9.3	12.3
Mean Serum E2 (pg/mL) on day of hCG	1236	1513
Mean treatment duration in days (range)	10.1 (5-15)	9.0 (5-12)
Clinical pregnancy* rate per attempt	21%	22%
Clinical pregnancy* rate per embryo transfer	26%	25%

* A clinical pregnancy was defined as a pregnancy during which a fetal sac (with or without heart activity) was visualized by ultrasound on day 34-36 after hCG administration.

For the 25 patients who had a clinical pregnancy (12 in Gonal-f® group; 13 in urofollitropin group), the outcome of the pregnancy is shown in Table 9.

Table 9: Pregnancy Outcome by Treatment Group in ART

Study 5533	Gonal-f® (n=12)	Urofollitropin (n=13)
Pregnancies not reaching term	33.3%	30.8%
Single births	41.7%	38.5%
Multiple births	25.0%	30.8%

Men:

The safety and efficacy of Gonal-f® administered concomitantly with hCG have been examined in three open-label clinical studies for induction of spermatogenesis in men with primary and secondary hypogonadotropic hypogonadism.

The three multicenter studies involved three to six months of pretreatment with chorionic gonadotropin for injection (Profasi®) to normalize serum testosterone levels, followed by 18 months of treatment with Gonal-f® and hCG. The objective of each study was induction of spermatogenesis (a sperm density of $\geq 1.5 \times 10^6$/mL).

Study 5844 enrolled 32 patients in six centers in the United Kingdom, France and Germany. The second trial, Study 6410, was conducted in Australia and enrolled 10 patients in two centers. Study 6793, conducted in 7 centers in the United States, was planned to enroll 32 patients. The interim data for the US study includes 30 of the planned 32 patients. For all 3 studies, a total of 72 patients were enrolled and received hCG and 56 of those patients entered the Gonal-f® treatment phase of the trials.

The populations enrolled in the three studies were similar: Study 5844 studied a naïve population who had had no prior treatment with gonadotropins; mean age was 25.9 (range 16 to 48) years, mean (± SD) testis volume was 2.0 ± 1.2 mL, and 12 of the 32 patients (37.5%) were anosmic. Thirty-one of the patients were Caucasian and one was Asian. In Study 6410, mean age was 36 (range 26 to 48) years, 6 and 1 of the 10 patients had previously been treated with gonadotropins and GnRH, respectively; mean testis volume was 4.5 ± 2.9 mL; and 2 of the 10 patients (20%) were anosmic. Seven patients were Caucasian and three were Asian. In the 30 patients reported in the interim analysis of Study 6793, the mean age was 30.1 (range 22 to 44) years; 4 and 3 of the 30 patients had been treated with gonadotropins and GnRH, respectively, in the past; mean testis volume was 4.4 ± 1.3 mL; and 10 of the 30 patients (33.3%) were anosmic. Twenty five of the patients were Caucasian, three were Asian, and one each of Moroccan and Indian ancestry. THE PRIMARY EFFICACY ENDPOINT OF ALL THREE STUDIES WAS THE ACHIEVEMENT OF A SPERM DENSITY $\geq 1.5 \times 10^6$/ML. THE STUDY RESULTS FOR THE PATIENTS TREATED WITH GONAL-F® AND HCG ARE SUMMARIZED IN TABLE 10.
[See table 10 at top of next page]
[See table 11 on next page]

Table 12: Pregnancy Outcome in Partners of Men Desiring Fertility

	Study 5844 (n=7)	Study 6410 (n=10)	Study 6793 (n=20) *
Pregnancy	6 (86%)	3 (30%)	3 (15%)
Pregnancy not reaching term	1 (14%)	1 (10%)	2 (10%)
Single births	5 (71%)	2 (20%)	1 (5%)

*Interim data

Of the 56 patients who received Gonal-f® in Studies 5844, 6410, and 6793, 12 pregnancies were achieved in 10 partners of the 37 patients who were seeking pregnancy and who currently had a partner during the studies. Thus, pregnancy (clinical and chemical) was documented to have been achieved by 27% of the patients' partners seeking pregnancy during the exposure period to Gonal-f® in the 3 trials. Eight pregnancies continued to term, and 8 healthy babies were born to 7 couples as a result of those studies.

INDICATIONS AND USAGE

Women: Gonal-f® (follitropin alfa for injection) is indicated for the induction of ovulation and pregnancy in the anovulatory infertile patient in whom the cause of infertility is functional and not due to primary ovarian failure. Gonal-f® is also indicated for the development of multiple follicles in the ovulatory patient participating in an Assisted Reproductive Technology (ART) program.

Selection of Patients:

1. Before treatment with Gonal-f® is instituted, a thorough gynecologic and endocrinologic evaluation must be performed. This should include an assessment of pelvic anatomy. Patients with tubal obstruction should receive Gonal-f® only if enrolled in an *in vitro* fertilization program.

2. Primary ovarian failure should be excluded by the determination of gonadotropin levels.

3. Appropriate evaluation should be performed to exclude pregnancy.

4. Patients in later reproductive life have a greater predisposition to endometrial carcinoma as well as a higher incidence of anovulatory disorders. A thorough diagnostic evaluation should always be performed in patients who demonstrate abnormal uterine bleeding or other signs of endometrial abnormalities before starting Gonal-f® therapy.

5. Evaluation of the partner's fertility potential should be included in the initial evaluation.

Men:

Gonal-f® (follitropin alfa for injection) is indicated for the induction of spermatogenesis in men with primary and secondary hypogonadotropic hypogonadism in whom the cause of infertility is not due to primary testicular failure.

Selection of Patients:

1. Before treatment with Gonal-f® is instituted for azoospermia, a thorough medical and endocrinologic evaluation must be performed.

2. Hypogonadotropic hypogonadism should be confirmed, and primary testicular failure should be excluded by the determination of gonadotropin levels.

3. Prior to Gonal-f® therapy for azoospermia in patients with hypogonadotropic hypogonadism, serum testosterone levels should be normalized.

CONTRAINDICATIONS

Gonal-f® (follitropin alfa for injection) is contraindicated in women and men who exhibit:

1. Prior hypersensitivity to recombinant FSH preparations or one of their excipients.

2. High levels of FSH indicating primary gonadal failure.

3. Uncontrolled thyroid or adrenal dysfunction.

4. Sex hormone dependent tumors of the reproductive tract and accessory organs.

5. An organic intracranial lesion such as a pituitary tumor.

And in women who exhibit:

6. Abnormal uterine bleeding of undetermined origin (see "Selection of Patients").

7. Ovarian cyst or enlargement of undetermined origin (see "Selection of Patients").

8. Pregnancy.

WARNINGS

Gonal-f® (follitropin alfa for injection) should only be used by physicians who are thoroughly familiar with infertility problems and their management.

Gonal-f® is a potent gonadotropic substance capable of causing Ovarian Hyperstimulation Syndrome (OHSS) in women with or without pulmonary or vascular complications. Gonadotropin therapy requires a certain time commitment by physicians and supportive health professionals, and requires the availability of appropriate monitoring facilities (see "Precautions/Laboratory Tests"). Safe and effective use of Gonal-f® in women requires monitoring of ovarian response with serum estradiol and vaginal ultrasound on a regular basis. The lowest effective dose should be used.

Overstimulation of the Ovary During FSH Therapy:

Ovarian Enlargement: Mild to moderate uncomplicated ovarian enlargement which may be accompanied by abdominal distention and/or abdominal pain occurs in approximately 20% of those treated with urofollitropin and hCG, and generally regresses without treatment within two or three weeks. Careful monitoring of ovarian response can further minimize the risk of overstimulation.

If the ovaries are abnormally enlarged on the last day of Gonal-f® therapy, hCG should not be administered in this course of therapy. This will reduce the chances of development of Ovarian Hyperstimulation Syndrome.

Table 10: Number of Men Receiving Gonal-f® Who Achieved a Sperm Density ≥1.5 × 10⁶/mL

Sperm Concentration ≥ 1.5×10^6/mL		Study 5844 (n=26)	Study 6410 (n=8)	Study 6793 (n=22)
	Yes	12 (46.2%)	5 (62.5%)	14 (63.6%)
	No	14 (53.8%)	3 (37.5%)	8 (36.4%)
95% Confidence Interval		(26.6%-66.6%)	(24.5%-91.5%)	(40.7%-82.8%)

*Interim data

THE TIME TO ACHIEVEMENT OF THE PRIMARY EFFICACY ENDPOINT IS SUMMARIZED IN TABLE 11.

Table 11: Time to Achievement of Sperm Density ≥1.5 × 10⁶/mL in Men Receiving Gonal-f®

		Study 5844 (n=26)	Study 6410 (n=8)	Study 6793 (n=22) *
Number of Men Achieving Sperm Concentration	n	12	5	14
Time (Months) to Sperm Concentration ≥ 1.5×10^6/mL	Median	12.4	9.1	6.8
	Range	(2.7–18.1)	(8.8–11.7)	(2.8–15.7)

*Interim data

Ovarian Hyperstimulation Syndrome (OHSS): OHSS is a medical event distinct from uncomplicated ovarian enlargement. Severe OHSS may progress rapidly (within 24 hours to several days) to become a serious medical event. It is characterized by an apparent dramatic increase in vascular permeability which can result in a rapid accumulation of fluid in the peritoneal cavity, thorax, and potentially, the pericardium. The early warning signs of development of OHSS are severe pelvic pain, nausea, vomiting, and weight gain. The following symptomatology has been seen with cases of OHSS: abdominal pain, abdominal distension, gastrointestinal symptoms including nausea, vomiting and diarrhea, severe ovarian enlargement, weight gain, dyspnea, and oliguria. Clinical evaluation may reveal hypovolemia, hemoconcentration, electrolyte imbalances, ascites, hemoperitoneum, pleural effusions, hydrothorax, acute pulmonary distress, and thromboembolic events (see "Pulmonary and Vascular Complications"). Transient liver function test abnormalities suggestive of hepatic dysfunction, which may be accompanied by morphologic changes on liver biopsy, have been reported in association with Ovarian Hyperstimulation Syndrome (OHSS).

OHSS occurred in 9 of 228 (3.9%) Gonal-f® treated women during ovulation induction clinical trials and of this number, 1 of 228 (0.4%) was classified as severe. In ART clinical studies, OHSS occurred in 0 of 116 (0.0%) Gonal-f® treated women. OHSS may be more severe and more protracted if pregnancy occurs. OHSS develops rapidly; therefore, patients should be followed for at least two weeks after hCG administration. Most often, OHSS occurs after treatment has been discontinued and reaches its maximum at about seven to ten days following treatment. Usually, OHSS resolves spontaneously with the onset of menses. If there is evidence that OHSS may be developing prior to hCG administration (see "Precautions/Laboratory Tests"), the hCG <u>must</u> be withheld.

If severe OHSS occurs, treatment <u>must</u> be stopped and the patient should be hospitalized.

A physician experienced in the management of this syndrome, or who is experienced in the management of fluid and electrolyte imbalances should be consulted.

Pulmonary and Vascular Complications:

Serious pulmonary conditions (e.g., atelectasis, acute respiratory distress syndrome and exacerbation of asthma) have been reported. In addition, thromboembolic events both in association with, and separate from Ovarian Hyperstimulation Syndrome have been reported. Intravascular thrombosis and embolism can result in reduced blood flow to critical organs or the extremities. Sequelae of such events have included venous thrombophlebitis, pulmonary embolism, pulmonary infarction, cerebral vascular occlusion (stroke), and arterial occlusion resulting in loss of limb. In rare cases, pulmonary complications and/or thromboembolic events have resulted in death.

Multiple Births:

Reports of multiple births have been associated with Gonal-f® treatment. In ovulation induction clinical trials, 12.3% of live births were multiple births in women receiving Gonal-f® and 14.5% of live births were multiple births in women receiving urofollitropin. In IVF/ET clinical trials, 44.0% of live births were multiple births in women receiving Gonal-f® and 41.0% of live births were multiple births in women receiving urofollitropin and is dependent on the number of embryos transferred. The patient should be advised of the potential risk of multiple births before starting treatment.

PRECAUTIONS

General:

Careful attention should be given to the diagnosis of infertility in candidates for Gonal-f® (follitropin alfa for injection) therapy (see "Indications and Usage/Selection of Patients").

Information for Patients:

Prior to therapy with Gonal-f®, patients should be informed of the duration of treatment and monitoring of their condition that will be required. The risks of ovarian hyperstimulation syndrome and multiple births in women (see **WARNINGS**) and other possible adverse reactions (see **"Adverse Reactions"**) should also be discussed.

A 'Patient's Information Leaflet' is provided for patients prescribed Gonal-f® Multi-Dose.

Laboratory Tests:

In most instances, treatment of women with Gonal-f® results only in follicular recruitment and development. In the absence of an endogenous LH surge, hCG is given when monitoring of the patient indicates that sufficient follicular development has occurred. This may be estimated by ultrasound alone or in combination with measurement of serum estradiol levels. The combination of both ultrasound and serum estradiol measurement are useful for monitoring the development of follicles, for timing of the ovulatory trigger, as well as for detecting ovarian enlargement and minimizing the risk of the Ovarian Hyperstimulation Syndrome and multiple gestation. It is recommended that the number of growing follicles be confirmed using ultrasonography because plasma estrogens do not give an indication of the size or number of follicles.

The clinical confirmation of ovulation, with the exception of pregnancy, is obtained by direct and indirect indices of progesterone production. The indices most generally used are as follows:

1. A rise in basal body temperature;

2. Increase in serum progesterone; and

3. Menstruation following a shift in basal body temperature.

When used in conjunction with the indices of progesterone production, sonographic visualization of the ovaries will assist in determining if ovulation has occurred. Sonographic evidence of ovulation may include the following:

1. Fluid in the cul-de-sac;

2. Ovarian stigmata;

3. Collapsed follicle; and

4. Secretory endometrium.

Accurate interpretation of the indices of follicle development and maturation require a physician who is experienced in the interpretation of these tests.

Drug Interactions:

No drug/drug interaction studies have been performed.

Carcinogenesis, Mutagenesis, Impairment of Fertility:

Long-term studies in animals have not been performed to evaluate the carcinogenic potential of Gonal-f®. However, follitropin alfa showed no mutagenic activity in a series of tests performed to evaluate its potential genetic toxicity including bacterial and mammalian cell mutation tests, a chromosomal aberration test and a micronucleus test.

Impaired fertility has been reported in rats, exposed to pharmacological doses of follitropin alfa (≥40 IU/kg/day) for extended periods, through reduced fecundity.

Pregnancy:

Pregnancy Category X. See CONTRAINDICATIONS.

ursing Mothers:
.s not known whether this drug is excreted in human k. Because many drugs are excreted in human milk and ause of the potential for serious adverse reactions in the rsing infant from Gonal-f®, a decision should be made .ether to discontinue nursing or to discontinue the drug, .ing into account the importance of the drug to the .ther.

diatric Use:
.fety and effectiveness in pediatric patients have not been .tablished.

OVERSE REACTIONS

'omen:
.he safety of Gonal-f® was examined in four clinical studies .at enrolled 691 patients into two studies for ovulation in-.uction (454 patients) and two studies for ART (237 pa-.ents).

.dverse events occurring in more than 10% of patients were .eadache, ovarian cyst, nausea, and upper respiratory tract .nfection in the U.S. ovulation induction study and head-.che in the U.S. ART study. Adverse events (without regard .o causality assessment) occurring in at least 2% of patients .re listed in Table 13 and Table 14.

Table 13: US Controlled Trial in Ovulation Induction, Study 5727

Body System Preferred Term	Gonal-f® Patients (%) Experiencing Events Treatment cycles = 288* n=118	Urofollitropin Patients (%) Experiencing Events Treatment cycles = 277* n= 114
Reproductive, Female		
Intermenstrual Bleeding	9.3%	4.4%
Breast Pain Female	4.2%	6.1%
Ovarian Hyperstimulation**	6.8%	3.5%
Dysmenorrhea	2.5%	6.1%
Ovarian Disorder	1.7%	2.6%
Cervix Lesion	2.5%	0.9%
Menstrual Disorder	2.5%	0.9%
Gastro-intestinal System		
Abdominal Pain	9.3%	12.3%
Nausea	13.6%	3.5%
Flatulence	6.8%	8.8%
Diarrhea	7.6%	3.5%
Vomiting	2.5%	2.6%
Dyspepsia	1.7%	3.5%
Central and Peripheral Nervous System		
Headache	22.0%	20.2%
Dizziness	2.5%	0.0%
Neoplasm		
Ovarian Cyst	15.3%	28.9%
Body as a Whole-General		
Pain	5.9%	6.1%
Back Pain	5.1%	1.8%
Influenza-like Symptoms	4.2%	2.6%
Fever	4.2%	1.8%
Respiratory System		
Upper Respiratory Tract Infection	11.9%	7.9%
Sinusitis	5.1%	5.3%
Pharyngitis	2.5%	3.5%
Coughing	1.7%	2.6%
Rhinitis	0.8%	2.6%
Skin and Appendages		
Acne	4.2%	2.6%
Psychiatric		
Emotional Lability	5.1%	2.6%
Urinary System		
Urinary Tract Infection	1.7%	4.4%
Resistance Mechanism		
Moniliasis Genital	2.5%	0.9%
Application Site		
Injection Site Pain	2.5%	0.9%

* up to 3 cycles of therapy
** Severe = 0.8% of 118 patients in Study 5727

Additional adverse events not listed in Table 13 that occurred in 1 to 2% of Gonal-f® treated patients in the US ovulation induction study included the following: leukor-rhea, vaginal hemorrhage, migraine, fatigue, asthma, ner-vousness, somnolence, and hypotension.

Table 14: US Controlled Trial in ART, Study 5533

Body System Preferred Term	Gonal-f® Patients (%) Experiencing Events n=59	Urofollitropin Patients (%) Experiencing Events n= 61
Reproductive, Female		
Intermenstrual Bleeding	3.6%	5.2%
Leukorrhea	1.7%	3.4%
Vaginal Hemorrhage	3.6%	3.4%
Gastro-intestinal System		
Nausea	5.4%	1.7%
Flatulence	3.6%	0.0%
Central and Peripheral Nervous System		
Headache	12.5%	3.4%
Body as a Whole-General		
Abdominal Pain	8.9%	3.4%
Pelvic Pain Female	7.1%	1.7%
Respiratory System		
Upper Respiratory Tract Infection	3.6%	1.7%
Metabolic and Nutritional		
Weight Increase	3.6%	0.0%

Additional adverse events not listed in Table 14 that occurred in 1 to 2% of Gonal-f® treated patients in the U.S. Assisted Reproductive Technology (ART) study included the following: D&C following delivery or abortion, dysmenor-rhea, vaginal hemorrhage, diarrhea, tooth disorder, vomit-ing, dizziness, paraesthesia, abdomen enlarged, chest pain, fatigue, dyspnea, anorexia, anxiety, somnolence, injection site inflammation, injection site reaction, pruritus, pruritus genital, myalgia, thirst, and palpitation.
TWO ADDITIONAL CLINICAL STUDIES (FOR OVULA-TION INDUCTION AND ART, RESPECTIVELY) WERE CONDUCTED IN EUROPE. THE SAFETY PROFILES FROM THESE TWO STUDIES WERE COMPARABLE TO THAT OF THE DATA PRESENTED ABOVE.
Gonal-f® Multi-Dose was examined in twenty-five healthy volunteers who received 300 IU each of Gonal-f® from single-dose ampules and multi-dose vials. Overall, both pre-sentations were well tolerated and local tolerability be-tween the two groups was comparable. Injection site inspec-tions revealed very rare local reactions (mild redness in one patient after single-dose injection and mild bruising in two subjects after multi-dose injection). Subjective assessments indicated minimal or mild transient pain in two and five subjects who received Gonal-f® single-dose and Gonal-f® Multi-Dose, respectively.
The following medical events have been reported subse-quent to pregnancies resulting from gonadotropins in con-trolled clinical studies:
1. Spontaneous Abortion
2. Ectopic Pregnancy
3. Premature Labor
4. Postpartum Fever
5. Congenital Abnormalities
Two incidents of congenital cardiac malformations have been reported in children born following pregnancies result-ing from treatment with Gonal-f® and hCG in Gonal-f® clin-ical studies 5642 and 5727. In addition, a pregnancy occur-ring in study 5533 following treatment with Gonal-f® and hCG was complicated by apparent failure of intrauterine growth and terminated by a suspected syndrome of congen-ital abnormalities. No specific diagnosis was made. The in-cidence does not exceed that found in the general popula-tion.
The following adverse reactions have been previously re-ported during menotropin therapy:
1. Pulmonary and vascular complications (see "Warnings"),
2. Adnexal torsion (as a complication of ovarian enlarge-ment),
3. Mild to moderate ovarian enlargement,
4. Hemoperitoneum
There have been infrequent reports of ovarian neoplasms, both benign and malignant, in women who have undergone multiple drug regimens for ovulation induction; however, a causal relationship has not been established.

Men:
The safety of Gonal-f® was examined in 3 clinical studies that enrolled 72 patients for induction of spermatogenesis and fertility of whom 56 patients received Gonal-f®. One hundred and twenty-three adverse events, including 7 seri-ous events, were reported in 34 of the 56 patients during Gonal-f® treatment.
In Study 5844, 21 adverse events, including 4 serious ad-verse events, were reported by 14 of the 26 patients (53.8%) treated with Gonal-f®. Events occurring in more than one patient were varicocele (4) and injection site reactions (4). The 4 serious adverse events were testicular surgery for

cryptorchidism, which existed prestudy, hemoptysis, an in-fected pilonidal cyst, and lymphadenopathy associated with an Epstein-Barr viral infection.
In Study 6410, 3 adverse events were reported in 2 of the 8 patients (24%) treated with Gonal-f®. One serious adverse event was reported, surgery for gynecomastia which existed at baseline.
In the interim analysis of Study 6793, 18 of 22 patients (81.8%) reported a total of 99 adverse events during Gonal-f® treatment. The most common events of possible, probable, or definite relationship to study drug therapy oc-curring in more than 2 patients were: acne (25 events in 13 patients; 59% of patients); breast pain (4 events in 3 pa-tients; 13.6% of patients); and fatigue, gynecomastia, and injection site pain (each of which was reported as 2 events by 2 patients; 9.1% of patients). Two serious adverse events (hospitalization for drug abuse and depression) were re-ported by a single patient in the interim analysis.
A total of 12,026 injections of Gonal-f® were administered by the 56 patients who received Gonal-f® in Studies 5844, 6410, and 6793 combined. The injections were well-tolerated, with no or mild reactions (redness, swelling, bruising and itching) reported by patients for 93.3% of in-jections. Moderate and severe reactions, consisting primar-ily of pain, were reported for 4.8% of injections, and no self-assessment was available for 1.9% of injections.

OVERDOSAGE

Aside from possible ovarian hyperstimulation and multiple gestations (see "Warnings"), there is no information on the consequences of acute overdosage with Gonal-f® (follitropin alfa for injection).

DOSAGE AND ADMINISTRATION

Each Gonal-f® Multi-Dose Vial delivers 450 IU or 1050 IU follitropin alfa, respectively.

Dosage:

Infertile Patients with oligo-anovulation:
The dose of Gonal-f® (follitropin alfa for injection) to stimu-late development of the follicle must be individualized for each patient.
The lowest dose consistent with the expectation of good re-sults should be used. Over the course of treatment, doses of Gonal-f® may range up to 300 IU per day depending on the individual patient response. Gonal-f® should be adminis-tered until adequate follicular development is indicated by serum estradiol and vaginal ultrasonography. A response is generally evident after 5 to 7 days. Subsequent monitoring intervals should be based on individual patient response.
It is recommended that the initial dose of the first cycle be 75 IU of Gonal-f® per day, ADMINISTERED SUBCUTANE-OUSLY. An incremental adjustment in dose of up to 37.5 IU may be considered after 14 days. Further dose increases of the same magnitude could be made, if necessary, every seven days. Treatment duration should not exceed 35 days unless an E2 rise indicates imminent follicular develop-ment. To complete follicular development and effect ovula-tion in the absence of an endogenous LH surge, chorionic gonadotropin, hCG, (5,000 USP units) should be given 1 day after the last dose of Gonal-f®. Chorionic gonadotropin should be withheld if the serum estradiol is greater than 2,000 pg/mL. If the ovaries are abnormally enlarged or ab-dominal pain occurs, Gonal-f® treatment should be discon-tinued, hCG should not be administered, and the patient should be advised not to have intercourse; this may reduce the chance of development of the Ovarian Hyperstimulation Syndrome and, should spontaneous ovulation occur, reduce the chance of multiple gestation. A follow-up visit should be conducted in the luteal phase.
The initial dose administered in the subsequent cycles should be individualized for each patient based on her re-sponse in the preceding cycle. Doses larger than 300 IU of FSH per day are not routinely recommended. As in the ini-tial cycle, 5,000 USP units of hCG must be given 1 day after the last dose of Gonal-f® to complete follicular development and induce ovulation. The precautions described above should be followed to minimize the chance of development of the Ovarian Hyperstimulation Syndrome.
The couple should be encouraged to have intercourse daily, beginning on the day prior to the administration of hCG un-til ovulation becomes apparent from the indices employed for the determination of progestational activity. Care should be taken to ensure insemination. In light of the indices and parameters mentioned, it should become obvious that, un-less a physician is willing to devote considerable time to these patients and be familiar with and conduct the neces-sary laboratory studies, he/she should not use Gonal-f®.

Assisted Reproductive Technologies:
As in the treatment of patients with oligo-anovulatory infer-tility, the dose of Gonal-f® to stimulate development of the follicle must be individualized for each patient. For Assisted Reproductive Technologies, therapy with Gonal-f® should be initiated in the early follicular phase (cycle day 2 or 3) at a

dose of 150 IU per day, until sufficient follicular development is attained. In most cases, therapy should not exceed ten days.

In patients undergoing ART, whose endogenous gonadotropin levels are suppressed, Gonal-f® should be initiated at a dose of 225 IU per day. Treatment should be continued until adequate follicular development is indicated as determined by ultrasound in combination with measurement of serum estradiol levels. Adjustments to dose may be considered after five days based on the patient's response; subsequently dosage should be adjusted no more frequently than every 3-5 days and by no more than 75-150 IU additionally at each adjustment. Doses greater than 450 IU per day are not recommended. Once adequate follicular development is evident, hCG (5,000 to 10,000 USP units) should be administered to induce final follicular maturation in preparation for oocyte retrieval. The administration of hCG must be withheld in cases where the ovaries are abnormally enlarged on the last day of therapy. This should reduce the chance of developing OHSS.

Male Patients with Hypogonadotropic Hypogonadism:

The dose of Gonal-f® (follitropin alfa for injection) to induce spermatogenesis must be individualized for each patient. Gonal-f® must be given in conjunction with hCG. Prior to concomitant therapy with Gonal-f® and hCG, pretreatment with hCG alone (1,000 to 2,250 USP units two to three times per week) is required. Treatment should continue for a period sufficient to achieve serum testosterone levels within the normal range. Such pretreatment may require 3 to 6 months and the dose of hCG may need to be increased to achieve normal serum testosterone levels.

After normal serum testosterone levels are reached, the recommended dose of Gonal-f® is 150 IU administered subcutaneously three times a week and the recommended dose of hCG is 1,000 USP units (or the dose required to maintain serum testosterone levels within the normal range) three times a week. The lowest dose of Gonal-f® which induces spermatogenesis should be utilized. If azoospermia persists, the dose of Gonal-f® may be increased to a maximum dose of 300 IU three times per week. Gonal-f® may need to be administered for up to 18 months to achieve adequate spermatogenesis.

Administration:

Multi-Dose 450 IU Vial:

Dissolve the contents of one Multi-Dose vial (450 IU) with 1 mL Bacteriostatic Water for Injection (0.9% benzyl alcohol), USP. Resulting concentration will be 600 IU/mL. Following reconstitution as directed, product will deliver the equivalent of six 75 IU doses.

Multi-Dose 1050 IU Vial:

Dissolve the contents of one Multi-Dose vial (1050 IU) with 2 mL Bacteriostatic Water for Injection (0.9% benzyl alcohol), USP. Resulting concentration will be 600 IU/mL. Following reconstitution as directed, product will deliver the equivalent of fourteen 75 IU doses. Patients should be instructed to use the accompanying syringes, calibrated in FSH units (IU FSH) for administration. The 27-gauge injection syringe (see figure below) has unit dose markings from 37.5 IU to 600 IU FSH for use with Gonal-f® Multi-Dose. Patients should be instructed to take a specific dose of Gonal-f® Multi-Dose. The doctor, nurse, or pharmacist should show the patient how to locate the syringe marking that corresponds to the prescribed dose.

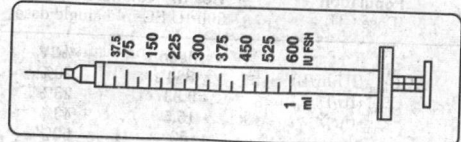

Patient Instructions for Use for Gonal-f® Multi-Dose Vial

Step 1: Mixing (reconstituting) Gonal-f® Multi-Dose Vial

1. Wash your hands with soap and water.
2. Using your thumb, flip off the plastic cap of the Gonal-f® Multi-Dose vial.
3. Wipe the top of the vial stopper with an alcohol swab.
4. Carefully twist the needle cap off the syringe labeled 'Bacteriostatic Water for Injection, USP'. Do not touch the needle or allow the needle to touch any surface.
5. Position the needle of the syringe of water in a straight, upright position over the **marked center circle** of the rubber stopper on the vial of Gonal-f® Multi-Dose powder. Keep the needle in a straight, upright position as you insert it through the center circle, or it may be difficult to depress the plunger. **Slowly** inject the water into the vial by depressing the syringe plunger. When all the water has been injected into the vial, withdraw the needle and safely dispose of it immediately in your needle container. Do not use this needle to inject your dose.

6. Do not shake the vial. If bubbles appear, wait a few moments for the bubbles to settle. The liquid drug should be clear.

Step 2: Preparing the Dose

1. Wipe the rubber stopper of the vial of Gonal-f® Multi-Dose liquid with an alcohol wipe.
2. Carefully pull the cap from the needle. Do not touch the needle or allow the needle to touch any surface. Firmly hold the vial of Gonal-f® Multi-Dose liquid on a flat surface, insert the needle through the marked center circle of the rubber stopper.
3. Keeping the needle in the vial, lift the vial and turn it upside down with the needle pointing toward the ceiling. With the needle tip in the liquid, slowly pull back the plunger until the syringe fills to slightly more than the mark for your prescribed dose. Next, keeping the needle in the vial, slowly adjust the plunger to your prescribed dose—this will clear away any air bubbles.
4. Check that you have the plunger set at your prescribed dose.
5. Remove the syringe needle from the vial.
6. Inject the prescribed dose as directed by the doctor.

Parenteral drug products should be inspected visually for particulate matter and discoloration prior to administration, whenever solution and container permit.

HOW SUPPLIED

Gonal-f® (follitropin alfa for injection) is supplied in a sterile, lyophilized form in multiple dose vials filled with 600 IU or 1200 IU in order to deliver 450 IU and 1050 IU FSH, respectively, after reconstitution with diluent (Bacteriostatic Water for injection, USP, containing 0.9% benzyl alcohol as a preservative). Each carton contains syringes with mounted 27G × 0.5 inch needle, calibrated in FSH units (IU FSH) which should be used for administration.

Lyophilized Multi-Dose vials may be stored refrigerated or at room temperature (2°-25°C/36°-77°F). Following reconstitution, the Multi-Dose vial may be stored refrigerated or at room temperature (2°-25°C/36°-77°F). Protect from light. Discard unused reconstituted solution after 28 days.

The following package combinations are available:
–1 vial Gonal-f® Multi-Dose 450 IU, 1 pre-filled syringe of Bacteriostatic Water for Injection, USP (0.9% benzyl alcohol), 1 mL and 5 syringes calibrated in FSH Units (IU FSH) for injection NDC 44087-9030-1
–1 vial Gonal-f® Multi-Dose 1050 IU, 1 pre-filled syringe of Bacteriostatic Water for Injection, USP (0.9% benzyl alcohol), 2 mL and 10 syringes calibrated in FSH Units (IU FSH) for injection NDC 44087-9070-1

Rx only

Manufactured for: EMD Serono, Inc., Rockland, MA 02370 U.S.A.

Revised: May 2009

Gonal-f® Multi-Dose

(follitropin alfa for injection)

Patient's Information Leaflet

This leaflet contains information about Gonal-f® Multi-Dose. This drug has been prescribed to you by your doctor for treating infertility. To help you prepare and use this medicine, you should read these instructions carefully and ask your doctor, nurse, or pharmacist to explain anything you do not understand. Keep this leaflet. You may want to read it again.

What is Gonal-f® Multi-Dose?

Gonal-f® Multi-Dose is an injectable hormone contained in a stoppered glass vial. The hormone in the vial is in the form of a white powder. The carton containing the vial of drug also contains a syringe labeled 'Bacteriostatic Water for Injection, USP'. This water must be mixed with the white powder in the vial to form a clear liquid solution for injection. Injection syringes for use with Gonal-f® Multi-Dose are also included in the carton. These injection syringes can only be used to administer Gonal-f® Multi-Dose. Gonal-f® Multi-Dose is only available with a prescription.

Gonal-f® Multi-Dose contains follitropin alfa, which is similar to the human hormone 'follicle stimulating hormone'; the abbreviation is 'FSH'. FSH belongs to the group of hormones associated with human reproduction. In women, FSH causes the ovaries to produce eggs. In men, FSH causes sperm production.

The hormone in Gonal-f® Multi-Dose is manufactured to meet standards for quality and purity. It cannot be taken by mouth since the acids in your stomach would destroy the hormone before it was absorbed into the body. Gonal-f® Multi-Dose is given as an injection usually every day in women and three times per week in men. It is prescribed to patients needing hormone replacement or supplementation to produce either eggs or sperm.

The Gonal-f® Multi-Dose 450 IU (33 µg) vial is filled with 600 IU of drug in order to deliver 450 IU in several smaller daily doses. This provides between 2 and 6 commonly prescribed daily doses.

The Gonal-f® Multi-Dose 1050 IU (77 µg) vial is filled with 1200 IU of drug in order to deliver 1050 IU in several smaller daily doses. This provides between 3 and 14 commonly prescribed daily doses.

Your doctor or nurse will tell you the number of units (IU FSH) of Gonal-f® to use each day and the number of days to use the same vial. It is common for a small amount of drug to be leftover in each vial that can not be retrieved with the syringe. This is normal. Any drug remaining in the vial after your treatment is complete should be discarded.

Your doctor, nurse, or pharmacist will show you how to inject the prescribed dose. Usual injection sites include the skin on the stomach, upper leg, or upper arm.

IMPORTANT

The Gonal-f® liquid solution may be stored refrigerated or at room temperature for a maximum of 28 days from the day the powder is mixed with the water. Do Not Freeze. Discard unused liquid solution after 28 days. Use only the prescribed dose. Call your doctor immediately should you accidentally inject more than the prescribed dose.

What are the uses of Gonal-f® Multi-Dose?

Doctors specializing in infertility or reproductive health prescribe Gonal-f® Multi-Dose to those patients trying to have a child but for a variety of reasons need medical assistance. After a thorough medical exam to determine your specific medical condition, your doctor may prescribe Gonal-f® Multi-Dose because you require hormone replacement or supplementation as part of your treatment program. Gonal-f® Multi-Dose can be used in women seeking pregnancy or in men with a rare condition that affects sperm production. Gonal-f® Multi-Dose may be one of several drugs prescribed to a patient as part of a treatment program.

IMPORTANT

Do NOT take Gonal-f® Multi-Dose if you have allergies to any of these materials:
• follitropin
• sucrose
• sodium phosphate
• benzyl alcohol
Do NOT take Gonal-f® Multi-Dose if you are pregnant or breast feeding.

Medical conditions you should tell your doctor about.

If you have any of the following conditions, make sure to tell your doctor before starting or continuing use of Gonal-f®:
• Abnormal bleeding from the uterus or vagina in women
• Swollen, enlarged or painful ovaries in women
• Cancer of the sex organs (uterus, ovaries, testes)
• Permanent damage to the male sex organs (testes)
• Uncontrolled thyroid or adrenal problems
• Cancer of the brain

How to Prepare Gonal-f® Multi-Dose for Use

See your doctor, nurse, or pharmacist to obtain training in the preparation and use of Gonal-f® Multi-Dose.

REVIEW THESE STEPS BEFORE YOU PREPARE OR ADMINISTER GONAL-F® MULTI-DOSE.

Getting ready

Make sure you have all the necessary items listed below before you begin.
• vial containing Gonal-f® Multi-Dose (white powder)
• single pre-filled syringe labeled 'Bacteriostatic Water for Injection, USP'
• 27-gauge injection syringe with unit dose markings from 37.5 IU to 600 IU FSH for use with the Gonal-f® Multi-Dose.
• alcohol wipes
• hard plastic or metal container (like an empty coffee can) suitable for safe disposal of used syringes and needles.

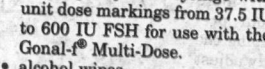

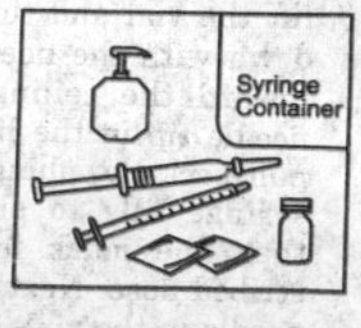

Syringe Container

Step 1: Mixing (reconstituting) the vial containing Gonal-f® Multi-Dose

• Wash your hands with soap and water.
• Using your thumb, flip off the plastic cap of the Gonal-f® Multi-Dose vial.
• Wipe the top of the vial stopper with an alcohol wipe.

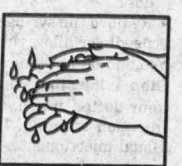

Carefully twist the needle cap off the syringe labeled 'Bacteriostatic Water for Injection, USP'. Do not touch the needle or allow the needle to touch any surface.

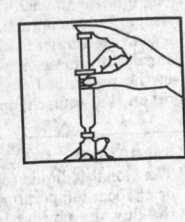

Position the needle of the syringe of water in a straight, upright position over the **marked center circle** of the rubber stopper on the vial of Gonal-f® Multi-Dose powder. Keep the needle in a straight, upright position as you insert it through the center circle, or it may be difficult to depress the plunger. **Slowly** inject the water into the vial by depressing the syringe plunger. The water and white powder will mix to form a clear liquid. When all the water has been injected into the vial, withdraw the needle and safely dispose of it immediately in your needle container. Do not use this needle to inject your dose.

• Do not shake the vial. If bubbles appear, wait a few moments for the bubbles to settle. The liquid drug should be clear.

IMPORTANT
Do not use the Gonal-f® Multi-Dose liquid solution if it contains any particles. Report this to your doctor, nurse, or pharmacist immediately.

Step 2: Determining your dose on the injection syringe
Your doctor will instruct you to take a specific dose of Gonal-f® Multi-Dose. Your doctor, nurse, or pharmacist should show you how to locate the syringe marking that corresponds to your prescribed dose (see illustration below).

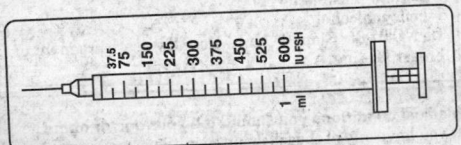

IMPORTANT
If your doctor or nurse instructs you to increase or decrease your dose for 1 or more days, find the correct dose marking on the injection syringe and make the change as directed. Contact your doctor or nurse if you have questions.

Step 3: Preparing your dose
• Wipe the rubber stopper of the vial of Gonal-f® Multi-Dose liquid with an alcohol wipe.
• Carefully pull the cap from the needle. Do not touch the needle or allow the needle to touch any surface. Firmly hold the vial of Gonal-f® Multi-Dose liquid on a flat surface, insert the needle through **the marked center** circle of the rubber stopper.
• Keeping the needle in the vial, lift the vial and turn it upside down with the needle pointing toward the ceiling. With the needle tip in the liquid, slowly pull back the plunger until the syringe fills to slightly more than the mark for your prescribed dose. Next, keeping the needle in the vial, slowly adjust the plunger to your prescribed dose—this will clear away any air bubbles.

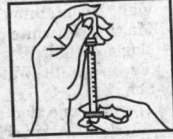

• Check that you have the plunger set at your prescribed dose.
• Remove the syringe needle from the vial. Do not touch the needle or allow the needle to touch any surface.
You should now be ready to prepare to receive the injection.

Step 4: Injecting your dose
Your doctor, nurse, or pharmacist should provide you with injection training. Inject the prescribed dose as directed. Usual injection sites include the skin on the stomach, upper arm, or upper leg. Change the injection location each day to

minimize discomfort. Dispose of all used syringes and needles safely in a container.

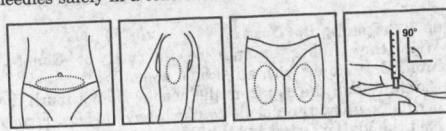

IMPORTANT
The injection syringes provided with Gonal-f® Multi-Dose are designed for use only with this product. Do NOT use the injection syringes to administer other drugs or hormones. All unused syringes should be discarded.

Step 5: Storing Your Vial of Gonal-f® Multi-Dose Between Uses
• After each use, the vial containing the Gonal-f® Multi-Dose liquid must be stored away from light and may be stored refrigerated or at room temperature between 36°–77° F (2°-25° C) for up to 28 days. Otherwise, the drug's potency can be reduced. Do not store the drug in the syringe.
• If you are traveling, keep the vial stored away from light and extreme temperatures. Do not freeze.
• Allow the liquid solution to adjust to room temperature prior to administering your injection.
• Check that the Gonal-f® liquid solution is clear. Do not use it if it contains any particles. Report this to your doctor, nurse or pharmacist immediately.

Are there any side effects associated with the use of Gonal-f® Multi-Dose?
Your doctor or staff member should review with you the risks and benefits of using Gonal-f® Multi-Dose. As with any medication, report any and all side effects, symptoms, or physical changes to your doctor.
The most common side effects are headache, ovarian cysts, upset stomach, and sinus infections in women and skin pimples, breast pain and growth, and tiredness in men. Needle injections may cause some discomfort.
Use of fertility drugs can be associated with fertilization of more than 1 egg. This can lead to complications for the mother and the birth of 2 or more babies. Pregnancy loss (miscarriage) is higher in women receiving fertility drugs than in women not taking fertility drugs.
Gonal-f® is a potent drug which should be used at the lowest dose expected to achieve the desired results. When used in women, your doctor should monitor your response often to avoid overdose which can lead to serious side effects including blood clots.

IMPORTANT
Contact your doctor if you take more than the prescribed amount of Gonal-f® or experience severe pain or bloating in the stomach or pelvic area, severe upset stomach, vomiting, and weight gain.

In rare cases, ovarian cancer has been reported in women receiving many courses of fertility drugs.

What should you do if you forget to take Gonal-f® Multi-Dose?
Do NOT take a double dose of Gonal-f®. Contact your doctor if you forget to take a dose of Gonal-f®.
Can you take Gonal-f® Multi-Dose with other medicines?
Inform your doctor and pharmacist if you are taking or have taken any other medicines, even those not requiring a prescription.
Where can more information about Gonal-f® Multi-Dose be obtained?
This leaflet is a summary of the important patient information about Gonal-f® Multi-Dose. If you have any questions or problems, talk to your doctor or other health care provider.
Gonal-f® Multi-Dose is manufactured and distributed by EMD Serono, Inc. You can also visit the Web site www.fertilitylifelines.com or contact EMD Serono at 1-866-538-7879.
© 2008 EMD Serono Inc.
N19Z0101C

GONAL-F® RFF PEN ℞
[gŏn-əl f]
(follitropin alfa injection)
*revised formulation female
For subcutaneous injection

DESCRIPTION
Gonal-f® RFF Pen (follitropin alfa injection) is a human follicle stimulating hormone (FSH) preparation of recombi-

nant DNA origin, which consists of two non-covalently linked, non-identical glycoproteins designated as the α-and β-subunits. The α-and β-subunits have 92 and 111 amino acids, respectively, and their primary and tertiary structures are indistinguishable from those of human follicle stimulating hormone. Recombinant human FSH production occurs in genetically modified Chinese Hamster Ovary (CHO) cells cultured in bioreactors. Purification by immunochromatography using an antibody specifically binding FSH results in a highly purified preparation with a consistent FSH isoform profile, and a high specific activity. The protein content is assessed by size exclusion high pressure liquid chromatography. The biological activity of follitropin alfa is determined by measuring the increase in ovary weight in female rats. The *in vivo* biological activity of follitropin alfa has been calibrated against the first International Standard for recombinant human follicle stimulating hormone established in 1995 by the Expert Committee on Biological Standards of the World Health Organization. Gonal-f® RFF Pen contains no luteinizing hormone (LH) activity. Based on available data derived from physicochemical tests and bioassays, follitropin alfa and follitropin beta, another recombinant follicle stimulating hormone product, are indistinguishable.
Gonal-f® RFF Pen is a disposable, prefilled drug delivery system intended for the subcutaneous injection of multiple and variable doses of a liquid formulation of follitropin alfa. Each Gonal-f® RFF Pen is filled with 415 IU (30 mcg), 568 IU (41 mcg), or 1026 IU (75 mcg) follitropin alfa to deliver at least 300 IU (22 mcg) in 0.5 mL, 450 IU (33 mcg) in 0.75 mL, or 900 IU (66 mcg) in 1.5 mL, respectively. Each Pen also contains 60 mg/mL sucrose, 3.0 mg/mL m-cresol, 1.1 mg/mL di-sodium hydrogen phosphate dihydrate, 0.45 mg/mL sodium dihydrogen phosphate monohydrate, 0.1 mg/mL methionine, 0.1 mg/mL Poloxamer 188. O-phosphoric acid and/or sodium hydroxide may be used for pH adjustment.
Under current storage conditions, Gonal-f® RFF Pen may contain up to 10% of oxidized follitropin alfa.
Therapeutic Class: Infertility

CLINICAL PHARMACOLOGY
Gonal-f® RFF Pen (follitropin alfa injection) stimulates ovarian follicular growth in women who do not have primary ovarian failure. FSH, the active component of Gonal-f® RFF Pen is the primary hormone responsible for follicular recruitment and development. In order to effect final maturation of the follicle and ovulation in the absence of an endogenous LH surge, human chorionic gonadotropin (hCG) must be given following the administration of Gonal-f® RFF Pen when monitoring of the patient indicates that sufficient follicular development has occurred. There is interpatient variability in response to FSH administration.

Pharmacokinetics
Single-dose pharmacokinetics of follitropin alfa were determined following subcutaneous administration of 300 IU Gonal-f® RFF Pen to 21 pre-menopausal healthy female volunteers who were pituitary down-regulated with a GnRH agonist.
The descriptive statistics for the pharmacokinetic parameters are presented in Table 1.

Table 1: Pharmacokinetic parameters of FSH following administration of Gonal-f® RFF Pen

Population Dose (IU)	Healthy Volunteers (n=21) 300 IU SC in a single dose	
	Mean	%CV
AUC_{last} (IU hr/L)	884	20%
C_{max} (IU/L)	9.83	23%
t_{max} (hr)	15.5	43%
$t_{1/2}$ (hr)	53	52%

Abbreviations are: C_{max}: peak concentration (above baseline); t_{max}: time of C_{max}; $t_{1/2}$: elimination half life

Absorption
The absorption rate of Gonal-f® RFF Pen following subcutaneous administration is slower than the elimination rate. Hence, the pharmacokinetics of Gonal-f® RFF Pen are absorption rate-limited.
Distribution
Human tissue or organ distribution of FSH has not been determined for Gonal-f® RFF Pen.
Metabolism/Excretion
FSH metabolism and excretion following administration of Gonal-f® RFF Pen have not been studied in humans.
Special populations: Safety, efficacy, and pharmacokinetics of Gonal-f® RFF Pen in patients with renal or hepatic insufficiency have not been established.
Drug-Drug Interactions: No drug-drug interaction studies have been conducted (see PRECAUTIONS).

CLINICAL STUDIES

The safety and efficacy of Gonal-f® RFF have been examined in two clinical studies: one study (Study 22240) for ovulation induction and one study (Study 21884) for Assisted Reproductive Technologies (ART).

1. Ovulation Induction (OI):
Study 22240 was a phase III, assessor-blind, randomized, comparative, multinational, multicenter study in oligo-anovulatory infertile women undergoing ovulation induction. Patients were randomized to either Gonal-f® RFF (n=83), administered subcutaneously, or a comparator recombinant human FSH. The use of insulin-sensitizing agents was allowed during the study. Efficacy was assessed using the mean ovulation rate in the first cycle of treatment. The cycle 1 ovulation rate (primary outcome) for Gonal-f® RFF is presented in Table 2. Additionally, this table includes cumulative secondary outcome results from cycle 1 through 3. Study 22240 was not powered to demonstrate differences in these secondary outcomes.

Table 2: Cumulative Ovulation and Clinical Pregnancy Rates in Ovulation Induction Study 22240

	n=83
Cumulative[a] Ovulation Rate	
Cycle 1	72%[b]
Cycle 2	89%[d]
Cycle 3	92%[d]
Cumulative[a] Clinical Pregnancy[c] Rate	
Cycle 1	28%[d]
Cycle 2	41%[d]
Cycle 3	45%[d]

a Cumulative rates were determined per patient over cycles 1, 2, and 3.
b Non-inferior to comparator recombinant human FSH based on a two-sided 95% confidence interval, intent-to-treat analysis.
c A clinical pregnancy was defined as a pregnancy during which a fetal sac (with or without heart activity) was visualized by ultrasound on day 34-36 after hCG administration.
d Secondary efficacy parameter. Study 22240 was not powered to demonstrate differences in this parameter.

2. Assisted Reproductive Technologies (ART):
Study 21884 was a phase III, assessor-blind, randomized, comparative, multinational, multicenter study in ovulatory, infertile women undergoing stimulation of multiple follicles for Assisted Reproductive Technologies (ART) after pituitary down-regulation with a GnRH agonist. Patients were randomized to either Gonal-f® RFF (n=237), administered subcutaneously, or a comparator recombinant human FSH. Randomization was stratified by insemination technique [conventional *in-vitro* fertilization (IVF) vs. intracytoplasmic sperm injection (ICSI)]. Efficacy was assessed using the mean number of fertilized oocytes the day after insemination. The initial doses of Gonal-f® RFF were 150 IU a day for patients < 35 years old and 225 IU for patients ≥ 35 years old. The maximal dose allowed for both age groups was 450 IU per day. Treatment outcomes for Gonal-f® RFF are summarized in Table 3.

Table 3: Treatment Outcomes in ART Study 21884

	value (n)
Mean number of 2PN oocytes per patient	6.3 (237)[a]
Mean number of 2PN oocytes per patient receiving IVF	6.1 (88)[b]
Mean number of 2PN oocytes per patient receiving ICSI	6.5 (132)[b]
Clinical pregnancy[c] rate per attempt	33.5% (218)[d]
Clinical pregnancy[c] rate per embryo transfer	35.8% (204)[d]
Mean treatment duration in days (range)	9.7 [3-21] (230)[d]

a Non-inferior to comparator recombinant human FSH based on a two-sided 95% confidence interval, intent-to-treat analysis.
b Study 21884 was not powered to demonstrate differences in subgroups.
c A clinical pregnancy was defined as a pregnancy during which a fetal sac (with or without heart activity) was visualized by ultrasound on day 35-42 after hCG administration.
d Secondary efficacy parameter. Study 21884 was not powered to demonstrate differences in this parameter.

INDICATIONS AND USAGE

Gonal-f® RFF Pen (follitropin alfa injection) is indicated for the induction of ovulation and pregnancy in the oligo-anovulatory infertile patient in whom the cause of infertility is functional and not due to primary ovarian failure. Gonal-f® RFF Pen is also indicated for the development of multiple follicles in the ovulatory patient participating in an Assisted Reproductive Technology (ART) program.

Selection of Patients:

1. Before treatment with Gonal-f® RFF Pen is instituted, a thorough gynecologic and endocrinologic evaluation must be performed. This should include an assessment of pelvic anatomy. Patients with tubal obstruction should receive Gonal-f® RFF Pen only if enrolled in an *in vitro* fertilization program.
2. Primary ovarian failure should be excluded by the determination of gonadotropin levels.
3. Appropriate evaluation should be performed to exclude pregnancy.
4. Patients in later reproductive life have a greater predisposition to endometrial carcinoma as well as a higher incidence of anovulatory disorders. A thorough diagnostic evaluation should always be performed in patients who demonstrate abnormal uterine bleeding or other signs of endometrial abnormalities before starting Gonal-f® RFF Pen therapy.
5. Evaluation of the partner's fertility potential should be included in the initial evaluation.

CONTRAINDICATIONS

Gonal-f® RFF Pen (follitropin alfa injection) is contraindicated in women who exhibit:

1. Prior hypersensitivity to recombinant FSH preparations or one of their excipients.
2. High levels of FSH indicating primary gonadal failure.
3. Uncontrolled thyroid or adrenal dysfunction.
4. Sex hormone dependent tumors of the reproductive tract and accessory organs.
5. An organic intracranial lesion such as a pituitary tumor.
6. Abnormal uterine bleeding of undetermined origin (see "Selection of Patients").
7. Ovarian cyst or enlargement of undetermined origin, not due to polycystic ovary syndrome (see "Selection of Patients").
8. Pregnancy.

WARNINGS

Gonal-f® RFF Pen (follitropin alfa injection) should only be used by physicians who are thoroughly familiar with infertility problems and their management.

Gonal-f® RFF Pen is a potent gonadotropic substance capable of causing Ovarian Hyperstimulation Syndrome (OHSS) in women with or without pulmonary or vascular complications. Gonadotropin therapy requires a certain time commitment by physicians and supportive health professionals, and requires the availability of appropriate monitoring facilities (see "Precautions/Laboratory Tests").

Safe and effective use of Gonal-f® RFF Pen in women requires monitoring of ovarian response with serum estradiol and vaginal ultrasound on a regular basis. The lowest effective dose should be used.

Overstimulation of the Ovary During FSH Therapy:

Ovarian Enlargement: Mild to moderate uncomplicated ovarian enlargement which may be accompanied by abdominal distention and/or abdominal pain occurs in approximately 20% of those treated with urofollitropin and hCG, and generally regresses without treatment within two or three weeks. Careful monitoring of ovarian response can further minimize the risk of overstimulation.

If the ovaries are abnormally enlarged on the last day of Gonal-f® RFF Pen therapy, hCG should not be administered in this course of therapy. This will reduce the chances of development of Ovarian Hyperstimulation Syndrome.

Ovarian Hyperstimulation Syndrome (OHSS): OHSS is a medical event distinct from uncomplicated ovarian enlargement. Severe OHSS may progress rapidly (within 24 hours to several days) to become a serious medical event. It is characterized by an apparent dramatic increase in vascular permeability which can result in a rapid accumulation of fluid in the peritoneal cavity, thorax, and potentially, the pericardium. The early warning signs of development of OHSS are severe pelvic pain, nausea, vomiting, and weight gain. The following symptomatology has been seen with cases of OHSS: abdominal pain, abdominal distension, gastrointestinal symptoms including nausea, vomiting and diarrhea, severe ovarian enlargement, weight gain, dyspnea, and oliguria. Clinical evaluation may reveal hypovolemia, hemoconcentration, electrolyte imbalances, ascites, hemoperitoneum, pleural effusions, hydrothorax, acute pulmonary distress, and thromboembolic events (see "Pulmonary and Vascular Complications"). Transient liver function test abnormalities suggestive of hepatic dysfunction, which may be accompanied by morphologic changes on liver biopsy, have been reported in association with Ovarian Hyperstimulation Syndrome (OHSS).

OHSS occurred in 6 of 83 (7.2%) Gonal-f® RFF trea women in Study 22240 (ovulation induction); none w classified as severe.

In Study 21884 (ART), OHSS occurred in 11 of 237 (4. Gonal-f® RFF treated women and 1 (0.42%) was classifiec severe. OHSS may be more severe and more protracte pregnancy occurs. OHSS develops rapidly; therefore, tients should be followed for at least two weeks after h administration. Most often, OHSS occurs after treatm has been discontinued and reaches its maximum at ab seven to ten days following treatment. Usually, OHSS solves spontaneously with the onset of menses. If there evidence that OHSS may be developing prior to hCG adm istration (see "Precautions / Laboratory Tests"), the h(must be withheld.

If severe OHSS occurs, treatment must be stopped and t patient should be hospitalized.

A physician experienced in the management of this sy drome, or who is experienced in the management of flu and electrolyte imbalances should be consulted.

Pulmonary and Vascular Complications:

Serious pulmonary conditions (e.g., atelectasis, acute resp ratory distress syndrome and exacerbation of asthma) ha been reported.

In addition, thromboembolic events both in associatic with, and separate from Ovarian Hyperstimulation Sy drome have been reported. Intravascular thrombosis an embolism can result in reduced blood flow to critical organ or the extremities. Sequelae of such events have include venous thrombophlebitis, pulmonary embolism, pulmonar infarction, cerebral vascular occlusion (stroke), and arteria occlusion resulting in loss of limb. In rare cases, pulmonar complications and/or thromboembolic events have resulte in death.

Multiple Births: Reports of multiple births have been asso ciated with Gonal-f® RFF treatment. In Study 22240 fo women receiving Gonal-f® RFF over three treatment cycles 20% of live births were multiple births. In Study 21884, 35.1% of live births were multiple births in women receiving Gonal-f® RFF. The rate of multiple births is dependent on the number of embryos transferred. The patient should be advised of the potential risk of multiple births before starting treatment.

PRECAUTIONS

General:

Careful attention should be given to the diagnosis of infertility in candidates for Gonal-f® RFF Pen (follitropin alfa injection) therapy (see "Indications and Usage/Selection of Patients").

Information for Patients:

Prior to therapy with Gonal-f® RFF Pen, patients should be informed of the duration of treatment and monitoring of their condition that will be required. The risks of Ovarian Hyperstimulation Syndrome and multiple births in women (see **WARNINGS**) and other possible adverse reactions (see "**Adverse Reactions**") should also be discussed.

A 'Patient's Information Leaflet' is provided for patients prescribed Gonal-f® RFF Pen.

Laboratory Tests:

In most instances, treatment of women with Gonal-f® RFF Pen results only in follicular recruitment and development. In the absence of an endogenous LH surge, hCG is given when monitoring of the patient indicates that sufficient follicular development has occurred.

This may be estimated by ultrasound alone or in combination with measurement of serum estradiol levels. The combination of both ultrasound and serum estradiol measurement are useful for monitoring the development of follicles, for timing of the ovulatory trigger, as well as for detecting ovarian enlargement and minimizing the risk of the Ovarian Hyperstimulation Syndrome and multiple gestation. It is recommended that the number of growing follicles be confirmed using ultrasonography because plasma estrogens do not give an indication of the size or number of follicles.

The clinical confirmation of ovulation, with the exception of pregnancy, is obtained by direct and indirect indices of progesterone production. The indices most generally used are as follows:

1. A rise in basal body temperature;
2. Increase in serum progesterone; and
3. Menstruation following a shift in basal body temperature.

When used in conjunction with the indices of progesterone production, sonographic visualization of the ovaries will assist in determining if ovulation has occurred. Sonographic evidence of ovulation may include the following:

1. Fluid in the cul-de-sac;
2. Ovarian stigmata;
3. Collapsed follicle; and
4. Secretory endometrium.

urate interpretation of the indices of follicle develop-
nt and maturation require a physician who is experi-
ed in the interpretation of these tests.

ug Interactions:
drug/drug interaction studies have been performed.

rcinogenesis, Mutagenesis, Impairment of Fertility:
ng-term studies in animals have not been performed to
aluate the carcinogenic potential of Gonal-f® RFF Pen.
wever, follitropin alfa showed no mutagenic activity in a
ies of tests performed to evaluate its potential genetic
cicity including, bacterial and mammalian cell mutation
ts, a chromosomal aberration test and a micronucleus
t.

paired fertility has been reported in rats, exposed to
armacological doses of follitropin alfa (≥40 IU/kg/day) for
tended periods, through reduced fecundity.

egnancy:
egnancy Category X. See CONTRAINDICATIONS.
rsing Mothers: It is not known whether this drug is ex-
eted in human milk. Because many drugs are excreted in
man milk and because of the potential for serious adverse
actions in the nursing infant from Gonal-f® RFF Pen, a
ecision should be made whether to discontinue nursing or
discontinue the drug, taking into account the importance
f the drug to the mother.

ediatric Use:
afety and effectiveness in pediatric patients have not been
stablished.

ADVERSE REACTIONS

he safety of Gonal-f® RFF was examined in two clinical
tudies [(one ovulation induction study (n=83) and one
tudy in ART (n=237)].
Adverse events (without regard to causality assessment) occurring in at least 2.0% of patients in Study 22240 (ovula-
ion induction) are listed in Table 4.

Table 4: Safety Profile in Ovulation Induction Study 22240

Body System Preferred Term	Patients (%) Experiencing Events Treatment cycles = 176* n=83†
Central and Peripheral Nervous System	
Headache	22 (26.5%)
Dizziness	2 (2.4%)
Migraine	3 (3.6%)
Gastro-intestinal System	
Abdominal Pain	10 (12.0%)
Nausea	3 (3.6%)
Flatulence	3 (3.6%)
Diarrhea	3 (3.6%)
Toothache	3 (3.6%)
Dyspepsia	2 (2.4%)
Constipation	2 (2.4%)
Stomatitis Ulcerative	2 (2.4%)
Neoplasm	
Ovarian Cyst	3 (3.6%)
Reproductive, Female	
Ovarian Hyperstimulation	6 (7.2%)
Breast Pain Female	5 (6.0%)
Vaginal Haemorrhage	5 (6.0%)
Gynecological-related pain	2 (2.4%)
Uterine haemorrhage	2 (2.4%)
Respiratory System	
Sinusitis	5 (6.0%)
Pharyngitis	6 (7.2%)
Rhinitis	6 (7.2%)
Coughing	2 (2.4%)
Application Site	
Injection Site Pain	4 (4.8%)
Injection Site Inflammation	2 (2.4%)
Body as a Whole-General	
Back Pain	3 (3.6%)
Pain	2 (2.4%)
Fever	2 (2.4%)
Hot Flushes	2 (2.4%)
Malaise	2 (2.4%)
Skin and Appendages	
Acne	3 (3.6%)
Urinary System	
Micturition Frequency	2 (2.4%)
Cystitis	2 (2.4%)
Resistance Mechanism	
Infection viral	2 (2.4%)

* up to 3 cycles of therapy
† total patients treated with Gonal-f® RFF

Headache occurred in greater than 20% of patients receiving Gonal-f® RFF in this study.

Adverse events (without regard to causality assessment) occurring in at least 2.0% of patients in Study 21884 (ART)
are listed in Table 5.

Table 5: Safety Profile in Assisted Reproductive Technologies Study 21884

Body System Preferred Term	Patients (%) Experiencing Events n=237†
Gastro-intestinal System	
Abdominal Pain	55 (23.2%)
Nausea	19 (8.0%)
Body as a Whole-General	
Abdomen Enlarged	33 (13.9%)
Pain	7 (3.0%)
Central and Peripheral Nervous System	
Headache	44 (18.6%)
Dizziness	5 (2.1%)
Application Site Disorders	
Injection site bruising	23 (9.7%)
Injection site pain	13 (5.5%)
Injection site inflammation	10 (4.2%)
Injection site reaction	10 (4.2%)
Application site edema	6 (2.5%)
Reproductive, Female	
Ovarian Hyperstimulation	11 (4.6%)
Intermenstrual Bleeding	9 (3.8%)

† total patients treated with Gonal-f® RFF

Headache and abdomen enlargement occurred in more than
10% of patients and abdominal pain occurred in more than
20% of patients.
The following medical events have been reported subsequent to pregnancies resulting from gonadotropin in controlled clinical studies:
1. Spontaneous Abortion
2. Ectopic Pregnancy
3. Premature Labor
4. Postpartum Fever
5. Congenital Abnormalities
There are no indications that use of gonadotropins during
ART is associated with an increased risk of congenital
malformations.
The following adverse reactions have been previously reported during Gonal-f® RFF therapy:
1. Pulmonary and vascular complications (see "WARN-
INGS"),
2. Adnexal torsion (as a complication of ovarian enlargement),
3. Mild to moderate ovarian enlargement,
4. Hemoperitoneum
There have been infrequent reports of ovarian neoplasms,
both benign and malignant, in women who have undergone
multiple drug regimens for ovulation induction; however, a
causal relationship has not been established.
Post Marketing Reports
During post-market surveillance, reports of hypersensitivity reactions including anaphylactoid reactions have been
reported with the use of Gonal-f® RFF.

OVERDOSAGE

Aside from possible ovarian hyperstimulation and multiple
gestations (see "WARNINGS"), there is no information on
the consequences of acute overdosage with Gonal-f® RFF
Pen (follitropin alfa injection).

DOSAGE AND ADMINISTRATION

The Gonal-f® RFF Pen delivery system delivers at least
300 IU, 450 IU, or 900 IU, equivalent to a maximum of four
75 IU injections, six 75 IU injections or twelve 75 IU injections, respectively. The minimum dose that can be set is
37.5 IU; the maximum dose that can be set is 300 IU (for
300 IU delivery system) or 450 IU (for 450 IU and 900 IU
delivery system).
Dosage:
Infertile Patients with Oligo-Anovulation: The dose of
Gonal-f® RFF Pen (follitropin alfa injection) to stimulate development of the follicle must be individualized for each patient.
The lowest dose consistent with the expectation of good results should be used. Over the course of treatment, doses of
Gonal-f® RFF Pen may range up to 300 IU per day depending on the individual patient response. Gonal-f® RFF Pen
should be administered until adequate follicular development is indicated by serum estradiol and vaginal ultrasonography. A response is generally evident after 5 to 7
days. Subsequent monitoring intervals should be based on
individual patient response.
It is recommended that the initial dose of the first cycle be
75 IU of Gonal-f® RFF Pen per day, administered subcuta-

neously. An incremental adjustment in dose of up to 37.5 IU
may be considered after 14 days. Further dose increases of
the same magnitude could be made, if necessary, every
seven days. Treatment duration should not exceed 35 days
unless an E2 rise indicates imminent follicular development. To complete follicular development and effect ovulation in the absence of an endogenous LH surge, chorionic
gonadotropin, hCG, should be given after the last dose of
Gonal-f® RFF Pen. Chorionic gonadotropin should be withheld if the serum estradiol is greater than 2,000 pg/mL. If
the ovaries are abnormally enlarged or abdominal pain occurs, Gonal-f® RFF Pen treatment should be discontinued,
hCG should not be administered, and the patient should be
advised not to have intercourse; this may reduce the chance
of development of the Ovarian Hyperstimulation Syndrome
and, should spontaneous ovulation occur, reduce the chance
of multiple gestation. A follow-up visit should be conducted
in the luteal phase.
The initial dose administered in the subsequent cycles
should be individualized for each patient based on her response in the preceding cycle. Doses larger than 300 IU of
FSH per day are not routinely recommended. As in the initial cycle, hCG must be given after the last dose of Gonal-f®
RFF Pen to complete follicular development and induce ovulation. The precautions described above should be followed
to minimize the chance of development of the Ovarian Hyperstimulation Syndrome.
The couple should be encouraged to have intercourse daily,
beginning on the day prior to the administration of hCG until ovulation becomes apparent from the indices employed
for the determination of progestational activity. Care should
be taken to ensure insemination. In light of the indices and
parameters mentioned, it should become obvious that, unless a physician is willing to devote considerable time to
these patients and be familiar with and conduct the necessary laboratory studies, he/she should not use Gonal-f® RFF
Pen.
Assisted Reproductive Technologies: As in the treatment
of patients with oligo-anovulatory infertility, the dose of
Gonal-f® RFF Pen to stimulate development of the follicle
must be individualized for each patient. For Assisted Reproductive Technologies, therapy with Gonal-f® RFF Pen
should be initiated in the early follicular phase (cycle day 2
or 3) at a dose of 150 IU per day administered subcutaneously, until sufficient follicular development is attained. In
most cases, therapy should not exceed ten days.
In patients undergoing ART under 35 years old, whose endogenous gonadotropin levels are suppressed, Gonal-f® RFF
Pen should be initiated at a dose of 150 IU per day. In patients 35 years old and older whose endogenous gonadotropin levels are suppressed, Gonal- f® RFF Pen should be initiated at a dose of 225 IU per day. Treatment should be
continued until adequate follicular development is indicated
as determined by ultrasound in combination with measurement of serum estradiol levels. Adjustments to dose may be
considered after five days based on the patient's response;
subsequently dosage should be adjusted no more frequently
than every 3-5 days and by no more than 75-150 IU additionally at each adjustment. Doses greater than 450 IU per
day are not recommended. Once adequate follicular development is evident, hCG should be administered to induce
final follicular maturation in preparation for oocyte retrieval. The administration of hCG must be withheld in
cases where the ovaries are abnormally enlarged on the last
day of therapy. This should reduce the chance of developing
OHSS.
Administration:
Administer subcutaneously in the abdomen as described in
the 'Patient's Information Leaflet' provided for patients prescribed Gonal-f® RFF Pen.
Patient Instructions for Use
*Make sure you have all the supplies listed below before
you begin.*
1. Gonal-f® RFF Pen
• Make sure the Gonal-f® RFF Pen is at room temperature
before using.
• Make sure the liquid in the Pen is clear. Do not use the
Gonal-f® RFF Pen if it contains any particles. Get a re-
placement from your doctor, nurse or pharmacist.

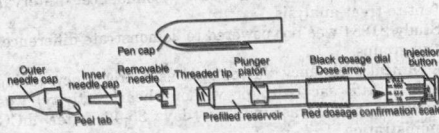

2. One new single-use, disposable administration needle
supplied with the Gonal-f® RFF Pen.
3. Alcohol wipes and gauze pad.
4. Safety container (hard plastic or metal container) to use
for safe disposal of used needles.
Before you start, wash your hands with soap and water. On
a clean surface, layout everything you need.

Preparing the Pen

Note: Read steps 1 through 7 prior to pulling the injection button on the pen. Do not pull the injection button until the dose is dialed and you are ready for injection.

1. Remove the protective Pen cap. Clean threaded tip of Pen with an alcohol swab.

2. Take a single-use disposable needle provided in the Gonal-f® RFF Pen carton. If the peel tab of the needle is damaged or loose, do not use it. Discard the needle and take a new one. Remove the peel tab from the outer needle cap.

3. With the tab removed, hold the outer needle cap firmly in one hand and hold the Pen firmly in the other hand. Press the threaded tip of the Gonal-f® RFF Pen into the open end of the needle cap and twist it clockwise until it is securely fixed.

4. Once the needle is securely attached, remove the outer needle cap by gently pulling it straight off. Do NOT remove the inner needle cap—leave it where it is. Do NOT throw away the outer needle cap—you will need it when you are ready to remove the needle following your injection.

Note: Use only the single-use disposable needles provided within the Gonal-f® RFF Pen carton or compatible needles distributed separately by EMD Serono, Inc.

Step 5 only needs to be performed before the first use of each new Pen; Otherwise, proceed to Step 6.

5. You must prime the Pen before the first use. You only need to prime the first time you use a new Pen. Do the following steps to get your Pen ready for use:

• Check to make sure the dose arrow is set at 37.5. If not, turn the dosage dial (black numbers) to align the dose arrow with 37.5.

• Pull out the injection button as far as it will go.

• Remove the inner needle cap and hold the Pen with the needle pointing upwards.

• Tap the drug reservoir gently with your finger so that any air bubbles rise up towards the needle. (If a few small air bubbles remain, do not worry; this is normal).

• Keep the needle pointing upright and push in the injection button completely. Stop pushing after you hear the first click. A small amount of liquid should come out of the needle indicating that the Pen is ready for use. The amount of liquid seen at the needle tip is part of the extra medicine from the Pen. If no liquid appears the first time, repeat these steps until liquid comes out of the needle tip.

• Replace the inner needle cap.

6. Select your prescribed dose by turning the dosage dial (black numbers) to the proper dose mark on the dial in front of the arrow mark. Carefully check the dosage dial before proceeding. Once you have set the dose correctly, load the Pen by pulling out the injection button straight as far as it will go. Do not twist the injection button while loading the Pen.

7. Check the red dosage confirmation scale on the injection button to ensure the correct dose has been loaded and that the accurate dose will be injected. The loaded dose is shown by the last mark (flat arrow) on the red dosage confirmation scale that is fully visible.

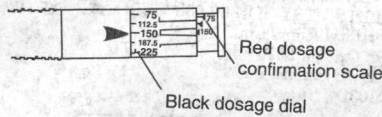

Red dosage confirmation scale

Black dosage dial

• If you accidentally pull out the injection button with an incorrect dose setting, do not inject. If the set dose is lower than the correct dose to be administered, you can turn the dosage dial to the correct dose and pull out the injection button again. If the set dose is higher than the dose to be administered, discard the dose by pushing all the liquid out into the safety container and repeat the previous steps for setting the dose.

Injecting the dose

Suitable injection sites on the stomach will be advised by your fertility specialist. Occasionally, your fertility specialist may suggest an alternative site.

[See figure at top of next column]

8. Clean the injection site with an alcohol swab and allow it to air dry.

9. Remove the inner needle cap from the needle on the Pen. Do not touch the needle or allow the needle to touch any surface.

10. To inject, insert the needle into the skin at a 90° angle and push the injection button—you will hear the button clicking. After the last click, allow the needle to remain in the skin for at least 5 seconds. This will ensure that you inject the full dose.

[See figure at top of next column]

11. After the injection is complete, keep the injection button pressed down and remove the needle out of your skin. Apply pressure using a gauze pad.

12. Each time you finish an injection, remove and discard the used needle as follows. Hold the Gonal-f® RFF Pen firmly by the drug reservoir. Carefully replace the outer

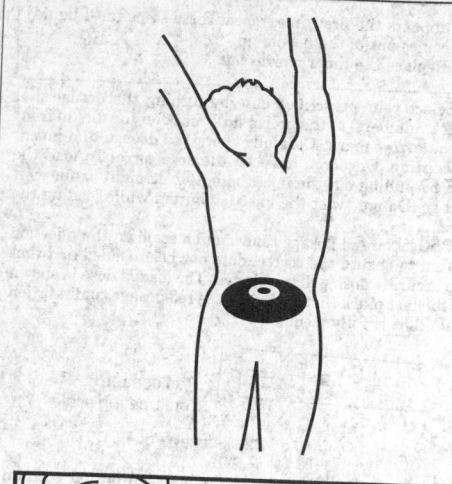

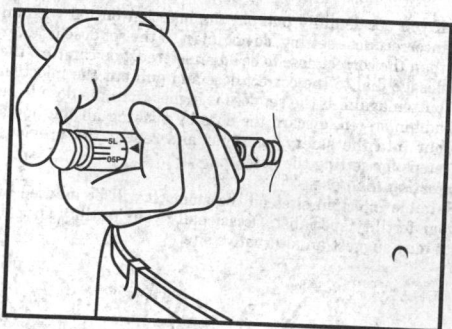

needle cap onto the needle. Gripping the outer needle cap firmly, remove the needle by unscrewing the Pen counter-clockwise and dispose of the needle in your safety container.

13. Replace the Pen cap and store properly. See "HOW SUPPLIED".

Parenteral drug products should be inspected visually for particulate matter and discoloration prior to administration, whenever solution and container permit.

HOW SUPPLIED

Gonal-f® RFF Pen (follitropin alfa injection) is a disposable, prefilled multiple-dose delivery system containing a sterile, ready-to-use liquid formulation of follitropin alfa. Each Gonal-f® RFF Pen is filled with 415 IU, 568 IU, or 1026 IU follitropin alfa to deliver a minimum total of 300 IU in 0.5 mL, 450 IU in 0.75 mL, or 900 IU in 1.5 mL, respectively. Each Pen is supplied in a carton containing 29G × 1/2 inch disposable needles to be used for administration.

The following package combinations are available:

NDC 44087-1113-1 - One Gonal-f® RFF Pen contains 415 IU to deliver a minimum total of 300 IU/0.5 mL and 5 single-use disposable 29G × ½" needles

NDC 44087-1112-1 - One Gonal-f® RFF Pen contains 568 IU to deliver a minimum total of 450 IU/0.75 mL and 7 single-use disposable 29G × ½" needles

NDC 44087-1114-1 - One Gonal-f® RFF Pen contains 1026 IU to deliver a minimum total of 900 IU/1.5 mL and 14 single-use disposable 29G × ½" needles

Store the Gonal-f® RFF Pen refrigerated (2°-8°C/36°-46°F) until dispensed. Upon dispensing, the patient may store the pen refrigerated (2°-8°C/36°-46°F) until the expiration date, or at room temperature (20°-25°C/68°-77°F) for up to three months or until the expiration date, whichever occurs first. After the first injection, the pen may be stored refrigerated (2°-8°C/36°-46°F) or at room temperature (20°-25°C/68°-77°F) for up to 28 days. Protect from light. Do not freeze. Discard unused material after 28 days.

Rx only

Manufactured for: EMD Serono, Inc., Rockland, MA 02370 U.S.A.

Revised: October 2009

PATIENT PACKAGE INSERT

Gonal-f® RFF Pen
(follitropin alfa injection)
*revised formulation female

PATIENT'S INFORMATION LEAFLET

Read the patient information before you start using the Gonal-f® RFF Pen. Read the patient information each time you get a refill, because there may be new information. This leaflet does not take the place of talking with your healthcare provider about your condition or treatment.

WHAT IS THE GONAL-F® RFF PEN?

The Gonal-f® RFF Pen is a prescription injectable medic provided in a device that contains the hormone follicle sti ulating hormone (FSH). FSH helps healthy ovaries to ma eggs in women.

WHAT ARE THE USES OF THE GONAL-F® RFF PEN?

Doctors specializing in infertility or reproductive heal prescribe the Gonal-f® RFF Pen to those patients needi medical assistance to have a child. After a thorough medic exam to determine your specific medical condition, your do tor may prescribe the Gonal-f® RFF Pen because you ne help with producing eggs or you need supplementation part of your treatment program. The Gonal-f® RFF Pen used only for women seeking pregnancy. The Gonal-f® RF Pen may be one of several drugs prescribed to you as part your treatment program.

Gonal-f® RFF Pen is used:

• in certain infertile women to help with ovulation (produ tion and release of a mature egg) and pregnancy. Gonal-RFF Pen will not help women whose ovaries no longe work because of a condition called primary ovarian fai ure.

• in women who are in an Assisted Reproductive Technol ogy (ART) program, such as in vitro fertilization, to hel their ovaries make more eggs.

WHO SHOULD NOT USE GONAL-F® RFF PEN?

Do not use the Gonal-f® RFF Pen if you:

• are allergic to recombinant human FSH products (see th end of this leaflet for a list of all the ingredients in the Gonal-f® RFF Pen)

• have primary ovarian failure (your ovaries no longe make eggs)

• are pregnant or think you may be pregnant

• have uncontrolled thyroid or adrenal problems

• have cancer in your female organs (ovaries, breast, uterus)

• have a pituitary tumor or other tumor in your brain

• have abnormal bleeding from your uterus or vagina

• have ovarian cysts or enlarged ovaries, not due to polycys tic ovary syndrome (PCOS)

TELL YOUR HEALTHCARE PROVIDER IF YOU ARE BREAST-FEEDING

It is not known if Gonal-f® RFF Pen passes into your milk.

CAN YOU USE THE GONAL-F® RFF PEN WITH OTHER MEDICINES?

Inform your doctor and pharmacist if you are taking or have taken any other medicines, including prescription and non-prescription medicines, vitamins, and herbal supplements. It is not known if Gonal-f® RFF Pen and other medicines can affect each other.

STORING THE GONAL-F® RFF PEN BEFORE THE FIRST USE

Store the Gonal-f® RFF Pen refrigerated (36°-46°F/2°-8°C) until dispensed. Upon dispensing, the Pen may be stored by the patient refrigerated (36°-46°F/2°-8°C) until the expiration date, or at room temperature (68°-77°F/20°-25°C) for up to three months or until the expiration date, whichever occurs first. Protect from light. Do not freeze.

HOW SHOULD I USE GONAL-F® RFF PEN?

• Use Gonal-f® RFF Pen exactly as prescribed. Your doctor will prescribe the dose that is right for you and your condition. Do not change the dose of Gonal-f® RFF Pen unless your doctor tells you to. Your doctor or healthcare provider will tell you the number of units (IU FSH) of Gonal-f® RFF Pen to use each day and the number of days to use the same Pen.

• Gonal-f® RFF Pen is given by an injection just under the skin (subcutaneous injection). Your doctor's office will teach you how to inject yourself. See the end of this leaflet for detailed instructions, "How do I prepare and use the Gonal-f® RFF Pen?" Do not inject Gonal-f® RFF Pen at home until your healthcare provider has taught you the correct way.

• Your condition must be closely monitored by your healthcare provider while you are using Gonal-f® RFF Pen. Your doctor may do regular ultrasound tests and blood tests to make sure that Gonal-f® RFF Pen is not making your ovaries too active (hyperstimulation) which can lead to rare, but serious side effects. Your doctor will decide if it is safe for you to continue with your fertility treatments based on the results of these tests.

• If you use too much Gonal-f® RFF Pen, call your doctor right away.

• Do not use Gonal-f® RFF Pen for a condition for which it was not prescribed. Do not give Gonal-f® RFF Pen to other people, even if they have the same symptoms you have.

WHAT ARE THE POSSIBLE SIDE EFFECTS OF THE GONAL-F® RFF PEN?

The most common side effects with the Gonal-f® RFF Pen are headache, stomach pain, stomach bloating, nausea, and ovarian hyperstimulation syndrome. Bruising, pain, and redness can happen at the injection site.

Gonal-f® RFF Pen and other FSH products can cause serious side effects including:

• **Ovarian Hyperstimulation Syndrome (OHSS).** OHSS causes fluid to suddenly build up in the stomach area, chest area, and heart area. Stop using Gonal-f RFF Pen and call your doctor right away if you get severe lower stomach area (pelvic) pain, nausea, vomiting, or weight gain.

Lung and blood vessel problems. FSH products may cause serious lung problems including fluid in the lungs, trouble breathing, and worsening of asthma. Blood vessel problems include blood clots and strokes.

Multiple births. FSH products can cause multiple births. Your healthcare provider will discuss your chances of multiple births.

These are not all the side effects of Gonal-f RFF Pen. As with any medication, report any and all side effects, symptoms, or physical changes to your healthcare provider.

WHAT SHOULD YOU DO IF YOU FORGET TO TAKE YOUR DOSE?

Do NOT double the dose of Gonal-f RFF Pen prescribed. Contact your doctor if you forget to take a dose of Gonal-f RFF Pen.

REVIEW THESE STEPS BEFORE YOU PREPARE OR ADMINISTER GONAL-F RFF PEN.

How do I prepare and use the Gonal-f RFF Pen?
Getting ready
Make sure you have all the supplies listed below before you begin.
1. Gonal-f RFF Pen
• Make sure the Gonal-f RFF Pen is at room temperature before using.
• Make sure the liquid in the Pen is clear. Do not use the Gonal-f RFF Pen if it contains any particles. Get a replacement from your doctor, nurse or pharmacist.

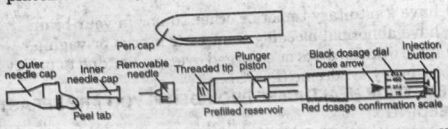

2. One new single-use, disposable administration needle supplied with the Gonal-f RFF Pen.
3. Alcohol wipes and gauze pad.
4. Safety container (hard plastic or metal container) to use for safe disposal of used needles.
Before you start, wash your hands with soap and water. On a clean surface, layout everything you need.

Preparing the Pen
Note: Read steps 1 through 7 prior to pulling the injection button on the pen. Do not pull the injection button until the dose is dialed and you are ready for injection.
1. Remove the protective pen cap. Clean threaded tip of pen with an alcohol swab.
2. Take a single-use disposable needle provided in the Gonal-f RFF Pen carton. If the peel tab of the needle is damaged or loose, do not use it. Discard the needle and take a new one. Remove the peel tab from the outer needle cap.
3. With the tab removed, hold the outer needle cap firmly in one hand and hold the pen firmly in the other hand. Press the threaded tip of the Gonal-f RFF Pen into the open end of the needle cap and twist it clockwise until it is securely fixed.
4. Once the needle is securely attached, remove the outer needle cap by gently pulling it straight off. Do NOT remove the inner needle cap—leave it where it is. Do NOT throw away the outer needle cap—you will need it when you are ready to remove the needle following your injection.
Note: Use only the single-use disposable needles provided within the Gonal-f RFF Pen carton or compatible needles distributed separately by EMD Serono, Inc.

This step only needs to be performed before the first use of each new pen; Otherwise, proceed to Step 6.
5. You must prime the Pen before the first use. You only need to prime the first time you use a new pen. Do the following steps to get your pen ready for use:
• Check to make sure the dose arrow is set at 37.5. If not, turn the dosage dial (black numbers) to align the dose arrow with 37.5.
• Pull out the injection button as far as it will go.
• Remove the inner needle cap and hold the Pen with the needle pointing upwards
• Tap the drug reservoir gently with your finger so that any air bubbles rise up towards the needle. (If a few small air bubbles remain, do not worry; this is normal).
• Keep the needle pointing upright and push in the injection button completely. Stop pushing after you hear the first click. A small amount of liquid should come out of the needle indicating that the pen is ready for use. The amount of liquid seen at the needle tip is part of the extra medicine from the Pen. If no liquid

appears the first time, repeat these steps until liquid comes out of the needle tip.
• Replace the inner needle cap.

6. Select your prescribed dose by turning the dosage dial (black numbers) to the proper dose mark on the dial in front of the arrow mark. Carefully check the dosage dial before proceeding. Once you have set the dose correctly, load the Pen by pulling out the injection button straight as far as it will go. Do not twist the injection button while loading the pen.
7. Check the red dosage confirmation scale on the injection button to ensure the correct dose has been loaded and that the accurate dose will be injected. The loaded dose is shown by the last mark (flat arrow) on the red dosage confirmation scale that is fully visible.

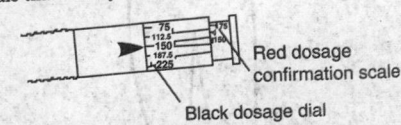

Red dosage confirmation scale

Black dosage dial

• If you accidentally pull out the injection button with an incorrect dose setting, do not inject. If the set dose is lower than the correct dose to be administered, you can turn the dosage dial to the correct dose and pull out the injection button again. If the set dose is higher than the dose to be administered, discard the dose by pushing all the liquid out into the safety container and repeat the previous steps for setting the dose.

Injecting the dose
Suitable injection sites on the stomach will be advised by your fertility specialist. Occasionally, your fertility specialist may suggest an alternative site.

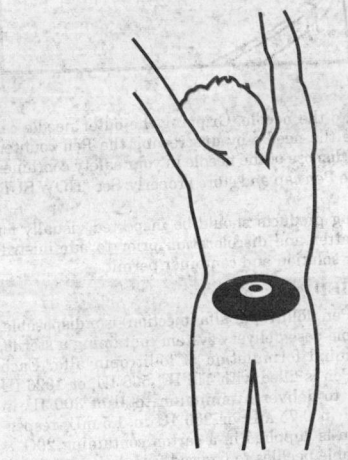

8. Clean the injection site with an alcohol swab and allow it to air dry.
9. Remove the inner needle cap from the needle on the Pen. Do not touch the needle or allow the needle to touch any surface.
10. To inject, insert the needle into the skin at a 90° angle and push the injection button—you will hear the button clicking. After the last click, allow the needle to remain in the skin for at least 5 seconds. This will ensure that you inject the full dose.

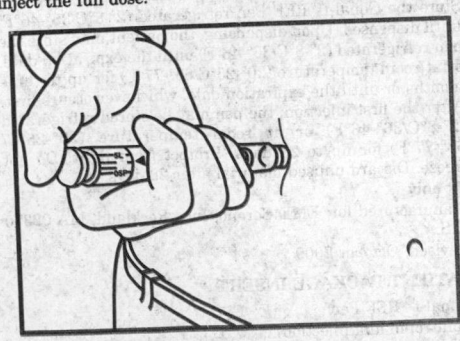

11. After the injection is complete, keep the injection button pressed down and remove the needle out of your skin. Apply pressure using a gauze pad.
12. Each time you finish an injection, remove and discard the used needle as follows. Hold the Gonal-f RFF Pen firmly by the drug reservoir. Carefully replace the outer needle cap onto the needle. Gripping the outer needle cap

firmly, remove the needle by unscrewing the Pen counter-clockwise and dispose of the needle in your safety container.
13. Replace the Pen cap and store properly. See the section "Storing the Gonal-f RFF Pen Between Uses".

If there is not enough medicine remaining in the Gonal-f RFF Pen.
• After several doses, you may not have enough Gonal-f RFF Pen remaining in the Pen to administer another full dose. The red dosage confirmation scale on the injection button enables you to check that the correct dose has been loaded. Dial your dose and pull out the injection button. It will go out only as far as the amount of drug that is left in the Pen. The amount of drug left in the Pen will be indicated by the last mark (flat arrow) on the red dosage confirmation scale that is fully visible. If this amount is lower than the set dose, the amount of Gonal-f RFF Pen left in the Pen is not enough to complete your full dose. If the loaded dose is not sufficient to complete your injection you have two options:
• Inject the partial dose (what is left in the Pen) and then immediately complete the dose with a new Gonal-f RFF Pen, remembering to measure out only what is required to complete your daily dose.
• Discard the Gonal-f RFF Pen and inject the full dose using a new Pen.
• It is common for a small amount of drug to be leftover in the Gonal-f RFF Pen. This is normal. Any drug remaining in the Gonal-f RFF Pen after your treatment is complete should be discarded.

Storing the Gonal-f RFF Pen Between Uses
• After each use, the Gonal-f RFF Pen must be stored away from light and may be stored refrigerated or at room temperature between 36°-77° F (2°-25° C) for up to 28 days.
• Do not store above 77°F (25°C).
• If you are traveling, keep the Gonal-f RFF Pen stored away from light and extreme temperatures. Do not freeze.
• Allow the liquid solution to adjust to room temperature prior to administering your injection.
• Check that the liquid is clear. Do not use if it contains any particles. Report this to your doctor, nurse or pharmacist immediately.
• Keep the Gonal-f RFF Pen and all medicines out of the reach of children.

What are the ingredients in Gonal-f RFF Pen?
Active ingredient: follitropin alfa (r-hFSH)
Inactive ingredients: sucrose, meta-cresol, di-sodium hydrogen phosphate dihydrate, sodium dihydrogen phosphate monohydrate, methionine, Poloxamer 188, O-phosphoric acid and/or sodium hydroxide

Where can more information about the Gonal-f RFF Pen be obtained? This leaflet is a summary of the important patient information about the Gonal-f RFF Pen. If you have any questions or problems, talk to your doctor or other health care provider.

The Gonal-f RFF Pen is manufactured and distributed by EMD Serono, Inc. You can also call toll free 1-866-LETS TRY (1-866-538-7879) or log on to www.fertilitylifelines.com.
Revised: October 2009
©2009 EMD Serono, Inc.
N19Z0103D

℞

NOVANTRONE®
(mitoXANTRONE for injection concentrate)

WARNING
NOVANTRONE® (mitoxantrone for injection concentrate) should be administered under the supervision of a physician experienced in the use of cytotoxic chemotherapy agents.
NOVANTRONE® should be given slowly into a freely flowing intravenous infusion. It must *never* be given subcutaneously, intramuscularly, or intra-arterially. Severe local tissue damage may occur if there is extravasation during administration. (See **ADVERSE REACTIONS, General,** Cutaneous and **DOSAGE AND ADMINISTRATION, Preparation and Administration Precautions).**
NOT FOR INTRATHECAL USE. Severe injury with permanent sequelae can result from intrathecal administration. (See **WARNINGS, General**)
Except for the treatment of acute nonlymphocytic leukemia, NOVANTRONE® therapy generally should not be given to patients with baseline neutrophil counts of less than 1,500 cells/mm³. In order to monitor the occurrence of bone marrow suppression, primarily neutropenia, which may be severe and result in infection, it is recommended that frequent peripheral blood cell counts be performed on all patients receiving NOVANTRONE®.

Cardiotoxicity:
Congestive heart failure (CHF), potentially fatal, may occur either during therapy with NOVANTRONE® or months to years after termination of therapy. Cardiotoxicity risk increases with cumulative NOVANTRONE dose and may occur whether or not cardiac risk factors are present. Presence or history of cardiovascular disease, radiotherapy to the mediastinal/pericardial area, previous therapy with other anthracyclines or anthracenediones, or use of other cardiotoxic drugs may increase this risk. In cancer patients, the risk of symptomatic CHF was estimated to be 2.6% for patients receiving up to a cumulative dose of 140 mg/m^2. To mitigate the cardiotoxicity risk with NOVANTRONE, prescribers should consider the following:

All Patients:
– All patients should be assessed for cardiac signs and symptoms by history, physical examination, and ECG prior to start of NOVANTRONE® therapy.
– All patients should have baseline quantitative evaluation of left ventricular ejection fraction (LVEF) using appropriate methodology (ex. Echocardiogram, multigated radionuclide angiography (MUGA), MRI, etc.).

Multiple Sclerosis Patients:
– MS patients with a baseline LVEF below the lower limit of normal should not be treated with NOVANTRONE®.
– MS patients should be assessed for cardiac signs and symptoms by history, physical examination and ECG prior to each dose.
– MS patients should undergo quantitative reevaluation of LVEF prior to each dose using the same methodology that was used to assess baseline LVEF. Additional doses of NOVANTRONE® should not be administered to multiple sclerosis patients who have experienced either a drop in LVEF to below the lower limit of normal or a clinically significant reduction in LVEF during NOVANTRONE® therapy.
– MS patients should not receive a cumulative NOVANTRONE dose greater than 140 mg/m^2.
– MS patients should undergo yearly quantitative LVEF evaluation after stopping NOVANTRONE to monitor for late occurring cardiotoxicity.

Secondary Leukemia:
NOVANTRONE® therapy in patients with MS and in patients with cancer increases the risk of developing secondary acute myeloid leukemia.

For additional information, see **WARNINGS** and **DOSAGE AND ADMINISTRATION**.

DESCRIPTION

NOVANTRONE® (mitoxantrone hydrochloride) is a synthetic antineoplastic anthracenedione for intravenous use. The molecular formula is $C_{22}H_{28}N_4O_6 \cdot 2HCl$ and the molecular weight is 517.41. It is supplied as a concentrate that MUST BE DILUTED PRIOR TO INJECTION. The concentrate is a sterile, nonpyrogenic, dark blue aqueous solution containing mitoxantrone hydrochloride equivalent to 2 mg/mL mitoxantrone free base, with sodium chloride (0.80% w/v), sodium acetate (0.005% w/v), and acetic acid (0.046% w/v) as inactive ingredients. The solution has a pH of 3.0 to 4.5 and contains 0.14 mEq of sodium per mL. The product does not contain preservatives. The chemical name is 1,4-dihydroxy-5,8-bis[[2-[(2-hydroxyethyl)amino]ethyl]amino]-9,10-anthracenedione dihydrochloride and the structural formula is:

CLINICAL PHARMACOLOGY

Mechanism of Action

Mitoxantrone, a DNA-reactive agent that intercalates into deoxyribonucleic acid (DNA) through hydrogen bonding, causes crosslinks and strand breaks. Mitoxantrone also interferes with ribonucleic acid (RNA) and is a potent inhibitor of topoisomerase II, an enzyme responsible for uncoiling and repairing damaged DNA. It has a cytocidal effect on both proliferating and nonproliferating cultured human cells, suggesting lack of cell cycle phase specificity.
NOVANTRONE® has been shown in vitro to inhibit B cell, T cell, and macrophage proliferation and impair antigen presentation, as well as the secretion of interferon gamma, TNFα, and IL-2.

Pharmacokinetics

Pharmacokinetics of mitoxantrone in patients following a single intravenous administration of NOVANTRONE can be characterized by a three-compartment model. The mean alpha half-life of mitoxantrone is 6 to 12 minutes, the mean beta half-life is 1.1 to 3.1 hours and the mean gamma (terminal or elimination) half-life is 23 to 215 hours (median approximately 75 hours). Pharmacokinetic studies have not been performed in humans receiving multiple daily dosing. Distribution to tissues is extensive: steady-state volume of distribution exceeds 1,000 L/m^2. Tissue concentrations of mitoxantrone appear to exceed those in the blood during the terminal elimination phase. In the healthy monkey, distribution to brain, spinal cord, eye, and spinal fluid is low.
In patients administered 15-90 mg/m^2 of NOVANTRONE intravenously, there is a linear relationship between dose and the area under the concentration-time curve (AUC). Mitoxantrone is 78% bound to plasma proteins in the observed concentration range of 26-455 ng/mL. This binding is independent of concentration and is not affected by the presence of phenytoin, doxorubicin, methotrexate, prednisone, prednisolone, heparin, or aspirin.

Metabolism and Elimination

Mitoxantrone is excreted in urine and feces as either unchanged drug or as inactive metabolites. In human studies, 11% and 25% of the dose were recovered in urine and feces, respectively, as either parent drug or metabolite during the 5-day period following drug administration. Of the material recovered in urine, 65% was unchanged drug. The remaining 35% was composed of monocarboxylic and dicarboxylic acid derivatives and their glucuronide conjugates. The pathways leading to the metabolism of NOVANTRONE have not been elucidated.

Special Populations

Gender
The effect of gender on mitoxantrone pharmacokinetics is unknown.

Geriatric
In elderly patients with breast cancer, the systemic mitoxantrone clearance was 21.3 L/hr/m^2, compared with 28.3 L/hr/m^2 and 16.2 L/hr/m^2 for non-elderly patients with nasopharyngeal carcinoma and malignant lymphoma, respectively.

Pediatric
Mitoxantrone pharmacokinetics in the pediatric population are unknown.

Race
The effect of race on mitoxantrone pharmacokinetics is unknown.

Renal Impairment
Mitoxantrone pharmacokinetics in patients with renal impairment are unknown.

Hepatic Impairment
Mitoxantrone clearance is reduced by hepatic impairment. Patients with severe hepatic dysfunction (bilirubin > 3.4 mg/dL) have an AUC more than three times greater than that of patients with normal hepatic function receiving the same dose. Patients with multiple sclerosis who have hepatic impairment should ordinarily not be treated with NOVANTRONE. Other patients with hepatic impairment should be treated with caution and dosage adjustment may be required.

Drug Interactions: In vitro drug interaction studies have demonstrated that mitoxantrone did not inhibit CYP450 1A2, 2A6, 2C9, 2C19, 2D6, 2E1, and 3A4 across a broad concentration range. The results of in vitro induction studies are inconclusive, but suggest that mitoxantrone may be a weak inducer of CYP450 2E1 activity.
Pharmacokinetic studies of the interaction of NOVANTRONE with concomitantly administered medications in humans have not been performed. The pathways leading to the metabolism of NOVANTRONE have not been elucidated. To date, post-marketing experience has not revealed any significant drug interactions in patients who have received NOVANTRONE for treatment of cancer. Information on drug interactions in patients with multiple sclerosis is limited.

CLINICAL TRIALS

Multiple Sclerosis

The safety and efficacy of NOVANTRONE in multiple sclerosis were assessed in two randomized, multicenter clinical studies.
One randomized, controlled study (Study 1) was conducted in patients with secondary progressive or progressive relapsing multiple sclerosis. Patients in this study demonstrated significant neurological disability based on the Kurtzke Expanded Disability Status Scale (EDSS). The EDSS is an ordinal scale with 0.5 point increments ranging from 0.0 to 10.0 (increasing score indicates worsening) and based largely on ambulatory impairment in its middle range (EDSS 4.5 to 7.5 points). Patients in this study had experienced a mean deterioration in EDSS of about 1.6 points over the 18 months prior to enrollment.
Patients were randomized to receive placebo, 5 mg/m^2 NOVANTRONE, or 12 mg/m^2 NOVANTRONE administered IV every 3 months for 2 years. High-dose methylprednisolone was administered to treat relapses. The intent-to-treat analysis cohort consisted of 188 patients; 149 completed the 2-year study. Patients were evaluated every 3 months, and clinical outcome was determined after 24 months. In addition, a subset of patients was assessed with magnetic resonance imaging (MRI) at baseline, Month 12, and Month 24. Neurologic assessments and MRI reviews were performed by evaluators blinded to study drug and clinical outcome, although the diagnosis of relapse and the decision to treat relapses with steroids were made by unblinded treating physicians. A multivariate analysis of five clinical variables (EDSS, Ambulation Index [AI], number of relapses requiring treatment with steroids, months to first relapse needing treatment with steroids, and Standard Neurological Status [SNS]) was used to determine primary efficacy. The AI is an ordinal scale ranging from 0 to 9 in one point increments to define progressive ambulatory impairment. The SNS provides an overall measure of neurologic impairment and disability, with scores ranging from 0 (normal neurologic examination) to 99 (worst possible score).
Results of Study 1 are summarized in Table 1.
[See table 1 above]
A second randomized, controlled study (Study 2) evaluated NOVANTRONE in combination with methylprednisolone (MP) and was conducted in patients with secondary progressive or worsening relapsing-remitting multiple sclerosis who had residual neurological deficit between relapses. All

Table 1 Efficacy Results at Month 24 Study 1

Primary Endpoints	Placebo (N = 64)	NOVANTRONE 5 mg/m^2 (N = 64)	NOVANTRONE 12 mg/m^2 (N = 60)	p-value Placebo vs 12 mg/m^2 NOVANTRONE
Primary efficacy multivariate analysis*	-	-	-	< 0.0001
Primary clinical variables analyzed:				
EDSS change** (mean)	0.23	−0.23	−0.13	0.0194
Ambulation Index change** (mean)	0.77	0.41	0.30	0.0306
Mean number of relapses per patient requiring corticosteroid treatment (adjusted for discontinuation)	1.20	0.73	0.40	0.0002
Months to first relapse requiring corticosteroid treatment (median [1st quartile])	14.2 [6.7]	NR [6.9]	NR [20.4]	0.0004
Standard Neurological Status change** (mean)	0.77	−0.38	−1.07	0.0269
MRI‡				
No. of patients with new Gd-enhancing lesions	5/32 (16%)	4/37 (11%)	0/31	0.022
Change in number of T2-weighted lesions, mean (n)**	1.94 (32)	0.68 (34)	0.29 (28)	0.027

NR = not reached within 24 months; MRI = magnetic resonance imaging.
* Wei-Lachin test.
** Month 24 value minus baseline.
‡ A subset of 110 patients was selected for MRI analysis. MRI results were not available for all patients at all time points.

Table 2 Efficacy Results Study 2

mary Endpoint	MP alone (N = 21)	NOV + MP (N = 21)	p-value
tients (%) without new Gd-enhancing lesions on MRIs (primary endpoint)*	5 (31%)	19 (90%)	0.001
condary Endpoints			
)SS change (Month 6 minus baseline)* (mean)	−0.1	−1.1	0.013
nualized relapse rate (mean per patient)	3.0	0.7	0.003
tients (%) without relapses	7 (33%)	14 (67%)	0.031

P = methylprednisolone; NOV + MP = NOVANTRONE plus methylprednisolone.
Results at Month 6, not including data for 5 withdrawals in the MP alone group.

Table 3 Response Rates, Time to Response, and Survival in U.S. and International Trials

rial	% Complete Response (CR)		Median Time to CR (days)		Survival (days)	
	NOV	DAUN	NOV	DAUN	NOV	DAUN
.S.	63 (62/98)	53 (54/102)	35	42	312	237
nternational	50 (56/112)	51 (62/123)	36	42	192	230

IOV = NOVANTRONE® + cytarabine
AUN = daunorubicin + cytarabine

patients had experienced at least two relapses with sequelae or neurological deterioration within the previous 12 months. The average deterioration in EDSS was 2.2 points during the previous 12 months. During the screening period, patients were treated with two monthly doses of 1 g of IV MP and underwent monthly MRI scans. Only patients who developed at least one new Gd-enhancing MRI lesion during the 2-month screening period were eligible for randomization. A total of 42 evaluable patients received monthly treatments of 1 g of IV MP alone (n = 21) or ~12 mg/m² of IV NOVANTRONE plus 1 g of IV MP (n = 21) (NOV + MP) for 6 months. Patients were evaluated monthly, and study outcome was determined after 6 months. The primary measure of effectiveness in this study was a comparison of the proportion of patients in each treatment group who developed no new Gd-enhancing MRI lesions at 6 months; these MRIs were assessed by a blinded panel. Additional outcomes were measured, including EDSS and number of relapses, but all clinical measures in this trial were assessed by an unblinded treating physician. Five patients, all in the MP alone arm, failed to complete the study due to lack of efficacy.

The results of this trial are displayed in Table 2.

[See table 2 above]

Advanced Hormone-Refractory Prostate Cancer

A multicenter Phase 2 trial of NOVANTRONE and low-dose prednisone (N + P) was conducted in 27 symptomatic patients with hormone-refractory prostate cancer. Using NPCP (National Prostate Cancer Project) criteria for disease response, there was one partial responder and 12 patients with stable disease. However, nine patients or 33% achieved a palliative response defined on the basis of reduction in analgesic use or pain intensity.

These findings led to the initiation of a randomized multicenter trial (CCI-NOV22) comparing the effectiveness of (N + P) to low-dose prednisone alone (P). Eligible patients were required to have metastatic or locally advanced disease that had progressed on standard hormonal therapy, a castrate serum testosterone level, and at least mild pain at study entry. NOVANTRONE was administered at a dose of 12 mg/m² by short IV infusion every 3 weeks. Prednisone was administered orally at a dose of 5 mg twice a day. Patients randomized to the prednisone arm were crossed over to the N + P arm if they progressed or if they were not improved after a minimum of 6 weeks of therapy with prednisone alone.

A total of 161 patients were randomized, 80 to the N + P arm and 81 to the P arm. The median NOVANTRONE dose administered was 12 mg/m² per cycle. The median cumulative NOVANTRONE dose administered was 73 mg/m² (range of 12 to 212 mg/m²).

A primary palliative response (defined as a 2-point decrease in pain intensity in a 6-point pain scale, associated with stable analgesic use, and lasting a minimum of 6 weeks) was achieved in 29% of patients randomized to N + P compared to 12% of patients randomized to P alone (p = 0.011). Two responders left the study after meeting primary response criterion for two consecutive cycles. For the purposes of this analysis, these two patients were assigned a response duration of zero days. A secondary palliative response was defined as a 50% or greater decrease in analgesic use, associated with stable pain intensity, and lasting a minimum of 6 weeks. An overall palliative response (defined as primary plus secondary responses) was achieved in 38% of patients randomized to N + P compared to 21% of patients randomized to P (p = 0.025).

The median duration of primary palliative response for patients randomized to N + P was 7.6 months compared to 2.1 months for patients randomized to P alone (p = 0.0009). The median duration of overall palliative response for patients randomized to N + P was 5.6 months compared to 1.9 months for patients randomized to P alone (p = 0.0004).

Time to progression was defined as a 1-point increase in pain intensity, or a > 25% increase in analgesic use, or evidence of disease progression on radiographic studies, or requirement for radiotherapy. The median time to progression for all patients randomized to N + P was 4.4 months compared to 2.3 months for all patients randomized to P alone (p = 0.0001). Median time to death was 11.3 months for all patients on the N + P arm compared to 10.8 months for all patients on P alone (p = 0.2324).

Forty-eight patients on the P arm crossed over to receive N + P. Of these, thirty patients had progressed on P, while 18 had stable disease on P. The median cycle of crossover was 5 cycles (range of 2 to 16 cycles). Time trends for pain intensity prior to crossover were significantly worse for patients who crossed over than for those who remained on P alone (p = 0.012). Nine patients (19%) demonstrated a palliative response on N + P after crossover. The median time to death for patients who crossed over to N + P was 12.7 months.

The clinical significance of a fall in prostate-specific antigen (PSA) concentrations after chemotherapy is unclear. On the CCI-NOV22 trial, a PSA fall of 50% or greater for two consecutive follow-up assessments after baseline was reported in 33% of all patients randomized to the N + P arm and 9% of all patients randomized to the P arm. These findings should be interpreted with caution since PSA responses were not defined prospectively. A number of patients were inevaluable for response, and there was an imbalance between treatment arms in the numbers of evaluable patients. In addition, PSA reduction did not correlate precisely with palliative response, the primary efficacy endpoint of this study. For example, among the 26 evaluable patients randomized to the N + P arm who had a ≥ 50% reduction in PSA, only 13 had a primary palliative response. Also, among 42 evaluable patients on this arm who did not have this reduction in PSA, 8 nonetheless had a primary palliative response.

Investigators at Cancer and Leukemia Group B (CALGB) conducted a Phase 3 comparative trial of NOVANTRONE plus hydrocortisone (N + H) versus hydrocortisone alone (H) in patients with hormone-refractory prostate cancer (CALGB 9182). Eligible patients were required to have metastatic disease that had progressed despite at least one hormonal therapy. Progression at study entry was defined on the basis of progressive symptoms, increases in measurable or osseous disease, or rising PSA levels. NOVANTRONE was administered intravenously at a dose of 14 mg/m² every 21 days and hydrocortisone was administered orally at a daily dose of 40 mg. A total of 242 subjects were randomized, 119 to the N + H arm and 123 to the H arm. There were no differences in survival between the two arms, with a median of 11.1 months in the N + H arm and 12 months in the H arm (p = 0.3298).

Using NPCP criteria for response, partial responses were achieved in 10 patients (8.4%) randomized to the N + H arm compared with 2 patients (1.6%) randomized to the H arm (p = 0.018). The median time to progression, defined by NPCP criteria, for patients randomized to the N + H arm was 7.3 months compared to 4.1 months for patients randomized to H alone (p = 0.0654).

Approximately 60% of patients on each arm required analgesics at baseline. Analgesic use was measured in this study using a 5-point scale. The best percent change from baseline in mean analgesic use was -17% for 61 patients with available data on the N + H arm, compared with +17% for 61 patients on H alone (p = 0.014). A time trend analysis for analgesic use in individual patients also showed a trend favoring the N + H arm over H alone but was not statistically significant.

Pain intensity was measured using the Symptom Distress Scale (SDS) Pain Item 2 (a 5-point scale). The best percent change from baseline in mean pain intensity was -14% for 37 patients with available data on the N + H arm, compared with +8% for 38 patients on H alone (p = 0.057). A time trend analysis for pain intensity in individual patients showed no difference between treatment arms.

Acute Nonlymphocytic Leukemia

In two large randomized multicenter trials, remission induction therapy for acute nonlymphocytic leukemia (ANLL) with NOVANTRONE 12 mg/m² daily for 3 days as a 10-minute intravenous infusion and cytarabine 100 mg/m² for 7 days given as a continuous 24-hour infusion was compared with daunorubicin 45 mg/m² daily by intravenous infusion for 3 days plus the same dose and schedule of cytarabine used with NOVANTRONE. Patients who had an incomplete antileukemic response received a second induction course in which NOVANTRONE or daunorubicin was administered for 2 days and cytarabine for 5 days using the same daily dosage schedule. Response rates and median survival information for both the U.S. and international multicenter trials are given in Table 3:

[See table 3 at left]

In these studies, two consolidation courses were administered to complete responders on each arm. Consolidation therapy consisted of the same drug and daily dosage used for remission induction, but only 5 days of cytarabine and 2 days of NOVANTRONE or daunorubicin were given. The first consolidation course was administered 6 weeks after the start of the final induction course if the patient achieved a complete remission. The second consolidation course was generally administered 4 weeks later. Full hematologic recovery was necessary for patients to receive consolidation therapy. For the U.S. trial, median granulocyte nadirs for patients receiving NOVANTRONE + cytarabine for consolidation courses 1 and 2 were 10/mm³ for both courses, and for those patients receiving daunorubicin + cytarabine nadirs were 170/mm³ and 260/mm³, respectively. Median platelet nadirs for patients who received NOVANTRONE + cytarabine for consolidation courses 1 and 2 were 17,000/mm³ and 14,000/mm³, respectively, and were 33,000/mm³ and 22,000/mm³ in courses 1 and 2 for those patients who received daunorubicin + cytarabine. The benefit of consolidation therapy in ANLL patients who achieve a complete remission remains controversial. However, in the only well-controlled prospective, randomized multicenter trials with NOVANTRONE in ANLL, consolidation therapy was given to all patients who achieved a complete remission. During consolidation in the U.S. study, two myelosuppression-related deaths occurred on the NOVANTRONE arm and one on the daunorubicin arm. However, in the international study there were eight deaths on the NOVANTRONE arm during consolidation which were related to the myelosuppression and none on the daunorubicin arm where less myelosuppression occurred.

INDICATIONS AND USAGE

NOVANTRONE is indicated for reducing neurologic disability and/or the frequency of clinical relapses in patients with secondary (chronic) progressive, progressive relapsing, or worsening relapsing-remitting multiple sclerosis (i.e., patients whose neurologic status is significantly abnormal between relapses). NOVANTRONE is not indicated in the treatment of patients with primary progressive multiple sclerosis.

The clinical patterns of multiple sclerosis in the studies were characterized as follows: secondary progressive and progressive relapsing disease were characterized by gradual increasing disability with or without superimposed clinical relapses, and worsening relapsing-remitting disease was characterized by clinical relapses resulting in a step-wise worsening of disability.

NOVANTRONE in combination with corticosteroids is indicated as initial chemotherapy for the treatment of patients with pain related to advanced hormone-refractory prostate cancer.

NOVANTRONE in combination with other approved drug(s) is indicated in the initial therapy of acute nonlymphocytic leukemia (ANLL) in adults. This category includes myelogenous, promyelocytic, monocytic, and erythroid acute leukemias.

CONTRAINDICATIONS

NOVANTRONE is contraindicated in patients who have demonstrated prior hypersensitivity to it.

WARNINGS

WHEN NOVANTRONE IS USED IN HIGH DOSES (> 14 mg/m²/d × 3 days) SUCH AS INDICATED FOR THE TREATMENT OF LEUKEMIA, SEVERE MYELOSUPPRESSION WILL OCCUR. THEREFORE, IT IS RECOMMENDED THAT NOVANTRONE BE ADMINISTERED ONLY BY PHYSICIANS EXPERIENCED IN THE CHEMOTHERAPY OF THIS DISEASE. LABORATORY AND SUPPORTIVE SERVICES MUST BE AVAILABLE FOR HEMATOLOGIC AND CHEMISTRY MONITORING AND ADJUNCTIVE THERAPIES, INCLUDING ANTIBIOTICS. BLOOD AND BLOOD PRODUCTS MUST BE AVAILABLE TO SUPPORT PATIENTS DURING THE EXPECTED PERIOD OF MEDULLARY HYPOPLASIA AND SEVERE MYELOSUPPRESSION. PARTICULAR CARE SHOULD BE GIVEN TO ASSURING FULL HEMATOLOGIC RECOVERY BEFORE UNDERTAKING CONSOLIDATION THERAPY (IF THIS TREATMENT IS USED) AND PATIENTS SHOULD BE MONITORED CLOSELY DURING THIS PHASE. NOVANTRONE ADMINISTERED AT ANY DOSE CAN CAUSE MYELOSUPPRESSION.

General

Patients with preexisting myelosuppression as the result of prior drug therapy should not receive NOVANTRONE unless it is felt that the possible benefit from such treatment warrants the risk of further medullary suppression.

The safety of NOVANTRONE (mitoxantrone for injection concentrate) in patients with hepatic insufficiency is not established (see **CLINICAL PHARMACOLOGY**).

Safety for use by routes other than intravenous administration has not been established.

NOVANTRONE is not indicated for subcutaneous, intramuscular, or intra-arterial injection. There have been reports of local/regional neuropathy, some irreversible, following intra-arterial injection.

NOVANTRONE must not be given by intrathecal injection. There have been reports of neuropathy and neurotoxicity, both central and peripheral, following intrathecal injection. These reports have included seizures leading to coma and severe neurologic sequelae, and paralysis with bowel and bladder dysfunction.

Topoisomerase II inhibitors, including NOVANTRONE, have been associated with the development of secondary acute myeloid leukemia and myelosuppression.

Cardiac Effects

Because of the possible danger of cardiac effects in patients previously treated with daunorubicin or doxorubicin, the benefit-to-risk ratio of NOVANTRONE therapy in such patients should be determined before starting therapy.

Functional cardiac changes including decreases in left ventricular ejection fraction (LVEF) and irreversible congestive heart failure can occur with NOVANTRONE. Cardiac toxicity may be more common in patients with prior treatment with anthracyclines, prior mediastinal radiotherapy, or with preexisting cardiovascular disease. Such patients should have regular cardiac monitoring of LVEF from the initiation of therapy. Cancer patients who received cumulative doses of 140 mg/m² either alone or in combination with other chemotherapeutic agents had a cumulative 2.6% probability of clinical congestive heart failure. In comparative oncology trials, the overall cumulative probability rate of moderate or severe decreases in LVEF at this dose was 13%.

Multiple Sclerosis

Changes in cardiac function may occur in patients with multiple sclerosis treated with NOVANTRONE. In one controlled trial (Study 1, see **CLINICAL TRIALS, Multiple Sclerosis**), two patients (2%) of 127 receiving NOVANTRONE, one receiving a 5 mg/m² dose and the other receiving the 12 mg/m² dose, had LVEF values that decreased to below 50%. An additional patient receiving 12 mg/m², who did not have LVEF measured, had a decrease in another echocardiographic measurement of ventricular function (fractional shortening) that led to discontinuation from the trial (see **ADVERSE REACTIONS, Multiple Sclerosis**). There were no reports of congestive heart failure in either controlled trial.

MS patients should be assessed for cardiac signs and symptoms by history, physical examination, ECG, and quantitative LVEF evaluation using appropriate methodology (ex. Echocardiogram, MUGA, MRI, etc.) prior to the start of NOVANTRONE therapy. MS patients with a baseline LVEF below the lower limit of normal should not be treated with NOVANTRONE. Subsequent LVEF and ECG evaluations are recommended if signs or symptoms of congestive heart failure develop and prior to every dose administered to MS patients. NOVANTRONE should not be administered to MS patients who experience a reduction in LVEF to below the lower limit of normal, to those who experience a clinically significant reduction in LVEF, or to those who have received a cumulative lifetime dose of 140 mg/m². MS patients should have yearly quantitative LVEF evaluation after stopping NOVANTRONE to monitor for late-occurring cardiotoxicity.

Leukemia

Acute congestive heart failure may occasionally occur in patients treated with NOVANTRONE for ANLL. In first-line comparative trials of NOVANTRONE + cytarabine vs daunorubicin + cytarabine in adult patients with previously untreated ANLL, therapy was associated with congestive heart failure in 6.5% of patients on each arm. A causal relationship between drug therapy and cardiac effects is difficult to establish in this setting since myocardial function is frequently depressed by the anemia, fever and infection, and hemorrhage that often accompany the underlying disease.

Hormone-Refractory Prostate Cancer

Functional cardiac changes such as decreases in LVEF and congestive heart failure may occur in patients with hormone-refractory prostate cancer treated with NOVANTRONE. In a randomized comparative trial of NOVANTRONE plus low-dose prednisone vs low-dose prednisone, 7 of 128 patients (5.5%) treated with NOVANTRONE had a cardiac event defined as any decrease in LVEF below the normal range, congestive heart failure (n = 3), or myocardial ischemia. Two patients had a prior history of cardiac disease. The total NOVANTRONE dose administered to patients with cardiac effects ranged from > 48 to 212 mg/m².

Among 112 patients evaluable for safety on the NOVANTRONE + hydrocortisone arm of the CALGB trial, 18 patients (19%) had a reduction in cardiac function, 5 patients (5%) had cardiac ischemia, and 2 patients (2%) experienced pulmonary edema. The range of total NOVANTRONE doses administered to these patients is not available.

Pregnancy

NOVANTRONE may cause fetal harm when administered to a pregnant woman. Women of childbearing potential should be advised to avoid becoming pregnant. Mitoxantrone is considered a potential human teratogen because of its mechanism of action and the developmental effects demonstrated by related agents. Treatment of pregnant rats during the organogenesis period of gestation was associated with fetal growth retardation at doses ≥ 0.1 mg/kg/day (0.01 times the recommended human dose on a mg/m² basis). When pregnant rabbits were treated during organogenesis, an increased incidence of premature delivery was observed at doses ≥ 0.1 mg/kg/day (0.01 times the recommended human dose on a mg/m² basis). No teratogenic effects were observed in these studies, but the maximum doses tested were well below the recommended human dose (0.02 and 0.05 times in rats and rabbits, respectively, on a mg/m² basis). There are no adequate and well-controlled studies in pregnant women. Women with multiple sclerosis who are biologically capable of becoming pregnant should have a pregnancy test prior to each dose, and the results should be known prior to administration of the drug. If this drug is used during pregnancy or if the patient becomes pregnant while taking this drug, the patient should be apprised of the potential risk to the fetus.

Secondary Leukemia

NOVANTRONE® therapy increases the risk of developing secondary leukemia in patients with cancer and in patients with multiple sclerosis.

In a study of patients with prostate cancer, acute myeloid leukemia occurred in 1% (5/487) of mitoxantrone-treated patients versus no cases in the control group (0/496) not receiving mitoxantrone at 4.7 years followup.

In a prospective, open-label, tolerability and safety monitoring study of NOVANTRONE® treated MS patients followed for up to five years (median of 2.8 years), leukemia occurred in 0.6% (3/509) of patients. Publications describe leukemia risks of 0.25% to 2.8% in cohorts of patients with MS treated with NOVANTRONE® and followed for varying periods of time. This leukemia risk exceeds the risk of leukemia in the general population. The most commonly reported types were acute promyelocytic leukemia and acute myelocytic leukemia.

In 1774 patients with breast cancer who received NOVANTRONE concomitantly with other cytotoxic agents and radiotherapy, the cumulative risk of developing treatment-related acute myeloid leukemia was estimated as 1.1% and 1.6% at 5 and 10 years, respectively. The second largest report involved 449 patients with breast cancer treated with NOVANTRONE, usually in combination with radiotherapy and/or other cytotoxic agents. In this study, the cumulative probability of developing secondary leukemia was estimated to be 2.2% at 4 years.

Secondary acute myeloid leukemia has also been reported in cancer patients treated with anthracyclines. NOVANTRONE is an anthracenedione, a related drug. T occurrence of secondary leukemia is more common when thracyclines are given in combination with DNA-damagi antineoplastic agents, when patients have been heavily p treated with cytotoxic drugs, or when doses of anthra clines have been escalated.

Symptoms of acute leukemia may include excessive bru ing, bleeding, and recurrent infections.

PRECAUTIONS

General

Therapy with NOVANTRONE should be accompanied close and frequent monitoring of hematologic and chemic laboratory parameters, as well as frequent patient observ tion.

Systemic infections should be treated concomitantly with just prior to commencing therapy with NOVANTRONE.

Information for Patients

NOVANTRONE may impart a blue-green color to the urin for 24 hours after administration, and patients should b advised to expect this during therapy. Bluish discoloratio of the sclera may also occur. Patients should be advised c the signs and symptoms of myelosuppression.

Patients with multiple sclerosis should be provided with th Patient Package Insert at the time that the decision is mad to treat with NOVANTRONE and prior to and in close tem poral proximity to each treatment. In addition, the physi cian should discuss the issues addressed in the Patien Package Insert with the patient.

Laboratory Tests

A complete blood count, including platelets, should be obtained prior to each course of NOVANTRONE and in the event that signs and symptoms of infection develop. Liver function tests should also be performed prior to each course of therapy. NOVANTRONE therapy in multiple sclerosis patients with abnormal liver function tests is not recommended because NOVANTRONE clearance is reduced by hepatic impairment and no laboratory measurement can predict drug clearance and dose adjustments.

In leukemia treatment, hyperuricemia may occur as a result of rapid lysis of tumor cells by NOVANTRONE. Serum uric acid levels should be monitored and hypouricemic therapy instituted prior to the initiation of antileukemic therapy.

Women with multiple sclerosis who are biologically capable of becoming pregnant, even if they are using birth control, should have a pregnancy test, and the results should be known, before receiving each dose of NOVANTRONE (see **WARNINGS, Pregnancy**).

Carcinogenesis, Mutagenesis, Impairment of Fertility

Carcinogenesis

Intravenous treatment of rats and mice, once every 21 days for 24 months, with NOVANTRONE resulted in an increased incidence of fibroma and external auditory canal tumors in rats at a dose of 0.03 mg/kg (0.02 fold the recommended human dose, on a mg/m² basis), and hepatocellular adenoma in male mice at a dose of 0.1 mg/kg (0.03 fold the recommended human dose, on a mg/m² basis). Intravenous treatment of rats, once every 21 days for 12 months with NOVANTRONE resulted in an increased incidence of external auditory canal tumors in rats at a dose of 0.3 mg/kg (0.15 fold the recommended human dose, on a mg/m² basis).

Mutagenesis

NOVANTRONE was clastogenic in the in vivo rat bone marrow assay. NOVANTRONE was also clastogenic in two in vitro assays; it induced DNA damage in primary rat hepatocytes and sister chromatid exchanges in Chinese hamster ovary cells. NOVANTRONE was mutagenic in bacterial and mammalian test systems (Ames/Salmonella and E. coli and L5178Y TK+/-mouse lymphoma).

Drug Interactions

Mitoxantrone and its metabolites are excreted in bile and urine, but it is not known whether the metabolic or excretory pathways are saturable, may be inhibited or induced, or if mitoxantrone and its metabolites undergo enterohepatic circulation. To date, post-marketing experience has not revealed any significant drug interactions in patients who have received NOVANTRONE for treatment of cancer. Information on drug interactions in patients with multiple sclerosis is limited.

Following concurrent administration of NOVANTRONE with corticosteroids, no evidence of drug interactions has been observed.

Special Populations

Hepatic Impairment

Patients with multiple sclerosis who have hepatic impairment should ordinarily not be treated with NOVANTRONE. NOVANTRONE should be administered with caution to other patients with hepatic impairment. In patients with severe hepatic impairment, the AUC is more than three times greater than the value observed in patients with normal hepatic function.

Pregnancy

Pregnancy Category D (see **WARNINGS**).

Table 4a Adverse Events of Any Intensity Occurring in ≥ 5% of Patients on Any Dose of NOVANTRONE and That Were Numerically Greater Than in the Placebo Group Study 1

	Percent of Patients		
Preferred Term	Placebo (N = 64)	5 mg/m² NOVANTRONE (N = 65)	12 mg/m² NOVANTRONE (N = 62)
Nausea	20	55	76
Alopecia	31	38	61
Menstrual disorder*	26	51	61
Amenorrhea*	3	28	43
Upper respiratory tract infection	52	51	53
Urinary tract infection	13	29	32
Stomatitis	8	15	19
Arrhythmia	8	6	18
Diarrhea	11	25	16
Urine abnormal	6	5	11
ECG abnormal	3	5	11
Constipation	6	14	10
Back pain	5	6	8
Sinusitis	2	3	6
Headache	5	6	6

Percentage of female patients.

Table 4b Laboratory Abnormalities Occurring in ≥ 5% of Patients* on Either Dose of NOVANTRONE and That Were More Frequent Than in the Placebo Group Study 1

	Percent of Patients		
Event	Placebo (N = 64)	5 mg/m² NOVANTRONE® (N = 65)	12 mg/m² NOVANTRONE® (N = 62)
Leukopenia[a]	0	9	19
Gamma-GT increased	3	3	15
SGOT increased	8	9	8
Granulocytopenia[b]	2	6	6
Anemia	2	9	6
SGPT increased	3	6	5

*Assessed using World Health Organization (WHO) toxicity criteria.
a. < 4000 cells/mm³
b. < 2000 cells/mm³

Table 5a Adverse Events of Any Intensity Occurring in > 5% of Patients* in the NOVANTRONE Group and Numerically More Frequent Than in the Control Group Study 2

	Percent of Patients	
Event	MP (n = 21)	N + MP (n = 21)
Amenorrhea[a]	0	53
Alopecia	0	33
Nausea	0	29
Asthenia	0	24
Pharyngitis/throat infection	5	19
Gastralgia/stomach burn/epigastric pain	5	14
Aphthosis	0	10
Cutaneous mycosis	0	10
Rhinitis	0	10
Menorrhagia[a]	0	7

N = NOVANTRONE, MP = methylprednisolone
*Assessed using National Cancer Institute (NCI) common toxicity criteria.
a. Percentage of female patients.

Table 5b Laboratory Abnormalities Occurring in > 5% of Patients* in the NOVANTRONE Group and Numerically More Frequent Than in the Control Group Study 2

	Percent of Patients	
Event	MP (n = 21)	N + MP (n = 21)
WBC low[a]	14	100
ANC low[b]	10	100
Lymphocytes low	43	95
Hemoglobin low	48	43
Platelets low[c]	0	33
SGOT high	5	15
SGPT high	10	15
Glucose high	5	10
Potassium low	0	10

N = NOVANTRONE, MP = methylprednisolone.
*Assessed using National Cancer Institute (NCI) common toxicity criteria.
a. < 4000 cells/mm³
b. < 1500 cells/mm³
c. < 100,000 cells/mm³

Nursing Mothers

NOVANTRONE is excreted in human milk and significant concentrations (18 ng/mL) have been reported for 28 days after the last administration. Because of the potential for serious adverse reactions in infants from NOVANTRONE, breast feeding should be discontinued before starting treatment.

Pediatric Use:

Safety and effectiveness in pediatric patients have not been established.

Geriatric Use:

Multiple Sclerosis: Clinical studies of Novantrone did not include sufficient numbers of patients aged 65 and over to determine whether they respond differently from younger patients. Other reported clinical experience has not identified differences in responses between the elderly and younger patients.

Hormone-Refractory Prostate Cancer: One hundred forty-six patients aged 65 and over and 52 younger patients (<65 years) have been treated with Novantrone in controlled clinical studies. These studies did not include sufficient numbers of younger patients to determine whether they respond differently from older patients. However, greater sensitivity of some older individuals cannot be ruled out.

Acute Nonlymphocytic Leukemia: Although definitive studies with Novantrone have not been performed in geriatric patients with ANLL, toxicity may be more frequent in the elderly. Elderly patients are more likely to have age-related comorbidities due to disease or disease therapy.

ADVERSE REACTIONS

Multiple Sclerosis

NOVANTRONE has been administered to 149 patients with multiple sclerosis in two randomized clinical trials, including 21 patients who received NOVANTRONE in combination with corticosteroids.

In Study 1, the proportion of patients who discontinued treatment due to an adverse event was 9.7% (n = 6) in the 12 mg/m² NOVANTRONE arm (leukopenia, depression, decreased LV function, bone pain and emesis, renal failure, and one discontinuation to prevent future complications from repeated urinary tract infections) compared to 3.1% (n = 2) in the placebo arm (hepatitis and myocardial infarction). The following clinical adverse experiences were significantly more frequent in the NOVANTRONE groups: nausea, alopecia, urinary tract infection, and menstrual disorders, including amenorrhea.

Table 4a summarizes clinical adverse events of all intensities occurring in ≥ 5% of patients in either dose group of NOVANTRONE and that were numerically greater on drug than on placebo in Study 1. The majority of these events were of mild to moderate intensity, and nausea was the only adverse event that occurred with severe intensity in more than one patient (three patients [5%] in the 12 mg/m² group). Of note, alopecia consisted of mild hair thinning. Two of the 127 patients treated with NOVANTRONE in Study 1 had decreased LVEF to below 50% at some point during the 2 years of treatment. An additional patient receiving 12 mg/m² did not have LVEF measured, but had another echocardiographic measure of ventricular function (fractional shortening) that led to discontinuation from the study.

[See table 4a above]

The proportion of patients experiencing any infection during Study 1 was 67% for the placebo group, 85% for the 5 mg/m² group, and 81% for the 12 mg/m² group. However, few of these infections required hospitalization: one placebo patient (tonsillitis), three 5 mg/m² patients (enteritis, urinary tract infection, viral infection), and four 12 mg/m² patients (tonsillitis, urinary tract infection [two], endometritis).

Table 4b summarizes laboratory abnormalities that occurred in ≥ 5% of patients in either NOVANTRONE dose group, and that were numerically more frequent than in the placebo group.

[See table 4b above]

There was no difference among treatment groups in the incidence or severity of hemorrhagic events.

In Study 2, NOVANTRONE was administered once a month. Clinical adverse events most frequently reported in the NOVANTRONE group included amenorrhea (53% of female patients), alopecia (33% of patients), nausea (29% of patients), and asthenia (24% of patients). Tables 5a and 5b respectively summarize adverse events and laboratory abnormalities occurring in > 5% of patients in the NOVANTRONE group and numerically more frequent than in the control group.

Leukopenia and neutropenia were reported in the N + MP group (see Table 5b). Neutropenia occurred within 3 weeks after NOVANTRONE administration and was always reversible. Only mild to moderate intensity infections were reported in 9 of 21 patients in the N +MP group and in 3 of 21 patients in the MP group; none of these required hospitalization. There was no difference among treatment groups in the incidence or severity of hemorrhagic events. There were no withdrawals from Study 2 for safety reasons.

Leukemia

NOVANTRONE has been studied in approximately 600 patients with acute non-lymphocytic leukemia (ANLL). Table 6 represents the adverse reaction experience in the large U.S. comparative study of mitoxantrone + cytarabine vs daunorubicin + cytarabine. Experience in the large international study was similar. A much wider experience in a variety of other tumor types revealed no additional important reactions other than cardiomyopathy (see **WARNINGS**). It should be appreciated that the listed adverse reaction categories include overlapping clinical symptoms related to the same condition, e.g., dyspnea, cough and pneumonia. In addition, the listed adverse reactions cannot all necessarily be attributed to chemotherapy as it is often impossible to distinguish effects of the drug and effects of the underlying disease. It is clear, however, that the combination of NOVANTRONE + cytarabine was responsible for nausea and vomiting, alopecia, mucositis/stomatitis, and myelosuppression.

Table 6 summarizes adverse reactions occurring in patients treated with NOVANTRONE + cytarabine in comparison with those who received daunorubicin + cytarabine for therapy of ANLL in a large multicenter randomized prospective U.S. trial.

Adverse reactions are presented as major categories and selected examples of clinically significant subcategories.

[See table 6 at top of next page]

Hormone-Refractory Prostate Cancer

Detailed safety information is available for a total of 353 patients with hormone-refractory prostate cancer treated with NOVANTRONE, including 274 patients who received NOVANTRONE in combination with corticosteroids.

Table 7 summarizes adverse reactions of all grades occurring in ≥ 5% of patients in Trial CCI-NOV22.

Table 7 Adverse Events of Any Intensity Occurring in ≥ 5% of Patients Trial CCI-NOV22

Event	N + P (n = 80) %	P (n = 81) %
Nausea	61	35
Fatigue	39	14
Alopecia	29	0
Anorexia	25	6
Constipation	16	14
Dyspnea	11	5
Nail bed changes	11	0
Edema	10	4
Systemic infection	10	7
Mucositis	10	0
UTI	9	4
Emesis	9	5
Pain	8	9
Fever	6	3
Hemorrhage/bruise	6	1
Anemia	5	3
Cough	5	0
Decreased LVEF	5	0
Anxiety/depression	5	3
Dyspepsia	5	6
Skin infection	5	3
Blurred vision	3	5

N = NOVANTRONE, P = prednisone.

No nonhematologic adverse events of Grade 3/4 were seen in > 5% of patients.

Table 8 summarizes adverse events of all grades occurring in ≥ 5% of patients in Trial CALGB 9182.

[See table 8 at top of next page]

General

Allergic Reaction

Hypotension, urticaria, dyspnea, and rashes have been reported occasionally. Anaphylaxis/anaphylactoid reactions have been reported rarely.

Cutaneous

Extravasation at the infusion site has been reported, which may result in erythema, swelling, pain, burning, and/or blue discoloration of the skin. Extravasation can result in tissue necrosis with resultant need for debridement and skin grafting. Phlebitis has also been reported at the site of the infusion.

Hematologic

Topoisomerase II inhibitors, including NOVANTRONE, in combination with other antineoplastic agents or alone, have been associated with the development of acute leukemia (see **WARNINGS**).

Leukemia

Myelosuppression is rapid in onset and is consistent with the requirement to produce significant marrow hypoplasia in order to achieve a response in acute leukemia. The incidences of infection and bleeding seen in the U.S. trial are consistent with those reported for other standard induction regimens.

Hormone-Refractory Prostate Cancer

In a randomized study where dose escalation was required for neutrophil counts greater than 1000/mm³, Grade 4 neutropenia (ANC < 500 /mm³) was observed in 54% of patients treated with NOVANTRONE + low-dose prednisone. In a separate randomized trial where patients were treated with 14 mg/m², Grade 4 neutropenia in 23% of patients treated with NOVANTRONE + hydrocortisone was observed. Neutropenic fever/infection occurred in 11% and 10% of patients receiving NOVANTRONE + corticosteroids, respectively, on the two trials. Platelets < 50,000/mm³ were noted in 4% and 3% of patients receiving NOVANTRONE + corticosteroids on these trials, and there was one patient death on NOVANTRONE + hydrocortisone due to intracranial hemorrhage after a fall.

Gastrointestinal

Nausea and vomiting occurred acutely in most patients and may have contributed to reports of dehydration, but were generally mild to moderate and could be controlled through the use of antiemetics. Stomatitis/mucositis occurred within 1 week of therapy.

Cardiovascular

Congestive heart failure, tachycardia, EKG changes including arrhythmias, chest pain, and asymptomatic decreases in left ventricular ejection fraction have occurred (See **WARNINGS**).

Pulmonary

Interstitial pneumonitis has been reported in cancer patients receiving combination chemotherapy that included NOVANTRONE.

Table 6 Adverse Events Occurring in ANLL Patients Receiving NOVANTRONE or Daunorubicin

Event	Induction [% pts entering induction] NOV N = 102	Induction [% pts entering induction] DAUN N = 102	Consolidation [% pts entering induction] NOV N = 55	Consolidation [% pts entering induction] DAUN N = 49
Cardiovascular				
CHF	26	28	11	24
Arrhythmias	5	6	0	0
Bleeding	3	3	4	4
GI	37	41	20	6
Petechiae/ecchymoses	16	12	2	2
Gastrointestinal	7	9	11	2
Nausea/vomiting	88	85	58	51
Diarrhea	72	67	31	31
Abdominal pain	47	47	18	8
Mucositis/stomatitis	15	9	9	4
Hepatic	29	33	18	8
Jaundice	10	11	14	2
Infections	3	8	7	0
UTI	66	73	60	43
Pneumonia	7	2	7	6
Sepsis	9	7	9	0
Fungal infections	34	36	31	18
Renal failure	15	13	9	6
Fever	8	6	0	2
Alopecia	78	71	24	18
Pulmonary	37	40	22	16
Cough	43	43	24	14
Dyspnea	13	9	9	2
CNS	18	20	6	0
Seizures	30	30	34	35
Headache	4	4	2	8
Eye	10	9	13	8
Conjunctivitis	7	6	2	4
	5	1	0	0

NOV = NOVANTRONE, DAUN = daunorubicin.

OVERDOSAGE

There is no known specific antidote for NOVANTRONE. Accidental overdoses have been reported. Four patients receiving 140-180 mg/m² as a single bolus injection died as a result of severe leukopenia with infection. Hematologic support and antimicrobial therapy may be required during prolonged periods of severe myelosuppression.

Although patients with severe renal failure have not been studied, NOVANTRONE is extensively tissue bound and it is unlikely that the therapeutic effect or toxicity would be mitigated by peritoneal or hemodialysis.

DOSAGE AND ADMINISTRATION

(See also **WARNINGS**)

Multiple Sclerosis

The recommended dosage of NOVANTRONE is 12 mg/m² given as a short (approximately 5 to 15 minutes) intravenous infusion every 3 months. Left ventricular ejection fraction (LVEF) should be evaluated by echocardiogram or MUGA prior to administration of the initial dose of NOVANTRONE and all subsequent doses. In addition, LVEF evaluations are recommended if signs or symptoms of congestive heart failure develop at any time during treatment with NOVANTRONE NOVANTRONE should not be administered to multiple sclerosis patients with an LVEF <50%, with a clinically significant reduction in LVEF, or to those who have received a cumulative lifetime dose of ≥ 140 mg/m².

Complete blood counts, including platelets, should be monitored prior to each course of NOVANTRONE and in the event that signs or symptoms of infection develop. NOVANTRONE generally should not be administered to multiple sclerosis patients with neutrophil counts less than 1500 cells/mm³. Liver function tests should also be monitored prior to each course. NOVANTRONE therapy in multiple sclerosis patients with abnormal liver function tests is not recommended because NOVANTRONE clearance is reduced by hepatic impairment and no laboratory measurement can predict drug clearance and dose adjustments.

Women with multiple sclerosis who are biologically capable of becoming pregnant, even if they are using birth control, should have a pregnancy test, and the results should be known, before receiving each dose of NOVANTRONE (see **WARNINGS, Pregnancy**).

Hormone-Refractory Prostate Cancer

Based on data from two Phase 3 comparative trials of NOVANTRONE plus corticosteroids versus corticosteroids alone, the recommended dosage of NOVANTRONE is 12 or 14 mg/m² given as a short intravenous infusion every 21 days.

Combination Initial Therapy for ANLL in Adults

For induction, the recommended dosage is 12 mg/m² of NOVANTRONE daily on Days 1-3 given as an intravenous infusion, and 100 mg/m² of cytarabine for 7 days given as a continuous 24-hour infusion on Days 1-7.

Most complete remissions will occur following the initial course of induction therapy. In the event of an incomplete antileukemic response, a second induction course may be given. NOVANTRONE should be given for 2 days and cytarabine for 5 days using the same daily dosage levels. If severe or life-threatening nonhematologic toxicity is observed during the first induction course, the second induction course should be withheld until toxicity resolves.

Consolidation therapy which was used in two large randomized multicenter trials consisted of NOVANTRONE, 12 mg/m² given by intravenous infusion daily on Days 1 and 2 and cytarabine, 100 mg/m² for 5 days given as a continuous 24-hour infusion on Days 1-5. The first course was given approximately 6 weeks after the final induction course; the second was generally administered 4 weeks after the first. Severe myelosuppression occurred. (See **CLINICAL PHARMACOLOGY**)

Hepatic Impairment

For patients with hepatic impairment, there is at present no laboratory measurement that allows for dose adjustment recommendations. (See **CLINICAL PHARMACOLOGY, Special Populations**, Hepatic Impairment)

Preparation and Administration Precautions

NOVANTRONE CONCENTRATE MUST BE DILUTED PRIOR TO USE.

Parenteral drug products should be inspected visually for particulate matter and discoloration prior to administration whenever solution and container permit.

The dose of NOVANTRONE should be diluted to at least 50 mL with either 0.9% Sodium Chloride Injection (USP) or 5% Dextrose Injection (USP). NOVANTRONE may be further diluted into Dextrose 5% in Water, Normal Saline or Dextrose 5% with Normal Saline and used immediately. DO NOT FREEZE.

NOVANTRONE should not be mixed in the same infusion as heparin since a precipitate may form. Because specific compatibility data are not available, it is recommended that NOVANTRONE not be mixed in the same infusion with other drugs. The diluted solution should be introduced slowly into the tubing as a freely running intravenous infusion of 0.9% Sodium Chloride Injection (USP) or 5% Dextrose Injection (USP) over a period of not less than 3 minutes. Unused infusion solutions should be discarded immediately in an appropriate fashion. In the case of multidose use, after penetration of the stopper, the remaining portion of the undiluted NOVANTRONE concentrate should

Table 8 Adverse Events of Any Intensity Occurring in ≥ 5 % of Patients Trial CALGB 9182

Event	N + H (n = 112)		H (n = 113)	
	n	%	n	%
creased WBC	96	87	4	4
normal granulocytes/bands	88	79	3	3
creased hemoglobin	83	75	42	39
normal lymphocytes count	78	72	27	25
in	45	41	44	39
normal platelet count	43	39	8	7
normal alkaline phosphatase	41	37	42	38
alaise/fatigue	37	34	16	14
yperglycemia	33	31	32	30
lema	31	30	15	14
ausea	28	26	9	8
norexia	24	22	16	14
bnormal BUN	24	22	22	20
bnormal Transaminase	22	20	16	14
lopecia	20	20	1	1
bnormal Cardiac function	19	18	0	0
nfection	18	17	4	4
Weight loss	18	17	13	12
yspnea	16	15	9	8
iarrhea	16	14	4	4
ever in absence of infection	15	14	7	6
Weight gain	15	14	16	15
Abnormal creatinine	14	13	11	10
Other gastrointestinal	13	14	11	11
Vomiting	12	11	6	5
Other neurologic	11	11	5	5
Hypocalcemia	11	10	5	5
Hematuria	10	11	5	6
Hyponatremia	9	9	3	3
Sweats	9	9	3	2
Other liver	9	9	2	2
Stomatitis	8	8	8	8
Cardiac dysrhythmia	8	7	1	3
Hypokalemia	7	7	3	4
Neuro/constipation	7	7	4	4
Neuro/motor disorder	7	7	2	2
Neuro/mood disorder	6	6	3	3
Skin disorder	6	6	4	4
Cardiac ischemia	5	5	1	0
Chills	5	5	0	3
Hemorrhage	5	5	3	3
Myalgias/arthralgias	5	5	3	3
Other kidney/bladder	5	6	3	4
Other endocrine	5	5	3	3
Other pulmonary	4	4	5	5
Hypertension	4	7	2	3
Impotence/libido	4	6	2	3
Proteinuria	3	5	2	3
Sterility				

N= NOVANTRONE, H= hydrocortisone

be stored not longer than 7 days between 15°-25°C (59°-77°F) or 14 days under refrigeration. DO NOT FREEZE. CONTAINS NO PRESERVATIVE.

Care in the administration of NOVANTRONE will reduce the chance of extravasation. NOVANTRONE should be administered into the tubing of a freely running intravenous infusion of 0.9% Sodium Chloride Injection, USP or 5% Dextrose Injection, USP. The tubing should be attached to a Butterfly needle or other suitable device and inserted preferably into a large vein. If possible, avoid veins over joints or in extremities with compromised venous or lymphatic drainage. Care should be taken to avoid extravasation at the infusion site and to avoid contact of NOVANTRONE with the skin, mucous membranes, or eyes. NOVANTRONE SHOULD NOT BE ADMINISTERED SUBCUTANEOUSLY. If any signs or symptoms of extravasation have occurred, including burning, pain, pruritis, erythema, swelling, blue discoloration, or ulceration, the injection or infusion should be immediately terminated and restarted in another vein. During intravenous administration of NOVANTRONE extravasation may occur with or without an accompanying stinging or burning sensation even if blood returns well on aspiration of the infusion needle. If it is known or suspected that subcutaneous extravasation has occurred, it is recommended that intermittent ice packs be placed over the area of extravasation and that the affected extremity be elevated. Because of the progressive nature of extravasation reactions, the area of injection should be frequently examined and surgery consultation obtained early if there is any sign of a local reaction.

Skin accidentally exposed to NOVANTRONE should be rinsed copiously with warm water and if the eyes are involved, standard irrigation techniques should be used immediately. The use of goggles, gloves, and protective gowns is recommended during preparation and administration of the drug.

Procedures for proper handling and disposal of anticancer drugs should be considered. Several guidelines on this subject have been published.[1-4] There is no general agreement that all of the procedures recommended in the guidelines are necessary or appropriate.

REFERENCES

1. NIOSH Alert: Preventing occupational exposures to antineoplastic and other hazardous drugs in healthcare settings. 2004. U.S. Department of Health and Human Services, Public Health Service, Centers for Disease Control and Prevention, National Institute for Occupational Safety and Health, DHHS (NIOSH) Publication No. 2004-165.
2. OSHA Technical Manual, TED 1-0.15A, Section VI: Chapter 2. Controlling Occupational Exposure to Hazardous Drugs. OSHA, 1999. http://www.osha.gov/dts/osta/otm_vi_2.html.
3. American Society of Health-System Pharmacists. (2006) ASHP Guidelines on Handling Hazardous Drugs.
4. Polovich, M., White, J.M., & Kelleher, L.O. (eds.) 2005. Chemotherapy and biotherapy guidelines and recommendations for practice (2nd ed.) Pittsburgh, PA: Oncology Nursing Society.

HOW SUPPLIED

NOVANTRONE® (mitoxantrone for injection concentrate) is a sterile aqueous solution containing mitoxantrone hydrochloride at a concentration equivalent to 2 mg mitoxantrone free base per mL supplied in vials for multidose use as follows:

NDC 44087-1520-1 - 20 mg/10 mL/multidose vial (2 mg/mL)

NOVANTRONE® (mitoxantrone for injection concentrate) should be stored between 15°-25°C (59°-77°F). DO NOT FREEZE.

Issue Date: June 2010

Manufactured for: EMD Serono, Inc. Rockland, MA 02370 USA

Marketed by:
(OSI)™ oncology
For oncology

Marketed by:
EMD Serono, Inc.
For multiple sclerosis

REBIF®
[rē'-bif]
(interferon beta-1a)

℞

DESCRIPTION

Rebif® (interferon beta-1a) is a purified 166 amino acid glycoprotein with a molecular weight of approximately 22,500 daltons. It is produced by recombinant DNA technology using genetically engineered Chinese Hamster Ovary cells into which the human interferon beta gene has been introduced. The amino acid sequence of Rebif® is identical to that of natural fibroblast derived human interferon beta. Natural interferon beta and interferon beta-1a (Rebif®) are glycosylated with each containing a single N-linked complex carbohydrate moiety.

Using a reference standard calibrated against the World Health Organization natural interferon beta standard (Second International Standard for Interferon, Human Fibroblast GB 23 902 531), Rebif® has a specific activity of approximately 270 million international units (MIU) of antiviral activity per mg of interferon beta-1a determined specifically by an in vitro cytopathic effect bioassay using WISH cells and Vesicular Stomatitis virus. Rebif® 8.8 mcg, 22 mcg and 44 mcg contain approximately 2.4 MIU, 6 MIU or 12 MIU, respectively, of antiviral activity using this method.

Rebif® (interferon beta-1a) is formulated as a sterile solution in a prefilled syringe intended for subcutaneous (sc) injection. Each 0.5 mL (0.5 cc) of Rebif® contains either 22 mcg or 44 mcg of interferon beta-1a, 2 or 4 mg albumin (human) USP, 27.3 mg mannitol USP, 0.4 mg sodium acetate, Water for Injection USP. Each 0.2 mL (0.2 cc) of Rebif® contains 8.8 mcg of interferon beta-1a, 0.8 mg albumin (human) USP, 10.9 mg mannitol USP, 0.16 mg sodium acetate, and Water for Injection USP.

CLINICAL PHARMACOLOGY

General

Interferons are a family of naturally occurring proteins that are produced by eukaryotic cells in response to viral infection and other biological inducers. Interferons possess immunomodulatory, antiviral and antiproliferative biological activities. They exert their biological effects by binding to specific receptors on the surface of cells. Three major groups of interferons have been distinguished: alpha, beta, and gamma. Interferons alpha and beta form the Type I interferons and interferon gamma is a Type II interferon. Type I interferons have considerably overlapping but also distinct biological activities. Interferon beta is produced naturally by various cell types including fibroblasts and macrophages. Binding of interferon beta to its receptors initiates a complex cascade of intracellular events that leads to the expression of numerous interferon-induced gene products and markers, including 2', 5'-oligoadenylate synthetase, beta 2-microglobulin and neopterin, which may mediate some of the biological activities. The specific interferon-induced proteins and mechanisms by which interferon beta-1a exerts its effects in multiple sclerosis have not been fully defined.

Pharmacokinetics

The pharmacokinetics of Rebif® (interferon beta-1a) in people with multiple sclerosis have not been evaluated. In healthy volunteer subjects, a single subcutaneous (sc) injection of 60 mcg of Rebif® (liquid formulation), resulted in peak serum concentration (C_{max}) of 5.1 ± 1.7 IU/mL (mean $\pm$ SD), with a median time of peak serum concentration (T_{max}) of 16 hours. The serum elimination half-life ($t_{1/2}$) was 69 ± 37 hours, and the area under the serum concentration versus time curve (AUC) from zero to 96 hours was 294 ± 81 IU•h/mL. Following every other day sc injections in healthy volunteer subjects, an increase in AUC of approximately 240% was observed, suggesting that accumulation of interferon beta-1a occurs after repeat administration. Total clearance is approximately 33-55 L/hour. There have been no observed gender-related effects on pharmacokinetic parameters. Pharmacokinetics of Rebif® in pediatric and geriatric patients or patients with renal or hepatic insufficiency have not been established.

Pharmacodynamics

Biological response markers (e.g., 2',5'-OAS activity, neopterin and beta 2-microglobulin) are induced by interferon beta-1a following parenteral doses administered to healthy volunteer subjects and to patients with multiple sclerosis.

Following a single sc administration of 60 mcg of Rebif® intracellular 2′,5′-OAS activity peaked between 12 to 24 hours and beta-2-microglobulin and neopterin serum concentrations showed a maximum at approximately 24 to 48 hours. All three markers remained elevated for up to four days. Administration of Rebif® 22 mcg three times per week (tiw) inhibited mitogen-induced release of pro-inflammatory cytokines (IFN-γ, IL-1, IL-6, TNF-α and TNF-β) by peripheral blood mononuclear cells that, on average, was near double that observed with Rebif® administered once per week (qw) at either 22 or 66 mcg.

The relationships between serum interferon beta-1a levels and measurable pharmacodynamic activities to the mechanism(s) by which Rebif® exerts its effects in multiple sclerosis are unknown. No gender-related effects on pharmacodynamic parameters have been observed.

CLINICAL STUDIES

Two multicenter studies evaluated the safety and efficacy of Rebif® in patients with relapsing-remitting multiple sclerosis.

Study 1 was a randomized, double-blind, placebo controlled study in patients with multiple sclerosis for at least one year, Kurtzke Expanded Disability Status Scale (EDSS) scores ranging from 0 to 5, and at least 2 acute exacerbations in the previous 2 years.(1) Patients with secondary progressive multiple sclerosis were excluded from the study. Patients received sc injections of either placebo (n = 187), Rebif® 22 mcg (n = 189), or Rebif® 44 mcg (n = 184) administered tiw for two years. Doses of study agents were progressively increased to their target doses during the first 4 to 8 weeks for each patient in the study (see **DOSAGE AND ADMINISTRATION**).

The primary efficacy endpoint was the number of clinical exacerbations. Numerous secondary efficacy endpoints were also evaluated and included exacerbation-related parameters, effects of treatment on progression of disability and magnetic resonance imaging (MRI)-related parameters. Progression of disability was defined as an increase in the EDSS score of at least 1 point sustained for at least 3 months. Neurological examinations were completed every 3 months, during suspected exacerbations, and coincident with MRI scans. All patients underwent proton density T2-weighted (PD/T2) MRI scans at baseline and every 6 months. A subset of 198 patients underwent PD/T2 and T1-weighted gadolinium-enhanced (Gd)-MRI scans monthly for the first 9 months. Of the 560 patients enrolled, 533 (95%) provided 2 years of data and 502 (90%) received 2 years of study agent.

Study results are shown in Table 1 and Figure 1. Rebif® at doses of 22 mcg and 44 mcg administered sc tiw significantly reduced the number of exacerbations per patient as compared to placebo. Differences between the 22 mcg and 44 mcg groups were not significant (p >0.05).

The exact relationship between MRI findings and the clinical status of patients is unknown. Changes in lesion area often do not correlate with changes in disability progression. The prognostic significance of the MRI findings in these studies has not been evaluated.

[See table above]

The time to onset of progression in disability sustained for three months was significantly longer in patients treated with Rebif® than in placebo-treated patients. The Kaplan-Meier estimates of the proportions of patients with sustained disability are depicted in Figure 1.

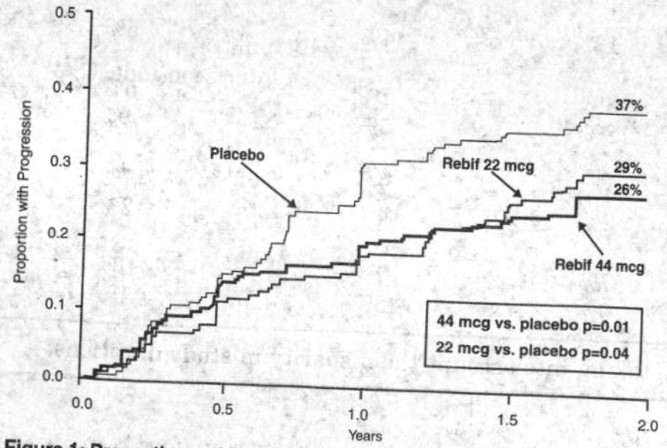

Figure 1: Proportions of Patients with Sustained Disability Progression

The safety and efficacy of treatment with Rebif® beyond 2 years have not been established.

Study 2 was a randomized, open-label, evaluator-blinded, active comparator study.(2) Patients with relapsing-remitting multiple sclerosis with EDSS scores ranging from 0 to 5.5, and at least 2 exacerbations in the previous 2 years were eligible for inclusion. Patients with secondary progressive multiple sclerosis were excluded from the study. Patients were randomized to treatment with Rebif® 44 mcg tiw by sc injection (n=339) or Avonex® 30 mcg qw by intramuscular (im) injection (n=338). Study duration was 48 weeks.

Table 1: Clinical and MRI Endpoints from Study 1

	Placebo	22 mcg tiw	44 mcg tiw
	n = 187	n = 189	n = 184
Exacerbation-related			
Mean number of exacerbations per patient over 2 years[1,2] (Percent reduction)	2.56	1.82** (29%)	1.73*** (32%)
Percent (%) of patients exacerbation-free at 2 years[3]	15%	25%*	32%***
Median time to first exacerbation (months)[1,4]	4.5	7.6**	9.6***
MRI			
Median percent (%) change of MRI PD-T2 lesion area at 2 years[5]	n = 172 11.0	n = 171 -1.2***	n = 171 -3.8***
Median number of active lesions per patient per scan (PD/T2; 6 monthly)[5]	2.25	0.75***	0.5***

* p<0.05 compared to placebo
** p<0.001 compared to placebo
*** p<0.0001 compared to placebo
(1) Intent-to-treat analysis
(2) Poisson regression model adjusted for center and time on study
(3) Logistic regression adjusted for center. Patients lost to follow-up prior to an exacerbation were excluded from this analysis (n = 185, 183, and 184 for the placebo, 22 mcg tiw, and 44 mcg tiw groups, respectively)
(4) Cox proportional hazard model adjusted for center
(5) ANOVA on ranks adjusted for center. Patients with missing scans were excluded from this analysis

The primary efficacy endpoint was the proportion of patients who remained exacerbation-free at 24 weeks. The principal secondary endpoint was the mean number per patient per scan of combined unique active MRI lesions through 24 weeks, defined as any lesion that was T1 active or T2 active. Neurological examinations were performed every three months by a neurologist blinded to treatment assignment. Patient visits were conducted monthly, and mid-month telephone contacts were made to inquire about potential exacerbations. If an exacerbation was suspected, the patient was evaluated with a neurological examination. MRI scans were performed monthly and analyzed in a treatment–blinded manner.

Patients treated with Rebif® 44 mcg sc tiw were more likely to remain relapse-free at 24 and 48 weeks than were patients treated with Avonex® 30 mcg im qw (Table 2). This study does not support any conclusion regarding effects on the accumulation of physical disability.

[See table 2 at top of next page]

The adverse reactions over 48 weeks were generally similar between the two treatment groups. Exceptions included injection site disorders (83% of patients on Rebif® vs. 28% of patients on Avonex®), hepatic function disorders (18% on Rebif® vs. 10% on Avonex®), and leukopenia (6% on Rebif® vs. <1% on Avonex®), which were observed with greater frequency in the Rebif® group compared to the Avonex® group.

INDICATIONS AND USAGE

Rebif® (interferon beta-1a) is indicated for the treatment of patients with relapsing forms of multiple sclerosis to decrease the frequency of clinical exacerbations and delay the accumulation of physical disability. Efficacy of Rebif® in chronic progressive multiple sclerosis has not been established.

CONTRAINDICATIONS

Rebif® (interferon beta-1a) is contraindicated in patients with a history of hypersensitivity to natural or recombinant interferon, human albumin, or any other component of the formulation.

WARNINGS

Depression and Suicide

Rebif® (interferon beta-1a) should be used with caution in patients with depression, a condition that is common in people with multiple sclerosis. Depression, suicidal ideation, and suicide attempts have been reported to occur with increased frequency in patients receiving interferon compounds, including Rebif®. In addition, there have been post-marketing reports of suicide in patients treated with Rebif®. Patients should be advised to report immediately any symptoms of depression and/or suicidal ideation to the prescribing physician. If a patient develops depression, cessation of treatment with Rebif® should be considered.

Hepatic Injury

Severe liver injury, including some cases of hepatic failure requiring liver transplantation, has been reported rarely in patients taking Rebif®. Symptoms of liver dysfunction began from one to six months following the initiation of Rebif®. If jaundice or other symptoms of liver dysfunction appear, treatment with Rebif® should be discontinued immediately due to the potential for rapid progression to liver failure.

Asymptomatic elevation of hepatic transaminases (particularly SGPT) is common with interferon therapy (see **ADVERSE REACTIONS**). Rebif® should be initiated with caution in patients with active liver disease, alcohol abuse, increased serum SGPT (> 2.5 times ULN), or a history of significant liver disease. Also, the potential risk of Rebif® used in combination with known hepatotoxic products should be considered prior to Rebif® administration, or when adding new agents to the regimen of patients already on Rebif®. Reduction of Rebif® dose should be considered if SGPT rises above 5 times the upper limit of normal. The dose may be gradually re-escalated when enzyme levels have normalized. (See **PRECAUTIONS:** Laboratory Tests and Drug Interactions; and **DOSAGE AND ADMINISTRATION**).

Anaphylaxis

Anaphylaxis has been reported as a rare complication of Rebif® use. Other allergic reactions have included skin rash and urticaria, and have ranged from mild to severe without a clear relationship to dose or duration of exposure. Several allergic reactions, some severe, have occurred after prolonged use.

Albumin (Human)

This product contains albumin, a derivative of human blood. Based on effective donor screening and product manufacturing processes, it carries an extremely remote risk for transmission of viral diseases. A theoretical risk for transmission of Creutzfeldt-Jakob disease (CJD) also is considered extremely remote. No cases of transmission of viral diseases or CJD have ever been identified for albumin.

PRECAUTIONS

General

Caution should be exercised when administering Rebif® to patients with pre-existing seizure disorders. Seizures have been associated with the use of beta interferons including Rebif®. Leukopenia and new or worsening thyroid abnormalities have developed in some patients treated with Rebif® (see **ADVERSE REACTIONS**). Regular monitoring for these conditions is recommended (see **PRECAUTIONS:** Laboratory Tests).

Information for Patients

All patients should be instructed to read the Rebif® Medication Guide supplied to them. Patients should be cautioned not to change the dosage or the schedule of administration without medical consultation.

Patients should be informed of the most common and the most severe adverse reactions associated with the use of Rebif® (see **WARNINGS** and **ADVERSE REACTIONS**). Patients should be advised of the symptoms associated with these conditions, and to report them to their physician.

Female patients should be cautioned about the abortifacient potential of Rebif® (see **PRECAUTIONS:** Pregnancy).

Patients should be instructed in the use of aseptic technique when administering Rebif®. Appropriate instruction for self-injection or injection by another person should be provided, including careful review of the Rebif® Medication Guide. If a patient is to self-administer Rebif®, the physical and cognitive ability of that patient to self-administer and properly dispose of syringes should be assessed. The initial injection should be performed under the supervision of an appropriately qualified health care professional. Patients should be advised of the importance of rotating sites of injection with each dose, to minimize the likelihood of severe injection site reactions or necrosis. A puncture-resistant container for disposal of used needles and syringes should be supplied to the patient along with instructions for safe disposal of full containers. Patients should be instructed in the technique and importance of proper syringe disposal and be cautioned against reuse of these items.

Laboratory Tests

In addition to those laboratory tests normally required for monitoring patients with multiple sclerosis, blood cell counts and liver function tests are recommended at regular intervals (1, 3, and 6 months) following introduction of Rebif® therapy and then periodically thereafter in the absence of clinical symptoms. Thyroid function tests are recommended every 6 months in patients with a history of thyroid dysfunction or as clinically indicated. Patients with myelosuppression may require more intensive monitoring of complete blood cell counts, with differential and platelet counts.

Drug Interactions

No formal drug interaction studies have been conducted with Rebif®. Due to its potential to cause neutropenia and lymphopenia, proper monitoring of patients is required if Rebif® is given in combination with myelosuppressive agents.

Also, the potential for hepatic injury should be considered when Rebif® is used in combination with other products associated with hepatic injury, or when new agents are added to the regimen of patients already on Rebif® (see **WARNINGS: Hepatic Injury**).

Immunization

In a nonrandomized prospective clinical study, 86 multiple sclerosis (MS) patients on Rebif® 44 mcg tiw for at least 6 months and 77 patients not receiving interferon received influenza vaccination. The proportion of patients achieving a positive antibody response (defined as a titer > 1:40 measured by a hemagglutination inhibition assay) was similar in the two groups (93% and 91%, respectively). The exact relationship of antibody titers to vaccine efficacy was not studied and is not known in patients receiving Rebif®. Therefore, while patients receiving Rebif® may receive concomitant vaccination, the overall effectiveness of such vaccination is unknown.

Carcinogenesis, Mutagenesis, Impairment of Fertility

Carcinogenesis: No carcinogenicity data for Rebif® are available in animals or humans.

Mutagenesis: Rebif® was not mutagenic when tested in the Ames bacterial test and in an *in vitro* cytogenetic assay in human lymphocytes in the presence and absence of metabolic activation.

Impairment of Fertility: No studies have been conducted to evaluate the effects of Rebif® on fertility in humans. In studies in normally cycling female cynomolgus monkeys given daily sc injections of Rebif® for six months at doses of up to 9 times the recommended weekly human dose (based on body surface area), no effects were observed on either menstrual cycling or serum estradiol levels. The validity of extrapolating doses used in animal studies to human doses is not established. In male monkeys, the same doses of Rebif® had no demonstrable adverse effects on sperm count, motility, morphology, or function.

Pregnancy Category C

Rebif® treatment has been associated with significant increases in embryolethal or abortifacient effects in cynomolgus monkeys administered doses approximately 2 times the cumulative weekly human dose (based on either body weight or surface area) either during the period of organogenesis (gestation day 21-89) or later in pregnancy. There were no fetal malformations or other evidence of teratogenesis noted in these studies. These effects are consistent with the abortifacient effects of other type I interferons. There are no adequate and well-controlled studies of Rebif® in pregnant women. However, in Studies 1 and 2, there were 2 spontaneous abortions observed and 5 fetuses carried to term among 7 women in the Rebif® groups. If a woman becomes pregnant or plans to become pregnant while taking Rebif®, she should be informed about the potential hazards to the fetus, and discontinuation of Rebif® should be considered.

Nursing Mothers

It is not known whether Rebif® is excreted in human milk. Because many drugs are excreted in human milk, caution should be exercised when Rebif® is administered to a nursing woman.

Pediatric Use: The safety and effectiveness of Rebif® in pediatric patients have not been studied.

Geriatric Use: Clinical studies of Rebif® did not include sufficient numbers of subjects aged 65 and over to determine whether they respond differently than younger subjects. In general, dose selection for an elderly patient should be cautious, usually starting at the low end of the dosing range, reflecting the greater frequency of decreased hepatic, renal or cardiac function, and of concomitant disease or other drug therapy.

ADVERSE REACTIONS

The most frequently reported serious adverse reactions with Rebif® were psychiatric disorders including depression and suicidal ideation or attempt (see **WARNINGS: Depression**).

Table 2: Clinical and MRI Results from Study 2

	Rebif®	Avonex®	Absolute Difference	Risk of relapse on Rebif® relative to Avonex®
	N=339	N=338		
Relapses Proportion of patients relapse-free at 24 weeks[1]	75%*	63%	12% (95% CI: 5%, 19%)	0.68 (95% CI: 0.54, 0.86)
Proportion of patients relapse-free at 48 weeks	62%**	52%	10% (95% CI: 2%, 17%)	0.81 (95% CI: 0.68, 0.96)
MRI (through 24 weeks) Median of the mean number of combined unique MRI lesions per patient per scan[2] (25th, 75th percentiles)	N=325 0.17* (0.00, 0.67)	N=325 0.33 (0.00, 1.25)		

* p <0.001, and
** p = 0.009, Rebif® compared to Avonex®
(1) Logistic regression model adjusted for treatment and center, intent to treat analysis
(2) Nonparametric ANCOVA model adjusted for treatment and center, with baseline combined unique lesions as the single covariate.

Table 3. Adverse Reactions and Laboratory Abnormalities in Study 1

Body System Preferred Term	Placebo tiw (n=187)	Rebif® 22 mcg tiw (n=189)	Rebif® 44 mcg tiw (n=184)
BODY AS A WHOLE	51%	56%	59%
Influenza-like symptoms	63%	65%	70%
Headache	36%	33%	41%
Fatigue	16%	25%	28%
Fever	5%	6%	13%
Rigors	5%	6%	8%
Chest Pain	1%	4%	5%
Malaise			
INJECTION SITE DISORDERS	39%	89%	92%
Injection Site Reaction	0%	1%	3%
Injection Site Necrosis			
CENTRAL & PERIPH NERVOUS SYSTEM DISORDERS	5%	7%	6%
Hypertonia	2%	5%	4%
Coordination Abnormal	2%	5%	4%
Convulsions			
ENDOCRINE DISORDERS	3%	4%	6%
Thyroid Disorder			
GASTROINTESTINAL SYSTEM DISORDERS	17%	22%	20%
Abdominal Pain	1%	1%	5%
Dry Mouth			
LIVER AND BILIARY SYSTEM DISORDERS	4%	20%	27%
SGPT Increased	4%	10%	17%
SGOT Increased	2%	4%	9%
Hepatic Function Abnormal	1%	3%	2%
Bilirubinaemia			
MUSCULO-SKELETAL SYSTEM DISORDERS	20%	25%	25%
Myalgia	20%	23%	25%
Back Pain	10%	15%	10%
Skeletal Pain			
HEMATOLOGIC DISORDERS	14%	28%	36%
Leukopenia	8%	11%	12%
Lymphadenopathy	2%	2%	8%
Thrombocytopenia	3%	3%	5%
Anemia			
PSYCHIATRIC DISORDERS	1%	4%	5%
Somnolence			5%
SKIN DISORDERS	3%	7%	4%
Rash Erythematous	2%	5%	
Rash Maculo-Papular			7%
URINARY SYSTEM DISORDERS	4%	2%	2%
Micturition Frequency	2%	4%	
Urinary Incontinence			13%
VISION DISORDERS	7%	7%	1%
Vision Abnormal	0%	3%	
Xerophthalmia			

The adverse reactions were generally similar in Studies 1 and 2, taking into account the disparity in study durations.

The incidence of depression of any severity in the Rebif®-treated groups and placebo-treated group was approximately 25%.

The most commonly reported adverse reactions were injection site disorders, influenza-like symptoms (headache, fatigue, fever, rigors, chest pain, back pain, myalgia), abdominal pain, depression, elevation of liver enzymes and hematologic abnormalities. The most frequently reported adverse reactions resulting in clinical intervention (e.g., discontinuation of Rebif®, adjustment in dosage, or the need for concomitant medication to treat an adverse reaction symptom) were injection site disorders, influenza-like symptoms, depression and elevation of liver enzymes (see **WARNINGS**).

In Study 1, 6 patients randomized to Rebif® 44 mcg tiw (3%), and 2 patients who received Rebif® 22 mcg tiw (1%) developed injection site necrosis during two years of therapy. Rebif® was continued in 7 patients and interrupted briefly in one patient. There was one report of injection site necrosis in Study 2 during 48 weeks of Rebif® treatment. All events resolved with conservative management.

The rates of adverse reactions and association with Rebif® in patients with relapsing-remitting multiple sclerosis are drawn from the placebo-controlled study (n = 560) and the active comparator-controlled study (n = 339).

The population encompassed an age range from 18 to 55 years. Nearly three-fourths of the patients were female, and more than 90% were Caucasian, largely reflecting the general demographics of the population of patients with multiple sclerosis.

Because clinical trials are conducted under widely varying conditions, adverse reaction rates observed in the clinical trials of Rebif® cannot be directly compared to rates in the clinical trials of other drugs and may not reflect the rates observed in practice.

Table 3 enumerates adverse events and laboratory abnormalities that occurred at an incidence that was at least 2% more in either Rebif® treated group than was observed in the placebo group.

[See table 3 on previous page]

Postmarketing Experience

In addition to adverse events reported from clinical trials, the following events have been reported during post-marketing use of Rebif®. Because these reactions were reported voluntarily from a population of uncertain size, the frequency or a causal relationship to Rebif can not be reliably determined.

Blood and Lymphatic System Disorders: Thrombotic thrombocytopenic purpura/hemolytic uremic syndrome (TTP/HUS).

Eye Disorders: Retinal vascular disorders (i.e. retinopathy, cotton wool spots or obstruction of retinal artery or vein).

Hepatobiliary Disorders: Rare cases of severe liver dysfunction, including hepatic failure requiring liver transplantation (**See WARNINGS: Hepatic Injury**).

Nervous System: Seizures (see PRECAUTIONS: General). Transient neurological symptoms (i.e., hypoesthesia, muscle spasm, paresthesia, difficulty walking, musculoskeletal stiffness) that mimic MS exacerbations of limited duration, temporally related to the injections and most prominent at the initiation of therapy. In some cases, these symptoms were associated with flu-like syndrome.

Psychiatric Disorders: suicide (**see WARNINGS: Depression and Suicide**).

Skin and Subcutaneous Tissue Disorders: Injection site abscesses, injection site infections, including cellulitis and necrosis requiring debridement, systemic antibiotic treatment and/or grafting; erythema multiforme, and Stevens-Johnson syndrome.

Immunogenicity

As with all therapeutic proteins, there is a potential for immunogenicity. In study 1, the presence of neutralizing antibodies (NAb) to Rebif® was determined by collecting and analyzing serum pre-study and at 6 month time intervals during the 2 years of the clinical trial. Serum NAb were detected in 59/189 (31%) and 45/184 (24%) of Rebif®-treated patients at the 22 mcg and 44 mcg tiw doses, respectively, at one or more times during the study. The clinical significance of the presence of NAb to Rebif® is unknown.

The data reflect the percentage of patients whose test results were considered positive for antibodies to Rebif® using an antiviral cytopathic effect assay, and are highly dependent on the sensitivity and specificity of the assay. Additionally, the observed incidence of NAb positivity in an assay may be influenced by several factors including sample handling, timing of sample collection, concomitant medications and underlying disease. For these reasons, comparison of the incidence of antibodies to Rebif® with the incidence of antibodies to other products may be misleading.

Anaphylaxis and other allergic reactions have been observed with the use of Rebif® (see **WARNINGS: Anaphylaxis**).

DRUG ABUSE AND DEPENDENCE

There is no evidence that abuse or dependence occurs with Rebif® therapy. However, the risk of dependence has not been systematically evaluated.

OVERDOSAGE

Safety of doses higher than 44 mcg sc tiw has not been adequately evaluated. The maximum amount of Rebif® that can be safely administered has not been determined.

DOSAGE AND ADMINISTRATION

Dosages of Rebif® shown to be safe and effective are 22 mcg and 44 mcg injected subcutaneously three times per week. Rebif® should be administered, if possible, at the same time (preferably in the late afternoon or evening) on the same three days (e.g., Monday, Wednesday, and Friday) at least 48 hours apart each week (see **CLINICAL STUDIES**). Generally, patients should be started at 20% of the prescribed dose tiw and increased over a 4-week period to the targeted dose, either 22 mcg or 44 mcg tiw (see Table 4). Following the administration of each dose, any residual product remaining in the syringe should be discarded in a safe and proper manner.

A Rebif® Titration Pack containing 6 doses of 8.8 mcg (0.2 mL) and 6 doses of 22 mcg (0.5 mL) is available for use during the titration period.

Table 4: Schedule for Patient Titration

	Recommended Titration (% of final dose)	Titration dose for Rebif® (22 mcg)	Titration dose for Rebif® (44 mcg)
Weeks 1-2	20%	4.4 mcg	8.8 mcg
Weeks 3-4	50%	11 mcg	22 mcg
Weeks 5+	100%	22 mcg	44 mcg

Leukopenia or elevated liver function tests may necessitate dose reduction or discontinuation of Rebif® administration until toxicity is resolved (see **WARNINGS: Hepatic Injury, PRECAUTIONS: General and ADVERSE REACTIONS**).

Rebif® is intended for use under the guidance and supervision of a physician. It is recommended that physicians or qualified medical personnel train patients in the proper technique for self-administering subcutaneous injections using the prefilled syringe. Patients should be advised to rotate sites for sc injections (see **PRECAUTIONS: Information for Patients**). Concurrent use of analgesics and/or antipyretics may help ameliorate flu-like symptoms on treatment days. Rebif® should be inspected visually for particulate matter and discoloration prior to administration.

Stability and Storage

Rebif® should be stored refrigerated between 2-8°C (36-46°F). DO NOT FREEZE. If a refrigerator is not available, Rebif® may be stored at or below 25° C/77° F for up to 30 days and away from heat and light.

Do not use beyond the expiration date printed on cartons. Rebif® contains no preservatives. Each syringe is intended for single use. Unused portions should be discarded.

HOW SUPPLIED

Rebif® is supplied as a sterile, preservative-free solution packaged in graduated, ready to use in 0.2 mL or 0.5 mL prefilled syringes with 29-gauge, 0.5 inch needle for subcutaneous injection. The following package presentations are available.

Rebif® (interferon beta-1a) Titration Pack, NDC 44087-8822-1

- Six Rebif® 8.8 mcg prefilled syringes and Six Rebif® 22 mcg prefilled syringe

Rebif® (interferon beta-1a) 22 mcg Prefilled syringe

- Twelve Rebif® 22 mcg prefilled syringes, NDC 44087-0022-3

Rebif® (interferon beta-1a) 44 mcg Prefilled syringe

- Twelve Rebif® 44 mcg prefilled syringes, NDC 44087-0044-3

RX only.

REFERENCES

1. PRISMS Study Group. Randomized double-blind placebo-controlled study of interferon β-1a in relapsing/remitting multiple sclerosis. Lancet 1998; 352: 1498-1504.
2. Panitch H. Goodin DS, Francis G, et al. Randomized, comparative study of interferon β-1a treatment regimens in MS. The EVIDENCE Trial. Neurology 2002 59:1496-1506.

Manufacturer: EMD Serono, Inc. Rockland, MA 02370 U.S. License # 1773

Co-Marketed by:
EMD Serono, Inc.
Rockland, MA 02370
Pfizer Inc.
New York, NY 10017
Revised: September 2009
*Avonex® is a registered trademark of Biogen Idec, Inc.
N6700101G

MEDICATION GUIDE

Medication Guide
Rebif® (Rē-bif)
Interferon beta-1a
(in-ter-feer-on beta-one-â)

Please read this leaflet carefully before you start to use Rebif® and each time your prescription is refilled since there may be new information. The information in this medication guide does not take the place of regularly talking with your doctor or healthcare professional.

What is the most important information I should know about Rebif®?

Rebif® will not cure multiple sclerosis (MS) but it has been shown to decrease the number of flare-ups and slow the occurrence of some of the physical disability that is common in people with MS. Rebif® can cause serious side effects, so before you start taking Rebif®, you should talk with your doctor about the possible benefits of Rebif® and its possible side effects to decide if Rebif® is right for you. Potential serious side effects include:

- **Depression.** Some patients treated with interferons, including Rebif®, have become seriously depressed (feeling sad). Some patients have thought about killing themselves and a few have committed suicide. Depression (a sinking of spirits or sadness) is not uncommon in people with multiple sclerosis. However, if you are feeling noticeably sadder or helpless, or feel like hurting yourself or others, you should tell a family member or friend right away and call your doctor as soon as possible. Your doctor may ask that you stop using Rebif®. You should also tell your doctor if you have ever had any mental illness, including depression, and if you take any medications for depression.
- **Liver problems.** Your liver may be affected by taking Rebif® and a few patients have developed severe liver injury. Your healthcare provider may ask you to have regular blood tests to make sure that your liver is working properly. If your skin or the whites of your eyes become yellow or if you are bruising easily you should call your doctor right away.
- **Risk to pregnancy.** If you become pregnant while taking Rebif® you should stop using Rebif® immediately and call your doctor. Rebif® may cause you to lose your baby (miscarry) or may cause harm to your unborn child. You and your doctor will need to decide whether the potential benefit of taking Rebif® is greater than the risks are to your unborn child.
- **Allergic reactions.** Some patients taking Rebif® have had severe allergic reactions leading to difficulty breathing, and loss of consciousness. Allergic reactions can happen after your first dose or may not happen until after you have taken Rebif® many times. Less severe allergic reactions such as itching, flushing or skin bumps can also happen at any time. If you think you are having an allergic reaction, stop using Rebif® immediately and call your doctor.
- **Injection site problems.** Rebif® may cause redness, pain or swelling at the place where an injection was given. Some patients have developed skin infections or areas of severe skin damage (necrosis) requiring treatment by a doctor. If one of your injection sites becomes swollen and painful or the area looks infected and it doesn't heal within a few days, you should call your doctor.

What is Rebif®?

Rebif® is a type of protein called beta interferon that occurs naturally in the body. It is used to treat relapsing forms of multiple sclerosis. It will not cure your MS but may decrease the number of flare-ups of the disease and slow the occurrence of some of the physical disability that is common in people with MS. MS is a life-long disease that affects your nervous system by destroying the protective covering (myelin) that surrounds your nerve fibers. The way Rebif® works in MS is not known.

Who should not take Rebif®?

Do not take Rebif® if you:

- have had an allergic reaction such as difficulty breathing, flushing or hives to another interferon beta or to human albumin.

If you have any of the following conditions or serious medical problems, you should tell your doctor *before* taking Rebif®:

- Depression (a sinking feeling or sadness), anxiety (feeling uneasy or fearful for no reason), or trouble sleeping
- Liver diseases
- Problems with your thyroid gland
- Blood problems such as bleeding or bruising easily and anemia (low red blood cells) or low white blood cells
- Epilepsy
- Are planning to become pregnant

Tell your doctor about all medicines you take, including prescription and non-prescription medicines, vitamins and herbal supplements. Rebif® and other medicines may affect each other causing serious side effects. Talk to your doctor before you take any new medicines.

How should I take Rebif®?

Rebif® is given by injection under the skin (subcutaneous injection) on the same three days a week (for example, Monday, Wednesday and Friday). Your injections should be at least 48 hours apart so it is best to take them the same time each day. Your doctor will tell you what dose of Rebif® to use, and may change the dose based on how your body responds. You should not change the dose without talking with your doctor.

If you miss a dose, you should take your next dose as soon as you remember or are able to take it, then skip the following day. **Do not take Rebif® on two consecutive days.** You should return to your regular schedule the following week. If you accidentally take more than your prescribed dose, or take it on two consecutive days, call your doctor right away. You should always follow your doctor's instructions and advice about how to take this medication. If your doctor feels that you, or a family member or friend may give you the injections then you and/or the other person should be trained by your doctor or healthcare provider in how to give an injection. Do not try to give yourself (or have another person give you) injections at home until you (or both of you)

Week of Use	Syringe to Use	Your Prescribed Dose	
		22 mcg	44 mcg
Weeks 1 and 2	8.8 mcg syringe	Use half of syringe	Use full syringe
Weeks 3 and 4	22 mcg syringe	Use half of syringe	Use full syringe
Weeks 5 and On	22 or 44 mcg syringe	Use full syringe depending on your prescribed dose: 22 or 44 mcg	

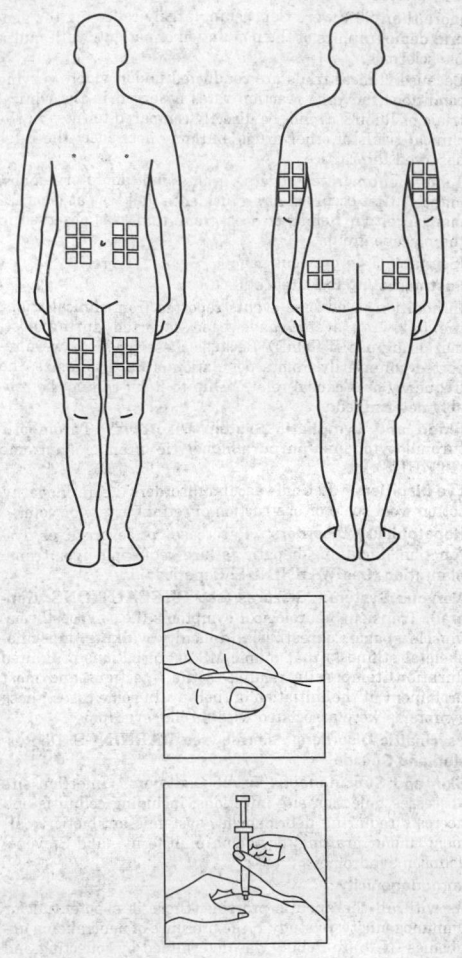

understand and are comfortable with how to prepare your dose and give the injections.

Always use a new, unopened, prefilled syringe of Rebif® for each injection. Never reuse syringes.

It is important that you change your injection site each time Rebif® is injected. This will lessen the chance of you having a serious skin reaction at the spot where you inject Rebif®. You should always avoid injecting Rebif® into an area of skin that is sore, reddened, infected or otherwise damaged. At the end of this leaflet there are detailed instructions on how to prepare and give an injection of Rebif®. You should become familiar with these instructions and follow your doctor's orders before injecting Rebif®.

What should I avoid while taking Rebif®?

• **Pregnancy.** You should avoid becoming pregnant while taking Rebif® until you have talked with your doctor. Rebif® can cause you to lose your baby (miscarry).

• **Breast feeding.** You should talk to your doctor if you are breast feeding an infant. It is not known if the interferon in Rebif® can be passed to an infant in mother's milk, and it is not known whether the drug could harm the infant if it is passed to an infant.

• Rebif® and other medicines may affect each other causing serious side effects. Talk to your doctor before you take any new medicines.

What are the possible side effects of Rebif®?

• **Flu-like symptoms.** Most patients have flu-like symptoms (fever, chills, sweating, muscle aches and tiredness). For many patients, these symptoms will lessen or go away over time. You should talk to your doctor about whether you should take an over the counter medication for pain or fever reduction before or after taking your dose of Rebif®.

• **Skin reactions.** Soreness, redness, pain, bruising or swelling may occur at the place of injection. (see: *"What is the most important information I should know about Rebif®?"*)

• **Depression and anxiety.** Some patients taking interferons have become very depressed and or anxious. There have been patients taking interferons who have had thoughts about killing themselves. If you feel sad or hopeless you should tell a friend or family member right away and call your doctor immediately. (see: *"What is the most important information I should know about Rebif®?"*)

• **Liver problems.** Your liver function may be affected. If you develop symptoms of changes in your liver, including yellowing of the skin and whites of the eyes and easy bruising, call your doctor immediately. (see: *"What is the most important information I should know about Rebif®?"*)

• **Blood problems.** You may have a drop in the levels of infection-fighting white blood cells, red blood cells or cells that help to form blood clots. If the drop in levels are severe, they can lessen your ability to fight infections, make you feel tired or sluggish or cause you to bruise or bleed easily.

• **Thyroid problems.** Your thyroid function may change. Symptoms of changes in the function of your thyroid include feeling cold or hot all the time, change in your weight (gain or loss) without a change in your diet or amount of exercise you are getting.

• **Allergic reactions.** Some patients have had hives, rash, skin bumps or itching while they were taking Rebif®. Other patients have had more serious allergic reactions such as difficulty breathing, or feeling light-headed. You should tell your doctor if you think you are having an allergic reaction. (see: *"What is the most important information I should know about Rebif®?"*)

Whether you experience any of these side effects or not, you and your doctor should periodically talk about your general health. Your doctor may want to monitor you more closely and ask you to have blood tests done more frequently.

Call your doctor for medical advice about side effects. You may report side effects to FDA at 1-800-FDA-1088.

Storage Conditions

Rebif® is packaged in prefilled syringes with needles already attached to the syringe.

Rebif® should be stored refrigerated between 2-8°C (36-46°F). DO NOT FREEZE. If a refrigerator is not available, Rebif® may be stored at or below 25°C/77°F for up to 30 days and away from heat and light.

General Information About Prescription Medicines

Medicines are sometimes prescribed for purposes other than those listed in a Medication Guide. This medication has

been prescribed for your particular medical condition. Do not use it for another condition or give this drug to anyone else. If you have any questions you should speak with your doctor or health care professional. You may also ask your doctor or pharmacist for a copy of the information provided to them with the product.

Keep this and all drugs out of the reach of children.

Instructions for Preparing and Giving Yourself an Injection of Rebif®

Before you begin, gather all of the supplies listed below:

• Rebif® prefilled syringe with 29 gauge needle. You may wish to remove your syringe from the refrigerator at least 30 minutes prior to use and let it adjust to room temperature so the liquid is not cold. Do not heat or microwave a syringe.

• Alcohol swabs (wipes) or cotton balls and rubbing alcohol

• Small adhesive bandage strip (if desired)

• Puncture resistant safety container for disposal of used syringes

• Antibacterial soap

• An over-the-counter pain or fever reducing medication, if your doctor has recommended that you take this prior to, at the same time, or after you give yourself Rebif® to help minimize the fever, chills, sweating and muscle aches (flu-like symptoms) that may occur.

When first starting treatment with Rebif®, your doctor may prescribe either the 22 mcg or 44 mcg dose of Rebif®. You should gradually increase the dose over 4 weeks, starting at 20% of the prescribed dose for the first 2 weeks, half-dose for the second 2 weeks (weeks 3 and 4), and then the full dose prescribed by your doctor.

A Rebif® Titration Pack containing 6 syringes with 8.8 mcg (0.2 mL) and 6 syringes with 22 mcg (0.5 mL) is available for use during the titration period. The following table explains how to use the Rebif® Titration Pack during the first four weeks to gradually increase your dose to 22 or 44 mcg. [See table above]

Preparing for an injection:

• Check the expiration date; **do not use if the medication is expired.** The expiration date is printed on the syringe, and carton.

• Be sure that the dose, either 8.8 mcg, 22 mcg or 44 mcg, described on the carton is the same as the dose prescribed by your doctor.

• Remove the Rebif® syringe from the plastic packaging. Keep the needle capped.

• Examine the contents of the syringe carefully. The liquid should be clear to slightly yellow. **Do not use if the liquid is cloudy, discolored or contains particles.**

• Choose the injection site. The best sites for giving yourself an injection are those areas with a layer of fat between the skin and muscle, like your thigh, the outer surface of your upper arm, your stomach or buttocks. Do not use the area near your navel or waistline. If you are very thin, use only the thigh and outer surface of the arm for injection. Use a different site each time you inject (thigh, hip, stomach or upper arm, see Figure below). Do not inject Rebif® into an area of your body where the skin is irritated, reddened, bruised, infected or abnormal in any way.

• Keep a record of the date and location of each injection.

• Wash your hands thoroughly with antibacterial soap before preparing to inject the medication.

• Clean the injection site with an alcohol swab (wipe) or cotton ball with rubbing alcohol using a circular motion. To avoid stinging, you should let your skin dry before you inject Rebif®.

[See first figure at top of next column]

Giving yourself an injection of Rebif®

• Remove the needle cap from the syringe needle.

• If your doctor has told you to use less than the full 0.5 mL dose, slowly push the plunger in until the amount of medication left in the syringe is the amount your doctor told you to use.

• Use your thumb and forefinger to pinch a pad of skin surrounding the cleaned injection site (see figure). Hold the syringe like a pencil with your other hand.

[See second figure at top of next column]

• While still pinching the skin, swiftly insert the needle like a dart at about a 90 degree angle (just under the skin) into the pad of tissue as shown.

[See third figure at top of next column]

• After the needle is in, remove the hand that you used to pinch your skin and inject the drug using a slow, steady

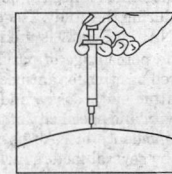

push on the plunger until all the medication is injected and the syringe is empty.

• Withdraw the needle and apply gentle pressure to the injection site with a dry cotton ball or sterile gauze. Applying a cold compress or ice pack to the injection site after injection may help reduce local skin reactions.

• Put a small adhesive bandage strip over the injection site, if desired.

• After 2 hours, check the injection site for redness, swelling, or tenderness. If you have a skin reaction and it doesn't clear up in a few days, contact your doctor or nurse.

Disposing of Needles and Syringes

• There are special state or local laws for properly disposing of used needles and syringes. Your doctor or health care professional will instruct you on how to discard your used syringe and needle and may provide you with a puncture resistant syringe disposal container called a Sharps container.

• Always keep your disposal container out of the reach of children.

• DO NOT throw the needle and syringe in the household trash or recycle.

This Medication Guide has been approved by the U.S. Food and Drug Administration.

Manufactured by:
EMD Serono, Inc.
Rockland, MA 02370
U.S. License 1773
Co-Marketed by:
EMD Serono, Inc.
Rockland, MA 02370
Pfizer Inc
New York, NY 10017

SEROSTIM®

℞

[sē-rō-stĭm]

[somatropin (rDNA origin) for injection]

DESCRIPTION

Serostim® [somatropin (rDNA origin) for injection] is a human growth hormone (hGH) produced by recombinant DNA technology. Serostim® has 191 amino acid residues and a molecular weight of 22,125 daltons. Its amino acid sequence and structure are identical to the dominant form of human pituitary GH. Serostim® is produced by a mammalian cell line (mouse C127) that has been modified by the addition of the hGH gene. Serostim® is secreted directly through the cell membrane into the cell-culture medium for collection and purification.

Serostim® is a highly purified preparation. Biological potency is determined by measuring the increase in the body weight induced in hypophysectomized rats.

Serostim® is available in 5 mg and 6 mg vials for single dose administration. Serostim® is also available in 4 mg and 8.8 mg vials for multi-dose administration. Each 4 mg vial contains 4.0 mg (approximately 12 IU) somatropin, 27.3 mg sucrose, 0.9 mg phosphoric acid. Each 5 mg vial contains 5.0 mg (approximately 15 IU) somatropin, 34.2 mg sucrose and 1.2 mg phosphoric acid. Each 6 mg vial contains 6.0 mg (approximately 18 IU) somatropin, 41.0 mg sucrose and 1.4 mg phosphoric acid. Each 8.8 mg vial contains 8.8 mg (approximately 26.4 IU) somatropin, 60.19 mg sucrose and 2.05 mg phosphoric acid. The pH is adjusted with sodium hydroxide or phosphoric acid to give a pH of 7.4 to 8.5 after reconstitution with Water for Injection, USP. The pH is adjusted with sodium hydroxide or phosphoric acid to give a pH of 6.5 to 8.5 after reconstitution with Bacteriostatic Water for Injection, USP (0.9% Benzyl Alcohol).

CLINICAL PHARMACOLOGY

Serostim® [somatropin (rDNA origin) for injection] is an anabolic and anticatabolic agent which exerts its influence by interacting with specific receptors on a variety of cell types including myocytes, hepatocytes, adipocytes, lymphocytes, and hematopoietic cells. Some, but not all of its effects, are mediated by insulin-like growth factor-I (IGF-I).

Human immunodeficiency virus (HIV)-associated wasting or cachexia, which commonly involves involuntary loss of lean body mass or body weight, is a metabolic disorder characterized by abnormalities of intermediary metabolism resulting in weight loss, inappropriate depletion of lean body mass (LBM), and paradoxical preservation of body fat. LBM includes primarily skeletal muscle, organ tissue, blood and blood constituents, and both intracellular and extracellular water. Depletion of LBM results in muscle weakness, organ failure, and death. Unlike nutritional intervention for HIV-associated wasting, in which supplemental calories are converted predominantly to body fat, Serostim® treatment resulted in a significant increase in LBM and a decrease in fat mass with a significant increase in body weight due to the dominant effect of LBM gain.

HIV-associated adipose redistribution syndrome (HARS) is characterized by abnormal accumulation of trunk fat, including visceral adipose tissue (VAT), in patients infected with HIV/acquired immune deficiency disorder (AIDS), the vast majority of whom have been treated with highly active antiretroviral therapy (HAART). VAT is comprised of the deep fat in the abdomen in the omental-mesenteric and retroperitoneal compartments. HARS, a subset of HIV lipodystrophy, is more specifically defined as maldistribution of body fat characterized by central fat accumulation (lipohypertrophy) with or without lipoatrophy (subcutaneous fat depletion primarily in the face and limbs). In HARS patients, fat may additionally accumulate in the upper body subcutaneous area such as the dorsocervical area (i.e., "buffalo hump"). These changes may be accompanied by metabolic disturbances including insulin resistance, glucose intolerance, and dyslipidemia, as well as belly image distress. Initial 12-week treatment with Serostim® resulted in decreases in VAT, trunk fat, and patient-reported belly appearance distress (see CLINICAL STUDIES). The clinical significance of these changes with respect to improved cardiovascular risk profile or compliance with HAART has not been studied.

Effects on Protein, Lipid, and Carbohydrate Metabolism:

A one-week study in 6 patients with HIV-associated wasting has shown that treatment with Serostim® 0.1 mg/kg/day improved nitrogen balance, increased protein-sparing lipid oxidation, and had little effect on overall carbohydrate metabolism.

Decreases in trunk fat and total body fat, and increases in lean body mass were observed during two double-blind, placebo-controlled studies wherein Serostim® vs. placebo were administered daily for 12 weeks to patients with HARS. (see CLINICAL STUDIES).

Effects on Nitrogen and Mineral Retention:

In the one-week study in 6 patients with HIV-associated wasting, treatment with Serostim® resulted in the retention of phosphorous, potassium, nitrogen, and sodium. The ratio of retained potassium and nitrogen during Serostim® therapy was consistent with retention of these elements in lean tissue.

Physical Performance:

Cycle ergometry work output and treadmill performance were examined in separate 12-week, placebo-controlled trials (see 'Clinical Studies'). In both studies, work output improved significantly in the group receiving Serostim® 0.1 mg/kg/day subcutaneously vs placebo. Isometric muscle performance, as measured by grip strength dynamometry, declined, probably as a result of a transient increase in tissue turgor known to occur with Serostim® therapy.

PHARMACOKINETICS

Subcutaneous Absorption: The absolute bioavailability of Serostim® [somatropin (rDNA origin) for injection] after subcutaneous administration of a formulation not equivalent to the marketed formulation was determined to be 70-90%. The t½ (Mean ± SD) after subcutaneous administration is significantly longer than that seen after intravenous administration in normal male volunteers down-regulated with somatostatin (3.94 ± 3.44 hrs. vs. 0.58 ± 0.08 hrs.), indicating that the subcutaneous absorption of the clinically tested formulation of the compound is slow and rate-limiting.

Distribution: The steady-state volume of distribution (Mean ± SD) following IV administration of Serostim® in healthy volunteers is 12.0 ± 1.08 L.

Metabolism: Although the liver plays a role in the metabolism of GH, GH is primarily cleaved in the kidney. GH undergoes glomerular filtration and, after cleavage within the renal cells, the peptides and amino acids are returned to the systemic circulation.

Elimination: The t½ (Mean ± SD) in nine patients with HIV-associated wasting with an average weight of 56.7 ± 6.8 kg, given a fixed dose of 6.0 mg recombinant hGH (r-hGH) subcutaneously was 4.28 ± 2.15 hrs. The renal clearance of r-hGH after subcutaneous administration in nine patients with HIV-associated wasting was 0.0015 ± 0.0037 L/h. No significant accumulation of r-hGH appears to occur after 6 weeks of dosing as indicated.

Special Populations:

Pediatric: Available evidence suggests that r-hGH clearances are similar in adults and children, but no pharmacokinetic studies have been conducted in children with HIV.

Gender: Biomedical literature indicates that a gender-related difference in the mean clearance of r-hGH could exist (clearance of r-hGH in males > clearance of r-hGH in females). However, no gender-based analysis is available in normal volunteers or patients infected with HIV.

Race: No data are available.

Renal Insufficiency: It has been reported that individuals with chronic renal failure tend to have decreased r-hGH clearance compared to normals, but there are no data on Serostim® use in the presence of renal insufficiency.

Hepatic Insufficiency: A reduction in r-hGH clearance has been noted in patients with severe liver dysfunction. However, the clinical significance of this in HIV+ patients is unknown.

CLINICAL STUDIES

HIV-Associated Wasting or Cachexia

The clinical efficacy of Serostim® [somatropin (rDNA origin) for injection] in HIV-associated wasting or cachexia was assessed in two placebo-controlled trials. All study subjects received concomitant antiretroviral therapy.

Clinical Trial 1: A 12-week, randomized, double-blind, placebo-controlled study followed by an open-label extension phase enrolled 178 patients with severe AIDS wasting taking nucleoside analogue therapy (pre-HAART era). The primary endpoint was body weight. Body composition was assessed using dual energy X-ray absorptiometry (DXA) and physical function was assessed by treadmill exercise testing. Patients meeting the inclusion/exclusion criteria were treated with either placebo or Serostim® 0.1 mg/kg daily. Ninety-six percent (96%) were male. The average baseline CD4 count/μL was 85. The results from one hundred forty (140) evaluable patients were analyzed (those completing the 12-week course of treatment and who were at least 80% compliant with study drug). After 12 weeks of therapy, the mean difference in weight increase between the Serostim®-treated group and the placebo-treated group was 1.6 kg (3.5 lb). Mean difference in lean body mass (LBM) change between the Serostim®-treated group and the placebo-treated group was 3.1 kg (6.8 lbs) as measured by DXA. Mean increase in weight and LBM, and mean decrease in body fat, were significantly greater in the Serostim®-treated group than in the placebo group (p=0.011, p<0.001, p<0.001, respectively) after 12 weeks of treatment (Figure 1). There were no significant changes with continued treatment beyond 12 weeks suggesting that the original gains of weight and LBM were maintained (Figure 1).

Treatment with Serostim® resulted in a significant increase in physical function as assessed by treadmill exercise testing. The median treadmill work output increased by 13% (p=0.039) at 12 weeks in the group receiving Serostim® (Figure 2). There was no improvement in the placebo-treated group at 12 weeks. Changes in treadmill performance were significantly correlated with changes in LBM.

Figure 1: Mean Changes in Body Composition

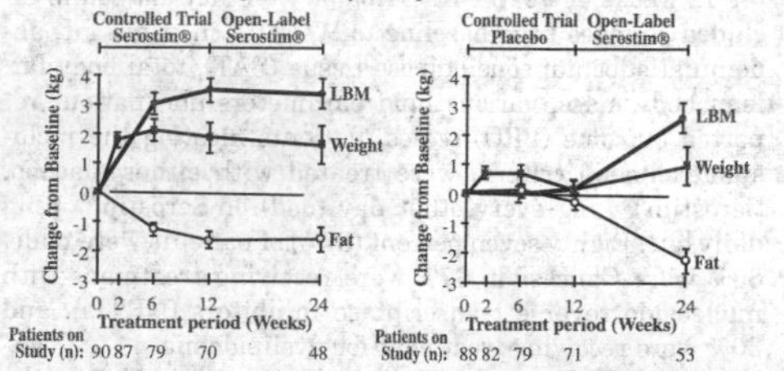

Figure 2: Median Treadmill Work Output

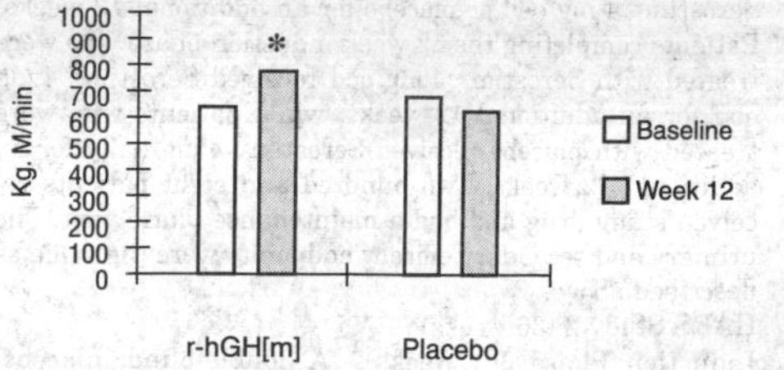

*p = 0.039

Clinical Trial 2: A 12-week, randomized, double-blind, placebo-controlled study enrolled 757 patients with HIV-associated wasting, or cachexia. The primary efficacy endpoint was physical function as measured by cycle ergometry work output. Body composition was assessed using bioelectrical impedance spectroscopy (BIS) and also by dual energy X-ray absorptiometry (DXA) at a subset of centers. Patients meeting the inclusion/exclusion criteria were treated with either placebo, approximately 0.1 mg/kg every other day (qod) of Serostim®, or approximately 0.1 mg/kg daily (qhs) of Serostim®. All results were analyzed in intent-to-treat populations (for cycle ergometry work output, n=670). Ninety-one percent (91%) were male and 88% were on HAART anti-retroviral therapy. The average baseline CD4 count/μL was 446. Six hundred forty-six patients (646) completed the 12-week study and continued in the Serostim® treatment extension phase of the trial.

Clinical Trial 2 results are summarized in Tables 1 and 2:

[See table 1 above]

[See table 2 at top of next page]

Table 1: Mean (Median) of Cycle Work Output (kJ) Response after 12 weeks of Treatment ITT Population

Cycle work output (kJ)	Placebo n=222	Half-Dose Serostim[b] n=230	Full-Dose Serostim[a] n=218
Baseline	25.92 (25.05)	27.79 (26.65)	27.57 (26.30)
Change from baseline	-0.05 (-0.25)	2.48 (2.30)	2.52 (2.40)
Percent change from baseline	0.2%	8.9%	9.1%
Difference from Placebo			
Mean (2-sided 95% C.I.)	-	2.53[c] (0.81, 4.25)	2.57[c](0.83, 4.31)
Median		2.55	2.65

(a) approximately 0.1 mg/kg daily
(b) approximately 0.1 mg/kg every other day
(c) p<0.01

The mean maximum cycle work output until exhaustion increased after 12 weeks by 2.57 kilojoules (kJ) in the Serostim® 0.1 mg/kg daily group (p<0.01) and by 2.53 kJ in the Serostim® 0.1 mg/kg every other day group (p<0.01) compared with placebo (Table 1). Cycle work output improved approximately 9% in both active treatment arms and decreased <1% in the placebo group. Lean body mass (LBM) and body weight (BW) increased, and fat mass decreased, in a dose-related fashion after treatment with Serostim® and placebo (Table 2). The LBM results obtained by BIS were confirmed with DXA.

Patients' perceptions of the impact of 12 weeks of treatment on their wasting symptoms as assessed by the Bristol-Meyers Anorexia/Cachexia Recovery Instrument improved with both doses of Serostim® in Clinical Trial 2.

Extension Phase: All patients (n=646) completing the 12-week placebo-controlled phase of Clinical Trial 2 continued Serostim® treatment into an extension phase. Five hundred and forty eight of these patients completed an additional 12 weeks of active treatment. In these patients, changes in cycle ergometry work output, LBM, BW, and fat mass either improved further or were maintained with continued Serostim® treatment.

HIV-Associated Adipose Redistribution Syndrome (HARS)
The clinical efficacy of Serostim® [somatropin (rDNA origin) for injection] for the treatment of patients with HARS was assessed in two double-blind, placebo-controlled studies. The inclusion and exclusion criteria were essentially identical in both studies. Patients with a history of diabetes, impaired fasting glucose or impaired glucose tolerance were excluded. Approximately 20% of the patients screened were excluded from study enrollment as a result of a diagnosis of diabetes or glucose intolerance. Study subjects received concomitant antiretroviral therapy and met the generally accepted criteria for excess central adipose tissue deposition assessed by anthropometric methodology (e.g., waist circumference, waist:hip ratio).

HARS Study 1 (24 weeks)
Induction Phase (12 weeks): A double-blind, placebo-controlled, parallel group study randomized 245 patients with HARS. The co-primary efficacy endpoints were change in visceral adipose tissue (VAT) and trunk:limb fat ratio after 12 weeks of treatment. Secondary efficacy endpoints included changes from baseline to Week 12 in trunk fat, abdominal subcutaneous adipose tissue (SAT), total body fat, lean body mass, various lipid parameters and patient reported outcome (PRO) scores. Patients meeting the inclusion/exclusion criteria were treated with either placebo, Serostim® 4 mg every other day (qod) or Serostim® 4 mg daily qhs. Eighty seven percent (87%) of patients were male, 80% were Caucasian, 97% were receiving treatment with nucleoside reverse transcriptase inhibitors (NRTIs), and 30% were receiving treatment for dyslipidemia.

Maintenance Phase (12 Weeks): Patients completing the 12-week induction phase who were treated with Serostim® 4 mg daily were rerandomized to therapy with either Serostim® 4 mg qod or placebo for an additional 12 weeks. Patients completing the 12 week induction phase who were treated with Serostim® 4 mg qod received Serostim® 4 mg qod for an additional 12 weeks, while patients who were treated with placebo received Serostim® 4 mg daily for an additional 12 weeks. Two hundred and eight patients received study drug and had a maintenance phase visit. The primary and secondary efficacy endpoints were the same as described above.

HARS Study 2 (36 weeks)
Induction Phase (12 Weeks): A double-blind, placebo-controlled, parallel group study randomized 326 patients with HARS. The primary efficacy endpoint was change in VAT after 12 weeks of treatment. The secondary endpoints were similar to those in HARS Study 1. Patients meeting the inclusion/exclusion criteria were treated with either placebo or Serostim® 4 mg daily qhs. Baseline demographic characteristics were very similar to Study 1.

Maintenance Phase (24 Weeks): Patients completing the 12-week induction phase were rerandomized to treatment with either Serostim® 2 mg qod or placebo for an additional 24 weeks. Two hundred fifty six patients received study drug and had a maintenance phase visit. The primary and secondary efficacy endpoints were the same as described above.

Induction Phase (Weeks 0-12) Results For Both Studies
The difference in the change from baseline to Week 12 in VAT (approximately -20 cm²) was statistically significant after treatment with Serostim® 4 mg qod vs. placebo in Study 1 (Table 3). As seen in Tables 3 and 4, the differences in the change from baseline to Week 12 in VAT (approximately -17-18 cm²) were also statistically significant after treatment with Serostim® 4 mg daily vs. placebo in both studies. The VAT response to treatment with Serostim® 4 mg qod vs. placebo in Study 1 was very similar to the response observed after treatment with Serostim® 4 mg daily (Table 3). Patients with the largest VAT levels at baseline manifested the largest reductions in VAT in response to Serostim® treatment (data not shown).
[See table 3 above]

Table 2: Mean (Median) Change from Baseline for Lean Body Mass, Fat Mass and Body Weight

	Placebo		Half-Dose Serostim[b]		Full-Dose Serostim[a]	
	n	Mean (Median)	n	Mean (Median)	n	Mean (Median)
Lean body mass (kg) (by BIS)	222	0.97 (0.67)	223	3.89 (3.65)	205	5.84 (5.47)
Fat mass (kg) (by DXA)	94	0.03 (0.01)	100	-1.25 (-1.23)	85	-1.72 (-1.51)
Body weight (kg)	247	0.69 (0.68)	257	2.18 (2.15)	253	2.79 (2.65)

(a) approximately 0.1 mg/kg daily
(b) approximately 0.1 mg/kg every other day

Table 3: HARS Study 1 Induction Phase – Mean Change from Baseline to Week 12 in Visceral Adipose Tissue (cm²)[a] by Treatment Group (Modified ITT Population with LOCF)

	Placebo n=57	Serostim® 4 mg qod n=58	Serostim® 4 mg daily n=61
Baseline (SE)[b]	133 (12)	130 (14)	138 (12)
Change from baseline (SE)[c]	-9 (6)	-28 (7)	-27 (6)
Difference from Placebo		-20 (-38, -2)	-18 (-35, -2)
for Change (95% CI)[c]		p=0.034	p=0.031

(a) Measured by computed tomography (CT) scan;
(b) Analysis of variance model with terms for treatment group, gender, and treatment-by-gender interaction;
(c) Analysis of covariance model with terms for treatment group, gender, and treatment-by-gender interaction, and baseline VAT as covariate;
(d) CI = confidence interval and SE = standard error

Table 5: HARS Study 2 Induction Phase – VAT (cm²)[a] Descriptive Statistics by Gender

	Female		Male	
Variable as Mean (SD)[b]	Placebo n=9	Serostim® 4 mg daily n=31	Placebo n=65	Serostim® 4 mg daily n=179
Baseline	77 (50)	87 (34)	143 (54)	144 (65)
Change from Baseline	-7 (44)	-7 (19)	2 (33)	-37 (39)

(a) Measured by computed tomography (CT) scan;
(b) SD = standard deviation

Table 4: HARS Study 2 Induction Phase – Mean Change from Baseline to Week 12 in Visceral Adipose Tissue (cm²)[a] by Treatment Group (Modified ITT Population with LOCF)

	Placebo n=74	Serostim® 4 mg daily n=210
Baseline (SE)[b]	110 (11)	116 (6)
Change from Baseline (SE)[c]	-12 (5)	-29 (3)
Difference from Placebo		-17 (-29, -5)
for Change (95% CI)[c]		p=0.005

(a) through (d) Same as Table 3

Subgroup analysis by gender revealed that women did not have a significant reduction in VAT in response to Serostim® 4 mg daily as indicated by the descriptive statistics by gender in Table 5 (only results from Study 2 are shown, but the results from Study 1 were similar).
[See table 5 above]
Improvements in some secondary body composition endpoints (trunk fat, abdominal SAT, total body fat, and lean body mass) were observed in both Serostim® dose groups regardless of gender. Although a greater response was observed with 4 mg daily dosing, this dose was associated with a higher rate of adverse events, dose reductions and study discontinuation (see PRECAUTIONS and ADVERSE REACTIONS). Improvements were not observed in other secondary endpoints including non-HDL cholesterol.

Maintenance Phase Results
In Study 2, VAT reaccumulated to the same extent in patients treated with Serostim® 2 mg qod and placebo. The maintenance phase results from Study 1 are summarized in Table 6. In patients initially treated with Serostim® 4 mg daily during the induction phase, rerandomization to Serostim® 4 mg qod (vs. placebo) resulted in less reaccumulation of VAT, trunk fat and total body fat.
[See table 6 at top of next page]

Patient Reported Outcomes
Belly appearance distress, belly size estimation and belly profile assessment (the essential PRO secondary efficacy endpoints) were measured using a validated PRO instrument, the Body Image Impact Module (BIIM) in both studies. Only results for belly appearance distress and belly size estimation are discussed in that the belly profile assessment was used to establish responder criteria for the belly appearance distress and the belly size estimation. Both Serostim® treatment groups manifested more improvement in belly appearance distress and belly size estimation than placebo-treated patients. Although a greater response was

observed with 4 mg daily dosing during the induction phase, this dose was associated with a higher rate of adverse events, dose reductions and study discontinuation (see PRECAUTIONS and ADVERSE REACTIONS). The improvements in belly appearance distress and belly size estimation were sustained during the maintenance phase of Study 1. The clinical significance of the changes described above in the HARS subsection of the CLINICAL STUDIES section with respect to improved cardiovascular risk profile or compliance with HAART has not been studied.

INDICATIONS AND USAGE
HIV-Associated Wasting or Cachexia
Serostim® [somatropin (rDNA origin) for injection] is indicated for the treatment of HIV patients with wasting or cachexia to increase lean body mass and body weight, and improve physical endurance. Concomitant antiretroviral therapy is necessary (see PRECAUTIONS).

CONTRAINDICATIONS
Growth hormone therapy should not be initiated in patients with acute critical illness due to complications following open heart or abdominal surgery, multiple accidental trauma or acute respiratory failure. Two placebo-controlled clinical trials in non-growth hormone deficient adult patients (n=522) with these conditions revealed a significant increase in mortality (41.9% vs. 19.3%) among somatropin-treated patients (doses 5.3-8 mg/day) compared to those receiving placebo (see WARNINGS).
Serostim® is contraindicated in patients with active neoplasia (either newly diagnosed or recurrent). Any anti-tumor therapy should be completed prior to starting therapy with Serostim®.
Serostim® [somatropin (rDNA origin) for injection] reconstituted with Bacteriostatic Water for Injection, USP (0.9% Benzyl Alcohol) should not be administered to patients with a known sensitivity to Benzyl Alcohol. (see WARNINGS).
Serostim® is contraindicated in patients with a known hypersensitivity to growth hormone.

WARNINGS
Benzyl Alcohol as a preservative in Bacteriostatic Water for Injection, USP has been associated with toxicity in newborns. If sensitivity to the diluent occurs, Serostim® [somatropin (rDNA origin) for injection] may be reconstituted with Sterile Water for Injection, USP. When Serostim® is reconstituted in this manner, the reconstituted solution should be used immediately and any unused portion should be discarded.
See CONTRAINDICATIONS for information regarding increased mortality in growth hormone-treated patients with

acute critical illnesses in intensive care units due to complications following open heart or abdominal surgery, multiple accidental trauma or acute respiratory failure. The safety of continuing growth hormone treatment in patients receiving replacement doses for approved indications who concurrently develop these illnesses has not been established. Therefore, the potential benefit of treatment continuation with growth hormone in patients developing acute critical illnesses should be weighed against the potential risk.

PRECAUTIONS

General

Serostim® [somatropin (rDNA origin) for injection] therapy should be carried out under the regular guidance of a physician who is experienced in the diagnosis and management of HIV infection. Inadequate nutritional intake, malabsorption and hypogonadism, which are common in individuals with HIV infection and which may contribute to catabolism and weight loss, should be diagnosed and treated.

There are limited data in women with HARS, especially those taking estrogen. The 47 women treated with Serostim®, 6 of whom were taking estrogen, showed no difference from placebo with respect to reduction in VAT after 12 weeks of induction treatment. It is well established that GH deficient women concomitantly treated with oral estrogen replacement therapy require substantially more rhGH to obtain comparable rhGH-related treatment effects. In addition, women with HARS have lower baseline VAT levels; lower baseline VAT levels have been demonstrated by several authors to predict a lesser reduction in VAT in response to treatment with rhGH.

HIV and Growth Hormone Considerations: In some experimental systems, recombinant human growth hormone (r-hGH) has been shown to potentiate HIV replication in vitro at concentrations ranging from 50-250 ng/ml. There was no increase in virus production when the antiretroviral agents, zidovudine, didanosine or lamivudine were added to the culture medium. Additional in vitro studies have shown that r-hGH does not interfere with the antiviral activity of zalcitabine or stavudine. In the controlled clinical trials, no significant growth hormone-associated increase in viral burden was observed. However, the protocol required all participants to be on concomitant antiretroviral therapy for the duration of the study. In view of the potential for acceleration of virus replication, it is recommended that HIV patients be maintained on antiretroviral therapy for the duration of Serostim® treatment.

Increased tissue turgor (swelling, particularly in the hands and feet) and musculoskeletal discomfort (pain, swelling and/or stiffness) may occur during treatment with Serostim®, but may resolve spontaneously, with analgesic therapy, or after reducing the frequency of dosing (see DOSAGE AND ADMINISTRATION).

Carpal tunnel syndrome may occur during treatment with Serostim®. If the symptoms of carpal tunnel syndrome do not resolve by decreasing the weekly number of doses of Serostim®, it is recommended that treatment be discontinued.

Patients should be informed that allergic reactions are possible and that prompt medical attention should be sought if an allergic reaction occurs. None of the 651 study participants with HIV-associated wasting treated with Serostim® for the first time developed detectable antibodies to growth hormone (> 4 pg binding). Patients were not rechallenged. None of the Serostim®-treated HARS study participants with available test results developed detectable antibodies to rhGH during the induction or maintenance phases of treatment.

Recombinant human growth hormone (rhGH) has been associated with acute pancreatitis.

Hyperglycemia may occur in HIV infected individuals due to a variety of reasons. In wasting patients, treatment with Serostim® 0.1 mg/kg daily and 0.1 mg/kg every other day for 12 weeks was associated with approximately 10 mg/dL and 6 mg/dL increases in mean fasting blood glucose concentrations, respectively. The increases occurred early in treatment. Patients with other risk factors for glucose intolerance should be monitored closely during Serostim® therapy. In HARS patients who had normal fasting glucose levels at screening, treatment with Serostim® 4 mg daily and 4 mg qod for 12 weeks (vs. placebo) was associated with approximately 7 and 6 mg/dL increases in mean fasting blood glucose concentrations, respectively. With respect to the induction phase, peak sugars on-study usually occurred early after initiation of Serostim® treatment, and, most often decreased spontaneously with continued Serostim® therapy or responded to dose reduction. Transient and occasionally sustained peak sugars between 100 and 126 mg/dL (and transient sugars in excess of 126 mg/dL) occurred in a substantial minority of patients (including patients with normal fasting blood glucose levels at baseline). Treatment with Serostim® 4 mg daily resulted in a greater number of glucose intolerance-related adverse reactions than treatment with Serostim® 4 mg qod (see ADVERSE REACTIONS). In HARS Study 2, hemoglobin A1c increased from a mean of 5.0% at baseline to 5.3% at Week 12 after treatment with Serostim® 4 mg daily, but it remained in the desirable range (less than 7.0%) in all patients. HARS patients are often insulin resistant and even glucose intolerant to some degree at baseline, and therefore are very susceptible to more overt glucose intolerance after treatment with large pharmacologic amounts of rhGH. Therefore, if HARS patients are treated with Serostim®, they should be very closely monitored for glucose intolerance.

Table 6: HARS Study 1 Maintenance Phase: Descriptive Statistics for Mean Changes from Week 12 to Week 24 in Various Body Composition Endpoints in Patients Randomized to Placebo vs. Serostim® 4 mg qod After 12 Weeks of Induction Therapy with Serostim® 4 mg Daily

Variable as Mean (SD)[c]		Placebo	Serostim® 4 mg qod
Visceral Adipose Tissue[a] (cm^2)	Week 12	138.7 (46.2) (n=25)	114.1 (75.0) (n=27)
	Change	17.7 (32.3) (n=25)	5.7 (41.4) (n=27)
Trunk Fat[b] (kg)	Week 12	8.3 (3.7) (n=27)	6.6 (3.3) (n=23)
	Change	1.2 (1.5) (n=27)	0.3 (1.2) (n=23)
Total Body Fat[b] (kg)	Week 12	13.9 (7.1) (n=27)	10.7 (5.5) (n=23)
	Change	1.3 (2.2) (n=27)	0.2 (1.9) (n=23)

(a) Measured by computed tomography (CT) scan;
(b) Assessed by dual energy X-Ray absorptiometry (DEXA) scan;
(c) SD = standard deviation

During safety surveillance of patients with HIV-associated wasting and HARS, cases of new onset impaired glucose tolerance, new onset type 2 diabetes mellitus and exacerbation of preexisting diabetes mellitus have been reported in patients receiving Serostim®. Some patients developed diabetic ketoacidosis and diabetic coma. In some patients, these conditions improved when Serostim® was discontinued, while in others, the glucose intolerance persisted. Some of these patients required initiation or adjustment of antidiabetic treatment while on Serostim®.

No cases of intracranial hypertension (IH) have been observed among patients treated with Serostim®. The syndrome of IH, with papilledema, visual changes, headache, and nausea and/or vomiting has been reported in a small number of children with growth failure treated with growth hormone products. Nevertheless, funduscopic evaluation of patients is recommended at the initiation and periodically during the course of Serostim® therapy.

Kaposi's sarcoma, lymphoma, and other malignancies are common in HIV+ individuals. There was no increase in the incidence of Kaposi's sarcoma, lymphoma, or in the progression of cutaneous Kaposi's sarcoma in clinical studies of Serostim®. Patients with internal KS lesions were excluded from the studies. Potential effects on other malignancies are unknown.

Information For Patients

Patients being treated with Serostim® should be informed of the potential benefits and risks associated with treatment. Patients should be instructed to contact their physician should they experience any side effects or discomfort during treatment with Serostim®.

It is recommended that Serostim® be administered using sterile, disposable syringes and needles. Patients should be thoroughly instructed in the importance of proper disposal and cautioned against any reuse of needles and syringes. An appropriate container for the disposal of used syringes and needles should be employed.

Patients should be instructed to rotate injection sites to avoid localized tissue atrophy.

Drug Interactions

Formal drug interaction studies have not been conducted. No data are available on drug interactions between Serostim® and HIV protease inhibitors or the non-nucleoside reverse transcriptase inhibitors.

Published *in vitro* data indicate that growth hormone may be an inducer of cytochrome P450 3A4. In clinical trials of HIV-infected patients with wasting or HARS who were receiving antiretroviral therapy, Serostim® did not adversely alter antiretroviral effectiveness, such as mean circulating levels of CD4 counts or HIV-1 RNA (viral load). When Serostim® is administered in combination with drugs known to be metabolized by CYP P450 3A4 hepatic enzymes, such as some antiretroviral drugs, it is advisable to monitor the clinical effectiveness of these drugs.

Somatropin inhibits 11β-hydroxysteroid dehydrogenase type 1 (11βHSD-1) in adipose/hepatic tissue and may significantly impact the metabolism of cortisol and cortisone. As a consequence, in patients treated with somatropin, previously undiagnosed primary (and secondary) hypoadrenalism may be unmasked requiring glucocorticoid replacement therapy. In addition, patients treated with glucocorticoid replacement therapy for previously diagnosed hypoadrenalism may require an increase in their maintenance or stress doses; this may be especially true for patients treated with cortisone acetate and prednisone since conversion of these drugs to their biologically active metabolites is dependent on the activity of the 11βHSD-1 enzyme.

Carcinogenesis, Mutagenesis, Impairment of Fertility

Long-term animal studies for carcinogenicity have not been performed with Serostim®. There is no evidence from animal studies to date of Serostim®-induced mutagenicity or impairment of fertility.

Pregnancy

Pregnancy Category B. Reproduction studies have been performed in rats and rabbits. Doses up to 5 to 10 times the human dose, based on body surface area, have revealed no evidence of impaired fertility or harm to the fetus due to Serostim®. There are, however, no adequate and well-controlled studies in pregnant women. Because animal reproduction studies are not always predictive of human response, this drug should be used during pregnancy only if clearly needed.

Nursing Women

It is not known whether Serostim® is excreted in human milk. Because many drugs are excreted in human milk, caution should be exercised when Serostim® is administered to a nursing woman.

Pediatric Use

In two small studies, 11 children with HIV-associated failure to thrive were treated subcutaneously with human growth hormone. In one study, five children (age range, 6 to 17 years) were treated with 0.04 mg/kg/day for 26 weeks. In a second study, six children (age range, 8 to 14 years) were treated with 0.07 mg/kg/day for 4 weeks. Treatment appeared to be well tolerated in both studies. The preliminary data collected on a limited number of patients with HIV-associated failure to thrive appear to be consistent with safety observations in growth hormone-treated adults with AIDS wasting.

Geriatric Use

Clinical studies with Serostim® did not include sufficient numbers of subjects aged 65 and over to determine whether they respond differently from younger subjects. Elderly patients may be more sensitive to growth hormone action, and may be more prone to develop adverse reactions. Thus, dose selection for an elderly patient should be cautious, usually starting at the low end of the dosing range.

ADVERSE REACTIONS

HIV-Associated Wasting or Cachexia

In the 12-week, placebo-controlled Clinical Trial 2, 510 patients were treated with Serostim® [somatropin (rDNA origin) for injection]. The most common adverse reactions judged to be associated with Serostim® were musculoskeletal discomfort and increased tissue turgor (swelling, particularly of the hands or feet), and were more frequently observed when Serostim® 0.1 mg/kg was administered on a daily basis (Table 7 and PRECAUTIONS). These symptoms were generally rated by investigators as mild to moderate in severity and often subsided with continued treatment or

Table 7: Controlled Clinical Trial 2 Adverse Events

Body System	Placebo	0.1 mg/kg qod Serostim®	0.1 mg/kg daily Serostim®
Preferred Term	Patients (n=247)	Patients (n=257)	Patients (n=253)
	%	%	%
Musculoskeletal System Disorders			
Arthralgia	11.3	24.5	36.4
Myalgia	11.7	17.9	30.4
Arthrosis	3.6	7.8	10.7
Gastro-Intestinal System Disorders			
Diarrhea	10.1	10.1	5.5
Nausea	4.9	5.4	9.1
Psychiatric Disorders			
Insomnia	6.1	3.9	5.9
Body As A Whole - General Disorders			
Edema Peripheral	2.8	11.3	26.1
Headache	9.3	10.1	12.6
Fatigue	4.5	3.5	5.1
Respiratory System Disorders			
Rhinitis	6.5	5.1	4.0
Upper Resp Tract Infection	5.7	4.3	3.6
Bronchitis	5.3	2.3	4.7
Endocrine Disorders			
Gynecomastia	0.4	3.5	5.5
Centr & Periph Nervous System Disorders			
Paresthesia	4.5	7.4	7.9
Hypoesthesia	2.4	1.6	5.1
Metabolic And Nutritional Disorders			
Edema Generalized	1.2	1.2	5.9

Table 8: Controlled HARS Studies 1 and 2 Combined - Adverse Events with >5% Incidence in Either Active Treatment Arm

System Organ Class	Placebo	Serostim® 4 mg qod[1]	Serostim® 4 mg daily
	Patients (n=159)	Patients (n=80)	Patients (n=326)
Preferred Term	%	%	%
Musculoskeletal and connective tissue disorders			
Arthralgia	11.9	27.8	37.1
Pain in extremity	3.8	5.0	19.3
Myalgia	3.8	2.5	12.6
Musculoskeletal stiffness	1.9	3.8	8.0
Joint stiffness	1.3	3.8	7.7
Joint swelling	0.6	5.0	6.1
General disorders and administration site conditions			
Edema peripheral	3.8	18.8	45.4
Fatigue	1.9	6.3	8.9
Nervous system disorders			
Hypoesthesia	0.6	8.8	15.0
Headache	3.1	3.8	14.1
Paraesthesia	2.5	12.5	11.0
Investigations (Laboratory Evaluations)			
Blood glucose increased[2]	2.5	3.8	13.8
Metabolism and nutrition disorders			
Hyperglycemia[2]	0.6	8.8	7.1
Fluid retention	0.6	2.5	5.2
Gastrointestinal disorders			
Nausea	2.5	1.3	6.1
Psychiatric disorders			
Insomnia	1.9	7.5	8.3
Infections and infestations			
Upper respiratory tract infection	5.0	10.0	5.2

[1] Study 22388 only
[2] similar terms were grouped together and reported below

dose reduction. Approximately 23% of patients receiving Serostim® 0.1 mg/kg daily and 11% of patients receiving 0.1 mg/kg every other day required dose reductions. Discontinuations as a result of adverse events occurred in 10.3% of patients receiving Serostim® 0.1 mg/kg daily and 6.6% of patients receiving 0.1 mg/kg every other day. The most common reasons for dose reduction and/or drug discontinuation were arthralgia, myalgia, edema, carpal tunnel syndrome, elevated glucose levels, and elevated triglyceride levels.

Clinical adverse events which occurred during the first 12 weeks of study in at least 5% of the patients in any one of the three treatment groups are listed below by treatment group, without regard to causality assessment.
[See table above]

Adverse events that occurred in 1% to less than 5% of trial participants receiving Serostim® during the first 12 weeks of Clinical Trial 2 thought to be related to Serostim® included dependent edema, periorbital edema, carpal tunnel syndrome, hyperglycemia and hypertriglyceridemia.

During the 12-week, placebo-controlled portion of Clinical Trial 2, the incidence of hyperglycemia reported as an adverse event was 3.6% for the placebo group, 1.9% for the 0.1 mg/kg qod group and 3.2% for the 0.1 mg/kg daily group. One case of diabetes mellitus was noted in the 0.1 mg/kg daily group during the first 12-weeks of therapy. In addition, during the extension phase of Clinical Trial 2, two patients converted from placebo to full dose Serostim®, and 1 patient converted from placebo to half-dose Serostim®, were discontinued because of the development of diabetes mellitus.

The types and incidences of adverse events reported during the Clinical Trial 2 extension phase were not different from, or greater in frequency than those observed during the 12-week, placebo-controlled portion of Clinical Trial 2.

HIV-Associated Adipose Redistribution Syndrome (HARS)
In the initial 12-week treatment periods of the two HARS, placebo-controlled clinical trials, 406 patients were treated with Serostim®. Clinical adverse events which occurred during the first 12 weeks of both studies combined in at least 5% of the patients in either of the two active treatment groups are listed by treatment group in Table 8, without regard to causality assessment. The most common adverse reactions judged to be associated with Serostim® were edema, arthralgia, pain in extremity, hypoesthesia, myalgia, and blood glucose increased, all of which were more frequently observed when Serostim® 4 mg was administered on a daily basis compared with alternate days. These symptoms were generally rated by investigators as mild to moderate in severity and often subsided with dose reduction. In addition, during the 12-week induction phase, 1) approximately 26% of patients receiving Serostim® 4 mg daily and 19% of patients receiving Serostim® 4 mg qod required dose reductions; and 2) discontinuations as a result of adverse events occurred in 13% of patients receiving Serostim® 4 mg daily and 5% of patients receiving Serostim® 4 mg qod. Once again, the most common reasons for dose reduction and/or drug discontinuation were peripheral edema, hyperglycemia (including blood glucose increased, blood glucose abnormal, and hyperglycemia), and arthralgia.
[See table 8 at left]

Glucose-Related Terms: Similar glucose-related adverse event terms (including hyperglycemia, blood glucose increased, blood glucose abnormal) were grouped together which resulted in a greater than 5% incidence in Serostim®-treated patients. During the initial 12-week treatment periods of HARS Studies 1 and 2, the incidence of glucose-related adverse events was 4% for the placebo group, 13% for the 4 mg qod group and 22% for the 4 mg daily group. No patients required treatment for hyperglycemia. Of the 23 patients who discontinued due to hyperglycemia during any phase of these studies, 13 were being treated with induction therapy with Serostim® 4 mg daily (and 9 of these 13 during the 12 week induction phases of HARS Studies 1 and 2). One of these patients whose baseline fasting blood glucose was 95 mg/dL demonstrated substantial hyperglycemia (384 mg/dL) 12 days after treatment with Serostim® 4 mg daily was begun; however, the patient was normoglycemic 1 month after Serostim® was discontinued without treatment for hyperglycemia. A second patient in HARS Study 2 whose fasting blood glucose was 89 mg/dL at baseline manifested a fasting blood glucose of 404 mg/dL 21 days after treatment with Serostim® 4 mg daily was begun. His last known fasting blood glucose 1 week after Serostim® had been discontinued was 224 mg/dL and then he was lost to follow-up. Whether sustained overt diabetes mellitus persisted is therefore unknown.

Breast-Related Terms: Similar breast-related adverse event terms (including nipple pain, gynecomastia, breast pain/mass/tenderness/swelling/edema/hypertrophy) were grouped together which resulted in a greater than 5% incidence in Serostim®-treated patients. The incidence of breast-related adverse event reports was 1% for the placebo group, 3% for the 4 mg qod group and 6% for the 4 mg daily group.

Adverse events that occurred in 1% to less than 5% of trial participants receiving Serostim® during the first 12 weeks of HARS Studies 1 and 2 thought to be related to Serostim® include carpal tunnel syndrome, tinel's sign and facial edema.

The adverse events reported for Serostim® 4 mg qod during the maintenance phase of HARS Study 1 (Week 12 to Week 24) were similar in frequency and quality to those observed after treatment with Serostim® 4 mg qod during the 12-week induction phase.

During safety surveillance of patients with HIV-associated wasting and HARS, cases of new onset impaired glucose tolerance, new onset type 2 diabetes mellitus and exacerbation of preexisting diabetes mellitus have been reported in patients receiving Serostim®. Some patients developed diabetic ketoacidosis and diabetic coma. In some patients, these conditions improved when Serostim® was discontinued, while in others the glucose intolerance persisted. Some of these patients required initiation or adjustment of antidiabetic treatment while on Serostim®.

OVERDOSAGE

Glucose intolerance can occur with overdosage. Long-term overdosage with growth hormone could result in signs and symptoms of acromegaly.

DOSAGE AND ADMINISTRATION

HIV-Associated Wasting or Cachexia
The usual starting dose of Serostim® [somatropin (rDNA origin) for injection] is 0.1 mg/kg subcutaneously (SC) daily (up to 6 mg). It should be administered SC daily at bedtime according to the following dosage recommendations:

Weight Range	Dose
>55kg (>121 lb)	6 mg* SC daily
45-55 kg (99-121 lb)	5 mg* SC daily
35-45 kg (75-99 lb)	4 mg* SC daily
<35 kg (<75 lb)	0.1 mg/kg SC daily

*Based on an approximate daily dosage of 0.1 mg/kg.

Serostim® 8.8 mg and Serostim® 4 mg with Bacteriostatic Water for Injection, USP (0.9% Benzyl Alcohol), multi-use vials, should be administered as per the above weight-based dosing table. Serostim® 5 or 6 mg with Sterile Water for Injection, USP, single use vials, should be administered to patients requiring 5 or 6 mg daily, respectively, as per the above weight-based dosing table.

Treatment with Serostim® 0.1 mg/kg every other day was associated with fewer side effects, and resulted in a similar improvement in work output, as compared with Serostim® 0.1 mg/kg daily. Therefore, a starting dose of Serostim® 0.1 mg/kg every other day should be considered in patients at increased risk for adverse effects related to recombinant human growth hormone therapy (i.e., glucose intolerance). In general, dose reductions (i.e., reducing the total daily dose or the number of doses per week) should be considered for side effects potentially related to recombinant human growth hormone therapy, which are unresponsive to symptom-directed treatment.

Most of the effect of Serostim® on work output and lean body mass was apparent after 12 weeks of treatment. The effect was maintained during an additional 12 weeks of therapy. There are no safety or efficacy data available from controlled studies in which patients were treated with Serostim® continuously for more than 48 weeks. There are no safety or efficacy data available from trials in which patients were treated intermittently with Serostim®.

Injection sites should be rotated to avoid local irritation.

Safety and effectiveness in pediatric patients with HIV have not been established.

Each vial of Serostim® 5 mg or 6 mg is reconstituted with 0.5 to 1 mL Sterile Water for Injection, USP. Each vial of Serostim® 8.8 mg is reconstituted in 1 to 2 mL of Bacteriostatic Water for Injection, USP (0.9% Benzyl Alcohol preserved) and each vial of Serostim® 4 mg is reconstituted in 0.5 to 1 mL of Bacteriostatic Water for Injection, USP (0.9% Benzyl Alcohol preserved). Approximately 10% mechanical loss can be associated with reconstitution and administration from multi-dose vials. For patients sensitive to this diluent, see WARNINGS.

To reconstitute Serostim®, inject the diluent into the vial of Serostim® aiming the liquid against the glass vial wall. Swirl the vial with a gentle rotary motion until contents are dissolved completely. The Serostim® solution should be clear immediately after reconstitution. **DO NOT INJECT** Serostim® if the reconstituted product is cloudy immediately after reconstitution or after refrigeration (2-8°C/36-46°F) for up to 14 days. Occasionally, after refrigeration, small colorless particles may be present in the Serostim® solution. This is not unusual for proteins like Serostim®.

STABILITY AND STORAGE

Before reconstitution: Vials of Serostim® and diluent should be stored at room temperature, (15°-30°C/59°-86°F). Expiration dates are stated on product labels.

After Reconstitution with Sterile Water for Injection, USP: The reconstituted solution should be used immediately and any unused portion should be discarded.

After Reconstitution with Bacteriostatic Water for Injection, USP (0.9% Benzyl Alcohol): The reconstituted solution should be stored under refrigeration (2-8°C/36-46°F) for up to 14 days.

Avoid freezing reconstituted vials of Serostim®.

HOW SUPPLIED

Serostim® can be administered using (1) a standard sterile, disposable syringe and needle, (2) a compatible Serostim® needle-free injection device or (3) a compatible Serostim® needle injection device. For proper use, refer to the Instructions for Use provided with the administration device.

Serostim® [somatropin (rDNA origin) for injection] is available in the following forms:

Serostim® vials containing 5 mg (approximately 15 IU) somatropin (mammalian-cell) with Sterile Water for Injection, USP. Package of 7 vials. NDC 44087-0005-7

Serostim® vials containing 6 mg (approximately 18 IU) somatropin (mammalian-cell) with Sterile Water for Injection, USP. Package of 7 vials. NDC 44087-0006-7

Serostim® vials containing 4 mg (approximately 12 IU) somatropin (mammalian-cell) with Bacteriostatic Water for Injection, USP (0.9% Benzyl Alcohol). Package of 7 vials. NDC 44087-0004-7

Serostim® vial containing 8.8 mg (approximately 26.4 IU) somatropin (mammalian-cell) with Bacteriostatic Water for Injection, USP (0.9% Benzyl Alcohol). Package of 1 vials. NDC 44087-0088-4

Manufactured for: EMD Serono, Inc., Rockland, MA 02370

Rx Only BX Rated

September 2007

EDUCATIONAL MATERIAL

Access the EMD Serono website www.emdserono.com for product, educational, and service information for practitioners and consumers.

To receive available educational and medical literature about EMD Serono products, or the conditions they treat, phone inquiries can be made by calling the U.S. Medical Information Group at (888) 275-7376 or (781) 982-9000.

Endo Pharmaceuticals

100 ENDO BOULEVARD
CHADDS FORD, PA 19317

Direct Inquiries to:
Pharmacovigilance – Serious Adverse Event Reporting
Phone: 800-462-3636
Fax: 408-501-1900 (LIDODERM Only)
Fax: 866-395-5312 (All Other Products)
Medical Information
Phone: 800-462-3636
Fax: 877-346-6394

DELATESTRYL® CIII ℞

[del-uh-tes-tril]

(Testosterone Enanthate Injection, USP)
Multiple Dose Vial

DESCRIPTION

DELATESTRYL® (Testosterone Enanthate Injection, USP) provides testosterone enanthate, a derivative of the primary endogenous androgen testosterone, for intramuscular administration. In their active form, androgens have a 17-beta-hydroxy group. Esterification of the 17-beta-hydroxy group increases the duration of action of testosterone; hydrolysis to free testosterone occurs *in vivo*. Each mL of sterile, colorless to pale yellow solution provides 200 mg testosterone enanthate in sesame oil with 5 mg chlorobutanol (chloral derivative) as a preservative.

Testosterone enanthate is designated chemically as androst-4-en-3-one, 17-[(1-oxoheptyl)-oxy]-, (17β)-. Structural formula:

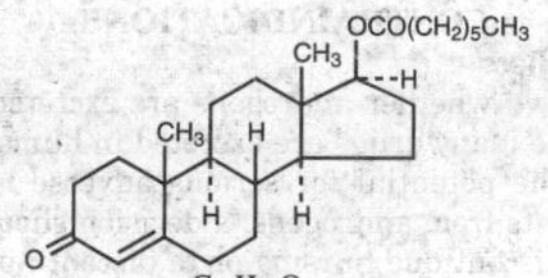

$C_{26}H_{40}O_3$
MW: 400.60

CLINICAL PHARMACOLOGY

Endogenous androgens are responsible for the normal growth and development of the male sex organs and for maintenance of secondary sex characteristics. These effects include growth and maturation of prostate, seminal vesicles, penis, and scrotum; development of male hair distribution, such as beard, pubic, chest, and axillary hair; laryngeal enlargement; vocal chord thickening; alterations in body musculature; and fat distribution.

Androgens also cause retention of nitrogen, sodium, potassium, and phosphorus, and decreased urinary excretion of calcium. Androgens have been reported to increase protein anabolism and decrease protein catabolism. Nitrogen balance is improved only when there is sufficient intake of calories and protein.

Androgens are responsible for the growth spurt of adolescence and for the eventual termination of linear growth which is brought about by fusion of the epiphyseal growth centers. In children, exogenous androgens accelerate linear growth rates but may cause a disproportionate advancement in bone maturation. Use over long periods may result in fusion of the epiphyseal growth centers and termination of the growth process. Androgens have been reported to stimulate the production of red blood cells by enhancing the production of erythropoietic stimulating factor.

During exogenous administration of androgens, endogenous testosterone release is inhibited through feedback inhibition of pituitary luteinizing hormone (LH). At large doses of exogenous androgens, spermatogenesis may also be suppressed through feedback inhibition of pituitary follicle stimulating hormone (FSH).

There is a lack of substantial evidence that androgens are effective in fractures, surgery, convalescence, and functional uterine bleeding.

PHARMACOKINETICS

Testosterone esters are less polar than free testosterone. Testosterone esters in oil injected intramuscularly are absorbed slowly from the lipid phase; thus testosterone enanthate can be given at intervals of two to four weeks.

Testosterone in plasma is 98 percent bound to a specific testosterone-estradiol binding globulin, and about two percent is free. Generally, the amount of this sex-hormone binding globulin (SHBG) in the plasma will determine the distribution of testosterone between free and bound forms, and the free testosterone concentration will determine its half-life.

About 90 percent of a dose of testosterone is excreted in the urine as glucuronic and sulfuric acid conjugates of testosterone and its metabolites; about six percent of a dose is excreted in the feces, mostly in the unconjugated form. Inactivation of testosterone occurs primarily in the liver. Testosterone is metabolized to various 17-keto steroids through two different pathways. There are considerable variations of the half-life of testosterone as reported in the literature, ranging from 10 to 100 minutes.

In responsive tissues, the activity of testosterone appears to depend on reduction to dihydrotestosterone (DHT), which binds to cytosol receptor proteins. The steroid-receptor complex is transported to the nucleus where it initiates transcription events and cellular changes related to androgen action.

INDICATIONS AND USAGE

Males

DELATESTRYL® (Testosterone Enanthate Injection, USP) is indicated for replacement therapy in conditions associated with a deficiency or absence of endogenous testosterone.

Primary hypogonadism (congenital or acquired)–Testicular failure due to cryptorchidism, bilateral torsion, orchitis, vanishing testis syndrome, or orchidectomy.

Hypogonadotropic hypogonadism (congenital or acquired)–Idiopathic gonadotropin or luteinizing hormone-releasing hormone (LHRH) deficiency, or pituitary-hypothalamic injury from tumors, trauma, or radiation. (Appropriate adrenal cortical and thyroid hormone replacement therapy are still necessary, however, and are actually of primary importance.)

If the above conditions occur prior to puberty, androgen replacement therapy will be needed during the adolescent years for development of secondary sexual characteristics. Prolonged androgen treatment will be required to maintain sexual characteristics in these and other males who develop testosterone deficiency after puberty.

Delayed puberty–DELATESTRYL® (Testosterone Enanthate Injection, USP) may be used to stimulate puberty in carefully selected males with clearly delayed puberty. These patients usually have a familial pattern of delayed puberty that is not secondary to a pathological disorder; puberty is expected to occur spontaneously at a relatively late date. Brief treatment with conservative doses may occasionally be justified in these patients if they do not respond to psychological support. The potential adverse effect on bone maturation should be discussed with the patient and parents prior to androgen administration. An X-ray of the hand and wrist to determine bone age should be obtained every six months to assess the effect of treatment on the epiphyseal centers (see **WARNINGS**).

Females

Metastatic mammary cancer–DELATESTRYL® (Testosterone Enanthate Injection, USP) may be used secondarily in women with advancing inoperable metastatic (skeletal) mammary cancer who are one to five years postmenopausal. Primary goals of therapy in these women include ablation of the ovaries. Other methods of counteracting estrogen activity are adrenalectomy, hypophysectomy, and/or antiestrogen therapy. This treatment has also been used in premenopausal women with breast cancer who have benefited from oophorectomy and are considered to have a hormone-responsive tumor. Judgment concerning androgen therapy should be made by an oncologist with expertise in this field.

CONTRAINDICATIONS

Androgens are contraindicated in men with carcinomas of the breast or with known or suspected carcinomas of the prostate and in women who are or may become pregnant. When administered to pregnant women, androgens cause virilization of the external genitalia of the female fetus. This virilization includes clitoromegaly, abnormal vaginal development, and fusion of genital folds to form a scrotal-like structure. The degree of masculinization is related to the amount of drug given and the age of the fetus and is most likely to occur in the female fetus when the drugs are given in the first trimester. If the patient becomes pregnant while taking androgens, she should be apprised of the potential hazard to the fetus.

This preparation is also contraindicated in patients with a history of hypersensitivity to any of its components.

WARNINGS

In patients with breast cancer and in immobilized patients, androgen therapy may cause hypercalcemia by stimulating osteolysis. In patients with cancer, hypercalcemia may indicate progression of bony metastasis. If hypercalcemia occurs, the drug should be discontinued and appropriate measures instituted.

Prolonged use of high doses of androgens has been associated with the development of peliosis hepatis and hepatic neoplasms including hepatocellular carcinoma (see **PRECAUTIONS, Carcinogenesis**). Peliosis hepatis can be a life-threatening or fatal complication.

If cholestatic hepatitis with jaundice appears or if liver function tests become abnormal, the androgen should be discontinued and the etiology should be determined. Drug-induced jaundice is reversible when the medication is discontinued.

Geriatric patients treated with androgens may be at an increased risk for the development of prostatic hypertrophy and prostatic carcinoma.

Due to sodium and water retention, edema with or without congestive heart failure may be a serious complication in patients with preexisting cardiac, renal, or hepatic disease. In addition to discontinuation of the drug, diuretic therapy may be required. If the administration of testosterone enanthate is restarted, a lower dose should be used.

Gynecomastia frequently develops and occasionally persists in patients being treated for hypogonadism.

Androgen therapy should be used cautiously in healthy males with delayed puberty. The effect on bone maturation should be monitored by assessing bone age of the wrist and hand every six months. In children, androgen treatment may accelerate bone maturation without producing compensatory gain in linear growth. This adverse effect may result in compromised adult stature. The younger the child the greater the risk of compromising final mature height.

PRECAUTIONS

General

Women should be observed for signs of virilization (deepening of the voice, hirsutism, acne, clitoromegaly, and menstrual irregularities). Discontinuation of drug therapy at the time of evidence of mild virilism is necessary to prevent irreversible virilization. Such virilization is usual following androgen use at high doses and is not prevented by concomitant use of estrogens. A decision may be made by the patient and the physician that some virilization will be tolerated during treatment for breast carcinoma.

Because androgens may alter serum cholesterol concentration, caution should be used when administering these drugs to patients with a history of myocardial infarction or coronary artery disease. Serial determinations of serum cholesterol should be made and therapy adjusted accordingly. A causal relationship between myocardial infarction and hypercholesterolemia has not been established.

Information for Patients

Male adolescent patients receiving androgens for delayed puberty should have bone development checked every six months.

The physician should instruct patients to report any of the following side effects of androgens:

Adult or adolescent males–too frequent or persistent erections of the penis.

Women–hoarseness, acne, changes in menstrual periods, or more facial hair.

All patients–any nausea, vomiting, changes in skin color, or ankle swelling.

Geriatric Use

Clinical studies of DELATESTRYL did not include sufficient numbers of subjects, aged 65 and older, to determine whether they respond differently from younger subjects. Testosterone replacement is not indicated in geriatric patients who have age-related hypogonadism only ("andropause"), because there is insufficient safety and efficacy information to support such use. Current studies do not assess whether testosterone use increases risks of prostate cancer, prostate hyperplasia, and cardiovascular disease in the geriatric population.

Intramuscular Administration

When properly given, injections of DELATESTRYL are well tolerated. Care should be taken to slowly inject the preparation deeply into the gluteal muscle, being sure to follow the usual precautions for intramuscular administration, such as the avoidance of intravascular injection. There have been rare postmarketing reports of transient reactions involving urge to cough, coughing fits, and respiratory distress immediately after the injection of DELATESTRYL, an oil-based depot preparation (see **DOSAGE AND ADMINISTRATION**).

Laboratory Tests

Women with disseminated breast carcinoma should have frequent determination of urine and serum calcium levels during the course of androgen therapy (see **WARNINGS**).

Periodic (every six months) X-ray examinations of bone age should be made during treatment of pre-pubertal males to determine the rate of bone maturation and the effects of androgen therapy on the epiphyseal centers.

Hemoglobin and hematocrit should be checked periodically for polycythemia in patients who are receiving high doses of androgens.

Drug Interactions

When administered concurrently, the following drugs may interact with androgens:

Anticoagulants, oral–C-17 substituted derivatives of testosterone, such as methandrostenolone, have been reported to decrease the anticoagulant requirement. Patients receiving oral anticoagulant therapy require close monitoring especially when androgens are started or stopped.

Antidiabetic drugs and insulin–In diabetic patients, the metabolic effects of androgens may decrease blood glucose and insulin requirements.

ACTH and corticosteroids–Enhanced tendency toward edema. Use caution when giving these drugs together, especially in patients with hepatic or cardiac disease.

Oxyphenbutazone–Elevated serum levels of oxyphenbutazone may result.

Drug/Laboratory Test Interferences

Androgens may decrease levels of thyroxine-binding globulin, resulting in decreased total T4 serum levels and increased resin uptake of T3 and T4. Free thyroid hormone levels remain unchanged, however, and there is no clinical evidence of thyroid dysfunction.

Carcinogenesis

Testosterone has been tested by subcutaneous injection and implantation in mice and rats. The implant induced cervical-uterine tumors in mice, which metastasized in some cases. There is suggestive evidence that injection of testosterone into some strains of female mice increases their susceptibility to hepatoma. Testosterone is also known to increase the number of tumors and decrease the degree of differentiation of chemically induced carcinomas of the liver in rats.

There are rare reports of hepatocellular carcinoma in patients receiving long-term therapy with androgens in high doses. Withdrawal of the drugs did not lead to regression of the tumors in all cases.

Geriatric patients treated with androgens may be at an increased risk for the development of prostatic hypertrophy and prostatic carcinoma.

Pregnancy: Teratogenic Effects

Category X (see **CONTRAINDICATIONS**).

Nursing Mothers

It is not known whether androgens are excreted in human milk. Because many drugs are excreted in human milk and because of the potential for serious adverse reactions in nursing infants from androgens, a decision should be made whether to discontinue nursing or to discontinue the drug, taking into account the importance of the drug to the mother.

Pediatric Use

Androgen therapy should be used very cautiously in pediatric patients and only by specialists who are aware of the adverse effects on bone maturation. Skeletal maturation must be monitored every six months by an X-ray of the hand and wrist (see **INDICATIONS AND USAGE**, and **WARNINGS**).

ADVERSE REACTIONS

Endocrine and Urogenital, Female–The most common side effects of androgen therapy are amenorrhea and other menstrual irregularities, inhibition of gonadotropin secretion, and virilization, including deepening of the voice and clitoral enlargement. The latter usually is not reversible after androgens are discontinued. When administered to a pregnant woman, androgens cause virilization of the external genitalia of the female fetus. *Male*–Gynecomastia, and excessive frequency and duration of penile erections. Oligospermia may occur at high dosages (see **CLINICAL PHARMACOLOGY**).

Skin and Appendages–Hirsutism, male pattern baldness, and acne.

Fluid and Electrolyte Disturbances–Retention of sodium, chloride, water, potassium, calcium (see **WARNINGS**), and inorganic phosphates.

Gastrointestinal–Nausea, cholestatic jaundice, alterations in liver function tests; rarely, hepatocellular neoplasms, peliosis hepatis (see **WARNINGS**).

Hematologic–Suppression of clotting factors II, V, VII, and X; bleeding in patients on concomitant anticoagulant therapy; polycythemia.

Nervous System–Increased or decreased libido, headache, anxiety, depression, and generalized paresthesia.

Metabolic–Increased serum cholesterol.

Miscellaneous–Rarely, anaphylactoid reactions; inflammation and pain at injection site.

DRUG ABUSE AND DEPENDENCE

DELATESTRYL® (Testosterone Enanthate Injection, USP) is classified as a controlled substance under the Anabolic Steroids Control Act of 1990 and has been assigned to Schedule III.

OVERDOSAGE

There have been no reports of acute overdosage with androgens.

DOSAGE AND ADMINISTRATION

Dosage and duration of therapy with DELATESTRYL® (Testosterone Enanthate Injection, USP) will depend on age, sex, diagnosis, patient's response to treatment, and appearance of adverse effects. When properly given, injections of DELATESTRYL are well tolerated. Care should be taken to inject the preparation deeply into the gluteal muscle, being sure to follow the usual precautions for intramuscular administration, such as the avoidance of intramuscular injection (see **PRECAUTIONS**).

In general, total doses above 400 mg per month are not required because of the prolonged action of the preparation. Injections more frequently than every two weeks are rarely indicated. NOTE: Use of a wet needle or wet syringe may cause the solution to become cloudy; however this does not affect the potency of the material. Parenteral drug products should be inspected visually for particulate matter and discoloration prior to administration, whenever solution and container permit. DELATESTRYL is a clear, colorless to pale yellow solution

Male hypogonadism: As replacement therapy, i.e., for eunuchism, the suggested dosage is 50 to 400 mg every 2 to 4 weeks.

In males with delayed puberty: Various dosage regimens have been used; some call for lower dosages initially with gradual increases as puberty progresses, with or without a decrease to maintenance levels. Other regimens call for higher dosage to induce pubertal changes and lower dosage for maintenance after puberty. The chronological and skeletal ages must be taken into consideration, both in determining the initial dose and in adjusting the dose. Dosage is within the range of 50 to 200 mg every 2 to 4 weeks for a limited duration, for example, 4 to 6 months. X-rays should be taken at appropriate intervals to determine the amount of bone maturation and skeletal development (see **INDICATIONS AND USAGE**, and **WARNINGS**).

Palliation of inoperable mammary cancer in women: A dosage of 200 to 400 mg every 2 to 4 weeks is recommended. Women with metastatic breast carcinoma must be followed closely because androgen therapy occasionally appears to accelerate the disease.

HOW SUPPLIED

DELATESTRYL® (Testosterone Enanthate Injection, USP) is available in 5 mL (200 mg/mL) multiple dose vials.

STORAGE

DELATESTRYL® (Testosterone Enanthate Injection, USP) should be stored at room temperature. Warming and rotating the vial between the palms of the hands will redissolve any crystals that may have formed during storage at low temperatures.

For Prescription Use Only
Manufactured for:
Indevus Pharmaceuticals, Inc.
Lexington, MA 02421
Manufactured by:
Sandoz Canada Inc.
Boucherville, QC, Canada J4B 7K8
Medical Inquiries:
877-263-2436
Made in Canada
Revised: July 2007

FROVA® ℞

[*frō-vă*]
(frovatriptan succinate)
Tablets

DESCRIPTION

FROVA (frovatriptan succinate) tablets contain frovatriptan succinate, a selective 5-hydroxy-tryptamine$_1$ (5-HT$_{1B/1D}$) receptor subtype agonist, as the active ingredient. Frovatriptan succinate is chemically designated as R-(+) 3-methylamino-6-carboxamido-1,2,3,4-tetrahydrocarbazole monosuccinate monohydrate and it has the following structure:

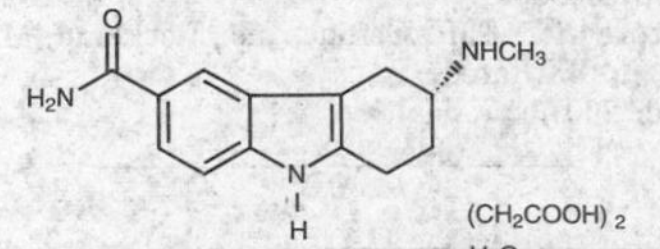

The empirical formula is $C_{14}H_{17}N_3O.C_4H_6O_4.H_2O$, representing a molecular weight of 379.4. Frovatriptan succinate is a white to off-white powder that is soluble in water. Each FROVA tablet for oral administration contains 3.91 mg frovatriptan succinate, equivalent to 2.5 mg of frovatriptan base. Each tablet also contains the inactive ingredients lactose NF, microcrystalline cellulose NF, colloidal silicon dioxide NF, sodium starch glycolate NF, magnesium stearate NF, hydroxypropylmethylcellulose USP, polyethylene glycol 3000 USP, triacetin USP, and titanium dioxide USP.

CLINICAL PHARMACOLOGY

Mechanism of Action

Frovatriptan is a 5-HT receptor agonist that binds with high affinity for 5-HT_{1B} and 5-HT_{1D} receptors. Frovatriptan has no significant effects on $GABA_A$ mediated channel activity and has no significant affinity for benzodiazepine binding sites.

Frovatriptan is believed to act on extracerebral, intracranial arteries and to inhibit excessive dilation of these vessels in migraine. In anesthetized dogs and cats, intravenous administration of frovatriptan produced selective constriction of the carotid vascular bed and had no effect on blood pressure (both species) or coronary resistance (in dogs).

Pharmacokinetics

Mean maximum blood concentrations (C_{max}) in patients are achieved approximately 2-4 hours after administration of a single oral dose of frovatriptan 2.5 mg. The absolute bioavailability of an oral dose of frovatriptan 2.5 mg in healthy subjects is about 20% in males and 30% in females. Food has no significant effect on the bioavailability of frovatriptan, but delays t_{max} by one hour.

Binding of frovatriptan to serum proteins is low (approximately 15%). Reversible binding to blood cells at equilibrium is approximately 60%, resulting in a blood:plasma ratio of about 2:1 in both males and females. The mean steady state volume of distribution of frovatriptan following intravenous administration of 0.8 mg is 4.2 L/kg in males and 3.0 L/kg in females.

In vitro, cytochrome P450 1A2 appears to be the principal enzyme involved in the metabolism of frovatriptan. Following administration of a single oral dose of radiolabeled frovatriptan 2.5 mg to healthy male and female subjects, 32% of the dose was recovered in urine and 62% in feces. Radiolabeled compounds excreted in urine were unchanged frovatriptan, hydroxylated frovatriptan, N-acetyl desmethyl frovatriptan, hydroxylated N-acetyl desmethyl frovatriptan and desmethyl frovatriptan, together with several other minor metabolites. Desmethyl frovatriptan has lower affinity for $5\text{-HT}_{1B/1D}$ receptors compared to the parent compound. The N-acetyl desmethyl metabolite has no significant affinity for 5-HT receptors. The activity of the other metabolites is unknown.

After an intravenous dose, mean clearance of frovatriptan was 220 and 130 mL/min in males and females, respectively. Renal clearance accounted for about 40% (82 mL/min) and 45% (60 mL/min) of total clearance in males and females, respectively. The mean terminal elimination half-life of frovatriptan in both males and females is approximately 26 hours.

The pharmacokinetics of frovatriptan are similar in migraine patients and healthy subjects.

Special Populations

Age:

Mean AUC of frovatriptan was 1.5- to 2-fold higher in healthy elderly subjects (age 65–77 years) compared to those in healthy younger subjects (age 21-37 years). There was no difference in t_{max} or $t_{1/2}$ between the two populations.

Gender:

There was no difference in the mean terminal elimination half-life of frovatriptan in males and females. Bioavailability was higher, and systemic exposure to frovatriptan was approximately 2-fold greater, in females than males, irrespective of age.

Renal Impairment:

Since less than 10% of FROVA is excreted in urine after an oral dose, it is unlikely that the exposure to frovatriptan will be affected by renal impairment. The pharmacokinetics of frovatriptan following a single oral dose of 2.5 mg was not different in patients with renal impairment (5 males and 6 females, creatinine clearance 16-73 mL/min) and in subjects with normal renal function.

Hepatic Impairment:

There is no clinical or pharmacokinetic experience with FROVA in patients with severe hepatic impairment. The AUC in subjects with mild (Child-Pugh 5-6) to moderate (Child-Pugh 7-9) hepatic impairment is about twice as high as the AUC in young, healthy subjects, but within the range found among normal elderly subjects.

Race:

The effect of race on the pharmacokinetics of frovatriptan has not been examined.

Drug Interactions (see also PRECAUTIONS, *Drug Interactions*)

Frovatriptan is not an inhibitor of human monoamine oxidase (MAO) enzymes or cytochrome P450 (isozymes 1A2, 2C9, 2C19, 2D6, 2E1, 3A4) *in vitro* at concentrations up to 250 to 500- fold higher than the highest blood concentrations observed in man at a dose of 2.5 mg. No induction of drug metabolizing enzymes was observed following multiple dosing of frovatriptan to rats or on addition to human hepatocytes *in vitro*. Although no clinical studies have been performed, it is unlikely that frovatriptan will affect the metabolism of co-administered drugs metabolized by these mechanisms.

Oral contraceptives:

Retrospective analysis of pharmacokinetic data from females across trials indicated that the mean C_{max} and AUC of frovatriptan are 30% higher in those subjects taking oral contraceptives compared to those not taking oral contraceptives.

Ergotamine:

The AUC and C_{max} of frovatriptan (2×2.5 mg dose) were reduced by approximately 25% when co-administered with ergotamine tartrate.

Propranolol:

Propranolol increased the AUC of frovatriptan 2.5 mg in males by 60% and in females by 29%. The C_{max} of frovatriptan was increased 23% in males and 16% in females in the presence of propranolol. The t_{max} as well as half-life of frovatriptan, though slightly longer in the females, were not affected by concomitant administration of propranolol.

Moclobemide:

The pharmacokinetic profile of frovatriptan was unaffected when a single oral dose of frovatriptan 2.5 mg was administered to healthy female subjects receiving the MAO-A inhibitor, moclobemide, at an oral dose of 150 mg bid for 8 days.

Clinical Trials

The efficacy of FROVA in the acute treatment of migraine headaches was demonstrated in five randomized, double-blind, placebo-controlled, outpatient trials. Two of these were dose-finding studies in which patients were randomized to receive doses of frovatriptan ranging from 0.5-40 mg. The three studies evaluating only one dose studied 2.5 mg. In these controlled short-term studies combined, patients were predominately female (88%) and Caucasian (94%) with a mean age of 42 years (range 18-69). Patients were instructed to treat a moderate to severe headache. Headache response, defined as a reduction in headache severity from moderate or severe pain to mild or no pain, was assessed for up to 24 hours after dosing. The associated symptoms nausea, vomiting, photophobia and phonophobia were also assessed. Maintenance of response was assessed for up to 24 hours post dose. In two of the trials a second dose of FROVA was provided after the initial treatment, to treat recurrence of the headache within 24 hours. Other medication, excluding other 5-HT_1 agonists and ergotamine containing compounds, was permitted from 2 hours after the first dose of FROVA. The frequency and time to use of additional medications were also recorded.

In all five placebo-controlled trials, the percentage of patients achieving a headache response 2 hours after treatment was significantly greater for those taking FROVA compared to those taking placebo (Table 1).

Lower doses of frovatriptan (1 mg or 0.5 mg) were not effective at 2 hours. Higher doses (5 mg to 40 mg) of frovatriptan showed no added benefit over 2.5 mg but did cause a greater incidence of adverse events.

Table 1 Percentage of Patients with Headache Response (Mild or No Headache) 2 Hours Following Treatment[a]

Trial	FROVA (frovatriptan 2.5 mg)	Placebo
1	42%* (n=90)	22% (n=91)
2	38%* (n=121)	25% (n=115)
3	39%* (n=187)	21% (n=99)
4	46%** (n=672)	27% (n=347)
5	37%** (n=438)	23% (n=225)

[a]ITT observed data, excludes patients who had missing data or were asleep;
*p<0.05,
**p<0.001 in comparison with placebo

Comparisons of drug performance based upon results obtained in different clinical trials are never reliable. Because trials are conducted at different times, with different samples of patients, by different investigators, employing different criteria and/or different interpretations of the same criteria, under different conditions (dose, dosing regimen, etc.), quantitative estimates of treatment response and the timing of response may be expected to vary considerably from study to study.

The estimated probability of achieving an initial headache response by 2 hours following treatment is depicted in Figure 1.

Figure 1
Estimated Probability of Achieving Initial Headache Response Within 2 Hours

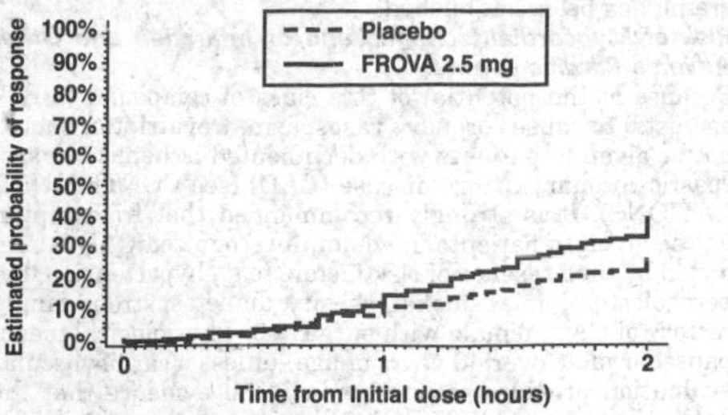

Figure 1 shows a Kaplan-Meier plot of the probability over time of obtaining headache response (no or mild pain) following treatment with frovatriptan 2.5 mg or placebo. The probabilities displayed are based on pooled data from four placebo-controlled trials described in Table 1 (Trials 1, 3, 4 and 5). Patients who did not achieve a response were censored at 24 hours.

In patients with migraine-associated nausea, photophobia and phonophobia at baseline there was a decreased incidence of these symptoms in FROVA treated patients compared to placebo. The estimated probability of patients taking a second dose or other medication for their migraine over the 24 hours following the initial dose of study treatment is summarized in Figure 2.

Figure 2
Estimated Probability of Patients Taking a Second Dose or Other Medication for Migraine Over the 24 Hours Following the Initial Dose of Study Treatment

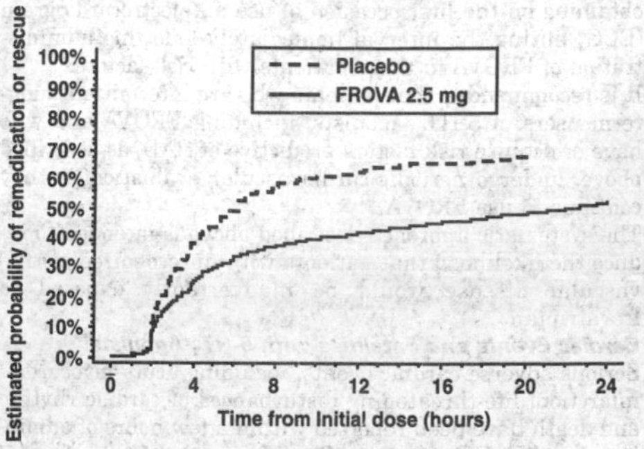

Figure 2 is a Kaplan-Meier plot showing the probability of patients taking a second dose or other medication for migraine over the 24 hours following the initial dose of study medication based on the data from four placebo-controlled trials described in Table 1 (Trials 1, 3, 4 and 5). The plot includes those patients who had a response to the initial dose and those who did not. The protocols did not permit remedication within 2 hours of the initial dose.

Efficacy was unaffected by a history of aura; gender; age, or concomitant medications commonly used by migraine patients FROVA.

INDICATIONS AND USAGE

FROVA is indicated for the acute treatment of migraine attacks with or without aura in adults.

FROVA is not intended for the prophylactic therapy of migraine or for use in the management of hemiplegic or basilar migraine (see CONTRAINDICATIONS). The safety and effectiveness of FROVA have not been established for cluster headache, which is present in an older, predominately male, population.

CONTRAINDICATIONS

FROVA should not be given to patients with ischemic heart disease (e.g. angina pectoris, history of myocardial infarction, or documented silent ischemia), or to patients who have symptoms or findings consistent with ischemic heart disease, coronary artery vasospasm, including Prinzmetal's variant angina or other significant underlying cardiovascular disease (see WARNINGS).

FROVA should not be given to patients with cerebrovascular syndromes including (but not limited to) strokes of any type as well as transient ischemic attacks.

FROVA should not be given to patients with peripheral vascular disease including (but is not limited to) ischemic bowel disease (see WARNINGS).

FROVA should not be given to patients with uncontrolled hypertension (see WARNINGS).

FROVA should not be administered to patients with hemiplegic or basilar migraine.

FROVA should not be used within 24 hours of treatment with another 5-HT_1 agonist, an ergotamine containing or ergot-type medication such as dihydroergotamine (DHE) or methysergide.

FROVA is contraindicated in patients who are hypersensitive to frovatriptan or any of the inactive ingredients in the tablets.

WARNINGS

FROVA should only be used where a clear diagnosis of migraine has been established.

Risk of Myocardial Ischemia and/or Infarction and Other Adverse Cardiac Events:

Because of the potential of this class of compound (5-HT_1 agonists) to cause coronary vasospasm, frovatriptan should not be given to patients with documented ischemic or vasospastic coronary artery disease (CAD) (see CONTRAINDICATIONS). It is strongly recommended that frovatriptan not be given to patients in whom unrecognized CAD is predicted by the presence of risk factors (e.g., hypertension, hypercholesterolemia, smoker, obesity, diabetes, strong family history of CAD, female with surgical or physiological menopause, or male over 40 years of age) unless a cardiovascular evaluation provides satisfactory clinical evidence that the patient is reasonably free of coronary artery and ischemic myocardial disease or other significant underlying cardiovascular disease. The sensitivity of cardiac diagnostic procedures to detect cardiovascular disease or predisposition to coronary artery vasospasm is modest, at best. If, during the cardiovascular evaluation, the patient's medical history, electrocardiographic, or other investigations reveal findings indicative of, or consistent with, coronary artery vasospasm or myocardial ischemia, frovatriptan should not be administered (see CONTRAINDICATIONS).

For patients with risk factors predictive of CAD, who are determined to have a satisfactory cardiovascular evaluation, it is strongly recommended that administration of the first dose of frovatriptan take place in the setting of a physician's office or similar medically staffed and equipped facility unless the patient has previously received frovatriptan. Because cardiac ischemia can occur in the absence of clinical symptoms, consideration should be given to obtaining on the first occasion of use an electrocardiogram (ECG) during the interval immediately following administration of FROVA in these patients with risk factors.

It is recommended that patients who are intermittent long-term users of 5-HT_1 agonists, including FROVA and who have or acquire risk factors predictive of CAD, as described above, undergo periodic cardiovascular evaluation as they continue to use FROVA.

The systematic approach described above is intended to reduce the likelihood that patients with unrecognized cardiovascular disease would be inadvertently exposed to frovatriptan.

Cardiac Events and Fatalities with 5-HT_1 Agonists:

Serious adverse cardiac events, including acute myocardial infarction, life-threatening disturbances of cardiac rhythm and death have been reported within a few hours of administration of 5-HT_1 agonists. Considering the extent of use of 5-HT_1 agonists in patients with migraine, the incidence of these events is extremely low.

Premarketing experience with frovatriptan:

Among more than 3000 patients with migraine who participated in premarketing clinical trials of FROVA no deaths or serious cardiac events were reported which were related to the use of FROVA.

Cerebrovascular Events and Fatalities with 5-HT_1 Agonists:

Cerebral hemorrhage, subarachnoid hemorrhage, stroke and other cerebrovascular events have been reported in patients treated with 5-HT_1 agonists; and some have resulted in fatalities. In a number of cases, it appears possible that the cerebrovascular events were primary, the agonist having been administered in the incorrect belief that the symptoms experienced were a consequence of migraine, when they were not. It should be noted that patients with migraine may be at increased risk of certain cerebrovascular events (e.g. stroke, hemorrhage, transient ischemic attack).

Other Vasospasm-Related Events:

5-HT_1 agonists may cause vasospastic reactions other than coronary artery spasm. Both peripheral vascular ischemia and colonic ischemia with abdominal pain and bloody diarrhea have been reported with 5-HT_1 agonists.

Effects on Blood Pressure:

In young healthy subjects, there were statistically significant increases in systolic and diastolic blood pressure after single doses of 80 mg frovatriptan (32 times the clinical dose) and above. These increases were transient, resolved spontaneously and were not clinically significant. At the recommended dose of 2.5 mg, transient changes in systolic blood pressure were recorded in some elderly subjects (65-77 years). Any increases were generally small, resolved spontaneously, and blood pressure remained within the normal range. Frovatriptan is contraindicated in patients with uncontrolled hypertension (see CONTRAINDICATIONS).

An 18% increase in mean pulmonary artery pressure was seen following dosing with another 5-HT_1 agonist in a study evaluating subjects undergoing cardiac catheterization.

Serotonin Syndrome:

The development of a potentially life-threatening serotonin syndrome may occur with triptans, including FROVA treatment, particularly during combined use with selective serotonin reuptake inhibitors (SSRIs) or serotonin norepinephrine reuptake inhibitors (SNRIs). If concomitant treatment with FROVA and an SSRI (e.g., fluoxetine, paroxetine, sertraline, fluvoxamine, citalopram, escitalopram) or SNRI (e.g., venlafaxine, duloxetine) is clinically warranted, careful observation of the patient is advised, particularly during treatment initiation and dose increases. Serotonin syndrome symptoms may include mental status changes (e.g., agitation hallucinations, coma), autonomic instability (e.g., tachycardia, labile blood pressure, hyperthermia), neuromuscular aberrations (e.g., hyperreflexia, incoordination) and/or gastrointestinal symptoms (e.g., nausea, vomiting, diarrhea). (See PRECAUTIONS – Drug Interactions).

PRECAUTIONS

General:

As with other 5-HT_1 agonists, sensations of pain, tightness, pressure and heaviness have been reported in the chest, throat, neck and jaw after treatment with FROVA. These events have not been associated with arrhythmias or ischemic ECG changes in clinical trials with FROVA. Because 5-HT_1 agonists may cause coronary vasospasm, patients who experience signs or symptoms suggestive of angina following dosing should be evaluated for the presence of CAD. Patients shown to have CAD and those with Prinzmetal's variant angina should not receive 5-HT_1 agonists (see CONTRAINDICATIONS). Patients who experience other symptoms or signs suggestive of decreased arterial flow, such as ischemic bowel syndrome or Raynaud's syndrome following the use of any 5-HT_1 agonist are candidates for further evaluation. If a patient has no response for the first migraine attack treated with FROVA, the diagnosis of migraine should be reconsidered before frovatriptan is administered to treat any subsequent attacks.

Hepatically Impaired Patients:

There is no clinical or pharmacokinetic experience with FROVA in patients with severe hepatic impairment. The AUC of frovatriptan in patients with mild (Child-Pugh 5-6) to moderate (Child-Pugh 7-9) hepatic impairment was about twice that of young, healthy subjects, but within the range observed in healthy elderly subjects and was considerably lower than the values attained with higher doses of frovatriptan (up to 40 mg), which were not associated with any serious adverse effects. Therefore, no dosage adjustment is necessary when FROVA is given to patients with mild to moderate hepatic impairment (see CLINICAL PHARMACOLOGY, Special Populations).

Binding to Melanin-Containing Tissues:

When pigmented rats were given a single oral dose of 5 mg/kg of radiolabeled frovatriptan, the radioactivity in the eye after 28 days was 87% of the value measured after 8 hours. This suggests that frovatriptan and/or its metabolites may bind to the melanin of the eye. Because there could be accumulation in melanin rich tissues over time, this raises the possibility that frovatriptan could cause toxicity in these tissues after extended use. However, no effects on the retina related to treatment with frovatriptan were noted in the toxicity studies. Although no systematic monitoring of ophthalmologic function was undertaken in clinical trials and no specific recommendations for ophthalmologic monitoring are made, prescribers should be aware of the possibility of long-term ophthalmologic effects.

Information for Patients

Physicians should instruct their patients to read the patient package insert before taking FROVA. See PATIENT INFORMATION at the end of this labeling for the text of the separate leaflet provided for patients.

Patients should be cautioned about the risk of serotonin syndrome with the use of FROVA or other triptans, especially during combined use with selective serotonin reuptake inhibitors (SSRIs) or serotonin norepinephrine reuptake inhibitors (SNRIs).

Laboratory Tests

No specific laboratory tests are recommended for monitoring patients prior to and/or after treatment with FROVA.

***Drug Interactions* (see also CLINICAL PHARMACOLOGY, *Drug Interactions*)**

Ergot-containing drugs have been reported to cause prolonged vasospastic reactions. Due to a theoretical risk of a pharmacodynamic interaction, use of ergotamine-containing or ergot-type medications (like dihydroergotamine or methysergide) and FROVA within 24 hours of each other should be avoided (see CONTRAINDICATIONS).

Concomitant use of other $5\text{-HT}_{1B/1D}$ agonists within 24 hours of FROVA treatment is not recommended (see CONTRAINDICATIONS).

Selective Serotonin Reuptake Inhibitors / Serotonin Norepinephrine Reuptake Inhibitors and Serotonin Syndrome: Cases of life-threatening serotonin syndrome have been reported during combined use of selective serotonin reuptake inhibitors (SSRIs) or serotonin norepinephrine reuptake inhibitors (SNRIs) and triptans. (See WARNINGS).

Drug/Laboratory Test Interactions

FROVA is not known to interfere with commonly employed clinical laboratory tests.

Carcinogenesis, Mutagenesis, Impairment of Fertility

Carcinogenesis: The carcinogenic potential of frovatriptan was evaluated in an 84-week study in mice (4, 13, and 40 mg/kg/day), a 104-week study in rats (8.5, 27 and 85 mg/kg/day), and a 26-week study in p53(+/-) transgenic mice (20, 62.5, 200, and 400 mg/kg/day). Although the maximum tolerated dose (MTD) was not achieved in the 84-week mouse study and in female rats, exposures at the highest doses studied were many fold greater than those achieved at the maximum recommended daily human dose (MRHD) of 7.5 mg. There were no increases in tumor incidence in the 84-week mouse study at doses producing 140 times the exposure achieved at the MRHD based on blood AUC comparisons. In the rat study, there was a statistically significant increase in the incidence of pituitary adenomas in males only at 85 mg/kg/day, a dose that produced 250 times the exposure achieved at the MRHD based on AUC comparisons. In the 26-week p53(+/-) transgenic mouse study, there was an increased incidence of subcutaneous sarcomas in females dosed at 200 and 400 mg/kg/day, or 390 and 630 times the human exposure based on AUC comparisons. The incidence of sarcomas was not increased at lower doses that achieved exposures 180 and 60 times the human exposure. These sarcomas were physically associated with subcutaneously implanted animal identification transponders. There were no other increases in tumor incidence of any type in any dose group. These sarcomas are not considered to be relevant to humans.

Mutagenesis: Frovatriptan was clastogenic in human lymphocyte cultures, in the absence of metabolic activation. In the bacterial reverse mutation assay (Ames test), frovatriptan produced an equivocal response in the absence of metabolic activation. No mutagenic or clastogenic activities were seen in an *in vitro* mouse lymphoma assay, an *in vivo* mouse bone marrow micronucleus test, or an *ex vivo* assay for unscheduled DNA synthesis in rat liver.

Impairment of Fertility: Male and female rats were dosed prior to and during mating, and up to implantation, at doses of 100, 500, and 1000 mg/kg/day (equivalent to approximately 130, 650, and 1300 times the MRHD on a mg/m^2 basis). At all dose levels there was an increase in the number of females that mated on the first day of pairing compared to control animals. This occurred in conjunction with a prolongation of the estrous cycle. In addition females had a decreased mean number of corpora lutea, and consequently a lower number of live fetuses per litter, which suggested a partial impairment of ovulation. There were no other fertility-related effects.

Pregnancy: Pregnancy Category C

When pregnant rats were administered frovatriptan during the period of organogenesis at oral doses of 100, 500 and 1000 mg/kg/day (equivalent to 130, 650 and 1300 times the maximum recommended human dose [MRHD] on a mg/m^2 basis) there were dose related increases in incidences of both litters and total numbers of fetuses with dilated ureters, unilateral and bilateral pelvic cavitation, hydronephrosis, and hydroureters. A no-effect dose for renal effects was not established. This signifies a syndrome of related effects on a specific organ in the developing embryo in all treated groups, which is consistent with a slight delay in fetal maturation. This delay was also indicated by a treatment related increased incidence of incomplete ossification of the sternebrae, skull and nasal bones in all treated groups. Slightly lower fetal weights and an increased incidence of early embryonic deaths in treated rats were observed; although not statistically significant compared to control, the latter effect occurred in both the embryo-fetal developmental study and in the prenatal-postnatal developmental study. There was no evidence of this latter effect at the lowest dose level studied, 100 mg/kg/day (equivalent to 130 times the MRHD on a mg/m^2 basis). When pregnant rabbits were dosed throughout organogenesis at doses up to 80 mg/kg/day (equivalent to 210 times the MRHD on a mg/m^2 basis) no effects on fetal development were observed. There are no adequate and well-controlled studies in pregnant women; therefore, frovatriptan should be used during pregnancy only if the potential benefit justifies the potential risk to the fetus.

Nursing Mothers

It is not known whether frovatriptan is excreted in human milk. Frovatriptan and/or its metabolites are excreted in the milk of lactating rats with the maximum concentration being four-fold higher than that seen in blood. Therefore, caution should be exercised when considering the administration of FROVA to a nursing woman.

Pediatric Use

Safety and effectiveness of FROVA in pediatric patients have not been established; therefore, FROVA is not recommended for use in patients under 18 years of age. Postmarketing experience with other triptans includes a limited number of reports that describe pediatric patients who have experienced clinically serious adverse events that are similar in nature to those reported rarely in adults.

Use in the Elderly

Mean blood concentrations of frovatriptan in elderly subjects were 1.5- to 2-times higher than those seen in younger adults (see CLINICAL PHARMACOLOGY, Special Populations). Because migraine occurs infrequently in the elderly, clinical experience with FROVA is limited in such patients.

ADVERSE REACTIONS

Serious cardiac events, including some that have been fatal, have occurred following use of 5-HT_1 agonists. These

events are extremely rare and most have been reported in patients with risk factors predictive of CAD. Events reported have included coronary artery vasospasm, transient myocardial ischemia, myocardial infarction, ventricular tachycardia and ventricular fibrillation (see CONTRAINDICATIONS, WARNINGS and PRECAUTIONS).

Incidence in Controlled Clinical Trials

Among 1554 patients treated with FROVA in four placebo-controlled trials (Trials 1, 3, 4 and 5 in Table 1), only 1% (16) patients withdrew because of treatment-emergent adverse events. In a long term, open-label study where patients were allowed to treat multiple migraine attacks with FROVA for up to 1 year, 5% (26/496) patients discontinued due to treatment-emergent adverse events.

The treatment-emergent adverse events that occurred most frequently following administration of frovatriptan 2.5 mg (i.e., in at least 2% of patients), and at an incidence ≥1% greater than with placebo, in the four placebo-controlled trials were dizziness, paresthesia, headache, dry mouth, fatigue, flushing, hot or cold sensation and chest pain.

Table 2 lists treatment-emergent adverse events reported within 48 hours of drug administration that occurred with frovatriptan 2.5 mg at an incidence of ≥ 2% and more often than on placebo, in the first attack in four placebo-controlled trials (Trials 1, 3, 4 and 5 in Table 1). These studies involved 2392 patients (1554 frovatriptan 2.5 mg and 838 placebo). The events cited reflect experience gained under closely monitored conditions of clinical trials in a highly selected patient population. In actual clinical practice or in other clinical trials, these incidence estimates may not apply, as the conditions of use, reporting behavior, and the kinds of patients treated may differ.

Table 2: Treatment-Emergent Adverse Events (Incidence ≥2% and Greater Than Placebo) of Patients in Four Placebo-Controlled Migraine Trials

Adverse events	Frovatriptan 2.5 mg (n=1554)	Placebo (n=838)
Central & peripheral nervous system		
Dizziness	8%	5%
Headache	4%	3%
Paresthesia	4%	2%
Gastrointestinal system disorders		
Mouth dry	3%	1%
Dyspepsia	2%	1%
Body as a whole – general disorders		
Fatigue	5%	2%
Hot or cold sensation	3%	2%
Chest pain	2%	1%
Musculo-skeletal		
Skeletal pain	3%	2%
Vascular		
Flushing	4%	2%

Other events that occurred at ≥2% on frovatriptan that were equally or more common in the placebo group were somnolence and nausea.

FROVA is generally well tolerated. The incidence of adverse events in clinical trials did not increase when up to 3 doses were used within 24 hours. The majority of adverse events were mild or moderate and transient. The incidence of adverse events in four placebo-controlled clinical trials was not affected by gender, age or concomitant medications commonly used by migraine patients. There were insufficient data to assess the impact of race on the incidence of adverse events.

Other Events Observed in Association with FROVA:

In the paragraphs that follow, the incidence of less commonly reported adverse events in four placebo-controlled trials are presented. Variability associated with adverse event reporting, the terminology used to describe adverse events etc, limit the value of the incidence estimates provided. The incidence of each adverse event is calculated as the number of patients reporting the event at least once divided by the number of patients who used FROVA. All adverse events reported within 48 hours of drug administration in the first attack in four placebo controlled trials involving 2392 patients (1554 frovatriptan 2.5 mg and 838 placebo) are included, except those already listed in Table 2, those too general to be informative, those not reasonably associated with the use of the drug and those which occurred at the same or a greater incidence in the placebo category. Events are further classified within body system categories and enumerated in order of decreasing frequency using the following definitions: frequent adverse events are those occurring in at least 1/100 patients, infrequent adverse events are those occurring in between 1/100 and 1/1000 patients, and rare adverse events are those occurring in fewer than 1/1000 patients.

Central and peripheral nervous system: Frequent: dysesthesia and hypoesthesia. Infrequent: tremor, hyperesthesia, migraine aggravated, involuntary muscle contractions, ver-

tigo, ataxia, abnormal gait and speech disorder. Rare: hypertonia, hypotonia, abnormal reflexes and tongue paralysis.

Gastrointestinal: Frequent: vomiting, abdominal pain and diarrhea. Infrequent: dysphagia, flatulence, constipation, anorexia, esophagospasm and saliva increased. Rare: change in bowel habits, cheilitis, eructation, gastroesophageal reflux, hiccup, peptic ulcer, salivary gland pain, stomatitis and toothache.

Body as a whole: Frequent: pain. Infrequent: asthenia, rigors, fever, hot flushes and malaise. Rare: feeling of relaxation, leg pain and edema mouth.

Psychiatric: Frequent: insomnia and anxiety. Infrequent: confusion, nervousness, agitation, euphoria, impaired concentration, depression, emotional lability, amnesia, thinking abnormal and depersonalization. Rare: depression aggravated, abnormal dreaming and personality disorder.

Musculoskeletal: Infrequent: myalgia, back pain, arthralgia, arthrosis, leg cramps and muscle weakness.

Respiratory: Frequent: sinusitis and rhinitis. Infrequent: pharyngitis, dyspnea, hyperventilation and laryngitis.

Vision disorders: Frequent: vision abnormal. Infrequent: eye pain, conjunctivitis and abnormal lacrimation.

Skin and appendages: Frequent: sweating increased. Infrequent: pruritis, and bullous eruption.

Hearing and vestibular disorders: Frequent: tinnitus. Infrequent: ear ache, and hyperacusis.

Heart rate and rhythm: Frequent: palpitation. Infrequent: tachycardia. Rare: bradycardia.

Metabolic and nutritional disorders: Infrequent: thirst and dehydration. Rare: hypocalcemia and hypoglycemia.

Special senses, other disorders: Infrequent: taste perversion.

Urinary system disorders: Infrequent: micturition frequency and polyuria. Rare: nocturia, renal pain and abnormal urine.

Cardiovascular disorders, general: Infrequent: abnormal ECG.

Platelet, bleeding and clotting disorders: Infrequent: epistaxis. Rare: purpura.

Autonomic nervous system: Rare: syncope.

Postmarketing Experience

Because these events are reported voluntarily from a population of uncertain size, it is not always possible to reliably estimate their frequency. Information is often incomplete so that a definite causal relationship to drug exposure can often not be established.

Central and peripheral nervous system: Seizure.

DRUG ABUSE AND DEPENDENCE

Although the abuse potential of FROVA has not been specifically assessed in clinical trials, no abuse of, tolerance to, withdrawal from, or drug-seeking behavior was observed in patients who received FROVA. The 5-HT₁ agonists, as a class, have not been associated with drug abuse.

OVERDOSAGE

There is no direct experience of any patient taking an overdose of FROVA. The maximum single dose of frovatriptan given to male and female patients with migraine was 40 mg (16 times the clinical dose) and the maximum single dose given to healthy male subjects was 100 mg (40 times the clinical dose) without significant adverse events.

As with other 5-HT₁ receptor agonists, there is no specific antidote for frovatriptan. The elimination half-life of frovatriptan is 26 hours, therefore if overdose occurs, the patient should be monitored closely for at least 48 hours and be given any necessary symptomatic treatment.

The effects of hemo- or peritoneal dialysis on blood concentrations of frovatriptan are unknown.

DOSAGE AND ADMINISTRATION

The recommended dose is a single tablet of FROVA (frovatriptan 2.5 mg) taken orally with fluids.

If the headache recurs after initial relief, a second tablet may be taken, providing there is an interval of at least 2 hours between doses. The total daily dose of frovatriptan should not exceed 3 tablets (3 × 2.5 mg per day).

There is no evidence that a second dose of frovatriptan is effective in patients who do not respond to a first dose of the drug for the same headache.

The safety of treating an average of more than 4 migraine attacks in a 30-day period has not been established.

HOW SUPPLIED

FROVA tablets, containing 2.5 mg of frovatriptan (base) as the succinate, are available as round, white, film-coated tablets debossed with 2.5 on one side and "E" on the other side.

The tablets are available in:

Blister card of 9 tablets, 1 blister card per carton (NDC 63481-025-09)

Store at controlled room temperature, 25°C (77°F) excursions permitted to 15-30°C (59°F-86°F) [see USP Controlled Room Temperature]. Protect from moisture.

U.S. Patent Nos 5,962,501, 5,827,871, 5,637,611 and 5,464,864 and 5,616,603.

Rx Only

Manufactured for:
Endo Pharmaceuticals Inc.
Chadds Ford, PA 19317

Manufactured by:
Almac Pharma Services Limited
Craigavon, BT63 5UA, UK

FROVA is a registered trademark of Vernalis Development Limited.

© 2007 Endo Pharmaceuticals Inc.   PX544-3 / April, 2007

PATIENT INFORMATION: The following wording is contained in a separate leaflet provided for patients.

PATIENT INFORMATION ABOUT

FROVA® (frovatriptan succinate) Tablets

Read this information before you start taking FROVA (FRO-va). Also, read the information each time you renew your prescription, in case anything has changed. This leaflet does not contain all of the information about FROVA. For further information or advice ask your doctor or pharmacist. You and your doctor should discuss FROVA before you start taking the medicine and at regular checkups.

What is FROVA?

FROVA is a prescription medicine used to treat migraine attacks in adults. It is in the class of drugs called selective serotonin receptor agonists.

FROVA should only be taken for a migraine headache. Do not use FROVA to treat headaches that might be caused by other conditions. Tell your doctor about your symptoms. Your doctor will decide if you have migraine headaches and if FROVA is for you.

There is more information about migraine at the end of this leaflet.

Who should not take FROVA?

Do not take FROVA if you:
- have uncontrolled high blood pressure
- have heart disease or a history of heart disease
- have hemiplegic or basilar migraine (if you are not sure about this, ask your doctor)
- have had a stroke
- have circulation (blood flow) problems
- have taken a similar drug (a serotonin receptor agonist) in the last 24 hours. These include sumatriptan (IMITREX®), naratriptan (AMERGE™), zolmitriptan (ZOMIG™), rizatriptan (MAXALT™), eletriptan hydrobromide (RELPAX®), or almotriptan (AXERT™).
- have taken ergotamine type medicines in the last 24 hours. These include BELLERGAL®, CAFERGOT®, ERGOMAR®, WIGRAINE®, DHE 45®, or SANSERT®
- have any allergic reaction to the tablet

What you should tell your doctor before and during treatment with FROVA?

To help your doctor decide if FROVA is right for you, tell your doctor if you:
- are pregnant, or planning to become pregnant
- are breast-feeding or plan to breast-feed
- have any history of chest pain, shortness of breath, or palpitations
- have any risk factors for heart disease, including
  - high blood pressure
  - diabetes
  - high cholesterol
  - overweight
  - smoking
  - a family history of heart disease
  - past menopause
  - male over 40 years old
- are taking any other medicines, including prescription and non-prescription medicines, and herbal supplements
- have any past or present medical problems
- have previous allergies to any medicine

Tell your doctor if you take
- propranolol
- selective serotonin reuptake inhibitors (SSRIs) or serotonin norepinephrine reuptake inhibitors (SNRIs), two types of drugs for depression or other disorders. Common SSRIs are CELEXA® (citalopram HBr), LEXAPRO® (escitalopram oxalate), PAXIL® (paroxetine), PROZAC®/SARAFEM® (fluoxetine), SYMBYAX® (olanzapine/fluoxetine), ZOLOFT® (sertraline), and fluvoxamine. Common SNRIs are CYMBALTA® (duloxetine) and EFFEXOR® (venlafaxine).

These medicines may affect how FROVA works, or FROVA may affect how these medicines work.

How should you take FROVA?

Take one FROVA tablet anytime after the start of your migraine headache. If your headache comes back after your first dose, you may take a second tablet after two (2) hours. Do not take more than three (3) FROVA tablets in a 24-hour period.

If you take too much medicine, contact your doctor, hospital emergency department, or poison control center right away.

What are the common side effects of FROVA?

The most common side effects associated with use of FROVA are:

- dizziness
- fatigue (tiredness)
- headache (other than a migraine headache)
- paresthesia (feeling of tingling)
- dry mouth
- flushing (hot flashes)
- feeling hot or cold
- chest pain
- dyspepsia (indigestion)
- skeletal pain (pain in joints or bones)

Tell your doctor about any symptoms that you develop while taking FROVA. If you feel dizziness or fatigue, take extra care or avoid driving and operating machinery.

In very rare cases, patients taking this class of medicines experience serious heart problems, stroke, or increased blood pressure. If you develop pain, tightness, heaviness, or pressure in your chest, throat, neck, or jaw, contact your doctor right away.

Also contact your doctor right away if you develop a rash or itching after taking FROVA. You may be allergic to this medicine.

What is a migraine and how does it differ from other headaches?

Migraine is an intense, throbbing headache that often affects one side of the head. It often includes nausea, vomiting, and sensitivity to light and sound. The pain and symptoms from a migraine headache may be worse than the pain and symptoms of a common headache. Migraine headaches usually last for hours or longer.

Some people have problems with vision (an aura) before they get a migraine headache. These include flashing lights, wavy lines, and dark spots.

Only your doctor can determine that your headache is a migraine headache, so it is important that you discuss all of your symptoms with your doctor.

LEXOPRO® / CELEXA® are registered trademarks of Forest Pharmaceuticals, Inc.

PAXIL® is a registered trademark of GlaxoSmithKline.

PROZAC® / SARAFEM® / SYMBYAX® / CYMBALTA® are registered trademarks of Eli Lilly and Company

ZOLOFT® is a registered trademark of Pfizer Pharmaceuticals.

EFFEXOR® is a registered trademark of Wyeth Pharmaceuticals.

FROVA is a registered trademark of Vernalis Development Limited.

© 2007 Endo Pharmaceuticals Inc.   PX544-3 / April, 2007
Shown in Product Identification Guide, page 308

LIDODERM®   ℞

[lī-dō-dĕrm]
(Lidocaine Patch 5%)
℞ only

DESCRIPTION

LIDODERM (lidocaine patch 5%) is comprised of an adhesive material containing 5% lidocaine, which is applied to a non-woven polyester felt backing and covered with a polyethylene terephthalate (PET) film release liner. The release liner is removed prior to application to the skin. The size of the patch is 10 cm × 14 cm.

Lidocaine is chemically designated as acetamide, 2-(diethylamino)-N-(2,6-dimethylphenyl), has an octanol: water partition ratio of 43 at pH 7.4, and has the following structure:

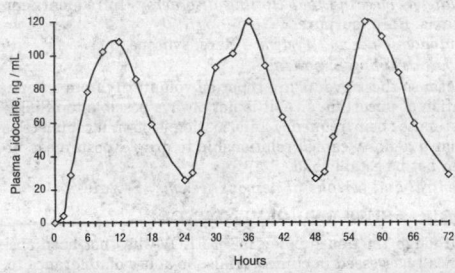

Each adhesive patch contains 700 mg of lidocaine (50 mg per gram adhesive) in an aqueous base. It also contains the following inactive ingredients: dihydroxyaluminum aminoacetate, disodium edetate, gelatin, glycerin, kaolin, methylparaben, polyacrylic acid, polyvinyl alcohol, propylene glycol, propylparaben, sodium carboxymethylcellulose, sodium polyacrylate, D-sorbitol, tartaric acid, and urea.

CLINICAL PHARMACOLOGY

Pharmacodynamics

Lidocaine is an amide-type local anesthetic agent and is suggested to stabilize neuronal membranes by inhibiting the ionic fluxes required for the initiation and conduction of impulses.

The penetration of lidocaine into intact skin after application of LIDODERM is sufficient to produce an analgesic effect, but less than the amount necessary to produce a complete sensory block.

Pharmacokinetics

Absorption: The amount of lidocaine systemically absorbed from LIDODERM is directly related to both the duration of application and the surface area over which it is applied. In a pharmacokinetic study, three LIDODERM patches were applied over an area of 420 cm² of intact skin on the back of normal volunteers for 12 hours. Blood samples were withdrawn for determination of lidocaine concentration during the application and for 12 hours after removal of patches. The results are summarized in Table 1. [See table 1 below]

When LIDODERM is used according to the recommended dosing instructions, only 3 ± 2% of the dose applied is expected to be absorbed. At least 95% (665 mg) of lidocaine will remain in a used patch. Mean peak blood concentration of lidocaine is about 0.13 µg/mL (about 1/10 of the therapeutic concentration required to treat cardiac arrhythmias). Repeated application of three patches simultaneously for 12 hours (recommended maximum daily dose), once per day for three days, indicated that the lidocaine concentration does not increase with daily use. The mean plasma pharmacokinetic profile for the 15 healthy volunteers is shown in Figure 1.

Figure 1

Mean lidocaine blood concentrations after three consecutive daily applications of three LIDODERM patches simultaneously for 12 hours per day in healthy volunteers (n = 15).

Distribution: When lidocaine is administered intravenously to healthy volunteers, the volume of distribution is 0.7 to 2.7 L/kg (mean 1.5 ± 0.6 SD, n = 15). At concentrations produced by application of LIDODERM, lidocaine is approximately 70% bound to plasma proteins, primarily alpha-1-acid glycoprotein. At much higher plasma concentrations (1 to 4 µg/mL of free base), the plasma protein binding of lidocaine is concentration dependent. Lidocaine crosses the placental and blood brain barriers, presumably by passive diffusion.

Metabolism: It is not known if lidocaine is metabolized in the skin. Lidocaine is metabolized rapidly by the liver to a number of metabolites, including monoethylglycinexylidide (MEGX) and glycinexylidide (GX), both of which have pharmacologic activity similar to, but less potent than that of lidocaine. A minor metabolite, 2,6-xylidine, has unknown pharmacologic activity but is carcinogenic in rats. The blood concentration of this metabolite is negligible following application of LIDODERM (lidocaine patch 5%). Following intravenous administration, MEGX and GX concentrations in serum range from 11 to 36% and from 5 to 11% of lidocaine concentrations, respectively.

Excretion: Lidocaine and its metabolites are excreted by the kidneys. Less than 10% of lidocaine is excreted unchanged. The half-life of lidocaine elimination from the plasma following IV administration is 81 to 149 minutes (mean 107 ± 22 SD, n = 15). The systemic clearance is 0.33 to 0.90 L/min (mean 0.64 ± 0.18 SD, n = 15).

CLINICAL STUDIES

Single-dose treatment with LIDODERM was compared to treatment with vehicle patch (without lidocaine), and to no

treatment (observation only) in a double-blind, crossover clinical trial with 35 post-herpetic neuralgia patients. Pain intensity and pain relief scores were evaluated periodically for 12 hours. LIDODERM performed statistically better than vehicle patch in terms of pain intensity from 4 to 12 hours.

Multiple-dose, two-week treatment with LIDODERM was compared to vehicle patch (without lidocaine) in a double-blind, crossover clinical trial of withdrawal-type design conducted in 32 patients, who were considered as responders to the open-label use of LIDODERM prior to the study. The constant type of pain was evaluated but not the pain induced by sensory stimuli (dysesthesia). Statistically significant differences favoring LIDODERM were observed in terms of time to exit from the trial (14 versus 3.8 days at p-value <0.001), daily average pain relief, and patient's preference of treatment. About half of the patients also took oral medication commonly used in the treatment of postherpetic neuralgia. The extent of use of concomitant medication was similar in the two treatment groups.

INDICATION AND USAGE

LIDODERM is indicated for relief of pain associated with post-herpetic neuralgia. It should be applied only to **intact skin**.

CONTRAINDICATIONS

LIDODERM is contraindicated in patients with a known history of sensitivity to local anesthetics of the amide type, or to any other component of the product.

WARNINGS

Accidental Exposure in Children

Even a *used* LIDODERM patch contains a large amount of lidocaine (at least 665 mg). The potential exists for a small child or a pet to suffer serious adverse effects from chewing or ingesting a new or used LIDODERM patch, although the risk with this formulation has not been evaluated. It is important for patients to **store and dispose of LIDODERM out of the reach of children, pets and others.** (See HANDLING AND DISPOSAL)

Excessive Dosing

Excessive dosing by applying LIDODERM to larger areas or for longer than the recommended wearing time could result in increased absorption of lidocaine and high blood concentrations, leading to serious adverse effects (see ADVERSE REACTIONS, Systemic Reactions). Lidocaine toxicity could be expected at lidocaine blood concentrations above 5 µg/mL. The blood concentration of lidocaine is determined by the rate of systemic absorption and elimination. Longer duration of application, application of more than the recommended number of patches, smaller patients, or impaired elimination may all contribute to increasing the blood concentration of lidocaine. With recommended dosing of LIDODERM, the average peak blood concentration is about 0.13 µg/mL, but concentrations higher than 0.25 µg/mL have been observed in some individuals.

PRECAUTIONS

General

Hepatic Disease: Patients with severe hepatic disease are at greater risk of developing toxic blood concentrations of lidocaine, because of their inability to metabolize lidocaine normally.

Allergic Reactions: Patients allergic to para-aminobenzoic acid derivatives (procaine, tetracaine, benzocaine, etc.) have not shown cross sensitivity to lidocaine. However, LIDODERM should be used with caution in patients with a history of drug sensitivities, especially if the etiologic agent is uncertain.

Non-intact Skin: Application to broken or inflamed skin, although not tested, may result in higher blood concentrations of lidocaine from increased absorption. LIDODERM is only recommended for use on intact skin.

External Heat Sources: Placement of external heat sources, such as heating pads or electric blankets, over LIDODERM patches is not recommended as this has not been evaluated and may increase plasma lidocaine levels.

Eye Exposure: The contact of LIDODERM with eyes, although not studied, should be avoided based on the findings of severe eye irritation with the use of similar products in animals. If eye contact occurs, immediately wash out the eye with water or saline and protect the eye until sensation returns.

Drug Interactions

Antiarrhythmic Drugs: LIDODERM should be used with caution in patients receiving Class I antiarrhythmic drugs (such as tocainide and mexiletine) since the toxic effects are additive and potentially synergistic.

Local Anesthetics: When LIDODERM is used concomitantly with other products containing local anesthetic agents, the amount absorbed from all formulations must be considered.

Carcinogenesis, Mutagenesis, Impairment of Fertility

Carcinogenesis: A minor metabolite, 2,6-xylidine, has been found to be carcinogenic in rats. The blood concentra-

---

Table 1 Absorption of lidocaine from LIDODERM

	Normal volunteers (n = 15, 12-hour wearing time)				
LIDODERM Patch	Application Site	Area (cm²)	Dose Absorbed (mg)	Cmax (µg/mL)	Tmax (hr)
3 patches (2100 mg)	Back	420	64 ± 32	0.13 ± 0.06	11 hr

---

tion of this metabolite is negligible following application of LIDODERM.

Mutagenesis: Lidocaine HCl is not mutagenic in Salmonella/mammalian microsome test nor clastogenic in chromosome aberration assay with human lymphocytes and mouse micronucleus test.

Impairment of Fertility: The effect of LIDODERM on fertility has not been studied.

Pregnancy

Teratogenic Effects: Pregnancy Category B. LIDODERM (lidocaine patch 5%) has not been studied in pregnancy. Reproduction studies with lidocaine have been performed in rats at doses up to 30 mg/kg subcutaneously and have revealed no evidence of harm to the fetus due to lidocaine. There are, however, no adequate and well-controlled studies in pregnant women. Because animal reproduction studies are not always predictive of human response, LIDODERM should be used during pregnancy only if clearly needed.

Labor and Delivery

LIDODERM has not been studied in labor and delivery. Lidocaine is not contraindicated in labor and delivery. Should LIDODERM be used concomitantly with other products containing lidocaine, total doses contributed by all formulations must be considered.

Nursing Mothers

LIDODERM has not been studied in nursing mothers. Lidocaine is excreted in human milk, and the milk:plasma ratio of lidocaine is 0.4. Caution should be exercised when LIDODERM is administered to a nursing woman.

Pediatric Use

Safety and effectiveness in pediatric patients have not been established.

ADVERSE REACTIONS

Application Site Reactions

During or immediately after treatment with LIDODERM (lidocaine patch 5%), the skin at the site of application may develop blisters, bruising, burning sensation, depigmentation, dermatitis, discoloration, edema, erythema, exfoliation, irritation, papules, petechia, pruritus, vesicles, or may be the locus of abnormal sensation. These reactions are generally mild and transient, resolving spontaneously within a few minutes to hours.

Allergic Reactions

Allergic and anaphylactoid reactions associated with lidocaine, although rare, can occur. They are characterized by angioedema, bronchospasm, dermatitis, dyspnea, hypersensitivity, laryngospasm, pruritus, shock, and urticaria. If they occur, they should be managed by conventional means. The detection of sensitivity by skin testing is of doubtful value.

Other Adverse Events

Due to the nature and limitation of spontaneous reports in postmarketing surveillance, causality has not been established for additional reported adverse events including: Asthenia, confusion, disorientation, dizziness, headache, hyperesthesia, hypoesthesia, lightheadedness, metallic taste, nausea, nervousness, pain exacerbated, paresthesia, somnolence, taste alteration, vomiting, visual disturbances such as blurred vision, flushing, tinnitus, and tremor.

Systemic (Dose-Related) Reactions

Systemic adverse reactions following appropriate use of LIDODERM are unlikely, due to the small dose absorbed (see CLINICAL PHARMACOLOGY, Pharmacokinetics). Systemic adverse effects of lidocaine are similar in nature to those observed with other amide local anesthetic agents, including CNS excitation and/or depression (light headedness, nervousness, apprehension, euphoria, confusion, dizziness, drowsiness, tinnitus, blurred or double vision, vomiting, sensations of heat, cold or numbness, twitching, tremors, convulsions, unconsciousness, respiratory depression and arrest. Excitatory CNS reactions may be brief or not occur at all, in which case the first manifestation may be drowsiness merging into unconsciousness. Cardiovascular manifestations may include bradycardia, hypotension and cardiovascular collapse leading to arrest.

OVERDOSAGE

Lidocaine overdose from cutaneous absorption is rare, but could occur. If there is any suspicion of lidocaine overdose (see ADVERSE REACTIONS, Systemic Reactions), drug blood concentration should be checked. The management of overdose includes close monitoring, supportive care, and symptomatic treatment. Dialysis is of negligible value in the treatment of acute overdose with lidocaine.

In the absence of massive topical overdose or oral ingestion, evaluation of symptoms of toxicity should include consideration of other etiologies for the clinical effects, or overdosage from other sources of lidocaine or other local anesthetics.

The oral LD_{50} of lidocaine HCl is 459 (346-773) mg/kg (as the salt) in non-fasted female rats and 214 (159-324) mg/kg (as the salt) in fasted female rats, which are equivalent to roughly 4000 mg and 2000 mg, respectively, in a 60 to 70 kg man based on the equivalent surface area dosage conversion factors between species.

DOSAGE AND ADMINISTRATION

Apply LIDODERM to intact skin to cover the most painful area. Apply up to three patches, only once for up to 12 hours within a 24-hour period. Patches may be cut into smaller sizes with scissors prior to removal of the release liner. (See HANDLING AND DISPOSAL) Clothing may be worn over the area of application. Smaller areas of treatment are recommended in a debilitated patient, or a patient with impaired elimination.

If irritation or a burning sensation occurs during application, remove the patch(es) and do not reapply until the irritation subsides.

When LIDODERM is used concomitantly with other products containing local anesthetic agents, the amount absorbed from all formulations must be considered.

HANDLING AND DISPOSAL

Hands should be washed after the handling of LIDODERM, and eye contact with LIDODERM should be avoided. Do not store patch outside the sealed envelope. Apply immediately after removal from the protective envelope. Fold used patches so that the adhesive side sticks to itself and safely discard used patches or pieces of cut patches where children and pets cannot get to them. LIDODERM should be kept out of the reach of children.

HOW SUPPLIED

LIDODERM (lidocaine patch 5%) is available as the following:

Carton of 30 patches, packaged into individual child-resistant envelopes.

NDC 63481-687-06

Store at 25°C (77°F); excursions permitted to 15°-30°C (59°-86°F). [See USP Controlled Room Temperature].

Manufactured for:

Endo Pharmaceuticals Inc.

Chadds Ford, Pennsylvania 19317

LIDODERM® is a Registered Trademark of Hind Health Care, Inc.

© 2010 Endo Pharmaceuticals

6524-12/March 2010

Shown in Product Identification Guide, page 308

OPANA®   Ⓒ Ⓡ
[ō-păn-a]
(oxymorphone hydrochloride)
tablets

HIGHLIGHTS OF PRESCRIBING INFORMATION

These highlights do not include all the information needed to use OPANA safely and effectively. See full prescribing information for OPANA.

OPANA (oxymorphone hydrochloride) tablets, CII
Initial U.S. Approval: 1959

————INDICATIONS AND USAGE————

OPANA is an opioid agonist indicated for the relief of moderate to severe acute pain where the use of an opioid is appropriate. (1)

————DOSAGE AND ADMINISTRATION————

• Titrate the dose based on individual response. (2.1)
• OPANA should be taken on an empty stomach, at least one hour prior to or two hours after eating. (2.2)
• Opioid-Naïve Patients: 10 to 20 mg orally every four to six hours. **Initiation of therapy with doses higher than 20 mg is not recommended.** If necessary, may be initiated with 5 mg (e.g., for renal or hepatic impairment, geriatric patients). (2)
• Conversion to OPANA: Follow recommendations for conversion from other opioids or parenteral oxymorphone. (2.2)
• Cessation of Therapy: Taper gradually. (2.4)

————DOSAGE FORMS AND STRENGTHS————

Tablets: 5 mg and 10 mg. (3)

————CONTRAINDICATIONS————

• Known hypersensitivity to oxymorphone, any other ingredients in OPANA, or morphine analogs (4)
• Respiratory depression in the absence of resuscitative equipment (4)
• Acute or severe bronchial asthma or hypercarbia (4)
• Paralytic ileus (4)
• Moderate or severe hepatic impairment (4)

————WARNINGS AND PRECAUTIONS————

• Respiratory depression: Increased risk in elderly, debilitated patients, and those suffering from conditions accompanied by hypoxia, hypercapnia, or decreased respiratory reserve. (5.1)
• Misuse, abuse, and diversion: OPANA is an opioid agonist and a Schedule II controlled substance with an abuse liability similar to morphine. (5.2)
• CNS effects: Additive CNS-depressive effects when used in conjunction with alcohol, other opioids, or illicit drugs. (5.3)
• Head injury: Effects may be markedly exaggerated. Administer with extreme caution. (5.4)

• Hypotensive effect: Increased risk with compromised ability to maintain blood pressure. Administer with caution to patients in circulatory shock. (5.5)
• Mild hepatic impairment: Use with caution and at lower doses due to higher plasma concentrations than in patients with normal hepatic function. (5.6)
• Prolonged gastric obstruction: May occur in patients with gastrointestinal obstruction, especially paralytic ileus. (5.8)
• Sphincter of Oddi: Administer with caution in patients with biliary tract disease. (5.9)
• Impaired mental/physical abilities: Caution must be used with potentially hazardous activities. (5.10)

————ADVERSE REACTIONS————

Adverse reactions (≥ 2% of patients): Nausea, pyrexia, somnolence, vomiting, pruritus, headache, dizziness, constipation, and confusion. (6.1)

To report SUSPECTED ADVERSE REACTIONS, contact Endo Pharmaceuticals Inc. at 1-800-462-3636 or FDA at 1-800-FDA-1088 or www.fda.gov/medwatch.

————DRUG INTERACTIONS————

• CNS depressants: Increased risk of respiratory depression, hypotension, profound sedation, coma or death. When combined therapy with CNS depressant is contemplated, the dose of one or both agents should be reduced. (7.1)
• Mixed agonist/antagonist opioids (i.e., pentazocine, nalbuphine, and butorphanol): May reduce analgesic effect and/or precipitate withdrawal symptoms. (7.2)
• Cimetidine: Combination use may precipitate confusion, disorientation, respiratory depression, apnea, seizures. (7.3)
• Anticholinergics: May result in urinary retention and/or severe constipation, which may lead to paralytic ileus. (7.4)
• Monoamine oxidase inhibitors (MAOIs): Potentiate the action of opioids. OPANA should not be used in patients taking MAOIs or within 14 days of stopping such treatment. (7.5)

————USE IN SPECIFIC POPULATIONS————

• Pregnancy: Based on animal data, may cause fetal harm. (8.1)
• Geriatric patients: OPANA should be used with caution in elderly patients. (8.5)

See 17 for PATIENT COUNSELING INFORMATION

Revised: 04/2010

FULL PRESCRIBING INFORMATION: CONTENTS*

1 INDICATIONS AND USAGE
2 DOSAGE AND ADMINISTRATION
  2.1 Individualization of Dosage
  2.2 Initiation of Therapy
  2.3 Maintenance of Therapy
  2.4 Cessation of Therapy
  2.5 Patients with Hepatic Impairment
  2.6 Patients with Renal Impairment
  2.7 Use with Central Nervous System Depressants
  2.8 Geriatric Patients
3 DOSAGE FORMS AND STRENGTHS
4 CONTRAINDICATIONS
5 WARNINGS AND PRECAUTIONS
  5.1 Respiratory Depression
  5.2 Misuse, Abuse, and Diversion of Opioids
  5.3 Additive CNS Depressant Effects
  5.4 Use in Patients with Head Injury and Increased Intracranial Pressure
  5.5 Hypotensive Effect
  5.6 Hepatic Impairment
  5.7 Special Risk Groups
  5.8 Gastrointestinal Effects
  5.9 Use in Pancreatic/Biliary Tract Disease
  5.10 Driving and Operating Machinery
6 ADVERSE REACTIONS
  6.1 Clinical Trials Experience
7 DRUG INTERACTIONS
  7.1 Use with CNS Depressants
  7.2 Interactions with Mixed Agonist/Antagonist Opioid Analgesics
  7.3 Cimetidine
  7.4 Anticholinergics
  7.5 MAO Inhibitors
8 USE IN SPECIFIC POPULATIONS
  8.1 Pregnancy
  8.2 Labor and Delivery
  8.3 Nursing Mothers
  8.4 Pediatric Use
  8.5 Geriatric Use
  8.6 Hepatic Impairment
  8.7 Renal Impairment
9 DRUG ABUSE AND DEPENDENCE
  9.1 Controlled Substance
  9.2 Abuse
  9.3 Dependence

*** Sections or subsections omitted from the full prescribing information are not listed**

FULL PRESCRIBING INFORMATION

1 INDICATIONS AND USAGE

OPANA is indicated for the relief of moderate to severe acute pain where the use of an opioid is appropriate.

2 DOSAGE AND ADMINISTRATION

Selection of patients for treatment with OPANA should be governed by the same principles that apply to the use of similar opioid analgesics *[see Indications and Usage (1)]*. Physicians should individualize treatment in every case *[see Dosage and Administration (2.1)]*, using non-opioid analgesics, opioids on an as needed basis, combination products, and chronic opioid therapy in a progressive plan of pain management such as outlined by the World Health Organization, the Agency for Healthcare Research and Quality, and the American Pain Society.

OPANA should be administered on an empty stomach, at least one hour prior to or two hours after eating *[see Clinical Pharmacology (12.3)]*

2.1 Individualization of Dosage

As with any opioid drug product, it is necessary to adjust the dosing regimen for each patient individually, taking into account the patient's prior analgesic treatment experience. In the selection of the initial dose of OPANA, attention should be given to the following:

- The total daily dose, potency and specific characteristics of the opioid the patient has been taking previously;
- The relative potency estimate used to calculate the equivalent oxymorphone dose needed;
- The patient's degree of opioid tolerance;
- The age, general condition, and medical status of the patient;
- Concurrent non-opioid analgesics and other medications;
- The type and severity of the patient's pain;
- The balance between pain control and adverse experiences;
- Risk factors for abuse or addiction, including a prior history of abuse or addiction.

Once therapy is initiated, frequently assess pain relief and other opioid effects. Titrate dose to adequate pain relief (generally mild or no pain). Patients who experience breakthrough pain may require dosage adjustment.

If signs of excessive opioid-related adverse experiences are observed, the next dose may be reduced. Adjust dosing to obtain an appropriate balance between pain relief and opioid-related adverse experiences. If significant adverse events occur before the therapeutic goal of mild or no pain is achieved, the events should be treated aggressively. Once adverse events are adequately managed, continue upward titration to an acceptable level of pain control.

During periods of changing analgesic requirements, including initial titration, frequent contact is recommended between physician, other members of the healthcare team, the patient, and the caregiver/family. Advise patients and family members of the potential common adverse reactions associated with changing opioid doses.

The dosing recommendations below, therefore, can only be considered as suggested approaches to what is actually a series of clinical decisions over time in the management of the pain of each individual patient.

2.2 Initiation of Therapy

Titrate dose to adequate pain relief (generally mild or no pain).

Opioid-Naïve Patients

Patients who have not been receiving opioid analgesics should be started on OPANA in a dosing range of 10 to 20 mg every four to six hours depending on the initial pain intensity. If deemed necessary to initiate therapy at a lower dose (e.g., for renal or hepatic impairment or for geriatric patients), patients may be started with OPANA 5 mg. The dose should be titrated based upon the individual patient's response to their initial dose of OPANA. This dose can then be adjusted to an acceptable level of analgesia taking into account the pain intensity and adverse reactions experienced by the patient.

Initiation of therapy with doses higher than 20 mg is not recommended because of potential serious adverse reactions *[see Clinical Studies (14.1)]*.

Conversion from Parenteral Oxymorphone to OPANA

Given OPANA's absolute oral bioavailability of approximately 10%, patients receiving parenteral oxymorphone may be converted to OPANA by administering 10 times the patient's total daily parenteral oxymorphone dose as OPANA, in four or six equally divided doses (e.g., [IV dose × 10] divided by 4 or 6). For example, approximately 10 mg of OPANA four times daily may be required to provide pain relief equivalent to a total daily IM dose of 4 mg oxymorphone. Due to patient variability with regard to opioid analgesic response, upon conversion patients should be closely monitored to ensure adequate analgesia and to minimize side effects.

Conversion from Other Oral Opioids to OPANA

For conversion from other opioids to OPANA, physicians and other healthcare professionals are advised to refer to published relative potency information, keeping in mind that conversion ratios are only approximate. In general, it is safest to start OPANA therapy by administering half of the calculated total daily dose of OPANA in 4 to 6 equally divided doses, every 4-6 hours. The initial dose of OPANA can be gradually adjusted until adequate pain relief and acceptable side effects have been achieved.

2.3 Maintenance of Therapy

During therapy, continual re-evaluation of the patient receiving OPANA is important, with special attention to the maintenance of pain control and the relative incidence of side effects associated with therapy. If the level of pain increases, effort should be made to identify the source of increased pain, while adjusting the dose *[see Dosage and Administration (2.1)]*.

2.4 Cessation of Therapy

When the patient no longer requires therapy with OPANA, doses should be tapered gradually to prevent signs and symptoms of withdrawal in the physically dependent patient *[see Drug Abuse and Dependence (9.3)]*.

2.5 Patients with Hepatic Impairment

OPANA is contraindicated in patients with moderate or severe hepatic impairment. Use OPANA with caution in patients with mild hepatic impairment, starting with the lowest dose (e.g., 5 mg) and titrating slowly while carefully monitoring side effects *[see Warnings and Precautions (5.6) and Clinical Pharmacology (12.3)]*.

2.6 Patients with Renal Impairment

There are 57% and 65% increases in oxymorphone bioavailability in patients with moderate and severe renal impairment, respectively; treated with extended-release oxymorphone tablets *[see Clinical Pharmacology (12.3)]*. Accordingly, OPANA should be administered cautiously and in reduced dosages to patients with creatinine clearance rates less than 50 mL/min.

2.7 Use with Central Nervous System Depressants

OPANA, like all opioid analgesics, should be started at 1/3 to 1/2 of the usual dose in patients who are concurrently receiving other central nervous system (CNS) depressants including sedatives or hypnotics, general anesthetics, phenothiazines, tranquilizers, and alcohol, because respiratory depression, hypotension and profound sedation, coma or death may result *[see Warnings and Precautions (5.3) and Drug Interactions (7.1)]*. When combined therapy with any of the above medications is considered, the dose of one or both agents should be reduced.

Although no specific interaction between oxymorphone and monoamine oxidase inhibitors has been observed, OPANA is not recommended for use in patients who have received MAO inhibitors within 14 days *[see Drug Interactions (7.5)]*.

2.8 Geriatric Patients

Exercise caution in the selection of the starting dose of OPANA for an elderly patient by starting at the low end of the dosing range (e.g., 5 mg) *[see Use in Specific Populations (8.5)]*.

3 DOSAGE FORMS AND STRENGTHS

The 5 mg dosage form is a blue, round, convex tablet debossed with E612 over 5 on one side and plain on the other. The 10 mg dosage form is a red, round, convex tablet debossed with E613 over 10 on one side and plain on the other.

4 CONTRAINDICATIONS

- OPANA is contraindicated in patients with a known hypersensitivity to oxymorphone or to any of the other ingredients in OPANA, or with known hypersensitivity to morphine analogs such as codeine.
- OPANA is contraindicated in patients with respiratory depression, except in monitored settings and in the presence of resuscitative equipment.
- OPANA is contraindicated in patients with acute or severe bronchial asthma or hypercarbia.
- OPANA is contraindicated in any patient who has or is suspected of having paralytic ileus *[see Warning and Precautions (5.8)]*.
- OPANA is contraindicated in patients with moderate or severe hepatic impairment *[see Warnings and Precautions (5.6)]*.

5 WARNINGS AND PRECAUTIONS

5.1 Respiratory Depression

Respiratory depression is the chief hazard of OPANA. Respiratory depression may occur more frequently in elderly or debilitated patients as well as in those suffering from conditions accompanied by hypoxia or hypercapnia, when even moderate therapeutic doses may dangerously decrease pulmonary ventilation.

Administer OPANA with extreme caution to patients with conditions accompanied by hypoxia, hypercapnia, or decreased respiratory reserve such as: asthma, chronic obstructive pulmonary disease or cor pulmonale, severe obesity, sleep apnea syndrome, myxedema, kyphoscoliosis, CNS depression, or coma. In these patients, even usual therapeutic doses of oxymorphone may decrease respiratory drive while simultaneously increasing airway resistance to the point of apnea. Consider alternative non-opioid analgesics and use OPANA only under careful medical supervision at the lowest effective dose in such patients.

5.2 Misuse, Abuse, and Diversion of Opioids

OPANA contains oxymorphone, a mu opioid agonist and a Schedule II controlled substance with an abuse liability similar to morphine. Opioid agonists are sought by drug abusers and people with addiction disorders and are subject to criminal diversion. Oxymorphone can be abused in a manner similar to other opioid agonists, legal or illicit. This issue should be considered when prescribing or dispensing oxymorphone in situations where the physician or pharmacist is concerned about an increased risk of misuse, abuse, or diversion.

OPANA tablets may be abused by crushing, chewing, snorting, or injecting the product. These practices pose a significant risk to the abuser that could result in overdose and death *[see Drug Abuse and Dependence (9)]*.

OPANA may be targeted for theft and diversion. Healthcare professionals should contact their State Medical Board, State Board of Pharmacy, or State Control Board for information on how to detect or prevent diversion of this product, and security requirements for storing and handling of OPANA.

Healthcare professionals should advise patients to store OPANA in a secure place, preferably locked and out of the reach of children and other non-caregivers.

Concerns about abuse, misuse, diversion and addiction should not prevent the proper management of pain.

5.3 Additive CNS Depressant Effects

The concomitant use of other CNS depressants including other opioids, general anesthetics, phenothiazines, other tranquilizers, sedatives, hypnotics, and alcohol with oxymorphone may produce increased depressant effects including hypoventilation, hypotension, profound sedation, coma and death *[see Drug Interactions (7.1)]*.

5.4 Use in Patients with Head Injury and Increased Intracranial Pressure

In the presence of head injury, intracranial lesions or a preexisting increase in intracranial pressure, the respiratory depressant effects of opioid analgesics and their potential to elevate cerebrospinal fluid pressure (resulting from vasodilation following CO_2 retention) may be markedly exaggerated. Furthermore, opioid analgesics can produce effects on papillary response and consciousness, which may obscure neurologic signs of further increases in intracranial pressure in patients with head injuries.

Administer OPANA with extreme caution in patients who may be particularly susceptible to the intracranial effects of CO_2 retention, such as those with evidence of increased intracranial pressure or impaired consciousness. Opioids may obscure the clinical course of a patient with a head injury and should be used only if clinically warranted.

5.5 Hypotensive Effect

OPANA, like all opioid analgesics, may cause severe hypotension in a patient whose ability to maintain blood pressure has been compromised by a depleted blood volume, or after concurrent administration with drugs such as phenothiazines or other agents that compromise vasomotor tone. Administer OPANA with caution to patients in circulatory shock, since vasodilation produced by the drug may further reduce cardiac output and blood pressure.

5.6 Hepatic Impairment

A study of extended-release oxymorphone tablets in patients with hepatic disease indicated greater plasma concentrations than in those with normal hepatic function *[see Clinical Pharmacology (12.3)]*. Use OPANA with caution in patients with mild impairment, starting with the lowest dose and titrating slowly while carefully monitoring for side effects *[see Dosage and Administration (2.2, 2.5)]*. OPANA is contraindicated in patients with moderate or severe hepatic impairment.

5.7 Special Risk Groups

Use OPANA with caution in the following conditions: adrenocortical insufficiency (e.g., Addison's disease), prostatic hypertrophy or urethral stricture, severe impairment of pulmonary or renal function, and toxic psychosis.

Opioids may aggravate convulsions in patients with convulsive disorders, and may induce or aggravate seizures in some clinical settings.

5.8 Gastrointestinal Effects

Opioids diminish propulsive peristaltic waves in the gastrointestinal tract. Monitor for decreased bowel motility in post-operative patients receiving opioids. The administration of OPANA may obscure the diagnosis or clinical course in patients with acute abdominal conditions. OPANA is contraindicated in patients with paralytic ileus.

5.9 Use in Pancreatic/Biliary Tract Disease

OPANA, like other opioids, may cause spasm of the sphincter of Oddi and should be used with caution in patients with biliary tract disease, including acute pancreatitis.

5.10 Driving and Operating Machinery

Opioid analgesics impair the mental and physical abilities needed to perform potentially hazardous activities such as driving a car or operating machinery.

6 ADVERSE REACTIONS

The following serious adverse reactions are discussed elsewhere in the labeling:

- Respiratory depression [see Warnings and Precautions (5.1)]
- Misuse and abuse [see Warnings and Precautions (5.2) and Drug Abuse and Dependence (9)]
- CNS depressant effects [see Warnings and Precautions (5.3)]

Because clinical trials are conducted under widely varying conditions, adverse reaction rates observed in the clinical trials of a drug cannot be directly compared to rates in the clinical trials of another drug and may not reflect the rates observed in clinical practice.

6.1 Clinical Trials Experience

A total of 591 patients were treated with OPANA in controlled clinical trials. The clinical trials consisted of patients with acute post-operative pain (n=557) and cancer pain (n=34) trials.

The following table lists adverse reactions that were reported in at least 2% of patients receiving OPANA in placebo-controlled trials (acute post-operative pain (N=557)).

Table 1: Adverse Reactions Reported in Placebo-Controlled Trials

MedDRA Preferred Term	OPANA (N=557)	Placebo (N=270)
Nausea	19%	12%
Pyrexia	14%	8%
Somnolence	9%	2%
Vomiting	9%	7%
Pruritus	8%	4%
Headache	7%	4%
Dizziness (Excluding Vertigo)	7%	2%
Constipation	4%	1%
Confusion	3%	<1%

The **common** (≥1%->10%) adverse drug reactions reported at least once by patients treated with OPANA in the clinical trials organized by MedDRA's (Medical Dictionary for Regulatory Activities) System Organ Class were and not represented in Table 1:

Cardiac disorders: tachycardia
Gastrointestinal disorders: dry mouth, abdominal distention, and flatulence
General disorders and administration site conditions: sweating increased
Nervous system disorders: anxiety and sedation
Respiratory, thoracic and mediastinal disorders: hypoxia
Vascular disorders: hypotension

Other **less common** adverse reactions known with opioid treatment that were seen <1% in the OPANA trials includes the following: Abdominal pain, ileus, diarrhea, agitation, disorientation, restlessness, feeling jittery, hypersensitivity, allergic reactions, bradycardia, central nervous system depression, depressed level of consciousness, lethargy, mental impairment, mental status changes, fatigue, depression, clamminess, flushing, hot flashes, dehydration, dermatitis, dyspepsia, dysphoria, edema, euphoric mood, hallucination, hypertension, insomnia, miosis, nervousness, palpitation, postural hypotension, syncope, dyspnea, respiratory depression, respiratory distress, respiratory rate decreased, oxygen saturation decreased, difficult micturition, urinary retention, urticaria, vision blurred, visual disturbances, weakness, appetite decreased, and weight decreased.

7 DRUG INTERACTIONS

7.1 Use with CNS Depressants

The concomitant use of other CNS depressants including sedatives, hypnotics, tranquilizers, general anesthetics, phenothiazines, other opioids, and alcohol may produce additive CNS depressant effects. OPANA, like all opioid analgesics, should be started at 1/3 to 1/2 of the usual dose in patients who are concurrently receiving other central nervous system depressants because respiratory depression, hypotension, and profound sedation, coma and death may result and titrated slowly as necessary for adequate pain relief. When combined therapy with any of the above medications is considered, the dose of one or both agents should be reduced [see Dosage and Administration (2.7) and Warnings and Precautions (5.3)].

7.2 Interactions with Mixed Agonist/Antagonist Opioid Analgesics

Agonist/antagonist analgesics (i.e., pentazocine, nalbuphine, butorphanol, and buprenorphine) should be administered with caution to a patient who has received or is receiving a course of therapy with a pure opioid agonist analgesic such as oxymorphone. In this situation, mixed agonist/antagonist analgesics may reduce the analgesic effect of oxymorphone and/or may precipitate withdrawal symptoms in these patients.

7.3 Cimetidine

CNS side effects have been reported (e.g., confusion, disorientation, respiratory depression, apnea, seizures) following coadministration of cimetidine with opioid analgesics; a causal relationship has not been established.

7.4 Anticholinergics

Anticholinergics or other medications with anticholinergic activity when used concurrently with opioid analgesics may result in increased risk of urinary retention and/or severe constipation, which may lead to paralytic ileus.

7.5 MAO Inhibitors

Opana is not recommended for use in patients who have received MAO inhibitors within 14 days, because severe and unpredictable potentiation by MAO inhibitors has been reported with opioid analgesics. No specific interaction between oxymorphone and monoamine oxidase inhibitors has been observed, but caution in the use of any opioid in patients taking this class of drugs is appropriate.

8 USE IN SPECIFIC POPULATIONS

8.1 Pregnancy

The safety of using oxymorphone in pregnancy has not been established with regard to possible adverse effects on fetal development. The use of OPANA in pregnancy, in nursing mothers, or in women of child-bearing potential requires that the possible benefits of the drug be weighted against the possible hazards to the mother and the child.

Teratogenic Effects
Pregnancy Category C

There are no adequate and well-controlled studies of oxymorphone in pregnant women. In animal studies, oxymorphone caused decreased fetal and pup weights, an increase in stillbirth, and a decrease in postnatal pup survival at maternal oxymorphone doses equivalent to 0.4 to 4 times the human daily dose of 120 mg (Based on body surface area). OPANA should be used during pregnancy only if the potential benefit justifies the potential risk to the fetus.

In embryo-fetal developmental toxicity studies, pregnant rats and rabbits received oxymorphone hydrochloride at doses up to about 2 times (rats) and 8 times (rabbits) total human daily dose of 120 mg (based on body surface area). No malformations occurred, but reduced fetal weights occurred at maternal doses of 0.8 (rat) and 4 (rabbit) times the total human daily dose of 120 mg (based on body surface area). There were no adverse developmental effects in rats that received 0.4 times or rabbits that received less than 4 times the total human dose. There were no effects of oxymorphone hydrochloride on intrauterine survival at doses in rats ≤2 times, or in rabbits at ≤8 times the human dose (see Non-teratogenic Effects, below). In a study conducted prior to the establishment of Good Laboratory Practices (GLP) and not according to current recommended methodology, a single subcutaneous injection of oxymorphone hydrochloride on gestation day 8 produced malformations in offspring of hamsters that received a dose equivalent to 10 times the total human daily dose of 120 mg (based on body surface area). This dose also produced 83% maternal lethality.

Non-teratogenic Effects
Oxymorphone hydrochloride administration to female rats during gestation in a pre- and postnatal developmental toxicity study reduced mean litter size (18%) at a dose of 25 mg/kg/day, attributed to an increase in the incidence of stillborn pups. An increase in neonatal death occurred at doses ≥5 mg/kg/day (0.4 times a total human daily dose of 120 mg, based on body surface area). Low pup birth weight, decreased post-natal weight gain, and reduced post-natal

survival of pups occurred following treatment of the dams with 25 mg/kg/day (about 2 times a total human daily dose of 120 mg, based on body surface area).

Prolonged use of opioid analgesics during pregnancy may cause fetal-neonatal physical dependence. Neonatal withdrawal may occur. Symptoms usually appear during the first days of life and may include convulsions, irritability, excessive crying, tremors, hyperactive reflexes, fever, vomiting, diarrhea, sneezing, yawning, and increased respiratory rate.

8.2 Labor and Delivery

Opioids cross the placenta and may produce respiratory depression in neonates. OPANA is not recommended for use in women during and immediately prior to labor, when use of shorter acting analgesics or other analgesic techniques are more appropriate. Occasionally, opioid analgesics may prolong labor through actions which temporarily reduce the strength, duration, and frequency of uterine contractions. However this effect is not consistent and may be offset by an increased rate of cervical dilatation, which tends to shorten labor. Neonates whose mothers received opioid analgesics during labor should be observed closely for signs of respiratory depression. A specific opioid antagonist, such as naloxone or nalmefene, should be available for reversal of opioid-induced respiratory depression in the neonate.

8.3 Nursing Mothers

It is not known whether oxymorphone is excreted in human milk. Because many drugs, including some opioids, are excreted in human milk, caution should be exercised when OPANA is administered to a nursing woman. Infants exposed to OPANA through breast milk should be monitored for excess sedation and respiratory depression. Withdrawal symptoms can occur in breast-fed infants when maternal administration of an opioid analgesic is stopped, or when breast-feeding is stopped.

8.4 Pediatric Use

Safety and effectiveness of OPANA in pediatric patients below the age of 18 years have not been established.

8.5 Geriatric Use

OPANA should be used with caution in elderly patients [see Clinical Pharmacology (12.3)].

Of the total number of subjects in clinical studies of OPANA, 31% were 65 and over, while 7% were 75 and over. No overall differences in effectiveness were observed between these subjects and younger subjects. There were several adverse events that were more frequently observed in subjects 65 and over compared to younger subjects. These adverse events included dizziness, somnolence, confusion, and nausea. In general, dose selection for elderly patients should be cautious, usually starting at the low end of the dosing range, reflecting the greater frequency of decreased hepatic, renal or cardiac function, and of concomitant disease or other drug therapy.

8.6 Hepatic Impairment

In a study of extended-release oxymorphone tablets, patients with mild hepatic impairment were shown to have an increase in bioavailability of 1.6 fold. OPANA should be used with caution in patients with mild impairment. These patients should be started with the lowest dose and titrated slowly while carefully monitoring for side effects. OPANA is contraindicated for patients with moderate and severe hepatic impairment [see Contraindications (4), Warnings and Precautions (5.6), and Dosage and Administration (2.5)].

8.7 Renal Impairment

In a study of extended-release oxymorphone tablets, patients with moderate to severe renal impairment were shown to have an increase in bioavailability ranging from 57-65% [see Clinical Pharmacology (12.3)]. Such patients should be started cautiously with lower doses of OPANA and titrated slowly while monitoring for side effects [see Dosage and Administration (2.6)].

9 DRUG ABUSE AND DEPENDENCE

9.1 Controlled Substance

OPANA contains oxymorphone, a mu opioid agonist and a Schedule II controlled substance with an abuse liability similar to morphine and other opioids. Oxymorphone can be abused and is subject to criminal diversion [see Warnings and Precautions (5.2)].

9.2 Abuse

All patients treated with opioids require careful monitoring for signs of abuse and addiction, since use of opioid analgesic products carries the risk of addiction even under appropriate medical use. Addiction is a primary, chronic, neurobiologic disease, with genetic, psychosocial, and environmental factors influencing its development and manifestations. Addiction is characterized by one or more of the following: impaired control over drug use, compulsive use, use for non-medical purposes, and continued use despite harm. Drug addiction is a treatable disease, utilizing a multidisciplinary approach, but relapse is common.

"Drug-seeking" behavior is very common to addicts and drug abusers. Drug-seeking tactics include emergency calls or visits near the end of office hours, refusal to undergo appropriate examination, testing or referral, repeated claims of loss of prescriptions, tampering with prescriptions, and reluctance to provide prior medical records or contact information for other treating physician(s). "Doctor shopping" (visiting multiple prescribers) to obtain additional prescriptions is common among drug abusers and people suffering from untreated addiction. Preoccupation with achieving adequate pain relief can be appropriate behavior in a patient with poor pain control.

Abuse and addiction are separate and distinct from physical dependence and tolerance. Physicians should be aware that addiction may not be accompanied by concurrent tolerance and symptoms of physical dependence in all addicts. In addition, abuse of opioids can occur in the absence of true addiction and is characterized by misuse for non-medical purposes, often in combination with other psychoactive substances. OPANA, like other opioids, may be diverted for non-medical use. Careful record-keeping of prescribing information, including quantity, frequency, and renewal requests is strongly advised.

OPANA is intended for oral use only. Abuse of OPANA poses a risk of overdose and death. This risk is increased with concurrent abuse of OPANA with alcohol and other substances. Parenteral drug abuse is commonly associated with transmission of infectious diseases such as hepatitis and HIV.

Proper assessment of the patient, proper prescribing practices, periodic re-evaluation of therapy, and proper dispensing and storage are appropriate measures that help to limit abuse of opioid drugs.

9.3 Dependence

Opioid analgesics may cause physical dependence. Physical dependence results in withdrawal symptoms after abrupt discontinuation of a drug or upon administration of an opioid antagonist or mixed opioid agonist/antagonist agent. Withdrawal also may be precipitated through the administration of drugs with opioid antagonist activity, e.g., naloxone, nalmefene, or mixed agonist/antagonist analgesics (pentazocine, butorphanol, buprenorphine, nalbuphine). Physical dependence may not occur to a clinically significant degree until after several days to weeks of continued opioid usage.

Tolerance is the need for increasing doses of opioids to maintain a defined effect such as analgesia (in the absence of disease progression or other external factors). The development of physical dependence and/or tolerance is not unusual during chronic opioid therapy.

OPANA should not be abruptly discontinued *[see Dosage and Administration (2.4)]*. If OPANA is abruptly discontinued in a physically-dependent patient, an abstinence syndrome may occur. Some or all of the following can characterize this syndrome: restlessness, lacrimation, rhinorrhea, yawning, perspiration, chills, myalgia, and mydriasis. Other symptoms also may develop, including: irritability, anxiety, backache, joint pain, weakness, abdominal cramps, insomnia, nausea, anorexia, vomiting, diarrhea, or increased blood pressure, respiratory rate, or heart rate.

Infants born to mothers physically dependent on opioids will also be physically dependent and may exhibit respiratory difficulties and withdrawal symptoms *[see Use in Specific Populations (8.1, 8.2)]*.

10 OVERDOSAGE

10.1 Symptoms

Acute overdosage with OPANA is characterized by respiratory depression (a decrease in respiratory rate and/or tidal volume, Cheyne-Stokes respiration, cyanosis), extreme somnolence progressing to stupor or coma, skeletal muscle flaccidity, cold and clammy skin, constricted pupils, and sometimes bradycardia and hypotension. In some cases, apnea, circulatory collapse, cardiac arrest, and death may occur.

OPANA may cause miosis, even in total darkness. Pinpoint pupils are a sign of opioid overdose but are not pathognomonic (e.g., pontine lesions of hemorrhagic or ischemic origin may produce similar findings). Marked mydriasis rather than miosis may be seen with hypoxia in overdose situations *[see Clinical Pharmacology (12.2)]*.

10.2 Treatment

In the treatment of OPANA overdosage, primary attention should be given to the re-establishment of a patent airway and institution of assisted or controlled ventilation. Supportive measures (including oxygen and vasopressors) should be employed in the management of circulatory shock and pulmonary edema accompanying overdose as indicated. Cardiac arrest or arrhythmias may require cardiac massage or defibrillation.

The opioid antagonist naloxone hydrochloride is a specific antidote against respiratory depression that may result from overdosage or unusual sensitivity to opioids including OPANA. Nalmefene is an alternative pure opioid antagonist, which may be administered as a specific antidote to respiratory depression resulting from opioid overdose. Since the duration of action of OPANA may exceed that of the antagonist, keep the patient under continued surveillance and administer repeated doses of the antagonist according to the antagonist labeling as needed to maintain adequate respiration.

In patients receiving OPANA, opioid antagonists should not be administered in the absence of clinically significant respiratory or circulatory depression. Administer opioid antagonists cautiously to persons who are known, or suspected to be, physically dependent on any opioid agonist including OPANA. In such cases, an abrupt or complete reversal of opioid effects may precipitate an acute abstinence syndrome. In an individual physically dependent on opioids, administration of the usual dose of the antagonist will precipitate an acute withdrawal syndrome. The severity of the withdrawal syndrome produced will depend on the degree of physical dependence and the dose of the antagonist administered. If respiratory depression is associated with muscular rigidity, administration of a neuromuscular blocking agent may be necessary to facilitate assisted or controlled ventilation. Muscular rigidity may also respond to opioid antagonist therapy.

11 DESCRIPTION

OPANA (oxymorphone hydrochloride) is a semi-synthetic opioid analgesic supplied in 5 mg and 10 mg tablet strengths for oral administration. The tablet strengths describe the amount of oxymorphone hydrochloride per tablet. The tablets contain the following inactive ingredients: lactose monohydrate, magnesium stearate, and pregelatinized starch. In addition, the 5 mg tablets contain FD&C blue No. 2 aluminum lake. The 10 mg tablets contain D&C red No. 30 aluminum lake.

Chemically, oxymorphone hydrochloride is 4, 5α-epoxy-3, 14-dihydroxy-17-methylmorphinan-6-one hydrochloride, a white or slightly off-white, odorless powder, which is sparingly soluble in alcohol and ether, but freely soluble in water. The molecular weight of oxymorphone hydrochloride is 337.80. The pK_a1 and pK_a2 of oxymorphone at 37°C are 8.17 and 9.54, respectively. The octanol/aqueous partition coefficient at 37°C and pH 7.4 is 0.98.

The structural formula for oxymorphone hydrochloride is as follows:

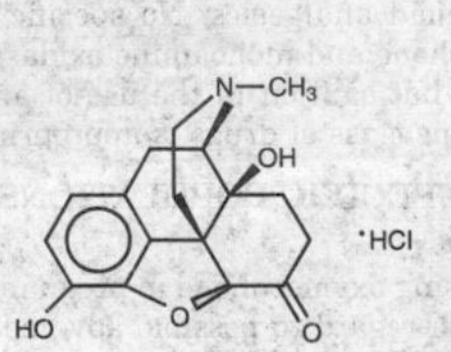

12 CLINICAL PHARMACOLOGY

12.1 Mechanism of Action

Oxymorphone, a pure opioid agonist, is relatively selective for the mu receptor, although it can interact with other opioid receptors at higher doses.

The precise mechanism of analgesia, the principal therapeutic action of oxymorphone, is unknown. Specific CNS opiate receptors and endogenous compounds with morphine-like activity have been identified throughout the brain and spinal cord and are likely to play a role in the expression and perception of analgesic effects.

12.2 Pharmacodynamics

Pharmacological effects of opioid agonists include analgesia, anxiolysis, euphoria, feelings of relaxation, respiratory depression, constipation, miosis, and cough suppression. Like all pure opioid agonist analgesics, with increasing doses there is increasing analgesia, unlike with mixed agonist/antagonists or non-opioid analgesics, where there is a limit to the analgesic effect with increasing doses. With pure opioid agonist analgesics, there is no defined maximum dose; the ceiling to analgesic effectiveness is imposed only by side effects, the more serious of which may include somnolence and respiratory depression.

Concentration-Efficacy Relationships

The minimum effective plasma concentration of oxymorphone for analgesia varies widely among patients, especially among patients who have been previously treated with potent agonist opioids. As a result, individually titrate patients to achieve a balance between therapeutic and adverse effects. The minimum effective analgesic concentration of oxymorphone for any individual patient may increase over time due to an increase in pain, progression of disease, development of a new pain syndrome and/or development of analgesic tolerance.

Concentration-Adverse Experience Relationships

There is a general relationship between increasing opioid plasma concentration and increasing frequency of adverse experiences such as nausea, vomiting, CNS effects, and respiratory depression.

As with all opioids, the dose of OPANA must be individualized *[see Dosage and Administration (2.2)]*. The effective analgesic dose for some patients will be too high to be tolerated by other patients.

Effects on the Central Nervous System (CNS)

The principal therapeutic action of oxymorphone is analgesia. In common with other opioids, oxymorphone causes respiratory depression, in part by a direct effect on the brainstem respiratory centers. The respiratory depression involves a reduction in the responsiveness of the brain stem respiratory centers to both increases in carbon dioxide tension and electrical stimulation. Opioids depress the cough reflex by direct effect on the cough center in the medulla. Antitussive effects may occur with doses lower than those usually required for analgesia. Oxymorphone causes miosis, even in total darkness. Pinpoint pupils are a sign of opioid overdose but are not pathognomonic (e.g., pontine lesions of hemorrhagic or ischemic origin may produce similar findings). Marked mydriasis rather than miosis may be seen with hypoxia in overdose situations *[see Overdosage (10.1)]*. Other therapeutic effects of oxymorphone include anxiolysis, euphoria and feelings of relaxation.

In addition to analgesia, the widely diverse effects of oxymorphone include drowsiness, changes in mood, decreased gastrointestinal motility, nausea, vomiting, and alterations of the endocrine and autonomic nervous system.

Effects on the Gastrointestinal Tract and on Other Smooth Muscle

Gastric, biliary and pancreatic secretions are decreased by oxymorphone. Oxymorphone causes a reduction in motility and is associated with an increase in tone in the antrum of the stomach and duodenum. Digestion of food in the small intestine is delayed and propulsive contractions are decreased. Propulsive peristaltic waves in the colon are decreased, while tone is increased to the point of spasm. The end result may be constipation. Oxymorphone can cause a marked increase in biliary tract pressure as a result of spasm of the sphincter of Oddi. Oxymorphone may also cause spasm of the sphincter of the urinary bladder.

Cardiovascular System Effects

Opioids produce peripheral vasodilation which may result in orthostatic hypotension. Release of histamine can occur and may contribute to opioid-induced hypotension. Manifestations of histamine release may include orthostatic hypotension, pruritus, flushing, red eyes, and sweating. Animal studies have shown that oxymorphone has a lower propensity to cause histamine release than other opioids.

Endocrine System Effects

Opioid agonists have been shown to have a variety of effects on the secretion of hormones. Opioids inhibit the secretion of ACTH, cortisol, and luteinizing hormone (LH) in humans. They also stimulate prolactin, growth hormone (GH) secretion, and pancreatic secretion of insulin and glucagon in humans and other species, rats and dogs. Thyroid stimulating hormone (TSH) has been shown to be both inhibited and stimulated by opioids.

Immune System Effects

Opioids have been shown to have a variety of effects on components of the immune system in *in vitro* and animal models. The clinical significance of these findings is unknown.

12.3 Pharmacokinetics

Absorption

The absolute oral bioavailability of oxymorphone is approximately 10%. Studies in healthy volunteers reveal predictable relationships between OPANA dosage and plasma oxymorphone concentrations.

Steady-state levels were achieved after three days of multiple dose administration. Under both single-dose and steady-state conditions, dose proportionality has been established for 5 mg, 10 mg and 20 mg doses of OPANA, for both peak plasma levels (Cmax) and extent of absorption (AUC) (see Table 2).

[See table 2 at top of next page]

Food Effect

After oral dosing with 40 mg of OPANA in healthy volunteers under fasting conditions or with a high-fat meal, the C_{max} and AUC were increased by approximately 38% in fed subjects relative to fasted subjects. As a result, OPANA should be dosed at least one hour prior to or two hours after eating *[see Dosage and Administration (2)]*.

Ethanol Effect

The effect of co-ingestion of alcohol with OPANA has not been evaluated. However, an *in vivo* study was performed to evaluate the effect of alcohol (40%, 20%, 4% and 0%) on the bioavailability of a single dose of 40 mg of extended-release oxymorphone tablets in healthy, fasted volunteers. Following concomitant administration of 240 mL of 40% ethanol the Cmax increased on average by 70% and up to 270% in individual subjects. Following the concomitant administration of 240 mL of 20% ethanol, the C_{max} increased on average by 31% and up to 260% in individual subjects. In some individuals there was also a decrease in oxymorphone peak plasma concentrations. No effect on the release of oxymorphone from the extended-release tablet was noted in an *in vitro* alcohol interaction study. The mechanism of the *in vivo* interaction is unknown. Therefore, avoid co-administration of oxymorphone and ethanol.

Distribution
Formal studies on the distribution of oxymorphone in various tissues have not been conducted. Oxymorphone is not extensively bound to human plasma proteins; binding is in the range of 10% to 12%.
Metabolism
Oxymorphone is highly metabolized, principally in the liver, and undergoes reduction or conjugation with glucuronic acid to form both active and inactive products. The two major metabolites of oxymorphone are oxymorphone-3-glucuronide and 6-OH-oxymorphone. The mean plasma AUC for oxymorphone-3-glucuronide is approximately 90-fold higher than the parent compound. The pharmacologic activity of the glucuronide metabolite has not been evaluated. 6-OH-oxymorphone has been shown in animal studies to have analgesic bioactivity. The mean plasma 6-OH-oxymorphone AUC is approximately 70% of the oxymorphone AUC following single oral doses but is essentially equivalent to the parent compound at steady-state.
Excretion
Because oxymorphone is extensively metabolized, <1% of the administered dose is excreted unchanged in the urine. On average, 33% to 38% of the administered dose is excreted in the urine as oxymorphone-3-glucuronide and 0.25% to 0.62% is excreted as 6-OH-oxymorphone in subjects with normal hepatic and renal function. In animals given radiolabeled oxymorphone, approximately 90% of the administered radioactivity was recovered within 5 days of dosing. The majority of oxymorphone-derived radioactivity was found in the urine and feces.
Pharmacokinetics in Special Populations
Elderly
The plasma levels of oxymorphone administered as an extended-release tablet were about 40% higher in elderly (≥65 years of age) than in younger subjects *[see Use in Specific Populations (8.5)]*.
Gender
The effect of gender on the pharmacokinetics of OPANA has not been studied. In a study with an extended-release formulation of oxymorphone, there was a consistent tendency for female subjects to have slightly higher AUC_{ss} and C_{max} values than male subjects. However, gender differences were not observed when AUCss and Cmax were adjusted by body weight.
Hepatic Impairment
The liver plays an important role in the pre-systemic clearance of orally administered oxymorphone. Accordingly, the bioavailability of orally administered oxymorphone may be markedly increased in patients with moderate to severe liver disease. The effect of hepatic impairment on the pharmacokinetics of OPANA has not been studied. However, in a study with an extended-release formulation of oxymorphone, the disposition of oxymorphone was compared in 6 patients with mild, 5 patients with moderate, and one patient with severe hepatic impairment, and 12 subjects with normal hepatic function. The bioavailability of oxymorphone was increased by 1.6-fold in patients with mild hepatic impairment and by 3.7-fold in patients with moderate hepatic impairment. In one patient with severe hepatic impairment, the bioavailability was increased by 12.2-fold. The half-life of oxymorphone was not significantly affected by hepatic impairment.
Renal Impairment
The effect of renal impairment on the pharmacokinetics of OPANA has not been studied. However, in a study with an extended-release formulation of oxymorphone, an increase of 26%, 57%, and 65% in oxymorphone bioavailability was observed in mild (creatinine clearance 51-80 mL/min; n=8), moderate (creatinine clearance 30-50 mL/min; n=8), and severe (creatinine clearance <30 mL/min; n=8) patients, respectively, compared to healthy controls.
Drug-Drug Interactions
In vitro studies revealed little to no biotransformation of oxymorphone to 6-OH-oxymorphone by any of the major cytochrome P450 (CYP P450) isoforms at therapeutically relevant oxymorphone plasma concentrations.
No inhibition of any of the major CYP P450 isoforms was observed when oxymorphone was incubated with human liver microsomes at concentrations of ≤50 µM. An inhibition of CYP 3A4 activity occurred at oxymorphone concentrations ≥150 µM. Therefore, it is not expected that oxymorphone, or its metabolites will act as inhibitors of any of the major CYP P450 enzymes *in vivo*.
Increases in the activity of the CYP 2C9 and CYP 3A4 isoforms occurred when oxymorphone was incubated with human hepatocytes. However, clinical drug interaction studies with OPANA ER showed no induction of CYP450 3A4 or 2C9 enzyme activity, indicating that no dose adjustment for CYP 3A4- or 2C9-mediated drug-drug interactions is required.

Table 2
Mean (±SD) OPANA Pharmacokinetic Parameters

Regimen	Dosage	C_{max} (ng/mL)	AUC (ng·hr/mL)	$T_{1/2}$ (hr)
Single Dose	5 mg	1.10±0.55	4.48±2.07	7.25±4.40
	10 mg	1.93±0.75	9.10±3.40	7.78±3.56
	20 mg	4.39±1.72	20.07±5.80	9.43±3.36
Multiple Dose[a]	5 mg	1.73±0.62	4.63±1.49	NA
	10 mg	3.51±0.91	10.19±3.34	NA
	20 mg	7.33±2.93	21.10±7.59	NA

NA = not applicable
[a] Results after 5 days of every 6 hours dosing.

13 NONCLINICAL TOXICOLOGY
13.1 Carcinogenesis, Mutagenesis, Impairment of Fertility
Carcinogenesis
Long-term studies have been completed to evaluate the carcinogenic potential of oxymorphone in both Sprague-Dawley rats and CD-1 mice. Oxymorphone was administered to Sprague-Dawley rats (2.5, 5, and 10 mg/kg/day in males and 5, 10, and 25 mg/kg/day in females) for 2 years by oral gavage. The systemic drug exposure (AUC ng•h/mL) at the 10 mg/kg/day dose in male rats was 0.34-fold and at the 25 mg/kg/day dose in female rats was 1.5-fold the human exposure at a dose of 260 mg/day. No evidence of carcinogenic potential was observed in rats. Oxymorphone was administered to CD-1 mice (10, 25, 75 and 150 mg/kg/day) for 2 years by oral gavage. The systemic drug exposure (AUC ng•h/mL) at the 150 mg/kg/day dose in mice was 14.5-fold (in males) and 17.3-fold (in females) times the human exposure at a dose of 260 mg/day. No evidence of carcinogenic potential was observed in mice.
Mutagenesis
Oxymorphone hydrochloride was not mutagenic when tested in the *in vitro* bacterial reverse mutation assay (Ames test) at concentrations of ≤5270 µg/plate, or in an *in vitro* mammalian cell chromosome aberration assay performed with human peripheral blood lymphocytes at concentrations ≤5000 µg/ml with or without metabolic activation. Oxymorphone hydrochloride tested positive in both the rat and mouse *in vivo* micronucleus assays. An increase in micronucleated polychromatic erythrocytes occurred in mice given doses of ≥250 mg/kg and in rats given doses of 20 and 40 mg/kg. A subsequent study demonstrated that oxymorphone hydrochloride was not aneugenic in mice following administration of up to 500 mg/kg. Additional studies indicate that the increased incidence of micronucleated polychromatic erythrocytes in rats may be secondary to increased body temperature following oxymorphone administration. Doses associated with increased micronucleated polychromatic erythrocytes also produce a marked, rapid increase in body temperature. Pretreatment of animals with sodium salicylate minimized the increase in body temperature and prevented the increase in micronucleated polychromatic erythrocytes after administration of 40 mg/kg oxymorphone.
Impairment of fertility
Oxymorphone did not affect reproductive function or sperm parameters in male rats at any dose tested (≤50 mg/kg/day). In female rats, an increase in the length of the estrus cycle and decrease in the mean number of viable embryos, implantation sites and corpora lutea were observed at doses of oxymorphone ≥10 mg/kg/day. The dose of oxymorphone associated with reproductive findings in female rats is 0.8 times a total human daily dose of 120 mg based on a body surface area. The dose of oxymorphone that produced no adverse effects on reproductive findings in female rats (i.e., NOAEL) is 0.4-times a total human daily dose of 120 mg based on body surface area.

14 CLINICAL STUDIES
The analgesic efficacy of OPANA has been evaluated in acute pain following orthopedic and abdominal surgeries.
14.1 Orthopedic Surgery
Two double-blind, placebo-controlled, dose-ranging studies in patients with acute moderate to severe pain following orthopedic surgery evaluated the doses of OPANA 10 mg and 20 mg, and 30 mg was included in one study. Both studies demonstrated that OPANA 20 mg provided greater analgesia as measured by total pain relief based on a weighted analysis over 8 hours using a 0-4 categorical, compared to placebo. OPANA 10 mg provided greater analgesia as compared to placebo in one of the two studies. There was no evidence of superiority of the 30 mg dose over the 20 mg dose. However, there was a high rate of naloxone use in patients receiving the OPANA 30 mg dose in the postoperative period *[see Dosage and Administration (2.2)]*.
14.2 Abdominal Surgery
In a randomized, double-blind, placebo-controlled, multiple-dose study, the efficacy of OPANA 10 mg and 20 mg was assessed in patients with moderate to severe acute pain following abdominal surgery. In this study, patients were dosed every 4 to 6 hours over a 48-hour treatment period. OPANA 10 and 20 mg provided greater analgesia, as measured by the mean average pain intensity on a 0-100 mm visual analog scale, over 48 hours, compared to placebo *[see Dosage and Administration (2.2)]*.

16 HOW SUPPLIED/STORAGE AND HANDLING
OPANA tablets are supplied as follows:
5 mg Tablet:
Blue, round, convex tablets debossed with E612 over 5 on one side and plain on the other.
Bottles of 100 tablets with child-resistant closure NDC 63481-612-70
Unit-Dose package of 100 tablets (5 blister cards of 20 tablets, not child-resistant, for hospital use only) NDC 63481-612-75
10 mg Tablet:
Red, round, convex tablets debossed with E613 over 10 on one side and plain on the other.
Bottles of 100 tablets with child-resistant closure NDC 63481-613-70
Unit-Dose package of 100 tablets (5 blister cards of 20 tablets, not child-resistant, for hospital use only) NDC 63481-613-75
OPANA may be targeted for theft and diversion. Healthcare professionals should contact their State Medical Board, State Board of Pharmacy, or State Control Board for information on how to detect or prevent diversion of this product, and security requirements for storing and handling of OPANA.
Healthcare professionals should advise patients to store OPANA in a secure place, preferably locked and out of the reach of children and other non-caregivers.
Store at 25°C (77°F); excursions permitted to 15°-30°C (59°-86°F). [See USP Controlled Room Temperature].
Dispense in tight container as defined in the USP, with a child-resistant closure (as required).
Advise patients to dispose of any unused tablets from a prescription by flushing them down the toilet as soon as they are no longer needed *[see Patient Counseling Information (17)]*.

17 PATIENT COUNSELING INFORMATION
- Advise patients that OPANA contains oxymorphone, which is a morphine-like pain reliever, and should be taken only as directed.
- Advise patients that OPANA is a potential drug of abuse. They should protect it from theft, and it should never be given to anyone other than the individual for whom it was prescribed.
- Advise patients to keep OPANA in a secure place out of the reach of children and pets. Accidental consumption especially in children may result in overdose or death. When OPANA is no longer needed, the unused tablets should be destroyed by flushing down the toilet.
- Advise patients to report episodes of breakthrough pain and adverse experiences occurring during therapy to their doctor. Individualization of dosage is essential to make optimal use of this medication.
- Advise patients not to adjust the dose of OPANA without consulting the prescriber.
- Advise patients that OPANA may cause drowsiness, dizziness, or lightheadedness and may impair mental and/or physical abilities required for the performance of potentially hazardous tasks, such as driving a car, operating machinery, etc.
- Advise patients that OPANA will add to the effect of alcohol and other CNS depressants (such as antihistamines, sedatives, hypnotics, tranquilizers, general anesthetics, phenothiazines, other opioids, and monoamine oxidase [MAO] inhibitors).
- Advise patients not to combine OPANA with alcohol or other central nervous system depressants (sleep aids, tranquilizers) except by the orders of the prescribing physician, because dangerous additive effects may occur, resulting in serious injury or death.
- Advise patients of the potential for severe constipation. Appropriate laxatives and/or stool softeners and other therapeutic approaches should be considered for use with the initiation of OPANA therapy.

- Advise women of childbearing potential who become or are planning to become pregnant to consult their physician regarding the effects of opioid analgesics and other drug use during pregnancy on themselves and their unborn child.
- Advise women of childbearing potential who become or are planning to become pregnant that safe use in pregnancy has not been established. Prolonged use of opioid analgesics during pregnancy may cause fetal-neonatal physical dependence, and neonatal withdrawal may occur.
- Advise patients that if they have been receiving treatment with OPANA for more than a few weeks and cessation of therapy is indicated, it may be appropriate to taper the OPANA dose, rather than abruptly discontinue it, due to the risk of precipitating withdrawal symptoms. Their physician can provide a dose schedule to accomplish a gradual discontinuation of the medication.

Manufactured for:
Endo Pharmaceuticals Inc., Chadds Ford, PA 19317
Manufactured by:
Novartis Consumer Health Inc., Lincoln, NE 68517
2005649/March 2010

Shown in Product Identification Guide, page 308

OPANA® ER Ⓒ℞
[O-pan-a ER]
(oxymorphone hydrochloride)
Tablet, Extended-Release

WARNING:
OPANA ER contains oxymorphone, which is a morphine-like opioid agonist and a Schedule II controlled substance, with an abuse liability similar to other opioid analgesics.
Oxymorphone can be abused in a manner similar to other opioid agonists, legal or illicit. This should be considered when prescribing or dispensing OPANA ER in situations where the physician or pharmacist is concerned about an increased risk of misuse, abuse, or diversion.
OPANA ER is an extended-release oral formulation of oxymorphone indicated for the management of moderate to severe pain when a continuous, around-the-clock opioid analgesic is needed for an extended period of time.
OPANA ER is NOT intended for use as an as needed analgesic.
OPANA ER Tablets are to be swallowed whole and are not to be broken, chewed, dissolved, or crushed. Taking broken, chewed, dissolved, or crushed OPANA ER Tablets leads to rapid release and absorption of a potentially fatal dose of oxymorphone.
Patients must not consume alcoholic beverages, or prescription or non-prescription medications containing alcohol, while on OPANA ER therapy. The co-ingestion of alcohol with OPANA ER may result in increased plasma levels and a potentially fatal overdose of oxymorphone.

DESCRIPTION

OPANA ER (oxymorphone hydrochloride) extended-release, is a semi-synthetic opioid analgesic supplied in 5 mg, 7.5 mg, 10 mg, 15 mg, 20 mg, 30 mg, and 40 mg tablet strengths for oral administration. The tablet strength describes the amount of oxymorphone hydrochloride per tablet. The tablets contain the following inactive ingredients: hypromellose, methylparaben, silicified microcrystalline cellulose, sodium stearyl fumarate, TIMERx®-N, titanium dioxide, and triacetin. The 5 mg, 10 mg, 15 mg, 20 mg, and 30 mg tablets also contain macrogol, and polysorbate 80. In addition, the 5 mg, 7.5 mg, and 30 mg tablets contain iron oxide red. The 7.5 mg tablets contain iron oxide black, and iron oxide yellow. The 10 mg tablets contain FD&C yellow No. 6. The 20 mg tablets contain FD&C blue No. 1, FD&C yellow No. 6, and D&C yellow No. 10. The 40 mg tablets contain FD&C yellow No. 6, D&C yellow No. 10, and lactose monohydrate.
Chemically, oxymorphone hydrochloride is 4, 5α-epoxy-3, 14-dihydroxy-17-methylmorphinan-6-one hydrochloride, a white or slightly off-white, odorless powder, which is sparingly soluble in alcohol and ether, but freely soluble in water. The molecular weight of oxymorphone hydrochloride is 337.80. The pK_a1 and pK_a2 of oxymorphone at 37°C are 8.17 and 9.54, respectively. The octanol/aqueous partition coefficient at 37°C and pH 7.4 is 0.98.
The structural formula for oxymorphone hydrochloride is as follows:

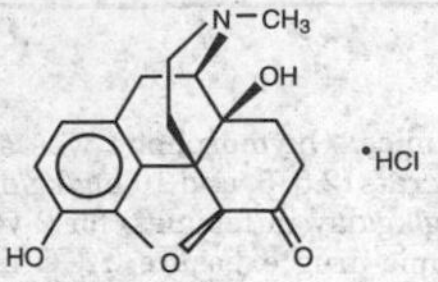

The tablet strengths, 5, 7.5, 10, 15, 20, 30, and 40 mg, describe the amount of oxymorphone hydrochloride per tablet.

CLINICAL PHARMACOLOGY

Oxymorphone is an opioid agonist whose principal therapeutic action is analgesia. Other members of the class known as opioid agonists include substances such as morphine, oxycodone, hydromorphone, fentanyl, codeine, hydrocodone, and tramadol. In addition to analgesia, other pharmacological effects of opioid agonists include anxiolysis, euphoria, feelings of relaxation, respiratory depression, constipation, miosis, and cough suppression. Like all pure opioid agonist analgesics, with increasing doses there is increasing analgesia, unlike with mixed agonist/antagonists or non-opioid analgesics, where there is a limit to the analgesic effect with increasing doses. With pure opioid agonist analgesics, there is no defined maximum dose; the ceiling to analgesic effectiveness is imposed only by side effects, the more serious of which may include somnolence and respiratory depression.

Central Nervous System
The precise mechanism of the analgesic action is unknown. However, specific CNS (central nervous system) opioid receptors for endogenous compounds with opioid-like activity have been identified throughout the brain and spinal cord and play a role in the analgesic effects of this drug. In addition, opioid receptors have also been identified within the PNS (peripheral nervous system). The role that these receptors play in these drugs' analgesic effects is unknown.
Opioids produce respiratory depression likely by direct action on brain stem respiratory centers. The respiratory depression involves a reduction in the responsiveness of the brain stem respiratory centers to both increases in carbon dioxide tension and electrical stimulation.
Opioids depress the cough reflex by direct effect on the cough center in the medulla oblongata. Antitussive effects may occur with doses lower than those usually required for analgesia. Opioids cause miosis, even in total darkness. Pinpoint pupils are a sign of opioid overdose but are not pathognomonic (e.g., pontine lesions of hemorrhagic or ischemic origin may produce similar findings). Marked mydriasis rather than miosis may be seen with hypoxia in overdose situations (see **OVERDOSAGE: Signs and Symptoms**).

Gastrointestinal Tract and Other Smooth Muscle
Opioids cause a reduction in motility associated with an increase in smooth muscle tone in the antrum of the stomach and duodenum. Digestion of food in the small intestine is delayed and propulsive contractions are decreased. Propulsive peristaltic waves in the colon are decreased, while tone may be increased to the point of spasm resulting in constipation. Other opioid-induced effects may include a reduction in gastric, biliary and pancreatic secretions, spasm of sphincter of Oddi, and transient elevations in serum amylase.

Table 1: Mean (±SD) OPANA ER Pharmacokinetic Parameters

Regimen	Dosage	C_{max} (ng/mL)	AUC (ng·hr/mL)	$T_{1/2}$ (hr)
Single Dose	5 mg	0.27±0.13	4.54±2.04	11.30±10.81
	10 mg	0.65±0.29	8.94±4.16	9.83±5.68
	20 mg	1.21±0.77	17.81±7.22	9.89±3.21
	40 mg	2.59±1.65	37.90±16.20	9.35±2.94
Multiple Dose[a]	5 mg	0.70±0.55	5.60±3.87	NA
	10 mg	1.24±0.56	9.77±3.52	NA
	20 mg	2.54±1.35	19.28±8.32	NA
	40 mg	4.47±1.91	36.98±13.53	NA

NA = not applicable
[a]Results after 5 days of every 12 hours dosing.

Cardiovascular System
Opioids produce peripheral vasodilation which may result in orthostatic hypotension. Release of histamine can occur and may contribute to opioid-induced hypotension. Manifestations of histamine release may include orthostatic hypotension, pruritus, flushing, red eyes, and sweating. Animal studies have shown that oxymorphone has a lower propensity to cause histamine release than other opioids.

Endocrine System
Opioids have been shown to have a variety of effects on the secretion of hormones. Opioids inhibit the secretion of ACTH, cortisol, and luteinizing hormone (LH) in humans. They also stimulate prolactin, growth hormone (GH) secretion, and pancreatic secretion of insulin and glucagon in humans and other species, rats and dogs. Thyroid stimulating hormone (TSH) has been shown to be both inhibited and stimulated by opioids.

Immune System
Opioids have been shown to have a variety of effects on components of the immune system in *in vitro* and animal models. The clinical significance of these findings is unknown.

Pharmacodynamics
Concentration-Efficacy Relationships
Studies in healthy volunteers reveal predictable relationships between OPANA ER dosage and plasma oxymorphone concentrations.
The minimum effective plasma concentration of oxymorphone for analgesia varies widely among patients, especially among patients who have been previously treated with agonist opioids. As a result, patients need to be individually titrated to achieve a balance between therapeutic and adverse effects. The minimum effective analgesic concentration of oxymorphone for any individual patient may increase over time due to an increase in pain, progression of disease, development of a new pain syndrome and/or potential development of analgesic tolerance.
Concentration-Adverse Experience Relationships
OPANA ER is associated with typical opioid-related adverse experiences. There is a general relationship between increasing opioid plasma concentration and increasing frequency of adverse experiences such as nausea, vomiting, CNS effects, and respiratory depression.
As with all opioids, the dose must be individualized (see **DOSAGE AND ADMINISTRATION**). The effective analgesic dose for some patients will be too high to be tolerated by other patients.

Pharmacokinetics
Absorption
The absolute oral bioavailability of oxymorphone is approximately 10%.
Steady-state levels are achieved after three days of multiple dose administration. Under both single-dose and steady-state conditions, dose proportionality has been established for the 5 mg, 10 mg, 20 mg, and 40 mg tablet strengths for both peak plasma levels (C_{max}) and extent of absorption (AUC) (Table 1).
[See table 1 below]
Food Effect
Two studies examined the effect of food on the bioavailability of single doses of 20 and 40 mg of OPANA ER in healthy volunteers. In both studies, after the administration of OPANA ER, the C_{max} was increased by approximately 50% in fed subjects compared to fasted subjects. A similar increase in Cmax was also observed with oxymorphone solution.
The AUC was unchanged in one study and increased by approximately 18% in the other study in fed subjects following the administration of OPANA ER. Examination of the AUC suggests that most of the difference between fed and fasting conditions occurs in the first four hours after dose administration. After oral dosing with a single dose of 40 mg, a peak oxymorphone plasma level of 2.8 ng/ml is achieved at 1 hour in fasted subjects and a peak of 4.25 ng/ml is achieved at 2 hours in fed subjects and that beyond the 12 hour time point, there is very little difference in the curves. As a result, OPANA ER should be dosed at least one hour prior to or two hours after eating (see **DOSAGE AND ADMINISTRATION**).
Ethanol Effect
In Vivo OPANA ER Formulation-Alcohol Interaction
Although *in vitro* studies have demonstrated that OPANA ER does not release oxymorphone more rapidly in 500 mL of 0.1N HCl solutions containing ethanol (4%, 20%, and 40%), there is an *in vivo* interaction with alcohol. An *in vivo* study examined the effect of alcohol (40%, 20%, 4% and 0%) on the bioavailability of a single dose of 40 mg of OPANA ER in healthy, fasted volunteers. The results showed that the oxymorphone mean AUC was 13% higher (not statistically significant) after co-administration of 240 mL of 40% alcohol. The AUC was essentially unaffected in subjects following the co-administration of OPANA ER and ethanol (240 mL of 20% or 4% ethanol).
There was a highly variable effect on C_{max} with concomitant administration of alcohol and OPANA ER. The change in

C_{max} ranged from a decrease of 50% to an increase of 270% across all conditions studied. Following concomitant administration of 240 mL of 40% ethanol the C_{max} increased on average by 70% and up to 270% in individual subjects. Following the concomitant administration of 240 mL of 20% ethanol, the C_{max} increased on average by 31% and up to 260% in individual subjects. Following the concomitant administration of 240 mL of 4% ethanol, the C_{max} increased 7% on average and by as much as 110% for individual subjects. After oral dosing with a single dose of 40 mg in fasted subjects, the mean peak oxymorphone plasma level is 2.4 ng/mL and the median T_{max} is 2 hours. Following co-administration of OPANA ER and alcohol (240 mL of 40% ethanol) in fasted subjects, the mean peak oxymorphone level is 3.9 ng/mL and the median T_{max} is 1.5 hours (range 0.75–6 hours).

Co-administration of oxymorphone and ethanol must be avoided.

Oxymorphone may be expected to have additive effects when used in conjunction with alcohol, other opioids, or illicit drugs that cause central nervous system depression because respiratory depression, hypotension, and profound sedation, coma, or death may result.

Distribution

Formal studies on the distribution of oxymorphone in various tissues have not been conducted. Oxymorphone is not extensively bound to human plasma proteins; binding is in the range of 10% to 12%.

Metabolism

Oxymorphone is highly metabolized principally in the liver and undergoes reduction or conjugation with glucuronic acid to form both active and inactive metabolites. The two major metabolites of oxymorphone are oxymorphone-3-glucuronide and 6-OH-oxymorphone. The mean plasma AUC for oxymorphone-3-glucuronide is approximately 90-fold higher than the parent compound. The pharmacologic activity of the glucuronide metabolite has not been evaluated. 6-OH-oxymorphone has been shown in animal studies to have analgesic bioactivity. The mean plasma 6-OH-oymorphone AUC is approximately 70% of the oxymorphone AUC following single oral doses, but is essentially equivalent to the parent compound at steady-state.

Excretion

Because oxymorphone is extensively metabolized, <1% of the administered dose is excreted unchanged in the urine. On average, 33% to 38% of the administered dose is excreted in the urine as oxymorphone-3-glucuronide and 0.25% to 0.62% excreted as 6-OH-oxymorphone in subjects with normal hepatic and renal function. In animals given radiolabeled oxymorphone, approximately 90% of the administered radioactivity was recovered within 5 days of dosing. The majority of oxymorphone-derived radioactivity was found in the urine and feces.

Special Populations

Elderly

The steady-state plasma concentrations of oxymorphone, 6-OH-oxymorphone, and oxymorphone-3-glucuronide are approximately 40% higher in elderly subjects (≥ 65 years of age) than in young subjects (18 to 40 years of age). On average, age greater than 65 years was associated with a 1.4-fold increase in oxymorphone AUC and a 1.5-fold increase in C_{max}. This observation does not appear related to a difference in body weight, metabolism, or excretion of oxymorphone (see **PRECAUTIONS: Geriatric Use**).

Gender

The effect of gender was evaluated following single- and multiple-doses of OPANA ER in male and female adult volunteers. There was a consistent tendency for female subjects to have slightly higher AUC_{ss} and C_{max} values than male subjects; however, gender differences were not observed when AUC_{ss} and C_{max} were adjusted by body weight.

Hepatic Impairment

The liver plays an important role in the pre-systemic clearance of orally administered oxymorphone. Accordingly, the bioavailability of orally administered oxymorphone may be markedly increased in patients with moderate to severe liver disease. The disposition of oxymorphone was compared in 6 patients with mild, 5 patients with moderate, and one patient with severe hepatic impairment and 12 subjects with normal hepatic function. The bioavailability of oxymorphone was increased by 1.6-fold in patients with mild hepatic impairment and by 3.7-fold in patients with moderate hepatic impairment. In one patient with severe hepatic impairment, the bioavailability was increased by 12.2-fold. The half-life of oxymorphone was not significantly affected by hepatic impairment (see **DOSAGE AND ADMINISTRATION: Patients with Hepatic Impairment**).

Renal Impairment

Data from a pharmacokinetic study involving 24 patients with renal dysfunction show an increase of 26%, 57%, and 65% in oxymorphone bioavailability in mild (creatinine clearance 51-80 mL/min; n=8), moderate (creatinine clearance 30-50 mL/min; n=8), and severe (creatinine clearance <30 mL/min; n=8) patients, respectively, compared to healthy controls.

Drug-Drug Interactions

In vitro studies revealed little to no biotransformation of oxymorphone to 6-OH-oxymorphone by any of the major cytochrome P450 (CYP P450) isoforms at therapeutically relevant oxymorphone plasma concentrations.

No inhibition of any of the major CYP P450 isoforms was observed when oxymorphone was incubated with human liver microsomes at concentrations of ≤ 50 μM. An inhibition of CYP3A4 activity occurred at oxymorphone concentrations ≥150 μM. Therefore, it is not expected that oxymorphone, or its metabolites will act as inhibitors of any of the major CYP P450 enzymes *in vivo*.

Increases in the activity of the CYP 2C9 and CYP 3A4 isoforms occurred when oxymorphone was incubated with human hepatocytes. However, clinical drug interaction studies with OPANA ER showed no induction of CYP450 3A4 or 2C9 enzyme activity, indicating that no dose adjustment for CYP 3A4- or 2C9-mediated drug-drug interactions is required.

CLINICAL TRIALS

The efficacy and safety of OPANA ER have been evaluated in double-blind, controlled clinical trials in opioid-naïve and opioid-experienced patients with moderate to severe pain including low back pain.

12-Week Study in Opioid-Naïve Patients with Low Back Pain

Patients with chronic low back pain who were suboptimally responsive to their current non-opioid therapy entered a 4-week, open-label dose titration phase. Patients initiated therapy with two days of treatment with OPANA ER 5 mg, every 12 hours. Thereafter, patients were titrated to a stabilized dose, at increments of 5-10 mg every 12 hours every 3-7 days. Of the patients who were able to stabilize within the Open-Label Titration Period, the mean±SD VAS score at Screening was 69.4±11.8 mm and at Baseline (beginning of Double-Blind Period) were 18.5±11.2 mm and 19.3±11.3 mm for the oxymorphone ER and placebo groups, respectively. Sixty three percent of the patients enrolled were able to titrate to a tolerable dose and were randomized into a 12-week double-blind treatment phase with placebo or their stabilized dose of OPANA ER. The mean±SD stabilized doses were 39.2±26.4 mg and 40.9±25.3 mg for the OPANA ER and placebo groups, respectively; total daily doses ranged from 10-140 mg. During the first 4 days of double-blind treatment patients were allowed an unlimited number of OPANA, an immediate-release (IR) formulation of oxymorphone, 5 mg tablets, every 4-6 hours as supplemental analgesia; thereafter the number of OPANA was limited to two tablets per day. This served as a tapering method to minimize opioid withdrawal symptoms in placebo patients. Sixty-eight percent of patients treated with OPANA ER completed the 12-week treatment compared to forty seven percent of patients treated with placebo. OPANA ER provided superior analgesia compared to placebo. The analgesic effect of OPANA ER was maintained throughout the double-blind treatment period in 89% of patients who completed the study. These patients reported a decrease, no change, or a ≤10 mm increase in VAS score from Day 7 until the end of the study.

A significantly higher proportion of OPANA ER patients (81.4%) had at least a 30% reduction in pain score from screening to study endpoint compared to placebo patients (51.7%). The proportion of patients with various degrees of improvement from screening to study endpoint is shown in Figure 1.

Figure 1: Percent Reduction in Average Pain Intensity from Screening to Final Visit

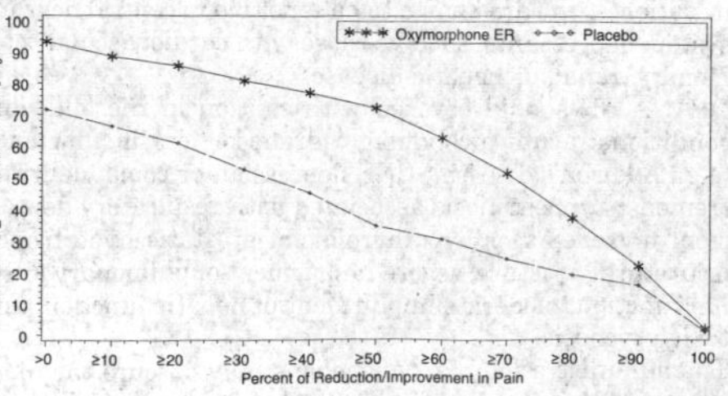

12-Week Study in Opioid-Experienced Patients with Low Back Pain

Patients currently on chronic opioid therapy entered a 4-week, open-label titration phase with OPANA ER dosed every 12 hours at an approximated equianalgesic dose of their pre-study opioid medication. Of the patients who were able to stabilize within the Open-Label Titration Period, the mean±SD VAS score at Screening was 69.5±17.0 mm and at Baseline (beginning of Double-Blind Period) were 23.9±12.1 mm and 22.2±10.8 mm for the oxymorphone ER and placebo groups, respectively. Stabilized patients entered a 12-week double-blind treatment phase with placebo or their stabilized dose of OPANA ER. The mean±SD stabilized doses were 80.9±59.3 mg and 93.3±61.3 mg for the OPANA ER and placebo groups, respectively; total daily doses ranged from 20-260 mg. During the first 4 days of double-blind treatment, patients were allowed an unlimited number of OPANA 5 mg tablets, every 4-6 hours as supplemental analgesia; thereafter the number of OPANA was limited to two tablets per day. This served as a tapering method to minimize opioid withdrawal symptoms in placebo patients. Fifty seven percent of patients were titrated to a stabilized dose within approximately 4 weeks of OPANA ER dose titration. Seventy percent of patients treated with OPANA ER and 26% of patients treated with placebo completed the 12-week treatment. OPANA ER provided superior analgesia compared to placebo. The analgesic effect of OPANA ER was maintained throughout the double-blind treatment period in 80% of patients who completed the study. These patients reported a decrease, no change, or a ≤10 mm increase in VAS score from Day 7 until the end of the study.

A significantly higher proportion of OPANA ER patients (79.7%) had at least a 30% reduction in pain score from screening to study endpoint compared to placebo patients (34.8%). Proportion of patients with various degrees of improvement from screening to study endpoint is shown in Figure 2.

Figure 2: Percent Reduction in Average Pain Intensity from Screening to Final Visit

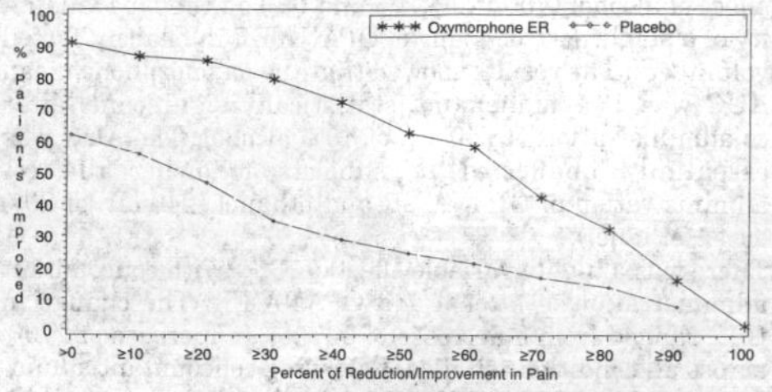

INDICATIONS AND USAGE

OPANA ER is indicated for the relief of moderate to severe pain in patients requiring continuous, around-the-clock opioid treatment for an extended period of time.

OPANA ER is not intended for use as an as needed analgesic.

OPANA ER is not indicated for pain in the immediate post-operative period (12-24 hours following surgery) for patients not previously taking opioids because of the risk of oversedation and respiratory depression requiring reversal with opioid antagonists.

OPANA ER is not indicated for pain in the post-operative period if the pain is mild or not expected to persist for an extended period of time.

CONTRAINDICATIONS

OPANA ER is contraindicated in patients with a known hypersensitivity to oxymorphone hydrochloride or to any of the other ingredients in OPANA ER, or with known hypersensitivity to morphine analogs such as codeine.

OPANA ER is not indicated for pain in the immediate post-operative period (the first 12-24 hours following surgery), or if the pain is mild, or not expected to persist for an extended period of time. OPANA ER is only indicated for post-operative use if the patient is already receiving the drug prior to surgery or if the post-operative pain is expected to be moderate or severe and persist for an extended period of time. Physicians should individualize treatment, moving from parenteral to oral analgesics as appropriate. (See American Pain Society guidelines).

OPANA ER is contraindicated in any situation where opioids are contraindicated such as: patients with respiratory depression (in the absence of resuscitative equipment or in unmonitored settings), and in patients with acute or severe bronchial asthma or hypercarbia.

OPANA ER, like all opioids, is contraindicated in any patient who has or is suspected of having paralytic ileus.

OPANA ER is contraindicated in patients with moderate and severe hepatic impairment (see **CLINICAL PHARMACOLOGY, PRECAUTIONS** and **DOSAGE AND ADMINISTRATION**).

WARNINGS

OPANA ER TABLETS are to be swallowed whole, and are not to be broken, chewed, crushed or dissolved. Taking broken, chewed, crushed or dissolved OPANA ER TABLETS could lead to the rapid release and absorption of a potentially fatal dose of oxymorphone.

Patients must not consume alcoholic beverages, or prescription or non-prescription medications containing al-

cohol, while on OPANA ER therapy. The co-ingestion of alcohol with OPANA ER may result in increased plasma levels and a potentially fatal overdose of oxymorphone.

Misuse, Abuse and Diversion of Opioids

OPANA ER contains oxymorphone, an opioid agonist similar to morphine, and is a Schedule II controlled substance. Opioid agonists have the potential for being abused and are sought by drug abusers and people with addiction disorders and are subject to criminal diversion.

Oxymorphone can be abused in a manner similar to other opioid agonists, legal or illicit. This should be considered when prescribing or dispensing OPANA ER in situations where the physician or pharmacist is concerned about an increased risk of misuse, abuse, or diversion.

OPANA ER tablets may be abused by crushing, chewing, snorting or injecting the product. These practices will result in the uncontrolled delivery of the opioid and pose a significant risk to the abuser that could result in overdose and death (see **WARNINGS** and **WARNINGS: Drug Abuse and Addiction**).

Concerns about abuse, addiction, and diversion should not prevent the proper management of pain.

Healthcare professionals should contact their State Professional Licensing Board, or State Controlled Substances Authority for information on how to prevent and detect abuse or diversion of this product.

Interactions with Alcohol and Drugs of Abuse

Oxymorphone may be expected to have additive effects when used in conjunction with alcohol, other opioids, or illicit drugs that cause central nervous system depression because respiratory depression, hypotension, and profound sedation or coma may result. An *in vivo* study examined the effect of alcohol (40%, 20%, 4% and 0%) on the bioavailability of a single dose of 40 mg of OPANA ER in healthy, fasted volunteers. The results showed that the oxymorphone mean AUC was 13% higher (not statistically significant) after co-administration of 240 mL of 40% alcohol. The AUC was essentially unaffected in subjects following the co-administration of OPANA ER and ethanol (240 mL of 20% or 4% ethanol).

There was a highly variable effect on C_{max} with concomitant administration of alcohol and OPANA ER. The change in C_{max} ranged from a decrease of 50% to an increase of 270% across all conditions studied. Following concomitant administration of 240 mL of 40% ethanol the C_{max} increased on average by 70%, and up to 270% in individual subjects. Following the concomitant administration of 240mL of 20% ethanol the C_{max} increased on average by 31% and up to 260% in individual subjects. Following the concomitant administration of 240 mL of 4% ethanol, the C_{max} increased by 7% on average and as much as 110% for individual subjects.

Drug Abuse and Addiction

Controlled Substance

OPANA ER contains oxymorphone, an opioid with an abuse liability similar to morphine and other opioid agonists and is a Schedule II controlled substance. OPANA ER and other opioids used in analgesia, can be abused and are subject to criminal diversion (see **WARNINGS: Misuse, Abuse and Diversion of Opioids**).

Drug addiction is characterized by a preoccupation with the procurement, hoarding, and abuse of drugs for non-medicinal purposes. Drug addiction is treatable, utilizing a multi-disciplinary approach, but relapse is common. "Drug seeking" behavior is very common to addicts and drug abusers. Drug-seeking tactics include emergency calls or visits near the end of office hours, refusal to undergo appropriate examination, testing or referral, repeated claims of loss of prescriptions, tampering with prescriptions and reluctance to provide prior medical records or contact information for other treating physician(s). "Doctor shopping" (visiting multiple prescribers) to obtain additional prescriptions is common among drug abusers and people suffering from untreated addiction. Preoccupation with achieving adequate pain relief can be appropriate behavior in a patient with poor pain control.

Abuse and addiction are separate and distinct from physical dependence and tolerance. Physicians should be aware that addiction may not be accompanied by concurrent tolerance and symptoms of physical dependence in all addicts. In addition, abuse of opioids can occur in the absence of true addiction and is characterized by misuse for non-medical purposes, often in combination with other psychoactive substances. OPANA ER, like other opioids, may be diverted for non-medical use. Careful record-keeping of prescribing information, including quantity, frequency, and renewal requests is strongly advised.

Abuse of OPANA ER poses a risk of overdose and death. This risk is increased with concurrent abuse of OPANA ER with alcohol and other substances. In addition, parenteral drug abuse is commonly associated with transmission of infectious disease such as hepatitis and HIV.

Proper assessment of the patient, proper prescribing practices, periodic re-evaluation of therapy, and proper dispensing and storage are appropriate measures that help to limit abuse of opioid drugs.

Infants born to mothers physically dependent on opioids will also be physically dependent and may exhibit respiratory difficulties and withdrawal symptoms (see **PRECAUTIONS: Usage in Pregnancy** and **PRECAUTIONS: Labor and Delivery**).

Respiratory Depression

Respiratory depression is the chief hazard of OPANA ER. Respiratory depression is a particular potential problem in elderly or debilitated patients as well as in those suffering from conditions accompanied by hypoxia or hypercapnia when even moderate therapeutic doses may dangerously decrease pulmonary ventilation.

OPANA ER should be administered with extreme caution to patients with conditions accompanied by hypoxia, hypercapnia, or decreased respiratory reserve such as: asthma, chronic obstructive pulmonary disease or cor pulmonale, severe obesity, sleep apnea syndrome, myxedema, kyphoscoliosis, CNS depression or coma. In these patients, even usual therapeutic doses of oxymorphone may decrease respiratory drive while simultaneously increasing airway resistance to the point of apnea. Alternative non-opioid analgesics should be considered, and oxymorphone should be employed only under careful medical supervision at the lowest effective dose in such patients.

Interactions with Other Central Nervous System Depressants

Patients receiving other opioid analgesics, general anesthetics, phenothiazines or other tranquilizers, sedatives, hypnotics, or other CNS depressants (including alcohol) concomitantly with oxymorphone may experience respiratory depression, hypotension, profound sedation, or coma (see **PRECAUTIONS: Drug-Drug Interactions**).

Head Injury and Increased Intracranial Pressure

In the presence of head injury, intracranial lesions or a pre-existing increase in intracranial pressure, the possible respiratory depressant effects of opioid analgesics and their potential to elevate cerebrospinal fluid pressure (resulting from vasodilation following CO_2 retention) may be markedly exaggerated. Furthermore, opioid analgesics can produce effects on pupillary response and consciousness, which may obscure neurologic signs of further increases in intracranial pressure in patients with head injuries.

Hypotensive Effect

OPANA ER, like all opioid analgesics, may cause severe hypotension in an individual whose ability to maintain blood pressure has been compromised by a depleted blood volume, or after concurrent administration with drugs such as phenothiazines or other agents which compromise vasomotor tone. OPANA ER, like all opioid analgesics, should be administered with caution to patients in circulatory shock, since vasodilation produced by the drug may further reduce cardiac output and blood pressure.

Hepatic Impairment

A study of OPANA ER in patients with hepatic disease indicated greater plasma concentrations than those with normal hepatic function (see **CLINICAL PHARMACOLOGY**). OPANA ER should be used with caution in patients with mild impairment. These patients should be started with the lowest dose and titrated slowly while carefully monitoring for side effects. OPANA ER is contraindicated for patients with moderate and severe hepatic impairment (see **CONTRAINDICATIONS, WARNINGS**, and **DOSAGE AND ADMINISTRATION**).

PRECAUTIONS

General

Opioid analgesics should be used with caution especially when combined with other drugs, and should be reserved for cases where the benefits of opioid analgesia outweigh the known potential risks of respiratory depression, altered mental state and postural hypotension. OPANA ER should be used with caution in elderly and debilitated patients and in patients who are known to be sensitive to central nervous system depressants, such as those with cardiovascular, pulmonary, renal, or hepatic disease.

OPANA ER should be used with caution in the following conditions: acute alcoholism; adrenocortical insufficiency (e.g., Addison's disease); CNS depression or coma; delirium tremens; kyphoscoliosis associated with respiratory depression; myxedema or hypothyroidism; prostatic hypertrophy or urethral stricture; severe impairment of pulmonary or renal function; moderate impairment of hepatic function; and toxic psychosis.

The administration of oxymorphone may obscure the diagnosis or clinical course in patients with acute abdominal conditions. Oxymorphone may aggravate convulsions in patients with convulsive disorders, and all opioids may induce or aggravate seizures in some clinical settings.

OPANA ER is intended for use in patients who require more than several days continuous treatment with an opioid analgesic.

Ambulatory Surgery and Post-Operative Use

OPANA ER is not indicated for pre-emptive analgesia (administration pre-operatively for the management of post-operative pain).

OPANA ER is not indicated for pain in the immediate post-operative period (12-24 hours following surgery) for patients not previously taking opioids because of the risk of oversedation and respiratory depression requiring reversal with opioid antagonists.

OPANA ER is not indicated for pain in the post-operative period if the pain is mild or not expected to persist for an extended period of time.

OPANA ER is only indicated for postoperative use in the patient if the patient is already receiving the drug prior to surgery or if the postoperative pain is expected to be moderate to severe and persist for an extended period of time. Physicians should individualize treatment, moving from parenteral to oral analgesics as appropriate (see American Pain Society guidelines).

Patients who are already receiving OPANA ER as part of ongoing analgesic therapy may be safely continued on the drug if appropriate dosage adjustments are made considering the procedure, other drugs given, and the temporary changes in physiology caused by the surgical intervention (see **DOSAGE AND ADMINISTRATION**).

OPANA ER, like other opioids, decreases bowel motility. Ileus is a common post-operative complication, especially after intra-abdominal surgery with opioid analgesia. Caution should be taken to monitor for decreased bowel motility in post-operative patients receiving opioids. Standard supportive therapy should be implemented.

Use in Pancreatic/Biliary Tract Disease

OPANA ER, like other opioids, may cause spasm of the sphincter of Oddi and should be used with caution in patients with biliary tract disease, including acute pancreatitis.

Physical Dependence and Tolerance

Physical dependence is the occurrence of withdrawal symptoms after abrupt discontinuation of a drug or upon administration of an opioid antagonist or mixed opioid agonist/antagonist agent. Tolerance is the need for increasing doses of opioids to maintain a defined effect such as analgesia (in the absence of disease progression or other external factors). The development of physical dependence and tolerance is not unusual during chronic opioid therapy.

If OPANA ER is abruptly discontinued in a physically-dependent patient, an abstinence syndrome may occur. Some or all of the following can characterize this syndrome: restlessness, lacrimation, rhinorrhea, yawning, perspiration, chills, myalgia, and mydriasis. Other symptoms also may develop, including: irritability, anxiety, backache, joint pain, weakness, abdominal cramps, insomnia, nausea, anorexia, vomiting, diarrhea, or increased blood pressure, respiratory rate, or heart rate.

In general, OPANA ER should not be abruptly discontinued. However, OPANA ER, like other opioids, can be safely discontinued without the development of withdrawal symptoms by slowly tapering the daily dose (see **DOSAGE AND ADMINISTRATION: Cessation of Therapy**).

Information for Patients/Caregivers

1. Patients should be advised that OPANA ER contains oxymorphone, a morphine-like pain reliever, and should be taken only as directed.

2. Patients should be advised that OPANA ER is designed to work properly only if swallowed whole. The extended-release tablets may release all their contents at once if broken, chewed or crushed, resulting in a risk of fatal overdose of oxymorphone.

3. Patients must not consume alcoholic beverages, or prescription or non-prescription medications containing alcohol, while on OPANA ER therapy. The co-ingestion of alcohol with OPANA ER may result in increased plasma levels and a potentially fatal overdose of oxymorphone.

4. Appropriate pain management requires changes in the dose to maintain best pain control. Patients should be advised of the need to contact their physician if pain control is inadequate, but not to change the dose of OPANA ER without consulting their physician.

5. Patients should be advised to report episodes of breakthrough pain and adverse experiences occurring during therapy to their doctor. Individualization of dosage is essential to make optimal use of this medication.

6. Patients should be cautioned that OPANA ER may cause drowsiness, dizziness, or lightheadedness, and may impair mental and/or physical abilities required for the performance of potentially hazardous tasks, such as driving a car, operating machinery, etc.

7. Patients should not combine OPANA ER with alcohol or other central nervous system depressants (sleep aids, tranquilizers) except by the orders of the prescribing physician, because additive effects may occur, resulting in serious injury or death.

8. Patients taking OPANA ER should be advised of the potential for severe constipation. Appropriate laxatives and/or stool softeners and other therapeutic approaches may be considered for use with the initiation of OPANA ER therapy.

9. Patients should be advised not to adjust the dose of OPANA ER without consulting the prescribing professional.
10. Patients should be advised that OPANA ER is a potential drug of abuse. They should protect it from theft, and it should never be given to anyone other than the individual for whom it was prescribed.
11. Women of childbearing potential who become, or are planning to become pregnant should be advised to consult their physician regarding the effects of opioid analgesics and other drug use during pregnancy on themselves and their unborn child.
12. If patients have been receiving treatment with OPANA ER for more than a few days to weeks and cessation of therapy is indicated, they should be counseled on the importance of safely tapering the dose and that abruptly discontinuing the medication could precipitate withdrawal symptoms. The physician should determine a dose schedule to accomplish a gradual discontinuation of the medication.
13. As with any potent opioid, misuse of OPANA ER may result in serious adverse events. Patients should be instructed to keep OPANA ER in a secure place out of the reach of children and pets. Accidental consumption especially in children can result in overdose or death. When OPANA ER is no longer needed, the unused tablets should be destroyed by flushing down the toilet.

Use in Drug and Alcohol Addiction
OPANA ER is not approved for use in detoxification or maintenance treatment of opioid addiction. However, the history of an addictive disorder does not necessarily preclude the use of this medication for the treatment of chronic pain. These patients will require intensive monitoring for signs of misuse, abuse, or addiction.

Drug-Drug Interactions
Oxymorphone is highly metabolized principally in the liver and undergoes reduction or conjugation with glucuronic acid to form both active and inactive metabolites (see **Pharmacokinetics: Metabolism**).

Use with CNS Depressants
The concomitant use of other CNS depressants including sedatives, hypnotics, tranquilizers, general anesthetics, phenothiazines, other opioids, and alcohol may produce additive CNS depressant effects. OPANA ER, like all opioid analgesics, should be started at 1/3 to 1/2 of the usual dose in patients who are concurrently receiving other central nervous system depressants including sedatives or hypnotics, general anesthetics, phenothiazines, tranquilizers, and alcohol because respiratory depression, hypotension, and profound sedation or coma may result, and titrated slowly as necessary for adequate pain relief.
Additive effects resulting in respiratory depression, hypotension, profound sedation or coma may result if these drugs are taken in combination with the usual doses of OPANA ER. No specific interaction between oxymorphone and monoamine oxidase inhibitors has been observed, but caution in the use of any opioid in patients taking this class of drugs is appropriate.
When combined therapy with any of the above medications is contemplated, the dose of one or both agents should be reduced (see **WARNINGS** and **DOSAGE AND ADMINISTRATION**).

Interactions with Mixed Agonist/Antagonist Opioid Analgesics
Agonist/antagonist analgesics (i.e., pentazocine, nalbuphine, butorphanol, or buprenorphine) should not be administered to patients who have received or are receiving a course of therapy with a pure opioid agonist analgesic, such as OPANA ER. In this situation, mixed agonist/antagonist analgesics may reduce the analgesic effect of OPANA ER and/or may precipitate withdrawal symptoms.

Other
Anticholinergics or other medications with anticholinergic activity when used concurrently with opioid analgesics may result in increased risk of urinary retention and/or severe constipation, which may lead to paralytic ileus.
In addition, CNS side effects have been reported (confusion, disorientation, respiratory depression, apnea, seizures) following coadministration of cimetidine with opioid analgesics; no clear-cut cause and effect relationship was established.

Carcinogenesis, Mutagenesis, Impairment of Fertility
Carcinogenesis: Long-term studies have been completed to evaluate the carcinogenic potential of oxymorphone in both Sprague-Dawley rats and CD-1 mice. Oxymorphone HCl was administered to Sprague-Dawley rats (2.5, 5, and 10 mg/kg/day in males and 5, 10, and 25 mg/kg/day in females) for 2 years by oral gavage. The systemic drug exposure (AUC ng•h/mL) at the 10 mg/kg/day in male rats was 0.34-fold and at the 25 mg/kg/day dose in female rats was 1.5-fold the human exposure at a dose of 260 mg/day. No evidence of carcinogenic potential was observed in rats. Oxymorphone HCl was administered to CD-1 mice (10, 25, 75 and 150 mg/kg/day) for 2 years by oral gavage. The systemic drug exposure (AUC ng•h/mL) at the 150 mg/kg/day dose in mice was 14.5-fold (in males) and 17.3-fold (in females) times the human exposure at a dose of 260 mg/day. No evidence of carcinogenic potential was observed in mice.
Mutagenesis: Oxymorphone hydrochloride was not mutagenic when tested in the *in vitro* bacterial reverse mutation assay (Ames test) at concentrations of ≤5270 μg/plate, or in an *in vitro* mammalian cell chromosome aberration assay performed with human peripheral blood lymphocytes at concentrations ≤5000 μg/ml with or without metabolic activation. Oxymorphone hydrochloride tested positive in both the rat and mouse *in vivo* micronucleus assays. An increase in micronucleated polychromatic erythrocytes occurred in mice given doses ≥250 mg/kg and in rats given doses of 20 and 40 mg/kg. A subsequent study demonstrated that oxymorphone hydrochloride was not aneugenic in mice following administration of up to 500 mg/kg. Additional studies indicate that the increased incidence of micronucleated polychromatic erythrocytes in rats may be secondary to increased body temperature following oxymorphone administration. Doses associated with increased micronucleated polychromatic erythrocytes also produce a marked, rapid increase in body temperature. Pretreatment of animals with sodium salicylate minimized the increase in body temperature and prevented the increase in micronucleated polychromatic erythrocytes after administration of 40 mg/kg oxymorphone.
Impairment of fertility: Oxymorphone hydrochloride did not affect reproductive function or sperm parameters in male rats at any dose tested (≤50 mg/kg/day). In female rats, an increase in the length of the estrus cycle and decrease in the mean number of viable embryos, implantation sites and corpora lutea were observed at doses of oxymorphone ≥10 mg/kg/day. The dose of oxymorphone associated with reproductive findings in female rats is 1.2-fold the human dose of 40 mg every 12 hours based on a body surface area. The dose of oxymorphone that produced no adverse effects on reproductive findings in female rats is 0.6-fold the human dose of 40 mg every 12 hours on a body surface area basis.

Pregnancy
The safety of using oxymorphone in pregnancy has not been established with regard to possible adverse effects on fetal development. The use of OPANA ER in pregnancy, in nursing mothers, or in women of child-bearing potential requires that the possible benefits of the drug be weighed against the possible hazards to the mother and the child (see **PRECAUTIONS**).

Teratogenic Effects
Pregnancy Category C
Oxymorphone hydrochloride administration did not cause malformations at any doses evaluated during developmental toxicity studies in rats (≤25 mg/kg/day) or rabbits (≤50 mg/kg/day). These doses are ~3-fold and ~12-fold the human dose of 40 mg every 12 hours, based on body surface area. There were no developmental effects in rats treated with 5 mg/kg/day or rabbits treated with 25 mg/kg/day. Fetal weights were reduced in rats and rabbits given doses of ≥10 mg/kg/day and 50 mg/kg/day, respectively. These doses are ~1.2-fold and ~6-fold the human dose of 40 mg every 12 hours based on body surface area, respectively. There were no effects of oxymorphone hydrochloride on intrauterine survival in rats at doses ≤25 mg/kg/day, or rabbits at ≤50 mg/kg/day in these studies (see Non-teratogenic Effects, below). In a study that was conducted prior to the establishment of Good Laboratory Practices (GLP) and not according to current recommended methodology, a single subcutaneous injection of oxymorphone hydrochloride on gestation day 8 was reported to produce malformations in offspring of hamsters that received 15.5-fold the human dose of 40 mg every 12 hours based on body surface area. This dose also produced 83% maternal lethality.
There are no adequate and well-controlled studies in pregnant women. OPANA ER should be used during pregnancy only if the potential benefit justifies the potential risk to the fetus.

Non-teratogenic Effects
Oxymorphone hydrochloride administration to female rats during gestation in a pre- and postnatal developmental toxicity study reduced mean litter size (18%) at a dose of 25 mg/kg/day, attributed to an increased incidence of stillborn pups. An increase in neonatal death occurred at ≥5 mg/kg/day. Post-natal survival of the pups was reduced throughout weaning following treatment of the dams with 25 mg/kg/day. Low pup birth weight and decreased postnatal weight gain occurred in pups born to oxymorphone-treated female rats given a dose of 25 mg/kg/day. This dose is ~3-fold higher than the human dose of 40 mg every 12 hours on a body surface area basis.
Prolonged use of opioid analgesics during pregnancy may cause fetal-neonatal physical dependence. Neonatal withdrawal may occur. Symptoms usually appear during the first days of life and may include convulsions, irritability, excessive crying, tremors, hyperactive reflexes, fever, vomiting, diarrhea, sneezing, yawning, and increased respiratory rate.

Labor and Delivery
Opioids cross the placenta and may produce respiratory depression and psycho-physiologic effects in neonates. OPANA ER is not recommended for use in women during and immediately prior to labor, when use of shorter acting analgesics or other analgesic techniques are more appropriate. Occasionally, opioid analgesics may prolong labor through actions which temporarily reduce the strength, duration and frequency of uterine contractions. However this effect is not consistent and may be offset by an increased rate of cervical dilatation, which tends to shorten labor. Neonates whose mothers received opioid analgesics during labor should be observed closely for signs of respiratory depression. A specific opioid antagonist, such as naloxone or nalmefene, should be available for reversal of opioid-induced respiratory depression in the neonate.

Nursing Mothers
It is not known whether oxymorphone is excreted in human milk. Because many drugs, including some opioids, are excreted in human milk, caution should be exercised when OPANA ER is administered to a nursing woman. Ordinarily, nursing should not be undertaken while a patient is receiving oxymorphone because of the possibility of sedation and/or respiratory depression in the infant.

Pediatric Use
Safety and effectiveness of OPANA ER in pediatric patients below the age of 18 years have not been established.

Geriatric Use
OPANA ER should be used with caution in elderly patients. The plasma levels of oxymorphone are about 40% higher in elderly (≥65 years of age) than in younger subjects (see **CLINICAL PHARMACOLOGY**). Elderly patients should initially receive smaller starting doses of oxymorphone and dose titration should proceed cautiously.
Of the total number of subjects in clinical studies of OPANA ER, 27 percent were 65 and over, while 9 percent were 75 and over. No overall differences in effectiveness were observed between these subjects and younger subjects. There were several adverse events that were more frequently observed in subjects 65 and over compared to younger subjects. These adverse events included dizziness, somnolence, confusion, and nausea.

Hepatic Impairment
A study of OPANA ER in patients with hepatic disease indicated greater plasma concentrations than those with normal hepatic function (see **CLINICAL PHARMACOLOGY**). OPANA ER should be used with caution in patients with mild impairment. These patients should be started with the lowest dose and titrated slowly while carefully monitoring for side effects. OPANA ER is contraindicated for patients with moderate and severe hepatic impairment (see **CONTRAINDICATIONS**, **WARNINGS**, and **DOSAGE AND ADMINISTRATION**).

Renal Impairment
In a study of OPANA ER, patients with moderate to severe renal impairment were shown to have an increase in bioavailability ranging from 57-65% (see **CLINICAL PHARMACOLOGY**). These patients should be started cautiously with lower doses of OPANA ER and titrated slowly while carefully monitored for side effects (see **DOSAGE AND ADMINISTRATION**).

Gender Differences
When normalized for body weight, gender differences were not observed (see **CLINICAL PHARMACOLOGY**). In clinical studies, the overall incidence rates for one or more adverse events were slightly higher among females than males for both OPANA ER subjects and placebo subjects.

ADVERSE REACTIONS

Tables 2 and 3 list the most frequently occurring adverse reactions (in at least 5% of patients) from the placebo-controlled trials in patients with low back pain.

Table 2: Treatment-Emergent Adverse Events Reported in ≥5% of Patients During the Open-Label Titration Period and Double-Blind Treatment Period by Preferred Term—Number (%) of Treated Patients (12-Week Study In Opioid-Naïve Patients with Low Back Pain)

	Open-Label Titration Period	Double-Blind Treatment Period	
	OPANA ER	OPANA ER	Placebo
Preferred Term	(N = 325)	(N = 105)	(N = 100)
Constipation	26.2%	6.7%	1.0%
Somnolence	19.1%	1.9%	0%
Nausea	18.2%	11.4%	9.0%
Dizziness	11.1%	4.8%	3.0%
Headache	10.5%	3.8%	2.0%
Pruritis	6.8%	2.9%	1.0%

Table 3. Treatment-Emergent Adverse Events Reported in ≥5% of Patients During the Open-Label Titration Period and Double-Blind Treatment Period by Preferred Term—Number (%) of Treated Patients (12-Week Study In Opioid-Experienced Patients with Low Back Pain)

	Open-Label Titration Period	Double-Blind Treatment Period	
	OPANA ER	OPANA ER	Placebo
Preferred Term	(N = 250)	(N = 70)	(N = 72)
Nausea	19.6%	2.9%	1.4%
Constipation	11.6%	5.7%	1.4%
Headache	11.6%	2.9%	0%
Somnolence	11.2%	2.9%	0%
Vomiting	8.8%	0%	1.4%
Pruritis	7.6%	0%	0%
Dizziness	6.4%	0%	0%

Adverse Reactions Reported in Placebo-Controlled Trials

The following table lists adverse reactions that were reported in at least 2% of patients in placebo-controlled trials (N=5)

Table 4: Adverse Reactions Reported in Placebo-Controlled Clinical Trials with Incidence ≥2% in Patients Receiving OPANA ER.

MedDRA Preferred Term	OPANA ER (N=1259)	Placebo (N=461)
Nausea	33.1%	13.2%
Constipation	27.6%	13.2%
Dizziness (Exc Vertigo)	17.8%	7.6%
Somnolence	17.2%	2.2%
Vomiting	15.6%	4.1%
Pruritus	15.2%	7.6%
Headache	12.2%	5.6%
Sweating increased	8.6%	8.7%
Dry mouth	6.4%	0.7%
Sedation	5.9%	7.6%
Diarrhea	4.3%	5.6%
Insomnia	4.0%	2.0%
Fatigue	3.9%	1.3%
Appetite decreased	2.9%	0.4%
Abdominal pain	2.5%	1.5%

Adverse Reactions Reported in All Clinical Trials

A total of 2011 patients were treated with OPANA ER in the Phase 2/3 controlled and open-label clinical trials. The clinical trials consisted of patients with moderate to severe chronic pain and post surgical pain.

The adverse reactions are presented in the following manner: most common, common, and less common adverse reactions.

The **most common** adverse drug reactions (≥10%) reported at least once by patients treated with OPANA ER in the clinical trials were nausea, constipation, dizziness (exc. vertigo), vomiting, pruritus, somnolence, headache, sweating increased, and sedation.

The **common** (≥1%-<10%) adverse drug reactions reported at least once by patients treated with OPANA ER in the clinical trials organized by MedDRA's (Medical Dictionary for Regulatory Activities) System Organ Class were:

Eye disorders: vision blurred

Gastrointestinal disorders: diarrhea, abdominal pain, dyspepsia

General disorders and administration site conditions: dry mouth, appetite decreased, fatigue, lethargy, weakness, pyrexia, dehydration, weight decreased, edema

Nervous system disorders: insomnia

Psychiatric disorders: anxiety, confusion, disorientation, restlessness, nervousness, depression

Respiratory, thoracic and mediastinal disorders: dyspnea

Vascular disorders: flushing and hypertension

Other **less common** adverse reactions known with opioid treatment that were seen <1% in the OPANA ER trials include the following in alphabetical order.

Abdominal distention, agitation, allergic reactions, bradycardia, central nervous system depression, clamminess, depressed level of consciousness, dermatitis, difficult micturition, dysphoria, euphoric mood, feeling jittery, hallucination, hot flashes, hypersensitivity, hypotension, hypoxia, ileus, mental impairment, mental status changes, miosis, oxygen saturation decreased, palpitation, postural hypotension, respiratory depression, respiratory distress, respiratory rate decreased, syncope, tachycardia, urinary retention, urticaria, and visual disturbances.

OVERDOSAGE

Signs and Symptoms

Acute overdosage with OPANA ER is characterized by respiratory depression (a decrease in respiratory rate and/or tidal volume, Cheyne-Stokes respiration, cyanosis), extreme somnolence progressing to stupor or coma, skeletal muscle flaccidity, cold and clammy skin, constricted pupils and sometimes bradycardia and hypotension. In severe overdosage, apnea, circulatory collapse, cardiac arrest and death may occur.

OPANA ER may cause miosis, even in total darkness. Pinpoint pupils are a sign of opioid overdose but are not pathognomonic (e.g., pontine lesions of hemorrhagic or ischemic origin may produce similar findings). Marked mydriasis rather than miosis may be seen with hypoxia in overdose situations (see **CLINICAL PHARMACOLOGY: Central Nervous System**).

Treatment

In the treatment of OPANA ER overdosage, primary attention should be given to the reestablishment of a patent airway and institution of assisted or controlled ventilation. Supportive measures (including oxygen and vasopressors) should be employed in the management of circulatory shock and pulmonary edema accompanying overdose as indicated. Cardiac arrest or arrhythmias may require cardiac massage or defibrillation. Elimination or evacuation of gastric contents may be necessary in order to eliminate unabsorbed drug. Before attempting treatment by gastric emptying or activated charcoal, care should be taken to secure the airway.

The opioid antagonist naloxone hydrochloride is a specific antidote against respiratory depression, which may result from overdosage or unusual sensitivity to opioids including OPANA ER. Therefore, an appropriate dose of naloxone hydrochloride should be administered (usual initial adult dose 0.4 mg-2 mg) preferably by the intravenous route and simultaneously with efforts at respiratory resuscitation. Nalmefene is an alternative pure opioid antagonist, which may be administered as a specific antidote to respiratory depression resulting from opioid overdose. Since the duration of action of OPANA ER may exceed that of the antagonist, the patient should be kept under continued surveillance and repeated doses of the antagonist should be administered according to the antagonist labeling as needed to maintain adequate respiration.

In patients receiving OPANA ER, opioid antagonists should not be administered in the absence of clinically significant respiratory or circulatory depression secondary to OPANA ER overdose. They should be administered cautiously to persons who are known, or suspected to be, physically dependent on any opioid agonist including OPANA ER. In such cases, an abrupt or complete reversal of opioid effects may precipitate an acute abstinence syndrome. In an individual physically dependent on opioids, administration of the usual dose of the antagonist will precipitate an acute withdrawal syndrome. The severity of the withdrawal syndrome produced will depend on the degree of physical dependence and the dose of the antagonist administered. If respiratory depression is associated with muscular rigidity, administration of a neuromuscular blocking agent may be necessary to facilitate assisted or controlled ventilation. Muscular rigidity may also respond to opioid antagonist therapy.

DOSAGE AND ADMINISTRATION

OPANA ER Tablets are to be swallowed whole and are not to be broken, chewed, dissolved, or crushed. Taking broken, chewed, dissolved, or crushed OPANA ER Tablets leads to rapid release and absorption of a potentially fatal dose of oxymorphone.

Patients must not consume alcoholic beverages, or prescription or non-prescription medications containing alcohol, while on OPANA ER therapy. The co-ingestion of alcohol with OPANA ER may result in increased plasma levels and a potentially fatal overdose of oxymorphone.

OPANA ER is an opioid agonist and a Schedule II controlled substance with an abuse liability similar to morphine and other opioids.

OPANA ER, like morphine and other opioids used in analgesia, can be abused and is subject to criminal diversion.

OPANA ER tablets are to be swallowed whole, and are not to be broken, chewed, crushed or dissolved. Taking broken, chewed, crushed or dissolved OPANA ER tablets leads to the rapid release and absorption of a potentially fatal dose of oxymorphone.

While symmetric (same dose AM and PM), around-the-clock, every 12 hours dosing is appropriate for the majority of patients, some patients may benefit from asymmetric (different dose given in AM than in PM) dosing, tailored to their pain pattern. It is usually appropriate to treat a patient with only one extended-release opioid for around-the-clock therapy.

Selection of patients for treatment with OPANA ER should be governed by the same principles that apply to the use of other extended-release opioid analgesics (see **INDICATIONS AND USAGE**). As with any opioid drug product, it is necessary to adjust the dosing regimen for each patient individually, taking into account the patient's prior analgesic treatment experience. Physicians should individualize treatment in every case (see **DOSAGE AND ADMINISTRATION**), using non-opioid analgesics, as needed opioids and/or combination products, and chronic opioid therapy in a progressive plan of pain management such as outlined by the World Health Organization, the American Pain Society and the Federation of State Medical Boards Model Guidelines. Healthcare professionals should follow appropriate pain management principles of careful assessment and ongoing monitoring (see **BOXED WARNING**).

In the selection of the initial dose of OPANA ER, attention should be given to the following:

1. The total daily dose, potency and specific characteristics of the opioid the patient has been taking previously;
2. The relative potency estimate used to calculate the equivalent oxymorphone dose needed;
3. The patient's degree of opioid tolerance;
4. The age, general condition, and medical status of the patient;
5. Concurrent non-opioid analgesic and other medications;
6. The type and severity of the patient's pain;
7. The balance between pain control and adverse experiences;
8. Risk factors for abuse, addiction or diversion, including a prior history of abuse, addiction or diversion.

The following dosing recommendations, therefore, can only be considered as suggested approaches to what is actually a series of clinical decisions over time in the management of the pain of each individual patient.

OPANA ER should be administered on an empty stomach, at least one hour prior to or two hours after eating.

Initiation of Therapy

Opioid-Naïve Patients

It is suggested that patients who are not opioid-experienced being initiated on chronic around-the-clock opioid therapy be started with OPANA ER 5 mg every 12 hours. Thereafter, it is recommended that the dose be individually titrated, preferably at increments of 5–10 mg every 12 hours every 3–7 days, to a level that provides adequate analgesia and minimizes side effects under the close supervision of the prescribing physician (see **CLINICAL TRIALS: 12-Week Study in Opioid-Naïve Patients with Low Back Pain**).

Opioid-Experienced Patients

Conversion from OPANA to OPANA ER

Patients receiving OPANA may be converted to OPANA ER by administering half the patient's total daily oral OPANA dose as OPANA ER, every 12 hours. For example, a patient receiving 40 mg/day OPANA may require 20 mg OPANA ER every 12 hours.

Conversion from Parenteral Oxymorphone to OPANA ER

Given the absolute oral bioavailability of approximately 10%, patients receiving parenteral oxymorphone may be converted to OPANA ER by administering 10 times the patient's total daily parenteral oxymorphone dose as OPANA ER in two equally divided doses (e.g., IV dose × 10/2). For example, approximately 20 mg of OPANA ER, every 12 hours, may be required to provide pain relief equivalent to a total daily dose of 4 mg of parenteral oxymorphone. Due to patient variability with regards to opioid analgesic response, upon conversion patients should be closely monitored to ensure adequate analgesia and to minimize side effects.

Conversion from Other Oral Opioids to OPANA ER

For conversion from other opioids to OPANA ER, physicians and other healthcare professionals are advised to refer to published relative potency information, keeping in mind that conversion ratios are only approximate. In general, it is safest to start the OPANA ER therapy by administering half of the calculated total daily dose of OPANA ER (see conversion ratio table below) in 2 divided doses, every 12 hours. The initial dose of OPANA ER can be gradually adjusted until adequate pain relief and acceptable side effects have been achieved. The following table provides approximate equivalent doses, which may be used as a guideline for conversion. **The conversion ratios and approximate equivalent doses in this conversion table are only to be used for the conversion from current opioid therapy to OPANA ER.** In a Phase 3 clinical trial with an open-label titration period, patients were converted from their current opioid to OPANA ER using the following table as a guide. In general, patients were able to successfully titrate to a stabilized dose of OPANA ER within 4 weeks (see **CLINICAL TRIALS: 12-Week Study in Opioid-Experienced Patients with Low Back Pain**). There is substantial patient variation in the relative potency of different opioid drugs and formulations.

CONVERSION RATIOS TO OPANA ER

Opioid	Approximate Equivalent Dose	Oral Conversion Ratio[a]
	Oral	
Oxymorphone	10 mg	1
Hydrocodone	20 mg	0.5
Oxycodone	20 mg	0.5
Methadone[b]	20 mg	0.5
Morphine	30 mg	0.333

[a]Ratio for conversion of oral opioid dose to approximate oxymorphone equivalent dose. Select opioid and multiply the dose by the conversion ratio to calculate the approximate oral oxymorphone equivalent.

- **The conversion ratios ad approximate equivalent doses in this conversion table are** only **to be used for the conversion from current opioid therapy to Opana ER.**
- Sum the total daily dose for the opioid and multiply by the conversion ratio to calculate the oxymorphone total daily dose.
- For patients on a regimen of mixed opioids, calculate the approximate oral oxymorphone dose for each opioid and sum the totals to estimate the total daily oxymorphone dose.
- The dose of OPANA ER can be gradually adjusted, preferably at increments of 10 mg every 12 hours every 3-7 days, until adequate pain relief and acceptable side effects have been achieved (see **Individualization of Dose**).

[b]It is extremely important to monitor all patients closely when converting from methadone to other opioid agonists. The ratio between methadone and other opioid agonists may vary widely as a function of previous dose exposure. Methadone has a long half-life and tends to accumulate in the plasma.

Individualization of Dose

Once therapy is initiated, pain relief and other opioid effects should be frequently assessed. In clinical practice, titration of the total daily OPANA ER dose should be based upon the amount of supplemental opioid utilization, severity of the patient's pain, and the patient's ability to tolerate the opioid. Patients should be titrated to generally mild or no pain with the regular use of no more than two doses of supplemental analgesia, i.e. "rescue," per 24 hours.

If signs of excessive opioid-related adverse experiences are observed, the next dose may be reduced. If this adjustment leads to inadequate analgesia, a supplemental dose of OPANA, another immediate-release opioid, or a non-opioid analgesic may be administered. Dose adjustments should be made to obtain an appropriate balance between pain relief and opioid-related adverse experiences. If significant adverse events occur before the therapeutic goal of mild or no pain is achieved, the events should be treated aggressively. Once adverse events are under control, upward titration should continue to an acceptable level of pain control.

During periods of changing analgesic requirements, including initial titration, frequent contact is recommended between physician, other members of the healthcare team, the patient and the caregiver/family. Patients and caregivers/family members should be advised of the potential side effects.

Patients with Hepatic Impairment

Patients with mild hepatic impairment should be started with the lowest dose and titrated slowly while carefully monitoring side effects. OPANA ER is contraindicated in patients with moderate and severe hepatic dysfunction (see **CLINICAL PHARMACOLOGY, CONTRAINDICATIONS** and **PRECAUTIONS**).

Patients with Renal Impairment

There are 57% and 65% increases in oxymorphone bioavailability in patients with moderate and severe renal impairment, respectively (see **CLINICAL PHARMACOLOGY** and **PRECAUTIONS**). Accordingly, in patients with creatinine clearance rate less than 50 mL/min, OPANA ER should be started with the lowest dose and titrated slowly while carefully monitoring side effects.

Use with CNS Depressants

OPANA ER, like all opioid analgesics, should be started at 1/3 to 1/2 of the usual dose in patients who are concurrently receiving other central nervous system depressants including sedatives or hypnotics, general anesthetics, phenothiazines, tranquilizers, and alcohol because respiratory depression, hypotension, and profound sedation or coma may result. No specific interaction between oxymorphone and monoamine oxidase inhibitors has been observed, but cau-

tion in the use of any opioid in patients taking this class of drugs is appropriate (see **PRECAUTIONS: General** and **PRECAUTIONS: Drug-Drug Interactions**).

Geriatrics

The steady-state plasma concentrations of oxymorphone are approximately 40% higher in elderly subjects than in young subjects (see **CLINICAL PHARMACOLOGY** and **PRECAUTIONS**). In general, caution should be exercised in the selection of the starting dose of OPANA ER for an elderly patient usually starting at the low end of the dosing range and slowly titrating to adequate analgesia.

Maintenance of Therapy and Supplemental Analgesia

The intent of the titration period is to establish a patient-specific every 12 hours dose that will maintain adequate analgesia with acceptable side effects for as long as pain relief is necessary. During titration and before a stable dose is achieved, OPANA or other immediate-release medications can be used as supplemental analgesia between dosings. Should pain recur, the dose can be incrementally increased to re-establish pain control. The method of therapy adjustment outlined above should be employed to re-establish pain control.

During chronic therapy with OPANA ER, the continued need for around-the-clock opioid therapy should be reassessed periodically.

Cessation of Therapy

When the patient no longer requires therapy with OPANA ER tablets, doses should be tapered gradually to prevent signs and symptoms of withdrawal in the physically dependent patient (see **CLINICAL TRIALS: 12-Week Study in Opioid-Naïve Patients with Low Back Pain** and **CLINICAL TRIALS: 12-Week Study in Opioid-Experienced Patients with Low Back Pain**).

SAFETY AND HANDLING

OPANA ER contains oxymorphone, which is a controlled substance. Oxymorphone is controlled under Schedule II of the Controlled Substances Act. Oxymorphone, like all opioids, is liable to diversion and misuse and should be handled accordingly. Patients and their families should be instructed to flush any OPANA ER tablets that are no longer needed.

OPANA ER may be targeted for theft and diversion. Healthcare professionals should contact their State Medical Board, State Board of Pharmacy or State Control Board for information on how to detect or prevent diversion of this product. Store at 25°C (77°F); excursions permitted to 15°-30°C (59°-86°F). [See USP Controlled Room Temperature].

Dispense in tight container as defined in the USP, with a child-resistant closure (as required).

HOW SUPPLIED

OPANA ER tablets are supplied as follows:

5 mg
Pink, octagon shape, film coated, convex tablets debossed with "5" on one side and plain on the other.
Bottles of 100 with child-resistant closure — NDC 63481-907-70
Unit-Dose package of 100 tablets (5 blister cards of 20 tablets, not child-resistant, for hospital use only) — NDC 63481-907-75

7.5 mg
Gray, octagon shape, film coated, convex tablets debossed with "7 ½" on one side and plain on the other.
Bottles of 100 with child-resistant closure — NDC 63481-522-70
Unit-Dose package of 100 tablets (5 blister cards of 20 tablets, not child-resistant, for hospital use only) — NDC 63481-522-75

10 mg
Light orange, octagon shape, film coated, convex tablets debossed with "10" on one side and plain on the other.
Bottles of 100 with child-resistant closure — NDC 63481-674-70
Unit-Dose package of 100 tablets (5 blister cards of 20 tablets, not child-resistant, for hospital use only) — NDC 63481-674-75

15 mg
White, octagon shape, film coated, convex tablets debossed with "15" on one side and plain on the other.
Bottles of 100 with child-resistant closure — NDC 63481-553-70
Unit-Dose package of 100 tablets (5 blister cards of 20 tablets, not child-resistant, for hospital use only) — NDC 63481-553-75

20 mg
Light green, octagon shape, film coated, convex tablets debossed with "20" on one side and plain on the other.
Bottles of 100 with child-resistant closure — NDC 63481-617-70
Unit-Dose package of 100 tablets (5 blister cards of 20 tablets, not child-resistant, for hospital use only) — NDC 63481-617-75

30 mg
Red, octagon shape, film coated, convex tablets debossed with "30" on one side and plain on the other.

Bottles of 100 with child-resistant closure — NDC 63481-571-70
Unit-Dose package of 100 tablets (5 blister cards of 20 tablets, not child-resistant, for hospital use only) — NDC 63481-571-75

40 mg
Yellow, octagon shape, film coated, convex tablets debossed with "40" on one side and plain on the other.
Bottles of 100 with child-resistant closure — NDC 63481-693-70
Unit-Dose package of 100 tablets (5 blister cards of 20 tablets, not child-resistant, for hospital use only) — NDC 63481-693-75

Rx Only
CAUTION
DEA Order Form Required.
Manufactured for:
Endo Pharmaceuticals Inc.
Chadds Ford, Pennsylvania 19317
Manufactured by:
Novartis Consumer Health Inc.
Lincoln, NE 68517
TIMERx®-N is a registered Trademark of Penwest Pharmaceuticals Co., Danbury, Connecticut and is used herein pursuant to a license agreement between Penwest and Endo Pharmaceuticals.
Copyright © Endo Pharmaceuticals Inc. 2008
2002862/February 2008

PATIENT INFORMATION

OPANA® ER (Ō-pan-a)
(Oxymorphone Hydrochloride)
Extended-Release Tablets
CII
Rx Only
OPANA ER Tablets, 5 mg
OPANA ER Tablets, 7.5 mg
OPANA ER Tablets, 10 mg
OPANA ER Tablets, 15 mg
OPANA ER Tablets, 20 mg
OPANA ER Tablets, 30 mg
OPANA ER Tablets, 40 mg

> **IMPORTANT: Keep OPANA ER in a safe place away from children. Accidental use by a child is a medical emergency and can result in death. If a child accidentally takes OPANA ER, get emergency help right away.**

Read the Patient Information that comes with OPANA ER before you start taking it and each time you get a new prescription. There may be new information. This information does not take the place of talking with your healthcare provider about your medical condition or your treatment. Share the important information in this leaflet with members of your household.

What Is the Most Important Information I Should Know About OPANA ER?
- **OPANA ER can cause trouble breathing (hypoventilation),** which can lead to death, if used differently than the way you were told to use it by your healthcare provider (see "What are the possible side effects of OPANA ER?").
- **Swallow OPANA ER tablets whole.** Do not break, crush, dissolve, or chew OPANA ER tablets before swallowing. **If a tablet is broken, crushed, dissolved, or chewed, the full 12 hour dose can be taken into your body all at once. This is very dangerous. You could die from an overdose of the medicine.** Use OPANA ER exactly the way your healthcare provider prescribes. If you cannot swallow tablets whole, tell your healthcare provider. You may need a different medicine.
- **Do not consume alcoholic beverages, or prescription or non-prescription medications containing alcohol, while taking Opana ER.**

What is OPANA ER?
- OPANA ER is a prescription medicine that contains the opioid (narcotic pain medicine) oxymorphone. OPANA ER is used to treat adults with constant pain (around the clock) that is moderate to severe and is expected to last for an extended period of time. **OPANA ER is not for occasional ("as needed") use.**
- **OPANA ER can cause physical dependence.** Do not stop taking OPANA ER all of a sudden if you have been taking it for more than a few days. You could become sick with uncomfortable withdrawal symptoms because your body has become use to the medicine. Talk to your healthcare provider about slowly stopping OPANA ER to avoid getting sick with withdrawal symptoms. Physical dependence is not the same as drug addiction. Your healthcare provider can tell you more about the differences between physical dependence and drug addiction.
- **OPANA ER is a controlled substance (CII)** because it contains a narcotic painkiller that can be a target for people

who abuse prescription medicines or street drugs. Keep your tablets in a safe place to protect them from being stolen. Never give your tablets to anyone else, even if they have the same symptoms you have. Selling or giving away this medicine may harm others, even causing death, and is against the law.

Who Should Not Take OPANA ER?

Do not take OPANA ER if:

- You had surgery within the past day (24 hours) and you were not taking OPANA ER before your surgery.
- Your pain is mild or will go away in a few days.
- Your pain can be controlled by the occasional use of other pain medicines.
- You are having an asthma attack or have severe asthma, trouble breathing, or lung problems.
- You have liver problems.
- You are allergic to OPANA ER or anything in it. See the end of this leaflet for a complete list of ingredients in OPANA ER.

You have had severe allergic reactions to other narcotic pain medicines (such as morphine or codeine medicines). A severe allergic reaction includes a severe rash, hives, breathing problems, or dizziness.

OPANA ER is not for children under 18 years of age.

What Should I Tell My Healthcare Provider Before Starting OPANA ER?

Tell your healthcare provider about all of your medical problems, especially if you:

- have trouble breathing or lung problems
- have a head injury or brain problems
- have liver or kidney problems
- have adrenal gland problems, such as Addison's disease
- have convulsions or seizures
- have thyroid problems
- have problems urinating or prostate problems
- have pancreas problems
- have a drinking problem or alcoholism
- have severe mental problems or hallucinations (see or hear things that are not really there)
- have past or present drug abuse or drug addiction problems
- **are pregnant or plan to become pregnant.** OPANA ER may harm your unborn baby.
- **are breastfeeding.** OPANA ER may pass through your milk and may harm your baby. You should not breastfeed while taking OPANA ER.

Tell your healthcare provider about all the medicines you take, including prescription and nonprescription medicines, vitamins, and herbal supplements. Some medicines may cause serious problems when taken with OPANA ER, especially if they cause sleepiness (like sleeping pills, anxiety medicines, antihistamines, or tranquilizers).

Do not take any new medicines while using OPANA ER until you have talked to your healthcare provider or pharmacist and they have told you it is safe.

Know the medicines you take. Keep a list of them to show your healthcare provider and pharmacist.

How Should I Take OPANA ER?

- **Follow your healthcare provider's directions exactly.** Your healthcare provider may change your dose based on your reactions to the medicine. Do not change your dose unless your healthcare provider tells you to change it. Do not take OPANA ER more often than prescribed.
- **Swallow OPANA ER tablets whole. Do not break, crush, dissolve, or chew OPANA ER tablets before swallowing. If a tablet is broken, crushed, dissolved, or chewed, the full 12 hour dose can be taken into your body all at once. This is very dangerous. You could die from an overdose of the medicine.** If you cannot swallow tablets whole, tell your healthcare provider. You may need a different medicine.
- Take OPANA ER every 12 hours or as instructed by your healthcare provider. OPANA ER should be taken on an empty stomach, at least one hour before or two hours after meals. Talk to your healthcare provider if you feel sick taking OPANA ER on an empty stomach.
- **If you miss a dose,** take it as soon as possible. If it is almost time for your next dose, skip the missed dose and go back to your regular dosing schedule. **Do not take 2 doses at once unless your healthcare provider tells you to.** If you are not sure about your dosing call your healthcare provider.
- **If you take too much OPANA ER or overdose,** call your local emergency number or poison control center right away.
- **Talk to your healthcare provider often about your pain. Your healthcare provider can** decide if you still need OPANA ER.
- If you have side effects that bother you or if you continue to have pain, call your healthcare provider.
- **Stopping OPANA ER.** If your healthcare provider decides you no longer need OPANA ER, ask how to slowly reduce the dose of your medicine so you don't get uncomfortable

(withdrawal) symptoms such as nausea, sweating, and pain. You should not stop taking OPANA ER all at once if you have been taking it for more than a few days without talking to your healthcare provider. OPANA ER can cause physical dependence. You can get sick with withdrawal symptoms if you stop OPANA ER all at once, because your body has become use to it.

After you stop taking OPANA ER, flush the unused tablets down the toilet. Safely dispose of OPANA ER out of the reach of children and pets.

What Should I Avoid While Taking OPANA ER?

- **Do not drive, operate heavy machinery, or participate in any other possibly dangerous activities** until you know how you react to this medicine. OPANA ER can make you sleepy. Ask your healthcare provider to tell you when it is okay to do these activities.
- **Do not drink alcohol while using OPANA ER. It may increase the chance of having dangerous side effects including overdose and death.**

What are the Possible Side Effects of OPANA ER?

OPANA ER can cause trouble breathing.

Call your healthcare provider or get medical help right away if:

- your breathing slows down
- you have shallow breathing (little chest movement with breathing)
- you feel faint, dizzy, confused, or have any other unusual symptoms

These can be signs that you have taken too much OPANA ER (overdose) or the dose is too high for you, which can be dangerous and lead to death if not treated.

OPANA ER can cause your blood pressure to drop. This can make you feel dizzy if you get up too fast from sitting or lying down. Low blood pressure is also more likely to happen if you are taking other medicines that can also lower your blood pressure.

OPANA ER can cause physical dependence. Your body will get used to OPANA ER if you take it more than a few days. You can get sick with withdrawal symptoms if you stop taking OPANA ER all at once. You can avoid getting sick with withdrawal symptoms by stopping OPANA ER slowly. Your healthcare provider will tell you how to do this.

There is a chance of abuse or addiction with OPANA ER. Abuse or addiction is different than a physical dependence. If you have abused prescription medicines, street drugs or alcohol in the past, you may have a higher chance of developing abuse or addiction again while using OPANA ER. If you have more concerns, talk to your healthcare provider for more information about abuse and addiction.

The most common side effects of OPANA ER are nausea, constipation, dizziness, vomiting, itching, sleepiness, headache, increased sweating, and sedation. Some of these side effects may decrease with continued use. Talk to your healthcare provider if you continue to have these side effects.

These are not all the possible side effects of OPANA ER. For a complete list, ask your healthcare provider or pharmacist. Constipation (decrease in the usual number of hard bowel movements) is a common side effect of opioid medicines, including OPANA ER. Talk to your healthcare provider or pharmacist about the use of laxatives (medicines to treat constipation) and stool softeners to prevent or treat constipation while taking OPANA ER.

How should I store OPANA ER?

- Store OPANA ER at room temperature between 59° to 86°F (15° to 30°C).
- Keep OPANA ER in a childproof container and store in a safe place to protect it from being stolen.
- **Keep OPANA ER out of the reach of children. Accidental overdose in children is an emergency and can result in death.**

General Information about OPANA ER

- Do not use OPANA ER for conditions for which it was not prescribed.
- Do not give OPANA ER to other people, even if they have the same symptoms you have. It may harm them, even causing death, and it is against the law.

This leaflet summarizes the most important information about OPANA ER. If you would like more information, talk with your healthcare provider. Also, you can ask your pharmacist or healthcare provider for information about OPANA ER that is written for healthcare professionals.

For additional information, please go to www.Endo.com or www.opana.com

What are the ingredients in OPANA ER?

Active Ingredient: oxymorphone hydrochloride

Inactive Ingredients: hypromellose, methylparaben, silicified microcrystalline cellulose, sodium stearyl fumarate, TIMERx®-N, titanium dioxide, and triacetin. The 5 mg, 10 mg, 15 mg, 20 mg, and 30 mg tablets also contain macrogol, and polysorbate 80. In addition, the 5 mg, 7.5 mg, and 30 mg tablets contain iron oxide red. The 7.5 mg tablets contain iron oxide black, and iron oxide yellow. The 10 mg tablets contain FD&C yellow No. 6. The 20 mg tablets contain

FD&C blue No. 1, FD&C yellow No. 6, and D&C yellow No. 10. The 40 mg tablets contain FD&C yellow No. 6, D&C yellow No.10, and lactose monohydrate.

CAUTION: Federal law prohibits dispensing without prescription.

Manufactured for:
Endo Pharmaceuticals Inc.
Chadds Ford, Pennsylvania 19317
Manufactured by:
Novartis Consumer Health Inc.
Lincoln, NE 68517
TIMERx®-N is a registered Trademark of Penwest Pharmaceuticals Co., Danbury, Connecticut and is used herein pursuant to a license agreement between Penwest and Endo Pharmaceuticals.
Copyright © Endo Pharmaceuticals Inc. 2008
2002861/February 2008
Shown in Product Identification Guide, page 309

PERCOCET® ⓒ Ⓡ

[perk′ ō-sĕt]

oxycodone hydrochloride and acetaminophen
tablet
Rx only

DESCRIPTION

Each tablet, for oral administration, contains oxycodone hydrochloride and acetaminophen in the following strengths:

Oxycodone Hydrochloride, USP   2.5 mg*
Acetaminophen, USP   325 mg
*2.5 mg oxycodone HCl is equivalent to 2.2409 mg of oxycodone.

Oxycodone Hydrochloride, USP   5 mg*
Acetaminophen, USP   325 mg
*5 mg oxycodone HCl is equivalent to 4.4815 mg of oxycodone.

Oxycodone Hydrochloride, USP   7.5 mg*
Acetaminophen, USP   325 mg
*7.5 mg oxycodone HCl is equivalent to 6.7228 mg of oxycodone.

Oxycodone Hydrochloride, USP   7.5 mg*
Acetaminophen, USP   500 mg
*7.5 mg oxycodone HCl is equivalent to 6.7228 mg of oxycodone.

Oxycodone Hydrochloride, USP   10 mg*
Acetaminophen, USP   325 mg
*10 mg oxycodone HCl is equivalent to 8.9637 mg of oxycodone.

Oxycodone Hydrochloride, USP   10 mg*
Acetaminophen, USP   650 mg
*10 mg oxycodone HCl is equivalent to 8.9637 mg of oxycodone.

All strengths of PERCOCET also contain the following inactive ingredients: Colloidal silicon dioxide, croscarmellose sodium, crospovidone, microcrystalline cellulose, povidone, pregelatinized cornstarch, and stearic acid. In addition, the 2.5 mg/325 mg strength contains FD&C Red No. 40 Aluminum Lake and the 5 mg/325 mg strength contains FD&C Blue No. 1 Aluminum Lake. The 7.5 mg/325 mg and the 7.5 mg/500 mg strengths contain FD&C Yellow No. 6 Aluminum Lake. The 10 mg/325 mg and the 10 mg/650 mg strengths contain D&C Yellow No. 10 Aluminum Lake.

Oxycodone, 14-hydroxydihydrocodeinone, is a semisynthetic opioid analgesic which occurs as a white, odorless, crystalline powder having a saline, bitter taste. The molecular formula for oxycodone hydrochloride is $C_{18}H_{21}NO_4 \cdot HCl$ and the molecular weight 351.83. It is derived from the opium alkaloid thebaine, and may be represented by the following structural formula:

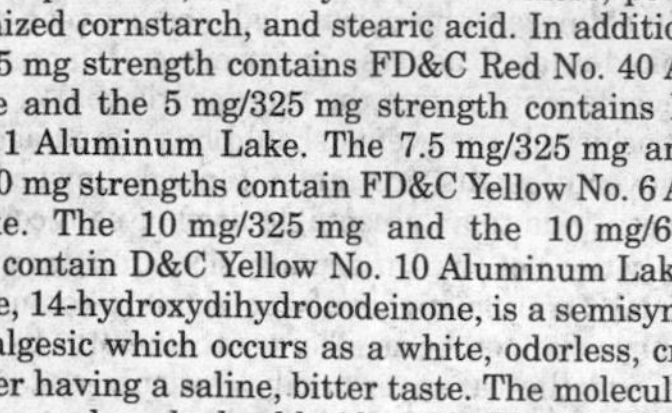

$C_{18}H_{21}NO_4 \cdot HCl$ MW 351.82

Acetaminophen, 4′-hydroxyacetanilide, is a non-opiate, non-salicylate analgesic and antipyretic which occurs as a white, odorless, crystalline powder, possessing a slightly bitter taste. The molecular formula for acetaminophen is $C_8H_9NO_2$ and the molecular weight is 151.17. It may be represented by the following structural formula:

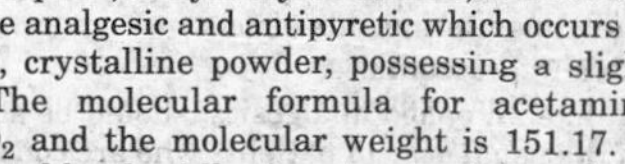

$C_8H_9NO_2$ MW 151.17

CLINICAL PHARMACOLOGY

Central Nervous System

Oxycodone is a semisynthetic pure opioid agonist whose principal therapeutic action is analgesia. Other pharmacological effects of oxycodone include anxiolysis, euphoria and feelings of relaxation. These effects are mediated by receptors (notably μ and κ) in the central nervous system for endogenous opioid-like compounds such as endorphins and enkephalins. Oxycodone produces respiratory depression through direct activity at respiratory centers in the brain stem and depresses the cough reflex by direct effect on the center of the medulla.

Acetaminophen is a non-opiate, non-salicylate analgesic and antipyretic. The site and mechanism for the analgesic effect of acetaminophen has not been determined. The antipyretic effect of acetaminophen is accomplished through the inhibition of endogenous pyrogen action on the hypothalamic heat-regulating centers.

Gastrointestinal Tract and Other Smooth Muscle

Oxycodone reduces motility by increasing smooth muscle tone in the stomach and duodenum. In the small intestine, digestion of food is delayed by decreases in propulsive contractions. Other opioid effects include contraction of biliary tract smooth muscle, spasm of the Sphincter of Oddi, increased ureteral and bladder sphincter tone, and a reduction in uterine tone.

Cardiovascular System

Oxycodone may produce a release of histamine and may be associated with orthostatic hypotension, and other symptoms, such as pruritus, flushing, red eyes, and sweating.

Pharmacokinetics

Absorption and Distribution

The mean absolute oral bioavailability of oxycodone in cancer patients was reported to be about 87%. Oxycodone has been shown to be 45% bound to human plasma proteins in vitro. The volume of distribution after intravenous administration is 211.9 ±186.6 L.

Absorption of acetaminophen is rapid and almost complete from the GI tract after oral administration. With overdosage, absorption is complete in 4 hours. Acetaminophen is relatively uniformly distributed throughout most body fluids. Binding of the drug to plasma proteins is variable; only 20% to 50% may be bound at the concentrations encountered during acute intoxication.

Metabolism and Elimination

A high portion of oxycodone is N-dealkylated to noroxycodone during first-pass metabolism. Oxymorphone, is formed by the O-demethylation of oxycodone. The metabolism of oxycodone to oxymorphone is catalyzed by CYP2D6. Free and conjugated noroxycodone, free and conjugated oxycodone, and oxymorphone are excreted in human urine following a single oral dose of oxycodone. Approximately 8% to 14% of the dose is excreted as free oxycodone over 24 hours after administration. Following a single, oral dose of oxycodone, the mean ± SD elimination half-life is 3.51 ± 1.43 hours.

Acetaminophen is metabolized in the liver via cytochrome P450 microsomal enzyme. About 80-85% of the acetaminophen in the body is conjugated principally with glucuronic acid and to a lesser extent with sulfuric acid and cysteine. After hepatic conjugation, 90 to 100% of the drug is recovered in the urine with in the first day.

About 4% of acetaminophen is metabolized via cytochrome P450 oxidase to a toxic metabolite which is further detoxified by conjugation with glutathione, present in a fixed amount. It is believed that the toxic metabolite NAPQI (N acetyl-p-benzoquinoneimine, N-acetylimidoquinone) is responsible for liver necrosis. High doses of acetaminophen may deplete the glutathione stores so that inactivation of the toxic metabolite is decreased. At high doses, the capacity of metabolic pathways for conjugation with glucuronic acid and sulfuric acid may be exceeded, resulting in increased metabolism of acetaminophen by alternate pathways.

INDICATIONS AND USAGE

PERCOCET is indicated for the relief of moderate to moderately severe pain.

CONTRAINDICATIONS

PERCOCET tablets should not be administered to patients with known hypersensitivity to oxycodone, acetaminophen, or any other component of this product.

Oxycodone is contraindicated in any situation where opioids are contraindicated including patients with significant respiratory depression (in unmonitored settings or the absence of resuscitative equipment) and patients with acute or severe bronchial asthma or hypercarbia. Oxycodone is contraindicated in the setting of suspected or known paralytic ileus.

WARNINGS

Misuse, Abuse and Diversion of Opioids

Oxycodone is an opioid agonist of the morphine-type. Such drugs are sought by drug abusers and people with addiction disorders and are subject to criminal diversion.

Oxycodone can be abused in a manner similar to other opioid agonists, legal or illicit. This should be considered when prescribing or dispensing PERCOCET tablets in situations where the physician or pharmacist is concerned about an increased risk of misuse, abuse, or diversion. Concerns about misuse, addiction, and diversion should not prevent the proper management of pain.

Healthcare professionals should contact their State Professional Licensing Board or State Controlled Substances Authority for information on how to prevent and detect abuse or diversion of this product.

Administration of PERCOCET (Oxycodone and Acetaminophen Tablets, USP) tablets should be closely monitored for the following potentially serious adverse reactions and complications:

Respiratory Depression

Respiratory depression is a hazard with the use of oxycodone, one of the active ingredients in PERCOCET tablets, as with all opioid agonists. Elderly and debilitated patients are at particular risk for respiratory depression as are non-tolerant patients given large initial doses of oxycodone or when oxycodone is given in conjunction with other agents that depress respiration. Oxycodone should be used with extreme caution in patients with acute asthma, chronic obstructive pulmonary disorder (COPD), cor pulmonale, or preexisting respiratory impairment. In such patients, even usual therapeutic doses of oxycodone may decrease respiratory drive to the point of apnea. In these patients alternative non-opioid analgesics should be considered, and opioids should be employed only under careful medical supervision at the lowest effective dose.

In case of respiratory depression, a reversal agent such as naloxone hydrochloride may be utilized (see OVERDOSAGE).

Head Injury and Increased Intracranial Pressure

The respiratory depressant effects of opioids include carbon dioxide retention and secondary elevation of cerebrospinal fluid pressure, and may be markedly exaggerated in the presence of head injury, other intracranial lesions or a preexisting increase in intracranial pressure. Oxycodone produces effects on pupillary response and consciousness which may obscure neurologic signs of worsening in patients with head injuries.

Hypotensive Effect

Oxycodone may cause severe hypotension particularly in individuals whose ability to maintain blood pressure has been compromised by a depleted blood volume, or after concurrent administration with drugs which compromise vasomotor tone such as phenothiazines. Oxycodone, like all opioid analgesics of the morphine-type, should be administered with caution to patients in circulatory shock, since vasodilation produced by the drug may further reduce cardiac output and blood pressure. Oxycodone may produce orthostatic hypotension in ambulatory patients.

Hepatotoxicity

Precaution should be taken in patients with liver disease. Hepatotoxicity and severe hepatic failure occurred in chronic alcoholics following therapeutic doses.

PRECAUTIONS

General

Opioid analgesics should be used with caution when combined with CNS depressant drugs, and should be reserved for cases where the benefits of opioid analgesia outweigh the known risks of respiratory depression, altered mental state, and postural hypotension.

Acute Abdominal Conditions

The administration of PERCOCET (Oxycodone and Acetaminophen Tablets, USP) or other opioids may obscure the diagnosis or clinical course in patients with acute abdominal conditions.

PERCOCET tablets should be given with caution to patients with CNS depression, elderly or debilitated patients, patients with severe impairment of hepatic, pulmonary, or renal function, hypothyroidism, Addison's disease, prostatic hypertrophy, urethral stricture, acute alcoholism, delirium tremens, kyphoscoliosis with respiratory depression, myxedema, and toxic psychosis.

PERCOCET tablets may obscure the diagnosis or clinical course in patients with acute abdominal conditions. Oxycodone may aggravate convulsions in patients with convulsive disorders, and all opioids may induce or aggravate seizures in some clinical settings.

Following administration of PERCOCET tablets, anaphylactic reactions have been reported in patients with a known hypersensitivity to codeine, a compound with a structure similar to morphine and oxycodone. The frequency of this possible cross-sensitivity is unknown.

Interactions with Other CNS Depressants

Patients receiving other opioid analgesics, general anesthetics, phenothiazines, other tranquilizers, centrally-acting anti-emetics, sedative-hypnotics or other CNS depressants (including alcohol) concomitantly with PERCOCET tablets may exhibit an additive CNS depression. When such combined therapy is contemplated, the dose of one or both agents should be reduced.

Interactions with Mixed Agonist/Antagonist Opioid Analgesics

Agonist/antagonist analgesics (i.e., pentazocine, nalbuphine, and butorphanol) should be administered with caution to a patient who has received or is receiving a course of therapy with a pure opioid agonist analgesic such as oxycodone. In this situation, mixed agonist/antagonist analgesics may reduce the analgesic effect of oxycodone and/or may precipitate withdrawal symptoms in these patients.

Ambulatory Surgery and Postoperative Use

Oxycodone and other morphine-like opioids have been shown to decrease bowel motility. Ileus is a common postoperative complication, especially after intra-abdominal surgery with use of opioid analgesia. Caution should be taken to monitor for decreased bowel motility in postoperative patients receiving opioids. Standard supportive therapy should be implemented.

Use in Pancreatic/Biliary Tract Disease

Oxycodone may cause spasm of the Sphincter of Oddi and should be used with caution in patients with biliary tract disease, including acute pancreatitis. Opioids like oxycodone may cause increases in the serum amylase level.

Tolerance and Physical Dependence

Tolerance is the need for increasing doses of opioids to maintain a defined effect such as analgesia (in the absence of disease progression or other external factors). Physical dependence is manifested by withdrawal symptoms after abrupt discontinuation of a drug or upon administration of an antagonist. Physical dependence and tolerance are not unusual during chronic opioid therapy.

The opioid abstinence or withdrawal syndrome is characterized by some or all of the following: restlessness, lacrimation, rhinorrhea, yawning, perspiration, chills, myalgia, and mydriasis. Other symptoms also may develop, including: irritability, anxiety, backache, joint pain, weakness, abdominal cramps, insomnia, nausea, anorexia, vomiting, diarrhea, or increased blood pressure, respiratory rate, or heart rate.

In general, opioids should not be abruptly discontinued (see DOSAGE AND ADMINISTRATION: Cessation of Therapy).

Information for Patients/Caregivers

The following information should be provided to patients receiving PERCOCET tablets by their physician, nurse, pharmacist, or caregiver:

1. Patients should be aware that PERCOCET tablets contain oxycodone, which is a morphine-like substance.
2. Patients should be instructed to keep PERCOCET tablets in a secure place out of the reach of children. In the case of accidental ingestions, emergency medical care should be sought immediately.
3. When PERCOCET tablets are no longer needed, the unused tablets should be destroyed by flushing down the toilet.
4. Patients should be advised not to adjust the medication dose themselves. Instead, they must consult with their prescribing physician.
5. Patients should be advised that PERCOCET tablets may impair mental and/or physical ability required for the performance of potentially hazardous tasks (e.g., driving, operating heavy machinery).
6. Patients should not combine PERCOCET tablets with alcohol, opioid analgesics, tranquilizers, sedatives, or other CNS depressants unless under the recommendation and guidance of a physician. When co-administered with another CNS depressant, PERCOCET tablets can cause dangerous additive central nervous system or respiratory depression, which can result in serious injury or death.
7. The safe use of PERCOCET tablets during pregnancy has not been established; thus, women who are planning to become pregnant or are pregnant should consult with their physician before taking PERCOCET tablets.
8. Nursing mothers should consult with their physicians about whether to discontinue nursing or discontinue PERCOCET tablets because of the potential for serious adverse reactions to nursing infants.
9. Patients who are treated with PERCOCET tablets for more than a few weeks should be advised not to abruptly discontinue the medication. Patients should consult with their physician for a gradual discontinuation dose schedule to taper off the medication.
10. Patients should be advised that PERCOCET tablets are a potential drug of abuse. They should protect it from theft, and it should never be given to anyone other than the individual for whom it was prescribed.

Laboratory Tests

Although oxycodone may cross-react with some drug urine tests, no available studies were found which determined the duration of detectability of oxycodone in urine drug screens. However, based on pharmacokinetic data, the approximate duration of detectability for a single dose of oxycodone is roughly estimated to be one to two days following drug exposure.

Urine testing for opiates may be performed to determine illicit drug use and for medical reasons such as evaluation of patients with altered states of consciousness or monitoring efficacy of drug rehabilitation efforts. The preliminary identification of opiates in urine involves the use of an immunoassay screening and thin-layer chromatography (TLC). Gas chromatography/mass spectrometry (GC/MS) may be utilized as a third-stage identification step in the medical investigational sequence for opiate testing after immunoassay and TLC. The identities of 6-keto opiates (e.g., oxycodone) can further be differentiated by the analysis of their methoxime-trimethylsilyl (MO-TMS) derivative.

Drug/Drug Interactions with Oxycodone

Opioid analgesics may enhance the neuromuscular-blocking action of skeletal muscle relaxants and produce an increase in the degree of respiratory depression.

Patients receiving CNS depressants such as other opioid analgesics, general anesthetics, phenothiazines, other tranquilizers, centrally-acting anti-emetics, sedative-hypnotics or other CNS depressants (including alcohol) concomitantly with PERCOCET tablets may exhibit an additive CNS depression. When such combined therapy is contemplated, the dose of one or both agents should be reduced. The concurrent use of anticholinergics with opioids may produce paralytic ileus.

Agonist/antagonist analgesics (i.e., pentazocine, nalbuphine, naltrexone, and butorphanol) should be administered with caution to a patient who has received or is receiving a pure opioid agonist such as oxycodone. These agonist/antagonist analgesics may reduce the analgesic effect of oxycodone or may precipitate withdrawal symptoms.

Drug/Drug Interactions with Acetaminophen

Alcohol, ethyl: Hepatotoxicity has occurred in chronic alcoholics following various dose levels (moderate to excessive) of acetaminophen.

Anticholinergics: The onset of acetaminophen effect may be delayed or decreased slightly, but the ultimate pharmacological effect is not significantly affected by anticholinergics.

Oral Contraceptives: Increase in glucuronidation resulting in increased plasma clearance and a decreased half-life of acetaminophen.

Charcoal (activated): Reduces acetaminophen absorption when administered as soon as possible after overdose.

Beta Blockers (Propanolol): Propanolol appears to inhibit the enzyme systems responsible for the glucuronidation and oxidation of acetaminophen. Therefore, the pharmacologic effects of acetaminophen may be increased.

Loop diuretics: The effects of the loop diuretic may be decreased because acetaminophen may decrease renal prostaglandin excretion and decrease plasma renin activity.

Lamotrigine: Serum lamotrigine concentrations may be reduced, producing a decrease in therapeutic effects.

Probenecid: Probenecid may increase the therapeutic effectiveness of acetaminophen slightly.

Zidovudine: The pharmacologic effects of zidovudine may be decreased because of enhanced non-hepatic or renal clearance of zidovudine.

Drug/Laboratory Test Interactions

Depending on the sensitivity/specificity and the test methodology, the individual components of PERCOCET (Oxycodone and Acetaminophen Tablets, USP) may cross-react with assays used in the preliminary detection of cocaine (primary urinary metabolite, benzoylecgonine) or marijuana (cannabinoids) in human urine. A more specific alternate chemical method must be used in order to obtain a confirmed analytical result. The preferred confirmatory method is gas chromatography/mass spectrometry (GC/MS). Moreover, clinical considerations and professional judgment should be applied to any drug-of-abuse test result, particularly when preliminary positive results are used.

Acetaminophen may interfere with home blood glucose measurement systems; decreases of >20% in mean glucose values may be noted. This effect appears to be drug, concentration and system dependent.

Carcinogenesis, Mutagenesis, Impairment of Fertility

Carcinogenesis

Animal studies to evaluate the carcinogenic potential of oxycodone and acetaminophen have not been performed.

Mutagenesis

The combination of oxycodone and acetaminophen has not been evaluated for mutagenicity. Oxycodone alone was negative in a bacterial reverse mutation assay (Ames), an *in vitro* chromosome aberration assay with human lymphocytes without metabolic activation and an *in vivo* mouse micronucleus assay. Oxycodone was clastogenic in the human lymphocyte chromosomal assay in the presence of metabolic activation and in the mouse lymphoma assay with or without metabolic activation.

Fertility

Animal studies to evaluate the effects of oxycodone on fertility have not been performed.

Pregnancy

Teratogenic Effects

Pregnancy Category C

Animal reproductive studies have not been conducted with PERCOCET. It is also not known whether PERCOCET can cause fetal harm when administered to a pregnant woman or can affect reproductive capacity. PERCOCET should not be given to a pregnant woman unless in the judgment of the physician, the potential benefits outweigh the possible hazards

Nonteratogenic Effects

Opioids can cross the placental barrier and have the potential to cause neonatal respiratory depression. Opioid use during pregnancy may result in a physically drug-dependent fetus. After birth, the neonate may suffer severe withdrawal symptoms.

Labor and Delivery

PERCOCET tablets are not recommended for use in women during and immediately prior to labor and delivery due to its potential effects on respiratory function in the newborn.

Nursing Mothers

Ordinarily, nursing should not be undertaken while a patient is receiving PERCOCET tablets because of the possibility of sedation and/or respiratory depression in the infant. Oxycodone is excreted in breast milk in low concentrations, and there have been rare reports of somnolence and lethargy in babies of nursing mothers taking an oxycodone/acetaminophen product. Acetaminophen is also excreted in breast milk in low concentrations.

Pediatric Use

Safety and effectiveness in pediatric patients have not been established.

Geriatric Use

Special precaution should be given when determining the dosing amount and frequency of PERCOCET tablets for geriatric patients, since clearance of oxycodone may be slightly reduced in this patient population when compared to younger patients.

Hepatic Impairment

In a pharmacokinetic study of oxycodone in patients with end-stage liver disease, oxycodone plasma clearance decreased and the elimination half-life increased. Care should be exercised when oxycodone is used in patients with hepatic impairment.

Renal Impairment

In a study of patients with end stage renal impairment, mean elimination half-life was prolonged in uremic patients due to increased volume of distribution and reduced clearance. Oxycodone should be used with caution in patients with renal impairment.

ADVERSE REACTIONS

Serious adverse reactions that may be associated with PERCOCET tablet use include respiratory depression, apnea, respiratory arrest, circulatory depression, hypotension, and shock (see OVERDOSAGE).

The most frequently observed non-serious adverse reactions include lightheadedness, dizziness, drowsiness or sedation, nausea, and vomiting. These effects seem to be more prominent in ambulatory than in nonambulatory patients, and some of these adverse reactions may be alleviated if the patient lies down. Other adverse reactions include euphoria, dysphoria, constipation, and pruritus.

Hypersensitivity reactions may include: Skin eruptions, urticarial, erythematous skin reactions. Hematologic reactions may include: Thrombocytopenia, neutropenia, pancytopenia, hemolytic anemia. Rare cases of agranulocytosis has likewise been associated with acetaminophen use. In high doses, the most serious adverse effect is a dose-dependent, potentially fatal hepatic necrosis. Renal tubular necrosis and hypoglycemic coma also may occur.

Other adverse reactions obtained from postmarketing experiences with PERCOCET tablets are listed by organ system and in decreasing order of severity and/or frequency as follows:

Body as a Whole

Anaphylactoid reaction, allergic reaction, malaise, asthenia, fatigue, chest pain, fever, hypothermia, thirst, headache, increased sweating, accidental overdose, non-accidental overdose

Cardiovascular

Hypotension, hypertension, tachycardia, orthostatic hypotension, bradycardia, palpitations, dysrhythmias

Central and Peripheral Nervous System

Stupor, tremor, paraesthesia, hypoaesthesia, lethargy, seizures, anxiety, mental impairment, agitation, cerebral edema, confusion, dizziness

Fluid and Electrolyte

Dehydration, hyperkalemia, metabolic acidosis, respiratory alkalosis

Gastrointestinal

Dyspepsia, taste disturbances, abdominal pain, abdominal distention, sweating increased, diarrhea, dry mouth, flatulence, gastrointestinal disorder, nausea, vomiting, pancreatitis, intestinal obstruction, ileus

Hepatic

Transient elevations of hepatic enzymes, increase in bilirubin, hepatitis, hepatic failure, jaundice, hepatotoxicity, hepatic disorder

Hearing and Vestibular

Hearing loss, tinnitus

Hematologic

Thrombocytopenia

Hypersensitivity

Acute anaphylaxis, angioedema, asthma, bronchospasm, laryngeal edema, urticaria, anaphylactoid reaction

Metabolic and Nutritional

Hypoglycemia, hyperglycemia, acidosis, alkalosis

Musculoskeletal

Myalgia, rhabdomyolysis

Ocular

Miosis, visual disturbances, red eye

Psychiatric

Drug dependence, drug abuse, insomnia, confusion, anxiety, agitation, depressed level of consciousness, nervousness, hallucination, somnolence, depression, suicide

Respiratory System

Bronchospasm, dyspnea, hyperpnea, pulmonary edema, tachypnea, aspiration, hypoventilation, laryngeal edema

Skin and Appendages

Erythema, urticaria, rash, flushing

Urogenital

Interstitial nephritis, papillary necrosis, proteinuria, renal insufficiency and failure, urinary retention

DRUG ABUSE AND DEPENDENCE

PERCOCET tablets are a Schedule II controlled substance. Oxycodone is a mu-agonist opioid with an abuse liability similar to morphine. Oxycodone, like morphine and other opioids used in analgesia, can be abused and is subject to criminal diversion.

Drug addiction is defined as an abnormal, compulsive use, use for non-medical purposes of a substance despite physical, psychological, occupational or interpersonal difficulties resulting from such use, and continued use despite harm or risk of harm. Drug addiction is a treatable disease, utilizing a multi-disciplinary approach, but relapse is common. Opioid addiction is relatively rare in patients with chronic pain but may be more common in individuals who have a past history of alcohol or substance abuse or dependence. Pseudoaddiction refers to pain relief seeking behavior of patients whose pain is poorly managed. It is considered an iatrogenic effect of ineffective pain management. The health care provider must assess continuously the psychological and clinical condition of a pain patient in order to distinguish addiction from pseudoaddiction and thus, be able to treat the pain adequately.

Physical dependence on a prescribed medication does not signify addiction. Physical dependence involves the occurrence of a withdrawal syndrome when there is sudden reduction or cessation in drug use or if an opiate antagonist is administered. Physical dependence can be detected after a few days of opioid therapy. However, clinically significant physical dependence is only seen after several weeks of relatively high dosage therapy. In this case, abrupt discontinuation of the opioid may result in a withdrawal syndrome. If the discontinuation of opioids is therapeutically indicated, gradual tapering of the drug over a 2-week period will prevent withdrawal symptoms. The severity of the withdrawal syndrome depends primarily on the daily dosage of the opioid, the duration of therapy and medical status of the individual.

The withdrawal syndrome of oxycodone is similar to that of morphine. This syndrome is characterized by yawning, anxiety, increased heart rate and blood pressure, restlessness, nervousness, muscle aches, tremor, irritability, chills alternating with hot flashes, salivation, anorexia, severe sneezing, lacrimation, rhinorrhea, dilated pupils, diaphoresis, piloerection, nausea, vomiting, abdominal cramps, diarrhea and insomnia, and pronounced weakness and depression. "Drug-seeking" behavior is very common in addicts and drug abusers. Drug-seeking tactics include emergency calls or visits near the end of office hours, refusal to undergo appropriate examination, testing or referral, repeated "loss" of prescriptions, tampering with prescriptions and reluctance to provide prior medical records or contact information for other treating physician(s). "Doctor Shopping" to obtain additional prescriptions is common among drug abusers and people suffering from untreated infection.

Abuse and addiction are separate and distinct from physical dependence and tolerance. Physicians should be aware that addiction may not be accompanied by concurrent tolerance and symptoms of physical dependence in all addicts. In addition, abuse of opioids can occur in the absence of true addiction and is characterized by misuse for non-medical purposes, often in combination with other psychoactive substances. Oxycodone, like other opioids, has been diverted for non-medical use. Careful record-keeping of prescribing information, including quantity, frequency, and renewal requests is strongly advised.

Proper assessment of the patient, proper prescribing practices, periodic re-evaluation of therapy, and proper dispensing and storage are appropriate measures that help to limit abuse of opioid drugs.

Like other opioid medications, PERCOCET tablets are subject to the Federal Controlled Substances Act. After chronic use, PERCOCET tablets should not be discontinued abruptly when it is thought that the patient has become physically dependent on oxycodone.

Interactions with Alcohol and Drugs of Abuse
Oxycodone may be expected to have additive effects when used in conjunction with alcohol, other opioids, or illicit drugs that cause central nervous system depression.

OVERDOSAGE
Signs and Symptoms
Serious overdose with PERCOCET (Oxycodone and Acetaminophen Tablets, USP) is characterized by signs and symptoms of opioid and acetaminophen overdose. Oxycodone overdosage can be manifested by respiratory depression (a decrease in respiratory rate and/or tidal volume, Cheyne-Stokes respiration, cyanosis), extreme somnolence progressing to stupor or coma, skeletal muscle flaccidity, cold and clammy skin, pupillary constriction (pupils may be dilated in the setting of hypoxia), and sometimes bradycardia and hypotension. In severe overdosage, apnea, circulatory collapse, cardiac arrest and death may occur.

In acute acetaminophen overdosage, dose-dependent, potentially fatal hepatic necrosis is the most serious adverse effect. Renal tubular necrosis, hypoglycemic coma and thrombocytopenia may also occur.

In adults, hepatic toxicity has rarely been reported with acute overdoses of less than 10 grams and fatalities with less than 15 grams. Plasma acetaminophen levels >300 mcg/ml at 4 hours post-ingestion were associated with hepatic damage in 90% of patients; minimal hepatic damage is anticipated if plasma levels at 4 hours are <120 mcg/ml or <30 mcg/ml at 12 hours after ingestion.

Importantly, young children seem to be more resistant than adults to the hepatotoxic effect of an acetaminophen overdose. Despite this, the measures outlined below should be initiated in any adult or child suspected of having ingested an acetaminophen overdose.

Early symptoms following a potentially hepatotoxic overdose may include: nausea, vomiting, diaphoresis and general malaise. Clinical and laboratory evidence of hepatic toxicity may not be apparent until 48 to 72 hours post-ingestion.

Treatment
Primary attention should be given to the reestablishment of adequate respiratory exchange through provision of a patent airway and the institution of assisted or controlled ventilation. Supportive measures (including oxygen, intravenous fluids, and vasopressors) should be employed in the management of circulatory shock and pulmonary edema accompanying overdose as indicated. Cardiac arrest or arrhythmias may require cardiac massage or defibrillation.

The opioid antagonist naloxone hydrochloride is a specific antidote against respiratory depression which may result from overdosage or unusual sensitivity to opioids including oxycodone. Therefore, an appropriate dose of naloxone hydrochloride should be administered (usual initial adult dose 0.4 mg-2 mg) preferably by the intravenous route, simultaneously with efforts at respiratory resuscitation. Since the duration of action of oxycodone may exceed that of the antagonist, the patient should be kept under continued surveillance and repeated doses of the antagonist should be administered as needed to maintain adequate respiration. Opioid antagonists should not be administered in the absence of clinically significant respiratory of circulatory depression secondary to oxycodone overdose. In patients who are physically dependent on any opioid agonist including oxycodone, an abrupt or complete reversal of opioid effects may precipitate an acute abstinence syndrome. The severity of the withdrawal syndrome produced will depend on the degree of physical dependence and the dose of the antagonist administered. Please see the prescribing information for the specific opioid antagonist for details of their proper use.

Gastric emptying and/or lavage may be useful in removing unabsorbed drug. This procedure is recommended as soon as possible after ingestion, even if the patient has vomited spontaneously. After lavage and/or emesis, administration of activated charcoal, as a slurry, is beneficial, if less than three hours have passed since ingestion. Charcoal adsorption should not be employed prior to lavage and emesis.

If an acetaminophen overdose is suspected, the stomach should be promptly emptied by lavage. A serum acetaminophen assay should be obtained as soon as possible, but no sooner than 4 hours following ingestion. Liver function studies should be obtained initially and repeated at 24-hour intervals. The antidote N-acetylcysteine (NAC) should be administered as early as possible, preferably within 16 hours of the overdose ingestion, but in any case within 24 hours. As a guide to treatment of acute ingestion, the acetaminophen level can be plotted against time since ingestion on a nomogram (Rumack-Matthew). The upper toxic line on the nomogram is equivalent to 200 mcg/ml at 4 hours while the lower line is equivalent to 50 mcg/ml at 12 hours. If serum level is above the lower line, and entire course of N-acetylcysteine treatment should be instituted. NAC therapy should be withheld if the acetaminophen level is below the lower line.

The toxicity of oxycodone and acetaminophen in combination is unknown.

DOSAGE AND ADMINISTRATION
Dosage should be adjusted according to the severity of the pain and the response of the patient. It may occasionally be necessary to exceed the usual dosage recommended below in cases of more severe pain or in those patients who have become tolerant to the analgesic effect of opioids. If pain is constant, the opioid analgesic should be given at regular intervals on an around-the-clock schedule. PERCOCET tablets are given orally.

Percocet 2.5 mg/325 mg
The usual adult dosage is one or 2 tablets every 6 hours. The total daily dose of acetaminophen should not exceed 4 grams.

Percocet 5 mg/325 mg; Percocet 7.5 mg/500 mg; Percocet 10 mg/650 mg
The usual adult dosage is one tablet every 6 hours as needed for pain. The total daily dose of acetaminophen should not exceed 4 grams.

Percocet 7.5 mg/325 mg; Percocet 10 mg/325 mg
The usual adult dosage is one tablet every 6 hours as needed for pain. The total daily dose of acetaminophen should not exceed 4 grams.

Strength	Maximal Daily Dose
Percocet 2.5 mg/325 mg	12 Tablets
Percocet 5 mg/325 mg	12 Tablets
Percocet 7.5 mg/325 mg	8 Tablets
Percocet 7.5 mg/500 mg	8 Tablets
Percocet 10 mg/325 mg	6 Tablets
Percocet 10 mg/650 mg	6 Tablets

Cessation of Therapy
In patients treated with PERCOCET tablets for more than a few weeks who no longer require therapy, doses should be tapered gradually to prevent signs and symptoms of withdrawal in the physically dependent patient.

HOW SUPPLIED
PERCOCET (Oxycodone and Acetaminophen Tablets, USP) is supplied as follows:
2.5 mg/325 mg
Pink, oval, tablet debossed with "PERCOCET" on one side and "2.5" on the other.
Bottles of 100   NDC 63481-627-70
5 mg/325 mg
Blue, round, tablet, debossed with "PERCOCET" and "5" on one side and bisect on the other.
Bottles of 100   NDC 63481-623-70
Bottles of 500   NDC 63481-623-85
Unit dose package of 100 tablets   NDC 63481-623-75
7.5 mg/325 mg
Peach, oval-shaped, tablet debossed with "PERCOCET" on one side and "7.5/325" on the other.
Bottles of 100   NDC 63481-628-70
7.5 mg/500 mg
Peach, capsule-shaped, tablet debossed with "PERCOCET" on one side and "7.5" on the other.
Bottles of 100   NDC 63481-621-70
10 mg/325 mg
Yellow, capsule-shaped, tablet debossed with "PERCOCET" on one side and "10/325" on the other.
Bottles of 100   NDC 63481-629-70
10 mg/650 mg
Yellow, oval, tablet debossed with "PERCOCET" on one side and "10" on the other.
Bottles of 100   NDC 63481-622-70
Store at 20° to 25°C (68° to 77°F). [see USP Controlled Room Temperature].
Dispense in a tight, light-resistant container as defined in the USP, with a child-resistant closure (as required).

DEA Order Form Required.
Manufactured for:
Endo Pharmaceuticals Inc.
Chadds Ford, Pennsylvania 19317
PERCOCET® is a Registered Trademark of Endo Pharmaceuticals Inc.
Copyright © Endo Pharmaceuticals Inc. 2006
Printed in U.S.A.   2000055/November, 2006
Shown in Product Identification Guide, page 309

PERCODAN®   C Ⅱ R
[perk 'o-dan]
(Oxycodone and Aspirin Tablets, USP)
Rx only

DESCRIPTION
Each PERCODAN Tablet contains:
Oxycodone Hydrochloride, USP   4.8355 mg[1]
Aspirin, USP   325 mg
PERCODAN Tablets also contain the following inactive ingredients: D&C Yellow 10, FD&C Yellow 6, microcrystalline cellulose and corn starch.
The oxycodone hydrochloride component is Morphinan-6-one, 4,5-epoxy-14-hydroxy-3-methoxy-17-methyl-, hydrochloride, (5a)-, a white to off-white, hygroscopic crystals or powder, odorless, soluble in water; slightly soluble in alcohol and is represented by the following structural formula:

$C_{18}H_{21}NO_4 \cdot HCl$ MW 351.82

The aspirin component is 2-(acetyloxy)-, Benzoic acid, a white crystal, commonly tabular or needle-like, or white, crystalline powder. Is odorless or has a faint odor. Is stable in dry air; in moist air it gradually hydrolyzes to salicylic and acetic acids. Slightly soluble in water; freely soluble in alcohol; soluble in chloroform and in ether; sparingly soluble in absolute ether and is represented by the following structural formula:

$C_9H_8O_4$ MW 180.16

14.8355 mg oxycodone HCl is equivalent to 4.3346 mg of oxycodone as the free base.

CLINICAL PHARMACOLOGY
Central Nervous System
Oxycodone is a semisynthetic pure opioid agonist whose principal therapeutic action is analgesia. Other pharmacological effects of oxycodone include anxiolysis, euphoria and feelings of relaxation. These effects are mediated by receptors (notably μ and κ) in the central nervous system for endogenous opioid-like compounds such as endorphins and enkephalins. Oxycodone produces respiratory depression through direct activity at respiratory centers in the brain stem and depresses the cough reflex by direct effect on the center of the medulla.

Aspirin (acetylsalicylic acid) works by inhibiting the body's production of prostaglandins, including prostaglandins involved in inflammation. Prostaglandins cause pain sensations by stimulating muscle contractions and dilating blood vessels throughout the body. In the CNS, aspirin works on the hypothalamus heat-regulating center to reduce fever, however, other mechanisms may be involved.

Gastrointestinal Tract and Other Smooth Muscle
Oxycodone reduces motility by increasing smooth muscle tone in the stomach and duodenum. In the small intestine, digestion of food is delayed by decreases in propulsive contractions. Other opioid effects include contraction of biliary tract smooth muscle, spasm of the Sphincter of Oddi, increased ureteral and bladder sphincter tone, and a reduction in uterine tone.

Aspirin can produce gastrointestinal injury (lesions, ulcers) through a mechanism that is not yet completely understood, but may involve a reduction in eicosanoid synthesis by the gastric mucosa. Decreased production of prostaglandins may compromise the defenses of the gastric mucosa and the activity of substances involved in tissue repair and ulcer healing.

Cardiovascular System

Oxycodone may produce a release of histamine and may be associated with orthostatic hypotension, and other symptoms, such as pruritus, flushing, red eyes, and sweating.

Platelet Aggregation

Aspirin affects platelet aggregation by irreversibly inhibiting prostaglandin cyclo-oxygenase. This effect lasts for the life of the platelet and prevents the formation of the platelet aggregating factor thromboxane A2. Nonacetylated salicylates do not inhibit this enzyme and have no effect on platelet aggregation. At somewhat higher doses, aspirin reversibly inhibits the formation of prostaglandin 12 (prostacyclin), which is an arterial vasodilator and inhibits platelet aggregation.

Pharmacokinetics

Absorption and Distribution

The mean absolute oral bioavailability of oxycodone in cancer patients was reported to be about 87%. Oxycodone has been shown to be 45% bound to human plasma proteins *in vitro*. The volume of distribution after intravenous administration is 211.9 ±186.6 L.

Aspirin is hydrolyzed primarily to salicylic acid in the gut wall and during first-pass metabolism through the liver. Salicylic acid is absorbed rapidly from the stomach, but most of the absorption occurs in the proximal small intestine. Following absorption, salicylate is distributed to most body tissues and fluids, including fetal tissues, breast milk, and the CNS. High concentrations are found in the liver and kidneys. Salicylate is variably bound to serum proteins, particularly albumin.

Metabolism and Elimination

A high portion of oxycodone is N-dealkylated to noroxycodone during first-pass metabolism. Oxymorphone, is formed by the O-demethylation of oxycodone. The metabolism of oxycodone to oxymorphone is catalyzed by CYP2D6. Free and conjugated noroxycodone, free and conjugated oxycodone, and oxymorphone are excreted in human urine following a single oral dose of oxycodone. Approximately 8% to 14% of the dose is excreted as free oxycodone over 24 hours after administration. Following a single, oral dose of oxycodone, the mean ± SD elimination half-life is 3.51 ± 1.43 hours.

The biotransformation of aspirin occurs primarily in the liver by the microsomal enzyme system. With a plasma half-life of approximately 15 minutes, aspirin is rapidly hydrolyzed to salicylate. At low doses, salicylate elimination follows first-order kinetics. The plasma half-life of salicylate is approximately 2 to 3 hours.

Approximately 10% of aspirin is excreted as unchanged salicylate in the urine. The major metabolites excreted in the urine are salicyluric acid (75%), salicyl phenolic glucuronide (10%), salicyl acyl glucuronide (5%), and gentisic and gentisuric acid (less than 1%) each. Eighty to 100% of a single dose is excreted in the urine within 24 to 72 hours.

INDICATIONS AND USAGE

PERCODAN tablets are indicated for the management of moderate to moderately severe pain.

CONTRAINDICATIONS

PERCODAN tablets are contraindicated in patients with known hypersensitivity to oxycodone or aspirin, and in any situation where opioids or aspirin are contraindicated. Aspirin is contraindicated for patients with hemophilia.

Reye Syndrome: Aspirin should not be used in children or teenagers for viral infections, with or without fever, because of the risk of Reye syndrome with concomitant use of aspirin in certain viral illnesses.

Allergy: Aspirin is contraindicated in patients with known allergy to nonsteroidal anti-inflammatory drug products and in patients with the syndrome of asthma, rhinitis, and nasal polyps. Aspirin may cause severe urticaria, angioedema, or bronchospasm (asthma).

Oxycodone is contraindicated in patients with known hypersensitivity to oxycodone. Oxycodone is contraindicated in any situation where opioids are contraindicated including patients with significant respiratory depression (in unmonitored settings or the absence of resuscitative equipment) and patients with acute or severe bronchial asthma or hypercarbia. Oxycodone is contraindicated in the setting of suspected or known paralytic ileus.

WARNINGS

Misuse and Abuse of Opioids

Oxycodone is an opioid agonist of the morphine-type. Such drugs are sought by drug abusers and people with addiction disorders and are subject to criminal diversion.

Oxycodone can be abused in a manner similar to other opioid agonists, legal or illicit. This should be considered when prescribing or dispensing PERCODAN tablets in situations where the physician or pharmacist is concerned about an increased risk of misuse, abuse, or diversion. Concerns about misuse, addiction, and diversion should not prevent the proper management of pain.

Healthcare professionals should contact their State Professional Licensing Board, or State Controlled Substances Authority for information on how to prevent and detect abuse or diversion of this product.

Administration of PERCODAN (Oxycodone and Aspirin Tablets, USP) tablets should be closely monitored for the following potentially serious adverse reactions and complications:

Respiratory Depression

Respiratory depression is a hazard with the use of oxycodone, one of the active ingredients in PERCODAN tablets, as with all opioid agonists. Elderly and debilitated patients are at particular risk for respiratory depression as are non-tolerant patients given large initial doses of oxycodone or when oxycodone is given in conjunction with other agents that depress respiration. Oxycodone should be used with extreme caution in patients with acute asthma, chronic obstructive pulmonary disorder (COPD), cor pulmonale, or preexisting respiratory impairment. In such patients, even usual therapeutic doses of oxycodone may decrease respiratory drive to the point of apnea. In these patients alternative non-opioid analgesics should be considered, and opioids should be employed only under careful medical supervision at the lowest effective dose.

In case of respiratory depression, a reversal agent such as naloxone hydrochloride may be utilized (see OVERDOSAGE).

Head Injury and Increased Intracranial Pressure

The respiratory depressant effects of opioids include carbon dioxide retention and secondary elevation of cerebrospinal fluid pressure, and may be markedly exaggerated in the presence of head injury, other intracranial lesions or a pre-existing increase in intracranial pressure. Oxycodone produces effects on pupillary response and consciousness which may obscure neurologic signs of worsening in patients with head injuries.

Hypotensive Effect

Oxycodone may cause severe hypotension particularly in individuals whose ability to maintain blood pressure has been compromised by a depleted blood volume, or after concurrent administration with drugs which compromise vasomotor tone such as phenothiazines. Oxycodone, like all opioid analgesics of the morphine-type, should be administered with caution to patients in circulatory shock, since vasodilation produced by the drug may further reduce cardiac output and blood pressure. Oxycodone may produce orthostatic hypotension in ambulatory patients.

Alcohol Warning

Patients who consume three or more alcoholic drinks every day should be counseled about the bleeding risks involved with chronic, heavy alcohol use while taking aspirin.

Coagulation Abnormalities

Even low doses of aspirin can inhibit platelet function leading to an increase in bleeding time. This can adversely affect patients with inherited (hemophilia) or acquired (liver disease or vitamin K deficiency) bleeding disorders.

GI Side Effects

GI side effects include stomach pain, heartburn, nausea, vomiting, and gross GI bleeding. Although minor upper GI symptoms, such as dyspepsia, are common and can occur anytime during therapy, physicians should remain alert for signs of ulceration and bleeding, even in the absence of previous GI symptoms. Physicians should inform patients about the signs and symptoms of GI side effects and what steps to take if they occur.

Peptic Ulcer Disease

Patients with a history of active peptic ulcer disease should avoid using aspirin, which can cause gastric mucosal irritation and bleeding.

PRECAUTIONS

General

Opioid analgesics should be used with caution when combined with CNS depressant drugs, and should be reserved for cases where the benefits of opioid analgesia outweigh the known risks of respiratory depression, altered mental state, and postural hypotension.

PERCODAN tablets should be given with caution to patients with CNS depression, elderly or debilitated patients, patients with severe impairment of hepatic, pulmonary, or renal function, hypothyroidism, Addison's disease, prostatic hypertrophy, urethral stricture, acute alcoholism, delirium tremens, kyphoscoliosis with respiratory depression, myxedema, and toxic psychosis.

PERCODAN tablets may obscure the diagnosis or clinical course in patients with acute abdominal conditions. Oxycodone may aggravate convulsions in patients with convulsive disorders, and all opioids may induce or aggravate seizures in some clinical settings.

Following administration of PERCODAN tablets, anaphylactic reactions have been reported in patients with a known hypersensitivity to codeine, a compound with a structure similar to morphine and oxycodone. The frequency of this possible cross-sensitivity is unknown.

Aspirin has been associated with elevated hepatic enzymes, blood urea nitrogen and serum creatinine, hyperkalemia, proteinuria, and prolonged bleeding time.

Hemorrhage

Aspirin may increase the likelihood of hemorrhage due to its effect on the gastric mucosa and platelet function (prolongation of bleeding time). Salicylates should be used with caution in the presence of peptic ulcer or coagulation abnormalities.

Pregnancy

Aspirin can cause fetal harm when administered to a pregnant woman. Salicylates readily cross the placenta and by inhibiting prostaglandin synthesis, may cause constriction of ductus arteriosus, resulting in pulmonary hypertension and increased fetal mortality and, possibly other untoward fetal effects. Aspirin use in pregnancy can also result in alteration in maternal and neonatal hemostasis mechanisms. Maternal aspirin use during later stages of pregnancy may cause low birth weight, increased incidence of intracranial hemorrhage in premature infants, stillbirths and neonatal death. The use of aspirin during pregnancy especially in the third trimester should be avoided. If PERCODAN tablets are used during pregnancy, or if the patient becomes pregnant while taking this drug, the patient should be apprised of the potential hazard to the fetus.

Renal Failure

Avoid aspirin in patients with severe renal failure (glomerular filtration rate less than 10 mL/minute).

Hepatic Insufficiency

Avoid aspirin in patients with severe hepatic insufficiency.

Interactions with Other CNS Depressants

Patients receiving other opioid analgesics, general anesthetics, phenothiazines, other tranquilizers, centrally-acting anti-emetics, sedative-hypnotics or other CNS depressants (including alcohol) concomitantly with PERCODAN tablets may exhibit an additive CNS depression. When such combined therapy is contemplated, the dose of one or both agents should be reduced.

Interactions with Mixed Agonist/Antagonist Opioid Analgesics

Agonist/antagonist analgesics (i.e., pentazocine, nalbuphine, and butorphanol) should be administered with caution to a patient who has received or is receiving a course of therapy with a pure opioid agonist analgesic such as oxycodone. In this situation, mixed agonist/antagonist analgesics may reduce the analgesic effect of oxycodone and/or may precipitate withdrawal symptoms in these patients.

Ambulatory Surgery and Postoperative Use

Oxycodone and other morphine-like opioids have been shown to decrease bowel motility. Ileus is a common postoperative complication, especially after intra-abdominal surgery with use of opioid analgesia. Caution should be taken to monitor for decreased bowel motility in postoperative patients receiving opioids. Standard supportive therapy should be implemented.

Use in Pancreatic/Biliary Tract Disease

Oxycodone may cause spasm of the sphincter of Oddi and should be used with caution in patients with biliary tract disease, including acute pancreatitis. Opioids like oxycodone may cause increases in the serum amylase level.

Tolerance and Physical Dependence

Tolerance is the need for increasing doses of opioids to maintain a defined effect such as analgesia (in the absence of disease progression or other external factors). Physical dependence is manifested by withdrawal symptoms after abrupt discontinuation of a drug or upon administration of an antagonist. Physical dependence and tolerance are not unusual during chronic opioid therapy.

The opioid abstinence or withdrawal syndrome is characterized by some or all of the following: restlessness, lacrimation, rhinorrhea, yawning, perspiration, chills, myalgia, and mydriasis. Other symptoms also may develop, including: irritability, anxiety, backache, joint pain, weakness, abdominal cramps, insomnia, nausea, anorexia, vomiting, diarrhea, or increased blood pressure, respiratory rate or heart rate.

In general, opioids should not be abruptly discontinued (see DOSAGE AND ADMINISTRATION: Cessation of Therapy).

Information for Patients/Caregivers

The following information should be provided to patients receiving PERCODAN tablets by their physician, nurse, pharmacist, or caregiver:

1. Patients should be aware that PERCODAN tablets contain oxycodone, which is a morphine-like substance.
2. Patients should be instructed to keep PERCODAN tablets in a secure place out of the reach of children. In the case of accidental ingestions, emergency medical care should be sought immediately.
3. When PERCODAN tablets are no longer needed, the unused tablets should be destroyed by flushing down the toilet.

4. Patients should be advised not to adjust the medication dose themselves. Instead, they must consult with their prescribing physician.

5. Patients should be advised that PERCODAN tablets may impair mental and/or physical ability required for the performance of potentially hazardous tasks (e.g., driving, operating heavy machinery).

6. Patients should not combine PERCODAN tablets with alcohol, opioid analgesics, tranquilizers, sedatives, or other CNS depressants unless under the recommendation and guidance of a physician. When co-administered with another CNS depressant, PERCODAN tablets can cause dangerous additive central nervous system or respiratory depression, which can result in serious injury or death.

7. The safe use of PERCODAN tablets during pregnancy has not been established; thus, women who are planning to become pregnant or are pregnant should consult with their physician before taking PERCODAN tablets.

8. Nursing mothers should consult with their physicians about whether to discontinue nursing or discontinue PERCODAN tablets because of the potential for serious adverse reactions to nursing infants.

9. Patients who are treated with PERCODAN tablets for more than a few weeks should be advised not to abruptly discontinue the medication. Patients should consult with their physician for a gradual discontinuation dose schedule to taper off the medication.

10. Patients should be advised that PERCODAN tablets are a potential drug of abuse. They should protect it from theft, and it should never be given to anyone other than the individual for whom it was prescribed.

11. Patients should be advised that PERCODAN tablets may cause or worsen constipation, as generally occurs with all opioids. They should discuss any past history of constipation with their prescribing physician so a management plan may be initiated.

Laboratory Tests

Although oxycodone may cross-react with some drug urine tests, no available studies were found which determined the duration of detectability of oxycodone in urine drug screens. However, based on pharmacokinetic data, the approximate duration of detectability for a single dose of oxycodone is roughly estimated to be one to two days following drug exposure.

Urine testing for opiates may be performed to determine illicit drug use and for medical reasons such as evaluation of patients with altered states of consciousness or monitoring efficacy of drug rehabilitation efforts. The preliminary identification of opiates in urine involves the use of an immunoassay screening and thin-layer chromatography (TLC). Gas chromatography/mass spectrometry (GC/MS) may be utilized as a third-stage identification step in the medical investigational sequence for opiate testing after immunoassay and TLC. The identities of 6-keto opiates (e.g., oxycodone) can further be differentiated by the analysis of their methoxime-trimethylsilyl (MO-TMS) derivative.

Drug/Drug Interactions with Oxycodone

Opioid analgesics may enhance the neuromuscular-blocking action of skeletal muscle relaxants and produce an increase in the degree of respiratory depression.

Patients receiving CNS depressants such as other opioid analgesics, general anesthetics, phenothiazines, other tranquilizers, centrally-acting anti-emetics, sedative-hypnotics or other CNS depressants (including alcohol) concomitantly with PERCODAN tablets may exhibit an additive CNS depression. When such combined therapy is contemplated, the dose of one or both agents should be reduced.

Agonist/antagonist analgesics (i.e., pentazocine, nalbuphine, naltrexone, and butorphanol) should be administered with caution to a patient who has received or is receiving a pure opioid agonist such as oxycodone. These agonist/antagonist analgesics may reduce the analgesic effect of oxycodone or may precipitate withdrawal symptoms.

Drug/Drug Interactions with Aspirin

Angiotensin Converting Enzyme (ACE) Inhibitors: The hyponatremic and hypotensive effects of ACE inhibitors may be diminished by the concomitant administration of aspirin due to its indirect effect on the renin-angiotensin conversion pathway.

Acetazolamide: Concurrent use of aspirin and acetazolamide can lead to high serum concentrations of acetazolamide (and toxicity) due to competition at the renal tubule for secretion.

Anticoagulant Therapy (Heparin and Warfarin): Patients on anticoagulation therapy are at increased risk for bleeding because of drug-drug interactions and the effect on platelets. Aspirin can displace warfarin from protein binding sites, leading to prolongation of both the prothrombin time and the bleeding time. Aspirin can increase the anticoagulant activity of heparin, increasing bleeding risk.

Anticonvulsants: Salicylate can displace protein-bound phenytoin and valproic acid, leading to a decrease in the to-

tal concentration of phenytoin and an increase in serum valproic acid levels.

Beta Blockers: The hypotensive effects of beta blockers may be diminished by the concomitant administration of aspirin due to inhibition of renal prostaglandins, leading to decreased renal blood flow, and salt and fluid retention.

Diuretics: The effectiveness of diuretics in patients with underlying renal or cardiovascular disease may be diminished by the concomitant administration of aspirin due to inhibition of renal prostaglandins, leading to decreased renal blood flow and salt and fluid retention.

Methotrexate: Aspirin may enhance the serious side and toxicity of methotrexate due to displacement from its plasma protein binding sites and/or reduced renal clearance.

Nonsteroidal Anti-inflammatory Drugs (NSAID's): The concurrent use of aspirin with other NSAID's should be avoided because this may increase bleeding or lead to decreased renal function. Aspirin may enhance the serious side effects and toxicity of ketorolac, due to displacement from its plasma protein binding sites and/or reduced renal clearance.

Oral Hypoglycemics Agents: Aspirin may increase the serum glucose-lowering action of insulin and sulfonylureas leading to hypoglycemia.

Uricosuric Agents: Salicylates antagonize the uricosuric action of probenecid or sulfinpyrazone.

Drug/Laboratory Test Interactions

Depending on the sensitivity/specificity and the test methodology, the individual components of PERCODAN tablets may cross-react with assays used in the preliminary detection of cocaine (primary urinary metabolite, benzoylecgonine) or marijuana (cannabinoids) in human urine. A more specific alternate chemical method must be used in order to obtain a confirmed analytical result. The preferred confirmatory method is gas chromatography/mass spectrometry (GC/MS). Moreover, clinical considerations and professional judgment should be applied to any drug-of-abuse test result, particularly when preliminary positive results are used.

Salicylates may increase the protein bound iodine (PBI) result by competing for the protein binding sites on prealbumin and possibly thyroid-binding globulins.

Carcinogenesis, Mutagenesis, Impairment of Fertility

Carcinogenesis

Animal studies to evaluate the carcinogenic potential of oxycodone and aspirin have not been performed.

Mutagenesis

The combination of oxycodone and aspirin has not been evaluated for mutagenicity. Oxycodone alone was negative in a bacterial reverse mutation assay (Ames), an *in vitro* chromosome aberration assay with human lymphocytes without metabolic activation and an *in vivo* mouse micronucleus assay. Oxycodone was clastogenic in the human lymphocyte chromosomal assay in the presence of metabolic activation and in the mouse lymphoma assay with or without metabolic activation. Aspirin induced chromosome aberrations in cultured human fibroblasts.

Fertility

Animal studies to evaluate the effects of oxycodone on fertility have not been performed. Aspirin has been shown to inhibit ovulation in rats.

Pregnancy

Teratogenic Effects

Oxycodone: *Pregnancy Category B*

Reproduction studies in rats and rabbits demonstrated that oral administration of oxycodone was not teratogenic or embryo-fetal toxic.

Aspirin: Pregnancy Category D (see PRECAUTIONS)

Salicylates readily cross the placenta and by inhibiting prostaglandin synthesis, may cause constriction of ductus arteriosus resulting in pulmonary hypertension and increased fetal mortality and, possibly other untoward fetal effects. Aspirin use in pregnancy can also result in alteration in maternal and neonatal hemostasis mechanisms. Maternal aspirin use during later stages of pregnancy may cause low birth weight, increased incidence of intracranial hemorrhage in premature infants, stillbirths and neonatal death. Use during pregnancy, especially in the third trimester, should be avoided.

Safe use of PERCODAN (Oxycodone and Aspirin Tablets, USP) in pregnancy has not been established relative to possible adverse effects on fetal development. Therefore, PERCODAN tablets should not be used in pregnant women unless, in the judgment of the physician, the potential benefits outweigh the possible hazards.

Nonteratogenic Effects

Opioids can cross the placental barrier and have the potential to cause neonatal respiratory depression. Opioid use during pregnancy may result in a physically drug-dependent fetus. After birth, the neonate may suffer severe withdrawal symptoms. Aspirin may produce anemia, ante- or postpartum hemorrhage, prolonged gestation and labor, and oligohydramnios.

Labor and Delivery

PERCODAN tablets are not recommended for use in women during and immediately prior to labor and delivery due to its potential effects on respiratory function in the newborn. Aspirin should be avoided one week prior to and during labor and delivery because it can result in excessive blood loss at delivery. Prolonged gestation and prolonged labor due to prostaglandin inhibition have been reported.

Nursing Mothers

Ordinarily, nursing should not be undertaken while a patient is receiving PERCODAN tablets because of the possibility of sedation and/or respiratory depression in the infant. Oxycodone is excreted in breast milk in low concentrations, and there have been rare reports of somnolence and lethargy in babies of nursing mothers taking an oxycodone/acetaminophen product. Salicylic acid has also been detected in breast milk. Adverse effects on platelet function in the nursing infant exposed to aspirin in breast milk may be a potential risk. Furthermore, the risk of **Reye Syndrome** caused by salicylate in breast milk is unknown. Because of the potential for serious adverse reactions in nursing infants, a decision should be made whether to discontinue nursing or to discontinue the drug, taking into account the potential benefits to the woman and the possible hazards to the nursing infant.

Pediatric Use

PERCODAN tablets should not be administered to pediatric patients. Reye Syndrome is a rare but serious disease which can follow flu or chicken pox in children and teenagers. While the cause of Reye Syndrome is unknown, some reports claim aspirin (or salicylates) may increase the risk of developing this disease.

Geriatric Use

Special precaution should be given when determining the dosing amount and frequency of PERCODAN tablets for geriatric patients, since clearance of oxycodone may be slightly reduced in this patient population when compared to younger patients.

Hepatic Impairment

In a pharmacokinetic study of oxycodone in patients with end-stage liver disease, oxycodone plasma clearance decreased and the elimination half-life increased. Care should be exercised when oxycodone is used in patients with hepatic impairment.

Renal Impairment

In a study of patients with end stage renal impairment, mean elimination half-life was prolonged in uremic patients due to increased volume of distribution and reduced clearance. Oxycodone should be used with caution in patients with renal impairment.

ADVERSE REACTIONS

Serious adverse reactions that may be associated with PERCODAN tablet use include respiratory depression, apnea, respiratory arrest, circulatory depression, hypotension, and shock (see OVERDOSAGE).

The most frequently observed non-serious adverse reactions include lightheadedness, dizziness, drowsiness or sedation, nausea, and vomiting. These effects seem to be more prominent in ambulatory than in nonambulatory patients, and some of these adverse reactions may be alleviated if the patient lies down. Other adverse reactions include euphoria, dysphoria, constipation and pruritus.

Aspirin may increase the likelihood of hemorrhage due to its effect on the gastric mucosa and platelet function. Furthermore, aspirin has the potential to cause anaphylaxis in hypersensitive patients as well as angioedema especially in patients with chronic urticaria.

Other adverse reactions due to aspirin use include anorexia, reversible hepatotoxicity, leukopenia, thrombocytopenia, purpura, decreased plasma iron concentration, and shortened erythrocyte survival time.

Other adverse reactions obtained from postmarketing experiences with PERCODAN tablets are listed by organ system and in decreasing order of severity and/or frequency as follows:

Body as a Whole

allergic reaction, malaise, asthenia, headache, anaphylaxis, fever, hypothermia, thirst, increased sweating, accident, accidental overdose, non-accidental overdose.

Cardiovascular

tachycardia, dysrhythmias, hypotension, orthostatic hypotension, bradycardia, palpitations

Central and Peripheral Nervous System

stupor, paresthesia, agitation, cerebral edema, coma, confusion, dizziness, headache, subdural or intracranial hemorrhage, lethargy, seizures, anxiety, mental impairment

Fluid and Electrolyte

dehydration, hyperkalemia, metabolic acidosis, respiratory alkalosis

Gastrointestinal

hemorrhagic gastric/duodenal ulcer, gastric/peptic ulcer, dyspepsia, abdominal pain, diarrhea, eructation, dry mouth, gastrointestinal bleeding, intestinal perforation, nausea, vomiting, transient elevations of hepatic enzymes, hepatitis, Reye syndrome, pancreatitis, intestinal obstruction, ileus

Hearing and Vestibular
hearing loss, tinnitus. Patients with high frequency loss may have difficulty perceiving tinnitus. In these patients, tinnitus cannot be used as a clinical indicator of salicylism.

Hematologic
unspecified hemorrhage, purpura, reticulocytosis, prolongation of prothrombin time, disseminated intravascular coagulation, ecchymosis, thrombocytopenia

Hypersensitivity
acute anaphylaxis, angioedema, asthma, bronchospasm, laryngeal edema, urticaria, anaphylactoid reaction

Metabolic and Nutritional
hypoglycemia, hyperglycemia, acidosis, alkalosis

Musculoskeletal
rhabdomyolysis

Ocular
miosis, visual disturbances, red eye

Psychiatric
drug dependence, drug abuse, somnolence, depression, nervousness, hallucination

Reproductive
prolonged pregnancy and labor, stillbirths, lower birth weight infants, antepartum and postpartum bleeding, closure of patent ductus arteriosis

Respiratory System
bronchospasm, dyspnea, hyperpnea, pulmonary edema, tachypnea, aspiration, hypoventilation, laryngeal edema

Skin and Appendages
urticaria, rash, flushing

Urogenital
interstitial nephritis, papillary necrosis, proteinuria, renal insufficiency and failure, urinary retention

OVERDOSAGE

Signs and Symptoms
Serious overdose with PERCODAN (Oxycodone and Aspirin Tablets, USP) is characterized by signs and symptoms of opioid and salicylate overdose. Oxycodone overdosage can be manifested by respiratory depression (a decrease in respiratory rate and/or tidal volume, Cheyne-Stokes respiration, cyanosis), extreme somnolence progressing to stupor or coma, skeletal muscle flaccidity, cold and clammy skin, pupillary constriction (pupils may be dilated in the setting of hypoxia), and sometimes bradycardia and hypotension. In severe overdosage, apnea, circulatory collapse, cardiac arrest and death may occur. Early signs of acute aspirin (salicylate) overdose including tinnitus occur at plasma concentrations approaching 200 mcg/mL. Plasma concentrations of aspirin above 300 mcg/mL are toxic. Severe toxic effects are associated with levels above 400 mcg/mL. A single lethal dose of aspirin in adults is not known with certainty but death may be expected at 30 g. For real or suspected overdose, a Poison Control Center should be contacted immediately.

In acute salicylate overdose, severe acid-base and electrolyte disturbances may occur and are complicated by hyperthermia and dehydration, and coma. Respiratory alkalosis occurs early while hyperventilation is present, but is quickly followed by metabolic acidosis. Serious symptoms such as depression, coma, and respiratory failure progress rapidly.

Salicylism (chronic salicylate toxicity) may be noted by symptoms such as dizziness, tinnitus, difficulty hearing, nausea, vomiting, diarrhea, and mental confusion. More severe salicylism may result in respiratory alkalosis.

Treatment
Primary attention should be given to the reestablishment of adequate respiratory exchange through provision of a patent airway and the institution of assisted or controlled ventilation. Supportive measures (including oxygen, intravenous fluids, and vasopressors) should be employed in the management of circulatory shock and pulmonary edema accompanying overdose as indicated. Cardiac arrest or arrhythmias may require cardiac massage or defibrillation. Treatment of acid-base disturbances and electrolyte disorders is also important. Because of the concern over salicylate toxicity, acid-base status should be followed closely with serial blood gas and serum pH determinations.

The opioid antagonist naloxone hydrochloride is a specific antidote against respiratory depression which may result from overdosage or unusual sensitivity to opioids including oxycodone. Therefore, an appropriate dose of naloxone hydrochloride should be administered (usual initial adult dose 0.4 mg-2 mg) preferably by the intravenous route, simultaneously with efforts at respiratory resuscitation. Since the duration of action of oxycodone may exceed that of the antagonist, the patient should be kept under continued surveillance and repeated doses of the antagonist should be administered as needed to maintain adequate respiration. Opioid antagonists should not be administered in the absence of clinically significant respiratory or circulatory depression secondary to oxycodone overdose. In patients who are physically dependent on any opioid agonist including

oxycodone, an abrupt or complete reversal of opioid effects may precipitate an acute abstinence syndrome. The severity of the withdrawal syndrome produced will depend on the degree of physical dependence and the dose of the antagonist administered. Please see the prescribing information for the specific opioid antagonist for details of their proper use.

Gastric emptying and/or lavage may be useful in removing unabsorbed drug. This procedure is recommended as soon as possible after ingestion, even if the patient has vomited spontaneously. After lavage and/or emesis, administration of activated charcoal, as a slurry, is beneficial, if less than three hours have passed since ingestion. Charcoal adsorption should not be employed prior to lavage and emesis.

In severe cases of salicylate overdose, hyperthermia and hypovolemia are the major immediate threats to life. Children should be sponged with tepid water. Replacement fluid should be administered intravenously and augmented with correction of acidosis. Plasma electrolytes and pH should be monitored to promote alkaline diuresis of salicylate if renal function is normal. Infusion of glucose may be required to control hypoglycemia. With more severe acute toxicity respiratory alkalosis may occur.

Hemodialysis and peritoneal dialysis can be performed to reduce the body content of aspirin. In patients with renal insufficiency or in cases of life-threatening salicylate intoxication dialysis is usually required. Exchange transfusion may be indicated in infants and young children.

In case of real or suspected overdose, a poison control center should be consulted for the treatment of salicylism.

The toxicity of oxycodone and aspirin in combination is unknown.

DOSAGE AND ADMINISTRATION

Dosage should be adjusted according to the severity of the pain and the response of the patient. It may occasionally be necessary to exceed the usual dosage recommended below in cases of more severe pain or in those patients who have become tolerant to the analgesic effect of opioids. If pain is constant, the opioid analgesic should be given at regular intervals on an around-the-clock schedule. PERCODAN tablets are given orally.

The usual dosage is one tablet every 6 hours as needed for pain. The maximum daily dose of aspirin should not exceed 4 grams or 12 tablets.

Cessation of Therapy
In patients treated with PERCODAN tablets for more than a few weeks who no longer require therapy, doses should be tapered gradually to prevent signs and symptoms of withdrawal in the physically dependent patient.

DRUG ABUSE AND DEPENDENCE

PERCODAN tablets are a Schedule II controlled substance. Oxycodone is a mu-agonist opioid with an abuse liability similar to morphine. Oxycodone, like morphine and other opioids used in analgesia, can be abused and is subject to criminal diversion.

Drug addiction is defined as an abnormal, compulsive use, use for non-medical purposes of a substance despite physical, psychological, occupational or interpersonal difficulties resulting from such use, and continued use despite harm or risk of harm. Drug addiction is a treatable disease, utilizing a multi-disciplinary approach, but relapse is common. Opioid addiction is relatively rare in patients with chronic pain but may be more common in individuals who have a past history of alcohol or substance abuse or dependence. Pseudoaddiction refers to pain relief seeking behavior of patients whose pain is poorly managed. It is considered an iatrogenic effect of ineffective pain management. The health care provider must assess continuously the psychological and clinical condition of a pain patient in order to distinguish addiction from pseudoaddiction and thus, be able to treat the pain adequately.

Physical dependence on a prescribed medication does not signify addiction. Physical dependence involves the occurrence of a withdrawal syndrome when there is sudden reduction or cessation in drug use or if an opiate antagonist is administered. Physical dependence can be detected after a few days of opioid therapy. However, clinically significant physical dependence is only seen after several weeks of relatively high dosage therapy. In this case, abrupt discontinuation of the opioid may result in a withdrawal syndrome. If the discontinuation of opioids is therapeutically indicated, gradual tapering of the drug over a 2-week period will prevent withdrawal symptoms. The severity of the withdrawal syndrome depends primarily on the daily dosage of the opioid, the duration of therapy and medical status of the individual.

The withdrawal syndrome of oxycodone is similar to that of morphine. This syndrome is characterized by yawning, anxiety, increased heart rate and blood pressure, restlessness, nervousness, muscle aches, tremor, irritability, chills alternating with hot flashes, salivation, anorexia, severe sneezing, lacrimation, rhinorrhea, dilated pupils, diaphoresis, piloerection, nausea, vomiting, abdominal cramps, diarrhea and insomnia, and pronounced weakness and depression.

"Drug-seeking" behavior is very common in addicts and drug abusers. Drug-seeking tactics include emergency calls or visits near the end of office hours, refusal to undergo appropriate examination, testing or referral, repeated "loss" of prescriptions, tampering with prescriptions and reluctance to provide prior medical records or contact information for other treating physician(s). "Doctor shopping" to obtain additional prescriptions is common among drug abusers and people suffering from untreated addiction.

Abuse and addiction are separate and distinct from physical dependence and tolerance. Physicians should be aware that addiction may not be accompanied by concurrent tolerance and symptoms of physical dependence in all addicts. In addition, abuse of opioids can occur in the absence of true addiction and is characterized by misuse for non-medical purposes, often in combination with other psychoactive substances. Oxycodone, like other opioids, has been diverted for non-medical use. Careful record-keeping of prescribing information, including quantity, frequency, and renewal requests is strongly advised.

Proper assessment of the patient, proper prescribing practices, periodic re-evaluation of therapy, and proper dispensing and storage are appropriate measures that help to limit abuse of opioid drugs.

Like other opioid medications, PERCODAN tablets are subject to the Federal Controlled Substances Act. After chronic use, PERCODAN tablets should not be discontinued abruptly when it is thought that the patient has become physically dependent on oxycodone.

Interactions with Alcohol and Drugs of Abuse
Oxycodone may be expected to have additive effects when used in conjunction with alcohol, other opioids, or illicit drugs that cause central nervous system depression.

HOW SUPPLIED

PERCODAN (Oxycodone and Aspirin Tablets, USP), tablets are supplied as a yellow round tablet, scored and debossed with "PERCODAN" on one side and plain on the other side. Available in:

Bottles of 100   NDC 63481-121-70

Store at 25°C (77°F); excursions permitted to 15°-30°C (59°-86°F). [See USP Controlled Room Temperature.]

Dispense in a tight, light-resistant container as defined in the USP, with a child-resistant closure (as required).

DEA Order Form Required.

Manufactured for:
Endo Pharmaceuticals Inc.
Chadds Ford, Pennsylvania 19317
PERCODAN® is a Registered Trademark of Endo Pharmaceuticals
© 2010 Endo Pharmaceuticals
Printed in U.S.A. 2005700/March 2010
Shown in Product Identification Guide, page 309

SUPPRELIN® LA ℞
[*Suh-Preh-Lin El-Ay*]
(histrelin acetate)
subcutaneous implant

HIGHLIGHTS OF PRESCRIBING INFORMATION
These highlights do not include all the information needed to use Supprelin® LA safely and effectively. See full prescribing information for Supprelin LA.
Supprelin LA (histrelin acetate) subcutaneous implant
Initial U.S. Approval: 2007

―――――――INDICATIONS AND USAGE―――――――
Supprelin LA is a gonadotropin releasing hormone (GnRH) agonist indicated for the treatment of children with central precocious puberty (CPP) (1).

―――――DOSAGE AND ADMINISTRATION―――――
The recommended dose of Supprelin LA is one implant every 12 months. The implant is inserted subcutaneously in the inner aspect of the upper arm and provides continuous release of histrelin for 12 months of hormonal therapy (2).

―――――DOSAGE FORMS AND STRENGTHS―――――
Supprelin LA is available as a 50 mg histrelin acetate subcutaneous implant which delivers approximately 65 mcg histrelin acetate per day over 12 months (3).

―――――――CONTRAINDICATIONS―――――――
• History of hypersensitivity to gonadotropin releasing hormone (GnRH) or GnRH analogs (4).
• Pregnancy: Supprelin LA can cause fetal harm when used during pregnancy (4).

―――――WARNINGS AND PRECAUTIONS―――――
Initial Agonistic Action: Initial transient increases of estradiol and/or testosterone may cause a temporary worsening of symptoms (5.1).

―――――――ADVERSE REACTIONS―――――――
• The most common adverse reaction is implant site reaction (51.1%), including complications related to the insertion or removal of the implant (6).
• Adverse events related to suppression of endogenous sex steroid secretion may occur (6.1).

To report SUSPECTED ADVERSE REACTIONS, contact Endo Pharmaceuticals Solutions Inc., at 1-800-462-3636 or FDA at 1-800-FDA-1088 or www.fda.gov/medwatch

——USE IN SPECIFIC POPULATIONS——

Use of Supprelin LA in children less than 2 years of age is not recommended (8.4).

See 17 for PATIENT COUNSELING INFORMATION and FDA-approved patient labeling

Revised: 08/2009

FULL PRESCRIBING INFORMATION: CONTENTS*

* Sections or subsections omitted from the full prescribing information are not listed

---

FULL PRESCRIBING INFORMATION

1   INDICATIONS AND USAGE

Supprelin LA (histrelin acetate) subcutaneous implant is indicated for the treatment of children with central precocious puberty (CPP).

Children with CPP (neurogenic or idiopathic) have an early onset of secondary sexual characteristics (earlier than 8 years of age in females and 9 years of age in males). They also show a significantly advanced bone age that can result in diminished adult height attainment.

Prior to initiation of treatment a clinical diagnosis of CPP should be confirmed by measurement of blood concentrations of total sex steroids, luteinizing hormone (LH) and follicle stimulating hormone (FSH) following stimulation with a GnRH analog, and assessment of bone age versus chronological age. Baseline evaluations should include height and weight measurements, diagnostic imaging of the brain (to rule out intracranial tumor), pelvic/testicular/adrenal ultrasound (to rule out steroid secreting tumors), human chorionic gonadotropin levels (to rule out a chorionic gonadotropin secreting tumor), and adrenal steroids to exclude congenital adrenal hyperplasia.

2   DOSAGE AND ADMINISTRATION

2.1   Recommended Dose

The recommended dose of Supprelin LA is one implant every 12 months. Each implant contains 50 mg histrelin acetate. The implant is inserted subcutaneously in the inner aspect of the upper arm and provides continuous release of histrelin (65 mcg/day) for 12 months of hormonal therapy. Supprelin LA should be removed after 12 months of therapy (the implant has been designed to allow for a few additional weeks of histrelin acetate release, in order to allow flexibility of medical appointments). At the time an implant is removed, another implant may be inserted to continue therapy. Discontinuation of Supprelin LA should be considered at the discretion of the physician and at the appropriate time point for the onset of puberty (approximately 11 years for females and 12 years for males).

2.2   Recommended Procedure

This procedure section is intended to provide guidance for the insertion and removal of Supprelin LA. The actual procedure used, however, is at the discretion of the qualified healthcare provider performing the procedure.

Insertion of a new implant can proceed using the following **Suggested Insertion Procedure**. If a previous Supprelin LA implant must first be removed, please see the **Suggested Removal Procedure** instructions below.

Suggested Insertion Procedure

The supplies necessary to insert the implant, including the Insertion Tool and local anesthetic, are provided in a separate Implantation Kit that is shipped along with the implant. Please note that the implant should be kept refrigerated (2-8° C) in its sealed vial, pouch, and carton, until needed for the procedure. Once removed from refrigeration, the vial containing the implant (still in its unopened pouch and carton) may remain at room temperature for up to 7 days, if necessary, before being used. If not used in that time, the packaged implant may again be properly refrigerated until the expiration date on the carton.

NOTE: The Implantation Kit is to be stored at room temperature and should *not* be refrigerated.

Insertion of the Supprelin LA implant is a surgical procedure. Sterile gloves and aseptic technique must be used to minimize any chance of infection.

Setting up the Sterile Field

Using proper aseptic technique, the sterilized components of the Implantation Kit needed for the insertion procedure, including the Insertion Tool, are to be carefully dispensed from their packaging onto the Sterile Field drape (*non-fenestrated*) provided. NOTE THAT THE KIT BOX AND ALL PACKAGING ARE NOT STERILE and should be kept off of the Sterile Field drape. DO NOT PLACE THE VIAL OF LOCAL ANESTHETIC OR THE VIAL CONTAINING THE IMPLANT ONTO THE DRAPE as the exterior surface of these vials is not sterile.

The implant vial should not be opened until just before the time of insertion. Open the vial by removing the metal band and carefully pour the sterile contents (implant and sterile saline) onto the Sterile Field drape. The implant can then be handled with sterile gloves or with the sterile mosquito clamp provided.

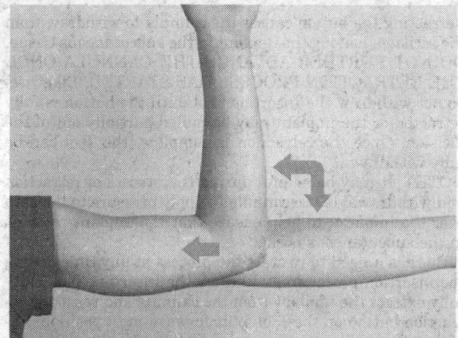

Preparing the Patient and the Insertion Site

The patient should be on his/her back, ideally with the arm least used (e.g., left arm for a right-handed person) positioned, either bent or extended, so that the physician has ready access to the inner aspect of the upper arm. Propping the arm with pillows may help the patient more easily hold the position. The suggested optimum site for subcutaneous insertion is approximately half-way between the shoulder and the elbow, in line with the crease between the biceps and triceps muscles.

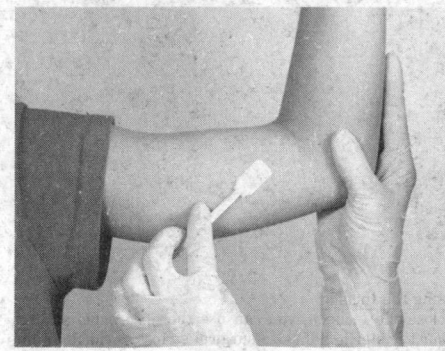

Antiseptic

Swab the insertion area with topical antiseptic, then overlay with the *fenestrated* Sterile Field drape provided, so that the opening is over the insertion site (for clarity of illustration, the following images do not show the drape).

[See figure at top of next column]

Anesthetic

The method of anesthesia utilized (i.e., local, conscious sedation, general) is at the discretion of the healthcare provider.

If local anesthesia is selected: a vial of sterile local anesthetic (note that the exterior of the vial is not sterile) has   or

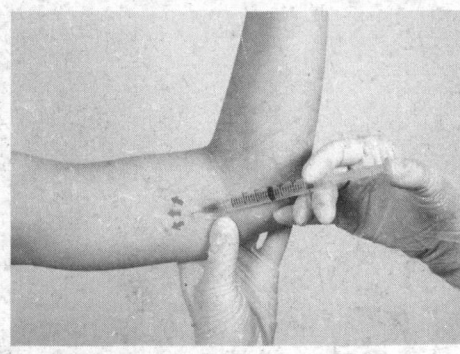

been provided along with a sterile hypodermic needle for injection. After determining the absence of known allergies to the anesthetic agent, inject anesthetic into the subcutaneous tissue, starting at the planned incision site, then infiltrating along the intended subcutaneous insertion path, up to the length of the implant (a little more than one inch). Local anesthesia may also be supplemented by the use of distraction techniques.

The following sections describe the suggested procedure for insertion of the implant using the Insertion Tool provided. The method of insertion used, however, is at the discretion of the healthcare provider performing the procedure.

Loading the Insertion Tool

The sterile Insertion Tool is comprised of a fixed handle attached to a retractable, beveltipped cannula, into the chamber of which the implant is to be placed for subcutaneous insertion. The cannula can be extended or retracted. The fully extended cannula contains a fixed piston upon which the implant, once inserted, rests. During the final step of the insertion procedure, the cannula will be retracted into the handle using the slide mechanism (green button), thereby exposing and leaving the implant to remain in the subcutaneous tissue.

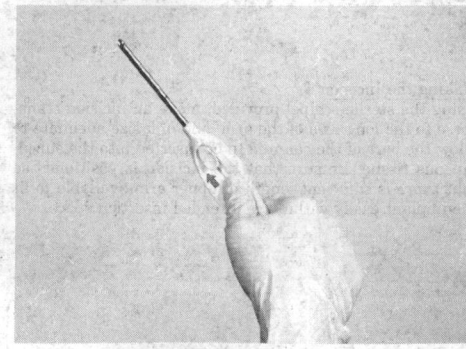

When first grasping the sterile Insertion Tool, confirm that the cannula is fully extended. Verify this by inspecting the position of the green retraction button. The button should be locked in position all the way forward, towards the cannula, farthest from the handle.

The implant can be picked up using sterile gloves or with the sterile mosquito clamp provided. Avoid bending or pinching the implant. Note that the implant may come out of its vial slightly curved after refrigerated storage. To help make the implant more symmetrical prior to loading into the Tool, you can roll the implant a few times (while wearing a sterile glove) between the fingers and thumb.

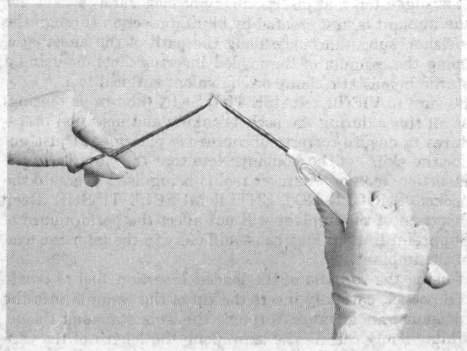

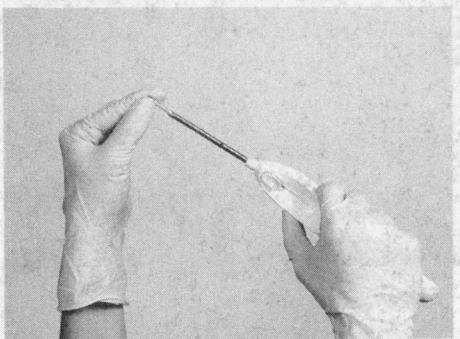

Insert the implant into the cannula of the Insertion Tool manually or using the mosquito clamp. When inserting the implant into the cannula, DO NOT FORCE the implant. If resistance is felt, the implant should be removed and manually manipulated or rolled as needed, and re-inserted into the cannula.

When fully inserted, the implant rests inside the cannula so that just the tip of the implant is visible at the beveled end of the cannula.

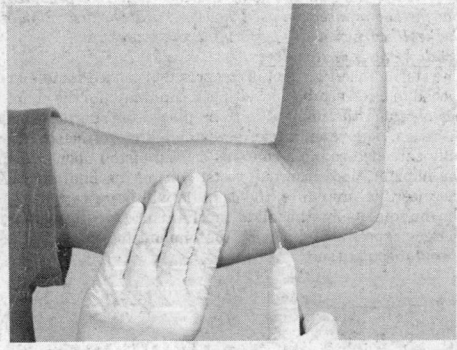

Making the Incision
Using the sterile scalpel provided, make an incision transverse to the long axis of the arm, and of a size adequate to allow the bore of the cannula to be inserted into the subcutaneous tissue. Be sure that the incision is positioned so that there is sufficient length of upper arm available to fit the implant easily within the intended insertion space.

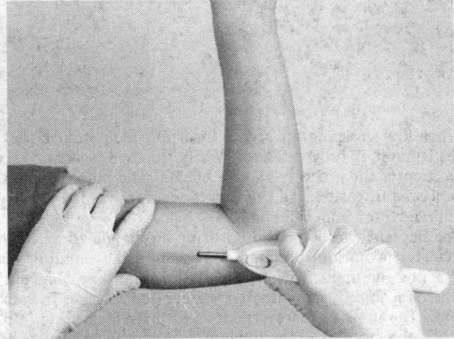

Inserting the Implant
It is suggested that insertion may be easier if a "pocket" for the implant is first created by blunt dissection through the incision, subcutaneously along the path of the anesthetic, using the cannula of the loaded Insertion Tool, or using a sterile hemostatic clamp or equivalent surgical tool.

Be sure to VISIBLY RAISE THE SKIN (known as tenting) at all times during the pocket-making and insertion procedures to ensure correct subcutaneous placement ("just under the skin") of the implant. Note that the cannula of the Insertion Tool, or whatever tool is being used to create the pocket, SHOULD NOT ENTER MUSCLE TISSUE. Deep insertion of the implant will not affect the performance of Supprelin LA, but may cause difficulty in the later removal of the implant.

If using the cannula of the loaded Insertion Tool to create the pocket, carefully insert the tip of the cannula into the incision and advance through the subcutaneous tissue, while visibly raising the skin along the length of the cannula up to, but no farther than, the inscribed black line on the cannula. DO NOT DEPRESS THE GREEN RETRAC-

TION BUTTON ON THE TOOL WHILE INSERTING OR ADVANCING THE TOOL INTO THE INCISION.
Pull the Tool back, almost to the beveled tip of the cannula, and advance the Tool forward again, so that the cannula reenters the pocket completely, but no farther than the inscribed black line. Be sure to keep the insertion path just immediately subcutaneous.

If another tool was used to create the pocket, now insert the loaded cannula of the Insertion Tool containing the implant through the incision, up to the inscribed black line.

Hold the Insertion Tool in place with the base against the patient's arm (if possible) as you carefully move your thumb to the green retraction button. Depress the button to release the locking mechanism, then slide the button back toward the handle until it stops, all the while holding the body of the Insertion Tool in place.

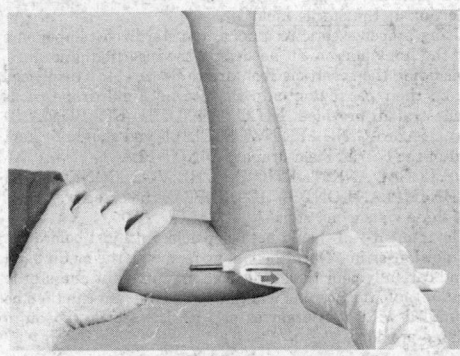

Retracting the button causes the cannula to withdraw from the incision, leaving the implant in the subcutaneous tissue. DO NOT FURTHER ADVANCE THE CANNULA ONCE THE RETRACTION PROCESS HAS STARTED. Likewise, do not withdraw the Insertion Tool until the button is fully retracted or the implant may be pulled partially out of the incision. Once the retraction is complete, the Tool can be fully withdrawn.

NOTE: It may be helpful during the process of retraction and withdrawal of the cannula to apply pressure to the skin over the implant, to help ensure that the implant remains in the subcutaneous pocket.

If there is a need to re-start the process at any time during the insertion procedure, withdraw the Insertion Tool, carefully extract the implant from the cannula and reset the retraction button on the Tool to its forward-most position. Examine the implant before reloading the implant into the Insertion Tool, and start again.

Placement of the implant should be confirmed by palpation. Note that the tip of a properly placed implant may not be visible through the incision.

After implantation, briefly cover the site with a sterile gauze pad and apply pressure to ensure hemostasis.

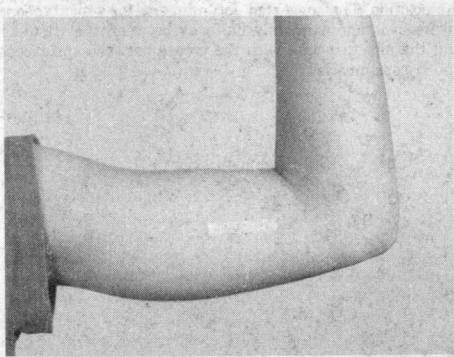

Closing the Incision
To close the incision, you can use the absorbable sutures and/or the sterile adhesive surgical strips provided. To improve adhesion of the strips, you can apply benzoin tincture antiseptic (provided) to the skin, and let it dry, before applying the adhesive strips.

Once closed, cover the incision site with sterile gauze pads and secure the dressing with the bandage provided.

Please provide the patient's parent or guardian with a Patient Information Leaflet, which includes information about the implant and instructions on proper care of the insertion site.

Suggested Removal Procedure
Supprelin LA should be removed after 12 months of therapy. Most of the supplies necessary to remove the implant, including the local anesthetic and the sterile mosquito clamp,

are provided in the Implantation Kit that is shipped along with a new Supprelin LA implant. Note that the Implantation Kit is to be stored at room temperature and must *not* be refrigerated. See the Suggested Insertion Procedure above for further instructions.

Removal of the Supprelin LA implant is a surgical procedure. Sterile gloves and aseptic technique must be used to minimize any chance of infection.

Setting up the Sterile Field
Using proper aseptic technique, the sterilized components of the Implantation Kit needed for the implant removal procedure are to be carefully dispensed from their packaging out onto the Sterile Field drape (non-fenestrated) provided. NOTE THAT THE KIT BOX AND ALL PACKAGING ARE NOT STERILE and should be kept off of the Sterile Field drape. DO NOT PLACE THE VIAL OF LOCAL ANESTHETIC ONTO THE DRAPE as the exterior surface of the vial is not sterile.

Preparing the Patient and the Site
The patient should be on his/her back, with the arm containing the implant positioned, either bent or extended, so that the physician has ready access to the inner aspect of the upper arm. Propping the arm with pillows may help the patient more easily hold the position.

The implant to be removed should first be located by palpating the inner aspect of the upper arm, near the incision from the prior year.

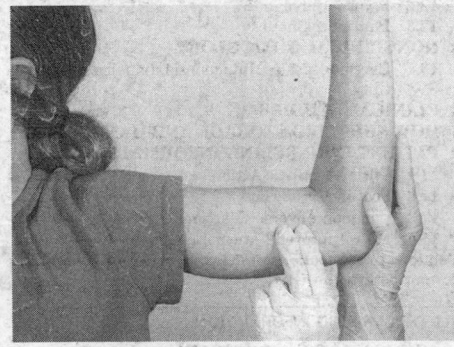

Generally, the previous implant is readily palpated. In the event the implant is difficult to locate, ultrasound may be used. If ultrasound fails to locate the implant, other imaging techniques such as CT or MRI may be used to locate it (plain films are not recommended as **the implant is not radiopaque**).

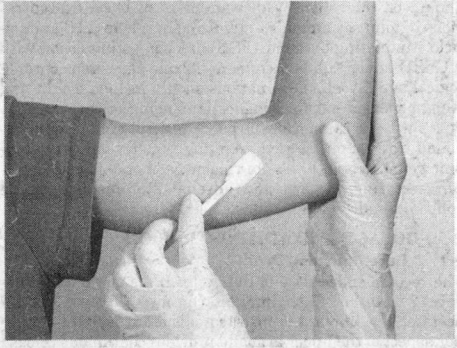

Antiseptic
Swab the area above and around the previous implant with topical antiseptic. Overlay the area with the *fenestrated* Sterile Field drape provided, so that the hole is over the previous insertion site (for clarity of illustration, the following images do not show the drape).
[See first figure at top of next page]

Anesthetic
The method of anesthesia utilized (i.e., local, conscious sedation, general) is at the discretion of the healthcare provider.

If local anesthesia is selected: a vial of sterile local anesthetic (note that the exterior of the vial is not sterile) has been provided along with a sterile hypodermic needle for injection. After determining the absence of known allergies to the anesthetic agent, inject anesthetic into the subcutaneous tissue at and around the site of the intended incision

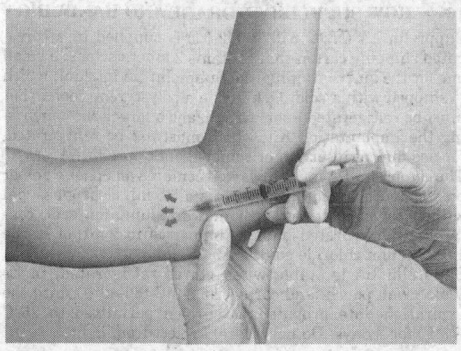

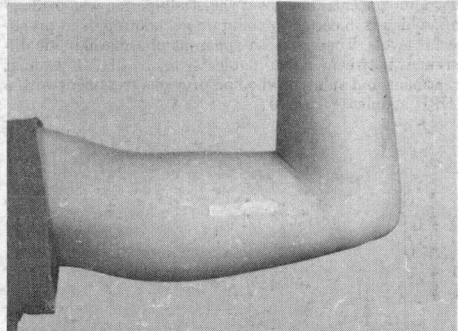

(the site of the previous implant). Local anesthesia may also be supplemented by the use of distraction techniques.

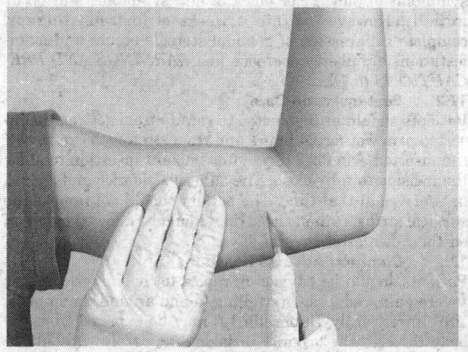

Making the Incision and Removing the Implant

Using the sterile scalpel provided, make an incision of a size adequate to allow the implant to be easily removed and, if a new implant will be inserted, large enough for the bore of the cannula of the Insertion Tool provided.

Generally, the tip of the implant will be visible through the incision, possibly covered by a pseudocapsule of tissue. In order to facilitate the removal of the implant, it may be necessary to palpate the head of the implant through the incision using your smallest finger, especially if the head of the implant is not readily visible. In addition, you may need to push down on the distal end of the implant and "massage it forward" towards the incision.

Carefully nick the pseudocapsule to reveal the polymer tip of the implant. It may be beneficial to insert the sterile mosquito clamp provided into the hole created in the pseudocapsule and expand by opening the clamp. Widening the opening of the pseudocapsule may ease the extraction of the implant.

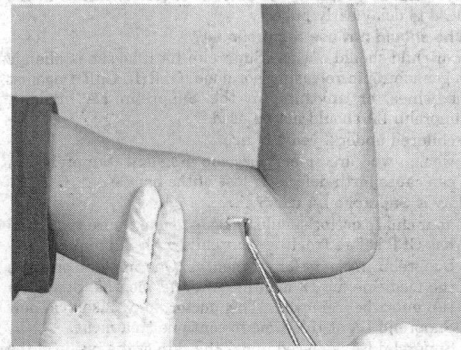

Gently but securely grasp the implant with the sterile mosquito clamp and extract the implant.

Dispose of the implant in a proper manner, treating it like any other bio-waste.

Briefly cover the site with a sterile gauze pad and apply pressure to ensure hemostasis.

If inserting a new implant, see the **Suggested Insertion Procedure** instructions provided above. Note that you can insert the new implant into the same "pocket" as the removed implant, or make a new incision at a different site in the same arm or in the contralateral arm.

If a new implant is not to be inserted, proceed to close the incision.

Closing the Incision

To close the incision, you can use the absorbable sutures and/or the sterile adhesive surgical strips provided. To improve adhesion of the strips, you can apply benzoin tincture antiseptic (provided) to the skin, and let it dry, before applying the adhesive strips.

Once closed, cover the incision site with sterile gauze pads and secure the dressing with the bandage provided.

3   DOSAGE FORMS AND STRENGTHS

Supprelin LA is a sterile, nonbiodegradable, diffusion-controlled, HYDRON® polymer reservoir drug delivery system designed to deliver histrelin acetate continuously for 12 months after subcutaneous implantation. The sterile implant contains 50 mg histrelin acetate and delivers approximately 65 mcg histrelin acetate per day over 12 months.

4   CONTRAINDICATIONS

Supprelin LA is contraindicated in patients who are hypersensitive to gonadotropin releasing hormone (GnRH) or GnRH agonist analogs.

Supprelin LA is contraindicated in females who are or may become pregnant while receiving the drug. Supprelin LA may cause fetal harm when administered to pregnant patients. If this drug is used during pregnancy, or if the patient becomes pregnant while taking this drug, the patient should be apprised of the potential hazard to a fetus. The possibility exists that spontaneous abortion may occur [see USE IN SPECIFIC POPULATIONS (8.1)].

5   WARNINGS AND PRECAUTIONS

5.1   Initial Agonistic Action

Supprelin LA, like other GnRH agonists, initially causes a transient increase in serum concentrations of estradiol in females and testosterone in both sexes during the first week of treatment. Patients may experience worsening of symptoms or onset of new symptoms during this period. However, within 4 weeks of histrelin therapy, suppression of gonadal steroids occurs and manifestations of puberty decrease.

5.2   Implant Insertion/Removal Procedure

Implant insertion is a surgical procedure and it is important that the insertion instructions are followed to avoid potential complications. The insertion and removal of the implant should be done aseptically. Proper surgical technique is critical in minimizing adverse events related to the insertion and the removal of the histrelin implant. On occasion, localizing and/or removal of implant products have been difficult and imaging techniques were used, including ultrasound, CT, or MRI (note: the histrelin implant is not radiopaque). Rare events of spontaneous extrusion of the implant have been observed in clinical trials. During Supprelin LA treatment, patients should be evaluated for evidence of clinical and biochemical suppression of CPP manifestations (see Section 5.3, Monitoring and Laboratory tests). Detailed instructions on the insertion and removal procedures of the implant are provided above [see DOSAGE AND ADMINISTRATION (2.2)].

5.3   Monitoring and Laboratory Tests

LH, FSH and estradiol or testosterone should be monitored at 1 month post implantation then every 6 months thereafter. Additionally, height (for calculation of height velocity) and bone age should be assessed every 6-12 months.

6   ADVERSE REACTIONS

6.1   Overall Adverse Reaction Profile

The most common adverse reactions with Supprelin LA involved the implant site. Local reactions after implant insertion include bruising, pain, soreness, erythema and swelling. During the early phase of therapy, gonadotropins and sex steroids rise above baseline because of the natural stimulatory effect of the drug. Therefore, an increase in clinical signs and symptoms may be observed [see WARNINGS AND PRECAUTIONS (5.1)].

6.2   Adverse Reactions in Clinical Trials

Because clinical trials are conducted under widely varying conditions, adverse reaction rates observed in the clinical trials of a drug cannot be directly compared to rates in the clinical trials of another drug and may not reflect the rates observed in practice.

The safety of Supprelin LA in children with CPP was evaluated in two single-arm clinical trials conducted in a total of 47 patients (44 females and 3 males) over a period of time ranging from 9 to 18 months. The most commonly reported adverse reaction was implant site reaction, which was reported by 24 of 47 (51.1%) patients. Implant site reaction includes discomfort, bruising, soreness, pain, tingling, itching, implant area protrusion and swelling. Two subjects experienced a serious adverse reaction: 1 subject who coincidentally had Stargardt's Disease experienced amblyopia and 1 subject had a benign pituitary tumor (pituitary adenoma). One subject discontinued the study due to an adverse reaction of infection at the implant site. There were no clinically meaningful findings in standard clinical hematology and chemistry tests and/or in vital signs. The incidence of implantation adverse events reported by more than 2 patients are summarized in Table 1.

Table 1: Incidence of implantation adverse reactions reported by ≥ 2 patients treated with Supprelin LA in both clinical trials

Adverse Reactions	N=47
	N (%)
Implant site reaction	24 (51.1)
Keloid scar	3 (6.4)
Scar	3 (6.4)
Suture related complication	3 (6.4)
Application site pain	2 (4.3)
Post procedural pain	2 (4.3)

The following adverse reactions were reported as possibly related or related in 1 patient each: wound infection, breast tenderness, dysmenorrhea, epistaxis, erythema, feeling cold, gynecomastia, headache, menorrhagia, migraine, mood swings, pituitary tumor benign, pruritus, weight increased, disease progression and influenza-like illness. The adverse reaction metrorrhagia was reported as possibly related or related in 2 patients.

7   DRUG INTERACTIONS

Overview: No formal drug-drug, drug-food, or drug-herb interaction studies were performed with Supprelin LA.

Drug-Laboratory Interactions: Therapy with Supprelin LA results in suppression of the pituitary-gonadal system. Results of diagnostic tests of pituitary gonadotropic and gonadal functions conducted during and after Supprelin LA therapy may be affected. Supprelin LA decreased mean serum insulin-like growth factor-1 (IGF-1) levels by approximately 11% in one study (Study 1). Supprelin LA increased the serum concentration of dehydroepiandrosterone (DHEA) in 8 of 36 patients in another study (Study 2).

8   USE IN SPECIFIC POPULATIONS

8.1   Pregnancy

Pregnancy category X [see CONTRAINDICATIONS (4)].

Supprelin LA is contraindicated in females who are, or may become, pregnant while receiving the drug. Supprelin LA can cause fetal harm when administered to a pregnant patient. The possibility exists that spontaneous abortion may occur.

Animal Data: Major fetal abnormalities were observed in rabbits at 3 times human therapeutic exposure but not in rats after administration of histrelin acetate throughout gestation. There was dose-related increased fetal mortality during organogenesis in both rats given 1, 3, 5 or 15 mcg/kg/day (at less than therapeutic exposures using body surface area comparisons, based on a 65 mcg per day human dose) and in rabbits at 20, 50 or 80 mcg/kg/day (at 3 times human exposure using body surface area comparisons, based on a 65 mcg/day dose in humans).

8.4   Pediatric Use

Safety and effectiveness in pediatric patients below the age of 2 years have not been established. The use of Supprelin LA in children under 2 years is not recommended.

10   OVERDOSAGE

There have been no reports of overdose in Supprelin LA clinical trials. High doses of histrelin acetate injection in animal studies were generally associated only with effects attributed to the expected pharmacology. The method of drug delivery makes accidental or intentional overdosage unlikely.

11   DESCRIPTION

Supprelin LA is a sterile, non-biodegradable, diffusion-controlled, HYDRON® polymer reservoir containing histrelin acetate, a synthetic nonapeptide analog of the naturally occurring gonadotropin releasing hormone (GnRH) possessing a greater potency than the natural sequence hormone. Supprelin LA is designed to deliver approximately 65 mcg histrelin acetate per day over 12 months.

The Supprelin LA implant looks like a small thin flexible tube and consists of a 50-mg histrelin acetate drug core inside a 3.5 cm by 3 mm, cylindrical, HYDRON® polymer reservoir (Figure 1).

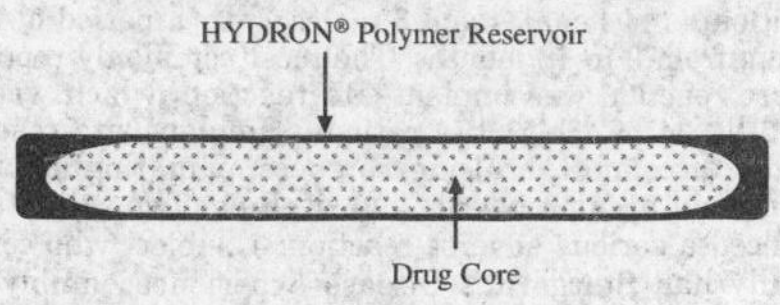

Figure 1. Supprelin LA Implant Diagram (not to scale)

The chemical name of histrelin acetate is: L-Pyroglutamyl-L-histidyl-L-tryptophyl-L-seryl-L-tyrosyl-N-benzyl-D-histidyl-L-leucyl-L-arginyl-L-proline N-ethylamide, acetate salt. The molecular formula for histrelin acetate is $C_{66}H_{86}N_{18}O_{12} \times 2\ CH_3COOH$ and its molecular weight is 1443.70 (or 1323.52 as free base). Histrelin is also chemically described as 5-oxo-L-prolyl-L-histidyl-L-tryptophyl-L-seryl-L-tyrosyl-Nt-benzyl-D-histidyl-L-leucyl-L-arginyl-N-ethyl-L-prolinamide diacetate. The chemical structure of the free base (histrelin) is represented below in Figure 2.

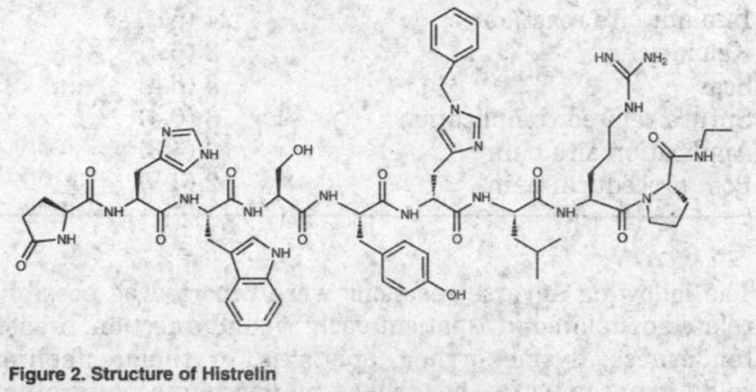

Figure 2. Structure of Histrelin

The drug core also contains the inactive ingredient stearic acid NF. The HYDRON® polymer (also known as a "hydrogel") reservoir is a hydrophilic cartridge composed of 2-hydroxyethyl methacrylate, 2-hydroxypropyl methacrylate, trimethylolpropane trimethacrylate, benzoin methyl ether, Perkadox-16, and Triton X-100. Each implant is packaged hydrated in a glass vial containing 2 mL of sterile 1.8% sodium chloride solution, so that it is primed for immediate release of the drug upon insertion.

A single use, sterile, Insertion Tool is provided along with the implant that can be used for the placement of the Supprelin LA implant into the subcutaneous tissue of the inner aspect of the upper arm. The Insertion Tool is enclosed in a sterile bag and is provided separately from the implant in the Implantation Kit [*see RECOMMENDED PROCEDURE (2.2)*].

12 CLINICAL PHARMACOLOGY

12.1 Mechanism of Action

Supprelin LA is a GnRH agonist and an inhibitor of gonadotropin secretion when given continuously. It delivers approximately 65 mcg histrelin acetate per day. Both animal and human studies indicate that following an initial stimulatory phase, chronic, subcutaneous administration of histrelin acetate desensitizes responsiveness of the pituitary gonadotropin which, in turn causes a reduction in ovarian and testicular steroidogenesis.

In humans, administration of histrelin acetate results in an initial increase in circulating levels of LH and FSH, leading to a transient increase in concentration of gonadal steroids (testosterone and dihydrotestosterone in males, and estrone and estradiol in premenopausal females). However, continuous administration of histrelin acetate causes a reversible down-regulation of the GnRH receptors in the pituitary gland and desensitization of the pituitary gonadotropes. These inhibitory effects result in decreased levels of LH and FSH.

12.2 Pharmacodynamics

Long-term treatment with histrelin acetate suppresses the LH response to GnRH causing LH levels to decrease to prepubertal levels within 1 month of treatment. As a result, serum concentrations of sex steroids (estrogen or testosterone) also decrease. Consequently, secondary sexual development ceases to progress in most patients. Additionally, linear growth velocity is slowed which improves the chance of attaining predicted adult height.

12.3 Pharmacokinetics

Pharmacokinetics of histrelin acetate after implantation of Supprelin LA was evaluated in a total of 47 children with CPP (11 subjects in Study 1 and 36 subjects in Study 2). Patients were examined at 4 weeks after implant insertion and a few times throughout the treatment period. Median serum histrelin concentrations remained above the limit of quantification for the treatment period. Histrelin acetate levels were sustained throughout the study period for most subjects (Figure 3). The median of maximum serum histrelin concentrations over the study period was 0.43 ng/mL, which is expected to maintain gonadotropins at prepubertal levels. There was no apparent pharmacokinetic difference between naïve subjects to a LHRH agonist treatment and subjects who had previous treatment with a LHRH agonist (Figure 3).

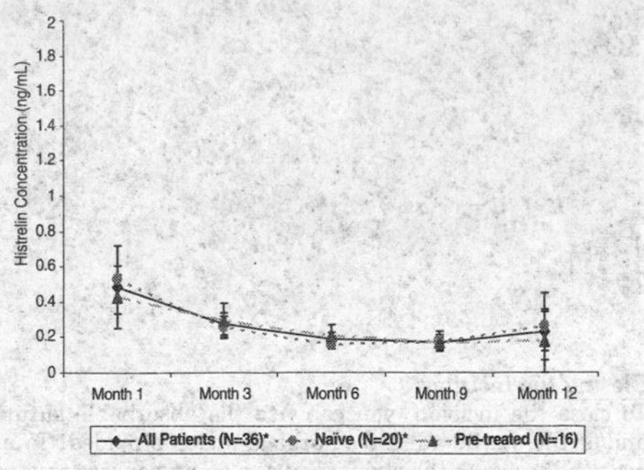

Figure 3. Mean and Standard Deviation of Serum Histrelin Concentrations (ng/mL) Results at Each Visit

13 NONCLINICAL TOXICOLOGY

13.1 Carcinogenesis, Mutagenesis, Impairment of Fertility

Carcinogenicity studies were conducted in rats for 2 years at doses of 5, 25 or 150 mcg/kg/day (up to 11 times human exposures using body surface area comparisons, based on a 65 mcg/day dose in humans) and in mice for 18 months at doses of 20, 200, or 2000 mcg/kg/day (at less than therapeutic exposure to 70 times human exposure using body surface area comparisons, based on a 65 mcg/day dose in humans). As seen with other GnRH agonists, histrelin injection administration was associated with an increase in tumors of hormonally responsive tissues. There was a significant increase in pituitary adenomas in rats at mid and high doses (2-11 times human exposure based on body surface area comparisons with a 65 mcg/day human dose). There was an increase in pancreatic islet-cell adenomas in treated female rats and a non-dose-related increase in testicular Leydig-cell tumors (highest incidence in the low-dose group). In mice, there was significant increase in mammary-gland adenocarcinomas in all treated females. In addition, there were increases in stomach papillomas in male rats given high doses, and an increase in histiocytic sarcomas in female mice at the highest dose.

Mutagenicity studies have not been performed with histrelin acetate. Saline extracts of implants with and without histrelin acetate were negative in a battery of genotoxicity studies. Fertility studies have been conducted in rats and monkeys given subcutaneous daily doses of histrelin acetate up to 180 mcg/kg/day (up to 13 and 30 times human exposure, respectively using body surface area comparisons, based on a 65 mcg/day human dose) for 6 months and full reversibility of fertility suppression was demonstrated. The development and reproductive performance of offspring from parents treated with histrelin acetate has not been investigated.

14 CLINICAL STUDIES

The efficacy of Supprelin LA in children with CPP has been evaluated in two single-arm, open label studies. Study 1 was conducted in 11 pretreated female patients, 3.7 to 11.0 years of age. Study 2 was conducted in 36 patients (33 females and 3 males), 4.5 to 11.6 years of age. Sixteen pretreated and 20 treatment-naïve patients were enrolled in Study 2. Baseline patient characteristics were typical of patients with CPP. Efficacy assessments were similar in both studies and included endpoints that measured the suppression of gonadotropins (luteinizing hormone and follicle stimulating hormone) and gonadal sex steroids (estrogen in girls and testosterone in boys, respectively) on treatment. Other assessments were clinical (evidence of stabilization or regression of signs of puberty) or gonadal steroid-dependent (bone age, linear growth). In Study 2, the primary measure of efficacy was LH suppression.

In Study 2, suppression of LH was induced in all treatment naïve subjects and maintained in all pretreated subjects at Month 1 after implantation and continued through Month 12 (suppression was defined as a peak LH < 4 mIU/mL following stimulation with the GnRH analog leuprolide acetate).

Secondary efficacy hormone assessments (FSH, estradiol and testosterone) and additional efficacy assessments (bone age advancement, linear growth, clinical progression of puberty) indicated stabilization of disease. Estradiol suppression was present in all 33 girls (100%) through Month 9 and 97% at Month 12. Testosterone suppression was maintained in the three pre-treated males participating in Study 2. The Supprelin LA effect on efficacy endpoints in the Study 1 was consistent with that observed in Study 2.

16 HOW SUPPLIED/STORAGE AND HANDLING

Supprelin LA (NDC 67979-002-01) is supplied in a corrugated shipping carton that contains 2 inner cartons: a small one for the vial containing the Supprelin LA implant, which is shipped with a cold pack inside a polystyrene cooler that must be refrigerated upon arrival, and a larger one comprising the Implantation Kit, which must *not* be refrigerated, for use during insertion or removal of Supprelin LA.

The Supprelin LA implant carton contains an opaque amber plastic pouch. Inside the pouch is a 3.5 mL clear glass vial with a Teflon-coated stopper and an aluminum seal, containing the hydrated implant immersed in 2 mL of sterile 1.8% sodium chloride solution.

Supprelin LA is stable when stored refrigerated, in its sealed vial, pouch, and carton, at 2-8°C (36-46°F) until the expiration date provided. Excursion permitted to 25°C (77°F) for 7 days. Do not freeze. Protect from light.

17 PATIENT COUNSELING INFORMATION

[*See FDA-Approved Patient Labeling (17.4)*]

17.1 Initial Agonistic Action

Patients should be advised that a transient worsening of symptoms of puberty or onset of new symptoms may occur initially. However, within 4 weeks of histrelin therapy, complete suppression of gonadal steroids occurs and manifestations of puberty decrease [*see WARNINGS AND PRECAUTIONS (5.1)*].

17.2 Post-insertion Care

Patients should be instructed to refrain from getting the inserted arm wet for 24 hours and from strenuous exertion of the inserted arm for 7 days after implant insertion to allow the incision to fully close. The adhesive elastic bandage can be removed at that time. The patient should not remove the surgical strips; rather, the strips should be allowed to fall off on their own after several days.

17.3 Common Adverse Reactions

Patients should be advised to report to their physician any severe pain, redness, or swelling in and around the implant site. Infrequently, Supprelin LA may be expelled from the body through the original incision site, rarely without the patient noticing. The patient should be instructed to monitor the incision site until it is healed. The patient should also return for routine checks of their condition and to ensure that Supprelin LA is present and functioning in his/her body [*see WARNINGS AND PRECAUTIONS (5.2)*].

17.4 FDA-Approved Patient Labeling

Supprelin® LA *[Suh-Preh-Lin El-Ay]*

(histrelin acetate) subcutaneous implant

Read the Patient Information that comes with Supprelin LA before your child begins treatment. This information does not take the place of talking with your child's doctor about their medical condition or treatment.

What is Supprelin LA?

Supprelin LA is an under-the-skin (subcutaneous) implant that contains the medicine histrelin, a gonadotropin releasing hormone (GnRH). Supprelin LA is used for treatment of children with central precocious puberty (CPP).

CPP makes puberty come early in girls (before 8 years of age) and in boys (before 9 years of age). Signs of early puberty include breast enlargement in girls and the appearance of hair in the genital area in boys and girls. Supprelin LA works by reducing the amount of sex hormones in the blood to delay early puberty.

Who should not use Supprelin LA?

Your child should not use Supprelin LA if he/she is allergic to gonadotropin releasing hormone (GnRH), GnRH agonist medicines, or anything in the Supprelin LA implant. Supprelin LA should not be used in:

- children under 2 years of age
- women who are or may become pregnant (Supprelin LA can cause birth defects or loss of the baby).

How is Supprelin LA used?

- Your child's doctor should do tests to make sure your child has CPP before treating your child with Supprelin LA.
- Supprelin LA lasts for 12 months. One implant provides the medicine for 12 months. After 12 months, Supprelin LA must be removed. The doctor may insert a new Supprelin LA at this time to continue treatment.
- Supprelin LA is placed under the skin of the inside of the upper arm. The doctor will temporarily numb the arm of your child, make a small cut, and then place Supprelin LA under the skin. The cut may be closed with stitches or surgical strips and covered with a pressure bandage.
- Your child should keep the arm clean and dry and should not swim or bathe for 24 hours. The bandage can be removed after 24 hours. Do not remove any surgical strips. They will fall off on their own in several days.
- Your child should avoid heavy play or exercise that uses the implanted arm for 7 days. After the cut has healed, your child can go back to his or her normal activities. The doctor will give you complete instructions.
- Keep all scheduled visits to the doctor. Your child's doctor will do regular exams and blood tests to check for signs of

puberty. Sometimes the doctor will have to do special examinations, such as ultrasound or MRI, if the Supprelin LA implant is difficult to find under your child's skin.

What are the possible side effects of Supprelin LA?

In the first few weeks of treatment, Supprelin LA can cause a brief increase in some hormones, and during this time you may notice more signs of puberty in your child, including light vaginal bleeding and breast enlargement in girls. Within 4 weeks of treatment, you should see signs in your child that puberty is stopping.

- The most common side effects of Supprelin LA are skin reactions at the place where the implant is inserted. Such reactions may include bruising, soreness, pain, tingling, itching, and swelling. They usually go away without treatment within 2 weeks. Call your child's doctor if your child has bleeding, redness or pain at the insertion site.
- Serious and life-threatening allergic reactions have happened with GnRH medicines (the type of medicine in Supprelin LA).

These may not be all the side effects of Supprelin LA. Ask your child's doctor for more information.

General information about Supprelin LA

This patient labeling summarizes the most important information about Supprelin LA. If you would like more information, talk with your doctor. You can ask your doctor or pharmacist for information about Supprelin LA that is written for health professionals.

Rx Only

For more information, call 1-800-462-3636 or visit www.supprelinla.com

Manufactured by: Endo Pharmaceuticals Solutions Inc., Chadds Ford, PA 19317

Supprelin® LA and HYDRON® are Registered Trademarks of Endo Pharmaceuticals.

©2009, Endo Pharmaceuticals

PK000033 Rev. 03 June 2009

Shown in Product Identification Guide, page 309

VALSTAR™ ℞

[val-star]

(valrubicin)

Sterile Solution For Intravesical Instillation

For Intravesical Use Only
Not for IV or IM Use
Rx Only

DESCRIPTION

Valrubicin (N-trifluoroacetyladriamycin-14-valerate), a semisynthetic analog of the anthra-cycline doxorubicin, is a cytotoxic agent with the chemical name, (2*S-cis*)-2-[1,2,3,4,6,11-hexahydro-2,5,12-trihydroxy-7-methoxy-6, 11-dioxo-4-[[2,3,6-trideoxy-3-[(trifluoroacetyl)amino]-α-L-*lyxo*-hexopyranosyl]oxyl]-2-naphthacenyl]-2-oxoethyl-pentanoate. Valrubicin is an orange or orange-red powder that is highly lipophilic, soluble in methylene chloride, ethanol, methanol and acetone, and relatively insoluble in water. Its chemical formula is $C_{34}H_{36}F_3NO_{13}$ and its molecular weight is 723.65. The chemical structure is shown in FIGURE 1.

FIGURE 1. Chemical Structure of Valrubicin

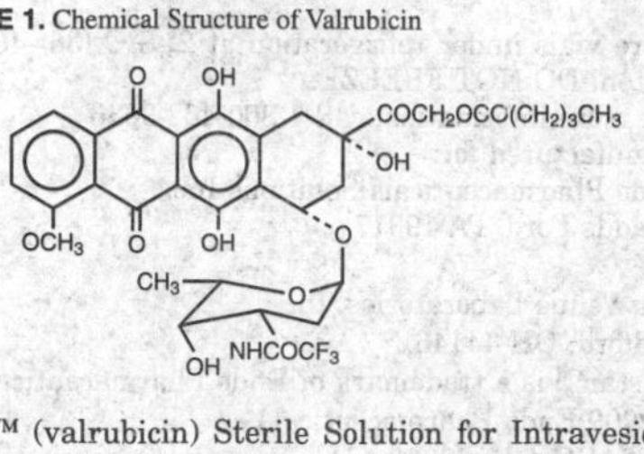

O
OH
COCH₂OCC(CH₂)₃CH₃
OH
OCH₃
O
OH
O
CH₃
O
NHCOCF₃
OH

VALSTAR™ (valrubicin) Sterile Solution for Intravesical Instillation is intended for intra-vesical administration in the urinary bladder. It is supplied as a nonaqueous solution that should be diluted before intravesical administration. Each vial of VALSTAR contains valrubicin at a concentration of 40 mg/mL in 50% polyoxyl castor oil/50% dehydrated alcohol, USP without preservatives or other additives. The solution is sterile and nonpyrogenic.

CLINICAL PHARMACOLOGY

Mechanism of Action: Valrubicin is an anthracycline that affects a variety of inter-related biological functions, most of which involve nucleic acid metabolism. It readily penetrates into cells, where it inhibits the incorporation of nucleosides into nucleic acids, causes extensive chromosomal damage, and arrests cell cycle in G_2. Although valrubicin does not bind strongly to DNA, a principal mechanism of its action, mediated by valrubicin metabolites, is interference with the normal DNA breaking-resealing action of DNA topoisomerase II.

Pharmacokinetics after Intravesical Administration of VALSTAR: When 800 mg VALSTAR was administered intravesically to patients with carcinoma *in situ*, VALSTAR penetrated into the bladder wall. The mean total anthracycline concentration measured in bladder tissue exceeded the levels causing 90% cytotoxicity to human bladder cells cultured *in vitro*. During the two-hour dose-retention period, the metabolism of VALSTAR to its major metabolites N-trifluoroacetyladriamycin and N-trifluoroacetyladriamycinol was negligible. After retention, the drug was almost completely excreted by voiding the instillate. Mean percent recovery of VALSTAR, N-trifluoroacetyladriamycin, and total anthracyclines in 14 urine samples from six patients was 98.6%, 0.4%, and 99.0% of the total administered drug, respectively. During the two-hour dose-retention period, only nanogram quantities of VALSTAR were absorbed into the plasma. VALSTAR metabolites N-trifluoroacetyladriamycin and N-trifluoroacetyladriamycinol were measured in blood.

Total systemic exposure to anthracyclines during and after intravesical administration of VALSTAR is dependent upon the condition of the bladder wall. The mean $AUC_{0\text{-}6\ hours}$ (total anthracyclines exposure) for an intravesical dose of 900 mg of VALSTAR administered 2 weeks after transurethral resection of bladder tumors (n=6) was 78 nmol/L•hr. In patients receiving 800 mg of VALSTAR 5 to 51 minutes after typical (n=8) and extensive (n=5) transurethral resection of bladder tumors (TURBs), the mean $AUC_{0\text{-}6\ hours}$ values for total anthracyclines were 409 and 788 nmol/L•hr, respectively. The $AUC_{0\text{-}6\ hours}$ total exposure to anthracyclines was 18,382 nmol/L•hr in one patient who experienced a perforated bladder following a transurethral resection that occurred 5 minutes before administration of an intravesical dose of 800 mg of VALSTAR. Administration of a comparable intravenous dose of VALSTAR (600 mg/m^2; n=2) as a 24-hour infusion resulted in an $AUC_{0\text{-}6\ hours}$ for total anthracyclines of 11,975 nmol/L•hr. These results are shown in FIGURE 2.

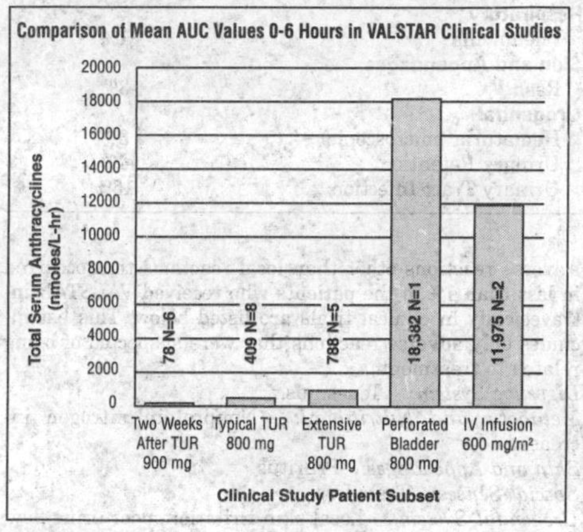

Comparison of Mean AUC Values 0-6 Hours in VALSTAR Clinical Studies
Total Serum Anthracyclines (nmoles/L-hr)
20000
18000
16000
14000
12000
10000
8000
6000
4000
2000
0
78 N=6
409 N=8
788 N=5
18,382 N=1
11,975 N=2
Two Weeks After TUR 900 mg
Typical TUR 800 mg
Extensive TUR 800 mg
Perforated Bladder 800 mg
IV Infusion 600 mg/m²
Clinical Study Patient Subset

FIGURE 2. Comparison of Mean AUC0-6 hours in VALSTAR Clinical Studies (N=number of patients)

The patient with a perforated bladder who received 800 mg of VALSTAR intravesically developed severe leukopenia and neutropenia approximately two weeks after drug administration. Systemic hematologic toxicity from VALSTAR was not seen after an intravesical dose of 800 mg of VALSTAR unless perforation of the urinary bladder occurred.

CLINICAL TRIALS

VALSTAR has been administered intravesically to a total of 230 patients with transitional cell carcinoma of the bladder, including 205 patients who received multiple weekly doses ranging from 200 to 900 mg. One hundred seventy-nine of the 205 patients received the approved dose and schedule of 800 mg weekly for multiple weeks.

In the 90 study patients with BCG-refractory carcinoma *in situ* (CIS), 70% had received at least 2 courses of BCG and 30% had received one course of BCG and at least one additional course of treatment with another agent(s) - e.g., mitomycin, thiotepa, or interferon. VALSTAR was administered beginning at least two weeks after transurethral resection and/or fulguration. After intravesical administration of VALSTAR, 16 patients (18%) had a complete response documented by bladder biopsies and cytology at 6 months following initiation of therapy. Median duration of response from start of treatment varied according to the method of analysis (13.5 months if measured to last bladder biopsy without tumor and 21 months if measured until time of documented recurrence). A retrospective analysis in the 16 patients with complete response to VALSTAR demonstrated that time to recurrence of their disease after treatment with VALSTAR was longer than time to recurrence after previous courses of intravesical therapy.

Of the 90 patients with BCG-refractory CIS, 11% (10 patients) developed metastatic or deeply-invasive bladder cancer during follow-up; four of these patients, none who underwent cystectomy, died with metastatic bladder cancer and six were found to have developed stage progression to deeply-invasive disease (T3), with lymph node involvement in one patient, at the time of cystectomy. It is difficult to ascertain to what extent the development of advanced bladder cancer in these patients was due to the delay in cystectomy required to receive treatment with VALSTAR (3 months was the time of follow-up to determine response), as cystectomy was often delayed or was never performed despite failure of treatment with VALSTAR. In the 10 patients documented to have invasive bladder cancer or metastatic disease, the delay between the time of treatment failure (when cystectomy should have been performed) and cystectomy or documentation of advanced bladder cancer was a median of 17.5 months.

INDICATIONS AND USAGE

VALSTAR is indicated for intravesical therapy of BCG-refractory carcinoma *in situ* (CIS) of the urinary bladder in patients for whom immediate cystectomy would be associated with unacceptable morbidity or mortality.

CONTRAINDICATIONS

VALSTAR is contraindicated in patients with known hypersensitivity to anthracyclines or polyoxyl castor oil.

Patients with concurrent urinary tract infections should not receive VALSTAR.

VALSTAR should not be administered to patients with a small bladder capacity, i.e., unable to tolerate a 75 mL instillation.

WARNINGS

Patients should be informed that VALSTAR has been shown to induce complete response in only about 1 in 5 patients with BCG-refractory CIS, and that delaying cystectomy could lead to development of metastatic bladder cancer, which is lethal. The exact risk of developing metastatic bladder cancer from such a delay may be difficult to assess (See CLINICAL TRIALS) but increases the longer cystectomy is delayed in the presence of persisting CIS. **If there is not a complete response of CIS to treatment after 3 months or if CIS recurs, cystectomy must be reconsidered.**

VALSTAR should not be administered to patients with a perforated bladder or to those in whom the integrity of the bladder mucosa has been compromised (see PRECAUTIONS and CLINICAL PHARMACOLOGY, Pharmacokinetics Figure 2).

In order to avoid possible dangerous systemic exposure to VALSTAR for the patients undergoing transurethral resection of the bladder, the status of the bladder should be evaluated before the intravesical instillation of drug. In case of bladder perforation, the administration of VALSTAR should be delayed until bladder integrity has been restored.

VALSTAR should be administered under the supervision of a physician experienced in the use of intravesical cancer chemotherapeutic agents.

PRECAUTIONS

General: Aseptic techniques must be used during administration of intravesical VALSTAR to avoid introducing contaminants into the urinary tract or traumatizing unduly the urinary mucosa.

Information for Patients: Patients should be informed that VALSTAR has been shown to induce complete responses in only about 1 in 5 patients, and that delaying cystectomy could lead to development of metastatic bladder cancer, which is lethal. They should discuss with their physician the relative risk of cystectomy versus the risk of metastatic bladder cancer (see CLINICAL TRIALS) and be aware that the risk increases the longer cystectomy is delayed in the presence of persisting CIS.

Patients should be informed that the major acute toxicities from VALSTAR are related to irritable bladder symptoms that may occur during instillation and retention of VALSTAR and for a limited period following voiding. For the first 24 hours following administration, red-tinged urine is typical. Patients should report prolonged irritable bladder symptoms or prolonged passage of red-colored urine immediately to their physician.

Women of childbearing potential should be advised not to become pregnant during treatment. Men should be advised to refrain from engaging in procreative activities while receiving therapy with VALSTAR. All patients of reproductive age should be advised to use an effective contraception method during the treatment period.

Irritable Bladder Symptoms: VALSTAR should be used with caution in patients with severe irritable bladder symptoms. Bladder spasm and spontaneous discharge of the intravesical instillate may occur; clamping of the urinary catheter is not advised and, if performed, should be executed under medical supervision and with caution.

Drug Interactions: Because systemic exposure to VALSTAR is negligible following intravesical administration, the potential for drug interactions is low. No drug interaction studies were conducted.

Carcinogenesis, Mutagenesis, Impairment of Fertility: The carcinogenic potential of VALSTAR has not been evaluated, but the drug does cause damage to DNA *in vitro*. VALSTAR was mutagenic in *in vitro* assays in *Salmonella typhimurium* and *Escherichia coli*. VALSTAR was clastogenic in the chromosomal aberration assay in CHO cells. Studies of the effects of VALSTAR on male or female fertility have not been done.

Pregnancy: Pregnancy Category C. Valrubicin can cause fetal harm if a pregnant woman is exposed to the drug systemically. Such exposure could occur after perforation of the urinary bladder during valrubicin therapy. Daily intravenous doses of 12 mg/kg (about one sixth of the recommended human intravesical dose on a mg/m² basis) given to rats during fetal development caused fetal malformations. A dose of 24 mg/kg (about one third the recommended human intravesical dose on a mg/m² basis) caused numerous, severe alterations in the skull and skeleton of the developing fetuses. This dose also caused an increase in fetal resorptions and a decrease in viable fetuses. Thus, valrubicin is embryo-toxic and teratogenic. There are no preclinical studies of the effects of intra-vesical valrubicin on fetal development and no adequate and well controlled studies of valrubicin in pregnant women. If valrubicin is used during pregnancy, or if the patient becomes pregnant while receiving this drug, the patient should be apprised of the potential hazard to the fetus. It should be used during pregnancy only if the potential benefit justifies the potential risk to the fetus. Women who might become pregnant should be advised to avoid doing so during therapy with VALSTAR.

Nursing Mothers: It is not known whether VALSTAR is excreted in human milk. Nevertheless, the drug is highly lipophilic and any exposure of infants to VALSTAR could pose serious health risks. Women should discontinue nursing before the initiation of VALSTAR therapy.

Pediatric Use: Safety and effectiveness in pediatric patients have not been established.

Geriatric Use: Because carcinoma *in situ* of the bladder generally occurs in older individuals, 85% of the patients enrolled in the clinical studies of VALSTAR were more than 60 years of age (49% of the patients were more than 70 years of age). In the primary efficacy studies, the mean age of the population was 69.5 years. There are no specific precautions regarding use of VALSTAR in geriatric patients who are otherwise in good health.

ADVERSE REACTIONS

Approximately 84% of patients who received intravesical VALSTAR in clinical studies experienced local adverse events, but approximately half of the patients reported irritable bladder symptoms prior to treatment. The local adverse reactions associated with VALSTAR usually occur during or shortly after instillation and resolve within 1 to 7 days after the instillate is removed from the bladder.

TABLE 1 displays the frequency of the local adverse experiences at baseline and during treatment among 170 patients who received 800 mg doses of VALSTAR™ (valrubicin) Sterile Solution for Intravesical Instillation in a multiple-cycle treatment regimen. Only 7 of 143 patients who were scheduled to receive six doses failed to receive all of the planned doses because of the occurrence of local bladder symptoms.

TABLE 1
Occurrence of Local Adverse Reactions Before and During Treatment with Intravesical VALSTAR (% of Patients)

Reaction	Before Treatment	Patients Who Received Multiple-Cycle Treatment Regimen at 800 mg/dose (N = 170) During 6-week Course of Treatment
ANY LOCAL BLADDER SYMPTOM	45%	88%
Urinary Frequency	30%	61%
Dysuria	11%	56%
Urinary Urgency	27%	57%
Bladder Spasm	3%	31%
Hematuria	11%	29%
Bladder Pain	6%	28%
Urinary Incontinence	7%	22%
Cystitis	4%	15%
Nocturia	2%	7%
Local Burning Symptoms – Procedure Related	0%	5%
Urethral Pain	0%	3%
Pelvic Pain	1%	1%
Hematuria (Gross)	0%	1%

Most systemic adverse events associated with use of VALSTAR have been mild in nature and self-limited, resolving within 24 hours after drug administration. TABLE 2 displays the adverse events other than local bladder symptoms that occurred in 1% or more of the 230 patients who received at least one dose of VALSTAR (200 to 900 mg) in a clinical trial. It cannot be determined whether these events are drug-related.

TABLE 2
Most Commonly Reported Systemic Adverse Reactions Following Intravesical Administration of VALSTAR (% of Patients)

Body System Preferred Term	All Patients Who Received VALSTAR (N = 230)
Body as a Whole	
Abdominal Pain	5%
Asthenia	4%
Back Pain	3%
Chest Pain	3%
Fever	2%
Headache	4%
Malaise	4%
Cardiovascular	
Vasodilation	2%
Digestive	
Diarrhea	3%
Flatulence	1%
Nausea	5%
Vomiting	2%
Hemic and Lymphatic	
Anemia	2%
Metabolic and Nutritional	
Hyperglycemia	1%
Peripheral Edema	1%
Musculoskeletal	
Myalgia	1%
Nervous	
Dizziness	3%
Respiratory	
Pneumonia	1%
Skin and Appendages	
Rash	3%
Urogenital	
Hematuria (microscopic)	3%
Urinary Retention	4%
Urinary Tract Infection	15%

Adverse reactions other than local reactions that occurred in less than 1% of the patients who received VALSTAR intravesically in clinical trials are listed below. This list includes only adverse reactions that were suspected of being related to treatment.

Digestive System: Tenesmus.
Metabolic and Nutritional: Nonprotein nitrogen increased.
Skin and Appendages: Pruritus.
Special Senses: Taste loss.
Urogenital System: Local skin irritation, poor urine flow, and urethritis.
Inadvertent paravenous extravasation of VALSTAR was not associated with skin ulceration or necrosis.

OVERDOSAGE

There is no known antidote for overdoses of VALSTAR. The primary anticipated complications of overdosage associated with intravesical administration would be consistent with irritable bladder symptoms.

Myelosuppression is possible if VALSTAR is inadvertently administered systemically or if significant systemic exposure occurs following intravesical administration (e.g., in patients with bladder rupture/perforation). The maximum tolerated dose in humans by either intraperitoneal or intravenous administration is 600 mg/m². Dose limiting toxicities are leukopenia and neutropenia, beginning within 1 week of dose administration, with nadirs by the second week, and recovery generally by the third week. If VALSTAR is administered when bladder rupture or perforation is suspected, weekly monitoring of complete blood counts should be performed for 3 weeks.

DOSAGE AND ADMINISTRATION

VALSTAR is recommended at a dose of 800 mg administered intravesically once a week for six weeks. Administration should be delayed at least two weeks after transurethral resection and/or fulguration. For each instillation, four 5 mL vials (200 mg valrubicin/5 mL vial) should be allowed to warm slowly to room temperature, but should not be heated. Twenty milliliters of VALSTAR should then be withdrawn from the four vials and diluted with 55 mL 0.9% Sodium Chloride Injection, USP providing 75 mL of a diluted VALSTAR solution. A urethral catheter should then be inserted into the patient's bladder under aseptic conditions, the bladder drained, and the diluted 75 mL VALSTAR solution instilled slowly via gravity flow over a period of several minutes. The catheter should then be withdrawn. The patient should retain the drug for two hours before voiding.

At the end of two hours, all patients should void. (Some patients will be unable to retain the drug for the full two hours.) Patients should be instructed to maintain adequate hydration following treatment.

Patients receiving VALSTAR for refractory carcinoma *in situ* must be monitored closely for disease recurrence or progression. Recommended evaluations include cystoscopy, biopsy, and urine cytology every 3 months.

Administration Precautions: As recommended with other cytotoxic agents, caution should be exercised in handling and preparing the solution of VALSTAR. Contact toxicity, common and severe with other anthracyclines, is not typical with VALSTAR and, when observed, has been mild. Skin reactions may occur with accidental exposure, and the use of gloves during dose preparation and administration is recommended. Irritation of the eye has also been reported with accidental exposure. If this happens, the eye should be flushed with water immediately and thoroughly.

VALSTAR sterile solution contains polyoxyl castor oil, which has been known to cause leaching of di(2-ethylhexyl) phthalate (DEHP) a hepatotoxic plasticizer, from polyvinyl chloride (PVC) bags and intravenous tubing. VALSTAR solutions should be prepared and stored in glass, polypropylene, or polyolefin containers and tubing. It is recommended that non-DEHP containing administration sets, such as those that are polyethylene-lined, be used.

Procedures for proper handling and disposal of anticancer drugs should be used.[1-7] Spills should be cleaned up with undiluted chlorine bleach.

Preparation for Administration: VALSTAR Sterile Solution for Intravesical Instillation is a clear red solution. It should be visually inspected for particulate matter and discoloration prior to administration. At temperatures below 4°C, polyoxyl castor oil may begin to form a waxy precipitate. If this happens, the vial should be warmed in the hand until the solution is clear. If particulate matter is still seen, VALSTAR should not be administered.

Stability: Unopened vials of VALSTAR are stable until the date indicated on the package when stored under refrigerated conditions at 2°-8°C (36°-46°F). Vials should not be heated. VALSTAR diluted in 0.9% Sodium Chloride Injection, USP for administration is stable for 12 hours at temperatures up to 25°C (77°F). Since compatibility data are not available, VALSTAR should not be mixed with other drugs.

HOW SUPPLIED

VALSTAR Sterile Solution for Intravesical Instillation is a clear red solution in polyoxyl castor oil/dehydrated alcohol, USP, containing 40 mg valrubicin per mL. VALSTAR Sterile Solution for Intravesical Instillation is available in single-use, clear glass vials, individually packaged in the following sizes:

NDC 67979-001-01	Carton of 4, 5 mL Single-Use Vials (200 mg/5 mL)
NDC 67979-001-02	Carton of 24, 5 mL Single-Use Vials (200 mg/5 mL)

Store vials under refrigeration at 2°-8°C (36°-46°F) in the carton. DO NOT FREEZE.
For more information, call 1-800-462-3636
Manufactured for:
Endo Pharmaceuticals Solutions Inc.
Chadds Ford, PA 19317
By:
Ben Venue Laboratories, Inc.
Bedford, OH 44146
Valstar™ is a trademark of Endo Pharmaceuticals.
© 2009 Endo Pharmaceuticals
109244 October 2009

REFERENCES

1. *Recommendations for the Safe Handling of Parenteral Antineoplastic Drugs*, NIH Publication No. 83-2621. For sale by the Superintendent of Documents, U.S. Government Printing Office, Washington, DC 20402.
2. "AMA Council Report, Guidelines for Handing Parenteral Antineoplastics." *JAMA*, 1985; 2.53(11): 1590-1592.
3. *National Study Commission on Cytotoxic Exposure-Recommendations for Handling Cytotoxic Agents*. Available from Louis P. Jeffrey, ScD., Chairman, National Study Commission on Cytotoxic Exposure, Massachusetts College of Pharmacy and Allied Health Sciences, 179 Longwood Avenue, Boston, Massachusetts 02115.
4. "Clinical Oncological Society of Australia, Guidelines and Recommendations for Safe Handling of Antineoplastic Agents." *Med J Australia*, 1983; 1:426-428.
5. Jones R.B., et al. "Safe Handling of Chemotherapeutic Agents: A Report from the Mount Sinai Medical Center." *CAA Cancer Journal for Clinicians*, 1983; (Sept/Oct): 258-263.

6. "American Society of Hospital Pharmacists Technical Assistance Bulletin on Handling Cytotoxic and Hazardous Drugs." *Am J. Hosp Pharm*, 1990; 47:1033-1049.
7. "Controlling Occupational Exposure to Hazardous Drugs." *(OSHA Work-Practice Guidelines), Am J Health-Syst Pharm*, 1996; 53:1669-1685.
Shown in Product Identification Guide, page 309

VANTAS®
[văn-tăs]
(histrelin implant)

DESCRIPTION

VANTAS® (histrelin implant) is a sterile, non-biodegradable, diffusion-controlled HYDRON® polymer reservoir containing histrelin acetate, a synthetic nonapeptide analog of the naturally occurring gonadotropin releasing hormone (GnRH), also known as luteinizing hormone releasing hormone (LH-RH), possessing a greater potency than the natural sequence hormone. VANTAS is designed to deliver approximately 50 µg histrelin per day over 12 months.

The VANTAS implant looks like a small thin flexible tube and consists of a 50-mg histrelin acetate drug core inside a 3.5 cm by 3 mm, cylindrical HYDRON® polymer reservoir (Figure A).

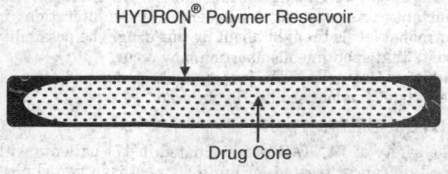

Figure A. VANTAS Implant diagram (not to scale)

Histrelin acetate is chemically described as: 5-oxo-L-prolyl-L-histidyl-L-tryptophyl-L-seryl-L-tyrosyl-Ntbenzyl-D-histidyl-L-leucyl-L-arginyl-N-ethyl-L-prolinamide acetate (salt) $[C_{66}H_{86}N_{18}O_{12}$ (1.7-2.8 moles) CH_3COOH, (0.6-7.0 moles) $H_2O]$, with the molecular weight of 1443.70 (or 1323.50 as histrelin base).

Histrelin acetate has the following structural formula:
[See chemical structure above]

The drug core also contains the inactive ingredient stearic acid NF. The HYDRON® polymer (also known as a "hydrogel") reservoir is a hydrophilic cartridge composed of 2-hydroxyethyl methacrylate, 2-hydroxypropyl methacrylate, trimethylolpropane trimethacrylate, benzoin methyl ether, Perkadox-16, and Triton X-100. Each implant is packaged hydrated in a glass vial containing 2 mL of sterile 1.8% sodium chloride solution. The implant is primed for immediate release of the drug upon insertion.

A single use, sterile Insertion Tool is provided along with the implant that may be used for the placement of the implant into the subcutaneous tissue of the inner aspect of the upper arm. The Insertion Tool is enclosed in a sterile bag and is provided separately from the implant in the Implantation Kit (see DOSAGE AND ADMINISTRATION: Recommended Procedure).

CLINICAL PHARMACOLOGY

Histrelin acetate, an LH-RH agonist, acts as a potent inhibitor of gonadotropin secretion when given continuously in therapeutic doses. Both animal and human studies indicate that following an initial stimulatory phase, chronic, subcutaneous administration of histrelin acetate desensitizes the responsiveness of the pituitary gonadotropin which, in turn, causes a reduction in testicular steroidogenesis.

In humans, administration of histrelin acetate results in an initial increase in circulating levels of luteinizing hormone (LH) and follicle-stimulating hormone (FSH), leading to a transient increase in concentration of gonadal steroids (testosterone and dihydrotestosterone in males). However, continuous administration of histrelin acetate results in decreased levels of LH and FSH. In males, testosterone is reduced to castrate levels. These decreases occur within 2 to 4 weeks after initiation of treatment.

Histrelin acetate is not active when given orally.

PHARMACOKINETICS

Absorption: Following subcutaneous insertion of one VANTAS implant in advanced prostate cancer patients (n = 17), peak serum concentrations of 1.10 ± 0.375 ng/mL (mean ± SD) occurred at a median of 12 hours. Continuous subcutaneous release was evident, as serum levels were sustained throughout the 52 week dosing period (see Figure 1). The mean serum histrelin concentration at the end of the 52 week treatment duration was 0.13 ± 0.065 ng/mL. When histrelin serum concentrations were measured following a second implant inserted after 52 weeks, the ob-

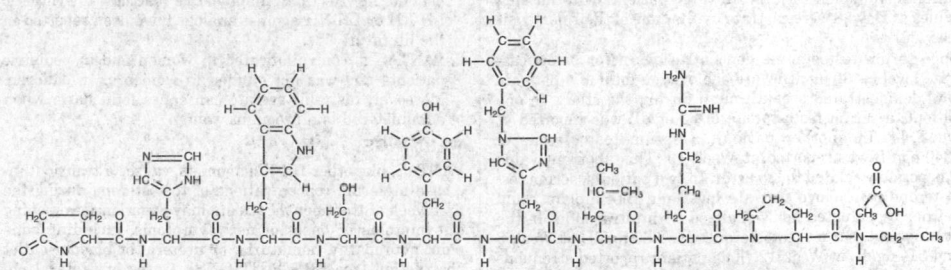

served serum concentrations over 8 weeks following the second implant were comparable to the same period following the first implant. The average rate of subcutaneous drug release from 41 implants assayed for residual drug content was 56.7 ± 7.71 µg/day, over the 52 week dosing period. The relative bioavailability for the VANTAS implant in prostate cancer patients with normal renal and hepatic function compared to a subcutaneous bolus dose in healthy male volunteers was 92%. Serum histrelin concentrations were proportional to dose after one, two or four 50 mg VANTAS implants (50, 100 or 200 mg as histrelin acetate) in 42 prostate cancer patients.

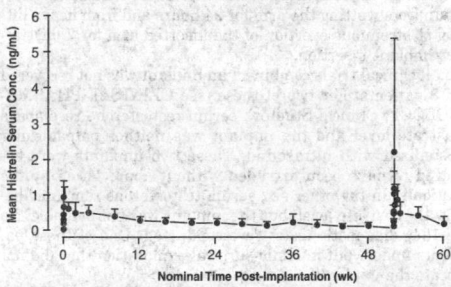

Figure 1: *Mean Serum Histrelin Concentration versus Time Profile for 17 Patients Following Insertion of First and Second VANTAS Implants. (Note that only four patients underwent intensive pharmacokinetic sampling during the first 96 hours following the second implant.)*

Distribution: The apparent volume of distribution of histrelin following a subcutaneous bolus dose (500 µg) in healthy volunteers was 58.4 ± 7.86 L. The fraction of drug unbound in plasma measured *in vitro* was 29.5% ± 8.9% (mean ± SD).

Metabolism: An *in vitro* drug metabolism study using human hepatocytes identified a single histrelin metabolite resulting from C-terminal dealkylation. Peptide fragments resulting from hydrolysis are also likely metabolites. Following a subcutaneous bolus dose in healthy volunteers the apparent clearance of histrelin was 179 ± 37.8 mL/min (mean ± SD) and the terminal half-life was 3.92 ± 1.01 hr (mean ± SD). The apparent clearance following a 50 mg (as histrelin acetate) VANTAS implant in 17 prostate cancer patients was 174 ± 56.5 mL/min (mean ± SD).

Excretion: No drug excretion study was conducted with VANTAS implants.

Special Populations:

Geriatrics: The majority (89.9%) of the 138 patients studied in the pivotal clinical trial were age 65 and over.

Pediatrics: The safety and efficacy of VANTAS in pediatric patients has not been established (see CONTRAINDICATIONS).

Race: When serum histrelin concentrations were compared for 7 Hispanic, 30 Black and 77 Caucasian patients, average serum histrelin concentrations were similar.

Renal Insufficiency: When average serum histrelin concentrations were compared between 42 prostate cancer patients with mild to severe renal impairment (CLcr: 15-60 mL/min) and 92 patients with no renal or hepatic impairment, levels were approximately 50% higher in those patients with renal impairment (0.392 ng/mL versus 0.264 ng/mL). These changes in exposure as a result of renal impairment are not considered to be clinically relevant. Therefore, no changes in drug dosing are warranted for these patient subpopulations.

Hepatic insufficiency: The influence of hepatic insufficiency on histrelin pharmacokinetics has not been adequately studied.

Drug-Drug Interactions: No pharmacokinetic-based drug-drug interaction studies were conducted with VANTAS.

CLINICAL STUDIES

In one open-label, multicenter, Phase 3 study (Study 1), 138 patients with prostate cancer were treated with a single VANTAS implant and were evaluated for at least 60 weeks.

Of these, 37 patients had Jewett stage C disease, 29 had stage D disease, and the remaining 72 patients had an elevated or rising serum PSA after definitive therapy for localized disease. Serum testosterone levels were assessed as the primary efficacy endpoint to evaluate both achievement and maintenance of castrate testosterone suppression, with treatment success being defined as a serum testosterone level ≤ 50 ng/dL. At Week 52, the study included the option for removal and insertion of a new implant, with evaluation for an additional 52 weeks (the "extension phase"). A total of 120 patients completed the initial 52-week treatment period. Reasons for discontinuation were: death (n=6), disease progression (n=5), implant expulsion (n=3), hospice placement (n=2), and patient request/no specific reason given (n=2). Of the 120 patients who successfully completed 52 weeks of treatment, 111 were evaluable for efficacy. A total of 113 patients underwent removal of the first implant and insertion of a second implant for another year of therapy.

In a subset of 17 patients, serum testosterone concentrations were measured within the first week following initial implantation. In these 17 patients, mean serum testosterone concentrations increased from 376.4 ng/dL at Baseline to 530.5 ng/dL on Day 2, then decreased to below baseline by Week 2, and to below the 50 ng/dL castrate threshold by Week 4 (see Figure 2). Serum testosterone concentrations remained below the castrate level in this subset for the entire treatment period.

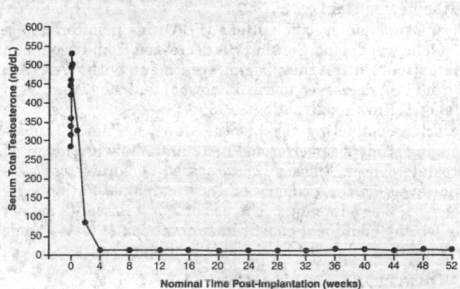

Figure 2: *Mean Serum Total Testosterone Concentrations for all PK Patients, n=17. (Note that in this group, sampling began minutes after insertion of VANTAS.)*

In the overall treatment group (n=138), mean serum testosterone was 388.3 ng/dL at Baseline. At the time of first assessment of testosterone (at the end of Week 1), the mean serum testosterone concentration was 382.8 ng/dL. At Week 2, mean serum testosterone was 92.2 ng/dL. At Week 4 it was 15 ng/dL. At Week 52, the final mean testosterone concentration was 14.3 ng/dL (see Figure 3).

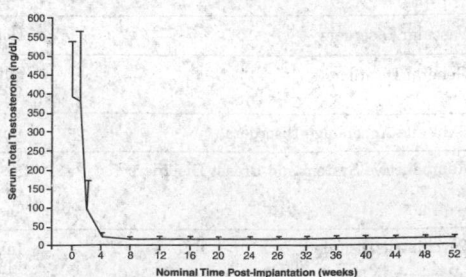

Figure 3. *Mean Serum Total Testosterone Concentrations (+SD) for All Patients (n=138) Who Received One VANTAS Implant. (Note that in this group, sampling began at the end of Week 1.)*

Of 138 patients who received an implant, one discontinued prior to Day 28 when the implant was expelled on Day 15. Three others did not have an efficacy measurement for the Day 28 visit. Otherwise serum testosterone was suppressed to below the castrate level (≤ 50 ng/dL) in all 134 evaluable patients (100%) on Day 28. All three patients with missing values at Day 28 were castrate by the time of their next visit (Day 56).

Once serum testosterone concentrations at or below castrate level (≤ 50 ng/dL) were achieved, a total of 4 patients (3%) demonstrated breakthrough during the study. In one patient, a serum testosterone of 63 ng/dL was reported at Week 44. In another patient, a serum testosterone of 3340 ng/dL was reported at Week 40. This aberrant value was possibly related to lab error. In two patients, serum testosterone rose above castrate level and the implant could neither be palpated nor visualized with ultrasound. In the first patient, serum testosterone was 669 ng/dL at Week 8 and 311 ng/dL at Week 12. This patient reported strenuous exertion after insertion of the implant and a large scab forming at the insertion site. The implant may have been expelled without the patient's appreciation of the event. The other patient developed erythema at the insertion site at Week 22 and was treated with oral antibiotics. At Week 26, the implant was not palpable and was not visualized with ultrasound. At Week 34, the serum testosterone rose to 135 ng/dL. The implant may have been expelled without the patient's appreciation of the event. A new implant was inserted.

Of 120 patients who completed 52 weeks of treatment, a total of 115 patients had a serum testosterone measurement at Week 52. Of these, all had serum testosterone ≤ 50 ng/dL. In patients without a Week 52 value, castrate levels were achieved by Day 28, were maintained up to Week 52, and remained below the castrate threshold after Week 52.

In all 18 patients who prematurely discontinued prior to Week 52 – except one (implant expulsion on Day 15) – castrate levels of serum testosterone were achieved by Day 28 and were maintained up to and including the time of withdrawal.

A total of 113 patients had a new implant inserted for a second year of therapy following removal of the first implant. Of this group, 68 patients had measurement of serum testosterone on Day 2 or Day 3 and on Day 7 after insertion of the second implant in order to assess for the "acute-on-chronic" phenomenon. No acute increase in serum testosterone was seen in any patient in this group following insertion of the new implant.

Serum prostate specific antigen (PSA) was monitored as a secondary endpoint. Serum PSA decreased from baseline in all patients after they began treatment with VANTAS. Serum PSA decreased to within normal limits by Week 24 in 103 of 111 evaluable patients (93%).

Prior to conducting the pivotal study, a Phase 2, dose-ranging study was performed in 42 patients with advanced prostate cancer. Efficacy was assessed by serum testosterone levels as the primary efficacy endpoint. Patients received 1, 2 or 4 implants. The use of 2 or 4 implants did not confer any additional benefit in suppression of testosterone beyond that produced by the single implant.

INDICATIONS AND USAGE

VANTAS is indicated in the palliative treatment of advanced prostate cancer.

CONTRAINDICATIONS

1. VANTAS is contraindicated in patients with hypersensitivity to GnRH, GnRH agonist analogs, or any of the components in VANTAS. Anaphylactic reactions to synthetic LH-RH or LH-RH agonist analogs have been reported in the literature.
2. VANTAS is contraindicated in women and in pediatric patients and was not studied in women or in children. Moreover, histrelin acetate can cause fetal harm when administered to a pregnant woman.

WARNINGS

VANTAS, like other LH-RH agonists, causes a transient increase in serum concentrations of testosterone during the first week of treatment. Patients may experience worsening of symptoms or onset of new symptoms, including bone pain, neuropathy, hematuria, or ureteral or bladder outlet obstruction (see PRECAUTIONS). Cases of ureteral obstruction and spinal cord compression, which may contribute to paralysis with or without fatal complications, have been reported with LH-RH agonists. If spinal cord compression or renal impairment develops, standard treatment of these complications should be instituted.

PRECAUTIONS

General: Patients with metastatic vertebral lesions and/or with urinary tract obstruction should be closely observed during the first few weeks of therapy (see WARNINGS).

Implant insertion is a surgical procedure. Careful adherence to the recommended Insertion and Removal Procedures (see DOSAGE AND ADMINISTRATION) is advised to minimize the potential for complications and for implant expulsion. In addition, patients should be instructed to refrain from wetting the arm for 24 hours and from heavy lifting or strenuous exertion of the inserted arm for 7 days after implant insertion.

In all clinical trials combined, an implant was not recovered in 8 patients. For two of these (see CLINICAL PHARMACOLOGY; Clinical Studies), serum testosterone rose above castrate level and the implant was neither palpable nor visualized with ultrasound. These two implants were believed to have been extruded without appreciation by the patients. In the other six, serum testosterone remained below the castrate level, but the implant was not palpable. No further diagnostic tests were conducted. One of these patients underwent in-clinic surgical exploration that did not locate the implant.

Information for Patients: An information leaflet for patients is included with the product and should be given to the patient.

Laboratory tests: Response to VANTAS should be monitored by measuring serum concentrations of testosterone and prostate-specific antigen periodically, especially if the anticipated clinical or biochemical response to treatment has not been achieved.

Results of testosterone determinations are dependent on assay methodology. It is advisable to be aware of the type and precision of the assay methodology to make appropriate clinical and therapeutic decisions.

Drug Interactions: See PHARMACOKINETICS.

Drug/Laboratory Test Interactions: Therapy with histrelin results in suppression of the pituitary-gonadal system. Results of diagnostic tests of pituitary gonadotropic and gonadal functions conducted during and after histrelin therapy may be affected.

Carcinogenesis, Mutagenesis, Impairment of Fertility: Carcinogenicity studies were conducted in rats for 2 years at doses of 5, 25 or 150 µg/kg/day (up to 15 times the human dose) and in mice for 18 months at doses of 20, 200, or 2000 µg/kg/day (up to 200 times the human dose). As seen with other LH-RH agonists, histrelin acetate injection administration was associated with an increase in tumors of hormonally responsive tissues. There was a significant increase in pituitary adenomas in rats. There was an increase in pancreatic islet-cell adenomas in treated female rats and a non-dose-related increase in testicular Leydig-cell tumors (highest incidence in the low-dose group). In mice, there was significant increase in mammary-gland adenocarcinomas in all treated females. In addition, there were increases in stomach papillomas in male rats given high doses, and an increase in histiocytic sarcomas in female mice at the highest dose.

Mutagenicity studies have not been performed with histrelin acetate. Saline extracts of implants with and without histrelin were negative in a battery of genotoxicity studies. Fertility studies have been conducted in rats and monkeys given subcutaneous daily doses of histrelin acetate, up to 180 µg/kg for 6 months, and full reversibility of fertility suppression was demonstrated. The development and reproductive performance of offspring from parents treated with histrelin acetate has not been investigated.

Pregnancy, Teratogenic Effects: Pregnancy Category X (see CONTRAINDICATIONS).

Major fetal abnormalities were observed in rabbits but not in rats after administration of histrelin acetate throughout gestation. There were increased fetal mortality and decreased fetal weights in rats and rabbits. The effects on fetal mortality are expected consequences of the alterations in hormonal levels brought about by this drug. The possibility exists that spontaneous abortion may occur.

Pediatric Use: VANTAS is contraindicated in pediatric patients and was not studied in children.

ADVERSE REACTIONS

The safety of VANTAS was evaluated in 171 patients with prostate cancer treated for up to 36 months in two clinical trials. The pivotal study (Study 1) consisted of 138 patients, while a separate supportive study (Study 2) consisted of 33 patients.

VANTAS, like other LH-RH analogs, caused a transient increase in serum testosterone concentrations during the first week of treatment. Therefore, potential exacerbations of signs and symptoms of the disease during the first few weeks of treatment are of concern in patients with vertebral metastases and/or urinary obstruction or hematuria. If these conditions are aggravated, it may lead to neurological problems such as weakness and/or paresthesia of the lower limbs or worsening of urinary symptoms (see WARNINGS and PRECAUTIONS).

In the first 12 months after initial insertion of the implant(s), an implant extruded through the incision site in eight of 171 patients in the clinical trials (see the Recommended Procedure for correct implant placement).

In the pivotal study (Study 1) a detailed evaluation for implant site reactions was conducted. Out of the 138 patients in the study, 19 patients (13.8%) experienced local or insertion site reactions. All these local site reactions were reported as mild in severity. The majority were associated with initial insertion or removal and insertion of a new implant, and began and resolved within the first two weeks following implant insertion. Reactions persisted in 4 (2.8%) patients. An additional 4 (2.8%) patients developed application-site reactions after the first two weeks following insertion.

Local reactions after implant insertion included bruising (7.2% of patients) and pain/soreness/tenderness (3.6% of patients). Other, less frequently reported, reactions included erythema (2.8% of patients) and swelling (0.7% of patients). In this study, two patients had events described as local infections/inflammations, one that resolved after treatment with oral antibiotics and the other without treatment.

Local reactions following insertion of a subsequent implant were comparable to those seen after initial insertion.

The following possibly or probably related systemic adverse events occurred during clinical trials of up to 24 months of treatment with VANTAS, and were reported in ≥ 2% of patients (Table 1).

[See table 1 at left]

Table 1: Incidence (%) of Possibly or Probably Related Systemic Adverse Events Reported by ≥ 2% of Patients Treated with VANTAS for up to 24 Months

Body System	Adverse Event	Number (%)
Vascular Disorders	Hot flashes*	112 (65.5%)
General Disorders	Fatigue	17 (9.9%)
	Weight increased	4 (2.3%)
Skin and Appendage Disorders	Implant site reaction	10 (5.8%)
Reproductive System and Breast Disorders	Erectile dysfunction*	6 (3.5%)
	Gynecomastia*	7 (4.1%)
	Testicular atrophy*	9 (5.3%)
Psychiatric Disorders	Insomnia	5 (2.9%)
	Libido decreased*	4 (2.3%)
Renal and Urinary Disorders	Renal impairment**	8 (4.7%)
Gastrointestinal Disorders	Constipation	6 (3.5%)
Nervous System Disorders	Headache	5 (2.9%)

*Expected pharmacological consequences of testosterone suppression.
** 5 of the 8 patients had a single occurrence of mild renal impairment (defined as creatinine clearance 30-<60 mL/min), which returned to a normal range by the next visit.

Hot flashes were the most common adverse event reported (65.5% of patients). In terms of severity, 2.3% of patients reported severe hot flashes, 25.4% of patients reported moderate hot flashes and 37.7% reported mild hot flashes. In addition, the following possibly or probably related systemic adverse events were reported by < 2% of patients using VANTAS in clinical studies.

Blood and Lymphatic System Disorders: Anemia

Cardiac Disorders: Palpitations, ventricular extrasystoles

Gastrointestinal Disorders: Abdominal discomfort, nausea

General Disorders: Feeling cold, lethargy, malaise, edema peripheral, pain, pain exacerbated, weakness, weight decreased

Hepatobiliary Disorders: Hepatic disorder

Injury, Poisoning and Procedural Complications: Stent occlusion

Laboratory Investigations: Aspartate aminotransferase increased, blood glucose increased, blood lactate dehydrogenase increased, blood testosterone increased, creatinine clearance decreased, prostatic acid phosphatase increased

Metabolism and Nutrition Disorders: Appetite increased, fluid retention, food craving, hypercalcaemia, hypercholesterolemia

Musculoskeletal and Connective Tissue Disorders: Arthralgia, back pain, back pain aggravated, bone pain, muscle twitching, myalgia, neck pain, pain in limb

Nervous System Disorders: Dizziness, tremor

Psychiatric Disorders: Depression, irritability

Renal and Urinary Disorders: Calculus renal, dysuria, hematuria aggravated, renal failure aggravated, urinary frequency, urinary frequency aggravated, urinary retention

Reproductive System and Breast Disorders: Breast pain, breast tenderness, genital pruritus male, gynecomastia aggravated, sexual dysfunction

Respiratory, Thoracic and Mediastinal Disorders: Dyspnea exertional

Skin and Subcutaneous Tissue Disorders: Contusion, hypotrichosis, night sweats, pruritus, sweating increased

Vascular Disorders: Flushing, hematoma

Changes in Bone Density: Decreased bone density has been reported in the medical literature in men who have had orchiectomy or who have been treated with an LH-RH agonist analog. It can be anticipated that long periods of medical castration in men will have effects on bone density.

Post-marketing

The following adverse reactions have been identified during post approval use of VANTAS. Because these reactions are reported voluntarily from a population of uncertain size, it is not always possible to reliably estimate their frequency or establish a causal relationship to drug exposure.

Pituitary Apoplexy: Rare cases of pituitary apoplexy (a clinical syndrome secondary to infarction of the pituitary gland) have been reported after the administration of gonadotropin-releasing hormone agonists. In a majority of these cases, a pituitary adenoma was diagnosed with a majority of pituitary apoplexy cases occurring within 2 weeks of the final dose, and some within the first hour. In these cases, pituitary apoplexy has presented as sudden headache, vomiting, visual changes, opthalmoplegia, altered mental status, and sometimes cardiovascular collapse. Immediate medical attention has been required.

Drug Induced Livery Injury: Post-marketing surveillance has identified drug induced liver injury potentially associated with VANTAS. Causality could not be established due to the associated use of confounding drugs that are known to cause liver injury; however, there was a strong temporal relationship between the indicated use of VANTAS and elevated liver enzymes.

OVERDOSAGE

Histrelin acetate injection of up to 200 µg/kg (rats, rabbits), or 2000 µg/kg (mice) resulted in no systemic toxicity. This represents 20 to 200 times the maximal recommended human dose of 10 µg/kg/day. Adverse event profiles were similar in patients receiving one, two or four VANTAS implants.

DOSAGE AND ADMINISTRATION

The recommended dose of VANTAS is one implant every 12 months. Each implant contains 50 mg histrelin acetate. The implant is inserted subcutaneously in the inner aspect of the upper arm and provides continuous release of histrelin (50 µg/day) for 12 months of hormonal therapy. VANTAS should be removed after 12 months of therapy (the implant has been designed to allow for a few additional weeks of histrelin release, in order to allow flexibility of medical appointments). At the time an implant is removed, another implant may be inserted to continue therapy (see Recommended Procedure below).

Recommended Procedure

This procedure section is intended to provide guidance for the insertion and removal of VANTAS. The actual procedure used, however, is at the discretion of the qualified healthcare provider performing the procedure.

Insertion of a new implant can proceed using the following **Suggested Insertion Procedure** . If a previous VANTAS implant must first be removed, please see the **Suggested Removal Procedure** instructions below.

Suggested Insertion Procedure

Many of the supplies necessary to insert the implant, including the Insertion Tool and local anesthetic, are provided in a separate Implantation Kit that is shipped along with the implant. Please note that the implant, in its sealed vial, pouch, and carton, must be kept refrigerated (2-8°C) until

needed for the procedure. Once removed from refrigeration, the vial containing the implant (still in its unopened pouch and carton) may remain at room temperature for up to 7 days, if necessary, before being used. If not used in that time, the packaged implant may again be properly refrigerated until the expiration date on the carton.

NOTE: The Implantation Kit is to be stored at room temperature and should *not* be refrigerated.

Insertion of the VANTAS implant is a surgical procedure. Sterile gloves and aseptic technique must be used to minimize any chance of infection.

Setting up the Sterile Field

Using proper aseptic technique, the sterilized components of the Implantation Kit needed for the insertion procedure, including the Insertion Tool, are to be carefully dispensed from their packaging onto the Sterile Field drape (*non*-fenestrated) provided. NOTE THAT THE KIT BOX AND ALL PACKAGING ARE NOT STERILE and should be kept off of the Sterile Field drape. DO NOT PLACE THE VIAL OF LOCAL ANESTHETIC OR THE VIAL CONTAINING THE IMPLANT ONTO THE DRAPE as the exterior surface of these vials is not sterile.

The implant vial should not be opened until just before the time of insertion. Open the vial by removing the metal band and carefully pour the sterile contents (implant and sterile saline) onto the Sterile Field drape. The implant can then be handled with sterile gloves or with the sterile mosquito clamp provided.

Preparing the Patient and the Insertion Site

The patient should be on his back, ideally with the arm least used (e.g., left arm for a right-handed person) positioned either bent or extended so that the physician has ready access to the inner aspect of the upper arm. Propping the arm with pillows may help the patient more easily hold the position. The suggested optimum site for subcutaneous insertion is approximately half-way between the shoulder and the elbow, in line with the crease between the biceps and triceps muscles.

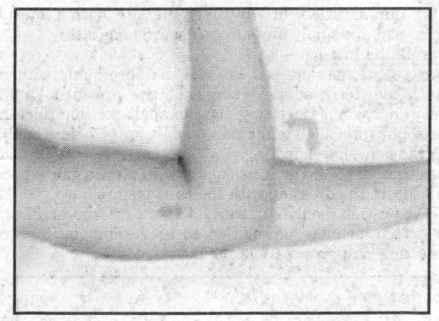

Antiseptic
Swab the insertion area with topical antiseptic, then overlay with the *fenestrated* Sterile Field drape provided, so that the opening is over the insertion site (for clarity of illustration, the following images do not show the drape).

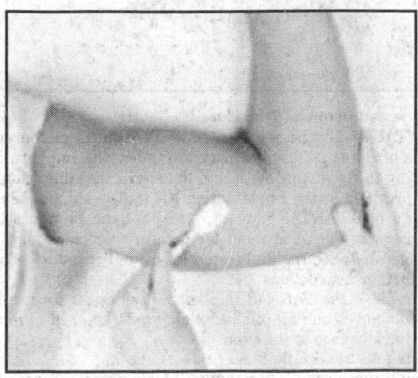

Anesthetic
The method of anesthesia utilized (i.e., local, conscious sedation, general) is at the discretion of the healthcare provider.

If local anesthesia is selected: a vial of sterile local anesthetic (note that the exterior of the vial is not sterile) has been provided along with a sterile hypodermic needle for injection. After determining the absence of known allergies to the anesthetic agent, inject anesthetic into the subcutaneous tissue, starting at the planned incision site, then infil-

trating along the intended subcutaneous insertion path, up to the length of the implant (a little more than one inch).

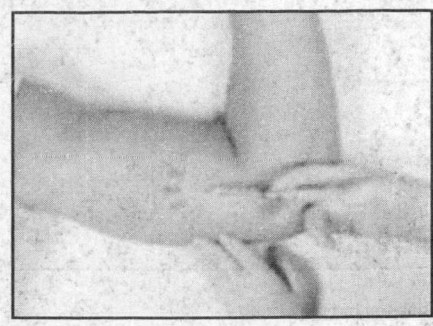

The following sections describe the suggested procedure for insertion of the implant using the Insertion Tool provided. The method of insertion used, however, is at the discretion of the healthcare provider performing the procedure.

Loading the Insertion Tool

The sterile Insertion Tool is comprised of a fixed handle attached to a retractable, bevel-tipped cannula, into the chamber of which the implant is placed for subcutaneous insertion. Inside the fully extended cannula, up to the level of the black marking, is a fixed piston upon which the implant rests. During the final step of the insertion procedure, the cannula will be retracted into the handle using the slide mechanism (green button), thereby exposing and leaving the implant to remain in the subcutaneous tissue.

When first grasping the sterile Insertion Tool, confirm that the cannula is fully extended. Verify this by inspecting the position of the green retraction button. The button should be locked in position all the way forward, towards the cannula, farthest from the handle.

The implant can be picked up using sterile gloves or with the sterile mosquito clamp provided. Avoid bending or pinching the implant. Note that the implant may come out of its vial slightly curved after refrigerated storage.

To help make the implant more symmetrical prior to loading into the Tool, you can roll the implant a few times (using a sterile glove) between the fingers and thumb.

Insert the implant into the cannula of the Insertion Tool manually or using the mosquito clamp. When inserting the implant into the cannula, DO NOT FORCE the implant. If resistance is felt, the implant should be removed and manually manipulated or rolled as needed, and re-inserted into the cannula.

When fully inserted, the implant rests inside the cannula so that just the tip of the or implant is visible at the beveled end of the cannula.

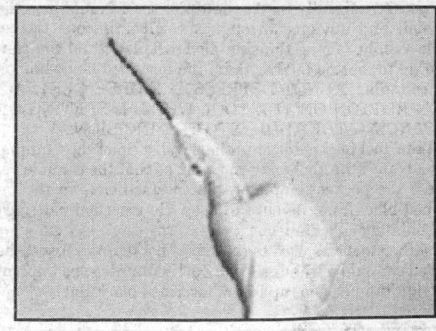

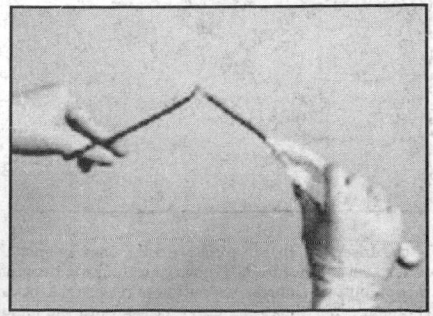

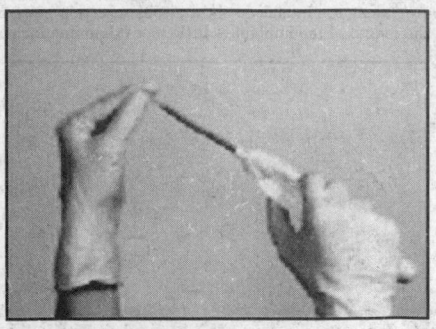

Making the Incision

Using the sterile scalpel provided, make an incision transverse to the long axis of the arm, and of a size adequate to allow the bore of the cannula to be inserted into the subcutaneous tissue.

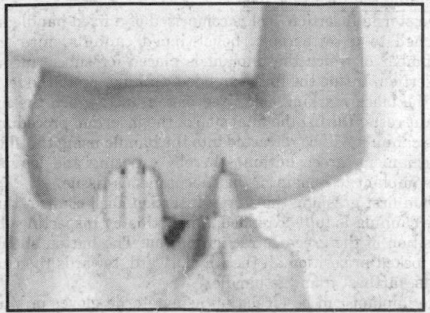

Inserting the Implant

It is suggested that insertion may be easier if a "pocket" for the implant is first created by blunt dissection through the incision, subcutaneously along the path of the anesthetic, using the cannula of the loaded Insertion Tool, or using a sterile hemostatic clamp or equivalent surgical tool.

Be sure to VISIBLY RAISE THE SKIN (known as tenting) at all times during the pocket-making and insertion procedures to ensure correct subcutaneous placement ("just under the skin") of the implant. Note that the cannula of the Insertion Tool, or whatever tool is being used to create the pocket, SHOULD NOT ENTER MUSCLE TISSUE. Deep insertion of the implant will not affect the performance of VANTAS, but may cause difficulty in the later removal of the implant.

If using the cannula of the loaded Insertion Tool to create the pocket, carefully insert the tip of the cannula into the incision and advance through the subcutaneous tissue, while visibly raising the skin along the length of the cannula up to, but no farther than, the inscribed black line on the cannula. DO NOT DEPRESS THE GREEN RETRACTION BUTTON ON THE TOOL WHILE INSERTING OR ADVANCING THE TOOL INTO THE INCISION.

Pull the Tool back, almost to the beveled tip of the cannula, and advance the Tool forward again, so that the cannula re-enters the pocket completely, but no farther than the inscribed black line. Be sure to keep the insertion path just immediately subcutaneous.

If another tool was used to create the pocket, now insert the loaded cannula of the Insertion Tool containing the implant through the incision, up to the inscribed black line.

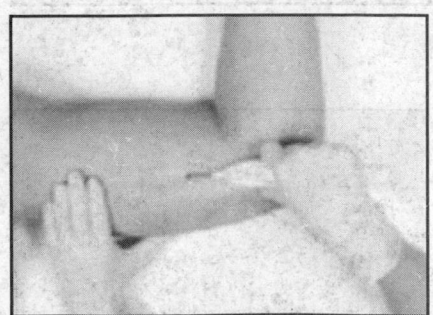

Hold the Insertion Tool in place with the base against the patient's arm as you carefully move your thumb to the green retraction button. Depress the button to release the locking mechanism, then slide the button back toward the handle

until it stops, all the while holding the body of the Insertion Tool in place.

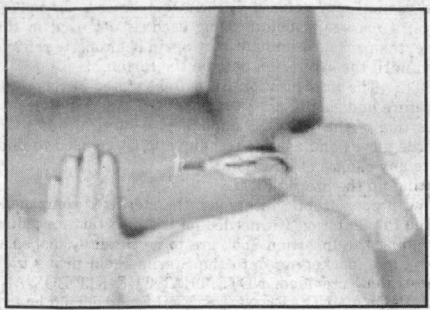

Retracting the button causes the cannula to withdraw from the incision, leaving the implant in the subcutaneous tissue. DO NOT FURTHER ADVANCE THE CANNULA ONCE THE RETRACTION PROCESS HAS STARTED. Likewise, do not withdraw the Insertion Tool until the button is fully retracted or the implant may be pulled partially out of the incision. Once the retraction is complete, the Tool can be fully withdrawn.

NOTE: It may be helpful during the process of retraction and withdrawal of the cannula to apply pressure to the skin over the implant, to help ensure that the implant remains in the subcutaneous pocket.

If there is a need to re-start the process at any time during the insertion procedure, withdraw the Insertion Tool, carefully extract the implant from the cannula and reset the retraction button on the Tool to its forward-most position. Examine the implant before reloading the implant into the Insertion Tool, and start again.

Placement of the implant should be confirmed by palpation. Note that the tip of a properly-placed implant may not be visible through the incision.

After implantation, briefly cover the site with a sterile gauze pad and apply pressure to ensure hemostasis.

Closing the Incision

To close the incision, you can use the absorbable sutures and/or the sterile adhesive surgical strips provided. To improve adhesion of the strips, you can apply benzoin tincture antiseptic (provided) to the skin, and let it dry, before applying the adhesive strips.

Once closed, cover the incision site with sterile gauze pads and secure the dressing with the bandage provided.

Please provide the patient with a Patient Information Leaflet, which includes information about the implant and instructions on proper care of the insertion site.

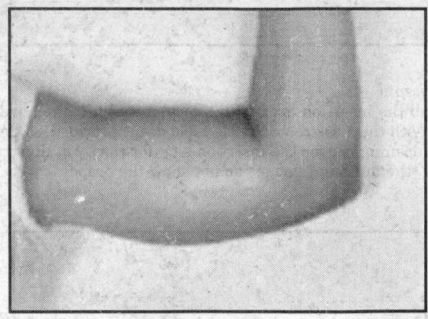

Suggested Removal Procedure

VANTAS should be removed after 12 months of therapy. Most of the supplies necessary to remove the implant, including the local anesthetic and the sterile mosquito clamp, are provided in the Implantation Kit that is shipped along with a new VANTAS implant. Note that the Implantation Kit is to be stored at room temperature and must not be refrigerated. See the **Suggested Insertion Procedure** above for further instructions.

Removal of the VANTAS implant is a surgical procedure. Sterile gloves and aseptic technique must be used to minimize any chance of infection.

Setting up the Sterile Field

Using proper aseptic technique, the sterilized components of the Implantation Kit needed for the implant removal procedure are to be carefully dispensed from their packaging onto the Sterile Field drape (non-fenestrated) provided. NOTE THAT THE KIT BOX AND ALL PACKAGING ARE NOT STERILE and should be kept off of the Sterile Field drape. DO NOT PLACE THE VIAL OF LOCAL ANESTHETIC ONTO THE DRAPE as the exterior surface of the vial is not sterile.

Preparing the Patient and the Site

The patient should be on his back, with the arm containing the implant positioned, either bent or extended, so that the

physician has ready access to the inner aspect of the upper arm. Propping the arm with pillows may help the patient more easily hold the position.

The implant to be removed should first be located by palpating the inner aspect of the upper arm, near the incision from the prior year.

Generally, the previous implant is readily palpated. In the event the implant is difficult to locate, ultrasound may be used. If ultrasound fails to locate the implant, other imaging techniques such as CT or MRI may be used to locate it (plain films are not recommended as **the implant is not radiopaque**).

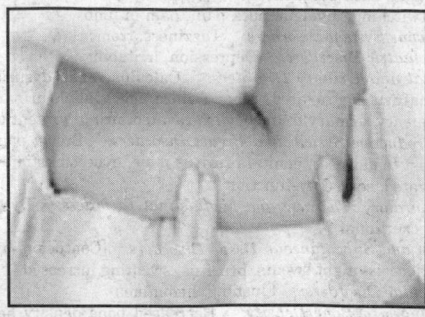

Antiseptic

Swab the area above and around the previous implant with topical antiseptic. Overlay the area with the *fenestrated* Sterile Field drape provided, so that the hole is over the previous insertion site (for clarity of illustration, the following images do not show the drape).

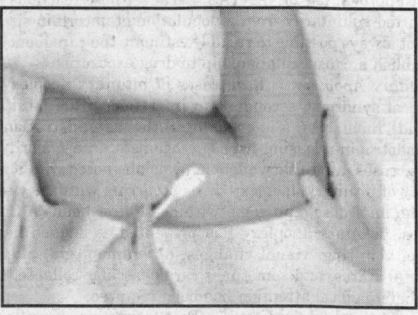

Anesthetic

The method of anesthesia utilized (i.e., local, conscious sedation, general) is at the discretion of the healthcare provider.

If local anesthesia is selected: a vial of sterile local anesthetic (note that the exterior of the vial is not sterile) has been provided along with a sterile hypodermic needle for injection. After determining the absence of known allergies to the anesthetic agent, inject anesthetic into the subcutaneous tissue at and around the site of the intended incision (the site of the previous implant).

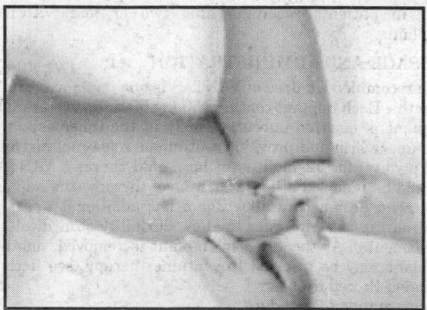

Making the Incision and Removing the Implant

Using the sterile scalpel provided, make an incision of a size adequate to allow the implant to be easily removed and, if a new implant will be inserted, large enough for the bore of the cannula of the Insertion Tool provided.

Generally, the tip of the implant will be visible through the incision, possibly covered by a pseudocapsule of tissue. In order to facilitate the removal of the implant, it may be necessary to palpate the head of the implant through the incision using your smallest finger, especially if the head of the implant is not readily visible. In addition, you may need to push down on the distal end of the implant and "massage it forward" toward the incision.

Carefully nick the pseudocapsule to reveal the polymer tip of the implant. It may be beneficial to insert the sterile mosquito clamp provided into the hole created in the pseudocapsule and expand by opening the clamp. Widening the opening of the pseudocapsule may ease the extraction of the implant.

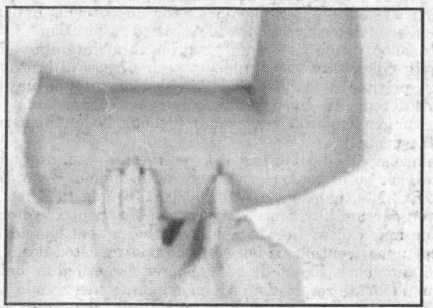

Gently but securely grasp the implant with the sterile mosquito clamp and extract the implant.

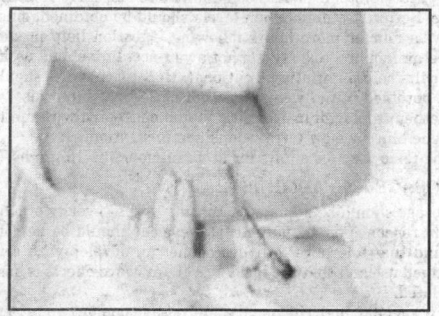

Dispose of the implant in a proper manner, treating it like any other biowaste.

Briefly cover the site with a sterile gauze pad and apply pressure to ensure hemostasis.

If inserting a new implant, see the **Suggested Insertion Procedure** instructions provided above. Note that you can insert the new implant into the same "pocket" as the removed implant, or make a new incision at a different site in the same arm or in the contralateral arm.

If a new implant is not to be inserted, proceed to close the incision.

Closing the Incision

To close the incision, you can use the absorbable sutures and/or the sterile adhesive surgical strips provided. To improve adhesion of the strips, you can apply benzoin tincture antiseptic (provided) to the skin, and let it dry, before applying the adhesive strips.

Once closed, cover the incision site with sterile gauze pads and secure the dressing with the bandage provided.

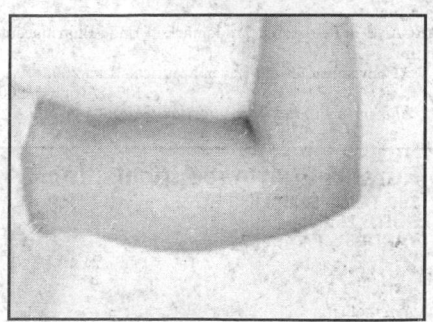

HOW SUPPLIED

VANTAS (NDC 67979-500-01) is supplied in a carton containing 2 inner cartons, one for the VANTAS implant and one for the VANTAS Implantation Kit:

The VANTAS implant carton contains a cold pack for refrigerated shipment and a small carton containing an amber plastic pouch. Inside the pouch is a glass vial with a Teflon-coated stopper and an aluminum seal, containing the implant immersed in 2 mL of sterile 1.8% sodium chloride solution.

Upon receipt, refrigerate the small carton containing the amber plastic pouch and glass vial (with the implant inside) until the day of insertion.

Store the implant refrigerated, 2-8°C (36-46°F), in the unopened glass vial with the sterile 1.8% sodium chloride solution, overwrapped in the amber plastic pouch and carton,

until the expiration date provided. Excursion permitted to 25°C (77°F) for 7 days. Protect from light. Do not freeze.

The VANTAS Implantation Kit, which should *not* be refrigerated, contains most of the equipment needed for insertion and removal.

Rx Only

For more information, call 1-800-462-3636 or visit www.vantasimplant.com.

VANTAS® and HYDRON® are Registered Trademarks of Endo Pharmaceuticals.

Manufactured by
Endo Pharmaceuticals Solutions Inc.
Chadds Ford, PA 19317
© 2010 Endo Pharmaceuticals
PK000003 Rev 05 February 2010

Shown in Product Identification Guide, page 309

ZYDONE®

[zī ''dōn]   Ⓒ ℞

(Hydrocodone Bitartrate and Acetaminophen Tablets, USP)

DESCRIPTION

ZYDONE (hydrocodone bitartrate and acetaminophen tablets) for oral administration, contain hydrocodone bitartrate and acetaminophen in the following strengths:

Hydrocodone Bitartrate, USP	5 mg
Acetaminophen, USP	400 mg
Hydrocodone Bitartrate, USP	7.5 mg
Acetaminophen, USP	400 mg
Hydrocodone Bitartrate, USP	10 mg
Acetaminophen, USP	400 mg

In addition, each tablet contains the following inactive ingredients: colloidal silicon dioxide, croscarmellose sodium, crospovidone, microcrystalline cellulose, povidone, pregelatinized starch, and stearic acid. The 5 mg/400 mg strength contains FD&C Yellow No. 10; 7.5 mg/400 mg contains FD&C Blue No. 2; and 10 mg/400 mg contains FD&C Red No. 40.

Zydone Tablets meet USP Dissolution Test 1.

Hydrocodone bitartrate is an opioid analgesic and antitussive and occurs as fine, white crystals or as a crystalline powder. It is affected by light. The chemical name is 4,5α-Epoxy-3-methoxy-17-methylmorphinan-6-one tartrate (1:1) hydrate (2:5). It has the following structural formula:

$$C_{18}H_{21}NO_3 \cdot C_4H_6O_6 \cdot 2\tfrac{1}{2}H_2O \qquad MW = 494.50$$

Acetaminophen, 4'-Hydroxyacetanilide, a slightly bitter, white, odorless, crystalline powder, is a non-opiate, non-salicylate analgesic and antipyretic. It has the following structural formula:

$$C_8H_9NO_2 \qquad MW = 151.17$$

CLINICAL PHARMACOLOGY

Hydrocodone is a semisynthetic opioid analgesic and antitussive with multiple actions qualitatively similar to those of codeine. Most of these involve the central nervous system and smooth muscle. The precise mechanism of action of hydrocodone and other opiates is not known, although it is believed to relate to the existence of opiate receptors in the central nervous system. In addition to analgesia, opioids may produce drowsiness, changes in mood and mental clouding.

The analgesic action of acetaminophen involves peripheral influences, but the specific mechanism is as yet undetermined. Antipyretic activity is mediated through hypothalamic heat-regulating centers. Acetaminophen inhibits prostaglandin synthetase. Therapeutic doses of acetaminophen have negligible effects on the cardiovascular or respiratory systems; however, toxic doses may cause circulatory failure and rapid, shallow breathing.

Pharmacokinetics

The behavior of the individual components is described below.

Hydrocodone: Following a 10 mg oral dose of hydrocodone administered to five adult male subjects, the mean peak concentration was 23.6 ± 5.2 ng/mL. Maximum serum levels were achieved at 1.3 ± 0.3 hours and the half-life was determined to be 3.8 ± 0.3 hours. Hydrocodone exhibits a complex pattern of metabolism including O-demethylation, N-demethylation and 6-keto reduction to the corresponding 6-α- and 6-β-hydroxymetabolites.

See **OVERDOSAGE** for toxicity information.

Acetaminophen: Acetaminophen is rapidly absorbed from the gastrointestinal tract and is distributed throughout most body tissues. The plasma half-life is 1.25 to 3 hours, but may be increased by liver damage and following overdosage. Elimination of acetaminophen is principally by liver metabolism (conjugation) and subsequent renal excretion of metabolites. Approximately 85% of an oral dose appears in the urine within 24 hours of administration, most as the glucuronide conjugate, with small amounts of other conjugates and unchanged drug.

See **OVERDOSAGE** for toxicity information.

INDICATIONS AND USAGE

ZYDONE (hydrocodone bitartrate and acetaminophen tablets) is indicated for the relief of moderate to moderately severe pain.

CONTRAINDICATIONS

ZYDONE tablets should not be administered to patients who have previously exhibited hypersensitivity to hydrocodone, acetaminophen, or any other component of this product.

Patients known to be hypersensitive to other opioids may exhibit cross-sensitivity to hydrocodone.

WARNINGS

Respiratory Depression

At high doses or in sensitive patients, hydrocodone may produce dose-related respiratory depression by acting directly on the brain stem respiratory center. Hydrocodone also affects the center that controls respiratory rhythm, and may produce irregular and periodic breathing.

Head Injury and Increased Intracranial Pressure

The respiratory depressant effects of opioids and their capacity to elevate cerebrospinal fluid pressure may be markedly exaggerated in the presence of head injury, other intracranial lesions or a preexisting increase in intracranial pressure. Furthermore, opioids produce adverse reactions which may obscure the clinical course of patients with head injuries.

Acute Abdominal Conditions

The administration of opioids may obscure the diagnosis or clinical course of patients with acute abdominal conditions.

PRECAUTIONS

General:

Special Risk Patients: As with any opioid analgesic agent, ZYDONE tablets should be used with caution in elderly or debilitated patients, and those with severe impairment of hepatic or renal function, hypothyroidism, Addison's disease, prostatic hypertrophy or urethral stricture. The usual precautions should be observed and the possibility of respiratory depression should be kept in mind.

Cough Reflex: Hydrocodone suppresses the cough reflex; as with all opioids, caution should be exercised when ZYDONE tablets are used postoperatively and in patients with pulmonary disease.

Information for Patients

Hydrocodone, like all opioids, may impair mental and/or physical abilities required for the performance of potentially hazardous tasks such as driving a car or operating machinery; patients should be cautioned accordingly.

Alcohol and other CNS depressants may produce an additive CNS depression, when taken with this combination product, and should be avoided.

Hydrocodone may be habit-forming. Patients should take the drug only for as long as it is prescribed, in the amounts prescribed, and no more frequently than prescribed.

Laboratory Tests

In patients with severe hepatic or renal disease, effects of therapy should be monitored with serial liver and/or renal function tests.

Drug Interactions

Patients receiving opioids, antihistamines, antipsychotics, antianxiety agents, or other CNS depressants (including alcohol) concomitantly with hydrocodone bitartrate and acetaminophen tablets may exhibit an additive CNS depression. When combined therapy is contemplated, the dose of one or both agents should be reduced.

The use of MAO inhibitors or tricyclic antidepressants with hydrocodone preparations may increase the effect of either the antidepressant or hydrocodone.

5 mg/400 mg Yellow, elongated octagonal, convex tablets debossed with "E" on one side and "5" on the other.	Bottles of 100	NDC 63481-668-70
7.5 mg/400 mg Blue, elongated octagonal, convex tablets debossed with "E" on one side and "7.5" on the other.	Bottles of 100	NDC 63481-669-70
10 mg/400 mg Red, elongated octagonal, convex tablets debossed with "E" on one side and "10" on the other.	Bottles of 100	NDC 63481-698-70

Drug/Laboratory Test Interactions

Acetaminophen may produce false-positive test results for urinary 5-hydroxyindoleacetic acid.

Carcinogenesis, Mutagenesis, Impairment of Fertility

No adequate studies have been conducted in animals to determine whether hydrocodone or acetaminophen have a potential for carcinogenesis, mutagenesis, or impairment of fertility.

Pregnancy

Teratogenic Effects; Pregnancy Category C: There are no adequate and well-controlled studies in pregnant women. ZYDONE tablets should be used during pregnancy only if the potential benefit justifies the potential risk to the fetus.

Nonteratogenic Effects: Babies born to mothers who have been taking opioids regularly prior to delivery will be physically dependent. The withdrawal signs include irritability and excessive crying, tremors, hyperactive reflexes, increased respiratory rate, increased stools, sneezing, yawning, vomiting, and fever. The intensity of the syndrome does not always correlate with the duration of maternal opioid use or dose. There is no consensus on the best method of managing withdrawal.

Labor and Delivery

As with all opioids, administration of this product to the mother shortly before delivery may result in some degree of respiratory depression in the newborn, especially if higher doses are used.

Nursing Mothers

Acetaminophen is excreted in breast milk in small amounts, but the significance of its effects on nursing infants is not known. It is not known whether hydrocodone is excreted in human milk. Because many drugs are excreted in human milk and because of the potential for serious adverse reactions in nursing infants from hydrocodone and acetaminophen, a decision should be made whether to discontinue nursing or to discontinue the drug, taking into account the importance of the drug to the mother.

Pediatric Use

Safety and effectiveness in the pediatric patients have not been established.

Geriatric Use

Clinical Studies of hydrocodone bitartrate and acetaminophen tablets did not include sufficient numbers of subjects aged 65 and over to determine whether they respond differently from younger subjects. Other reported clinical experience has not identified differences in responses between the elderly and younger patients. In general, dose selection for an elderly patient should be cautious, usually starting at the low end of the dosing range, reflecting the grater frequency of decreased hepatic, renal, or cardiac function, and of concomitant disease or other drug therapy.

Hydrocodone and the major metabolites of acetaminophen are known to be substantially excreted by the kidney. Thus the risk of toxic reactions may be greater in patients with impaired renal function due to the accumulation of the parent compound and/or metabolites in the plasma. Because elderly patients are more likely to have decreased renal function, care should be taken in dose selection, and it may be useful to monitor renal function.

Hydrocodone may cause confusion and over-sedation in the elderly; elderly patients generally should be started on low doses of hydrocodone bitartrate and acetaminophen tablets and observed closely.

ADVERSE REACTIONS

The most frequently reported adverse reactions are lightheadedness, dizziness, sedation, nausea and vomiting. These effects seem to be more prominent in ambulatory than in non-ambulatory patients, and some of these adverse reactions may be alleviated if the patient lies down. Other adverse reactions include:

Central Nervous System: Drowsiness, mental clouding, lethargy, impairment of mental and physical performance, anxiety, fear, dysphoria, psychic dependence, mood changes.

Gastrointestinal System: Prolonged administration of ZYDONE (hydrocodone bitartrate and acetaminophen tablets) may produce constipation.

Genitourinary System: Ureteral spasm, spasm of vesical sphincters and urinary retention have been reported with opiates.

Respiratory Depression: Hydrocodone bitartrate may produce dose-related respiratory depression by acting directly on brain stem respiratory center (see **OVERDOSAGE**).

Special Senses: Cases of hearing impairment or permanent loss have been reported predominantly in patients with chronic overdose.

Dermatological: Skin rash, pruritus.

The following adverse drug events may be borne in mind as potential effects of acetaminophen: allergic reactions, rash, thrombocytopenia, agranulocytosis.

Potential effects of high dosage are listed in the **OVERDOSAGE** section.

DRUG ABUSE AND DEPENDENCE

Controlled Substance

ZYDONE tablets are classified as a Schedule III controlled substance.

Abuse and Dependence

Psychic dependence, physical dependence, and tolerance may develop upon repeated administration of opioids; therefore, this product should be prescribed and administered with caution. However, psychic dependence is unlikely to develop when hydrocodone bitartrate and acetaminophen tablets are used for a short time for the treatment of pain. Physical dependence, the condition in which continued administration of the drug is required to prevent the appearance of a withdrawal syndrome, assumes clinically significant proportions only after several weeks of continued opioid use, although some mild degree of physical dependence may develop after a few days of opioid therapy. Tolerance, in which increasingly large doses are required in order to produce the same degree of analgesia, is manifested initially by a shortened duration of analgesic effect, and subsequently by decreases in the intensity of analgesia. The rate of development of tolerance varies among patients.

OVERDOSAGE

Following an acute overdosage, toxicity may result from hydrocodone or acetaminophen.

Signs and Symptoms

Hydrocodone: Serious overdose with hydrocodone is characterized by respiratory depression (a decrease in respiratory rate and/or tidal volume, Cheyne-Stokes respiration, cyanosis) extreme somnolence progressing to stupor or coma, skeletal muscle flaccidity, cold and clammy skin, and sometimes bradycardia and hypotension. In severe overdosage, apnea, circulatory collapse, cardiac arrest and death may occur.

Acetaminophen: In acetaminophen overdosage: dose-dependent, potentially fatal hepatic necrosis is the most serious adverse effect. Renal tubular necrosis, hypoglycemic coma and thrombocytopenia may also occur.

Early symptoms following a potentially hepatotoxic overdose may include: nausea, vomiting, diaphoresis and general malaise. Clinical and laboratory evidence of hepatic toxicity may not be apparent until 48 to 72 hours postingestion.

In adults, hepatic toxicity has rarely been reported with acute overdose of less than 10 grams or fatalities with less than 15 grams.

Treatment

A single or multiple overdose with hydrocodone and acetaminophen is a potentially lethal polydrug overdose, and consultation with a regional poison control center is recommended.

Immediate treatment includes support of cardiorespiratory function and measures to reduce drug absorption. Vomiting should be induced mechanically, or with syrup of ipecac, if the patient is alert (adequate pharyngeal and laryngeal reflexes). Oral activated charcoal (1 g/kg) should follow gastric emptying. The first dose should be accompanied by an appropriate cathartic. If repeated doses are used, the cathartic might be included with alternate doses as required. Hypotension is usually hypovolemic and should respond to fluids. Vasopressors and other supportive measures should be employed as indicated. A cuffed endotracheal tube should be inserted before gastric lavage of the unconscious patient and, when necessary, to provide assisted respiration. Meticulous attention should be given to maintaining adequate pulmonary ventilation. In severe cases of intoxication, pertitoneal dialysis, or preferably hemodialysis may be considered. If hypoprothrombinemia occurs due to acetaminophen overdose, vitamin K should be administered intravenously.

Naloxone, an opioid antagonist, can reverse respiratory depression and coma associated with opioid overdose. NARCAN® (naloxone hydrochloride) 0.4 mg to 2 mg is given parenterally. Since the duration of action of hydrocodone may exceed that of naloxone, the patient should be kept under continuous surveillance and repeated doses of the antagonist should be administered as needed to maintain adequate respiration. An opioid antagonist should not be administered in the absence of clinically significant respiratory or cardiovascular depression.

If the dose of acetaminophen may have exceeded 140 mg/kg, acetylcysteine should be administered as early as possible. Serum acetaminophen levels should be obtained, since levels four or more hours following ingestion help predict acetaminophen toxicity. Do not await acetaminophen assay results before initiating treatment. Hepatic enzymes should be obtained initially, and repeated at 24-hour intervals. Methemoglobinemia over 30% should be treated with methylene blue by slow intravenous administration.

The toxic dose for adults for acetaminophen is 10 grams.

DOSAGE AND ADMINISTRATION

Dosage should be adjusted according to the severity of pain and response of the patient. However, it should be kept in mind that tolerance to hydrocodone can develop with continued use and that the incidence of untoward effects is dose related.

5 mg/400 mg: The usual adult dose is one or two tablets every four to six hours as needed for pain. The total daily dosage should not exceed eight tablets.

7.5 mg/400 mg: The usual adult dosage is one tablet every four to six hours as needed for pain. The total daily dosage should not exceed six tablets.

10 mg/400 mg: The usual adult dosage is one tablet every four to six hours as needed for pain. The total daily dosage should not exceed six tablets.

HOW SUPPLIED

ZYDONE (hydrocodone bitartrate and acetaminophen tablets, USP) is supplied as follows:
[See table at top left]
Store at 25°C (77°F); excursions permitted to 15°–30°C (59°–86°F). [See USP Controlled Room Temperature].
Dispense in a tight, light-resistant container as defined in the USP, with a child-resistant closure (as required).
A Schedule III Opioid. Oral prescription where permitted by State law.
ZYDONE® is a Registered Trademark of Endo Pharmaceuticals Inc.
NARCAN® is Registered Trademark of Endo Pharmaceuticals Inc.

Copyright © Endo Pharmaceuticals Inc. 2003
413742/August, 2003
Shown in Product Identification Guide, page 309

Eurand Pharmaceuticals, Inc.

790 TOWNSHIP LINE RD
SUITE 250
YARDLEY, PA 19067

Tel: 267-759-9400
Fax: 215-968-2941

ZENPEP®

[ZEN-pep]
(pancrelipase)
Delayed Release Capsules

℞

HIGHLIGHTS OF PRESCRIBING INFORMATION

These highlights do not include all the information needed to use ZENPEP safely and effectively. See full **prescribing information for ZENPEP.**
ZENPEP® (pancrelipase) delayed release capsules
Initial U.S. Approval: 2009
——————INDICATIONS AND USAGE——————
ZENPEP® is a combination of porcine-derived lipases, proteases, and amylases indicated for the treatment of exocrine

pancreatic insufficiency due to cystic fibrosis, or other conditions (1)

DOSAGE AND ADMINISTRATION

Dosage
ZENPEP is not interchangeable with any other pancrelipase product.

Infants (up to 12 months)
- Infants may be given 2,000 to 4,000 lipase units per 120 mL of formula or per breast-feeding. (2.1)
- Do not mix ZENPEP capsule contents directly into formula or breast milk prior to administration. (2.2)

Children Older than 12 Months and Younger than 4 Years
- Enzyme dosing should begin with 1,000 lipase units/kg of body weight per meal to a maximum of 2,500 lipase units/kg of body weight per meal (or less than or equal to 10,000 lipase units/kg of body weight per day), or less than 4,000 lipase units/g fat ingested per day. (2.1)

Children 4 Years and Older and Adults
- Enzyme dosing should begin with 500 lipase units/kg of body weight per meal to a maximum of 2,500 lipase units/kg of body weight per meal (or less than or equal to 10,000 lipase units/kg of body weight per day), or less than 4,000 lipase units/g fat ingested per day. (2.1)

Limitations on Dosing
- Dosing should not exceed the recommended maximum dosage set forth by the Cystic Fibrosis Foundation Consensus Conferences Guidelines (2.1)

Administration
- ZENPEP should be swallowed whole. For infants or patients unable to swallow intact capsules, the contents may be sprinkled on soft acidic food, e.g., applesauce. (2.2)

DOSAGE FORMS AND STRENGTHS
- Capsules: 5,000 USP units of lipase; 17,000 USP units of protease; 27,000 USP units of amylase. Capsules have a white opaque cap and body, printed with "EURAND 5" (3)
- Capsules: 10,000 USP units of lipase; 34,000 USP units of protease; 55,000 USP units of amylase. Capsules have a yellow opaque cap and white opaque body, printed with "EURAND 10" (3)
- Capsules: 15,000 USP units of lipase; 51,000 USP units of protease; 82,000 USP units of amylase. Capsules have a red opaque cap and white opaque body, printed with "EURAND 15" (3)
- Capsules: 20,000 USP units of lipase; 68,000 USP units of protease; 109,000 USP units of amylase. Capsules have a green opaque cap and white opaque body, printed with "EURAND 20" (3)

CONTRAINDICATIONS
None (4)

WARNINGS AND PRECAUTIONS
- Fibrosing colonopathy is associated with high-dose use of pancreatic enzyme replacement. Exercise caution when doses of ZENPEP exceed 2,500 lipase units/kg of body weight per meal (or greater than 10,000 lipase units/kg of body weight per day). (5.1)
- To avoid irritation of oral mucosa, do not chew ZENPEP or retain in the mouth. (5.2)
- Exercise caution when prescribing ZENPEP to patients with gout, renal impairment, or hyperuricemia. (5.3)
- There is theoretical risk of viral transmission with all pancreatic enzyme products including ZENPEP. (5.4)
- Exercise caution when administering pancrelipase to a patient with a known allergy to proteins of porcine origin. (5.5)

ADVERSE REACTIONS
- The most common adverse events (≥6% of patients treated with ZENPEP) are abdominal pain, flatulence, headache, cough, decreased weight, early satiety, and contusion. (6.1)
- There is no postmarketing experience with this formulation of Zenpep (6.2)

To report SUSPECTED ADVERSE REACTIONS, contact EURAND Pharmaceuticals, Inc. at 1-800-716-6507 or FDA at 1-800-FDA-1088 or www.fda.gov/medwatch

USE IN SPECIFIC POPULATIONS
Pediatric Patients:
- The safety and effectiveness of ZENPEP were assessed in pediatric patients, ages 1 to 17 years. (8.4)
- The safety and efficacy of pancreatic enzyme products with different formulations of pancrelipase in pediatric patients have been described in the medical literature and through clinical experience. (8.4)

See 17 for PATIENT COUNSELING INFORMATION and Medication Guide.

Revised: April 2010

FULL PRESCRIBING INFORMATION: CONTENTS*
*Sections or subsections omitted from the full prescribing information are not listed

---

FULL PRESCRIBING INFORMATION

1 INDICATIONS AND USAGE
ZENPEP® (pancrelipase) is indicated for the treatment of exocrine pancreatic insufficiency due to cystic fibrosis or other conditions.

2 DOSAGE AND ADMINISTRATION
2.1 Dosage
ZENPEP is not interchangeable with other pancrelipase products.

ZENPEP is orally administered. Therapy should be initiated at the lowest recommended dose and gradually increased. The dosage of ZENPEP should be individualized based on clinical symptoms, the degree of steatorrhea present, and the fat content of the diet (see Limitations on Dosing below).

Dosage recommendations for pancreatic enzyme replacement therapy were published following the Cystic Fibrosis Foundation Consensus Conferences.[1, 2, 3] ZENPEP should be administered in a manner consistent with the recommendations of the Conferences provided in the following paragraphs. Patients may be dosed on a fat ingestion-based or actual body weight-based dosing scheme.

Infants (up to 12 months)
Infants may be given 2,000 to 4,000 lipase units per 120 mL of formula or per breast-feeding. Do not mix ZENPEP capsule contents directly into formula or breast milk prior to administration *[see Dosage and Administration (2.2)]*.

Children Older than 12 Months and Younger than 4 Years
Enzyme dosing should begin with 1,000 lipase units/kg of body weight per meal for children less than age 4 years to a maximum of 2,500 lipase units/kg of body weight per meal (or less than or equal to 10,000 lipase units/kg of body weight per day), or less than 4,000 lipase units/g fat ingested per day.

Children 4 Years and Older and Adults
Enzyme dosing should begin with 500 lipase units/kg of body weight per meal for those older than age 4 years to a maximum of 2,500 lipase units/kg of body weight per meal (or less than or equal to 10,000 lipase units/kg of body weight per day), or less than 4,000 lipase units/g fat ingested per day.

Usually, half of the prescribed ZENPEP dose for an individualized full meal should be given with each snack. The total daily dose should reflect approximately three meals plus two or three snacks per day.

Enzyme doses expressed as lipase units/kg of body weight per meal should be decreased in older patients because they weigh more but tend to ingest less fat per kilogram of body weight.

Limitations on Dosing
Dosing should not exceed the recommended maximum dosage set forth by the Cystic Fibrosis Foundation Consensus Conferences Guidelines.[1, 2, 3]

If symptoms and signs of steatorrhea persist, the dosage may be increased by a healthcare professional. Patients should be instructed not to increase the dosage on their own. There is great inter-individual variation in response to enzymes; thus, a range of doses is recommended. Changes in dosage may require an adjustment period of several days. If doses are to exceed 2,500 lipase units/kg of body weight per meal, further investigation is warranted.

Doses greater than 2,500 lipase units/kg of body weight per meal (or greater than 10,000 lipase units/kg of body weight per day) should be used with caution and only if they are documented to be effective by 3-day fecal fat measures that indicate a significantly improved coefficient of fat absorption. Doses greater than 6000 lipase units/kg of body weight per meal have been associated with colonic strictures, indicative of fibrosing colonopathy, in children with cystic fibrosis less than 12 years of age *[see Warnings and Precautions (5.1)]*. Patients currently receiving higher doses than 6,000 lipase units/kg of body weight per meal should be examined and the dosage either immediately decreased or titrated downward to a lower range.

2.2 Administration
ZENPEP should always be taken as prescribed by a healthcare professional.

Infants (up to 12 months)
ZENPEP should be administered to infants immediately prior to each feeding, using a dosage of 2,000 to 4,000 lipase units per 120 mL of formula or per breast-feeding. Contents of the capsule may be administered with a small amount of applesauce, or other acidic food with a pH of 4.5 or less (e.g., commercially available preparations of bananas, or pears). Contents of the capsule may also be administered directly to the mouth. Administration should be followed by breast milk or formula. Contents of the capsule **should not** be mixed directly into formula or breast milk as this may diminish efficacy. Care should be taken to ensure that ZENPEP is not crushed or chewed or retained in the mouth, to avoid irritation of the oral mucosa.

Children and Adults
ZENPEP should be taken during meals or snacks, with sufficient fluid. **ZENPEP capsules and capsule contents should not be crushed or chewed.** Capsules should be swallowed whole.

For patients who are unable to swallow intact capsules, the capsules may be carefully opened and the contents sprinkled on small amounts of acidic soft food of pH 4.5 or less (e.g., commercially available preparations of bananas, pears and applesauce).

The ZENPEP-soft food mixture should be swallowed immediately without crushing or chewing, and followed with water or juice to ensure complete ingestion. Care should be taken to ensure that no drug is retained in the mouth.

3 DOSAGE FORMS AND STRENGTHS
The active ingredient in ZENPEP evaluated in clinical trials is lipase. ZENPEP is dosed by lipase units.

ZENPEP is available in 4 color coded capsule strengths. Other active ingredients include protease and amylase. Each ZENPEP capsule strength contains the specified amounts of lipase, protease, and amylase.

Capsules of all strengths have a blue radial print on the capsule body and are colored as follows:
- 5,000 USP units of lipase; 17,000 USP units of protease; 27,000 USP units of amylase capsules have a white opaque cap and white opaque body, printed with "EURAND 5"
- 10,000 USP units of lipase; 34,000 USP units of protease; 55,000 USP units of amylase capsules have a yellow opaque cap and white opaque body, printed with "EURAND 10"
- 15,000 USP units of lipase; 51,000 USP units of protease; 82,000 USP units of amylase capsules have a red opaque cap and white opaque body, printed with "EURAND 15"
- 20,000 USP units of lipase; 68,000 USP units of protease; 109,000 USP units of amylase capsules have a green opaque cap and white opaque body, printed with "EURAND 20"

4 CONTRAINDICATIONS
None.

5 WARNINGS AND PRECAUTIONS
5.1 Fibrosing Colonopathy
Fibrosing colonopathy has been reported following treatment with different pancreatic enzyme products. Fibrosing colonopathy is a rare serious adverse reaction initially described in association with high-dose pancreatic enzyme use, usually with use over a prolonged period of time and most commonly reported in pediatric patients with cystic fibrosis. The underlying mechanism of fibrosing colonopathy remains unknown. *Doses of pancreatic enzyme products exceeding 6000 lipase units/kg of body weight per meal have been associated with colonic strictures in children less than 12 years of age.*[1] Patients with fibrosing colonopathy should be closely monitored because some patients may be at risk of progressing to stricture formation. It is uncertain whether regression of fibrosing colonopathy occurs. It is generally recommended, unless clinically indicated, that enzyme doses should be less than 2,500 lipase units/kg of body weight per meal (or less than 10,000 lipase units/kg of body weight per day) or less than 4,000 lipase units/g fat ingested per day *[see Dosage and Administration (2.1)]*.

Doses greater than 2,500 lipase units/kg of body weight per meal (or greater than 10,000 lipase units/kg of body weight per day) should be used with caution and only if they are documented to be effective by 3-day fecal fat measures that indicate a significantly improved coefficient of fat absorption. Patients receiving higher doses than 6,000 lipase units/kg of body weight per meal should be examined and the dosage either immediately decreased or titrated downward to a lower range.

5.2 Potential for Irritation to Oral Mucosa

Care should be taken to ensure that no drug is retained in the mouth. ZENPEP should not be crushed or chewed or mixed in foods having a pH greater than 4.5. These actions can disrupt the protective enteric coating resulting in early release of enzymes, irritation of oral mucosa, and/or loss or enzyme activity *[see Dosage and Administration (2.2) and Patient Counseling Information (17.4)]*. For patients who are unable to swallow intact capsules, the capsules may be carefully opened and the contents added to a small amount of acidic soft food with a pH of 4.5 or less, such as applesauce. The Zenpep-soft food mixture should be swallowed immediately and followed with water or juice to ensure complete ingestion.

5.3 Potential for Risk of Hyperuricemia

Caution should be exercised when prescribing ZENPEP to patients with gout, renal impairment, or hyperuricemia. Porcine-derived pancreatic enzyme products contain purines that may increase blood uric acid levels.

5.4 Potential Viral Exposure from the Product Source

ZENPEP is sourced from pancreatic tissue from swine used for food consumption. Although the risk that ZENPEP will transmit an infectious agent to humans has been reduced by testing for certain viruses during manufacturing and by inactivating certain viruses during manufacturing, there is a theoretical risk for transmission of viral disease, including diseases caused by novel or unidentified viruses. Thus, the presence of porcine viruses that might infect humans cannot be definitely excluded. However, no cases of transmission of an infectious illness associated with the use of porcine pancreatic extracts have been reported.

5.5 Allergic Reactions

Caution should be exercised when administering pancrelipase to a patient with a known allergy to proteins of porcine origin. Rarely, severe allergic reactions including anaphylaxis, asthma, hives, and pruritus, have been reported with other pancreatic enzyme products with different formulations of the same active ingredient (pancrelipase). The risks and benefits of continued ZENPEP treatment in patients with severe allergy should be taken into consideration with the overall clinical needs of the patient.

6 ADVERSE REACTIONS

The most serious adverse reactions reported with different pancreatic enzyme products of the same active ingredient (pancrelipase) include fibrosing colonopathy, hyperuricemia and allergic reactions *[see Warnings and Precautions, (5)]*

6.1 Clinical Trials Experience

Because clinical trials are conducted under widely varying conditions, adverse reaction rates observed in the clinical trials of a drug cannot be directly compared to the rates in the clinical trials of another drug and may not reflect the rates observed in clinical practice.

The short-term safety of ZENPEP was assessed in two clinical trials conducted in 53 patients, ages 1 to 23 years, with exocrine pancreatic insufficiency (EPI) due to CF. In both studies, ZENPEP was administered in doses of approximately 5,000 lipase units per kilogram per day, for lengths of treatment ranging from 19 to 42 days. The population was nearly evenly distributed in gender, and approximately 96% of patients were Caucasian.

Study 1 was a randomized, double-blind, placebo-controlled, 2-treatment, crossover study of 34 patients, ages 7 to 23 years, with EPI due to CF. In this study, patients were randomized to receive ZENPEP at individually titrated doses (not to exceed 2,500 lipase units per kilogram per meal) or matching placebo for 6 to 7 days of treatment, followed by crossover to the alternate treatment for an additional 6 to 7 days. The mean exposure to ZENPEP during this study, including titration period and open label transition, was 30 days.

The incidence of adverse events (regardless of causality) was similar during double blind ZENPEP treatment (56%) and placebo treatment (50%). The most common adverse events reported during the study were gastrointestinal complaints, which were reported more commonly during placebo treatment (41%) than during ZENPEP treatment (32%), and headache, which was reported more commonly during ZENPEP treatment (15%) than during placebo treatment (0). The type and incidence of adverse events were similar in children (7-11 years), adolescents (12-16 years), and adults (greater than 18 years).

Because clinical trials are conducted under controlled conditions, the observed adverse event rates may not reflect the rates observed in clinical practice.

Table 1 enumerates treatment-emergent adverse events that occurred in at least 2 patients (greater than or equal to 6%) treated with either ZENPEP or placebo in Study 1. Adverse events were classified by Medical Dictionary for Regulatory Activities (MedDRA) terminology.

Table 1: Treatment-Emergent Adverse Events Occurring in at least 2 Patients (greater than or equal to 6%) During Treatment Period and Crossover Treatment Period of the Placebo-Controlled, Crossover Clinical Study of ZENPEP (Study 1)

MedDRA Primary System Organ Class Preferred Term	ZENPEP (N=34) %	Placebo (N=32) %
Gastrointestinal Disorders		
Abdominal pain	*6 (18%)*	*9 (28%)*
Flatulence	2 (6%)	3 (9%)
Nervous System Disorders		
Headache	5 (15%)	0
Injury, Poisoning and Procedural Complications		
Contusion	2 (6%)	0
Investigations		
Weight decreased	2 (6%)	2 (6%)
Respiratory, Thoracic and Mediastinal Disorders		
Cough	2 (6%)	0
General Disorders and Administration Site Conditions		
Early Satiety	2 (6%)	0

Study 2 was an open-label, uncontrolled study of 19 patients, ages 1 to 6 years, with EPI due to CF. After a 4-14 days screening period on the current PEP, patients in Study 2 received ZENPEP at individually titrated doses ranging between 2,300 and 10,000 lipase units per kg body weight per day, with a mean of approximately 5000 lipase units per kg body weight per day (not to exceed 2,500 lipase units per kilogram per meal) for 14 days. There was no comparator treatment, and adverse events were collected on patient diary entries and at each study visit.

The most commonly reported adverse events were gastrointestinal, including abdominal pain and steatorrhea, and were similar in type and frequency to those reported in the double-blind, placebo-controlled trial (Study 1).

6.2 Postmarketing Experience

There is no postmarketing experience with this formulation of ZENPEP.

Delayed- and immediate-release pancreatic enzyme products with different formulations of the same active ingredient (pancrelipase) have been used for the treatment of patients with exocrine pancreatic insufficiency due to cystic fibrosis and other conditions, such as chronic pancreatitis. The long-term safety profile of these products has been described in the medical literature. The most serious adverse events include fibrosing colonopathy, distal intestinal obstruction syndrome (DIOS), recurrence of pre-existing carcinoma, and severe allergic reactions including anaphylaxis, asthma, hives, and pruritus. The most commonly reported adverse events are gastrointestinal disorders, including abdominal pain, diarrhea, flatulence, constipation and nausea, and skin disorders, including pruritus, urticaria and rash. In general, pancreatic enzyme products have a well defined and favorable risk-benefit profile in exocrine pancreatic insufficiency.

7 DRUG INTERACTIONS

No drug interactions have been identified. No formal interaction studies have been conducted.

8 USE IN SPECIFIC POPULATIONS

8.1 Pregnancy

Teratogenic effects

Pregnancy Category C: Animal reproduction studies have not been conducted with pancrelipase. It is also not known whether pancrelipase can cause fetal harm when administered to a pregnant woman or can affect reproduction capacity. ZENPEP should be given to a pregnant woman only if clearly needed. The risk and benefit of pancrelipase should be considered in the context of the need to provide adequate nutritional support to a pregnant woman with exocrine pancreatic insufficiency. Adequate caloric intake during pregnancy is important for normal maternal weight gain and fetal growth. Reduced maternal weight gain and malnutrition can be associated with adverse pregnancy outcomes.

8.3 Nursing Mothers

It is not known whether this drug is excreted in human milk. Because many drugs are excreted in human milk, caution should be exercised when ZENPEP is administered to a nursing woman. The risk and benefit of pancrelipase should be considered in the context of the need to provide adequate nutritional support to a nursing mother with exocrine pancreatic insufficiency.

8.4 Pediatric Use

The short-term safety and effectiveness of ZENPEP were assessed in 2 clinical studies in pediatric patients, ages 1 to 17 years, with EPI due to CF.

Study 1 was a randomized, double-blind, placebo-controlled, crossover study in 34 patients 26 of whom were children, including 8 children aged 7 to 11 years, and 18 adolescents aged 12 to 17 patients.. The safety and efficacy in pediatric patients in this study were similar to adult patients *[see Adverse Reactions (6.1) and Clinical studies (14)]*.

Study 2 was an open-label, single arm study in 19 patients, ages 1 to 6 years, with EPI due to CF. When patient regimen was switched from their usual PEP regimen to ZENPEP at similar doses, patients showed similar control of their clinical symptoms.

The safety and efficacy of pancreatic enzyme products with different formulations of pancrelipase consisting of the same active ingredient (lipases, proteases, and amylases) for treatment of children with exocrine pancreatic insufficiency due to cystic fibrosis has been described in the medical literature and through clinical experience.

Dosing of pediatric patients should be in accordance with recommended guidance from the Cystic Fibrosis Foundation Consensus Conferences *[see Dosage and Administration (2.1)]*. Doses of other pancreatic enzyme products exceeding 6,000 lipase units/kg of body weight per meal have been associated with fibrosing colonopathy and colonic strictures in children less than 12 years of age *[see Warnings and Precautions (5.1)]*.

10 OVERDOSAGE

In Study 1, a 10 year-old patient was administered a dose of 10,856 lipase units per kg body weight of ZENPEP for a period of one day. The patient did not experience any adverse events as a result of the dose increase, nor did this patient experience any adverse events during a 44-day follow-up period. No abnormalities from analyses of safety labs (chemistry, hematology, urinalysis or uric acid) were noted.

Chronic high doses of pancreatic enzyme products have been associated with fibrosing colonopathy and colonic strictures *[see Dosage and Administration (2.1) and Warnings and Precautions (5.1)]*. High doses of pancreatic enzyme products have been associated with hyperuricosuria and hyperuricemia, and should be used with caution in patients with a history of hyperuricemia, gout, or renal impairment *[see Warnings and Precautions (5.3)]*.

11 DESCRIPTION

ZENPEP is a pancreatic enzyme preparation consisting of pancrelipase, an extract derived from porcine pancreatic glands. Pancrelipase contains multiple enzyme classes, including porcine-derived lipases, proteases, and amylases.

Pancrelipase is a cream-colored powder. It is miscible in water and practically insoluble or insoluble in alcohol and ether.

Each capsule for oral administration contains enteric-coated beads (1.8-1.9mm for 5,000 USP units of lipase, 2.2-2.5mm for 10,000, 15,000 and 20,000 USP units of lipase).

The active ingredient evaluated in clinical trials is lipase. ZENPEP is dosed by lipase units.

Other active ingredients include protease and amylase.

Inactive ingredients in ZENPEP include colloidal silicon dioxide, croscarmellose sodium, hydrogenated castor oil, hypromellose phthalate, magnesium stearate, microcrystalline cellulose, talc, and triethyl citrate and are contained in hypromellose capsules. The imprinting ink on the capsules contains dehydrated alcohol, FD&C Blue #2 aluminum lake C.I. 73015-E132, isopropyl alcohol, n-butyl alcohol, propylene glycol, shellac and strong ammonia solution.

5,000 USP units of lipase; 17,000 USP units of protease; 27,000 USP units of amylase. Capsules have a white opaque cap and a white opaque body with imprint "EURAND 5". The shells contain carnauba wax or talc, carrageenan, hypromellose, potassium chloride, titanium oxide, and water.

10,000 USP units of lipase; 34,000 USP units of protease; 55,000 USP units of amylase. Capsules have a yellow opaque cap and a white opaque body with imprint "EURAND 10". The shells contain carnauba wax or talc, carrageenan, hypromellose, potassium chloride, titanium oxide, water and yellow ferric oxide.

15,000 USP units of lipase; 51,000 USP units of protease; 82,000 USP units of amylase. Capsules have a red opaque cap and a white opaque body with imprint "EURAND 15".

The shells contain carnauba wax or talc, carrageenan, hypromellose, potassium chloride, red ferric oxide, titanium oxide, and water.

20,000 USP units of lipase; 68,000 USP units of protease; 109,000 USP units of amylase. Capsules have a green opaque cap and a white opaque body with imprint "EURAND 20". The shells contain carnauba wax or talc, carrageenan, FD&C Blue #2, hypromellose, potassium chloride, titanium oxide, water, and yellow ferric oxide.

12 CLINICAL PHARMACOLOGY

12.1 Mechanism of Action

The pancreatic enzymes in ZENPEP catalyze the hydrolysis of fats to monoglycerol, glycerol and fatty acids, protein into peptides and amino acids, and starch into dextrins and short chain sugars in the duodenum and proximal small intestine, thereby acting like digestive enzymes physiologically secreted by the pancreas.

12.3 Pharmacokinetics

The pancreatic enzymes in ZENPEP are enteric-coated to minimize destruction or inactivation in gastric acid. ZENPEP is designed to release most of the enzymes in vivo at pH greater than 5.5. Pancreatic enzymes are not absorbed from the gastrointestinal tract in any appreciable amount.

13 NONCLINICAL TOXICOLOGY

13.1 Carcinogenesis, Mutagenesis and Impairment of Fertility

Carcinogenicity, genetic toxicology, and animal fertility studies have not been performed.

14 CLINICAL STUDIES

The short-term safety and efficacy of ZENPEP were evaluated in 2 studies conducted in 53 patients, ages 1 to 23 years, with exocrine pancreatic insufficiency (EPI) associated with cystic fibrosis (CF).

Study 1, was a randomized, double-blind, placebo-controlled, crossover study of 34 patients, ages 7 to 23 years, with EPI due to CF. The final analysis population was limited to 32 patients, who completed both double-blind treatment periods, and were included in the efficacy analysis population. Patients were randomized to receive ZENPEP or matching placebo for 6 to 7 days of treatment, followed by crossover to the alternate treatment for an additional 6 to 7 days. The mean dose during the controlled treatment periods ranged from a mean dose of 3,900 lipase units per kilogram per day to 5,700 lipase units per kilogram per day. All patients consumed a high-fat diet (greater than or equal to 100 grams of fat per day) during the treatment period.

The primary efficacy endpoint was the mean difference in the coefficient of fat absorption (CFA) between ZENPEP and placebo treatment. The CFA was determined by a 72-hour stool collection during both treatments, when both fat excretion and fat ingestion were measured. Each patient's CFA during placebo treatment was used as their no-treatment CFA value.

Mean CFA was 88% with ZENPEP treatment compared to 63% with placebo treatment. The mean difference in CFA was 26 percentage points in favor of ZENPEP treatment with 95% Confidence Interval of (19, 32) and p≤0.001. Subgroup analyses of the CFA results showed that mean change in CFA was greater in patients with lower no-treatment (placebo) CFA values than in patients with higher no-treatment (placebo) CFA values. There were similar responses to ZENPEP by age and gender.

Study 2, was an open-label, uncontrolled study of 19 patients, ages 1 to 6 years (mean age 4 years), with EPI due to CF. Approximately half of the patients were ages 1 to 3 years. Study 2 compared a measurement of fat malabsorption, spot fecal fat testing, before (while receiving therapy with another commercial PEP) and after oral administration of Zenpep capsules with each meal or snack.

All patients in Study 2 were transitioned to ZENPEP from their usual PEP treatment. After a 4-14 days screening period on the current PEP, patients in Study 2 received ZENPEP at individually titrated doses ranging between 2,300 and 10,000 lipase units per kg body weight per day, with a mean of approximately 5000 lipase units per kg body weight per day (not to exceed 2,500 lipase units per kilogram per meal) for 14 days. There was no wash-out period. Overall, patients showed similar control of fat malabsorption by spot fecal fat testing when switched to ZENPEP treatment at similar doses.

15 REFERENCES

1. Borowitz DS, Grand RJ, Durie PR, et al. Use of pancreatic enzyme supplements for patients with cystic fibrosis in the context of fibrosing colonopathy. *Journal of Pediatrics.* 1995; 127: 681-684.

2. Borowitz DS, Baker RD, Stallings V. Consensus report on nutrition for pediatric patients with cystic fibrosis. *Journal of Pediatric Gastroenterology Nutrition.* 2002 Sep; 35: 246-259.

3. Stallings VA, Start LJ, Robinson KA, et al. Evidence-based practice recommendations for nutrition-related management of children and adults with cystic fibrosis and pancreatic insufficiency: results of a systematic review. *Journal of the American Dietetic Association.* 2008; 108: 832-839.

4. Smyth RL, Ashby D, O'Hea U, et al. Fibrosing colonopathy in cystic fibrosis: results of a case-control study.9 *Lancet.* 1995; 346: 1247-1251.

5. FitzSimmons SC, Burkhart GA, Borowitz DS, et al. High-dose pancreatic-enzyme supplements and fibrosing colonopathy in children with cystic fibrosis. *New England Journal of Medicine.* 1997; 336: 1283-1289

16 HOW SUPPLIED/STORAGE AND HANDLING

ZENPEP® (pancrelipase) Delayed-Release Capsules

5,000 USP units of lipase; 17,000 USP units of protease; 27,000 units of amylase.

Each ZENPEP capsule is available as a two piece hypromellose capsule with white opaque cap and white body with a blue radial print and printed with "EURAND 5", *that contains* 1.8-1.9mm enteric-coated beads. Capsules are supplied in bottles of:

- 12 capsules (NDC 42865-100-01)
- 100 capsules (NDC 42865-100-02)

ZENPEP® (pancrelipase) Delayed-Release Capsules

10,000 USP units of lipase; 34,000 units of protease; 55,000 units of amylase.

Each ZENPEP capsule is available as a two piece hypromellose capsule with yellow opaque cap and white body with a blue radial print and printed with "EURAND 10", that contains 2.2-2.5mm enteric-coated beads. Capsules are supplied in bottles of:

- 12 capsules (NDC 42865-101-01)
- 100 capsules (NDC 42865-101-02)

ZENPEP® (pancrelipase) Delayed-Release Capsules

15,000 USP units of lipase; 51,000 units of protease; 82,000 units of amylase.

Each ZENPEP capsule is available as a two piece hypromellose capsule with red opaque cap and white body with a blue radial print and printed with "EURAND 15", that contains 2.2-2.5mm enteric-coated beads. Capsules are supplied in bottles of:

- 12 capsules (NDC 42865-102-01)
- 100 capsules (NDC 42865-102-02)

ZENPEP® (pancrelipase) Delayed-Release Capsules

20,000 USP units of lipase; 68,000 units of protease; 109,000 units of amylase.

Each ZENPEP capsule is available as a two piece hypromellose capsule with green opaque cap and white body with a blue radial print and printed with "EURAND 20", that contains 2.2-2.5mm enteric-coated beads. Capsules are supplied in bottles of:

- 12 capsules (NDC 42865-103-01)
- 100 capsules (NDC 42865-103-02)
- 500 capsules (NDC 42865-103-04)

Storage and Handling

Avoid excessive heat. Store at room temperature (68-77°F; 20-25°C), brief excursions permitted to 15-40°C (59-104°F). Protect from moisture. AFTER OPENING, KEEP BOTTLE TIGHTLY CLOSED between uses to PROTECT FROM MOISTURE.

Dispense in tight container (USP).

Keep out of reach of children.

DO NOT CRUSH ZENPEP delayed-release capsules.

17 PATIENT COUNSELING INFORMATION

See Medication Guide

17.1 Dosing and Administration

- Instruct patients and caregivers that ZENPEP should only be taken as directed by their healthcare professional. Patients should be advised that the total daily dose should not exceed 10,000 lipase units/kg body weight/day unless clinically indicated. This needs to be especially emphasized for patients eating multiple snacks and meals per day. Patients should be informed that if a dose is missed, the next dose should be taken with the next meal or snack as directed. Doses should not be doubled. *[see Dosage and Administration (2)].*

- Instruct patients and caregivers that ZENPEP should always be taken with food. Patients should be advised that ZENPEP delayed-release capsules must not be crushed or chewed as doing so could cause early release of enzymes and/or loss of enzymatic activity. Patients should swallow the intact capsules with adequate amounts of liquid at mealtimes. If necessary, the capsules contents can also be sprinkled on soft acidic foods. *[see Dosage and Administration (2)].*

- Instruct patients to notify their healthcare professional if they are pregnant or are thinking of becoming pregnant during treatment with ZENPEP. *[see Use in Specific Populations (8.1).]*

17.2 Fibrosing Colonopathy

Advise patients and caregivers to follow dosing instructions carefully, as doses of pancreatic enzyme products exceeding 6,000 lipase units/kg of body weight per meal (10,000 lipase units/kg body weight/day) have been associated with colonic strictures in children below the age of 12 years. *[see Dosage and Administration (2)].*

17.3 Allergic Reactions

Advise patients and caregivers to contact their healthcare professional immediately if allergic reactions to ZENPEP develop. *[see Warnings and Precautions (5.5)].*

ZENPEP® is subject of US Patent No. 7,658,918.

Manufactured by: Eurand S.p.A.
Via Martin Luther King, 13
20060, Pessano con Bornago
Milan, Italy
Marketed by:
Eurand Pharmaceuticals, Inc.
790 Township Line Road, Suite 250
Yardley, PA 19067
For further information, please call Eurand Medical Information Department toll-free at 1-800-716-6507.
©2010 Eurand Pharmaceuticals, Inc.
PKG-1028
04/10 rev. 1

MEDICATION GUIDE
ZENPEP® (ZEN-pep)
(pancrelipase)
Delayed-Release Capsules

Read this Medication Guide before you start taking ZENPEP and each time you get a refill. There may be new information. This information does not take the place of talking to your doctor about your medical condition or treatment.

What is the most important information I should know about ZENPEP?

- ZENPEP may increase your chance of having a rare bowel disorder called fibrosing colonopathy. This condition is serious and may require surgery. The risk of having this condition may be reduced by following the dosing instructions that your healthcare professional gave you. **Call your healthcare professional right away if you have any unusual or severe:**
- Stomach area (abdominal) pain
- Bloating
- Trouble passing stool (having bowel movements)
- Nausea, vomiting, or diarrhea

Take ZENPEP exactly as prescribed. Do not take more or less ZENPEP than directed by your healthcare professional.

What is ZENPEP?

ZENPEP is a prescription medicine for people who cannot digest food normally because their pancreas does not make enough enzymes. ZENPEP may help your body use fats, proteins and sugars from food.

ZENPEP contains a mixture of digestive enzymes including lipases, proteases, and amylases from pig pancreas.

ZENPEP is safe and effective in children.

What should I tell my doctor before taking ZENPEP?

Before taking ZENPEP, tell your doctor about all your medical conditions, including if you

- are allergic to pork (pig) products.
- have a history of blockage of your intestines, or scarring or thickening of your bowel wall (fibrosing colonopathy)
- have gout, kidney disease, or high blood uric acid (hyperuricemia)
- have trouble swallowing capsules
- have any other medical condition
- are pregnant or plan to become pregnant. It is not known if ZENPEP will harm your unborn baby. Talk to your doctor if you are pregnant or plan to become pregnant.
- are breast-feeding or plan to breast-feed. It is not known if ZENPEP passes into your breast milk. You and your doctor should decide if you will take ZENPEP or breastfeed.

Tell your doctor about all the medicines you take, including prescription and nonprescription medicines, vitamins, and dietary or herbal supplements. Know the medicines you take. Keep a list of them and show it to your doctor and pharmacist when you get a new medicine.

How should I take ZENPEP? Take ZENPEP exactly as your doctor tells you.

- Do not take more capsules in a day than the number your doctor tells you. (total daily dose).
- Always take ZENPEP with a meal or snack. If you eat a lot of meals or snacks in a day, be careful not to go over your total daily dose.
- **Do not crush or chew the ZENPEP capsules or its contents, and do not hold the capsule or contents in your mouth.** Crushing, chewing or holding the ZENPEP Capsules in your mouth may cause irritation in your mouth or change the way ZENPEP works in your body.

Giving ZENPEP to children and adults

- Swallow ZENPEP capsules whole and take them with enough liquid to swallow them right away.
- If you have trouble swallowing capsules, open the capsules and sprinkle the beads on a small amount of acidic food such as applesauce, pureed bananas or pears. Ask your doctor about other foods you can mix with ZENPEP.

- If you sprinkle ZENPEP on food, swallow it right after you mix it. Do not store ZENPEP that is mixed with food.
- Swallow the ZENPEP and food mixture right away followed with water or juice. Make sure the medicine is swallowed completely.
- If you forget to take ZENPEP, call your healthcare professional or wait until your next meal and take your usual number of capsules. **Do not make up for missed doses.** Take your next dose at the usual time.

Giving ZENPEP to infants (children up to 12 months):

1. Give ZENPEP right before each feeding of formula or breast milk.
2. Do not mix ZENPEP capsule contents directly into formula or breast milk.
3. Open the capsules and sprinkle the contents on a small amount of applesauce, pureed bananas or pears. These foods should be the kind found in baby food jars that you buy at the store, or other food recommended by your doctor. You may also sprinkle the contents directly into your child's mouth.
4. If you sprinkle the ZENPEP on food, give the ZENPEP and food mixture to your child right away.
5. Give your child enough liquid to completely swallow the ZENPEP contents or the ZENPEP and food mixture.
6. Look in your child's mouth to make sure that all of the medicine has been swallowed.

What are possible side effects of ZENPEP?
ZENPEP may cause serious side effects, including:
See "What is the most important information I should know about ZENPEP?"

- Worsening of swollen, painful joints (gout) caused by an increase in your blood uric acid levels
- **Allergic reactions** including trouble with breathing, skin rashes, or swollen lips.

Call your doctor right away if you have any of these symptoms.

The most common side effects of ZENPEP include
- Pain in your belly
- Gas
- Headache

Other Possible Side Effects
ZENPEP and other pancreatic enzyme products are made from the pancreas of pigs, the same pigs people eat as pork. These pigs may carry viruses. Although it has never been reported, it may be possible for a person to get a viral infection from taking pancreatic enzyme products that come from pigs.
Tell your doctor if you have any side effect that bothers you or does not go away.
These are not all the possible side effects of ZENPEP. For more information, ask your doctor or pharmacist.
Call your doctor for medical advice about side effects. You may report side effects to FDA at 1-800-FDA-1088.
You may also report side effects to Eurand Pharmaceuticals, Inc. at 1-800-716-6507

How do I store ZENPEP?
- Store ZENPEP at room temperature (68° to 77°F; 20°C to 25°C). Avoid heat.
- After opening the bottle, keep it closed tightly between doses
- DO NOT eat or throw away the packet (desiccant) in your medicine bottle. This packet will protect your medicine from moisture.
- Store ZENPEP in a dry place.

Keep ZENPEP and all medicines out of the reach of children.

General information about ZENPEP
Medicines are sometimes prescribed for purposes other than those listed in a Medication Guide. Do not use ZENPEP for a condition for which it was not prescribed. Do not give ZENPEP to other people, even if they have the same symptoms you have. It may harm them.
This Medication Guide summarizes the most important information about ZENPEP. If you would like more information, talk with your doctor. You can ask your pharmacist or doctor for information about ZENPEP that is written for health professionals. For more information, go to www.ZENPEP.com or call 1-888-ZENPEP1 (1-888-936-7371).

What are the ingredients in ZENPEP?
Active ingredient: lipase, protease, amylase
Inactive ingredients: colloidal silicon dioxide, croscarmellose sodium, hydrogenated castor oil, hypromellose phthalate, magnesium stearate, microcrystalline cellulose, talc, and triethyl citrate in hypromellose capsules. The imprinting ink on the capsules contains dehydrated alcohol, FD&C Blue #2 aluminum lake C.I. 73015-E132, isopropyl alcohol, n-butyl alcohol, propylene glycol, shellac and strong ammonia solution.
ZENPEP® is subject of US Patent No. 7,658,918.
Manufactured by: Eurand S.p.A.
Via Martin Luther King, 13
20060, Pessano con Bornago
Milan, Italy

Marketed by:
Eurand Pharmaceuticals, Inc.
790 Township Line Road, Suite 250
Yardley, PA 19067
©2010 Eurand Pharmaceuticals, Inc.
This Medication Guide has been approved by the U.S. Food and Drug Administration.
Issued April 2010
PKG-1046
04/10 rev. 1

Fleet Laboratories
Division of C. B. Fleet Company, Incorporated
LYNCHBURG, VA 24502

Direct Inquiries to:
Sherrie McNamara, RN, MSN, MBA
Director of Medical Affairs and Global Pharmacovigilance Coordinator
1-866-255-6960
www.fleetlabs.com

FLEET® GLYCERIN LAXATIVES: OTC
FLEET® SUPPOSITORIES, FLEET® BABYLAX® AND FLEET® PEDIA-LAX® SUPPOSITORIES AND FLEET® LIQUID GLYCERIN SUPPOSITORIES
A HYPEROSMOTIC LAXATIVE

COMPOSITION

FLEET® Pedia-Lax® and Babylax® Liquid Glycerin Suppositories—Each rectal applicator delivers 2.8 g of glycerin.
FLEET® Liquid Glycerin Suppositories for Adults and Children 6 years of age and over—Each rectal applicator delivers 5.4 g of glycerin.
FLEET® Glycerin Suppositories for Adults—Each suppository contains 2 g of glycerin.
FLEET® Pedia-Lax® Glycerin Suppositories for Children 2 years to under 6—Each suppository contains 1 g of glycerin.

ACTIONS AND USES

Glycerin is a hyperosmotic laxative, given rectally, which usually produces a bowel movement within 15 minutes to 1 hour. Hyperosmotic laxatives encourage bowel movements by drawing water into the bowel from surrounding tissues. This produces a softer stool mass and increased bowel action. These products are used for fast, predictable relief of occasional constipation. However, rectal irritation may occur with its use.

INFORMATION FOR PATIENT

WARNINGS

This product may cause rectal discomfort or a burning sensation.

GENERAL LAXATIVE WARNINGS

Do not use a laxative product when nausea, vomiting or abdominal pain is present unless directed by a physician. If you notice a sudden change in bowel habits that persists over a period of 2 weeks, consult a physician before using a laxative. Rectal bleeding or failure to have a bowel movement after 1 hour of using this laxative product may indicate a serious condition. Discontinue use and consult a physician. Laxative products should not be used longer than 1 week unless directed by a physician.
Keep this and all drugs out of the reach of children. In case of accidental overdose or ingestion, seek professional assistance or contact a Poison Control Center right away.

DOSAGE AND ADMINISTRATION

FLEET® Pedia-Lax® and Babylax® Liquid Glycerin Suppositories—Children 2 to under 6 years: only 1 suppository per 24 hours or as directed by a physician. Children under 2 years: Consult a physician.
Positions for using the liquid suppository:
- **Left-side position:** Place child on left side with knees bent, and arms resting comfortably.
- **Knee-chest position:** Have child kneel, then lower head and chest forward until left side of face is resting on surface with left arm folded comfortably.
REMOVE ORANGE PROTECTIVE SHIELD FROM TIP BEFORE INSERTING. Hold the unit upright, grasping the bulb with fingers. Grasp the orange protective shield with the other hand; pull gently to remove.
- With steady pressure, gently insert tip into rectum with a slight side-to side movement, with tip pointing toward navel. Insertion may be easier if child receiving the liquid suppository bears down, as if having a bowel movement. This helps relax the muscles around the anus.
- **DISCONTINUE USE IF RESISTANCE IS ENCOUNTERED. FORCING THE TIP INTO RECTUM CAN CAUSE INJURY.**
- Squeeze bulb until nearly all liquid is gone. It is not necessary to empty the bulb completely, as it contains more liquid than needed. A small amount of liquid will remain in the bulb after squeezing.
- Remove tip from rectum and discard the bulb. The liquid suppository will usually cause a bowel movement after 15 minutes but may take up to 1 hour. Do not allow child to retain liquid suppository for more than 1 hour.
- Stop using this product and consult a doctor if your child doesn't have a bowel movement within 1 hour of using this product.

FLEET® Liquid Glycerin Suppositories for Adults and Children 6 years of age and older: only 1 suppository per 24 hours or as directed by a physician. Children 2 years to under 6 use Fleet® Pedia-Lax® or Fleet® Babylax® Liquid Glycerin Suppositories. Children under 2 years, consult a physician.
Positions for using the liquid suppository:
- **Left-side position:** Lie on left side with knee bent, and arms resting comfortably.
- **Knee-chest position:** Kneel, then lower head and chest forward until left side of face is resting on surface with left arm folded comfortably.
REMOVE ORANGE PROTECTIVE SHIELD FROM TIP BEFORE INSERTING. Hold the unit upright, grasping the bulb with fingers. Grasp the orange protective shield with the other hand; pull gently to remove.
- With steady pressure, gently insert tip into rectum with a slight side-to side movement, with tip pointing toward navel. Insertion may be easier if person receiving the liquid suppository bears down, as if having a bowel movement. This helps relax the muscles around the anus.
- **DISCONTINUE USE IF RESISTANCE IS ENCOUNTERED. FORCING THE TIP INTO RECTUM CAN CAUSE INJURY.**
- Squeeze bulb until nearly all liquid is gone. It is not necessary to empty the bulb completely, as it contains more liquid than needed. A small amount of liquid will remain in the bulb after squeezing.
- Remove tip from rectum and discard the bulb. The liquid suppository will usually cause a bowel movement after 15 minutes but may take up to 1 hour. Do not retain liquid suppository for more than 1 hour.
- Stop using this product and consult a doctor if you don't have a bowel movement within 1 hour of using this product.

FLEET® Glycerin Suppositories—Adults and Children 6 years of age and older: only 1 suppository per 24 hours or as directed by a physician.
Positions for using the suppository:
- **Left-side position:** Lie on left side with knee bent, and arms resting comfortably.
- **Knee-chest position:** Kneel, then lower head and chest forward until left side of face is resting on surface with left arm folded comfortably.
  - Insert one suppository fully into the rectum. The suppository need not melt completely to produce laxative action.
  - The suppository will usually cause a bowel movement after 15 minutes but may take up to 1 hour.
  - Do not retain suppository for more than 1 hour.
  - Stop using this product and consult a doctor if you don't have a bowel movement within 1 hour of using this product.
Store the container tightly closed and keep away from excessive heat.

FLEET® Pedia-Lax® Glycerin Suppositories—Children 2 to under 6 years: only 1 suppository per 24 hours or as directed by a physician.
Children under 2 years: Consult a physician.
Positions for using the suppository:
- **Left-side position:** Place child on left side with knees bent, and arms resting comfortably.
- **Knee-chest position:** Have child kneel, then lower head and chest forward until left side of face is resting on surface with left arm folded comfortably.
  - Insert one suppository fully into the rectum. The suppository need not melt completely to produce laxative action.
  - The suppository will usually cause a bowel movement after 15 minutes but may take up to 1 hour. Do not allow child to retain suppository for more than 1 hour.
  - Stop using this product and consult a doctor if your child doesn't have a bowel movement within 1 hour of using this product.
Store the container tightly closed and keep away from excessive heat.

HOW SUPPLIED

FLEET® Pedia-Lax® and Babylax® Liquid Glycerin Suppositories for children 2 to under 6 years—Each box contains 6 child rectal applicators (4 mL each).
FLEET® Liquid Glycerin Suppositories for Adults and Children 6 years of age and over—Each box contains 4 adult rectal applicators (7.5 mL each).
FLEET® Glycerin Suppositories—Available in jars of 12, 24, 50 and 100 adult suppositories.
FLEET® Pedia-Lax® Glycerin Suppositories—Available in jars of 12.
IS THIS PRODUCT OTC? Yes.
QUESTIONS? Call 1-866-255-6960 or visit www.fleetlabs.com or www.pedia-lax.com.

FLEET® BISACODYL LAXATIVES: ENEMA, TABLETS, AND SUPPOSITORIES
A STIMULANT LAXATIVE

COMPOSITION

Latex-free FLEET® Bisacodyl Enema - 10 mg bisacodyl enema solution in a 37-mL ready-to-use squeeze bottle with a 2 inch, pre-lubricated Comfortip®. It is disposable after a single use.
FLEET® Stimulant Laxative Tablets - Enteric-coated 5 mg bisacodyl each tablet.
FLEET® Laxative Suppositories - 10 mg bisacodyl each suppository.

ACTION AND USES

Bisacodyl is a stimulant laxative given either orally or rectally, acting directly on the colonic mucosa where it stimulates sensory nerve endings to produce parasympathetic reflexes resulting in increased peristaltic contractions of the colon. The contact action of the drug is restricted to the colon, and motility in the small intestine is not appreciably influenced. FLEET® Stimulant Laxative Tablets usually work within 6–12 hours. FLEET® Bisacodyl Suppositories produce a bowel movement within 15 minutes to 1 hour, and the latex-free FLEET® Bisacodyl Enema produces a bowel movement within 5–20 minutes. Bisacodyl is useful as a laxative for relief of occasional constipation and in bowel cleansing in preparation for x-ray or endoscopic examination. Bisacodyl may be used as a laxative in postoperative, antepartum, or postpartum care or in preparation for delivery under guidance of a healthcare professional.
Store at temperatures not above 86°F (30°C)
WARNINGS: Do not administer Fleet® Bisacodyl Enema to children under 12 years of age.

GENERAL LAXATIVE WARNINGS
INFORMATION FOR PATIENT

Do not use a laxative product when nausea, vomiting or abdominal pain is present unless directed by a physician. If you notice a sudden change in bowel habits that persists over a period of 2 weeks, consult a physician before using a laxative. Rectal bleeding or failure to have a bowel movement after use of a laxative may indicate a serious condition. Discontinue use and consult a physician. Laxative products should not be used longer than 1 week unless directed by a physician. As with any drug, if you are pregnant or nursing a baby, seek the advice of a healthcare professional before using this product. All bisacodyl products may cause abdominal discomfort, faintness and mild cramps. Rectal products may also cause rectal burning.
Keep this and all drugs out of the reach of children. In case of accidental overdose or ingestion, seek professional assistance or contact a Poison Control Center right away.

DOSAGE AND ADMINISTRATION
Enema
SHAKE BEFORE USING.
Dosage:
Adults and children 12 years of age and over: Use one 1.25 fl. oz. bottle (30-mL delivered dose) as a single daily dose.
Children under 12 years of age: DO NOT USE.
Positions for using this enema:
• **Left-side position:** Lie on left side with knee bent, and arms resting comfortably.
• **Knee-chest position:** Kneel, then lower head and chest forward until left side of face is resting on surface with left arm folded comfortably.
Fleet® Bisacodyl Enema should be used at room temperature.
How to use this enema:
• **REMOVE ORANGE PROTECTIVE SHIELD FROM ENEMA COMFORTIP® BEFORE INSERTING.**
• With steady pressure, gently insert enema tip into rectum with a slight side-to side movement, with tip pointing toward navel. Insertion may be easier if person receiving enema bears down, as if having a bowel movement. This helps relax the muscles around the anus.
• **DO NOT FORCE THE ENEMA TIP INTO RECTUM AS THIS CAN CAUSE INJURY.**

• Squeeze bottle until nearly all liquid is gone. It is not necessary to empty the bottle completely, as it contains more liquid than needed. A small amount of liquid will remain in the bottle after squeezing.
• Remove Comfortip® from rectum and discard bottle.
• Maintain position until urge to evacuate is strong (usually 5 to 20 minutes). Do not retain enema solution for more than 20 minutes.
• Stop using this product and consult a doctor if you don't have a bowel movement within 20 minutes of using this product.
The diaphragm at the base of the tube prevents reflux and assures controlled flow of the enema solution.
IMPORTANT: FLEET® Bisacodyl Enema IS NOT INTENDED FOR ORAL CONSUMPTION in any dosage size.
PROFESSIONAL ADMINISTRATION
FLEET® Bisacodyl Enema should not be used in children under 12 years of age. Careful consideration of the use of enemas in children in general is recommended. Proper and safe use of FLEET® enemas also requires that the products be administered according to the directions. Healthcare professionals should remember when administering the product to gently insert the enema into the rectum with the tip pointing toward the navel. Insertion may be made easier by having the patient bear down as if having a bowel movement. Care during insertion is necessary due to lack of sensory innervation of the rectum and due to the possibility of bowel perforation. Once inserted, squeeze the bottle until nearly all the liquid is expelled. If resistance is encountered on insertion of the nozzle or in administering the solution, the procedure should be discontinued. **Forcing the enema can result in perforation and/or abrasion of the rectum.**
Tablets
Adults and children 12 years of age and over: Take 1 to 3 tablets (usually 2) in a single dose once daily.
Children 6 to under 12 years of age: Take 1 tablet once daily.
Expect results in 6–12 hours if taken at bedtime or within 6 hours if taken before breakfast. Swallow tablets whole. Do not chew or crush tablets. Do not administer tablets within 1 hour after taking an antacid, milk, or milk products.
Children under 6 years of age: Consult a physician.
Suppositories
Adults and children 12 years of age and over: Use 1 suppository once daily. Remove foil wrapper. Lie on your side and, with pointed end first, insert the suppository towards the navel and well up into the rectum. Make sure the suppository touches the bowel wall.
Children 6 to under 12 years of age: One-half of one 10 mg. suppository once daily.
Children under 6 years of age: Consult a physician.

HOW SUPPLIED
Enema
FLEET® Bisacodyl Enema is supplied in a 1.25 fl. oz. (37-mL) ready-to-use squeeze bottle.
Tablets
FLEET® Stimulant Laxative Tablets are supplied in cartons of 25 tablets (5 mg bisacodyl in each tablet) wrapped in a foil seal.
Suppositories
FLEET® Bisacodyl Suppositories are supplied in cartons of 4 individually foil-wrapped suppositories (10 mg bisacodyl in each suppository).
IS THIS PRODUCT OTC? Yes.
QUESTIONS? Call 1-866-255-6960 or visit www.fleetlabs.com

FLEET® ENEMA, A SALINE LAXATIVE — OTC
FLEET® ENEMA EXTRA®, A SALINE LAXATIVE
FLEET® PEDIA-LAX® ENEMA, A SALINE LAXATIVE, FLEET® ENEMA FOR CHILDREN, A SALINE LAXATIVE

FLEET® enemas are designed for quick, convenient administration by nurse, patient or parent according to instructions. Each is disposable after a single use.

COMPOSITION
FLEET® ENEMA: Each **latex-free** FLEET® Enema unit, with a 2 inch, pre-lubricated Comfortip®, contains 4.5 fl. oz. (133 mL) of enema solution in a ready-to-use squeeze bottle. Each enema unit delivers a dose of 118 mL, which contains 19 g monobasic sodium phosphate monohydrate and 7 g dibasic sodium phosphate heptahydrate. Each Fleet® Enema 118 mL delivered dose contains 4.4 grams sodium.
FLEET® ENEMA EXTRA®: Each **latex-free** FLEET® Enema EXTRA® unit, with a 2 inch, pre-lubricated Comfortip®, contains 7.8 fl. oz. (230 mL) of enema solution in a ready-to-use squeeze bottle. Each enema unit delivers a dose of 197 mL, which contains 19 g monobasic sodium phosphate monohydrate and 7 g dibasic sodium phosphate heptahydrate. Each Fleet® Enema EXTRA® 197 mL delivered dose contains 4.4 grams sodium.
Fleet® Pedia-Lax® Enema and FLEET® ENEMA FOR CHILDREN: Each **latex-free** Fleet® Pedia-Lax® Enema and

FLEET® Enema for Children unit, with a 2 inch, pre-lubricated Comfortip®, contains 2.25 fl. oz. (66 mL) of enema solution in a ready-to-use squeeze bottle. Each enema unit delivers a dose of 59 mL, which contains 9.5 g monobasic sodium phosphate monohydrate and 3.5 g dibasic sodium phosphate heptahydrate. Each Fleet® Enema for Children and Fleet® Pedia-Lax® Enema 59 mL delivered dose contains 2.2 grams sodium.

ELEMENTAL AND ELECTROLYTIC CONTENT (Fleet® Enema, Fleet® Pedia-Lax® Enema and Fleet® Enema for Children)

mEq Phosphate (PO₄) per mL	4.15
mEq Sodium (Na) per mL	1.61
mg Sodium (Na) per mL	37
mmole Phosphorus (P) per mL	1.38

ELEMENTAL AND ELECTROLYTIC CONTENT (Fleet® Enema EXTRA®)

mEq Phosphate (PO₄) per mL	2.484
mEq Sodium (Na) per mL	0.961
mg Sodium (Na) per mL	22.1
mmole Phosphorus (P) per mL	0.828

ACTION AND USES

FLEET® Enema, FLEET® Enema EXTRA® Fleet® Pedia-Lax® Enema and FLEET® Enema for Children are useful as laxatives in the relief of occasional constipation and as part of a bowel cleansing regimen in preparing the colon for surgery, x-ray or endoscopic examination.
When used as directed, FLEET® Enema, FLEET® Enema EXTRA®, Fleet® Pedia-Lax® Enema and FLEET® Enema for Children provide thorough yet safe cleansing action and induce complete emptying of the left colon, usually within 1 to 5 minutes, without pain or spasm.
INFORMATION FOR PATIENT
WARNINGS
Using more than one enema in 24 hours can be harmful.
AFTER THE ENEMA SOLUTION IS ADMINISTERED, THE RETENTION TIME SHOULD NOT EXCEED 10 MINUTES. IF THE RETENTION TIME EXCEEDS 10 MINUTES OR THERE IS NO RETURN OF ENEMA SOLUTION, CONTACT A PHYSICIAN IMMEDIATELY, AS ELECTROLYTE DISTURBANCES AND CONSEQUENT SERIOUS SIDE EFFECTS COULD OCCUR.
DO NOT USE ANY FLEET® ENEMA IN CHILDREN UNDER 2 YEARS OF AGE.
DO NOT ADMINISTER THE 4.5 FL. OZ. ADULT SIZE OR THE 7.8 FL.OZ. EXTRA® SIZE TO CHILDREN UNDER 12 YEARS OF AGE.
DO NOT ADMINISTER A FULL 2.25 FL. OZ. CHILDREN'S SIZE TO CHILDREN UNDER 5 YEARS OF AGE. FOR CHILDREN 2 TO UNDER 5 YEARS, USE ONE-HALF BOTTLE OF 2.25 FL. OZ. CHILDREN'S SIZE. (SEE **DOSAGE AND ADMINISTRATION**).
IMPORTANT: FLEET® Enema (Adult size), FLEET® Enema EXTRA®, Fleet® Pedia-Lax® Enema and Fleet® Enema for Children ARE NOT INTENDED FOR ORAL CONSUMPTION in any dosage size.
When using any of these Fleet® enemas, patient may experience anal discomfort.

GENERAL LAXATIVE WARNINGS

Do not use laxative products when nausea, vomiting or abdominal pain is present unless directed by a physician. If you notice a sudden change in bowel habits that persists over a period of 2 weeks, consult a physician. Fleet® enemas should be administered according to the instructions for use and handling. Stop use if resistance is encountered as forced administration of the enema may cause injury. Stop using this product and consult a doctor if you have rectal bleeding following the use of this product as this may indicate a serious condition. Failure to have bowel movement within 30 minutes of using this product may also indicate a serious condition. Discontinue use and consult a physician. Stop use and ask a doctor if you have any symptoms that your body is losing more fluids than you are drinking. This is called dehydration. Early symptoms of dehydration include feeling thirsty, dizziness, urinating less often than normal and vomiting. Laxative products should not be used longer than 1 week unless directed by a physician. As with any drug, if you are pregnant or nursing a baby, seek the advice of a healthcare professional before using this product. As sodium phosphate may pass into the breast milk, it is advised that breast milk is expressed and discarded for at least 24 hours after receiving the Fleet® enema.
Keep this and all drugs out of the reach of children. In case of accidental overdose or ingestion, seek professional assistance or contact a Poison Control Center right away.

PROFESSIONAL USE INFORMATION
CONTRAINDICATIONS
Do not use in patients with
• Congestive heart failure
• Clinically significant impairment of renal function
• Known or suspected gastrointestinal obstruction
• Megacolon (congenital or acquired)

- Paralytic ileus
- Perforation
- Active inflammatory bowel disease
- Imperforate anus
- Dehydration
- Generally in all cases where absorption capacity is increased or elimination capacity is decreased
- Children under 2 years of age
- Hypersensitivity to active ingredients or to any of the excipients of the product

PRECAUTIONS

Use with caution in patients
- With impaired renal function
- Taking medications known to affect renal perfusion or function, or hydration status
- With pre-existing electrolyte disturbances or who are taking diuretics or other medications which may affect electrolyte levels
- Who are taking medications known to prolong the QT interval
- Ascites
- With a colostomy
- In children 2-11 years of age
- 65 or older and under a doctor's care for any medical condition
- Who are pregnant or nursing a baby

Patients with conditions that may predispose to dehydration or those taking medications which may decrease glomerular filtration rate, such as diuretics, angiotensin converting enzyme inhibitors (ACE-Is), angiotensin receptor blockers (ARBs), or non-steroidal anti-inflammatory drugs (NSAIDs), should be assessed for hydration status prior to use and managed appropriately.

Fleet® Pedia-Lax® Enema and Fleet® Enema for Children should be used with caution in children of any age. Careful consideration of the use of enemas in children in general is recommended.

Careful consideration of the use of sodium phosphates enemas in the elderly with co-morbidities is also recommended. See PROFESSIONAL USE WARNINGS. In those cases where complications have been reported, elderly patients with co-morbidities are often involved.

Since FLEET® enemas contain sodium phosphates, in all patients there is a risk of elevated serum levels of sodium and phosphate and decreased levels of calcium and potassium, and consequently hypernatremia, hyperphosphatemia, hypocalcemia and hypokalemia may occur which could result in metabolic acidosis, tetany, renal failure, QT prolongation and/or, in more severe cases, multi-organ failure, cardiac arrhythmia/arrest and death. This is of particular concern in children with megacolon or any other condition where there is retention of enema solution, and in patients with co-morbidities, particularly gastrointestinal, renal and neurological disorders. If any patient develops vomiting and/or signs of dehydration, measure post-administration labs (phosphate, calcium, potassium, sodium, creatinine, GFR and BUN.)

SINCE FLEET® BRAND ENEMAS ARE AVAILABLE IN ADULT, ADULT EXTRA, AND CHILDREN'S SIZES, PRESCRIBE CAREFULLY.

DRUG INTERACTIONS

NO OTHER SODIUM PHOSPHATES PREPARATIONS INCLUDING SODIUM PHOSPHATES ORAL SOLUTION OR TABLETS SHOULD BE GIVEN CONCOMITANTLY.

Electrolyte disturbances and hypovolemia from purgation may be exacerbated by inadequate oral fluid intake, nausea, vomiting, loss of appetite, or use of diuretics, angiotensin converting enzyme inhibitors (ACE-Is), angiotensin receptor blockers (ARBs), non-steroidal anti-inflammatory drugs (NSAIDs), and lithium or other medications that may affect electrolyte levels, and may result in metabolic acidosis, tetany, renal failure, QT prolongation and, in more severe cases, multi-organ failure, cardiac arrhythmia/arrest and death.

As hypernatremia is associated with lower lithium levels, concomitant use of Fleet® enemas and lithium therapy could lead to a fall in serum lithium levels with a lessening of effectiveness.

POSSIBLE SIDE EFFECTS

Hypersensitivity
Pruritis
Dehydration
Hyperphosphatemia
Hypocalcemia
Hypokalemia
Hypernatremia
Metabolic Acidosis
Nausea
Vomiting
Abdominal Pain
Abdominal Distension
Diarrhea
Gastrointestinal Pain
Chills
Blistering
Stinging

Anal Discomfort
Protalgia

HYDRATION

Additional liquids by mouth are recommended.

Encourage patients to drink large amounts of clear liquids to prevent dehydration. Inadequate fluid intake when using any effective purgative may lead to excessive fluid loss, possibly producing dehydration and hypovolemia.

OVERDOSAGE OR RETENTION

Overdosage (more than one enema in a 24 hour period), no return of enema solution, retention time greater than 10 minutes or failure to have a bowel movement within 30 minutes of enema use may lead to severe electrolyte disturbances, including hypernatremia, hyperphosphatemia, hypocalcemia, and hypokalemia, as well as dehydration and hypovolemia, with attendant signs and symptoms of these disturbances (such as metabolic acidosis, renal failure, and tetany), QT prolongation and/or, in more severe cases, multi-organ failure, cardiac arrhythmia/arrest and death. The patient who has taken an overdose or who has retained the product for more than 10 minutes should be monitored carefully. If any patient develops vomiting and/or signs of dehydration, measure post-procedure labs (phosphate, calcium, potassium, sodium, creatinine, GFR and BUN.) **Treatment of electrolyte imbalance may require immediate medical intervention with appropriate electrolyte and fluid replacement therapy.**

DOSAGE AND ADMINISTRATION

Dosage: FLEET® Enema (Adult size) and FLEET® Enema EXTRA®:

Use only 1 enema per 24 hours.

Do not use more unless directed by a doctor. See Warnings. Do not use if taking another sodium phosphates product.

adults and children 12 years and older	one bottle
children 2 to 11 years	use Fleet® Pedia-Lax® Enema or FLEET® Enema for Children (See below)
children under 2 years	**DO NOT USE**

How to use this enema:
- **REMOVE ORANGE PROTECTIVE SHIELD FROM ENEMA COMFORTIP® BEFORE INSERTING.**
- With steady pressure, gently insert enema tip into rectum with a slight side-to-side movement, with tip pointing toward navel. Insertion may be easier if person receiving enema bears down, as if having a bowel movement. This helps relax the muscles around the anus.
- **DO NOT FORCE THE ENEMA TIP INTO RECTUM AS THIS CAN CAUSE INJURY.**
- Squeeze bottle until nearly all liquid is gone. It is not necessary to empty the bottle completely, as it contains more liquid than needed.
- Remove Comfortip® from rectum and maintain position until urge to evacuate is strong (usually 1 to 5 minutes). Do not retain enema solution for more than 10 minutes.

Positions for using this enema:
- **Left-side position:** Lie on left side with knee bent, and arms resting comfortably.
- **Knee-chest position:** Kneel, then lower head and chest forward until left side of face is resting on surface with left arm folded comfortably.

The diaphragm at base of tube prevents reflux and assures controlled flow of the enema solution. Fleet® Enema should be used at room temperature.

Dosage: Fleet® Pedia-Lax® Enema and FLEET® Enema for Children:

Use only 1 enema per 24 hours.

Do not use more unless directed by a doctor. See Warnings. Do not use if child is taking another sodium phosphates product.

children 5 to 11 years	one bottle or as directed by a doctor
children 2 to under 5 years	one-half bottle (see below) or as directed by a doctor
children under 2 years	**DO NOT USE**

One-half bottle preparation: Unscrew cap and remove 2 Tablespoons of liquid with a measuring spoon. Replace cap and follow DIRECTIONS on back of carton.

How to use this enema:
- **REMOVE ORANGE PROTECTIVE SHIELD FROM ENEMA COMFORTIP® BEFORE INSERTING.**
- With steady pressure, gently insert enema tip into rectum with a slight side-to-side movement, with tip pointing toward navel. Insertion may be easier if child receiving enema bears down, as if having a bowel movement. This helps relax the muscles around the anus.
- **DO NOT FORCE THE ENEMA TIP INTO RECTUM AS THIS CAN CAUSE INJURY.**
- Squeeze bottle until nearly all liquid is gone. It is not necessary to empty the bottle completely, as it contains more liquid than needed.
- Remove Comfortip® from rectum and keep child in position until urge to evacuate is strong (usually 1 to 5 minutes). Do not allow child to retain enema solution for more than 10 minutes.

Positions for using this enema:
- **Left-side position:** Place child on left side with knees bent, and arms resting comfortably.
- **Knee-chest position:** Have child kneel, then lower head and chest forward until left side of face is resting on surface with left arm folded comfortably.

The diaphragm at base of tube prevents reflux and assures controlled flow of the enema solution. Fleet® Pedia-Lax® Enema and FLEET® Enema for Children should be used at room temperature.

PROFESSIONAL DOSAGE AND ADMINISTRATION

Administration of more than one enema in 24 hours can be harmful. In those cases where complications have been reported, overdoses are often involved.

NO OTHER SODIUM PHOSPHATES PREPARATIONS INCLUDING SODIUM PHOSPHATES ORAL SOLUTION OR TABLETS SHOULD BE GIVEN CONCOMITANTLY.

FLEET® Enema (Adult size) and FLEET® Enema EXTRA® should not be used in children under 12 years of age. In those cases where complications have been reported, infants and young children are often involved. Fleet® Pedia-Lax® Enema and FLEET® Enema for Children should be used with caution in children of any age. Careful consideration of the use of enemas in children in general is recommended.

Careful consideration of the use of sodium phosphates enemas in the elderly with co-morbidities is also recommended. See PROFESSIONAL USE WARNINGS. In those cases where complications have been reported, elderly patients with co-morbidities are often involved.

See **DOSAGE AND ADMINISTRATION** for dosing detail. Proper and safe use of FLEET® Enemas also requires that the products be administered according to the Directions. Healthcare professionals should remember when administering the product to gently insert the enema into the rectum with the tip pointing toward the navel. Insertion may be made easier by having the patient bear down as if having a bowel movement. Care during insertion is necessary due to lack of sensory innervation of the rectum and due to possibility of bowel perforation. Once inserted, squeeze the bottle until nearly all the liquid is expelled. If resistance is encountered on insertion of the nozzle or in administering the solution, the procedure should be discontinued. **Forcing the enema can result in perforation and/or abrasion of the rectum.**

If an enema containing phosphate or sodium is not advised, consider using FLEET® Bisacodyl Enema.

HOW SUPPLIED

FLEET® Enema is supplied in a 4.5 fl. oz. (133-mL) ready-to-use squeeze bottle. Fleet® Enema EXTRA® is supplied in a 7.8 fl. oz. (230-mL) ready-to-use squeeze bottle. Fleet® Pedia-Lax® Enema and Fleet® Enema for Children are supplied in a 2.25 fl. oz. (66 mL) ready-to-use squeeze bottle. **QUESTIONS?** Call 1-866-255-6960 or visit www.fleetlabs.com

---

FLEET® MINERAL OIL ENEMA   OTC
A LUBRICANT LAXATIVE

COMPOSITION

Latex-free FLEET® Mineral Oil Enema unit, with a 2-inch, pre-lubricated Comfortip®, delivers 118 mL of mineral oil, 100%, in a ready-to-use squeeze bottle. FLEET® Mineral Oil Enema is sodium-free. The unit is disposable after a single use.

ACTION AND USES

FLEET® Mineral Oil Enema serves to soften and lubricate hard stools, easing their passage without irritating the mucosa. Results approximate a normal bowel movement in that only the rectum, sigmoid, and part or all of the descending colon are evacuated. FLEET® Mineral Oil Enema is indicated for relief of fecal impaction; is valuable in relief of occasional constipation when straining must be avoided (in hypertension, coronary occlusion, proctologic procedures, or postoperative care); is indicated for removal of barium sulfate residues from the colon after barium administration and is indicated for obtaining the laxative benefits of mineral oil while avoiding possible untoward effects of oral administration such as (1) interference with intestinal absorption of fat-soluble vitamins A, D, E and K and other nutrients, (2) danger of systemic absorption, or (3) possible risk of lipid pneumonia due to aspiration. It is generally effective in 2 to 15 minutes.

WARNINGS

DO NOT ADMINISTER TO CHILDREN UNDER 2 YEARS OF AGE.

GENERAL LAXATIVE WARNINGS
INFORMATION FOR PATIENT

Do not use laxative products when nausea, vomiting or abdominal pain is present unless directed by a physician. If you notice a sudden change in bowel habits that persists over a period of 2 weeks, consult a physician before using a laxative. Rectal bleeding or failure to have a bowel movement after use of a laxative may indicate a serious condition. Discontinue use and consult a physician. Laxative products should not be used longer than 1 week unless directed by a physician. As with any drug, if you are pregnant or nursing a baby, seek the advice of a healthcare professional before using this product.
Keep this and all drugs out of the reach of children. In case of accidental overdose or ingestion, seek professional assistance or contact a Poison Control Center right away.

DOSAGE AND ADMINISTRATION

Use only 1 enema per 24 hours.

Adults & children 12 years of age and over	1 bottle
Children 2 to 11 years of age	One-half bottle
Children under 2 years of age	DO NOT USE

Positions for using this enema:
• **Left-side position:** Lie on left side with knee bent, and arms resting comfortably.
• **Knee-chest position:** Kneel, then lower head and chest forward until left side of face is resting on surface with left arm folded comfortably.
REMOVE ORANGE PROTECTIVE SHIELD FROM ENEMA COMFORTIP® BEFORE INSERTING.
• With steady pressure, gently insert enema tip into rectum with a slight side-to side movement, with tip pointing toward navel. Insertion may be easier if person receiving enema bears down, as if having a bowel movement. This helps relax the muscles around the anus.
• **DISCONTINUE USE IF RESISTANCE IS ENCOUNTERED. FORCING THE TIP INTO RECTUM CAN CAUSE INJURY**
• Squeeze bottle until nearly all liquid is gone. It is not necessary to empty the bottle completely, as it contains more liquid than needed. A small amount of liquid will remain in the bottle after squeezing.
• Remove tip from rectum and discard bottle. The enema will usually cause a bowel movement within 2 to 15 minutes. Do not retain liquid for more than 15 minutes.
• Stop using this product and consult a doctor if you don't have a bowel movement within 15 minutes of using this product.
The diaphragm at base of tube prevents reflux and assures controlled flow of the enema solution. The enema should be used at room temperature.

PROFESSIONAL DOSAGE AND ADMINISTRATION

FLEET® Mineral Oil Enema should not be used in children under 2 years of age and should be used with caution in children of any age. In general, careful consideration of the use of enemas in children is recommended.
Proper and safe use of FLEET® Mineral Oil Enema also requires that the product be administered according to the Directions. Healthcare professionals should remember when administering the product to gently insert the enema into the rectum with the tip pointing toward the navel. Insertion may be made easier by having the patient bear down as if having a bowel movement. Care during insertion is necessary due to lack of sensory innervation of the rectum and due to the possibility of bowel perforation. Once inserted, squeeze the bottle until nearly all the liquid is expelled. If resistance is encountered on insertion of the nozzle or in administering the solution, the procedure should be discontinued. **Forcing the enema can result in perforation and/or abrasion of the rectum.**

HOW SUPPLIED

FLEET® Mineral Oil Enema is supplied in 4.5 fl. oz. (133-mL) ready-to-use squeeze bottle.
IS THIS PRODUCT OTC? Yes.
QUESTIONS? Call 1-866-255-6960 or visit www.fleetlabs.com

FLEET® PEDIA-LAX® DOCUSATE SODIUM LIQUID STOOL SOFTENER
Stool softener laxative

DRUG FACTS

Active ingredient (in each tablespoon – 15 mL)	**Purpose**
Docusate sodium 50 mg	Stool softener

USES
• to help prevent dry, hard stools
• to relieve occasional constipation

DESCRIPTION

Docusate sodium is a stool softener laxative, given orally, which usually produces a bowel movement within 12 to 72 hours. Stool softener laxatives penetrate and soften the stool, thereby promoting bowel movement.

INFORMATION FOR PATIENT
DRUG INTERACTION PRECAUTION: Do not give this product to child if child is presently taking mineral oil, unless directed by a doctor.

WARNINGS

Ask a doctor before using any laxative if your child has
• abdominal pain, nausea or vomiting
• a sudden change in bowel habits lasting more than 2 weeks
• already used a laxative for more than 1 week
Stop using this product and consult your doctor if your child has
• rectal bleeding
• no bowel movement within 72 hours of using this product
These symptoms may be signs of a serious condition.
Keep this and all drugs out of the reach of children. In case of overdose, get medical help or contact a Poison Control Center right away.

DIRECTIONS

Doses may be taken as a single daily dose or in divided doses in a 24-hour period.
Doses must be given in a 6-8 ounce glass of milk or juice, to prevent throat irritation.
Each tablespoon (15 mL) contains 13 mg sodium.

Dosing Chart

Age	Starting Dose	Maximum Dose per Day (24 hours)
Children 2 to 11 years	1–3 tablespoons	3 tablespoons
Children under 2	Ask a doctor	Ask a doctor

Inactive ingredients: citric acid, edetate disodium, FD&C Red #3, flavor, methylparaben, polyethylene glycol, povidone, propylene glycol, propylparaben, sodium citrate, sorbitol, sucralose, water, zanthan gum, xylitol.

HOW SUPPLIED

4 fl.oz. (118 mL) bottles with child-resistant cap, and sealed for your protection. Fruit punch flavor.
Is this product OTC?
Yes.
QUESTIONS? Call 1-866-255-6960 or visit www.Pedia-Lax.com

FLEET® PEDIA-LAX® MAGNESIUM HYDROXIDE CHEWABLE TABLETS   OTC
Saline laxative

DRUG FACTS

Active ingredient (in each tablet):	**Purpose**
Magnesium hydroxide 400 mg	Saline laxative

USE
• to relieve occasional constipation

DESCRIPTION

Magnesium hydroxide is a saline laxative, given orally, which usually produces a bowel movement within 30 minutes to 6 hours. Saline laxatives increase water in the intestine thereby promoting bowel movement.

INFORMATION FOR PATIENT
WARNINGS

Ask a physician before using this product if child has a magnesium-restricted diet or kidney disease.
Ask a doctor before using any laxative if your child has
• abdominal pain, nausea or vomiting
• a sudden change in bowel habits lasting more than 2 weeks
• already used a laxative for more than 1 week
Stop using this product and consult a doctor if your child has
• rectal bleeding
• no bowel movement within 6 hours of taking this product
These symptoms may be signs of a serious condition.
Keep this and all drugs out of the reach of children. In case of overdose, get medical help or contact a Poison Control Center right away.

DIRECTIONS

Doses may be taken as a single daily dose or in divided doses in a 24-hour period. **Have child drink a full glass (8 fluid ounces) of liquid with each dose.**
Each tablet contains 170 mg magnesium.

Dosing Chart

Age	Starting Dose	Maximum Dose per Day (24 hours)
Children 6 to 11 years	3–6 tablets	6 tablets
Children 2 to 5 years	1–3 tablets	3 tablets
Children under 2	Ask a doctor	Ask a doctor

Inactive ingredients: colloidal silicon dioxide, FD&C Red #40 aluminum lake, flavor, magnesium stearate, maltodextrin, mannitol, sorbitol, stearic acid, sucralose

HOW SUPPLIED

30 Pedia-Lax Chewable Tablets per bottle with child-resistant cap, sealed for your protection. Watermelon flavor.
Is this product OTC?
Yes.
QUESTIONS?
Call 1-866-255-6960 or visit www.Pedia-Lax.com

FLEET® PEDIA-LAX® SENNA   OTC
QUICK DISSOLVE STRIPS
Stimulant laxative

DRUG FACTS

Active ingredient (in each strip)	**Purpose**
Standardized Sennosides 8.6 mg	Stimulant laxative

USE
• to relieve occasional constipation

DESCRIPTION

Senna is a stimulant laxative, given orally, which usually produces a bowel movement within 6 to 12 hours. Stimulant laxatives promote bowel movement by one or more direct actions on the intestine.

INFORMATION FOR PATIENT
WARNINGS

Ask a physician before using this product if child is taking non-steroidal anti-inflammatory drugs (NSAIDs).
Ask a doctor before using any laxative if your child has
• abdominal pain, nausea, or vomiting
• a sudden change in bowel habits lasting more than 2 weeks
• already used a laxative for more than 1 week
Stop using this product and consult a doctor if your child has
• rectal bleeding
• no bowel movement within 12 hours of taking this product
These symptoms may be signs of a serious condition.
Keep this and all drugs out of the reach of children. In case of overdose, get medical help or contact a Poison Control Center right away.

DIRECTIONS

Dosing Chart

Age	Starting Dose	Maximum Dose per Day
Children 6 to 11 years	2 strips	Do not exceed 4 strips in 24 hours
Children 2 to 5 years	1 strip	Do not exceed 2 strips in 24 hours
Children under 2	Ask a doctor	Ask a doctor

Place quick dissolve strip on child's tongue or have child place on the tongue. Allow strip to dissolve. Encourage child to drink plenty of liquids.

Inactive ingredients: butylated hydroxytoluene, FD&C Red #40, flavor, hydroxypropyl methylcellulose, malic acid, methylparaben, polydextrose, polyethylene oxide, simethicone, sodium bicarbonate, sucralose, white ink.

HOW SUPPLIED

12 individually-wrapped Pedia-Lax Quick Dissolve Strips per carton. Grape flavor.

Other Information: Color of strips may vary. Store at controlled room temperature 59°–86°F (15°–30°C).

Is this product OTC?

Yes.

QUESTIONS?

Call 1-866-255-6960 or
visit www.Pedia-Lax.com

FLEET® PREP KIT 3   OTC
Bowel Evacuant

COMPOSITION

FLEET® Prep Kit 3 contains:
1. FLEET® Phospho-soda® Oral Saline Laxative—1.5 fl. oz. (45 mL). Active Ingredients: Each Tablespoon (15 mL) contains monobasic sodium phosphate monohydrate 7.2 g and dibasic sodium phosphate heptahydrate 2.7 g. Natural ginger-lemon flavoring.
2. FLEET® Bisacodyl Tablets—4 laxative tablets. Active Ingredient: Each enteric-coated tablet contains 5 mg bisacodyl.
3. FLEET® Bisacodyl Enema 1.25 fl. oz. (37 mL)—1 laxative enema. Active Ingredient: Each 30-mL delivered dose contains 10 mg bisacodyl USP.
4. 1 Patient Instruction Sheet.
5. 1 Patient Information Sheet.

FLEET® Prep Kit 3 should not be used in children under 18 years of age.

PHARMACOKINETICS

Caswell M, Thompson WO, Kanapka JA, Galt DJB. The time course and effect on serum electrolytes of oral sodium phosphates solution in healthy male and female volunteers. Can J Clin Pharmacol 14(3):e260-e274, 2007 http://www.cjcp.ca/pdf/CJCP07005e260_e274.pdf

Each recommended dose (1.5 fl. oz.) (45 mL) of FLEET® Phospho-soda® oral saline laxative contains 5004 mg sodium.

ACTIONS AND USES

Bowel Cleansing System

INDICATIONS

For use as part of a bowel cleansing regimen in preparing the colon for surgery, x-ray or endoscopic examination.

PROFESSIONAL USE INFORMATION
WARNINGS

RENAL DISEASE AND ACUTE PHOSPHATE NEPHROPATHY: There have been rare, but serious reports of acute phosphate nephropathy (also known as nephrocalcinosis) in patients who received oral sodium phosphates products (solution and tablets) for bowel cleansing prior to colonoscopy or other medical procedures. Some cases resulted in permanent impairment of renal function, with some patients requiring long term dialysis and/or kidney transplant. The time to onset is typically within days; however, in some cases, the diagnosis of these events has been delayed up to several months after the ingestion of these products. While some cases occurred in patients without identifiable risk factors, patients at increased risk of acute phosphate nephropathy may include those with increased age, hypovolemia, increased bowel transit time (such as bowel obstruction), active colitis, or baseline kidney disease, and those using medicines that affect renal perfusion or function (such as diuretics, angiotensin converting enzyme [ACE] inhibitors, angiotensin receptor blockers [ARBs], and possibly nonsteroidal anti-inflammatory drugs [NSAIDs]). Patients at increased risk should be assessed for hydration status prior to use of purgative preparations and managed appropriately. See PRECAUTIONS. It is important to use the dose and dosing regimen as recommended.

ELECTROLYTE DISORDERS: Administration of sodium phosphate products prior to colonoscopy for colon cleansing or other medical procedures has resulted in fatalities due to significant fluid shifts, severe electrolyte abnormalities, and cardiac arrhythmias. These fatalities have been observed in elderly patients, in patients with renal insufficiency, in patients with bowel perforation, and in patients who misused or overdosed sodium phosphate products. The benefit/risk ratio of Fleet® Prep Kit 3 needs to be carefully considered before initiating treatment in this at-risk population. Special attention should be taken when prescribing Fleet® Prep Kit 3 to any patient with regard to known contraindications and risks, the importance of adequate hydration and, in at-risk populations (see below), the importance of also obtaining baseline and post-treatment serum electrolyte levels, and blood urea nitrogen and creatinine levels.

In all patients there is a risk of elevated serum levels of sodium and phosphate and decreased serum levels of calcium and potassium; consequently, hypernatremia, hyperphosphatemia, hypocalcemia, hypokalemia, and acidosis may occur.

CARDIAC ARRHYTHMIAS: There have been rare, but serious, reports of arrhythmias associated with the use of sodium phosphate products. Fleet® Prep Kit 3 should be used with caution in patients with prolonged QT interval, patients with a history of uncontrolled arrhythmias, and patients with a recent history of a myocardial infarction. Predose and post-colonoscopy ECGs should be considered in patients with high risk of serious cardiac arrhythmias.

OTHER IMPORTANT SAFETY INFORMATION:

Renal Impact: Sodium phosphate is known to be substantially excreted by the kidney, and the risk of adverse reactions with sodium phosphates may be greater in patients with impaired renal function. Since elderly patients are more likely to have impaired renal function, consider performing baseline and post-procedure labs (phosphate, calcium, potassium, sodium, creatinine, GFR and BUN) in these patients (see WARNINGS).

Hypersensitivity Reactions: There have been reports of hypersensitivity reactions (e.g., rash, urticaria, pruritus, tongue edema, throat tightness, and paresthesia of the lips) associated with the use of marketed sodium phosphates products.

Aphthoid Lesions: Single or multiple aphthoid-like punctiform lesions located in the rectosigmoid region have been observed by endoscopy. These were either lymphoid follicles or discrete inflammatory infiltrates or epithelial congestions/changes revealed by the colonic preparation. These abnormalities are not clinically significant and disappear spontaneously without any treatment.

Absorption of Medications: During the intake of Fleet® Prep Kit 3 the absorption of drugs from the gastrointestinal tract may be delayed or even completely prevented. The efficacy of regularly taken oral drugs (e.g. oral contraceptives, antiepileptic drugs, diabetic medications, antibiotics) may be reduced or completely absent.

Concomitant Medications: NO OTHER SODIUM PHOSPHATES PREPARATIONS INCLUDING SODIUM PHOSPHATES-BASED ENEMAS OR TABLETS SHOULD BE GIVEN CONCOMITANTLY.

CONTRAINDICATIONS

Do not use in patients with
• Biopsy proven acute phosphate nephropathy
• Congestive heart failure
• Clinically significant impairment of renal function
• Ascites
• Known or suspected gastrointestinal obstruction
• Megacolon (congenital or acquired)
• Perforation
• Hyperparathyroidism
• Ileus
• Active inflammatory bowel disease; Crohn's disease; ulcerative colitis.

Do not use
• In children under the age of 18 years
• When abdominal pain, nausea, or vomiting are present
• If there is a hypersensitivity to the active ingredients or any of the excipients

PRECAUTIONS

Use with caution in patients who are
• Elderly
• Debilitated

• Taking medications known to affect renal perfusion or function, or hydration status
• Taking medications known to prolong the QT interval
• Taking parathyroid hormone medications
• On a low-salt diet
• Pregnant or nursing a baby

And in patients with
• Heart disease
• Arrhythmia
• Cardiomyopathy
• Recent myocardial infarction
• Unstable angina
• Prolonged QT interval
• An increased risk for underlying renal impairment
• An increased risk for, or pre-existing, electrolyte disturbances, including patients with
  • Dehydration
  • Inability to take adequate oral fluid
  • Hypertension or other conditions in which the patients are taking products that affect electrolytes or may result in dehydration (see Hydration information below)
  • Gastric retention, hypomotility disorders, history of gastric bypass/stapling surgery; or
  • Colitis
• A colostomy or ileostomy

In at-risk patients, including elderly patients, the benefit/risk ratio of Fleet® Prep Kit 3 needs to be carefully considered before initiating treatment. Consider obtaining baseline and post-procedure serum sodium, potassium, calcium, chloride, bicarbonate, phosphate, blood urea nitrogen and creatinine values. If any patient develops vomiting and/or signs of dehydration, measure post-procedure labs (phosphate, calcium, potassium, sodium, creatinine, GFR and BUN.)

Patients with electrolyte abnormalities such as hypernatremia, hyperphosphatemia, hypokalemia, or hypocalcemia should have their electrolytes corrected before use of Fleet® Prep Kit 3.

Bisacodyl products may cause abdominal discomfort, faintness, and cramps. FLEET® Bisacodyl Tablets should be swallowed whole. Do not prescribe to patients who cannot swallow without chewing unless directed by a physician. Store at temperatures not above 86°F (30°C)

HYDRATION

Additional liquids by mouth are recommended with all bowel cleansing dosages. Encourage patients to drink large amounts of clear liquids before and during the bowel preparation process, and after the procedure, in order to prevent dehydration. Before the procedure, the patient should begin drinking plenty of clear liquids, such as 36 to 48 fl. oz. of a carbohydrate-electrolyte solution; during the preparation the patient should drink a minimum of 72 fl. oz. of clear liquids; during the procedure it is recommended that intravenous fluids (500-1,000 mL) be administered; and after the procedure the patient should drink as much liquid as possible to help prevent dehydration. Inadequate fluid intake when using any effective purgative may lead to excessive fluid loss, possibly producing dehydration and hypovolemia. Dehydration and hypovolemia from purgation may be exacerbated by inadequate oral liquid intake, nausea, vomiting, loss of appetite, or use of diuretics, ACE-Is, ARBs, NSAIDs, and lithium or other medications that may affect electrolyte levels, and may be associated with acute renal failure. There have been reports of acute renal failure associated with bowel purgatives. Drinking large amounts of clear liquids (at least 72 fl. oz. during the bowel preparation process) also helps ensure that your patient's bowel will be clean for the procedure. Instruct the patient to contact a physician if there is no bowel movement after six hours as electrolyte imbalance can occur. (See OVERDOSAGE OR NO BOWEL MOVEMENT below).

OVERDOSAGE OR NO BOWEL MOVEMENT

Overdosage (including shorter time intervals between doses than recommended) or no bowel movement may lead to severe electrolyte disturbances, including hypernatremia, hyperphosphatemia, hypocalcemia, and hypokalemia, as well as dehydration and hypovolemia, with attendant signs and symptoms of these disturbances (such as metabolic acidosis, renal failure, and tetany). Certain severe electrolyte disturbances may lead to cardiac arrhythmia and death. The patient who has taken an overdose or who fails to have a bowel movement after six hours should be monitored carefully. Patients experiencing overdose or no bowel movement have presented the following symptoms; dehydration, hypotension, tachycardia, bradycardia, tachypnoea, cardiac arrest, shock, respiratory failure, dyspnoea, convulsions, ileus paralytic, anxiety, and pain. Overdoses or no bowel movement can also lead to elevated serum levels of sodium and phosphate and decreased levels of calcium and potassium.

In those cases, hypernatremia, hyperphosphatemia, hypocalcemia and hypokalemia may occur with resulting metabolic acidosis, renal failure, tetany and in severe cases, multi-organ failure, cardiac arrhythmia and death. **Treatment of electrolyte imbalance may require immediate medical intervention with appropriate electrolyte and fluid replacement therapy.**

INFORMATION FOR PATIENT

The patient should be instructed to open and read directions and patient information sheet at least two (2) days in advance of the examination.

Instruct the patient to use this product for bowel cleansing only as directed by a doctor, to discuss with the doctor the patient's health and warnings about use of this product for bowel cleansing, to follow the special directions from the doctor exactly and to take only the dose the doctor has recommended. The patient should be instructed to drink plenty of clear liquids before beginning the bowel preparation process; consider recommending the patient consume 36–48 fl. oz. of a carbohydrate-electrolyte solution in the six hours before the first dose is taken. During the bowel preparation process, the patient should be instructed to drink as much extra clear liquids as they can to replace the fluids lost during bowel movements: minimum 72 fl. oz. The patient should be instructed to drink as much liquid as possible after the procedure to help prevent dehydration.

WARNINGS FOR PATIENTS

DO NOT EXCEED RECOMMENDED DOSE UNLESS DIRECTED BY A PHYSICIAN. SERIOUS SIDE EFFECTS MAY OCCUR FROM EXCESS DOSAGE. IF THERE IS NO BOWEL MOVEMENT AFTER SIX HOURS, CONTACT A PHYSICIAN, AS ELECTROLYTE IMBALANCE AND CONSEQUENT SERIOUS SIDE EFFECTS COULD OCCUR.

During bowel preparation you will lose significant amounts of fluid. THIS IS NORMAL. It is very important that you replace this fluid to prevent dehydration. Early symptoms of dehydration include feeling thirsty, dizziness, urinating less often than normal, or vomiting. These symptoms may be signs of serious problems. Drink as much extra liquids as you can to help replace the fluids you are losing during bowel movements. Drinking large amounts of clear liquids also helps ensure that your bowel will be clean for the examination or procedure.

DO NOT TAKE MORE THAN 45 ML (1.5 FL. OZ.) OF FLEET® PHOSPHO-SODA® PER DOSE. NEVER TAKE MORE THAN 1 BOTTLE AT ONE TIME.

Swallow Fleet® Bisacodyl Tablets whole; do not chew tablets unless directed by a physician. Do not take tablets within one hour after taking antacids, milk, or milk products.

DO NOT USE if you have congestive heart failure, if you have serious kidney problems, or in children under 18 years of age. Ask a doctor before use if you are under a doctor's care for any medical condition, are on a low-salt diet or are pregnant or nursing a baby. Ask a doctor or pharmacist before use if you are taking any other prescription or non-prescription drugs. Ask a doctor before using any laxative if you have abdominal (belly) pain, nausea, or vomiting, have a change in your daily bowel movements that lasts more than 2 weeks, or have already used another laxative daily for constipation for more than 1 week. Stop using this product and consult a doctor if you have any rectal bleeding, do not have a bowel movement within 6 hours of taking this product or have any symptoms that your body is losing more fluids than you are drinking. This is called dehydration. Early symptoms of dehydration include feeling thirsty, dizziness, urinating less often than normal, or vomiting. These symptoms may be signs of serious problems.

Keep this and all drugs out of the reach of children. In case of accidental overdose or ingestion, seek professional assistance or contact a Poison Control Center right away.

PATIENT SAFETY INFORMATION GUIDE
FLEET® Prep Kit 3

This Patient Safety Information Guide should be shared with your patient before your patient uses FLEET® Prep Kit 3. The Patient Safety Information Guide should not take the place of any discussion between doctor and patient about the patient's medical condition or treatment. Encourage your patient to ask you questions about FLEET® Prep Kit 3.

What is the most important information I should know about FLEET® Prep Kit 3?

FLEET® Prep Kit 3 can cause serious side effects, including:
Serious kidney problems. Rare, but serious kidney problems can happen in people who take medicines made with sodium phosphate, including FLEET® Prep

---

Kit 3, to clean your colon before a colonoscopy or other medical procedures. These kidney problems can sometimes lead to kidney failure, the need for dialysis for a long time or kidney transplant. These problems often happen within a few days, but sometimes may happen several months after taking FLEET® Prep Kit 3.

Conditions that can make you more at risk for having serious kidney problems with FLEET® Prep Kit 3 include if you:
• lose too much body fluid (dehydration)
• have slow moving bowel
• have bowel blocked with stool (constipation)
• have severe stomach pain or bloating
• have any disease that causes bowel irritation (colitis)
• have kidney disease
• have heart failure
• take water pills or non-steroidal anti-inflammatory drugs (NSAIDS)

Your age may also affect your risk for having kidney problems with FLEET® Prep Kit 3.

Before you start taking FLEET® Prep Kit 3, tell your doctor if you:
• have kidney problems
• take any medicines for blood pressure, heart disease, or kidney disease.

Severe fluid loss (dehydration). People who take medicines that contain sodium phosphate can have severe loss of body fluid, with severe changes in body salts in the blood, and abnormal heart rhythms. These problems can lead to death.

Tell your doctor if you have any of these symptoms of loss of too much body fluid (dehydration) while taking FLEET® Prep Kit 3:
• vomiting
• dizziness
• urinating less often than normal
• headache

See "What are the possible side effects of FLEET® Prep Kit 3?" for more information about side effects.

What is FLEET® Prep Kit 3?

FLEET® Prep Kit 3 is a medicine used in adults 18 years or older, to clean your colon before a colonoscopy or other medical procedure. FLEET® Prep Kit 3 cleans your colon by causing you to have diarrhea. Cleaning your colon helps your doctor see the inside of your colon more clearly during the colonoscopy or other medical procedure.

It is not known if FLEET® Prep Kit 3 is safe and works in children under age 18.

Who should not take FLEET® Prep Kit 3?

Do not take FLEET® Prep Kit 3 if:
• you have had a kidney biopsy that shows you have kidney problems because of too much phosphate
• you are allergic to sodium phosphate salts, bisacodyl or any of the ingredients in FLEET® Prep Kit 3

What should I tell my doctor before taking FLEET® Prep Kit 3?

Before taking FLEET® Prep Kit 3, tell your doctor about all your medical conditions, including if you have:
• any of the medical conditions listed in the section "What is the most important information I should know about FLEET® Prep Kit 3?"
• irritation of the bowel (colitis). FLEET® Prep Kit 3 can cause symptoms of irritable bowel disease to flare-up.
• damage to your bowel
• problems with abnormal heart beat
• had a recent heart attack or have other heart problems
• symptoms of too much body fluid loss (dehydration) including vomiting, dizziness, urinating less often than normal, or headache
• had stomach surgery
• a history of seizures
• if you drink alcohol
• are on a low salt diet
• are pregnant. It is not known if FLEET® Prep Kit 3 will harm your unborn baby.

Tell your doctor about all the medicines you take, including prescription and non-prescription medicines, vitamins, and herbal supplements. Any medicine that you take close to the time that you take FLEET® Prep Kit 3 may not work as well. Especially tell your doctor if you take:
• water pills (diuretics)
• medicines for blood pressure or heart problems
• medicines for kidney damage
• medicines for pain, such as aspirin or a non-steroidal anti-inflammatory drug (NSAID)
• a medicine for seizures
• a laxative for constipation in the last 7 days. You should not take another medicine that contains sodium phosphate while you take FLEET® Prep Kit 3.

Ask your doctor if you are not sure if your medicine is listed above.

Know the medicines you take. Keep a list of your medicines to show your doctor or pharmacist when you get a new prescription.

How should I take FLEET® Prep Kit 3?
• take FLEET® Prep Kit 3 exactly as prescribed by your doctor.
• **It is important for you to drink clear liquids before, during, and after taking FLEET® Prep Kit 3. This may help prevent kidney damage. Examples of clear liquids** are water, flavored water, lemonade (no pulp), ginger ale, or apple juice. Do not drink any liquids colored purple or red.
• Follow the detailed instructions enclosed.

Tell your doctor if you have any of these symptoms while taking FLEET® Prep Kit 3:
• vomiting, dizziness, or if you urinate less often than normal. These may be signs that you have lost too much fluid while taking FLEET® Prep Kit 3.
• trouble drinking clear fluids
• severe stomach cramping, bloating, nausea, or headache

If you take too much FLEET® Prep Kit 3, call your doctor or get medical help right away.

What should I avoid while taking FLEET® Prep Kit 3?
• You should not take other laxatives or enemas made with sodium phosphate while taking FLEET® Prep Kit 3.
• You should not use FLEET® Prep Kit 3 if you have already used it or any other sodium phosphate product for colon cleansing in the last 7 days.

What are the possible side effects of FLEET® Prep Kit 3?

FLEET® Prep Kit 3 can cause serious side effects, including:
• See "What is the most important information I should know about FLEET® Prep Kit 3?"
• Seizures or fainting (black-outs). People who take a medicine that contains sodium phosphate, such as FLEET® Prep Kit 3, can have seizures or faint (become unconscious) even if they have not had seizures before. Tell your doctor right away if you have a seizure or faint while taking FLEET® Prep Kit 3.
• abnormal heart beat (arrhythmias)
• changes in your blood levels of calcium, phosphate, potassium, sodium

The most common side effects of FLEET® Prep Kit 3 are:
• bloating
• stomach area (abdominal) pain
• nausea
• vomiting
• cramping
• fainting

These are not all the possible side effects of FLEET® Prep Kit 3. For more information, ask your doctor or pharmacist.

Call your doctor for medical advice about side effects. You may report side effects to FDA at 1- 800-FDA-1088.

How do I store FLEET® Prep Kit 3?
• Store FLEET® Prep Kit 3 at room temperature, between 59° F to 86° F (15° C to 30° C).
• Keep FLEET® Prep Kit 3 and all medicines out of the reach of children.

DOSAGE AND ADMINISTRATION

SEE PATIENT INSTRUCTION SHEET FOR 18-, AND 24-HOUR PREPARATION SCHEDULE IN EACH KIT. The patient should open and read the enclosed directions, patient information sheet and carton labels at least 48 hours in advance of examination.

Fleet® Prep Kit 3 or any of the sodium phosphates-based bowel preparations should not be used for colon cleansing within seven (7) days of previous administration.

FLEET® PREP KIT 3 SHOULD NOT BE USED IN CHILDREN UNDER 18 YEARS OF AGE.

Additional patient instruction and information sheets are available by calling 1-866-255-6960

HOW SUPPLIED

See "Description" for contents of each kit.
Shipping Unit: 48 FLEET® Prep Kits per case.

For additional information, see individual listings under FLEET® Bisacodyl Laxatives.

IS THIS PRODUCT OTC? Yes.
QUESTIONS? Call 1-866-255-6960

Forest Pharmaceuticals, Inc.
(Subsidiary of Forest Laboratories, Inc.)
13600 SHORELINE DRIVE
ST. LOUIS, MO 63045

Direct Inquiries to:
Medical Information and
Communications
Forest Pharmaceuticals, Inc.
13600 Shoreline Drive
St. Louis, MO 63045
(800) 678-1605

AEROCHAMBER PLUS FLOW-VU™
Anti-Static Valved Holding Chamber
MOUTPIECE
LARGE MASK

℞

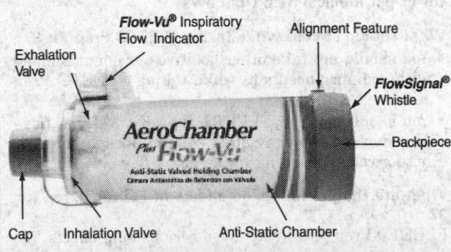

MOUTHPIECE CHAMBER

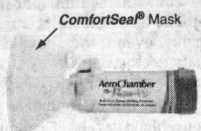

LARGE MASK CHAMBER

INDICATIONS FOR USE
This product is intended to be used by patients who are under the care or treatment of a physician or licensed healthcare professional. The device is intended to be used by these patients to administer aerosolized medication from most pressurized Metered Dose Inhalers. The intended environments for use include the home, hospitals and clinics.

INSTRUCTIONS FOR USE

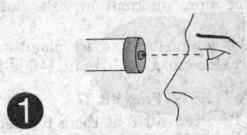

❶

Carefully examine the product for damage, missing parts or foreign objects. Remove any foreign objects prior to use. The product should be replaced IMMEDIATELY if there are any damaged or missing parts. If necessary, use the Metered Dose Inhaler (MDI) alone until a replacement is obtained. If the patient's symptoms worsen, please seek immediate medical attention.

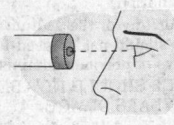

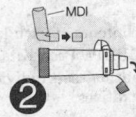

❷

Remove cap(s) from the MDI and chamber (if applicable).

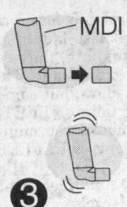

❸

Shake the MDI immediately before each use as per the instructions supplied with the MDI.

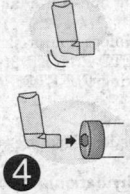

❹

Insert the MDI into the backpiece of the chamber.

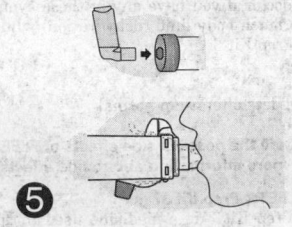

❺

Put mouthpiece into mouth and close lips around it to ensure an effective seal. The **Flow-Vu®** Inspiratory Flow Indicator only moves if the patient has a good seal.
Apply mask to face and ensure an effective seal. The **Flow-Vu®** Inspiratory Flow Indicator only moves if the patient has a good seal.

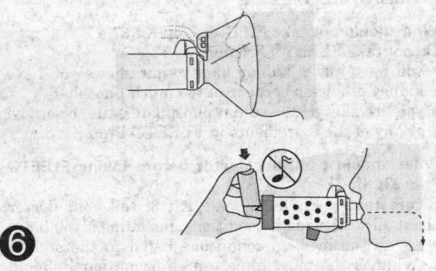

❻

Breathe out gently and depress the MDI at the beginning of a slow inhalation. Use the **Flow-Vu®** Indicator to assist in the coordination of this maneuver. Breathe in slowly and deeply through the mouth until a full breath has been taken. Hold breath for 5–10 seconds, if possible. Otherwise, keep lips tight on the mouthpiece to maintain seal for 2–3 breaths after the MDI is depressed. *Slow down inhalation if you hear the **FlowSignal®** Whistle sound.* **Administer one (1) puff at a time.**
Breathe out gently and depress the MDI at the beginning of a slow inhalation. Use the **Flow-Vu®** Indicator to assist in the coordination of this maneuver. Maintain seal for 5–6 breaths after the MDI is depressed. *Slow down inhalation if you hear the **FlowSignal®** Whistle sound.* **Administer one (1) puff at a time.**

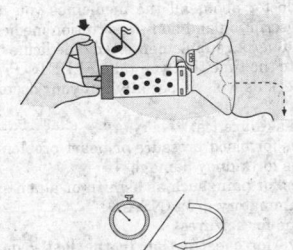

❼

Follow instructions supplied with the MDI on how long to wait before repeating steps 3–6 as prescribed.

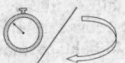

CLEANING INSTRUCTIONS FOR MASK AND MOUTHPIECE CHAMBERS
THIS PRODUCT CAN BE USED RIGHT OUT OF THE PACKAGE AND THEN CLEANED WEEKLY.

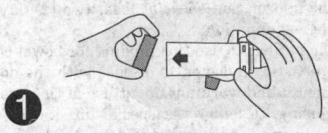

❶

Remove the Backpiece only. Do not tamper with valve during cleaning or disassemble the product beyond what is recommended or damage may result. For mask product, do not remove mask.

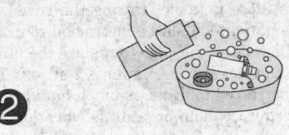

❷

Soak the parts for 15 minutes in a mild solution of liquid dish detergent and lukewarm clean water. Agitate gently.

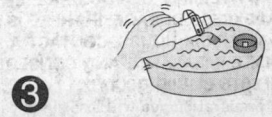

❸

Rinse parts in clean water.

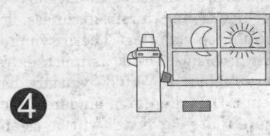

❹

Shake out excess water from the parts and allow to air dry in a vertical position. Ensure parts are dry before reassembly.

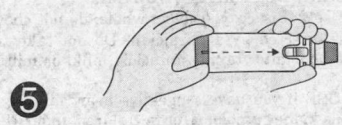

❺

To reassemble, center the Alignment Feature on the Backpiece with the **Flow-Vu®** Indicator, as shown. Press firmly to attach the Backpiece. For mouthpiece models, the protective cap should always be placed on the mouthpiece when the product is not in use.

Notes:
- Storage and operating range 5° C-40° C (41° F-104° F) at 15 to 95% relative humidity.
- Product may need to be replaced after 12 months of use. Environmental conditions, storage and proper cleaning can affect product life span.
- THIS PRODUCT CONTAINS NO LATEX.
- Do not share this medical device.
- Clarity of the chamber is a result of the properties of the **StatBan®** anti-static material.
- If you notice medication build-up in your chamber, wash the inside of the chamber gently with a soft cloth.

Cautions:
- **To ensure proper performance this product should only be cleaned according to these instructions.**
- **Do not leave the chamber unattended with children.**
- **Federal (USA) law restricts the sale of this device on or by the order of a physician.**
℞ Only

Distributed by:
Forest Pharmaceuticals, Inc.
Subsidiary of Forest Laboratories, Inc.
St. Louis, MO 63045
Monaghan Medical Corporation, 5 Latour Ave., Suite 1600, Plattsburgh, NY 12901
© 2009 Monaghan Medical Corporation. ™ and ® are trademarks and registered trademarks used under license by Forest Pharmaceuticals, Inc. Printed in USA. Covered by one or more of the following patents # 5,645,049; 5,848,588; 5,988,160; 6,293,279; 6,345,617; 6,435,177; 6,904,908 and patents pending. RMC 16416 Revision: 01/10
Shown in Product Identification Guide, page 309

BYSTOLIC®
[bi-STOL-ik]
(nebivolol)
tablets
℞

HIGHLIGHTS OF PRESCRIBING INFORMATION
These highlights do not include all the information needed to use Bystolic safely and effectively. See full prescribing information for Bystolic tablets.
Bystolic® (nebivolol) tablets
Initial U.S. Approval: 2007

—INDICATIONS AND USAGE—
BYSTOLIC is a beta-adrenergic blocking agent indicated for the treatment of:
• Hypertension (1.1)

—DOSAGE AND ADMINISTRATION—
Can be taken with and without food. Individualize to the needs of the patient and monitor during up-titration. (2)
• Hypertension: Most patients start at 5 mg once daily. Dose can be increased at 2-week intervals up to 40 mg. (2.1)

—DOSAGE FORMS AND STRENGTHS—
Tablets: 2.5, 5, 10, 20 mg (3)

—CONTRAINDICATIONS—
• Severe bradycardia (4)
• Heart block greater than first degree (4)
• Patients with cardiogenic shock (4)
• Decompensated cardiac failure (4)
• Sick sinus syndrome (unless a permanent pacemaker is in place) (4)
• Patients with severe hepatic impairment (Child-Pugh >B) (4)
• Hypersensitive to any component of this product (4)

—WARNINGS AND PRECAUTIONS—
• Acute exacerbation of coronary artery disease upon cessation of therapy: Do not abruptly discontinue (5.1)
• Diabetes: Monitor glucose as β-blockers may mask symptoms of hypoglycemia (5.6)

—ADVERSE REACTIONS—
Most common adverse reactions (6.1):
• Headache, fatigue
To report SUSPECTED ADVERSE REACTIONS, Contact Forest Laboratories, Inc. at 1-800-678-1605 or FDA at 1-800-FDA-1088 or www.fda.gov/medwatch.

—DRUG INTERACTIONS—
• CYP2D6 enzyme inhibitors may increase nebivolol levels (7.1)
• Reserpine or clonidine may produce excessive reduction of sympathetic activity. (7.2)
• Both digitalis glycosides and β-blockers slow atrioventricular conduction and decrease heart rate. Concomitant use can increase the risk of bradycardia. (7.3)
• Verapamil- or diltiazem-type calcium channel blockers may cause excessive reductions in heart rate, blood pressure, and cardiac contractility. (7.4)
See 17 for PATIENT COUNSELING INFORMATION and FDA-approved patient labeling

Revised: 02/2010

FULL PRESCRIBING INFORMATION

1. INDICATIONS AND USAGE
1.1 Hypertension
BYSTOLIC is indicated for the treatment of hypertension [see Clinical Studies (14.1)]. BYSTOLIC may be used alone or in combination with other antihypertensive agents [see Drug Interactions (7)].

2. DOSAGE AND ADMINISTRATION
2.1 Hypertension
The dose of BYSTOLIC must be individualized to the needs of the patient. For most patients, the recommended starting dose is 5 mg once daily, with or without food, as monotherapy or in combination with other agents. For patients requiring further reduction in blood pressure, the dose can be increased at 2-week intervals up to 40 mg. A more frequent dosing regimen is unlikely to be beneficial.

Renal Impairment
In patients with severe renal impairment (ClCr less than 30 mL/min) the recommended initial dose is 2.5 mg once daily; titrate up slowly if needed. BYSTOLIC has not been studied in patients receiving dialysis [see Clinical Pharmacology (12.4)].

Hepatic Impairment
In patients with moderate hepatic impairment, the recommended initial dose is 2.5 mg once daily; titrate up slowly if needed. BYSTOLIC has not been studied in patients with severe hepatic impairment and therefore it is not recommended in that population [see Clinical Pharmacology (12.4)].

2.2 Subpopulations
Geriatric Patients
It is not necessary to adjust the dose in the elderly [see use in Specific Populations (8.5)].
CYP2D6 Polymorphism
No dose adjustments are necessary for patients who are CYP2D6 poor metabolizers. The clinical effect and safety profile observed in poor metabolizers were similar to those of extensive metabolizers [see Clinical Pharmacology (12.3)].

3. DOSAGE FORMS AND STRENGTHS
BYSTOLIC is available as tablets for oral administration containing nebivolol hydrochloride equivalent to 2.5, 5, 10, and 20 mg of nebivolol.
BYSTOLIC tablets are triangular-shaped, biconvex, unscored, differentiated by color and are engraved with "FL" on one side and the number of mg (2½, 5, 10, or 20) on the other side.

4. CONTRAINDICATIONS
Bystolic is contraindicated in the following conditions:
• Severe bradycardia
• Heart block greater than first degree
• Patients with cardiogenic shock
• Decompensated cardiac failure
• Sick sinus syndrome (unless a permanent pacemaker is in place)
• Patients with severe hepatic impairment (Child-Pugh >B)
• Patients who are hypersensitive to any component of this product.

5. WARNINGS AND PRECAUTIONS
5.1 Abrupt Cessation of Therapy
Do not abruptly discontinue BYSTOLIC therapy in patients with coronary artery disease. Severe exacerbation of angina, myocardial infarction and ventricular arrhythmias have been reported in patients with coronary artery disease following the abrupt discontinuation of therapy with β-blockers. Myocardial infarction and ventricular arrhythmias may occur with or without preceding exacerbation of the angina pectoris. Caution patients without overt coronary artery disease against interruption or abrupt discontinuation of therapy. As with other β-blockers, when discon-

tinuation of BYSTOLIC is planned, carefully observe and advise patients to minimize physical activity. Taper BYSTOLIC over 1 to 2 weeks when possible. If the angina worsens or acute coronary insufficiency develops, re-start BYSTOLIC promptly, at least temporarily.
5.2 Angina and Acute Myocardial Infarction
BYSTOLIC was not studied in patients with angina pectoris or who had a recent MI.
5.3 Bronchospastic Diseases
In general, patients with bronchospastic diseases should not receive β-blockers.
5.4 Anesthesia and Major Surgery
Because beta-blocker withdrawal has been associated with an increased risk of MI and chest pain, patients already on beta-blockers should generally continue treatment throughout the perioperative period. If BYSTOLIC is to be continued perioperatively, monitor patients closely when anesthetic agents which depress myocardial function, such as ether, cyclopropane, and trichloroethylene, are used. If β-blocking therapy is withdrawn prior to major surgery, the impaired ability of the heart to respond to reflex adrenergic stimuli may augment the risks of general anesthesia and surgical procedures.
The β-blocking effects of BYSTOLIC can be reversed by β-agonists, e.g., dobutamine or isoproterenol. However, such patients may be subject to protracted severe hypotension. Additionally, difficulty in restarting and maintaining the heartbeat has been reported with β-blockers.
5.5 Diabetes and Hypoglycemia
β-blockers may mask some of the manifestations of hypoglycemia, particularly tachycardia. Nonselective β-blockers may potentiate insulin-induced hypoglycemia and delay recovery of serum glucose levels. It is not known whether nebivolol has these effects. Advise patients subject to spontaneous hypoglycemia and diabetic patients receiving insulin or oral hypoglycemic agents about these possibilities.
5.6 Thyrotoxicosis
β-blockers may mask clinical signs of hyperthyroidism, such as tachycardia. Abrupt withdrawal of β-blockers may be followed by an exacerbation of the symptoms of hyperthyroidism or may precipitate a thyroid storm.
5.7 Peripheral Vascular Disease
β-blockers can precipitate or aggravate symptoms of arterial insufficiency in patients with peripheral vascular disease.
5.8 Non-dihydropyridine Calcium Channel Blockers
Because of significant negative inotropic and chronotropic effects in patients treated with β-blockers and calcium channel blockers of the verapamil and diltiazem type, monitor the ECG and blood pressure in patients treated concomitantly with these agents.
5.9 Use with CYP2D6 Inhibitors
Nebivolol exposure increases with inhibition of CYP2D6 [see Drug Interactions (7)]. The dose of BYSTOLIC may need to be reduced.
5.10 Impaired Renal Function
Renal clearance of nebivolol is decreased in patients with severe renal impairment. BYSTOLIC has not been studied in patients receiving dialysis [see Clinical Pharmacology (12.4) and Dosage and Administration (2.1)].
5.11 Impaired Hepatic Function
Metabolism of nebivolol is decreased in patients with moderate hepatic impairment. BYSTOLIC has not been studied in patients with severe hepatic impairment [see Clinical Pharmacology (12.4) and Dosage and Administration (2.1)].
5.12 Risk of Anaphylactic Reactions
While taking β-blockers, patients with a history of severe anaphylactic reactions to a variety of allergens may be more reactive to repeated accidental, diagnostic, or therapeutic challenge. Such patients may be unresponsive to the usual doses of epinephrine used to treat allergic reactions.
5.13 Pheochromocytoma
In patients with known or suspected pheochromocytoma, initiate an α-blocker prior to the use of any β-blocker.

6. ADVERSE REACTIONS
6.1 Clinical Studies Experience
BYSTOLIC has been evaluated for safety in patients with hypertension and in patients with heart failure. The observed adverse reaction profile was consistent with the pharmacology of the drug and the health status of the patients in the clinical trials. Adverse reactions reported for each of these patient populations are provided below. Excluded are adverse reactions considered too general to be informative and those not reasonably associated with the use of the drug because they were associated with the condition being treated or are very common in the treated population.
The data described below reflect worldwide clinical trial exposure to BYSTOLIC in 6545 patients, including 5038 patients treated for hypertension and the remaining 1507 subjects treated for other cardiovascular diseases. Doses ranged from 0.5 mg to 40 mg. Patients received BYSTOLIC for up to 24 months, with over 1900 patients treated for at least 6 months, and approximately 1300 patients for more than one year.
HYPERTENSION: In placebo-controlled clinical trials comparing BYSTOLIC with placebo, discontinuation of therapy due to adverse reactions was reported in 2.8% of patients treated with nebivolol and 2.2% of patients given placebo. The most common adverse reactions that led to dis-

continuation of BYSTOLIC were headache (0.4%), nausea (0.2%) and bradycardia (0.2%).

Table 1 lists treatment-emergent adverse reactions that were reported in three 12-week, placebo-controlled monotherapy trials involving 1597 hypertensive patients treated with either 5 mg, 10 mg, or 20-40 mg of BYSTOLIC and 205 patients given placebo and for which the rate of occurrence was at least 1% of patients treated with nebivolol and greater than the rate for those treated with placebo in at least one dose group.

[See table below]

Listed below are other reported adverse reactions with an incidence of at least 1% in the more than 4300 patients treated with BYSTOLIC in controlled or open-label trials except for those already appearing in **Table 1**, terms too general to be informative, minor symptoms, or adverse reactions unlikely to be attributable to drug because they are common in the population. These adverse reactions were in most cases observed at a similar frequency in placebo-treated patients in the controlled studies.

Body as a whole: asthenia.
Gastrointestinal System Disorders: abdominal pain
Metabolic and Nutritional Disorders: hypercholesterolemia
Nervous System Disorders: paraesthesia

6.2   Laboratory Abnormalities
In controlled monotherapy trials of hypertensive patients, BYSTOLIC was associated with an increase in BUN, uric acid, triglycerides and a decrease in HDL cholesterol and platelet count.

6.3   Postmarketing Experience
The following adverse reactions have been identified from spontaneous reports of BYSTOLIC received worldwide and have not been listed elsewhere. These adverse reactions have been chosen for inclusion due to a combination of seriousness, frequency of reporting or potential causal connection to BYSTOLIC. Adverse reactions common in the population have generally been omitted. Because these adverse reactions were reported voluntarily from a population of uncertain size, it is not possible to estimate their frequency or establish a causal relationship to BYSTOLIC exposure: abnormal hepatic function (including increased AST, ALT and bilirubin), acute pulmonary edema, acute renal failure, atrioventricular block (both second and third degree), bronchospasm, erectile dysfunction, hypersensitivity (including urticaria, allergic vasculitis and rare reports of angioedema), myocardial infarction, pruritus, psoriasis, Raynaud's phenomenon, peripheral ischemia/claudication, somnolence, syncope, thrombocytopenia, various rashes and skin disorders, vertigo, and vomiting.

7.   DRUG INTERACTIONS
7.1   CYP2D6 Inhibitors
Use caution when BYSTOLIC is co-administered with CYP2D6 inhibitors (quinidine, propafenone, fluoxetine, paroxetine, etc.) *[see Clinical Pharmacology (12.5)].*
7.2   Hypotensive Agents
Do not use BYSTOLIC with other β-blockers. Closely monitor patients receiving catecholamine-depleting drugs, such as reserpine or guanethidine, because the added β-blocking action of BYSTOLIC may produce excessive reduction of sympathetic activity. In patients who are receiving BYSTOLIC and clonidine, discontinue BYSTOLIC for several days before the gradual tapering of clonidine.
7.3   Digitalis Glycosides
Both digitalis glycosides and β-blockers slow atrioventricular conduction and decrease heart rate. Concomitant use can increase the risk of bradycardia.
7.4   Calcium Channel Blockers
BYSTOLIC can exacerbate the effects of myocardial depressants or inhibitors of AV conduction, such as certain calcium antagonists (particularly of the phenylalkylamine [verapamil] and benzothiazepine [diltiazem] classes), or antiarrhythmic agents, such as disopyramide.

8.   USE IN SPECIFIC POPULATIONS
8.1   Pregnancy: Teratogenic Effects. Category C:
Decreased pup body weights occurred at 1.25 and 2.5 mg/kg in rats, when exposed during the perinatal period (late gestation, parturition and lactation). At 5 mg/kg and higher doses (1.2 times the MRHD), prolonged gestation, dystocia and reduced maternal care were produced with corresponding increases in late fetal deaths and stillbirths and decreased birth weight, live litter size and pup survival. Insufficient numbers of pups survived at 5 mg/kg to evaluate the offspring for reproductive performance.

In studies in which pregnant rats were given nebivolol during organogenesis, reduced fetal body weights were observed at maternally toxic doses of 20 and 40 mg/kg/day (5 and 10 times the MRHD), and small reversible delays in sternal and thoracic ossification associated with the reduced fetal body weights and a small increase in resorption occurred at 40 mg/kg/day (10 times the MRHD). No adverse effects on embryo-fetal viability, sex, weight or morphology were observed in studies in which nebivolol was given to pregnant rabbits at doses as high as 20 mg/kg/day (10 times the MRHD).

8.2   Labor and Delivery
Nebivolol caused prolonged gestation and dystocia at doses ≥ 5 mg/kg in rats (1.2 times the MRHD). These effects were associated with increased fetal deaths and stillborn pups,

and decreased birth weight, live litter size and pup survival rate, events that occurred only when nebivolol was given during the perinatal period (late gestation, parturition and lactation).

No studies of nebivolol were conducted in pregnant women. Use BYSTOLIC during pregnancy only if the potential benefit justifies the potential risk to the fetus.
8.3   Nursing Mothers
Studies in rats have shown that nebivolol or its metabolites cross the placental barrier and are excreted in breast milk. It is not known whether this drug is excreted in human milk.

Because of the potential for β-blockers to produce serious adverse reactions in nursing infants, especially bradycardia, BYSTOLIC is not recommended during nursing.
8.4   Pediatric Use
Safety and effectiveness in pediatric patients have not been established. Pediatric studies in ages newborn to 18 years old have not been conducted because of incomplete characterization of developmental toxicity and possible adverse effects on long-term fertility *[see Nonclinical Toxicology (13.1)].*
8.5   Geriatric Use
Of the 2800 patients in the U.S. sponsored placebo-controlled clinical hypertension studies, 478 patients were 65 years of age or older. No overall differences in efficacy or in the incidence of adverse events were observed between older and younger patients.
8.6   Heart Failure
In a placebo-controlled trial of 2128 patients (1067 BYSTOLIC, 1061 placebo) over 70 years of age with chronic heart failure receiving a maximum dose of 10 mg per day for a median of 20 months, no worsening of heart failure was reported with nebivolol compared to placebo. However, if heart failure worsens consider discontinuation of BYSTOLIC.

10.   OVERDOSAGE
In clinical trials and worldwide postmarketing experience there were reports of BYSTOLIC overdose. The most common signs and symptoms associated with BYSTOLIC overdosage are bradycardia and hypotension. Other important adverse reactions reported with BYSTOLIC overdose include cardiac failure, dizziness, hypoglycemia, fatigue and vomiting. Other adverse reactions associated with β-blocker overdose include bronchospasm and heart block.

The largest known ingestion of BYSTOLIC worldwide involved a patient who ingested up to 500 mg of BYSTOLIC along with several 100 mg tablets of acetylsalicylic acid in a suicide attempt. The patient experienced hyperhydrosis, pallor, depressed level of consciousness, hypokinesia, hypotension, sinus bradycardia, hypoglycemia, hypokalemia, respiratory failure and vomiting. The patient recovered.

Because of extensive drug binding to plasma proteins, hemodialysis is not expected to enhance nebivolol clearance. If overdose occurs, provide general supportive and specific symptomatic treatment. Based on expected pharmacologic actions and recommendations for other β-blockers, consider the following general measures, including stopping BYSTOLIC, when clinically warranted:

Bradycardia: Administer IV atropine. If the response is inadequate, isoproterenol or another agent with positive chronotropic properties may be given cautiously. Under some circumstances, transthoracic or transvenous pacemaker placement may be necessary.

Hypotension: Administer IV fluids and vasopressors. Intravenous glucagon may be useful.

Heart Block (second or third degree): Monitor and treat with isoproterenol infusion. Under some circumstances, transthoracic or transvenous pacemaker placement may be necessary.

Congestive Heart Failure: Initiate therapy with digitalis glycoside and diuretics. In certain cases, consider the use of inotropic and vasodilating agents.

Bronchospasm: Administer bronchodilator therapy such as a short acting inhaled β2-agonist and/or aminophylline.

Hypoglycemia: Administer IV glucose. Repeated doses of IV glucose or possibly glucagon may be required.

Supportive measures should continue until clinical stability is achieved. The half-life of low doses of nebivolol is 12-19 hours.

Call the National Poison Control Center (800-222-1222) for the most current information on β-blocker overdose treatment.

11.   DESCRIPTION
The chemical name for the active ingredient in BYSTOLIC (nebivolol) tablets is (1RS,1'RS)-1,1'-[(2RS,2'SR)-bis(6-fluoro-3,4-dihydro-2H-1-benzopyran-2-yl)]-2,2'-iminodiethanol hydrochloride. Nebivolol is a racemate composed of d-Nebivolol and l-Nebivolol with the stereochemical designations of [SRRR]-nebivolol and [RSSS]-nebivolol, respec-

Table 1. Treatment-Emergent Adverse Reactions with an Incidence (over 6 weeks) ≥ 1% in BYSTOLIC-Treated Patients and at a Higher Frequency than Placebo-Treated Patients

System Organ Class – Preferred Term	Placebo (n = 205) (%)	Nebivolol 5 mg (n = 459) (%)	Nebivolol 10 mg (n = 461) (%)	Nebivolol 20-40 mg (n = 677) (%)
Cardiac Disorders				
Bradycardia	0	0	0	1
Gastrointestinal Disorders				
Diarrhea	2	2	2	3
Nausea	0	1	3	2
General Disorders				
Fatigue	1	2	2	5
Chest pain	0	0	1	1
Peripheral edema	0	1	1	1
Nervous System Disorders				
Headache	6	9	6	7
Dizziness	2	2	3	4
Psychiatric Disorders				
Insomnia	0	1	1	1
Respiratory Disorders				
Dyspnea	0	0	1	1
Skin and subcutaneous Tissue Disorders				
Rash	0	0	1	1

tively. Nebivolol's molecular formula is ($C_{22}H_{25}F_2NO_4$•HCl) with the following structural formula:

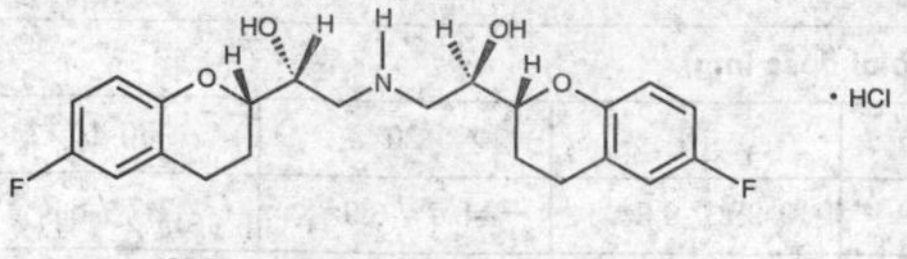

SRRR - or d-nebivolol hydrochloride

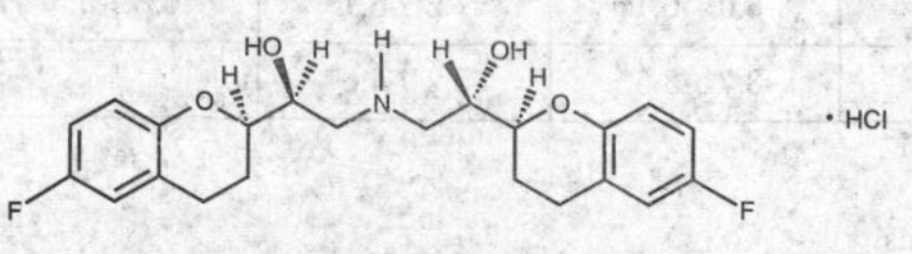

RSSS - or l-nebivolol hydrochloride

MW: 441.90 g/mol

Nebivolol hydrochloride is a white to almost white powder that is soluble in methanol, dimethylsulfoxide, and N,N-dimethylformamide, sparingly soluble in ethanol, propylene glycol, and polyethylene glycol, and very slightly soluble in hexane, dichloromethane, and methylbenzene.

BYSTOLIC as tablets for oral administration contains nebivolol hydrochloride equivalent to 2.5, 5, 10, and 20 mg of nebivolol base. In addition, BYSTOLIC contains the following inactive ingredients: colloidal silicon dioxide, croscarmellose sodium, D&C Red #27 Lake, FD&C Blue #2 Lake, FD&C Yellow #6 Lake, hypromellose, lactose monohydrate, magnesium stearate, microcrystalline cellulose, pregelatinized starch, polysorbate 80, and sodium lauryl sulfate.

12. CLINICAL PHARMACOLOGY

Nebivolol is a β-adrenergic receptor blocking agent. In extensive metabolizers (most of the population) and at doses less than or equal to 10 mg, nebivolol is preferentially β_1 selective. In poor metabolizers and at higher doses, nebivolol inhibits both β_1- and β_2-adrenergic receptors. Nebivolol lacks intrinsic sympathomimetic and membrane stabilizing activity at therapeutically relevant concentrations. At clinically relevant doses, BYSTOLIC does not demonstrate α_1-adrenergic receptor blockade activity. Various metabolites, including glucuronides, contribute to β-blocking activity.

12.1 Mechanism of Action

The mechanism of action of the antihypertensive response of BYSTOLIC has not been definitively established. Possible factors that may be involved include: (1) decreased heart rate, (2) decreased myocardial contractility, (3) diminution of tonic sympathetic outflow to the periphery from cerebral vasomotor centers, (4) suppression of renin activity and (5) vasodilation and decreased peripheral vascular resistance.

12.3 Pharmacokinetics

Nebivolol is metabolized by a number of routes, including glucuronidation and hydroxylation by CYP2D6. The active isomer (d-nebivolol) has an effective half-life of about 12 hours in CYP2D6 extensive metabolizers (most people), and 19 hours in poor metabolizers and exposure to d-nebivolol is substantially increased in poor metabolizers. This has less importance than usual, however, because the metabolites, including the hydroxyl metabolite and glucuronides (the predominant circulating metabolites), contribute to β-blocking activity.

Plasma levels of d–nebivolol increase in proportion to dose in EMs and PMs for doses up to 20mg. Exposure to l-nebivolol is higher than to d-nebivolol but l-nebivolol contributes little to the drug's activity as d-nebivolol's beta receptor affinity is > 1000-fold higher than l-nebivolol. For the same dose, PMs attain a 5-fold higher C_{max} and 10-fold higher AUC of d-nebivolol than do EMs. d-Nebivolol accumulates about 1.5-fold with repeated once-daily dosing in EMs.

Absorption

Absorption of BYSTOLIC is similar to an oral solution. The absolute bioavailability has not been determined.

Mean peak plasma nebivolol concentrations occur approximately 1.5 to 4 hours post-dosing in EMs and PMs.

Food does not alter the pharmacokinetics of nebivolol. Under fed conditions, nebivolol glucuronides are slightly reduced. BYSTOLIC may be administered without regard to meals.

Distribution

The in vitro human plasma protein binding of nebivolol is approximately 98%, mostly to albumin, and is independent of nebivolol concentrations.

Metabolism

Nebivolol is predominantly metabolized via direct glucuronidation of parent and to a lesser extent via N-dealkylation and oxidation via cytochrome P450 2D6. Its stereospecific metabolites contribute to the pharmacologic activity *[see Drug Interactions (7)]*.

Elimination

After a single oral administration of 14C-nebivolol, 38% of the dose was recovered in urine and 44% in feces for EMs and 67% in urine and 13% in feces for PMs. Essentially all nebivolol was excreted as multiple oxidative metabolites or their corresponding glucuronide conjugates.

12.4 Special Populations

Hepatic Disease

d-Nebivolol peak plasma concentration increased 3-fold, exposure (AUC) increased 10-fold, and the apparent clearance decreased by 86% in patients with moderate hepatic impairment (Child-Pugh Class B). No formal studies have been performed in patients with severe hepatic impairment and nebivolol should be contraindicated for these patients *[see Dosage and Administration (2)]*.

Renal Disease

The apparent clearance of nebivolol was unchanged following a single 5 mg dose of BYSTOLIC in patients with mild renal impairment (ClCr 50 to 80 mL/min, n=7), and it was reduced negligibly in patients with moderate (ClCr 30 to 50 mL/min, n=9), but clearance was reduced by 53% in patients with severe renal impairment (ClCr <30 mL/min, n=5). No studies have been conducted in patients on dialysis *[see Dosage and Administration (2)]*.

12.5 Drug-Drug Interactions

Drugs that inhibit CYP2D6 can be expected to increase plasma levels of nebivolol. When BYSTOLIC is co-administered with an inhibitor or an inducer of this enzyme, monitor patients closely and adjust the nebivolol dose according to blood pressure response. *In vitro* studies have demonstrated that at therapeutically relevant concentrations, d- and l-nebivolol do not inhibit any cytochrome P450 pathways.

Digoxin: Concomitant administration of BYSTOLIC (10 mg once daily) and digoxin (0.25 mg once daily) for 10 days in 14 healthy adult individuals resulted in no significant changes in the pharmacokinetics of digoxin or nebivolol *[see Drug Interactions (7)]*.

Warfarin: Administration of BYSTOLIC (10 mg once daily for 10 days) led to no significant changes in the pharmacokinetics of nebivolol or R- or S-warfarin following a single 10 mg dose of warfarin. Similarly, nebivolol has no significant effects on the anticoagulant activity of warfarin, as assessed by Prothrombin time and INR profiles from 0 to 144 hours after a single 10 mg warfarin dose in 12 healthy adult volunteers.

Diuretics: No pharmacokinetic interactions were observed in healthy adults between nebivolol (10 mg daily for 10 days) and furosemide (40 mg single dose), hydrochlorothiazide (25 mg once daily for 10 days), or spironolactone (25 mg once daily for 10 days).

Ramipril: Concomitant administration of BYSTOLIC (10 mg once daily) and ramipril (5 mg once daily) for 10 days in 15 healthy adult volunteers produced no pharmacokinetic interactions.

Losartan: Concomitant administration of BYSTOLIC (10 mg single dose) and losartan (50 mg single dose) in 20 healthy adult volunteers did not result in pharmacokinetic interactions.

Fluoxetine: Fluoxetine, a CYP2D6 inhibitor, administered at 20 mg per day for 21 days prior to a single 10 mg dose of nebivolol to 10 healthy adults, led to an 8-fold increase in the AUC and 3-fold increase in C_{max} for d-nebivolol *[see Drug Interactions (7)]*.

Histamine-2 Receptor Antagonists: The pharmacokinetics of nebivolol (5 mg single dose) were not affected by the co-administration of ranitidine (150 mg twice daily). Cimetidine (400 mg twice daily) causes a 23% increase in the plasma levels of d-nebivolol.

Charcoal: The pharmacokinetics of nebivolol (10 mg single dose) were not affected by repeated co-administration (4, 8, 12, 16, 22, 28, 36, and 48 hours after nebivolol administration) of activated charcoal (Actidose-Aqua®).

Sidenafil: The co-administration of nebivolol and sildenafil decreased AUC and C_{max} of sildenafil by 21 and 23% respectively. The effect on the C_{max} and AUC for d-nebivolol was also small (< 20%). The effect on vital signs (e.g., pulse and blood pressure) was approximately the sum of the effects of sildenafil and nebivolol.

Other Concomitant Medications: Utilizing population pharmacokinetic analyses, derived from hypertensive patients, the following drugs were observed not to have an effect on the pharmacokinetics of nebivolol: acetaminophen, acetylsalicylic acid, atorvastatin, esomeprazole, ibuprofen, levothyroxine sodium, metformin, sildenafil, simvastatin, or tocopherol.

Protein Binding: No meaningful changes in the extent of *in vitro* binding of nebivolol to human plasma proteins were noted in the presence of high concentrations of diazepam, digoxin, diphenylhydantoin, enalapril, hydrochlorothiazide, imipramine, indomethacin, propranolol, sulfamethazine, tolbutamide, or warfarin. Additionally, nebivolol did not significantly alter the protein binding of the following drugs: diazepam, digoxin, diphenylhydantoin, hydrochlorothiazide, imipramine, or warfarin at their therapeutic concentrations.

13. NONCLINICAL TOXICOLOGY

13.1 Carcinogenesis, Mutagenesis, and Impairment of Fertility

In a two-year study of nebivolol in mice, a statistically significant increase in the incidence of testicular Leydig cell hyperplasia and adenomas was observed at 40 mg/kg/day (5 times the maximally recommended human dose of 40 mg on a mg/m^2 basis). Similar findings were not reported in mice administered doses equal to approximately 0.3 or 1.2 times the maximum recommended human dose. No evidence of a tumorigenic effect was observed in a 24-month study in Wistar rats receiving doses of nebivolol 2.5, 10 and 40 mg/kg/day (equivalent to 0.6, 2.4, and 10 times the maximally recommended human dose). Co-administration of dihydrotestosterone reduced blood LH levels and prevented the Leydig cell hyperplasia, consistent with an indirect LH-mediated effect of nebivolol in mice and not thought to be clinically relevant in man.

A randomized, double-blind, placebo- and active-controlled, parallel-group study in healthy male volunteers was conducted to determine the effects of nebivolol on adrenal function, luteinizing hormone, and testosterone levels. This study demonstrated that 6 weeks of daily dosing with 10 mg of nebivolol had no significant effect on ACTH-stimulated mean serum cortisol $AUC_{0\text{-}120\ min}$, serum LH, or serum total testosterone.

Effects on spermatogenesis were seen in male rats and mice at ≥ 40 mg/kg/day (10 and 5 times the MRHD, respectively). For rats the effects on spermatogenesis were not reversed and may have worsened during a four week recovery period. The effects of nebivolol on sperm in mice, however, were partially reversible.

Mutagenesis: Nebivolol was not genotoxic when tested in a battery of assays (Ames, *in vitro* mouse lymphoma $TK^{+/-}$, *in vitro* human peripheral lymphocyte chromosome aberration, *in vivo* Drosophila melanogaster sex-linked recessive lethal, and *in vivo* mouse bone marrow micronucleus tests).

14. CLINICAL STUDIES

14.1 Hypertension

The antihypertensive effectiveness of BYSTOLIC as monotherapy has been demonstrated in three randomized, double-blind, multi-center, placebo-controlled trials at doses ranging from 1.25 to 40 mg for 12 weeks (Studies 1, 2, and 3). A fourth placebo-controlled trial demonstrated additional antihypertensive effects of BYSTOLIC at doses ranging from 5 to 20 mg when administered concomitantly with up to two other antihypertensive agents (ACE inhibitors, angiotensin II receptor antagonists, and thiazide diuretics) in patients with inadequate blood pressure control.

The three monotherapy trials included a total of 2016 patients (1811 BYSTOLIC, 205 placebo) with mild to moderate hypertension who had baseline diastolic blood pressures (DBP) of 95 to 109 mmHg. Patients received either BYSTOLIC or placebo once daily for twelve weeks. Two of these monotherapy trials (Studies 1 and 2) studied 1716 patients in the general hypertensive population with a mean age of 54 years, 55% males, 26% non-Caucasians, 7% diabetics and 6% genotyped as PMs. The third monotherapy trial (Study 3) studied 300 Black patients with a mean age of 51 years, 45% males, 14% diabetics, and 3% as PMs.

Placebo-subtracted blood pressure reductions by dose for each study are presented in **Table 3**. Most studies showed increasing response to doses above 5 mg.

[See table 3 at top of next page]

Study 4 enrolled 669 patients with a mean age of 54 years, 55% males, 54% Caucasians, 29% Blacks, 15% Hispanics, 1% Asians, 14% diabetics, and 5% PMs. BYSTOLIC, 5 mg to 20 mg, administered once daily concomitantly with stable doses of up to two other antihypertensive agents (ACE inhibitors, angiotensin II receptor antagonists, and thiazide diuretics) resulted in significant additional antihypertensive effects over placebo compared to baseline blood pressure.

Effectiveness was similar in subgroups analyzed by age and sex. Effectiveness was established in Blacks, but as monotherapy the magnitude of effect was somewhat less than in Caucasians.

The blood pressure lowering effect of BYSTOLIC was seen within two weeks of treatment and was maintained over the 24-hour dosing interval.

16. HOW SUPPLIED/STORAGE AND HANDLING

BYSTOLIC is available as tablets for oral administration containing nebivolol hydrochloride equivalent to 2.5, 5, 10, and 20 mg of nebivolol.

BYSTOLIC tablets are triangular-shaped, biconvex, unscored, differentiated by color and are engraved with **"FL"** on one side and the number of mg (2½, 5, 10, or 20) on the other side. BYSTOLIC tablets are supplied in the following strengths and package configurations:

[See second table on next page]

Store at 20° to 25°C (68° to 77°F). [See USP for Controlled Room Temperature.]

Dispense in a tight, light-resistant container as defined in the USP using a child-resistant closure.

17 PATIENT COUNSELING INFORMATION

See FDA-Approved Patient Labeling (17.2).

17.1 Patient Advice

Advise patients to take BYSTOLIC regularly and continuously, as directed. BYSTOLIC can be taken with or without food. If a dose is missed, take the next scheduled dose only (without doubling it). Do not interrupt or discontinue BYSTOLIC without consulting the physician.

Patients should know how they react to this medicine before they operate automobiles, use machinery, or engage in other tasks requiring alertness.

Advise patients to consult a physician if any difficulty in breathing occurs, or if they develop signs or symptoms of worsening congestive heart failure such as weight gain or increasing shortness of breath, or excessive bradycardia.

Caution patients subject to spontaneous hypoglycemia, or diabetic patients receiving insulin or oral hypoglycemic agents, that β-blockers may mask some of the manifestations of hypoglycemia, particularly tachycardia.

17.2 FDA-Approved Patient Labeling

PATIENT INFORMATION

BYSTOLIC® (bi-STOL-ik) (nebivolol) Tablets

Read the Patient Information that comes with BYSTOLIC before you start taking it and each time you get a refill. There may be new information. This information does not take the place of talking with your doctor about your medical condition or your treatment. If you have any questions about BYSTOLIC, ask your doctor or pharmacist.

WHAT IS BYSTOLIC?

BYSTOLIC is a kind of prescription medicine called a "beta-blocker". BYSTOLIC treats:
• High blood pressure (hypertension)
BYSTOLIC can lower blood pressure when used by itself and with other medicines.
BYSTOLIC is not approved for children less than 18 years of age.

WHO SHOULD NOT TAKE BYSTOLIC?

Do not take BYSTOLIC if you:
• Have heart failure and are in the ICU or need medicines to keep up your blood circulation
• Have a slow heartbeat or your heart skips beats (irregular heartbeat)
• Have severe liver damage
• Are allergic to any ingredient in BYSTOLIC. The active ingredient is nebivolol. See the end of this leaflet for a list of ingredients.

WHAT SHOULD I TELL MY DOCTOR BEFORE TAKING BYSTOLIC?

Tell your doctor about all of your medical problems, including if you:
• Have asthma or other lung problems (such as bronchitis or emphysema)
• Have problems with blood flow in your feet and legs (peripheral vascular disease) BYSTOLIC can make symptoms of blood flow problems worse.
• Have diabetes and take medicine to control blood sugar
• Have thyroid problems
• Have liver or kidney problems
• Had allergic reactions to medications or have allergies
• Have a condition called pheochromocytoma
• Are pregnant or trying to become pregnant. It is not known if BYSTOLIC is safe for your unborn baby. Talk with your doctor about the best way to treat high blood pressure while you are pregnant.
• Are breastfeeding. It is not known if BYSTOLIC passes into your breast milk. You should not breastfeed while using BYSTOLIC.
• Are scheduled for surgery and will be given anesthetic agents

Tell your doctor about all the medicines you take. Include prescription and non-prescription medicines, vitamins, and herbal products. BYSTOLIC and certain other medicines can affect each other and cause serious side effects.

Keep a list of all the medicines you take. Show this list to your doctor and pharmacist before you start a new medicine.

HOW SHOULD I TAKE BYSTOLIC?

• **Do not suddenly stop taking BYSTOLIC. You could have chest pain or a heart attack.** If your doctor decides to stop BYSTOLIC, your doctor may slowly lower your dose over time before stopping it completely.
• **Take BYSTOLIC every day exactly as your doctor tells you.** Your doctor will tell you how much BYSTOLIC to take and how often. Your doctor may start with a low dose and raise it over time.
• Do not stop taking BYSTOLIC or change your dose without talking with your doctor.
• Take BYSTOLIC with or without food.
• If you miss a dose, take your dose as soon as you remember, unless it is close to the time to take your next dose. Do

not take 2 doses at the same time. Take your next dose at the usual time.
• If you take too much BYSTOLIC, call your doctor or poison control center right away.

WHAT ARE POSSIBLE SIDE EFFECTS OF BYSTOLIC?

• Low blood pressure and feeling dizzy. If you feel dizzy, sit or lie down and tell your doctor right away.
• Tiredness
• Slow heartbeat
• Headache
• Leg swelling due to fluid retention (edema). Tell your doctor if you gain weight or have trouble breathing while taking BYSTOLIC.

Tell your doctor if you have any side effects that bother you or don't go away.

HOW SHOULD I STORE BYSTOLIC?

• Store BYSTOLIC between 68° to 77°F (20°-25°C).
• Safely throw away BYSTOLIC that is out of date or no longer needed.
• Keep BYSTOLIC and all medicines out of the reach of children.

GENERAL INFORMATION ABOUT BYSTOLIC

Doctors sometimes prescribe medicines for conditions not included in the patient information leaflets.
• Only use BYSTOLIC for the medical problem it was prescribed for.
• Do not give BYSTOLIC to other people, even if they have the same symptoms. It may harm them.

This leaflet summarizes the most important information about BYSTOLIC. For more information:
• Talk with your doctor.
• Ask your doctor or pharmacist for information about BYSTOLIC that is written for healthcare professionals.
• Visit www.BYSTOLIC.com on the web or call 1-800-678-1605.

WHAT IS IN BYSTOLIC?

Active Ingredient: Nebivolol

Inactive Ingredients: colloidal silicon dioxide, croscarmellose sodium, D&C Red #27 Lake, FD&C Blue #2 Lake, FD&C Yellow #6 Lake, hypromellose, lactose monohydrate, magnesium stearate, microcrystalline cellulose, pregelatinized starch, polysorbate 80, and sodium lauryl sulfate

Forest Pharmaceuticals, Inc.
Subsidiary of Forest Laboratories, Inc.
St. Louis, MO 63045, USA

Table 3. Placebo-Subtracted Least-Square Mean Reductions in Trough Sitting Systolic/Diastolic Blood Pressure (SiSBP/SiDBP mmHg) by Dose in Studies with Once Daily BYSTOLIC

	Nebivolol dose (mg)					
	1.25	2.5	5.0	10	20	30-40
Study 1	-6.6*/-5.1*	-8.5*/-5.6*	-8.1*/-5.5*	-9.2*/-6.3*	-8.7*/-6.9*	-11.7*/-8.3*
Study 2			-3.8/-3.2*	-3.1/-3.9*	-6.3*/-4.5*	
Study 3¶		-1.5/-2.9	-2.6/-4.9*	-6.0*/-6.1*	-7.2*/-6.1*	-6.8*/-5.5*
Study 4^			-5.7*/-3.3*	-3.7*/-3.5*	-6.2*/-4.6*	

* p<0.05 based on pair-wise comparison vs. placebo
¶ Study enrolled only African Americans.
^ Study on top of one or two other antihypertensive medications.

BYSTOLIC

Tablet Strength	Package Configuration	NDC #	Tablet Color
2.5 mg	Bottle of 30	0456-1402-30	Light Blue
	Bottle of 100	0456-1402-01	
	10 × 10 Unit Dose	0456-1402-63	
5 mg	Bottle of 30	0456-1405-30	Beige
	Bottle of 100	0456-1405-01	
	10 × 10 Unit Dose	0456-1405-63	
10 mg	Bottle of 30	0456-1410-30	Pinkish-Purple
	Bottle of 100	0456-1410-01	
	10 × 10 Unit Dose	0456-1410-63	
20 mg	Bottle of 30	0456-1420-30	Light Blue
	Bottle of 100	0456-1420-01	
	10 × 10 Unit Dose	0456-1420-63	

Licensed from Mylan Laboratories, Inc.
Under license from Janssen Pharmaceutica N.V., Beerse, Belgium
Actidose-Aqua® is a registered trademark of Paddock Laboratories, Inc.
Rev. 02/10
© 2010 Forest Laboratories, Inc.

Shown in Product Identification Guide, page 309

CERVIDIL®

℞

[ser-vĭ-dĭl]

Brand of dinoprostone vaginal insert

Rx only

DESCRIPTION

Dinoprostone vaginal insert is a thin, flat, polymeric slab which is rectangular in shape with rounded corners contained within the pouch of an off-white knitted polyester retrieval system. Each slab is buff colored, semitransparent and contains 10 mg of dinoprostone in a hydrogel insert. An integral part of the knitted polyester retrieval system is a long tape designed to aid retrieval at the end of the dosing interval or earlier if clinically indicated. The finished product is a controlled release formulation which has been found to release dinoprostone *in vivo* at a rate of approximately 0.3 mg/hr.

The chemical name for dinoprostone (commonly known as prostaglandin E_2 or PGE_2) is 11α, 15S-dihydroxy-9-oxo-prosta-5Z,13E-dien-1-oic acid and the structural formula is represented below:

The molecular formula is $C_{20}H_{32}O_5$ and its molecular weight is 352.5. Dinoprostone occurs as a white to off-white crystalline powder. It has a melting point within the range of 65° to 69°C. Dinoprostone is soluble in ethanol and in 25% ethanol in water. Each insert contains 10 mg of dinoprostone in 241 mg of a cross-linked polyethylene oxide/

urethane polymer which is a semi-opaque, beige colored, flat rectangular slab measuring 29 mm by 9.5 mm and 0.8 mm in thickness. The insert and its retrieval system, made of polyester yarn, are non-toxic and when placed in a moist environment, absorb water, swell, and release dinoprostone.

CLINICAL PHARMACOLOGY

Dinoprostone (PGE_2) is a naturally-occurring biomolecule. It is found in low concentrations in most tissues of the body and functions as a local hormone (1-3). As with any local hormone, it is very rapidly metabolized in the tissues of synthesis (the half-life estimated to be 2.5-5 minutes). The rate limiting step for inactivation is regulated by the enzyme 15-hydroxyprostaglandin dehydrogenase (PGDH) (1,4). Any PGE_2 that escapes local inactivation is rapidly cleared to the extent of 95% on the first pass through the pulmonary circulation (1,2).

In pregnancy, PGE_2 is secreted continuously by the fetal membranes and placenta and plays an important role in the final events leading to the initiation of labor (1,2). It is known that PGE_2 stimulates the production of $PGF_{2\alpha}$ which in turn sensitizes the myometrium to endogenous or exogenously administered oxytocin. Although PGE_2 is capable of initiating uterine contractions and may interact with oxytocin to increase uterine contractility, the available evidence indicates that, in the concentrations found during the early part of labor, PGE_2 plays an important role in cervical ripening without affecting uterine contractions (5-7). This distinction serves as the basis for considering cervical ripening and induction of labor, usually by the use of oxytocin (8-10), as two separate processes.

PGE_2 plays an important role in the complex set of biochemical and structural alterations involved in cervical ripening. Cervical ripening involves a marked relaxation of the cervical smooth muscle fibers of the uterine cervix which must be transformed from a rigid structure to a softened, yielding and dilated configuration to allow passage of the fetus through the birth canal (11-13). This process involves activation of the enzyme collagenase which is responsible for digestion of some of the structural collagen network of the cervix (1, 14). This is associated with a concomitant increase in the amount of hydrophilic glycosaminoglycan, hyaluronic acid and a decrease in dermatan sulfate (1). Failure of the cervix to undergo these natural physiologic changes, usually assessed by the method described by Bishop (15,16), prior to the onset of effective uterine contractions, results in an unfavourable outcome for successful vaginal delivery and may result in fetal compromise. It is estimated that in approximately 5% of pregnancies the cervix does not ripen normally (17). In an additional 10-11% of pregnancies, labor must be induced for medical or obstetric reasons prior to the time of cervical ripening (17).

The delivery rate of PGE_2 *in vivo* is about 0.3 mg/hour over a period of 12 hours. The controlled release of PGE_2 from the hydrogel insert is an attempt to provide sufficient quantities of PGE_2 to the local receptors to satisfy hormonal requirements. In the majority of patients, these local effects are manifested by changes in the consistency, dilatation and effacement of the cervix as measured by the Bishop score. Although some patients experience uterine hyperstimulation as a result of direct PGE_2- or $PGF_{2\alpha}$-, mediated sensitization of the myometrium to oxytocin, systemic effects of PGE_2 are rarely encountered. The insert is fitted with a biocompatible retrieval system which facilitates removal at the conclusion of therapy or in the event of an adverse reaction. No correlation could be established between PGE_2 release and plasma concentrations of PGE_m. The relative contributions of endogenously and exogenously released PGE_2 to the plasma levels of the metabolite PGE_m could not be determined. Moreover, it is uncertain as to whether the measured concentrations of PGE_m reflect the natural progression of PGE_m concentrations in blood as birth approaches or to what extent the measured concentrations following PGE_2 administration represent an increase over basal levels that might be measured in control patients.

INDICATIONS AND USAGE

Cervidil Vaginal Insert (dinoprostone, 10 mg) is indicated for the initiation and/or continuation of cervical ripening in patients at or near term in whom there is a medical or obstetrical indication for the induction of labor.

CONTRAINDICATIONS

Cervidil is contraindicated in:

- Patients with known hypersensitivity to prostaglandins.
- Patients in whom there is clinical suspicion or definite evidence of fetal distress where delivery is not imminent.
- Patients with unexplained vaginal bleeding during this pregnancy.
- Patients in whom there is evidence or strong suspicion of marked cephalopelvic disproportion.
- Patients in whom oxytocic drugs are contraindicated or when prolonged contraction of the uterus may be detrimental to fetal safety or uterine integrity, such as previous cesarean section or major uterine surgery (see **PRECAUTIONS** and **ADVERSE REACTIONS**).
- Patients already receiving intravenous oxytocic drugs.
- Multipara with 6 or more previous term pregnancies.

Table 1 Total Cervidil–Treated Drug Related Adverse Events

	Controlled Studies[1] Active	Placebo
Uterine hyperstimulation with fetal distress	2.8%	0.3%
Uterine hyperstimulation without fetal distress	4.7%	0%
Fetal Distress without uterine hyperstimulation	3.8%	1.2%
N	320	338
	STUDY 101-801[2] Active	**Placebo**
Uterine hyperstimulation with fetal distress	2.9%	0%
Uterine hyperstimulation without fetal distress	2.0%	0%
Fetal Distress without uterine hyperstimulation	2.9%	1.0%
N	102	104

[1] Controlled Studies (with and without retrieval system)
[2] Controlled Study (with retrieval system)

WARNINGS

For hospital use only

Cervidil should be administered only by trained obstetrical personnel in a hospital setting with appropriate obstetrical care facilities.

Women aged 30 years or older, those with complications during pregnancy and those with a gestational age over 40 weeks have been shown to have an increased risk of postpartum disseminated intravascular coagulation. In addition, these factors may further increase the risk associated with labor induction (See **ADVERSE REACTIONS**, Postmarketing surveillance). Therefore, in these women, use of dinoprostone should be undertaken with caution. Measures should be applied to detect as soon as possible an evolving fibrinolysis in the immediate post-partum period.

The Clinician should be alert that use of dinoprostone may result in inadvertent disruption and subsequent embolization of antigenic tissue causing in rare circumstances the development of Anaphylactoid Syndrome of Pregnancy (Amniotic Fluid Embolism).

PRECAUTIONS

1. General Precautions: Since prostaglandins potentiate the effect of oxytocin, Cervidil must be removed before oxytocin administration is initiated and the patient's uterine activity carefully monitored for uterine hyperstimulation. If uterine hyperstimulation is encountered or if labor commences, the vaginal insert should be removed. Cervidil should also be removed prior to amniotomy.

Cervidil is contraindicated when prolonged contraction of the uterus may be detrimental to fetal safety and uterine integrity. Therefore, Cervidil should not be administered to patients with a history of previous cesarean section or uterine surgery given the potential risk for uterine rupture and associated obstetrical complications, including the need for hysterectomy and the occurrence of fetal or neonatal death. Caution should be exercised in the administration of Cervidil for cervical ripening in patients with ruptured membranes, in cases of non-vertex or non-singleton presentation, and in patients with a history of previous uterine hypertony, glaucoma, or a history of childhood asthma, even though there have been no asthma attacks in adulthood.

Uterine activity, fetal status and the progression of cervical dilatation and effacement should be carefully monitored whenever the dinoprostone vaginal insert is in place. With any evidence of uterine hyperstimulation, sustained uterine contractions, fetal distress, or other fetal or maternal adverse reactions, the vaginal insert should be removed.

An increased risk of post-partum disseminated intravascular coagulation has been described in patients whose labor was induced by physiologic means, either with dinoprostone or oxytocin.

2. Drug Interactions: Cervidil may augment the activity of oxytocic agents and their concomitant use is not recommended. A dosing interval of at least 30 minutes is recommended for the sequential use of oxytocin following the removal of the dinoprostone vaginal insert. No other drug interactions have been identified.

3. Carcinogenesis, Mutagenesis, Impairment of Fertility: Long-term carcinogenicity and fertility studies have not been conducted with Cervidil (dinoprostone) Vaginal Insert. No evidence of mutagenicity has been observed with prostaglandin E_2 in the Unscheduled DNA Synthesis Assay, the Micronucleus Test, or Ames Assay.

4. Pregnancy, Teratogenic Effects:

Pregnancy Category C.

Prostaglandin E_2 has produced an increase in skeletal anomalies in rats and rabbits. No effect would be expected clinically, when used as indicated, since Cervidil (dinoprostone) Vaginal Insert is administered after the period of organogenesis. Prostaglandin E_2 has been shown to be embryotoxic in rats and rabbits, and any dose that produces sustained increased uterine tone could put the embryo or fetus at risk.

5. Pediatric Use: The safety and efficacy of Cervidil has been established in women of a reproductive age and women who are pregnant. Although safety and efficacy has not been established in pediatric patients, safety and efficacy are expected to be the same for adolescents.

ADVERSE REACTIONS

Cervidil is well tolerated. In placebo-controlled trials in which 658 women were entered and 320 received active therapy (218 without retrieval system, 102 with retrieval system), the following events were reported.

[See table above]

Drug related fever, nausea, vomiting, diarrhea, and abdominal pain were noted in less than 1% of patients who received Cervidil.

In study 101-801 (with the retrieval system) cases of hyperstimulation reversed within 2 to 13 minutes of removal of the product. Tocolytics were required in one of the five cases. In cases of fetal distress, when product removal was thought advisable there was a return to normal rhythm and no neonatal sequelae.

Five minute Apgar scores were 7 or above in 98.2% (646/658) of studied neonates whose mothers received Cervidil.

In a report of a 3 year pediatric follow-up study in 121 infants, 51 of whose mothers received Cervidil, there were no deleterious effects on physical examination or psychomotor evaluation (18).

Post-marketing surveillance:

Immune System Disorders: Hypersensitivity

Blood and lymphatic system disorders: Disseminated Intravascular Coagulation (See Warnings Section)

Reproductive system: Reports of uterine rupture have been reported in association with use of Cervidil some required a hysterectomy and some resulted in subsequent fetal or neonatal death.

Vascular Disorders: Hypotension

Pregnancy, Puerperium and Perinatal Conditions: Amniotic fluid embolism

DRUG ABUSE AND DEPENDENCE

No drug abuse or dependence has been seen with the use of Cervidil.

OVERDOSAGE

Cervidil is used as a single dosage in a single application. Overdosage is usually manifested by uterine hyperstimulation which may be accompanied by fetal distress, and is usually responsive to removal of the insert. Other treatment must be symptomatic since, to date, clinical experience with prostaglandin antagonists is insufficient.

The use of beta-adrenergic agents should be considered in the event of undesirable increased uterine activity.

DOSAGE AND ADMINISTRATION

The dosage of dinoprostone in the vaginal insert is 10 mg designed to be released at approximately 0.3 mg/hour over a 12 hour period. Cervidil should be removed upon onset of active labor or 12 hours after insertion.

Table 2 Efficacy of Cervidil in Double Blind Studies

Parameter	Study #	Primip/Nullip		Multip		P-Value
		Cervidil	Placebo	Cervidil	Placebo	
Treatment Success*	101-103 (N=81)	65%	28%	87%	29%	<0.001
	101-003 (N=371)	68%	24%	77%	24%	<0.001
	101-801 (N=206)	72%	48%	55%	41%	0.003
Time to Delivery (hours) Average Median	101-103 (N=81)	33.7	48.6	14.0	28.6	0.001
		25.7	34.5	12.3	24.6	
Average Median	101-801 (N=206)	31.1	51.8	52.3	45.9	<0.001
		25.5	37.2	20.8	27.4	
Time to Onset of Labor (hrs) Average Median	101-103 (N=81)	19.9	39.4	6.8	22.4	<0.001
		12.0	19.2	6.9	18.3	

*Treatment success was defined as Bishop score increase at 12 hours of ≥ 3, vaginal delivery within 12 hours or Bishop score at 12 hours ≥ 6. These studies were not designed with the power to show differences in cesarean section rates between Cervidil and placebo groups and none were noted.

Cervidil is supplied in an individually wrapped aluminium/polyethylene package with a "tear mark" on one side of the package. The package should only be opened by tearing the aluminium package along the tear mark. The package should never be opened with scissors or other sharp objects which may compromise or cut the knitted polyester pouch that serves as the retrieval system for the polymeric slab. Cervidil must be kept frozen until use, and is administered by placing one unit transversely in the posterior fornix of the vagina immediately after removal from its foil package. The insertion of the vaginal insert does not require sterile conditions. The vaginal insert must not be used without its retrieval system. There is no need for previous warming of the product. A minimal amount of water-miscible lubricant may be used to assist insertion of Cervidil. Care should be taken not to permit excess contact or coating with the lubricant which could prevent optimal swelling and release of dinoprostone from the vaginal insert. Patients should remain in the recumbent position for 2 hours following insertion, but thereafter may be ambulatory. If the patient is ambulatory, care should be taken to ensure the vaginal insert remains in place. If uterine hyperstimulation is encountered or if labor commences, the vaginal insert should be removed. Cervidil should also be removed prior to amniotomy.

Upon removal of Cervidil, it is essential to ensure that the slab has been removed, as it will continue delivering the active ingredient. This is accomplished by visualizing the knitted polyester retrieval system and confirming that it contains the slab. In the rare instance that the slab is not contained within the polyester retrieval system, a vaginal exam should be performed to remove the slab.

HOW SUPPLIED
Cervidil (NDC 0456-4123-63) contains 10 mg dinoprostone. The product is wound and enclosed in an aluminium/polyethylene pack.
Store in a freezer: between -20°C and -10°C (-4°F and 14°F). Cervidil is packed in foil and is stable when stored in a freezer for a period of three years. Vaginal inserts exposed to high humidity will absorb moisture from the air and thereby alter the release characteristics of dinoprostone. Once used, the vaginal insert should be discarded.

CLINICAL STUDIES
[See table above]

REFERENCES
1. Physiology of Labor In: Williams Obstetrics. Eds. Pritchard, J. A., MacDonald, P. C., and Gant, N.F. Appleton-Century-Crofts, Conn, Pp 295-321, (1985).
2. Rall, T. W. and Schliefer, L. S. Oxytocin, prostaglandin, ergot alkaloids, and other drugs; tocolytics agents, In: The Pharmacological Basis of Therapeutics. Eds. Gilman, A.G., Goodman, L.S., Rall, T.W., and Murad, F. MacMillan, Publ. Co., New York, Pp. 926-945, (1985).
3. Casey, M.L. and MacDonald, P.C. The initiation of labor in women: Regulation of phospholipid and arachidonic acid metabolism and of prostaglandin production. Semin. Perinat. 10:270-275, (1986).
4. Casey, M.L., MacDonald, P.C. and Mitchell, M.D. Stimulation of Prostaglandin E₂ production in amnion cells in culture by a substance(s) in human fetal urine. Biochem. Biophys. Res. Comm. 114:1056, (1983).
5. Olson, C.M., Lye, S.J., Skinner, K. and Challis, J.R.G. Prostanoid concentrations in maternal/fetal plasma and amniotic fluid and intrauterine tissue prostanoid output in relation to myometrial contractility during the onset of Endocrinology, 116: 389-397, (1985).
6. Ledger, W.L., Ellwood, D.A., and Taylor, M.J. Cervical softening in late pregnant sheep by infusion of Prostaglandin E₂ into cervical artery. J. Reprod. Fert. 69, 511-515, (1983).
7. Olson, D.M., Lye, S.J., Skinner, K. and Challis, J.R.G. Early changes in prostaglandin concentrations in ovine maternal and fetal plasma, amniotic fluid and from dispersed cells of intrauterine tissues before the onset of ACTH-induced pre-term labor. J. Reprod. Fert., 71: 45-55, (1984).
8. Caldero-Garcia, R. and Posiero, J. Oxytocin and the contractility of the human uterus, Ann, N. Y. Acad. Sci. 75: 813, (1959).
9. Posiero, J. and Noriega-Guerra, L. Dose-response relationships in uterine effects of oxytocin infusion. Oxytocin. Eds., Caldero-Garcia, R. and Heller, J. Pergamon Press, New York, (1961).
10. Cibils, L. Enhancement of induction of labor. In: Risks in the Practice of Modern Obstetrics. Aldjem, S. Ed. Mosby Publishing, St. Louis, (1972).
11. Bryman, I., Lindblom, B., and Norstrom, A. Extreme sensitivity of cervical musculature to prostaglandin E₂ in early pregnancy. Lancet, 2:1471, (1982).
12. Thiery, M. Induction of labor with prostaglandins. In: Human Parturition. Eds. Keirse, M.J.N.C., Anderson, A.B.M., and Gravenhorst, J.B. Martinus Nijhoff Publ., Boston, 155-164, (1979).
13. Thiery, M. and Amy, J.J. Induction of labor with prostaglandins. In: Advances in Prostaglandin Research. Prostaglandin and Reproduction, Karim, S.M.M., Ed., MTP, Lancaster, Pp. 149-228, (1975).
14. MacLennan, A.H., Katz, M., and Creasey, R. The morphologic characteristics of cervical ripening induced by the hormones relaxin and prostaglandin F₂ in a rabbit model. Am. J. Obstet. Gynecol. 152:910696, (1985).
15. Bishop, E. Elective induction of labor. Obstet & Gynecol, 5: 519-527, (1955).
16. Bishop, E. Pelvic scoring for elective induction. Obstet & Gynecol. 24: 266-268, (1969).
17. Thiery, M. Preinduction cervical ripening. In: Obstetrics and Gynecology Annual, Vol. 12, Ed. Wynn, R. M. Appleton-Century-Crofts, New York, Pp. 103-146, (1983).
18. MacKenzie, I.; Information on File: Controlled Therapeutics (Scotland).
19. De Abajo FJ et al. Labor induction with dinoprostone or oxytocin and postpartum disseminated intravascular coagulation: a hospital-based case-control study. Am J Obs Gynecol, 2004, 191: 1637-1643.

Mfg by:
Controlled Therapeutics
East Kilbride, Scotland, G74 5PB
Made in the U.K.
Distributed by:
FOREST PHARMACEUTICALS, INC.
Subsidiary of Forest Laboratories, Inc.
St. Louis, MO 63045 USA
Rev. 04/10   RMC 226
Shown in Product Identification Guide, page 309

LEXAPRO
[lĕks'ă-prō]
(escitalopram oxalate)
tablet for oral use
LEXAPRO
(escitalopram oxalate)
solution for oral use

HIGHLIGHTS OF PRESCRIBING INFORMATION
These highlights do not include all the information needed to use LEXAPRO safely and effectively. See full prescribing information for LEXAPRO.

LEXAPRO (escitalopram oxalate) tablet for oral use
LEXAPRO (escitalopram oxalate) solution for oral use
Initial U.S. Approval: 2002

> **WARNING:** Suicidality and Antidepressant Drugs
> *See full prescribing information for complete boxed warning.*
> Increased risk of suicidal thinking and behavior in children, adolescents and young adults taking antidepressants for major depressive disorder (MDD) and other psychiatric disorders. Lexapro is not approved for use in pediatric patients less than 12 years of age (5.1).

——RECENT MAJOR CHANGES——
Indication and Usage, Major Depressive Disorder (1.1)	03/2009
Dosage and Administration, Major Depressive Disorder (2.1)	03/2009
Warnings and Precautions, Serotonin Syndrome or Neuroleptic Malignant Syndrome (NMS)-like Reactions (5.2)	01/2009
Warnings and Precaution, Hyponatremia (5.6)	03/2008
Warnings and Precautions, Abnormal Bleeding (5.7)	03/2008

——INDICATIONS AND USAGE——
Lexapro® is a selective serotonin reuptake inhibitor (SSRI) indicated for:
- Acute and Maintenance Treatment of Major Depressive Disorder (MDD) in adults and adolescents aged 12-17 years (1.1)
- Acute Treatment of Generalized Anxiety Disorder (GAD) in adults (1.2)

——DOSAGE AND ADMINISTRATION——
Lexapro should generally be administered once daily, morning or evening with or without food (2.1, 2.2).

Indication	Recommended Dose
MDD (2.1)	
Adolescents (2.1)	Initial: 10 mg once daily Recommended: 10 mg once daily Maximum: 20 mg once daily
Adults (2.1)	Initial: 10 mg once daily Recommended: 10 mg once daily Maximum: 20 mg once daily
GAD (2.2)	
Adults (2.2)	Initial: 10 mg once daily Recommended: 10 mg once daily

- No additional benefits seen at 20 mg/day dose (2.1).
- 10 mg/day is the recommended dose for most elderly patients and patients with hepatic impairment (2.3).
- No dosage adjustment for patients with mild or moderate renal impairment. Use caution in patients with severe renal impairment (2.3).
- Discontinuing Lexapro: A gradual dose reduction is recommended (2.4).

——DOSAGE FORMS AND STRENGTHS——
- Tablets: 5 mg, 10 mg (scored) and 20 mg (scored) (3.1)
- Oral solution: 1 mg per mL (3.2)

——CONTRAINDICATIONS——
- Monoamine Oxidase Inhibitors: Do not use with an MAOI or within 14 days of stopping an MAOI. Allow 14 days after stopping Lexapro before starting an MAOI (4.1, 5.10).
- Pimozide: Do not use concomitantly (4.2, 7.10).
- Known hypersensitivity to escitalopram or citalopram or any of the inactive ingredients (4.3).

——WARNINGS AND PRECAUTIONS——
- Clinical Worsening/Suicide Risk: Monitor for clinical worsening, suicidality and unusual change in behavior, especially during the initial few months of therapy or at times of dose changes (5.1).
- Serotonin Syndrome or Neuroleptic Malignant Syndrome (NMS)-like Reactions: Manage with immediate discontinuation and continuing monitoring (5.2).
- Discontinuation of Treatment with Lexapro: A gradual reduction in dose rather than abrupt cessation is recommended whenever possible (5.3).
- Seizures: Prescribe with care in patients with a history of seizure (5.4).
- Activation of Mania/Hypomania: Use cautiously in patients with a history of mania (5.5).
- Hyponatremia: Can occur in association with SIADH (5.6).
- Abnormal Bleeding: Use caution in concomitant use with NSAIDs, aspirin, warfarin or other drugs that affect coagulation (5.7).

℞

- Interference with Cognitive and Motor Performance: Use caution when operating machinery (5.8).
- Use in Patients with Concomitant Illness: Use caution in patients with diseases or conditions that produce altered metabolism or hemodynamic responses (5.9).

———————ADVERSE REACTIONS———————

Most commonly observed adverse reactions (incidence ≥ 5% and at least twice the incidence of placebo patients) are: insomnia, ejaculation disorder (primarily ejaculatory delay), nausea, sweating increased, fatigue and somnolence, decreased libido, and anorgasmia (6.1).

To report SUSPECTED ADVERSE REACTIONS, contact Forest Laboratories Inc. at 1-800-678-1605, or FDA at 1-800-FDA-1088 or www.fda.gov/medwatch

———————DRUG INTERACTIONS———————

Concomitant use with SSRIs, SNRIs or Tryptophan is not recommended (7.1).
Use caution when concomitant use with drugs that affect Hemostasis (NSAIDs, Aspiring, Warfarin) (7.6).

———USE IN SPECIFIC POPULATIONS———

Pregnancy: Use only if the potential benefit justifies the potential risk to the fetus (8.1).
Nursing Mothers: Caution should be exercised when administered to a nursing woman (8.3)
Pediatric Use: Safety and effectiveness of Lexapro has not been established in pediatric MDD patients less than 12 years of age (8.4).

See 17 for PATIENT COUNSELING INFORMATION and Medication Guide

Revised: 03/2009

FULL PRESCRIBING INFORMATION

WARNINGS: SUICIDALITY AND ANTIDEPRESSANT DRUGS

Antidepressants increased the risk compared to placebo of suicidal thinking and behavior (suicidality) in children, adolescents, and young adults in short-term studies of major depressive disorder (MDD) and other psychiatric disorders. Anyone considering the use of Lexapro or any other antidepressant in a child, adolescent, or young adult must balance this risk with the clinical need. Short-term studies did not show an increase in the risk of suicidality with antidepressants compared to placebo in adults beyond age 24; there was a reduction in risk with antidepressants compared to placebo in adults aged 65 and older. Depression and certain other psychiatric disorders are themselves associated with increases in the risk of suicide. Patients of all ages who are started on antidepressant therapy should be monitored appropriately and observed closely for clinical worsening, suicidality, or unusual changes in behavior. Families and caregivers should be advised of the need for close observation and communication with the prescriber. Lexapro is not approved for use in pediatric patients less than 12 years of age.

[See Warnings and Precautions: Clinical Worsening and Suicide Risk (5.1), Patient Counseling Information: Information for Patients (17.1), and Used in Specific Populations: Pediatric Use (8.4)].

---

1   INDICATIONS AND USAGE

1.1   Major Depressive Disorder

Lexapro (escitalopram) is indicated for the acute and maintenance treatment of major depressive disorder in adults and in adolescents 12 to 17 years of age [see *Clinical Studies* (14.1)].

A major depressive episode (DSM-IV) implies a prominent and relatively persistent (nearly every day for at least 2 weeks) depressed or dysphoric mood that usually interferes with daily functioning, and includes at least five of the following nine symptoms: depressed mood, loss of interest in usual activities, significant change in weight and/or appetite, insomnia or hypersomnia, psychomotor agitation or retardation, increased fatigue, feelings of guilt or worthlessness, slowed thinking or impaired concentration, a suicide attempt or suicidal ideation.

1.2   Generalized Anxiety Disorder

Lexapro is indicated for the acute treatment of Generalized Anxiety Disorder (GAD) in adults [see *Clinical Studies* (14.2)].

Generalized Anxiety Disorder (DSM-IV) is characterized by excessive anxiety and worry (apprehensive expectation) that is persistent for at least 6 months and which the person finds difficult to control. It must be associated with at least 3 of the following symptoms: restlessness or feeling keyed up or on edge, being easily fatigued, difficulty concentrating or mind going blank, irritability, muscle tension, and sleep disturbance.

2   DOSAGE AND ADMINISTRATION

Lexapro should be administered once daily, in the morning or evening, with or without food.

2.1   Major Depressive Disorder
Initial Treatment
Adolescents
The recommended dose of Lexapro is 10 mg once daily. A flexible-dose trial of Lexapro (10 to 20 mg/day) demonstrated the effectiveness of Lexapro [see *Clinical Studies* (14.1)]. If the dose is increased to 20 mg, this should occur after a minimum of three weeks.
Adults
The recommended dose of Lexapro is 10 mg once daily. A fixed-dose trial of Lexapro demonstrated the effectiveness of both 10 mg and 20 mg of Lexapro, but failed to demonstrate a greater benefit of 20 mg over 10 mg [see *Clinical Studies* (14.1)]. If the dose is increased to 20 mg, this should occur after a minimum of one week.
Maintenance Treatment
It is generally agreed that acute episodes of major depressive disorder require several months or longer of sustained pharmacological therapy beyond response to the acute episode. Systematic evaluation of continuing Lexapro 10 or 20 mg/day in adults patients with major depressive disorder who responded while taking Lexapro during an 8-week, acute-treatment phase demonstrated a benefit of such maintenance treatment [see Clinical Studies (14.1)]. Nevertheless, the physician who elects to use Lexapro for extended periods should periodically re-evaluate the long-term usefulness of the drug for the individual patient. Patients should be periodically reassessed to determine the need for maintenance treatment.

2.2   Generalized Anxiety Disorder
Initial Treatment
Adults
The recommended starting dose of Lexapro is 10 mg once daily. If the dose is increased to 20 mg, this should occur after a minimum of one week.
Maintenance Treatment
Generalized anxiety disorder is recognized as a chronic condition. The efficacy of Lexapro in the treatment of GAD beyond 8 weeks has not been systematically studied. The physician who elects to use Lexapro for extended periods should periodically re-evaluate the long-term usefulness of the drug for the individual patient.

2.3   Special Populations
10 mg/day is the recommended dose for most elderly patients and patients with hepatic impairment.
No dosage adjustment is necessary for patients with mild or moderate renal impairment. Lexapro should be used with caution in patients with severe renal impairment.

2.4   Discontinuation of Treatment with Lexapro
Symptoms associated with discontinuation of Lexapro and other SSRIs and SNRIs have been reported [see *Warnings and Precautions (5.3)*]. Patients should be monitored for these symptoms when discontinuing treatment. A gradual reduction in the dose rather than abrupt cessation is recommended whenever possible. If intolerable symptoms occur following a decrease in the dose or upon discontinuation of treatment, then resuming the previously prescribed dose may be considered. Subsequently, the physician may continue decreasing the dose but at a more gradual rate.

2.5   Switching Patients To or From a Monoamine Oxidase Inhibitor
At least 14 days should elapse between discontinuation of an MAOI and initiation of Lexapro therapy. Similarly, at least 14 days should be allowed after stopping Lexapro before starting an MAOI [see *Contraindications (4.1) and Warnings and Precautions (5.10)*].

3   DOSAGE FORMS AND STRENGTHS

3.1   Tablets
Lexapro tablets are film-coated, round tablets containing escitalopram oxalate in strengths equivalent to 5 mg, 10 mg and 20 mg escitalopram base. The 10 and 20 mg tablets are scored. Imprinted with "FL" on one side and either "5", "10", or "20" on the other side according to their respective strengths.
3.2   Oral Solution
Lexapro oral solution contains escitalopram oxalate equivalent to 1 mg/mL escitalopram base.

4   CONTRAINDICATIONS
4.1   Monoamine oxidase inhibitors (MAOIs)
Concomitant use in patients taking monoamine oxidase inhibitors (MAOIs) is contraindicated [see *Warnings and Precautions (5.10)*].
4.2   Pimozide
Concomitant use in patients taking pimozide is contraindicated [see *Drug Interactions (7.10)*].
4.3   Hypersensitivity to escitalopram or citalopram
Lexapro is contraindicated in patients with a hypersensitivity to escitalopram or citalopram or any of the inactive ingredients in Lexapro.

5   WARNINGS AND PRECAUTIONS
5.1   Clinical Worsening and Suicide Risk
Patients with major depressive disorder (MDD), both adult and pediatric, may experience worsening of their depression

and/or the emergence of suicidal ideation and behavior (suicidality) or unusual changes in behavior, whether or not they are taking antidepressant medications, and this risk may persist until significant remission occurs. Suicide is a known risk of depression and certain other psychiatric disorders, and these disorders themselves are the strongest predictors of suicide. There has been a long-standing concern, however, that antidepressants may have a role in inducing worsening of depression and the emergence of suicidality in certain patients during the early phases of treatment. Pooled analyses of short-term placebo-controlled trials of antidepressant drugs (SSRIs and others) showed that these drugs increase the risk of suicidal thinking and behavior (suicidality) in children, adolescents, and young adults (ages 18-24) with major depressive disorder (MDD) and other psychiatric disorders. Short-term studies did not show an increase in the risk of suicidality with antidepressants compared to placebo in adults beyond age 24; there was a reduction with antidepressants compared to placebo in adults aged 65 and older.

The pooled analyses of placebo-controlled trials in children and adolescents with MDD, obsessive compulsive disorder (OCD), or other psychiatric disorders included a total of 24 short-term trials of 9 antidepressant drugs in over 4400 patients. The pooled analyses of placebo-controlled trials in adults with MDD or other psychiatric disorders included a total of 295 short-term trials (median duration of 2 months) of 11 antidepressant drugs in over 77,000 patients. There was considerable variation in risk of suicidality among drugs, but a tendency toward an increase in the younger patients for almost all drugs studied. There were differences in absolute risk of suicidality across the different indications, with the highest incidence in MDD. The risk differences (drug vs. placebo), however, were relatively stable within age strata and across indications. These risk differences (drug-placebo difference in the number of cases of suicidality per 1000 patients treated) are provided in Table 1.

TABLE 1

Age Range	Drug-Placebo Difference in Number of Cases of Suicidality per 1000 Patients Treated
	Increases Compared to Placebo
<18	14 additional cases
18-24	5 additional cases
	Decreases Compared to Placebo
25-64	1 fewer case
≥65	6 fewer cases

No suicides occurred in any of the pediatric trials. There were suicides in the adult trials, but the number was not sufficient to reach any conclusion about drug effect on suicide.

It is unknown whether the suicidality risk extends to longer-term use, i.e., beyond several months. However, there is substantial evidence from placebo-controlled maintenance trials in adults with depression that the use of antidepressants can delay the recurrence of depression.

All patients being treated with antidepressants for any indication should be monitored appropriately and observed closely for clinical worsening, suicidality, and unusual changes in behavior, especially during the initial few months of a course of drug therapy, or at times of dose changes, either increases or decreases.

The following symptoms, anxiety, agitation, panic attacks, insomnia, irritability, hostility, aggressiveness, impulsivity, akathisia (psychomotor restlessness), hypomania, and mania, have been reported in adult and pediatric patients being treated with antidepressants for major depressive disorder as well as for other indications, both psychiatric and nonpsychiatric. Although a causal link between the emergence of such symptoms and either the worsening of depression and/or the emergence of suicidal impulses has not been established, there is concern that such symptoms may represent precursors to emerging suicidality.

Consideration should be given to changing the therapeutic regimen, including possibly discontinuing the medication, in patients whose depression is persistently worse, or who are experiencing emergent suicidality or symptoms that might be precursors to worsening depression or suicidality, especially if these symptoms are severe, abrupt in onset, or were not part of the patient's presenting symptoms.

If the decision has been made to discontinue treatment, medication should be tapered, as rapidly as is feasible, but with recognition that abrupt discontinuation can be associated with certain symptoms [see Dosage and Administration (2.4)].

Families and caregivers of patients being treated with antidepressants for major depressive disorder or other indications, both psychiatric and nonpsychiatric, should be alerted about the need to monitor patients for the emergence of agitation, irritability, unusual changes in behavior, and the other symptoms described above, as well as the emergence of suicidality, and to report such symptoms immediately to health care providers. Such monitoring should include daily observation by families and caregivers [see also Patient Counseling Information (17.1)]. Prescriptions for Lexapro should be written for the smallest quantity of tablets consistent with good patient management, in order to reduce the risk of overdose.

Screening Patients for Bipolar Disorder

A major depressive episode may be the initial presentation of bipolar disorder. It is generally believed (though not established in controlled trials) that treating such an episode with an antidepressant alone may increase the likelihood of precipitation of a mixed/manic episode in patients at risk for bipolar disorder. Whether any of the symptoms described above represent such a conversion is unknown. However, prior to initiating treatment with an antidepressant, patients with depressive symptoms should be adequately screened to determine if they are at risk for bipolar disorder; such screening should include a detailed psychiatric history, including a family history of suicide, bipolar disorder, and depression. It should be noted that Lexapro is not approved for use in treating bipolar depression.

5.2   Serotonin Syndrome or Neuroleptic Malignant Syndrome (NMS)-like Reactions

The development of a potentially life-threatening serotonin syndrome or Neuroleptic Malignant Syndrome (NMS)-like reactions have been reported with SNRIs and SSRIs alone, including Lexapro treatment, but particularly with concomitant use of serotonergic drugs (including triptans) with drugs which impair metabolism of serotonin (including MAOIs), or with antipsychotics or other dopamine antagonists. Serotonin syndrome symptoms may include mental status changes (e.g., agitation, hallucinations, coma), autonomic instability (e.g., tachycardia, labile blood pressure, hyperthermia), neuromuscular aberrations (e.g., hyperreflexia, incoordination) and/or gastrointestinal symptoms (e.g., nausea, vomiting, diarrhea). Serotonin syndrome, in its most severe form can resemble neuroleptic malignant syndrome, which includes hyperthermia, muscle rigidity, autonomic instability with possible rapid fluctuation of vital signs, and mental status changes. Patients should be monitored for the emergence of serotonin syndrome or NMS-like signs and symptoms.

The concomitant use of Lexapro with MAOIs intended to treat depression is contraindicated. If concomitant treatment of Lexapro with a 5-hydroxytryptamine receptor agonist (triptan) is clinically warranted, careful observation of the patient is advised, particularly during treatment initiation and dose increases.

The concomitant use of Lexapro with serotonin precursors (such as tryptophan) is not recommended. Treatment with Lexapro and any concomitant serotonergic or antidopaminergic agents, including antipsychotics, should be discontinued immediately if the above events occur and supportive symptomatic treatment should be initiated.

5.3   Discontinuation of Treatment with Lexapro

During marketing of Lexapro and other SSRIs and SNRIs (serotonin and norepinephrine reuptake inhibitors), there have been spontaneous reports of adverse events occurring upon discontinuation of these drugs, particularly when abrupt, including the following: dysphoric mood, irritability, agitation, dizziness, sensory disturbances (e.g., paresthesias such as electric shock sensations), anxiety, confusion, headache, lethargy, emotional lability, insomnia, and hypomania. While these events are generally self-limiting, there have been reports of serious discontinuation symptoms.

Patients should be monitored for these symptoms when discontinuing treatment with Lexapro. A gradual reduction in the dose rather than abrupt cessation is recommended whenever possible. If intolerable symptoms occur following a decrease in the dose or upon discontinuation of treatment, then resuming the previously prescribed dose may be considered. Subsequently, the physician may continue decreasing the dose but at a more gradual rate [see Dosage and Administration (2.4)].

5.4   Seizures

Although anticonvulsant effects of racemic citalopram have been observed in animal studies, Lexapro has not been systematically evaluated in patients with a seizure disorder. These patients were excluded from clinical studies during the product's premarketing testing. In clinical trials of Lexapro, cases of convulsion have been reported in association with Lexapro treatment. Like other drugs effective in the treatment of major depressive disorder, Lexapro should be introduced with care in patients with a history of seizure disorder.

5.5   Activation of Mania/Hypomania

In placebo-controlled trials of Lexapro in major depressive disorder, activation of mania/hypomania was reported in

one (0.1%) of 715 patients treated with Lexapro and in none of the 592 patients treated with placebo. One additional case of hypomania has been reported in association with Lexapro treatment. Activation of mania/hypomania has also been reported in a small proportion of patients with major affective disorders treated with racemic citalopram and other marketed drugs effective in the treatment of major depressive disorder. As with all drugs effective in the treatment of major depressive disorder, Lexapro should be used cautiously in patients with a history of mania.

5.6   Hyponatremia

Hyponatremia may occur as a result of treatment with SSRIs and SNRIs, including Lexapro. In many cases, this hyponatremia appears to be the result of the syndrome of inappropriate antidiuretic hormone secretion (SIADH), and was reversible when Lexapro was discontinued. Cases with serum sodium lower than 110 mmol/L have been reported. Elderly patients may be at greater risk of developing hyponatremia with SSRIs and SNRIs. Also, patients taking diuretics or who are otherwise volume depleted may be at greater risk [see Geriatric Use (8.5)]. Discontinuation of Lexapro should be considered in patients with symptomatic hyponatremia and appropriate medical intervention should be instituted.

Signs and symptoms of hyponatremia include headache, difficulty concentrating, memory impairment, confusion, weakness, and unsteadiness, which may lead to falls. Signs and symptoms associated with more severe and/or acute cases have included hallucination, syncope, seizure, coma, respiratory arrest, and death.

5.7   Abnormal Bleeding

SSRIs and SNRIs, including Lexapro, may increase the risk of bleeding events. Concomitant use of aspirin, nonsteroidal anti-inflammatory drugs, warfarin, and other anticoagulants may add to the risk. Case reports and epidemiological studies (case-control and cohort design) have demonstrated an association between use of drugs that interfere with serotonin reuptake and the occurrence of gastrointestinal bleeding. Bleeding events related to SSRIs and SNRIs use have ranged from ecchymoses, hematomas, epistaxis, and petechiae to life-threatening hemorrhages.

Patients should be cautioned about the risk of bleeding associated with the concomitant use of Lexapro and NSAIDs, aspirin, or other drugs that affect coagulation.

5.8   Interference with Cognitive and Motor Performance

In a study in normal volunteers, Lexapro 10 mg/day did not produce impairment of intellectual function or psychomotor performance. Because any psychoactive drug may impair judgment, thinking, or motor skills, however, patients should be cautioned about operating hazardous machinery, including automobiles, until they are reasonably certain that Lexapro therapy does not affect their ability to engage in such activities.

5.9   Use in Patients with Concomitant Illness

Clinical experience with Lexapro in patients with certain concomitant systemic illnesses is limited. Caution is advisable in using Lexapro in patients with diseases or conditions that produce altered metabolism or hemodynamic responses.

Lexapro has not been systematically evaluated in patients with a recent history of myocardial infarction or unstable heart disease. Patients with these diagnoses were generally excluded from clinical studies during the product's premarketing testing.

In subjects with hepatic impairment, clearance of racemic citalopram was decreased and plasma concentrations were increased. The recommended dose of Lexapro in hepatically impaired patients is 10 mg/day [see Dosage and Administration (2.3)].

Because escitalopram is extensively metabolized, excretion of unchanged drug in urine is a minor route of elimination. Until adequate numbers of patients with severe renal impairment have been evaluated during chronic treatment with Lexapro, however, it should be used with caution in such patients [see Dosage and Administration (2.3)].

5.10   Potential for Interaction with Monoamine Oxidase Inhibitors

In patients receiving serotonin reuptake inhibitor drugs in combination with a monoamine oxidase inhibitor (MAOI), there have been reports of serious, sometimes fatal, reactions including hyperthermia, rigidity, myoclonus, autonomic instability with possible rapid fluctuations of vital signs, and mental status changes that include extreme agitation progressing to delirium and coma. These reactions have also been reported in patients who have recently discontinued SSRI treatment and have been started on an MAOI. Some cases presented with features resembling neuroleptic malignant syndrome. Furthermore, limited animal data on the effects of combined use of SSRIs and MAOIs suggest that these drugs may act synergistically to elevate blood pressure and evoke behavioral excitation. Therefore, it is recommended that Lexapro should not be used in combination with an MAOI, or within 14 days of discontinuing treatment with an MAOI. Similarly, at least 14 days should be allowed after stopping Lexapro before starting an MAOI. Serotonin syndrome has been reported in two patients who were concomitantly receiving linezolid, an antibiotic which is a reversible non-selective MAOI.

6 ADVERSE REACTIONS

6.1 Clinical Trials Experience

Because clinical studies are conducted under widely varying conditions, adverse reaction rates observed in the clinical studies of a drug cannot be directly compared to rates in the clinical studies of another drug and may not reflect the rates observed in practice.

Clinical Trial Data Sources

Pediatrics (6-17 years)

Adverse events were collected in 576 pediatric patients (286 Lexapro, 290 placebo) with major depressive disorder in double-blind placebo-controlled studies. Safety and effectiveness of Lexapro in pediatric patients less than 12 years of age has not been established.

Adults

Adverse events information for Lexapro was collected from 715 patients with major depressive disorder who were exposed to escitalopram and from 592 patients who were exposed to placebo in double-blind, placebo-controlled trials. An additional 284 patients with major depressive disorder were newly exposed to escitalopram in open-label trials. The adverse event information for Lexapro in patients with GAD was collected from 429 patients exposed to escitalopram and from 427 patients exposed to placebo in double-blind, placebo-controlled trials.

Adverse events during exposure were obtained primarily by general inquiry and recorded by clinical investigators using terminology of their own choosing. Consequently, it is not possible to provide a meaningful estimate of the proportion of individuals experiencing adverse events without first grouping similar types of events into a smaller number of standardized event categories. In the tables and tabulations that follow, standard World Health Organization (WHO) terminology has been used to classify reported adverse events.

The stated frequencies of adverse reactions represent the proportion of individuals who experienced, at least once, a treatment-emergent adverse event of the type listed. An event was considered treatment-emergent if it occurred for the first time or worsened while receiving therapy following baseline evaluation.

Adverse Events Associated with Discontinuation of Treatment

Major Depressive Disorder

Pediatrics (6-17 years)

Adverse events were associated with discontinuation of 3.5% of 286 patients receiving Lexapro and 1% of 290 patients receiving placebo. The most common adverse event (incidence at least 1% for Lexapro and greater than placebo) associated with discontinuation was insomnia (1% Lexapro, 0% placebo).

Adults

Among the 715 depressed patients who received Lexapro in placebo-controlled trials, 6% discontinued treatment due to an adverse event, as compared to 2% of 592 patients receiving placebo. In two fixed-dose studies, the rate of discontinuation for adverse events in patients receiving 10 mg/day Lexapro was not significantly different from the rate of discontinuation for adverse events in patients receiving placebo. The rate of discontinuation for adverse events in patients assigned to a fixed dose of 20 mg/day Lexapro was 10%, which was significantly different from the rate of discontinuation for adverse events in patients receiving 10 mg/day Lexapro (4%) and placebo (3%). Adverse events that were associated with the discontinuation of at least 1% of patients treated with Lexapro, and for which the rate was at least twice that of placebo, were nausea (2%) and ejaculation disorder (2% of male patients).

Generalized Anxiety Disorder

Adults

Among the 429 GAD patients who received Lexapro 10-20 mg/day in placebo-controlled trials, 8% discontinued treatment due to an adverse event, as compared to 4% of 427 patients receiving placebo. Adverse events that were associated with the discontinuation of at least 1% of patients treated with Lexapro, and for which the rate was at least twice the placebo rate, were nausea (2%), insomnia (1%), and fatigue (1%).

Incidence of Adverse Reactions in Placebo-Controlled Clinical Trials

Major Depressive Disorder

Pediatrics (6-17 years)

The overall profile of adverse reactions in pediatric patients was generally similar to that seen in adult studies, as shown in Table 2. However, the following adverse reactions (excluding those which appear in Table 2 and those for which the coded terms were uninformative or misleading)

were reported at an incidence of at least 2% for Lexapro and greater than placebo: back pain, urinary tract infection, vomiting, and nasal congestion.

Adults

The most commonly observed adverse reactions in Lexapro patients (incidence of approximately 5% or greater and approximately twice the incidence in placebo patients) were insomnia, ejaculation disorder (primarily ejaculatory delay), nausea, sweating increased, fatigue, and somnolence.

Table 2 enumerates the incidence, rounded to the nearest percent, of treatment-emergent adverse events that occurred among 715 depressed patients who received Lexapro at doses ranging from 10 to 20 mg/day in placebo-controlled trials. Events included are those occurring in 2% or more of patients treated with Lexapro and for which the incidence in patients treated with Lexapro was greater than the incidence in placebo-treated patients.

TABLE 2 Treatment-Emergent Adverse Reactions observed with a frequency of ≥ 2% and greater than placebo for Major Depressive Disorder

Adverse Reaction	Lexapro	Placebo
	(N=715) %	(N=592) %
Autonomic Nervous System Disorders		
Dry Mouth	6%	5%
Sweating Increased	5%	2%
Central & Peripheral Nervous System Disorders		
Dizziness	5%	3%
Gastrointestinal Disorders		
Nausea	15%	7%
Diarrhea	8%	5%
Constipation	3%	1%
Indigestion	3%	1%
Abdominal Pain	2%	1%
General		
Influenza-like Symptoms	5%	4%
Fatigue	5%	2%
Psychiatric Disorders		
Insomnia	9%	4%
Somnolence	6%	2%
Appetite Decreased	3%	1%
Libido Decreased	3%	1%
Respiratory System Disorders		
Rhinitis	5%	4%
Sinusitis	3%	2%
Urogenital		
Ejaculation Disorder[1,2]	9%	<1%
Impotence[2]	3%	<1%
Anorgasmia[3]	2%	<1%

[1] Primarily ejaculatory delay.
[2] Denominator used was for males only (N=225 Lexapro; N=188 placebo).
[3] Denominator used was for females only (N=490 Lexapro; N=404 placebo).

Generalized Anxiety Disorder

Adults

The most commonly observed adverse reactions in Lexapro patients (incidence of approximately 5% or greater and approximately twice the incidence in placebo patients) were nausea, ejaculation disorder (primarily ejaculatory delay), insomnia, fatigue, decreased libido, and anorgasmia.

Table 3 enumerates the incidence, rounded to the nearest percent of treatment-emergent adverse events that occurred

among 429 GAD patients who received Lexapro 10 to 20 mg/day in placebo-controlled trials. Events included are those occurring in 2% or more of patients treated with Lexapro and for which the incidence in patients treated with Lexapro was greater than the incidence in placebo-treated patients.

TABLE 3 Treatment-Emergent Adverse Reactions observed with a frequency of ≥ 2% and greater than placebo for Generalized Anxiety Disorder

Adverse Reactions	Lexapro	Placebo
	(N=429) %	(N=427) %
Autonomic Nervous System Disorders		
Dry Mouth	9%	5%
Sweating Increased	4%	1%
Central & Peripheral Nervous System Disorders		
Headache	24%	17%
Paresthesia	2%	1%
Gastrointestinal Disorders		
Nausea	18%	8%
Diarrhea	8%	6%
Constipation	5%	4%
Indigestion	3%	2%
Vomiting	3%	1%
Abdominal Pain	2%	1%
Flatulence	2%	1%
Toothache	2%	0%
General		
Fatigue	8%	2%
Influenza-like Symptoms	5%	4%
Musculoskeletal System Disorder		
Neck/Shoulder Pain	3%	1%
Psychiatric Disorders		
Somnolence	13%	7%
Insomnia	12%	6%
Libido Decreased	7%	2%
Dreaming Abnormal	3%	2%
Appetite Decreased	3%	1%
Lethargy	3%	1%
Respiratory System Disorders		
Yawning	2%	1%
Urogenital		
Ejaculation Disorder[1,2]	14%	2%
Anorgasmia[3]	6%	<1%
Menstrual Disorder	2%	1%

[1] Primarily ejaculatory delay.
[2] Denominator used was for males only (N=182 Lexapro; N=195 placebo).
[3] Denominator used was for females only (N=247 Lexapro; N=232 placebo).

Dose Dependency of Adverse Reactions

The potential dose dependency of common adverse reactions (defined as an incidence rate of ≥5% in either the 10 mg or 20 mg Lexapro groups) was examined on the basis of the combined incidence of adverse reactions in two fixed-dose trials. The overall incidence rates of adverse events in

10 mg Lexapro-treated patients (66%) was similar to that of the placebo-treated patients (61%), while the incidence rate in 20 mg/day Lexapro-treated patients was greater (86%). Table 4 shows common adverse reactions that occurred in the 20 mg/day Lexapro group with an incidence that was approximately twice that of the 10 mg/day Lexapro group and approximately twice that of the placebo group.

TABLE 4 Incidence of Common Adverse Reactions in Patients with Major Depressive Disorder

Adverse Reaction	Placebo	10 mg/day	20 mg/day
	(N=311)	Lexapro	Lexapro
		(N=310)	(N=125)
Insomnia	4%	7%	14%
Diarrhea	5%	6%	14%
Dry Mouth	3%	4%	9%
Somnolence	1%	4%	9%
Dizziness	2%	4%	7%
Sweating Increased	<1%	3%	8%
Constipation	1%	3%	6%
Fatigue	2%	2%	6%
Indigestion	1%	2%	6%

Male and Female Sexual Dysfunction with SSRIs
Although changes in sexual desire, sexual performance, and sexual satisfaction often occur as manifestations of a psychiatric disorder, they may also be a consequence of pharmacologic treatment. In particular, some evidence suggests that SSRIs can cause such untoward sexual experiences.
Reliable estimates of the incidence and severity of untoward experiences involving sexual desire, performance, and satisfaction are difficult to obtain, however, in part because patients and physicians may be reluctant to discuss them. Accordingly, estimates of the incidence of untoward sexual experience and performance cited in product labeling are likely to underestimate their actual incidence.

TABLE 5 Incidence of Sexual Side Effects in Placebo-Controlled Clinical Trials

Adverse Event	Lexapro	Placebo
	In Males Only	
	(N=407)	(N=383)
Ejaculation Disorder (primarily ejaculatory delay)	12%	1%
Libido Decreased	6%	2%
Impotence	2%	<1%
	In Females Only	
	(N=737)	(N=636)
Libido Decreased	3%	1%
Anorgasmia	3%	<1%

There are no adequately designed studies examining sexual dysfunction with escitalopram treatment.
Priapism has been reported with all SSRIs.
While it is difficult to know the precise risk of sexual dysfunction associated with the use of SSRIs, physicians should routinely inquire about such possible side effects.
Vital Sign Changes
Lexapro and placebo groups were compared with respect to (1) mean change from baseline in vital signs (pulse, systolic blood pressure, and diastolic blood pressure) and (2) the incidence of patients meeting criteria for potentially clinically significant changes from baseline in these variables. These analyses did not reveal any clinically important changes in vital signs associated with Lexapro treatment. In addition, a comparison of supine and standing vital sign measures in subjects receiving Lexapro indicated that Lexapro treatment is not associated with orthostatic changes.

Weight Changes
Patients treated with Lexapro in controlled trials did not differ from placebo-treated patients with regard to clinically important change in body weight.
Laboratory Changes
Lexapro and placebo groups were compared with respect to (1) mean change from baseline in various serum chemistry, hematology, and urinalysis variables, and (2) the incidence of patients meeting criteria for potentially clinically significant changes from baseline in these variables. These analyses revealed no clinically important changes in laboratory test parameters associated with Lexapro treatment.
ECG Changes
Electrocardiograms from Lexapro (N=625), racemic citalopram (N=351), and placebo (N=527) groups were compared with respect to (1) mean change from baseline in various ECG parameters and (2) the incidence of patients meeting criteria for potentially clinically significant changes from baseline in these variables. These analyses revealed (1) a decrease in heart rate of 2.2 bpm for Lexapro and 2.7 bpm for racemic citalopram, compared to an increase of 0.3 bpm for placebo and (2) an increase in QTc interval of 3.9 msec for Lexapro and 3.7 msec for racemic citalopram, compared to 0.5 msec for placebo. Neither Lexapro nor racemic citalopram were associated with the development of clinically significant ECG abnormalities.
Other Reactions Observed During the Premarketing Evaluation of Lexapro
Following is a list of treatment-emergent adverse events, as defined in the introduction to the **ADVERSE REACTIONS** section, reported by the 1428 patients treated with Lexapro for periods of up to one year in double-blind or open-label clinical trials during its premarketing evaluation. The listing does not include those events already listed in **Tables 2 & 3**, those events for which a drug cause was remote and at a rate less than 1% or lower than placebo, those events which were so general as to be uninformative, and those events reported only once which did not have a substantial probability of being acutely life threatening. Events are categorized by body system. Events of major clinical importance are described in the Warnings and Precautions section (5).
Cardiovascular—hypertension, palpitation.
Central and Peripheral Nervous System Disorders—light-headed feeling, migraine.
Gastrointestinal Disorders—abdominal cramp, heartburn, gastroenteritis.
General—allergy, chest pain, fever, hot flushes, pain in limb.
Metabolic and Nutritional Disorders—increased weight.
Musculoskeletal System Disorders—arthralgia, myalgia jaw stiffness.
Psychiatric Disorders—appetite increased, concentration impaired, irritability.
Reproductive Disorders/Female—menstrual cramps, menstrual disorder.
Respiratory System Disorders—bronchitis, coughing, nasal congestion, sinus congestion, sinus headache.
Skin and Appendages Disorders—rash.
Special Senses—vision blurred, tinnitus.
Urinary System Disorders—urinary frequency, urinary tract infection.
6.2   Post-Marketing Experience
Adverse Reactions Reported Subsequent to the Marketing of Escitalopram
The following additional adverse reactions have been identified from spontaneous reports of escitalopram received worldwide. These adverse reactions have been chosen for inclusion because of a combination of seriousness, frequency of reporting, or potential causal connection to escitalopram and have not been listed elsewhere in labeling. However, because these adverse reactions were reported voluntarily from a population of uncertain size, it is not always possible to reliably estimate their frequency or establish a causal relationship to drug exposure. These events include:
Blood and Lymphatic System Disorders: anemia, agranulocytis, aplastic anemia, hemolytic anemia, idiopathic thrombocytopenia purpura, leukopenia, thrombocytopenia.
Cardiac Disorders: atrial fibrillation, bradycardia, cardiac failure, myocardial infarction, tachycardia, torsade de pointes, ventricular arrhythmia, ventricular tachycardia.
Ear and labyrinth disorders: vertigo
Endocrine Disorders: diabetes mellitus, hyperprolactinemia, SIADH.
Eye Disorders: diplopia, glaucoma, mydriasis, visual disturbance.
Gastrointestinal Disorder: dysphagia, gastrointestinal hemorrhage, gastroesophageal reflux, pancreatitis, rectal hemorrhage.
General Disorders and Administration Site Conditions: abnormal gait, asthenia, edema, fall, feeling abnormal, malaise.
Hepatobiliary Disorders: fulminant hepatitis, hepatic failure, hepatic necrosis, hepatitis.

Immune System Disorders: allergic reaction, anaphylaxis.
Investigations: bilirubin increased, decreased weight, electrocardiogram QT prolongation, hepatic enzymes increased, hypercholesterolemia, INR increased, prothrombin decreased.
Metabolism and Nutrition Disorders: hyperglycemia, hypoglycemia, hypokalemia, hyponatremia.
Musculoskeletal and Connective Tissue Disorders: muscle cramp, muscle stiffness, muscle weakness, rhabdomyolysis.
Nervous System Disorders: akathisia, amnesia, ataxia, choreoathetosis, cerebrovascular accident, dysarthria, dyskinesia, dystonia, extrapyramidal disorders, grand mal seizures (or convulsions), hypoaesthesia, myoclonus, nystagmus, Parkinsonism, restless legs, seizures, syncope, tardive dyskinesia, tremor.
Pregnancy, Puerperium and Perinatal Conditions: spontaneous abortion.
Psychiatric Disorders: acute psychosis, aggression, agitation, anger, anxiety, apathy, completed suicide, confusion, depersonalization, depression aggravated, delirium, delusion, disorientation, feeling unreal, hallucinations (visual and auditory), mood swings, nervousness, nightmare, panic reaction, paranoia, restlessness, self-harm or thoughts of self-harm, suicide attempt, suicidal ideation, suicidal tendency.
Renal and Urinary Disorders: acute renal failure, dysuria, urinary retention.
Reproductive System and Breast Disorders: menorrhagia, priapism.
Respiratory, Thoracic and Mediastinal Disorders: dyspnea, epistaxis, pulmonary embolism, pulmonary hypertension of the newborn.
Skin and Subcutaneous Tissue Disorders: alopecia, angioedema, dermatitis, ecchymosis, erythema multiforme, photosensitivity reaction, Stevens Johnson Syndrome, toxic epidermal necrolysis, urticaria.
Vascular Disorders: deep vein thrombosis, flushing, hypertensive crisis, hypotension, orthostatic hypotension, phlebitis, thrombosis.

7   DRUG INTERACTIONS
7.1   Serotonergic Drugs
Based on the mechanism of action of SNRIs and SSRIs including Lexapro, and the potential for serotonin syndrome, caution is advised when Lexapro is coadministered with other drugs that may affect the serotonergic neurotransmitter systems, such as triptans, linezolid (an antibiotic which is a reversible non-selective MAOI), lithium, tramadol, or St. John's Wort [see Warnings and Precautions (5.2)]. The concomitant use of Lexapro with other SSRIs, SNRIs or tryptophan is not recommended.
7.2   Triptans
There have been rare postmarketing reports of serotonin syndrome with use of an SSRI and a triptan. If concomitant treatment of Lexapro with a triptan is clinically warranted, careful observation of the patient is advised, particularly during treatment initiation and dose increases [see Warnings and Precautions (5.2)].
7.3   CNS Drugs
Given the primary CNS effects of escitalopram, caution should be used when it is taken in combination with other centrally acting drugs.
7.4   Alcohol
Although Lexapro did not potentiate the cognitive and motor effects of alcohol in a clinical trial, as with other psychotropic medications, the use of alcohol by patients taking Lexapro is not recommended.
7.5   Monoamine Oxidase Inhibitors (MAOIs)
[see Contraindications (4.1) and Warnings and Precautions (5.10)].
7.6   Drugs That Interfere With Hemostasis (NSAIDs, Aspirin, Warfarin, etc.)
Serotonin release by platelets plays an important role in hemostasis. Epidemiological studies of the case-control and cohort design that have demonstrated an association between use of psychotropic drugs that interfere with serotonin reuptake and the occurrence of upper gastrointestinal bleeding have also shown that concurrent use of an NSAID or aspirin may potentiate the risk of bleeding. Altered anticoagulant effects, including increased bleeding, have been reported when SSRIs and SNRIs are coadministered with warfarin. Patients receiving warfarin therapy should be carefully monitored when Lexapro is initiated or discontinued.
7.7   Cimetidine
In subjects who had received 21 days of 40 mg/day racemic citalopram, combined administration of 400 mg/day cimetidine for 8 days resulted in an increase in citalopram AUC and C_{max} of 43% and 39%, respectively. The clinical significance of these findings is unknown.
7.8   Digoxin
In subjects who had received 21 days of 40 mg/day racemic citalopram, combined administration of citalopram and digoxin (single dose of 1 mg) did not significantly affect the pharmacokinetics of either citalopram or digoxin.

7.9 Lithium

Coadministration of racemic citalopram (40 mg/day for 10 days) and lithium (30 mmol/day for 5 days) had no significant effect on the pharmacokinetics of citalopram or lithium. Nevertheless, plasma lithium levels should be monitored with appropriate adjustment to the lithium dose in accordance with standard clinical practice. Because lithium may enhance the serotonergic effects of escitalopram, caution should be exercised when Lexapro and lithium are coadministered.

7.10 Pimozide and Celexa

In a controlled study, a single dose of pimozide 2 mg co-administered with racemic citalopram 40 mg given once daily for 11 days was associated with a mean increase in QTc values of approximately 10 msec compared to pimozide given alone. Racemic citalopram did not alter the mean AUC or C_{max} of pimozide. The mechanism of this pharmacodynamic interaction is not known.

7.11 Sumatriptan

There have been rare postmarketing reports describing patients with weakness, hyperreflexia, and incoordination following the use of an SSRI and sumatriptan. If concomitant treatment with sumatriptan and an SSRI (e.g., fluoxetine, fluvoxamine, paroxetine, sertraline, citalopram, escitalopram) is clinically warranted, appropriate observation of the patient is advised.

7.12 Theophylline

Combined administration of racemic citalopram (40 mg/day for 21 days) and the CYP1A2 substrate theophylline (single dose of 300 mg) did not affect the pharmacokinetics of theophylline. The effect of theophylline on the pharmacokinetics of citalopram was not evaluated.

7.13 Warfarin

Administration of 40 mg/day racemic citalopram for 21 days did not affect the pharmacokinetics of warfarin, a CYP3A4 substrate. Prothrombin time was increased by 5%, the clinical significance of which is unknown.

7.14 Carbamazepine

Combined administration of racemic citalopram (40 mg/day for 14 days) and carbamazepine (titrated to 400 mg/day for 35 days) did not significantly affect the pharmacokinetics of carbamazepine, a CYP3A4 substrate. Although trough citalopram plasma levels were unaffected, given the enzyme-inducing properties of carbamazepine, the possibility that carbamazepine might increase the clearance of escitalopram should be considered if the two drugs are coadministered.

7.15 Triazolam

Combined administration of racemic citalopram (titrated to 40 mg/day for 28 days) and the CYP3A4 substrate triazolam (single dose of 0.25 mg) did not significantly affect the pharmacokinetics of either citalopram or triazolam.

7.16 Ketoconazole

Combined administration of racemic citalopram (40 mg) and ketoconazole (200 mg), a potent CYP3A4 inhibitor, decreased the C_{max} and AUC of ketoconazole by 21% and 10%, respectively, and did not significantly affect the pharmacokinetics of citalopram.

7.17 Ritonavir

Combined administration of a single dose of ritonavir (600 mg), both a CYP3A4 substrate and a potent inhibitor of CYP3A4, and escitalopram (20 mg) did not affect the pharmacokinetics of either ritonavir or escitalopram.

7.18 CYP3A4 and -2C19 Inhibitors

In vitro studies indicated that CYP3A4 and -2C19 are the primary enzymes involved in the metabolism of escitalopram. However, coadministration of escitalopram (20 mg) and ritonavir (600 mg), a potent inhibitor of CYP3A4, did not significantly affect the pharmacokinetics of escitalopram. Because escitalopram is metabolized by multiple enzyme systems, inhibition of a single enzyme may not appreciably decrease escitalopram clearance.

7.19 Drugs Metabolized by Cytochrome P4502D6

In vitro studies did not reveal an inhibitory effect of escitalopram on CYP2D6. In addition, steady state levels of racemic citalopram were not significantly different in poor metabolizers and extensive CYP2D6 metabolizers after multiple-dose administration of citalopram, suggesting that coadministration, with escitalopram, of a drug that inhibits CYP2D6, is unlikely to have clinically significant effects on escitalopram metabolism. However, there are limited in vivo data suggesting a modest CYP2D6 inhibitory effect for escitalopram, i.e., coadministration of escitalopram (20 mg/day for 21 days) with the tricyclic antidepressant desipramine (single dose of 50 mg), a substrate for CYP2D6, resulted in a 40% increase in C_{max} and a 100% increase in AUC of desipramine. The clinical significance of this finding is unknown. Nevertheless, caution is indicated in the coadministration of escitalopram and drugs metabolized by CYP2D6.

7.20 Metoprolol

Administration of 20 mg/day Lexapro for 21 days in healthy volunteers resulted in a 50% increase in C_{max} and 82% increase in AUC of the beta-adrenergic blocker metoprolol (given in a single dose of 100 mg). Increased metoprolol plasma levels have been associated with decreased cardioselectivity. Coadministration of Lexapro and metoprolol had no clinically significant effects on blood pressure or heart rate.

7.21 Electroconvulsive Therapy (ECT)

There are no clinical studies of the combined use of ECT and escitalopram.

8 USE IN SPECIFIC POPULATIONS

8.1 Pregnancy

Pregnancy Category C

In a rat embryo/fetal development study, oral administration of escitalopram (56, 112, or 150 mg/kg/day) to pregnant animals during the period of organogenesis resulted in decreased fetal body weight and associated delays in ossification at the two higher doses (approximately $\geq$ 56 times the maximum recommended human dose [MRHD] of 20 mg/day on a body surface area [mg/m^2] basis). Maternal toxicity (clinical signs and decreased body weight gain and food consumption), mild at 56 mg/kg/day, was present at all dose levels. The developmental no-effect dose of 56 mg/kg/day is approximately 28 times the MRHD on a mg/m^2 basis. No teratogenicity was observed at any of the doses tested (as high as 75 times the MRHD on a mg/m^2 basis).

When female rats were treated with escitalopram (6, 12, 24, or 48 mg/kg/day) during pregnancy and through weaning, slightly increased offspring mortality and growth retardation were noted at 48 mg/kg/day which is approximately 24 times the MRHD on a mg/m^2 basis. Slight maternal toxicity (clinical signs and decreased body weight gain and food consumption) was seen at this dose. Slightly increased offspring mortality was also seen at 24 mg/kg/day. The no-effect dose was 12 mg/kg/day which is approximately 6 times the MRHD on a mg/m^2 basis.

In animal reproduction studies, racemic citalopram has been shown to have adverse effects on embryo/fetal and postnatal development, including teratogenic effects, when administered at doses greater than human therapeutic doses.

In two rat embryo/fetal development studies, oral administration of racemic citalopram (32, 56, or 112 mg/kg/day) to pregnant animals during the period of organogenesis resulted in decreased embryo/fetal growth and survival and an increased incidence of fetal abnormalities (including cardiovascular and skeletal defects) at the high dose. This dose was also associated with maternal toxicity (clinical signs, decreased body weight gain). The developmental no-effect dose was 56 mg/kg/day. In a rabbit study, no adverse effects on embryo/fetal development were observed at doses of racemic citalopram of up to 16 mg/kg/day. Thus, teratogenic effects of racemic citalopram were observed at a maternally toxic dose in the rat and were not observed in the rabbit.

When female rats were treated with racemic citalopram (4.8, 12.8, or 32 mg/kg/day) from late gestation through weaning, increased offspring mortality during the first 4 days after birth and persistent offspring growth retardation were observed at the highest dose. The no-effect dose was 12.8 mg/kg/day. Similar effects on offspring mortality and growth were seen when dams were treated throughout gestation and early lactation at doses $\geq$ 24 mg/kg/day. A no-effect dose was not determined in that study.

There are no adequate and well-controlled studies in pregnant women; therefore, escitalopram should be used during pregnancy only if the potential benefit justifies the potential risk to the fetus.

Pregnancy-Nonteratogenic Effects

Neonates exposed to Lexapro and other SSRIs or SNRIs, late in the third trimester, have developed complications requiring prolonged hospitalization, respiratory support, and tube feeding. Such complications can arise immediately upon delivery. Reported clinical findings have included respiratory distress, cyanosis, apnea, seizures, temperature instability, feeding difficulty, vomiting, hypoglycemia, hypotonia, hypertonia, hyperreflexia, tremor, jitteriness, irritability, and constant crying. These features are consistent with either a direct toxic effect of SSRIs and SNRIs or, possibly, a drug discontinuation syndrome. It should be noted that, in some cases, the clinical picture is consistent with serotonin syndrome [see Warnings and Precautions (5.2)].

Infants exposed to SSRIs in late pregnancy may have an increased risk for persistent pulmonary hypertension of the newborn (PPHN). PPHN occurs in 1—2 per 1000 live births in the general population and is associated with substantial neonatal morbidity and mortality. In a retrospective, case-control study of 377 women whose infants were born with PPHN and 836 women whose infants were born healthy, the risk for developing PPHN was approximately six-fold higher for infants exposed to SSRIs after the 20th week of gestation compared to infants who had not been exposed to antidepressants during pregnancy. There is currently no corroborative evidence regarding the risk for PPHN following exposure to SSRIs in pregnancy; this is the first study that has investigated the potential risk. The study did not include enough cases with exposure to individual SSRIs to determine if all SSRIs posed similar levels of PPHN risk. When treating a pregnant woman with Lexapro during the third trimester, the physician should carefully consider both the potential risks and benefits of treatment [see Dosage and Administration (2.1)]. Physicians should note that in a prospective longitudinal study of 201 women with a history of major depression who were euthymic at the beginning of pregnancy, women who discontinued antidepressant medication during pregnancy were more likely to experience a relapse of major depression than women who continued antidepressant medication.

8.2 Labor and Delivery

The effect of Lexapro on labor and delivery in humans is unknown.

8.3 Nursing Mothers

Escitalopram is excreted in human breast milk. Limited data from women taking 10-20 mg escitalopram showed that exclusively breast-fed infants receive approximately 3.9% of the maternal weight-adjusted dose of escitalopram and 1.7% of the maternal weight-adjusted dose of desmethylcitalopram. There were two reports of infants experiencing excessive somnolence, decreased feeding, and weight loss in association with breastfeeding from a racemic citalopram-treated mother; in one case, the infant was reported to recover completely upon discontinuation of racemic citalopram by its mother and, in the second case, no follow-up information was available. Caution should be exercised and breastfeeding infants should be observed for adverse reactions when Lexapro is administered to a nursing woman.

8.4 Pediatric Use

Safety and effectiveness of Lexapro has not been established in pediatric patients (less than 12 years of age) with Major Depressive Disorder. Safety and effectiveness of Lexapro has been established in adolescents (12 to 17 years of age) for the treatment of major depressive disorder [see Clinical Studies (14.1)]. Although maintenance efficacy in adolescent patients with Major Depressive Disorder has not been systematically evaluated, maintenance efficacy can be extrapolated from adult data along with comparisons of escitalopram pharmacokinetic parameters in adults and adolescent patients.

Safety and effectiveness of Lexapro has not been established in pediatric patients less than 18 years of age with Generalized Anxiety Disorder.

8.5 Geriatric Use

Approximately 6% of the 1144 patients receiving escitalopram in controlled trials of Lexapro in major depressive disorder and GAD were 60 years of age or older; elderly patients in these trials received daily doses of Lexapro between 10 and 20 mg. The number of elderly patients in these trials was insufficient to adequately assess for possible differential efficacy and safety measures on the basis of age. Nevertheless, greater sensitivity of some elderly individuals to effects of Lexapro cannot be ruled out.

SSRIs and SNRIs, including Lexapro, have been associated with cases of clinically significant hyponatremia in elderly patients, who may be at greater risk for this adverse event [see Hyponatremia (5.6)].

In two pharmacokinetic studies, escitalopram half-life was increased by approximately 50% in elderly subjects as compared to young subjects and C_{max} was unchanged [see Clinical Pharmacology (12.3)]. 10 mg/day is the recommended dose for elderly patients [see Dosage and Administration (2.3)].

Of 4422 patients in clinical studies of racemic citalopram, 1357 were 60 and over, 1034 were 65 and over, and 457 were 75 and over. No overall differences in safety or effectiveness were observed between these subjects and younger subjects, and other reported clinical experience has not identified differences in responses between the elderly and younger patients, but again, greater sensitivity of some elderly individuals cannot be ruled out.

9 DRUG ABUSE AND DEPENDENCE

9.2 Abuse and Dependence

Physical and Psychological Dependence

Animal studies suggest that the abuse liability of racemic citalopram is low. Lexapro has not been systematically studied in humans for its potential for abuse, tolerance, or physical dependence. The premarketing clinical experience with Lexapro did not reveal any drug-seeking behavior. However, these observations were not systematic and it is not possible to predict on the basis of this limited experience the extent to which a CNS-active drug will be misused, diverted, and/or abused once marketed. Consequently, physicians should carefully evaluate Lexapro patients for history of drug abuse and follow such patients closely, observing them for signs of misuse or abuse (e.g., development of tolerance, incrementations of dose, drug-seeking behavior).

10 OVERDOSAGE

10.1 Human Experience

In clinical trials of escitalopram, there were reports of escitalopram overdose, including overdoses of up to 600 mg, with no associated fatalities. During the postmarketing evaluation of escitalopram, Lexapro overdoses involving overdoses of over 1000 mg have been reported. As with other SSRIs, a fatal outcome in a patient who has taken an overdose of escitalopram has been rarely reported.

Symptoms most often accompanying escitalopram overdose, alone or in combination with other drugs and/or alcohol, included convulsions, coma, dizziness, hypotension, insomnia, nausea, vomiting, sinus tachycardia, somnolence, and ECG changes (including QT prolongation and very rare cases of torsade de pointes). Acute renal failure has been very rarely reported accompanying overdose.

10.2 Management of Overdose

Establish and maintain an airway to ensure adequate ventilation and oxygenation. Gastric evacuation by lavage and use of activated charcoal should be considered. Careful observation and cardiac and vital sign monitoring are recommended, along with general symptomatic and supportive care. Due to the large volume of distribution of escitalopram, forced diuresis, dialysis, hemoperfusion, and exchange transfusion are unlikely to be of benefit. There are no specific antidotes for Lexapro.

In managing overdosage, consider the possibility of multiple-drug involvement. The physician should consider contacting a poison control center for additional information on the treatment of any overdose.

11 DESCRIPTION

Lexapro® (escitalopram oxalate) is an orally administered selective serotonin reuptake inhibitor (SSRI). Escitalopram is the pure S-enantiomer (single isomer) of the racemic bicyclic phthalane derivative citalopram. Escitalopram oxalate is designated S-(+)-1-[3-(dimethyl-amino)propyl]-1-(*p*-fluorophenyl)-5-phthalancarbonitrile oxalate with the following structural formula:

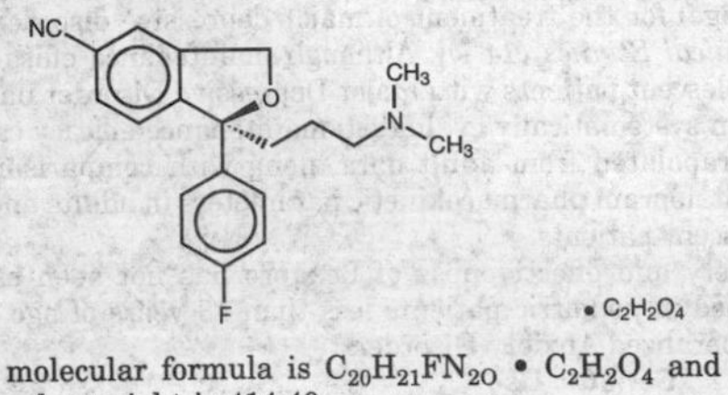

The molecular formula is $C_{20}H_{21}FN_{2O}$ • $C_2H_2O_4$ and the molecular weight is 414.40.

Escitalopram oxalate occurs as a fine, white to slightly-yellow powder and is freely soluble in methanol and dimethyl sulfoxide (DMSO), soluble in isotonic saline solution, sparingly soluble in water and ethanol, slightly soluble in ethyl acetate, and insoluble in heptane.

Lexapro (escitalopram oxalate) is available as tablets or as an oral solution.

Lexapro tablets are film-coated, round tablets containing escitalopram oxalate in strengths equivalent to 5 mg, 10 mg, and 20 mg escitalopram base. The 10 and 20 mg tablets are scored. The tablets also contain the following inactive ingredients: talc, croscarmellose sodium, microcrystalline cellulose/colloidal silicon dioxide, and magnesium stearate. The film coating contains hypromellose, titanium dioxide, and polyethylene glycol.

Lexapro oral solution contains escitalopram oxalate equivalent to 1 mg/mL escitalopram base. It also contains the following inactive ingredients: sorbitol, purified water, citric acid, sodium citrate, malic acid, glycerin, propylene glycol, methylparaben, propylparaben, and natural peppermint flavor.

12 CLINICAL PHARMACOLOGY

12.1 Mechanism of Action

The mechanism of antidepressant action of escitalopram, the S-enantiomer of racemic citalopram, is presumed to be linked to potentiation of serotonergic activity in the central nervous system (CNS) resulting from its inhibition of CNS neuronal reuptake of serotonin (5-HT).

12.2 Pharmacodynamics

In vitro and *in vivo* studies in animals suggest that escitalopram is a highly selective serotonin reuptake inhibitor (SSRI) with minimal effects on norepinephrine and dopamine neuronal reuptake. Escitalopram is at least 100-fold more potent than the R-enantiomer with respect to inhibition of 5-HT reuptake and inhibition of 5-HT neuronal firing rate. Tolerance to a model of antidepressant effect in rats was not induced by long-term (up to 5 weeks) treatment with escitalopram. Escitalopram has no or very low affinity for serotonergic ($5\text{-}HT_{1\text{-}7}$) or other receptors including alpha- and beta-adrenergic, dopamine ($D_{1\text{-}5}$), histamine ($H_{1\text{-}3}$), muscarinic ($M_{1\text{-}5}$), and benzodiazepine receptors. Escitalopram also does not bind to, or has low affinity for, various ion channels including Na^+, K^+, Cl^-, and Ca^{++} channels. Antagonism of muscarinic, histaminergic, and adrenergic receptors has been hypothesized to be associated with various anticholinergic, sedative, and cardiovascular side effects of other psychotropic drugs.

12.3 Pharmacokinetics

The single- and multiple-dose pharmacokinetics of escitalopram are linear and dose-proportional in a dose range of 10 to 30 mg/day. Biotransformation of escitalopram is mainly hepatic, with a mean terminal half-life of about 27-32 hours. With once-daily dosing, steady state plasma concentrations are achieved within approximately one week. At steady state, the extent of accumulation of escitalopram in plasma in young healthy subjects was 2.2-2.5 times the plasma concentrations observed after a single dose. The tablet and the oral solution dosage forms of escitalopram oxalate are bioequivalent.

Absorption and Distribution

Following a single oral dose (20 mg tablet or solution) of escitalopram, peak blood levels occur at about 5 hours. Absorption of escitalopram is not affected by food.

The absolute bioavailability of citalopram is about 80% relative to an intravenous dose, and the volume of distribution of citalopram is about 12 L/kg. Data specific on escitalopram are unavailable.

The binding of escitalopram to human plasma proteins is approximately 56%.

Metabolism and Elimination

Following oral administrations of escitalopram, the fraction of drug recovered in the urine as escitalopram and S-demethylcitalopram (S-DCT) is about 8% and 10%, respectively. The oral clearance of escitalopram is 600 mL/min, with approximately 7% of that due to renal clearance.

Escitalopram is metabolized to S-DCT and S-didemethylcitalopram (S-DDCT). In humans, unchanged escitalopram is the predominant compound in plasma. At steady state, the concentration of the escitalopram metabolite S-DCT in plasma is approximately one-third that of escitalopram. The level of S-DDCT was not detectable in most subjects. *In vitro* studies show that escitalopram is at least 7 and 27 times more potent than S-DCT and S-DDCT, respectively, in the inhibition of serotonin reuptake, suggesting that the metabolites of escitalopram do not contribute significantly to the antidepressant actions of escitalopram. S-DCT and S-DDCT also have no or very low affinity for serotonergic ($5\text{-}HT_{1\text{-}7}$) or other receptors including alpha- and beta-adrenergic, dopamine ($D_{1\text{-}5}$), histamine ($H_{1\text{-}3}$), muscarinic ($M_{1\text{-}5}$), and benzodiazepine receptors. S-DCT and S-DDCT also do not bind to various ion channels including Na^+, K^+, Cl^-, and Ca^{++} channels.

In vitro studies using human liver microsomes indicated that CYP3A4 and CYP2C19 are the primary isozymes involved in the N-demethylation of escitalopram.

Population Subgroups

Age

Adolescents—In a single dose study of 10 mg escitalopram, AUC of escitalopram decreased by 19%, and C_{max} increased by 26% in healthy adolescent subjects (12 to 17 years of age) compared to adults. Following multiple dosing of 40 mg/day citalopram, escitalopram elimination half-life, steady-state C_{max} and AUC were similar in patients with MDD (12 to 17 years of age) compared to adult patients. No adjustment of dosage is needed in adolescent patients.

Elderly—Escitalopram pharmacokinetics in subjects ≥ 65 years of age were compared to younger subjects in a single-dose and a multiple-dose study. Escitalopram AUC and half-life were increased by approximately 50% in elderly subjects, and C_{max} was unchanged. 10 mg is the recommended dose for elderly patients [*see Dosage and Administration (2.3)*].

Gender—Based on data from single- and multiple-dose studies measuring escitalopram in elderly, young adults, and adolescents, no dosage adjustment on the basis of gender is needed.

Reduced hepatic function—Citalopram oral clearance was reduced by 37% and half-life was doubled in patients with reduced hepatic function compared to normal subjects. 10 mg is the recommended dose of escitalopram for most hepatically impaired patients [*see Dosage and Administration (2.3)*].

Reduced renal function—In patients with mild to moderate renal function impairment, oral clearance of citalopram was reduced by 17% compared to normal subjects. No adjustment of dosage for such patients is recommended. No information is available about the pharmacokinetics of escitalopram in patients with severely reduced renal function (creatinine clearance < 20 mL/min).

Drug-Drug Interactions

In vitro enzyme inhibition data did not reveal an inhibitory effect of escitalopram on CYP3A4, -1A2, -2C9, -2C19, and -2E1. Based on *in vitro* data, escitalopram would be expected to have little inhibitory effect on *in vivo* metabolism mediated by these cytochromes. While *in vivo* data to address this question are limited, results from drug interaction studies suggest that escitalopram, at a dose of 20 mg, has no 3A4 inhibitory effect and a modest 2D6 inhibitory effect. See *Drug Interactions (7.18)* for more detailed information on available drug interaction data.

13 NONCLINICAL TOXICOLOGY

13.1 Carcinogenesis, Mutagenesis, Impairment of Fertility

Carcinogenesis

Racemic citalopram was administered in the diet to NMRI/BOM strain mice and COBS WI strain rats for 18 and 24 months, respectively. There was no evidence for carcinogenicity of racemic citalopram in mice receiving up to 240 mg/kg/day. There was an increased incidence of small intestine carcinoma in rats receiving 8 or 24 mg/kg/day racemic citalopram. A no-effect dose for this finding was not established. The relevance of these findings to humans is unknown.

Mutagenesis

Racemic citalopram was mutagenic in the *in vitro* bacterial reverse mutation assay (Ames test) in 2 of 5 bacterial strains (Salmonella TA98 and TA1537) in the absence of metabolic activation. It was clastogenic in the *in vitro* Chinese hamster lung cell assay for chromosomal aberrations in the presence and absence of metabolic activation. Racemic citalopram was not mutagenic in the *in vitro* mammalian forward gene mutation assay (HPRT) in mouse lymphoma cells or in a coupled *in vitro/in vivo* unscheduled DNA synthesis (UDS) assay in rat liver. It was not clastogenic in the *in vitro* chromosomal aberration assay in human lymphocytes or in two *in vivo* mouse micronucleus assays.

Impairment of Fertility

When racemic citalopram was administered orally to 16 male and 24 female rats prior to and throughout mating and gestation at doses of 32, 48, and 72 mg/kg/day, mating was decreased at all doses, and fertility was decreased at doses ≥ 32 mg/kg/day. Gestation duration was increased at 48 mg/kg/day.

13.2 Animal Toxicology and/or Pharmacology

Retinal Changes in Rats

Pathologic changes (degeneration/atrophy) were observed in the retinas of albino rats in the 2-year carcinogenicity study with racemic citalopram. There was an increase in both incidence and severity of retinal pathology in both male and female rats receiving 80 mg/kg/day. Similar findings were not present in rats receiving 24 mg/kg/day of racemic citalopram for two years, in mice receiving up to 240 mg/kg/day of racemic citalopram for 18 months, or in dogs receiving up to 20 mg/kg/day of racemic citalopram for one year.

Additional studies to investigate the mechanism for this pathology have not been performed, and the potential significance of this effect in humans has not been established.

Cardiovascular Changes in Dogs

In a one-year toxicology study, 5 of 10 beagle dogs receiving oral racemic citalopram doses of 8 mg/kg/day died suddenly between weeks 17 and 31 following initiation of treatment. Sudden deaths were not observed in rats at doses of racemic citalopram up to 120 mg/kg/day, which produced plasma levels of citalopram and its metabolites demethylcitalopram and didemethylcitalopram (DDCT) similar to those observed in dogs at 8 mg/kg/day. A subsequent intravenous dosing study demonstrated that in beagle dogs, racemic DDCT caused QT prolongation, a known risk factor for the observed outcome in dogs.

14 CLINICAL STUDIES

14.1 Major Depressive Disorder

Adolescents

The efficacy of Lexapro as an acute treatment for major depressive disorder in adolescent patients was established in an 8-week, flexible-dose, placebo-controlled study that compared Lexapro 10-20 mg/day to placebo in outpatients 12 to 17 years of age inclusive who met DSM-IV criteria for major depressive disorder. The primary outcome was change from baseline to endpoint in the Children's Depression Rating Scale - Revised (CDRS-R). In this study, Lexapro showed statistically significant greater mean improvement compared to placebo on the CDRS-R.

The efficacy of Lexapro in the acute treatment of major depressive disorder in adolescents was established, in part, on the basis of extrapolation from the 8-week, flexible-dose, placebo-controlled study with racemic citalopram 20-40 mg/day. In this outpatient study in children and adolescents 7 to 17 years of age who met DSM-IV criteria for major depressive disorder, citalopram treatment showed statistically significant greater mean improvement from baseline, compared to placebo, on the CDRS-R; the positive results for this trial largely came from the adolescent subgroup.

Two additional flexible-dose, placebo-controlled MDD studies (one Lexapro study in patients ages 7 to 17 and one citalopram study in adolescents) did not demonstrate efficacy. Although maintenance efficacy in adolescent patients has not been systematically evaluated, maintenance efficacy can be extrapolated from adult data along with comparisons of escitalopram pharmacokinetic parameters in adults and adolescent patients.

Adults

The efficacy of Lexapro as a treatment for major depressive disorder was established in three, 8-week, placebo-controlled studies conducted in outpatients between 18 and

65 years of age who met DSM-IV criteria for major depressive disorder. The primary outcome in all three studies was change from baseline to endpoint in the Montgomery Asberg Depression Rating Scale (MADRS).

A fixed-dose study compared 10 mg/day Lexapro and 20 mg/day Lexapro to placebo and 40 mg/day citalopram. The 10 mg/day and 20 mg/day Lexapro treatment groups showed statistically significant greater mean improvement compared to placebo on the MADRS. The 10 mg and 20 mg Lexapro groups were similar on this outcome measure.

In a second fixed-dose study of 10 mg/day Lexapro and placebo, the 10 mg/day Lexapro treatment group showed statistically significant greater mean improvement compared to placebo on the MADRS.

In a flexible-dose study, comparing Lexapro, titrated between 10 and 20 mg/day, to placebo and citalopram, titrated between 20 and 40 mg/day, the Lexapro treatment group showed statistically significant greater mean improvement compared to placebo on the MADRS.

Analyses of the relationship between treatment outcome and age, gender, and race did not suggest any differential responsiveness on the basis of these patient characteristics. In a longer-term trial, 274 patients meeting (DSM-IV) criteria for major depressive disorder, who had responded during an initial 8-week, open-label treatment phase with Lexapro 10 or 20 mg/day, were randomized to continuation of Lexapro at their same dose, or to placebo, for up to 36 weeks of observation for relapse. Response during the open-label phase was defined by having a decrease of the MADRS total score to ≤ 12. Relapse during the double-blind phase was defined as an increase of the MADRS total score to ≥ 22, or discontinuation due to insufficient clinical response. Patients receiving continued Lexapro experienced a statistically significant longer time to relapse compared to those receiving placebo.

14.2 Generalized Anxiety Disorder

The efficacy of Lexapro in the acute treatment of Generalized Anxiety Disorder (GAD) was demonstrated in three, 8-week, multicenter, flexible-dose, placebo-controlled studies that compared Lexapro 10-20 mg/day to placebo in adult outpatients between 18 and 80 years of age who met DSM-IV criteria for GAD. In all three studies, Lexapro showed statistically significant greater mean improvement compared to placebo on the Hamilton Anxiety Scale (HAM-A).

There were too few patients in differing ethnic and age groups to adequately assess whether or not Lexapro has differential effects in these groups. There was no difference in response to Lexapro between men and women.

16 HOW SUPPLIED/STORAGE AND HANDLING
16.1 Tablets
5 mg Tablets:
Bottle of 100   NDC # 0456-2005-01
White to off-white, round, non-scored, film-coated. Imprint "FL" on one side of the tablet and "5" on the other side.
10 mg Tablets:
Bottle of 100   NDC # 0456-2010-01
10 × 10 Unit Dose   NDC # 0456-2010-63
White to off-white, round, scored, film-coated. Imprint on scored side with "F" on the left side and "L" on the right side. Imprint on the non-scored side with "10".
20 mg Tablets:
Bottle of 100   NDC # 0456-2020-01
10 × 10 Unit Dose   NDC # 0456-2020-63
White to off-white, round, scored, film-coated. Imprint on scored side with "F" on the left side and "L" on the right side. Imprint on the non-scored side with "20".

16.2 Oral Solution
5 mg/5 mL, peppermint flavor (240 mL) NDC # 0456-2101-08
Storage and Handling
Store at 25°C (77°F); excursions permitted to 15-30°C (59-86°F).

17 PATIENT COUNSELING INFORMATION
See FDA-approved Medication Guide
17.1 Information for Patients
Physicians are advised to discuss the following issues with patients for whom they prescribe Lexapro.
General Information about Medication Guide
Prescribers or other health professionals should inform patients, their families, and their caregivers about the benefits and risks associated with treatment with Lexapro and should counsel them in its appropriate use. A patient Medication Guide about "Antidepressant Medicines, Depression and other Serious Mental Illness, and Suicidal Thoughts or Actions" is available for Lexapro. The prescriber or health professional should instruct patients, their families, and their caregivers to read the Medication Guide and should assist them in understanding its contents. Patients should be given the opportunity to discuss the contents of the Medication Guide and to obtain answers to any questions they may have. The complete text of the Medication Guide is reprinted at the end of this document.

Patients should be advised of the following issues and asked to alert their prescriber if these occur while taking Lexapro.
Clinical Worsening and Suicide Risk
Patients, their families, and their caregivers should be encouraged to be alert to the emergence of anxiety, agitation, panic attacks, insomnia, irritability, hostility, aggressiveness, impulsivity, akathisia (psychomotor restlessness), hypomania, mania, other unusual changes in behavior, worsening of depression, and suicidal ideation, especially early during antidepressant treatment and when the dose is adjusted up or down. Families and caregivers of patients should be advised to look for the emergence of such symptoms on a day-to-day basis, since changes may be abrupt. Such symptoms should be reported to the patient's prescriber or health professional, especially if they are severe, abrupt in onset, or were not part of the patient's presenting symptoms. Symptoms such as these may be associated with an increased risk for suicidal thinking and behavior and indicate a need for very close monitoring and possibly changes in the medication [see Warnings and Precautions (5.1)].
Serotonin Syndrome
Patients should be cautioned about the risk of serotonin syndrome with the concomitant use of Lexapro and triptans, tramadol or other serotonergic agents [see Warnings and Precautions (5.2)].
Abnormal Bleeding
Patients should be cautioned about the concomitant use of Lexapro and NSAIDs, aspirin, warfarin, or other drugs that affect coagulation since combined use of psychotropic drugs that interfere with serotonin reuptake and these agents has been associated with an increased risk of bleeding [see Warnings and Precautions (5.7)].
Concomitant Medications
Since escitalopram is the active isomer of racemic citalopram (Celexa), the two agents should not be coadministered. Patients should be advised to inform their physician if they are taking, or plan to take, any prescription or over-the-counter drugs, as there is a potential for interactions.
Continuing the Therapy Prescribed
While patients may notice improvement with Lexapro therapy in 1 to 4 weeks, they should be advised to continue therapy as directed.
Interference with Psychomotor Performance
Because psychoactive drugs may impair judgment, thinking, or motor skills, patients should be cautioned about operating hazardous machinery, including automobiles, until they are reasonably certain that Lexapro therapy does not affect their ability to engage in such activities.
Alcohol
Patients should be told that, although Lexapro has not been shown in experiments with normal subjects to increase the mental and motor skill impairments caused by alcohol, the concomitant use of Lexapro and alcohol in depressed patients is not advised.
Pregnancy and Breast Feeding
Patients should be advised to notify their physician if they
• become pregnant or intend to become pregnant during therapy.
• are breastfeeding an infant.
Need for Comprehensive Treatment Program
Lexapro is indicated as an integral part of a total treatment program for MDD that may include other measures (psychological, educational, social) for patients with this syndrome. Drug treatment may not be indicated for all adolescents with this syndrome. Safety and effectiveness of Lexapro in MDD has not been established in pediatrics patients less than 12 years of age. Antidepressants are not intended for use in the adolescent who exhibits symptoms secondary to environmental factors and/or other primary psychiatric disorders. Appropriate educational placement is essential and psychosocial intervention is often helpful. When remedial measures alone are insufficient, the decision to prescribe antidepressant medication will depend upon the physician's assessment of the chronicity and severity of the patient's symptoms.

17.2 FDA-Approved Medication Guide
MEDICATION GUIDE
Lexapro® (escitalopram oxalate) Tablets/Oral Solution
Antidepressant Medicines, Depression and other Serious Mental Illnesses, and Suicidal Thoughts or Actions
Read the Medication Guide that comes with you or your family member's antidepressant medicine. This Medication Guide is only about the risk of suicidal thoughts and actions with antidepressant medicines. **Talk to your, or your family member's, healthcare provider about:**
• all risks and benefits of treatment with antidepressant medicines
• all treatment choices for depression or other serious mental illness
What is the most important information I should know about antidepressant medicines, depression and other serious mental illnesses, and suicidal thoughts or actions?
1. **Antidepressant medicines may increase suicidal thoughts or actions in some children, teenagers, and young adults within the first few months of treatment.**

2. **Depression and other serious mental illnesses are the most important causes of suicidal thoughts and actions.** Some people may have a particularly high risk of having suicidal thoughts or actions. These include people who have (or have a family history of) bipolar illness (also called manic-depressive illness) or suicidal thoughts or actions.
3. **How can I watch for and try to prevent suicidal thoughts and actions in myself or a family member?**
• Pay close attention to any changes, especially sudden changes, in mood, behaviors, thoughts, or feelings. This is very important when an antidepressant medicine is started or when the dose is changed.
• Call the healthcare provider right away to report new or sudden changes in mood, behavior, thoughts, or feelings.
• Keep all follow-up visits with the healthcare provider as scheduled. Call the healthcare provider between visits as needed, especially if you have concerns about symptoms.
Call a healthcare provider right away if you or your family member has any of the following symptoms, especially if they are new, worse, or worry you:
• thoughts about suicide or dying
• attempts to commit suicide
• new or worse depression
• new or worse anxiety
• feeling very agitated or restless
• panic attacks
• trouble sleeping (insomnia)
• new or worse irritability
• acting aggressive, being angry, or violent
• acting on dangerous impulses
• an extreme increase in activity and talking (mania)
• other unusual changes in behavior or mood
Call your doctor for medical advice about side effects. You may report side effects to FDA at 1-800-FDA-1088
What else do I need to know about antidepressant medicines?
• **Never stop an antidepressant medicine without first talking to a healthcare provider.** Stopping an antidepressant medicine suddenly can cause other symptoms.
• **Antidepressants are medicines used to treat depression and other illnesses.** It is important to discuss all the risks of treating depression and also the risks of not treating it. Patients and their families or other caregivers should discuss all treatment choices with the healthcare provider, not just the use of antidepressants.
• **Antidepressant medicines have other side effects.** Talk to the healthcare provider about the side effects of the medicine prescribed for you or your family member.
• **Antidepressant medicines can interact with other medicines.** Know all of the medicines that you or your family member takes. Keep a list of all medicines to show the healthcare provider. Do not start new medicines without first checking with your healthcare provider.
• **Not all antidepressant medicines prescribed for children are FDA approved for use in children.** Talk to your child's healthcare provider for more information.
This Medication Guide has been approved by the U.S. Food and Drug Administration for all antidepressants.
Forest Pharmaceuticals, Inc.
Subsidiary of Forest Laboratories, Inc.
St. Louis, MO 63045 USA
Licensed from H. Lundbeck A/S
© 2009 Forest Laboratories, Inc.
Rev. 01/09
Revised: 03/2009
Shown in Product Identification Guide, page 309

NAMENDA® TABLETS/ORAL SOLUTION ℞
[nă-mĕn-dă]
(memantine hydrochloride)
Rx Only

DESCRIPTION
Namenda® (memantine hydrochloride) is an orally active NMDA receptor antagonist. The chemical name for memantine hydrochloride is 1-amino-3,5-dimethyladamantane hydrochloride with the following structural formula:

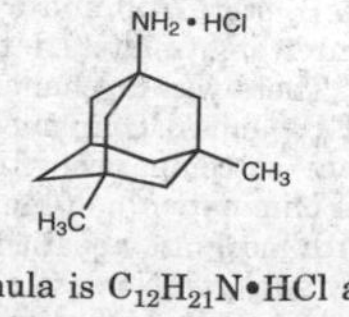

The molecular formula is $C_{12}H_{21}N \cdot HCl$ and the molecular weight is 215.76.
Memantine HCl occurs as a fine white to off-white powder and is soluble in water. Namenda is available as tablets or as an oral solution. Namenda is available for oral administration as capsule-shaped, film-coated tablets containing

5 mg and 10 mg of memantine hydrochloride. The tablets also contain the following inactive ingredients: microcrystalline cellulose/colloidal silicon dioxide, talc, croscarmellose sodium, and magnesium stearate. In addition the following inactive ingredients are also present as components of the film coat: hypromellose, titanium dioxide, polyethylene glycol 400, FD&C yellow #6 and FD&C blue #2 (5 mg tablets), and hypromellose, titanium dioxide, macrogol/polyethylene glycol 400 and iron oxide black (10 mg tablets). Namenda oral solution contains memantine hydrochloride in a strength equivalent to 2 mg of memantine hydrochloride in each mL. The oral solution also contains the following inactive ingredients: sorbitol solution (70%), methyl paraben, propylparaben, propylene glycol, glycerin, natural peppermint flavor #104, citric acid, sodium citrate, and purified water.

CLINICAL PHARMACOLOGY

Mechanism of Action and Pharmacodynamics

Persistent activation of central nervous system N-methyl-D-aspartate (NMDA) receptors by the excitatory amino acid glutamate has been hypothesized to contribute to the symptomatology of Alzheimer's disease. Memantine is postulated to exert its therapeutic effect through its action as a low to moderate affinity uncompetitive (open-channel) NMDA receptor antagonist which binds preferentially to the NMDA receptor-operated cation channels. There is no evidence that memantine prevents or slows neurodegeneration in patients with Alzheimer's disease.

Memantine showed low to negligible affinity for GABA, benzodiazepine, dopamine, adrenergic, histamine and glycine receptors and for voltage-dependent Ca^{2+}, Na^{+} or K^{+} channels. Memantine also showed antagonistic effects at the $5HT_3$ receptor with a potency similar to that for the NMDA receptor and blocked nicotinic acetylcholine receptors with one-sixth to one-tenth the potency.

In vitro studies have shown that memantine does not affect the reversible inhibition of acetylcholinesterase by donepezil, galantamine, or tacrine.

Pharmacokinetics

Memantine is well absorbed after oral administration and has linear pharmacokinetics over the therapeutic dose range. It is excreted predominantly in the urine, unchanged, and has a terminal elimination half life of about 60-80 hours.

Absorption and Distribution

Following oral administration memantine is highly absorbed with peak concentrations reached in about 3-7 hours. Food has no effect on the absorption of memantine. The mean volume of distribution of memantine is 9-11 L/kg and the plasma protein binding is low (45%).

Metabolism and Elimination

Memantine undergoes partial hepatic metabolism. About 48% of administered drug is excreted unchanged in urine; the remainder is converted primarily to three polar metabolites which possess minimal NMDA receptor antagonistic activity: the N-glucuronide conjugate, 6-hydroxy memantine, and 1-nitroso-deaminated memantine. A total of 74% of the administered dose is excreted as the sum of the parent drug and the N-glucuronide conjugate. The hepatic microsomal CYP450 enzyme system does not play a significant role in the metabolism of memantine. Memantine has a terminal elimination half-life of about 60-80 hours. Renal clearance involves active tubular secretion moderated by pH dependent tubular reabsorption.

Special Populations

Renal Impairment: Memantine pharmacokinetics were evaluated following single oral administration of 20 mg memantine HCl in 8 subjects with mild renal impairment (creatinine clearance, CLcr, >50–80 mL/min), 8 subjects with moderate renal impairment (CLcr 30–49 mL/min), 7 subjects with severe renal impairment (CLcr 5–29 mL/min) and 8 healthy subjects (CLcr > 80 mL/min) matched as closely as possible by age, weight and gender to the subjects with renal impairment. Mean $AUC_{0-\infty}$ increased by 4%, 60%, and 115% in subjects with mild, moderate, and severe renal impairment, respectively, compared to healthy subjects. The terminal elimination half-life increased by 18%, 41%, and 95% in subjects with mild, moderate, and severe renal impairment, respectively, compared to healthy subjects.

No dosage adjustment is recommended for patients with mild and moderate renal impairment. Dosage should be reduced in patients with severe renal impairment (See DOSAGE AND ADMINISTRATION).

Hepatic Impairment: Memantine pharmacokinetics were evaluated following the administration of single oral doses of 20 mg in 8 subjects with moderate hepatic impairment (Child-Pugh Class B, score 7-9) and 8 subjects who were age-, gender-, and weight-matched to the hepatically-impaired subjects. There was no change in memantine exposure (based on C_{max} and AUC) in subjects with moderate hepatic impairment as compared with healthy subjects. However, terminal elimination half-life increased by about 16% in subjects with moderate hepatic impairment as compared with healthy subjects. No dose adjustment is recommended for patients with mild and moderate hepatic impairment. Memantine should be administered with caution to patients with severe hepatic impairment as the pharmacokinetics of memantine have not been evaluated in that population.

Elderly: The pharmacokinetics of Namenda in young and elderly subjects are similar.

Gender: Following multiple dose administration of Namenda 20 mg b.i.d., females had about 45% higher exposure than males, but there was no difference in exposure when body weight was taken into account.

Drug-Drug Interactions

Substrates of Microsomal Enzymes: *In vitro* studies indicated that at concentrations exceeding those associated with efficacy, memantine does not induce the cytochrome P450 isozymes CYP1A2, CYP2C9, CYP2E1 and CYP3A4/5. In addition, *in vitro* studies have shown that memantine produces minimal inhibition of CYP450 enzymes CYP1A2, CYP2A6, CYP2C9, CYP2D6, CYP2E1, and CYP3A4. These data indicate that no pharmacokinetic interactions with drugs metabolized by these enzymes are expected.

Inhibitors of Microsomal Enzymes: Since memantine undergoes minimal metabolism, with the majority of the dose excreted unchanged in urine, an interaction between memantine and drugs that are inhibitors of CYP450 enzymes is unlikely. Coadministration of Namenda with the AChE inhibitor donepezil HCl does not affect the pharmacokinetics of either compound.

Drugs Eliminated via Renal Mechanisms: Memantine is eliminated in part by tubular secretion. *In vivo* studies have shown that multiple doses of the diuretic hydrochlorothiazide/triamterene (HCTZ/TA) did not affect the AUC of memantine at steady state. Memantine did not affect the bioavailability of TA, and decreased AUC and C_{max} of HCTZ by about 20%. Coadministration of memantine with the antihyperglycemic drug Glucovance® (glyburide and metformin HCl) did not affect the pharmacokinetics of memantine, metformin and glyburide. Memantine did not modify the serum glucose lowering effects of Glucovance®, indicating the absence of a pharmacodynamic interaction.

Drugs that make the urine alkaline: The clearance of memantine was reduced by about 80% under alkaline urine conditions at pH 8. Therefore, alterations of urine pH towards the alkaline state may lead to an accumulation of the drug with a possible increase in adverse effects. Drugs that alkalinize the urine (e.g. carbonic anhydrase inhibitors, sodium bicarbonate) would be expected to reduce renal elimination of memantine.

Drugs highly bound to plasma proteins: Because the plasma protein binding of memantine is low (45%), an interaction with drugs that are highly bound to plasma proteins, such as warfarin and digoxin, is unlikely.

CLINICAL TRIALS

The effectiveness of Namenda (memantine hydrochloride) as a treatment for patients with moderate to severe Alzheimer's disease was demonstrated in 2 randomized, double-blind, placebo-controlled clinical studies (Studies 1 and 2) conducted in the United States that assessed both cognitive function and day to day function. The mean age of patients participating in these two trials was 76 with a range of 50-93 years. Approximately 66% of patients were female and 91% of patients were Caucasian.

A third study (Study 3), carried out in Latvia, enrolled patients with severe dementia, but did not assess cognitive function as a planned endpoint.

Study Outcome Measures: In each U.S. study, the effectiveness of Namenda was determined using both an instrument designed to evaluate overall function through caregiver-related assessment, and an instrument that measures cognition. Both studies showed that patients on Namenda experienced significant improvement on both measures compared to placebo.

Day-to-day function was assessed in both studies using the modified Alzheimer's disease Cooperative Study - Activities of Daily Living inventory (ADCS-ADL). The ADCS-ADL consists of a comprehensive battery of ADL questions used to measure the functional capabilities of patients. Each ADL item is rated from the highest level of independent performance to complete loss. The investigator performs the inventory by interviewing a caregiver familiar with the behavior of the patient. A subset of 19 items, including ratings of the patient's ability to eat, dress, bathe, telephone, travel, shop, and perform other household chores has been validated for the assessment of patients with moderate to severe dementia. This is the modified ADCS-ADL, which has a scoring range of 0 to 54, with the lower scores indicating greater functional impairment.

The ability of Namenda to improve cognitive performance was assessed in both studies with the Severe Impairment Battery (SIB), a multi-item instrument that has been validated for the evaluation of cognitive function in patients with moderate to severe dementia. The SIB examines selected aspects of cognitive performance, including elements of attention, orientation, language, memory, visuospatial ability, construction, praxis, and social interaction. The SIB scoring range is from 0 to 100, with lower scores indicating greater cognitive impairment.

Study 1 (Twenty-Eight-Week Study)

In a study of 28 weeks duration, 252 patients with moderate to severe probable Alzheimer's disease (diagnosed by DSM-IV and NINCDS-ADRDA criteria, with Mini-Mental State Examination scores ≥3 and ≤14 and Global Deterioration Scale Stages 5-6) were randomized to Namenda or placebo. For patients randomized to Namenda, treatment was initiated at 5 mg once daily and increased weekly by 5 mg/day in divided doses to a dose of 20 mg/day (10 mg twice a day).

Effects on the ADCS-ADL:

Figure 1 shows the time course for the change from baseline in the ADCS-ADL score for patients in the two treatment groups completing the 28 weeks of the study. At 28 weeks of treatment, the mean difference in the ADCS-ADL change scores for the Namenda-treated patients compared to the patients on placebo was 3.4 units. Using an analysis based on all patients and carrying their last study observation forward (LOCF analysis), Namenda treatment was statistically significantly superior to placebo.

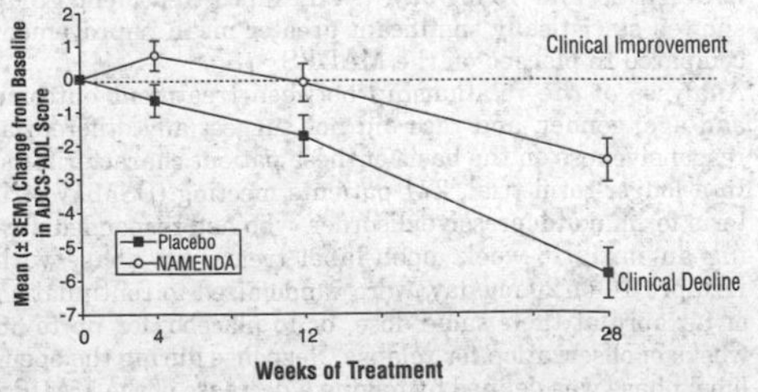

Figure 1: Time course of the change from baseline in ADCS-ADL score for patients completing 28 weeks of treatment.

Figure 2 shows the cumulative percentages of patients from each of the treatment groups who had attained at least the change in the ADCS-ADL shown on the X axis.

The curves show that both patients assigned to Namenda and placebo have a wide range of responses and generally show deterioration (a negative change in ADCS-ADL compared to baseline), but that the Namenda group is more likely to show a smaller decline or an improvement. (In a cumulative distribution display, a curve for an effective treatment would be shifted to the left of the curve for placebo, while an ineffective or deleterious treatment would be superimposed upon or shifted to the right of the curve for placebo.)

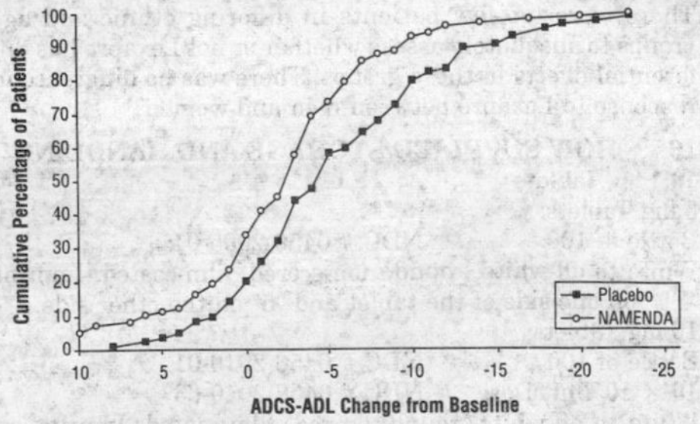

Figure 2: Cumulative percentage of patients completing 28 weeks of double-blind treatment with specified changes from baseline in ADCS-ADL scores.

Effects on the SIB:

Figure 3 shows the time course for the change from baseline in SIB score for the two treatment groups over the 28 weeks of the study. At 28 weeks of treatment, the mean difference in the SIB change scores for the Namenda-treated patients compared to the patients on placebo was 5.7 units. Using an LOCF analysis, Namenda treatment was statistically significantly superior to placebo.

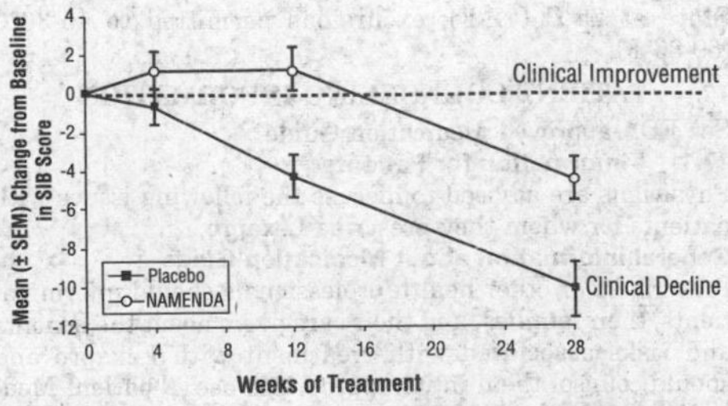

Figure 3: Time course of the change from baseline in SIB score for patients completing 28 weeks of treatment.

Figure 4 shows the cumulative percentages of patients from each treatment group who had attained at least the measure of change in SIB score shown on the X axis.

The curves show that both patients assigned to Namenda and placebo have a wide range of responses and generally show deterioration, but that the Namenda group is more likely to show a smaller decline or an improvement.

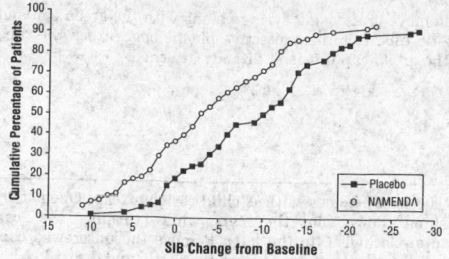

Figure 4: Cumulative percentage of patients completing 28 weeks of double-blind treatment with specified changes from baseline in SIB scores.

Study 2 (Twenty-Four-Week Study)

In a study of 24 weeks duration, 404 patients with moderate to severe probable Alzheimer's disease (diagnosed by NINCDS-ADRDA criteria, with Mini-Mental State Examination scores ≥5 and ≤14) who had been treated with donepezil for at least 6 months and who had been on a stable dose of donepezil for the last 3 months were randomized to Namenda or placebo while still receiving donepezil. For patients randomized to Namenda, treatment was initiated at 5 mg once daily and increased weekly by 5 mg/day in divided doses to a dose of 20 mg/day (10 mg twice a day).

Effects on the ADCS-ADL:

Figure 5 shows the time course for the change from baseline in the ADCS-ADL score for the two treatment groups over the 24 weeks of the study. At 24 weeks of treatment, the mean difference in the ADCS-ADL change scores for the Namenda/donepezil treated patients (combination therapy) compared to the patients on placebo/donepezil (monotherapy) was 1.6 units. Using an LOCF analysis, Namenda/donepezil treatment was statistically significantly superior to placebo/donepezil.

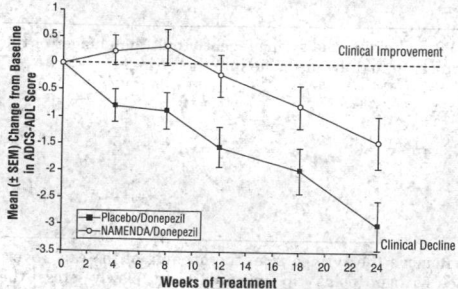

Figure 5: Time course of the change from baseline in ADCS-ADL score for patients completing 24 weeks of treatment.

Figure 6 shows the cumulative percentages of patients from each of the treatment groups who had attained at least the measure of improvement in the ADCS-ADL shown on the X axis.

The curves show that both patients assigned to Namenda/donepezil and placebo/donepezil have a wide range of responses and generally show deterioration, but that the Namenda/donepezil group is more likely to show a smaller decline or an improvement.

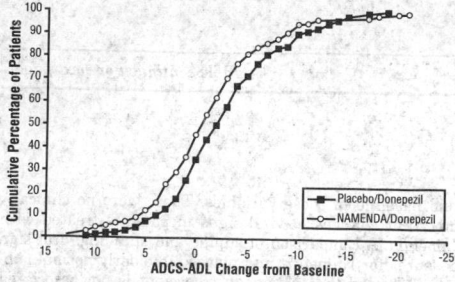

Figure 6: Cumulative percentage of patients completing 24 weeks of double-blind treatment with specified changes from baseline in ADCS-ADL scores.

Effects on the SIB:

Figure 7 shows the time course for the change from baseline in SIB score for the two treatment groups over the 24 weeks of the study. At 24 weeks of treatment, the mean difference in the SIB change scores for the Namenda/donepezil-treated patients compared to the patients on placebo/donepezil was 3.3 units. Using an LOCF analysis, Namenda/donepezil

treatment was statistically significantly superior to placebo/donepezil.

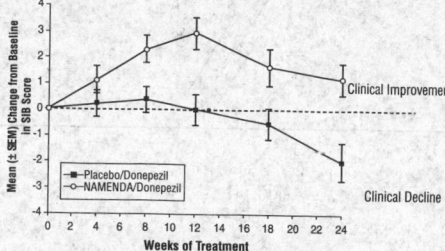

Figure 7: Time course of the change from baseline in SIB score for patients completing 24 weeks of treatment.

Figure 8 shows the cumulative percentages of patients from each treatment group who had attained at least the measure of improvement in SIB score shown on the X axis. The curves show that both patients assigned to Namenda/donepezil and placebo/donepezil have a wide range of responses, but that the Namenda/donepezil group is more likely to show an improvement or a smaller decline.

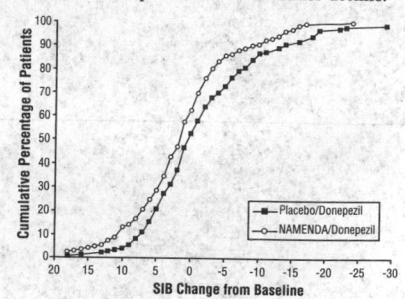

Figure 8: Cumulative percentage of patients completing 24 weeks of double-blind treatment with specified changes from baseline in SIB scores.

Study 3 (Twelve-Week Study)

In a double-blind study of 12 weeks duration, conducted in nursing homes in Latvia, 166 patients with dementia according to DSM-III-R, a Mini-Mental State Examination score of <10, and Global Deterioration Scale staging of 5 to 7 were randomized to either Namenda or placebo. For patients randomized to Namenda, treatment was initiated at 5 mg once daily and increased to 10 mg once daily after 1 week. The primary efficacy measures were the care dependency subscale of the Behavioral Rating Scale for Geriatric Patients (BGP), a measure of day-to-day function, and a Clinical Global Impression of Change (CGI-C), a measure of overall clinical effect. No valid measure of cognitive function was used in this study. A statistically significant treatment difference at 12 weeks that favored Namenda over placebo was seen on both primary efficacy measures. Because the patients entered were a mixture of Alzheimer's disease and vascular dementia, an attempt was made to distinguish the two groups and all patients were later designated as having either vascular dementia or Alzheimer's disease, based on their scores on the Hachinski Ischemic Scale at study entry. Only about 50% of the patients had computerized tomography of the brain. For the subset designated as having Alzheimer's disease, a statistically significant treatment effect favoring Namenda over placebo at 12 weeks was seen on both the BGP and CGI-C.

INDICATIONS AND USAGE

Namenda (memantine hydrochloride) is indicated for the treatment of moderate to severe dementia of the Alzheimer's type.

CONTRAINDICATIONS

Namenda (memantine hydrochloride) is contraindicated in patients with known hypersensitivity to memantine hydrochloride or to any excipients used in the formulation.

PRECAUTIONS

Information for Patients and Caregivers: Caregivers should be instructed in the recommended administration (twice per day for doses above 5 mg) and dose escalation (minimum interval of one week between dose increases).

Neurological Conditions

Seizures: Namenda has not been systematically evaluated in patients with a seizure disorder. In clinical trials of Namenda, seizures occurred in 0.2% of patients treated with Namenda and 0.5% of patients treated with placebo.

Genitourinary Conditions

Conditions that raise urine pH may decrease the urinary elimination of memantine resulting in increased plasma levels of memantine.

Special Populations

Hepatic Impairment

Namenda undergoes partial hepatic metabolism, with about 48% of administered dose excreted in urine as unchanged drug or as the sum of parent drug and the N-glucuronide conjugate (74%). No dosage adjustment is needed in patients with mild or moderate hepatic impairment. Namenda should be administered with caution to patients with severe hepatic impairment.

Renal Impairment

No dosage adjustment is needed in patients with mild or moderate renal impairment. A dosage reduction is recommended in patients with severe renal impairment (see CLINICAL PHARMACOLOGY and DOSAGE AND ADMINISTRATION).

Drug-Drug Interactions

N-methyl-D-aspartate (NMDA) antagonists: The combined use of Namenda with other NMDA antagonists (amantadine, ketamine, and dextromethorphan) has not been systematically evaluated and such use should be approached with caution.

Effects of Namenda on substrates of microsomal enzymes: In vitro studies conducted with marker substrates of CYP450 enzymes (CYP1A2, -2A6, -2C9, -2D6, -2E1, -3A4) showed minimal inhibition of these enzymes by memantine. In addition, in vitro studies indicate that at concentrations exceeding those associated with efficacy, memantine does not induce the cytochrome P450 isozymes CYP1A2, CYP2C9, CYP2E1 and CYP3A4/5. No pharmacokinetic interactions with drugs metabolized by these enzymes are expected.

Effects of inhibitors and/or substrates of microsomal enzymes on Namenda: Memantine is predominantly renally eliminated, and drugs that are substrates and/or inhibitors of the CYP450 system are not expected to alter the metabolism of memantine.

Acetylcholinesterase (AChE) inhibitors: Coadministration of Namenda with the AChE inhibitor donepezil HCl did not affect the pharmacokinetics of either compound. In a 24-week controlled clinical study in patients with moderate to severe Alzheimer's disease, the adverse event profile observed with a combination of memantine and donepezil was similar to that of donepezil alone.

Drugs eliminated via renal mechanisms: Because memantine is eliminated in part by tubular secretion, coadministration of drugs that use the same renal cationic system, including hydrochlorothiazide (HCTZ), triamterene (TA), metformin, cimetidine, ranitidine, quinidine, and nicotine, could potentially result in altered plasma levels of both agents. However, coadministration of Namenda and HCTZ/TA did not affect the bioavailability of either memantine or TA, and the bioavailability of HCTZ decreased by 20%. In addition, coadministration of memantine with the antihyperglycemic drug Glucovance® (glyburide and metformin HCl) did not affect the pharmacokinetics of memantine, metformin and glyburide. Furthermore, memantine did not modify the serum glucose lowering effect of Glucovance®.

Drugs that make the urine alkaline: The clearance of memantine was reduced by about 80% under alkaline urine conditions at pH 8. Therefore, alterations of urine pH towards the alkaline condition may lead to an accumulation of the drug with a possible increase in adverse effects. Urine pH is altered by diet, drugs (e.g. carbonic anhydrase inhibitors, sodium bicarbonate) and clinical state of the patient (e.g. renal tubular acidosis or severe infections of the urinary tract). Hence, memantine should be used with caution under these conditions.

Carcinogenesis, Mutagenesis and Impairment of Fertility

There was no evidence of carcinogenicity in a 113-week oral study in mice at doses up to 40 mg/kg/day (10 times the maximum recommended human dose [MRHD] on a mg/m² basis). There was also no evidence of carcinogenicity in rats orally dosed at up to 40 mg/kg/day for 71 weeks followed by 20 mg/kg/day (20 and 10 times the MRHD on a mg/m² basis, respectively) through 128 weeks.

Memantine produced no evidence of genotoxic potential when evaluated in the in vitro S. typhimurium or E. coli reverse mutation assay, an in vitro chromosomal aberration test in human lymphocytes, an in vivo cytogenetics assay for chromosome damage in rats, and the in vivo mouse micronucleus assay. The results were equivocal in an in vitro gene mutation assay using Chinese hamster V79 cells.

No impairment of fertility or reproductive performance was seen in rats administered up to 18 mg/kg/day (9 times the MRHD on a mg/m² basis) orally from 14 days prior to mating through gestation and lactation in females, or for 60 days prior to mating in males.

Pregnancy

Pregnancy Category B: Memantine given orally to pregnant rats and pregnant rabbits during the period of organogenesis was not teratogenic up to the highest doses tested (18 mg/kg/day in rats and 30 mg/kg/day in rabbits, which are 9 and 30 times, respectively, the maximum recommended human dose [MRHD] on a mg/m² basis). Slight maternal toxicity, decreased pup weights and an increased incidence of non-ossified cervical vertebrae were seen at an oral dose of 18 mg/kg/day in a study in which rats were given oral memantine beginning pre-mating and continuing through the postpartum period. Slight maternal toxicity and decreased pup weights were also seen at this dose in a study in which rats were treated from day 15 of gestation through the post-partum period. The no-effect dose for these effects was 6 mg/kg, which is 3 times the MRHD on a mg/m^2 basis.

There are no adequate and well-controlled studies of memantine in pregnant women. Memantine should be used during pregnancy only if the potential benefit justifies the potential risk to the fetus.

Nursing Mothers

It is not known whether memantine is excreted in human breast milk. Because many drugs are excreted in human milk, caution should be exercised when memantine is administered to a nursing mother.

Pediatric Use

There are no adequate and well-controlled trials documenting the safety and efficacy of memantine in any illness occurring in children.

ADVERSE REACTIONS

The experience described in this section derives from studies in patients with Alzheimer's disease and vascular dementia.

Adverse Events Leading to Discontinuation: In placebo-controlled trials in which dementia patients received doses of Namenda up to 20 mg/day, the likelihood of discontinuation because of an adverse event was the same in the Namenda group as in the placebo group. No individual adverse event was associated with the discontinuation of treatment in 1% or more of Namenda-treated patients and at a rate greater than placebo.

Adverse Events Reported in Controlled Trials: The reported adverse events in Namenda (memantine hydrochloride) trials reflect experience gained under closely monitored conditions in a highly selected patient population. In actual practice or in other clinical trials, these frequency estimates may not apply, as the conditions of use, reporting behavior and the types of patients treated may differ. Table 1 lists treatment-emergent signs and symptoms that were reported in at least 2% of patients in placebo-controlled dementia trials and for which the rate of occurrence was greater for patients treated with Namenda than for those treated with placebo. No adverse event occurred at a frequency of at least 5% and twice the placebo rate.

Table 1: Adverse Events Reported in Controlled Clinical Trials in at Least 2% of Patients Receiving Namenda and at a Higher Frequency than Placebo-treated Patients.

Body System Adverse Event	Placebo (N = 922) %	Namenda (N = 940) %
Body as a Whole		
Fatigue	1	2
Pain	1	3
Cardiovascular System		
Hypertension	2	4
Central and Peripheral Nervous System		
Dizziness	5	7
Headache	3	6
Gastrointestinal System		
Constipation	3	5
Vomiting	2	3
Musculoskeletal System		
Back pain	2	3
Psychiatric Disorders		
Confusion	5	6
Somnolence	2	3
Hallucination	2	3
Respiratory System		
Coughing	3	4
Dyspnea	1	2

Other adverse events occurring with an incidence of at least 2% in Namenda-treated patients but at a greater or equal rate on placebo were agitation, fall, inflicted injury, urinary incontinence, diarrhea, bronchitis, insomnia, urinary tract infection, influenza-like symptoms, abnormal gait, depression, upper respiratory tract infection, anxiety, peripheral edema, nausea, anorexia, and arthralgia.

The overall profile of adverse events and the incidence rates for individual adverse events in the subpopulation of patients with moderate to severe Alzheimer's disease were not different from the profile and incidence rates described above for the overall dementia population.

Vital Sign Changes: Namenda and placebo groups were compared with respect to (1) mean change from baseline in vital signs (pulse, systolic blood pressure, diastolic blood pressure, and weight) and (2) the incidence of patients meeting criteria for potentially clinically significant changes from baseline in these variables. There were no clinically important changes in vital signs in patients treated with Namenda. A comparison of supine and standing vital sign measures for Namenda and placebo in elderly normal subjects indicated that Namenda treatment is not associated with orthostatic changes.

Laboratory Changes: Namenda and placebo groups were compared with respect to (1) mean change from baseline in various serum chemistry, hematology, and urinalysis variables and (2) the incidence of patients meeting criteria for potentially clinically significant changes from baseline in these variables. These analyses revealed no clinically important changes in laboratory test parameters associated with Namenda treatment.

ECG Changes: Namenda and placebo groups were compared with respect to (1) mean change from baseline in var-

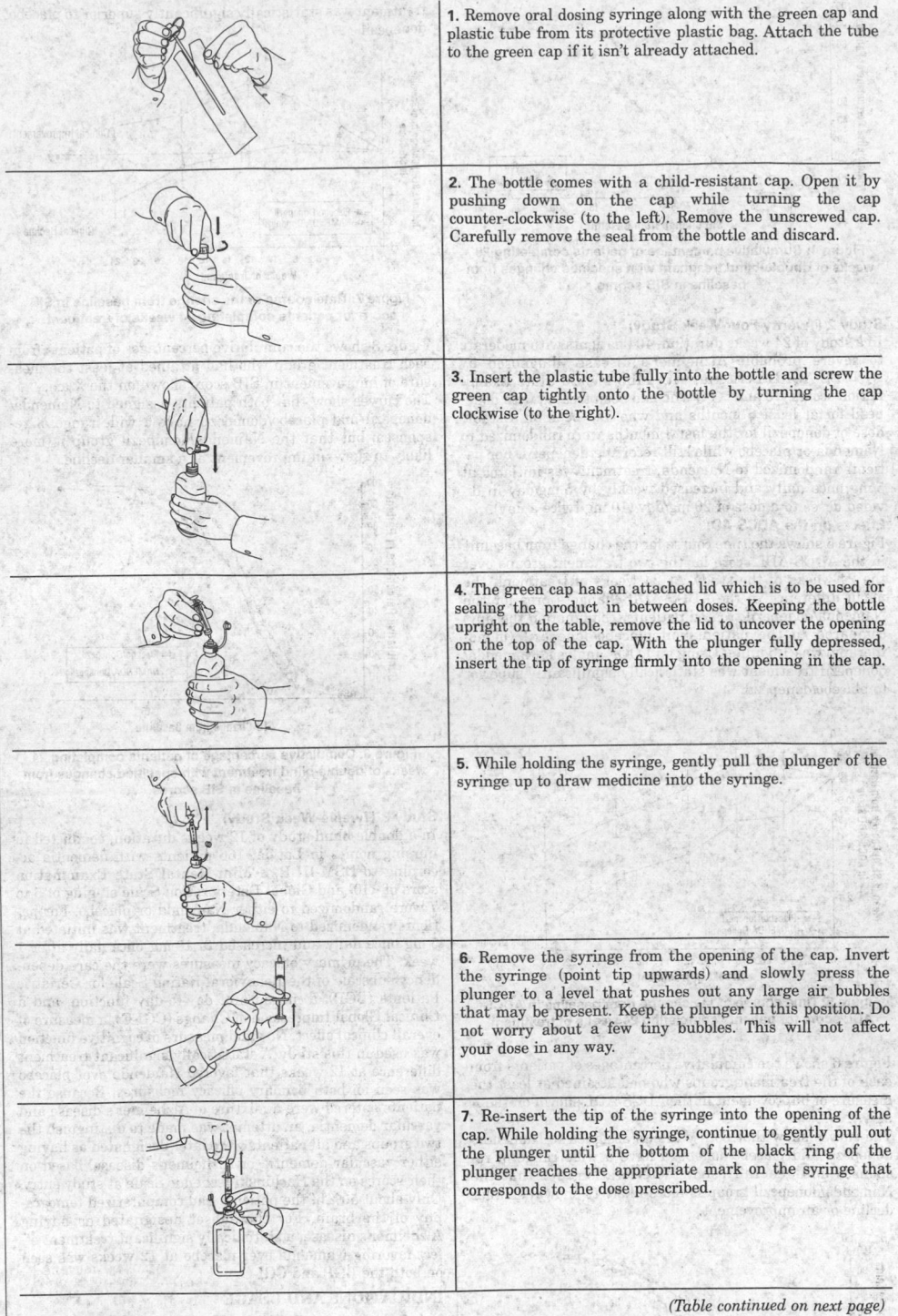

1. Remove oral dosing syringe along with the green cap and plastic tube from its protective plastic bag. Attach the tube to the green cap if it isn't already attached.

2. The bottle comes with a child-resistant cap. Open it by pushing down on the cap while turning the cap counter-clockwise (to the left). Remove the unscrewed cap. Carefully remove the seal from the bottle and discard.

3. Insert the plastic tube fully into the bottle and screw the green cap tightly onto the bottle by turning the cap clockwise (to the right).

4. The green cap has an attached lid which is to be used for sealing the product in between doses. Keeping the bottle upright on the table, remove the lid to uncover the opening on the top of the cap. With the plunger fully depressed, insert the tip of syringe firmly into the opening in the cap.

5. While holding the syringe, gently pull the plunger of the syringe up to draw medicine into the syringe.

6. Remove the syringe from the opening of the cap. Invert the syringe (point tip upwards) and slowly press the plunger to a level that pushes out any large air bubbles that may be present. Keep the plunger in this position. Do not worry about a few tiny bubbles. This will not affect your dose in any way.

7. Re-insert the tip of the syringe into the opening of the cap. While holding the syringe, continue to gently pull out the plunger until the bottom of the black ring of the plunger reaches the appropriate mark on the syringe that corresponds to the dose prescribed.

(Table continued on next page)

ious ECG parameters and (2) the incidence of patients meeting criteria for potentially clinically significant changes from baseline in these variables. These analyses revealed no clinically important changes in ECG parameters associated with Namenda treatment.

Other Adverse Events Observed During Clinical Trials
Namenda has been administered to approximately 1350 patients with dementia, of whom more than 1200 received the maximum recommended dose of 20 mg/day. Patients received Namenda treatment for periods of up to 884 days, with 862 patients receiving at least 24 weeks of treatment and 387 patients receiving 48 weeks or more of treatment. Treatment emergent signs and symptoms that occurred during 8 controlled clinical trials and 4 open-label trials were recorded as adverse events by the clinical investigators using terminology of their own choosing. To provide an overall estimate of the proportion of individuals having similar types of events, the events were grouped into a smaller number of standardized categories using WHO terminology, and event frequencies were calculated across all studies. All adverse events occurring in at least two patients are included, except for those already listed in Table 1, WHO terms too general to be informative, minor symptoms or events unlikely to be drug-caused, e.g., because they are common in the study population. Events are classified by body system and listed using the following definitions: frequent adverse events - those occurring in at least 1/100 patients; infrequent adverse events - those occurring in 1/100 to 1/1000 patients. These adverse events are not necessarily related to Namenda treatment and in most cases were observed at a similar frequency in placebo-treated patients in the controlled studies.

Body as a Whole: *Frequent:* syncope. *Infrequent:* hypothermia, allergic reaction.
Cardiovascular System: *Frequent:* cardiac failure. *Infrequent:* angina pectoris, bradycardia, myocardial infarction, thrombophlebitis, atrial fibrillation, hypotension, cardiac arrest, postural hypotension, pulmonary embolism, pulmonary edema.
Central and Peripheral Nervous System: *Frequent:* transient ischemic attack, cerebrovascular accident, vertigo, ataxia, hypokinesia. *Infrequent:* paresthesia, convulsions, extrapyramidal disorder, hypertonia, tremor, aphasia, hypoesthesia, abnormal coordination, hemiplegia, hyperkinesia, involuntary muscle contractions, stupor, cerebral hemorrhage, neuralgia, ptosis, neuropathy.
Gastrointestinal System: *Infrequent:* gastroenteritis, diverticulitis, gastrointestinal hemorrhage, melena, esophageal ulceration.
Hemic and Lymphatic Disorders: *Frequent:* anemia. *Infrequent:* leukopenia.
Metabolic and Nutritional Disorders: *Frequent:* increased alkaline phosphatase, decreased weight. *Infrequent:* dehydration, hyponatremia, aggravated diabetes mellitus.
Psychiatric Disorders: *Frequent:* aggressive reaction. *Infrequent:* delusion, personality disorder, emotional lability, nervousness, sleep disorder, libido increased, psychosis, amnesia, apathy, paranoid reaction, thinking abnormal, crying abnormal, appetite increased, paroniria, delirium, depersonalization, neurosis, suicide attempt.
Respiratory System: *Frequent:* pneumonia. *Infrequent:* apnea, asthma, hemoptysis.
Skin and Appendages: *Frequent:* rash. *Infrequent:* skin ulceration, pruritus, cellulitis, eczema, dermatitis, erythematous rash, alopecia, urticaria.
Special Senses: *Frequent:* cataract, conjunctivitis. *Infrequent:* macula lutea degeneration, decreased visual acuity, decreased hearing, tinnitus, blepharitis, blurred vision, corneal opacity, glaucoma, conjunctival hemorrhage, eye pain, retinal hemorrhage, xerophthalmia, diplopia, abnormal lacrimation, myopia, retinal detachment.
Urinary System: *Frequent:* frequent micturition. *Infrequent:* dysuria, hematuria, urinary retention.
Events Reported Subsequent to the Marketing of Namenda, both US and Ex-US
Although no causal relationship to memantine treatment has been found, the following adverse events have been reported to be temporally associated with memantine treatment and are not described elsewhere in labeling: aspiration pneumonia, asthenia, atrioventricular block, bone fracture, carpal tunnel syndrome, cerebral infarction, chest pain, cholelithiasis, claudication, colitis, deep venous thrombosis, depressed level of consciousness (including loss of consciousness and rare reports of coma), dyskinesia, dysphagia, encephalopathy, gastritis, gastroesophageal reflux, grand mal convulsions, intracranial hemorrhage, hepatitis (including increased ALT and AST and hepatic failure), hyperglycemia, hyperlipidemia, hypoglycemia, ileus, increased INR, impotence, lethargy, malaise, myoclonus, neu-

(continued)

8. Remove the syringe from the bottle and swallow the **Oral Solution** directly from the syringe. **Do not mix with any other liquid.**

9. After use, reseal the bottle by snapping the attached lid closed.

10. Rinse the empty syringe by inserting the open end of the syringe into a glass of water, pulling the plunger out to draw in water, and pushing the plunger in to remove the water. Repeat several times. Allow the syringe to air dry.

roleptic malignant syndrome, acute pancreatitis, Parkinsonism, acute renal failure (including increased creatinine and renal insufficiency), prolonged QT interval, restlessness, sepsis, Stevens-Johnson syndrome, suicidal ideation, sudden death, supraventricular tachycardia, tachycardia, tardive dyskinesia, thrombocytopenia, and hallucinations (both visual and auditory).

ANIMAL TOXICOLOGY

Memantine induced neuronal lesions (vacuolation and necrosis) in the multipolar and pyramidal cells in cortical layers III and IV of the posterior cingulate and retrosplenial neocortices in rats, similar to those which are known to occur in rodents administered other NMDA receptor antagonists. Lesions were seen after a single dose of memantine. In a study in which rats were given daily oral doses of memantine for 14 days, the no-effect dose for neuronal necrosis was 6 times the maximum recommended human dose on a mg/m² basis. In a juvenile toxicology study conducted in rats, treatment with memantine was associated with degenerative changes in the anterior ventral thalamus and lateral mammillary bodies. The relevance of these changes to humans is unknown.

DRUG ABUSE AND DEPENDENCE

Controlled Substance Class: Memantine HCl is not a controlled substance.
Physical and Psychological Dependence: Memantine HCl is a low to moderate affinity uncompetitive NMDA antagonist that did not produce any evidence of drug-seeking behavior or withdrawal symptoms upon discontinuation in 2,504 patients who participated in clinical trials at therapeutic doses. Post marketing data, outside the U.S., retrospectively collected, has provided no evidence of drug abuse or dependence.

OVERDOSAGE

Signs and symptoms associated with memantine overdosage in clinical trials and from worldwide marketing experience include agitation, confusion, ECG changes, loss of consciousness, psychosis, restlessness, slowed movement, somnolence, stupor, unsteady gait, visual hallucinations, vertigo, vomiting, and weakness. The largest known ingestion of memantine worldwide was 2.0 grams in a patient who took memantine in conjunction with unspecified antidiabetic medications. The patient experienced coma, diplopia, and agitation, but subsequently recovered.
Because strategies for the management of overdose are continually evolving, it is advisable to contact a poison control center to determine the latest recommendations for the management of an overdose of any drug.
As in any cases of overdose, general supportive measures should be utilized, and treatment should be symptomatic. Elimination of memantine can be enhanced by acidification of urine.

DOSAGE AND ADMINISTRATION

The dosage of Namenda (memantine hydrochloride) shown to be effective in controlled clinical trials is 20 mg/day. The recommended starting dose of Namenda is 5 mg once daily. The recommended target dose is 20 mg/day. The dose should be increased in 5 mg increments to 10 mg/day (5 mg twice a day), 15 mg/day (5 mg and 10 mg as separate doses), and 20 mg/day (10 mg twice a day). The minimum recommended interval between dose increases is one week.

Namenda can be taken with or without food.
Patients/caregivers should be instructed on how to use the Namenda Oral Solution dosing device. They should be made aware of the patient instruction sheet that is enclosed with the product. Patients/caregivers should be instructed to address any questions on the usage of the solution to their physician or pharmacist.
Doses in Special Populations
A target dose of 5 mg BID is recommended in patients with severe renal impairment (creatinine clearance of 5–29 mL/min based on the Cockroft-Gault equation):
For males: CLcr = [140-age (years)] • Weight (kg)/[72 • serum creatinine (mg/dL)]
For females: CLcr = 0.85 • [140-age (years)] • Weight (kg)/[72 • serum creatinine (mg/dL)]
HOW SUPPLIED
5 mg Tablet:

Bottle of 60	NDC #0456-3205-60
10 × 10 Unit Dose	NDC #0456-3205-63

The capsule-shaped, film-coated tablets are tan, with the strength (5) debossed on one side and FL on the other.
10 mg Tablet:

Bottle of 60	NDC #0456-3210-60
10 × 10 Unit Dose	NDC #0456-3210-63

The capsule-shaped, film-coated tablets are gray, with the strength (10) debossed on one side and FL on the other.
Titration Pak:
PVC/Aluminum Blister package containing 49 tablets. 28 × 5 mg and 21 × 10 mg tablets.
NDC #0456-3200-14
The 5 mg capsule-shaped, film-coated tablets are tan, with the strength (5) debossed on one side and FL on the other. The 10 mg capsule-shaped, film-coated tablets are gray, with the strength (10) debossed on one side and FL on the other.
Oral Solution:
The dosage recommendations for oral solution are the same as those for tablets. The oral solution is clear, alcohol-free, sugar-free, and peppermint flavored.
2 mg/mL Oral Solution (10 mg = 5 mL)
12 fl. oz. (360 mL) bottle   NDC #0456-3202-12
Store at 25°C (77°F); excursions permitted to 15-30°C (59-86°F) [see USP Controlled Room Temperature].
Forest Pharmaceuticals, Inc.
Subsidiary of Forest Laboratories, Inc.
St. Louis, MO 63045
Licensed from Merz Pharmaceuticals GmbH
Rev. 04/07
© 2007 Forest Laboratories, Inc.

PATIENT INSTRUCTIONS FOR NAMENDA® Oral Solution

Follow the directions below to use your Namenda® Oral Solution dosing device.
IMPORTANT: Read these instructions before using Namenda® Oral Solution.
[See table on previous page and above]
Shown in Product Identification Guide, page 309

Genentech, Inc.
A Member of the Roche Group
1 DNA WAY
SOUTH SAN FRANCISCO, CA 94080-4990

Contact:
Genentech, Inc.
A Member of the Roche Group
1 DNA Way
South San Francisco, CA 94080-4990
(650) 225-1000
www.gene.com
For Medical Information
Contact
1-800-821-8590
www.gene.com/gene/contact/
For Customer Service
Contact
1-800-551-2231
For Reimbursement Support
Contact
1-866-422-2377

ACTEMRA®   Rx
[AC-TEM-RA]
(tocilizumab)
Injection, for intravenous infusion

HIGHLIGHTS OF PRESCRIBING INFORMATION
These highlights do not include all the information needed to use ACTEMRA safely and effectively. See full prescribing information for ACTEMRA.
ACTEMRA® (tocilizumab)
Injection, for intravenous infusion
Initial U.S. Approval: 2010

WARNING: RISK OF SERIOUS INFECTIONS
See full prescribing information for complete boxed warning.
- **Serious infections leading to hospitalization or death including tuberculosis (TB), bacterial, invasive fungal, viral, and other opportunistic infections have occurred in patients receiving ACTEMRA. (5.1)**
- **If a serious infection develops, interrupt ACTEMRA until the infection is controlled. (5.1)**
- **Perform test for latent TB; if positive, start treatment for TB prior to starting ACTEMRA. (5.1)**
- **Monitor all patients for active TB during treatment, even if initial latent TB test is negative. (5.1)**

INDICATIONS AND USAGE
ACTEMRA® (tocilizumab) is an interleukin-6 (IL-6) receptor inhibitor indicated for treatment of:
Rheumatoid Arthritis (1)
- Adult patients with moderately to severely active rheumatoid arthritis who have had an inadequate response to one or more TNF antagonist therapies.

DOSAGE AND ADMINISTRATION
Rheumatoid Arthritis (2.1)
ACTEMRA may be used alone or in combination with methotrexate or other DMARDs.

Recommended Adult Dosage Every 4 Weeks

Patients who have had an inadequate response to one or more TNF antagonists	When used in combination with DMARDs or as monotherapy the recommended starting dose is 4 mg/kg followed by an increase to 8 mg/kg based on clinical response.

- It is recommended that ACTEMRA not be initiated in patients with an absolute neutrophil count (ANC) below 2000/mm³, platelet count below 100,000/mm³, or who have ALT or AST above 1.5 times the upper limit of normal (ULN). (2.1, 5.3)
- ACTEMRA doses exceeding 800 mg per infusion are not recommended. (2.1, 12.3)
Administration (2.2)
- Dilute to 100 mL in 0.9% Sodium Chloride for intravenous infusion using aseptic technique.
- Administer as a single intravenous drip infusion over 1 hour; do not administer as bolus or push.
Dose Modifications (2.3)
- Recommended for management of certain dose-related laboratory changes including elevated liver enzymes, neutropenia, and thrombocytopenia.

DOSAGE FORMS AND STRENGTHS
Single-use vials of ACTEMRA (20 mg/mL):
- 80 mg/4 mL (3)
- 200 mg/10 mL (3)
- 400 mg/20 mL (3)

CONTRAINDICATIONS
- None (4)

WARNINGS AND PRECAUTIONS
- Serious Infections—do not administer ACTEMRA during an active infection, including localized infections. If a serious infection develops, interrupt ACTEMRA until the infection is controlled. (5.1)
- Gastrointestinal (GI) perforation—use with caution in patients who may be at increased risk. (5.2)
- Laboratory monitoring—recommended due to potential consequences of treatment-related changes in neutrophils, platelets, lipids, and liver function tests. (2.3, 5.3)
- Anaphylaxis or serious hypersensitivity reactions have occurred. (5.5)
- Live vaccines—should not be given with ACTEMRA. (5.8, 7.3)

ADVERSE REACTIONS
Most common adverse reactions (incidence ≥ 5%): upper respiratory tract infections, nasopharyngitis, headache, hypertension, increased ALT. (6.1)
To report SUSPECTED ADVERSE REACTIONS, contact Genentech at 1-888-835-2555 or FDA at 1-800-FDA-1088 or www.fda.gov/medwatch

USE IN SPECIFIC POPULATIONS
- **Pregnancy:** Based on animal data, may cause fetal harm. Pregnancy registry available. (8.1)

See 17 for PATIENT COUNSELING INFORMATION and the FDA-approved Medication Guide

               Issued: 01/2010

FULL PRESCRIBING INFORMATION: CONTENTS*
WARNING: RISK OF SERIOUS INFECTIONS
1   **INDICATIONS AND USAGE**
2   **DOSAGE AND ADMINISTRATION**
    2.1   Rheumatoid Arthritis
    2.2   General Considerations for Administration
    2.3   Dosage Modifications
3   **DOSAGE FORMS AND STRENGTHS**
4   **CONTRAINDICATIONS**
5   **WARNINGS AND PRECAUTIONS**
    5.1   Serious Infections
    5.2   Gastrointestinal Perforations
    5.3   Laboratory Parameters
    5.4   Immunosuppression
    5.5   Hypersensitivity Reactions
    5.6   Demyelinating Disorders
    5.7   Active Hepatic Disease and Hepatic Impairment
    5.8   Vaccinations
6   **ADVERSE REACTIONS**
    6.1   Clinical Trials Experience
7   **DRUG INTERACTIONS**
    7.1   Other Drugs for Treatment of Rheumatoid Arthritis
    7.2   Interactions with CYP450 Substrates
    7.3   Live Vaccines
8   **USE IN SPECIFIC POPULATIONS**
    8.1   Pregnancy
    8.3   Nursing Mothers
    8.4   Pediatric Use
    8.5   Geriatric Use
    8.6   Hepatic Impairment
    8.7   Renal Impairment
9   **DRUG ABUSE AND DEPENDENCE**
10   **OVERDOSAGE**
11   **DESCRIPTION**
12   **CLINICAL PHARMACOLOGY**
    12.1   Mechanism of Action
    12.2   Pharmacodynamics
    12.3   Pharmacokinetics
13   **NONCLINICAL TOXICOLOGY**
    13.1   Carcinogenesis, Mutagenesis, Impairment of Fertility
14   **CLINICAL STUDIES**
16   **HOW SUPPLIED/STORAGE AND HANDLING**
17   **PATIENT COUNSELING INFORMATION**
    17.1   Patient Counseling
    17.2   Medication Guide
* Sections or subsections omitted from the full prescribing information are not listed

---

FULL PRESCRIBING INFORMATION

WARNING: RISK OF SERIOUS INFECTIONS
Patients treated with ACTEMRA are at increased risk for developing serious infections that may lead to hospitalization or death *[see Warnings and Precautions (5.1), Adverse Reactions (6.1)]*. Most patients who developed these infections were taking concomitant immunosuppressants such as methotrexate or corticosteroids.
If a serious infection develops, interrupt ACTEMRA until the infection is controlled.
Reported infections include:
- Active tuberculosis, which may present with pulmonary or extrapulmonary disease. Patients should be tested for latent tuberculosis before ACTEMRA use and during therapy. Treatment for latent infection should be initiated prior to ACTEMRA use.
- Invasive fungal infections, including candidiasis, aspergillosis, and pneumocystis. Patients with invasive fungal infections may present with disseminated, rather than localized, disease.
- Bacterial, viral and other infections due to opportunistic pathogens.

The risks and benefits of treatment with ACTEMRA should be carefully considered prior to initiating therapy in patients with chronic or recurrent infection.
Patients should be closely monitored for the development of signs and symptoms of infection during and after treatment with ACTEMRA, including the possible development of tuberculosis in patients who tested negative for latent tuberculosis infection prior to initiating therapy *[see Warnings and Precautions (5.1)]*.

---

1   INDICATIONS AND USAGE
ACTEMRA® (tocilizumab) is indicated for the treatment of adult patients with moderately to severely active rheumatoid arthritis who have had an inadequate response to one or more TNF antagonist therapies.

2   DOSAGE AND ADMINISTRATION
2.1   Rheumatoid Arthritis
ACTEMRA may be used as monotherapy or concomitantly with methotrexate or other DMARDs. The recommended dose of ACTEMRA for adult patients given once every 4 weeks as a 60-minute single intravenous drip infusion is:

Recommended Adult Dosage Every 4 Weeks

Patients who have had an inadequate response to one or more TNF antagonists	When used in combination with DMARDs or as monotherapy the recommended starting dose is 4 mg/kg followed by an increase to 8 mg/kg based on clinical response.

- ACTEMRA has not been studied and its use should be avoided in combination with biological DMARDs such as TNF antagonists, IL-1R antagonists, anti-CD20 monoclonal antibodies and selective co-stimulation modulators because of the possibility of increased immunosuppression and increased risk of infection.
- It is recommended that ACTEMRA not be initiated in patients with an absolute neutrophil count (ANC) below 2000/mm³, platelet count below 100,000/mm³, or who have ALT or AST above 1.5 times the upper limit of normal (ULN).
- Reduction of dose from 8 mg/kg to 4 mg/kg is recommended for management of certain dose-related laboratory changes including elevated liver enzymes, neutropenia, and thrombocytopenia *[see Dosage and Administration (2.3), Warnings and Precautions (5.3), and Adverse Reactions (6.1)]*.
- Doses exceeding 800 mg per infusion are not recommended *[see Clinical Pharmacology (12.3)]*.
2.2   General Considerations for Administration
ACTEMRA for intravenous infusion should be diluted to 100 mL by a healthcare professional using aseptic technique as follows:
1. From a 100 mL infusion bag or bottle, withdraw a volume of 0.9% Sodium Chloride Injection, USP, equal to the volume of the ACTEMRA solution required for the patient's dose.
2. Slowly add ACTEMRA for intravenous infusion from each vial into the infusion bag or bottle. To mix the solution, gently invert the bag to avoid foaming.
3. Parenteral drug products should be inspected visually for particulate matter and discoloration prior to administration, whenever solution and container permit. If particulates and discolorations are noted, the product should not be used. Fully diluted ACTEMRA solutions are compatible with polypropylene, polyethylene and polyvinyl chloride infusion bags and polypropylene, polyethylene and glass infusion bottles.
4. The fully diluted ACTEMRA solutions for infusion may be stored at 2°-8°C (36°-46°F) or room temperature for up to 24 hours and should be protected from light. ACTEMRA solutions do not contain preservatives; therefore, unused product remaining in the vials should not be used.

---

5. Allow the fully diluted ACTEMRA solution to reach room temperature prior to infusion.

6. The infusion should be administered over 60 minutes, and must be administered with an infusion set. Do not administer as an intravenous push or bolus.

7. ACTEMRA should not be infused concomitantly in the same intravenous line with other drugs. No physical or biochemical compatibility studies have been conducted to evaluate the co-administration of ACTEMRA with other drugs.

2.3   Dosage Modifications

ACTEMRA treatment should be interrupted if a patient develops a serious infection until the infection is controlled. [See table at right]

3   DOSAGE FORMS AND STRENGTHS

Single-use vials of ACTEMRA (20 mg/mL):
- 80 mg/4 mL
- 200 mg/10 mL
- 400 mg/20 mL

4   CONTRAINDICATIONS

None

5   WARNINGS AND PRECAUTIONS

5.1   Serious Infections

Serious and sometimes fatal infections due to bacterial, mycobacterial, invasive fungal, viral, protozoal, or other opportunistic pathogens have been reported in patients receiving immunosuppressive agents including ACTEMRA for rheumatoid arthritis. The most common serious infections included pneumonia, urinary tract infection, cellulitis, herpes zoster, gastroenteritis, diverticulitis, sepsis and bacterial arthritis [see Adverse Reactions (6.1)]. Among opportunistic infections, tuberculosis, cryptococcus, aspergillosis, candidiasis, and pneumocystosis were reported with ACTEMRA. Other serious infections, not reported in clinical studies, may also occur (e.g., histoplasmosis, coccidioidomycosis, listeriosis). Patients have presented with disseminated rather than localized disease, and were often taking concomitant immunosuppressants such as methotrexate or corticosteroids which in addition to rheumatoid arthritis may predispose them to infections.

ACTEMRA should not be administered in patients with an active infection, including localized infections. The risks and benefits of treatment should be considered prior to initiating ACTEMRA in patients:
- with chronic or recurrent infection;
- who have been exposed to tuberculosis;
- with a history of serious or an opportunistic infection;
- who have resided or traveled in areas of endemic tuberculosis or endemic mycoses; or
- with underlying conditions that may predispose them to infection.

Patients should be closely monitored for the development of signs and symptoms of infection during and after treatment with ACTEMRA, as signs and symptoms of acute inflammation may be lessened due to suppression of the acute phase reactants [see Dosage and Administration (2.3), Adverse Reactions (6.1), and Patient Counseling Information (17.1)].

ACTEMRA should be interrupted if a patient develops a serious infection, an opportunistic infection, or sepsis. A patient who develops a new infection during treatment with ACTEMRA should undergo a prompt and complete diagnostic workup appropriate for an immunocompromised patient, appropriate antimicrobial therapy should be initiated, and the patient should be closely monitored.

Tuberculosis

Patients should be evaluated for tuberculosis risk factors and tested for latent infection prior to initiating ACTEMRA. Anti-tuberculosis therapy should also be considered prior to initiation of ACTEMRA in patients with a past history of latent or active tuberculosis in whom an adequate course of treatment cannot be confirmed, and for patients with a negative test for latent tuberculosis but having risk factors for tuberculosis infection. Consultation with a physician with expertise in the treatment of tuberculosis is recommended to aid in the decision whether initiating anti-tuberculosis therapy is appropriate for an individual patient.

Patients should be closely monitored for the development of signs and symptoms of tuberculosis including patients who tested negative for latent tuberculosis infection prior to initiating therapy.

It is recommended that patients be screened for latent tuberculosis infection prior to starting ACTEMRA. The incidence of tuberculosis in worldwide clinical development programs is 0.1%. Patients with latent tuberculosis should be treated with standard antimycobacterial therapy before initiating ACTEMRA.

Viral Reactivation

Viral reactivation has been reported with immunosuppressive biologic therapies and cases of herpes zoster exacerbation were observed in clinical studies with ACTEMRA. No

Liver Enzyme Abnormalities [see Warnings and Precautions (5.3)]:

Lab Value	Recommendation
> 1 to 3× ULN	Dose modify concomitant DMARDs if appropriate For persistent increases in this range, reduce ACTEMRA dose to 4 mg/kg or interrupt ACTEMRA until ALT/AST have normalized
> 3 to 5× ULN (confirmed by repeat testing)	Interrupt ACTEMRA dosing until < 3× ULN and follow recommendations above for >1 to 3× ULN For persistent increases > 3× ULN, discontinue ACTEMRA
> 5× ULN	Discontinue ACTEMRA

Low Absolute Neutrophil Count (ANC) [see Warnings and Precautions (5.3)]:

Lab Value (cells/mm³)	Recommendation
ANC > 1000	Maintain dose
ANC 500 to 1000	Interrupt ACTEMRA dosing When ANC > 1000 cells/mm³ resume ACTEMRA at 4 mg/kg and increase to 8 mg/kg as clinically appropriate
ANC < 500	Discontinue ACTEMRA

Low Platelet Count [see Warnings and Precautions (5.3)]:

Lab Value (cells/mm³)	Recommendation
50,000 to 100,000	Interrupt ACTEMRA dosing When platelet count is > 100,000 cells/mm³ resume ACTEMRA at 4 mg/kg and increase to 8 mg/kg as clinically appropriate
< 50,000	Discontinue ACTEMRA

cases of Hepatitis B reactivation were observed in the trials; however patients who screened positive for hepatitis were excluded.

5.2   Gastrointestinal Perforations

Events of gastrointestinal perforation have been reported in clinical trials, primarily as complications of diverticulitis. ACTEMRA should be used with caution in patients who may be at increased risk for gastrointestinal perforation. Patients presenting with new onset abdominal symptoms should be evaluated promptly for early identification of gastrointestinal perforation [see Adverse Reactions (6.1)].

5.3   Laboratory Parameters

Neutrophils

Treatment with ACTEMRA was associated with a higher incidence of neutropenia. Infections have been uncommonly reported in association with treatment-related neutropenia in long-term extension studies and postmarketing clinical experience.

–It is not recommended to initiate ACTEMRA treatment in patients with a low neutrophil count i.e., absolute neutrophil count (ANC) <2000/mm³. In patients who develop an absolute neutrophil count <500/mm³ treatment is not recommended.

–Neutrophils should be monitored every 4 to 8 weeks [see Clinical Pharmacology (12.2)]. For recommended modifications based on ANC results see Dosage and Administration (2.3).

Platelets

Treatment with ACTEMRA was associated with a reduction in platelet counts. Treatment-related reduction in platelets was not associated with serious bleeding events in clinical trials [see Adverse Reactions (6.1)].

–It is not recommended to initiate ACTEMRA treatment in patients with a platelet count below 100,000/mm³. In patients who develop a platelet count <50,000/mm³ treatment is not recommended.

–Platelets should be monitored every 4 to 8 weeks. For recommended modifications based on platelet counts see Dosage and Administration (2.3).

Liver Function Tests

Treatment with ACTEMRA was associated with a higher incidence of transaminase elevations. These elevations did not result in apparent permanent or clinically evident hepatic injury in clinical trials [see Adverse Reactions (6.1)]. Increased frequency and magnitude of these elevations was observed when potentially hepatotoxic drugs (e.g., MTX) were used in combination with ACTEMRA.

In one case, a patient who had received ACTEMRA 8 mg/kg monotherapy without elevations in transaminases experienced elevation in AST to above 10× ULN and elevation in ALT to above 16× ULN when MTX was initiated in combination with ACTEMRA. Transaminases normalized when both treatments were held, but elevations recurred when MTX and ACTEMRA were restarted at lower doses. Elevations resolved when MTX and ACTEMRA were discontinued.

–It is not recommended to initiate ACTEMRA treatment in patients with elevated transaminases ALT or AST > 1.5× ULN. In patients who develop elevated ALT or AST > 5× ULN treatment is not recommended.

–ALT and AST levels should be monitored every 4 to 8 weeks. When clinically indicated, other liver function tests such as bilirubin should be considered. For recommended modifications based on transaminases see Dosage and Administration (2.3).

Lipids

Treatment with ACTEMRA was associated with increases in lipid parameters such as total cholesterol, triglycerides, LDL cholesterol, and/or HDL cholesterol [see Adverse Reactions (6.1)].

–Assessment of lipid parameters should be performed approximately 4 to 8 weeks following initiation of ACTEMRA therapy, then at approximately 6 month intervals.

–Patients should be managed according to clinical guidelines [e.g., National Cholesterol Educational Program (NCEP)] for the management of hyperlipidemia.

5.4   Immunosuppression

The impact of treatment with ACTEMRA on the development of malignancies is not known but malignancies were observed in clinical studies [see Adverse Reactions (6.1)]. ACTEMRA is an immunosuppressant, and treatment with immunosuppressants may result in an increased risk of malignancies.

5.5   Hypersensitivity Reactions

Serious hypersensitivity reactions, including anaphylaxis, have been reported in association with infusion of ACTEMRA [see Adverse Reactions (6.1)]. Appropriate medical treatment should be available for immediate use in the event of an anaphylactic reaction during administration of ACTEMRA.

5.6   Demyelinating Disorders

The impact of treatment with ACTEMRA on demyelinating disorders is not known, but multiple sclerosis and chronic inflammatory demyelinating polyneuropathy were reported rarely in clinical studies. Patients should be closely monitored for signs and symptoms potentially indicative of demyelinating disorders. Prescribers should exercise caution in considering the use of ACTEMRA in patients with preexisting or recent onset demyelinating disorders.

5.7   Active Hepatic Disease and Hepatic Impairment

Treatment with ACTEMRA is not recommended in patients with active hepatic disease or hepatic impairment [see Adverse Reactions (6.1), Use in Specific Populations (8.6)].

5.8   Vaccinations

Live vaccines should not be given concurrently with ACTEMRA as clinical safety has not been established. No data are available on the secondary transmission of infection from persons receiving live vaccines to patients receiving ACTEMRA. No data are available on the effectiveness of vaccination in patients receiving ACTEMRA. Because IL-6 inhibition may interfere with the normal immune response to new antigens, patients should be brought up to date on all recommended vaccinations, except for live vaccines, prior to initiation of therapy with ACTEMRA.

6 ADVERSE REACTIONS

Because clinical studies are conducted under widely varying conditions, adverse reaction rates observed in the clinical studies of a drug cannot be directly compared to rates in the clinical studies of another drug and may not predict the rates observed in a broader patient population in clinical practice.

The ACTEMRA data described below includes 5 double-blind, controlled, multicenter studies. In these studies, patients received doses of ACTEMRA 8 mg/kg monotherapy (288 patients), ACTEMRA 8 mg/kg in combination with DMARDs (including methotrexate) (1582 patients), or ACTEMRA 4 mg/kg in combination with methotrexate (774 patients).

The all exposure population includes all patients in registration studies who received at least one dose of ACTEMRA. Of the 4009 patients in this population, 3577 received treatment for at least 6 months, 3296 for at least one year; 2806 received treatment for at least 2 years and 1222 for 3 years. All patients in these studies had moderately to severely active rheumatoid arthritis. The study population had a mean age of 52 years, 82% were female and 74% were Caucasian.

6.1 Clinical Trials Experience

The most common serious adverse reactions were serious infections *[see Warnings and Precautions (5.1)]*. The most commonly reported adverse reactions in controlled studies up to 6 months (occurring in ≥ 5% of patients treated with ACTEMRA monotherapy or in combination with DMARDs) were upper respiratory tract infections, nasopharyngitis, headache, hypertension and increased ALT.

The proportion of patients who discontinued treatment due to any adverse reactions during the double-blind, placebo-controlled studies was 5% for patients taking ACTEMRA and 3% for placebo-treated patients. The most common adverse reactions that required discontinuation of ACTEMRA were increased hepatic transaminase values (per protocol requirement) and serious infections.

Overall Infections

In the 6-month, controlled clinical studies, the rate of infections in the ACTEMRA monotherapy group was 119 events per 100 patient-years and was similar in the methotrexate monotherapy group. The rate of infections in the 4 mg/kg and 8 mg/kg ACTEMRA plus DMARD group was 133 and 127 events per 100 patient-years, respectively, compared to 112 events per 100 patient-years in the placebo plus DMARD group. The most commonly reported infections (5% to 8% of patients) were upper respiratory tract infections and nasopharyngitis.

The overall rate of infections with ACTEMRA in the all exposure population was 108 events per 100 patient-years.

Serious Infections

In the 6-month, controlled clinical studies, the rate of serious infections in the ACTEMRA monotherapy group was 3.6 per 100 patient-years compared to 1.5 per 100 patient-years in the methotrexate group. The rate of serious infections in the 4 mg/kg and 8 mg/kg ACTEMRA plus DMARD group was 4.4 and 5.3 events per 100 patient-years, respectively, compared to 3.9 events per 100 patient-years in the placebo plus DMARD group.

In the all-exposure population, the overall rate of serious infections was 4.7 events per 100 patient-years. The most common serious infections included pneumonia, urinary tract infection, cellulitis, herpes zoster, gastroenteritis, diverticulitis, sepsis and bacterial arthritis. The overall rate of fatal serious infections was 0.13 per 100 patient-years. Cases of opportunistic infections have been reported *[see Warnings and Precautions (5.1)]*.

Gastrointestinal Perforations

During the 6-month, controlled clinical trials, the overall rate of gastrointestinal perforation was 0.26 events per 100 patient-years with ACTEMRA therapy.

In the all-exposure population, the overall rate of gastrointestinal perforation was 0.28 events per 100 patient-years. Reports of gastrointestinal perforation were primarily reported as complications of diverticulitis including generalized purulent peritonitis, lower GI perforation, fistula and abscess. Most patients who developed gastrointestinal perforations were taking concomitant nonsteroidal anti-inflammatory medications (NSAIDs), corticosteroids, or methotrexate *[see Warnings and Precautions (5.2)]*. The relative contribution of these concomitant medications versus ACTEMRA to the development of GI perforations is not known.

Infusion Reactions

In the 6-month, controlled clinical studies, adverse events associated with the infusion (occurring during or within 24 hours of the start of infusion) were reported in 8% and 7% of patients in the 4 mg/kg and 8 mg/kg ACTEMRA plus DMARD group, respectively, compared to 5% of patients in the placebo plus DMARD group. The most frequently reported event on the 4 mg/kg and 8 mg/kg dose during the infusion was hypertension (1% for both doses), while the most frequently reported event occurring within 24 hours of finishing an infusion were headache (1% for both doses) and skin reactions (1% for both doses), including rash, pruritus and urticaria. These events were not treatment limiting.

Clinically significant hypersensitivity reactions (e.g., anaphylactoid and anaphylactic reactions) associated with ACTEMRA and requiring treatment discontinuation were reported 0.1% (3/2644) in the 6-month, controlled trials and in 0.2% (9/4009) in the all-exposure population. These reactions were generally observed during the second to fourth infusion of ACTEMRA. Appropriate medical treatment should be available for immediate use in the event of a serious hypersensitivity reaction *[see Warnings and Precautions (5.5)]*.

Laboratory Tests

Neutrophils

In the 6-month, controlled clinical studies, decreases in neutrophil counts below 1000/mm^3 occurred in 1.8% and 3.4% of patients in the 4 mg/kg and 8 mg/kg ACTEMRA plus DMARD group, respectively, compared to 0.1% of patients in the placebo plus DMARD group. Approximately half of the instances of ANC below 1000/mm^3 occurred within 8 weeks of starting therapy. Decreases in neutrophil counts below 500/mm^3 occurred in 0.4% and 0.3% of patients in the 4 mg/kg and 8 mg/kg ACTEMRA plus DMARD, respectively, compared to 0.1% of patients in the placebo plus DMARD group. There was no clear relationship between decreases in neutrophils below 1000/mm^3 and the occurrence of serious infections.

In the all-exposure population, the pattern and incidence of decreases in neutrophil counts remained consistent with what was seen in the 6-month controlled clinical studies *[see Warnings and Precautions (5.3)]*.

Platelets

In the 6-month, controlled clinical studies, decreases in platelet counts below 100,000/mm^3 occurred in 1.3% and 1.7% of patients on 4 mg/kg and 8 mg/kg ACTEMRA plus DMARD, respectively, compared to 0.5% of patients on placebo plus DMARD, without associated bleeding events.

In the all-exposure population, the pattern and incidence of decreases in platelet counts remained consistent with what was seen in the 6-month controlled clinical studies *[see Warnings and Precautions (5.3)]*.

Liver Function Tests

Liver enzyme abnormalities are summarized in Table 1. In patients experiencing liver enzyme elevation, modification of treatment regimen, such as reduction in the dose of concomitant DMARD, interruption of ACTEMRA, or reduction in ACTEMRA dose, resulted in decrease or normalization of liver enzymes *[see Dosage and Administration (2.3)]*. These elevations were not associated with clinically relevant increases in direct bilirubin, nor were they associated with clinical evidence of hepatitis or hepatic insufficiency *[see Warnings and Precautions (5.3)]*.

[See table 1 at bottom left]

Table 1 Incidence of Liver Enzyme Abnormalities in the 6-Month Controlled Period of Studies I-V*

	ACTEMRA 8 mg/kg MONOTHERAPY N = 288 (%)	Methotrexate N = 284 (%)	ACTEMRA 4 mg/kg + DMARDs N = 774 (%)	ACTEMRA 8 mg/kg + DMARDs N = 1582 (%)	Placebo + DMARDs N = 1170 (%)
AST (U/L)					
> ULN to 3× ULN	22	26	34	41	17
> 3× ULN to 5× ULN	0.3	2	1	2	0.3
> 5× ULN	0.7	0.4	0.1	0.2	< 0.1
ALT (U/L)					
> ULN to 3× ULN	36	33	45	48	23
> 3× ULN to 5× ULN	1	4	5	5	1
> 5× ULN	0.7	1	1.3	1.5	0.3

ULN = Upper Limit of Normal

*For a description of these studies, see Section 14, Clinical Studies

Lipids

Elevations in lipid parameters (total cholesterol, LDL, HDL, triglycerides) were first assessed at 6 weeks following initiation of ACTEMRA in the controlled 6-month clinical trials. Increases were observed at this time point and remained stable thereafter. Increases in triglycerides to levels above 500 mg/dL were rarely observed. Changes in other lipid parameters from baseline to week 24 were evaluated and are summarized below:

–Mean LDL increased by 13 mg/dL in the TCZ 4 mg/kg+DMARD arm, 20 mg/dL in the TCZ 8 mg/kg+DMARD, and 25 mg/dL in TCZ 8 mg/kg monotherapy.

–Mean HDL increased by 3 mg/dL in the TCZ 4 mg/kg+DMARD arm, 5 mg/dL in the TCZ 8 mg/kg+DMARD, and 4 mg/dL in TCZ 8 mg/kg monotherapy.

–Mean LDL/HDL ratio increased by an average of 0.14 in the TCZ 4 mg/kg+DMARD arm, 0.15 in the TCZ 8 mg/kg+DMARD, and 0.26 in TCZ 8 mg/kg monotherapy.

–ApoB/ApoA1 ratios were essentially unchanged in ACTEMRA-treated patients.

Elevated lipids responded to lipid lowering agents.

Immunogenicity

In the 6-month, controlled clinical studies, a total of 2876 patients have been tested for anti-tocilizumab antibodies. Forty-six patients (2%) developed positive anti-tocilizumab antibodies, of whom 5 had an associated, medically significant, hypersensitivity reaction leading to withdrawal. Thirty patients (1%) developed neutralizing antibodies.

The data reflect the percentage of patients whose test results were positive for antibodies to tocilizumab in specific assays. The observed incidence of antibody positivity in an assay is highly dependent on several factors, including assay sensitivity and specificity, assay methodology, sample handling, timing of sample collection, concomitant medication, and underlying disease. For these reasons, comparison of the incidence of antibodies to tocilizumab with the incidence of antibodies to other products may be misleading.

Malignancies

During the 6-month, controlled period of the studies, 15 malignancies were diagnosed in patients receiving ACTEMRA, compared to 8 malignancies in patients in the control groups. Exposure-adjusted incidence was similar in the ACTEMRA groups (1.32 events per 100 patient-years) and in the placebo plus DMARD group (1.37 events per 100 patient-years).

In the all-exposure population, the rate of malignancies remained consistent (1.10 events per 100 patient-years) with the rate observed in the 6-month, controlled period *[see Warnings and Precautions (5.4)]*.

Other Adverse Reactions

Adverse reactions occurring in 2% or more of patients on 4 or 8 mg/kg ACTEMRA plus DMARD and at least 1% greater than that observed in patients on placebo plus DMARD are summarized in Table 2.

[See table 2 at top of next page]

7 DRUG INTERACTIONS

7.1 Other Drugs for Treatment of Rheumatoid Arthritis

Population pharmacokinetic analyses did not detect any effect of methotrexate, non-steroidal anti-inflammatory drugs or corticosteroids on tocilizumab clearance.

Concomitant administration of a single dose of 10 mg/kg ACTEMRA with 10-25 mg MTX once weekly had no clinically significant effect on MTX exposure.

ACTEMRA has not been studied in combination with biological DMARDs such as TNF antagonists *[see Dosage and Administration (2.1)]*.

7.2 Interactions with CYP450 Substrates

Cytochrome P450s in the liver are down-regulated by infection and inflammation stimuli including cytokines such as IL-6. Inhibition of IL-6 signaling in RA patients treated with tocilizumab may restore CYP450 activities to higher levels than those in the absence of tocilizumab leading to increased metabolism of drugs that are CYP450 substrates. In vitro studies showed that tocilizumab has the potential to affect expression of multiple CYP enzymes including CYP1A2, CYP2B6, CYP2C9, CYP2C19, CYP2D6 and CYP3A4. Its effects on CYP2C8 or transporters is unknown.

In vivo studies with omeprazole, metabolized by CYP2C19 and CYP3A4, and simvastatin, metabolized by CYP3A4, showed up to a 28% and 57% decrease in exposure one week following a single dose of ACTEMRA, respectively. The effect of tocilizumab on CYP enzymes may be clinically relevant for CYP450 substrates with narrow therapeutic index, where the dose is individually adjusted. Upon initiation or discontinuation of ACTEMRA, in patients being treated with these types of medicinal products, therapeutic monitoring of effect (e.g., warfarin) or drug concentration (e.g., cyclosporine or theophylline) should be performed and the individual dose of the medicinal product adjusted as needed. Prescribers should exercise caution when ACTEMRA is co-administered with CYP3A4 substrate drugs where decrease in effectiveness is undesirable, e.g., oral contraceptives, lovastatin, atorvastatin, etc. The effect of tocilizumab on CYP450 enzyme activity may persist for several weeks after stopping therapy *[see Clinical Pharmacology (12.3)].*

7.3   Live Vaccines
Live vaccines should not be given concurrently with ACTEMRA *[see Warnings and Precautions (5.8)].*

8   USE IN SPECIFIC POPULATIONS
8.1   Pregnancy
Teratogenic Effects. Pregnancy Category C. There are no adequate and well-controlled studies in pregnant women. ACTEMRA should be used during pregnancy only if the potential benefit justifies the potential risk to the fetus.
An embryo-fetal developmental toxicity study was performed in which pregnant cynomolgus monkeys were treated intravenously with tocilizumab (daily doses of 2, 10, or 50 mg/kg from gestation day 20-50) during organogenesis. Although there was no evidence for a teratogenic/dysmorphogenic effect at any dose, tocilizumab produced an increase in the incidence of abortion/embryo-fetal death at 10 mg/kg and 50 mg/kg doses (1.25 and 6.25 times the human dose of 8 mg/kg every 4 weeks based on a mg/kg comparison).
Nonteratogenic Effects. Testing of a murine analogue of tocilizumab in mice did not yield any evidence of harm to offspring during the pre- and postnatal development phase when dosed at 50 mg/kg intravenously with treatment every three days from implantation until day 21 after delivery (weaning). There was no evidence for any functional impairment of the development and behavior, learning ability, immune competence and fertility of the offspring.
Pregnancy Registry: To monitor the outcomes of pregnant women exposed to ACTEMRA, a pregnancy registry has been established. Physicians are encouraged to register patients and pregnant women are encouraged to register themselves by calling 1-877-311-8972.

8.3   Nursing Mothers
It is not known whether tocilizumab is excreted in human milk or absorbed systemically after ingestion. Because many drugs are excreted in human milk, and because of the potential for serious adverse reactions in nursing infants from ACTEMRA, a decision should be made whether to discontinue nursing or to discontinue the drug, taking into account the importance of the drug to the mother.

8.4   Pediatric Use
Safety and effectiveness of ACTEMRA in pediatric patients have not been established.

8.5   Geriatric Use
Of the 2644 patients who received ACTEMRA in Studies I to V *[see Clinical Studies (14)],* a total of 435 rheumatoid arthritis patients were 65 years of age and older, including 50 patients 75 years and older. The frequency of serious infection among ACTEMRA treated subjects 65 years of age and older was higher than those under the age of 65. As there is a higher incidence in infections in the elderly population in general, caution should be used when treating the elderly.

8.6   Hepatic Impairment
The safety and efficacy of ACTEMRA have not been studied in patients with hepatic impairment, including patients with positive HBV and HCV serology *[see Warnings and Precautions (5.7)].*

8.7   Renal Impairment
No dose adjustment is required in patients with mild renal impairment. ACTEMRA has not been studied in patients with moderate to severe renal impairment *[see Clinical Pharmacology (12.3)].*

9   DRUG ABUSE AND DEPENDENCE
No studies on the potential for ACTEMRA to cause dependence have been performed. However, there is no evidence from the available data that ACTEMRA treatment results in dependence.

10   OVERDOSAGE
There are limited data available on overdoses with ACTEMRA. One case of accidental overdose was reported in which a patient with multiple myeloma received a dose of 40 mg/kg. No adverse drug reactions were observed. No serious adverse drug reactions were observed in healthy vol-

Table 2 Adverse Reactions Occurring in at Least 2% or More of Patients on 4 or 8 mg/kg ACTEMRA plus DMARD and at Least 1% Greater Than That Observed in Patients on Placebo plus DMARD

Preferred Term	6 Month Phase 3 Controlled Study Population				
	ACTEMRA 8 mg/kg MONOTHERAPY N = 288 (%)	Methotrexate N = 284 (%)	ACTEMRA 4 mg/kg + DMARDs N = 774 (%)	ACTEMRA 8 mg/kg + DMARDs N = 1582 (%)	Placebo + DMARDs N = 1170 (%)
Upper Respiratory Tract Infection	7	5	6	8	6
Nasopharyngitis	7	6	4	6	4
Headache	7	2	6	5	3
Hypertension	6	2	4	4	3
ALT increased	6	4	3	3	1
Dizziness	3	1	2	3	2
Bronchitis	3	2	3	3	2
Rash	2	1	4	3	1
Mouth Ulceration	2	2	1	2	1
Abdominal Pain Upper	2	2	3	3	2
Gastritis	1	2	1	2	1
Transaminase increased	1	5	2	2	1

unteers who received single doses of up to 28 mg/kg, although all 5 patients at the highest dose of 28 mg/kg developed dose-limiting neutropenia.
In case of an overdose, it is recommended that the patient be monitored for signs and symptoms of adverse reactions. Patients who develop adverse reactions should receive appropriate symptomatic treatment.

11   DESCRIPTION
ACTEMRA (tocilizumab) is a recombinant humanized anti-human interleukin 6 (IL-6) receptor monoclonal antibody of the immunoglobulin IgG1κ (gamma 1, kappa) subclass with a typical H_2L_2 polypeptide structure. Each light chain and heavy chain consists of 214 and 448 amino acids, respectively. The four polypeptide chains are linked intra- and inter-molecularly by disulfide bonds. ACTEMRA has a molecular weight of approximately 148 kDa.
ACTEMRA is supplied as a sterile, preservative-free solution for intravenous (IV) infusion at a concentration of 20 mg/mL. ACTEMRA is a colorless to pale yellow liquid, with a pH of about 6.5. Single-use vials are available containing 80 mg/4 mL, 200 mg/10 mL, or 400 mg/20 mL of ACTEMRA. Injectable solutions of ACTEMRA are formulated in an aqueous solution containing disodium phosphate dodecahydrate and sodium dihydrogen phosphate dehydrate (as a 15 mmol/L phosphate buffer), polysorbate 80 (0.5 mg/mL), and sucrose (50 mg/mL).

12   CLINICAL PHARMACOLOGY
12.1   Mechanism of Action
Tocilizumab binds specifically to both soluble and membrane-bound IL-6 receptors (sIL-6R and mIL-6R), and has been shown to inhibit IL-6-mediated signaling through these receptors. IL-6 is a pleiotropic pro-inflammatory cytokine produced by a variety of cell types including T- and B-cells, lymphocytes, monocytes and fibroblasts. IL-6 has been shown to be involved in diverse physiological processes such as T-cell activation, induction of immunoglobulin secretion, initiation of hepatic acute phase protein synthesis, and stimulation of hematopoietic precursor cell proliferation and differentiation. IL-6 is also produced by synovial and endothelial cells leading to local production of IL-6 in joints affected by inflammatory processes such as rheumatoid arthritis.

12.2   Pharmacodynamics
In clinical studies with the 4 mg/kg and 8 mg/kg doses of ACTEMRA, decreases in levels of C-reactive protein (CRP) to within normal ranges were seen as early as week 2. Changes in pharmacodynamic parameters were observed (i.e., decreases in rheumatoid factor, erythrocyte sedimentation rate, serum amyloid A and increases in hemoglobin) with both doses, however the greatest improvements were observed with 8 mg/kg ACTEMRA.
In healthy subjects administered ACTEMRA in doses from 2 to 28 mg/kg, absolute neutrophil counts decreased to the nadir 3 to 5 days following ACTEMRA administration. Thereafter, neutrophils recovered towards baseline in a dose dependent manner. Rheumatoid arthritis patients

demonstrated a similar pattern of absolute neutrophil counts following ACTEMRA administration *[see Warnings and Precautions (5.3)].*

12.3   Pharmacokinetics
The pharmacokinetics characterized in healthy subjects and RA patients suggested that PK is similar between the two populations. The clearance (CL) of tocilizumab decreased with increased doses. At the 10 mg/kg single dose in RA patients, mean CL was 0.29 ± 0.10 mL/hr/kg and mean apparent terminal $t_{1/2}$ was 151 ± 59 hours (6.3 days).
The pharmacokinetics of tocilizumab were determined using a population pharmacokinetic analysis of 1793 rheumatoid arthritis patients treated with ACTEMRA 4 and 8 mg/kg every 4 weeks for 24 weeks.
The pharmacokinetic parameters of tocilizumab did not change with time. A more than dose-proportional increase in area under the curve (AUC) and trough concentration (C_{min}) was observed for doses of 4 and 8 mg/kg every 4 weeks. Maximum concentration (C_{max}) increased dose-proportionally. At steady-state, predicted AUC and C_{min} were 2.7 and 6.5-fold higher at 8 mg/kg as compared to 4 mg/kg, respectively.
For doses of ACTEMRA 4 mg/kg given every 4 weeks, the predicted mean (± SD) steady-state AUC, C_{min} and C_{max} of tocilizumab were 13000 ± 5800 mcg•h/mL, 1.49 ± 2.13 mcg/mL, and 88.3 ± 41.4 mcg/mL, respectively. The accumulation ratios for AUC and C_{max} were 1.11 and 1.02, respectively. The accumulation ratio was higher for C_{min} (1.96). Steady-state was reached following the first administration for C_{max} and AUC, respectively, and after 16 weeks C_{min}.
For doses of ACTEMRA 8 mg/kg given every 4 weeks, the predicted mean (± SD) steady-state AUC, C_{min} and C_{max} of tocilizumab were 35000 ± 15500 mcg•h/mL, 9.74 ± 10.5 mcg/mL, and 183 ± 85.6 mcg/mL, respectively. The accumulation ratios for AUC and C_{max} were 1.22 and 1.06, respectively. The accumulation ratio was higher for C_{min} (2.35). Steady-state was reached following the first administration and after 8 and 20 weeks for C_{max}, AUC, and C_{min}, respectively. Tocilizumab AUC, C_{min} and C_{max} increased with increase of body weight. At body weight ≥ 100 kg, the predicted mean (± SD) steady-state AUC, C_{min} and C_{max} of tocilizumab were 55500 ± 14100 mcg•h/mL, 19.0 ± 12.0 mcg/mL, and 269 ± 57 mcg/mL, respectively, which are higher than mean exposure values for the patient population. Therefore, ACTEMRA doses exceeding 800 mg per infusion are not recommended *[see Dosage and Administration (2.1)].*

Distribution
Following intravenous dosing, tocilizumab undergoes biphasic elimination from the circulation. In rheumatoid arthritis patients the central volume of distribution was 3.5 L and the peripheral volume of distribution was 2.9 L, resulting in a volume of distribution at steady state of 6.4 L.

Elimination
The total clearance of tocilizumab is concentration-dependent and is the sum of the linear clearance and the nonlinear clearance. The linear clearance was estimated to

Table 3 ACR Response at 6 Months in Active and Placebo Controlled Trials (Percent of Patients)

	Study I		Study II			Study III			Study IV		Study V		
Response Rate Week 24	MTX N=284	ACTEMRA 8 mg/kg N=286	Placebo + MTX N=393	ACTEMRA 4 mg/kg + MTX N=399	ACTEMRA 8 mg/kg + MTX N=398	Placebo + MTX N=204	ACTEMRA 4 mg/kg + MTX N=213	ACTEMRA 8 mg/kg + MTX N=205	Placebo + DMARDs N=413	ACTEMRA 8 mg/kg + DMARDs N=803	Placebo + MTX N=158	ACTEMRA 4 mg/kg + MTX N=161	ACTEMRA 8 mg/kg + MTX N=170
ACR20													
Responders Weighted Difference %[a] (95% CI)[b]	53%	70% 19 (11, 27)	27%	51% 23 (17, 29)	56% 29 (23, 35)	27%	48% 23 (15, 32)	59% 32 (23, 41)	25%	61% 35 (30, 40)	10%	30% 25 (15, 36)	50% 46 (36, 56)
ACR50													
Responders Weighted Difference %[a] (95% CI)[b]	34%	44% 12 (4, 20)	10%	25% 15 (9, 20)	32% 22 (16, 28)	11%	32% 21 (13, 29)	44% 33 (25, 41)	9%	38% 28 (23, 33)	4%	17% 15 (5, 25)	29% 31 (21, 41)
ACR70													
Responders Weighted Difference %[a] (95% CI)[b]	15%	28% 14 (7, 22)	2%	11% 8 (3, 13)	13% 10 (5, 15)	2%	12% 11 (4, 18)	22% 20 (12, 27)	3%	21% 17 (13, 21)	1%	5% 4 (-6, 13)	12% 12 (3, 22)

[a]The weighted difference is the difference between ACTEMRA and Placebo response rates, adjusted for site (and disease duration for Study I only).
[b]CI: 95% confidence interval of the weighted difference

Table 4 Components of ACR Response at 6 Months

	Study III						Study V					
	ACTEMRA 4 mg/kg + MTX N=213		ACTEMRA 8 mg/kg + MTX N=205		Placebo + MTX N=204		ACTEMRA 4 mg/kg + MTX N=161		ACTEMRA 8 mg/kg + MTX N=170		Placebo + MTX N=158	
Component (mean)	Baseline	Week 24[a]	Baseline	Week 24[a]	Baseline	Week 24	Baseline	Week 24[a]	Baseline	Week 24[a]	Baseline	Week 24
Number of tender joints (0-68)	33	19 -7.0 (-10.0, -4.1)	32	14.5 -9.6 (-12.6, -6.7)	33	25	31	21 -10.8 (-14.6, -7.1)	32	17 -15.1 (-18.8, -11.4)	30	30
Number of swollen joints (0-66)	20	10 -4.2 (-6.1, -2.3)	19.5	8 -6.2 (-8.1, -4.2)	21	15	19.5	13 -6.2 (-9.0, -3.5)	19	11 -7.2 (-9.9, -4.5)	19	18
Pain[b]	61	33 -11.0 (-17.0, -5.0)	60	30 -15.8 (-21.7, -9.9)	57	43	63.5	43 -12.4 (-22.1, -2.1)	65	33 -23.9 (-33.7, -14.1)	64	48
Patient global assessment[b]	66	34 -10.9 (-17.1, -4.8)	65	31 -14.9 (-20.9, -8.9)	64	45	70	46 -10.0 (-20.3, 0.3)	70	36 -17.4 (-27.8, -7.0)	71	51
Physician global assessment[b]	64	26 -5.6 (-10.5, -0.8)	64	23 -9.0 (-13.8, -4.2)	64	32	66.5	39 -10.5 (-18.6, -2.5)	66	28 -18.2 (-26.3, -10.0)	67.5	43
Disability index (HAQ)[c]	1.64	1.01 -0.18 (-0.34, -0.02)	1.55	0.96 -0.21 (-0.37, -0.05)	1.55	1.21	1.67	1.39 -0.25 (-0.42, -0.09)	1.75	1.34 -0.34 (-0.51, -0.17)	1.70	1.58
CRP (mg/dL)	2.79	1.17 -1.30 (-2.0, -0.59)	2.61	0.25 -2.156 (-2.86, -1.46)	2.36	1.89	3.11	1.77 -1.34 (-2.5, -0.15)	2.80	0.28 -2.52 (-3.72, -1.32)	3.705	3.06

[a]Data shown is mean at week 24, difference in adjusted mean change from baseline compared with placebo + MTX at week 24 and 95% confidence interval for that difference
[b]Visual analog scale: 0 = best, 100 = worst
[c]Health Assessment Questionnaire: 0 = best, 3 = worst; 20 questions; 8 categories: dressing and grooming, arising, eating, walking, hygiene, reach, grip, and activities

be 12.5 mL/h in the population pharmacokinetic analysis. The concentration-dependent nonlinear clearance plays a major role at low tocilizumab concentrations. Once the nonlinear clearance pathway is saturated, at higher tocilizumab concentrations, clearance is mainly determined by the linear clearance.

The $t_{1/2}$ of tocilizumab is concentration-dependent. The concentration-dependent apparent $t_{1/2}$ is up to 11 days for 4 mg/kg and up to 13 days for 8 mg/kg every 4 weeks at steady-state.

Pharmacokinetics in Special Populations
Population pharmacokinetic analyses in adult rheumatoid arthritis patients showed that age, gender and race did not affect the pharmacokinetics of tocilizumab. Linear clearance was found to increase with body size. The body weight-based dose (8 mg/kg) resulted in approximately 86% higher exposure in patients who are greater than 100 kg in comparison to patients who are less than 60 kg.

Hepatic Impairment
No formal study of the effect of hepatic impairment on the pharmacokinetics of tocilizumab was conducted.

Renal Impairment
No formal study of the effect of renal impairment on the pharmacokinetics of tocilizumab was conducted.
Most patients in the population pharmacokinetic analysis had normal renal function or mild renal impairment. Mild renal impairment (creatinine clearance < 80 mL/min and

$\geq$ 50 mL/min based on Cockcroft-Gault) did not impact the pharmacokinetics of tocilizumab. No dose adjustment is required in patients with mild renal impairment.
Drug Interactions
In vitro data suggested that IL-6 reduced mRNA expression for several CYP450 isoenzymes including CYP1A2, CYP2B6, CYP2C9, CYP2C19, CYP2D6 and CYP3A4, and this reduced expression was reversed by co-incubation with tocilizumab at clinically relevant concentrations. Accordingly, inhibition of IL-6 signaling in RA patients treated with tocilizumab may restore CYP450 activities to higher levels than those in the absence of tocilizumab leading to increased metabolism of drugs that are CYP450 substrates. Its effect on CYP2C8 or transporters (e.g., P-gp) is unknown. This is clinically relevant for CYP450 substrates with a narrow therapeutic index, where the dose is individually adjusted. Upon initiation of ACTEMRA, in patients being treated with these types of medicinal products, therapeutic monitoring of the effect (e.g., warfarin) or drug concentration (e.g., cyclosporine or theophylline) should be performed and the individual dose of the medicinal product adjusted as needed. Caution should be exercised when ACTEMRA is coadministered with drugs where decrease in effectiveness is undesirable, e.g., oral contraceptives (CYP3A4 substrates) *[see Drug Interactions (7.2)]*.
Simvastatin
Simvastatin is a CYP3A4 and OATP1B1 substrate. In 12 RA patients, not treated with ACTEMRA, receiving 40 mg

simvastatin, exposures of simvastatin and its metabolite, simvastatin acid, was 4- to 10-fold and 2-fold higher, respectively, than the exposures observed in healthy subjects. One week following administration of a single infusion of ACTEMRA (10 mg/kg), exposure of simvastatin and simvastatin acid decreased by 57% and 39%, respectively, to exposures that were similar or slightly higher than those observed in healthy subjects. Exposures of simvastatin and simvastatin acid increased upon withdrawal of ACTEMRA in RA patients. Selection of a particular dose of simvastatin in RA patients should take into account the potentially lower exposures that may result after initiation of ACTEMRA (due to normalization of CYP3A4) or higher exposures after discontinuation of ACTEMRA.
Omeprazole
Omeprazole is a CYP2C19 and CYP3A4 substrate. In RA patients receiving 10 mg omeprazole, exposure to omeprazole was approximately 2 fold higher than that observed in healthy subjects. In RA patients receiving 10 mg omeprazole, before and one week after ACTEMRA infusion (8 mg/kg), the omeprazole AUC_{inf} decreased by 12% for poor (N=5) and intermediate metabolizers (N=5) and by 28% for extensive metabolizers (N=8) and were slightly higher than those observed in healthy subjects.
Dextromethorphan
Dextromethorphan is a CYP2D6 and CYP3A4 substrate. In 13 RA patients receiving 30 mg dextromethorphan, expo-

sure to dextromethorphan was comparable to that in healthy subjects. However, exposure to its metabolite, dextrorphan (a CYP3A4 substrate), was a fraction of that observed in healthy subjects. One week following administration of a single infusion of ACTEMRA (8 mg/kg), dextromethorphan exposure was decreased by approximately 5%. However, a larger decrease (29%) in dextrorphan levels was noted after ACTEMRA infusion.

13 NONCLINICAL TOXICOLOGY

13.1 Carcinogenesis, Mutagenesis, Impairment of Fertility

Carcinogenesis. No long-term animal studies have been performed to establish the carcinogenicity potential of tocilizumab.

Mutagenesis. Tocilizumab was negative in the in vitro Ames bacterial reverse mutation assay and the in vitro chromosomal aberrations assay using human peripheral blood lymphocytes.

Impairment of Fertility. Fertility studies conducted in male and female mice using a murine analogue of tocilizumab showed no impairment of fertility.

14 CLINICAL STUDIES

The efficacy and safety of ACTEMRA was assessed in five randomized, double-blind, multicenter studies in patients > 18 years with active rheumatoid arthritis diagnosed according to American College of Rheumatology (ACR) criteria. Patients had at least 8 tender and 6 swollen joints at baseline. ACTEMRA was given intravenously every 4 weeks as monotherapy (Study I), in combination with methotrexate (MTX) (Studies II and III) or other disease-modifying anti-rheumatic drugs (DMARDs) (Study IV) in patients with an inadequate response to those drugs, or in combination with MTX in patients with an inadequate response to TNF antagonists (Study V).

Study I evaluated patients with moderate to severe active rheumatoid arthritis who had not been treated with MTX within 6 months prior to randomization, or who had not discontinued previous methotrexate treatment as a result of clinically important toxic effects or lack of response. In this study, 67% of patients were MTX-naïve, and over 40% of patients had rheumatoid arthritis < 2 years. Patients received ACTEMRA 8 mg/kg monotherapy or MTX alone (dose titrated over 8 weeks from 7.5 mg to a maximum of 20 mg weekly). The primary endpoint was the proportion of ACTEMRA patients who achieved an ACR20 response at Week 24.

Study II is an ongoing 2-year study with a planned interim analysis at week 24 that evaluated patients with moderate to severe active rheumatoid arthritis who had an inadequate clinical response to MTX. Patients received ACTEMRA 8 mg/kg, ACTEMRA 4 mg/kg, or placebo every four weeks, in combination with MTX (10 to 25 mg weekly). The primary endpoint at week 24 was the proportion of patients who achieved an ACR20 response.

Study III evaluated patients with moderate to severe active rheumatoid arthritis who had an inadequate clinical response to MTX. Patients received ACTEMRA 8 mg/kg, ACTEMRA 4 mg/kg, or placebo every four weeks, in combination with MTX (10 to 25 mg weekly). The primary endpoint was the proportion of patients who achieved an ACR20 response at week 24.

Study IV evaluated patients who had an inadequate response to their existing therapy, including one or more DMARDs. Patients received ACTEMRA 8 mg/kg or placebo every four weeks, in combination with the stable DMARDs. The primary endpoint was the proportion of patients who achieved an ACR20 response at week 24.

Study V evaluated patients with moderate to severe active rheumatoid arthritis who had an inadequate clinical response or were intolerant to one or more TNF antagonist therapies. The TNF antagonist therapy was discontinued prior to randomization. Patients received ACTEMRA 8 mg/kg, ACTEMRA 4 mg/kg, or placebo every four weeks, in combination with MTX (10 to 25 mg weekly). The primary endpoint was the proportion of patients who achieved an ACR20 response at week 24.

Clinical Response

The percentages of ACTEMRA-treated patients achieving ACR20, 50 and 70 responses are shown in Table 3. In all studies, patients treated with 8 mg/kg ACTEMRA had statistically significant ACR20, ACR50, and ACR70 response rates versus MTX- or placebo-treated patients at week 24. Patients treated with ACTEMRA at a dose of 4 mg/kg in patients with inadequate response to DMARDs or TNF antagonist therapy had lower response rates compared to patients treated with ACTEMRA 8 mg/kg.

[See table 3 at top of previous page]

The results of the components of the ACR response criteria for Studies III and V are shown in **Table 4**. Similar results to Study III were observed in Studies I, II and IV.

[See table 4 on previous page]

The percent of ACR20 responders by visit for Study III is shown in **Figure 1**. Similar responses were observed in studies I, II, IV, and V.

Figure 1 Percent of ACR20 Responders by Visit for Study III (Inadequate Response to MTX)*

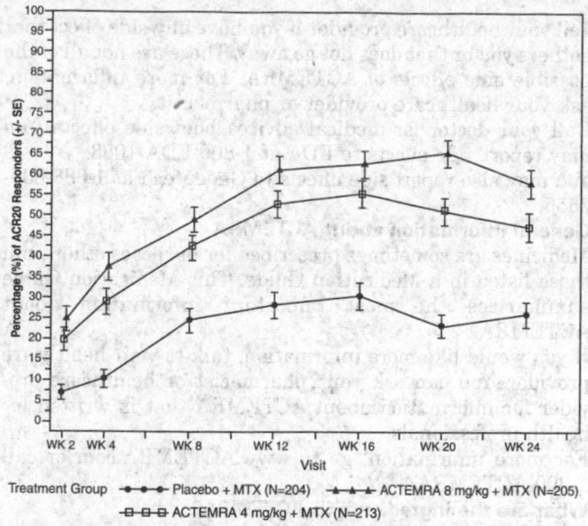
Percentage (%) of ACR20 Responders (+/- SE)
Visit
WK 2
WK 4
WK 8
WK 12
WK 16
WK 20
WK 24
Treatment Group
Placebo + MTX (N=204)
ACTEMRA 8 mg/kg + MTX (N=205)
ACTEMRA 4 mg/kg + MTX (N=213)

*The same patients may not have responded at each timepoint.

16 HOW SUPPLIED/STORAGE AND HANDLING

ACTEMRA (tocilizumab) is supplied in single-use vials as a preservative-free, sterile concentrate (20 mg/mL) solution for intravenous infusion. The following packaging configurations are available:

Individually packaged, single-use vials:
NDC 50242-135-01 providing 80 mg/4 mL
NDC 50242-136-01 providing 200 mg/10 mL
NDC 50242-137-01 providing 400 mg/20 mL
Box of 4 single-use vials:
NDC 50242-135-04 providing 80 mg/4 mL
NDC 50242-136-04 providing 200 mg/10 mL
NDC 50242-137-04 providing 400 mg/20 mL

Storage and Stability: Do not use beyond expiration date on the container. ACTEMRA must be refrigerated at 2°C to 8°C (36°F to 46°F). Do not freeze. Protect the vials from light by storage in the original package until time of use. Parenteral drug products should be inspected visually for particulate matter and discoloration prior to administration, whenever solution and container permit. If visibly opaque particles, discoloration or other foreign particles are observed, the solution should not be used.

17 PATIENT COUNSELING INFORMATION

17.1 Patient Counseling

Patients should be advised of the potential benefits and risks of ACTEMRA. Physicians should instruct their patients to read the Medication Guide before starting ACTEMRA therapy.

- **Infections:**
  Inform patients that ACTEMRA may lower their resistance to infections. Instruct the patient of the importance of contacting their doctor immediately when symptoms suggesting infection appear in order to assure rapid evaluation and appropriate treatment.
- **Gastrointestinal Perforation:**
  Inform patients that some patients who have been treated with ACTEMRA have had serious side effects in the stomach and intestines. Instruct the patient of the importance of contacting their doctor immediately when symptoms of severe, persistent abdominal pain appear to assure rapid evaluation and appropriate treatment.

17.2 Medication Guide

MEDICATION GUIDE
ACTEMRA® (AC-TEM-RA)
(tocilizumab)

Read this Medication Guide before you start ACTEMRA and before each infusion. There may be new information. This Medication Guide does not take the place of talking with your healthcare provider about your medical condition or your treatment.

What is the most important information I should know about ACTEMRA?

ACTEMRA can cause serious side effects including:

1. Serious Infections

ACTEMRA is a medicine that affects your immune system. ACTEMRA can lower the ability of your immune system to fight infections. Some people have serious infections while taking ACTEMRA, including tuberculosis (TB), and infections caused by bacteria, fungi, or viruses that can spread throughout the body. Some people have died from these infections.

- Your doctor should test you for TB before starting ACTEMRA.
- Your doctor should monitor you closely for signs and symptoms of TB during treatment with ACTEMRA.

You should not start taking ACTEMRA if you have any kind of infection unless your healthcare provider says it is okay.

Before starting ACTEMRA, tell your healthcare provider if you:

- think you have an infection or have symptoms of an infection such as:
  - fever, sweating, or chills
  - muscle aches
  - cough
  - shortness of breath
  - blood in phlegm
  - weight loss
  - warm, red, or painful skin or sores on your body
  - diarrhea or stomach pain
  - burning when you urinate or urinating more often than normal
  - feel very tired
- are being treated for an infection
- get a lot of infections or have infections that keep coming back
- have diabetes, HIV, or a weak immune system. People with these conditions have a higher chance for infections.
- have TB, or have been in close contact with someone with TB
- live or have lived, or have traveled to certain parts of the country (such as the Ohio and Mississippi River valleys and the Southwest) where there is an increased chance for getting certain kinds of fungal infections (histoplasmosis, coccidiomycosis, or blastomycosis). These infections may happen or become more severe if you use ACTEMRA. Ask your healthcare provider, if you do not know if you have lived in an area where these infections are common.
- have or have had hepatitis B.

After starting ACTEMRA, call your healthcare provider right away if you have any symptoms of an infection. ACTEMRA can make you more likely to get infections or make worse any infection that you have.

2. Tears (perforation) of the stomach or intestines.

- Before taking ACTEMRA, tell your healthcare provider if you have had diverticulitis (inflammation in parts of the large intestine) or ulcers in your stomach or intestines. Some people taking ACTEMRA get tears in their stomach or intestine. This happens most often in people who also take nonsteroidal anti-inflammatory drugs (NSAIDs), corticosteroids, or methotrexate.
- Tell your healthcare provider right away if you have fever and stomach-area pain that does not go away, and a change in your bowel habits.

3. Changes in certain laboratory test results. Your healthcare provider should do blood tests before you start receiving ACTEMRA and every 4 to 8 weeks during treatment to check for the following side effects of ACTEMRA:

- **low neutrophil count.** Neutrophils are white blood cells that help the body fight off bacterial infections.
- **low platelet count.** Platelets are blood cells that help with blood clotting and stop bleeding.
- **increase in certain liver function tests.**

You should not receive ACTEMRA if your neutrophil or platelet counts are too low or your liver function tests are too high.

Your healthcare provider may stop your ACTEMRA treatment for a period of time or change your dose of medicine if needed because of changes in these blood test results.

You may also have changes in other laboratory tests, such as your blood cholesterol levels. Your healthcare provider should do blood tests to check your cholesterol levels 4 to 8 weeks after you start receiving ACTEMRA, and then every 6 months after that. Normal cholesterol levels are important to good heart health.

4. Cancer.

ACTEMRA may decrease the activity of your immune system. Medicines that affect the immune system may increase your risk of certain cancers. Tell your healthcare provider if you have ever had any type of cancer.

See "What are the possible side effects with ACTEMRA?" for more information about side effects.

What is ACTEMRA?

ACTEMRA is a prescription medicine called an Interleukin-6 (IL-6) receptor inhibitor. ACTEMRA is used to treat adults with moderately to severely active rheumatoid arthritis (RA) after at least one other medicine called a Tumor Necrosis Factor (TNF) antagonist has been used and did not work well.

It is not known if ACTEMRA is safe and effective in children.

What should I tell my healthcare provider before receiving ACTEMRA?

ACTEMRA may not be right for you. Before starting ACTEMRA, tell your healthcare provider if you:

- have an infection. See "What is the most important information I should know about ACTEMRA?"
- have liver problems
- have any stomach-area (abdominal) pain or been diagnosed with diverticulitis or ulcers in your stomach or intestines

- have or had a condition that affects your nervous system, such as multiple sclerosis
- have recently received or are scheduled to receive a vaccine. People who take ACTEMRA should not receive live vaccines. People taking ACTEMRA can receive non-live vaccines
- plan to have surgery or a medical procedure
- have any other medical conditions
- plan to become pregnant or are pregnant. It is not known if ACTEMRA will harm your unborn baby.

  Pregnancy Registry: Genentech has a registry for pregnant women who take ACTEMRA. The purpose of this registry is to check the health of the pregnant mother and her baby. If you are pregnant or become pregnant while taking ACTEMRA, talk to your healthcare provider about how you can join this pregnancy registry or you may contact the registry at 1-877-311-8972 to enroll.
- plan to breast-feed or are breast-feeding. You and your healthcare provider should decide if you will take ACTEMRA or breast-feed. You should not do both.

Tell your healthcare provider about all of the medicines you take, including prescription and non-prescription medicines, vitamins and herbal supplements. ACTEMRA and other medicines may affect each other causing side effects. Especially tell your healthcare provider if you take:
- any other medicines to treat your RA. You should not take etanercept (Enbrel®), adalimumab (Humira®), infliximab (Remicade®), rituximab (Rituxan®), abatacept (Orencia®), anakinra (Kineret®), certolizumab (Cimzia®), or golimumab (Simponi®), while you are taking ACTEMRA. Taking ACTEMRA with these medicines may increase your risk of infection.
- medicines that affect the way certain liver enzymes work. Ask your healthcare provider if you are not sure if your medicine is one of these.

Know the medicines you take. Keep a list of them to show to your healthcare provider and pharmacist when you get a new medicine.

How will I receive ACTEMRA?
- You will receive ACTEMRA from a healthcare provider through a needle placed in a vein in your arm (IV or intravenous infusion). The infusion will take about 1 hour to give you the full dose of medicine.
- You will receive a dose of ACTEMRA about every 4 weeks.
- If you miss a scheduled dose of ACTEMRA, ask your healthcare provider when to schedule your next infusion.
- While taking ACTEMRA, you may continue to use other medicines that help treat your rheumatoid arthritis such as methotrexate, non-steroidal anti-inflammatory drugs (NSAIDs) and prescription steroids, as instructed by your healthcare provider.
- Keep all of your follow-up appointments and get your blood tests as ordered by your healthcare provider.

What are the possible side effects with ACTEMRA?
ACTEMRA can cause serious side effects, including:
- See "What is the most important information I should know about ACTEMRA?"
- **Hepatitis B infection in people who carry the virus in their blood.** If you are a carrier of the hepatitis B virus (a virus that affects the liver), the virus may become active while you use ACTEMRA. This happens with other biologic medicines used to treat RA. Your doctor may do blood tests before you start treatment with ACTEMRA and while you are using ACTEMRA. Tell your healthcare provider if you have any of the following symptoms of a possible hepatitis B infection:

• feel very tired	• chills
• skin or eyes look yellow	• stomach discomfort
• little or no appetite	• muscle aches
• vomiting	• dark urine
• clay-colored bowel movements	• skin rash
• fevers	

- **Nervous system problems.** Multiple Sclerosis has been diagnosed rarely in people who take ACTEMRA. It is not known what effect ACTEMRA may have on some nervous system disorders.
- **Allergic Reactions.** Serious allergic reactions can happen with ACTEMRA. These reactions may not happen with your first infusion, and may happen with future infusions of ACTEMRA. Tell your healthcare provider right away if you have any of the following signs of a serious allergic reaction:

- shortness of breath or trouble breathing
- skin rash
- swelling of the lips, tongue, or face
- chest pain
- feeling dizzy or faint

Common side effects of ACTEMRA include:

• upper respiratory tract infections (common cold, sinus infections)	• increased blood pressure (hypertension)
• headache	

Tell your healthcare provider if you have any side effect that bothers you or that does not go away. These are not all of the possible side effects of ACTEMRA. For more information, ask your healthcare provider or pharmacist.
Call your doctor for medical advice about side effects. You may report side effects to FDA at 1-800-FDA-1088.
You may also report side effects to Genentech at 1-888-835-2555.

General information about ACTEMRA
Medicines are sometimes prescribed for purposes other than those listed in a Medication Guide. This Medication Guide summarizes the most important information about ACTEMRA.
If you would like more information, talk to your healthcare provider. You can ask your pharmacist or healthcare provider for information about ACTEMRA that is written for health professionals.
For more information, go to www.ACTEMRA.com or call 1-800-ACTEMRA.

What are the ingredients in ACTEMRA?
Active ingredient: tocilizumab
Inactive ingredients: sucrose, polysorbate 80, disodium phosphate dodecahydrate, sodium dihydrogen phosphate dihydrate.
This Medication Guide has been approved by the U.S. Food and Drug Administration.
ACTEMRA is a registered trademark of Chugai Seiyaku Kabushiki Kaisha Corp., a member of the Roche Group.
Genentech, Inc.
A Member of the Roche Group
1 DNA Way
South San Francisco, CA 94080-4990
US License No. 1048
10094884_01
AAI_4877533_PI_062009_N_5
AAI_4877533_MG_062009_N_5
PI Issued: January 2010
© 2010 Genentech, Inc. All rights reserved.
Shown in Product Identification Guide, page 309

Gilead Sciences, Inc.
333 LAKESIDE DRIVE
FOSTER CITY, CA 94404

For Product Information:
1-800-445-3235, press option 2
medicalinformation@gilead.com
To Report Adverse Events:
1-800-445-3235, press option 3
For Business Operations and Contract Compliance:
1-800-445-3235, press option 8

ATRIPLA®

ATRIPLA® is co-marketed by Bristol-Myers Squibb and Gilead Sciences. Please see Bristol-Myers Squibb & Gilead Sciences, LLC for full prescribing information.
Shown in Product Identification Guide, page 309

CAYSTON®   ℞
[kay-stun]
(aztreonam for inhalation solution)

HIGHLIGHTS OF PRESCRIBING INFORMATION
These highlights do not include all the information needed to use CAYSTON safely and effectively. See full prescribing information for CAYSTON.
CAYSTON® (aztreonam for inhalation solution)
Initial U.S. Approval: 1986
To reduce the development of drug-resistant bacteria and maintain the effectiveness of CAYSTON and other antibacterial drugs, CAYSTON should be used only to treat patients with cystic fibrosis (CF) known to have *Pseudomonas aeruginosa* in the lungs.

──────INDICATIONS AND USAGE──────
CAYSTON is a monobactam antibacterial indicated to improve respiratory symptoms in cystic fibrosis (CF) patients with *Pseudomonas aeruginosa*. Safety and effectiveness have not been established in pediatric patients below the age of 7 years, patients with FEV₁ <25% or >75% predicted, or patients colonized with *Burkholderia cepacia*. (1)

──────DOSAGE AND ADMINISTRATION──────
- Administer one dose (one single use vial and one ampule of diluent) 3 times a day for 28 days. (2.1)
- Use dose immediately after reconstitution. (2.2)
- Administer only with the Altera® Nebulizer System. Do not administer with any other type of nebulizer. (2.3)

──────DOSAGE FORMS AND STRENGTHS──────
- Lyophilized aztreonam (75 mg/vial) (3)
- Diluent (0.17% sodium chloride): 1 mL/ampule (3)

──────CONTRAINDICATIONS──────
- Do not administer to patients with a known allergy to aztreonam. (4)

──────WARNINGS AND PRECAUTIONS──────
- Allergic reaction to CAYSTON was seen in clinical trials. Stop treatment if an allergic reaction occurs. Use caution when CAYSTON is administered to patients with a known allergic reaction to beta-lactams. (5.1)
- Bronchospasm has been reported with CAYSTON. Stop treatment if chest tightness develops during nebulizer use. (5.2)

──────ADVERSE REACTIONS──────
- Common adverse reactions (more than 5%) occurring more frequently in CAYSTON patients are cough, nasal congestion, wheezing, pharyngolaryngeal pain, pyrexia, chest discomfort, abdominal pain and vomiting. (6.1)
To report SUSPECTED ADVERSE REACTIONS, contact Gilead Sciences, Inc. at 1-800-GILEAD5, option 3 or FDA at 1-800-FDA-1088 or www.fda.gov/medwatch.
See 17 for PATIENT COUNSELING INFORMATION and FDA-approved patient labeling

                                            Revised: 02/2010

FULL PRESCRIBING INFORMATION: CONTENTS*

FULL PRESCRIBING INFORMATION

1   INDICATIONS AND USAGE
CAYSTON® is indicated to improve respiratory symptoms in cystic fibrosis (CF) patients with *Pseudomonas aeruginosa*. Safety and effectiveness have not been established in pediatric patients below the age of 7 years, patients with FEV₁ <25% or >75% predicted, or patients colonized with *Burkholderia cepacia* [see Clinical Studies (14)].
To reduce the development of drug-resistant bacteria and maintain the effectiveness of CAYSTON and other antibacterial drugs, CAYSTON should be used only to treat patients with CF known to have *Pseudomonas aeruginosa* in the lungs.

2   DOSAGE AND ADMINISTRATION
2.1   Dosing Information
The recommended dose of CAYSTON for both adults and pediatric patients 7 years of age and older is one single-use vial (75 mg of aztreonam) reconstituted with 1 mL of sterile diluent administered 3 times a day for a 28-day course (followed by 28 days off CAYSTON therapy). Dosage is not based on weight or adjusted for age. Doses should be taken at least 4 hours apart.
CAYSTON is administered by inhalation using an Altera® Nebulizer System. Patients should use a bronchodilator before administration of CAYSTON.
2.2   Instructions for CAYSTON Reconstitution
CAYSTON should be administered immediately after reconstitution. Do not reconstitute CAYSTON until ready to administer a dose.

Take one amber glass vial containing CAYSTON and one diluent ampule from the carton. To open the glass vial, carefully remove the metal ring by pulling the tab and remove the gray rubber stopper. Twist the tip off the diluent ampule and squeeze the liquid into the glass vial. Replace the rubber stopper, then gently swirl the vial until contents have completely dissolved.
The empty vial, stopper, and diluent ampule should be disposed of properly upon completion of dosing.

2.3 Instructions for CAYSTON Administration

CAYSTON is administered by inhalation using an Altera Nebulizer System. CAYSTON should not be administered with any other nebulizer. CAYSTON should not be mixed with any other drugs in the Altera Nebulizer Handset.
CAYSTON is not for intravenous or intramuscular administration.
Patients should use a bronchodilator before administration of CAYSTON. Short-acting bronchodilators can be taken between 15 minutes and 4 hours prior to each dose of CAYSTON. Alternatively, long-acting bronchodilators can be taken between 30 minutes and 12 hours prior to administration of CAYSTON. For patients taking multiple inhaled therapies, the recommended order of administration is as follows: bronchodilator, mucolytics, and lastly, CAYSTON.
To administer CAYSTON, pour the reconstituted solution into the handset of the nebulizer system. Turn the unit on. Place the mouthpiece of the handset in your mouth and breathe normally only through your mouth. Administration typically takes between 2 and 3 minutes. Further patient instructions on how to administer CAYSTON are provided in the FDA-approved patient labeling. Instructions on testing nebulizer functionality and cleaning the handset are provided in the Instructions for Use included with the nebulizer system.

3 DOSAGE FORMS AND STRENGTHS

A dose of CAYSTON consists of a single-use vial of sterile, lyophilized aztreonam (75 mg) reconstituted with a 1 mL ampule of sterile diluent (0.17% sodium chloride). Reconstituted CAYSTON is administered by inhalation.

4 CONTRAINDICATIONS

CAYSTON is contraindicated in patients with a known allergy to aztreonam.

5 WARNINGS AND PRECAUTIONS

5.1 Allergic Reactions

Severe allergic reactions have been reported following administration of aztreonam for injection to patients with no known history of exposure to aztreonam. In addition, allergic reaction with facial rash, facial swelling, and throat tightness was reported with CAYSTON in clinical trials. If an allergic reaction to CAYSTON occurs, stop administration of CAYSTON and initiate treatment as appropriate.
Caution is advised when administering CAYSTON to patients if they have a history of beta-lactam allergy, although patients with a known beta-lactam allergy have received CAYSTON in clinical trials and no severe allergic reactions were reported. A history of allergy to beta-lactam antibiotics, such as penicillins, cephalosporins, and/or carbapenems, may be a risk factor, since cross-reactivity may occur.

5.2 Bronchospasm

Bronchospasm is a complication associated with nebulized therapies, including CAYSTON. Reduction of 15% or more in forced expiratory volume in 1 second (FEV_1) immediately following administration of study medication after pretreatment with a bronchodilator was observed in 3% of patients treated with CAYSTON.

5.3 Decreases in FEV_1 After 28-Day Treatment Cycle

In clinical trials, patients with increases in FEV_1 during a 28-day course of CAYSTON were sometimes treated for pulmonary exacerbations when FEV_1 declined after the treatment period. Healthcare providers should consider a patient's baseline FEV_1 measured prior to CAYSTON therapy and the presence of other symptoms when evaluating whether post-treatment changes in FEV_1 are caused by a pulmonary exacerbation.

5.4 Development of Drug-Resistant Bacteria

Prescribing CAYSTON in the absence of known *Pseudomonas aeruginosa* infection in patients with CF is unlikely to provide benefit and increases the risk of development of drug-resistant bacteria.

6 ADVERSE REACTIONS

6.1 Clinical Trials Experience

Because clinical trials are conducted under widely varying conditions, adverse reaction rates observed in the clinical trials of drugs cannot be directly compared to rates in the clinical trials of another drug and may not reflect the rates observed in practice.
The safety of CAYSTON was evaluated in 344 patients from two placebo-controlled trials and one open-label follow-on trial. In controlled trials, 146 patients with CF received 75 mg CAYSTON 3 times a day for 28 days.
Table 1 displays adverse reactions reported in more than 5% of patients treated with CAYSTON 3 times a day in placebo-controlled trials. The listed adverse reactions occurred more frequently in CAYSTON-treated patients than in placebo-treated patients.

Table 1. Adverse Reactions Reported in more than 5% of Patients Treated with CAYSTON in the Placebo-Controlled Trials

Event (Preferred Term)	Placebo (N = 160) n (%)	CAYSTON 75 mg 3 times a day (N = 146) n (%)
Cough	82 (51%)	79 (54%)
Nasal congestion	19 (12%)	23 (16%)
Wheezing	16 (10%)	23 (16%)
Pharyngolaryngeal pain	17 (11%)	18 (12%)
Pyrexia	9 (6%)	19 (13%)
Chest discomfort	10 (6%)	11 (8%)
Abdominal Pain	8 (5%)	10 (7%)
Vomiting	7 (4%)	9 (6%)

Adverse reactions that occurred in less than 5% of patients treated with CAYSTON were bronchospasm (3%) [*see Warnings and Precautions (5.2)*] and rash (2%).

7 DRUG INTERACTIONS

No formal clinical studies of drug interactions with CAYSTON have been conducted.

8 USE IN SPECIFIC POPULATIONS

8.1 Pregnancy

Pregnancy Category B

No reproductive toxicology studies have been conducted with CAYSTON. However, studies were conducted with aztreonam for injection. Aztreonam has been shown to cross the placenta and enter fetal circulation. No evidence of embryo or fetotoxicity or teratogenicity has been shown in studies with pregnant rats and rabbits. In rats receiving aztreonam for injection during late gestation and lactation, no drug induced changes in maternal, fetal or neonatal parameters were observed. These animal reproduction and developmental toxicity studies used parenteral routes of administration that would provide systemic exposures far in excess of the average peak plasma levels measured in humans following CAYSTON therapy.
No adequate and well-controlled studies of aztreonam for injection or CAYSTON in pregnant women have been conducted. Because animal reproduction studies are not always predictive of human response, CAYSTON should be used during pregnancy only if clearly needed.

8.3 Nursing Mothers

Following administration of aztreonam for injection, aztreonam is excreted in human milk at concentrations that are less than one percent of those determined in simultaneously obtained maternal serum. Peak plasma concentrations of aztreonam following administration of CAYSTON (75 mg) are approximately 1% of peak concentrations observed following IV aztreonam (500 mg). Therefore, use of CAYSTON during breastfeeding is unlikely to pose a risk to infants.

8.4 Pediatric Use

Patients 7 years and older were included in clinical trials with CAYSTON. Fifty-five patients under 18 years of age received CAYSTON in placebo-controlled trials. No dose adjustments were made for pediatric patients. Pyrexia was more commonly reported in pediatric patients than in adult patients. Safety and effectiveness in pediatric patients below the age of 7 years have not been established.

8.5 Geriatric Use

Clinical trials of CAYSTON did not include CAYSTON-treated patients aged 65 years of age and older to determine whether they respond differently from younger patients.

8.6 Use in Patients with Renal Impairment

Aztreonam is known to be excreted by the kidney. Placebo-controlled clinical trials with CAYSTON excluded patients with abnormal baseline renal function (defined as serum creatinine greater than 2 times the upper limit of normal range). Given the low systemic exposure of aztreonam following administration of CAYSTON, clinically relevant accumulation of aztreonam is unlikely to occur in patients with renal impairment. Therefore, CAYSTON may be administered to patients with mild, moderate and severe renal impairment with no dosage adjustment.

10 OVERDOSAGE

No overdoses have been reported with CAYSTON in clinical trials to date. In clinical trials, 225 mg doses of CAYSTON via inhalation were associated with higher rates of drug-related respiratory adverse reactions, particularly cough. Since the peak plasma concentration of aztreonam following administration of CAYSTON (75 mg) is approximately 0.6 mcg/mL, compared to a serum concentration of 54 mcg/mL following administration of aztreonam for injection (500 mg), no systemic safety issues associated with CAYSTON overdose are anticipated.

11 DESCRIPTION

A dose of CAYSTON consists of a 2 mL amber glass vial containing lyophilized aztreonam (75 mg) and lysine (46.7 mg), and a low-density polyethylene ampule containing 1 mL sterile diluent (0.17% sodium chloride). The reconstituted solution is for inhalation. The formulation contains no preservatives or arginine.
The active ingredient in CAYSTON is aztreonam, a monobactam antibacterial. The monobactams are structurally different from beta- lactam antibiotics (e.g., penicillins, cephalosporins, carbapenems) due to a monocyclic nucleus. This nucleus contains several side chains; sulfonic acid in the 1-position activates the nucleus, an aminothiazolyl oxime side chain in the 3-position confers specificity for aerobic Gram-negative bacteria including *Pseudomonas spp.*, and a methyl group in the 4-position enhances beta-lactamase stability.
Aztreonam is designated chemically as (Z)-2-[[[(2-amino-4-thiazolyl)[[(2S,3S)-2-methyl-4-oxo-1-sulfo-3-azetidinyl] carbamoyl]methylene]amino]oxy]-2-methylpropionic acid. The structural formula is presented below:

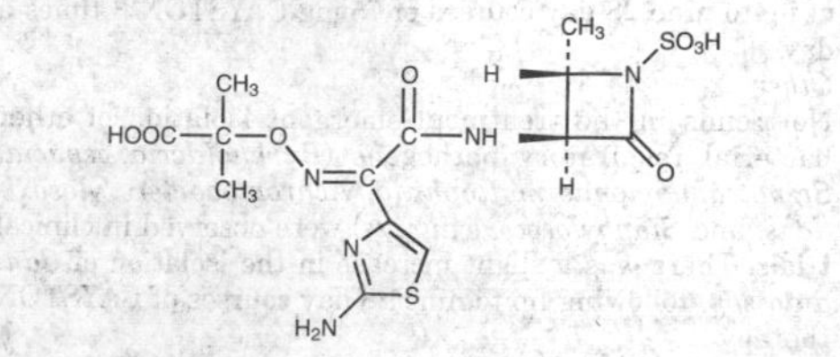

CAYSTON is a white to off-white powder. CAYSTON is sterile, hygroscopic, and light sensitive. Once reconstituted with the supplied diluent, the pH range is 4.5 to 6.0.

12 CLINICAL PHARMACOLOGY

12.1 Mechanism of Action

Aztreonam is an antibacterial drug [*see Clinical Pharmacology (12.4)*].

12.3 Pharmacokinetics

Sputum Concentrations

Sputum aztreonam concentrations exhibited considerable variability between patients receiving CAYSTON (75 mg) in clinical trials. The mean sputum concentration 10 minutes following the first dose of CAYSTON (n = 195 patients with CF) was 726 mcg/g. Mean sputum concentrations of aztreonam in patients receiving CAYSTON 3 times a day for 28 days were 984 mcg/g, 793 mcg/g, and 715 mcg/g 10 minutes after dose administration on Days 0, 14, and 28, respectively, indicating no accumulation of aztreonam in sputum.

Plasma Concentrations

Plasma aztreonam concentrations exhibited considerable variability between patients receiving CAYSTON (75 mg) in the clinical trials. The mean plasma concentration one hour following the first dose of CAYSTON (at approximately the peak plasma concentration) was 0.59 mcg/mL. Mean peak plasma concentrations in patients receiving CAYSTON 3 times a day for 28 days were 0.55 mcg/mL, 0.67 mcg/mL, and 0.65 mcg/mL on Days 0, 14, and 28, respectively, indicating no systemic accumulation of aztreonam. In contrast, the serum concentration of aztreonam following administration of aztreonam for injection (500 mg) is approximately 54 mcg/mL.

Absorption

Evaluation of plasma and urine aztreonam concentrations following administration of CAYSTON indicates low systemic absorption of aztreonam. Approximately 10% of the total CAYSTON dose is excreted in the urine as unchanged drug, as compared to 60–65% following intravenous administration of aztreonam for injection.

Distribution

The protein binding of aztreonam in serum is approximately 56% and is independent of dose.

Metabolism

Following intramuscular administration of aztreonam for injection 500 mg every 8 hours for 7 days, approximately 6% of the dose was excreted as a microbiologically inactive open β-lactam ring hydrolysis product in an 8-hour urine collection on the last day of multiple dosing.

Excretion

The elimination half-life of aztreonam from plasma is approximately 2.1 hours following administration of CAYSTON to adult patients with CF, similar to what has been reported for aztreonam for injection. Approximately

10% of the total CAYSTON dose is excreted in the urine as unchanged drug. Systemically absorbed aztreonam is eliminated about equally by active tubular secretion and glomerular filtration. Following administration of a single intravenous dose of radiolabeled aztreonam for injection, about 12% of the dose was recovered in the feces.

12.4 Microbiology

Mechanism of Action

Aztreonam exhibits activity *in vitro* against Gram-negative aerobic pathogens including *P. aeruginosa*. Aztreonam binds to penicillin-binding proteins of susceptible bacteria, which leads to inhibition of bacterial cell wall synthesis and death of the cell. Aztreonam activity is not decreased in the presence of CF lung secretions.

Susceptibility Testing

A single sputum sample from a patient with CF may contain multiple morphotypes of *P. aeruginosa* and each morphotype may have a different level of *in vitro* susceptibility to aztreonam. There are no *in vitro* susceptibility test interpretive criteria for isolates of *P. aeruginosa* obtained from the sputum of CF patients.[1]

Development of Resistance

No changes in the susceptibility of *P. aeruginosa* to aztreonam were observed following a 28-day course of CAYSTON in the placebo-controlled trials.

Cross-Resistance

No cross-resistance to other classes of antibiotics, including aminoglycosides, quinolones, and beta-lactams, was observed following a 28-day course of CAYSTON in the Phase 3 placebo-controlled trials or in an open-label follow-on trial of up to nine 28-day courses of 75 mg CAYSTON 3 times a day.

Other

No trends in the treatment-emergent isolation of other bacterial respiratory pathogens (*Burkholderia cepacia, Stenotrophomonas maltophilia, Achromobacter xylosoxidans,* and *Staphylococcus aureus*) were observed in clinical trials. There was a slight increase in the isolation of *Candida spp.* following up to nine 28-day courses of CAYSTON therapy.

13 NONCLINICAL TOXICOLOGY

13.1 Carcinogenesis, Mutagenesis, Impairment of Fertility

A 104-week rat inhalation toxicology study to assess the carcinogenic potential of aztreonam demonstrated no drug-related increase in the incidence of tumors. Rats were exposed to aztreonam for up to 4 hours per day. Peak plasma levels of aztreonam averaging approximately 6.8 mcg/mL were measured in rats at the highest dose level. This is approximately 12-fold higher than the average peak plasma level measured in humans following CAYSTON therapy.

Genetic toxicology studies performed *in vitro* demonstrated that aztreonam did not induce structural chromosome aberrations in CHO cells and did not induce mutations at the TK locus in mouse lymphoma L5178Y $TK^{+/-}$ cells. Likewise, genetic toxicology studies performed *in vivo* did not reveal evidence of mutagenic potential.

Aztreonam did not impair the fertility of rats when administered at doses that would provide systemic exposures far in excess of peak plasma levels measured in humans following CAYSTON therapy.

14 CLINICAL STUDIES

CAYSTON was evaluated over a period of 28 days of treatment in a randomized, double-blind, placebo-controlled, multicenter trial that enrolled patients with CF and *P. aeruginosa*. This trial was designed to evaluate improvement in respiratory symptoms. Patients 7 years of age and older and with FEV_1 of 25% to 75% predicted were enrolled. All patients received CAYSTON or placebo on an outpatient basis administered with the Altera Nebulizer System. All patients were required to take a dose of an inhaled bronchodilator (beta-agonist) prior to taking a dose of CAYSTON or placebo. Patients were receiving standard care for CF, including drugs for obstructive airway diseases.

The trial enrolled 164 patients with CF and *P. aeruginosa*. The mean age was 30 years, and the mean baseline FEV_1 % predicted was 55%; 43% were females and 96% were Caucasian. These patients were randomized in a 1:1 ratio to receive either CAYSTON (75 mg) or volume-matched placebo administered by inhalation 3 times a day for 28 days. Patients were required to have been off antibiotics for at least 28 days before treatment with study drug. The primary efficacy endpoint was improvement in respiratory symptoms on the last day of treatment with CAYSTON or placebo. Respiratory symptoms were also assessed two weeks after the completion of treatment with CAYSTON or placebo. Changes in respiratory symptoms were assessed using a questionnaire that asks patients to report on symptoms like cough, wheezing, and sputum production.

Improvement in respiratory symptoms was noted for CAYSTON-treated patients relative to placebo-treated patients on the last day of drug treatment. Statistically significant improvements were seen in both adult and pediatric patients, but were substantially smaller in adult patients. Two weeks after completion of treatment, a difference in respiratory symptoms between treatment groups was still present, though the difference was smaller.

Pulmonary function, as measured by FEV_1 (L), increased from baseline in patients treated with CAYSTON (see Figure 1). The treatment difference at Day 28 between CAYSTON-treated and placebo-treated patients for percent change in FEV_1 (L) was statistically significant at 10% (95% CI: 6%, 14%). Improvements in FEV_1 were comparable between adult and pediatric patients. Two weeks after completion of drug treatment, the difference in FEV_1 between CAYSTON and placebo groups had decreased to 6% (95% CI: 2%, 9%).

Figure 1. Adjusted Mean Percent Change in FEV_1 from Baseline to Study End (Days 0–42).

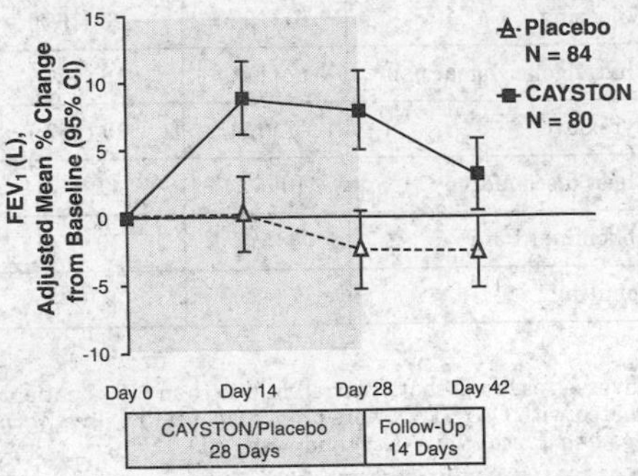

15 REFERENCES

1. Clinical and Laboratory Standards Institute (CLSI). Methods for Dilution Antimicrobial Susceptibility Tests for Bacteria that Grow Aerobically—Eighth Edition; Approved Standard. CLSI Document M7-A8. CLSI, Wayne, PA 19087. January, 2009.

16 HOW SUPPLIED/STORAGE AND HANDLING

Each kit for a 28-day course of CAYSTON contains 84 sterile vials of CAYSTON and 88 ampules of sterile diluent packed in 2 cartons, each carton containing a 14-day supply. The four additional diluent ampules are provided in case of spillage.

Package Configuration	Dosage Strength	NDC No.
28-Day Kit	75 mg	61958-0901-1

CAYSTON vials and diluent ampules should be stored in the refrigerator at 2 °C to 8 °C (36 °F to 46 °F) until needed. Once removed from the refrigerator, CAYSTON and diluent may be stored at room temperature (up to 25 °C/77 °F) for up to 28 days. Do not separate the CAYSTON vials from the diluent ampules. CAYSTON should be protected from light. Do not use CAYSTON if it has been stored at room temperature for more than 28 days. Do not use CAYSTON beyond the expiration date stamped on the vial. Do not use diluent beyond the expiration date embossed on the ampule.

CAYSTON should be used immediately upon reconstitution. Do not reconstitute more than one dose at a time.

Do not use diluent or reconstituted CAYSTON if it is cloudy or if there are particles in the solution.

17 PATIENT COUNSELING INFORMATION

See FDA-Approved Patient Labeling

Patients should be advised that CAYSTON is for inhalation use only and that CAYSTON should only be administered using the Altera Nebulizer System. Patients should be instructed only to reconstitute CAYSTON with the provided diluent and not mix other drugs with CAYSTON in the Altera Nebulizer System.

Patients should be advised to complete the full 28-day course of CAYSTON even if they are feeling better. Inform the patient that if they miss a dose, they should take all 3 daily doses as long as the doses are at least 4 hours apart.

Patients should be advised to use a bronchodilator prior to administration of CAYSTON. Patients taking several inhaled medications should be advised to use the medications in the following order of administration: bronchodilator, mucolytics, and lastly, CAYSTON.

Patients should be advised to tell their doctor if they have new or worsening symptoms. Patients who believe they are experiencing an allergic reaction to CAYSTON should be advised to contact their doctor immediately.

Patients should be counseled that antibacterial drugs including CAYSTON should only be used to treat bacterial infections. They do not treat viral infection (e.g., the common cold). When CAYSTON is prescribed to treat a bacterial infection, patients should be told that although it is common to feel better early in the course of therapy, the medication should be taken as directed. Skipping doses or not completing the full course of therapy may (1) decrease the effectiveness of the immediate treatment and (2) increase the likelihood that bacteria will develop resistance and will not be treatable by CAYSTON or other antibacterial drugs in the future.

Manufactured by: Gilead Sciences, Inc., Foster City, CA 94404

50-814-GS-000

FDA-Approved Patient Labeling

Patient Information

CAYSTON® (kay-stun)

(aztreonam for inhalation solution)

Read this Patient Information before you start taking CAYSTON and each time you get a refill. This information does not take the place of talking with your doctor about your medical condition or your treatment.

What is CAYSTON?

CAYSTON is a prescription inhaled antibiotic. CAYSTON is used to improve breathing symptoms in people with cystic fibrosis (CF) who have *Pseudomonas aeruginosa (P. aeruginosa)* in their lungs.

CAYSTON is only for infections caused by bacteria. It is not for infections caused by viruses, such as the common cold.

CAYSTON is used only with the Altera® Nebulizer System.

It is not known if CAYSTON is safe and effective in children under the age of 7.

Who should not take CAYSTON?

Do not take CAYSTON if you are allergic to aztreonam (AZACTAM®).

What should I tell my doctor before taking CAYSTON?

Before taking CAYSTON, tell your doctor if you:

- are allergic to any antibiotics.
- are pregnant or plan to become pregnant.
- are breast-feeding or plan to breast feed. Talk to your doctor about the best way to breast feed your baby if you take CAYSTON.

Tell your doctor about all the medicine you take, including prescription and non-prescription medicines, vitamins and herbal supplements.

Know the medicines you take. Keep a list of them to show your doctor and pharmacist when you get a new medicine.

How should I take CAYSTON?

- Take CAYSTON exactly as prescribed by your doctor.
- The dose of CAYSTON for both adults and children 7 years of age and older is one vial of CAYSTON, mixed with one ampule of saline (diluent) 3 times a day.
- Doses of CAYSTON should be taken at least 4 hours apart (for example: morning, after school, and before bed).
- CAYSTON should be taken for 28 days.
- CAYSTON is taken as a breathing treatment (inhalation) with the Altera Nebulizer System. Do not use any other nebulizer for your CAYSTON treatment.
- You should use an inhaled bronchodilator (a type of medicine used to relax and open your airways) before taking a dose of CAYSTON. If you do not have an inhaled bronchodilator, ask your doctor to prescribe one for you.
- If you are taking several medicines or treatments to treat your cystic fibrosis, you should take your medicines or other treatments in this order:
  - 1)bronchodilator
  - 2)mucolytics (medicines to help clear mucus from your lungs)
  - 3)CAYSTON
- You should take CAYSTON as prescribed, in courses of 28 days on CAYSTON, followed by at least 28 days off CAYSTON, as directed by your doctor.
- Do not mix CAYSTON with any other medicines in your Altera Nebulizer System.
- Do not mix CAYSTON with the saline until right before you are ready to use it. Do not mix more than one dose of CAYSTON at a time.
- Each treatment should take about 2 to 3 minutes.
- If you miss a dose of CAYSTON, you can still take all 3 daily doses as long as they are at least 4 hours apart.
- It is important for you to finish taking the full 28-day course of CAYSTON even if you are feeling better. If you skip doses or do not finish the full 28-day course of CAYSTON, your infection may not be fully treated and CAYSTON may not work as well as a treatment for infections in the future.
- See the end of this Patient Information leaflet for the Patient Instructions for Use on how to take CAYSTON the right way.

What are the possible side effects of CAYSTON?
CAYSTON can cause serious side effects, including:
- **Severe allergic reactions. Stop your treatment with CAYSTON and call your doctor right away if you have any symptoms of an allergic reaction, including:**
  - Rash or swelling of your face
  - Throat tightness
- **Trouble breathing right after treatment with CAYSTON (bronchospasm).** To decrease the chance of this happening, be sure to use your inhaled bronchodilator medicine before each treatment with CAYSTON. See "How should I take CAYSTON?"

Common side effects of CAYSTON include:
- Cough
- Nasal congestion
- Wheezing
- Sore throat
- Fever. Fever may be more common in children than in adults.
- Chest discomfort
- Stomach area (abdominal) pain
- Vomiting

Tell your doctor if you have any new or worsening symptoms while taking CAYSTON. Tell your doctor about any side effect that bothers you or that does not go away.

These are not all the possible side effects of CAYSTON. For more information, ask your doctor or pharmacist.

Call your doctor for medical advice about side effects. You may report side effects to FDA at 1-800-FDA-1088.

How should I store CAYSTON?
- Each CAYSTON kit contains enough vials of CAYSTON and ampules of saline for 28 days of treatment. There are 4 extra saline ampules in case some saline spills.
- Always keep your CAYSTON and saline together.
- Store CAYSTON and saline in the refrigerator at 36 °F to 46 °F (2 °C to 8 °C) until needed.
- When you remove CAYSTON and saline from the refrigerator, they may be stored at room temperature (less than 77 °F) for up to 28 days. Do not use any CAYSTON that has been stored at room temperature for more than 28 days.
- Keep CAYSTON away from light.
- Do not use CAYSTON after the expiration date on the vial. Do not use the saline after the expiration date on the ampule.

Keep CAYSTON and all medicines out of the reach of children.

General information about CAYSTON
Medicines are sometimes prescribed for purposes other than those listed in a Patient Information leaflet. Do not use CAYSTON for a condition for which it was not prescribed. Do not give CAYSTON to other people, even if they have the same symptoms that you have. It may harm them.

This Patient Information leaflet summarizes the most important information about CAYSTON. If you would like more information, talk with your doctor. You can ask your pharmacist or doctor for information about CAYSTON that is written for health professionals. For more information, call 1-877-7CAYSTON (1-877-722-9786).

What are the ingredients in CAYSTON?
Active ingredient: aztreonam
Inactive ingredient: sodium chloride (diluent)

Patient Instructions for Use
CAYSTON®
(aztreonam for inhalation solution)
Be sure that you read, understand and follow the Patient Instructions for Use below for the right way to take CAYSTON. If you have any questions, ask your doctor or pharmacist.

You will need the following supplies (Figure 1):
- 1 amber colored CAYSTON vial
- 1 ampule of saline (diluent)
- Altera Nebulizer System

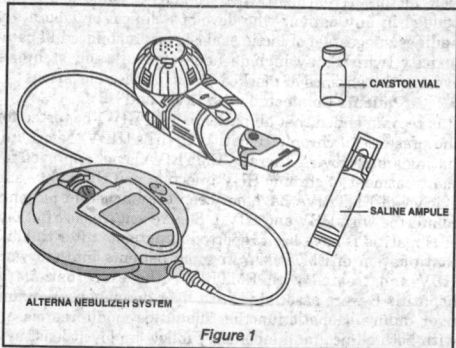

ALTERA NEBULIZER SYSTEM
Figure 1

Check to make sure that your Altera Nebulizer System works properly before starting your treatment with

CAYSTON. See the manufacturer's instructions for use that comes with your Altera Nebulizer System. This should have complete information about how to put together (assemble), prepare, use, and care for your Altera Nebulizer System.

Step 1 Preparing your CAYSTON for inhalation
- 1. Mix (reconstitute) CAYSTON with the saline only when ready to take a dose. Take one amber vial of CAYSTON and one ampule of saline from the carton. Separate the saline ampules by gently pulling apart.
- 2. Look at the ampule of saline. If it looks cloudy do not use it. Throw away this ampule and get another ampule of saline.
- 3. Gently tap the vial so that the powder settles to the bottom of the vial. This helps you get the proper dose of medicine. Open the amber drug vial by lifting up the metal flap on the top (Figure 2) and pulling down (Figure 3) to carefully remove the entire metal ring from the vial (Figure 4). Safely dispose of the ring in household garbage. Carefully remove the rubber stopper.

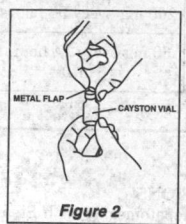
METAL FLAP / CAYSTON VIAL
Figure 2

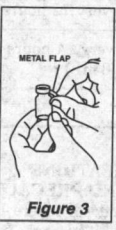
METAL FLAP
Figure 3

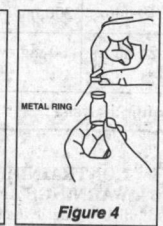
METAL RING
Figure 4

- 4. Open the ampule of saline by twisting off the tip. Squeeze out the contents completely into the vial (Figure 5). Next, close the vial with the rubber stopper and gently swirl the vial until the powder has completely dissolved and the liquid is clear.

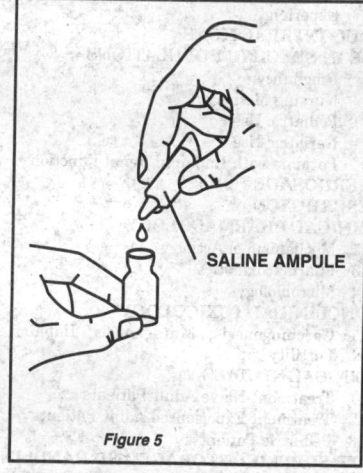
SALINE AMPULE
Figure 5

- 5. After mixing CAYSTON with the saline, check to make sure the diluted medicine is clear. If it is cloudy or has particles in it, do not use this medicine. Throw away this dose of medicine and start over again with a new vial of CAYSTON and a new ampule of saline.
- 6. Use CAYSTON right away after you mix with the saline.

Step 2 Taking your CAYSTON treatment
See the manufacturer's instructions for use that comes with your Altera Nebulizer System for complete instructions on taking a treatment, and how to clean and disinfect your Altera Nebulizer Handset.
- 7. Make sure the handset is on a flat, stable surface.
- 8. Remove the rubber stopper from the vial, then pour all of the mixed CAYSTON and saline into the Medication Reservoir of the handset (Figure 6). Be sure to completely empty the vial, gently tapping the vial against the side of the Medication Reservoir if necessary. Close the Medication Reservoir (Figure 7).
[See figure 7 at top of next column]
- 9. Begin your treatment by sitting in a relaxed, upright position. Hold the handset level, and place the Mouthpiece in your mouth. Close your lips around the Mouthpiece (Figure 8).
[See figure 8 in next column]
- 10. Breathe in and out normally (inhale and exhale) through the Mouthpiece. Avoid breathing through your nose. Continue to inhale and exhale comfortably until the treatment is finished.

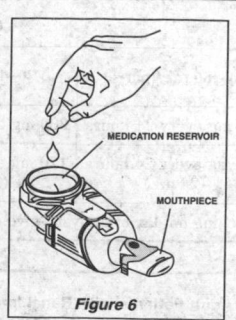
MEDICATION RESERVOIR
MOUTHPIECE
Figure 6

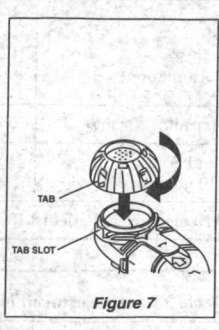
TAB
TAB SLOT
Figure 7

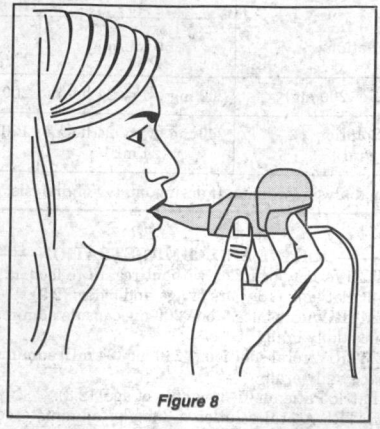
Figure 8

- 11. The empty vial, stopper and saline ampule should be disposed of in household garbage upon completion of dosing.

Manufactured by: Gilead Sciences, Inc., Foster City, CA 94404
CAYSTON is a trademark of Gilead Sciences, Inc. All other trademarks referenced herein are the property of their respective owners.
© 2010 Gilead Sciences, Inc. All rights reserved.
50-814-GS-000

Shown in Product Identification Guide, page 309

EMTRIVA® CAPSULES AND ORAL SOLUTION ℞
[ĕm-trĭvă]
(emtricitabine)
capsule for oral use

EMTRIVA
(emtricitabine)
solution for oral use

HIGHLIGHTS OF PRESCRIBING INFORMATION
These highlights do not include all the information needed to use EMTRIVA safely and effectively. See full prescribing information for EMTRIVA.
EMTRIVA (emtricitabine) capsule for oral use
EMTRIVA (emtricitabine) solution for oral use
Initial U.S. Approval: 2003

WARNINGS: LACTIC ACIDOSIS/SEVERE HEPATO-MEGALY WITH STEATOSIS and POST TREATMENT EXACERBATION OF HEPATITIS B
See full prescribing information for complete boxed warning.
- Lactic acidosis and severe hepatomegaly with steatosis, including fatal cases, have been reported with the use of nucleoside analogs. (5.1)
- Emtriva is not approved for the treatment of chronic Hepatitis B virus (HBV) infection. Severe acute exacerbations of Hepatitis B have been reported in patients who have discontinued EMTRIVA. Hepatic function should be monitored closely in patients coinfected with HIV-1 and HBV. If appropriate, initiation of anti-Hepatitis B therapy may be warranted. (5.2)

———**INDICATIONS AND USAGE**———
EMTRIVA, a nucleoside analog HIV-1 reverse transcriptase inhibitor, is indicated in combination with other antiretroviral agents for the treatment of HIV-1 infection. (1)

Formulation	Creatinine Clearance (mL/min)			
	≥50 mL/min	30–49 mL/min	15–29 mL/min	<15 mL/min or on hemodialysis*
Capsule (200 mg)	200 mg every 24 hours	200 mg every 48 hours	200 mg every 72 hours	200 mg every 96 hours
Oral Solution (10 mg/mL)	240 mg every 24 hours (24 mL)	120 mg every 24 hours (12 mL)	80 mg every 24 hours (8 mL)	60 mg every 24 hours (6 mL)

*Hemodialysis Patients: If dosing on day of dialysis, give dose after dialysis.

Table 1 Dose Adjustment in Adult Patients with Renal Impairment

Formulation	Creatinine Clearance (mL/min)			
	≥50 mL/min	30–49 mL/min	15–29 mL/min	<15 mL/min or on hemodialysis*
Capsule (200 mg)	200 mg every 24 hours	200 mg every 48 hours	200 mg every 72 hours	200 mg every 96 hours
Oral Solution (10 mg/mL)	240 mg every 24 hours (24 mL)	120 mg every 24 hours (12 mL)	80 mg every 24 hours (8 mL)	60 mg every 24 hours (6 mL)

*Hemodialysis Patients: If dosing on day of dialysis, give dose after dialysis.

---DOSAGE AND ADMINISTRATION---
• EMTRIVA may be taken without regard to food. (2.1)
• Adult Patients (18 years of age and older) (2.2):
  • EMTRIVA capsules: one 200 mg capsule administered once daily orally.
  • EMTRIVA oral solution: 240 mg (24 mL) administered once daily orally.
• Pediatric Patients (0–3 months of age) (2.3):
  • EMTRIVA oral solution: 3 mg/kg administered once daily orally.
• Pediatric Patients (3 months through 17 years) (2.4):
  • EMTRIVA oral solution: 6 mg/kg up to a maximum of 240 mg (24 mL) administered once daily orally.
  • EMTRIVA capsules: for children weighing more than 33 kg who can swallow an intact capsule, one 200 mg capsule administered once daily orally.
• Dose interval adjustment in adult patients with renal impairment (2.5):
[See first table above]

---DOSAGE FORMS AND STRENGTHS---
• Capsules: 200 mg (3)
• Oral solution: 10 mg per mL (3)

---CONTRAINDICATIONS---
EMTRIVA is contraindicated in patients with previously demonstrated hypersensitivity to any of the components of the products. (4)

---WARNINGS AND PRECAUTIONS---
• Products with same active ingredient: Do not use with other emtricitabine-containing products (e.g., ATRIPLA and TRUVADA). (5.3)
• Redistribution/accumulation of body fat: Observed in patients receiving antiretroviral therapy. (5.5)
• Immune reconstitution syndrome: May necessitate further evaluation and treatment. (5.6)

---ADVERSE REACTIONS---
Most common adverse reactions (incidence ≥10%) are headache, diarrhea, nausea, fatigue, dizziness, depression, insomnia, abnormal dreams, rash, abdominal pain, asthenia, increased cough, and rhinitis. Skin hyperpigmentation was very common (≥10%) in pediatric patients. (6)
To report SUSPECTED ADVERSE REACTIONS, contact Gilead Sciences, Inc. at 1-800-GILEAD-5 or FDA at 1-800-FDA-1088 or www.fda.gov/medwatch

---USE IN SPECIFIC POPULATIONS---
• Nursing mothers: Women infected with HIV should be instructed not to breast feed. (8.3)
• Pediatrics: Dose adjustment based on age and weight. (2.3, 2.4, 12.3)
See 17 for PATIENT COUNSELING INFORMATION and FDA-approved patient labeling

Revised: 05/2008

FULL PRESCRIBING INFORMATION: CONTENTS*
WARNINGS: LACTIC ACIDOSIS/SEVERE HEPATOMEGALY WITH STEATOSIS AND POST TREATMENT EXACERBATION OF HEPATITIS B
1 INDICATIONS AND USAGE
2 DOSAGE AND ADMINISTRATION
  2.1 Recommended Dose
  2.2 Adult Patients (18 years of age and older)
  2.3 Pediatric Patients (0–3 months of age)
  2.4 Pediatric Patients (3 months through 17 years)
  2.5 Dose Adjustment in Adult Patients with Renal Impairment
3 DOSAGE FORMS AND STRENGTHS

4 CONTRAINDICATIONS
5 WARNINGS AND PRECAUTIONS
  5.1 Lactic Acidosis/Severe Hepatomegaly with Steatosis
  5.2 Patients Coinfected with HIV-1 and HBV
  5.3 Coadministration with Related Products
  5.4 New Onset or Worsening Renal Impairment
  5.5 Fat Redistribution
  5.6 Immune Reconstitution Syndrome
6 ADVERSE REACTIONS
  6.1 Adverse Reactions from Clinical Trials Experience
7 DRUG INTERACTIONS
8 USE IN SPECIFIC POPULATIONS
  8.1 Pregnancy
  8.3 Nursing Mothers
  8.4 Pediatric Use
  8.5 Geriatric Use
  8.6 Patients with Impaired Renal Function
10 OVERDOSAGE
11 DESCRIPTION
12 CLINICAL PHARMACOLOGY
  12.1 Mechanism of Action
  12.3 Pharmacokinetics
  12.4 Microbiology
13 NONCLINICAL TOXICOLOGY
  13.1 Carcinogenesis, Mutagenesis, Impairment of Fertility
14 CLINICAL STUDIES
  14.1 Treatment-Naive Adult Patients
  14.2 Treatment-Experienced Adult Patients
  14.3 Pediatric Patients
16 HOW SUPPLIED/STORAGE AND HANDLING
17 PATIENT COUNSELING INFORMATION
  17.1 Information for Patients
  17.2 FDA-Approved Patient Labeling
* Sections or subsections omitted from the full prescribing information are not listed

FULL PRESCRIBING INFORMATION

WARNINGS: LACTIC ACIDOSIS/SEVERE HEPATOMEGALY WITH STEATOSIS AND POST TREATMENT EXACERBATION OF HEPATITIS B
Lactic acidosis and severe hepatomegaly with steatosis, including fatal cases, have been reported with the use of nucleoside analogs alone or in combination with other antiretrovirals [See Warnings and Precautions (5.1)].
EMTRIVA is not approved for the treatment of chronic hepatitis B virus (HBV) infection and the safety and efficacy of EMTRIVA have not been established in patients coinfected with HBV and HIV-1. Severe acute exacerbations of hepatitis B have been reported in patients who have discontinued EMTRIVA. Hepatic function should be monitored closely with both clinical and laboratory follow-up for at least several months in patients who are coinfected with HIV-1 and HBV and discontinue EMTRIVA. If appropriate, initiation of anti-hepatitis B therapy may be warranted [See Warnings and Precautions (5.2)].

1 INDICATIONS AND USAGE
EMTRIVA® is indicated in combination with other antiretroviral agents for the treatment of HIV-1 infection. Additional important information regarding the use of EMTRIVA for the treatment of HIV-1 Infection:
• EMTRIVA should not be coadministered with ATRIPLA®, TRUVADA®, or lamivudine-containing products [See Warnings and Precautions (5.3)].
• In treatment-experienced patients, the use of EMTRIVA should be guided by laboratory testing and treatment history [See Clinical Pharmacology (12.4)].

2 DOSAGE AND ADMINISTRATION
2.1 Recommended Dose
EMTRIVA may be taken without regard to food.
2.2 Adult Patients (18 years of age and older)
• EMTRIVA capsules: one 200 mg capsule administered once daily orally.
• EMTRIVA oral solution: 240 mg (24 mL) administered once daily orally.
2.3 Pediatric Patients (0–3 months of age)
• EMTRIVA oral solution: 3 mg/kg administered once daily orally.
2.4 Pediatric Patients (3 months through 17 years)
• EMTRIVA oral solution: 6 mg/kg up to a maximum of 240 mg (24 mL) administered once daily orally.
• EMTRIVA capsules: for children weighing more than 33 kg who can swallow an intact capsule, one 200 mg capsule administered once daily orally.
2.5 Dose Adjustment in Adult Patients with Renal Impairment
Significantly increased drug exposures were seen when EMTRIVA was administered to patients with renal impairment [See Clinical Pharmacology (12.3)]. Therefore, the dosing interval or dose of EMTRIVA should be adjusted in patients with baseline creatinine clearance <50 mL/min using the following guidelines (see Table 1). The safety and effectiveness of these dose adjustment guidelines have not been clinically evaluated. Therefore, clinical response to treatment and renal function should be closely monitored in these patients.
[See table 1 at left]
Although there are insufficient data to recommend a specific dose adjustment of EMTRIVA in pediatric patients with renal impairment, a reduction in the dose and/or an increase in the dosing interval similar to adjustments for adults should be considered.

3 DOSAGE FORMS AND STRENGTHS
EMTRIVA is available as capsules and oral solution.
EMTRIVA capsules, containing 200 mg of emtricitabine, are size 1 hard gelatin capsules with a blue cap and white body, printed with "200 mg" in black on the cap and "GILEAD" and the corporate logo in black on the body.
EMTRIVA oral solution is a clear, orange to dark orange liquid containing 10 mg of emtricitabine per mL.

4 CONTRAINDICATIONS
EMTRIVA is contraindicated in patients with previously demonstrated hypersensitivity to any of the components of the products.

5 WARNINGS AND PRECAUTIONS
5.1 Lactic Acidosis/Severe Hepatomegaly with Steatosis
Lactic acidosis and severe hepatomegaly with steatosis, including fatal cases, have been reported with the use of nucleoside analogs alone or in combination, including emtricitabine and other antiretrovirals. A majority of these cases have been in women. Obesity and prolonged nucleoside exposure may be risk factors. Particular caution should be exercised when administering nucleoside analogs to any patient with known risk factors for liver diseases; however, cases have also been reported in patients with no known risk factors. Treatment with EMTRIVA should be suspended in any patient who develops clinical or laboratory findings suggestive of lactic acidosis or pronounced hepatotoxicity (which may include hepatomegaly and steatosis even in the absence of marked transaminase elevations).
5.2 Patients Coinfected with HIV-1 and HBV
It is recommended that all patients with HIV-1 be tested for the presence of chronic Hepatitis B virus (HBV) before initiating antiretroviral therapy. EMTRIVA is not approved for the treatment of chronic HBV infection and the safety and efficacy of EMTRIVA have not been established in patients coinfected with HBV and HIV-1. Severe acute exacerbations of Hepatitis B have been reported in patients after the discontinuation of EMTRIVA. In some patients infected with HBV and treated with EMTRIVA, the exacerbations of hepatitis B were associated with liver decompensation and liver failure. Hepatic function should be monitored closely with both clinical and laboratory follow-up for at least several months in patients who are coinfected with HIV-1 and HBV and discontinue EMTRIVA. If appropriate, initiation of anti-Hepatitis B therapy may be warranted.

5.3 Coadministration with Related Products

EMTRIVA is a component of TRUVADA (a fixed-dose combination of emtricitabine and tenofovir disoproxil fumarate) and ATRIPLA (a fixed-dose combination of efavirenz, emtricitabine, and tenofovir disoproxil fumarate). EMTRIVA should not be coadministered with TRUVADA or ATRIPLA. Due to similarities between emtricitabine and lamivudine, EMTRIVA should not be coadministered with other drugs containing lamivudine, including Combivir (lamivudine/zidovudine), Epivir or Epivir-HBV (lamivudine), Epzicom (abacavir sulfate/lamivudine), or Trizivir (abacavir sulfate/lamivudine/zidovudine).

5.4 New Onset or Worsening Renal Impairment

Emtricitabine is principally eliminated by the kidney. Reduction of the dosage of EMTRIVA is recommended for patients with impaired renal function [See Dosage and Administration (2.5) and Clinical Pharmacology (12.3)].

5.5 Fat Redistribution

Redistribution/accumulation of body fat including central obesity, dorsocervical fat enlargement (buffalo hump), peripheral wasting, facial wasting, breast enlargement, and "cushingoid appearance" have been observed in patients receiving antiretroviral therapy. The mechanism and long-term consequences of these events are currently unknown. A causal relationship has not been established.

5.6 Immune Reconstitution Syndrome

Immune reconstitution syndrome has been reported in patients treated with combination antiretroviral therapy, including EMTRIVA. During the initial phase of combination antiretroviral treatment, patients whose immune system responds may develop an inflammatory response to indolent or residual opportunistic infections [such as Mycobacterium avium infection, cytomegalovirus, Pneumocystis jirovecii pneumonia (PCP), or tuberculosis], which may necessitate further evaluation and treatment.

6 ADVERSE REACTIONS

The following adverse reactions are discussed in other sections of the labeling:

- Lactic acidosis/severe hepatomegaly with steatosis [See Boxed Warning, Warnings and Precautions (5.1)].
- Severe acute exacerbations of Hepatitis B [See Boxed Warning, Warnings and Precautions (5.2)].
- Immune reconstitution syndrome [See Warnings and Precautions (5.6)]

6.1 Adverse Reactions from Clinical Trials Experience

Adult Patients

More than 2,000 adult patients with HIV-1 infection have been treated with EMTRIVA alone or in combination with other antiretroviral agents for periods of 10 days to 200 weeks in clinical trials.

Because clinical trials are conducted under widely varying conditions, adverse reaction rates observed in the clinical trials of a drug cannot be directly compared to rates in the clinical trials of another drug and may not reflect the rates observed in practice.

The most common adverse reactions (incidence ≥10%, any severity) identified from any of the 3 large controlled clinical trials include headache, diarrhea nausea, fatigue, dizziness, depression, insomnia, abnormal dreams, rash, abdominal pain, asthenia, increased cough, and rhinitis.

Studies 301A and 303 - Treatment Emergent Adverse Reactions: The most common adverse reactions that occurred in patients receiving EMTRIVA with other antiretroviral agents in clinical studies 301A and 303 were headache, diarrhea, nausea, and rash, which were generally of mild to moderate severity. Approximately 1% of patients discontinued participation in the clinical studies due to these events. All adverse reactions were reported with similar frequency in EMTRIVA and control treatment groups with the exception of skin discoloration which was reported with higher frequency in the EMTRIVA treated group.

Skin discoloration, manifested by hyperpigmentation on the palms and/or soles was generally mild and asymptomatic. The mechanism and clinical significance are unknown.

A summary of EMTRIVA treatment emergent clinical adverse reactions in studies 301A and 303 is provided in Table 2.

[See table 2 at right]

Studies 301A and 303 - Laboratory Abnormalities:

Laboratory abnormalities in these studies occurred with similar frequency in the EMTRIVA and comparator groups. A summary of Grade 3 and 4 laboratory abnormalities is provided in Table 3 below.

[See table 3 at right]

Study 934 - Treatment Emergent Adverse Reactions: In Study 934, 511 antiretroviral-naïve patients received either VIREAD + EMTRIVA administered in combination with efavirenz (N=257) or zidovudine/lamivudine administered in combination with efavirenz (N=254). Adverse reactions observed in this study were generally consistent with those seen in previous studies in treatment-experienced or treatment-naïve patients (Table 4).

Table 2 Selected Treatment-Emergent Adverse Reactions (All Grades, Regardless of Causality) Reported in ≥3% of EMTRIVA-Treated Patients in Either Study 301A or 303 (0–48 Weeks)

	303		301A	
	EMTRIVA + ZDV/d4T + NNRTI/PI (N=294)	Lamivudine + ZDV/d4T + NNRTI/PI (N=146)	EMTRIVA + didanosine + efavirenz (N=286)	Stavudine + didanosine + efavirenz (N=285)
Body as a Whole				
Abdominal pain	8%	11%	14%	17%
Asthenia	16%	10%	12%	17%
Headache	13%	6%	22%	25%
Digestive System				
Diarrhea	23%	18%	23%	32%
Dyspepsia	4%	5%	8%	12%
Nausea	18%	12%	13%	23%
Vomiting	9%	7%	9%	12%
Musculoskeletal				
Arthralgia	3%	4%	5%	6%
Myalgia	4%	4%	6%	3%
Nervous System				
Abnormal dreams	2%	<1%	11%	19%
Depressive disorders	6%	10%	9%	13%
Dizziness	4%	5%	25%	26%
Insomnia	7%	3%	16%	21%
Neuropathy/peripheral neuritis	4%	3%	4%	13%
Paresthesia	5%	7%	6%	12%
Respiratory				
Increased cough	14%	11%	14%	8%
Rhinitis	18%	12%	12%	10%
Skin				
Rash event*	17%	14%	30%	33%

*Rash event includes rash, pruritus, maculopapular rash, urticaria, vesiculobullous rash, pustular rash, and allergic reaction.

Table 3 Treatment-Emergent Grade 3/4 Laboratory Abnormalities Reported in ≥1% of EMTRIVA-Treated Patients in Either Study 301A or 303

	303		301A	
	EMTRIVA + ZDV/d4T + NNRTI/PI (N=294)	Lamivudine + ZDV/d4T + NNRTI/PI (N=146)	EMTRIVA + Didanosine + Efavirenz (N=286)	Stavudine + Didanosine + Efavirenz (N=285)
Percentage with grade 3 or grade 4 laboratory abnormality	31%	28%	34%	38%
ALT (>5.0 × ULN*)	2%	1%	5%	6%
AST (>5.0 × ULN)	3%	<1%	6%	9%
Bilirubin (>2.5 × ULN)	1%	2%	<1%	<1%
Creatine kinase (>4.0 × ULN)	11%	14%	12%	11%
Neutrophils (<750 mm³)	5%	3%	5%	7%
Pancreatic amylase (>2.0 × ULN)	2%	2%	<1%	1%
Serum amylase (>2.0 × ULN)	2%	2%	5%	10%
Serum glucose (<40 or >250 mg/dL)	3%	3%	2%	3%
Serum lipase (>2.0 × ULN)	<1%	<1%	1%	2%
Triglycerides (>750 mg/dL)	10%	8%	9%	6%

* ULN = Upper limit of normal

Table 4 Selected Treatment-Emergent Adverse Reactions* (Grades 2–4) Reported in ≥5% in Any Treatment Group in Study 934 (0–144 Weeks)

	TDF[†] + EMTRIVA + EFV	AZT/3TC + EFV
	N=257	N=254
Gastrointestinal Disorder		
Diarrhea	9%	5%
Nausea	9%	7%
Vomiting	2%	5%
General Disorders and Administration Site Condition		
Fatigue	9%	8%
Infections and Infestations		
Sinusitis	8%	4%
Upper respiratory tract infections	8%	5%
Nasopharyngitis	5%	3%
Nervous System Disorders		
Headache	6%	5%
Dizziness	8%	7%
Psychiatric Disorders		
Depression	9%	7%
Insomnia	5%	7%
Skin and Subcutaneous Tissue Disorders		
Rash event[‡]	7%	9%

*Frequencies of adverse reactions are based on all treatment-emergent adverse events, regardless of relationship to study drug.
†From Weeks 96 to 144 of the study, patients received TRUVADA with efavirenz in place of VIREAD + EMTRIVA with efavirenz.
‡Rash event includes rash, exfoliative rash, rash generalized, rash macular, rash maculo-papular, rash pruritic, and rash vesicular.

Study 934 – Laboratory Abnormalities: Significant laboratory abnormalities observed in this study are shown in Table 5.

Table 5 Significant Laboratory Abnormalities Reported in ≥1% of Patients in Any Treatment Group in Study 934 (0–144 Weeks)

	TDF* + EMTRIVA + EFV	AZT/3TC + EFV
	N=257	N=254
Any ≥ Grade 3 Laboratory Abnormality	30%	26%
Fasting Cholesterol (>240 mg/dL)	22%	24%
Creatine Kinase (M: >990 U/L) (F: >845 U/L)	9%	7%
Serum Amylase (>175 U/L)	8%	4%
Alkaline Phosphatase (>550 U/L)	1%	0%
AST (M: >180 U/L) (F: >170 U/L)	3%	3%
ALT (M: >215 U/L) (F: >170 U/L)	2%	3%
Hemoglobin (<8.0 mg/dL)	0%	4%
Hyperglycemia (>250 mg/dL)	2%	1%
Hematuria (>75 RBC/HPF)	3%	2%
Glycosuria (3+)	<1%	1%

(continued from Table 5):

Neutrophils (<750/mm³)	3%	5%
Fasting Triglycerides (>750 mg/dL)	4%	2%

*From Weeks 96 to 144 of the study, patients received TRUVADA with efavirenz in place of VIREAD + EMTRIVA with efavirenz.

Pediatric Patients
Assessment of adverse reactions is based on data from Study 203, an open label, uncontrolled study of 116 HIV-1-infected pediatric patients who received emtricitabine through 48 weeks. The adverse reaction profile in pediatric patients was generally comparable to that observed in clinical studies of EMTRIVA in adult patients *[See Adverse Reactions (6.1)]*. Hyperpigmentation was more frequent in children. Additional adverse reactions identified from this study include anemia.
Selected treatment-emergent adverse events, regardless of causality, reported in patients during 48 weeks of treatment were the following: infection (44%), hyperpigmentation (32%), increased cough (28%), vomiting (23%), otitis media (23%), rash (21%), rhinitis (20%), diarrhea (20%), fever (18%), pneumonia (15%), gastroenteritis (11%), abdominal pain (10%), and anemia (7%). Treatment-emergent grade 3/4 laboratory abnormalities were experienced by 9% of pediatric patients, including amylase >2.0 × ULN (n=4), neutrophils <750/mm³ (n=3), ALT >5 × ULN (n=2), elevated CPK (>4 × ULN) (n=2) and one patient each with elevated bilirubin (>3.0 × ULN), elevated GGT (>10 × ULN), elevated lipase (>2.5 × ULN), decreased hemoglobin (<7 g/dL), and decreased glucose (<40 mg/dL).

7 DRUG INTERACTIONS
The potential for drug interactions with EMTRIVA has been studied in combination with zidovudine, indinavir, stavudine, famciclovir, and tenofovir disoproxil fumarate. There were no clinically significant drug interactions for any of these drugs Drug interactions studies are described elsewhere in the labeling *[See Clinical Pharmacology (12.3)]*

8 USE IN SPECIFIC POPULATIONS
8.1 Pregnancy
Pregnancy Category B
The incidence of fetal variations and malformations was not increased in embryofetal toxicity studies performed with emtricitabine in mice at exposures (AUC) approximately 60-fold higher and in rabbits at approximately 120-fold higher than human exposures at the recommended daily dose. There are, however, no adequate and well-controlled studies in pregnant women. Because animal reproduction studies are not always predictive of human response, EMTRIVA should be used during pregnancy only if clearly needed.
Antiretroviral Pregnancy Registry: To monitor fetal outcomes of pregnant women exposed to EMTRIVA, an Antiretroviral Pregnancy Registry has been established. Healthcare providers are encouraged to register patients by calling 1–800–258–4263.
8.3 Nursing Mothers
Nursing Mothers: The Centers for Disease Control and Prevention recommend that HIV-1-infected mothers not breast-feed their infants to avoid risking postnatal transmission of HIV-1. It is not known whether emtricitabine is excreted in human milk. Because of both the potential for HIV-1 transmission and the potential for serious adverse reactions in nursing infants, **mothers should be instructed not to breast-feed if they are receiving EMTRIVA.**
8.4 Pediatric Use
The safety and efficacy of emtricitabine in patients between 3 months and 21 years of age is supported by data from three open-label, non-randomized clinical studies in which emtricitabine was administered to 169 HIV-1 infected treatment-naive and experienced (defined as virologically suppressed on a lamivudine containing regimen for which emtricitabine was substituted for lamivudine) subjects *[See Clinical Studies (14.3)]*.
The pharmacokinetics of emtricitabine were studied in 20 neonates born to HIV-1-positive mothers *[See Clinical Studies (14.3)]*. All neonates were HIV-1 negative at the end of the study; the efficacy of emtricitabine in preventing or treating HIV-1 could not be determined.
8.5 Geriatric Use
Clinical studies of EMTRIVA did not include sufficient numbers of subjects aged 65 years and over to determine whether they respond differently from younger subjects. In general, dose selection for the elderly patient should be cautious, keeping in mind the greater frequency of decreased hepatic, renal, or cardiac function, and of concomitant disease or other drug therapy.
8.6 Patients with Impaired Renal Function
It is recommended that the dose or dosing interval for EMTRIVA be modified in patients with creatinine clearance <50 mL/min or in patients who require dialysis *[See Dosage and Administration (2.5)]*.

10 OVERDOSAGE
There is no known antidote for EMTRIVA. Limited clinical experience is available at doses higher than the therapeutic dose of EMTRIVA. In one clinical pharmacology study single doses of emtricitabine 1200 mg were administered to 11 patients. No severe adverse reactions were reported.
The effects of higher doses are not known. If overdose occurs the patient should be monitored for signs of toxicity, and standard supportive treatment applied as necessary.
Hemodialysis treatment removes approximately 30% of the emtricitabine dose over a 3-hour dialysis period starting within 1.5 hours of emtricitabine dosing (blood flow rate of 400 mL/min and a dialysate flow rate of 600 mL/min). It is not known whether emtricitabine can be removed by peritoneal dialysis.

11 DESCRIPTION
EMTRIVA is the brand name of emtricitabine, a synthetic nucleoside analog with activity against human immunodeficiency virus type 1 (HIV-1) reverse transcriptase.
The chemical name of emtricitabine is 5-fluoro-1-(2R,5S)-[2-(hydroxymethyl)-1,3-oxathiolan-5-yl]cytosine. Emtricitabine is the (-) enantiomer of a thio analog of cytidine, which differs from other cytidine analogs in that it has a fluorine in the 5-position.
It has a molecular formula of $C_8H_{10}FN_3O_3S$ and a molecular weight of 247.24. It has the following structural formula:

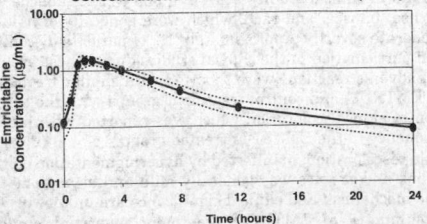

Emtricitabine is a white to off-white powder with a solubility of approximately 112 mg/mL in water at 25 °C. The log P for emtricitabine is -0.43 and the pKa is 2.65.
EMTRIVA is available as capsules or as an oral solution. EMTRIVA capsules are for oral administration. Each capsule contains 200 mg of emtricitabine and the inactive ingredients, crospovidone, magnesium stearate, microcrystalline cellulose, and povidone.
EMTRIVA oral solution is for oral administration. One milliliter (1 mL) of EMTRIVA oral solution contains 10 mg of emtricitabine in an aqueous solution with the following inactive ingredients: cotton candy flavor, FD&C yellow No. 6, edetate disodium, methylparaben, and propylparaben (added as preservatives), sodium phosphate (monobasic), propylene glycol, water, and xylitol (added as a sweetener). Sodium hydroxide and hydrochloric acid may be used to adjust pH.

12 CLINICAL PHARMACOLOGY
12.1 Mechanism of Action
Emtricitabine is an antiviral drug. *[See Clinical Pharmacology (12.4)]*
12.3 Pharmacokinetics
Adult Subjects
The pharmacokinetics of emtricitabine were evaluated in healthy volunteers and HIV-1-infected individuals. Emtricitabine pharmacokinetics are similar between these populations.
Figure 1 shows the mean steady-state plasma emtricitabine concentration-time profile in 20 HIV-1-infected subjects receiving EMTRIVA capsules.

Figure 1 Mean (±95% CI) Steady-State Plasma Emtricitabine Concentrations in HIV-1-Infected Adults (N=20)

Absorption
Emtricitabine is rapidly and extensively absorbed following oral administration with peak plasma concentrations occurring at 1–2 hours post-dose. Following multiple dose oral administration of EMTRIVA capsules to 20 HIV-1-infected subjects, the (mean ± SD) steady-state plasma emtricitabine peak concentration (C_{max}) was 1.8 ± 0.7 μg/mL and the area-under the plasma concentration-time curve over a 24-hour dosing interval (AUC) was 10.0 ± 3.1 μg•hr/mL. The mean steady state plasma trough concentration at 24 hours post-dose was 0.09 μg/mL. The mean absolute bioavailability of EMTRIVA capsules was 93% while the mean absolute bioavailability of EMTRIVA oral solution was 75%. The relative bioavailability of EMTRIVA oral solution was approximately 80% of EMTRIVA capsules. The multiple dose pharmacokinetics of emtricitabine are dose proportional over a dose range of 25–200 mg.

Distribution

In vitro binding of emtricitabine to human plasma proteins was <4% and independent of concentration over the range of 0.02–200 μg/mL. At peak plasma concentration, the mean plasma to blood drug concentration ratio was ~1.0 and the mean semen to plasma drug concentration ratio was ~4.0.

Metabolism

In vitro studies indicate that emtricitabine is not an inhibitor of human CYP450 enzymes. Following administration of ^{14}C-emtricitabine, complete recovery of the dose was achieved in urine (~86%) and feces (~14%). Thirteen percent (13%) of the dose was recovered in urine as three putative metabolites. The biotransformation of emtricitabine includes oxidation of the thiol moiety to form the 3'-sulfoxide diastereomers (~9% of dose) and conjugation with glucuronic acid to form 2'-O-glucuronide (~4% of dose). No other metabolites were identifiable.

Elimination

The plasma emtricitabine half-life is approximately 10 hours. The renal clearance of emtricitabine is greater than the estimated creatinine clearance, suggesting elimination by both glomerular filtration and active tubular secretion. There may be competition for elimination with other compounds that are also renally eliminated.

Effects of Food on Oral Absorption

EMTRIVA capsules and oral solution may be taken with or without food. Emtricitabine systemic exposure (AUC) was unaffected while C_{max} decreased by 29% when EMTRIVA capsules were administered with food (an approximately 1000 kcal high-fat meal). Emtricitabine systemic exposure (AUC) and C_{max} were unaffected when 200 mg EMTRIVA oral solution was administered with either a high-fat or low-fat meal.

Special Populations

Race, Gender

The pharmacokinetics of emtricitabine were similar in adult male and female patients and no pharmacokinetic differences due to race have been identified.

Pediatric Patients

The pharmacokinetics of emtricitabine at steady state were determined in 77 HIV-1-infected children, and the pharmacokinetic profile was characterized in four age groups (Table 6). The emtricitabine exposure achieved in children receiving a daily dose of 6 mg/kg up to a maximum of 240 mg oral solution or a 200 mg capsule is similar to exposures achieved in adults receiving a once-daily dose of 200 mg. The pharmacokinetics of emtricitabine were studied in 20 neonates born to HIV-1-positive mothers. Each mother received prenatal and intrapartum combination antiretroviral therapy. Neonates received up to 6 weeks of zidovudine prophylactically after birth. The neonates were administered two short courses of emtricitabine oral solution (each 3 mg/kg once daily × 4 days) during the first 3 months of life. The AUC observed in neonates who received a daily dose of 3 mg/kg of emtricitabine was similar to the AUC observed in pediatric patients ≥3 months to 17 years who received a daily dose of emtricitabine as a 6 mg/kg oral solution up to 240 mg or as a 200 mg capsule (Table 6).

[See table 6 at right]

Geriatric Patients

The pharmacokinetics of emtricitabine have not been fully evaluated in the elderly.

Patients with Impaired Renal Function

The pharmacokinetics of emtricitabine are altered in patients with renal impairment [See Warnings and Precautions (5.4)]. In adult patients with creatinine clearance <50 mL/min or with end-stage renal disease (ESRD) requiring dialysis, C_{max} and AUC of emtricitabine were increased due to a reduction in renal clearance (Table 7). It is recommended that the dosing interval for EMTRIVA be modified in adult patients with creatinine clearance <50 mL/min or in adult patients with ESRD who require dialysis [See Dosage and Administration (2.5)]. The effects of renal impairment on emtricitabine pharmacokinetics in pediatric patients are not known.

[See table 7 at right]

Hemodialysis: Hemodialysis treatment removes approximately 30% of the emtricitabine dose over a 3-hour dialysis period starting within 1.5 hours of emtricitabine dosing (blood flow rate of 400 mL/min and a dialysate flow rate of 600 mL/min). It is not known whether emtricitabine can be removed by peritoneal dialysis.

Patients with Hepatic Impairment

The pharmacokinetics of emtricitabine have not been studied in patients with hepatic impairment, however, emtricitabine is not metabolized by liver enzymes, so the impact of liver impairment should be limited.

Assessment of Drug Interactions

At concentrations up to 14-fold higher than those observed in vivo, emtricitabine did not inhibit in vitro drug metabolism mediated by any of the following human CYP isoforms: CYP1A2, CYP2A6, CYP2B6, CYP2C9, CYP2C19, CYP2D6, and CYP3A4. Emtricitabine did not inhibit the enzyme responsible for glucuronidation (uridine-5'-

Table 6 Mean ± SD Pharmacokinetic Parameters by Age Groups for Pediatric Patients and Neonates Receiving EMTRIVA Capsules or Oral Solution

Age	HIV-1-exposed Neonates	HIV-1-infected Pediatric Patients			
	0–3 mo (N=20)*	3–24 mo (N=14)	25 mo–6 yr (N=19)	7–12 yr (N=17)	13–17 yr (N=27)
Formulation					
Capsule (n)	0	0	0	10	26
Oral Solution (n)	20	14	19	7	1
Dose (mg/kg)†	3.1 (2.9–3.4)	6.1 (5.5–6.8)	6.1 (5.6–6.7)	5.6 (3.1–6.6)	4.4 (1.8–7.0)
Cmax (μg/mL)	1.6 ± 0.6	1.9 ± 0.6	1.9 ± 0.7	2.7 ± 0.8	2.7 ± 0.9
AUC (μg•hr/mL)	11.0 ± 4.2	8.7 ± 3.2	9.0 ± 3.0	12.6 ± 3.5	12.6 ± 5.4
T1/2 (hr)	12.1 ± 3.1	8.9 ± 3.2	11.3 ± 6.4	8.2 ± 3.2	8.9 ± 3.3

*Two pharmacokinetic evaluations were conducted in 20 neonates over the first 3 months of life. Median (range) age of infant on day of pharmacokinetic evaluation was 26 (5–81) days.
†Mean (range)

Table 7 Mean ± SD Pharmacokinetic Parameters in Adult Patients with Varying Degrees of Renal Function

Creatinine Clearance (mL/min)	>80 (N=6)	50–80 (N=6)	30–49 (N=6)	<30 (N=5)	ESRD* <30 (N=5)
Baseline creatinine clearance (mL/min)	107 ± 21	59.8 ± 6.5	40.9 ± 5.1	22.9 ± 5.3	8.8 ± 1.4
Cmax (μg/mL)	2.2 ± 0.6	3.8 ± 0.9	3.2 ± 0.6	2.8 ± 0.7	2.8 ± 0.5
AUC (μg•hr/mL)	11.8 ± 2.9	19.9 ± 1.2	25.1 ± 5.7	33.7 ± 2.1	53.2 ± 9.9
CL/F (mL/min)	302 ± 94	168 ± 10	138 ± 28	99 ± 6	64 ± 12
CLr (mL/min)	213 ± 89	121 ± 39	69 ± 32	30 ± 11	NA†

* ESRD patients requiring dialysis
† NA = Not Applicable

Table 8 Drug Interactions: Change in Pharmacokinetic Parameters for Emtricitabine in the Presence of the Coadministered Drug*

Coadministered Drug	Dose of Coadministered Drug (mg)	Emtricitabine Dose (mg)	N	% Change of Emtricitabine Pharmacokinetic Parameters† (90% CI)		
				Cmax	AUC	Cmin
Tenofovir DF	300 once daily × 7 days	200 once daily × 7 days	17	⇔	⇔	↑ 20 (↑ 12 to ↑ 29)
Zidovudine	300 twice daily × 7 days	200 once daily × 7 days	27	⇔	⇔	⇔
Indinavir	800 × 1	200 × 1	12	⇔	⇔	NA
Famciclovir	500 × 1	200 × 1	12	⇔	⇔	NA
Stavudine	40 × 1	200 × 1	6	⇔	⇔	NA

* All interaction studies conducted in healthy volunteers.
† ↑ = Increase; ↓ = Decrease; ⇔ = No Effect; NA = Not Applicable

disphosphoglucuronyl transferase). Based on the results of these in vitro experiments and the known elimination pathways of emtricitabine, the potential for CYP mediated interactions involving emtricitabine with other medicinal products is low.

EMTRIVA has been evaluated in healthy volunteers in combination with tenofovir disoproxil fumarate (DF), zidovudine, indinavir, famciclovir, and stavudine. Tables 8 and 9 summarize the pharmacokinetic effects of coadministered drug on emtricitabine pharmacokinetics and effects of emtricitabine on the pharmacokinetics of coadministered drug.

[See table 8 above]
[See table 9 at top of next page]

12.4   Microbiology

Mechanism of Action

Emtricitabine, a synthetic nucleoside analog of cytidine, is phosphorylated by cellular enzymes to form emtricitabine 5'-triphosphate. Emtricitabine 5'-triphosphate inhibits the activity of the HIV-1 reverse transcriptase by competing with the natural substrate deoxycytidine 5'-triphosphate and by being incorporated into nascent viral DNA which re-

sults in chain termination. Emtricitabine 5'-triphosphate is a weak inhibitor of mammalian DNA polymerase α, β, ε, and mitochondrial DNA polymerase γ.

Antiviral Activity

The antiviral activity in cell culture of emtricitabine against laboratory and clinical isolates of HIV-1 was assessed in lymphoblastoid cell lines, the MAGI-CCR5 cell line, and peripheral blood mononuclear cells. The 50% effective concentration (EC$_{50}$) value for emtricitabine was in the range of 0.0013–0.64 μM (0.0003–0.158 μg/mL). In drug combination studies of emtricitabine with nucleoside reverse transcriptase inhibitors (abacavir, lamivudine, stavudine, tenofovir, zalcitabine, zidovudine), non-nucleoside reverse transcriptase inhibitors (delavirdine, efavirenz, nevirapine), and protease inhibitors (amprenavir, nelfinavir, ritonavir, saquinavir), additive to synergistic effects were observed. Emtricitabine displayed antiviral activity in cell culture against HIV-1 clades A, B, C, D, E, F, and G (EC$_{50}$ values ranged from 0.007–0.075 μM) and showed strain specific activity against HIV-2 (EC$_{50}$ values ranged from 0.007–1.5 μM).

The in vivo activity of emtricitabine was evaluated in two clinical trials in which 101 patients were administered

Table 9 Drug Interactions: Change in Pharmacokinetic Parameters for Coadministered Drug in the Presence of Emtricitabine*

Coadministered Drug	Dose of Coadministered Drug (mg)	Emtricitabine Dose (mg)	N	% Change of Coadministered Drug Pharmacokinetic Parameters[†] (90% CI)		
				C_{max}	AUC	C_{min}
Tenofovir DF	300 once daily × 7 days	200 once daily × 7 days	17	⇔	⇔	⇔
Zidovudine	300 twice daily × 7 days	200 once daily × 7 days	27	↑ 17 (↑ 0 to ↑ 38)	↑ 13 (↑ 5 to ↑ 20)	⇔
Indinavir	800 × 1	200 × 1	12	⇔	⇔	NA
Famciclovir	500 × 1	200 × 1	12	⇔	⇔	NA
Stavudine	40 × 1	200 × 1	6	⇔	⇔	NA

* All interaction studies conducted in healthy volunteers.
† ↑ = Increase; ↓ = Decrease; ⇔ = No Effect; NA = Not Applicable

Table 10 Outcomes of Randomized Treatment at Week 48 and 144 (Study 934)

Outcomes	Week 48		Week 144	
	EMTRIVA +TDF +EFV (N=244)	AZT/3TC +EFV (N=243)	EMTRIVA +TDF +EFV (N=227)*	AZT/3TC +EFV (N=229)*
Responder[†]	84%	73%	71%	58%
Virologic failure[‡]	2%	4%	3%	6%
Rebound	1%	3%	2%	5%
Never suppressed	0%	0%	0%	0%
Change in antiretroviral regimen	1%	1%	1%	1%
Death	<1%	1%	1%	1%
Discontinued due to adverse event	4%	9%	5%	12%
Discontinued for other reasons[§]	10%	14%	20%	22%

*Patients who were responders at Week 48 or Week 96 (HIV-1 RNA <400 copies/mL) but did not consent to continue study after Week 48 or Week 96 were excluded from analysis.
†Patients achieved and maintained confirmed HIV-1 RNA <400 copies/mL through Weeks 48 and 144.
‡Includes confirmed viral rebound and failure to achieve confirmed <400 copies/mL through Weeks 48 and 144.
§Includes lost to follow-up, patient withdrawal, noncompliance, protocol violation and other reasons.

25–400 mg a day of EMTRIVA as monotherapy for 10–14 days. A dose-related antiviral effect was observed, with a median decrease from baseline in plasma HIV-1 RNA of 1.3 $\log_{10}$ at a dose of 25 mg once daily and 1.7 $\log_{10}$ to 1.9 $\log_{10}$ at a dose of 200 mg once daily or twice daily.

Resistance
Emtricitabine-resistant isolates of HIV-1 have been selected in cell culture and in vivo. Genotypic analysis of these isolates showed that the reduced susceptibility to emtricitabine was associated with a substitution in the HIV-1 reverse transcriptase gene at codon 184 which resulted in an amino acid substitution of methionine by valine or isoleucine (M184V/I).

Emtricitabine-resistant isolates of HIV-1 have been recovered from some patients treated with emtricitabine alone or in combination with other antiretroviral agents. In a clinical study of treatment-naive patients treated with EMTRIVA, didanosine, and efavirenz [See Clinical Studies (14.1)], viral isolates from 37.5% of patients with virologic failure showed reduced susceptibility to emtricitabine. Genotypic analysis of these isolates showed that the resistance was due to M184V/I substitutions in the HIV-1 reverse transcriptase gene.

In a clinical study of treatment-naive patients treated with either EMTRIVA, VIREAD, and efavirenz or zidovudine/lamivudine and efavirenz [See Clinical Studies (14.1)], resistance analysis was performed on HIV-1 isolates from all confirmed virologic failure patients with >400 copies/mL of HIV-1 RNA at Week 144 or early discontinuation. Development of efavirenz resistance-associated substitutions occurred most frequently and was similar between the treatment arms. The M184V amino acid substitution, associated with resistance to EMTRIVA and lamivudine, was observed in 2/19 analyzed patient isolates in the EMTRIVA + VIREAD group and in 10/29 analyzed patient isolates in the lamivudine/zidovudine group. Through 144 weeks of Study 934, no patients have developed a detectable K65R substitution in their HIV-1 as analyzed through standard genotypic analysis.

Cross Resistance
Cross-resistance among certain nucleoside analog reverse transcriptase inhibitors has been recognized. Emtricitabine-resistant isolates (M184V/I) were cross-resistant to lamivudine and zalcitabine but retained sensitivity in cell culture to didanosine, stavudine, tenofovir, zidovudine, and NNRTIs (delavirdine, efavirenz, and nevirapine). HIV-1 isolates containing the K65R substitution, selected in vivo by abacavir, didanosine, tenofovir, and zalcitabine, demonstrated reduced susceptibility to inhibition by emtricitabine. Viruses harboring substitutions conferring reduced susceptibility to stavudine and zidovudine (M41L, D67N, K70R, L210W, T215Y/F, K219Q/E) or didanosine (L74V) remained sensitive to emtricitabine. HIV-1 containing the K103N substitution associated with resistance to NNRTIs was susceptible to emtricitabine.

13 NONCLINICAL TOXICOLOGY

13.1 Carcinogenesis, Mutagenesis, Impairment of Fertility

In long-term oral carcinogenicity studies of emtricitabine, no drug-related increases in tumor incidence were found in mice at doses up to 750 mg/kg/day (26 times the human systemic exposure at the therapeutic dose of 200 mg/day) or in rats at doses up to 600 mg/kg/day (31 times the human systemic exposure at the therapeutic dose).

Emtricitabine was not genotoxic in the reverse mutation bacterial test (Ames test), mouse lymphoma or mouse micronucleus assays.

Emtricitabine did not affect fertility in male rats at approximately 140-fold or in male and female mice at approximately 60-fold higher exposures (AUC) than in humans given the recommended 200 mg daily dose. Fertility was normal in the offspring of mice exposed daily from before birth (in utero) through sexual maturity at daily exposures (AUC) of approximately 60-fold higher than human exposures at the recommended 200 mg daily dose.

14 CLINICAL STUDIES

14.1 Treatment-Naive Adult Patients

Study 934
Data through 144 weeks are reported for Study 934, a randomized, open-label, active-controlled multicenter study comparing EMTRIVA + VIREAD administered in combination with efavirenz versus zidovudine/lamivudine fixed-dose combination administered in combination with efavirenz in 511 antiretroviral-naive patients. From Weeks 96 to 144 of the study, patients received emtricitabine + tenofovir disoproxil fumarate (tenofovir DF) with efavirenz in place of EMTRIVA + tenofovir DF with efavirenz. Patients had a mean age of 38 years (range 18–80), 86% were male, 59% were Caucasian and 23% were Black. The mean baseline CD4$^+$ cell count was 245 cells/mm^3 (range 2–1191) and median baseline plasma HIV-1 RNA was 5.01 $\log_{10}$ copies/mL (range 3.56–6.54). Patients were stratified by baseline CD4$^+$ cell count (< or ≥200 cells/mm^3); 41% had CD4$^+$ cell counts <200 cells/mm^3 and 51% of patients had baseline viral loads >100,000 copies/mL. Treatment outcomes through 48 and 144 weeks for those patients who did not have efavirenz resistance at baseline are presented in Table 10.

[See table 10 at left]

Through Week 48, 84% and 73% of patients in the EMTRIVA + tenofovir DF group and the zidovudine/lamivudine group, respectively, achieved and maintained HIV-1 RNA <400 copies/mL (71% and 58% through Week 144). The difference in the proportion of patients who achieved and maintained HIV-1 RNA <400 copies/mL through 48 weeks largely results from the higher number of discontinuations due to adverse events and other reasons in the zidovudine/lamivudine group in this open-label study. In addition, 80% and 70% of patients in the EMTRIVA + tenofovir DF group and the zidovudine/lamivudine group, respectively, achieved and maintained HIV-1 RNA <50 copies/mL through Week 48 (64% and 56% through Week 144). The mean increase from baseline in CD4$^+$ cell count was 190 cells/mm^3 in the EMTRIVA + tenofovir DF group and 158 cells/mm^3 in the zidovudine/lamivudine group at Week 48 (312 and 271 cells/mm^3 at Week 144).

Through 48 weeks, 7 patients in the EMTRIVA + tenofovir DF group and 5 patients in the zidovudine/lamivudine group experienced a new CDC Class C event (10 and 6 patients through 144 weeks).

Study 301A
Study 301A was a 48 week double-blind, active-controlled multicenter study comparing EMTRIVA (200 mg once daily) administered in combination with didanosine and efavirenz versus stavudine, didanosine and efavirenz in 571 antiretroviral naive adult patients. Patients had a mean age of 36 years (range 18–69), 85% were male, 52% Caucasian, 16% African-American and 26% Hispanic. Patients had a mean baseline CD4$^+$ cell count of 318 cells/mm^3 (range 5–1317) and a median baseline plasma HIV-1 RNA of 4.9 $\log_{10}$ copies/mL (range 2.6–7.0). Thirty-eight percent of patients had baseline viral loads >100,000 copies/mL and 31% had CD4$^+$ cell counts <200 cells/mL. Treatment outcomes are presented in Table 11 below.

Table 11 Outcomes of Randomized Treatment at Week 48 (Study 301A)

Outcomes	EMTRIVA + Didanosine + Efavirenz (N=286)	Stavudine + Didanosine + Efavirenz (N=285)
Responder*	81% (78%)	68% (59%)
Virologic Failure[†]	3%	11%
Death	0%	<1%
Study Discontinuation Due to Adverse Event	7%	13%
Study Discontinuation for Other Reasons[‡]	9%	8%

*Patients achieved and maintained confirmed HIV RNA <400 copies/mL (<50 copies/mL) through Week 48.
†Includes patients who failed to achieve virologic suppression or rebounded after achieving virologic suppression.
‡Includes lost to follow-up, patient withdrawal, non-compliance, protocol violation and other reasons.

The mean increase from baseline in CD4$^+$ cell count was 168 cells/mm^3 for the EMTRIVA arm and 134 cells/mm^3 for the stavudine arm.

Through 48 weeks in the EMTRIVA group, 5 patients (1.7%) experienced a new CDC Class C event, compared to 7 patients (2.5%) in the stavudine group.

14.2 Treatment-Experienced Adult Patients

Study 303

Study 303 was a 48 week, open-label, active-controlled multicenter study comparing EMTRIVA (200 mg once daily) to lamivudine, in combination with stavudine or zidovudine and a protease inhibitor or NNRTI in 440 adult patients who were on a lamivudine-containing triple-antiretroviral drug regimen for at least 12 weeks prior to study entry and had HIV-1 RNA ≤400 copies/mL.

Patients were randomized 1:2 to continue therapy with lamivudine (150 mg twice daily) or to switch to EMTRIVA (200 mg once daily). All patients were maintained on their stable background regimen. Patients had a mean age of 42 years (range 22–80), 86% were male, 64% Caucasian, 21% African-American and 13% Hispanic. Patients had a mean baseline CD4$^+$ cell count of 527 cells/mm^3 (range 37–1909), and a median baseline plasma HIV-1 RNA of 1.7 log$_{10}$ copies/mL (range 1.7–4.0).

The median duration of prior antiretroviral therapy was 27.6 months. Treatment outcomes are presented in Table 12 below.

Table 12 Outcomes of Randomized Treatment at Week 48 (Study 303)

Outcomes	EMTRIVA + ZDV/d4T + NNRTI/PI (N=294)	Lamivudine + ZDV/d4T + NNRTI/PI (N=146)
Responder*	77% (67%)	82% (72%)
Virologic Failure[†]	7%	8%
Death	0%	<1%
Study Discontinuation Due to Adverse Event	4%	0%
Study Discontinuation for Other Reasons[‡]	12%	10%

*Patients achieved and maintained confirmed HIV RNA <400 copies/mL (<50 copies/mL) through Week 48.
[†]Includes patients who failed to achieve virologic suppression or rebounded after achieving virologic suppression.
[‡]Includes lost to follow-up, patient withdrawal, non-compliance, protocol violation and other reasons.

The mean increase from baseline in CD4$^+$ cell count was 29 cells/mm^3 for the EMTRIVA arm and 61 cells/mm^3 for the lamivudine arm.

Through 48 weeks, in the EMTRIVA group 2 patients (0.7%) experienced a new CDC Class C event, compared to 2 patients (1.4%) in the lamivudine group.

14.3 Pediatric Patients

In three open-label, non-randomized clinical studies, emtricitabine was administered to 169 HIV-1 infected treatment-naive and experienced (defined as virologically suppressed on a lamivudine containing regimen for which emtricitabine was substituted for lamivudine) patients between 3 months and 21 years of age. Patients received once-daily EMTRIVA oral solution (6 mg/kg to a maximum of 240 mg/day) or EMTRIVA capsules (a single 200 mg capsule once daily) in combination with at least two other antiretroviral agents.

Patients had a mean age of 7.9 years (range 0.3–21), 49% were male, 15% Caucasian, 61% Black and 24% Hispanic. Patients had a median baseline HIV-1 RNA of 4.6 log$_{10}$ copies/mL (range 1.7–6.4) and a mean baseline CD4$^+$ cell count of 745 cells/mm^3 (range 2–2650). Through 48 weeks of therapy, the overall proportion of patients who achieved and sustained an HIV-1 RNA <400 copies/mL was 86%, and <50 copies/mL was 73%. The mean increase from baseline in CD4$^+$ cell count was 232 cells/mm^3 (-945, +1512). The adverse reaction profile observed during these clinical trials was similar to that of adult patients, with the exception of the occurrence of anemia and higher frequency of hyperpigmentation in children [See Adverse Reactions (6)].

The pharmacokinetics of emtricitabine were studied in 20 neonates born to HIV-1-positive mothers. Each mother received prenatal and intrapartum combination antiretroviral therapy. Neonates received up to 6 weeks of zidovudine prophylactically after birth. The neonates were administered two short courses of emtricitabine oral solution (each 3 mg/kg once daily × 4 days) during the first 3 months of life. Emtricitabine exposures in neonates were similar to the exposures achieved in patients >3 months to 17 years [See Clinical Pharmacology (12.3)]. During the two short dosing periods on emtricitabine there were no safety issues

identified in the treated neonates. All neonates were HIV-1 negative at the end of the study; the efficacy of emtricitabine in preventing or treating HIV-1 could not be determined.

16 HOW SUPPLIED/STORAGE AND HANDLING

Capsules

The size 1 hard gelatin capsules with a blue cap and white body contain 200 mg of emtricitabine, are printed with "200 mg" in black on the cap and "GILEAD" and the corporate logo in black on the body, and are available in unit of use bottles (closed with induction sealed child-resistant closures) of:

• 30 capsules (NDC 61958–0601–1).

Store at 25 °C (77 °F); excursions permitted to 15 °C–30 °C (59 °F–86 °F)

Oral Solution

The oral solution is a clear, orange to dark orange liquid, contains 10 mg/mL of emtricitabine, and is available in unit of use plastic, amber bottles (closed with child resistant closures and packaged with a marked dosing cup) of:

• 170 mL (NDC 61958–0602–1).

Store refrigerated, 2–8 °C (36–46 °F). Emtriva oral solution should be used within 3 months if stored by the patient at 25 °C (77 °F); excursions permitted to 15–30 °C (59–86 °F).

17 PATIENT COUNSELING INFORMATION

See FDA-approved patient labeling (17.2)

17.1 Information for Patients

Patients should be advised that:

• EMTRIVA is not a cure for HIV-1 infection and patients may continue to experience illnesses associated with HIV-1 infection, including opportunistic infections. Patients should remain under the care of a physician when using EMTRIVA.

• The use of EMTRIVA has not been shown to reduce the risk of transmission of HIV-1 to others through sexual contact or blood contamination.

• The long term effects of EMTRIVA are unknown.

• EMTRIVA capsules and oral solution are for oral ingestion only.

• It is important to take EMTRIVA with combination therapy on a regular dosing schedule to avoid missing doses.

• Lactic acidosis and severe hepatomegaly with steatosis, including fatal cases, have been reported. Treatment with EMTRIVA should be suspended in any patient who develops clinical symptoms suggestive of lactic acidosis or pronounced hepatotoxicity (including nausea, vomiting, unusual or unexpected stomach discomfort, and weakness) [See Warnings and Precautions (5.1)].

• Patients with HIV-1 should be tested for Hepatitis B virus (HBV) before initiating antiretroviral therapy.

• Severe acute exacerbations of Hepatitis B have been reported in patients who are coinfected with HBV and HIV-1 and have discontinued EMTRIVA.

• EMTRIVA should not be coadministered with other drugs containing lamivudine, including Combivir (lamivudine/ zidovudine), Epivir or Epivir-HBV (lamivudine), Epzicom (abacavir sulfate/lamivudine), or Trizivir (abacavir sulfate/lamivudine/zidovudine) [See Warnings and Precautions (5.3)].

• Dose or dosing interval of EMTRIVA may need adjustment in patients with renal impairment [See Dosage and Administration (2.5)].

17.2 FDA-Approved Patient Labeling

EMTRIVA® (em-treev'-ah) capsules

EMTRIVA oral solution

Generic name: emtricitabine (em tri SIT uh bean)

Read the Patient Information that comes with EMTRIVA before you start using it and each time you get a refill. There may be new information. This information does not take the place of talking to your healthcare provider about your medical condition or treatment.

You should stay under a healthcare provider's care when taking EMTRIVA. **Do not change or stop your medicine without first talking with your healthcare provider.** Talk to your healthcare provider or pharmacist if you have any questions about EMTRIVA.

What is the most important information I should know about EMTRIVA?

• Some people who have taken medicines like EMTRIVA (a nucleoside analog) have developed a serious condition called lactic acidosis (buildup of an acid in the blood). Lactic acidosis can be a medical emergency and may need to be treated in the hospital. Call your healthcare provider right away if you get the following signs of lactic acidosis.

• You feel very weak or tired.

• You have unusual (not normal) muscle pain.

• You have trouble breathing.

• You have stomach pain with nausea and vomiting.

• You feel cold, especially in your arm and legs.

• You feel dizzy or lightheaded.

• You have a fast or irregular heartbeat.

• **Some people who have taken medicines like EMTRIVA have developed serious liver problems called hepatotox-**

icity, with liver enlargement (hepatomegaly) and fat in the liver (steatosis). **Call your healthcare provider right away if you get the following signs of liver problems.**

• Your skin or the white part of your eyes turns yellow (jaundice).

• Your urine turns dark.

• Your bowel movements (stools) turn light in color.

• You don't feel like eating food for several days or longer.

• You feel sick to your stomach (nausea).

• You have lower stomach area (abdominal) pain.

• **You may be more likely to get lactic acidosis or liver problems if you are female, very overweight (obese), or have been taking nucleoside analog medicines, like EMTRIVA, for a long time.**

• **If you are also infected with the Hepatitis B Virus (HBV),** you need close medical follow-up for several months after stopping treatment with EMTRIVA. Follow-up includes medical exams and blood tests to check for HBV that is getting worse. **Patients with HBV infection, who take EMTRIVA and then stop it, may get "flare-ups" of their hepatitis. A "flare-up" is when the disease suddenly returns in a worse way than before.**

What is EMTRIVA?

EMTRIVA is a type of medicine called an HIV-1 (human immunodeficiency virus) nucleoside reverse transcriptase inhibitor (NRTI). EMTRIVA is always used with other anti-HIV-1 medicines to treat people with HIV-1 infection. **EMTRIVA is for adults and children, but has not been studied fully in adults over age 65.**

HIV infection destroys CD4$^+$ T cells, which are important to the immune system. The immune system helps fight infection. After a large number of T cells are destroyed, acquired immune deficiency syndrome (AIDS) develops.

EMTRIVA helps to block HIV-1 reverse transcriptase, a chemical in your body (enzyme) that is needed for HIV-1 to multiply. EMTRIVA may lower the amount of HIV-1 in the blood (viral load). EMTRIVA may also help to increase the number of T cells called CD4$^+$ cells. Lowering the amount of HIV-1 in the blood lowers the chance of death or infections that happen when your immune system is weak (opportunistic infections).

EMTRIVA does not cure HIV-1 infection or AIDS. The long-term effects of EMTRIVA are not known at this time. People taking EMTRIVA may still get opportunistic infections or other conditions that happen with HIV-1 infection. Opportunistic infections are infections that develop because the immune system is weak. Some of these conditions are pneumonia, herpes virus infections, and *Mycobacterium avium complex* (MAC) infections. **It is very important that you see your healthcare provider regularly while taking EMTRIVA.**

EMTRIVA does not lower your chance of passing HIV-1 to other people through sexual contact, sharing needles, or being exposed to your blood. For your health and the health of others, it is important to always practice safer sex by using a latex or polyurethane condom or other barrier to lower the chance of sexual contact with semen, vaginal secretions, or blood. Never use or share dirty needles.

Who should not take EMTRIVA?

• Do not take EMTRIVA if you are allergic to EMTRIVA or any of its ingredients. The active ingredient is emtricitabine. See the end of this leaflet for a complete list of ingredients.

• Do not take EMTRIVA if you are already taking ATRIPLA®, TRUVADA®, Combivir, Epivir, Epivir-HBV, Epzicom, or Trizivir because these medicines contain the same or similar active ingredients.

What should I tell my healthcare provider before taking EMTRIVA?

Tell your healthcare provider

• **If you are pregnant or planning to become pregnant.** We do not know if EMTRIVA can harm your unborn child. You and your healthcare provider will need to decide if EMTRIVA is right for you. If you use EMTRIVA while you are pregnant, talk to your healthcare provider about how you can be on the EMTRIVA Antiviral Pregnancy Registry.

• **If you are breast-feeding.** You should not breast feed if you are HIV-positive because of the chance of passing the HIV virus to your baby. Also, it is not known if EMTRIVA can pass into your breast milk and if it can harm your baby. If you are a woman who has or will have a baby, talk with your healthcare provider about the best way to feed your baby.

• **If you have kidney problems.** You may need to take EMTRIVA less often.

• **If you have any liver problems including Hepatitis B Virus infection.**

• **Tell your healthcare provider about all your medical conditions.**

• **Tell your healthcare provider about all the medicines you take** such as prescription and non-prescription medicines and dietary supplements. Keep a complete list of all the medicines that you take. Make a new list when medicines are added or stopped. Give copies of this list to all of your healthcare providers and pharmacist **every** time you visit or fill a prescription.

How should I take EMTRIVA?

- Take EMTRIVA by mouth exactly as your healthcare provider prescribed it. Follow the directions from your healthcare provider, exactly as written on the label.
- Dosing in adults: The usual dose of EMTRIVA is 1 capsule once a day.
- Dosing in children: The child's doctor will calculate the right dose of EMTRIVA (oral solution or capsule) based on the child's weight.
- EMTRIVA is always used with other anti-HIV-1 medicines.
- EMTRIVA may be taken with or without a meal. Food does not affect how EMTRIVA works.
- If you forget to take EMTRIVA, take it as soon as you remember that day. **Do not** take more than 1 dose of EMTRIVA in a day. **Do not** take 2 doses at the same time. Call your healthcare provider or pharmacist if you are not sure what to do. **It is important that you do not miss any doses of EMTRIVA or your other anti-HIV-1 medicines.**
- When your EMTRIVA supply starts to run low, get more from your healthcare provider or pharmacy. This is very important because the amount of virus in your blood may increase if the medicine is stopped for even a short time. The virus may develop resistance to EMTRIVA and become harder to treat.
- Stay under a healthcare provider's care when taking EMTRIVA. Do not change your treatment or stop treatment without first talking with your healthcare provider.
- If you take too much EMTRIVA, call your local poison control center or emergency room right away.

What should I avoid while taking EMTRIVA?

- **Do not breast-feed.** See "What should I tell my healthcare provider before taking EMTRIVA?" Talk with your healthcare provider about the best way to feed your baby.
- Avoid doing things that can spread HIV-1 infection since EMTRIVA doesn't stop you from passing the HIV-1 infection to others.
- **Do not share needles or other injection equipment.**
- **Do not share personal items that can have blood or body fluids on them, like toothbrushes or razor blades.**
- **Do not have any kind of sex without protection.** Always practice safer sex by using a latex or polyurethane condom or other barrier to reduce the chance of sexual contact with semen, vaginal secretions, or blood.

What are the possible side effects of EMTRIVA?

EMTRIVA may cause the following serious side effects (See "What is the most important information I should know about EMTRIVA?"):

- **lactic acidosis** (buildup of an acid in the blood). Lactic acidosis can be a medical emergency and may need to be treated in the hospital. **Call your doctor right away if you get signs of lactic acidosis.** (See "What is the most important information I should know about EMTRIVA?")
- **serious liver problems (hepatotoxicity)**, with liver enlargement (hepatomegaly) and fat in the liver (steatosis). Call your healthcare provider right away if you get any signs of liver problems. (See "What is the most important information I should know about EMTRIVA?")
- **"flare-ups"** of Hepatitis B Virus infection, in which the disease suddenly returns in a worse way than before, can occur if you stop taking EMTRIVA. EMTRIVA is not for the treatment of Hepatitis B Virus (HBV) infection.

Other side effects with EMTRIVA when used with other anti-HIV-1 medicines Include:

- Changes in body fat have been seen in some patients taking EMTRIVA and other anti-HIV-1 medicines. These changes may include increased amount of fat in the upper back and neck ("buffalo hump"), breast, and around the main part of your body (trunk). Loss of fat from the legs, arms and face may also happen. The cause and long term health effects of these conditions are not known at this time.

The most common side effects of EMTRIVA used with other anti-HIV-1 medicines are headache, diarrhea, and nausea. Other side effects include allergic reaction, dizziness, sleeping problems, abnormal dreams, vomiting, indigestion, stomach pain, pain, weakness and rash. Skin discoloration may also happen with EMTRIVA.

There have been other side effects in patients taking EMTRIVA. However, these side effects may have been due to other medicines that patients were taking or to HIV-1 itself. Some of these side effects can be serious.

This list of side effects is **not** complete. If you have questions about side effects, ask your healthcare provider or pharmacist. You should report any new or continuing symptoms to your healthcare provider right away. Your healthcare provider may be able to help you manage these side effects.

How do I store EMTRIVA?

- Keep EMTRIVA and all other medicines out of reach of children.

- Store EMTRIVA capsules between 59 °F and 86 °F (15 °C to 30 °C).
- Store EMTRIVA oral solution in a refrigerator between 36 °F and 46 °F (2–8 °C). Do not freeze. Alternatively, the product may be stored at room temperature for up to 3 months and any remaining solution in the bottle must be discarded after the 3 months.
- Do not keep your medicine in places that are too hot or cold.
- Do not keep medicine that is out of date or that you no longer need. If you throw any medicines away make sure that children will not find them.

General information about EMTRIVA:

Medicines are sometimes prescribed for conditions that are not mentioned in patient information leaflets. Do not use EMTRIVA for a condition for which it was not prescribed. Do not give EMTRIVA to other people, even if they have the same symptoms you have. It may harm them.

This leaflet summarizes the most important information about EMTRIVA. If you would like more information, talk with your doctor. You can ask your healthcare provider or pharmacist for information about EMTRIVA that is written for health professionals. For more information, you may also call 1-800-GILEAD5.

What are the ingredients of EMTRIVA?

Active Ingredient: emtricitabine

Inactive Ingredients for EMTRIVA capsules: crospovidone, magnesium stearate, microcrystalline cellulose, and povidone.

Inactive Ingredients for EMTRIVA oral solution: Cotton candy flavor, FD&C yellow No. 6, edetate disodium, methylparaben and propylparaben, sodium phosphate (monobasic), propylene glycol, water, and xylitol. Sodium hydroxide and hydrochloric acid may be used to adjust pH.

℞ Only

May 2008

EMTRIVA, TRUVADA, and VIREAD are trademarks of Gilead Sciences, Inc. ATRIPLA is a trademark of Bristol-Myers Squibb & Gilead Sciences, LLC. All other trademarks referenced herein are the property of their respective owners.

21-500-896-GS-014

Revised: 05/2008   Distributed by: Gilead Sciences, Inc.

Shown in Product Identification Guide, page 309

HEPSERA® Tablets   ℞

[hep-SER-rah]
(adefovir dipivoxil)
tablet for oral use

HIGHLIGHTS OF PRESCRIBING INFORMATION
These highlights do not include all the information needed to use HEPSERA safely and effectively. See full prescribing information for HEPSERA.
HEPSERA (adefovir dipivoxil) tablet for oral use
Initial U.S. Approval: 2002

> **WARNING: SEVERE ACUTE EXACERBATIONS OF HEPATITIS, NEPHROTOXICITY, HIV RESISTANCE, LACTIC ACIDOSIS AND SEVERE HEPATOMEGALY WITH STEATOSIS**
> *See full prescribing information for complete boxed warning.*
> - Severe acute exacerbations of hepatitis may occur in patients who discontinue HEPSERA. Monitor hepatic function closely in these patients. (5.1)
> - Chronic use of HEPSERA may result in nephrotoxicity in patients at risk of renal dysfunction or having underlying renal dysfunction. Monitor renal function closely in these patients. Dose adjustment may be required. (5.2)
> - HIV resistance may emerge in chronic hepatitis B patients with unrecognized or untreated HIV infection. (5.3)
> - Lactic acidosis and severe hepatomegaly with steatosis, including fatal cases, have been reported with the use of nucleoside analogues. (5.4)

———RECENT MAJOR CHANGES———

Warnings and Precautions	
Nephrotoxicity (5.2)	10/2009
Coadministration with Other Products (5.5)	10/2009

———INDICATIONS AND USAGE———
HEPSERA is a nucleotide analogue indicated for the treatment of chronic hepatitis B in patients ≥12 years of age. (1)

———DOSAGE AND ADMINISTRATION———
- One tablet containing 10 mg adefovir dipivoxil once daily orally with or without food. (2.1)
- Dose adjustment in renal impairment for adults (2.2)

[See table at top of next page]
- No dose recommendations for (2.1):
  - Non-hemodialysis patients with creatinine clearance <10mL/min.
  - Adolescent patients with renal impairment.

———DOSAGE FORMS AND STRENGTHS———
Tablets: 10 mg (3)

———CONTRAINDICATIONS———
HEPSERA is contraindicated in patients with previously demonstrated hypersensitivity to any of the components of the product. (4)

———WARNINGS AND PRECAUTIONS———
- Severe acute exacerbations of hepatitis: Monitor hepatic function closely at repeated intervals for at least several months in patients who discontinue HEPSERA. (5.1)
- Nephrotoxicity: Monitor renal function during therapy for all patients, particularly those with pre-existing or other risks for renal impairment. Dose adjustment may be required. (5.2)
- HIV Resistance: Offer HIV testing to all patients prior to initiating HEPSERA. Untreated HIV may result in HIV resistance. (5.3)
- Lactic acidosis and severe hepatomegaly with steatosis: If suspected, suspend treatment. (5.4)
- Coadministration with Other Products: Do not administer HEPSERA concurrently with VIREAD or other tenofovir-containing products. (5.5)
- Clinical Resistance: For patients with lamivudine-resistant HBV use adefovir dipivoxil in combination with lamivudine. For all patients, consider modifying treatment in case serum HBV DNA remains above 1000 copies/mL with continued treatment. (5.6)

———ADVERSE REACTIONS———
Most common adverse reaction (>10%) in compensated disease patients is asthenia and in pre- and post-transplantation lamivudine-resistant liver disease patients is increased creatinine. (6)
To report SUSPECTED ADVERSE REACTIONS, contact Gilead at (1-800-GILEAD-5) or FDA at 1-800-FDA-1088 or www.fda.gov/medwatch

———DRUG INTERACTIONS———
- Co-administration with drugs that reduce renal function or compete for active tubular secretion may increase serum concentrations of adefovir or the co-administered drug. Monitor for HEPSERA associated adverse events. (7)

———USE IN SPECIFIC POPULATIONS———
- Pregnancy: No human data. Pregnancy registry available. (8.1)
- Nursing Mothers: Unknown if present in human milk (8.3)
- Pediatrics: Not recommended in children <12 years of age. (8.4, 2.1, 14.4)
- Renal Impairment: Dose adjustment may be required. (2.2)

See 17 for PATIENT COUNSELING INFORMATION and FDA-approved patient labeling

Revised: 10/2009

FULL PRESCRIBING INFORMATION: CONTENTS*

FULL PRESCRIBING INFORMATION

	Creatinine Clearance (mL/min)*			
	≥50	30–49	10–29	Hemodialysis Patients
Recommended dose and dosing interval	10 mg every 24 hours	10 mg every 48 hours	10 mg every 72 hours	10 mg every 7 days following dialysis

* Creatinine clearance calculated by Cockcroft-Gault method using lean or ideal body weight.

Table 1. Dosing Interval Adjustment of HEPSERA in Adult Patients with Renal Impairment

	Creatinine Clearance (mL/min)*			
	≥50	30–49	10–29	Hemodialysis Patients
Recommended dose and dosing interval	10 mg every 24 hours	10 mg every 48 hours	10 mg every 72 hours	10 mg every 7 days following dialysis

* Creatinine clearance calculated by Cockcroft-Gault method using lean or ideal body weight.

> **WARNING: SEVERE ACUTE EXACERBATIONS OF HEPATITIS, NEPHROTOXICITY, HIV RESISTANCE, LACTIC ACIDOSIS AND SEVERE HEPATOMEGALY WITH STEATOSIS**
>
> Severe acute exacerbations of hepatitis have been reported in patients who have discontinued anti-Hepatitis B therapy including HEPSERA. Hepatic function should be monitored closely with both clinical and laboratory follow-up for at least several months in patients who discontinue anti-Hepatitis B therapy. If appropriate, resumption of anti-Hepatitis B therapy may be warranted *[see Warnings and Precautions (5.1)]*.
>
> In patients at risk of or having underlying renal dysfunction, chronic administration of HEPSERA may result in nephrotoxicity. These patients should be monitored closely for renal function and may require dose adjustment *[see Warnings and Precautions (5.2) and Dosage and Administration (2.2)]*.
>
> HIV resistance may emerge in chronic hepatitis B patients with unrecognized or untreated Human Immunodeficiency Virus (HIV) infection treated with anti-hepatitis B therapies, such as therapy with HEPSERA, that may have activity against HIV *[see Warnings and Precautions (5.3)]*.
>
> Lactic acidosis and severe hepatomegaly with steatosis, including fatal cases, have been reported with the use of nucleoside analogs alone or in combination with other antiretrovirals *[see Warnings and Precautions (5.4)]*.

1 INDICATIONS AND USAGE

HEPSERA is indicated for the treatment of chronic hepatitis B in patients 12 years of age and older with evidence of active viral replication and either evidence of persistent elevations in serum aminotransferases (ALT or AST) or histologically active disease.

This indication is based on histological, virological, biochemical, and serological responses in adult patients with HBeAg+ and HBeAg-chronic hepatitis B with compensated liver function, and with clinical evidence of lamivudine-resistant hepatitis B virus with either compensated or decompensated liver function.

For patients 12 to <18 years of age, the indication is based on virological and biochemical responses in patients with HBeAg+ chronic hepatitis B virus infection with compensated liver function.

2 DOSAGE AND ADMINISTRATION

2.1 Chronic Hepatitis B

The recommended dose of HEPSERA in chronic hepatitis B patients for patients ≥12 years of age with adequate renal function is 10 mg, once daily, taken orally, without regard to food. The optimal duration of treatment is unknown. HEPSERA is not recommended for use in children less than 12 years of age.

2.2 Dose Adjustment in Renal Impairment

Significantly increased drug exposures were seen when HEPSERA was administered to adult patients with renal impairment *[see Warnings and Precautions (5.2) and Clinical Pharmacology (12.3)]*. Therefore, the dosing interval of HEPSERA should be adjusted in adult patients with baseline creatinine clearance <50 mL/min using the following suggested guidelines (see Table 1). The safety and effectiveness of these dosing interval adjustment guidelines have not been clinically evaluated.

Additionally, it is important to note that these guidelines were derived from data in patients with pre-existing renal impairment at baseline. They may not be appropriate for patients in whom renal insufficiency evolves during treatment with HEPSERA. Therefore, clinical response to treatment and renal function should be closely monitored in these patients.

[See table 1 above]

The pharmacokinetics of adefovir have not been evaluated in non-hemodialysis patients with creatinine clearance <10 mL/min; therefore, no dosing recommendation is available for these patients.

No clinical data are available to make dosing recommendations in adolescent patients with renal insufficiency *[see Warnings and Precautions (5.2)]*.

3 DOSAGE FORMS AND STRENGTHS

HEPSERA is available as tablets. Each tablet contains 10 mg of adefovir dipivoxil. The tablets are white and debossed with "10" and "GILEAD" on one side and the stylized figure of a liver on the other side.

4 CONTRAINDICATIONS

HEPSERA is contraindicated in patients with previously demonstrated hypersensitivity to any of the components of the product.

5 WARNINGS AND PRECAUTIONS

5.1 Exacerbation of Hepatitis after Discontinuation of Treatment

Severe acute exacerbation of hepatitis has been reported in patients who have discontinued anti-hepatitis B therapy, including therapy with HEPSERA. Hepatic function should be monitored at repeated intervals with both clinical and laboratory follow-up for at least several months in patients who discontinue HEPSERA. If appropriate, resumption of anti-hepatitis B therapy may be warranted.

In clinical trials of HEPSERA, exacerbations of hepatitis (ALT elevations 10 times the upper limit of normal or greater) occurred in up to 25% of patients after discontinuation of HEPSERA. These events were identified in studies GS-98-437 and GS-98-438 (N=492). Most of these events occurred within 12 weeks of drug discontinuation. These exacerbations generally occurred in the absence of HBeAg seroconversion, and presented as serum ALT elevations in addition to re-emergence of viral replication. In the HBeAg-positive and HBeAg-negative studies in patients with compensated liver function, the exacerbations were not generally accompanied by hepatic decompensation. However, patients with advanced liver disease or cirrhosis may be at higher risk for hepatic decompensation. Although most events appear to have been self-limited or resolved with re-initiation of treatment, severe hepatitis exacerbations, including fatalities, have been reported. Therefore, patients should be closely monitored after stopping treatment.

5.2 Nephrotoxicity

Nephrotoxicity characterized by a delayed onset of gradual increases in serum creatinine and decreases in serum phosphorus was historically shown to be the treatment-limiting toxicity of adefovir dipivoxil therapy at substantially higher doses in HIV-infected patients (60 and 120 mg daily) and in chronic hepatitis B patients (30 mg daily). Chronic administration of HEPSERA (10 mg once daily) may result in delayed nephrotoxicity. The overall risk of nephrotoxicity in patients with adequate renal function is low. However, this is of special importance in patients at risk of or having underlying renal dysfunction and patients taking concomitant nephrotoxic agents such as cyclosporine, tacrolimus, aminoglycosides, vancomycin and non-steroidal anti-inflammatory drugs *[see Adverse Reactions (6.2) and Clinical Pharmacology (12.3)]*. It is recommended that creatinine clearance is calculated in all patients prior to initiating therapy with HEPSERA.

It is important to monitor renal function for all patients during treatment with HEPSERA, particularly for those with pre-existing or other risks for renal impairment. Patients with renal insufficiency at baseline or during treatment may require dose adjustment *[see Dosage and Administration (2.2)]*. The risks and benefits of HEPSERA treatment should be carefully evaluated prior to discontinuing HEPSERA in a patient with treatment-emergent nephrotoxicity.

Pediatric Patients

The efficacy and safety of HEPSERA have not been studied in patients less than 18 years of age with different degrees of renal impairment and no data are available to make dosage recommendations in these patients *[see Dosage and Administration (2.2)]*. Caution should be exercised when prescribing HEPSERA to adolescents with underlying renal dysfunction, and renal function in these patients should be closely monitored.

5.3 HIV Resistance

Prior to initiating HEPSERA therapy, HIV antibody testing should be offered to all patients. Treatment with anti-hepatitis B therapies, such as HEPSERA, that have activity against HIV in a chronic hepatitis B patient with unrecognized or untreated HIV infection may result in emergence of HIV resistance. HEPSERA has not been shown to suppress HIV RNA in patients; however, there are limited data on the use of HEPSERA to treat patients with chronic hepatitis B co-infected with HIV.

5.4 Lactic Acidosis/Severe Hepatomegaly with Steatosis

Lactic acidosis and severe hepatomegaly with steatosis, including fatal cases, have been reported with the use of nucleoside analogs alone or in combination with antiretrovirals.

A majority of these cases have been in women. Obesity and prolonged nucleoside exposure may be risk factors. Particular caution should be exercised when administering nucleoside analogs to any patient with known risk factors for liver disease; however, cases have also been reported in patients with no known risk factors. Treatment with HEPSERA should be suspended in any patient who develops clinical or laboratory findings suggestive of lactic acidosis or pronounced hepatotoxicity (which may include hepatomegaly and steatosis even in the absence of marked transaminase elevations).

5.5 Coadministration with Other Products

HEPSERA should not be used concurrently with VIREAD (tenofovir disoproxil fumarate) or tenofovir disoproxil fumarate-containing products including TRUVADA (emtricitabine/tenofovir disoproxil fumarate combination tablet) and ATRIPLA (efavirenz/emtricitabine/tenofovir disoproxil fumarate combination tablet).

5.6 Clinical Resistance

Resistance to adefovir dipivoxil can result in viral load rebound which may result in exacerbation of hepatitis B and, in the setting of diminished hepatic function, lead to liver decompensation and possible fatal outcome.

In order to reduce the risk of resistance in patients with lamivudine resistant HBV, adefovir dipivoxil should be used in combination with lamivudine and not as adefovir dipivoxil monotherapy.

In order to reduce the risk of resistance in all patients receiving adefovir dipivoxil monotherapy, a modification of treatment should be considered if serum HBV DNA remains above 1000 copies/mL with continued treatment.

Long-term (144 week) data from Study 438 (n=124) show that patients with HBV DNA levels greater than 1000 copies/mL at Week 48 of treatment with HEPSERA were at greater risk of developing resistance than patients with serum HBV DNA levels below 1000 copies/mL at Week 48 of therapy.

6 ADVERSE REACTIONS

The following adverse reactions are discussed in other sections of the labeling:

- Severe acute exacerbations of Hepatitis *[see Boxed Warning, Warnings and Precautions (5.1)]*
- Nephrotoxicity *[see Boxed Warning, Warnings and Precautions (5.2)]*

6.1 Clinical Trials Experience

Because clinical trials are conducted under widely varying conditions, adverse reaction rates observed in the clinical trials of a drug cannot be directly compared to rates in the clinical trials of another drug and may not reflect the rates observed in practice.

Clinical and laboratory evidence of exacerbations of hepatitis have occurred after discontinuation of treatment with HEPSERA.

Adverse reactions to HEPSERA identified from placebo-controlled and open label studies include the following: asthenia, headache, abdominal pain, diarrhea, nausea, dyspepsia, flatulence, increased creatinine, and hypophosphatemia.

The incidence of these adverse reactions in studies 437 and 438, where 522 patients with chronic hepatitis B and compensated liver disease received double-blind treatment with HEPSERA (n=294) or placebo (n=228) for 48 weeks is presented in Table 2. Patients who received open-label HEPSERA for up to 240 weeks in Study 438 reported adverse reactions similar in nature and severity to those reported in the first 48 weeks.

Table 2 Adverse Reactions (Grades 1–4) Reported in ≥3% of All HEPSERA-Treated Patients in Pooled Studies 437–438 Studies (0–48 Weeks)*

Adverse Reaction	HEPSERA 10mg (N=294)	Placebo (N=228)
Asthenia	13%	14%
Headache	9%	10%
Abdominal Pain	9%	11%
Nausea	5%	8%
Flatulence	4%	4%
Diarrhea	3%	4%
Dyspepsia	3%	2%

*In these studies, the overall incidence of adverse reactions with HEPSERA was similar to that reported with placebo. The incidence of adverse reactions is derived from treatment-related events as identified by the study investigators.

No patients treated with HEPSERA developed a confirmed serum creatinine increase ≥0.5 mg/dL or confirmed phosphorus decrease ≤2 mg/dL from baseline by Week 48. By Week 96, 2% of HEPSERA-treated patients, by Kaplan-Meier estimate, had increases in serum creatinine ≥0.5 mg/dL from baseline (no placebo-controlled results were available for comparison beyond Week 48). For patients who chose to continue HEPSERA for up to 240 weeks in Study 438, 4 of 125 patients (3%) had a confirmed increase of 0.5 mg/dL from baseline. The creatinine elevation resolved in 1 patient who permanently discontinued treatment and remained stable in 3 patients who continued treatment. For 65 patients who chose to continue HEPSERA for up to 240 weeks in Study 437, 6 had a confirmed increase in serum creatinine of ≥0.5 mg/dL from baseline with 2 patients discontinuing from the study due to the elevated serum creatinine concentration. *See Adverse Reactions (6.2)* for changes in serum creatinine in patients with underlying renal insufficiency at baseline.

6.2 Special Risk Patients

Pre- and Post-Liver Transplantation Patients

Additional adverse reactions observed from an open-label study (Study 435) in pre- and post-liver transplantation patients with chronic hepatitis B and lamivudine-resistant hepatitis B administered HEPSERA once daily for up to 203 weeks include: abnormal renal function, renal failure, vomiting, rash, and pruritus.

Changes in renal function occurred in pre-and post-liver transplantation patients with risk factors for renal dysfunction, including concomitant use of cyclosporine and tacrolimus, renal insufficiency at baseline, hypertension, diabetes, and on-study transplantation. Therefore, the contributory role of HEPSERA to these changes in renal function is difficult to assess.

Increases in serum creatinine ≥0.3 mg/dL from baseline were observed in 37% and 53% of pre-liver transplantation patients by Weeks 48 and 96, respectively, by Kaplan-Meier estimates. Increases in serum creatinine ≥0.3 mg/dL from baseline were observed in 32% and 51% of post-liver transplantation patients by Weeks 48 and 96, respectively, by Kaplan-Meier estimates. Serum phosphorus values <2 mg/dL were observed in 3/226 (1.3%) of pre-liver transplantation patients and in 6/241 (2.5%) of post-liver transplantation patients by last study visit. Four percent (19 of 467) of patients discontinued treatment with HEPSERA due to renal adverse events.

6.3 Pediatric Patients

Assessment of adverse reactions is based on a placebo-controlled study (Study 518) in which 173 pediatric patients aged 2 to <18 years with chronic hepatitis B and compensated liver disease received double-blind treatment with HEPSERA (n=115), or placebo (n=58) for 48 weeks *[see Clinical Studies (14.4) and Use In Specific Populations (8.4)]*.

The safety profile of HEPSERA in patients ≥12 to <18 years of age (n=56) was similar to that observed in adults. No pediatric patients treated with HEPSERA developed a confirmed serum creatinine increase ≥ 0.5 mg/dL or confirmed phosphorus decrease to <2 mg/dL from baseline by Week 48.

6.4 Post-Marketing Experience

In addition to adverse reaction reports from clinical trials, the following possible adverse reactions have also been identified during post-approval use of adefovir dipivoxil. Because these events have been reported voluntarily from a population of unknown size, estimates of frequency cannot be made.

Metabolism and Nutrition Disorders: hypophosphatemia

Gastrointestinal Disorders: pancreatitis

Musculoskeletal System and Connective Tissue Disorders: myopathy, osteomalacia (both associated with proximal renal tubulopathy)

Renal and Urinary Disorders: renal failure, Fanconi syndrome, proximal renal tubulopathy

7 DRUG INTERACTIONS

Since adefovir is eliminated by the kidney, coadministration of HEPSERA with drugs that reduce renal function or compete for active tubular secretion may increase serum concentrations of either adefovir and/or these co-administered drugs *[see Clinical Pharmacology (12.3)]*.

Patients should be monitored closely for adverse events when HEPSERA is co-administered with drugs that are excreted renally or with other drugs known to affect renal function *[see Warnings and Precautions (5.2)]*.

HEPSERA should not be administered in combination with VIREAD *[see Warnings and Precautions (5.5)]*.

8 USE IN SPECIFIC POPULATIONS

8.1 Pregnancy

Teratogenic Effects: Pregnancy Category C

There are no adequate and well-controlled studies of HEPSERA in pregnant women. Chronic hepatitis B is a serious condition that requires treatment. HEPSERA should be used during pregnancy only if the potential benefit to the mother justifies the potential risk to the fetus.

Reproduction studies with oral administration of adefovir dipivoxil to pregnant rats and rabbits showed no evidence of embryotoxicity or teratogenicity at systemic exposures equivalent to 23 times (rats) and 40 times (rabbits) that achieved in humans at the therapeutic dose. However, embryotoxicity and an increased incidence of fetal malformations (anasarca, depressed eye bulge, umbilical hernia and kinked tail) occurred when adefovir was administered intravenously to pregnant rats at 38 times the human therapeutic exposure. These adverse reproductive effects did not occur following an intravenous dose where exposure was 12 times the human therapeutic exposure.

Because animal reproduction studies are not always predictive of human response, HEPSERA should be used during pregnancy only if clearly needed and after careful consideration of the risks and benefits *[see Nonclinical Toxicology (13.2)]*.

Pregnancy Registry

To monitor fetal outcomes of pregnant women exposed to HEPSERA, a pregnancy registry has been established. Healthcare providers are encouraged to register patients by calling 1-800-258-4263.

8.2 Labor and Delivery

There are no studies in pregnant women and no data on the effect of HEPSERA on transmission of HBV from mother to infant. Therefore, appropriate infant immunizations should be used to prevent neonatal acquisition of hepatitis B virus.

8.3 Nursing Mothers

It is not known whether adefovir is excreted in human milk. Because many drugs are excreted into human milk and because of the potential for serious adverse reactions in nursing infants from HEPSERA, a decision should be made whether to discontinue nursing or to discontinue drug, taking into account the importance of the drug to the mother.

8.4 Pediatric Use

Pediatric patients 12 to <18 years: The safety, efficacy, and pharmacokinetics of HEPSERA in pediatric patients (aged ≥12 to <18 years) were evaluated in a double-blind, randomized, placebo-controlled study (GS-US-103-518, Study 518) in 83 pediatric patients with chronic hepatitis B and compensated liver disease. The proportion of patients treated with HEPSERA who achieved the primary efficacy endpoint of serum HBV DNA <1,000 copies/mL and normal ALT levels at the end of 48 weeks blinded treatment was significantly greater (23%) when compared to placebo-treated patients (0%). *[see Clinical Studies (14.4), Dosage And Administration (2) and Adverse Reactions (6.3)]*.

Pediatric patients 2 to <12 years: Patients 2 to <12 years of age were also evaluated in Study 518. The efficacy of adefovir dipivoxil was not significantly different from placebo in patients less than 12 years of age.

Hepsera is not recommended for use in children below 12 years of age.

8.5 Geriatric Use

Clinical studies of HEPSERA did not include sufficient numbers of patients aged 65 and over to determine whether they respond differently from younger patients. In general, caution should be exercised when prescribing to elderly patients since they have greater frequency of decreased renal or cardiac function due to concomitant disease or other drug therapy.

8.6 Patients with Impaired Renal Function

It is recommended that the dosing interval for HEPSERA be modified in adult patients with baseline creatinine clearance <50 mL/min. The pharmacokinetics of adefovir have not been evaluated in non-hemodialysis patients with creatinine clearance <10 mL/min or in adolescent patients with renal insufficiency; therefore, no dosing recommendations are available for these patients. *[see Dosage And Administration (2.2) and Warning And Precautions (5.2)]*.

10 OVERDOSAGE

Doses of adefovir dipivoxil 500 mg daily for 2 weeks and 250 mg daily for 12 weeks have been associated with gastrointestinal side effects. If overdose occurs the patient must be monitored for evidence of toxicity, and standard supportive treatment applied as necessary.

Following a 10 mg single dose of HEPSERA, a four-hour hemodialysis session removed approximately 35% of the adefovir dose.

11 DESCRIPTION

HEPSERA® is the tradename for adefovir dipivoxil, a diester prodrug of adefovir. Adefovir is an acyclic nucleotide analog with activity against human hepatitis B virus (HBV).

The chemical name of adefovir dipivoxil is 9-[2-[[bis[(pivaloyloxy)methoxy]-phosphinyl]-methoxy]ethyl]adenine. It has a molecular formula of $C_{20}H_{32}N_5O_8P$, a molecular weight of 501.48 and the following structural formula:

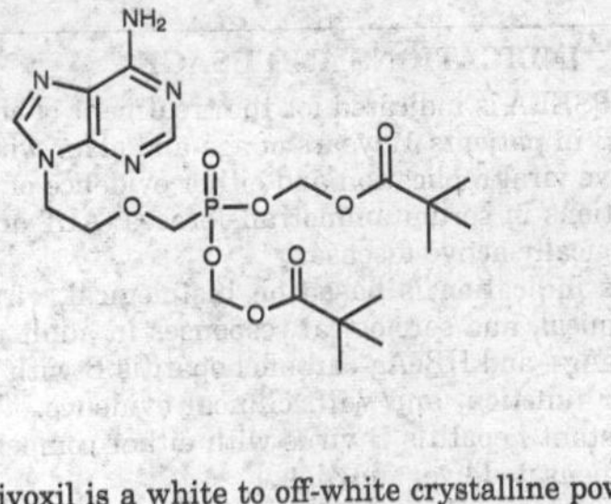

Adefovir dipivoxil is a white to off-white crystalline powder with an aqueous solubility of 19 mg/mL at pH 2.0 and 0.4 mg/mL at pH 7.2. It has an octanol/aqueous phosphate buffer (pH 7) partition coefficient (log p) of 1.91.

HEPSERA tablets are for oral administration. Each tablet contains 10 mg of adefovir dipivoxil and the following inactive ingredients: croscarmellose sodium, lactose monohydrate, magnesium stearate, pregelatinized starch, and talc.

12 CLINICAL PHARMACOLOGY

12.1 Mechanism of Action

Adefovir is an antiviral drug. *[see Clinical Pharmacology (12.4)]*.

12.3 Pharmacokinetics

Adult Subjects

The pharmacokinetics of adefovir have been evaluated in healthy volunteers and patients with chronic hepatitis B. Adefovir pharmacokinetics are similar between these populations.

Absorption

Adefovir dipivoxil is a diester prodrug of the active moiety adefovir. Based on a cross study comparison, the approximate oral bioavailability of adefovir from HEPSERA is 59%.

Following oral administration of a 10 mg single dose of HEPSERA to chronic hepatitis B patients (N=14), the peak adefovir plasma concentration (C_{max}) was 18.4 ± 6.26 ng/mL (mean ± SD) and occurred between 0.58

and 4.00 hours (median=1.75 hours) post dose. The adefovir area under the plasma concentration-time curve ($AUC_{0-\infty}$) was 220 ± 70.0 ng•h/mL. Plasma adefovir concentrations declined in a biexponential manner with a terminal elimination half-life of 7.48 ± 1.65 hours.

The pharmacokinetics of adefovir in subjects with adequate renal function were not affected by once daily dosing of 10 mg HEPSERA over seven days. The impact of long-term once daily administration of 10 mg HEPSERA on adefovir pharmacokinetics has not been evaluated.

Effects of Food on Oral Absorption

Adefovir exposure was unaffected when a 10 mg single dose of HEPSERA was administered with food (an approximately 1000 kcal high-fat meal). HEPSERA may be taken without regard to food.

Distribution

In vitro binding of adefovir to human plasma or human serum proteins is ≤4% over the adefovir concentration range of 0.1 to 25 μg/mL. The volume of distribution at steady-state following intravenous administration of 1.0 or 3.0 mg/kg/day is 392 ± 75 and 352 ± 9 mL/kg, respectively.

Metabolism and Elimination

Following oral administration, adefovir dipivoxil is rapidly converted to adefovir. Forty-five percent of the dose is recovered as adefovir in the urine over 24 hours at steady state following 10 mg oral doses of HEPSERA. Adefovir is renally excreted by a combination of glomerular filtration and active tubular secretion *[see Drug Interactions (7) and Clinical Pharmacology (12.3)]*.

Assessment of Drug Interactions

Adefovir dipivoxil is rapidly converted to adefovir in vivo. At concentrations substantially higher (>4000-fold) than those observed in vivo, adefovir did not inhibit any of the common human CYP450 enzymes, CYP1A2, CYP2C9, CYP2C19, CYP2D6, and CYP3A4. Adefovir is not a substrate for these enzymes. However, the potential for adefovir to induce CYP450 enzymes is unknown. Based on the results of these in vitro experiments and the renal elimination pathway of adefovir, the potential for CYP450 mediated interactions involving adefovir as an inhibitor or substrate with other medicinal products is low.

The pharmacokinetics of adefovir have been evaluated in healthy adult volunteers following multiple dose administration of HEPSERA (10 mg once daily) in combination with lamivudine (100 mg once daily) (N=18), trimethoprim/sulfamethoxazole (160/800 mg twice daily) (N=18), acetaminophen (1000 mg four times daily) (N=20), ibuprofen (800 mg three times daily) (N=18), and enteric coated didanosine (400 mg) (N=21). The pharmacokinetics of adefovir have also been evaluated in post-liver transplantation patients following multiple dose administration of HEPSERA (10 mg once daily) in combination with tacrolimus (N=16). The pharmacokinetics of adefovir have been evaluated in healthy volunteers following single dose pegylated interferon α-2a (PEG-IFN) (180 μg) (N=15).

Adefovir did not alter the pharmacokinetics of lamivudine, trimethoprim/sulfamethoxazole, acetaminophen, ibuprofen, enteric coated didanosine (didanosine EC), or tacrolimus. The evaluation of the effect of adefovir on the pharmacokinetics of pegylated interferon α-2a was inconclusive due to the high variability of pegylated interferon alpha-2a.

The pharmacokinetics of adefovir were unchanged when HEPSERA was coadministered with lamivudine, trimethoprim/sulfamethoxazole, acetaminophen, didanosine EC, tacrolimus (based on cross study comparison), and pegylated interferon α-2a. When HEPSERA was coadministered with ibuprofen (800 mg three times daily) increases in adefovir C_{max} (33%), AUC (23%) and urinary recovery were observed. This increase appears to be due to higher oral bioavailability, not a reduction in renal clearance of adefovir.

Apart from lamivudine, trimethoprim/sulfamethoxazole, and acetaminophen, the effects of co-administration of HEPSERA with drugs that are excreted renally, or other drugs known to affect renal function have not been evaluated.

The effect of adefovir on cyclosporine concentrations is not known.

No drug interaction studies have been performed in adolescent patients aged ≥12 years to <18 years.

Special Populations

Gender

The pharmacokinetics of adefovir were similar in male and female patients.

Race

The pharmacokinetics of adefovir have been shown to be comparable in Caucasians and Asians. Pharmacokinetic data are not available for other racial groups.

Geriatric Patients

Pharmacokinetic studies have not been conducted in the elderly.

Pediatric Patients

The pharmacokinetics of adefovir were assessed from drug plasma concentrations in 53 HBeAg positive hepatitis B pediatric patients with compensated liver disease. The exposure of adefovir following a 48 week daily treatment with adefovir dipivoxil 10 mg tablet in pediatric patients aged ≥ 12 to <18 years (C_{max} = 23.3 ng/ml and AUC_{0-24} = 248.8 ng•h/ml) was comparable to that observed in adult patients.

Renal Impairment

In adults with moderately or severely impaired renal function or with end-stage renal disease (ESRD) requiring hemodialysis, C_{max}, AUC, and half-life ($T_{1/2}$) were increased compared to adults with normal renal function. It is recommended that the dosing interval of HEPSERA be modified in these patients *[see Dosage and Administration (2.2)]*.

The pharmacokinetics of adefovir in non-chronic hepatitis B patients with varying degrees of renal impairment are described in Table 3. In this study, subjects received a 10 mg single dose of HEPSERA.

[See table above]

Table 3. Pharmacokinetic Parameters (Mean ± SD) of Adefovir in Patients with Varying Degrees of Renal Function

Renal Function Group	Unimpaired	Mild	Moderate	Severe
Baseline creatinine clearance (mL/min)	>80 (N=7)	50–80 (N=8)	30–49 (N=7)	10–29 (N=10)
C_{max} (ng/mL)	17.8 ± 3.22	22.4 ± 4.04	28.5 ± 8.57	51.6 ± 10.3
$AUC_{0-\infty}$ (ng•h/mL)	201 ± 40.8	266 ± 55.7	455 ± 176	1240 ± 629
CL/F (mL/min)	469 ± 99.0	356 ± 85.6	237 ± 118	91.7 ± 51.3
CL_{renal} (mL/min)	231 ± 48.9	148 ± 39.3	83.9 ± 27.5	37.0 ± 18.4

A four-hour period of hemodialysis removed approximately 35% of the adefovir dose. The effect of peritoneal dialysis on adefovir removal has not been evaluated.

The pharmacokinetics of adefovir have not been studied in adolescent patients with renal dysfunction *[see Use in Specific Populations (8.4)]*.

Hepatic Impairment

The pharmacokinetics of adefovir following a 10 mg single dose of HEPSERA have been studied in non-chronic hepatitis B patients with hepatic impairment. There were no substantial alterations in adefovir pharmacokinetics in patients with moderate and severe hepatic impairment compared to unimpaired patients. No change in HEPSERA dosing is required in patients with hepatic impairment.

12.4 Microbiology

Mechanism of Action

Adefovir is an acyclic nucleotide analog of adenosine monophosphate which is phosphorylated to the active metabolite adefovir diphosphate by cellular kinases. Adefovir diphosphate inhibits HBV DNA polymerase (reverse transcriptase) by competing with the natural substrate deoxyadenosine triphosphate and by causing DNA chain termination after its incorporation into viral DNA. The inhibition constant (K_i) for adefovir diphosphate for HBV DNA polymerase was 0.1 μM. Adefovir diphosphate is a weak inhibitor of human DNA polymerases α and γ with K_i values of 1.18 μM and 0.97 μM, respectively.

Antiviral Activity

The concentration of adefovir that inhibited 50% of viral DNA synthesis (EC_{50}) in HBV transfected human hepatoma cell lines ranged from 0.2 to 2.5 μM. The combination of adefovir with lamivudine showed additive anti-HBV activity.

Resistance

Clinical isolates with genotypic changes conferring reduced susceptibility in cell culture to nucleoside analog reverse transcriptase inhibitors for the treatment of HBV infection have been observed. Long-term resistance analyses performed by genotyping samples from all adefovir dipivoxil-treated patients with detectable serum HBV DNA demonstrated that amino acid substitutions rtN236T and rtA181T/V have been observed in association with adefovir resistance. In cell culture, the rtN236T substitution demonstrated 4- to 14-fold, the rtA181V substitution 2.5- to 4.2-fold, and the rtA181T substitution 1.3- to 1.9-fold reduced susceptibility to adefovir.

In HBeAg-positive nucleoside-naïve patient isolates (Study GS-98-437, N=171), no adefovir resistance-associated substitutions were observed at Week 48. Sixty-five patients continued on long term treatment after a median duration on adefovir dipivoxil of 235 weeks (range 110–279 weeks). Isolates from 16 of 38 (42%) patients developed adefovir resistance-associated substitutions in the setting of virologic failure (confirmed increase of ≥1 log_{10} HBV DNA copies/mL above nadir or never suppressed below 10^3 copies/mL). The substitutions included rtN236T (n=2), rtA181V (n=4), rtA181T (n=3), rtA181T+rtN236T (n=5), and rtA181V+rtN236T (n=2). In HBeAg-negative nucleoside-naïve patients (Study GS-98-438), isolates from 30 patients were identified with adefovir resistance-associated substitutions with a cumulative probability of 0%, 3%, 11%, 19%, and 30% at 48, 96, 144, 192, and 240 weeks, respectively. Of those 30 patients, 22 had a confirmed increase of ≥1 log_{10} HBV DNA copies/mL above nadir or never achieved HBV DNA levels below 10^3 copies/mL; an additional 8 patients had adefovir resistance-associated substitutions without virologic failure. In addition, the long term (4 to 5 years) development of resistance to adefovir dipivoxil was significantly lower in patients who had serum HBV DNA below the limit of quantification (less than 1,000 copies/mL) at Week 48 as compared to patients who had serum HBV DNA above 1,000 copies/mL at Week 48.

In an open-label study of pre- and post-liver transplantation patients (Study GS-98-435), isolates from 129 patients with clinical evidence of lamivudine-resistant hepatitis B virus at baseline were evaluated for adefovir resistance-associated substitutions. The incidence of adefovir resistance-associated (rtN236T or rtA181T/V) substitutions was 0% at 48 weeks. Isolates from four patients developed the rtN236T substitution after 72 weeks of adefovir dipivoxil therapy. Development of the rtN236T substitution was associated with serum HBV DNA rebound. All 4 patients who developed the rtN236T substitution in their HBV had discontinued lamivudine therapy before the development of genotypic resistance and all 4 lost the lamivudine resistance-associated substitutions present at baseline. In a study of 35 HIV/HBV co-infected patients with lamivudine-resistant HBV (Study 460i) who added adefovir dipivoxil to lamivudine, no adefovir resistance-associated substitutions were observed in HBV isolates from 15/35 patients tested up to 144 weeks of therapy.

Clinical resistance in pediatric patients

In a Phase 3 pediatric Study GS-US-103-518, HBV isolates from 49 of 56 pediatric subjects (aged 12 to 17 years) had serum HBV DNA >169 copies/mL and were evaluated for adefovir resistance-associated substitutions. rtN236T and/or rtA181V adefovir resistance-associated substitutions were not observed at Week 48. However, the rtA181T substitution was present in baseline and Week 48 isolates from 2 pediatric patients.

Cross-resistance

Recombinant HBV variants containing lamivudine-resistance-associated substitutions (rtL180M, rtM204I, rtM204V, rtL180M + rtM204V, rtV173L + rtL180M + rtM204V) were susceptible to adefovir in cell culture. Adefovir dipivoxil has also demonstrated anti-HBV activity (median reduction in serum HBV DNA of 4.1 log_{10} copies/mL) in patients with HBV containing lamivudine-resistance-associated substitutions (Study 435). Adefovir also demonstrated in cell culture activity against HBV variants with entecavir resistance-associated substitutions (rtT184G, rtS202I, rtM250V). HBV variants with DNA polymerase substitutions rtT128N and rtR153Q or rtW153Q associated with resistance to hepatitis B virus immunoglobulin were susceptible to adefovir in cell culture.

HBV variants expressing the adefovir resistance-associated substitution rtN236T showed no change in susceptibility to entecavir in cell culture, and a 2- to 3-fold decrease in lamivudine susceptibility. HBV mutants with the adefovir resistance-associated substitution rtA181V showed a range of decreased susceptibilities to lamivudine of 1- to 14-fold and a 12-fold decrease in susceptibility to entecavir. In patients whose HBV expressed the rtA181V substitution (n=2) or the rtN236T substitution (n=3), a reduction in serum HBV DNA of 2.4 to 3.1 and 2.0 to 5.1 log_{10} copies/mL, respectively, was observed when treatment with lamivudine was added to treatment with adefovir dipivoxil.

13 NONCLINICAL TOXICOLOGY

13.1 Carcinogenesis, Mutagenesis, Impairment of Fertility

Long-term oral carcinogenicity studies of adefovir dipivoxil in mice and rats were carried out at exposures up to approximately 10 times (mice) and 4 times (rats) those observed in humans at the therapeutic dose for HBV infection. In both mouse and rat studies, adefovir dipivoxil was negative for carcinogenic findings. Adefovir dipivoxil was mutagenic in the in vitro mouse lymphoma cell assay (with or without metabolic activation). Adefovir induced chromosomal aberrations in the in vitro human peripheral blood lymphocyte

Table 4. Histological Response at Week 48*

	Study 437		Study 438	
	HEPSERA 10 mg (N=168)	Placebo (N=161)	HEPSERA 10 mg (N=121)	Placebo (N=57)
Improvement†	53%	25%	64%	35%
No Improvement	37%	67%	29%	63%
Missing/Unassessable Data	10%	7%	7%	2%

*Intent-to-Treat population (patients with ≥1 dose of study drug) with assessable baseline biopsies.
†Histological improvement defined as ≥2 point decrease in the Knodell necro-inflammatory score with no worsening of the Knodell fibrosis score.

Table 5. Changes in Ishak Fibrosis Score at Week 48

	Study 437		Study 438	
Number of Adequate Biopsy Pairs	HEPSERA 10 mg (N=152)	Placebo (N=149)	HEPSERA 10 mg (N=113)	Placebo (N=56)
Ishak Fibrosis Score Improved*	34%	19%	34%	14%
Unchanged	55%	60%	62%	50%
Worsened*	11%	21%	4%	36%

*Change of 1 point or more in Ishak Fibrosis Score.

Table 6. Change in Serum HBV DNA, ALT Normalization, and HBeAg Seroconversion at Week 48

	Study 437		Study 438	
	HEPSERA 10 mg (N=171)	Placebo (N=167)	HEPSERA 10 mg (N=123)	Placebo (N=61)
Mean change ± SD in serum HBV DNA from baseline ($\log_{10}$ copies/mL)	−3.57 ± 1.64	−0.98 ± 1.32	−3.65 ± 1.14	−1.32 ± 1.25
ALT normalization	48%	16%	72%	29%
HBeAg seroconversion	12%	6%	NA*	NA*

*Patients with HBeAg-negative disease cannot undergo HBeAg seroconversion.

assay without metabolic activation. Adefovir dipivoxil was not clastogenic in the in vivo mouse micronucleus assay and adefovir was not mutagenic in the Ames bacterial reverse mutation assay using *S. typhimurium* and *E. coli* strains in the presence or absence of metabolic activation. In reproductive toxicology studies, no evidence of impaired fertility was seen in male or female rats at systemic exposure approximately 19 times that achieved in humans at the therapeutic dose.

13.2   Animal Toxicology and/or Pharmacology
Toxicology Studies
Animal reproduction studies were conducted in rats and rabbits with orally administered adefovir dipivoxil and intravenously administered adefovir.
In rats and rabbits, no embryotoxicity or teratogenicity was shown from oral administration of adefovir dipivoxil at maternal doses producing systemic exposures approximately 23 times (rats) and 40 times (rabbits) that achieved in humans at the therapeutic dose of 10 mg/day.
When pregnant rats were administered intravenous adefovir at maternally toxic doses associated with systemic exposure 38 times that in humans, embryotoxicity and an increased incidence of fetal malformations (anasarca, depressed eye bulge, umbilical hernia, and kinked tail) were observed. No adverse effects on development were seen with intravenous adefovir administered to pregnant rats at a systemic exposure 12 times that in humans.
Animal Toxicology Studies
Renal tubular nephropathy characterized by histological alterations and/or increases in BUN and serum creatinine was the primary dose-limiting toxicity associated with administration of adefovir dipivoxil in animals. Nephrotoxicity was observed in animals at systemic exposures approximately 3–10 times higher than those in humans at the recommended therapeutic dose of 10 mg/day.

14   CLINICAL STUDIES
14.1   Studies 437 and 438 (Pivotal Studies)
HBeAg-Positive Chronic Hepatitis B
Study 437 was a randomized, double-blind, placebo-controlled, three-arm study in patients with HBeAg-positive

chronic hepatitis B that allowed for a comparison between placebo and HEPSERA. The median age of patients was 33 years. Seventy-four percent were male, 59% were Asian, 36% were Caucasian, and 24% had prior interferon-α treatment. At baseline, patients had a median total Knodell Histology Activity Index (HAI) score of 10, a median serum HBV DNA level as measured by the Roche Amplicor Monitor polymerase chain reaction (PCR) assay (LLOQ = 1000 copies/mL) of $8.36 \log_{10}$ copies/mL and a median ALT level of 2.3 times the upper limit of normal.
HBeAg-Negative (Anti-HBe Positive/HBV DNA Positive) Chronic Hepatitis B
Study 438 was a randomized, double-blind, placebo-controlled study in patients who were HBeAg-negative at screening, and anti-HBe positive. The median age of patients was 46 years. Eighty-three percent were male, 66% were Caucasian, 30% were Asian and 41% had prior interferon-α treatment. At baseline, the median total Knodell HAI score was 10, the median serum HBV DNA level as measured by the Roche Amplicor Monitor PCR assay (LLOQ = 1000 copies/mL) was $7.08 \log_{10}$ copies/mL, and the median ALT was 2.3 times the upper limit of normal.
The primary efficacy endpoint in both studies was histological improvement at Week 48; results of which are shown in Table 4.
[See table 4 above]
Table 5 illustrates the changes in Ishak Fibrosis Score by treatment group.
[See table 5 above]
At Week 48, improvement was seen with respect to mean change in serum HBV DNA ($\log_{10}$ copies/mL), normalization of ALT, and HBeAg seroconversion as compared to placebo in patients receiving HEPSERA (Table 6).
[See table 6 above]
Treatment Beyond 48 Weeks
In Study 437, continued treatment with HEPSERA to 72 weeks resulted in continued maintenance of mean reductions in serum HBV DNA observed at Week 48. An increase

in the proportion of patients with ALT normalization was also observed in Study 437. The effect of continued treatment with HEPSERA on seroconversion is unknown.
In Study 438, patients who received HEPSERA during the first 48 weeks were re-randomized in a blinded manner to continue on HEPSERA or receive placebo for an additional 48 weeks. At Week 96, 50 of 70 (71%) of patients who continued treatment with HEPSERA had undetectable HBV DNA levels (<1000 copies/mL), and 47 of 64 (73%) of patients had ALT normalization. HBV DNA and ALT levels returned towards baseline in most patients who stopped treatment with HEPSERA.
From 141 eligible patients, there were 125 (89%) patients in Study 438 who chose to continue HEPSERA for up to 192 weeks or 240 weeks (4 years or 5 years). As these patients had already received HEPSERA for at least 48 weeks and appeared to be experiencing a benefit, they are not necessarily representative of patients initiating HEPSERA. Of these patients, 89/125 (71%) and 47/70 (67%) had an undetectable HBV DNA level (<1000 copies/mL) at Week 192 and Week 240, respectively. Of the patients who had an elevated ALT at baseline, 77/104 (74%) and 42/64 (66%) had a normal ALT at Week 192 and Week 240, respectively. Six (5%) patients experienced HBsAg loss.
14.2   Study 435 (Pre- and Post-Liver Transplantation Patients)
HEPSERA was also evaluated in an open-label, uncontrolled study of 467 chronic hepatitis B patients pre- (N=226) and post- (N=241) liver transplantation with clinical evidence of lamivudine-resistant hepatitis B virus (Study 435). At baseline, 60% of pre-liver transplantation patients were classified as Child-Pugh-Turcotte score of Class B or C. The median baseline HBV DNA as measured by the Roche Amplicor Monitor PCR assay (LLOQ = 1000 copies/mL) was 7.4 and $8.2 \log_{10}$ copies/mL, and the median baseline ALT was 1.8 and 2.0 times the upper limit of normal in pre- and post-liver transplantation patients, respectively. Results of this study are displayed in Table 5. Treatment with HEPSERA resulted in a similar reduction in serum HBV DNA regardless of the patterns of lamivudine-resistant HBV DNA polymerase mutations at baseline. The significance of the efficacy results listed in Table 7 as they relate to clinical outcomes is not known.
[See table 7 at top of next page]
14.3   Study 461 (Clinical Evidence of Lamivudine Resistance)
In Study 461, a double-blind, active controlled study in 59 chronic hepatitis B patients with clinical evidence of lamivudine-resistant hepatitis B virus, patients were randomized to receive either HEPSERA monotherapy or HEPSERA in combination with lamivudine 100 mg or lamivudine 100 mg alone. At Week 48, the mean ± SD decrease in serum HBV DNA as measured by the Roche Amplicor Monitor PCR assay (LLOQ = 1000 copies/mL) was $4.00 \pm 1.41 \log_{10}$ copies/mL for patients treated with HEPSERA and $3.46 \pm 1.10 \log_{10}$ copies/mL for patients treated with HEPSERA in combination with lamivudine. There was a mean decrease in serum HBV DNA of $0.31 \pm 0.93 \log_{10}$ copies/mL in patients receiving lamivudine alone. ALT normalized in 47% of patients treated with HEPSERA, in 53% of patients treated with HEPSERA in combination with lamivudine, and 5% of patients treated with lamivudine alone. The significance of these findings as they relate to clinical outcomes is not known.
14.4   Study 518 (Pediatric Study)
Study 518 was a double-blind, placebo-controlled, study in which 173 pediatric patients (ages 2 to <18 years) with chronic hepatitis B (CHB) infection and elevated ALT were randomized 2:1 (115 receiving adefovir dipivoxil and 58 receiving placebo). Randomization was stratified by prior treatment and age 2 to <7 years old (cohort 1), 7 to <12 years old (cohort 2), and 12 to <18 years old (cohort 3). All patients in cohort 3 received via 10 mg tablet formulation; all patients in cohorts 1 and 2 received an investigational suspension formulation (0.3 mg/kg/day cohort 1, 0.25 mg/kg/day cohort 2) once daily. The primary efficacy endpoint was HBV DNA <1000 copies/mL plus normalization of ALT at the end of Week 48.
In cohort 3 (n=83), significantly more patients treated with HEPSERA achieved the primary efficacy endpoint at the end of 48 weeks of blinded treatment (23%) when compared to placebo-treated patients (0%). The proportion of patients from cohorts 1 and 2 who responded to treatment with adefovir dipivoxil was not statistically significant when compared to the placebo arm, although the adefovir plasma concentrations in these patients were comparable to those observed in older patients. Overall, 22 of 115 (19%) of pediatric patients who received adefovir dipivoxil vs. 1 of 58 (2%) of placebo treated patients responded to treatment by Week 48 [see Adverse Reactions (6.3), Use In Special Populations (8.4) and Clinical Pharmacology (12.3, 12.4)].

16   HOW SUPPLIED/STORAGE AND HANDLING
HEPSERA is available as tablets. Each tablet contains 10 mg of adefovir dipivoxil. The tablets are white and de-

bossed with "10" and "GILEAD" on one side and the stylized figure of a liver on the other side. They are packaged as follows: Bottles of 30 tablets (NDC 61958-0501-1) containing desiccant (silica gel) and closed with a child-resistant closure.

Store in original container at 25 °C (77 °F), excursions permitted to 15–30 °C (59–86 °F) (see USP Controlled Room Temperature).

Do not use if seal over bottle opening is broken or missing.

17   PATIENT COUNSELING INFORMATION

17.1   Instructions for Safe Use
See FDA-approved patient labeling

- Physicians should inform patients of the potential risks and benefits of HEPSERA and of alternative modes of therapy.
- Physicians should instruct their patients to
  - –Read the Patient Package Insert before starting HEPSERA therapy.
  - –Follow a regular dosing schedule to avoid missing doses.
  - –Immediately report any severe abdominal pain, muscle pain, yellowing of the eyes, dark urine, pale stools, and/or loss in appetite.
  - –Inform their doctor or pharmacist if they develop any unusual symptom(s), or if any known symptom persists or worsens.
- Patients should remain under the care of a physician when using HEPSERA.
- Patients should be advised that
  - –The optimal duration of HEPSERA treatment and the relationship between treatment response and long-term outcomes such as hepatocellular carcinoma or decompensated cirrhosis are not known.
  - –Patients should not discontinue Hepsera without first informing their physician *[See Warnings and Precautions. (5.1)]*
  - –Routine laboratory monitoring and follow-up with a physician is important during HEPSERA therapy.
  - –Obtaining HIV antibody testing prior to starting HEPSERA is important *[See Warnings and Precautions. (5.3)]*
  - –HEPSERA should not be administered concurrently with VIREAD or TRUVADA or ATRIPLA *[See Warnings and Precautions. (5.5)]*
  - –Lamivudine-resistant patients should use HEPSERA in combination with lamivudine and not as HEPSERA monotherapy *[See Warnings and Precautions. (5.6)]*

17.2   Pregnancy and Breastfeeding

- Physicians should inform women of childbearing age about the risks associated with exposure to HEPSERA during pregnancy.
- Patients should inform their physician if they become pregnant while using HEPSERA.
- Pregnant patients using HEPSERA should be informed about the HEPSERA pregnancy registry and offered the opportunity to enroll.
- Patients should be informed that it is not known whether HEPSERA is excreted into human milk or if it can harm a nursing infant. Therefore, a decision should be made whether to discontinue breastfeeding or drug.

Manufactured for: Gilead Sciences, Inc.

Foster City, CA 94404

HEPSERA® is a trademark of Gilead Sciences, Inc.

©2009 Gilead Sciences, Inc.

FDA-Approved Patient Labeling

PATIENT INFORMATION

HEPSERA® (hep-SER-rah)

Generic Name: (adefovir dipivoxil) tablets

Read this information carefully before you start taking HEPSERA. Read and check for new information each time you get more HEPSERA. This information does not take the place of talking with your doctor about your medical condition or your treatment.

What is the most important information I should know about HEPSERA?

- **1.Some people who stop taking HEPSERA get a very serious hepatitis.** This usually happens within 12 weeks after stopping. You will need to have regular blood tests to check for liver function and hepatitis B virus levels if you stop taking HEPSERA.
- **2.HEPSERA may cause a severe kidney problem called nephrotoxicity.** It usually happens in people that already have a kidney problem, but it can happen to anyone that uses HEPSERA. You will need to have regular blood tests to check for kidney function while you are taking HEPSERA.
- **3.If you get or have HIV that isn't being treated with medicines, HEPSERA may increase the chances your HIV infection cannot be helped with usual HIV medicines.** This can happen if you get or have HIV and don't know it, or if your HIV is not being treated while you are taking

Table 7. Efficacy in Pre- and Post-Liver Transplantation Patients at Week 48

Efficacy Parameter*	Pre-Liver Transplantation (N=226)	Post-Liver Transplantation (N=241)
Mean change ± SD in HBV DNA from baseline (log$_{10}$ copies/mL)	−3.7 ± 1.6 (n=117)	−4.0 ± 1.6 (n=164)
Proportion with undetectable HBV DNA (< 1000 copies/mL)†	77/109 (71%)	64/159 (40%)
Stable or improved Child-Pugh-Turcotte score	86/90 (96%)	107/115 (93%)
Normalization of:‡ ALT	61/82 (74%)	56/110 (51%)
Albumin	43/54 (80%)	21/26 (81%)
Bilirubin	38/68 (58%)	29/38 (76%)
Prothrombin time	39/46 (85%)	5/9 (56%)

*Data are missing for 29% (HBV DNA) and 37% to 45% (CPT Score, Normalization of ALT, Albumin, Bilirubin, and PT) of total patients enrolled in the study.

†Denominator is the number of patients with serum HBV DNA ≥1000 copies/mL at baseline using the Roche Amplicor Monitor PCR Assay (LLOQ = 1000 copies/mL) and non-missing value at Week 48.

‡Denominator is patients with abnormal values at baseline and non-missing value at Week 48.

HEPSERA. You should get an HIV test before you start taking HEPSERA and anytime after that when there's a chance you were exposed to HIV.

- **4.Some people who have taken medicines like HEPSERA that are called nucleoside or nucleotide analogs have developed a serious condition called lactic acidosis** (build up of an acid in the blood). Lactic acidosis is a medical emergency and must be treated in the hospital. **Call your doctor right away if you get any of the following signs of lactic acidosis:**
  - You feel very weak or tired.
  - You have unusual (not normal) muscle pain.
  - You have trouble breathing.
  - You have stomach pain with nausea and vomiting.
  - You feel cold, especially in your arms and legs.
  - You feel dizzy or lightheaded.
  - You have a fast or irregular heartbeat.

Some people who have taken medicines like HEPSERA have developed serious liver problems called hepatotoxicity, with liver enlargement (hepatomegaly) and fat in the liver (steatosis). Call your doctor right away if you get any of the following signs of liver problems.
  - Your skin or the white part of your eyes turns yellow (jaundice).
  - Your urine turns dark.
  - Your bowel movements (stools) turn light in color.
  - You don't feel like eating food for several days or longer.
  - You feel sick to your stomach (nausea).
  - You have lower stomach pain.

You may be more likely to get lactic acidosis or serious liver problems if you are very overweight (obese) or have been taking nucleoside analog medicines [Atripla® (efavirenz plus emtricitabine plus tenofovir disoproxil fumarate), Combivir (zidovudine plus lamivudine), Emtriva® (emtricitabine), Epivir, Epivir-HBV (lamivudine), Epzicom (abacavir plus lamivudine), Hivid (zalcitabine), Retrovir (zidovudine), Trizivir (zidovudine plus lamivudine plus abacavir), Truvada® (emtricitabine plus tenofovir disoproxil fumarate), Videx (didanosine), Viread® (tenofovir disoproxil fumarate), Zerit (stavudine), and Ziagen (abacavir)] for a long time.

What is HEPSERA?

HEPSERA is a medicine used to treat patients at least 12 years of age with continuing (chronic) infections with active hepatitis B virus. HEPSERA has not been studied in adults over the age of 65 and is not recommended for use in children less than 12 years of age.

- HEPSERA will not cure your chronic hepatitis B.
- HEPSERA may help lower the amount of hepatitis B virus in your body.
- HEPSERA may lower the ability of the virus to multiply and infect new liver cells.
- We do not know if HEPSERA will reduce your chances of getting liver cancer or liver damage (cirrhosis) from chronic hepatitis B.
- We do not know how long HEPSERA may help your hepatitis. Sometimes viruses change in your body and medicines no longer work. This is called drug resistance.
- HEPSERA does not stop you from spreading hepatitis B virus to others by sex or sharing needles. So practice safe sex and needle use.

Who should not take HEPSERA?

- Do not take HEPSERA if you are allergic to any of the ingredients in HEPSERA. The active ingredient in

HEPSERA is adefovir dipivoxil. See the end of this leaflet for a complete list of all the ingredients in HEPSERA.

- Do not take HEPSERA if you are already taking VIREAD, TRUVADA or ATRIPLA.

Tell your doctor if:

- **You are pregnant.** We do not know if HEPSERA can harm your unborn child. You and your doctor will need to decide if HEPSERA is right for you. If you take HEPSERA and you are pregnant, talk to your doctor about how you can join the HEPSERA pregnancy registry.
- **You are breast-feeding.** We do not know if HEPSERA can pass into your milk and if it can harm your baby. You will need to choose either to breast feed or take HEPSERA, but not both.
- **You have kidney problems now or had them before.** Your dose and schedule of HEPSERA may be reduced. Blood tests will need to be done regularly to see how your kidneys are working.

Tell your doctor about all the medicines you take, including prescription and non-prescription medicines, vitamins, and herbal supplements. Some medicines may affect how HEPSERA works, **especially medicines that affect how your kidneys work.** HEPSERA can affect how your other medicines work. Your dose of HEPSERA and the other medicines may be changed. **Do not take any other medicines while you are taking HEPSERA, unless your doctor has told you it is okay.**

How should I take HEPSERA?

- Your doctor will tell you how much HEPSERA to take.
- Your doctor will tell you when and how often to take HEPSERA.
- Take HEPSERA the same time each day that your doctor tells you. If you forget to take HEPSERA, take it as soon as you remember that day. Do not take more than 1 dose of HEPSERA in a day. Do not take 2 doses at the same time. Call your doctor or pharmacist if you are not sure what to do.
- **Do not** change your dose of HEPSERA or stop HEPSERA without talking to your doctor. Your hepatitis may get worse if you change doses or stop.
- You may take HEPSERA with or without food.
- When your HEPSERA supply gets low, call your doctor or pharmacy for a refill. **Do not run out of HEPSERA.**
- If you take too much HEPSERA, call your local poison control center or emergency room right away.

Some patients get worse or very serious hepatitis B symptoms when they stop taking HEPSERA (see, "What is the most important information I should know about HEPSERA?"). We don't know how long you should use HEPSERA. You and your doctor will need to decide when it is best for you to stop taking HEPSERA. After you stop taking HEPSERA, your doctor will still need to check your health and take blood tests to check your liver for a few months.

What should I avoid while taking HEPSERA?

Avoid doing things that can spread hepatitis B virus since HEPSERA doesn't stop you from passing the infection to others.
- Do not share needles or other injection equipment.
- Do not share personal items that can have blood or body fluids on them, like toothbrushes or razor blades.
- Do not have any kind of sex without protection. Practice "safe sex" using condoms and dental dams.

What are the possible side effects of HEPSERA?

HEPSERA can cause the following serious side effects: (see, "What is the most important information I should know about HEPSERA?")

1. **1.a very serious hepatitis if you stop taking it.**
2. **2.a severe kidney problem called nephrotoxicity.**
3. **3.increase your chance of developing a form of HIV that cannot be treated with usual HIV medicines**
4. **4.lactic acidosis and liver problems.**

The most common side effects of HEPSERA are weakness, headache, stomach pain, nausea, flatulence (intestinal gas), diarrhea, indigestion and changes in the way the kidneys work. Additional side effects in liver transplant patients with chronic hepatitis B are vomiting, rash and itching. Some patients with liver transplants also had undesirable effects on their kidneys, including failure of the kidneys. Other side effects reported since HEPSERA has been marketed include kidney failure, damage to kidney cells, muscle pain or weakness and weakening of the bone, which could cause them to break (both associated with kidney problems), and inflammation of the pancreas.

These are not all of the possible side effects of HEPSERA. For more information, ask your doctor or pharmacist.

General information about the safe and effective use of HEPSERA:

Medicines are sometimes prescribed for conditions not mentioned in patient information leaflets. Do not use HEPSERA for a condition for which it was not prescribed. Do not give HEPSERA to other people, even if they have the same symptoms that you have.

This leaflet summarizes the most important information about HEPSERA. If you would like more information, talk with your doctor. You can ask your doctor or pharmacist for information about HEPSERA that is written for health professionals.

HEPSERA Tablets should be stored at room temperature and should be stored in their original container.

Do not use if seal over bottle opening is broken or missing.

What are the Ingredients of HEPSERA?

Active Ingredient: adefovir dipivoxil

Inactive Ingredients: croscarmellose sodium, lactose monohydrate, magnesium stearate, pregelatinized starch, and talc

Manufactured for: Gilead Sciences, Inc.

Foster City, CA 94404

VIREAD®, EMTRIVA®, and TRUVADA® are trademarks of Gilead Sciences, Inc. ATRIPLA® is a trademark of Bristol-Myers Squibb & Gilead Sciences, LLC. Other brands listed are the trademarks of their respective owners.

©2009 Gilead Sciences, Inc.

21-449-GS-011

Shown in Product Identification Guide, page 309

LETAIRIS®   ℞

[le-TAIR-is]
(ambrisentan)
Tablets Tor Oral Use

HIGHLIGHTS OF PRESCRIBING INFORMATION
These highlights do not include all the information needed to use LETAIRIS® tablets safely and effectively. See full prescribing information for LETAIRIS.

LETAIRIS (ambrisentan) tablets for oral use
Initial U.S. Approval: 2007

> **WARNING: POTENTIAL LIVER INJURY AND CONTRAINDICATION IN PREGNANCY**
> *See full prescribing information for complete boxed warning.*
> - Elevations of liver aminotransferases (ALT, AST) have been reported with LETAIRIS and serious liver injury has been reported with related drugs.
> - Monitor liver aminotransferases monthly and discontinue LETAIRIS if >5 × ULN or if elevations are accompanied by bilirubin >2 × ULN or by signs or symptoms of liver dysfunction.
> - May cause fetal harm if taken during pregnancy (4.1).
> - Must exclude pregnancy before the start of treatment (2.2).
> - Prevent pregnancy during treatment and for one month after stopping treatment by the use of two acceptable methods of contraception unless the patient has had a tubal sterilization or chooses to use a Copper T 380A IUD or LNg 20 IUS, in which case no additional contraception is needed (2.2, 5.5).

———RECENT MAJOR CHANGES———
- Boxed Warning 05/2009
- Dosage and Administration, Women of Childbearing Potential (2.2) 05/2009
- Contraindications, Pregnancy Category X (4.1) 05/2009
- Warnings and Precautions, Hematological Changes (5.2) 08/2009
- Warnings and Precautions, Decreased Sperm Counts (5.4) 07/2009
- Warnings and Precautions, Prescribing and Distribution Program for LETAIRIS (5.5) 05/2009

- Deleted: Warnings and Precautions, Co-administration of LETAIRIS and Cyclosporine A (5.4) 08/2009
- Deleted: Warnings and Precautions, Co-administration of LETAIRIS with Strong CYP3A and 2C19 Inhibitors (5.5) 08/2009

———INDICATIONS AND USAGE———
LETAIRIS is an endothelin receptor antagonist indicated for the treatment of pulmonary arterial hypertension (WHO Group 1) in patients with WHO Class II or III symptoms to improve exercise capacity and delay clinical worsening (1).

———DOSAGE AND ADMINISTRATION———
- Initiate treatment at 5 mg once daily with or without food, and consider increasing the dose to 10 mg once daily if 5 mg is tolerated (2.1).
- Treat women of childbearing potential only after a negative pregnancy test and treat only women who are using two acceptable methods of contraception unless the patient has had a tubal sterilization or chooses to use a Copper T 380A IUD or LNg 20 IUS, in which case no additional contraception is needed. Obtain monthly pregnancy tests (2.2, 5.5).
- Not recommended in patients with moderate or severe hepatic impairment (2.3).

———DOSAGE FORMS AND STRENGTHS———
- 5 mg and 10 mg film-coated, unscored tablets (3).

———CONTRAINDICATIONS———
- Do not administer LETAIRIS to a pregnant woman because it can cause fetal harm (4.1).

———WARNINGS AND PRECAUTIONS———
- Decreases in hemoglobin have been observed within the first few weeks; measure hemoglobin at initiation, at 1 month, and periodically thereafter (5.2).
- Fluid retention may require intervention (5.3).
- Decreases in sperm count have been observed in patients taking endothelin receptor antagonists (5.4).

———ADVERSE REACTIONS———
- Most common placebo-adjusted adverse reactions are peripheral edema, nasal congestion, sinusitis, flushing, palpitations, nasopharyngitis, abdominal pain, and constipation (6.1).
- Fluid retention was identified as an adverse reaction during postapproval use of LETAIRIS (6.2).

To report SUSPECTED ADVERSE REACTIONS, contact Gilead Sciences, Inc. at (1-800-GILEAD5, Option 3) or FDA at 1-800-FDA-1088 or www.fda.gov/medwatch.

———DRUG INTERACTIONS———
- No clinically significant interactions of LETAIRIS with warfarin, sildenafil, tadalafil, omeprazole (CYP2C19 inhibitor), ketoconazole (strong CYP3A inhibitor), digoxin, ethinylestradiol, or norethindrone have been observed (7.2).
- Other potential interactions are not well characterized, but, based on *in vitro* data, interactions with P-glycoprotein (P-gp), the Organic Anion Transport Protein (OATP), and uridine 5′-diphosphate glucuronosyltransferases (UGTs) would be expected (7.3).

———USE IN SPECIFIC POPULATIONS———
- Pregnancy Category X: LETAIRIS is contraindicated in pregnant women (4.1 and 8.1).
- Nursing mothers: Breastfeeding while receiving LETAIRIS is not recommended (8.3).

See 17 for PATIENT COUNSELING INFORMATION and Medication Guide

Revised: 08/2009

FULL PRESCRIBING INFORMATION: CONTENTS*
WARNING: POTENTIAL LIVER INJURY
CONTRAINDICATION: PREGNANCY

* Sections or subsections omitted from the full prescribing information are not listed

FULL PRESCRIBING INFORMATION

> **WARNING: POTENTIAL LIVER INJURY**
> LETAIRIS (ambrisentan) can cause elevation of liver aminotransferases (ALT and AST) to at least 3 times the upper limit of normal (ULN). LETAIRIS treatment was associated with aminotransferase elevations >3 × ULN in 0.8% of patients in 12-week trials and 2.8% of patients including long-term open-label trials out to one year. One case of aminotransferase elevations >3 × ULN has been accompanied by bilirubin elevations >2 × ULN. Because these changes are a marker for potentially serious liver injury, serum aminotransferase levels (and bilirubin if aminotransferase levels are elevated) must be measured prior to initiation of treatment and then monthly.
> In the post-marketing period with another endothelin receptor antagonist (ERA), bosentan, rare cases of unexplained hepatic cirrhosis were reported after prolonged (>12 months) therapy. In at least one case with bosentan, a late presentation (after >20 months of treatment) included pronounced elevations in aminotransferases and bilirubin levels accompanied by non-specific symptoms, all of which resolved slowly over time after discontinuation of the suspect drug. This case reinforces the importance of strict adherence to the monthly monitoring schedule for the duration of treatment.
> Elevations in aminotransferases require close attention. LETAIRIS should generally be avoided in patients with elevated aminotransferases (>3 × ULN) at baseline because monitoring liver injury may be more difficult. If liver aminotransferase elevations are accompanied by clinical symptoms of liver injury (such as nausea, vomiting, fever, abdominal pain, jaundice, or unusual lethargy or fatigue) or increases in bilirubin >2 × ULN, treatment should be stopped. There is no experience with the re-introduction of LETAIRIS in these circumstances.
> **CONTRAINDICATION: PREGNANCY**
> LETAIRIS is very likely to produce serious birth defects if used by pregnant women, as this effect has been seen consistently when it is administered to animals *[see Contraindications (4.1)]*. Pregnancy must therefore be excluded before the initiation of treatment with LETAIRIS and prevented during treatment and for one month after stopping treatment by the use of two acceptable methods of contraception unless the patient has had a tubal sterilization or chooses to use a Copper T 380A IUD or LNg 20 IUS, in which case no additional contraception is needed. Obtain monthly pregnancy tests.
> Because of the risks of liver injury and birth defects, LETAIRIS is available only through a special restricted distribution program called the LETAIRIS Education and Access Program (LEAP), by calling 1-866-664-LEAP (5327). Only prescribers and pharmacies registered with LEAP may prescribe and distribute LETAIRIS. In addition, LETAIRIS may be dispensed only to patients who are enrolled in and meet all conditions of LEAP *[see Warnings and Precautions (5.5)]*.

1 INDICATIONS AND USAGE

LETAIRIS is indicated for the treatment of pulmonary arterial hypertension (WHO Group 1) in patients with WHO Class II or III symptoms to improve exercise capacity and delay clinical worsening.

2 DOSAGE AND ADMINISTRATION

2.1 Adult Dosage

Initiate treatment at 5 mg once daily with or without food, and consider increasing the dose to 10 mg once daily if 5 mg is tolerated.

Tablets may be administered with or without food. Tablets should not be split, crushed, or chewed. Doses higher than 10 mg once daily have not been studied in patients with pulmonary arterial hypertension (PAH). Liver function tests should be measured prior to initiation and during treatment with LETAIRIS [see Warnings and Precautions (5.1)].

2.2 Women of Childbearing Potential

Treat women of childbearing potential only after a negative pregnancy test and treat only women who are using two acceptable methods of contraception unless the patient has had a tubal sterilization or chooses to use a Copper T 380A IUD or LNg 20 IUS, in which case no additional contraception is needed. Pregnancy tests should be obtained monthly in women of childbearing potential taking LETAIRIS [see Contraindications (4.1) and Warnings and Precautions (5.5)].

2.3 Pre-existing Hepatic Impairment

LETAIRIS is not recommended in patients with moderate or severe hepatic impairment [see Use in Specific Populations (8.7)]. There is no information on the use of LETAIRIS in patients with mild hepatic impairment; however, exposure to ambrisentan may be increased in these patients.

3 DOSAGE FORMS AND STRENGTHS

LETAIRIS is available as 5 mg and 10 mg film-coated, unscored tablets.

4 CONTRAINDICATIONS

4.1 Pregnancy Category X

LETAIRIS may cause fetal harm when administered to a pregnant woman. Ambrisentan was teratogenic at oral doses of ≥15 mg/kg/day in rats and ≥7 mg/kg/day in rabbits; it was not studied at lower doses. In both species, there were abnormalities of the lower jaw and hard and soft palate, malformation of the heart and great vessels, and failure of formation of the thymus and thyroid. Teratogenicity is a class effect of endothelin receptor antagonists. There are no data on the use of LETAIRIS in pregnant women.

LETAIRIS is contraindicated in women who are or may become pregnant. If this drug is used during pregnancy, or if the patient becomes pregnant while taking this drug, the patient should be apprised of the potential hazard to a fetus. Pregnancy must be excluded before the initiation of treatment with LETAIRIS and prevented during treatment and for one month after stopping treatment by the use of two acceptable methods of contraception. If the patient has had a tubal sterilization or chooses to use a Copper T 380A IUD or LNg 20 IUS for pregnancy prevention, no additional contraception is needed [see Dosage and Administration (2.2), and Warnings and Precautions (5.5)].

5 WARNINGS AND PRECAUTIONS

5.1 Potential Liver Injury
(see BOXED WARNING)

Treatment with endothelin receptor antagonists has been associated with dose-dependent liver injury manifested primarily by elevation of serum aminotransferases (ALT or AST), but sometimes accompanied by abnormal liver function (elevated bilirubin). The combination of aminotransferases greater than 3-times the upper limit of normal (>3 × ULN) and total bilirubin >2 × ULN is a marker for potentially serious hepatic injury.

Liver function tests were closely monitored in all clinical studies with LETAIRIS. For all LETAIRIS-treated patients (N=483), the 12-week incidence of aminotransferases >3 × ULN was 0.8% and >8 × ULN was 0.2%. For placebo-treated patients, the 12-week incidence of aminotransferases >3 × ULN was 2.3% and >8 × ULN was 0.0%. The 1-year rate of aminotransferase elevations >3 × ULN with LETAIRIS was 2.8% and >8 × ULN was 0.5%. One case of aminotransferase elevations >3 × ULN has been accompanied by bilirubin elevations >2 × ULN.

Liver chemistries must be measured prior to initiation of LETAIRIS and at least every month thereafter. If there are aminotransferase elevations >3 × ULN and ≤5 × ULN, they should be re-measured. If the confirmed level is >3 × ULN and ≤5 × ULN, reduce the daily dose or interrupt treatment and continue to monitor every two weeks until the levels are <3 × ULN. If there are aminotransferase elevations >5 × ULN and ≤8 × ULN, LETAIRIS should be discontinued and monitoring should continue until the levels are <3 × ULN. LETAIRIS can then be re-initiated with more frequent measurement of aminotransferase levels. If there are aminotransferase elevations >8 × ULN, treatment should be stopped and re-initiation should not be considered.

LETAIRIS is not recommended in patients with elevated aminotransferases (>3 × ULN) at baseline because monitoring liver injury may be more difficult. If aminotransferase elevations are accompanied by clinical symptoms of liver injury (such as anorexia, nausea, vomiting, fever, malaise, fatigue, right upper quadrant abdominal discomfort, itching, or jaundice) or increases in bilirubin >2 × ULN, LETAIRIS treatment should be stopped. There is no experience with the re-introduction of LETAIRIS in these circumstances.

5.2 Hematological Changes

Decreases in hemoglobin concentration and hematocrit have followed administration of other endothelin receptor antagonists and were observed in clinical studies with LETAIRIS. These decreases were observed within the first few weeks of treatment with LETAIRIS, and stabilized thereafter. The mean decrease in hemoglobin from baseline to end of treatment for those patients receiving LETAIRIS in the 12-week placebo-controlled studies was 0.8 g/dL. Marked decreases in hemoglobin (>15% decrease from baseline resulting in a value below the lower limit of normal) were observed in 7% of all patients receiving LETAIRIS (and 10% of patients receiving 10 mg) compared to 4% of patients receiving placebo. The cause of the decrease in hemoglobin is unknown, but it does not appear to result from hemorrhage or hemolysis.

Measure hemoglobin prior to initiation of LETAIRIS, at one month, and periodically thereafter. Initiation of LETAIRIS therapy is not recommended for patients with clinically significant anemia. If a clinically significant decrease in hemoglobin is observed and other causes have been excluded, consider discontinuing LETAIRIS.

5.3 Fluid Retention

Peripheral edema is a known class effect of endothelin receptor antagonists, and is also a clinical consequence of PAH and worsening PAH. In the placebo-controlled studies, there was an increased incidence of peripheral edema in patients treated with doses of 5 or 10 mg LETAIRIS compared to placebo [see Adverse Reactions (6)]. Most edema was mild to moderate in severity, and it occurred with greater frequency and severity in elderly patients.

In addition, there have been post-marketing reports of fluid retention in patients with pulmonary hypertension, occurring within weeks after starting LETAIRIS. Patients required intervention with a diuretic, fluid management, or, in some cases, hospitalization for decompensating heart failure.

If clinically significant fluid retention develops, with or without associated weight gain, further evaluation should be undertaken to determine the cause, such as LETAIRIS or underlying heart failure, and the possible need for specific treatment or discontinuation of LETAIRIS therapy.

5.4 Decreased Sperm Counts

In a 6-month study of another endothelin receptor antagonist, bosentan, 25 male patients with WHO functional class III and IV PAH and normal baseline sperm count were evaluated for effects on testicular function. There was a decline in sperm count of at least 50% in 25% of the patients after 3 or 6 months of treatment with bosentan. One patient developed marked oligospermia at 3 months and the sperm count remained low with 2 follow-up measurements over the subsequent 6 weeks. Bosentan was discontinued and after 2 months the sperm count had returned to baseline levels. In 22 patients who completed 6 months of treatment, sperm count remained within the normal range and no changes in sperm morphology, sperm motility, or hormone levels were observed. Based on these findings and preclinical data [see Nonclinical Toxicology (13.1)] from endothelin receptor antagonists, it cannot be excluded that endothelin receptor antagonists such as LETAIRIS have an adverse effect on spermatogenesis.

5.5 Prescribing and Distribution Program for LETAIRIS

Because of the risks of liver injury and birth defects, LETAIRIS is available only through a special restricted distribution program called the LETAIRIS Education and Access Program (LEAP). Only prescribers and pharmacies registered with LEAP may prescribe and distribute LETAIRIS. In addition, LETAIRIS may be dispensed only to patients who are enrolled in and meet all conditions of LEAP.

To enroll in LEAP, prescribers must complete the LEAP Prescriber Enrollment and Agreement Form indicating agreement to (see LEAP Prescriber Enrollment and Agreement Form for full prescribing physician agreement):

• Read the Prescribing Information (PI) and Medication Guide for LETAIRIS.
• Enroll all patients in LEAP and re-enroll patients after the first 12 months of treatment and annually thereafter.
• Review the LETAIRIS Medication Guide and patient education brochure(s) with every patient.
• Educate patients on the risks of LETAIRIS, including the risks of hepatotoxicity and teratogenicity [see Boxed Warning].

• Educate and counsel women of childbearing potential to use highly reliable contraception during LETAIRIS treatment and for one month after stopping treatment. If the patient has had a tubal sterilization or chooses to use a Copper T 380A IUD or LNg 20 IUS for pregnancy prevention, no additional contraception is needed. Women who do not choose one of these methods should always use two acceptable forms of contraception—one hormone method and one barrier method, or two barrier methods where one method is the male condom.
Acceptable hormone methods include: progesterone injectables, progesterone implants, combination oral contraceptives, transdermal patch, and vaginal ring.
Acceptable barrier methods include: diaphragm (with spermicide), cervical cap (with spermicide), and the male condom.
Partner's vasectomy must be used along with a hormone method or a barrier method [see Boxed Warning, Contraindications (4.1)].
• Order and review liver function tests (including aminotransferases and bilirubin) prior to initiation of LETAIRIS treatment and monthly during treatment.
• For women of childbearing potential, order and review a pregnancy test prior to initiation of LETAIRIS treatment and monthly during treatment.
• Counsel patients who fail to comply with the program requirements.
• Notify LEAP of any adverse events, including liver injury, or if any patient becomes pregnant during LETAIRIS treatment.

6 ADVERSE REACTIONS

6.1 Clinical Trials Experience

See Boxed Warning for discussion of potential liver injury and Warnings and Precautions (5.2) for discussion of hematological changes.

Because clinical trials are conducted under widely varying conditions, adverse reaction rates observed in the clinical trials of a drug cannot be directly compared to rates in the clinical trials of another drug and may not reflect the rates observed in practice.

Safety data for LETAIRIS were obtained from two 12-week, placebo-controlled studies in patients with PAH (ARIES-1 and ARIES-2) and four nonplacebo-controlled studies in 483 patients with PAH who were treated with doses of 1, 2.5, 5, or 10 mg once daily. The exposure to LETAIRIS in these studies ranged from 1 day to 4 years (N=418 for at least 6 months and N=343 for at least 1 year).

In ARIES-1 and ARIES-2, a total of 261 patients received LETAIRIS at doses of 2.5, 5, or 10 mg once daily and 132 patients received placebo. The adverse events that occurred in >3% of the patients receiving LETAIRIS and were more frequent on LETAIRIS than placebo are shown in Table 1.
[See table 1 at top of next page]

Most adverse drug reactions were mild to moderate and only nasal congestion was dose-dependent. Fewer patients receiving LETAIRIS had adverse events related to liver function tests compared to placebo.

Few notable differences in the incidence of adverse drug reactions were observed for patients by age or sex. Peripheral edema was similar in younger patients (<65 years) receiving LETAIRIS (14%; 29/205) or placebo (13%; 13/104), and was greater in elderly patients (≥65 years) receiving LETAIRIS (29%; 16/56) compared to placebo (4%; 1/28). The results of such subgroup analyses must be interpreted cautiously.

The incidence of treatment discontinuations due to adverse events other than those related to pulmonary hypertension during the clinical trials in patients with pulmonary arterial hypertension was similar for LETAIRIS (2%; 5/261 patients) and placebo (2%; 3/132 patients). The incidence of patients with serious adverse events other than those related to pulmonary hypertension during the clinical trials in patients with pulmonary arterial hypertension was similar for placebo (7%; 9/132 patients) and for LETAIRIS (5%; 13/261 patients).

6.2 Postmarketing Experience

The following adverse reactions were identified during postapproval use of LETAIRIS: Fluid retention [see Warnings and Precautions (5.3)], heart failure (associated with fluid retention), hypersensitivity (e.g., angioedema, rash), and anemia.

Because these reactions were reported voluntarily from a population of uncertain size, it is not possible to reliably estimate the frequency or establish a causal relationship to drug exposure.

7 DRUG INTERACTIONS

7.1 In vitro studies

Studies with human liver tissue indicate that ambrisentan is metabolized by CYP3A, CYP2C19, uridine 5'-diphosphate glucuronosyltransferases (UGTs), 1A9S, 2B7S, and 1A3S. In vitro studies suggest that ambrisentan is a substrate of the Organic Anion Transport Protein (OATP), and a substrate but not an inhibitor of P-gp.

Table 1 Adverse Events in >3% of PAH Patients Receiving LETAIRIS and More Frequent than Placebo

Adverse event	Placebo (N=132) n (%)	LETAIRIS (N=261) n (%)	Placebo-adjusted (%)
Peripheral edema	14 (11)	45 (17)	6
Nasal congestion	2 (2)	15 (6)	4
Sinusitis	0 (0)	8 (3)	3
Flushing	1 (1)	10 (4)	3
Palpitations	3 (2)	12 (5)	3
Nasopharyngitis	1 (1)	9 (3)	2
Abdominal pain	1 (1)	8 (3)	2
Constipation	2 (2)	10 (4)	2
Dyspnea	4 (3)	11 (4)	1
Headache	18 (14)	38 (15)	1

Note: This table includes all adverse events >3% incidence in the combined LETAIRIS treatment group and more frequent than in the placebo group, with a difference of ≥1% between the LETAIRIS and placebo groups.

7.2 In vivo studies

Co-administration of ambrisentan with the following drugs does not result in clinically relevant changes in ambrisentan exposure:

- Ketoconazole
- Omeprazole
- Sildenafil
- Tadalafil

Co-administration of ambrisentan does not change the exposure to the following drugs:

- Warfarin
- Digoxin
- Sildenafil
- Tadalafil
- Ethinylestradiol/Norethindrone

In a clinical study in healthy subjects, steady state dosing with ambrisentan 10 mg did not significantly affect the single-dose pharmacokinetics of the ethinylestradiol or norethindrone components of a combined oral contraceptive (Ortho-Novum 1/35). Based on this pharmacokinetic study, ambrisentan would not be expected to affect significantly the exposure to other estrogen- or progestin-based contraceptives.

7.3 Unknown

The drug interaction potential of ambrisentan is not fully characterized because in vivo drug interaction studies have not been conducted with the following types of drugs: strong inducers of CYP3A and 2C19 (rifampin), inducers of UGTs and P-gp (rifampin), strong inhibitors of the transporters P-gp (cyclosporine A) and OATP (cyclosporine A, rifampin, ritonavir). Because ritonavir, cyclosporine A and rifampin can impact the above enzymes and transporters involved in the disposition of ambrisentan, clinically significant changes in the exposure to ambrisentan cannot be excluded.

8   USE IN SPECIFIC POPULATIONS

8.1   Pregnancy

Pregnancy Category X [see Contraindications (4.1)].

8.3   Nursing Mothers

It is not known whether ambrisentan is excreted in human milk. Breastfeeding while receiving LETAIRIS is not recommended. A preclinical study in rats has shown decreased survival of newborn pups (mid and high doses) and effects on testicle size and fertility of pups (high dose) following maternal treatment with ambrisentan from late gestation through weaning. Doses tested were $17\times$, $51\times$, and $170\times$ (low, mid, high dose, respectively) the maximum oral human dose of 10 mg on a mg/mm^2 basis.

8.4   Pediatric Use

Safety and effectiveness of LETAIRIS in pediatric patients have not been established.

8.5   Geriatric Use

In the two placebo-controlled clinical studies of LETAIRIS, 21% of patients were ≥65 years old and 5% were ≥75 years old. The elderly (age ≥65 years) showed less improvement in walk distances with LETAIRIS than younger patients did, but the results of such subgroup analyses must be interpreted cautiously. Peripheral edema was more common in the elderly than in younger patients.

8.6   Renal Impairment

The impact of renal impairment on the pharmacokinetics of ambrisentan has been examined using a population pharmacokinetic approach in PAH patients with creatinine clearances ranging between 20 and 150 mL/min. There was no significant impact of mild or moderate renal impairment on exposure to ambrisentan [see Clinical Pharmacology (12.3)]. Dose adjustment of LETAIRIS in patients with mild or moderate renal impairment is therefore not required. There is no information on the exposure to ambrisentan in patients with severe renal impairment.

The impact of hemodialysis on the disposition of ambrisentan has not been investigated.

8.7   Hepatic Impairment

The influence of pre-existing hepatic impairment on the pharmacokinetics of ambrisentan has not been evaluated. Because there is in vitro and in vivo evidence of significant metabolic and biliary contribution to the elimination of ambrisentan, hepatic impairment would be expected to have significant effects on the pharmacokinetics of ambrisentan [see Clinical Pharmacology (12.3)]. LETAIRIS is not recommended in patients with moderate or severe hepatic impairment. There is no information on the use of LETAIRIS in patients with mild pre-existing impaired liver function; however, exposure to ambrisentan may be increased in these patients [see Dosage and Administration (2.3)].

10   OVERDOSAGE

There is no experience with overdosage of LETAIRIS. The highest single dose of LETAIRIS administered to healthy volunteers was 100 mg and the highest daily dose administered to patients with PAH was 10 mg once daily. In healthy volunteers, single doses of 50 mg and 100 mg (5 to 10 times the maximum recommended dose) were associated with headache, flushing, dizziness, nausea, and nasal congestion. Massive overdosage could potentially result in hypotension that may require intervention.

11   DESCRIPTION

LETAIRIS is the brand name for ambrisentan, an endothelin receptor antagonist that is selective for the endothelin type-A (ET$_A$) receptor. The chemical name of ambrisentan is (+)-(2S)-2-[(4,6-dimethylpyrimidin-2-yl)oxy]-3-methoxy-3,3-diphenylpropanoic acid. It has a molecular formula of C$_{22}$H$_{22}$N$_2$O$_4$ and a molecular weight of 378.42. It contains a single chiral center determined to be the (S) configuration and has the following structural formula:

Figure 1 Ambrisentan Structural Formula

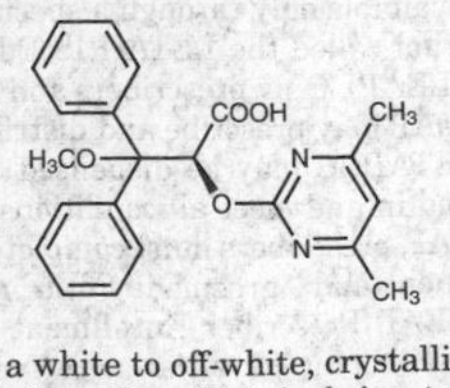

Ambrisentan is a white to off-white, crystalline solid. It is a carboxylic acid with a pKa of 4.0. Ambrisentan is practically insoluble in water and in aqueous solutions at low pH. Solubility increases in aqueous solutions at higher pH. In the solid state ambrisentan is very stable, is not hygroscopic, and is not light sensitive.

LETAIRIS is available as 5 mg and 10 mg film-coated tablets for once-daily oral administration. The tablets include the following inactive ingredients: croscarmellose sodium, lactose monohydrate, magnesium stearate and microcrystalline cellulose. The tablets are film-coated with a coating material containing FD&C Red #40 aluminum lake, lecithin, polyethylene glycol, polyvinyl alcohol, talc, and titanium dioxide. Each square, pale pink LETAIRIS tablet contains 5 mg of ambrisentan. Each oval, deep pink LETAIRIS tablet contains 10 mg of ambrisentan. LETAIRIS tablets are unscored.

12   CLINICAL PHARMACOLOGY

12.1   Mechanism of Action

Endothelin-1 (ET-1) is a potent autocrine and paracrine peptide. Two receptor subtypes, ET$_A$ and ET$_B$, mediate the effects of ET-1 in the vascular smooth muscle and endothelium. The primary actions of ET$_A$ are vasoconstriction and cell proliferation, while the predominant actions of ET$_B$ are vasodilation, antiproliferation, and ET-1 clearance.

In patients with PAH, plasma ET-1 concentrations are increased as much as 10-fold and correlate with increased mean right atrial pressure and disease severity. ET-1 and ET-1 mRNA concentrations are increased as much as 9-fold in the lung tissue of patients with PAH, primarily in the endothelium of pulmonary arteries. These findings suggest that ET-1 may play a critical role in the pathogenesis and progression of PAH.

Ambrisentan is a high affinity (K$_i$=0.011 nM) ET$_A$ receptor antagonist with a high selectivity for the ET$_A$ versus ET$_B$ receptor (>4000-fold). The clinical impact of high selectivity for ET$_A$ is not known.

12.2   Pharmacodynamics

Cardiac Electrophysiology

In a randomized, positive- and placebo-controlled, parallel-group study, healthy subjects received either LETAIRIS 10 mg daily followed by a single dose of 40 mg, placebo followed by a single dose of moxifloxacin 400 mg, or placebo alone. LETAIRIS 10 mg daily had no significant effect on the QTc interval. The 40 mg dose of LETAIRIS increased mean QTc at t$_{max}$ by 5 ms with an upper 95% confidence limit of 9 ms. For patients receiving LETAIRIS 5–10 mg daily and not taking metabolic inhibitors, no significant QT prolongation is expected.

12.3   Pharmacokinetics

The pharmacokinetics of ambrisentan (S-ambrisentan) in healthy subjects are dose proportional. The absolute bioavailability of ambrisentan is not known. Ambrisentan is rapidly absorbed with peak concentrations occurring approximately 2 hours after oral administration in healthy subjects and PAH patients. Food does not affect its bioavailability. In vitro studies indicate that ambrisentan is a substrate of P-gp. Ambrisentan is highly bound to plasma proteins (99%). The elimination of ambrisentan is predominantly by non-renal pathways, but the relative contributions of metabolism and biliary elimination have not been well characterized. In plasma, the AUC of 4-hydroxymethyl ambrisentan accounts for approximately 4% relative to parent ambrisentan AUC. The in vivo inversion of S-ambrisentan to R-ambrisentan is negligible. The mean oral clearance of ambrisentan is 38 mL/min and 19 mL/min in healthy subjects and in PAH patients, respectively. Although ambrisentan has a 15-hour terminal half-life, the mean trough concentration of ambrisentan at steady-state is about 15% of the mean peak concentration and the accumulation factor is about 1.2 after long-term daily dosing, indicating that the effective half-life of ambrisentan is about 9 hours.

Ambrisentan is metabolized by CYP3A, CYP2C19 and uridine 5'-diphosphate glucuronosyltransferases (UGTs) 1A9S, 2B7S, and 1A3S. In vitro studies suggest that ambrisentan is a substrate of the Organic Anion Transport Protein (OATP), and a substrate but not an inhibitor of P-gp. Drug interactions might be expected because of these factors; however, clinically relevant interactions with drugs utilizing these metabolic pathways have not been demonstrated [see Drug Interactions (7)].

13   NONCLINICAL TOXICOLOGY

13.1   Carcinogenesis, Mutagenesis, Impairment of Fertility

Oral carcinogenicity studies of up to two years duration were conducted at starting doses of 10, 30, and 60 mg/kg/day in rats (8 to 48 times the maximum recommended human dose [MRHD] on a mg/m^2 basis) and at 50, 150 and 250 mg/kg/day in mice (28 to 140 times the MRHD). In the rat study, the high and mid-dose male and female groups had their doses lowered to 40 and 20 mg/kg/day, respectively, in week 51 because of effects on survival. The high dose males and females were taken off drug completely in weeks 69 and 93, respectively. The only evidence of ambrisentan-related carcinogenicity was a positive trend in male rats, for the combined incidence of benign basal cell tumor and basal cell carcinoma of skin/subcutis in the mid-dose group (high-dose group excluded from analysis), and the occurrence of mammary fibroadenomas in males in the high-dose group. In the mouse study, high dose male and female groups had their doses lowered to 150 mg/kg/day in week 39 and were taken off drug completely in week 96 (males) or week 76 (females). In mice, ambrisentan was not associated with excess tumors in any dosed group.

Positive findings of clastogenicity were detected, at drug concentrations producing moderate to high toxicity, in the chromosome aberration assay in cultured human lymphocytes. There was no evidence for genetic toxicity of ambrisentan when tested in vitro in bacteria (Ames test) or in vivo in rats (micronucleus assay, unscheduled DNA synthesis assay).

The development of testicular tubular atrophy and impaired fertility has been linked to the chronic administration of endothelin receptor antagonists in rodents. Testicular tubular degeneration was observed in rats treated with ambrisentan for two years at doses ≥10 mg/kg/day (8-fold MRHD). Increased incidences of testicular findings were also observed in mice treated for two years at doses ≥50 mg/kg/day (28-fold MRHD). Effects on sperm count, sperm morphology, mating performance and fertility were observed in fertility studies in which male rats were treated with ambrisentan at oral doses of 300 mg/kg/day (236-fold MRHD). At doses of ≥10 mg/kg/day, observations of testicular histopathology in the absence of fertility and sperm effects were also present.

14 CLINICAL STUDIES

14.1 Pulmonary Arterial Hypertension (PAH)

Two 12-week, randomized, double-blind, placebo-controlled, multicenter studies were conducted in 393 patients with PAH (WHO Group 1). The two studies were identical in design except for the doses of LETAIRIS and the geographic region of the investigational sites. ARIES-1 compared once-daily doses of 5 mg and 10 mg LETAIRIS to placebo, while ARIES-2 compared once-daily doses of 2.5 mg and 5 mg LETAIRIS to placebo. In both studies, LETAIRIS or placebo was added to current therapy, which could have included a combination of anticoagulants, diuretics, calcium channel blockers, or digoxin, but not epoprostenol, treprostinil, iloprost, bosentan, or sildenafil. The primary study endpoint was 6-minute walk distance. In addition, clinical worsening, WHO functional class, dyspnea, and SF-36® Health Survey were assessed.

Patients had idiopathic PAH (64%) or PAH associated with connective tissue disease (32%), HIV infection (3%), or anorexigen use (1%). There were no patients with PAH associated with congenital heart disease.

Patients had WHO functional class I (2%), II (38%), III (55%), or IV (5%) symptoms at baseline. The mean age of patients was 50 years, 79% of patients were female, and 77% were Caucasian.

Submaximal Exercise Capacity

Results of the 6-minute walk distance at 12 weeks for the ARIES-1 and ARIES-2 studies are shown in Table 2 and Figure 2.

[See table 2 at right]

Figure 2 Mean Change in 6-minute Walk Distance

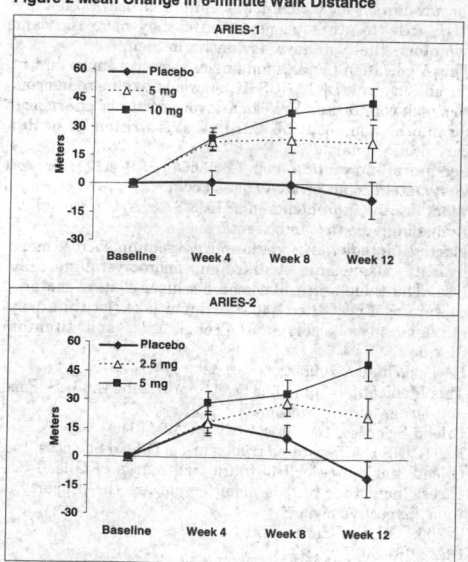

Mean change from baseline in 6-minute walk distance in the placebo and LETAIRIS groups. Values are expressed as mean ± standard error of the mean.

In both studies, treatment with LETAIRIS resulted in a significant improvement in 6-minute walk distance for each dose of LETAIRIS and the improvements increased with dose. An increase in 6-minute walk distance was observed after 4 weeks of treatment with LETAIRIS, with a dose-response observed after 12 weeks of treatment. Improvements in walk distance with LETAIRIS were smaller for elderly patients (age ≥65) than younger patients and for patients with secondary PAH than for patients with idiopathic PAH. The results of such subgroup analyses must be interpreted cautiously.

Table 2 Changes from Baseline in 6-Minute Walk Distance (meters)

	ARIES-1			ARIES-2		
	Placebo (N=67)	5 mg (N=67)	10 mg (N=67)	Placebo (N=65)	2.5 mg (N=64)	5 mg (N=63)
Baseline	342 ± 73	340 ± 77	342 ± 78	343 ± 86	347 ± 84	355 ± 84
Mean change from baseline	-8 ± 79	23 ± 83	44 ± 63	-10 ± 94	22 ± 83	49 ± 75
Placebo-adjusted mean change from baseline	–	31	51	–	32	59
Placebo-adjusted median change from baseline	–	27	39	–	30	45
p-value*	–	0.008	<0.001	–	0.022	<0.001

Mean ± standard deviation
* p-values are Wilcoxon rank sum test comparisons of LETAIRIS to placebo at Week 12 stratified by idiopathic PAH and non-idiopathic PAH patients

Table 3 Time to Clinical Worsening

	ARIES-1		ARIES-2	
	Placebo (N=67)	LETAIRIS (N=134)	Placebo (N=65)	LETAIRIS (N=127)
Clinical worsening, no. (%)	7 (10%)	4 (3%)	13 (22%)	8 (6%)
Hazard ratio	–	0.28	–	0.30
p-value, Fisher exact test	–	0.044	–	0.006
p-value, Log-rank test	–	0.030	–	0.005

Intention-to-treat population
Note: Patients may have had more than one reason for clinical worsening.
Nominal p-values

The effects of LETAIRIS on walk distances at trough drug levels are not known. Because only once daily dosing was studied in the clinical trials, the efficacy and safety of more frequent dosing regimens for LETAIRIS are not known. If exercise capacity is not sustained throughout the day in a patient, consider other PAH treatments that have been studied with more frequent dosing regimens.

Clinical Worsening

Time to clinical worsening of PAH was defined as the first occurrence of death, lung transplantation, hospitalization for PAH, atrial septostomy, study withdrawal due to the addition of other PAH therapeutic agents or study withdrawal due to early escape. Early escape was defined as meeting two or more of the following criteria: a 20% decrease in the 6-minute walk distance; an increase in WHO functional class; worsening right ventricular failure; rapidly progressing cardiogenic, hepatic, or renal failure; or refractory systolic hypotension. The clinical worsening events during the 12-week treatment period of the LETAIRIS clinical trials are shown in Table 3 and Figure 3.

[See table 3 above]

There was a significant delay in the time to clinical worsening for patients receiving LETAIRIS compared to placebo. Results in subgroups such as the elderly were also favorable.

[See figure 3 in next column]

14.2 Long-term Treatment of PAH

The long-term follow-up of the patients who were treated with LETAIRIS in the two pivotal studies and their open-label extension (N=383) shows that 95% were still alive at one year and 94% were still receiving LETAIRIS monotherapy. These uncontrolled observations do not allow comparison with a group not given LETAIRIS and cannot be used to determine the long-term effect of LETAIRIS.

14.3 Use in Patients with Prior Endothelin Receptor Antagonist (ERA) Related Liver Function Abnormalities

In an uncontrolled, open-label study, 36 patients who had previously discontinued endothelin receptor antagonists (ERAs: bosentan, an investigational drug, or both) due to aminotransferase elevations >3 × upper limit of normal (ULN) were treated with LETAIRIS. Prior elevations were predominantly moderate, with 64% of the ALT elevations <5 × ULN, but 9 patients had elevations >8 × ULN. Eight patients had been re-challenged with bosentan and/or the investigational ERA and all eight had a recurrence of aminotransferase abnormalities that required discontinuation of ERA therapy. All patients had to have normal aminotransferase levels on entry to this study. Twenty-five of the 36 patients were also receiving prostanoid and/or phosphodiesterase type 5 (PDE5) inhibitor therapy. Two patients

Figure 3 Time to Clinical Worsening

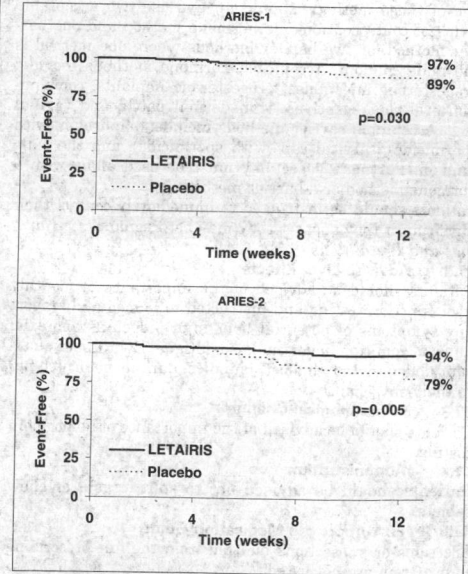

Time from randomization to clinical worsening with Kaplan-Meier estimates of the proportions of failures in ARIES-1 and ARIES-2.
p-values shown are the log-rank comparisons of LETAIRIS to placebo stratified by idiopathic PAH and non-idiopathic PAH patients

discontinued early (including one of the patients with a prior 8 × ULN elevation). Of the remaining 34 patients, one patient experienced a mild aminotransferase elevation at 12 weeks on LETAIRIS 5 mg that resolved with decreasing the dosage to 2.5 mg, and that did not recur with later escalations to 10 mg. With a median follow-up of 13 months and with 50% of patients increasing the dose of LETAIRIS to 10 mg, no patients were discontinued for aminotransferase elevations. While the uncontrolled study design does not provide information about what would have occurred with re-administration of previously used ERAs or show that LETAIRIS led to fewer aminotransferase elevations than would have been seen with those drugs, the study indicates that LETAIRIS may be tried in patients who have experienced asymptomatic aminotransferase elevations on other ERAs after aminotransferase levels have returned to normal.

Package Configuration	Tablet Strength	NDC No.	Description of Tablet; Debossed on Tablet; Size
30 count blister	5 mg	61958-0801-2	Square convex; pale pink; "5" on side 1 and "GSI" on side 2; 6.6 mm Square
30 count blister	10 mg	61958-0802-2	Oval convex; deep pink; "10" on side 1 and "GSI" on side 2; 9.8 mm × 4.9 mm Oval

16 HOW SUPPLIED/STORAGE AND HANDLING

Because of the risk of liver injury and birth defects, LETAIRIS may be prescribed only through the LETAIRIS Education and Access Program (LEAP) by calling 1-866-664-LEAP (5327) or by logging on to www.letairis.com. Adverse events can also be reported directly via this number. LETAIRIS film-coated, unscored tablets are supplied as follows:

[See table above]

℞ only

Store at 25 °C (77 °F); excursions permitted to 15–30 °C (59–86 °F) [see USP controlled room temperature]. Store LETAIRIS in its original packaging.

17 PATIENT COUNSELING INFORMATION

As a part of patient counseling, doctors must review the LETAIRIS Medication Guide with every patient [see FDA-Approved Medication Guide (17.5)].

17.1 Importance of Preventing Pregnancy

Patients should be advised that LETAIRIS may cause fetal harm. LETAIRIS treatment should only be initiated in women of childbearing potential following a negative pregnancy test.

Women of childbearing potential should be informed of the importance of monthly pregnancy tests and the need to use highly reliable contraception during LETAIRIS treatment and for one month after stopping treatment. If the patient has had a tubal sterilization or chooses to use a Copper T 380A IUD or LNg 20 IUS for pregnancy prevention, no additional contraception is needed. Women who do not choose one of these methods should always use two acceptable forms of contraception–one hormone method and one barrier method, or two barrier methods where one method is the male condom. Acceptable hormone methods include: progesterone injectables, progesterone implants, combination oral contraceptives, transdermal patch, and vaginal ring. Acceptable barrier methods include: diaphragm (with spermicide), cervical cap (with spermicide), and the male condom. Partner's vasectomy must be used along with a hormone method or a barrier method.

Patients should be instructed to immediately contact their physician if they suspect they may be pregnant [see Warnings and Precautions (5.5)].

17.2 Adverse Liver Effects

Patients should be advised of the importance of monthly liver function testing and instructed to immediately report any symptoms of potential liver injury (such as anorexia, nausea, vomiting, fever, malaise, fatigue, right upper quadrant abdominal discomfort, jaundice, dark urine or itching) to their physician.

17.3 Hematological Change

Patients should be advised of the importance of hemoglobin testing.

17.4 Administration

Patients should be advised not to split, crush, or chew tablets.

17.5 FDA-Approved Medication Guide

*Sections or subsections omitted from the full prescribing information are not listed.

Gilead Sciences, Inc., Foster City, CA 94404

Revised August 2009

LETAIRIS is a registered trademark of Gilead Sciences, Inc. Gilead and the Gilead logo are trademarks of Gilead Sciences, Inc. Other brands noted herein are the property of their respective owners.

© 2009 Gilead Sciences, Inc.

GS22-081-005

Medication Guide

LETAIRIS® (le-TAIR-is)

Tablets

(ambrisentan)

Read this Medication Guide before you start taking LETAIRIS and each time you get a refill. There may be new information. This Medication Guide does not take the place of talking with your doctor about your medical condition or your treatment.

What is the most important information I should know about LETAIRIS?

• Possible liver injury.

LETAIRIS can cause liver injury. You must have a blood test to check your liver function before you start LETAIRIS and each month after that. Your doctor will order these blood tests. (See "What are the possible effects of LETAIRIS?" for information about the signs of liver problems.) **Tell your doctor if you have had moderate or severe liver problems, including liver problems while taking other medicines.**

• Serious birth defects.

LETAIRIS can cause serious birth defects if taken during pregnancy. Women must not be pregnant when they start taking LETAIRIS or become pregnant during treatment. Women who are able to get pregnant must have a negative pregnancy test before beginning treatment with LETAIRIS and each month during treatment. Your doctor will decide when to do the test, depending on your menstrual cycle.

Women who are able to get pregnant must use two acceptable forms of birth control at the same time, during LETAIRIS treatment and for one month after stopping LETAIRIS. Talk with your doctor or gynecologist (a doctor who specializes in female reproduction) to find out about how to prevent pregnancy. **Do not have unprotected sex. Tell your doctor right away if you miss a menstrual period or think you may be pregnant.**

LETAIRIS is available only through a restricted program called the LETAIRIS Education and Access Program (LEAP). To receive LETAIRIS, you must talk to your doctor, understand the benefits and risks of LETAIRIS, and agree to all of the instructions in the LEAP program.

What is LETAIRIS?

LETAIRIS is a prescription medicine to treat pulmonary arterial hypertension (PAH), which is high blood pressure in the arteries of your lungs.

LETAIRIS can improve your ability to exercise and it can help slow down the worsening of your physical condition and symptoms.

Who should not take LETAIRIS?

Do not take LETAIRIS if:

• **you are pregnant, plan to become pregnant, or become pregnant during treatment with LETAIRIS. LETAIRIS can cause serious birth defects.** (See "What is the important information I should know about LETAIRIS?") Serious birth defects from LETAIRIS happen early in pregnancy.

• **your blood tests show possible liver injury.**

Tell your doctor about all your medical conditions and all the medicines you take including prescription and nonprescription medicines. LETAIRIS and other medicines may affect each other causing side effects. Do not start any new medicines until you check with your doctor.

LETAIRIS has not been studied in children.

How should I take LETAIRIS?

LETAIRIS will be mailed to you by a specialty pharmacy. Your doctor will give you complete details.

• Take LETAIRIS exactly as your doctor tells you. Do not stop taking LETAIRIS unless your doctor tells you.

• You can take LETAIRIS with or without food.

• Do not split, crush or chew LETAIRIS tablets.

• It will be easier to remember to take LETAIRIS if you take it at the same time each day.

• If you take more than your regular dose of LETAIRIS, call your doctor right away.

• If you miss a dose, take it as soon as you remember that day. Take your next dose at the regular time. Do not take two doses at the same time to make up for a missed dose.

• During treatment your doctor will test your blood for signs of side effects to your liver and red blood cells.

What should I avoid while taking LETAIRIS?

• **Do not get pregnant** while taking LETAIRIS. (See the serious birth defects section of "What is the most important information I should know about LETAIRIS?") If you miss a menstrual period, or think you might be pregnant, call your doctor right away.

• **Breastfeeding is not recommended** while taking LETAIRIS. It is not known if LETAIRIS can pass through your milk and harm your baby.

What are the possible side effects of LETAIRIS?

Serious side effects of LETAIRIS include:

• **Possible liver injury.** (See "What is the most important information I should know about LETAIRIS?") Call your doctor right away if you have any of these symptoms of liver problems: loss of appetite, nausea, vomiting, fever, unusual tiredness, abdominal (stomach area) pain, yellowing of the skin or the whites of your eyes (jaundice), dark urine, or itching.

• **Serious birth defects.** (See "What is the most important information I should know about LETAIRIS?")

• **Swelling all over the body** (fluid retention) can happen within weeks after starting LETAIRIS. Tell your doctor right away if you have any unusual weight gain, tiredness, or trouble breathing while taking LETAIRIS. These may be symptoms of a serious health problem. You may need to be treated with medicine or need to go to the hospital.

• **Sperm count reduction.** Reduced sperm counts have been observed in some men taking a drug similar to LETAIRIS, an effect which might impair their ability to father a child. Tell your doctor if remaining fertile is important to you.

The most common side effects of LETAIRIS are:

• Lowering of red blood cell count
• Swelling of hands, legs, ankles and feet (peripheral edema)
• Stuffy nose (nasal congestion)
• Inflamed nasal passages (sinusitis)
• Hot flashes or getting red in the face (flushing)
• Feeling your heart beat (palpitations)
• Red and sore throat and nose
• Stomach pain
• Constipation
• Shortness of breath
• Headache

Allergic reactions (rash, swelling of the face, lips, mouth, tongue, or throat which may cause difficulty in swallowing or breathing) have been reported infrequently.

Tell your doctor if you have any side effect that bothers you or that does not go away. These are not all of the possible side effects of LETAIRIS. For more information, ask your doctor or pharmacist.

Call your doctor for medical advice about side effects. You may report side effects to FDA at 1-800-FDA-1088.

How should I store LETAIRIS?

Store LETAIRIS at 59 °F to 86 °F (15 °C to 30 °C), in the package it comes in.

Keep LETAIRIS and all medicines out of the reach of children.

General information about LETAIRIS

Medicines are sometimes prescribed for purposes other than those listed in a Medication Guide. Do not use LETAIRIS for a condition for which it was not prescribed. Do not give LETAIRIS to other people, even if they have the same symptoms that you have. It may harm them.

This Medication Guide summarizes the most important information about LETAIRIS. If you would like more information, ask your doctor. You can ask your doctor or pharmacist for information about LETAIRIS that is written for healthcare professionals.

For more information, call 1-866-664-LEAP (5327) or visit www.letairis.com or www.gilead.com.

What are the ingredients in LETAIRIS?

Active ingredient: ambrisentan

Inactive Ingredients: croscarmellose sodium, lactose monohydrate, magnesium stearate and microcrystalline cellulose. The tablets are film-coated with a coating material containing FD&C Red #40 aluminum lake, lecithin, polyethylene glycol, polyvinyl alcohol, talc, and titanium dioxide.

Revised August 2009

This Medication Guide has been approved by the U.S. Food and Drug Administration.

Gilead Sciences, Inc., Foster City, CA 94404

LETAIRIS is a registered trademark of Gilead Sciences, Inc. Gilead and the Gilead logo are trademarks of Gilead Sciences, Inc. Other brands noted herein are the property of their respective owners.

© 2009 Gilead Sciences, Inc.

GS22-081-005

Shown in Product Identification Guide, page 309

RANEXA ℞

[rAn-ex-α]

(ranolazine)

Extended-Release Tablets

HIGHLIGHTS OF PRESCRIBING INFORMATION

These highlights do not include all the information needed to use Ranexa safely and effectively. See full prescribing information for Ranexa.

Ranexa (ranolazine) extended-release tablets

Initial U.S. Approval: 2006

RECENT MAJOR CHANGES

Indications and Usage (1)   11/2008
Contraindications (4)   11/2008

INDICATIONS AND USAGE

Ranexa is indicated for the treatment of chronic angina. (1)

DOSAGE AND ADMINISTRATION

500 mg twice daily and increase to 1000 mg twice daily, based on clinical symptoms (2.1)

DOSAGE FORMS AND STRENGTHS

Extended-release tablets: 500 mg, 1000 mg (3)

CONTRAINDICATIONS

- Use with strong CYP3A inhibitors (e.g., ketoconazole, clarithromycin, nelfinavir) (4, 7.1)
- Use with CYP3A inducers (e.g., rifampin, phenobarbital) (4, 7.1)
- Use in patients with clinically significant hepatic impairment (4, 8.6)

WARNINGS AND PRECAUTIONS

- QT interval prolongation: Can occur with ranolazine. Little data available on high doses, long exposure, use with QT interval-prolonging drugs, or potassium channel variants causing prolonged QT interval. (5.1)

ADVERSE REACTIONS

Most common adverse reactions (> 4% and more common than with placebo) are dizziness, headache, constipation, nausea. (6.1)

To report SUSPECTED ADVERSE REACTIONS, contact Gilead Sciences, Inc.,, at 1-800-GILEAD-5 or FDA at 1-800-FDA-1088 or www.fda.gov/medwatch.

DRUG INTERACTIONS

- CYP3A inhibitors: Do not use Ranexa with strong CYP3A inhibitors. With moderate 3A inhibitors (e.g., diltiazem, verapamil, erythromycin), limit maximum dose of Ranexa to 500 mg twice daily. (7.1)
- CYP3A inducers: Do not use Ranexa with CYP3A inducers. (7.1)
- P-gp inhibitors (e.g., cyclosporine): May need to lower Ranexa dose based on clinical response. (7.1)
- Drugs transported by P-gp or metabolized by CYP2D6 (e.g., digoxin, tricyclic antidepressants): May need reduced doses of these drugs when used with Ranexa. (7.2)

See 17 for PATIENT COUNSELING INFORMATION

Revised: 09/2009

FULL PRESCRIBING INFORMATION

1 INDICATIONS AND USAGE

Ranexa is indicated for the treatment of chronic angina. Ranexa may be used with beta-blockers, nitrates, calcium channel blockers, anti-platelet therapy, lipid-lowering therapy, ACE inhibitors, and angiotensin receptor blockers.

2 DOSAGE AND ADMINISTRATION

2.1 Dosing Information

Initiate Ranexa dosing at 500 mg twice daily and increase to 1000 mg twice daily, as needed, based on clinical symptoms. Take Ranexa with or without meals. Swallow Ranexa tablets whole; do not crush, break, or chew.

The maximum recommended daily dose of Ranexa is 1000 mg twice daily.

If a dose of Ranexa is missed, take the prescribed dose at the next scheduled time; do not double the next dose.

2.2 Dose Modification

Dose adjustments may be needed when Ranexa is taken in combination with certain other drugs [see Drug Interactions (7.1)]. Limit the maximum dose of Ranexa to 500 mg twice daily in patients on diltiazem, verapamil, and other moderate CYP3A inhibitors. Down-titrate Ranexa based on clinical response in patients concomitantly treated with P-gp inhibitors, such as cyclosporine.

3 DOSAGE FORMS AND STRENGTHS

Ranexa is supplied as film-coated, oblong-shaped, extended-release tablets in the following strengths:

- 500 mg tablets are light orange, with GSI500 on one side
- 1000 mg tablets are pale yellow, with GSI1000 on one side

4 CONTRAINDICATIONS

Ranexa is contraindicated in patients:

- Taking strong inhibitors of CYP3A [see Drug Interactions (7.1)]
- Taking inducers of CYP3A [see Drug Interactions (7.1)]
- With clinically significant hepatic impairment [see Use in Specific Populations (8.6)]

5 WARNINGS AND PRECAUTIONS

5.1 QT Interval Prolongation

Ranolazine blocks I_{Kr} and prolongs the QTc interval in a dose-related manner.

Clinical experience in an acute coronary syndrome population did not show an increased risk of proarrhythmia or sudden death [see Clinical Studies (14.2)]. However, there is little experience with high doses (> 1000 mg twice daily) or exposure, other QT-prolonging drugs, or potassium channel variants resulting in a long QT interval.

6 ADVERSE REACTIONS

6.1 Clinical Trial Experience

Because clinical trials are conducted under widely varying conditions, adverse reaction rates observed in the clinical trials of a drug cannot be directly compared to rates in the clinical trials of another drug and may not reflect the rates observed in practice.

A total of 2,018 patients with chronic angina were treated with ranolazine in controlled clinical trials. Of the patients treated with Ranexa, 1,026 were enrolled in three double-blind, placebo-controlled, randomized studies (CARISA, ERICA, MARISA) of up to 12 weeks duration. In addition, upon study completion, 1,251 patients received treatment with Ranexa in open-label, long-term studies; 1,227 patients were exposed to Ranexa for more than 1 year, 613 patients for more than 2 years, 531 patients for more than 3 years, and 326 patients for more than 4 years.

At recommended doses, about 6% of patients discontinued treatment with Ranexa because of an adverse event in controlled studies in angina patients compared to about 3% on placebo. The most common adverse events that led to discontinuation more frequently on Ranexa than placebo were dizziness (1.3% versus 0.1%), nausea (1% versus 0%), asthenia, constipation, and headache (each about 0.5% versus 0%). Doses above 1000 mg twice daily are poorly tolerated. In controlled clinical trials of angina patients, the most frequently reported treatment-emergent adverse reactions (> 4% and more common on Ranexa than on placebo) were dizziness (6.2%), headache (5.5%), constipation (4.5%), and nausea (4.4%). Dizziness may be dose-related. In open-label, long-term treatment studies, a similar adverse reaction profile was observed.

The following additional adverse reactions occurred at an incidence of 0.5 to 2.0% in patients treated with Ranexa and were more frequent than the incidence observed in placebo-treated patients:

Cardiac Disorders–bradycardia, palpitations
Ear and Labyrinth Disorders–tinnitus, vertigo
Gastrointestinal Disorders–abdominal pain, dry mouth, vomiting
General Disorders and Administrative Site Adverse Events–peripheral edema
Respiratory, Thoracic, and Mediastinal Disorders–dyspnea
Vascular Disorders–hypotension, orthostatic hypotension

Other (< 0.5%) but potentially medically important adverse reactions observed more frequently with Ranexa than placebo treatment in all controlled studies included: angioedema, renal failure, eosinophilia, blurred vision, confusional state, hematuria, hypoesthesia, paresthesia, tremor, pulmonary fibrosis, thrombocytopenia, leukopenia, and pancytopenia.

A large clinical trial in acute coronary syndrome patients was unsuccessful in demonstrating a benefit for Ranexa, but there was no apparent proarrhythmic effect in these high-risk patients [see Clinical Trials (14.2)].

Laboratory Abnormalities

Ranexa produces small reductions in hemoglobin A1c. Ranexa is not a treatment for diabetes.

Ranexa produces elevations of serum creatinine by 0.1 mg/dL, regardless of previous renal function. The elevation has a rapid onset, shows no signs of progression during long-term therapy, is reversible after discontinuation of Ranexa, and is not accompanied by changes in BUN. In healthy volunteers, Ranexa 1000 mg twice daily had no effect upon the glomerular filtration rate. The elevated creatinine levels are likely due to a blockage of creatinine's tubular secretion by ranolazine or one of its metabolites.

7 DRUG INTERACTIONS

7.1 Effects of Other Drugs on Ranolazine

Ranolazine is primarily metabolized by CYP3A and is a substrate of P-glycoprotein (P-gp).

CYP3A Inhibitors

Do not use Ranexa with strong CYP3A inhibitors, including ketoconazole, itraconazole, clarithromycin, nefazodone, nelfinavir, ritonavir, indinavir, and saquinavir. Ketoconazole (200 mg twice daily) increases average steady-state plasma concentrations of ranolazine 3.2-fold [see Contraindications (4)].

Limit the dose of Ranexa to 500 mg twice daily in patients on moderate CYP3A inhibitors, including diltiazem, verapamil, aprepitant, erythromycin, fluconazole, and grapefruit juice or grapefruit-containing products. Diltiazem (180–360 mg daily) and verapamil (120 mg three times daily) increase ranolazine steady-state plasma concentrations about 2-fold [see Dosage and Administration (2.2)].

Weak CYP3A inhibitors such as simvastatin (20 mg once daily) and cimetidine (400 mg three times daily) do not increase the exposure to ranolazine in healthy volunteers.

P-gp Inhibitors

Down-titrate Ranexa based on clinical response in patients concomitantly treated with P-gp inhibitors, such as cyclosporine [see Dosage and Administration (2.2)].

CYP3A and P-gp Inducers

Avoid co-administration of Ranexa and CYP3A inducers such as rifampin, rifabutin, rifapentin, phenobarbital, phenytoin, carbamazepine, and St. John's wort. Rifampin (600 mg once daily) decreases the plasma concentration of ranolazine (1000 mg twice daily) by approximately 95% by induction of CYP3A and, probably, P-gp.

CYP2D6 Inhibitors

The potent CYP2D6 inhibitor, paroxetine (20 mg once daily), increases ranolazine concentrations 1.2-fold. No dose adjustment of Ranexa is required in patients treated with CYP2D6 inhibitors.

Digoxin

Digoxin (0.125 mg) does not significantly alter ranolazine levels.

7.2 Effects of Ranolazine on Other Drugs

In vitro studies indicate that ranolazine and its O-demethylated metabolite are weak inhibitors of CYP3A, moderate inhibitors of CYP2D6 and moderate P-gp inhibitors. Ranolazine and its most abundant metabolites are not known to inhibit the metabolism of substrates for CYP 1A2, 2C8, 2C9, 2C19, or 2E1 in human liver microsomes, suggesting that ranolazine is unlikely to alter the pharmacokinetics of drugs metabolized by these enzymes.

Drugs Metabolized by CYP3A

The plasma levels of simvastatin, a CYP3A substrate, and its active metabolite are each increased about 2-fold in healthy subjects receiving simvastatin (80 mg once daily) and Ranexa (1000 mg twice daily). Dose adjustments of simvastatin are not required when Ranexa is co-administered with simvastatin.

The pharmacokinetics of diltiazem is not affected by ranolazine in healthy volunteers receiving diltiazem 60 mg three times daily and Ranexa 1000 mg twice daily.

Drugs Transported by P-gp

Ranexa (1000 mg twice daily) causes a 1.5-fold elevation of digoxin plasma concentrations. The dose of digoxin may have to be adjusted.

Drugs Metabolized by CYP2D6

Ranolazine or its metabolites partially inhibit CYP2D6. There are no studies of concomitant use of Ranexa with other drugs metabolized by CYP2D6, such as tricyclic antidepressants and antipsychotics, but lower doses of CYP2D6 substrates may be required.

8 USE IN SPECIFIC POPULATIONS

8.1 Pregnancy

Pregnancy Category C

In animal studies, ranolazine at exposures 1.5 (rabbit) to 2 (rat) times the usual human exposure caused maternal toxicity and misshapen sternebrae and reduced ossification in offspring. These doses in rats and rabbits were associated with an increased maternal mortality rate *[see Reproductive Toxicology Studies (13.3)]*. There are no adequate well-controlled studies in pregnant women. Ranexa should be used during pregnancy only when the potential benefit to the patient justifies the potential risk to the fetus.

8.3 Nursing Mothers

It is not known whether ranolazine is excreted in human milk. Because many drugs are excreted in human milk and because of the potential for serious adverse reactions from ranolazine in nursing infants, decide whether to discontinue nursing or to discontinue Ranexa, taking into account the importance of the drug to the mother.

8.4 Pediatric Use

Safety and effectiveness have not been established in pediatric patients.

8.5 Geriatric Use

Of the chronic angina patients treated with Ranexa in controlled studies, 496 (48%) were ≥ 65 years of age, and 114 (11%) were ≥ 75 years of age. No overall differences in efficacy were observed between older and younger patients. There were no differences in safety for patients ≥ 65 years compared to younger patients, but patients ≥ 75 years of age on ranolazine, compared to placebo, had a higher incidence of adverse events, serious adverse events, and drug discontinuations due to adverse events. In general, dose selection for an elderly patient should usually start at the low end of the dosing range, reflecting the greater frequency of decreased hepatic, renal, or cardiac function, and of concomitant disease, or other drug therapy.

8.6 Use in Patients with Hepatic Impairment

Ranexa is contraindicated in patients with clinically significant hepatic impairment. Plasma concentrations of ranolazine were increased by 30% in patients with mild (Child-Pugh Class A) and by 60% in patients with moderate (Child-Pugh Class B) hepatic impairment. This was not enough to account for the 3-fold increase in QT prolongation seen in patients with mild to severe hepatic impairment *[see Contraindications (4)]*.

8.7 Use in Patients with Renal Impairment

In patients with varying degrees of renal impairment, ranolazine plasma levels increased up to 50%. The pharmacokinetics of ranolazine has not been assessed in patients on dialysis.

8.8 Use in Patients with Heart Failure

Heart failure (NYHA Class I to IV) had no significant effect on ranolazine pharmacokinetics. Ranexa had minimal effects on heart rate and blood pressure in patients with angina and heart failure NYHA Class I to IV. No dose adjustment of Ranexa is required in patients with heart failure.

8.9 Use in Patients with Diabetes Mellitus

A population pharmacokinetic evaluation of data from angina patients and healthy subjects showed no effect of diabetes on ranolazine pharmacokinetics. No dose adjustment is required in patients with diabetes.

Ranexa produces small reductions in HbA1c in patients with diabetes, the clinical significance of which is unknown. Ranexa should not be considered a treatment for diabetes.

10 OVERDOSAGE

High oral doses of ranolazine produce dose-related increases in dizziness, nausea, and vomiting. High intravenous exposure also produces diplopia, paresthesia, confusion, and syncope. In addition to general supportive measures, continuous ECG monitoring may be warranted in the event of overdose.

Since ranolazine is about 62% bound to plasma proteins, hemodialysis is unlikely to be effective in clearing ranolazine.

11 DESCRIPTION

Ranexa (ranolazine) is available as a film-coated, nonscored, extended-release tablet for oral administration.

Ranolazine is a racemic mixture, chemically described as 1-piperazineacetamide, *N*-(2,6-dimethylphenyl)-4-[2-hydroxy-3-(2-methoxyphenoxy)propyl]-, (±)-. It has an empirical formula of $C_{24}H_{33}N_3O_4$, a molecular weight of 427.54 g/mole, and the following structural formula:

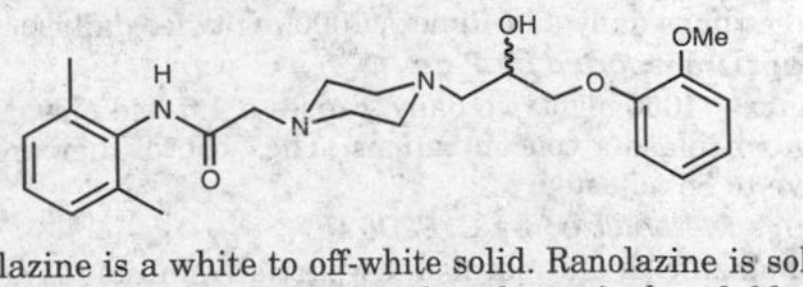

Ranolazine is a white to off-white solid. Ranolazine is soluble in dichloromethane and methanol; sparingly soluble in tetrahydrofuran, ethanol, acetonitrile, and acetone; slightly soluble in ethyl acetate, isopropanol, toluene, and ethyl ether; and very slightly soluble in water.

Ranexa tablets contain 500 mg or 1000 mg of ranolazine and the following inactive ingredients: carnauba wax, hypromellose, magnesium stearate, methacrylic acid copolymer (Type C), microcrystalline cellulose, polyethylene glycol, sodium hydroxide, and titanium dioxide. Additional inactive ingredients for the 500 mg tablet include polyvinyl alcohol, talc, Iron Oxide Yellow, and Iron Oxide Red; additional inactive ingredients for the 1000 mg tablet include lactose monohydrate, triacetin, and Iron Oxide Yellow.

12 CLINICAL PHARMACOLOGY

12.1 Mechanism of Action

The mechanism of action of ranolazine's antianginal effects has not been determined. Ranolazine has anti-ischemic and antianginal effects that do not depend upon reductions in heart rate or blood pressure. It does not affect the rate-pressure product, a measure of myocardial work, at maximal exercise. Ranolazine at therapeutic levels can inhibit the cardiac late sodium current (I_{Na}). However, the relationship of this inhibition to angina symptoms is uncertain.

The QT prolongation effect of ranolazine on the surface electrocardiogram is the result of inhibition of I_{Kr}, which prolongs the ventricular action potential.

12.2 Pharmacodynamics

Hemodynamic Effects

Patients with chronic angina treated with Ranexa in controlled clinical studies had minimal changes in mean heart rate (< 2 bpm) and systolic blood pressure (< 3 mm Hg). Similar results were observed in subgroups of patients with CHF NYHA Class I or II, diabetes, or reactive airway disease, and in elderly patients.

Electrocardiographic Effects

Dose and plasma concentration-related increases in the QTc interval *[see Warnings and Precautions (5.1)]*, reductions in T wave amplitude, and, in some cases, notched T waves, have been observed in patients treated with Ranexa. These effects are believed to be caused by ranolazine and not by its metabolites. The relationship between the change in QTc and ranolazine plasma concentrations is linear, with a slope of about 2.6 msec/1000 ng/mL, through exposures corresponding to doses several-fold higher than the maximum recommended dose of 1000 mg twice daily. The variable blood levels attained after a given dose of ranolazine give a wide range of effects on QTc. At T_{max} following repeat dosing at 1000 mg twice daily, the mean change in QTc is about 6 msec, but in the 5% of the population with the highest plasma concentrations, the prolongation of QTc is at least 15 msec. In subjects with mild or moderate hepatic impairment, the relationship between plasma level of ranolazine and QTc is much steeper *[see Contraindications (4)]*.

Age, weight, gender, race, heart rate, congestive heart failure, diabetes, and renal impairment did not alter the slope of the QTc-concentration relationship of ranolazine.

No proarrhythmic effects were observed on 7-day Holter recordings in 3,162 acute coronary syndrome patients treated with Ranexa. There was a significantly lower incidence of arrhythmias (ventricular tachycardia, bradycardia, supraventricular tachycardia, and new atrial fibrillation) in patients treated with Ranexa (80%) versus placebo (87%), including ventricular tachycardia ≥ 3 beats (52% versus 61%). However, this difference in arrhythmias did not lead to a reduction in mortality, a reduction in arrhythmia hospitalization, or a reduction in arrhythmia symptoms.

12.3 Pharmacokinetics

Ranolazine is extensively metabolized in the gut and liver and its absorption is highly variable. For example, at a dose of 1000 mg twice daily, the mean steady-state C_{max} was 2600 ng/mL with 95% confidence limits of 400 and 6100 ng/mL. The pharmacokinetics of the (+) R- and (-) S-enantiomers of ranolazine are similar in healthy volunteers. The apparent terminal half-life of ranolazine is 7 hours. Steady state is generally achieved within 3 days of twice-daily dosing with Ranexa. At steady state over the dose range of 500 to 1000 mg twice daily, C_{max} and $AUC_{0-\tau}$ increase slightly more than proportionally to dose, 2.2- and 2.4-fold, respectively. With twice-daily dosing, the trough:peak ratio of the ranolazine plasma concentration is 0.3 to 0.6. The pharmacokinetics of ranolazine is unaffected by age, gender, or food.

Absorption and Distribution

After oral administration of Ranexa, peak plasma concentrations of ranolazine are reached between 2 and 5 hours. After oral administration of ^{14}C-ranolazine as a solution, 73% of the dose is systemically available as ranolazine or metabolites. The bioavailability of ranolazine from Ranexa tablets relative to that from a solution of ranolazine is 76%. Because ranolazine is a substrate of P-gp, inhibitors of P-gp may increase the absorption of ranolazine.

Food (high-fat breakfast) has no important effect on the C_{max} and AUC of ranolazine. Therefore, Ranexa may be taken without regard to meals. Over the concentration range of 0.25 to 10 µg/mL, ranolazine is approximately 62% bound to human plasma proteins.

Metabolism and Excretion

Ranolazine is metabolized mainly by CYP3A and, to a lesser extent, by CYP2D6. Following a single oral dose of ranolazine solution, approximately 75% of the dose is excreted in urine and 25% in feces. Ranolazine is metabolized rapidly and extensively in the liver and intestine; less than 5% is excreted unchanged in urine and feces. The pharmacologic activity of the metabolites has not been well characterized. After dosing to steady state with 500 mg to 1500 mg twice daily, the four most abundant metabolites in plasma have AUC values ranging from about 5 to 33% that of ranolazine, and display apparent half-lives ranging from 6 to 22 hours.

13 NONCLINICAL TOXICOLOGY

13.1 Carcinogenesis, Mutagenesis, Impairment of Fertility

Ranolazine tested negative for genotoxic potential in the following assays: Ames bacterial mutation assay, Saccharomyces assay for mitotic gene conversion, chromosomal aberrations assay in Chinese hamster ovary (CHO) cells, mammalian CHO/HGPRT gene mutation assay, and mouse and rat bone marrow micronucleus assays.

There was no evidence of carcinogenic potential in mice or rats. The highest oral doses used in the carcinogenicity studies were 150 mg/kg/day for 21 months in rats (900 mg/m^2/day) and 50 mg/kg/day for 24 months in mice (150 mg/m^2/day). These maximally tolerated doses are 0.8 and 0.1 times, respectively, the maximum recommended human dose (MRHD) of 2 grams on a surface area basis. A published study reported that ranolazine promoted tumor formation and progression to malignancy when given to transgenic APC (min/+) mice at a dose of 30 mg/kg twice daily *[see References (15)]*. The clinical significance of this finding is unclear.

13.3 Reproductive Toxicology Studies

Animal reproduction studies with ranolazine were conducted in rats and rabbits.

There was an increased incidence of misshapen sternebrae and reduced ossification of pelvic and cranial bones in fetuses of pregnant rats dosed at 400 mg/kg/day (2 times the MRHD on a surface area basis). Reduced ossification of sternebrae was observed in fetuses of pregnant rabbits dosed at 150 mg/kg/day (1.5 times the MRHD on a surface area basis). These doses in rats and rabbits were associated with an increased maternal mortality rate.

14 CLINICAL STUDIES

14.1 Chronic Stable Angina

CARISA (Combination Assessment of Ranolazine In Stable Angina) was a study in 823 chronic angina patients randomized to receive 12 weeks of treatment with twice-daily Ranexa 750 mg, 1000 mg, or placebo, who also continued on daily doses of atenolol 50 mg, amlodipine 5 mg, or diltiazem CD 180 mg. Sublingual nitrates were used in this study as needed.

In this trial, statistically significant ($p < 0.05$) increases in modified Bruce treadmill exercise duration and time to angina were observed for each Ranexa dose versus placebo, at both trough (12 hours after dosing) and peak (4 hours after dosing) plasma levels, with minimal effects on blood pressure and heart rate. The changes versus placebo in exercise parameters are presented in Table 1. Exercise treadmill results showed no increase in effect on exercise at the 1000 mg dose compared to the 750 mg dose.

Table 1 Exercise Treadmill Results (CARISA)

	Mean Difference from Placebo (sec)	
Study	**CARISA (N = 791)**	
Ranexa Twice-daily Dose	**750 mg**	**1000 mg**
Exercise Duration		
Trough	24*	24*
Peak	34†	26*
Time to Angina		
Trough	30*	26*
Peak	38†	38†
Time to 1 mm ST-Segment Depression		
Trough	20	21
Peak	41†	35†

* p-value ≤ 0.05
† p-value ≤ 0.005

The effects of Ranexa on angina frequency and nitroglycerin use are shown in Table 2.

[See table 2 at top of next page]

Table 2 Angina Frequency and Nitroglycerin Use (CARISA)

		Placebo	Ranexa 750 mg*	Ranexa 1000 mg*
Angina Frequency (attacks/week)	N	258	272	261
	Mean	3.3	2.5	2.1
	p-value vs placebo	—	0.006	< 0.001
Nitroglycerin Use (doses/week)	N	252	262	244
	Mean	3.1	2.1	1.8
	p-value vs placebo	—	0.016	< 0.001

* Twice daily

Table 3 Angina Frequency and Nitroglycerin Use (ERICA)

		Placebo	Ranexa*
Angina Frequency (attacks/week)	N	281	277
	Mean	4.3	3.3
	Median	2.4	2.2
Nitroglycerin Use (doses/week)	N	281	277
	Mean	3.6	2.7
	Median	1.7	1.3

*1000 mg twice daily

Tolerance to Ranexa did not develop after 12 weeks of therapy. Rebound increases in angina, as measured by exercise duration, have not been observed following abrupt discontinuation of Ranexa.

Ranexa has been evaluated in patients with chronic angina who remained symptomatic despite treatment with the maximum dose of an antianginal agent. In the ERICA (Efficacy of Ranolazine In Chronic Angina) trial, 565 patients were randomized to receive an initial dose of Ranexa 500 mg twice daily or placebo for 1 week, followed by 6 weeks of treatment with Ranexa 1000 mg twice daily or placebo, in addition to concomitant treatment with amlodipine 10 mg once daily. In addition, 45% of the study population also received long-acting nitrates. Sublingual nitrates were used as needed to treat angina episodes. Results are shown in Table 3. Statistically significant decreases in angina attack frequency (p = 0.028) and nitroglycerin use (p = 0.014) were observed with Ranexa compared to placebo. These treatment effects appeared consistent across age and use of long-acting nitrates.
[See table 3 above]

Gender
Effects on angina frequency and exercise tolerance were considerably smaller in women than in men. In CARISA, the improvement in Exercise Tolerance Test (ETT) in females was about 33% of that in males at the 1000 mg twice-daily dose level. In ERICA, where the primary endpoint was angina attack frequency, the mean reduction in weekly angina attacks was 0.3 for females and 1.3 for males.
Race
There were insufficient numbers of non-Caucasian patients to allow for analyses of efficacy or safety by racial subgroup.
14.2   Lack of Benefit in Acute Coronary Syndrome
In a large (n = 6,560) placebo-controlled trial (MERLIN-TIMI 36) in patients with acute coronary syndrome, there was no benefit shown on outcome measures. However, the study is somewhat reassuring regarding proarrhythmic risks, as ventricular arrhythmias were less common on ranolazine *[see Clinical Pharmacology (12.2)]*, and there was no difference between Ranexa and placebo in the risk of all-cause mortality (relative risk ranolazine:placebo 0.99 with an upper 95% confidence limit of 1.22).

15   REFERENCES
M.A. Suckow et al. The anti-ischemia agent ranolazine promotes the development of intestinal tumors in APC (min/+) mice. Cancer Letters 209(2004):165–9.

16   HOW SUPPLIED/STORAGE AND HANDLING
Ranexa is supplied as film-coated, oblong-shaped, extended-release tablets in the following strengths:
• 500 mg tablets are light orange, with GSI500 on one side
• 1000 mg tablets are pale yellow, with GSI1000 on one side
Ranexa (ranolazine) extended-release tablets are available in:

	Strength	NDC
Unit-of-Use Bottle (60 Tablets)	500 mg	61958-1001-1
Unit-of-Use Bottle (60 Tablets)	1000 mg	61958-1002-1

Store Ranexa tablets at 25 °C (77 °F) with excursions permitted to 15 ° to 30 °C (59 ° to 86 °F).

17   PATIENT COUNSELING INFORMATION
To ensure safe and effective use of Ranexa, the following information and instructions should be communicated to the patient when appropriate.
Patients should be advised:
• that Ranexa will not abate an acute angina episode
• to inform their physician of any other medications when taken concurrently with Ranexa, including over-the-counter medications
• that Ranexa may produce changes in the electrocardiogram (QTc interval prolongation)
• to inform their physician of any personal or family history of QTc prolongation, congenital long QT syndrome, or if they are receiving drugs that prolong the QTc interval such as Class Ia (e.g., quinidine) or Class III (e.g., dofetilide, sotalol, amiodarone) antiarrhythmic agents, erythromycin, and certain antipsychotics (e.g., thioridazine, ziprasidone)
• that Ranexa should not be used in patients who are receiving drugs that are strong CYP3A inhibitors (e.g., ketoconazole, clarithromycin, nefazodone, ritonavir)
• that initiation of treatment with Ranexa should be avoided during administration of inducers of CYP3A (e.g., rifampin, rifabutin, rifapentin, barbiturates, carbamazepine, phenytoin, St. John's wort)
• to inform their physician if they are receiving drugs that are moderate CYP3A inhibitors (e.g., diltiazem, verapamil, erythromycin) or P-gp inhibitors (e.g., cyclosporine)
• that grapefruit juice or grapefruit products should be limited when taking Ranexa
• that Ranexa should generally not be used in patients with clinically significant liver impairment
• that doses of Ranexa higher than 1000 mg twice daily should not be used
• that if a dose is missed, the usual dose should be taken at the next scheduled time. The next dose should not be doubled
• that Ranexa may be taken with or without meals
• that Ranexa tablets should be swallowed whole and not crushed, broken, or chewed
• to contact their physician if they experience fainting spells while taking Ranexa

• that Ranexa may cause dizziness and lightheadedness; therefore, patients should know how they react to this drug before they operate an automobile, or machinery, or engage in activities requiring mental alertness or coordination
Manufactured for:
Gilead Sciences, Inc.
Foster City, CA 94404 USA
Ranexa is a registered U.S. trademark of Gilead, Palo Alto, Inc.
©2009 Gilead Sciences, Inc.
21-526-GS-007 Sept 2009
Shown in Product Identification Guide, page 309

TRUVADA®   ℞
[*tru-VAH-dah*]
(emtricitabine/tenofovir disoproxil fumarate)
Tablets

HIGHLIGHTS OF PRESCRIBING INFORMATION
These highlights do not include all the information needed to use TRUVADA safely and effectively. See full prescribing information for TRUVADA.
TRUVADA® (emtricitabine/tenofovir disoproxil fumarate) tablets
Initial U.S. Approval: 2004

> **WARNINGS: LACTIC ACIDOSIS/SEVERE HEPATO-MEGALY WITH STEATOSIS and POST TREATMENT ACUTE EXACERBATION OF HEPATITIS B**
> *See full prescribing information for complete boxed warning.*
> • Lactic acidosis and severe hepatomegaly with steatosis, including fatal cases, have been reported with the use of nucleoside analogs, including VIREAD, a component of TRUVADA. (5.1)
> • TRUVADA is not approved for the treatment of chronic hepatitis B virus (HBV) infection. Severe acute exacerbations of hepatitis B have been reported in patients coinfected with HIV-1 and HBV who have discontinued TRUVADA. Hepatic function should be monitored closely in these patients. If appropriate, initiation of anti-hepatitis B therapy may be warranted. (5.2)

————RECENT MAJOR CHANGES————

Warnings and Precautions
New Onset or Worsening Renal Impairment (5,3) 11/2009

————INDICATIONS AND USAGE————
TRUVADA, a combination of EMTRIVA and VIREAD, both nucleoside analog HIV-1 reverse transcriptase inhibitors, is indicated in combination with other antiretroviral agents for the treatment of HIV-1 infection in adults. (1)

————DOSAGE AND ADMINISTRATION————
• Recommended dose: One tablet (containing 200 mg of emtricitabine and 300 mg of tenofovir disoproxil fumarate) once daily taken orally with or without food. (2.1)
• Dose recommended in renal impairment:
Creatinine clearance 30–49 mL/min: 1 tablet every 48 hours. (2.2)
CrCl <30 mL/min or hemodialysis: Do not use TRUVADA. (2.2)

————DOSAGE FORMS AND STRENGTHS————
Tablets: 200 mg of emtricitabine and 300 mg of tenofovir disoproxil fumarate. (3)

————CONTRAINDICATIONS————
None. (4)

————WARNINGS AND PRECAUTIONS————
• New onset or worsening renal impairment: Can include acute renal failure and Fanconi syndrome. Assess creatinine clearance (CrCl) before initiating treatment with TRUVADA. Monitor CrCl and serum phosphorus in patients at risk. Avoid administering Truvada with concurrent or recent use of nephrotoxic drugs. (5.3)
• Coadministration with Other Products: Do not use with drugs containing emtricitabine or tenofovir disoproxil fumarate including ATRIPLA, EMTRIVA, VIREAD; or with drugs containing lamivudine. Do not administer in combination with HEPSERA. (5.4)
• Decreases in bone mineral density (BMD): Consider monitoring BMD in patients with a history of pathologic fracture or who are at risk for osteopenia. (5.5)
• Redistribution/accumulation of body fat: Observed in patients receiving antiretroviral therapy. (5.6)
• Immune reconstitution syndrome: May necessitate further evaluation and treatment. (5.7)
• Triple nucleoside-only regimens: Early virologic failure has been reported in HIV-infected patients. Monitor carefully and consider treatment modification. (5.8)

————ADVERSE REACTIONS————
Most common adverse reactions (incidence ≥10%) are diarrhea, nausea, fatigue, headache, dizziness, depression, insomnia, abnormal dreams, and rash. (6)

Table 1 Dosage Adjustment for Patients with Altered Creatinine Clearance

	Creatinine Clearance (mL/min)*		
	≥50	30–49	<30 (Including Patients Requiring Hemodialysis)
Recommended Dosing Interval	Every 24 hours	Every 48 hours	TRUVADA should not be administered.

*Calculated using ideal (lean) body weight

To report SUSPECTED ADVERSE REACTIONS, contact Gilead Sciences, Inc. at 1-800-GILEAD-5 or FDA at 1-800-FDA-1088 or www.fda.gov/medwatch

DRUG INTERACTIONS

- Didanosine: Tenofovir disoproxil fumarate increases didanosine concentrations. Use with caution and monitor for evidence of didanosine toxicity (e.g., pancreatitis, neuropathy) when coadministered. Consider dose reductions or discontinuations of didanosine if warranted. (7.1)
- Atazanavir: Coadministration decreases atazanavir concentrations and increases tenofovir concentrations. Use atazanavir with TRUVADA only with ritonavir; monitor for evidence of tenofovir toxicity. (7.2)
- Lopinavir/ritonavir: Coadministration increases tenofovir concentrations. Monitor for evidence of tenofovir toxicity. (7.2)

USE IN SPECIFIC POPULATIONS

- Pregnancy: pregnancy registry available: Enroll patients by calling 1-800-258-4263.
- Nursing mothers: Women infected with HIV should be instructed not to breast feed. (8.3)
- Pediatrics: Safety and efficacy not established in patients less than 18 years of age. (8.4)

See 17 for PATIENT COUNSELING INFORMATION and FDA-approved patient labeling

Revised: 11/2009

FULL PRESCRIBING INFORMATION: CONTENTS*
WARNINGS: LACTIC ACIDOSIS/SEVERE HEPATOMEGALY WITH STEATOSIS AND POST TREATMENT ACUTE EXACERBATION OF HEPATITIS B
1 **INDICATIONS AND USAGE**
2 **DOSAGE AND ADMINISTRATION**
  2.1 Recommended Dose
  2.2 Dose Adjustment for Renal Impairment
3 **DOSAGE FORMS AND STRENGTHS**
4 **CONTRAINDICATIONS**
5 **WARNINGS AND PRECAUTIONS**
  5.1 Lactic Acidosis/Severe Hepatomegaly with Steatosis
  5.2 Patients Coinfected with HIV-1 and HBV
  5.3 New Onset or Worsening Renal Impairment
  5.4 Coadministration with Other Products
  5.5 Decreases in Bone Mineral Density
  5.6 Fat Redistribution
  5.7 Immune Reconstitution Syndrome
  5.8 Early Virologic Failure
6 **ADVERSE REACTIONS**
  6.1 Adverse Reactions from Clinical Trials Experience
  6.2 Postmarketing Experience
7 **DRUG INTERACTIONS**
  7.1 Didanosine
  7.2 Atazanavir
  7.3 Lopinavir/Ritonavir
  7.4 Drugs Affecting Renal Function
8 **USE IN SPECIFIC POPULATIONS**
  8.1 Pregnancy
  8.3 Nursing Mothers
  8.4 Pediatric Use
  8.5 Geriatric Use
  8.6 Patients with Impaired Renal Function
10 **OVERDOSAGE**
11 **DESCRIPTION**
12 **CLINICAL PHARMACOLOGY**
  12.1 Mechanism of Action
  12.3 Pharmacokinetics
  12.4 Microbiology
13 **NONCLINICAL TOXICOLOGY**
  13.1 Carcinogenesis, Mutagenesis, Impairment of Fertility
  13.2 Animal Toxicology and/or Pharmacology
14 **CLINICAL STUDIES**
  14.1 Study 934
16 **HOW SUPPLIED/STORAGE AND HANDLING**
17 **PATIENT COUNSELING INFORMATION AND FDA-APPROVED PATIENT LABELING**
* Sections or subsections omitted from the full prescribing information are not listed

FULL PRESCRIBING INFORMATION

WARNINGS: LACTIC ACIDOSIS/SEVERE HEPATOMEGALY WITH STEATOSIS AND POST TREATMENT ACUTE EXACERBATION OF HEPATITIS B

Lactic acidosis and severe hepatomegaly with steatosis, including fatal cases, have been reported with the use of nucleoside analogs, including VIREAD, a component of TRUVADA, in combination with other antiretrovirals [See Warnings and Precautions (5.1)]. TRUVADA is not approved for the treatment of chronic hepatitis B virus (HBV) infection and the safety and efficacy of TRUVADA have not been established in patients coinfected with HBV and HIV-1. Severe acute exacerbations of hepatitis B have been reported in patients who are coinfected with HBV and HIV-1 and have discontinued TRUVADA. Hepatic function should be monitored closely with both clinical and laboratory follow-up for at least several months in patients who are coinfected with HIV-1 and HBV and discontinue TRUVADA. If appropriate, initiation of anti-hepatitis B therapy may be warranted [See Warnings and Precautions (5.2)].

1 INDICATIONS AND USAGE

TRUVADA®, a combination of EMTRIVA® and VIREAD®, is indicated in combination with other antiretroviral agents (such as non-nucleoside reverse transcriptase inhibitors or protease inhibitors) for the treatment of HIV-1 infection in adults.

The following points should be considered when initiating therapy with TRUVADA for the treatment of HIV-1 infection:

- It is not recommended that TRUVADA be used as a component of a triple nucleoside regimen.
- TRUVADA should not be coadministered with ATRIPLA®, EMTRIVA, VIREAD or lamivudine-containing products [See Warnings and Precautions (5.4)].
- In treatment experienced patients, the use of TRUVADA should be guided by laboratory testing and treatment history [See Clinical Pharmacology (12.4)].

2 DOSAGE AND ADMINISTRATION

2.1 Recommended Dose
The dose of TRUVADA is one tablet (containing 200 mg of emtricitabine and 300 mg of tenofovir disoproxil fumarate) once daily taken orally with or without food.

2.2 Dose Adjustment for Renal Impairment
Significantly increased drug exposures occurred when EMTRIVA or VIREAD were administered to subjects with moderate to severe renal impairment [see EMTRIVA or VIREAD Package Insert]. Therefore, the dosing interval of TRUVADA should be adjusted in patients with baseline creatinine clearance 30–49 mL/min using the recommendations in Table 1. These dosing interval recommendations are based on modeling of single-dose pharmacokinetic data in non-HIV infected subjects. The safety and effectiveness of these dosing interval adjustment recommendations have not been clinically evaluated in patients with moderate renal impairment, therefore clinical response to treatment and renal function should be closely monitored in these patients [See Warnings and Precautions (5.3)].

No dose adjustment is necessary for patients with mild renal impairment (creatinine clearance 50–80 mL/min). Routine monitoring of calculated creatinine clearance and serum phosphorus should be performed in patients with mild renal impairment [See Warnings and Precautions (5.3)].

[See table 1 above]

3 DOSAGE FORMS AND STRENGTHS

TRUVADA is available as tablets. Each tablet contains 200 mg of emtricitabine and 300 mg of tenofovir disoproxil fumarate (which is equivalent to 245 mg of tenofovir disoproxil). The tablets are blue, capsule-shaped, film-coated, debossed with "GILEAD" on one side and with "701" on the other side.

4 CONTRAINDICATIONS
None.

5 WARNINGS AND PRECAUTIONS

5.1 Lactic Acidosis/Severe Hepatomegaly with Steatosis
Lactic acidosis and severe hepatomegaly with steatosis, including fatal cases, have been reported with the use of nucleoside analogs, including VIREAD, a component of TRUVADA, in combination with other antiretrovirals. A majority of these cases have been in women. Obesity and prolonged nucleoside exposure may be risk factors. Particular caution should be exercised when administering nucleoside analogs to any patient with known risk factors for liver disease; however, cases have also been reported in patients with no known risk factors. Treatment with TRUVADA should be suspended in any patient who develops clinical or laboratory findings suggestive of lactic acidosis or pronounced hepatotoxicity (which may include hepatomegaly and steatosis even in the absence of marked transaminase elevations).

5.2 Patients Coinfected with HIV-1 and HBV
It is recommended that all patients with HIV-1 be tested for the presence of chronic hepatitis B virus (HBV) before initiating antiretroviral therapy. TRUVADA is not approved for the treatment of chronic HBV infection and the safety and efficacy of TRUVADA have not been established in patients coinfected with HBV and HIV-1. Severe acute exacerbations of hepatitis B have been reported in patients who are coinfected with HBV and HIV-1 and have discontinued TRUVADA. In some patients infected with HBV and treated with EMTRIVA, the exacerbations of hepatitis B were associated with liver decompensation and liver failure. Patients who are coinfected with HIV-1 and HBV should be closely monitored with both clinical and laboratory follow up for at least several months after stopping treatment with Truvada. If appropriate, initiation of anti-hepatitis B therapy may be warranted.

5.3 New Onset or Worsening Renal Impairment
Emtricitabine and tenofovir are principally eliminated by the kidney. Renal impairment, including cases of acute renal failure and Fanconi syndrome (renal tubular injury with severe hypophosphatemia), has been reported with the use of VIREAD [See Adverse Reactions (6.2)].

It is recommended that creatinine clearance be calculated in all patients prior to initiating therapy and as clinically appropriate during therapy with TRUVADA. Routine monitoring of calculated creatinine clearance and serum phosphorus should be performed in patients at risk for renal impairment, including patients who have previously experienced renal events while receiving HEPSERA.

Dosing interval adjustment of TRUVADA and close monitoring of renal function are recommended in all patients with creatinine clearance 30–49 mL/min, [See Dosage and Administration (2.2)]. No safety or efficacy data are available in patients with renal impairment who received TRUVADA using these dosing guidelines, so the potential benefit of TRUVADA therapy should be assessed against the potential risk of renal toxicity. TRUVADA should not be administered to patients with creatinine clearance <30 mL/min or patients requiring hemodialysis.

TRUVADA should be avoided with concurrent or recent use of a nephrotoxic agent.

5.4 Coadministration with Other Products
TRUVADA is a fixed-dose combination of emtricitabine and tenofovir disoproxil fumarate. TRUVADA should not be coadministered with ATRIPLA, EMTRIVA, or VIREAD. Due to similarities between emtricitabine and lamivudine, TRUVADA should not be coadministered with other drugs containing lamivudine, including Combivir (lamivudine/zidovudine), Epivir or Epivir-HBV (lamivudine), Epzicom (abacavir sulfate/lamivudine), or Trizivir (abacavir sulfate/lamivudine/zidovudine).

TRUVADA should not be administered with HEPSERA® (adefovir dipivoxil).

5.5 Decreases in Bone Mineral Density
Bone mineral density (BMD) monitoring should be considered for HIV-1 infected patients who have a history of pathologic bone fracture or are at risk for osteopenia. Although the effect of supplementation with calcium and vitamin D was not studied, such supplementation may be beneficial for all patients. If bone abnormalities are suspected then appropriate consultation should be obtained.
Tenofovir Disoproxil Fumarate: In a 144-week study of treatment-naive subjects, decreases in BMD were seen at the lumbar spine and hip in both arms of the study. At Week 144, there was a significantly greater mean percentage decrease from baseline in BMD at the lumbar spine in subjects receiving VIREAD + lamivudine + efavirenz compared with subjects receiving stavudine + lamivudine + efavirenz. Changes in BMD at the hip were similar between the two treatment groups. In both groups, the majority of the reduction in BMD occurred in the first 24–48 weeks of the study and this reduction was sustained through 144 weeks.

Twenty-eight percent of VIREAD-treated subjects vs. 21% of the comparator subjects lost at least 5% of BMD at the spine or 7% of BMD at the hip. Clinically relevant fractures (excluding fingers and toes) were reported in 4 subjects in the VIREAD group and 6 subjects in the comparator group. Tenofovir disoproxil fumarate was associated with significant increases in biochemical markers of bone metabolism (serum bone-specific alkaline phosphatase, serum osteocalcin, serum C-telopeptide, and urinary N-telopeptide), suggesting increased bone turnover. Serum parathyroid hormone levels and 1,25 Vitamin D levels were also higher in subjects receiving VIREAD. The effects of VIREAD-associated changes in BMD and biochemical markers on long-term bone health and future fracture risk are unknown. For additional information, please consult the VIREAD prescribing information.

Cases of osteomalacia (associated with proximal renal tubulopathy and which may contribute to fractures) have been reported in association with the use of VIREAD [See Adverse Reactions (6.2)].

5.6   Fat Redistribution
Redistribution/accumulation of body fat including central obesity, dorsocervical fat enlargement (buffalo hump), peripheral wasting, facial wasting, breast enlargement, and "cushingoid appearance" have been observed in patients receiving antiretroviral therapy. The mechanism and long-term consequences of these events are currently unknown. A causal relationship has not been established.

5.7   Immune Reconstitution Syndrome
Immune reconstitution syndrome has been reported in patients treated with combination antiretroviral therapy, including TRUVADA. During the initial phase of combination antiretroviral treatment, patients whose immune system responds may develop an inflammatory response to indolent or residual opportunistic infections [such as Mycobacterium avium infection, cytomegalovirus, Pneumocystis jirovecii pneumonia (PCP), or tuberculosis], which may necessitate further evaluation and treatment.

5.8   Early Virologic Failure
Clinical studies in HIV-infected subjects have demonstrated that certain regimens that only contain three nucleoside reverse transcriptase inhibitors (NRTI) are generally less effective than triple drug regimens containing two NRTIs in combination with either a non-nucleoside reverse transcriptase inhibitor or a HIV-1 protease inhibitor. In particular, early virological failure and high rates of resistance substitutions have been reported. Triple nucleoside regimens should therefore be used with caution. Patients on a therapy utilizing a triple nucleoside-only regimen should be carefully monitored and considered for treatment modification.

6   ADVERSE REACTIONS
The following adverse reactions are discussed in other sections of the labeling:
- Lactic Acidosis/Severe Hepatomegaly with Steatosis [See Boxed Warning, Warnings and Precautions (5.1)].
- Severe Acute Exacerbations of hepatitis B [See Boxed Warning, Warnings and Precautions (5.2)].
- New Onset or Worsening Renal Impairment [See Warnings and Precautions (5.3)].
- Decreases in Bone Mineral Density [See Warnings and Precautions (5.5)].
- Immune Reconstitution Syndrome [See Warnings and Precautions (5.7)].

6.1   Adverse Reactions from Clinical Trials Experience
Because clinical trials are conducted under widely varying conditions, adverse reaction rates observed in the clinical trials of a drug cannot be directly compared to rates in the clinical trials of another drug and may not reflect the rates observed in practice.

The most common adverse reactions (incidence ≥10%, any severity) occurring in Study 934, an active-controlled clinical study of efavirenz, emtricitabine, and tenofovir disoproxil fumarate, include diarrhea, nausea, fatigue, headache, dizziness, depression, insomnia, abnormal dreams, and rash. See also Table 2 for the frequency of treatment-emergent adverse reactions (Grade 2–4) occurring in ≥5% of subjects treated with efavirenz, emtricitabine, and tenofovir disoproxil fumarate in this study.

Skin discoloration, manifested by hyperpigmentation on the palms and/or soles was generally mild and asymptomatic. The mechanism and clinical significance are unknown.

Study 934 - Treatment Emergent Adverse Reactions: In Study 934, 511 antiretroviral-naive subjects received either VIREAD + EMTRIVA administered in combination with efavirenz (N=257) or zidovudine/lamivudine administered in combination with efavirenz (N=254). Adverse reactions observed in this study were generally consistent with those seen in other studies in treatment-experienced or treatment-naive subjects receiving VIREAD and/or EMTRIVA (Table 2).

Table 2 Selected Treatment-Emergent Adverse Reactions* (Grades 2–4) Reported in ≥5% in Any Treatment Group in Study 934 (0–144 Weeks)

	FTC + TDF + EFV†	AZT/3TC + EFV
	N=257	N=254
Gastrointestinal Disorder		
Diarrhea	9%	5%
Nausea	9%	7%
Vomiting	2%	5%
General Disorders and Administration Site Condition		
Fatigue	9%	8%
Infections and Infestations		
Sinusitis	8%	4%
Upper respiratory tract infections	8%	5%
Nasopharyngitis	5%	3%
Nervous System Disorders		
Headache	6%	5%
Dizziness	8%	7%
Psychiatric Disorders		
Depression	9%	7%
Insomnia	5%	7%
Skin and Subcutaneous Tissue Disorders		
Rash event‡	7%	9%

* Frequencies of adverse reactions are based on all treatment-emergent adverse events, regardless of relationship to study drug.

† From Weeks 96 to 144 of the study, subjects received TRUVADA with efavirenz in place of VIREAD + EMTRIVA with efavirenz.

‡ Rash event includes rash, exfoliative rash, rash generalized, rash macular, rash maculo-papular, rash pruritic, and rash vesicular.

Laboratory Abnormalities: Laboratory abnormalities observed in this study were generally consistent with those seen in other studies of VIREAD and/or EMTRIVA (Table 3).

Table 3 Significant Laboratory Abnormalities Reported in ≥1% of Subjects in Any Treatment Group in Study 934 (0–144 Weeks)

	FTC + TDF + EFV*	AZT/3TC + EFV
	N=257	N=254
Any ≥ Grade 3 Laboratory Abnormality	30%	26%
Fasting Cholesterol (>240 mg/dL)	22%	24%
Creatine Kinase (M: >990 U/L) (F: >845 U/L)	9%	7%
Serum Amylase (>175 U/L)	8%	4%
Alkaline Phosphatase (>550 U/L)	1%	0%
AST (M: >180 U/L) (F: >170 U/L)	3%	3%
ALT (M: >215 U/L) (F: >170 U/L)	2%	3%
Hemoglobin (<8.0 mg/dL)	0%	4%
Hyperglycemia (>250 mg/dL)	2%	1%
Hematuria (>75 RBC/HPF)	3%	2%
Glycosuria (≥3+)	<1%	1%
Neutrophils (<750/mm³)	3%	5%
Fasting Triglycerides (>750 mg/dL)	4%	2%

* From Weeks 96 to 144 of the study, subjects received TRUVADA with efavirenz in place of VIREAD + EMTRIVA with efavirenz.

In addition to the events described above for Study 934, other adverse reactions that occurred in at least 5% of subjects receiving EMTRIVA or VIREAD with other antiretroviral agents in clinical trials include anxiety, arthralgia, increased cough, dyspepsia, fever, myalgia, pain, abdominal pain, back pain, paresthesia, peripheral neuropathy (including peripheral neuritis and neuropathy), pneumonia, and rhinitis.

In addition to the laboratory abnormalities described above for Study 934, Grade 3/4 elevations of bilirubin (>2.5 × ULN), pancreatic amylase (>2.0 × ULN), serum glucose (<40 or >250 mg/dL), and serum lipase (>2.0 × ULN) occurred in up to 3% of subjects treated with EMTRIVA or VIREAD with other antiretroviral agents in clinical trials.

6.2   Postmarketing Experience
The following adverse reactions have been identified during postapproval use of VIREAD. No additional adverse reactions have been identified during postapproval use of EMTRIVA. Because postmarketing reactions are reported voluntarily from a population of uncertain size, it is not always possible to reliably estimate their frequency or establish a causal relationship to drug exposure.
Immune System Disorders
allergic reaction, including angioedema
Metabolism and Nutrition Disorders
lactic acidosis, hypokalemia, hypophosphatemia
Respiratory, Thoracic, and Mediastinal Disorders
dyspnea
Gastrointestinal Disorders
pancreatitis, increased amylase, abdominal pain
Hepatobiliary Disorders
hepatic steatosis, hepatitis, increased liver enzymes (most commonly AST, ALT gamma GT)
Skin and Subcutaneous Tissue Disorders
rash
Musculoskeletal and Connective Tissue Disorders
rhabdomyolysis, osteomalacia (manifested as bone pain and which may contribute to fractures), muscular weakness, myopathy
Renal and Urinary Disorders
acute renal failure, renal failure, acute tubular necrosis, Fanconi syndrome, proximal renal tubulopathy, interstitial nephritis (including acute cases), nephrogenic diabetes insipidus, renal insufficiency, increased creatinine, proteinuria, polyuria
General Disorders and Administration Site Conditions
asthenia

The following adverse reactions, listed under the body system headings above, may occur as a consequence of proximal renal tubulopathy: rhabdomyolysis, osteomalacia, hypokalemia, muscular weakness, myopathy, hypophosphatemia.

7   DRUG INTERACTIONS
No drug interaction studies have been conducted using TRUVADA tablets. Drug interaction studies have been conducted with emtricitabine and tenofovir disoproxil fumarate, the components of TRUVADA. This section describes clinically relevant drug interactions observed with emtricitabine and tenofovir disoproxil fumarate [See Clinical Pharmacology (12.3)].

7.1   Didanosine
Coadministration of TRUVADA and didanosine should be undertaken with caution and patients receiving this combination should be monitored closely for didanosine-associated adverse reactions. Didanosine should be discontinued in patients who develop didanosine-associated adverse reactions.

When tenofovir disoproxil fumarate was administered with didanosine the C_{max} and AUC of didanosine administered as either the buffered or enteric-coated formulation increased significantly [See Clinical Pharmacology (12.3)]. The mechanism of this interaction is unknown. Higher didanosine concentrations could potentiate didanosine-associated adverse reactions, including pancreatitis, and neuropathy. Suppression of CD4+ cell counts has been observed in patients receiving tenofovir DF with didanosine 400 mg daily. In adults weighing >60 kg, the didanosine dose should be reduced to 250 mg when it is coadministered with TRUVADA. Data are not available to recommend a dose adjustment of didanosine for patients weighing <60 kg. When coadministered, TRUVADA and Videx EC may be taken under fasted conditions or with a light meal (<400 kcal, 20% fat). Coadministration of didanosine buffered tablet formulation with TRUVADA should be under fasted conditions.

Table 4 Single Dose Pharmacokinetic Parameters for Emtricitabine and Tenofovir in Adults*

	Emtricitabine	Tenofovir
Fasted Oral Bioavailability[†] (%)	92 (83.1–106.4)	25 (NC–45.0)
Plasma Terminal Elimination Half-Life[†] (hr)	10 (7.4–18.0)	17 (12.0–25.7)
C_{max}[‡] (µg/mL)	1.8 ± 0.72[§]	0.30 ± 0.09
AUC[‡] (µg•hr/mL)	10.0 ± 3.12[§]	2.29 ± 0.69
CL/F[‡] (mL/min)	302 ± 94	1043 ± 115
CL_{renal}[‡] (mL/min)	213 ± 89	243 ± 33

* NC = Not calculated
† Median (range)
‡ Mean (± SD)
§ Data presented as steady state values.

Table 5 Drug Interactions: Changes in Pharmacokinetic Parameters for Emtricitabine in the Presence of the Coadministered Drug*

Coadministered Drug	Dose of Coadministered Drug (mg)	Emtricitabine Dose (mg)	N	% Change of Emtricitabine Pharmacokinetic Parameters[†] (90% CI)		
				C_{max}	AUC	C_{min}
Tenofovir DF	300 once daily × 7 days	200 once daily × 7 days	17	⇔	⇔	↑ 20 (↑ 12 to ↑ 29)
Zidovudine	300 twice daily × 7 days	200 once daily × 7 days	27	⇔	⇔	⇔
Indinavir	800 × 1	200 × 1	12	⇔	⇔	NA
Famciclovir	500 × 1	200 × 1	12	⇔	⇔	NA
Stavudine	40 × 1	200 × 1	6	⇔	⇔	NA

* All interaction studies conducted in healthy volunteers.
† ↑ = Increase; ↓ = Decrease; ⇔ = No Effect; NA = Not Applicable

7.2 Atazanavir

Atazanavir has been shown to increase tenofovir concentrations *[See Clinical Pharmacology (12.3)]*. The mechanism of this interaction is unknown. Patients receiving atazanavir and TRUVADA should be monitored for TRUVADA-associated adverse reactions. TRUVADA should be discontinued in patients who develop TRUVADA-associated adverse reactions.

Tenofovir decreases the AUC and C_{min} of atazanavir *[See Clinical Pharmacology (12.3)]*. When coadministered with TRUVADA, it is recommended that atazanavir 300 mg is given with ritonavir 100 mg. Atazanavir without ritonavir should not be coadministered with TRUVADA.

7.3 Lopinavir/Ritonavir

Lopinavir/ritonavir has been shown to increase tenofovir concentrations *[See Clinical Pharmacology (12.3)]*. The mechanism of this interaction is unknown. Patients receiving lopinavir/ritonavir and TRUVADA should be monitored for TRUVADA-associated adverse reactions. TRUVADA should be discontinued in patients who develop TRUVADA-associated adverse reactions.

7.4 Drugs Affecting Renal Function

Emtricitabine and tenofovir are primarily excreted by the kidneys by a combination of glomerular filtration and active tubular secretion *[See Clinical Pharmacology (12.3)]*. No drug-drug interactions due to competition for renal excretion have been observed; however, coadministration of TRUVADA with drugs that are eliminated by active tubular secretion may increase concentrations of emtricitabine, tenofovir, and/or the coadministered drug. Some examples include, but are not limited to, acyclovir, adefovir dipivoxil, cidofovir, ganciclovir, valacyclovir, and valganciclovir. Drugs that decrease renal function may increase concentrations of emtricitabine and/or tenofovir.

8 USE IN SPECIFIC POPULATIONS

8.1 Pregnancy

Pregnancy Category B
Emtricitabine: The incidence of fetal variations and malformations was not increased in embryofetal toxicity studies performed with emtricitabine in mice at exposures (AUC) approximately 60-fold higher and in rabbits at approximately 120-fold higher than human exposures at the recommended daily dose.

Tenofovir Disoproxil Fumarate: Reproduction studies have been performed in rats and rabbits at doses up to 14 and 19 times the human dose based on body surface area comparisons and revealed no evidence of impaired fertility or harm to the fetus due to tenofovir.

There are, however, no adequate and well-controlled studies in pregnant women. Because animal reproduction studies are not always predictive of human response, TRUVADA should be used during pregnancy only if clearly needed.

Antiretroviral Pregnancy Registry: To monitor fetal outcomes of pregnant women exposed to TRUVADA, an Antiretroviral Pregnancy Registry has been established. Healthcare providers are encouraged to register patients by calling 1-800-258-4263.

8.3 Nursing Mothers

Nursing Mothers: The Centers for Disease Control and Prevention recommend that HIV-1 infected mothers not breast-feed their infants to avoid risking postnatal transmission of HIV-1. Studies in rats have demonstrated that tenofovir is secreted in milk. It is not known whether tenofovir is excreted in human milk. It is not known whether emtricitabine is excreted in human milk. Because of both the potential for HIV-1 transmission and the potential for serious adverse reactions in nursing infants, **mothers should be instructed not to breast-feed if they are receiving TRUVADA.**

8.4 Pediatric Use

Truvada is not recommended for patients less than 18 years of age because it is a fixed-dose combination tablet containing a component, VIREAD, for which safety and efficacy have not been established in this age group.

8.5 Geriatric Use

Clinical studies of EMTRIVA or VIREAD did not include sufficient numbers of subjects aged 65 and over to determine whether they respond differently from younger subjects. In general, dose selection for the elderly patients should be cautious, keeping in mind the greater frequency of decreased hepatic, renal, or cardiac function, and of concomitant disease or other drug therapy.

8.6 Patients with Impaired Renal Function

It is recommended that the dosing interval for TRUVADA be modified in patients with creatinine clearance 30–49 mL/min. TRUVADA should not be used in patients with creatinine clearance <30 mL/min and in patients with end-stage renal disease requiring dialysis *[See Dosage and Administration (2.2)]*.

10 OVERDOSAGE

If overdose occurs the patient must be monitored for evidence of toxicity, and standard supportive treatment applied as necessary.

Emtricitabine: Limited clinical experience is available at doses higher than the therapeutic dose of EMTRIVA. In one clinical pharmacology study single doses of emtricitabine 1200 mg were administered to 11 subjects. No severe adverse reactions were reported.

Hemodialysis treatment removes approximately 30% of the emtricitabine dose over a 3-hour dialysis period starting within 1.5 hours of emtricitabine dosing (blood flow rate of 400 mL/min and a dialysate flow rate of 600 mL/min). It is not known whether emtricitabine can be removed by peritoneal dialysis.

Tenofovir Disoproxil Fumarate: Limited clinical experience at doses higher than the therapeutic dose of VIREAD 300 mg is available. In one study, 600 mg tenofovir disoproxil fumarate was administered to 8 subjects orally for 28 days, and no severe adverse reactions were reported. The effects of higher doses are not known.

Tenofovir is efficiently removed by hemodialysis with an extraction coefficient of approximately 54%. Following a single 300 mg dose of VIREAD, a four-hour hemodialysis session removed approximately 10% of the administered tenofovir dose.

11 DESCRIPTION

TRUVADA tablets are fixed dose combination tablets containing emtricitabine and tenofovir disoproxil fumarate. EMTRIVA is the brand name for emtricitabine, a synthetic nucleoside analog of cytidine. Tenofovir disoproxil fumarate (tenofovir DF) is converted in vivo to tenofovir, an acyclic nucleoside phosphonate (nucleotide) analog of adenosine 5'-monophosphate. Both emtricitabine and tenofovir exhibit inhibitory activity against HIV-1 reverse transcriptase.

Emtricitabine: The chemical name of emtricitabine is 5-fluoro-1-(2R,5S)-[2-(hydroxymethyl)-1,3-oxathiolan-5-yl]cytosine. Emtricitabine is the (-) enantiomer of a thio analog of cytidine, which differs from other cytidine analogs in that it has a fluorine in the 5-position.
It has a molecular formula of $C_8H_{10}FN_3O_3S$ and a molecular weight of 247.24. It has the following structural formula:

Emtricitabine is a white to off-white crystalline powder with a solubility of approximately 112 mg/mL in water at 25 °C. The partition coefficient (log p) for emtricitabine is -0.43 and the pKa is 2.65.

Tenofovir Disoproxil Fumarate: Tenofovir disoproxil fumarate is a fumaric acid salt of the bis-isopropoxycarbonyloxymethyl ester derivative of tenofovir. The chemical name of tenofovir disoproxil fumarate is 9-[(R)-2 [[bis[[(isopropoxycarbonyl)oxy]-methoxy] phosphinyl]methoxy]propyl]adenine fumarate (1:1). It has a molecular formula of $C_{19}H_{30}N_5O_{10}P • C_4H_4O_4$ and a molecular weight of 635.52. It has the following structural formula:

Tenofovir disoproxil fumarate is a white to off-white crystalline powder with a solubility of 13.4 mg/mL in water at 25 °C. The partition coefficient (log p) for tenofovir disoproxil is 1.25 and the pKa is 3.75. All dosages are expressed in terms of tenofovir disoproxil fumarate except where otherwise noted.

TRUVADA tablets are for oral administration. Each film-coated tablet contains 200 mg of emtricitabine and 300 mg of tenofovir disoproxil fumarate, (which is equivalent to 245 mg of tenofovir disoproxil), as active ingredients. The tablets also include the following inactive ingredients: croscarmellose sodium, lactose monohydrate, magnesium stearate, microcrystalline cellulose, and pregelatinized starch (gluten free). The tablets are coated with Opadry II Blue Y-30-10701, which contains FD&C Blue #2 aluminum lake, hydroxypropyl methylcellulose 2910, lactose monohydrate, titanium dioxide, and triacetin.

12 CLINICAL PHARMACOLOGY

For additional information on Mechanism of Action, Antiviral Activity, Resistance and Cross Resistance, please consult the EMTRIVA and VIREAD prescribing information.

12.1 Mechanism of Action

TRUVADA is a fixed-dose combination of antiviral drugs emtricitabine and tenofovir disoproxil fumarate. *[See Clinical Pharmacology (12.4)]*.

IMPORTANT NOTICE: Updated drug information is sent bi-monthly via the PDR® Update Insert. For *monthly* email updates, register at PDR.net.

12.3 Pharmacokinetics

TRUVADA: One TRUVADA tablet was bioequivalent to one EMTRIVA capsule (200 mg) plus one VIREAD tablet (300 mg) following single-dose administration to fasting healthy subjects (N=39).

Emtricitabine: The pharmacokinetic properties of emtricitabine are summarized in Table 4. Following oral administration of EMTRIVA, emtricitabine is rapidly absorbed with peak plasma concentrations occurring at 1–2 hours post-dose. In vitro binding of emtricitabine to human plasma proteins is <4% and is independent of concentration over the range of 0.02–200 μg/mL. Following administration of radiolabelled emtricitabine, approximately 86% is recovered in the urine and 13% is recovered as metabolites. The metabolites of emtricitabine include 3′-sulfoxide diastereomers and their glucuronic acid conjugate. Emtricitabine is eliminated by a combination of glomerular filtration and active tubular secretion. Following a single oral dose of EMTRIVA, the plasma emtricitabine half-life is approximately 10 hours.

Tenofovir Disoproxil Fumarate: The pharmacokinetic properties of tenofovir disoproxil fumarate are summarized in Table 4. Following oral administration of VIREAD, maximum tenofovir serum concentrations are achieved in 1.0 ± 0.4 hour. In vitro binding of tenofovir to human plasma proteins is <0.7% and is independent of concentration over the range of 0.01–25 μg/mL. Approximately 70–80% of the intravenous dose of tenofovir is recovered as unchanged drug in the urine. Tenofovir is eliminated by a combination of glomerular filtration and active tubular secretion. Following a single oral dose of VIREAD, the terminal elimination half-life of tenofovir is approximately 17 hours.

[See table 4 at top of previous page]

Effects of Food on Oral Absorption

TRUVADA may be administered with or without food. Administration of TRUVADA following a high fat meal (784 kcal; 49 grams of fat) or a light meal (373 kcal; 8 grams of fat) delayed the time of tenofovir C_{max} by approximately 0.75 hour. The mean increases in tenofovir AUC and C_{max} were approximately 35% and 15%, respectively, when administered with a high fat or light meal, compared to administration in the fasted state. In previous safety and efficacy studies, VIREAD (tenofovir) was taken under fed conditions. Emtricitabine systemic exposures (AUC and C_{max}) were unaffected when TRUVADA was administered with either a high fat or a light meal.

Special Populations

Race

Emtricitabine: No pharmacokinetic differences due to race have been identified following the administration of EMTRIVA.

Tenofovir Disoproxil Fumarate: There were insufficient numbers from racial and ethnic groups other than Caucasian to adequately determine potential pharmacokinetic differences among these populations following the administration of VIREAD.

Gender

Emtricitabine and Tenofovir Disoproxil Fumarate: Emtricitabine and tenofovir pharmacokinetics are similar in male and female subjects.

Pediatric and Geriatric Patients

Pharmacokinetic studies of tenofovir have not been performed in pediatric subjects (<18 years). Pharmacokinetics of emtricitabine and tenofovir have not been fully evaluated in the elderly (>65 years).

Patients with Impaired Renal Function

The pharmacokinetics of emtricitabine and tenofovir are altered in subjects with renal impairment *[See Warnings and Precautions (5.3)]*. In subjects with creatinine clearance <50 mL/min, C_{max} and $AUC_{0-\infty}$ of emtricitabine and tenofovir were increased. It is recommended that the dosing interval for TRUVADA be modified in patients with creatinine clearance 30–49 mL/min. TRUVADA should not be used in patients with creatinine clearance <30 mL/min and in patients with end-stage renal disease requiring dialysis *[See Dosage and Administration (2.2)]*.

Patients with Hepatic Impairment

The pharmacokinetics of tenofovir following a 300 mg dose of VIREAD have been studied in non-HIV infected subjects with moderate to severe hepatic impairment. There were no substantial alterations in tenofovir pharmacokinetics in subjects with hepatic impairment compared with unimpaired subjects. The pharmacokinetics of TRUVADA or emtricitabine have not been studied in subjects with hepatic impairment; however, emtricitabine is not significantly metabolized by liver enzymes, so the impact of liver impairment should be limited.

Assessment of Drug Interactions

The steady state pharmacokinetics of emtricitabine and tenofovir were unaffected when emtricitabine and tenofovir disoproxil fumarate were administered together versus each agent dosed alone.

Table 6 Drug Interactions: Changes in Pharmacokinetic Parameters for Coadministered Drug in the Presence of Emtricitabine*

Coadministered Drug	Dose of Coadministered Drug (mg)	Emtricitabine Dose (mg)	N	% Change of Coadministered Drug Pharmacokinetic Parameters[†] (90% CI)		
				C_{max}	AUC	C_{min}
Tenofovir DF	300 once daily × 7 days	200 once daily × 7 days	17	⇔	⇔	⇔
Zidovudine	300 twice daily × 7 days	200 once daily × 7 days	27	↑ 17 (↑ 0 to ↑ 38)	↑ 13 (↑ 5 to ↑ 20)	⇔
Indinavir	800 × 1	200 × 1	12	⇔	⇔	NA
Famciclovir	500 × 1	200 × 1	12	⇔	⇔	NA
Stavudine	40 × 1	200 × 1	6	⇔	⇔	NA

* All interaction studies conducted in healthy volunteers.
† ↑ = Increase; ↓ = Decrease; ⇔ = No Effect; NA = Not Applicable

Table 7 Drug Interactions: Changes in Pharmacokinetic Parameters for Tenofovir* in the Presence of the Coadministered Drug

Coadministered Drug	Dose of Coadministered Drug (mg)	N	% Change of Tenofovir Pharmacokinetic Parameters[†] (90% CI)		
			C_{max}	AUC	C_{min}
Abacavir	300 once	8	⇔	⇔	NC
Atazanavir‡	400 once daily × 14 days	33	↑ 14 (↑ 8 to ↑ 20)	↑ 24 (↑ 21 to ↑ 28)	↑ 22 (↑ 15 to ↑ 30)
Didanosine (enteric-coated)	400 once	25	⇔	⇔	⇔
Didanosine (buffered)	250 or 400 once daily × 7 days	14	⇔	⇔	⇔
Efavirenz	600 once daily × 14 days	29	⇔	⇔	⇔
Emtricitabine	200 once daily × 7 days	17	⇔	⇔	⇔
Entecavir	1 mg once daily × 10 days	28	⇔	⇔	⇔
Indinavir	800 three times daily × 7 days	13	↑ 14 (↓ 3 to ↑ 33)	⇔	⇔
Lamivudine	150 twice daily × 7 days	15	⇔	⇔	⇔
Lopinavir/Ritonavir	400/100 twice daily × 14 days	24	⇔	↑ 32 (↑ 25 to ↑ 38)	↑ 51 (↑ 37 to ↑ 66)
Nelfinavir	1250 twice daily × 14 days	29	⇔	⇔	⇔
Saquinavir/Ritonavir	1000/100 twice daily × 14 days	35	⇔	⇔	↑ 23 (↑ 16 to ↑ 30)
Tacrolimus	0.05 mg/kg twice daily × 7 days	21	↑ 13) (↑ 1 to ↑ 27)	⇔	⇔

* Patients received VIREAD 300 mg once daily.
† Increase = ↑; Decrease = ↓; No Effect = ⇔; NC = Not Calculated
‡ Reyataz Prescribing Information

In vitro and clinical pharmacokinetic drug-drug interaction studies have shown that the potential for CYP mediated interactions involving emtricitabine and tenofovir with other medicinal products is low.

No clinically significant drug interactions have been observed between emtricitabine and famciclovir, indinavir, stavudine, tenofovir disoproxil fumarate, and zidovudine (see Tables 5 and 6). Similarly, no clinically significant drug interactions have been observed between tenofovir disoproxil fumarate and abacavir, efavirenz, emtricitabine, entecavir, indinavir, lamivudine, lopinavir/ritonavir, methadone, nelfinavir, oral contraceptives, ribavirin, saquinavir/ritonavir, and tacrolimus in studies conducted in healthy volunteers (see Tables 7 and 8).

[See table 5 on previous page]
[See table 6 above]
[See table 7 above]
[See table 8 at top of next page]

Following multiple dosing to HIV-negative subjects receiving either chronic methadone maintenance therapy or oral contraceptives, or single doses of ribavirin, steady state tenofovir pharmacokinetics were similar to those observed in previous studies, indicating lack of clinically significant drug interactions between these agents and VIREAD. Coadministration of tenofovir disoproxil fumarate with didanosine results in changes in the pharmacokinetics of didanosine that may be of clinical significance. Table 9 summarizes the effects of tenofovir disoproxil fumarate on the pharmacokinetics of didanosine. Concomitant dosing of tenofovir disoproxil fumarate with didanosine buffered tablets or enteric-coated capsules significantly increases the C_{max} and AUC of didanosine. When didanosine 250 mg enteric-coated capsules were administered with tenofovir disoproxil fumarate, systemic exposures of didanosine were similar to those seen with the 400 mg enteric-coated capsules alone under fasted conditions. The mechanism of this interaction is unknown. See *Drug Interactions (7.1)* regarding use of didanosine with VIREAD.

[See table 9 at top of page 1177]

12.4 Microbiology

Mechanism of Action

Emtricitabine: Emtricitabine, a synthetic nucleoside analog of cytidine, is phosphorylated by cellular enzymes to

Table 8 Drug Interactions: Changes in Pharmacokinetic Parameters for Coadministered Drug in the Presence of Tenofovir

Coadministered Drug	Dose of Coadministered Drug (mg)	N	% Change of Coadministered Drug Pharmacokinetic Parameters* (90% CI)		
			C_{max}	AUC	C_{min}
Abacavir	300 once	8	↑ 12 (↓ 1 to ↑ 26)	⇔	NA
Atazanavir[†]	400 once daily × 14 days	34	↓ 21 (↓ 27 to ↓ 14)	↓ 25 (↓ 30 to ↓ 19)	↓ 40 (↓ 48 to ↓ 32)
Atazanavir[†]	Atazanavir/Ritonavir 300/100 once daily × 42 days	10	↓ 28 (↓ 50 to ↑ 5)	↓25[‡] (↓ 42 to ↓ 3)	↓ 23[‡] (↓ 46 to ↑ 10)
Efavirenz	600 once daily × 14 days	30	⇔	⇔	⇔
Emtricitabine	200 once daily × 7 days	17	⇔	⇔	↑ 20 (↑ 12 to ↑ 29)
Indinavir	800 three times daily × 7 days	12	↓ 11 (↓ 30 to ↑ 12)	⇔	⇔
Entecavir	1 mg once daily × 10 days	28	⇔	↑ 13 (↑ 11 to ↑ 15)	
Lamivudine	150 twice daily × 7 days	15	↓ 24 (↓ 34 to ↓ 12)	⇔	⇔
Lopinavir Ritonavir	Lopinavir/Ritonavir 400/100 twice daily × 14 days	24	⇔ ⇔	⇔ ⇔	⇔ ⇔
Methadone[§]	40–110 once daily × 14 days[¶]	13	⇔	⇔	⇔
Nelfinavir M8 metabolite	1250 twice daily × 14 days	29	⇔ ⇔	⇔ ⇔	⇔ ⇔
Oral Contraceptives[#]	Ethinyl Estradiol/ Norgestimate (Ortho-Tricyclen) Once daily × 7 days	20	⇔	⇔	⇔
Ribavirin	600 once	22	⇔	⇔	NA
Saquinavir Ritonavir	Saquinavir/Ritonavir 1000/100 twice daily × 14 days	32	↑ 22 (↑ 6 to ↑ 41)	↑ 29[b] (↑ 12 to ↑ 48) ⇔	↑ 47[b] (↑ 23 to ↑ 76) ↑ 23 (↑ 3 to ↑ 46)
Tacrolimus	0.05 mg/kg twice daily × 7 days	21	⇔	⇔	⇔

* Increase = ↑; Decrease = ↓; No Effect = ⇔; NA = Not Applicable
† Reyataz Prescribing Information
‡ In HIV-infected subjects, addition of tenofovir DF to atazanavir 300 mg plus ritonavir 100 mg, resulted in AUC and C_{min} values of atazanavir that were 2.3 and 4-fold higher than the respective values observed for atazanavir 400 mg when given alone.
§ R-(active), S- and total methadone exposures were equivalent when dosed alone or with VIREAD.
¶ Individual subjects were maintained on their stable methadone dose. No pharmacodynamic alterations (opiate toxicity or withdrawal signs or symptoms) were reported.
# Ethinyl estradiol and 17-deacetyl norgestimate (pharmacologically active metabolite) exposures were equivalent when dosed alone or with VIREAD.
Þ Increases in AUC and C_{min} are not expected to be clinically relevant; hence no dose adjustments are required when tenofovir DF and ritonavir-boosted saquinavir are coadministered.

form emtricitabine 5′-triphosphate. Emtricitabine 5′-triphosphate inhibits the activity of the HIV-1 reverse transcriptase (RT) by competing with the natural substrate deoxycytidine 5′-triphosphate and by being incorporated into nascent viral DNA which results in chain termination. Emtricitabine 5′-triphosphate is a weak inhibitor of mammalian DNA polymerase α, β, ε and mitochondrial DNA polymerase γ.
Tenofovir Disoproxil Fumarate: Tenofovir disoproxil fumarate is an acyclic nucleoside phosphonate diester analog of adenosine monophosphate. Tenofovir disoproxil fumarate requires initial diester hydrolysis for conversion to tenofovir and subsequent phosphorylations by cellular enzymes to form tenofovir diphosphate. Tenofovir diphosphate inhibits the activity of HIV-1 RT by competing with the natural substrate deoxyadenosine 5′-triphosphate and, after incorporation into DNA, by DNA chain termination. Tenofovir diphosphate is a weak inhibitor of mamma-

lian DNA polymerases α, β, and mitochondrial DNA polymerase γ.
Antiviral Activity
Emtricitabine and Tenofovir Disoproxil Fumarate: In combination studies evaluating the cell culture antiviral activity of emtricitabine and tenofovir together, synergistic antiviral effects were observed.
Emtricitabine: The antiviral activity of emtricitabine against laboratory and clinical isolates of HIV-1 was assessed in lymphoblastoid cell lines, the MAGI-CCR5 cell line, and peripheral blood mononuclear cells. The 50% effective concentration (EC_{50}) values for emtricitabine were in the range of 0.0013–0.64 µM (0.0003–0.158 µg/mL). In drug combination studies of emtricitabine with nucleoside reverse transcriptase inhibitors (abacavir, lamivudine, stavudine, zalcitabine, zidovudine), non-nucleoside reverse transcriptase inhibitors (delavirdine, efavirenz, nevirapine), and protease inhibitors (amprenavir, nelfinavir, ritonavir, saquinavir), additive to synergistic effects were observed.

Emtricitabine displayed antiviral activity in cell culture against HIV-1 clades A, B, C, D, E, F, and G (EC_{50} values ranged from 0.007–0.075 µM) and showed strain specific activity against HIV-2 (EC_{50} values ranged from 0.007–1.5 µM).
Tenofovir Disoproxil Fumarate: The antiviral activity of tenofovir against laboratory and clinical isolates of HIV-1 was assessed in lymphoblastoid cell lines, primary monocyte/macrophage cells and peripheral blood lymphocytes. The EC_{50} values for tenofovir were in the range of 0.04–8.5 µM. In drug combination studies of tenofovir with nucleoside reverse transcriptase inhibitors (abacavir, didanosine, lamivudine, stavudine, zalcitabine, zidovudine), non-nucleoside reverse transcriptase inhibitors (delavirdine, efavirenz, nevirapine), and protease inhibitors (amprenavir, indinavir, nelfinavir, ritonavir, saquinavir), additive to synergistic effects were observed. Tenofovir displayed antiviral activity in cell culture against HIV-1 clades A, B, C, D, E, F, G and O (EC_{50} values ranged from 0.5–2.2 µM) and showed strain specific activity against HIV-2 (EC_{50} values ranged from 1.6 µM to 5.5 µM).
Resistance
Emtricitabine and Tenofovir Disoproxil Fumarate: HIV-1 isolates with reduced susceptibility to the combination of emtricitabine and tenofovir have been selected in cell culture. Genotypic analysis of these isolates identified the M184V/I and/or K65R amino acid substitutions in the viral RT.
In a clinical study of treatment-naive subjects [*Study 934, see Clinical Studies (14.1)*], resistance analysis was performed on HIV-1 isolates from all confirmed virologic failure subjects with >400 copies/mL of HIV-1 RNA at Week 144 or early discontinuation. Development of efavirenz resistance-associated substitutions occurred most frequently and was similar between the treatment arms. The M184V amino acid substitution, associated with resistance to EMTRIVA and lamivudine, was observed in 2/19 analyzed subjects isolates in the EMTRIVA + VIREAD group and in 10/29 analyzed subjects isolates in the zidovudine/lamivudine group. Through 144 weeks of Study 934, no subjects have developed a detectable K65R substitution in their HIV-1 as analyzed through standard genotypic analysis.
Emtricitabine: Emtricitabine-resistant isolates of HIV-1 have been selected in cell culture and in vivo. Genotypic analysis of these isolates showed that the reduced susceptibility to emtricitabine was associated with a substitution in the HIV-1 RT gene at codon 184 which resulted in an amino acid substitution of methionine by valine or isoleucine (M184V/I).
Tenofovir Disoproxil Fumarate: HIV-1 isolates with reduced susceptibility to tenofovir have been selected in cell culture. These viruses expressed a K65R substitution in RT and showed a 2–4 fold reduction in susceptibility to tenofovir.
In treatment-naive subjects, isolates from 8/47 (17%) analyzed subjects developed the K65R substitution in the VIREAD arm through 144 weeks; 7 occurred in the first 48 weeks of treatment and 1 at Week 96. In treatment-experienced subjects, 14/304 (5%) isolates from subjects failing VIREAD through Week 96 showed >1.4 fold (median 2.7) reduced susceptibility to tenofovir. Genotypic analysis of the resistant isolates showed a substitution in the HIV-1 RT gene resulting in the K65R amino acid substitution.
Cross Resistance
Emtricitabine and Tenofovir Disoproxil Fumarate: Cross-resistance among certain nucleoside reverse transcriptase inhibitors (NRTIs) has been recognized. The M184V/I and/or K65R substitutions selected in cell culture by the combination of emtricitabine and tenofovir are also observed in some HIV-1 isolates from subjects failing treatment with tenofovir in combination with either lamivudine or emtricitabine, and either abacavir or didanosine. Therefore, cross-resistance among these drugs may occur in patients whose virus harbors either or both of these amino acid substitutions.
Emtricitabine: Emtricitabine-resistant isolates (M184V/I) were cross-resistant to lamivudine and zalcitabine but retained susceptibility in cell culture to didanosine, stavudine, tenofovir, zidovudine, and NNRTIs (delavirdine, efavirenz, and nevirapine). HIV-1 isolates containing the K65R substitution, selected in vivo by abacavir, didanosine, tenofovir, and zalcitabine, demonstrated reduced susceptibility to inhibition by emtricitabine. Viruses harboring substitutions conferring reduced susceptibility to stavudine and zidovudine (M41L, D67N, K70R, L210W, T215Y/F, K219Q/E), or didanosine (L74V) remained sensitive to emtricitabine. HIV-1 containing the K103N substitution associated with resistance to NNRTIs was susceptible to emtricitabine.
Tenofovir Disoproxil Fumarate: HIV-1 isolates from patients (N=20) whose HIV-1 expressed a mean of 3 zidovudine-associated RT amino acid substitutions (M41L, D67N, K70R, L210W, T215Y/F, or K219Q/E/N) showed a 3.1-fold decrease in the susceptibility to tenofovir. Subjects

whose virus expressed an L74V substitution without zidovudine resistance associated substitutions (N=8) had reduced response to VIREAD. Limited data are available for patients whose virus expressed a Y115F substitution (N=3), Q151M substitution (N=2), or T69 insertion (N=4), all of whom had a reduced response.

13 NONCLINICAL TOXICOLOGY

13.1 Carcinogenesis, Mutagenesis, Impairment of Fertility

Emtricitabine: In long-term oral carcinogenicity studies of emtricitabine, no drug-related increases in tumor incidence were found in mice at doses up to 750 mg/kg/day (26 times the human systemic exposure at the therapeutic dose of 200 mg/day) or in rats at doses up to 600 mg/kg/day (31 times the human systemic exposure at the therapeutic dose).

Emtricitabine was not genotoxic in the reverse mutation bacterial test (Ames test), mouse lymphoma or mouse micronucleus assays.

Emtricitabine did not affect fertility in male rats at approximately 140-fold or in male and female mice at approximately 60-fold higher exposures (AUC) than in humans given the recommended 200 mg daily dose. Fertility was normal in the offspring of mice exposed daily from before birth (in utero) through sexual maturity at daily exposures (AUC) of approximately 60-fold higher than human exposures at the recommended 200 mg daily dose.

Tenofovir Disoproxil Fumarate: Long-term oral carcinogenicity studies of tenofovir disoproxil fumarate in mice and rats were carried out at exposures up to approximately 16 times (mice) and 5 times (rats) those observed in humans at the therapeutic dose for HIV-1 infection. At the high dose in female mice, liver adenomas were increased at exposures 16 times that in humans. In rats, the study was negative for carcinogenic findings at exposures up to 5 times that observed in humans at the therapeutic dose.

Tenofovir disoproxil fumarate was mutagenic in the in vitro mouse lymphoma assay and negative in an in vitro bacterial mutagenicity test (Ames test). In an in vivo mouse micronucleus assay, tenofovir disoproxil fumarate was negative when administered to male mice.

There were no effects on fertility, mating performance or early embryonic development when tenofovir disoproxil fumarate was administered to male rats at a dose equivalent to 10 times the human dose based on body surface area comparisons for 28 days prior to mating and to female rats for 15 days prior to mating through day seven of gestation. There was, however, an alteration of the estrous cycle in female rats.

13.2 Animal Toxicology and/or Pharmacology

Tenofovir and tenofovir disoproxil fumarate administered in toxicology studies to rats, dogs and monkeys at exposures (based on AUCs) greater than or equal to 6-fold those observed in humans caused bone toxicity. In monkeys the bone toxicity was diagnosed as osteomalacia. Osteomalacia observed in monkeys appeared to be reversible upon dose reduction or discontinuation of tenofovir. In rats and dogs, the bone toxicity manifested as reduced bone mineral density. The mechanism(s) underlying bone toxicity is unknown.

Evidence of renal toxicity was noted in 4 animal species. Increases in serum creatinine, BUN, glycosuria, proteinuria, phosphaturia, and/or calciuria and decreases in serum phosphate were observed to varying degrees in these animals. These toxicities were noted at exposures (based on AUCs) 2–20 times higher than those observed in humans. The relationship of the renal abnormalities, particularly the phosphaturia, to the bone toxicity is not known.

14 CLINICAL STUDIES

Clinical Study 934 supports the use of TRUVADA tablets for the treatment of HIV-1 infection. Additional data in support of the use of TRUVADA are derived from Study 903, in which lamivudine and tenofovir disoproxil fumarate (tenofovir DF) were used in combination in treatment-naive adults, and clinical Study 303 in which emtricitabine and lamivudine demonstrated comparable efficacy, safety and resistance patterns as part of multidrug regimens. For additional information about these studies, please consult the prescribing information for tenofovir DF and emtricitabine.

14.1 Study 934

Data through 144 weeks are reported for Study 934, a randomized, open-label, active-controlled multicenter study comparing emtricitabine + tenofovir DF administered in combination with efavirenz versus zidovudine/lamivudine fixed-dose combination administered in combination with efavirenz in 511 antiretroviral-naive subjects. From Weeks 96 to 144 of the study, subjects received TRUVADA with efavirenz in place of emtricitabine + tenofovir DF with efavirenz. Subjects had a mean age of 38 years (range 18–80), 86% were male, 59% were Caucasian and 23% were Black. The mean baseline CD4+ cell count was 245 cells/mm³ (range 2–1191) and median baseline plasma HIV-1 RNA was 5.01 log₁₀ copies/mL (range 3.56–6.54). Subjects were stratified by baseline CD4+ cell count (< or ≥200 cells/

mm³); 41% had CD4+ cell counts <200 cells/mm³ and 51% of subjects had baseline viral loads >100,000 copies/mL. Treatment outcomes through 48 and 144 weeks for those subjects who did not have efavirenz resistance at baseline are presented in Table 10.

[See table 10 above]

Through Week 48, 84% and 73% of subjects in the emtricitabine + tenofovir DF group and the zidovudine/lamivudine group, respectively, achieved and maintained HIV-1 RNA <400 copies/mL (71% and 58% through Week 144). The difference in the proportion of subjects who achieved and maintained HIV-1 RNA <400 copies/mL through 48 weeks largely results from the higher number of discontinuations due to adverse events and other reasons in the zidovudine/lamivudine group in this open-label study. In addition, 80% and 70% of subjects in the emtricitabine + tenofovir DF group and the zidovudine/lamivudine group, respectively, achieved and maintained HIV-1 RNA <50 copies/mL through Week 48 (64% and 56% through Week 144). The mean increase from baseline in CD4+ cell count was 190 cells/mm³ in the emtricitabine + tenofovir DF group and 158 cells/mm³ in the zidovudine/lamivudine group at Week 48 (312 and 271 cells/mm³ at Week 144). Through 48 weeks, 7 subjects in the emtricitabine + tenofovir DF group and 5 subjects in the zidovudine/lamivudine group experienced a new CDC Class C event (10 and 6 subjects through 144 weeks).

Table 9 Drug Interactions: Pharmacokinetic Parameters for Didanosine in the Presence of VIREAD

Didanosine* Dose (mg)/ Method of Administration*	VIREAD Method of Administration*	N	% Difference (90% CI) vs. Didanosine 400 mg Alone, Fasted†	
			Cmax	AUC
Buffered tablets				
400 once daily‡ × 7 days	Fasted 1 hour after didanosine	14	↑ 28 (↑ 11 to ↑ 48)	↑ 44 (↑ 31 to ↑ 59)
Enteric coated capsules				
400 once, fasted	With food, 2 hours after didanosine	26	↑ 48 (↑ 25 to ↑ 76)	↑ 48 (↑ 31 to ↑ 67)
400 once, with food	Simultaneously with didanosine	26	↑ 64 (↑ 41 to ↑ 89)	↑ 60 (↑ 44 to ↑ 79)
250 once, fasted	With food, 2 hours after didanosine	28	↓ 10 (↓ 22 to ↑ 3)	⇔
250 once, fasted	Simultaneously with didanosine	28	⇔	↑ 14 (0 to ↑ 31)
250 once, with food	Simultaneously with didanosine	28	↓ 29 (↓ 39 to ↓ 18)	↓ 11 (↓ 23 to ↑ 2)

* Administration with food was with a light meal (~373 kcal, 20% fat).
† Increase = ↑; Decrease = ↓; No Effect = ⇔
‡ Includes 4 subjects weighing <60 kg receiving ddI 250 mg.

Table 10 Outcomes of Randomized Treatment at Week 48 and 144 (Study 934)

Outcomes	At Week 48		At Week 144	
	FTC + TDF + EFV (N=244)	AZT/3TC + EFV (N=243)	FTC + TDF + EFV (N=227)*	AZT/3TC + EFV (N=229)*
Responder†	84%	73%	71%	58%
Virologic failure‡	2%	4%	3%	6%
Rebound	1%	3%	2%	5%
Never suppressed	0%	0%	0%	0%
Change in antiretroviral regimen	1%	1%	1%	1%
Death	<1%	1%	1%	1%
Discontinued due to adverse event	4%	9%	5%	12%
Discontinued for other reasons§	10%	14%	20%	22%

* Subjects who were responders at Week 48 or Week 96 (HIV-1 RNA <400 copies/mL) but did not consent to continue study after Week 48 or Week 96 were excluded from analysis.
† Subjects achieved and maintained confirmed HIV-1 RNA <400 copies/mL through Weeks 48 and 144.
‡ Includes confirmed viral rebound and failure to achieve confirmed <400 copies/mL through Weeks 48 and 144.
§ Includes lost to follow-up, subject withdrawal, noncompliance, protocol violation and other reasons.

16 HOW SUPPLIED/STORAGE AND HANDLING

The blue, capsule-shaped, film-coated, tablets contain 200 mg of emtricitabine and 300 mg of tenofovir disoproxil fumarate (which is equivalent to 245 mg of tenofovir disoproxil), are debossed with "GILEAD" on one side and with "701" on the other side, and are available in unit of use bottles (containing a dessicant [silica gel canister or sachet] and closed with a child-resistant closure) of:
• 30 tablets (NDC 61958-0701-1)
Store at 25 °C (77 °F), excursions permitted to 15–30 °C (59–86 °F) (see USP Controlled Room Temperature).
• Keep container tightly closed
• Dispense only in original container
• Do not use if seal over bottle opening is broken or missing.

17 PATIENT COUNSELING INFORMATION AND FDA-APPROVED PATIENT LABELING

Information for Patients

Patients should be advised that:
• TRUVADA is not a cure for HIV-1 infection and patients may continue to experience illnesses associated with HIV-1 infection, including opportunistic infections. Patients should remain under the care of a physician when using TRUVADA.
• The use of TRUVADA has not been shown to reduce the risk of transmission of HIV-1 to others through sexual contact or blood contamination. Patients should be ad-

vised to continue to practice safer sex and to use latex or polyurethane condoms to lower the chance of sexual contact with any body fluids such as semen, vaginal secretions or blood. Patients should be advised never to re-use or share needles.

- The long term effects of TRUVADA are unknown.
- TRUVADA tablets are for oral ingestion only.
- It is important to take TRUVADA with combination therapy on a regular dosing schedule to avoid missing doses.
- Lactic acidosis and severe hepatomegaly with steatosis, including fatal cases, have been reported. Treatment with TRUVADA should be suspended in any patients who develop clinical symptoms suggestive of lactic acidosis or pronounced hepatotoxicity (including nausea, vomiting, unusual or unexpected stomach discomfort, and weakness) [See Warnings and Precautions (5.1)].
- All patients with HIV-1 should be tested for hepatitis B virus (HBV) before initiating antiretroviral therapy.
- Severe acute exacerbations of hepatitis B have been reported in patients who are coinfected with HBV and HIV-1 and have discontinued TRUVADA.
- Renal impairment, including cases of acute renal failure and Fanconi syndrome, has been reported in association with the use of VIREAD. TRUVADA should be avoided with concurrent or recent use of a nephrotoxic agent [See Warnings and Precautions (5.3)]. Dosing interval of TRUVADA may need adjustment in patients with renal impairment [See Dosage and Administration (2.1)].
- TRUVADA should not be coadministered with ATRIPLA, EMTRIVA, or VIREAD; or with drugs containing lamivudine, including Combivir (lamivudine/zidovudine), Epivir or Epivir-HBV (lamivudine), Epzicom (abacavir sulfate/lamivudine), or Trizivir (abacavir sulfate/lamivudine/zidovudine) [See Warnings and Precautions (5.4)].
- TRUVADA should not be administered with HEPSERA [See Warnings and Precautions (5.4)].
- Decreases in bone mineral density have been observed with the use of VIREAD. Bone monitoring should be considered in patients who have a history of pathologic bone fracture or at risk for osteopenia [See Warnings and Precautions (5.5)].

FDA-Approved Patient Labeling
TRUVADA® (tru-VAH-dah) tablets
Generic name: emtricitabine and tenofovir disoproxil fumarate (em tri SIT uh bean and te NOE' fo veer dye soe PROX il FYOU mar ate)
Read the Patient Information that comes with TRUVADA before you start taking it and each time you get a refill. There may be new information. This information does not take the place of talking to your healthcare provider about your medical condition or treatment. You should stay under a healthcare provider's care when taking TRUVADA. **Do not change or stop your medicine without first talking with your healthcare provider.** Talk to your healthcare provider or pharmacist if you have any questions about TRUVADA.
What is the most important information I should know about TRUVADA?
- **Some people who have taken medicine like TRUVADA (nucleoside analogs) have developed a serious condition called lactic acidosis** (build up of an acid in the blood). Lactic acidosis can be a medical emergency and may need to be treated in the hospital. **Call your healthcare provider right away if you get the following signs or symptoms of lactic acidosis:**
  - You feel very weak or tired.
  - You have unusual (not normal) muscle pain.
  - You have trouble breathing.
  - You have stomach pain with nausea and vomiting.
  - You feel cold, especially in your arms and legs.
  - You feel dizzy or lightheaded.
  - You have a fast or irregular heartbeat.
- **Some people who have taken medicines like TRUVADA have developed serious liver problems called hepatotoxicity,** with liver enlargement (hepatomegaly) and fat in the liver (steatosis). **Call your healthcare provider right away if you get the following signs or symptoms of liver problems:**
  - Your skin or the white part of your eyes turns yellow (jaundice).
  - Your urine turns dark.
  - Your bowel movements (stools) turn light in color.
  - You don't feel like eating food for several days or longer.
  - You feel sick to your stomach (nausea).
  - You have lower stomach area (abdominal) pain.
- **You may be more likely to get lactic acidosis or liver problems** if you are female, very overweight (obese), or have been taking nucleoside analog medicines, like TRUVADA, for a long time.
- **If you are also infected with the hepatitis B virus (HBV),** you need close medical follow-up for several months after stopping treatment with TRUVADA. Follow-up includes medical exams and blood tests to check for HBV that could be getting worse. **Patients with hepatitis B virus infection, who take TRUVADA and then stop it, may get

"flare-ups" of their hepatitis. A "flare-up" is when the disease suddenly returns in a worse way than before.**
What is TRUVADA?
TRUVADA is a type of medicine called an HIV-1 (human immunodeficiency virus) nucleoside analog reverse transcriptase inhibitor (NRTI). TRUVADA contains 2 medicines, EMTRIVA® (emtricitabine) and VIREAD® (tenofovir disoproxil fumarate, or tenofovir DF) combined in one pill. TRUVADA is always used with other anti-HIV-1 medicines to treat people with HIV-1 infection. TRUVADA is for adults age 18 and older. TRUVADA has not been studied in children under age 18 or adults over age 65.
HIV infection destroys CD4+ T cells, which are important to the immune system. The immune system helps fight infection. After a large number of T cells are destroyed, acquired immune deficiency syndrome (AIDS) develops.
TRUVADA helps block HIV-1 reverse transcriptase, a chemical in your body (enzyme) that is needed for HIV-1 to multiply. TRUVADA lowers the amount of HIV-1 in the blood (viral load). TRUVADA may also help to increase the number of T cells (CD4+ cells). Lowering the amount of HIV-1 in the blood lowers the chance of death or infections that happen when your immune system is weak (opportunistic infections).
TRUVADA does not cure HIV-1 infection or AIDS. The long-term effects of TRUVADA are not known at this time. People taking TRUVADA may still get opportunistic infections or other conditions that happen with HIV-1 infection. Opportunistic infections are infections that develop because the immune system is weak. Some of these conditions are pneumonia, herpes virus infections, and *Mycobacterium avium complex* (MAC) infection. **It is very important that you see your healthcare provider regularly while taking TRUVADA.**
TRUVADA does not lower your chance of passing HIV-1 to other people through sexual contact, sharing needles, or being exposed to your blood. For your health and the health of others, it is important to always practice safer sex by using a latex or polyurethane condom or other barrier to lower the chance of sexual contact with semen, vaginal secretions, or blood. Never use or share dirty needles.
Who should not take TRUVADA?
- Do not take TRUVADA if you are allergic to TRUVADA or any of its ingredients. The active ingredients of TRUVADA are emtricitabine and tenofovir DF. See the end of this leaflet for a complete list of ingredients.
- Do not take TRUVADA if you are already taking ATRIPLA®, Combivir (lamivudine/zidovudine), EMTRIVA, Epivir or Epivir-HBV (lamivudine), Epzicom (abacavir sulfate/lamivudine), Trizivir (abacavir sulfate/lamivudine/zidovudine), or VIREAD because these medicines contain the same or similar active ingredients.
- Do not take TRUVADA to treat your HIV infection if you are also taking HEPSERA® to treat your HBV infection.
What should I tell my healthcare provider before taking TRUVADA?
Tell your healthcare provider if you:
- **are pregnant or planning to become pregnant.** We do not know if TRUVADA can harm your unborn child. You and your healthcare provider will need to decide if TRUVADA is right for you. If you use TRUVADA while you are pregnant, talk to your healthcare provider about how you can be on the TRUVADA Antiviral Pregnancy Registry.
- **are breast-feeding.** You should not breast feed if you are HIV-positive because of the chance of passing the HIV virus to your baby. Also, it is not known if TRUVADA can pass into your breast milk and if it can harm your baby. If you are a woman who has or will have a baby, talk with your healthcare provider about the best way to feed your baby.
- **have kidney problems or are undergoing kidney dialysis treatment.**
- **have bone problems.**
- **have liver problems including hepatitis B virus infection.**
Tell your healthcare provider about all the medicines you take, including prescription and non-prescription medicines, vitamins, and herbal supplements. Especially tell your healthcare provider if you take:
- Videx, Videx EC (didanosine). Tenofovir DF (a component of TRUVADA) may increase the amount of Videx in your blood. **You may need to be followed more carefully if you are taking TRUVADA and Videx together.** Also, the dose of didanosine may need to be reduced.
- Reyataz (atazanavir sulfate) or Kaletra (lopinavir/ritonavir). These medicines may increase the amount of tenofovir DF (a component of TRUVADA) in your blood, which could result in more side effects. You may need to be followed more carefully if you are taking TRUVADA and Reyataz or Kaletra together. TRUVADA may decrease the amount of Reyataz in your blood. If you are taking TRUVADA and Reyataz together, you should also be taking Norvir (ritonavir).
Keep a complete list of all the medicines that you take. Make a new list when medicines are added or stopped. Give

copies of this list to all of your healthcare providers and pharmacist **every** time you visit your healthcare provider or fill a prescription.
How should I take TRUVADA?
- Take TRUVADA exactly as your healthcare provider prescribed it. Follow the directions from your healthcare provider, exactly as written on the label.
- The usual dose of TRUVADA is 1 tablet once a day. TRUVADA is always used with other anti-HIV-1 medicines. If you have kidney problems, you may need to take TRUVADA less often.
- TRUVADA may be taken with or without a meal. Food does not affect how TRUVADA works. Take TRUVADA at the same time each day.
- If you forget to take TRUVADA, take it as soon as you remember that day. **Do not** take more than 1 dose of TRUVADA in a day. **Do not** take 2 doses at the same time. Call your healthcare provider or pharmacist if you are not sure what to do. **It is important that you do not miss any doses of TRUVADA or your anti-HIV-1 medicines.**
- When your TRUVADA supply starts to run low, get more from your healthcare provider or pharmacy. This is very important because the amount of virus in your blood may increase if the medicine is stopped for even a short time. The virus may develop resistance to TRUVADA and become harder to treat.
- Do not change your dose or stop taking TRUVADA without first talking with your healthcare provider. Stay under a healthcare provider's care when taking TRUVADA.
- If you take too much TRUVADA, call your local poison control center or emergency room right away.
What should I avoid while taking TRUVADA?
- **Do not breast-feed.** See "What should I tell my healthcare provider before taking TRUVADA?"
- **Avoid doing things that can spread HIV infection** since TRUVADA does not stop you from passing the HIV infection to others.
  - **Do not share needles or other injection equipment.**
  - **Do not share personal items that can have blood or body fluids on them, like toothbrushes or razor blades.**
  - **Do not have any kind of sex without protection.** Always practice safer sex by using a latex or polyurethane condom or other barrier to reduce the chance of sexual contact with semen, vaginal secretions, or blood.
- ATRIPLA, Combivir (lamivudine/zidovudine), EMTRIVA, Epivir or Epivir-HBV (lamivudine), Epzicom (abacavir sulfate/lamivudine), Trizivir (abacavir sulfate/lamivudine/zidovudine), or VIREAD. **TRUVADA should not be used with these medicines.**
- TRUVADA should not be used with HEPSERA.
What are the possible side effects of TRUVADA?
TRUVADA may cause the following serious side effects (see "What is the most important information I should know about TRUVADA?"):
- **Lactic acidosis** (buildup of an acid in the blood). Lactic acidosis can be a medical emergency and may need to be treated in the hospital. **Call your doctor right away if you get signs of lactic acidosis.** (See "What is the most important information I should know about TRUVADA?")
- **Serious liver problems (hepatotoxicity),** with liver enlargement (hepatomegaly) and fat in the liver (steatosis). Call your healthcare provider right away if you get any signs of liver problems. (See "What is the most important information I should know about TRUVADA?")
- **"Flare-ups" of hepatitis B virus infection,** in which the disease suddenly returns in a worse way than before, can occur if you stop taking TRUVADA. Your healthcare provider will monitor your condition for several months after stopping TRUVADA if you have both HIV-1 and HBV infection. TRUVADA is not approved for the treatment of hepatitis B virus infection. If you have advanced liver disease and stop treatment with TRUVADA, the "flare-up" of hepatitis B may cause your liver function to decline.
- **Kidney problems.** If you have had kidney problems in the past or take other medicines that can cause kidney problems, your healthcare provider should do regular blood tests to check your kidneys.
- **Changes in bone mineral density (thinning bones).** Laboratory tests show changes in the bones of patients treated with VIREAD, a component of TRUVADA. Some HIV patients treated with VIREAD developed thinning of the bones (osteopenia) which could lead to fractures. If you have had bone problems in the past, your healthcare provider may need to do tests to check your bone mineral density or may prescribe medicines to help your bone mineral density. Additionally, bone pain and softening of the bone (which may contribute to fractures) may occur as a consequence of kidney problems.
Other side effects with TRUVADA when used with other anti-HIV-1 medicines include:
- Changes in body fat have been seen in some patients taking TRUVADA and other anti-HIV-1 medicines. These changes may include increased amount of fat in the upper back and neck ("buffalo hump"), breast, and around the main part of your body (trunk). Loss of fat from the legs, arms and face may also happen. The cause and long term health effect of these conditions are not known at this time.

- In some patients with advanced HIV infection (AIDS), signs and symptoms of inflammation from previous infections may occur soon after anti-HIV treatment is started. It is believed that these symptoms are due to an improvement in the body's immune response, enabling the body to fight infections that may have been present with no obvious symptoms. If you notice any symptoms of infection, please inform your doctor immediately.

The most common side effects of EMTRIVA or VIREAD when used with other anti-HIV-1 medicines are: diarrhea, dizziness, nausea, headache, fatigue, abnormal dreams, sleeping problems, rash, depression, and vomiting. Additional side effects are lactic acidosis, kidney problems (including decline or failure of kidney function), inflammation of the pancreas, inflammation of the liver, allergic reaction (including swelling of the face, lips, tongue, or throat), shortness of breath, pain, fatty liver, stomach pain, weakness, indigestion, intestinal gas, and high volume of urine and thirst caused by kidney problems. Muscle pain and muscle weakness, bone pain, and softening of the bone (which may contribute to fractures) as a consequence of kidney problems have been reported. Skin discoloration (small spots or freckles) may also happen with TRUVADA.

These are not all the side effects of TRUVADA. If you have questions about side effects, ask your healthcare provider. Report any new or continuing symptoms to your healthcare provider right away. Your healthcare provider may be able to help you manage these side effects.

How do I store TRUVADA?

- **Keep TRUVADA and all other medicines out of reach of children.**
- Store TRUVADA at room temperature 77 °F (25 °C).
- Keep TRUVADA in its original container and keep the container tightly closed.
- Do not keep medicine that is out of date or that you no longer need. If you throw any medicines away make sure that children will not find them.

General information about TRUVADA:

Medicines are sometimes prescribed for conditions that are not mentioned in patient information leaflets. Do not use TRUVADA for a condition for which it was not prescribed. Do not give TRUVADA to other people, even if they have the same symptoms you have. It may harm them.

This leaflet summarizes the most important information about TRUVADA. If you would like more information, talk with your healthcare provider. You can ask your healthcare provider or pharmacist for information about TRUVADA that is written for health professionals. For more information, you may also call 1-800-GILEAD-5 or access the TRUVADA website at www.TRUVADA.com.

Do not use TRUVADA if seal over bottle opening is broken or missing.

What are the ingredients of TRUVADA?

Active Ingredients: emtricitabine and tenofovir disoproxil fumarate

Inactive Ingredients: Croscarmellose sodium, lactose monohydrate, magnesium stearate, microcrystalline cellulose, and pregelatinized starch (gluten free). The tablets are coated with Opadry II Blue Y-30-10701 containing FD&C Blue #2 aluminum lake, hydroxypropyl methylcellulose 2910, lactose monohydrate, titanium dioxide, and triacetin.

℞ Only
November 2009
TRUVADA, EMTRIVA, HEPSERA and VIREAD are registered trademarks of Gilead Sciences, Inc. ATRIPLA is a trademark of Bristol-Myers Squibb & Gilead Sciences, LLC. All other trademarks referenced herein are the property of their respective owners.

21-752-GS-023

Shown in Product Identification Guide, page 309

VIREAD® ℞
[VEER-ee-ad]
(tenofovir disoproxil fumarate)
Tablets

HIGHLIGHTS OF PRESCRIBING INFORMATION
These highlights do not include all the information needed to use VIREAD safely and effectively. See full prescribing information for VIREAD.
VIREAD® (tenofovir disoproxil fumarate) tablets
Initial U.S. Approval: 2001

WARNINGS: LACTIC ACIDOSIS/SEVERE HEPATO-MEGALY WITH STEATOSIS and POST TREATMENT EXACERBATION OF HEPATITIS
See full prescribing information for complete boxed warning.
- **Lactic acidosis and severe hepatomegaly with steatosis, including fatal cases, have been reported with the use of nucleoside analogs, including VIREAD. (5.1)**

- **Severe acute exacerbations of hepatitis have been reported in HBV-infected patients who have discontinued anti-hepatitis B therapy, including VIREAD. Hepatic function should be monitored closely in these patients. If appropriate, resumption of anti-hepatitis B therapy may be warranted. (5.2)**

---RECENT MAJOR CHANGES---

Indications and Usage	
Chronic Hepatitis B (1.2)	10/2009
Dosage and Administration (2.1, 2.2, 2.3)	03/2010
Warnings and Precautions	
New Onset or Worsening Renal Impairment (5.3)	10/2009
Decreases in Bone Mineral Density (5.6)	03/2010

---INDICATIONS AND USAGE---
VIREAD is a nucleotide analog HIV-1 reverse transcriptase and HBV polymerase inhibitor.
Viread is indicated in combination with other antiretroviral agents for the treatment of HIV-1 infection in adults and adolescents. (1)
Viread is indicated for the treatment of chronic hepatitis B in adults. (1)

---DOSAGE AND ADMINISTRATION---
- Recommended dose for the treatment of HIV or chronic hepatitis B in adults: 300 mg once daily taken orally without regard to food. (2.1)
- Recommended dose for the treatment of HIV in adolescents (≥12 years of age and ≥35 kg): 300 mg once daily taken orally without regard to food. (2.2)
- Dose recommended in renal impairment in adults:
  Creatinine clearance 30–49 mL/min: 300 mg every 48 hours. (2.3)
  Creatinine clearance 10–29 mL/min: 300 mg every 72 to 96 hours. (2.3)
  Hemodialysis: 300 mg every 7 days or after approximately 12 hours of dialysis. (2.3)

---DOSAGE FORMS AND STRENGTHS---
Tablets: 300 mg. (3)

---CONTRAINDICATIONS---
None. (4)

---WARNINGS AND PRECAUTIONS---
- New onset or worsening renal impairment: Can include acute renal failure and Fanconi syndrome. Assess creatinine clearance (CrCl) before initiating treatment with VIREAD. Monitor CrCl and serum phosphorus in patients at risk. Avoid administering VIREAD with concurrent or recent use of nephrotoxic drugs. (5.3)
- Coadministration with Other Products: Do not use with other tenofovir-containing products (e.g., ATRIPLA and TRUVADA). Do not administer in combination with HEPSERA. (5.4)
- HIV testing: HIV antibody testing should be offered to all HBV-infected patients before initiating therapy with VIREAD. VIREAD should only be used as part of an appropriate antiretroviral combination regimen in HIV-infected patients with or without HBV coinfection. (5.5)
- Decreases in bone mineral density (BMD): Observed in HIV-infected patients. Consider assessment of BMD in patients with a history of pathologic fracture or other risk factors for osteoporosis or bone loss. (5.6)
- Redistribution/accumulation of body fat: Observed in HIV-infected patients receiving antiretroviral combination therapy. (5.7)
- Immune reconstitution syndrome: Observed in HIV-infected patients. May necessitate further evaluation and treatment. (5.8)
- Triple nucleoside-only regimens: Early virologic failure has been reported in HIV-infected patients. Monitor carefully and consider treatment modification. (5.9)

---ADVERSE REACTIONS---
In HIV-infected patients: Most common adverse reactions (incidence ≥10%, Grades 2–4) are rash, diarrhea, headache, pain, depression, asthenia, and nausea. (6)
In HBV-infected patients: Most common adverse reaction (all grades) was nausea (9%). (6)

To report SUSPECTED ADVERSE REACTIONS, contact Gilead Sciences, Inc. at 1-800-GILEAD-5 or FDA at 1-800-FDA-1088 or www.fda.gov/medwatch

---DRUG INTERACTIONS---
- Didanosine: Coadministration increases didanosine concentrations. Use with caution and monitor for evidence of didanosine toxicity (e.g., pancreatitis, neuropathy). Consider dose reductions or discontinuations of didanosine if warranted. (7.1)
- Atazanavir: Coadministration decreases atazanavir concentrations and increases tenofovir concentrations. Use atazanavir with VIREAD only with additional ritonavir; monitor for evidence of tenofovir toxicity. (7.2)

- Lopinavir/ritonavir: Coadministration increases tenofovir concentrations. Monitor for evidence of tenofovir toxicity. (7.3)

---USE IN SPECIFIC POPULATIONS---
- Pregnancy: Pregnancy registry available. Enroll patients by calling 1-800-258-4263.
- Nursing mothers: Women infected with HIV should be instructed not to breast feed. (8.3)
- Safety and efficacy not established in patients less than 12 years of age. (8.4)

See 17 for PATIENT COUNSELING INFORMATION and FDA-approved patient labeling

Revised: 03/2010

FULL PRESCRIBING INFORMATION: CONTENTS *
WARNINGS: LACTIC ACIDOSIS/SEVERE HEPATOMEGALY WITH STEATOSIS AND POST TREATMENT EXACERBATION OF HEPATITIS
1 INDICATIONS AND USAGE
  1.1 HIV-1 Infection
  1.2 Chronic Hepatitis B
2 DOSAGE AND ADMINISTRATION
  2.1 Recommended Dose in Adults
  2.2 Recommended Dose in Adolescents (≥12 Years of Age and ≥35 kg)
  2.3 Dose Adjustment for Renal Impairment
3 DOSAGE FORMS AND STRENGTHS
4 CONTRAINDICATIONS
5 WARNINGS AND PRECAUTIONS
  5.1 Lactic Acidosis/Severe Hepatomegaly with Steatosis
  5.2 Exacerbation of Hepatitis after Discontinuation of Treatment
  5.3 New Onset or Worsening Renal Impairment
  5.4 Coadministration with Other Products
  5.5 Patients Coinfected with HIV-1 and HBV
  5.6 Decreases in Bone Mineral Density
  5.7 Fat Redistribution
  5.8 Immune Reconstitution Syndrome
  5.9 Early Virologic Failure
6 ADVERSE REACTIONS
  6.1 Adverse Reactions from Clinical Trials Experience
  6.2 Postmarketing Experience
7 DRUG INTERACTIONS
  7.1 Didanosine
  7.2 Atazanavir
  7.3 Lopinavir/Ritonavir
  7.4 Drugs Affecting Renal Function
8 USE IN SPECIFIC POPULATIONS
  8.1 Pregnancy
  8.3 Nursing Mothers
  8.4 Pediatric Use
  8.5 Geriatric Use
  8.6 Patients with Impaired Renal Function
10 OVERDOSAGE
11 DESCRIPTION
12 CLINICAL PHARMACOLOGY
  12.1 Mechanism of Action
  12.3 Pharmacokinetics
  12.4 Microbiology
13 NONCLINICAL TOXICOLOGY
  13.1 Carcinogenesis, Mutagenesis, Impairment of Fertility
  13.2 Animal Toxicology and/or Pharmacology
14 CLINICAL STUDIES
  14.1 Clinical Efficacy in Patients with HIV-1 Infection
  14.2 Clinical Efficacy in Patients with Chronic Hepatitis B
16 HOW SUPPLIED/STORAGE AND HANDLING
17 PATIENT COUNSELING INFORMATION AND FDA-APPROVED PATIENT LABELING
* Sections or subsections omitted from the full prescribing information are not listed

FULL PRESCRIBING INFORMATION

WARNINGS: LACTIC ACIDOSIS/SEVERE HEPATO-MEGALY WITH STEATOSIS AND POST TREATMENT EXACERBATION OF HEPATITIS
Lactic acidosis and severe hepatomegaly with steatosis, including fatal cases, have been reported with the use of nucleoside analogs, including VIREAD, in combination with other antiretrovirals *[See Warnings and Precautions (5.1)]*.
Severe acute exacerbations of hepatitis have been reported in HBV-infected patients who have discontinued anti-hepatitis B therapy, including VIREAD. Hepatic function should be monitored closely with both clinical and laboratory follow-up for at least several months in patients who discontinue anti-hepatitis B therapy, in-

cluding VIREAD. If appropriate, resumption of anti-hepatitis B therapy may be warranted [See Warnings and Precautions (5.2)].

1 INDICATIONS AND USAGE

1.1 HIV-1 Infection

VIREAD® is indicated in combination with other antiretro-viral agents for the treatment of HIV-1 infection in adults and adolescents.

The following points should be considered when initiating therapy with VIREAD for the treatment of HIV-1 infection:
- VIREAD should not be used in combination with TRUVADA® or ATRIPLA® [See Warnings and Precautions (5.4)].

1.2 Chronic Hepatitis B

VIREAD is indicated for the treatment of chronic hepatitis B in adults.

The following points should be considered when initiating therapy with VIREAD for the treatment of HBV infection:
- This indication is based primarily on data from treatment of nucleoside-treatment-naïve subjects and a smaller number of subjects who had previously received lamivu-dine or adefovir. Subjects were adults with HBeAg-positive and HBeAg-negative chronic hepatitis B with compensated liver disease [See Clinical Efficacy in Patients with Chronic Hepatitis B (14.2)].
- The numbers of subjects in clinical trials who had lamivudine- or adefovir-associated substitutions at base-line were too small to reach conclusions of efficacy [See Microbiology (12.4), Clinical Efficacy in Patients with Chronic Hepatitis B (14.2)].
- VIREAD has not been evaluated in patients with decompensated liver disease.

2 DOSAGE AND ADMINISTRATION

2.1 Recommended Dose in Adults

For the treatment of HIV-1 or chronic hepatitis B: The dose is one 300 mg VIREAD tablet once daily taken orally, without regard to food.

In the treatment of chronic hepatitis B, the optimal duration of treatment is unknown.

2.2 Recommended Dose in Adolescents (≥12 Years of Age and ≥35 kg)

For the treatment of HIV-1 in adolescents with body weight ≥35 kg (≥77 lb): The dose is one 300 mg VIREAD tablet once daily taken orally, without regard to food.

2.3 Dose Adjustment for Renal Impairment

Significantly increased drug exposures occurred when VIREAD was administered to subjects with moderate to severe renal impairment [See Clinical Pharmacology (12.3)]. Therefore, the dosing interval of VIREAD should be adjusted in patients with baseline creatinine clearance <50 mL/min using the recommendations in Table 1. These dosing interval recommendations are based on modeling of single-dose pharmacokinetic data in non-HIV and non-HBV infected subjects with varying degrees of renal impairment, including end-stage renal disease requiring hemodialysis. The safety and effectiveness of these dosing interval adjustment recommendations have not been clinically evaluated in patients with moderate or severe renal impairment, therefore clinical response to treatment and renal function should be closely monitored in these patients [See Warnings and Precautions (5.3)].

No dose adjustment is necessary for patients with mild renal impairment (creatinine clearance 50–80 mL/min). Routine monitoring of calculated creatinine clearance and serum phosphorus should be performed in patients with mild renal impairment [See Warnings and Precautions (5.3)].

[See table 1 below]

The pharmacokinetics of tenofovir have not been evaluated in non-hemodialysis patients with creatinine clearance <10 mL/min; therefore, no dosing recommendation is available for these patients.

No data are available to make dose recommendations in adolescent patients with renal impairment.

3 DOSAGE FORMS AND STRENGTHS

VIREAD is available as tablets. Each tablet contains 300 mg of tenofovir disoproxil fumarate, which is equivalent to 245 mg of tenofovir disoproxil. The tablets are almond-shaped, light blue, film-coated, and debossed with "GILEAD" and "4331" on one side and with "300" on the other side.

4 CONTRAINDICATIONS

None.

5 WARNINGS AND PRECAUTIONS

5.1 Lactic Acidosis/Severe Hepatomegaly with Steatosis

Lactic acidosis and severe hepatomegaly with steatosis, including fatal cases, have been reported with the use of nucleoside analogs, including VIREAD, in combination with other antiretrovirals. A majority of these cases have been in women. Obesity and prolonged nucleoside exposure may be risk factors. Particular caution should be exercised when administering nucleoside analogs to any patient with known risk factors for liver disease; however, cases have also been reported in patients with no known risk factors. Treatment with VIREAD should be suspended in any patient who develops clinical or laboratory findings suggestive of lactic acidosis or pronounced hepatotoxicity (which may include hepatomegaly and steatosis even in the absence of marked transaminase elevations).

5.2 Exacerbation of Hepatitis after Discontinuation of Treatment

Discontinuation of anti-HBV therapy, including VIREAD, may be associated with severe acute exacerbations of hepatitis. Patients infected with HBV who discontinue VIREAD should be closely monitored with both clinical and laboratory follow-up for at least several months after stopping treatment. If appropriate, resumption of anti-hepatitis B therapy may be warranted.

5.3 New Onset or Worsening Renal Impairment

Tenofovir is principally eliminated by the kidney. Renal impairment, including cases of acute renal failure and Fanconi syndrome (renal tubular injury with severe hypophosphatemia), has been reported with the use of VIREAD [See Adverse Reactions (6.2)].

It is recommended that creatinine clearance be calculated in all patients prior to initiating therapy and as clinically appropriate during therapy with VIREAD. Routine monitoring of calculated creatinine clearance and serum phosphorus should be performed in patients at risk for renal impairment, including patients who have previously experienced renal events while receiving HEPSERA.

Dosing interval adjustment of VIREAD and close monitoring of renal function are recommended in all patients with creatinine clearance <50 mL/min [See Dosage and Administration (2.3)]. No safety or efficacy data are available in patients with renal impairment who received VIREAD using these dosing guidelines, so the potential benefit of VIREAD therapy should be assessed against the potential risk of renal toxicity.

VIREAD should be avoided with concurrent or recent use of a nephrotoxic agent.

5.4 Coadministration with Other Products

VIREAD should not be used in combination with the fixed-dose combination products TRUVADA or ATRIPLA since tenofovir disoproxil fumarate is a component of these products.

VIREAD should not be administered in combination with HEPSERA® (adefovir dipivoxil) [See Drug Interactions (7.4)].

5.5 Patients Coinfected with HIV-1 and HBV

Due to the risk of development of HIV-1 resistance, VIREAD should only be used in HIV-1 and HBV coinfected patients as part of an appropriate antiretroviral combination regimen.

HIV-1 antibody testing should be offered to all HBV-infected patients before initiating therapy with VIREAD. It is also recommended that all patients with HIV-1 be tested for the presence of chronic hepatitis B before initiating treatment with VIREAD.

5.6 Decreases in Bone Mineral Density

Assessment of bone mineral density (BMD) should be considered for adults and adolescents who have a history of pathologic bone fracture or other risk factors for osteoporosis or bone loss. Although the effect of supplementation with calcium and vitamin D was not studied, such supplementa-tion may be beneficial for all patients. If bone abnormalities are suspected then appropriate consultation should be obtained.

In HIV-1 infected adult subjects treated with VIREAD in Study 903 through 144 weeks, decreases from baseline in BMD were seen at the lumbar spine and hip in both arms of the study. At Week 144, there was a significantly greater mean percentage decrease from baseline in BMD at the lumbar spine in subjects receiving VIREAD + lamivudine + efavirenz (-2.2% ± 3.9) compared with subjects receiving stavudine + lamivudine + efavirenz (-1.0% ± 4.6). Changes in BMD at the hip were similar between the two treatment groups (-2.8% ± 3.5 in the VIREAD group vs. -2.4% ± 4.5 in the stavudine group). In both groups, the majority of the reduction in BMD occurred in the first 24–48 weeks of the study and this reduction was sustained through Week 144. Twenty-eight percent of VIREAD-treated subjects vs. 21% of the stavudine-treated subjects lost at least 5% of BMD at the spine or 7% of BMD at the hip. Clinically relevant fractures (excluding fingers and toes) were reported in 4 subjects in the VIREAD group and 6 subjects in the stavudine group. In addition, there were significant increases in biochemical markers of bone metabolism (serum bone-specific alkaline phosphatase, serum osteocalcin, serum C-telopeptide, and urinary N-telopeptide) in the VIREAD group relative to the stavudine group, suggesting increased bone turnover. Serum parathyroid hormone levels and 1,25 Vitamin D levels were also higher in the VIREAD group. Except for bone specific alkaline phosphatase, these changes resulted in values that remained within the normal range.

In a clinical study of HIV-1 infected adolescent subjects (Study 321), bone effects were similar to adult subjects. Under normal circumstances BMD increases rapidly in adolescents. In this study, the mean rate of bone gain was less in the VIREAD-treated group compared to the placebo group. Six VIREAD treated adolescents and one placebo treated adolescent had significant (>4%) lumbar spine BMD loss in 48 weeks. Among 28 subjects receiving 96 weeks of VIREAD, Z-scores declined by -0.341 for lumbar spine and -0.458 for total body. Skeletal growth (height) appeared to be unaffected. Markers of bone turnover in VIREAD-treated adolescents suggest increased bone turnover, consistent with the effects observed in adults.

The effects of VIREAD-associated changes in BMD and biochemical markers on long-term bone health and future fracture risk are unknown.

Cases of osteomalacia (associated with proximal renal tubulopathy and which may contribute to fractures) have been reported in association with the use of VIREAD [See Adverse Reactions (6.2)].

The bone effects of VIREAD have not been studied in patients with chronic HBV infection.

5.7 Fat Redistribution

In HIV-infected patients redistribution/accumulation of body fat including central obesity, dorsocervical fat enlargement (buffalo hump), peripheral wasting, facial wasting, breast enlargement, and "cushingoid appearance" have been observed in patients receiving combination antiretroviral therapy. The mechanism and long-term consequences of these events are currently unknown. A causal relationship has not been established.

5.8 Immune Reconstitution Syndrome

Immune reconstitution syndrome has been reported in HIV-infected patients treated with combination antiretroviral therapy, including VIREAD. During the initial phase of combination antiretroviral treatment, patients whose immune system responds may develop an inflammatory response to indolent or residual opportunistic infections [such as Mycobacterium avium infection, cytomegalovirus, Pneumocystis jirovecii pneumonia (PCP), or tuberculosis], which may necessitate further evaluation and treatment.

5.9 Early Virologic Failure

Clinical studies in HIV-infected subjects have demonstrated that certain regimens that only contain three nucleoside reverse transcriptase inhibitors (NRTI) are generally less effective than triple drug regimens containing two NRTIs in combination with either a non-nucleoside reverse transcriptase inhibitor or a HIV-1 protease inhibitor. In particular, early virological failure and high rates of resistance substitutions have been reported. Triple nucleoside regimens should therefore be used with caution. Patients on a therapy utilizing a triple nucleoside-only regimen should be carefully monitored and considered for treatment modification.

6 ADVERSE REACTIONS

The following adverse reactions are discussed in other sections of the labeling:
- Lactic Acidosis/Severe Hepatomegaly with Steatosis [See Boxed Warning, Warnings and Precautions (5.1)].
- Severe Acute Exacerbation of Hepatitis [See Boxed Warning, Warnings and Precautions (5.2)].

Table 1 Dosage Adjustment for Patients with Altered Creatinine Clearance

	Creatinine Clearance (mL/min)*			
	≥50	30–49	10–29	Hemodialysis Patients
Recommended 300 mg Dosing Interval	Every 24 hours	Every 48 hours	Every 72 to 96 hours	Every 7 days or after a total of approximately 12 hours of dialysis†

* Calculated using ideal (lean) body weight.

† Generally once weekly assuming three hemodialysis sessions a week of approximately 4 hours duration. VIREAD should be administered following completion of dialysis.

- New Onset or Worsening Renal Impairment *[See Warnings and Precautions (5.3)]*.
- Decreases in Bone Mineral Density *[See Warnings and Precautions (5.6)]*.
- Immune Reconstitution Syndrome *[See Warnings and Precautions (5.8)]*.

6.1   Adverse Reactions from Clinical Trials Experience
Because clinical trials are conducted under widely varying conditions, adverse reaction rates observed in the clinical trials of a drug cannot be directly compared to rates in the clinical trials of another drug and may not reflect the rates observed in practice.
Clinical Trials in Adult Patients with HIV-1 Infection
More than 12,000 subjects have been treated with VIREAD alone or in combination with other antiretroviral medicinal products for periods of 28 days to 215 weeks in clinical trials and expanded access studies. A total of 1,544 subjects have received VIREAD 300 mg once daily in clinical trials; over 11,000 subjects have received VIREAD in expanded access studies.
The most common adverse reactions (incidence ≥10%, Grades 2–4) identified from any of the 3 large controlled clinical trials include rash, diarrhea, headache, pain, depression, asthenia, and nausea.
Treatment-Naïve Patients
Study 903 - Treatment-Emergent Adverse Reactions: The most common adverse reactions seen in a double-blind comparative controlled study in which 600 treatment-naïve subjects received VIREAD (N=299) or stavudine (N=301) in combination with lamivudine and efavirenz for 144 weeks (Study 903) were mild to moderate gastrointestinal events and dizziness.
Mild adverse reactions (Grade 1) were common with a similar incidence in both arms, and included dizziness, diarrhea, and nausea. Selected treatment-emergent moderate to severe adverse reactions are summarized in Table 2.

Table 2 Selected Treatment-Emergent Adverse Reactions* (Grades 2–4) Reported in ≥5% in Any Treatment Group in Study 903 (0–144 Weeks)

	VIREAD + 3TC + EFV	d4T + 3TC + EFV
	N=299	N=301
Body as a Whole		
Headache	14%	17%
Pain	13%	12%
Fever	8%	7%
Abdominal pain	7%	12%
Back pain	9%	8%
Asthenia	6%	7%
Digestive System		
Diarrhea	11%	13%
Nausea	8%	9%
Dyspepsia	4%	5%
Vomiting	5%	9%
Metabolic Disorders		
Lipodystrophy†	1%	8%
Musculoskeletal		
Arthralgia	5%	7%
Myalgia	3%	5%
Nervous System		
Depression	11%	10%
Insomnia	5%	8%
Dizziness	3%	6%
Peripheral neuropathy‡	1%	5%
Anxiety	6%	6%
Respiratory		
Pneumonia	5%	5%
Skin and Appendages		
Rash event§	18%	12%

* Frequencies of adverse reactions are based on all treatment-emergent adverse events, regardless of relationship to study drug.
† Lipodystrophy represents a variety of investigator-described adverse events not a protocol-defined syndrome.
‡ Peripheral neuropathy includes peripheral neuritis and neuropathy.
§ Rash event includes rash, pruritus, maculopapular rash, urticaria, vesiculobullous rash, and pustular rash.

Laboratory Abnormalities: With the exception of fasting cholesterol and fasting triglyceride elevations that were more common in the stavudine group (40% and 9%) com-
pared with VIREAD (19% and 1%) respectively, laboratory abnormalities observed in this study occurred with similar frequency in the VIREAD and stavudine treatment arms. A summary of Grade 3 and 4 laboratory abnormalities is provided in Table 3.

Table 3 Grade 3/4 Laboratory Abnormalities Reported in ≥1% of VIREAD-Treated Subjects in Study 903 (0–144 Weeks)

	VIREAD + 3TC + EFV	d4T + 3TC + EFV
	N=299	N=301
Any ≥ Grade 3 Laboratory Abnormality	36%	42%
Fasting Cholesterol (>240 mg/dL)	19%	40%
Creatine Kinase (M: >990 U/L; F: >845 U/L)	12%	12%
Serum Amylase (>175 U/L)	9%	8%
AST (M: >180 U/L; F: >170 U/L)	5%	7%
ALT (M: >215 U/L; F: >170 U/L)	4%	5%
Hematuria (>100 RBC/HPF)	7%	7%
Neutrophils (<750/mm³)	3%	1%
Fasting Triglycerides (>750 mg/dL)	1%	9%

Study 934 - Treatment Emergent Adverse Reactions: In Study 934, 511 antiretroviral-naïve subjects received either VIREAD + EMTRIVA® administered in combination with efavirenz (N=257) or zidovudine/lamivudine administered in combination with efavirenz (N=254). Adverse reactions observed in this study were generally consistent with those seen in previous studies in treatment-experienced or treatment-naïve subjects (Table 4).

Table 4 Selected Treatment-Emergent Adverse Reactions* (Grades 2–4) Reported in ≥5% in Any Treatment Group in Study 934 (0–144 Weeks)

	VIREAD† + FTC + EFV	AZT/3TC + EFV
	N=257	N=254
Gastrointestinal Disorder		
Diarrhea	9%	5%
Nausea	9%	7%
Vomiting	2%	5%
General Disorders and Administration Site Condition		
Fatigue	9%	8%
Infections and Infestations		
Sinusitis	8%	4%
Upper respiratory tract infections	8%	5%
Nasopharyngitis	5%	3%
Nervous System Disorders		
Headache	6%	5%
Dizziness	8%	7%
Psychiatric Disorders		
Depression	9%	7%
Insomnia	5%	7%
Skin and Subcutaneous Tissue Disorders		
Rash event‡	7%	9%

* Frequencies of adverse reactions are based on all treatment-emergent adverse events, regardless of relationship to study drug.
† From Weeks 96 to 144 of the study, subjects received TRUVADA with efavirenz in place of VIREAD + EMTRIVA with efavirenz.

‡ Rash event includes rash, exfoliative rash, rash generalized, rash macular, rash maculo-papular, rash pruritic, and rash vesicular.

Laboratory Abnormalities: Laboratory abnormalities observed in this study were generally consistent with those seen in previous studies (Table 5).

Table 5 Significant Laboratory Abnormalities Reported in ≥1% of Subjects in Any Treatment Group in Study 934 (0–144 Weeks)

	VIREAD* + FTC + EFV	AZT/3TC + EFV
	N=257	N=254
Any ≥ Grade 3 Laboratory Abnormality	30%	26%
Fasting Cholesterol (>240 mg/dL)	22%	24%
Creatine Kinase (M: >990 U/L; F: >845 U/L)	9%	7%
Serum Amylase (>175 U/L)	8%	4%
Alkaline Phosphatase (>550 U/L)	1%	0%
AST (M: >180 U/L; F: >170 U/L)	3%	3%
ALT (M: >215 U/L; F: >170 U/L)	2%	3%
Hemoglobin (<8.0 mg/dL)	0%	4%
Hyperglycemia (>250 mg/dL)	2%	1%
Hematuria (>75 RBC/HPF)	3%	2%
Glycosuria (≥3+)	<1%	1%
Neutrophils (<750/mm³)	3%	5%
Fasting Triglycerides (>750 mg/dL)	4%	2%

* From Weeks 96 to 144 of the study, subjects received TRUVADA with efavirenz in place of VIREAD + EMTRIVA with efavirenz.

Treatment-Experienced Patients
Treatment-Emergent Adverse Reactions: The adverse reactions seen in treatment experienced subjects were generally consistent with those seen in treatment naïve subjects including mild to moderate gastrointestinal events, such as nausea, diarrhea, vomiting, and flatulence. Less than 1% of subjects discontinued participation in the clinical studies due to gastrointestinal adverse reactions (Study 907).
A summary of moderate to severe, treatment-emergent adverse reactions that occurred during the first 48 weeks of Study 907 is provided in Table 6.
[See table 6 at top of next page]
Laboratory Abnormalities: Laboratory abnormalities observed in this study occurred with similar frequency in the VIREAD and placebo-treated groups. A summary of Grade 3 and 4 laboratory abnormalities is provided in Table 7.
[See table 7 on next page]
Clinical Trials in Adolescent Patients with HIV-1 Infection
Assessment of adverse reactions is based on one randomized trial (Study 321) in 87 HIV-1 infected adolescent subjects (12 to <18 years of age) who received treatment with VIREAD (N=45) or placebo (N=42) in combination with other antiretroviral agents for 48 weeks. The adverse reactions observed in adolescent subjects who received treatment with VIREAD were consistent with those observed in clinical trials in adults.
Bone effects observed in adolescent subjects were consistent with those observed in adult clinical trials *[See Warnings and Precautions (5.6)]*.
Clinical Trials in Adult Patients with Chronic Hepatitis B
Treatment-Emergent Adverse Reactions: In controlled clinical trials in subjects with chronic hepatitis B (0102 and 0103), more subjects treated with VIREAD during the 48-week double-blind period experienced nausea: 9% with VIREAD versus 2% with HEPSERA. Other treatment-emergent adverse reactions reported in >5% of subjects treated with VIREAD included: abdominal pain, diarrhea, headache, dizziness, fatigue, nasopharyngitis, back pain and skin rash.

No significant change in the tolerability profile (frequency, nature, or severity of adverse reactions) was observed in subjects continuing treatment with VIREAD for up to 96 weeks in these studies.

Laboratory Abnormalities: A summary of Grade 3 and 4 laboratory abnormalities is provided in Table 8.

Table 8. Grade 3/4 Laboratory Abnormalities Reported in ≥1% of VIREAD-Treated Subjects in Studies 0102 and 0103 (0–48 Weeks)

	VIREAD (N=426)	HEPSERA (N=215)
Any ≥ Grade 3 Laboratory Abnormality	19%	13%
Creatine Kinase (M: >990U/L; F: >845 U/L)	2%	3%
Serum Amylase (>175 U/L)	4%	1%
Glycosuria (≥3+)	3%	<1%
AST (M: >180 U/L; F: >170 U/L)	4%	4%
ALT (M: >215 U/L; F: >170 U/L)	10%	6%

The overall incidence of on-treatment ALT elevations (defined as serum ALT >2 × baseline and >10 × ULN, with or without associated symptoms) was similar between VIREAD (2.6%) and HEPSERA (2%). ALT elevations generally occurred within the first 4–8 weeks of treatment and were accompanied by decreases in HBV DNA levels. No subject had evidence of decompensation. ALT flares typically resolved within 4 to 8 weeks without changes in study medication.

Grade 3/4 laboratory abnormalities were similar in nature and frequency in subjects continuing treatment for up to 96 weeks in these studies.

6.2   Postmarketing Experience

The following adverse reactions have been identified during postapproval use of VIREAD. Because postmarketing reactions are reported voluntarily from a population of uncertain size, it is not always possible to reliably estimate their frequency or establish a causal relationship to drug exposure.

Immune System Disorders
allergic reaction, including angioedema
Metabolism and Nutrition Disorders
lactic acidosis, hypokalemia, hypophosphatemia
Respiratory, Thoracic, and Mediastinal Disorders
dyspnea
Gastrointestinal Disorders
pancreatitis, increased amylase, abdominal pain
Hepatobiliary Disorders
hepatic steatosis, hepatitis, increased liver enzymes (most commonly AST, ALT gamma GT)
Skin and Subcutaneous Tissue Disorders
rash
Musculoskeletal and Connective Tissue Disorders
rhabdomyolysis, osteomalacia (manifested as bone pain and which may contribute to fractures), muscular weakness, myopathy
Renal and Urinary Disorders
acute renal failure, renal failure, acute tubular necrosis, Fanconi syndrome, proximal renal tubulopathy, interstitial nephritis (including acute cases), nephrogenic diabetes insipidus, renal insufficiency, increased creatinine, proteinuria, polyuria
General Disorders and Administration Site Conditions
asthenia
The following adverse reactions, listed under the body system headings above, may occur as a consequence of proximal renal tubulopathy: rhabdomyolysis, osteomalacia, hypokalemia, muscular weakness, myopathy, hypophosphatemia.

7   DRUG INTERACTIONS

This section describes clinically relevant drug interactions with VIREAD. Drug interactions studies are described elsewhere in the labeling *[See Clinical Pharmacology (12.3)].*

7.1   Didanosine

Coadministration of VIREAD and didanosine should be undertaken with caution and patients receiving this combination should be monitored closely for didanosine-associated adverse reactions. Didanosine should be discontinued in patients who develop didanosine-associated adverse reactions. When administered with VIREAD, C_{max} and AUC of didanosine (administered as either the buffered or enteric-coated formulation) increased significantly *[See Clinical*

Table 6 Selected Treatment-Emergent Adverse Reactions* (Grades 2–4) Reported in ≥3% in Any Treatment Group in Study 907 (0–48 Weeks)

	VIREAD (N=368) (Week 0–24)	Placebo (N=182) (Week 0–24)	VIREAD (N=368) (Week 0–48)	Placebo Crossover to VIREAD (N=170) (Week 24–48)
Body as a Whole				
Asthenia	7%	6%	11%	1%
Pain	7%	7%	12%	4%
Headache	5%	5%	8%	2%
Abdominal pain	4%	3%	7%	6%
Back pain	3%	3%	4%	2%
Chest pain	3%	1%	3%	2%
Fever	2%	2%	4%	2%
Digestive System				
Diarrhea	11%	10%	16%	11%
Nausea	8%	5%	11%	7%
Vomiting	4%	1%	7%	5%
Anorexia	3%	2%	4%	1%
Dyspepsia	3%	2%	4%	2%
Flatulence	3%	1%	4%	1%
Respiratory				
Pneumonia	2%	0%	3%	2%
Nervous System				
Depression	4%	3%	8%	4%
Insomnia	3%	2%	4%	4%
Peripheral neuropathy†	3%	3%	5%	2%
Dizziness	1%	3%	3%	1%
Skin and Appendage				
Rash event‡	5%	4%	7%	1%
Sweating	3%	2%	3%	1%
Musculoskeletal				
Myalgia	3%	3%	4%	1%
Metabolic				
Weight loss	2%	1%	4%	2%

* Frequencies of adverse reactions are based on all treatment-emergent adverse events, regardless of relationship to study drug.
† Peripheral neuropathy includes peripheral neuritis and neuropathy.
‡ Rash event includes rash, pruritus, maculopapular rash, urticaria, vesiculobullous rash, and pustular rash.

Table 7 Grade 3/4 Laboratory Abnormalities Reported in ≥1% of VIREAD-Treated Subjects in Study 907 (0–48 Weeks)

	VIREAD (N=368) (Week 0–24)	Placebo (N=182) (Week 0–24)	VIREAD (N=368) (Week 0–48)	Placebo Crossover to VIREAD (N=170) (Week 24–48)
Any ≥ Grade 3 Laboratory Abnormality	25%	38%	35%	34%
Triglycerides (>750 mg/dL)	8%	13%	11%	9%
Creatine Kinase (M: >990 U/L; F: >845 U/L)	7%	14%	12%	12%
Serum Amylase (>175 U/L)	6%	7%	7%	6%
Glycosuria (≥3+)	3%	3%	3%	2%
AST (M: >180 U/L; F: >170 U/L)	3%	3%	4%	5%
ALT (M: >215 U/L; F: >170 U/L)	2%	2%	4%	5%
Serum Glucose (>250 U/L)	2%	4%	3%	3%
Neutrophils (<750/mm³)	1%	1%	2%	1%

Pharmacology (12.3)]. The mechanism of this interaction is unknown. Higher didanosine concentrations could potentiate didanosine-associated adverse reactions, including pancreatitis and neuropathy. Suppression of CD4⁺ cell counts has been observed in patients receiving tenofovir disoproxil fumarate (tenofovir DF) with didanosine 400 mg daily.
In patients weighing >60 kg, the didanosine dose should be reduced to 250 mg when it is coadministered with VIREAD. Data are not available to recommend a dose adjustment of didanosine for adult or pediatric patients weighing <60 kg. When coadministered, VIREAD and didanosine EC may be taken under fasted conditions or with a light meal (<400 kcal, 20% fat). Coadministration of didanosine buffered tablet formulation with VIREAD should be under fasted conditions.

7.2   Atazanavir

Atazanavir has been shown to increase tenofovir concentrations *[See Clinical Pharmacology (12.3)].* The mechanism of this interaction is unknown. Patients receiving atazanavir and VIREAD should be monitored for VIREAD-associated adverse reactions. VIREAD should be discontinued in patients who develop VIREAD-associated adverse reactions. VIREAD decreases the AUC and C_{min} of atazanavir *[See Clinical Pharmacology (12.3)].* When coadministered with VIREAD, it is recommended that atazanavir 300 mg is given with ritonavir 100 mg. Atazanavir without ritonavir should not be coadministered with VIREAD.

7.3   Lopinavir/Ritonavir

Lopinavir/ritonavir has been shown to increase tenofovir concentrations *[See Clinical Pharmacology (12.3)].* The mechanism of this interaction is unknown. Patients receiving lopinavir/ritonavir and VIREAD should be monitored for VIREAD-associated adverse reactions. VIREAD should be discontinued in patients who develop VIREAD-associated adverse reactions.

7.4 Drugs Affecting Renal Function

Since tenofovir is primarily eliminated by the kidneys [See Clinical Pharmacology (12.3)], coadministration of VIREAD with drugs that reduce renal function or compete for active tubular secretion may increase serum concentrations of tenofovir and/or increase the concentrations of other renally eliminated drugs. Some examples include, but are not limited to cidofovir, acyclovir, valacyclovir, ganciclovir, and valganciclovir. Drugs that decrease renal function may also increase serum concentrations of tenofovir.

In the treatment of chronic hepatitis B, VIREAD should not be administered in combination with HEPSERA (adefovir dipivoxil).

8 USE IN SPECIFIC POPULATIONS

8.1 Pregnancy

Pregnancy Category B

Reproduction studies have been performed in rats and rabbits at doses up to 14 and 19 times the human dose based on body surface area comparisons and revealed no evidence of impaired fertility or harm to the fetus due to tenofovir. There are, however, no adequate and well-controlled studies in pregnant women. Because animal reproduction studies are not always predictive of human response, VIREAD should be used during pregnancy only if clearly needed.

Antiretroviral Pregnancy Registry: To monitor fetal outcomes of pregnant women exposed to VIREAD, an Antiretroviral Pregnancy Registry has been established. Healthcare providers are encouraged to register patients by calling 1-800-258-4263.

8.3 Nursing Mothers

Nursing Mothers: The Centers for Disease Control and Prevention recommend that HIV-1-infected mothers not breast-feed their infants to avoid risking postnatal transmission of HIV-1. Studies in rats have demonstrated that tenofovir is secreted in milk. It is not known whether tenofovir is excreted in human milk. Because of both the potential for HIV-1 transmission and the potential for serious adverse reactions in nursing infants, **mothers should be instructed not to breast-feed if they are receiving VIREAD.**

8.4 Pediatric Use

Adolescent Patients

The safety of VIREAD in adolescent patients aged 12 to <18 years is supported by data from one randomized study in which VIREAD was administered to HIV-1 infected treatment-experienced subjects. In this study, the pharmacokinetic profile of VIREAD was similar to that found to be safe and effective in adult clinical trials.

In Study 321, 87 treatment-experienced subjects 12 to <18 years of age were treated with VIREAD (N=45) or placebo (N=42) in combination with an optimized background regimen (OBR) for 48 weeks. The mean baseline CD4 cell count was 374 cells/mm^3 and the mean baseline plasma HIV-1 RNA was 4.6 log$_{10}$ copies/mL. At baseline, 90% of subjects harbored NRTI resistance-associated substitutions in their HIV-1 isolates. Overall, the trial failed to show a difference in virologic response between the VIREAD and placebo treatment groups. Subgroup analyses suggest the lack of difference in virologic response may be attributable to imbalances between treatment arms in baseline viral susceptibility to VIREAD and OBR.

Although changes in HIV-1 RNA in these highly treatment-experienced adolescent subjects were less than anticipated, the comparability of the pharmacokinetic and safety data to that observed in adults supports the use of VIREAD in patients ≥12 years of age who weigh ≥35 kg and whose HIV-1 isolate is expected to be sensitive to VIREAD. [See Warnings and Precautions (5.6), Adverse Reactions (6.1), and Clinical Pharmacology (12.3)].

Safety and effectiveness in patients less than 12 years of age have not been established.

8.5 Geriatric Use

Clinical studies of VIREAD did not include sufficient numbers of subjects aged 65 and over to determine whether they respond differently from younger subjects. In general, dose selection for the elderly patient should be cautious, keeping in mind the greater frequency of decreased hepatic, renal, or cardiac function, and of concomitant disease or other drug therapy.

8.6 Patients with Impaired Renal Function

It is recommended that the dosing interval for VIREAD be modified in patients with creatinine clearance <50 mL/min or in patients with ESRD who require dialysis [See Dosage and Administration (2.3), Clinical Pharmacology (12.3)].

10 OVERDOSAGE

Limited clinical experience at doses higher than the therapeutic dose of VIREAD 300 mg is available. In Study 901, 600 mg tenofovir disoproxil fumarate was administered to 8

Table 9 Pharmacokinetic Parameters (Mean ± SD) of Tenofovir* in Subjects with Varying Degrees of Renal Function

Baseline Creatinine Clearance (mL/min)	>80 (N=3)	50–80 (N=10)	30–49 (N=8)	12–29 (N=11)
C_{max} (µg/mL)	0.34 ± 0.03	0.33 ± 0.06	0.37 ± 0.16	0.60 ± 0.19
$AUC_{0-\infty}$ (µg•hr/mL)	2.18 ± 0.26	3.06 ± 0.93	6.01 ± 2.50	15.98 ± 7.22
CL/F (mL/min)	1043.7 ± 115.4	807.7 ± 279.2	444.4 ± 209.8	177.0 ± 97.1
CL_{renal} (mL/min)	243.5 ± 33.3	168.6 ± 27.5	100.6 ± 27.5	43.0 ± 31.2

* 300 mg, single dose of VIREAD

Table 10 Drug Interactions: Changes in Pharmacokinetic Parameters for Tenofovir* in the Presence of the Coadministered Drug

Coadministered Drug	Dose of Coadministered Drug (mg)	N	% Change of Tenofovir Pharmacokinetic Parameters[†] (90% CI)		
			C_{max}	AUC	C_{min}
Abacavir	300 once	8	⇔	⇔	NC
Atazanavir[‡]	400 once daily × 14 days	33	↑ 14 (↑ 8 to ↑ 20)	↑ 24 (↑ 21 to ↑ 28)	↑ 22 (↑ 15 to ↑ 30)
Didanosine (enteric-coated)	400 once	25	⇔	⇔	⇔
Didanosine (buffered)	250 or 400 once daily × 7 days	14	⇔	⇔	⇔
Efavirenz	600 once daily × 14 days	29	⇔	⇔	⇔
Emtricitabine	200 once daily × 7 days	17	⇔	⇔	⇔
Entecavir	1 mg once daily × 10 days	28	⇔	⇔	⇔
Indinavir	800 three times daily × 7 days	13	↑ 14 (↓ 3 to ↑ 33)	⇔	⇔
Lamivudine	150 twice daily × 7 days	15	⇔	⇔	⇔
Lopinavir/Ritonavir	400/100 twice daily × 14 days	24	⇔	↑ 32 (↑ 25 to ↑ 38)	↑ 51 (↑ 37 to ↑ 66)
Nelfinavir	1250 twice daily × 14 days	29	⇔	⇔	⇔
Saquinavir/Ritonavir	1000/100 twice daily × 14 days	35	⇔	⇔	↑ 23 (↑ 16 to ↑ 30)
Tacrolimus	0.05 mg/kg twice daily × 7 days	21	↑ 13 (↑ 1 to ↑ 27)	⇔	⇔

* Subjects received VIREAD 300 mg once daily.
† Increase = ↑; Decrease = ↓; No Effect = ⇔; NC = Not Calculated
‡ Reyataz Prescribing Information

subjects orally for 28 days. No severe adverse reactions were reported. The effects of higher doses are not known.

If overdose occurs the patient must be monitored for evidence of toxicity, and standard supportive treatment applied as necessary.

Tenofovir is efficiently removed by hemodialysis with an extraction coefficient of approximately 54%. Following a single 300 mg dose of VIREAD, a four-hour hemodialysis session removed approximately 10% of the administered tenofovir dose.

11 DESCRIPTION

VIREAD is the brand name for tenofovir disoproxil fumarate (a prodrug of tenofovir) which is a fumaric acid salt of bis-isopropoxycarbonyloxymethyl ester derivative of tenofovir. In vivo tenofovir disoproxil fumarate is converted to tenofovir, an acyclic nucleoside phosphonate (nucleotide) analog of adenosine 5'-monophosphate. Tenofovir exhibits activity against HIV-1 reverse transcriptase.

The chemical name of tenofovir disoproxil fumarate is 9-[(R)-2-[[bis[[(isopropoxycarbonyl)oxy]methoxy]phosphinyl]methoxy]propyl]adenine fumarate (1:1). It has a molecular formula of $C_{19}H_{30}N_5O_{10}P \cdot C_4H_4O_4$ and a molecular weight of 635.52. It has the following structural formula:

Tenofovir disoproxil fumarate is a white to off-white crystalline powder with a solubility of 13.4 mg/mL in distilled water at 25 °C. It has an octanol/phosphate buffer (pH 6.5) partition coefficient (log p) of 1.25 at 25 °C.

VIREAD tablets are for oral administration. Each tablet contains 300 mg of tenofovir disoproxil fumarate, which is equivalent to 245 mg of tenofovir disoproxil, and the following inactive ingredients: croscarmellose sodium, lactose monohydrate, magnesium stearate, microcrystalline cellulose, and pregelatinized starch. The tablets are coated with Opadry II Y–30–10671–A, which contains FD&C blue #2 aluminum lake, hydroxypropyl methylcellulose 2910, lactose monohydrate, titanium dioxide, and triacetin.

Table 11 Drug Interactions: Changes in Pharmacokinetic Parameters for Coadministered Drug in the Presence of VIREAD

Coadministered Drug	Dose of Coadministered Drug (mg)	N	% Change of Coadministered Drug Pharmacokinetic Parameters* (90% CI)		
			C_{max}	AUC	C_{min}
Abacavir	300 once	8	↑ 12 (↓ 1 to ↑ 26)	⇔	NA
Atazanavir[†]	400 once daily × 14 days	34	↓ 21 (↓ 27 to ↓ 14)	↓ 25 (↓ 30 to ↓ 19)	↓ 40 (↓ 48 to ↓ 32)
Atazanavir[†]	Atazanavir/ Ritonavir 300/100 once daily × 42 days	10	↓ 28 (↓ 50 to ↑ 5)	↓ 25[‡] (↓ 42 to ↓ 3)	↓ 23[‡] (↓ 46 to ↑ 10)
Efavirenz	600 once daily × 14 days	30	⇔	⇔	⇔
Emtricitabine	200 once daily × 7 days	17	⇔	⇔	↑ 20 (↑ 12 to ↑ 29)
Entecavir	1 mg once daily × 10 days	28	⇔	↑ 13 (↑ 11 to ↑ 15)	⇔
Indinavir	800 three times daily × 7 days	12	↓ 11 (↓ 30 to ↑ 12)	⇔	⇔
Lamivudine	150 twice daily × 7 days	15	↓ 24 (↓ 34 to ↓ 12)	⇔	⇔
Lopinavir Ritonavir	Lopinavir/Ritonavir 400/100 twice daily × 14 days	24	⇔	⇔	⇔
Methadone[§]	40–110 once daily × 14 days[¶]	13	⇔	⇔	⇔
Nelfinavir M8 metabolite	1250 twice daily × 14 days	29	⇔ ⇔	⇔ ⇔	⇔ ⇔
Oral Contraceptives[#]	Ethinyl Estradiol/ Norgestimate (Ortho-Tricyclen) once daily × 7 days	20	⇔	⇔	⇔
Ribavirin	600 once	22	⇔	⇔	NA
Saquinavir Ritonavir	Saquinavir/Ritonavir 1000/100 twice daily × 14 days	32	↑ 22 (↑ 6 to ↑ 41) ⇔	↑ 29[Þ] (↑ 12 to ↑ 48) ⇔	↑ 47[Þ] (↑ 23 to ↑ 76) ↑ 23 (↑ 3 to ↑ 46)
Tacrolimus	0.05 mg/kg twice daily × 7 days	21	⇔	⇔	⇔

* Increase = ↑; Decrease = ↓; No Effect = ⇔; NA = Not Applicable
† Reyataz Prescribing Information
‡ In HIV-infected subjects, addition of tenofovir DF to atazanavir 300 mg plus ritonavir 100 mg, resulted in AUC and C_{min} values of atazanavir that were 2.3- and 4-fold higher than the respective values observed for atazanavir 400 mg when given alone.
§ R-(active), S- and total methadone exposures were equivalent when dosed alone or with VIREAD.
¶ Individual subjects were maintained on their stable methadone dose. No pharmacodynamic alterations (opiate toxicity or withdrawal signs or symptoms) were reported.
# Ethinyl estradiol and 17-deacetyl norgestimate (pharmacologically active metabolite) exposures were equivalent when dosed alone or with VIREAD.
Þ Increases in AUC and C_{min} are not expected to be clinically relevant; hence no dose adjustments are required when tenofovir DF and ritonavir-boosted saquinavir are coadministered.

In this insert, all dosages are expressed in terms of tenofovir disoproxil fumarate except where otherwise noted.

12 CLINICAL PHARMACOLOGY

12.1 Mechanism of Action
Tenofovir disoproxil fumarate is an antiviral drug [See Clinical Pharmacology (12.4)].

12.3 Pharmacokinetics
The pharmacokinetics of tenofovir disoproxil fumarate have been evaluated in healthy volunteers and HIV-1 infected individuals. Tenofovir pharmacokinetics are similar between these populations.

Absorption
VIREAD is a water soluble diester prodrug of the active ingredient tenofovir. The oral bioavailability of tenofovir from VIREAD in fasted subjects is approximately 25%. Following oral administration of a single dose of VIREAD 300 mg to HIV-1 infected subjects in the fasted state, maximum serum concentrations (C_{max}) are achieved in 1.0 ± 0.4 hrs. C_{max} and AUC values are 0.30 ± 0.09 µg/mL and 2.29 ± 0.69 µg•hr/mL, respectively.

The pharmacokinetics of tenofovir are dose proportional over a VIREAD dose range of 75 to 600 mg and are not affected by repeated dosing.

Distribution
In vitro binding of tenofovir to human plasma or serum proteins is less than 0.7 and 7.2%, respectively, over the tenofovir concentration range 0.01 to 25 µg/mL. The volume of distribution at steady-state is 1.3 ± 0.6 L/kg and 1.2 ± 0.4 L/kg, following intravenous administration of tenofovir 1.0 mg/kg and 3.0 mg/kg.

Metabolism and Elimination
In vitro studies indicate that neither tenofovir disoproxil nor tenofovir are substrates of CYP enzymes.
Following IV administration of tenofovir, approximately 70–80% of the dose is recovered in the urine as unchanged tenofovir within 72 hours of dosing. Following single dose, oral administration of VIREAD, the terminal elimination half-life of tenofovir is approximately 17 hours. After multiple oral doses of VIREAD 300 mg once daily (under fed conditions), 32 ± 10% of the administered dose is recovered in urine over 24 hours.

Tenofovir is eliminated by a combination of glomerular filtration and active tubular secretion. There may be competition for elimination with other compounds that are also renally eliminated.

Effects of Food on Oral Absorption
Administration of VIREAD following a high-fat meal (~700 to 1000 kcal containing 40 to 50% fat) increases the oral bioavailability, with an increase in tenofovir $AUC_{0-\infty}$ of approximately 40% and an increase in C_{max} of approximately 14%. However, administration of VIREAD with a light meal did not have a significant effect on the pharmacokinetics of tenofovir when compared to fasted administration of the drug. Food delays the time to tenofovir C_{max} by approximately 1 hour. C_{max} and AUC of tenofovir are 0.33 ± 0.12 µg/mL and 3.32 ± 1.37 µg•hr/mL following multiple doses of VIREAD 300 mg once daily in the fed state, when meal content was not controlled.

Special Populations
Race: There were insufficient numbers from racial and ethnic groups other than Caucasian to adequately determine potential pharmacokinetic differences among these populations.
Gender: Tenofovir pharmacokinetics are similar in male and female subjects.
Pediatric Patients: Steady-state pharmacokinetics of tenofovir were evaluated in 8 HIV-1 infected adolescent subjects (12 to <18 years). Mean (± SD) C_{max} and AUC_{tau} are 0.38 ± 0.13 µg/mL and 3.39 ± 1.22 µg•hr/mL, respectively. Tenofovir exposure achieved in adolescent subjects receiving oral daily doses of VIREAD 300 mg was similar to exposures achieved in adults receiving once-daily doses of VIREAD 300 mg.
Pharmacokinetic studies have not been performed in pediatric subjects <12 years of age.
Geriatric Patients: Pharmacokinetic studies have not been performed in the elderly (>65 years).
Patients with Impaired Renal Function: The pharmacokinetics of tenofovir are altered in subjects with renal impairment [See Warnings and Precautions (5.3)]. In subjects with creatinine clearance <50 mL/min or with end-stage renal disease (ESRD) requiring dialysis, C_{max}, and $AUC_{0-\infty}$ of tenofovir were increased (Table 9). It is recommended that the dosing interval for VIREAD be modified in patients with creatinine clearance <50 mL/min or in patients with ESRD who require dialysis [See Dosage and Administration (2.3)].
[See table 9 at top of previous page]
Tenofovir is efficiently removed by hemodialysis with an extraction coefficient of approximately 54%. Following a single 300 mg dose of VIREAD, a four-hour hemodialysis session removed approximately 10% of the administered tenofovir dose.
Patients with Hepatic Impairment: The pharmacokinetics of tenofovir following a 300 mg single dose of VIREAD have been studied in non-HIV infected subjects with moderate to severe hepatic impairment. There were no substantial alterations in tenofovir pharmacokinetics in subjects with hepatic impairment compared with unimpaired subjects. No change in VIREAD dosing is required in patients with hepatic impairment.
Assessment of Drug Interactions
At concentrations substantially higher (~300-fold) than those observed in vivo, tenofovir did not inhibit in vitro drug metabolism mediated by any of the following human CYP isoforms: CYP3A4, CYP2D6, CYP2C9, or CYP2E1. However, a small (6%) but statistically significant reduction in metabolism of CYP1A substrate was observed. Based on the results of in vitro experiments and the known elimination pathway of tenofovir, the potential for CYP mediated interactions involving tenofovir with other medicinal products is low [See Clinical Pharmacology (12.3)].
VIREAD has been evaluated in healthy volunteers in combination with abacavir, atazanavir, didanosine, efavirenz, emtricitabine, entecavir, indinavir, lamivudine, lopinavir/ritonavir, methadone, nelfinavir, oral contraceptives, ribavirin, saquinavir/ritonavir, and tacrolimus. Tables 10 and 11 summarize pharmacokinetic effects of coadministered drug on tenofovir pharmacokinetics and effects of VIREAD on the pharmacokinetics of coadministered drug.
[See table 10 on previous page]
Following multiple dosing to HIV- and HBV-negative subjects receiving either chronic methadone maintenance therapy or oral contraceptives, or single doses of ribavirin, steady state tenofovir pharmacokinetics were similar to those observed in previous studies, indicating lack of clinically significant drug interactions between these agents and VIREAD.
[See table 11 at left]
Table 12 summarizes the drug interaction between VIREAD and didanosine. Coadministration of VIREAD and didanosine should be undertaken with caution [See Drug Interactions (7.1)]. When administered with multiple doses of VIREAD, the C_{max} and AUC of didanosine 400 mg increased significantly. The mechanism of this interaction is unknown. When didanosine 250 mg enteric-coated capsules were administered with VIREAD, systemic exposures to didanosine were similar to those seen with the 400 mg enteric-coated capsules alone under fasted conditions.
[See table 12 at top of next page]

12.4 Microbiology

Mechanism of Action

Tenofovir disoproxil fumarate is an acyclic nucleoside phosphonate diester analog of adenosine monophosphate. Tenofovir disoproxil fumarate requires initial diester hydrolysis for conversion to tenofovir and subsequent phosphorylations by cellular enzymes to form tenofovir diphosphate, an obligate chain terminator. Tenofovir diphosphate inhibits the activity of HIV-1 reverse transcriptase and HBV polymerase by competing with the natural substrate deoxyadenosine 5′-triphosphate and, after incorporation into DNA, by DNA chain termination. Tenofovir diphosphate is a weak inhibitor of mammalian DNA polymerases α, β, and mitochondrial DNA polymerase γ.

Activity against HIV

Antiviral Activity

The antiviral activity of tenofovir against laboratory and clinical isolates of HIV-1 was assessed in lymphoblastoid cell lines, primary monocyte/macrophage cells and peripheral blood lymphocytes. The EC_{50} (50% effective concentration) values for tenofovir were in the range of 0.04 µM to 8.5 µM. In drug combination studies of tenofovir with nucleoside reverse transcriptase inhibitors (abacavir, didanosine, lamivudine, stavudine, zalcitabine, zidovudine), non-nucleoside reverse transcriptase inhibitors (delavirdine, efavirenz, nevirapine), and protease inhibitors (amprenavir, indinavir, nelfinavir, ritonavir, saquinavir), additive to synergistic effects were observed. Tenofovir displayed antiviral activity in cell culture against HIV-1 clades A, B, C, D, E, F, G, and O (EC_{50} values ranged from 0.5 µM to 2.2 µM) and strain specific activity against HIV-2 (EC_{50} values ranged from 1.6 µM to 5.5 µM).

Resistance

HIV-1 isolates with reduced susceptibility to tenofovir have been selected in cell culture. These viruses expressed a K65R substitution in reverse transcriptase and showed a 2–4 fold reduction in susceptibility to tenofovir.

In Study 903 of treatment-naïve subjects (VIREAD + lamivudine + efavirenz versus stavudine + lamivudine + efavirenz) *[See Clinical Studies (14.1)]*, genotypic analyses of isolates from subjects with virologic failure through Week 144 showed development of efavirenz and lamivudine resistance-associated substitutions to occur most frequently and with no difference between the treatment arms. The K65R substitution occurred in 8/47 (17%) analyzed patient isolates on the VIREAD arm and in 2/49 (4%) analyzed patient isolates on the stavudine arm. Of the 8 subjects whose virus developed K65R in the VIREAD arm through 144 weeks, 7 of these occurred in the first 48 weeks of treatment and one at Week 96. Other substitutions resulting in resistance to VIREAD were not identified in this study.

In Study 934 of treatment-naïve subjects (VIREAD + EMTRIVA + efavirenz versus zidovudine (AZT)/lamivudine (3TC) + efavirenz) *[See Clinical Studies (14.1)]*, genotypic analysis performed on HIV-1 isolates from all confirmed virologic failure subjects with >400 copies/mL of HIV-1 RNA at Week 144 or early discontinuation showed development of efavirenz resistance-associated substitutions occurred most frequently and was similar between the two treatment arms. The M184V substitution, associated with resistance to EMTRIVA and lamivudine, was observed in 2/19 analyzed subject isolates in the VIREAD + EMTRIVA group and in 10/29 analyzed subject isolates in the zidovudine/lamivudine group. Through 144 weeks of Study 934, no subjects have developed a detectable K65R substitution in their HIV-1 as analyzed through standard genotypic analysis.

Cross Resistance

Cross-resistance among certain reverse transcriptase inhibitors has been recognized. The K65R substitution selected by tenofovir is also selected in some HIV-1 infected subjects treated with abacavir, didanosine, or zalcitabine. HIV-1 isolates with this mutation also show reduced susceptibility to emtricitabine and lamivudine. Therefore, cross-resistance among these drugs may occur in patients whose virus harbors the K65R substitution. HIV-1 isolates from subjects (N=20) whose HIV-1 expressed a mean of 3 zidovudine-associated reverse transcriptase substitutions (M41L, D67N, K70R, L210W, T215Y/F, or K219Q/E/N), showed a 3.1-fold decrease in the susceptibility to tenofovir. In Studies 902 and 907 conducted in treatment-experienced subjects (VIREAD + Standard Background Therapy (SBT) compared to Placebo + SBT) *[See Clinical Studies (14.1)]*, 14/304 (5%) of the VIREAD-treated subjects with virologic failure through Week 96 had >1.4-fold (median 2.7-fold) reduced susceptibility to tenofovir. Genotypic analysis of the baseline and failure isolates showed the development of the K65R substitution in the HIV-1 reverse transcriptase gene.

The virologic response to VIREAD therapy has been evaluated with respect to baseline viral genotype (N=222) in treatment-experienced subjects participating in Studies 902 and 907.

In these clinical studies, 94% of the participants evaluated had baseline HIV-1 isolates expressing at least one NRTI mutation. These included resistance substitutions associated with zidovudine (M41L, D67N, K70R, L210W, T215Y/F, or K219Q/E/N), the abacavir/emtricitabine/lamivudine resistance-associated substitution (M184V), and others. In addition the majority of participants evaluated had substitutions associated with either PI or NNRTI use. Virologic responses for subjects in the genotype substudy were similar to the overall study results.

Table 12 Drug Interactions: Pharmacokinetic Parameters for Didanosine in the Presence of VIREAD

Didanosine Dose (mg)/ Method of Administration	VIREAD Method of Administration*	N	% Difference (90% CI) vs. Didanosine 400 mg Alone, Fasted†	
			C_{max}	AUC
Buffered Tablets				
400 once daily‡ × 7 days	Fasted 1 hour after didanosine	14	↑ 28 (↑ 11 to ↑ 48)	↑ 44 (↑ 31 to ↑ 59)
Enteric coated capsules				
400 once, fasted	With food, 2 hours after didanosine	26	↑ 48 (↑ 25 to ↑ 76)	↑ 48 (↑ 31 to ↑ 67)
400 once, with food	Simultaneously with didanosine	26	↑ 64 (↑ 41 to ↑ 89)	↑ 60 (↑ 44 to ↑ 79)
250 once, fasted	With food, 2 hours after didanosine	28	↓ 10 (↓ 22 to ↑ 3)	⇔
250 once, fasted	Simultaneously with didanosine	28	⇔	↑ 14 (0 to ↑ 31)
250 once, with food	Simultaneously with didanosine	28	↓ 29 (↓ 39 to ↓ 18)	↓ 11 (↓ 23 to ↑ 2)

* Administration with food was with a light meal (~373 kcal, 20% fat).
† Increase = ↑; Decrease = ↓; No Effect = ⇔
‡ Includes 4 subjects weighing <60 kg receiving ddI 250 mg.

Several exploratory analyses were conducted to evaluate the effect of specific substitutions and substitutional patterns on virologic outcome. Because of the large number of potential comparisons, statistical testing was not conducted. Varying degrees of cross-resistance of VIREAD to pre-existing zidovudine resistance-associated substitutions were observed and appeared to depend on the number of specific substitutions. VIREAD-treated subjects whose HIV-1 expressed 3 or more zidovudine resistance-associated substitutions that included either the M41L or L210W reverse transcriptase substitution showed reduced responses to VIREAD therapy; however, these responses were still improved compared with placebo. The presence of the D67N, K70R, T215Y/F, or K219Q/E/N substitution did not appear to affect responses to VIREAD therapy. Subjects whose virus expressed an L74V substitution without zidovudine resistance associated substitutions (N=8) had reduced response to VIREAD. Limited data are available for subjects whose virus expressed a Y115F substitution (N=3), Q151M substitution (N=2), or T69 insertion (N=4), all of whom had a reduced response.

In the protocol defined analyses, virologic response to VIREAD was not reduced in subjects with HIV-1 that expressed the abacavir/emtricitabine/lamivudine resistance-associated M184V substitution. HIV-1 RNA responses among these subjects were durable through Week 48.

Studies 902 and 907 Phenotypic Analyses

The virologic response to VIREAD therapy has been evaluated with respect to baseline phenotype (N=100) in treatment-experienced subjects participating in two controlled trials. Phenotypic analysis of baseline HIV-1 from subjects in these studies demonstrated a correlation between baseline susceptibility to VIREAD and response to VIREAD therapy. Table 13 summarizes the HIV-1 RNA response by baseline VIREAD susceptibility.

Table 13 HIV-1 RNA Response at Week 24 by Baseline VIREAD Susceptibility (Intent-To-Treat)*

Baseline VIREAD Susceptibility†	Change in HIV-1 RNA‡ (N)
<1	-0.74 (35)
>1 and ≤3	-0.56 (49)
>3 and ≤4	-0.3 (7)
>4	-0.12 (9)

* Tenofovir susceptibility was determined by recombinant phenotypic Antivirogram assay (Virco).
† Fold change in susceptibility from wild-type.
‡ Average HIV-1 RNA change from baseline through Week 24 ($DAVG_{24}$) in log_{10} copies/mL.

Activity against HBV

Antiviral Activity

The antiviral activity of tenofovir against HBV was assessed in the HepG2 2.2.15 cell line. The EC_{50} values for tenofovir ranged from 0.14 to 1.5 µM, with CC_{50} (50% cytotoxicity concentration) values >100 µM. In cell culture combination antiviral activity studies of tenofovir with the nucleoside anti-HBV reverse transcriptase inhibitors emtricitabine, entecavir, lamivudine and telbivudine, no antagonistic activity was observed.

Resistance

Cumulative VIREAD genotypic resistance analysis of paired pre-treatment and on-treatment isolates was performed using an as-treated analysis. Subjects remaining viremic with HBV DNA >400 copies/mL at the last evaluable study visit after 96 weeks of cumulative treatment (16%[26/160] of HBeAg positive subjects in Study 103 and 3% [8/234] of HBeAg negative subjects in Study 102) were evaluated for genotypic resistance. These 34 subjects with viremia were primarily treatment-naïve and received VIREAD for up to 96 weeks; of these, 65% (17/26) of HBeAg-positive and 13% (1/8) of HBeAg-negative subjects had a baseline viral load of >9 log_{10} copies/mL.

In addition, 16 of the 84 HBeAg-positive subjects who received 48 weeks of HEPSERA and then switched to VIREAD for up to 48 weeks, and 18 of 53 Hepsera treatment-experienced subjects from an ongoing Phase 2 study who received up to 48 weeks of VIREAD monotherapy and who had plasma HBV DNA >400 copies/mL, were included in the resistance analysis. Subjects in the Phase 2 study were previously treated for 24 to 96 weeks with HEPSERA for chronic HBV infection and had plasma HBV DNA levels ≥ 1,000 copies/mL at screening.

In the three VIREAD-treatment studies, paired genotypic data were obtained for 55 of 68 viremic subjects. No specific amino acid substitutions in the HBV reverse transcriptase domain occurred at a sufficient frequency to be associated with resistance to VIREAD (genotypic or phenotypic analyses).

In the three VIREAD-treatment studies, prior to treatment with VIREAD, 13 and 10 subjects had HBV harboring adefovir resistance-associated substitutions (rtA181T/V and/or rtN236T) or lamivudine resistance-associated substitution (rtM204I/V), respectively. Following up to 96 weeks of VIREAD treatment, 11 of the 13 subjects with adefovir-resistant HBV and 8 of the 10 subjects with lamivudine-resistant HBV achieved virologic suppression (HBV DNA <400 copies/mL). Two of the 4 subjects harboring both the rtA181T/V and rtN236T substitutions remained viremic following 24 weeks of VIREAD monotherapy.

Cross Resistance

Cross-resistance has been observed among HBV reverse transcriptase inhibitors.

In cell based assays, HBV strains expressing the rtV173L, rtL180M, and rtM204I/V substitutions associated with resistance to lamivudine and telbivudine showed a susceptibility to tenofovir ranging from 0.7 to 3.4-fold that of wild type virus. The rtL180M and rtM204I/V double substitutions conferred 3.4-fold reduced susceptibility to tenofovir. HBV strains expressing the rtL180M, rtT184G, rtS202G/I, rtM204V, and rtM250V substitutions associated with resistance to entecavir showed a susceptibility to tenofovir rang-

Table 14 Outcomes of Randomized Treatment at Week 48 and 144 (Study 903)

Outcomes	At Week 48		At Week 144	
	VIREAD+3TC +EFV (N=299)	d4T+3TC +EFV (N=301)	VIREAD+3TC +EFV (N=299)	d4T+3TC +EFV (N=301)
Responder*	79%	82%	68%	62%
Virologic failure†	6%	4%	10%	8%
Rebound	5%	3%	8%	7%
Never suppressed	0%	1%	0%	0%
Added an antiretroviral agent	1%	1%	2%	1%
Death	<1%	1%	<1%	2%
Discontinued due to adverse event	6%	6%	8%	13%
Discontinued for other reasons‡	8%	7%	14%	15%

* Subjects achieved and maintained confirmed HIV-1 RNA <400 copies/mL through Week 48 and 144.
† Includes confirmed viral rebound and failure to achieve confirmed <400 copies/mL through Week 48 and 144.
‡ Includes lost to follow-up, subject's withdrawal, noncompliance, protocol violation and other reasons.

Table 15 Outcomes of Randomized Treatment at Week 48 and 144 (Study 934)

Outcomes	At Week 48		At Week 144	
	FTC +VIREAD +EFV (N=244)	AZT/3TC +EFV (N=243)	FTC +VIREAD +EFV (N=227)*	AZT/3TC +EFV (N=229)*
Responder†	84%	73%	71%	58%
Virologic failure‡	2%	4%	3%	6%
Rebound	1%	3%	2%	5%
Never suppressed	0%	0%	0%	0%
Change in antiretroviral regimen	1%	1%	1%	1%
Death	<1%	1%	1%	1%
Discontinued due to adverse event	4%	9%	5%	12%
Discontinued for other reasons§	10%	14%	20%	22%

* Subjects who were responders at Week 48 or Week 96 (HIV-1 RNA <400 copies/mL) but did not consent to continue study after Week 48 or Week 96 were excluded from analysis.
† Subjects achieved and maintained confirmed HIV-1 RNA <400 copies/mL through Weeks 48 and 144.
‡ Includes confirmed viral rebound and failure to achieve confirmed <400 copies/mL through Weeks 48 and 144.
§ Includes lost to follow-up, subject withdrawal, noncompliance, protocol violation and other reasons.

ing from 0.6 to 6.9-fold that of wild type virus. An HBV strain expressing rtL180M, rtT184G, rtS202I and rtM204V together had a 6.9-fold reduction in susceptibility to tenofovir.
HBV strains expressing the adefovir resistance-associated substitutions rtA181V and/or rtN236T showed reductions in susceptibility to tenofovir ranging from 2.9 to 10-fold that of wild type virus.
Strains containing the rtA181T substitution showed changes in susceptibility to tenofovir ranging from 0.9 to 1.5-fold that of wild type virus.

13 NONCLINICAL TOXICOLOGY
13.1 Carcinogenesis, Mutagenesis, Impairment of Fertility
Long-term oral carcinogenicity studies of tenofovir disoproxil fumarate in mice and rats were carried out at exposures up to approximately 16 times (mice) and 5 times (rats) those observed in humans at the therapeutic dose for HIV-1 infection. At the high dose in female mice, liver adenomas were increased at exposures 16 times that in humans. In rats, the study was negative for carcinogenic findings at exposures up to 5 times that observed in humans at the therapeutic dose.
Tenofovir disoproxil fumarate was mutagenic in the in vitro mouse lymphoma assay and negative in an in vitro bacterial mutagenicity test (Ames test). In an in vivo mouse micronucleus assay, tenofovir disoproxil fumarate was negative when administered to male mice.
There were no effects on fertility, mating performance or early embryonic development when tenofovir disoproxil fumarate was administered to male rats at a dose equivalent to 10 times the human dose based on body surface area comparisons for 28 days prior to mating and to female rats

for 15 days prior to mating through day seven of gestation. There was, however, an alteration of the estrous cycle in female rats.

13.2 Animal Toxicology and/or Pharmacology
Tenofovir and tenofovir disoproxil fumarate administered in toxicology studies to rats, dogs, and monkeys at exposures (based on AUCs) greater than or equal to 6 fold those observed in humans caused bone toxicity. In monkeys the bone toxicity was diagnosed as osteomalacia. Osteomalacia observed in monkeys appeared to be reversible upon dose reduction or discontinuation of tenofovir. In rats and dogs, the bone toxicity manifested as reduced bone mineral density. The mechanism(s) underlying bone toxicity is unknown.
Evidence of renal toxicity was noted in 4 animal species. Increases in serum creatinine, BUN, glycosuria, proteinuria, phosphaturia, and/or calciuria and decreases in serum phosphate were observed to varying degrees in these animals. These toxicities were noted at exposures (based on AUCs) 2–20 times higher than those observed in humans. The relationship of the renal abnormalities, particularly the phosphaturia, to the bone toxicity is not known.

14 CLINICAL STUDIES
14.1 Clinical Efficacy in Patients with HIV-1 Infection
Treatment-Naïve Adult Patients
Study 903
Data through 144 weeks are reported for Study 903, a double-blind, active-controlled multicenter study comparing VIREAD (300 mg once daily) administered in combination with lamivudine and efavirenz versus stavudine (d4T), lamivudine, and efavirenz in 600 antiretroviral-naïve subjects. Subjects had a mean age of 36 years (range 18–64), 74% were male, 64% were Caucasian and 20% were Black. The mean baseline CD4+ cell count was 279 cells/mm3

(range 3–956) and median baseline plasma HIV-1 RNA was 77,600 copies/mL (range 417–5,130,000). Subjects were stratified by baseline HIV-1 RNA and CD4+ cell count. Forty-three percent of subjects had baseline viral loads >100,000 copies/mL and 39% had CD4+ cell counts <200 cells/mm3. Treatment outcomes through 48 and 144 weeks are presented in Table 14.
[See table 14 at left]
Achievement of plasma HIV-1 RNA concentrations of less than 400 copies/mL at Week 144 was similar between the two treatment groups for the population stratified at baseline on the basis of HIV-1 RNA concentration (> or ≤100,000 copies/mL) and CD4+ cell count (< or ≥200 cells/mm3). Through 144 weeks of therapy, 62% and 58% of subjects in the VIREAD and stavudine arms, respectively achieved and maintained confirmed HIV-1 RNA <50 copies/mL. The mean increase from baseline in CD4+ cell count was 263 cells/mm3 for the VIREAD arm and 283 cells/mm3 for the stavudine arm.
Through 144 weeks, 11 subjects in the VIREAD group and 9 subjects in the stavudine group experienced a new CDC Class C event.
Study 934
Data through 144 weeks are reported for Study 934, a randomized, open-label, active-controlled multicenter study comparing emtricitabine + VIREAD administered in combination with efavirenz versus zidovudine/lamivudine fixed-dose combination administered in combination with efavirenz in 511 antiretroviral-naïve subjects. From Weeks 96 to 144 of the study, subjects received a fixed-dose combination of emtricitabine and tenofovir DF with efavirenz in place of emtricitabine + VIREAD with efavirenz. Subjects had a mean age of 38 years (range 18–80), 86% were male, 59% were Caucasian and 23% were Black. The mean baseline CD4+ cell count was 245 cells/mm3 (range 2–1191) and median baseline plasma HIV-1 RNA was 5.01 log10 copies/mL (range 3.56–6.54). Subjects were stratified by baseline CD4+ cell count (< or ≥200 cells/mm3); 41% had CD4+ cell counts <200 cells/mm3 and 51% of subjects had baseline viral loads >100,000 copies/mL. Treatment outcomes through 48 and 144 weeks for those subjects who did not have efavirenz resistance at baseline are presented in Table 15.
[See table 15 at left]
Through Week 48, 84% and 73% of subjects in the emtricitabine + VIREAD group and the zidovudine/lamivudine group, respectively, achieved and maintained HIV-1 RNA <400 copies/mL (71% and 58% through Week 144). The difference in the proportion of subjects who achieved and maintained HIV-1 RNA <400 copies/mL through 48 weeks largely results from the higher number of discontinuations due to adverse events and other reasons in the zidovudine/lamivudine group in this open-label study. In addition, 80% and 70% of subjects in the emtricitabine + VIREAD group and the zidovudine/lamivudine group, respectively, achieved and maintained HIV-1 RNA <50 copies/mL through Week 48 (64% and 56% through Week 144). The mean increase from baseline in CD4+ cell count was 190 cells/mm3 in the EMTRIVA + VIREAD group and 158 cells/mm3 in the zidovudine/lamivudine group at Week 48 (312 and 271 cells/mm3 at Week 144).
Through 48 weeks, 7 subjects in the emtricitabine + VIREAD group and 5 subjects in the zidovudine/lamivudine group experienced a new CDC Class C event (10 and 6 subjects through 144 weeks).
Treatment-Experienced Adult Patients
Study 907
Study 907 was a 24-week, double-blind placebo-controlled multicenter study of VIREAD added to a stable background regimen of antiretroviral agents in 550 treatment-experienced subjects. After 24 weeks of blinded study treatment, all subjects continuing on study were offered open-label VIREAD for an additional 24 weeks. Subjects had a mean baseline CD4+ cell count of 427 cells/mm3 (range 23–1385), median baseline plasma HIV-1 RNA of 2340 (range 50–75,000) copies/mL, and mean duration of prior HIV-1 treatment was 5.4 years. Mean age of the subjects was 42 years, 85% were male and 69% were Caucasian, 17% Black and 12% Hispanic.
Changes from baseline in log10 copies/mL plasma HIV-1 RNA levels over time up to Week 48 are presented below in Figure 1.
[See figure 1 at top of next column]
The percent of subjects with HIV-1 RNA <400 copies/mL and outcomes of subjects through 48 weeks are summarized in Table 16.
[See table 16 at top of next page]
At 24 weeks of therapy, there was a higher proportion of subjects in the VIREAD arm compared to the placebo arm with HIV-1 RNA <50 copies/mL (19% and 1%, respectively). Mean change in absolute CD4+ cell counts by Week 24 was +11 cells/mm3 for the VIREAD group and -5 cells/mm3 for the placebo group. Mean change in absolute CD4+ cell counts by Week 48 was +4 cells/mm3 for the VIREAD group.

Figure 1 Mean Change from Baseline in Plasma HIV-1 RNA (log₁₀ copies/mL) Through Week 48 (Study 907; All Available Data)†

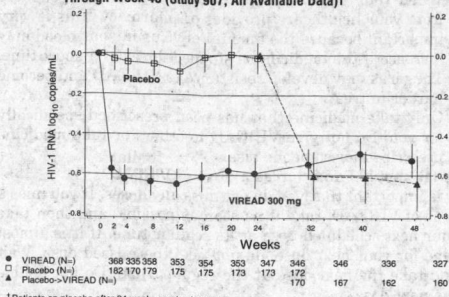

VIREAD (N=)	368 335 358	353	354	353	347	346	346	336	327
Placebo (N=)	182 170 179	175	175	173	173	172			
Placebo->VIREAD (N=)						170	167	162	160

† Patients on placebo after 24 weeks received VIREAD.

Through Week 24, one subject in the VIREAD group and no subjects in the placebo arm experienced a new CDC Class C event.

14.2 Clinical Efficacy in Patients with Chronic Hepatitis B

HBeAg-Negative Chronic Hepatitis B

Study 0102 was a Phase 3, randomized, double-blind, active-controlled study of VIREAD 300 mg compared to HEPSERA 10 mg in 375 HBeAg- (anti-HBe+) subjects with compensated liver function, the majority of whom were nucleoside-naïve. The mean age of subjects was 44 years, 77% were male, 25% were Asian, 65% were Caucasian, 17% had previously received alpha-interferon therapy and 18% were nucleoside-experienced (16% had prior lamivudine experience). At baseline, subjects had a mean Knodell necroinflammatory score of 7.8; mean plasma HBV DNA was 6.9 log₁₀ copies/mL; and mean serum ALT was 140 U/L.

HBeAg-Positive Chronic Hepatitis B

Study 0103 was a Phase 3, randomized, double-blind, active-controlled study of VIREAD 300 mg compared to HEPSERA 10 mg in 266 HBeAg+ nucleoside-naïve subjects with compensated liver function. The mean age of subjects was 34 years, 69% were male, 36% were Asian, 52% were Caucasian, 16% had previously received alpha-interferon therapy, and <5% were nucleoside experienced. At baseline, subjects had a mean Knodell necroinflammatory score of 8.4; mean plasma HBV DNA was 8.7 log₁₀ copies /mL; and mean serum ALT was 147 U/L.

The primary data analysis was conducted after all subjects reached 48 weeks of treatment and results are summarized below.

The primary efficacy endpoint in both studies was complete response to treatment defined as HBV DNA <400 copies/mL and Knodell necroinflammatory score improvement of at least 2 points, without worsening in Knodell fibrosis at Week 48 (Table 17).

[See table 17 at right]

Treatment beyond 48 Weeks

In Studies 0102 (HBeAg-negative) and 0103 (HBeAg-positive), subjects rolled over with no interruption in treatment to open-label VIREAD through Week 96 after receiving double-blind treatment for 48 weeks (either VIREAD or HEPSERA). At Week 72 or thereafter, emtricitabine could be added to VIREAD in subjects who had detectable HBV DNA.

In Study 0102, 90% of subjects who were randomized to VIREAD completed 96 weeks of treatment. Among subjects randomized to VIREAD followed by open-label treatment with VIREAD, 89% had undetectable HBV DNA (< 400 copies/mL), and 71% had ALT normalization at Week 96. In the group of subjects randomized to HEPSERA followed by open-label treatment with VIREAD, 88% completed 96 weeks of treatment; 96% of this cohort had undetectable HBV DNA (< 400 copies/mL) and 71% had ALT normalization at Week 96. Emtricitabine was added to VIREAD in 2 (<1%) subjects initially randomized to VIREAD and none of those randomized to HEPSERA. No subject in either treatment group experienced HBsAg loss/seroconversion through Week 96.

In Study 0103, 82% of subjects randomized to VIREAD completed 96 weeks of treatment. Among subjects randomized to VIREAD, 81% had undetectable HBV DNA (< 400 copies/mL), 64% had ALT normalization, 27% had HBeAg loss (23% seroconversion to anti-HBe antibody), and 5% had HBsAg loss (4% seroconversion to anti-HBs antibody) through Week 96. Among subjects randomized to HEPSERA followed by up to 48 weeks of open-label treatment with VIREAD, 92% of subjects completed 96 weeks of treatment; 76% had undetectable HBV DNA (< 400 copies/mL), 67% had ALT normalization, 24% had HBeAg loss (21% seroconversion to anti-HBe antibody), and 6% experienced HBsAg loss (5% seroconversion to anti-HBs antibody) through Week 96. Emtricitabine was added to VIREAD in 15 (9%) subjects randomized to VIREAD, and in 13 (14%) subjects randomized to HEPSERA.

Table 16 Outcomes of Randomized Treatment (Study 907)

| Outcomes | 0–24 weeks | | 0–48 weeks | 24–48 weeks |
	VIREAD (N=368)	Placebo (N=182)	VIREAD (N=368)	Placebo Crossover to VIREAD (N=170)
HIV-1 RNA <400 copies/mL*	40%	11%	28%	30%
Virologic failure†	53%	84%	61%	64%
Discontinued due to adverse event	3%	3%	5%	5%
Discontinued for other reasons‡	3%	3%	5%	1%

* Subjects with HIV-1 RNA <400 copies/mL and no prior study drug discontinuation at Week 24 and 48 respectively.
† Subjects with HIV-1 RNA ≥400 copies/mL efficacy failure or missing HIV-1 RNA at Week 24 and 48 respectively.
‡ Includes lost to follow-up, subject withdrawal, noncompliance, protocol violation and other reasons.

Table 17 Histological, Virological, Biochemical, and Serological Response at Week 48

| | 0102 (HBeAg-) | | 0103 (HBeAg+) | |
	VIREAD (N=250)	HEPSERA (N=125)	VIREAD (N=176)	HEPSERA (N=90)
Complete Response	71%	49%	67%	12%
Histology Histological Response*	72%	69%	74%	68%
HBV DNA <400 copies/mL (<69 IU/mL)	93%	63%	76%	13%
ALT Normalized ALT†	76%	77%	68%	54%
Serology HBeAg Loss/Seroconversion	NA‡	NA‡	20%/19%	16%/16%
HBsAg Loss/Seroconversion	0/0	0/0	3%/1%	0/0

* Knodell necroinflammatory score improvement of at least 2 points without worsening in Knodell fibrosis.
† The population used for analysis of ALT normalization included only subjects with ALT above ULN at baseline.
‡ NA = Not Applicable

Across the combined HBV treatment studies, the number of subjects with lamivudine- or adefovir-resistance associated substitutions at baseline was too small to establish efficacy in this subgroup.

16 HOW SUPPLIED/STORAGE AND HANDLING

The almond-shaped, light blue, film-coated tablets contain 300 mg of tenofovir disoproxil fumarate, which is equivalent to 245 mg of tenofovir disoproxil, are debossed with "GILEAD" and "4331" on one side and with "300" on the other side, and are available in unit of use bottles (containing a desiccant [silica gel canister or sachet] and closed with a child-resistant closure) of:

• 30 tablets (NDC 61958–0401–1)

Store at 25 °C (77 °F), excursions permitted to 15–30 °C (59–86 °F) (see USP Controlled Room Temperature).

Do not use if seal over bottle opening is broken or missing.

17 PATIENT COUNSELING INFORMATION AND FDA-APPROVED PATIENT LABELING

Information for Patients

Patients should be advised that:

• VIREAD is not a cure for HIV-1 infection and patients may continue to experience illnesses associated with HIV-1 infection, including opportunistic infections. Patients should remain under the care of a physician when using VIREAD.

• The use of VIREAD has not been shown to reduce the risk of transmission of HIV-1 or HBV to others through sexual contact or blood contamination. Patients should be advised to continue to practice safer sex and to use latex or polyurethane condoms to lower the chance of sexual contact with any body fluids such as semen, vaginal secretions or blood. Patients should be advised never to re-use or share needles.

• The long term effects of VIREAD are unknown.

• VIREAD Tablets are for oral ingestion only.

• VIREAD should not be discontinued without first informing their physician.

• If you have HIV-1 infection, with or without HBV coinfection, it is important to take VIREAD with combination therapy.

• It is important to take VIREAD on a regular dosing schedule and to avoid missing doses.

• Lactic acidosis and severe hepatomegaly with steatosis, including fatal cases, have been reported. Treatment with

VIREAD should be suspended in any patient who develops clinical symptoms suggestive of lactic acidosis or pronounced hepatotoxicity (including nausea, vomiting, unusual or unexpected stomach discomfort, and weakness) *[See Warnings and Precautions (5.1)].*

• Patients with HIV-1 should be tested for Hepatitis B virus (HBV) before initiating antiretroviral therapy *[See Warnings and Precautions (5.5)].*

• Severe acute exacerbations of hepatitis have been reported in patients who are infected with HBV and have discontinued VIREAD *[See Warnings and Precautions (5.2)].*

• In patients with chronic hepatitis B, it is important to obtain HIV antibody testing prior to initiating VIREAD *[See Warnings and Precautions (5.5)].*

• Renal impairment, including cases of acute renal failure and Fanconi syndrome, has been reported. VIREAD should be avoided with concurrent or recent use of a nephrotoxic agent *[See Warnings and Precautions (5.3)].* Dosing interval of VIREAD may need adjustment in patients with renal impairment *[See Dosage and Administration (2.3)].*

• VIREAD should not be coadministered with the fixed-dose combination products TRUVADA and ATRIPLA since it is a component of these products *[See Warnings and Precautions (5.4)].*

• VIREAD should not be administered in combination with HEPSERA *[See Warnings and Precautions (5.4)].*

• Decreases in bone mineral density have been observed with the use of VIREAD in patients with HIV. Bone mineral density monitoring should be considered in patients who have a history of pathologic bone fracture or at risk for osteopenia *[See Warnings and Precautions (5.6)].*

• In the treatment of chronic hepatitis B, the optimal duration of treatment is unknown. The relationship between response and long-term prevention of outcomes such as hepatocellular carcinoma is not known.

FDA-APPROVED PATIENT LABELING

VIREAD® (VEER ee ad) Tablets

Generic Name: tenofovir disoproxil fumarate (te NOF fo veer dye soe PROX il FYOU-mar-ate)

Read this leaflet carefully before you start taking VIREAD. Also, read it each time you get your VIREAD prescription refilled, in case something has changed. This information does not take the place of talking with your healthcare provider when you start this medicine and at check ups. You should stay under a healthcare provider's care when taking VIREAD. Do not change or stop your medicine without first talking with your healthcare provider. Talk to your healthcare provider if you have any questions about VIREAD.

What is the most important information I should know about VIREAD?

• **Some people who have taken medicine like VIREAD (nucleoside analogs) have developed a serious condition called lactic acidosis** (build up of an acid in the blood). Lactic acidosis can be a medical emergency and may need to be treated in the hospital. **Call your healthcare provider right away if you get the following signs or symptoms of lactic acidosis.**
  • You feel very weak or tired.
  • You have unusual (not normal) muscle pain.
  • You have trouble breathing.
  • You have stomach pain with nausea and vomiting.
  • You feel cold, especially in your arms and legs.
  • You feel dizzy or lightheaded.
  • You have a fast or irregular heartbeat.
• **Some people who have taken medicines like VIREAD have developed serious liver problems called hepatotoxicity,** with liver enlargement (hepatomegaly) and fat in the liver (steatosis). **Call your healthcare provider right away if you get the following signs or symptoms of liver problems.**
  • Your skin or the white part of your eyes turns yellow (jaundice).
  • Your urine turns dark.
  • Your bowel movements (stools) turn light in color.
  • You don't feel like eating food for several days or longer.
  • You feel sick to your stomach (nausea).
  • You have lower stomach area (abdominal) pain.
• **You may be more likely to get lactic acidosis or liver problems** if you are female, very overweight (obese), or have been taking nucleoside analog medicines, like VIREAD, for a long time.

If you are infected with the Hepatitis B Virus (HBV), you need close medical follow-up for several months after stopping treatment with VIREAD. Follow-up includes medical exams and blood tests to check for HBV that could be getting worse. **Patients with Hepatitis B Virus infection, who take VIREAD and then stop it, may get "flare-ups" of their hepatitis. A "flare-up" is when the disease suddenly returns in a worse way than before.**

What is VIREAD and how does it work?
VIREAD is a type of medicine called an HIV nucleotide analog reverse transcriptase inhibitor (NRTI) and an HBV polymerase inhibitor.

Use in the Treatment of HIV-1 Infection:
VIREAD is a treatment for Human Immunodeficiency Virus (HIV) infection in adults and adolescents age 12 years and older and weighing at least 35 kg (77 lb). VIREAD is always used in combination with other anti-HIV-1 medicines to treat people with HIV-1 infection.
HIV infection destroys CD4+ T cells, which are important to the immune system. After a large number of T cells are destroyed, acquired immune deficiency syndrome (AIDS) develops.
VIREAD helps to block HIV-1 reverse transcriptase, a chemical in your body (enzyme) that is needed for HIV-1 to multiply. VIREAD lowers the amount of HIV-1 in the blood (called viral load) and may help to increase the number of T cells (called CD4+ cells). Lowering the amount of HIV-1 in the blood lowers the chance of death or infections that happen when your immune system is weak (opportunistic infections).

Use in the Treatment of Chronic Hepatitis B:
VIREAD is also used to treat chronic hepatitis B (an infection with hepatitis B virus [HBV]) in adults age 18 years and older. VIREAD works by interfering with the normal working of an enzyme (HBV DNA polymerase) that is essential for the HBV virus to reproduce itself. VIREAD may help lower the amount of hepatitis B virus in your body by lowering the ability of the virus to multiply and infect new liver cells.
We do not know how long VIREAD may help your hepatitis. Sometimes viruses change in your body and medicines no longer work. This is called drug resistance.
Viread may improve the condition of your liver; but we do not know if VIREAD will reduce your chances of getting liver damage (cirrhosis) or liver cancer from chronic hepatitis B.

Does VIREAD cure HIV-1 or AIDS?
VIREAD does not cure HIV-1 infection or AIDS. The long-term effects of VIREAD are not known at this time. People taking VIREAD may still get opportunistic infections or other conditions that happen with HIV-1 infection. Opportunistic infections are infections that develop because the

immune system is weak. Some of these conditions are pneumonia, herpes virus infections, and *Mycobacterium avium* complex (MAC) infections.

Does VIREAD reduce the risk of passing HIV-1 or HBV to others?
VIREAD does not reduce the risk of passing HIV-1 or HBV to others through sexual contact or blood contamination. Continue to practice safe sex and do not use or share dirty needles. Do not share personal items that can have blood or body fluids on them like toothbrushes or razor blades. A shot (vaccine) is available to protect people at risk for becoming infected with HBV.

Who should not take VIREAD?
Together with your healthcare provider, you need to decide whether VIREAD is right for you.
Do not take VIREAD if
• you are allergic to VIREAD or any of its ingredients
• you are already taking TRUVADA® or ATRIPLA® because VIREAD is one of the active ingredients in TRUVADA and ATRIPLA
• you are currently taking HEPSERA®

What should I tell my healthcare provider before taking VIREAD?
Tell your healthcare provider
• *If you are pregnant or planning to become pregnant:* The effects of VIREAD on pregnant women or their unborn babies are not known. You and your healthcare provider will need to decide if VIREAD is right for you. If you use VIREAD while you are pregnant, talk to your healthcare provider about how you can be on the VIREAD Antiviral Pregnancy Registry.
• *If you are breast-feeding:* You should not breastfeed if you are taking VIREAD. It is not known whether VIREAD is passed to the infant in breast milk; and whether it could harm your baby. Do not breast-feed if you have HIV. If your baby does not already have HIV, there is a chance that the baby can get HIV through breast-feeding. Talk with your healthcare provider about the best way to feed your baby.
• If you have kidney or bone problems
• If you have liver problems including Hepatitis B Virus infection
• If you have HIV-1 Infection
• Tell your healthcare provider about all your medical conditions

TELL YOUR HEALTHCARE PROVIDER ABOUT ALL THE MEDICINES YOU TAKE, INCLUDING PRESCRIPTION AND NON-PRESCRIPTION MEDICINES AND DIETARY SUPPLEMENTS. ESPECIALLY TELL YOUR HEALTHCARE PROVIDER IF YOU TAKE:
• VIDEX, VIDEX EC (DIDANOSINE). VIREAD MAY INCREASE THE AMOUNT OF VIDEX IN YOUR BLOOD. YOU MAY NEED TO BE FOLLOWED MORE CAREFULLY IF YOU ARE TAKING VIDEX AND VIREAD TOGETHER. IF YOU ARE TAKING VIDEX AND VIREAD TOGETHER YOUR HEALTHCARE PROVIDER MAY NEED TO REDUCE YOUR DOSE OF VIDEX.
• REYATAZ (ATAZANAVIR SULFATE) OR KALETRA (LOPINAVIR/RITONAVIR). THESE MEDICINES MAY INCREASE THE AMOUNT OF VIREAD IN YOUR BLOOD, WHICH COULD RESULT IN MORE SIDE EFFECTS. YOU MAY NEED TO BE FOLLOWED MORE CAREFULLY IF YOU ARE TAKING VIREAD AND REYATAZ OR KALETRA TOGETHER. VIREAD MAY DECREASE THE AMOUNT OF REYATAZ IN YOUR BLOOD. IF YOU ARE TAKING VIREAD AND REYATAZ TOGETHER YOU SHOULD ALSO BE TAKING NORVIR (RITONAVIR).
KEEP A COMPLETE LIST OF ALL THE MEDICINES THAT YOU TAKE. MAKE A NEW LIST WHEN MEDICINES ARE ADDED OR STOPPED. GIVE COPIES OF THIS LIST TO ALL OF YOUR HEALTHCARE PROVIDERS **EVERY** TIME YOU VISIT YOUR HEALTHCARE PROVIDER OR FILL A PRESCRIPTION.

How should I take VIREAD?
• Stay under a healthcare provider's care when taking VIREAD. Do not change your treatment or stop treatment without first talking with your healthcare provider.
• Take VIREAD exactly as your healthcare provider prescribed it. Follow the directions from your healthcare provider, exactly as written on the label. Set up a dosing schedule and follow it carefully.
• If you are taking VIREAD to treat your HIV or if you have both HIV and HBV infection and are taking VIREAD, always take VIREAD in combination with other anti-HIV medicines. VIREAD and other products like VIREAD may be less likely to work in the future if you are not taking VIREAD with other anti-HIV medicines because you may develop resistance to those medicines.
• Talk to your doctor about taking an HIV test before you start treatment with VIREAD for chronic hepatitis B.
• The usual dose of VIREAD is 1 tablet once a day. If you have kidney problems, your healthcare provider may recommend that you take VIREAD less frequently.

• VIREAD may be taken with or without a meal.
• When your VIREAD supply starts to run low, get more from your healthcare provider or pharmacy. This is very important because the amount of virus in your blood may increase if the medicine is stopped for even a short time. The virus may develop resistance to VIREAD and become harder to treat.
• Only take medicine that has been prescribed specifically for you. Do not give VIREAD to others or take medicine prescribed for someone else.

What should I do if I miss a dose of VIREAD?
It is important that you do not miss any doses. If you miss a dose of VIREAD, take it as soon as possible and then take your next scheduled dose at its regular time. If it is almost time for your next dose, do not take the missed dose. Wait and take the next dose at the regular time. Do not double the next dose.

What happens if I take too much VIREAD?
If you suspect that you took more than the prescribed dose of VIREAD, contact your local poison control center or emergency room right away.
As with all medicines, VIREAD should be kept out of reach of children.

What should I avoid while taking VIREAD?
• Do not breast-feed. See "What should I tell my healthcare provider before taking VIREAD?"

What are the possible side effects of VIREAD? (see also "What is the most important information I should know about VIREAD")
• Clinical studies in patients with HIV-1: The most common side effects of VIREAD are: rash, headache, pain, diarrhea, depression, weakness, and nausea. Less common side effects include vomiting, dizziness, and intestinal gas.
  Clinical studies in patients with chronic hepatitis B: The most common side effect of VIREAD is nausea. Less common side effects include abdominal pain, diarrhea, headache, dizziness, fatigue, common cold symptoms such as sore throat and runny nose, back pain, and skin rash.
• Marketing experience: Other side effects reported since VIREAD has been marketed include: lactic acidosis, kidney problems (including decline or failure of kidney function), inflammation of the pancreas, inflammation of the liver, allergic reactions (including itching, or swelling of the face, lips, tongue or throat), shortness of breath, stomach pain, and high volume of urine and thirst caused by kidney problems. Muscle pain and muscle weakness, bone pain, and softening of the bone (which may contribute to fractures) as a consequence of kidney problems have been reported.
• Some patients treated with VIREAD have had kidney problems. If you have had kidney problems in the past or need to take another drug that can cause kidney problems, your healthcare provider may need to perform additional blood tests.
• Laboratory tests show changes in the bones of patients treated with VIREAD. Some HIV patients treated with VIREAD developed thinning of the bones (osteopenia) which could lead to fractures. If you have had bone problems in the past, your healthcare provider may need to perform additional tests or may suggest additional medication. Additionally, bone pain and softening of the bone (which may contribute to fractures) may occur as a consequence of kidney problems.
• Changes in body fat have been seen in some patients taking anti-HIV-1 medicine. These changes may include increased amount of fat in the upper back and neck ("buffalo hump"), breast, and around the main part of your body (trunk). Loss of fat from the legs, arms and face may also happen. The cause and long term health effects of these conditions are not known at this time.
• In some patients with advanced HIV infection (AIDS), signs and symptoms of inflammation from previous infections may occur soon after anti-HIV treatment is started. It is believed that these symptoms are due to an improvement in the body's immune response, enabling the body to fight infections that may have been present with no obvious symptoms. If you notice any symptoms of infection, please inform your doctor immediately.
• After stopping treatment with VIREAD, some patients with HBV have had symptoms or blood tests showing that their hepatitis has gotten worse ("flare-ups"). Therefore, your doctor should check your health, which may include blood tests, for at least several months after stopping treatment with VIREAD. Tell your doctor right away about any new or unusual symptoms that you notice after stopping treatment.
• If you have HBV infection or HIV and HBV infection together, you may have a "flare-up" of Hepatitis B, in which the disease suddenly returns in a worse way than before if you stop taking VIREAD. Do not stop taking VIREAD without your doctor's advice. After stopping VIREAD, tell your doctor immediately about any new, unusual, or worsening symptoms that you notice after stopping treatment.

After you stop taking VIREAD, your doctor will still need to check your health and take blood tests to check your liver for several months.

- There have been other side effects in patients taking VIREAD. However, these side effects may have been due to other medicines that patients were taking or to the illness itself. Some of these side effects can be serious.
- This list of side effects is **not** complete. If you have questions about side effects, ask your healthcare provider. You should report any new or continuing symptoms to your healthcare provider right away. Your healthcare provider may be able to help you manage these side effects.

How do I store VIREAD?

- Keep VIREAD and all other medications out of reach of children.
- Store VIREAD at room temperature 77 °F (25 °C). It should remain stable until the expiration date printed on the label.
- Do not keep your medicine in places that are too hot or cold.
- Do not keep medicine that is out of date or that you no longer need. If you throw any medicines away make sure that children will not find them.

General advice about prescription medicines:
TALK TO YOUR HEALTHCARE PROVIDER IF YOU HAVE ANY QUESTIONS ABOUT THIS MEDICINE OR YOUR CONDITION. MEDICINES ARE SOMETIMES PRESCRIBED FOR PURPOSES OTHER THAN THOSE LISTED IN A PATIENT INFORMATION LEAFLET. IF YOU HAVE ANY CONCERNS ABOUT THIS MEDICINE, ASK YOUR HEALTHCARE PROVIDER. YOUR HEALTH-CARE PROVIDER OR PHARMACIST CAN GIVE YOU IN-FORMATION ABOUT THIS MEDICINE THAT WAS WRITTEN FOR HEALTH CARE PROFESSIONALS. DO NOT USE THIS MEDICINE FOR A CONDITION FOR WHICH IT WAS NOT PRESCRIBED. DO NOT SHARE THIS MEDICINE WITH OTHER PEOPLE.
DO NOT USE IF SEAL OVER BOTTLE OPENING IS BROKEN OR MISSING.

What are the ingredients of VIREAD?
Active Ingredient: tenofovir disoproxil fumarate
Inactive Ingredients: croscarmellose sodium, lactose monohydrate, magnesium stearate, microcrystalline cellulose, and pregelatinized starch. The tablets are coated with Opadry II Y–30–10671–A, which contains FD&C blue #2 aluminum lake, hydroxypropyl methylcellulose 2910, lactose monohydrate, titanium dioxide, and triacetin.
March 2010
VIREAD, EMTRIVA, HEPSERA and TRUVADA are registered trademarks of Gilead Sciences, Inc. ATRIPLA is a trademark of Bristol-Myers Squibb & Gilead Sciences, LLC. All other trademarks referenced herein are the property of their respective owners.
21-356-GS-025 24032010
Shown in Product Identification Guide, page 309

GlaxoSmithKline
FIVE MOORE DRIVE
RESEARCH TRIANGLE PARK, NC 27709

For all inquiries, including adverse event and quality assurance reporting, contact the GSK Response Center at 1-888-825-5249.
For updates to the product information listed below, also consult www.gsk.com.

ADVAIR DISKUS™ 100/50   ℞
[ad' vair disk' us]
(fluticasone propionate 100mcg and salmeterol 50 mcg inhalation powder)

ADVAIR DISKUS™ 250/50
(fluticasone propionate 250 mcg and salmeterol 50 mcg inhalation powder)

ADVAIR DISKUS™ 500/50
(fluticasone propionate 500 mcg and salmeterol 50 mcg inhalation powder)
FOR ORAL INHALATION

HIGHLIGHTS OF PRESCRIBING INFORMATION
These highlights do not include all the information needed to use ADVAIR DISKUS safely and effectively. See full prescribing information for ADVAIR DISKUS.
ADVAIR DISKUS 100/50
(fluticasone propionate 100 mcg and salmeterol 50 mcg inhalation powder)
ADVAIR DISKUS 250/50
(fluticasone propionate 250 mcg and salmeterol 50 mcg inhalation powder)

ADVAIR DISKUS 500/50
(fluticasone propionate 500 mcg and salmeterol 50 mcg inhalation powder)
FOR ORAL INHALATION
Initial U.S. Approval: 2000

WARNING: ASTHMA-RELATED DEATH
See full prescribing information for complete boxed warning.

- **Long-acting beta₂-adrenergic agonists (LABAs), such as salmeterol, one of the active ingredients in ADVAIR DISKUS, increase the risk of asthma-related death.** A US study showed an increase in asthma-related deaths in patients receiving salmeterol (13 deaths out of 13,176 patients treated for 28 weeks on salmeterol versus 3 out of 13,179 patients on placebo). Currently available data are inadequate to determine whether concurrent use of inhaled corticosteroids or other long-term asthma control drugs mitigates the increased risk of asthma-related death from LABAs. Available data from controlled clinical trials suggest that LABAs increase the risk of asthma-related hospitalization in pediatric and adolescent patients. (5.1)
- **When treating patients with asthma, only prescribe ADVAIR DISKUS for patients not adequately controlled on a long-term asthma control medication, such as an inhaled corticosteroid, or whose disease severity clearly warrants initiation of treatment with both an inhaled corticosteroid and a LABA. Once asthma control is achieved and maintained, assess the patient at regular intervals and step down therapy (e.g., discontinue ADVAIR DISKUS) if possible without loss of asthma control and maintain the patient on a long-term asthma control medication, such as an inhaled corticosteroid. Do not use ADVAIR DISKUS for patients whose asthma is adequately controlled on low- or medium-dose inhaled corticosteroids. (1.1, 5.1)**

INDICATIONS AND USAGE
ADVAIR DISKUS is a combination product containing a corticosteroid and a LABA indicated for:
- Treatment of asthma in patients aged 4 years and older. (1.1)
- Maintenance treatment of airflow obstruction and reducing exacerbations in patients with chronic obstructive pulmonary disease (COPD). (1.2)
Important limitation:
- Not indicated for the relief of acute bronchospasm. (1.1, 1.2)

DOSAGE AND ADMINISTRATION
For oral inhalation only.
- Treatment of asthma in patients ≥12 years: 1 inhalation of ADVAIR DISKUS 100/50, 250/50, or 500/50 twice daily. Starting dosage is based on asthma severity. (2.1)
- Treatment of asthma in patients aged 4 to 11 years: 1 inhalation of ADVAIR DISKUS 100/50 twice daily. (2.1)
- Maintenance treatment of COPD: 1 inhalation of ADVAIR DISKUS 250/50 twice daily. (2.2)

DOSAGE FORMS AND STRENGTHS
DISKUS device containing a combination of fluticasone propionate (100, 250, or 500 mcg) and salmeterol (50 mcg) as an oral inhalation powder. (3)

CONTRAINDICATIONS
- Primary treatment of status asthmaticus or acute episodes of asthma or COPD requiring intensive measures. (4)
- Severe hypersensitivity to milk proteins. (4)

WARNINGS AND PRECAUTIONS
- Asthma-related death: LABAs increase the risk. Prescribe only for recommended patient populations. (5.1)
- Deterioration of disease and acute episodes: Do not initiate in acutely deteriorating asthma or to treat acute symptoms. (5.2)
- Use with additional LABA: Do not use in combination because of risk of overdose. (5.3)
- Localized infections: *Candida albicans* infection of the mouth and throat may occur. Monitor patients periodically for signs of adverse effects on the oral cavity. Advise patients to rinse the mouth following inhalation. (5.4)

- Pneumonia: Increased risk in patients with COPD. Monitor patients for signs and symptoms of pneumonia. (5.5)
- Immunosuppression: Potential worsening of infections (e.g., existing tuberculosis, fungal, bacterial, viral, or parasitic infection; or ocular herpes simplex). Use with caution in patients with these infections. More serious or even fatal course of chickenpox or measles can occur in susceptible patients. (5.6)
- Transferring patients from systemic corticosteroids: Risk of impaired adrenal function when transferring from oral steroids. Taper patients slowly from systemic corticosteroids if transferring to ADVAIR DISKUS. (5.7)
- Hypercorticism and adrenal suppression: May occur with very high dosages or at the regular dosage in susceptible individuals. If such changes occur, discontinue ADVAIR DISKUS slowly. (5.8)
- Strong cytochrome P450 3A4 inhibitors (e.g., ritonavir): Risk of increased systemic corticosteroid and cardiovascular effects. Use not recommended with ADVAIR DISKUS. (5.9)
- Paradoxical bronchospasm: Discontinue ADVAIR DISKUS and institute alternative therapy if paradoxical bronchospasm occurs. (5.10)
- Patients with cardiovascular or central nervous system disorders: Use with caution because of beta-adrenergic stimulation. (5.12)
- Decreases in bone mineral density: Assess bone mineral density initially and periodically thereafter. (5.13)
- Effects on growth: Monitor growth of pediatric patients. (5.14)
- Glaucoma and cataracts: Close monitoring is warranted. (5.15)
- Metabolic effects: Be alert to eosinophilic conditions, hypokalemia, and hyperglycemia. (5.16, 5.18)
- Coexisting conditions: Use with caution in patients with convulsive disorders, thyrotoxicosis, diabetes mellitus, and ketoacidosis. (5.17)

ADVERSE REACTIONS
Most common adverse reactions (incidence ≥3%) are:
- Asthma: upper respiratory tract infection or inflammation, pharyngitis, dysphonia, oral candidiasis, bronchitis, cough, headaches, nausea and vomiting. (6.1)
- COPD: pneumonia, oral candidiasis, throat irritation, dysphonia, viral respiratory infections, headaches, musculoskeletal pain. (6.2)

To report SUSPECTED ADVERSE REACTIONS, contact GlaxoSmithKline at 1-888-825-5249 or FDA at 1-800-FDA-1088 or www.fda.gov/medwatch

DRUG INTERACTIONS
- Strong cytochrome P450 3A4 inhibitors (e.g., ritonavir): Use not recommended. May cause systemic corticosteroid and cardiovascular effects. (7.1)
- Monoamine oxidase inhibitors and tricyclic antidepressants: Use with extreme caution. May potentiate effect of salmeterol on vascular system. (7.2)
- Beta-blockers: Use with caution. May block bronchodilatory effects of beta-agonists and produce severe bronchospasm. (7.3)
- Diuretics: Use with caution. Electrocardiographic changes and/or hypokalemia associated with nonpotassium-sparing diuretics may worsen with concomitant beta-agonists. (7.4)

USE IN SPECIFIC POPULATIONS
Hepatic impairment: Monitor patients for signs of increased drug exposure. (8.6)

See 17 for PATIENT COUNSELING INFORMATION and MEDICATION GUIDE.

Revised: 06/2010

FULL PRESCRIBING INFORMATION

WARNING: ASTHMA-RELATED DEATH

Long-acting beta$_2$-adrenergic agonists (LABAs), such as salmeterol, one of the active ingredients in ADVAIR DISKUS®, increase the risk of asthma-related death. Data from a large placebo-controlled US study that compared the safety of salmeterol (SEREVENT® Inhalation Aerosol) or placebo added to usual asthma therapy showed an increase in asthma-related deaths in patients receiving salmeterol (13 deaths out of 13,176 patients treated for 28 weeks on salmeterol versus 3 out of 13,179 patients on placebo). Currently available data are inadequate to determine whether concurrent use of inhaled corticosteroids or other long-term asthma control drugs mitigates the increased risk of asthma-related death from LABAs. Available data from controlled clinical trials suggest that LABAs increase the risk of asthma-related hospitalization in pediatric and adolescent patients.

Therefore, when treating patients with asthma, physicians should only prescribe ADVAIR DISKUS for patients not adequately controlled on a long-term asthma control medication, such as an inhaled corticosteroid, or whose disease severity clearly warrants initiation of treatment with both an inhaled corticosteroid and a LABA. Once asthma control is achieved and maintained, assess the patient at regular intervals and step down therapy (e.g., discontinue ADVAIR DISKUS) if possible without loss of asthma control and maintain the patient on a long-term asthma control medication, such as an inhaled corticosteroid. Do not use ADVAIR DISKUS for patients whose asthma is adequately controlled on low- or medium-dose inhaled corticosteroids [see Warnings and Precautions (5.1)].

1 INDICATIONS AND USAGE

1.1 Treatment of Asthma

ADVAIR DISKUS is indicated for the treatment of asthma in patients aged 4 years and older.

Long-acting beta$_2$-adrenergic agonists (LABAs), such as salmeterol, one of the active ingredients in ADVAIR DISKUS, increase the risk of asthma-related death. Available data from controlled clinical trials suggest that LABAs increase the risk of asthma-related hospitalization in pediatric and adolescent patients [see Warnings and Precautions (5.1)]. Therefore, when treating patients with asthma, physicians should only prescribe ADVAIR DISKUS for patients not adequately controlled on a long-term asthma control medication, such as an inhaled corticosteroid, or whose disease severity clearly warrants initiation of treatment with both an inhaled corticosteroid and a LABA. Once asthma control is achieved and maintained, assess the patient at regular intervals and step down therapy (e.g., discontinue ADVAIR DISKUS) if possible without loss of asthma control and maintain the patient on a long-term asthma control medication, such as an inhaled corticosteroid. Do not use ADVAIR DISKUS for patients whose asthma is adequately controlled on low- or medium-dose inhaled corticosteroids.

Important Limitation of Use: ADVAIR DISKUS is NOT indicated for the relief of acute bronchospasm.

1.2 Maintenance Treatment of Chronic Obstructive Pulmonary Disease

ADVAIR DISKUS 250/50 is indicated for the twice-daily maintenance treatment of airflow obstruction in patients with chronic obstructive pulmonary disease (COPD), including chronic bronchitis and/or emphysema. ADVAIR DISKUS 250/50 is also indicated to reduce exacerbations of COPD in patients with a history of exacerbations. ADVAIR DISKUS 250/50 twice daily is the only approved dosage for the treatment of COPD because an efficacy advantage of the higher strength ADVAIR DISKUS 500/50 over ADVAIR DISKUS 250/50 has not been demonstrated.

Important Limitation of Use: ADVAIR DISKUS is NOT indicated for the relief of acute bronchospasm.

2 DOSAGE AND ADMINISTRATION

ADVAIR DISKUS should be administered twice daily every day by the orally inhaled route only. After inhalation, the patient should rinse the mouth with water without swallowing [see Patient Counseling Information (17.4)].

More frequent administration or a higher number of inhalations (more than 1 inhalation twice daily) of the prescribed strength of ADVAIR DISKUS is not recommended as some patients are more likely to experience adverse effects with higher doses of salmeterol. Patients using ADVAIR DISKUS should not use additional LABAs for any reason. [See Warnings and Precautions (5.3, 5.12).]

2.1 Asthma

If asthma symptoms arise in the period between doses, an inhaled, short-acting beta$_2$-agonist should be taken for immediate relief.

Adult and Adolescent Patients Aged 12 Years and Older: For patients aged 12 years and older, the dosage is 1 inhalation twice daily (morning and evening, approximately 12 hours apart).

The recommended starting dosages for ADVAIR DISKUS for patients aged 12 years and older are based upon patients' asthma severity.

The maximum recommended dosage is ADVAIR DISKUS 500/50 twice daily.

Improvement in asthma control following inhaled administration of ADVAIR DISKUS can occur within 30 minutes of beginning treatment, although maximum benefit may not be achieved for 1 week or longer after starting treatment. Individual patients will experience a variable time to onset and degree of symptom relief.

For patients who do not respond adequately to the starting dosage after 2 weeks of therapy, replacing the current strength of ADVAIR DISKUS with a higher strength may provide additional improvement in asthma control.

If a previously effective dosage regimen of ADVAIR DISKUS fails to provide adequate improvement in asthma control, the therapeutic regimen should be reevaluated and additional therapeutic options (e.g., replacing the current strength of ADVAIR DISKUS with a higher strength, adding additional inhaled corticosteroid, initiating oral corticosteroids) should be considered.

Pediatric Patients Aged 4 to 11 Years: For patients with asthma aged 4 to 11 years who are not controlled on an inhaled corticosteroid, the dosage is 1 inhalation of ADVAIR DISKUS 100/50 twice daily (morning and evening, approximately 12 hours apart).

2.2 Chronic Obstructive Pulmonary Disease

The recommended dosage for patients with COPD is 1 inhalation of ADVAIR DISKUS 250/50 twice daily (morning and evening, approximately 12 hours apart).

If shortness of breath occurs in the period between doses, an inhaled, short-acting beta$_2$-agonist should be taken for immediate relief.

3 DOSAGE FORMS AND STRENGTHS

Disposable purple device with 60 blisters containing a combination of fluticasone propionate (100, 250, or 500 mcg) and salmeterol (50 mcg) as an oral inhalation powder formulation. An institutional pack containing 14 blisters is also available.

4 CONTRAINDICATIONS

The use of ADVAIR DISKUS is contraindicated in the following conditions:

- Primary treatment of status asthmaticus or other acute episodes of asthma or COPD where intensive measures are required
- Severe hypersensitivity to milk proteins [see Warnings and Precautions (5.11), Description (11)]

5 WARNINGS AND PRECAUTIONS

5.1 Asthma-Related Death

LABAs, such as salmeterol, one of the active ingredients in ADVAIR DISKUS, increase the risk of asthma-related death. Currently available data are inadequate to determine whether concurrent use of inhaled corticosteroids or other long-term asthma control drugs mitigates the increased risk of asthma-related death from LABAs. Available data from controlled clinical trials suggest that LABAs increase the risk of asthma-related hospitalization in pediatric and adolescent patients. Therefore, when treating patients with asthma, physicians should only prescribe ADVAIR DISKUS for patients not adequately controlled on a long-term asthma-control medication, such as an inhaled corticosteroid, or whose disease severity clearly warrants initiation of treatment with both an inhaled corticosteroid and a LABA. Once asthma control is achieved and maintained, assess the patient at regular intervals and step down therapy (e.g., discontinue ADVAIR DISKUS) if possible without loss of asthma control and maintain the patient on a long-term asthma control medication, such as an inhaled corticosteroid. Do not use ADVAIR DISKUS for patients whose asthma is adequately controlled on low- or medium-dose inhaled corticosteroids.

A large, placebo-controlled US study that compared the safety of salmeterol with placebo, each added to usual asthma therapy, showed an increase in asthma-related deaths in patients receiving salmeterol. The Salmeterol Multi-center Asthma Research Trial (SMART) that enrolled LABA-naive patients with asthma to assess the safety of salmeterol (SEREVENT® Inhalation Aerosol) 42 mcg twice daily over 28 weeks compared with placebo when added to usual asthma therapy. A planned interim analysis was conducted when approximately half of the intended number of patients had been enrolled (N = 26,355), which led to premature termination of the study. The results of the interim analysis showed that patients receiving salmeterol were at increased risk for fatal asthma events (see Table 1 and Figure 1). In the total population, a higher rate of asthma-related death occurred in patients treated with salmeterol than those treated with placebo (0.10% versus 0.02%, relative risk: 4.37 [95% CI: 1.25, 15.34]).

Post-hoc subpopulation analyses were performed. In Caucasians, asthma-related death occurred at a higher rate in patients treated with salmeterol than in patients treated with placebo (0.07% versus 0.01%, relative risk: 5.82 [95% CI: 0.70, 48.37]). In African Americans also, asthma-related death occurred at a higher rate in patients treated with salmeterol than those treated with placebo (0.31% versus 0.04%, relative risk: 7.26 [95% CI: 0.89, 58.94]). Although the relative risks of asthma-related death were similar in Caucasians and African Americans, the estimate of excess deaths in patients treated with salmeterol was greater in African Americans because there was a higher overall rate of asthma-related death in African American patients (see Table 1). Given the similar basic mechanisms of action of beta$_2$-agonists, the findings seen in the SMART study are considered a class effect.

Post-hoc analyses in pediatric patients aged 12 to 18 years were also performed. Pediatric patients accounted for approximately 12% of patients in each treatment arm. Respiratory-related death or life-threatening experience occurred at a similar rate in the salmeterol group (0.12% [2/1,653]) and the placebo group (0.12% [2/1,622]; relative risk: 1.0 [95% CI: 0.1, 7.2]). All-cause hospitalization, however, was increased in the salmeterol group (2% [35/1,653]) versus the placebo group (<1% [16/1,622]; relative risk: 2.1 [95% CI: 1.1, 3.7]).

The data from the SMART study are not adequate to determine whether concurrent use of inhaled corticosteroids, such as fluticasone propionate, the other active ingredient in ADVAIR DISKUS, or other long-term asthma control therapy mitigates the risk of asthma-related death.

[See table 1 at top of next page]

[See figure 1 at top of next column]

A 16-week clinical study performed in the United Kingdom, the Salmeterol Nationwide Surveillance (SNS) study, showed results similar to the SMART study. In the SNS

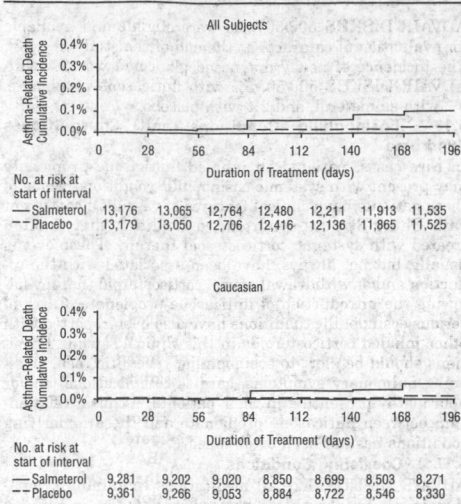

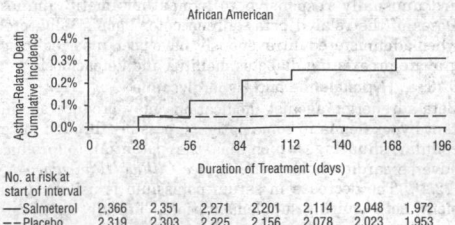

Figure 1. Cumulative Incidence of Asthma-Related Deaths in the 28-Week Salmeterol Multi-center Asthma Research Trial (SMART), by Duration of Treatment

Table 1. Asthma-Related Deaths in the 28-Week Salmeterol Multi-center Asthma Research Trial (SMART)

	Salmeterol n (%[a])	Placebo n (%[a])	Relative Risk[b] (95% Confidence Interval)	Excess Deaths Expressed per 10,000 Patients[c] (95% Confidence Interval)
Total Population[d]				
Salmeterol: N = 13,176	13 (0.10%)		4.37 (1.25, 15.34)	8 (3, 13)
Placebo: N = 13,179		3 (0.02%)		
Caucasian				
Salmeterol: N = 9,281	6 (0.07%)		5.82 (0.70, 48.37)	6 (1, 10)
Placebo: N = 9,361		1 (0.01%)		
African American				
Salmeterol: N = 2,366	7 (0.31%)		7.26 (0.89, 58.94)	27 (8, 46)
Placebo: N = 2,319		1 (0.04%)		

[a]Life-table 28-week estimate, adjusted according to the patients' actual lengths of exposure to study treatment to account for early withdrawal of patients from the study.
[b]Relative risk is the ratio of the rate of asthma-related death in the salmeterol group and the rate in the placebo group. The relative risk indicates how many more times likely an asthma-related death occurred in the salmeterol group than in the placebo group in a 28-week treatment period.
[c]Estimate of the number of additional asthma-related deaths in patients treated with salmeterol in SMART, assuming 10,000 patients received salmeterol for a 28-week treatment period. Estimate calculated as the difference between the salmeterol and placebo groups in the rates of asthma-related death multiplied by 10,000.
[d]The Total Population includes the following ethnic origins listed on the case report form: Caucasian, African American, Hispanic, Asian, and "Other." In addition, the Total Population includes those patients whose ethnic origin was not reported. The results for Caucasian and African American subpopulations are shown above. No asthma-related deaths occurred in the Hispanic (salmeterol n = 996, placebo n = 999), Asian (salmeterol n = 173, placebo n = 149), or "Other" (salmeterol n = 230, placebo n = 224) subpopulations. One asthma-related death occurred in the placebo group in the subpopulation whose ethnic origin was not reported (salmeterol n = 130, placebo n = 127).

study, the rate of asthma-related death was numerically, though not statistically significantly, greater in patients with asthma treated with salmeterol (42 mcg twice daily) than those treated with albuterol (180 mcg 4 times daily) added to usual asthma therapy.

The SNS and SMART studies enrolled patients with asthma. No studies have been conducted that were primarily designed to determine whether the rate of death in patients with COPD is increased by LABAs.

5.2 Deterioration of Disease and Acute Episodes
ADVAIR DISKUS should not be initiated in patients during rapidly deteriorating or potentially life-threatening episodes of asthma or COPD. ADVAIR DISKUS has not been studied in patients with acutely deteriorating asthma or COPD. The initiation of ADVAIR DISKUS in this setting is not appropriate.

Serious acute respiratory events, including fatalities, have been reported when salmeterol, a component of ADVAIR DISKUS, has been initiated in patients with significantly worsening or acutely deteriorating asthma. In most cases, these have occurred in patients with severe asthma (e.g., patients with a history of corticosteroid dependence, low pulmonary function, intubation, mechanical ventilation, frequent hospitalizations, previous life-threatening acute asthma exacerbations) and in some patients with acutely deteriorating asthma (e.g., patients with significantly increasing symptoms; increasing need for inhaled, short-acting beta2-agonists; decreasing response to usual medications; increasing need for systemic corticosteroids; recent emergency room visits; deteriorating lung function). However, these events have occurred in a few patients with less severe asthma as well. It was not possible from these reports to determine whether salmeterol contributed to these events.

Increasing use of inhaled, short-acting beta2-agonists is a marker of deteriorating asthma. In this situation, the patient requires immediate reevaluation with reassessment of the treatment regimen, giving special consideration to the possible need for replacing the current strength of ADVAIR DISKUS with a higher strength, adding additional inhaled corticosteroid, or initiating systemic corticosteroids. Patients should not use more than 1 inhalation twice daily (morning and evening) of ADVAIR DISKUS.

ADVAIR DISKUS should not be used for the relief of acute symptoms, i.e., as rescue therapy for the treatment of acute episodes of bronchospasm. An inhaled, short-acting beta2-agonist, not ADVAIR DISKUS, should be used to relieve acute symptoms such as shortness of breath. When prescribing ADVAIR DISKUS, the physician must also provide the patient with an inhaled, short-acting beta2-agonist (e.g., albuterol) for treatment of acute symptoms, despite regular twice-daily (morning and evening) use of ADVAIR DISKUS.

When beginning treatment with ADVAIR DISKUS, patients who have been taking oral or inhaled, short-acting beta2-agonists on a regular basis (e.g., 4 times a day) should be instructed to discontinue the regular use of these drugs.

5.3 Excessive Use of ADVAIR DISKUS and Use With Other Long-Acting Beta2-Agonists
As with other inhaled drugs containing beta2-adrenergic agents, ADVAIR DISKUS should not be used more often than recommended, at higher doses than recommended, or in conjunction with other medications containing LABAs, as an overdose may result. Clinically significant cardiovascular effects and fatalities have been reported in association with excessive use of inhaled sympathomimetic drugs. Patients using ADVAIR DISKUS should not use an additional LABA (e.g., salmeterol, formoterol fumarate, arformoterol tartrate) for any reason, including prevention of exercise-induced bronchospasm (EIB) or the treatment of asthma or COPD.

5.4 Local Effects
In clinical studies, the development of localized infections of the mouth and pharynx with *Candida albicans* has occurred in patients treated with ADVAIR DISKUS. When such an infection develops, it should be treated with appropriate local or systemic (i.e., oral antifungal) therapy while treatment with ADVAIR DISKUS continues, but at times therapy with ADVAIR DISKUS may need to be interrupted. Patients should rinse the mouth after inhalation of ADVAIR DISKUS.

5.5 Pneumonia
Physicians should remain vigilant for the possible development of pneumonia in patients with COPD as the clinical features of pneumonia and exacerbations frequently overlap.

Lower respiratory tract infections, including pneumonia, have been reported in patients with COPD following the inhaled administration of corticosteroids, including fluticasone propionate and ADVAIR DISKUS. In 2 replicate 12-month studies of 1,579 patients with COPD, there was a higher incidence of pneumonia reported in patients receiving ADVAIR DISKUS 250/50 (7%) than in those receiving salmeterol 50 mcg (3%). The incidence of pneumonia in the patients treated with ADVAIR DISKUS was higher in patients over 65 years of age (9%) compared with the incidence in patients less than 65 years of age (4%). [See Adverse Reactions (6.2), Use in Specific Populations (8.5).]

In a 3-year study of 6,184 patients with COPD, there was a higher incidence of pneumonia reported in patients receiving ADVAIR DISKUS 500/50 compared with placebo (16% with ADVAIR DISKUS 500/50, 14% with fluticasone propionate 500 mcg, 11% with salmeterol 50 mcg, and 9% with placebo). Similar to what was seen in the 1-year studies with ADVAIR DISKUS 250/50, the incidence of pneumonia was higher in patients over 65 years of age (18% with ADVAIR DISKUS 500/50 versus 10% with placebo) compared with patients less than 65 years of age (14% with ADVAIR DISKUS 500/50 versus 8% with placebo). [See Adverse Reactions (6.2), Use in Specific Populations (8.5).]

5.6 Immunosuppression
Persons who are using drugs that suppress the immune system are more susceptible to infections than healthy indi-

viduals. Chickenpox and measles, for example, can have a more serious or even fatal course in susceptible children or adults using corticosteroids. In such children or adults who have not had these diseases or been properly immunized, particular care should be taken to avoid exposure. How the dose, route, and duration of corticosteroid administration affect the risk of developing a disseminated infection is not known. The contribution of the underlying disease and/or prior corticosteroid treatment to the risk is also not known. If a patient is exposed to chickenpox, prophylaxis with varicella zoster immune globulin (VZIG) may be indicated. If a patient is exposed to measles, prophylaxis with pooled intramuscular immunoglobulin (IG) may be indicated. (See the respective package inserts for complete VZIG and IG prescribing information.) If chickenpox develops, treatment with antiviral agents may be considered.

Inhaled corticosteroids should be used with caution, if at all, in patients with active or quiescent tuberculosis infections of the respiratory tract; untreated systemic fungal, bacterial, viral, or parasitic infections; or ocular herpes simplex.

5.7 Transferring Patients From Systemic Corticosteroid Therapy
Particular care is needed for patients who have been transferred from systemically active corticosteroids to inhaled corticosteroids because deaths due to adrenal insufficiency have occurred in patients with asthma during and after transfer from systemic corticosteroids to less systemically available inhaled corticosteroids. After withdrawal from systemic corticosteroids, a number of months are required for recovery of hypothalamic-pituitary-adrenal (HPA) function.

Patients who have been previously maintained on 20 mg or more per day of prednisone (or its equivalent) may be most susceptible, particularly when their systemic corticosteroids have been almost completely withdrawn. During this period of HPA suppression, patients may exhibit signs and symptoms of adrenal insufficiency when exposed to trauma, surgery, or infection (particularly gastroenteritis) or other conditions associated with severe electrolyte loss. Although ADVAIR DISKUS may provide control of asthma symptoms during these episodes, in recommended doses it supplies less than normal physiological amounts of glucocorticoid systemically and does NOT provide the mineralocorticoid activity that is necessary for coping with these emergencies. During periods of stress or a severe asthma attack, patients who have been withdrawn from systemic corticosteroids should be instructed to resume oral corticosteroids (in large doses) immediately and to contact their physicians for further instruction. These patients should also be instructed to carry a warning card indicating that they may need supplementary systemic corticosteroids during periods of stress or a severe asthma attack.

Patients requiring oral corticosteroids should be weaned slowly from systemic corticosteroid use after transferring to ADVAIR DISKUS. Prednisone reduction can be accomplished by reducing the daily prednisone dose by 2.5 mg on a weekly basis during therapy with ADVAIR DISKUS. Lung function (mean forced expiratory volume in 1 second [FEV1] or morning peak expiratory flow [PEF]), beta-agonist use, and asthma symptoms should be carefully monitored during withdrawal of oral corticosteroids. In addition to monitoring asthma signs and symptoms, patients should be observed for signs and symptoms of adrenal insufficiency, such as fatigue, lassitude, weakness, nausea and vomiting, and hypotension.

Transfer of patients from systemic corticosteroid therapy to inhaled corticosteroids or ADVAIR DISKUS may unmask conditions previously suppressed by the systemic corticosteroid therapy (e.g., rhinitis, conjunctivitis, eczema, arthritis, eosinophilic conditions). Some patients may experience symptoms of systemically active corticosteroid withdrawal (e.g., joint and/or muscular pain, lassitude, depression) despite maintenance or even improvement of respiratory function.

5.8 Hypercorticism and Adrenal Suppression

Fluticasone propionate, a component of ADVAIR DISKUS, will often help control asthma symptoms with less suppression of HPA function than therapeutically equivalent oral doses of prednisone. Since fluticasone propionate is absorbed into the circulation and can be systemically active at higher doses, the beneficial effects of ADVAIR DISKUS in minimizing HPA dysfunction may be expected only when recommended dosages are not exceeded and individual patients are titrated to the lowest effective dose. A relationship between plasma levels of fluticasone propionate and inhibitory effects on stimulated cortisol production has been shown after 4 weeks of treatment with fluticasone propionate inhalation aerosol. Since individual sensitivity to effects on cortisol production exists, physicians should consider this information when prescribing ADVAIR DISKUS.

Because of the possibility of systemic absorption of inhaled corticosteroids, patients treated with ADVAIR DISKUS should be observed carefully for any evidence of systemic corticosteroid effects. Particular care should be taken in observing patients postoperatively or during periods of stress for evidence of inadequate adrenal response.

It is possible that systemic corticosteroid effects such as hypercorticism and adrenal suppression (including adrenal crisis) may appear in a small number of patients, particularly when fluticasone propionate is administered at higher than recommended doses over prolonged periods of time. If such effects occur, the dosage of ADVAIR DISKUS should be reduced slowly, consistent with accepted procedures for reducing systemic corticosteroids and for management of asthma symptoms.

5.9 Drug Interactions With Strong Cytochrome P450 3A4 Inhibitors

The use of strong cytochrome P450 3A4 (CYP3A4) inhibitors (e.g., ritonavir, atazanavir, clarithromycin, indinavir, itraconazole, nefazodone, nelfinavir, saquinavir, ketoconazole, telithromycin) with ADVAIR DISKUS is not recommended because increased systemic corticosteroid and increased cardiovascular adverse effects may occur [see Drug interactions (7.1), Clinical Pharmacology (12.3)].

5.10 Paradoxical Bronchospasm and Upper Airway Symptoms

As with other inhaled medications, ADVAIR DISKUS can produce paradoxical bronchospasm, which may be life threatening. If paradoxical bronchospasm occurs following dosing with ADVAIR DISKUS, it should be treated immediately with an inhaled, short-acting bronchodilator; ADVAIR DISKUS should be discontinued immediately; and alternative therapy should be instituted. Upper airway symptoms of laryngeal spasm, irritation, or swelling, such as stridor and choking, have been reported in patients receiving fluticasone propionate and salmeterol.

5.11 Immediate Hypersensitivity Reactions

Immediate hypersensitivity reactions may occur after administration of ADVAIR DISKUS, as demonstrated by cases of urticaria, angioedema, rash, and bronchospasm. There have been reports of anaphylactic reactions in patients with severe milk protein allergy; therefore, patients with severe milk protein allergy should not take ADVAIR DISKUS [see Contraindications (4)].

5.12 Cardiovascular and Central Nervous System Effects

Excessive beta-adrenergic stimulation has been associated with seizures, angina, hypertension or hypotension, tachycardia with rates up to 200 beats/min, arrhythmias, nervousness, headache, tremor, palpitation, nausea, dizziness, fatigue, malaise, and insomnia [see Overdosage (10)]. Therefore, ADVAIR DISKUS, like all products containing sympathomimetic amines, should be used with caution in patients with cardiovascular disorders, especially coronary insufficiency, cardiac arrhythmias, and hypertension.

Salmeterol, a component of ADVAIR DISKUS, can produce a clinically significant cardiovascular effect in some patients as measured by pulse rate, blood pressure, and/or symptoms. Although such effects are uncommon after administration of salmeterol at recommended doses, if they occur, the drug may need to be discontinued. In addition, beta-agonists have been reported to produce ECG changes, such as flattening of the T wave, prolongation of the QTc interval,

and ST segment depression. The clinical significance of these findings is unknown. Large doses of inhaled or oral salmeterol (12 to 20 times the recommended dose) have been associated with clinically significant prolongation of the QTc interval, which has the potential for producing ventricular arrhythmias. Fatalities have been reported in association with excessive use of inhaled sympathomimetic drugs.

5.13 Reduction in Bone Mineral Density

Decreases in bone mineral density (BMD) have been observed with long-term administration of products containing inhaled corticosteroids. The clinical significance of small changes in BMD with regard to long-term consequences such as fracture is unknown. Patients with major risk factors for decreased bone mineral content, such as prolonged immobilization, family history of osteoporosis, postmenopausal status, tobacco use, advanced age, poor nutrition, or chronic use of drugs that can reduce bone mass (e.g., anticonvulsants, oral corticosteroids) should be monitored and treated with established standards of care. Since patients with COPD often have multiple risk factors for reduced BMD, assessment of BMD is recommended prior to initiating ADVAIR DISKUS and periodically thereafter. If significant reductions in BMD are seen and ADVAIR DISKUS is still considered medically important for that patient's COPD therapy, use of medication to treat or prevent osteoporosis should be strongly considered.

2-Year Fluticasone Propionate Study: A 2-year study of 160 patients (females aged 18 to 40 years, males 18 to 50) with asthma receiving CFC-propelled fluticasone propionate inhalation aerosol 88 or 440 mcg twice daily demonstrated no statistically significant changes in BMD at any time point (24, 52, 76, and 104 weeks of double-blind treatment) as assessed by dual-energy x-ray absorptiometry at lumbar regions L1 through L4.

3-Year Bone Mineral Density Study: Effects of treatment with ADVAIR DISKUS 250/50 or salmeterol 50 mcg on BMD at the L_1-L_4 lumbar spine and total hip were evaluated in 186 patients with COPD (aged 43 to 87 years) in a 3-year double-blind study. Of those enrolled, 108 patients (72 males and 36 females) were followed for the entire 3 years. BMD evaluations were conducted at baseline and at 6-month intervals. Conclusions cannot be drawn from this study regarding BMD decline in patients treated with ADVAIR DISKUS versus salmeterol due to the inconsistency of treatment differences across gender and between lumbar spine and total hip.

In this study there were 7 non-traumatic fractures reported in 5 patients treated with ADVAIR DISKUS and 1 non-traumatic fracture in 1 patient treated with salmeterol. None of the non-traumatic fractures occurred in the vertebrae, hip, or long bones.

3-Year Survival Study: Effects of treatment with ADVAIR DISKUS 500/50, fluticasone propionate 500 mcg, salmeterol 50 mcg, or placebo on BMD was evaluated in a subset of 658 patients (females and males aged 40 to 80 years) with COPD in the 3-year survival study. BMD evaluations were conducted at baseline and at 48, 108, and 158 weeks. Conclusions cannot be drawn from this study because of the large number of drop outs (>50%) before the end of the follow-up and the maldistribution of covariates among the treatment groups that can affect BMD.

Fracture risk was estimated for the entire population of patients with COPD in the survival study (N = 6,184). The probability of a fracture over 3 years was 6.3% for ADVAIR DISKUS, 5.4% for fluticasone propionate, 5.1% for salmeterol, and 5.1% for placebo.

5.14 Effect on Growth

Orally inhaled corticosteroids may cause a reduction in growth velocity when administered to pediatric patients. Monitor the growth of pediatric patients receiving ADVAIR DISKUS routinely (e.g., via stadiometry). To minimize the systemic effects of orally inhaled corticosteroids, including ADVAIR DISKUS, titrate each patient's dose to the lowest dosage that effectively controls his/her symptoms. [See Dosage and Administration (2.1), Use in Specific Populations (8.4).]

5.15 Glaucoma and Cataracts

Glaucoma, increased intraocular pressure, and cataracts have been reported in patients with asthma and COPD following the long-term administration of inhaled corticosteroids, including fluticasone propionate, a component of ADVAIR DISKUS. Therefore, close monitoring is warranted in patients with a change in vision or with a history of increased intraocular pressure, glaucoma, and/or cataracts. Effects of treatment with ADVAIR DISKUS 500/50, fluticasone propionate 500 mcg, salmeterol 50 mcg, or placebo on development of cataracts or glaucoma was evaluated in a subset of 658 patients with COPD in the 3-year survival study. Ophthalmic examinations were conducted at baseline and at 48, 108, and 158 weeks. Conclusions about cataracts cannot be drawn from this study because the high incidence of cataracts at baseline (61% to 71%) resulted in an inadequate number of patients treated with

ADVAIR DISKUS 500/50 who were eligible and available for evaluation of cataracts at the end of the study (n = 53). The incidence of newly diagnosed glaucoma was 2% with ADVAIR DISKUS 500/50, 5% with fluticasone propionate, 0% with salmeterol, and 2% with placebo.

5.16 Eosinophilic Conditions and Churg-Strauss Syndrome

In rare cases, patients on inhaled fluticasone propionate may present with systemic eosinophilic conditions. Some of these patients have clinical features of vasculitis consistent with Churg-Strauss syndrome, a condition that is often treated with systemic corticosteroid therapy. These events usually, but not always, have been associated with the reduction and/or withdrawal of oral corticosteroid therapy following the introduction of fluticasone propionate. Cases of serious eosinophilic conditions have also been reported with other inhaled corticosteroids in this clinical setting. Physicians should be alert to eosinophilia, vasculitic rash, worsening pulmonary symptoms, cardiac complications, and/or neuropathy presenting in their patients. A causal relationship between fluticasone propionate and these underlying conditions has not been established.

5.17 Coexisting Conditions

ADVAIR DISKUS, like all medications containing sympathomimetic amines, should be used with caution in patients with convulsive disorders or thyrotoxicosis and in those who are unusually responsive to sympathomimetic amines. Doses of the related beta$_2$-adrenoceptor agonist albuterol, when administered intravenously, have been reported to aggravate preexisting diabetes mellitus and ketoacidosis.

5.18 Hypokalemia and Hyperglycemia

Beta-adrenergic agonist medications may produce significant hypokalemia in some patients, possibly through intracellular shunting, which has the potential to produce adverse cardiovascular effects [see Clinical Pharmacology (12.2)]. The decrease in serum potassium is usually transient, not requiring supplementation. Clinically significant changes in blood glucose and/or serum potassium were seen infrequently during clinical studies with ADVAIR DISKUS at recommended doses.

6 ADVERSE REACTIONS

LABAs, such as salmeterol, one of the active ingredients in ADVAIR DISKUS, increase the risk of asthma-related death. Data from a large placebo-controlled US study that compared the safety of salmeterol (SEREVENT Inhalation Aerosol) or placebo added to usual asthma therapy showed an increase in asthma-related deaths in patients receiving salmeterol [see Warnings and Precautions (5.1)]. Currently available data are inadequate to determine whether concurrent use of inhaled corticosteroids or other long-term asthma control drugs mitigates the increased risk of asthma-related death from LABA. Available data from controlled clinical trials suggest that LABA increase the risk of asthma-related hospitalization in pediatric and adolescent patients.

Systemic and local corticosteroid use may result in the following:

- *Candida albicans* infection [see Warnings and Precautions (5.4)]
- Pneumonia in patients with COPD [see Warnings and Precautions (5.5)]
- Immunosuppression [see Warnings and Precautions (5.6)]
- Hypercorticism and adrenal suppression [see Warnings and Precautions (5.8)]
- Growth effects [see Warnings and Precautions (5.14)]
- Glaucoma and cataracts [see Warnings and Precautions (5.15)]

Because clinical trials are conducted under widely varying conditions, adverse reaction rates observed in the clinical trials of a drug cannot be directly compared with rates in the clinical trials of another drug and may not reflect the rates observed in practice.

6.1 Clinical Trials Experience in Asthma

Adult and Adolescent Patients Aged 12 Years and Older: The incidence of adverse reactions associated with ADVAIR DISKUS in Table 2 is based upon 2 placebo-controlled, 12-week, US clinical studies (Studies 1 and 2). A total of 705 adolescent and adult patients (349 females and 356 males) previously treated with salmeterol or inhaled corticosteroids were treated twice daily with ADVAIR DISKUS (100/50- or 250/50-mcg doses), fluticasone propionate inhalation powder (100- or 250-mcg doses), salmeterol inhalation powder 50 mcg, or placebo. The average duration of exposure was 60 to 79 days in the active treatment groups compared with 42 days in the placebo group.

[See table 2 at top of next page]

The types of adverse reactions and events reported in Study 3, a 28-week, non-US clinical study of 503 patients previously treated with inhaled corticosteroids who were treated twice daily with ADVAIR DISKUS 500/50, fluticasone propionate inhalation powder 500 mcg and salmeterol inhalation powder 50 mcg used concurrently, or fluticasone propionate inhalation powder 500 mcg, were similar to those reported in Table 2.

Additional Adverse Reactions: Other adverse reactions not previously listed, whether considered drug-related or not by the investigators, that were reported more frequently by patients with asthma treated with ADVAIR DISKUS compared with patients treated with placebo include the following: lymphatic signs and symptoms; muscle injuries; fractures; wounds and lacerations; contusions and hematomas; ear signs and symptoms; nasal signs and symptoms; nasal sinus disorders; keratitis and conjunctivitis; dental discomfort and pain; gastrointestinal signs and symptoms; oral ulcerations; oral discomfort and pain; lower respiratory signs and symptoms; pneumonia; muscle stiffness, tightness, and rigidity; bone and cartilage disorders; sleep disorders; compressed nerve syndromes; viral infections; pain; chest symptoms; fluid retention; bacterial infections; unusual taste; viral skin infections; skin flakiness and acquired ichthyosis; disorders of sweat and sebum.

Pediatric Patients Aged 4 to 11 Years: The safety data for pediatric patients aged 4 to 11 years is based upon 1 US trial of 12 weeks' treatment duration. A total of 203 patients (74 females and 129 males) who were receiving inhaled corticosteroids at study entry were randomized to either ADVAIR DISKUS 100/50 or fluticasone propionate inhalation powder 100 mcg twice daily. Common adverse reactions (≥3% and greater than placebo) seen in the pediatric patients but not reported in the adult and adolescent clinical trials include: throat irritation and ear, nose, and throat infections.

Laboratory Test Abnormalities: Elevation of hepatic enzymes was reported in ≥1% of patients in clinical trials. The elevations were transient and did not lead to discontinuation from the studies. In addition, there were no clinically relevant changes noted in glucose or potassium.

6.2   Clinical Trials Experience in Chronic Obstructive Pulmonary Disease

Short-Term (6 Months to 1 Year) Trials: The short-term safety data are based on exposure to ADVAIR DISKUS 250/50 twice daily in one 6-month and two 1-year clinical trials. In the 6-month trial, a total of 723 adult patients (266 females and 457 males) were treated twice daily with ADVAIR DISKUS 250/50, fluticasone propionate inhalation powder 250 mcg, salmeterol inhalation powder, or placebo. The mean age of the patients was 64, and the majority (93%) was Caucasian. In this trial, 70% of the patients treated with ADVAIR DISKUS reported an adverse reaction compared with 64% on placebo. The average duration of exposure to ADVAIR DISKUS 250/50 was 141.3 days compared with 131.6 days for placebo. The incidence of adverse reactions in the 6-month study is shown in Table 3.

[See table 3 at right]

In the two 1-year studies, ADVAIR DISKUS 250/50 was compared with salmeterol in 1,579 patients (863 males and 716 females). The mean age of the patients was 65, and the majority (94%) was Caucasian. To be enrolled, all of the patients had to have had a COPD exacerbation in the previous 12 months. In this trial, 88% of the patients treated with ADVAIR DISKUS and 86% of the patients treated with salmeterol reported an adverse event. The most common events that occurred with a frequency of >5% and more frequently in the patients treated with ADVAIR DISKUS were nasopharyngitis, upper respiratory tract infection, nasal congestion, back pain, sinusitis, dizziness, nausea, pneumonia, candidiasis, and dysphonia. Overall, 55 (7%) of the patients treated with ADVAIR DISKUS and 25 (3%) of the patients treated with salmeterol developed pneumonia. The incidence of pneumonia was higher in patients over 65 years of age, 9% in the patients treated with ADVAIR DISKUS compared with 4% in the patients treated with ADVAIR DISKUS less than 65 years of age. In the patients treated with salmeterol, the incidence of pneumonia was the same (3%) in both age-groups. [See Warnings and Precautions (5.5), Use in Specific Populations (8.5).]

Long-Term (3-Year) Trial: The safety of ADVAIR DISKUS 500/50 was evaluated in a randomized, double-blind, placebo-controlled, multicenter, international, 3-year study in 6,184 adult patients with COPD (4,684 males and 1,500 females). The mean age of the patients was 65, and the majority (82%) was Caucasian. The distribution of adverse events was similar to that seen in the 1-year trials with ADVAIR DISKUS 250/50. In addition, pneumonia was reported in a significantly increased number of patients treated with ADVAIR DISKUS 500/50 and fluticasone propionate 500 mcg (16% and 14%, respectively) compared with patients treated with salmeterol 50 mcg or placebo (11% and 9%, respectively). When adjusted for time on treatment, the rates of pneumonia were 84 and 88 events per 1,000 treatment-years in the groups treated with fluticasone propionate 500 mcg and with ADVAIR DISKUS 500/50, respectively, compared with 52 events per 1,000 treatment-years in the salmeterol and placebo groups. Similar to what was seen in the 1-year studies with ADVAIR

Table 2. Adverse Reactions With ≥3% Incidence With ADVAIR DISKUS in Adult and Adolescent Patients With Asthma

Adverse Event	ADVAIR DISKUS 100/50 (N = 92) %	ADVAIR DISKUS 250/50 (N = 84) %	Fluticasone Propionate 100 mcg (N = 90) %	Fluticasone Propionate 250 mcg (N = 84) %	Salmeterol 50 mcg (N = 180) %	Placebo (N = 175) %
Ear, nose, & throat						
Upper respiratory tract infection	27	21	29	25	19	14
Pharyngitis	13	10	7	12	8	6
Upper respiratory inflammation	7	6	7	8	8	5
Sinusitis	4	5	6	1	3	4
Hoarseness/dysphonia	5	2	2	4	<1	<1
Oral candidiasis	1	4	2	2	0	0
Lower respiratory						
Viral respiratory infections	4	4	4	10	6	3
Bronchitis	2	8	1	2	2	2
Cough	3	6	0	0	3	2
Neurology						
Headaches	12	13	14	8	10	7
Gastrointestinal						
Nausea & vomiting	4	6	3	4	1	1
Gastrointestinal discomfort & pain	4	1	0	2	1	1
Diarrhea	4	2	2	2	1	2
Viral gastrointestinal infections	3	0	3	1	2	2
Non-site specific						
Candidiasis unspecified site	3	0	1	4	0	1
Musculoskeletal						
Musculoskeletal pain	4	2	1	5	3	3

Table 3. Overall Adverse Reactions With ≥3% Incidence With ADVAIR DISKUS 250/50 in Patients With Chronic Obstructive Pulmonary Disease Associated With Chronic Bronchitis

Adverse Event	ADVAIR DISKUS 250/50 (N = 178) %	Fluticasone Propionate 250 mcg (N = 183) %	Salmeterol 50 mcg (N = 177) %	Placebo (N = 185) %
Ear, nose, & throat				
Candidiasis mouth/throat	10	6	3	1
Throat irritation	8	5	4	7
Hoarseness/dysphonia	5	3	<1	0
Sinusitis	3	8	5	3
Lower respiratory				
Viral respiratory infections	6	4	3	3
Neurology				
Headaches	16	11	10	12
Dizziness	4	<1	3	2
Non-site specific				
Fever	4	3	0	3
Malaise & fatigue	3	2	2	3
Musculoskeletal				
Musculoskeletal pain	9	8	12	9
Muscle cramps & spasms	3	3	1	1

DISKUS 250/50, the incidence of pneumonia was higher in patients over 65 years of age (18% with ADVAIR DISKUS 500/50 versus 10% with placebo) compared with patients less than 65 years of age (14% with ADVAIR DISKUS 500/50 versus 8% with placebo). [See Warnings and Precautions (5.5), Use in Specific Populations (8.5).]

Additional Adverse Reactions: Other adverse reactions not previously listed, whether considered drug-related or not by the investigators, that were reported more frequently by patients with COPD treated with ADVAIR DISKUS compared with patients treated with placebo include the following: syncope; ear, nose, and throat infections; ear signs and symptoms; laryngitis; nasal congestion/blockage; nasal sinus disorders; pharyngitis/throat infection; hypothyroidism; dry eyes; eye infections; gastrointestinal signs and symptoms; oral lesions; abnormal liver function tests; bacterial infections; edema and swelling; viral infections.

Laboratory Abnormalities: There were no clinically relevant changes in these trials. Specifically, no increased reporting of neutrophilia or changes in glucose or potassium was noted.

6.3   Postmarketing Experience

In addition to adverse events reported from clinical trials, the following events have been identified during worldwide use of any formulation of ADVAIR, fluticasone propionate, and/or salmeterol regardless of indication. Because they are reported voluntarily from a population of unknown size, estimates of frequency cannot be made. These events have been chosen for inclusion due to either their seriousness, frequency of reporting, or causal connection to ADVAIR DISKUS, fluticasone propionate, and/or salmeterol or a combination of these factors.

Cardiac Disorders: Arrhythmias (including atrial fibrillation, extrasystoles, supraventricular tachycardia), ventricular tachycardia.

Endocrine Disorders: Cushing's syndrome, Cushingoid features, growth velocity reduction in children/adolescents, hypercorticism.

Eye Disorders: Glaucoma.

Gastrointestinal Disorders: Abdominal pain, dyspepsia, xerostomia.

Immune System Disorders: Immediate and delayed hypersensitivity reaction (including very rare anaphylactic reaction). Very rare anaphylactic reaction in patients with severe milk protein allergy.

Metabolic and Nutrition Disorders: Hyperglycemia, weight gain.

Musculoskeletal, Connective Tissue, and Bone Disorders: Arthralgia, cramps, myositis, osteoporosis.

Nervous System Disorders: Paresthesia, restlessness.

Psychiatric Disorders: Agitation, aggression, depression. Behavioral changes, including hyperactivity and irritability, have been reported very rarely and primarily in children.

Reproductive System and Breast Disorders: Dysmenorrhea.

Respiratory, Thoracic, and Mediastinal Disorders: Chest congestion; chest tightness; dyspnea; facial and oropharyngeal edema, immediate bronchospasm; paradoxical bronchospasm; tracheitis; wheezing; reports of upper respiratory symptoms of laryngeal spasm, irritation, or swelling such as stridor or choking.

Skin and Subcutaneous Tissue Disorders: Ecchymoses, photodermatitis.

Vascular Disorders: Pallor.

7 DRUG INTERACTIONS

ADVAIR DISKUS has been used concomitantly with other drugs, including short-acting beta2-agonists, methylxanthines, and intranasal corticosteroids, commonly used in patients with asthma or COPD, without adverse drug reactions. No formal drug interaction studies have been performed with ADVAIR DISKUS.

7.1 Inhibitors of Cytochrome P450 3A4

Fluticasone propionate and salmeterol, the individual components of ADVAIR DISKUS, are substrates of CYP3A4. The use of strong CYP3A4 inhibitors (e.g., ritonavir, atazanavir, clarithromycin, indinavir, itraconazole, nefazodone, nelfinavir, saquinavir, ketoconazole, telithromycin) with ADVAIR DISKUS is not recommended because increased systemic corticosteroid and increased cardiovascular adverse effects may occur.

Ritonavir: Fluticasone Propionate: A drug interaction study with fluticasone propionate aqueous nasal spray in healthy subjects has shown that ritonavir (a strong CYP3A4 inhibitor) can significantly increase plasma fluticasone propionate exposure, resulting in significantly reduced serum cortisol concentrations [see Clinical Pharmacology (12.3)]. During postmarketing use, there have been reports of clinically significant drug interactions in patients receiving fluticasone propionate and ritonavir, resulting in systemic corticosteroid effects including Cushing's syndrome and adrenal suppression.

Ketoconazole: Fluticasone Propionate: Coadministration of orally inhaled fluticasone propionate (1,000 mcg) and ketoconazole (200 mg once daily) resulted in increased plasma fluticasone propionate exposure and reduced plasma cortisol area under the curve (AUC), but had no effect on urinary excretion of cortisol.

Salmeterol: In a drug interaction study in 20 healthy subjects, coadministration of inhaled salmeterol (50 mcg twice daily) and oral ketoconazole (400 mg once daily) for 7 days resulted in greater systemic exposure to salmeterol (AUC increased 16-fold and C_{max} increased 1.4-fold). Three (3) subjects were withdrawn due to beta2-agonist side effects (2 with prolonged QTc and 1 with palpitations and sinus tachycardia). Although there was no statistical effect on the mean QTc, coadministration of salmeterol and ketoconazole was associated with more frequent increases in QTc duration compared with salmeterol and placebo administration.

7.2 Monoamine Oxidase Inhibitors and Tricyclic Antidepressants

ADVAIR DISKUS should be administered with extreme caution to patients being treated with monoamine oxidase inhibitors or tricyclic antidepressants, or within 2 weeks of discontinuation of such agents, because the action of salmeterol, a component of ADVAIR DISKUS, on the vascular system may be potentiated by these agents.

7.3 Beta-Adrenergic Receptor Blocking Agents

Beta-blockers not only block the pulmonary effect of beta-agonists, such as salmeterol, a component of ADVAIR DISKUS, but may also produce severe bronchospasm in patients with reversible obstructive airways disease. Therefore, patients with asthma or COPD should not normally be treated with beta-blockers. However, under certain circumstances, there may be no acceptable alternatives to the use of beta-adrenergic blocking agents for these patients; cardioselective beta-blockers could be considered, although they should be administered with caution.

7.4 Diuretics

The ECG changes and/or hypokalemia that may result from the administration of nonpotassium-sparing diuretics (such as loop or thiazide diuretics) can be acutely worsened by beta-agonists, especially when the recommended dose of the beta-agonist is exceeded. Although the clinical relevance of these effects is not known, caution is advised in the coadministration of beta-agonists with nonpotassium-sparing diuretics.

8 USE IN SPECIFIC POPULATIONS

8.1 Pregnancy

Teratogenic Effects: Pregnancy Category C. There are no adequate and well-controlled studies with ADVAIR DISKUS in pregnant women. ADVAIR DISKUS was teratogenic in mice and not in rats, although it lowered fetal weight in rats. Fluticasone propionate alone was teratogenic in mice, rats, and rabbits, and salmeterol alone was teratogenic in rabbits and not in rats. From the reproduction toxicity studies in mice and rats, no evidence of enhanced toxicity was seen using combinations of fluticasone propionate and salmeterol when compared with toxicity data from the components administered separately. ADVAIR DISKUS should be used during pregnancy only if the potential benefit justifies the potential risk to the fetus.

ADVAIR DISKUS: In the mouse reproduction assay, fluticasone propionate by the subcutaneous route at a dose approximately 3/5 the maximum recommended human daily inhalation dose (MRHD) on an mg/m^2 basis combined with oral salmeterol at a dose approximately 410 times the MRHD on an mg/m^2 basis produced cleft palate, fetal death, increased implantation loss, and delayed ossification. These observations are characteristic of glucocorticoids. No developmental toxicity was observed at combination doses of fluticasone propionate subcutaneously up to approximately 1/6 the MRHD on an mg/m^2 basis and oral doses of salmeterol up to approximately 55 times the MRHD on an mg/m^2 basis. In rats, combining fluticasone propionate subcutaneously at a dose equivalent to the MRHD on an mg/m^2 basis and an oral dose of salmeterol at approximately 810 times the MRHD on an mg/m^2 basis produced decreased fetal weight, umbilical hernia, delayed ossification, and changes in the occipital bone. No such effects were seen when combining fluticasone propionate subcutaneously at a dose less than the MRHD on an mg/m^2 basis and an oral dose of salmeterol at approximately 80 times the MRHD on an mg/m^2 basis.

Fluticasone Propionate: Subcutaneous studies in mice at a dose less than the MRHD on an mg/m^2 basis and in rats at a dose equivalent to the MRHD on an mg/m^2 basis revealed fetal toxicity characteristic of potent corticosteroid compounds, including embryonic growth retardation, omphalocele, cleft palate, and retarded cranial ossification. In rabbits, fetal weight reduction and cleft palate were observed at a subcutaneous dose less than the MRHD on an mg/m^2 basis. However, no teratogenic effects were reported at oral doses up to approximately 5 times the MRHD on an mg/m^2 basis. No fluticasone propionate was detected in the plasma in this study, consistent with the established low bioavailability following oral administration [see Clinical Pharmacology (12.3)].

Experience with oral corticosteroids since their introduction in pharmacologic, as opposed to physiologic, doses suggests that rodents are more prone to teratogenic effects from corticosteroids than humans. In addition, because there is a natural increase in corticosteroid production during pregnancy, most women will require a lower exogenous corticosteroid dose and many will not need corticosteroid treatment during pregnancy.

Salmeterol: No teratogenic effects occurred in rats at oral doses approximately 160 times the MRHD on an mg/m^2 basis. In pregnant Dutch rabbits administered oral doses approximately 50 times the MRHD based on comparison of the AUCs, salmeterol exhibited fetal toxic effects characteristically resulting from beta-adrenoceptor stimulation. These included precocious eyelid openings, cleft palate, sternebral fusion, limb and paw flexures, and delayed ossification of the frontal cranial bones. No such effects occurred at an oral dose approximately 20 times the MRHD based on comparison of the AUCs.

New Zealand White rabbits were less sensitive since only delayed ossification of the frontal cranial bones was seen at an oral dose approximately 1,600 times the MRHD on an mg/m^2 basis. Extensive use of other beta-agonists has provided no evidence that these class effects in animals are relevant to their use in humans.

8.2 Labor and Delivery

There are no well-controlled human studies that have investigated effects of ADVAIR DISKUS on preterm labor or labor at term. Because of the potential for beta-agonist interference with uterine contractility, use of ADVAIR DISKUS during labor should be restricted to those patients in whom the benefits clearly outweigh the risks.

8.3 Nursing Mothers

Plasma levels of salmeterol, a component of ADVAIR DISKUS, after inhaled therapeutic doses are very low. In rats, salmeterol xinafoate is excreted in the milk. There are no data from controlled trials on the use of salmeterol by nursing mothers. It is not known whether fluticasone propionate, a component of ADVAIR DISKUS, is excreted in human breast milk. However, other corticosteroids have been detected in human milk. Subcutaneous administration to lactating rats of tritiated fluticasone propionate resulted in measurable radioactivity in milk.

Since there are no data from controlled trials on the use of ADVAIR DISKUS by nursing mothers, a decision should be made whether to discontinue nursing or to discontinue ADVAIR DISKUS, taking into account the importance of ADVAIR DISKUS to the mother.

Caution should be exercised when ADVAIR DISKUS is administered to a nursing woman.

8.4 Pediatric Use

Use of ADVAIR DISKUS 100/50 in patients aged 4 to 11 years is supported by extrapolation of efficacy data from older patients and by safety and efficacy data from a study of ADVAIR DISKUS 100/50 in children with asthma aged 4 to 11 years [see Adverse Reactions (6.1), Clinical Studies (14.1)]. The safety and effectiveness of ADVAIR DISKUS in children with asthma less than 4 years of age have not been established.

Inhaled corticosteroids, including fluticasone propionate, a component of ADVAIR DISKUS, may cause a reduction in growth velocity in children and adolescents [see Warnings and Precautions (5.14)]. The growth of pediatric patients receiving orally inhaled corticosteroids, including ADVAIR DISKUS, should be monitored.

A 52-week placebo-controlled study to assess the potential growth effects of fluticasone propionate inhalation powder (FLOVENT® ROTADISK®) at 50 and 100 mcg twice daily was conducted in the US in 325 prepubescent children (244 males and 81 females) aged 4 to 11 years. The mean growth velocities at 52 weeks observed in the intent-to-treat population were 6.32 cm/year in the placebo group (N = 76), 6.07 cm/year in the 50-mcg group (N = 98), and 5.66 cm/year in the 100-mcg group (N = 89). An imbalance in the proportion of children entering puberty between groups and a higher dropout rate in the placebo group due to poorly controlled asthma may be confounding factors in interpreting these data. A separate subset analysis of children who remained prepubertal during the study revealed growth rates at 52 weeks of 6.10 cm/year in the placebo group (n = 57), 5.91 cm/year in the 50-mcg group (n = 74), and 5.67 cm/year in the 100-mcg group (n = 79). In children aged 8.5 years, the mean age of children in this study, the range for expected growth velocity is: boys – 3rd percentile = 3.8 cm/year, 50th percentile = 5.4 cm/year, and 97th percentile = 7.0 cm/year; girls – 3rd percentile = 4.2 cm/year, 50th percentile = 5.7 cm/year, and 97th percentile = 7.3 cm/year. The clinical relevance of these growth data is not certain.

If a child or adolescent on any corticosteroid appears to have growth suppression, the possibility that he/she is particularly sensitive to this effect of corticosteroids should be considered. The potential growth effects of prolonged treatment should be weighed against the clinical benefits obtained. To minimize the systemic effects of orally inhaled corticosteroids, including ADVAIR DISKUS, each patient should be titrated to the lowest strength that effectively controls his/her asthma [see Dosage and Administration (2.1)].

8.5 Geriatric Use

Clinical studies of ADVAIR DISKUS for asthma did not include sufficient numbers of patients aged 65 years and older to determine whether older patients with asthma respond differently than younger patients.

Of the total number of patients in clinical studies receiving ADVAIR DISKUS for COPD, 1,621 were aged 65 years or older and 379 were aged 75 years or older. Patients with COPD aged 65 years and older had a higher incidence of serious adverse events compared with patients less than 65 years of age. Although the distribution of adverse events was similar in the 2 age-groups, patients over 65 years of age experienced more severe events. In two 1-year studies, the excess risk of pneumonia that was seen in patients treated with ADVAIR DISKUS compared with those treated with salmeterol was greater in patients over 65 years of age than in patients less than 65 years of age [see Adverse Reactions (6.2)]. As with other products containing beta2-agonists, special caution should be observed when using ADVAIR DISKUS in geriatric patients who have concomitant cardiovascular disease that could be adversely affected by beta2-agonists. Based on available data for ADVAIR DISKUS or its active components, no adjustment of dosage of ADVAIR DISKUS in geriatric patients is warranted.

No relationship between fluticasone propionate systemic exposure and age was observed in 57 patients with COPD (aged 40 to 82 years) given 250 or 500 mcg twice daily.

8.6 Hepatic Impairment

Formal pharmacokinetic studies using ADVAIR DISKUS have not been conducted in patients with hepatic impairment. However, since both fluticasone propionate and salmeterol are predominantly cleared by hepatic metabolism, impairment of liver function may lead to accumulation of fluticasone propionate and salmeterol in plasma. Therefore, patients with hepatic disease should be closely monitored.

8.7 Renal Impairment

Formal pharmacokinetic studies using ADVAIR DISKUS have not been conducted in patients with renal impairment.

10 OVERDOSAGE

No human overdosage data has been reported for ADVAIR DISKUS.

No deaths occurred in rats given an inhaled single-dose combination of salmeterol 3.6 mg/kg (approximately 290 and 140 times the MRHD for adults and children, respectively, on an mg/m^2 basis) and 1.9 mg/kg of fluticasone propionate (approximately 15 and 35 times the MRHD for adults and children, respectively, on an mg/m^2 basis).

Fluticasone Propionate: Chronic overdosage with fluticasone propionate may result in signs/symptoms of hypercorticism [see Warnings and Precautions (5.7)]. Inhalation by healthy volunteers of a single dose of 4,000 mcg of fluticasone propionate inhalation powder or single doses of 1,760 or 3,520 mcg of fluticasone propionate CFC inhalation aerosol was well tolerated. Fluticasone propionate given by inhalation aerosol at dosages of 1,320 mcg twice daily for 7 to 15 days to healthy human volunteers was also well tolerated. Repeat oral doses up to 80 mg daily for 10 days in healthy volunteers and repeat oral doses up to 20 mg daily for 42 days in patients were well tolerated. Adverse reactions were of mild or moderate severity, and incidences were similar in active and placebo treatment groups.

No deaths were seen in mice given an oral dose of 1,000 mg/kg (4,100 and 9,600 times the MRHD dose for adults and children, respectively, on an mg/m^2 basis). No deaths were seen in rats given an oral dose of 1,000 mg/kg (8,100 and 19,200 times the MRHD for adults and children, respectively, on an mg/m^2 basis).

Salmeterol: The expected signs and symptoms with overdosage of salmeterol are those of excessive beta-adrenergic stimulation and/or occurrence or exaggeration of any of the following: seizures, angina, hypertension or hypotension, tachycardia with rates up to 200 beats/min, arrhythmias, nervousness, headache, tremor, muscle cramps, dry mouth, palpitation, nausea, dizziness, fatigue, malaise, and insomnia. Overdosage with salmeterol can lead to clinically significant prolongation of the QTc interval, which can produce ventricular arrhythmias. Other signs of overdosage may include hypokalemia and hyperglycemia.

As with all sympathomimetic medications, cardiac arrest and even death may be associated with abuse of salmeterol. Treatment consists of discontinuation of salmeterol together with appropriate symptomatic therapy. The judicious use of a cardioselective beta-receptor blocker may be considered, bearing in mind that such medication can produce bronchospasm. There is insufficient evidence to determine if dialysis is beneficial for overdosage of salmeterol. Cardiac monitoring is recommended in cases of overdosage.

No deaths were seen in rats given salmeterol at an inhalation dose of 2.9 mg/kg (approximately 240 and 110 times the MRHD for adults and children, respectively, on an mg/m^2 basis) and in dogs at an inhalation dose of 0.7 mg/kg (approximately 190 and 90 times the MRHD for adults and children, respectively, on an mg/m^2 basis). By the oral route, no deaths occurred in mice at 150 mg/kg (approximately 6,100 and 2,900 times the MRHD for adults and children, respectively, on an mg/m^2 basis) and in rats at 1,000 mg/kg (approximately 81,000 and 38,000 times the MRHD for adults and children, respectively, on an mg/m^2 basis).

11 DESCRIPTION

ADVAIR DISKUS 100/50, ADVAIR DISKUS 250/50, and ADVAIR DISKUS 500/50 are combinations of fluticasone propionate and salmeterol xinafoate.

One active component of ADVAIR DISKUS is fluticasone propionate, a corticosteroid having the chemical name S-(fluoromethyl) 6α,9-difluoro-11β,17-dihydroxy-16α-methyl-3-oxoandrosta-1,4-diene-17β-carbothioate, 17-propionate and the following chemical structure:

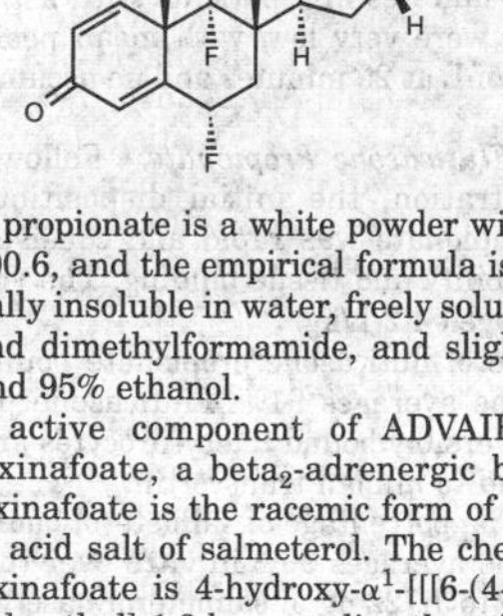

Fluticasone propionate is a white powder with a molecular weight of 500.6, and the empirical formula is $C_{25}H_{31}F_3O_5S$. It is practically insoluble in water, freely soluble in dimethyl sulfoxide and dimethylformamide, and slightly soluble in methanol and 95% ethanol.

The other active component of ADVAIR DISKUS is salmeterol xinafoate, a beta$_2$-adrenergic bronchodilator. Salmeterol xinafoate is the racemic form of the 1-hydroxy-2-naphthoic acid salt of salmeterol. The chemical name of salmeterol xinafoate is 4-hydroxy-α^1-[[[6-(4-phenylbutoxy)hexyl]amino]methyl]-1,3-benzenedimethanol, 1-hydroxy-2-naphthalenecarboxylate, and it has the following chemical structure:

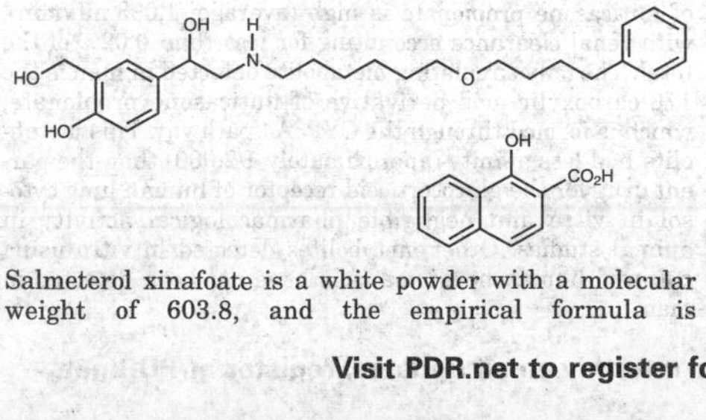

Salmeterol xinafoate is a white powder with a molecular weight of 603.8, and the empirical formula is

$C_{25}H_{37}NO_4 \bullet C_{11}H_8O_3$. It is freely soluble in methanol; slightly soluble in ethanol, chloroform, and isopropanol; and sparingly soluble in water.

ADVAIR DISKUS 100/50, ADVAIR DISKUS 250/50, and ADVAIR DISKUS 500/50 are specially designed plastic devices containing a double-foil blister strip of a powder formulation of fluticasone propionate and salmeterol xinafoate intended for oral inhalation only. Each blister on the double-foil strip within the device contains 100, 250, or 500 mcg of microfine fluticasone propionate and 72.5 mcg of microfine salmeterol xinafoate salt, equivalent to 50 mcg of salmeterol base, in 12.5 mg of formulation containing lactose (which contains milk proteins). Each blister contains 1 complete dose of both medications. After a blister containing medication is opened by activating the device, the medication is dispersed into the airstream created by the patient inhaling through the mouthpiece.

Under standardized in vitro test conditions, ADVAIR DISKUS delivers 93, 233, and 465 mcg of fluticasone propionate and 45 mcg of salmeterol base per blister from ADVAIR DISKUS 100/50, 250/50, and 500/50, respectively, when tested at a flow rate of 60 L/min for 2 seconds. In adult patients with obstructive lung disease and severely compromised lung function (mean FEV$_1$ 20% to 30% of predicted), mean peak inspiratory flow (PIF) through a DISKUS inhalation device was 82.4 L/min (range, 46.1 to 115.3 L/min). Inhalation profiles for adolescent (N = 13, aged 12 to 17 years) and adult (N = 17, aged 18 to 50 years) patients with asthma inhaling maximally through the DISKUS device show mean PIF of 122.2 L/min (range: 81.6 to 152.1 L/min). Inhalation profiles for pediatric patients with asthma inhaling maximally through the DISKUS device show a mean PIF of 75.5 L/min (range: 49.0 to 104.8 L/min) for the 4-year-old patient set (N = 20) and 7-year-old patient set (N = 20). The mean PIF for age 6 (range: 82.8 to 125.6 L/min) for the 8-year-old patient set (N = 20). The actual amount of drug delivered to the lung will depend on patient factors, such as inspiratory flow profile.

12 CLINICAL PHARMACOLOGY

12.1 Mechanism of Action

ADVAIR DISKUS: Since ADVAIR DISKUS contains both fluticasone propionate and salmeterol, the mechanisms of action described below for the individual components apply to ADVAIR DISKUS. These drugs represent 2 classes of medications (a synthetic corticosteroid and a selective LABA) that have different effects on clinical and physiological indices.

Fluticasone Propionate: Fluticasone propionate is a synthetic trifluorinated corticosteroid with potent anti-inflammatory activity. In vitro assays using human lung cytosol preparations have established fluticasone propionate as a human glucocorticoid receptor agonist with an affinity 18 times greater than dexamethasone, almost twice that of beclomethasone-17-monopropionate (BMP), the active metabolite of beclomethasone dipropionate, and over 3 times that of budesonide. Data from the McKenzie vasoconstrictor assay in man are consistent with these results.

Inflammation is an important component in the pathogenesis of asthma. Corticosteroids have been shown to inhibit multiple cell types (e.g., mast cells, eosinophils, basophils, lymphocytes, macrophages, neutrophils) and mediator production or secretion (e.g., histamine, eicosanoids, leukotrienes, cytokines) involved in the asthmatic response. These anti-inflammatory actions of corticosteroids contribute to their efficacy in asthma.

Inflammation is also a component in the pathogenesis of COPD. In contrast to asthma, however, the predominant inflammatory cells in COPD include neutrophils, CD8+ T-lymphocytes, and macrophages. The effects of corticosteroids in the treatment of COPD are not well defined and inhaled corticosteroids and fluticasone propionate when used apart from ADVAIR DISKUS are not indicated for the treatment of COPD.

Salmeterol Xinafoate: Salmeterol is a selective LABA. In vitro studies show salmeterol to be at least 50 times more selective for beta$_2$-adrenoceptors than albuterol. Although beta$_2$-adrenoceptors are the predominant adrenergic receptors in bronchial smooth muscle and beta$_1$-adrenoceptors are the predominant receptors in the heart, there are also beta$_2$-adrenoceptors in the human heart comprising 10% to 50% of the total beta-adrenoceptors. The precise function of these receptors has not been established, but their presence raises the possibility that even highly selective beta$_2$-agonists may have cardiac effects.

The pharmacologic effects of beta$_2$-adrenoceptor agonist drugs, including salmeterol, are at least in part attributable to stimulation of intracellular adenyl cyclase, the enzyme that catalyzes the conversion of adenosine triphosphate (ATP) to cyclic-3′,5′-adenosine monophosphate (cyclic AMP). Increased cyclic AMP levels cause relaxation of bronchial smooth muscle and inhibition of release of mediators of immediate hypersensitivity from cells, especially from mast cells.

In vitro tests show that salmeterol is a potent and long-lasting inhibitor of the release of mast cell mediators, such as histamine, leukotrienes, and prostaglandin D$_2$, from human lung. Salmeterol inhibits histamine-induced plasma protein extravasation and inhibits platelet-activating factor-induced eosinophil accumulation in the lungs of guinea pigs when administered by the inhaled route. In humans, single doses of salmeterol administered via inhalation aerosol attenuate allergen-induced bronchial hyper-responsiveness.

12.2 Pharmacodynamics

ADVAIR DISKUS: Healthy Subjects: Cardiovascular Effects: Since systemic pharmacodynamic effects of salmeterol are not normally seen at the therapeutic dose, higher doses were used to produce measurable effects. Four (4) studies were conducted in healthy adult subjects: (1) a single-dose crossover study using 2 inhalations of ADVAIR DISKUS 500/50, fluticasone propionate powder 500 mcg and salmeterol powder 50 mcg given concurrently, or fluticasone propionate powder 500 mcg given alone, (2) a cumulative dose study using 50 to 400 mcg of salmeterol powder given alone or as ADVAIR DISKUS 500/50, (3) a repeat-dose study for 11 days using 2 inhalations twice daily of ADVAIR DISKUS 250/50, fluticasone propionate powder 250 mcg, or salmeterol powder 50 mcg, and (4) a single-dose study using 5 inhalations of ADVAIR DISKUS 100/50, fluticasone propionate powder 100 mcg alone, or placebo. In these studies no significant differences were observed in the pharmacodynamic effects of salmeterol (pulse rate, blood pressure, QTc interval, potassium, and glucose) whether the salmeterol was given as ADVAIR DISKUS, concurrently with fluticasone propionate from separate inhalers, or as salmeterol alone. The systemic pharmacodynamic effects of salmeterol were not altered by the presence of fluticasone propionate in ADVAIR DISKUS. The potential effect of salmeterol on the effects of fluticasone propionate on the HPA axis was also evaluated in these studies.

HPA Axis Effects: No significant differences across treatments were observed in 24-hour urinary cortisol excretion and, where measured, 24-hour plasma cortisol AUC. The systemic pharmacodynamic effects of fluticasone propionate were not altered by the presence of salmeterol in ADVAIR DISKUS in healthy subjects.

Asthma: Adults and Adolescent Patients: Cardiovascular Effects: In clinical studies with ADVAIR DISKUS in adult and adolescent patients aged 12 years and older with asthma, no significant differences were observed in the systemic pharmacodynamic effects of salmeterol (pulse rate, blood pressure, QTc interval, potassium, and glucose) whether the salmeterol was given alone or as ADVAIR DISKUS. In 72 adolescent and adult patients with asthma given either ADVAIR DISKUS 100/50 or ADVAIR DISKUS 250/50, continuous 24-hour electrocardiographic monitoring was performed after the first dose and after 12 weeks of therapy, and no clinically significant dysrhythmias were noted.

HPA Axis Effects: In a 28-week study in adolescent and adult patients with asthma, ADVAIR DISKUS 500/50 twice daily was compared with the concurrent use of salmeterol powder 50 mcg plus fluticasone propionate powder 500 mcg from separate inhalers or fluticasone propionate powder 500 mcg alone. No significant differences across treatments were observed in serum cortisol AUC after 12 weeks of dosing or in 24-hour urinary cortisol excretion after 12 and 28 weeks.

In a 12-week study in adolescent and adult patients with asthma, ADVAIR DISKUS 250/50 twice daily was compared with fluticasone propionate powder 250 mcg alone, salmeterol powder 50 mcg alone, and placebo. For most patients, the ability to increase cortisol production in response to stress, as assessed by 30-minute cosyntropin stimulation, remained intact with ADVAIR DISKUS. One patient (3%) who received ADVAIR DISKUS 250/50 had an abnormal response (peak serum cortisol <18 mcg/dL) after dosing, compared with 2 patients (6%) who received placebo, 2 patients (6%) who received fluticasone propionate 250 mcg, and no patients who received salmeterol.

In a repeat-dose, 3-way crossover study, 1 inhalation twice daily of ADVAIR DISKUS 100/50, FLOVENT® DISKUS® 100 mcg (fluticasone propionate inhalation powder, 100 mcg), or placebo was administered to 20 adolescent and adult patients with asthma. After 28 days of treatment, geometric mean serum cortisol AUC over 12 hours showed no significant difference between ADVAIR DISKUS and FLOVENT DISKUS or between either active treatment and placebo.

Pediatric Patients: HPA Axis Effects: In a 12-week study in patients with asthma aged 4 to 11 years who were receiving inhaled corticosteroids at study entry, ADVAIR DISKUS 100/50 twice daily was compared with fluticasone propionate inhalation powder 100 mcg administered twice daily via the DISKUS. The values for 24-hour urinary cortisol excretion at study entry and after 12 weeks of treatment were similar within each treatment group. After 12 weeks, 24-hour urinary cortisol excretion was also similar between the 2 groups.

Chronic Obstructive Pulmonary Disease: Cardiovascular Effects: In clinical studies with ADVAIR DISKUS in patients with COPD, no significant differences were seen in pulse rate, blood pressure, potassium, and glucose between ADVAIR DISKUS, the individual components of ADVAIR DISKUS, and placebo. In a study of ADVAIR DISKUS 250/50, 8 patients (2 [1.1%] in the group given ADVAIR DISKUS 250/50, 1 [0.5%] in the fluticasone propionate 250-mcg group, 3 [1.7%] in the salmeterol group, and 2 [1.1%] in the placebo group) had QTc intervals >470 msec at least 1 time during the treatment period. Five (5) of these 8 patients had a prolonged QTc interval at baseline.

In a 24-week study, 130 patients with COPD received continuous 24-hour electrocardiographic monitoring prior to the first dose and after 4 weeks of twice-daily treatment with either ADVAIR DISKUS 500/50, fluticasone propionate powder 500 mcg, salmeterol powder 50 mcg, or placebo. No significant differences in ventricular or supraventricular arrhythmias and heart rate were observed among the groups treated with ADVAIR DISKUS 500/50, the individual components, or placebo. One (1) subject in the fluticasone propionate group experienced atrial flutter/atrial fibrillation, and 1 subject in the group given ADVAIR DISKUS 500/50 experienced heart block. There were 3 cases of nonsustained ventricular tachycardia (1 each in the placebo, salmeterol, and fluticasone propionate 500-mcg treatment groups).

In 24-week clinical studies in patients with COPD, the incidence of clinically significant electrocardiogram (ECG) abnormalities (myocardial ischemia, ventricular hypertrophy, clinically significant conduction abnormalities, clinically significant arrhythmias) was lower for patients who received salmeterol (1%, 9 of 688 patients who received either salmeterol 50 mcg or ADVAIR DISKUS) compared with placebo (3%, 10 of 370 patients).

No significant differences with salmeterol 50 mcg alone or in combination with fluticasone propionate as ADVAIR DISKUS 500/50 were observed on pulse rate and systolic and diastolic blood pressure in a subset of patients with COPD who underwent 12-hour serial vital sign measurements after the first dose (N = 183) and after 12 weeks of therapy (N = 149). Median changes from baseline in pulse rate and systolic and diastolic blood pressure were similar to those seen with placebo.

HPA Axis Effects: Short-cosyntropin stimulation testing was performed both at Day 1 and Endpoint in 101 patients with COPD receiving twice-daily ADVAIR DISKUS 250/50, fluticasone propionate powder 250 mcg, salmeterol powder 50 mcg, or placebo. For most patients, the ability to increase cortisol production in response to stress, as assessed by short cosyntropin stimulation, remained intact with ADVAIR DISKUS 250/50. One (1) patient (3%) who received ADVAIR DISKUS 250/50 had an abnormal stimulated cortisol response (peak cortisol <14.5 mcg/dL assessed by high-performance liquid chromatography) after dosing, compared with 2 patients (9%) who received fluticasone propionate 250 mcg, 2 patients (7%) who received salmeterol 50 mcg, and 1 patient (4%) who received placebo following 24 weeks of treatment or early discontinuation from study.

After 36 weeks of dosing, serum cortisol concentrations in a subset of patients with COPD (n = 83) were 22% lower in patients receiving ADVAIR DISKUS 500/50 and 21% lower in patients receiving fluticasone propionate 500 mcg than in patients receiving placebo.

Other Fluticasone Propionate Products: Asthma: HPA Axis Effects: In clinical trials with fluticasone propionate inhalation powder using doses up to and including 250 mcg twice daily, occasional abnormal short cosyntropin tests (peak serum cortisol <18 mcg/dL assessed by radioimmunoassay) were noted both in patients receiving fluticasone propionate and in patients receiving placebo. The incidence of abnormal tests at 500 mcg twice daily was greater than placebo. In a 2-year study carried out with the DISKHALER® inhalation device in 64 patients with mild, persistent asthma (mean FEV$_1$ 91% of predicted) randomized to fluticasone propionate 500 mcg twice daily or placebo, no patient receiving fluticasone propionate had an abnormal response to 6-hour cosyntropin infusion (peak serum cortisol <18 mcg/dL). With a peak cortisol threshold of <35 mcg/dL, 1 patient receiving fluticasone propionate (4%) had an abnormal response at 1 year; repeat testing at 18 months and 2 years was normal. Another patient receiving fluticasone propionate (5%) had an abnormal response at 2 years. No patient on placebo had an abnormal response at 1 or 2 years.

Chronic Obstructive Pulmonary Disease: HPA Axis Effects: After 4 weeks of dosing, the steady-state fluticasone propionate pharmacokinetics and serum cortisol levels were described in a subset of patients with COPD (n = 86) randomized to twice-daily fluticasone propionate inhalation powder via the DISKUS 500 mcg, fluticasone propionate inhalation powder 250 mcg, or placebo. Serial serum corti-

sol concentrations were measured across a 12-hour dosing interval. Serum cortisol concentrations following 250- and 500-mcg twice-daily dosing were 10% and 21% lower than placebo, respectively, indicating a dose-dependent increase in systemic exposure to fluticasone propionate.

Other Salmeterol Xinafoate Products: Asthma: Cardiovascular Effects: Inhaled salmeterol, like other beta-adrenergic agonist drugs, can produce dose-related cardiovascular effects and effects on blood glucose and/or serum potassium *[see Warnings and Precautions (5.12, 5.18)]*. The cardiovascular effects (heart rate, blood pressure) associated with salmeterol occur with similar frequency, and are of similar type and severity, as those noted following albuterol administration.

The effects of rising doses of inhaled salmeterol and standard inhaled doses of albuterol were studied in volunteers and in patients with asthma. Salmeterol doses up to 84 mcg administered as inhalation aerosol resulted in heart rate increases of 3 to 16 beats/min, about the same as albuterol dosed at 180 mcg by inhalation aerosol (4 to 10 beats/min). Adolescent and adult patients receiving 50-mcg doses of salmeterol inhalation powder (N = 60) underwent continuous electrocardiographic monitoring during two 12-hour periods after the first dose and after 1 month of therapy, and no clinically significant dysrhythmias were noted.

Concomitant Use of ADVAIR DISKUS With Other Respiratory Medications: Short-Acting Beta$_2$-Agonists: In clinical trials with patients with asthma, the mean daily need for albuterol by 166 adult and adolescent patients aged 12 years and older using ADVAIR DISKUS was approximately 1.3 inhalations/day, and ranged from 0 to 9 inhalations/day. Five percent (5%) of patients using ADVAIR DISKUS in these trials averaged 6 or more inhalations per day over the course of the 12-week trials. No increase in frequency of cardiovascular adverse reactions was observed among patients who averaged 6 or more inhalations per day.

In a COPD clinical trial, the mean daily need for albuterol for patients using ADVAIR DISKUS 250/50 was 4.1 inhalations/day. Twenty-six percent (26%) of patients using ADVAIR DISKUS 250/50 averaged 6 or more inhalations per day over the course of the 24-week trial. No increase in frequency of cardiovascular adverse reactions was observed among patients who averaged 6 or more inhalations of albuterol per day.

Methylxanthines: The concurrent use of intravenously or orally administered methylxanthines (e.g., aminophylline, theophylline) by adult and adolescent patients aged 12 years and older receiving ADVAIR DISKUS has not been completely evaluated. In clinical trials with patients with asthma, 39 patients receiving ADVAIR DISKUS 100/50, 250/50, or 500/50 twice daily concurrently with a theophylline product had adverse event rates similar to those in 304 patients receiving ADVAIR DISKUS without theophylline. Similar results were observed in patients receiving salmeterol 50 mcg plus fluticasone propionate 500 mcg twice daily concurrently with a theophylline product (n = 39) or without theophylline (n = 132).

In a COPD clinical trial, 17 patients receiving ADVAIR DISKUS 250/50 twice daily concurrently with a theophylline product had adverse event rates similar to those in 161 patients receiving ADVAIR DISKUS without theophylline. Based on the available data, the concomitant administration of methylxanthines with ADVAIR DISKUS did not alter the observed adverse event profile.

Fluticasone Propionate Nasal Spray: In adult and adolescent patients aged 12 years and older taking ADVAIR DISKUS in clinical trials, no difference in the profile of adverse events or HPA axis effects was noted between patients who were taking FLONASE® (fluticasone propionate) Nasal Spray, 50 mcg concurrently (n = 46) and those who were not (n = 130).

12.3 Pharmacokinetics

Absorption: Fluticasone Propionate: Healthy Subjects: Fluticasone propionate acts locally in the lung; therefore, plasma levels do not predict therapeutic effect. Studies using oral dosing of labeled and unlabeled drug have demonstrated that the oral systemic bioavailability of fluticasone propionate is negligible (<1%), primarily due to incomplete absorption and presystemic metabolism in the gut and liver. In contrast, the majority of the fluticasone propionate delivered to the lung is systemically absorbed.

Following administration of ADVAIR DISKUS to healthy adult subjects, peak plasma concentrations of fluticasone propionate were achieved in 1 to 2 hours. In a single-dose crossover study, a higher-than-recommended dose of ADVAIR DISKUS was administered to 14 healthy adult subjects. Two (2) inhalations of the following treatments were administered: ADVAIR DISKUS 500/50, fluticasone propionate powder 500 mcg and salmeterol powder 50 mcg given concurrently, and fluticasone propionate powder 500 mcg alone. Mean peak plasma concentrations of fluticasone propionate averaged 107, 94, and 120 pg/mL, respectively, indicating no significant changes in systemic exposures of fluticasone propionate.

In 15 healthy subjects, systemic exposure to fluticasone propionate from 4 inhalations of ADVAIR® HFA 230/21 (fluticasone propionate 230 mcg and salmeterol 21 mcg) Inhalation Aerosol (920/84 mcg) and 2 inhalations of ADVAIR DISKUS 500/50 (1,000/100 mcg) were similar between the 2 inhalers (i.e., 799 versus 832 pg•hr/mL, respectively), but approximately half the systemic exposure from 4 inhalations of fluticasone propionate CFC inhalation aerosol 220 mcg (880 mcg, AUC = 1,543 pg•hr/mL). Similar results were observed for peak fluticasone propionate plasma concentrations (186 and 182 pg/mL from ADVAIR HFA and ADVAIR DISKUS, respectively, and 307 pg/mL from the fluticasone propionate CFC inhalation aerosol). Absolute bioavailability of fluticasone propionate was 5.3% and 5.5% following administration of ADVAIR HFA and ADVAIR DISKUS, respectively.

Asthma and COPD Patients: Peak steady-state fluticasone propionate plasma concentrations in adult patients with asthma (N = 11) ranged from undetectable to 266 pg/mL after a 500-mcg twice-daily dose of fluticasone propionate inhalation powder using the DISKUS device. The mean fluticasone propionate plasma concentration was 110 pg/mL.

Full pharmacokinetic profiles were obtained from 9 female and 16 male patients with asthma given fluticasone propionate inhalation powder 500 mcg twice daily using the DISKUS device and from 14 female and 43 male patients with COPD given 250 or 500 mcg twice daily. No overall differences in fluticasone propionate pharmacokinetics were observed.

Peak steady-state fluticasone propionate plasma concentrations in patients with COPD averaged 53 pg/mL (range: 19.3 to 159.3 pg/mL) after treatment with 250 mcg twice daily (N = 30) and 84 pg/mL (range: 24.3 to 197.1 pg/mL) after treatment with 500 mcg twice daily (N = 27) via the fluticasone propionate DISKUS device. In another study in patients with COPD, peak steady-state fluticasone propionate plasma concentrations averaged 115 pg/mL (range: 52.6 to 366.0 pg/mL) after treatment with 500 mcg twice daily via the fluticasone propionate DISKUS device (N = 15) and 105 pg/mL (range: 22.5 to 299.0 pg/mL) via ADVAIR DISKUS (N = 24).

Salmeterol Xinafoate: Healthy Subjects: Salmeterol xinafoate, an ionic salt, dissociates in solution so that the salmeterol and 1-hydroxy-2-naphthoic acid (xinafoate) moieties are absorbed, distributed, metabolized, and eliminated independently. Salmeterol acts locally in the lung; therefore, plasma levels do not predict therapeutic effect.

Following administration of ADVAIR DISKUS to healthy adult subjects, peak plasma concentrations of salmeterol were achieved in about 5 minutes.

In 15 healthy subjects receiving ADVAIR HFA 230/21 Inhalation Aerosol (920/84 mcg) and ADVAIR DISKUS 500/50 (1,000/100 mcg), systemic exposure to salmeterol was higher (317 versus 169 pg•hr/mL) and peak salmeterol concentrations were lower (196 versus 223 pg/mL) following ADVAIR HFA compared with ADVAIR DISKUS, although pharmacodynamic results were comparable.

Asthma Patients: Because of the small therapeutic dose, systemic levels of salmeterol are low or undetectable after inhalation of recommended doses (50 mcg of salmeterol inhalation powder twice daily). Following chronic administration of an inhaled dose of 50 mcg of salmeterol inhalation powder twice daily, salmeterol was detected in plasma within 5 to 45 minutes in 7 patients with asthma; plasma concentrations were very low, with mean peak concentrations of 167 pg/mL at 20 minutes and no accumulation with repeated doses.

Distribution: Fluticasone Propionate: Following intravenous administration, the initial disposition phase for fluticasone propionate was rapid and consistent with its high lipid solubility and tissue binding. The volume of distribution averaged 4.2 L/kg.

The percentage of fluticasone propionate bound to human plasma proteins averages 91%. Fluticasone propionate is weakly and reversibly bound to erythrocytes and is not significantly bound to human transcortin.

Salmeterol: The percentage of salmeterol bound to human plasma proteins averages 96% in vitro over the concentration range of 8 to 7,722 ng of salmeterol base per milliliter, much higher concentrations than those achieved following therapeutic doses of salmeterol.

Metabolism: Fluticasone Propionate: The total clearance of fluticasone propionate is high (average, 1,093 mL/min), with renal clearance accounting for less than 0.02% of the total. The only circulating metabolite detected in man is the 17β-carboxylic acid derivative of fluticasone propionate, which is formed through the CYP3A4 pathway. This metabolite had less affinity (approximately 1/2,000) than the parent drug for the glucocorticoid receptor of human lung cytosol in vitro and negligible pharmacological activity in animal studies. Other metabolites detected in vitro using cultured human hepatoma cells have not been detected in man.

Salmeterol: Salmeterol base is extensively metabolized by hydroxylation, with subsequent elimination predominantly in the feces. No significant amount of unchanged salmeterol base was detected in either urine or feces.
An in vitro study using human liver microsomes showed that salmeterol is extensively metabolized to α-hydroxysalmeterol (aliphatic oxidation) by CYP3A4. Ketoconazole, a strong inhibitor of CYP3A4, essentially completely inhibited the formation of α-hydroxysalmeterol in vitro.
Elimination: *Fluticasone Propionate:* Following intravenous dosing, fluticasone propionate showed polyexponential kinetics and had a terminal elimination half-life of approximately 7.8 hours. Less than 5% of a radiolabeled oral dose was excreted in the urine as metabolites, with the remainder excreted in the feces as parent drug and metabolites. Terminal half-life estimates of fluticasone propionate for ADVAIR HFA, ADVAIR DISKUS, and fluticasone propionate CFC inhalation aerosol were similar and averaged 5.6 hours.
Salmeterol: In 2 healthy adult subjects who received 1 mg of radiolabeled salmeterol (as salmeterol xinafoate) orally, approximately 25% and 60% of the radiolabeled salmeterol was eliminated in urine and feces, respectively, over a period of 7 days. The terminal elimination half-life was about 5.5 hours (1 volunteer only).
The xinafoate moiety has no apparent pharmacologic activity. The xinafoate moiety is highly protein bound (>99%) and has a long elimination half-life of 11 days. No terminal half-life estimates were calculated for salmeterol following administration of ADVAIR DISKUS.
Special Populations: A population pharmacokinetic analysis was performed for fluticasone propionate and salmeterol utilizing data from 9 controlled clinical trials that included 350 patients with asthma aged 4 to 77 years who received treatment with ADVAIR DISKUS, the combination of HFA-propelled fluticasone propionate and salmeterol inhalation aerosol (ADVAIR HFA), fluticasone propionate inhalation powder (FLOVENT DISKUS), HFA-propelled fluticasone propionate inhalation aerosol (FLOVENT® HFA), or CFC-propelled fluticasone propionate inhalation aerosol. The population pharmacokinetic analyses for fluticasone propionate and salmeterol showed no clinically relevant effects of age, gender, race, body weight, body mass index, or percent of predicted FEV_1 on apparent clearance and apparent volume of distribution.
Age: When the population pharmacokinetic analysis for fluticasone propionate was divided into subgroups based on fluticasone propionate strength, formulation, and age (adolescents/adults and children), there were some differences in fluticasone propionate exposure. Higher fluticasone propionate exposure from ADVAIR DISKUS 100/50 compared with FLOVENT DISKUS 100 mcg was observed in adolescents and adults (ratio 1.52 [90% CI: 1.08, 2.13]). However, in clinical studies of up to 12 weeks' duration comparing ADVAIR DISKUS 100/50 and FLOVENT DISKUS 100 mcg in adolescents and adults, no differences in systemic effects of corticosteroid treatment (e.g., HPA axis effects) were observed. Similar fluticasone propionate exposure was observed from ADVAIR DISKUS 500/50 and FLOVENT DISKUS 500 mcg (ratio 0.83 [90% CI: 0.65, 1.07]) in adolescents and adults.
Steady-state systemic exposure to salmeterol when delivered as ADVAIR DISKUS 100/50, ADVAIR DISKUS 250/50, or ADVAIR HFA 115/21 (fluticasone propionate 115 mcg and salmeterol 21 mcg) Inhalation Aerosol was evaluated in 127 patients aged 4 to 57 years. The geometric mean AUC was 325 pg•hr/mL (90% CI: 309, 341) in adolescents and adults. The population pharmacokinetic analysis included 160 patients with asthma aged 4 to 11 years who received ADVAIR DISKUS 100/50 or FLOVENT DISKUS 100 mcg. Higher fluticasone propionate exposure (AUC) was observed in children from ADVAIR DISKUS 100/50 compared with FLOVENT DISKUS 100 mcg (ratio 1.20 [90% CI: 1.06, 1.37]). Higher fluticasone propionate exposure (AUC) from ADVAIR DISKUS 100/50 was observed in children compared with adolescents and adults (ratio 1.63 [90% CI: 1.35, 1.96]). However, in clinical studies of up to 12 weeks' duration comparing ADVAIR DISKUS 100/50 and FLOVENT DISKUS 100 mcg in both adolescents and adults and in children, no differences in systemic effects of corticosteroid treatment (e.g., HPA axis effects) were observed.
Exposure to salmeterol was higher in children compared with adolescents and adults who received ADVAIR DISKUS 100/50 (ratio 1.23 [90% CI: 1.10, 1.38]). However, in clinical studies of up to 12 weeks' duration with ADVAIR DISKUS 100/50 in both adolescents and adults and in children, no differences in systemic effects of $beta_2$-agonist treatment (e.g., cardiovascular effects, tremor) were observed.
Gender: The population pharmacokinetic analysis involved 202 males and 148 females with asthma who received fluticasone propionate alone or in combination with salmeterol and showed no gender differences for fluticasone propionate pharmacokinetics.
The population pharmacokinetic analysis involved 76 males and 51 females with asthma who received salmeterol in combination with fluticasone propionate and showed no gender differences for salmeterol pharmacokinetics.
Hepatic and Renal Impairment: Formal pharmacokinetic studies using ADVAIR DISKUS have not been conducted in patients with hepatic or renal impairment. However, since both fluticasone propionate and salmeterol are predominantly cleared by hepatic metabolism, impairment of liver function may lead to accumulation of fluticasone propionate and salmeterol in plasma. Therefore, patients with hepatic disease should be closely monitored.
Drug Interactions: In the repeat- and single-dose studies, there was no evidence of significant drug interaction in systemic exposure between fluticasone propionate and salmeterol when given as ADVAIR DISKUS. The population pharmacokinetic analysis from 9 controlled clinical trials in 350 patients with asthma showed no significant effects on fluticasone propionate or salmeterol pharmacokinetics following co-administration with $beta_2$-agonists, corticosteroids, antihistamines, or theophyllines.
Inhibitors of Cytochrome P450 3A4: Ritonavir: Fluticasone Propionate: Fluticasone propionate is a substrate of CYP3A4. Coadministration of fluticasone propionate and the strong CYP3A4 inhibitor ritonavir is not recommended based upon a multiple-dose, crossover drug interaction study in 18 healthy subjects. Fluticasone propionate aqueous nasal spray (200 mcg once daily) was coadministered for 7 days with ritonavir (100 mg twice daily). Plasma fluticasone propionate concentrations following fluticasone propionate aqueous nasal spray alone were undetectable (<10 pg/mL) in most subjects, and when concentrations were detectable peak levels (C_{max}) averaged 11.9 pg/mL (range: 10.8 to 14.1 pg/mL) and $AUC_{(0-\tau)}$ averaged 8.43 pg•hr/mL (range: 4.2 to 18.8 pg•hr/mL). Fluticasone propionate C_{max} and $AUC_{(0-\tau)}$ increased to 318 pg/mL (range: 110 to 648 pg/mL) and 3,102.6 pg•hr/mL (range: 1,207.1 to 5,662.0 pg•hr/mL), respectively, after coadministration of ritonavir with fluticasone propionate aqueous nasal spray. This significant increase in plasma fluticasone propionate exposure resulted in a significant decrease (86%) in serum cortisol AUC.
Ketoconazole: Fluticasone Propionate: In a placebo-controlled, crossover study in 8 healthy adult volunteers, coadministration of a single dose of orally inhaled fluticasone propionate (1,000 mcg) with multiple doses of ketoconazole (200 mg) to steady state resulted in increased plasma fluticasone propionate exposure, a reduction in plasma cortisol AUC, and no effect on urinary excretion of cortisol.
Salmeterol: In a placebo-controlled, crossover drug interaction study in 20 healthy male and female subjects, coadministration of salmeterol (50 mcg twice daily) and the strong CYP3A4 inhibitor ketoconazole (400 mg once daily) for 7 days resulted in a significant increase in plasma salmeterol exposure as determined by a 16-fold increase in AUC (ratio with and without ketoconazole 15.76 [90% CI: 10.66, 23.31]) mainly due to increased bioavailability of the swallowed portion of the dose. Peak plasma salmeterol concentrations were increased by 1.4-fold (90% CI: 1.23, 1.68). Three (3) out of 20 subjects (15%) were withdrawn from salmeterol and ketoconazole coadministration due to beta-agonist–meiated systemic effects (2 with QTc prolongation and 1 with palpitations and sinus tachycardia). Coadministration of salmeterol and ketoconazole did not result in a clinically significant effect on mean heart rate, mean blood potassium, or mean blood glucose. Although there was no statistical effect on the mean QTc, coadministration of salmeterol and ketoconazole was associated with more frequent increases in QTc duration compared with salmeterol and placebo administration.
Erythromycin: Fluticasone Propionate: In a multiple-dose drug interaction study, coadministration of orally inhaled fluticasone propionate (500 mcg twice daily) and erythromycin (333 mg 3 times daily) did not affect fluticasone propionate pharmacokinetics.
Salmeterol: In a repeat-dose study in 13 healthy subjects, concomitant administration of erythromycin (a moderate CYP3A4 inhibitor) and salmeterol inhalation aerosol resulted in a 40% increase in salmeterol C_{max} at steady state (ratio with and without erythromycin 1.4 [90% CI: 0.96, 2.03], p = 0.12), a 3.6-beat/min increase in heart rate ([95% CI: 0.19, 7.03], p<0.04), a 5.8-msec increase in QTc interval ([95% CI: -6.14, 17.77], p = 0.34), and no change in plasma potassium.

13 NONCLINICAL TOXICOLOGY

13.1 Carcinogenesis, Mutagenesis, Impairment of Fertility

Fluticasone Propionate: Fluticasone propionate demonstrated no tumorigenic potential in mice at oral doses up to 1,000 mcg/kg (approximately 4 and 10 times the MRHD for adults and children, respectively, on an mg/m^2 basis) for 78 weeks or in rats at inhalation doses up to 57 mcg/kg (less than and approximately equivalent to the MRHD for adults and children, respectively, on an mg/m^2 basis) for 104 weeks.
Fluticasone propionate did not induce gene mutation in prokaryotic or eukaryotic cells in vitro. No significant clastogenic effect was seen in cultured human peripheral lymphocytes in vitro or in the in vivo mouse micronucleus test.
No evidence of impairment of fertility was observed in reproductive studies conducted in rats at subcutaneous doses up to 50 mcg/kg (less than the MRHD on an mg/m^2 basis). Prostate weight was significantly reduced.
Salmeterol: In an 18-month carcinogenicity study in CD-mice, salmeterol at oral doses of 1.4 mg/kg and above (approximately 20 times the MRHD for adults and children based on comparison of the plasma AUCs) caused a dose-related increase in the incidence of smooth muscle hyperplasia, cystic glandular hyperplasia, leiomyomas of the uterus, and ovarian cysts. No tumors were seen at 0.2 mg/kg (approximately 3 times the MRHD for adults and children based on comparison of the AUCs).
In a 24-month oral and inhalation carcinogenicity study in Sprague Dawley rats, salmeterol caused a dose-related increase in the incidence of mesovarian leiomyomas and ovarian cysts at doses of 0.68 mg/kg and above (approximately 55 and 25 times the MRHD for adults and children, respectively, on an mg/m^2 basis). No tumors were seen at 0.21 mg/kg (approximately 15 and 8 times the MRHD for adults and children, respectively, on an mg/m^2 basis). These findings in rodents are similar to those reported previously for other beta-adrenergic agonist drugs. The relevance of these findings to human use is unknown.
Salmeterol produced no detectable or reproducible increases in microbial and mammalian gene mutation in vitro. No clastogenic activity occurred in vitro in human lymphocytes or in vivo in a rat micronucleus test. No effects on fertility were identified in rats treated with salmeterol at oral doses up to 2 mg/kg (approximately 160 times the MRHD for adults on an mg/m^2 basis).

13.2 Animal Toxicology and/or Pharmacology

Preclinical: Studies in laboratory animals (minipigs, rodents, and dogs) have demonstrated the occurrence of cardiac arrhythmias and sudden death (with histologic evidence of myocardial necrosis) when beta-agonists and methylxanthines are administered concurrently. The clinical relevance of these findings is unknown.
Reproductive Toxicology Studies: *ADVAIR DISKUS:* In mice, combining 150 mcg/kg subcutaneously of fluticasone propionate (less than the MRHD on an mg/m^2 basis) with 10 mg/kg orally of salmeterol (approximately 410 times the MRHD on an mg/m^2 basis) produced cleft palate, fetal death, increased implantation loss, and delayed ossification. No such effects were observed at combination subcutaneous doses up to 40 mcg/kg subcutaneously of fluticasone propionate (less than the MRHD on an mg/m^2 basis) and up to 1.4 mg/kg orally doses of salmeterol (approximately 55 times the MRHD on an mg/m^2 basis).
In rats, combining 100 mcg/kg subcutaneously of fluticasone propionate (equivalent to the MRHD on an mg/m^2 basis) and 10 mg/kg orally of salmeterol (approximately 810 times the MRHD on an mg/m^2 basis) produced decreased fetal weight, umbilical hernia, delayed ossification, and changes in the occipital bone. No such effects were observed at combination doses up to 30 mcg/kg subcutaneously of fluticasone propionate (less than the MRHD on an mg/m^2 basis) and up to 1 mg/kg orally of salmeterol (approximately 80 times the MRHD on an mg/m^2 basis).
Fluticasone Propionate: Subcutaneous studies in the mouse and rat at 45 and 100 mcg/kg (less than and equivalent to the MRHD on an mg/m^2 basis), respectively, revealed fetal toxicity characteristic of potent corticosteroid compounds, including embryonic growth retardation, omphalocele, cleft palate, and retarded cranial ossification.
In the rabbit, fetal weight reduction and cleft palate were observed at a subcutaneous dose of 4 mcg/kg (less than the MRHD on an mg/m^2 basis). However, no teratogenic effects were reported at oral doses up to 300 mcg/kg (approximately 5 times the MRHD on an mg/m^2 basis) of fluticasone propionate. No fluticasone propionate was detected in the plasma in this study, consistent with the established low bioavailability following oral administration *[see Clinical Pharmacology (12.3)]*.
Fluticasone propionate crossed the placenta following subcutaneous administration to mice and rats and oral administration to rabbits.
Salmeterol: No teratogenic effects occurred in rats at oral doses up to 2 mg/kg (approximately 160 times the MRHD on an mg/m^2 basis).
In Dutch rabbits administered oral doses of 1 mg/kg and above (approximately 50 times and above the MRHD based on comparison of the AUCs), salmeterol exhibited fetal toxic effects characteristically resulting from beta-adrenoceptor stimulation. These included precocious eyelid openings, cleft palate, sternebral fusion, limb and paw flexures, and delayed ossification of the frontal cranial bones. No such effects occurred at an oral dose of 0.6 mg/kg (approximately

Table 5. Peak Expiratory Flow Results for Patients With Asthma Previously Treated With Either Inhaled Corticosteroids or Salmeterol (Study 1)

Efficacy Variable[a]	ADVAIR DISKUS 100/50 (N = 87)	Fluticasone Propionate 100 mcg (N = 85)	Salmeterol 50 mcg (N = 86)	Placebo (N = 77)
AM PEF (L/min)				
Baseline	393	374	369	382
Change from baseline	53	17	-2	-24
PM PEF (L/min)				
Baseline	418	390	396	398
Change from baseline	35	18	-7	-13

[a]Change from baseline = change from baseline at Endpoint (last available data).

20 times the MRHD based on comparison of the AUCs). New Zealand White rabbits were less sensitive since only delayed ossification of the frontal bones was seen at an oral dose of 10 mg/kg (approximately 1,600 times the MRHD on an mg/m² basis).

Salmeterol crossed the placenta following oral administration to mice and rats.

14 CLINICAL STUDIES
14.1 Asthma

Adult and Adolescent Patients Aged 12 Years and Older: In clinical trials comparing ADVAIR DISKUS with its individual components, improvements in most efficacy endpoints were greater with ADVAIR DISKUS than with the use of either fluticasone propionate or salmeterol alone. In addition, clinical trials showed similar results between ADVAIR DISKUS and the concurrent use of fluticasone propionate plus salmeterol at corresponding doses from separate inhalers.

Studies Comparing ADVAIR DISKUS to Fluticasone Propionate Alone or Salmeterol Alone: Three (3) double-blind, parallel-group clinical trials were conducted with ADVAIR DISKUS in 1,208 adolescent and adult patients (≥12 years, baseline FEV_1 63% to 72% of predicted normal) with asthma that was not optimally controlled on their current therapy. All treatments were inhalation powders given as 1 inhalation from the DISKUS device twice daily, and other maintenance therapies were discontinued.

Study 1: Clinical Trial With ADVAIR DISKUS 100/50: This placebo-controlled, 12-week, US study compared ADVAIR DISKUS 100/50 with its individual components, fluticasone propionate 100 mcg and salmeterol 50 mcg. The study was stratified according to baseline asthma maintenance therapy; patients were using either inhaled corticosteroids (N = 250) (daily doses of beclomethasone dipropionate 252 to 420 mcg; flunisolide 1,000 mcg; fluticasone propionate inhalation aerosol 176 mcg; or triamcinolone acetonide 600 to 1,000 mcg) or salmeterol (N = 106). Baseline FEV_1 measurements were similar across treatments: ADVAIR DISKUS 100/50, 2.17 L; fluticasone propionate 100 mcg, 2.11 L; salmeterol, 2.13 L; and placebo, 2.15 L.

Predefined withdrawal criteria for lack of efficacy, an indicator of worsening asthma, were utilized for this placebo-controlled study. Worsening asthma was defined as a clinically important decrease in FEV_1 or PEF, increase in use of VENTOLIN® (albuterol, USP) Inhalation Aerosol, increase in night awakenings due to asthma, emergency intervention or hospitalization due to asthma, or requirement for asthma medication not allowed by the protocol. As shown in Table 4, statistically significantly fewer patients receiving ADVAIR DISKUS 100/50 were withdrawn due to worsening asthma compared with fluticasone propionate, salmeterol, and placebo.

Table 4. Percent of Patients Withdrawn Due to Worsening Asthma in Patients Previously Treated With Either Inhaled Corticosteroids or Salmeterol (Study 1)

ADVAIR DISKUS 100/50 (N = 87)	Fluticasone Propionate 100 mcg (N = 85)	Salmeterol 50 mcg (N = 86)	Placebo (N = 77)
3%	11%	35%	49%

The FEV_1 results are displayed in Figure 2. Because this trial used predetermined criteria for worsening asthma, which caused more patients in the placebo group to be withdrawn, FEV_1 results at Endpoint (last available FEV_1 result) are also provided. Patients receiving ADVAIR DISKUS 100/50 had significantly greater improvements in FEV_1 (0.51 L, 25%) compared with fluticasone propionate 100 mcg (0.28 L, 15%), salmeterol (0.11 L, 5%), and placebo (0.01 L, 1%). These improvements in FEV_1 with ADVAIR

DISKUS were achieved regardless of baseline asthma maintenance therapy (inhaled corticosteroids or salmeterol).

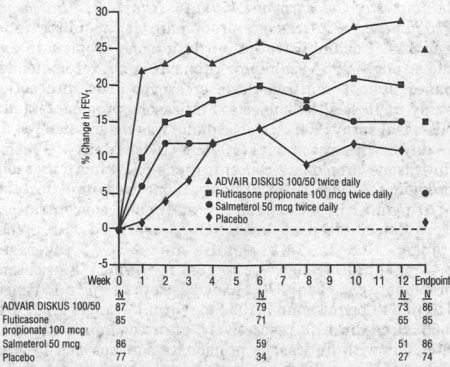
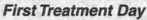

Figure 2. Mean Percent Change From Baseline in FEV_1 in Patients With Asthma Previously Treated With Either Inhaled Corticosteroids or Salmeterol (Study 1)

The effect of ADVAIR DISKUS 100/50 on morning and evening PEF endpoints is shown in Table 5.
[See table above]

The subjective impact of asthma on patients' perception of health was evaluated through use of an instrument called the Asthma Quality of Life Questionnaire (AQLQ) (based on a 7-point scale where 1 = maximum impairment and 7 = none). Patients receiving ADVAIR DISKUS 100/50 had clinically meaningful improvements in overall asthma-specific quality of life as defined by a difference between groups of ≥0.5 points in change from baseline AQLQ scores (difference in AQLQ score of 1.25 compared with placebo).

Study 2: Clinical Trial With ADVAIR DISKUS 250/50: This placebo-controlled, 12-week, US study compared ADVAIR DISKUS 250/50 with its individual components, fluticasone propionate 250 mcg and salmeterol 50 mcg, in 349 patients with asthma using inhaled corticosteroids (daily doses of beclomethasone dipropionate 462 to 672 mcg; flunisolide 1,250 to 2,000 mcg; fluticasone propionate inhalation aerosol 440 mcg; or triamcinolone acetonide 1,100 to 1,600 mcg). Baseline FEV_1 measurements were similar across treatments: ADVAIR DISKUS 250/50, 2.23 L; fluticasone propionate 250 mcg, 2.12 L; salmeterol, 2.20 L; and placebo, 2.19 L.

Efficacy results in this study were similar to those observed in Study 1. Patients receiving ADVAIR DISKUS 250/50 had significantly greater improvements in FEV_1 (0.48 L, 23%) compared with fluticasone propionate 250 mcg (0.25 L, 13%), salmeterol (0.05 L, 4%), and placebo (decrease of 0.11 L, decrease of 5%). Statistically significantly fewer patients receiving ADVAIR DISKUS 250/50 were withdrawn from this study for worsening asthma (4%) compared with fluticasone propionate (22%), salmeterol (38%), and placebo (62%). In addition, ADVAIR DISKUS 250/50 was superior to fluticasone propionate, salmeterol, and placebo for improvements in morning and evening PEF. Patients receiving ADVAIR DISKUS 250/50 also had clinically meaningful improvements in overall asthma-specific quality of life as described in Study 1 (difference in AQLQ score of 1.29 compared with placebo).

Study 3: Clinical Trial With ADVAIR DISKUS 500/50: This 28-week, non-US study compared ADVAIR DISKUS 500/50 with fluticasone propionate 500 mcg alone and concurrent therapy (salmeterol 50 mcg plus fluticasone propionate 500 mcg administered from separate inhalers) twice daily in 503 patients with asthma using inhaled corticosteroids (daily doses of beclomethasone dipropionate 1,260 to 1,680 mcg; budesonide 1,500 to 2,000 mcg; flunisolide 1,500 to 2,000 mcg; or fluticasone propionate inhalation aerosol 660 to 880 mcg [750 to 1,000 mcg

inhalation powder]). The primary efficacy parameter, morning PEF, was collected daily for the first 12 weeks of the study. The primary purpose of weeks 13 to 28 was to collect safety data.

Baseline PEF measurements were similar across treatments: ADVAIR DISKUS 500/50, 359 L/min; fluticasone propionate 500 mcg, 351 L/min; and concurrent therapy, 345 L/min. Morning PEF improved significantly with ADVAIR DISKUS 500/50 compared with fluticasone propionate 500 mcg over the 12-week treatment period. Improvements in morning PEF observed with ADVAIR DISKUS 500/50 were similar to improvements observed with concurrent therapy.

Onset of Action and Progression of Improvement in Asthma Control: The onset of action and progression of improvement in asthma control were evaluated in the 2 placebo-controlled US trials. Following the first dose, the median time to onset of clinically significant bronchodilatation (≥15% improvement in FEV_1) in most patients was seen within 30 to 60 minutes. Maximum improvement in FEV_1 generally occurred within 3 hours, and clinically significant improvement was maintained for 12 hours (see Figure 3). Following the initial dose, predose FEV_1 relative to Day 1 baseline improved markedly over the first week of treatment and continued to improve over the 12 weeks of treatment in both studies. No diminution in the 12-hour bronchodilator effect was observed with either ADVAIR DISKUS 100/50 (Figures 3 and 4) or ADVAIR DISKUS 250/50 as assessed by FEV_1 following 12 weeks of therapy.

First Treatment Day

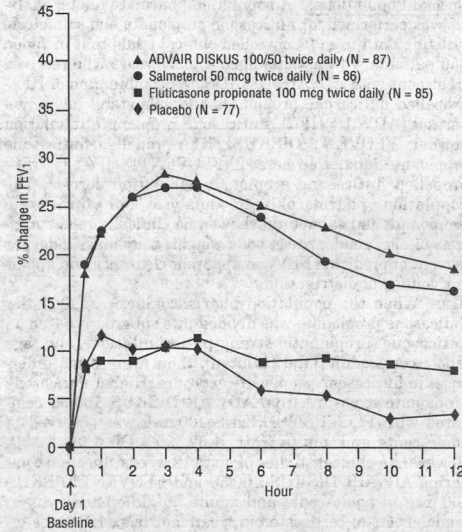

Figure 3. Percent Change in Serial 12-hour FEV_1 in Patients With Asthma Previously Using Either Inhaled Corticosteroids or Salmeterol (Study 1)

Last Treatment Day (Week 12)

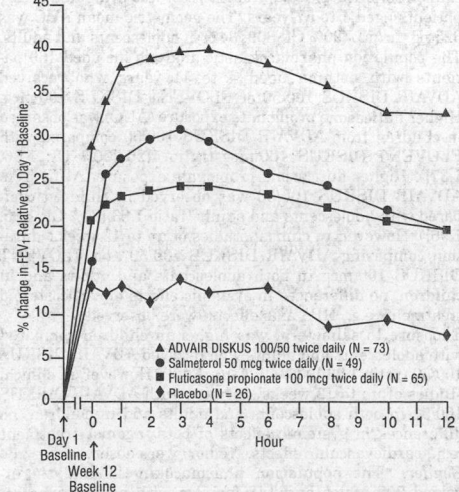

Figure 4. Percent Change in Serial 12-hour FEV_1 in Patients With Asthma Previously Using Either Inhaled Corticosteroids or Salmeterol (Study 1)

Reduction in asthma symptoms, use of rescue VENTOLIN Inhalation Aerosol, and improvement in morning and evening PEF also occurred within the first day of treatment with ADVAIR DISKUS, and continued to improve over the 12 weeks of therapy in both studies.

Pediatric Patients: In a 12-week US study, ADVAIR DISKUS 100/50 twice daily was compared with fluticasone propionate inhalation powder 100 mcg twice daily in 203 children with asthma aged 4 to 11 years. At study entry, the children were symptomatic on low doses of inhaled corticosteroids (beclomethasone dipropionate 252 to 336 mcg/day; budesonide 200 to 400 mcg/day; flunisolide 1,000 mcg/day; triamcinolone acetonide 600 to 1,000 mcg/day; or fluticasone propionate 88 to 250 mcg/day). The primary objective of this study was to determine the safety of ADVAIR DISKUS 100/50 compared with fluticasone propionate inhalation powder 100 mcg in this age-group; however, the study also included secondary efficacy measures of pulmonary function. Morning predose FEV_1 was obtained at baseline and Endpoint (last available FEV_1 result) in children aged 6 to 11 years. In patients receiving ADVAIR DISKUS 100/50, FEV_1 increased from 1.70 L at baseline (N = 79) to 1.88 L at Endpoint (N = 69) compared with an increase from 1.65 L at baseline (N = 83) to 1.77 L at Endpoint (N = 75) in patients receiving fluticasone propionate 100 mcg.

The findings of this study, along with extrapolation of efficacy data from patients aged 12 years and older, support the overall conclusion that ADVAIR DISKUS 100/50 is efficacious in the treatment of asthma in patients aged 4 to 11 years.

14.2 Chronic Obstructive Pulmonary Disease

The efficacy of ADVAIR DISKUS 250/50 and ADVAIR DISKUS 500/50 in the treatment of patients with COPD was evaluated in 6 randomized, double-blind, parallel-group clinical trials in adult patients aged 40 years and older. These trials were primarily designed to evaluate the efficacy of ADVAIR DISKUS on lung function (3 trials), exacerbations (2 trials), and survival (1 trial).

Lung Function: Two of the 3 clinical trials primarily designed to evaluate the efficacy of ADVAIR DISKUS on lung function were conducted in 1,414 patients with COPD associated with chronic bronchitis. In these 2 trials, all the patients had a history of cough productive of sputum that was not attributable to another disease process on most days for at least 3 months of the year for at least 2 years. The trials were randomized, double-blind, parallel-group, 24-week treatment duration. One trial evaluated the efficacy of ADVAIR DISKUS 250/50 compared with its components fluticasone propionate 250 mcg and salmeterol 50 mcg and with placebo, and the other trial evaluated the efficacy of ADVAIR DISKUS 500/50 compared with its components fluticasone propionate 500 mcg and salmeterol 50 mcg and with placebo. Study treatments were inhalation powders given as 1 inhalation from the DISKUS device twice daily. Maintenance COPD therapies were discontinued, with the exception of theophylline. The patients had a mean prebronchodilator FEV_1 of 41% and 20% reversibility at study entry. Percent reversibility was calculated as 100 times (FEV_1 post-albuterol minus FEV_1 pre-albuterol)/FEV_1 pre-albuterol.

Improvements in lung function (as defined by predose and postdose FEV_1) were significantly greater with ADVAIR DISKUS than with fluticasone propionate, salmeterol, or placebo. The improvement in lung function with ADVAIR DISKUS 500/50 was similar to the improvement seen with ADVAIR DISKUS 250/50.

Figures 5 and 6 display predose and 2-hour postdose, respectively, FEV_1 results for the study with ADVAIR DISKUS 250/50. To account for patient withdrawals during the study, FEV_1 at Endpoint (last evaluable FEV_1) was evaluated. Patients receiving ADVAIR DISKUS 250/50 had significantly greater improvements in predose FEV_1 at Endpoint (165 mL, 17%) compared with salmeterol 50 mcg (91 mL, 9%) and placebo (1 mL, 1%), demonstrating the contribution of fluticasone propionate to the improvement in lung function with ADVAIR DISKUS (Figure 5). Patients receiving ADVAIR DISKUS 250/50 had significantly greater improvements in postdose FEV_1 at Endpoint (281 mL, 27%) compared with fluticasone propionate 250 mcg (147 mL, 14%) and placebo (58 mL, 6%), demonstrating the contribution of salmeterol to the improvement in lung function with ADVAIR DISKUS (Figure 6).

[See figure 5 at top of next column]

[See figure 6 in next column]

The third trial was a 1-year study that evaluated ADVAIR DISKUS 500/50, fluticasone propionate 500 mcg, salmeterol 50 mcg, and placebo in 1,465 patients. The patients had an established history of COPD and exacerbations, a pre-bronchodilator FEV_1 <70% of predicted at study entry, and 8.3% reversibility. The primary endpoint was the comparison of pre-bronchodilator FEV_1 in the groups receiving ADVAIR DISKUS 500/50 or placebo. Patients treated with ADVAIR DISKUS 500/50 had greater improvements in

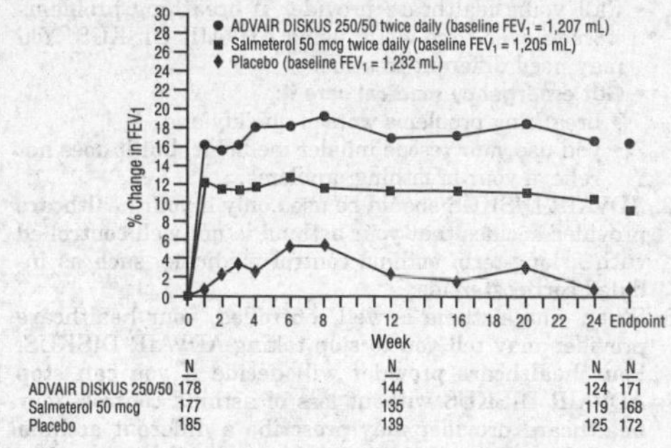

Figure 5. Predose FEV_1: Mean Percent Change From Baseline in Patients With Chronic Obstructive Pulmonary Disease

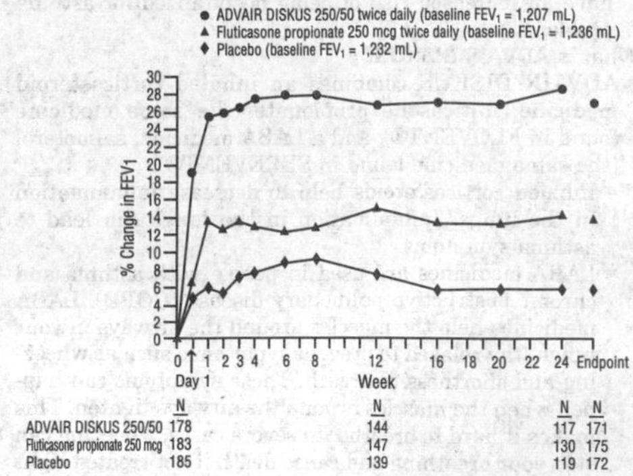

Figure 6. Two-Hour Postdose FEV_1: Mean Percent Changes From Baseline Over Time in Patients With Chronic Obstructive Pulmonary Disease

FEV_1 (113 mL, 10%) compared with fluticasone propionate 500 mcg (7 mL, 2%), salmeterol (15 mL, 2%), and placebo (-60 mL, -3%).

Exacerbations: Two studies were primarily designed to evaluate the effect of ADVAIR DISKUS 250/50 on exacerbations. In these 2 studies, exacerbations were defined as worsening of 2 or more major symptoms (dyspnea, sputum volume, and sputum purulence) or worsening of any 1 major symptom together with any 1 of the following minor symptoms: sore throat, colds (nasal discharge and/or nasal congestion), fever without other cause, and increased cough or wheeze for at least 2 consecutive days. COPD exacerbations were considered of moderate severity if treatment with systemic corticosteroids and/or antibiotics was required and were considered severe if hospitalization was required.

Exacerbations were also evaluated as a secondary outcome in the 1- and 3-year trials with ADVAIR DISKUS 500/50. There was not a symptomatic definition of exacerbation in these 2 trials. Exacerbations were defined in terms of severity requiring treatment with antibiotics and/or systemic corticosteroids (moderately severe) or requiring hospitalization (severe).

The 2 exacerbation trials with ADVAIR DISKUS 250/50 were identical studies designed to evaluate the effect of ADVAIR DISKUS 250/50 and salmeterol 50 mcg, each given twice daily, on exacerbations of COPD over a 12-month period. A total of 1,579 patients had an established history of COPD (but no other significant respiratory disorders). Patients had a pre-bronchodilator FEV_1 of 33% of predicted, a mean reversibility of 23% at baseline, and a history of ≥1 COPD exacerbation in the previous year that was moderate or severe. All patients were treated with ADVAIR DISKUS 250/50 twice daily during a 4-week run-in period prior to being assigned study treatment with twice-daily ADVAIR DISKUS 250/50 or salmeterol 50 mcg. In both studies, treatment with ADVAIR DISKUS 250/50 resulted in a significantly lower annual rate of moderate/severe COPD exacerbations compared with salmeterol (30.5% reduction [95% CI: 17.0, 41.8], p<0.001) in the first study and (30.4% reduction [95% CI: 16.9, 41.7], p<0.001) in the second study. Patients treated with ADVAIR DISKUS 250/50 also had a significantly lower annual rate of exacerbations requiring treatment with oral corticosteroids compared with patients treated with salmeterol (39.7% reduction [95% CI: 22.8, 52.9], p <0.001) in the first study and (34.3% reduction [95% CI: 18.6, 47.0], p<0.001) in the second study. Secondary endpoints including pulmonary function and symptom scores improved more in patients treated with ADVAIR DISKUS 250/50 than with salmeterol 50 mcg in both studies.

Exacerbations were evaluated in the 1- and the 3-year trials with ADVAIR DISKUS 500/50 as 1 of the secondary efficacy endpoints. In the 1-year trial, the group receiving ADVAIR DISKUS 500/50 had a significantly lower rate of moderate and severe exacerbations compared with placebo (25.4% reduction compared with placebo [95% CI: 13.5, 35.7]) but not when compared with its components (7.5% reduction compared with fluticasone propionate [95% CI: -7.3, 20.3] and 7% reduction compared with salmeterol [95% CI: -8.0, 19.9]). In the 3-year trial, the group receiving ADVAIR DISKUS 500/50 had a significantly lower rate of moderate and severe exacerbations compared with each of the other treatment groups (25.1% reduction compared with placebo [95% CI: 18.6, 31.1], 9.0% reduction compared with fluticasone propionate [95% CI: 1.2, 16.2], and 12.2% reduction compared with salmeterol [95% CI: 4.6, 19.2]).

There were no studies conducted to directly compare the efficacy of ADVAIR DISKUS 250/50 with ADVAIR DISKUS 500/50 on exacerbations. Across studies, the reduction in exacerbations seen with ADVAIR DISKUS 500/50 was not greater than the reduction in exacerbations seen with ADVAIR DISKUS 250/50.

Survival: A 3-year multicenter, international study evaluated the efficacy of ADVAIR DISKUS 500/50 compared with fluticasone propionate 500 mcg, salmeterol 50 mcg, and placebo on survival in 6,112 patients with COPD. During the study patients were permitted usual COPD therapy with the exception of other inhaled corticosteroids and long-acting bronchodilators. The patients were aged 40 to 80 years with an established history of COPD, a pre-bronchodilator FEV_1 <60% of predicted at study entry, and <10% of predicted reversibility. Each patient who withdrew from double-blind treatment for any reason was followed for the full 3-year study period to determine survival status. The primary efficacy endpoint was all-cause mortality. Survival with ADVAIR DISKUS 500/50 was not significantly improved compared with placebo or the individual components (all-cause mortality rate 12.6% ADVAIR DISKUS versus 15.2% placebo). The rates for all-cause mortality were 13.5% and 16.0% in the groups treated with salmeterol 50 mcg and fluticasone propionate 500 mcg, respectively. Secondary outcomes, including pulmonary function (post-bronchodilator FEV_1), improved with ADVAIR DISKUS 500/50, salmeterol, and fluticasone propionate 500/50 compared with placebo.

16 HOW SUPPLIED/STORAGE AND HANDLING

ADVAIR DISKUS 100/50 is supplied as a disposable purple device containing 60 blisters. The DISKUS inhalation device is packaged within a plastic-coated, moisture-protective foil pouch (NDC 0173-0695-00). ADVAIR DISKUS 100/50 is also supplied in an institutional pack of 1 disposable purple device containing 14 blisters. The DISKUS inhalation device is packaged within a plastic-coated, moisture-protective foil pouch (NDC 0173-0695-04).

ADVAIR DISKUS 250/50 is supplied as a disposable purple device containing 60 blisters. The DISKUS inhalation device is packaged within a plastic-coated, moisture-protective foil pouch (NDC 0173-0696-00). ADVAIR DISKUS 250/50 is also supplied in an institutional pack of 1 disposable purple device containing 14 blisters. The DISKUS inhalation device is packaged within a plastic-coated, moisture-protective foil pouch (NDC 0173-0696-04).

ADVAIR DISKUS 500/50 is supplied as a disposable purple device containing 60 blisters. The DISKUS inhalation device is packaged within a plastic-coated, moisture-protective foil pouch (NDC 0173-0697-00). ADVAIR DISKUS 500/50 is also supplied in an institutional pack of 1 disposable purple device containing 14 blisters. The DISKUS inhalation device is packaged within a plastic-coated, moisture-protective foil pouch (NDC 0173-0697-04).

Store at controlled room temperature (see USP), 20° to 25°C (68° to 77°F), in a dry place away from direct heat or sunlight. Keep out of reach of children. The DISKUS inhalation device is not reusable. The device should be discarded 1 month after removal from the moisture-protective foil overwrap pouch or after all blisters have been used (when the dose indicator reads "0"), whichever comes first. Do not attempt to take the device apart.

17 PATIENT COUNSELING INFORMATION

See FDA-approved Medication Guide.

17.1 Asthma-Related Death

Patients with asthma should be informed that salmeterol, one of the active ingredients in ADVAIR DISKUS, increases the risk of asthma-related death and may increase the risk of asthma-related hospitalization in pediatric and adolescent patients. They should also be informed that currently available data are inadequate to determine whether concurrent use of inhaled corticosteroids or other long-term asthma control drugs mitigates the increased risk of asthma-related death from LABAs.

17.2 Not for Acute Symptoms

ADVAIR DISKUS is not meant to relieve acute asthma symptoms or exacerbations of COPD and extra doses should not be used for that purpose. Acute symptoms should be treated with an inhaled, short-acting beta$_2$-agonist such as albuterol. (The physician should provide the patient with such medication and instruct the patient in how it should be used.)

Patients should be instructed to notify their physician immediately if they experience any of the following:
- Decreasing effectiveness of inhaled, short-acting beta$_2$-agonists
- Need for more inhalations than usual of inhaled, short-acting beta$_2$-agonists
- Significant decrease in lung function as outlined by the physician

Patients should not stop therapy with ADVAIR DISKUS without physician/provider guidance since symptoms may recur after discontinuation.

17.3   Do Not Use Additional Long-Acting Beta$_2$-Agonists
When patients are prescribed ADVAIR DISKUS, other LABAs for asthma and COPD should not be used.

17.4   Risks Associated With Corticosteroid Therapy
Local Effects: Patients should be advised that localized infections with *Candida albicans* occurred in the mouth and pharynx in some patients. If oropharyngeal candidiasis develops, it should be treated with appropriate local or systemic (i.e., oral) antifungal therapy while still continuing therapy with ADVAIR DISKUS, but at times therapy with ADVAIR DISKUS may need to be temporarily interrupted under close medical supervision. Rinsing the mouth after inhalation is advised.

Pneumonia: Patients with COPD have a higher risk of pneumonia and should be instructed to contact their healthcare provider if they develop symptoms of pneumonia.

Immunosuppression: Patients who are on immunosuppressant doses of corticosteroids should be warned to avoid exposure to chickenpox or measles and, if exposed, to consult their physician without delay. Patients should be informed of potential worsening of existing tuberculosis, fungal, bacterial, viral, or parasitic infections, or ocular herpes simplex.

Hypercorticism and Adrenal Suppression: Patients should be advised that ADVAIR DISKUS may cause systemic corticosteroid effects of hypercorticism and adrenal suppression. Additionally, patients should be instructed that deaths due to adrenal insufficiency have occurred during and after transfer from systemic corticosteroids. Patients should taper slowly from systemic corticosteroids if transferring to ADVAIR DISKUS.

Reduction in Bone Mineral Density: Patients who are at an increased risk for decreased BMD should be advised that the use of corticosteroids may pose an additional risk.

Reduced Growth Velocity: Patients should be informed that orally inhaled corticosteroids, including fluticasone propionate, a component of ADVAIR DISKUS, may cause a reduction in growth velocity when administered to pediatric patients. Physicians should closely follow the growth of children and adolescents taking corticosteroids by any route.

Ocular Effects: Long-term use of inhaled corticosteroids may increase the risk of some eye problems (cataracts or glaucoma); regular eye examinations should be considered.

17.5   Risks Associated With Beta-Agonist Therapy
Patients should be informed of adverse effects associated with beta$_2$-agonists, such as palpitations, chest pain, rapid heart rate, tremor, or nervousness.

ADVAIR, ADVAIR DISKUS, DISKHALER, DISKUS, FLONASE, FLOVENT, ROTADISK, SEREVENT, and VENTOLIN are registered trademarks of GlaxoSmithKline.
GlaxoSmithKline
Research Triangle Park, NC 27709
©2010, GlaxoSmithKline. All rights reserved.
June 2010
ADD: 8PI

MEDICATION GUIDE
ADVAIR [ad ' vair] DISKUS® 100/50
(fluticasone propionate 100 mcg and salmeterol 50 mcg inhalation powder)
ADVAIR DISKUS® 250/50
(fluticasone propionate 250 mcg and salmeterol 50 mcg inhalation powder)
ADVAIR DISKUS® 500/50
(fluticasone propionate 500 mcg and salmeterol 50 mcg inhalation powder)
Read the Medication Guide that comes with ADVAIR DISKUS before you start using it and each time you get a refill. There may be new information. This Medication Guide does not take the place of talking to your healthcare provider about your medical condition or treatment.

What is the most important information I should know about ADVAIR DISKUS?
ADVAIR DISKUS can cause serious side effects, including:
1. **People with asthma who take long-acting beta$_2$-adrenergic agonist (LABA) medicines, such as salmeterol (one of the medicines in ADVAIR DISKUS), have an increased risk of death from asthma problems.** It is not known whether fluticasone propionate, the other medicine in ADVAIR DISKUS, reduces the risk of death from asthma problems seen with salmeterol.

- Call your healthcare provider if breathing problems worsen over time while using ADVAIR DISKUS. You may need different treatment.
- **Get emergency medical care if:**
  - breathing problems worsen quickly and
  - you use your rescue inhaler medicine, but it does not relieve your breathing problems.
2. ADVAIR DISKUS should be used only if your healthcare provider decides that your asthma is not well controlled with a long-term asthma control medicine, such as inhaled corticosteroids.
3. When your asthma is well controlled, your healthcare provider may tell you to stop taking ADVAIR DISKUS. Your healthcare provider will decide if you can stop ADVAIR DISKUS without loss of asthma control. Your healthcare provider may prescribe a different asthma control medicine for you, such as an inhaled corticosteriod.
4. Children and adolescents who take LABA medicines may have an increased risk of being hospitalized for asthma problems.

What is ADVAIR DISKUS?
- ADVAIR DISKUS combines an inhaled corticosteroid medicine, fluticasone propionate (the same medicine found in FLOVENT®), and a LABA medicine, salmeterol (the same medicine found in SEREVENT®).
  - Inhaled corticosteroids help to decrease inflammation in the lungs. Inflammation in the lungs can lead to asthma symptoms.
  - LABA medicines are used in people with asthma and chronic obstructive pulmonary disease (COPD). LABA medicines help the muscles around the airways in your lungs stay relaxed to prevent symptoms, such as wheezing and shortness of breath. These symptoms can happen when the muscles around the airways tighten. This makes it hard to breathe. In severe cases, wheezing can stop your breathing and cause death if not treated right away.
- ADVAIR DISKUS is used for asthma and COPD as follows:

Asthma:
ADVAIR DISKUS is used to control symptoms of asthma and to prevent symptoms such as wheezing in adults and children aged 4 years and older.
ADVAIR DISKUS contains salmeterol (the same medicine found in SEREVENT). LABA medicines, such as salmeterol, increase the risk of death from asthma problems.
ADVAIR DISKUS is not for adults and children with asthma who:
- are well controlled with an asthma control medicine, such as a low to medium dose of an inhaled corticosteroid medicine
- have sudden asthma symptoms

COPD:
COPD is a chronic lung disease that includes chronic bronchitis, emphysema, or both. ADVAIR DISKUS 250/50 is used long term, 2 times each day to help improve lung function for better breathing in adults with COPD. ADVAIR DISKUS 250/50 has been shown to decrease the number of flare-ups and worsening of COPD symptoms (exacerbations).

Who should not use ADVAIR DISKUS?
Do not use ADVAIR DISKUS:
- to treat sudden, severe symptoms of asthma or COPD and
- if you have a severe allergy to milk proteins. Ask your doctor if you are not sure.

What should I tell my healthcare provider before using ADVAIR DISKUS?
Tell your healthcare provider about all of your health conditions, including if you:
- **have heart problems**
- **have high blood pressure**
- **have seizures**
- **have thyroid problems**
- **have diabetes**
- **have liver problems**
- **have osteoporosis**
- **have an immune system problem**
- **are pregnant or planning to become pregnant.** It is not known if ADVAIR DISKUS may harm your unborn baby.
- **are breastfeeding.** It is not known if ADVAIR DISKUS passes into your milk and if it can harm your baby.
- **are allergic to any of the ingredients in ADVAIR DISKUS, any other medicines, or food products.** See the end of this Medication Guide for a complete list of the ingredients in ADVAIR DISKUS.

are exposed to chickenpox or measles
Tell your healthcare provider about all the medicines you take including prescription and non-prescription medicines, vitamins, and herbal supplements. ADVAIR DISKUS and certain other medicines may interact with each other. This may cause serious side effects. Especially, tell your healthcare provider if you take ritonavir. The anti-HIV medicines

NORVIR® (ritonavir capsules) Soft Gelatin, NORVIR (ritonavir oral solution), and KALETRA® (lopinavir/ritonavir) Tablets contain ritonavir.
Know the medicines you take. Keep a list and show it to your healthcare provider and pharmacist each time you get a new medicine.

How do I use ADVAIR DISKUS?
See the step-by-step instructions for using ADVAIR DISKUS at the end of this Medication Guide. Do not use ADVAIR DISKUS unless your healthcare provider has taught you and you understand everything. Ask your healthcare provider or pharmacist if you have any questions.
- Children should use ADVAIR DISKUS with an adult's help, as instructed by the child's healthcare provider.
- Use ADVAIR DISKUS exactly as prescribed. **Do not use ADVAIR DISKUS more often than prescribed.** ADVAIR DISKUS comes in 3 strengths. Your healthcare provider has prescribed the one that is best for your condition.
- The usual dosage of ADVAIR DISKUS is 1 inhalation 2 times each day (morning and evening). The 2 doses should be about 12 hours apart. Rinse your mouth with water after using ADVAIR DISKUS.
- If you take more ADVAIR DISKUS than your doctor has prescribed, get medical help right away if you have any unusual symptoms, such as worsening shortness of breath, chest pain, increased heart rate, or shakiness.
- If you miss a dose of ADVAIR DISKUS, just skip that dose. Take your next dose at your usual time. Do not take 2 doses at one time.
- Do not use a spacer device with ADVAIR DISKUS.
- Do not breathe into ADVAIR DISKUS.
- **While you are using ADVAIR DISKUS 2 times each day, do not use other medicines that contain a LABA for any reason.** Ask your healthcare provider or pharmacist if any of your other medicines are LABA medicines.
- Do not stop using ADVAIR DISKUS or other asthma medicines unless told to do so by your healthcare provider because your symptoms might get worse. Your healthcare provider will change your medicines as needed.
- ADVAIR DISKUS does not relieve sudden symptoms. Always have a rescue inhaler medicine with you to treat sudden symptoms. If you do not have an inhaled, short-acting bronchodilator, call your healthcare provider to have one prescribed for you.
- Call your healthcare provider or get medical care right away if:
  - your breathing problems worsen with ADVAIR DISKUS
  - you need to use your rescue inhaler medicine more often than usual
  - your rescue inhaler medicine does not work as well for you at relieving symptoms
  - you need to use 4 or more inhalations of your rescue inhaler medicine for 2 or more days in a row
  - you use 1 whole canister of your rescue inhaler medicine in 8 weeks' time
  - your peak flow meter results decrease. Your healthcare provider will tell you the numbers that are right for you.
  - you have asthma and your symptoms do not improve after using ADVAIR DISKUS regularly for 1 week

What are the possible side effects with ADVAIR DISKUS?
ADVAIR DISKUS can cause serious side effects, including:
- See "What is the most important information I should know about ADVAIR DISKUS?"
- **serious allergic reactions.** Call your healthcare provider or get emergency medical care if you get any of the following symptoms of a serious allergic reaction:
  - rash
  - hives
  - swelling of the face, mouth, and tongue
  - breathing problems
- **sudden breathing problems immediately after inhaling your medicine**
- **effects on heart**
  - increased blood pressure
  - a fast and irregular heartbeat
  - chest pain
- **effects on nervous system**
  - tremor
  - nervousness
- **reduced adrenal function (may result in loss of energy)**
- **changes in blood (sugar, potassium, certain types of white blood cells)**
- **weakened immune system and a higher chance of infections**
- **lower bone mineral density.** This may be a problem for people who already have a higher chance of low bone density (osteoporosis).
- **eye problems including glaucoma and cataracts.** You should have regular eye exams while using ADVAIR DISKUS.
- **slowed growth in children.** A child's growth should be checked often.
- **pneumonia.** People with COPD have a higher chance of getting pneumonia. ADVAIR DISKUS may increase the

chance of getting pneumonia. Call your healthcare provider if you notice any of the following symptoms:
• increase in mucus (sputum) production
• change in mucus color
• fever
• chills
• increased cough
• increased breathing problems

Common side effects of ADVAIR DISKUS include:
Asthma:
• upper respiratory tract infection
• throat irritation
• hoarseness and voice changes
• thrush in the mouth and throat
• bronchitis
• cough
• headache
• nausea and vomiting
In children with asthma, infections in the ear, nose, and throat are common.
COPD:
• thrush in the mouth and throat
• throat irritation
• hoarseness and voice changes
• viral respiratory infections
• headache
• muscle and bone pain
Tell your healthcare provider about any side effect that bothers you or that does not go away.
These are not all the side effects with ADVAIR DISKUS. Ask your healthcare provider or pharmacist for more information.
Call your doctor for medical advice about side effects. You may report side effects to FDA at 1-800-FDA-1088 or 1-800-332-1088.

How do I store ADVAIR DISKUS?
• Store ADVAIR DISKUS at room temperature between 68° to 77° F (20° to 25° C). Keep in a dry place away from heat and sunlight.
• Safely discard ADVAIR DISKUS 1 month after you remove it from the foil pouch, or after the dose indicator reads "0", whichever comes first.
• Keep ADVAIR DISKUS and all medicines out of the reach of children.

General Information about ADVAIR DISKUS
Medicines are sometimes prescribed for purposes not mentioned in a Medication Guide. Do not use ADVAIR DISKUS for a condition for which it was not prescribed. Do not give your ADVAIR DISKUS to other people, even if they have the same condition that you have. It may harm them.
This Medication Guide summarizes the most important information about ADVAIR DISKUS. If you would like more information, talk with your healthcare provider or pharmacist. You can ask your healthcare provider or pharmacist for information about ADVAIR DISKUS that was written for healthcare professionals. You can also contact the company that makes ADVAIR DISKUS (toll free) at 1-888-825-5249 or at www.advair.com.

What are the ingredients in ADVAIR DISKUS?
Active ingredients: fluticasone propionate, salmeterol xinafoate
Inactive ingredient: lactose (contains milk proteins)

Instructions for Using ADVAIR DISKUS
Follow the instructions below for using your ADVAIR DISKUS. **You will breathe in (inhale) the medicine from the DISKUS®.** If you have any questions, ask your healthcare provider or pharmacist.

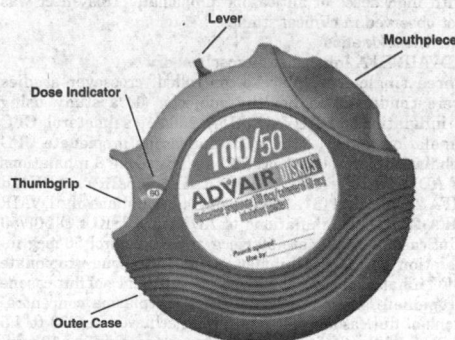

Take ADVAIR DISKUS out of the box and foil pouch. Write the "Pouch opened" and "Use by" dates on the label on top of the DISKUS. **The "Use by" date is 1 month from date of opening the pouch.**
• The DISKUS will be in the closed position when the pouch is opened.
• The **dose indicator** on the top of the DISKUS tells you how many doses are left. The dose indicator number will

decrease each time you use the DISKUS. After you have used 55 doses from the DISKUS, the numbers 5 to 0 will appear in **red** to warn you that there are only a few doses left *(see Figure 1)*. If you are using a "sample" DISKUS, the numbers 5 to 0 will appear in red after 9 doses.

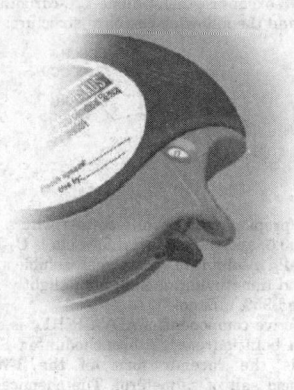

Figure 1

Taking a dose from the DISKUS requires the following 3 simple steps: Open, Click, Inhale.
1. OPEN
Hold the DISKUS in one hand and put the thumb of your other hand on the **thumbgrip**. Push your thumb away from you as far as it will go until the mouthpiece appears and snaps into position *(see Figure 2)*.

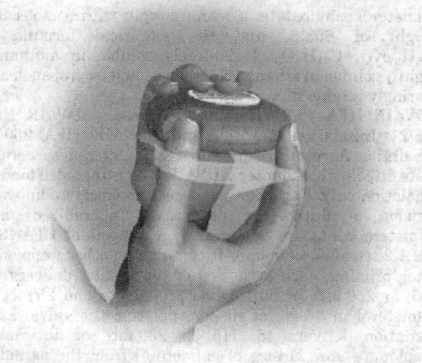

Figure 2

2. CLICK
Hold the DISKUS in a level, flat position with the mouthpiece towards you. Slide the **lever** away from you as far as it will go until it **clicks** *(see Figure 3)*. The DISKUS is now ready to use.

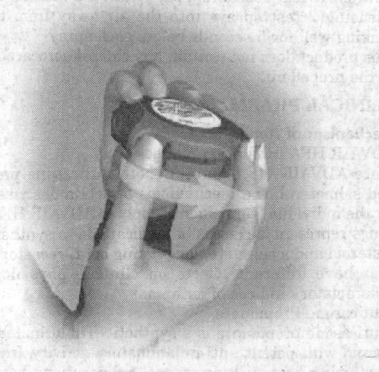

Figure 3

Every time the **lever** is pushed back, a dose is ready to be inhaled. This is shown by a decrease in numbers on the dose counter. **To avoid releasing or wasting doses once the DISKUS is ready:**
• **Do not close the DISKUS.**
• **Do not tilt the DISKUS.**
• **Do not play with the lever.**
• **Do not move the lever more than once.**
3. INHALE
Before inhaling your dose from the DISKUS, breathe out (exhale) fully while holding the DISKUS level and away from your mouth *(see Figure 4)*. **Remember, never breathe out into the DISKUS mouthpiece.**

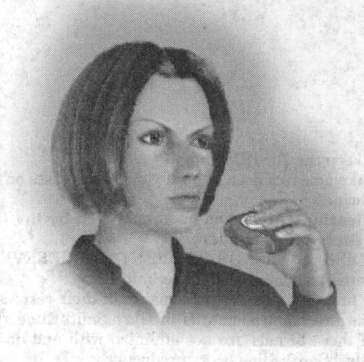

Figure 4

Put the mouthpiece to your lips *(see Figure 5)*. Breathe in quickly and deeply through the DISKUS. Do not breathe in through your nose.

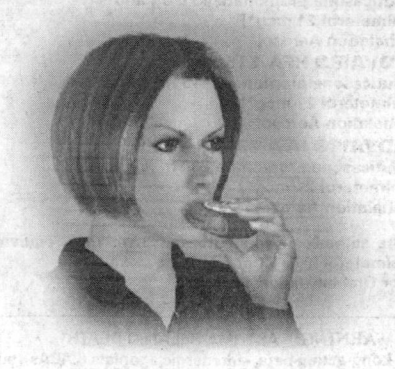

Figure 5

Remove the DISKUS from your mouth. Hold your breath for about 10 seconds, or for as long as is comfortable. Breathe out slowly.
The DISKUS delivers your dose of medicine as a very fine powder. Most patients can taste or feel the powder. Do not use another dose from the DISKUS if you do not feel or taste the medicine.
Rinse your mouth with water after breathing-in the medicine. Spit the water out. Do not swallow.
4. Close the DISKUS when you are finished taking a dose so that the DISKUS will be ready for you to take your next dose. Put your thumb on the thumbgrip and slide the thumbgrip back towards you as far as it will go *(see Figure 6)*. The DISKUS will click shut. The lever will automatically return to its original position. The DISKUS is now ready for you to take your next scheduled dose, due in about 12 hours. (Repeat steps 1 to 4.)
[See figure at top of next column]
Remember:
• Never breathe into the DISKUS.
• Never take the DISKUS apart.
• Always ready and use the DISKUS in a level, flat position.
• Do not use the DISKUS with a spacer device.
• After each dose, rinse your mouth with water and spit the water out. Do not swallow.
• Never wash the mouthpiece or any part of the DISKUS. **Keep it dry.**

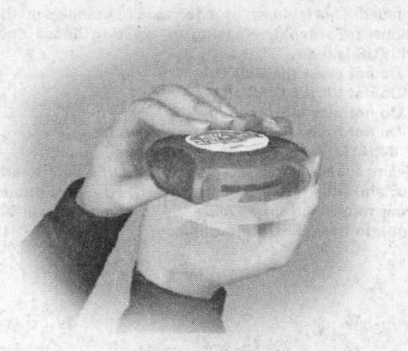

Figure 6

- Always keep the DISKUS in a dry place.
- Never take an extra dose, even if you did not taste or feel the medicine.

This Medication Guide has been approved by the U.S. Food and Drug Administration.
ADVAIR DISKUS, DISKUS, FLOVENT, and SEREVENT are registered trademarks of GlaxoSmithKline.
The other brands listed are trademarks of their respective owners and are not trademarks of GlaxoSmithKline. The makers of these brands are not affiliated with and do not endorse GlaxoSmithKline or its products.
GlaxoSmithKline
Research Triangle Park, NC 27709
©2010, GlaxoSmithKline. All rights reserved.
June 2010
ADD:6MG

ADVAIR® HFA 45/21 ℞

[ad' vair]
(fluticasone propionate 45 mcg and salmeterol 21 mcg*)
Inhalation Aerosol
ADVAIR® HFA 115/21
(fluticasone propionate 115 mcg and salmeterol 21 mcg*)
Inhalation Aerosol
ADVAIR® HFA 230/21
(fluticasone propionate 230 mcg and salmeterol 21 mcg*)
Inhalation Aerosol

*As salmeterol xinafoate salt 30.45 mcg, equivalent to salmeterol base 21 mcg
For Oral Inhalation Only

WARNING: ASTHMA-RELATED DEATH
Long-acting beta$_2$-adrenergic agonists (LABAs), such as salmeterol, one of the active ingredients in ADVAIR HFA, increase the risk of asthma-related death. Data from a large placebo-controlled US study that compared the safety of salmeterol (SEREVENT® Inhalation Aerosol) or placebo added to usual asthma therapy showed an increase in asthma-related deaths in patients receiving salmeterol (13 deaths out of 13,176 patients treated for 28 weeks on salmeterol versus 3 deaths out of 13,179 patients on placebo). Currently available data are inadequate to determine whether concurrent use of inhaled corticosteroids or other long-term asthma control drugs mitigates the increased risk of asthma-related death from LABAs. Available data from controlled clinical trials suggest that LABAs increase the risk of asthma-related hospitalization in pediatric and adolescent patients.
Therefore, when treating patients with asthma, physicians should only prescribe ADVAIR HFA for patients not adequately controlled on a long-term asthma control medication, such as an inhaled corticosteroid, or whose disease severity clearly warrants initiation of treatment with both an inhaled corticosteroid and a LABA. Once asthma control is achieved and maintained, assess the patient at regular intervals and step down therapy (e.g., discontinue ADVAIR HFA) if possible without loss of asthma control and maintain the patient on a long-term asthma control medication, such as an inhaled corticosteroid. Do not use ADVAIR HFA for patients whose asthma is adequately controlled on low- or medium-dose inhaled corticosteroids (see WARNINGS).

DESCRIPTION

ADVAIR HFA 45/21 Inhalation Aerosol, ADVAIR HFA 115/21 Inhalation Aerosol, and ADVAIR HFA 230/21 Inhalation Aerosol are combinations of fluticasone propionate and salmeterol xinafoate.
One active component of ADVAIR HFA is fluticasone propionate, a corticosteroid having the chemical name S-(fluoromethyl) 6α,9-difluoro-11β,17-dihydroxy-16α-methyl-3-oxoandrosta-1,4-diene-17β-carbothioate, 17-propionate and the following chemical structure:

Fluticasone propionate is a white powder with a molecular weight of 500.6, and the empirical formula is $C_{25}H_{31}F_3O_5S$. It is practically insoluble in water, freely soluble in dimethyl sulfoxide and dimethylformamide, and slightly soluble in methanol and 95% ethanol.
The other active component of ADVAIR HFA is salmeterol xinafoate, a beta$_2$-adrenergic bronchodilator. Salmeterol xinafoate is the racemic form of the 1-hydroxy-2-naphthoic acid salt of salmeterol. The chemical name of salmeterol xinafoate is 4-hydroxy-α^1-[[[6-(4-phenylbutoxy)hexyl]amino]methyl]-1,3-benzenedimethanol, 1-hydroxy-2-naphthalenecarboxylate, and it has the following chemical structure:

Salmeterol xinafoate is a white powder with a molecular weight of 603.8, and the empirical formula is $C_{25}H_{37}NO_4 \cdot C_{11}H_8O_3$. It is freely soluble in methanol; slightly soluble in ethanol, chloroform, and isopropanol; and sparingly soluble in water.
ADVAIR HFA 45/21 Inhalation Aerosol, ADVAIR HFA 115/21 Inhalation Aerosol, and ADVAIR HFA 230/21 Inhalation Aerosol are pressurized metered-dose aerosol units fitted with a counter. ADVAIR HFA is intended for oral inhalation only. Each unit contains a microcrystalline suspension of fluticasone propionate (micronized) and salmeterol xinafoate (micronized) in propellant HFA-134a (1,1,1,2-tetrafluoroethane). It contains no other excipients.
After priming, each actuation of the inhaler delivers 50, 125, or 250 mcg of fluticasone propionate and 25 mcg of salmeterol in 75 mg of suspension from the valve. Each actuation delivers 45, 115, or 230 mcg of fluticasone propionate and 21 mcg of salmeterol from the actuator. Twenty-one micrograms (21 mcg) of salmeterol base is equivalent to 30.45 mcg of salmeterol xinafoate. The actual amount of drug delivered to the lung may depend on patient factors, such as the coordination between the actuation of the device and inspiration through the delivery system.
Each 8-g canister contains 60 inhalations. Each 12-g canister provides 120 inhalations.
ADVAIR HFA should be primed before using for the first time by releasing 4 test sprays into the air away from the face, shaking well for 5 seconds before each spray. In cases where the inhaler has not been used for more than 4 weeks or when it has been dropped, prime the inhaler again by releasing 2 test sprays into the air away from the face, shaking well for 5 seconds before each spray.
This product does not contain any chlorofluorocarbon (CFC) as the propellant.

CLINICAL PHARMACOLOGY

Mechanism of Action
ADVAIR HFA Inhalation Aerosol
Since ADVAIR HFA contains both fluticasone propionate and salmeterol, the mechanisms of action described below for the individual components apply to ADVAIR HFA. These drugs represent 2 classes of medications (a synthetic corticosteroid and a selective, long-acting beta$_2$-receptor agonist) that have different effects on clinical, physiologic, and inflammatory indices of asthma.
Fluticasone Propionate
Fluticasone propionate is a synthetic trifluorinated corticosteroid with potent anti-inflammatory activity. In vitro assays using human lung cytosol preparations have established fluticasone propionate as a human glucocorticoid receptor agonist with an affinity 18 times greater than dexamethasone, almost twice that of beclomethasone-17-

monopropionate (BMP), the active metabolite of beclomethasone dipropionate, and over 3 times that of budesonide. Data from the McKenzie vasoconstrictor assay in man are consistent with these results.
Inflammation is an important component in the pathogenesis of asthma. Corticosteroids have been shown to inhibit multiple cell types (e.g., mast cells, eosinophils, basophils, lymphocytes, macrophages, neutrophils) and mediator production or secretion (e.g., histamine, eicosanoids, leukotrienes, cytokines) involved in the asthmatic response. These anti-inflammatory actions of corticosteroids contribute to their efficacy in asthma.
Salmeterol Xinafoate
Salmeterol is a long-acting beta$_2$-adrenergic agonist (LABA). In vitro studies and in vivo pharmacologic studies demonstrate that salmeterol is selective for beta$_2$-adrenoceptors compared with isoproterenol, which has approximately equal agonist activity on beta$_1$- and beta$_2$-adrenoceptors. In vitro studies show salmeterol to be at least 50 times more selective for beta$_2$-adrenoceptors than albuterol. Although beta$_2$-adrenoceptors are the predominant adrenergic receptors in bronchial smooth muscle and beta$_1$-adrenoceptors are the predominant receptors in the heart, there are also beta$_2$-adrenoceptors in the human heart comprising 10% to 50% of the total beta-adrenoceptors. The precise function of these receptors has not been established, but their presence raises the possibility that even selective beta$_2$-agonists may have cardiac effects.
The pharmacologic effects of beta$_2$-adrenoceptor agonist drugs, including salmeterol, are at least in part attributable to stimulation of intracellular adenyl cyclase, the enzyme that catalyzes the conversion of adenosine triphosphate (ATP) to cyclic-3',5'-adenosine monophosphate (cyclic AMP). Increased cyclic AMP levels cause relaxation of bronchial smooth muscle and inhibition of release of mediators of immediate hypersensitivity from cells, especially from mast cells.
In vitro tests show that salmeterol is a potent and long-lasting inhibitor of the release of mast cell mediators, such as histamine, leukotrienes, and prostaglandin D_2, from human lung. Salmeterol inhibits histamine-induced plasma protein extravasation and inhibits platelet-activating factor–induced eosinophil accumulation in the lungs of guinea pigs when administered by the inhaled route. In humans, single doses of salmeterol administered via inhalation aerosol attenuate allergen-induced bronchial hyper-responsiveness.
Preclinical
In animals and humans, propellant HFA-134a was found to be rapidly absorbed and rapidly eliminated, with an elimination half-life of 3 to 27 minutes in animals and 5 to 7 minutes in humans. Time to maximum plasma concentration (T_{max}) and mean residence time are both extremely short, leading to a transient appearance of HFA-134a in the blood with no evidence of accumulation.
Propellant HFA-134a is devoid of pharmacological activity except at very high doses in animals (i.e., 380 to 1,300 times the maximum human exposure based on comparisons of area under the plasma concentration versus time curve [AUC] values), primarily producing ataxia, tremors, dyspnea, or salivation. These events are similar to effects produced by the structurally related CFCs, which have been used extensively in metered-dose inhalers. In drug interaction studies in male and female dogs, there was a slight increase in the salmeterol-related effect on heart rate (a known effect of beta$_2$-agonists) when given in combination with high doses of fluticasone propionate. This effect was not observed in clinical studies.
Pharmacokinetics
ADVAIR HFA Inhalation Aerosol
Three single-dose, placebo-controlled, crossover studies were conducted in healthy subjects: (1) a study using 4 inhalations of ADVAIR HFA 230/21, salmeterol CFC inhalation aerosol 21 mcg, or fluticasone propionate CFC inhalation aerosol 220 mcg, (2) a study using 8 inhalations of ADVAIR HFA 45/21, ADVAIR HFA 115/21, or ADVAIR HFA 230/21, and (3) a study using 4 inhalations of ADVAIR HFA 230/21; 2 inhalations of ADVAIR DISKUS® 500/50 (fluticasone propionate 500 mcg and salmeterol 50 mcg inhalation powder); 4 inhalations of fluticasone propionate CFC inhalation aerosol 220 mcg; or 1,010 mcg of fluticasone propionate given intravenously. Peak plasma concentrations of fluticasone propionate were achieved in 0.33 to 1.5 hours and those of salmeterol were achieved in 5 to 10 minutes.
Peak plasma concentrations of fluticasone propionate (N = 20 subjects) following 8 inhalations of ADVAIR HFA 45/21, ADVAIR HFA 115/21, and ADVAIR HFA 230/21 averaged 41, 108, and 173 pg/mL, respectively. Peak plasma salmeterol concentrations ranged from 220 to 470 pg/mL. Systemic exposure (N = 20 subjects) from 4 inhalations of ADVAIR HFA 230/21 was 53% of the value from the individual inhaler for fluticasone propionate CFC inhalation

aerosol and 42% of the value from the individual inhaler for salmeterol CFC inhalation aerosol. Peak plasma concentrations from ADVAIR HFA for fluticasone propionate (86 versus 120 pg/mL) and salmeterol (170 versus 510 pg/mL) were significantly lower compared with individual inhalers.

In 15 healthy subjects, systemic exposure to fluticasone propionate from 4 inhalations of ADVAIR HFA 230/21 (920/84 mcg) and 2 inhalations of ADVAIR DISKUS 500/50 (1,000/100 mcg) were similar between the 2 inhalers (i.e., 799 versus 832 pg•hr/mL, respectively) but approximately half the systemic exposure from 4 inhalations of fluticasone propionate CFC inhalation aerosol 220 mcg (880 mcg, AUC = 1,543 pg•hr/mL). Similar results were observed for peak fluticasone propionate plasma concentrations (186 and 182 pg/mL from ADVAIR HFA and ADVAIR DISKUS, respectively, and 307 pg/mL from the fluticasone propionate CFC inhalation aerosol). Systemic exposure to salmeterol was higher (317 versus 169 pg•hr/mL) and peak salmeterol concentrations were lower (196 versus 223 pg/mL) following ADVAIR HFA compared with ADVAIR DISKUS, although pharmacodynamic results were comparable.

Absolute bioavailability of fluticasone propionate from ADVAIR HFA in 15 healthy subjects was 5.3%. Terminal half-life estimates of fluticasone propionate for ADVAIR HFA, ADVAIR DISKUS, and fluticasone propionate CFC inhalation aerosol were similar and averaged 5.6 hours. No terminal half-life estimates were calculated for salmeterol. A double-blind crossover study was conducted in 13 adult patients with asthma to evaluate the steady-state pharmacokinetics of fluticasone propionate and salmeterol following administration of 2 inhalations of ADVAIR HFA 115/21 twice daily or 1 inhalation of ADVAIR DISKUS 250/50 twice daily for 4 weeks. Systemic exposure (AUC) to fluticasone propionate was similar for ADVAIR HFA (274 pg•hr/mL [95% CI: 150, 502]) and ADVAIR DISKUS (338 pg•hr/mL [95% CI: 197, 581]). Systemic exposure to salmeterol was also similar for ADVAIR HFA (53 pg•hr/mL [95% CI: 17, 164]) and ADVAIR DISKUS (70 pg•hr/mL [95% CI: 19, 254]).

Special Populations
Hepatic and Renal Impairment
Formal pharmacokinetic studies using ADVAIR HFA have not been conducted to examine gender differences or in special populations, such as elderly patients or patients with hepatic or renal impairment. However, since both fluticasone propionate and salmeterol are predominantly cleared by hepatic metabolism, impairment of liver function may lead to accumulation of fluticasone propionate and salmeterol in plasma. Therefore, patients with hepatic disease should be closely monitored.

Drug Interactions
In repeat- and single-dose studies, there was no evidence of significant drug interaction on systemic exposure to fluticasone propionate and salmeterol when given alone or in combination via the DISKUS. Similar definitive studies have not been performed with ADVAIR HFA.

Fluticasone Propionate
Absorption
Fluticasone propionate acts locally in the lung; therefore, plasma levels do not predict therapeutic effect. Studies using oral dosing of labeled and unlabeled drug have demonstrated that the oral systemic bioavailability of fluticasone propionate is negligible (<1%), primarily due to incomplete absorption and presystemic metabolism in the gut and liver. In contrast, the majority of the fluticasone propionate delivered to the lung is systemically absorbed.

Distribution
Following intravenous administration, the initial disposition phase for fluticasone propionate was rapid and consistent with its high lipid solubility and tissue binding. The volume of distribution averaged 4.2 L/kg.
The percentage of fluticasone propionate bound to human plasma proteins averages 99%. Fluticasone propionate is weakly and reversibly bound to erythrocytes and is not significantly bound to human transcortin.

Metabolism
The total clearance of fluticasone propionate is high (average, 1,093 mL/min), with renal clearance accounting for less than 0.02% of the total. The only circulating metabolite detected in man is the 17β-carboxylic acid derivative of fluticasone propionate, which is formed through the cytochrome P450 3A4 (CYP34A) pathway. This metabolite had less affinity (approximately 1/2,000) than the parent drug for the glucocorticoid receptor of human lung cytosol in vitro and negligible pharmacological activity in animal studies. Other metabolites detected in vitro using cultured human hepatoma cells have not been detected in man.

Elimination
Following intravenous dosing, fluticasone propionate showed polyexponential kinetics and had a terminal elimination half-life of approximately 7.8 hours. Less than 5% of a radiolabeled oral dose was excreted in the urine as metabolites, with the remainder excreted in the feces as parent drug and metabolites.

Special Populations
Gender
In 19 male and 33 female patients with asthma, systemic exposure was similar from 2 inhalations of fluticasone propionate CFC inhalation aerosol 44, 110, and 220 mcg twice daily.

Drug Interactions
Fluticasone propionate is a substrate of CYP3A4. Coadministration of fluticasone propionate and the strong CYP3A4 inhibitor ritonavir is not recommended based upon a multiple-dose, crossover drug interaction study in 18 healthy subjects. Fluticasone propionate aqueous nasal spray (200 mcg once daily) was coadministered for 7 days with ritonavir (100 mg twice daily). Plasma fluticasone propionate concentrations following fluticasone propionate aqueous nasal spray alone were undetectable (<10 pg/mL) in most subjects, and when concentrations were detectable, peak levels (C_{max}) averaged 11.9 pg/mL (range: 10.8 to 14.1 pg/mL) and $AUC_{(0-\tau)}$ averaged 8.43 pg•hr/mL (range: 4.2 to 18.8 pg•hr/mL). Fluticasone propionate C_{max} and $AUC_{(0-\tau)}$ increased to 318 pg/mL (range: 110 to 648 pg/mL) and 3,102.6 pg•hr/mL (range: 1,207.1 to 5,662.0 pg•hr/mL), respectively, after coadministration of ritonavir with fluticasone propionate aqueous nasal spray. This significant increase in systemic fluticasone propionate exposure resulted in a significant decrease (86%) in serum cortisol AUC.
Caution should be exercised when other strong CYP3A4 inhibitors are coadministered with fluticasone propionate. In a drug interaction study, coadministration of orally inhaled fluticasone propionate (1,000 mcg) and ketoconazole (200 mg once daily) resulted in increased systemic fluticasone propionate exposure and reduced plasma cortisol AUC, but had no effect on urinary excretion of cortisol. In another multiple-dose drug interaction study, coadministration of orally inhaled fluticasone propionate (500 mcg twice daily) and erythromycin (333 mg 3 times daily) did not affect fluticasone propionate pharmacokinetics.

Salmeterol Xinafoate
Salmeterol xinafoate, an ionic salt, dissociates in solution so that the salmeterol and 1-hydroxy-2-naphthoic acid (xinafoate) moieties are absorbed, distributed, metabolized, and excreted independently. Salmeterol acts locally in the lung; therefore, plasma levels do not predict therapeutic effect.

Absorption
Because of the small therapeutic dose, systemic levels of salmeterol are low or undetectable after inhalation of recommended dosages (42 mcg of salmeterol inhalation aerosol twice daily). Following chronic administration of an inhaled dosage of 42 mcg twice daily, salmeterol was detected in plasma within 5 to 10 minutes in 6 patients with asthma; plasma concentrations were very low, with mean peak concentrations of 150 pg/mL and no accumulation with repeated doses.

Distribution
The percentage of salmeterol bound to human plasma proteins averages 96% in vitro over the concentration range of 8 to 7,722 ng of salmeterol base per milliliter, much higher concentrations than those achieved following therapeutic doses of salmeterol.

Metabolism
Salmeterol base is extensively metabolized by hydroxylation, with subsequent elimination predominantly in the feces. No significant amount of unchanged salmeterol base was detected in either urine or feces.
An in vitro study using human liver microsomes showed that salmeterol is extensively metabolized to α-hydroxysalmeterol (aliphatic oxidation) by CYP3A4. Ketoconazole, a strong inhibitor of CYP3A4, essentially completely inhibited the formation of α-hydroxysalmeterol in vitro.

Elimination
In 2 healthy adult subjects who received 1 mg of radiolabeled salmeterol (as salmeterol xinafoate) orally, approximately 25% and 60% of the radiolabeled salmeterol was eliminated in urine and feces, respectively, over a period of 7 days. The terminal elimination half-life was about 5.5 hours (1 volunteer only).
The xinafoate moiety has no apparent pharmacologic activity. The xinafoate moiety is highly protein bound (>99%) and has a long elimination half-life of 11 days.

Drug Interactions
Salmeterol is a substrate of CYP3A4.
Inhibitors of Cytochrome P450 3A4: Ketoconazole
In a placebo-controlled, crossover drug interaction study in 20 healthy male and female subjects, coadministration of salmeterol (50 mcg twice daily) and the strong CYP3A4 inhibitor ketoconazole (400 mg once daily) for 7 days resulted in a significant increase in plasma salmeterol exposure as determined by a 16-fold increase in AUC (ratio with and without ketoconazole 15.76; 90% CI: 10.66, 23.31) mainly due to increased bioavailability of the swallowed portion of the dose. Peak plasma salmeterol concentrations were in-

creased by 1.4-fold (90% CI: 1.23, 1.68). Three (3) out of 20 subjects (15%) were withdrawn from salmeterol and ketoconazole coadministration due to beta-agonist–mediated systemic effects (2 with QTc prolongation and 1 with palpitations and sinus tachycardia). Coadministration of salmeterol and ketoconazole did not result in a clinically significant effect on mean heart rate, mean blood potassium, or mean blood glucose. Although there was no statistical effect on the mean QTc, coadministration of salmeterol and ketoconazole was associated with more frequent increases in QTc duration compared with salmeterol and placebo administration. Due to the potential increased risk of cardiovascular adverse events, the concomitant use of salmeterol with strong CYP3A4 inhibitors (e.g., ketoconazole, ritonavir, atazanavir, clarithromycin, indinavir, itraconazole, nefazodone, nelfinavir, saquinavir, telithromycin) is not recommended.

Erythromycin
In a repeat-dose study in 13 healthy subjects, concomitant administration of erythromycin (a moderate CYP3A4 inhibitor) and salmeterol inhalation aerosol resulted in a 40% increase in salmeterol C_{max} at steady state (ratio with and without erythromycin 1.4; 90% CI: 0.96, 2.03; p = 0.12), a 3.6-beat/min increase in heart rate (95% CI: 0.19, 7.03; p<0.04), a 5.8-msec increase in QTc interval (95% CI: -6.14, 17.77; p = 0.34), and no change in plasma potassium.

Pharmacodynamics
ADVAIR HFA Inhalation Aerosol
Since systemic pharmacodynamic effects of salmeterol are not normally seen at the therapeutic dose, higher doses were used to produce measurable effects. Four placebo-controlled, crossover studies were conducted in healthy subjects: (1) a cumulative-dose study using 42 to 336 mcg of salmeterol CFC inhalation aerosol given alone or as ADVAIR HFA 115/21, (2) a single-dose study using 4 inhalations of ADVAIR HFA 230/21, salmeterol CFC inhalation aerosol 21 mcg, or fluticasone propionate CFC inhalation aerosol 220 mcg, (3) a single-dose study using 8 inhalations of ADVAIR HFA 45/21, ADVAIR HFA 115/21, or ADVAIR HFA 230/21, and (4) a single-dose study using 4 inhalations of ADVAIR HFA 230/21; 2 inhalations of ADVAIR DISKUS 500/50; 4 inhalations of fluticasone propionate CFC inhalation aerosol 220 mcg; or 1,010 mcg of fluticasone propionate given intravenously. In these studies pulse rate, blood pressure, QTc interval, glucose, and/or potassium were measured. Comparable or lower effects were observed for ADVAIR HFA compared with ADVAIR DISKUS or salmeterol alone. The effect of salmeterol on pulse rate and potassium was not altered by the presence of different amounts of fluticasone propionate in ADVAIR HFA. The potential effect of salmeterol on the effects of fluticasone propionate on the hypothalamic-pituitary-adrenal (HPA) axis was also evaluated in 3 of these studies. Compared with fluticasone propionate CFC inhalation aerosol, ADVAIR HFA had less effect on 24-hour urinary cortisol excretion and less or comparable effect on 24-hour serum cortisol. In these crossover studies in healthy subjects, ADVAIR HFA and ADVAIR DISKUS had similar effects on urinary and serum cortisol.
In clinical studies with ADVAIR HFA in patients with asthma, systemic pharmacodynamic effects of salmeterol (pulse rate, blood pressure, QTc interval, potassium, and glucose) were similar to or slightly lower in patients treated with ADVAIR HFA compared with patients treated with salmeterol CFC inhalation aerosol 21 mcg. In 61 adolescent and adult patients with asthma given ADVAIR HFA (45/21 or 115/21 mcg), continuous 24-hour electrocardiographic monitoring was performed after the first dose and after 12 weeks of twice-daily therapy, and no clinically significant dysrhythmias were noted.
A 4-way crossover study in 13 patients with asthma compared pharmacodynamics at steady state following 4 weeks of twice-daily treatment with 2 inhalations of ADVAIR HFA 115/21, 1 inhalation of ADVAIR DISKUS 250/50 mcg, 2 inhalations of fluticasone propionate HFA inhalation aerosol 110 mcg, and placebo. No significant differences in serum cortisol AUC were observed between active treatments and placebo. Mean 12-hour serum cortisol AUC ratios comparing active treatment with placebo ranged from 0.9 to 1.2. No statistically or clinically significant increases in heart rate or QTc interval were observed for any active treatment compared with placebo.
In a 12-week study (see CLINICAL TRIALS: Studies Comparing ADVAIR HFA With Fluticasone Propionate Alone or Salmeterol Alone: *Study 3*) in patients with asthma, ADVAIR HFA 115/21 was compared with the individual components, fluticasone propionate CFC inhalation aerosol 110 mcg and salmeterol CFC inhalation aerosol 21 mcg, and placebo. All treatments were administered as 2 inhalations twice daily. After 12 weeks of treatment with these therapeutic doses, the geometric mean ratio of urinary cortisol excretion compared with baseline was 0.9 for ADVAIR HFA and fluticasone propionate and 1.0 for placebo and salmeterol. In addition, the ability to increase cortisol pro-

duction in response to stress, as assessed by 30-minute cosyntropin stimulation in 23 to 32 patients per treatment group, remained intact for the majority of patients and was similar across treatments. Three patients who received ADVAIR HFA 115/21 had an abnormal response (peak serum cortisol <18 mcg/dL) after dosing, compared with 1 patient who received placebo, 2 patients who received fluticasone propionate 110 mcg, and 1 patient who received salmeterol.

In another 12-week study (see CLINICAL TRIALS: Studies Comparing ADVAIR HFA With Fluticasone Propionate Alone or Salmeterol Alone: *Study 4*) in patients with asthma, ADVAIR HFA 230/21 (2 inhalations twice daily) was compared with ADVAIR DISKUS 500/50 (1 inhalation twice daily) and fluticasone propionate CFC inhalation aerosol 220 mcg (2 inhalations twice daily). The geometric mean ratio of 24-hour urinary cortisol excretion at week 12 compared with baseline was 0.9 for all 3 treatment groups.

Fluticasone Propionate

In clinical trials with fluticasone propionate inhalation powder using dosages up to and including 250 mcg twice daily, occasional abnormal short cosyntropin tests (peak serum cortisol <18 mcg/dL) were noted both in patients receiving fluticasone propionate and in patients receiving placebo. The incidence of abnormal tests at 500 mcg twice daily was greater than placebo. In a 2-year study carried out in 64 patients with mild, persistent asthma (mean FEV_1 91% of predicted) randomized to fluticasone propionate 500 mcg twice daily or placebo, no patient receiving fluticasone propionate had an abnormal response to 6-hour cosyntropin infusion (peak serum cortisol <18 mcg/dL). With a peak cortisol threshold of <35 mcg/dL, 1 patient receiving fluticasone propionate (4%) had an abnormal response at 1 year; repeat testing at 18 months and 2 years was normal. Another patient receiving fluticasone propionate (5%) had an abnormal response at 2 years. No patient on placebo had an abnormal response at 1 or 2 years.

Salmeterol Xinafoate

Inhaled salmeterol, like other beta-adrenergic agonist drugs, can produce dose-related cardiovascular effects and effects on blood glucose and/or serum potassium in some patients (see PRECAUTIONS). The cardiovascular effects (heart rate, blood pressure) associated with salmeterol occur with similar frequency, and are of similar type and severity, as those noted following albuterol administration.

The effects of rising inhaled doses of salmeterol and standard inhaled doses of albuterol were studied in volunteers and in patients with asthma. Salmeterol doses up to 84 mcg resulted in heart rate increases of 3 to 16 beats/min, about the same as albuterol dosed at 180 mcg by inhalation aerosol (4 to 10 beats/min). In 2 double-blind asthma studies, patients receiving either 42 mcg of salmeterol inhalation aerosol twice daily (n = 81) or 180 mcg of albuterol inhalation aerosol 4 times daily (n = 80) underwent continuous electrocardiographic monitoring during four 24-hour periods; no clinically significant dysrhythmias were noted.

Studies in laboratory animals (minipigs, rodents, and dogs) have demonstrated the occurrence of cardiac arrhythmias and sudden death (with histologic evidence of myocardial necrosis) when beta-agonists and methylxanthines are administered concurrently. The clinical significance of these findings is unknown.

CLINICAL TRIALS

ADVAIR HFA has been studied in patients with asthma aged 12 years and older. ADVAIR HFA has not been studied in patients less than 12 years of age or in patients with chronic obstructive pulmonary disease (COPD). In clinical trials comparing ADVAIR HFA Inhalation Aerosol with the individual components, improvements in most efficacy endpoints were greater with ADVAIR HFA than with the use of either fluticasone propionate or salmeterol alone. In addition, clinical trials showed comparable results between ADVAIR HFA and ADVAIR DISKUS.

Studies Comparing ADVAIR HFA With Fluticasone Propionate Alone or Salmeterol Alone

Four (4) double-blind, parallel-group clinical trials were conducted with ADVAIR HFA in 1,517 adolescent and adult patients (≥12 years, mean baseline forced expiratory volume in 1 second [FEV_1] 65% to 75% of predicted normal) with asthma that was not optimally controlled on their current therapy. All metered-dose inhaler treatments were inhalation aerosols given as 2 inhalations twice daily, and other maintenance therapies were discontinued.

Study 1: Clinical Trial With ADVAIR HFA 45/21 Inhalation Aerosol

This placebo-controlled 12-week US study compared ADVAIR HFA 45/21 with fluticasone propionate CFC inhalation aerosol 44 mcg or salmeterol CFC inhalation aerosol 21 mcg, each given as 2 inhalations twice daily. The primary efficacy endpoints were predose FEV_1 and withdrawals due to worsening asthma. This study was stratified according to baseline asthma therapy: patients using beta-agonists (al-

buterol alone [n = 142], salmeterol [n = 84], or inhaled corticosteroids [n = 134] [daily doses of beclomethasone dipropionate 252 to 336 mcg; budesonide 400 to 600 mcg; flunisolide 1,000 mcg; fluticasone propionate inhalation aerosol 176 mcg; fluticasone propionate inhalation powder 200 mcg; or triamcinolone acetonide 600 to 800 mcg]). Baseline FEV_1 measurements were similar across treatments: ADVAIR HFA 45/21, 2.29 L; fluticasone propionate 44 mcg, 2.20 L; salmeterol, 2.33 L; and placebo, 2.27 L.

Predefined withdrawal criteria for lack of efficacy, an indicator of worsening asthma, were utilized for this placebo-controlled study. Worsening asthma was defined as a clinically important decrease in FEV_1 or peak expiratory flow (PEF), increase in use of VENTOLIN® (albuterol, USP) Inhalation Aerosol, increase in night awakenings due to asthma, emergency intervention or hospitalization due to asthma, or requirement for asthma medication not allowed by the protocol. As shown in Table 1, statistically significantly fewer patients receiving ADVAIR HFA 45/21 were withdrawn due to worsening asthma compared with salmeterol and placebo. Fewer patients receiving ADVAIR HFA 45/21 were withdrawn due to worsening asthma compared with fluticasone propionate 44 mcg; however, the difference was not statistically significant.

Table 1. Percent of Patients Withdrawn Due to Worsening Asthma in Patients Previously Treated With Beta$_2$-Agonists (Albuterol or Salmeterol) or Inhaled Corticosteroids (Study 1)

ADVAIR HFA 45/21 (n = 92)	Fluticasone Propionate CFC Inhalation Aerosol 44 mcg (n = 89)	Salmeterol CFC Inhalation Aerosol 21 mcg (n = 92)	Placebo HFA Inhalation Aerosol (n = 87)
2%	8%	25%	28%

The FEV_1 results are displayed in Figure 1. Because this trial used predetermined criteria for worsening asthma, which caused more patients in the placebo group to be withdrawn, FEV_1 results at Endpoint (last available FEV_1 result) are also provided. Patients receiving ADVAIR HFA 45/21 had significantly greater improvements in FEV_1 (0.58 L, 27%) compared with fluticasone propionate 44 mcg (0.36 L, 18%), salmeterol (0.25 L, 12%), and placebo (0.14 L, 5%). These improvements in FEV_1 with ADVAIR HFA 45/21 were achieved regardless of baseline asthma therapy (albuterol alone, salmeterol, or inhaled corticosteroids).

[See figure 1 at next column]

The effect of ADVAIR HFA 45/21 on the secondary efficacy parameters, including morning and evening PEF, usage of VENTOLIN Inhalation Aerosol, and asthma symptoms over 24 hours on a scale of 0 to 5 is shown in Table 2.

[See table 2 above]

The subjective impact of asthma on patients' perceptions of health was evaluated through use of an instrument called the Asthma Quality of Life Questionnaire (AQLQ) (based on a 7-point scale where 1 = maximum impairment and 7 = none). Patients receiving ADVAIR HFA 45/21 had clinically meaningful improvements in overall asthma-specific quality of life as defined by a difference between groups of

Table 2. Secondary Efficacy Variable Results for Patients Previously Treated With Beta$_2$-Agonists (Albuterol or Salmeterol) or Inhaled Corticosteroids (Study 1)

Efficacy Variable[a]	ADVAIR HFA 45/21 (n = 92)	Fluticasone Propionate CFC Inhalation Aerosol 44 mcg (n = 89)	Salmeterol CFC Inhalation Aerosol 21 mcg (n = 92)	Placebo HFA Inhalation Aerosol (n = 87)
AM PEF (L/min)				
Baseline	377	369	381	382
Change from baseline	58	27	25	1
PM PEF (L/min)				
Baseline	397	387	402	407
Change from baseline	48	20	16	3
Use of VENTOLIN Inhalation Aerosol (inhalations/day)				
Baseline	3.1	2.4	2.7	2.7
Change from baseline	-2.1	-0.4	-0.8	0.2
Asthma symptom score/day				
Baseline	1.8	1.6	1.7	1.7
Change from baseline	-1.0	-0.3	-0.4	0

[a]Change from baseline = change from baseline at Endpoint (last available data).

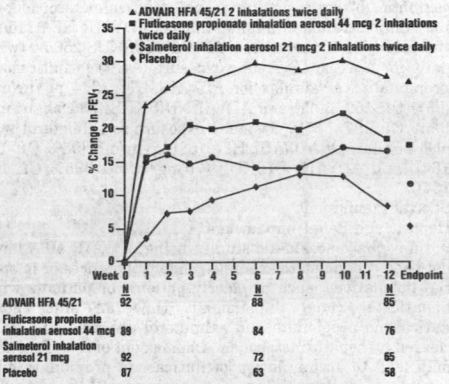

Figure 1. Mean Percent Change From Baseline in FEV_1 in Patients Previously Treated With Either Beta$_2$-Agonists (Albuterol or Salmeterol) or Inhaled Corticosteroids (Study 1)

≥0.5 points in change from baseline AQLQ scores (difference in AQLQ score of 1.14 [95% CI: 0.85, 1.44] compared with placebo).

Study 2: Clinical Trial With ADVAIR HFA 45/21 Inhalation Aerosol

This active-controlled 12-week US study compared ADVAIR HFA 45/21 with fluticasone propionate CFC inhalation aerosol 44 mcg and salmeterol CFC inhalation aerosol 21 mcg, each given as 2 inhalations twice daily, in 283 patients using as-needed albuterol alone. The primary efficacy endpoint was predose FEV_1. Baseline FEV_1 measurements were similar across treatments: ADVAIR HFA 45/21, 2.37 L; fluticasone propionate 44 mcg, 2.31 L; and salmeterol, 2.34 L.

Efficacy results in this study were similar to those observed in Study 1. Patients receiving ADVAIR HFA 45/21 had significantly greater improvements in FEV_1 (0.69 L, 33%) compared with fluticasone propionate 44 mcg (0.51 L, 25%) and salmeterol (0.47 L, 22%).

Study 3: Clinical Trial With ADVAIR HFA 115/21 Inhalation Aerosol

This placebo-controlled 12-week US study compared ADVAIR HFA 115/21 with fluticasone propionate CFC inhalation aerosol 110 mcg or salmeterol CFC inhalation aerosol 21 mcg, each given as 2 inhalations twice daily, in 365 patients using inhaled corticosteroids (daily doses of beclomethasone dipropionate 378 to 840 mcg; budesonide 800 to 1,200 mcg; flunisolide 1,250 to 2,000 mcg; fluticasone propionate inhalation aerosol 440 to 660 mcg; fluticasone propionate inhalation powder 400 to 600 mcg; or triamcinolone acetonide 900 to 1,600 mcg). The primary efficacy endpoints were predose FEV_1 and withdrawals due to worsening asthma. Baseline FEV_1 measurements were similar across treatments: ADVAIR HFA 115/21, 2.23 L; fluticasone propionate 110 mcg, 2.18 L; salmeterol, 2.22 L; and placebo, 2.17 L.

Efficacy results in this study were similar to those observed in Studies 1 and 2. Patients receiving ADVAIR HFA 115/21 had significantly greater improvements in FEV_1 (0.41 L, 20%) compared with fluticasone propionate 110 mcg (0.19 L, 9%), salmeterol (0.15 L, 8%), and placebo (-0.12 L, -6%). Significantly fewer patients receiving ADVAIR HFA 115/21 were withdrawn from this study for worsening asthma (7%) compared with salmeterol (24%) and placebo (54%). Fewer patients receiving ADVAIR HFA 115/21 were withdrawn due to worsening asthma (7%) compared with fluticasone propionate 110 mcg (11%); however, the difference was not statistically significant.

Study 4: Clinical Trial With ADVAIR HFA 230/21 Inhalation Aerosol

This active-controlled 12-week non-US study compared ADVAIR HFA 230/21 with fluticasone propionate CFC inhalation aerosol 220 mcg, each given as 2 inhalations twice daily, and with ADVAIR DISKUS 500/50 given as 1 inhalation twice daily in 509 patients using inhaled corticosteroids (daily doses of beclomethasone dipropionate CFC inhalation aerosol 1,500 to 2,000 mcg; budesonide 1,500 to 2,000 mcg; flunisolide 1,500 to 2,000 mcg; fluticasone propionate inhalation aerosol 660 to 880 mcg; or fluticasone propionate inhalation powder 750 to 1,000 mcg). The primary efficacy endpoint was morning PEF.

Baseline morning PEF measurements were similar across treatments: ADVAIR HFA 230/21, 327 L/min; ADVAIR DISKUS 500/50, 341 L/min; and fluticasone propionate 220 mcg, 345 L/min. As shown in Figure 2, morning PEF improved significantly with ADVAIR HFA 230/21 compared with fluticasone propionate 220 mcg over the 12-week treatment period. Improvements in morning PEF observed with ADVAIR HFA 230/21 were similar to improvements observed with ADVAIR DISKUS 500/50.

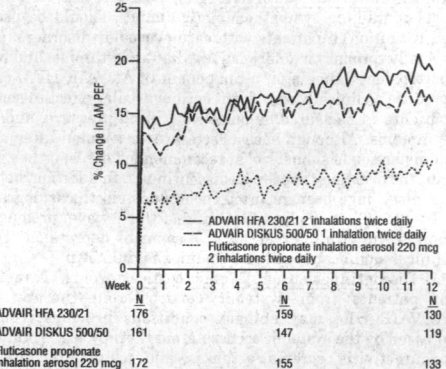

Figure 2. Mean Percent Change From Baseline in Morning Peak Expiratory Flow in Patients Previously Treated With Inhaled Corticosteroids (Study 4)

One-Year Safety Study
Clinical Trial With ADVAIR HFA 45/21, 115/21, and 230/21 Inhalation Aerosol

This 1-year open-label non-US study evaluated the safety of ADVAIR HFA 45/21, 115/21, and 230/21 given as 2 inhalations twice daily in 325 patients. This study was stratified into 3 groups according to baseline asthma therapy: patients using short-acting beta$_2$-agonists alone (n = 42), salmeterol (n = 91), or inhaled corticosteroids (n = 277). Patients treated with short-acting beta$_2$-agonists alone, salmeterol, or low doses of inhaled corticosteroids with or without concurrent salmeterol received ADVAIR HFA 45/21. Patients treated with moderate doses of inhaled corticosteroids with or without concurrent salmeterol received ADVAIR HFA 115/21. Patients treated with high doses of inhaled corticosteroids with or without concurrent salmeterol received ADVAIR HFA 230/21. Baseline FEV$_1$ measurements ranged from 2.3 to 2.6 L.

Improvements in FEV$_1$ (0.17 to 0.35 L at 4 weeks) were seen across all 3 treatments and were sustained throughout the 52-week treatment period. Few patients (3%) were withdrawn due to worsening asthma over 1 year.

Onset of Action and Progression of Improvement in Asthma Control

The onset of action and progression of improvement in asthma control were evaluated in 2 placebo-controlled US trials and 1 active-controlled US trial. Following the first dose, the median time to onset of clinically significant bronchodilatation (≥15% improvement in FEV$_1$) in most patients was seen within 30 to 60 minutes. Maximum improvement in FEV$_1$ occurred within 4 hours, and clinically significant improvement was maintained for 12 hours (see Figure 3).

Following the initial dose, predose FEV$_1$ relative to day 1 baseline improved markedly over the first week of treatment and continued to improve over the 12 weeks of treatment in all 3 studies.

No diminution in the 12-hour bronchodilator effect was observed with either ADVAIR HFA 45/21 (Figures 3 and 4) or ADVAIR HFA 230/21 as assessed by FEV$_1$ following 12 weeks of therapy.

First Treatment Day

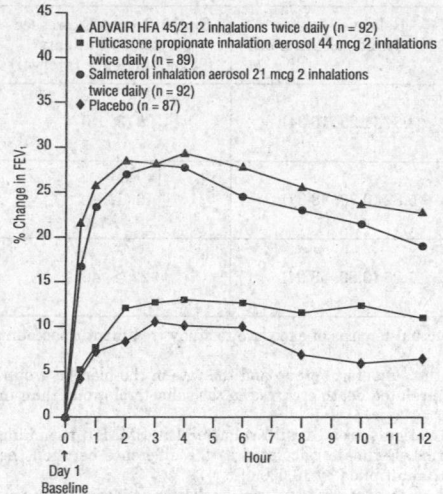

Figure 3. Percent Change in Serial 12-Hour FEV$_1$ in Patients Previously Using Either Beta$_2$-Agonists (Albuterol or Salmeterol) or Inhaled Corticosteroids (Study 1)

Last Treatment Day (Week 12)

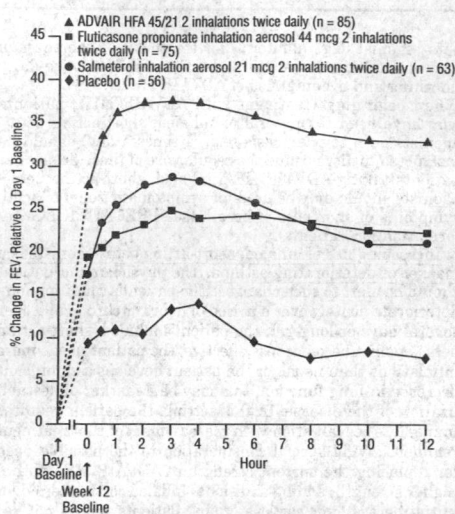

Figure 4. Percent Change in Serial 12-Hour FEV1 in Patients Previously Using Either Beta2-Agonists (Albuterol or Salmeterol) or Inhaled Corticosteroids (Study 1)

Reduction in asthma symptoms and use of rescue VENTOLIN Inhalation Aerosol and improvement in morning and evening PEF also occurred within the first day of treatment with ADVAIR HFA, and continued to improve over the 12 weeks of therapy in all 3 studies.

INDICATIONS AND USAGE

ADVAIR HFA is indicated for the treatment of asthma in patients aged 12 years and older.

LABAs, such as salmeterol, one of the active ingredients in ADVAIR HFA, increase the risk of asthma-related death. Available data from controlled clinical trials suggest that LABAs increase the risk of asthma-related hospitalization in pediatric and adolescent patients (see WARNINGS). Therefore, when treating patients with asthma, physicians should only prescribe ADVAIR HFA for patients not adequately controlled on a long-term asthma control medication, such as an inhaled corticosteroid, or whose disease severity clearly warrants initiation of treatment with both an inhaled corticosteroid and a LABA. Once asthma control is achieved and maintained, assess the patient at regular intervals and step down therapy (e.g., discontinue ADVAIR HFA) if possible without loss of asthma control and maintain the patient on a long-term asthma control medication, such as an inhaled corticosteroid. Do not use ADVAIR HFA for patients whose asthma is adequately controlled on low- or medium-dose inhaled corticosteroids.

ADVAIR HFA is NOT indicated for the relief of acute bronchospasm.

CONTRAINDICATIONS

ADVAIR HFA is contraindicated in the primary treatment of status asthmaticus or other acute episodes of asthma where intensive measures are required.

Hypersensitivity to any of the ingredients of these preparations contraindicates their use.

WARNINGS
Asthma-Related Death

LABAs, such as salmeterol, one of the active ingredients in ADVAIR HFA, increase the risk of asthma-related death. Currently available data are inadequate to determine whether concurrent use of inhaled corticosteroids or other long-term asthma control drugs mitigates the increased risk of asthma-related death from LABAs. Available data from controlled clinical trials suggest that LABAs increase the risk of asthma-related hospitalization in pediatric and adolescent patients. Therefore, when treating patients with asthma, physicians should only prescribe ADVAIR HFA for patients not adequately controlled on a long-term asthma control medication such as an inhaled corticosteroid, or whose disease severity clearly warrants initiation of treatment with both an inhaled corticosteroid and a LABA. Once asthma control is achieved and maintained, assess the patient at regular intervals and step down therapy (e.g., discontinue ADVAIR HFA) if possible without loss of asthma control and maintain the patient on a long-term asthma control medication, such as an inhaled corticosteroid. Do not use ADVAIR HFA for patients whose asthma is adequately controlled on low- or medium-dose inhaled corticosteroids.

A large placebo-controlled US study that compared the safety of salmeterol with placebo, each added to usual asthma therapy, showed an increase in asthma-related deaths in patients receiving salmeterol. The Salmeterol Multi-center Asthma Research Trial (SMART) was a randomized, double-blind study that enrolled LABA-naive patients with asthma to assess the safety of salmeterol (SEREVENT Inhalation Aerosol) 42 mcg twice daily over 28 weeks compared with placebo when added to usual asthma therapy. A planned interim analysis was conducted when approximately half of the intended number of patients had been enrolled (N = 26,355), which led to premature termination of the study. The results of the interim analysis showed that patients receiving salmeterol were at increased risk for fatal asthma events (see Table 3 and Figure 5). In the total population, a higher rate of asthma-related death occurred in patients treated with salmeterol than those treated with placebo (0.10% versus 0.02%; relative risk: 4.37 [95% CI: 1.25, 15.34]).

Post-hoc subpopulation analyses were performed. In Caucasians, asthma-related death occurred at a higher rate in patients treated with salmeterol than in patients treated with placebo (0.07% versus 0.01%; relative risk: 5.82 [95% CI: 0.70, 48.37]). In African Americans also, asthma-related death occurred at a higher rate in patients treated with salmeterol than those treated with placebo (0.31% versus 0.04%; relative risk: 7.26 [95% CI: 0.89, 58.94]). Although the relative risks of asthma-related death were similar in Caucasians and African Americans, the estimate of excess deaths in patients treated with salmeterol was greater in African Americans because there was a higher overall rate of asthma-related death in African American patients (see Table 3). Given the similar basic mechanisms of action of beta$_2$-agonists, the findings seen in the SMART study are considered a class effect.

Post-hoc analyses in pediatric patients aged 12 to 18 years were also performed. Pediatric patients accounted for approximately 12% of patients in each treatment arm. Respiratory-related death or life-threatening experience occurred at a similar rate in the salmeterol group (0.12% [2/1,653]) and the placebo group (0.12% [2/1,622]; relative risk: 1.0 [95% CI: 0.1, 7.2]). All-cause hospitalization, however, was increased in the salmeterol group (2% [35/1,653]) versus the placebo group (<1% [16/1,622]; relative risk: 2.1 [95% CI: 1.1, 3.7]).

The data from the SMART study are not adequate to determine whether concurrent use of inhaled corticosteroids, such as fluticasone propionate, the other active ingredient in ADVAIR HFA, or other long-term asthma-control therapy mitigates the risk of asthma-related death.

[See table 3 at top of next page]
[See figure 5 on next page]

A 16-week clinical study performed in the United Kingdom, the Salmeterol Nationwide Surveillance (SNS) study, showed results similar to the SMART study. In the SNS study, the rate of asthma-related death was numerically, though not statistically significantly, greater in patients with asthma treated with salmeterol (42 mcg twice daily) than those treated with albuterol (180 mcg 4 times daily) added to usual asthma therapy.

The following additional WARNINGS about ADVAIR HFA should be noted.

1. ADVAIR HFA should not be initiated in patients during rapidly deteriorating or potentially life-threatening episodes of asthma. Serious acute respiratory events, including fatalities, have been reported both in the United States and worldwide when salmeterol, a component of ADVAIR HFA, has been initiated in patients with significantly worsening or acutely deteriorating asthma. In most cases, these have occurred in patients with severe asthma (e.g., patients with

Table 3: Asthma-Related Deaths in the 28-Week Salmeterol Multi-center Asthma Research Trial (SMART)

	Salmeterol n (%[a])	Placebo n (%[a])	Relative Risk[b] (95% Confidence Interval)	Excess Deaths Expressed per 10,000 Patients[c] (95% Confidence Interval)
Total Population[d]				
Salmeterol: N = 13,176	13 (0.10%)		4.37 (1.25, 15.34)	8 (3, 13)
Placebo: N = 13,179		3 (0.02%)		
Caucasian				
Salmeterol: N = 9,281	6 (0.07%)		5.82 (0.70, 48.37)	6 (1, 10)
Placebo: N = 9,361		1 (0.01%)		
African American				
Salmeterol: N = 2,366	7 (0.31%)		7.26 (0.89, 58.94)	27 (8, 46)
Placebo: N = 2,319		1 (0.04%)		

[a]Life-table 28-week estimate, adjusted according to the patients' actual lengths of exposure to study treatment to account for early withdrawal of patients from the study.

[b]Relative risk is the ratio of the rate of asthma-related death in the salmeterol group and the rate in the placebo group. The relative risk indicates how many more times likely an asthma-related death occurred in the salmeterol group than in the placebo group in a 28-week treatment period.

[c]Estimate of the number of additional asthma-related deaths in patients treated with salmeterol in SMART, assuming 10,000 patients received salmeterol for a 28-week treatment period. Estimate calculated as the difference between the salmeterol and placebo groups in the rates of asthma-related death multiplied by 10,000.

[d]The Total Population includes the following ethnic origins listed on the case report form: Caucasian, African American, Hispanic, Asian, and "Other." In addition, the Total Population includes those patients whose ethnic origin was not reported. The results for Caucasian and African American subpopulations are shown above. No asthma-related deaths occurred in the Hispanic (salmeterol n = 996, placebo n = 999), Asian (salmeterol n = 173, placebo n = 149), or "Other" (salmeterol n = 230, placebo n = 224) subpopulations. One asthma-related death occurred in the placebo group in the subpopulation whose ethnic origin was not reported (salmeterol n = 130, placebo n = 127).

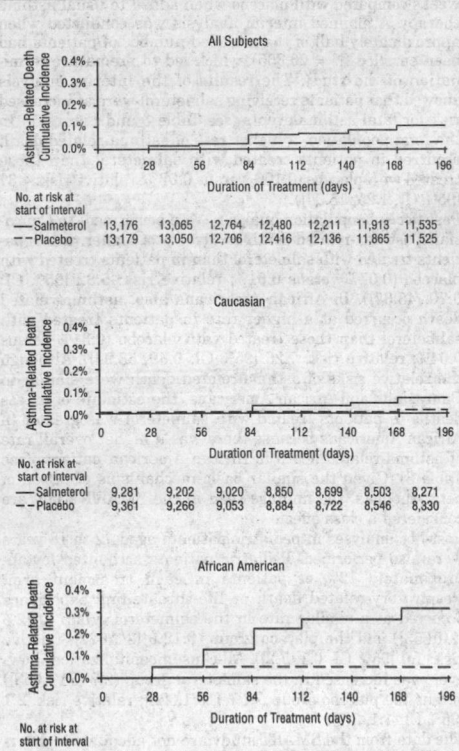

Figure 5. Cumulative Incidence of Asthma-Related Deaths in the 28-Week Salmeterol Multi-center Asthma Research Trial (SMART), by Duration of Treatment

a history of corticosteroid dependence, low pulmonary function, intubation, mechanical ventilation, frequent hospitalizations, previous life-threatening acute asthma exacerbations) and/or in some patients in whom asthma has been acutely deteriorating (e.g., unresponsive to usual medications; increasing need for inhaled, short-acting beta$_2$-agonists; increasing need for systemic corticosteroids; significant increase in symptoms; recent emergency room visits; sudden or progressive deterioration in pulmonary function). However, they have occurred in a few patients with less severe asthma as well. It was not possible from these reports to determine whether salmeterol contributed to these events.

2. ADVAIR HFA should not be used to treat acute symptoms. An inhaled, short-acting beta$_2$-agonist, not ADVAIR HFA, should be used to relieve acute symptoms of shortness of breath. When prescribing ADVAIR HFA, the physician must also provide the patient with an inhaled, short-acting beta$_2$-agonist (e.g., albuterol) for treatment of shortness of breath that occurs acutely, despite regular twice-daily (morning and evening) use of ADVAIR HFA.

When beginning treatment with ADVAIR HFA, patients who have been taking oral or inhaled, short-acting beta$_2$-agonists on a regular basis (e.g., 4 times a day) should be instructed to discontinue the regular use of these drugs. For patients taking ADVAIR HFA, inhaled, short-acting beta$_2$-agonists should only be used for symptomatic relief of acute symptoms of shortness of breath (see PRECAUTIONS: Information for Patients).

3. Increasing use of inhaled, short-acting beta$_2$-agonists is a marker of deteriorating asthma. The physician and patient should be alert to such changes. The patient's condition may deteriorate acutely over a period of hours or chronically over several days or longer. If the patient's inhaled, short-acting beta$_2$-agonist becomes less effective, the patient needs more inhalations than usual, or the patient develops a significant decrease in lung function, this may be a marker of destabilization of the disease. In this setting, the patient requires immediate reevaluation with reassessment of the treatment regimen, giving special consideration to the possible need for replacing the current strength of ADVAIR HFA with a higher strength, adding additional inhaled corticosteroid, or initiating systemic corticosteroids. Patients should not use more than 2 inhalations twice daily (morning and evening) of ADVAIR HFA.

4. ADVAIR HFA should not be used for transferring patients from systemic corticosteroid therapy. Particular care is needed for patients who have been transferred from systemically active corticosteroids to inhaled corticosteroids because deaths due to adrenal insufficiency have occurred in patients with asthma during and after transfer from systemic corticosteroids to less systemically available inhaled corticosteroids. After withdrawal from systemic corticosteroids, a number of months are required for recovery of HPA function.

Patients who have been previously maintained on 20 mg or more per day of prednisone (or its equivalent) may be most susceptible, particularly when their systemic corticosteroids have been almost completely withdrawn. During this period of HPA suppression, patients may exhibit signs and symptoms of adrenal insufficiency when exposed to trauma, surgery, or infection (particularly gastroenteritis) or other conditions associated with severe electrolyte loss. Although inhaled corticosteroids may provide control of asthma symptoms during these episodes, in recommended doses they supply less than normal physiologic amounts of glucocorticoid (cortisol) systemically and do NOT provide the mineralocorticoid activity that is necessary for coping with these emergencies.

During periods of stress or a severe asthma attack, patients who have been withdrawn from systemic corticosteroids should be instructed to resume oral corticosteroids (in large doses) immediately and to contact their physicians for further instruction. These patients should also be instructed to carry a warning card indicating that they may need supplementary systemic corticosteroids during periods of stress or a severe asthma attack.

5. ADVAIR HFA should not be used in conjunction with an inhaled LABA. Patients who are receiving ADVAIR HFA twice daily should not use additional salmeterol or other LABAs (e.g., formoterol) for prevention of exercise-induced bronchospasm (EIB) or the treatment of asthma. Additional benefit would not be gained from using supplemental salmeterol or formoterol for prevention of EIB since ADVAIR HFA already contains an inhaled LABA.

6. The recommended dosage should not be exceeded. ADVAIR HFA should not be used more often or at higher doses than recommended. Fatalities have been reported in association with excessive use of inhaled sympathomimetic drugs. Large doses of inhaled or oral salmeterol (12 to 20 times the recommended dose) have been associated with clinically significant prolongation of the QTc interval, which has the potential for producing ventricular arrhythmias.

7. Paradoxical bronchospasm. As with other inhaled asthma medications, ADVAIR HFA can produce paradoxical bronchospasm, which may be life threatening. If paradoxical bronchospasm occurs following dosing with ADVAIR HFA, it should be treated immediately with an inhaled, short-acting bronchodilator; ADVAIR HFA should be discontinued immediately; and alternative therapy should be instituted.

8. Immediate hypersensitivity reactions. Immediate hypersensitivity reactions may occur after administration of ADVAIR HFA, as demonstrated by cases of urticaria, angioedema, rash, and bronchospasm.

9. Upper airway symptoms. Symptoms of laryngeal spasm, irritation, or swelling, such as stridor and choking, have been reported in patients receiving fluticasone propionate and salmeterol, components of ADVAIR HFA.

10. Cardiovascular disorders. ADVAIR HFA, like all products containing sympathomimetic amines, should be used with caution in patients with cardiovascular disorders, especially coronary insufficiency, cardiac arrhythmias, and hypertension. Salmeterol, a component of ADVAIR HFA, can produce a clinically significant cardiovascular effect in some patients as measured by pulse rate, blood pressure, and/or symptoms. Although such effects are uncommon after administration of salmeterol at recommended doses, if they occur, the drug may need to be discontinued. In addition, beta-agonists have been reported to produce electrocardiogram (ECG) changes, such as flattening of the T wave, prolongation of the QTc interval, and ST segment depression. The clinical significance of these findings is unknown.

11. Discontinuation of systemic corticosteroids. Transfer of patients from systemic corticosteroid therapy to ADVAIR HFA may unmask conditions previously suppressed by the systemic corticosteroid therapy, e.g., rhinitis, conjunctivitis, eczema, arthritis, and eosinophilic conditions.

12. Immunosuppression. Persons who are using drugs that suppress the immune system are more susceptible to infections than healthy individuals. Chickenpox and measles, for example, can have a more serious or even fatal course in susceptible children or adults using corticosteroids. In such children or adults who have not had these diseases or been properly immunized, particular care should be taken to avoid exposure. How the dose, route, and duration of corticosteroid administration affect the risk of developing a disseminated infection is not known. The contribution of the underlying disease and/or prior corticosteroid treatment to the risk is also not known. If exposed to chickenpox, prophylaxis with varicella zoster immune globulin (VZIG) may be indicated. If exposed to measles, prophylaxis with pooled intramuscular immunoglobulin (IG) may be indicated. (See the respective package inserts for complete VZIG and IG prescribing information.) If chickenpox develops, treatment with antiviral agents may be considered.

13. Pneumonia. Lower respiratory tract infections, including pneumonia, have been reported in patients with COPD following the inhaled administration of corticosteroids, including fluticasone propionate and ADVAIR DISKUS. In 2 replicate 12-month studies of 1,579 patients with COPD, there was a higher incidence of pneumonia reported in patients receiving ADVAIR DISKUS 250/50 (7%) than in those receiving salmeterol 50 mcg (3%). The incidence of pneumonia in the patients treated with ADVAIR DISKUS was higher in patients over 65 years of age (9%) compared with the incidence in patients less than 65 years of age (4%).

In a 3-year study of 6,184 patients with COPD, there was a higher incidence of pneumonia reported in patients receiving ADVAIR DISKUS 500/50 compared with placebo (16% with ADVAIR DISKUS 500/50, 14% with fluticasone propionate 500 mcg, 11% with salmeterol 50 mcg, and 9% with placebo). Similar to what was seen in the 1-year studies with ADVAIR DISKUS 250/50, the incidence of pneumonia was higher in patients over 65 years of age (18% with ADVAIR DISKUS 500/50 versus 10% with placebo) compared with patients less than 65 years of age (14% with ADVAIR DISKUS 500/50 versus 8% with placebo).

14. Potential drug interactions with CYP3A4 inhibitors. Both fluticasone propionate and salmeterol are substrates of CYP3A4.

Fluticasone Propionate: A drug interaction study in healthy subjects has shown that ritonavir (a strong CYP3A4 inhibitor) can significantly increase systemic fluticasone propionate exposure (AUC), resulting in significantly reduced serum cortisol concentrations (see CLINICAL PHARMACOLOGY: Pharmacokinetics: *Fluticasone Propionate: Drug Interactions* and PRECAUTIONS: Drug Interactions: *Inhibitors of Cytochrome P450*). During postmarketing use, there have been reports of clinically significant drug interactions in patients receiving fluticasone propionate and ritonavir, resulting in systemic corticosteroid effects including Cushing's syndrome and adrenal suppression. Therefore, coadministration of fluticasone propionate and ritonavir is not recommended unless the potential benefit to the patient outweighs the risk of systemic corticosteroid side effects.

Salmeterol: Because of the potential for drug interactions and the potential for increased risk of cardiovascular adverse events, the concomitant use of ADVAIR HFA with strong CYP 3A4 inhibitors (e.g., ketoconazole, ritonavir, atazanavir, clarithromycin, indinavir, itraconazole, nefazodone, nelfinavir, saquinavir, telithromycin) is not recommended (see CLINICAL PHARMACOLOGY: Pharmacokinetics: *Salmeterol Xinafoate: Drug Interactions*).

PRECAUTIONS
General
Cardiovascular Effects
Cardiovascular and central nervous system effects seen with all sympathomimetic drugs (e.g., increased blood pressure, heart rate, excitement) can occur after use of salmeterol, a component of ADVAIR HFA, and may require discontinuation of ADVAIR HFA. ADVAIR HFA, like all medications containing sympathomimetic amines, should be used with caution in patients with cardiovascular disorders, especially coronary insufficiency, cardiac arrhythmias, and hypertension; in patients with convulsive disorders or thyrotoxicosis; and in patients who are unusually responsive to sympathomimetic amines.

As has been described with other beta-adrenergic agonist bronchodilators, clinically significant changes in ECGs have been seen infrequently in individual patients in controlled clinical studies with ADVAIR HFA and salmeterol. Clinically significant changes in systolic and/or diastolic blood pressure and pulse rate have been seen infrequently in individual patients in controlled clinical studies with salmeterol, a component of ADVAIR HFA.

Metabolic and Other Effects
Long-term use of orally inhaled corticosteroids may affect normal bone metabolism, resulting in a loss of bone mineral density. In patients with major risk factors for decreased bone mineral content, such as tobacco use, advanced age, sedentary lifestyle, poor nutrition, family history of osteoporosis, or chronic use of drugs that can reduce bone mass (e.g., anticonvulsants, corticosteroids), ADVAIR HFA may pose an additional risk.

Doses of the related beta$_2$-adrenoceptor agonist albuterol, when administered intravenously, have been reported to aggravate preexisting diabetes mellitus and ketoacidosis. Beta-adrenergic agonist medications may produce significant hypokalemia in some patients, possibly through intracellular shunting, which has the potential to produce adverse cardiovascular effects. The decrease in serum potassium is usually transient, not requiring supplementation.

Clinically significant changes in blood glucose and/or serum potassium were seen infrequently during clinical studies with ADVAIR HFA at recommended doses.

During withdrawal from oral corticosteroids, some patients may experience symptoms of systemically active corticosteroid withdrawal (e.g., joint and/or muscular pain, lassitude, depression), despite maintenance or even improvement of respiratory function.

Fluticasone propionate, a component of ADVAIR HFA, will often help control asthma symptoms with less suppression of HPA function than therapeutically equivalent oral doses of prednisone. Since fluticasone propionate is absorbed into the circulation and can be systemically active at higher doses, the beneficial effects of ADVAIR HFA in minimizing HPA dysfunction may be expected only when recommended dosages are not exceeded and individual patients are titrated to the lowest effective dose. A relationship between plasma levels of fluticasone propionate and inhibitory effects on stimulated cortisol production has been shown after 4 weeks of treatment with fluticasone propionate inhalation aerosol. Since individual sensitivity to effects on cortisol production exists, physicians should consider this information when prescribing ADVAIR HFA.

Because of the possibility of systemic absorption of inhaled corticosteroids, patients treated with ADVAIR HFA should be observed carefully for any evidence of systemic corticosteroid effects. Particular care should be taken in observing patients postoperatively or during periods of stress for evidence of inadequate adrenal response.

It is possible that systemic corticosteroid effects such as hypercorticism and adrenal suppression (including adrenal

crisis) may appear in a small number of patients, particularly when fluticasone propionate is administered at higher than recommended doses over prolonged periods of time. If such effects occur, the dosage of ADVAIR HFA should be reduced slowly, consistent with accepted procedures for reducing systemic corticosteroids and for management of asthma. A reduction of growth velocity in children and adolescents may occur as a result of poorly controlled asthma or from the therapeutic use of corticosteroids, including inhaled corticosteroids (see PRECAUTIONS: Pediatric Use). The effects of long-term treatment of children and adolescents with inhaled corticosteroids, including fluticasone propionate, on final adult height are not known. Patients should be maintained on the lowest strength of ADVAIR HFA that effectively controls their asthma.

The long-term effects of ADVAIR HFA in human subjects are not fully known. In particular, the effects resulting from chronic use of fluticasone propionate on developmental or immunologic processes in the mouth, pharynx, trachea, and lung are unknown. Some patients received inhaled fluticasone propionate on a continuous basis in a clinical study for up to 4 years. In clinical studies with patients treated for 2 years with inhaled fluticasone propionate, no apparent differences in the type or severity of adverse reactions were observed after long- versus short-term treatment.

Glaucoma, increased intraocular pressure, and cataracts have been reported in patients following the long-term administration of inhaled corticosteroids, including fluticasone propionate, a component of ADVAIR HFA.

Lower respiratory tract infections, including pneumonia, have been reported following the inhaled administration of corticosteroids, including fluticasone propionate, a component of ADVAIR HFA.

In clinical studies with ADVAIR HFA, the development of localized infections of the pharynx with *Candida albicans* has occurred. When such an infection develops, it should be treated with appropriate local or systemic (e.g., oral antifungal) therapy while remaining on treatment with ADVAIR HFA, but at times therapy with ADVAIR HFA may need to be interrupted.

Inhaled corticosteroids should be used with caution, if at all, in patients with active or quiescent tuberculosis infections of the respiratory tract; untreated systemic fungal, bacterial, viral, or parasitic infections; or ocular herpes simplex.

Eosinophilic Conditions
In rare cases, patients on inhaled fluticasone propionate, a component of ADVAIR HFA, may present with systemic eosinophilic conditions, with some patients presenting with clinical features of vasculitis consistent with Churg-Strauss syndrome, a condition that is often treated with systemic corticosteroid therapy. These events usually, but not always, have been associated with the reduction and/or withdrawal of oral corticosteroid therapy following the introduction of fluticasone propionate. Cases of serious eosinophilic conditions have also been reported with other inhaled corticosteroids in this clinical setting. Physicians should be alert to eosinophilia, vasculitic rash, worsening pulmonary symptoms, cardiac complications, and/or neuropathy presenting in their patients. A causal relationship between fluticasone propionate and these underlying conditions has not been established (see ADVERSE REACTIONS: Observed During Clinical Practice: *Eosinophilic Conditions*).

Information for Patients: Patients should be instructed to read the Medication Guide, which is supplied as a tear-off leaflet from this document, with each new prescription and refill.
Patients being treated with ADVAIR HFA should receive the following information and instructions. This information is intended to aid them in the safe and effective use of this medication. It is not a disclosure of all possible adverse or intended effects. It is important that patients understand how to use ADVAIR HFA in relation to other asthma medications they are taking.

1. **Patients should be informed that salmeterol, one of the active ingredients in ADVAIR HFA, has been associated with an increased risk of asthma-related death and increases the risk of asthma-related hospitalization in pediatric and adolescent patients.** They should also be informed that currently available data are inadequate to determine whether concurrent use of inhaled corticosteroids or other long-term asthma control drugs mitigates the increased risk of asthma-related death from LABAs.
2. ADVAIR HFA is not meant to relieve acute asthma symptoms and extra doses should not be used for that purpose. Acute symptoms should be treated with an inhaled, short-acting beta$_2$-agonist such as albuterol. The physician should provide the patient with such medication and instruct the patient in how it should be used.
3. The physician should be notified immediately if any of the following signs of seriously worsening asthma occur:
   - decreasing effectiveness of inhaled, short-acting beta$_2$-agonists;

   - need for more inhalations than usual of inhaled, short-acting beta$_2$-agonists;
   - significant decrease in lung function as outlined by the physician.
4. Patients should not stop therapy with ADVAIR HFA without physician/provider guidance since symptoms may recur after discontinuation.
5. Patients should be cautioned regarding common adverse effects associated with beta$_2$-agonists, such as palpitations, chest pain, rapid heart rate, tremor, or nervousness.
6. Long-term use of inhaled corticosteroids, including fluticasone propionate, a component of ADVAIR HFA, may increase the risk of some eye problems (cataracts or glaucoma). Regular eye examinations should be considered.
7. When patients are prescribed ADVAIR HFA, other medications for asthma should be used only as directed by the physician.
8. Patients who are pregnant or nursing should contact the physician about the use of ADVAIR HFA.
9. Patients should use ADVAIR HFA at regular intervals as directed. Results of clinical trials indicated significant improvement may occur within the first 30 minutes of taking the first dose; however, the full benefit may not be achieved until treatment has been administered for 1 week or longer. The patient should not use more than the prescribed dosage but should contact the physician if symptoms do not improve or if the condition worsens.
10. The bronchodilation from a single dose of ADVAIR HFA may last up to 12 hours or longer. The recommended dosage (2 inhalations twice daily, morning and evening) should not be exceeded. Patients who are receiving ADVAIR HFA twice daily should not use salmeterol or other inhaled LABAs (e.g., formoterol) for prevention of EIB or treatment of asthma.
11. Patients should be warned to avoid exposure to chickenpox or measles and, if they are exposed to consult the physician without delay.
12. Prime the inhaler before using for the first time by releasing 4 test sprays into the air away from the face, shaking well for 5 seconds before each spray. In cases where the inhaler has not been used for more than 4 weeks or when it has been dropped, prime the inhaler again by releasing 2 test sprays into the air away from the face, shaking well for 5 seconds before each spray.
13. After inhalation, rinse the mouth with water and spit out. Do not swallow.
14. Clean the inhaler at least once a week after the evening dose. Keeping the canister and plastic actuator clean is important to prevent medicine buildup. (See the cleaning instructions in the "How to use your ADVAIR HFA" section of the Medication Guide tear-off leaflet.)
15. Use ADVAIR HFA only with the actuator supplied with the product. When the counter reads 020, contact the pharmacist for a refill of medication or consult the physician to determine whether a prescription refill is needed. Discard the inhaler when the counter reads 000. Never try to alter the numbers or remove the counter from the metal canister.
16. For important summary information and instructions for the proper use of ADVAIR HFA, the patient should carefully read and follow the Medication Guide tear-off leaflet.

Drug Interactions
ADVAIR HFA has been used concomitantly with other drugs, including short-acting beta$_2$-agonists, methylxanthines, and intranasal corticosteroids, commonly used in patients with asthma, without adverse drug reactions. No formal drug interaction studies have been performed with ADVAIR HFA.

Short-Acting Beta$_2$-Agonists
In three 12-week US clinical trials, the mean daily need for additional beta$_2$-agonist use in 277 patients receiving ADVAIR HFA was approximately 1.2 inhalations/day and ranged from 0 to 9 inhalations/day. Two percent (2%) of patients receiving ADVAIR HFA in these trials averaged 6 or more inhalations per day over the course of the 12-week trials. No increase in frequency of cardiovascular events was observed among patients who averaged 6 or more inhalations per day.

Methylxanthines
The concurrent use of intravenously or orally administered methylxanthines (e.g., aminophylline, theophylline) by patients receiving ADVAIR HFA has not been completely evaluated. In five 12-week clinical trials (3 US and 2 non-US), 45 patients receiving ADVAIR HFA 45/21, 115/21, or 230/21 twice daily concurrently with a theophylline product had adverse event rates similar to those in 577 patients receiving ADVAIR HFA without theophylline.

Fluticasone Propionate Nasal Spray
In patients receiving ADVAIR HFA in three 12-week US clinical trials, no difference in the profile of adverse events

or HPA axis effects was noted between patients receiving FLONASE® (fluticasone propionate) Nasal Spray, 50 mcg concurrently (n = 89) and those who were not (n = 192).

Monoamine Oxidase Inhibitors and Tricyclic Antidepressants

ADVAIR HFA should be administered with extreme caution to patients being treated with monoamine oxidase inhibitors or tricyclic antidepressants, or within 2 weeks of discontinuation of such agents, because the action of salmeterol, a component of ADVAIR HFA, on the vascular system may be potentiated by these agents.

Beta-Adrenergic Receptor Blocking Agents

Beta-blockers not only block the pulmonary effect of beta-agonists, such as salmeterol, a component of ADVAIR HFA, but may produce severe bronchospasm in patients with asthma. Therefore, patients with asthma should not normally be treated with beta-blockers. However, under certain circumstances, there may be no acceptable alternatives to the use of beta-adrenergic blocking agents in patients with asthma. In this setting, cardioselective beta-blockers could be considered, although they should be administered with caution.

Diuretics

The ECG changes and/or hypokalemia that may result from the administration of nonpotassium-sparing diuretics (such as loop or thiazide diuretics) can be acutely worsened by beta-agonists, especially when the recommended dose of the beta-agonist is exceeded. Although the clinical significance of these effects is not known, caution is advised in the coadministration of beta-agonists with nonpotassium-sparing diuretics.

Inhibitors of Cytochrome P450

Fluticasone propionate and salmeterol are substrates of CYP3A4.

Fluticasone propionate

A drug interaction study with fluticasone propionate aqueous nasal spray in healthy subjects has shown that ritonavir (a strong CYP3A4 inhibitor) can significantly increase plasma fluticasone propionate exposure, resulting in significantly reduced serum cortisol concentrations (see CLINICAL PHARMACOLOGY: Pharmacokinetics: *Fluticasone Propionate: Drug Interactions*). During post-marketing use, there have been reports of clinically significant drug interactions in patients receiving fluticasone propionate and ritonavir, resulting in systemic corticosteroid effects including Cushing's syndrome and adrenal suppression. Therefore, coadministration of fluticasone propionate and ritonavir is not recommended unless the potential benefit to the patient outweighs the risk of systemic corticosteroid side effects.

In a placebo-controlled, crossover study in 8 healthy adult volunteers, coadministration of a single dose of orally inhaled fluticasone propionate (1,000 mcg) with multiple doses of ketoconazole (200 mg) to steady state resulted in increased systemic fluticasone propionate exposure, a reduction in plasma cortisol AUC, and no effect on urinary excretion of cortisol.

Salmeterol

In a drug interaction study in 20 healthy subjects, coadministration of inhaled salmeterol (50 mcg twice daily) and oral ketoconazole (400 mg once daily) for 7 days resulted in greater systemic exposure to salmeterol (AUC increased 16-fold and C_{max} increased 1.4-fold). Three (3) subjects were withdrawn due to beta$_2$-agonist side effects (2 with prolonged QTc and 1 with palpitations and sinus tachycardia). Although there was no statistical effect on the mean QTc, coadministration of salmeterol and ketoconazole was associated with more frequent increases in QTc duration compared with salmeterol and placebo administration. Due to the potential increased risk of cardiovascular adverse events, the concomitant use of salmeterol with strong CYP 3A4 inhibitors (e.g., ketoconazole, ritonavir, atazanavir, clarithromycin, indinavir, itraconazole, nefazodone, nelfinavir, saquinavir, telithromycin) is not recommended (see CLINICAL PHARMACOLOGY: Pharmacokinetics: *Salmeterol Xinafoate: Drug Interactions*).

Carcinogenesis, Mutagenesis, Impairment of Fertility

Fluticasone Propionate

Fluticasone propionate demonstrated no tumorigenic potential in mice at oral doses up to 1,000 mcg/kg (approximately 4 times the maximum recommended human daily inhalation dose [MRHD] on an mcg/m^2 basis) for 78 weeks or in rats at inhalation doses up to 57 mcg/kg (less than the MRHD on an mcg/m^2 basis) for 104 weeks.

Fluticasone propionate did not induce gene mutation in prokaryotic or eukaryotic cells in vitro. No significant clastogenic effect was seen in cultured human peripheral lymphocytes in vitro or in the mouse micronucleus test.

No evidence of impairment of fertility was observed in reproductive studies conducted in male and female rats at subcutaneous doses up to 50 mcg/kg (less than the MRHD on an mcg/m^2 basis). Prostate weight was significantly reduced at a subcutaneous dose of 50 mcg/kg.

Salmeterol

In an 18-month oral carcinogenicity study in CD-mice, salmeterol at oral doses of 1.4 mg/kg and above (approximately 10 times the MRHD based on comparison of the AUCs) caused a dose-related increase in the incidence of smooth muscle hyperplasia, cystic glandular hyperplasia, leiomyomas of the uterus, and ovarian cysts. The incidence of leiomyosarcomas was not statistically significant. No tumors were seen at 0.2 mg/kg (approximately 2 times the MRHD for adults based on comparison of the AUCs).

In a 24-month oral and inhalation carcinogenicity study in Sprague Dawley rats, salmeterol caused a dose-related increase in the incidence of mesovarian leiomyomas and ovarian cysts at doses of 0.68 mg/kg and above (approximately 65 times the MRHD on an mg/m^2 basis). No tumors were seen at 0.21 mg/kg (approximately 20 times the MRHD on an mg/m^2 basis). These findings in rodents are similar to those reported previously for other beta-adrenergic agonist drugs. The relevance of these findings to human use is unknown.

Salmeterol produced no detectable or reproducible increases in microbial and mammalian gene mutation in vitro. No clastogenic activity occurred in vitro in human lymphocytes or in vivo in a rat micronucleus test. No effects on fertility were identified in male and female rats treated with salmeterol at oral doses up to 2 mg/kg (approximately 190 times the MRHD on an mg/m^2 basis).

Pregnancy

Teratogenic Effects

ADVAIR HFA Inhalation Aerosol

Pregnancy Category C. From the reproduction toxicity studies in mice and rats, no evidence of enhanced toxicity was seen using combinations of fluticasone propionate and salmeterol compared with toxicity data from the components administered separately. In mice combining 150 mcg/kg subcutaneously of fluticasone propionate (less than the MRHD on an mcg/m^2 basis) with 10 mg/kg orally of salmeterol (approximately 480 times the MRHD on an mg/m^2 basis) were teratogenic. Cleft palate, fetal death, increased implantation loss and delayed ossification was seen. These observations are characteristic of glucocorticoids. No developmental toxicity was observed at combination doses up to 40 mcg/kg subcutaneously of fluticasone propionate (less than the MRHD on an mcg/m^2 basis) and up to 1.4 mg/kg orally of salmeterol (approximately 70 times the MRHD on an mg/m^2 basis). In rats, no teratogenicity was observed at combination doses up to 30 mcg/kg subcutaneously of fluticasone propionate (less than the MRHD on an mcg/m^2 basis) and up to 1 mg/kg of salmeterol (approximately 95 times the MRHD on an mg/m^2 basis). Combining 100 mcg/kg subcutaneously of fluticasone propionate (equivalent to the MRHD on an mcg/m^2 basis) with 10 mg/kg orally of salmeterol (approximately 970 times the MRHD on an mg/m^2 basis) produced maternal toxicity, decreased placental weight, decreased fetal weight, umbilical hernia, delayed ossification, and changes in the occipital bone.

There are no adequate and well-controlled studies with ADVAIR HFA in pregnant women. ADVAIR HFA should be used during pregnancy only if the potential benefit justifies the potential risk to the fetus.

Fluticasone Propionate

Pregnancy Category C. Subcutaneous studies in the mouse and rat at 45 and 100 mcg/kg, respectively (less than and equivalent to, respectively, the MRHD on an mcg/m^2 basis), revealed fetal toxicity characteristic of potent corticosteroid compounds, including embryonic growth retardation, omphalocele, cleft palate, and retarded cranial ossification. No teratogenicity was seen in rats at inhalation doses up to 68.7 mcg/kg (less than the MRHD on an mcg/m^2 basis).

In the rabbit, fetal weight reduction and cleft palate were observed at a subcutaneous dose of 4 mcg/kg (less than the MRHD on an mcg/m^2 basis). However, no teratogenic effects were reported at oral doses up to 300 mcg/kg (approximately 5 times the MRHD on an mcg/m^2 basis) of fluticasone propionate. No fluticasone propionate was detected in the plasma in this study, consistent with the established low bioavailability following oral administration (see CLINICAL PHARMACOLOGY: Pharmacokinetcs: *Fluticasone Propionate: Absorption*).

Fluticasone propionate crossed the placenta following administration of a subcutaneous dose of 100 mcg/kg to mice (less than the MRHD on an mcg/m^2 basis), a subcutaneous or an oral dose of 100 mcg/kg to rats (equivalent to the MRHD on an mcg/m^2 basis), and an oral dose of 300 mcg/kg to rabbits (approximately 5 times the MRHD on an mcg/m^2 basis).

There are no adequate and well-controlled studies in pregnant women. ADVAIR HFA should be used during pregnancy only if the potential benefit justifies the potential risk to the fetus.

Experience with oral corticosteroids since their introduction in pharmacologic, as opposed to physiologic, doses suggests that rodents are more prone to teratogenic effects from corticosteroids than humans. In addition, because there is a natural increase in corticosteroid production during pregnancy, most women will require a lower exogenous corticosteroid dose and many will not need corticosteroid treatment during pregnancy.

Salmeterol

Pregnancy Category C. No teratogenic effects occurred in rats at oral doses up to 2 mg/kg (approximately 190 times the MRHD on an mg/m^2 basis). In pregnant Dutch rabbits administered oral doses of 1 mg/kg and above (approximately 25 times the MRHD based on the comparison of the AUCs), salmeterol exhibited fetal toxic effects characteristically resulting from beta-adrenoceptor stimulation. These included precocious eyelid openings, cleft palate, sternebral fusion, limb and paw flexures, and delayed ossification of the frontal cranial bones. No significant effects occurred at an oral dose of 0.6 mg/kg (approximately 10 times the MRHD based on comparison of the AUCs).

New Zealand White rabbits were less sensitive since only delayed ossification of the frontal cranial bones was seen at an oral dose of 10 mg/kg (approximately 1,900 times the MRHD on an mg/m^2 basis). Extensive use of other beta-agonists has provided no evidence that these class effects in animals are relevant to their use in humans.

Salmeterol xinafoate crossed the placenta following oral administration of 10 mg/kg to mice and rats (approximately 480 and 970 times, respectively, the MRHD on an mg/m^2 basis).

There are no adequate and well-controlled studies with salmeterol in pregnant women. Salmeterol should be used during pregnancy only if the potential benefit justifies the potential risk to the fetus.

Use in Labor and Delivery

There are no well-controlled human studies that have investigated effects of ADVAIR HFA on preterm labor or labor at term. Because of the potential for beta-agonist interference with uterine contractility, use of ADVAIR HFA for management of asthma during labor should be restricted to those patients in whom the benefits clearly outweigh the risks.

Nursing Mothers

Plasma levels of salmeterol, a component of ADVAIR HFA, after inhaled therapeutic doses are very low. In rats, salmeterol xinafoate is excreted in the milk. There are no data from controlled trials on the use of salmeterol by nursing mothers. It is not known whether fluticasone propionate, a component of ADVAIR HFA, is excreted in human breast milk. However, other corticosteroids have been detected in human milk. Subcutaneous administration to lactating rats of 10 mcg/kg tritiated fluticasone propionate (less than the MRHD on an mcg/m^2 basis) resulted in measurable radioactivity in milk.

Since there are no data from controlled trials on the use of ADVAIR HFA by nursing mothers, a decision should be made whether to discontinue nursing or to discontinue ADVAIR HFA, taking into account the importance of ADVAIR HFA to the mother.

Caution should be exercised when ADVAIR HFA is administered to a nursing woman.

Pediatric Use

Thirty-eight (38) patients aged 12 to 17 years were treated with ADVAIR HFA in US pivotal clinical trials. Patients in this age-group demonstrated efficacy results similar to those observed in patients aged 18 years and older. There were no obvious differences in the type or frequency of adverse events reported in this age-group compared with patients aged 18 years and older.

The safety and effectiveness of ADVAIR HFA in children less than 12 years have not been established.

Controlled clinical studies have shown that inhaled corticosteroids may cause a reduction in growth in pediatric patients. In these studies, the mean reduction in growth velocity was approximately 1 cm/year (range: 0.3 to 1.8 cm/year) and appears to depend upon dose and duration of exposure. This effect was observed in the absence of laboratory evidence of HPA axis suppression, suggesting that growth velocity is a more sensitive indicator of systemic corticosteroid exposure in pediatric patients than some commonly used tests of HPA axis function. The long-term effects of this reduction in growth velocity associated with orally inhaled corticosteroids, including the impact on final adult height, are unknown. The potential for "catch-up" growth following discontinuation of treatment with orally inhaled corticosteroids has not been adequately studied. The effects on growth velocity of treatment with orally inhaled corticosteroids for over 1 year, including the impact on final adult height, are unknown. The growth of children and adolescents receiving orally inhaled corticosteroids, including ADVAIR HFA, should be monitored. If a child or adolescent on any corticosteroid appears to have growth suppression, the possibility that he/she is particularly sensitive to this effect of corticosteroids should be considered. The potential growth effects of prolonged treatment should be weighed against the clinical benefits obtained and the risks associated with alternative therapies. To minimize the systemic effects of orally inhaled corticosteroids, including

ADVAIR HFA, each patient should be titrated to the lowest strength that effectively controls his/her asthma (see DOSAGE AND ADMINISTRATION).

Geriatric Use
Of the total number of patients in clinical studies treated with ADVAIR HFA, 41 were aged 65 years or older and 21 were aged 75 years or older. No overall differences in safety were observed between these patients and younger patients, and other reported clinical experience, including studies of the individual components, has not identified differences in responses between the elderly and younger patients, but greater sensitivity of some older individuals cannot be ruled out. As with other products containing beta$_2$-agonists, special caution should be observed when using ADVAIR HFA in geriatric patients who have concomitant cardiovascular disease that could be adversely affected by beta$_2$-agonists. Based on available data for ADVAIR HFA or its active components, no adjustment of dosage of ADVAIR HFA in geriatric patients is warranted.

ADVERSE REACTIONS
LABAs, such as salmeterol, one of the active ingredients in ADVAIR HFA, increase the risk of asthma-related death. Data from a large placebo-controlled US study that compared the safety of salmeterol (SEREVENT Inhalation Aerosol) or placebo added to usual asthma therapy showed an increase in asthma-related deaths in patients receiving salmeterol (see WARNINGS). Currently available data are inadequate to determine whether concurrent use of inhaled corticosteroids or other long-term asthma control drugs mitigates the increased risk of asthma-related death from LABAs. Available data from controlled clinical trials suggest that LABAs increase the risk of asthma-related hospitalization in pediatric and adolescent patients.

The incidence of common adverse events in Table 4 is based upon 2 placebo-controlled, 12-week, US clinical studies (Studies 1 and 3) and 1 active-controlled, 12-week, US clinical study (Study 2). A total of 1,008 adolescent and adult patients with asthma (556 females and 452 males) previously treated with albuterol alone, salmeterol, or inhaled corticosteroids were treated twice daily with 2 inhalations of ADVAIR HFA 45/21 or ADVAIR HFA 115/21, fluticasone propionate CFC inhalation aerosol (44- or 110-mcg doses), salmeterol CFC inhalation aerosol 21 mcg, or placebo HFA inhalation aerosol.
[See table 4 at right]

Table 4 includes all events (whether considered drug-related or nondrug-related by the investigator) that occurred at a rate of 3% or greater in any of the groups receiving ADVAIR HFA and were more common than in the placebo group. In considering these data, differences in average duration of exposure should be taken into account. These adverse reactions were mostly mild to moderate in severity.

Other adverse events that occurred in the groups receiving ADVAIR HFA in these studies with an incidence of 1% to 3% and that occurred at a greater incidence than with placebo were:

Cardiovascular
Tachycardia, arrhythmias, myocardial infarction.
Drug Interaction, Overdose, and Trauma
Postoperative complications, wounds and lacerations, soft tissue injuries, poisoning and toxicity, pressure-induced disorder.
Ear, Nose, and Throat
Ear, nose, and throat infection; ear signs and symptoms; rhinorrhea/postnasal drip; epistaxis; nasal congestion/blockage; laryngitis; unspecified oropharyngeal plaques; dryness of nose.
Endocrine and Metabolic
Weight gain.
Eye
Allergic eye disorders, eye edema and swelling.
Gastrointestinal
Gastrointestinal discomfort and pain, dental discomfort and pain, candidiasis mouth/throat, hyposalivation, gastrointestinal infections, disorders of hard tissue of teeth, hemorrhoids, gastrointestinal gaseous symptoms, abdominal discomfort and pain, constipation, oral abnormalities.
Musculoskeletal
Arthralgia and articular rheumatism, muscle cramps and spasms, musculoskeletal inflammation, bone and skeletal pain.
Neurology
Sleep disorders, migraines.
Non-Site Specific
Allergies and allergic reactions, viral infections, bacterial infections, candidiasis unspecified site, congestion, inflammation.
Reproduction
Bacterial reproductive infections.
Respiratory
Lower respiratory signs and symptoms, lower respiratory infections, lower respiratory hemorrhage.

Table 4. Overall Adverse Events With ≥3% Incidence in US Controlled Clinical Trials With ADVAIR HFA Inhalation Aerosol in Patients With Asthma

Adverse Events	ADVAIR HFA		Fluticasone Propionate CFC Inhalation Aerosol		Salmeterol CFC Inhalation Aerosol	Placebo HFA Inhalation Aerosol
	45/21 (n = 187) %	115/21 (n = 94) %	44 mcg (n = 186) %	110 mcg (n = 91) %	21 mcg (n = 274) %	(n = 176) %
Ear, nose, & throat						
Upper respiratory tract infection	16	24	13	15	17	13
Throat irritation	9	7	12	13	9	7
Upper respiratory inflammation	4	4	3	7	5	3
Hoarseness/dysphonia	3	1	2	0	1	0
Lower respiratory						
Viral respiratory infections	3	5	4	5	3	4
Neurology						
Headaches	21	15	24	16	20	11
Dizziness	4	1	1	0	<1	0
Gastrointestinal						
Nausea & vomiting	5	3	4	2	2	3
Viral gastrointestinal infections	4	2	2	0	1	2
Gastrointestinal signs & symptoms	3	2	2	1	1	1
Non-site specific						
Pain	3	1	2	1	2	2
Musculoskeletal						
Musculoskeletal pain	5	7	8	2	4	4
Muscle pain	4	1	1	1	3	<1
Drug interaction, overdose, & trauma						
Muscle injuries	3	0	2	1	3	2
Reproduction						
Menstruation symptoms	5	3	1	1	<1	<1
Psychiatry						
Intoxication & hangover	3	0	0	0	0	0
Average duration of exposure (days)	81.3	78.6	79.9	74.6	71.4	56.3

Skin
Eczema, dermatitis and dermatosis.
Urology
Urinary infections.
Rare cases of immediate and delayed hypersensitivity reactions, including rash and other rare events of angioedema and bronchospasm, have been reported.
The incidence of common adverse events reported in Study 4, a 12-week, non-US clinical study of 509 patients previously treated with inhaled corticosteroids who were treated twice daily with 2 inhalations of ADVAIR HFA 230/21, fluticasone propionate CFC inhalation aerosol 220 mcg, or 1 inhalation of ADVAIR DISKUS 500/50 was similar to the incidences reported in Table 4.
Observed During Clinical Practice
In addition to adverse events reported from clinical trials, the following events have been identified during worldwide use of any formulation of ADVAIR, fluticasone propionate, and/or salmeterol regardless of indication. Because they are reported voluntarily from a population of unknown size, estimates of frequency cannot be made. These events have been chosen for inclusion due to either their seriousness, frequency of reporting, or causal connection to ADVAIR, fluticasone propionate, and/or salmeterol or a combination of these factors.
In extensive US and worldwide postmarketing experience with salmeterol, a component of ADVAIR HFA, serious exacerbations of asthma, including some that have been fatal, have been reported. In most cases, these have occurred in patients with severe asthma and/or in some patients in whom asthma has been acutely deteriorating (see WARNINGS), but they have also occurred in a few patients with less severe asthma. It was not possible from these reports to determine whether salmeterol contributed to these events.
Cardiovascular
Arrhythmias (including atrial fibrillation, extrasystoles, supraventricular tachycardia), hypertension, ventricular tachycardia.
Ear, Nose, and Throat
Aphonia, earache, facial and oropharyngeal edema, paranasal sinus pain, rhinitis, throat soreness and irritation, tonsillitis.
Endocrine and Metabolic
Cushing's syndrome, Cushingoid features, growth velocity reduction in children/adolescents, hypercorticism, hyperglycemia, osteoporosis.

Eye
Cataracts, glaucoma.
Gastrointestinal
Dyspepsia, xerostomia.
Hepatobiliary Tract and Pancreas
Abnormal liver function tests.
Musculoskeletal
Back pain, myositis.
Neurology
Paresthesia, restlessness.
Non-Site Specific
Fever, immediate and delayed hypersensitivity reaction, pallor.
Psychiatry
Agitation, aggression, anxiety, depression. Behavioral changes, including hyperactivity and irritability, have been reported very rarely and primarily in children.
Respiratory
Asthma; asthma exacerbation; chest congestion; chest tightness; cough; dyspnea; immediate bronchospasm; influenza; paradoxical bronchospasm; tracheitis; wheezing; pneumonia; reports of upper respiratory symptoms of laryngeal spasm, irritation, or swelling; stridor; choking.
Skin
Contact dermatitis, contusions, ecchymoses, photodermatitis, pruritus.
Urogenital
Dysmenorrhea, irregular menstrual cycle, pelvic inflammatory disease, vaginal candidiasis, vaginitis, vulvovaginitis.
Eosinophilic Conditions
In rare cases, patients on inhaled fluticasone propionate, a component of ADVAIR HFA, may present with systemic eosinophilic conditions, with some patients presenting with clinical features of vasculitis consistent with Churg-Strauss syndrome, a condition that is often treated with systemic corticosteroid therapy. These events usually, but not always, have been associated with the reduction and/or withdrawal of oral corticosteroid therapy following the introduction of fluticasone propionate. Cases of serious eosinophilic conditions have also been reported with other inhaled corticosteroids in this clinical setting. While ADVAIR HFA should not be used for transferring patients from systemic corticosteroid therapy, physicians should be alert to eosinophilia, vasculitic rash, worsening pulmonary symptoms, cardiac complications, and/or neuropathy presenting in their patients.

A causal relationship between fluticasone propionate and these underlying conditions has not been established (see PRECAUTIONS: General: *Eosinophilic Conditions*).

OVERDOSAGE

ADVAIR HFA Inhalation Aerosol

No deaths occurred in rats given a single-dose combination of salmeterol 3.6 mg/kg and fluticasone propionate 1.9 mg/kg given as the inhalation powder (approximately 290 and 15 times, respectively, the MRHD on an mg/m^2 basis).

Fluticasone Propionate

Chronic overdosage with fluticasone propionate may result in signs/symptoms of hypercorticism (see PRECAUTIONS: General: *Metabolic and Other Effects*). Inhalation by healthy volunteers of a single dose of 4,000 mcg of fluticasone propionate inhalation powder or single doses of 1,760 or 3,520 mcg of fluticasone propionate CFC inhalation aerosol was well tolerated. Fluticasone propionate given by inhalation aerosol at dosages of 1,320 mcg twice daily for 7 to 15 days to healthy human volunteers was also well tolerated. Repeat oral doses up to 80 mg daily for 10 days in healthy volunteers and repeat oral doses up to 20 mg daily for 42 days in patients were well tolerated. Adverse reactions were of mild or moderate severity, and incidences were similar in active and placebo treatment groups. In mice the oral median lethal dose was >1,000 mg/kg (>4,400 times the MRHD on an mg/m^2 basis). In rats the subcutaneous median lethal dose was >1,000 mg/kg (>8,800 times the MRHD on an mg/m^2 basis).

Salmeterol

The expected signs and symptoms with overdosage of salmeterol are those of excessive beta-adrenergic stimulation and/or occurrence or exaggeration of any of the signs and symptoms listed under ADVERSE REACTIONS, e.g., seizures, angina, hypertension or hypotension, tachycardia with rates up to 200 beats/min, arrhythmias, nervousness, headache, tremor, muscle cramps, dry mouth, palpitation, nausea, dizziness, fatigue, malaise, insomnia. Overdosage with salmeterol may be expected to result in exaggeration of the pharmacologic adverse effects associated with beta-adrenoceptor agonists, including tachycardia and/or arrhythmia, tremor, headache, and muscle cramps. Overdosage with salmeterol can lead to clinically significant prolongation of the QTc interval, which can produce ventricular arrhythmias. Other signs of overdosage may include hypokalemia and hyperglycemia.

As with all sympathomimetic medications, cardiac arrest and even death may be associated with abuse of salmeterol. Treatment consists of discontinuation of salmeterol together with appropriate symptomatic therapy. The judicious use of a cardioselective beta-receptor blocker may be considered, bearing in mind that such medication can produce bronchospasm. There is insufficient evidence to determine if dialysis is beneficial for overdosage of salmeterol. Cardiac monitoring is recommended in cases of overdosage.

No deaths were seen in rats given salmeterol at an inhalation dose of 2.9 mg/kg (approximately 280 times the MRHD on an mg/m^2 basis) and in dogs at an inhalation dose of 0.7 mg/kg (approximately 230 times the MRHD on an mg/m^2 basis). By the oral route, no deaths occurred in mice at 150 mg/kg (approximately 7,200 times the MRHD on an mg/m^2 basis) and in rats at 1,000 mg/kg (approximately 97,000 times the MRHD on an mg/m^2 basis).

DOSAGE AND ADMINISTRATION

ADVAIR HFA should be administered by the orally inhaled route only in patients aged 12 years and older. ADVAIR HFA should not be used for transferring patients from systemic corticosteroid therapy. ADVAIR HFA has not been studied in patients less than 12 years of age or in patients with COPD.

LABAs, such as salmeterol, one of the active ingredients in ADVAIR HFA, increase the risk of asthma-related death. Available data from controlled clinical trials suggest that LABAs increase the risk of asthma-related hospitalization in pediatric and adolescent patients (see WARNINGS). Therefore, when treating patients with asthma, physicians should only prescribe ADVAIR HFA for patients not adequately controlled on a long-term asthma control medication, such as an inhaled corticosteroid, or whose disease severity clearly warrants initiation of treatment with both an inhaled corticosteroid and a LABA. Once asthma control is achieved and maintained, assess the patient at regular intervals and step down therapy (e.g., discontinue ADVAIR HFA) if possible without loss of asthma control and maintain the patient on a long-term asthma control medication, such as an inhaled corticosteroid. Do not use ADVAIR HFA for patients whose asthma is adequately controlled on low- or medium-dose inhaled corticosteroids.

ADVAIR HFA is available in 3 strengths, ADVAIR HFA 45/21 Inhalation Aerosol, ADVAIR HFA 115/21 Inhalation Aerosol, and ADVAIR HFA 230/21 Inhalation Aerosol, containing 45, 115, and 230 mcg of fluticasone propionate, respectively, and 21 mcg of salmeterol per inhalation.

ADVAIR HFA should be administered as 2 inhalations twice daily every day. More frequent administration (more than twice daily) or a higher number of inhalations (more than 2 inhalations twice daily) of the prescribed strength of ADVAIR HFA is not recommended as some patients are more likely to experience adverse effects with higher doses of salmeterol. The safety and efficacy of ADVAIR HFA when administered in excess of recommended doses have not been established.

If symptoms arise in the period between doses, an inhaled, short-acting beta$_2$-agonist should be taken for immediate relief.

Patients who are receiving ADVAIR HFA twice daily should not use additional salmeterol or other inhaled LABAs (e.g., formoterol) for prevention of EIB or for any other reason.

For patients aged 12 years and older, the dosage is 2 inhalations twice daily (morning and evening, approximately 12 hours apart).

The recommended starting dosages for ADVAIR HFA are based upon patients' current asthma therapy.

The maximum recommended dosage is 2 inhalations of ADVAIR HFA 230/21 twice daily.

Improvement in asthma control following inhaled administration of ADVAIR HFA can occur within 30 minutes of beginning treatment, although maximum benefit may not be achieved for 1 week or longer after starting treatment. Individual patients will experience a variable time to onset and degree of symptom relief.

For patients who do not respond adequately to the starting dosage after 2 weeks of therapy, replacing the current strength of ADVAIR HFA with a higher strength may provide additional improvement in asthma control.

If a previously effective dosage regimen of ADVAIR HFA fails to provide adequate improvement in asthma control, the therapeutic regimen should be reevaluated and additional therapeutic options, e.g., replacing the current strength of ADVAIR HFA with a higher strength, adding additional inhaled corticosteroid, initiating oral corticosteroids, should be considered.

ADVAIR HFA should be primed before using for the first time by releasing 4 test sprays into the air away from the face, shaking well for 5 seconds before each spray. In cases where the inhaler has not been used for more than 4 weeks or when it has been dropped, prime the inhaler again by releasing 2 test sprays into the air away from the face, shaking well for 5 seconds before each spray.

Geriatric Use

In studies where geriatric patients (aged 65 years or older, see PRECAUTIONS: Geriatric Use) have been treated with ADVAIR HFA, efficacy and safety did not differ from that in younger patients. Based on available data for ADVAIR HFA and its active components, no dosage adjustment is recommended.

HOW SUPPLIED

ADVAIR HFA 45/21 Inhalation Aerosol is supplied in 12-g pressurized aluminum canisters containing 120 metered actuations in boxes of 1 (NDC 0173-0715-20) and 8-g pressurized aluminum canisters containing 60 metered actuations in institutional pack boxes of 1 (NDC 0173-0715-22).

ADVAIR HFA 115/21 Inhalation Aerosol is supplied in 12-g pressurized aluminum canisters containing 120 metered actuations in boxes of 1 (NDC 0173-0716-20) and 8-g pressurized aluminum canisters containing 60 metered actuations in institutional pack boxes of 1 (NDC 0173-0716-22).

ADVAIR HFA 230/21 Inhalation Aerosol is supplied in 12-g pressurized aluminum canisters containing 120 metered actuations in boxes of 1 (NDC 0173-0717-20) and 8-g pressurized aluminum canisters containing 60 metered actuations in institutional pack boxes of 1 (NDC 0173-0717-22).

Each canister is fitted with a counter, supplied with a purple actuator with a light purple strapcap, and sealed in a plastic-coated, moisture-protective foil pouch with a desiccant that should be discarded when the pouch is opened. Each canister is packaged with a Medication Guide leaflet. **The purple actuator supplied with ADVAIR HFA Inhalation Aerosol should not be used with any other product canisters, and actuators from other products should not be used with an ADVAIR HFA Inhalation Aerosol canister.**

The correct amount of medication in each actuation cannot be assured after the counter reads 000, even though the canister is not completely empty and will continue to operate. The inhaler should be discarded when the counter reads 000.

Keep out of reach of children. Avoid spraying in eyes.

Contents Under Pressure: Do not puncture. Do not use or store near heat or open flame. Exposure to temperatures above 120°F may cause bursting. Never throw container into fire or incinerator.

Store at 25°C (77°F); excursions permitted to 15°-30°C (59°-86°F). Store the inhaler with the mouthpiece down. For best results, the inhaler should be at room temperature before use. SHAKE WELL FOR 5 SECONDS BEFORE USING.

ADVAIR HFA Inhalation Aerosol does not contain chlorofluorocarbons (CFCs) as the propellant.

ADVAIR, ADVAIR DISKUS, FLONASE, and VENTOLIN are registered trademarks of GlaxoSmithKline.

GlaxoSmithKline
Research Triangle Park, NC 27709
©2010, GlaxoSmithKline. All rights reserved.
June 2010
ADH:6PI
PHARMACIST—DETACH HERE AND GIVE MEDICATION GUIDE TO PATIENT

MEDICATION GUIDE

ADVAIR® HFA [*ad' vair*] 45/21 Inhalation Aerosol (fluticasone propionate 45 mcg and salmeterol 21 mcg)
ADVAIR® HFA 115/21 Inhalation Aerosol (fluticasone propionate 115 mcg and salmeterol 21 mcg)
ADVAIR® HFA 230/21 Inhalation Aerosol (fluticasone propionate 230 mcg and salmeterol 21 mcg)
Read the Medication Guide that comes with ADVAIR HFA Inhalation Aerosol before you start using it and each time you get a refill. There may be new information. This Medication Guide does not take the place of talking to your healthcare provider about your medical condition or treatment.

What is the most important information I should know about ADVAIR HFA?
ADVAIR HFA can cause serious side effects, including:
1. **People with asthma who take long-acting beta$_2$-adrenergic agonist (LABA) medicines, such as salmeterol (one of the medicines in ADVAIR HFA), have an increased risk of death from asthma problems.** It is not known whether fluticasone propionate, the other medicine in ADVAIR HFA, reduces the risk of death from asthma problems seen with salmeterol.
   - **Call your healthcare provider if breathing problems worsen over time while using ADVAIR HFA.** You may need different treatment.
   - **Get emergency medical care if:**
     - breathing problems worsen quickly and
     - you use your rescue inhaler medicine, but it does not relieve your breathing problems.
2. ADVAIR HFA should be used only if your healthcare provider decides that your asthma is not well controlled with a long-term asthma control medicine, such as inhaled corticosteroids.
3. When your asthma is well controlled, your healthcare provider may tell you to stop taking ADVAIR HFA. Your healthcare provider will decide if you can stop ADVAIR HFA without loss of asthma control. Your healthcare provider may prescribe a different long-term asthma control medicine for you, such as an inhaled corticosteroid.
4. Children and adolescents who take LABA medicines may have an increased risk of being hospitalized for asthma problems.

What is ADVAIR HFA?
- ADVAIR HFA combines an inhaled corticosteroid medicine, fluticasone propionate (the same medicine found in FLOVENT®), and a LABA medicine, salmeterol (the same medicine found in SEREVENT®).
  - Inhaled corticosteroids help to decrease inflammation in the lungs. Inflammation in the lungs can lead to asthma symptoms.
  - LABA medicines are used in people with asthma and chronic obstructive pulmonary disease (COPD). LABA medicines help the muscles around the airways in your lungs stay relaxed to prevent symptoms, such as wheezing and shortness of breath. These symptoms can happen when the muscles around the airways tighten. This makes it hard to breathe. In severe cases, wheezing can stop your breathing and cause death if not treated right away.
- ADVAIR HFA is used to control symptoms of asthma and to prevent symptoms such as wheezing in adults and children aged 12 years and older.
- ADVAIR HFA contains salmeterol (the same medicine found in SEREVENT). LABA medicines, such as salmeterol, increase the risk of death from asthma problems.
ADVAIR HFA is not for adults and children with asthma who are well controlled with an asthma control medicine, such as a low to medium dose of an inhaled corticosteroid medicine.

Who should not use ADVAIR HFA?
Do not use ADVAIR HFA:
- to treat sudden, severe symptoms of asthma and
- if you are allergic to any of the ingredients in ADVAIR HFA. See the end of this Medication Guide for a list of ingredients in ADVAIR HFA.

What should I tell my healthcare provider before using ADVAIR HFA?
Tell your healthcare provider about all of your health conditions, including if you:
- have heart problems

- have high blood pressure
- have seizures
- have thyroid problems
- have diabetes
- have liver problems
- have osteoporosis
- have an immune system problem
- **are pregnant or planning to become pregnant.** It is not known if ADVAIR HFA may harm your unborn baby.
- **are breastfeeding.** It is not known if ADVAIR HFA passes into your milk and if it can harm your baby.
- **are allergic to ADVAIR HFA or any other medicines**
- **are exposed to chickenpox or measles**

Tell your healthcare provider about all the medicines you take including prescription and non-prescription medicines, vitamins, and herbal supplements. ADVAIR HFA and certain other medicines may interact with each other. This may cause serious side effects. Especially, tell your healthcare provider if you take ritonavir. The anti-HIV medicines NORVIR® (ritonavir capsules) Soft Gelatin, NORVIR (ritonavir oral solution), and KALETRA® (lopinavir/ritonavir) Tablets contain ritonavir.

Know the medicines you take. Keep a list and show it to your healthcare provider and pharmacist each time you get a new medicine.

How do I use ADVAIR HFA?
See the step-by-step instructions for using ADVAIR HFA at the end of this Medication Guide. Do not use ADVAIR HFA unless your healthcare provider has taught you and you understand everything. Ask your healthcare provider or pharmacist if you have any questions.

- Use ADVAIR HFA exactly as prescribed. **Do not use ADVAIR HFA more often than prescribed.** ADVAIR HFA comes in 3 strengths. Your healthcare provider has prescribed the one that is best for your condition.
- The usual dosage of ADVAIR HFA is 2 inhalations 2 times each day (morning and evening). The 2 doses should be about 12 hours apart. Rinse your mouth with water after using ADVAIR HFA.
- If you miss a dose of ADVAIR HFA, just skip that dose. Take your next dose at your usual time. Do not take 2 doses at one time.
- **While you are using ADVAIR HFA 2 times each day, do not use other medicines that contain a LABA for any reason.** Ask your healthcare provider or pharmacist if any of your other medicines are LABA medicines.
- Do not stop using ADVAIR HFA or other asthma medicines unless told to do so by your healthcare provider because your symptoms might get worse. Your healthcare provider will change your medicines as needed.
- ADVAIR HFA does not relieve sudden symptoms. Always have a rescue inhaler medicine with you to treat sudden symptoms. If you do not have an inhaled, short-acting bronchodilator, call your healthcare provider to have one prescribed for you.
- Call your healthcare provider or get medical care right away if:
  - your breathing problems worsen with ADVAIR HFA
  - you need to use your rescue inhaler medicine more often than usual
  - your rescue inhaler medicine does not work as well for you at relieving symptoms
  - you need to use 4 or more inhalations of your rescue inhaler medicine for 2 or more days in a row
  - you use 1 whole canister of your rescue inhaler medicine in 8 weeks' time
  - your peak flow meter results decrease. Your healthcare provider will tell you the numbers that are right for you.
  - you have asthma and your symptoms do not improve after using ADVAIR HFA regularly for 1 week

What are the possible side effects with ADVAIR HFA?
ADVAIR HFA can cause serious side effects, including:
- See "What is the most important information I should know about ADVAIR HFA?"
- **serious allergic reactions.** Call your healthcare provider or get emergency medical care if you get any of the following symptoms of a serious allergic reaction:
  - rash
  - hives
  - swelling of the face, mouth, and tongue
  - breathing problems
- **sudden breathing problems immediately after inhaling your medicine**
- **effects on heart**
  - increased blood pressure
  - a fast and irregular heartbeat
  - chest pain
- **effects on nervous system**
  - tremor
  - nervousness
- **reduced adrenal function (may result in loss of energy)**
- **changes in blood (sugar, potassium, certain types of white blood cells)**

- **weakened immune system and a higher chance of infections**
- **lower bone mineral density.** This may be a problem for people who already have a higher chance of low bone density (osteoporosis).
- **eye problems including glaucoma and cataracts.** You should have regular eye exams while using ADVAIR HFA.
- **slowed growth in children.** A child's growth should be checked often.
- **throat tightness**
- **pneumonia.** ADVAIR HFA contains the same medicine found in ADVAIR DISKUS®. ADVAIR DISKUS is used to treat people with asthma and people with chronic obstructive pulmonary disease (COPD). People with COPD have a higher chance of getting pneumonia. ADVAIR DISKUS may increase the chance of getting pneumonia. ADVAIR HFA has not been studied in people with COPD. Call your healthcare provider if you notice any of the following symptoms:
  - increase in mucus (sputum) production
  - change in mucus color
  - fever
  - chills
  - increased cough
  - increased breathing problems

Common side effects of ADVAIR HFA include:
- upper respiratory tract infection
- headache
- throat irritation
- musculoskeletal pain
- nausea and vomiting

Tell your healthcare provider about any side effect that bothers you or that does not go away.

These are not all the side effects with ADVAIR HFA. Ask your healthcare provider or pharmacist for more information.

Call your doctor for medical advice about side effects. You may report side effects to FDA at 1-800-FDA-1088 or 1-800-332-1088.

How do I store ADVAIR HFA?
- Store at room temperature with the mouthpiece down.
- **Contents Under Pressure:** Do not puncture. Do not use or store near heat or open flame. Exposure to temperatures above 120°F may cause bursting.
- Do not throw into fire or an incinerator.
- Keep ADVAIR HFA and all medicines out of the reach of children.

General Information About ADVAIR HFA
Medicines are sometimes prescribed for purposes not mentioned in a Medication Guide. Do not use ADVAIR HFA for a condition for which it was not prescribed. Do not give your ADVAIR HFA to other people, even if they have the same condition that you have. It may harm them.

This Medication Guide summarizes the most important information about ADVAIR HFA. If you would like more information, talk with your healthcare provider or pharmacist. You can ask your healthcare provider or pharmacist for information about ADVAIR HFA that was written for healthcare professionals. You can also contact the company that makes ADVAIR HFA (toll free) at 1-888-825-5249 or at www.advair.com.

What are the ingredients in ADVAIR HFA?
Active ingredients: fluticasone propionate, salmeterol xinafoate
Inactive ingredient: propellant HFA-134a

How to use your ADVAIR HFA
The parts of your ADVAIR HFA
There are 2 main parts to your ADVAIR HFA inhaler—the metal canister that holds the medicine and the purple plastic actuator that sprays the medicine from the canister (see Figure 1).

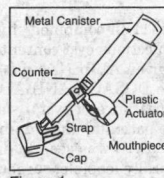

Figure 1

The inhaler also has a cap that covers the mouthpiece of the actuator. The strap on the cap will stay attached to the actuator.

Do not use the actuator with a canister of medicine from any other inhaler. Do not use an ADVAIR HFA canister with an actuator from any other inhaler.
The canister has a counter to show how many sprays of medicine you have left. The number shows through a window in the back of the actuator.

The counter starts at 124, or at 064 if you have a sample or institutional canister. The number will count down by 1 each time you spray the inhaler. The counter will stop counting at 000.
Never try to change the numbers or take the counter off the metal canister. The counter cannot be reset, and it is permanently attached to the canister.
Before using your ADVAIR HFA:
Take the inhaler out of the foil pouch. Safely throw away the foil pouch and the drying packet that comes inside the pouch. The counter should read 124, or 064 if you have a sample or institutional canister.
The inhaler should be at room temperature before you use it.
Check each time to make sure the canister fits firmly in the plastic actuator. Also look into the mouthpiece to make sure there are no foreign objects there, especially if the strap is no longer attached to the actuator or if the cap is not being used to cover the mouthpiece.
Priming your ADVAIR HFA:
Before you use ADVAIR HFA for the first time, you must prime the inhaler so that you will get the right amount of medicine when you use it. To prime the inhaler, take the cap off the mouthpiece and shake the inhaler well for 5 seconds. Then spray it 1 time into the air away from your face. Shake and spray the inhaler like this 3 more times to finish priming it. **Avoid spraying in eyes.** The counter should now read 120, or 060 if you have a sample or institutional canister.
You must prime your inhaler again if you have not used it in more than 4 weeks or if you have dropped it. Take the cap off the mouthpiece, shake the inhaler well for 5 seconds, and spray it into the air away from your face. Shake and spray the inhaler like this 1 more time to finish priming it.
Instructions for taking a dose from your ADVAIR HFA:
Read through the 7 steps below before using ADVAIR HFA. If you have any questions, ask your doctor or pharmacist.
1. Take the cap off the mouthpiece of the actuator. **Shake the inhaler well** for 5 seconds before each spray.
2. Hold the inhaler with the mouthpiece down (see Figure 2). **Breathe out through your mouth** and push as much air from your lungs as you can. Put the mouthpiece in your mouth and close your lips around it.

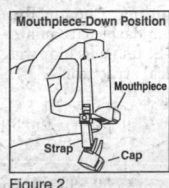

Figure 2

3. **Push the top of the canister all the way down while you breathe in deeply and slowly through your mouth** (see Figure 3). Right after the spray comes out, take your finger off the canister. After you have breathed in all the way, take the inhaler out of your mouth and close your mouth.

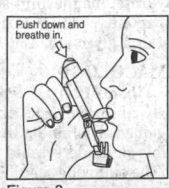

Figure 3

4. **Hold your breath as long as you can,** up to 10 seconds, then breathe normally.
5. Wait about 30 seconds and **shake** the inhaler again for 5 seconds. Repeat steps 2 through 4.
6. After you finish taking this medicine, rinse your mouth with water. Spit out the water. Do not swallow it.
7. Put the cap back on the mouthpiece after every time you use the inhaler, and make sure it snaps firmly into place.
When to replace your ADVAIR HFA:
- **When the counter reads 020,** you should refill your prescription or ask your doctor if you need another prescription for ADVAIR HFA.
- **Throw the inhaler away** when the counter reads 000. You should not keep using the inhaler when the counter reads 000 because you will not receive the right amount of medicine.
- **Do not use the inhaler** after the expiration date, which is on the packaging it comes in.
How to clean your ADVAIR HFA:
Clean the inhaler at least once a week after your evening dose. It is important to keep the canister and plastic actuator clean so the medicine will not build-up and block the spray.

1. Take the cap off the mouthpiece. The strap on the cap will stay attached to the actuator. Do not take the canister out of the plastic actuator.
2. Use a dry cotton swab to clean the small circular opening where the medicine sprays out of the canister. Carefully twist the swab in a circular motion to take off any medicine (see Figure 4).

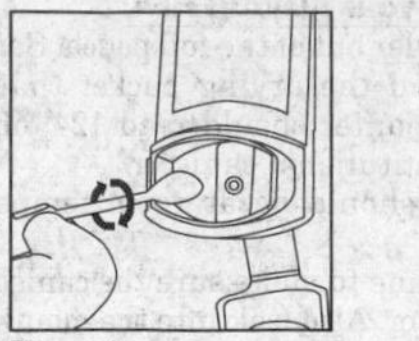

Figure 4

3. Wipe the inside of the mouthpiece with a clean tissue dampened with water. Let the actuator air-dry overnight.
4. Put the cap back on the mouthpiece after the actuator has dried.

This Medication Guide has been approved by the U.S. Food and Drug Administration.

ADVAIR, ADVAIR DISKUS, FLOVENT, and SEREVENT are registered trademarks of GlaxoSmithKline.

The other brands listed are trademarks of their respective owners and are not trademarks of GlaxoSmithKline. The makers of these brands are not affiliated with and do not endorse GlaxoSmithKline or its products.

GlaxoSmithKline
Research Triangle Park, NC 27709
©2010, GlaxoSmithKline. All rights reserved.
June 2010
ADH:6MG

ALBENZA® ℞

[ăl-ben' ză]
(albendazole)
Tablets

DESCRIPTION

ALBENZA (albendazole) is an orally administered broad-spectrum anthelmintic. Chemically, it is methyl 5-(propylthio)-2-benzimidazolecarbamate. Its molecular formula is $C_{12}H_{15}N_3O_2S$. Its molecular weight is 265.34. It has the following chemical structure:

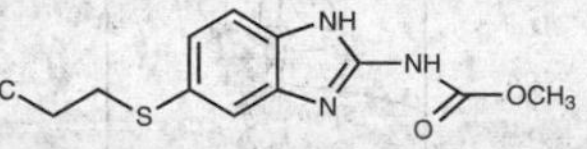

Albendazole is a white to off-white powder. It is soluble in dimethylsulfoxide, strong acids, and strong bases. It is slightly soluble in methanol, chloroform, ethyl acetate, and acetonitrile. Albendazole is practically insoluble in water. Each white to off-white, film-coated tablet contains 200 mg of albendazole.

Inactive ingredients consist of: carnauba wax, hypromellose, lactose monohydrate, magnesium stearate, microcrystalline cellulose, povidone, sodium lauryl sulfate, sodium saccharin, sodium starch glycolate, and starch.

CLINICAL PHARMACOLOGY

Pharmacokinetics: ***Absorption and Metabolism:*** Albendazole is poorly absorbed from the gastrointestinal tract due to its low aqueous solubility. Albendazole concentrations are negligible or undetectable in plasma as it is rapidly converted to the sulfoxide metabolite prior to reaching the systemic circulation. The systemic anthelmintic activity has been attributed to the primary metabolite, albendazole sulfoxide. Oral bioavailability appears to be enhanced when albendazole is coadministered with a fatty meal (estimated fat content 40 g) as evidenced by higher (up to 5-fold on average) plasma concentrations of albendazole sulfoxide as compared to the fasted state.

Maximal plasma concentrations of albendazole sulfoxide are typically achieved 2 to 5 hours after dosing and are on average 1.31 mcg/mL (range 0.46 to 1.58 mcg/mL) following oral doses of albendazole (400 mg) in 6 hydatid disease patients, when administered with a fatty meal. Plasma concentrations of albendazole sulfoxide increase in a dose-proportional manner over the therapeutic dose range following ingestion of a fatty meal (fat content 43.1 g). The mean apparent terminal elimination half-life of albendazole sulfoxide typically ranges from 8 to 12 hours in 25 normal subjects, as well as in 14 hydatid and 8 neurocysticercosis patients.

Following 4 weeks of treatment with albendazole (200 mg three times daily), 12 patients' plasma concentrations of albendazole sulfoxide were approximately 20% lower than those observed during the first half of the treatment period, suggesting that albendazole may induce its own metabolism.

Distribution: Albendazole sulfoxide is 70% bound to plasma protein and is widely distributed throughout the body; it has been detected in urine, bile, liver, cyst wall, cyst fluid, and cerebral spinal fluid (CSF). Concentrations in plasma were 3- to 10-fold and 2- to 4-fold higher than those simultaneously determined in cyst fluid and CSF, respectively. Limited in vitro and clinical data suggest that albendazole sulfoxide may be eliminated from cysts at a slower rate than observed in plasma.

Metabolism and Excretion: Albendazole is rapidly converted in the liver to the primary metabolite, albendazole sulfoxide, which is further metabolized to albendazole sulfone and other primary oxidative metabolites that have been identified in human urine. Following oral administration, albendazole has not been detected in human urine. Urinary excretion of albendazole sulfoxide is a minor elimination pathway with less than 1% of the dose recovered in the urine. Biliary elimination presumably accounts for a portion of the elimination as evidenced by biliary concentrations of albendazole sulfoxide similar to those achieved in plasma.

Special Populations: ***Patients with Impaired Renal Function:*** The pharmacokinetics of albendazole in patients with impaired renal function have not been studied. However, since renal elimination of albendazole and its primary metabolite, albendazole sulfoxide, is negligible, it is unlikely that clearance of these compounds would be altered in these patients.

Biliary Effects: In patients with evidence of extrahepatic obstruction (n = 5), the systemic availability of albendazole sulfoxide was increased, as indicated by a 2-fold increase in maximum serum concentration and a 7-fold increase in area under the curve. The rate of absorption/conversion and elimination of albendazole sulfoxide appeared to be prolonged with mean T_{max} and serum elimination half-life values of 10 hours and 31.7 hours, respectively. Plasma concentrations of parent albendazole were measurable in only 1 of 5 patients.

Pediatrics: Following single-dose administration of 200 mg to 300 mg (approximately 10 mg/kg) albendazole to 3 fasted and 2 fed pediatric patients with hydatid cyst disease (age range 6 to 13 years), albendazole sulfoxide pharmacokinetics were similar to those observed in fed adults.

Elderly Patients: Although no studies have investigated the effect of age on albendazole sulfoxide pharmacokinetics, data in 26 hydatid cyst patients (up to 79 years) suggest pharmacokinetics similar to those in young healthy subjects.

Microbiology: The principal mode of action for albendazole is by its inhibitory effect on tubulin polymerization which results in the loss of cytoplasmic microtubules. In the specified treatment indications albendazole appears to be active against the larval forms of the following organisms:

Echinococcus granulosus
Taenia solium

INDICATIONS AND USAGE

ALBENZA is indicated for the treatment of the following infections:

Neurocysticercosis: ALBENZA is indicated for the treatment of parenchymal neurocysticercosis due to active lesions caused by larval forms of the pork tapeworm, *Taenia solium*.

Lesions considered responsive to albendazole therapy appear as nonenhancing cysts with no surrounding edema on contrast-enhanced computerized tomography. Clinical studies in patients with lesions of this type demonstrate a 74% to 88% reduction in number of cysts; 40% to 70% of albendazole-treated patients showed resolution of all active cysts.

Hydatid Disease: ALBENZA is indicated for the treatment of cystic hydatid disease of the liver, lung, and peritoneum, caused by the larval form of the dog tapeworm, *Echinococcus granulosus*.

This indication is based on combined clinical studies which demonstrated non-infectious cyst contents in approximately 80-90% of patients given ALBENZA for 3 cycles of therapy of 28 days each (see DOSAGE AND ADMINISTRATION). Clinical cure (disappearance of cysts) was seen in approximately 30% of these patients, and improvement (reduction in cyst diameter of ≥25%) was seen in an additional 40%.

NOTE: When medically feasible, surgery is considered the treatment of choice for hydatid disease. When administering ALBENZA in the pre- or post-surgical setting, optimal killing of cyst contents is achieved when 3 courses of therapy have been given.

NOTE: The efficacy of albendazole in the therapy of alveolar hydatid disease caused by *Echinococcus multilocularis* has not been clearly demonstrated in clinical studies.

CONTRAINDICATIONS

ALBENZA is contraindicated in patients with known hypersensitivity to the benzimidazole class of compounds or any components of ALBENZA.

WARNINGS

Rare fatalities associated with the use of ALBENZA have been reported due to granulocytopenia or pancytopenia (see PRECAUTIONS). Albendazole has been shown to cause bone marrow suppression, aplastic anemia, and agranulocytosis in patients with and without underlying hepatic dysfunction. Blood counts should be monitored at the beginning of each 28-day cycle of therapy, and every 2 weeks while on therapy with albendazole in all patients. Patients with liver disease, including hepatic echinococcosis, appear to be more at risk for bone marrow suppression leading to pancytopenia, aplastic anemia, agranulocytosis, and leukopenia attributable to albendazole and warrant closer monitoring of blood counts. Albendazole should be discontinued in all patients if clinically significant decreases in blood cell counts occur.

Albendazole should not be used in pregnant women except in clinical circumstances where no alternative management is appropriate. Patients should not become pregnant for at least 1 month following cessation of albendazole therapy. If a patient becomes pregnant while taking this drug, albendazole should be discontinued immediately. If pregnancy occurs while taking this drug, the patient should be apprised of the potential hazard to the fetus.

PRECAUTIONS

General: Patients being treated for neurocysticercosis should receive appropriate steroid and anticonvulsant therapy as required. Oral or intravenous corticosteroids should be considered to prevent cerebral hypertensive episodes during the first week of anticysticeral therapy.

Pre-existing neurocysticercosis may also be uncovered in patients treated with albendazole for other conditions. Patients may experience neurological symptoms (e.g. seizures, increased intracranial pressure and focal signs) as a result of an inflammatory reaction caused by death of the parasite within the brain. Symptoms may occur soon after treatment; appropriate steroid and anticonvulsant therapy should be started immediately.

Cysticercosis may, in rare cases, involve the retina. Before initiating therapy for neurocysticercosis, the patient should be examined for the presence of retinal lesions. If such lesions are visualized, the need for anticysticeral therapy should be weighed against the possibility of retinal damage caused by albendazole-induced changes to the retinal lesion.

Information for Patients: Patients should be advised that:

- Some people, particularly young children, may experience difficulties swallowing the tablets whole. In young children, the tablets should be crushed or chewed and swallowed with a drink of water.
- Albendazole may cause fetal harm, therefore, women of childbearing age should begin treatment after a negative pregnancy test.
- Women of childbearing age should be cautioned against becoming pregnant while on albendazole or within 1 month of completing treatment.
- During albendazole therapy, because of the possibility of harm to the liver or bone marrow, routine (every 2 weeks) monitoring of blood counts and liver function tests should take place.
- Albendazole should be taken with food.

Laboratory Tests: ***White Blood Cell Count:*** Albendazole has been shown to cause occasional (less than 1% of treated patients) reversible reductions in total white blood cell count. Rarely, more significant reductions may be encountered including granulocytopenia, agranulocytosis, or pancytopenia. Blood counts should be performed at the start of each 28-day treatment cycle and every 2 weeks during each 28-day cycle in all patients. Patients with liver disease, including hepatic echinococcosis, appear to be more at risk of bone marrow suppression and warrant closer monitoring of blood counts (see WARNINGS). Albendazole should be discontinued in all patients if clinically significant decreases in blood cell counts occur.

Liver Function: In clinical trials, treatment with albendazole has been associated with mild to moderate elevations of hepatic enzymes in approximately 16% of patients. These elevations have generally returned to normal upon discontinuation of therapy. There have also been case reports of acute liver failure of uncertain causality and hepatitis (see ADVERSE REACTIONS).

Liver function tests (transaminases) should be performed before the start of each treatment cycle and at least every 2 weeks during treatment. If hepatic enzymes exceed twice the upper limit of normal, consideration should be given to discontinuing albendazole therapy based on individual patient circumstances. Restarting albendazole treatment in patients whose hepatic enzymes have normalized off treatment is an individual decision that should take into account the risk/benefit of further albendazole usage. Laboratory tests should be performed frequently if albendazole treatment is restarted.

Patients with abnormal liver function test results are at increased risk for hepatotoxicity and bone marrow suppression (see WARNINGS). Therapy should be discontinued if liver enzymes are significantly increased or if clinically significant decreases in blood cell counts occur.

Theophylline: Although single doses of albendazole have been shown not to inhibit theophylline metabolism (see Drug Interactions), albendazole does induce cytochrome P450 1A in human hepatoma cells. Therefore, it is recommended that plasma concentrations of theophylline be monitored during and after treatment with ALBENZA.

Drug Interactions: *Dexamethasone:* Steady-state trough concentrations of albendazole sulfoxide were about 56% higher when 8 mg dexamethasone was coadministered with each dose of albendazole (15 mg/kg/day) in 8 neurocysticercosis patients.

Praziquantel: In the fed state, praziquantel (40 mg/kg) increased mean maximum plasma concentration and area under the curve of albendazole sulfoxide by about 50% in healthy subjects (n = 10) compared with a separate group of subjects (n = 6) given albendazole alone. Mean T_{max} and mean plasma elimination half-life of albendazole sulfoxide were unchanged. The pharmacokinetics of praziquantel were unchanged following coadministration with albendazole (400 mg).

Cimetidine: Albendazole sulfoxide concentrations in bile and cystic fluid were increased (about 2-fold) in hydatid cyst patients treated with cimetidine (10 mg/kg/day) (n = 7) compared with albendazole (20 mg/kg/day) alone (n = 12). Albendazole sulfoxide plasma concentrations were unchanged 4 hours after dosing.

Theophylline: The pharmacokinetics of theophylline (aminophylline 5.8 mg/kg infused over 20 minutes) were unchanged following a single oral dose of albendazole (400 mg) in 6 healthy subjects.

Carcinogenesis, Mutagenesis, Impairment of Fertility: Long-term carcinogenicity studies were conducted in mice and rats. In the mouse study, albendazole was administered in the diet at doses of 25, 100, and 400 mg/kg/day (0.1, 0.5, and 2 times the recommended human dose based on body surface area in mg/m², respectively) for 108 weeks. In the rat study, albendazole was administered in the diet at doses of 3.5, 7, and 20 mg/kg/day (0.04, 0.08, and 0.21 times the recommended human dose based on body surface area in mg/m², respectively) for 117 weeks. There was no evidence of increased incidence of tumors in the treated mice and rats when compared to the control group.

In genotoxicity tests, albendazole was found negative in an Ames Salmonella/Microsome Plate mutation assay with and without metabolic activation or with and without pre-incubation, cell-mediated Chinese Hamster Ovary chromosomal aberration test and in vivo mouse micronucleus test. In the *in vitro* BALB/3T3 cells transformation assay, albendazole produced weak activity in the presence of metabolic activation while no activity was found in the absence of metabolic activation.

Albendazole did not adversely affect male or female fertility in the rat at an oral dose of 30 mg/kg/day (0.32 times the recommended human dose based on body surface area in mg/m²).

Pregnancy: *Teratogenic Effects:* Pregnancy Category C. Albendazole has been shown to be teratogenic (to cause embryotoxicity and skeletal malformations) in pregnant rats and rabbits. The teratogenic response in the rat was shown at oral doses of 10 and 30 mg/kg/day (0.10 times and 0.32 times the recommended human dose based on body surface area in mg/m², respectively) during gestation days 6 to 15 and in pregnant rabbits at oral doses of 30 mg/kg/day (0.60 times the recommended human dose based on body surface area in mg/m²) administered during gestation days 7 to 19. In the rabbit study, maternal toxicity (33% mortality) was noted at 30 mg/kg/day. In mice, no teratogenic effects were observed at oral doses up to 30 mg/kg/day (0.16 times the recommended human dose based on body surface area in mg/m²), administered during gestation days 6 to 15. There are no adequate and well-controlled studies of albendazole administration in pregnant women. Albendazole should be used during pregnancy only if the potential benefit justifies the potential risk to the fetus (see WARNINGS).

Nursing Mothers: Albendazole is excreted in animal milk. It is not known whether it is excreted in human milk. Because many drugs are excreted in human milk, caution should be exercised when albendazole is administered to a nursing woman.

Pediatric Use: Experience in children under the age of 6 years is limited. In hydatid disease, infection in infants and young children is uncommon, but no problems have been encountered in those who have been treated. In neurocysticercosis, infection is more frequently encountered. In 5 published studies involving pediatric patients as young as 1 year, no significant problems were encountered, and the efficacy appeared similar to the adult population.

Geriatric Use: Experience in patients 65 years of age or older is limited. The number of patients treated for either hydatid disease or neurocysticercosis is limited, but no problems associated with an older population have been observed.

Indication	Patient Weight	Dose	Duration
Hydatid Disease	60 kg or greater	400 mg twice daily, with meals	28-day cycle followed by a 14-day albendazole-free interval, for a total of 3 cycles
	less than 60 kg	15 mg/kg/day given in divided doses twice daily with meals (maximum total daily dose 800 mg)	
	NOTE: When administering ALBENZA in the pre- or post-surgical setting, optimal killing of cyst contents is achieved when 3 courses of therapy have been given.		
Neurocysticercosis	60 kg or greater	400 mg twice daily, with meals	8-30 days
	less than 60 kg	15 mg/kg/day given in divided doses twice daily with meals (maximum total daily dose 800 mg)	

ADVERSE REACTIONS

The adverse event profile of albendazole differs between hydatid disease and neurocysticercosis. Adverse events occurring with a frequency of ≥1% in either disease are described in the table below.

These symptoms were usually mild and resolved without treatment. Treatment discontinuations were predominantly due to leukopenia (0.7%) or hepatic abnormalities (3.8% in hydatid disease). The following incidence reflects events that were reported by investigators to be at least possibly or probably related to albendazole.

Adverse Event Incidence ≥1% in Hydatid Disease and Neurocysticercosis

Adverse Event	Hydatid Disease	Neurocysticercosis
Abnormal Liver Function Tests	15.6	<1.0
Abdominal Pain	6.0	0
Nausea/Vomiting	3.7	6.2
Headache	1.3	11.0
Dizziness/Vertigo	1.2	<1.0
Raised Intracranial Pressure	0	1.5
Meningeal Signs	0	1.0
Reversible Alopecia	1.6	<1.0
Fever	1.0	0

The following adverse events were observed at an incidence of <1%:

Blood and Lymphatic System Disorders: Leukopenia. There have been rare reports of granulocytopenia, pancytopenia, agranulocytosis, or thrombocytopenia (see WARNINGS). Patients with liver disease, including hepatic echinococcosis, appear to be more at risk of bone marrow suppression (see WARNINGS and PRECAUTIONS).

Immune System Disorders: Hypersensitivity reactions, including rash and urticaria.

Postmarketing Adverse Reactions: In addition to adverse events reported from clinical trials, the following events have been identified during world-wide post-approval use of ALBENZA. Because they are reported voluntarily from a population of unknown size, estimates of frequency cannot be made. These events have been chosen for inclusion due to a combination of their seriousness, frequency of reporting, or potential causal connection to ALBENZA.

Blood and Lymphatic System Disorders: Aplastic anemia, bone marrow suppression, neutropenia.

Hepatobiliary Disorders: Elevations of hepatic enzymes, hepatitis, acute liver failure.

Skin and Subcutaneous Tissue Disorders: Erythema multiforme, Stevens-Johnson syndrome.

Renal and Urinary Disorders: Acute renal failure.

OVERDOSAGE

Significant toxicity and mortality were shown in male and female mice at doses exceeding 5,000 mg/kg; in rats, at estimated doses between 1,300 and 2,400 mg/kg; in hamsters, at doses exceeding 10,000 mg/kg; and in rabbits, at estimated doses between 500 and 1,250 mg/kg. In the animals, symptoms were demonstrated in a dose-response relationship and included diarrhea, vomiting, tachycardia, and respiratory distress.

One overdosage has been reported with ALBENZA in a patient who took at least 16 grams over 12 hours. No untoward effects were reported. In case of overdosage, symptomatic therapy and general supportive measures are recommended.

DOSAGE AND ADMINISTRATION

Dosing of ALBENZA will vary, depending upon which of the following parasitic infections is being treated. In young children, the tablets should be crushed or chewed and swallowed with a drink of water.

[See table above]

Patients being treated for neurocysticercosis should receive appropriate steroid and anticonvulsant therapy as required. Oral or intravenous corticosteroids should be considered to prevent cerebral hypertensive episodes during the first week of treatment.

HOW SUPPLIED

ALBENZA is supplied as 200 mg, white to off-white, circular, biconvex, bevel-edged, film-coated TILTAB tablets in bottles of 112.

NDC 0007-5500-40 Bottles of 112

Store between 20° and 25°C (68° and 77°F).

ALBENZA and TILTAB are registered trademarks of GlaxoSmithKline.

GlaxoSmithKline

Research Triangle Park, NC 27709

©2009, GlaxoSmithKline. All rights reserved.

June 2009 ALB:8PI

ALKERAN® ℞

[ăl′kə-ran]

(melphalan hydrochloride)

for Injection

> **WARNING**
> Melphalan should be administered under the supervision of a qualified physician experienced in the use of cancer chemotherapeutic agents. Severe bone marrow suppression with resulting infection or bleeding may occur. Controlled trials comparing intravenous (IV) to oral melphalan have shown more myelosuppression with the IV formulation. Hypersensitivity reactions, including anaphylaxis, have occurred in approximately 2% of patients who received the IV formulation. Melphalan is leukemogenic in humans. Melphalan produces chromosomal aberrations in vitro and in vivo and, therefore, should be considered potentially mutagenic in humans.

DESCRIPTION

Melphalan, also known as L-phenylalanine mustard, phenylalanine mustard, L-PAM, or L-sarcolysin, is a phenylalanine derivative of nitrogen mustard. Melphalan is a bifunctional alkylating agent that is active against selected human neoplastic diseases. It is known chemically as 4-[bis(2-chloroethyl)amino]-L-phenylalanine. The molecular formula is $C_{13}H_{18}Cl_2N_2O_2$ and the molecular weight is 305.20. The structural formula is:

$(ClCH_2CH_2)_2N$—⬡—CH_2—$\overset{NH_2}{\underset{H}{C}}$—COOH

Melphalan is the active L-isomer of the compound and was first synthesized in 1953 by Bergel and Stock; the D-isomer, known as medphalan, is less active against certain animal tumors, and the dose needed to produce effects on chromosomes is larger than that required with the L-isomer. The racemic (DL-) form is known as merphalan or sarcolysin. Melphalan is practically insoluble in water and has a pKa_1 of ~2.5.

ALKERAN for Injection is supplied as a sterile, nonpyrogenic, freeze-dried powder. Each single-use vial contains melphalan hydrochloride equivalent to 50 mg melphalan and 20 mg povidone. ALKERAN for Injection is reconstituted using the sterile diluent provided. Each vial of sterile diluent contains sodium citrate 0.2 g, propylene glycol 6.0 mL, ethanol (96%) 0.52 mL, and Water for Injection to a total of 10 mL. ALKERAN for Injection is administered intravenously.

CLINICAL PHARMACOLOGY

Melphalan is an alkylating agent of the bischloroethylamine type. As a result, its cytotoxicity appears to be related to the extent of its interstrand cross-linking with DNA, probably by binding at the N^7 position of guanine. Like other bifunctional alkylating agents, it is active against both resting and rapidly dividing tumor cells.

Pharmacokinetics: The pharmacokinetics of melphalan after IV administration has been extensively studied in adult patients. Following injection, drug plasma concentrations declined rapidly in a biexponential manner with distribution phase and terminal elimination phase half-lives of approximately 10 and 75 minutes, respectively. Estimates of average total body clearance varied among studies, but typical values of approximately 7 to 9 mL/min/kg (250 to 325 mL/min/m²) were observed. One study has reported that on repeat dosing of 0.5 mg/kg every 6 weeks, the clearance of melphalan decreased from 8.1 mL/min/kg after the first course, to 5.5 mL/min/kg after the third course, but did not decrease appreciably after the third course. Mean (±SD) peak melphalan plasma concentrations in myeloma patients given IV melphalan at doses of 10 or 20 mg/m² were 1.2 ± 0.4 and 2.8 ± 1.9 mcg/mL, respectively.

The steady-state volume of distribution of melphalan is 0.5 L/kg. Penetration into cerebrospinal fluid (CSF) is low. The extent of melphalan binding to plasma proteins ranges from 60% to 90%. Serum albumin is the major binding protein, while α_1-acid glycoprotein appears to account for about 20% of the plasma protein binding. Approximately 30% of the drug is (covalently) irreversibly bound to plasma proteins. Interactions with immunoglobulins have been found to be negligible.

Melphalan is eliminated from plasma primarily by chemical hydrolysis to monohydroxymelphalan and dihydroxymelphalan. Aside from these hydrolysis products, no other melphalan metabolites have been observed in humans. Although the contribution of renal elimination to melphalan clearance appears to be low, one study noted an increase in the occurrence of severe leukopenia in patients with elevated BUN after 10 weeks of therapy.

Clinical Trial: A randomized trial compared prednisone plus IV melphalan to prednisone plus oral melphalan in the treatment of myeloma. As discussed below, overall response rates at week 22 were comparable; however, because of changes in trial design, conclusions as to the relative activity of the 2 formulations after week 22 are impossible to make.

Both arms received oral prednisone starting at 0.8 mg/kg/day with doses tapered over 6 weeks. Melphalan doses in each arm were:

Arm 1: Oral melphalan 0.15 mg/kg/day × 7 followed by 0.05 mg/kg/day when WBC began to rise.

Arm 2: IV melphalan 16 mg/m² q 2 weeks × 4 (over 6 weeks) followed by the same dose every 4 weeks.

Doses of melphalan were adjusted according to the following criteria:

Table 1. Criteria for Dosage Adjustment in a Randomized Clinical Trial

WBC/mm³	Platelets	Percent of Full Dose
≥4,000	≥100,000	100
≥3,000	≥75,000	75
≥2,000	≥50,000	50
<2,000	<50,000	0

One hundred seven patients were randomized to the oral melphalan arm and 203 patients to the IV melphalan arm. More patients had a poor-risk classification (58% versus 44%) and high tumor load (51% versus 34%) on the oral compared to the IV arm ($P<0.04$). Response rates at week 22 are shown in the following table:

Table 2. Response Rates at Week 22

Initial Arm	Evaluable Patients	Responders n (%)	P
Oral melphalan	100	44 (44%)	P>0.2
IV melphalan	195	74 (38%)	

Because of changes in protocol design after week 22, other efficacy parameters such as response duration and survival cannot be compared.

Severe myelotoxicity (WBC ≤1,000 and/or platelets ≤25,000) was more common in the IV melphalan arm (28%) than in the oral melphalan arm (11%).

An association was noted between poor renal function and myelosuppression; consequently, an amendment to the protocol required a 50% reduction in IV melphalan dose if the BUN was ≥30 mg/dL. The rate of severe leukopenia in the IV arm in the patients with BUN over 30 mg/dL decreased from 50% (8/16) before protocol amendment to 11% (3/28) ($P = 0.01$) after the amendment.

Before the dosing amendment, there was a 10% (8/77) incidence of drug-related death in the IV arm. After the dosing amendment, this incidence was 3% (3/108). This compares to an overall 1% (1/100) incidence of drug-related death in the oral arm.

INDICATIONS AND USAGE

ALKERAN for Injection is indicated for the palliative treatment of patients with multiple myeloma for whom oral therapy is not appropriate.

CONTRAINDICATIONS

Melphalan should not be used in patients whose disease has demonstrated prior resistance to this agent. Patients who have demonstrated hypersensitivity to melphalan should not be given the drug.

WARNINGS

ALKERAN for Injection may cause local tissue damage should extravasation occur, and consequently it should not be administered by direct injection into a peripheral vein. It is recommended that ALKERAN for Injection be administered by injecting slowly into a fast-running IV infusion via an injection port, or via a central venous line (see DOSAGE AND ADMINISTRATION: Administration Precautions).

Melphalan should be administered in carefully adjusted dosage by or under the supervision of experienced physicians who are familiar with the drug's actions and the possible complications of its use.

As with other nitrogen mustard drugs, excessive dosage will produce marked bone marrow suppression. Bone marrow suppression is the most significant toxicity associated with ALKERAN for Injection in most patients. Therefore, the following tests should be performed at the start of therapy and prior to each subsequent dose of ALKERAN: platelet count, hemoglobin, white blood cell count, and differential. Thrombocytopenia and/or leukopenia are indications to withhold further therapy until the blood counts have sufficiently recovered. Frequent blood counts are essential to determine optimal dosage and to avoid toxicity. Dose adjustment on the basis of blood counts at the nadir and day of treatment should be considered.

Hypersensitivity reactions including anaphylaxis have occurred in approximately 2% of patients who received the IV formulation (see ADVERSE REACTIONS). These reactions usually occur after multiple courses of treatment. Treatment is symptomatic. The infusion should be terminated immediately, followed by the administration of volume expanders, pressor agents, corticosteroids, or antihistamines at the discretion of the physician. If a hypersensitivity reaction occurs, IV or oral melphalan should not be readministered since hypersensitivity reactions have also been reported with oral melphalan.

Carcinogenesis: Secondary malignancies, including acute nonlymphocytic leukemia, myeloproliferative syndrome, and carcinoma, have been reported in patients with cancer treated with alkylating agents (including melphalan). Some patients also received other chemotherapeutic agents or radiation therapy. Precise quantitation of the risk of acute leukemia, myeloproliferative syndrome, or carcinoma is not possible. Published reports of leukemia in patients who have received melphalan (and other alkylating agents) suggest that the risk of leukemogenesis increases with chronicity of treatment and with cumulative dose. In one study, the 10-year cumulative risk of developing acute leukemia or myeloproliferative syndrome after oral melphalan therapy was 19.5% for cumulative doses ranging from 730 to 9,652 mg. In this same study, as well as in an additional study, the 10-year cumulative risk of developing acute leukemia or myeloproliferative syndrome after oral melphalan therapy was less than 2% for cumulative doses under

600 mg. This does not mean that there is a cumulative dose below which there is no risk of the induction of secondary malignancy. The potential benefits from melphalan therapy must be weighed on an individual basis against the possible risk of the induction of a second malignancy.

Adequate and well-controlled carcinogenicity studies have not been conducted in animals. However, intraperitoneal (IP) administration of melphalan in rats (5.4 to 10.8 mg/m²) and in mice (2.25 to 4.5 mg/m²) 3 times per week for 6 months followed by 12 months post-dose observation produced peritoneal sarcoma and lung tumors, respectively.

Mutagenesis: Melphalan has been shown to cause chromatid or chromosome damage in humans. Intramuscular administration of melphalan at 6 and 60 mg/m² produced structural aberrations of the chromatid and chromosomes in bone marrow cells of Wistar rats.

Impairment of Fertility: Melphalan causes suppression of ovarian function in premenopausal women, resulting in amenorrhea in a significant number of patients. Reversible and irreversible testicular suppression have also been reported.

Pregnancy: Pregnancy Category D. Melphalan may cause fetal harm when administered to a pregnant woman. While adequate animal studies have not been conducted with IV melphalan, oral (6 to 18 mg/m²/day for 10 days) and IP (18 mg/m²) administration in rats was embryolethal and teratogenic. Malformations resulting from melphalan included alterations of the brain (underdevelopment, deformation, meningocele, and encephalocele) and eye (anophthalmia and microphthalmos), reduction of the mandible and tail, as well as hepatocele (exomphaly). There are no adequate and well-controlled studies in pregnant women. If this drug is used during pregnancy, or if the patient becomes pregnant while taking this drug, the patient should be apprised of the potential hazard to the fetus. Women of childbearing potential should be advised to avoid becoming pregnant.

PRECAUTIONS

General: In all instances where the use of ALKERAN for Injection is considered for chemotherapy, the physician must evaluate the need and usefulness of the drug against the risk of adverse events. Melphalan should be used with extreme caution in patients whose bone marrow reserve may have been compromised by prior irradiation or chemotherapy or whose marrow function is recovering from previous cytotoxic therapy.

Dose reduction should be considered in patients with renal insufficiency receiving IV melphalan. In one trial, increased bone marrow suppression was observed in patients with BUN levels ≥30 mg/dL. A 50% reduction in the IV melphalan dose decreased the incidence of severe bone marrow suppression in the latter portion of this study.

Administration of live vaccines to immunocompromised patients should be avoided.

Information for Patients: Patients should be informed that the major acute toxicities of melphalan are related to bone marrow suppression, hypersensitivity reactions, gastrointestinal toxicity, and pulmonary toxicity. The major long-term toxicities are related to infertility and secondary malignancies. Patients should never be allowed to take the drug without close medical supervision and should be advised to consult their physicians if they experience skin rash, signs or symptoms of vasculitis, bleeding, fever, persistent cough, nausea, vomiting, amenorrhea, weight loss, or unusual lumps/masses. Women of childbearing potential should be advised to avoid becoming pregnant.

Laboratory Tests: Periodic complete blood counts with differentials should be performed during the course of treatment with melphalan. At least 1 determination should be obtained prior to each dose. Patients should be observed closely for consequences of bone marrow suppression, which include severe infections, bleeding, and symptomatic anemia (see WARNINGS).

Drug Interactions: The development of severe renal failure has been reported in patients treated with a single dose of IV melphalan followed by standard oral doses of cyclosporine. Cisplatin may affect melphalan kinetics by inducing renal dysfunction and subsequently altering melphalan clearance. IV melphalan may also reduce the threshold for BCNU lung toxicity. When nalidixic acid and IV melphalan are given simultaneously, the incidence of severe hemorrhagic necrotic enterocolitis has been reported to increase in pediatric patients.

Carcinogenesis, Mutagenesis, Impairment of Fertility: See WARNINGS section.

Pregnancy: *Teratogenic Effects:* Pregnancy Category D: See WARNINGS section.

Nursing Mothers: It is not known whether this drug is excreted in human milk. IV melphalan should not be given to nursing mothers.

Pediatric Use: The safety and effectiveness in pediatric patients have not been established.

Geriatric Use: Clinical studies of ALKERAN for Injection did not include sufficient numbers of subjects aged 65 and over to determine whether they respond differently from younger subjects. Other reported clinical experience has not identified differences in responses between the elderly and younger patients. In general, dose selection for an elderly patient should be cautious, usually starting at the low end of the dosing range, reflecting the greater frequency of decreased hepatic, renal, or cardiac function, and of concomitant disease or other drug therapy.

ADVERSE REACTIONS
(SEE OVERDOSAGE)

The following information on adverse reactions is based on data from both oral and IV administration of melphalan as a single agent, using several different dose schedules for treatment of a wide variety of malignancies.

Hematologic: The most common side effect is bone marrow suppression leading to leukopenia, thrombocytopenia, and anemia. White blood cell count and platelet count nadirs usually occur 2 to 3 weeks after treatment, with recovery in 4 to 5 weeks after treatment. Irreversible bone marrow failure has been reported.

Gastrointestinal: Gastrointestinal disturbances such as nausea and vomiting, diarrhea, and oral ulceration occur infrequently. Hepatic disorders ranging from abnormal liver function tests to clinical manifestations such as hepatitis and jaundice have been reported. Hepatic veno-occlusive disease has been reported.

Hypersensitivity: Acute hypersensitivity reactions including anaphylaxis were reported in 2.4% of 425 patients receiving ALKERAN for Injection for myeloma (see WARNINGS). These reactions were characterized by urticaria, pruritus, edema, skin rashes, and in some patients, tachycardia, bronchospasm, dyspnea, and hypotension. These patients appeared to respond to antihistamine and corticosteroid therapy. If a hypersensitivity reaction occurs, IV or oral melphalan should not be readministered since hypersensitivity reactions have also been reported with oral melphalan. Cardiac arrest has also been reported rarely in association with such reports.

Miscellaneous: Other reported adverse reactions include skin hypersensitivity, skin ulceration at injection site, skin necrosis rarely requiring skin grafting, maculopapular rashes, vasculitis, alopecia, hemolytic anemia, allergic reaction, pulmonary fibrosis (including fatal outcomes), and interstitial pneumonitis. Temporary significant elevation of the blood urea has been seen in the early stages of therapy in patients with renal damage. Subjective and transient sensation of warmth and/or tingling.

OVERDOSAGE

Overdoses resulting in death have been reported. Overdoses, including doses up to 290 mg/m^2, have produced the following symptoms: severe nausea and vomiting, decreased consciousness, convulsions, muscular paralysis, and cholinomimetic effects. Severe mucositis, stomatitis, colitis, diarrhea, and hemorrhage of the gastrointestinal tract occur at high doses (>100 mg/m^2). Elevations in liver enzymes and veno-occlusive disease occur infrequently. Significant hyponatremia caused by an associated inappropriate secretion of ADH syndrome has been observed. Nephrotoxicity and adult respiratory distress syndrome have been reported rarely. The principal toxic effect is bone marrow suppression. Hematologic parameters should be closely followed for 3 to 6 weeks. An uncontrolled study suggests that administration of autologous bone marrow or hematopoietic growth factors (i.e., sargramostim, filgrastim) may shorten the period of pancytopenia. General supportive measures together with appropriate blood transfusions and antibiotics should be instituted as deemed necessary by the physician. This drug is not removed from plasma to any significant degree by hemodialysis or hemoperfusion. A pediatric patient survived a 254-mg/m^2 overdose treated with standard supportive care.

DOSAGE AND ADMINISTRATION

The usual IV dose is 16 mg/m^2. Dosage reduction of up to 50% should be considered in patients with renal insufficiency (BUN ≥30 mg/dL) (see PRECAUTIONS: General). The drug is administered as a single infusion over 15 to 20 minutes. Melphalan is administered at 2-week intervals for 4 doses, then, after adequate recovery from toxicity, at 4-week intervals. Available evidence suggests about one third to one half of the patients with multiple myeloma show a favorable response to the drug. Experience with oral melphalan suggests that repeated courses should be given since improvement may continue slowly over many months, and the maximum benefit may be missed if treatment is abandoned prematurely. Dose adjustment on the basis of blood cell counts at the nadir and day of treatment should be considered.

Administration Precautions: As with other toxic compounds, caution should be exercised in handling and preparing the solution of ALKERAN. Skin reactions associated with accidental exposure may occur. The use of gloves is recommended. If the solution of ALKERAN contacts the skin or mucosa, immediately wash the skin or mucosa thoroughly with soap and water. Procedures for proper handling and disposal of anticancer drugs should be considered. Several guidelines on this subject have been published.[1-8] There is no general agreement that all of the procedures recommended in the guidelines are necessary or appropriate.

Parenteral drug products should be visually inspected for particulate matter and discoloration prior to administration whenever solution and container permit. If either occurs, do not use this product.

Care should be taken to avoid possible extravasation of melphalan and in cases of poor peripheral venous access, consideration should be given to use of a central venous line (see WARNINGS).

Preparation for Administration/Stability

1. ALKERAN for Injection must be reconstituted by rapidly injecting 10 mL of the supplied diluent directly into the vial of lyophilized powder using a sterile needle (20-gauge or larger needle diameter) and syringe. Immediately shake vial vigorously until a clear solution is obtained. This provides a 5-mg/mL solution of melphalan. Rapid addition of the diluent followed by immediate vigorous shaking is important for proper dissolution.

2. **Immediately** dilute the dose to be administered in 0.9% Sodium Chloride Injection, USP, to a concentration not greater than 0.45 mg/mL.

3. Administer the diluted product over a minimum of 15 minutes.

4. Complete administration within 60 minutes of reconstitution.

The time between reconstitution/dilution and administration of ALKERAN should be kept to a minimum because reconstituted and diluted solutions of ALKERAN are unstable. Over as short a time as 30 minutes, a citrate derivative of melphalan has been detected in reconstituted material from the reaction of ALKERAN with Sterile Diluent for ALKERAN. Upon further dilution with saline, nearly 1% label strength of melphalan hydrolyzes every 10 minutes. A precipitate forms if the reconstituted solution is stored at 5°C. DO NOT REFRIGERATE THE RECONSTITUTED PRODUCT.

HOW SUPPLIED

ALKERAN for Injection is supplied in a carton containing one single-use clear glass vial of freeze-dried melphalan hydrochloride equivalent to 50 mg melphalan and one 10-mL clear glass vial of sterile diluent (NDC 0173-0130-93).

Store at controlled room temperature 15° to 30°C (59° to 86°F) and protect from light.

REFERENCES

1. ONS Clinical Practice Committee. Cancer Chemotherapy Guidelines and Recommendations for Practice. Pittsburgh, PA: Oncology Nursing Society;1999:32-41.
2. Recommendations for the safe handling of parenteral antineoplastic drugs. Washington, DC: Division of Safety, Clinical Center Pharmacy Department and Cancer Nursing Services, National Institutes of Health; 1992. US Dept of Health and Human Services. Public Health Service publication NIH 92-2621.
3. AMA Council on Scientific Affairs. Guidelines for handling parenteral antineoplastics. *JAMA*. 1985;253:1590-1591.
4. National Study Commission on Cytotoxic Exposure. Recommendations for handling cytotoxic agents. 1987. Available from Louis P. Jeffrey, Chairman, National Study Commission on Cytotoxic Exposure. Massachusetts College of Pharmacy and Allied Health Sciences, 179 Longwood Avenue, Boston, MA 02115.
5. Clinical Oncological Society of Australia. Guidelines and recommendations for safe handling of antineoplastic agents. *Med J Australia.* 1983;1:426-428.
6. Jones RB, Frank R, Mass T. Safe handling of chemotherapeutic agents: a report from the Mount Sinai Medical Center. *CA-A Cancer J for Clin.* 1983;33:258-263.
7. American Society of Hospital Pharmacists. ASHP technical assistance bulletin on handling cytotoxic and hazardous drugs. *Am J Hosp Pharm.* 1990;47:1033-1049.
8. Controlling Occupational Exposure to Hazardous Drugs. (OSHA Work-Practice Guidelines.) *Am J Health-Syst Pharm.* 1996;53:1669-1685.

ALKERAN is registered trademark of GlaxoSmithKline.
ALKERAN and Diluent manufactured by:
GlaxoSmithKline
Research Triangle Park, NC 27709
©2008, GlaxoSmithKline. All rights reserved.
October 2008 ALJ:4PI

ALKERAN®
[ăl' kə-ran]
(melphalan)
Tablets

℞

DESCRIPTION

ALKERAN (melphalan), also known as L-phenylalanine mustard, phenylalanine mustard, L-PAM, or L-sarcolysin, is a phenylalanine derivative of nitrogen mustard. Melphalan is a bifunctional alkylating agent which is active against selective human neoplastic diseases. It is known chemically as 4-[bis(2-chloroethyl)amino]-*L*-phenylalanine. The molecular formula is $C_{13}H_{18}Cl_2N_2O_2$ and the molecular weight is 305.20. The structural formula is:

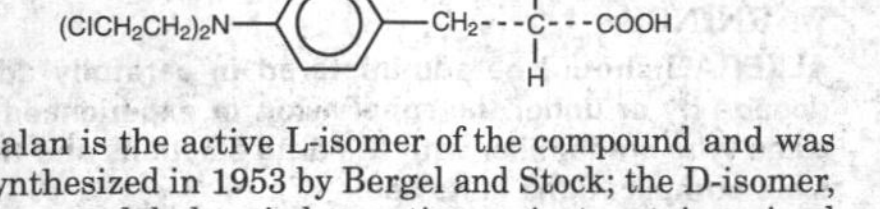

$$(ClCH_2CH_2)_2N \!-\!\bigcirc\!-\! CH_2\!-\!\underset{\underset{H}{|}}{\overset{\overset{NH_2}{|}}{C}}\!-\! COOH$$

Melphalan is the active L-isomer of the compound and was first synthesized in 1953 by Bergel and Stock; the D-isomer, known as medphalan, is less active against certain animal tumors, and the dose needed to produce effects on chromosomes is larger than that required with the L-isomer. The racemic (DL-) form is known as merphalan or sarcolysin. Melphalan is practically insoluble in water and has a pKa_1 of ~2.5.

ALKERAN (melphalan) is available in tablet form for oral administration. Each film-coated tablet contains 2 mg melphalan and the inactive ingredients colloidal silicon dioxide, crospovidone, hypromellose, macrogol/PEG 400, magnesium stearate, microcrystalline cellulose, and titanium dioxide.

CLINICAL PHARMACOLOGY

Melphalan is an alkylating agent of the bischloroethylamine type. As a result, its cytotoxicity appears to be related to the extent of its interstrand cross-linking with DNA, probably by binding at the N^7 position of guanine. Like other bifunctional alkylating agents, it is active against both resting and rapidly dividing tumor cells.

Pharmacokinetics: The pharmacokinetics of ALKERAN after oral administration has been extensively studied in adult patients. Plasma melphalan levels are highly variable after oral dosing, both with respect to the time of the first appearance of melphalan in plasma (range approximately 0 to 6 hours) and to the peak plasma concentration (C_{max}) (range 70 to 4,000 ng/mL, depending upon the dose) achieved. These results may be due to incomplete intestinal absorption, a variable "first pass" hepatic metabolism, or to rapid hydrolysis. Five patients were studied after both oral and intravenous (IV) dosing with 0.6 mg/kg as a single bolus dose by each route. The areas under the plasma concentration-time curves (AUC) after oral administration averaged 61% ± 26% (± standard deviation [SD]; range 25% to 89%) of those following IV administration. In 18 patients given a single oral dose of 0.6 mg/kg of ALKERAN, the terminal elimination plasma half-life ($t_{1/2}$) of parent drug was 1.5 ± 0.83 hours. The 24-hour urinary excretion of parent drug in these patients was 10% ± 4.5%, suggesting that renal clearance is not a major route of elimination of parent drug. In a separate study in 18 patients given single oral doses of 0.2 to 0.25 mg/kg of ALKERAN, C_{max} and AUC, when dose adjusted to a dose of 14 mg, were (mean ± SD) 212 ± 74 ng/mL and 498 ± 137 ng•hr/mL, respectively. Elimination phase t½ in these patients was approximately 1 hour and the median t_{max} was 1 hour.

One study using universally labeled ^{14}C-melphalan, found substantially less radioactivity in the urine of patients given the drug by mouth (30% of administered dose in 9 days) than in the urine of those given it intravenously (35% to 65% in 7 days). Following either oral or IV administration, the pattern of label recovery was similar, with the majority being recovered in the first 24 hours. Following oral administration, peak radioactivity occurred in plasma at 2 hours and then disappeared with a half-life of approximately 160 hours. In 1 patient where parent drug (rather than just radiolabel) was determined, the melphalan half-disappearance time was 67 minutes.

The steady-state volume of distribution of melphalan is 0.5 L/kg. Penetration into cerebrospinal fluid (CSF) is low. The extent of melphalan binding to plasma proteins ranges from 60% to 90%. Serum albumin is the major binding protein, while α_1-acid glycoprotein appears to account for about 20% of the plasma protein binding. Approximately 30% of melphalan is (covalently) irreversibly bound to plasma proteins. Interactions with immunoglobulins have been found to be negligible.

Melphalan is eliminated from plasma primarily by chemical hydrolysis to monohydroxymelphalan and dihydroxymelphalan. Aside from these hydrolysis products, no other melphalan metabolites have been observed in humans. Although the contribution of renal elimination to melphalan clearance appears to be low, one pharmacokinetic study showed a significant positive correlation between the elimination rate constant for melphalan and renal function and a significant negative correlation between renal function and the area under the plasma melphalan concentration/time curve.

INDICATIONS AND USAGE

ALKERAN Tablets are indicated for the palliative treatment of multiple myeloma and for the palliation of non-resectable epithelial carcinoma of the ovary.

CONTRAINDICATIONS

ALKERAN should not be used in patients whose disease has demonstrated a prior resistance to this agent. Patients who have demonstrated hypersensitivity to melphalan should not be given the drug.

WARNINGS

ALKERAN should be administered in carefully adjusted dosage by or under the supervision of experienced physicians who are familiar with the drug's actions and the possible complications of its use.

As with other nitrogen mustard drugs, excessive dosage will produce marked bone marrow suppression. Bone marrow suppression is the most significant toxicity associated with ALKERAN in most patients. Therefore, the following tests should be performed at the start of therapy and prior to each subsequent course of ALKERAN: platelet count, hemoglobin, white blood cell count, and differential. Thrombocytopenia and/or leukopenia are indications to withhold further therapy until the blood counts have sufficiently recovered. Frequent blood counts are essential to determine optimal dosage and to avoid toxicity (see PRECAUTIONS: Laboratory Tests). Dose adjustment on the basis of blood counts at the nadir and day of treatment should be considered.

Hypersensitivity reactions, including anaphylaxis, have occurred rarely (see ADVERSE REACTIONS). These reactions have occurred after multiple courses of treatment and have recurred in patients who experienced a hypersensitivity reaction to IV ALKERAN. If a hypersensitivity reaction occurs, oral or IV ALKERAN should not be readministered.

Carcinogenesis: Secondary malignancies, including acute nonlymphocytic leukemia, myeloproliferative syndrome, and carcinoma have been reported in patients with cancer treated with alkylating agents (including melphalan). Some patients also received other chemotherapeutic agents or radiation therapy. Precise quantitation of the risk of acute leukemia, myeloproliferative syndrome, or carcinoma is not possible. Published reports of leukemia in patients who have received melphalan (and other alkylating agents) suggest that the risk of leukemogenesis increases with chronicity of treatment and with cumulative dose. In one study, the 10-year cumulative risk of developing acute leukemia or myeloproliferative syndrome after melphalan therapy was 19.5% for cumulative doses ranging from 730 mg to 9,652 mg. In this same study, as well as in an additional study, the 10-year cumulative risk of developing acute leukemia or myeloproliferative syndrome after melphalan therapy was less than 2% for cumulative doses under 600 mg. This does not mean that there is a cumulative dose below which there is no risk of the induction of secondary malignancy. The potential benefits from melphalan therapy must be weighed on an individual basis against the possible risk of the induction of a second malignancy.

Adequate and well-controlled carcinogenicity studies have not been conducted in animals. However, i.p. administration of melphalan in rats (5.4 to 10.8 mg/m²) and in mice (2.25 to 4.5 mg/m²) 3 times per week for 6 months followed by 12 months post-dose observation produced peritoneal sarcoma and lung tumors, respectively.

Mutagenesis: ALKERAN has been shown to cause chromatid or chromosome damage in humans. Intramuscular administration of ALKERAN at 6 and 60 mg/m² produced structural aberrations of the chromatid and chromosomes in bone marrow cells of Wistar rats.

Impairment of Fertility: ALKERAN causes suppression of ovarian function in premenopausal women, resulting in amenorrhea in a significant number of patients. Reversible and irreversible testicular suppression have also been reported.

Pregnancy: Pregnancy Category D. ALKERAN may cause fetal harm when administered to a pregnant woman.

Melphalan was embryolethal and teratogenic in rats following oral (6 to 18 mg/m²/day for 10 days) and intraperitoneal (18 mg/m²) administration. Malformations resulting from melphalan included alterations of the brain (underdevelopment, deformation, meningocele, and encephalocele) and eye (anophthalmia and microphthalmos), reduction of the mandible and tail, as well as hepatocele (exomphaly).

There are no adequate and well-controlled studies in pregnant women. If this drug is used during pregnancy, or if the patient becomes pregnant while taking this drug, the patient should be apprised of the potential hazard to the fetus. Women of childbearing potential should be advised to avoid becoming pregnant.

PRECAUTIONS

General: In all instances where the use of ALKERAN is considered for chemotherapy, the physician must evaluate the need and usefulness of the drug against the risk of adverse events. ALKERAN should be used with extreme caution in patients whose bone marrow reserve may have been compromised by prior irradiation or chemotherapy, or whose marrow function is recovering from previous cytotoxic therapy. If the leukocyte count falls below 3,000 cells/mcL, or the platelet count below 100,000 cells/mcL, ALKERAN should be discontinued until the peripheral blood cell counts have recovered.

A recommendation as to whether or not dosage reduction should be made routinely in patients with renal insufficiency cannot be made because:

a) There is considerable inherent patient-to-patient variability in the systemic availability of melphalan in patients with normal renal function.

b) Only a small amount of the administered dose appears as parent drug in the urine of patients with normal renal function.

Patients with azotemia should be closely observed, however, in order to make dosage reductions, if required, at the earliest possible time.

Administration of live vaccines to immunocompromised patients should be avoided.

Information for Patients: Patients should be informed that the major toxicities of ALKERAN are related to bone marrow suppression, hypersensitivity reactions, gastrointestinal toxicity, and pulmonary toxicity. The major long-term toxicities are related to infertility and secondary malignancies. Patients should never be allowed to take the drug without close medical supervision and should be advised to consult their physician if they experience skin rash, vasculitis, bleeding, fever, persistent cough, nausea, vomiting, amenorrhea, weight loss, or unusual lumps/masses. Women of childbearing potential should be advised to avoid becoming pregnant.

Laboratory Tests: Periodic complete blood counts with differentials should be performed during the course of treatment with ALKERAN. At least one determination should be obtained prior to each treatment course. Patients should be observed closely for consequences of bone marrow suppression, which include severe infections, bleeding, and symptomatic anemia (see WARNINGS).

Drug Interactions: There are no known drug/drug interactions with oral ALKERAN.

Carcinogenesis, Mutagenesis, Impairment of Fertility: See WARNINGS section.

Pregnancy: *Teratogenic Effects:* Pregnancy Category D: See WARNINGS section.

Nursing Mothers: It is not known whether this drug is excreted in human milk. ALKERAN should not be given to nursing mothers.

Pediatric Use: The safety and effectiveness of ALKERAN in pediatric patients have not been established.

Geriatric Use: Clinical studies of ALKERAN Tablets did not include sufficient numbers of subjects aged 65 and over to determine whether they respond differently from younger subjects. Other reported clinical experience has not identified differences in responses between the elderly and younger patients. In general, dose selection for an elderly patient should be cautious, usually starting at the low end of the dosing range, reflecting the greater frequency of decreased hepatic, renal, or cardiac function, and of concomitant disease or other drug therapy.

ADVERSE REACTIONS

Hematologic: The most common side effect is bone marrow suppression leading to leukopenia, thrombocytopenia, and anemia. Although bone marrow suppression frequently occurs, it is usually reversible if melphalan is withdrawn early enough. However, irreversible bone marrow failure has been reported.

Gastrointestinal: Nausea, vomiting, diarrhea, and oral ulceration occur. Hepatic disorders ranging from abnormal liver function tests to clinical manifestations such as hepatitis and jaundice have been reported.

Miscellaneous: Other reported adverse reactions include: pulmonary fibrosis (including fatal outcomes) and interstitial pneumonitis, skin hypersensitivity, maculopapular

rashes, vasculitis, alopecia, and hemolytic anemia. Allergic reactions, including urticaria, edema, skin rashes, and rare anaphylaxis, have occurred after multiple courses of treatment. Cardiac arrest has also been reported rarely in association with such reports.

OVERDOSAGE

Overdoses, including doses up to 50 mg/day for 16 days, have been reported. Immediate effects are likely to be vomiting, ulceration of the mouth, diarrhea, and hemorrhage of the gastrointestinal tract. The principal toxic effect is bone marrow suppression. Hematologic parameters should be closely followed for 3 to 6 weeks. An uncontrolled study suggests that administration of autologous bone marrow or hematopoietic growth factors (i.e., sargramostim, filgrastim) may shorten the period of pancytopenia. General supportive measures, together with appropriate blood transfusions and antibiotics, should be instituted as deemed necessary by the physician. This drug is not removed from plasma to any significant degree by hemodialysis.

DOSAGE AND ADMINISTRATION

Multiple Myeloma: The usual oral dose is 6 mg (3 tablets) daily. The entire daily dose may be given at one time. The dose is adjusted, as required, on the basis of blood counts done at approximately weekly intervals. After 2 to 3 weeks of treatment, the drug should be discontinued for up to 4 weeks, during which time the blood count should be followed carefully. When the white blood cell and platelet counts are rising, a maintenance dose of 2 mg daily may be instituted. Because of the patient-to-patient variation in melphalan plasma levels following oral administration of the drug, several investigators have recommended that the dosage of ALKERAN be cautiously escalated until some myelosuppression is observed in order to assure that potentially therapeutic levels of the drug have been reached.

Other dosage regimens have been used by various investigators. Osserman and Takatsuki have used an initial course of 10 mg/day for 7 to 10 days. They report that maximal suppression of the leukocyte and platelet counts occurs within 3 to 5 weeks and recovery within 4 to 8 weeks. Continuous maintenance therapy with 2 mg/day is instituted when the white blood cell count is greater than 4,000 cells/mcL and the platelet count is greater than 100,000 cells/mcL. Dosage is adjusted to between 1 and 3 mg/day depending upon the hematological response. It is desirable to try to maintain a significant degree of bone marrow depression so as to keep the leukocyte count in the range of 3,000 to 3,500 cells/mcL.

Hoogstraten et al have started treatment with 0.15 mg/kg/day for 7 days. This is followed by a rest period of at least 14 days, but it may be as long as 5 to 6 weeks. Maintenance therapy is started when the white blood cell and platelet counts are rising. The maintenance dose is 0.05 mg/kg/day or less and is adjusted according to the blood count.

Available evidence suggests that about one third to one half of the patients with multiple myeloma show a favorable response to oral administration of the drug.

One study by Alexanian et al has shown that the use of ALKERAN in combination with prednisone significantly improves the percentage of patients with multiple myeloma who achieve palliation. One regimen has been to administer courses of ALKERAN at 0.25 mg/kg/day for 4 consecutive days (or, 0.20 mg/kg/day for 5 consecutive days) for a total dose of 1 mg/kg/course. These 4- to 5-day courses are then repeated every 4 to 6 weeks if the granulocyte count and the platelet count have returned to normal levels.

It is to be emphasized that response may be very gradual over many months; it is important that repeated courses or continuous therapy be given since improvement may continue slowly over many months, and the maximum benefit may be missed if treatment is abandoned too soon. In patients with moderate to severe renal impairment, currently available pharmacokinetic data do not justify an absolute recommendation on dosage reduction to those patients, but it may be prudent to use a reduced dose initially.

Epithelial Ovarian Cancer: One commonly employed regimen for the treatment of ovarian carcinoma has been to administer ALKERAN at a dose of 0.2 mg/kg daily for 5 days as a single course. Courses are repeated every 4 to 5 weeks depending upon hematologic tolerance.

Administration Precautions: Procedures for proper handling and disposal of anticancer drugs should be considered. Several guidelines on this subject have been published.[1-8] There is no general agreement that all of the procedures recommended in the guidelines are necessary or appropriate.

HOW SUPPLIED

ALKERAN is supplied as white, film-coated, round, biconvex tablets containing 2 mg melphalan in amber glass bottles with child-resistant closures. One side is engraved with "GX EH3" and the other side is engraved with an "A." Bottle of 50 (NDC 0173-0045-35).

Store in a refrigerator, 2° to 8°C (36° to 46°F). Protect from light.

REFERENCES

1. ONS Clinical Practice Committee. Cancer Chemotherapy Guidelines and Recommendations for Practice. Pittsburgh, PA: Oncology Nursing Society;1999:32-41.
2. Recommendations for the safe handling of parenteral antineoplastic drugs. Washington, DC: Division of Safety, Clinical Center Pharmacy Department and Cancer Nursing Services, National Institutes of Health; 1992. US Dept of Health and Human Services. Public Health Service publication NIH 92-2621.
3. AMA Council on Scientific Affairs. Guidelines for handling parenteral antineoplastics. *JAMA.* 1985;253:1590-1591.
4. National Study Commission on Cytotoxic Exposure. Recommendations for handling cytotoxic agents. 1987. Available from Louis P. Jeffrey, Chairman, National Study Commission on Cytotoxic Exposure. Massachusetts College of Pharmacy and Allied Health Sciences, 179 Longwood Avenue, Boston, MA 02115.
5. Clinical Oncological Society of Australia. Guidelines and recommendations for safe handling of antineoplastic agents. *Med J Australia.* 1983;1:426-428.
6. Jones RB, Frank R, Mass T. Safe handling of chemotherapeutic agents: a report from the Mount Sinai Medical Center. *CA-A Cancer J for Clin.* 1983;33:258-263.
7. American Society of Hospital Pharmacists. ASHP technical assistance bulletin on handling cytotoxic and hazardous drugs. *Am J Hosp Pharm.* 1990;47:1033-1049.
8. Controlling Occupational Exposure to Hazardous Drugs. (OSHA Work-Practice Guidelines.) *Am J Health-Syst Pharm.* 1996;53:1669-1685.

ALKERAN is registered trademark of GlaxoSmithKline.
GlaxoSmithKline
Research Triangle Park, NC 27709
©2008, GlaxoSmithKline. All rights reserved.
October 2008 ALT:2PI

ALTABAX®

[awl'tə-bax]
(retapamulin ointment), 1%

HIGHLIGHTS OF PRESCRIBING INFORMATION
These highlights do not include all the information needed to use ALTABAX safely and effectively. See full prescribing information for ALTABAX.
ALTABAX (retapamulin ointment), 1%
For Dermatological use only
Initial U.S. Approval: 2007

INDICATIONS AND USAGE
• ALTABAX, a pleuromutilin antibacterial, is indicated for the topical treatment of impetigo due to *Staphylococcus aureus* (methicillin-susceptible isolates only) or *Streptococcus pyogenes* in patients aged 9 months or older. (1)

DOSAGE AND ADMINISTRATION
• Apply a thin layer of ALTABAX to the affected area (up to 100 cm² in total area in adults or 2% total body surface area in pediatric patients aged 9 months or older) twice daily for 5 days. (2)
• The treated layer may be covered with a sterile bandage or gauze dressing if desired. (2)

DOSAGE FORMS AND STRENGTHS
10 mg retapamulin/1g of ointment in 5, 10, 15, and 30 gram tubes. (3)

CONTRAINDICATIONS
None. (4)

WARNINGS AND PRECAUTIONS
• Discontinue in the event of sensitization or severe local irritation. (5.1)
• Not intended for ingestion. Not for intraoral, intranasal, ophthalmic, or intravaginal use. (5.2)

ADVERSE REACTIONS
The most common drug-related adverse reaction was application site irritation (≤2% of patients). (6)
To report SUSPECTED ADVERSE REACTIONS, contact GlaxoSmithKline at 1-888-825-5249 or FDA at 1-800-FDA-1088 or www.fda.gov/medwatch.
See 17 for PATIENT COUNSELING INFORMATION
Revised: 07/2010

FULL PRESCRIBING INFORMATION: CONTENTS*
1 **INDICATIONS AND USAGE**
2 **DOSAGE AND ADMINISTRATION**
3 **DOSAGE FORMS AND STRENGTHS**
4 **CONTRAINDICATIONS**
5 **WARNINGS AND PRECAUTIONS**
  5.1 Local Irritation
  5.2 Not for Systemic or Mucosal Use
  5.3 Potential for Microbial Overgrowth
6 **ADVERSE REACTIONS**
  6.1 Clinical Studies Experience
7 **DRUG INTERACTIONS**
8 **USE IN SPECIFIC POPULATIONS**
  8.1 Pregnancy
  8.3 Nursing Mothers
  8.4 Pediatric Use
  8.5 Geriatric Use
10 **OVERDOSAGE**
11 **DESCRIPTION**
12 **CLINICAL PHARMACOLOGY**
  12.1 Mechanism of Action
  12.2 Pharmacodynamics
  12.3 Pharmacokinetics
  12.4 Microbiology
13 **NONCLINICAL TOXICOLOGY**
  13.1 Carcinogenesis, Mutagenesis, Impairment of Fertility
14 **CLINICAL STUDIES**
15 **REFERENCES**
16 **HOW SUPPLIED/STORAGE AND HANDLING**
17 **PATIENT COUNSELING INFORMATION**
* Sections or subsections omitted from the full prescribing information are not listed

---

FULL PRESCRIBING INFORMATION

1 INDICATIONS AND USAGE
ALTABAX® is indicated for use in adults and pediatric patients aged 9 months and older for the topical treatment of impetigo (up to 100 cm² in total area in adults or 2% total body surface area in pediatric patients aged 9 months or older) due to *Staphylococcus aureus* (methicillin-susceptible isolates only) or *Streptococcus pyogenes* [see Clinical Studies (14)].
To reduce the development of drug-resistant bacteria and maintain the effectiveness of ALTABAX and other antibacterial drugs, ALTABAX should be used only to treat or prevent infections that are proven or strongly suspected to be caused by susceptible bacteria.

2 DOSAGE AND ADMINISTRATION
A thin layer of ALTABAX should be applied to the affected area (up to 100 cm² in total area in adults or 2% total body surface area in pediatric patients aged 9 months or older) twice daily for 5 days. The treated area may be covered with a sterile bandage or gauze dressing if desired [see Patient Counseling Information (17)].

3 DOSAGE FORMS AND STRENGTHS
10 mg retapamulin/1g of ointment in 5, 10, 15, and 30 gram tubes

4 CONTRAINDICATIONS
None.

5 WARNINGS AND PRECAUTIONS
5.1 Local Irritation
In the event of sensitization or severe local irritation from ALTABAX, usage should be discontinued, the ointment wiped off, and appropriate alternative therapy for the infection instituted [see Patient Counseling Information (17)].
5.2 Not for Systemic or Mucosal Use
ALTABAX is not intended for ingestion or for oral, intranasal, ophthalmic, or intravaginal use. ALTABAX has not been evaluated for use on mucosal surfaces [see Patient Counseling Information (17)]. Epistaxis has been reported with the use of ALTABAX on nasal mucosa.
5.3 Potential for Microbial Overgrowth
The use of antibiotics may promote the selection of nonsusceptible organisms. Should superinfection occur during therapy, appropriate measures should be taken.
Prescribing ALTABAX in the absence of a proven or strongly suspected bacterial infection is unlikely to provide benefit to the patient and increases the risk of the development of drug-resistant bacteria.

6 ADVERSE REACTIONS
6.1 Clinical Studies Experience
The safety profile of ALTABAX was assessed in 2,115 adult and pediatric patients ≥9 months who used at least one dose from a 5-day, twice a day regimen of retapamulin ointment. Control groups included 819 adult and pediatric patients who used at least one dose of the active control (oral cephalexin), 172 patients who used an active topical comparator (not available in the US), and 71 patients who used placebo.
Adverse events rated by investigators as drug-related occurred in 5.5% (116/2,115) of patients treated with retapamulin ointment, 6.6% (54/819) of patients receiving cephalexin, and 2.8% (2/71) of patients receiving placebo. The most common drug-related adverse events (≥1% of patients) were application site irritation (1.4%) in the retapamulin group, diarrhea (1.7%) in the cephalexin group, and application site pruritus (1.4%) and application site paresthesia (1.4%) in the placebo group.
Because clinical studies are conducted under varying conditions, adverse reaction rates observed in the clinical studies of a drug cannot be directly compared to rates in the clinical studies of another drug and may not reflect the rates observed in practice. The adverse reaction information from the clinical studies does, however, provide a basis for identifying the adverse events that appear to be related to drug use and for approximating rates.
Adults
The adverse events, regardless of attribution, reported in at least 1% of adults (18 years of age and older) who received ALTABAX are listed in Table 1.

Table 1. Adverse Events Reported by ≥1% of Adult Patients Treated With ALTABAX in Phase 3 Clinical Studies

Adverse Event	ALTABAX N = 1,527 %	Cephalexin N = 698 %
Headache	2.0	2.0
Application site irritation	1.6	<1.0
Diarrhea	1.4	2.3
Nausea	1.2	1.9
Nasopharyngitis	1.2	<1.0
Creatinine phosphokinase increased	<1.0	1.0

Pediatrics
The adverse events, regardless of attribution, reported in at least 1% of pediatric patients aged 9 months to 17 years who received ALTABAX are listed in Table 2.
[See table 2 above]
Other Adverse Events
Application site pain, erythema, and contact dermatitis were reported in less than 1% of patients in clinical studies.

Table 2. Adverse Events Reported by ≥1% in Pediatric Patients Aged 9 Months to 17 Years Treated With ALTABAX in Phase 3 Clinical Studies

Adverse Event	ALTABAX N = 588 %	Cephalexin N = 121 %	Placebo N = 64 %
Application site pruritus	1.9	0	0
Diarrhea	1.7	5.0	0
Nasopharyngitis	1.5	1.7	0
Pruritus	1.5	1.0	1.6
Eczema	1.0	0	0
Headache	1.2	1.7	0
Pyrexia	1.2	<1.0	1.6

7 DRUG INTERACTIONS
Co-administration of oral ketoconazole 200 mg twice daily increased retapamulin geometric mean AUC$_{(0-24)}$ and C$_{max}$ by 81% after topical application of retapamulin ointment, 1% on the abraded skin of healthy adult males. Due to low systemic exposure to retapamulin following topical application in patients, dosage adjustments for retapamulin are unnecessary when co-administered with CYP3A4 inhibitors, such as ketoconazole. Based on in vitro P450 inhibition

studies and the low systemic exposure observed following topical application of ALTABAX, retapamulin is unlikely to affect the metabolism of other P450 substrates.

The effect of concurrent application of ALTABAX and other topical products to the same area of skin has not been studied.

8 USE IN SPECIFIC POPULATIONS

8.1 Pregnancy

Pregnancy Category B

Effects on embryo-fetal development were assessed in pregnant rats given 50, 150, or 450 mg/kg/day by oral gavage on days 6 to 17 postcoitus. Maternal toxicity (decreased body weight gain and food consumption) and developmental toxicity (decreased fetal body weight and delayed skeletal ossification) were evident at doses ≥150 mg/kg/day. There were no treatment-related malformations observed in fetal rats.

Retapamulin was given as a continuous intravenous infusion to pregnant rabbits at dosages of 2.4, 7.2, or 24 mg/kg/day from day 7 to 19 of gestation. Maternal toxicity (decreased body weight gain, food consumption, and abortions) was demonstrated at dosages ≥7.2 mg/kg/day (8-fold the estimated maximum achievable human exposure, based on AUC, at 7.2 mg/kg/day). There was no treatment-related effect on embryo-fetal development.

There are no adequate and well-controlled studies in pregnant women. Because animal reproduction studies are not always predictive of human response, ALTABAX should be used in pregnancy only when the potential benefits outweigh the potential risk.

8.3 Nursing Mothers

It is not known whether retapamulin is excreted in human milk. Because many drugs are excreted in human milk, caution should be exercised when ALTABAX is administered to a nursing woman. The safe use of retapamulin during breast-feeding has not been established.

8.4 Pediatric Use

The safety and effectiveness of ALTABAX in the treatment of impetigo have been established in pediatric patients 9 months to 17 years of age. Use of ALTABAX in pediatric patients is supported by evidence from adequate and well-controlled studies of ALTABAX in which 588 pediatric patients received at least one dose of retapamulin ointment, 1% *[see Adverse Reactions (6), Clinical Studies (14)]*. The magnitude of efficacy and the safety profile of ALTABAX in pediatric patients 9 months and older were similar to those in adults.

The safety and effectiveness of ALTABAX in pediatric patients younger than 9 months of age have not been established.

8.5 Geriatric Use

Of the total number of patients in the adequate and well-controlled studies of ALTABAX, 234 patients were 65 years of age and older, of whom 114 patients were 75 years of age and older. No overall differences in effectiveness or safety were observed between these patients and younger adult patients.

10 OVERDOSAGE

Overdosage with ALTABAX has not been reported. Any signs or symptoms of overdose, either topically or by accidental ingestion, should be treated symptomatically consistent with good clinical practice.

There is no known antidote for overdoses of ALTABAX.

11 DESCRIPTION

ALTABAX contains retapamulin, a semisynthetic pleuromutilin antibiotic. The chemical name of retapamulin is acetic acid, [[(3-*exo*)-8-methyl-8-azabicyclo[3.2.1]oct-3-yl]thio]-, (3a*S*,4*R*,5*S*,6*S*,8*R*,9*R*,9a*R*,10*R*)-6-ethenyldecahydro-5-hydroxy-4,6,9,10-tetramethyl-1-oxo-3a,9-propano-3a*H*-cyclopentacycloocten-8-yl ester. Retapamulin, a white to pale-yellow crystalline solid, has a molecular formula of $C_{30}H_{47}NO_4S$, and a molecular weight of 517.78. The chemical structure is:

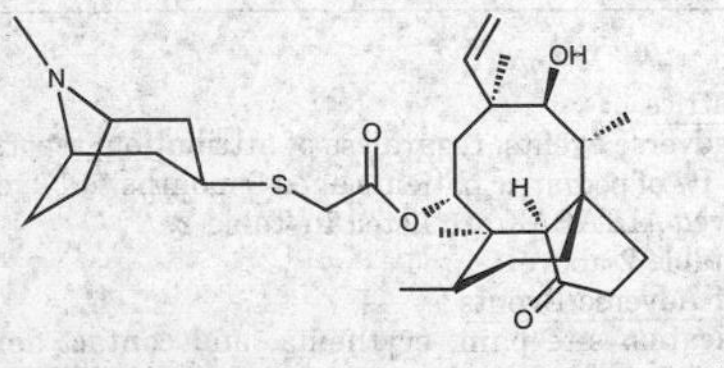

Each gram of ointment for dermatological use contains 10 mg of retapamulin in white petrolatum.

12 CLINICAL PHARMACOLOGY

12.1 Mechanism of Action

ALTABAX is an antibacterial agent *[see Clinical Pharmacology (12.4)]*.

12.2 Pharmacodynamics

In post-hoc analyses of manually over-read 12-lead ECGs from healthy subjects (N = 103), no significant effects on QT/QTc intervals were observed after topical application of retapamulin ointment on intact and abraded skin. Due to the low systemic exposure to retapamulin with topical application, QT prolongation in patients is unlikely *[see Clinical Pharmacology (12.3)]*.

12.3 Pharmacokinetics

Absorption

In a study of healthy adult subjects, retapamulin ointment, 1% was applied once daily to intact skin (800 cm^2 surface area) and to abraded skin (200 cm^2 surface area) under occlusion for up to 7 days. Systemic exposure following topical application of retapamulin through intact and abraded skin was low. Three percent of blood samples obtained on Day 1 after topical application to intact skin had measurable retapamulin concentrations (lower limit of quantitation 0.5 ng/mL); thus C_{max} values on Day 1 could not be determined. Eighty-two percent of blood samples obtained on Day 7 after topical application to intact skin and 97% and 100% of blood samples obtained after topical application to abraded skin on Days 1 and 7, respectively, had measurable retapamulin concentrations. The median C_{max} value in plasma after application to 800 cm^2 of intact skin was 3.5 ng/mL on Day 7 (range 1.2 to 7.8 ng/mL). The median C_{max} value in plasma after application to 200 cm^2 of abraded skin was 11.7 ng/mL on Day 1 (range 5.6 to 22.1 ng/mL) and 9.0 ng/mL on Day 7 (range 6.7 to 12.8 ng/mL).

Plasma samples were obtained from 380 adult patients and 136 pediatric patients (aged 2-17 years) who were receiving topical treatment with ALTABAX topically twice daily. Eleven percent had measurable retapamulin concentrations (lower limit of quantitation 0.5 ng/mL), of which the median concentration was 0.8 ng/mL. The maximum measured retapamulin concentration in adults was 10.7 ng/mL and in pediatric patients was 18.5 ng/mL.

Distribution

Retapamulin is approximately 94% bound to human plasma proteins, and the protein binding is independent of concentration. The apparent volume of distribution of retapamulin has not been determined in humans.

Metabolism

In vitro studies with human hepatocytes showed that the main routes of metabolism were mono-oxygenation and di-oxygenation. In vitro studies with human liver microsomes demonstrated that retapamulin is extensively metabolized to numerous metabolites, of which the predominant routes of metabolism were mono-oxygenation and N-demethylation. The major enzyme responsible for metabolism of retapamulin in human liver microsomes was cytochrome P450 3A4 (CYP3A4).

Elimination

Retapamulin elimination in humans has not been investigated due to low systemic exposure after topical application.

12.4 Microbiology

Retapamulin is a semisynthetic derivative of the compound pleuromutilin, which is isolated through fermentation from *Clitopilus passeckerianus* (formerly *Pleurotus passeckerianus*). In vitro activity of retapamulin against isolates of *Staphylococcus aureus* as well as *Streptococcus pyogenes* has been demonstrated.

Antimicrobial Mechanism of Action

Retapamulin selectively inhibits bacterial protein synthesis by interacting at a site on the 50S subunit of the bacterial ribosome through an interaction that is different from that of other antibiotics. This binding site involves ribosomal protein L3 and is in the region of the ribosomal P site and peptidyl transferase center. By virtue of binding to this site, pleuromutilins inhibit peptidyl transfer, block P-site interactions, and prevent the normal formation of active 50S ribosomal subunits. Retapamulin is bacteriostatic against *Staphylococcus aureus* and *Streptococcus pyogenes* at the retapamulin in vitro minimum inhibitory concentration (MIC) for these organisms. At concentrations 1,000× the in vitro MIC, retapamulin is bactericidal against these same organisms. Retapamulin demonstrates no in vitro target-specific cross-resistance with other classes of antibiotics.

Mechanisms of Decreased Susceptibility to Retapamulin

In vitro, 2 mechanisms that cause reduced susceptibility to retapamulin have been identified, specifically, mutations in ribosomal protein L3 or the presence of an efflux mechanism. Decreased susceptibility of *S. aureus* to retapamulin (highest retapamulin MIC was 2 mcg/mL) develops slowly in vitro via multistep mutations in L3 after serial passage in sub-inhibitory concentrations of retapamulin. There was no apparent treatment-associated reduction in susceptibility to retapamulin in the Phase 3 clinical program. The clinical significance of these findings is not known.

Other

Based on in vitro broth microdilution susceptibility testing, no differences were observed in susceptibility of *S. aureus* to retapamulin whether the isolates were methicillin-resistant or methicillin-susceptible. Retapamulin susceptibility did not correlate with clinical success rates in patients with methicillin-resistant *S. aureus*. The reason for this is not known but may have been influenced by the presence of particular strains of *S. aureus* possessing certain virulence factors, such as Panton-Valentine Leukocidin (PVL). In the case of treatment failure associated with *S. aureus* (regardless of methicillin susceptibility), the presence of strains possessing additional virulence factors (such as PVL) should be considered.

Retapamulin has been shown to be active against the following microorganisms, both in vitro and in clinical trials *[see Indications and Usage (1)]*.

Aerobic and Facultative Gram-Positive Bacteria

Staphylococcus aureus (methicillin-susceptible isolates only)

Streptococcus pyogenes

Susceptibility Testing

The clinical microbiology laboratory should provide cumulative results of the in vitro susceptibility test results for antimicrobial drugs used in local hospitals and practice areas to the physician as periodic reports that describe the susceptibility profile of nosocomial and community-acquired pathogens. These reports should aid the physician in selecting the most effective antimicrobial.

Susceptibility Testing Techniques

Dilution Techniques

Quantitative methods can be used to determine the minimum inhibitory concentration (MIC) of retapamulin that will inhibit the growth of the bacteria being tested. The MIC provides an estimate of the susceptibility of bacteria to retapamulin. The MIC should be determined using a standardized procedure.[1,2] Standardized procedures are based on a dilution method (broth or agar) or equivalent with standardized inoculum concentrations and standardized concentrations of retapamulin powder.

Diffusion Techniques

Quantitative methods that require measurement of zone diameters also provide reproducible estimates of the susceptibility of bacteria to antimicrobial compounds. One such standardized procedure requires the use of standardized inoculum concentrations.[2,3] This procedure uses paper disks impregnated with 2 mcg of retapamulin to test the susceptibility of microorganisms to retapamulin.

Susceptibility Test Interpretive Criteria

In vitro susceptibility test interpretive criteria for retapamulin have not been determined for this topical antimicrobial. The relation of the in vitro MIC and/or disk diffusion susceptibility test results to clinical efficacy of retapamulin against the bacteria tested should be monitored.

Quality Control Parameters for Susceptibility Testing

In vitro susceptibility test quality control parameters were developed for retapamulin so that laboratories that test the susceptibility of bacterial isolates to retapamulin can determine if the susceptibility test is performing correctly. Standardized dilution techniques and diffusion methods require the use of laboratory control microorganisms to monitor the technical aspects of the laboratory procedures. Standard retapamulin powder should provide the following MIC and a 2 mcg retapamulin disk should produce the following zone diameters with the indicated quality control strains in Table 3.

[See table 3 at top of next page]

13 NONCLINICAL TOXICOLOGY

13.1 Carcinogenesis, Mutagenesis, Impairment of Fertility

Long-term studies in animals to evaluate carcinogenic potential have not been conducted with retapamulin.

Retapamulin showed no genotoxicity when evaluated in vitro for gene mutation and/or chromosomal effects in the mouse lymphoma cell assay, in cultured human peripheral blood lymphocytes, or when evaluated in vivo in a rat micronucleus test.

No evidence of impaired fertility was found in male or female rats given retapamulin 50, 150, or 450 mg/kg/day orally.

14 CLINICAL STUDIES

ALTABAX was evaluated in a placebo-controlled study that enrolled adult and pediatric patients 9 months of age and older for treatment of impetigo up to 100 cm^2 in total area (up to 10 lesions) or a total body surface area not exceeding 2%. The majority of patients enrolled (164/210, 78%) were under the age of 13. The study was a double-blind, randomized, multi-center, parallel-group comparison of the safety of ALTABAX and placebo ointment, both applied twice daily for 5 days. The study was randomized 2 ALTABAX to 1 placebo patient. Patients with underlying skin disease (e.g., preexisting eczematous dermatitis) or skin trauma, with clinical evidence of secondary infection were excluded from these studies. In addition, patients with any systemic signs and symptoms of infection (such as fever) were excluded from the study. Clinical success was defined as the absence of treated lesions, or treated lesions had become dry without crusts with or without erythema compared to baseline, or had improved (defined as a decline in the size of the affected area, number of lesions or both) such that no further antimicrobial therapy was required. The intent-to-treat clinical

Table 3. Acceptable Quality Control Ranges for Retapamulin

Microorganism	MIC Range (mcg/mL)	Disk Diffusion Zone Diameter (mm)
Staphylococcus aureus ATCC 29213	0.06-0.25	NA
Staphylococcus aureus ATCC 25923	NA	23-30
Streptococcus pneumoniae ATCC 49619	0.06-0.5[a]	13-19[b]

NA = Not applicable.
[a] This quality control range is applicable using cation-adjusted Mueller-Hinton broth with 2-5% lysed horse blood.
[b] This quality control limit is applicable using Mueller-Hinton agar with 5% sheep blood.

Table 4. Clinical Response at End of Therapy and at Follow-Up by Analysis Population

Analysis Population	ALTABAX		Placebo		Difference in Success Rates (%)	95% CI (%)
	n/N	Success Rate (%)	n/N	Success Rate (%)		
End of Therapy						
PPC	111/124	89.5	33/62	53.2	36.3	(22.8, 49.8)
ITTC	119/139	85.6	37/71	52.1	33.5	(20.5, 46.5)
PPB	96/107	89.7	26/52	50.0	39.7	(25.0, 54.5)
ITTB	101/114	88.6	28/57	49.1	39.5	(25.2, 53.7)
Follow-Up						
PPC	98/119	82.4	25/58	43.1	39.2	(24.8, 53.7)
ITTC	105/139	75.5	28/71	39.4	36.1	(22.7, 49.5)
PPB	86/102	84.3	18/48	37.5	46.8	(31.4, 62.2)
ITTB	91/114	79.8	19/57	33.3	46.5	(32.2, 60.8)

n = number with clinical success outcome, N = number in analysis population, PPC = Clinical Per Protocol Population, ITTC = Clinical Intent to Treat Population, PPB = Bacteriological Per Protocol Population, ITTB = Bacteriological Intent to Treat Population

Table 5. Clinical Response at End of Therapy and Follow-Up for Patients With Staphylococcus aureus and Streptococcus pyogenes at Baseline in the Per Protocol Bacteriological Population (PPB)

Pathogen	ALTABAX		Placebo	
	n/N	Success Rate (%)	n/N	Success Rate (%)
End of Therapy				
Staphylococcus aureus (Methicillin-susceptible)	79/88	89.8	25/48	52.1
Streptococcus pyogenes	29/32	90.6	3/7	42.9
Follow-Up				
Staphylococcus aureus (Methicillin-susceptible)	71/84	84.5	19/44	43.2
Streptococcus pyogenes	29/32	90.6	2/6	33.3

n/N = number of clinical successes/number of pathogens isolated at baseline.

(ITTC) population consisted of all randomized patients who took at least 1 dose of study medication. The clinical per protocol (PPC) population included all ITTC patients who satisfied the inclusion/exclusion criteria and subsequently adhered to the protocol. The intent-to-treat bacteriological (ITTB) population consisted of all randomized patients who took at least one dose of study medication and had a pathogen identified at study entry. The bacteriological per protocol (PPB) population included all ITTB patients who satisfied the inclusion/exclusion criteria and subsequently adhered to the protocol.
The following table describes the results for clinical response at end of therapy (2 days after treatment) and follow-up (9 days after treatment), by analysis population:
[See table 4 above]
The following table describes the clinical success at end of therapy and follow-up by baseline pathogen:
[See table 5 above]
Examination of age and gender subgroups did not identify differences in response to ALTABAX among these groups. The majority of patients entered into this study were classified as White/Caucasian or of Asian heritage; when response rates by racial subgroups were viewed across studies, differences in response to ALTABAX were not identified.

15 REFERENCES
1. Clinical and Laboratory Standards Institute (CLSI) Methods for Dilution Antimicrobial Susceptibility Tests for Bacteria that Grow Aerobically. Approved Standard. CLSI Document M7-A7. CLSI, Wayne, PA, Jan. 2006.
2. Clinical and Laboratory Standards Institute (CLSI). Performance Standards for Antimicrobial Susceptibility Testing – 17th Informational Standard. M100-S17. CLSI, Wayne, PA, Jan. 2007.
3. Clinical and Laboratory Standards Institute (CLSI). Performance Standards for Antimicrobial Disk Susceptibility Tests. Approved Standard. CLSI Document M2-A9. CLSI, Wayne, PA, Jan. 2006.

16 HOW SUPPLIED/STORAGE AND HANDLING
ALTABAX is supplied in 5 gram, 10 gram, 15, and 30 gram tubes.
NDC 0007-5180-05 (5 gram tube)
NDC 0007-5180-10 (10 gram tube)
NDC 0007-5180-22 (15 gram tube)
NDC 0007-5180-25 (30 gram tube)
Store at 25°C (77°F) with excursions permitted to 15°-30°C (59°-86°F).

17 PATIENT COUNSELING INFORMATION
Patients using ALTABAX and/or their guardians should receive the following information and instructions:
- Use ALTABAX as directed by the healthcare practitioner. As with any topical medication, patients and caregivers should wash their hands after application if the hands are not the area for treatment.
- ALTABAX is for external use only. Do not swallow ALTABAX or use it in the eyes, on the mouth or lips, inside the nose, or inside the female genital area.
- The treated area may be covered by a sterile bandage or gauze dressing, if desired. This may also be helpful for infants and young children who accidentally touch or lick the lesion site. A bandage will protect the treated area and avoid accidental transfer of ointment to the eyes or other areas.
- Use the medication for the full time recommended by the healthcare practitioner, even though symptoms may have improved.
- Notify the healthcare practitioner if there is no improvement in symptoms within 3 to 4 days after starting use of ALTABAX.
- ALTABAX may cause reactions at the site of application of the ointment. Inform the healthcare practitioner if the area of application worsens in irritation, redness, itching, burning, swelling, blistering, or oozing.

ALTABAX is a registered trademark of GlaxoSmithKline.
GlaxoSmithKline
Research Triangle Park, NC 27709
©2010, GlaxoSmithKline. All rights reserved.
June 2010
ALX:3PI

AMERGE®
[ə-merj′]
(naratriptan hydrochloride)
Tablets

DESCRIPTION
AMERGE Tablets contain naratriptan as the hydrochloride, which is a selective 5-hydroxytryptamine$_1$ receptor subtype agonist. Naratriptan hydrochloride is chemically designated as N-methyl-3-(1-methyl-4-piperidinyl)-1H-indole-5-ethanesulfonamide monohydrochloride, and it has the following structure:

The empirical formula is $C_{17}H_{25}N_3O_2S \bullet HCl$, representing a molecular weight of 371.93. Naratriptan hydrochloride is a white to pale yellow powder that is readily soluble in water. Each AMERGE Tablet for oral administration contains 1.11 or 2.78 mg of naratriptan hydrochloride equivalent to 1 or 2.5 mg of naratriptan, respectively. Each tablet also contains the inactive ingredients croscarmellose sodium; hypromellose; lactose; magnesium stearate; microcrystalline cellulose; triacetin; titanium dioxide, iron oxide yellow (2.5-mg tablet only), and indigo carmine aluminum lake (FD&C Blue No. 2) (2.5-mg tablet only) for coloring.

CLINICAL PHARMACOLOGY
Mechanism of Action
Naratriptan binds with high affinity to 5-HT$_{1D}$ and 5-HT$_{1B}$ receptors and has no significant affinity or pharmacological activity at 5-HT$_{2-4}$ receptor subtypes or at adrenergic α$_1$, α$_2$, or β; dopaminergic D$_1$ or D$_2$; muscarinic; or benzodiazepine receptors.
The therapeutic activity of naratriptan in migraine is generally attributed to its agonist activity at 5-HT$_{1D/1B}$ receptors. Two current theories have been proposed to explain the efficacy of 5-HT$_{1D/1B}$ receptor agonists in migraine. One theory suggests that activation of 5-HT$_{1D/1B}$ receptors located on intracranial blood vessels, including those on the arteriovenous anastomoses, leads to vasoconstriction, which is correlated with the relief of migraine headache. The other hypothesis suggests that activation of 5-HT$_{1D/1B}$ receptors on sensory nerve endings in the trigeminal system results in the inhibition of pro-inflammatory neuropeptide release.
In the anesthetized dog, naratriptan has been shown to reduce the carotid arterial blood flow with little or no effect on arterial blood pressure or total peripheral resistance. While the effect on blood flow was selective for the carotid arterial bed, increases in vascular resistance of up to 30% were seen in the coronary arterial bed. Naratriptan has also been shown to inhibit trigeminal nerve activity in rat and cat. In 10 human subjects with suspected coronary artery disease (CAD) undergoing coronary artery catheterization, there was a 1% to 10% reduction in coronary artery diameter following subcutaneous injection of 1.5 mg of naratriptan.

Table 1. Percentage of Adult Patients With Headache Response (Mild or No Headache) 4 Hours Following Treatment

	Placebo	AMERGE 1.0 mg	AMERGE 2.5 mg
Study 1	34% (n = 122)	50%[a] (n = 117)	60%[a] (n = 127)
Study 2	27% (n = 104)	52%[a] (n = 208)	66%[ab] (n = 199)
Study 3	32% (n = 169)	54%[a] (n = 166)	65%[a] (n = 167)

[a]p<0.05 in comparison with placebo.
[b]p<0.05 in comparison with 1 mg.

Pharmacokinetics

Naratriptan tablets are well absorbed, with about 70% oral bioavailability. Following administration of a 2.5-mg tablet orally, the peak concentrations are obtained in 2 to 3 hours. After administration of 1- or 2.5-mg tablets, the C_{max} is somewhat (about 50%) higher in women (not corrected for milligram-per-kilogram dose) than in men. During a migraine attack, absorption was slower, with a T_{max} of 3 to 4 hours. Food does not affect the pharmacokinetics of naratriptan. Naratriptan displays linear kinetics over the therapeutic dose range.

The steady-state volume of distribution of naratriptan is 170 L. Plasma protein binding is 28% to 31% over the concentration range of 50 to 1,000 ng/mL.

Naratriptan is predominantly eliminated in urine, with 50% of the dose recovered unchanged and 30% as metabolites in urine. In vitro, naratriptan is metabolized by a wide range of cytochrome P450 isoenzymes into a number of inactive metabolites.

The mean elimination half-life of naratriptan is 6 hours. The systemic clearance of naratriptan is 6.6 mL/min/kg. The renal clearance (220 mL/min) exceeds glomerular filtration rate, indicating active tubular secretion. Repeat administration of naratriptan tablets does not result in drug accumulation.

Special Populations

Age

A small decrease in clearance (approximately 26%) was observed in healthy elderly subjects (65 to 77 years) compared to younger patients, resulting in slightly higher exposure (see PRECAUTIONS).

Race

The effect of race on the pharmacokinetics of naratriptan has not been examined.

Renal Impairment

Clearance of naratriptan was reduced by 50% in patients with moderate renal impairment (creatinine clearance: 18 to 39 mL/min) compared to the normal group. Decrease in clearances resulted in an increase of mean half-life from 6 hours (healthy) to 11 hours (range: 7 to 20 hours). The mean C_{max} increased by approximately 40%. The effects of severe renal impairment (creatinine clearance: ≤15 mL/min) on the pharmacokinetics of naratriptan has not been assessed (see CONTRAINDICATIONS and DOSAGE AND ADMINISTRATION).

Hepatic Impairment

Clearance of naratriptan was decreased by 30% in patients with moderate hepatic impairment (Child-Pugh grade A or B). This resulted in an approximately 40% increase in the half-life (range: 8 to 16 hours). The effects of severe hepatic impairment (Child-Pugh grade C) on the pharmacokinetics of naratriptan have not been assessed (see CONTRAINDICATIONS and DOSAGE AND ADMINISTRATION).

Drug Interactions

In normal volunteers, coadministration of single doses of naratriptan tablets and alcohol did not result in substantial modification of naratriptan pharmacokinetic parameters.

From population pharmacokinetic analyses, coadministration of naratriptan and fluoxetine, beta-blockers, or tricyclic antidepressants did not affect the clearance of naratriptan.

Naratriptan does not inhibit monoamine oxidase (MAO) enzymes and is a poor inhibitor of P450; metabolic interactions between naratriptan and drugs metabolized by P450 or MAO are therefore unlikely.

Oral Contraceptives

Oral contraceptives reduced clearance by 32% and volume of distribution by 22%, resulting in slightly higher concentrations of naratriptan. Hormone replacement therapy had no effect on pharmacokinetics in older female patients.

Smoking increased the clearance of naratriptan by 30%.

CLINICAL TRIALS

The efficacy of AMERGE Tablets in the acute treatment of migraine headaches was evaluated in 6 randomized, double-blind, placebo-controlled studies of which 4 used the recommended dosing regimen and were conducted as outpatient trials. Three of these studies enrolled adult patients who were predominantly female (86%) and Caucasian (96%) with a mean age of 41 (range: 18 to 65). One study enrolled adolescents with a mean age of 14 (range: 12 to 17). In the adolescent study, 54% of the patients were female and 89% were Caucasian. In all studies, patients were instructed to treat at least 1 moderate to severe headache. Headache response, defined as a reduction in headache severity from moderate or severe pain to mild or no pain, was assessed up to 4 hours after dosing. Associated symptoms such as nausea, vomiting, photophobia, and phonophobia were also assessed. Maintenance of response was assessed for up to 24 hours postdose. A second dose of AMERGE Tablets or other medication was allowed 4 to 24 hours after the initial treatment for recurrent headache. The frequency and time to use of these additional treatments were also determined.

In all 3 trials in adults utilizing the recommended dosage regimen and outpatient use, the percentage of patients achieving headache response 4 hours after treatment, the primary outcome measure, was significantly greater among patients receiving AMERGE compared to those who received placebo. In all studies, response to 2.5 mg was numerically greater than response to 1 mg and in the largest of the 3 studies, there was a statistically significant greater percentage of patients with headache response at 4 hours in the 2.5-mg group compared to the 1-mg group. The results are summarized in Table 1.

[See table 1 above]

In the single study in adolescents, there were no statistically significant differences between any of the treatment groups. The headache response rates at 4 hours (n) were 65% (n = 74), 67% (n = 78), and 64% (n = 70) for placebo, 1-mg, and 2.5-mg groups, respectively.

Comparisons of drug performance based upon results obtained in different clinical trials are never reliable. Because studies are conducted at different times, with different samples of patients, by different investigators, employing different criteria and/or different interpretations of the same criteria, under different conditions (dose, dosing regimen, etc.), quantitative estimates of treatment response and the timing of response may be expected to vary considerably from study to study.

The estimated probability of achieving an initial headache response in adults over the 4 hours following treatment is depicted in Figure 1.

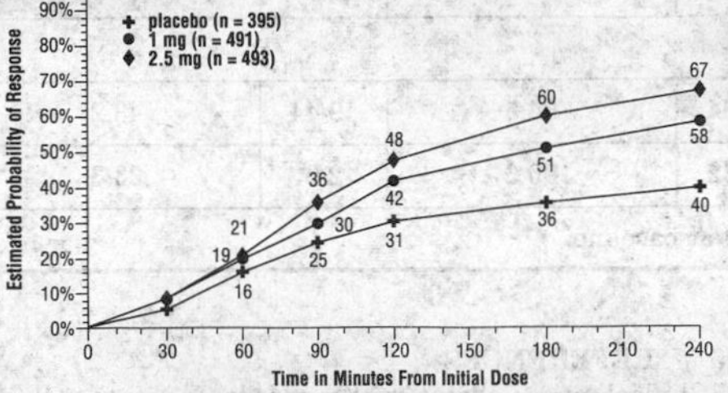

Figure 1. Estimated Probability of Achieving Initial Headache Response Within 4 Hours[a]

[a]The figure shows the probability over time of obtaining headache response (no or mild pain) following treatment with AMERGE Tablets. The averages displayed are based on pooled data from the 3 controlled clinical trials providing evidence of efficacy (Studies 1, 2, and 3). In this Kaplan-Meier plot, patients not achieving response within 240 minutes were censored at 240 minutes.

For patients with migraine-associated nausea, photophobia, and phonophobia at baseline, there was a lower incidence of these symptoms 4 hours following administration of 1- and 2.5-mg AMERGE Tablets compared to placebo.

Four to 24 hours following the initial dose of study treatment, patients were allowed to use additional treatment for pain relief in the form of a second dose of study treatment or other medication. The estimated probability of patients taking a second dose or other medication for migraine over the 24 hours following the initial dose of study treatment is summarized in Figure 2.

[See figure 2 at top of next column]

There is no evidence that doses of 5 mg provide a greater effect than 2.5 mg. There was no evidence to suggest that treatment with AMERGE was associated with an increase

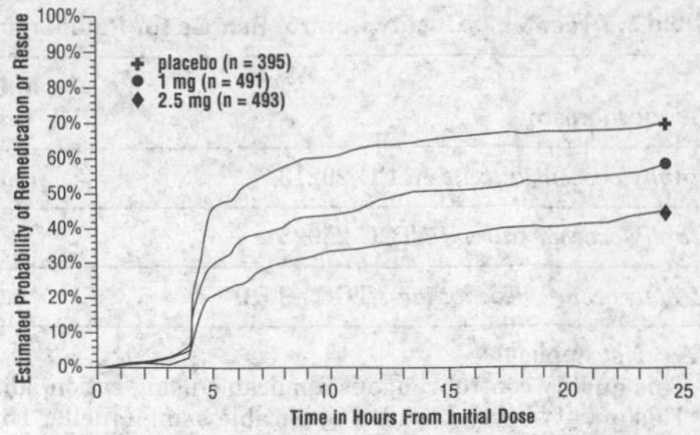

Figure 2. Estimated Probability of Patients Taking a Second Dose of AMERGE Tablets or Other Medication for Migraine Over the 24 Hours Following the Initial Dose of Study Treatment[a]

[a]Kaplan-Meier plot based on data obtained in the 3 controlled clinical trials (Studies 1, 2, and 3) providing evidence of efficacy with patients not using additional treatments censored at 24 hours. The plot also includes patients who had no response to the initial dose. Remedication was discouraged prior to 4 hours postdose.

in the severity or frequency of migraine attacks. The efficacy of AMERGE Tablets was unaffected by presence of aura; gender, age, or weight of the patient; oral contraceptive use; or concomitant use of common migraine prophylactic drugs (e.g., beta-blockers, calcium channel blockers, tricyclic antidepressants). There was insufficient data to assess the impact of race on efficacy.

INDICATIONS AND USAGE

AMERGE Tablets are indicated for the acute treatment of migraine attacks with or without aura in adults.

AMERGE Tablets are not intended for the prophylactic therapy of migraine or for use in the management of hemiplegic or basilar migraine (see CONTRAINDICATIONS). Safety and effectiveness of AMERGE Tablets have not been established for cluster headache, which is present in an older, predominantly male population.

CONTRAINDICATIONS

AMERGE Tablets should not be given to patients with history, symptoms, or signs of ischemic cardiac, cerebrovascular, or peripheral vascular syndromes. In addition, patients with other significant underlying cardiovascular diseases should not receive AMERGE Tablets. Ischemic cardiac syndromes include, but are not limited to, angina pectoris of any type (e.g., stable angina of effort, vasospastic forms of angina such as the Prinzmetal variant), all forms of myocardial infarction, and silent myocardial ischemia. Cerebrovascular syndromes include, but are not limited to, strokes of any type as well as transient ischemic attacks. Peripheral vascular disease includes, but is not limited to, ischemic bowel disease (see WARNINGS).

Because AMERGE Tablets may increase blood pressure, they should not be given to patients with uncontrolled hypertension (see WARNINGS).

AMERGE Tablets are contraindicated in patients with severe renal impairment (creatinine clearance, <15 mL/min) (see CLINICAL PHARMACOLOGY and DOSAGE AND ADMINISTRATION).

AMERGE Tablets are contraindicated in patients with severe hepatic impairment (Child-Pugh grade C) (see CLINICAL PHARMACOLOGY and DOSAGE AND ADMINISTRATION).

AMERGE Tablets should not be administered to patients with hemiplegic or basilar migraine.

AMERGE Tablets should not be used within 24 hours of treatment with another 5-HT_1 agonist, an ergotamine-containing or ergot-type medication like dihydroergotamine or methysergide.

AMERGE Tablets are contraindicated in patients with hypersensitivity to naratriptan or any of the components.

WARNINGS

AMERGE Tablets should only be used where a clear diagnosis of migraine has been established.

Risk of Myocardial Ischemia and/or Infarction and Other Adverse Cardiac Events

Because of the potential of this class of compounds (5-$HT_{1B/1D}$ agonists) to cause coronary vasospasm, naratriptan should not be given to patients with documented ischemic or vasospastic coronary artery disease (CAD) (see CONTRAINDICATIONS). It is strongly recommended that 5-HT_1 agonists (including naratriptan) not be given to patients in whom unrecognized CAD is predicted by the presence of risk factors (e.g., hypertension, hypercholesterolemia, smoker, obesity, diabetes, strong family history of CAD, female with surgical or physiological menopause, male over 40 years of age) unless a cardiovascular evaluation provides satisfactory clinical evidence that the patient is reasonably free of coronary artery and ischemic myocardial disease or other significant underlying cardiovascular disease. The sensitivity of cardiac diagnostic procedures to detect cardiovascular disease or predisposition to coronary artery vasospasm is modest, at best. If, during the cardiovascular evaluation, the patient's medical his-

tory, electrocardiographic, or other investigations reveal findings indicative of, or consistent with, coronary artery vasospasm or myocardial ischemia, naratriptan should not be administered (see CONTRAINDICATIONS).

For patients with risk factors predictive of CAD, who are determined to have a satisfactory cardiovascular evaluation, it is strongly recommended that administration of the first dose of naratriptan take place in the setting of a physician's office or similar medically staffed and equipped facility. Because cardiac ischemia can occur in the absence of clinical symptoms, consideration should be given to obtaining on the first occasion of use an electrocardiogram (ECG) during the interval immediately following administration of AMERGE Tablets, in these patients with risk factors.

It is recommended that patients who are intermittent long-term users of 5-HT$_1$ agonists, including AMERGE Tablets, and who have or acquire risk factors predictive of CAD, as described above, undergo periodic cardiovascular evaluation as they continue to use AMERGE Tablets.

The systematic approach described above is intended to reduce the likelihood that patients with unrecognized cardiovascular disease will be inadvertently exposed to naratriptan.

Cardiac Events and Fatalities Associated With 5-HT$_1$ Agonists

Naratriptan can cause coronary artery vasospasm (see CLINICAL PHARMACOLOGY). Serious adverse cardiac events, including acute myocardial infarction, life-threatening disturbances of cardiac rhythm, and death have been reported within a few hours following the administration of 5-HT$_1$ agonists. Considering the extent of use of 5-HT$_1$ agonists in patients with migraine, the incidence of these events is extremely low.

Premarketing Experience With AMERGE Tablets

Among approximately 3,500 patients with migraine who participated in premarketing clinical trials of naratriptan tablets, 4 patients treated with single oral doses of naratriptan ranging from 1 to 10 mg experienced asymptomatic ischemic ECG changes with at least 1, who took 7.5 mg, likely due to coronary vasospasm.

Cerebrovascular Events and Fatalities With 5-HT$_1$ Agonists

Cerebral hemorrhage, subarachnoid hemorrhage, stroke, and other cerebrovascular events have been reported in patients treated with 5-HT$_1$ agonists, and some have resulted in fatalities. In a number of cases, it appears possible that the cerebrovascular events were primary, the agonist having been administered in the incorrect belief that the symptoms experienced were a consequence of migraine, when they were not. It should be noted that patients with migraine may be at increased risk of certain cerebrovascular events (e.g., stroke, hemorrhage, transient ischemic attack).

Other Vasospasm-Related Events

5-HT$_1$ agonists may cause vasospastic reactions other than coronary artery spasm. Both peripheral vascular ischemia and colonic ischemia with abdominal pain and bloody diarrhea have been reported with naratriptan.

Serotonin Syndrome

The development of a potentially life-threatening serotonin syndrome may occur with triptans, including treatment with AMERGE, particularly during combined use with selective serotonin reuptake inhibitors (SSRIs) or serotonin norepinephrine reuptake inhibitors (SNRIs). If concomitant treatment with naratriptan and an SSRI (e.g., fluoxetine, paroxetine, sertraline, fluvoxamine, citalopram, escitalopram) or SNRI (e.g., venlafaxine, duloxetine) is clinically warranted, careful observation of the patient is advised, particularly during treatment initiation and dose increases. Serotonin syndrome symptoms may include mental status changes (e.g., agitation, hallucinations, coma), autonomic instability (e.g., tachycardia, labile blood pressure, hyperthermia), neuromuscular aberrations (e.g., hyperreflexia, incoordination), and/or gastrointestinal symptoms (e.g., nausea, vomiting, diarrhea).

Increase in Blood Pressure

In healthy volunteers, dose-related increases in systemic blood pressure have been observed after administration of up to 20 mg of oral naratriptan. At the recommended doses, the elevations are generally small, although an increase of systolic pressure of 32 mmHg was seen in 1 patient following a single 2.5-mg dose. The effect may be more pronounced in the elderly and hypertensive patients. A patient who was mildly hypertensive (the baseline blood pressure was 150/98) experienced a significant increase in blood pressure to 204/144 mmHg 225 minutes after administration of a 10-mg oral dose. Significant elevation in blood pressure, including hypertensive crisis, has been reported on rare occasions in patients receiving 5-HT$_1$ agonists with and without a history of hypertension. Naratriptan is contraindicated in patients with uncontrolled hypertension (see CONTRAINDICATIONS).

An 18% increase in mean pulmonary artery pressure and an 8% increase in mean aortic pressure was seen following dosing with 1.5 mg of subcutaneous naratriptan in a study evaluating 10 subjects with suspected CAD undergoing cardiac catheterization.

Hypersensitivity

Hypersensitivity (anaphylaxis/anaphylactoid) reactions may occur in patients receiving naratriptan. Such reactions can be life threatening or fatal. In general, hypersensitivity reactions to drugs are more likely to occur in individuals with a history of sensitivity to multiple allergens (see CONTRAINDICATIONS).

PRECAUTIONS

General

Chest discomfort (including pain, pressure, heaviness, tightness) has been reported after administration of 5-HT$_1$ agonists, including AMERGE Tablets. These events have not been associated with arrhythmias or ischemic ECG changes in clinical trials with AMERGE Tablets. Because naratriptan may cause coronary artery vasospasm, patients who experience signs or symptoms suggestive of angina following naratriptan should be evaluated for the presence of CAD or a predisposition to Prinzmetal variant angina before receiving additional doses of naratriptan, and should be monitored electrocardiographically if dosing is resumed and similar symptoms recur. Similarly, patients who experience other symptoms or signs suggestive of decreased arterial flow, such as ischemic bowel syndrome or Raynaud syndrome following naratriptan administration should be evaluated for atherosclerosis or predisposition to vasospasm (see CONTRAINDICATIONS and WARNINGS).

AMERGE Tablets should also be administered with caution to patients with diseases that may alter the absorption, metabolism, or excretion of drugs, such as impaired renal or hepatic function (see CLINICAL PHARMACOLOGY, CONTRAINDICATIONS, and DOSAGE AND ADMINISTRATION).

Care should be taken to exclude other potentially serious neurological conditions before treating headache in patients not previously diagnosed with migraine or who experience a headache that is atypical for them. There have been rare reports where patients received 5-HT$_1$ agonists for severe headaches that were subsequently shown to have been secondary to an evolving neurologic lesion (see WARNINGS).

For a given attack, if a patient has no response to the first dose of AMERGE, the diagnosis of migraine should be reconsidered before administration of a second dose.

Overuse of acute migraine treatments has been associated with the exacerbation of headache (medication overuse headache) in susceptible patients. Withdrawal of the treatment may be necessary.

Binding to Melanin-Containing Tissues

In rats treated with a single oral dose (10 mg/kg) of radiolabeled naratriptan, the elimination half-life of radioactivity from the eye was 90 days, suggesting that naratriptan and/or its metabolites may bind to the melanin of the eye. Because there could be accumulation in melanin-rich tissues over time, this raises the possibility that naratriptan could cause toxicity in these tissues after extended use. Although no systematic monitoring of ophthalmologic function was undertaken in clinical trials, and no specific recommendations for ophthalmologic monitoring are offered, prescribers should be aware of the possibility of long-term ophthalmologic effects.

Changes in the Precorneal Tear Film

Dogs receiving oral naratriptan showed transient changes in the precorneal tear film. Corneal stippling was seen at the lowest dose tested, 1 mg/kg/day, and occurred intermittently from day 1 throughout the first 2 to 3 weeks of treatment. Although a no-effect dose was not established, the exposure at the lowest dose tested was approximately 5 times the human exposure after a 5-mg oral dose.

Information for Patients

See PATIENT INFORMATION at the end of the full prescribing information for the text of the separate leaflet provided for patients.

Patients should be cautioned about the risk of serotonin syndrome with the use of naratriptan or other triptans, especially during combined use with SSRIs or SNRIs.

Laboratory Tests

No specific laboratory tests are recommended for monitoring patients prior to and/or after treatment with AMERGE Tablets.

Drug Interactions

Selective Serotonin Reuptake Inhibitors/Serotonin Norepinephrine Reuptake Inhibitors and Serotonin Syndrome

Cases of life-threatening serotonin syndrome have been reported during combined use of SSRIs or SNRIs and triptans (see WARNINGS).

Ergot-Containing Drugs

Ergot-containing drugs have been reported to cause prolonged vasospastic reactions. Because there is a theoretical basis that these effects may be additive, use of ergotamine-containing or ergot-type medications (like dihydroergotamine or methysergide) and naratriptan within 24 hours is contraindicated (see CONTRAINDICATIONS).

Other 5-HT$_1$ Agonists

The administration of naratriptan with other 5-HT$_1$ agonists has not been evaluated in migraine patients. Because their vasospastic effects may be additive, coadministration of naratriptan and other 5-HT$_1$ agonists within 24 hours of each other is not recommended (see CONTRAINDICATIONS).

Drug/Laboratory Test Interactions

AMERGE Tablets are not known to interfere with commonly employed clinical laboratory tests.

Carcinogenesis, Mutagenesis, Impairment of Fertility

Carcinogenesis

Lifetime carcinogenicity studies, 104 weeks in duration, were carried out in mice and rats by oral gavage. There was no evidence of an increase in tumors related to naratriptan administration in mice receiving up to 200 mg/kg/day. That dose was associated with a plasma area-under-the-curve (AUC) exposure that was 110 times the exposure in humans receiving the maximum recommended daily dose of 5 mg. Two rat studies were conducted, 1 using a standard diet and the other a nitrite-supplemented diet (naratriptan can be nitrosated in vitro to form a mutagenic product that has been detected in the stomachs of rats fed a high nitrite diet). Doses of 5, 20, and 90 mg/kg were associated with week 13 AUC exposures that in the standard diet study were 7, 40, and 236 times, respectively, and in the nitrite-supplemented diet study were 7, 29, and 180 times, respectively, the exposure attained in humans given the maximum recommended daily dose of 5 mg. In both studies, there was an increase in the incidence of thyroid follicular hyperplasia in high-dose males and females and in thyroid follicular adenomas in high-dose males. In the standard diet study only, there was also an increase in the incidence of benign c-cell adenomas in the thyroid of high-dose males and females. The exposures achieved at the no-effect dose for thyroid tumors were 40 (standard diet) and 29 (nitrite-supplemented diet) times the exposure achieved in humans receiving the maximum recommended daily dose of 5 mg. In the nitrite-supplemented diet study only, the incidence of benign lymphocytic thymoma was increased in all treated groups of females. It was not determined if the nitrosated product is systemically absorbed. However, no changes were seen in the stomachs of rats in that study.

Mutagenesis

Naratriptan was not mutagenic when tested in 2 gene mutation assays, the Ames test and the in vitro thymidine locus mouse lymphoma assay. It was not clastogenic in 2 cytogenetics assays, the in vitro human lymphocyte assay and the in vivo mouse micronucleus assay. Naratriptan can be nitrosated in vitro to form a mutagenic product (WHO nitrosation assay) that has been detected in the stomachs of rats fed a nitrite-supplemented diet.

Impairment of Fertility

In a reproductive toxicity study in which male and female rats were dosed prior to and throughout the mating period with 10, 60, 170, or 340 mg/kg/day (plasma exposures [AUC] approximately 11, 70, 230, and 470 times, respectively, the human exposure at the maximum recommended daily dose [MRDD] of 5 mg), there was a treatment-related decrease in the number of females exhibiting normal estrous cycles at doses of 170 mg/kg/day or greater and an increase in preimplantation loss at 60 mg/kg/day or greater. In high-dose group males, testicular/epididymal atrophy accompanied by spermatozoa depletion reduced mating success and may have contributed to the observed preimplantation loss. The exposures achieved at the no-effect doses for preimplantation loss, anestrus, and testicular effects were approximately 11, 70, and 230 times, respectively, the exposures in humans receiving the MRDD.

In a study in which rats were dosed orally with 10, 60, or 340 mg/kg/day for 6 months, changes in the female reproductive tract including atrophic or cystic ovaries and anestrus were seen at the high dose. The exposure at the no-effect dose of 60 mg/kg was approximately 85 times the exposure in humans receiving the MRDD.

Pregnancy

Pregnancy Category C. There are no adequate and well-controlled studies in pregnant women; therefore, naratriptan should be used during pregnancy only if the potential benefit justifies the potential risk to the fetus.

To monitor fetal outcomes of pregnant women exposed to AMERGE, GlaxoSmithKline maintains a Naratriptan Pregnancy Registry. Healthcare providers are encouraged to register patients by calling (800) 336-2176.

In reproductive toxicity studies in rats and rabbits, oral administration of naratriptan was associated with developmental toxicity (embryolethality, fetal abnormalities, pup mortality, offspring growth retardation) at doses producing maternal plasma drug exposures as low as 11 and 2.5 times, respectively, the exposure in humans receiving the MRDD of 5 mg.

Table 2. Treatment-Emergent Adverse Events Reported by at Least 2% of Patients in Placebo-Controlled Migraine Trials

Adverse Event Type	Placebo (n = 498)	AMERGE 1 mg (n = 627)	AMERGE 2.5 mg (n = 627)
Atypical sensation	1%	2%	4%
Paresthesias (all types)	<1%	1%	2%
Gastrointestinal	5%	6%	7%
Nausea	4%	4%	5%
Neurological	3%	4%	7%
Dizziness	1%	1%	2%
Drowsiness	<1%	1%	2%
Malaise/fatigue	1%	2%	2%
Pain and pressure sensation	2%	2%	4%
Throat/neck symptoms	1%	1%	2%

When pregnant rats were administered naratriptan during the period of organogenesis at doses of 10, 60, or 340 mg/kg/day, there was a dose-related increase in embryonic death, with a statistically significant difference at the highest dose, and incidences of fetal structural variations (incomplete/irregular ossification of skull bones, sternebrae, ribs) were increased at all doses. The maternal plasma exposures (AUC) at these doses were approximately 11, 70, and 470 times the exposure in humans at the MRDD. The high dose was maternally toxic, as evidenced by decreased maternal body weight gain during gestation. A no-effect dose for developmental toxicity in rats exposed during organogenesis was not established.

When doses of 1, 5, or 30 mg/kg/day were given to pregnant Dutch rabbits throughout organogenesis, the incidence of a specific fetal skeletal malformation (fused sternebrae) was increased at the high dose, and increased incidences of embryonic death and fetal variations (major blood vessel variations, supernumerary ribs, incomplete skeletal ossification) were observed at all doses (4, 20, and 120 times, respectively, the MRDD on a body surface area basis). Maternal toxicity (decreased body weight gain) was evident at the high dose in this study. In a similar study in New Zealand White rabbits (1, 5, or 30 mg/kg/day throughout organogenesis), decreased fetal weights and increased incidences of fetal skeletal variations were observed at all doses (maternal exposures equivalent to 2.5, 19, and 140 times exposure in humans receiving the MRDD), while maternal body weight gain was reduced at 5 mg/kg or greater. A no-effect dose for developmental toxicity in rabbits exposed during organogenesis was not established.

When female rats were treated with 10, 60, or 340 mg/kg/day during late gestation and lactation, offspring behavioral impairment (tremors) and decreased offspring viability and growth were observed at doses of 60 mg/kg or greater, while maternal toxicity occurred only at the highest dose. Maternal exposures at the no-effect dose for developmental effects in this study were approximately 11 times the exposure in humans receiving the MRDD.

Nursing Mothers
Naratriptan-related material is excreted in the milk of rats. Therefore, caution should be exercised when considering the administration of AMERGE Tablets to a nursing woman.

Pediatric Use
Safety and effectiveness of AMERGE Tablets in pediatric patients (younger than 18 years) have not been established. One randomized, placebo-controlled clinical trial evaluating oral naratriptan (0.25 to 2.5 mg) in pediatric patients aged 12 to 17 years evaluated a total of 300 adolescent migraineurs. This study did not establish the efficacy of oral naratriptan compared to placebo in the treatment of migraine in adolescents (see CLINICAL TRIALS). Adverse events observed in this clinical trial were similar in nature to those reported in clinical trials in adults.

Geriatric Use
The use of AMERGE Tablets in elderly patients is not recommended.
Naratriptan is known to be substantially excreted by the kidney, and the risk of adverse reactions to this drug may be greater in elderly patients who have reduced renal function. In addition, elderly patients are more likely to have decreased hepatic function; they are at higher risk for CAD; and blood pressure increases may be more pronounced in the elderly. Clinical studies of AMERGE Tablets did not include patients over 65 years of age.

ADVERSE REACTIONS
Serious cardiac events, including some that have been fatal, have occurred following the use of 5-HT₁ agonists. These events are extremely rare and most have been reported in patients with risk factors predictive of CAD. Events reported have included coronary artery vasospasm, transient myocardial ischemia, myocardial infarction, ven-

tricular tachycardia, and ventricular fibrillation (see **CONTRAINDICATIONS, WARNINGS, and PRECAUTIONS)**.

Incidence in Controlled Clinical Trials
The most common adverse events were paresthesias, dizziness, drowsiness, malaise/fatigue, and throat/neck symptoms, which occurred at a rate of 2% and at least 2 times placebo rate. Since patients treated only 1 to 3 headaches in the controlled clinical trials, the opportunity for discontinuation of therapy in response to an adverse event was limited. In a long-term, open-label study where patients were allowed to treat multiple migraine attacks for up to 1 year, 15 patients (3.6%) discontinued treatment due to adverse events.

Table 2 lists adverse events that occurred in 5 placebo-controlled clinical trials of approximately 1,752 exposures to placebo and AMERGE Tablets in adult migraine patients. The events cited reflect experience gained under closely monitored conditions of clinical trials in a highly selected patient population. In actual clinical practice or in other clinical trials, these frequency estimates may not apply, as the conditions of use, reporting behavior, and the kinds of patients treated may differ. Only events that occurred at a frequency of 2% or more in the group treated with AMERGE Tablets 2.5 mg and were more frequent in that group than in the placebo group are included in Table 2. From this table, it appears that many of these adverse events are dose related.

[See table 2 above]
One event (vomiting) present in more than 1% of patients receiving AMERGE Tablets occurred more frequently on placebo than on naratriptan 2.5 mg.

AMERGE Tablets are generally well tolerated. Most adverse reactions were mild and transient.

The incidence of adverse events in placebo-controlled clinical trials was not affected by age or weight of the patients, duration of headache prior to treatment, presence of aura, use of prophylactic medications, or tobacco use. There was insufficient data to assess the impact of race on the incidence of adverse events.

Other Events Observed in Association With the Administration of AMERGE Tablets
In the paragraphs that follow, the frequencies of less commonly reported adverse clinical events are presented. Because the reports include events observed in open and uncontrolled studies, the role of AMERGE Tablets in their causation cannot be reliably determined. Furthermore, variability associated with adverse event reporting, the terminology used to describe adverse events, etc., limit the value of the quantitative frequency estimates provided. Event frequencies are calculated as the number of patients reporting an event divided by the total number of patients (n = 3,557) exposed to oral naratriptan doses up to 10 mg. All reported events are included except those already listed in the previous table, those too general to be informative, and those not reasonably associated with the use of the drug. Events are further classified within body system categories and enumerated in order of decreasing frequency using the following definitions: frequent adverse events are those occurring in at least 1/100 patients, infrequent adverse events are those occurring in 1/100 to 1/1,000 patients, and rare adverse events are those occurring in fewer than 1/1,000 patients.

Atypical Sensations
Frequent were warm/cold temperature sensations. Infrequent were feeling strange and burning/stinging sensation.
Cardiovascular
Infrequent were palpitations, increased blood pressure, tachyarrhythmias, and abnormal ECG (PR prolongation, QT$_c$ prolongation, ST/T wave abnormalities, premature ventricular contractions, atrial flutter, or atrial fibrillation), and syncope. Rare were bradycardia, varicosities, hypotension, and heart murmurs.

Ear, Nose, and Throat
Frequent were ear, nose, and throat infections. Infrequent were phonophobia, sinusitis, upper respiratory inflammation, and tinnitus. Rare were allergic rhinitis; labyrinthitis; ear, nose, and throat hemorrhage; and hearing difficulty.
Endocrine and Metabolic
Infrequent were thirst and polydipsia, dehydration, and fluid retention. Rare were hyperlipidemia, hypercholesterolemia, hypothyroidism, hyperglycemia, glycosuria and ketonuria, and parathyroid neoplasm.
Eye
Frequent was photophobia. Infrequent was blurred vision. Rare were eye pain and discomfort, sensation of eye pressure, eye hemorrhage, dry eyes, difficulty focusing, and scotoma.
Gastrointestinal
Frequent were hyposalivation and vomiting. Infrequent were dyspeptic symptoms, diarrhea, gastrointestinal discomfort and pain, gastroenteritis, and constipation. Rare were abnormal liver function tests, abnormal bilirubin levels, hemorrhoids, gastritis, esophagitis, salivary gland inflammation, oral itching and irritation, regurgitation and reflux, and gastric ulcers.
Hematological Disorders
Infrequent was increased white cells. Rare were thrombocytopenia, quantitative red cell or hemoglobin defects, anemia, and purpura.
Lower Respiratory Tract
Infrequent were bronchitis, cough, and pneumonia. Rare were tracheitis, asthma, pleuritis, and airway constriction and obstruction.
Musculoskeletal
Infrequent were muscle pain, arthralgia and articular rheumatism, muscle cramps and spasms, joint and muscle stiffness, tightness, and rigidity. Rare were bone and skeletal pain.
Neurological
Frequent was vertigo. Infrequent were tremors, cognitive function disorders, sleep disorders, and disorders of equilibrium. Rare were compressed nerve syndromes, confusion, sedation, hyperesthesia, coordination disorders, paralysis of cranial nerves, decreased consciousness, dreams, altered sense of taste, neuralgia, neuritis, aphasia, hypoesthesia, motor retardation, muscle twitching and fasciculation, psychomotor restlessness, and convulsions.
Non-Site Specific
Infrequent were chills and/or fever, descriptions of odor or taste, edema and swelling, allergies, and allergic reactions. Rare were spasms and mobility disorders.
Pain and Pressure Sensations
Frequent were pressure/tightness/heaviness sensations.
Psychiatry
Infrequent were anxiety, depressive disorders, and detachment. Rare were aggression and hostility, agitation, hallucinations, panic, and hyperactivity.
Reproduction
Rare were lumps of female reproductive tract, breast inflammation, inflammation of vagina, inflammation of fallopian tube, breast discharge, endometrium disorders, decreased libido, and lumps of breast.
Skin
Infrequent were sweating, skin rashes, pruritus, and urticaria. Rare were skin erythema, dermatitis and dermatosis, hair loss and alopecia, pruritic skin rashes, acne and folliculitis, allergic skin reactions, macular skin/rashes, skin photosensitivity, photodermatitis, skin flakiness, and dry skin.
Urology
Infrequent were bladder inflammation and polyuria and diuresis. Rare were urinary tract hemorrhage, urinary urgency, pyelitis, and urinary incontinence.

Observed During Clinical Practice
The following section enumerates potentially important adverse events that have occurred in clinical practice and that have been reported spontaneously to various surveillance systems. The events enumerated represent reports arising from both domestic and nondomestic use of naratriptan. These events do not include those already listed in the AD-VERSE REACTIONS section above. Because the reports cite events reported spontaneously from worldwide postmarketing experience, frequency of events and the role of naratriptan in their causation cannot be reliably determined.
Cardiovascular
Angina, myocardial infarction (see WARNINGS).
Gastrointestinal
Colonic ischemia (see WARNINGS).
Lower Respiratory
Dyspnea.
Miscellaneous
Hypersensitivity, including anaphylaxis/anaphylactoid reactions, in some cases severe (e.g., circulatory collapse) (see WARNINGS).

Neurologic

Cerebral vascular accident, including transient ischemic attack, subarachnoid hemorrhage, and cerebral infarction (see WARNINGS); serotonin syndrome.

DRUG ABUSE AND DEPENDENCE

In one clinical study enrolling 12 subjects, all of whom had experience using oral opiates and other psychoactive drugs, AMERGE Tablets produced less intense subjective responses ordinarily associated with many drugs of abuse than did codeine (30 to 90 mg).

OVERDOSAGE

A patient who was mildly hypertensive experienced a significant increase in blood pressure after administration of a 10-mg dose starting at 30 minutes (baseline value of 150/98 to 204/144 mmHg 225 minutes). This event resolved after treatment with antihypertensive therapy. Oral administration of 25 mg of naratriptan in 1 healthy young male subject increased blood pressure from 120/67 mmHg pretreatment up to 191/113 mmHg at approximately 6 hours postdose and resulted in adverse events including lightheadedness, tension in the neck, tiredness, and loss of coordination. Blood pressure returned to near baseline by 8 hours after dosing without any pharmacological intervention.

Another subject experienced asymptomatic ischemic ECG changes likely due to coronary artery vasospasm approximately 2 hours following a 7.5-mg oral dose.

The elimination half-life of naratriptan is about 6 hours (see CLINICAL PHARMACOLOGY), and therefore monitoring of patients after overdose with AMERGE Tablets should continue for at least 24 hours or while symptoms or signs persist. There is no specific antidote to naratriptan. Standard supportive treatment should be applied as required. If the patient presents with chest pain or other symptoms consistent with angina pectoris, ECG monitoring should be performed for evidence of ischemia. It is unknown what effect hemodialysis or peritoneal dialysis has on the serum concentrations of naratriptan.

DOSAGE AND ADMINISTRATION

In controlled clinical trials, single doses of 1 and 2.5 mg of AMERGE Tablets taken with fluid were effective for the acute treatment of migraines in adults. A greater proportion of patients had headache response following a 2.5-mg dose than following a 1-mg dose (see CLINICAL TRIALS). Individuals may vary in response to doses of AMERGE Tablets. The choice of dose should therefore be made on an individual basis, weighing the possible benefit of the 2.5-mg dose with the potential for a greater risk of adverse events. If the headache returns or if the patient has only partial response, the dose may be repeated once after 4 hours, for a maximum dose of 5 mg in a 24-hour period. There is evidence that doses of 5 mg do not provide a greater effect than 2.5 mg.

The safety of treating, on average, more than 4 headaches in a 30-day period has not been established.

Renal Impairment

The use of AMERGE is contraindicated in patients with severe renal impairment (creatinine clearance, <15 mL/min) because of decreased clearance of the drug (see CONTRAINDICATIONS and CLINICAL PHARMACOLOGY). In patients with mild to moderate renal impairment, the maximum daily dose should not exceed 2.5 mg over a 24-hour period and a lower starting dose should be considered.

Hepatic Impairment

The use of AMERGE is contraindicated in patients with severe hepatic impairment (Child-Pugh grade C) because of decreased clearance (see CONTRAINDICATIONS and CLINICAL PHARMACOLOGY). In patients with mild or moderate hepatic impairment, the maximum daily dose should not exceed 2.5 mg over a 24-hour period and a lower starting dose should be considered (see CLINICAL PHARMACOLOGY).

HOW SUPPLIED

AMERGE Tablets 1 and 2.5 mg of naratriptan (base) as the hydrochloride. AMERGE Tablets, 1 mg, are white, D-shaped, film-coated tablets debossed with "GX CE3" on one side in blister packs of 9 tablets (NDC 0173-0561-00). AMERGE Tablets, 2.5 mg, are green, D-shaped, film-coated tablets debossed with "GX CE5" on one side in blister packs of 9 tablets (NDC 0173-0562-00).

Store at controlled room temperature, 20° to 25°C (68° to 77°F) (see USP).

This product's prescribing information may have been updated. Please refer to www.gsk.com for the most current version.

GlaxoSmithKline
Research Triangle Park, NC 27709
©2010, GlaxoSmithKline. All rights reserved.
February 2010
AMG:2PI

PATIENT INFORMATION

The following wording is contained in a separate leaflet provided for patients.

Information for the Patient
AMERGE® (naratriptan hydrochloride) Tablets
Read this leaflet carefully before you start to take AMERGE Tablets. Keep the leaflet for reference because it gives you a summary of important information about AMERGE Tablets.

Read the leaflet that comes with each refill of your prescription because there may be new information.

This leaflet does not have all the information about AMERGE Tablets. Ask your healthcare provider for more information or advice.

What are AMERGE Tablets?
AMERGE is a kind of medicine called a triptan. You should take it only if you have a prescription.

AMERGE is used to relieve your migraine. It is **not** used to prevent attacks or reduce the number of attacks you have. Use AMERGE only to treat an actual migraine attack.

The decision to use AMERGE Tablets is one that you and your healthcare provider should make together, based on your personal needs and health.

Talk with your healthcare provider before taking AMERGE Tablets

1. **Risk factors for heart disease to tell your healthcare provider:**
   Tell your healthcare provider if you have risk factors for heart disease such as:
   ◦ high blood pressure
   ◦ high cholesterol
   ◦ being overweight
   ◦ diabetes
   ◦ smoking
   ◦ strong family history of heart disease
   ◦ you are postmenopausal
   ◦ you are a male over 40 years of age
   If you do have risk factors for heart disease, your healthcare provider should check you for heart disease to see if AMERGE is right for you.
   Most of the people who have taken AMERGE Tablets have not had any serious side effects. Rarely, deaths and/or serious heart problems have been reported with this kind of medicine. Usually, these deaths and/or serious heart problems happened in people with heart disease. It was not clear whether the medicine had anything to do with these deaths and/or serious heart problems.

2. **Important questions to ask yourself before you take AMERGE Tablets:**
   If the answer to any of the following questions is **YES** or if you do not know the answer, then please talk with your healthcare provider before you take AMERGE Tablets.
   ◦ Are you pregnant? Do you think you might be pregnant? Are you trying to become pregnant? Are you not using adequate contraception? Are you breastfeeding?
   ◦ Do you have any chest pain, heart disease, shortness of breath, or irregular heartbeats? Have you had a heart attack?
   ◦ Do you have risk factors for heart disease (see list above)?
   ◦ Have you had a stroke, a mini-stroke (also called a transient ischemic attack or TIA), or Raynaud syndrome?
   ◦ Do you have high blood pressure?
   ◦ Have you ever had to stop taking this or any other medicine because of an allergy or other problems?
   ◦ Are you taking any other migraine medicines, including other triptans such as IMITREX® (sumatriptan/sumatriptan succinate)? Are you taking any medicines containing ergotamine, dihydroergotamine, or methysergide?
   ◦ Are you taking any medicine for depression or other health problems such as a selective serotonin reuptake inhibitor (SSRI) or serotonin norepinephrine reuptake inhibitor (SNRI)? Common SSRIs are citalopram HBr (CELEXA®), escitalopram oxalate (LEXAPRO®), paroxetine (PAXIL®), fluoxetine (PROZAC®/SARAFEM®), olanzapine/fluoxetine (SYMBYAX®), sertraline (ZOLOFT®), and fluvoxamine. Common SNRIs are duloxetine (CYMBALTA®) and venlafaxine (EFFEXOR®).
   ◦ Have you had, or do you have, any disease of the kidney or liver?
   ◦ Is this headache different from your usual migraine attacks?
   Remember, if you answered **YES** to any of the above questions, then talk with your healthcare provider about it.

Important points about AMERGE Tablets

1. **The use of AMERGE Tablets during pregnancy:**
   Do not take AMERGE Tablets if you are pregnant, think you might be pregnant, are trying to become pregnant, or are not using adequate contraception unless you have talked with your healthcare provider about this.

2. **How to take AMERGE Tablets:**
   For adults, the usual dose is a single tablet taken whole

with liquids. You can take it at any time after the headache starts. If you need more relief because you only got a partial response or your headache came back after the first tablet, you can take a second tablet 4 hours after the first tablet, but not sooner.
For any attack, if you have no response to the first tablet, do not take a second tablet without first talking with your healthcare provider. Do not take more than a total of 2 AMERGE Tablets in any 24-hour period.
If you have kidney or liver disease, take as directed by your healthcare provider.

3. **Caution for activities requiring alertness:**
   You may feel drowsy or dizzy because of your migraine or treatment with AMERGE Tablets. Use caution for activities requiring alertness (like driving or using machines).

4. **What to do if you take an overdose:**
   If you have taken more medicine than has been prescribed for you, contact either your healthcare provider, hospital emergency department, or nearest poison control center right away.

5. **How to store your medicine:**
   Keep your medicine in a safe place where children cannot reach it. It may be harmful to children.
   Store your medicine away from heat and light. Do not store at temperatures above 77°F (25°C).
   The expiration date of your medicine is printed on the packaging. If your medicine has expired, throw it away. If your healthcare provider decides to stop your treatment, do not keep any leftover medicine unless your healthcare provider tells you to.

Some possible side effects of AMERGE Tablets

- Some patients feel pain or tightness in the chest or throat when using AMERGE Tablets. If this happens to you, tell your healthcare provider before taking any more AMERGE Tablets. If the chest pain, tightness, or pressure is severe or does not go away, call your healthcare provider right away.
- Call your healthcare provider right away if you have sudden and/or severe abdominal pain after you take AMERGE Tablets.
- Some people may have a reaction called serotonin syndrome when they take certain kinds of medicines for depression called SSRIs or SNRIs while they are taking AMERGE Tablets. Symptoms may include confusion, hallucinations, fast heartbeat, feeling faint, fever, sweating, muscle spasm, difficulty walking, and/or diarrhea. Call your healthcare provider right away if you have any of these symptoms after taking AMERGE Tablets.
- Shortness of breath; wheeziness; heart throbbing; swelling of eyelids, face, or lips; or a skin rash, skin lumps, or hives happens rarely. If it happens to you, then tell your healthcare provider right away. Do not take any more AMERGE Tablets unless your healthcare provider tells you to.
- Some people may feel tingling, heat, flushing (redness of face lasting a short time), heaviness, or pressure after taking AMERGE Tablets. A few people may feel drowsy, dizzy, tired, or sick. If you have any of these symptoms, tell your healthcare provider at your next visit.
- If you feel unwell in any other way or have any symptoms that you do not understand, you should contact your healthcare provider right away.

AMERGE, IMITREX, and PAXIL are registered trademarks of GlaxoSmithKline. The other brands listed are trademarks of their respective owners and are not trademarks of GlaxoSmithKline. The makers of these brands are not affiliated with and do not endorse GlaxoSmithKline or its products.

GlaxoSmithKline
Research Triangle Park, NC 27709
©2010, GlaxoSmithKline. All rights reserved.
February 2010
AMG:2PIL

AMOXIL® ℞
[ə-mäx′ ĭl]
(amoxicillin)
Capsules, Tablets, Chewable Tablets, and Powder for Oral Suspension

To reduce the development of drug-resistant bacteria and maintain the effectiveness of AMOXIL (amoxicillin) and other antibacterial drugs, AMOXIL should be used only to treat or prevent infections that are proven or strongly suspected to be caused by bacteria.

DESCRIPTION

Formulations of AMOXIL contain amoxicillin, a semisynthetic antibiotic, an analog of ampicillin, with a broad spectrum of bactericidal activity against many grampositive and gram-negative microorganisms. Chemically, it is (2S,5R,6R)-6-[(R)-(-)-2-amino-2-(p-hydroxyphenyl)acetamido]-3,3-dimethyl-7-oxo-4-thia-1-azabicyclo[3.2.0]heptane-2-carboxylic acid trihydrate. It may be represented structurally as:
[See chemical structure at top of next page]
The amoxicillin molecular formula is $C_{16}H_{19}N_3O_5S \bullet 3H_2O$, and the molecular weight is 419.45.
Capsules and powder for oral suspension of AMOXIL are intended for oral administration.

Capsules

Each capsule of AMOXIL, with royal blue opaque cap and pink opaque body, contains 500 mg amoxicillin as the trihydrate. The cap and body of the 500-mg capsule are imprinted with AMOXIL and 500. Inactive ingredients: D&C Red No. 28, FD&C Blue No. 1, FD&C Red No. 40, gelatin, magnesium stearate, and titanium dioxide.

Powder for Oral Suspension

Each 5 mL of reconstituted suspension contains 250 mg, or 400 mg amoxicillin as the trihydrate. Each 5 mL of the 250-mg reconstituted suspension contains 0.15 mEq (3.36 mg) of sodium; each 5 mL of the 400-mg reconstituted suspension contains 0.19 mEq (4.33 mg) of sodium.

Pediatric Drops for Oral Suspension

Each mL of reconstituted suspension contains 50 mg amoxicillin as the trihydrate and 0.03 mEq (0.69 mg) of sodium.

Amoxicillin trihydrate for oral suspension 250 mg/5 mL (or 50 mg/mL), and 400 mg/5 mL are bubble-gum-flavored pink suspensions. Inactive ingredients: FD&C Red No. 3, flavorings, silica gel, sodium benzoate, sodium citrate, sucrose, and xanthan gum.

CLINICAL PHARMACOLOGY

Amoxicillin is stable in the presence of gastric acid and is rapidly absorbed after oral administration. The effect of food on the absorption of amoxicillin from the tablets and suspension of AMOXIL has been partially investigated. The 400-mg and 875-mg formulations have been studied only when administered at the start of a light meal. However, food effect studies have not been performed with the 200-mg and 500-mg formulations. Amoxicillin diffuses readily into most body tissues and fluids, with the exception of brain and spinal fluid, except when meninges are inflamed. The half-life of amoxicillin is 61.3 minutes. Most of the amoxicillin is excreted unchanged in the urine; its excretion can be delayed by concurrent administration of probenecid. In blood serum, amoxicillin is approximately 20% protein-bound.

Orally administered doses of 250-mg and 500-mg amoxicillin capsules result in average peak blood levels 1 to 2 hours after administration in the range of 3.5 mcg/mL to 5.0 mcg/mL and 5.5 mcg/mL to 7.5 mcg/mL, respectively.

Mean amoxicillin pharmacokinetic parameters from an open, two-part, single-dose crossover bioequivalence study in 27 adults comparing 875 mg of AMOXIL with 875 mg of AUGMENTIN® (amoxicillin/clavulanate potassium) showed that the 875-mg tablet of AMOXIL produces an $AUC_{0-\infty}$ of 35.4 ± 8.1 mcg•hr/mL and a C_{max} of 13.8 ± 4.1 mcg/mL. Dosing was at the start of a light meal following an overnight fast.

Orally administered doses of amoxicillin suspension, 125 mg/5 mL and 250 mg/5 mL, result in average peak blood levels 1 to 2 hours after administration in the range of 1.5 mcg/mL to 3.0 mcg/mL and 3.5 mcg/mL to 5.0 mcg/mL, respectively.

Oral administration of single doses of 400-mg chewable tablets and 400 mg/5 mL suspension of AMOXIL to 24 adult volunteers yielded comparable pharmacokinetic data:

Dose[a]	$AUC_{0-\infty}$ (mcg•hr/mL)	C_{max} (mcg/mL)[b]
Amoxicillin	Amoxicillin (±S.D.)	Amoxicillin (±S.D.)
400 mg (5 mL of suspension)	17.1 (3.1)	5.92 (1.62)
400 mg (1 chewable tablet)	17.9 (2.4)	5.18 (1.64)

[a] Administered at the start of a light meal.
[b] Mean values of 24 normal volunteers. Peak concentrations occurred approximately 1 hour after the dose.

Detectable serum levels are observed up to 8 hours after an orally administered dose of amoxicillin. Following a 1-gram dose and utilizing a special skin window technique to determine levels of the antibiotic, it was noted that therapeutic levels were found in the interstitial fluid. Approximately 60% of an orally administered dose of amoxicillin is excreted in the urine within 6 to 8 hours.

Microbiology

Amoxicillin is similar to ampicillin in its bactericidal action against susceptible organisms during the stage of active multiplication. It acts through the inhibition of biosynthesis

of cell wall mucopeptide. Amoxicillin has been shown to be active against most strains of the following microorganisms, both in vitro and in clinical infections as described in the INDICATIONS AND USAGE section.

Aerobic Gram-Positive Microorganisms

Enterococcus faecalis
Staphylococcus spp.* (β-lactamase–negative strains only)
Streptococcus pneumoniae
Streptococcus spp. (α- and β-hemolytic strains only)

* Staphylococci which are susceptible to amoxicillin but resistant to methicillin/oxacillin should be considered as resistant to amoxicillin.

Aerobic Gram-Negative Microorganisms

Escherichia coli (β-lactamase–negative strains only)
Haemophilus influenzae (β-lactamase–negative strains only)
Neisseria gonorrhoeae (β-lactamase–negative strains only)
Proteus mirabilis (β-lactamase–negative strains only)

Helicobacter

Helicobacter pylori

Susceptibility Tests

Dilution Techniques

Quantitative methods are used to determine antimicrobial minimum inhibitory concentrations (MICs). These MICs provide estimates of the susceptibility of bacteria to antimicrobial compounds. The MICs should be determined using a standardized procedure. Standardized procedures are based on a dilution method[1] (broth or agar) or equivalent with standardized inoculum concentrations and standardized concentrations of **ampicillin** powder. Ampicillin is sometimes used to predict susceptibility of *S. pneumoniae* to amoxicillin; however, some intermediate strains have been shown to be susceptible to amoxicillin. Therefore, *S. pneumoniae* susceptibility should be tested using amoxicillin powder. The MIC values should be interpreted according to the following criteria:

For Gram-Positive Aerobes:

Enterococcus

MIC (mcg/mL)	Interpretation
≤ 8	Susceptible (S)
≥ 16	Resistant (R)

Staphylococcus[a]

MIC (mcg/mL)	Interpretation
≤ 0.25	Susceptible (S)
≥ 0.5	Resistant (R)

Streptococcus (except *S. pneumoniae*)

MIC (mcg/mL)	Interpretation
≤ 0.25	Susceptible (S)
0.5 to 4	Intermediate (I)
≥ 8	Resistant (R)

S. pneumoniae[b] from non-meningitis sources.
(**Amoxicillin** powder should be used to determine susceptibility.)

MIC (mcg/mL)	Interpretation
≤ 2	Susceptible (S)
4	Intermediate (I)
≥ 8	Resistant (R)

NOTE: These interpretive criteria are based on the recommended doses for respiratory tract infections.

For Gram-Negative Aerobes:

Enterobacteriaceae

MIC (mcg/mL)	Interpretation
≤ 8	Susceptible (S)
16	Intermediate (I)
≥ 32	Resistant (R)

H. influenzae[c]

MIC (mcg/mL)	Interpretation
≤ 1	Susceptible (S)
2	Intermediate (I)
≥ 4	Resistant (R)

[a] Staphylococci which are susceptible to amoxicillin but resistant to methicillin/oxacillin should be considered as resistant to amoxicillin.
[b] These interpretive standards are applicable only to broth microdilution susceptibility tests using cation-adjusted Mueller-Hinton broth with 2-5% lysed horse blood.
[c] These interpretive standards are applicable only to broth microdilution test with *H. influenzae* using *Haemophilus* Test Medium (HTM).[1]

A report of "Susceptible" indicates that the pathogen is likely to be inhibited if the antimicrobial compound in the blood reaches the concentrations usually achievable. A report of "Intermediate" indicates that the result should be considered equivocal, and, if the microorganism is not fully susceptible to alternative, clinically feasible drugs, the test should be repeated. This category implies possible clinical applicability in body sites where the drug is physiologically concentrated or in situations where high dosage of drug can be used. This category also provides a buffer zone, which prevents small uncontrolled technical factors from causing major discrepancies in interpretation. A report of "Resistant" indicates that the pathogen is not likely to be inhibited if the antimicrobial compound in the blood reaches the concentrations usually achievable; other therapy should be selected.

Standardized susceptibility test procedures require the use of laboratory control microorganisms to control the technical aspects of the laboratory procedures. Standard **ampicillin** powder should provide the following MIC values:

Microorganism	MIC Range (mcg/mL)
E. coli ATCC 25922	2 to 8
E. faecalis ATCC 29212	0.5 to 2
H. influenzae ATCC 49247[d]	2 to 8
S. aureus ATCC 29213	0.25 to 1

Using **amoxicillin** to determine susceptibility:

Microorganism	MIC Range (mcg/mL)
S. pneumoniae ATCC 49619[e]	0.03 to 0.12

[d] This quality control range is applicable to only *H. influenzae* ATCC 49247 tested by a broth microdilution procedure using HTM.[1]

[e] This quality control range is applicable to only *S. pneumoniae* ATCC 49619 tested by the broth microdilution procedure using cation-adjusted Mueller-Hinton broth with 2-5% lysed horse blood.

Diffusion Techniques

Quantitative methods that require measurement of zone diameters also provide reproducible estimates of the susceptibility of bacteria to antimicrobial compounds. One such standardized procedure[2] requires the use of standardized inoculum concentrations. This procedure uses paper disks impregnated with 10 mcg ampicillin to test the susceptibility of microorganisms, except *S. pneumoniae*, to amoxicillin. Interpretation involves correlation of the diameter obtained in the disk test with the MIC for **ampicillin**.

Reports from the laboratory providing results of the standard single-disk susceptibility test with a 10-mcg ampicillin disk should be interpreted according to the following criteria:

For Gram-Positive Aerobes:

Enterococcus

Zone Diameter (mm)	Interpretation
≥ 17	Susceptible (S)
≤ 16	Resistant (R)

Staphylococcus[f]

Zone Diameter (mm)	Interpretation
≥ 29	Susceptible (S)
≤ 28	Resistant (R)

β-hemolytic streptococci

Zone Diameter (mm)	Interpretation
≥ 26	Susceptible (S)
19 to 25	Intermediate (I)
≤ 18	Resistant (R)

NOTE: For streptococci (other than β-hemolytic streptococci and *S. pneumoniae*), an ampicillin MIC should be determined.

S. pneumoniae

S. pneumoniae should be tested using a 1-mcg oxacillin disk. Isolates with oxacillin zone sizes of ≥ 20 mm are susceptible to amoxicillin. An amoxicillin MIC should be determined on isolates of *S. pneumoniae* with oxacillin zone sizes of ≤ 19 mm.

For Gram-Negative Aerobes:

Enterobacteriaceae

Zone Diameter (mm)	Interpretation
≥ 17	Susceptible (S)
14 to 16	Intermediate (I)
≤ 13	Resistant (R)

H. influenzae[g]

Zone Diameter (mm)	Interpretation
≥ 22	Susceptible (S)
19 to 21	Intermediate (I)
≤ 18	Resistant (R)

[f] Staphylococci which are susceptible to amoxicillin but resistant to methicillin/oxacillin should be considered as resistant to amoxicillin.

[g] These interpretive standards are applicable only to disk diffusion susceptibility tests with *H. influenzae* using Haemophilus Test Medium (HTM).[2]

Interpretation should be as stated above for results using dilution techniques.

As with standard dilution techniques, disk diffusion susceptibility test procedures require the use of laboratory control microorganisms. The 10-mcg ampicillin disk should provide the following zone diameters in these laboratory test quality control strains:

Microorganism		Zone diameter (mm)
E. coli	ATCC 25922	16 to 22
H. influenzae	ATCC 49247[h]	13 to 21
S. aureus	ATCC 25923	27 to 35

Using 1-mcg oxacillin disk:

Microorganism		Zone diameter (mm)
S. pneumoniae	ATCC 49619[i]	8 to 12

[h] This quality control range is applicable to only *H. influenzae* ATCC 49247 tested by a disk diffusion procedure using HTM.[2]
[i] This quality control range is applicable to only *S. pneumoniae* ATCC 49619 tested by a disk diffusion procedure using Mueller-Hinton agar supplemented with 5% sheep blood and incubated in 5% CO_2.

Susceptibility Testing for *Helicobacter pylori*
In vitro susceptibility testing methods and diagnostic products currently available for determining minimum inhibitory concentrations (MICs) and zone sizes have not been standardized, validated, or approved for testing *H. pylori* microorganisms.

Culture and susceptibility testing should be obtained in patients who fail triple therapy. If clarithromycin resistance is found, a non-clarithromycin-containing regimen should be used.

INDICATIONS AND USAGE
AMOXIL is indicated in the treatment of infections due to susceptible (ONLY β-lactamase–negative) strains of the designated microorganisms in the conditions listed below:

Infections of the ear, nose, and throat—due to *Streptococcus* spp. (α- and β-hemolytic strains only), *S. pneumoniae, Staphylococcus* spp., or *H. influenzae.*

Infections of the genitourinary tract—due to *E. coli, P. mirabilis,* or *E. faecalis.*

Infections of the skin and skin structure—due to *Streptococcus* spp. (α- and β-hemolytic strains only), *Staphylococcus* spp., or *E. coli.*

Infections of the lower respiratory tract—due to *Streptococcus* spp. (α- and β-hemolytic strains only), *S. pneumoniae, Staphylococcus* spp., or *H. influenzae.*

Gonorrhea, acute uncomplicated (ano-genital and urethral infections)—due to *N. gonorrhoeae* (males and females).

H. pylori eradication to reduce the risk of duodenal ulcer recurrence

Triple Therapy
AMOXIL/clarithromycin/lansoprazole
AMOXIL, in combination with clarithromycin plus lansoprazole as triple therapy, is indicated for the treatment of patients with *H. pylori* infection and duodenal ulcer disease (active or 1-year history of a duodenal ulcer) to eradicate *H. pylori.* Eradication of *H. pylori* has been shown to reduce the risk of duodenal ulcer recurrence. (See CLINICAL STUDIES and DOSAGE AND ADMINISTRATION.)

Dual Therapy
AMOXIL/lansoprazole
AMOXIL, in combination with lansoprazole delayed-release capsules as dual therapy, is indicated for the treatment of patients with *H. pylori* infection and duodenal ulcer disease (active or 1-year history of a duodenal ulcer) **who are either allergic or intolerant to clarithromycin or in whom resistance to clarithromycin is known or suspected.** (See the clarithromycin package insert, MICROBIOLOGY.) Eradication of *H. pylori* has been shown to reduce the risk of duodenal ulcer recurrence. (See CLINICAL STUDIES and DOSAGE AND ADMINISTRATION.)

To reduce the development of drug-resistant bacteria and maintain the effectiveness of AMOXIL and other antibacterial drugs, AMOXIL should be used only to treat or prevent infections that are proven or strongly suspected to be caused by susceptible bacteria. When culture and susceptibility information are available, they should be considered in selecting or modifying antibacterial therapy. In the absence of such data, local epidemiology and susceptibility patterns may contribute to the empiric selection of therapy. Indicated surgical procedures should be performed.

CONTRAINDICATIONS
A history of allergic reaction to any of the penicillins is a contraindication.

WARNINGS
SERIOUS AND OCCASIONALLY FATAL HYPERSENSITIVITY (ANAPHYLACTIC) REACTIONS HAVE BEEN REPORTED IN PATIENTS ON PENICILLIN THERAPY. ALTHOUGH ANAPHYLAXIS IS MORE FREQUENT FOLLOWING PARENTERAL THERAPY, IT HAS OCCURRED IN PATIENTS ON ORAL PENICILLINS. THESE REACTIONS ARE MORE LIKELY TO OCCUR IN INDIVIDUALS WITH A HISTORY OF PENICILLIN HYPERSENSITIVITY AND/OR A HISTORY OF SENSITIVITY TO MULTIPLE ALLERGENS. THERE HAVE BEEN REPORTS OF INDIVIDUALS WITH A HISTORY OF PENICILLIN HYPERSENSITIVITY WHO HAVE EXPERIENCED SEVERE REACTIONS WHEN TREATED WITH CEPHALOSPORINS. BEFORE INITIATING THERAPY WITH AMOXIL, CAREFUL INQUIRY SHOULD BE MADE CONCERNING PREVIOUS HYPERSENSITIVITY REACTIONS TO PENICILLINS, CEPHALOSPORINS, OR OTHER ALLERGENS. IF AN ALLERGIC REACTION OCCURS, AMOXIL SHOULD BE DISCONTINUED AND APPROPRIATE THERAPY INSTITUTED. SERIOUS ANAPHYLACTIC REACTIONS REQUIRE IMMEDIATE EMERGENCY TREATMENT WITH EPINEPHRINE. OXYGEN, INTRAVENOUS STEROIDS, AND AIRWAY MANAGEMENT, INCLUDING INTUBATION, SHOULD ALSO BE ADMINISTERED AS INDICATED.

Clostridium difficile associated diarrhea (CDAD) has been reported with use of nearly all antibacterial agents, including AMOXIL, and may range in severity from mild diarrhea to fatal colitis. Treatment with antibacterial agents alters the normal flora of the colon leading to overgrowth of *C. difficile.*

C. difficile produces toxins A and B which contribute to the development of CDAD. Hypertoxin producing strains of *C. difficile* cause increased morbidity and mortality, as these infections can be refractory to antimicrobial therapy and may require colectomy. CDAD must be considered in all patients who present with diarrhea following antibiotic use. Careful medical history is necessary since CDAD has been reported to occur over two months after the administration of antibacterial agents.

If CDAD is suspected or confirmed, ongoing antibiotic use not directed against *C. difficile* may need to be discontinued. Appropriate fluid and electrolyte management, protein supplementation, antibiotic treatment of *C. difficile,* and surgical evaluation should be instituted as clinically indicated.

PRECAUTIONS
General
The possibility of superinfections with mycotic or bacterial pathogens should be kept in mind during therapy. If superinfections occur, amoxicillin should be discontinued and appropriate therapy instituted.

A high percentage of patients with mononucleosis who receive ampicillin develop an erythematous skin rash. Thus, ampicillin-class antibiotics should not be administered to patients with mononucleosis.

Prescribing AMOXIL in the absence of a proven or strongly suspected bacterial infection or a prophylactic indication is unlikely to provide benefit to the patient and increases the risk of the development of drug-resistant bacteria.

Phenylketonurics
Each 200-mg chewable tablet of AMOXIL contains 1.82 mg phenylalanine; each 400-mg chewable tablet contains 3.64 mg phenylalanine. The suspensions of AMOXIL do not contain phenylalanine and can be used by phenylketonurics.

Laboratory Tests
As with any potent drug, periodic assessment of renal, hepatic, and hematopoietic function should be made during prolonged therapy.

All patients with gonorrhea should have a serologic test for syphilis at the time of diagnosis. Patients treated with amoxicillin should have a follow-up serologic test for syphilis after 3 months.

Drug Interactions
Probenecid decreases the renal tubular secretion of amoxicillin. Concurrent use of amoxicillin and probenecid may result in increased and prolonged blood levels of amoxicillin.

Abnormal prolongation of prothrombin time (increased international normalized ratio [INR]) has been reported rarely in patients receiving amoxicillin and oral anticoagulants. Appropriate monitoring should be undertaken when anticoagulants are prescribed concurrently. Adjustments in the dose of oral anticoagulants may be necessary to maintain the desired level of anticoagulation.

Chloramphenicol, macrolides, sulfonamides, and tetracyclines may interfere with the bactericidal effects of penicillin. This has been demonstrated in vitro; however, the clinical significance of this interaction is not well documented.

In common with other antibiotics, AMOXIL may affect the gut flora, leading to lower estrogen reabsorption and reduced efficacy of combined oral estrogen/progesterone contraceptives.

Drug/Laboratory Test Interactions
High urine concentrations of ampicillin may result in false-positive reactions when testing for the presence of glucose in urine using CLINITEST®, Benedict's Solution, or Fehling's Solution. Since this effect may also occur with amoxicillin, it is recommended that glucose tests based on enzymatic glucose oxidase reactions (such as CLINISTIX®) be used.

Following administration of ampicillin to pregnant women, a transient decrease in plasma concentration of total conjugated estriol, estriol-glucuronide, conjugated estrone, and estradiol has been noted. This effect may also occur with amoxicillin.

Carcinogenesis, Mutagenesis, Impairment of Fertility
Long-term studies in animals have not been performed to evaluate carcinogenic potential. Studies to detect mutagenic potential of amoxicillin alone have not been conducted; however, the following information is available from tests on a 4:1 mixture of amoxicillin and potassium clavulanate (AUGMENTIN). AUGMENTIN was non-mutagenic in the Ames bacterial mutation assay, and the yeast gene conversion assay. AUGMENTIN was weakly positive in the mouse lymphoma assay, but the trend toward increased mutation frequencies in this assay occurred at doses that were also associated with decreased cell survival. AUGMENTIN was negative in the mouse micronucleus test, and in the dominant lethal assay in mice. Potassium clavulanate alone was tested in the Ames bacterial mutation assay and in the mouse micronucleus test, and was negative in each of these assays. In a multi-generation reproduction study in rats, no impairment of fertility or other adverse reproductive effects were seen at doses up to 500 mg/kg (approximately 3 times the human dose in mg/m²).

Pregnancy
Teratogenic Effects
Pregnancy Category B. Reproduction studies have been performed in mice and rats at doses up to 10 times the human dose and have revealed no evidence of impaired fertility or harm to the fetus due to amoxicillin. There are, however, no adequate and well-controlled studies in pregnant women. Because animal reproduction studies are not always predictive of human response, this drug should be used during pregnancy only if clearly needed.

Labor and Delivery
Oral ampicillin-class antibiotics are poorly absorbed during labor. Studies in guinea pigs showed that intravenous administration of ampicillin slightly decreased the uterine tone and frequency of contractions but moderately increased the height and duration of contractions. However, it is not known whether use of amoxicillin in humans during labor or delivery has immediate or delayed adverse effects on the fetus, prolongs the duration of labor, or increases the likelihood that forceps delivery or other obstetrical intervention or resuscitation of the newborn will be necessary.

Nursing Mothers
Penicillins have been shown to be excreted in human milk. Amoxicillin use by nursing mothers may lead to sensitization of infants. Caution should be exercised when amoxicillin is administered to a nursing woman.

Pediatric Use
Because of incompletely developed renal function in neonates and young infants, the elimination of amoxicillin may be delayed. Dosing of AMOXIL should be modified in pediatric patients 12 weeks or younger (≤ 3 months). (See DOSAGE AND ADMINISTRATION: Neonates and Infants.)

Geriatric Use

An analysis of clinical studies of AMOXIL was conducted to determine whether subjects aged 65 and over respond differently from younger subjects. Of the 1,811 subjects treated with capsules of AMOXIL, 85% were < 60 years old, 15% were ≥ 61 years old and 7% were ≥ 71 years old. This analysis and other reported clinical experience have not identified differences in responses between the elderly and younger patients, but a greater sensitivity of some older individuals cannot be ruled out.

This drug is known to be substantially excreted by the kidney, and the risk of toxic reactions to this drug may be greater in patients with impaired renal function. Because elderly patients are more likely to have decreased renal function, care should be taken in dose selection, and it may be useful to monitor renal function.

Information for Patients

AMOXIL may be taken every 8 hours or every 12 hours, depending on the strength of the product prescribed.

Patients should be counseled that antibacterial drugs, including AMOXIL, should only be used to treat bacterial infections. They do not treat viral infections (e.g., the common cold). When AMOXIL is prescribed to treat a bacterial infection, patients should be told that although it is common to feel better early in the course of therapy, the medication should be taken exactly as directed. Skipping doses or not completing the full course of therapy may: (1) decrease the effectiveness of the immediate treatment, and (2) increase the likelihood that bacteria will develop resistance and will not be treatable by AMOXIL or other antibacterial drugs in the future.

Diarrhea is a common problem caused by antibiotics which usually ends when the antibiotic is discontinued. Some times after starting treatment with antibiotics, patients can develop watery and bloody stools (with or without stomach cramps and fever) even as late as 2 or more months after having taken the last dose of the antibiotic. If this occurs, patients should contact their physician as soon as possible.

ADVERSE REACTIONS

As with other penicillins, it may be expected that untoward reactions will be essentially limited to sensitivity phenomena. They are more likely to occur in individuals who have previously demonstrated hypersensitivity to penicillins and in those with a history of allergy, asthma, hay fever, or urticaria. The following adverse reactions have been reported as associated with the use of penicillins:

Infections and Infestations

Mucocutaneous candidiasis.

Gastrointestinal

Nausea, vomiting, diarrhea, black hairy tongue, and hemorrhagic/pseudomembranous colitis.

Onset of pseudomembranous colitis symptoms may occur during or after antibiotic treatment. (See WARNINGS.)

Hypersensitivity Reactions

Anaphylaxis (See WARNING)

Serum sickness–like reactions, erythematous maculopapular rashes, erythema multiforme, Stevens-Johnson syndrome, exfoliative dermatitis, toxic epidermal necrolysis, acute generalized exanthematous pustulosis, hypersensitivity vasculitis and urticaria have been reported.

NOTE: These hypersensitivity reactions may be controlled with antihistamines and, if necessary, systemic corticosteroids. Whenever such reactions occur, amoxicillin should be discontinued unless, in the opinion of the physician, the condition being treated is life-threatening and amenable only to amoxicillin therapy.

Liver

A moderate rise in AST (SGOT) and/or ALT (SGPT) has been noted, but the significance of this finding is unknown. Hepatic dysfunction including cholestatic jaundice, hepatic cholestasis and acute cytolytic hepatitis have been reported.

Renal

Crystalluria has also been reported (see OVERDOSAGE).

Hemic and Lymphatic Systems

Anemia, including hemolytic anemia, thrombocytopenia, thrombocytopenic purpura, eosinophilia, leukopenia, and agranulocytosis have been reported during therapy with penicillins. These reactions are usually reversible on discontinuation of therapy and are believed to be hypersensitivity phenomena.

Central Nervous System

Reversible hyperactivity, agitation, anxiety, insomnia, confusion, convulsions, behavioral changes, and/or dizziness have been reported rarely.

Miscellaneous

Tooth discoloration (brown, yellow, or gray staining) has been rarely reported. Most reports occurred in pediatric patients. Discoloration was reduced or eliminated with brushing or dental cleaning in most cases.

Combination Therapy with Clarithromycin and Lansoprazole

In clinical trials using combination therapy with amoxicillin plus clarithromycin and lansoprazole, and amoxicillin plus lansoprazole, no adverse reactions peculiar to these drug combinations were observed. Adverse reactions that have occurred have been limited to those that had been previously reported with amoxicillin, clarithromycin, or lansoprazole.

Triple Therapy

Amoxicillin/Clarithromycin/Lansoprazole

The most frequently reported adverse events for patients who received triple therapy were diarrhea (7%), headache (6%), and taste perversion (5%). No treatment-emergent adverse events were observed at significantly higher rates with triple therapy than with any dual therapy regimen.

Dual Therapy

Amoxicillin/Lansoprazole

The most frequently reported adverse events for patients who received amoxicillin three times daily plus lansoprazole three times daily dual therapy were diarrhea (8%) and headache (7%). No treatment-emergent adverse events were observed at significantly higher rates with amoxicillin three times daily plus lansoprazole three times daily dual therapy than with lansoprazole alone.

For more information on adverse reactions with clarithromycin or lansoprazole, refer to their package inserts, ADVERSE REACTIONS.

OVERDOSAGE

In case of overdosage, discontinue medication, treat symptomatically, and institute supportive measures as required. If the overdosage is very recent and there is no contraindication, an attempt at emesis or other means of removal of drug from the stomach may be performed. A prospective study of 51 pediatric patients at a poison-control center suggested that overdosages of less than 250 mg/kg of amoxicillin are not associated with significant clinical symptoms and do not require gastric emptying.[3]

Interstitial nephritis resulting in oliguric renal failure has been reported in a small number of patients after overdosage with amoxicillin.

Crystalluria, in some cases leading to renal failure, has also been reported after amoxicillin overdosage in adult and pediatric patients. In case of overdosage, adequate fluid intake and diuresis should be maintained to reduce the risk of amoxicillin crystalluria.

Renal impairment appears to be reversible with cessation of drug administration. High blood levels may occur more readily in patients with impaired renal function because of decreased renal clearance of amoxicillin. Amoxicillin may be removed from circulation by hemodialysis.

DOSAGE AND ADMINISTRATION

Capsules, chewable tablets, and oral suspensions of AMOXIL may be given without regard to meals. The 400-mg suspension, 400-mg chewable tablet, and the 875-mg tablet have been studied only when administered at the start of a light meal. However, food effect studies have not been performed with the 200-mg and 500-mg formulations.

Neonates and Infants Aged ≤ 12 Weeks (≤ 3 Months)

Due to incompletely developed renal function affecting elimination of amoxicillin in this age group, the recommended upper dose of AMOXIL is 30 mg/kg/day divided q12h. [See table at left]

After reconstitution, the required amount of suspension should be placed directly on the child's tongue for swallowing. Alternate means of administration are to add the required amount of suspension to formula, milk, fruit juice, water, ginger ale, or cold drinks. These preparations should then be taken immediately. To be certain the child is receiving full dosage, such preparations should be consumed in entirety.

Adults and Pediatric Patients > 3 Months:			
Infection	Severity[a]	Usual Adult Dose	Usual Dose for Children > 3 Months[b]
Ear/Nose/Throat	Mild/Moderate	500 mg every 12 hours or 250 mg every 8 hours	25 mg/kg/day in divided doses every 12 hours or 20 mg/kg/day in divided doses every 8 hours
	Severe	875 mg every 12 hours or 500 mg every 8 hours	45 mg/kg/day in divided doses every 12 hours or 40 mg/kg/day in divided doses every 8 hours
Lower Respiratory Tract	Mild/Moderate or Severe	875 mg every 12 hours or 500 mg every 8 hours	45 mg/kg/day in divided doses every 12 hours or 40 mg/kg/day in divided doses every 8 hours
Skin/Skin Structure	Mild/Moderate	500 mg every 12 hours or 250 mg every 8 hours	25 mg/kg/day in divided doses every 12 hours or 20 mg/kg/day in divided doses every 8 hours
	Severe	875 mg every 12 hours or 500 mg every 8 hours	45 mg/kg/day in divided doses every 12 hours or 40 mg/kg/day in divided doses every 8 hours
Genitourinary Tract	Mild/Moderate	500 mg every 12 hours or 250 mg every 8 hours	25 mg/kg/day in divided doses every 12 hours or 20 mg/kg/day in divided doses every 8 hours
	Severe	875 mg every 12 hours or 500 mg every 8 hours	45 mg/kg/day in divided doses every 12 hours or 40 mg/kg/day in divided doses every 8 hours
Gonorrhea Acute, uncomplicated ano-genital and urethral infections in males and females		3 grams as single oral dose	Prepubertal children: 50 mg/kg AMOXIL, combined with 25 mg/kg probenecid as a single dose. NOTE: SINCE PROBENECID IS CONTRAINDICATED IN CHILDREN UNDER 2 YEARS, DO NOT USE THIS REGIMEN IN THESE CASES.

[a] Dosing for infections caused by less susceptible organisms should follow the recommendations for severe infections.
[b] The children's dosage is intended for individuals whose weight is less than 40 kg. Children weighing 40 kg or more should be dosed according to the adult recommendations.

All patients with gonorrhea should be evaluated for syphilis. (See PRECAUTIONS: Laboratory Tests.)

Larger doses may be required for stubborn or severe infections.

General

It should be recognized that in the treatment of chronic urinary tract infections, frequent bacteriological and clinical appraisals are necessary. Smaller doses than those recommended above should not be used. Even higher doses may be needed at times. In stubborn infections, therapy may be required for several weeks. It may be necessary to continue clinical and/or bacteriological follow-up for several months after cessation of therapy. Except for gonorrhea, treatment should be continued for a minimum of 48 to 72 hours beyond the time that the patient becomes asymptomatic or evidence of bacterial eradication has been obtained. It is recommended that there be at least 10 days' treatment for any infection caused by *Streptococcus pyogenes* to prevent the occurrence of acute rheumatic fever.

H. pylori Eradication to Reduce the Risk of Duodenal Ulcer Recurrence

Triple Therapy

AMOXIL/clarithromycin/lansoprazole

The recommended adult oral dose is 1 gram AMOXIL, 500 mg clarithromycin, and 30 mg lansoprazole, all given twice daily (q12h) for 14 days. (See INDICATIONS AND USAGE.)

Dual Therapy

AMOXIL/lansoprazole

The recommended adult oral dose is 1 gram AMOXIL and 30 mg lansoprazole, each given three times daily (q8h) for 14 days. (See INDICATIONS AND USAGE.)

Please refer to clarithromycin and lansoprazole full prescribing information for CONTRAINDICATIONS and WARNINGS, and for information regarding dosing in elderly and renally impaired patients.

Dosing Recommendations for Adults with Impaired Renal Function

Patients with impaired renal function do not generally require a reduction in dose unless the impairment is severe. Severely impaired patients with a glomerular filtration rate of < 30 mL/min. should not receive the 875-mg tablet. Patients with a glomerular filtration rate of 10 to 30 mL/min. should receive 500 mg or 250 mg every 12 hours, depending on the severity of the infection. Patients with a less than 10 mL/min. glomerular filtration rate should receive 500 mg or 250 mg every 24 hours, depending on severity of the infection.

Hemodialysis patients should receive 500 mg or 250 mg every 24 hours, depending on severity of the infection. They should receive an additional dose both during and at the end of dialysis.

There are currently no dosing recommendations for pediatric patients with impaired renal function.

Directions for Mixing Oral Suspension

Prepare suspension at time of dispensing as follows: Tap bottle until all powder flows freely. Add approximately 1/3 of the total amount of water for reconstitution (see table below) and shake vigorously to wet powder. Add remainder of the water and again shake vigorously.

250 mg/5 mL

Bottle Size	Amount of Water Required for Reconstitution
100 mL	74 mL
150 mL	111 mL

Each teaspoonful (5 mL) will contain 250 mg amoxicillin.

400 mg/5 mL

Bottle Size	Amount of Water Required for Reconstitution
100 mL	71 mL

Each teaspoonful (5 mL) will contain 400 mg amoxicillin.

Directions for Mixing Pediatric Drops

Prepare pediatric drops at time of dispensing as follows: Add the required amount of water (see table below) to the bottle and shake vigorously. Each mL of suspension will then contain amoxicillin trihydrate equivalent to 50 mg amoxicillin.

Bottle Size	Amount of Water Required for Reconstitution
30 mL	23 mL

NOTE: SHAKE BOTH ORAL SUSPENSION AND PEDIATRIC DROPS WELL BEFORE USING. Keep bottle tightly closed. Any unused portion of the reconstituted suspension must be discarded after 14 days. Refrigeration preferable, but not required.

HOW SUPPLIED

Capsules of AMOXIL

Each capsule contains 500 mg amoxicillin as the trihydrate.

500 mg Capsule

NDC 0029-6007-32	Bottles of 500

AMOXIL for Oral Suspension

Each 5 mL of reconstituted bubble-gum-flavored suspension contains 250, or 400 mg amoxicillin as the trihydrate.

250 mg/5 mL

NDC 0029-6009-23	100-mL bottle
NDC 0029-6009-22	150-mL bottle

400 mg/5 mL

NDC 0029-6049-59	100-mL bottle

Pediatric Drops of AMOXIL for Oral Suspension

Each mL of bubble-gum-flavored reconstituted suspension contains 50 mg amoxicillin as the trihydrate.

NDC 0029-6038-39	30-mL bottle

Store at or below 20°C (68°F)
- 500-mg capsules
- 250-mg unreconstituted powder

Store at or below 25°C (77°F)
- 400-mg unreconstituted powder

Dispense in a tight container.

CLINICAL STUDIES

H. pylori Eradication to Reduce the Risk of Duodenal Ulcer Recurrence

Randomized, double-blind clinical studies performed in the United States in patients with *H. pylori* and duodenal ulcer disease (defined as an active ulcer or history of an ulcer within 1 year) evaluated the efficacy of lansoprazole in combination with amoxicillin capsules and clarithromycin tablets as triple 14-day therapy, or in combination with amoxicillin capsules as dual 14-day therapy, for the eradication of *H. pylori*. Based on the results of these studies, the safety and efficacy of 2 different eradication regimens were established:

Triple Therapy

Amoxicillin 1 gram twice daily/clarithromycin 500 mg twice daily/lansoprazole 30 mg twice daily.

Dual Therapy

Amoxicillin 1 gram three times daily/lansoprazole 30 mg three times daily.

All treatments were for 14 days. *H. pylori* eradication was defined as 2 negative tests (culture and histology) at 4 to 6 weeks following the end of treatment.

Triple therapy was shown to be more effective than all possible dual therapy combinations. Dual therapy was shown to be more effective than both monotherapies. Eradication of *H. pylori* has been shown to reduce the risk of duodenal ulcer recurrence.

H. pylori Eradication Rates–Triple Therapy
(amoxicillin/clarithromycin/lansoprazole)
Percent of Patients Cured [95% Confidence Interval]
(Number of Patients)

Study	Triple Therapy	Triple Therapy
	Evaluable Analysis[a]	Intent-to-Treat Analysis[b]
Study 1	92[c] [80.0-97.7] (n = 48)	86[c] [73.3-93.5] (n = 55)
Study 2	86[d] [75.7-93.6] (n = 66)	83[d] [72.0-90.8] (n = 70)

[a] This analysis was based on evaluable patients with confirmed duodenal ulcer (active or within 1 year) and *H. pylori* infection at baseline defined as at least 2 of 3 positive endoscopic tests from CLOtest®, (Delta West Ltd., Bentley, Australia), histology, and/or culture. Patients were included in the analysis if they completed the study. Additionally, if patients dropped out of the study due to an adverse event related to the study drug, they were included in the analysis as failures of therapy.

[b] Patients were included in the analysis if they had documented *H. pylori* infection at baseline as defined above and had a confirmed duodenal ulcer (active or within 1 year). All dropouts were included as failures of therapy.

[c] (P < 0.05) versus lansoprazole/amoxicillin and lansoprazole/clarithromycin dual therapy.

[d] (P < 0.05) versus clarithromycin/amoxicillin dual therapy.

H. pylori Eradication Rates–Dual Therapy
(amoxicillin/lansoprazole)
Percent of Patients Cured [95% Confidence Interval]
(Number of Patients)

Study	Dual Therapy	Dual Therapy
	Evaluable Analysis[a]	Intent-to-Treat Analysis[b]
Study 1	77[c] [62.5-87.2] (n = 51)	70[c] [56.8-81.2] (n = 60)
Study 2	66[d] [51.9-77.5] (n = 58)	61[d] [48.5-72.9] (n = 67)

[a] This analysis was based on evaluable patients with confirmed duodenal ulcer (active or within 1 year) and *H. pylori* infection at baseline defined as at least 2 of 3 positive endoscopic tests from CLOtest®, histology and/or culture. Patients were included in the analysis if they completed the study. Additionally, if patients dropped out of the study due to an adverse event related to the study drug, they were included in the analysis as failures of therapy.

[b] Patients were included in the analysis if they had documented *H. pylori* infection at baseline as defined above and had a confirmed duodenal ulcer (active or within 1 year). All dropouts were included as failures of therapy.

[c] (P < 0.05) versus lansoprazole alone.

[d] (P < 0.05) versus lansoprazole alone or amoxicillin alone.

REFERENCES

1. National Committee for Clinical Laboratory Standards. Methods for Dilution Antimicrobial Susceptibility Tests for Bacteria that Grow Aerobically – Fourth Edition; Approved Standard NCCLS Document M7-A4, Vol. 17, No. 2. NCCLS, Wayne, PA, January 1997.
2. National Committee for Clinical Laboratory Standards. Performance Standards for Antimicrobial Disk Susceptibility Tests – Sixth Edition; Approved Standard NCCLS Document M2-A6, Vol. 17, No. 1. NCCLS, Wayne, PA, January 1997.
3. Swanson-Biearman B, Dean BS, Lopez G, Krenzelok EP. The effects of penicillin and cephalosporin ingestions in children less than six years of age. *Vet Hum Toxicol.* 1988;30:66-67.

AMOXIL and AUGMENTIN are registered trademarks of GlaxoSmithKline. The following are registered trademarks of their respective owners: CLINITEST and CLINISTIX/Bayer Corporation; CLOtest/Kimberly-Clark Corporation.

GlaxoSmithKline
Research Triangle Park, NC 27709
September 2009   AMX:33PI

ARGATROBAN   ℞

[är-ga' trō-ban]
Injection

DESCRIPTION

Argatroban is a synthetic direct thrombin inhibitor derived from L-arginine. The chemical name for Argatroban is 1-[5-[(aminoiminomethyl)amino]-1-oxo-2-[[(1,2,3,4-tetrahydro-3-methyl-8-quinolinyl)sulfonyl]amino]pentyl]-4-methyl-2-piperidinecarboxylic acid, monohydrate. Argatroban has 4 asymmetric carbons. One of the asymmetric carbons has an R configuration (stereoisomer Type I) and an S configuration (stereoisomer Type II). Argatroban consists of a mixture of R and S stereoisomers at a ratio of approximately 65:35.

The molecular formula of Argatroban is $C_{23}H_{36}N_6O_5S \cdot H_2O$. Its molecular weight is 526.66. The structural formula is shown below:

[See chemical structure at top of next column]

Argatroban is a white, odorless crystalline powder that is freely soluble in glacial acetic acid, slightly soluble in ethanol, and insoluble in acetone, ethyl acetate, and ether. Argatroban Injection is a sterile clear, colorless to pale yellow, slightly viscous solution. Argatroban is available in

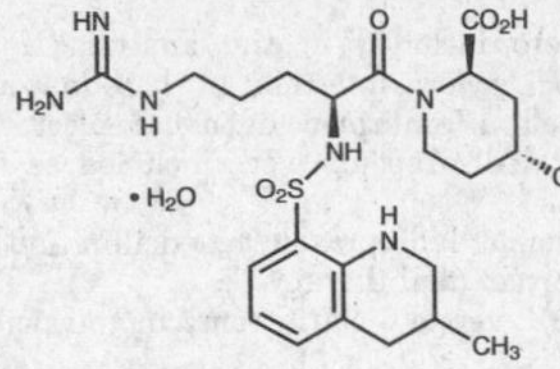

250-mg (in 2.5-mL) single-use amber vials, with gray flip-top caps. Each mL of sterile, nonpyrogenic solution contains 100 mg Argatroban. Inert ingredients: 750 mg D-sorbitol, 1,000 mg dehydrated alcohol.

CLINICAL PHARMACOLOGY

Mechanism of Action: Argatroban is a direct thrombin inhibitor that reversibly binds to the thrombin active site. Argatroban does not require the co-factor antithrombin III for antithrombotic activity. Argatroban exerts its anticoagulant effects by inhibiting thrombin-catalyzed or -induced reactions, including fibrin formation; activation of coagulation factors V, VIII, and XIII; activation of protein C; and platelet aggregation.

Argatroban is highly selective for thrombin with an inhibitory constant (K_i) of 0.04 μM. At therapeutic concentrations, Argatroban has little or no effect on related serine proteases (trypsin, factor Xa, plasmin, and kallikrein).

Argatroban is capable of inhibiting the action of both free and clot-associated thrombin.

Argatroban does not interact with heparin-induced antibodies. Evaluation of sera in 12 healthy subjects and 8 patients who received multiple doses of Argatroban did not reveal antibody formation to Argatroban (see CLINICAL STUDIES).

Pharmacokinetics: ***Distribution:*** Argatroban distributes mainly in the extracellular fluid as evidenced by an apparent steady-state volume of distribution of 174 mL/kg (12.18 L in a 70-kg adult). Argatroban is 54% bound to human serum proteins, with binding to albumin and α_1-acid glycoprotein being 20% and 34%, respectively.

Metabolism: The main route of Argatroban metabolism is hydroxylation and aromatization of the 3-methyltetrahydroquinoline ring in the liver. The formation of each of the 4 known metabolites is catalyzed in vitro by the human liver microsomal cytochrome P450 enzymes CYP3A4/5. The primary metabolite (M1) exerts 3- to 5-fold weaker anticoagulant effects than Argatroban. Unchanged Argatroban is the major component in plasma. The plasma concentrations of M1 range between 0% and 20% of that of the parent drug. The other metabolites (M2 to M4) are found only in very low quantities in the urine and have not been detected in plasma or feces. These data, together with the lack of effect of erythromycin (a potent CYP3A4/5 inhibitor) on Argatroban pharmacokinetics, suggest that CYP3A4/5-mediated metabolism is not an important elimination pathway in vivo.

Total body clearance is approximately 5.1 mL/kg/min (0.31 L/kg/hr) for infusion doses up to 40 mcg/kg/min. The terminal elimination half-life of Argatroban ranges between 39 and 51 minutes.

There is no interconversion of the 21–(R):21–(S) diastereoisomers. The plasma ratio of these diastereoisomers is unchanged by metabolism or hepatic impairment, remaining constant at 65:35 (± 2%).

Excretion: Argatroban is excreted primarily in the feces, presumably through biliary secretion. In a study in which ^{14}C-Argatroban (5 mcg/kg/min) was infused for 4 hours into healthy subjects, approximately 65% of the radioactivity was recovered in the feces within 6 days of the start of infusion with little or no radioactivity subsequently detected. Approximately 22% of the radioactivity appeared in the urine within 12 hours of the start of infusion. Little or no additional urinary radioactivity was subsequently detected. Average percent recovery of unchanged drug, relative to total dose, was 16% in urine and at least 14% in feces.

Pharmacokinetic/Pharmacodynamic Relationship: When Argatroban is administered by continuous infusion, anticoagulant effects and plasma concentrations of Argatroban follow similar, predictable temporal response profiles, with low intersubject variability. Immediately upon initiation of Argatroban infusion, anticoagulant effects are produced as plasma Argatroban concentrations begin to rise. Steady-state levels of both drug and anticoagulant effect are typically attained within 1 to 3 hours and are maintained until the infusion is discontinued or the dosage adjusted. Steady-state plasma Argatroban concentrations increase proportionally with dose (for infusion doses up to 40 mcg/kg/min in healthy subjects) and are well correlated with steady-state anticoagulant effects. For infusion doses up to 40 mcg/kg/min, Argatroban increases in a dose-dependent fashion, the activated partial thromboplastin time (aPTT), the activated clotting time (ACT), the prothrombin time (PT), the International Normalized Ratio (INR), and the thrombin time (TT) in healthy volunteers and cardiac patients. Representative steady-state plasma Argatroban concentrations and anticoagulant effects are shown below for Argatroban infusion doses up to 10 mcg/kg/min (see Figure 1).

Figure 1. Relationship at Steady State Between Argatroban Dose, Plasma Argatroban Concentration and Anticoagulant Effect

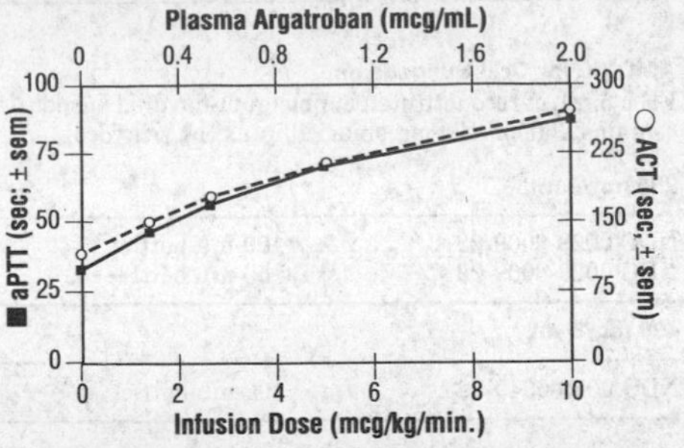

Effect on International Normalized Ratio (INR): Because Argatroban is a direct thrombin inhibitor, co-administration of Argatroban and warfarin produces a combined effect on the laboratory measurement of the INR. However, concurrent therapy, compared to warfarin monotherapy, exerts no additional effect on vitamin K–dependent factor Xa activity.

The relationship between INR on co-therapy and warfarin alone is dependent on both the dose of Argatroban and the thromboplastin reagent used. This relationship is influenced by the International Sensitivity Index (ISI) of the thromboplastin. Data for 2 commonly utilized thromboplastins with ISI values of 0.88 (Innovin, Dade) and 1.78 (Thromboplastin C Plus, Dade) are presented in Figure 2 for an Argatroban dose of 2 mcg/kg/min. Thromboplastins with higher ISI values than shown result in higher INRs on combined therapy of warfarin and Argatroban. These data are based on results obtained in normal individuals (see PRECAUTIONS, Drug Interactions and DOSAGE AND ADMINISTRATION, Conversion to Oral Anticoagulant Therapy).

Figure 2. INR Relationship of Argatroban Plus Warfarin Versus Warfarin Alone

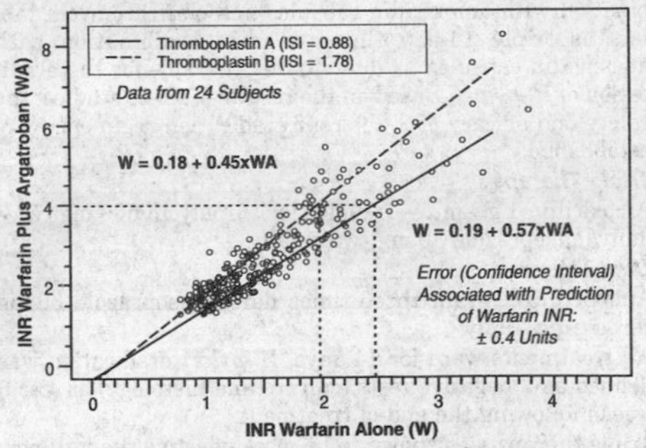

Figure 2 demonstrates the relationship between INR for warfarin alone and INR for warfarin co-administered with Argatroban at a dose of 2 mcg/kg/min. To calculate INR for warfarin alone (INR_W), based on INR for co-therapy of warfarin and Argatroban (INR_{WA}), when the Argatroban dose is 2 mcg/kg/min, use the equation next to the appropriate curve. Example: At a dose of 2 mcg/kg/min and an INR performed with Thromboplastin A, the equation 0.19 + 0.57 (INR_{WA}) = INR_W would allow a prediction of the INR on warfarin alone (INR_W). Thus, using an INR_{WA} value of 4.0 obtained on combined therapy: $INR_W = 0.19 + 0.57\ (4) = 2.47$ as the value for INR on warfarin alone. The error (confidence interval) associated with a prediction is ± 0.4 units. Similar linear relationships and prediction errors exist for Argatroban at a dose of 1 mcg/kg/min. Thus, for Argatroban doses of 1 or 2 mcg/kg/min, INR_W can be predicted from INR_{WA}. For Argatroban doses greater than 2 mcg/kg/min, the error associated with predicting INR_W from INR_{WA} is ± 1. Thus, INR_W cannot be reliably predicted from INR_{WA} at doses greater than 2 mcg/kg/min.

SPECIAL POPULATIONS

Renal Impairment: No dosage adjustment is necessary in patients with renal dysfunction. The effect of renal disease on the pharmacokinetics of Argatroban was studied in 6 subjects with normal renal function (mean Clcr = 95 ± 16 mL/min) and in 18 subjects with mild (mean Clcr = 64 ± 10 mL/min), moderate (mean Clcr = 41 ± 5.8 mL/min), and severe (mean Clcr = 5 ± 7 mL/min) renal impairment. The pharmacokinetics and pharmacodynamics of Argatroban at dosages up to 5 mcg/kg/min were not significantly affected by renal dysfunction.

Use of Argatroban was evaluated in a study of 12 patients with stable end-stage renal disease undergoing chronic intermittent hemodialysis. Argatroban was administered at a rate of 2 to 3 mcg/kg/min (begun at least 4 hours prior to dialysis) or as a bolus dose of 250 mcg/kg at the start of dialysis followed by a continuous infusion of 2 mcg/kg/min. Although these regimens did not achieve the goal of maintaining ACT values at 1.8 times the baseline value throughout most of the hemodialysis period, the hemodialysis sessions were successfully completed with both of these regimens. The mean ACTs produced in this study ranged from 1.39 to 1.82 times baseline, and the mean aPTTs ranged from 1.96 to 3.4 times baseline. When Argatroban was administered as a continuous infusion of 2 mcg/kg/min prior to and during a 4-hour hemodialysis session, approximately 20% was cleared through dialysis.

Hepatic Impairment: The dosage of Argatroban should be decreased in patients with hepatic impairment (see PRECAUTIONS and DOSAGE AND ADMINISTRATION). Patients with hepatic impairment were not studied in percutaneous coronary intervention (PCI) trials. At a dose of 2.5 mcg/kg/min, hepatic impairment is associated with decreased clearance and increased elimination half-life of Argatroban (to 1.9 mL/kg/min and 181 minutes, respectively, for patients with a Child-Pugh score >6).

Gender: Gender has not been shown to significantly affect Argatroban pharmacokinetics or pharmacodynamics (e.g., aPTT).

Age: ***Adult:*** Age has not been shown to significantly affect Argatroban pharmacokinetics or pharmacodynamics (e.g., aPTT).

Pediatric: Argatroban clearance is decreased in seriously ill pediatric patients. Pharmacokinetic parameters of Argatroban were characterized in a population pharmacokinetic/pharmacodynamic analysis with sparse data from 15 seriously ill pediatric patients. Clearance in pediatric patients (0.16 L/hr/kg) was 50% lower compared to healthy adults (0.31 L/hr/kg). Four pediatric patients with elevated bilirubin (secondary to cardiac complications or hepatic impairment) had, on average, 80% lower clearance (0.03 L/hr/kg) when compared to pediatric patients with normal bilirubin levels. (See PRECAUTIONS, Pediatric Use.)

Drug-Drug Interactions: ***Digoxin:*** In 12 healthy volunteers, intravenous infusion of Argatroban (2 mcg/kg/min) over 5 days (study days 11 to 15) did not affect the steady-state pharmacokinetics of oral digoxin (0.375 mg daily for 15 days).

Erythromycin: In 10 healthy subjects, orally administered erythromycin (a potent inhibitor of CYP3A4/5) at 500 mg four times daily for 7 days had no effect on the pharmacokinetics of Argatroban at a dose of 1 mcg/kg/min for 5 hours. These data suggest oxidative metabolism by CYP3A4/5 is not an important elimination pathway in vivo for Argatroban.

CLINICAL STUDIES

Heparin-Induced Thrombocytopenia: Heparin-induced thrombocytopenia (HIT) is a potentially serious, immune-mediated complication of heparin therapy that is strongly associated with subsequent venous and arterial thrombosis. Whereas initial treatment of HIT is to discontinue administration of all heparin, patients may require anticoagulation for prevention and treatment of thromboembolic events.

The conclusion that Argatroban is an effective treatment for heparin-induced thrombocytopenia (HIT) and heparin-induced thrombocytopenia and thrombosis syndrome (HITTS) is based upon the data from an historically controlled efficacy and safety study (Study 1) and a follow-on efficacy and safety study (Study 2). These studies were comparable with regard to study design, study objectives, dosing regimens as well as study outline, conduct, and monitoring.

In these studies, 568 adult patients were treated with Argatroban and 193 adult patients made up the historical control group. Patients were required to have a clinical diagnosis of heparin-induced thrombocytopenia, either without thrombosis (HIT) or with thrombosis (HITTS) and be males or non-pregnant females between the age of 18 and 80 years old. HIT/HITTS was defined by a fall in platelet count to less than 100,000/μL or a 50% decrease in platelets after the initiation of heparin therapy with no apparent explanation other than HIT. Patients with HITTS also had presence of an arterial or venous thrombosis documented by appropriate imaging techniques or supported by clinical evidence such as acute myocardial infarction, stroke, pulmonary embolism, or other clinical indications of vascular occlusion. Patients who required anticoagulation with documented histories of positive HIT antibody test were also eligible in the absence of thrombocytopenia or heparin challenge (e.g., patients with latent disease).

Patients with documented unexplained aPTT >200% of control at baseline, documented coagulation disorder or bleeding diathesis unrelated to HITTS, a lumbar puncture within the past 7 days or a history of previous aneurysm, hemorrhagic stroke, or recent thrombotic stroke, within the past 6 months, unrelated to HITTS were excluded from these studies.

The initial dose of Argatroban was 2 mcg/kg/min, not to exceed 10 mcg/kg/min. Two hours after the start of the Argatroban infusion, an aPTT level was obtained and dose adjustments were made to achieve a steady-state aPTT value that was 1.5 to 3.0 times the baseline value, not to exceed 100 seconds. In Study 1, the mean aPTT level for HIT patients was 38 seconds prior to start of Argatroban infusion. At first assessment,* during the Argatroban infusion, mean aPTT level for HIT patients was 64 seconds. Overall the mean aPTT level during the Argatroban infusion for HIT patients was 62.5 seconds. In Study 1, the mean aPTT level for HITTS patients was 34 seconds prior to start of Argatroban infusion. At first assessment,* during the Argatroban infusion, mean aPTT level for HITTS patients was 70 seconds. Overall, the mean aPTT level during the Argatroban infusion for HITTS patients was 64.5 seconds (see DOSAGE AND ADMINISTRATION). (*First assessment was defined as occurring at least 2 hours post-infusion start time.)

The primary efficacy analysis was based on a comparison of event rates for a composite endpoint that included death (all causes), amputation (all causes) or new thrombosis during the treatment and follow-up period (study days 0 to 37). Secondary analyses included evaluation of the event rates for the components of the composite endpoint as well as time-to-event analyses.

In Study 1, 304 patients were enrolled having active HIT (129/304, 42%), active HITTS (144/304, 47%), or latent disease (31/304, 10%). Among the 193 historical controls, 139 (72%) had active HIT, 46 (24%) had active HITTS, and 8 (4%) had latent disease. Within each group, those with active HIT and those with latent disease were analyzed together. Positive laboratory confirmation of HIT/HITTS by the heparin-induced platelet aggregation test or serotonin release assay was demonstrated in 174 of 304 (57%) Argatroban-treated patients (i.e., in 80 with HIT or latent disease and 94 with HITTS) and in 149 of 193 (77%) historical controls (i.e., in 119 with HIT or latent disease and 30 with HITTS). The test results for the remainder of the patients and controls were either negative or not determined.

A categorical analysis showed a significant improvement in the composite outcome in patients with HIT and HITTS treated with Argatroban versus those in the historical control group (see Table 1). The components of the composite endpoint are shown in Table 2.

[See table 1 at top right]
[See table 2 at right]

Table 1. Efficacy Results of Study 1: Composite Endpoint*

Parameter, N (%)	HIT Control n = 147	HIT Argatroban n = 160	HITTS Control n = 46	HITTS Argatroban n = 144	HIT/HITTS Control n = 193	HIT/HITTS Argatroban n = 304
Composite Endpoint	57 (38.8)	41 (25.6)	26 (56.5)	63 (43.8)	83 (43.0)	104 (34.2)

*Death (all causes), amputation (all causes), or new thrombosis within 37-day study period.

Table 2. Efficacy Results of Study 1: Components of the Composite Endpoint, Ranked by Severity*

Parameter, N (%)	HIT Control n = 147	HIT Argatroban n = 160	HITTS Control n = 46	HITTS Argatroban n = 144	HIT/HITTS Control n = 193	HIT/HITTS Argatroban n = 304
Death	32 (21.8)	27 (16.9)	13 (28.3)	26 (18.1)	45 (23.3)	53 (17.4)
Amputation	3 (2.0)	3 (1.9)	4 (8.7)	16 (11.1)	7 (3.6)	19 (6.2)
New Thrombosis	22 (15.0)	11 (6.9)	9 (19.6)	21 (14.6)	31 (16.1)	32 (10.5)

*Reported as the most severe outcome among the components of composite endpoint (severity ranking: death > amputation > new thrombosis); patients may have had multiple outcomes.

Time-to-event analyses showed significant improvements in the time-to-first event in patients with HIT or HITTS treated with Argatroban versus those in the historical control group. The between-group differences in the proportion of patients who remained free of death, amputation, or new thrombosis were statistically significant in favor of Argatroban by these analyses ($p = 0.007$ in patients with HIT and $p = 0.018$ in patients with HITTS, according to log-rank test).

A time-to-event analysis for the composite endpoint is shown in Figure 3 for patients with HIT and Figure 4 for patients with HITTS.

STUDY 1

Figure 3. Time-to-First Event for the Composite Efficacy Endpoint: HIT Patients

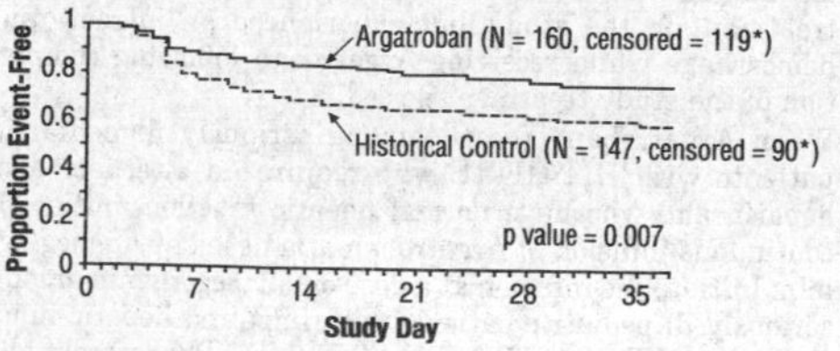

*Censored indicates no clinical endpoint (defined as death, amputation, or new thrombosis) was observed during the follow-up period (maximum period of follow-up was 37 days).

[See figure 4 at top of next column]

In Study 2, 264 patients were enrolled, having either HIT (125/264, 47.3%) or HITTS (139/264, 52.7%), and then treated with Argatroban. Categorical analysis demonstrated significant improvement in the composite efficacy outcome for Argatroban-treated patients, versus the same historical control group from Study 1, among patients having HIT (25.6% vs. 38.8%), patients having HITTS (41.0% vs. 56.5%), and patients having either HIT or HITTS (33.7% vs. 43.0%). Time-to-event analyses showed significant improvements in the time-to-first event in patients with HIT or HITTS treated with Argatroban versus those in the historical control group. The between-group differences in the proportion of patients who remained free of death, amputation, or new thrombosis were statistically significant in favor of Argatroban.

STUDY 1

Figure 4. Time-to-First Event for the Composite Efficacy Endpoint: HITTS Patients

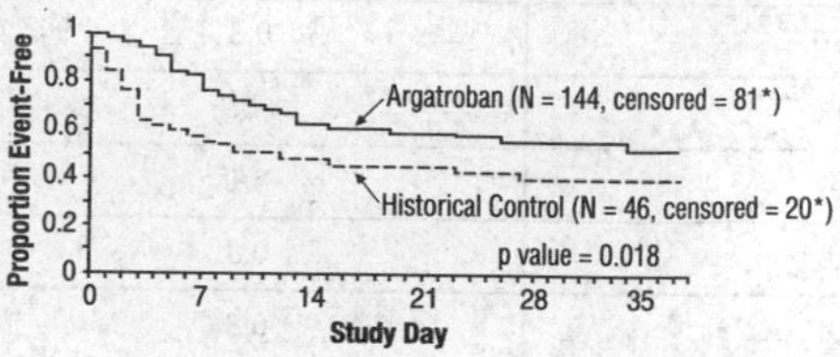

*Censored indicates no clinical endpoint (defined as death, amputation, or new thrombosis) was observed during the follow-up period (maximum period of follow-up was 37 days).

Anticoagulant Effect: In Study 1, the mean (± SE) dose of Argatroban administered was 2.0 ± 0.1 mcg/kg/min in the HIT arm and 1.9 ± 0.1 mcg/kg/min in the HITTS arm. Seventy-six percent of patients with HIT and 81% of patients with HITTS achieved a target aPTT at least 1.5-fold greater than the baseline aPTT at the first assessment occurring on average at 4.6 hours (HIT) and 3.9 hours (HITTS) following initiation of Argatroban therapy.

No enhancement of aPTT response was observed in subjects receiving repeated administration of Argatroban.

Platelet Count Recovery: In Study 1, the majority of patients, 53% of those with HIT and 58% of those with HITTS, had a recovery of platelet count by day 3. Platelet Count Recovery was defined as an increase in platelet count to >100,000/μL or to at least 1.5-fold greater than the baseline count (platelet count at study initiation) by day 3 of the study.

Percutaneous Coronary Intervention (PCI) in HIT/HITTS Patients: In 3 similarly designed trials, Argatroban was administered to 91 patients with current or previous clinical diagnosis of HIT/HITTS or heparin-dependent antibodies, who underwent a total of 112 percutaneous coronary interventions (PCIs) including percutaneous transluminal coronary angioplasty (PTCA), coronary stent placement, or atherectomy.

Among the 91 patients undergoing their first PCI with Argatroban, notable ongoing or recent medical history included myocardial infarction (n = 35), unstable angina (n = 23), and chronic angina (n = 34). There were 33 females and 58 males. The average age was 67.6 years (median 70.7, range 44 to 86), and the average weight was 82.5 kg (median 81.0 kg, range 49 to 141).

Due to the history or presence of the heparin-dependent antibody or HIT/HITTS, these patients required alternative anticoagulation. Twenty-one of the 91 patients had a repeat PCI using Argatroban an average of 150 days after their initial PCI. Seven of 91 patients received glycoprotein IIb/IIIa inhibitors. Safety and efficacy were assessed against historical control populations.

Per protocol, all patients received oral aspirin (325 mg) 2 to 24 hours prior to the interventional procedure. After venous or arterial sheaths were in place, anticoagulation was initiated with a bolus of Argatroban of 350 mcg/kg via a large-bore IV line or through the venous sheath over 3 to 5 minutes. Simultaneously, a maintenance infusion of 25 mcg/kg/min was initiated to achieve a therapeutic activated clotting time (ACT) of 300 to 450 seconds. If necessary to achieve this therapeutic range, the maintenance infusion dose was titrated (15 to 40 mcg/kg/min) and/or an additional bolus dose of 150 mcg/kg could be given. Each patient's ACT was checked 5 to 10 minutes following the bolus dose. The ACT was checked as clinically indicated thereafter. Arterial and venous sheaths were removed no sooner than 2 hours after discontinuation of Argatroban and when the ACT was less than 160 seconds.

If a patient required anticoagulation after the procedure, Argatroban could be continued, but at a lower infusion dose between 2.5 and 5 mcg/kg/min. An aPTT was drawn 2 hours after this dose reduction and the dose of Argatroban then adjusted as clinically indicated (not to exceed 10 mcg/kg/min), to reach an aPTT between 1.5 and 3 times baseline value (not to exceed 100 seconds).

Ninety-one patients were treated with Argatroban on their first PCI, and 21 patients were reexposed to Argatroban on subsequent PCIs. In 92 of the 112 interventions (82%), the patient received the initial bolus of 350 mcg/kg and an initial infusion dose of 25 mcg/kg/min. The majority of patients did not require additional bolus dosing during the PCI procedure. The mean value for the initial ACT measurement after the start of dosing for all interventions was 379 sec (median 338 sec; 5th percentile-95th percentile 238 to 675 sec). The mean ACT value per intervention over all measurements taken during the procedure was 416 sec (median 390 sec; 5th percentile-95th percentile 261 to 698 sec). About 65% of patients had ACTs within the recommended range of 300 to 450 seconds throughout the procedure. The investigators did not achieve anticoagulation within the recommended range in about 23% of patients. However, in this small sample, patients with ACTs below 300 seconds did not have more coronary thrombotic events, and patients with ACTs over 450 seconds did not have higher bleeding rates.

Acute procedural success was defined as lack of death, emergent coronary artery bypass graft (CABG), or Q-wave myocardial infarction. Acute procedural success was reported in 98.2% of patients who underwent PCIs with Argatroban anticoagulation compared with 94.3% of historical control patients anticoagulated with heparin (p = NS). Among the 112 interventions, 2 patients had emergency CABGs, 3 had repeat PTCAs, 4 had non-Q-wave myocardial infarctions, 3 had myocardial ischemia, 1 had an abrupt closure, and 1 had an impending closure (some patients may have experienced more than 1 event). No patients died. Two patients had protocol-defined major bleeding, 1 of which was retroperitoneal and the other gastrointestinal. Minor bleeding, defined as spontaneous and observed with hemoglobin decreasing >3g/dL or with no bleeding site and hemoglobin decreasing >4g/dL, occurred in 4.5% of interventions.

Additional Information: ***Cardiac Therapy:*** The safety and effectiveness of Argatroban for cardiac indications outside of percutaneous coronary intervention in patients with HIT have not been established.

Reexposure and Lack of Antibody Formation: Plasma from 12 healthy volunteers treated with Argatroban over 6 days showed no evidence of neutralizing antibodies. Repeated administration of Argatroban to more than 40 patients was tolerated with no loss of anticoagulant activity. No change in the dose is required.

INDICATIONS AND USAGE

Argatroban is indicated as an anticoagulant for prophylaxis or treatment of thrombosis in patients with heparin-induced thrombocytopenia.

Table 3. Major and Minor Hemorrhagic Adverse Events in HIT/HITTS Patients

Major Hemorrhagic Events*

	Argatroban-treated Patients (Study 1 and Study 2) (n = 568) %	Historical Control (n = 193) %
Overall bleeding	5.3	6.7
Gastrointestinal	2.3	1.6
Genitourinary and hematuria	0.9	0.5
Decrease in hemoglobin and hematocrit	0.7	0
Multisystem hemorrhage and DIC	0.5	1
Limb and BKA stump	0.5	0
Intracranial hemorrhage	0[†]	0.5

Minor Hemorrhagic Events*

	Argatroban-treated Patients (Study 1 and Study 2) (n = 568) %	Historical Control (n = 193) %
Gastrointestinal	14.4	18.1
Genitourinary and hematuria	11.6	0.8
Decrease in hemoglobin and hematocrit	10.4	0
Groin	5.4	3.1
Hemoptysis	2.9	0.8
Brachial	2.4	0.8

* Patients may have experienced more than 1 adverse event.
† One patient experienced intracranial hemorrhage 4 days after discontinuation of Argatroban and following therapy with urokinase and oral anticoagulation.
DIC = disseminated intravascular coagulation.
BKA = below-the-knee amputation.

Argatroban is indicated as an anticoagulant in patients with or at risk for heparin-induced thrombocytopenia undergoing percutaneous coronary intervention (PCI).

CONTRAINDICATIONS
Argatroban is contraindicated in patients with overt major bleeding, or in patients hypersensitive to this product or any of its components (see WARNINGS).

WARNINGS
Argatroban is intended for intravenous administration. All parenteral anticoagulants should be discontinued before administration of Argatroban.
Hemorrhage: Hemorrhage can occur at any site in the body in patients receiving Argatroban. An unexplained fall in hematocrit, a fall in blood pressure, or any other unexplained symptom should lead to consideration of a hemorrhagic event. Argatroban should be used with extreme caution in disease states and other circumstances in which there is an increased danger of hemorrhage. These include severe hypertension; immediately following lumbar puncture; spinal anesthesia; major surgery, especially involving the brain, spinal cord, or eye; hematologic conditions associated with increased bleeding tendencies such as congenital or acquired bleeding disorders and gastrointestinal lesions such as ulcerations.

PRECAUTIONS
Hepatic Impairment: Caution should be exercised when administering Argatroban to patients with hepatic impairment by starting with a lower dose and carefully titrating until the desired level of anticoagulation is achieved. Achievement of steady state aPTT levels may take longer and require more Argatroban dose adjustments in patients with hepatic impairment compared to patients with normal hepatic function (see PRECAUTIONS, Pediatric Use). Also, upon cessation of Argatroban infusion in the hepatically impaired patient, full reversal of anticoagulant effects may require longer than 4 hours due to decreased clearance and increased elimination half-life of Argatroban (see DOSAGE AND ADMINISTRATION). Use of high doses of Argatroban in PCI patients with clinically significant hepatic disease or AST/ALT levels ≥3 times the upper limit of normal should be avoided. Such patients were not studied in PCI trials.
Laboratory Tests: Anticoagulation effects associated with Argatroban infusion at doses up to 40 mcg/kg/min correlate with increases of the activated partial thromboplastin time (aPTT).

Although other global clot-based tests including prothrombin time (PT), the International Normalized Ratio (INR), and thrombin time (TT) are affected by Argatroban, the therapeutic ranges for these tests have not been identified for Argatroban therapy. Plasma Argatroban concentrations also correlate well with anticoagulant effects (see CLINICAL PHARMACOLOGY).
In clinical trials in PCI, the activated clotting time (ACT) was used for monitoring Argatroban anticoagulant activity during the procedure.
The concomitant use of Argatroban and warfarin results in prolongation of the PT and INR beyond that produced by warfarin alone. Alternative approaches for monitoring concurrent Argatroban and warfarin therapy are described in a subsequent section (see DOSAGE AND ADMINISTRATION).
Drug Interactions: **Heparin:** Since heparin is contraindicated in patients with heparin-induced thrombocytopenia, the co-administration of Argatroban and heparin is unlikely for this indication. However, if Argatroban is to be initiated after cessation of heparin therapy, allow sufficient time for heparin's effect on the aPTT to decrease prior to initiation of Argatroban therapy.
Aspirin/Acetaminophen: Pharmacokinetic or pharmacodynamic drug-drug interactions have not been demonstrated between Argatroban and concomitantly administered aspirin (162.5 mg orally given 26 and 2 hours prior to initiation of Argatroban 1 mcg/kg/min over 4 hours) or acetaminophen (1,000 mg orally given 12, 6, and 0 hours prior to, and 6 and 12 hours subsequent to, initiation of Argatroban 1.5 mcg/kg/min over 18 hours).
Oral Anticoagulant Agents: Pharmacokinetic drug-drug interactions between Argatroban and warfarin (7.5 mg single oral dose) have not been demonstrated. However, the concomitant use of Argatroban and warfarin (5 to 7.5 mg initial oral dose, followed by 2.5 to 6 mg/day orally for 6 to 10 days) results in prolongation of the prothrombin time (PT) and International Normalized Ratio (INR) (see CLINICAL PHARMACOLOGY and DOSAGE AND ADMINISTRATION).
Thrombolytic Agents: The safety and effectiveness of Argatroban with thrombolytic agents have not been established (see ADVERSE REACTIONS, *Intracranial Bleeding*).
Glycoprotein IIb/IIIa Antagonists: The safety and effectiveness of Argatroban with glycoprotein IIb/IIIa antagonists have not been established.

Co-Administration: Concomitant use of Argatroban with antiplatelet agents, thrombolytics, and other anticoagulants may increase the risk of bleeding (see WARNINGS). Drug-drug interactions have not been observed between Argatroban and digoxin or erythromycin (see CLINICAL PHARMACOLOGY, Drug-Drug Interactions).
Carcinogenesis, Mutagenesis, Impairment of Fertility: No long-term studies in animals have been performed to evaluate the carcinogenic potential of Argatroban.
Argatroban was not genotoxic in the Ames test, the Chinese hamster ovary cell (CHO/HGPRT) forward mutation test, the Chinese hamster lung fibroblast chromosome aberration test, the rat hepatocyte, and WI-38 human fetal lung cell unscheduled DNA synthesis (UDS) tests, or the mouse micronucleus test.
Argatroban at intravenous doses up to 27 mg/kg/day (0.3 times the recommended maximum human dose based on body surface area) was found to have no effect on fertility and reproductive performance of male and female rats.
Pregnancy: *Teratogenic Effects:* Pregnancy Category B. Teratology studies have been performed in rats with intravenous doses up to 27 mg/kg/day (0.3 times the recommended maximum human dose based on body surface area) and rabbits at intravenous doses up to 10.8 mg/kg/day (0.2 times the recommended maximum human dose based on body surface area) and have revealed no evidence of impaired fertility or harm to the fetus due to Argatroban. There are, however, no adequate and well-controlled studies in pregnant women. Because animal reproduction studies are not always predictive of human response, this drug should be used during pregnancy only if clearly needed.
Nursing Mothers: Experiments in rats show that Argatroban is detected in milk. It is not known whether this drug is excreted in human milk. Because many drugs are excreted in human milk and because of the potential for serious adverse reactions in nursing infants from Argatroban, a decision should be made whether to discontinue nursing or to discontinue the drug, taking into account the importance of the drug to the mother.
Geriatric Use: In the clinical studies of adult patients with HIT or HITTS, the effectiveness of Argatroban was not affected by age.
Pediatric Use: The safety and effectiveness of Argatroban, including the appropriate anticoagulation goals and duration of therapy, have not been established among pediatric patients.
Argatroban was studied among 18 seriously ill pediatric patients who required an alternative to heparin anticoagulation. Most patients were diagnosed with HIT or suspected HIT. Age ranges of patients were <6 months, n = 8; six months to <8 years, n = 6; 8 to 16 years, n = 4. All patients had serious underlying conditions and were receiving multiple concomitant medications. Thirteen patients received Argatroban solely as a continuous infusion (no bolus dose). Dosing was initiated in the majority of these 13 patients at 1 mcg/kg/min. Dosing was titrated as needed to achieve and maintain an aPTT of 1.5 to 3 times the baseline value. Most patients required multiple dose adjustments to maintain anticoagulation parameters within the desired range. During the 30-day study period, thrombotic events occurred during Argatroban administration to two patients and following Argatroban discontinuation in three other patients. Major bleeding occurred among two patients; one patient experienced an intracranial hemorrhage after 4 days of Argatroban therapy in the setting of sepsis and thrombocytopenia. Another patient completed 14 days of Argatroban treatment in the study, but experienced an intracranial hemorrhage while receiving Argatroban following completion of the study treatment period.
When Argatroban is used among seriously ill pediatric patients with HIT/HITTS who require an alternative to heparin and who have normal hepatic function, initiate a continuous infusion of Argatroban at a dose of 0.75 mcg/kg/min. Initiate the infusion at a dose of 0.2 mcg/kg/min among seriously ill pediatric patients with impaired hepatic function (see CLINICAL PHARMACOLOGY, Pharmacokinetics). Check the aPTT two hours after the initiation of the Argatroban infusion and adjust the dose to achieve the target aPTT. These dose recommendations are based upon a goal of aPTT prolongation of 1.5 to 3 times the baseline value and avoidance of an aPTT >100 seconds. Increments of 0.1 to 0.25 mcg/kg/min for pediatric patients with normal hepatic function and increments of 0.05 mcg/kg/min or lower for pediatric patients with impaired hepatic function may be considered but dose selection must take into account multiple factors including the current Argatroban dose, the current aPTT, target aPTT, and the clinical status of the patient. These dose recommendations are based upon a goal of aPTT prolongation of 1.5 to 3 times the baseline value and avoidance of an aPTT >100 seconds.

ADVERSE REACTIONS
Adverse Events Reported in HIT/HITTS Patients: The following safety information is based on all 568 patients

treated with Argatroban in Study 1 and Study 2. The safety profile of the patients from these studies is compared with that of 193 historical controls in which the adverse events were collected retrospectively. The adverse events reported in this section include all events regardless of relationship to treatment. Adverse events are separated into hemorrhagic and non-hemorrhagic events.

Major bleeding was defined as bleeding that was overt and associated with a hemoglobin decrease ≥2 g/dL, that led to a transfusion of ≥2 units, or that was intracranial, retroperitoneal, or into a major prosthetic joint. Minor bleeding was overt bleeding that did not meet the criteria for major bleeding.

Table 3 gives an overview of the most frequently observed hemorrhagic events, presented separately by major and minor bleeding, sorted by decreasing occurrence among Argatroban-treated HIT/HITTS patients.

[See table 3 at top of previous page]

Table 4 gives an overview of the most frequently observed non-hemorrhagic events sorted by decreasing frequency of occurrence (≥2%) among Argatroban-treated HIT/HITTS patients.

[See table 4 at right]

Adverse Events Reported in HIT/HITTS Patients Undergoing PCI: The following safety information is based on 91 patients initially treated with Argatroban and 21 patients subsequently re-exposed to Argatroban for a total of 112 PCIs with Argatroban anticoagulation. The adverse events reported in this section include all events regardless of relationship to treatment. Adverse events are separated into hemorrhagic (Table 5) and non-hemorrhagic (Table 6) events.

Major bleeding was defined as bleeding that was overt and associated with a hemoglobin decrease ≥5 g/dL, that led to a transfusion of ≥2 units, or that was intracranial, retroperitoneal, or into a major prosthetic joint.

The rate of major bleeding events and intracranial hemorrhage in the PCI trials was 1.8% and in the placebo arm of the EPILOG trial (placebo plus standard dose, weight-adjusted heparin) was 3.1%.

Table 4. Non-hemorrhagic Adverse Events in HIT/HITTS Patients*

	Argatroban-treated Patients (Study 1 and Study 2) (n = 568) %	Historical Control (n = 193) %
Dyspnea	8.1	8.8
Hypotension	7.2	2.6
Fever	6.9	2.1
Diarrhea	6.2	1.6
Sepsis	6.0	12.4
Cardiac arrest	5.8	3.1
Nausea	4.8	0.5
Ventricular tachycardia	4.8	3.1
Pain	4.6	3.1
Urinary tract infection	4.6	5.2
Vomiting	4.2	0
Infection	3.7	3.6
Pneumonia	3.3	9.3
Atrial fibrillation	3.0	11.4
Coughing	2.8	1.6
Abnormal renal function	2.8	4.7
Abdominal pain	2.6	1.6
Cerebrovascular disorder	2.3	4.1

*Patients may have experienced more than 1 adverse event.

Table 5. Major and Minor Hemorrhagic Adverse Events in HIT/HITTS Patients Undergoing PCI

Major Hemorrhagic Events*	Argatroban-treated Patients (n = 112)[†] %
Retroperitoneal	0.9
Gastrointestinal	0.9
Intracranial	0

Minor Hemorrhagic Events*	Argatroban-treated Patients (n = 112)[†] %
Groin (bleeding or hematoma)	3.6
Gastrointestinal (includes hematemesis)	2.6
Genitourinary (includes hematuria)	1.8
Decrease in hemoglobin and/or hematocrit	1.8
CABG (coronary arteries)	1.8
Access site	0.9
Hemoptysis	0.9
Other	0.9

* Patients may have experienced more than 1 adverse event.
[†] 91 patients who underwent 112 interventions.
CABG = coronary artery bypass graft.

Table 6 gives an overview of the most frequently observed non-hemorrhagic events (>2%), sorted by decreasing frequency of occurrence among Argatroban-treated PCI patients.

Table 6. Non-hemorrhagic Adverse Events* in HIT/HITTS Patients Undergoing PCI

	Argatroban Procedures* (n = 112)[†] %	Controls (n = 2226)[‡] %
Chest pain	15.2	9.3
Hypotension	10.7	10.3
Back pain	8.0	13.7
Nausea	7.1	11.5
Vomiting	6.3	6.8
Headache	5.4	5.5
Bradycardia	4.5	3.5
Abdominal pain	3.6	2.2
Fever	3.6	<0.5
Myocardial infarction	3.6	NR[§]

* Patients may have experienced more than 1 adverse event.

[†] 91 patients who underwent 112 interventions.

[‡] Controls from EPIC (Evaluation of c7E3 Fab in the Prevention of Ischemic Complications), EPILOG (Evaluation in PTCA to Improve Long-Term Outcome with Abciximab GP IIb/IIIa Blockade Study) and CAPTURE (Chimeric 7E3 Antiplatelet Therapy in Unstable angina Refractory to standard treatment) trials. Source: ReoPro® Prescribing Information.

[§] NR = not reported.

There were 22 serious adverse events in 17 PCI patients (19.6% in 112 interventions). The types of events, which are listed regardless of relationship to treatment, are shown in Table 7. Table 7 lists the serious adverse events occurring in Argatroban-treated HIT/HITTS patients undergoing PCI.

Table 7. Serious Adverse Events in HIT/HITTS Patients Undergoing PCI*

Coded Term	Argatroban Procedures[†] (n = 112)
Chest pain	1 (0.9%)
Fever	1 (0.9%)
Retroperitoneal hemorrhage	1 (0.9%)
Angina pectoris	2 (1.8%)
Aortic stenosis	1 (0.9%)
Coronary thrombosis	2 (1.8%)
Arterial thrombosis	1 (0.9%)
Myocardial infarction	4 (3.5%)
Myocardial ischemia	2 (1.8%)
Occlusion coronary	2 (1.8%)
Gastrointestinal hemorrhage	1 (0.9%)
Gastrointestinal disorder (GERD)	1 (0.9%)
Cerebrovascular disorder	1 (0.9%)
Lung edema	1 (0.9%)
Vascular disorder	1 (0.9%)

* Individual events may also have been reported elsewhere (see Table 5 and 6).

[†] 91 patients underwent 112 procedures. Some patients may have experienced more than 1 event.

Adverse Events Reported in Other Populations: *Intracranial Bleeding:* The overall frequency of intracranial bleeding among patients with acute myocardial infarction receiving both Argatroban and thrombolytic therapy (streptokinase or tissue plasminogen activator) was 1% (8 out of

810 patients). Intracranial bleeding was not observed in 317 subjects or patients who did not receive concomitant thrombolysis (see PRECAUTIONS, Drug Interactions).

Intracranial bleeding was also observed in a prospective, placebo-controlled study of Argatroban in patients who had onset of acute stroke within 12 hours of study entry. Symptomatic intracranial hemorrhage was reported in 5 of 117 patients (4.3%) who received Argatroban at 1.0 to 3.0 mcg/kg/min and in none of the 54 patients who received placebo. Asymptomatic intracranial hemorrhage occurred in 5 (4.3%) and 2 (3.7%) of the patients, respectively.

Allergic Reactions: 156 allergic reactions or suspected allergic reactions were observed in 1,127 individuals who were treated with Argatroban in clinical pharmacology studies or for various clinical indications. About 95% (148/156) of these reactions occurred in patients who concomitantly received thrombolytic therapy (e.g., streptokinase) for acute myocardial infarction and/or contrast media for coronary angiography.

Allergic reactions or suspected allergic reactions in populations other than HIT/HITTS patients include (in descending order of frequency*):
• Airway reactions (coughing, dyspnea): 10% or more
• Skin reactions (rash, bullous eruption): 1 to <10%
• General reactions (vasodilation): 1 to 10%
*The CIOMS (Council for International Organization of Medical Sciences) III standard categories are used for classification of frequencies.

OVERDOSAGE

Symptoms/Treatment: Excessive anticoagulation, with or without bleeding, may be controlled by discontinuing Argatroban or by decreasing the Argatroban infusion dosage (see WARNINGS). In clinical studies at therapeutic levels, anticoagulation parameters generally return to baseline within 2 to 4 hours after discontinuation of the drug. Reversal of anticoagulant effect may take longer in patients with hepatic impairment.

No specific antidote to Argatroban is available; if life-threatening bleeding occurs and excessive plasma levels of Argatroban are suspected, Argatroban should be discontinued immediately, aPTT and other coagulation tests should be determined. Symptomatic and supportive therapy should be provided to the patient (see WARNINGS). When Argatroban was administered as a continuous infusion (2 mcg/kg/min) prior to and during a 4-hour hemodialysis session, approximately 20% of Argatroban was cleared through dialysis.

Single intravenous doses of Argatroban at 200, 124, 150, and 200 mg/kg were lethal to mice, rats, rabbits, and dogs, respectively. The symptoms of acute toxicity were loss of righting reflex, tremors, clonic convulsions, paralysis of hind limbs, and coma.

DOSAGE AND ADMINISTRATION

Each 2.5-mL vial contains 250 mg of Argatroban; and, as supplied, is a concentrated drug (100 mg/mL), which must be diluted 100-fold prior to infusion. Argatroban should not be mixed with other drugs prior to dilution in a suitable intravenous fluid.

Preparation for Intravenous Administration: Argatroban should be diluted in 0.9% Sodium Chloride Injection, 5% Dextrose Injection, or Lactated Ringer's Injection to a final concentration of 1 mg/mL. The contents of each 2.5-mL vial should be diluted 100-fold by mixing with 250 mL of diluent. Use 250 mg (2.5 mL) per 250 mL of diluent or 500 mg (5 mL) per 500 mL of diluent. The constituted solution must be mixed by repeated inversion of the diluent bag for 1 minute. Upon preparation, the solution may show slight but brief haziness due to the formation of microprecipitates that rapidly dissolve upon mixing. The pH of the intravenous solution prepared as recommended is 3.2 to 7.5.

Heparin-Induced Thrombocytopenia (HIT/HITTS): *Initial Dosage:* Before administering Argatroban, discontinue heparin therapy and obtain a baseline aPTT. The recommended initial dose of Argatroban for adult patients without hepatic impairment is 2 mcg/kg/min, administered as a continuous infusion (see Table 8).

Table 8. Recommended Doses and Infusion Rates for 2 mcg/kg/min Dose of Argatroban for Patients With HIT/HITTS (Without Hepatic Impairment) (1 mg/mL Final Concentration)

Body Weight (kg)	Dose (mcg/min)	Infusion Rate (mL/hr)
50	100	6
60	120	7
70	140	8
80	160	10
90	180	11
100	200	12
110	220	13
120	240	14
130	260	16
140	280	17

Monitoring Therapy: In general, therapy with Argatroban is monitored using the aPTT. Tests of anticoagulant effects (including the aPTT) typically attain steady-state levels within one to three hours following initiation of Argatroban. Dose adjustment may be required to attain the target aPTT. Check the aPTT two hours after initiation of therapy and any dose change to confirm that the patient has attained the desired therapeutic range.

Dosage Adjustment: After the initial dose of Argatroban, the dose can be adjusted as clinically indicated (not to exceed 10 mcg/kg/min), until the steady-state aPTT is 1.5 to 3 times the initial baseline value (not to exceed 100 seconds) (see CLINICAL STUDIES for mean values of aPTT obtained after initial doses of Argatroban).

Percutaneous Coronary Interventions (PCI) in HIT/HITTS Patients: *Initial Dosage:* An infusion of Argatroban should be started at 25 mcg/kg/min and a bolus of 350 mcg/kg administered via a large bore intravenous (IV) line over 3 to 5 minutes (see Table 9). Activated clotting time (ACT) should be checked 5 to 10 minutes after the bolus dose is completed. The procedure may proceed if the ACT is greater than 300 seconds.

Dosage Adjustment: If the ACT is less than 300 seconds, an additional IV bolus dose of 150 mcg/kg should be administered, the infusion dose increased to 30 mcg/kg/min, and the ACT checked 5 to 10 minutes later (see Table 9). If the ACT is greater than 450 seconds, the infusion rate should be decreased to 15 mcg/kg/min, and the ACT checked 5 to 10 minutes later (see Table 9). Once a therapeutic ACT (between 300 and 450 seconds) has been achieved, this infusion dose should be continued for the duration of the procedure. [See table 9 below]

In case of dissection, impending abrupt closure, thrombus formation during the procedure, or inability to achieve or maintain an ACT over 300 seconds, additional bolus doses of 150 mcg/kg may be administered and the infusion dose increased to 40 mcg/kg/min. The ACT should be checked after each additional bolus or change in the rate of infusion.

Monitoring therapy: Therapy with Argatroban is monitored using ACT. ACTs should be obtained before dosing, 5 to 10 minutes after bolus dosing and after change in the infusion rate, and at the end of the PCI procedure. Additional ACTs should be drawn about every 20 to 30 minutes during a prolonged procedure.

Continued Anticoagulation after PCI: If a patient requires anticoagulation after the procedure, Argatroban may be continued, but at a lower infusion dose [see DOSAGE AND ADMINISTRATION, Heparin-Induced Thrombocytopenia (HIT/HITTS)].

Dosing in Special Populations: *Hepatic Impairment:* For adult patients with heparin-induced thrombocytopenia with hepatic impairment, the initial dose of Argatroban should be reduced. For adult patients with moderate hepatic impairment, an initial dose of 0.5 mcg/kg/min is recommended, based on the approximate 4-fold decrease in Argatroban clearance relative to those with normal hepatic function. The aPTT should be monitored closely, and the dosage should be adjusted as clinically indicated (see PRECAUTIONS).

Hepatic Impairment in HIT/HITTS Patients Undergoing PCI: Carefully titrate Argatroban until the desired level of anticoagulation is achieved (see PRECAUTIONS, Hepatic Impairment).

Renal Impairment: No dosage adjustment is necessary in patients with renal impairment (see SPECIAL POPULATIONS, Renal Impairment).

Pediatric HIT/HITTS Patients: Initial Argatroban infusion doses are lower for seriously ill pediatric patients compared to adults with normal hepatic function (see PRECAUTIONS, Pediatric Use).

Monitoring Therapy: In general, therapy with Argatroban is monitored using the aPTT. Tests of anticoagulant effects (including the aPTT) typically attain steady-state levels within one to three hours following initiation of Argatroban in patients without hepatic impairment (see PRECAUTIONS, Hepatic Impairment). Dose adjustment may be required to attain the target aPTT. Check the aPTT two hours after initiation of therapy and after any dose change to confirm that the patient has attained the desired therapeutic range.

Dosage Adjustment: See PRECAUTIONS, Pediatric Use.

CONVERSION TO ORAL ANTICOAGULANT THERAPY

Initiating Oral Anticoagulant Therapy: Once the decision is made to initiate oral anticoagulant therapy, recognize the potential for combined effects on INR with co-administration of Argatroban and warfarin. A loading dose of warfarin should not be used. Initiate therapy using the expected daily dose of warfarin. To avoid prothrombotic effects and to ensure continuous anticoagulation when initiating warfarin, it is suggested that Argatroban and warfarin therapy be overlapped. There are insufficient data available to recommend the duration of the overlap.

Co-Administration of Warfarin and Argatroban at Doses Up to 2 mcg/kg/min: Use of Argatroban with warfarin results in prolongation of INR beyond that produced by warfarin alone. To avoid prothrombotic effects and to ensure continuous anticoagulation when initiating warfarin, it is suggested that warfarin be co-administered before discontinuing Argatroban. There are insufficient data available to recommend the duration of the co-administration. The previously established relationship between INR and bleeding risk is altered. The combination of Argatroban and warfarin does not cause further reduction in the vitamin K–dependent factor Xa activity than that which is seen with warfarin alone. The relationship between INR obtained on

Table 9. Recommended Doses and Infusion Rates of Argatroban for Patients Undergoing PCI (Without Hepatic Impairment) (1 mg/mL Final Concentration)

Body Weight (kg)	For ACT 300-450 seconds Initial Dosage* 25 mcg/kg/min			If ACT <300 seconds Dosage Adjustment† 30 mcg/kg/min			If ACT >450 seconds Dosage Adjustment 15 mcg/kg/min	
	Bolus Dose (mcg)	Infusion Dose (mcg/min)	Infusion Rate (mL/hr)	Bolus Dose (mcg)	Infusion Dose (mcg/min)	Infusion Rate (mL/hr)	Infusion Dose (mcg/min)	Infusion Rate (mL/hr)
50	17500	1250	75	7500	1500	90	750	45
60	21000	1500	90	9000	1800	108	900	54
70	24500	1750	105	10500	2100	126	1050	63
80	28000	2000	120	12000	2400	144	1200	72
90	31500	2250	135	13500	2700	162	1350	81
100	35000	2500	150	15000	3000	180	1500	90
110	38500	2750	165	16500	3300	198	1650	99
120	42000	3000	180	18000	3600	216	1800	108
130	45500	3250	195	19500	3900	234	1950	117
140	49000	3500	210	21000	4200	252	2100	126

NOTE: 1 mg = 1000 mcg; 1 kg = 2.2 lbs
* Initial IV bolus dose of 350 mcg/kg should be administered.
† Additional IV bolus dose of 150 mcg/kg should be administered if ACT <300 seconds.

combined therapy and INR obtained on warfarin alone is dependent on both the dose of Argatroban and the thromboplastin reagent used. The INR value on warfarin alone (INR$_W$) can be calculated from the INR value on combination Argatroban and warfarin therapy (see CLINICAL PHARMACOLOGY, Figure 2 explanation and PRECAUTIONS, Drug Interactions).

INR should be measured daily while Argatroban and warfarin are co-administered. In general, with doses of Argatroban up to 2 mcg/kg/min, Argatroban can be discontinued when the INR is >4 on combined therapy. After Argatroban is discontinued, repeat the INR measurement in 4 to 6 hours. If the repeat INR is below the desired therapeutic range, resume the infusion of Argatroban and repeat the procedure daily until the desired therapeutic range on warfarin alone is reached.

Co-Administration of Warfarin and Argatroban at Doses Greater than 2 mcg/kg/min: For doses greater than 2 mcg/kg/min, the relationship of INR between warfarin alone to the INR on warfarin plus Argatroban is less predictable. In this case, in order to predict the INR on warfarin alone, temporarily reduce the dose of Argatroban to a dose of 2 mcg/kg/min. Repeat the INR on Argatroban and warfarin 4 to 6 hours after reduction of the Argatroban dose and follow the process outlined above for administering Argatroban at doses up to 2 mcg/kg/min.

STABILITY/COMPATIBILITY

Argatroban is a clear, colorless to pale yellow, slightly viscous solution. If the solution is cloudy, or if an insoluble precipitate is noted, the vial should be discarded.

Solutions prepared as recommended are stable at 25°C (77°F), with excursions permitted to 15° to 30°C (59° to 86°F) in ambient indoor light for 24 hours; therefore, light-resistant measures such as foil protection for intravenous lines are unnecessary. Solutions are physically and chemically stable for up to 96 hours when protected from light and stored at controlled room temperature, 20° to 25°C (68° to 77°F) (see USP), or at refrigerated conditions, 5° ± 3°C (41° ± 5°F). Prepared solutions should not be exposed to direct sunlight. No significant potency losses have been noted following simulated delivery of the solution through intravenous tubing.

HOW SUPPLIED

Argatroban Injection is supplied in 2.5-mL solution in single-use vials at the concentration of 100 mg/mL. Each vial contains 250 mg of Argatroban.

NDC 0007-4407-01   (Package of 1)

Storage: Store the vials in original cartons at room temperature [25°C (77°F), with excursions permitted to 15° to 30°C (59° to 86°F)]. Do not freeze. Retain in the original carton to protect from light.

Manufactured, Distributed, and Marketed by **GlaxoSmithKline**

Research Triangle Park, NC 27709

©2009, GlaxoSmithKline. All rights reserved.

March 2009 ARG:11PI

ARIXTRA®   ℞

[ə-rix' trə]

(fondaparinux sodium)

Solution for subcutaneous injection

HIGHLIGHTS OF PRESCRIBING INFORMATION

These highlights do not include all the information needed to use ARIXTRA safely and effectively. See full prescribing information for ARIXTRA.

ARIXTRA (fondaparinux sodium) Solution for subcutaneous injection

Initial U.S. Approval: 2001

WARNING: SPINAL/EPIDURAL HEMATOMAS

Epidural or spinal hematomas may occur in patients who are anticoagulated with low molecular weight heparins (LMWH), heparinoids, or fondaparinux sodium and are receiving neuraxial anesthesia or undergoing spinal puncture. These hematomas may result in long-term or permanent paralysis. Consider these risks when scheduling patients for spinal procedures. Factors that can increase the risk of developing epidural or spinal hematomas in these patients include:

• use of indwelling epidural catheters

• concomitant use of other drugs that affect hemostasis, such as non-steroidal anti-inflammatory drugs (NSAIDs), platelet inhibitors, or other anticoagulants

• a history of traumatic or repeated epidural or spinal puncture

• a history of spinal deformity or spinal surgery

Monitor patients frequently for signs and symptoms of neurologic impairment. If neurologic compromise is noted, urgent treatment is necessary.

Consider the benefit and risks before neuraxial intervention in patients anticoagulated or to be anticoagulated for thromboprophylaxis. *[See Warnings and Precautions (5.5) and Drug Interactions (7).]*

———RECENT MAJOR CHANGES———

Boxed Warning	01/2010
Dosage and Administration, Hepatic Impairment (2.4)	08/2009

———INDICATIONS AND USAGE———

ARIXTRA is a Factor Xa inhibitor (anticoagulant) indicated for:

• Prophylaxis of deep vein thrombosis (DVT) in patients undergoing hip fracture surgery (including extended prophylaxis), hip replacement surgery, knee replacement surgery, or abdominal surgery. (1.1)

• Treatment of DVT or acute pulmonary embolism (PE) when administered in conjunction with warfarin. (1.2, 1.3)

———DOSAGE AND ADMINISTRATION———

• Prophylaxis of deep vein thrombosis: ARIXTRA 2.5 mg subcutaneously once daily after hemostasis has been established. The initial dose should be given no earlier than 6 to 8 hours after surgery and continued for 5 to 9 days. For patients undergoing hip fracture surgery, extended prophylaxis up to 24 additional days is recommended. (2.1, 2.2)

• Treatment of deep vein thrombosis and pulmonary embolism: ARIXTRA 5 mg (body weight <50 kg), 7.5 mg (50 to 100 kg), or 10 mg (>100 kg) subcutaneously once daily. Treatment should continue for at least 5 days until INR 2 to 3 achieved with warfarin sodium. (2.3)

Do not use as intramuscular injection. For subcutaneous use, do not mix with other injections or infusions.

———DOSAGE FORMS AND STRENGTHS———

Single-dose, prefilled syringes containing 2.5 mg, 5 mg, 7.5 mg, or 10 mg of fondaparinux. (3)

———CONTRAINDICATIONS———

ARIXTRA is contraindicated in the following conditions: (4)

• Severe renal impairment (creatinine clearance <30 mL/min) in prophylaxis or treatment of venous thromboembolism.

• Active major bleeding.

• Bacterial endocarditis.

• Thrombocytopenia associated with a positive *in vitro* test for anti-platelet antibody in the presence of fondaparinux sodium.

• Body weight <50 kg (venous thromboembolism prophylaxis only).

———WARNINGS AND PRECAUTIONS———

• Use with caution in patients who have conditions or are taking concomitant medications that increase risk of hemorrhage. (5.1)

• Bleeding risk is increased in renal impairment and in patients with low body weight <50 kg. (5.2, 5.3)

• Thrombocytopenia can occur with administration of ARIXTRA. (5.4)

• Periodic routine complete blood counts (including platelet counts), serum creatinine level, and stool occult blood tests are recommended (5.6)

• The packaging (needle guard) contains dry natural rubber and may cause allergic reactions in latex sensitive individuals (5.7)

———ADVERSE REACTIONS———

The most common adverse reactions associated with the use of ARIXTRA are bleeding complications. (6.1) Mild local irritation (injection site bleeding, rash, and pruritus) may occur following subcutaneous injection. (6.2)

Anemia, insomnia, increased wound drainage, hypokalemia, dizziness, hypotension, confusion, bullous eruption, hematoma, post-operative hemorrhage, and purpura may occur. (6.4)

To report SUSPECTED ADVERSE REACTIONS, contact GlaxoSmithKline at 1-888-825-5249 or FDA at 1-800-FDA-1088 or www.fda.gov/medwatch.

———DRUG INTERACTIONS———

Discontinue agents that may enhance the risk of hemorrhage prior to initiation of therapy with ARIXTRA unless essential. If co-administration is necessary, monitor patients closely for hemorrhage. (7)

———USE IN SPECIFIC POPULATIONS———

• Safety and effectiveness of ARIXTRA in pediatric patients have not been established. Because the risk for bleeding during treatment with ARIXTRA is increased in adults who weigh <50 kg, bleeding may be a particular safety concern for use of ARIXTRA in the pediatric population. (4, 5.3)

• Because elderly patients are more likely to have reduced renal function, ARIXTRA should be used with caution in these patients. (8.5)

• The risk of bleeding is increased with reduced renal or hepatic function. (8.6, 8.7)

Revised: 03/2010

See 17 for PATIENT COUNSELING INFORMATION and FDA-approved patient labeling

Revised: 03/2010

FULL PRESCRIBING INFORMATION: CONTENTS*

FULL PRESCRIBING INFORMATION

WARNING: SPINAL/EPIDURAL HEMATOMAS

Epidural or spinal hematomas may occur in patients who are anticoagulated with low molecular weight heparins (LMWH), heparinoids, or fondaparinux sodium and are receiving neuraxial anesthesia or undergoing spinal puncture. These hematomas may result in long-term or permanent paralysis. Consider these risks when scheduling patients for spinal procedures. Factors that can increase the risk of developing epidural or spinal hematomas in these patients include:

• use of indwelling epidural catheters

- concomitant use of other drugs that affect hemostasis, such as non-steroidal anti-inflammatory drugs (NSAIDs), platelet inhibitors, or other anticoagulants
- a history of traumatic or repeated epidural or spinal puncture
- a history of spinal deformity or spinal surgery

Monitor patients frequently for signs and symptoms of neurologic impairment. If neurologic compromise is noted, urgent treatment is necessary.

Consider the benefit and risks before neuraxial intervention in patients anticoagulated or to be anticoagulated for thromboprophylaxis. *[See Warnings and Precautions (5.5) and Drug Interactions (7).]*

1 INDICATIONS AND USAGE

1.1 Prophylaxis of Deep Vein Thrombosis
ARIXTRA® is indicated for the prophylaxis of deep vein thrombosis (DVT), which may lead to pulmonary embolism (PE):
- in patients undergoing hip fracture surgery, including extended prophylaxis;
- in patients undergoing hip replacement surgery;
- in patients undergoing knee replacement surgery;
- in patients undergoing abdominal surgery who are at risk for thromboembolic complications.

1.2 Treatment of Acute Deep Vein Thrombosis
ARIXTRA is indicated for the treatment of acute deep vein thrombosis when administered in conjunction with warfarin sodium.

1.3 Treatment of Acute Pulmonary Embolism
ARIXTRA is indicated for the treatment of acute pulmonary embolism when administered in conjunction with warfarin sodium when initial therapy is administered in the hospital.

2 DOSAGE AND ADMINISTRATION

Do not mix other medications or solutions with ARIXTRA. Administer ARIXTRA only subcutaneously.

2.1 Deep Vein Thrombosis Prophylaxis Following Hip Fracture, Hip Replacement, and Knee Replacement Surgery
In patients undergoing hip fracture, hip replacement, or knee replacement surgery, the recommended dose of ARIXTRA is 2.5 mg administered by subcutaneous injection once daily after hemostasis has been established. Administer the initial dose no earlier than 6 to 8 hours after surgery. Administration of ARIXTRA earlier than 6 hours after surgery increases the risk of major bleeding. The usual duration of therapy is 5 to 9 days; up to 11 days of therapy was administered in clinical trials.

In patients undergoing hip fracture surgery, an extended prophylaxis course of up to 24 additional days is recommended. In patients undergoing hip fracture surgery, a total of 32 days (peri-operative and extended prophylaxis) was administered in clinical trials. *[See Warnings and Precautions (5.6), Adverse Reactions (6), and Clinical Studies (14).]*

2.2 Deep Vein Thrombosis Prophylaxis Following Abdominal Surgery
In patients undergoing abdominal surgery, the recommended dose of ARIXTRA is 2.5 mg administered by subcutaneous injection once daily after hemostasis has been established. Administer the initial dose no earlier than 6 to 8 hours after surgery. Administration of ARIXTRA earlier than 6 hours after surgery increases the risk of major bleeding. The usual duration of administration is 5 to 9 days, and up to 10 days of ARIXTRA was administered in clinical trials.

2.3 Deep Vein Thrombosis and Pulmonary Embolism Treatment
In patients with acute symptomatic DVT and in patients with acute symptomatic PE, the recommended dose of ARIXTRA is 5 mg (body weight <50 kg), 7.5 mg (body weight 50 to 100 kg), or 10 mg (body weight >100 kg) by subcutaneous injection once daily (ARIXTRA treatment regimen). Initiate concomitant treatment with warfarin sodium as soon as possible, usually within 72 hours. Continue treatment with ARIXTRA for at least 5 days and until a therapeutic oral anticoagulant effect is established (INR 2 to 3). The usual duration of administration of ARIXTRA is 5 to 9 days; up to 26 days of ARIXTRA injection was administered in clinical trials. *[See Warnings and Precautions (5.6), Adverse Reactions (6), and Clinical Studies (14).]*

2.4 Hepatic Impairment
No dose adjustment is recommended in patients with mild to moderate hepatic impairment, based upon single-dose pharmacokinetic data. Pharmacokinetic data are not available for patients with severe hepatic impairment. Patients with hepatic impairment may be particularly vulnerable to bleeding during ARIXTRA therapy. Observe these patients closely for signs and symptoms of bleeding. *[See Clinical Pharmacology (12.4).]*

2.5 Instructions for Use
ARIXTRA Injection is provided in a single-dose, prefilled syringe affixed with an automatic needle protection system. ARIXTRA is administered by subcutaneous injection. It must not be administered by intramuscular injection. ARIXTRA is intended for use under a physician's guidance. Patients may self-inject only if their physician determines that it is appropriate and the patients are trained in subcutaneous injection techniques.

Prior to administration, visually inspect ARIXTRA to ensure the solution is clear and free of particulate matter.

To avoid the loss of drug when using the prefilled syringe, do not expel the air bubble from the syringe before the injection. Administration should be made in the fatty tissue, alternating injection sites (e.g., between the left and right anterolateral or the left and right posterolateral abdominal wall).

To administer ARIXTRA:

1. Wipe the surface of the injection site with an alcohol swab.
2. Twist the plunger cap and remove it (Figure 1).

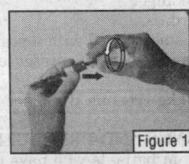

Figure 1

3. Hold the syringe with either hand and use your other hand to twist the rigid needle guard (covers the needle) counter-clockwise. Pull the rigid needle guard straight off the needle (Figure 2). Discard the needle guard.
4. Do not try to remove the air bubbles from the syringe before giving the injection.
5. Pinch a fold of skin at the injection site between your thumb and forefinger and hold it throughout the injection.
6. Hold the syringe with your thumb on the top pad of the plunger rod and your next 2 fingers on the finger grips on the syringe barrel. Pay attention to avoid sticking yourself with the exposed needle (Figure 3).

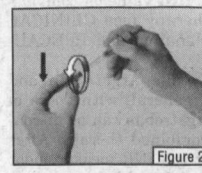

Figure 2

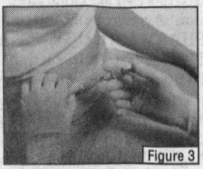

Figure 3

7. Insert the full length of the syringe needle perpendicularly into the skin fold held between the thumb and forefinger (Figure 4).
8. Push the plunger rod firmly with your thumb as far as it will go. This will ensure you have injected all the contents of the syringe (Figure 5).

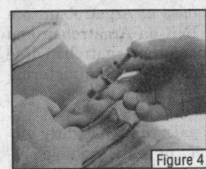

Figure 4

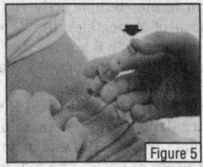

Figure 5

9. When you have injected all the contents of the syringe, the plunger should be released. The plunger will then rise automatically while the needle withdraws from the skin and retracts into the security sleeve. Discard the syringe into the sharps container.
10. You will know that the syringe has worked when:
- The needle is pulled back into the security sleeve and the white safety indicator appears above the blue upper body.
- You may also hear or feel a soft click when the plunger rod is released fully.

3 DOSAGE FORMS AND STRENGTHS
Single-dose, prefilled syringes containing either 2.5 mg, 5 mg, 7.5 mg, or 10 mg of fondaparinux.

4 CONTRAINDICATIONS
ARIXTRA is contraindicated in the following conditions:
- Severe renal impairment (creatinine clearance [CrCl] <30 mL/min). *[See Warnings and Precautions (5.2) and Use in Specific Populations (8.6).]*
- Active major bleeding.
- Bacterial endocarditis.
- Thrombocytopenia associated with a positive *in vitro* test for anti-platelet antibody in the presence of fondaparinux sodium.
- Body weight <50 kg (venous thromboembolism [VTE] prophylaxis only) *[see Warnings and Precautions (5.3)].*

5 WARNINGS AND PRECAUTIONS
5.1 Hemorrhage
Use ARIXTRA with extreme caution in conditions with increased risk of hemorrhage, such as congenital or acquired bleeding disorders, active ulcerative and angiodysplastic gastrointestinal disease, hemorrhagic stroke, uncontrolled arterial hypertension, diabetic retinopathy, or shortly after brain, spinal, or ophthalmological surgery. Isolated cases of elevated aPTT temporally associated with bleeding events have been reported following administration of ARIXTRA (with or without concomitant administration of other anticoagulants) *[See Adverse Reactions (6.5)].*

Do not administer agents that enhance the risk of hemorrhage with ARIXTRA unless essential for the management of the underlying condition, such as vitamin K antagonists for the treatment of VTE. If co-administration is essential, closely monitor patients for signs and symptoms of bleeding. Do not administer the initial dose of ARIXTRA earlier than 6 to 8 hours after surgery. Administration earlier than 6 hours after surgery increases risk of major bleeding *[see Dosage and Administration (2) and Adverse Reactions (6.1)].*

5.2 Renal Impairment and Bleeding Risk
ARIXTRA increases the risk of bleeding in patients with impaired renal function due to reduced clearance *[see Clinical Pharmacology (12.4)].*

The incidence of major bleeding by renal function status reported in clinical trials of patients receiving ARIXTRA for VTE surgical prophylaxis is provided in Table 1. In these patient populations, the following is recommended:
- Do not use ARIXTRA for VTE prophylaxis and treatment in patients with CrCl <30 mL/min *[see Contraindications (4)].*
- Use ARIXTRA with caution in patients with CrCl 30 to 50 mL/min.

[See table 1 at left]

Table 1. Incidence of Major Bleeding in Patients Treated With ARIXTRA by Renal Function Status for Surgical Prophylaxis and Treatment of Deep Vein Thrombosis (DVT) and Pulmonary Embolism (PE)

Population	Timing of Dose	Degree of Renal Impairment			
		Normal % (n/N)	Mild % (n/N)	Moderate % (n/N)	Severe % (n/N)
CrCl (mL/min)		≥80	≥50-<80	≥30-<50	<30
Orthopedic surgery[a]	Overall	1.6% (25/1,565)	2.4% (31/1,288)	3.8% (19/504)	4.8% (4/83)
	6-8 hours after surgery	1.8% (16/905)	2.2% (15/675)	2.3% (6/265)	0% (0/40)
Abdominal surgery	Overall	2.1% (13/606)	3.6% (22/613)	6.7% (12/179)	7.1% (1/14)
	6-8 hours after surgery	2.1% (10/467)	3.3% (16/481)	5.8% (8/137)	7.7% (1/13)
DVT and PE Treatment		0.4% (4/1,132)	1.6% (12/733)	2.2% (7/318)	7.3% (4/55)

CrCl = creatinine clearance.
[a] Hip fracture, hip replacement, and knee replacement surgery prophylaxis.

Assess renal function periodically in patients receiving ARIXTRA. Discontinue the drug immediately in patients who develop severe renal impairment while on therapy. After discontinuation of ARIXTRA, its anticoagulant effects may persist for 2 to 4 days in patients with normal renal function (i.e., at least 3 to 5 half-lives). The anticoagulant effects of ARIXTRA may persist even longer in patients with renal impairment [see Clinical Pharmacology (12.4)].

5.3 Body Weight <50 Kg and Bleeding Risk

ARIXTRA increases the risk for bleeding in patients who weigh less than 50 kg, compared to patients with higher weights. In patients who weigh less than 50 kg:

- Do not administer ARIXTRA as prophylactic therapy for patients undergoing hip fracture, hip replacement, or knee replacement surgery and abdominal surgery [see Contraindications (4)].
- Use ARIXTRA with caution in the treatment of PE and DVT.

During the randomized clinical trials of VTE prophylaxis in the peri-operative period following hip fracture, hip replacement, or knee replacement surgery and abdominal surgery, major bleeding occurred at a higher rate among patients with a body weight <50 kg compared to those with a body weight >50 kg (5.4% versus 2.1% in patients undergoing hip fracture, hip replacement, or knee replacement surgery; 5.3% versus 3.3% in patients undergoing abdominal surgery).

5.4 Thrombocytopenia

Thrombocytopenia can occur with the administration of ARIXTRA. Thrombocytopenia of any degree should be monitored closely. Discontinue ARIXTRA if the platelet count falls below 100,000/mm^3. Moderate thrombocytopenia (platelet counts between 100,000/mm^3 and 50,000/mm^3) occurred at a rate of 3.0% in patients given ARIXTRA 2.5 mg in the peri-operative hip fracture, hip replacement, or knee replacement surgery and abdominal surgery clinical trials. Severe thrombocytopenia (platelet counts less than 50,000/mm^3) occurred at a rate of 0.2% in patients given ARIXTRA 2.5 mg in these clinical trials. During extended prophylaxis, no cases of moderate or severe thrombocytopenia were reported.

Moderate thrombocytopenia occurred at a rate of 0.5% in patients given the ARIXTRA treatment regimen in the DVT and PE treatment clinical trials. Severe thrombocytopenia occurred at a rate of 0.04% in patients given the ARIXTRA treatment regimen in the DVT and PE treatment clinical trials.

Isolated occurrences of thrombocytopenia with thrombosis that manifested similar to heparin-induced thrombocytopenia have been reported with the use of ARIXTRA in postmarketing experience. [See Adverse Reactions (6.5).]

5.5 Neuraxial Anesthesia and Post-operative Indwelling Epidural Catheter Use

Spinal or epidural hematomas, which may result in long-term or permanent paralysis, can occur with the use of anticoagulants and neuraxial (spinal/epidural) anesthesia or spinal puncture. The risk of these events may be higher with post-operative use of indwelling epidural catheters or concomitant use of other drugs affecting hemostasis such as NSAIDs [see Boxed Warning]. In the postmarketing experience, epidural or spinal hematoma has been reported in association with the use of ARIXTRA by subcutaneous (SC) injection. Monitor patients undergoing these procedures for signs and symptoms of neurologic impairment. Consider the potential risks and benefits before neuraxial intervention in patients anticoagulated or who may be anticoagulated for thromboprophylaxis.

5.6 Monitoring: Laboratory Tests

Routine coagulation tests such as Prothrombin Time (PT) and Activated Partial Thromboplastin Time (aPTT) are relatively insensitive measures of the activity of ARIXTRA and international standards of heparin or LMWH are not calibrators to measure anti-Factor Xa activity of ARIXTRA. If unexpected changes in coagulation parameters or major bleeding occur during therapy with ARIXTRA, discontinue ARIXTRA. In postmarketing experience, isolated occurrences of aPTT elevations have been reported following administration of ARIXTRA [see Adverse Reactions (6.5)].

Periodic routine complete blood counts (including platelet count), serum creatinine level, and stool occult blood tests are recommended during the course of treatment with ARIXTRA.

The anti-Factor Xa activity of fondaparinux sodium can be measured by anti-Xa assay using the appropriate calibrator (fondaparinux). The activity of fondaparinux sodium is expressed in milligrams (mg) of the fondaparinux and cannot be compared with activities of heparin or low molecular weight heparins. [See Clinical Pharmacology (12.2, 12.3).]

5.7 Latex

The packaging (needle guard) of the prefilled syringe of ARIXTRA contains dry natural latex rubber that may cause allergic reactions in latex sensitive individuals.

Table 2. Bleeding Across Randomized, Controlled Hip Fracture, Hip Replacement, and Knee Replacement Surgery Studies

	Peri-Operative Prophylaxis (Day 1 to Day 7 ± 1 post-surgery)		Extended Prophylaxis (Day 8 to Day 28 ± 2 post-surgery)	
	ARIXTRA	Enoxaparin Sodium[a, b]	ARIXTRA	Placebo
	2.5 mg SC once daily N = 3,616	N = 3,956	2.5 mg SC once daily N = 327	SC once daily N = 329
Major bleeding[c]	96 (2.7%)	75 (1.9%)	8 (2.4%)	2 (0.6%)
Hip fracture	18/831 (2.2%)	19/842 (2.3%)	8/327 (2.4%)	2/329 (0.6%)
Hip replacement	67/2,268 (3.0%)	55/2,597 (2.1%)	—	—
Knee replacement	11/517 (2.1%)	1/517 (0.2%)	—	—
Fatal bleeding	0 (0.0%)	1 (<0.1%)	0 (0.0%)	0 (0.0%)
Non-fatal bleeding at critical site	0 (0.0%)	1 (<0.1%)	0 (0.0%)	0 (0.0%)
Re-operation due to bleeding	12 (0.3%)	10 (0.3%)	2 (0.6%)	2 (0.6%)
BI ≥2[d]	84 (2.3%)	63 (1.6%)	6 (1.8%)	0 (0.0%)
Minor bleeding[e]	109 (3.0%)	116 (2.9%)	5 (1.5%)	2 (0.6%)

[a] Enoxaparin sodium dosing regimen: 30 mg every 12 hours or 40 mg once daily.
[b] Not approved for use in patients undergoing hip fracture surgery.
[c] Major bleeding was defined as clinically overt bleeding that was (1) fatal, (2) bleeding at critical site (e.g. intracranial, retroperitoneal, intraocular, pericardial, spinal, or into adrenal gland), (3) associated with re-operation at operative site, or (4) with a bleeding index (BI) ≥2.
[d] BI ≥2: Overt bleeding associated only with a bleeding index (BI) ≥2 calculated as [number of whole blood or packed red blood cell units transfused + [(pre-bleeding) – (post-bleeding)] hemoglobin (g/dL) values].
[e] Minor bleeding was defined as clinically overt bleeding that was not major.

6 ADVERSE REACTIONS

The most serious adverse reactions reported with ARIXTRA are bleeding complications and thrombocytopenia [see Warnings and Precautions (5)].

Because clinical trials are conducted under widely varying conditions, adverse reaction rates observed in the clinical trials of a drug cannot be directly compared to rates in the clinical trials of another drug and may not reflect the rates observed in practice.

The adverse reaction information below is based on data from 8,877 patients exposed to ARIXTRA in controlled trials of hip fracture, hip replacement, major knee, or abdominal surgeries, and DVT and PE treatment. These trials consisted of the following:

- 2 peri-operative dose-response trials (n = 989)
- 4 active-controlled peri-operative VTE prophylaxis trials with enoxaparin sodium (n = 3,616), an extended VTE prophylaxis trial (n = 327), and an active-controlled trial with dalteparin sodium (n = 1,425)
- a dose-response trial (n = 111) and an active-controlled trial with enoxaparin sodium in DVT treatment (n = 1,091)
- an active-controlled trial with heparin in PE treatment (n = 1,092)

6.1 Hemorrhage

During administration of ARIXTRA, the most common adverse reactions were bleeding complications [see Warnings and Precautions (5.1)].

Hip Fracture, Hip Replacement, and Knee Replacement Surgery: The rates of major bleeding events reported during the hip fracture, hip replacement, or knee replacement surgery clinical trials with ARIXTRA 2.5 mg are provided in Table 2.

[See table 2 above]

A separate analysis of major bleeding across all randomized, controlled, peri-operative, prophylaxis clinical studies of hip fracture, hip replacement, or knee replacement surgery according to the time of the first injection of ARIXTRA after surgical closure was performed in patients who received ARIXTRA only post-operatively. In this analysis, the incidences of major bleeding were as follows: <4 hours was 4.8% (5/104), 4 to 6 hours was 2.3% (28/1,196), 6 to 8 hours was 1.9% (38/1,965). In all studies, the majority (≥75%) of the major bleeding events occurred during the first 4 days after surgery.

Abdominal Surgery: In a randomized study of patients undergoing abdominal surgery, ARIXTRA 2.5 mg once daily (n = 1,433) was compared with dalteparin 5,000 IU once daily (n = 1,425). Bleeding rates are shown in Table 3.

Table 3. Bleeding in the Abdominal Surgery Study

	ARIXTRA 2.5 mg SC once daily	Dalteparin Sodium 5,000 IU SC once daily
	N = 1,433	N = 1,425
Major bleeding[a]	49 (3.4%)	34 (2.4%)
Fatal bleeding	2 (0.1%)	2 (0.1%)
Non-fatal bleeding at critical site	0 (0.0%)	0 (0.0%)
Other non-fatal major bleeding		
Surgical site	38 (2.7%)	26 (1.8%)
Non-surgical site	9 (0.6%)	6 (0.4%)
Minor bleeding[b]	31 (2.2%)	23 (1.6%)

[a] Major bleeding was defined as bleeding that was (1) fatal, (2) bleeding at the surgical site leading to intervention, (3) non-surgical bleeding at a critical site (e.g. intracranial, retroperitoneal, intraocular, pericardial, spinal, or into adrenal gland), or leading to an intervention, and/or with a bleeding index (BI) ≥2.
[b] Minor bleeding was defined as clinically overt bleeding that was not major.

The rates of major bleeding according to the time interval following the first ARIXTRA injection were as follows: <6 hours was 3.4% (9/263) and 6 to 8 hours was 2.9% (32/1112).

Treatment of Deep Vein Thrombosis and Pulmonary Embolism: The rates of bleeding events reported during the DVT and PE clinical trials with the ARIXTRA injection treatment regimen are provided in Table 4.

[See table 4 at top of next page]

6.2 Local Reactions

Local irritation (injection site bleeding, rash, and pruritus) may occur following subcutaneous injection of ARIXTRA.

6.3 Elevations of Serum Aminotransferases

In the peri-operative prophylaxis randomized clinical trials of 7 ± 2 days, asymptomatic increases in aspartate (AST) and alanine (ALT) aminotransferase levels greater than 3 times the upper limit of normal were reported in 1.7% and 2.6% of patients, respectively, during treatment with ARIXTRA 2.5 mg once daily versus 3.2% and 3.9% of patients, respectively, during treatment with enoxaparin

Table 4. Bleeding[a] in Deep Vein Thrombosis and Pulmonary Embolism Treatment Studies

	ARIXTRA N = 2,294	Enoxaparin Sodium N = 1,101	Heparin aPTT adjusted IV N = 1,092
Major bleeding[b]	28 (1.2%)	13 (1.2%)	12 (1.1%)
Fatal bleeding	3 (0.1%)	0 (0.0%)	1 (0.1%)
Non-fatal bleeding at a critical site	3 (0.1%)	0 (0.0%)	2 (0.2%)
Intracranial bleeding	3 (0.1%)	0 (0.0%)	1 (0.1%)
Retro-peritoneal bleeding	0 (0.0%)	0 (0.0%)	1 (0.1%)
Other clinically overt bleeding[c]	22 (1.0%)	13 (1.2%)	10 (0.9%)
Minor bleeding[d]	70 (3.1%)	33 (3.0%)	57 (5.2%)

[a] Bleeding rates are during the study drug treatment period (approximately 7 days). Patients were also treated with vitamin K antagonists initiated within 72 hours after the first study drug administration.
[b] Major bleeding was defined as clinically overt: –and/or contributing to death – and/or in a critical organ including intracranial, retroperitoneal, intraocular, spinal, pericardial, or adrenal gland – and/or associated with a fall in hemoglobin level ≥2 g/dL – and/or leading to a transfusion ≥2 units of packed red blood cells or whole blood.
[c] Clinically overt bleeding with a 2 g/dL fall in hemoglobin and/or leading to transfusion of PRBC or whole blood ≥2 units.
[d] Minor bleeding was defined as clinically overt bleeding that was not major.

Table 5. Adverse Reactions Across Randomized, Controlled, Hip Fracture Surgery, Hip Replacement Surgery, and Knee Replacement Surgery Studies

Adverse Reactions	Peri-Operative Prophylaxis (Day 1 to Day 7 ± 1 post-surgery)		Extended Prophylaxis (Day 8 to Day 28 ± 2 post-surgery)	
	ARIXTRA 2.5 mg SC once daily	Enoxaparin Sodium[a, b]	ARIXTRA 2.5 mg SC once daily	Placebo SC once daily
	N = 3,616	N = 3,956	N = 327	N = 329
Anemia	707 (19.6%)	670 (16.9%)	5 (1.5%)	4 (1.2%)
Insomnia	179 (5.0%)	214 (5.4%)	3 (0.9%)	1 (0.3%)
Wound drainage increased	161 (4.5%)	184 (4.7%)	2 (0.6%)	0 (0.0%)
Hypokalemia	152 (4.2%)	164 (4.1%)	0 (0.0%)	0 (0.0%)
Dizziness	131 (3.6%)	165 (4.2%)	2 (0.6%)	0 (0.0%)
Purpura	128 (3.5%)	137 (3.5%)	0 (0.0%)	0 (0.0%)
Hypotension	126 (3.5%)	125 (3.2%)	1 (0.3%)	0 (0.0%)
Confusion	113 (3.1%)	132 (3.3%)	4 (1.2%)	1 (0.3%)
Bullous eruption[c]	112 (3.1%)	102 (2.6%)	0 (0.0%)	1 (0.3%)
Hematoma	103 (2.8%)	109 (2.8%)	7 (2.1%)	1 (0.3%)
Post-operative hemorrhage	85 (2.4%)	69 (1.7%)	2 (0.6%)	2 (0.6%)

[a] Enoxaparin sodium dosing regimen: 30 mg every 12 hours or 40 mg once daily.
[b] Not approved for use in patients undergoing hip fracture surgery.
[c] Localized blister coded as bullous eruption.

sodium 30 mg every 12 hours or 40 mg once daily enox-aparin sodium. These elevations are reversible and rarely associated with increases in bilirubin. In the extended prophylaxis clinical trial, no significant differences in AST and ALT levels between ARIXTRA 2.5 mg and placebo-treated patients were observed.

In the DVT and PE treatment clinical trials, asymptomatic increases in AST and ALT levels greater than 3 times the upper limit of normal of the laboratory reference range were reported in 0.7% and 1.3% of patients, respectively, during treatment with ARIXTRA. In comparison, these increases were reported in 4.8% and 12.3% of patients, respectively, in the DVT treatment trial during treatment with enoxaparin sodium 1 mg/kg every 12 hours and in 2.9% and 8.7% of patients, respectively, in the PE treatment trial during treatment with aPTT adjusted heparin.

Since aminotransferase determinations are important in the differential diagnosis of myocardial infarction, liver disease, and pulmonary emboli, elevations that might be caused by drugs like ARIXTRA should be interpreted with caution.

6.4 Other Adverse Reactions
Other adverse reactions that occurred during treatment with ARIXTRA in clinical trials with patients undergoing hip fracture, hip replacement, or knee replacement surgery are provided in Table 5.

[See table 5 above]
Adverse reactions in the abdominal surgery study and in the VTE treatment trials generally occurred at lower rates than in the hip and knee surgery trials described above. The most common adverse reaction in the abdominal surgery trial was post-operative wound infection (4.9%), and the most common adverse reaction in the VTE treatment trials was epistaxis (1.3%).

6.5 Postmarketing Experience
The following adverse reactions have been identified during post-approval use of ARIXTRA. Because these reactions are reported voluntarily from a population of uncertain size, it is not always possible to reliably estimate their frequency or establish a causal relationship to drug exposure.
Isolated occurrences of thrombocytopenia with thrombosis that manifested similar to heparin-induced thrombocytopenia have been reported in the postmarketing experience and isolated cases of elevated aPTT temporally associated with bleeding events have been reported following administration of ARIXTRA (with or without concomitant administration of other anticoagulants) [see Warnings and Precautions (5.4)].

7 DRUG INTERACTIONS
In clinical studies performed with ARIXTRA, the concomitant use of oral anticoagulants (warfarin), platelet inhibitors (acetylsalicylic acid), NSAIDs (piroxicam), and digoxin did not significantly affect the pharmacokinetics/pharmacodynamics of fondaparinux sodium. In addition, ARIXTRA neither influenced the pharmacodynamics of warfarin, acetylsalicylic acid, piroxicam, and digoxin, nor the pharmacokinetics of digoxin at steady state.
Agents that may enhance the risk of hemorrhage should be discontinued prior to initiation of therapy with ARIXTRA unless these agents are essential. If co-administration is necessary, monitor patients closely for hemorrhage. [See Warnings and Precautions (5.1).] In an in vitro study in human liver microsomes, inhibition of CYP2A6 hydroxylation of coumarin by fondaparinux (200 micromolar i.e., 350 mg/L) was 17 to 28%. Inhibition of the other isozymes evaluated (CYPs 1A2, 2C9, 2C19, 2D6, 3A4, and 3E1) was 0 to 16%. Since fondaparinux does not markedly inhibit CYP450s (CYP1A2, CYP2A6, CYP2C9, CYP2C19, CYP2D6, CYP2E1, or CYP3A4) in vitro, fondaparinux sodium is not expected to significantly interact with other drugs in vivo by inhibition of metabolism mediated by these isozymes.
Since fondaparinux sodium does not bind significantly to plasma proteins other than ATIII, no drug interactions by protein-binding displacement are expected.

8 USE IN SPECIFIC POPULATIONS
8.1 Pregnancy
Pregnancy Category B. Reproduction studies have been performed in pregnant rats at subcutaneous doses up to 10 mg/kg/day (about 32 times the recommended human dose based on body surface area) and pregnant rabbits at subcutaneous doses up to 10 mg/kg/ day (about 65 times the recommended human dose based on body surface area) and have revealed no evidence of impaired fertility or harm to the fetus due to fondaparinux sodium. There are, however, no adequate and well-controlled studies in pregnant women. Because animal reproduction studies are not always predictive of human response, ARIXTRA should be used during pregnancy only if clearly needed.

8.3 Nursing Mothers
Fondaparinux sodium was found to be excreted in the milk of lactating rats. However, it is not known whether this drug is excreted in human milk. Because many drugs are excreted in human milk, caution should be exercised when ARIXTRA is administered to a nursing mother.

8.4 Pediatric Use
Safety and effectiveness of ARIXTRA in pediatric patients have not been established. Because risk for bleeding during treatment with ARIXTRA is increased in adults who weigh <50 kg, bleeding may be a particular safety concern for use of ARIXTRA in the pediatric population [see Warnings and Precautions (5.3)].

8.5 Geriatric Use
In clinical trials the efficacy of ARIXTRA in the elderly (65 years or older) was similar to that seen in patients younger than 65 years; however, serious adverse events increased with age. Exercise caution when using ARIXTRA in elderly patients, paying particular attention to dosing directions and concomitant medications (especially anti-platelet medication). [See Warnings and Precautions (5.1).]
Fondaparinux sodium is substantially excreted by the kidney, and the risk of adverse reactions to ARIXTRA may be greater in patients with impaired renal function. Because elderly patients are more likely to have decreased renal function, assess renal function prior to ARIXTRA administration. [See Contraindications (4), Warnings and Precautions (5.2), and Clinical Pharmacology (12.4).] In the peri-operative hip fracture, hip replacement, or knee replacement surgery clinical trials with patients receiving ARIXTRA 2.5 mg, serious adverse events increased with age for patients receiving ARIXTRA. The incidence of major bleeding in clinical trials of ARIXTRA by age is provided in Table 6.

[See table 6 at top of next page]

8.6 Renal Impairment
Patients with impaired renal function are at increased risk of bleeding due to reduced clearance of ARIXTRA [see Contraindications (4) and Warnings and Precautions (5.2)]. Assess renal function periodically in patients receiving ARIXTRA. Discontinue ARIXTRA immediately in patients who develop severe renal impairment while on therapy. After discontinuation of ARIXTRA, its anticoagulant effects may persist for 2 to 4 days in patients with normal renal function (i.e., at least 3 to 5 half-lives). The anticoagulant effects of ARIXTRA may persist even longer in patients with renal impairment [see Clinical Pharmacology (12.4)].

8.7 Hepatic Impairment
Following a single, subcutaneous dose of 7.5 mg of ARIXTRA in patients with moderate hepatic impairment (Child-Pugh Category B) compared to subjects with normal liver function, changes from baseline in aPTT, PT/INR, and antithrombin III were similar in the two groups. However, a higher incidence of hemorrhage was observed in subjects with moderate hepatic impairment than in normal subjects,

especially mild hematomas at the blood sampling or injection site. The pharmacokinetics of fondaparinux have not been studied in patients with severe hepatic impairment. [See Dosage and Administration (2.4) and Clinical Pharmacology (12.4).]

10 OVERDOSAGE

There is no known antidote for ARIXTRA. Overdose of ARIXTRA may lead to hemorrhagic complications. Discontinue treatment and initiate appropriate therapy if bleeding complications associated with overdosage occur.

Data obtained in patients undergoing chronic intermittent hemodialysis suggest that clearance of ARIXTRA can increase by 20% during hemodialysis.

11 DESCRIPTION

ARIXTRA (fondaparinux sodium) Injection is a sterile solution containing fondaparinux sodium. It is a synthetic and specific inhibitor of activated Factor X (Xa). Fondaparinux sodium is methyl O-2-deoxy-6-O-sulfo-2-(sulfoamino)-α-D-glucopyranosyl-(1→4)-O-β-D-glucopyra-nuronosyl-(1→4)-O-2-deoxy-3,6-di-O-sulfo-2-(sulfoamino)-α-D-glucopyranosyl-(1→4)-O-2-O-sulfo-α-L-idopyranuronosyl-(1→4)-2-deoxy-6-O-sulfo-2-(sulfoamino)-α-D-glucopyranoside, decasodium salt.

The molecular formula of fondaparinux sodium is $C_{31}H_{43}N_3Na_{10}O_{49}S_8$ and its molecular weight is 1728. The structural formula is provided below:

ARIXTRA is supplied as a sterile, preservative-free injectable solution for subcutaneous use.

Each single-dose, prefilled syringe of ARIXTRA, affixed with an automatic needle protection system, contains 2.5 mg of fondaparinux sodium in 0.5 mL, 5.0 mg of fondaparinux sodium in 0.4 mL, 7.5 mg of fondaparinux sodium in 0.6 mL, or 10.0 mg of fondaparinux sodium in 0.8 mL of an isotonic solution of sodium chloride and water for injection. The final drug product is a clear and colorless to slightly yellow liquid with a pH between 5.0 and 8.0.

12 CLINICAL PHARMACOLOGY

12.1 Mechanism of Action

The antithrombotic activity of fondaparinux sodium is the result of antithrombin III (ATIII)-mediated selective inhibition of Factor Xa. By selectively binding to ATIII, fondaparinux sodium potentiates (about 300 times) the innate neutralization of Factor Xa by ATIII. Neutralization of Factor Xa interrupts the blood coagulation cascade and thus inhibits thrombin formation and thrombus development. Fondaparinux sodium does not inactivate thrombin (activated Factor II) and has no known effect on platelet function. At the recommended dose, fondaparinux sodium does not affect fibrinolytic activity or bleeding time.

12.2 Pharmacodynamics

Anti-Xa Activity: The pharmacodynamics/pharmacokinetics of fondaparinux sodium are derived from fondaparinux plasma concentrations quantified via anti-Factor Xa activity. Only fondaparinux can be used to calibrate the anti-Xa assay. (The international standards of heparin or LMWH are not appropriate for this use.) As a result, the activity of fondaparinux sodium is expressed as milligrams (mg) of the fondaparinux calibrator. The anti-Xa activity of the drug increases with increasing drug concentration, reaching maximum values in approximately three hours.

12.3 Pharmacokinetics

Absorption: Fondaparinux sodium administered by subcutaneous injection is rapidly and completely absorbed (absolute bioavailability is 100%). Following a single subcutaneous dose of fondaparinux sodium 2.5 mg in young male subjects, C_{max} of 0.34 mg/L is reached in approximately 2 hours. In patients undergoing treatment with fondaparinux sodium injection 2.5 mg, once daily, the peak steady-state plasma concentration is, on average, 0.39 to 0.50 mg/L and is reached approximately 3 hours post-dose. In these patients, the minimum steady-state plasma concentration is 0.14 to 0.19 mg/L. In patients with symptomatic deep vein thrombosis and pulmonary embolism undergoing treatment with fondaparinux sodium injection 5 mg (body weight <50 kg), 7.5 mg (body weight 50 to 100 kg), and 10 mg (body weight >100 kg) once daily, the body-weight-adjusted doses provide similar mean steady-state peaks and minimum plasma concentrations across all body weight categories. The mean peak steady-state plasma concentration is in the range of 1.20 to 1.26 mg/L. In these patients, the mean minimum steady-state plasma concentration is in the range of 0.46 to 0.62 mg/L.

Distribution: In healthy adults, intravenously or subcutaneously administered fondaparinux sodium distributes mainly in blood and only to a minor extent in extravascular fluid as evidenced by steady state and non-steady state

Table 6. Incidence of Major Bleeding in Patients Treated With ARIXTRA by Age

	Age		
	<65 years % (n/N)	65 to 74 years % (n/N)	≥75 years % (n/N)
Orthopedic surgery[a]	1.8% (23/1,253)	2.2% (24/1,111)	2.7% (33/1,277)
Extended prophylaxis	1.9% (1/52)	1.4% (1/71)	2.9% (6/204)
Abdominal surgery	3.0% (19/644)	3.2% (16/507)	5.0% (14/282)
DVT and PE treatment	0.6% (7/1,151)	1.6% (9/560)	2.1% (12/583)

[a] Includes hip fracture, hip replacement, and knee replacement surgery prophylaxis.

Table 7. Efficacy of ARIXTRA in the Peri-operative Prophylaxis of Thromboembolic Events Following Hip Fracture Surgery

Endpoint	Peri-operative Prophylaxis (Day 1 to Day 7 ± 2 post-surgery)			
	ARIXTRA 2.5 mg SC once daily		Enoxaparin Sodium 40 mg SC once daily	
	n/N[a]	% (95% CI)	n/N[a]	% (95% CI)
VTE	52/626	8.3%[b] (6.3, 10.8)	119/624	19.1% (16.1, 22.4)
All DVT	49/624	7.9%[b] (5.9, 10.2)	117/623	18.8% (15.8, 22.1)
Proximal DVT	6/650	0.9%[b] (0.3, 2.0)	28/646	4.3% (2.9, 6.2)
Symptomatic PE	3/831	0.4%[c] (0.1, 1.1)	3/840	0.4% (0.1, 1.0)

[a] N = all evaluable hip fracture surgery patients. Evaluable patients were those who were treated and underwent the appropriate surgery (i.e., hip fracture surgery of the upper third of the femur), with an adequate efficacy assessment up to Day 11.
[b] P value versus enoxaparin sodium <0.001.
[c] P value versus enoxaparin sodium: NS.

apparent volume of distribution of 7 to 11 L. Similar fondaparinux distribution occurs in patients undergoing elective hip surgery or hip fracture surgery. In vitro, fondaparinux sodium is highly (at least 94%) and specifically bound to antithrombin III (ATIII) and does not bind significantly to other plasma proteins (including platelet Factor 4 [PF4]) or red blood cells.

Metabolism: In vivo metabolism of fondaparinux has not been investigated since the majority of the administered dose is eliminated unchanged in urine in individuals with normal kidney function.

Elimination: In individuals with normal kidney function, fondaparinux is eliminated in urine mainly as unchanged drug. In healthy individuals up to 75 years of age, up to 77% of a single subcutaneous or intravenous fondaparinux dose is eliminated in urine as unchanged drug in 72 hours. The elimination half-life is 17 to 21 hours.

12.4 Special Populations

Renal Impairment: Fondaparinux elimination is prolonged in patients with renal impairment since the major route of elimination is urinary excretion of unchanged drug. In patients undergoing prophylaxis following elective hip surgery or hip fracture surgery, the total clearance of fondaparinux is approximately 25% lower in patients with mild renal impairment (CrCl 50 to 80 mL/min), approximately 40% lower in patients with moderate renal impairment (CrCl 30 to 50 mL/min), and approximately 55% lower in patients with severe renal impairment (<30 mL/min) compared to patients with normal renal function. A similar relationship between fondaparinux clearance and extent of renal impairment was observed in DVT treatment patients. [See Contraindications (4) and Warnings and Precautions (5.2).]

Hepatic Impairment: Following a single, subcutaneous dose of 7.5 mg of ARIXTRA in patients with moderate hepatic impairment (Child-Pugh Category B), C_{max} and AUC were decreased by 22% and 39%, respectively, compared to subjects with normal liver function. The changes from baseline in pharmacodynamic parameters, such as aPTT, PT/INR, and antithrombin III, were similar in normal subjects and in patients with moderate hepatic impairment. Based on these data, no dosage adjustment is recommended in these patients. However, a higher incidence of hemorrhage was observed in subjects with moderate hepatic impairment than in normal subjects [see Use in Specific Populations (8.7)]. The pharmacokinetics of fondaparinux have not been studied in patients with severe hepatic impairment. [See Dosage and Administration (2.4).]

Pediatric: The pharmacokinetics of fondaparinux have not been investigated in pediatric patients. [See Contraindica-

tions (4), Warnings and Precautions (5.3), and Pediatric Use (8.4).]

Geriatric: Fondaparinux elimination is prolonged in patients older than 75 years. In studies evaluating fondaparinux sodium 2.5 mg prophylaxis in hip fracture surgery or elective hip surgery, the total clearance of fondaparinux was approximately 25% lower in patients older than 75 years as compared to patients younger than 65 years. A similar relationship between fondaparinux clearance and age was observed in DVT treatment patients. [See Use in Specific Populations (8.5).]

Patients Weighing Less Than 50 kg: Total clearance of fondaparinux sodium is decreased by approximately 30% in patients weighing less than 50 kg [see Dosage and Administration (2.3) and Contraindications (4)].

Gender: The pharmacokinetic properties of fondaparinux sodium are not significantly affected by gender.

Race: Pharmacokinetic differences due to race have not been studied prospectively. However, studies performed in Asian (Japanese) healthy subjects did not reveal a different pharmacokinetic profile compared to Caucasian healthy subjects. Similarly, no plasma clearance differences were observed between black and Caucasian patients undergoing orthopedic surgery.

13 NONCLINICAL TOXICOLOGY

13.1 Carcinogenesis, Mutagenesis, Impairment of Fertility

No long-term studies in animals have been performed to evaluate the carcinogenic potential of fondaparinux sodium. Fondaparinux sodium was not genotoxic in the Ames test, the mouse lymphoma cell (L5178Y/TK[+/-]) forward mutation test, the human lymphocyte chromosome aberration test, the rat hepatocyte unscheduled DNA synthesis (UDS) test, or the rat micronucleus test.

At subcutaneous doses up to 10 mg/kg/day (about 32 times the recommended human dose based on body surface area), fondaparinux sodium was found to have no effect on fertility and reproductive performance of male and female rats.

14 CLINICAL STUDIES

14.1 Prophylaxis of Thromboembolic Events Following Hip Fracture Surgery

In a randomized, double-blind, clinical trial in patients undergoing hip fracture surgery, ARIXTRA 2.5 mg SC once daily was compared to enoxaparin sodium 40 mg SC once daily, which is not approved for use in patients undergoing hip fracture surgery. A total of 1,711 patients were randomized and 1,673 were treated. Patients ranged in age from 17 to 101 years (mean age 77 years) with 25% men and 75% women. Patients were 99% Caucasian, 1% other races.

Table 8. Efficacy of ARIXTRA Injection in the Extended Prophylaxis of Thromboembolic Events Following Hip Fracture Surgery

	Extended Prophylaxis (Day 8 to Day 28 ± 2 post-surgery)			
	ARIXTRA 2.5 mg SC once daily		Placebo SC once daily	
Endpoint	n/Nª	% (95% CI)	n/Nª	% (95% CI)
VTE	3/208	1.4%[b] (0.3, 4.2)	77/220	35.0% (28.7, 41.7)
All DVT	3/208	1.4%[b] (0.3, 4.2)	74/218	33.9% (27.7, 40.6)
Proximal DVT	2/221	0.9%[b] (0.1, 3.2)	35/222	15.8% (11.2, 21.2)
Symptomatic VTE (all)	1/326	0.3%[c] (0.0, 1.7)	9/330	2.7% (1.3, 5.1)
Symptomatic PE	0/326	0.0%[d] (0.0, 1.1)	3/330	0.9% (0.2, 2.6)

[a] N = all randomized evaluable hip fracture surgery patients. Evaluable patients were those who were treated in the post-randomization period, with an adequate efficacy assessment for up to 24 days following randomization.
[b] P value versus placebo <0.001.
[c] P value versus placebo = 0.021.
[d] P value versus placebo = NS.

Table 9. Efficacy of ARIXTRA in the Prophylaxis of Thromboembolic Events Following Hip Replacement Surgery

	Study 1 n/Nª % (95% CI)		Study 2 n/Nª % (95% CI)	
Endpoint	ARIXTRA 2.5 mg SC once daily	Enoxaparin Sodium 30 mg SC every 12 hr	ARIXTRA 2.5 mg SC once daily	Enoxaparin Sodium 40 mg SC once daily
VTE[b]	48/787 6.1%[c] (4.5, 8.0)	66/797 8.3% (6.5, 10.4)	37/908 4.1%[e] (2.9, 5.6)	85/919 9.2% (7.5, 11.3)
All DVT	44/784 5.6%[d] (4.1, 7.5)	65/796 8.2% (6.4, 10.3)	36/908 4.0%[e] (2.8, 5.4)	83/918 9.0% (7.3, 11.1)
Proximal DVT	14/816 1.7%[c] (0.9, 2.9)	10/830 1.2% (0.6, 2.2)	6/922 0.7%[f] (0.2, 1.4)	23/927 2.5% (1.6, 3.7)
Symptomatic PE	5/1,126 0.4%[c] (0.1, 1.0)	1/1,128 0.1% (0.0, 0.5)	2/1,129 0.2%[c] (0.0, 0.6)	2/1,123 0.2% (0.0, 0.6)

[a] N = all evaluable hip replacement surgery patients. Evaluable patients were those who were treated and underwent the appropriate surgery (i.e., hip replacement surgery), with an adequate efficacy assessment up to Day 11.
[b] VTE was a composite of documented DVT and/or documented symptomatic PE reported up to Day 11.
[c] P value versus enoxaparin sodium: NS.
[d] P value versus enoxaparin sodium in study 1: <0.05.
[e] P value versus enoxaparin sodium in study 2: <0.001.
[f] P value versus enoxaparin sodium in study 2: <0.01.

Table 10. Efficacy of ARIXTRA in the Prophylaxis of Thromboembolic Events Following Knee Replacement Surgery

	ARIXTRA 2.5 mg SC once daily		Enoxaparin Sodium 30 mg SC every 12 hours	
Endpoint	n/Nª	% (95% CI)	n/Nª	% (95% CI)
VTE[b]	45/361	12.5%[c] (9.2, 16.3)	101/363	27.8% (23.3, 32.7)
All DVT	45/361	12.5%[c] (9.2, 16.3)	98/361	27.1% (22.6, 32.0)
Proximal DVT	9/368	2.4%[d] (1.1, 4.6)	20/372	5.4% (3.3, 8.2)
Symptomatic PE	1/517	0.2%[d] (0.0, 1.1)	4/517	0.8% (0.2, 2.0)

[a] N = all evaluable knee replacement surgery patients. Evaluable patients were those who were treated and underwent the appropriate surgery (i.e., knee replacement surgery), with an adequate efficacy assessment up to Day 11.
[b] VTE was a composite of documented DVT and/or documented symptomatic PE reported up to Day 11.
[c] P value versus enoxaparin sodium <0.001.
[d] P value versus enoxaparin sodium: NS.

Patients with multiple traumas affecting more than one organ system, serum creatinine level more than 2 mg/dL (180 micromol/L), or platelet count less than 100,000/mm³ were excluded from the trial. ARIXTRA was initiated after surgery in 88% of patients (mean 6 hours) and enoxaparin sodium was initiated after surgery in 74% of patients (mean 18 hours). For both drugs, treatment was continued for 7 ± 2 days. The primary efficacy endpoint, venous thromboembolism (VTE), was a composite of documented deep vein thrombosis (DVT) and/or documented symptomatic pulmonary embolism (PE) reported up to Day 11. The efficacy data are provided in Table 7 and demonstrate that under the con-

ditions of the trial ARIXTRA was associated with a VTE rate of 8.3% compared with a VTE rate of 19.1% for enoxaparin sodium for a relative risk reduction of 56% (95% CI: 39%, 70%; P <0.001). Major bleeding episodes occurred in 2.2% of patients receiving ARIXTRA and 2.3% of enoxaparin sodium patients [see Adverse Reactions (6.1)].
[See table 7 on previous page]

14.2   Extended Prophylaxis of Thromboembolic Events Following Hip Fracture Surgery
In a noncomparative, unblinded manner, 737 patients undergoing hip fracture surgery were initially treated during the peri-operative period with ARIXTRA 2.5 mg once daily

for 7 ± 1 days. Eighty-one (81) of the 737 patients were not eligible for randomization into the 3-week double-blind period. Three hundred twenty-six (326) patients and 330 patients were randomized to receive ARIXTRA 2.5 mg once daily or placebo, respectively, in or out of the hospital for 21 ± 2 days. Patients ranged in age from 23 to 96 years (mean age 75 years) and were 29% men and 71% women. Patients were 99% Caucasian and 1% other races. Patients with multiple traumas affecting more than one organ system or serum creatinine level more than 2 mg/dL (180 micromol/L) were excluded from the trial. The primary efficacy endpoint, venous thromboembolism (VTE), was a composite of documented deep vein thrombosis (DVT) and/or documented symptomatic pulmonary embolism (PE) reported for up to 24 days following randomization. The efficacy data are provided in Table 8 and demonstrate that extended prophylaxis with ARIXTRA was associated with a VTE rate of 1.4% compared with a VTE rate of 35.0% for placebo for a relative risk reduction of 95.9% (95% CI = [98.7; 87.1], P <0.0001). Major bleeding rates during the 3-week extended prophylaxis period for ARIXTRA occurred in 2.4% of patients receiving ARIXTRA and 0.6% of placebo-treated patients [see Adverse Reactions (6.1)].
[See table 8 at left]

14.3   Prophylaxis of Thromboembolic Events Following Hip Replacement Surgery
In 2 randomized, double-blind, clinical trials in patients undergoing hip replacement surgery, ARIXTRA 2.5 mg SC once daily was compared to either enoxaparin sodium 30 mg SC every 12 hours (Study 1) or to enoxaparin sodium 40 mg SC once a day (Study 2). In Study 1, a total of 2,275 patients were randomized and 2,257 were treated. Patients ranged in age from 18 to 92 years (mean age 65 years) with 48% men and 52% women. Patients were 94% Caucasian, 4% black, <1% Asian, and 2% others. In Study 2, a total of 2,309 patients were randomized and 2,273 were treated. Patients ranged in age from 24 to 97 years (mean age 65 years) with 42% men and 58% women. Patients were 99% Caucasian, and 1% other races. Patients with serum creatinine level more than 2 mg/dL (180 micromol/L), or platelet count less than 100,000/mm³ were excluded from both trials. In Study 1, ARIXTRA was initiated 6 ± 2 hours (mean 6.5 hours) after surgery in 92% of patients and enoxaparin sodium was initiated 12 to 24 hours (mean 20.25 hours) after surgery in 97% of patients. In Study 2, ARIXTRA was initiated 6 ± 2 hours (mean 6.25 hours) after surgery in 86% of patients and enoxaparin sodium was initiated 12 hours before surgery in 78% of patients. The first post-operative enoxaparin sodium dose was given within 12 hours after surgery in 60% of patients and 12 to 24 hours after surgery in 35% of patients with a mean of 13 hours. For both studies, both study treatments were continued for 7 ± 2 days. The efficacy data are provided in Table 9. Under the conditions of Study 1, ARIXTRA was associated with a VTE rate of 6.1% compared with a VTE rate of 8.3% for enoxaparin sodium for a relative risk reduction of 26% (95% CI: -11%, 53%; P = NS). Under the conditions of Study 2, fondaparinux sodium was associated with a VTE rate of 4.1% compared with a VTE rate of 9.2% for enoxaparin sodium for a relative risk reduction of 56% (95% CI: 33%, 73%; P <0.001). For the 2 studies combined, the major bleeding episodes occurred in 3.0% of patients receiving ARIXTRA and 2.1% of enoxaparin sodium patients [see Adverse Reactions (6.1)].
[See table 9 at left]

14.4   Prophylaxis of Thromboembolic Events Following Knee Replacement Surgery
In a randomized, double-blind, clinical trial in patients undergoing knee replacement surgery (i.e., surgery requiring resection of the distal end of the femur or proximal end of the tibia), ARIXTRA 2.5 mg SC once daily was compared to enoxaparin sodium 30 mg SC every 12 hours. A total of 1,049 patients were randomized and 1,034 were treated. Patients ranged in age from 19 to 94 years (mean age 68 years) with 41% men and 59% women. Patients were 88% Caucasian, 8% black, <1% Asian, and 3% others. Patients with serum creatinine level more than 2 mg/dL (180 micromol/L), or platelet count less than 100,000/mm³ were excluded from the trial. ARIXTRA was initiated 6 ± 2 hours (mean 6.25 hours) after surgery in 94% of patients, and enoxaparin sodium was initiated 12 to 24 hours (mean 21 hours) after surgery in 96% of patients. For both drugs, treatment was continued for 7 ± 2 days. The efficacy data are provided in Table 10 and demonstrate that under the conditions of the trial, ARIXTRA was associated with a VTE rate of 12.5% compared with a VTE rate of 27.8% for enoxaparin sodium for a relative risk reduction of 55% (95% CI: 36%, 70%; P <0.001). Major bleeding episodes occurred in 2.1% of patients receiving ARIXTRA and 0.2% of enoxaparin sodium patients [see Adverse Reactions (6.1)].
[See table 10 at left]

14.5   Prophylaxis of Thromboembolic Events Following Abdominal Surgery in Patients at Risk for Thromboembolic Complications
Abdominal surgery patients at risk included the following: Those undergoing surgery under general anesthesia lasting longer than 45 minutes who are older than 60 years with or

without additional risk factors; and those undergoing surgery under general anesthesia lasting longer than 45 minutes who are older than 40 years with additional risk factors. Risk factors included neoplastic disease, obesity, chronic obstructive pulmonary disease, inflammatory bowel disease, history of deep vein thrombosis (DVT) or pulmonary embolism (PE), or congestive heart failure.

In a randomized, double-blind, clinical trial in patients undergoing abdominal surgery, ARIXTRA 2.5 mg SC once daily started postoperatively was compared to dalteparin sodium 5,000 IU SC once daily, with one 2,500 IU SC preoperative injection and a 2,500 IU SC first postoperative injection. A total of 2,927 patients were randomized and 2,858 were treated. Patients ranged in age from 17 to 93 years (mean age 65 years) with 55% men and 45% women. Patients were 97% Caucasian, 1% black, 1% Asian, and 1% others. Patients with serum creatinine level more than 2 mg/dL (180 micromol/L), or platelet count less than 100,000/mm³ were excluded from the trial. Sixty-nine percent (69%) of study patients underwent cancer-related abdominal surgery. Study treatment was continued for 7 ± 2 days. The efficacy data are provided in Table 11 and demonstrate that prophylaxis with ARIXTRA was associated with a VTE rate of 4.6% compared with 6.1% for dalteparin sodium (P = NS).

[See table 11 at right]

14.6   Treatment of Deep Vein Thrombosis

In a randomized, double-blind, clinical trial in patients with a confirmed diagnosis of acute symptomatic DVT without PE, ARIXTRA 5 mg (body weight <50 kg), 7.5 mg (body weight 50 to 100 kg), or 10 mg (body weight >100 kg) SC once daily (ARIXTRA treatment regimen) was compared to enoxaparin sodium 1 mg/kg SC every 12 hours. Almost all patients started study treatment in hospital. Approximately 30% of patients in both groups were discharged home from the hospital while receiving study treatment. A total of 2,205 patients were randomized and 2,192 were treated. Patients ranged in age from 18 to 95 years (mean age 61 years) with 53% men and 47% women. Patients were 97% Caucasian, 2% black, and 1% other races. Patients with serum creatinine level more than 2 mg/dL (180 micromol/L), or platelet count less than 100,000/mm³ were excluded from the trial. For both groups, treatment continued for at least 5 days with a treatment duration range of 7 ± 2 days, and both treatment groups received vitamin K antagonist therapy initiated within 72 hours after the first study drug administration and continued for 90 ± 7 days, with regular dose adjustments to achieve an INR of 2 to 3. The primary efficacy endpoint was confirmed, symptomatic, recurrent VTE reported up to Day 97. The efficacy data are provided in Table 12.

[See table 12 at right]

During the initial treatment period, 18 (1.6%) of patients treated with fondaparinux sodium and 10 (0.9%) of patients treated with enoxaparin sodium had a VTE endpoint (95% CI for the treatment difference [fondaparinux sodium-enoxaparin sodium] for VTE rates: -0.2%; 1.7%).

14.7   Treatment of Pulmonary Embolism

In a randomized, open-label, clinical trial in patients with a confirmed diagnosis of acute symptomatic PE, with or without DVT, ARIXTRA 5 mg (body weight <50 kg), 7.5 mg (body weight 50 to 100 kg), or 10 mg (body weight >100 kg) SC once daily (ARIXTRA treatment regimen) was compared to heparin IV bolus (5,000 USP units) followed by a continuous IV infusion adjusted to maintain 1.5 to 2.5 times aPTT control value. Patients with a PE requiring thrombolysis or surgical thrombectomy were excluded from the trial. All patients started study treatment in hospital. Approximately 15% of patients were discharged home from the hospital while receiving ARIXTRA therapy. A total of 2,213 patients were randomized and 2,184 were treated. Patients ranged in age from 18 to 97 years (mean age 62 years) with 44% men and 56% women. Patients were 94% Caucasian, 5% black, and 1% other races. Patients with serum creatinine level more than 2 mg/dL (180 micromol/L), or platelet count less than 100,000/mm³ were excluded from the trial. For both groups, treatment continued for at least 5 days with a treatment duration range 7 ± 2 days, and both treatment groups received vitamin K antagonist therapy initiated within 72 hours after the first study drug administration and continued for 90 ± 7 days, with regular dose adjustments to achieve an INR of 2 to 3. The primary efficacy endpoint was confirmed, symptomatic, recurrent VTE reported up to Day 97. The efficacy data are provided in Table 13.

[See table 13 at right]

During the initial treatment period, 12 (1.1%) of patients treated with fondaparinux sodium and 19 (1.7%) of patients treated with heparin had a VTE endpoint (95% CI for the treatment difference [fondaparinux sodium-heparin] for VTE rates: -1.6%; 0.4%).

16   HOW SUPPLIED/STORAGE AND HANDLING

ARIXTRA Injection is available in the following strengths and package sizes:

Table 11. Efficacy of ARIXTRA In Prophylaxis of Thromboembolic Events Following Abdominal Surgery

Endpoint	ARIXTRA 2.5 mg SC once daily		Dalteparin Sodium 5,000 IU SC once daily	
	n/N[a]	% (95% CI)	n/N[a]	% (95% CI)
VTE[b]	47/1,027	4.6%[c] (3.4, 6.0)	62/1,021	6.1% (4.7, 7.7)
All DVT	43/1,024	4.2% (3.1, 5.6)	59/1,018	5.8% (4.4, 7.4)
Proximal DVT	5/1,076	0.5% (0.2, 1.1)	5/1,077	0.5% (0.2, 1.1)
Symptomatic VTE	6/1,465	0.4% (0.2, 0.9)	5/1,462	0.3% (0.1, 0.8)

[a] N = all evaluable abdominal surgery patients. Evaluable patients were those who were randomized and had an adequate efficacy assessment up to Day 10; non-treated patients and patients who did not undergo surgery did not get a VTE assessment.
[b] VTE was a composite of venogram positive DVT, symptomatic DVT, non-fatal PE and/or fatal PE reported up to Day 10.
[c] P value versus dalteparin sodium: NS.

Table 12. Efficacy of ARIXTRA in the Treatment of Deep Vein Thrombosis (All Randomized)

Endpoint	ARIXTRA 5, 7.5, or 10 mg SC once daily N = 1,098		Enoxaparin Sodium 1 mg/kg SC every 12 hours N = 1,107	
	n	% (95% CI)	n	% (95% CI)
Total VTE[a]	43	3.9% (2.8, 5.2)	45	4.1% (3.0, 5.4)
DVT only	18	1.6% (1.0, 2.6)	28	2.5% (1.7, 3.6)
Non-fatal PE	20	1.8% (1.1, 2.8)	12	1.1% (0.6, 1.9)
Fatal PE	5	0.5% (0.1, 1.1)	5	0.5% (0.1, 1.1)

[a] VTE was a composite of symptomatic recurrent non-fatal VTE or fatal PE reported up to Day 97. The 95% confidence interval for the treatment difference for total VTE was: (-1.8% to 1.5%).

Table 13. Efficacy of ARIXTRA in the Treatment of Pulmonary Embolism (All Randomized)

Endpoint	ARIXTRA 5, 7.5, or 10 mg SC once daily N = 1,103		Heparin aPTT adjusted IV N = 1,110	
	n	% (95% CI)	n	% (95% CI)
Total VTE[a]	42	3.8% (2.8, 5.1)	56	5.0% (3.8, 6.5)
DVT only	12	1.1% (0.6, 1.9)	17	1.5% (0.9, 2.4)
Non-fatal PE	14	1.3% (0.7, 2.1)	24	2.2% (1.4, 3.2)
Fatal PE	16	1.5% (0.8, 2.3)	15	1.4% (0.8, 2.2)

[a] VTE was a composite of symptomatic recurrent non-fatal VTE or fatal PE reported up to Day 97. The 95% confidence interval for the treatment difference for total VTE was: (-3.0% to 0.5%).

2.5 mg ARIXTRA in 0.5 mL single-dose prefilled syringe, affixed with a 27-gauge × ½-inch needle and an automatic needle protection system with blue plunger rod.

| NDC 0007-3230-02 | 2 Single Unit Syringes |
| NDC 0007-3230-11 | 10 Single Unit Syringes |

5 mg ARIXTRA in 0.4 mL single-dose prefilled syringe, affixed with a 27-gauge × ½-inch needle and an automatic needle protection system with orange plunger rod.

| NDC 0007-3232-02 | 2 Single Unit Syringes |
| NDC 0007-3232-11 | 10 Single Unit Syringes |

7.5 mg ARIXTRA in 0.6 mL single-dose prefilled syringe, affixed with a 27-gauge × ½-inch needle and an automatic needle protection system with magenta plunger rod.

| NDC 0007-3234-02 | 2 Single Unit Syringes |
| NDC 0007-3234-11 | 10 Single Unit Syringes |

10 mg ARIXTRA in 0.8 mL single-dose prefilled syringe, affixed with a 27-gauge × ½-inch needle and an automatic needle protection system with violet plunger rod.

| NDC 0007-3236-02 | 2 Single Unit Syringes |
| NDC 0007-3236-11 | 10 Single Unit Syringes |

Store at 25°C (77°F); excursions permitted to 15–30°C (59–86°F).

17   PATIENT COUNSELING INFORMATION

See FDA-Approved Patient Labeling (17.2)

17.1   Patient Advice

If the patients have had neuraxial anesthesia or spinal puncture, and particularly if they are taking concomitant NSAIDS, platelet inhibitors, or other anticoagulants, they should be informed to watch for signs and symptoms of spinal or epidural hematomas, such as tingling, numbness (especially in the lower limbs) and muscular weakness. If any of these symptoms occur, the patients should contact his or her physician immediately.

The use of aspirin and other NSAIDS may enhance the risk of hemorrhage. Their use should be discontinued prior to ARIXTRA therapy whenever possible; if co-administration is essential, the patient's clinical and laboratory status should be closely monitored. [See Drug Interactions (7).]

If patients must self-administer ARIXTRA (e.g., if ARIXTRA is used at home), they should be advised of the following:

• ARIXTRA should be given by subcutaneous injection. Patients must be instructed in the proper technique for administration.

Instructions for self-administration

The different parts of ARIXTRA safety syringe are:

1. Rigid needle guard
2. Cap
3. Plunger
4. Finger-grip
5. Security sleeve

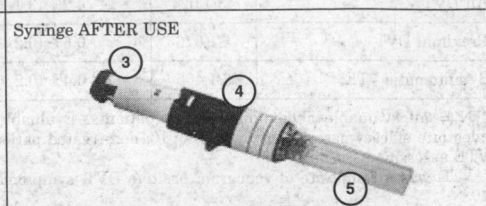

Syringe BEFORE USE

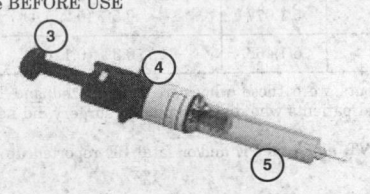

Syringe AFTER USE

1. Wash your hands thoroughly with soap and water. Towel dry.

2. Sit or lie down in a comfortable position. Choose a spot on the lower stomach area (abdomen), at least 2 inches below your belly button (Figure A). Change (alternate) between using the left and right side of the lower abdomen for each injection. If you have any questions talk to your nurse or doctor.

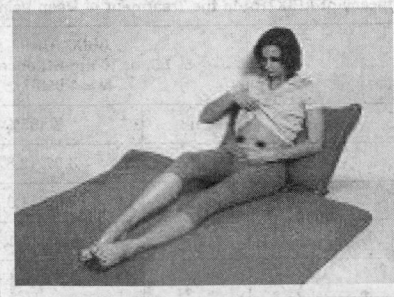

Figure A.

3. Clean the injection area with an alcohol swab.

4. Hold the security sleeve firmly in one hand. Pull off the cap that protects the plunger (Figure B). Discard the plunger cap.

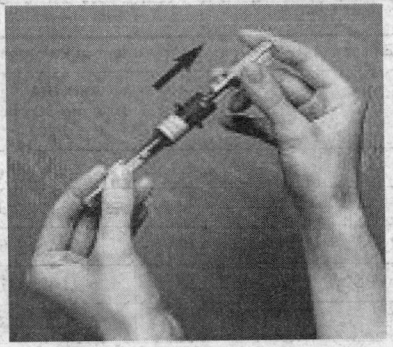

Figure B.

5. Remove the needle guard, by first twisting it and then pulling it in a straight line away from the body of the syringe (Figure C). Discard the needle guard.

To prevent infection, do not touch the needle or let it come in contact with any surface before the injection. A small air bubble in the syringe is normal. To be sure that you do not lose any medicine from the syringe, do not try to remove air bubbles from the syringe before giving the injection.

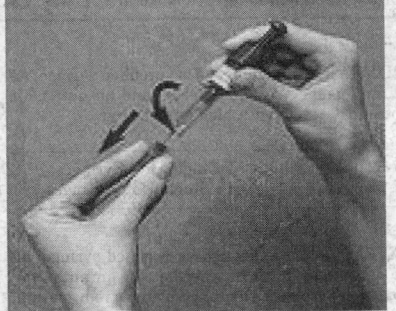

Figure C.

(Table continued on next page)

- As with all anticoagulants, the most important risk with ARIXTRA administration is bleeding. Patients should be counseled on signs and symptoms of possible bleeding.
- It may take them longer than usual to stop bleeding.
- They may bruise and/or bleed more easily when they are treated with ARIXTRA.
- They should report any unusual bleeding, bruising, or signs of thrombocytopenia (such as a rash of dark red spots under the skin) to their physician *[see Warnings and Precautions (5.1, 5.4)]*.
- To tell their physicians and dentists they are taking ARIXTRA and/or any other product known to affect bleeding before any surgery is scheduled and before any new drug is taken *[see Warnings and Precautions (5.1)]*.

- To tell their physicians and dentists of all medications they are taking, including those obtained without a prescription, such as aspirin or other NSAIDs. *[See Drug Interactions (7)]*.

Keep out of the reach of children.

17.2   FDA-Approved Patient Labeling

Patient labeling is provided as a tear-off leaflet at the end of this full prescribing information.

ARIXTRA is a registered trademark of GlaxoSmithKline.
GlaxoSmithKline
Research Triangle Park, NC 27709
©2010, GlaxoSmithKline. All rights reserved.
March 2010
ARX:7PI

PHARMACIST-DETACH HERE AND GIVE INSTRUCTIONS TO PATIENT

PATIENT INFORMATION

ARIXTRA® (Ah-RIX-trah)
fondaparinux sodium injection

Read the Patient Information that comes with ARIXTRA before you start taking it and each time you get a refill. There may be new information. This information does not take the place of talking with your doctor about your medical condition or your treatment. If you have any questions about ARIXTRA, ask your doctor or pharmacist.

What is the most important information I should know about ARIXTRA?

Certain medical procedures involving the spine, such as an epidural (pain medication given through the spine), spinal anesthesia, or spinal puncture, may be used during your hospital stay. If you need any of these procedures while receiving ARIXTRA, heparins, heparinoids, or low-molecular weight heparins (anticoagulants), you may be at risk for having a blood clot (hematoma) in or around your spine. This type of clot is very serious, as it can cause long-term and possibly permanent paralysis (loss of the ability to move). If you receive ARIXTRA after an epidural or spinal anesthetic is used, as the anesthesia for your surgery, your doctor will watch you closely for problems with feeling (sensation) and being able to move. Tell your doctor right away if you have any of these signs and symptoms, especially in your legs and feet:
- tingling
- numbness
- muscle weakness

Because the risk of bleeding may be higher, tell your doctor before taking ARIXTRA if you:
- are also taking certain other medicines that affect blood clotting such as aspirin, an NSAID (for example, ibuprofen or naproxen), clopidogrel, or warfarin sodium.
- have bleeding problems.
- had problems in the past with pain medication given through the spine.
- have had surgery to your spine.
- have a spinal deformity.

What is ARIXTRA?

ARIXTRA is a prescription medicine that "thins your blood" (also known as an anticoagulant). ARIXTRA is used to:
- help prevent blood clots from forming in patients who have had certain surgeries of the hip, knee, or the stomach area (abdominal surgery)
- treat people who have blood clots in their legs or blood clots that travel to their lungs

It is not known if ARIXTRA is safe and effective for use in children younger than 18 years of age.

Who should not take ARIXTRA?

Do not take ARIXTRA if you have:
- certain kidney problems
- active bleeding problems
- an infection in your heart
- low platelet counts and if you test positive for a certain antibody while you are taking ARIXTRA.

People who weigh less than 110 pounds (50 kg) should not use ARIXTRA to prevent blood clots from forming after surgery.

What should I tell my doctor before taking ARIXTRA?

Tell your doctor about all of your medical conditions, including if you:
- have had any bleeding problems (such as stomach ulcers)
- have had a stroke
- have had recent surgeries, including eye surgery
- have diabetic eye disease
- have kidney problems
- have uncontrolled high blood pressure
- have a latex allergy. The packaging (needle guard) for ARIXTRA contains dry natural rubber.
- are pregnant. It is not known if ARIXTRA will harm your unborn baby. If you are pregnant, talk to your doctor about the best way for you to prevent or treat blood clots.
- are breast-feeding. It is not known if ARIXTRA passes into breast milk.

Tell your doctor about all the medicines you take including prescriptions and non-prescription medicines, vitamins, and herbal supplements. Some medicines can increase your risk of bleeding. Especially tell your doctor if you take:
- aspirin
- NSAIDS (such as ibuprofen or naproxen)
- other blood thinner medicines, such as clopidogrel or warfarin

See "What is the most important information I should know about ARIXTRA?" Do not start taking any new medicines without first talking to your doctor.

Know the medicines you take. Tell all your doctors and dentist that you take ARIXTRA, especially if you need to have any kind of surgery or a dental procedure. Keep a list of your medicines and show it to all your doctors and pharmacist before you start a new medicine.

Instructions for self-administration *(continued)*

6. Gently pinch the skin that has been cleaned to make a fold. Hold the fold between the thumb and the forefinger of one hand during the entire injection (Figure D).

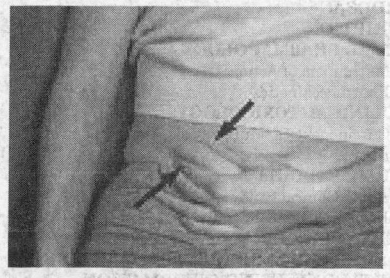

Figure D.

7. Hold the syringe firmly in your other hand using the finger grip. Insert the full length of the needle directly up and down (at an angle of 90°) into the skin fold (Figure E).

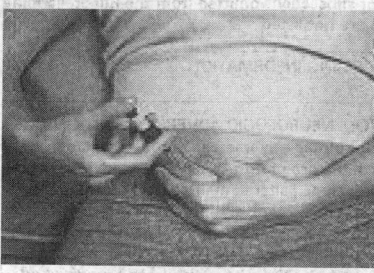

Figure E.

8. Inject all of the medicine in the syringe by pressing down on the plunger as far as it goes. This will activate the automatic needle protection system (Figure F).

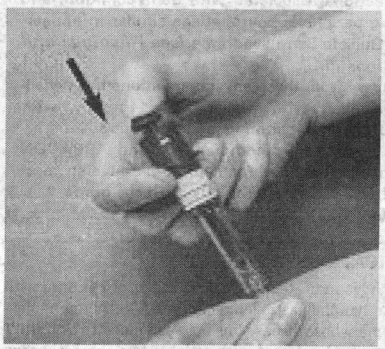

Figure F.

9. Release the plunger. The needle will withdraw automatically from the skin, and pull back (retract) into the security sleeve where it will be locked (Figure G).

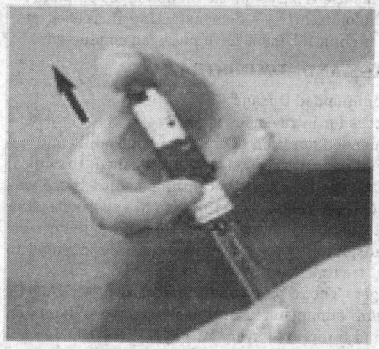

Figure G.

Follow the instructions given to you by your nurse or doctor about the right way to throw away used syringes and needles. There may be state laws about the right way to dispose of used syringes, needles, and disposal containers.

How should I take ARIXTRA?
• Take ARIXTRA exactly as prescribed by your doctor.
• ARIXTRA is given by injection under the skin (subcutaneous injection). See "How should I give an injection of ARIXTRA?"
• If your doctor tells you that you may give yourself injections of ARIXTRA at home, you will be shown how to give the injections first before you do them on your own.
• Tell your doctor if you have any bleeding or bruising while taking ARIXTRA.
• If you miss a dose of ARIXTRA, take your dose as soon as you remember. Do not take 2 doses at the same time.
• If you take too much ARIXTRA, call your doctor right away.
• Do not use ARIXTRA if:
  • the solution appears discolored (the solution should normally appear clear),
  • you see any particles in the solution, or
  • the syringe is damaged.

What are possible side effects of ARIXTRA?
ARIXTRA can cause serious side effects. See "What is the most important information I should know about ARIXTRA?"
• Severe **bleeding**
  Certain conditions can increase your risk for severe bleeding, including:
  -some bleeding problems
  -some gastrointestinal problems including ulcers
  -some types of strokes
  -uncontrolled high blood pressure
  -diabetic eye disease
  -soon after brain, spine, or eye surgery
  • **Certain kidney problems can also increase your risk of bleeding with ARIXTRA.** Your doctor may check your kidney function while you are taking ARIXTRA.
  • **People undergoing surgery who weigh less than 110 pounds.** See "Who should not take ARIXTRA?"
  • **Low blood platelets.** Low blood platelets can happen when you take ARIXTRA. Platelets are blood cells that

help your blood to clot normally. Your doctor may check your platelet counts while you take ARIXTRA.
You may bruise or bleed more easily while taking ARIXTRA, and it may take longer than usual for bleeding to stop.
Tell your doctor if you have any of these signs or symptoms of bleeding while taking ARIXTRA.
-any bleeding
-bruising
-rash of dark red spots under the skin
• **Allergic reactions.** See "What should I tell my doctor before taking ARIXTRA?"
Other side effects include:
• **Injection site reactions.** Bleeding, rash, and itching can happen at the place where you inject ARIXTRA.
• **Low red blood cell counts (anemia).** Your doctor may check your red blood cell counts while you are taking ARIXTRA.
• **Increased liver enzyme test results.** Your doctor may check your liver function while you are taking ARIXTRA.
• **Sleep problems (insomnia).**
These are not all the possible side effects of ARIXTRA. Call your doctor if you have any side effects that bother you or don't go away.
Call your doctor for medical advice about side effects. You may report side effects to the FDA at 1-800-FDA-1088.
How should I store ARIXTRA?
Store ARIXTRA at room temperature 59°F to 86°F (15°C to 30°C). Do not freeze.
Safely, throw away ARIXTRA that is out of date or no longer needed.
Keep ARIXTRA and all medicines out of the reach of children.
General information about ARIXTRA
Medicines are sometimes prescribed for purposes other than those described in patient information leaflets. Do not use ARIXTRA for a condition for which it was not prescribed. Do not give ARIXTRA to other people. It may harm them.
This leaflet summarizes the most important information about ARIXTRA. If you would like more information, talk with your doctor. You can ask your doctor or pharmacist for information about ARIXTRA that is written for healthcare professionals. For more information about ARIXTRA, go to www.ARIXTRA.com or call 1-888-825-5249.
What are the ingredients in ARIXTRA?
Active Ingredient: fondaparinux sodium
Inactive Ingredients: sodium chloride and water for injection
How should I give an injection of ARIXTRA?
ARIXTRA is injected into a skin fold of the lower stomach area (abdomen). Do not inject ARIXTRA into muscle. Usually a doctor or nurse will give this injection to you. In some cases you may be taught how to do this yourself. Be sure that you read, understand, and follow the step-by-step instructions in this leaflet, on how to give yourself an injection of ARIXTRA.
[See table on previous page and at left]
ARIXTRA is a registered trademark of GlaxoSmithKline.
GlaxoSmithKline
Research Triangle Park, NC 27709
©2010, GlaxoSmithKline. All rights reserved.
Revised: January 2010
ARX:3PIL

ARRANON® ℞
[air' ə-non]
(nelarabine)
Injection

HIGHLIGHTS OF PRESCRIBING INFORMATION
These highlights do not include all the information needed to use ARRANON safely and effectively. See full prescribing information for ARRANON.
ARRANON (nelarabine) Injection
Initial U.S. Approval: 2005

> **WARNING: NEUROLOGIC ADVERSE REACTIONS**
> *See full prescribing information for complete boxed warning.*
> **Severe neurologic adverse reactions have been reported with the use of ARRANON. These adverse reactions have included altered mental states including severe somnolence, central nervous system effects including convulsions, and peripheral neuropathy ranging from numbness and paresthesias to motor weakness and paralysis. There have also been reports of adverse reactions associated with demyelination, and ascending peripheral neuropathies similar in appearance to Guillain-Barré syndrome. (5.1)**
> **Full recovery from these adverse reactions has not always occurred with cessation of therapy with ARRANON. Close monitoring for neurologic adverse reactions is strongly recommended, and ARRANON**

should be discontinued for neurologic adverse reactions of NCI Common Toxicity Criteria grade 2 or greater. (5.1)

INDICATIONS AND USAGE

ARRANON is a nucleoside metabolic inhibitor indicated for the treatment of patients with T-cell acute lymphoblastic leukemia and T-cell lymphoblastic lymphoma whose disease has not responded to or has relapsed following treatment with at least two chemotherapy regimens. This use is based on the induction of complete responses. Randomized trials demonstrating increased survival or other clinical benefit have not been conducted. (1)

DOSAGE AND ADMINISTRATION

- Adult dose: 1,500 mg/m^2 administered intravenously over 2 hours on days 1, 3, and 5 repeated every 21 days. (2.1)
- Pediatric dose: 650 mg/m^2 administered intravenously over 1 hour daily for 5 consecutive days repeated every 21 days. (2.1)
- Discontinue treatment for ≥grade 2 neurologic reactions. (2.2)
- Dosage may be delayed for hematologic reactions (2.2)
- Take measures to prevent hyperuricemia. (2.4)

DOSAGE FORMS AND STRENGTHS

250 mg/50 mL (5 mg/mL) vial (3)

CONTRAINDICATIONS

None.

WARNINGS AND PRECAUTIONS

- Severe neurologic reactions have been reported. Monitor for signs and symptoms of neurologic toxicity. (5.1)
- Hematologic Reactions: Complete blood counts including platelets should be monitored regularly. (5.2)
- Fetal harm can occur if administered to a pregnant woman. Women should be advised not to become pregnant when taking ARRANON. (5.3)

ADVERSE REACTIONS

The most common (≥ 20%) adverse reactions were:
- Adult: anemia, thrombocytopenia, neutropenia, nausea, diarrhea, vomiting, constipation, fatigue, pyrexia, cough, and dyspnea (6.1)
- Pediatric: anemia, neutropenia, thrombocytopenia, and leukopenia (6.1)

The most common (>10%) neurological adverse reactions were:
- Adult: somnolence, dizziness, peripheral neurologic disorders, hypoesthesia, headache, and paresthesia (6.1)
- Pediatric: headache and peripheral neurologic disorders (6.1)

To report SUSPECTED ADVERSE REACTIONS, contact GlaxoSmithKline at 1-888-825-5249 or FDA at 1-800-FDA-1088 or www.fda.gov/medwatch.

DRUG INTERACTIONS

Administration in combination with adenosine deaminase inhibitors, such as pentostatin, is not recommended. (7, 12.3)

USE IN SPECIFIC POPULATIONS

- Renal Impairment: Closely monitor patients with moderate or severe renal impairment for toxicities. (8.6)
- Hepatic Impairment: Closely monitor patients with severe hepatic impairment for toxicities. (8.7)

Revised: December 2009
ARR:1PI

See 17 for PATIENT COUNSELING INFORMATION and FDA-approved patient labeling

Revised: 12/2009

FULL PRESCRIBING INFORMATION

> **WARNING: NEUROLOGIC ADVERSE REACTIONS**
> Severe neurologic adverse reactions have been reported with the use of ARRANON. These adverse reactions have included altered mental states including severe somnolence, central nervous system effects including convulsions, and peripheral neuropathy ranging from numbness and paresthesias to motor weakness and paralysis. There have also been reports of adverse reactions associated with demyelination, and ascending peripheral neuropathies similar in appearance to Guillain-Barré syndrome [see Warnings and Precautions (5.1)].
> Full recovery from these adverse reactions has not always occurred with cessation of therapy with ARRANON. Close monitoring for neurologic adverse reactions is strongly recommended, and ARRANON should be discontinued for neurologic adverse reactions of NCI Common Toxicity Criteria grade 2 or greater [see Warnings and Precautions (5.1)].

1   INDICATIONS AND USAGE

ARRANON® is indicated for the treatment of patients with T-cell acute lymphoblastic leukemia and T-cell lymphoblastic lymphoma whose disease has not responded to or has relapsed following treatment with at least two chemotherapy regimens. This use is based on the induction of complete responses. Randomized trials demonstrating increased survival or other clinical benefit have not been conducted.

2   DOSAGE AND ADMINISTRATION

2.1   Recommended Dosage

This product is for intravenous use only.

The recommended duration of treatment for adult and pediatric patients has not been clearly established. In clinical trials, treatment was generally continued until there was evidence of disease progression, the patient experienced unacceptable toxicity, the patient became a candidate for bone marrow transplant, or the patient no longer continued to benefit from treatment.

Adult Dosage: The recommended adult dose of ARRANON is 1,500 mg/m^2 administered intravenously over 2 hours on days 1, 3, and 5 repeated every 21 days. ARRANON is administered undiluted.

Pediatric Dosage: The recommended pediatric dose of ARRANON is 650 mg/m^2 administered intravenously over 1 hour daily for 5 consecutive days repeated every 21 days. ARRANON is administered undiluted.

2.2   Dosage Modification

ARRANON administration should be discontinued for neurologic adverse reactions of NCI Common Toxicity Criteria grade 2 or greater. Dosage may be delayed for other toxicity including hematologic toxicity. [See Boxed Warning and Warnings and Precautions (5.1, 5.2).]

2.3   Adjustment of Dose in Special Populations

ARRANON has not been studied in patients with renal or hepatic dysfunction [see Use in Specific Populations (8.6, 8.7)]. No dose adjustment is recommended for patients with a creatinine clearance (CL$_{cr}$) ≥50 mL/min [see Clinical Pharmacology (12.3)]. There are insufficient data to support a dose recommendation for patients with a CL$_{cr}$ <50 mL/min.

2.4   Prevention of Hyperuricemia

Appropriate measures (e.g., hydration, urine alkalinization, and prophylaxis with allopurinol) must be taken to prevent hyperuricemia [see Warnings and Precautions (5.4)].

2.5   Instructions for Handling, Preparation, and Administration

Handling: ARRANON is a cytotoxic agent. Caution should be used during handling and preparation. Use of gloves and other protective clothing to prevent skin contact is recommended. Proper aseptic technique should be used. Guidelines for proper handling and disposal of anticancer drugs have been published.[1-4]

Preparation and Administration: Do not dilute ARRANON prior to administration. The appropriate dose of ARRANON is transferred into polyvinylchloride (PVC) infusion bags or glass containers and administered as a two-hour infusion in adult patients and as a one-hour infusion in pediatric patients.

Prior to administration, inspect the drug product visually for particulate matter and discoloration.

Stability: ARRANON Injection is stable in polyvinylchloride (PVC) infusion bags and glass containers for up to 8 hours at up to 30° C.

3   DOSAGE FORMS AND STRENGTHS

250 mg/50 mL (5 mg/mL) vial

4   CONTRAINDICATIONS

None.

5   WARNINGS AND PRECAUTIONS

5.1   Neurologic Adverse Reactions

Neurotoxicity is the dose-limiting toxicity of nelarabine. Patients undergoing therapy with ARRANON should be closely observed for signs and symptoms of neurologic toxicity [see Boxed Warning and Dosage and Administration (2.2)]. Common signs and symptoms of nelarabine-related neurotoxicity include somnolence, confusion, convulsions, ataxia, paresthesias, and hypoesthesia. Severe neurologic toxicity can manifest as coma, status epilepticus, craniospinal demyelination, or ascending neuropathy similar in presentation to Guillain-Barré syndrome.

Patients treated previously or concurrently with intrathecal chemotherapy or previously with craniospinal irradiation may be at increased risk for neurologic adverse events.

5.2   Hematologic Adverse Reactions

Leukopenia, thrombocytopenia, anemia, and neutropenia, including febrile neutropenia have been associated with nelarabine therapy. Complete blood counts including platelets should be monitored regularly [see Dosage and Administration (2.2) and Adverse Reactions (6.1)].

5.3   Pregnancy

Pregnancy Category D

ARRANON can cause fetal harm when administered to a pregnant woman.

Nelarabine administered during the period of organogenesis caused increased incidences of fetal malformations, anomalies, and variations in rabbits (see Use in Specific Populations (8.1)).

There are no adequate and well-controlled studies of ARRANON in pregnant women. If this drug is used during pregnancy, or if the patient becomes pregnant while taking this drug, the patient should be apprised of the potential hazard to the fetus. Women of child-bearing potential should be advised to avoid becoming pregnant while receiving treatment with ARRANON.

5.4   Hyperuricemia

Patients receiving ARRANON should receive intravenous hydration according to standard medical practice for the management of hyperuricemia in patients at risk for tumor lysis syndrome. Consideration should be given to the use of allopurinol in patients at risk of hyperuricemia [see Dosage and Administration (2.4)].

5.5   Vaccinations

Administration of live vaccines to immunocompromised patients should be avoided.

6   ADVERSE REACTIONS

The following serious adverse reactions are discussed in greater detail in other sections of the label:
- Neurologic [see Boxed Warning and Warnings and Precautions (5.1)]
- Hematologic [see Warnings and Precautions (5.2)]
- Hyperuricemia [see Warnings and Precautions (5.4)]

6.1   Clinical Trials Experience

Because clinical trials are conducted under widely varying conditions, adverse reaction rates observed in the clinical trials of a drug cannot be directly compared to rates in the clinical trials of another drug and may not reflect the rates observed in practice.

ARRANON was studied in 459 patients in Phase I and Phase II clinical trials.

Adults: The safety profile of ARRANON is based on data from 103 adult patients treated with the recommended dose and schedule in 2 studies: an adult T-cell acute lymphoblastic leukemia (T-ALL)/T-cell lymphoblastic lymphoma (T-LBL) study and an adult chronic lymphocytic leukemia study.

The most common adverse reactions in adults, regardless of causality, were fatigue; gastrointestinal (GI) disorders (nausea, diarrhea, vomiting, and constipation); hematologic disorders (anemia, neutropenia, and thrombocytopenia); respiratory disorders (cough and dyspnea); nervous system disorders (somnolence and dizziness); and pyrexia.

The most common adverse reactions in adults, by System Organ Class, regardless of causality, including severe or life threatening adverse reactions (NCI Common Toxicity Criteria grade 3 or grade 4) and fatal adverse reactions (grade 5) are shown in Table 1.

Table 1. Most Commonly Reported (≥5% Overall) Adverse Reactions Regardless of Causality in Adult Patients Treated with 1,500 mg/m² of ARRANON Administered Intravenously Over 2 Hours on Days 1, 3, and 5 Repeated Every 21 Days

System Organ Class Preferred Term	Percentage of Patients (N = 103)		
	Toxicity Grade		
	Grade 3	Grade 4 and 5[a]	All Grades
	%	%	%
Blood and Lymphatic System Disorders			
Anemia	20	14	99
Thrombocytopenia	37	22	86
Neutropenia	14	49	81
Febrile neutropenia	9	1	12
Cardiac Disorders			
Sinus tachycardia	1	0	8
Gastrointestinal Disorders			
Nausea	0	0	41
Diarrhea	1	0	22
Vomiting	1	0	22
Constipation	1	0	21
Abdominal pain	1	0	9
Stomatitis	1	0	8
Abdominal distension	0	0	6
General Disorders and Administration Site Conditions			
Fatigue	10	2	50
Pyrexia	5	0	23
Asthenia	0	1	17
Edema, peripheral	0	0	15
Edema	0	0	11
Pain	3	0	11
Rigors	0	0	8
Gait, abnormal	0	0	6
Chest pain	0	0	5
Non-cardiac chest pain	0	1	5
Infections			
Infection	2	1	9
Pneumonia	4	1	8
Sinusitis	1	0	7
Hepatobiliary Disorders			
AST increased	1	0	6
Metabolism and Nutrition Disorders			
Anorexia	0	0	9
Dehydration	3	1	7
Hyperglycemia	1	0	6
Musculoskeletal and Connective Tissue Disorders			
Myalgia	1	0	13
Arthralgia	1	0	9
Back pain	0	0	8
Muscular weakness	5	0	8
Pain in extremity	1	0	7
Nervous System Disorders (see Table 2)			
Psychiatric Disorders			
Confusional state	2	0	8
Insomnia	0	0	7
Depression	1	0	6
Respiratory, Thoracic, and Mediastinal Disorders			
Cough	0	0	25
Dyspnea	4	2	20
Pleural effusion	5	1	10
Epistaxis	0	0	8
Dyspnea, exertional	0	0	7
Wheezing	0	0	5
Vascular Disorders			
Petechiae	2	0	12
Hypotension	1	1	8

[a] Five patients had a fatal adverse reaction. Fatal adverse reactions included hypotension (n = 1), respiratory arrest (n = 1), pleural effusion/pneumothorax (n = 1), pneumonia (n = 1), and cerebral hemorrhage/coma/leukoencephalopathy (n = 1).

Other Adverse Events: Blurred vision was also reported in 4% of adult patients. There was a single report of biopsy confirmed progressive multifocal leukoencephalopathy in the adult patient population.

Neurologic Adverse Reactions: Nervous system adverse reactions, regardless of drug relationship, were reported for 76% of adult patients across the Phase I and Phase II studies. The most common neurologic adverse reactions (≥2%) in adult patients, regardless of causality, including all grades (NCI Common Toxicity Criteria) are shown in Table 2.

[See table below]

One patient had a fatal neurologic adverse reaction, cerebral hemorrhage/coma/leukoencephalopathy.

Most nervous system adverse reactions in the adult patients were evaluated as grade 1 or 2. The additional grade 3 adverse reactions in adult patients, regardless of causality, were aphasia, convulsion, hemiparesis, and loss of consciousness, each reported in 1 patient (1%). The additional grade 4 adverse reactions, regardless of causality, were cerebral hemorrhage, coma, intracranial hemorrhage, leukoencephalopathy, and metabolic encephalopathy, each reported in one patient (1%).

The other neurologic adverse reactions, regardless of causality, reported as grade 1, 2, or unknown in adult patients were abnormal coordination, burning sensation, disturbance in attention, dysarthria, hyporeflexia, neuropathic pain, nystagmus, peroneal nerve palsy, sciatica, sensory disturbance, sinus headache, and speech disorder, each reported in one patient (1%).

Pediatrics: The safety profile for children is based on data from 84 pediatric patients treated with the recommended dose and schedule in a T-cell acute lymphoblastic leukemia (T-ALL)/T-cell lymphoblastic lymphoma (T-LBL) treatment study.

The most common adverse reactions in pediatric patients, regardless of causality, were hematologic disorders (anemia, leukopenia, neutropenia, and thrombocytopenia). Of the non-hematologic adverse reactions in pediatric patients, the most frequent adverse reactions reported were headache, increased transaminase levels, decreased blood potassium, decreased blood albumin, increased blood bilirubin, and vomiting.

Table 2. Neurologic Adverse Reactions (≥2%) Regardless of Causality in Adult Patients Treated with 1,500 mg/m² of ARRANON Administered Intravenously Over 2 Hours on Days 1, 3, and 5 Repeated Every 21 Days

Nervous System Disorders Preferred Term	Percentage of Patients (N = 103)				
	Grade 1 %	Grade 2 %	Grade 3 %	Grade 4 %	All Grades %
Somnolence	20	3	0	0	23
Dizziness	14	8	0	0	21
Peripheral neurologic disorders, any adverse reaction	8	12	2	0	21
Neuropathy	0	4	0	0	4
Peripheral neuropathy	2	2	1	0	5
Peripheral motor neuropathy	3	3	1	0	7
Peripheral sensory neuropathy	7	6	0	0	13
Hypoesthesia	5	10	2	0	17
Headache	11	3	1	0	15
Paresthesia	11	4	0	0	15
Ataxia	1	6	2	0	9
Depressed level of consciousness	4	1	0	1	6
Tremor	2	3	0	0	5
Amnesia	2	1	0	0	3
Dysgeusia	2	1	0	0	3
Balance disorder	1	1	0	0	2
Sensory loss	0	2	0	0	2

The most common adverse reactions in pediatric patients, by System Organ Class, regardless of causality, including severe or life threatening adverse reactions (NCI Common Toxicity Criteria grade 3 or grade 4) and fatal adverse reactions (grade 5) are shown in Table 3.

Table 3. Most Commonly Reported (≥5% Overall) Adverse Reactions Regardless of Causality in Pediatric Patients Treated with 650 mg/m² of ARRANON Administered Intravenously Over 1 Hour Daily for 5 Consecutive Days Repeated Every 21 Days

System Organ Class Preferred Term	Percentage of Patients (N = 84)		
	Toxicity Grade		
	Grade 3 %	Grade 4 and 5[a] %	All Grades %
Blood and Lymphatic System Disorders			
Anemia	45	10	95
Neutropenia	17	62	94
Thrombocytopenia	27	32	88
Leukopenia	14	7	38
Hepatobiliary Disorders			
Transaminases increased	4	0	12
Blood albumin decreased	5	0	10
Blood bilirubin increased	7	2	10
Metabolic/Laboratory			
Blood potassium decreased	4	2	11
Blood calcium decreased	1	1	8
Blood creatinine increased	0	0	6
Blood glucose decreased	4	0	6
Blood magnesium decreased	2	0	6
Nervous System Disorders (see Table 4)			
Gastrointestinal Disorders			
Vomiting	0	0	10
General Disorders & Administration Site Conditions			
Asthenia	1	0	6
Infections & Infestations			
Infection	2	1	5

[a] Three patients had a fatal adverse reaction. Fatal adverse reactions included neutropenia and pyrexia (n = 1), status epilepticus/seizure (n = 1), and fungal pneumonia (n = 1).

Neurologic Adverse Reactions: Nervous system adverse reactions, regardless of drug relationship, were reported for 42% of pediatric patients across the Phase I and Phase II studies. The most common neurologic adverse reactions (≥2%) in pediatric patients, regardless of causality, including all grades (NCI Common Toxicity Criteria) are shown in Table 4.
[See table 4 at right]
The other grade 3 neurologic adverse reaction in pediatric patients, regardless of causality, was hypertonia reported in 1 patient (1%).
The additional grade 4 neurologic adverse reactions, regardless of causality, were 3rd nerve paralysis, and 6th nerve paralysis, each reported in 1 patient (1%).
The other neurologic adverse reactions, regardless of causality, reported as grade 1, 2, or unknown in pediatric patients were dysarthria, encephalopathy, hydrocephalus, hyporeflexia, lethargy, mental impairment, paralysis, and sensory loss, each reported in 1 patient (1%).

6.2 Postmarketing Experience
The following adverse reactions have been identified during post-approval use of ARRANON. Because these reactions are reported voluntarily from a population of uncertain size, it is not always possible to reliably estimate their frequency or establish a causal relationship to drug exposure.

Table 4. Neurologic Adverse Reactions (≥2%) Regardless of Causality in Pediatric Patients Treated with 650 mg/m² of ARRANON Administered Intravenously Over 1 Hour Daily for 5 Consecutive Days Repeated Every 21 Days

Nervous System Disorders Preferred Term	Percentage of Patients (N = 84)				
	Grade 1 %	Grade 2 %	Grade 3 %	Grade 4 and 5[a] %	All Grades %
Headache	8	2	4	2	17
Peripheral neurologic disorders, any adverse reaction	1	4	7	0	12
Peripheral neuropathy	0	4	2	0	6
Peripheral motor neuropathy	1	0	2	0	4
Peripheral sensory neuropathy	0	0	6	0	6
Somnolence	1	4	1	1	7
Hypoesthesia	1	1	4	0	6
Seizures	0	0	0	6	6
Convulsions	0	0	0	3	4
Grand mal convulsions	0	0	0	1	1
Status epilepticus	0	0	0	1	1
Motor dysfunction	1	1	1	0	4
Nervous system disorder	1	2	0	0	4
Paresthesia	0	2	1	0	4
Tremor	1	2	0	0	4
Ataxia	1	0	1	0	2

[a] One (1) patient had a fatal neurologic adverse reaction, status epilepticus.

Infections and Infestations: Fatal opportunistic infections. Metabolism and Nutrition Disorders: Tumor lysis syndrome.
Nervous System Disorders: Demyelination and ascending peripheral neuropathies similar in appearance to Guillain-Barré syndrome.

7 DRUG INTERACTIONS
Administration of nelarabine in combination with adenosine deaminase inhibitors, such as pentostatin, is not recommended [see Clinical Pharmacology (12.3)].

8 USE IN SPECIFIC POPULATIONS
8.1 Pregnancy
Pregnancy Category D [see Warnings and Precautions (5.3)]
ARRANON can cause fetal harm when administered to a pregnant woman. Nelarabine administered to rabbits during the period of organogenesis caused increased incidences of fetal malformations, anomalies, and variations at doses ≥360 mg/m²/day (8-hour IV infusion; approximately ¼ the adult dose compared on a mg/m² basis), which was the lowest dose tested. Cleft palate was seen in rabbits given 3,600 mg/m²/day (approximately 2-fold the adult dose), absent pollices (digits) in rabbits given ≥1,200 mg/m²/day (approximately ¾ the adult dose), while absent gall bladder, absent accessory lung lobes, fused or extra sternebrae and delayed ossification was seen at all doses. Maternal body weight gain and fetal body weights were reduced in rabbits given 3,600 mg/m²/day (approximately 2-fold the adult dose), but could not account for the increased incidence of malformations seen at this or lower administered doses.
There are no adequate and well-controlled studies of ARRANON in pregnant women. If this drug is used during pregnancy, or if the patient becomes pregnant while taking this drug, the patient should be apprised of the potential hazard to the fetus. Women of child-bearing potential should be advised to avoid becoming pregnant while receiving treatment with ARRANON.
8.3 Nursing Mothers
It is not known whether nelarabine or ara-G are excreted in human milk. Because many drugs are excreted in human milk and because of the potential for serious adverse reactions in nursing infants from ARRANON, a decision should be made whether to discontinue nursing or to discontinue the drug, taking into account the importance of the drug to the mother.
8.4 Pediatric Use
The safety and effectiveness of ARRANON has been established in pediatric patients [see Dosage and Administration (2.1) and Clinical Studies (14.2].
8.5 Geriatric Use
Clinical studies of ARRANON did not include sufficient numbers of patients aged 65 and over to determine whether they respond differently from younger patients. In an exploratory analysis, increasing age, especially age 65 years and older, appeared to be associated with increased rates of neurologic adverse reactions. Because elderly patients are more likely to have decreased renal function, care should be taken in dose selection, and it may be useful to monitor renal function.
8.6 Renal Impairment
Ara-G clearance decreased as renal function decreased [see Clinical Pharmacology (12.3)]. Because the risk of adverse reactions to this drug may be greater in patients with moderate (CL_cr 30 to 50 mL/min) or severe (CL_cr <30 mL/min) renal impairment, these patients should be closely monitored for toxicities when treated with ARRANON [see Dosage and Administration (2.3)].
8.7 Hepatic Impairment
The influence of hepatic impairment on the pharmacokinetics of nelarabine has not been evaluated. Because the risk of adverse reactions to this drug may be greater in patients with severe hepatic impairment (total bilirubin >3 times upper limit of normal), these patients should be closely monitored for toxicities when treated with ARRANON.

10 OVERDOSAGE
There is no known antidote for overdoses of ARRANON. It is anticipated that overdosage would result in severe neurotoxicity (possibly including paralysis, coma), myelosuppression, and potentially death. In the event of overdose, supportive care consistent with good clinical practice should be provided.
Nelarabine has been administered in clinical trials up to a dose of 2,900 mg/m² on days 1, 3, and 5 to 2 adult patients. At a dose of 2,200 mg/m² given on days 1, 3, and 5 every 21 days, 2 patients developed a significant grade 3 ascending sensory neuropathy. MRI evaluations of the 2 patients demonstrated findings consistent with a demyelinating process in the cervical spine.

11 DESCRIPTION
ARRANON (nelarabine) is a pro-drug of the cytotoxic deoxyguanosine analogue, 9-β-D-arabinofuranosylguanine (ara-G).
The chemical name for nelarabine is 2-amino-9-β-D-arabinofuranosyl-6-methoxy-9H-purine. It has the molecular formula $C_{11}H_{15}N_5O_5$ and a molecular weight of 297.27.
Nelarabine has the following structural formula:
[See chemical structure at top of next column]
Nelarabine is slightly soluble to soluble in water and melts with decomposition between 209° and 217° C.
ARRANON Injection is supplied as a clear, colorless, sterile solution in glass vials. Each vial contains 250 mg of nelarabine (5 mg nelarabine per mL) and the inactive ingre-

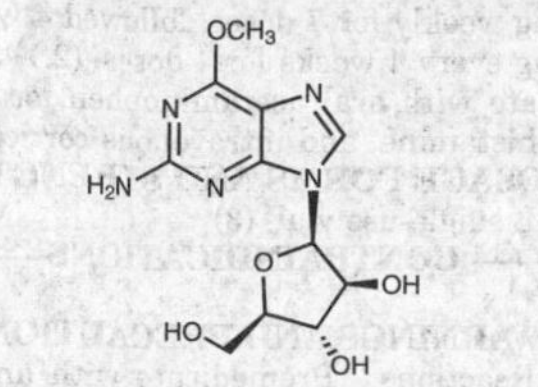

dient sodium chloride (4.5 mg per mL) in 50 mL Water for Injection, USP. ARRANON is intended for intravenous infusion.

Hydrochloric acid and sodium hydroxide may have been used to adjust the pH. The solution pH ranges from 5.0 to 7.0.

12 CLINICAL PHARMACOLOGY

12.1 Mechanism of Action

Nelarabine is a pro-drug of the deoxyguanosine analogue 9-β-*D*-arabinofuranosylguanine (ara-G), a nucleoside metabolic inhibitor. Nelarabine is demethylated by adenosine deaminase (ADA) to ara-G, mono-phosphorylated by deoxyguanosine kinase and deoxycytidine kinase, and subsequently converted to the active 5′-triphosphate, ara-GTP. Accumulation of ara-GTP in leukemic blasts allows for incorporation into deoxyribonucleic acid (DNA), leading to inhibition of DNA synthesis and cell death. Other mechanisms may contribute to the cytotoxic and systemic toxicity of nelarabine.

12.3 Pharmacokinetics

Absorption: Following intravenous administration of nelarabine to adult patients with refractory leukemia or lymphoma, plasma ara-G C_{max} values generally occurred at the end of the nelarabine infusion and were generally higher than nelarabine C_{max} values, suggesting rapid and extensive conversion of nelarabine to ara-G. Mean plasma nelarabine and ara-G C_{max} values were 5.0 ± 3.0 μg/mL and 31.4 ± 5.6 μg/mL, respectively, after a 1,500 mg/m^2 nelarabine dose infused over 2 hours in adult patients. The area under the concentration-time curve (AUC) of ara-G is 37 times higher than that for nelarabine on Day 1 after nelarabine IV infusion of 1,500 mg/m^2 dose (162 ± 49 μg.h/mL versus 4.4 ± 2.2 μg.h/mL, respectively). Comparable C_{max} and AUC values were obtained for nelarabine between Days 1 and 5 at the nelarabine adult dosage of 1,500 mg/m^2, indicating that nelarabine does not accumulate after multiple-dosing. There are not enough ara-G data to make a comparison between Day 1 and Day 5. After a nelarabine adult dose of 1,500 mg/m^2, intracellular C_{max} for ara-GTP appeared within 3 to 25 hours on Day 1. Exposure (AUC) to intracellular ara-GTP was 532 times higher than that for nelarabine and 14 times higher than that for ara-G (2,339 ± 2,628 μg.h/mL versus 4.4 ± 2.2 μg.h/mL and 162 ± 49 μg.h/mL, respectively). Because the intracellular levels of ara-GTP were so prolonged, its elimination half-life could not be accurately estimated.

Distribution: Nelarabine and ara-G are extensively distributed throughout the body. For nelarabine, V_{SS} values were 197 ± 216 L/m^2 in adult patients. For ara-G, V_{SS}/F values were 50 ± 24 L/m^2 in adult patients.

Nelarabine and ara-G are not substantially bound to human plasma proteins (<25%) in vitro, and binding is independent of nelarabine or ara-G concentrations up to 600 μM.

Metabolism: The principal route of metabolism for nelarabine is O-demethylation by adenosine deaminase to form ara-G, which undergoes hydrolysis to form guanine. In addition, some nelarabine is hydrolyzed to form methylguanine, which is O-demethylated to form guanine. Guanine is N-deaminated to form xanthine, which is further oxidized to yield uric acid.

Excretion: Nelarabine and ara-G are partially eliminated by the kidneys. Mean urinary excretion of nelarabine and ara-G was 6.6 ± 4.7% and 27 ± 15% of the administered dose, respectively, in 28 adult patients over the 24 hours after nelarabine infusion on Day 1. Renal clearance averaged 24 ± 23 L/h for nelarabine and 6.2 ± 5.0 L/h for ara-G in 21 adult patients. Combined Phase 1 pharmacokinetic data at nelarabine doses of 199 to 2,900 mg/m^2 (n = 66 adult patients) indicate that the mean clearance (CL) of nelarabine is 197 ± 189 L/h/m^2 on Day 1. The apparent clearance of ara-G (CL/F) is 10.5 ± 4.5 L/h/m^2 on Day 1. Nelarabine and ara-G are rapidly eliminated from plasma with a mean half-life of 18 minutes and 3.2 hours, respectively, in adult patients.

Pediatrics: No pharmacokinetic data are available in pediatric patients at the once daily 650 mg/m^2 nelarabine dosage. Combined Phase 1 pharmacokinetic data at nelarabine doses of 104 to 2,900 mg/m^2 indicate that the mean clearance (CL) of nelarabine is about 30% higher in pediatric patients than in adult patients (259 ± 409 L/h/m^2 versus 197 ± 189 L/h/m^2, respectively) (n = 66 adults, n = 22 pediatric patients) on Day 1. The apparent clearance of ara-G (CL/F) is comparable between the two groups (10.5 ± 4.5 L/h/m^2 in adult patients and 11.3 ± 4.2 L/h/m^2 in pediatric patients) on Day 1. Nelarabine and ara-G are extensively distributed throughout the body. For nelarabine, V_{SS} values were 213 ± 358 L/m^2 in pediatric patients. For ara-G, V_{SS}/F values were 33 ± 9.3 L/m^2 in pediatric patients. Nelarabine and ara-G are rapidly eliminated from plasma in pediatric patients, with a half-life of 13 minutes and 2 hours, respectively.

Effect of Age: Age has no effect on the pharmacokinetics of nelarabine or ara-G in adults. Decreased renal function, which is more common in the elderly, may reduce ara-G clearance *[see Use in Specific Populations (8.5)]*.

Effect of Gender: Gender has no effect on nelarabine or ara-G pharmacokinetics.

Effect of Race: In general, nelarabine mean clearance and volume of distribution values tend to be higher in Whites (n = 63) than in Blacks (by about 10%) (n = 15). The opposite is true for ara-G; mean apparent clearance and volume of distribution values tend to be lower in Whites than in Blacks (by about 15-20%). No differences in safety or effectiveness were observed between these groups.

Effect of Renal Impairment: The pharmacokinetics of nelarabine and ara-G have not been specifically studied in renally impaired or hemodialyzed patients. Nelarabine is excreted by the kidney to a small extent (5 to 10% of the administered dose). Ara-G is excreted by the kidney to a greater extent (20 to 30% of the administered nelarabine dose). In the combined Phase 1 studies, patients were categorized into 3 groups: normal with CL_{cr} >80 mL/min (n = 67), mild with CL_{cr} = 50-80 mL/min (n = 15), and moderate with CL_{cr} <50 mL/min (n = 3). The mean apparent clearance (CL/F) of ara-G was about 15% and 40% lower in patients with mild and moderate renal impairment, respectively, than in patients with normal renal function *[see Use in Specific Populations (8.6) and Dosage and Administration (2.3)]*. No differences in safety or effectiveness were observed.

Effect of Hepatic Impairment: The influence of hepatic impairment on the pharmacokinetics of nelarabine has not been evaluated *[see Use in Specific Populations (8.7)]*.

Drug Interactions: *Cytochrome P450:* Nelarabine and ara-G did not significantly inhibit the activities of the human hepatic cytochrome P450 isoenzymes 1A2, 2A6, 2B6, 2C8, 2C9, 2C19, 2D6, or 3A4 in vitro at concentrations of nelarabine and ara-G up to 100 μM.

Fludarabine: Administration of fludarabine 30 mg/m^2 as a 30-minute infusion 4 hours before a 1,200 mg/m^2 infusion of nelarabine did not affect the pharmacokinetics of nelarabine, ara-G, or ara-GTP in 12 patients with refractory leukemia.

Pentostatin: There is in vitro evidence that pentostatin is a strong inhibitor of adenosine deaminase. Inhibition of adenosine deaminase may result in a reduction in the conversion of the pro-drug nelarabine to its active moiety and consequently in a reduction in efficacy of nelarabine and/or change in adverse reaction profile of either drug *[see Drug Interactions (7)]*.

13 NONCLINICAL TOXICOLOGY

13.1 Carcinogenesis, Mutagenesis, Impairment of Fertility

Carcinogenicity testing of nelarabine has not been done. However, nelarabine was mutagenic when tested in vitro in L5178Y/TK mouse lymphoma cells with and without metabolic activation. No studies have been conducted in animals to assess genotoxic potential or effects on fertility. The effect on human fertility is unknown.

14 CLINICAL STUDIES

The safety and efficacy of ARRANON were evaluated in two open-label, single-arm, multicenter studies.

14.1 Adult Clinical Study

The safety and efficacy of ARRANON in adult patients were studied in a clinical trial which included 39 treated patients, 28 who had T-cell acute lymphoblastic leukemia (T-ALL) or T-cell lymphoblastic lymphoma (T-LBL) that had relapsed following or was refractory to at least two prior induction regimens. A 1,500 mg/m^2 dose of ARRANON was administered intravenously over 2 hours on days 1, 3, and 5 repeated every 21 days. Patients who experienced signs or symptoms of grade 2 or greater neurologic toxicity on therapy were to be discontinued from further therapy with ARRANON. Seventeen patients had a diagnosis of T-ALL and 11 had a diagnosis of T-LBL. For patients with ≥2 prior inductions, the age range was 16-65 years (mean 34 years) and most patients were male (82%) and Caucasian (61%). Patients with central nervous system (CNS) disease were not eligible.

Complete response (CR) in this study was defined as bone marrow blast counts ≤5%, no other evidence of disease, and full recovery of peripheral blood counts. Complete response without complete hematologic recovery (CR*) was also assessed. The results of the study for patients who had received ≥2 prior inductions are shown in Table 5.

Table 5. Efficacy Results in Adult Patients With ≥2 Prior Inductions Treated with 1,500 mg/m^2 of ARRANON Administered Intravenously Over 2 Hours on Days 1, 3, and 5 Repeated Every 21 Days

	N = 28
CR plus CR* % (n) [95% CI]	21% (6) [8%, 41%]
CR % (n) [95% CI]	18% (5) [6%, 37%]
CR* % (n) [95% CI]	4% (1) [0%, 18%]
Duration of CR plus CR* (range in weeks)[a]	4 to 195+
Median overall survival (weeks) [95% CI]	20.6 weeks [10.4, 36.4]

CR = Complete response
CR* = Complete response without hematologic recovery
[a] Does not include 1 patient who was transplanted (duration of response was 156+ weeks).

The mean number of days on therapy was 56 days (range of 10 to 136 days). Time to CR plus CR* ranged from 2.9 to 11.7 weeks.

14.2 Pediatric Clinical Study

The safety and efficacy of ARRANON in pediatric patients were studied in a clinical trial which included patients 21 years of age and younger, who had relapsed or refractory T-cell acute lymphoblastic leukemia (T-ALL) or T-cell lymphoblastic lymphoma (T-LBL). Eighty-four (84) patients, 39 of whom had received two or more prior induction regimens, were treated with 650 mg/m^2/day of ARRANON administered intravenously over 1 hour daily for 5 consecutive days repeated every 21 days (see Table 6). Patients who experienced signs or symptoms of grade 2 or greater neurologic toxicity on therapy were to be discontinued from further therapy with ARRANON.

Table 6. Pediatric Clinical Study - Patient Allocation

Patient Population	N
Patients treated at 650 mg/m^2/day × 5 days every 21 days.	84
Patients with T-ALL or T-LBL with two or more prior induction treated at 650 mg/m^2/day × 5 days every 21 days.	39
Patients with T-ALL or T-LBL with one prior induction treated at 650 mg/m^2/day × 5 days every 21 days.	31

The 84 patients ranged in age from 2.5-21.7 years (overall mean, 11.9 years), 52% were 3 to 12 years of age and most were male (74%) and Caucasian (62%). The majority (77%) of patients had a diagnosis of T-ALL.

Complete response (CR) in this study was defined as bone marrow blast counts ≤5%, no other evidence of disease, and full recovery of peripheral blood counts. Complete response without full hematologic recovery (CR*) was also assessed as a meaningful outcome in this heavily pretreated population. Duration of response is reported from date of response to date of relapse, and may include subsequent stem cell transplant. Efficacy results are presented in Table 7.

Table 7. Efficacy Results in Patients 21 Years of Age and Younger at Diagnosis With ≥2 Prior Inductions Treated with 650 mg/m^2 of ARRANON Administered Intravenously Over 1 Hour Daily for 5 Consecutive Days Repeated Every 21 Days

	N = 39
CR plus CR* % (n) [95% CI]	23% (9) [11%, 39%]
CR % (n) [95% CI]	13% (5) [4%, 27%]
CR* % (n) [95% CI]	10% (4) [3%, 24%]
Duration of CR plus CR* (range in weeks)[a]	3.3 to 9.3
Median overall survival (weeks) [95% CI]	13.1 [8.7, 17.4]

CR = Complete response
CR* = Complete response without hematologic recovery
[a] Does not include 5 patients who were transplanted or had subsequent systemic chemotherapy (duration of response in these 5 patients was 4.7 to 42.1 weeks).

The mean number of days on therapy was 46 days (range of 7 to 129 days). Median time to CR plus CR* was 3.4 weeks (95% CI: 3.0, 3.7).

15 REFERENCES

1. Preventing Occupational Exposures to Antineoplastic and Other Hazardous Drugs in Health Care Settings. NIOSH Alert 2004-165.
2. OSHA Technical Manual, TED 1-0.15A, Section VI: Chapter 2. Controlling Occupational Exposure to Hazardous Drugs. OSHA, 1999. http://www.osha.gov/dts/osta/otm/otm_vi/otm_vi_2.html
3. American Society of Health-System Pharmacists. ASHP Guidelines on Handling Hazardous Drugs. *Am J Health-Syst Pharm.* 2006;63:1172-1193.
4. Polovich M, White JM, Kelleher LO (eds.) 2005. Chemotherapy and Biotherapy Guidelines and Recommendations for Practice. (2nd ed) Pittsburgh, PA: Oncology Nursing Society.

16 HOW SUPPLIED/STORAGE AND HANDLING

ARRANON Injection is supplied as a clear, colorless, sterile solution in Type I, clear glass vials with a gray butyl rubber (latex-free) stopper and a red snap-off aluminum seal. Each vial contains 250 mg of nelarabine (5 mg nelarabine per mL) and the inactive ingredient sodium chloride (4.5 mg per mL) in 50 mL Water for Injection, USP. Vials are available in the following carton size: NDC 0007-4401-06 (package of 6)

Store at 25° C (77° F); excursions permitted to 15° to 30° C (59° to 86° F) [see USP Controlled Room Temperature].

17 PATIENT COUNSELING INFORMATION

Patient labeling is provided as a tear-off leaflet at the end of this full prescribing information. However, inform the patients of the following:

- Since patients receiving nelarabine therapy may experience somnolence, they should be cautioned about operating hazardous machinery, including automobiles.
- Patients should be instructed to contact their physician if they experience new or worsening symptoms of peripheral neuropathy *(see Boxed Warning, Warnings and Precautions (5.1), and Dosage and Administration (2.3)]*. These signs and symptoms include: tingling or numbness in fingers, hands, toes, or feet; difficulty with the fine motor coordination tasks such as buttoning clothing; unsteadiness while walking; weakness arising from a low chair; weakness in climbing stairs; increased tripping while walking over uneven surfaces.
- Patients should be instructed that seizures have been known to occur in patients who receive nelarabine. If a seizure occurs, the physician administering ARRANON should be promptly informed.
- Patients who develop fever or signs of infection while on therapy should notify their physician promptly.
- Patients should be advised to use effective contraceptive measures to prevent pregnancy and to avoid breast-feeding during treatment with ARRANON.

ARRANON is a registered trademark of GlaxoSmithKline.
GlaxoSmithKline
Research Triangle Park, NC 27709
©2009, GlaxoSmithKline. All rights reserved.
PHARMACIST-DETACH HERE AND GIVE INSTRUCTIONS TO PATIENT

PATIENT INFORMATION LEAFLET

ARRANON® (AIR-ra-non)
Nelarabine Injection

Read the Patient Information that comes with ARRANON before you or your child start treatment with ARRANON. Read the information you get each time before each treatment with ARRANON. There may be new information. This information does not take the place of talking with the doctor about your or your child's medical condition or treatment. Talk to your or your child's doctor, if you have any questions.

What is the most important information I should know about ARRANON?

ARRANON may cause serious nervous system problems including:

- extreme sleepiness
- seizures
- coma
- numbness and tingling in the hands, fingers, feet, or toes (peripheral neuropathy)
- weakness and paralysis

Call the doctor right away if you or your child has the following symptoms:

- seizures
- numbness and tingling in the hands, fingers, feet, or toes
- problems with fine motor skills such as buttoning clothes
- unsteadiness while walking
- increased tripping while walking
- weakness when getting out of a chair or walking up stairs

These symptoms may not go away even when treatment with ARRANON is stopped.

What is ARRANON?
ARRANON is an anti-cancer medicine used to treat adults and children who have:

- T-cell acute lymphoblastic leukemia
- T-cell lymphoblastic lymphoma

What should you tell the doctor before you or your child starts ARRANON?
Tell the doctor about all health conditions you or your child have, including if you or your child:

- have any nervous system problems.
- have kidney problems.
- are breast-feeding or plan to breast-feed. It is not known whether ARRANON passes through breast milk. You should not breast-feed during treatment with ARRANON.
- are pregnant or plan to become pregnant. ARRANON may harm an unborn baby. You should use effective birth control to avoid getting pregnant. Talk with your doctor about your choices.

Tell the doctor about all the medicines you or your child take, including prescription and nonprescription medicines, vitamins, and herbal supplements.

How is ARRANON given?
ARRANON is an intravenous medicine. This means it is given through a tube in your vein.

What should you or your child avoid during treatment with ARRANON?

- You or your child should not drive or operate dangerous machines. ARRANON may cause sleepiness.
- You or your child should not receive vaccines made with live germs during treatment with ARRANON.

What are the possible side effects of ARRANON?
ARRANON may cause serious nervous system problems. See "What is the most important information I should know about ARRANON?"

ARRANON may also cause:

- decreased blood counts such as low red blood cells, low white blood cells, and low platelets. Blood tests should be done regularly to check blood counts. Call the doctor right away if you or your child:
  - is more tired than usual, pale, or has trouble breathing
  - has a fever or other signs of an infection
  - bruises easy or has any unusual bleeding
- stomach area problems such as nausea, vomiting, diarrhea, and constipation
- headache
- sleepiness
- blurry eyesight

These are not all the side effects associated with ARRANON. Ask your doctor or pharmacist for more information.

General Advice about ARRANON
This leaflet summarizes important information about ARRANON. If you have questions or problems, talk with your or your child's doctor. You can ask your doctor or pharmacist for information about ARRANON that is written for healthcare providers or it is available at www.GSK.com.
ARRANON is a registered trademark of GlaxoSmithKline.
GlaxoSmithKline
Research Triangle Park, NC 27709
©2009, GlaxoSmithKline. All rights reserved.
December 2009
ARR:1PIL

ARZERRA ℞

[ar-zer-ra]
(ofatumumab)
Injection, for intravenous infusion

HIGHLIGHTS OF PRESCRIBING INFORMATION

These highlights do not include all the information needed to use ARZERRA safely and effectively. See full prescribing information for ARZERRA.
ARZERRA (ofatumumab)
Injection, for intravenous infusion
Initial U.S. Approval: 2009

———INDICATIONS AND USAGE———
ARZERRA™ (ofatumumab) is a CD20-directed cytolytic monoclonal antibody indicated for the treatment of patients with chronic lymphocytic leukemia (CLL) refractory to fludarabine and alemtuzumab. The effectiveness of ARZERRA is based on the demonstration of durable objective responses. No data demonstrate an improvement in disease related symptoms or increased survival with ARZERRA. (1, 14)

———DOSAGE AND ADMINISTRATION———

- Dilute and administer as an intravenous infusion. Do not administer as an intravenous push or bolus. (2.1)
- Recommended dose and schedule is 12 doses administered as follows:
  - 300 mg initial dose, followed 1 week later by

- 2,000 mg weekly for 7 doses, followed 4 weeks later by
- 2,000 mg every 4 weeks for 4 doses. (2.1)
- Premedicate with oral acetaminophen, oral or intravenous antihistamine, and intravenous corticosteroid. (2.4)

———DOSAGE FORMS AND STRENGTHS———
100 mg/5 mL single-use vial. (3)

———CONTRAINDICATIONS———
None. (4)

———WARNINGS AND PRECAUTIONS———

- Infusion Reactions: Premedicate with an intravenous corticosteroid (as appropriate), an oral analgesic, and an oral or intravenous antihistamine. Monitor patients closely during infusions. Interrupt infusion if infusion reactions occur. (2.3, 2.4, 5.1)
- Cytopenias: Monitor blood counts at regular intervals for neutropenia and thrombocytopenia. (5.2)
- Progressive Multifocal Leukoencephalopathy (PML): Monitor neurologic function and discontinue ARZERRA if PML is suspected. (5.3)
- Hepatitis B Reactivation: Screen high-risk patients. Discontinue ARZERRA in patients who develop viral hepatitis or reactivation of viral hepatitis. (5.4)

———ADVERSE REACTIONS———
Most common adverse reactions (≥10%) were neutropenia, pneumonia, pyrexia, cough, diarrhea, anemia, fatigue, dyspnea, rash, nausea, bronchitis, and upper respiratory tract infections. (6)

To report SUSPECTED ADVERSE REACTIONS, contact GlaxoSmithKline at 1-888-825-5249 or FDA at 1-800-FDA-1088 or www.fda.gov/medwatch.

———USE IN SPECIFIC POPULATIONS———

- Pregnancy: Based on animal data, may cause fetal harm. (8.1)
- Nursing mothers: Published data suggest that consumption of breast milk does not result in substantial absorption of maternal antibodies into circulation. (8.3)

See 17 for PATIENT COUNSELING INFORMATION
Revised: 07/2010

FULL PRESCRIBING INFORMATION

1 INDICATIONS AND USAGE

ARZERRA™ (ofatumumab) is indicated for the treatment of patients with chronic lymphocytic leukemia (CLL) refractory to fludarabine and alemtuzumab.

The effectiveness of ARZERRA is based on the demonstration of durable objective responses *[see Clinical Studies (14)]*. No data demonstrate an improvement in disease related symptoms or increased survival with ARZERRA.

2 DOSAGE AND ADMINISTRATION

2.1 Recommended Dosage Regimen

- Do not administer as an intravenous push or bolus.
- Premedicate before each infusion *[see Dosage and Administration (2.4)]*.
- Administer with in-line filter supplied with product. The recommended dose and schedule is 12 doses administered as follows:
- 300 mg initial dose (Dose 1), followed 1 week later by
- 2,000 mg weekly for 7 doses (Doses 2 through 8), followed 4 weeks later by
- 2,000 mg every 4 weeks for 4 doses (Doses 9 through 12)

2.2 Administration

Prepare all doses in 1,000 mL of 0.9% Sodium Chloride Injection, USP *[see Dosage and Administration (2.5)]*.

- Dose 1: Initiate infusion at a rate of 3.6 mg/hour (12 mL/hour).
- Dose 2: Initiate infusion at a rate of 24 mg/hour (12 mL/hour).
- Doses 3 through 12: Initiate infusion at a rate of 50 mg/hour (25 mL/hour).

In the absence of infusional toxicity, the rate of infusion may be increased every 30 minutes as described in Table 1. Do not exceed the infusion rates in Table 1.
[See table above]

2.3 Dose Modification

- Interrupt infusion for infusion reactions of any severity *[see Warnings and Precautions (5.1)]*.
- For Grade 4 infusion reactions, do not resume the infusion.
- For Grade 1, 2, or 3 infusion reaction, if the infusion reaction resolves or remains less than or equal to Grade 2, resume infusion with the following modifications according to the initial Grade of the infusion reaction.
  - Grade 1 or 2: Infuse at one-half of the previous infusion rate.
  - Grade 3: Infuse at a rate of 12 mL/hour.
- After resuming the infusion, the infusion rate may be increased according to Table 1 above, based on patient tolerance.

2.4 Premedication

- Premedicate 30 minutes to 2 hours prior to each dose with oral acetaminophen 1,000 mg (or equivalent), oral or intravenous antihistamine (cetirizine 10 mg or equivalent), and intravenous corticosteroid (prednisolone 100 mg or equivalent).
- Do not reduce corticosteroid dose for Doses 1, 2, and 9.
- Corticosteroid dose may be reduced as follows for Doses 3 through 8 and 10 through 12:
  - Doses 3 through 8: Gradually reduce corticosteroid dose with successive infusions if a Grade 3 or greater infusion reaction did not occur with the preceding dose.
  - Doses 10 through 12: Administer prednisolone 50 mg to 100 mg or equivalent if a Grade 3 or greater infusion reaction did not occur with Dose 9.

2.5 Preparation and Administration

- Do not shake product.
- Inspect parenteral drug products visually for particulate matter and discoloration prior to administration. ARZERRA should be a colorless solution and may contain a small amount of visible translucent-to-white, amorphous, ofatumumab particles. The solution should not be used if discolored or cloudy, or if foreign particulate matter is present.

Preparation of Solution:

- 300-mg dose: Withdraw and discard 15 mL from a 1,000-mL polyolefin bag of 0.9% Sodium Chloride Injection, USP. Withdraw 5 mL from each of 3 vials of ARZERRA and add to the bag. Mix diluted solution by gentle inversion.
- 2,000-mg dose: Withdraw and discard 100 mL from a 1,000-mL bag of 0.9% Sodium Chloride Injection, USP. Withdraw 5 mL from each of 20 vials of ARZERRA and add to the bag. Mix diluted solution by gentle inversion.
- Store diluted solution between 2° to 8°C (36° to 46°F).

Administration Instructions:

- Do not mix ARZERRA with, or administer as an infusion with, other medicinal products.
- Administer using an infusion pump, the in-line filter provided with the product, and polyvinyl chloride (PVC) administration sets.
- Flush the intravenous line with 0.9% Sodium Chloride Injection, USP before and after each dose.
- Start infusion within 12 hours of preparation.
- Discard prepared solution after 24 hours.

3 DOSAGE FORMS AND STRENGTHS

100 mg/5 mL single-use vial.

4 CONTRAINDICATIONS

None.

Table 1. Infusion Rates for ARZERRA

Interval After Start of Infusion (min)	Dose 1[a] (mL/hour)	Dose 2[b] (mL/hour)	Doses 3 - 12[b] (mL/hour)
0 - 30	12	12	25
31 - 60	25	25	50
61 - 90	50	50	100
91 - 120	100	100	200
>120	200	200	400

[a] Dose 1 = 300 mg (0.3 mg/mL)
[b] Doses 2 and 3 - 12 = 2,000 mg (2 mg/mL)

5 WARNINGS AND PRECAUTIONS

5.1 Infusion Reactions

ARZERRA can cause serious infusion reactions manifesting as bronchospasm, dyspnea, laryngeal edema, pulmonary edema, flushing, hypertension, hypotension, syncope, cardiac ischemia/infarction, back pain, abdominal pain, pyrexia, rash, urticaria, and angioedema. Infusion reactions occur more frequently with the first 2 infusions *[see Adverse Reactions (6.1)]*.

Premedicate with acetaminophen, an antihistamine, and a corticosteroid *[see Dosage and Administration (2.1, 2.4)]*. Interrupt infusion for infusion reactions of any severity. Institute medical management for severe infusion reactions including angina or other signs and symptoms of myocardial ischemia *[see Dosage and Administration (2.3)]*.

In a study of patients with moderate to severe chronic obstructive pulmonary disease, an indication for which ARZERRA is not approved, 2 of 5 patients developed Grade 3 bronchospasm during infusion.

5.2 Cytopenias

Prolonged (≥1 week) severe neutropenia and thrombocytopenia can occur with ARZERRA. Monitor complete blood counts (CBC) and platelet counts at regular intervals during therapy, and increase the frequency of monitoring in patients who develop Grade 3 or 4 cytopenias.

5.3 Progressive Multifocal Leukoencephalopathy

Progressive multifocal leukoencephalopathy (PML), including fatal PML, can occur with ARZERRA. Consider PML in any patient with new onset of or changes in pre-existing neurological signs or symptoms. Discontinue ARZERRA if PML is suspected, and initiate evaluation for PML including consultation with a neurologist, brain MRI, and lumbar puncture.

5.4 Hepatitis B Reactivation

Hepatitis B reactivation, including fulminant hepatitis and death, occurs with other monoclonal antibodies directed against CD20. Screen patients at high risk of hepatitis B virus (HBV) infection before initiation of ARZERRA. Closely monitor carriers of hepatitis B for clinical and laboratory signs of active HBV infection during treatment with ARZERRA and for 6 to 12 months following the last infusion of ARZERRA. Discontinue ARZERRA in patients who develop viral hepatitis or reactivation of viral hepatitis, and institute appropriate treatment. Insufficient data exist regarding the safety of administration of ARZERRA in patients with active hepatitis.

5.5 Intestinal Obstruction

Obstruction of the small intestine can occur in patients receiving ARZERRA. Perform a diagnostic evaluation if obstruction is suspected.

5.6 Immunizations

The safety of immunization with live viral vaccines during or following administration of ARZERRA has not been studied. Do not administer live viral vaccines to patients who have recently received ARZERRA. The ability to generate an immune response to any vaccine following administration of ARZERRA has not been studied.

6 ADVERSE REACTIONS

The following serious adverse reactions are discussed in greater detail in other sections of the labeling:

- Infusion Reactions *[see Warnings and Precautions (5.1)]*
- Cytopenias *[see Warnings and Precautions (5.2)]*
- Progressive Multifocal Leukoencephalopathy *[see Warnings and Precautions (5.3)]*
- Hepatitis B Reactivation *[see Warnings and Precautions (5.4)]*
- Intestinal Obstruction *[see Warnings and Precautions (5.5)]*

The most common adverse reactions (≥10%) in Study 1 were neutropenia, pneumonia, pyrexia, cough, diarrhea, anemia, fatigue, dyspnea, rash, nausea, bronchitis, and upper respiratory tract infections.

The most common serious adverse reactions in Study 1 were infections (including pneumonia and sepsis), neutropenia, and pyrexia. Infections were the most common adverse reactions leading to drug discontinuation in Study 1.

6.1 Clinical Trials Experience

Because clinical trials are conducted under widely varying conditions, adverse reaction rates observed in the clinical trials of a drug cannot be directly compared to rates in the clinical trials of another drug and may not reflect the rates observed in practice.

The safety of monotherapy with ARZERRA was evaluated in 181 patients with relapsed or refractory CLL in 2 open-label, non-randomized, single-arm studies. In these studies, ARZERRA was administered at 2,000 mg beginning with the second dose for 11 doses (Study 1 [n = 154]) or 3 doses (Study 2 [n = 27]).

The data described in Table 2 and other sections below are derived from 154 patients in Study 1. All patients received 2,000 mg weekly from the second dose onward. Ninety percent of patients received at least 8 infusions of ARZERRA and 55% received all 12 infusions. The median age was 63 years (range: 41 to 86 years), 72% were male, and 97% were White.

[See table 2 at top of next page]

Infusion Reactions: Infusion reactions occurred in 44% of patients on the day of the first infusion (300 mg), 29% on the day of the second infusion (2,000 mg), and less frequently during subsequent infusions.

Infections: A total of 108 patients (70%) experienced bacterial, viral, or fungal infections. A total of 45 patients (29%) experienced ≥Grade 3 infections, of which 19 (12%) were fatal. The proportion of fatal infections in the fludarabine- and alemtuzumab-refractory group was 17%.

Neutropenia: Of 108 patients with normal neutrophil counts at baseline, 45 (42%) developed ≥Grade 3 neutropenia. Nineteen (18%) developed Grade 4 neutropenia. Some patients experienced new onset Grade 4 neutropenia >2 weeks in duration.

6.2 Immunogenicity

There is a potential for immunogenicity with therapeutic proteins such as ofatumumab. Serum samples from patients with CLL in Study 1 were tested by enzyme-linked immunosorbent assay (ELISA) for anti-ofatumumab antibodies during and after the 24-week treatment period. Results were negative in 46 patients after the 8th infusion and in 33 patients after the 12th infusion.

Immunogenicity assay results are highly dependent on several factors including assay sensitivity and specificity, assay methodology, sample handling, timing of sample collection, concomitant medications, and underlying disease. For these reasons, comparison of incidence of antibodies to ARZERRA with the incidence of antibodies to other products may be misleading.

7 DRUG INTERACTIONS

No formal drug-drug interaction studies have been conducted with ARZERRA.

8 USE IN SPECIFIC POPULATIONS

8.1 Pregnancy

Pregnancy Category C: There are no adequate or well-controlled studies of ofatumumab in pregnant women. A reproductive study in pregnant cynomolgus monkeys that received ofatumumab at doses up to 3.5 times the recommended human dose of ofatumumab did not demonstrate maternal toxicity or teratogenicity. Ofatumumab crossed the placental barrier, and fetuses exhibited depletion of peripheral B cells and decreased spleen and placental weights. ARZERRA should be used during pregnancy only if the potential benefit to the mother justifies the potential risk to the fetus.

There are no human or animal data on the potential short-term and long-term effects of perinatal B-cell depletion in

Table 2. Incidence of All Adverse Reactions Occurring in ≥5% of Patients in Study 1 and in the Fludarabine- and Alemtuzumab-Refractory Subset of Study 1 (MedDRA 9.0)

Body System/Adverse Event	Total Population (n = 154)		Fludarabine- and Alemtuzumab-Refractory (n = 59)	
	All Grades %	Grade ≥3 %	All Grades %	Grade ≥3 %
Infections and infestations				
Pneumonia[a]	23	14	25	15
Upper respiratory tract infection	11	0	3	0
Bronchitis	11	<1	19	2
Sepsis[b]	8	8	10	10
Nasopharyngitis	8	0	8	0
Herpes zoster	6	1	7	2
Sinusitis	5	2	3	2
Blood and lymphatic system disorders				
Anemia	16	5	17	8
Psychiatric disorders				
Insomnia	7	0	10	0
Nervous system disorders				
Headache	6	0	7	0
Cardiovascular disorders				
Hypertension	5	0	8	0
Hypotension	5	0	3	0
Tachycardia	5	<1	7	2
Respiratory, thoracic, and mediastinal disorders				
Cough	19	0	19	0
Dyspnea	14	2	19	5
Gastrointestinal disorders				
Diarrhea	18	0	19	0
Nausea	11	0	12	0
Skin and subcutaneous tissue disorders				
Rash[c]	14	<1	17	2
Urticaria	8	0	5	0
Hyperhidrosis	5	0	5	0
Musculoskeletal and connective tissue disorders				
Back pain	8	1	12	2
Muscle spasms	5	0	3	0
General disorders and administration site conditions				
Pyrexia	20	3	25	5
Fatigue	15	0	15	0
Edema peripheral	9	<1	8	2
Chills	8	0	10	0

[a] Pneumonia includes pneumonia, lung infection, lobar pneumonia, and bronchopneumonia.
[b] Sepsis includes sepsis, neutropenic sepsis, bacteremia, and septic shock.
[c] Rash includes rash, rash macular, and rash vesicular.

offspring following in-utero exposure to ofatumumab. Ofatumumab does not bind normal human tissues other than B lymphocytes. It is not known if binding occurs to unique embryonic or fetal tissue targets. In addition, the kinetics of B-lymphocyte recovery are unknown in offspring with B-cell depletion [see Nonclinical Toxicology (13.3)].

8.3 Nursing Mothers
It is not known whether ofatumumab is secreted in human milk; however human IgG is secreted in human milk. Pub-lished data suggest that neonatal and infant consumption of breast milk does not result in substantial absorption of these maternal antibodies into circulation. Because the ef-fects of local gastrointestinal and limited systemic exposure to ofatumumab are unknown, caution should be exercised when ARZERRA is administered to a nursing woman.

8.4 Pediatric Use
Safety and effectiveness of ARZERRA have not been estab-lished in children.

8.5 Geriatric Use
Clinical studies of ARZERRA did not include sufficient num-bers of subjects aged 65 and over to determine whether they respond differently from younger subjects [see Clinical Pharmacology (12.3)].

8.6 Renal Impairment
No formal studies of ARZERRA in patients with renal im-pairment have been conducted [see Clinical Pharmacology (12.3)].

8.7 Hepatic Impairment
No formal studies of ARZERRA in patients with hepatic im-pairment have been conducted.

10 OVERDOSAGE
No data are available regarding overdosage with ARZERRA.

11 DESCRIPTION
ARZERRA (ofatumumab) is an IgG1κ human monoclonal antibody with a molecular weight of approximately 149 kDa. The antibody was generated via transgenic mouse and hybridoma technology and is produced in a recombi-nant murine cell line (NS0) using standard mammalian cell cultivation and purification technologies.
ARZERRA is a sterile, colorless, preservative-free liquid concentrate for intravenous administration. ARZERRA is supplied at a concentration of 20 mg/mL in 10 mL single-use vials. Each single-use vial contains 100 mg ofatumumab in 5 mL of solution. Inactive ingredients include: 8.55 mg/mL sodium citrate and 0.195 mg/mL citric acid monohydrate as buffering agents, 5.85 mg/mL sodium chlo-ride as an isotonic agent, and Water for Injection, USP as the solvent. The pH is 6.5.

12 CLINICAL PHARMACOLOGY
12.1 Mechanism of Action
Ofatumumab binds specifically to both the small and large extracellular loops of the CD20 molecule. The CD20 mole-cule is expressed on normal B lymphocytes (pre-B- to ma-ture B-lymphocyte) and on B-cell CLL. The CD20 molecule is not shed from the cell surface and is not internalized fol-lowing antibody binding.
The Fab domain of ofatumumab binds to the CD20 molecule and the Fc domain mediates immune effector functions to result in B-cell lysis in vitro. Data suggest that possible mechanisms of cell lysis include complement-dependent cy-totoxicity and antibody-dependent, cell-mediated cytotoxic-ity.

12.2 Pharmacodynamics
In patients with CLL refractory to fludarabine and alemtu-zumab, the median decrease in circulating CD19-positive B cells was 91% (n = 50) with the 8th infusion and 85% (n = 32) with the 12th infusion. The time to recovery of lymphocytes, including CD19-positive B cells, to normal levels has not been determined.

12.3 Pharmacokinetics
Pharmacokinetic data were obtained from 146 patients with refractory CLL who received a 300-mg initial dose followed by 7 weekly and 4 monthly infusions of 2,000 mg. The C_{max} and $AUC_{(0-\infty)}$ after the 8th infusion in Study 1 were approx-imately 40% and 60% higher than after the 4th infusion in Study 2. The mean volume of distribution at steady-state (V_{ss}) values ranged from 1.7 to 5.1 L. Ofatumumab is elim-inated through both a target-independent route and a B cell-mediated route. Ofatumumab exhibited dose-dependent clearance in the dose range of 100 to 2,000 mg. Due to the depletion of B cells, the clearance of ofatumumab decreased substantially after subsequent infusions compared to the first infusion. The mean clearance between the 4th and 12th infusions was approximately 0.01 L/hr and exhibited large inter-subject variability with CV% greater than 50%. The mean $t_{1/2}$ between the 4th and 12th infusions was approxi-mately 14 days (range: 2.3 to 61.5 days).
Special Populations: Cross-study analyses were performed on data from patients with a variety of conditions, including 162 patients with CLL, who received multiple infusions of ARZERRA as a single agent at doses ranging from 100 to 2,000 mg. The effects of various covariates (e.g., body size [weight, height, body surface area], age, gender, baseline creatinine clearance) on ofatumumab pharmacokinetics were assessed in a population pharmacokinetic analysis.
Body Weight: Volume of distribution and clearance in-creased with body weight. However, this increase was not clinically significant. No dosage adjustment is recom-mended based on body weight.
Age: Age did not significantly influence ofatumumab phar-macokinetics in patients ranging from 21 to 86 years of age. No pharmacokinetic data are available in pediatric pa-tients.
Gender: Gender had a modest effect on ofatumumab phar-macokinetics (14% to 25% lower clearance and volume of distribution in female patients compared to male patients) in a cross-study population analysis (41% of the patients in

Carton Contents	NDC
3 single-use vials with 2 filters	NDC 0173-0808-02
10 single-use vials with 2 filters	NDC 0173-0808-05

this analysis were male and 59% were female). These effects are not considered clinically important, and no dosage adjustment is recommended.

Renal Impairment: Creatinine clearance at baseline did not have a clinically important effect on ofatumumab pharmacokinetics in patients with calculated creatinine clearance values ranging from 33 to 287 mL/min.

13 NONCLINICAL TOXICOLOGY

13.1 Carcinogenesis, Mutagenesis, Impairment of Fertility

No carcinogenicity or mutagenicity studies of ofatumumab have been conducted. In a repeat-dose toxicity study, no tumorigenic or unexpected mitogenic responses were noted in cynomolgus monkeys treated for 7 months with up to 3.5 times the human dose of ofatumumab. Effects on male and female fertility have not been evaluated in animal studies.

13.3 Reproductive and Developmental Toxicology

Pregnant cynomolgus monkeys dosed with 0.7 or 3.5 times the human dose of ofatumumab weekly during the period of organogenesis (gestation days 20 to 50) had no maternal toxicity or teratogenicity. Both dose levels of ofatumumab depleted circulating B cells in the dams, with signs of initial B cell recovery 50 days after the final dose. Following Caesarean section at gestational day 100, fetuses from ofatumumab-treated dams exhibited decreases in mean peripheral B-cell counts (decreased to approximately 10% of control values), splenic B-cell counts (decreased to approximately 15 to 20% of control values), and spleen weights (decreased by 15% for the low-dose and by 30% for the high-dose group, compared to control values). Fetuses from treated dams exhibiting anti-ofatumumab antibody responses had higher B cell counts and higher spleen weights compared to the fetuses from other treated dams, indicating partial recovery in those animals developing anti-ofatumumab antibodies. When compared to control animals, fetuses from treated dams in both dose groups had a 10% decrease in mean placental weights. A 15% decrease in mean thymus weight compared to the controls was also observed in fetuses from dams treated with 3.5 times the human dose of ofatumumab. The biological significance of decreased placental and thymic weights is unknown.

The kinetics of B-lymphocyte recovery and the potential long-term effects of perinatal B-cell depletion in offspring from ofatumumab-treated dams have not been studied in animals.

14 CLINICAL STUDIES

Study 1 was a single-arm, multicenter study in 154 patients with relapsed or refractory CLL. ARZERRA was administered by intravenous infusion according to the following schedule: 300 mg (Week 0), 2,000 mg weekly for 7 infusions (Weeks 1 through 7), and 2,000 mg every 4 weeks for 4 infusions (Weeks 12 through 24). Patients with CLL refractory to fludarabine and alemtuzumab (n = 59) comprised the efficacy population. Drug refractoriness was defined as failure to achieve at least a partial response to, or disease progression within 6 months of, the last dose of fludarabine or alemtuzumab. The main efficacy outcome was durable objective tumor response rate. Objective tumor responses were determined using the 1996 National Cancer Institute Working Group (NCIWG) Guidelines for CLL.

In patients with CLL refractory to fludarabine and alemtuzumab, the median age was 64 years (range: 41 to 86 years), 75% were male, and 95% were White. The median number of prior therapies was 5; 93% received prior alkylating agents, 59% received prior rituximab, and all received prior fludarabine and alemtuzumab. Eighty-eight percent of patients received at least 8 infusions of ARZERRA and 54% received 12 infusions.

The investigator-determined overall response rate in patients with CLL refractory to fludarabine and alemtuzumab was 42% (99% CI: 26, 60) with a median duration of response of 6.5 months (95% CI: 5.8, 8.3). There were no complete responses. Anti-tumor activity was also observed in additional patients in Study 1 and in a multicenter, open-label, dose-escalation study (Study 2) conducted in patients with relapsed or refractory CLL.

16 HOW SUPPLIED/STORAGE AND HANDLING

ARZERRA (ofatumumab) is a sterile, colorless, preservative-free liquid concentrate (20 mg/mL) for dilution and intravenous administration provided in single-use glass vials with a latex-free rubber stopper and an aluminum overseal. Each vial contains 100 mg ofatumumab in 5 mL of solution.

ARZERRA is available as follows:
[See table above]

Store ARZERRA refrigerated between 2° to 8°C (36° to 46°F). Do not freeze. Vials should be protected from light.

17 PATIENT COUNSELING INFORMATION

Advise patients to contact a healthcare professional for any of the following:

- Signs and symptoms of infusion reactions including fever, chills, rash, or breathing problems within 24 hours of infusion *[see Warnings and Precautions (5.1) and Adverse Reactions (6.1)]*
- Bleeding, easy bruising, petechiae, pallor, worsening weakness, or fatigue *[see Warnings and Precautions (5.2)]*
- Signs of infections including fever and cough *[see Warnings and Precautions (5.2) and Adverse Reactions (6.1)]*
- New neurological symptoms such as confusion, dizziness or loss of balance, difficulty talking or walking, or vision problems *[see Warnings and Precautions (5.3)]*
- Symptoms of hepatitis including worsening fatigue or yellow discoloration of skin or eyes *[see Warnings and Precautions (5.4)]*
- New or worsening abdominal pain or nausea *[see Warnings and Precautions (5.5)]*
- Pregnancy or nursing *[see Use in Specific Populations (8.1, 8.3)]*

Advise patients of the need for:

- Periodic monitoring for blood counts *[see Warnings and Precautions (5.2)]*
- Avoiding vaccination with live viral vaccines *[see Warnings and Precautions (5.6)]*

Manufactured by:
GLAXO GROUP LIMITED
Greenford, Middlesex, UB6 0NN, United Kingdom
U.S. Lic. 1809
Distributed by:
GlaxoSmithKline
Research Triangle Park, NC 27709
©2009, GlaxoSmithKline. All rights reserved.
October 2009
ARZ:1PI

AUGMENTIN® ℞
[ăg-mint′ in]
(amoxicillin/clavulanate potassium)
Powder for Oral Suspension and Chewable Tablets

To reduce the development of drug-resistant bacteria and maintain the effectiveness of AUGMENTIN (amoxicillin/clavulanate potassium) and other antibacterial drugs, AUGMENTIN should be used only to treat or prevent infections that are proven or strongly suspected to be caused by bacteria.

DESCRIPTION

AUGMENTIN is an oral antibacterial combination consisting of the semisynthetic antibiotic amoxicillin and the β-lactamase inhibitor, clavulanate potassium (the potassium salt of clavulanic acid). Amoxicillin is an analog of ampicillin, derived from the basic penicillin nucleus, 6-aminopenicillanic acid. The amoxicillin molecular formula is $C_{16}H_{19}N_3O_5S \cdot 3H_2O$, and the molecular weight is 419.46. Chemically, amoxicillin is $(2S,5R,6R)$-6-[(R)-(-)-2-Amino-2-(p-hydroxyphenyl)acetamido]-3,3-dimethyl-7-oxo-4-thia-1-azabicyclo[3.2.0]heptane-2-carboxylic acid trihydrate and may be represented structurally as:

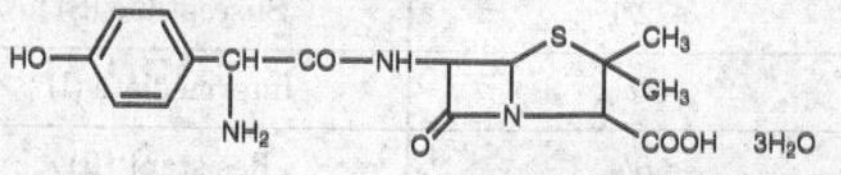

Clavulanic acid is produced by the fermentation of *Streptomyces clavuligerus*. It is a β-lactam structurally related to the penicillins and possesses the ability to inactivate a wide variety of β-lactamases by blocking the active sites of these enzymes. Clavulanic acid is particularly active against the clinically important plasmid-mediated β-lactamases frequently responsible for transferred drug resistance to penicillins and cephalosporins. The clavulanate potassium molecular formula is $C_8H_8KNO_5$, and the molecular weight is 237.25. Chemically, clavulanate potassium is potassium (Z)-($2R$,$5R$)-3-(2-hydroxyethylidene)-7-oxo-4-oxa-1-azabicyclo[3.2.0]-heptane-2-carboxylate and may be represented structurally as:

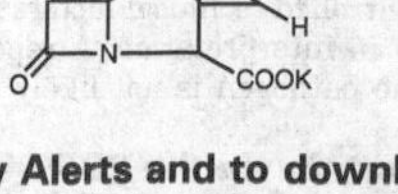

Inactive Ingredients

Powder for Oral Suspension—Colloidal silicon dioxide, flavorings (see HOW SUPPLIED), xanthan gum, and 1 or more of the following: Aspartame[a], hypromellose, mannitol, silica gel, silicon dioxide, and sodium saccharin. Chewable Tablets—Colloidal silicon dioxide, flavorings (see HOW SUPPLIED), magnesium stearate, mannitol, and 1 or more of the following: Aspartame[a], D&C Yellow No. 10, FD&C Red No. 40, glycine, sodium saccharin and succinic acid.

[a] See PRECAUTIONS—Information for the Patient.

Each 125-mg chewable tablet and each 5 mL of reconstituted 125 mg/5 mL oral suspension of AUGMENTIN contains 0.16 mEq of potassium. Each 250-mg chewable tablet and each 5 mL of reconstituted 250 mg/5 mL oral suspension of AUGMENTIN contains 0.32 mEq potassium. Each 200-mg chewable tablet and each 5 mL of reconstituted 200 mg/5 mL oral suspension of AUGMENTIN contains 0.14 mEq potassium. Each 400-mg chewable tablet and each 5 mL of reconstituted 400 mg/5 mL oral suspension of AUGMENTIN contains 0.29 mEq of potassium.

CLINICAL PHARMACOLOGY

Amoxicillin and clavulanate potassium are well absorbed from the gastrointestinal tract after oral administration of AUGMENTIN. Dosing in the fasted or fed state has minimal effect on the pharmacokinetics of amoxicillin. While AUGMENTIN can be given without regard to meals, absorption of clavulanate potassium when taken with food is greater relative to the fasted state. In 1 study, the relative bioavailability of clavulanate was reduced when AUGMENTIN was dosed at 30 and 150 minutes after the start of a high-fat breakfast. The safety and efficacy of AUGMENTIN have been established in clinical trials where AUGMENTIN was taken without regard to meals.

Oral administration of single doses of 400-mg chewable tablets of AUGMENTIN and 400 mg/5 mL suspension to 28 adult volunteers yielded comparable pharmacokinetic data:
[See table at top of next page]

Oral administration of 5 mL of 250 mg/5 mL suspension of AUGMENTIN or the equivalent dose of 10 mL of 125 mg/5 mL suspension of AUGMENTIN provides average peak serum concentrations approximately 1 hour after dosing of 6.9 mcg/mL for amoxicillin and 1.6 mcg/mL for clavulanic acid. The areas under the serum concentration curves obtained during the first 4 hours after dosing were 12.6 mcg.hr/mL for amoxicillin and 2.9 mcg.hr/mL for clavulanic acid when 5 mL of 250 mg/5 mL suspension of AUGMENTIN or equivalent dose of 10 mL of 125 mg/5 mL suspension of AUGMENTIN was administered to adult volunteers. One 250-mg chewable tablet of AUGMENTIN or two 125-mg chewable tablets of AUGMENTIN are equivalent to 5 mL of 250 mg/5 mL suspension of AUGMENTIN and provide similar serum levels of amoxicillin and clavulanic acid.

Amoxicillin serum concentrations achieved with AUGMENTIN are similar to those produced by the oral administration of equivalent doses of amoxicillin alone. The half-life of amoxicillin after the oral administration of AUGMENTIN is 1.3 hours and that of clavulanic acid is 1.0 hour. Time above the minimum inhibitory concentration of 1.0 mcg/mL for amoxicillin has been shown to be similar after corresponding every 12 hours and every 8 hours dosing regimens of AUGMENTIN in adults and children.

Approximately 50% to 70% of the amoxicillin and approximately 25% to 40% of the clavulanic acid are excreted unchanged in urine during the first 6 hours after administration of 10 mL of 250 mg/5 mL suspension of AUGMENTIN. Concurrent administration of probenecid delays amoxicillin excretion but does not delay renal excretion of clavulanic acid.

Neither component in AUGMENTIN is highly protein-bound; clavulanic acid has been found to be approximately 25% bound to human serum and amoxicillin approximately 18% bound.

Amoxicillin diffuses readily into most body tissues and fluids with the exception of the brain and spinal fluid. The results of experiments involving the administration of clavulanic acid to animals suggest that this compound, like amoxicillin, is well distributed in body tissues.

Two hours after oral administration of a single 35 mg/kg dose of suspension of AUGMENTIN to fasting children, average concentrations of 3.0 mcg/mL of amoxicillin and 0.5 mcg/mL of clavulanic acid were detected in middle ear effusions.

Microbiology

Amoxicillin is a semisynthetic antibiotic with a broad spectrum of bactericidal activity against many gram-positive and gram-negative microorganisms. Amoxicillin is, however, susceptible to degradation by β-lactamases, and therefore, the spectrum of activity does not include organisms which produce these enzymes. Clavulanic acid is a β-lactam, structurally related to the penicillins, which pos-

Dose[a]	AUC$_{0-\infty}$ (mcg.hr/mL)		C$_{max}$ (mcg/mL)[b]	
(amoxicillin/clavulanate potassium)	amoxicillin (±S.D.)	clavulanate potassium (±S.D.)	amoxicillin (±S.D.)	clavulanate potassium (±S.D.)
400/57 mg (5 mL of suspension)	17.29 ± 2.28	2.34 ± 0.94	6.94 ± 1.24	1.10 ± 0.42
400/57 mg (1 chewable tablet)	17.24 ± 2.64	2.17 ± 0.73	6.67 ± 1.37	1.03 ± 0.33

[a] Administered at the start of a light meal.
[b] Mean values of 28 normal volunteers. Peak concentrations occurred approximately 1 hour after the dose.

sesses the ability to inactivate a wide range of β-lactamase enzymes commonly found in microorganisms resistant to penicillins and cephalosporins. In particular, it has good activity against the clinically important plasmid-mediated β-lactamases frequently responsible for transferred drug resistance.

The formulation of amoxicillin and clavulanic acid in AUGMENTIN protects amoxicillin from degradation by β-lactamase enzymes and effectively extends the antibiotic spectrum of amoxicillin to include many bacteria normally resistant to amoxicillin and other β-lactam antibiotics. Thus, AUGMENTIN possesses the distinctive properties of a broad-spectrum antibiotic and a β-lactamase inhibitor.

Amoxicillin/clavulanic acid has been shown to be active against most strains of the following microorganisms, both in vitro and in clinical infections as described in INDICATIONS AND USAGE.

Gram-Positive Aerobes
Staphylococcus aureus (β-lactamase and non–β-lactamase–producing)[c]
[c] Staphylococci which are resistant to methicillin/oxacillin must be considered resistant to amoxicillin/clavulanic acid.

Gram-Negative Aerobes
Enterobacter species (Although most strains of *Enterobacter* species are resistant in vitro, clinical efficacy has been demonstrated with AUGMENTIN in urinary tract infections caused by these organisms.)
Escherichia coli (β-lactamase and non–β-lactamase–producing)
Haemophilus influenzae (β-lactamase and non–β-lactamase–producing)
Klebsiella species (All known strains are β-lactamase–producing.)
Moraxella catarrhalis (β-lactamase and non–β-lactamase–producing)
The following in vitro data are available, **but their clinical significance is unknown.**
Amoxicillin/clavulanic acid exhibits in vitro minimal inhibitory concentrations (MICs) of 2 mcg/mL or less against most (≥ 90%) strains of *Streptococcus pneumoniae*[d]; MICs of 0.06 mcg/mL or less against most (≥ 90%) strains of *Neisseria gonorrhoeae*; MICs of 4 mcg/mL or less against most (≥ 90%) strains of staphylococci and anaerobic bacteria; MICs of 8 mcg/mL or less against most (≥ 90%) strains of other listed organisms. However, with the exception of organisms shown to respond to amoxicillin alone, the safety and effectiveness of amoxicillin/clavulanic acid in treating clinical infections due to these microorganisms have not been established in adequate and well-controlled clinical trials.
[d] Because amoxicillin has greater in vitro activity against *S. pneumoniae* than does ampicillin or penicillin, the majority of *S. pneumoniae* strains with intermediate susceptibility to ampicillin or penicillin are fully susceptible to amoxicillin.

Gram-Positive Aerobes
Enterococcus faecalis[e]
Staphylococcus epidermidis (β-lactamase and non–β-lactamase–producing)
Staphylococcus saprophyticus (β-lactamase and non–β-lactamase–producing)
Streptococcus pneumoniae[e, f]
Streptococcus pyogenes[e, f]
viridans group[e, f]

Gram-Negative Aerobes
Eikenella corrodens (β-lactamase and non–β-lactamase–producing)
Neisseria gonorrhoeae[e] (β-lactamase and non–β-lactamase–producing)
Proteus mirabilis[e] (β-lactamase and non–β-lactamase–producing)

Anaerobic Bacteria
Bacteroides species, including *Bacteroides fragilis* (β-lactamase and non–β-lactamase–producing)
Fusobacterium species (β-lactamase and non–β-lactamase–producing)
Peptostreptococcus species[f]

[e] Adequate and well-controlled clinical trials have established the effectiveness of amoxicillin alone in treating certain clinical infections due to these organisms.
[f] These are non–β-lactamase–producing organisms, and therefore, are susceptible to amoxicillin alone.

Susceptibility Testing
Dilution Techniques
Quantitative methods are used to determine antimicrobial MICs. These MICs provide estimates of the susceptibility of bacteria to antimicrobial compounds. The MICs should be determined using a standardized procedure. Standardized procedures are based on a dilution method[1] (broth or agar) or equivalent with standardized inoculum concentrations and standardized concentrations of amoxicillin/clavulanate potassium powder.
The recommended dilution pattern utilizes a constant amoxicillin/clavulanate potassium ratio of 2 to 1 in all tubes with varying amounts of amoxicillin. MICs are expressed in terms of the amoxicillin concentration in the presence of clavulanic acid at a constant 2 parts amoxicillin to 1 part clavulanic acid. The MIC values should be interpreted according to the following criteria:

RECOMMENDED RANGES FOR AMOXICILLIN/ CLAVULANIC ACID SUSCEPTIBILITY TESTING

For Gram-Negative Enteric Aerobes:

MIC (mcg/mL)	Interpretation
≤ 8/4	Susceptible (S)
16/8	Intermediate (I)
≥ 32/16	Resistant (R)

For *Staphylococcus*[g] and *Haemophilus* species:

MIC (mcg/mL)	Interpretation
≤ 4/2	Susceptible (S)
≥ 8/4	Resistant (R)

[g] Staphylococci which are susceptible to amoxicillin/clavulanic acid but resistant to methicillin/oxacillin must be considered as resistant.

For *S. pneumoniae* from non-meningitis sources:
Isolates should be tested using amoxicillin/clavulanic acid and the following criteria should be used:

MIC (mcg/mL)	Interpretation
≤ 2/1	Susceptible (S)
4/2	Intermediate (I)
≥ 8/4	Resistant (R)

Note: These interpretive criteria are based on the recommended doses for respiratory tract infections.
A report of "Susceptible" indicates that the pathogen is likely to be inhibited if the antimicrobial compound in the blood reaches the concentration usually achievable. A report of "Intermediate" indicates that the result should be considered equivocal, and, if the microorganism is not fully susceptible to alternative, clinically feasible drugs, the test should be repeated. This category implies possible clinical applicability in body sites where the drug is physiologically concentrated or in situations where high dosage of drug can be used. This category also provides a buffer zone that prevents small uncontrolled technical factors from causing major discrepancies in interpretation. A report of "Resistant" indicates that the pathogen is not likely to be inhibited if

the antimicrobial compound in the blood reaches the concentrations usually achievable; other therapy should be selected.
Standardized susceptibility test procedures require the use of laboratory control microorganisms to control the technical aspects of the laboratory procedures. Standard amoxicillin/clavulanate potassium powder should provide the following MIC values:

Microorganism	MIC Range (mcg/mL)[h]
E. coli ATCC 25922	2 to 8
E. coli ATCC 35218	4 to 16
E. faecalis ATCC 29212	0.25 to 1.0
H. influenzae ATCC 49247	2 to 16
S. aureus ATCC 29213	0.12 to 0.5
S. pneumoniae ATCC 49619	0.03 to 0.12

[h] Expressed as concentration of amoxicillin in the presence of clavulanic acid at a constant 2 parts amoxicillin to 1 part clavulanic acid.

Diffusion Techniques
Quantitative methods that require measurement of zone diameters also provide reproducible estimates of the susceptibility of bacteria to antimicrobial compounds. One such standardized procedure[2] requires the use of standardized inoculum concentrations. This procedure uses paper disks impregnated with 30 mcg of amoxicillin/clavulanate potassium (20 mcg amoxicillin plus 10 mcg clavulanate potassium) to test the susceptibility of microorganisms to amoxicillin/clavulanic acid.
Reports from the laboratory providing results of the standard single-disk susceptibility test with a 30-mcg amoxicillin/clavulanate potassium (20 mcg amoxicillin plus 10 mcg clavulanate potassium) disk should be interpreted according to the following criteria:

RECOMMENDED RANGES FOR AMOXICILLIN/ CLAVULANIC ACID SUSCEPTIBILITY TESTING

For *Staphylococcus*[i] species and *H. influenzae*[j]:

Zone Diameter (mm)	Interpretation
≥ 20	Susceptible (S)
≤ 19	Resistant (R)

For Other Organisms Except *S. pneumoniae*[k] and *N. gonorrhoeae*[l]:

Zone Diameter (mm)	Interpretation
≥ 18	Susceptible (S)
14 to 17	Intermediate (I)
≤ 13	Resistant (R)

[i] Staphylococci which are resistant to methicillin/oxacillin must be considered as resistant to amoxicillin/clavulanic acid.
[j] A broth microdilution method should be used for testing *H. influenzae*. Beta-lactamase–negative, ampicillin-resistant strains must be considered resistant to amoxicillin/clavulanic acid.
[k] Susceptibility of *S. pneumoniae* should be determined using a 1-mcg oxacillin disk. Isolates with oxacillin zone sizes of ≥ 20 mm are susceptible to amoxicillin/clavulanic acid. An amoxicillin/clavulanic acid MIC should be determined on isolates of *S. pneumoniae* with oxacillin zone sizes of ≤ 19 mm.
[l] A broth microdilution method should be used for testing *N. gonorrhoeae* and interpreted according to penicillin breakpoints.

Interpretation should be as stated above for results using dilution techniques. Interpretation involves correlation of the diameter obtained in the disk test with the MIC for amoxicillin/clavulanic acid.
As with standardized dilution techniques, diffusion methods require the use of laboratory control microorganisms that are used to control the technical aspects of the laboratory procedures. For the diffusion technique, the 30-mcg amoxicillin/clavulanate potassium (20 mcg amoxicillin plus 10 mcg clavulanate potassium) disk should provide the following zone diameters in these laboratory quality control strains:

Microorganism	Zone Diameter (mm)
E. coli ATCC 25922	19 to 25 mm
E. coli ATCC 35218	18 to 22 mm
S. aureus ATCC 25923	28 to 36 mm

INDICATIONS AND USAGE

AUGMENTIN is indicated in the treatment of infections caused by susceptible strains of the designated organisms in the conditions listed below:

Lower Respiratory Tract Infections – caused by β-lactamase–producing strains of *H. influenzae* and *M. catarrhalis*.

Otitis Media – caused by β-lactamase–producing strains of *H. influenzae* and *M. catarrhalis*.

Sinusitis – caused by β-lactamase–producing strains of *H. influenzae* and *M. catarrhalis*.

Skin and Skin Structure Infections – caused by β-lactamase–producing strains of *S. aureus, E. coli,* and *Klebsiella* spp.

Urinary Tract Infections – caused by β-lactamase–producing strains of *E. coli, Klebsiella* spp. and *Enterobacter* spp.

While AUGMENTIN is indicated only for the conditions listed above, infections caused by ampicillin-susceptible organisms are also amenable to treatment with AUGMENTIN due to its amoxicillin content. Therefore, mixed infections caused by ampicillin-susceptible organisms and β-lactamase–producing organisms susceptible to AUGMENTIN should not require the addition of another antibiotic. Because amoxicillin has greater in vitro activity against *S. pneumoniae* than does ampicillin or penicillin, the majority of *S. pneumoniae* strains with intermediate susceptibility to ampicillin or penicillin are fully susceptible to amoxicillin and AUGMENTIN. (See Microbiology.)

To reduce the development of drug-resistant bacteria and maintain the effectiveness of AUGMENTIN and other antibacterial drugs, AUGMENTIN should be used only to treat or prevent infections that are proven or strongly suspected to be caused by susceptible bacteria. When culture and susceptibility information are available, they should be considered in selecting or modifying antibacterial therapy. In the absence of such data, local epidemiology and susceptibility patterns may contribute to the empiric selection of therapy. Bacteriological studies, to determine the causative organisms and their susceptibility to AUGMENTIN, should be performed together with any indicated surgical procedures.

CONTRAINDICATIONS

AUGMENTIN is contraindicated in patients with a history of allergic reactions to any penicillin. It is also contraindicated in patients with a previous history of cholestatic jaundice/hepatic dysfunction associated with AUGMENTIN.

WARNINGS

SERIOUS AND OCCASIONALLY FATAL HYPERSENSITIVITY (ANAPHYLACTIC) REACTIONS HAVE BEEN REPORTED IN PATIENTS ON PENICILLIN THERAPY. THESE REACTIONS ARE MORE LIKELY TO OCCUR IN INDIVIDUALS WITH A HISTORY OF PENICILLIN HYPERSENSITIVITY AND/OR A HISTORY OF SENSITIVITY TO MULTIPLE ALLERGENS. THERE HAVE BEEN REPORTS OF INDIVIDUALS WITH A HISTORY OF PENICILLIN HYPERSENSITIVITY WHO HAVE EXPERIENCED SEVERE REACTIONS WHEN TREATED WITH CEPHALOSPORINS. BEFORE INITIATING THERAPY WITH AUGMENTIN, CAREFUL INQUIRY SHOULD BE MADE CONCERNING PREVIOUS HYPERSENSITIVITY REACTIONS TO PENICILLINS, CEPHALOSPORINS, OR OTHER ALLERGENS. IF AN ALLERGIC REACTION OCCURS, AUGMENTIN SHOULD BE DISCONTINUED AND THE APPROPRIATE THERAPY INSTITUTED. **SERIOUS ANAPHYLACTIC REACTIONS REQUIRE IMMEDIATE EMERGENCY TREATMENT WITH EPINEPHRINE. OXYGEN, INTRAVENOUS STEROIDS, AND AIRWAY MANAGEMENT, INCLUDING INTUBATION, SHOULD ALSO BE ADMINISTERED AS INDICATED.**

Clostridium difficile associated diarrhea (CDAD) has been reported with use of nearly all antibacterial agents, including AUGMENTIN, and may range in severity from mild diarrhea to fatal colitis. Treatment with antibacterial agents alters the normal flora of the colon leading to overgrowth of *C. difficile.*

C. difficile produces toxins A and B which contribute to the development of CDAD. Hypertoxin producing strains of *C. difficile* cause increased morbidity and mortality, as these infections can be refractory to antimicrobial therapy and may require colectomy. CDAD must be considered in all patients who present with diarrhea following antibiotic use. Careful medical history is necessary since CDAD has been reported to occur over two months after the administration of antibacterial agents.

If CDAD is suspected or confirmed, ongoing antibiotic use not directed against *C. difficile* may need to be discontinued. Appropriate fluid and electrolyte management, protein supplementation, antibiotic treatment of *C. difficile,* and surgical evaluation should be instituted as clinically indicated. AUGMENTIN should be used with caution in patients with evidence of hepatic dysfunction. Hepatic toxicity associated with the use of AUGMENTIN is usually reversible. On rare occasions, deaths have been reported (less than 1 death reported per estimated 4 million prescriptions worldwide). These have generally been cases associated with serious underlying diseases or concomitant medications. (See CONTRAINDICATIONS and ADVERSE REACTIONS—Liver.)

PRECAUTIONS

General

While AUGMENTIN possesses the characteristic low toxicity of the penicillin group of antibiotics, periodic assessment of organ system functions, including renal, hepatic, and hematopoietic function, is advisable during prolonged therapy.

A high percentage of patients with mononucleosis who receive ampicillin develop an erythematous skin rash. Thus, ampicillin-class antibiotics should not be administered to patients with mononucleosis.

The possibility of superinfections with mycotic or bacterial pathogens should be kept in mind during therapy. If superinfections occur (usually involving *Pseudomonas* or *Candida*), the drug should be discontinued and/or appropriate therapy instituted.

Prescribing AUGMENTIN in the absence of a proven or strongly suspected bacterial infection or a prophylactic indication is unlikely to provide benefit to the patient and increases the risk of the development of drug-resistant bacteria.

Information for the Patient

AUGMENTIN may be taken every 8 hours or every 12 hours, depending on the strength of the product prescribed. Each dose should be taken with a meal or snack to reduce the possibility of gastrointestinal upset. Many antibiotics can cause diarrhea. If diarrhea is severe or lasts more than 2 or 3 days, call your doctor.

Diarrhea is a common problem caused by antibiotics which usually ends when the antibiotic is discontinued. Sometimes after starting treatment with antibiotics, patients can develop watery and bloody stools (with or without stomach cramps and fever) even as late as 2 or more months after having taken the last dose of the antibiotic. If this occurs, patients should contact their physician as soon as possible.

Keep suspension refrigerated. Shake well before using. When dosing a child with the suspension (liquid) of AUGMENTIN, use a dosing spoon or medicine dropper. Be sure to rinse the spoon or dropper after each use. Bottles of suspension of AUGMENTIN may contain more liquid than required. Follow your doctor's instructions about the amount to use and the days of treatment your child requires. Discard any unused medicine.

Patients should be counseled that antibacterial drugs including AUGMENTIN, should only be used to treat bacterial infections. They do not treat viral infections (e.g., the common cold). When AUGMENTIN is prescribed to treat a bacterial infection, patients should be told that although it is common to feel better early in the course of therapy, the medication should be taken exactly as directed. Skipping doses or not completing the full course of therapy may: (1) decrease the effectiveness of the immediate treatment, and (2) increase the likelihood that bacteria will develop resistance and will not be treatable by AUGMENTIN or other antibacterial drugs in the future.

Phenylketonurics

Each 200-mg chewable tablet of AUGMENTIN contains 2.1 mg phenylalanine; each 400-mg chewable tablet contains 4.2 mg phenylalanine; each 5 mL of either the 200 mg/5 mL or 400 mg/5 mL oral suspension contains 7 mg phenylalanine. The other products of AUGMENTIN do not contain phenylalanine and can be used by phenylketonurics. Contact your physician or pharmacist.

Drug Interactions

Probenecid decreases the renal tubular secretion of amoxicillin. Concurrent use with AUGMENTIN may result in increased and prolonged blood levels of amoxicillin. Co-administration of probenecid cannot be recommended.

Abnormal prolongation of prothrombin time (increased international normalized ratio [INR]) has been reported rarely in patients receiving amoxicillin and oral anticoagulants. Appropriate monitoring should be undertaken when anticoagulants are prescribed concurrently. Adjustments in the dose of oral anticoagulants may be necessary to maintain the desired level of anticoagulation.

The concurrent administration of allopurinol and ampicillin increases substantially the incidence of rashes in patients receiving both drugs as compared to patients receiving ampicillin alone. It is not known whether this potentiation of ampicillin rashes is due to allopurinol or the hyperuricemia

present in these patients. There are no data with AUGMENTIN and allopurinol administered concurrently. In common with other broad-spectrum antibiotics, AUGMENTIN may reduce the efficacy of oral contraceptives.

Drug/Laboratory Test Interactions

Oral administration of AUGMENTIN will result in high urine concentrations of amoxicillin. High urine concentrations of ampicillin may result in false-positive reactions when testing for the presence of glucose in urine using CLINITEST®, Benedict's Solution, or Fehling's Solution. Since this effect may also occur with amoxicillin and therefore AUGMENTIN, it is recommended that glucose tests based on enzymatic glucose oxidase reactions (such as CLINISTIX®) be used.

Following administration of ampicillin to pregnant women, a transient decrease in plasma concentration of total conjugated estriol, estriol-glucuronide, conjugated estrone, and estradiol has been noted. This effect may also occur with amoxicillin and therefore AUGMENTIN.

Carcinogenesis, Mutagenesis, Impairment of Fertility

Long-term studies in animals have not been performed to evaluate carcinogenic potential.

Mutagenesis

The mutagenic potential of AUGMENTIN was investigated in vitro with an Ames test, a human lymphocyte cytogenetic assay, a yeast test and a mouse lymphoma forward mutation assay, and in vivo with mouse micronucleus tests and a dominant lethal test. All were negative apart from the in vitro mouse lymphoma assay where weak activity was found at very high, cytotoxic concentrations.

Impairment of Fertility

AUGMENTIN at oral doses of up to 1,200 mg/kg/day (5.7 times the maximum human dose, 1,480 mg/m²/day, based on body surface area) was found to have no effect on fertility and reproductive performance in rats, dosed with a 2:1 ratio formulation of amoxicillin:clavulanate.

Pregnancy

Teratogenic Effects

Pregnancy (Category B). Reproduction studies performed in pregnant rats and mice given AUGMENTIN at oral dosages up to 1,200 mg/kg/day, equivalent to 7,200 and 4,080 mg/m²/day, respectively (4.9 and 2.8 times the maximum human oral dose based on body surface area), revealed no evidence of harm to the fetus due to AUGMENTIN. There are, however, no adequate and well-controlled studies in pregnant women. Because animal reproduction studies are not always predictive of human response, this drug should be used during pregnancy only if clearly needed.

Labor and Delivery

Oral ampicillin-class antibiotics are generally poorly absorbed during labor. Studies in guinea pigs have shown that intravenous administration of ampicillin decreased the uterine tone, frequency of contractions, height of contractions, and duration of contractions. However, it is not known whether the use of AUGMENTIN in humans during labor or delivery has immediate or delayed adverse effects on the fetus, prolongs the duration of labor, or increases the likelihood that forceps delivery or other obstetrical intervention or resuscitation of the newborn will be necessary. In a single study in women with premature rupture of fetal membranes, it was reported that prophylactic treatment with AUGMENTIN may be associated with an increased risk of necrotizing enterocolitis in neonates.

Nursing Mothers

Ampicillin-class antibiotics are excreted in the milk; therefore, caution should be exercised when AUGMENTIN is administered to a nursing woman.

Pediatric Use

Because of incompletely developed renal function in neonates and young infants, the elimination of amoxicillin may be delayed. Dosing of AUGMENTIN should be modified in pediatric patients younger than 12 weeks (3 months). (See DOSAGE AND ADMINISTRATION—Pediatric.)

ADVERSE REACTIONS

AUGMENTIN is generally well tolerated. The majority of side effects observed in clinical trials were of a mild and transient nature and less than 3% of patients discontinued therapy because of drug-related side effects. From the original premarketing studies, where both pediatric and adult patients were enrolled, the most frequently reported adverse effects were diarrhea/loose stools (9%), nausea (3%), skin rashes and urticaria (3%), vomiting (1%) and vaginitis (1%). The overall incidence of side effects, and in particular diarrhea, increased with the higher recommended dose. Other less frequently reported reactions include: Abdominal discomfort, flatulence, and headache.

In pediatric patients (aged 2 months to 12 years), 1 US/Canadian clinical trial was conducted which compared 45/6.4 mg/kg/day (divided every 12 hours) of AUGMENTIN for 10 days versus 40/10 mg/kg/day (divided every 8 hours) of AUGMENTIN for 10 days in the treatment of acute otitis media. A total of 575 patients were enrolled, and only the suspension formulations were used in this trial. Overall, the adverse event profile seen was comparable to that noted above; however, there were differences in the rates of diarrhea, skin rashes/urticaria, and diaper area rashes. (See CLINICAL STUDIES.)

The following adverse reactions have been reported for ampicillin-class antibiotics:

Gastrointestinal
Diarrhea, nausea, vomiting, indigestion, gastritis, stomatitis, glossitis, black "hairy" tongue, mucocutaneous candidiasis, enterocolitis, and hemorrhagic/pseudomembranous colitis. Onset of pseudomembranous colitis symptoms may occur during or after antibiotic treatment. (See WARNINGS.)

Hypersensitivity Reactions
Skin rashes, pruritus, urticaria, angioedema, serum sickness–like reactions (urticaria or skin rash accompanied by arthritis, arthralgia, myalgia, and frequently fever), erythema multiforme (rarely Stevens-Johnson syndrome), acute generalized exanthematous pustulosis, hypersensitivity vasculitis, and an occasional case of exfoliative dermatitis (including toxic epidermal necrolysis) have been reported. These reactions may be controlled with antihistamines and, if necessary, systemic corticosteroids. Whenever such reactions occur, the drug should be discontinued, unless the opinion of the physician dictates otherwise. Serious and occasional fatal hypersensitivity (anaphylactic) reactions can occur with oral penicillin. (See WARNINGS.)

Liver
A moderate rise in AST (SGOT) and/or ALT (SGPT) has been noted in patients treated with ampicillin-class antibiotics, but the significance of these findings is unknown. Hepatic dysfunction, including hepatitis and cholestatic jaundice, (See CONTRAINDICATIONS), increases in serum transaminases (AST and/or ALT), serum bilirubin and/or alkaline phosphatase, has been infrequently reported with AUGMENTIN. It has been reported more commonly in the elderly, in males, or in patients on prolonged treatment. The histologic findings on liver biopsy have consisted of predominantly cholestatic, hepatocellular, or mixed cholestatic-hepatocellular changes. The onset of signs/symptoms of hepatic dysfunction may occur during or several weeks after therapy has been discontinued. The hepatic dysfunction, which may be severe, is usually reversible. On rare occasions, deaths have been reported (less than 1 death reported per estimated 4 million prescriptions worldwide). These have generally been cases associated with serious underlying diseases or concomitant medications.

Renal
Interstitial nephritis and hematuria have been reported rarely. Crystalluria has also been reported (see OVERDOSAGE).

Hemic and Lymphatic Systems
Anemia, including hemolytic anemia, thrombocytopenia, thrombocytopenic purpura, eosinophilia, leukopenia, and agranulocytosis have been reported during therapy with penicillins. These reactions are usually reversible on discontinuation of therapy and are believed to be hypersensitivity phenomena. A slight thrombocytosis was noted in less than 1% of the patients treated with AUGMENTIN. There have been reports of increased prothrombin time in patients receiving AUGMENTIN and anticoagulant therapy concomitantly.

Central Nervous System
Agitation, anxiety, behavioral changes, confusion, convulsions, dizziness, insomnia, and reversible hyperactivity have been reported rarely.

Miscellaneous
Tooth discoloration (brown, yellow, or gray staining) has been rarely reported. Most reports occurred in pediatric patients. Discoloration was reduced or eliminated with brushing or dental cleaning in most cases.

OVERDOSAGE
Following overdosage, patients have experienced primarily gastrointestinal symptoms including stomach and abdominal pain, vomiting, and diarrhea. Rash, hyperactivity, or drowsiness have also been observed in a small number of patients.

In the case of overdosage, discontinue AUGMENTIN, treat symptomatically, and institute supportive measures as required. If the overdosage is very recent and there is no contraindication, an attempt at emesis or other means of removal of drug from the stomach may be performed. A prospective study of 51 pediatric patients at a poison center suggested that overdosages of less than 250 mg/kg of amoxicillin are not associated with significant clinical symptoms and do not require gastric emptying.[3]

Interstitial nephritis resulting in oliguric renal failure has been reported in a small number of patients after overdosage with amoxicillin.

Crystalluria, in some cases leading to renal failure, has also been reported after amoxicillin overdosage in adult and pediatric patients. In case of overdosage, adequate fluid intake and diuresis should be maintained to reduce the risk of amoxicillin crystalluria.

Renal impairment appears to be reversible with cessation of drug administration. High blood levels may occur more readily in patients with impaired renal function because of decreased renal clearance of both amoxicillin and clavulanate. Both amoxicillin and clavulanate are removed from the circulation by hemodialysis.

DOSAGE AND ADMINISTRATION
Dosage
Pediatric Patients
Based on the amoxicillin component, AUGMENTIN should be dosed as follows:

Neonates and infants aged < 12 weeks (3 months)
Due to incompletely developed renal function affecting elimination of amoxicillin in this age group, the recommended dose of AUGMENTIN is 30 mg/kg/day divided every 12 hours, based on the amoxicillin component. Clavulanate elimination is unaltered in this age group. Experience with the 200 mg/5 mL formulation in this age group is limited and, thus, use of the 125 mg/5 mL oral suspension is recommended.

Patients aged 12 weeks (3 months) and older

INFECTIONS	DOSING REGIMEN	
	q12h[a]	q8h
	200 mg/5 mL or 400 mg/5 mL oral suspension[b]	125 mg/5 mL or 250 mg/5 mL oral suspension
Otitis media[c], sinusitis, lower respiratory tract infections, and more severe infections	45 mg/kg/day q12h	40 mg/kg/day q8h
Less severe infections	25 mg/kg/day q12h	20 mg/kg/day q8h

[a] The q12h regimen is recommended as it is associated with significantly less diarrhea. (See CLINICAL STUDIES.) However, the q12h formulations (200 and 400 mg) contain aspartame and should not be used by phenylketonurics.
[b] Each strength of suspension of AUGMENTIN is available as a chewable tablet for use by older children.
[c] Duration of therapy studied and recommended for acute otitis media is 10 days.

Pediatric Patients Weighing 40 kg and More
Should be dosed according to the following adult recommendations: The usual adult dose is one 500-mg tablet of AUGMENTIN every 12 hours or one 250-mg tablet of AUGMENTIN every 8 hours. For more severe infections and infections of the respiratory tract, the dose should be one 875-mg tablet of AUGMENTIN every 12 hours or one 500-mg tablet of AUGMENTIN every 8 hours. Among adults treated with 875 mg every 12 hours, significantly fewer experienced severe diarrhea or withdrawals with diarrhea versus adults treated with 500 mg every 8 hours. For detailed adult dosage recommendations, please see complete prescribing information for tablets of AUGMENTIN.

Hepatically impaired patients should be dosed with caution and hepatic function monitored at regular intervals. (See WARNINGS.)

Adults
Adults who have difficulty swallowing may be given the 125 mg/5 mL or 250 mg/5 mL suspension in place of the 500-mg tablet. The 200 mg/5 mL suspension or the 400 mg/5 mL suspension may be used in place of the 875-mg tablet. See dosage recommendations above for children weighing 40 kg or more.

The 250-mg tablet of AUGMENTIN and the 250-mg chewable tablet do not contain the same amount of clavulanic acid (as the potassium salt). The 250-mg tablet of AUGMENTIN contains 125 mg of clavulanic acid, whereas the 250-mg chewable tablet contains 62.5 mg of clavulanic acid. Therefore, the 250-mg tablet of AUGMENTIN and the 250-mg chewable tablet should not be substituted for each other, as they are not interchangeable.

Due to the different amoxicillin to clavulanic acid ratios in the 250-mg tablet of AUGMENTIN (250/125) versus the 250-mg chewable tablet of AUGMENTIN (250/62.5), the 250-mg tablet of AUGMENTIN should not be used until the child weighs at least 40 kg and more.

Directions for Mixing Oral Suspension
Prepare a suspension at time of dispensing as follows: Tap bottle until all the powder flows freely. Add approximately 2/3 of the total amount of water for reconstitution (see table below) and shake vigorously to suspend powder. Add remainder of the water and again shake vigorously.

AUGMENTIN 125 mg/5 mL Suspension

Bottle Size	Amount of Water Required for Reconstitution
75 mL	67 mL
100 mL	90 mL
150 mL	134 mL

Each teaspoonful (5 mL) will contain 125 mg amoxicillin and 31.25 mg of clavulanic acid as the potassium salt.

AUGMENTIN 200 mg/5 mL Suspension

Bottle Size	Amount of Water Required for Reconstitution
50 mL	50 mL
75 mL	75 mL
100 mL	95 mL

Each teaspoonful (5 mL) will contain 200 mg amoxicillin and 28.5 mg of clavulanic acid as the potassium salt.

AUGMENTIN 250 mg/5 mL Suspension

Bottle Size	Amount of Water Required for Reconstitution
75 mL	65 mL
100 mL	87 mL
150 mL	130 mL

Each teaspoonful (5 mL) will contain 250 mg amoxicillin and 62.5 mg of clavulanic acid as the potassium salt.

AUGMENTIN 400 mg/5 mL Suspension

Bottle Size	Amount of Water Required for Reconstitution
50 mL	50 mL
75 mL	70 mL
100 mL	90 mL

Each teaspoonful (5 mL) will contain 400 mg amoxicillin and 57.0 mg of clavulanic acid as the potassium salt.

Note: SHAKE ORAL SUSPENSION WELL BEFORE USING.
Reconstituted suspension must be stored under refrigeration and discarded after 10 days.

Administration
AUGMENTIN may be taken without regard to meals; however, absorption of clavulanate potassium is enhanced when AUGMENTIN is administered at the start of a meal. To minimize the potential for gastrointestinal intolerance, AUGMENTIN should be taken at the start of a meal.

HOW SUPPLIED
AUGMENTIN 125 mg/5 mL for Oral Suspension: Each 5 mL of reconstituted banana-flavored suspension contains 125 mg amoxicillin and 31.25 mg clavulanic acid as the potassium salt.
NDC 0029-6085-39   75 mL bottle
NDC 0029-6085-23   100 mL bottle
NDC 0029-6085-22   150 mL bottle
AUGMENTIN 200 mg/5 mL for Oral Suspension: Each 5 mL of reconstituted orange-flavored suspension contains 200 mg amoxicillin and 28.5 mg clavulanic acid as the potassium salt.
NDC 0029-6087-29   50 mL bottle
NDC 0029-6087-39   75 mL bottle
NDC 0029-6087-51   100 mL bottle
AUGMENTIN 250 mg/5 mL for Oral Suspension: Each 5 mL of reconstituted orange-flavored suspension contains 250 mg amoxicillin and 62.5 mg clavulanic acid as the potassium salt.
NDC 0029-6090-39   75 mL bottle

NDC 0029-6090-23 100 mL bottle
NDC 0029-6090-22 150 mL bottle

AUGMENTIN 400 mg/5 mL for Oral Suspension: Each 5 mL of reconstituted orange-flavored suspension contains 400 mg amoxicillin and 57 mg clavulanic acid as the potassium salt.

NDC 0029-6092-29 50 mL bottle
NDC 0029-6092-39 75 mL bottle
NDC 0029-6092-51 100 mL bottle

AUGMENTIN 125-mg Chewable Tablets: Each mottled yellow, round, lemon-lime-flavored tablet, debossed with BMP 189, contains 125 mg amoxicillin as the trihydrate and 31.25 mg clavulanic acid as the potassium salt.

NDC 0029-6073-47 carton of 30 tablets

AUGMENTIN 200-mg Chewable Tablets: Each mottled pink, round, biconvex, cherry-banana-flavored tablet contains 200 mg amoxicillin as the trihydrate and 28.5 mg clavulanic acid as the potassium salt.

NDC 0029-6071-12 carton of 20 tablets

AUGMENTIN 250-mg Chewable Tablets: Each mottled yellow, round, lemon-lime-flavored tablet, debossed with BMP 190, contains 250 mg amoxicillin as the trihydrate and 62.5 mg clavulanic acid as the potassium salt.

NDC 0029-6074-47 carton of 30 tablets

AUGMENTIN 400-mg Chewable Tablets: Each mottled pink, round, biconvex, cherry-banana-flavored tablet contains 400 mg amoxicillin as the trihydrate and 57.0 mg clavulanic acid as the potassium salt.

NDC 0029-6072-12 carton of 20 tablets

AUGMENTIN is Also Supplied as:

AUGMENTIN 250-mg Tablets (250 mg amoxicillin/125 mg clavulanic acid):

NDC 0029-6075-27 bottles of 30
NDC 0029-6075-31 100 Unit Dose tablets

AUGMENTIN 500-mg Tablets (500 mg amoxicillin/125 mg clavulanic acid):

NDC 0029-6080-12 bottles of 20
NDC 0029-6080-31 100 Unit Dose tablets

AUGMENTIN 875-mg Tablets (875 mg amoxicillin/125 mg clavulanic acid):

NDC 0029-6086-12 bottles of 20
NDC 0029-6086-21 100 Unit Dose tablets

Store tablets and dry powder at or below 25°C (77°F). Dispense in original containers. Store reconstituted suspension under refrigeration. Discard unused suspension after 10 days.

CLINICAL STUDIES

In pediatric patients (aged 2 months to 12 years), 1 US/Canadian clinical trial was conducted which compared 45/6.4 mg/kg/day (divided every 12 hours) of AUGMENTIN for 10 days versus 40/10 mg/kg/day (divided every 8 hours) of AUGMENTIN for 10 days in the treatment of acute otitis media. Only the suspension formulations were used in this trial. A total of 575 patients were enrolled, with an even distribution among the 2 treatment groups and a comparable number of patients were evaluable (i.e., ≥ 84%) per treatment group. Strict otitis media-specific criteria were required for eligibility and a strong correlation was found at the end of therapy and follow-up between these criteria and physician assessment of clinical response. The clinical efficacy rates at the end of therapy visit (defined as 2-4 days after the completion of therapy) and at the follow-up visit (defined as 22-28 days post-completion of therapy) were comparable for the 2 treatment groups, with the following cure rates obtained for the evaluable patients: At end of therapy, 87.2% (n = 265) and 82.3% (n = 260) for 45 mg/kg/day every 12 hours and 40 mg/kg/day every 8 hours, respectively. At follow-up, 67.1% (n = 249) and 68.7% (n = 243) for 45 mg/kg/day every 12 hours and 40 mg/kg/day every 8 hours, respectively.

The incidence of diarrhea[a] was significantly lower in patients in the every 12 hours treatment group compared to patients who received the every 8 hours regimen (14.3% and 34.3%, respectively). In addition, the number of patients with either severe diarrhea or who were withdrawn with diarrhea was significantly lower in the every 12 hours treatment group (3.1% and 7.6% for the every 12 hours/10 day and every 8 hours/10 day, respectively). In the every 12 hours treatment group, 3 patients (1.0%) were withdrawn with an allergic reaction, while 1 patient (0.3%) in the every 8 hours group was withdrawn for this reason. The number of patients with a candidal infection of the diaper area was 3.8% and 6.2% for the every 12 hours and every 8 hours groups, respectively.

It is not known if the finding of a statistically significant reduction in diarrhea with the oral suspensions dosed every 12 hours, versus suspensions dosed every 8 hours, can be extrapolated to the chewable tablets. The presence of mannitol in the chewable tablets may contribute to a different diarrhea profile. The every 12 hours oral suspensions are sweetened with aspartame only.

[a] Diarrhea was defined as either: (a) 3 or more watery or 4 or more loose/watery stools in 1 day; OR (b) 2 watery stools per day or 3 loose/watery stools per day for 2 consecutive days.

REFERENCES

1. National Committee for Clinical Laboratory Standards. Methods for Dilution Antimicrobial Susceptibility Tests for Bacteria That Grow Aerobically – Third Edition. Approved Standard NCCLS Document M7-A3, Vol. 13, No. 25. NCCLS, Villanova, PA, Dec. 1993.
2. National Committee for Clinical Laboratory Standards. Performance Standard for Antimicrobial Disk Susceptibility Tests – Fifth Edition. Approved Standard NCCLS Document M2-A5, Vol. 13, No. 24. NCCLS, Villanova, PA, Dec. 1993.
3. Swanson-Biearman B, Dean BS, Lopez G, Krenzelok EP. The effects of penicillin and cephalosporin ingestions in children less than six years of age. *Vet Hum Toxicol* 1988;30:66-67.

AUGMENTIN is a registered trademark of GlaxoSmithKline.
CLINITEST is a registered trademark of Miles, Inc.
CLINISTIX is a registered trademark of Bayer Corporation.

GlaxoSmithKline
Research Triangle Park, NC 27709
©2009, GlaxoSmithKline All rights reserved.
September 2009 AUP:18PI

AUGMENTIN® ℞

[äg-mint' in]
(amoxicillin/clavulanate potassium)
Tablets

To reduce the development of drug-resistant bacteria and maintain the effectiveness of AUGMENTIN (amoxicillin/clavulanate potassium) and other antibacterial drugs, AUGMENTIN should be used only to treat or prevent infections that are proven or strongly suspected to be caused by bacteria.

DESCRIPTION

AUGMENTIN is an oral antibacterial combination consisting of the semisynthetic antibiotic amoxicillin and the β-lactamase inhibitor, clavulanate potassium (the potassium salt of clavulanic acid). Amoxicillin is an analog of ampicillin, derived from the basic penicillin nucleus, 6-aminopenicillanic acid. The amoxicillin molecular formula is $C_{16}H_{19}N_3O_5S \bullet 3H_2O$, and the molecular weight is 419.46. Chemically, amoxicillin is (2*S*,5*R*,6*R*)-6-[(*R*)-(-)-2-Amino-2-(*p*-hydroxyphenyl)acetamido]-3,3-dimethyl-7-oxo-4-thia-1-azabicyclo[3.2.0]heptane-2-carboxylic acid trihydrate and may be represented structurally as:

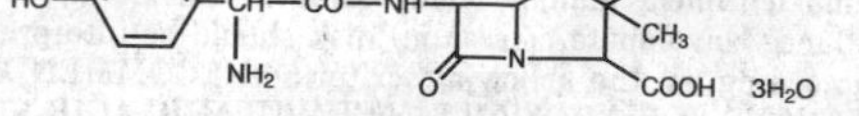

Clavulanic acid is produced by the fermentation of *Streptomyces clavuligerus*. It is a β-lactam structurally related to the penicillins and possesses the ability to inactivate a wide variety of β-lactamases by blocking the active sites of these enzymes. Clavulanic acid is particularly active against the clinically important plasmid-mediated β-lactamases frequently responsible for transferred drug resistance to penicillins and cephalosporins. The clavulanate potassium molecular formula is $C_8H_8KNO_5$, and the molecular weight is 237.25. Chemically, clavulanate potassium is potassium (*Z*)-(2*R*, 5*R*)-3-(2-hydroxyethylidene)-7-oxo-4-oxa-1-azabicyclo [3.2.0]-heptane-2-carboxylate, and may be represented structurally as:

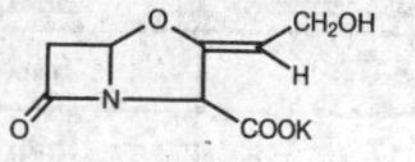

Inactive Ingredients

Colloidal silicon dioxide, hypromellose, magnesium stearate, microcrystalline cellulose, polyethylene glycol, sodium starch glycolate, and titanium dioxide.

Each tablet of AUGMENTIN contains 0.63 mEq potassium.

CLINICAL PHARMACOLOGY

Amoxicillin and clavulanate potassium are well absorbed from the gastrointestinal tract after oral administration of AUGMENTIN. Dosing in the fasted or fed state has minimal effect on the pharmacokinetics of amoxicillin. While AUGMENTIN can be given without regard to meals, absorption of clavulanate potassium when taken with food is greater relative to the fasted state. In 1 study, the relative bioavailability of clavulanate was reduced when AUGMENTIN was dosed at 30 and 150 minutes after the start of a high-fat breakfast. The safety and efficacy of AUGMENTIN have been established in clinical trials where AUGMENTIN was taken without regard to meals.

[See table at top of next page]

Amoxicillin serum concentrations achieved with AUGMENTIN are similar to those produced by the oral administration of equivalent doses of amoxicillin alone. The half-life of amoxicillin after the oral administration of AUGMENTIN is 1.3 hours and that of clavulanic acid is 1.0 hour.

Approximately 50% to 70% of the amoxicillin and approximately 25% to 40% of the clavulanic acid are excreted unchanged in urine during the first 6 hours after administration of a single 250-mg or 500-mg tablet of AUGMENTIN. Concurrent administration of probenecid delays amoxicillin excretion but does not delay renal excretion of clavulanic acid.

Neither component in AUGMENTIN is highly protein-bound; clavulanic acid has been found to be approximately 25% bound to human serum and amoxicillin approximately 18% bound.

Amoxicillin diffuses readily into most body tissues and fluids with the exception of the brain and spinal fluid. The results of experiments involving the administration of clavulanic acid to animals suggest that this compound, like amoxicillin, is well distributed in body tissues.

Microbiology

Amoxicillin is a semisynthetic antibiotic with a broad spectrum of bactericidal activity against many gram-positive and gram-negative microorganisms. Amoxicillin is, however, susceptible to degradation by β-lactamases, and therefore, the spectrum of activity does not include organisms which produce these enzymes. Clavulanic acid is a β-lactam, structurally related to the penicillins, which possesses the ability to inactivate a wide range of β-lactamase enzymes commonly found in microorganisms resistant to penicillins and cephalosporins. In particular, it has good activity against the clinically important plasmid-mediated β-lactamases frequently responsible for transferred drug resistance.

The formulation of amoxicillin and clavulanic acid in AUGMENTIN protects amoxicillin from degradation by β-lactamase enzymes and effectively extends the antibiotic spectrum of amoxicillin to include many bacteria normally resistant to amoxicillin and other β-lactam antibiotics. Thus, AUGMENTIN possesses the properties of a broad-spectrum antibiotic and a β-lactamase inhibitor.

Amoxicillin/clavulanic acid has been shown to be active against most strains of the following microorganisms, both in vitro and in clinical infections as described in INDICATIONS AND USAGE.

Gram-Positive Aerobes

Staphylococcus aureus (β-lactamase and non–β-lactamase–producing)[c]

[c] Staphylococci which are resistant to methicillin/oxacillin must be considered resistant to amoxicillin/clavulanic acid.

Gram-Negative Aerobes

Enterobacter species (Although most strains of *Enterobacter* species are resistant in vitro, clinical efficacy has been demonstrated with AUGMENTIN in urinary tract infections caused by these organisms.)

Escherichia coli (β-lactamase and non–β-lactamase–producing)

Haemophilus influenzae (β-lactamase and non–β-lactamase–producing)

Klebsiella species (All known strains are β-lactamase–producing.)

Moraxella catarrhalis (β-lactamase and non–β-lactamase–producing)

The following in vitro data are available, **but their clinical significance is unknown.**

Amoxicillin/clavulanic acid exhibits in vitro minimal inhibitory concentrations (MICs) of 2 mcg/mL or less against most (≥ 90%) strains of *Streptococcus pneumoniae*[d]; MICs of 0.06 mcg/mL or less against most (≥ 90%) strains of *Neisseria gonorrhoeae*; MICs of 4 mcg/mL or less against most (≥ 90%) strains of staphylococci and anaerobic bacteria; and MICs of 8 mcg/mL or less against most (≥ 90%) strains of other listed organisms. However, with the exception of organisms shown to respond to amoxicillin alone, the safety and effectiveness of amoxicillin/clavulanic acid in treating clinical infections due to these microorganisms have not been established in adequate and well-controlled clinical trials.

[d] Because amoxicillin has greater in vitro activity against *S. pneumoniae* than does ampicillin or penicillin, the majority of *S. pneumoniae* strains with intermediate susceptibility to ampicillin or penicillin are fully susceptible to amoxicillin.

Gram-Positive Aerobes

Enterococcus faecalis[e]

Staphylococcus epidermidis (β-lactamase and non–β-lactamase–producing)

Staphylococcus saprophyticus (β-lactamase and non–β-lactamase–producing)

Streptococcus pneumoniae[e f]

Streptococcus pyogenes[e f]

viridans group *Streptococcus*[e f]

Gram-Negative Aerobes

Eikenella corrodens (β-lactamase and non–β-lactamase–producing)

Neisseria gonorrhoeae[e] (β-lactamase and non–β-lactamase–producing)

Proteus mirabilis[e] (β-lactamase and non–β-lactamase–producing)

Anaerobic Bacteria

Bacteroides species, including *Bacteroides fragilis* (β-lactamase and non–β-lactamase–producing)

Fusobacterium species (β-lactamase and non–β-lactamase–producing)

Peptostreptococcus species[f]

[e] Adequate and well-controlled clinical trials have established the effectiveness of amoxicillin alone in treating certain clinical infections due to these organisms.

[f] These are non–β-lactamase–producing organisms, and therefore, are susceptible to amoxicillin alone.

Susceptibility Testing

Dilution Techniques

Quantitative methods are used to determine antimicrobial MICs. These MICs provide estimates of the susceptibility of bacteria to antimicrobial compounds. The MICs should be determined using a standardized procedure. Standardized procedures are based on a dilution method[1] (broth or agar) or equivalent with standardized inoculum concentrations and standardized concentrations of amoxicillin/clavulanate potassium powder.

The recommended dilution pattern utilizes a constant amoxicillin/clavulanate potassium ratio of 2 to 1 in all tubes with varying amounts of amoxicillin. MICs are expressed in terms of the amoxicillin concentration in the presence of clavulanic acid at a constant 2 parts amoxicillin to 1 part clavulanic acid. The MIC values should be interpreted according to the following criteria: RECOMMENDED RANGES FOR AMOXICILLIN/CLAVULANIC ACID SUSCEPTIBILITY TESTING

For Gram-Negative Enteric Aerobes:

MIC (mcg/mL)	Interpretation
≤ 8/4	Susceptible (S)
16/8	Intermediate (I)
≥ 32/16	Resistant (R)

For *Staphylococcus*[g] and *Haemophilus* species:

MIC (mcg/mL)	Interpretation
≤ 4/2	Susceptible (S)
≥ 8/4	Resistant (R)

[g] Staphylococci which are susceptible to amoxicillin/clavulanic acid but resistant to methicillin/oxacillin must be considered as resistant.

For *S. pneumoniae* from non-meningitis sources:

Isolates should be tested using amoxicillin/clavulanic acid and the following criteria should be used:

MIC (mcg/mL)	Interpretation
≤ 2/1	Susceptible (S)
4/2	Intermediate (I)
≥ 8/4	Resistant (R)

NOTE: These interpretive criteria are based on the recommended doses for respiratory tract infections.

A report of "Susceptible" indicates that the pathogen is likely to be inhibited if the antimicrobial compound in the blood reaches the concentration usually achievable. A report of "Intermediate" indicates that the result should be considered equivocal, and, if the microorganism is not fully susceptible to alternative, clinically feasible drugs, the test should be repeated. This category implies possible clinical applicability in body sites where the drug is physiologically concentrated or in situations where high dosage of drug can be used. This category also provides a buffer zone, which prevents small uncontrolled technical factors from causing major discrepancies in interpretation. A report of "Resistant" indicates that the pathogen is not likely to be inhibited if the antimicrobial compound in the blood reaches the concentrations usually achievable; other therapy should be selected.

Mean[a] amoxicillin and clavulanate potassium pharmacokinetic parameters are shown in the table below:

Dose[b] and regimen	AUC$_{0-24}$ (mcg•hr/mL)		C$_{max}$ (mcg/mL)	
amoxicillin/clavulanate potassium	amoxicillin (±S.D.)	clavulanate potassium (±S.D.)	amoxicillin (±S.D.)	clavulanate potassium (±S.D.)
250/125 mg q8h	26.7 ± 4.56	12.6 ± 3.25	3.3 ± 1.12	1.5 ± 0.70
500/125 mg q12h	33.4 ± 6.76	8.6 ± 1.95	6.5 ± 1.41	1.8 ± 0.61
500/125 mg q8h	53.4 ± 8.87	15.7 ± 3.86	7.2 ± 2.26	2.4 ± 0.83
875/125 mg q12h	53.5 ± 12.31	10.2 ± 3.04	11.6 ± 2.78	2.2 ± 0.99

[a] Mean values of 14 normal volunteers (n = 15 for clavulanate potassium in the low-dose regimens). Peak concentrations occurred approximately 1.5 hours after the dose.

[b] Administered at the start of a light meal.

Standardized susceptibility test procedures require the use of laboratory control microorganisms to control the technical aspects of the laboratory procedures. Standard amoxicillin/clavulanate potassium powder should provide the following MIC values:

Microorganism	MIC Range (mcg/mL)[h]
Escherichia coli ATCC 25922	2 to 8
Escherichia coli ATCC 35218	4 to 16
Enterococcus faecalis ATCC 29212	0.25 to 1.0
Haemophilus influenzae ATCC 49247	2 to 16
Staphylococcus aureus ATCC 29213	0.12 to 0.5
Streptococcus pneumoniae ATCC 49619	0.03 to 0.12

[h] Expressed as concentration of amoxicillin in the presence of clavulanic acid at a constant 2 parts amoxicillin to 1 part clavulanic acid.

Diffusion Techniques

Quantitative methods that require measurement of zone diameters also provide reproducible estimates of the susceptibility of bacteria to antimicrobial compounds. One such standardized procedure[2] requires the use of standardized inoculum concentrations. This procedure uses paper disks impregnated with 30 mcg of amoxicillin/clavulanate potassium (20 mcg amoxicillin plus 10 mcg clavulanate potassium) to test the susceptibility of microorganisms to amoxicillin/clavulanic acid.

Reports from the laboratory providing results of the standard single-disk susceptibility test with a 30-mcg amoxicillin/clavulanate acid (20 mcg amoxicillin plus 10 mcg clavulanate potassium) disk should be interpreted according to the following criteria: RECOMMENDED RANGES FOR AMOXICILLIN/CLAVULANIC ACID SUSCEPTIBILITY TESTING

For *Staphylococcus*[i] species and *H. influenzae*[j]:

Zone Diameter (mm)	Interpretation
≥ 20	Susceptible (S)
≤ 19	Resistant (R)

For Other Organisms Except *S. pneumoniae*[k] and *N. gonorrhoeae*[l]:

Zone Diameter (mm)	Interpretation
≥ 18	Susceptible (S)
14 to 17	Intermediate (I)
≤ 13	Resistant (R)

[i] Staphylococci which are resistant to methicillin/oxacillin must be considered as resistant to amoxicillin/clavulanic acid.

[j] A broth microdilution method should be used for testing *H. influenzae*. Beta-lactamase–negative, ampicillin-resistant strains must be considered resistant to amoxicillin/clavulanic acid.

[k] Susceptibility of *S. pneumoniae* should be determined using a 1-mcg oxacillin disk. Isolates with oxacillin zone sizes of ≥20 mm are susceptible to amoxicillin/clavulanic acid. An amoxicillin/clavulanic acid MIC should be determined on isolates of *S. pneumoniae* with oxacillin zone sizes of ≤19 mm.

[l] A broth microdilution method should be used for testing *N. gonorrhoeae* and interpreted according to penicillin breakpoints.

Interpretation should be as stated above for results using dilution techniques. Interpretation involves correlation of the diameter obtained in the disk test with the MIC for amoxicillin/clavulanic acid.

As with standardized dilution techniques, diffusion methods require the use of laboratory control microorganisms that are used to control the technical aspects of the laboratory procedures. For the diffusion technique, the 30-mcg amoxicillin/clavulanate potassium (20-mcg amoxicillin plus 10-mcg clavulanate potassium) disk should provide the following zone diameters in these laboratory quality control strains:

Microorganism	Zone Diameter (mm)
Escherichia coli ATCC 25922	19 to 25
Escherichia coli ATCC 35218	18 to 22
Staphylococcus aureus ATCC 25923	28 to 36

INDICATIONS AND USAGE

AUGMENTIN is indicated in the treatment of infections caused by susceptible strains of the designated organisms in the conditions listed below:

Lower Respiratory Tract Infections

– caused by β-lactamase–producing strains of *H. influenzae* and *M. catarrhalis*.

Otitis Media

– caused by β-lactamase–producing strains of *H. influenzae* and *M. catarrhalis*.

Sinusitis

– caused by β-lactamase–producing strains of *H. influenzae* and *M. catarrhalis*.

Skin and Skin Structure Infections

– caused by β-lactamase–producing strains of *S. aureus*, *E. coli*, and *Klebsiella* spp.

Urinary Tract Infections

– caused by β-lactamase–producing strains of *E. coli*, *Klebsiella* spp., and *Enterobacter* spp.

While AUGMENTIN is indicated only for the conditions listed above, infections caused by ampicillin-susceptible organisms are also amenable to treatment with AUGMENTIN due to its amoxicillin content; therefore, mixed infections caused by ampicillin-susceptible organisms and β-lactamase–producing organisms susceptible to AUGMENTIN should not require the addition of another antibiotic. Because amoxicillin has greater in vitro activity against *S. pneumoniae* than does ampicillin or penicillin, the majority of *S. pneumoniae* strains with intermediate susceptibility to ampicillin or penicillin are fully susceptible to amoxicillin and AUGMENTIN. (See Microbiology.)

To reduce the development of drug-resistant bacteria and maintain the effectiveness of AUGMENTIN and other antibacterial drugs, AUGMENTIN should be used only to treat or prevent infections that are proven or strongly suspected to be caused by susceptible bacteria. When culture and susceptibility information are available, they should be considered in selecting or modifying antibacterial therapy. In the absence of such data, local epidemiology and susceptibility patterns may contribute to the empiric selection of therapy. Bacteriological studies, to determine the causative organisms and their susceptibility to AUGMENTIN, should be performed together with any indicated surgical procedures.

CONTRAINDICATIONS

AUGMENTIN is contraindicated in patients with a history of allergic reactions to any penicillin. It is also contraindicated in patients with a previous history of cholestatic jaundice/hepatic dysfunction associated with AUGMENTIN.

WARNINGS

SERIOUS AND OCCASIONALLY FATAL HYPERSENSITIVITY (ANAPHYLACTIC) REACTIONS HAVE BEEN REPORTED IN PATIENTS ON PENICILLIN THERAPY. THESE REACTIONS ARE MORE LIKELY TO OCCUR IN INDIVIDUALS WITH A HISTORY OF PENICILLIN HYPERSENSITIVITY AND/OR A HISTORY OF SENSITIVITY TO MULTIPLE ALLERGENS. THERE HAVE BEEN REPORTS OF INDIVIDUALS WITH A HISTORY OF PENICILLIN HYPERSENSITIVITY WHO HAVE EXPERIENCED SEVERE REACTIONS WHEN TREATED WITH CEPHALOSPORINS. BEFORE INITIATING THERAPY WITH AUGMENTIN, CAREFUL INQUIRY SHOULD BE MADE CONCERNING PREVIOUS HYPERSENSITIVITY REACTIONS TO PENICILLINS, CEPHALOSPORINS, OR OTHER ALLERGENS. IF AN ALLERGIC REACTION OCCURS, AUGMENTIN SHOULD BE DISCONTINUED AND THE APPROPRIATE THERAPY INSTITUTED. SERIOUS ANAPHYLACTIC REACTIONS REQUIRE IMMEDIATE EMERGENCY TREATMENT WITH EPINEPHRINE. OXYGEN, INTRAVENOUS STEROIDS, AND AIRWAY MANAGEMENT, INCLUDING INTUBATION, SHOULD ALSO BE ADMINISTERED AS INDICATED.

Clostridium difficile associated diarrhea (CDAD) has been reported with use of nearly all antibacterial agents, including AUGMENTIN, and may range in severity from mild diarrhea to fatal colitis. Treatment with antibacterial agents alters the normal flora of the colon leading to overgrowth of *C. difficile.*

C. difficile produces toxins A and B which contribute to the development of CDAD. Hypertoxin producing strains of *C. difficile.* cause increased morbidity and mortality, as these infections can be refractory to antimicrobial therapy and may require colectomy. CDAD must be considered in all patients who present with diarrhea following antibiotic use. Careful medical history is necessary since CDAD has been reported to occur over two months after the administration of antibacterial agents.

If CDAD is suspected or confirmed, ongoing antibiotic use not directed against *C. difficile.* may need to be discontinued. Appropriate fluid and electrolyte management, protein supplementation, antibiotic treatment of *C. difficile*, and surgical evaluation should be instituted as clinically indicated.

AUGMENTIN should be used with caution in patients with evidence of hepatic dysfunction. Hepatic toxicity associated with the use of AUGMENTIN is usually reversible. On rare occasions, deaths have been reported (less than 1 death reported per estimated 4 million prescriptions worldwide). These have generally been cases associated with serious underlying diseases or concomitant medications. (See CONTRAINDICATIONS and ADVERSE REACTIONS: Liver.)

PRECAUTIONS

General

While AUGMENTIN possesses the characteristic low toxicity of the penicillin group of antibiotics, periodic assessment of organ system functions, including renal, hepatic, and hematopoietic function, is advisable during prolonged therapy.

A high percentage of patients with mononucleosis who receive ampicillin develop an erythematous skin rash. Thus, ampicillin-class antibiotics should not be administered to patients with mononucleosis.

The possibility of superinfections with mycotic or bacterial pathogens should be kept in mind during therapy. If superinfections occur (usually involving *Pseudomonas* or *Candida*), the drug should be discontinued and/or appropriate therapy instituted.

Prescribing AUGMENTIN in the absence of a proven or strongly suspected bacterial infection or a prophylactic indication is unlikely to provide benefit to the patient and increases the risk of the development of drug-resistant bacteria.

Drug Interactions

Probenecid decreases the renal tubular secretion of amoxicillin. Concurrent use with AUGMENTIN may result in increased and prolonged blood levels of amoxicillin. Co-administration of probenecid cannot be recommended.

Abnormal prolongation of prothrombin time (increased international normalized ratio [INR]) has been reported rarely in patients receiving amoxicillin and oral anticoagulants. Appropriate monitoring should be undertaken when anticoagulants are prescribed concurrently. Adjustments in the dose of oral anticoagulants may be necessary to maintain the desired level of anticoagulation.

The concurrent administration of allopurinol and ampicillin increases substantially the incidence of rashes in patients receiving both drugs as compared to patients receiving ampicillin alone. It is not known whether this potentiation of ampicillin rashes is due to allopurinol or the hyperuricemia present in these patients. There are no data with AUGMENTIN and allopurinol administered concurrently.

In common with other broad-spectrum antibiotics, AUGMENTIN may reduce the efficacy of oral contraceptives.

Drug/Laboratory Test Interactions

Oral administration of AUGMENTIN will result in high urine concentrations of amoxicillin. High urine concentrations of ampicillin may result in false-positive reactions when testing for the presence of glucose in urine using CLINITEST®, Benedict's Solution, or Fehling's Solution. Since this effect may also occur with amoxicillin and therefore AUGMENTIN, it is recommended that glucose tests based on enzymatic glucose oxidase reactions (such as CLINISTIX®) be used.

Following administration of ampicillin to pregnant women, a transient decrease in plasma concentration of total conjugated estriol, estriol-glucuronide, conjugated estrone and estradiol has been noted. This effect may also occur with amoxicillin and therefore AUGMENTIN.

Information for Patients

Patients should be counseled that antibacterial drugs including AUGMENTIN, should only be used to treat bacterial infections. They do not treat viral infections (e.g., the common cold). When AUGMENTIN is prescribed to treat a bacterial infection, patients should be told that although it is common to feel better early in the course of therapy, the medication should be taken exactly as directed. Skipping doses or not completing the full course of therapy may: (1) decrease the effectiveness of the immediate treatment, and (2) increase the likelihood that bacteria will develop resistance and will not be treatable by AUGMENTIN or other antibacterial drugs in the future.

Diarrhea is a common problem caused by antibiotics which usually ends when the antibiotic is discontinued. Sometimes after starting treatment with antibiotics, patients can develop watery and bloody stools (with or without stomach cramps and fever) even as late as two or more months after having taken the last dose of the antibiotic. If this occurs, patients should contact their physician as soon as possible.

Carcinogenesis, Mutagenesis, Impairment of Fertility

Long-term studies in animals have not been performed to evaluate carcinogenic potential.

Mutagenesis

The mutagenic potential of AUGMENTIN was investigated in vitro with an Ames test, a human lymphocyte cytogenetic assay, a yeast test and a mouse lymphoma forward mutation assay, and in vivo with mouse micronucleus tests and a dominant lethal test. All were negative apart from the in vitro mouse lymphoma assay where weak activity was found at very high, cytotoxic concentrations.

Impairment of Fertility

AUGMENTIN at oral doses of up to 1,200 mg/kg/day (5.7 times the maximum human dose, 1,480 mg/m²/day, based on body surface area) was found to have no effect on fertility and reproductive performance in rats, dosed with a 2:1 ratio formulation of amoxicillin:clavulanate.

Pregnancy

Teratogenic Effects

Pregnancy (Category B). Reproduction studies performed in pregnant rats and mice given AUGMENTIN at oral dosages up to 1,200 mg/kg/day, equivalent to 7,200 and 4,080 mg/m²/day, respectively (4.9 and 2.8 times the maximum human oral dose based on body surface area), revealed no evidence of harm to the fetus due to AUGMENTIN. There are, however, no adequate and well-controlled studies in pregnant women. Because animal reproduction studies are not always predictive of human response, this drug should be used during pregnancy only if clearly needed.

Labor and Delivery

Oral ampicillin-class antibiotics are generally poorly absorbed during labor. Studies in guinea pigs have shown that intravenous administration of ampicillin decreased the uterine tone, frequency of contractions, height of contractions, and duration of contractions; however, it is not known whether the use of AUGMENTIN in humans during labor or delivery has immediate or delayed adverse effects on the fetus, prolongs the duration of labor, or increases the likelihood that forceps delivery or other obstetrical intervention or resuscitation of the newborn will be necessary. In a single study in women with premature rupture of fetal membranes, it was reported that prophylactic treatment with AUGMENTIN may be associated with an increased risk of necrotizing enterocolitis in neonates.

Nursing Mothers

Ampicillin-class antibiotics are excreted in the milk; therefore, caution should be exercised when AUGMENTIN is administered to a nursing woman.

Pediatric Use

Pediatric patients weighing 40 kg or more should be dosed according to the adult recommendations (see DOSAGE AND ADMINISTRATION: Pediatric Patients). Safety and effectiveness of AUGMENTIN Tablets in pediatric patients weighing less than 40 kg have not been established. (See prescribing information for AUGMENTIN Powder for Oral Suspension and Chewable Tablets.)

Geriatric Use

An analysis of clinical studies of AUGMENTIN was conducted to determine whether subjects aged 65 and over respond differently from younger subjects. Of the 3,119 patients in this analysis, 68% were <65 years old, 32% were ≥65 years old and 14% were ≥75 years old. This analysis and other reported clinical experience have not identified differences in responses between the elderly and younger patients, but a greater sensitivity of some older individuals cannot be ruled out.

This drug is known to be substantially excreted by the kidney, and the risk of toxic reactions to this drug may be greater in patients with impaired renal function. Because elderly patients are more likely to have decreased renal function, care should be taken in dose selection, and it may be useful to monitor renal function.

ADVERSE REACTIONS

AUGMENTIN is generally well tolerated. The majority of side effects observed in clinical trials were of a mild and transient nature and less than 3% of patients discontinued therapy because of drug-related side effects. The most frequently reported adverse effects were diarrhea/loose stools (9%), nausea (3%), skin rashes and urticaria (3%), vomiting (1%) and vaginitis (1%). The overall incidence of side effects, and in particular diarrhea, increased with the higher recommended dose. Other less frequently reported reactions include: Abdominal discomfort, flatulence, and headache.

The following adverse reactions have been reported for ampicillin-class antibiotics:

Gastrointestinal

Diarrhea, nausea, vomiting, indigestion, gastritis, stomatitis, glossitis, black "hairy" tongue, mucocutaneous candidiasis, enterocolitis, and hemorrhagic/pseudomembranous colitis. Onset of pseudomembranous colitis symptoms may occur during or after antibiotic treatment. (See WARNINGS.)

Hypersensitivity Reactions

Skin rashes, pruritus, urticaria, angioedema, serum sickness–like reactions (urticaria or skin rash accompanied by arthritis, arthralgia, myalgia, and frequently fever), erythema multiforme (rarely Stevens-Johnson syndrome), acute generalized exanthematous pustulosis, hypersensitivity vasculitis, and an occasional case of exfoliative dermatitis (including toxic epidermal necrolysis) have been reported. These reactions may be controlled with antihistamines and, if necessary, systemic corticosteroids. Whenever such reactions occur, the drug should be discontinued, unless the opinion of the physician dictates otherwise. Serious and occasional fatal hypersensitivity (anaphylactic) reactions can occur with oral penicillin. (See WARNINGS.)

Liver

A moderate rise in AST (SGOT) and/or ALT (SGPT) has been noted in patients treated with ampicillin-class antibiotics but the significance of these findings is unknown. Hepatic dysfunction, including hepatitis and cholestatic jaundice, [see CONTRAINDICATIONS], increases in serum transaminases (AST and/or ALT), serum bilirubin, and/or alkaline phosphatase, has been infrequently reported with AUGMENTIN. It has been reported more commonly in the elderly, in males, or in patients on prolonged treatment. The histologic findings on liver biopsy have consisted of predominantly cholestatic, hepatocellular, or mixed cholestatic-hepatocellular changes. The onset of signs/symptoms of hepatic dysfunction may occur during or several weeks after therapy has been discontinued. The hepatic dysfunction, which may be severe, is usually reversible. On rare occasions, deaths have been reported (less than 1 death reported per estimated 4 million prescriptions worldwide). These have generally been cases associated with serious underlying diseases or concomitant medications.

Renal

Interstitial nephritis and hematuria have been reported rarely. Crystalluria has also been reported (see OVERDOSAGE).

Hemic and Lymphatic Systems

Anemia, including hemolytic anemia, thrombocytopenia, thrombocytopenic purpura, eosinophilia, leukopenia, and agranulocytosis have been reported during therapy with penicillins. These reactions are usually reversible on discontinuation of therapy and are believed to be hypersensitivity phenomena. A slight thrombocytosis was noted in less than 1% of the patients treated with AUGMENTIN. There have been reports of increased prothrombin time in patients receiving AUGMENTIN and anticoagulant therapy concomitantly.

Central Nervous System

Agitation, anxiety, behavioral changes, confusion, convulsions, dizziness, insomnia, and reversible hyperactivity have been reported rarely.

Miscellaneous

Tooth discoloration (brown, yellow, or gray staining) has been rarely reported. Most reports occurred in pediatric patients. Discoloration was reduced or eliminated with brushing or dental cleaning in most cases.

OVERDOSAGE

Following overdosage, patients have experienced primarily gastrointestinal symptoms including stomach and abdominal pain, vomiting, and diarrhea. Rash, hyperactivity, or drowsiness have also been observed in a small number of patients.

In the case of overdosage, discontinue AUGMENTIN, treat symptomatically, and institute supportive measures as required. If the overdosage is very recent and there is no contraindication, an attempt at emesis or other means of removal of drug from the stomach may be performed. A prospective study of 51 pediatric patients at a poison center suggested that overdosages of less than 250 mg/kg of amoxicillin are not associated with significant clinical symptoms and do not require gastric emptying.[3]

Interstitial nephritis resulting in oliguric renal failure has been reported in a small number of patients after overdosage with amoxicillin.

Crystalluria, in some cases leading to renal failure, has also been reported after amoxicillin overdosage in adult and pediatric patients. In case of overdosage, adequate fluid intake and diuresis should be maintained to reduce the risk of amoxicillin crystalluria.

Renal impairment appears to be reversible with cessation of drug administration. High blood levels may occur more readily in patients with impaired renal function because of decreased renal clearance of both amoxicillin and clavulanate. Both amoxicillin and clavulanate are removed from the circulation by hemodialysis. (See DOSAGE AND ADMINISTRATION for recommended dosing for patients with impaired renal function.)

DOSAGE AND ADMINISTRATION

Since both the 250-mg and 500-mg tablets of AUGMENTIN contain the same amount of clavulanic acid (125 mg, as the potassium salt), two 250-mg tablets of AUGMENTIN are not equivalent to one 500-mg tablet of AUGMENTIN; therefore, two 250-mg tablets of AUGMENTIN should not be substituted for one 500-mg tablet of AUGMENTIN.

Dosage
Adults

The usual adult dose is one 500-mg tablet of AUGMENTIN every 12 hours or one 250-mg tablet of AUGMENTIN every 8 hours. For more severe infections and infections of the respiratory tract, the dose should be one 875-mg tablet of AUGMENTIN every 12 hours or one 500-mg tablet of AUGMENTIN every 8 hours.

Patients with impaired renal function do not generally require a reduction in dose unless the impairment is severe. Severely impaired patients with a glomerular filtration rate of <30 mL/min. should not receive the 875-mg tablet. Patients with a glomerular filtration rate of 10 to 30 mL/min. should receive 500 mg or 250 mg every 12 hours, depending on the severity of the infection. Patients with a less than 10 mL/min. glomerular filtration rate should receive 500 mg or 250 mg every 24 hours, depending on severity of the infection.

Hemodialysis patients should receive 500 mg or 250 mg every 24 hours, depending on severity of the infection. They should receive an additional dose both during and at the end of dialysis.

Hepatically impaired patients should be dosed with caution and hepatic function monitored at regular intervals. (See WARNINGS.)

Pediatric Patients

Pediatric patients weighing 40 kg or more should be dosed according to the adult recommendations.

Due to the different amoxicillin to clavulanic acid ratios in the 250-mg tablet of AUGMENTIN (250/125) versus the 250-mg chewable tablet of AUGMENTIN (250/62.5), the 250-mg tablet of AUGMENTIN should not be used until the pediatric patient weighs at least 40 kg or more.

Administration

AUGMENTIN may be taken without regard to meals; however, absorption of clavulanate potassium is enhanced when AUGMENTIN is administered at the start of a meal. To minimize the potential for gastrointestinal intolerance, AUGMENTIN should be taken at the start of a meal.

HOW SUPPLIED

AUGMENTIN 250-mg Tablets

Each white oval filmcoated tablet, debossed with AUGMENTIN on 1 side and 250/125 on the other side, contains 250 mg amoxicillin as the trihydrate and 125 mg clavulanic acid as the potassium salt.
NDC 0029-6075-27   bottles of 30
NDC 0029-6075-31   Unit Dose (10×10) 100 tablets

AUGMENTIN 500-mg Tablets

Each white oval filmcoated tablet, debossed with AUGMENTIN on 1 side and 500/125 on the other side, contains 500 mg amoxicillin as the trihydrate and 125 mg clavulanic acid as the potassium salt.
NDC 0029-6080-12   bottles of 20
NDC 0029-6080-31   Unit Dose (10×10) 100 tablets

AUGMENTIN 875-mg Tablets

Each scored white capsule-shaped tablet, debossed with AUGMENTIN 875 on 1 side and scored on the other side, contains 875 mg amoxicillin as the trihydrate and 125 mg clavulanic acid as the potassium salt.
NDC 0029-6086-12   bottles of 20
NDC 0029-6086-21   Unit Dose (10×10) 100 tablets

AUGMENTIN is Also Supplied as:
AUGMENTIN 125 mg/5 mL (125 mg amoxicillin/31.25 mg clavulanic acid) For Oral Suspension:
NDC 0029-6085-39   75 mL bottle
NDC 0029-6085-23   100 mL bottle
NDC 0029-6085-22   150 mL bottle
AUGMENTIN 200 mg/5 mL (200 mg amoxicillin/28.5 mg clavulanic acid) For Oral Suspension:
NDC 0029-6087-29   50 mL bottle
NDC 0029-6087-39   75 mL bottle
NDC 0029-6087-51   100 mL bottle
AUGMENTIN 250 mg/5 mL (250 mg amoxicillin/62.5 mg clavulanic acid) For Oral Suspension:
NDC 0029-6090-39   75 mL bottle
NDC 0029-6090-23   100 mL bottle
NDC 0029-6090-22   150 mL bottle
AUGMENTIN 400 mg/5 mL (400 mg amoxicillin/57 mg clavulanic acid) For Oral Suspension:
NDC 0029-6092-29   50 mL bottle
NDC 0029-6092-39   75 mL bottle
NDC 0029-6092-51   100 mL bottle
AUGMENTIN 125 mg (125 mg amoxicillin/31.25 mg clavulanic acid) Chewable Tablets:
NDC 0029-6073-47   carton of 30 (5×6) tablets
AUGMENTIN 200 mg (200 mg amoxicillin/28.5 mg clavulanic acid) Chewable Tablets:
NDC 0029-6071-12   carton of 20 tablets
AUGMENTIN 250 mg (250 mg amoxicillin/62.5 mg clavulanic acid) Chewable Tablets:
NDC 0029-6074-47   carton of 30 (5×6) tablets
AUGMENTIN 400 mg (400 mg amoxicillin/57.0 mg clavulanic acid) Chewable Tablets:
NDC 0029-6072-12   carton of 20 tablets
Store tablets and dry powder at or below 25°C (77°F). Dispense in original container.

CLINICAL STUDIES

Data from 2 pivotal studies in 1,191 patients treated for either lower respiratory tract infections or complicated urinary tract infections compared a regimen of 875-mg tablets of AUGMENTIN every 12 hours to 500-mg tablets of AUGMENTIN dosed every 8 hours (584 and 607 patients, respectively). Comparable efficacy was demonstrated between the every 12 hours and every 8 hours dosing regimens. There was no significant difference in the percentage of adverse events in each group. The most frequently reported adverse event was diarrhea; incidence rates were similar for the 875-mg every 12 hours and 500-mg every 8 hours dosing regimens (14.9% and 14.3%, respectively); however, there was a statistically significant difference ($P < 0.05$) in rates of severe diarrhea or withdrawals with diarrhea between the regimens: 1.0% for 875-mg every 12 hours dosing versus 2.5% for the 500-mg every 8 hours dosing.

In 1 of these pivotal studies, 629 patients with either pyelonephritis or a complicated urinary tract infection (i.e., patients with abnormalities of the urinary tract that predispose to relapse of bacteriuria following eradication) were randomized to receive either 875-mg tablets of AUGMENTIN every 12 hours or 500-mg tablets of AUGMENTIN every 8 hours in the following distribution:

	875 mg q12h	500 mg q8h
Pyelonephritis	173 patients	188 patients
Complicated UTI	135 patients	133 patients
Total patients	308	321

The number of bacteriologically evaluable patients was comparable between the 2 dosing regimens. AUGMENTIN produced comparable bacteriological success rates in patients assessed 2 to 4 days immediately following end of therapy. The bacteriologic efficacy rates were comparable at 1 of the follow-up visits (5 to 9 days post-therapy) and at a late post-therapy visit (in the majority of cases, this was 2 to 4 weeks post-therapy), as seen in the table below:

	875 mg q12h	500 mg q8h
2 to 4 days	81%, n = 58	80%, n = 54
5 to 9 days	58.5%, n = 41	51.9%, n = 52
2 to 4 weeks	52.5%, n = 101	54.8%, n = 104

As noted before, though there was no significant difference in the percentage of adverse events in each group, there was a statistically significant difference in rates of severe diarrhea or withdrawals with diarrhea between the regimens.

REFERENCES

1. National Committee for Clinical Laboratory Standards. Methods for Dilution Antimicrobial Susceptibility Tests for Bacteria that Grow Aerobically - Third Edition. Approved Standard NCCLS Document M7-A3, Vol. 13, No. 25. NCCLS, Villanova, PA, December 1993.
2. National Committee for Clinical Laboratory Standards. Performance Standards for Antimicrobial Disk Susceptibility Tests - Fifth Edition. Approved Standard NCCLS Document M2-A5, Vol. 13, No. 24. NCCLS, Villanova, PA, December 1993.
3. Swanson-Biearman B, Dean BS, Lopez G, Krenzelok EP. The effects of penicillin and cephalosporin ingestions in children less than six years of age. *Vet Hum Toxicol.* 1988;30:66-67.

AUGMENTIN is a registered trademark of GlaxoSmithKline.
CLINITEST is a registered trademark of Miles, Inc.
CLINISTIX is a registered trademark of Bayer Corporation.
GlaxoSmithKline
Research Triangle Park, NC 27709
September 2009   AUT:17PI

AUGMENTIN ES-600®   ℞
[ăg-mint' in]
(amoxicillin/clavulanate potassium)
Powder for Oral Suspension

To reduce the development of drug-resistant bacteria and maintain the effectiveness of AUGMENTIN ES-600 (amoxicillin/clavulanate potassium) and other antibacterial drugs, AUGMENTIN ES-600 should be used only to treat or prevent infections that are proven or strongly suspected to be caused by bacteria.

DESCRIPTION

AUGMENTIN ES-600 is an oral antibacterial combination consisting of the semisynthetic antibiotic amoxicillin and the β-lactamase inhibitor, clavulanate potassium (the potassium salt of clavulanic acid). Amoxicillin is an analog of ampicillin, derived from the basic penicillin nucleus, 6-aminopenicillanic acid. The amoxicillin molecular formula is $C_{16}H_{19}N_3O_5S \bullet 3H_2O$, and the molecular weight is 419.46. Chemically, amoxicillin is $(2S,5R,6R)$-6-[(R)-(-)-2-Amino-2-(p-hydroxyphenyl)acetamido]-3,3-dimethyl-7-oxo-4-thia-1-azabicyclo[3.2.0]heptane-2-carboxylic acid trihydrate and may be represented structurally as:

Clavulanic acid is produced by the fermentation of *Streptomyces clavuligerus*. It is a β-lactam structurally related to the penicillins and possesses the ability to inactivate a wide variety of β-lactamases by blocking the active sites of these enzymes. Clavulanic acid is particularly active against the clinically important plasmid-mediated β-lactamases frequently responsible for transferred drug resistance to penicillins and cephalosporins. The clavulanate potassium molecular formula is $C_8H_8KNO_5$ and the molecular weight is 237.25. Chemically, clavulanate potassium is potassium (Z)-$(2R,5R)$-3-(2-hydroxyethylidene)-7-oxo-4-oxa-1-azabicyclo[3.2.0]-heptane-2-carboxylate and may be represented structurally as:

Inactive Ingredients
Powder for Oral Suspension—Colloidal silicon dioxide, strawberry cream flavor, xanthan gum, aspartame[a], sodium carboxymethylcellulose, and silicon dioxide.
[a] See PRECAUTIONS–Information for the Patient/Phenylketonurics.
Each 5 mL of reconstituted 600 mg/5 mL oral suspension of AUGMENTIN ES-600 contains 0.23 mEq potassium.

CLINICAL PHARMACOLOGY

The pharmacokinetics of amoxicillin and clavulanate were determined in a study of 19 pediatric patients, 8 months to 11 years, given AUGMENTIN ES-600 at an amoxicillin dose of 45 mg/kg every 12 hours with a snack or meal. The mean plasma amoxicillin and clavulanate pharmacokinetic parameter values are listed in Table 1.
[See table 1 at top of next page]

The effect of food on the oral absorption of AUGMENTIN ES-600 has not been studied.

Approximately 50% to 70% of the amoxicillin and approximately 25% to 40% of the clavulanic acid are excreted unchanged in urine during the first 6 hours after administration of 10 mL of 250 mg/5 mL suspension of AUGMENTIN. Concurrent administration of probenecid delays amoxicillin excretion but does not delay renal excretion of clavulanic acid.

Neither component in AUGMENTIN ES-600 is highly protein-bound; clavulanic acid has been found to be approximately 25% bound to human serum and amoxicillin approximately 18% bound.

Oral administration of a single dose of AUGMENTIN ES-600 at 45 mg/kg (based on the amoxicillin component) to pediatric patients, 9 months to 8 years, yielded the following pharmacokinetic data for amoxicillin in plasma and middle ear fluid (MEF) (Table 2).

[See table 2 at right]

Dose administered immediately prior to eating.

Amoxicillin diffuses readily into most body tissues and fluids with the exception of the brain and spinal fluid. The results of experiments involving the administration of clavulanic acid to animals suggest that this compound, like amoxicillin, is well distributed in body tissues.

Microbiology

Amoxicillin is a semisynthetic antibiotic with a broad spectrum of bactericidal activity against many gram-positive and gram-negative microorganisms. Amoxicillin is, however, susceptible to degradation by β-lactamases, and therefore, its spectrum of activity does not include organisms which produce these enzymes. Clavulanic acid is a β-lactam, structurally related to penicillin, which possesses the ability to inactivate a wide range of β-lactamase enzymes commonly found in microorganisms resistant to penicillins and cephalosporins. In particular, it has good activity against the clinically important plasmid-mediated β-lactamases frequently found responsible for transferred drug resistance.

The clavulanic acid component of AUGMENTIN ES-600 protects amoxicillin from degradation by β-lactamase enzymes and effectively extends the antibiotic spectrum of amoxicillin to include many bacteria normally resistant to amoxicillin and other β-lactam antibiotics. Thus, AUGMENTIN ES-600 possesses the distinctive properties of a broad-spectrum antibiotic and a β-lactamase inhibitor.

Amoxicillin/clavulanic acid has been shown to be active against most isolates of the following microorganisms, both in vitro and in clinical infections as described in the INDICATIONS AND USAGE section.

Aerobic Gram-Positive Microorganisms

Streptococcus pneumoniae (including isolates with penicillin MICs ≤ 2 mcg/mL)

Aerobic Gram-Negative Microorganisms

Haemophilus influenzae (including β-lactamase–producing isolates)

Moraxella catarrhalis (including β-lactamase–producing isolates)

The following in vitro data are available, **but their clinical significance is unknown.**

At least 90% of the following microorganisms exhibit in vitro minimum inhibitory concentrations (MICs) less than or equal to the susceptible breakpoint for amoxicillin/clavulanic acid. However, the safety and efficacy of amoxicillin/clavulanic acid in treating infections due to these microorganisms have not been established in adequate and well-controlled trials.

Aerobic Gram-Positive Microorganisms

Staphylococcus aureus (including β-lactamase–producing isolates)

NOTE: Staphylococci which are resistant to methicillin/oxacillin must be considered resistant to amoxicillin/clavulanic acid.

Streptococcus pyogenes

NOTE: S. pyogenes do not produce β-lactamase, and therefore, are susceptible to amoxicillin alone. Adequate and well-controlled clinical trials have established the effectiveness of amoxicillin alone in treating certain clinical infections due to S. pyogenes.

Susceptibility Test Methods

When available, the clinical microbiology laboratory should provide cumulative results of in vitro susceptibility test results for antimicrobial drugs used in local hospitals and practice areas to the physician as periodic reports that describe the susceptibility profile of nosocomial and community-acquired pathogens. These reports should aid the physician in selecting the most effective antimicrobial.

Dilution Technique

Quantitative methods are used to determine antimicrobial minimum inhibitory concentrations (MICs). These MICs provide estimates of the susceptibility of bacteria to antimicrobial compounds. The MICs should be determined using a standardized procedure.[1,2] Standardized procedures are based on dilution methods (broth for *S. pneumoniae* and *H.*

influenzae) or equivalent with standardized inoculum concentration and standardized concentrations of amoxicillin/clavulanate potassium powder.

The recommended dilution pattern utilizes a constant amoxicillin/clavulanate potassium ratio of 2 to 1 in all tubes with varying amounts of amoxicillin. MICs are expressed in terms of the amoxicillin concentration in the presence of clavulanic acid at a constant 2 parts amoxicillin to 1 part clavulanic acid. The MIC values should be interpreted according to criteria provided in Table 3.

Diffusion Technique

Quantitative methods that require measurement of zone diameters also provides reproducible estimates of the susceptibility of bacteria to antimicrobials. One such standardized technique requires the use of a standardized inoculum concentration.[2,3] This procedure uses paper disks impregnated with 30 mcg amoxicillin/clavulanate potassium (20 mcg amoxicillin plus 10 mcg clavulanate potassium) to test susceptibility of microorganisms to amoxicillin/clavulanate potassium. Disk diffusion zone sizes should be interpreted according to criteria provided in Table 3.

[See table 3 above]

NOTE: Susceptibility of *S. pneumoniae* should be determined using a 1-mcg oxacillin disk. Isolates with oxacillin zone sizes of ≥ 20 mm are susceptible to amoxicillin/clavulanic acid. An amoxicillin/clavulanic acid MIC should be determined on isolates of *S. pneumoniae* with oxacillin zone sizes of ≤ 19 mm.

NOTE: β-lactamase–negative, ampicillin-resistant *H. influenzae* isolates must be considered resistant to amoxicillin/clavulanic acid.

A report of S ("Susceptible") indicates that the antimicrobial is likely to inhibit growth of the pathogen if the antimicrobial compound in the blood reaches the concentration usually achievable. A report of I ("Intermediate") indicates that the result should be considered equivocal, and, if the microorganism is not fully susceptible to alternative, clinically feasible antimicrobials, the test should be repeated. This category implies possible clinical applicability in body sites where the drug is physiologically concentrated or in situations where high doses of antimicrobial can be used. This category also provides a buffer zone that prevents small uncontrolled technical factors from causing major discrepancies in interpretation. A report of R ("Resistant") indicates that the antimicrobial is not likely to inhibit growth of the pathogen if the antimicrobial compound in the blood reaches the concentration usually achievable; other therapy should be selected.

Standardized susceptibility test procedures require the use of quality control microorganisms to determine the performance of the test procedures.[1-3] Standard amoxicillin/clavulanate potassium powder should provide the MIC ranges for the quality control organisms in Table 4. For the disk diffusion technique, the 30 mcg-amoxicillin/clavulanate potassium disk should provide the zone diameter ranges for the quality control organisms in Table 4.

[See table 4 at top of next page]

INDICATIONS AND USAGE

AUGMENTIN ES-600 is indicated for the treatment of pediatric patients with recurrent or persistent acute otitis media due to *S. pneumoniae* (penicillin MICs ≤ 2 mcg/mL), *H. influenzae* (including β-lactamase–producing strains), or *M. catarrhalis* (including β-lactamase–producing strains) characterized by the following risk factors:

- antibiotic exposure for acute otitis media within the preceding 3 months, and either of the following:
  - age ≤ 2 years
  - daycare attendance

[See CLINICAL PHARMACOLOGY, Microbiology.]

NOTE: Acute otitis media due to *S. pneumoniae* alone can be treated with amoxicillin. AUGMENTIN ES-600 is not indicated for the treatment of acute otitis media due to *S. pneumoniae* with penicillin MIC ≥ 4 mcg/mL.

Therapy may be instituted prior to obtaining the results from bacteriological studies when there is reason to believe the infection may involve both *S. pneumoniae* (penicillin MIC ≤ 2 mcg/mL) and the β-lactamase–producing organisms listed above.

Table 1. Mean (±SD) Plasma Amoxicillin and Clavulanate Pharmacokinetic Parameter Values Following Administration of 45 mg/kg of AUGMENTIN ES-600 Every 12 Hours to Pediatric Patients

Parameter[a]	Amoxicillin	Clavulanate
C_{max} (mcg/mL)	15.7 ± 7.7	1.7 ± 0.9
T_{max} (hr)	2.0 (1.0–4.0)	1.1 (1.0–4.0)
AUC_{0-t} (mcg•hr/mL)	59.8 ± 20.0	4.0 ± 1.9
$T_{1/2}$ (hr)	1.4 ± 0.3	1.1 ± 0.3
CL/F (L/hr/kg)	0.9 ± 0.4	1.1 ± 1.1

[a] Arithmetic mean ± standard deviation, except T_{max} values which are medians (ranges).

Table 2. Amoxicillin Concentrations in Plasma and Middle Ear Fluid Following Administration of 45 mg/kg of AUGMENTIN ES-600 to Pediatric Patients

Timepoint		Amoxicillin concentration in plasma (mcg/mL)	Amoxicillin concentration in MEF (mcg/mL)
1 hour	Mean	7.7	3.2
	Median	9.3	3.5
	range	1.5–14.0	0.2–5.5
		(n = 5)	(n = 4)
2 hour	mean	15.7	3.3
	median	13.0	2.4
	range	11.0–25.0	1.9–6
		(n = 7)	(n = 5)
3 hour	mean	13.0	5.8
	median	12.0	6.5
	range	5.5–21.0	3.9–7.4
		(n = 5)	(n = 5)

Table 3. Susceptibility Test Result Interpretive Criteria for Amoxicillin/Clavulanate Potassium

Pathogen	Minimum Inhibitory Concentration (mcg/mL)			Disk Diffusion (Zone Diameter in mm)		
	S	I	R	S	I	R
Streptococcus pneumoniae	≤ 2/1	4/2	≥ 8/4	Not applicable (NA)		
Haemophilus influenzae	≤ 4/2	NA	≥ 8/4	≥ 20	NA	≤ 19

Table 4. Acceptable Quality Control Ranges for Amoxicillin/Clavulanate Potassium

Quality Control Organism	Minimum Inhibitory Concentration Range (mcg/mL)	Disk Diffusion (Zone Diameter Range in mm)
Escherichia coli ATCC®[a] 35218[b] (*H. influenzae* quality control)	4/2 to 16/8	17 to 22
Haemophilus influenzae ATCC 49247	2/1 to 16/8	15 to 23
Streptococcus pneumoniae ATCC 49619	0.03/0.016 to 0.12/0.06	NA

[a] ATCC is a trademark of the American Type Culture Collection.
[b] When using *Haemophilus* Test Medium (HTM).

To reduce the development of drug-resistant bacteria and maintain the effectiveness of AUGMENTIN ES-600 and other antibacterial drugs, AUGMENTIN ES-600 should be used only to treat or prevent infections that are proven or strongly suspected to be caused by susceptible bacteria. When culture and susceptibility information are available, they should be considered in selecting or modifying antibacterial therapy. In the absence of such data, local epidemiology and susceptibility patterns may contribute to the empiric selection of therapy.

CONTRAINDICATIONS

AUGMENTIN ES-600 is contraindicated in patients with a history of allergic reactions to any penicillin. It is also contraindicated in patients with a previous history of cholestatic jaundice/hepatic dysfunction associated with AUGMENTIN.

WARNINGS

SERIOUS AND OCCASIONALLY FATAL HYPERSENSITIVITY (ANAPHYLACTIC) REACTIONS HAVE BEEN REPORTED IN PATIENTS ON PENICILLIN THERAPY. THESE REACTIONS ARE MORE LIKELY TO OCCUR IN INDIVIDUALS WITH A HISTORY OF PENICILLIN HYPERSENSITIVITY AND/OR A HISTORY OF SENSITIVITY TO MULTIPLE ALLERGENS. THERE HAVE BEEN REPORTS OF INDIVIDUALS WITH A HISTORY OF PENICILLIN HYPERSENSITIVITY WHO HAVE EXPERIENCED SEVERE REACTIONS WHEN TREATED WITH CEPHALOSPORINS. BEFORE INITIATING THERAPY WITH AUGMENTIN ES-600, CAREFUL INQUIRY SHOULD BE MADE CONCERNING PREVIOUS HYPERSENSITIVITY REACTIONS TO PENICILLINS, CEPHALOSPORINS, OR OTHER ALLERGENS. IF AN ALLERGIC REACTION OCCURS, AUGMENTIN ES-600 SHOULD BE DISCONTINUED AND THE APPROPRIATE THERAPY INSTITUTED. **SERIOUS ANAPHYLACTIC REACTIONS REQUIRE IMMEDIATE EMERGENCY TREATMENT WITH EPINEPHRINE. OXYGEN, INTRAVENOUS STEROIDS, AND AIRWAY MANAGEMENT, INCLUDING INTUBATION, SHOULD ALSO BE ADMINISTERED AS INDICATED.**

Clostridium difficile associated diarrhea (CDAD) has been reported with use of nearly all antibacterial agents, including AUGMENTIN ES-600, and may range in severity from mild diarrhea to fatal colitis. Treatment with antibacterial agents alters the normal flora of the colon leading to overgrowth of *C. difficile*.

C. difficile produces toxins A and B which contribute to the development of CDAD. Hypertoxin producing strains of *C. difficile* cause increased morbidity and mortality, as these infections can be refractory to antimicrobial therapy and may require colectomy. CDAD must be considered in all patients who present with diarrhea following antibiotic use. Careful medical history is necessary since CDAD has been reported to occur over two months after the administration of antibacterial agents.

If CDAD is suspected or confirmed, ongoing antibiotic use not directed against *C. difficile* may need to be discontinued. Appropriate fluid and electrolyte management, protein supplementation, antibiotic treatment of *C. difficile*, and surgical evaluation should be instituted as clinically indicated.

AUGMENTIN ES-600 should be used with caution in patients with evidence of hepatic dysfunction. Hepatic toxicity associated with the use of amoxicillin/clavulanate potassium is usually reversible. On rare occasions, deaths have been reported (less than 1 death reported per estimated 4 million prescriptions worldwide). These have generally been cases associated with serious underlying diseases or concomitant medications. (See CONTRAINDICATIONS and ADVERSE REACTIONS—Liver.)

PRECAUTIONS

General

While amoxicillin/clavulanate possesses the characteristic low toxicity of the penicillin group of antibiotics, periodic assessment of organ system functions, including renal, hepatic, and hematopoietic function, is advisable if therapy is for longer than the drug is approved for administration.

A high percentage of patients with mononucleosis who receive ampicillin develop an erythematous skin rash. Thus, ampicillin-class antibiotics should not be administered to patients with mononucleosis.

The possibility of superinfections with mycotic or bacterial pathogens should be kept in mind during therapy. If superinfections occur (usually involving *Pseudomonas* or *Candida*), the drug should be discontinued and/or appropriate therapy instituted.

Prescribing AUGMENTIN ES-600 in the absence of a proven or strongly suspected bacterial infection or a prophylactic indication is unlikely to provide benefit to the patient and increases the risk of the development of drug-resistant bacteria.

Information for the Patient

AUGMENTIN ES-600 should be taken every 12 hours with a meal or snack to reduce the possibility of gastrointestinal upset. If diarrhea develops and is severe or lasts more than 2 or 3 days, call your doctor.

Diarrhea is a common problem caused by antibiotics which usually ends when the antibiotic is discontinued. Sometimes after starting treatment with antibiotics, patients can develop watery and bloody stools (with or without stomach cramps and fever) even as late as 2 or more months after having taken the last dose of the antibiotic. If this occurs, patients should contact their physician as soon as possible.

Keep suspension refrigerated. Shake well before using. When dosing a child with the suspension (liquid) of AUGMENTIN ES-600, use a dosing spoon or medicine dropper. Be sure to rinse the spoon or dropper after each use. Bottles of suspension of AUGMENTIN ES-600 may contain more liquid than required. Follow your doctor's instructions about the amount to use and the days of treatment your child requires. Discard any unused medicine.

Patients should be counseled that antibacterial drugs, including AUGMENTIN ES-600, should only be used to treat bacterial infections. They do not treat viral infections (e.g., the common cold). When AUGMENTIN ES-600 is prescribed to treat a bacterial infection, patients should be told that although it is common to feel better early in the course of therapy, the medication should be taken exactly as directed. Skipping doses or not completing the full course of therapy may: (1) decrease the effectiveness of the immediate treatment, and (2) increase the likelihood that bacteria will develop resistance and will not be treatable by AUGMENTIN ES-600 or other antibacterial drugs in the future.

Phenylketonurics

Each 5 mL of the 600 mg/5 mL suspension of AUGMENTIN ES-600 contains 7 mg phenylalanine.

Drug Interactions

Probenecid decreases the renal tubular secretion of amoxicillin. Concurrent use with AUGMENTIN ES-600 may result in increased and prolonged blood levels of amoxicillin. Co-administration of probenecid cannot be recommended.

Abnormal prolongation of prothrombin time (increased international normalized ratio [INR]) has been reported rarely in patients receiving amoxicillin and oral anticoagulants. Appropriate monitoring should be undertaken when anticoagulants are prescribed concurrently. Adjustments in the dose of oral anticoagulants may be necessary to maintain the desired level of anticoagulation.

The concurrent administration of allopurinol and ampicillin increases substantially the incidence of rashes in patients receiving both drugs as compared to patients receiving ampicillin alone. It is not known whether this potentiation of ampicillin rashes is due to allopurinol or the hyperuricemia present in these patients. There are no data with AUGMENTIN ES-600 and allopurinol administered concurrently.

In common with other broad-spectrum antibiotics, amoxicillin/clavulanate may reduce the efficacy of oral contraceptives.

Drug/Laboratory Test Interactions

Oral administration of AUGMENTIN will result in high urine concentrations of amoxicillin. High urine concentrations of ampicillin may result in false-positive reactions when testing for the presence of glucose in urine using CLINITEST®, Benedict's Solution, or Fehling's Solution. Since this effect may also occur with amoxicillin and therefore AUGMENTIN ES-600, it is recommended that glucose tests based on enzymatic glucose oxidase reactions (such as CLINISTIX®) be used.

Following administration of ampicillin to pregnant women, a transient decrease in plasma concentration of total conjugated estriol, estriol-glucuronide, conjugated estrone, and estradiol has been noted. This effect may also occur with amoxicillin and therefore AUGMENTIN ES-600.

Carcinogenesis, Mutagenesis, Impairment of Fertility

Long-term studies in animals have not been performed to evaluate carcinogenic potential. The mutagenic potential of AUGMENTIN was investigated in vitro with an Ames test, a human lymphocyte cytogenetic assay, a yeast test, and a mouse lymphoma forward mutation assay, and in vivo with mouse micronucleus tests and a dominant lethal test. All were negative apart from the in vitro mouse lymphoma assay where weak activity was found at very high, cytotoxic concentrations. AUGMENTIN at oral doses of up to 1,200 mg/kg/day (5.7 times the maximum adult human dose based on body surface area) was found to have no effect on fertility and reproductive performance in rats, dosed with a 2:1 ratio formulation of amoxicillin:clavulanate.

Pregnancy

Teratogenic Effects

Pregnancy (Category B). Reproduction studies performed in pregnant rats and mice given AUGMENTIN at oral dosages up to 1,200 mg/kg/day (4.9 and 2.8 times the maximum adult human oral dose based on body surface area, respectively), revealed no evidence of harm to the fetus due to AUGMENTIN. There are, however, no adequate and well-controlled studies in pregnant women. Because animal reproduction studies are not always predictive of human response, this drug should be used during pregnancy only if clearly needed.

Labor and Delivery

Oral ampicillin-class antibiotics are generally poorly absorbed during labor. Studies in guinea pigs have shown that intravenous administration of ampicillin decreased the uterine tone, frequency of contractions, height of contractions, and duration of contractions. However, it is not known whether the use of AUGMENTIN in humans during labor or delivery has immediate or delayed adverse effects on the fetus, prolongs the duration of labor, or increases the likelihood that forceps delivery or other obstetrical intervention or resuscitation of the newborn will be necessary. In a single study in women with premature rupture of fetal membranes, it was reported that prophylactic treatment with AUGMENTIN may be associated with an increased risk of necrotizing enterocolitis in neonates.

Nursing Mothers

Ampicillin-class antibiotics are excreted in human milk; therefore, caution should be exercised when AUGMENTIN is administered to a nursing woman.

Pediatric Use

Safety and efficacy of AUGMENTIN ES-600 in infants younger than 3 months have not been established. Safety and efficacy of AUGMENTIN ES-600 have been demonstrated for treatment of acute otitis media in infants and children 3 months to 12 years (see Description of Clinical Studies).

The safety and effectiveness of AUGMENTIN ES–600 have been established for the treatment of pediatric patients (3 months to 12 years) with acute bacterial sinusitis. This use is supported by evidence from adequate and well-controlled studies of AUGMENTIN XR™ Extended Release Tablets in adults with acute bacterial sinusitis, studies of AUGMENTIN ES-600 in pediatric patients with acute otitis media, and by similar pharmacokinetics of amoxicillin and clavulanate in pediatric patients taking AUGMENTIN ES-600 (see CLINICAL PHARMACOLOGY) and adults taking AUGMENTIN XR.

ADVERSE REACTIONS

AUGMENTIN ES-600 is generally well tolerated. The majority of side effects observed in pediatric clinical trials of acute otitis media were either mild or moderate, and transient in nature; 4.4% of patients discontinued therapy because of drug-related side effects. The most commonly reported side effects with probable or suspected relationship to AUGMENTIN ES-600 were contact dermatitis, i.e., diaper rash (3.5%), diarrhea (2.9%), vomiting (2.2%), moniliasis (1.4%), and rash (1.1%). The most common adverse experiences leading to withdrawal that were of probable or suspected relationship to AUGMENTIN ES-600 were diarrhea (2.5%) and vomiting (1.4%).

The following adverse reactions have been reported for ampicillin-class antibiotics:

Gastrointestinal

Diarrhea, nausea, vomiting, indigestion, gastritis, stomatitis, glossitis, black "hairy" tongue, mucocutaneous candidiasis, enterocolitis, and hemorrhagic/pseudomembranous colitis. Onset of pseudomembranous colitis symptoms may occur during or after antibiotic treatment. (See WARNINGS.)

Hypersensitivity Reactions

Skin rashes, pruritus, urticaria, angioedema, serum sickness–like reactions (urticaria or skin rash accompanied by arthritis, arthralgia, myalgia, and frequently fever), erythema multiforme (rarely Stevens-Johnson syndrome), acute generalized exanthematous pustulosis, hypersensitivity vasculitis, and an occasional case of exfoliative dermatitis (including toxic epidermal necrolysis) have been reported. These reactions may be controlled with antihistamines and, if necessary, systemic corticosteroids. Whenever such reactions occur, the drug should be discontinued, unless the opinion of the physician dictates otherwise. Serious and occasional fatal hypersensitivity (anaphylactic) reactions can occur with oral penicillin. (See WARNINGS.)

Liver

A moderate rise in AST (SGOT) and/or ALT (SGPT) has been noted in patients treated with ampicillin-class antibiotics, but the significance of these findings is unknown. Hepatic dysfunction, including hepatitis and cholestatic jaundice, (See CONTRAINDICATIONS.) increases in serum transaminases (AST and/or ALT), serum bilirubin, and/or alkaline phosphatase, has been infrequently reported with AUGMENTIN. It has been reported more commonly in the elderly, in males, or in patients on prolonged treatment. The histologic findings on liver biopsy have consisted of predominantly cholestatic, hepatocellular, or mixed cholestatic-hepatocellular changes. The onset of signs/symptoms of hepatic dysfunction may occur during or several weeks after therapy has been discontinued. The hepatic dysfunction, which may be severe, is usually reversible. On rare occasions, deaths have been reported (less than 1 death reported per estimated 4 million prescriptions worldwide). These have generally been cases associated with serious underlying diseases or concomitant medications.

Renal

Interstitial nephritis and hematuria have been reported rarely. Crystalluria has also been reported (see OVERDOSAGE).

Hemic and Lymphatic Systems

Anemia, including hemolytic anemia, thrombocytopenia, thrombocytopenic purpura, eosinophilia, leukopenia, and agranulocytosis have been reported during therapy with penicillins. These reactions are usually reversible on discontinuation of therapy and are believed to be hypersensitivity phenomena. A slight thrombocytosis was noted in less than 1% of the patients treated with AUGMENTIN. There have been reports of increased prothrombin time in patients receiving AUGMENTIN and anticoagulant therapy concomitantly.

Central Nervous System

Agitation, anxiety, behavioral changes, confusion, convulsions, dizziness, insomnia, and reversible hyperactivity have been reported rarely.

Miscellaneous

Tooth discoloration (brown, yellow, or gray staining) has been rarely reported. Most reports occurred in pediatric patients. Discoloration was reduced or eliminated with brushing or dental cleaning in most cases.

OVERDOSAGE

Following overdosage, patients have experienced primarily gastrointestinal symptoms including stomach and abdominal pain, vomiting, and diarrhea. Rash, hyperactivity, or drowsiness have also been observed in a small number of patients.

In the case of overdosage, discontinue AUGMENTIN ES-600, treat symptomatically, and institute supportive measures as required. If the overdosage is very recent and there is no contraindication, an attempt at emesis or other means of removal of drug from the stomach may be performed. A prospective study of 51 pediatric patients at a poison control center suggested that overdosages of less than 250 mg/kg of amoxicillin are not associated with significant clinical symptoms and do not require gastric emptying.[4]

Interstitial nephritis resulting in oliguric renal failure has been reported in a small number of patients after overdosage with amoxicillin.

Crystalluria, in some cases leading to renal failure, has also been reported after amoxicillin overdosage in adult and pediatric patients. In case of overdosage, adequate fluid intake and diuresis should be maintained to reduce the risk of amoxicillin crystalluria.

Renal impairment appears to be reversible with cessation of drug administration. High blood levels may occur more readily in patients with impaired renal function because of decreased renal clearance of both amoxicillin and clavulanate. Both amoxicillin and clavulanate are removed from the circulation by hemodialysis.

Table 5. Bacteriologic Eradication Rates in the Per Protocol Population

Pathogen	Bacteriologic Eradication on Therapy		
	n/N	%	95% CI[a]
All *S. pneumoniae*	121/123	98.4	(94.3, 99.8)
S. pneumoniae with penicillin MIC = 2 mcg/mL	19/19	100	(82.4, 100.0)
S. pneumoniae with penicillin MIC = 4 mcg/mL	12/14	85.7	(57.2, 98.2)
H. influenzae	75/81	92.6	(84.6, 97.2)
M. catarrhalis	11/11	100	(71.5, 100.0)

[a] CI = confidence intervals; 95% CIs are not adjusted for multiple comparisons.

DOSAGE AND ADMINISTRATION

AUGMENTIN ES-600, 600 mg/5 mL, does not contain the same amount of clavulanic acid (as the potassium salt) as any of the other suspensions of AUGMENTIN. AUGMENTIN ES-600 contains 42.9 mg of clavulanic acid per 5 mL, whereas the 200 mg/5 mL suspension of AUGMENTIN contains 28.5 mg of clavulanic acid per 5 mL and the 400 mg/5 mL suspension contains 57 mg of clavulanic acid per 5 mL. Therefore, the 200 mg/5 mL and 400 mg/5 mL suspensions of AUGMENTIN should *not* be substituted for AUGMENTIN ES-600, as they are not interchangeable.

Dosage

Pediatric patients 3 months and older

Based on the amoxicillin component (600 mg/5 mL), the recommended dose of AUGMENTIN ES-600 is 90 mg/kg/day divided every 12 hours, administered for 10 days (see chart below).

Body Weight (kg)	Volume of AUGMENTIN ES-600 providing 90 mg/kg/day
8	3.0 mL twice daily
12	4.5 mL twice daily
16	6.0 mL twice daily
20	7.5 mL twice daily
24	9.0 mL twice daily
28	10.5 mL twice daily
32	12.0 mL twice daily
36	13.5 mL twice daily

Pediatric patients weighing 40 kg and more

Experience with AUGMENTIN ES-600 (600 mg/5 mL formulation) in this group is not available.

Adults

Experience with AUGMENTIN ES-600 (600 mg/5 mL formulation) in adults is not available and adults who have difficulty swallowing should not be given AUGMENTIN ES-600 (600 mg/5 mL) in place of the 500-mg or 875-mg tablet of AUGMENTIN.

Hepatically impaired patients should be dosed with caution and hepatic function monitored at regular intervals. (See WARNINGS.)

Directions for Mixing Oral Suspension

Prepare a suspension at time of dispensing as follows: Tap bottle until all the powder flows freely. Add approximately 2/3 of the total amount of water for reconstitution (see table below) and shake vigorously to suspend powder. Add remainder of the water and again shake vigorously.

AUGMENTIN ES-600 (600 mg/5 mL Suspension)

Bottle Size	Amount of Water Required for Reconstitution
75 mL	70 mL
125 mL	110 mL
200 mL	180 mL

Each teaspoonful (5 mL) will contain 600 mg amoxicillin as the trihydrate and 42.9 mg of clavulanic acid as the potassium salt.

NOTE: SHAKE ORAL SUSPENSION WELL BEFORE USING.

Information for the Pharmacist

For patients who wish to alter the taste of AUGMENTIN ES-600, immediately after reconstitution 1 drop of FLAVORx™ (apple, banana cream, bubble gum, cherry, or watermelon flavor) may be added for every 5 mL of AUGMENTIN ES-600. The resulting suspension is stable for 10 days under refrigeration. Other than the 5 flavors listed above, GlaxoSmithKline has not evaluated the stability of AUGMENTIN ES-600 when mixed with other flavors distributed by FLAVORx.

Administration

To minimize the potential for gastrointestinal intolerance, AUGMENTIN ES-600 should be taken at the start of a meal. Absorption of clavulanate potassium may be enhanced when AUGMENTIN ES-600 is administered at the start of a meal.

HOW SUPPLIED

AUGMENTIN ES-600, 600 mg/5 mL, for Oral Suspension

Each 5 mL of reconstituted strawberry cream-flavored suspension contains 600 mg amoxicillin and 42.9 mg clavulanic acid as the potassium salt.

NDC 0029-6094-40	75 mL bottle
NDC 0029-6094-46	125 mL bottle
NDC 0029-6094-25	200 mL bottle

STORAGE

Store reconstituted suspension under refrigeration. Discard unused suspension after 10 days. Store dry powder for oral suspension at or below 25°C (77°F). Dispense in original container.

DESCRIPTION OF CLINICAL STUDIES

Two clinical studies were conducted in pediatric patients with acute otitis media.

A non-comparative, open-label study assessed the bacteriologic and clinical efficacy of AUGMENTIN ES-600 (90/6.4 mg/kg/day, divided every 12 hours) for 10 days in 521 pediatric patients (3 to 50 months) with acute otitis media. The primary objective was to assess bacteriological response in children with acute otitis media due to *S. pneumoniae* with amoxicillin/clavulanic acid MICs of 4 mcg/mL. The study sought the enrollment of patients with the following risk factors: Failure of antibiotic therapy for acute otitis media in the previous 3 months, history of recurrent episodes of acute otitis media, ≤ 2 years, or daycare attendance. Prior to receiving AUGMENTIN ES-600, all patients had tympanocentesis to obtain middle ear fluid for bacteriological evaluation. Patients from whom *S. pneumoniae* (alone or in combination with other bacteria) was isolated had a second tympanocentesis 4 to 6 days after the start of therapy. Clinical assessments were planned for all patients during treatment (4-6 days after starting therapy), as well as 2-4 days post-treatment and 15-18 days post-treatment. Bacteriological success was defined as the absence of the pretreatment pathogen from the on-therapy tympanocentesis specimen. Clinical success was defined as improvement or resolution of signs and symptoms. Clinical failure was defined as lack of improvement or worsening of signs and/or symptoms at any time following at least 72 hours of AUGMENTIN ES-600 (amoxicillin/clavulanate potassium); patients who received an additional systemic antibacterial drug for otitis media after 3 days of therapy were considered clinical failures. Bacteriological eradication on therapy (day 4-6 visit) in the per protocol population is summarized in Table 5.

[See table 5 above]

Clinical assessments were made in the per protocol population 2-4 days post-therapy and 15-18 days post-therapy. Patients who responded to therapy 2-4 days post-therapy were followed for 15-18 days post-therapy to assess them for acute otitis media. Nonresponders at 2-4 days post-therapy were considered failures at the latter timepoint.

Table 6. Clinical Assessments in the Per Protocol Population (Includes *S. pneumoniae* Patients With Penicillin MICs = 2 or 4 mcg/mL[a])

Pathogen	2-4 Days Post-Therapy (Primary Endpoint)		
	n/N	%	95% CI[b]
All *S. pneumoniae*	122/137	89.1	(82.6, 93.7)
S. pneumoniae with penicillin MIC = 2 mcg/mL	17/20	85.0	(62.1, 96.8)
S. pneumoniae with penicillin MIC = 4 mcg/mL	11/14	78.6	(49.2, 95.3)
H. influenzae	141/162	87.0	(80.9, 91.8)
M. catarrhalis	22/26	84.6	(65.1, 95.6)
	15-18 Days Post-Therapy[c] (Secondary Endpoint)		
	N/N	%	95% CI[†]
All *S. pneumoniae*	95/136	69.9	(61.4, 77.4)
S. pneumoniae with penicillin MIC = 2 mcg/mL	11/20	55.0	(31.5, 76.9)
S. pneumoniae with penicillin MIC = 4 mcg/mL	5/14	35.7	(12.8, 64.9)
H. influenzae	106/156	67.9	(60.0, 75.2)
M. catarrhalis	14/25	56.0	(34.9, 75.6)

[a] *S. pneumoniae* strains with penicillin MICs of 2 or 4 mcg/mL are considered resistant to penicillin.
[b] CI = confidence intervals; 95% CIs are not adjusted for multiple comparisons.
[c] Clinical assessments at 15-18 days post-therapy may have been confounded by viral infections and new episodes of acute otitis media with time elapsed post-treatment.

[See table above]
In the intent-to-treat analysis, overall clinical outcomes at 2-4 days and 15-18 days post-treatment in patients with *S. pneumoniae* with penicillin MIC = 2 mcg/mL and 4 mcg/mL were 29/41 (71%) and 17/41 (41.5%), respectively.
In the intent-to-treat population of 521 patients, the most frequently reported adverse events were vomiting (6.9%), fever (6.1%), contact dermatitis (i.e., diaper rash) (6.1%), upper respiratory tract infection (4.0%), and diarrhea (3.8%). Protocol-defined diarrhea (i.e., 3 or more watery stools in one day or 2 watery stools per day for 2 consecutive days as recorded on diary cards) occurred in 12.9% of patients.
A double-blind, randomized, clinical study compared AUGMENTIN ES-600 (90/6.4 mg/kg/day, divided every 12 hours) to AUGMENTIN (45/6.4 mg/kg/day, divided every 12 hours) for 10 days in 450 pediatric patients (3 months to 12 years) with acute otitis media. The primary objective of the study was to compare the safety of AUGMENTIN ES-600 to AUGMENTIN. There was no statistically significant difference between treatments in the proportion of patients with 1 or more adverse events. The most frequently reported adverse events for AUGMENTIN ES-600 and the comparator of AUGMENTIN were coughing (11.9% versus 6.8%), vomiting (6.5% versus 7.7%), contact dermatitis (i.e., diaper rash, 6.0% versus 4.8%), fever (5.5% versus 3.9%), and upper respiratory infection (3.0% versus 9.2%), respectively. The frequencies of protocol-defined diarrhea with AUGMENTIN ES-600 (11.1%) and AUGMENTIN (9.4%) were similar (95% confidence interval on difference: -4.2% to 7.7%). Only 2 patients in the group treated with AUGMENTIN ES-600 and 1 patient in the group treated with AUGMENTIN were withdrawn due to diarrhea.

REFERENCES

1. National Committee for Clinical Laboratory Standards. Methods for Dilution Antimicrobial Susceptibility Tests for Bacteria That Grow Aerobically – Sixth Edition; Approved Standard, NCCLS Document M7-A6, Vol. 23, No. 2, NCCLS, Wayne, PA, January 2003.
2. National Committee for Clinical Laboratory Standards for Antimicrobial Susceptibility Testing: Fourteenth Informational Supplement; Approved Standard, NCCLS Document 100-S14, Vol. 24, No. 1, NCCLS, Wayne, PA, January 2004.
3. National Committee for Clinical Laboratory Standards. Performance Standards for Antimicrobial Disk Susceptibility Tests – Eighth Edition; Approved Standard, NCCLS Document M2-A8, Vol. 23, No. 1, NCCLS, Wayne, PA, January 2003.
4. Swanson-Biearman B, Dean BS, Lopez G, Krenzelok EP. The effects of penicillin and cephalosporin ingestions in children less than six years of age. *Vet Hum Toxicol.* 1988;30:66-67.

AUGMENTIN ES-600 is a registered trademark of GlaxoSmithKline.
AUGMENTIN XR is a trademark of GlaxoSmithKline.
CLINITEST is a registered trademark of Miles, Inc.
CLINISTIX is a registered trademark of Bayer Corporation.
FLAVORx is a trademark of FLAVORx, Inc.
GlaxoSmithKline
Research Triangle Park, NC 27709
©2009, GlaxoSmithKline. All rights reserved.
September 2009   AUE:14PI

AUGMENTIN XR®   ℞

[äg-mint' in]
(amoxicillin/clavulanate potassium)
Extended Release Tablets

To reduce the development of drug-resistant bacteria and maintain the effectiveness of AUGMENTIN XR (amoxicillin/clavulanate potassium) and other antibacterial drugs, AUGMENTIN XR should be used only to treat or prevent infections that are proven or strongly suspected to be caused by bacteria.

DESCRIPTION

AUGMENTIN XR is an oral antibacterial combination consisting of the semisynthetic antibiotic amoxicillin (present as amoxicillin trihydrate and amoxicillin sodium) and the β-lactamase inhibitor clavulanate potassium (the potassium salt of clavulanic acid). Amoxicillin is an analog of ampicillin, derived from the basic penicillin nucleus 6-aminopenicillanic acid. The amoxicillin trihydrate molecular formula is $C_{16}H_{19}N_3O_5S \cdot 3H_2O$, and the molecular weight is 419.45. Chemically, amoxicillin trihydrate is (2*S*,5*R*,6*R*)-6-[(*R*)-(-)-2-Amino-2-(*p*-hydroxyphenyl)acetamido]-3,3-dimethyl-7-oxo-4-thia-1-azabicyclo[3.2.0]heptane-2-carboxylic acid trihydrate and may be represented structurally as:

The amoxicillin sodium molecular formula is $C_{16}H_{18}N_3NaO_5S$, and the molecular weight is 387.39. Chemically, amoxicillin sodium is [2*S*-[2α,5α,6β(*S**)]]-6-[[Amino(4-hydroxyphenyl)acetyl]amino]-3,3-dimethyl-7-oxo-4-thia-1-azabicyclo[3.2.0]heptane-2-carboxylic acid monosodium salt and may be represented structurally as:

Clavulanic acid is produced by the fermentation of *Streptomyces clavuligerus*. It is a β-lactam structurally related to the penicillins and possesses the ability to inactivate a wide variety of β-lactamases by blocking the active sites of these enzymes. Clavulanic acid is particularly active against the clinically important plasmid-mediated β-lactamases frequently responsible for transferred drug resistance to penicillins and cephalosporins. The clavulanate potassium molecular formula is $C_8H_8KNO_5$, and the molecular weight is 237.25. Chemically, clavulanate potassium is potassium (*Z*)-(2*R*,5*R*)-3-(2-hydroxyethylidene)-7-oxo-4-oxa-1-azabicyclo[3.2.0]-heptane-2-carboxylate, and may be represented structurally as:

Inactive Ingredients

Citric acid, colloidal silicon dioxide, hypromellose, magnesium stearate, microcrystalline cellulose, polyethylene glycol, sodium starch glycolate, titanium dioxide, and xanthan gum.
Each tablet of AUGMENTIN XR contains 12.6 mg (0.32 mEq) of potassium and 29.3 mg (1.27 mEq) of sodium.

CLINICAL PHARMACOLOGY

Amoxicillin and clavulanate potassium are well absorbed from the gastrointestinal tract after oral administration of AUGMENTIN XR.
AUGMENTIN XR is an extended-release formulation which provides sustained plasma concentrations of amoxicillin. Amoxicillin systemic exposure achieved with AUGMENTIN XR is similar to that produced by the oral administration of equivalent doses of amoxicillin alone. In a study of healthy adult volunteers, the pharmacokinetics of AUGMENTIN XR were compared when administered in a fasted state, at the start of a standardized meal (612 kcal, 89.3 g carb, 24.9 g fat, and 14.0 g protein), or 30 minutes after a high-fat meal. When the systemic exposure to both amoxicillin and clavulanate is taken into consideration, AUGMENTIN XR is optimally administered at the start of a standardized meal. Absorption of amoxicillin is decreased in the fasted state. AUGMENTIN XR is not recommended to be taken with a high-fat meal, because clavulanate absorption is decreased. The pharmacokinetics of the components of AUGMENTIN XR following administration of two AUGMENTIN XR tablets at the start of a standardized meal are presented in Table 1.

Table 1. Mean (SD) Pharmacokinetic Parameters for Amoxicillin and Clavulanate Following Oral Administration of Two AUGMENTIN XR Tablets (2,000 mg/125 mg) to Healthy Adult Volunteers (n = 55) Fed a Standardized Meal

Parameter (units)	Amoxicillin	Clavulanate
$AUC_{(0-inf)}$ (mcg•hr/mL)	71.6 (16.5)	5.29 (1.55)
C_{max} (mcg/mL)	17.0 (4.0)	2.05 (0.80)
T_{max} (hours)[a]	1.50 (1.00-6.00)	1.03 (0.75-3.00)
$T_{1/2}$ (hours)	1.27 (0.20)	1.03 (0.17)

[a] Median (range).

The half-life of amoxicillin after the oral administration of AUGMENTIN XR is approximately 1.3 hours, and that of clavulanate is approximately 1.0 hour.
Clearance of amoxicillin is predominantly renal, with approximately 60% to 80% of the dose being excreted unchanged in urine, whereas clearance of clavulanate has both a renal (30% to 50%) and a non-renal component.
Concurrent administration of probenecid delays amoxicillin excretion but does not delay renal excretion of clavulanate. In a study of adults, the pharmacokinetics of amoxicillin and clavulanate were not affected by administration of an antacid (MAALOX®), either simultaneously with or 2 hours after AUGMENTIN XR.
Neither component in AUGMENTIN XR is highly protein-bound; clavulanate has been found to be approximately 25% bound to human serum and amoxicillin approximately 18% bound.

Amoxicillin diffuses readily into most body tissues and fluids, with the exception of the brain and spinal fluid. The results of experiments involving the administration of clavulanic acid to animals suggest that this compound, like amoxicillin, is well distributed in body tissues.

Microbiology

Amoxicillin is a semisynthetic antibiotic with a broad spectrum of bactericidal activity against many gram-positive and gram-negative microorganisms. Amoxicillin is, however, susceptible to degradation by β-lactamases, and therefore, its spectrum of activity does not include organisms which produce these enzymes. Clavulanic acid is a β-lactam, structurally related to penicillin, which possesses the ability to inactivate a wide range of β-lactamase enzymes commonly found in microorganisms resistant to penicillins and cephalosporins. In particular, it has good activity against the clinically important plasmid-mediated β-lactamases frequently found responsible for transferred drug resistance.

The clavulanic acid component of AUGMENTIN XR protects amoxicillin from degradation by β-lactamase enzymes and effectively extends the antibiotic spectrum of amoxicillin to include many bacteria normally resistant to amoxicillin and other β-lactam antibiotics.

Amoxicillin/clavulanic acid has been shown to be active against most isolates of the following microorganisms, both in vitro and in clinical infections as described in the INDICATIONS AND USAGE section.

Aerobic Gram-Positive Microorganisms

Streptococcus pneumoniae (including isolates with penicillin MICs ≤ 2 mcg/mL)

Staphylococcus aureus (including β-lactamase–producing isolates)

NOTE: Staphylococci which are resistant to methicillin/oxacillin must be considered resistant to amoxicillin/clavulanic acid.

Aerobic Gram-Negative Microorganisms

Haemophilus influenzae (including β-lactamase–producing isolates)

Moraxella catarrhalis (including β-lactamase–producing isolates)

Haemophilus parainfluenzae (including β-lactamase–producing isolates)

Klebsiella pneumoniae (all known isolates are β-lactamase–producing)

The following in vitro data are available, **but their clinical significance is unknown.**

At least 90% of the following microorganisms exhibit in vitro minimum inhibitory concentrations (MICs) less than or equal to the susceptible breakpoint for amoxicillin/clavulanic acid.[1,2] However, the safety and efficacy of amoxicillin/clavulanic acid in treating infections due to these microorganisms have not been established in adequate and well-controlled trials.

Aerobic Gram-Positive Microorganisms

Streptococcus pyogenes

Anaerobic Microorganisms

Bacteroides fragilis (including β-lactamase–producing isolates)

Fusobacterium nucleatum (including β-lactamase–producing isolates)

Peptostreptococcus magnus

Peptostreptococcus micros

NOTE: *S. pyogenes, P. magnus,* and *P. micros* do not produce β-lactamase, and therefore, are susceptible to amoxicillin alone. Adequate and well-controlled clinical trials have established the effectiveness of amoxicillin alone in treating certain clinical infections due to *S. pyogenes.*

Susceptibility Test Methods

When available, the clinical microbiology laboratory should provide cumulative results of in vitro susceptibility test results for antimicrobial drugs used in local hospitals and practice areas to the physician as periodic reports that describe the susceptibility profile of nosocomial and community-acquired pathogens. These reports should aid the physician in selecting the most effective antimicrobial.

Dilution Technique

Quantitative methods are used to determine antimicrobial minimum inhibitory concentrations (MICs). These MICs provide estimates of the susceptibility of bacteria to antimicrobial compounds. The MICs should be determined using a standardized procedure.[1,3] Standardized procedures are based on dilution methods (broth or agar; broth for *S. pneumoniae* and *H. influenzae*) or equivalent with standardized inoculum concentration and standardized concentrations of amoxicillin/clavulanate potassium powder.

The recommended dilution pattern utilizes a constant amoxicillin/clavulanate potassium ratio of 2 to 1 in all tubes with varying amounts of amoxicillin. MICs are expressed in terms of the amoxicillin concentration in the presence of clavulanic acid at a constant 2 parts amoxicillin to 1 part clavulanic acid. The MIC values should be interpreted according to criteria provided in Table 2.

Table 2. Susceptibility Test Result Interpretive Criteria for Amoxicillin/Clavulanate Potassium

Pathogen	Minimum Inhibitory Concentration (mcg/mL)			Disk Diffusion (Zone Diameter in mm)		
	S	I	R	S	I	R
Haemophilus spp.	≤ 4/2	Not applicable (NA)	≥ 8/4	≥ 20	NA	≤ 19
Klebsiella pneumoniae	≤ 8/4	16/8	≥ 32/16	≥ 18	14 to 17	≤ 13
Staphylococcus spp.	≤ 4/2	NA	≥ 8/4	≥ 20	NA	≤ 19
Streptococcus pneumoniae	≤ 2/1	4/2	≥ 8/4	NA		

Table 3. Acceptable Quality Control Ranges for Amoxicillin/Clavulanate Potassium

Quality Control Organism	Minimum Inhibitory Concentration Range (mcg/mL)	Disk Diffusion (Zone Diameter Range in mm)
Escherichia coli ATCC®[a] 35218[b] (*H. influenzae* quality control)	4/2 to 16/8	17 to 22
Escherichia coli ATCC 25922	2/1 to 8/4	18 to 24
Haemophilus influenzae ATCC 49247	2/1 to 16/8	15 to 23
Staphylococcus aureus ATCC 29213	0.12/0.06 to 0.5/0.25	Not applicable (NA)
Staphylococcus aureus ATCC 25923	NA	28 to 36
Streptococcus pneumoniae ATCC 49619	0.03/0.015 to 0.12/0.06	NA

[a] ATCC is a trademark of the American Type Culture Collection.
[b] When using *Haemophilus* Test Medium (HTM).

Diffusion Technique

Quantitative methods that require measurement of zone diameters also provide reproducible estimates of the susceptibility of bacteria to antimicrobials. One such standardized technique requires the use of a standardized inoculum concentration.[1,4] This procedure uses paper disks impregnated with 30 mcg amoxicillin/clavulanate potassium (20 mcg amoxicillin plus 10 mcg clavulanate potassium) to test susceptibility of microorganisms to amoxicillin/clavulanate potassium. Disk diffusion zone sizes should be interpreted according to criteria provided in Table 2.

[See table 2 above]

NOTE: Susceptibility of *S. pneumoniae* should be determined using a 1-mcg oxacillin disk. Isolates with oxacillin zone sizes of ≥ 20 mm are susceptible to amoxicillin/clavulanate acid. An amoxicillin/clavulanate acid MIC should be determined on isolates of *S. pneumoniae* with oxacillin zone sizes of ≤ 19 mm.

NOTE: β-lactamase–negative, ampicillin-resistant *H. influenzae* isolates must be considered resistant to amoxicillin/clavulanic acid.

A report of S ("Susceptible") indicates that the antimicrobial is likely to inhibit growth of the pathogen if the antimicrobial compound in the blood reaches the concentration usually achievable. A report of I ("Intermediate") indicates that the result should be considered equivocal, and, if the microorganism is not fully susceptible to alternative, clinically feasible antimicrobials, the test should be repeated. This category implies possible clinical applicability in body sites where the drug is physiologically concentrated or in situations where high doses of antimicrobial can be used. This category also provides a buffer zone that prevents small uncontrolled technical factors from causing major discrepancies in interpretation. A report of R ("Resistant") indicates that the antimicrobial is not likely to inhibit growth of the pathogen if the antimicrobial compound in the blood reaches the concentration usually achievable; other therapy should be selected.

Standardized susceptibility test procedures require the use of quality control microorganisms to determine the performance of the test procedures.[1,3,4] Standard amoxicillin/clavulanate potassium powder should provide the MIC ranges for the quality control organisms in Table 3. For the disk diffusion technique, the 30 mcg amoxicillin/clavulanate potassium disk should provide the zone diameter ranges for the quality control organisms in Table 3.

[See table 3 above]

INDICATIONS AND USAGE

AUGMENTIN XR Extended Release Tablets are indicated for the treatment of patients with community-acquired pneumonia or acute bacterial sinusitis due to confirmed, or suspected β-lactamase–producing pathogens (i.e., *H. influenzae, M. catarrhalis, H. parainfluenzae, K. pneumoniae,* or methicillin-susceptible *S. aureus*) and *S. pneumoniae* with reduced susceptibility to penicillin (i.e., penicillin MICs = 2 mcg/mL). AUGMENTIN XR is not indicated for the treatment of infections due to *S. pneumoniae* with penicillin MICs ≥ 4 mcg/mL. Data are limited with regard to infections due to *S. pneumoniae* with penicillin MICs ≥ 4 mcg/mL (see CLINICAL STUDIES).

Of the common epidemiological risk factors for patients with resistant pneumococcal infections, only age > 65 years was studied. Patients with other common risk factors for resistant pneumococcal infections (e.g., alcoholism, immunesuppressive illness, and presence of multiple co-morbid conditions) were not studied.

In patients with community-acquired pneumonia in whom penicillin-resistant *S. pneumoniae* is suspected, bacteriological studies should be performed to determine the causative organisms and their susceptibility when AUGMENTIN XR is prescribed.

Acute bacterial sinusitis or community-acquired pneumonia due to a penicillin-susceptible strain of *S. pneumoniae* plus a β-lactamase–producing pathogen can be treated with another AUGMENTIN® (amoxicillin/clavulanate potassium) product containing lower daily doses of amoxicillin (i.e., 500 mg every 8 hours or 875 mg every 12 hours). Acute bacterial sinusitis or community-acquired pneumonia due to *S. pneumoniae* alone can be treated with amoxicillin.

To reduce the development of drug-resistant bacteria and maintain the effectiveness of AUGMENTIN XR and other antibacterial drugs, AUGMENTIN XR should be used only to treat or prevent infections that are proven or strongly suspected to be caused by susceptible bacteria. When culture and susceptibility information are available, they should be considered in selecting or modifying antibacterial therapy. In the absence of such data, local epidemiology and susceptibility patterns may contribute to the empiric selection of therapy.

CONTRAINDICATIONS

AUGMENTIN XR is contraindicated in patients with a history of allergic reactions to any penicillin. It is also contraindicated in patients with a previous history of cholestatic jaundice/hepatic dysfunction associated with treatment with amoxicillin/clavulanate potassium.

AUGMENTIN XR is contraindicated in patients with severe renal impairment (creatinine clearance < 30 mL/min.) and in hemodialysis patients.

WARNINGS

SERIOUS AND OCCASIONALLY FATAL HYPERSENSITIVITY (ANAPHYLACTIC) REACTIONS HAVE BEEN REPORTED IN PATIENTS ON PENICILLIN THERAPY. THESE REACTIONS ARE MORE LIKELY TO OCCUR IN INDIVIDUALS WITH A HISTORY OF PENICILLIN HYPERSENSITIVITY AND/OR A HISTORY OF SENSITIVITY TO MULTIPLE ALLERGENS. THERE HAVE BEEN REPORTS OF INDIVIDUALS WITH A HISTORY OF PENICILLIN HYPERSENSITIVITY WHO HAVE EXPERIENCED SEVERE REACTIONS WHEN TREATED WITH CEPHALOSPORINS. BEFORE INITIATING THERAPY WITH AUGMENTIN XR, CAREFUL INQUIRY SHOULD

BE MADE CONCERNING PREVIOUS HYPERSENSITIVITY REACTIONS TO PENICILLINS, CEPHALOSPORINS, OR OTHER ALLERGENS. IF AN ALLERGIC REACTION OCCURS, AUGMENTIN XR SHOULD BE DISCONTINUED AND THE APPROPRIATE THERAPY INSTITUTED. **SERIOUS ANAPHYLACTIC REACTIONS REQUIRE IMMEDIATE EMERGENCY TREATMENT WITH EPINEPHRINE. OXYGEN, INTRAVENOUS STEROIDS, AND AIRWAY MANAGEMENT, INCLUDING INTUBATION, SHOULD ALSO BE ADMINISTERED AS INDICATED.**

Clostridium difficile associated diarrhea (CDAD) has been reported with use of nearly all antibacterial agents, including AUGMENTIN XR, and may range in severity from mild diarrhea to fatal colitis. Treatment with antibacterial agents alters the normal flora of the colon leading to overgrowth of *C. difficile*.

C. difficile produces toxins A and B which contribute to the development of CDAD. Hypertoxin producing strains of *C. difficile* cause increased morbidity and mortality, as these infections can be refractory to antimicrobial therapy and may require colectomy. CDAD must be considered in all patients who present with diarrhea following antibiotic use. Careful medical history is necessary since CDAD has been reported to occur over two months after the administration of antibacterial agents.

If CDAD is suspected or confirmed, ongoing antibiotic use not directed against *C. difficile* may need to be discontinued. Appropriate fluid and electrolyte management, protein supplementation, antibiotic treatment of *C. difficile*, and surgical evaluation should be instituted as clinically indicated.

AUGMENTIN XR should be used with caution in patients with evidence of hepatic dysfunction. Hepatic toxicity associated with the use of amoxicillin/clavulanate potassium is usually reversible. On rare occasions, deaths have been reported (less than 1 death reported per estimated 4 million prescriptions worldwide). These have generally been cases associated with serious underlying diseases or concomitant medications (see CONTRAINDICATIONS and ADVERSE REACTIONS—Liver).

PRECAUTIONS

General

While amoxicillin/clavulanate potassium possesses the characteristic low toxicity of the penicillin group of antibiotics, periodic assessment of organ system functions, including renal, hepatic, and hematopoietic function, is advisable if therapy is for longer than the drug is approved for administration.

A high percentage of patients with mononucleosis who receive ampicillin develop an erythematous skin rash. Thus, ampicillin-class antibiotics should not be administered to patients with mononucleosis.

The possibility of superinfections with mycotic or bacterial pathogens should be kept in mind during therapy. If superinfections occur (usually involving *Pseudomonas* spp. or *Candida* spp.), the drug should be discontinued and/or appropriate therapy instituted.

Prescribing AUGMENTIN XR in the absence of a proven or strongly suspected bacterial infection or a prophylactic indication is unlikely to provide benefit to the patient and increases the risk of the development of drug-resistant bacteria.

Information for Patients

AUGMENTIN XR should be taken every 12 hours with a meal or snack to reduce the possibility of gastrointestinal upset. If diarrhea develops and is severe or lasts more than 2 or 3 days, call your doctor.

Diarrhea is a common problem caused by antibiotics which usually ends when the antibiotic is discontinued. Sometimes after starting treatment with antibiotics, patients can develop watery and bloody stools (with or without stomach cramps and fever) even as late as 2 or more months after having taken the last dose of the antibiotic. If this occurs, patients should contact their physician as soon as possible.

Patients should be counseled that antibacterial drugs, including AUGMENTIN XR, should only be used to treat bacterial infections. They do not treat viral infections (e.g., the common cold). When AUGMENTIN XR is prescribed to treat a bacterial infection, patients should be told that although it is common to feel better early in the course of therapy, the medication should be taken exactly as directed. Skipping doses or not completing the full course of therapy may: (1) decrease the effectiveness of the immediate treatment, and (2) increase the likelihood that bacteria will develop resistance and will not be treatable by AUGMENTIN XR or other antibacterial drugs in the future.

Discard any unused medicine.

Drug Interactions

Probenecid decreases the renal tubular secretion of amoxicillin. Concurrent use with AUGMENTIN XR may result in increased and prolonged blood levels of amoxicillin. Coadministration of probenecid cannot be recommended.

Abnormal prolongation of prothrombin time (increased international normalized ratio [INR]) has been reported rarely in patients receiving amoxicillin and oral anticoagulants. Appropriate monitoring should be undertaken when anticoagulants are prescribed concurrently. Adjustments in the dose of oral anticoagulants may be necessary to maintain the desired level of anticoagulation. The concurrent administration of allopurinol and ampicillin increases substantially the incidence of rashes in patients receiving both drugs as compared to patients receiving ampicillin alone. It is not known whether this potentiation of ampicillin rashes is due to allopurinol or the hyperuricemia present in these patients. In controlled clinical trials of AUGMENTIN XR, 25 patients received concomitant allopurinol and AUGMENTIN XR. No rashes were reported in these patients. However, this sample size is too small to allow for any conclusions to be drawn regarding the risk of rashes with concomitant AUGMENTIN XR and allopurinol use.

In common with other broad-spectrum antibiotics, AUGMENTIN XR may reduce the efficacy of oral contraceptives.

Drug/Laboratory Test Interactions

Oral administration of AUGMENTIN XR will result in high urine concentrations of amoxicillin. High urine concentrations of ampicillin may result in false-positive reactions when testing for the presence of glucose in urine using CLINITEST®, Benedict's Solution, or Fehling's Solution. Since this effect may also occur with amoxicillin and therefore AUGMENTIN XR, it is recommended that glucose tests based on enzymatic glucose oxidase reactions (such as CLINISTIX®) be used.

Following administration of ampicillin to pregnant women, a transient decrease in plasma concentration of total conjugated estriol, estriol-glucuronide, conjugated estrone, and estradiol has been noted. This effect may also occur with amoxicillin, and therefore, AUGMENTIN XR.

Carcinogenesis, Mutagenesis, Impairment of Fertility

Long-term studies in animals have not been performed to evaluate carcinogenic potential. The mutagenic potential of AUGMENTIN was investigated in vitro with an Ames test, a human lymphocyte cytogenetic assay, a yeast test, and a mouse lymphoma forward mutation assay, and in vivo with mouse micronucleus tests and a dominant lethal test. All were negative apart from the in vitro mouse lymphoma assay, where weak activity was found at very high, cytotoxic concentrations. AUGMENTIN at oral doses of up to 1,200 mg/kg/day (1.9 times the maximum human dose of amoxicillin and 15 times the maximum human dose of clavulanate based on body surface area) was found to have no effect on fertility and reproductive performance in rats dosed with a 2:1 ratio formulation of amoxicillin: clavulanate.

Pregnancy

Teratogenic Effects

Pregnancy Category B. Reproduction studies performed in pregnant rats and mice given AUGMENTIN at oral doses up to 1,200 mg/kg/day revealed no evidence of harm to the fetus due to AUGMENTIN. In terms of body surface area, the doses in rats were 1.6 times the maximum human oral dose of amoxicillin and 13 times the maximum human dose for clavulanate. For mice, these doses were 0.9 and 7.4 times the maximum human oral dose of amoxicillin and clavulanate, respectively. There are, however, no adequate and well-controlled studies in pregnant women. Because animal reproduction studies are not always predictive of human response, this drug should be used during pregnancy only if clearly needed.

Labor and Delivery

Oral ampicillin-class antibiotics are generally poorly absorbed during labor. Studies in guinea pigs have shown that intravenous administration of ampicillin decreased the uterine tone, frequency of contractions, height of contractions, and duration of contractions. However, it is not known whether the use of AUGMENTIN XR in humans during labor or delivery has immediate or delayed adverse effects on the fetus, prolongs the duration of labor, or increases the likelihood that forceps delivery or other obstetrical intervention or resuscitation of the newborn will be necessary. In a single study in women with premature rupture of fetal membranes, it was reported that prophylactic treatment with AUGMENTIN may be associated with an increased risk of necrotizing enterocolitis in neonates.

Nursing Mothers

Ampicillin-class antibiotics are excreted in the milk; therefore, caution should be exercised when AUGMENTIN XR is administered to a nursing woman.

Pediatric Use

Safety and effectiveness in pediatric patients younger than 16 years have not been established.

Geriatric Use

Of the total number of subjects in clinical studies of AUGMENTIN XR, 18.4% were 65 years or older and 7.2% were 75 years or older. No overall differences in safety and effectiveness were observed between these subjects and younger subjects, and other clinical experience has not reported differences in responses between the elderly and younger patients, but a greater sensitivity of some older individuals cannot be ruled out.

This drug is known to be substantially excreted by the kidney, and the risk of dose-dependent toxic reactions to this drug may be greater in patients with impaired renal function. Because elderly patients are more likely to have decreased renal function, it may be useful to monitor renal function.

Each tablet of AUGMENTIN XR contains 29.3 mg (1.27 mEq) of sodium.

ADVERSE REACTIONS

In clinical trials, 5,643 patients have been treated with AUGMENTIN XR. The majority of side effects observed in clinical trials were of a mild and transient nature; 2% of patients discontinued therapy because of drug-related side effects. The most frequently reported adverse effects which were suspected or probably drug-related were diarrhea (14.5%), vaginal mycosis (3.3%) nausea (2.1%), and loose stools (1.6%). AUGMENTIN XR had a higher rate of diarrhea which required corrective therapy (3.8% versus 2.6% for AUGMENTIN XR and all comparators, respectively).

The following adverse reactions have been reported for ampicillin-class antibiotics:

Gastrointestinal

Diarrhea, nausea, vomiting, indigestion, gastritis, stomatitis, glossitis, black "hairy" tongue, mucocutaneous candidiasis, enterocolitis, and hemorrhagic/pseudomembranous colitis. Onset of pseudomembranous colitis symptoms may occur during or after antibiotic treatment (see WARNINGS).

Hypersensitivity Reactions

Skin rashes, pruritus, urticaria, angioedema, serum sickness-like reactions (urticaria or skin rash accompanied by arthritis, arthralgia, myalgia, and frequently fever), erythema multiforme (rarely Stevens-Johnson syndrome), acute generalized exanthematous pustulosis, hypersensitivity vasculitis, and an occasional case of exfoliative dermatitis (including toxic epidermal necrolysis) have been reported. Whenever such reactions occur, the drug should be discontinued, unless the opinion of the physician dictates otherwise. Serious and occasional fatal hypersensitivity (anaphylactic) reactions can occur with oral penicillin (see WARNINGS).

Liver

A moderate rise in AST (SGOT) and/or ALT (SGPT) has been noted in patients treated with ampicillin-class antibiotics, but the significance of these findings is unknown. Hepatic dysfunction, including hepatitis and cholestatic jaundice, (see CONTRAINDICATIONS), increases in serum transaminases (AST and/or ALT), serum bilirubin, and/or alkaline phosphatase, has been infrequently reported with AUGMENTIN or AUGMENTIN XR. It has been reported more commonly in the elderly, in males, or in patients on prolonged treatment. The histologic findings on liver biopsy have consisted of predominantly cholestatic, hepatocellular, or mixed cholestatic-hepatocellular changes. The onset of signs/symptoms of hepatic dysfunction may occur during or several weeks after therapy has been discontinued. The hepatic dysfunction, which may be severe, is usually reversible. On rare occasions, deaths have been reported (less than 1 death reported per estimated 4 million prescriptions worldwide). These have generally been cases associated with serious underlying diseases or concomitant medications.

Renal

Interstitial nephritis and hematuria have been reported rarely. Crystalluria has also been reported (see OVERDOSAGE).

Hemic and Lymphatic Systems

Anemia, including hemolytic anemia, thrombocytopenia, thrombocytopenic purpura, eosinophilia, leukopenia, and agranulocytosis have been reported during therapy with penicillins. These reactions are usually reversible on discontinuation of therapy and are believed to be hypersensitivity phenomena. There have been reports of increased prothrombin time in patients receiving AUGMENTIN and anticoagulant therapy concomitantly.

Central Nervous System

Agitation, anxiety, behavioral changes, confusion, convulsions, dizziness, headache, insomnia, and reversible hyperactivity have been reported rarely.

Miscellaneous

Tooth discoloration (brown, yellow, or gray staining) has been rarely reported. Most reports occurred in pediatric patients. Discoloration was reduced or eliminated with brushing or dental cleaning in most cases.

OVERDOSAGE

Following overdosage, patients have experienced primarily gastrointestinal symptoms including stomach and abdominal pain, vomiting, and diarrhea. Rash, hyperactivity, or drowsiness have also been observed in a small number of patients.

In the case of overdosage, discontinue AUGMENTIN XR, treat symptomatically, and institute supportive measures as required. If the overdosage is very recent and there is no contraindication, an attempt at emesis or other means of removal of drug from the stomach may be performed. A prospective study of 51 pediatric patients at a poison control center suggested that overdosages of less than 250 mg/kg of amoxicillin are not associated with significant clinical symptoms and do not require gastric emptying.[5]

Interstitial nephritis resulting in oliguric renal failure has been reported in a small number of patients after overdosage with amoxicillin.

Crystalluria, in some cases leading to renal failure, has also been reported after amoxicillin overdosage in adult and pediatric patients. In case of overdosage, adequate fluid intake and diuresis should be maintained to reduce the risk of amoxicillin crystalluria.

Renal impairment appears to be reversible with cessation of drug administration. High blood levels may occur more readily in patients with impaired renal function because of decreased renal clearance of both amoxicillin and clavulanate. Both amoxicillin and clavulanate are removed from the circulation by hemodialysis (see DOSAGE AND ADMINISTRATION).

DOSAGE AND ADMINISTRATION

AUGMENTIN XR should be taken at the start of a meal to enhance the absorption of amoxicillin and to minimize the potential for gastrointestinal intolerance. Absorption of the amoxicillin component is decreased when AUGMENTIN XR is taken on an empty stomach (see CLINICAL PHARMACOLOGY).

The recommended dose of AUGMENTIN XR is 4,000 mg/250 mg daily according to the following table:

Indication	Dose	Duration
Acute bacterial sinusitis	2 tablets q12h	10 days
Community-acquired pneumonia	2 tablets q12h	7-10 days

Tablets of AUGMENTIN (250 mg or 500 mg) CANNOT be used to provide the same dosages as AUGMENTIN XR Extended Release Tablets. This is because AUGMENTIN XR contains 62.5 mg of clavulanic acid, while the AUGMENTIN 250-mg and 500-mg tablets each contain 125 mg of clavulanic acid. In addition, the Extended Release Tablet provides an extended time course of plasma amoxicillin concentrations compared to immediate-release Tablets. Thus, two AUGMENTIN 500-mg tablets are not equivalent to one AUGMENTIN XR tablet.

Scored AUGMENTIN XR Extended Release Tablets are available for greater convenience for adult patients who have difficulty swallowing. The scored tablet is not intended to reduce the dosage of medication taken; as stated in the table above, the recommended dose of AUGMENTIN XR is two tablets twice a day (every 12 hours).

Renally Impaired Patients

The pharmacokinetics of AUGMENTIN XR have not been studied in patients with renal impairment. AUGMENTIN XR is contraindicated in patients with a creatinine clearance of < 30 mL/min. and in hemodialysis patients (see CONTRAINDICATIONS).

Hepatically Impaired Patients

Hepatically impaired patients should be dosed with caution and hepatic function monitored at regular intervals (see WARNINGS).

Pediatric Use

Safety and effectiveness in pediatric patients younger than 16 years have not been established.

Geriatric Use

No dosage adjustment is required for the elderly (see PRECAUTIONS, Geriatric Use).

HOW SUPPLIED

AUGMENTIN XR Extended Release Tablets

Each white, oval film-coated bilayer scored tablet, debossed with AUGMENTIN XR, contains amoxicillin trihydrate and amoxicillin sodium equivalent to a total of 1,000 mg of amoxicillin and clavulanate potassium equivalent to 62.5 mg of clavulanic acid.

NDC 0029-6096-48   Bottles of 28 (7 day XR pack)
NDC 0029-6096-60   Bottles of 40 (10 day XR pack)

STORAGE

Store tablets at or below 25°C (77°F). Dispense in original container.

CLINICAL STUDIES

Acute Bacterial Sinusitis

Adults with a diagnosis of acute bacterial sinusitis (ABS) were evaluated in 3 clinical studies. In one study, 363 patients were randomized to receive either AUGMENTIN XR 2,000 mg/125 mg orally every 12 hours or levofloxacin

Clinical Outcome for ABS

Penicillin MICs of S. pneumoniae Isolates	Intent-To-Treat			Clinically Evaluable		
	n/N[a]	%	95% CI[b]	n/N[a]	%	95% CI[b]
All S. pneumoniae	344/370	93.0	—	318/326	97.5	—
MIC ≥ 2.0 mcg/mL[c]	35/36	97.2	85.5, 99.9	30/31	95.8	83.3, 99.9
MIC = 2.0 mcg/mL	23/24	95.8	78.9, 99.9	19/20	95.0	75.1, 99.9
MIC ≥ 4.0 mcg/mL[d]	12/12	100	73.5, 100	11/11	100	71.5, 100
H. influenzae	265/305	86.9	—	242/259	93.4	—
M. catarrhalis	94/105	89.5	—	86/90	95.6	—

[a] n/N = patients with pathogen eradicated or presumed eradicated/total number of patients.
[b] Confidence limits calculated using exact probabilities.
[c] S. pneumoniae strains with penicillin MICs of ≥ 2 mcg/mL are considered resistant to penicillin.
[d] Includes one patient each with S. pneumoniae penicillin MICs of 8 and 16 mcg/mL.

Clinical Outcome for CAP due to S. pneumoniae

Penicillin MICs of S. pneumoniae Isolates	Intent-To-Treat			Clinically Evaluable		
	n/N[a]	%	95% CI[b]	n/N[a]	%	95% CI[b]
All S. pneumoniae	318/367	86.6	—	275/297	92.6	—
MIC ≥ 2.0 mcg/mL[c]	30/35	85.7	69.7, 95.2	24/25	96.0	79.6, 99.9
MIC = 2.0 mcg/mL	22/24	91.7	73.0, 99.0	18/18	100	81.5, 100
MIC ≥ 4.0 mcg/mL[d]	8/11	72.7	39.0, 94.0	6/7	85.7	42.1, 99.6

[a] n/N = patients with pathogen eradicated or presumed eradicated/total number of patients.
[b] Confidence limits calculated using exact probabilities.
[c] S. pneumoniae strains with penicillin MICs of ≥ 2 mcg/mL are considered resistant to penicillin.
[d] Includes one patient each with S. pneumoniae penicillin MICs of 8 and 16 mcg/mL in the Intent-To-Treat group only.

500 mg orally daily for 10 days in a double-blind, multicenter, prospective trial. These patients were clinically and radiologically evaluated at the test of cure (day 17-28) visit. The combined clinical and radiological responses were 83.7% for AUGMENTIN XR and 84.3% for levofloxacin at the test of cure visit in clinically evaluable patients (95% CI for the treatment difference = -9.4, 8.3). The clinical response rates at the test of cure were 87.0% and 88.6%, respectively.

The other 2 trials were non-comparative, multicenter studies designed to assess the bacteriological and clinical efficacy of AUGMENTIN XR (2,000 mg/125 mg orally every 12 hours for 10 days) in the treatment of 2288 patients with ABS. Evaluation timepoints were the same as in the prior study. Patients underwent maxillary sinus puncture for culture prior to receiving study medication. At test of cure, the clinical success rates were 87.5% and 86.6% (intention-to-treat) and 92.5% and 92.1% (per protocol populations). Patients with acute bacterial sinusitis due to S. pneumoniae with reduced susceptibility to penicillin were accrued through enrollment in these 2 open-label non-comparative clinical trials. Microbiologic eradication rates for key pathogens in these studies are shown in the following table:

[See first table above]

Community-Acquired Pneumonia

Four randomized, controlled, double-blind clinical studies and one non-comparative study were conducted in adults with community-acquired pneumonia (CAP). In comparative studies, 904 patients received AUGMENTIN XR at a dose of 2,000 mg/125 mg orally every 12 hours for 7 or 10 days. In the non-comparative study to assess both clinical and bacteriological efficacy, 1,122 patients received AUGMENTIN XR 2,000 mg/125 mg orally every 12 hours for 7 days. In the 4 comparative studies, the combined clinical success rate at test of cure ranged from 86.3% to 94.7% in clinically evaluable patients who received AUGMENTIN XR; in the non-comparative study, the clinical success rate was 85.6%.

Data on the efficacy of AUGMENTIN XR in the treatment of community-acquired pneumonia due to S. pneumoniae with reduced susceptibility to penicillin were accrued from the 4 controlled clinical studies and the 1 non-comparative study. The majority of these cases were accrued from the non-comparative study.

[See second table above]

Safety

In 2 randomized, double-blind, multicenter studies, AUGMENTIN XR (2,000 mg/125 mg orally every 12 hours, n = 577) was compared to AUGMENTIN (875 mg/125 mg orally every 12 hours, n = 570), administered for 7 days for the treatment of community-acquired pneumonia. Adverse events, regardless of relationship to test drug, were reported by 44.4% of patients who received AUGMENTIN XR (versus 46.3% in comparator group). Treatment-related adverse events were reported in 21.7% of patients who received AUGMENTIN XR (versus 21.2% in comparator group); most were mild and transient in nature. Adverse events which led to withdrawal were reported by 2.8% of patients who received AUGMENTIN XR (versus 5.3% in comparator group). In each group, the most frequently reported adverse events were diarrhea (14.4% versus 13.0%, p = 0.47), nausea (3.5 % versus 4.4%), and headache (3.5% versus 3.2%). Only 2 patients (0.3%) who received AUGMENTIN XR and 3 patients (0.5%) in the comparator group withdrew due to diarrhea. Serious adverse events considered suspected or probably related to test drug were reported in 0.3% of patients (versus 0.5% in comparator).

REFERENCES

1. Clinical and Laboratory Standards Institute (CLSI) (formerly the National Committee for Clinical Laboratory Standards). Performance Standards for Antimicrobial Susceptibility Testing – Fifteenth Informational Supplement. CSLI Document M100-S15. CLSI, Wayne, PA, 2005.
2. Clinical and Laboratory Standards Institute (CLSI) (formerly the National Committee for Clinical Laboratory Standards). Methods for Antimicrobial Susceptibility Testing of Anaerobic Bacteria – Sixth Edition. Approved Standard CSLI Document M11-A6, Vol. 24, No. 2. CLSI, Wayne, PA, 2004.
3. Clinical and Laboratory Standards Institute (CLSI) (formerly the National Committee for Clinical Laboratory Standards). Methods for Dilution Antimicrobial Susceptibility Tests for Bacteria that Grow Aerobically – Sixth Edition. Approved Standard CLSI Document M7-A6, Vol. 23, No. 2. CLSI, Wayne, PA, 2003.
4. Clinical and Laboratory Standards Institute (CLSI) (formerly the National Committee for Clinical Laboratory Standards). Performance Standards for Antimicrobial Disk Susceptibility Tests – Eighth Edition. Approved Standard CLSI Document M2-A8, Vol. 23, No. 1. CLSI, Wayne, PA, 2003.
5. Swanson-Biearman B, Dean BS, Lopez G, Krenzelok EP. The effects of penicillin and cephalosporin ingestions in children less than six years of age. Vet Hum Toxicol 1988; 30: 66-67.

AUGMENTIN XR and AUGMENTIN are registered trademarks of GlaxoSmithKline.
MAALOX is a registered trademark of Novartis Consumer Health, Inc.

GlaxoSmithKline
Research Triangle Park, NC 27709
©2009, GlaxoSmithKline. All rights reserved.
September 2009

AUX:10PI

AVANDAMET® ℞
[ə-van' də-met]
(rosiglitazone maleate andmetformin hydrochloride) Tablets

HIGHLIGHTS OF PRESCRIBING INFORMATION
These highlights do not include all the information needed to use AVANDAMET safely and effectively. See full prescribing information for AVANDAMET.
AVANDAMET (rosiglitazone maleate and metformin hydrochloride) Tablets
Initial U.S. Approval: 2002

WARNINGS
See full prescribing information for complete boxed warning.
Rosiglitazone maleate: CONGESTIVE HEART FAILURE AND MYOCARDIAL ISCHEMIA

- Thiazolidinediones, including rosiglitazone, cause or exacerbate heart failure in some patients (5.2). After initiation of AVANDAMET, and after dose increases, observe patients carefully for signs and symptoms of heart failure (including excessive, rapid weight gain, dyspnea, and/or edema). If these signs and symptoms develop, the heart failure should be managed according to current standards of care. Furthermore, discontinuation or dose reduction must be considered. (5.2)
- AVANDAMET is not recommended in patients with symptomatic heart failure. Initiation of AVANDAMET in patients with established NYHA Class III or IV heart failure is contraindicated. (4, 5.2)
- A meta-analysis of 42 studies (mean duration 6 months; 14,237 total patients), most of which compared rosiglitazone to placebo, showed rosiglitazone to be associated with an increased risk of myocardial ischemic events. Three other studies (mean duration 41 months; 14,067 total patients), comparing rosiglitazone to some other approved oral antidiabetic agents or placebo, have not confirmed or excluded this risk. Available data on the risk of myocardial ischemia are inconclusive. (5.3)
Metformin hydrochloride: LACTIC ACIDOSIS
- Lactic acidosis can occur due to metformin accumulation. The risk increases with conditions such as sepsis, dehydration, excess alcohol intake, hepatic insufficiency, renal impairment and acute congestive heart failure. (5.1)
- Symptoms include malaise, myalgias, respiratory distress, increasing somnolence and nonspecific abdominal distress. Laboratory abnormalities include low pH, increased anion gap and elevated blood lactate. (5.1)
- If acidosis is suspected, discontinue AVANDAMET and hospitalize the patient immediately. (5.1)

RECENT MAJOR CHANGES

Boxed Warning	12/2008
Indications and Usage, Important Limitations of Use (1.1)	12/2008
Warnings and Precautions, Cardiac Failure (5.2)	12/2008
Warnings and Precautions, Myocardial Ischemia (5.3)	12/2008
Warnings and Precautions, Coadministration of Rosiglitazone with Insulin (5.4)	12/2008
Warnings and and Precautions, Edema (5.5)	12/2008

INDICATIONS AND USAGE

AVANDAMET is indicated as an adjunct to diet and exercise to improve glycemic control in adults with type 2 diabetes mellitus when treatment with both rosiglitazone and metformin is appropriate.
Important Limitations of Use:
- Should not be used in patients with type 1 diabetes or for the treatment of diabetic ketoacidosis. (1.1)
- Use with nitrates is not recommended. (1.1, 5.3)
- Coadministration with insulin is not recommended. (1.1, 5.4)

DOSAGE AND ADMINISTRATION

- Individualize the starting dose based on the patient's current regimen. (2.1)
- Dose increases should be accompanied by careful monitoring for adverse events related to fluid retention. (2.1)
- Give in divided doses with meals with gradual dose escalation to reduce the gastrointestinal side effects. (2.2)
- Do not exceed the maximum recommended daily dose of 8 mg rosiglitazone and 2,000 mg metformin. (2.3)
- Do not initiate if the patient exhibits clinical evidence of active liver disease or increased serum transaminase levels. (2.4)

DOSAGE FORMS AND STRENGTHS

Oval, film-coated tablets containing rosiglitazone/metformin hydrochloride: 2 mg/500 mg, 4 mg/500 mg, 2 mg/1,000 mg, and 4 mg/1,000 mg (3)

CONTRAINDICATIONS

- Initiation in patients with established NYHA Class III or IV heart failure. (4)
- Use in significant renal disease or renal dysfunction. (4)
- Use in acute or chronic metabolic acidosis. (4)
- Use in patients undergoing radiologic studies involving intravascular administration of iodinated contrast materials. (4, 5.1)

WARNINGS AND PRECAUTIONS

- Fluid retention, which may exacerbate or lead to heart failure, may occur. Combination use with insulin and use in congestive heart failure NYHA Class I and II may increase risk of other cardiovascular effects. (5.2, 5.3, 5.5)
- Increased risk of myocardial ischemic events has been observed in a meta-analysis of 42 clinical trials of rosiglitazone (incidence rate 2% versus 1.5%). (5.3)
- Use with nitrates is not recommended. (5.3)
- Coadministration with insulin is not recommended. (1.1, 5.3, 5.4)
- Assess renal function before starting therapy and at least annually. (5.1)
- Avoid use in patients with evidence of hepatic disease. (2.4, 5.1)
- Warn patients against excessive alcohol intake. (5.1)
- Promptly evaluate patients who develop laboratory abnormalities or clinical illness for evidence of ketoacidosis or lactic acidosis. (5.1)
- Dose-related edema (5.5), weight gain (5.6), and anemia (5.10) may occur.
- Macular edema has been reported. (5.8)
- Increased incidence of bone fracture in female patients. (5.9)
- Measure hematologic parameters annually. (5.10)
- There have been no clinical studies establishing conclusive evidence of macrovascular risk reduction with AVANDAMET or any other antidiabetic drug. (5.3)

ADVERSE REACTIONS

The most common adverse reactions (≥10%) include nausea/vomiting, diarrhea, headache, and dyspepsia. (6.1)
To report SUSPECTED ADVERSE REACTIONS, contact GlaxoSmithKline at 1-888-825-5249 or FDA at 1-800-FDA-1088 or www.fda.gov/medwatch

---

DRUG INTERACTIONS

- Inhibitors of CYP2C8 (e.g., gemfibrozil) may increase rosiglitazone levels. (7.1)
- Inducers of CYP2C8 (e.g., rifampin) may decrease rosiglitazone levels. (7.1)
- Cationic drugs eliminated by renal tubular secretion; use with caution. (7.2)

USE IN SPECIFIC POPULATIONS

- Do not use during pregnancy. No human or animal data. (8.1)
- Safety and effectiveness in children under 18 years have not been established. (8.4)
- Because reduced renal function is associated with increasing age, use with caution in elderly patients. (8.5)

Revised: December 2008
AVM:18PI

See 17 for PATIENT COUNSELING INFORMATION and FDA-approved Medication Guide.

FULL PRESCRIBING INFORMATION: CONTENTS*
WARNINGS
*Sections or subsections omitted from the full prescribing information are not listed.

FULL PRESCRIBING INFORMATION

WARNINGS
Rosiglitazone maleate: CONGESTIVE HEART FAILURE AND MYOCARDIAL ISCHEMIA

- Thiazolidinediones, including rosiglitazone, cause or exacerbate congestive heart failure in some patients *[see Warnings and Precautions (5.2)]*. After initiation of AVANDAMET, and after dose increases, observe patients carefully for signs and symptoms of heart failure (including excessive, rapid weight gain, dyspnea, and/or edema). If these signs and symptoms develop, the heart failure should be managed according to current standards of care. Furthermore, discontinuation or dose reduction of AVANDAMET must be considered.
- AVANDAMET is not recommended in patients with symptomatic heart failure. Initiation of AVANDAMET in patients with established NYHA Class III or IV heart failure is contraindicated. *[See Contraindications (4) and Warnings and Precautions (5.2).]*
- A meta-analysis of 42 clinical studies (mean duration 6 months; 14,237 total patients), most of which compared rosiglitazone to placebo, showed rosiglitazone to be associated with an increased risk of myocardial ischemic events such as angina or myocardial infarction. Three other studies (mean duration 41 months; 14,067 total patients), comparing rosiglitazone to some other approved oral antidiabetic agents or placebo, have not confirmed or excluded this risk. In their entirety, the available data on the risk of myocardial ischemia are inconclusive. *[See Warnings and Precautions (5.3).]*
Metformin hydrochloride: LACTIC ACIDOSIS
- Lactic acidosis is a rare, but serious complication that can occur due to metformin accumulation. The risk increases with conditions such as sepsis, dehydration, excess alcohol intake, hepatic insufficiency, renal impairment, and acute congestive heart failure. *[See Warnings and Precautions (5.1).]*
- Symptoms include malaise, myalgias, respiratory distress, increasing somnolence, and nonspecific abdominal distress. Laboratory abnormalities include low pH, increased anion gap and elevated blood lactate. *[See Warnings and Precautions (5.1).]*
- If acidosis is suspected, discontinue AVANDAMET and hospitalize the patient immediately *[see Warnings and Precautions (5.1)]*.

---

1   INDICATIONS AND USAGE

AVANDAMET is indicated as an adjunct to diet and exercise to improve glycemic control in adults with type 2 diabetes mellitus when treatment with both rosiglitazone and metformin is appropriate. *[See Clinical Studies (14).]*

1.1 Important Limitations of Use

- Due to its mechanism of action, rosiglitazone is active only in the presence of endogenous insulin. Therefore, AVANDAMET should not be used in patients with type 1 diabetes.
- The use of AVANDAMET with nitrates is not recommended [see Warnings and Precautions (5.3)].
- Coadministration of AVANDAMET with insulin is not recommended [see Warnings and Precautions (5.4)].

2 DOSAGE AND ADMINISTRATION

The dosage of antidiabetic therapy with AVANDAMET should be individualized on the basis of effectiveness and tolerability. The risk-benefit of initiating monotherapy versus dual therapy with AVANDAMET should be considered.

2.1 Starting Dose

AVANDAMET is generally given in divided doses with meals.

All patients should start the rosiglitazone component of AVANDAMET at the lowest recommended dose. Further increases in the dose of rosiglitazone should be accompanied by careful monitoring for adverse events related to fluid retention [see **Boxed Warning** and Warnings and Precautions (5.5)].

Patients Inadequately Controlled With Diet and Exercise: If therapy with a combination tablet containing rosiglitazone and metformin is considered appropriate for a patient with type 2 diabetes mellitus inadequately controlled with diet and exercise alone, the recommended starting dose of AVANDAMET is 2 mg/500 mg administered once or twice daily. For patients with HbA1c >11% or fasting plasma glucose (FPG) >270 mg/dL, a starting dose of 2 mg/500 mg twice daily may be considered. The dose of AVANDAMET may be increased in increments of 2 mg/500 mg per day given in divided doses if patients are not adequately controlled after 4 weeks. The maximum dose of AVANDAMET is 8 mg/2,000 mg per day.

Patients Inadequately Controlled With Rosiglitazone or Metformin Monotherapy: If therapy with a combination tablet containing rosiglitazone and metformin is considered appropriate for a patient with type 2 diabetes mellitus inadequately controlled on rosiglitazone or metformin monotherapy, then the selection of the dose of AVANDAMET should be based on the patient's current doses of rosiglitazone and/or metformin.

For patients inadequately controlled on metformin monotherapy, the usual starting dose of AVANDAMET is 4 mg rosiglitazone (total daily dose) plus the dose of metformin already being taken (see Table 1).

For patients inadequately controlled on rosiglitazone monotherapy, the usual starting dose of AVANDAMET is 1,000 mg metformin (total daily dose) plus the dose of rosiglitazone already being taken (see Table 1).

When switching from combination therapy of rosiglitazone plus metformin as separate tablets, the usual starting dose of AVANDAMET is the dose of rosiglitazone and metformin already being taken.

Table 1. AVANDAMET Starting Dose for Patients Treated with Metformin and/or Rosiglitazone

PRIOR THERAPY	Usual AVANDAMET Starting Dose	
Total daily dose	Tablet strength	Number of tablets
Metformin*		
1,000 mg/day	2 mg/500 mg	1 tablet twice a day
2,000 mg/day	2 mg/1,000 mg	1 tablet twice a day
Rosiglitazone		
4 mg/day	2 mg/500 mg	1 tablet twice a day
8 mg/day	4 mg/500 mg	1 tablet twice a day

*For patients on doses of metformin between 1,000 and 2,000 mg/day, initiation of AVANDAMET requires individualization of therapy.

2.2 Dose Titration

AVANDAMET is generally given in divided doses with meals, with gradual dose escalation. This reduces gastrointestinal side effects (largely due to metformin) and permits determination of the minimum effective dose for the individual patient.

Sufficient time should be given to assess adequacy of therapeutic response. FPG should be used initially to determine the therapeutic response to AVANDAMET. If additional glycemic control is needed, the daily dose of AVANDAMET may be increased by increments of 4 mg rosiglitazone and/or 500 mg metformin.

After an increase in metformin dosage, dose titration is recommended if patients are not adequately controlled after 1

to 2 weeks. After an increase in rosiglitazone dosage, dose titration is recommended if patients are not adequately controlled after 8 to 12 weeks.

2.3 Maximum Dose

The maximum recommended total daily dose of AVANDAMET is 8 mg rosiglitazone (taken as 4 mg twice daily) and 2,000 mg metformin (taken as 1,000 mg twice daily).

2.4 Specific Patient Populations

Renal Impairment: Any dosage adjustment should be based on a careful assessment of renal function. Generally, elderly, debilitated, and malnourished patients should not be titrated to the maximum dose of AVANDAMET. Monitoring of renal function is necessary to aid in prevention of metformin-associated lactic acidosis, particularly in the elderly [see Warnings and Precautions (5.1)].

Hepatic Impairment: Liver enzymes should be measured prior to initiating treatment with AVANDAMET. Therapy with AVANDAMET should not be initiated if the patient exhibits clinical evidence of active liver disease or increased serum transaminase levels (ALT >2.5× upper limit of normal at start of therapy). After initiation of AVANDAMET, liver enzymes should be monitored periodically per the clinical judgment of the healthcare professional [see Warnings and Precautions (5.7) and Clinical Pharmacology (12.3)].

Geriatric: The initial and maintenance dosing of AVANDAMET should be conservative in patients with advanced age, due to the potential for decreased renal function in this population.

Pediatric: Safety and effectiveness of AVANDAMET in pediatric patients have not been established. AVANDAMET and rosiglitazone are not recommended for use in pediatric patients.

Pregnancy: AVANDAMET is not recommended for use in pregnancy.

3 DOSAGE FORMS AND STRENGTHS

Each film-coated oval tablet contains rosiglitazone as the maleate and metformin hydrochloride as follows:

- 2 mg/500 mg – pale pink, debossed with gsk on one side and 2/500 on the other
- 4 mg/500 mg – orange, debossed with gsk on one side and 4/500 on the other
- 2 mg/1,000 mg – yellow, debossed with gsk on one side and 2/1000 on the other
- 4 mg/1,000 mg – pink, debossed with gsk on one side and 4/1000 on the other

4 CONTRAINDICATIONS

- Initiation in patients with established New York Heart Association (NYHA) Class III or IV heart failure [see Boxed Warning].
- Use in patients with renal disease or renal dysfunction (e.g., as suggested by serum creatinine levels ≥1.5 mg/dL [males], ≥1.4 mg/dL [females], or abnormal creatinine clearance), which may also result from conditions such as cardiovascular collapse (shock), acute myocardial infarction, and septicemia [see Warnings and Precautions (5.1)].
- Use in patients with acute or chronic metabolic acidosis, including diabetic ketoacidosis, with or without coma.
- Use in patients undergoing radiologic studies involving intravascular administration of iodinated contrast materials, because use of such products may result in acute alteration of renal function. AVANDAMET should be temporarily discontinued in these patients. [See Warnings and Precautions (5.1).]

5 WARNINGS AND PRECAUTIONS

5.1 Lactic Acidosis

Incidence and Management: Lactic acidosis is a rare, but serious, metabolic complication that can occur due to metformin accumulation during treatment with AVANDAMET; when it occurs, it is fatal in approximately 50% of cases. Lactic acidosis may also occur in association with a number of pathophysiologic conditions, including diabetes mellitus, and whenever there is significant tissue hypoperfusion and hypoxemia. Lactic acidosis is characterized by elevated blood lactate levels (>5 mmol/L), decreased blood pH, electrolyte disturbances with an increased anion gap, and an increased lactate/pyruvate ratio. When metformin is implicated as the cause of lactic acidosis, metformin plasma levels >5 mcg/mL are generally found.

The reported incidence of lactic acidosis in patients receiving metformin is very low (approximately 0.03 cases/1,000 patient years of exposure, with approximately 0.015 fatal cases/1,000 patient years of exposure). Reported cases have occurred primarily in diabetic patients with significant renal insufficiency, including both intrinsic renal disease and renal hypoperfusion, often in the setting of multiple concomitant medical/surgical problems and multiple concomitant medications. Patients with congestive heart failure requiring pharmacologic management, in particular those with unstable or acute congestive heart failure who are at risk of hypoperfusion and hypoxemia, are at increased risk of lactic acidosis. The risk of lactic acidosis increases with the degree of renal dysfunction and the patient's age. The

risk of lactic acidosis may, therefore, be significantly decreased by regular monitoring of renal function in patients taking AVANDAMET and by use of the minimum effective dose of AVANDAMET. In particular, treatment of the elderly should be accompanied by careful monitoring of renal function.

Treatment with AVANDAMET should not be initiated in patients ≥80 years of age unless measurement of creatinine clearance demonstrates that renal function is not reduced, as these patients are more susceptible to developing lactic acidosis. In addition, AVANDAMET should be promptly withheld in the presence of any condition associated with hypoxemia, dehydration, or sepsis. Because impaired hepatic function may significantly limit the ability to clear lactate, AVANDAMET should generally be avoided in patients with clinical or laboratory evidence of hepatic disease. Patients should be cautioned against excessive alcohol intake, either acute or chronic, when taking AVANDAMET, since alcohol potentiates the effects of metformin on lactate metabolism. In addition, AVANDAMET should be temporarily discontinued prior to any intravascular radiocontrast study and for any surgical procedure.

The onset of lactic acidosis often is subtle, and accompanied only by nonspecific symptoms such as malaise, myalgias, respiratory distress, increasing somnolence, and nonspecific abdominal distress. There may be associated hypothermia, hypotension, and resistant bradyarrhythmias with more marked acidosis. The patient and the patient's physician must be aware of the possible importance of such symptoms and the patient should be instructed to notify the physician immediately if they occur. AVANDAMET should be withdrawn until the situation is clarified. Serum electrolytes, ketones, blood glucose and, if indicated, blood pH, lactate levels, and even blood metformin levels may be useful. Once a patient is stabilized on any dose level of AVANDAMET, gastrointestinal symptoms, which are common during initiation of therapy, are unlikely to be drug related. Later occurrence of gastrointestinal symptoms could be due to lactic acidosis or other serious disease.

Levels of fasting venous plasma lactate above the upper limit of normal but less than 5 mmol/L in patients taking AVANDAMET do not necessarily indicate impending lactic acidosis and may be explainable by other mechanisms, such as poorly controlled diabetes or obesity, vigorous physical activity or technical problems in sample handling.

Lactic acidosis should be suspected in any diabetic patient with metabolic acidosis lacking evidence of ketoacidosis (ketonuria and ketonemia).

Lactic acidosis is a medical emergency that must be treated in a hospital setting. In a patient with lactic acidosis who is taking AVANDAMET, the drug should be discontinued immediately and general supportive measures promptly instituted. Because metformin is dialyzable (with a clearance of up to 170 mL/min under good hemodynamic conditions), prompt hemodialysis is recommended to correct the acidosis and remove the accumulated metformin. Such management often results in prompt reversal of symptoms and recovery [see Contraindications (4)].

Factors That May Predispose Patients to Lactic Acidosis: Assessment of Renal Function: Metformin is known to be substantially excreted by the kidney, and the risk of metformin accumulation and lactic acidosis increases with the degree of impairment of renal function. Thus, patients with serum creatinine levels above the upper limit of normal for their age should not receive AVANDAMET. In patients with advanced age, AVANDAMET should be carefully titrated to establish the minimum dose for adequate glycemic effect, because aging is associated with reduced renal function. [See Dosage and Administration (2.4) and Use in Specific Populations (8.5).]

Before initiation of therapy with AVANDAMET and at least annually thereafter, renal function should be assessed and verified as normal. In patients in whom development of renal dysfunction is anticipated, renal function should be assessed more frequently and AVANDAMET discontinued if evidence of renal impairment is present.

Medications That Affect Renal Function: Concomitant medication(s) that may affect renal function or result in significant hemodynamic change or may interfere with the disposition of metformin, such as cationic drugs that are eliminated by renal tubular secretion [see Drug Interactions (7.2) and Clinical Pharmacology (12.4)], should be used with caution.

Hypoxic States: Cardiovascular collapse (shock) from whatever cause, acute congestive heart failure, acute myocardial infarction, and other conditions characterized by hypoxemia have been associated with lactic acidosis and may also cause prerenal azotemia. When such events occur in patients receiving AVANDAMET, the drug should be promptly discontinued.

Radiologic Studies With Intravascular Iodinated Contrast Materials: Intravascular contrast studies with iodinated materials can lead to acute alteration of renal function and have been associated with lactic acidosis in patients receiving metformin [see Contraindications (4)]. Therefore, in patients in whom any such study is planned, AVANDAMET should be temporarily discontinued at the time of or prior to the procedure, and withheld for 48 hours subsequent to the procedure and reinstituted only after renal function has been re-evaluated and found to be normal.

Surgical Procedures: Use of AVANDAMET should be temporarily suspended for any surgical procedure (except minor procedures not associated with restricted intake of food and fluids) and should not be restarted until the patient's oral intake has resumed and renal function has been evaluated as normal.

Alcohol Intake: Alcohol potentiates the effect of metformin on lactate metabolism. Patients, therefore, should be warned against excessive alcohol intake, acute or chronic, while receiving AVANDAMET.

Change in Clinical Status of Patients With Previously Controlled Diabetes: A patient with type 2 diabetes previously well-controlled on AVANDAMET who develops laboratory abnormalities or clinical illness (especially vague and poorly defined illness) should be evaluated promptly for evidence of ketoacidosis or lactic acidosis. Evaluation should include serum electrolytes and ketones, blood glucose and, if indicated, blood pH, lactate, pyruvate, and metformin levels. If acidosis of either form occurs, AVANDAMET must be stopped immediately and other appropriate corrective measures initiated.

[See also Warnings and Precautions (5.7).]

5.2 Cardiac Failure

Rosiglitazone, like other thiazolidinediones, alone or in combination with other antidiabetic agents, can cause fluid retention, which may exacerbate or lead to heart failure. Patients should be observed for signs and symptoms of heart failure. If these signs and symptoms develop, the heart failure should be managed according to current standards of care. Furthermore, discontinuation or dose reduction of rosiglitazone must be considered *[see **Boxed Warning**]*.

Patients with congestive heart failure (CHF) NYHA Class I and II treated with rosiglitazone have an increased risk of cardiovascular events. A 52-week, double-blind, placebo-controlled echocardiographic study was conducted in 224 patients with type 2 diabetes mellitus and NYHA Class I or II CHF (ejection fraction ≤45%) on background antidiabetic and CHF therapy. An independent committee conducted a blinded evaluation of fluid-related events (including congestive heart failure) and cardiovascular hospitalizations according to predefined criteria (adjudication). Separate from the adjudication, other cardiovascular adverse events were reported by investigators. Although no treatment difference in change from baseline of ejection fractions was observed, more cardiovascular adverse events were observed with rosiglitazone treatment compared to placebo during the 52-week study. (See Table 2.)

Table 2. Emergent Cardiovascular Adverse Events in Patients With Congestive Heart Failure (NYHA Class I and II) Treated With Rosiglitazone or Placebo (in Addition to Background Antidiabetic and CHF Therapy)

Events	Rosiglitazone	Placebo
	N = 110 n (%)	N = 114 n (%)
Adjudicated		
Cardiovascular deaths	5 (5%)	4 (4%)
CHF worsening	7 (6%)	4 (4%)
– with overnight hospitalization	5 (5%)	4 (4%)
– without overnight hospitalization	2 (2%)	0 (0%)
New or worsening edema	28 (25%)	10 (9%)
New or worsening dyspnea	29 (26%)	19 (17%)
Increases in CHF medication	36 (33%)	20 (18%)
Cardiovascular hospitalization*	21 (19%)	15 (13%)
Investigator-reported, non-adjudicated		
Ischemic adverse events	10 (9%)	5 (4%)
– Myocardial infarction	5 (5%)	2 (2%)
– Angina	6 (5%)	3 (3%)

*Includes hospitalization for any cardiovascular reason.

Initiation of AVANDAMET in patients with established NYHA Class III or IV heart failure is contraindicated. AVANDAMET is not recommended in patients with symptomatic heart failure. *[See **Boxed Warning**.]*

Patients experiencing acute coronary syndromes have not been studied in controlled clinical trials. In view of the potential for development of heart failure in patients having an acute coronary event, initiation of AVANDAMET is not recommended for patients experiencing an acute coronary event, and discontinuation of AVANDAMET during this acute phase should be considered.

Patients with NYHA Class III and IV cardiac status (with or without CHF) have not been studied in controlled clinical trials. AVANDAMET is not recommended in patients with NYHA Class III and IV cardiac status.

5.3 Myocardial Ischemia

Meta-Analysis of Myocardial Ischemia in a Group of 42 Clinical Trials of Rosiglitazone: A meta-analysis was conducted retrospectively to assess cardiovascular adverse events reported across 42 double-blind, randomized, controlled clinical trials (mean duration 6 months).[1] These studies had been conducted to assess glucose-lowering efficacy in type 2 diabetes, and prospectively planned adjudication of cardiovascular events had not occurred in the trials. Some trials were placebo-controlled and some used active oral antidiabetic drugs as controls. Placebo-controlled studies included monotherapy trials (monotherapy with rosiglitazone versus placebo monotherapy) and add-on trials (rosiglitazone or placebo, added to sulfonylurea, metformin, or insulin). Active control studies included monotherapy trials (monotherapy with rosiglitazone versus sulfonylurea or metformin monotherapy) and add-on trials (rosiglitazone plus sulfonylurea or rosiglitazone plus metformin, versus sulfonylurea plus metformin). A total of 14,237 patients were included (8,604 in treatment groups containing rosiglitazone, 5,633 in comparator groups), with 4,143 patient-years of exposure to rosiglitazone and 2,675 patient-years of exposure to comparator. Myocardial ischemic events included angina pectoris, angina pectoris aggravated, unstable angina, cardiac arrest, chest pain, coronary artery occlusion, dyspnea, myocardial infarction, coronary thrombosis, myocardial ischemia, coronary artery disease, and coronary artery disorder. In this analysis, an increased risk of myocardial ischemia with rosiglitazone versus pooled comparators was observed (2% rosiglitazone versus 1.5% comparators, odds ratio 1.4, 95% confidence interval [CI] 1.1, 1.8). An increased risk of myocardial ischemic events with rosiglitazone was observed in the placebo-controlled studies, but not in the active-controlled studies. (See Figure 1.)

A greater increased risk of myocardial ischemic events was observed in studies where rosiglitazone was added to insulin (2.8% for rosiglitazone plus insulin versus 1.4% for placebo plus insulin, [OR 2.1, 95% CI 0.9, 5.1]). This increased risk reflects a difference of 3 events per 100 patient-years (95% CI −0.1, 6.3) between treatment groups. *[See Warnings and Precautions (5.4).]*

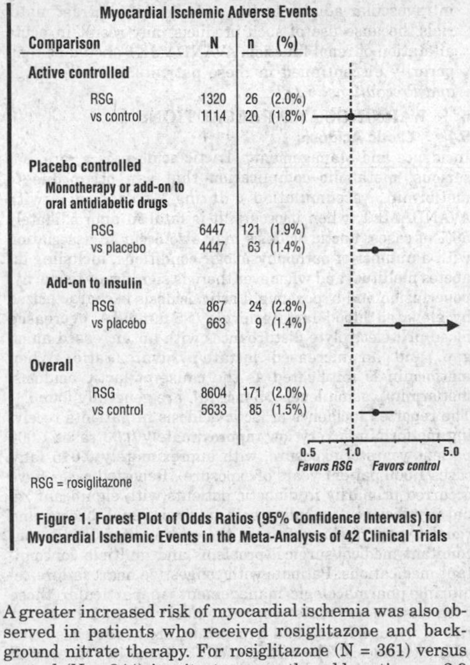
Myocardial Ischemic Adverse Events
Comparison
N
n (%)
Active controlled
RSG 1320 26 (2.0%)
vs control 1114 20 (1.8%)
Placebo controlled
Monotherapy or add-on to oral antidiabetic drugs
RSG 6447 121 (1.9%)
vs placebo 4447 63 (1.4%)
Add-on to insulin
RSG 867 24 (2.8%)
vs placebo 663 9 (1.4%)
Overall
RSG 8604 171 (2.0%)
vs control 5633 85 (1.5%)
0.5
1.0
5.0
Favors RSG
Favors control

RSG = rosiglitazone

Figure 1. Forest Plot of Odds Ratios (95% Confidence Intervals) for Myocardial Ischemic Events in the Meta-Analysis of 42 Clinical Trials

A greater increased risk of myocardial ischemia was also observed in patients who received rosiglitazone and background nitrate therapy. For rosiglitazone (N = 361) versus control (N = 244) in nitrate users, the odds ratio was 2.9 (95% CI 1.4, 5.9), while for non-nitrate users (about 14,000 patients total), the odds ratio was 1.3 (95% CI 0.9, 1.7). This increased risk represents a difference of 12 myocardial ischemic events per 100 patient years (95% CI 3.3, 21.4). Most of the nitrate users had established coronary heart disease. Among patients with known coronary heart disease who were not on nitrate therapy, an increased risk of myocardial ischemic events for rosiglitazone versus comparator was not demonstrated.

Myocardial Ischemic Events in Large Long-Term Prospective Randomized Controlled Trials of Rosiglitazone: Data from 3 other large long-term prospective randomized controlled clinical trials of rosiglitazone were assessed separately from the meta-analysis. These 3 trials include a total of 14,067 patients (treatment groups containing rosiglitazone N = 6,311, comparator groups N = 7,756), with patient-year exposure of 21,803 patient-years for rosiglitazone and 25,998 patient-years for comparator. Duration of follow-up exceeded 3 years in each study. ADOPT (A Diabetes Outcomes Progression Trial) was a 4- to 6-year randomized, active-controlled study in recently diagnosed patients with type 2 diabetes naïve to drug therapy. It was an efficacy and general safety trial that was designed to examine the durability of rosiglitazone as monotherapy (N = 1,456) for glycemic control in type 2 diabetes, with comparator arms of sulfonylurea monotherapy (N = 1,441) and metformin monotherapy (N = 1,454). DREAM (Diabetes Reduction Assessment with Rosiglitazone and Ramipril Medication, published report[2]) was a 3- to 5-year randomized, placebo-controlled study in patients with impaired glucose tolerance and/or impaired fasting glucose. It had a 2×2 factorial design, intended to evaluate the effect of rosiglitazone, and separately of ramipril (an angiotensin converting enzyme inhibitor [ACEI]), on progression to overt diabetes. In DREAM, 2,635 patients were in treatment groups containing rosiglitazone, and 2,634 were in treatment groups not containing rosiglitazone. Interim results have been published[3] for RECORD (Rosiglitazone Evaluated for Cardiac Outcomes and Regulation of Glycemia in Diabetes), an ongoing open-label, 6-year cardiovascular outcomes study in patients with type 2 diabetes with an average treatment duration of 3.75 years. RECORD includes patients who have failed metformin or sulfonylurea monotherapy; those who have failed metformin are randomized to receive either add-on rosiglitazone or add-on sulfonylurea, and those who have failed sulfonylurea are randomized to receive either add-on rosiglitazone or add-on metformin. In RECORD, a total of 2,220 patients are receiving add-on rosiglitazone, and 2,227 patients are on one of the add-on regimens not containing rosiglitazone.

For these 3 trials, analyses were performed using a composite of major adverse cardiovascular events (myocardial infarction, cardiovascular death, or stroke), referred to hereafter as MACE. This endpoint differed from the meta-analysis's broad endpoint of myocardial ischemic events, more than half of which were angina. Myocardial infarction included adjudicated fatal and nonfatal myocardial infarction plus sudden death. As shown in Figure 2, the results for the 3 endpoints (MACE, MI, and Total Mortality) were not statistically significantly different between rosiglitazone and comparators.

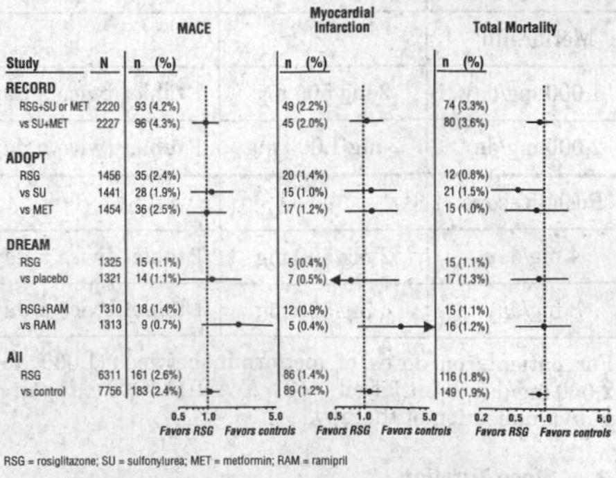
MACE
Myocardial Infarction
Total Mortality
Study N n (%) n (%) n (%)
RECORD
RSG+SU or MET 2220 93 (4.2%) 49 (2.2%) 74 (3.3%)
vs SU+MET 2227 96 (4.3%) 45 (2.0%) 80 (3.6%)
ADOPT
RSG 1456 35 (2.4%) 20 (1.4%) 12 (0.8%)
vs SU 1441 28 (1.9%) 15 (1.0%) 21 (1.5%)
vs MET 1454 36 (2.5%) 17 (1.2%) 15 (1.0%)
DREAM
RSG 1325 15 (1.1%) 5 (0.4%) 15 (1.1%)
vs placebo 1321 14 (1.1%) 7 (0.5%) 17 (1.3%)
RSG+RAM 1310 18 (1.4%) 12 (0.9%) 15 (1.1%)
vs RAM 1313 9 (0.7%) 5 (0.4%) 16 (1.2%)
All
RSG 6311 161 (2.6%) 86 (1.4%) 116 (1.8%)
vs control 7756 183 (2.4%) 89 (1.2%) 149 (1.9%)
0.5 1.0 5.0
Favors RSG Favors controls
0.5 1.0 5.0
Favors RSG Favors controls
0.2 0.5 1.0 5.0
Favors RSG Favors controls

RSG = rosiglitazone; SU = sulfonylurea; MET = metformin; RAM = ramipril

Figure 2. Hazard Ratios for the Risk of MACE (Myocardial Infarction, Cardiovascular Death, or Stroke), Myocardial Infarction, and Total Mortality With Rosiglitazone Compared With a Control Group

In preliminary analyses of the DREAM trial, the incidence of cardiovascular events was higher among subjects who received rosiglitazone in combination with ramipril than among subjects who received ramipril alone, as illustrated in Figure 2. This finding was not confirmed in ADOPT and RECORD (active-controlled trials in patients with diabetes) in which 30% and 40% of patients respectively, reported ACE-inhibitor use at baseline.

In their entirety, the available data on the risk of myocardial ischemia with rosiglitazone use are inconclusive. Definitive conclusions regarding this risk await completion of an adequately-designed cardiovascular outcome study.

There have been no clinical studies establishing conclusive evidence of macrovascular risk reduction with AVANDAMET or any other antidiabetic drug.

5.4 Congestive Heart Failure and Myocardial Ischemia During Coadministration of Rosiglitazone With Insulin

In studies in which rosiglitazone was added to insulin, rosiglitazone increased the risk of congestive heart failure and myocardial ischemia. (See Table 3.) Coadministration of AVANDAMET and insulin is not recommended. *[See Indications and Usage (1.1) and Warnings and Precautions (5.3).]*

In five, 26-week, controlled, randomized, double-blind trials which were included in the meta-analysis *[see Warnings and Precautions (5.3)]*, patients with type 2 diabetes mellitus were randomized to coadministration of rosiglitazone and insulin (N = 867) or insulin (N = 663). In these 5 trials, rosiglitazone was added to insulin. These trials included patients with long-standing diabetes (median duration of 12 years) and a high prevalence of pre-existing medical conditions, including peripheral neuropathy, retinopathy, ischemic heart disease, vascular disease, and congestive heart failure. The total number of patients with emergent congestive heart failure was 21 (2.4%) and 7 (1.1%) in the rosiglitazone plus insulin and insulin groups, respectively. The total number of patients with emergent myocardial ischemia was 24 (2.8%) and 9 (1.4%) in the rosiglitazone plus insulin and insulin groups, respectively (OR 2.1 [95% CI 0.9, 5.1]). Although the event rate for congestive heart failure and myocardial ischemia was low in the studied population, consistently the event rate was 2-fold or higher with coadministration of rosiglitazone and insulin. These cardiovascular events were noted at both the 4 mg and 8 mg daily doses of rosiglitazone. (See Table 3.)

Table 3. Occurrence of Cardiovascular Events in 5 Controlled Trials of Addition of Rosiglitazone to Established Insulin Treatment

Event*	Rosiglitazone + Insulin (N = 867) n (%)	Insulin (N = 663) n (%)
Congestive heart failure	21 (2.4%)	7 (1.1%)
Myocardial ischemia	24 (2.8%)	9 (1.4%)
Composite of cardiovascular death, myocardial infarction, or stroke	10 (1.2%)	5 (0.8%)
Stroke	5 (0.6%)	4 (0.6%)
Myocardial infarction	4 (0.5%)	1 (0.2%)
Cardiovascular death	4 (0.5%)	1 (0.2%)
All deaths	6 (0.7%)	1 (0.2%)

*Events are not exclusive; i.e., a patient with a cardiovascular death due to a myocardial infarction would be counted in 4 event categories (myocardial ischemia; cardiovascular death, myocardial infarction or stroke; myocardial infarction; cardiovascular death).

In a sixth, 24-week, controlled, randomized, double-blind trial of rosiglitazone and insulin coadministration, insulin was added to AVANDAMET (N = 161) and compared to insulin plus placebo (N = 158), after a single-blind 8-week run-in with AVANDAMET. Patients with edema requiring pharmacologic therapy and those with congestive heart failure were excluded at baseline and during the run-in period. In the group receiving AVANDAMET plus insulin, there was one myocardial ischemic event and one sudden death. No myocardial ischemia was observed in the insulin group, and no congestive heart failure was reported in either treatment group.

5.5 Edema

AVANDAMET should be used with caution in patients with edema. In a clinical study in healthy volunteers who received rosiglitazone 8 mg once daily for 8 weeks, there was a statistically significant increase in median plasma volume compared to placebo. Since thiazolidinediones, including rosiglitazone, can cause fluid retention, which can exacerbate or lead to congestive heart failure, AVANDAMET should be used with caution in patients at risk for heart failure. Patients should be monitored for signs and symptoms of heart failure *[see **Boxed Warning**, Warnings and Precautions (5.2), and Patient Counseling Information (17.1)].*

In controlled clinical trials of patients with type 2 diabetes, mild to moderate edema was reported in patients treated

Table 4. Weight Changes (kg) From Baseline at Endpoint During Clinical Trials [Median (25th, 75th, Percentile)]

Monotherapy

Duration	Control Group		Rosiglitazone 4 mg	Rosiglitazone 8 mg
26 weeks	Placebo	-0.9 (-2.8, 0.9) N = 210	1.0 (0.9, 3.6) N = 436	3.1 (1.1, 5.8) N = 439
52 weeks	Sulfonylurea	2.0 (0, 4.0) N = 173	2.0 (-0.6, 4.0) N = 150	2.6 (0, 5.3) N = 157

Combination Therapy

Duration	Control Group		Rosiglitazone + Control Therapy	
			Rosiglitazone 4 mg	Rosiglitazone 8 mg
24–26 weeks	Sulfonylurea	0 (-1.0, 1.3) N = 1,155	2.2 (0.5, 4.0) N = 613	3.5 (1.4, 5.9) N = 841
26 weeks	Metformin	-1.4 (-3.2, 0.2) N = 175	0.8 (-1.0, 2.6) N = 100	2.1 (0, 4.3) N = 184
26 weeks	Insulin	0.9 (-0.5, 2.7) N = 162	4.1 (1.4, 6.3) N = 164	5.4 (3.4, 7.3) N = 150

AVANDAMET in Patients With Inadequate Control on Diet and Exercise

Duration	Control Group		AVANDAMET
32 weeks	Metformin	-2.2 (-5.5, -0.5) N = 123	0.05 kg (-3.45, 3.0) N = 136
	Rosiglitazone	1.7 (-1.2, 4.5) N = 136	

AVANDAMET + Insulin

Duration	Control Group	AVANDAMET + Insulin
24 weeks	Insulin	2.6 kg (0.3, 4.8) N = 145	3.3 kg (1.5, 6.0) N = 147

with rosiglitazone, and may be dose-related. Patients with ongoing edema were more likely to have adverse events associated with edema if started on combination therapy with insulin and rosiglitazone *[see Adverse Reactions (6.1)]*. The use of AVANDAMET in combination with insulin is not recommended. *[See Warnings and Precautions (5.4).]*

5.6 Weight Gain

Dose-related weight gain was seen with rosiglitazone alone and rosiglitazone together with other hypoglycemic agents (see Table 4). No overall change in median weight was observed with AVANDAMET in drug-naïve patients. The mechanism of weight gain with rosiglitazone is unclear but probably involves a combination of fluid retention and fat accumulation.

[See table 4 above]

In a 4- to 6-year, monotherapy, comparative trial (ADOPT) in patients recently diagnosed with type 2 diabetes not previously treated with antidiabetic medication, the median weight change (25th, 75th percentiles) from baseline at 4 years was 3.5 kg (0.0, 8.1) for rosiglitazone, 2.0 kg (-1.0, 4.8) for glyburide, and -2.4 kg (-5.4, 0.5) for metformin.

In postmarketing experience with rosiglitazone alone or in combination with other hypoglycemic agents, there have been rare reports of unusually rapid increases in weight and increases in excess of that generally observed in clinical trials. Patients who experience such increases should be assessed for fluid accumulation and volume-related events such as excessive edema and congestive heart failure *[see Boxed Warning]*.

5.7 Hepatic Effects

Metformin: Since impaired hepatic function has been associated with some cases of lactic acidosis, AVANDAMET should generally be avoided in patients with clinical or laboratory evidence of hepatic disease.

Rosiglitazone: Liver enzymes should be measured prior to the initiation of therapy with AVANDAMET in all patients and periodically thereafter per the clinical judgment of the healthcare professional. Therapy with AVANDAMET should not be initiated in patients with increased baseline liver enzyme levels (ALT >2.5× upper limit of normal). Patients with mildly elevated liver enzymes (ALT levels ≤2.5× upper limit of normal) at baseline or during therapy with AVANDAMET should be evaluated to determine the cause of the liver enzyme elevation. Initiation of, or continuation of, therapy with AVANDAMET in patients with mild liver enzyme elevations should proceed with caution and include close clinical follow-up, including more frequent liver enzyme monitoring, to determine if the liver enzyme elevations resolve or worsen. If at any time ALT levels increase to >3× the upper limit of normal in patients on therapy with

AVANDAMET, liver enzyme levels should be rechecked as soon as possible. If ALT levels remain >3× the upper limit of normal, therapy with AVANDAMET should be discontinued. If any patient develops symptoms suggesting hepatic dysfunction, which may include unexplained nausea, vomiting, abdominal pain, fatigue, anorexia, and/or dark urine, liver enzymes should be checked. The decision whether to continue the patient on therapy with AVANDAMET should be guided by clinical judgment pending laboratory evaluations. If jaundice is observed, drug therapy should be discontinued.

In addition, if the presence of hepatic disease or hepatic dysfunction of sufficient magnitude to predispose to lactic acidosis is confirmed, therapy with AVANDAMET should be discontinued.

5.8 Macular Edema

Macular edema has been reported in postmarketing experience in some diabetic patients who were taking rosiglitazone or another thiazolidinedione. Some patients presented with blurred vision or decreased visual acuity, but some patients appear to have been diagnosed on routine ophthalmologic examination. Most patients had peripheral edema at the time macular edema was diagnosed. Some patients had improvement in their macular edema after discontinuation of their thiazolidinedione. Patients with diabetes should have regular eye exams by an ophthalmologist, per the Standards of Care of the American Diabetes Association. Additionally, any diabetic who reports any kind of visual symptom should be promptly referred to an ophthalmologist, regardless of the patient's underlying medications or other physical findings. *[See Adverse Reactions (6.3).]*

5.9 Fractures

In a 4- to 6-year comparative study (ADOPT) of glycemic control with monotherapy in drug-naïve patients recently diagnosed with type 2 diabetes mellitus, an increased incidence of bone fracture was noted in female patients taking rosiglitazone. Over the 4- to 6-year period, the incidence of bone fracture in females was 9.3% (60/645) for rosiglitazone versus 3.5% (21/605) for glyburide and 5.1% (30/590) for metformin. This increased incidence was noted after the first year of treatment and persisted during the course of the study. The majority of the fractures in the women who received rosiglitazone occurred in the upper arm, hand, and foot. These sites of fracture are different from those usually associated with postmenopausal osteoporosis (e.g., hip or spine). No increase in fracture rates was observed in men treated with rosiglitazone. The risk of fracture should be considered in the care of patients, especially female patients, treated with rosiglitazone, and attention given to assessing and maintaining bone health according to current standards of care.

Table 5. Adverse Events (≥5% for AVANDAMET) Reported by Patients With Inadequate Glycemic Control on Diet and Exercise in a 32-week Double-Blind Clinical Trial of AVANDAMET

	AVANDAMET	Metformin	Rosiglitazone
	N = 155	N = 154	N = 159
Preferred term	%	%	%
Nausea/vomiting	16	13	8
Diarrhea	14	21	7
Headache	11	12	10
Dyspepsia	10	8	9
Upper respiratory tract infection	9	7	8
Dizziness	8	3	5
Edema	6	3	7
Nasopharyngitis	6	5	4
Abdominal pain	5	6	7
Arthralgia	5	3	7
Loose stools	5	6	1
Constipation	5	4	6

Table 6. Adverse Events (≥5% for Rosiglitazone Plus Metformin) Reported by Patients in 26-week Double-blind Clinical Trials of Rosiglitazone Added to Metformin Therapy

	Rosiglitazone + Metformin	Rosiglitazone	Placebo	Metformin
	N = 338	N = 2,526	N = 601	N = 225
Preferred term	%	%	%	%
Upper respiratory tract infection	16.0	9.9	8.7	8.9
Diarrhea	12.7	2.3	3.3	15.6
Injury	8.0	7.6	4.3	7.6
Anemia	7.1	1.9	0.7	2.2
Headache	6.5	5.9	5.0	8.9
Sinusitis	6.2	3.2	4.5	5.3
Fatigue	5.9	3.6	5.0	4.0
Back pain	5.0	4.0	3.8	4.0
Viral infection	5.0	3.2	4.0	3.6
Arthralgia	5.0	3.0	4.0	2.2

5.10 Hematologic Effects
Decreases in mean hemoglobin and hematocrit occurred in a dose-related fashion in adult patients treated with rosiglitazone [see Adverse Reactions (6.2)]. The observed changes may be related to the increased plasma volume observed with treatment with rosiglitazone and may be dose-related. The decrease in hemoglobin was seen more frequently in combination rosiglitazone and metformin therapy than in rosiglitazone therapy alone. Vitamin B_{12} deficiency may contribute to the observed reductions in hemoglobin [see Warnings and Precautions (5.11)]. Initial and periodic monitoring of hematologic parameters (e.g., hemoglobin/hematocrit and red blood cell indices) should be performed, at least on an annual basis.

5.11 Vitamin B_{12} Levels
In controlled clinical trials of metformin of 29 weeks' duration, a decrease to subnormal levels of previously normal serum vitamin B_{12} levels, without clinical manifestations, was observed in approximately 7% of patients. Such decrease, possibly due to interference with B_{12} absorption from the B_{12}-intrinsic factor complex, is, however, very rarely associated with anemia and appears to be rapidly reversible with discontinuation of metformin or vitamin B_{12} supplementation. Certain individuals (those with inadequate vitamin B_{12} or calcium intake or absorption) appear to be predisposed to developing subnormal vitamin B_{12} levels. In these patients, routine serum vitamin B_{12} measurements at 2- to 3-year intervals may be useful. Vitamin B_{12} deficiency should be excluded if megaloblastic anemia is suspected. [See Warnings and Precautions (5.10).]

5.12 Diabetes and Blood Glucose Control
Periodic fasting blood glucose and HbA1c measurements should be performed to monitor therapeutic response.

When a patient stabilized on any diabetic regimen is exposed to stress such as fever, trauma, infection, or surgery, a temporary loss of glycemic control may occur. At such times, it may be necessary to withhold AVANDAMET and temporarily administer insulin. AVANDAMET may be reinstituted after the acute episode is resolved.

Hypoglycemia does not occur in patients receiving metformin alone under usual circumstances of use but could occur when caloric intake is deficient, when strenuous exercise is not compensated by caloric supplementation, or during concomitant use with hypoglycemic agents (such as sulfonylureas or insulin) or ethanol. Elderly, debilitated or malnourished patients, and those with adrenal or pituitary insufficiency or alcohol intoxication are particularly susceptible to hypoglycemic effects. Hypoglycemia may be difficult to recognize in the elderly and in people who are taking β-adrenergic blocking drugs.

Patients receiving rosiglitazone in combination with other hypoglycemic agents may be at risk for hypoglycemia, and a reduction in the dose of the concomitant agent may be necessary.

5.13 Ovulation
Therapy with rosiglitazone, like other thiazolidinediones, may result in ovulation in some premenopausal anovulatory women. As a result, these patients may be at an increased risk for pregnancy while taking AVANDAMET [see Use in Specific Populations (8.1)]. Thus, adequate contraception in premenopausal women should be recommended. This possible effect has not been specifically investigated in clinical studies; therefore, the frequency of this occurrence is not known.

Although hormonal imbalance has been seen in preclinical studies [see Nonclinical Toxicology (13.1)], the clinical significance of this finding is not known. If unexpected menstrual dysfunction occurs, the benefits of continued therapy with AVANDAMET should be reviewed.

6 ADVERSE REACTIONS
6.1 Clinical Trial Experience
Because clinical trials are conducted under widely varying conditions, adverse reaction rates observed in the clinical trials of a drug cannot be directly compared to rates in the clinical trials of another drug and may not reflect the rates observed in practice.

Patients With Inadequate Glycemic Control on Diet and Exercise: Table 5 summarizes the incidence and types of adverse reactions without regard to causality reported in a controlled, 32-week double-blind clinical trial of AVANDAMET in patients with inadequate glycemic control on diet and exercise (N = 468).

[See table 5 at left]

Mild (no intervention required) to moderate (minor intervention required) symptomatic hypoglycemia was reported by 18/155 (12%) of patients treated with AVANDAMET, 14/154 (9%) with metformin, and 13/159 (8%) with rosiglitazone. Approximately half of these episodes were accompanied by a simultaneous capillary glucose measurement, and the rate of confirmed hypoglycemia (blood glucose ≤50 mg/dL) was low in this clinical study: 0.6% (1/155) for AVANDAMET, 1.3% (2/154) for metformin and 0% with rosiglitazone. No hypoglycemic episode led to withdrawal with AVANDAMET treatment, and no patients required medical intervention due to hypoglycemia.

The incidence of edema was 6% on AVANDAMET compared to 7% on rosiglitazone and 3% on metformin.

The incidence of anemia was 4% in patients treated with AVANDAMET compared to either rosiglitazone (2%) or metformin (0%).

Patients Inadequately Controlled on Rosiglitazone Monotherapy: The incidence and types of adverse events reported in controlled, 26-week clinical trials of rosiglitazone administered in combination with metformin 2,500 mg/day in comparison to adverse reactions reported in association with rosiglitazone and metformin monotherapies are shown in Table 6. Overall, the types of adverse reactions without regard to causality reported when rosiglitazone was used in combination with metformin were similar to those reported during monotherapy with rosiglitazone.

[See table 6 at left]

Reports of hypoglycemia in patients treated with rosiglitazone added to maximum metformin therapy in double-blind studies were more frequent (3.0%) than in patients treated with rosiglitazone (0.6%) or metformin monotherapies (1.3%) or placebo (0.2%). Overall, anemia and edema were generally mild to moderate in severity and usually did not require discontinuation of treatment with rosiglitazone.

Edema was reported in 4.8% of patients receiving rosiglitazone compared to 1.3% on placebo, and 2.2% on metformin monotherapy and 4.4% on rosiglitazone in combination with maximum doses of metformin.

Reports of anemia (7.1%) were greater in patients treated with rosiglitazone added to metformin compared to monotherapy with rosiglitazone. Lower pre-treatment hemoglobin/hematocrit levels in patients enrolled in the metformin and rosiglitazone combination therapy clinical trials may have contributed to the higher reporting rate of anemia in these studies [see Adverse Reactions (6.2)].

Combination with Insulin: The incidence of hypoglycemia (confirmed by fingerstick blood glucose concentration ≤50 mg/dL) was 14% for patients on AVANDAMET plus insulin compared to 10% for patients on insulin monotherapy.

The incidence of edema was 7% when insulin was added to AVANDAMET compared to 3% with insulin monotherapy. This trial excluded patients with pre-existing heart failure or new or worsening edema on AVANDAMET therapy. However, in 26-week double-blind, fixed-dose studies of rosiglitazone added to insulin, edema was reported with higher frequency (rosiglitazone in combination with insulin, 14.7%; insulin, 5.4%) [see Warnings and Precautions (5.4).]

In studies in which rosiglitazone was added to insulin, rosiglitazone increased the risk of congestive heart failure and myocardial ischemia [see Warnings and Precautions (5.4)].

In a study in which insulin was added to AVANDAMET, no myocardial ischemia was observed in the insulin group (N = 158), and no congestive heart failure was reported in either group. There was one myocardial ischemic event and one sudden death in the group receiving AVANDAMET plus insulin (N = 161). [See Warnings and Precautions (5.4).]

The incidence of anemia was 2% for AVANDAMET in combination with insulin compared to 1% for insulin monotherapy.

A long-term, 4- to 6-year study (ADOPT) compared the use of rosiglitazone (n = 1,456), glyburide (n = 1,441), and metformin (n = 1,454) as monotherapy in patients recently diagnosed with type 2 diabetes who were not previously treated with antidiabetic medication. Table 7 presents adverse reactions without regard to causality; rates are expressed per 100 patient-years (PY) exposure to account for the differences in exposure to study medication across the 3 treatment groups.

In ADOPT, fractures were reported in a greater number of women treated with rosiglitazone (9.3%, 2.7/100 patient-years) compared to glyburide (3.5%, 1.3/100 patient-years) or metformin (5.1%, 1.5/100 patient-years). The majority of the fractures in the women who received rosiglitazone were reported in the upper arm, hand, and foot. *[See Warnings and Precautions (5.9).]* The observed incidence of fractures for male patients was similar among the 3 treatment groups.

[See table 7 at right]

Table 7. On-Therapy Adverse Events (≥5 Events/100 Patient-Years [PY]) in Any Treatment Group Reported in a 4- to 6-Year Clinical Trial of Rosiglitazone as Monotherapy (ADOPT)

	Rosiglitazone	Glyburide	Metformin
	N = 1,456	N = 1,441	N = 1,454
	PY = 4,954	PY = 4,244	PY = 4,906
Nasopharyngitis	6.3	6.9	6.6
Back pain	5.1	4.9	5.3
Arthralgia	5.0	4.8	4.2
Hypertension	4.4	6.0	6.1
Upper respiratory tract infection	4.3	5.0	4.7
Hypoglycemia	2.9	13.0	3.4
Diarrhea	2.5	3.2	6.8

6.2 Laboratory Abnormalities

Hematologic: Decreases in mean hemoglobin and hematocrit occurred in a dose-related fashion in adult patients treated with rosiglitazone (mean decreases in individual studies as much as 1.0 gram/dL hemoglobin and as much as 3.3% hematocrit). The changes occurred primarily during the first 3 months following initiation of rosiglitazone therapy or following an increase in rosiglitazone dose. The time course and magnitude of decreases were similar in patients treated with a combination of rosiglitazone and other hypoglycemic agents or monotherapy with rosiglitazone. Pretreatment levels of hemoglobin and hematocrit were lower in patients in metformin combination studies and may have contributed to the higher reporting rate of anemia. In a single study in pediatric patients, decreases in hemoglobin and hematocrit (mean decreases of 0.29 g/dL and 0.95%, respectively) were reported with rosiglitazone. White blood cell counts also decreased slightly in adult patients treated with rosiglitazone. Decreases in hematologic parameters may be related to increased plasma volume observed with rosiglitazone treatment.

In controlled clinical trials of metformin of 29 weeks' duration, a decrease to subnormal levels of previously normal serum vitamin B_{12} levels, without clinical manifestations, was observed in approximately 7% of patients. Such a decrease, possibly due to interference with B_{12} absorption from the B_{12}-intrinsic factor complex, is, however, very rarely associated with anemia and appears to be rapidly reversible with discontinuation of metformin metformin or vitamin B_{12} supplementation.

Lipids: Changes in serum lipids have been observed following treatment with rosiglitazone in adults *[see Clinical Pharmacology (12.2)]*.

Serum Transaminase Levels: In pre-approval clinical studies in 4,598 patients treated with rosiglitazone encompassing approximately 3,600 patient years of exposure, and in a long-term 4- to 6-year study in 1,456 patients treated with rosiglitazone (4,954 patient-years exposure), there was no evidence of drug-induced hepatotoxicity.

In pre-approval controlled trials, 0.2% of patients treated with rosiglitazone had reversible elevations in ALT >3× the upper limit of normal compared to 0.2% on placebo and 0.5% on active comparators. The ALT elevations in patients treated with rosiglitazone were reversible. Hyperbilirubinemia was found in 0.3% of patients treated with rosiglitazone compared with 0.9% treated with placebo and 1% in patients treated with active comparators. In pre-approval clinical trials, there were no cases of idiosyncratic drug reactions leading to hepatic failure. *[see Warnings and Precautions (5.7)]*.

In the 4- to 6-year ADOPT trial, patients treated with rosiglitazone (4,954 patient-years exposure), glyburide (4,244 patient-years exposure) or metformin (4,906 patient-years exposure) as monotherapy, had the same rate of ALT increase to >3× upper limit of normal (0.3 per 100 patient-years exposure).

6.3 Postmarketing Experience

In addition to adverse reactions reported from clinical trials, the events described below have been identified during post-approval use of AVANDAMET or its individual components. Because these events are reported voluntarily from a population of unknown size, it is not possible to reliably estimate their frequency or to always establish a causal relationship to drug exposure.

In patients receiving thiazolidinedione therapy, serious adverse events with or without a fatal outcome, potentially related to volume expansion (e.g., congestive heart failure, pulmonary edema, and pleural effusions) have been reported *[see **Boxed Warning** and Warnings and Precautions (5.2)]*.

There are postmarketing reports with rosiglitazone of hepatitis, hepatic enzyme elevations to 3 or more times the upper limit of normal, and hepatic failure with and without fatal outcome, although causality has not been established. There are postmarketing reports with rosiglitazone of rash, pruritus, urticaria, angioedema, anaphylactic reaction, Stevens-Johnson syndrome, and new onset or worsening diabetic macular edema with decreased visual acuity *[see Warnings and Precautions (5.8)]*.

(See also GLUCOPHAGE® prescribing information.)

7 DRUG INTERACTIONS

7.1 Drugs Metabolized by Cytochrome P450

An inhibitor of CYP2C8 (e.g., gemfibrozil) may increase the AUC of rosiglitazone and an inducer of CYP2C8 (e.g., rifampin) may decrease the AUC of rosiglitazone. Therefore, if an inhibitor or an inducer of CYP2C8 is started or stopped during treatment with rosiglitazone, changes in diabetes treatment may be needed based upon clinical response. *[See Clinical Pharmacology (12.4).]*

7.2 Cationic Drugs

Although drug interactions for metformin with cationic drugs (e.g., amiloride, digoxin, morphine, procainamide, quinidine, quinine, ranitidine, triamterene, trimethoprim, and vancomycin) remain theoretical (except for cimetidine), careful patient monitoring and dose adjustment of AVANDAMET and/or the interfering drug is recommended in patients who are taking cationic medications that are excreted via the proximal renal tubular secretory system. *[See Warnings and Precautions (5.1) and Clinical Pharmacology (12.4).]*

7.3 Drugs That Produce Hyperglycemia

When drugs that produce hyperglycemia which may lead to loss of glycemic control are administered to a patient receiving AVANDAMET, the patient should be closely observed to maintain adequate glycemic control. *[See Clinical Pharmacology (12.4).]*

8 USE IN SPECIFIC POPULATIONS

8.1 Pregnancy

Pregnancy Category C.

All pregnancies have a background risk of birth defects, loss, or other adverse outcome regardless of drug exposure. This background risk is increased in pregnancies complicated by hyperglycemia and may be decreased with good metabolic control. It is essential for patients with diabetes or history of gestational diabetes to maintain good metabolic control before conception and throughout pregnancy. Careful monitoring of glucose control is essential in such patients. Most experts recommend that insulin monotherapy be used during pregnancy to maintain blood glucose levels as close to normal as possible. AVANDAMET should not be used during pregnancy.

Human Data: There are no adequate and well-controlled studies with AVANDAMET or its individual components in pregnant women. Rosiglitazone has been reported to cross the human placenta and be detectable in fetal tissue. The clinical significance of these findings is unknown.

Animal Studies: No animal studies have been conducted with AVANDAMET. The following data are based on findings in studies performed with rosiglitazone or metformin individually.

Rosiglitazone: There was no effect on implantation or the embryo with rosiglitazone treatment during early pregnancy in rats, but treatment during mid-late gestation was associated with fetal death and growth retardation in both rats and rabbits. Teratogenicity was not observed at doses up to 3 mg/kg in rats and 100 mg/kg in rabbits (approximately 20 and 75 times human AUC at the maximum recommended human daily dose of the rosiglitazone component of AVANDAMET, respectively). Rosiglitazone caused placental pathology in rats (3 mg/kg/day). Treatment of rats during gestation through lactation reduced litter size, neonatal viability, and postnatal growth, with growth retardation reversible after puberty. For effects on the placenta, embryo/fetus, and offspring, the no-effect dose was 0.2 mg/kg/day in rats and 15 mg/kg/day in rabbits. These no-effect levels are approximately 4 times human AUC at the maximum recommended human daily dose of the rosiglitazone component of AVANDAMET. Rosiglitazone reduced the number of uterine implantations and live offspring when juvenile female rats were treated at 40 mg/kg/day from 27 days of age through to sexual maturity (approximately 68 times human AUC at the maximum recommended daily dose). The no-effect level was 2 mg/kg/day (approximately 4 times human AUC at the maximum recommended daily dose). There was no effect on pre- or post-natal survival or growth.

Metformin: Metformin was not teratogenic in rats and rabbits at doses up to 600 mg/kg/day. This represents an exposure of about 2 and 6 times the maximum recommended human daily dose of 2,000 mg based on body surface area comparisons for rats and rabbits, respectively. Determination of fetal concentrations demonstrated a partial placental barrier to metformin.

8.2 Labor And Delivery

The effect of AVANDAMET or its components on labor and delivery in humans is unknown.

8.3 Nursing Mothers

No studies have been conducted with AVANDAMET. In studies performed with the individual components, both rosiglitazone-related material and metformin were detectable in milk from lactating rats. It is not known whether rosiglitazone or metformin is excreted in human milk. Because many drugs are excreted in human milk, AVANDAMET should not be administered to a nursing woman.

8.4 Pediatric Use

Safety and effectiveness of AVANDAMET in pediatric patients have not been established. AVANDAMET and rosiglitazone are not indicated for use in pediatric patients.

8.5 Geriatric Use

Metformin is known to be substantially excreted by the kidney and because the risk of serious adverse reactions to the drug is greater in patients with impaired renal function, AVANDAMET should only be used in patients with normal renal function *[see Contraindications (4), Warnings and Precautions (5.1), and Clinical Pharmacology (12.3)]*. Because reduced renal function is associated with increasing age, AVANDAMET should be used with caution in elderly patients. Care should be taken in dose selection and should be based on careful and regular monitoring of renal function. Generally, elderly patients should not be titrated to the maximum dose of AVANDAMET *[see Dosage and Administration (2.4) and Warnings and Precautions (5.1)]*.

10 OVERDOSAGE

Rosiglitazone: Limited data are available with regard to overdosage in humans. In clinical studies in volunteers, rosiglitazone has been administered at single oral doses of up to 20 mg and was well tolerated. In the event of an overdose, appropriate supportive treatment should be initiated as dictated by the patient's clinical status.

Metformin: Hypoglycemia has not been seen with ingestion of up to 85 grams of metformin, although lactic acidosis has occurred in such circumstances *[see Warnings and Precautions (5.1)]*. Metformin is dialyzable with a clearance of up to 170 mL/min under good hemodynamic conditions. Therefore, hemodialysis may be useful for removal of accumulated metformin from patients in whom metformin overdosage is suspected.

11 DESCRIPTION

AVANDAMET contains 2 oral antidiabetic drugs: rosiglitazone maleate and metformin hydrochloride.

Table 8. Summary of Mean* Lipid Changes in a 32-Week Study of AVANDAMET in Patients with Type 2 Diabetes Mellitus Who Have Inadequate Glycemic Control on Diet and Exercise

	AVANDAMET $N^\dagger$ = 132	Rosiglitazone $N^\dagger$ = 128	Metformin $N^\dagger$ = 117
Total Cholesterol (mg/dL)			
Baseline (mean)	200.4	198.4	201.6
% Change from baseline (mean)	-2.2%	5.3%	-9.0%
LDL (mg/dL)			
Baseline (mean)	113.8	114.6	116.0
% Change from baseline (mean)	-0.2%	4.5%	-10.7%
HDL (mg/dL)			
Baseline (mean)	42.6	42.8	42.9
% Change from baseline (mean)	5.8%	3.1%	0.0%
Triglycerides (mg/dL)			
Baseline (mean)	180.3	166.6	175.7
% Change from baseline (mean)	-18.7%	-4.8%	-15.4%

* Data presented as geometric means throughout table.
† N = number of subjects with a baseline and end of treatment value.

Rosiglitazone maleate is an oral antidiabetic agent, which acts primarily by increasing insulin sensitivity. Rosiglitazone improves glycemic control while reducing circulating insulin levels. Rosiglitazone maleate is not chemically or functionally related to the sulfonylureas, the biguanides, or the alpha-glucosidase inhibitors. Chemically, rosiglitazone maleate is (±)-5-[[4-[2-(methyl-2-pyridinylamino)ethoxy]phenyl]methyl]-2,4-thiazolidine-dione, (Z)-2-butenedioate (1:1) with a molecular weight of 473.52 (357.44 free base). The molecule has a single chiral center and is present as a racemate. Due to rapid interconversion, the enantiomers are functionally indistinguishable. The molecular formula is $C_{18}H_{19}N_3O_3S \bullet C_4H_4O_4$. Rosiglitazone maleate is a white to off-white solid with a melting point range of 122° to 123°C. The pK_a values of rosiglitazone maleate are 6.8 and 6.1. It is readily soluble in ethanol and a buffered aqueous solution with pH of 2.3; solubility decreases with increasing pH in the physiological range. The structural formula of rosiglitazone maleate is:

Metformin hydrochloride (N,N-dimethylimidodicarbonimidic diamide hydrochloride) is not chemically or pharmacologically related to any other classes of oral antidiabetic agents. Metformin hydrochloride is a white to off-white crystalline compound with a molecular formula of $C_4H_{11}N_5 \bullet HCl$ and a molecular weight of 165.63. Metformin hydrochloride is freely soluble in water and is practically insoluble in acetone, ether, and chloroform. The pK_a of metformin is 12.4. The pH of a 1% aqueous solution of metformin hydrochloride is 6.68. The structural formula of metformin hydrochloride is:

AVANDAMET is available for oral administration as film-coated tablets containing rosiglitazone maleate and metformin hydrochloride equivalent to: 2 mg rosiglitazone with 500 mg metformin hydrochloride (2 mg/500 mg), 4 mg rosiglitazone with 500 mg metformin hydrochloride (4 mg/500 mg), 2 mg rosiglitazone with 1,000 mg metformin hydrochloride (2 mg/1,000 mg), and 4 mg rosiglitazone with 1,000 mg metformin hydrochloride (4 mg/1,000 mg). Inactive ingredients are: Hypromellose 2910, lactose monohydrate, magnesium stearate, microcrystalline cellulose, polyethylene glycol 400, povidone 29-32, sodium starch glycolate, titanium dioxide, and 1 or more of the following: Red and yellow iron oxides.

12   CLINICAL PHARMACOLOGY
12.1   Mechanism Of Action
AVANDAMET: AVANDAMET combines 2 antidiabetic agents with different mechanisms of action to improve glycemic control in patients with type 2 diabetes: Rosiglitazone, a member of the thiazolidinedione class, and metformin, a member of the biguanide class. Thiazolidinediones are insulin sensitizing agents that act primarily by enhancing peripheral glucose utilization, whereas biguanides act primarily by decreasing endogenous hepatic glucose production.

Rosiglitazone: Rosiglitazone improves glycemic control by improving insulin sensitivity. Rosiglitazone is a highly selective and potent agonist for the peroxisome proliferator–activated receptor-gamma (PPARγ). In humans, PPAR receptors are found in key target tissues for insulin action such as adipose tissue, skeletal muscle, and liver. Activation of PPARγ nuclear receptors regulates the transcription of insulin-responsive genes involved in the control of glucose production, transport, and utilization. In addition, PPARγ-responsive genes also participate in the regulation of fatty acid metabolism.

Insulin resistance is a common feature characterizing the pathogenesis of type 2 diabetes. The antidiabetic activity of rosiglitazone has been demonstrated in animal models of type 2 diabetes in which hyperglycemia and/or impaired glucose tolerance is a consequence of insulin resistance in target tissues. Rosiglitazone reduces blood glucose concentrations and reduces hyperinsulinemia in the ob/ob obese mouse, db/db diabetic mouse, and fa/fa fatty Zucker rat.

In animal models, the antidiabetic activity of rosiglitazone was shown to be mediated by increased sensitivity to insulin's action in the liver, muscle, and adipose tissue. Pharmacologic studies in animal models indicate that rosiglitazone improves sensitivity to insulin in muscle and adipose tissue and inhibits hepatic gluconeogenesis. The expression of the insulin-regulated glucose transporter GLUT-4 was increased in adipose tissue. Rosiglitazone did not induce hypoglycemia in animal models of type 2 diabetes and/or impaired glucose tolerance.

Metformin: Metformin is an antidiabetic agent, which improves glucose tolerance in patients with type 2 diabetes, lowering both basal and postprandial plasma glucose. Its pharmacologic mechanisms of action are different from other classes of oral antidiabetic agents. Metformin decreases hepatic glucose production, decreases intestinal absorption of glucose, and increases peripheral glucose uptake and utilization. Unlike sulfonylureas, metformin does not produce hypoglycemia in either patients with type 2 diabetes or normal subjects except in special circumstances [see Warnings and Precautions (5.12)] and does not cause hyperinsulinemia. With metformin therapy, insulin secretion remains unchanged while fasting insulin levels and day-long plasma insulin response may actually decrease.

12.2   Pharmacodynamics
In all 26-week controlled trials, across the recommended dose range, rosiglitazone as monotherapy was associated with increases in total cholesterol, LDL-cholesterol and HDL-cholesterol and decreases in free fatty acids.

The lipid profiles of AVANDAMET as well as rosiglitazone and metformin monotherapies in patients who have inadequate glycemic control on diet and exercise are shown in Table 8.
[See table 8 above]

The pattern of LDL, HDL, and total cholesterol changes following therapy with rosiglitazone added to metformin was generally similar to those seen with rosiglitazone monotherapy, and a small decrease in mean triglycerides was observed with the combination therapy.

12.3   Pharmacokinetics
Absorption: AVANDAMET: In a bioequivalence and dose proportionality study of AVANDAMET 4 mg/500 mg, both the rosiglitazone component and the metformin component were bioequivalent to coadministered 4 mg rosiglitazone tablet and 500 mg metformin tablet under fasted conditions (see Table 9). In this study, dose proportionality of rosiglitazone in the combination formulations of 1 mg/500 mg and 4 mg/500 mg was demonstrated.
[See table 9 at top of next page]
Administration of AVANDAMET 4 mg/500 mg with food resulted in no change in overall exposure (AUC) for either rosiglitazone or metformin. However, there were decreases in C_{max} of both components (22% for rosiglitazone and 15% for metformin, respectively) and a delay in T_{max} of both components (1.5 hours for rosiglitazone and 0.5 hours for metformin, respectively). These changes are not likely to be clinically significant. The pharmacokinetics of both the rosiglitazone component and the metformin component of AVANDAMET when taken with food were similar to the pharmacokinetics of rosiglitazone and metformin when administered concomitantly as separate tablets with food.

Absorption: Rosiglitazone: The absolute bioavailability of rosiglitazone is 99%. Peak plasma concentrations are observed about 1 hour after dosing. Maximum plasma concentration (C_{max}) and the area under the curve (AUC) of rosiglitazone increase in a dose-proportional manner over the therapeutic dose range.

Absorption: Metformin: The absolute bioavailability of a 500 mg metformin tablet given under fasting conditions is approximately 50% to 60%. Studies using single oral doses of metformin tablets of 500 mg to 1,500 mg, and 850 mg to 2,550 mg, indicate that there is a lack of dose proportionality with increasing doses, which is due to decreased absorption rather than an alteration in elimination.

Distribution: Rosiglitazone: The mean (CV%) oral volume of distribution (V_{ss}/F) of rosiglitazone is approximately 17.6 (30%) liters, based on a population pharmacokinetic analysis. Rosiglitazone is approximately 99.8% bound to plasma proteins, primarily albumin.

Distribution: Metformin: The apparent volume of distribution (V/F) of metformin following single oral doses of 850 mg metformin averaged 654 ± 358 L. Metformin is negligibly bound to plasma proteins. Metformin partitions into erythrocytes, most likely as a function of time. At usual clinical doses and dosing schedules of metformin, steady-state plasma concentrations of metformin are reached within 24 to 48 hours and are generally <1 mcg/mL. During controlled clinical trials, maximum metformin plasma levels did not exceed 5 mcg/mL, even at maximum doses.

Metabolism and Excretion: Rosiglitazone: Rosiglitazone is extensively metabolized with no unchanged drug excreted in the urine. The major routes of metabolism were N-demethylation and hydroxylation, followed by conjugation with sulfate and glucuronic acid. All the circulating metabolites are considerably less potent than parent and, therefore, are not expected to contribute to the insulin-sensitizing activity of rosiglitazone. In vitro data demonstrate that rosiglitazone is predominantly metabolized by Cytochrome P450 (CYP) isoenzyme 2C8, with CYP2C9 contributing as a minor pathway. Following oral or intravenous administration of [14C]rosiglitazone maleate, approximately 64% and 23% of the dose was eliminated in the urine and in the feces, respectively. The plasma half-life of [14C]related material ranged from 103 to 158 hours. The elimination half-life is 3 to 4 hours and is independent of dose.

Metabolism and Excretion: Metformin: Intravenous single-dose studies in normal subjects demonstrate that metformin is excreted unchanged in the urine and does not undergo hepatic metabolism (no metabolites have been identified in humans) nor biliary excretion. Renal clearance is approximately 3.5 times greater than creatinine clearance which indicates that tubular secretion is the major route of metformin elimination. Following oral administration, approximately 90% of the absorbed drug is eliminated via the renal route within the first 24 hours, with a plasma elimination half-life of approximately 6.2 hours. In blood, the elimination half-life is approximately 17.6 hours, suggesting that the erythrocyte mass may be a compartment of distribution.

Special Populations: Renal Impairment: In subjects with decreased renal function (based on measured creatinine clearance), the plasma and blood half-life of metformin is prolonged and the renal clearance is decreased in proportion to the decrease in creatinine clearance [see Warnings and Precautions (5.1) and GLUCOPHAGE prescribing information]. Since metformin is contraindicated in patients with renal impairment, administration of AVANDAMET is contraindicated in these patients.

Hepatic Impairment: Unbound oral clearance of rosiglitazone was significantly lower in patients with moderate to severe liver disease (Child-Pugh Class B/C) compared to healthy subjects. As a result, unbound C_{max} and AUC_{0-inf} were increased 2- and 3-fold, respectively. Elimination half-life for rosiglitazone was about 2 hours longer in patients with liver disease, compared to healthy subjects. Therapy with AVANDAMET should not be initiated if the patient exhibits clinical evidence of active liver disease or increased serum transaminase levels (ALT >2.5× upper limit of normal) at baseline *[see Warnings and Precautions (5.7)].*

No pharmacokinetic studies of metformin have been conducted in subjects with hepatic insufficiency.

Geriatric: Results of the population pharmacokinetics analysis (N = 716 <65 years; N = 331 ≥65 years) showed that age does not significantly affect the pharmacokinetics of rosiglitazone. However, limited data from controlled pharmacokinetic studies of metformin in healthy elderly subjects suggest that total plasma clearance of metformin is decreased, the half-life is prolonged, and C_{max} is increased, compared to healthy young subjects. From these data, it appears that the change in metformin pharmacokinetics with aging is primarily accounted for by a change in renal function *[see Use in Specific Populations (8.5) and GLUCOPHAGE prescribing information].* Metformin treatment and therefore treatment with AVANDAMET should not be initiated in patients ≥80 years of age unless measurement of creatinine clearance demonstrates that renal function is not reduced *[see Dosage and Administration (2) and Warnings and Precautions (5.1)].*

Gender: Results of the population pharmacokinetics analysis showed that the mean oral clearance of rosiglitazone in female patients (N = 405) was approximately 6% lower compared to male patients of the same body weight (N = 642). In rosiglitazone and metformin combination studies, efficacy was demonstrated with no gender differences in glycemic response.

Metformin pharmacokinetic parameters did not differ significantly between normal subjects and patients with type 2 diabetes when analyzed according to gender (males = 19, females = 16). Similarly, in controlled clinical studies in patients with type 2 diabetes, the antihyperglycemic effect of metformin tablets was comparable in males and females.

Race: Results of a population pharmacokinetic analysis including subjects of white, black, and other ethnic origins indicate that race has no influence on the pharmacokinetics of rosiglitazone.

No studies of metformin pharmacokinetic parameters according to race have been performed. In controlled clinical studies of metformin in patients with type 2 diabetes, the antihyperglycemic effect was comparable in whites (N = 249), blacks (N = 51), and Hispanics (N = 24).

Pediatric: No pharmacokinetic data from studies in pediatric subjects are available for AVANDAMET.

12.4 Drug-Drug Interactions

Rosiglitazone: *Drugs That Inhibit, Induce, or are Metabolized by Cytochrome P450:* In vitro drug metabolism studies suggest that rosiglitazone does not inhibit any of the major P450 enzymes at clinically relevant concentrations. In vitro data demonstrate that rosiglitazone is predominantly metabolized by CYP2C8, and to a lesser extent, 2C9. *[See Drug Interactions (7.1).]*

Rosiglitazone (4 mg twice daily) was shown to have no clinically relevant effect on the pharmacokinetics of nifedipine and oral contraceptives (ethinyl estradiol and norethindrone), which are predominantly metabolized by CYP3A4.

Gemfibrozil: Concomitant administration of gemfibrozil (600 mg twice daily), an inhibitor of CYP2C8, and rosiglitazone (4 mg once daily) for 7 days increased rosiglitazone AUC by 127%, compared to the administration of rosiglitazone (4 mg once daily) alone. Given the potential for dose-related adverse events with rosiglitazone, a decrease in the dose of rosiglitazone may be needed when gemfibrozil is introduced. *[See Drug Interactions (7.1).]*

Rifampin: Rifampin administration (600 mg once a day), an inducer of CYP2C8, for 6 days is reported to decrease rosiglitazone AUC by 66%, compared to the administration of rosiglitazone (8 mg) alone. *[See Drug Interactions (7.1).]*

Metformin: *Cationic Drugs:* Cationic drugs (e.g., amiloride, digoxin, morphine, procainamide, quinidine, quinine, ranitidine, triamterene, trimethoprim, and vancomycin) that are eliminated by renal tubular secretion theoretically have the potential for interaction with metformin by competing for common renal tubular transport systems. Such interaction between metformin and oral cimetidine has been observed in normal healthy volunteers in both single- and multiple-dose, metformin-cimetidine drug interaction studies, with a 60% increase in peak metformin plasma and whole blood concentrations and a 40% increase in plasma and whole blood metformin AUC. There was no change in elimination half-life in the single-dose study. Metformin had no effect on cimetidine pharmacokinetics.

Table 9. Mean (SD) Pharmacokinetic Parameters for Rosiglitazone and Metformin

		Pharmacokinetic Parameter			
Regimen	N	AUC_{0-inf} (ng.h/mL)	C_{max} (ng/mL)	T_{max} * (h)	$T_{1/2}$ (h)
Rosiglitazone					
A	25	1,442 (324)	242 (70)	0.95 (0.48-2.47)	4.26 (1.18)
B	25	1,398 (340)	254 (69)	0.57 (0.43-2.58)	3.95 (0.81)
C	24	349 (91)	63.0 (15.0)	0.57 (0.47-1.45)	3.87 (0.88)
Metformin					
A	25	7,116 (2,096)	1,106 (329)	2.97 (1.02-4.02)	3.46 (0.96)
B	25	7,413 (1,838)	1,135 (253)	2.50 (1.03-3.98)	3.36 (0.54)
C	24	6,945 (2,045)	1,080 (327)	2.97 (1.00-5.98)	3.35 (0.59)

*Median and range presented for T_{max}.
Regimen A = 4 mg/500 mg AVANDAMET; Regimen B = 4 mg rosiglitazone tablet + 500 mg metformin tablet; Regimen C = 1 mg/500 mg AVANDAMET

[See Warnings and Precautions (5.1) and Drug Interactions (7.2).]

Furosemide: A single-dose, metformin-furosemide drug interaction study in healthy subjects demonstrated that pharmacokinetic parameters of both compounds were affected by coadministration. Furosemide increased the metformin plasma and blood C_{max} by 22% and blood AUC by 15%, without any significant change in metformin renal clearance. When administered with metformin, the C_{max} and AUC of furosemide were 31% and 12% smaller, respectively, than when administered alone, and the terminal half-life was decreased by 32%, without any significant change in furosemide renal clearance. No information is available about the interaction of metformin and furosemide when coadministered chronically.

Nifedipine: A single-dose, metformin-nifedipine drug interaction study in normal healthy volunteers demonstrated that coadministration of nifedipine increased plasma metformin C_{max} and AUC by 20% and 9%, respectively, and increased the amount excreted in the urine. T_{max} and half-life were unaffected. Nifedipine appears to enhance the absorption of metformin. Metformin had minimal effects on nifedipine.

Other: Certain drugs tend to produce hyperglycemia and may lead to loss of glycemic control. These drugs include thiazides and other diuretics, corticosteroids, phenothiazines, thyroid products, estrogens, oral contraceptives, phenytoin, nicotinic acid, sympathomimetics, calcium channel blocking drugs, and isoniazid.

In healthy volunteers, the pharmacokinetics of metformin and propranolol and metformin and ibuprofen were not affected when coadministered in single-dose interaction studies.

Metformin is negligibly bound to plasma proteins and is therefore, less likely to interact with highly protein-bound drugs such as salicylates, sulfonamides, chloramphenicol, and probenecid.

13 NONCLINICAL TOXICOLOGY

13.1 Carcinogenesis, Mutagenesis, Impairment Of Fertility

No animal studies have been conducted with AVANDAMET. The following data are based on findings in studies performed with rosiglitazone or metformin individually.

Rosiglitazone: A 2-year carcinogenicity study was conducted in Charles River CD-1 mice at doses of 0.4, 1.5, and 6 mg/kg/day in the diet (highest dose equivalent to approximately 12 times human AUC at the maximum recommended human daily dose of the rosiglitazone component of AVANDAMET). Sprague-Dawley rats were dosed for 2 years by oral gavage at doses of 0.05, 0.3, and 2 mg/kg/day (highest dose equivalent to approximately 10 and 20 times human AUC at the maximum recommended human daily dose of the rosiglitazone component of AVANDAMET for male and female rats, respectively).

Rosiglitazone was not carcinogenic in the mouse. There was an increase in incidence of adipose hyperplasia in the mouse at doses ≥1.5 mg/kg/day (approximately 2 times human AUC at the maximum recommended human daily dose of the rosiglitazone component of AVANDAMET). In rats, there was a significant increase in the incidence of benign adipose tissue tumors (lipomas) at doses ≥0.3 mg/kg/day (approximately 2 times human AUC at the maximum recommended human daily dose of the rosiglitazone component of AVANDAMET). These proliferative changes in both species are considered due to the persistent pharmacological overstimulation of adipose tissue.

Rosiglitazone was not mutagenic or clastogenic in the in vitro bacterial assays for gene mutation, the in vitro chromosome aberration test in human lymphocytes, the in vivo mouse micronucleus test, and the in vivo/in vitro rat UDS assay. There was a small (about 2-fold) increase in mutation in the in vitro mouse lymphoma assay in the presence of metabolic activation.

Rosiglitazone had no effects on mating or fertility of male rats given up to 40 mg/kg/day (approximately 116 times human AUC at the maximum recommended human daily dose of the rosiglitazone component of AVANDAMET). Rosiglitazone altered estrous cyclicity (2 mg/kg/day) and reduced fertility (40 mg/kg/day) of female rats in association with lower plasma levels of progesterone and estradiol (approximately 20 and 200 times human AUC at the maximum recommended human daily dose of the rosiglitazone component of AVANDAMET, respectively). No such effects were noted at 0.2 mg/kg/day (approximately 3 times human AUC at the maximum recommended human daily dose of the rosiglitazone component of AVANDAMET). In juvenile rats dosed from 27 days of age through to sexual maturity (at up to 40 mg/kg/day), there was no effect on male reproductive performance, or on estrous cyclicity, mating performance or pregnancy incidence in females (approximately 68 times human AUC at the maximum recommended daily dose of rosiglitazone). In monkeys, rosiglitazone (0.6 and 4.6 mg/kg/day; approximately 3 and 15 times human AUC at the maximum recommended human daily dose of the rosiglitazone component of AVANDAMET, respectively) diminished the follicular phase rise in serum estradiol with consequential reduction in the luteinizing hormone surge, lower luteal phase progesterone levels, and amenorrhea. The mechanism for these effects appears to be direct inhibition of ovarian steroidogenesis.

Metformin: Long-term carcinogenicity studies have been performed in rats (dosing duration of 104 weeks) and mice (dosing duration of 91 weeks) at doses up to and including 900 mg/kg/day and 1,500 mg/kg/day, respectively. These doses are both approximately 4 times the maximum recommended human daily dose of 2,000 mg of the metformin component of AVANDAMET based on body surface area comparisons. No evidence of carcinogenicity with metformin was found in either male or female mice. Similarly, there was no tumorigenic potential observed with metformin in male rats. There was, however, an increased incidence of benign stromal uterine polyps in female rats treated with 900 mg/kg/day.

There was no evidence of mutagenic potential of metformin in the following in vitro tests: Ames test (*S. typhimurium*), gene mutation test (mouse lymphoma cells), or chromosomal aberrations test (human lymphocytes). Results in the in vivo mouse micronucleus test were also negative.

Fertility of male or female rats was unaffected by metformin when administrated at doses as high as 600 mg/kg/day,

Table 10. Glycemic Parameters in a 32-Week Study of AVANDAMET in Patients With Type 2 Diabetes Mellitus Inadequately Controlled With Diet and Exercise

	AVANDAMET	Rosiglitazone	Metformin
Mean Final Dose	7.2 mg/1,799 mg	7.7 mg	1,847 mg
N	152	155	150
FPG (mg/dL)			
Baseline (mean)	201	194	199
Change from baseline (mean)	-74	-47	-51
Difference between AVANDAMET and monotherapy (adjusted mean)		-22*	-22*
% of patients with ≥30 mg/dL decrease from baseline	86%	68%	64%
HbA1c (%)			
Baseline (mean)	8.9%	8.8%	8.8%
Change from baseline (mean)	-2.3%	-1.6%	-1.8%
Difference between AVANDAMET and monotherapy (adjusted mean)		-0.6*	-0.4*
% of patients with HbA1c ≥0.7% decrease from baseline	92%	79%	84%
% of Patients with HbA1c <7.0%	77%	58%	57%

*$p<0.001$ AVANDAMET compared to rosiglitazone or metformin.

Table 11. Glycemic Parameters in a 26-Week Study of Rosiglitazone Added to Metformin Therapy

	Metformin	Rosiglitazone 4 mg once daily + metformin	Rosiglitazone 8 mg once daily + metformin
N	113	116	110
FPG (mg/dL)			
Baseline (mean)	214	215	220
Change from baseline (mean)	6	-33	-48
Difference from metformin alone (adjusted mean)		-40*	-53*
% of patients with ≥30 mg/dL decrease from baseline	20%	45%	61%
HbA1c (%)			
Baseline (mean)	8.6	8.9	8.9
Change from baseline (mean)	0.5	-0.6	-0.8
Difference from metformin alone (adjusted mean)		-1.0*	-1.2*
% of patients with HbA1c ≥0.7% decrease from baseline	11%	45%	52%

*$p<0.0001$ compared to metformin.

which is approximately 3 times the maximum recommended human daily dose of the metformin component of AVANDAMET based on body surface area comparisons.

13.2 Animal Toxicology
Heart weights were increased in mice (3 mg/kg/day), rats (5 mg/kg/day), and dogs (2 mg/kg/day) with rosiglitazone treatments (approximately 5, 22, and 2 times human AUC at the maximum recommended human daily dose of the rosiglitazone component of AVANDAMET, respectively). Effects in juvenile rats were consistent with those seen in adults. Morphometric measurement indicated that there was hypertrophy in cardiac ventricular tissues, which may be due to increased heart work as a result of plasma volume expansion.

14 CLINICAL STUDIES
14.1 Patients Who Have Inadequate Glycemic Control on Diet and Exercise
In a 32-week, randomized, double-blind clinical trial, 468 patients with type 2 diabetes mellitus inadequately controlled with diet and exercise alone (mean baseline FPG 198 mg/dL and mean baseline HbA1c 8.8%) were randomized to AVANDAMET 2 mg/500 mg, rosiglitazone 4 mg, or metformin 500 mg. Doses were increased at 4-week intervals up to a maximum of 8 mg/2,000 mg for AVANDAMET, 8 mg for rosiglitazone, and 2,000 mg for metformin to reach a target mean daily glucose of ≤110 mg/dL. Following the initial dosage level, AVANDAMET, rosiglitazone, and

metformin were all administered as twice daily regimens. Statistically significant improvements in FPG and HbA1c were observed in patients treated with AVANDAMET compared to either rosiglitazone or metformin alone (see Table 10). However, when considering the choice of therapy for drug-naïve patients, the risk-benefit of initiating monotherapy or dual therapy should be considered.
[See table 10 above]
Patients screened in the double-blind clinical trial described above with HbA1c >11% or FPG >270 mg/dL were not eligible for blinded treatment but were treated with open-label AVANDAMET (4 mg/1,000 mg up to a maximum dose of 8 mg/2,000 mg). Treatment with AVANDAMET reduced mean HbA1c from a baseline of 11.8% to 7.8% and mean FPG from a baseline of 305 mg/dL to 166 mg/dL. Given the lack of direct comparators in this evaluation, determination of the exact contribution of rosiglitazone and metformin as well as diet and exercise, to the observed improvement in glycemic control is not possible.

14.2 Patients Previously Treated With Metformin
AVANDAMET was not studied in patients previously treated with metformin monotherapy; however, the combination of rosiglitazone and metformin was compared to rosiglitazone and metformin monotherapies in clinical trials. Bioequivalence between AVANDAMET and coadministered rosiglitazone tablets and metformin tablets has been demonstrated [see Clinical Pharmacology (12.3)].

A total of 670 patients with type 2 diabetes participated in two 26-week, randomized, double-blind, placebo/active-controlled studies designed to assess the efficacy of rosiglitazone in combination with metformin. Rosiglitazone, administered in either once-daily or twice-daily dosing regimens, was added to the therapy of patients who were inadequately controlled on 2.5 grams/day of metformin.
In one study, patients inadequately controlled on 2.5 grams/day of metformin (mean baseline FPG 216 mg/dL and mean baseline HbA1c 8.8%) were randomized to receive rosiglitazone 4 mg once daily, rosiglitazone 8 mg once daily, or placebo in addition to metformin. A statistically significant improvement in FPG and HbA1c was observed in patients treated with the combinations of metformin and rosiglitazone 4 mg once daily and rosiglitazone 8 mg once daily, versus patients continued on metformin alone (see Table 11).
[See table 11 at left]
In a second 26-week study, patients with type 2 diabetes inadequately controlled on 2.5 grams/day of metformin who were randomized to receive the combination of rosiglitazone 4 mg twice daily and metformin (N = 105) showed a statistically significant improvement in glycemic control with a mean treatment effect for FPG of –56 mg/dL and a mean treatment effect for HbA1c of –0.8% over metformin alone. The combination of metformin and rosiglitazone resulted in lower levels of FPG and HbA1c than either agent alone.

15 REFERENCES
1. Food and Drug Administration Briefing Document. Joint meeting of the Endocrinologic and Metabolic Drugs and Drug Safety and Risk Management Advisory Committees. July 30, 2007.
2. DREAM Trial Investigators. Effect of rosiglitazone on the frequency of diabetes in patients with impaired glucose tolerance or impaired fasting glucose: a randomised controlled trial. Lancet 2006;368:1096-1105.
3. Home PD, Pocock SJ, Beck-Nielsen H, et al. Rosiglitazone evaluated for cardiovascular outcomes – an interim analysis. NEJM 2007;357:1-11.
4. Park JY, Kim KA, Kang MH, et al. Effect of rifampin on the pharmacokinetics of rosiglitazone in healthy subjects. Clin Pharmacol Ther 2004;75:157-162.

16 HOW SUPPLIED/STORAGE AND HANDLING
Each film-coated oval tablet contains rosiglitazone as the maleate and metformin hydrochloride as follows:
2 mg/500 mg – pale pink, tablet, debossed with gsk on one side and 2/500 on the other.
4 mg/500 mg – orange, tablet, debossed with gsk on one side and 4/500 on the other.
2 mg/1,000 mg – yellow, tablet, debossed with gsk on one side and 2/1000 on the other.
4 mg/1,000 mg – pink, tablet, debossed with gsk on one side and 4/1000 on the other.
2 mg/500 mg bottles of 60: NDC 0007-3167-18
4 mg/500 mg bottles of 60: NDC 0007-3168-18
2 mg/1,000 mg bottles of 60: NDC 0007-3163-18
4 mg/1,000 mg bottles of 60: NDC 0007-3164-18
Store at 25°C (77°F); excursions permitted to 15° to 30°C (59° to 86°F). Dispense in a tight, light-resistant container.

17 PATIENT COUNSELING INFORMATION
See FDA-approved Medication Guide (17.2).
17.1 Patient Advice
Patients should be informed of the following:
• The risks of lactic acidosis, its symptoms, and conditions that predispose to its development, as noted in the WARNINGS and PRECAUTIONS sections, should be explained to patients. Patients should be advised to discontinue AVANDAMET immediately and to promptly notify their health practitioner if unexplained hyperventilation, myalgia, malaise, unusual somnolence, or other nonspecific symptoms occur. Once a patient is stabilized on any dose level of AVANDAMET, gastrointestinal symptoms, which are common during initiation of metformin therapy, are unlikely to be drug related. Later occurrence of gastrointestinal symptoms could be due to lactic acidosis or other serious disease.
• Avoid excessive alcohol intake, either acute or chronic, while receiving AVANDAMET.
• AVANDAMET is not recommended for patients with symptoms of heart failure.
• Patients with more severe heart failure (NYHA Class III or IV) cannot start AVANDAMET as the risks exceed any potential benefits in such patients.
• Results of a set of clinical studies suggest that treatment with rosiglitazone is associated with an increased risk for myocardial ischemic events, such as angina or myocardial infarction (heart attack), especially in patients taking insulin or nitrates. Because this risk has not been confirmed or excluded in different long-term trials, definitive conclusions regarding this risk await completion of an adequately-designed cardiovascular outcome study.
• AVANDAMET is not recommended for patients who are taking insulin.

- AVANDAMET is not recommended for patients who are taking nitrates.
- There are multiple medications available to treat type 2 diabetes. The benefits and risks of each available diabetes medication should be taken into account when choosing a particular diabetes medication for a given patient.
- There have been no clinical studies establishing conclusive evidence of macrovascular risk reduction with AVANDAMET or any other oral antidiabetic drug.
- Management of type 2 diabetes should include diet control. Caloric restriction, weight loss, and exercise are essential for the proper treatment of the diabetic patient because they help improve insulin sensitivity. This is important not only in the primary treatment of type 2 diabetes but also in maintaining the efficacy of drug therapy.
- It is important to adhere to dietary instructions and to regularly have blood glucose, glycosylated hemoglobin (HbA1c), renal function, and hematologic parameters tested. It can take 2 weeks to see a reduction in blood glucose and 2 to 3 months to see the full effect of AVANDAMET.
- Blood will be drawn to check their liver function prior to the start of therapy and periodically thereafter per the clinical judgment of the healthcare professional. Patients with unexplained symptoms of nausea, vomiting, abdominal pain, fatigue, anorexia, or dark urine should immediately report these symptoms to their physician.
- Patients who experience an unusually rapid increase in weight or edema or who develop shortness of breath or other symptoms of heart failure while on AVANDAMET should immediately report these symptoms to their physician.
- Therapy with AVANDAMET, like other thiazolidinediones, may result in ovulation in some premenopausal anovulatory women. As a result, these patients may be at an increased risk for pregnancy while taking AVANDAMET. Thus, adequate contraception in premenopausal women should be recommended. This possible effect has not been specifically investigated in clinical studies so the frequency of this occurrence is not known.

17.2   FDA-Approved Medication Guide
See separate leaflet.
AVANDAMET and AVANDIA are registered trademarks of GlaxoSmithKline.
GLUCOPHAGE is a registered trademark of Merck Santé S.A.S. (an associate of Merck KGaA of Darmstadt, Germany; licensed to Bristol-Myers Squibb Company).
GlaxoSmithKline
Research Triangle Park, NC 27709
©2008, GlaxoSmithKline. All rights reserved.

MEDICATION GUIDE
AVANDAMET® (ah-VAN-duh-met)
Rosiglitazone Maleate and Metformin Hydrochloride Tablets
Read this Medication Guide carefully before you start taking AVANDAMET and each time you get a refill. There may be new information. This information does not take the place of talking with your doctor about your medical condition or your treatment. If you have any questions about AVANDAMET, ask your doctor or pharmacist.

What is the most important information I should know about AVANDAMET?
AVANDAMET is a prescription medicine to treat adults with diabetes. It helps to control high blood sugar. (See "What is AVANDAMET?"). Each AVANDAMET tablet contains two different diabetes medicines, one is called rosiglitazone and the other is called metformin. It is important that you take AVANDAMET exactly how it is prescribed by your doctor to best treat your diabetes.
AVANDAMET may cause serious side effects, including:

New or worse heart failure
- Rosiglitazone, one of the medicines in AVANDAMET, can cause your body to keep extra fluid (fluid retention), which leads to swelling (edema) and weight gain. Extra body fluid can make some heart problems worse or lead to heart failure. Heart failure means your heart does not pump blood well enough.
- If you have severe heart failure, you cannot start AVANDAMET.
- If you have heart failure with symptoms (such as shortness of breath or swelling), even if these symptoms are not severe, AVANDAMET may not be right for you.

Call your doctor right away if you have any of the following:
- swelling or fluid retention, especially in the ankles or legs
- shortness of breath or trouble breathing, especially when you lie down
- an unusually fast increase in weight
- unusual tiredness

Other heart problems
Rosiglitazone, one of the medicines in AVANDAMET may raise the risk of heart problems related to reduced blood flow to the heart. These include possible increases in the risk of heart-related chest pain (angina) or "heart attack"

(myocardial infarction). This risk seemed to be higher in people who took rosiglitazone with insulin or with nitrate medicines. Most people who take insulin or nitrate medicines should not also take AVANDAMET.
- If you have chest pain or a feeling of chest pressure, get medical help right away, no matter what diabetes medicines you are taking.
- People with diabetes have a greater risk for heart problems. It is important to work with your doctor to manage other conditions, such as high blood pressure or high cholesterol.

Lactic acidosis
Metformin, one of the medicines in AVANDAMET, can cause a rare but serious condition called lactic acidosis (a build-up of an acid in the blood) that can cause death. Lactic acidosis is a medical emergency and must be treated in the hospital. Most people who have had lactic acidosis with metformin have other things that, combined with the metformin, led to the lactic acidosis. Tell your doctor if you have any of the following, because you have a higher chance for getting lactic acidosis with AVANDAMET if you:
- have kidney problems or your kidneys are affected by certain X-ray tests that use injectable dye. People with kidney problems should not take AVANDAMET.
- have liver problems
- drink alcohol very often, or drink a lot of alcohol in short-term "binge" drinking
- get dehydrated (lose a large amount of body fluids). This can happen if you are sick with a fever, vomiting or diarrhea. Dehydration can also happen when you sweat a lot with activity or exercise and do not drink enough fluids.
- have surgery
- have a heart attack, severe infection, or stroke
- are 80 years of age or older, and your kidneys are not working properly

The best way to keep from having a problem with lactic acidosis from metformin is to tell your doctor if you have any of the problems in the list above. Your doctor may decide to stop your AVANDAMET for a while if you have any of these things.
Lactic acidosis can be hard to diagnose early, because the early symptoms could seem like the symptoms of many other health problems besides lactic acidosis. You should call your doctor right away if you get the following symptoms, which could be signs of lactic acidosis:
- you feel very weak or tired
- you have unusual (not normal) muscle pain
- you have stomach pains
- you have trouble breathing
- you feel dizzy or lightheaded
- you have a slow or irregular heartbeat

AVANDAMET can have other serious side effects. Be sure to read the section below "What are possible side effects of AVANDAMET?".

What is AVANDAMET?
AVANDAMET contains two prescription medicines for treating diabetes, rosiglitazone maleate (AVANDIA) and metformin hydrochloride. AVANDAMET is used, with diet and exercise, to treat adults with type 2 ("adult-onset" or "non-insulin dependent") diabetes ("high blood sugar"). Metformin works mainly by decreasing the production of sugar by your liver. Rosiglitazone helps your body respond better to its natural insulin and does not cause your body to make more insulin. These medicines work together to help control your blood sugar. AVANDAMET may be used alone or with other diabetes medicines.
- For AVANDAMET to work best, it is very important to exercise, lose extra weight, and follow the diet recommended by your doctor.
- AVANDAMET has not been studied enough in children under 18 years of age to know if it is safe or effective in children.
- AVANDAMET is not for people with type 1 diabetes mellitus or to treat a condition called diabetic ketoacidosis.

Who should not take AVANDAMET?
Do not take AVANDAMET if you:
- have kidney problems. Before you take AVANDAMET and while you take it, your doctor should test your blood to check for signs of kidney problems.
- have a condition known as metabolic acidosis, including diabetic ketoacidosis.
- are going to have an x-ray procedure with an injection of dyes (contrast agents) in your vein with a needle. Talk to your doctor about when to stop AVANDAMET and when to start it again.

Many people with heart failure should not start taking AVANDAMET. See "What should I tell my doctor before taking AVANDAMET?"

What should I tell my doctor before taking AVANDAMET?
Before starting AVANDAMET, ask your doctor about what the choices are for diabetes medicines, and what the expected benefits and possible risks are for you in particular.
Before taking AVANDAMET, tell your doctor about all your medical conditions, including if you:

- have heart problems or heart failure
- have kidney problems
- have type 1 ("juvenile") diabetes or had diabetic ketoacidosis. These conditions should be treated with insulin.
- are going to have dye injected into a vein for an X-ray, CAT scan, heart study, or other type of scanning
- drink a lot of alcohol (all the time or short binge drinking).
- develop a serious condition such as a heart attack, severe infection, or a stroke.
- are 80 years old or older. People who are over 80 years old should not take AVANDAMET unless their kidney function is checked and it is normal.
- have a type of diabetic eye disease called macular edema (swelling of the back of the eye).
- have liver problems. Your doctor should do blood tests to check your liver before you start taking AVANDAMET and during treatment as needed.
- had liver problems while taking REZULIN® (troglitazone), another medicine for diabetes.
- are pregnant or plan to become pregnant. AVANDAMET should not be used during pregnancy. It is not known if AVANDAMET can harm your unborn baby. You and your doctor should talk about the best way to control your diabetes during pregnancy. If you are a premenopausal woman (before the "change of life") who does not have regular monthly periods, AVANDAMET may increase your chances of becoming pregnant. Talk to your doctor about birth control choices while taking AVANDAMET. Tell your doctor right away if you become pregnant while taking AVANDAMET.
- are breast-feeding or planning to breast-feed. It is not known if AVANDAMET passes into breast milk. You should not use AVANDAMET while breast-feeding.

Tell your doctor about all the medicines you take including prescription and non-prescription medicines, vitamins or herbal supplements. AVANDAMET and certain other medicines can affect each other and may lead to serious side effects including high blood sugar or low blood sugar, or heart problems. Your doctor may need to change your dose of AVANDAMET or your other medicines. Especially tell your doctor if you take:
- insulin.
- nitrate medicines such as nitroglycerin or isosorbide to treat a type of chest pain called angina.
- any medicines for high blood pressure, high cholesterol or heart failure, or for prevention of heart disease or stroke.

Know the medicines you take. Keep a list of all your medicines and show it to your doctor and pharmacist before you start a new medicine. They will tell you if it is okay to take AVANDAMET with other medicines.

How should I take AVANDAMET?
- Take AVANDAMET exactly as prescribed. Your doctor may need to change your dose until your blood sugar is better controlled.
- AVANDAMET should be taken by mouth and with meals.
- AVANDAMET may be prescribed alone or with other diabetes medicines. This will depend on how well your blood sugar is controlled.
- It can take 2 weeks for AVANDAMET to start lowering your blood sugar. It may take 2 to 3 months to see the full effect on your blood sugar level.
- If you miss a dose of AVANDAMET, take it as soon as you remember, unless it is time to take your next dose. Take your next dose at the usual time. Do not take double doses to make up for a missed dose.
- If you take too much AVANDAMET, call your doctor or poison control center right away.
- Test your blood sugar regularly as your doctor tells you.
- Diet and exercise can help your body use its blood sugar better. It is important to stay on your recommended diet, lose extra weight, and get regular exercise while taking AVANDAMET.
- Your doctor should do blood tests to check your liver and kidneys before you start AVANDAMET and during treatment as needed. Your doctor should also do regular blood sugar tests (for example, "A1C") to monitor your response to AVANDAMET.

There may be times when you will need to stop taking AVANDAMET for a short time. Tell your doctor if you:
- are sick with severe vomiting, diarrhea or fever, or if you drink a much lower amount of liquid than normal.
- are going to have dye injected into a vein for an X-ray, CAT scan, heart study or other type of scanning.
- plan to have surgery.

What should I avoid while taking AVANDAMET?
Do not drink a lot of alcohol while taking AVANDAMET. This means you should not "binge drink", and you should not drink a lot of alcohol on a regular basis. Drinking a lot of alcohol can increase the chance of getting lactic acidosis.

What are possible side effects of AVANDAMET?
AVANDAMET may cause serious side effects, including:
- **Weight gain.** Rosiglitazone, one of the medicines in AVANDAMET, can cause weight gain from fluid retention

or extra body fat. Metformin, the other medicine in AVANDAMET, can cause weight loss. There is little change in weight with AVANDAMET. Weight gain can be a serious problem for people with certain conditions including heart problems. See "What is the most important information I should know about AVANDAMET?"

• **Liver problems.** It is important for your liver to be working normally when you take AVANDAMET. Your doctor should do blood tests to check your liver before you start taking AVANDAMET and during treatment as needed. Call your doctor right away if you have unexplained symptoms such as:
  ◦ nausea or vomiting
  ◦ stomach pain
  ◦ unusual or unexplained tiredness
  ◦ loss of appetite
  ◦ dark urine
  ◦ yellowing of your skin or the whites of your eyes.

• **Macular edema** (a diabetic eye disease with swelling in the back of the eye). Tell your doctor right away if you have any changes in your vision. Your doctor should check your eyes regularly. Very rarely, some people have experienced vision changes due to swelling in the back of the eye while taking rosiglitazone, one of the medicines in AVANDAMET.

• **Fractures (broken bones)**, usually in the hand, upper arm or foot, in women. Talk to your doctor for advice on how to keep your bones healthy.

• **Low red blood cell count (anemia).**

• **Low blood sugar (hypoglycemia).** Lightheadedness, dizziness, shakiness or hunger may indicate that your blood sugar is too low. This can happen if you skip meals, if you use another medicine that lowers blood sugar, or if you have certain medical problems. Call your doctor if low blood sugar levels are a problem for you.

• **Ovulation** (release of egg from an ovary in a woman) leading to pregnancy. Ovulation may happen in premenopausal women who do not have regular monthly periods. This can increase the chance of pregnancy. See "What should I tell my doctor before taking AVANDAMET?".

Common side effects of AVANDAMET include:

• **Diarrhea, nausea, and upset stomach.** These side effects usually happen during the first few weeks of treatment. Taking AVANDAMET with food can help lessen these side effects. If you have unusual or unexpected stomach problems, talk with your doctor. Stomach problems that start up later during treatment with AVANDAMET may be a sign of something more serious and should be discussed with your doctor.

• **Cold-like symptoms**
• **Headache**
• **Joint aches**
• **Dizziness**

Call your doctor for medical advice about side effects. You may report side effects to FDA at 1-800-FDA-1088.

How should I store AVANDAMET?

• Store AVANDAMET at room temperature, 59° to 86°F (15° to 30°C).
• Keep AVANDAMET in the container it comes in. Keep the container closed tightly.
• Safely, throw away AVANDAMET that is out of date or no longer needed.

Keep AVANDAMET and all medicines out of the reach of children.

General information about AVANDAMET

Medicines are sometimes prescribed for purposes other than those listed in a Patient Medication Guide. Do not use AVANDAMET for a condition for which it was not prescribed. Do not give AVANDAMET to other people, even if they have the same symptoms you have. It may harm them. This Medication Guide summarizes important information about AVANDAMET. If you would like more information, talk with your doctor. You can ask your doctor or pharmacist for information about AVANDAMET that is written for healthcare professionals. For more information, call 1-888-825-5249 or go to the website www.avandamet.com.

What are the ingredients in AVANDAMET?

Active Ingredients: Rosiglitazone maleate and metformin hydrochloride

Inactive Ingredients: Hypromellose 2910, lactose monohydrate, magnesium stearate, microcrystalline cellulose, polyethylene glycol 400, povidone 29-32, sodium starch glycolate, titanium dioxide, and 1 or more of the following: Red and yellow iron oxides.

Always check to make sure that the medicine you are taking is the correct one. AVANDAMET tablets are oval and look like this:

• 2 mg/500 mg strength tablets – pale pink, printed with "gsk" on one side and "2/500" on the other.
• 4 mg/500 mg strength tablets – orange, printed with "gsk" on one side and "4/500" on the other.
• 2 mg/1,000 mg strength tablets – yellow, printed with "gsk" on one side and "2/1000" on the other
• 4 mg/1,000 mg strength tablets – pink, printed with "gsk" on one side and "4/1000" on the other

AVANDAMET and AVANDIA are registered trademarks of GlaxoSmithKline.
GLUCOPHAGE is a registered trademark of Merck Santé S.A.S., an associate of Merck KGaA of Darmstadt, Germany. Licensed to Bristol-Myers Squibb Company.
REZULIN is a registered trademark of Parke-Davis Pharmaceuticals Ltd.

This Medication Guide has been approved by the U.S. Food and Drug Administration.
GlaxoSmithKline
Research Triangle Park, NC 27709
©2008, GlaxoSmithKline. All rights reserved.
December 2008
AVM:1MG

AVANDARYL®

[ə-van' də-ril]
(rosiglitazone maleate and glimepiride)
Tablets

℞

HIGHLIGHTS OF PRESCRIBING INFORMATION
These highlights do not include all the information needed to use AVANDARYL safely and effectively. See full prescribing information for AVANDARYL.
AVANDARYL® (rosiglitazone maleate and glimepiride) Tablets
Initial U.S. Approval: 2005

WARNING: CONGESTIVE HEART FAILURE AND MYOCARDIAL ISCHEMIA
See full prescribing information for complete boxed warning.

• Thiazolidinediones, including rosiglitazone, cause or exacerbate congestive heart failure in some patients (5.2). After initiation of AVANDARYL, and after dose increases, observe patients carefully for signs and symptoms of heart failure (including excessive, rapid weight gain, dyspnea, and/or edema). If these signs and symptoms develop, the heart failure should be managed according to current standards of care. Furthermore, discontinuation or dose reduction of AVANDARYL must be considered.

• AVANDARYL is not recommended in patients with symptomatic heart failure. Initiation of AVANDARYL in patients with established NYHA Class III or IV heart failure is contraindicated. (4, 5.2)

• A meta-analysis of 42 clinical studies (mean duration 6 months; 14,237 total patients), most of which compared rosiglitazone to placebo, showed rosiglitazone to be associated with an increased risk of myocardial ischemic events such as angina or myocardial infarction. Three other studies (mean duration 41 months; 14,067 total patients), comparing rosiglitazone to some other approved oral antidiabetic agents or placebo, have not confirmed or excluded this risk. In their entirety, the available data on the risk of myocardial ischemia are inconclusive. (5.3)

——————RECENT MAJOR CHANGES——————
Warnings and Precautions, Hemolytic
Anemia (5.12)   12/2009

——————INDICATIONS AND USAGE——————
AVANDARYL is indicated as an adjunct to diet and exercise to improve glycemic control in adults with type 2 diabetes when treatment with both rosiglitazone and glimepiride is appropriate.
Important Limitations of Use:
• Should not be used in patients with type 1 diabetes or for the treatment of diabetic ketoacidosis. (1.1, 4)
• Use with nitrates is not recommended. (1.1, 5.3)
• Coadministration with insulin is not recommended. (1.1, 5.4)

——————DOSAGE AND ADMINISTRATION——————
• Individualize the starting dose based on the patient's current regimen. (2.1)
• Dose increases should be accompanied by careful monitoring for adverse events related to fluid retention. (2.2)
• Do not exceed the maximum recommended daily dose of 8 mg rosiglitazone and 4 mg glimepiride. (2.3)
• Do not initiate if the patient exhibits clinical evidence of active liver disease or increased serum transaminase levels. (2.4)

——————DOSAGE FORMS AND STRENGTHS——————
Rounded triangular tablets containing rosiglitazone/glimepiride: 4 mg/1 mg, 4 mg/2 mg, 4 mg/4 mg, 8 mg/2 mg, and 8 mg/4 mg (3)

——————CONTRAINDICATIONS——————
• Initiation in patients with established NYHA Class III or IV heart failure. (4)

——————WARNINGS AND PRECAUTIONS——————
• One sulfonylurea has been shown to increase cardiovascular mortality; consider this risk when prescribing any sulfonylurea. (5.1)
• Fluid retention, which may exacerbate or lead to heart failure, may occur. Combination use with insulin and use in congestive heart failure NYHA Class I and II may increase risk of other cardiovascular effects. (5.2, 5.4)

• Increased risk of myocardial ischemic events has been observed in a meta-analysis of 42 clinical trials of rosiglitazone (incidence rate 2% versus 1.5%). (5.3)
• Use with insulin or nitrates is not recommended. (1.2, 5.3)
• Severe hypoglycemia may occur. Use particular care in elderly or debilitated patients and those with adrenal, pituitary, renal or hepatic insufficiency. (5.5)
• Dose-related edema (5.6), weight gain (5.7), and anemia (5.11) may occur.
• Macular edema has been reported. (5.9)
• Increased incidence of bone fracture in female patients. (5.10)
• The glimepiride component may cause hemolytic anemia in patients with glucose 6-phosphate dehydrogenase (G6PD) deficiency. Consider a non-sulfonylurea alternative in these patients. (5.12)
• There have been no clinical studies establishing conclusive evidence of macrovascular risk reduction with AVANDARYL or any other antidiabetic drug. (5.3)

——————ADVERSE REACTIONS——————
Common adverse reactions (≥5%) reported in clinical trials for AVANDARYL without regard to causality were headache, hypoglycemia, and nasopharyngitis. (6.1)
To report SUSPECTED ADVERSE REACTIONS, contact GlaxoSmithKline at 1-888-825-5249 or FDA at 1-800-FDA-1088 or www.fda.gov/medwatch.

——————DRUG INTERACTIONS——————
• Inhibitors of CYP2C8 (e.g., gemfibrozil) may increase rosiglitazone levels. (7.1)
• Inducers of CYP2C8 (e.g., rifampin) may decrease rosiglitazone levels. (7.1)
• Monitor patients for loss of control with drugs that cause hyperglycemia. (7.2)

——————USE IN SPECIFIC POPULATIONS——————
• Do not use during pregnancy. No human or animal data. (8.1)
• Safety and effectiveness in children under 18 years have not been established. (8.4)
• Elderly patients may be particularly susceptible to hypoglycemic effects. (8.5)

Revised: December 2009
AVR:10PI
See 17 for PATIENT COUNSELING INFORMATION and Medication Guide

Revised: 11/2009

FULL PRESCRIBING INFORMATION: CONTENTS*
WARNING: CONGESTIVE HEART FAILURE AND MYOCARDIAL ISCHEMIA

*** Sections or subsections omitted from the full prescribing information are not listed**

FULL PRESCRIBING INFORMATION

WARNING: CONGESTIVE HEART FAILURE AND MYOCARDIAL ISCHEMIA

- **Thiazolidinediones, including rosiglitazone, cause or exacerbate congestive heart failure in some patients *[see Warnings and Precautions (5.2)]*. After initiation of AVANDARYL, and after dose increases, observe patients carefully for signs and symptoms of heart failure (including excessive, rapid weight gain, dyspnea, and/or edema). If these signs and symptoms develop, the heart failure should be managed according to current standards of care. Furthermore, discontinuation or dose reduction of AVANDARYL must be considered.**
- **AVANDARYL is not recommended in patients with symptomatic heart failure. Initiation of AVANDARYL in patients with established NYHA Class III or IV heart failure is contraindicated. *[See Contraindications (4) and Warnings and Precautions (5.2).]***
- **A meta-analysis of 42 clinical studies (mean duration 6 months; 14,237 total patients), most of which compared rosiglitazone to placebo, showed rosiglitazone to be associated with an increased risk of myocardial ischemic events such as angina or myocardial infarction. Three other studies (mean duration 41 months; 14,067 total patients), comparing rosiglitazone to some other approved oral antidiabetic agents or placebo, have not confirmed or excluded this risk. In their entirety, the available data on the risk of myocardial ischemia are inconclusive. *[See Warnings and Precautions (5.3).]***

1 INDICATIONS AND USAGE

AVANDARYL is indicated as an adjunct to diet and exercise to improve glycemic control in adults with type 2 diabetes mellitus when treatment with both rosiglitazone and glimepiride is appropriate. *[See Clinical Studies (14).]*

1.1 Important Limitations of Use

- Due to its mechanism of action, rosiglitazone is active only in the presence of endogenous insulin. Therefore, AVANDARYL should not be used in patients with type 1 diabetes or for the treatment of diabetic ketoacidosis.
- The use of AVANDARYL with nitrates is not recommended.
- The coadministration of AVANDARYL and insulin is not recommended.

2 DOSAGE AND ADMINISTRATION

Therapy with AVANDARYL should be individualized for each patient. The risk-benefit of initiating monotherapy versus dual therapy with AVANDARYL should be considered. No studies have been performed specifically examining the safety and efficacy of AVANDARYL in patients previously treated with other oral hypoglycemic agents and switched to AVANDARYL. Any change in therapy of type 2 diabetes should be undertaken with care and appropriate monitoring as changes in glycemic control can occur. *[See Indications and Usage (1).]*

2.1 Starting Dose

The recommended starting dose is 4 mg/1 mg administered once daily with the first meal of the day. For adults already treated with a sulfonylurea or a thiazolidinedione, a starting dose of 4 mg/2 mg may be considered.

All patients should start the rosiglitazone component of AVANDARYL at the lowest recommended dose. Further increases in the dose of rosiglitazone should be accompanied by careful monitoring for adverse events related to fluid retention *[see **Boxed Warning** and Warnings and Precautions (5.6)]*.

When switching from combination therapy of rosiglitazone plus glimepiride as separate tablets, the usual starting dose of AVANDARYL is the dose of rosiglitazone and glimepiride already being taken.

2.2 Dose Titration

Dose increases should be individualized according to the glycemic response of the patient. Patients who may be more sensitive to glimepiride *[see Warnings and Precautions (5.5)]*, including the elderly, debilitated, or malnourished, and those with renal, hepatic, or adrenal insufficiency, should be carefully titrated to avoid hypoglycemia. If hypoglycemia occurs during up-titration of the dose or while maintained on therapy, a dosage reduction of the glimepiride component of AVANDARYL may be considered. Increases in the dose of rosiglitazone should be accompanied by careful monitoring for adverse events related to fluid retention *[see **Boxed Warning** and Warnings and Precautions (5.6)]*.

For **adults previously treated with thiazolidinedione monotherapy** and switched to AVANDARYL, dose titration of the glimepiride component of AVANDARYL is recommended if patients are not adequately controlled after 1 to 2 weeks. The glimepiride component may be increased in no more than 2 mg increments. After an increase in the dosage of the glimepiride component, dose titration of AVANDARYL is recommended if patients are not adequately controlled after 1 to 2 weeks.

For **adults previously treated with sulfonylurea monotherapy** and switched to AVANDARYL, it may take 2 weeks to see a reduction in blood glucose and 2 to 3 months to see the full effect of the rosiglitazone component. Therefore, dose titration of the rosiglitazone component of AVANDARYL is recommended if patients are not adequately controlled after 8 to 12 weeks. Patients should be observed carefully (1 to 2 weeks) for hypoglycemia when being transferred from longer half-life sulfonylureas (e.g., chlorpropamide) to AVANDARYL due to potential overlapping of drug effect. After an increase in the dosage of the rosiglitazone component, dose titration of AVANDARYL is recommended if patients are not adequately controlled after 2 to 3 months.

2.3 Maximum Dose

The maximum recommended daily dose is 8 mg rosiglitazone and 4 mg glimepiride.

2.4 Specific Patient Populations

Elderly and Malnourished Patients and Those With Renal, Hepatic, or Adrenal Insufficiency: In elderly, debilitated, or malnourished patients, or in patients with renal, hepatic, or adrenal insufficiency, the starting dose, dose increments, and maintenance dosage of AVANDARYL should be conservative to avoid hypoglycemic reactions. *[See Warnings and Precautions (5.5) and Clinical Pharmacology (12.3).]*

Hepatic Impairment: Liver enzymes should be measured prior to initiating treatment with AVANDARYL. Therapy with AVANDARYL should not be initiated if the patient exhibits clinical evidence of active liver disease or increased serum transaminase levels (ALT >2.5× upper limit of normal at start of therapy). After initiation of AVANDARYL, liver enzymes should be monitored periodically per the clinical judgment of the healthcare professional. *[See Warnings and Precautions (5.8) and Clinical Pharmacology (12.3).]*

Pregnancy and Lactation: AVANDARYL should not be used during pregnancy or in nursing mothers.

Pediatric Use: Safety and effectiveness of AVANDARYL in pediatric patients have not been established. AVANDARYL and its components, rosiglitazone and glimepiride, are not recommended for use in pediatric patients.

3 DOSAGE FORMS AND STRENGTHS

Each rounded triangular tablet contains rosiglitazone maleate and glimepiride as follows:

- 4 mg/1 mg – yellow, gsk debossed on one side and 4/1 on the other.
- 4 mg/2 mg – orange, gsk debossed on one side and 4/2 on the other.
- 4 mg/4 mg – pink, gsk debossed on one side and 4/4 on the other.
- 8 mg/2 mg – pale pink, gsk debossed on one side and 8/2 on the other.
- 8 mg/4 mg – red, gsk debossed on one side and 8/4 on the other.

4 CONTRAINDICATIONS

Initiation of AVANDARYL in patients with established New York Heart Association (NYHA) Class III or IV heart failure is contraindicated *[see **Boxed Warning**]*.

5 WARNINGS AND PRECAUTIONS

5.1 Increased Risk of Cardiovascular Mortality for Sulfonylurea Drugs

The administration of oral hypoglycemic drugs has been reported to be associated with increased cardiovascular mortality as compared to treatment with diet alone or diet plus insulin. This warning is based on the study conducted by the University Group Diabetes Program (UGDP), a long-term, prospective clinical trial designed to evaluate the effectiveness of glucose-lowering drugs in preventing or delaying vascular complications in patients with non-insulin-dependent diabetes. The study involved 823 patients who were randomly assigned to one of four treatment groups (*Diabetes* 1970;19[Suppl. 2]:747-830). UGDP reported that patients treated for 5 to 8 years with diet plus a fixed dose of tolbutamide (1.5 grams per day) had a rate of cardiovascular mortality approximately 2½ times that of patients treated with diet alone. A significant increase in total mortality was not observed, but the use of tolbutamide was discontinued based on the increase in cardiovascular mortality, thus limiting the opportunity for the study to show an increase in overall mortality. Despite controversy regarding the interpretation of these results, the findings of the UGDP study provide an adequate basis for this warning. The patient should be informed of the potential risks and advantages of glimepiride-containing tablets and of alternative modes of therapy.

Although only one drug in the sulfonylurea class (tolbutamide) was included in this study, it is prudent from a safety standpoint to consider that this warning may also apply to other oral hypoglycemic drugs in this class, in view of their close similarities in mode of action and chemical structure.

5.2 Cardiac Failure With Rosiglitazone

Rosiglitazone, like other thiazolidinediones, alone or in combination with other antidiabetic agents, can cause fluid retention, which may exacerbate or lead to heart failure. Patients should be observed for signs and symptoms of heart failure. If these signs and symptoms develop, the heart failure should be managed according to current standards of care. Furthermore, discontinuation or dose reduction of rosiglitazone must be considered *[see **Boxed Warning**]*.

Patients with congestive heart failure (CHF) NYHA Class I and II treated with rosiglitazone have an increased risk of cardiovascular events. A 52-week, double-blind, placebo-controlled echocardiographic study was conducted in 224 patients with type 2 diabetes mellitus and NYHA Class I or II CHF (ejection fraction ≤45%) on background antidiabetic and CHF therapy. An independent committee conducted a blinded evaluation of fluid-related events (including congestive heart failure) and cardiovascular hospitalizations according to predefined criteria (adjudication). Separate from the adjudication, other cardiovascular adverse events were reported by investigators. Although no treatment difference in change from baseline of ejection fractions was observed, more cardiovascular adverse events were observed with rosiglitazone treatment compared to placebo during the 52-week study. (See Table 1.)

[See table at top of next page]

Initiation of AVANDARYL in patients with established NYHA Class III or IV heart failure is contraindicated. AVANDARYL is not recommended in patients with symptomatic heart failure. *[See **Boxed Warning**.]*

Patients experiencing acute coronary syndromes have not been studied in controlled clinical trials. In view of the potential for development of heart failure in patients having an acute coronary event, initiation of AVANDARYL is not recommended for patients experiencing an acute coronary event, and discontinuation of AVANDARYL during this acute phase should be considered.

Patients with NYHA Class III and IV cardiac status (with or without CHF) have not been studied in controlled clinical trials. AVANDARYL is not recommended in patients with NYHA Class III and IV cardiac status.

5.3 Myocardial Ischemia With Rosiglitazone

Meta-Analysis of Myocardial Ischemia in a Group of 42 Clinical Trials: A meta-analysis was conducted retrospectively to assess cardiovascular adverse events reported across 42 double-blind, randomized, controlled clinical trials (mean duration 6 months).[1] These studies had been conducted to assess glucose-lowering efficacy in type 2 diabetes, and prospectively planned adjudication of cardiovascular events had not occurred in the trials. Some trials were placebo-controlled and some used active oral antidiabetic drugs as controls. Placebo-controlled studies included monotherapy trials (monotherapy with rosiglitazone versus placebo monotherapy) and add-on trials (rosiglitazone or placebo, added to sulfonylurea, metformin, or insulin). Active control studies included monotherapy trials (monotherapy with rosiglitazone versus sulfonylurea or metformin monotherapy) and add-on trials (rosiglitazone plus sulfonylurea or rosiglitazone plus metformin, versus sulfonylurea plus metformin). A total of 14,237 patients were included (8,604 in treatment groups containing rosiglitazone, 5,633 in comparator groups), with 4,143 patient-years of exposure to rosiglitazone and 2,675 patient-years of exposure to comparator. Myocardial ischemic events included angina pectoris, angina pectoris aggravated, unstable angina, cardiac arrest, chest pain, coronary artery occlusion, dyspnea, myocardial infarction, coronary thrombosis, myocardial ischemia, coronary artery disease, and coronary artery disorder. In this analysis, an increased risk of myocardial ischemia with rosiglitazone versus pooled comparators was observed (2% rosiglitazone versus 1.5% comparators, odds ratio 1.4, 95% confidence interval [CI] 1.1, 1.8). An increased risk of myocardial ischemic events with rosiglitazone was observed in

Table 1. Emergent Cardiovascular Adverse Events in Patients With Congestive Heart Failure (NYHA Class I and II) Treated With Rosiglitazone or Placebo (in Addition to Background Antidiabetic and CHF Therapy)

Events	Rosiglitazone	Placebo
	N = 110 n (%)	N = 114 n (%)
Adjudicated		
Cardiovascular deaths	5 (5%)	4 (4%)
CHF worsening	7 (6%)	4 (4%)
– with overnight hospitalization	5 (5%)	4 (4%)
– without overnight hospitalization	2 (2%)	0 (0%)
New or worsening edema	28 (25%)	10 (9%)
New or worsening dyspnea	29 (26%)	19 (17%)
Increases in CHF medication	36 (33%)	20 (18%)
Cardiovascular hospitalization*	21 (19%)	15 (13%)
Investigator-reported, non-adjudicated		
Ischemic adverse events	10 (9%)	5 (4%)
– Myocardial infarction	5 (5%)	2 (2%)
– Angina	6 (5%)	3 (3%)

*Includes hospitalization for any cardiovascular reason.

the placebo-controlled studies, but not in the active-controlled studies. (See Figure 1.)

A greater increased risk of myocardial ischemic events was observed in studies where rosiglitazone was added to insulin (2.8% for rosiglitazone plus insulin versus 1.4% for placebo plus insulin, [OR 2.1, 95% CI 0.9, 5.1]). This increased risk reflects a difference of 3 events per 100 patient-years (95% CI -0.1, 6.3) between treatment groups. [See Warnings and Precautions (5.4).]

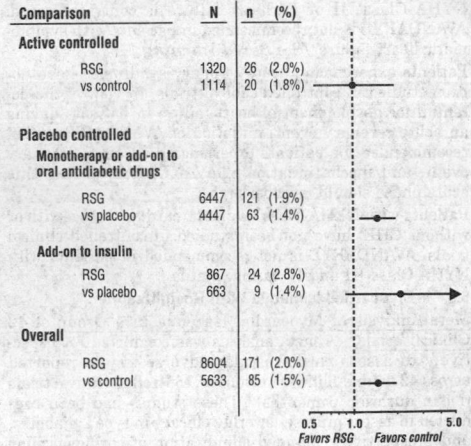

Myocardial Ischemic Adverse Events

Comparison	N	n	(%)
Active controlled			
RSG	1320	26	(2.0%)
vs control	1114	20	(1.8%)
Placebo controlled			
Monotherapy or add-on to oral antidiabetic drugs			
RSG	6447	121	(1.9%)
vs placebo	4447	63	(1.4%)
Add-on to insulin			
RSG	867	24	(2.8%)
vs placebo	663	9	(1.4%)
Overall			
RSG	8604	171	(2.0%)
vs control	5633	85	(1.5%)

0.5   1.0   5.0
Favors RSG Favors control

RSG = rosiglitazone

Figure 1. Forest Plot of Odds Ratios (95% Confidence Intervals) for Myocardial Ischemic Events in the Meta-Analysis of 42 Clinical Trials

A greater increased risk of myocardial ischemia was also observed in patients who received rosiglitazone and background nitrate therapy. For rosiglitazone (N = 361) versus control (N = 244) in nitrate users, the odds ratio was 2.9 (95% CI 1.4, 5.9), while for non-nitrate users (about 14,000 patients total), the odds ratio was 1.3 (95% CI 0.9, 1.7). This increased risk represents a difference of 12 myocardial ischemic events per 100 patient-years (95% CI 3.3, 21.4). Most of the nitrate users had established coronary heart disease. Among patients with known coronary heart disease who were not on nitrate therapy, an increased risk of myocardial ischemic events for rosiglitazone versus comparator was not demonstrated.

Myocardial Ischemic Events in Large, Long-Term, Prospective, Randomized, Controlled Trials of Rosiglitazone: Data from 3 other large, long-term, prospective, randomized, controlled clinical trials of rosiglitazone were assessed separately from the meta-analysis. These 3 trials include a total of 14,067 patients (treatment groups containing rosiglitazone N = 6,311, comparator groups N = 7,756), with

patient-year exposure of 21,803 patient-years for rosiglitazone and 25,998 patient-years for comparator. Duration of follow-up exceeded 3 years in each study. ADOPT (A Diabetes Outcomes Progression Trial) was a 4- to 6-year randomized, active-controlled study in recently diagnosed patients with type 2 diabetes naïve to drug therapy. It was an efficacy and general safety trial that was designed to examine the durability of rosiglitazone as monotherapy (N = 1,456) for glycemic control in type 2 diabetes, with comparator arms of sulfonylurea monotherapy (N = 1,441) and metformin monotherapy (N = 1,454). DREAM (Diabetes Reduction Assessment with Rosiglitazone and Ramipril Medication, published report[2]) was a 3- to 5-year randomized, placebo-controlled study in patients with impaired glucose tolerance and/or impaired fasting glucose. It had a 2×2 factorial design, intended to evaluate the effect of rosiglitazone, and separately of ramipril (an angiotensin converting enzyme inhibitor [ACEI]), on progression to overt diabetes. In DREAM, 2,635 patients were in treatment groups containing rosiglitazone, and 2,634 were in treatment groups not containing rosiglitazone. Interim results have been published[3] for RECORD (Rosiglitazone Evaluated for Cardiac Outcomes and Regulation of Glycemia in Diabetes), an ongoing open-label, 6-year cardiovascular outcomes study in patients with type 2 diabetes with an average treatment duration of 3.75 years. RECORD includes patients who have failed metformin or sulfonylurea monotherapy; those who have failed metformin are randomized to receive either add-on rosiglitazone or add-on sulfonylurea, and those who have failed sulfonylurea are randomized to receive either add-on rosiglitazone or add-on metformin. In RECORD, a total of 2,220 patients are receiving add-on rosiglitazone, and 2,227 patients are on one of the add-on regimens not containing rosiglitazone.

For these 3 trials, analyses were performed using a composite of major adverse cardiovascular events (myocardial infarction, cardiovascular death, or stroke), referred to hereafter as MACE. This endpoint differed from the meta-analysis's broad endpoint of myocardial ischemic events, more than half of which were angina. Myocardial infarction included adjudicated fatal and nonfatal myocardial infarction plus sudden death. As shown in Figure 2, the results for the 3 endpoints (MACE, MI, and Total Mortality) were not statistically significantly different between rosiglitazone and comparators.

[See figure 2 at top of next column]

In preliminary analyses of the DREAM trial, the incidence of cardiovascular events was higher among subjects who received rosiglitazone in combination with ramipril than among subjects who received ramipril alone, as illustrated in Figure 2. This finding was not confirmed in ADOPT and RECORD (active-controlled trials in patients with diabetes) in which 30% and 40% of patients respectively, reported ACE-inhibitor use at baseline.

In their entirety, the available data on the risk of myocardial ischemia with rosiglitazone use are inconclusive. Definitive conclusions regarding this risk await completion of an adequately-designed cardiovascular outcome study.

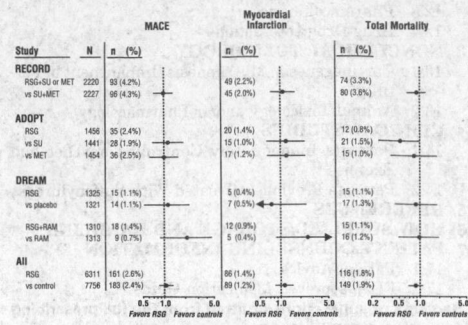

Study	N	n (%)			Myocardial Infarction n (%)			Total Mortality n (%)
RECORD								
RSG+SU or MET	2220	93 (4.2%)			49 (2.2%)			74 (3.3%)
vs SU+MET	2227	96 (4.3%)			45 (2.0%)			80 (3.6%)
ADOPT								
RSG	1456	35 (2.4%)			20 (1.4%)			12 (0.8%)
vs SU	1441	28 (1.9%)			15 (1.0%)			21 (1.5%)
vs MET	1454	36 (2.5%)			17 (1.2%)			15 (1.0%)
DREAM								
RSG	1325	15 (1.1%)			5 (0.4%)			15 (1.1%)
vs placebo	1321	14 (1.1%)			7 (0.5%)			17 (1.3%)
RSG+RAM	1310	18 (1.4%)			12 (0.9%)			15 (1.1%)
vs RAM	1313	9 (0.7%)			5 (0.4%)			16 (1.2%)
All								
RSG	6311	161 (2.6%)			86 (1.4%)			116 (1.8%)
vs control	7756	183 (2.4%)			89 (1.2%)			149 (1.9%)

0.5 1.0 5.0   0.5 1.0 5.0   0.2 1.0 5.0
Favors RSG Favors controls

RSG = rosiglitazone, SU = sulfonylurea; MET = metformin; RAM = ramipril

Figure 2. Hazard Ratios for the Risk of MACE (Myocardial Infarction, Cardiovascular Death, or Stroke), Myocardial Infarction, and Total Mortality With Rosiglitazone Compared With a Control Group

There have been no clinical studies establishing conclusive evidence of macrovascular risk reduction with AVANDARYL or any other antidiabetic drug.

5.4 Congestive Heart Failure and Myocardial Ischemia During Coadministration of Rosiglitazone With Insulin

In studies in which rosiglitazone was added to insulin, rosiglitazone increased the risk of congestive heart failure and myocardial ischemia. (See Table 2.) Coadministration of AVANDARYL and insulin is not recommended. [See Indications and Usage (1.1) and Warnings and Precautions (5.3).]

In five, 26-week, controlled, randomized, double-blind trials which were included in the meta-analysis [see Warnings and Precautions (5.3)], patients with type 2 diabetes mellitus were randomized to coadministration of rosiglitazone and insulin (N = 867) or insulin (N = 663). In these 5 trials, rosiglitazone was added to insulin. These trials included patients with long-standing diabetes (median duration of 12 years) and a high prevalence of pre-existing medical conditions, including peripheral neuropathy, retinopathy, ischemic heart disease, vascular disease, and congestive heart failure. The total number of patients with emergent congestive heart failure was 21 (2.4%) and 7 (1.1%) in the rosiglitazone plus insulin and insulin groups, respectively. The total number of patients with emergent myocardial ischemia was 24 (2.8%) and 9 (1.4%) in the rosiglitazone plus insulin and insulin groups, respectively (OR 2.1 [95% CI 0.9, 5.1]). Although the event rate for congestive heart failure and myocardial ischemia was low in the studied population, consistently the event rate was 2-fold or higher with coadministration of rosiglitazone and insulin. These cardiovascular events were noted at the 4 mg and 8 mg daily doses of rosiglitazone. (See Table 2.)

[See table 2 at top of next page]

In a sixth, 24-week, controlled, randomized, double-blind trial of rosiglitazone and insulin coadministration, insulin was added to AVANDAMET® (rosiglitazone maleate and metformin HCl) (N = 161) and compared to insulin plus placebo (N = 158), after a single-blind 8-week run-in with AVANDAMET. Patients with edema requiring pharmacologic therapy and those with congestive heart failure were excluded at baseline and during the run-in period. In the group receiving AVANDAMET plus insulin, there was one myocardial ischemic event and one sudden death. No myocardial ischemia was observed in the insulin group, and no congestive heart failure was reported in either treatment group.

5.5 Hypoglycemia

AVANDARYL is a combination tablet containing rosiglitazone and glimepiride, a sulfonylurea. All sulfonylurea drugs are capable of producing severe hypoglycemia. Proper patient selection, dosage, and instructions are important to avoid hypoglycemic episodes. Elderly patients are particularly susceptible to hypoglycemic action of glucose-lowering drugs. Debilitated or malnourished patients, and those with adrenal, pituitary, renal, or hepatic insufficiency are particularly susceptible to the hypoglycemic action of glucose-lowering drugs. A starting dose of 1 mg glimepiride, as contained in AVANDARYL 4 mg/1 mg, followed by appropriate dose titration is recommended in these patients. [See Clinical Pharmacology (12.3).] Hypoglycemia may be difficult to recognize in the elderly and in people who are taking beta-adrenergic blocking drugs or other sympatholytic agents. Hypoglycemia is more likely to occur when caloric intake is deficient, after severe or prolonged exercise, when alcohol is ingested, or when more than one glucose-lowering drug is used.

Patients receiving rosiglitazone in combination with a sulfonylurea may be at risk for hypoglycemia, and a reduction in the dose of the sulfonylurea may be necessary [see Dosage and Administration (2.2)].

5.6 Edema

AVANDARYL should be used with caution in patients with edema. In a clinical study in healthy volunteers who received 8 mg of rosiglitazone once daily for 8 weeks, there was a statistically significant increase in median plasma volume compared to placebo.

Since thiazolidinediones, including rosiglitazone, can cause fluid retention, which can exacerbate or lead to congestive heart failure, AVANDARYL should be used with caution in patients at risk for heart failure. Patients should be monitored for signs and symptoms of heart failure [see *Boxed Warning, Warnings and Precautions (5.2), and Patient Counseling Information (17.1)*].

In controlled clinical trials of patients with type 2 diabetes, mild to moderate edema was reported in patients treated with rosiglitazone, and may be dose-related. Patients with ongoing edema were more likely to have adverse events associated with edema if started on combination therapy with insulin and rosiglitazone [see *Adverse Reactions (6.1)*]. The use of AVANDARYL in combination with insulin is not recommended [see *Warnings and Precautions (5.4)*].

5.7 Weight Gain

Dose-related weight gain was seen with AVANDARYL, rosiglitazone alone, and rosiglitazone together with other hypoglycemic agents (see Table 3). The mechanism of weight gain is unclear but probably involves a combination of fluid retention and fat accumulation.

[See table 3 at right]

In a 4- to 6-year, monotherapy, comparative trial (ADOPT) in patients recently diagnosed with type 2 diabetes not previously treated with antidiabetic medication, the median weight change (25th, 75th percentiles) from baseline at 4 years was 3.5 kg (0.0, 8.1) for rosiglitazone, 2.0 kg (-1.0, 4.8) for glyburide, and -2.4 kg (-5.4, 0.5) for metformin.

In postmarketing experience with rosiglitazone alone or in combination with other hypoglycemic agents, there have been rare reports of unusually rapid increases in weight and increases in excess of that generally observed in clinical trials. Patients who experience such increases should be assessed for fluid accumulation and volume-related events such as excessive edema and congestive heart failure [see *Boxed Warning*].

5.8 Hepatic Effects

With sulfonylureas, including glimepiride, there may be an elevation of liver enzyme levels in rare cases. In isolated instances, impairment of liver function (e.g., with cholestasis and jaundice), as well as hepatitis (which may also lead to liver failure) have been reported.

Liver enzymes should be measured prior to the initiation of therapy with AVANDARYL in all patients and periodically thereafter per the clinical judgment of the healthcare professional. Therapy with AVANDARYL should not be initiated in patients with increased baseline liver enzyme levels (ALT >2.5× upper limit of normal). Patients with mildly elevated liver enzymes (ALT levels ≤2.5× upper limit of normal) at baseline or during therapy with AVANDARYL should be evaluated to determine the cause of the liver enzyme elevation. Initiation of, or continuation of, therapy with AVANDARYL in patients with mild liver enzyme elevations should proceed with caution and include close clinical follow-up, including more frequent liver enzyme monitoring, to determine if the liver enzyme elevations resolve or worsen. If at any time ALT levels increase to >3× the upper limit of normal in patients on therapy with AVANDARYL, liver enzyme levels should be rechecked as soon as possible. If ALT levels remain >3× the upper limit of normal, therapy with AVANDARYL should be discontinued.

If any patient develops symptoms suggesting hepatic dysfunction, which may include unexplained nausea, vomiting, abdominal pain, fatigue, anorexia, and/or dark urine, liver enzymes should be checked. The decision whether to continue the patient on therapy with AVANDARYL should be guided by clinical judgment pending laboratory evaluations. If jaundice is observed, drug therapy should be discontinued.

5.9 Macular Edema

Macular edema has been reported in postmarketing experience in some diabetic patients who were taking rosiglitazone or another thiazolidinedione. Some patients presented with blurred vision or decreased visual acuity, but some patients appear to have been diagnosed on routine ophthalmologic examination. Most patients had peripheral edema at the time macular edema was diagnosed. Some patients had improvement in their macular edema after discontinuation of their thiazolidinedione. Patients with diabetes should have regular eye exams by an ophthalmologist, per the Standards of Care of the American Diabetes Association. Additionally, any diabetic who reports any kind of visual symptom should be promptly referred to an ophthalmologist, regardless of the patient's underlying medications or other physical findings. [See *Adverse Reactions (6.3)*.]

5.10 Fractures

In a 4- to 6-year comparative study (ADOPT) of glycemic control with monotherapy in drug-naïve patients recently diagnosed with type 2 diabetes mellitus, an increased incidence of bone fracture was noted in female patients taking rosiglitazone. Over the 4- to 6-year period, the incidence of

bone fracture in females was 9.3% (60/645) for rosiglitazone versus 3.5% (21/605) for glyburide and 5.1% (30/590) for metformin. This increased incidence was noted after the first year of treatment and persisted during the course of the study. The majority of the fractures in the women who received rosiglitazone occurred in the upper arm, hand, and foot. These sites of fracture are different from those usually associated with postmenopausal osteoporosis (e.g., hip or spine). No increase in fracture rates was observed in men treated with rosiglitazone. The risk of fracture should be considered in the care of patients, especially female patients, treated with rosiglitazone, and attention given to assessing and maintaining bone health according to current standards of care.

5.11 Hematologic Effects

Decreases in hemoglobin and hematocrit occurred in a dose-related fashion in adult patients treated with rosiglitazone [see *Adverse Reactions (6.2)*]. The observed changes may be related to the increased plasma volume observed with treatment with rosiglitazone.

5.12 Hemolytic Anemia

Treatment of patients with glucose 6-phosphate dehydrogenase (G6PD) deficiency with sulfonylurea agents can lead to hemolytic anemia. Because glimepiride, a component of AVANDARYL, belongs to the class of sulfonylurea agents, caution should be used in patients with G6PD deficiency and a non-sulfonylurea alternative should be considered. In post-marketing experience, hemolytic anemia has also been reported in patients receiving sulfonylureas who did not have known G6PD deficiency [see *Adverse Reactions (6.1)*].

5.13 Diabetes and Blood Glucose Control

When a patient stabilized on any antidiabetic regimen is exposed to stress such as fever, trauma, infection, or surgery, a temporary loss of glycemic control may occur. At such times, it may be necessary to withhold AVANDARYL and temporarily administer insulin. AVANDARYL may be reinstituted after the acute episode is resolved.

Periodic fasting glucose and HbA1c measurements should be performed to monitor therapeutic response.

5.14 Ovulation

Therapy with rosiglitazone, like other thiazolidinediones, may result in ovulation in some premenopausal anovulatory women. As a result, these patients may be at an increased risk for pregnancy while taking rosiglitazone [see *Use in Specific Populations (8.1)*]. Thus, adequate contraception in premenopausal women should be recommended. This possible effect has not been specifically investigated in clinical studies; therefore the frequency of this occurrence is not known.

Although hormonal imbalance has been seen in preclinical studies [see *Nonclinical Toxicology (13.1)*], the clinical significance of this finding is not known. If unexpected menstrual dysfunction occurs, the benefits of continued therapy with AVANDARYL should be reviewed.

6 ADVERSE REACTIONS

6.1 Clinical Trial Experience

Because clinical trials are conducted under widely varying conditions, adverse reaction rates observed in the clinical trials of a drug cannot be directly compared to rates in the clinical trials of another drug and may not reflect the rates observed in practice.

Table 2. Occurrence of Cardiovascular Events in 5 Controlled Trials of Addition of Rosiglitazone to Established Insulin Treatment

Event*	Rosiglitazone + Insulin (N = 867) n (%)	Insulin (N = 663) n (%)
Congestive heart failure	21 (2.4%)	7 (1.1%)
Myocardial ischemia	24 (2.8%)	9 (1.4%)
Composite of cardiovascular death, myocardial infarction, or stroke	10 (1.2%)	5 (0.8%)
Stroke	5 (0.6%)	4 (0.6%)
Myocardial infarction	4 (0.5%)	1 (0.2%)
Cardiovascular death	4 (0.5%)	1 (0.2%)
All deaths	6 (0.7%)	1 (0.2%)

*Events are not exclusive; i.e., a patient with a cardiovascular death due to a myocardial infarction would be counted in 4 event categories (myocardial ischemia; cardiovascular death, myocardial infarction or stroke; myocardial infarction; cardiovascular death).

Table 3. Weight Changes (kg) From Baseline at Endpoint During Clinical Trials [Median (25th, 75th, Percentile)]

Monotherapy

Duration	Control Group		Rosiglitazone 4 mg	Rosiglitazone 8 mg
26 weeks	Placebo	-0.9 (-2.8, 0.9) N = 210	1.0 (-0.9, 3.6) N = 436	3.1 (1.1, 5.8) N = 439
52 weeks	Sulfonylurea	2.0 (0, 4.0) N = 173	2.0 (-0.6, 4.0) N = 150	2.6 (0, 5.3) N = 157

Combination Therapy

Duration	Control Group		Rosiglitazone + Control Therapy	
			Rosiglitazone 4 mg	Rosiglitazone 8 mg
24-26 weeks	Sulfonylurea	0 (-1.0, 1.3) N = 1,155	2.2 (0.5, 4.0) N = 613	3.5 (1.4, 5.9) N = 841
26 weeks	Metformin	-1.4 (-3.2, 0.2) N = 175	0.8 (-1.0, 2.6) N = 100	2.1 (0, 4.3) N = 184
26 weeks	Insulin	0.9 (-0.5, 2.7) N = 162	4.1 (1.4, 6.3) N = 164	5.4 (3.4, 7.3) N = 150

AVANDARYL in Patients With Inadequate Control on Diet and Exercise

Duration	Control Group		AVANDARYL 4 mg/4 mg	AVANDARYL 8 mg/4 mg
28 weeks	Glimepiride	1.1 (-1.1, 3.2) N = 222	2.2 (0, 4.5) N = 221	2.9 (0, 5.8) N = 217
	Rosiglitazone	0.9 (-1.4, 3.2) N = 228		

Table 4. Adverse Events (≥5% in Any Treatment Group) Reported by Patients With Inadequate Glycemic Control on Diet and Exercise in a 28-Week Double-Blind Clinical Trial of AVANDARYL

Preferred Term	Glimepiride Monotherapy	Rosiglitazone Monotherapy	AVANDARYL 4 mg/4 mg	AVANDARYL 8 mg/4 mg
	N = 222	N = 230	N = 224	N = 218
	%	%	%	%
Headache	2.3	6.1	3.1	6.0
Nasopharyngitis	3.6	5.2	4.0	4.6
Hypertension	3.6	5.2	3.1	2.3
Hypoglycemia*	4.1	0.4	3.6	5.5

*As documented by symptoms and a fingerstick blood glucose measurement of <50 mg/dL.

Table 5. On-Therapy Adverse Events (≥5 Events/100 Patient-Years [PY]) in Any Treatment Group Reported in a 4- to 6-Year Clinical Trial of Rosiglitazone as Monotherapy (ADOPT)

	Rosiglitazone	Glyburide	Metformin
	N = 1,456	N = 1,441	N = 1,454
	PY = 4,954	PY = 4,244	PY = 4,906
Nasopharyngitis	6.3	6.9	6.6
Back pain	5.1	4.9	5.3
Arthralgia	5.0	4.8	4.2
Hypertension	4.4	6.0	6.1
Upper respiratory tract infection	4.3	5.0	4.7
Hypoglycemia	2.9	13.0	3.4
Diarrhea	2.5	3.2	6.8

Patients With Inadequate Glycemic Control on Diet and Exercise: Table 4 summarizes adverse events occurring at a frequency of ≥5% in any treatment group in the 28-week double-blind trial of AVANDARYL in patients with type 2 diabetes mellitus inadequately controlled on diet and exercise. Patients in this trial were started on AVANDARYL 4 mg/1 mg, rosiglitazone 4 mg, or glimepiride 1 mg. Doses could be increased at 4-week intervals to reach a maximum total daily dose of either 4 mg/4 mg or 8 mg/4 mg for AVANDARYL, 8 mg for rosiglitazone monotherapy, or 4 mg for glimepiride monotherapy.
[See table 4 above]
Hypoglycemia was reported to be generally mild to moderate in intensity and none of the reported events of hypoglycemia resulted in withdrawal from the study. Hypoglycemia requiring parenteral treatment (i.e., intravenous glucose or glucagon injection) was observed in 3 (0.7%) patients treated with AVANDARYL.
Edema was reported by 3.2% of patients on AVANDARYL, 3.0% on rosiglitazone alone, and 2.3% on glimepiride alone. Congestive heart failure was observed in 1 (0.2%) patient treated with AVANDARYL and in 1 (0.4%) patient treated with rosiglitazone monotherapy.
Patients Treated With Rosiglitazone Added to Sulfonylurea Monotherapy and Other Experience With Rosiglitazone or Glimepiride: Studies utilizing rosiglitazone in combination with a sulfonylurea provide support for the use of AVANDARYL. Adverse event data from these trials, in addition to adverse events reported with the use of rosiglitazone and glimepiride therapy, are presented below.
Rosiglitazone: The most common adverse experiences with rosiglitazone monotherapy (≤5%) were upper respiratory tract infection, injury, and headache. Overall, the types of adverse experiences reported when rosiglitazone was added to a sulfonylurea were similar to those during monotherapy with rosiglitazone. In controlled combination therapy studies with sulfonylureas, mild to moderate hypoglycemic symptoms, which appear to be dose-related, were reported. Few patients were withdrawn for hypoglycemia (<1%) and few episodes of hypoglycemia were considered to be severe (<1%).
Events of anemia and edema tended to be reported more frequently at higher doses, and were generally mild to moderate in severity and usually did not require discontinuation of treatment with rosiglitazone.
Edema was reported by 4.8% of patients receiving rosiglitazone compared to 1.3% on placebo, and 1.0% on sulfonylurea monotherapy. The reporting rate of edema was higher for rosiglitazone 8 mg added to a sulfonylurea

(12.4%) compared to other combinations, with the exception of insulin. Anemia was reported by 1.9% of patients receiving rosiglitazone compared to 0.7% on placebo, 0.6% on sulfonylurea monotherapy, and 2.3% on rosiglitazone in combination with a sulfonylurea. Overall, the types of adverse experiences reported when rosiglitazone was added to a sulfonylurea were similar to those during monotherapy with rosiglitazone.
In 26-week double-blind, fixed-dose studies, edema was reported with higher frequency in the rosiglitazone plus insulin combination trials (insulin, 5.4%; and rosiglitazone in combination with insulin, 14.7%). Reports of new onset or exacerbation of congestive heart failure occurred at rates of 1% for insulin alone, and 2% (4 mg) and 3% (8 mg) for insulin in combination with rosiglitazone [see **Boxed Warning** and Warnings and Precautions (5.4)].
Glimepiride: Hypoglycemia: The incidence of hypoglycemia with glimepiride, as documented by blood glucose values <60 mg/dL, ranged from 0.9% to 1.7% in 2 large, well-controlled, 1-year studies. In patients treated with glimepiride in US placebo-controlled trials (N = 746), adverse events, other than hypoglycemia, considered to be possibly or probably related to study drug that occurred in more than 1% of patients included dizziness (1.7%), asthenia (1.6%), headache (1.5%), and nausea (1.1%).
• *Gastrointestinal Reactions:* Vomiting, gastrointestinal pain, and diarrhea have been reported, but the incidence in placebo-controlled trials was less than 1%. In rare cases, there may be an elevation of liver enzyme levels. In isolated instances, impairment of liver function (e.g., with cholestasis and jaundice), as well as hepatitis, which may also lead to liver failure have been reported with sulfonylureas, including glimepiride.
• *Dermatologic Reactions:* Allergic skin reactions, e.g., pruritus, erythema, urticaria, and morbilliform or maculopapular eruptions, occur in less than 1% of treated patients. These may be transient and may disappear despite continued use of glimepiride. If those hypersensitivity reactions persist or worsen, the drug should be discontinued. Porphyria cutanea tarda, photosensitivity reactions, and allergic vasculitis have been reported with sulfonylureas, including glimepiride.
• *Hematologic Reactions:* Leukopenia, agranulocytosis, thrombocytopenia, hemolytic anemia [see Warnings and Precautions (5.12)], aplastic anemia, and pancytopenia have been reported with sulfonylureas, including glimepiride.
• *Metabolic Reactions:* Hepatic porphyria reactions and disulfiram-like reactions have been reported with sulfo-

nylureas, including glimepiride. Cases of hyponatremia have been reported with glimepiride and all other sulfonylureas, most often in patients who are on other medications or have medical conditions known to cause hyponatremia or increase release of antidiuretic hormone. The syndrome of inappropriate antidiuretic hormone (SIADH) secretion has been reported with certain other sulfonylureas, including glimepiride, and it has been suggested that certain sulfonylureas may augment the peripheral (antidiuretic) action of ADH and/or increase release of ADH.
• *Other Reactions:* Changes in accommodation and/or blurred vision may occur with the use of glimepiride. This is thought to be due to changes in blood glucose, and may be more pronounced when treatment is initiated. This condition is also seen in untreated diabetic patients, and may actually be reduced by treatment. In placebo-controlled trials of glimepiride, the incidence of blurred vision was placebo, 0.7%, and glimepiride, 0.4%.
• *Human Ophthalmology Data:* Ophthalmic examinations were carried out in more than 500 subjects during long-term studies of glimepiride using the methodology of Taylor and West and Laties et al. No significant differences were seen between glimepiride and glyburide in the number of subjects with clinically important changes in visual acuity, intraocular tension, or in any of the 5 lens-related variables examined. Ophthalmic examinations were carried out during long-term studies using the method of Chylack et al. No significant or clinically meaningful differences were seen between glimepiride and glipizide with respect to cataract progression by subjective LOCS II grading and objective image analysis systems, visual acuity, intraocular pressure, and general ophthalmic examination [see Nonclinical Toxicology (13.2)].
Long-Term Trial of Rosiglitazone as Monotherapy: A 4- to 6-year study (ADOPT) compared the use of rosiglitazone (n = 1,456), glyburide (n = 1,441), and metformin (n = 1,454) as monotherapy in patients recently diagnosed with type 2 diabetes who were not previously treated with antidiabetic medication. Table 5 presents adverse reactions without regard to causality; rates are expressed per 100 patient-years (PY) exposure to account for the differences in exposure to study medication across the 3 treatment groups.
In ADOPT, fractures were reported in a greater number of women treated with rosiglitazone (9.3%, 2.7/100 patient-years) compared to glyburide (3.5%, 1.3/100 patient-years) or metformin (5.1%, 1.5/100 patient-years). The majority of the fractures in the women who received rosiglitazone were reported in the upper arm, hand, and foot. [See Warnings and Precautions (5.10).] The observed incidence of fractures for male patients was similar among the 3 treatment groups.
[See table 5 at left]
6.2 Laboratory Abnormalities
Rosiglitazone: Hematologic: Decreases in mean hemoglobin and hematocrit occurred in a dose-related fashion in adult patients treated with rosiglitazone (mean decreases in individual studies as much as 1.0 g/dL hemoglobin and as much as 3.3% hematocrit). The changes occurred primarily during the first 3 months following initiation of therapy with rosiglitazone or following a dose increase in rosiglitazone. The time course and magnitude of decreases were similar in patients treated with a combination of rosiglitazone and other hypoglycemic agents or monotherapy with rosiglitazone. White blood cell counts also decreased slightly in adult patients treated with rosiglitazone. Decreases in hematologic parameters may be related to increased plasma volume observed with treatment with rosiglitazone.
Lipids: Changes in serum lipids have been observed following treatment with rosiglitazone in adults [see Clinical Pharmacology (12.2)].
Serum Transaminase Levels: In pre-approval clinical studies in 4,598 patients treated with rosiglitazone encompassing approximately 3,600 patient-years of exposure, there was no evidence of drug-induced hepatotoxicity.
In pre-approval controlled trials, 0.2% of patients treated with rosiglitazone had reversible elevations in ALT >3× the upper limit of normal compared to 0.2% on placebo and 0.5% on active comparators. The ALT elevations in patients treated with rosiglitazone were reversible. Hyperbilirubinemia was found in 0.3% of patients treated with rosiglitazone compared with 0.9% treated with placebo and 1% in patients treated with active comparators. In pre-approval clinical trials, there were no cases of idiosyncratic drug reactions leading to hepatic failure. [See Warnings and Precautions (5.8).]
In the 4- to 6-year ADOPT trial, patients treated with rosiglitazone (4,954 patient-years exposure), glyburide (4,244 patient-years exposure) or metformin (4,906 patient-years exposure) as monotherapy had the same rate of ALT increase to >3× upper limit of normal (0.3 per 100 patient-years exposure).
6.3 Postmarketing Experience
In addition to adverse reactions reported from clinical trials, the events described below have been identified during

post-approval use of AVANDARYL or its individual components. Because these events are reported voluntarily from a population of unknown size, it is not possible to reliably estimate their frequency or to always establish a causal relationship to drug exposure.

In patients receiving thiazolidinedione therapy, serious adverse events with or without a fatal outcome, potentially related to volume expansion (e.g., congestive heart failure, pulmonary edema, and pleural effusions) have been reported *[see **Boxed Warning** and Warnings and Precautions (5.2)]*.

There are postmarketing reports with rosiglitazone of hepatitis, hepatic enzyme elevations to 3 or more times the upper limit of normal, and hepatic failure with and without fatal outcome, although causality has not been established.

There are postmarketing reports with rosiglitazone of rash, pruritus, urticaria, angioedema, anaphylactic reaction, Stevens-Johnson syndrome, and new onset or worsening diabetic macular edema with decreased visual acuity *[see Warnings and Precautions (5.9)]*.

7 DRUG INTERACTIONS

7.1 Drugs Metabolized by Cytochrome P450

An inhibitor of CYP2C8 (e.g., gemfibrozil) may increase the AUC of rosiglitazone and an inducer of CYP2C8 (e.g., rifampin) may decrease the AUC of rosiglitazone. Therefore, if an inhibitor or an inducer of CYP2C8 is started or stopped during treatment with rosiglitazone, changes in diabetes treatment may be needed based upon clinical response. *[See Clinical Pharmacology (12.4).]*

A potential interaction between oral miconazole and oral hypoglycemic agents leading to severe hypoglycemia has been reported. Whether this interaction also occurs with the IV, topical, or vaginal preparations of miconazole is not known. Potential interactions of glimepiride with other drugs metabolized by cytochrome P450 2C9 also include phenytoin, diclofenac, ibuprofen, naproxen, and mefenamic acid. *[See Clinical Pharmacology (12.4).]*

7.2 Drugs That Produce Hyperglycemia

Certain drugs tend to produce hyperglycemia and may lead to loss of control. These drugs include the thiazides and other diuretics, corticosteroids, phenothiazines, thyroid products, estrogens, oral contraceptives, phenytoin, nicotinic acid, sympathomimetics, and isoniazid. When these drugs are administered to a patient receiving glimepiride, the patient should be closely observed for loss of control. When these drugs are withdrawn from a patient receiving glimepiride, the patient should be observed closely for hypoglycemia.

8 USE IN SPECIFIC POPULATIONS

8.1 Pregnancy

Pregnancy Category C.

All pregnancies have a background risk of birth defects, loss, or other adverse outcome regardless of drug exposure. This background risk is increased in pregnancies complicated by hyperglycemia and may be decreased with good metabolic control. It is essential for patients with diabetes or history of gestational diabetes to maintain good metabolic control before conception and throughout pregnancy. Careful monitoring of glucose control is essential in such patients. Most experts recommend that insulin monotherapy be used during pregnancy to maintain blood glucose levels as close to normal as possible. AVANDARYL should not be used during pregnancy.

Human Data: There are no adequate and well-controlled studies with AVANDARYL or its individual components in pregnant women. Rosiglitazone has been reported to cross the human placenta and be detectable in fetal tissue. The clinical significance of these findings is unknown.

Animal Studies: No animal studies have been conducted with AVANDARYL. The following data are based on findings in studies performed with rosiglitazone or glimepiride individually.

Rosiglitazone: There was no effect on implantation or the embryo with rosiglitazone treatment during early pregnancy in rats, but treatment during mid-late gestation was associated with fetal death and growth retardation in both rats and rabbits. Teratogenicity was not observed at doses up to 3 mg/kg in rats and 100 mg/kg in rabbits (approximately 20 and 75 times human AUC at the maximum recommended human daily dose, respectively). Rosiglitazone caused placental pathology in rats (3 mg/kg/day). Treatment of rats during gestation through lactation reduced litter size, neonatal viability, and postnatal growth, with growth retardation reversible after puberty. For effects on the placenta, embryo/fetus, and offspring, the no-effect dose was 0.2 mg/kg/day in rats and 15 mg/kg/day in rabbits. These no-effect levels are approximately 4 times human AUC at the maximum recommended human daily dose. Rosiglitazone reduced the number of uterine implantations and live offspring when juvenile female rats were treated at 40 mg/kg/day from 27 days of age through to sexual maturity (approximately 68 times human AUC at the maximum recommended daily dose). The no-effect level was 2 mg/kg/day (approximately 4 times human AUC at the maximum recommended daily dose). There was no effect on pre- or post-natal survival or growth.

Glimepiride: Glimepiride did not produce teratogenic effects in rats exposed orally up to 4,000 mg/kg body weight (approximately 4,000 times the maximum recommended human dose based on surface area) or in rabbits exposed up to 32 mg/kg body weight (approximately 60 times the maximum recommended human dose based on surface area). Glimepiride has been shown to be associated with intrauterine fetal death in rats when given in doses as low as 50 times the human dose based on surface area and in rabbits when given in doses as low as 0.1 times the human dose based on surface area. This fetotoxicity, observed only at doses inducing maternal hypoglycemia, has been similarly noted with other sulfonylureas, and is believed to be directly related to the pharmacologic (hypoglycemic) action of glimepiride.

In some studies in rats, offspring of dams exposed to high levels of glimepiride during pregnancy and lactation developed skeletal deformities consisting of shortening, thickening, and bending of the humerus during the postnatal period. Significant concentrations of glimepiride were observed in the serum and breast milk of the dams as well as in the serum of the pups. These skeletal deformations were determined to be the result of nursing from mothers exposed to glimepiride. Prolonged severe hypoglycemia (4 to 10 days) has been reported in neonates born to mothers who were receiving a sulfonylurea drug at the time of delivery. This has been reported more frequently with the use of agents with prolonged half-lives.

8.2 Labor and Delivery

The effect of AVANDARYL or its components on labor and delivery in humans is unknown.

8.3 Nursing Mothers

No studies have been conducted with AVANDARYL. It is not known whether rosiglitazone or glimepiride is excreted in human milk. Because many drugs are excreted in human milk, AVANDARYL should not be administered to a nursing woman.

Rosiglitazone: Drug-related material was detected in milk from lactating rats.

Glimepiride: In rat reproduction studies, significant concentrations of glimepiride were observed in the serum and breast milk of the dams, as well as in the serum of the pups. Although it is not known whether glimepiride is excreted in human milk, other sulfonylureas are excreted in human milk.

8.4 Pediatric Use

Safety and effectiveness of AVANDARYL in pediatric patients have not been established. AVANDARYL and its components, rosiglitazone and glimepiride, are not indicated for use in pediatric patients.

8.5 Geriatric Use

Rosiglitazone: Results of the population pharmacokinetic analysis showed that age does not significantly affect the pharmacokinetics of rosiglitazone *[see Clinical Pharmacology (12.3)]*. Therefore, no dosage adjustments are required for the elderly. In controlled clinical trials, no overall differences in safety and effectiveness between older (≥65 years) and younger (<65 years) patients were observed.

Glimepiride: In US clinical studies of glimepiride, 608 of 1,986 patients were 65 and older. No overall differences in safety or effectiveness were observed between these subjects and younger subjects, but greater sensitivity of some older individuals cannot be ruled out.

Comparison of glimepiride pharmacokinetics in type 2 diabetes patients ≤65 years (N = 49) and those >65 years (N = 42) was performed in a study using a dosing regimen of 6 mg daily. There were no significant differences in glimepiride pharmacokinetics between the 2 age groups *[see Clinical Pharmacology (12.3)]*.

The drug is known to be substantially excreted by the kidney, and the risk of toxic reactions to this drug may be greater in patients with impaired renal function. Because elderly patients are more likely to have decreased renal function, care should be taken in dose selection, and it may be useful to monitor renal function.

Elderly patients are particularly susceptible to hypoglycemic action of glucose-lowering drugs. In elderly, debilitated, or malnourished patients, or in patients with renal, hepatic or adrenal insufficiency, the starting dose, dose increments, and maintenance dosage should be conservative based upon blood glucose levels prior to and after initiation of treatment to avoid hypoglycemic reactions. Hypoglycemia may be difficult to recognize in the elderly and in people who are taking beta-adrenergic blocking drugs or other sympatholytic agents *[see Dosage and Administration (2.4), Warnings and Precautions (5.5), and Clinical Pharmacology (12.3)]*.

10 OVERDOSAGE

Rosiglitazone: Limited data are available with regard to overdosage in humans. In clinical studies in volunteers, rosiglitazone has been administered at single oral doses of up to 20 mg and was well tolerated. In the event of an overdose, appropriate supportive treatment should be initiated as dictated by the patient's clinical status.

Glimepiride: Overdosage of sulfonylureas, including glimepiride, can produce hypoglycemia. Mild hypoglycemic symptoms without loss of consciousness or neurologic findings should be treated aggressively with oral glucose and adjustments in drug dosage and/or meal patterns. Close monitoring should continue until the physician is assured that the patient is out of danger. Severe hypoglycemic reactions with coma, seizure, or other neurological impairment occur infrequently, but constitute medical emergencies requiring immediate hospitalization. If hypoglycemic coma is diagnosed or suspected, the patient should be given a rapid IV injection of concentrated (50%) glucose solution. This should be followed by a continuous infusion of a more dilute (10%) glucose solution at a rate that will maintain the blood glucose level above 100 mg/dL. Patients should be closely monitored for a minimum of 24 to 48 hours, because hypoglycemia may recur after apparent clinical recovery.

11 DESCRIPTION

AVANDARYL contains 2 oral antidiabetic drugs used in the management of type 2 diabetes: rosiglitazone maleate and glimepiride.

Rosiglitazone maleate is an oral antidiabetic agent which acts primarily by increasing insulin sensitivity. Rosiglitazone maleate is not chemically or functionally related to the sulfonylureas, the biguanides, or the alpha-glucosidase inhibitors. Chemically, rosiglitazone maleate is (±)-5-[[4-[2-(methyl-2-pyridinylamino) ethoxy]phenyl] methyl]-2,4-thiazolidinedione, (*Z*)-2-butenedioate (1:1) with a molecular weight of 473.52 (357.44 free base). The molecule has a single chiral center and is present as a racemate. Due to rapid interconversion, the enantiomers are functionally indistinguishable. The molecular formula is $C_{18}H_{19}N_3O_3S{\bullet}C_4H_4O_4$. Rosiglitazone maleate is a white to off-white solid with a melting point range of 122° to 123°C. The pK_a values of rosiglitazone maleate are 6.8 and 6.1. It is readily soluble in ethanol and a buffered aqueous solution with pH of 2.3; solubility decreases with increasing pH in the physiological range. The structural formula of rosiglitazone maleate is:

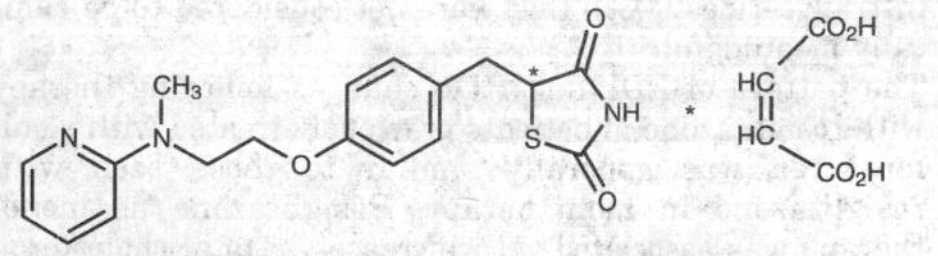

Glimepiride is an oral antidiabetic drug of the sulfonylurea class. Glimepiride is a white to yellowish-white, crystalline, odorless to practically odorless powder. Chemically, glimepiride is 1-[[p-[2-(3-ethyl-4-methyl-2-oxo-3-pyrroline-1-carboxamido)ethyl]phenyl]sulfonyl]-3-(trans-4-methylcyclohexyl)urea with a molecular weight of 490.62. The molecular formula for glimepiride is $C_{24}H_{34}N_4O_5S$. Glimepiride is practically insoluble in water. The structural formula of glimepiride is:

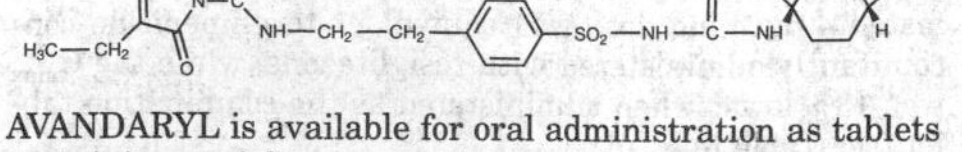

AVANDARYL is available for oral administration as tablets containing rosiglitazone maleate and glimepiride, respectively, in the following strengths (expressed as rosiglitazone maleate/glimepiride): 4 mg/1 mg, 4 mg/2 mg, 4 mg/4 mg, 8 mg/2 mg, and 8 mg/4 mg. Each tablet contains the following inactive ingredients: Hypromellose 2910, lactose monohydrate, macrogol (polyethylene glycol), magnesium stearate, microcrystalline cellulose, sodium starch glycolate, titanium dioxide, and 1 or more of the following: Yellow, red, or black iron oxides.

12 CLINICAL PHARMACOLOGY

12.1 Mechanism of Action

AVANDARYL combines 2 antidiabetic agents with different mechanisms of action to improve glycemic control in patients with type 2 diabetes: Rosiglitazone maleate, a member of the thiazolidinedione class, and glimepiride, a member of the sulfonylurea class. Thiazolidinediones are insulin-sensitizing agents that act primarily by enhancing peripheral glucose utilization, whereas sulfonylureas act primarily by stimulating release of insulin from functioning pancreatic beta cells.

Rosiglitazone: Rosiglitazone improves glycemic control by improving insulin sensitivity. Rosiglitazone is a highly selective and potent agonist for the peroxisome proliferator-activated receptor-gamma (PPARγ). In humans, PPAR receptors are found in key target tissues for insulin action such as adipose tissue, skeletal muscle, and liver. Activation of PPARγ nuclear receptors regulates the transcription of insulin-responsive genes involved in the control of glucose production, transport, and utilization. In addition, PPARγ-responsive genes also participate in the regulation of fatty acid metabolism.

Insulin resistance is a common feature characterizing the pathogenesis of type 2 diabetes. The antidiabetic activity of rosiglitazone has been demonstrated in animal models of type 2 diabetes in which hyperglycemia and/or impaired glucose tolerance is a consequence of insulin resistance in target tissues. Rosiglitazone reduces blood glucose concentrations and reduces hyperinsulinemia in the ob/ob obese mouse, db/db diabetic mouse, and fa/fa fatty Zucker rat.

In animal models, the antidiabetic activity of rosiglitazone was shown to be mediated by increased sensitivity to insulin's action in the liver, muscle, and adipose tissues. Pharmacologic studies in animal models indicate that rosiglitazone improves sensitivity to insulin in muscle and adipose tissue and inhibits hepatic gluconeogenesis. The expression of the insulin-regulated glucose transporter GLUT-4 was increased in adipose tissue. Rosiglitazone did not induce hypoglycemia in animal models of type 2 diabetes and/or impaired glucose tolerance.

Glimepiride: The primary mechanism of action of glimepiride in lowering blood glucose appears to be dependent on stimulating the release of insulin from functioning pancreatic beta cells. In addition, extrapancreatic effects may also play a role in the activity of sulfonylureas such as glimepiride. This is supported by both preclinical and clinical studies demonstrating that glimepiride administration can lead to increased sensitivity of peripheral tissues to insulin. These findings are consistent with the results of a long-term, randomized, placebo-controlled trial in which glimepiride therapy improved postprandial insulin/C-peptide responses and overall glycemic control without producing clinically meaningful increases in fasting insulin/C-peptide levels. However, as with other sulfonylureas, the mechanism by which glimepiride lowers blood glucose during long-term administration has not been clearly established.

12.2 Pharmacodynamics

The lipid profiles of rosiglitazone and glimepiride in a clinical trial of patients with inadequate glycemic control on diet and exercise were consistent with the known profile of each monotherapy. AVANDARYL was associated with increases in HDL and LDL (3% to 4% for each) and decreases in triglycerides (-4%), that were not considered to be clinically meaningful.

The pattern of LDL and HDL changes following therapy with rosiglitazone in patients previously treated with a sulfonylurea was generally similar to those seen with rosiglitazone in monotherapy. Rosiglitazone as monotherapy was associated with increases in total cholesterol, LDL, and HDL and decreases in free fatty acids. The changes in triglycerides during therapy with rosiglitazone were variable and were generally not statistically different from placebo or glyburide controls.

12.3 Pharmacokinetics

In a bioequivalence study of AVANDARYL 4 mg/4 mg, the area under the curve (AUC) and maximum concentration (C_{max}) of rosiglitazone following a single dose of the combination tablet were bioequivalent to rosiglitazone 4 mg concomitantly administered with glimepiride 4 mg under fasted conditions. The AUC of glimepiride following a single fasted 4 mg/4 mg dose was equivalent to glimepiride concomitantly administered with rosiglitazone, while the C_{max} was 13% lower when administered as the combination tablet (see Table 6).

[See table 6 below]

The rate and extent of absorption of both the rosiglitazone component and glimepiride component of AVANDARYL when taken with food were equivalent to the rate and extent of absorption of rosiglitazone and glimepiride when administered concomitantly as separate tablets with food.

Absorption: The AUC and C_{max} of glimepiride increased in a dose-proportional manner following administration of AVANDARYL 4 mg/1 mg, 4 mg/2 mg, and 4 mg/4 mg. Administration of AVANDARYL in the fed state resulted in no change in the overall exposure of rosiglitazone; however, the C_{max} of rosiglitazone decreased by 32% compared to the fasted state. There was an increase in both AUC (19%) and C_{max} (55%) of glimepiride in the fed state compared to the fasted state.

Rosiglitazone: The absolute bioavailability of rosiglitazone is 99%. Peak plasma concentrations are observed about 1 hour after dosing. The C_{max} and AUC of rosiglitazone increase in a dose-proportional manner over the therapeutic dose range.

Glimepiride: After oral administration, glimepiride is completely (100%) absorbed from the gastrointestinal tract. Studies with single oral doses in normal subjects and with multiple oral doses in patients with type 2 diabetes have shown significant absorption of glimepiride within 1 hour after administration and C_{max} at 2 to 3 hours.

Distribution: *Rosiglitazone:* The mean (CV%) oral volume of distribution (V_{ss}/F) of rosiglitazone is approximately 17.6 (30%) liters, based on a population pharmacokinetic analysis. Rosiglitazone is approximately 99.8% bound to plasma proteins, primarily albumin.

Glimepiride: After intravenous (IV) dosing in normal subjects, the volume of distribution (Vd) was 8.8 L (113 mL/kg), and the total body clearance (CL) was 47.8 mL/min. Protein binding was greater than 99.5%.

Metabolism and Excretion: *Rosiglitazone:* Rosiglitazone is extensively metabolized with no unchanged drug excreted in the urine. The major routes of metabolism were N-demethylation and hydroxylation, followed by conjugation with sulfate and glucuronic acid. All the circulating metabolites are considerably less potent than parent and, therefore, are not expected to contribute to the insulin-sensitizing activity of rosiglitazone. In vitro data demonstrate that rosiglitazone is predominantly metabolized by cytochrome P450 (CYP) isoenzyme 2C8, with CYP2C9 contributing as a minor pathway. Following oral or IV administration of $[^{14}C]$rosiglitazone maleate, approximately 64% and 23% of the dose was eliminated in the urine and in the feces, respectively. The plasma half-life of $[^{14}C]$related material ranged from 103 to 158 hours. The elimination half-life is 3 to 4 hours and is independent of dose.

Glimepiride: Glimepiride is completely metabolized by oxidative biotransformation after either an IV or oral dose. The major metabolites are the cyclohexyl hydroxy methyl derivative (M1) and the carboxyl derivative (M2). Cytochrome P450 2C9 has been shown to be involved in the biotransformation of glimepiride to M1. M1 is further metabolized to M2 by one or several cytosolic enzymes. M1, but not M2, possesses about ⅓ of the pharmacological activity as compared to its parent in an animal model; however, whether the glucose-lowering effect of M1 is clinically meaningful is not clear.

When $[^{14}C]$glimepiride was given orally, approximately 60% of the total radioactivity was recovered in the urine in 7 days and M1 (predominant) and M2 accounted for 80 to 90% of that recovered in the urine. Approximately 40% of the total radioactivity was recovered in feces and M1 and M2 (predominant) accounted for about 70% of that recovered in feces. No parent drug was recovered from urine or feces. After IV dosing in patients, no significant biliary excretion of glimepiride or its M1 metabolite has been observed.

Special Populations: No pharmacokinetic data are available for AVANDARYL in the following special populations. Information is provided for the individual components of AVANDARYL.

Gender: Rosiglitazone: Results of the population pharmacokinetics analysis showed that the mean oral clearance of rosiglitazone in female patients (N = 405) was approximately 6% lower compared to male patients of the same body weight (N = 642). Combination therapy with rosiglitazone and sulfonylureas improved glycemic control in both males and females with a greater therapeutic response observed in females. For a given body mass index (BMI), females tend to have a greater fat mass than males. Since the molecular target of rosiglitazone, PPARγ, is expressed in adipose tissues, this differentiating characteristic may account, at least in part, for the greater response to rosiglitazone in combination with sulfonylureas in females. Since therapy should be individualized, no dose adjustments are necessary based on gender alone.

- *Glimepiride:* There were no differences between males and females in the pharmacokinetics of glimepiride when adjustment was made for differences in body weight.

Geriatric: Rosiglitazone: Results of the population pharmacokinetics analysis (N = 716 <65 years; N = 331 ≥65 years) showed that age does not significantly affect the pharmacokinetics of rosiglitazone.

- *Glimepiride:* Comparison of glimepiride pharmacokinetics in type 2 diabetes patients 65 years and younger with those older than 65 years was performed in a study using a dosing regimen of 6 mg daily. There were no significant differences in glimepiride pharmacokinetics between the 2 age groups. The mean AUC at steady state for the older patients was about 13% lower than that for the younger patients; the mean weight-adjusted clearance for the older patients was about 11% higher than that for the younger patients. *[See Use in Specific Populations (8.5).]*

Hepatic Impairment: Therapy with AVANDARYL should not be initiated if the patient exhibits clinical evidence of active liver disease or increased serum transaminase levels (ALT >2.5× upper limit of normal) at baseline *[see Warnings and Precautions (5.8)]*.

- *Rosiglitazone:* Unbound oral clearance of rosiglitazone was significantly lower in patients with moderate to severe liver disease (Child-Pugh Class B/C) compared to healthy subjects. As a result, unbound C_{max} and $AUC_{0\text{-}inf}$ were increased 2- and 3-fold, respectively. Elimination half-life for rosiglitazone was about 2 hours longer in patients with liver disease, compared to healthy subjects.
- *Glimepiride:* No studies of glimepiride have been conducted in patients with hepatic insufficiency.

Race: Rosiglitazone: Results of a population pharmacokinetic analysis including subjects of white, black, and other ethnic origins indicate that race has no influence on the pharmacokinetics of rosiglitazone.

- *Glimepiride:* No pharmacokinetic studies to assess the effects of race have been performed, but in placebo-controlled studies of glimepiride in patients with type 2 diabetes, the antihyperglycemic effect was comparable in whites (N = 536), blacks (N = 63), and Hispanics (N = 63).

Renal Impairment: Rosiglitazone: There are no clinically relevant differences in the pharmacokinetics of rosiglitazone in patients with mild to severe renal impairment or in hemodialysis-dependent patients compared to subjects with normal renal function.

- *Glimepiride:* A single-dose glimepiride, open-label study was conducted in 15 patients with renal impairment. Glimepiride (3 mg) was administered to 3 groups of patients with different levels of mean creatinine clearance (CL_{cr}); (Group I, CL_{cr} = 77.7 mL/min, N = 5), (Group II, CL_{cr} = 27.7 mL/min, N = 3), and (Group III, CL_{cr} = 9.4 mL/min, N = 7). Glimepiride was found to be well tolerated in all 3 groups. The results showed that glimepiride serum levels decreased as renal function decreased. However, M1 and M2 serum levels (mean AUC values) increased 2.3 and 8.6 times from Group I to Group III. The apparent terminal half-life ($T_{1/2}$) for glimepiride did not change, while the half-lives for M1 and M2 increased as renal function decreased. Mean urinary excretion of M1 plus M2 as percent of dose, however, decreased (44.4%, 21.9%, and 9.3% for Groups I to III). A multiple-dose titration study was also conducted in 16 type 2 diabetes patients with renal impairment using doses ranging from 1 to 8 mg daily for 3 months. The results were consistent with those observed after single doses. All patients with a CL_{cr} less than 22 mL/min had adequate control of their glucose levels with a dosage regimen of only 1 mg daily. The results from this study suggest that a starting dose of 1 mg glimepiride, as contained in AVANDARYL 4 mg/1 mg, may be given to type 2 diabetes patients with kidney disease, and the dose may be titrated based on fasting glucose levels.

Table 6. Pharmacokinetic Parameters for Rosiglitazone and Glimepiride (N = 28)

	Rosiglitazone		Glimepiride	
Parameter (Units)	Regimen A	Regimen B	Regimen A	Regimen B
$AUC_{0\text{-}inf}$ (ng.hr/mL)	1,259 (833-2,060)	1,253 (756-2,758)	1,052 (643-2,117)	1,101 (648-2,555)
$AUC_{0\text{-}t}$ (ng.hr/mL)	1,231 (810-2,019)	1,224 (744-2,654)	944 (511-1,898)	1,038 (606-2,337)
C_{max} (ng/mL)	257 (157-352)	251 (77.3-434)	151 (63.2-345)	173 (70.5-329)
$T_{1/2}$ (hr)	3.53 (2.60-4.57)	3.54 (2.10-5.03)	7.63 (4.42-12.4)	5.08 (1.80-11.31)
T_{max} (hr)	1.00 (0.48-3.02)	0.98 (0.48-5.97)	3.02 (1.50-8.00)	2.53 (1.00-8.03)

AUC = area under the curve; C_{max}= maximum concentration; $T_{1/2}$ = terminal half-life; T_{max} = time of maximum concentration.

Regimen A = AVANDARYL 4 mg/4 mg tablet; Regimen B = Concomitant dosing of a rosiglitazone 4 mg tablet AND a glimepiride 4 mg tablet.

Data presented as geometric mean (range), except $T_{1/2}$ which is presented as arithmetic mean (range) and T_{max}, which is presented as median (range).

Pediatric: No pharmacokinetic data from studies in pediatric subjects are available for AVANDARYL.

• *Rosiglitazone:* Pharmacokinetic parameters of rosiglitazone in pediatric patients were established using a population pharmacokinetic analysis with sparse data from 96 pediatric patients in a single pediatric clinical trial including 33 males and 63 females with ages ranging from 10 to 17 years (weights ranging from 35 to 178.3 kg). Population mean CL/F and V/F of rosiglitazone were 3.15 L/hr and 13.5 L, respectively. These estimates of CL/F and V/F were consistent with the typical parameter estimates from a prior adult population analysis.

• *Glimepiride:* The pharmacokinetics of glimepiride (1 mg) were evaluated in a single-dose study conducted in 30 type 2 diabetic patients (male = 7; female = 23) between ages 10 and 17 years. The mean AUC_{0-last} (338.8 ± 203.1 ng.hr/mL), C_{max} (102.4 ± 47.7 ng/mL), and $T_{1/2}$ (3.1 ± 1.7 hours) were comparable to those previously reported in adults (AUC_{0-last} 315.2 ± 95.9 ng.hr/mL, C_{max} 103.2 ± 34.3 ng/mL, and $T_{1/2}$ 5.3 ± 4.1 hours).

12.4 Drug-Drug Interactions

Single oral doses of glimepiride in 14 healthy adult subjects had no clinically significant effect on the steady-state pharmacokinetics of rosiglitazone. No clinically significant reductions in glimepiride AUC and C_{max} were observed after repeat doses of rosiglitazone (8 mg once daily) for 8 days in healthy adult subjects.

Rosiglitazone: *Drugs That Inhibit, Induce or are Metabolized by Cytochrome P450:* In vitro drug metabolism studies suggest that rosiglitazone does not inhibit any of the major P450 enzymes at clinically relevant concentrations. In vitro data demonstrate that rosiglitazone is predominantly metabolized by CYP2C8, and to a lesser extent, 2C9. *[See Drug Interactions (7.1).]*

Rosiglitazone (4 mg twice daily) was shown to have no clinically relevant effect on the pharmacokinetics of nifedipine and oral contraceptives (ethinyl estradiol and norethindrone), which are predominantly metabolized by CYP3A4.

Gemfibrozil: Concomitant administration of gemfibrozil (600 mg twice daily), an inhibitor of CYP2C8, and rosiglitazone (4 mg once daily) for 7 days increased rosiglitazone AUC by 127%, compared to the administration of rosiglitazone (4 mg once daily) alone. Given the potential for dose-related adverse events with rosiglitazone, a decrease in the dose of rosiglitazone may be needed when gemfibrozil is introduced *[see Drug Interactions (7.1)].*

Rifampin: Rifampin administration (600 mg once a day), an inducer of CYP2C8, for 6 days is reported to decrease rosiglitazone AUC by 66%, compared to the administration of rosiglitazone (8 mg) alone *[see Drug Interactions (7.1)].*[4]

Glyburide: Rosiglitazone (2 mg twice daily) taken concomitantly with glyburide (3.75 to 10 mg/day) for 7 days did not alter the mean steady-state 24-hour plasma glucose concentrations in diabetic patients stabilized on glyburide therapy. Repeat doses of rosiglitazone (8 mg once daily) for 8 days in healthy adult Caucasian subjects caused a decrease in glyburide AUC and C_{max} of approximately 30%. In Japanese subjects, glyburide AUC and C_{max} slightly increased following coadministration of rosiglitazone.

Digoxin: Repeat oral dosing of rosiglitazone (8 mg once daily) for 14 days did not alter the steady-state pharmacokinetics of digoxin (0.375 mg once daily) in healthy volunteers.

Warfarin: Repeat dosing with rosiglitazone had no clinically relevant effect on the steady-state pharmacokinetics of warfarin enantiomers.

Additional pharmacokinetic studies demonstrated no clinically relevant effect of acarbose, ranitidine, or metformin on the pharmacokinetics of rosiglitazone.

Glimepiride: The hypoglycemic action of sulfonylureas may be potentiated by certain drugs, including nonsteroidal anti-inflammatory drugs (NSAIDs) and other drugs that are highly protein bound, such as salicylates, sulfonamides, chloramphenicol, coumarins, probenecid, monoamine oxidase inhibitors, and beta-adrenergic blocking agents. When these drugs are administered to a patient receiving glimepiride, the patient should be observed closely for hypoglycemia. When these drugs are withdrawn from a patient receiving glimepiride, the patient should be observed closely for loss of glycemic control.

Certain drugs tend to produce hyperglycemia and may lead to loss of control. These drugs include the thiazides and other diuretics, corticosteroids, phenothiazines, thyroid products, estrogens, oral contraceptives, phenytoin, nicotinic acid, sympathomimetics, and isoniazid. When these drugs are administered to a patient receiving glimepiride, the patient should be closely observed for loss of control. When these drugs are withdrawn from a patient receiving glimepiride, the patient should be observed closely for hypoglycemia.

Drugs Metabolized by Cytochrome P450: A potential interaction between oral miconazole and oral hypoglycemic agents leading to severe hypoglycemia has been reported. Whether this interaction also occurs with the IV, topical, or vaginal preparations of miconazole is not known. There is a potential interaction of glimepiride with inhibitors (e.g., fluconazole) and inducers (e.g., rifampicin) of cytochrome P450 2C9.

Aspirin: Coadministration of aspirin (1 g three times daily) and glimepiride led to a 34% decrease in the mean glimepiride AUC and, therefore, a 34% increase in the mean CL/F. The mean C_{max} had a decrease of 4%. Blood glucose and serum C-peptide concentrations were unaffected and no hypoglycemic symptoms were reported.

H₂-Receptor Antagonists: Coadministration of either cimetidine (800 mg once daily) or ranitidine (150 mg twice daily) with a single 4-mg oral dose of glimepiride did not significantly alter the absorption and disposition of glimepiride, and no differences were seen in hypoglycemic symptomatology.

Beta-Blockers: Concomitant administration of propranolol (40 mg three times daily) and glimepiride significantly increased C_{max}, AUC, and $T_{1/2}$ of glimepiride by 23%, 22%, and 15%, respectively, and it decreased CL/F by 18%. The recovery of M1 and M2 from urine, however, did not change. The pharmacodynamic responses to glimepiride were nearly identical in normal subjects receiving propranolol and placebo. Pooled data from clinical trials in patients with type 2 diabetes showed no evidence of clinically significant adverse interactions with uncontrolled concurrent administration of beta-blockers. However, if beta-blockers are used, caution should be exercised and patients should be warned about the potential for hypoglycemia.

Warfarin: Concomitant administration of glimepiride tablets (4 mg once daily) did not alter the pharmacokinetic characteristics of R- and S-warfarin enantiomers following administration of a single dose (25 mg) of racemic warfarin to healthy subjects. No changes were observed in warfarin plasma protein binding. Glimepiride treatment did result in a slight, but statistically significant, decrease in the pharmacodynamic response to warfarin. The reductions in mean area under the prothrombin time (PT) curve and maximum PT values during glimepiride treatment were very small (3.3% and 9.9%, respectively) and are unlikely to be clinically important.

ACE Inhibitors: The responses of serum glucose, insulin, C-peptide, and plasma glucagon to 2 mg glimepiride were unaffected by coadministration of ramipril (an ACE inhibitor) 5 mg once daily in normal subjects. No hypoglycemic symptoms were reported.

Other: Although no specific interaction studies were performed, pooled data from clinical trials showed no evidence of clinically significant adverse interactions with uncontrolled concurrent administration of aspirin and other salicylates, H₂-receptor antagonists, ACE inhibitors, calcium-channel blockers, estrogens, fibrates, NSAIDs, HMG CoA reductase inhibitors, sulfonamides, or thyroid hormone.

13 NONCLINICAL TOXICOLOGY

13.1 Carcinogenesis, Mutagenesis, Impairment of Fertility

No animal studies have been conducted with AVANDARYL. The following data are based on findings in studies performed with rosiglitazone or glimepiride alone.

Rosiglitazone: *Carcinogenesis:* A 2-year carcinogenicity study was conducted in Charles River CD-1 mice at doses of 0.4, 1.5, and 6 mg/kg/day in the diet (highest dose equivalent to approximately 12 times human AUC at the maximum recommended human daily dose). Sprague-Dawley rats were dosed for 2 years by oral gavage at doses of 0.05 mg/kg/day, 0.3 mg/kg/day, and 2 mg/kg/day (highest dose equivalent to approximately 10 and 20 times human AUC at the maximum recommended human daily dose for male and female rats, respectively).

Rosiglitazone was not carcinogenic in the mouse. There was an increase in incidence of adipose hyperplasia in the mouse at doses ≥1.5 mg/kg/day (approximately 2 times human AUC at the maximum recommended human daily dose). In rats, there was a significant increase in the incidence of benign adipose tissue tumors (lipomas) at doses ≥0.3 mg/kg/day (approximately 2 times human AUC at the maximum recommended human daily dose). These proliferative changes in both species are considered due to the persistent pharmacological overstimulation of adipose tissue.

Mutagenesis: Rosiglitazone was not mutagenic or clastogenic in the in vitro bacterial assays for gene mutation, the in vitro chromosome aberration test in human lymphocytes, the in vivo mouse micronucleus test, and the in vivo/in vitro rat UDS assay. There was a small (about 2-fold) increase in mutation in the in vitro mouse lymphoma assay in the presence of metabolic activation.

Impairment of Fertility: Rosiglitazone had no effects on mating or fertility of male rats given up to 40 mg/kg/day (approximately 116 times human AUC at the maximum recommended human daily dose). Rosiglitazone altered estrous cyclicity (2 mg/kg/day) and reduced fertility (40 mg/kg/day) of female rats in association with lower plasma levels of progesterone and estradiol (approximately 20 and 200 times human AUC at the maximum recommended human daily dose, respectively). No such effects were noted at 0.2 mg/kg/day (approximately 3 times human AUC at the maximum recommended human daily dose). In juvenile rats dosed from 27 days of age through to sexual maturity (at up to 40 mg/kg/day), there was no effect on male reproductive performance, or on estrous cyclicity, mating performance or pregnancy incidence in females (approximately 68 times human AUC at the maximum recommended daily dose). In monkeys, rosiglitazone (0.6 and 4.6 mg/kg/day; approximately 3 and 15 times human AUC at the maximum recommended human daily dose, respectively) diminished the follicular phase rise in serum estradiol with consequential reduction in the luteinizing hormone surge, lower luteal phase progesterone levels, and amenorrhea. The mechanism for these effects appears to be direct inhibition of ovarian steroidogenesis.

Glimepiride: *Carcinogenesis:* Studies in rats at doses of up to 5,000 parts per million (ppm) in complete feed (approximately 340 times the maximum recommended human dose, based on surface area) for 30 months showed no evidence of carcinogenesis. In mice, administration of glimepiride for 24 months resulted in an increase in benign pancreatic adenoma formation which was dose-related and is thought to be the result of chronic pancreatic stimulation. The no-effect dose for adenoma formation in mice in this study was 320 ppm in complete feed, or 46 to 54 mg/kg body weight/day. This is about 35 times the maximum human recommended dose based on surface area.

Mutagenesis: Glimepiride was non-mutagenic in a battery of in vitro and in vivo mutagenicity studies (Ames test, somatic cell mutation, chromosomal aberration, unscheduled DNA synthesis, mouse micronucleus test).

Impairment of Fertility: There was no effect of glimepiride on male mouse fertility in animals exposed up to 2,500 mg/kg body weight (>1,700 times the maximum recommended human dose based on surface area). Glimepiride had no effect on the fertility of male and female rats administered up to 4,000 mg/kg body weight (approximately 4,000 times the maximum recommended human dose based on surface area).

13.2 Animal Toxicology and/or Pharmacology

Rosiglitazone: Heart weights were increased in mice (3 mg/kg/day), rats (5 mg/kg/day), and dogs (2 mg/kg/day) with rosiglitazone treatments (approximately 5, 22, and 2 times human AUC at the maximum recommended human daily dose, respectively). Effects in juvenile rats were consistent with those seen in adults. Morphometric measurement indicated that there was hypertrophy in cardiac ventricular tissues, which may be due to increased heart work as a result of plasma volume expansion.

Glimepiride: Reduced serum glucose values and degranulation of the pancreatic beta cells were observed in beagle dogs exposed to glimepiride 320 mg/kg/day for 12 months (approximately 1,000 times the recommended human dose based on surface area). No evidence of tumor formation was observed in any organ. One female and one male dog developed bilateral subcapsular cataracts. Non-GLP studies indicated that glimepiride was unlikely to exacerbate cataract formation. Evaluation of the co-cataractogenic potential of glimepiride in several diabetic and cataract rat models was negative and there was no adverse effect of glimepiride on bovine ocular lens metabolism in organ culture *[see Adverse Reactions (6.1)].*

14 CLINICAL STUDIES

14.1 Patients Inadequately Controlled on Diet and Exercise

In a 28-week, randomized, double-blind clinical trial, 901 patients with type 2 diabetes inadequately controlled with diet and exercise alone (baseline mean fasting plasma glucose [FPG] 211 mg/dL and baseline mean HbA1c 9.1%) were started on AVANDARYL 4 mg/1 mg, rosiglitazone 4 mg, or glimepiride 1 mg. Doses could be increased at 4-week intervals to reach a target mean daily glucose of ≤110 mg/dL. Patients who received AVANDARYL were randomized to 1 of 2 titration schemes differing in the maximum total daily dose (4 mg/4 mg or 8 mg/4 mg). The maximum total daily dose was 8 mg for rosiglitazone monotherapy and 4 mg for glimepiride monotherapy. All treatments were administered as a once daily regimen. Improvements in FPG and HbA1c were observed in patients treated with AVANDARYL compared to either rosiglitazone or glimepiride alone (see Table 7).

[See table 7 at top of next page]

Treatment with AVANDARYL resulted in statistically significant improvements in FPG and HbA1c compared with each of the monotherapies. However, when considering choice of therapy for drug-naïve patients, the risk-benefit of initiating monotherapy or dual therapy should be considered. In particular, the risk of hypoglycemia and weight gain with dual therapy should be taken into account. *[See Warnings and Precautions (5.5, 5.7) and Adverse Reactions (6.1).]*

Table 7. Glycemic Parameters in a 28-Week Study of AVANDARYL in Patients with Type 2 Diabetes Mellitus Inadequately Controlled on Diet and Exercise

	Glimepiride	Rosiglitazone	AVANDARYL 4 mg/4 mg	AVANDARYL 8 mg/4 mg
Mean Final Dose	3.5 mg	7.5 mg	4.0 mg/3.2 mg	6.8 mg/2.9 mg
N	221	227	221	214
FPG (mg/dL) [mean (SD)]				
Baseline	211 (70)	212 (66)	207 (58)	214 (61)
Change from baseline	-42 (66)	-57 (58)	-70 (57)	-80 (57)
Treatment difference between				
– AVANDARYL and glimepiride	—	—	-30*	-37*
– AVANDARYL and rosiglitazone	—	—	-16*	-23*
% of patients with ≥30 mg/dL decrease from baseline	56%	64%	77%	85%
HbA1c (%) [mean (SD)]				
Baseline	9.0 (1.3)	9.1 (1.3)	9.0 (1.3)	9.2 (1.4)
Change from baseline	-1.7 (1.4)	-1.8 (1.5)	-2.4 (1.4)	-2.5 (1.4)
Treatment difference between				
– AVANDARYL and glimepiride	—	—	-0.6*	-0.7*
– AVANDARYL and rosiglitazone	—	—	-0.7*	-0.8*
% of patients with ≥0.7% decrease from baseline	82%	76%	93%	93%
% of patients at HbA1c Target <7.0%[†]	49%	46%	75%	72%

* Least squared means, p<0.0001 compared to monotherapy.
† Response is related to baseline HbA1c.

14.2 Patients Previously Treated With Sulfonylureas

The safety and efficacy of rosiglitazone added to a sulfonylurea have been studied in clinical trials in patients with type 2 diabetes inadequately controlled on sulfonylureas alone. No clinical trials have been conducted with the fixed-dose combination of AVANDARYL in patients inadequately controlled on a sulfonylurea or who have initially responded to rosiglitazone alone and require additional glycemic control.

A total of 3,457 patients with type 2 diabetes participated in ten 24- to 26-week randomized, double-blind, placebo/active-controlled studies and one 2-year double-blind, active-controlled study in elderly patients designed to assess the efficacy and safety of rosiglitazone in combination with a sulfonylurea. Rosiglitazone 2 mg, 4 mg, or 8 mg daily, was administered either once daily (3 studies) or in divided doses twice daily (7 studies), to patients inadequately controlled on a submaximal or maximal dose of sulfonylurea.

In these studies, the combination of rosiglitazone 4 mg or 8 mg daily (administered as single or twice daily divided doses) and a sulfonylurea significantly reduced FPG and HbA1c compared to placebo plus sulfonylurea or further up-titration of the sulfonylurea. Table 8 shows pooled data for 8 studies in which rosiglitazone added to sulfonylurea was compared to placebo plus sulfonylurea.

[See table at top of next page]

One of the 24- to 26-week studies included patients who were inadequately controlled on maximal doses of glyburide and switched to 4 mg of rosiglitazone daily as monotherapy; in this group, loss of glycemic control was demonstrated, as evidenced by increases in FPG and HbA1c.

In a 2-year double-blind study, elderly patients (aged 59 to 89 years) on half-maximal sulfonylurea (glipizide 10 mg twice daily) were randomized to the addition of rosiglitazone (N = 115, 4 mg once daily to 8 mg as needed) or to continued up-titration of glipizide (N = 110), to a maximum of 20 mg twice daily. Mean baseline FPG and HbA1c were 157 mg/dL and 7.72%, respectively, for the rosiglitazone plus glipizide arm and 159 mg/dL and 7.65%, respectively, for the glipizide up-titration arm. Loss of glycemic control (FPG ≥180 mg/dL) occurred in a significantly lower proportion of patients (2%) on rosiglitazone plus glipizide compared to patients in the glipizide up-titration arm (28.7%). About 78% of the patients on combination therapy completed the 2 years of therapy while only 51% completed on glipizide monotherapy. The effect of combination therapy on FPG and HbA1c was durable over the 2-year study period, with patients achieving a mean of 132 mg/dL for FPG and a mean of 6.98% for HbA1c compared to no change on the glipizide arm.

15 REFERENCES

1. Food and Drug Administration Briefing Document. Joint meeting of the Endocrinologic and Metabolic Drugs and Drug Safety and Risk Management Advisory Committees. July 30, 2007.
2. DREAM Trial Investigators. Effect of rosiglitazone on the frequency of diabetes in patients with impaired glucose tolerance or impaired fasting glucose: a randomised controlled trial. *Lancet* 2006;368:1096-1105.
3. Home PD, Pocock SJ, Beck-Nielsen H, et al. Rosiglitazone evaluated for cardiovascular outcomes – an interim analysis. *NEJM* 2007;357:1-11.
4. Park JY, Kim KA, Kang MH, et al. Effect of rifampin on the pharmacokinetics of rosiglitazone in healthy subjects. *Clin Pharmacol Ther* 2004;75:157-162.

16 HOW SUPPLIED/STORAGE AND HANDLING

Each rounded triangular tablet contains rosiglitazone as the maleate and glimepiride as follows:

4 mg/1 mg – yellow, gsk debossed on one side and 4/1 on the other.

4 mg/2 mg – orange, gsk debossed on one side and 4/2 on the other.

4 mg/4 mg – pink, gsk debossed on one side and 4/4 on the other.

8 mg/2 mg – pale pink, gsk debossed on one side and 8/2 on the other.

8 mg/4 mg – red, gsk debossed on one side and 8/4 on the other.

4 mg/1 mg bottles of 30: NDC 0007-3151-13
4 mg/2 mg bottles of 30: NDC 0007-3152-13
4 mg/4 mg bottles of 30: NDC 0007-3153-13
8 mg/2 mg bottles of 30: NDC 0007-3148-13
8 mg/4 mg bottles of 30: NDC 0007-3149-13

Store at 25°C (77°F); excursions permitted to 15° to 30°C (59° to 86°F). Dispense in a tight, light-resistant container.

17 PATIENT COUNSELING INFORMATION

See FDA-approved Medication Guide (17.2).

17.1 Patient Advice

Patients should be informed of the following:

- AVANDARYL is not recommended in patients with symptoms of heart failure.
- Patients with more severe heart failure (NYHA Class 3 or 4) must not start AVANDARYL as the risks exceed any potential benefits in such patients.
- Results of a set of clinical studies suggest that treatment with rosiglitazone is associated with an increased risk for myocardial ischemic events, such as angina or myocardial infarction (heart attack), especially in patients taking insulin or nitrates. Because this risk has not been confirmed or excluded in different long-term trials, definitive conclusions regarding this risk await completion of an adequately-designed cardiovascular outcome study.
- AVANDARYL is not recommended for patients who are taking insulin or nitrates.
- There are multiple medications available to treat type 2 diabetes. The benefits and risks of each available diabetes medication should be taken into account when choosing a particular diabetes medication for a given patient.
- Management of type 2 diabetes should include diet control. Caloric restriction, weight loss, and exercise are essential for the proper treatment of the diabetic patient because they help improve insulin sensitivity. This is important not only in the primary treatment of type 2 diabetes, but also in maintaining the efficacy of drug therapy.
- There have been no clinical studies establishing conclusive evidence of macrovascular risk reduction with AVANDARYL or any other antidiabetic drug.
- It is important to adhere to dietary instructions and to regularly have blood glucose and glycosylated hemoglobin (HbA1c) tested. It can take 2 weeks to see a reduction in blood glucose and 2 to 3 months to see the full effect of AVANDARYL.
- The risks of hypoglycemia, its symptoms and treatment, and conditions that predispose to its development should be explained to patients and their family members.
- Blood will be drawn to check their liver function prior to the start of therapy and periodically thereafter per the clinical judgment of the healthcare professional. Patients with unexplained symptoms of nausea, vomiting, abdominal pain, fatigue, anorexia, or dark urine should immediately report these symptoms to their physician.
- Patients who experience an unusually rapid increase in weight or edema or who develop shortness of breath or other symptoms of heart failure while on AVANDARYL should immediately report these symptoms to their physician.
- AVANDARYL should be taken with the first meal of the day.
- Therapy with rosiglitazone, like other thiazolidinediones, may result in ovulation in some premenopausal anovulatory women. As a result, these patients may be at an increased risk for pregnancy while taking AVANDARYL. Thus, adequate contraception in premenopausal women should be recommended. This possible effect has not been specifically investigated in clinical studies so the frequency of this occurrence is not known.

17.2 FDA-Approved Medication Guide

See separate leaflet.

AVANDARYL and AVANDAMET are registered trademarks of GlaxoSmithKline.

GlaxoSmithKline
Research Triangle Park, NC 27709

©2009, GlaxoSmithKline. All rights reserved.

MEDICATION GUIDE

AVANDARYL® (ah-VAN-duh-ril)
(rosiglitazone maleate and glimepiride) Tablets

Read this Medication Guide carefully before you start taking AVANDARYL and each time you get a refill. There may be new information. This information does not take the place of talking with your doctor about your medical condition or your treatment. If you have any questions about AVANDARYL, ask your doctor or pharmacist.

What is the most important information I should know about AVANDARYL?

AVANDARYL is a prescription medicine to treat adults with diabetes. It helps to control high blood sugar. (See "What is AVANDARYL?"). Each AVANDARYL tablet contains two different diabetes medicines, one is called rosiglitazone and the other is called glimepiride. It is important that you take AVANDARYL exactly how it is prescribed by your doctor to best treat your diabetes.

AVANDARYL may cause serious side effects, including:

New or worse heart failure

- Rosiglitazone, one of the two drugs that make up AVANDARYL, can cause your body to keep extra fluid (fluid retention), which leads to swelling (edema) and weight gain. Extra body fluid can make some heart problems worse or lead to heart failure. Heart failure means your heart does not pump blood well enough.
- If you have severe heart failure, you cannot start AVANDARYL.
- If you have heart failure with symptoms (such as shortness of breath or swelling), even if these symptoms are not severe, AVANDARYL may not be right for you.

Call your doctor right away if you have any of the following:

- swelling or fluid retention, especially in the ankles or legs
- shortness of breath or trouble breathing, especially when you lie down
- an unusually fast increase in weight
- unusual tiredness

Other heart problems

Rosiglitazone, one of the medicines in AVANDARYL, may raise the risk of heart problems related to reduced blood flow to the heart. These include possible increases in the risk of heart-related chest pain (angina) or "heart attack" (myocardial infarction). This risk seemed to be higher in people who took rosiglitazone with insulin or with nitrate medicines. Most people who take insulin or nitrate medicines should not also take AVANDARYL.

• If you have chest pain or a feeling of chest pressure, get medical help right away, no matter what diabetes medicines you are taking.

• People with diabetes have a greater risk for heart problems. It is important to work with your doctor to manage other conditions, such as high blood pressure or high cholesterol.

AVANDARYL can have other serious side effects. Be sure to read the section "What are possible side effects of AVANDARYL?".

What is AVANDARYL?

AVANDARYL contains 2 prescription medicines to treat diabetes, rosiglitazone maleate (AVANDIA) and glimepiride (AMARYL). AVANDARYL is used with diet and exercise to treat adults with type 2 ("adult-onset" or "non-insulin dependent") diabetes mellitus ("high blood sugar").

Glimepiride can help your body release more of its own insulin. Rosiglitazone can help your body respond better to the insulin made in your body and does not cause your body to make more insulin. These medicines can work together to help control your blood sugar.

• For AVANDARYL to work best, it is important to exercise, lose extra weight, and follow the diet recommended for your diabetes.

• AVANDARYL has not been studied in children under 18 years of age to know if it is safe and effective in children.

• AVANDARYL is not for people with type 1 diabetes mellitus or to treat a condition called diabetic ketoacidosis.

Who should not take AVANDARYL?

Many people with heart failure should not start taking AVANDARYL (see "What should I tell my doctor before starting AVANDARYL?").

What should I tell my doctor before starting AVANDARYL?

Before starting AVANDARYL, ask your doctor about what the choices are for diabetes medicines and what the expected benefits and possible risks are for you in particular. Before taking AVANDARYL, tell your doctor about all your medical conditions, including if you:

• **have heart problems or heart failure.**

• **have type 1 ("juvenile") diabetes or had diabetic keto-acidosis.** These conditions should be treated with insulin and should not be treated with AVANDARYL.

• **have a type of diabetic eye disease called macular edema** (swelling of the back of the eye).

• **have liver problems.** Your doctor should do blood tests to check your liver before you start taking AVANDARYL and during treatment as needed.

• **had liver problems while taking REZULIN® (troglitazone),** another medicine for diabetes.

• **have kidney problems.** If people with kidney problems use AVANDARYL, they may need a lower dose of the medication.

• **have glucose 6-phosphate dehydrogenase (G6PD) deficiency.** This condition runs in families. People with G6PD deficiency who take glimepiride (one of the medicines in AVANDARYL) may develop hemolytic anemia (fast breakdown of red blood cells).

• **are pregnant or plan to become pregnant.** AVANDARYL should not be used during pregnancy. It is not known if AVANDARYL can harm your unborn baby. You and your doctor should talk about the best way to control your diabetes during pregnancy. If you are a premenopausal woman (before the "change of life") who does not have regular monthly periods, AVANDARYL may increase your chances of becoming pregnant. Talk to your doctor about birth control choices while taking AVANDARYL. Tell your doctor right away if you become pregnant while taking AVANDARYL.

• **are breast-feeding or planning to breast-feed.** It is not known if AVANDARYL passes into breast milk. You should not use AVANDARYL while breast-feeding.

Tell your doctor about all the medicines you take including prescription and non-prescription medicines, vitamins or herbal supplements. AVANDARYL and certain other medicines can affect each other and may lead to serious side effects including high blood sugar or low blood sugar, or heart problems. Especially tell your doctor if you take:

• **insulin.**

• **nitrate medicines** such as nitroglycerin or isosorbide to treat a type of chest pain called angina.

• **any medicines for high blood pressure, high cholesterol or heart failure, or for prevention of heart disease or stroke.**

Table 8. Glycemic Parameters in 24- to 26-Week Combination Studies of Rosiglitazone Plus Sulfonylurea

Twice Daily Divided Dosing (5 Studies)	Sulfonylurea	Rosiglitazone 2 mg twice daily + sulfonylurea	Sulfonylurea	Rosiglitazone 4 mg twice daily + sulfonylurea
N	397	497	248	346
FPG (mg/dL)				
Baseline (mean)	204	198	188	187
Change from baseline (mean)	11	-29	8	-43
Difference from sulfonylurea alone (adjusted mean)		-42*		-53*
% of patients with ≥30 mg/dL decrease from baseline	17%	49%	15%	61%
HbA1c (%)				
Baseline (mean)	9.4	9.5	9.3	9.6
Change from baseline (mean)	0.2	-1.0	0.0	-1.6
Difference from sulfonylurea alone (adjusted mean)	—	-1.1*	—	-1.4*
% of patients with ≥0.7% decrease from baseline	21%	60%	23%	75%

Once Daily Dosing (3 Studies)	Sulfonylurea	Rosiglitazone 4 mg once daily + sulfonylurea	Sulfonylurea	Rosiglitazone 8 mg once daily + sulfonylurea
N	172	172	173	176
FPG (mg/dL)				
Baseline (mean)	198	206	188	192
Change from baseline (mean)	17	-25	17	-43
Difference from sulfonylurea alone (adjusted mean)	—	-47*	—	-66*
% of patients with ≥30 mg/dL decrease from baseline	17%	48%	19%	55%
HbA1c (%)				
Baseline (mean)	8.6	8.8	8.9	8.9
Change from baseline (mean)	0.4	-0.5	0.1	-1.2
Difference from sulfonylurea alone (adjusted mean)	—	-0.9*	—	-1.4*
% of patients with ≥0.7% decrease from baseline	11%	36%	20%	68%

* p<0.0001 compared to sulfonylurea alone.

Know the medicines you take. Keep a list of all your medicines and show it to your doctor and pharmacist before you start a new medicine. They will tell you if it is okay to take AVANDARYL with other medicines.

How should I take AVANDARYL?

• Take AVANDARYL exactly as prescribed. Your doctor may need to change your dose until your blood sugar is better controlled.

• Take AVANDARYL by mouth one time each day with your first main meal.

• It usually takes a few days for AVANDARYL to start lowering your blood sugar. It may take 2 to 3 months to see the full effect on your blood sugar level.

• If you miss a dose of AVANDARYL, take it as soon as you remember unless it is time to take your next dose. Take your next dose at the usual time. Do not take double doses to make up for a missed dose.

• If you take too much AVANDARYL, call your doctor or poison control center right away.

• Test your blood sugar regularly as your doctor tells you.

• Your doctor should do blood tests to check your liver before you start taking AVANDARYL and during treatment as needed. Your doctor should also do regular blood sugar tests (for example, "A1c") to monitor your response to AVANDARYL.

• Call your doctor if you get sick, get injured, get an infection, or have surgery. AVANDARYL may not control your blood sugar levels during these times. Your doctor may need to stop AVANDARYL for a short time and give you insulin to control your blood sugar level.

What are possible side effects of AVANDARYL?

AVANDARYL may cause serious side effects, including:

• **Low blood sugar (hypoglycemia).** Lightheadedness, dizziness, shakiness or hunger may mean that your blood sugar is too low. This can happen if you skip meals, drink alcohol, use another medicine that lowers blood sugar, exercise (particularly hard or long), or if you have certain medical problems. Call your doctor if you have low blood sugar.

• **Weight gain.** AVANDARYL can cause weight gain from fluid retention or extra body fat. Weight gain can be a serious problem for people with certain conditions including heart problems. See "What is the most important information I should know about AVANDARYL?".

• **Liver problems.** It is important for your liver to be working normally when you take AVANDARYL. Your doctor should do blood tests to check your liver before you start taking AVANDARYL and during treatment as needed. Call your doctor right away if you have unexplained symptoms such as:
  • nausea or vomiting
  • stomach pain
  • unusual or unexplained tiredness
  • loss of appetite
  • dark urine

- yellowing of your skin or the whites of your eyes.
- **Macular edema** (a diabetic eye disease with swelling in the back of the eye). Tell your doctor right away if you have any changes in your vision. Your doctor should check your eyes regularly. Some people have had vision changes due to swelling in the back of the eye while taking rosiglitazone, one of the medicines in AVANDARYL.
- **Fractures (broken bones)**, usually in the hand, upper arm or foot, in females. Talk to your doctor for advice on how to keep your bones healthy.
- **Low red blood cell count (anemia)**.
- **Ovulation** (release of egg from an ovary in women) leading to pregnancy. Ovulation may happen in premenopausal women who do not have regular monthly periods. This can increase the chance of pregnancy. See "What should I tell my doctor before taking AVANDARYL?".

Common side effects with AVANDARYL include cold-like symptoms and headache.

Call your doctor for medical advice about side effects. You may report side effects to FDA at 1-800-FDA-1088.

How should I store AVANDARYL?
- Store AVANDARYL at room temperature, 59° to 86° F (15° to 30° C). Keep AVANDARYL in the container it comes in. Keep the container closed tightly.
- Safely, throw away AVANDARYL that is out of date or no longer needed.

Keep AVANDARYL and all medicines out of the reach of children.

General information about AVANDARYL
Medicines are sometimes prescribed for purposes other than those listed in a Medication Guide. Do not use AVANDARYL for a condition for which it was not prescribed. Do not give AVANDARYL to other people, even if they have the same symptoms you have. It may harm them.

This Medication Guide summarizes important information about AVANDARYL. If you would like more information, talk with your doctor. You can ask your doctor or pharmacist for information about AVANDARYL that is written for healthcare professionals. For more information, call 1-888-825-5249 or go to the website www.avandaryl.com.

What are the ingredients in AVANDARYL?
Active Ingredients: Rosiglitazone maleate and glimepiride.
Inactive Ingredients: Hypromellose 2910, lactose monohydrate, macrogol (polyethylene glycol), magnesium stearate, microcrystalline cellulose, sodium starch glycolate, titanium dioxide, triacetin, and 1 or more of the following: Yellow, red, or black iron oxides.

Always check to make sure that the medicine you are taking is the correct one. AVANDARYL tablets are triangles with rounded corners and look like this:
4 mg/1 mg strength tablets – yellow with "gsk" on one side and "4/1" on the other.
4 mg/2 mg strength tablets – orange with "gsk" on one side and "4/2" on the other.
4 mg/4 mg strength tablets – pink with "gsk" on one side and "4/4" on the other.
8 mg/2 mg strength tablets – pale pink with "gsk" on one side and "8/2" on the other.
8 mg/4 mg strength tablets – red with "gsk" on one side and "8/4" on the other.

AVANDARYL and AVANDIA are registered trademarks of GlaxoSmithKline.
The following are registered trademarks of their respective owners: AMARYL/AVENTIS Pharmaceuticals Inc.; REZULIN/Parke-Davis Pharmaceuticals Ltd.
This Medication Guide has been approved by the U.S. Food and Drug Administration.
GlaxoSmithKline
Research Triangle Park, NC 27709
©2009, GlaxoSmithKline. All rights reserved.
December 2009
AVR:2MG

AVANDIA®
[ə-van'dē-ə]
(rosiglitazone maleate)
Tablets   ℞

HIGHLIGHTS OF PRESCRIBING INFORMATION
These highlights do not include all the information needed to use AVANDIA safely and effectively. See full prescribing information for AVANDIA.
AVANDIA® (rosiglitazone maleate) Tablets
Initial U.S. Approval: 1999

WARNING: CONGESTIVE HEART FAILURE AND MYOCARDIAL ISCHEMIA
See full prescribing information for complete boxed warning.
- Thiazolidinediones, including rosiglitazone, cause or exacerbate congestive heart failure in some patients (5.1). After initiation of AVANDIA, and after dose in-

creases, observe patients carefully for signs and symptoms of heart failure (including excessive, rapid weight gain, dyspnea, and/or edema). If these signs and symptoms develop, the heart failure should be managed according to current standards of care. Furthermore, discontinuation or dose reduction of AVANDIA must be considered.
- AVANDIA is not recommended in patients with symptomatic heart failure. Initiation of AVANDIA in patients with established NYHA Class III or IV heart failure is contraindicated. (4, 5.1)
- A meta-analysis of 42 clinical studies (mean duration 6 months; 14,237 total patients), most of which compared AVANDIA to placebo, showed AVANDIA to be associated with an increased risk of myocardial ischemic events such as angina or myocardial infarction. Three other studies (mean duration 41 months; 14,067 total patients), comparing AVANDIA to some other approved oral antidiabetic agents or placebo, have not confirmed or excluded this risk. In their entirety, the available data on the risk of myocardial ischemia are inconclusive. (5.2)

———INDICATIONS AND USAGE———
AVANDIA is a thiazolidinedione antidiabetic agent indicated as an adjunct to diet and exercise to improve glycemic control in adults with type 2 diabetes mellitus. (1)
Important Limitations of Use:
- AVANDIA should not be used in patients with type 1 diabetes mellitus or for the treatment of diabetic ketoacidosis. (1.2)
- Coadministration of AVANDIA and insulin is not recommended. (1.2, 5.3)
- Use of AVANDIA with nitrates is not recommended. (1.2, 5.2)

———DOSAGE AND ADMINISTRATION———
- Start at 4 mg daily in single or divided doses; do not exceed 8 mg daily. (2)
- Dose increases should be accompanied by careful monitoring for adverse events related to fluid retention. (2)
- Do not initiate AVANDIA if the patient exhibits clinical evidence of active liver disease or increased serum transaminase levels. (2.4)

———DOSAGE FORMS AND STRENGTHS———
Pentagonal, film-coated tablets in the following strengths:
- 2 mg, 4 mg, and 8 mg (3)

———CONTRAINDICATIONS———
Initiation of AVANDIA in patients with established NYHA Class III or IV heart failure is contraindicated. (4)

———WARNINGS AND PRECAUTIONS———
- Fluid retention, which may exacerbate or lead to heart failure, may occur. Combination use with insulin and use in congestive heart failure NYHA Class I and II may increase risk of other cardiovascular effects. (5.1, 5.3)
- Increased risk of myocardial ischemic events has been observed in a meta-analysis of 42 clinical trials (incidence rate 2% versus 1.5%). (5.2)
- Use of AVANDIA with nitrates is not recommended. (1.2, 5.2)
- Coadministration of AVANDIA and insulin is not recommended. (1.2, 5.3)
- Dose-related edema (5.4), weight gain (5.5), and anemia (5.9) may occur.
- Macular edema has been reported. (5.7)
- Increased incidence of bone fracture in female patients. (5.8)
- There have been no clinical studies establishing conclusive evidence of macrovascular risk reduction with AVANDIA or any other oral antidiabetic drug. (5.2)

———ADVERSE REACTIONS———
Common adverse reactions (>5%) reported in clinical trials without regard to causality were upper respiratory tract infection, injury, and headache. (6.1)
To report SUSPECTED ADVERSE REACTIONS, contact GlaxoSmithKline at 1-888-825-5249 or FDA at 1-800-FDA-1088 or www.fda.gov/medwatch.

———DRUG INTERACTIONS———
Inhibitors of CYP2C8 (e.g., gemfibrozil) may increase rosiglitazone levels; inducers of CYP2C8 (e.g., rifampin) may decrease rosiglitazone levels. (7.1)
See 17 for PATIENT COUNSELING INFORMATION and FDA-approved Medication Guide.

Revised: February 2009
AVD:28PI

FULL PRESCRIBING INFORMATION: CONTENTS*

FULL PRESCRIBING INFORMATION

WARNING: CONGESTIVE HEART FAILURE AND MYOCARDIAL ISCHEMIA
- Thiazolidinediones, including rosiglitazone, cause or exacerbate congestive heart failure in some patients [see Warnings and Precautions (5.1)]. After initiation of AVANDIA, and after dose increases, observe patients carefully for signs and symptoms of heart failure (including excessive, rapid weight gain, dyspnea, and/or edema). If these signs and symptoms develop, the heart failure should be managed according to current standards of care. Furthermore, discontinuation or dose reduction of AVANDIA must be considered.
- AVANDIA is not recommended in patients with symptomatic heart failure. Initiation of AVANDIA in patients with established NYHA Class III or IV heart failure is contraindicated. [See Contraindications (4) and Warnings and Precautions (5.1).]
- A meta-analysis of 42 clinical studies (mean duration 6 months; 14,237 total patients), most of which compared AVANDIA to placebo, showed AVANDIA to be associated with an increased risk of myocardial ischemic events such as angina or myocardial infarction. Three other studies (mean duration 41 months; 14,067 total patients), comparing AVANDIA to some other approved oral antidiabetic agents or placebo, have not confirmed or excluded this risk. In their entirety, the available data on the risk of myocardial ischemia are inconclusive. [See Warnings and Precautions (5.2).]

1   INDICATIONS AND USAGE

1.1   Monotherapy and Combination Therapy
AVANDIA is indicated as an adjunct to diet and exercise to improve glycemic control in adults with type 2 diabetes mellitus.

1.2   Important Limitations of Use
- Due to its mechanism of action, AVANDIA is active only in the presence of endogenous insulin. Therefore, AVANDIA

should not be used in patients with type 1 diabetes mellitus or for the treatment of diabetic ketoacidosis.
- The coadministration of AVANDIA and insulin is not recommended.
- The use of AVANDIA with nitrates is not recommended.

2 DOSAGE AND ADMINISTRATION

The management of antidiabetic therapy should be individualized. All patients should start AVANDIA at the lowest recommended dose. Further increases in the dose of AVANDIA should be accompanied by careful monitoring for adverse events related to fluid retention *[see Boxed Warning and Warnings and Precautions (5.1)]*.

AVANDIA may be administered at a starting dose of 4 mg either as a single daily dose or in 2 divided doses. For patients who respond inadequately following 8 to 12 weeks of treatment, as determined by reduction in fasting plasma glucose (FPG), the dose may be increased to 8 mg daily as monotherapy or in combination with metformin, sulfonylurea, or sulfonylurea plus metformin. Reductions in glycemic parameters by dose and regimen are described under *Clinical Studies (14.1)*. AVANDIA may be taken with or without food.

The total daily dose of AVANDIA should not exceed 8 mg.

2.1 Monotherapy

The usual starting dose of AVANDIA is 4 mg administered either as a single dose once daily or in divided doses twice daily. In clinical trials, the 4-mg twice-daily regimen resulted in the greatest reduction in FPG and hemoglobin A1c (HbA1c).

2.2 Combination With Sulfonylurea or Metformin

When AVANDIA is added to existing therapy, the current dose(s) of the agent(s) can be continued upon initiation of therapy with AVANDIA.

Sulfonylurea: When used in combination with sulfonylurea, the usual starting dose of AVANDIA is 4 mg administered as either a single dose once daily or in divided doses twice daily. If patients report hypoglycemia, the dose of the sulfonylurea should be decreased.

Metformin: The usual starting dose of AVANDIA in combination with metformin is 4 mg administered as either a single dose once daily or in divided doses twice daily. It is unlikely that the dose of metformin will require adjustment due to hypoglycemia during combination therapy with AVANDIA.

2.3 Combination With Sulfonylurea Plus Metformin

The usual starting dose of AVANDIA in combination with a sulfonylurea plus metformin is 4 mg administered as either a single dose once daily or in divided doses twice daily. If patients report hypoglycemia, the dose of the sulfonylurea should be decreased.

2.4 Specific Patient Populations

Renal Impairment: No dosage adjustment is necessary when AVANDIA is used as monotherapy in patients with renal impairment. Since metformin is contraindicated in such patients, concomitant administration of metformin and AVANDIA is also contraindicated in patients with renal impairment.

Hepatic Impairment: Liver enzymes should be measured prior to initiating treatment with AVANDIA. Therapy with AVANDIA should not be initiated if the patient exhibits clinical evidence of active liver disease or increased serum transaminase levels (ALT >2.5× upper limit of normal at start of therapy). After initiation of AVANDIA, liver enzymes should be monitored periodically per the clinical judgment of the healthcare professional. *[See Warnings and Precautions (5.6) and Clinical Pharmacology (12.3).]*

Pediatric: Data are insufficient to recommend pediatric use of AVANDIA *[see Use in Specific Populations (8.4)]*.

3 DOSAGE FORMS AND STRENGTHS

Pentagonal film-coated TILTAB® tablet contains rosiglitazone as the maleate as follows:
- 2 mg - pink, debossed with SB on one side and 2 on the other
- 4 mg - orange, debossed with SB on one side and 4 on the other
- 8 mg - red-brown, debossed with SB on one side and 8 on the other

4 CONTRAINDICATIONS

Initiation of AVANDIA in patients with established New York Heart Association (NYHA) Class III or IV heart failure is contraindicated *[see Boxed Warning]*.

5 WARNINGS AND PRECAUTIONS

5.1 Cardiac Failure

AVANDIA, like other thiazolidinediones, alone or in combination with other antidiabetic agents, can cause fluid retention, which may exacerbate or lead to heart failure. Patients should be observed for signs and symptoms of heart failure. If these signs and symptoms develop, the heart failure should be managed according to current standards of care. Furthermore, discontinuation or dose reduction of rosiglitazone must be considered *[see Boxed Warning]*.

Patients with congestive heart failure (CHF) NYHA Class I and II treated with AVANDIA have an increased risk of cardiovascular events. A 52-week, double-blind, placebo-controlled echocardiographic study was conducted in 224 patients with type 2 diabetes mellitus and NYHA Class I or II CHF (ejection fraction ≤45%) on background antidiabetic and CHF therapy. An independent committee conducted a blinded evaluation of fluid-related events (including congestive heart failure) and cardiovascular hospitalizations according to predefined criteria (adjudication). Separate from the adjudication, other cardiovascular adverse events were reported by investigators. Although no treatment difference in change from baseline of ejection fractions was observed, more cardiovascular adverse events were observed following treatment with AVANDIA compared to placebo during the 52-week study. (See Table 1.)

Table 1. Emergent Cardiovascular Adverse Events in Patients With Congestive Heart Failure (NYHA Class I and II) Treated With AVANDIA or Placebo (in Addition to Background Antidiabetic and CHF Therapy)

Events	AVANDIA	Placebo
	N = 110 n (%)	N = 114 n (%)
Adjudicated		
Cardiovascular deaths	5 (5%)	4 (4%)
CHF worsening	7 (6%)	4 (4%)
— with overnight hospitalization	5 (5%)	4 (4%)
— without overnight hospitalization	2 (2%)	0 (0%)
New or worsening edema	28 (25%)	10 (9%)
New or worsening dyspnea	29 (26%)	19 (17%)
Increases in CHF medication	36 (33%)	20 (18%)
Cardiovascular hospitalization*	21 (19%)	15 (13%)
Investigator-reported, non-adjudicated		
Ischemic adverse events	10 (9%)	5 (4%)
— Myocardial infarction	5 (5%)	2 (2%)
— Angina	6 (5%)	3 (3%)

*Includes hospitalization for any cardiovascular reason.

Initiation of AVANDIA in patients with established NYHA Class III or IV heart failure is contraindicated. AVANDIA is not recommended in patients with symptomatic heart failure. *[See Boxed Warning.]*

Patients experiencing acute coronary syndromes have not been studied in controlled clinical trials. In view of the potential for development of heart failure in patients having an acute coronary event, initiation of AVANDIA is not recommended for patients experiencing an acute coronary event, and discontinuation of AVANDIA during this acute phase should be considered.

Patients with NYHA Class III and IV cardiac status (with or without CHF) have not been studied in controlled clinical trials. AVANDIA is not recommended in patients with NYHA Class III and IV cardiac status.

5.2 Myocardial Ischemia

Meta-Analysis of Myocardial Ischemia in a Group of 42 Clinical Trials: A meta-analysis was conducted retrospectively to assess cardiovascular adverse events reported across 42 double-blind, randomized, controlled clinical trials (mean duration 6 months).[1] These studies had been conducted to assess glucose-lowering efficacy in type 2 diabetes, and prospectively planned adjudication of cardiovascular events had not occurred in the trials. Some trials were placebo-controlled and some used active oral antidiabetic drugs as controls. Placebo-controlled studies included monotherapy trials (monotherapy with AVANDIA versus placebo monotherapy) and add-on trials (AVANDIA or placebo, added to sulfonylurea, metformin, or insulin). Active control studies included monotherapy trials (monotherapy with AVANDIA versus sulfonylurea or metformin monotherapy) and add-on trials (AVANDIA plus sulfonylurea or AVANDIA plus metformin, versus sulfonylurea plus metformin). A total of 14,237 patients were included (8,604 in treatment groups containing AVANDIA, 5,633 in comparator groups), with 4,143 patient-years of exposure to AVANDIA and 2,675 patient-years of exposure to comparator. Myocardial ischemic events included angina pectoris, angina pectoris aggravated, unstable angina, cardiac arrest, chest pain, coronary artery occlusion, dyspnea, myocardial infarction, coronary thrombosis, myocardial ischemia, coronary artery disease, and coronary artery disorder. In this analysis, an increased risk of myocardial ischemia with AVANDIA versus pooled comparators was observed (2% AVANDIA versus 1.5% comparators, odds ratio 1.4, 95% confidence interval [CI] 1.1, 1.8). An increased risk of myocardial ischemic events with AVANDIA was observed in the placebo-controlled studies, but not in the active-controlled studies. (See Figure 1.)

A greater increased risk of myocardial ischemic events was observed in studies where AVANDIA was added to insulin (2.8% for AVANDIA plus insulin versus 1.4% for placebo plus insulin, [OR 2.1, 95% CI 0.9, 5.1]). This increased risk reflects a difference of 3 events per 100 patient-years (95% CI -0.1, 6.3) between treatment groups. *[See Warnings and Precautions (5.3).]*

Figure 1. Forest Plot of Odds Ratios (95% Confidence Intervals) for Myocardial Ischemic Events in the Meta-Analysis of 42 Clinical Trials

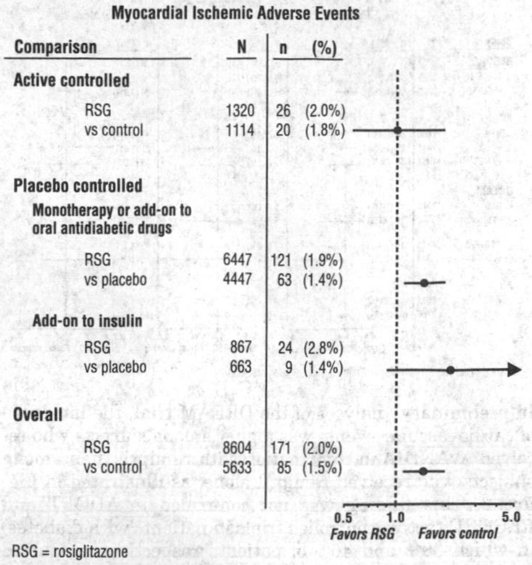

Myocardial Ischemic Adverse Events
Comparison
N
n (%)
Active controlled
RSG 1320 26 (2.0%)
vs control 1114 20 (1.8%)
Placebo controlled
Monotherapy or add-on to oral antidiabetic drugs
RSG 6447 121 (1.9%)
vs placebo 4447 63 (1.4%)
Add-on to insulin
RSG 867 24 (2.8%)
vs placebo 663 9 (1.4%)
Overall
RSG 8604 171 (2.0%)
vs control 5633 85 (1.5%)
0.5
1.0
5.0
Favors RSG
Favors control
RSG = rosiglitazone

A greater increased risk of myocardial ischemia was also observed in patients who received AVANDIA and background nitrate therapy. For AVANDIA (N = 361) versus control (N = 244) in nitrate users, the odds ratio was 2.9 (95% CI 1.4, 5.9), while for non-nitrate users (about 14,000 patients total), the odds ratio was 1.3 (95% CI 0.9, 1.7). This increased risk represents a difference of 12 myocardial ischemic events per 100 patient-years (95% CI 3.3, 21.4). Most of the nitrate users had established coronary heart disease. Among patients with known coronary heart disease who were not on nitrate therapy, an increased risk of myocardial ischemic events for AVANDIA versus comparator was not demonstrated.

Myocardial Ischemic Events in Large, Long-Term, Prospective, Randomized, Controlled Trials of AVANDIA: Data from 3 other large, long-term, prospective, randomized, controlled clinical trials of AVANDIA were assessed separately from the meta-analysis. These 3 trials include a total of 14,067 patients (treatment groups containing AVANDIA N = 6,311, comparator groups N = 7,756), with patient-year exposure of 21,803 patient-years for AVANDIA and 25,998 patient-years for comparator. Duration of follow-up exceeded 3 years in each study. ADOPT (A Diabetes Outcomes Progression Trial) was a 4- to 6-year randomized, active-controlled study in recently diagnosed patients with type 2 diabetes naïve to drug therapy. It was an efficacy and general safety trial that was designed to examine the durability of AVANDIA as monotherapy (N = 1,456) for glycemic control in type 2 diabetes, with comparator arms of sulfonylurea monotherapy (N = 1,441) and metformin monotherapy (N = 1,454). DREAM (Diabetes Reduction Assessment with Rosiglitazone and Ramipril Medication, published report[2]) was a 3- to 5-year randomized, placebo-controlled study in patients with impaired glucose tolerance and/or impaired fasting glucose. It had a 2×2 factorial design, intended to evaluate the effect of AVANDIA, and separately of ramipril (an angiotensin converting enzyme inhibitor [ACEI]), on progression to overt diabetes. In DREAM, 2,635 patients were in treatment groups containing AVANDIA, and 2,634 were in treatment groups not containing AVANDIA. Interim results have been published[3] for RECORD (Rosiglitazone Evaluated for Cardiac Outcomes and Regulation of Glycemia in Diabetes), an ongoing open-label, 6-year cardiovascular outcomes study in patients with type 2 diabetes with an average treatment duration of 3.75 years. RECORD includes patients who have failed metformin or sulfonylurea monotherapy; those who have failed metformin are randomized to receive either add-on AVANDIA or add-on sulfonylurea, and those who have failed sulfonylurea are randomized to receive either add-on AVANDIA or add-on metformin. In RECORD, a total of 2,220 patients are receiving add-on AVANDIA, and 2,227 patients are on one of the add-on regimens not containing AVANDIA.

For these 3 trials, analyses were performed using a composite of major adverse cardiovascular events (myocardial infarction, cardiovascular death, or stroke), referred to hereafter as MACE. This endpoint differed from the meta-analysis' broad endpoint of myocardial ischemic events, more than half of which were angina. Myocardial infarction included adjudicated fatal and nonfatal myocardial infarction plus sudden death. As shown in Figure 2, the results for the 3 endpoints (MACE, MI, and Total Mortality) were not statistically significantly different between AVANDIA and comparators.

Figure 2. Hazard Ratios for the Risk of MACE (Myocardial Infarction, Cardiovascular Death, or Stroke), Myocardial Infarction, and Total Mortality With AVANDIA Compared With a Control Group

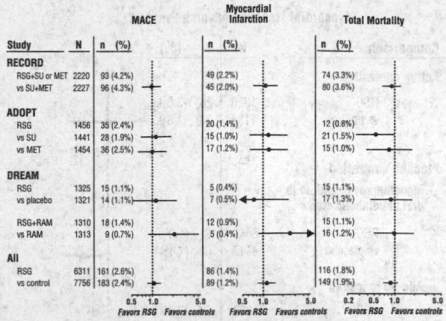

RSG = rosiglitazone; SU = sulfonylurea; MET = metformin; RAM = ramipril

In preliminary analyses of the DREAM trial, the incidence of cardiovascular events was higher among subjects who received AVANDIA in combination with ramipril than among subjects who received ramipril alone, as illustrated in Figure 2. This finding was not confirmed in ADOPT and RECORD (active-controlled trials in patients with diabetes) in which 30% and 40% of patients respectively, reported ACE-inhibitor use at baseline.

In their entirety, the available data on the risk of myocardial ischemia are inconclusive. Definitive conclusions regarding this risk await completion of an adequately-designed cardiovascular outcome study.

There have been no clinical studies establishing conclusive evidence of macrovascular risk reduction with AVANDIA or any other oral antidiabetic drug.

5.3 Congestive Heart Failure and Myocardial Ischemia During Coadministration of AVANDIA With Insulin

In studies in which AVANDIA was added to insulin, AVANDIA increased the risk of congestive heart failure and myocardial ischemia. (See Table 2.) Coadministration of AVANDIA and insulin is not recommended. *[See Indications and Usage (1.2) and Warnings and Precautions (5.1, 5.2).]*

In five, 26-week, controlled, randomized, double-blind trials which were included in the meta-analysis *[see Warnings and Precautions (5.2)]*, patients with type 2 diabetes mellitus were randomized to coadministration of AVANDIA and insulin (N = 867) or insulin (N = 663). In these 5 trials, AVANDIA was added to insulin. These trials included patients with long-standing diabetes (median duration of 12

years) and a high prevalence of pre-existing medical conditions, including peripheral neuropathy, retinopathy, ischemic heart disease, vascular disease, and congestive heart failure. The total number of patients with emergent congestive heart failure was 21 (2.4%) and 7 (1.1%) in the AVANDIA plus insulin and insulin groups, respectively. The total number of patients with emergent myocardial ischemia was 24 (2.8%) and 9 (1.4%) in the AVANDIA plus insulin and insulin groups, respectively (OR 2.1 [95% CI 0.9, 5.1]). Although the event rate for congestive heart failure and myocardial ischemia was low in the studied population, consistently the event rate was 2-fold or higher with coadministration of AVANDIA and insulin. These cardiovascular events were noted at both the 4 mg and 8 mg daily doses of AVANDIA. (See Table 2.)

Table 2. Occurrence of Cardiovascular Events in 5 Controlled Trials of Addition of AVANDIA to Established Insulin Treatment

Event*	AVANDIA + Insulin (n = 867) n (%)	Insulin (n = 663) n (%)
Congestive heart failure	21 (2.4%)	7 (1.1%)
Myocardial ischemia	24 (2.8%)	9 (1.4%)
Composite of cardiovascular death, myocardial infarction, or stroke	10 (1.2%)	5 (0.8%)
Stroke	5 (0.6%)	4 (0.6%)
Myocardial infarction	4 (0.5%)	1 (0.2%)
Cardiovascular death	4 (0.5%)	1 (0.2%)
All deaths	6 (0.7%)	1 (0.2%)

*Events are not exclusive; i.e., a patient with a cardiovascular death due to a myocardial infarction would be counted in 4 event categories (myocardial ischemia; cardiovascular death, myocardial infarction or stroke; myocardial infarction; cardiovascular death).

In a sixth, 24-week, controlled, randomized, double-blind trial of AVANDIA and insulin coadministration, insulin was added to AVANDAMET® (rosiglitazone maleate and metformin HCl) (n = 161) and compared to insulin plus placebo (n = 158), after a single-blind 8-week run-in with AVANDAMET. Patients with edema requiring pharmacologic therapy and those with congestive heart failure were excluded at baseline and during the run-in period. In the group receiving AVANDAMET plus insulin, there was one myocardial ischemic event and one sudden death. No myocardial ischemia was observed in the insulin group, and no congestive heart failure was reported in either treatment group.

5.4 Edema

AVANDIA should be used with caution in patients with edema. In a clinical study in healthy volunteers who received 8 mg of AVANDIA once daily for 8 weeks, there was a statistically significant increase in median plasma volume compared to placebo.

Since thiazolidinediones, including rosiglitazone, can cause fluid retention, which can exacerbate or lead to congestive heart failure, AVANDIA should be used with caution in patients at risk for heart failure. Patients should be monitored for signs and symptoms of heart failure *[see Boxed Warning, Warnings and Precautions (5.1), and Patient Counseling Information (17.1)]*.

In controlled clinical trials of patients with type 2 diabetes, mild to moderate edema was reported in patients treated with AVANDIA, and may be dose related. Patients with ongoing edema were more likely to have adverse events associated with edema if started on combination therapy with insulin and AVANDIA *[see Adverse Reactions (6.1)]*.

5.5 Weight Gain

Dose-related weight gain was seen with AVANDIA alone and in combination with other hypoglycemic agents (Table 3). The mechanism of weight gain is unclear but probably involves a combination of fluid retention and fat accumulation.

In postmarketing experience, there have been reports of unusually rapid increases in weight and increases in excess of that generally observed in clinical trials. Patients who experience such increases should be assessed for fluid accumulation and volume-related events such as excessive edema and congestive heart failure *[see Boxed Warning]*. [See table 3 at bottom left]

In a 4- to 6-year, monotherapy, comparative trial (ADOPT) in patients recently diagnosed with type 2 diabetes not previously treated with antidiabetic medication *[see Clinical Studies (14.1)]*, the median weight change (25th, 75th percentiles) from baseline at 4 years was 3.5 kg (0.0, 8.1) for AVANDIA, 2.0 kg (-1.0, 4.8) for glyburide, and -2.4 kg (-5.4, 0.5) for metformin.

In a 24-week study in pediatric patients aged 10 to 17 years treated with AVANDIA 4 to 8 mg daily, a median weight gain of 2.8 kg (25th, 75th percentiles: 0.0, 5.8) was reported.

5.6 Hepatic Effects

Liver enzymes should be measured prior to the initiation of therapy with AVANDIA in all patients and periodically thereafter per the clinical judgment of the healthcare professional. Therapy with AVANDIA should not be initiated in patients with increased baseline liver enzyme levels (ALT >2.5× upper limit of normal). Patients with mildly elevated liver enzymes (ALT levels ≤2.5× upper limit of normal) at baseline or during therapy with AVANDIA should be evaluated to determine the cause of the liver enzyme elevation. Initiation of, or continuation of, therapy with AVANDIA in patients with mild liver enzyme elevations should proceed with caution and include close clinical follow-up, including liver enzyme monitoring, to determine if the liver enzyme elevations resolve or worsen. If at any time ALT levels increase to >3× the upper limit of normal in patients on therapy with AVANDIA, liver enzyme levels should be rechecked as soon as possible. If ALT levels remain >3× the upper limit of normal, therapy with AVANDIA should be discontinued.

If any patient develops symptoms suggesting hepatic dysfunction, which may include unexplained nausea, vomiting, abdominal pain, fatigue, anorexia and/or dark urine, liver enzymes should be checked. The decision whether to continue the patient on therapy with AVANDIA should be guided by clinical judgment pending laboratory evaluations. If jaundice is observed, drug therapy should be discontinued. *[See Adverse Reactions (6.2, 6.3).]*

5.7 Macular Edema

Macular edema has been reported in postmarketing experience in some diabetic patients who were taking AVANDIA or another thiazolidinedione. Some patients presented with blurred vision or decreased visual acuity, but some patients appear to have been diagnosed on routine ophthalmologic examination. Most patients had peripheral edema at the time macular edema was diagnosed. Some patients had improvement in their macular edema after discontinuation of their thiazolidinedione. Patients with diabetes should have regular eye exams by an ophthalmologist, per the Standards of Care of the American Diabetes Association. Additionally, any diabetic who reports any kind of visual symptom should be promptly referred to an ophthalmologist, regardless of the patient's underlying medications or other physical findings. *[See Adverse Reactions (6.1).]*

5.8 Fractures

In a 4- to 6-year comparative study (ADOPT) of glycemic control with monotherapy in drug-naïve patients recently diagnosed with type 2 diabetes mellitus, an increased incidence of bone fracture was noted in female patients taking AVANDIA. Over the 4- to 6-year period, the incidence of bone fracture in females was 9.3% (60/645) for AVANDIA versus 3.5% (21/605) for glyburide and 5.1% (30/590) for metformin. This increased incidence was noted after the first year of treatment and persisted during the course of the study. The majority of the fractures in the women who received AVANDIA occurred in the upper arm, hand, and foot. These sites of fracture are different from those usually associated with postmenopausal osteoporosis (e.g., hip or

Table 3. Weight Changes (kg) From Baseline at Endpoint During Clinical Trials

	Duration	Control Group	Control Group Median (25th, 75th percentile)	AVANDIA 4 mg Median (25th, 75th percentile)	AVANDIA 8 mg Median (25th, 75th percentile)
Monotherapy					
	26 weeks	placebo	-0.9 (-2.8, 0.9) N = 210	1.0 (-0.9, 3.6) N = 436	3.1 (1.1, 5.8) N = 439
	52 weeks	sulfonylurea	2.0 (0, 4.0) N = 173	2.0 (-0.6, 4.0) N = 150	2.6 (0, 5.3) N = 157
Combination therapy					
Sulfonylurea	24-26 weeks	sulfonylurea	0 (-1.0, 1.3) N = 1,155	2.2 (0.5, 4.0) N = 613	3.5 (1.4, 5.9) N = 841
Metformin	26 weeks	metformin	-1.4 (-3.2, 0.2) N = 175	0.8 (-1.0, 2.6) N = 100	2.1 (0, 4.3) N = 184
Insulin	26 weeks	insulin	0.9 (-0.5, 2.7) N = 162	4.1 (1.4, 6.3) N = 164	5.4 (3.4, 7.3) N = 150
Sulfonylurea + metformin	26 weeks	sulfonylurea + metformin	0.2 (-1.2, 1.6) N = 272	2.5 (0.8, 4.6) N = 275	4.5 (2.4, 7.3) N = 276

spine). No increase in fracture rates was observed in men treated with AVANDIA. The risk of fracture should be considered in the care of patients, especially female patients, treated with AVANDIA, and attention given to assessing and maintaining bone health according to current standards of care.

5.9 Hematologic Effects

Decreases in mean hemoglobin and hematocrit occurred in a dose-related fashion in adult patients treated with AVANDIA *[see Adverse Reactions (6.2)]*. The observed changes may be related to the increased plasma volume observed with treatment with AVANDIA.

5.10 Diabetes and Blood Glucose Control

Patients receiving AVANDIA in combination with other hypoglycemic agents may be at risk for hypoglycemia, and a reduction in the dose of the concomitant agent may be necessary.

Periodic fasting blood glucose and HbA1c measurements should be performed to monitor therapeutic response.

5.11 Ovulation

Therapy with AVANDIA, like other thiazolidinediones, may result in ovulation in some premenopausal anovulatory women. As a result, these patients may be at an increased risk for pregnancy while taking AVANDIA *[see Use in Specific Populations (8.1)]*. Thus, adequate contraception in premenopausal women should be recommended. This possible effect has not been specifically investigated in clinical studies; therefore, the frequency of this occurrence is not known. Although hormonal imbalance has been seen in preclinical studies *[see Nonclinical Toxicology (13.1)]*, the clinical significance of this finding is not known. If unexpected menstrual dysfunction occurs, the benefits of continued therapy with AVANDIA should be reviewed.

6 ADVERSE REACTIONS

6.1 Clinical Trial Experience

Adult: In clinical trials, approximately 9,900 patients with type 2 diabetes have been treated with AVANDIA.

Short-Term Trials of AVANDIA as Monotherapy and in Combination With Other Hypoglycemic Agents: The incidence and types of adverse events reported in short-term clinical trials of AVANDIA as monotherapy are shown in Table 4. [See table 4 at right]

Overall, the types of adverse reactions without regard to causality reported when AVANDIA was used in combination with a sulfonylurea or metformin were similar to those during monotherapy with AVANDIA.

Events of anemia and edema tended to be reported more frequently at higher doses, and were generally mild to moderate in severity and usually did not require discontinuation of treatment with AVANDIA.

In double-blind studies, anemia was reported in 1.9% of patients receiving AVANDIA as monotherapy compared to 0.7% on placebo, 0.6% on sulfonylureas, and 2.2% on metformin. Reports of anemia were greater in patients treated with a combination of AVANDIA and metformin (7.1%) and with a combination of AVANDIA and a sulfonylurea plus metformin (6.7%) compared to monotherapy with AVANDIA or in combination with a sulfonylurea (2.3%). Lower pretreatment hemoglobin/hematocrit levels in patients enrolled in the metformin combination clinical trials may have contributed to the higher reporting rate of anemia in these studies *[see Adverse Reactions (6.2)]*.

In clinical trials, edema was reported in 4.8% of patients receiving AVANDIA as monotherapy compared to 1.3% on placebo, 1.0% on sulfonylureas, and 2.2% on metformin. The reporting rate of edema was higher for AVANDIA 8 mg in sulfonylurea combinations (12.4%) compared to other combinations, with the exception of insulin. Edema was reported in 14.7% of patients receiving AVANDIA in the insulin combination trials compared to 5.4% on insulin alone. Reports of new onset or exacerbation of congestive heart failure occurred at rates of 1% for insulin alone, and 2% (4 mg) and 3% (8 mg) for insulin in combination with AVANDIA *[see Boxed Warning and Warnings and Precautions (5.3)]*.

In controlled combination therapy studies with sulfonylureas, mild to moderate hypoglycemic symptoms, which appear to be dose related, were reported. Few patients were withdrawn for hypoglycemia (<1%) and few episodes of hypoglycemia were considered to be severe (<1%). Hypoglycemia was the most frequently reported adverse event in the fixed-dose insulin combination trials, although few patients withdrew for hypoglycemia (4 of 408 for AVANDIA plus insulin and 1 of 203 for insulin alone). Rates of hypoglycemia, confirmed by capillary blood glucose concentration ≤50 mg/dL, were 6% for insulin alone and 12% (4 mg) and 14% (8 mg) for insulin in combination with AVANDIA. *[See Warnings and Precautions (5.10).]*

Long-Term Trial of AVANDIA as Monotherapy: A 4- to 6-year study (ADOPT) compared the use of AVANDIA (n = 1,456), glyburide (n = 1,441), and metformin (n = 1,454) as monotherapy in patients recently diagnosed with type 2 diabetes who were not previously treated with antidiabetic

medication. Table 5 presents adverse reactions without regard to causality; rates are expressed per 100 patient-years (PY) exposure to account for the differences in exposure to study medication across the 3 treatment groups.

In ADOPT, fractures were reported in a greater number of women treated with AVANDIA (9.3%, 2.7/100 patient-years) compared to glyburide (3.5%, 1.3/100 patient-years) or metformin (5.1%, 1.5/100 patient-years). The majority of the fractures in the women who received rosiglitazone were reported in the upper arm, hand, and foot. *[See Warnings and Precautions (5.7).]* The observed incidence of fractures for male patients was similar among the 3 treatment groups.

Table 4. Adverse Events (≥5% in Any Treatment Group) Reported by Patients in Short-Term* Double-Blind Clinical Trials With AVANDIA as Monotherapy

Preferred Term	AVANDIA Monotherapy	Placebo	Metformin	Sulfonylureas[†]
	N = 2,526	N = 601	N = 225	N = 626
	%	%	%	%
Upper respiratory tract infection	9.9	8.7	8.9	7.3
Injury	7.6	4.3	7.6	6.1
Headache	5.9	5.0	8.9	5.4
Back pain	4.0	3.8	4.0	5.0
Hyperglycemia	3.9	5.7	4.4	8.1
Fatigue	3.6	5.0	4.0	1.9
Sinusitis	3.2	4.5	5.3	3.0
Diarrhea	2.3	3.3	15.6	3.0
Hypoglycemia	0.6	0.2	1.3	5.9

* Short-term trials ranged from 8 weeks to 1 year.
[†] Includes patients receiving glyburide (N = 514), gliclazide (N = 91), or glipizide (N = 21).

Table 5. On-Therapy Adverse Events (≥5 Events/100 Patient-Years [PY]) in Any Treatment Group Reported in a 4- to 6-Year Clinical Trial of AVANDIA as Monotherapy (ADOPT)

	AVANDIA N = 1,456 PY = 4,954	Glyburide N = 1,441 PY = 4,244	Metformin N = 1,454 PY = 4,906
Nasopharyngitis	6.3	6.9	6.6
Back pain	5.1	4.9	5.3
Arthralgia	5.0	4.8	4.2
Hypertension	4.4	6.0	6.1
Upper respiratory tract infection	4.3	5.0	4.7
Hypoglycemia	2.9	13.0	3.4
Diarrhea	2.5	3.2	6.8

Pediatric: AVANDIA has been evaluated for safety in a single, active-controlled trial of pediatric patients with type 2 diabetes in which 99 were treated with AVANDIA and 101 were treated with metformin. The most common adverse reactions (>10%) without regard to causality for either AVANDIA or metformin were headache (17% versus 14%), nausea (4% versus 11%), nasopharyngitis (3% versus 12%), and diarrhea (1% versus 13%). In this study, one case of diabetic ketoacidosis was reported in the metformin group. In addition, there were 3 patients in the rosiglitazone group who had FPG of ~300 mg/dL, 2+ ketonuria, and an elevated anion gap.

6.2 Laboratory Abnormalities

Hematologic: Decreases in mean hemoglobin and hematocrit occurred in a dose-related fashion in adult patients treated with AVANDIA (mean decreases in individual studies as much as 1.0 g/dL hemoglobin and as much as 3.3% hematocrit). The changes occurred primarily during the first 3 months following initiation of therapy with AVANDIA or following a dose increase in AVANDIA. The time course and magnitude of decreases were similar in patients treated with a combination of AVANDIA and other hypoglycemic agents or monotherapy with AVANDIA. Pre-treatment levels of hemoglobin and hematocrit were lower in patients in metformin combination studies and may have contributed to the higher reporting rate of anemia. In a single study in

pediatric patients, decreases in hemoglobin and hematocrit (mean decreases of 0.29 g/dL and 0.95%, respectively) were reported. Small decreases in hemoglobin and hematocrit have also been reported in pediatric patients treated with AVANDIA. White blood cell counts also decreased slightly in adult patients treated with AVANDIA. Decreases in hematologic parameters may be related to increased plasma volume observed with treatment with AVANDIA.

Lipids: Changes in serum lipids have been observed following treatment with AVANDIA in adults *[see Clinical Pharmacology (12.2)]*. Small changes in serum lipid parameters were reported in children treated with AVANDIA for 24 weeks.

Serum Transaminase Levels: In pre-approval clinical studies in 4,598 patients treated with AVANDIA (3,600 patient-years of exposure) and in a long-term 4- to 6-year study in 1,456 patients treated with AVANDIA (4,954 patient-years exposure), there was no evidence of drug-induced hepatotoxicity.

In pre-approval controlled trials, 0.2% of patients treated with AVANDIA had elevations in ALT >3× the upper limit of normal compared to 0.2% on placebo and 0.5% on active comparators. The ALT elevations in patients treated with AVANDIA were reversible. Hyperbilirubinemia was found in 0.3% of patients treated with AVANDIA compared with 0.9% treated with placebo and 1% in patients treated with active comparators. In pre-approval clinical trials, there were no cases of idiosyncratic drug reactions leading to hepatic failure. *[See Warnings and Precautions (5.6).]*

In the 4- to 6-year ADOPT trial, patients treated with AVANDIA (4,954 patient-years exposure), glyburide (4,244 patient-years exposure), or metformin (4,906 patient-years exposure), as monotherapy, had the same rate of ALT increase to >3× upper limit of normal (0.3 per 100 patient-years exposure).

6.3 Postmarketing Experience

In addition to adverse reactions reported from clinical trials, the events described below have been identified during post-approval use of AVANDIA. Because these events are reported voluntarily from a population of unknown size, it is not possible to reliably estimate their frequency or to always establish a causal relationship to drug exposure.

In patients receiving thiazolidinedione therapy, serious adverse events with or without a fatal outcome, potentially related to volume expansion (e.g., congestive heart failure, pulmonary edema, and pleural effusions) have been reported *[see Boxed Warning and Warnings and Precautions (5.1)]*.

There are postmarketing reports with AVANDIA of hepatitis, hepatic enzyme elevations to 3 or more times the upper limit of normal, and hepatic failure with and without fatal outcome, although causality has not been established.

There are postmarketing reports with AVANDIA of rash, pruritus, urticaria, angioedema, anaphylactic reaction, Stevens-Johnson syndrome, and new onset or worsening diabetic macular edema with decreased visual acuity *[see Warnings and Precautions (5.7)]*.

7 DRUG INTERACTIONS

7.1 CYP2C8 Inhibitors and Inducers

An inhibitor of CYP2C8 (e.g., gemfibrozil) may increase the AUC of rosiglitazone and an inducer of CYP2C8 (e.g., rifampin) may decrease the AUC of rosiglitazone. Therefore, if an inhibitor or an inducer of CYP2C8 is started or stopped during treatment with rosiglitazone, changes in diabetes treatment may be needed based upon clinical response. [See Clinical Pharmacology (12.4).]

8 USE IN SPECIFIC POPULATIONS

8.1 Pregnancy

Pregnancy Category C.

All pregnancies have a background risk of birth defects, loss, or other adverse outcome regardless of drug exposure. This background risk is increased in pregnancies complicated by hyperglycemia and may be decreased with good metabolic control. It is essential for patients with diabetes or history of gestational diabetes to maintain good metabolic control before conception and throughout pregnancy. Careful monitoring of glucose control is essential in such patients. Most experts recommend that insulin monotherapy be used during pregnancy to maintain blood glucose levels as close to normal as possible.

Human Data: Rosiglitazone has been reported to cross the human placenta and be detectable in fetal tissue. The clinical significance of these findings is unknown. There are no adequate and well-controlled studies in pregnant women. AVANDIA should not be used during pregnancy.

Animal Studies: There was no effect on implantation or the embryo with rosiglitazone treatment during early pregnancy in rats, but treatment during mid-late gestation was associated with fetal death and growth retardation in both rats and rabbits. Teratogenicity was not observed at doses up to 3 mg/kg in rats and 100 mg/kg in rabbits (approximately 20 and 75 times human AUC at the maximum recommended human daily dose, respectively). Rosiglitazone caused placental pathology in rats (3 mg/kg/day). Treatment of rats during gestation through lactation reduced litter size, neonatal viability, and postnatal growth, with growth retardation reversible after puberty. For effects on the placenta, embryo/fetus, and offspring, the no-effect dose was 0.2 mg/kg/day in rats and 15 mg/kg/day in rabbits. These no-effect levels are approximately 4 times human AUC at the maximum recommended human daily dose. Rosiglitazone reduced the number of uterine implantations and live offspring when juvenile female rats were treated at 40 mg/kg/day from 27 days of age through to sexual maturity (approximately 68 times human AUC at the maximum recommended daily dose). The no-effect level was 2 mg/kg/day (approximately 4 times human AUC at the maximum recommended daily dose). There was no effect on pre- or post-natal survival or growth.

8.2 Labor and Delivery

The effect of rosiglitazone on labor and delivery in humans is not known.

8.3 Nursing Mothers

Drug-related material was detected in milk from lactating rats. It is not known whether AVANDIA is excreted in human milk. Because many drugs are excreted in human milk, AVANDIA should not be administered to a nursing woman.

8.4 Pediatric Use

After placebo run-in including diet counseling, children with type 2 diabetes mellitus, aged 10 to 17 years and with a baseline mean body mass index (BMI) of 33 kg/m², were randomized to treatment with 2 mg twice daily of AVANDIA (n = 99) or 500 mg twice daily of metformin (n = 101) in a 24-week, double-blind clinical trial. As expected, FPG decreased in patients naïve to diabetes medication (n = 104)

and increased in patients withdrawn from prior medication (usually metformin) (n = 90) during the run-in period. After at least 8 weeks of treatment, 49% of patients treated with AVANDIA and 55% of metformin-treated patients had their dose doubled if FPG >126 mg/dL. For the overall intent-to-treat population, at week 24, the mean change from baseline in HbA1c was -0.14% with AVANDIA and -0.49% with metformin. There was an insufficient number of patients in this study to establish statistically whether these observed mean treatment effects were similar or different. Treatment effects differed for patients naïve to therapy with antidiabetic drugs and for patients previously treated with antidiabetic therapy (Table 6).

[See table 6 below]

Treatment differences depended on baseline BMI or weight such that the effects of AVANDIA and metformin appeared more closely comparable among heavier patients. The median weight gain was 2.8 kg with rosiglitazone and 0.2 kg with metformin [see Warnings and Precautions (5.4)]. Fifty-four percent of patients treated with rosiglitazone and 32% of patients treated with metformin gained ≥2 kg, and 33% of patients treated with rosiglitazone and 7% of patients treated with metformin gained ≥5 kg on study.

Adverse events observed in this study are described in Adverse Reactions (6.1).

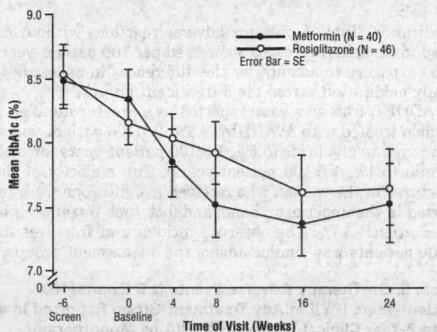

Figure 3. Mean HbA1c Over Time in a 24-Week Study of AVANDIA and Metformin in Pediatric Patients — Drug-Naïve Subgroup

8.5 Geriatric Use

Results of the population pharmacokinetic analysis showed that age does not significantly affect the pharmacokinetics of rosiglitazone [see Clinical Pharmacology (12.3)]. Therefore, no dosage adjustments are required for the elderly. In controlled clinical trials, no overall differences in safety and effectiveness between older (≥65 years) and younger (<65 years) patients were observed.

10 OVERDOSAGE

Limited data are available with regard to overdosage in humans. In clinical studies in volunteers, AVANDIA has been administered at single oral doses of up to 20 mg and was well-tolerated. In the event of an overdose, appropriate supportive treatment should be initiated as dictated by the patient's clinical status.

11 DESCRIPTION

AVANDIA (rosiglitazone maleate) is an oral antidiabetic agent which acts primarily by increasing insulin sensitivity. AVANDIA improves glycemic control while reducing circulating insulin levels.

Rosiglitazone maleate is not chemically or functionally related to the sulfonylureas, the biguanides, or the alpha-glucosidase inhibitors.

Chemically, rosiglitazone maleate is (±)-5-[[4-[2-(methyl-2-pyridinylamino)ethoxy]phenyl]methyl]-2,4-thiazolidinedione, (Z)-2-butenedioate (1:1) with a molecular weight of 473.52 (357.44 free base). The molecule has a single chiral center and is present as a racemate. Due to rapid interconversion, the enantiomers are functionally indistinguishable. The structural formula of rosiglitazone maleate is:

The molecular formula is $C_{18}H_{19}N_3O_3S \cdot C_4H_4O_4$. Rosiglitazone maleate is a white to off-white solid with a melting point range of 122° to 123°C. The pKa values of rosiglitazone maleate are 6.8 and 6.1. It is readily soluble in ethanol and a buffered aqueous solution with pH of 2.3; solubility decreases with increasing pH in the physiological range.

Each pentagonal film-coated TILTAB tablet contains rosiglitazone maleate equivalent to rosiglitazone, 2 mg, 4 mg, or 8 mg, for oral administration. Inactive ingredients are: Hypromellose 2910, lactose monohydrate, magnesium stearate, microcrystalline cellulose, polyethylene glycol 3000, sodium starch glycolate, titanium dioxide, triacetin, and 1 or more of the following: Synthetic red and yellow iron oxides and talc.

12 CLINICAL PHARMACOLOGY

12.1 Mechanism of Action

Rosiglitazone, a member of the thiazolidinedione class of antidiabetic agents, improves glycemic control by improving insulin sensitivity. Rosiglitazone is a highly selective and potent agonist for the peroxisome proliferator-activated receptor-gamma (PPARγ). In humans, PPAR receptors are found in key target tissues for insulin action such as adipose tissue, skeletal muscle, and liver. Activation of PPARγ nuclear receptors regulates the transcription of insulin-responsive genes involved in the control of glucose production, transport, and utilization. In addition, PPARγ-responsive genes also participate in the regulation of fatty acid metabolism.

Insulin resistance is a common feature characterizing the pathogenesis of type 2 diabetes. The antidiabetic activity of rosiglitazone has been demonstrated in animal models of type 2 diabetes in which hyperglycemia and/or impaired glucose tolerance is a consequence of insulin resistance in target tissues. Rosiglitazone reduces blood glucose concentrations and reduces hyperinsulinemia in the ob/ob obese mouse, db/db diabetic mouse, and fa/fa fatty Zucker rat.

In animal models, the antidiabetic activity of rosiglitazone was shown to be mediated by increased sensitivity to insulin's action in the liver, muscle, and adipose tissues. Pharmacological studies in animal models indicate that rosiglitazone inhibits hepatic gluconeogenesis. The expression of the insulin-regulated glucose transporter GLUT-4 was increased in adipose tissue. Rosiglitazone did not induce hypoglycemia in animal models of type 2 diabetes and/or impaired glucose tolerance.

12.2 Pharmacodynamics

Patients with lipid abnormalities were not excluded from clinical trials of AVANDIA. In all 26-week controlled trials, across the recommended dose range, AVANDIA as monotherapy was associated with increases in total cholesterol, LDL, and HDL and decreases in free fatty acids. These changes were statistically significantly different from placebo or glyburide controls (Table 7).

Increases in LDL occurred primarily during the first 1 to 2 months of therapy with AVANDIA and LDL levels remained elevated above baseline throughout the trials. In contrast, HDL continued to rise over time. As a result, the LDL/HDL ratio peaked after 2 months of therapy and then appeared to decrease over time. Because of the temporal nature of lipid changes, the 52-week glyburide-controlled study is most pertinent to assess long-term effects on lipids. At baseline, week 26, and week 52, mean LDL/HDL ratios were 3.1, 3.2, and 3.0, respectively, for AVANDIA 4 mg twice daily. The corresponding values for glyburide were 3.2, 3.1, and 2.9. The differences in change from baseline between AVANDIA and glyburide at week 52 were statistically significant.

Table 6. Week 24 FPG and HbA1c Change From Baseline Last-Observation-Carried Forward in Children With Baseline HbA1c >6.5%

	Naïve Patients		Previously-Treated Patients	
	Metformin	Rosiglitazone	Metformin	Rosiglitazone
	N = 40	N = 45	N = 43	N = 32
FPG (mg/dL)				
Baseline (mean)	170	165	221	205
Change from baseline (mean)	-21	-11	-33	-5
Adjusted treatment difference* (rosiglitazone–metformin)[†] (95% CI)		8 (-15, 30)		21 (-9, 51)
% of patients with ≥30 mg/dL decrease from baseline	43%	27%	44%	28%
HbA1c (%)				
Baseline (mean)	8.3	8.2	8.8	8.5
Change from baseline (mean)	-0.7	-0.5	-0.4	0.1
Adjusted treatment difference* (rosiglitazone–metformin)[†] (95% CI)		0.2 (-0.6, 0.9)		0.5 (-0.2, 1.3)
% of patients with ≥0.7% decrease from baseline	63%	52%	54%	31%

* Change from baseline means are least squares means adjusting for baseline HbA1c, gender, and region.
† Positive values for the difference favor metformin.

The pattern of LDL and HDL changes following therapy with AVANDIA in combination with other hypoglycemic agents were generally similar to those seen with AVANDIA in monotherapy.

The changes in triglycerides during therapy with AVANDIA were variable and were generally not statistically different from placebo or glyburide controls.

[See table 7 at right]

12.3 Pharmacokinetics

Maximum plasma concentration (C_{max}) and the area under the curve (AUC) of rosiglitazone increase in a dose-proportional manner over the therapeutic dose range (Table 8). The elimination half-life is 3 to 4 hours and is independent of dose.

Table 8. Mean (SD) Pharmacokinetic Parameters for Rosiglitazone Following Single Oral Doses (N = 32)

Parameter	1 mg Fasting	2 mg Fasting	8 mg Fasting	8 mg Fed
$AUC_{0\text{-}inf}$ [ng•hr/mL]	358 (112)	733 (184)	2,971 (730)	2,890 (795)
C_{max} [ng/mL]	76 (13)	156 (42)	598 (117)	432 (92)
Half-life [hr]	3.16 (0.72)	3.15 (0.39)	3.37 (0.63)	3.59 (0.70)
CL/F* [L/hr]	3.03 (0.87)	2.89 (0.71)	2.85 (0.69)	2.97 (0.81)

*CL/F = Oral clearance.

Absorption: The absolute bioavailability of rosiglitazone is 99%. Peak plasma concentrations are observed about 1 hour after dosing. Administration of rosiglitazone with food resulted in no change in overall exposure (AUC), but there was an approximately 28% decrease in C_{max} and a delay in T_{max} (1.75 hours). These changes are not likely to be clinically significant; therefore, AVANDIA may be administered with or without food.

Distribution: The mean (CV%) oral volume of distribution (Vss/F) of rosiglitazone is approximately 17.6 (30%) liters, based on a population pharmacokinetic analysis. Rosiglitazone is approximately 99.8% bound to plasma proteins, primarily albumin.

Metabolism: Rosiglitazone is extensively metabolized with no unchanged drug excreted in the urine. The major routes of metabolism were N-demethylation and hydroxylation, followed by conjugation with sulfate and glucuronic acid. All the circulating metabolites are considerably less potent than parent and, therefore, are not expected to contribute to the insulin-sensitizing activity of rosiglitazone.

In vitro data demonstrate that rosiglitazone is predominantly metabolized by Cytochrome P450 (CYP) isoenzyme 2C8, with CYP2C9 contributing as a minor pathway.

Excretion: Following oral or intravenous administration of [^{14}C]rosiglitazone maleate, approximately 64% and 23% of the dose was eliminated in the urine and in the feces, respectively. The plasma half-life of [^{14}C]related material ranged from 103 to 158 hours.

Population Pharmacokinetics in Patients With Type 2 Diabetes: Population pharmacokinetic analyses from 3 large clinical trials including 642 men and 405 women with type 2 diabetes (aged 35 to 80 years) showed that the pharmacokinetics of rosiglitazone are not influenced by age, race, smoking, or alcohol consumption. Both oral clearance (CL/F) and oral steady-state volume of distribution (Vss/F) were shown to increase with increases in body weight. Over the weight range observed in these analyses (50 to 150 kg), the range of predicted CL/F and Vss/F values varied by <1.7-fold and <2.3-fold, respectively. Additionally, rosiglitazone CL/F was shown to be influenced by both weight and gender, being lower (about 15%) in female patients.

Special Populations: *Geriatric:* Results of the population pharmacokinetic analysis (n = 716 <65 years; n = 331 ≥65 years) showed that age does not significantly affect the pharmacokinetics of rosiglitazone.

Gender: Results of the population pharmacokinetics analysis showed that the mean oral clearance of rosiglitazone in female patients (n = 405) was approximately 6% lower compared to male patients of the same body weight (n = 642).

As monotherapy and in combination with metformin, AVANDIA improved glycemic control in both males and females. In metformin combination studies, efficacy was demonstrated with no gender differences in glycemic response. In monotherapy studies, a greater therapeutic response was observed in females; however, in more obese patients, gender differences were less evident. For a given body mass index (BMI), females tend to have a greater fat mass than males. Since the molecular target PPARγ is expressed in adipose tissues, this differentiating characteristic may account, at least in part, for the greater response to AVANDIA in females. Since therapy should be individualized, no dose adjustments are necessary based on gender alone.

Hepatic Impairment: Unbound oral clearance of rosiglitazone was significantly lower in patients with moderate to severe liver disease (Child-Pugh Class B/C) compared to healthy subjects. As a result, unbound C_{max} and $AUC_{0\text{-}inf}$ were increased 2- and 3-fold, respectively. Elimination half-life for rosiglitazone was about 2 hours longer in patients with liver disease, compared to healthy subjects. Therapy with AVANDIA should not be initiated if the patient exhibits clinical evidence of active liver disease or increased serum transaminase levels (ALT >2.5× upper limit of normal) at baseline *[see Warnings and Precautions (5.6)]*.

Pediatric: Pharmacokinetic parameters of rosiglitazone in pediatric patients were established using a population pharmacokinetic analysis with sparse data from 96 pediatric patients in a single pediatric clinical trial including 33 males and 63 females with ages ranging from 10 to 17 years (weights ranging from 35 to 178.3 kg). Population mean CL/F and V/F of rosiglitazone were 3.15 L/hr and 13.5 L, respectively. These estimates of CL/F and V/F were consistent with the typical parameter estimates from a prior adult population analysis.

Renal Impairment: There are no clinically relevant differences in the pharmacokinetics of rosiglitazone in patients with mild to severe renal impairment or in hemodialysis-dependent patients compared to subjects with normal renal function. No dosage adjustment is therefore required in such patients receiving AVANDIA. Since metformin is contraindicated in patients with renal impairment, coadministration of metformin with AVANDIA is contraindicated in these patients.

Race: Results of a population pharmacokinetic analysis including subjects of Caucasian, black, and other ethnic origins indicate that race has no influence on the pharmacokinetics of rosiglitazone.

12.4 Drug-Drug Interactions

Drugs That Inhibit, Induce, or are Metabolized by Cytochrome P450: In vitro drug metabolism studies suggest that rosiglitazone does not inhibit any of the major P450 enzymes at clinically relevant concentrations. In vitro data demonstrate that rosiglitazone is predominantly metabolized by CYP2C8, and to a lesser extent, 2C9. AVANDIA (4 mg twice daily) was shown to have no clinically relevant effect on the pharmacokinetics of nifedipine and oral contraceptives (ethinyl estradiol and norethindrone), which are predominantly metabolized by CYP3A4.

Gemfibrozil: Concomitant administration of gemfibrozil (600 mg twice daily), an inhibitor of CYP2C8, and rosiglitazone (4 mg once daily) for 7 days increased rosiglitazone AUC by 127%, compared to the administration of rosiglitazone (4 mg once daily) alone. Given the potential for dose-related adverse events with rosiglitazone, a decrease in the dose of rosiglitazone may be needed when gemfibrozil is introduced *[see Drug Interactions (7.1)]*.

Rifampin: Rifampin administration (600 mg once a day), an inducer of CYP2C8, for 6 days is reported to decrease rosiglitazone AUC by 66%, compared to the administration of rosiglitazone (8 mg) alone *[see Drug Interactions (7.1)]*.[4]

Glyburide: AVANDIA (2 mg twice daily) taken concomitantly with glyburide (3.75 to 10 mg/day) for 7 days did not alter the mean steady-state 24-hour plasma glucose concentrations in diabetic patients stabilized on glyburide therapy. Repeat doses of AVANDIA (8 mg once daily) for 8 days in healthy adult Caucasian subjects caused a decrease in glyburide AUC and C_{max} of approximately 30%. In Japanese subjects, glyburide AUC and C_{max} slightly increased following coadministration of AVANDIA.

Glimepiride: Single oral doses of glimepiride in 14 healthy adult subjects had no clinically significant effect on the steady-state pharmacokinetics of AVANDIA. No clinically significant reductions in glimepiride AUC and C_{max} were observed after repeat doses of AVANDIA (8 mg once daily) for 8 days in healthy adult subjects.

Metformin: Concurrent administration of AVANDIA (2 mg twice daily) and metformin (500 mg twice daily) in healthy volunteers for 4 days had no effect on the steady-state pharmacokinetics of either metformin or rosiglitazone.

Acarbose: Coadministration of acarbose (100 mg three times daily) for 7 days in healthy volunteers had no clinically relevant effect on the pharmacokinetics of a single oral dose of AVANDIA.

Digoxin: Repeat oral dosing of AVANDIA (8 mg once daily) for 14 days did not alter the steady-state pharmacokinetics of digoxin (0.375 mg once daily) in healthy volunteers.

Warfarin: Repeat dosing with AVANDIA had no clinically relevant effect on the steady-state pharmacokinetics of warfarin enantiomers.

Ethanol: A single administration of a moderate amount of alcohol did not increase the risk of acute hypoglycemia in type 2 diabetes mellitus patients treated with AVANDIA.

Ranitidine: Pretreatment with ranitidine (150 mg twice daily for 4 days) did not alter the pharmacokinetics of either single oral or intravenous doses of rosiglitazone in healthy volunteers. These results suggest that the absorption of oral rosiglitazone is not altered in conditions accompanied by increases in gastrointestinal pH.

Table 7. Summary of Mean Lipid Changes in 26-Week Placebo-Controlled and 52-Week Glyburide-Controlled Monotherapy Studies

	Placebo-Controlled Studies Week 26			Glyburide-Controlled Study Week 26 and Week 52			
	Placebo	AVANDIA		Glyburide Titration		AVANDIA 8 mg	
		4 mg daily*	8 mg daily*	Wk 26	Wk 52	Wk 26	Wk 52
Free fatty acids							
N	207	428	436	181	168	166	145
Baseline (mean)	18.1	17.5	17.9	26.4	26.4	26.9	26.6
% Change from baseline (mean)	+0.2%	-7.8%	-14.7%	-2.4%	-4.7%	-20.8%	-21.5%
LDL							
N	190	400	374	175	160	161	133
Baseline (mean)	123.7	126.8	125.3	142.7	141.9	142.1	142.1
% Change from baseline (mean)	+4.8%	+14.1%	+18.6%	-0.9%	-0.5%	+11.9%	+12.1%
HDL							
N	208	429	436	184	170	170	145
Baseline (mean)	44.1	44.4	43.0	47.2	47.7	48.4	48.3
% Change from baseline (mean)	+8.0%	+11.4%	+14.2%	+4.3%	+8.7%	+14.0%	+18.5%

*Once daily and twice daily dosing groups were combined.

13 NONCLINICAL TOXICOLOGY

13.1 Carcinogenesis, Mutagenesis, Impairment of Fertility

Carcinogenesis: A 2-year carcinogenicity study was conducted in Charles River CD-1 mice at doses of 0.4, 1.5, and 6 mg/kg/day in the diet (highest dose equivalent to approximately 12 times human AUC at the maximum recommended human daily dose). Sprague-Dawley rats were dosed for 2 years by oral gavage at doses of 0.05, 0.3, and 2 mg/kg/day (highest dose equivalent to approximately 10 and 20 times human AUC at the maximum recommended human daily dose for male and female rats, respectively). Rosiglitazone was not carcinogenic in the mouse. There was an increase in incidence of adipose hyperplasia in the mouse at doses ≥1.5 mg/kg/day (approximately 2 times human AUC at the maximum recommended human daily dose). In rats, there was a significant increase in the incidence of benign adipose tissue tumors (lipomas) at doses ≥0.3 mg/kg/day (approximately 2 times human AUC at the maximum recommended human daily dose). These proliferative changes in both species are considered due to the persistent pharmacological overstimulation of adipose tissue.

Mutagenesis: Rosiglitazone was not mutagenic or clastogenic in the in vitro bacterial assays for gene mutation, the in vitro chromosome aberration test in human lymphocytes, the in vivo mouse micronucleus test, and the in vivo/in vitro rat UDS assay. There was a small (about 2-fold) increase in mutation in the in vitro mouse lymphoma assay in the presence of metabolic activation.

Impairment of Fertility: Rosiglitazone had no effects on mating or fertility of male rats given up to 40 mg/kg/day (approximately 116 times human AUC at the maximum recommended human daily dose). Rosiglitazone altered estrous cyclicity (2 mg/kg/day) and reduced fertility (40 mg/kg/day) of female rats in association with lower plasma levels of progesterone and estradiol (approximately 20 and 200 times human AUC at the maximum recommended human daily dose, respectively). No such effects were noted at 0.2 mg/kg/day (approximately 3 times human AUC at the maximum recommended human daily dose). In juvenile rats dosed from 27 days of age through to sexual maturity (at up to 40 mg/kg/day), there was no effect on male reproductive performance, or on estrous cyclicity, mating performance or pregnancy incidence in females (approximately 68 times human AUC at the maximum recommended human daily dose). In monkeys, rosiglitazone (0.6 and 4.6 mg/kg/day; approximately 3 and 15 times human AUC at the maximum recommended human daily dose, respectively) diminished the follicular phase rise in serum estradiol with consequential reduction in the luteinizing hormone surge, lower luteal phase progesterone levels, and amenorrhea. The mechanism for these effects appears to be direct inhibition of ovarian steroidogenesis.

13.2 Animal Toxicology

Heart weights were increased in mice (3 mg/kg/day), rats (5 mg/kg/day), and dogs (2 mg/kg/day) with rosiglitazone treatments (approximately 5, 22, and 2 times human AUC at the maximum recommended human daily dose, respectively). Effects in juvenile rats were consistent with those seen in adults. Morphometric measurement indicated that there was hypertrophy in cardiac ventricular tissues, which may be due to increased heart work as a result of plasma volume expansion.

14 CLINICAL STUDIES

14.1 Monotherapy

In clinical studies, treatment with AVANDIA resulted in an improvement in glycemic control, as measured by FPG and HbA1c, with a concurrent reduction in insulin and C-peptide. Postprandial glucose and insulin were also reduced. This is consistent with the mechanism of action of AVANDIA as an insulin sensitizer.

The maximum recommended daily dose is 8 mg. Dose-ranging studies suggested that no additional benefit was obtained with a total daily dose of 12 mg.

Short-Term Clinical Studies: A total of 2,315 patients with type 2 diabetes, previously treated with diet alone or antidiabetic medication(s), were treated with AVANDIA as monotherapy in 6 double-blind studies, which included two 26-week placebo-controlled studies, one 52-week glyburide-controlled study, and 3 placebo-controlled dose-ranging studies of 8 to 12 weeks duration. Previous antidiabetic medication(s) were withdrawn and patients entered a 2 to 4 week placebo run-in period prior to randomization.

Two 26-week, double-blind, placebo-controlled trials, in patients with type 2 diabetes (n = 1,401) with inadequate glycemic control (mean baseline FPG approximately 228 mg/dL [101 to 425 mg/dL] and mean baseline HbA1c 8.9% [5.2% to 16.2%]), were conducted. Treatment with AVANDIA produced statistically significant improvements in FPG and HbA1c compared to baseline and relative to placebo. Data from one of these studies are summarized in Table 9.

[See table 9 below]

When administered at the same total daily dose, AVANDIA was generally more effective in reducing FPG and HbA1c when administered in divided doses twice daily compared to once daily doses. However, for HbA1c, the difference between the 4 mg once daily and 2 mg twice daily doses was not statistically significant.

Long-Term Clinical Studies: Long-term maintenance of effect was evaluated in a 52-week, double-blind, glyburide-controlled trial in patients with type 2 diabetes. Patients were randomized to treatment with AVANDIA 2 mg twice daily (N = 195) or AVANDIA 4 mg twice daily (N = 189) or glyburide (N = 202) for 52 weeks. Patients receiving glyburide were given an initial dosage of either 2.5 mg/day or 5.0 mg/day. The dosage was then titrated in 2.5 mg/day increments over the next 12 weeks, to a maximum dosage of 15.0 mg/day in order to optimize glycemic control. Thereafter, the glyburide dose was kept constant.

The median titrated dose of glyburide was 7.5 mg. All treatments resulted in a statistically significant improvement in glycemic control from baseline (Figure 4 and Figure 5). At the end of week 52, the reduction from baseline in FPG and HbA1c was -40.8 mg/dL and -0.53% with AVANDIA 4 mg twice daily; -25.4 mg/dL and -0.27% with AVANDIA 2 mg twice daily; and -30.0 mg/dL and -0.72% with glyburide. For HbA1c, the difference between AVANDIA 4 mg twice daily and glyburide was not statistically significant at week 52. The initial fall in FPG with glyburide was greater than with AVANDIA; however, this effect was less durable over time. The improvement in glycemic control seen with AVANDIA 4 mg twice daily at week 26 was maintained through week 52 of the study.

Figure 4. Mean FPG Over Time in a 52-Week Glyburide-Controlled Study

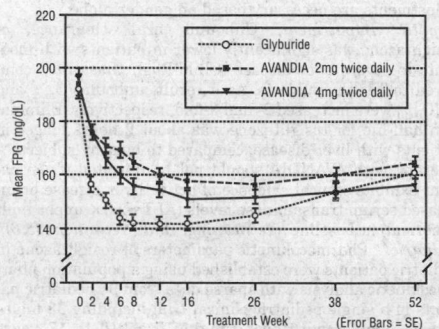

[See figure at top of next column]

Hypoglycemia was reported in 12.1% of glyburide-treated patients versus 0.5% (2 mg twice daily) and 1.6% (4 mg twice daily) of patients treated with AVANDIA. The improvements in glycemic control were associated with a mean weight gain of 1.75 kg and 2.95 kg for patients treated with 2 mg and 4 mg twice daily of AVANDIA, respectively, versus 1.9 kg in glyburide-treated patients. In patients treated with AVANDIA, C-peptide, insulin, pro-insulin, and pro-insulin split products were significantly reduced in a dose-ordered fashion, compared to an increase in the glyburide-treated patients.

A Diabetes Outcome Progression Trial (ADOPT) was a multicenter, double-blind, controlled trial (N = 4,351) conducted over 4 to 6 years to compare the safety and efficacy of AVANDIA, metformin, and glyburide monotherapy in pa-

Figure 5. Mean HbA1c Over Time in a 52-Week Glyburide-Controlled Study

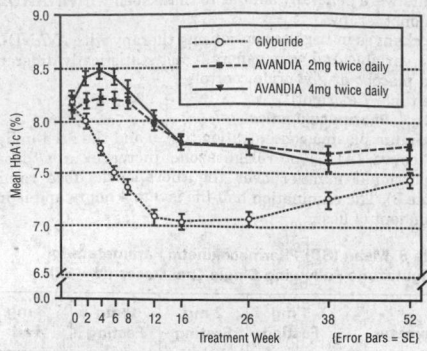

tients recently diagnosed with type 2 diabetes mellitus (≤3 years) inadequately controlled with diet and exercise. The mean age of patients in this trial was 57 years and the majority of patients (83%) had no known history of cardiovascular disease. The mean baseline FPG and HbA1c were 152 mg/dL and 7.4%, respectively. Patients were randomized to receive either AVANDIA 4 mg once daily, glyburide 2.5 mg once daily, or metformin 500 mg once daily, and doses were titrated to optimal glycemic control up to a maximum of 4 mg twice daily for AVANDIA, 7.5 mg once daily for glyburide, and 1,000 mg twice daily for metformin. The primary efficacy outcome was time to consecutive FPG >180 mg/dL after at least 6 weeks of treatment at the maximum tolerated dose of study medication or time to inadequate glycemic control, as determined by an independent adjudication committee.

The cumulative incidence of the primary efficacy outcome at 5 years was 15% with AVANDIA, 21% with metformin, and 34% with glyburide (hazard ratio 0.68 [95% CI 0.55, 0.85] versus metformin, HR 0.37 [95% CI 0.30, 0.45] versus glyburide).

Cardiovascular and adverse event data (including effects on body weight and bone fracture) from ADOPT for AVANDIA, metformin, and glyburide are described in *Warnings and Precautions (5.2, 5.5, and 5.8)* and *Adverse Reactions (6.1)*, respectively. As with all medications, efficacy results must be considered together with safety information to assess the potential benefit and risk for an individual patient.

14.2 Combination With Metformin or Sulfonylurea

The addition of AVANDIA to either metformin or sulfonylurea resulted in significant reductions in hyperglycemia compared to either of these agents alone. These results are consistent with an additive effect on glycemic control when AVANDIA is used as combination therapy.

Combination With Metformin: A total of 670 patients with type 2 diabetes participated in two 26-week, randomized, double-blind, placebo/active-controlled studies designed to assess the efficacy of AVANDIA in combination with metformin. AVANDIA, administered in either once daily or twice daily dosing regimens, was added to the therapy of patients who were inadequately controlled on a maximum dose (2.5 grams/day) of metformin.

In one study, patients inadequately controlled on 2.5 grams/day of metformin (mean baseline FPG 216 mg/dL and mean baseline HbA1c 8.8%) were randomized to receive 4 mg of AVANDIA once daily, 8 mg of AVANDIA once daily, or placebo in addition to metformin. A statistically significant improvement in FPG and HbA1c was observed in patients treated with the combinations of metformin and 4 mg of AVANDIA once daily and 8 mg of AVANDIA once daily, versus patients continued on metformin alone (Table 10).

[See table 10 at top of next page]

In a second 26-week study, patients with type 2 diabetes inadequately controlled on 2.5 grams/day of metformin who were randomized to receive the combination of AVANDIA 4 mg twice daily and metformin (N = 105) showed a statistically significant improvement in glycemic control with a mean treatment effect for FPG of -56 mg/dL and a mean treatment effect for HbA1c of -0.8% over metformin alone. The combination of metformin and AVANDIA resulted in lower levels of FPG and HbA1c than either agent alone. Patients who were inadequately controlled on a maximum dose (2.5 grams/day) of metformin and who were switched to monotherapy with AVANDIA demonstrated loss of glycemic control, as evidenced by increases in FPG and HbA1c. In this group, increases in LDL and VLDL were also seen.

Combination With a Sulfonylurea: A total of 3,457 patients with type 2 diabetes participated in ten 24- to 26-week randomized, double-blind, placebo/active-controlled studies and one 2-year double-blind, active-controlled study in elderly patients designed to assess the efficacy and safety of AVANDIA in combination with a sulfonylurea. AVANDIA 2 mg, 4 mg, or 8 mg daily was administered, either once

Table 9. Glycemic Parameters in a 26-Week Placebo-Controlled Trial

		AVANDIA		AVANDIA	
	Placebo	4 mg once daily	2 mg twice daily	8 mg once daily	4 mg twice daily
	N = 173	N = 180	N = 186	N = 181	N = 187
FPG (mg/dL)					
Baseline (mean)	225	229	225	228	228
Change from baseline (mean)	8	-25	-35	-42	-55
Difference from placebo (adjusted mean)	-	-31*	-43*	-49*	-62*
% of patients with ≥30 mg/dL decrease from baseline	19%	45%	54%	58%	70%
HbA1c (%)					
Baseline (mean)	8.9	8.9	8.9	8.9	9.0
Change from baseline (mean)	0.8	-0.1	-0.1	-0.3	-0.7
Difference from placebo (adjusted mean)	-	-0.8*	-0.9*	-1.1*	-1.5*
% of patients with ≥0.7% decrease from baseline	9%	28%	29%	39%	54%

*p<0.0001 compared to placebo.

daily (3 studies) or in divided doses twice daily (7 studies), to patients inadequately controlled on a submaximal or maximal dose of sulfonylurea.

In these studies, the combination of AVANDIA 4 mg or 8 mg daily (administered as single or twice daily divided doses) and a sulfonylurea significantly reduced FPG and HbA1c compared to placebo plus sulfonylurea or further up-titration of the sulfonylurea. Table 11 shows pooled data for 8 studies in which AVANDIA added to sulfonylurea was compared to placebo plus sulfonylurea.

[See table 11 at right]

One of the 24- to 26-week studies included patients who were inadequately controlled on maximal doses of glyburide and switched to 4 mg of AVANDIA daily as monotherapy; in this group, loss of glycemic control was demonstrated, as evidenced by increases in FPG and HbA1c.

In a 2-year double-blind study, elderly patients (aged 59 to 89 years) on half-maximal sulfonylurea (glipizide 10 mg twice daily) were randomized to the addition of AVANDIA (n = 115, 4 mg once daily to 8 mg as needed) or to continued up-titration of glipizide (n = 110), to a maximum of 20 mg twice daily. Mean baseline FPG and HbA1c were 157 mg/dL and 7.72%, respectively, for the AVANDIA plus glipizide arm and 159 mg/dL and 7.65%, respectively, for the glipizide up-titration arm. Loss of glycemic control (FPG ≥180 mg/dL) occurred in a significantly lower proportion of patients (2%) on AVANDIA plus glipizide compared to patients in the glipizide up-titration arm (28.7%). About 78% of the patients on combination therapy completed the 2 years of therapy while only 51% completed on glipizide monotherapy. The effect of combination therapy on FPG and HbA1c was durable over the 2-year study period, with patients achieving a mean of 132 mg/dL for FPG and a mean of 6.98% for HbA1c compared to no change on the glipizide arm.

14.3 Combination With Sulfonylurea Plus Metformin

In two 24- to 26-week, double-blind, placebo-controlled, studies designed to assess the efficacy and safety of AVANDIA in combination with sulfonylurea plus metformin, AVANDIA 4 mg or 8 mg daily, was administered in divided doses twice daily, to patients inadequately controlled on submaximal (10 mg) and maximal (20 mg) doses of glyburide and maximal dose of metformin (2 g/day). A statistically significant improvement in FPG and HbA1c was observed in patients treated with the combinations of sulfonylurea plus metformin and 4 mg of AVANDIA and 8 mg of AVANDIA versus patients continued on sulfonylurea plus metformin, as shown in Table 12.

[See table 12 at top of next page]

15 REFERENCES

1. Food and Drug Administration Briefing Document. Joint meeting of the Endocrinologic and Metabolic Drugs and Drug Safety and Risk Management Advisory Committees. July 30, 2007.
2. DREAM Trial Investigators. Effect of rosiglitazone on the frequency of diabetes in patients with impaired glucose tolerance or impaired fasting glucose: a randomised controlled trial. *Lancet* 2006;368:1096-1105.
3. Home PD, Pocock SJ, Beck-Nielsen H, et al. Rosiglitazone evaluated for cardiovascular outcomes – an interim analysis. *NEJM* 2007;357:1-11.
4. Park JY, Kim KA, Kang MH, et al. Effect of rifampin on the pharmacokinetics of rosiglitazone in healthy subjects. *Clin Pharmacol Ther* 2004;75:157-162.

16 HOW SUPPLIED/STORAGE AND HANDLING

Each pentagonal film-coated TILTAB tablet contains rosiglitazone as the maleate as follows: 2 mg–pink, debossed with SB on one side and 2 on the other; 4 mg–orange, debossed with SB on one side and 4 on the other; 8 mg–red-brown, debossed with SB on one side and 8 on the other.

2 mg bottles of 60:	NDC 0029-3158-18
4 mg bottles of 30:	NDC 0029-3159-13
4 mg bottles of 90:	NDC 0029-3159-00
8 mg bottles of 30:	NDC 0029-3160-13
8 mg bottles of 90:	NDC 0029-3160-59

Store at 25°C (77°F); excursions 15° to 30°C (59° to 86°F). Dispense in a tight, light-resistant container.

17 PATIENT COUNSELING INFORMATION

17.1 Patient Advice

Patients should be informed of the following:
- AVANDIA is not recommended for patients with symptoms of heart failure.
- Patients with more severe heart failure (NYHA Class 3 or 4) cannot start AVANDIA as the risks exceed any potential benefits in such patients.
- Results of a set of clinical studies suggest that treatment with AVANDIA is associated with an increased risk for myocardial ischemic events, such as angina or myocardial infarction (heart attack), especially in patients taking insulin or nitrates. Because this risk has not been confirmed or excluded in different long-term trials, definitive conclusions regarding this risk await completion of an adequately-designed cardiovascular outcome study.

- AVANDIA is not recommended for patients who are taking nitrates or insulin.
- There are multiple medications available to treat type 2 diabetes. The benefits and risks of each available diabetes medication should be taken into account when choosing a particular diabetes medication for a given patient.
- There have been no clinical studies establishing conclusive evidence of macrovascular risk reduction with AVANDIA or any other oral antidiabetic drug.
- Management of type 2 diabetes should include diet control. Caloric restriction, weight loss, and exercise are essential for the proper treatment of the diabetic patient because they help improve insulin sensitivity. This is important not only in the primary treatment of type 2 diabetes, but in maintaining the efficacy of drug therapy.
- It is important to adhere to dietary instructions and to regularly have blood glucose and glycosylated hemoglobin

tested. It can take 2 weeks to see a reduction in blood glucose and 2 to 3 months to see the full effect of AVANDIA.
- Blood will be drawn to check their liver function prior to the start of therapy and periodically thereafter per the clinical judgment of the healthcare professional. Patients with unexplained symptoms of nausea, vomiting, abdominal pain, fatigue, anorexia, or dark urine should immediately report these symptoms to their physician.
- Patients who experience an unusually rapid increase in weight or edema or who develop shortness of breath or other symptoms of heart failure while on AVANDIA should immediately report these symptoms to their physician.
- AVANDIA can be taken with or without meals.
- When using AVANDIA in combination with other hypoglycemic agents, the risk of hypoglycemia, its symptoms and

Table 10. Glycemic Parameters in a 26-Week Combination Study of AVANDIA Plus Metformin

	Metformin	AVANDIA 4 mg once daily + metformin	AVANDIA 8 mg once daily + metformin
	N = 113	N = 116	N = 110
FPG (mg/dL)			
Baseline (mean)	214	215	220
Change from baseline (mean)	6	-33	-48
Difference from metformin alone (adjusted mean)	-	-40*	-53*
% of patients with ≥30 mg/dL decrease from baseline	20%	45%	61%
HbA1c (%)			
Baseline (mean)	8.6	8.9	8.9
Change from baseline (mean)	0.5	-0.6	-0.8
Difference from metformin alone (adjusted mean)	-	-1.0*	-1.2*
% of patients with ≥0.7% decrease from baseline	11%	45%	52%

*p<0.0001 compared to metformin.

Table 11. Glycemic Parameters in 24- to 26-Week Combination Studies of AVANDIA Plus Sulfonylurea

Twice Daily Divided Dosing (5 Studies)	Sulfonylurea	AVANDIA 2 mg twice daily + sulfonylurea	Sulfonylurea	AVANDIA 4 mg twice daily + sulfonylurea
	N = 397	N = 497	N = 248	N = 346
FPG (mg/dL)				
Baseline (mean)	204	198	188	187
Change from baseline (mean)	11	-29	8	-43
Difference from sulfonylurea alone (adjusted mean)	-	-42*	-	-53*
% of patients with ≥30 mg/dL decrease from baseline	17%	49%	15%	61%
HbA1c (%)				
Baseline (mean)	9.4	9.5	9.3	9.6
Change from baseline (mean)	0.2	-1.0	0.0	-1.6
Difference from sulfonylurea alone (adjusted mean)	-	-1.1*	-	-1.4*
% of patients with ≥0.7% decrease from baseline	21%	60%	23%	75%
Once Daily Dosing (3 Studies)	Sulfonylurea	AVANDIA 4 mg once daily + sulfonylurea	Sulfonylurea	AVANDIA 8 mg once daily + sulfonylurea
	N = 172	N = 172	N = 173	N = 176
FPG (mg/dL)				
Baseline (mean)	198	206	188	192
Change from baseline (mean)	17	-25	17	-43
Difference from sulfonylurea alone (adjusted mean)	-	-47*	-	-66*
% of patients with ≥30 mg/dL decrease from baseline	17%	48%	19%	55%
HbA1c (%)				
Baseline (mean)	8.6	8.8	8.9	8.9
Change from baseline (mean)	0.4	-0.5	0.1	-1.2
Difference from sulfonylurea alone (adjusted mean)	-	-0.9*	-	-1.4*
% of patients with ≥0.7% decrease from baseline	11%	36%	20%	68%

*p<0.0001 compared to sulfonylurea alone.

Table 12. Glycemic Parameters in a 26-Week Combination Study of AVANDIA Plus Sulfonylurea and Metformin

	Sulfonylurea + metformin	AVANDIA 2 mg twice daily + sulfonylurea + metformin	AVANDIA 4 mg twice daily + sulfonylurea + metformin
	N = 273	N = 276	N = 277
FPG (mg/dL)			
Baseline (mean)	189	190	192
Change from baseline (mean)	14	-19	-40
Difference from sulfonylurea plus metformin (adjusted mean)	-	-30*	-52*
% of patients with ≥30 mg/dL decrease from baseline	16%	46%	62%
HbA1c (%)			
Baseline (mean)	8.7	8.6	8.7
Change from baseline (mean)	0.2	-0.4	-0.9
Difference from sulfonylurea plus metformin (adjusted mean)	-	-0.6*	-1.1*
% of patients with ≥0.7% decrease from baseline	16%	39%	63%

*p<0.0001 compared to placebo.

treatment, and conditions that predispose to its development should be explained to patients and their family members.

• Therapy with AVANDIA, like other thiazolidinediones, may result in ovulation in some premenopausal anovulatory women. As a result, these patients may be at an increased risk for pregnancy while taking AVANDIA. Thus, adequate contraception in premenopausal women should be recommended. This possible effect has not been specifically investigated in clinical studies so the frequency of this occurrence is not known.

17.2   FDA-Approved Medication Guide
See separate leaflet.
AVANDIA and TILTAB are registered trademarks of GlaxoSmithKline.
GlaxoSmithKline
Research Triangle Park, NC 27709
©2009, GlaxoSmithKline. All rights reserved.

MEDICATION GUIDE
AVANDIA® (ah-VAN-dee-a)
rosiglitazone maleate tablets
Read this Medication Guide carefully before you start taking AVANDIA and each time you get a refill. There may be new information. This information does not take the place of talking with your doctor about your medical condition or your treatment. If you have any questions about AVANDIA, ask your doctor or pharmacist.

What is the most important information I should know about AVANDIA?
AVANDIA is a prescription medicine to treat adults with diabetes. It helps to control high blood sugar. (See "What is AVANDIA?"). It is important that you take AVANDIA exactly how it is prescribed by your doctor to best treat your diabetes.
AVANDIA may cause serious side effects, including:
New or worse heart failure
• AVANDIA can cause your body to keep extra fluid (fluid retention), which leads to swelling (edema) and weight gain. Extra body fluid can make some heart problems worse or lead to heart failure. Heart failure means your heart does not pump blood well enough.
• If you have severe heart failure, you cannot start AVANDIA.
• If you have heart failure with symptoms (such as shortness of breath or swelling), even if these symptoms are not severe, AVANDIA may not be right for you.
Call your doctor right away if you have any of the following:
• swelling or fluid retention, especially in the ankles or legs
• shortness of breath or trouble breathing, especially when you lie down
• an unusually fast increase in weight
• unusual tiredness
Other heart problems
AVANDIA may raise the risk of heart problems related to reduced blood flow to the heart. These include possible increases in the risk of heart-related chest pain (angina) or "heart attack" (myocardial infarction). This risk seemed to be higher in people who took AVANDIA with insulin or with nitrate medicines. Most people who take insulin or nitrate medicines should not also take AVANDIA.
• If you have chest pain or a feeling of chest pressure, get medical help right away, no matter what diabetes medicines you are taking.

• People with diabetes have a greater risk for heart problems. It is important to work with your doctor to manage other conditions, such as high blood pressure or high cholesterol.
AVANDIA can have other serious side effects. Be sure to read the section below "What are possible side effects of AVANDIA?".
What is AVANDIA?
AVANDIA is a prescription medicine used with diet and exercise to treat adults with type 2 ("adult-onset" or "non-insulin dependent") diabetes mellitus ("high blood sugar"). AVANDIA helps to control high blood sugar. AVANDIA may be used alone or with other diabetes medicines. AVANDIA can help your body respond better to insulin made in your body. AVANDIA does not cause your body to make more insulin.
• For AVANDIA to work best, it is very important to exercise, lose extra weight, and follow the diet recommended by your doctor.
• AVANDIA has not been studied enough in children under 18 years of age to know if it is safe or effective in children.
• AVANDIA is not for people with type 1 diabetes mellitus or to treat a condition called diabetic ketoacidosis.
Who should not take AVANDIA?
Many people with heart failure should not start taking AVANDIA. See "What should I tell my doctor before taking AVANDIA?".
What should I tell my doctor before taking AVANDIA?
Before starting AVANDIA, ask your doctor about what the choices are for diabetes medicines, and what the expected benefits and possible risks are for you in particular.
Before taking AVANDIA, tell your doctor about all your medical conditions, including if you:
• **have heart problems or heart failure.**
• **have type 1 ("juvenile") diabetes or had diabetic keto-acidosis.** These conditions should be treated with insulin.
• **have a type of diabetic eye disease called macular edema** (swelling of the back of the eye).
• **have liver problems.** Your doctor should do blood tests to check your liver before you start taking AVANDIA and during treatment as needed.
• **had liver problems while taking REZULIN® (troglitazone), another medicine for diabetes.**
• **are pregnant or plan to become pregnant.** AVANDIA should not be used during pregnancy. It is not known if AVANDIA can harm your unborn baby. You and your doctor should talk about the best way to control your diabetes during pregnancy. If you are a premenopausal woman (before the "change of life") who does not have regular monthly periods, AVANDIA may increase your chances of becoming pregnant. Talk to your doctor about birth control choices while taking AVANDIA. Tell your doctor right away if you become pregnant while taking AVANDIA.
• **are breast-feeding or planning to breast-feed.** It is not known if AVANDIA passes into breast milk. You should not use AVANDIA while breast-feeding.
Tell your doctor about all the medicines you take including prescription and non-prescription medicines, vitamins or herbal supplements. AVANDIA and certain other medicines can affect each other and may lead to serious side effects including high or low blood sugar, or heart problems. Especially tell your doctor if you take:
• **insulin.**

• **nitrate medicines** such as nitroglycerin or isosorbide to treat a type of chest pain called angina.
• **any medicines for high blood pressure, high cholesterol or heart failure, or for prevention of heart disease or stroke.**
Know the medicines you take. Keep a list of your medicines and show it to your doctor and pharmacist before you start a new medicine. They will tell you if it is alright to take AVANDIA with other medicines.
How should I take AVANDIA?
• Take AVANDIA exactly as prescribed. Your doctor will tell you how many tablets to take and how often. The usual daily starting dose is 4 mg a day taken one time each day or 2 mg taken two times each day. Your doctor may need to adjust your dose until your blood sugar is better controlled.
• AVANDIA may be prescribed alone or with other diabetes medicines. This will depend on how well your blood sugar is controlled.
• Take AVANDIA with or without food.
• It can take 2 weeks for AVANDIA to start lowering blood sugar. It may take 2 to 3 months to see the full effect on your blood sugar level.
• If you miss a dose of AVANDIA, take it as soon as you remember, unless it is time to take your next dose. Take your next dose at the usual time. Do not take double doses to make up for a missed dose.
• If you take too much AVANDIA, call your doctor or poison control center right away.
• Test your blood sugar regularly as your doctor tells you.
• Diet and exercise can help your body use its blood sugar better. It is important to stay on your recommended diet, lose extra weight, and get regular exercise while taking AVANDIA.
• Your doctor should do blood tests to check your liver before you start AVANDIA and during treatment as needed. Your doctor should also do regular blood sugar tests (for example, "A1C") to monitor your response to AVANDIA.
What are possible side effects of AVANDIA?
AVANDIA may cause serious side effects including:
• **New or worse heart failure.** See "What is the most important information I should know about AVANDIA?".
• **Other heart problems.** AVANDIA may increase the risk of heart problems related to reduced blood flow to the heart. These include possible increases in the risk of heart-related chest pain (angina) or "heart attack" (myocardial infarction). See "What is the most important information I should know about AVANDIA?".
• **Swelling (edema).** AVANDIA can cause swelling due to fluid retention. See "What is the most important information I should know about AVANDIA?".
• **Weight gain.** AVANDIA can cause weight gain that may be due to fluid retention or extra body fat. Weight gain can be a serious problem for people with certain conditions including heart problems. See "What is the most important information I should know about AVANDIA?".
• **Liver problems.** It is important for your liver to be working normally when you take AVANDIA. Your doctor should do blood tests to check your liver before you start taking AVANDIA and during treatment as needed. Call your doctor right away if you have unexplained symptoms such as:
  • nausea or vomiting
  • stomach pain
  • unusual or unexplained tiredness
  • loss of appetite
  • dark urine
  • yellowing of your skin or the whites of your eyes.
• **Macular edema** (a diabetic eye disease with swelling in the back of the eye). Tell your doctor right away if you have any changes in your vision. Your doctor should check your eyes regularly. Very rarely, some people have experienced vision changes due to swelling in the back of the eye while taking AVANDIA.
• **Fractures (broken bones)**, usually in the hand, upper arm or foot, in females. Talk to your doctor for advice on how to keep your bones healthy.
• **Low red blood cell count (anemia).**
• **Low blood sugar (hypoglycemia).** Lightheadedness, dizziness, shakiness or hunger may mean that your blood sugar is too low. This can happen if you skip meals, if you use another medicine that lowers blood sugar, or if you have certain medical problems. Call your doctor if low blood sugar levels are a problem for you.
• **Ovulation** (release of egg from an ovary in a woman) leading to pregnancy. Ovulation may happen in premenopausal women who do not have regular monthly periods. This can increase the chance of pregnancy. See "What should I tell my doctor before taking AVANDIA?".
The most common side effects of AVANDIA reported in clinical trials included cold-like symptoms and headache.
Call your doctor for medical advice about side effects. You may report side effects to FDA at 1-800-FDA-1088.
How should I store AVANDIA?
• Store AVANDIA at room temperature, 59° to 86°F (15° to 30°C). Keep AVANDIA in the container it comes in.
• Safely, throw away AVANDIA that is out of date or no longer needed.
• Keep AVANDIA and all medicines out of the reach of children.

General information about AVANDIA

Medicines are sometimes prescribed for purposes other than those listed in a Medication Guide. Do not use AVANDIA for a condition for which it was not prescribed. Do not give AVANDIA to other people, even if they have the same symptoms you have. It may harm them.

This Medication Guide summarizes important information about AVANDIA. If you would like more information, talk with your doctor. You can ask your doctor or pharmacist for information about AVANDIA that is written for healthcare professionals. You can also find out more about AVANDIA by calling 1-888-825-5249 or visiting the website www.avandia.com.

What are the ingredients in AVANDIA?

Active Ingredient: Rosiglitazone maleate.

Inactive Ingredients: Hypromellose 2910, lactose monohydrate, magnesium stearate, microcrystalline cellulose, polyethylene glycol 3000, sodium starch glycolate, titanium dioxide, triacetin, and 1 or more of the following: Synthetic red and yellow iron oxides and talc.

Always check to make sure that the medicine you are taking is the correct one. AVANDIA tablets are triangles with rounded corners and look like this:

2 mg strength tablets — pink with "SB" on one side and "2" on the other.

4 mg strength tablets — orange with "SB" on one side and "4" on the other.

8 mg strength tablets — red-brown with "SB" on one side and "8" on the other.

AVANDIA is a registered trademark of GlaxoSmithKline.

REZULIN is a registered trademark of Parke-Davis Pharmaceuticals Ltd.

This Medication Guide has been approved by the U.S. Food and Drug Administration.

GlaxoSmithKline

Research Triangle Park, NC 27709

©2008, GlaxoSmithKline. All rights reserved.

October 2008 AVD:4MG

AVODART®

[av' ō dart]

(dutasteride)

Soft Gelatin Capsules

Rx

HIGHLIGHTS OF PRESCRIBING INFORMATION

These highlights do not include all the information needed to use AVODART safely and effectively. See full prescribing information for AVODART.

AVODART (dutasteride) Soft Gelatin Capsules

Initial U.S. Approval: 2001

RECENT MAJOR CHANGES

Warnings and Precautions, Effects on Prostate-Specific Antigen (PSA) and the Use of PSA in Prostate Cancer Detection (5.3) 6/2010

INDICATIONS AND USAGE

AVODART, a 5α-reductase inhibitor, is indicated for the treatment of symptomatic benign prostatic hyperplasia (BPH) in men with an enlarged prostate to: (1.1)
• improve symptoms,
• reduce the risk of acute urinary retention, and
• reduce the risk of the need for BPH-related surgery.

AVODART in combination with the alpha-blocker tamsulosin is indicated for the treatment of symptomatic BPH in men with an enlarged prostate. (1.2)

DOSAGE AND ADMINISTRATION

Monotherapy: 0.5 mg once daily. (2.1)

Combination with tamsulosin: 0.5 mg once daily and tamsulosin 0.4 mg once daily. (2.2)

Dosing considerations: Swallow whole. May take with or without food. (2)

DOSAGE FORMS AND STRENGTHS

0.5-mg soft gelatin capsules (3)

CONTRAINDICATIONS

• Pregnancy and women of childbearing potential. (4, 5.1, 8.1)
• Pediatric patients. (4)
• Patients with previously demonstrated, clinically significant hypersensitivity (e.g., serious skin reactions, angioedema) to AVODART or other 5α-reductase inhibitors. (4)

WARNINGS AND PRECAUTIONS

• Women who are pregnant or may become pregnant should not handle AVODART Capsules. (5.1, 8.1)
• Patients should be assessed to rule out other urological diseases, including prostate cancer, prior to prescribing AVODART. (5.2)
• AVODART reduces total serum prostate-specific antigen (PSA) concentration by approximately 50%. Any confirmed increases in PSA levels from nadir while on AVODART should be evaluated for the presence of prostate cancer. (5.3)
• Patients should not donate blood until 6 months after their last dose. (5.4)

ADVERSE REACTIONS

The most common adverse reactions, reported in ≥1% of patients treated with AVODART and more commonly than in patients treated with placebo, are impotence, decreased libido, ejaculation disorders, and breast disorders. (6.1)

To report SUSPECTED ADVERSE REACTIONS, contact GlaxoSmithKline at 1-888-825-5249 or FDA at 1-800-FDA-1088 or www.fda.gov/medwatch.

DRUG INTERACTIONS

Use with caution in patients taking potent, chronic CYP3A4 enzyme inhibitors (e.g., ritonavir). (7)

See 17 for PATIENT COUNSELING INFORMATION and FDA-approved patient labeling

Revised: 06/2010

FULL PRESCRIBING INFORMATION

1 INDICATIONS AND USAGE

1.1 Monotherapy

AVODART® (dutasteride) Soft Gelatin Capsules are indicated for the treatment of symptomatic benign prostatic hyperplasia (BPH) in men with an enlarged prostate to:
• improve symptoms,
• reduce the risk of acute urinary retention (AUR), and
• reduce the risk of the need for BPH-related surgery.

1.2 Combination With Alpha-Blocker

AVODART in combination with the alpha-blocker tamsulosin is indicated for the treatment of symptomatic BPH in men with an enlarged prostate.

2 DOSAGE AND ADMINISTRATION

The capsules should be swallowed whole and not chewed or opened, as contact with the capsule contents may result in irritation of the oropharyngeal mucosa. AVODART may be administered with or without food.

2.1 Monotherapy

The recommended dose of AVODART is 1 capsule (0.5 mg) taken once daily.

2.2 Combination With Alpha-Blocker

The recommended dose of AVODART is 1 capsule (0.5 mg) taken once daily and tamsulosin 0.4 mg taken once daily.

2.3 Dosage Adjustment in Specific Populations

No dose adjustment is necessary for patients with renal impairment or for the elderly [see Clinical Pharmacology (12.3)]. Due to the absence of data in patients with hepatic impairment, no dosage recommendation can be made [see Specific Populations (8.7) and Clinical Pharmacology (12.3)].

3 DOSAGE FORMS AND STRENGTHS

0.5 mg, opaque, dull yellow, gelatin capsules imprinted with "GX CE2" in red ink on one side.

4 CONTRAINDICATIONS

AVODART is contraindicated for use in:
• Pregnancy. Dutasteride inhibits the activity of 5α-reductase, which prevents conversion of testosterone to dihydrotestosterone, a hormone necessary for normal development of male genitalia. In animal reproduction and developmental toxicity studies, dutasteride inhibited development of male fetus external genitalia. Therefore, AVODART may cause fetal harm when administered to a pregnant woman. If AVODART is used during pregnancy or if the patient becomes pregnant while taking AVODART, the patient should be apprised of the potential hazard to the fetus [see Warnings and Precautions (5.1), Use in Specific Populations (8.1)].
• Women of childbearing potential [see Warnings and Precautions (5.1), Use in Specific Populations (8.1)].
• Pediatric patients [see Use in Specific Populations (8.4)].
• Patients with previously demonstrated, clinically significant hypersensitivity (e.g., serious skin reactions, angioedema) to AVODART or other 5α-reductase inhibitors.

5 WARNINGS AND PRECAUTIONS

5.1 Exposure of Women—Risk to Male Fetus

AVODART Capsules should not be handled by a woman who is pregnant or who may become pregnant. Dutasteride is absorbed through the skin and could result in unintended fetal exposure. If a woman who is pregnant or who may become pregnant comes in contact with leaking dutasteride capsules, the contact area should be washed immediately with soap and water [see Use in Specific Populations (8.1)].

5.2 Evaluation for Other Urological Diseases

Lower urinary tract symptoms of BPH can be indicative of other urological diseases, including prostate cancer. Patients should be assessed to rule out prostate cancer and other urological diseases prior to treatment with AVODART and periodically thereafter. Patients with a large residual urinary volume and/or severely diminished urinary flow may not be good candidates for 5α-reductase inhibitor therapy and should be carefully monitored for obstructive uropathy.

5.3 Effects on Prostate-Specific Antigen (PSA) and the Use of PSA in Prostate Cancer Detection

Dutasteride reduces total serum PSA concentration by approximately 40% following 3 months of treatment and by approximately 50% following 6, 12, and 24 months of treatment. This decrease is predictable over the entire range of PSA values, although it may vary in individual patients. Therefore, for interpretation of serial PSAs in a man taking AVODART, a new baseline PSA concentration should be established after 3 to 6 months of treatment, and this new value should be used to assess potentially cancer-related changes in PSA. To interpret an isolated PSA value in a man treated with AVODART for 6 months or more, the PSA value should be doubled for comparison with normal values in untreated men. Any confirmed increases in PSA levels from nadir while on AVODART may signal the presence of prostate cancer and should be carefully evaluated, even if those values are still within the normal range for men not taking a 5-alpha reductase inhibitor.

The free-to-total PSA ratio (percent free PSA) remains constant at Month 12, even under the influence of AVODART. If clinicians elect to use percent free PSA as an aid in the detection of prostate cancer in men receiving AVODART, no adjustment to its value appears necessary.

Coadminstration of tamsulosin with dutasteride resulted in similar changes to total PSA as dutasteride monotherapy.

5.4 Blood Donation

Men being treated with dutasteride should not donate blood until at least 6 months have passed following their last dose. The purpose of this deferred period is to prevent administration of dutasteride to a pregnant female transfusion recipient.

5.5 Effect on Semen Characteristics

The effects of dutasteride 0.5 mg/day on semen characteristics were evaluated in normal volunteers aged 18 to 52 (n = 27 dutasteride, n = 23 placebo) throughout 52 weeks of treatment and 24 weeks of post-treatment follow-up. At 52 weeks, the mean percent reduction from baseline in total sperm count, semen volume, and sperm motility were 23%, 26%, and 18%, respectively, in the dutasteride group when

Table 1. Adverse Reactions Reported in ≥1% of Subjects Over a 24-Month Period and More Frequently in the Group Receiving AVODART Than the Placebo Group (Randomized, Double-Blind, Placebo-Controlled Studies Pooled) by Time of Onset

	Adverse Reaction Time of Onset			
Adverse Reactions AVODART (n) Placebo (n)	Month 0-6 (n = 2,167) (n = 2,158)	Month 7-12 (n = 1,901) (n = 1,922)	Month 13-18 (n = 1,725) (n = 1,714)	Month 19-24 (n = 1,605) (n = 1,555)
Impotence				
AVODART	4.7%	1.4%	1.0%	0.8%
Placebo	1.7%	1.5%	0.5%	0.9%
Decreased libido				
AVODART	3.0%	0.7%	0.3%	0.3%
Placebo	1.4%	0.6%	0.2%	0.1%
Ejaculation disorders				
AVODART	1.4%	0.5%	0.5%	0.1%
Placebo	0.5%	0.3%	0.1%	0.0%
Breast disorders[a]				
AVODART	0.5%	0.8%	1.1%	0.6%
Placebo	0.2%	0.3%	0.3%	0.1%

[a] Includes breast tenderness and breast enlargement.

Table 2. Adverse Reactions Reported Over a 24-Month Period in ≥1% of Subjects in Any Treatment Group (CombAT) by Time of Onset

	Adverse Reaction Time of Onset			
Adverse Reactions Combination (n)[a] AVODART (n) Tamsulosin (n)	Month 0-6 (n = 1,610) (n = 1,623) (n = 1,611)	Month 7-12 (n = 1,524) (n = 1,547) (n = 1,542)	Month 13-18 (n = 1,424) (n = 1,457) (n = 1,468)	Month 19-24 (n = 1,345) (n = 1,378) (n = 1,363)
Impotence				
Combination	5.5%	1.2%	0.8%	0.3%
AVODART	3.9%	1.2%	0.6%	0.7%
Tamsulosin	2.7%	0.8%	0.4%	0.4%
Decreased libido				
Combination	4.5%	0.9%	0.4%	<0.1%
AVODART	3.3%	0.6%	0.7%	0.2%
Tamsulosin	1.9%	0.6%	0.4%	0.2%
Ejaculation disorders				
Combination	7.6%	1.6%	0.4%	<0.1%
AVODART	1.1%	0.6%	0.1%	0.1%
Tamsulosin	2.2%	0.5%	0.4%	0.1%
Breast disorders[b]				
Combination	1.0%	1.1%	0.7%	0.3%
AVODART	0.9%	1.0%	0.8%	0.5%
Tamsulosin	0.4%	0.4%	0.2%	0.1%
Dizziness				
Combination	1.1%	0.4%	0.2%	0.0%
AVODART	0.4%	0.2%	<0.1%	<0.1%
Tamsulosin	0.9%	0.5%	0.3%	0.1%

[a] Combination = AVODART 0.5 mg once daily plus tamsulosin 0.4 mg once daily.
[b] Includes breast tenderness and breast enlargement.

adjusted for changes from baseline in the placebo group. Sperm concentration and sperm morphology were unaffected. After 24 weeks of follow-up, the mean percent change in total sperm count in the dutasteride group remained 23% lower than baseline. While mean values for all semen parameters at all time-points remained within the normal ranges and did not meet predefined criteria for a clinically significant change (30%), 2 subjects in the dutasteride group had decreases in sperm count of greater than 90% from baseline at 52 weeks, with partial recovery at the 24-week follow-up. The clinical significance of dutasteride's effect on semen characteristics for an individual patient's fertility is not known.

6   ADVERSE REACTIONS
6.1   Clinical Trials Experience
Because clinical trials are conducted under widely varying conditions, adverse reaction rates observed in the clinical trials of a drug cannot be directly compared to rates in the clinical trial of another drug and may not reflect the rates observed in practice.

Monotherapy:
• The most common adverse reactions reported in subjects receiving AVODART were impotence, decreased libido, breast disorders (including breast enlargement and tenderness), and ejaculation disorders.
• Study withdrawal due to adverse reactions occurred in 4% of subjects receiving AVODART and 3% of subjects receiv-

ing placebo. The most common adverse reaction leading to study withdrawal was impotence (1%).

Over 4,300 male subjects with BPH were randomly assigned to receive placebo or 0.5-mg daily doses of AVODART in 3 identical 2-year, placebo-controlled, double-blind, Phase 3 treatment studies, each with 2-year open-label extensions. During the double-blind treatment period, 2,167 male subjects were exposed to AVODART, including 1,772 exposed for 1 year and 1,510 exposed for 2 years. When including the open-label extensions, 1,009 male subjects were exposed to AVODART for 3 years and 812 were exposed for 4 years. The population was aged 47 to 94 years (mean age, 66 years) and greater than 90% Caucasian. Table 1 summarizes clinical adverse reactions reported in at least 1% of subjects receiving AVODART and at a higher incidence than subjects receiving placebo.

[See table 1 above]

Long-Term Treatment (Up to 4 Years):   There is no evidence of increased drug-related sexual adverse reactions (impotence, decreased libido, and ejaculation disorder) or breast disorders with increased duration of treatment. The relationship between long-term use of AVODART and male breast neoplasia is currently unknown.

Combination with Alpha-Blocker Therapy (CombAT):
• The most common adverse reactions reported in subjects receiving combination therapy (AVODART plus tamsu-

losin) were impotence, decreased libido, breast disorders (including breast enlargement and tenderness), ejaculation disorders, and dizziness. Over 2 years of treatment, drug-related ejaculation disorders occurred more frequently in subjects receiving combination therapy (9%) compared to AVODART (2%) or tamsulosin (3%) as monotherapy.
• Study withdrawal due to adverse reactions occurred in 5% of subjects receiving combination therapy (AVODART plus tamsulosin) and 3% of subjects receiving AVODART or tamsulosin as monotherapy. The most common adverse reaction leading to study withdrawal in subjects receiving combination therapy was impotence (1%).

Over 4,800 male subjects with BPH were randomly assigned to receive either 0.5-mg AVODART, 0.4-mg tamsulosin, or combination therapy (0.5-mg AVODART plus 0.4-mg tamsulosin) administered once daily in a 4-year double-blind study. Adverse reaction information over the first 2 years of treatment is presented below; information for years 2 to 4 is not yet available. During the first 2 years, 1,623 subjects received monotherapy with AVODART; 1,611 subjects received monotherapy with tamsulosin; and 1,610 subjects received combination therapy. The population was aged 49 to 88 years (mean age, 66 years) and 88% Caucasian. Table 2 summarizes adverse reactions reported in at least 1% of subjects in any treatment group.

[See table 2 at left]

Cardiac Failure: In CombAT, after 4 years of treatment, the incidence of the composite term cardiac failure in the combination therapy group (12/1,610; 0.7%) was higher than in either monotherapy group: AVODART, 2/1,623 (0.1%) and tamsulosin, 9/1,611 (0.6%). Composite cardiac failure was also examined in a separate 4-year placebo-controlled trial evaluating AVODART in men at risk for development of prostate cancer. The incidence of cardiac failure in subjects taking AVODART was 0.6% (26/4,105) compared to 0.4% (15/4,126) in subjects on placebo. A majority of subjects with cardiac failure in both studies had comorbidities associated with an increased risk of cardiac failure. Therefore, the clinical significance of the numerical imbalances in cardiac failure is unknown. No causal relationship between AVODART, alone or in combination with tamsulosin, and cardiac failure has been established. No imbalance was observed in the incidence of overall cardiovascular adverse events in either study.

6.2   Postmarketing Experience
The following adverse reactions have been identified during postapproval use of AVODART. Because these reactions are reported voluntarily from a population of uncertain size, it is not always possible to reliably estimate their frequency or establish a causal relationship to drug exposure. These reactions have been chosen for inclusion due to a combination of their seriousness, frequency of reporting, or potential causal connection to AVODART.

Immune System Disorders: Hypersensitivity reactions, including rash, pruritus, urticaria, localized edema, serious skin reactions, and angioedema.

7   DRUG INTERACTIONS
7.1   Cytochrome P450 3A Inhibitors
Dutasteride is extensively metabolized in humans by the CYP3A4 and CYP3A5 isoenzymes. The effect of potent CYP3A4 inhibitors on dutasteride has not been studied. Because of the potential for drug-drug interactions, use caution when prescribing AVODART to patients taking potent, chronic CYP3A4 enzyme inhibitors (e.g., ritonavir) [see Clinical Pharmacology (12.3)].

7.2   Alpha-Adrenergic Blocking Agents
The administration of AVODART in combination with tamsulosin or terazosin has no effect on the steady-state pharmacokinetics of either alpha-adrenergic blocker. The effect of administration of tamsulosin or terazosin on dutasteride pharmacokinetic parameters has not been evaluated.

7.3   Calcium Channel Antagonists
Coadministration of verapamil or diltiazem decreases dutasteride clearance and leads to increased exposure to dutasteride. The change in dutasteride exposure is not considered to be clinically significant. No dose adjustment is recommended [see Clinical Pharmacology (12.3)].

7.4   Cholestyramine
Administration of a single 5-mg dose of AVODART followed 1 hour later by 12 g of cholestyramine does not affect the relative bioavailability of dutasteride [see Clinical Pharmacology (12.3)].

7.5   Digoxin
AVODART does not alter the steady-state pharmacokinetics of digoxin when administered concomitantly at a dose of 0.5 mg/day for 3 weeks [see Clinical Pharmacology (12.3)].

7.6   Warfarin
Concomitant administration of AVODART 0.5 mg/day for 3 weeks with warfarin does not alter the steady-state phar-

macokinetics of the S- or R-warfarin isomers or alter the effect of warfarin on prothrombin time *[see Clinical Pharmacology (12.3)]*.

8 USE IN SPECIFIC POPULATIONS

8.1 Pregnancy

Pregnancy Category X. *[See Contraindications (4)]*. AVODART is contraindicated for use in women of childbearing potential and during pregnancy. AVODART is a 5α-reductase inhibitor that prevents conversion of testosterone to dihydrotestosterone (DHT), a hormone necessary for normal development of male genitalia. In animal reproduction and developmental toxicity studies, dutasteride inhibited normal development of external genitalia in male fetuses. Therefore, AVODART may cause fetal harm when administered to a pregnant woman. If AVODART is used during pregnancy or if the patient becomes pregnant while taking AVODART, the patient should be apprised of the potential hazard to the fetus.

Abnormalities in the genitalia of male fetuses is an expected physiological consequence of inhibition of the conversion of testosterone to 5α-dihydrotestosterone (DHT) by 5α-reductase inhibitors. These results are similar to observations in male infants with genetic 5α-reductase deficiency.

Dutasteride is absorbed through the skin. To avoid potential fetal exposure, women who are pregnant or may become pregnant should not handle AVODART Soft Gelatin Capsules. If contact is made with leaking capsules, the contact area should be washed immediately with soap and water. Dutasteride is secreted into male semen. The highest measured semen concentration of dutasteride in treated men was 14 ng/mL. Assuming exposure of a 50-kg woman to 5 mL of semen and 100% absorption, the woman's dutasteride concentration would be about 0.175 ng/mL. This concentration is more than 100 times less than concentrations producing abnormalities of male genitalia in animal studies. Dutasteride is highly protein bound in human semen (>96%), which may reduce the amount of dutasteride available for vaginal absorption *[see Warnings and Precautions (5.1)]*.

In an embryo-fetal development study in female rats, oral administration of dutasteride at doses 10 times less than the maximum recommended human dose (MRHD) resulted in abnormalities of male genitalia in the fetus, and nipple development, hypospadias, and distended preputial glands in male offspring. An increase in stillborn pups was observed at 111 times the MRHD, and reduced fetal body weight was observed at doses ≥15 times the MRHD. Increased incidences of skeletal variations considered to be delays in ossification associated with reduced body weight were observed at doses ≥56 times the MRHD. Abnormalities of male genitalia were also observed in an oral pre- and post-natal development study in rats and in 2 embryo-fetal studies in rabbits at one-third the MRHD.

In an embryo-fetal development study, pregnant rhesus monkeys were exposed intravenously to a dutasteride blood level comparable to the dutasteride concentration found in human semen. The development of male external genitalia of monkey offspring was not adversely affected. Reduction of fetal adrenal weights, reduction in fetal prostate weights, and increases in fetal ovarian and testis weights were observed in monkeys *[see Nonclinical Toxicology (13.3)]*.

8.3 Nursing Mothers

AVODART should not be used by nursing women. It is not known whether dutasteride is excreted in human milk.

8.4 Pediatric Use

AVODART is contraindicated for use in pediatric patients. Safety and effectiveness in pediatric patients have not been established.

8.5 Geriatric Use

Of 2,167 male subjects treated with AVODART in 3 clinical studies, 60% were 65 and over and 15% were 75 and over. No overall differences in safety or efficacy were observed between these subjects and younger subjects. Other reported clinical experience has not identified differences in responses between the elderly and younger patients *[see Clinical Pharmacology (12.3)]*.

8.6 Renal Impairment

No dose adjustment is necessary for AVODART in patients with renal impairment *[see Clinical Pharmacology (12.3)]*.

8.7 Hepatic Impairment

The effect of hepatic impairment on dutasteride pharmacokinetics has not been studied. Because dutasteride is extensively metabolized, exposure could be higher in hepatically impaired patients. However, in a clinical study where 60 subjects received 5 mg (10 times the therapeutic dose) daily for 24 weeks, no additional adverse events were observed compared with those observed at the therapeutic dose of 0.5 mg *[see Clinical Pharmacology (12.3)]*.

10 OVERDOSAGE

In volunteer studies, single doses of dutasteride up to 40 mg (80 times the therapeutic dose) for 7 days have been administered without significant safety concerns. In a clinical study, daily doses of 5 mg (10 times the therapeutic dose) were administered to 60 subjects for 6 months with no additional adverse effects to those seen at therapeutic doses of 0.5 mg.

There is no specific antidote for dutasteride. Therefore, in cases of suspected overdosage symptomatic and supportive treatment should be given as appropriate, taking the long half-life of dutasteride into consideration.

11 DESCRIPTION

AVODART is a synthetic 4-azasteroid compound that is a selective inhibitor of both the type 1 and type 2 isoforms of steroid 5α-reductase, an intracellular enzyme that converts testosterone to DHT.

Dutasteride is chemically designated as (5α,17β)-N-{2,5 bis(trifluoromethyl)phenyl}-3-oxo-4-azaandrost-1-ene-17-carboxamide. The empirical formula of dutasteride is $C_{27}H_{30}F_6N_2O_2$, representing a molecular weight of 528.5 with the following structural formula:

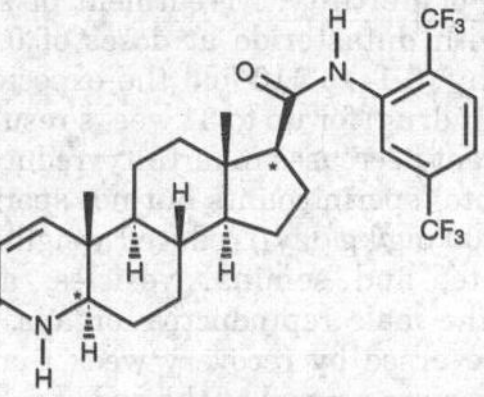

Dutasteride is a white to pale yellow powder with a melting point of 242° to 250°C. It is soluble in ethanol (44 mg/mL), methanol (64 mg/mL), and polyethylene glycol 400 (3 mg/mL), but it is insoluble in water.

Each AVODART Soft Gelatin Capsule, administered orally, contains 0.5 mg of dutasteride dissolved in a mixture of mono-di-glycerides of caprylic/capric acid and butylated hydroxytoluene. The inactive excipients in the capsule shell are gelatin (from certified BSE-free bovine sources), glycerin, and ferric oxide (yellow). The soft gelatin capsules are printed with edible red ink.

12 CLINICAL PHARMACOLOGY

12.1 Mechanism of Action

Dutasteride inhibits the conversion of testosterone to dihydrotestosterone (DHT). DHT is the androgen primarily responsible for the initial development and subsequent enlargement of the prostate gland. Testosterone is converted to DHT by the enzyme 5α-reductase, which exists as 2 isoforms, type 1 and type 2. The type 2 isoenzyme is primarily active in the reproductive tissues, while the type 1 isoenzyme is also responsible for testosterone conversion in the skin and liver.

Dutasteride is a competitive and specific inhibitor of both type 1 and type 2 5α-reductase isoenzymes, with which it forms a stable enzyme complex. Dissociation from this complex has been evaluated under in vitro and in vivo conditions and is extremely slow. Dutasteride does not bind to the human androgen receptor.

12.2 Pharmacodynamics

Effect on 5α-Dihydrotestosterone and Testosterone: The maximum effect of daily doses of dutasteride on the reduction of DHT is dose dependent and is observed within 1 to 2 weeks. After 1 and 2 weeks of daily dosing with dutasteride 0.5 mg, median serum DHT concentrations were reduced by 85% and 90%, respectively. In patients with BPH treated with dutasteride 0.5 mg/day for 4 years, the median decrease in serum DHT was 94% at 1 year, 93% at 2 years, and 95% at both 3 and 4 years. The median increase in serum testosterone was 19% at both 1 and 2 years, 26% at 3 years, and 22% at 4 years, but the mean and median levels remained within the physiologic range.

In patients with BPH treated with 5 mg/day of dutasteride or placebo for up to 12 weeks prior to transurethral resection of the prostate, mean DHT concentrations in prostatic tissue were significantly lower in the dutasteride group compared with placebo (784 and 5,793 pg/g, respectively, $P<0.001$). Mean prostatic tissue concentrations of testosterone were significantly higher in the dutasteride group compared with placebo (2,073 and 93 pg/g, respectively, $P<0.001$).

Adult males with genetically inherited type 2 5α-reductase deficiency also have decreased DHT levels. These 5α-reductase deficient males have a small prostate gland throughout life and do not develop BPH. Except for the associated urogenital defects present at birth, no other clinical abnormalities related to 5α-reductase deficiency have been observed in these individuals.

Effects on Other Hormones: In healthy volunteers, 52 weeks of treatment with dutasteride 0.5 mg/day (n = 26) resulted in no clinically significant change compared with placebo (n = 23) in sex hormone-binding globulin, estradiol, luteinizing hormone, follicle-stimulating hormone, thyroxine (free T4), and dehydroepiandrosterone. Statistically significant, baseline-adjusted mean increases compared with placebo were observed for total testosterone at 8 weeks (97.1 ng/dL, $P<0.003$) and thyroid-stimulating hormone at 52 weeks (0.4 mcIU/mL, $P<0.05$). The median percentage changes from baseline within the dutasteride group were 17.9% for testosterone at 8 weeks and 12.4% for thyroid-stimulating hormone at 52 weeks. After stopping dutasteride for 24 weeks, the mean levels of testosterone and thyroid-stimulating hormone had returned to baseline in the group of subjects with available data at the visit. In patients with BPH treated with dutasteride in a large randomized, double-blind, placebo-controlled study, there was a median percent increase in luteinizing hormone of 12% at 6 months and 19% at both 12 and 24 months.

Other Effects: Plasma lipid panel and bone mineral density were evaluated following 52 weeks of dutasteride 0.5 mg once daily in healthy volunteers. There was no change in bone mineral density as measured by dual energy x-ray absorptiometry compared with either placebo or baseline. In addition, the plasma lipid profile (i.e., total cholesterol, low density lipoproteins, high density lipoproteins, and triglycerides) was unaffected by dutasteride. No clinically significant changes in adrenal hormone responses to ACTH stimulation were observed in a subset population (n = 13) of the 1-year healthy volunteer study.

12.3 Pharmacokinetics

Absorption: Following administration of a single 0.5-mg dose of a soft gelatin capsule, time to peak serum concentrations (T_{max}) of dutasteride occurs within 2 to 3 hours. Absolute bioavailability in 5 healthy subjects is approximately 60% (range, 40% to 94%). When the drug is administered with food, the maximum serum concentrations were reduced by 10% to 15%. This reduction is of no clinical significance.

Distribution: Pharmacokinetic data following single and repeat oral doses show that dutasteride has a large volume of distribution (300 to 500 L). Dutasteride is highly bound to plasma albumin (99.0%) and alpha-1 acid glycoprotein (96.6%).

In a study of healthy subjects (n = 26) receiving dutasteride 0.5 mg/day for 12 months, semen dutasteride concentrations averaged 3.4 ng/mL (range, 0.4 to 14 ng/mL) at 12 months and, similar to serum, achieved steady-state concentrations at 6 months. On average, at 12 months 11.5% of serum dutasteride concentrations partitioned into semen.

Metabolism and Elimination: Dutasteride is extensively metabolized in humans. In vitro studies showed that dutasteride is metabolized by the CYP3A4 and CYP3A5 isoenzymes. Both of these isoenzymes produced the 4′-hydroxydutasteride, 6-hydroxydutasteride, and the 6,4′-dihydroxydutasteride metabolites. In addition, the 15-hydroxydutasteride metabolite was formed by CYP3A4. Dutasteride is not metabolized in vitro by human cytochrome P450 isoenzymes CYP1A2, CYP2A6, CYP2B6, CYP2C8, CYP2C9, CYP2C19, CYP2D6, and CYP2E1. In human serum following dosing to steady state, unchanged dutasteride, 3 major metabolites (4′-hydroxydutasteride, 1,2-dihydrodutasteride, and 6-hydroxydutasteride), and 2 minor metabolites (6,4′-dihydroxydutasteride and 15-hydroxydutasteride), as assessed by mass spectrometric response, have been detected. The absolute stereochemistry of the hydroxyl additions in the 6 and 15 positions is not known. In vitro, the 4′-hydroxydutasteride and 1,2-dihydrodutasteride metabolites are much less potent than dutasteride against both isoforms of human 5α-reductase. The activity of 6β-hydroxydutasteride is comparable to that of dutasteride.

Dutasteride and its metabolites were excreted mainly in feces. As a percent of dose, there was approximately 5% unchanged dutasteride (~1% to ~15%) and 40% as dutasteride-related metabolites (~2% to ~90%). Only trace amounts of unchanged dutasteride were found in urine (<1%). Therefore, on average, the dose unaccounted for approximated 55% (range, 5% to 97%).

The terminal elimination half-life of dutasteride is approximately 5 weeks at steady state. The average steady-state serum dutasteride concentration was 40 ng/mL following 0.5 mg/day for 1 year. Following daily dosing, dutasteride serum concentrations achieve 65% of steady-state concentration after 1 month and approximately 90% after 3 months. Due to the long half-life of dutasteride, serum concentrations remain detectable (greater than 0.1 ng/mL) for up to 4 to 6 months after discontinuation of treatment.

Specific Populations: *Pediatric:* Dutasteride pharmacokinetics have not been investigated in subjects younger than 18 years.

Geriatric: No dose adjustment is necessary in the elderly. The pharmacokinetics and pharmacodynamics of dutasteride were evaluated in 36 healthy male subjects aged between 24 and 87 years following administration of a single 5-mg dose of dutasteride. In this single-dose study, dutasteride half-life increased with age (approximately 170 hours in men aged 20 to 49 years, approximately 260 hours in men aged 50 to 69 years, and approximately 300 hours in men older than 70 years). Of 2,167 men treated with dutasteride in the 3 pivotal studies, 60% were age 65 and over and 15% were age 75 and over. No overall differences in safety or efficacy were observed between these patients and younger patients.

Gender: AVODART is contraindicated in pregnancy and women of childbearing potential and is not indicated for use in other women *[see Contraindications (4), Warnings and Precautions (5.1)]*. The pharmacokinetics of dutasteride in women have not been studied.

Race: The effect of race on dutasteride pharmacokinetics has not been studied.

Renal Impairment: The effect of renal impairment on dutasteride pharmacokinetics has not been studied. However, less than 0.1% of a steady-state 0.5-mg dose of dutasteride is recovered in human urine, so no adjustment in dosage is anticipated for patients with renal impairment.

Hepatic Impairment: The effect of hepatic impairment on dutasteride pharmacokinetics has not been studied. Because dutasteride is extensively metabolized, exposure could be higher in hepatically impaired patients.

Drug Interactions: No clinical drug interaction studies have been performed to evaluate the impact of CYP3A enzyme inhibitors on dutasteride pharmacokinetics. However, based on in vitro data, blood concentrations of dutasteride may increase in the presence of inhibitors of CYP3A4/5 such as ritonavir, ketoconazole, verapamil, diltiazem, cimetidine, troleandomycin, and ciprofloxacin. Dutasteride does not inhibit the in vitro metabolism of model substrates for the major human cytochrome P450 isoenzymes (CYP1A2, CYP2C9, CYP2C19, CYP2D6, and CYP3A4) at a concentration of 1,000 ng/mL, 25 times greater than steady-state serum concentrations in humans.

Alpha-Adrenergic Blocking Agents: In a single-sequence, crossover study in healthy volunteers, the administration of tamsulosin or terazosin in combination with AVODART had no effect on the steady-state pharmacokinetics of either alpha-adrenergic blocker. Although the effect of administration of tamsulosin or terazosin on dutasteride pharmacokinetic parameters was not evaluated, the percent change in DHT concentrations was similar for AVODART alone compared with the combination treatment.

Calcium Channel Antagonists: In a population pharmacokinetics analysis, a decrease in clearance of dutasteride was noted when coadministered with the CYP3A4 inhibitors verapamil (-37%, n = 6) and diltiazem (-44%, n = 5). In contrast, no decrease in clearance was seen when amlodipine, another calcium channel antagonist that is not a CYP3A4 inhibitor, was coadministered with dutasteride (+7%, n = 4). The decrease in clearance and subsequent increase in exposure to dutasteride in the presence of verapamil and diltiazem is not considered to be clinically significant. No dose adjustment is recommended.

Cholestyramine: Administration of a single 5-mg dose of AVODART followed 1 hour later by 12 g cholestyramine did not affect the relative bioavailability of dutasteride in 12 normal volunteers.

Digoxin: In a study of 20 healthy volunteers, AVODART did not alter the steady-state pharmacokinetics of digoxin when administered concomitantly at a dose of 0.5 mg/day for 3 weeks.

Warfarin: In a study of 23 healthy volunteers, 3 weeks of treatment with AVODART 0.5 mg/day did not alter the steady-state pharmacokinetics of the S- or R-warfarin isomers or alter the effect of warfarin on prothrombin time when administered with warfarin.

Other Concomitant Therapy: Although specific interaction studies were not performed with other compounds, approximately 90% of the subjects in the 3 Phase 3 pivotal efficacy studies receiving AVODART were taking other medications concomitantly. No clinically significant adverse interactions could be attributed to the combination of AVODART and concurrent therapy when AVODART was coadministered with anti-hyperlipidemics, angiotensin-converting enzyme (ACE) inhibitors, beta-adrenergic blocking agents, calcium channel blockers, corticosteroids, diuretics, nonsteroidal anti-inflammatory drugs (NSAIDs), phosphodiesterase Type V inhibitors, and quinolone antibiotics.

13 NONCLINICAL TOXICOLOGY

13.1 Carcinogenesis, Mutagenesis, Impairment of Fertility

Carcinogenesis: A 2-year carcinogenicity study was conducted in B6C3F1 mice at doses of 3, 35, 250, and 500 mg/kg/day for males and 3, 35, and 250 mg/kg/day for females; an increased incidence of benign hepatocellular adenomas was noted at 250 mg/kg/day (290-fold the expected clinical exposure to a 0.5-mg daily dose) in females only. Two of the 3 major human metabolites have been detected in mice. The exposure to these metabolites in mice is either lower than in humans or is not known.

In a 2-year carcinogenicity study in Han Wistar rats, at doses of 1.5, 7.5, and 53 mg/kg/day for males and 0.8, 6.3, and 15 mg/kg/day for females, there was an increase in Leydig cell adenomas in the testes at 53 mg/kg/day (135-fold the expected clinical exposure). An increased incidence of Leydig cell hyperplasia was present at 7.5 mg/kg/day (52-fold the expected clinical exposure) and 53 mg/kg/day in male rats. A positive correlation between proliferative changes in the Leydig cells and an increase in circulating luteinizing hormone levels has been demonstrated with 5α-reductase inhibitors and is consistent with an effect on the hypothalamic-pituitary-testicular axis following 5α-reductase inhibition. At tumorigenic doses in rats, luteinizing hormone levels in rats were increased by 167%. In this study, the major human metabolites were tested for carcinogenicity at approximately 1 to 3 times the expected clinical exposure.

Mutagenesis: Dutasteride was tested for genotoxicity in a bacterial mutagenesis assay (Ames test), a chromosomal aberration assay in CHO cells, and a micronucleus assay in rats. The results did not indicate any genotoxic potential of the parent drug. Two major human metabolites were also negative in either the Ames test or an abbreviated Ames test.

Impairment of Fertility: Treatment of sexually mature male rats with dutasteride at doses of 0.05, 10, 50, and 500 mg/kg/day (0.1- to 110-fold the expected clinical exposure of parent drug) for up to 31 weeks resulted in dose- and time-dependent decreases in fertility; reduced cauda epididymal (absolute) sperm counts but not sperm concentration (at 50 and 500 mg/kg/day); reduced weights of the epididymis, prostate, and seminal vesicles; and microscopic changes in the male reproductive organs. The fertility effects were reversed by recovery week 6 at all doses, and sperm counts were normal at the end of a 14-week recovery period. The 5α-reductase–related changes consisted of cytoplasmic vacuolation of tubular epithelium in the epididymides and decreased cytoplasmic content of epithelium, consistent with decreased secretory activity in the prostate and seminal vesicles. The microscopic changes were no longer present at recovery week 14 in the low-dose group and were partly recovered in the remaining treatment groups. Low levels of dutasteride (0.6 to 17 ng/mL) were detected in the serum of untreated female rats mated to males dosed at 10, 50, or 500 mg/kg/day for 29 to 30 weeks.

In a fertility study in female rats, oral administration of dutasteride at doses of 0.05, 2.5, 12.5, and 30 mg/kg/day resulted in reduced litter size, increased embryo resorption and feminization of male fetuses (decreased anogenital distance) at doses of ≥2.5 mg/kg/day (2- to 10-fold the clinical exposure of parent drug in men). Fetal body weights were also reduced at ≥0.05 mg/kg/day in rats (<0.02-fold the human exposure).

13.2 Animal Toxicology

Central Nervous System Toxicology Studies: In rats and dogs, repeated oral administration of dutasteride resulted in some animals showing signs of non-specific, reversible, centrally-mediated toxicity without associated histopathological changes at exposure 425- and 315-fold the expected clinical exposure (of parent drug), respectively.

13.3 Reproductive and Developmental Toxicity

In an intravenous embryo-fetal development study in the rhesus monkey (12/group), administration of dutasteride at 400, 780, 1,325, or 2,010 ng/day on gestation days 20 to 100 did not adversely affect development of male external genitalia. Reduction of fetal adrenal weights, reduction in fetal prostate weights, and increases in fetal ovarian and testis weights were observed in monkeys treated with the highest dose. Based on the highest measured semen concentration of dutasteride in treated men (14 ng/mL), these doses represent 0.8 to 16 times based on blood levels of parent drug (32 to 186 times based on a ng/kg daily dose) the potential maximum exposure of a 50-kg human female to 5 mL semen daily from a dutasteride-treated man, assuming 100% absorption. Dutasteride is highly bound to proteins in human semen (>96%), potentially reducing the amount of dutasteride available for vaginal absorption.

In an embryo-fetal development study in female rats, oral administration of dutasteride at doses of 0.05, 2.5, 12.5, and 30 mg/kg/day resulted in feminization of male fetuses (decreased anogenital distance) and male offspring (nipple development, hypospadias, and distended preputial glands) at all doses (0.07- to 111-fold the expected male clinical exposure). An increase in stillborn pups was observed at 30 mg/kg/day, and reduced fetal body weight was observed at doses ≥2.5 mg/kg/day (15- to 111-fold the expected clinical exposure). Increased incidences of skeletal variations considered to be delays in ossification associated with reduced body weight were observed at doses of 12.5 and 30 mg/kg/day (56- to 111-fold the expected clinical exposure).

In an oral pre- and post-natal development study in rats, dutasteride doses of 0.05, 2.5, 12.5, or 30 mg/kg/day were administered. Unequivocal evidence of feminization of the genitalia (i.e., decreased anogenital distance, increased incidence of hypospadias, nipple development) of F1 generation male offspring occurred at doses ≥2.5 mg/kg/day (14- to 90-fold the expected clinical exposure in men). At a daily dose of 0.05 mg/kg/day (0.05-fold the expected clinical exposure), evidence of feminization was limited to a small, but statistically significant, decrease in anogenital distance. Doses of 2.5 to 30 mg/kg/day resulted in prolonged gestation in the parental females and a decrease in time to vaginal patency for female offspring and a decrease in prostate and seminal vesicle weights in male offspring. Effects on newborn startle response were noted at doses greater than or equal to 12.5 mg/kg/day. Increased stillbirths were noted at 30 mg/kg/day.

In the rabbit, embryo-fetal study doses of 30, 100, and 200 mg/kg (28- to 93-fold the expected clinical exposure in men) were administered orally on days 7 to 29 of pregnancy to encompass the late period of external genitalia development. Histological evaluation of the genital papilla of fetuses revealed evidence of feminization of the male fetus at all doses. A second embryo-fetal study in rabbits at doses of 0.05, 0.4, 3.0, and 30 mg/kg/day (0.3- to 53-fold the expected clinical exposure) also produced evidence of feminization of the genitalia in male fetuses at all doses. It is not known whether rabbits or rhesus monkeys produce any of the major human metabolites.

14 CLINICAL STUDIES

14.1 Monotherapy

AVODART 0.5 mg/day (n = 2,167) or placebo (n = 2,158) was evaluated in male subjects with BPH in three 2-year multicenter, placebo-controlled, double-blind studies, each with 2-year open-label extensions (n = 2,340). More than 90% of the study population was Caucasian. Subjects were at least 50 years of age with a serum PSA ≥1.5 ng/mL and <10 ng/mL and BPH diagnosed by medical history and physical examination, including enlarged prostate (≥30 cc) and BPH symptoms that were moderate to severe according to the American Urological Association Symptom Index (AUA-SI). Most of the 4,325 subjects randomly assigned to receive either dutasteride or placebo completed 2 years of double-blind treatment (70% and 67%, respectively). Most of the 2,340 subjects in the study extensions completed 2 additional years of open-label treatment (71%).

Effect on Symptom Scores: Symptoms were quantified using the AUA-SI, a questionnaire that evaluates urinary symptoms (incomplete emptying, frequency, intermittency, urgency, weak stream, straining, and nocturia) by rating on a 0 to 5 scale for a total possible score of 35. The baseline AUA-SI score across the 3 studies was approximately 17 units in both treatment groups.

Subjects receiving dutasteride achieved statistically significant improvement in symptoms versus placebo by Month 3 in 1 study and by Month 12 in the other 2 pivotal studies. At Month 12, the mean decrease from baseline in AUA-SI symptom scores across the 3 studies pooled was -3.3 units for dutasteride and -2.0 units for placebo with a mean difference between the 2 treatment groups of -1.3 (range, -1.1 to -1.5 units in each of the 3 studies, $P<0.001$) and was consistent across the 3 studies. At Month 24, the mean decrease from baseline was -3.8 units for dutasteride and -1.7 units for placebo with a mean difference of -2.1 (range, -1.9 to -2.2 units in each of the 3 studies, $P<0.001$). See Figure 1.

The improvement in BPH symptoms seen during the first 2 years of double-blind treatment was maintained throughout an additional 2 years of open-label extension studies.

These studies were prospectively designed to evaluate effects on symptoms based on prostate size at baseline. In men with prostate volumes ≥40 cc, the mean decrease was -3.8 units for dutasteride and -1.6 units for placebo, with a mean difference between the 2 treatment groups of -2.2 at Month 24. In men with prostate volumes <40 cc, the mean decrease was -3.7 units for dutasteride and -2.2 units for placebo, with a mean difference between the 2 treatment groups of -1.5 at Month 24.

Figure 1. AUA-SI Score[a] Change from Baseline (Randomized, Double-Blind, Placebo-Controlled Studies Pooled)

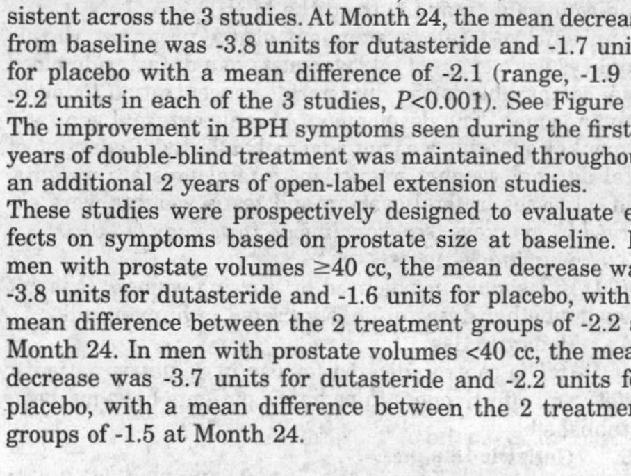

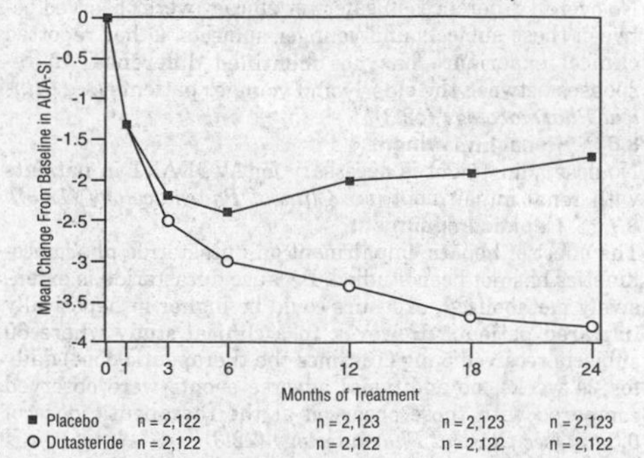
Mean Change From Baseline in AUA-SI
0
-0.5
-1
-1.5
-2
-2.5
-3
-3.5
-4
0 1 3 6 12 18 24
Months of Treatment
■ Placebo n = 2,122 n = 2,123 n = 2,123 n = 2,123
O Dutasteride n = 2,122 n = 2,122 n = 2,122 n = 2,122

[a] AUA-SI score ranges from 0 to 35.

Effect on Acute Urinary Retention and the Need for Surgery: Efficacy was also assessed after 2 years of treatment by the incidence of AUR requiring catheterization and BPH-related urological surgical intervention. Compared with placebo, AVODART was associated with a statistically significantly lower incidence of AUR (1.8% for AVODART vs. 4.2% for placebo, $P<0.001$; 57% reduction in risk, [95% CI: 38% to 71%]) and with a statistically significantly lower incidence of surgery (2.2% for AVODART vs. 4.1% for placebo, $P<0.001$; 48% reduction in risk, [95% CI: 26% to 63%]). See Figures 2 and 3.

Figure 2. Percent of Subjects Developing Acute Urinary Retention Over a 24-Month Period (Randomized, Double-Blind, Placebo-Controlled Studies Pooled)

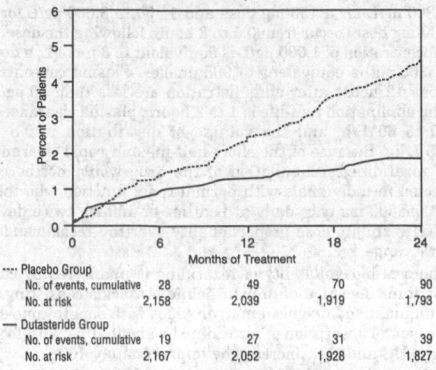

---- Placebo Group				
No. of events, cumulative	28	49	70	90
No. at risk	2,158	2,039	1,919	1,793
— Dutasteride Group				
No. of events, cumulative	19	27	31	39
No. at risk	2,167	2,052	1,928	1,827

Figure 3. Percent of Subjects Having Surgery for Benign Prostatic Hyperplasia Over a 24-Month Period (Randomized, Double-Blind, Placebo-Controlled Studies Pooled)

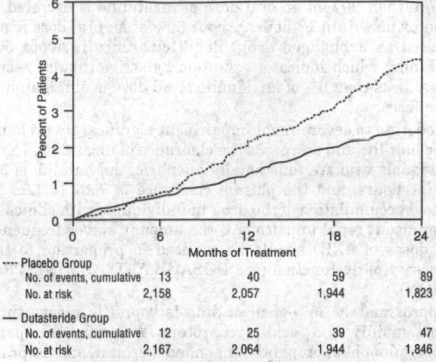

---- Placebo Group				
No. of events, cumulative	13	40	59	89
No. at risk	2,158	2,057	1,944	1,823
— Dutasteride Group				
No. of events, cumulative	12	25	39	47
No. at risk	2,167	2,064	1,944	1,846

Effect on Prostate Volume: A prostate volume of at least 30 cc measured by transrectal ultrasound was required for study entry. The mean prostate volume at study entry was approximately 54 cc.

Statistically significant differences (AVODART versus placebo) were noted at the earliest post-treatment prostate volume measurement in each study (Month 1, Month 3, or Month 6) and continued through Month 24. At Month 12, the mean percent change in prostate volume across the 3 studies pooled was -24.7% for dutasteride and -3.4% for placebo; the mean difference (dutasteride minus placebo) was -21.3% (range, -21.0% to -21.6% in each of the 3 studies, $P<0.001$). At Month 24, the mean percent change in prostate volume across the 3 studies pooled was -26.7% for dutasteride and -2.2% for placebo with a mean difference of -24.5% (range, -24.0% to -25.1% in each of the 3 studies, $P<0.001$). See Figure 4. The reduction in prostate volume seen during the first 2 years of double-blind treatment was maintained throughout an additional 2 years of open-label extension studies.

Figure 4. Prostate Volume Percent Change from Baseline (Randomized, Double-Blind, Placebo-Controlled Studies Pooled)

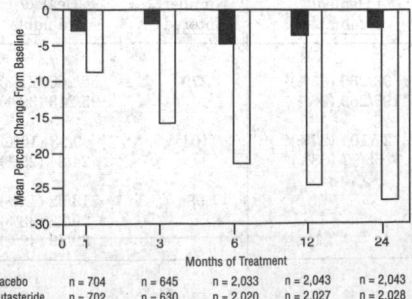

■ Placebo	n = 704	n = 645	n = 2,033	n = 2,043	n = 2,043
□ Dutasteride	n = 702	n = 630	n = 2,020	n = 2,027	n = 2,028

Effect on Maximum Urine Flow Rate: A mean peak urine flow rate (Q_{max}) of ≤15 mL/sec was required for study entry. Q_{max} was approximately 10 mL/sec at baseline across the 3 pivotal studies.

Differences between the 2 groups were statistically significant from baseline at Month 3 in all 3 studies and were maintained through Month 12. At Month 12, the mean increase in Q_{max} across the 3 studies pooled was 1.6 mL/sec for AVODART and 0.7 mL/sec for placebo; the mean difference (dutasteride minus placebo) was 0.8 mL/sec (range, 0.7 to 1.0 mL/sec in each of the 3 studies, $P<0.001$). At Month 24, the mean increase in Q_{max} was 1.8 mL/sec for dutasteride and 0.7 mL/sec for placebo, with a mean difference of 1.1 mL/sec (range, 1.0 to 1.2 mL/sec in each of the 3 studies, $P<0.001$). See Figure 5. The increase in maximum urine flow rate seen during the first 2 years of double-blind treatment was maintained throughout an additional 2 years of open-label extension studies.

Figure 5. Q_{max} Change from Baseline (Randomized, Double-Blind, Placebo-Controlled Studies Pooled)

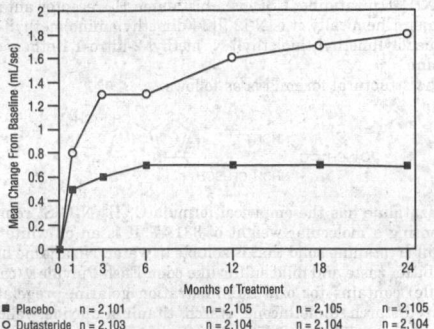

■ Placebo	n = 2,101		n = 2,105	n = 2,105	n = 2,105
○ Dutasteride	n = 2,103		n = 2,104	n = 2,104	n = 2,104

Summary of Clinical Studies: Data from 3 large, well-controlled efficacy studies demonstrate that treatment with AVODART (0.5 mg once daily) reduces the risk of both AUR and BPH-related surgical intervention relative to placebo, improves BPH-related symptoms, decreases prostate volume, and increases maximum urinary flow rates. These data suggest that AVODART arrests the disease process of BPH in men with an enlarged prostate.

14.2   Combination With Alpha-Blocker Therapy (CombAT)

The efficacy of combination therapy (AVODART 0.5 mg/day plus tamsulosin 0.4 mg/day, n = 1,610) was compared with AVODART alone (n = 1,623) or tamsulosin alone (n = 1,611) in a 4-year multicenter, randomized, double-blind study. Study entry criteria were similar to the Phase 3 monotherapy efficacy trials described above in section 14.1. The results presented below are from data collected following 2 years of treatment in the 4-year study. Eighty-eight percent (88%) of the enrolled study population was Caucasian. Approximately 52% of subjects had previous exposure to 5α-reductase inhibitor or alpha-blocker treatment. The primary efficacy endpoint evaluated during the first 2 years of treatment was change in international prostate symptom score (IPSS). Most of the 4,844 subjects randomly assigned to receive combination, AVODART, or tamsulosin completed 2 years of double-blind treatment (79%, 80%, and 78%, respectively).

Effect on Symptom Score: Symptoms were quantified using the first 7 questions of the IPSS (identical to the AUA-SI). The baseline score was approximately 16.4 units for each treatment group. Combination therapy was statistically superior to each of the monotherapy treatments in decreasing symptom score at Month 24. This difference was seen by Month 9 and continued through Month 24. At Month 24, the mean change from baseline (±SD) in IPSS symptom scores was -6.2 (±7.14) for combination, -4.9 (±6.81) for AVODART, and -4.3 (±7.01) for tamsulosin, with a mean difference between combination and AVODART of -1.3 units ($P<0.001$; [95% CI: -1.69, -0.86]), and between combination and tamsulosin of -1.8 units ($P<0.001$; [95% CI: -2.23, -1.40]). See Figure 6.
[See figure 6 at top of next column]

Effect on Maximum Urine Flow Rate: The baseline Q_{max} was approximately 10.7 mL/sec for each treatment group. Combination therapy was statistically superior to each of the monotherapy treatments in increasing Q_{max} at Month 24. This difference was seen by Month 6 and continued through Month 24. At Month 24, the mean increase from baseline (±SD) in Q_{max} was 2.4 (±5.26) mL/sec for combination, 1.9 (±5.10) mL/sec for AVODART, and 0.9 (±4.57) mL/sec for tamsulosin, with a mean difference between combination and AVODART of 0.5 mL/sec ($P = 0.003$; [95% CI: 0.17, 0.84]), and between combination and tamsulosin of 1.5 mL/sec ($P<0.001$; [95% CI: 1.19, 1.86]). See Figure 7.
[See figure 7 in next column]

Figure 6. International Prostate Symptom Score Change from Baseline (CombAT study)

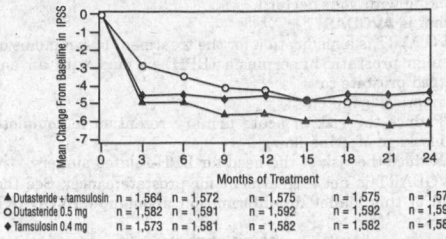

▲ Dutasteride + tamsulosin	n = 1,564	n = 1,572	n = 1,575	n = 1,575	n = 1,575
○ Dutasteride 0.5 mg	n = 1,582	n = 1,591	n = 1,592	n = 1,592	n = 1,592
◆ Tamsulosin 0.4 mg	n = 1,573	n = 1,581	n = 1,582	n = 1,582	n = 1,582

Figure 7. Q_{max} Change from Baseline (CombAT study)

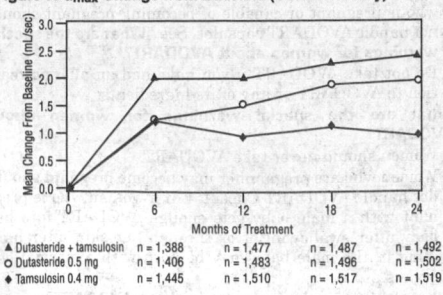

▲ Dutasteride + tamsulosin	n = 1,388	n = 1,477	n = 1,487	n = 1,492
○ Dutasteride 0.5 mg	n = 1,406	n = 1,483	n = 1,496	n = 1,502
◆ Tamsulosin 0.4 mg	n = 1,445	n = 1,510	n = 1,517	n = 1,519

Effect on Prostate Volume: The mean prostate volume at study entry was approximately 55 cc. At Month 24, the mean percent change from baseline (±SD) in prostate volume was -26.9% (±22.57) for combination therapy, -28.0% (±24.88) for AVODART, and 0% (±31.14) for tamsulosin, with a mean difference between combination and AVODART of 1.1% (P = NS; [95% CI: -0.6, 2.8]), and between combination and tamsulosin of -26.9% ($P<0.001$; [95% CI: -28.9, -24.9]).

16   HOW SUPPLIED/STORAGE AND HANDLING

AVODART Soft Gelatin Capsules 0.5 mg are oblong, opaque, dull yellow, gelatin capsules imprinted with "GX CE2" with red edible ink on one side packaged in bottles of 30 (NDC 0173-0712-15) and 90 (NDC 0173-0712-04) with child-resistant closures.

Store at 25°C (77°F); excursions permitted to 15-30°C (59-86°F) [see USP Controlled Room Temperature].

Dutasteride is absorbed through the skin. AVODART Capsules should not be handled by women who are pregnant or who may become pregnant because of the potential for absorption of dutasteride and the subsequent potential risk to a developing male fetus [see Warnings and Precautions (5.1)].

17   PATIENT COUNSELING INFORMATION

See FDA-Approved Patient Labeling.

17.1   Exposure of Women—Risk to Male Fetus

Physicians should inform patients that AVODART Capsules should not be handled by a woman who is pregnant or who may become pregnant because of the potential for absorption of dutasteride and the subsequent potential risk to a developing male fetus. Dutasteride is absorbed through the skin and could result in unintended fetal exposure. If a pregnant woman or woman of childbearing potential comes in contact with leaking AVODART Capsules, the contact area should be washed immediately with soap and water [see Warnings and Precautions (5.1), Specific Populations (8.1)].

17.2   Blood Donation

Physicians should inform men treated with AVODART that they should not donate blood until at least 6 months following their last dose to prevent pregnant women from receiving dutasteride through blood transfusion [see Warnings and Precautions (5.4)]. Serum levels of dutasteride are detectable for 4 to 6 months after treatment ends [see Clinical Pharmacology (12.3)].

GlaxoSmithKline
Research Triangle Park, NC 27709
Manufactured by Catalent Pharma Solutions, Beinheim, France for
GlaxoSmithKline, Research Triangle Park, NC 27709
©2010, GlaxoSmithKline. All rights reserved.
June 2010
AVT:5PI

PHARMACIST-DETACH HERE AND GIVE INSTRUCTIONS TO PATIENT

PATIENT INFORMATION
AVODART® (dutasteride) Soft Gelatin Capsules
AVODART is for use by men only.
Read this information carefully before you start taking AVODART. Read the information you get with AVODART

each time you refill your prescription. There may be new information. This information does not take the place of talking with your doctor.

What is AVODART?

AVODART is a medication for the treatment of symptoms of benign prostatic hyperplasia (BPH) in men with an enlarged prostate to:

- Improve symptoms
- Reduce the risk of acute urinary retention (a complete blockage of urine flow)
- Reduce the risk of the need for BPH-related surgery

AVODART is not a treatment for prostate cancer. See the end of this leaflet for information about how AVODART works.

Who should NOT take AVODART?

- Women and children should not take AVODART. A woman who is pregnant or capable of becoming pregnant should not handle AVODART capsules. See **"What are the special warnings for women about AVODART?"**
- Do not take AVODART if you have had an allergic reaction to AVODART or any of its ingredients.

What are the special warnings for women about AVODART?

- Women should never take AVODART.
- Women who are pregnant or may become pregnant should not handle AVODART Capsules. If a woman who is pregnant with a male baby gets enough AVODART into her body after swallowing it or through her skin after handling it, the male baby may be born with abnormal sex organs.

What are the special precautions about AVODART?

- Men treated with AVODART should not donate blood until at least 6 months after their final dose to prevent giving AVODART to a pregnant female through a blood transfusion.
- Tell your doctor if you have liver problems. AVODART may not be right for you.

How should I take AVODART?

- Take 1 AVODART capsule once a day.
- Swallow the capsule whole because the contents of the capsule may irritate your lips, mouth, or throat.
- You can take AVODART with or without food.
- If you miss a dose, you may take it later that day. Do not make up the missed dose by taking 2 doses the next day.
- You may find it helpful to take AVODART at the same time every day to help you remember to take your dose.

What are the possible side effects of AVODART?

Possible side effects are impotence (trouble getting or keeping an erection), a decrease in libido (sex drive), enlarged breasts, a decrease in the amount of semen released during sex, and allergic reactions such as rash, itching, hives, and swelling of the lips or face. These events occurred infrequently.

Talk to your doctor about these and other possible side effects. Call your doctor for medical advice about side effects. You may report side effects to FDA at 1-800-FDA-1088.

How should I store AVODART?

AVODART is a soft gelatin capsule that may become soft and leak or may stick to other capsules if kept at high temperatures. Store AVODART capsules at room temperature of 77°F (25°C) or lower.

If your capsules are cracked or leaking, don't use them, and contact your pharmacist.

General information about AVODART.

- Do not use AVODART for a condition for which it was not prescribed.
- Do not share your AVODART.
- Ask your doctor about how often you should return for a visit to check your BPH.
- A blood test called PSA (prostate-specific antigen) is sometimes used to detect prostate cancer. AVODART will reduce the amount of PSA measured in your blood. Your doctor is aware of this effect and can still use PSA to detect prostate cancer in you. Increases in your PSA levels from their lowest point while on treatment with AVODART (even if the PSA values are in the normal range) should be evaluated by your physician.
- If you have questions about AVODART, ask your doctor or pharmacist. They can show you detailed information about AVODART that was written for healthcare professionals.

How does AVODART work?

Prostate growth is caused by a hormone in the blood called dihydrotestosterone (DHT). AVODART lowers DHT production in the body, leading to shrinkage of the enlarged prostate in most men. Just as your prostate became large over a long period of time, reducing the size of your prostate and improving your symptoms will take time. While some men have fewer problems and symptoms after 3 months of treatment with AVODART, a treatment period of at least 6 months is usually necessary to see if AVODART will work for you. Studies have shown that treatment with AVODART

for 2 years reduces the risk of complete blockage of urine flow (acute urinary retention) and/or the need for surgery for benign prostatic hyperplasia.

GlaxoSmithKline
Research Triangle Park, NC 27709
Manufactured by Catalent Pharma Solutions
Beinheim, France for
GlaxoSmithKline
Research Triangle Park, NC 27709
©2010, GlaxoSmithKline. All rights reserved.
June 2010
AVT:2PIL

AXID® ℞
[ax' ĭd]
(nizatidine)
Capsules, USP

DESCRIPTION

AXID® (nizatidine, USP) is a histamine H_2-receptor antagonist. Chemically, it is N-[2-[[[2-[(dimethylamino)methyl]-4-thiazolyl]methyl]thio]ethyl]-N′-methyl-2-nitro-1,1-ethenediamine.

The structural formula is as follows:

Nizatidine has the empirical formula $C_{12}H_{21}N_5O_2S_2$ representing a molecular weight of 331.47. It is an off-white to buff crystalline solid that is soluble in water. Nizatidine has a bitter taste and mild sulfur-like odor. Each Pulvule® (capsule) contains for oral administration gelatin, pregelatinized starch, dimethicone, starch, titanium dioxide, yellow iron oxide, 150 mg (0.45 mmol) of nizatidine, and other inactive ingredients. The 150 mg Pulvule also contains magnesium stearate.

CLINICAL PHARMACOLOGY

AXID is a competitive, reversible inhibitor of histamine at the histamine H_2-receptors, particularly those in the gastric parietal cells.

Antisecretory Activity: 1. Effects on Acid Secretion: AXID significantly inhibited nocturnal gastric acid secretion for up to 12 hours. AXID also significantly inhibited gastric acid secretion stimulated by food, caffeine, betazole, and pentagastrin (Table 1).

Table 1. Effect of Oral AXID on Gastric Acid Secretion

	Time After Dose (h)	% Inhibition of Gastric Acid Output by Dose (mg)				
		20-50	75	100	150	300
Nocturnal	Up to 10	57		73		90
Betazole	Up to 3		93		100	90
Pentagastrin	Up to 6		25		64	67
Meal	Up to 4	41	64		98	97
Caffeine	Up to 3		73		85	96

2. Effects on Other Gastrointestinal Secretions:
Pepsin: Oral administration of 75 to 300 mg of AXID did not affect pepsin activity in gastric secretions. Total pepsin output was reduced in proportion to the reduced volume of gastric secretions.
Intrinsic Factor: Oral administration of 75 to 300 mg of AXID increased betazole-stimulated secretion of intrinsic factor.

Serum Gastrin: AXID had no effect on basal serum gastrin. No rebound of gastrin secretion was observed when food was ingested 12 hours after administration of AXID.
3. Other Pharmacologic Actions:
a. Hormones: AXID was not shown to affect the serum concentrations of gonadotropins, prolactin, growth hormone, antidiuretic hormone, cortisol, triiodothyronine, thyroxin, testosterone, 5α-dihydrotestosterone, androstenedione, or estradiol.
b. AXID had no demonstrable antiandrogenic action.
4. Pharmacokinetics: The absolute oral bioavailability of nizatidine exceeds 70%. Peak plasma concentrations (700 to 1,800 µg/L for a 150-mg dose and 1,400 to 3,600 µg/L for a 300-mg dose) occur from 0.5 to 3 hours following the dose. A concentration of 1,000 µg/L is equivalent to 3 µmol/L; a dose of 300 mg is equivalent to 905 µmoles. Plasma concentrations 12 hours after administration are less than 10 µg/L. The elimination half-life is 1 to 2 hours, plasma clearance is 40 to 60 L/h, and the volume of distribution is 0.8 to 1.5 L/kg. Because of the short half-life and rapid clearance of nizatidine, accumulation of the drug would not be expected in individuals with normal renal function who take either 300 mg once daily at bedtime or 150 mg twice daily. AXID exhibits dose proportionality over the recommended dose range.

The oral bioavailability of nizatidine is unaffected by concomitant ingestion of propantheline. Antacids consisting of aluminum and magnesium hydroxides with simethicone decrease the absorption of nizatidine by about 10%. With food, the AUC and C_{max} increase by approximately 10%.

In humans, less than 7% of an oral dose is metabolized as N2-monodes-methylnizatidine, an H_2-receptor antagonist, which is the principal metabolite excreted in the urine. Other likely metabolites are the N2-oxide (less than 5% of the dose) and the S-oxide (less than 6% of the dose).

More than 90% of an oral dose of nizatidine is excreted in the urine within 12 hours. About 60% of an oral dose is excreted as unchanged drug. Renal clearance is about 500 mL/min, which indicates excretion by active tubular secretion. Less than 6% of an administered dose is eliminated in the feces.

Moderate to severe renal impairment significantly prolongs the half-life and decreases the clearance of nizatidine. In individuals who are functionally anephric, the half-life is 3.5 to 11 hours, and the plasma clearance is 7 to 14 L/h. To avoid accumulation of the drug in individuals with clinically significant renal impairment, the amount and/or frequency of doses of AXID should be reduced in proportion to the severity of dysfunction (see DOSAGE AND ADMINISTRATION).

Approximately 35% of nizatidine is bound to plasma protein, mainly to α_1-acid glycoprotein. Warfarin, diazepam, acetaminophen, propantheline, phenobarbital, and propranolol did not affect plasma protein binding of nizatidine in vitro.

Clinical Trials: 1. Active Duodenal Ulcer: In multicenter, double-blind, placebo-controlled studies in the United States, endoscopically diagnosed duodenal ulcers healed more rapidly following administration of AXID, 300 mg h.s. or 150 mg b.i.d., than with placebo (Table 2). Lower doses, such as 100 mg h.s., had slightly lower effectiveness.
[See table 2 below]
2. Maintenance of Healed Duodenal Ulcer:
Treatment with a reduced dose of AXID has been shown to be effective as maintenance therapy following healing of active duodenal ulcers. In multicenter, double-blind, placebo-controlled studies conducted in the United States, 150 mg of AXID taken at bedtime resulted in a significantly lower incidence of duodenal ulcer recurrence in patients treated for up to 1 year (Table 3).

Table 2. Healing Response of Ulcers to AXID

	AXID					
	300 mg h.s.		150 mg b.i.d.		Placebo	
	Number Entered	Healed/ Evaluable	Number Entered	Healed/ Evaluable	Number Entered	Healed/ Evaluable
STUDY 1						
Week 2			276	93/265 (35%)*	279	55/260 (21%)
Week 4				198/259 (76%)*		95/243 (39%)
STUDY 2						
Week 2	108	24/103 (23%)*	106	27/101 (27%)*	101	9/93 (10%)
Week 4		65/97 (67%)*		66/97 (68%)*		24/84 (29%)
STUDY 3						
Week 2	92	22/90 (24%)†			98	13/92 (14%)
Week 4		52/85 (61%)*				29/88 (33%)
Week 8		68/83 (82%)*				39/79 (49%)

*$P<0.01$ as compared with placebo.
†$P<0.05$ as compared with placebo.

IMPORTANT NOTICE: Updated drug information is sent bi-monthly via the PDR® Update Insert. For *monthly* email updates, register at PDR.net.

Table 3. Percentage of Ulcers Recurring by 3, 6, and 12 Months in Double-Blind Studies Conducted in the United States

Month	AXID, 150 mg h.s.	Placebo
3	13% (28/208)*	40% (82/204)
6	24% (45/188)*	57% (106/187)
12	34% (57/166)*	64% (112/175)

*$P<0.001$ as compared with placebo.

3. Gastroesophageal Reflux Disease (GERD):
In 2 multicenter, double-blind, placebo-controlled clinical trials performed in the United States and Canada, AXID was more effective than placebo in improving endoscopically diagnosed esophagitis and in healing erosive and ulcerative esophagitis.

In patients with erosive or ulcerative esophagitis, 150 mg b.i.d. of AXID given to 88 patients compared with placebo in 98 patients in Study 1 yielded a higher healing rate at 3 weeks (16% vs 7%) and at 6 weeks (32% vs 16%, $P<0.05$). Of 99 patients on AXID and 94 patients on placebo, Study 2 at the same dosage yielded similar results at 6 weeks (21% vs 11%, $P<0.05$) and at 12 weeks (29% vs 13%, $P<0.01$).

In addition, relief of associated heartburn was greater in patients treated with AXID. Patients treated with AXID consumed fewer antacids than did patients treated with placebo.

4. Active Benign Gastric Ulcer:
In a multicenter, double-blind, placebo-controlled study conducted in the United States and Canada, endoscopically diagnosed benign gastric ulcers healed significantly more rapidly following administration of nizatidine than of placebo (Table 4).

Table 4

Week	Treatment	Healing Rate	vs. Placebo p-value*
4	Niz 300 mg h.s.	52/153 (34%)	0.342
	Niz 150 mg b.i.d.	65/151 (43%)	0.022
	Placebo	48/151 (32%)	
8	Niz 300 mg h.s.	99/153 (65%)	0.011
	Niz 150 mg b.i.d.	105/151 (70%)	<0.001
	Placebo	78/151 (52%)	

*P-values are one-sided, obtained by Chi-square test, and not adjusted for multiple comparisons.

In a multicenter, double-blind, comparator-controlled study in Europe, healing rates for patients receiving nizatidine (300 mg h.s. or 150 mg b.i.d.) were equivalent to rates for patients receiving a comparator drug, and statistically superior to historical placebo control rates.

INDICATIONS AND USAGE

AXID is indicated for up to 8 weeks for the treatment of active duodenal ulcer. In most patients, the ulcer will heal within 4 weeks.

AXID is indicated for maintenance therapy for duodenal ulcer patients, at a reduced dosage of 150 mg h.s. after healing of an active duodenal ulcer. The consequences of continuous therapy with AXID for longer than 1 year are not known.

AXID is indicated for up to 12 weeks for the treatment of endoscopically diagnosed esophagitis, including erosive and ulcerative esophagitis, and associated heartburn due to GERD.

AXID is indicated for up to 8 weeks for the treatment of active benign gastric ulcer. Before initiating therapy, care should be taken to exclude the possibility of malignant gastric ulceration.

CONTRAINDICATION

AXID is contraindicated in patients with known hypersensitivity to the drug. Because cross sensitivity in this class of compounds has been observed, H_2- receptor antagonists, including AXID should not be administered to patients with a history of hypersensitivity to other H_2- receptor antagonists.

PRECAUTIONS
General:
1. Symptomatic response to nizatidine therapy does not preclude the presence of gastric malignancy.

2. Because nizatidine is excreted primarily by the kidney, dosage should be reduced in patients with moderate to severe renal insufficiency (see DOSAGE AND ADMINISTRATION).

3. Pharmacokinetic studies in patients with hepatorenal syndrome have not been done. Part of the dose of nizatidine is metabolized in the liver. In patients with normal renal function and uncomplicated hepatic dysfunction, the disposition of nizatidine is similar to that in normal subjects.

Laboratory Tests: False-positive tests for urobilinogen with Multistix® may occur during therapy with nizatidine.

Drug Interactions: No interactions have been observed between AXID and theophylline, chlordiazepoxide, lorazepam, lidocaine, phenytoin, and warfarin. AXID does not inhibit the cytochrome P-450-linked drug-metabolizing enzyme system; therefore, drug interactions mediated by inhibition of hepatic metabolism are not expected to occur. In patients given very high doses (3,900 mg) of aspirin daily, increases in serum salicylate levels were seen when nizatidine, 150 mg b.i.d., was administered concurrently.

Carcinogenesis, Mutagenesis, Impairment of Fertility: A 2-year oral carcinogenicity study in rats with doses as high as 500 mg/kg/day (about 80 times the recommended daily therapeutic dose) showed no evidence of a carcinogenic effect. There was a dose-related increase in the density of enterochromaffin-like (ECL) cells in the gastric oxyntic mucosa. In a 2-year study in mice, there was no evidence of a carcinogenic effect in male mice; although hyperplastic nodules of the liver were increased in the high-dose males as compared with placebo. Female mice given the high dose of AXID (2,000 mg/kg/day, about 330 times the human dose) showed marginally statistically significant increases in hepatic carcinoma and hepatic nodular hyperplasia with no numerical increase seen in any of the other dose groups. The rate of hepatic carcinoma in the high-dose animals was within the historical control limits seen for the strain of mice used. The female mice were given a dose larger than the maximum tolerated dose, as indicated by excessive (30%) weight decrement as compared with concurrent controls and evidence of mild liver injury (transaminase elevations). The occurrence of a marginal finding at high dose only in animals given an excessive and somewhat hepatotoxic dose, with no evidence of a carcinogenic effect in rats, male mice, and female mice (given up to 360 mg/kg/day, about 60 times the human dose), and a negative mutagenicity battery are not considered evidence of a carcinogenic potential for AXID.

AXID was not mutagenic in a battery of tests performed to evaluate its potential genetic toxicity, including bacterial mutation tests, unscheduled DNA synthesis, sister chromatid exchange, mouse lymphoma assay, chromosome aberration tests, and a micronucleus test.

In a 2-generation, perinatal and postnatal fertility study in rats, doses of nizatidine up to 650 mg/kg/day produced no adverse effects on the reproductive performance of parental animals or their progeny.

Pregnancy: *Teratogenic Effects:* Pregnancy Category B. Oral reproduction studies in pregnant rats at doses up to 1500 mg/kg/day (9000 mg/m²/day, 40.5 times the recommended human dose based on body surface area) and in pregnant rabbits at doses up to 275 mg/kg/day (3245 mg/m²/day, 14.6 times the recommended human dose based on body surface area) have revealed no evidence of impaired fertility or harm to the fetus due to nizatidine. There are, however, no adequate and well-controlled studies in pregnant women. Because animal reproduction studies are not always predictive of human response, this drug should be used during pregnancy only if clearly needed.

Nursing Mothers: Studies conducted in lactating women have shown that 0.1% of the administered oral dose of nizatidine is secreted in human milk in proportion to plasma concentrations. Because of the growth depression in pups reared by lactating rats treated with nizatidine, a decision should be made whether to discontinue nursing or discontinue the drug, taking into account the importance of the drug to the mother.

Pediatric Use: Safety and effectiveness in pediatric patients have not been established.

Geriatric Use: Of the 955 patients in clinical studies who were treated with nizatidine, 337 (35.3%) were 65 and older. No overall differences in safety or effectiveness were observed between these and younger subjects. Other reported clinical experience has not identified differences in responses between the elderly and younger patients, but greater sensitivity of some older individuals cannot be ruled out.

This drug is known to be substantially excreted by the kidney, and the risk of toxic reactions to this drug may be greater in patients with impaired renal function. Because elderly patients are more likely to have decreased renal function, care should be taken in dose selection, and it may be useful to monitor renal function (see DOSAGE AND ADMINISTRATION).

ADVERSE REACTIONS

Worldwide, controlled clinical trials of nizatidine included over 6,000 patients given nizatidine in studies of varying durations. Placebo-controlled trials in the United States and Canada included over 2,600 patients given nizatidine and over 1,700 given placebo. Among the adverse events in these placebo-controlled trials, anemia (0.2% vs 0%) and urticaria (0.5% vs 0.1%) were significantly more common in the nizatidine group.

Incidence in Placebo-Controlled Clinical Trials in the United States and Canada:
Table 5 lists adverse events that occurred at a frequency of 1% or more among nizatidine-treated patients who participated in placebo-controlled trials. The cited figures provide some basis for estimating the relative contribution of drug and nondrug factors to the side effect incidence rate in the population studied.

Table 5. Incidence of Treatment-Emergent Adverse Events in Placebo-Controlled Clinical Trials in the United States and Canada

Body System/Adverse Event*	Nizatidine (N=2,694)	Placebo (N=1,729)
Body as a Whole		
Headache	16.6	15.6
Abdominal pain	7.5	12.5
Pain	4.2	3.8
Asthenia	3.1	2.9
Back pain	2.4	2.6
Chest pain	2.3	2.1
Infection	1.7	1.1
Fever	1.6	2.3
Surgical procedure	1.4	1.5
Injury, accident	1.2	0.9
Digestive		
Diarrhea	7.2	6.9
Nausea	5.4	7.4
Flatuence	4.9	5.4
Vomiting	3.6	5.6
Dyspepsia	3.6	4.4
Constipation	2.5	3.8
Dry mouth	1.4	1.3
Nausea and vomiting	1.2	1.9
Anorexia	1.2	1.6
Gastrointestinal disorder	1.1	1.2
Tooth disorder	1.0	0.8
Musculoskeletal		
Myalgia	1.7	1.5
Nervous		
Dizziness	4.6	3.8
Insomnia	2.7	3.4
Abnormal dreams	1.9	1.9
Somnolence	1.9	1.6
Anxiety	1.6	1.4
Nervousness	1.1	0.8
Respiratory		
Rhinitis	9.8	9.6
Pharyngitis	3.3	3.1
Sinusitis	2.4	2.1
Cough, increased	2.0	2.0
Skin and Appendages		
Rash	1.9	2.1
Pruritis	1.7	1.3
Special Senses		
Amblyopia	1.0	0.9

*Events reported by at least 1% of nizatidine-treated patients are included.

A variety of less common events were also reported; it was not possible to determine whether these were caused by nizatidine.

Hepatic: Hepatocellular injury, evidenced by elevated liver enzyme tests (SGOT [AST], SGPT [ALT], or alkaline phosphatase), occurred in some patients and was possibly or probably related to nizatidine. In some cases there was marked elevation of SGOT, SGPT enzymes (greater than 500 IU/L) and, in a single instance, SGPT was greater than 2,000 IU/L. The overall rate of occurrences of elevated liver enzymes and elevations to 3 times the upper limit of normal, however, did not significantly differ from the rate of liver enzyme abnormalities in placebo-treated patients. All abnormalities were reversible after discontinuation of AXID. Since market introduction, hepatitis and jaundice have been reported. Rare cases of cholestatic or mixed hepatocellular and cholestatic injury with jaundice have been reported with reversal of the abnormalities after discontinuation of AXID.

Cardiovascular: In clinical pharmacology studies, short episodes of asymptomatic ventricular tachycardia occurred in 2 individuals administered AXID and in 3 untreated subjects.

CNS: Rare cases of reversible mental confusion have been reported.

Endocrine: Clinical pharmacology studies and controlled clinical trials showed no evidence of antiandrogenic activity due to AXID. Impotence and decreased libido were reported with similar frequency by patients who received AXID and by those given placebo. Rare reports of gynecomastia occurred.

Hematologic: Anemia was reported significantly more frequently in nizatidine- than in placebo-treated patients. Fatal thrombocytopenia was reported in a patient who was treated with AXID and another H$_2$-receptor antagonist. On previous occasions, this patient had experienced thrombocytopenia while taking other drugs. Rare cases of thrombocytopenic purpura have been reported.

Integumental: Sweating and urticaria were reported significantly more frequently in nizatidine- than in placebo-treated patients. Rash and exfoliative dermatitis were also reported. Vasculitis has been reported rarely.

Hypersensitivity: As with other H$_2$-receptor antagonists, rare cases of anaphylaxis following administration of nizatidine have been reported. Rare episodes of hypersensitivity reactions (eg, bronchospasm, laryngeal edema, rash, and eosinophilia) have been reported.

Body as a Whole: Serum sickness-like reactions have occurred rarely in conjunction with nizatidine use.

Genitourinary: Reports of impotence have occurred.

Other: Hyperuricemia unassociated with gout or nephrolithiasis was reported. Eosinophilia, fever, and nausea related to nizatidine administration have been reported.

OVERDOSAGE

Overdoses of AXID have been reported rarely. The following is provided to serve as a guide should such an overdose be encountered.

Signs and Symptoms: There is little clinical experience with overdosage of AXID in humans. Test animals that received large doses of nizatidine have exhibited cholinergic-type effects, including lacrimation, salivation, emesis, miosis, and diarrhea. Single oral doses of 800 mg/kg in dogs and of 1,200 mg/kg in monkeys were not lethal. Intravenous median lethal doses in the rat and mouse were 301 mg/kg and 232 mg/kg respectively.

Treatment: To obtain up-to-date information about the treatment of overdose, a good resource is your certified Regional Poison Control Center. Telephone numbers of certified poison control centers are listed in the *Physicians' Desk Reference (PDR)*. In managing overdosage, consider the possibility of multiple drug overdoses, interaction among drugs, and unusual drug kinetics in your patient.

If overdosage occurs, use of activated charcoal, emesis, or lavage should be considered along with clinical monitoring and supportive therapy. The ability of hemodialysis to remove nizatidine from the body has not been conclusively demonstrated; however, due to its large volume of distribution, nizatidine is not expected to be efficiently removed from the body by this method.

DOSAGE AND ADMINISTRATION

Active Duodenal Ulcer: The recommended oral dosage for adults is 300 mg once daily at bedtime. An alternative dosage regimen is 150 mg twice daily.

Maintenance of Healed Duodenal Ulcer: The recommended oral dosage for adults is 150 mg once daily at bedtime.

Gastroesophageal Reflux Disease: The recommended oral dosage in adults for the treatment of erosions, ulcerations, and associated heartburn is 150 mg twice daily.

Active Benign Gastric Ulcer: The recommended oral dosage is 300 mg given either as 150 mg twice daily or 300 mg once daily at bedtime. Prior to treatment, care should be taken to exclude the possibility of malignant gastric ulceration.

Dosage Adjustment for Patients With Moderate to Severe Renal Insufficiency: The dose for patients with renal dysfunction should be reduced as follows:

Table 6. Active Duodenal Ulcer, GERD and Benign Gastric Ulcer

C$_{cr}$	Dose
25 - 50 mL/min	150 mg daily
<20 mL/min	150 mg every other day

Maintenance Therapy	
C$_{cr}$	Dose
25 - 50 mL/min	150 mg every other day
<20 mL/min	150 mg every 3 days

Some elderly patients may have creatinine clearances of less than 50 mL/min, and, based on pharmacokinetic data in patients with renal impairment, the dose for such patients should be reduced accordingly. The clinical effects of this dosage reduction in patients with renal failure have not been evaluated.

HOW SUPPLIED

AXID® Pulvules®* are available in:
The 150-mg Pulvules are imprinted with "150" on the opaque dark yellow cap and "AXID" and "Reliant" on the opaque pale yellow body, using black ink. They are available as follows:
Bottles of 60   NDC 65726-144-15
*Pulvules® (filled gelatin capsules, Lilly)
Store at controlled room temperature 20° to 25°C (68° to 77°F) in a tightly closed container [see USP].
The USP defines controlled room temperature as: A temperature maintained thermostatically that encompasses the usual and customary working environment of 20° to 25°C (68° to 77°F); that results in a mean kinetic temperature calculated to be not more than 25°C; and that allows for excursions between 15° and 30°C (59° and 86°F) that are experienced in pharmacies, hospitals, and warehouses.
Distributed by:
GlaxoSmithKline
Research Triangle Park, NC 27709
©2008, GlaxoSmithKline. All rights reserved.
July 2008
AXD:1PI

BACTROBAN CREAM® ℞
[bac' trō ban]
(mupirocin calcium cream, 2%)
For Dermatologic Use

DESCRIPTION

BACTROBAN CREAM (mupirocin calcium cream), 2% contains the dihydrate crystalline calcium hemi-salt of the antibiotic mupirocin. Chemically, it is ($\alpha E,2S,3R,4R,5S$)-5-[($2S,3S,4S,5S$)-2,3-Epoxy-5-hydroxy-4-methylhexyl]tetrahydro-3,4-dihydroxy-β-methyl-2H-pyran-2-crotonic acid, ester with 9-hydroxynonanoic acid, calcium salt (2:1), dihydrate.
The molecular formula of mupirocin calcium is ($C_{26}H_{43}O_9$)$_2$Ca•2H$_2$O, and the molecular weight is 1075.3. The molecular weight of mupirocin free acid is 500.6. The structural formula of mupirocin calcium is:

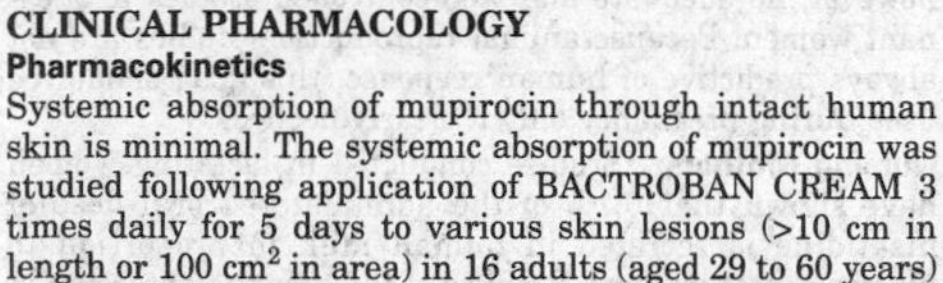

BACTROBAN CREAM is a white cream that contains 2.15% w/w mupirocin calcium (equivalent to 2.0% mupirocin free acid) in an oil and water-based emulsion. The inactive ingredients are benzyl alcohol, cetomacrogol 1000, cetyl alcohol, mineral oil, phenoxyethanol, purified water, stearyl alcohol, and xanthan gum.

CLINICAL PHARMACOLOGY
Pharmacokinetics
Systemic absorption of mupirocin through intact human skin is minimal. The systemic absorption of mupirocin was studied following application of BACTROBAN CREAM 3 times daily for 5 days to various skin lesions (>10 cm in length or 100 cm² in area) in 16 adults (aged 29 to 60 years) and 10 children (aged 3 to 12 years). Some systemic absorption was observed as evidenced by the detection of the metabolite, monic acid, in urine. Data from this study indicated more frequent occurrence of percutaneous absorption in children (90% of patients) compared to adults (44% of patients); however, the observed urinary concentrations in children (0.07-1.3 mcg/mL [1 pediatric patient had no detectable level]) are within the observed range (0.08-10.03 mcg/mL [9 adults had no detectable level]) in the adult population. In general, the degree of percutaneous absorption following multiple dosing appears to be minimal in adults and children. Any mupirocin reaching the systemic circulation is rapidly metabolized, predominantly to inactive monic acid, which is eliminated by renal excretion.
Microbiology
Mupirocin is an antibacterial agent produced by fermentation using the organism *Pseudomonas fluorescens*. It is active against a wide range of gram-positive bacteria including methicillin-resistant *Staphylococcus aureus* (MRSA). It is also active against certain gram-negative bacteria. Mupirocin inhibits bacterial protein synthesis by reversibly and specifically binding to bacterial isoleucyl

transfer-RNA synthetase. Due to this unique mode of action, mupirocin demonstrates no in vitro cross-resistance with other classes of antimicrobial agents.
Resistance occurs rarely; however, when mupirocin resistance does occur, it appears to result from the production of a modified isoleucyl-tRNA synthetase. High-level plasmid-mediated resistance (MIC >1024 mcg/mL) has been reported in some strains of *Staphylococcus aureus* and coagulase-negative staphylococci.
Mupirocin is bactericidal at concentrations achieved by topical application. The minimum bactericidal concentration (MBC) against relevant pathogens is generally 8-fold to 30-fold higher than the minimum inhibitory concentration (MIC). In addition, mupirocin is highly protein bound (>97%), and the effect of wound secretions on the MICs of mupirocin has not been determined.
Mupirocin has been shown to be active against most strains of *S. aureus* and *Streptococcus pyogenes*, both in vitro and in clinical studies. (See INDICATIONS AND USAGE.) The following in vitro data are available, BUT THEIR CLINICAL SIGNIFICANCE IS UNKNOWN. Mupirocin is active against most strains of *Staphylococcus epidermidis* and *Staphylococcus saprophyticus*.

INDICATIONS AND USAGE

BACTROBAN CREAM is indicated for the treatment of secondarily infected traumatic skin lesions (up to 10 cm in length or 100 cm² in area) due to susceptible strains of *S.aureus* and *S. pyogenes*.

CONTRAINDICATIONS

BACTROBAN CREAM is contraindicated in patients with known hypersensitivity to any of the constituents of the product.

WARNINGS

Avoid contact with the eyes.
In the case of a sensitization or severe local irritation from BACTROBAN CREAM, usage should be discontinued, and appropriate alternative therapy for the infection instituted.

PRECAUTIONS
General
As with other antibacterial products, prolonged use may result in overgrowth of nonsusceptible microorganisms, including fungi. (See DOSAGE AND ADMINISTRATION.)
BACTROBAN CREAM is not formulated for use on mucosal surfaces.

Information for Patients
• Use this medication only as directed by your healthcare provider. It is for external use only. Avoid contact with the eyes.
• The treated area may be covered by gauze dressing if desired.
• Report to your healthcare provider any signs of local adverse reactions. The medication should be stopped and your healthcare provider contacted if irritation, severe itching, or rash occurs.
• If no improvement is seen in 3 to 5 days, contact your healthcare provider.

Drug Interactions
The effect of the concurrent application of topical mupirocin calcium cream and other topical products has not been studied.

Carcinogenesis, Mutagenesis, Impairment of Fertility
Long-term studies in animals to evaluate carcinogenic potential of mupirocin calcium have not been conducted.
Results of the following studies performed with mupirocin calcium or mupirocin sodium in vitro and in vivo did not indicate a potential for mutagenicity: Rat primary hepatocyte unscheduled DNA synthesis, sediment analysis for DNA strand breaks, *Salmonella* reversion test (Ames), *Escherichia coli* mutation assay, metaphase analysis of human lymphocytes, mouse lymphoma assay, and bone marrow micronuclei assay in mice.
Fertility studies were performed in rats with mupirocin administered subcutaneously at doses up to 49 times a human topical dose of 1 gram/day (approximately 20 mg mupirocin per day) on a mg/m² basis and revealed no evidence of impaired fertility from mupirocin sodium.

Pregnancy
Teratogenic Effects: Pregnancy Category B. Teratology studies have been performed in rats and rabbits with mupirocin administered subcutaneously at doses up to 78 and 154 times, respectively, a human topical dose of 1 gram/day (approximately 20 mg mupirocin per day) on a mg/m² basis and revealed no evidence of harm to the fetus due to mupirocin. There are, however, no adequate and well-controlled studies in pregnant women. Because animal reproduction studies are not always predictive of human response, this drug should be used during pregnancy only if clearly needed.

Nursing Mothers
It is not known whether this drug is excreted in human milk. Because many drugs are excreted in human milk, caution should be exercised when BACTROBAN CREAM is administered to a nursing woman.

Pediatric Use
The safety and effectiveness of BACTROBAN CREAM have been established in the age groups 3 months to 16 years. Use of BACTROBAN CREAM in these age groups is supported by evidence from adequate and well-controlled studies of BACTROBAN CREAM in adults with additional data from 93 pediatric patients studied as part of the pivotal trials in adults. (See CLINICAL STUDIES.)

Geriatric Use
In 2 well-controlled studies, 30 patients older than 65 years were treated with BACTROBAN CREAM. No overall difference in the efficacy or safety of BACTROBAN CREAM was observed in this patient population when compared to that observed in younger patients.

ADVERSE REACTIONS

In 2 randomized, double-blind, double-dummy trials, 339 patients were treated with topical BACTROBAN CREAM plus oral placebo. Adverse events thought to be possibly or probably drug-related occurred in 28 (8.3%) patients. The incidence of those events that were reported in at least 1% of patients enrolled in these trials were: Headache (1.7%), rash, and nausea (1.1% each).

Other adverse events thought to be possibly or probably drug-related which occurred in less than 1% of patients were: Abdominal pain, burning at application site, cellulitis, dermatitis, dizziness, pruritus, secondary wound infection, and ulcerative stomatitis.

In a supportive study in the treatment of secondarily infected eczema, 82 patients were treated with BACTROBAN CREAM. The incidence of adverse events thought to be possibly or probably drug-related was as follows: Nausea (4.9%), headache, and burning at application site (3.6% each), pruritus (2.4%) and 1 report each of abdominal pain, bleeding secondary to eczema, pain secondary to eczema, hives, dry skin, and rash.

OVERDOSAGE

Intravenous infusions of 252 mg, as well as single oral doses of 500 mg of mupirocin, have been well tolerated in healthy adult subjects. There is no information regarding overdose of BACTROBAN CREAM.

DOSAGE AND ADMINISTRATION

A small amount of BACTROBAN CREAM should be applied to the affected area 3 times daily for 10 days. The area treated may be covered with gauze dressing if desired. Patients not showing a clinical response within 3 to 5 days should be re-evaluated.

CLINICAL STUDIES

The efficacy of topical BACTROBAN CREAM for the treatment of secondarily infected traumatic skin lesions (e.g., lacerations, sutured wounds, and abrasions not more than 10 cm in length or 100 cm^2 in total area) was compared to that of oral cephalexin in 2 randomized, double-blind, double-dummy clinical trials. Clinical efficacy rates at follow-up in the per protocol populations (adults and pediatric patients included) were 96.1% for BACTROBAN CREAM (n = 231) and 93.1% for oral cephalexin (n = 219). Pathogen eradication rates at follow-up in the per protocol populations were 100% for both BACTROBAN CREAM and oral cephalexin.

Pediatrics
There were 93 pediatric patients aged 2 weeks to 16 years enrolled per protocol in the secondarily infected skin lesion studies, although only 3 were less than 2 years of age in the population treated with BACTROBAN CREAM. Patients were randomized to either 10 days of topical BACTROBAN CREAM 3 times daily or 10 days of oral cephalexin (250 mg 4 times daily for patients >40 kg or 25 mg/kg/day oral suspension in 4 divided doses for patients ≤ 40 kg). Clinical efficacy at follow-up (7 to 12 days post-therapy) in the per protocol populations was 97.7% (43/44) for BACTROBAN CREAM and 93.9% (46/49) for cephalexin. Only 1 adverse event (headache) was thought to be possibly or probably related to drug therapy with BACTROBAN CREAM in the intent-to-treat pediatric population of 70 children (1.4%).

HOW SUPPLIED

BACTROBAN CREAM is supplied in 15-gram and 30-gram tubes.
NDC 0029-1527-22 (15-gram tube)
NDC 0029-1527-25 (30-gram tube)
Store at or below 25°C (77°F). Do not freeze.
GlaxoSmithKline
Research Triangle Park, NC 27709
BACTROBAN CREAM is a registered trademark of GlaxoSmithKline.
©2005, GlaxoSmithKline. All rights reserved.
May 2005 BB:L7B

BACTROBAN NASAL® ℞

[*bac' trō ban*]
(mupirocin calcium ointment, 2%)
for intranasal use only

DESCRIPTION

BACTROBAN NASAL (mupirocin calcium ointment, 2%) contains the dihydrate crystalline calcium hemi-salt of the antibiotic mupirocin. Chemically, it is (α*E*,2*S*,3*R*,4*R*,5*S*)-5-[(2*S*,3*S*,4*S*,5*S*)-2,3-Epoxy-5-hydroxy-4-methylhexyl]-tetrahydro-3,4-dihydroxy-β-methyl-2*H*-pyran-2-crotonic acid, ester with 9-hydroxynonanoic acid, calcium salt (2:1), dihydrate.

The molecular formula of mupirocin calcium is $(C_{26}H_{43}O_9)_2Ca \bullet 2H_2O$, and the molecular weight is 1075.3. The molecular weight of mupirocin free acid is 500.6. The structural formula of mupirocin calcium is:

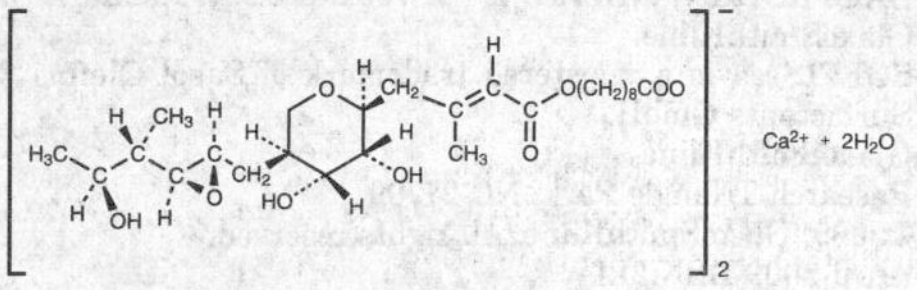

BACTROBAN NASAL is a white to off-white ointment that contains 2.15% w/w mupirocin calcium (equivalent to 2.0% pure mupirocin free acid) in a soft white ointment base. The inactive ingredients are paraffin and a mixture of glycerin esters (SOFTISAN® 649).

CLINICAL PHARMACOLOGY

Pharmacokinetics: Following single or repeated intranasal applications of 0.2 gram of BACTROBAN NASAL 3 times daily for 3 days to 5 healthy **adult** male subjects, no evidence of systemic absorption of mupirocin was demonstrated. The dosage regimen used in this study was for pharmacokinetic characterization only. (See DOSAGE AND ADMINISTRATION for proper clinical dosing information.)

In this study, the concentrations of mupirocin in urine and of monic acid in urine and serum were below the limit of determination of the assay for up to 72 hours after the applications. The lowest levels of determination of the assay used were 50 ng/mL of mupirocin in urine, 75 ng/mL of monic acid in urine, and 10 ng/mL of monic acid in serum. Based on the detectable limit of the urine assay for monic acid, one can extrapolate that a mean of 3.3% (range: 1.2 to 5.1%) of the applied dose could be systemically absorbed from the nasal mucosa of **adults**.

Data from a report of a pharmacokinetic study in neonates and premature infants indicate that, unlike in adults, significant systemic absorption occurred following intranasal administration of BACTROBAN NASAL in this population. **At this time, the pharmacokinetic properties of mupirocin following intranasal application of BACTROBAN NASAL have not been adequately characterized in neonates or other children less than 12 years of age, and in addition, the safety of the product in children less than 12 years of age has not been established.**

The effect of the concurrent application of intranasal mupirocin calcium ointment, 2% with other intranasal products has not been studied. (See PRECAUTIONS, Drug Interactions.)

Following intravenous or oral administration, mupirocin is rapidly metabolized. The principal metabolite, monic acid, demonstrates no antibacterial activity. In a study conducted in 7 healthy adult male subjects, the elimination half-life after intravenous administration of mupirocin was 20 to 40 minutes for mupirocin and 30 to 80 minutes for monic acid. Monic acid is predominantly eliminated by renal excretion. The pharmacokinetics of mupirocin has not been studied in individuals with renal insufficiency.

Microbiology: Mupirocin is an antibacterial agent produced by fermentation using the organism *Pseudomonas fluorescens*. Mupirocin inhibits bacterial protein synthesis by reversibly and specifically binding to bacterial isoleucyl transfer-RNA synthetase. Due to this mode of action, mupirocin demonstrates no in vitro cross-resistance with other classes of antimicrobial agents.

When mupirocin resistance does occur, it appears to result from the production of a modified isoleucyl-tRNA synthetase. High-level plasmid-mediated resistance (MIC >1,024 mcg/mL) has been reported in some strains of *Staphylococcus aureus* and coagulase-negative staphylococci.

Mupirocin is bactericidal at concentrations achieved topically by intranasal administration. However, the minimum bactericidal concentration (MBC) against relevant intranasal pathogens is generally 8-fold to 30-fold higher than the minimum inhibitory concentration (MIC). In addition, mupirocin is highly protein bound (>97%), and the effect of nasal secretions on the MICs of intranasally applied mupirocin has not been determined.

Mupirocin has been shown to be active against most strains of methicillin-resistant *S. aureus*, both in vitro and in clinical studies of the eradication of nasal colonization. BACTROBAN NASAL only has established clinical utility in nasal eradication as part of a comprehensive program to curtail institutional outbreaks of infections with methicillin-resistant *S. aureus*. (See INDICATIONS AND USAGE.)

The following in vitro data are available, **but their clinical significance is unknown**. Mupirocin exhibits in vitro MICs of 1 mcg/mL or less against most (>90%) strains of methicillin-susceptible *S. aureus*; however, the safety and effectiveness of mupirocin calcium in eradicating nasal colonization of and preventing subsequent infections due to methicillin-susceptible *S. aureus* have not been established.

INDICATIONS AND USAGE

BACTROBAN NASAL is indicated for the eradication of nasal colonization with methicillin-resistant *S. aureus* in adult patients and health care workers as part of a comprehensive infection control program to reduce the risk of infection among patients at high risk of methicillin-resistant *S. aureus* infection during institutional outbreaks of infections with this pathogen.

NOTE:

1. There are insufficient data at this time to establish that this product is safe and effective as part of an intervention program to prevent autoinfection of high-risk patients from their own nasal colonization with *S. aureus*.
2. There are insufficient data at this time to recommend use of BACTROBAN NASAL for general prophylaxis of any infection in any patient population.
3. Greater than 90% of subjects/patients in clinical trials had eradication of nasal colonization 2 to 4 days after therapy was completed. Approximately 30% recolonization was reported in 1 domestic study within 4 weeks after completion of therapy. These eradication rates were clinically and statistically superior to those reported in subjects/patients in the vehicle-treated arms of the adequate and well-controlled studies. Those treated with vehicle had eradication rates of 5% to 30% at 2 to 4 days post-therapy with 85% to 100% recolonization within 4 weeks.

All adequate and well-controlled trials of this product were vehicle-controlled; therefore, no data from direct, head-to-head comparisons with other products are available at this time.

CONTRAINDICATIONS

BACTROBAN NASAL is contraindicated in patients with known hypersensitivity to any of the constituents of the product.

WARNINGS

AVOID CONTACT WITH THE EYES. Application of BACTROBAN NASAL to the eye under testing conditions has caused severe symptoms such as burning and tearing. These symptoms resolved within days to weeks after discontinuation of the ointment.

In the event of a sensitization or severe local irritation from BACTROBAN NASAL, usage should be discontinued.

PRECAUTIONS

General: As with other antibacterial products, prolonged use may result in overgrowth of nonsusceptible microorganisms, including fungi. (See DOSAGE AND ADMINISTRATION.)

Information for Patients: Patients should be given the following instructions:

- Apply approximately one-half of the ointment from the single-use tube directly into 1 nostril and the other half into the other nostril;
- Avoid contact of the medication with the eyes;
- Discard the tube after using, do not re-use;
- Press the sides of the nose together and gently massage after application to spread the ointment throughout the inside of the nostrils; and
- Discontinue usage of the medication and call your healthcare practitioner if sensitization or severe local irritation occurs.

Drug Interactions: The effect of the concurrent application of intranasal mupirocin calcium and other intranasal products has not been studied. Until further information is known, mupirocin calcium ointment, 2% should not be applied concurrently with any other intranasal products.

Carcinogenesis, Mutagenesis, Impairment of Fertility: Long-term studies in animals to evaluate carcinogenic potential of mupirocin calcium have not been conducted.

Results of the following studies performed with mupirocin calcium or mupirocin sodium in vitro and in vivo did not indicate a potential for mutagenicity: Rat primary hepatocyte unscheduled DNA synthesis, sediment analysis for DNA strand breaks, *Salmonella* reversion test (Ames), *Escherichia coli* mutation assay, metaphase analysis of human lymphocytes, mouse lymphoma assay, and bone marrow micronuclei assay in mice.

Reproduction studies were performed in rats with mupirocin administered subcutaneously at doses up to **40** times the human intranasal dose (approximately 20 mg mupirocin per day) on a mg/m^2 basis and revealed no evidence of impaired fertility from mupirocin sodium.

Pregnancy: ***Teratogenic Effects: Pregnancy Category B:*** Reproduction studies have been performed in rats and rabbits with mupirocin administered subcutaneously at doses up to 65 and 130 times, respectively, the human intranasal dose (approximately 20 mg mupirocin per day) on a mg/m^2 basis and revealed no evidence of harm to the fetus due to mupirocin. There are, however, no adequate and well-controlled studies in pregnant women. Because animal reproduction studies are not always predictive of human response, this drug should be used during pregnancy only if clearly needed.

Nursing Mothers: It is not known whether this drug is excreted in human milk. Because many drugs are excreted in human milk, caution should be exercised when BACTROBAN NASAL is administered to a nursing woman.

Pediatric Use: Safety in children under the age of 12 years has not been established. (See CLINICAL PHARMACOLOGY.)

ADVERSE REACTIONS

Clinical Trials: In clinical trials, 210 domestic and 2,130 foreign adult subjects/patients received BACTROBAN NASAL ointment. Less than 1% of domestic or foreign subjects and patients in clinical trials were withdrawn due to adverse events.

The most frequently reported adverse events in foreign clinical trials were as follows: Rhinitis (1.0%), taste perversion (0.8%), pharyngitis (0.5%).

In domestic clinical trials, 17% (36/210) of adults treated with BACTROBAN NASAL ointment reported adverse events thought to be at least possibly drug-related. The incidence of adverse events that were reported in at least 1% of adults enrolled in domestic clinical trials were as follows:

ADVERSE EVENTS (≥1% INCIDENCE)-ADULTS IN US TRIALS

	% of Subjects/Patients Experiencing Event BACTROBAN NASAL (n=210)
Headache	9%
Rhinitis	6%
Respiratory disorder, including upper respiratory tract congestion	5%
Pharyngitis	4%
Taste perversion	3%
Burning/stinging	2%
Cough	2%
Pruritus	1%

The following events thought possibly drug-related were reported in less than 1% of adults enrolled in domestic clinical trials: Blepharitis, diarrhea, dry mouth, ear pain, epistaxis, nausea, and rash.

All adequate and well-controlled clinical trials have been performed using BACTROBAN NASAL ointment, 2% in 1 arm and the vehicle ointment in the other arm of the study. No adequate and well-controlled safety data are available from direct, head-to-head comparative studies of this product and other products for this indication.

OVERDOSAGE

Following single or repeated intranasal applications of BACTROBAN NASAL to adults, no evidence for systemic absorption of mupirocin was obtained. Intravenous infusions of 252 mg, as well as single oral doses of 500 mg of mupirocin, have been well tolerated in healthy adult subjects. There is no information regarding local overdose of BACTROBAN NASAL or regarding oral ingestion of the nasal ointment formulation.

DOSAGE AND ADMINISTRATION

(See INDICATIONS AND USAGE.)

Adults (12 years of age and older): Approximately one-half of the ointment from the single-use tube should be applied into 1 nostril and the other half into the other nostril twice daily (morning and evening) for 5 days.

After application, the nostrils should be closed by pressing together and releasing the sides of the nose repetitively for approximately 1 minute. This will spread the ointment throughout the nares.

The single-use 1.0 gram tube will deliver a total of approximately 0.5 grams of the ointment (approximately 0.25 grams/nostril).

The tube should be discarded after usage; it should not be re-used.

The safety and effectiveness of applications of this medication for greater than 5 days have not been established. There are no human clinical or pre-clinical animal data to support the use of this product in a chronic manner or in manners other than those described in this package insert. Until further information is known, BACTROBAN NASAL should not be applied concurrently with any other intranasal products.

HOW SUPPLIED

BACTROBAN NASAL is supplied in 1.0-gram tubes.
NDC 0029-1526-11 (package of 10 single-tube cartons).
Store between 20° and 25°C (68° and 77°F); excursions permitted to 15°-30°C (59°-86°F). Do not refrigerate.

REFERENCE

1. Clinical and Laboratory Standards Institute (CLSI). Methods for Dilution Antimicrobial Susceptibility Tests for Bacteria That Grow Aerobically. Approved Standard. CLSI Document M7-A7. CLSI, Wayne, PA, January 2006.

BACTROBAN NASAL is a registered trademark of GlaxoSmithKline.
SOFTISAN is a registered trademark of Sasol Olefins & Surfactants GmbH.
GlaxoSmithKline
Research Triangle Park, NC 27709
©2009, GlaxoSmithKline. All rights reserved.
April 2009 BBN:2PI

BACTROBAN OINTMENT® ℞

[bac' trō ban]
(mupirocin ointment, 2%)
For Dermatologic Use

DESCRIPTION

Each gram of BACTROBAN OINTMENT (mupirocin ointment, 2%) contains 20 mg mupirocin in a bland water miscible ointment base (polyethylene glycol ointment, N.F.) consisting of polyethylene glycol 400 and polyethylene glycol 3350. Mupirocin is a naturally occurring antibiotic. The chemical name is (*E*)-(2*S*,3*R*,4*R*,5*S*)-5-[(2*S*,3*S*,4*S*,5*S*)-2,3-Epoxy-5-hydroxy-4-methylhexyl]tetrahydro-3,4-dihydroxy-β-methyl-2*H*-pyran-2-crotonic acid, ester with 9-hydroxynonanoic acid. The molecular formula of mupirocin is $C_{26}H_{44}O_9$, and the molecular weight is 500.63. The chemical structure is:

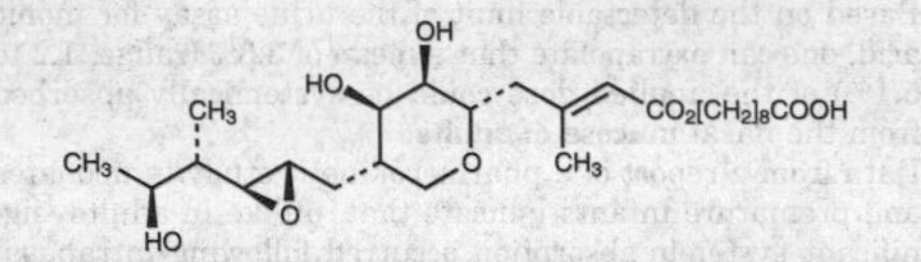

CLINICAL PHARMACOLOGY

Application of ^{14}C-labeled mupirocin ointment to the lower arm of normal male subjects followed by occlusion for 24 hours showed no measurable systemic absorption (<1.1 nanogram mupirocin per milliliter of whole blood). Measurable radioactivity was present in the stratum corneum of these subjects 72 hours after application.

Following intravenous or oral administration, mupirocin is rapidly metabolized. The principal metabolite, monic acid, is eliminated by renal excretion, and demonstrates no antibacterial activity. In a study conducted in 7 healthy adult male subjects, the elimination half-life after intravenous administration of mupirocin was 20 to 40 minutes for mupirocin and 30 to 80 minutes for monic acid. The pharmacokinetics of mupirocin has not been studied in individuals with renal insufficiency.

Microbiology: Mupirocin is an antibacterial agent produced by fermentation using the organism *Pseudomonas fluorescens*. It is active against a wide range of gram-positive bacteria including methicillin-resistant *Staphylococcus aureus* (MRSA). It is also active against certain gram-negative bacteria. Mupirocin inhibits bacterial protein synthesis by reversibly and specifically binding to bacterial isoleucyl transfer-RNA synthetase. Due to this unique mode of action, mupirocin demonstrates no in vitro cross-resistance with other classes of antimicrobial agents.

Resistance occurs rarely. However, when mupirocin resistance does occur, it appears to result from the production of a modified isoleucyl-tRNA synthetase. High-level plasmid-mediated resistance (MIC >1024 mcg/mL) has been reported in some strains of *S. aureus* and coagulase-negative staphylococci.

Mupirocin is bactericidal at concentrations achieved by topical administration. However, the minimum bactericidal concentration (MBC) against relevant pathogens is generally 8-fold to 30-fold higher than the minimum inhibitory concentration (MIC). In addition, mupirocin is highly protein-bound (>97%), and the effect of wound secretions on the MICs of mupirocin has not been determined.

Mupirocin has been shown to be active against most strains of *S. aureus* and *Streptococcus pyogenes*, both in vitro and in clinical studies (see INDICATIONS AND USAGE). The following in vitro data are available, BUT THEIR CLINICAL SIGNIFICANCE IS UNKNOWN. Mupirocin is active against most strains of *Staphylococcus epidermidis* and *Staphylococcus saprophyticus*.

INDICATIONS AND USAGE

BACTROBAN OINTMENT is indicated for the topical treatment of impetigo due to: *S. aureus* and *S. pyogenes*.

CONTRAINDICATIONS

This drug is contraindicated in individuals with a history of sensitivity reactions to any of its components.

WARNINGS

BACTROBAN OINTMENT is not for ophthalmic use.

PRECAUTIONS

If a reaction suggesting sensitivity or chemical irritation should occur with the use of BACTROBAN OINTMENT, treatment should be discontinued and appropriate alternative therapy for the infection instituted.

As with other antibacterial products, prolonged use may result in overgrowth of nonsusceptible organisms, including fungi.

BACTROBAN OINTMENT is not formulated for use on mucosal surfaces. Intranasal use has been associated with isolated reports of stinging and drying. A paraffin-based formulation — BACTROBAN NASAL® (mupirocin calcium ointment) — is available for intranasal use.

Polyethylene glycol can be absorbed from open wounds and damaged skin and is excreted by the kidneys. In common with other polyethylene glycol-based ointments, BACTROBAN OINTMENT should not be used in conditions where absorption of large quantities of polyethylene glycol is possible, especially if there is evidence of moderate or severe renal impairment.

Information for Patients: Use this medication only as directed by your healthcare provider. It is for external use only. Avoid contact with the eyes. The medication should be stopped and your healthcare practitioner contacted if irritation, severe itching, or rash occurs.

If impetigo has not improved in 3 to 5 days, contact your healthcare practitioner.

Drug Interactions: The effect of the concurrent application of BACTROBAN OINTMENT and other drug products has not been studied.

Carcinogenesis, Mutagenesis, Impairment of Fertility: Long-term studies in animals to evaluate carcinogenic potential of mupirocin have not been conducted.

Results of the following studies performed with mupirocin calcium or mupirocin sodium in vitro and in vivo did not indicate a potential for genotoxicity: Rat primary hepatocyte unscheduled DNA synthesis, sediment analysis for DNA strand breaks, *Salmonella* reversion test (Ames), *Escherichia coli* mutation assay, metaphase analysis of human lymphocytes, mouse lymphoma assay, and bone marrow micronuclei assay in mice.

Reproduction studies were performed in male and female rats with mupirocin administered subcutaneously at doses up to 14 times a human topical dose (approximately 60 mg mupirocin per day) on a mg/m^2 basis and revealed no evidence of impaired fertility and reproductive performance from mupirocin.

Pregnancy: ***Teratogenic Effects:*** Reproduction studies have been performed in rats and rabbits with mupirocin administered subcutaneously at doses up to 22 and 43 times, respectively, the human topical dose (approximately 60 mg mupirocin per day) on a mg/m^2 basis and revealed no evidence of harm to the fetus due to mupirocin. There are, however, no adequate and well-controlled studies in pregnant women. Because animal studies are not always predictive of human response, this drug should be used during pregnancy only if clearly needed.

Nursing Mothers: It is not known whether this drug is excreted in human milk. Because many drugs are excreted in human milk, caution should be exercised when BACTROBAN OINTMENT is administered to a nursing woman.

Pediatric Use: The safety and effectiveness of BACTROBAN OINTMENT have been established in the age range of 2 months to 16 years. Use of BACTROBAN OINTMENT in these age groups is supported by evidence from adequate and well-controlled studies of BACTROBAN OINTMENT in impetigo in pediatric patients studied as a part of the pivotal clinical trials (see CLINICAL STUDIES).

ADVERSE REACTIONS

The following local adverse reactions have been reported in connection with the use of BACTROBAN OINTMENT: Burning, stinging, or pain in 1.5% of patients; itching in 1% of patients; rash, nausea, erythema, dry skin, tenderness, swelling, contact dermatitis, and increased exudate in less than 1% of patients. Systemic reactions to BACTROBAN OINTMENT have occurred rarely.

DOSAGE AND ADMINISTRATION

A small amount of BACTROBAN OINTMENT should be applied to the affected area 3 times daily. The area treated may be covered with a gauze dressing if desired. Patients not showing a clinical response within 3 to 5 days should be re-evaluated.

CLINICAL STUDIES

The efficacy of topical BACTROBAN OINTMENT in impetigo was tested in 2 studies. In the first, patients with impetigo were randomized to receive either BACTROBAN OINTMENT or vehicle placebo 3 times daily for 8 to 12 days. Clinical efficacy rates at end of therapy in the evaluable populations (adults and pediatric patients included) were 71% for BACTROBAN OINTMENT (n = 49) and 35% for vehicle placebo (n = 51). Pathogen eradication rates in the evaluable populations were 94% for BACTROBAN OINTMENT and 62% for vehicle placebo. There were no side effects reported in the group receiving BACTROBAN OINTMENT.

In the second study, patients with impetigo were randomized to receive either BACTROBAN OINTMENT 3 times daily or 30 to 40 mg/kg oral erythromycin ethylsuccinate per day (this was an unblinded study) for 8 days. There was a follow-up visit 1 week after treatment ended. Clinical efficacy rates at the follow-up visit in the evaluable populations (adults and pediatric patients included) were 93% for BACTROBAN OINTMENT (n = 29) and 78.5% for erythromycin (n = 28). Pathogen eradication rates in the evaluable patient populations were 100% for both test groups. There were no side effects reported in the group receiving BACTROBAN OINTMENT.

Pediatrics: There were 91 pediatric patients aged 2 months to 15 years in the first study described above. Clinical efficacy rates at end of therapy in the evaluable populations were 78% for BACTROBAN OINTMENT (n = 42) and 36% for vehicle placebo (n = 49). In the second study described above, all patients were pediatric except 2 adults in the group receiving BACTROBAN OINTMENT. The age range of the pediatric patients was 7 months to 13 years. The clinical efficacy rate for BACTROBAN OINTMENT (n = 27) was 96%, and for erythromycin it was unchanged (78.5%).

HOW SUPPLIED

BACTROBAN OINTMENT is supplied in 22-gram tubes.
NDC 0029-1525-44 (22-gram tube)
Store at controlled room temperature 20° to 25°C (68° to 77°F).
GlaxoSmithKline
Research Triangle Park, NC 27709
BACTROBAN OINTMENT and BACTROBAN NASAL are registered trademarks of GlaxoSmithKline.
©2005, GlaxoSmithKline. All rights reserved.
MAY 2005   BC:L13C

BECONASE AQ®
[be′kō-nāz]
(beclomethasone dipropionate, monohydrate)
Nasal Spray, 42 mcg
For Intranasal Use Only
SHAKE WELL BEFORE USE

DESCRIPTION

Beclomethasone dipropionate, monohydrate, the active component of BECONASE AQ Nasal Spray, is an anti-inflammatory steroid having the chemical name 9-chloro-11β,17,21-trihydroxy-16β-methylpregna-1,4-diene-3,20-dione 17,21-dipropionate, monohydrate and the following chemical structure:

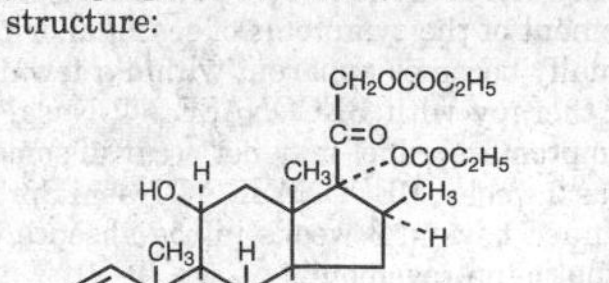

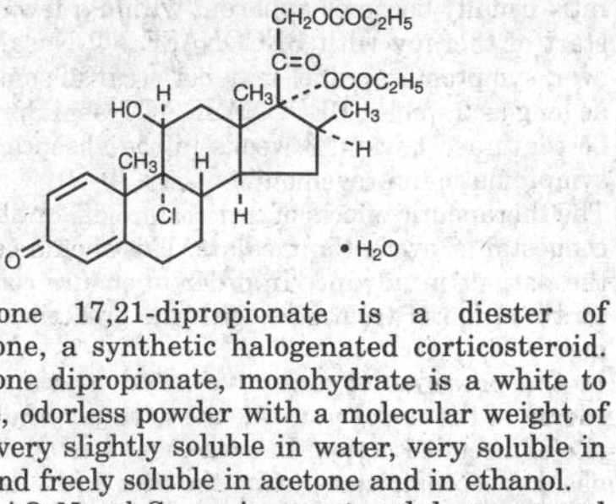

Beclomethasone 17,21-dipropionate is a diester of beclomethasone, a synthetic halogenated corticosteroid. Beclomethasone dipropionate, monohydrate is a white to creamy-white, odorless powder with a molecular weight of 539.06. It is very slightly soluble in water, very soluble in chloroform, and freely soluble in acetone and in ethanol.

BECONASE AQ Nasal Spray is a metered-dose, manual pump spray unit containing a microcrystalline suspension of beclomethasone dipropionate, monohydrate equivalent to 42 mcg of beclomethasone dipropionate, calculated on the dried basis, in an aqueous medium containing microcrystalline cellulose, carboxymethylcellulose sodium, dextrose, benzalkonium chloride, polysorbate 80, and 0.25% v/w phenylethyl alcohol. The pH through expiry is 5.0 to 6.8.

After initial priming (6 actuations), each actuation of the pump delivers from the nasal adapter 100 mg of suspension containing beclomethasone dipropionate, monohydrate equivalent to 42 mcg of beclomethasone dipropionate. If the pump is not used for 7 days, it should be primed until a fine spray appears. Each 25-g bottle of BECONASE AQ Nasal Spray provides 180 metered sprays.

CLINICAL PHARMACOLOGY
Mechanism of Action

Following topical administration, beclomethasone dipropionate produces anti-inflammatory and vasoconstrictor effects. The mechanisms responsible for the anti-inflammatory action of beclomethasone dipropionate are unknown. Corticosteroids have been shown to have a wide range of effects on multiple cell types (e.g., mast cells, eosinophils, neutrophils, macrophages, and lymphocytes) and mediators (e.g., histamine, eicosanoids, leukotrienes, and cytokines) involved in inflammation. The direct relationship of these findings to the effects of beclomethasone dipropionate on allergic rhinitis symptoms is not known. Biopsies of nasal mucosa obtained during clinical studies showed no histopathologic changes when beclomethasone dipropionate was administered intranasally.

Beclomethasone dipropionate is a pro-drug with weak glucocorticoid receptor binding affinity. It is hydrolyzed via esterase enzymes to its active metabolite beclomethasone-17-monopropionate (B-17-MP), which has high topical anti-inflammatory activity.

Pharmacokinetics
Absorption

Beclomethasone dipropionate is sparingly soluble in water. When given by nasal inhalation in the form of an aqueous or aerosolized suspension, the drug is deposited primarily in the nasal passages. The majority of the drug is eventually swallowed. Following intranasal administration of aqueous beclomethasone dipropionate, the systemic absorption was assessed by measuring the plasma concentrations of its active metabolite B-17-MP, for which the absolute bioavailability following intranasal administration is 44% (43% of the administered dose came from the swallowed portion and only 1% of the total dose was bioavailable from the nose). The absorption of unchanged beclomethasone dipropionate following oral and intranasal dosing was undetectable (plasma concentrations <50 pg/mL).

Distribution

The tissue distribution at steady state for beclomethasone dipropionate is moderate (20 L) but more extensive for B-17-MP (424 L). There is no evidence of tissue storage of beclomethasone dipropionate or its metabolites. Plasma protein binding is moderately high (87%).

Metabolism

Beclomethasone dipropionate is cleared very rapidly from the systemic circulation by metabolism mediated via esterase enzymes that are found in most tissues. The main product of metabolism is the active metabolite (B-17-MP). Minor inactive metabolites, beclomethasone-21-monopropionate (B-21-MP) and beclomethasone (BOH), are also formed, but these contribute little to systemic exposure.

Elimination

The elimination of beclomethasone dipropionate and B-17-MP after intravenous administration are characterized by high plasma clearance (150 and 120 L/hour) with corresponding terminal elimination half-lives of 0.5 and 2.7 hours. Following oral administration of tritiated beclomethasone dipropionate, approximately 60% of the dose was excreted in the feces within 96 hours, mainly as free and conjugated polar metabolites. Approximately 12% of the dose was excreted as free and conjugated polar metabolites in the urine. The renal clearance of beclomethasone dipropionate and its metabolites is negligible.

Pharmacodynamics

The effects of beclomethasone dipropionate on hypothalamic-pituitary-adrenal (HPA) function have been evaluated in adult volunteers by other routes of administration. Studies with beclomethasone dipropionate by the intranasal route may demonstrate that there is more or that there is less absorption by this route of administration. There was no suppression of early morning plasma cortisol concentrations when beclomethasone dipropionate was administered in a dose of 1,000 mcg/day for 1 month as an oral aerosol or for 3 days by intramuscular injection. However, partial suppression of plasma cortisol concentrations was observed when beclomethasone dipropionate was administered in doses of 2,000 mcg/day either by oral aerosol or intramuscular injection. Immediate suppression of plasma cortisol concentrations was observed after single doses of 4,000 mcg of beclomethasone dipropionate. Suppression of HPA function (reduction of early morning plasma cortisol levels) has been reported in adult patients who received 1,600-mcg daily doses of oral beclomethasone dipropionate for 1 month. In clinical studies using beclomethasone dipropionate aerosol intranasally, there was no evidence of

adrenal insufficiency. The effect of BECONASE AQ Nasal Spray on HPA function was not evaluated but would not be expected to differ from intranasal beclomethasone dipropionate aerosol.

In 1 study in children with asthma, the administration of inhaled beclomethasone at recommended daily doses for at least 1 year was associated with a reduction in nocturnal cortisol secretion. The clinical significance of this finding is not clear. It reinforces other evidence, however, that topical beclomethasone may be absorbed in amounts that can have systemic effects and that physicians should be alert for evidence of systemic effects, especially in chronically treated patients (see PRECAUTIONS).

INDICATIONS AND USAGE

BECONASE AQ Nasal Spray is indicated for the relief of the symptoms of seasonal or perennial allergic and nonallergic (vasomotor) rhinitis.

Results from 2 clinical trials have shown that significant symptomatic relief was obtained within 3 days. However, symptomatic relief may not occur in some patients for as long as 2 weeks. BECONASE AQ Nasal Spray should not be continued beyond 3 weeks in the absence of significant symptomatic improvement. BECONASE AQ Nasal Spray should not be used in the presence of untreated localized infection involving the nasal mucosa.

BECONASE AQ Nasal Spray is also indicated for the prevention of recurrence of nasal polyps following surgical removal.

Clinical studies have shown that treatment of the symptoms associated with nasal polyps may have to be continued for several weeks or more before a therapeutic result can be fully assessed. Recurrence of symptoms due to polyps can occur after stopping treatment, depending on the severity of the disease.

CONTRAINDICATIONS

Hypersensitivity to any of the ingredients of this preparation contraindicates its use.

WARNINGS

The replacement of a systemic corticosteroid with BECONASE AQ Nasal Spray can be accompanied by signs of adrenal insufficiency.

Careful attention must be given when patients previously treated for prolonged periods with systemic corticosteroids are transferred to BECONASE AQ Nasal Spray. This is particularly important in those patients who have associated asthma or other clinical conditions where too rapid a decrease in systemic corticosteroids may cause a severe exacerbation of their symptoms.

If recommended doses of intranasal beclomethasone are exceeded or if individuals are particularly sensitive or predisposed by virtue of recent systemic steroid therapy, symptoms of hypercorticism may occur, including very rare cases of menstrual irregularities, acneiform lesions, cataracts, and cushingoid features. If such changes occur, BECONASE AQ Nasal Spray should be discontinued slowly consistent with accepted procedures for discontinuing oral steroid therapy.

Persons who are using drugs that suppress the immune system are more susceptible to infections than healthy individuals. Chickenpox and measles, for example, can have a more serious or even fatal course in susceptible children or adults using corticosteroids. In children or adults who have not had these diseases or been properly immunized, particular care should be taken to avoid exposure. How the dose, route, and duration of corticosteroid administration affect the risk of developing a disseminated infection is not known. The contribution of the underlying disease and/or prior corticosteroid treatment to the risk is also not known. If exposed to chickenpox, prophylaxis with varicella zoster immune globulin (VZIG) may be indicated. If exposed to measles, prophylaxis with pooled intramuscular immunoglobulin (IG) may be indicated. (See the respective package inserts for complete VZIG and IG prescribing information.) If chickenpox develops, treatment with antiviral agents may be considered.

Avoid spraying in eyes.

PRECAUTIONS
General

Intranasal corticosteroids may cause a reduction in growth velocity when administered to pediatric patients (see PRECAUTIONS: Pediatric Use).

During withdrawal from oral corticosteroids, some patients may experience symptoms of withdrawal, e.g., joint and/or muscular pain, lassitude, and depression.

Rarely, immediate hypersensitivity reactions may occur after the intranasal administration of beclomethasone (see ADVERSE REACTIONS).

Rare instances of nasal septum perforation have been spontaneously reported.

Rare instances of wheezing, cataracts, glaucoma, and increased intraocular pressure have been reported following the intranasal use of beclomethasone dipropionate.

In clinical studies with beclomethasone dipropionate administered intranasally, the development of localized infections of the nose and pharynx with *Candida albicans* has occurred only rarely. When such an infection develops, it may require treatment with appropriate local therapy and discontinuation of treatment with BECONASE AQ Nasal Spray.

If persistent nasopharyngeal irritation occurs, it may be an indication for stopping BECONASE AQ Nasal Spray.

Beclomethasone dipropionate is absorbed into the circulation. Use of excessive doses of BECONASE AQ Nasal Spray may suppress HPA function.

Intranasal corticosteroids should be used with caution, if at all, in patients with active or quiescent tuberculous infections of the respiratory tract, untreated local or systemic fungal or bacterial infections, systemic viral or parasitic infections, or ocular herpes simplex.

For BECONASE AQ Nasal Spray to be effective in the treatment of nasal polyps, the spray must be able to enter the nose. Therefore, treatment of nasal polyps with BECONASE AQ Nasal Spray should be considered adjunctive therapy to surgical removal and/or the use of other medications that will permit effective penetration of BECONASE AQ Nasal Spray into the nose. Nasal polyps may recur after any form of treatment.

As with any long-term treatment, patients using BECONASE AQ Nasal Spray over several months or longer should be examined periodically for possible changes in the nasal mucosa.

Because of the inhibitory effect of corticosteroids on wound healing, patients who have experienced recent nasal septal ulcers, nasal surgery, or nasal trauma should not use a nasal corticosteroid until healing has occurred.

Although systemic effects have been minimal with recommended doses, this potential increases with excessive doses. Therefore, larger than recommended doses should be avoided.

Information for Patients

Patients being treated with BECONASE AQ Nasal Spray should receive the following information and instructions. This information is intended to aid them in the safe and effective use of this medication. It is not a disclosure of all possible adverse or intended effects.

Patients should use BECONASE AQ Nasal Spray at regular intervals since its effectiveness depends on its regular use. The patient should take the medication as directed. It is not acutely effective, and the prescribed dosage should not be increased. Instead, nasal vasoconstrictors or oral antihistamines may be needed until the effects of BECONASE AQ Nasal Spray are fully manifested. One to 2 weeks may pass before full relief is obtained. The patient should contact the physician if symptoms do not improve, if the condition worsens, or if sneezing or nasal irritation occurs.

For the proper use of BECONASE AQ Nasal Spray and to attain maximum improvement, the patient should read and follow carefully the patient's instructions accompanying the product.

Persons who are using immunosuppressant doses of corticosteroids should be warned to avoid exposure to chickenpox or measles. Patients should also be advised that if they are exposed, medical advice should be sought without delay.

Carcinogenesis, Mutagenesis, Impairment of Fertility

The carcinogenicity of beclomethasone dipropionate was evaluated in rats that were exposed for a total of 95 weeks, 13 weeks at inhalation doses up to 0.4 mg/kg and the remaining 82 weeks at combined oral and inhalation doses up to 2.4 mg/kg. There was no evidence of carcinogenicity in this study at the highest dose, approximately 60 times the maximum recommended daily intranasal dose in adults on a mg/m^2 basis or approximately 35 times the maximum recommended daily intranasal dose in children on a mg/m^2 basis.

Beclomethasone dipropionate did not induce gene mutation in bacterial cells or mammalian Chinese hamster ovary (CHO) cells in vitro. No significant clastogenic effect was seen in cultured CHO cells in vitro or in the mouse micronucleus test in vivo.

In rats, beclomethasone dipropionate caused decreased conception rates at an oral dose of 16 mg/kg (approximately 390 times the maximum recommended daily intranasal dose in adults on a mg/m^2 basis). There was no significant effect of beclomethasone dipropionate on fertility in rats at oral doses of 1.6 mg/kg (approximately 40 times the maximum recommended daily intranasal dose in adults on a mg/m^2 basis). Inhibition of the estrous cycle in dogs was observed following oral dosing at 0.5 mg/kg (approximately 40 times the maximum recommended daily intranasal dose in adults on a mg/m^2 basis). No inhibition of the estrous cycle in dogs was seen following 12 months' exposure at an estimated inhalation dose of 0.33 mg/kg (approximately 25 times the maximum recommended daily intranasal dose in adults on a mg/m^2 basis).

Pregnancy

Teratogenic Effects

Pregnancy Category C. Like other corticosteroids, beclomethasone dipropionate was teratogenic and embryocidal in the mouse and rabbit at a subcutaneous dose of 0.1 mg/kg in mice or 0.025 mg/kg in rabbits (approximately equal to the maximum recommended daily intranasal dose in adults on a mg/m^2 basis). No teratogenicity or embryocidal effects were seen in rats when exposed to an inhalation dose of 0.1 mg/kg plus oral doses of up to 10 mg/kg per day for a combined dose of 10.1 mg/kg (approximately 240 times the maximum recommended daily intranasal dose in adults on a mg/m^2 basis).

There are no adequate and well-controlled studies in pregnant women. Beclomethasone dipropionate should be used during pregnancy only if the potential benefit justifies the potential risk to the fetus.

Nonteratogenic Effects

Hypoadrenalism may occur in infants born of mothers receiving corticosteroids during pregnancy. Such infants should be carefully observed.

Nursing Mothers

It is not known whether beclomethasone dipropionate is excreted in human milk. Because other corticosteroids are excreted in human milk, caution should be exercised when BECONASE AQ Nasal Spray is administered to a nursing woman.

Pediatric Use

The safety and effectiveness of BECONASE AQ Nasal Spray have been established in children aged 6 years and above through evidence from extensive clinical use in adult and pediatric patients. The safety and effectiveness of BECONASE AQ Nasal Spray in children below 6 years of age have not been established.

Controlled clinical studies have shown that intranasal corticosteroids may cause a reduction in growth velocity in pediatric patients. This effect has been observed in the absence of laboratory evidence of HPA axis suppression, suggesting that growth velocity is a more sensitive indicator of systemic corticosteroid exposure in pediatric patients than some commonly used tests of HPA axis function. The long-term effects of this reduction in growth velocity associated with intranasal corticosteroids, including the impact on final adult height, are unknown. The potential for "catch-up" growth following discontinuation of treatment with intranasal corticosteroids has not been adequately studied. The growth of pediatric patients receiving intranasal corticosteroids, including BECONASE AQ Nasal Spray, should be monitored routinely (e.g., via stadiometry). The potential growth effects of prolonged treatment should be weighed against the clinical benefits obtained and the risks/benefits of treatment alternatives. To minimize the systemic effects of intranasal corticosteroids, including BECONASE AQ Nasal Spray, each patient should be titrated to the lowest dose that effectively controls his/her symptoms.

In a double-blind, controlled trial, 100 children between the ages of 6 and 9½ years with allergic rhinitis were randomized to receive aqueous intranasal beclomethasone dipropionate 168 mcg twice daily or placebo for 1 year. As measured by stadiometry, children who received beclomethasone dipropionate grew more slowly than those who received placebo. A difference in mean change in height was observed within 1 month of drug initiation. At the end of 12 months, the beclomethasone dipropionate-treated group had a growth velocity on average of 4.75 cm/year compared to 6.20 cm/year in the placebo group (p<0.01). While the placebo group had an expected distribution of growth velocity, approximately 50% of the beclomethasone dipropionate-treated children grew below the 10th percentile. In children 7.3 years of age, the mean age of children in this study, the range for expected growth velocity is: boys – 3rd percentile = 4.1 cm/year, 50th percentile = 5.8 cm/year, and 97th percentile = 7.5 cm/year; girls – 3rd percentile = 4.3 cm/year, 50th percentile = 5.9 cm/year, and 97th percentile = 7.5 cm/year. The potential reversibility of the reduction in growth velocity was not studied. No significant differences were observed between the 2 groups for mean basal plasma cortisol or ACTH-stimulated plasma cortisol levels.

Geriatric Use

Clinical studies of BECONASE AQ Nasal Spray did not include sufficient numbers of subjects aged 65 and over to determine whether they respond differently from younger subjects. Other reported clinical experience has not identified differences in responses between the elderly and younger patients. In general, dose selection for an elderly patient should be cautious, starting at the low end of the dosing range, reflecting the greater frequency of decreased hepatic, renal, or cardiac function, and of concomitant disease or other drug therapy.

ADVERSE REACTIONS

In general, side effects in clinical studies have been primarily associated with irritation of the nasal mucous membranes.

Adverse reactions reported in controlled clinical trials and open studies in patients treated with BECONASE AQ Nasal Spray are described below.

Mild nasopharyngeal irritation following the use of beclomethasone aqueous nasal spray has been reported in up to 24% of patients treated, including occasional sneezing attacks (about 4%) occurring immediately following use of the spray. In patients experiencing these symptoms, none had to discontinue treatment. The incidence of transient irritation and sneezing was approximately the same in the group of patients who received placebo in these studies, implying that these complaints may be related to vehicle components of the formulation.

Fewer than 5 per 100 patients reported headache, nausea, or lightheadedness following the use of BECONASE AQ Nasal Spray. Fewer than 3 per 100 patients reported nasal stuffiness, nosebleeds, rhinorrhea, or tearing eyes.

Rare cases of ulceration of the nasal mucosa and instances of nasal septum perforation have been spontaneously reported (see PRECAUTIONS).

Reports of dryness and irritation of the nose and throat and unpleasant taste and smell have been received. There are rare reports of loss of taste and smell.

Rare instances of wheezing, cataracts, glaucoma, and increased intraocular pressure have been reported following the use of intranasal beclomethasone dipropionate (see PRECAUTIONS).

Rare cases of immediate and delayed hypersensitivity reactions, including anaphylactoid/anaphylactic reactions, urticaria, angioedema, rash, and bronchospasm, have been reported following the oral and intranasal inhalation of beclomethasone dipropionate.

Cases of growth suppression have been reported for intranasal corticosteroids, including BECONASE AQ (see PRECAUTIONS: Pediatric Use).

OVERDOSAGE

When used at excessive doses, systemic corticosteroid effects such as hypercorticism and adrenal suppression may appear. If such changes occur, BECONASE AQ Nasal Spray should be discontinued slowly consistent with accepted procedures for discontinuing oral steroid therapy. No deaths occurred when beclomethasone dipropionate was given as single oral doses of 3,000 mg/kg to mice (approximately 36,000 times the maximum recommended daily intranasal dose in adults on a mg/m^2 basis, or approximately 21,000 times the maximum recommended daily intranasal dose in children on a mg/m^2 basis) and 2,000 mg/kg to rats (approximately 48,000 times the maximum recommended daily intranasal dose in adults or approximately 29,000 times the maximum recommended daily intranasal dose in children on a mg/m^2 basis). One bottle of BECONASE AQ Nasal Spray contains beclomethasone dipropionate, monohydrate equivalent to 10.5 mg of beclomethasone dipropionate; therefore, acute overdosage is unlikely.

DOSAGE AND ADMINISTRATION

Adults and Children 12 Years of Age and Older

The usual dosage is 1 or 2 nasal inhalations (42 to 84 mcg) in each nostril twice a day (total dose, 168 to 336 mcg/day).

Children 6 to 12 Years of Age

Patients should be started with 1 nasal inhalation in each nostril twice daily; patients not adequately responding to 168 mcg or those with more severe symptoms may use 336 mcg (2 inhalations in each nostril). Once adequate control is achieved, the dosage should be decreased to 84 mcg (1 spray in each nostril) twice daily. BECONASE AQ Nasal Spray is *not* recommended for children below 6 years of age. The maximum total daily dosage should not exceed 2 sprays in each nostril twice daily (336 mcg/day).

In patients who respond to BECONASE AQ Nasal Spray, an improvement of the symptoms of seasonal or perennial rhinitis usually becomes apparent within a few days after the start of therapy with BECONASE AQ Nasal Spray. However, symptomatic relief may not occur in some patients for as long as 2 weeks. BECONASE AQ Nasal Spray should not be continued beyond 3 weeks in the absence of significant symptomatic improvement.

The therapeutic effects of corticosteroids, unlike those of decongestants, are not immediate. This should be explained to the patient in advance in order to ensure cooperation and continuation of treatment with the prescribed dosage regimen.

In the presence of excessive nasal mucous secretion or edema of the nasal mucosa, the drug may fail to reach the site of intended action. In such cases it is advisable to use a nasal vasoconstrictor during the first 2 to 3 days of therapy with BECONASE AQ Nasal Spray.

Directions for Use

Illustrated Patient's Instructions for Use accompany each package of BECONASE AQ Nasal Spray.

HOW SUPPLIED

BECONASE AQ Nasal Spray, 42 mcg is supplied in an amber glass bottle fitted with a metering atomizing pump and nasal adapter in a box of 1 (NDC 0173-0388-79) with patient's instructions for use. Each bottle contains 25 g of suspension and will provide 180 metered sprays.

The correct amount of medication in each spray cannot be assured after 180 sprays even though the bottle is not completely empty. The bottle should be discarded when the labeled number of actuations has been used.

Store between 15° and 30°C (59° and 86°F).
GlaxoSmithKline
Research Triangle Park, NC 27709
April 2005 RL-2182

PHARMACIST—DETACH HERE AND GIVE INSTRUCTIONS TO PATIENT

BECONASE AQ ®

(beclomethasone dipropionate, monohydrate)
Nasal Spray, 42mcg
For Intranasal Use Only. SHAKE WELL BEFORE USE.
Patient's Instructions for Use
Shake the suspension spray bottle well before using it. Read complete instructions carefully and use only as directed.
To Use:
1. Remove the safety clip and the plastic dust cap from the nasal applicator (Figure 1).

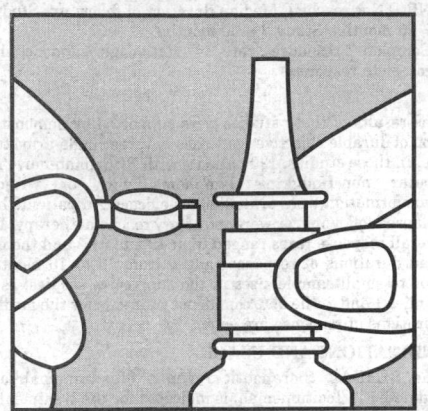

Figure 1

2. The very first time the spray is used, prime the pump into the air by pressing downward on the white collar, using your forefinger and middle finger while supporting the base of the bottle with your thumb. When you prime the pump for the first time, press down and release the pump 6 times or until a fine spray appears (Figure 2).
The pump is now ready for use. If the pump is not used for 7 days, prime until a fine spray appears.

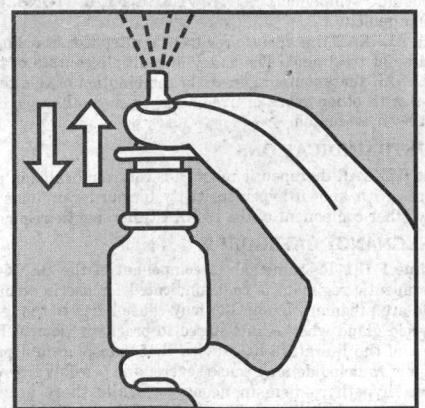

Figure 2

3. Gently blow your nose to clear your nostrils. Close 1 nostril. Tilt your head forward slightly and, keeping the bottle upright, carefully insert the nasal applicator into the other nostril (Figure 3).
[See figure at top of next column]
4. For each spray, press firmly downward once on the white collar, using your forefinger and middle finger while supporting the base of the bottle with your thumb. Avoid spraying in eyes. Breathe gently inward through the nostril.
5. Breathe out through your mouth.
6. Repeat steps 5 through 7 in the other nostril.
7. Replace the plastic dust cap and safety clip.
8. **DISCARD THE BOTTLE AFTER** the date calculated by your doctor or pharmacist. The correct amount of medication in

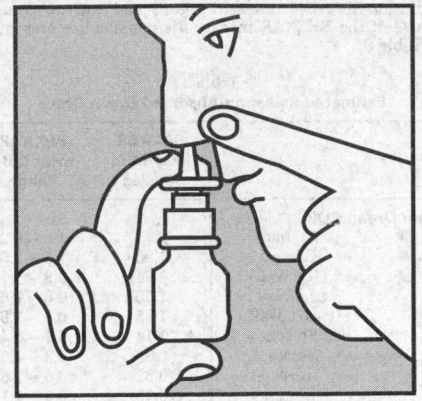

Figure 3

each spray cannot be assured after 180 sprays even though the bottle is not completely empty. Discard the bottle after 180 sprays. Before the discard date you should consult your doctor to see if a refill is needed. Do not take extra doses or stop taking BECONASE AQ Nasal Spray without consulting your doctor.

Cleansing: To clean the nasal applicator, remove the plastic dust cap and safety clip and then press gently upward on the white collar to free the nasal applicator. Wash the applicator and dust cap with cold water. Dry and replace with the plastic dust cap and safety clip back in position.
If the nasal applicator becomes blocked, remove the dust cap, unscrew the complete pump mechanism, and soak the pump in warm water for a few minutes. Rinse with cold water, dry, refit to bottle, and reprime the pump.

Caution: BECONASE AQ Nasal Spray is not intended to give rapid relief of your nasal symptoms. BECONASE AQ Nasal Spray controls the underlying disorders responsible for your attacks, so it is important that you use it regularly at the times recommended by your doctor. The full benefit of BECONASE AQ Nasal Spray may take a few days to develop.

Storage: Store between 15° and 30°C (59°and 86°F).

GlaxoSmithKline
Research Triangle Park, NC 27709
April 2005 RL-2182

BEXXAR®   ℞
[bex'ar]
(Tositumomab and Iodine I 131 Tositumomab)

WARNINGS
Hypersensitivity Reactions, including Anaphylaxis: Serious hypersensitivity reactions, including some with fatal outcome, have been reported with the BEXXAR therapeutic regimen. Medications for the treatment of severe hypersensitivity reactions should be available for immediate use. Patients who develop severe hypersensitivity reactions should have infusions of the BEXXAR therapeutic regimen discontinued and receive medical attention (see **WARNINGS**).
Prolonged and Severe Cytopenias: The majority of patients who received the BEXXAR therapeutic regimen experienced severe thrombocytopenia and neutropenia. The BEXXAR therapeutic regimen should not be administered to patients with >25% lymphoma marrow involvement and/or impaired bone marrow reserve (see **WARNINGS** and **ADVERSE REACTIONS**).
Pregnancy Category X: The BEXXAR therapeutic regimen can cause fetal harm when administered to a pregnant woman.
Special requirements: The BEXXAR therapeutic regimen (Tositumomab and Iodine I 131 Tositumomab) contains a radioactive component and should be administered only by physicians and other health care professionals qualified by training in the safe use and handling of therapeutic radionuclides. The BEXXAR therapeutic regimen should be administered only by physicians who are in the process of being or have been certified by GlaxoSmithKline in dose calculation and administration of the BEXXAR therapeutic regimen.

DESCRIPTION
The BEXXAR therapeutic regimen (Tositumomab and Iodine I 131 Tositumomab) is an anti-neoplastic radioimmu-

notherapeutic monoclonal antibody-based regimen composed of the monoclonal antibody, Tositumomab, and the radiolabeled monoclonal antibody, Iodine I 131 Tositumomab.
Tositumomab
Tositumomab is a murine IgG_{2a} lambda monoclonal antibody directed against the CD20 antigen, which is found on the surface of normal and malignant B lymphocytes. Tositumomab is produced in an antibiotic-free culture of mammalian cells and is composed of two murine gamma 2a heavy chains of 451 amino acids each and two lambda light chains of 220 amino acids each. The approximate molecular weight of Tositumomab is 150 kD.
Tositumomab is supplied as a sterile, pyrogen-free, clear to opalescent, colorless to slightly yellow, preservative-free liquid concentrate. It is supplied at a nominal concentration of 14 mg/mL Tositumomab in 35 mg and 225 mg single-use vials. The formulation contains 10% (w/v) maltose, 145 mM sodium chloride, 10 mM phosphate, and Water for Injection, USP. The pH is approximately 7.2.
Iodine I 131 Tositumomab
Iodine I 131 Tositumomab is a radio-iodinated derivative of Tositumomab that has been covalently linked to Iodine-131. Unbound radio-iodine and other reactants have been removed by chromatographic purification steps. Iodine I 131 Tositumomab is supplied as a sterile, clear, preservative-free liquid for IV administration. The dosimetric dosage form is supplied at nominal protein and activity concentrations of 0.1 mg/mL and 0.61 mCi/mL (at date of calibration), respectively. The therapeutic dosage form is supplied at nominal protein and activity concentrations of 1.1 mg/mL and 5.6 mCi/mL (at date of calibration), respectively. The formulation for the dosimetric and the therapeutic dosage forms contains 4.4%–6.6% (w/v) povidone, 1–2 mg/mL maltose (dosimetric dose) or 9–15 mg/mL maltose (therapeutic dose), 8.5–9.5 mg/mL sodium chloride, and 0.9–1.3 mg/mL ascorbic acid. The pH is approximately 7.0.
BEXXAR Therapeutic Regimen
The BEXXAR therapeutic regimen is administered in two discrete steps: the dosimetric and therapeutic steps. Each step consists of a sequential infusion of Tositumomab followed by Iodine I 131 Tositumomab. The therapeutic step is administered 7–14 days after the dosimetric step. The BEXXAR therapeutic regimen is supplied in two distinct package configurations as follows:
BEXXAR Dosimetric Packaging
- A carton containing two single-use 225 mg vials and one single-use 35 mg vial of Tositumomab supplied by McKesson BioServices and
- A package containing a single-use vial of Iodine I 131 Tositumomab (0.61 mCi/mL at calibration), supplied by MDS Nordion.
BEXXAR Therapeutic Packaging
- A carton containing two single-use 225 mg vials and one single-use 35 mg vial of Tositumomab, supplied by McKesson BioServices and
- A package containing one or two single-use vials of Iodine I 131 Tositumomab (5.6 mCi/mL at calibration), supplied by MDS Nordion.
Physical/Radiochemical Characteristics of Iodine-131
Iodine-131 decays with beta and gamma emissions with a physical half-life of 8.04 days. The principal beta emission has a mean energy of 191.6 keV and the principal gamma emission has an energy of 364.5 keV (Ref 1).
External Radiation: The specific gamma ray constant for Iodine-131 is 2.2 R/millicurie hour at 1 cm. The first half-value layer is 0.24 cm lead (Pb) shielding. A range of values is shown in Table 1 for the relative attenuation of the radiation emitted by this radionuclide that results from interposition of various thicknesses of Pb. To facilitate control of the radiation exposure from this radionuclide, the use of a 2.55 cm thickness of Pb will attenuate the radiation emitted by a factor of about 1,000.

Table 1
Radiation Attenuation by Lead Shielding

Shield Thickness (Pb) cm	Attenuation Factor
0.24	0.5
0.89	10^{-1}
1.60	10^{-2}
2.55	10^{-3}
3.7	10^{-4}

The fraction of Iodine-131 radioactivity that remains in the vial after the date of calibration is calculated as follows:
Fraction of remaining radioactivity of Iodine-131 after x days = $2^{-(x/8.04)}$.
Physical decay is presented in Table 2.

Table 2
Physical Decay Chart: Iodine-131: Half-Life 8.04 Days

Days	Fraction Remaining
0*	1.000
1	0.917
2	0.842
3	0.772
4	0.708
5	0.650
6	0.596
7	0.547
8	0.502
9	0.460
10	0.422
11	0.387
12	0.355
13	0.326
14	0.299

*(Calibration day)

CLINICAL PHARMACOLOGY

General Pharmacology
Tositumomab binds specifically to the CD20 (human B-lymphocyte–restricted differentiation antigen, Bp 35 or B1) antigen. This antigen is a transmembrane phosphoprotein expressed on pre-B lymphocytes and at higher density on mature B lymphocytes (Ref. 2). The antigen is also expressed on >90% of B-cell non-Hodgkin's lymphomas (NHL) (Ref. 3). The recognition epitope for Tositumomab is found within the extracellular domain of the CD20 antigen. CD20 does not shed from the cell surface and does not internalize following antibody binding (Ref. 4).

Mechanism of Action: Possible mechanisms of action of the BEXXAR therapeutic regimen include induction of apoptosis (Ref. 5), complement-dependent cytotoxicity (CDC) (Ref. 6), and antibody-dependent cellular cytotoxicity (ADCC) (Ref. 5) mediated by the antibody. Additionally, cell death is associated with ionizing radiation from the radioisotope.

Pharmacokinetics/Pharmacodynamics
The phase 1 study of Iodine I 131 Tositumomab determined that a 475 mg predose of unlabeled antibody decreased splenic targeting and increased the terminal half-life of the radiolabeled antibody. The median blood clearance following administration of 485 mg of Tositumomab in 110 patients with NHL was 68.2 mg/hr (range: 30.2–260.8 mg/hr). Patients with high tumor burden, splenomegaly, or bone marrow involvement were noted to have a faster clearance, shorter terminal half-life, and larger volume of distribution. The total body clearance, as measured by total body gamma camera counts, was dependent on the same factors noted for blood clearance. Patient-specific dosing, based on total body clearance, provided a consistent radiation dose, despite variable pharmacokinetics, by allowing each patient's administered activity to be adjusted for individual patient variables. The median total body effective half-life, as measured by total body gamma camera counts, in 980 patients with NHL was 67 hours (range: 28–115 hours).

Elimination of Iodine-131 occurs by decay (see Table 2) and excretion in the urine. Urine was collected for 49 dosimetric doses. After 5 days, the whole body clearance was 67% of the injected dose. Ninety-eight percent of the clearance was accounted for in the urine.

Administration of the BEXXAR therapeutic regimen results in sustained depletion of circulating CD20 positive cells. The impact of administration of the BEXXAR therapeutic regimen on circulating CD20 positive cells was assessed in two clinical studies, one conducted in chemotherapy naïve patients and one in heavily pretreated patients. The assessment of circulating lymphocytes did not distinguish normal from malignant cells. Consequently, assessment of recovery of normal B cell function was not directly assessed. At seven weeks, the median number of circulating CD20 positive cells was zero (range: 0–490 cells/mm^3). Lymphocyte recovery began at approximately 12 weeks following treatment. Among patients who had CD20 positive cell counts recorded at baseline and at 6 months, 8 of 58 (14%) chemotherapy naïve patients had CD20 positive cell counts below normal limits at six months and 6 of 19 (32%) heavily pretreated patients had CD20 positive cell counts below normal limits at six months. There was no consistent effect of the BEXXAR therapeutic regimen on post-treatment serum IgG, IgA, or IgM levels.

Radiation Dosimetry
Estimations of radiation-absorbed doses for Iodine I 131 Tositumomab were performed using sequential whole body images and the MIRDOSE 3 software program. Patients with apparent thyroid, stomach, or intestinal imaging were selected for organ dosimetry analyses. The estimated radiation-absorbed doses to organs and marrow from a course of the BEXXAR therapeutic regimen are presented in Table 3.

Table 3
Estimated Radiation-Absorbed Organ Doses

	BEXXAR mGy/MBq Median	BEXXAR mGy/MBq Range
From Organ ROIs		
Thyroid	2.71	1.4 – 6.2
Kidneys	1.96	1.5 – 2.5
ULI Wall	1.34	0.8 – 1.7
LLI Wall	1.30	0.8 – 1.6
Heart Wall	1.25	0.5 – 1.8
Spleen	1.14	0.7 – 5.4
Testes	0.83	0.3 – 1.3
Liver	0.82	0.6 – 1.3
Lungs	0.79	0.5 – 1.1
Red Marrow	0.65	0.5 – 1.1
Stomach Wall	0.40	0.2 – 0.8
From Whole Body ROIs		
Urine Bladder Wall	0.64	0.6 – 0.9
Bone Surfaces	0.41	0.4 – 0.6
Pancreas	0.31	0.2 – 0.4
Gall Bladder Wall	0.29	0.2 – 0.3
Adrenals	0.28	0.2 – 0.3
Ovaries	0.25	0.2 – 0.3
Small Intestine	0.23	0.2 – 0.3
Thymus	0.22	0.1 – 0.3
Uterus	0.20	0.2 – 0.2
Muscle	0.18	0.1 – 0.2
Breasts	0.16	0.1 – 0.2
Skin	0.13	0.1 – 0.2
Brain	0.13	0.1 – 0.2
Total Body	0.24	0.2 – 0.3

CLINICAL STUDIES
The efficacy of the BEXXAR therapeutic regimen was evaluated in 2 studies conducted in patients with low-grade, transformed low-grade, or follicular large-cell lymphoma. Determination of clinical benefit of the BEXXAR therapeutic regimen was based on evidence of durable responses without evidence of an effect on survival. All patients had received prior treatment without an objective response or had progression of disease following treatment. Patients were required to have a granulocyte count >1500 cells/mm^3, a platelet count ≥100,000/mm^3, an average of ≤25% of the intratrabecular marrow space involved by lymphoma, and no evidence of progressive disease arising in a field irradiated with >3500 cGy within 1 year of completion of irradiation.

Study 1 was a multicenter, single-arm study of 40 patients whose disease had not responded to or had progressed after at least four doses of Rituximab therapy. The median age was 57 (range: 35–78); the median time from diagnosis to protocol entry was 50 months (range: 12–170); and the median number of prior chemotherapy regimens was 4 (range: 1–11). The efficacy outcome data from this study, as determined by an independent panel that reviewed patient records and radiologic studies, are summarized in Table 4. Among the forty patients in the study, twenty-four patients had disease that did not respond to their last treatment with Rituximab, 11 patients had disease that responded to Rituximab for less than 6 months, and five patients had disease that responded to Rituximab, with a duration of response of 6 months or greater. Overall, 35 of the 40 patients met the definition of "Rituximab refractory", defined as no response or a response of less than 6 months duration. In this subset of patients the overall objective response was 63% (95% confidence interval 45%, 79%) with a median duration of 25 months (range of 4 – 38+ months). The complete response in this subset of patients was 29% (95% CI of 15%, 46%) with a median duration of response not yet reached (range of 4 – 38+ months).

Study 2 was a multicenter, single arm, open-label study of 60 chemotherapy refractory patients. The median age was 60 (range 38–82), the median time from diagnosis to protocol entry was 53 months (range: 9–334), and the median number of prior chemotherapy regimens was 4 (range 2–13). Fifty-three patients had not responded to prior therapy and 7 patients had responded with a duration of response of <6 months. The efficacy outcome data from this study, as determined by an independent panel that reviewed patient records and radiologic studies are also summarized in Table 4. Investigators continued to follow eight patients with complete response after the last independent review panel assessment. The updated duration of ongoing response as per investigators was reported to range from 42 to 85 months.

Table 4: Efficacy Outcomes in BEXXAR Clinical Studies

	Study 1 (n = 40)	Study 2 (n = 60)
Overall Response		
Rate	68%	47%
95% CI[a]	(51%, 81%)	(34%, 60%)
Response Duration (mos)		
Median	16	12
95% CI[a]	(10, NR[b])	(7, 47)
Range	1+ to 38+	2 to 47
Complete Response[c]		
Rate	33%	20%
95% CI[a]	(19%, 49%)	(11%, 32%)
Complete response[c] duration (mos)		
Median	NR[b]	47
95% CI[a]	(15, NR)	(47, NR)
Range	4 to 38+	9 to 47

[a] CI = Confidence Interval
[b] NR = Not reached, Median duration of follow up: Study 1 = 26 months; Study 2 = 30 months
[c] Complete response rate = Pathologic and clinical complete responses

The results of these studies were supported by demonstration of durable objective responses in three single-arm studies. In these studies, 130 patients with Rituximab-naïve follicular non-Hodgkin's lymphoma with or without transformation were evaluated for efficacy. All patients had relapsed following, or were refractory to, chemotherapy. The overall response rates ranged from 49% to 64% and the median durations of response ranged from 13 to 16 months. Due to small sample sizes in the supportive studies, as in studies 1 and 2, the 95% confidence intervals for the median durations of response are wide.

INDICATIONS AND USAGE
The BEXXAR therapeutic regimen (Tositumomab and Iodine I 131 Tositumomab) is indicated for the treatment of patients with CD20 antigen-expressing relapsed or refractory, low grade, follicular, or transformed non-Hodgkin's lymphoma, including patients with Rituximab-refractory non-Hodgkin's lymphoma. Determination of the effectiveness of the BEXXAR therapeutic regimen is based on overall response rates in patients whose disease is refractory to chemotherapy alone or to chemotherapy and Rituximab. The effects of the BEXXAR therapeutic regimen on survival are not known.

The BEXXAR therapeutic regimen is not indicated for the initial treatment of patients with CD20 positive non-Hodgkin's lymphoma. (See ADVERSE REACTIONS, Immunogenicity.)

The BEXXAR therapeutic regimen is intended as a single course of treatment. The safety of multiple courses of the BEXXAR therapeutic regimen, or combination of this regimen with other forms of irradiation or chemotherapy, has not been evaluated.

CONTRAINDICATIONS
The BEXXAR therapeutic regimen is contraindicated in patients with known hypersensitivity to murine proteins or any other component of the BEXXAR therapeutic regimen.

PREGNANCY CATEGORY X
Iodine I 131 Tositumomab (a component of the BEXXAR therapeutic regimen) is contraindicated for use in women who are pregnant. Iodine-131 may cause harm to the fetal thyroid gland when administered to pregnant women. Review of the literature has shown that transplacental passage of radioiodide may cause severe, and possibly irreversible, hypothyroidism in neonates. While there are no adequate and well-controlled studies of the BEXXAR therapeutic regimen in pregnant animals or humans, use of the BEXXAR therapeutic regimen in women of childbearing age should be deferred until the possibility of pregnancy has been ruled out. If the patient becomes pregnant while being treated with the BEXXAR therapeutic regimen, the patient should be apprised of the potential hazard to the fetus (see BOXED WARNING, Pregnancy Category X).

WARNINGS
Prolonged and Severe Cytopenias (see BOXED WARNINGS; ADVERSE REACTIONS, Hematologic Events): The most common adverse reactions associated with the BEXXAR therapeutic regimen were severe or life-threatening cytopenias (NCI CTC grade 3 or 4) with 71% of the 230 patients enrolled in clinical studies experiencing grade 3 or 4 cytopenias. These consisted primarily of grade 3 or 4 thrombocytopenia (53%) and grade 3 or 4 neutropenia

(63%). The time to nadir was 4 to 7 weeks and the duration of cytopenias was approximately 30 days. Thrombocytopenia, neutropenia, and anemia persisted for more than 90 days following administration of the BEXXAR therapeutic regimen in 16 (7%), 15 (7%), and 12 (5%) patients respectively (this includes patients with transient recovery followed by recurrent cytopenia). Due to the variable nature in the onset of cytopenias, complete blood counts should be obtained weekly for 10–12 weeks. The sequelae of severe cytopenias were commonly observed in the clinical studies and included infections (45% of patients), hemorrhage (12%), a requirement for growth factors (12% G- or GM-CSF; 7% Epoetin alfa) and blood product support (15% platelet transfusions; 16% red blood cell transfusions). Prolonged cytopenias may also influence subsequent treatment decisions.

The safety of the BEXXAR therapeutic regimen has not been established in patients with >25% lymphoma marrow involvement, platelet count <100,000 cells/mm^3 or neutrophil count <1,500 cells/mm^3.

Hypersensitivity Reactions Including Anaphylaxis (see BOXED WARNINGS; ADVERSE REACTIONS, Hypersensitivity Reactions and Immunogenicity): Serious hypersensitivity reactions, including some with fatal outcome, were reported during and following administration of the BEXXAR therapeutic regimen. Emergency supplies including medications for the treatment of hypersensitivity reactions, e.g., epinephrine, antihistamines and corticosteroids, should be available for immediate use in the event of an allergic reaction during administration of the BEXXAR therapeutic regimen. Patients who have received murine proteins should be screened for human anti-mouse antibodies (HAMA). Patients who are positive for HAMA may be at increased risk of anaphylaxis and serious hypersensitivity reactions during administration of the BEXXAR therapeutic regimen.

Secondary Malignancies: Myelodysplastic syndrome (MDS) and/or acute leukemia were reported in 10% (24/230) of patients enrolled in the clinical studies and 3% (20/765) of patients included in expanded access programs, with median follow-up of 39 and 27 months, respectively. Among the 44 reported cases, the median time to development of MDS/ leukemia was 31 months following treatment; however, the cumulative rate continues to increase.

Additional non-hematological malignancies were also reported in 54 of the 995 patients enrolled in clinical studies or included in the expanded access program. Approximately half of these were non-melanomatous skin cancers. The remainder, which occurred in 2 or more patients, included colorectal cancer (7), head and neck cancer (6), breast cancer (5), lung cancer (4), bladder cancer (4), melanoma (3), and gastric cancer (2). The relative risk of developing secondary malignancies in patients receiving the BEXXAR therapeutic regimen over the background rate in this population cannot be determined, due to the absence of controlled studies (see **ADVERSE REACTIONS**).

Pregnancy Category X: (see **BOXED WARNINGS; CONTRAINDICATIONS**).

Hypothyroidism: Administration of the BEXXAR therapeutic regimen may result in hypothyroidism (see **ADVERSE REACTIONS, Hypothyroidism**). Thyroid-blocking medications should be initiated at least 24 hours before receiving the dosimetric dose and continued until 14 days after the therapeutic dose (see **DOSAGE and ADMINISTRATION**). All patients must receive thyroid-blocking agents; any patient who is unable to tolerate thyroid-blocking agents should not receive the BEXXAR therapeutic regimen. Patients should be evaluated for signs and symptoms of hypothyroidism and screened for biochemical evidence of hypothyroidism annually.

PRECAUTIONS

Radionuclide Precautions: Iodine I 131 Tositumomab is radioactive. Care should be taken, consistent with the institutional radiation safety practices and applicable federal guidelines, to minimize exposure of medical personnel and other patients.

Renal Function: Iodine I 131 Tositumomab and Iodine-131 are excreted primarily by the kidneys. Impaired renal function may decrease the rate of excretion of the radiolabeled iodine and increase patient exposure to the radioactive component of the BEXXAR therapeutic regimen. There are no data regarding the safety of administration of the BEXXAR therapeutic regimen in patients with impaired renal function.

Immunization: The safety of immunization with live viral vaccines following administration of the BEXXAR therapeutic regimen has not been studied. The ability of patients who have received the BEXXAR therapeutic regimen to generate a primary or anamnestic humoral response to any vaccine has not been studied.

Information for Patients: Prior to administration of the BEXXAR therapeutic regimen, patients should be advised that they will have a radioactive material in their body for several days upon their release from the hospital or clinic. After discharge, patients should be provided with both oral and written instructions for minimizing exposure of family members, friends and the general public. Patients should be given a copy of the written instructions for use as a reference for the recommended precautionary actions.

The pregnancy status of women of childbearing potential should be assessed and these women should be advised of the potential risks to the fetus (see **CONTRAINDICATIONS**). Women who are breastfeeding should be instructed to discontinue breastfeeding and should be apprised of the resultant potential harmful effects to the infant if these instructions are not followed.

Patients should be advised of the potential risk of toxic effects on the male and female gonads following the BEXXAR therapeutic regimen, and be instructed to use effective contraceptive methods during treatment and for 12 months following the administration of the BEXXAR therapeutic regimen.

Patients should be informed of the risks of hypothyroidism and be advised of the importance of compliance with thyroid blocking agents and need for life-long monitoring.

Patients should be informed of the possibility of developing a HAMA immune response and that HAMA may affect the results of *in vitro* and *in vivo* diagnostic tests as well as results of therapies that rely on murine antibody technology.

Patients should be informed of the risks of cytopenias and symptoms associated with cytopenia, the need for frequent monitoring for up to 12 weeks after treatment, and the potential for persistent cytopenias beyond 12 weeks.

Patients should be informed that MDS, secondary leukemia, and solid tumors have also been observed in patients receiving the BEXXAR therapeutic regimen.

Due to lack of controlled clinical studies, and high background incidence in the heavily pretreated patient population, the relative risk of development of myelodysplastic syndrome/acute leukemia and solid tumors due to the BEXXAR therapeutic regimen cannot be determined.

Laboratory Monitoring: A complete blood count (CBC) with differential and platelet count should be obtained prior to, and at least weekly following administration of the BEXXAR therapeutic regimen. Weekly monitoring of blood counts should continue for a minimum of 10 weeks or, if persistent, until severe cytopenias have completely resolved. More frequent monitoring is indicated in patients with evidence of moderate or more severe cytopenias (see **BOXED WARNINGS** and **WARNINGS**). Thyroid stimulating hormone (TSH) level should be monitored before treatment and annually thereafter. Serum creatinine levels should be measured immediately prior to administration of the BEXXAR therapeutic regimen.

Drug Interactions: No formal drug interaction studies have been performed. Due to the frequent occurrence of severe and prolonged thrombocytopenia, the potential benefits of medications that interfere with platelet function and/or anticoagulation should be weighed against the potential increased risk of bleeding and hemorrhage.

Drug/Laboratory Test Interactions: Administration of the BEXXAR therapeutic regimen may result in the development of HAMA. The presence of HAMA may affect the accuracy of the results of *in vitro* and *in vivo* diagnostic tests and may affect the toxicity profile and efficacy of therapeutic agents that rely on murine antibody technology. Patients who are HAMA positive may be at increased risk for serious allergic reactions and other side effects if they undergo *in vivo* diagnostic testing or treatment with murine monoclonal antibodies.

Carcinogenesis, Mutagenesis, Impairment of Fertility: No long-term animal studies have been performed to establish the carcinogenic or mutagenic potential of the BEXXAR therapeutic regimen or to determine its effects on fertility in males or females. However, radiation is a potential carcinogen and mutagen. Administration of the BEXXAR therapeutic regimen results in delivery of a significant radiation dose to the testes. The radiation dose to the ovaries has not been established. There have been no studies to evaluate whether administration of the BEXXAR therapeutic regimen causes hypogonadism, premature menopause, azoospermia and/or mutagenic alterations to germ cells. There is a potential risk that the BEXXAR therapeutic regimen may cause toxic effects on the male and female gonads. Effective contraceptive methods should be used during treatment and for 12 months following administration of the BEXXAR therapeutic regimen.

Pregnancy Category X: (**See CONTRAINDICATIONS; WARNINGS.**)

Nursing Mothers: Radioiodine is excreted in breast milk and may reach concentrations equal to or greater than maternal plasma concentrations. Immunoglobulins are also known to be excreted in breast milk. The absorption potential and potential for adverse effects of the monoclonal antibody component (Tositumomab) in the infant are not known. Therefore, formula feedings should be substituted for breast feedings before starting treatment. Women should be advised to discontinue nursing.

Pediatric Use: The safety and effectiveness of the BEXXAR therapeutic regimen in children have not been established.

Geriatric Use: Clinical studies of the BEXXAR therapeutic regimen did not include sufficient numbers of patients aged 65 and over to determine whether they respond differently from younger patients. In clinical studies, 230 patients received the BEXXAR therapeutic regimen at the recommended dose. Of these, 27% (61 patients) were age 65 or older and 4% (10 patients) were age 75 or older. Across all studies, the overall response rate was lower in patients age 65 and over (41% vs. 61%) and the duration of responses was shorter (10 months vs. 16 months); however, these findings are primarily derived from 2 of the 5 studies. While the incidence of severe hematologic toxicity was lower, the duration of severe hematologic toxicity was longer in those age 65 or older as compared to patients less than 65 years of age. Due to the limited experience greater sensitivity of some older individuals cannot be ruled out.

ADVERSE REACTIONS

The most serious adverse reactions observed in the clinical trials were severe and prolonged cytopenias and the sequelae of cytopenias which included infections (sepsis) and hemorrhage in thrombocytopenic patients, allergic reactions (bronchospasm and angioedema), secondary leukemia and myelodysplasia (see **BOXED WARNINGS** and **WARNINGS**).

The most common adverse reactions occurring in the clinical trials included neutropenia, thromobocytopenia, and anemia that are both prolonged and severe. Less common but severe adverse reactions included pneumonia, pleural effusion and dehydration.

Data regarding adverse events were primarily obtained in 230 patients with non-Hodgkin's lymphoma enrolled in five clinical trials using the recommended dose and schedule. Patients had a median follow-up of 39 months and 79% of the patients were followed at least 12 months for survival and selected adverse events. Patients had a median of 3 prior chemotherapy regimens, a median age of 55 years, 60% male, 27% had transformation to a higher grade histology, 29% were intermediate grade and 2% high grade histology (IWF) and 68% had Ann Arbor stage IV disease. Patients enrolled in these studies were not permitted to have prior hematopoietic stem cell transplantation or irradiation to more than 25% of the red marrow. In the expanded access program, which included 765 patients, data regarding clinical serious adverse events and HAMA and TSH levels were used to supplement the characterization of delayed adverse events (see **ADVERSE REACTIONS, Hypothyroidism, Secondary Leukemia and Myelodysplastic Syndrome, Immunogenicity**).

Because clinical trials are conducted under widely varying conditions, adverse reaction rates observed in the clinical trials of a drug cannot be directly compared to rates in the clinical trials of another drug and may not reflect the rates observed in practice. The adverse reaction information from clinical trials does, however, provide a basis for identifying the adverse events that appear to be related to drug use and for approximating rates.

Hematologic Events: Hematologic toxicity was the most frequently observed adverse event in clinical trials with the BEXXAR therapeutic regimen (Table 6). Sixty-three (27%) of 230 patients received one or more hematologic supportive care measures following the therapeutic dose: 12% received G-CSF; 7% received Epoetin alfa; 15% received platelet transfusions; and 16% received packed red blood cell transfusions. Twenty-eight (12%) patients experienced hemorrhagic events; the majority were mild to moderate.

Infectious Events: One hundred and four of the 230 (45%) patients experienced one or more adverse events possibly related to infection. The majority were viral (e.g., rhinitis, pharyngitis, flu symptoms, or herpes) or other minor infections. Twenty of 230 (9%) patients experienced infections that were considered serious because the patient was hospitalized to manage the infection. Documented infections included pneumonia, bacteremia, septicemia, bronchitis, and skin infections.

Hypersensitivity Reactions: Fourteen patients (6%) experienced one or more of the following adverse events: allergic reaction, face edema, injection site hypersensitivity, anaphylactic reaction, laryngismus, and serum sickness. In the post-marketing setting, severe hypersensitivity reactions, including fatal anaphylaxis have been reported.

Gastrointestinal Toxicity: Eighty-seven patients (38%) experienced one or more gastrointestinal adverse events, including nausea, emesis, abdominal pain, and diarrhea. These events were temporally related to the infusion of the antibody. Nausea, vomiting, and abdominal pain were often reported within days of infusion, whereas diarrhea was generally reported days to weeks after infusion.

Infusional Toxicity: A constellation of symptoms, including fever, rigors or chills, sweating, hypotension, dyspnea, bronchospasm, and nausea, have been reported during or within

48 hours of infusion. Sixty-seven patients (29%) reported fever, rigors/chills, or sweating within 14 days following the dosimetric dose. Although all patients in the clinical studies received pretreatment with acetaminophen and an antihistamine, the value of premedication in preventing infusion-related toxicity was not evaluated in any of the clinical studies. Infusional toxicities were managed by slowing and/or temporarily interrupting the infusion. Symptomatic management was required in more severe cases. Adjustment of the rate of infusion to control adverse reactions occurred in 16 patients (7%); seven patients required adjustments for only the dosimetric infusion, two required adjustments for only the therapeutic infusion, and seven required adjustments for both the dosimetric and the therapeutic infusions. Adjustments included reduction in the rate of infusion by 50%, temporary interruption of the infusion, and in 2 patients, infusion was permanently discontinued.

Table 5 lists clinical adverse events that occurred in ≥5% of patients. Table 6 provides a detailed description of the hematologic toxicity.

Table 5
Incidence of Clinical Adverse Experiences Regardless of Relationship to Study Drug Occurring in ≥5% of the Patients Treated with BEXXAR Therapeutic Regimen[a] (N = 230)

Body System Preferred Term	All Grades	Grade 3/4
Total	**(96%)**	**(48%)**
Non-Hematologic AEs		
Body as a Whole	81%	12%
Asthenia	46%	2%
Fever	37%	2%
Infection[b]	21%	<1%
Pain	19%	1%
Chills	18%	1%
Headache	16%	0%
Abdominal pain	15%	3%
Back pain	8%	1%
Chest pain	7%	0%
Neck pain	6%	1%
Cardiovascular System	26%	3%
Hypotension	7%	1%
Vasodilatation	5%	0%
Digestive System	56%	9%
Nausea	36%	3%
Vomiting	15%	1%
Anorexia	14%	0%
Diarrhea	12%	0%
Constipation	6%	1%
Dyspepsia	6%	<1%
Endocrine System	7%	0%
Hypothyroidism	7%	0%
Metabolic and Nutritional Disorders	21%	3%
Peripheral edema	9%	0%
Weight loss	6%	<1%
Musculoskeletal System	23%	3%
Myalgia	13%	<1%
Arthralgia	10%	1%
Nervous System	26%	3%
Dizziness	5%	0%
Somnolence	5%	0%
Respiratory System	44%	8%
Cough increased	21%	1%
Pharyngitis	12%	0%
Dyspnea	11%	3%
Rhinitis	10%	0%
Pneumonia	6%	0%
Skin and Appendages	44%	5%
Rash	17%	<1%
Pruritus	10%	0%
Sweating	8%	<1%

[a] Excludes laboratory derived hematologic adverse events (see Table 6).
[b] The COSTART term for infection includes a subset of infections (e.g., upper respiratory infection). Other terms are mapped to preferred terms (e.g., pneumonia and sepsis). For a more inclusive summary see ADVERSE REACTIONS, Infectious Events.

[See table below]

Delayed Adverse Reactions
Delayed adverse reactions, including hypothyroidism, HAMA, and myelodysplasia/leukemia, were assessed in 230 patients included in clinical studies and 765 patients included in expanded access programs. The entry characteristics of patients included from the expanded access programs were similar to the characteristics of patients enrolled in the clinical studies, except that the median number of prior chemotherapy regimens was fewer (2 vs. 3) and the proportion with low-grade histology was higher (77% vs. 70%) in patients from the expanded access programs.

Secondary Leukemia and Myelodysplastic Syndrome (MDS): There were 44 cases of MDS/secondary leukemia reported among 995 (4.0%) patients included in clinical studies and expanded access programs, with a median follow-up of 29 months. The overall incidence of MDS/secondary leukemia among the 230 patients included in the clinical studies was 10% (24/230), with a median follow-up of 39 months and a median time to development of 34 months. The cumulative incidence of MDS/secondary leukemia in this patient population was 4.7% at 2 years and 15% at 5 years. The incidence of MDS/secondary leukemia among the 765 patients in the expanded access programs was 3% (20/765), with a median follow-up of 27 months and a median time to development of MDS of 31 months. The cumulative incidence of MDS/secondary leukemia in this patient population was 1.6% at 2 years and 6% at 5 years.

Secondary Malignancies: Of the 995 patients in clinical studies and the expanded access programs, there were 65 reports of second malignancies in 54 patients, excluding secondary leukemias. The most common included non-melanomatous skin cancers (26), colorectal cancer (7), head and neck cancer (6), breast cancer (5), lung cancer (4), bladder cancer (4), melanoma (3), and gastric cancer (2). Some of these events included recurrence of an earlier diagnosis of cancer.

Hypothyroidism: Of the 230 patients in the clinical studies, 203 patients did not have elevated TSH upon study entry. Of these, 137 patients had at least one post-treatment TSH value available and were not taking thyroid hormonal treatment upon study entry. With a median follow up period of 46 months, the incidence of hypothyroidism based on elevated TSH or initiation of thyroid replacement therapy in these patients was 18% with a median time to development of hypothyroidism of 16 months. The cumulative incidences of hypothyroidism at 2 and 5 years in these 137 patients were 11% and 19% respectively. New events have been observed up to 90 months post-treatment.

Of the 765 patients in the expanded access programs, 670 patients did not have elevated TSH upon study entry. Of these, 455 patients had at least one post-treatment TSH value available and were not taking thyroid hormonal treatment upon study entry. With a median follow up period of 33 months, the incidence of hypothyroidism based on elevated TSH or initiation of thyroid replacement therapy in these 455 patients was 13% with a median time to development of hypothyroidism of 15 months. The cumulative incidences of hypothyroidism at 2 and 5 years in these patients were 9% and 17%, respectively.

Immunogenicity: One percent (11/989) of the chemotherapy-relapsed or refractory patients included in the clinical studies or the expanded access program had a positive serology for HAMA prior to treatment and six patients had no baseline assessment for HAMA. Of the 230 patients in the clinical studies, 220 patients were seronegative for HAMA prior to treatment, and 219 had at least one post-treatment HAMA value obtained. With a median observation period of 6 months, a total of 23 patients (11%) became seropositive for HAMA post-treatment. The median time of HAMA development was 6 months. The cumulative incidences of HAMA seropositivity at 6 months, 12 months, and 18 months were 6%, 17% and 21% respectively.

Of the 765 patients in the expanded access programs, 758 patients were seronegative for HAMA prior to treatment, and 569 patients had at least one post-treatment HAMA value obtained. With a median observation period of 7 months, a total of 57 patients (10%) became seropositive for HAMA post-treatment. The median time of HAMA development was 5 months. The cumulative incidences of HAMA seropositivity at 6 months, 12 months, and 18 months were 7%, 12% and 13%, respectively.

In a study of 76 previously untreated patients with low-grade non-Hodgkin's lymphoma who received the BEXXAR therapeutic regimen, the incidence of conversion to HAMA seropositivity was 70%, with a median time to development of HAMA of 27 days.

The data reflect the percentage of patients whose test results were considered positive for HAMA in an ELISA assay that detects antibodies to the Fc portion of IgG$_1$ murine immunoglobulin and are highly dependent on the sensitivity and specificity of the assay. Additionally, the observed incidence of antibody positivity in an assay may be influenced by several factors including sample handling, concomitant medications, and underlying disease. For these reasons, comparison of the incidence of HAMA in patients treated with the BEXXAR therapeutic regimen with the incidence of HAMA in patients treated with other products may be misleading.

OVERDOSAGE
The maximum dose of the BEXXAR therapeutic regimen that was administered in clinical trials was 88 cGy. Three patients were treated with a total body dose of 85 cGy of Iodine I 131 Tositumomab in a dose escalation study. Two of the 3 patients developed Grade 4 toxicity of 5 weeks duration with subsequent recovery. In addition, accidental overdose of the BEXXAR therapeutic regimen occurred in one patient at a total body dose of 88 cGy. The patient developed Grade 3 hematologic toxicity of 18 days duration. Patients who receive an accidental overdose of Iodine I 131 Tositumomab should be monitored closely for cytopenias and radiation related toxicity. The effectiveness of hematopoietic stem cell transplantation as a supportive care measure for marrow injury has not been studied; however, the timing of such support should take into account the pharmacokinetics of the BEXXAR therapeutic regimen and decay rate of the Iodine-131 in order to minimize the possibility of irradiation of infused hematopoietic stem cells.

DOSAGE AND ADMINISTRATION
Recommended Dose
The BEXXAR therapeutic regimen consists of four components administered in two discrete steps: the dosimetric step, followed 7–14 days later by a therapeutic step.
Note: The safety of the BEXXAR therapeutic regimen was established only in the setting of patients receiving thyroid blocking agents and premedication to ameliorate/prevent infusion reactions (see **Concomitant Medications**).
Dosimetric step
• Tositumomab 450 mg intravenously in 50 ml 0.9% Sodium Chloride over 60 minutes. Reduce the rate of infu-

Table 6
Hematologic Toxicity[a] (N = 230)

Endpoint	Values
Platelets	
Median nadir (cells/mm^3)	43,000
Per patient incidence[a] platelets <50,000/mm^3	53% (n = 123)
Median[b] duration of platelets <50,000/mm^3 (days)	32
Grade 3/4 without recovery to Grade 2, N (%)	16 (7%)
Per patient incidence[c] platelets <25,000/mm^3	21% (n = 47)
ANC	
Median nadir (cells/mm^3)	690
Per patient incidence[a] ANC<1,000 cells/mm^3	63% (n = 145)
Median[b] duration of ANC<1,000 cells/mm^3 (days)	31
Grade 3/4 without recovery to Grade 2, N (%)	15 (7%)
Per patient incidence[c] ANC<500 cells/mm^3	25% (n = 57)
Hemoglobin	
Median nadir (gm/dL)	10
Per patient incidence[a] <8 gm/dL	29% (n = 66)
Median[b] duration of hemoglobin <8.0 gm/dL (days)	23
Grade 3/4 without recovery to Grade 2, N (%)	12 (5%)
Per patient incidence[c] hemoglobin <6.5 gm/dL	5% (n = 11)

[a] Grade 3/4 toxicity was assumed if patient was missing 2 or more weeks of hematology data between Week 5 and Week 9.
[b] Duration of Grade 3/4 of 1,000+ days (censored) was assumed for those patients with undocumented Grade 3/4 and no hematologic data on or after Week 9.
[c] Grade 4 toxicity was assumed if patient had documented Grade 3 toxicity and was missing 2 or more weeks of hematology data between Week 5 and Week 9.

sion by 50% for mild to moderate infusional toxicity; interrupt infusion for severe infusional toxicity. After complete resolution of severe infusional toxicity, infusion may be resumed with a 50% reduction in the rate of infusion.

- Iodine I 131 Tositumomab (containing 5.0 mCi Iodine-131 and 35 mg Tositumomab) intravenously in 30 ml 0.9% Sodium Chloride over 20 minutes. Reduce the rate of infusion by 50% for mild to moderate infusional toxicity; interrupt infusion for severe infusional toxicity. After complete resolution of severe infusional toxicity, infusion may be resumed with a 50% reduction in the rate of infusion.

Therapeutic step

Note: Do not administer the therapeutic step if biodistribution is altered (see **Assessment of Biodistribution of Iodine I 131 Tositumomab**).

- Tositumomab 450 mg intravenously in 50 ml 0.9% Sodium Chloride over 60 minutes. Reduce the rate of infusion by 50% for mild to moderate infusional toxicity; interrupt infusion for severe infusional toxicity. After complete resolution of severe infusional toxicity, infusion may be resumed with a 50% reduction in the rate of infusion.
- Iodine I 131 Tositumomab (see **CALCULATION OF IODINE-131 ACTIVITY FOR THE THERAPEUTIC DOSE**). Reduce the rate of infusion by 50% for mild to moderate infusional toxicity; interrupt infusion for severe infusional toxicity. After complete resolution of severe infusional toxicity, infusion may be resumed with a 50% reduction in the rate of infusion.
  - Patients with ≥150,000 platelets/mm^3: The recommended dose is the activity of Iodine-131 calculated to deliver 75 cGy total body irradiation and 35 mg Tositumomab, administered intravenously over 20 minutes.
  - Patients with NCI Grade 1 thrombocytopenia (platelet counts ≥100,000 but <150,000 platelets/mm^3): The recommended dose is the activity of Iodine-131 calculated to deliver 65 cGy total body irradiation and 35 mg Tositumomab, administered intravenously over 20 minutes.

Concomitant Medications: The safety of the BEXXAR therapeutic regimen was established in studies in which all patients received the following concurrent medications:

- Thyroid protective agents: Saturated solution of potassium iodide (SSKI) 4 drops orally t.i.d.; Lugol's solution 20 drops orally t.i.d.; or potassium iodide tablets 130 mg orally q.d. Thyroid protective agents should be initiated at least 24 hours prior to administration of the Iodine I 131 Tositumomab dosimetric dose and continued until 2 weeks after administration of the Iodine I 131 Tositumomab therapeutic dose.

  Patients should not receive the dosimetric dose of Iodine I 131 Tositumomab if they have not yet received at least three doses of SSKI, three doses of Lugol's solution, or one dose of 130 mg potassium iodide tablet (at least 24 hours prior to the dosimetric dose).
- Acetaminophen 650 mg orally and diphenhydramine 50 mg orally 30 minutes prior to administration of Tositumomab in the dosimetric and therapeutic steps.

The BEXXAR therapeutic regimen is administered via an IV tubing set with an in-line 0.22 micron filter. **THE SAME IV TUBING SET AND FILTER MUST BE USED THROUGHOUT THE ENTIRE DOSIMETRIC OR THERAPEUTIC STEP. A CHANGE IN FILTER CAN RESULT IN LOSS OF DRUG.**

Figure 1 shows an overview of the dosing schedule.

[See figure 1 at top of next column]

PREPARATION OF THE BEXXAR THERAPEUTIC REGIMEN GENERAL

Read all directions thoroughly and assemble all materials before preparing the dose for administration.

The Iodine I 131 Tositumomab dosimetric and therapeutic doses should be measured by a suitable radioactivity calibration system immediately prior to administration. The dose calibrator must be operated in accordance with the manufacturer's specifications and quality control for the measurement of Iodine-131.

All supplies for preparation and administration of the BEXXAR therapeutic regimen should be sterile. Use appropriate aseptic technique and radiation precautions for the preparation of the components of the BEXXAR therapeutic regimen.

Waterproof gloves should be utilized in the preparation and administration of the product. Iodine I 131 Tositumomab doses should be prepared, assayed, and administered by personnel who are licensed to handle and/or administer radionuclides. Appropriate shielding should be used during preparation and administration of the product.

Restrictions on patient contact with others and release from the hospital must follow all applicable federal, state, and institutional regulations.

Figure 1
Dosing Schedule

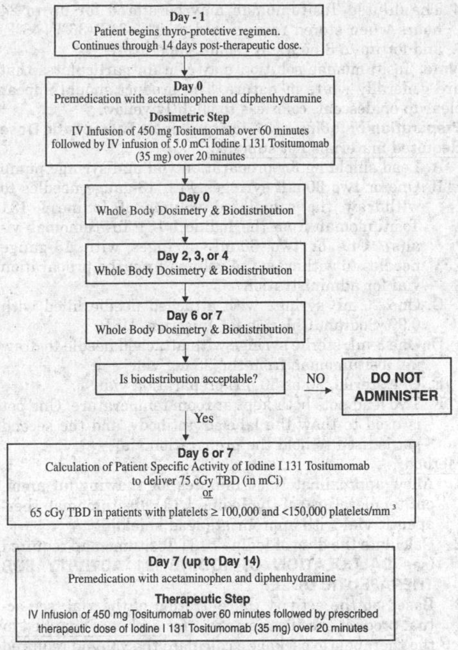

Day - 1
Patient begins thyro-protective regimen.
Continues through 14 days post-therapeutic dose.
Day 0
Premedication with acetaminophen and diphenhydramine
Dosimetric Step
IV Infusion of 450 mg Tositumomab over 60 minutes followed by IV infusion of 5.0 mCi Iodine I 131 Tositumomab (35 mg) over 20 minutes
Day 0
Whole Body Dosimetry & Biodistribution
Day 2, 3, or 4
Whole Body Dosimetry & Biodistribution
Day 6 or 7
Whole Body Dosimetry & Biodistribution
Is biodistribution acceptable?
NO
DO NOT ADMINISTER
Yes
Day 6 or 7
Calculation of Patient Specific Activity of Iodine I 131 Tositumomab to deliver 75 cGy TBD (in mCi)
or
65 cGy TBD in patients with platelets ≥ 100,000 and <150,000 platelets/mm 3
Day 7 (up to Day 14)
Premedication with acetaminophen and diphenhydramine
Therapeutic Step
IV infusion of 450 mg Tositumomab over 60 minutes followed by prescribed therapeutic dose of Iodine I 131 Tositumomab (35 mg) over 20 minutes

Preparation for the Dosimetric Step

Tositumomab Dose

Required materials not supplied:

A. One 50 mL syringe with attached 18-gauge needle (to withdraw 450 mg of Tositumomab from two vials each containing 225 mg Tositumomab)
B. One 50 mL bag of sterile 0.9% Sodium Chloride for Injection, USP
C. One 50 mL syringe for drawing up 32 mL of saline for disposal from the 50 mL bag of sterile 0.9% Sodium Chloride for Injection, USP

Method:

1. Withdraw and dispose of 32 mL of saline from a 50 mL bag of sterile 0.9% Sodium Chloride for Injection, USP.
2. Withdraw the entire contents from each of the two 225 mg vials (a total of 450 mg Tositumomab in 32 mL) and transfer to the infusion bag containing 18 mL of 0.9% Sodium Chloride for Injection, USP to yield a final volume of 50 mL.
3. Gently mix the solution by inverting/rotating the bag. DO NOT SHAKE.
4. The diluted Tositumomab may be stored for up to 24 hours when stored refrigerated at 2°C–8°C (36°F–46°F) and for up to 8 hours at room temperature.

Note: Tositumomab solution may contain particulates that are generally white in nature. The product should appear clear to opalescent, colorless to slightly yellow.

Preparation of Iodine I 131 Tositumomab Dosimetric Dose

Required materials not supplied:

A. Lead shielding for preparation vial and syringe pump
B. One 30 mL syringe with 18-gauge needle to withdraw the calculated volume of Iodine I 131 Tositumomab from the Iodine I 131 Tositumomab vial. One 60 mL syringe with 18-gauge needle to withdraw the volume from the preparation vial for administration
C. One 20 mL syringe with attached needle, filled with 0.9% Sodium Chloride for Injection, USP
D. One 3 mL syringe with attached needle to withdraw Tositumomab from 35 mg vial
E. One sterile, 30 or 50 mL preparation vial
F. Two lead pots, both kept at room temperature. One pot is used to thaw the labeled antibody and the second pot is used to hold the preparation vial

Method:

1. Allow approximately 60 minutes for thawing (at ambient temperature) of the Iodine I 131 Tositumomab dosimetric vial with appropriate lead shielding.
2. Based on the activity concentration of the vial (see actual product specification sheet for the vial supplied in the dosimetric package), calculate the volume required for an Iodine I 131 Tositumomab activity of 5.0 mCi.
3. Withdraw the calculated volume from the Iodine I 131 Tositumomab vial.
4. Transfer this volume to the shielded preparation vial.
5. Assay the dose to ensure that the appropriate activity (mCi) has been prepared.
   a. If the assayed dose is 5.0 mCi (±10%) proceed with step 6.
   b. If the assayed dose does not contain 5.0 mCi (±10%) recalculate the activity concentration of the Iodine I 131 Tositumomab at this time, based on the volume and the activity in the preparation vial. Recalculate the volume required for an Iodine I 131 Tositumomab activity of 5.0 mCi. Using the same 30 mL syringe, add or subtract the appropriate volume from the Iodine I 131 Tositumomab vial so that the preparation vial contains the volume required for an Iodine I 131 Tositumomab activity of 5.0 mCi (±10%). Reassay the preparation vial and proceed with step 6.
6. Calculate the amount of Tositumomab contained in the solution of Iodine I 131 Tositumomab in the shielded preparation vial, based on the volume and protein concentration (see actual product specification sheet supplied in the dosimetric package).
7. If the shielded preparation vial contains less than 35 mg, calculate the amount of additional Tositumomab needed to yield a total of 35 mg protein. Calculate the volume needed from the 35 mg vial of Tositumomab, based on the protein concentration. Withdraw the calculated volume of Tositumomab from the 35 mg vial of Tositumomab, and transfer this volume to the shielded preparation vial. The preparation vial should now contain a total of 35 mg of Tositumomab.
8. Using the 20 mL syringe containing 0.9% Sodium Chloride for Injection, USP, add a sufficient quantity to the shielded preparation vial to yield a final volume of 30 mL. Gently mix the solutions.
9. Withdraw the entire contents from the preparation vial into a 60 mL syringe using a large bore needle (18-gauge).
10. Assay and record the activity.

Administration of the Dosimetric Step

Required materials not supplied: For questions about required materials call the BEXXAR Service Center at 1-877-423-9927.

A. IV Filter set (0.22 micron filter), 15 inch with injection site (port) and luer lock
B. One Primary IV infusion set
C. One 100 mL bag of sterile 0.9% Sodium Chloride for Injection, USP
D. Two Secondary IV infusion sets
E. One IV Extension set, 30 inch luer lock
F. One 3-way stopcock
G. One 50 mL bag of sterile 0.9% Sodium Chloride for Injection, USP
H. One Infusion pump for Tositumomab infusion
I. One Syringe Pump for Iodine I 131 Tositumomab infusion
J. Lead shielding for use in the administration of the dosimetric dose

Tositumomab Infusion:

(See Figure 1 in the ***"Workbook for Dosimetry Methodology and Administration Set-Up"*** for diagrammatic illustration of the configuration of the infusion set components.)

1. Attach a primary IV infusion set (Item B) to the 0.22 micron in-line filter set (Item A) and the 100 mL bag of sterile 0.9% Sodium Chloride for Injection, USP (Item C).
2. After priming the primary IV infusion set (Item B) and IV filter set (Item A), connect the infusion bag containing 450 mg Tositumomab (50 mL) via a secondary IV infusion set (Item D) to the primary IV infusion set (Item B) at a port distal to the 0.22 micron in-line filter. Infuse Tositumomab over 60 minutes.
3. After completion of the Tositumomab infusion, disconnect the secondary IV infusion set (Item D) and flush the primary IV infusion set (Item B) and the in-line IV filter set (Item A) with sterile 0.9% Sodium Chloride for Injection, USP. Discard the Tositumomab bag and secondary IV infusion set.

Iodine I 131 Tositumomab Dosimetric Infusion:

(See Figure 2 in the ***"Workbook for Dosimetry Methodology and Administration Set-Up"*** for diagrammatic illustration of the configuration of the infusion set components.)

1. Appropriate shielding should be used in the administration of the dosimetric dose.
2. The dosimetric dose is delivered in a 60 mL syringe.
3. Connect the extension set (Item E) to the 3-way stopcock (Item F).
4. Connect the 50 mL bag of sterile 0.9% Sodium Chloride for Injection, USP (Item G) to a secondary IV infusion set (Item D) and connect the infusion set to the 3-way stopcock (Item F). Prime the secondary IV infusion set (Item D) and the extension set (Item E). Connect the extension set (Item E) to a port in the primary IV infusion set (Item B), distal to the filter.

   (**Note: You must** use the same primary infusion set (Item B) and IV filter set (Item A) with pre-wetted filter that was used for the Tositumomab infusion. A change in filter can result in loss of up to 7% of the Iodine I 131 Tositumomab dose.)
5. Attach the syringe filled with the Iodine I 131 Tositumomab to the 3-way stopcock (Item F).

6. Set syringe pump to deliver the entire 5.0 mCi (35 mg) dose of Iodine I 131 Tositumomab over 20 minutes.
7. After completion of the infusion of Iodine I 131 Tositumomab, close the stopcock (Item F) to the syringe. Flush the extension set (Item E) and the secondary IV infusion set (Item D) with 0.9% Sodium Chloride for Injection, USP from the 50 mL bag (Item G).
8. After the flush, disconnect the extension set (Item E), 3-way stopcock (Item F) and syringe. Disconnect the primary IV infusion set (Item B) and in-line filter set (Item A). Determine the combined residual activity of the syringe and infusion set components (stopcock, extension set, primary infusion set and in-line filter set) by assaying these items in a suitable radioactivity calibration system immediately following completion of administration of all components of the dosimetric step. Calculate and record the dose delivered to the patient by subtracting the residual activity in the syringe and the infusion set components from the activity of Iodine I 131 Tositumomab in the syringe prior to infusion.
9. Discard all materials used to deliver the Iodine I 131 Tositumomab (e.g., syringes, vials, inline filter set, extension set and infusion sets) in accordance with local, state, and federal regulations governing radioactive and biohazardous waste.

Determination of Dose for the Therapeutic Step (see Calculation of Iodine-131 Activity for Therapeutic Dose): The method for determining and calculating the patient-specific dose of Iodine-131 activity (mCi) to be administered in the therapeutic step is described below. The derived values obtained in steps 3 and 4 and calculation of the therapeutic dose as described in step 6 may be determined manually [see **"Workbook for Dosimetry Methodology and Administration Set-Up"**] or calculated automatically using the GlaxoSmithKline proprietary software program [BEXXAR Patient Management Templates]. To receive training and to obtain the "BEXXAR Patient Management Templates" call the BEXXAR Service Center at 1-877-423-9927. For assistance with either manual or automated calculations call the BEXXAR Service Center at 1-877-423-9927.

1. Following infusion of the Iodine I 131 Tositumomab dosimetric dose, obtain total body gamma camera counts and whole body images at the following timepoints:
   a. Within one hour of infusion and prior to urination
   b. 2–4 days after infusion of the dosimetric dose, following urination
   c. 6–7 days after infusion of the dosimetric dose, following urination
2. Assess biodistribution. If biodistribution is altered, the therapeutic step should not be administered.
3. Determine total body residence time (see Graph 1, "Determination of Residence Time", in the "Workbook for Dosimetry Methodology and Administration Set-Up").
4. Determine activity hours (see Table 2, **"Determination of Activity Hours"**, in the **"Workbook for Dosimetry Methodology and Administration Set-Up"**), according to gender. Use actual patient mass (in kg) or maximum effective mass (in kg) whichever is lower (see Table 1, **"Determination of Maximum Effective Mass"**, in the **"Workbook for Dosimetry Methodology and Administration Set-Up"**).
5. Determine whether the desired total body dose should be reduced (to 65 cGy) due to a platelet count of 100,000 to <150,000 cells/mm^3.
6. Based on the total body residence time and activity hours, calculate the Iodine-131 activity (mCi) to be administered to deliver the therapeutic dose of 65 or 75 cGy.

The following equation is used to calculate the activity of Iodine-131 required for delivery of the desired total body dose of radiation.

$$\text{Iodine-131 Activity (mCI)} = \frac{\text{Activity Hours (mCi hr)}}{\text{Residence Time (hr)}} \times \frac{\text{Desired Total Body Dose (cGy)}}{75\text{ cGy}}$$

Preparation for the Therapeutic Step

Tositumomab Dose

Required materials not supplied:

A. One 50 mL syringe with attached 18-gauge needle (to withdraw 450 mg of Tositumomab from two vials each containing 225 mg Tositumomab)
B. One 50 mL bag of sterile 0.9% Sodium Chloride for Injection, USP
C. One 50 mL syringe for drawing up 32 mL of saline for disposal from the 50 mL bag of sterile 0.9% Sodium Chloride for Injection, USP

Method:

1. Withdraw and dispose of 32 mL of saline from a 50 mL bag of sterile 0.9% Sodium Chloride for Injection, USP.
2. Withdraw the entire contents from each of the two 225 mg vials (a total of 450 mg Tositumomab in 32 mL) and transfer to the infusion bag containing 18 mL of 0.9% Sodium Chloride for Injection, USP to yield a final volume of 50 mL.
3. Gently mix the solutions by inverting/rotating the bag. DO NOT SHAKE.
4. The diluted Tositumomab may be stored for up to 24 hours when stored refrigerated at 2°C–8°C (36°F–46°F) and for up to 8 hours at room temperature.

Note: Tositumomab solution may contain particulates that are generally white in nature. The product should appear clear to opalescent, colorless to slightly yellow.

Preparation of Iodine I 131 Tositumomab Therapeutic Dose

Required materials not supplied:

A. Lead shielding for preparation vial and syringe pump
B. One or two 30 mL syringes with 18-gauge needles to withdraw the calculated volume of Iodine I 131 Tositumomab from the Iodine I 131 Tositumomab vial(s). One or two 60 mL syringes with 18-gauge needles to withdraw the volume from the preparation vial for administration
C. One 20 mL syringe with attached needle filled with 0.9% Sodium Chloride for Injection, USP
D. One 3 mL sterile syringe with attached needle to draw up Tositumomab from the 35 mg vial
E. One sterile, 30 or 50 mL preparation vial
F. Two lead pots both kept at room temperature. One pot is used to thaw the labeled antibody, and the second pot is used to hold the preparation vial

Method:

1. Allow approximately 60 minutes for thawing (at ambient temperature) of the Iodine I 131 Tositumomab therapeutic vial with appropriate lead shielding.
2. Calculate the dose of Iodine I 131 Tositumomab required (see **CALCULATION OF IODINE-131 ACTIVITY FOR THERAPEUTIC DOSE**).
3. Based on the activity concentration of the vial (see actual product specification sheet for each vial supplied in the therapeutic package), calculate the volume required for the Iodine I 131 Tositumomab activity required for the therapeutic dose.
4. Using one or more 30 mL syringes with an 18-gauge needle, withdraw the calculated volume from the Iodine I 131 Tositumomab vial.
5. Transfer this volume to the shielded preparation vial.
6. Assay the dose to ensure that the appropriate activity (mCi) has been prepared.
   a. If the assayed dose is the calculated dose (±10%) needed for the therapeutic step, proceed with step 7.
   b. If the assayed dose does not contain the desired dose (±10%), re-calculate the activity concentration of the Iodine I 131 Tositumomab at this time, based on the volume and the activity in the preparation vial. Recalculate the volume required for an Iodine I 131 Tositumomab activity for the therapeutic dose. Using the same 30 mL syringe, add or subtract the appropriate volume from the Iodine I 131 Tositumomab vial so that the preparation vial contains the volume required for the Iodine I 131 Tositumomab activity required for the therapeutic dose. Re-assay the preparation vial. Proceed to step 7.
7. Calculate the amount of Tositumomab protein contained in the solution of Iodine I 131 Tositumomab in the shielded preparation vial, based on the volume and protein concentration (see product specification sheet).
8. If the shielded preparation vial contains less than 35 mg, calculate the amount of additional Tositumomab needed to yield a total of 35 mg protein. Calculate the volume needed from the 35 mg vial of Tositumomab, based on the protein concentration. Withdraw the calculated volume of Tositumomab from the 35 mg vial of Tositumomab, and transfer this volume to the shielded preparation vial. The preparation vial should now contain a total of 35 mg of Tositumomab.
   Note: If the dose of Iodine I 131 Tositumomab requires the use of 2 vials of Iodine I 131 Tositumomab or the entire contents of a single vial of Iodine I 131 Tositumomab, there may be no need to add protein from the 35 mg vial of Tositumomab.
9. Using the 20 mL syringe containing 0.9% Sodium Chloride for Injection, USP, add a sufficient volume (if needed) to the shielded preparation vial to yield a final volume of 30 mL. Gently mix the solution.
10. Withdraw the entire volume from the preparation vial into a one or more sterile 60 mL syringes using a large bore needle (18-gauge).
11. Assay and record the activity.

Administration of the Therapeutic Step

Note: Restrictions on patient contact with others and release from the hospital must follow all applicable federal, state, and institutional regulations.

Required materials not supplied: For questions about required materials call the BEXXAR Service Center at 1-877-423-9927.

A. One IV Filter set (0.22 micron, filter), 15 inch with injection site (port) and luer lock
B. One Primary IV infusion set
C. One 100 mL bag of sterile 0.9% Sodium Chloride for Injection, USP
D. Two Secondary IV infusion sets
E. One IV extension set, 30 inch luer lock
F. One 3-way stopcock
G. One 50 mL bag of sterile 0.9% Sodium Chloride for Injection, USP
H. One Infusion pump for Tositumomab infusion
I. One Syringe Pump for Iodine I 131 Tositumomab infusion
J. Lead shielding for use in the administration of the therapeutic dose

Tositumomab Infusion:

(See Figure 1 in the **"Workbook for Dosimetry Methodology and Administration Set-Up"** for diagrammatic illustration of the configuration of the infusion set components.)

1. Attach a primary IV infusion set (Item B) to the 0.22 micron in-line filter set (Item A) and a 100 mL bag of sterile 0.9% Sodium Chloride for Injection, USP (Item C).
2. After priming the primary IV infusion set (Item B) and filter set (Item A), connect the infusion bag containing 450 mg Tositumomab (50 mL) via a secondary IV infusion set (Item D) to the primary IV infusion set (Item B) at a port distal to the 0.22 micron in-line filter. Infuse Tositumomab over 60 minutes.
3. After completion of the Tositumomab infusion, disconnect the secondary IV infusion set (Item D) and flush the primary IV infusion set (Item B) and the IV filter set (Item A) with sterile 0.9% Sodium Chloride for Injection, USP. Discard the Tositumomab bag and secondary IV infusion set.

Iodine I 131 Tositumomab Therapeutic Infusion:

(See Figure 2 in the **"Workbook for Dosimetry Methodology and Administration Set-Up"** for diagrammatic illustration of the configuration of the infusion set components.)

1. Appropriate shielding should be used in the administration of the therapeutic dose.
2. The therapeutic dose is delivered in one or more 60 mL syringes.
3. Connect the extension set (Item E) to the 3-way stopcock (Item F).
4. Connect the 50 mL bag of sterile 0.9% Sodium Chloride for Injection, USP (Item G) to a secondary IV infusion set (Item D) and connect the infusion set to the 3-way stopcock (Item F). Prime the secondary IV infusion set (Item D) and the extension set (Item E). Connect the extension set (Item E) to a port in the primary IV infusion set (Item B), distal to the filter.
   (**Note:** You **must** use the same primary infusion set (Item B) and IV filter set (Item A) with pre-wetted filter that was used for the Tositumomab infusion. A change in filter can result in loss of up to 7% of the Iodine I 131 Tositumomab dose.)
5. Attach the syringe filled with the Iodine I 131 Tositumomab to the 3-way stopcock (Item F).
6. Set syringe pump to deliver the entire therapeutic dose of Iodine I 131 Tositumomab over 20 minutes. (**Note:** If more than one syringe is required, remove the syringe and repeat steps 5 and 6.)
7. After completion of the infusion of Iodine I 131 Tositumomab, close the stopcock (Item F) to the syringe. Flush the secondary IV infusion set (Item D) and the extension set (Item E) with 0.9% Sodium Chloride from the 50 mL bag of sterile, 0.9% Sodium Chloride for Injection, USP (Item G).
8. After the flush, disconnect the extension set (Item E), 3-way stopcock (Item F) and syringe. Disconnect the primary IV infusion set (Item B) and in-line filter set (Item A). Determine the combined residual activity of the syringe(s) and infusion set components (stopcock, extension set, primary infusion set and in-line filter set) by assaying these items in a suitable radioactivity calibration system immediately following completion of administration of all components of the therapeutic step. Calculate and record the dose delivered to the patient by subtracting the residual activity in the syringe and infusion set components from the activity of Iodine I 131 Tositumomab in the syringe prior to infusion.
9. Discard all materials used to deliver the Iodine I 131 Tositumomab (e.g., syringes, vials, inline filter set, extension set and infusion sets) in accordance with local, state, and federal regulations governing radioactive and biohazardous waste.

DOSIMETRY

The following sections describe the procedures for image acquisition for collection of dosimetry data, interpretation of biodistribution images, calculation of residence time, and calculation of activity hours. Please read all sections carefully.

IMAGE ACQUISITION AND INTERPRETATION

Gamma Camera and Dose Calibrator Procedures

Manufacturer-specific quality control procedures should be followed for the gamma camera/computer system, the collimator, and the dose calibrator. Less than 20% variance between maximum and minimum pixel count values in the useful field of view is acceptable on Iodine-131 intrinsic flood fields and variability <10% is preferable. Iodine-131-specific camera uniformity corrections are strongly recommended, rather than applying lower energy correction to the Iodine-131 window. Camera extrinsic uniformity should be assessed at least monthly using ^{99m}Tc or ^{57}Co as a source with imaging at the appropriate window.

Additional (non-routine) quality control procedures are required. To assure the accuracy and precision of the patient total body counts, the gamma camera must undergo validation and daily quality control on each day it is used to collect patient images.

Use the same setup and region of interest (ROI) for calibration, determination of background, and whole body patient studies.

Gamma Camera Set-Up

The **same** camera, collimator, scanning speed, energy window, and setup must be used for all studies. The gamma camera must be capable of whole body imaging and have a large or extra large field of view with a digital interface. It must be equipped with a parallel-hole collimator rated to at least 364 keV by the manufacturer with a septal penetration for Iodine-131 of <7%. The camera and computer must be set up for scanning as follows:

- Parallel hole collimator rated to at least 364 keV with a septal penetration for Iodine-131 of <7%
- Symmetric window (20–25%) centered on the 364 keV photo peak of Iodine-131 (314–414 keV)
- Matrix: appropriate whole body matrix
- Scanning speed: 10–30 cm/minute

Counts from Calibrated Source for Quality Control

Camera sensitivity for Iodine-131 must be determined each day. Determination of the gamma camera's sensitivity is obtained by scanning a calibrated activity of Iodine-131 (e.g., 200–250 µCi in at least 20 mL of saline within a sealed pharmaceutical vial). The radioactivity of the Iodine-131 source is first determined using a NIST-traceable-calibrated clinical dose calibrator at the Iodine-131 setting.

Background Counts

The background count is obtained from a scan with no radioactive source. This should be obtained following the count of the calibrated source and just prior to obtaining the patient count.

If abnormally high background counts are measured, the source should be identified and, if possible, removed. If abnormally low background counts are measured, the camera energy window setting and collimator should be verified before repeating the background counts.

The counts per µCi are obtained by dividing the background-corrected source count by the calibrated activity for that day. For a specific camera and collimator, the counts per µCi should be relatively constant. When values vary more than 10% from the established ratio, the reason for the discrepancy should be ascertained and corrected and the source count repeated.

Patient Total Body Counts

The source and background counts are obtained first and the camera sensitivity (i.e., constant counting efficiency) is established prior to obtaining the patient count. The same rectangular region of interest (ROI) must be used for the whole body counts, the quality control counts of the radioactive source, and the background counts.

Acquire anterior and posterior whole body images for gamma camera counts. For any particular patient, the same gamma camera must be used for all scans. To obtain proper counts, extremities must be included in the images, and arms should not cross over the body. The scans should be centered on the midline of the patient. Record the time of the start of the radiolabeled dosimetric infusion and the time of the start of each count acquisition.

Gamma camera counts will be obtained at the three imaging timepoints:

- **Count 1:** ***Within an hour of end of the infusion*** of the Iodine I 131 Tositumomab dosimetric dose prior to patient voiding.
- **Count 2:** Two to 4 days after administration of the Iodine I 131 Tositumomab dosimetric dose and immediately following patient voiding.
- **Count 3:** Six to 7 days after the administration of the Iodine I 131 Tositumomab dosimetric dose and immediately following patient voiding.

Assessment of Biodistribution of Iodine I 131 Tositumomab

The biodistribution of Iodine I 131 Tositumomab should be assessed by determination of total body residence time and by visual examination of whole body camera images from the first image taken at the time of Count 1 (within an hour of the end of the infusion) and from the second image taken at the time of Count 2 (at 2 to 4 days after administration). To resolve ambiguities, an evaluation of the third image at the time of Count 3 (6 to 7 days after administration) may be necessary. If either of these methods indicates that the biodistribution is altered, the Iodine I 131 Tositumomab therapeutic dose should not be administered.

Expected Biodistribution

- On the first imaging timepoint: Most of the activity is in the blood pool (heart and major blood vessels) and the uptake in normal liver and spleen is less than in the heart.
- On the second and third imaging timepoints: The activity in the blood pool decreases significantly and there is decreased accumulation of activity in normal liver and spleen. Images may show uptake by thyroid, kidney, and urinary bladder and minimal uptake in the lungs. Tumor uptake in soft tissues and in normal organs is seen as areas of increased intensity.

Results Indicating Altered Biodistribution

- On the first imaging timepoint: If the blood pool is not visualized or if there is diffuse, intense tracer uptake in the liver and/or spleen or uptake suggestive of urinary obstruction the biodistribution is altered. Diffuse lung uptake greater than that of blood pool on the first day represents altered biodistribution.
- On the second and third imaging timepoints: Uptake suggestive of urinary obstruction and diffuse lung uptake greater than that of the blood pool represent altered biodistribution.
- Total body residence times of less than 50 hours and more than 150 hours.

CALCULATION OF IODINE-131 ACTIVITY FOR THE THERAPEUTIC DOSE

There are two options for calculation of the Iodine-131 activity for the therapeutic dose. The derived values and calculation of the therapeutic dose may be determined manually [see **"Workbook for Dosimetry Methodology and Administration Set-Up"**] or calculated automatically using the GlaxoSmithKline proprietary software program [BEXXAR Patient Management Templates]. The following describes in greater detail the stepwise method for manual determination of the Iodine-131 activity for the therapeutic dose.

Residence Time (hr)

For each timepoint, calculate the background corrected total body count at each timepoint (defined as the geometric mean). The following equation is used:

$$\text{Geometric mean of counts} = \sqrt{(C_A - C_{BA})(C_P - C_{BP})}$$

In this equation, C_A = the anterior counts, C_{BA} = the anterior background counts, C_P = the posterior counts, and C_{BP} = the posterior background counts.

Once the geometric mean of the counts has been calculated for each of the 3 timepoints, the % injected activity remaining for each timepoint is calculated by dividing the geometric mean of the counts from that timepoint by the geometric mean of the counts from Day 0 and multiplying by 100.

The residence time (h) is then determined by plotting the time from the start of infusion and the % injected activity values for the 3 imaging timepoints on Graph 1 (see Worksheet **"Determination of Residence Time"** in the **"Workbook for Dosimetry Methodology and Administration Set-Up"** supplied with Dosimetric Dose Packaging). A best-fit line is then drawn from 100% (the pre-plotted Day 0 value) through the other 2 plotted points (if the line does not intersect the two points, one point must lie above the best-fit line and one point must lie below the best-fit line). The residence time (h) is read from the x-axis of the graph at the point where the fitted line intersects with the horizontal 37% injected activity line.

Activity Hours (mCi hr)

In order to determine the activity hours (mCi hr), look up the patient's maximum effective mass derived from the patient's sex and height (see Worksheet **"Determination of Maximum Effective Mass"** in the **"Workbook for Dosimetry Methodology and Administration Set-Up"** supplied with Dosimetric Dose Packaging). If the patient's actual weight is less than the maximum effective mass, the actual weight should be used in the activity hours table (see Worksheet **"Determination of Activity Hours"** in the **"Workbook for Dosimetry Methodology and Administration Set-Up"** supplied with Dosimetric Dose Packaging). If the patient's actual weight is greater than the maximum effective mass, the mass from the worksheet for **"Determination of Maximum Effective Mass"** should be used.

Calculation of Iodine-131 Activity for the Therapeutic Dose

The following equation is used to calculate the activity of Iodine-131 required for delivery of the desired total body dose of radiation.

$$\text{Iodine-131 Activity (mCI)} = \frac{\text{Activity Hours (mCi hr)}}{\text{Residence Time (hr)}} \times \frac{\text{Desired Total Body Dose (cGy)}}{75 \text{ cGy}}$$

HOW SUPPLIED

TOSITUMOMAB DOSIMETRIC PACKAGING

The components of the dosimetric step will be shipped **ONLY** to individuals who are participating in the certification program or have been certified in the preparation and administration of the BEXXAR therapeutic regimen. The components are shipped from separate sites; when ordering, ensure that the components are scheduled to arrive on the same day. The components of the Tositumomab Dosimetric Step include:

1. Tositumomab: Two single-use 225 mg vials (16.1 mL) and one single-use 35 mg vial (2.5 mL) of Tositumomab at a protein concentration of 14 mg/mL supplied by McKesson BioServices.
   NDC 0007-3260-31
2. Iodine I 131 Tositumomab: A single-use vial of Iodine I 131 Tositumomab within a lead pot, supplied by MDS Nordion. Each single-use vial contains not less than 20 mL of Iodine I 131 Tositumomab at nominal protein and activity concentrations of 0.1 mg/mL and 0.61 mCi/mL (at calibration), respectively. (Refer to the product specification sheet for the lot-specific protein concentration, activity concentration, total activity and expiration date.)
   NDC 0007-3261-01

TOSITUMOMAB THERAPEUTIC PACKAGING

The components of the therapeutic step will be shipped **ONLY** to individuals who are participating in the certification program or have been certified in the preparation and administration of the BEXXAR therapeutic regimen for an individual patient who has completed the Dosimetric Step. The components of the therapeutic step are shipped from separate sites; when ordering, ensure that the components are scheduled to arrive on the same day. The components of the Tositumomab Therapeutic Step include:

1. Tositumomab: Two single-use 225 mg vials (16.1 mL) and one single-use 35 mg vial (2.5 mL) of Tositumomab at a protein concentration of 14 mg/mL supplied by McKesson BioServices.
   NDC 0007-3260-36
2. Iodine I 131 Tositumomab: One or two single-use vials of Iodine I 131 Tositumomab within a lead pot(s), supplied by MDS Nordion. Each single-use vial contains not less than 20 mL of Iodine I 131 Tositumomab at nominal protein and activity concentrations of 1.1 mg/mL and 5.6 mCi/mL (at calibration), respectively. Refer to the product specification sheet for the lot-specific protein concentration, activity concentration, total activity and expiration date.
   NDC 0007-3262-01

STABILITY AND STORAGE

TOSITUMOMAB

Vials of Tositumomab (35 mg and 225 mg) should be stored refrigerated at 2°C-8°C (36°F-46°F) prior to dilution. Do not use beyond expiration date. Protect from strong light. **DO NOT SHAKE.** Do not freeze. Discard any unused portions left in the vial.

Solutions of diluted Tositumomab are stable for up to 24 hours when stored refrigerated at 2°C-8°C (36°F-46°F) and for up to 8 hours at room temperature. However, it is recommended that the diluted solution be stored refrigerated at 2°C-8°C (36°F-46°F) prior to administration because it does not contain preservatives. Any unused portion must be discarded. Do not freeze solutions of diluted Tositumomab.

IODINE I 131 TOSITUMOMAB

Store frozen in the original lead pots. The lead pot containing the product must be stored in a freezer at a temperature of −20°C or below until it is removed for thawing prior to administration to the patient. Do not use beyond the expiration date on the label of the lead pot. Thawed dosimetric and therapeutic doses of Iodine I 131 Tositumomab are stable for up to 8 hours at 2°C-8°C (36°F-46°F) or at room temperature. Solutions of Iodine I 131 Tositumomab diluted for infusion contain no preservatives and should be stored refrigerated at 2°C-8°C (36°F-46°F) prior to administration (do not freeze). Any unused portion must be discarded according to federal and state laws.

REFERENCES

1. Weber DA, Eckman KF, Dillman LT, Ryman JC. In: MIRD: radionuclide data and decay schemes. New York: Society of Nuclear Medicine Inc. 1989:229.
2. Tedder T, Boyd A, Freedman A, Nadler L, Schlossman S. The B cell surface molecule is functionally linked with B cell activation and differentiation. J Immunol 1985;135(2):973–979.
3. Anderson, KC, Bates MP, Slaughenhoupt BL, Pinkus GS, Schlossman SF, Nadler LM. Expression of human B cell-associated antigens on leukemias and lymphomas: a model of human B cell differentiation. Blood 1984;63(6): 1424–1433.
4. Press OW, Howell-Clark J, Anderson S, Bernstein I. Retention of B-cell-specific monoclonal antibodies by human lymphoma cells. Blood 1994;83:1390–7.

5. Cardarelli PM, Quinn M, Buckman D, Fang Y, Colcher D, King DJ, Bebbington C, et al. Binding to CD20 by anti-B1 antibody or F(ab′)(2) is sufficient for induction of apoptosis in B-cell lines. Cancer Immunol Immunother 2002 Mar;51(1):15–24.
6. Stashenko P, Nadler LM, Hardy R, Schlossman SF. Characterization of a human B lymphocyte-specific antigen. J Immunol 1980;125:1678–85.

U.S. Lic. 1727
GlaxoSmithKline
Research Triangle Park, NC 27709
BEXXAR is a registered trademark of GlaxoSmithKline.
©2005, GlaxoSmithKline. All rights reserved.
October 2005   RL-2245

BOOSTRIX®   ℞

[*boos′ trix*]

(Tetanus Toxoid, Reduced Diphtheria Toxoid and Acellular Pertussis Vaccine, Adsorbed)

HIGHLIGHTS OF PRESCRIBING INFORMATION

These highlights do not include all the information needed to use BOOSTRIX safely and effectively. See full prescribing information for BOOSTRIX.

BOOSTRIX® (Tetanus Toxoid, Reduced Diphtheria Toxoid and Acellular Pertussis Vaccine, Adsorbed)
Suspension for Intramuscular Injection
Initial U.S. Approval: 2005

——————— RECENT MAJOR CHANGES ———————

Indications and Usage (1)	12/2008
Warnings and Precautions (5.2)	12/2008

——————— INDICATIONS AND USAGE ———————
BOOSTRIX is a vaccine indicated for active booster immunization against tetanus, diphtheria, and pertussis as a single dose. BOOSTRIX is approved for use in individuals 10 through 64 years of age. (1)

——————— DOSAGE AND ADMINISTRATION ———————
A single intramuscular injection (0.5 mL). (2.2)

——————— DOSAGE FORMS AND STRENGTHS ———————
Suspension for injection in 0.5 mL single-dose vials or syringes. (3)

——————— CONTRAINDICATIONS ———————
• Severe allergic reaction (e.g., anaphylaxis) to any component of BOOSTRIX. (4.1)
• Encephalopathy (e.g., coma, decreased level of consciousness, prolonged seizures) within 7 days of administration of a previous pertussis antigen-containing vaccine. (4.2)

——————— WARNINGS AND PRECAUTIONS ———————
• If Guillain-Barré syndrome occurs within 6 weeks of receipt of a prior vaccine containing tetanus toxoid, the decision to give BOOSTRIX should be based on potential benefits and risks. (5.1)
• If progressive or unstable neurologic disorders exist, consider risks and benefits of vaccination. (5.2)
• Persons who experienced an Arthus-type hypersensitivity reaction following a prior dose of a tetanus toxoid-containing vaccine should not receive BOOSTRIX unless at least 10 years have elapsed since the last dose of a tetanus toxoid-containing vaccine. (5.3)
• The needleless prefilled syringes contain dry natural latex rubber and may cause allergic reactions. (5.4)

——————— ADVERSE REACTIONS ———————
• Common solicited adverse events (≥15%) in adolescents were pain, redness, and swelling at the injection site, increase in arm circumference of injected arm, headache, fatigue, and gastrointestinal symptoms. (6.1)
• Common solicited adverse events (≥15%) in adults were pain, redness, and swelling at the injection site, headache, fatigue, and gastrointestinal symptoms. (6.1)

To report SUSPECTED ADVERSE REACTIONS, contact GlaxoSmithKline at 1-888-825-5249 or VAERS at 1-800-822-7967 or www.vaers.hhs.gov.

——————— DRUG INTERACTIONS ———————
• Lower levels for antibodies to the pertussis antigens FHA and pertactin were observed when BOOSTRIX was administered concomitantly with an inactivated influenza vaccine as compared to BOOSTRIX alone. (7.1)
• Do not mix BOOSTRIX with any other vaccine in the same syringe or vial. (7.1)

——————— USE IN SPECIFIC POPULATIONS ———————
• Safety and effectiveness of BOOSTRIX have not been established in pregnant women, nursing mothers, and children younger than 10 years of age. (8.1, 8.3, 8.4)
• Register women who receive BOOSTRIX while pregnant in the pregnancy registry by calling 1-888-452-9622. (8.1)

Revised: August 2009
BTX:9PI

See 17 for PATIENT COUNSELING INFORMATION
                                        Revised: 03/2010

FULL PRESCRIBING INFORMATION: CONTENTS*

FULL PRESCRIBING INFORMATION

1   INDICATIONS AND USAGE

BOOSTRIX® is indicated for active booster immunization against tetanus, diphtheria, and pertussis as a single dose in individuals 10 through 64 years of age.

2   DOSAGE AND ADMINISTRATION

2.1   Preparation for Administration
Shake vigorously to obtain a homogeneous, turbid, white suspension before administration. Do not use if resuspension does not occur with vigorous shaking. Inspect BOOSTRIX visually for particulate matter, discoloration, or cracks in the vial or syringe prior to administration. If any of these conditions exist, the vaccine should not be administered. BOOSTRIX should not be combined through reconstitution or mixed with any other vaccine.
Do not administer this product intravenously, intradermally, or subcutaneously.

2.2   Dose
BOOSTRIX is administered as a single 0.5-mL intramuscular injection into the deltoid muscle of the upper arm.
There are no data to support repeat administration of BOOSTRIX.
Five years should elapse between the last dose of the recommended series of Diphtheria and Tetanus Toxoids and Acellular Pertussis Vaccine Adsorbed (DTaP) and/or Tetanus and Diphtheria Toxoids Adsorbed For Adult Use (Td) vaccine and the administration of BOOSTRIX.

2.3   Additional Dosing Information
Primary Series: The use of BOOSTRIX as a primary series or to complete the primary series for diphtheria, tetanus, or pertussis has not been studied.

Wound Management: Clinicians should refer to guidelines for tetanus prophylaxis in routine wound management.[1] Individuals who have completed a primary series against tetanus and who sustain wounds which are minor and uncomplicated should receive a booster dose of a tetanus toxoid-containing vaccine only if they have not received tetanus toxoid within the preceding 10 years. In case of tetanus-prone injury (e.g., wounds contaminated with dirt, feces, soil, and saliva; puncture wounds; avulsions; and wounds resulting from missiles, crushing, burns, and frostbite) in an individual who is in need of tetanus toxoid, BOOSTRIX can be used as an alternative to Td vaccine in patients for whom the pertussis component is also indicated.

---

3   DOSAGE FORMS AND STRENGTHS

BOOSTRIX is a suspension for injection available in 0.5-mL single-dose vials and prefilled TIP-LOK® syringes. See *Description (11)* for the complete listing of ingredients.

4   CONTRAINDICATIONS
4.1   Hypersensitivity
A severe allergic reaction (e.g., anaphylaxis) after a previous dose of any tetanus toxoid-, diphtheria toxoid-, or pertussis antigen-containing vaccine or any component of this vaccine is a contraindication to administration of BOOSTRIX[2,3] *[see Description (11)]*. Because of the uncertainty as to which component of the vaccine might be responsible, none of the components should be administered. Alternatively, such individuals may be referred to an allergist for evaluation if immunization with any of these components is considered.

4.2   Encephalopathy
Encephalopathy (e.g., coma, decreased level of consciousness, prolonged seizures) within 7 days of administration of a previous dose of a pertussis antigen-containing vaccine that is not attributable to another identifiable cause is a contraindication to administration of any pertussis antigen-containing vaccine, including BOOSTRIX.[2,3]

5   WARNINGS AND PRECAUTIONS
5.1   Guillain-Barré Syndrome and Brachial Neuritis
If Guillain-Barré syndrome has occurred within 6 weeks of receipt of a prior vaccine containing tetanus toxoid, the decision to give BOOSTRIX or any vaccine containing tetanus toxoid should be based on careful consideration of the potential benefits and possible risks. A review by the Institute of Medicine (IOM) found evidence for a causal relationship between receipt of tetanus toxoid and both brachial neuritis and Guillain-Barré syndrome.[4]

5.2   Progressive or Unstable Neurologic Disorders
Progressive neurologic disorder, uncontrolled epilepsy, progressive encephalopathy or unstable neurological conditions (e.g., cerebrovascular events and acute encephalopathic conditions) are considered reasons to defer Tdap (Tetanus Toxoid, Reduced Diphtheria Toxoid and Acellular Pertussis Vaccine, Adsorbed) vaccination. In these situations, administration of any pertussis antigen-containing vaccine, including BOOSTRIX, should be based on careful consideration of the potential benefits and possible risks.[2,3]

5.3   Arthus-Type Hypersensitivity
Persons who experienced an Arthus-type hypersensitivity reaction following a prior dose of a tetanus toxoid-containing vaccine usually have a high serum tetanus antitoxin level and should not receive BOOSTRIX or other tetanus toxoid-containing vaccines unless at least 10 years have elapsed since the last dose of tetanus toxoid-containing vaccine.

5.4   Latex
The tip cap and the rubber plunger of the needleless prefilled syringes contain dry natural latex rubber that may cause allergic reactions in latex sensitive individuals. The vial stopper is latex-free.

5.5   Altered Immunocompetence
As with any vaccine, if administered to immunosuppressed persons, including individuals receiving immunosuppressive therapy, the expected immune response may not be obtained.

5.6   Preventing and Managing Allergic Vaccine Reactions
Prior to administration, the healthcare provider should review the immunization history for possible vaccine sensitivity and previous vaccination-related adverse reactions to allow an assessment of benefits and risks. Epinephrine and other appropriate agents used for the control of immediate allergic reactions must be immediately available should an acute anaphylactic reaction occur.

6   ADVERSE REACTIONS
6.1   Clinical Trials Experience
Because clinical trials are conducted under widely varying conditions, adverse reaction rates observed in the clinical trials of a vaccine cannot be directly compared to rates in the clinical trials of another vaccine, and may not reflect the rates observed in practice. As with any vaccine, there is the possibility that broad use of BOOSTRIX could reveal adverse reactions not observed in clinical trials.
In clinical studies, 3,608 adolescents and 2,972 adults were vaccinated with a single dose of BOOSTRIX. Of these adults, 1,450 were vaccinated with BOOSTRIX in a coadministration study with influenza vaccine *[see Clinical Studies (14.4)]*. An additional 1,092 adolescents 10 to 18 years of age received a non-US formulation of BOOSTRIX (formulated to contain 0.5 mg aluminum per dose) in non-US clinical studies.
In a randomized, observer-blinded, controlled study in the US, 3,080 adolescents 10 to 18 years of age received a single dose of BOOSTRIX and 1,034 received the control Td vaccine, manufactured by MassBioLogics. There were no substantive differences in demographic characteristics be-

tween the vaccine groups. Among BOOSTRIX and control vaccine recipients, approximately 75% were 10 to 14 years of age and approximately 25% were 15 to 18 years of age. Approximately 98% of participants in this study had received the recommended series of 4 or 5 doses of either Diphtheria and Tetanus Toxoids and Pertussis Vaccine Adsorbed (DTwP) or a combination of DTwP and DTaP in childhood. Subjects were monitored for solicited adverse events using standardized diary cards (day 0-14). Unsolicited adverse events were monitored for the 31-day period following vaccination (day 0-30). Subjects were also monitored for 6 months post-vaccination for non-routine medical visits, visits to an emergency room, onset of new chronic illness, and serious adverse events. Information regarding late onset adverse events was obtained via a telephone call 6 months following vaccination. At least 97% of subjects completed the 6-month follow-up evaluation.

In a study conducted in Germany, BOOSTRIX was administered to 319 children 10 to 12 years of age previously vaccinated with 5 doses of acellular pertussis antigen-containing vaccines; 193 of these subjects had previously received 5 doses of INFANRIX® (Diphtheria and Tetanus Toxoids and Acellular Pertussis Vaccine Adsorbed). Adverse events were recorded on diary cards during the 15 days following vaccination. Unsolicited adverse events that occurred within 31 days of vaccination (day 0-30) were recorded on the diary card or verbally reported to the investigator. Subjects were monitored for 6 months post-vaccination for physician office visits, emergency room visits, onset of new chronic illness, and serious adverse events. The 6-month follow-up evaluation, conducted via telephone interview, was completed by 90% of subjects.

A randomized, observer-blinded study in adults, conducted in the US, evaluated the safety of BOOSTRIX compared with ADACEL® (Tetanus Toxoid, Reduced Diphtheria Toxoid and Acellular Pertussis Vaccine Adsorbed), a US-licensed Tdap vaccine, manufactured by Sanofi Pasteur SA. Vaccines were administered as a single-dose booster to adults 19 to 64 years of age (N = 2,284). There were no substantive differences in demographic characteristics between the vaccine groups. Subjects were monitored for solicited adverse events using standardized diary cards (day 0-14). Unsolicited adverse events were monitored for the 31-day period following vaccination (day 0-30). Subjects were also monitored for 6 months post-vaccination for serious adverse events, visits to an emergency room, hospitalizations, and onset of new chronic illness. Approximately 95% of subjects completed the 6-month follow-up evaluation.

Solicited Adverse Events in the US Adolescent Safety Study: Table 1 presents the solicited local adverse reactions and general adverse events within 15 days of vaccination with BOOSTRIX or Td vaccine for the total vaccinated cohort.

The primary safety endpoint was the incidence of grade 3 pain (spontaneously painful and/or prevented normal activity) at the injection site within 15 days of vaccination. Grade 3 pain was reported in 4.6% of those who received BOOSTRIX compared with 4.0% of those who received the Td vaccine. The difference in rate of grade 3 pain was within the pre-defined clinical limit for non-inferiority (upper limit of the 95% CI for the difference [BOOSTRIX minus Td] ≤4%).

Table 1. Rates of Solicited Local Adverse Reactions or General Adverse Events Within the 15-day[a] Post-Vaccination Period in Individuals 10 to 18 Years of Age (Total Vaccinated Cohort)

	BOOSTRIX (N = 3,032) %	Td (N = 1,013) %
Local		
Pain, any[b]	75.3	71.7
Pain, grade 2 or 3[b]	51.2	42.5
Pain, grade 3[c]	4.6	4.0
Redness, any	22.5	19.8
Redness, >20 mm	4.1	3.9
Redness, ≥50 mm	1.7	1.6
Swelling, any	21.1	20.1
Swelling, >20 mm	5.3	4.9
Swelling, ≥50 mm	2.5	3.2
Arm circumference increase, >5 mm[d]	28.3	29.5
Arm circumference increase, >20 mm[d]	2.0	2.2
Arm circumference increase, >40 mm[d]	0.5	0.3
General		
Fever, ≥99.5°F (37.5°C)[e]	13.5	13.1
Fever, >100.4°F (38.0°C)[e]	5.0	4.7
Fever, >102.2°F (39.0°C)[e]	1.4	1.0
Headache, any	43.1	41.5
Headache, grade 2 or 3[b]	15.7	12.7
Headache, grade 3	3.7	2.7
Fatigue, any	37.0	36.7
Fatigue, grade 2 or 3	14.4	12.9
Fatigue, grade 3	3.7	3.2
Gastrointestinal symptoms, any[f]	26.0	25.8
Gastrointestinal symptoms, grade 2 or 3[f]	9.8	9.7
Gastrointestinal symptoms, grade 3[f]	3.0	3.2

Td = Tetanus and Diphtheria Toxoids Adsorbed For Adult Use manufactured by MassBioLogics.
N = Number of subjects in the total vaccinated cohort with local/general symptoms sheets completed.
Grade 2 = Local: painful when limb moved; General: interfered with normal activity.
Grade 3 = Local: spontaneously painful and/or prevented normal activity; General: prevented normal activity.
[a]Day of vaccination and the next 14 days.
[b]Statistically significantly higher (P <0.05) following BOOSTRIX as compared to Td vaccine.
[c]Grade 3 injection site pain following BOOSTRIX was not inferior to Td vaccine (upper limit of two-sided 95% CI for the difference [BOOSTRIX minus Td] in the percentage of subjects ≤4%).
[d]Mid-upper region of the vaccinated arm.
[e]Oral temperatures or axillary temperatures.
[f]Gastrointestinal symptoms included nausea, vomiting, diarrhea and/or abdominal pain.

Unsolicited Adverse Events in the US Adolescent Safety Study: The incidence of unsolicited adverse events reported in the 31 days after vaccination was comparable between the 2 groups (25.4% and 24.5% for BOOSTRIX and Td vaccine, respectively).

Solicited Adverse Events in the German Adolescent Safety Study: Table 2 presents the rates of solicited local adverse reactions and fever within 15 days of vaccination for those subjects who had previously been vaccinated with 5 doses of INFANRIX. No cases of whole arm swelling were reported. Two individuals (2/193) reported large injection site swelling (range 110 to 200 mm diameter), in one case associated with grade 3 pain. Neither individual sought medical attention. These episodes were reported to resolve without sequelae within 5 days.

Table 2. Rates of Solicited Adverse Events Reported Within the 15-day[a] Post-Vaccination Period Following Administration of BOOSTRIX in Individuals 10 to 12 Years of Age Who Had Previously Received 5 Doses of INFANRIX

	BOOSTRIX (N = 193) %
Pain, any	62.2
Pain, grade 2 or 3	33.2
Pain, grade 3	5.7
Redness, any	47.7
Redness, >20 mm	15.0
Redness, ≥50 mm	10.9
Swelling, any	38.9
Swelling, >20 mm	17.6
Swelling, ≥50 mm	14.0
Fever, ≥99.5°F (37.5°C)[b]	8.8
Fever, >100.4°F (38.0°C)[b]	4.1
Fever, >102.2°F (39.0°C)[b]	1.0

N = Number of subjects with local/general symptoms sheets completed.
Grade 2 = Painful when limb moved.
Grade 3 = Spontaneously painful and/or prevented normal activity.
[a]Day of vaccination and the next 14 days.
[b]Oral temperatures or axillary temperatures.

Solicited Adverse Events in the US Adult Safety Study: Table 3 presents solicited local adverse reactions and general adverse events within 15 days of vaccination with BOOSTRIX or the comparator Tdap vaccine for the total vaccinated cohort.

Table 3. Rates of Solicited Local Adverse Reactions or General Adverse Events Within the 15-day[a] Post-Vaccination Period in Adults (Total Vaccinated Cohort)

	BOOSTRIX (N = 1,480) %	Tdap (N = 741) %
Local		
Pain, any	61.0	69.2
Pain, grade 2 or 3	35.1	44.4
Pain, grade 3	1.6	2.3
Redness, any	21.1	27.1
Redness, >20 mm	4.0	6.2
Redness, ≥50 mm	1.6	2.3
Swelling, any	17.6	25.6
Swelling, >20 mm	3.9	6.3
Swelling, ≥50 mm	1.4	2.8
General		
Fever, ≥99.5°F (37.5°C)[b]	5.5	8.0
Fever, >100.4°F (38.0°C)[b]	1.0	1.5
Fever, >102.2°F (39.0°C)[b]	0.1	0.4
Headache, any	30.1	31.0
Headache, grade 2 or 3	11.1	10.5
Headache, grade 3	2.2	1.5
Fatigue, any	28.1	28.9
Fatigue, grade 2 or 3	9.1	9.4
Fatigue, grade 3	2.5	1.2
Gastrointestinal symptoms, any[c]	15.9	17.5
Gastrointestinal symptoms, grade 2 or 3[c]	4.3	5.7
Gastrointestinal symptoms, grade 3[c]	1.2	1.3
	1.2	1.3

Tdap = Tetanus Toxoid, Reduced Diphtheria Toxoid and Acellular Pertussis Vaccine Adsorbed, a US-licensed Tdap vaccine, manufactured by Sanofi Pasteur SA.
N = Number of subjects in the total vaccinated cohort with local/general symptoms sheets completed.
Grade 2 = Local: painful when limb moved; General: interfered with normal activity.
Grade 3 = Local/General: prevented normal activity.
[a]Day of vaccination and the next 14 days.
[b]Oral temperatures.
[c]Gastrointestinal symptoms included nausea, vomiting, diarrhea, and/or abdominal pain.

Table 4. Antibody Responses to Tetanus and Diphtheria Toxoids Following BOOSTRIX as Compared With Td Vaccine in Individuals 10 to 18 Years of Age (ATP Cohort for Immunogenicity)

	N	% ≥0.1 IU/mL (95% CI)	% ≥1.0 IU/mL (95% CI)	% BR[a] (95% CI)
Anti-Tetanus				
BOOSTRIX	2,469-2,516			
Pre-vaccination		97.7 (97.1, 98.3)	36.8 (34.9, 38.7)	—
Post-vaccination		100 (99.8, 100)[b]	99.5 (99.1, 99.7)[c]	89.7 (88.4, 90.8)[b]
Td	817-834			
Pre-vaccination		96.8 (95.4, 97.9)	39.9 (36.5, 43.4)	—
Post-vaccination		100 (99.6, 100)	99.8 (99.1, 100)	92.5 (90.5, 94.2)
Anti-Diphtheria				
BOOSTRIX	2,463-2,515			
Pre-vaccination		85.8 (84.3, 87.1)	17.1 (15.6, 18.6)	—
Post-vaccination		99.9 (99.7, 100)[b]	97.3 (96.6, 97.9)[c]	90.6 (89.4, 91.7)[b]
Td	814-834			
Pre-vaccination		84.8 (82.1, 87.2)	19.5 (16.9, 22.4)	—
Post-vaccination		99.9 (99.3, 100)	99.3 (98.4, 99.7)	95.9 (94.4, 97.2)

Td manufactured by MassBioLogics.
ATP = according-to-protocol; CI = Confidence Interval; BR = booster response.
[a]Booster response: In subjects with pre-vaccination <0.1 IU/mL, post-vaccination concentration ≥0.4 IU/mL. In subjects with pre-vaccination concentration ≥0.1 IU/mL, an increase of at least 4 times the pre-vaccination concentration.
[b]Seroprotection rate or booster response rate to BOOSTRIX was non-inferior to Td (upper limit of two-sided 95% CI on the difference for Td minus BOOSTRIX ≤10%).
[c]Non-inferiority criteria not prospectively defined for this endpoint.

Unsolicited Adverse Events in the US Adult Safety Study:
The incidence of unsolicited adverse events reported in the 31 days after vaccination was comparable between the 2 groups (17.8% and 22.2% for BOOSTRIX and Tdap vaccine, respectively).

Serious Adverse Events (SAEs): In the US and German adolescent safety studies, no serious adverse events were reported to occur within 31 days of vaccination. During the 6-month extended safety evaluation period, no serious adverse events that were of potential autoimmune origin or new onset and chronic in nature were reported to occur. In non-US adolescent studies in which serious adverse events were monitored for up to 37 days, one subject was diagnosed with insulin-dependent diabetes 20 days following administration of BOOSTRIX. No other serious adverse events of potential autoimmune origin or that were new onset and chronic in nature were reported to occur in these studies. In the US adult safety study, serious adverse events were reported to occur during the entire study period (0-6 months) by 1.4% and 1.7% of subjects who received BOOSTRIX and the comparator Tdap vaccine, respectively. During the 6-month extended safety evaluation period, no serious adverse events of a neuroinflammatory nature or with information suggesting an autoimmune etiology were reported in subjects who received BOOSTRIX.

6.2 Postmarketing Experience
In addition to reports in clinical trials, worldwide voluntary reports of adverse events received for BOOSTRIX in persons 10 to 64 years of age since market introduction of this vaccine are listed below. This list includes serious events or events which have causal connection to components of this or other vaccines or drugs. Because these events are reported voluntarily from a population of uncertain size, it is not possible to reliably estimate their frequency or establish a causal relationship to the vaccine.
Blood and Lymphatic System Disorders: Lymphadenitis, lymphadenopathy.
Cardiac Disorders: Myocarditis.
General Disorders and Administration Site Conditions: Extensive swelling of the injected limb, injection site induration, injection site inflammation, injection site mass, injection site pruritus, injection site nodule, injection site warmth, local reaction.
Musculoskeletal and Connective Tissue Disorders: Arthralgia, back pain, myalgia.
Nervous System Disorders: Convulsion, encephalitis, facial palsy, paraesthesia.
Skin and Subcutaneous Tissue Disorders: Exanthem, Henoch-Schönlein purpura, rash, urticaria.

7 DRUG INTERACTIONS
7.1 Concomitant Immunizations
BOOSTRIX was administered concomitantly with FLUARIX® (Influenza Virus Vaccine) in a clinical study [see Clinical Studies (14.4)]. Lower geometric mean antibody concentrations (GMCs) for antibodies to the pertussis antigens filamentous hemagglutinin (FHA) and pertactin were observed when BOOSTRIX was administered concomitantly with FLUARIX as compared with BOOSTRIX alone.
There are no immunogenicity or safety data to assess the concomitant use of BOOSTRIX with other vaccines.
When BOOSTRIX is administered concomitantly with other injectable vaccines, they should be given with separate syringes and at different injection sites. BOOSTRIX should not be mixed with any other vaccine in the same syringe or vial.
Tetanus Immune Globulin, if needed, should be given at a separate site, with a separate needle and syringe.

7.2 Immunosuppressive Therapies
Immunosuppressive therapies, including irradiation, antimetabolites, alkylating agents, cytotoxic drugs, and corticosteroids (used in greater than physiologic doses), may reduce the immune response to BOOSTRIX.

8 USE IN SPECIFIC POPULATIONS
8.1 Pregnancy
Pregnancy Category C
Animal reproduction studies have not been conducted with BOOSTRIX. It is also not known whether BOOSTRIX can cause fetal harm when administered to a pregnant woman or can affect reproduction capacity. BOOSTRIX should be given to a pregnant woman only if clearly needed.
Animal fertility studies have not been conducted with BOOSTRIX. In a developmental toxicity study, the effect of BOOSTRIX on embryo-fetal and pre-weaning development was evaluated in pregnant rats. Animals were administered INFANRIX prior to gestation and BOOSTRIX during the period of organogenesis (gestation days 6, 8, 11) and later in pregnancy (gestation day 15), 0.1 mL/rat/occasion (a 45-fold increase compared with the human dose of BOOSTRIX on a body weight basis), by intramuscular injection. No adverse effect on pregnancy and lactation parameters, embryo-fetal or pre-weaning development was observed. There were no fetal malformations or other evidence of teratogenesis noted in this study.
Pregnancy Exposure Registry: Healthcare providers are encouraged to register pregnant women who receive BOOSTRIX in the GlaxoSmithKline vaccination pregnancy registry by calling 1-888-452-9622.

8.3 Nursing Mothers
It is not known whether BOOSTRIX is excreted in human milk. Because many drugs are excreted in human milk, caution should be exercised when BOOSTRIX is administered to a nursing woman.
8.4 Pediatric Use
BOOSTRIX is not indicated for use in children younger than 10 years of age. Safety and effectiveness of BOOSTRIX in this age group have not been established.
8.5 Geriatric Use
BOOSTRIX is not indicated for use in individuals older than 64 years of age. Clinical studies of BOOSTRIX did not include sufficient numbers of subjects older than 65 years to determine whether they respond differently from younger subjects.

11 DESCRIPTION
BOOSTRIX (Tetanus Toxoid, Reduced Diphtheria Toxoid and Acellular Pertussis Vaccine, Adsorbed) is a noninfectious, sterile, vaccine for intramuscular administration. It contains tetanus toxoid, diphtheria toxoid, and pertussis antigens (inactivated pertussis toxin [PT] and formaldehyde-treated filamentous hemagglutinin [FHA] and pertactin). The antigens are the same as those in INFANRIX, but BOOSTRIX is formulated with reduced quantities of these antigens.
Tetanus toxin is produced by growing Clostridium tetani in a modified Latham medium derived from bovine casein. The diphtheria toxin is produced by growing Corynebacterium diphtheriae in Fenton medium containing a bovine extract. The bovine materials used in these extracts are sourced from countries which the United States Department of Agriculture (USDA) has determined neither have nor are at risk of bovine spongiform encephalopathy (BSE). Both toxins are detoxified with formaldehyde, concentrated by ultrafiltration, and purified by precipitation, dialysis, and sterile filtration.
The acellular pertussis antigens (PT, FHA, and pertactin) are isolated from Bordetella pertussis culture grown in modified Stainer-Scholte liquid medium. PT and FHA are isolated from the fermentation broth; pertactin is extracted from the cells by heat treatment and flocculation. The antigens are purified in successive chromatographic and precipitation steps. PT is detoxified using glutaraldehyde and formaldehyde. FHA and pertactin are treated with formaldehyde.
Each antigen is individually adsorbed onto aluminum hydroxide. Each 0.5-mL dose is formulated to contain 5 Lf of tetanus toxoid, 2.5 Lf of diphtheria toxoid, 8 mcg of inactivated PT, 8 mcg of FHA, and 2.5 mcg of pertactin (69 kiloDalton outer membrane protein).
Tetanus and diphtheria toxoid potency is determined by measuring the amount of neutralizing antitoxin in previously immunized guinea pigs. The potency of the acellular pertussis components (inactivated PT and formaldehyde-treated FHA and pertactin) is determined by enzyme-linked immunosorbent assay (ELISA) on sera from previously immunized mice.
Each 0.5-mL dose also contains 4.5 mg of NaCl, aluminum adjuvant (not more than 0.39 mg aluminum by assay), ≤100 mcg of residual formaldehyde, and ≤100 mcg of polysorbate 80 (Tween 80).

12 CLINICAL PHARMACOLOGY
12.1 Mechanism of Action
Tetanus: Tetanus is a condition manifested primarily by neuromuscular dysfunction caused by a potent exotoxin released by C. tetani. Protection against disease is due to the development of neutralizing antibodies to the tetanus toxin. A serum tetanus antitoxin level of at least 0.01 IU/mL, measured by neutralization assays, is considered the minimum protective level.[5,6] A level ≥0.1 IU/mL has been considered as protective.[7]
Diphtheria: Diphtheria is an acute toxin-mediated infectious disease caused by toxigenic strains of C. diphtheriae. Protection against disease is due to the development of neutralizing antibodies to the diphtheria toxin. A serum diphtheria antitoxin level of 0.01 IU/mL is the lowest level giving some degree of protection; a level of 0.1 IU/mL is regarded as protective.[8]
Pertussis: Pertussis (whooping cough) is a disease of the respiratory tract caused by B. pertussis. The role of the different components produced by B. pertussis in either the pathogenesis of, or the immunity to, pertussis is not well understood.

13 NONCLINICAL TOXICOLOGY
13.1 Carcinogenesis, Mutagenesis, Impairment of Fertility
BOOSTRIX has not been evaluated for carcinogenic or mutagenic potential, or for impairment of fertility.

Table 7. Antibody Responses to Tetanus and Diphtheria Toxoids Following One Dose of BOOSTRIX as Compared With the Control Tdap Vaccine in Adults 19 to 64 Years of Age (ATP Cohort for Immunogenicity)

	N	% ≥0.1 IU/mL (95% CI)	% ≥1.0 IU/mL (95% CI)
Anti-Tetanus			
BOOSTRIX	1,445-1,447		
Pre-vaccination		95.9 (94.8, 96.9)	71.9 (69.5, 74.2)
Post-vaccination		99.6 (99.1, 99.8)[a]	98.3 (97.5, 98.9)[a]
Tdap	727-728		
Pre-vaccination		97.2 (95.8, 98.3)	74.7 (71.4, 77.8)
Post-vaccination		100 (95.5, 100)	99.3 (98.4, 99.8)
Anti-Diphtheria			
BOOSTRIX	1,440-1,444		
Pre-vaccination		85.2 (83.3, 87.0)	23.7 (21.5, 26.0)
Post-vaccination		98.2 (97.4, 98.8)[a]	87.9 (86.1, 89.5)[b]
Tdap	720-727		
Pre-vaccination		89.2 (86.7, 91.3)	26.5 (23.3, 29.9)
Post-vaccination		98.6 (97.5, 99.3)	92.0 (89.8, 93.9)

Tdap = Tetanus Toxoid, Reduced Diphtheria Toxoid and Acellular Pertussis Vaccine, Adsorbed manufactured by Sanofi Pasteur SA.
ATP = according-to-protocol; CI = Confidence Interval.
[a]Seroprotection rates for BOOSTRIX were non-inferior to the comparator Tdap vaccine (lower limit of 95% CI on the difference of BOOSTRIX minus Tdap ≥-10%).
[b]Non-inferiority criteria not prospectively defined for this endpoint.

Table 8. GMCs and Booster Responses for the Pertussis Antigens Following One Dose of BOOSTRIX in Adults 19 to 64 Years of Age (ATP Cohort for Immunogenicity)

	N	GMC EL.U./mL	% BR[a] (95% CI)
BOOSTRIX	1,419-1,444		
Anti-PT		63.6	77.2 (74.9, 79.3)[b]
Anti-FHA		624.4	96.9 (95.8, 97.7)[c]
Anti-pertactin		401.0	93.2 (91.8, 94.4)[c]

GMC = geometric mean antibody concentration; ATP = according-to-protocol; BR = booster response; CI = Confidence Interval.
[a]Booster response: In initially seronegative subjects (<5 EL.U./mL), post-vaccination antibody concentrations ≥20 EL.U./mL. In initially seropositive subjects with pre-vaccination antibody concentrations ≥5 EL.U./mL and <20 EL.U./mL, an increase of at least 4 times the pre-vaccination antibody concentration. In initially seropositive subjects with pre-vaccination antibody concentrations ≥20 EL.U./mL, an increase of at least 2 times the pre-vaccination antibody concentration.
[b]The PT antigen booster response lower limit of the 95% CI did not exceed the pre-defined limit of 80%.
[c]The FHA and pertactin antigens booster response lower limit of the 95% CI exceeded the pre-defined limit of 80%.

14 CLINICAL STUDIES
The efficacy of the tetanus and diphtheria toxoid components of BOOSTRIX is based on the immunogenicity of the individual antigens compared to US-licensed vaccines using established serologic correlates of protection. The efficacy of the pertussis components of BOOSTRIX was evaluated by comparison of the immune response of adolescents and adults following a single dose of BOOSTRIX to the immune response of infants following a 3-dose primary series of INFANRIX. In addition, the ability of BOOSTRIX to induce a booster response to each of the antigens was evaluated.

14.1 Efficacy of INFANRIX
The efficacy of a 3-dose primary series of INFANRIX in infants has been assessed in 2 clinical studies: A prospective efficacy trial conducted in Germany employing a household contact study design and a double-blind, randomized, active Diphtheria and Tetanus Toxoids (DT)-controlled trial conducted in Italy sponsored by the National Institutes of Health (NIH) (for details see INFANRIX prescribing information). Serological data from a subset of infants immunized with INFANRIX in the household contact study were compared with the sera of adolescents and adults immunized with BOOSTRIX [see Clinical Studies (14.2, 14.3)]. In the household contact study, the protective efficacy of INFANRIX, in infants, against WHO-defined pertussis (21 days or more of paroxysmal cough with infection confirmed by culture and/or serologic testing) was calculated to be 89% (95% CI: 77%, 95%). When the definition of pertussis was expanded to include clinically milder disease, with infection confirmed by culture and/or serologic testing, the efficacy of INFANRIX against ≥7 days of any cough was 67% (95% CI: 52%, 78%) and against ≥7 days of paroxysmal cough was 81% (95% CI: 68%, 89%) (for details see INFANRIX prescribing information).

14.2 Immunological Evaluation in Adolescents
In a multicenter, randomized, controlled study conducted in the United States, the immune responses to each of the antigens contained in BOOSTRIX were evaluated in sera obtained approximately 1 month after administration of a single dose of vaccine to adolescent subjects (10 to 18 years of age). Of the subjects enrolled in this study, approximately 76% were 10 to 14 years of age and 24% were 15 to 18 years of age. Approximately 98% of participants in this study had received the recommended series of 4 or 5 doses of either DTwP or a combination of DTwP and DTaP in childhood. The racial/ethnic demographics were as follows: Caucasian 85.8%, Black 5.7%, Hispanic 5.6%, Oriental 0.8%, and other 2.1%.
Response to Tetanus and Diphtheria Toxoids: The antibody responses to the tetanus and diphtheria toxoids of BOOSTRIX compared with Td vaccine are shown in Table 4. One month after a single dose, anti-tetanus and antidiphtheria seroprotective rates (≥0.1 IU/mL) and booster response rates were comparable between BOOSTRIX and the control Td vaccine.
[See table at top of previous page]

Response to Pertussis Antigens: The booster response rates of adolescents to the pertussis antigens are shown in Table 5. For each of the pertussis antigens the lower limit of the two-sided 95% CI for the percentage of subjects with a booster response exceeded the pre-defined lower limit of 80% for demonstration of an acceptable booster response.

Table 5. Booster Responses to the Pertussis Antigens Following BOOSTRIX in Individuals 10 to 18 Years of Age (ATP Cohort for Immunogenicity)

	N	BOOSTRIX % BR[a] (95% CI)
Anti-PT	2,677	84.5 (83.0, 85.9)
Anti-FHA	2,744	95.1 (94.2, 95.9)
Anti-pertactin	2,752	95.4 (94.5, 96.1)

ATP = according-to-protocol; CI = Confidence Interval; BR = booster response.
[a]Booster response: In initially seronegative subjects (<5 EL.U./mL), post-vaccination antibody concentrations ≥20 EL.U./mL. In initially seropositive subjects with pre-vaccination antibody concentrations ≥5 EL.U./mL and <20 EL.U./mL, an increase of at least 4 times the pre-vaccination antibody concentration. In initially seropositive subjects with pre-vaccination antibody concentrations ≥20 EL.U./mL, an increase of at least 2 times the pre-vaccination antibody concentration.

The GMCs to each of the pertussis antigens 1 month following a single dose of BOOSTRIX in the US adolescent study (N = 2,941-2,979) were compared with the GMCs of infants following a 3-dose primary series of INFANRIX administered at 3, 4, and 5 months of age (N = 631-2,884). Table 6 presents the results for the total immunogenicity cohort in both studies (vaccinated subjects with serology data available for at least one pertussis antigen; the majority of subjects in the study of INFANRIX had anti-PT serology data only). These infants were a subset of those who formed the cohort for the German household contact study in which the efficacy of INFANRIX was demonstrated [see Clinical Studies (14.1)]. Although a serologic correlate of protection for pertussis has not been established, anti-PT, anti-FHA, and anti-pertactin antibody concentrations of adolescents 1 month after a single dose of BOOSTRIX were non-inferior to those of infants following a primary vaccination series with INFANRIX.

Table 6. Ratio of GMCs to Pertussis Antigens Following One Dose of BOOSTRIX in Individuals 10 to 18 Years of Age as Compared With 3 Doses of INFANRIX in Infants (Total Immunogenicity Cohort)

	GMC Ratio: BOOSTRIX/INFANRIX (95% CI)
Anti-PT	1.90 (1.82, 1.99)[a]
Anti-FHA	7.35 (6.85, 7.89)[a]
Anti-pertactin	4.19 (3.73, 4.71)[a]

GMC = geometric mean antibody concentration, measured in arbitrary ELISA units; CI = Confidence Interval.
Number of subjects for BOOSTRIX GMC evaluation: Anti-PT = 2,941, anti-FHA = 2,979, and anti-pertactin = 2,978.
Number of subjects for INFANRIX GMC evaluation: Anti-PT = 2,884, anti-FHA = 685, and anti-pertactin = 631.
[a]GMC following BOOSTRIX was non-inferior to GMC following INFANRIX (lower limit of 95% CI for the GMC ratio of BOOSTRIX/INFANRIX >0.67).

14.3 Immunological Evaluation in Adults
A multicenter, randomized, observer-blinded study, conducted in the United States, evaluated the immunogenicity of BOOSTRIX compared with the licensed comparator Tdap vaccine (Sanofi Pasteur SA). Vaccines were administered as a single-dose booster to adults 19 to 64 years of age (N = 2,284), who had not received a tetanus-diphtheria booster within 5 years. The immune responses to each of the antigens contained in BOOSTRIX were evaluated in sera obtained approximately 1 month after administration. Approximately 33% of patients were 19 to 29 years of age, 33% were 30 to 49 years of age and 34% were 50 to 64 years of age. Among subjects in the combined vaccine groups, 62% were female; 84% of subjects were Caucasian, 8% Black, 1% Asian, and 7% were of other racial groups.
Response to Tetanus and Diphtheria Toxoids: The antibody responses to the tetanus and diphtheria toxoids of

BOOSTRIX compared with the control Tdap vaccine are shown in Table 7. One month after a single dose, anti-tetanus and anti-diphtheria seroprotective rates (≥0.1 IU/mL) were comparable between BOOSTRIX and the control Tdap vaccine.

[See table 7 at top of previous page]

Response to Pertussis Antigens: The GMCs and booster response rates to the pertussis antigens are shown in Table 8. For the FHA and pertactin antigens, the lower limit of the 95% CI for the booster responses exceeded the pre-defined limit of 80% demonstrating an acceptable booster response following BOOSTRIX. The PT antigen booster response lower limit of the 95% CI (74.9%) did not exceed the pre-defined limit of 80%.

[See table 8 on previous page]

The GMCs to each of the pertussis antigens 1 month following a single dose of BOOSTRIX in the US adult study were compared with the GMCs of infants following a 3-dose primary series of INFANRIX administered at 3, 4, and 5 months of age. Table 9 presents the results for the total immunogenicity cohort in both studies (vaccinated subjects with serology data available for at least one pertussis antigen). These infants were a subset of those who formed the cohort for the German household contact study in which the efficacy of INFANRIX was demonstrated *[see Clinical Studies (14.1)]*. Although a serologic correlate of protection for pertussis has not been established, anti-PT, anti-FHA, and anti-pertactin antibody concentrations of adults 1 month after a single dose of BOOSTRIX were non-inferior to those of infants following a primary vaccination series with INFANRIX.

Table 9. Ratio of GMCs to Pertussis Antigens Following One Dose of BOOSTRIX in Adults 19 to 64 Years of Age as Compared With 3 Doses of INFANRIX in Infants (Total Immunogenicity Cohort)

	GMC Ratio: BOOSTRIX/INFANRIX (95% CI)
Anti-PT	1.39 (1.32, 1.47)[a]
Anti-FHA	7.46 (6.86, 8.12)[a]
Anti-pertactin	3.56 (3.10, 4.08)[a]

GMC = geometric mean antibody concentration; CI = Confidence Interval.

Number of subjects for BOOSTRIX GMC evaluation: Anti-PT = 1,460, anti-FHA = 1,472, and anti-pertactin = 1,473.

Number of subjects for INFANRIX GMC evaluation: Anti-PT = 2,884, anti-FHA = 685, and anti-pertactin = 631.

[a]BOOSTRIX was non-inferior to INFANRIX (lower limit of 95% CI for the GMC ratio of BOOSTRIX/INFANRIX ≥0.67).

14.4 Concomitant Vaccine Administration

The concomitant use of BOOSTRIX and FLUARIX was evaluated in a multicenter, open-label, randomized, controlled study of 1,497 adults 19 to 64 years of age. In one group, subjects received BOOSTRIX and FLUARIX concurrently (n = 748). The other group received FLUARIX at the first visit, then 1 month later received BOOSTRIX (n = 749). Sera was obtained prior to and 1 month following concomitant or separate administration of BOOSTRIX and/or FLUARIX, as well as 1 month after the separate administration of FLUARIX.

Immune responses following concurrent administration of BOOSTRIX and FLUARIX were non-inferior to separate administration for diphtheria (seroprotection defined as ≥0.1 IU/mL), tetanus (seroprotection defined as ≥0.1 IU/mL and based on concentrations ≥1.0 IU/mL), pertussis toxin (PT) antigen (anti-PT GMC) and influenza antigens (percent of subjects with hemagglutination-inhibition [HI] antibody titer ≥1:40 and ≥4-fold rise in HI titer). Non-inferiority criteria were not met for the anti-pertussis antigens FHA and pertactin. The lower limit of the 95% CI of the GMC ratio was 0.64 for anti-FHA and 0.60 for anti-pertactin and the pre-specified limit was ≥0.67.

15 REFERENCES

1. Centers for Disease Control. Diphtheria, tetanus, and pertussis: Recommendations for vaccine use and other preventive measures — Recommendations of the Immunization Practices Advisory Committee (ACIP). *MMWR* 1991;40(RR-10):1-28.
2. Centers for Disease Control and Prevention. Preventing tetanus, diphtheria and pertussis among adults: Use of tetanus toxoid, reduced diphtheria toxoid and acellular pertussis vaccine: Recommendations of the Advisory Committee on Immunization Practices (ACIP) and Recommendation of ACIP, supported by the Healthcare Infection Control Practices Advisory Committee (HICPAC), for Use of Tdap Among Health-Care Personnel. *MMWR* 2006;55(RR-17):1-37.
3. Centers for Disease Control and Prevention. Preventing tetanus, diphtheria and pertussis among adolescents: Use of tetanus toxoid, reduced diphtheria toxoid and acellular pertussis vaccine: Recommendations of the Advisory Committee on Immunization Practices (ACIP). *MMWR* 2006;55(RR-3):1-43.
4. Institute of Medicine (IOM). Stratton KR, Howe CJ, Johnston RB, eds. *Adverse events associated with childhood vaccines. Evidence bearing on causality.* Washington, DC: National Academy Press; 1994.
5. Wassilak SGF, Roper MH, Kretsinger K, and Orenstein WA. Tetanus Toxoid. In: Plotkin SA, Orenstein WA, and Offit PA, eds. *Vaccines*. 5th ed. Saunders; 2008:805-839.
6. Department of Health and Human Services, Food and Drug Administration. Biological products; Bacterial vaccines and toxoids; Implementation of efficacy review; Proposed rule. *Federal Register* December 13, 1985;50(240):51002-51117.
7. Centers for Disease Control and Prevention. General Recommendations on Immunization. Recommendations of the Advisory Committee on Immunization Practices (ACIP). *MMWR* 2006;55(RR-15):1-48.
8. Vitek CR and Wharton M. Diphtheria Toxoid. In: Plotkin SA, Orenstein WA, and Offit PA, eds. *Vaccines*. 5th ed. Saunders; 2008:139-156.

16 HOW SUPPLIED/STORAGE AND HANDLING

BOOSTRIX is available in 0.5-mL single-dose vials and disposable prefilled TIP-LOK syringes.

Single-Dose Vials

NDC 58160-842-11 (package of 10)

Single-Dose Prefilled Disposable TIP-LOK Syringes (packaged without needles)

NDC 58160-842-32 (package of 1)

NDC 58160-842-46 (package of 5)

Store refrigerated between 2° and 8°C (36° and 46°F). Do not freeze. Discard if the vaccine has been frozen.

17 PATIENT COUNSELING INFORMATION

The patient, parent, or guardian should be:

- informed of the potential benefits and risks of immunization with BOOSTRIX.
- informed about the potential for adverse reactions that have been temporally associated with administration of BOOSTRIX or other vaccines containing similar components.
- instructed to report any adverse events to their healthcare provider.
- given the Vaccine Information Statements, which are required by the National Childhood Vaccine Injury Act of 1986 to be given prior to immunization. These materials are available free of charge at the Centers for Disease Control and Prevention (CDC) website (www.cdc.gov/vaccines).

BOOSTRIX, FLUARIX, INFANRIX, and TIP-LOK are registered trademarks of GlaxoSmithKline. ADACEL is a registered trademark of Sanofi Pasteur Limited.

Manufactured by **GlaxoSmithKline Biologicals**
Rixensart, Belgium, US License 1617, and
Novartis Vaccines and Diagnostics GmbH & Co. KG
Marburg, Germany, US License 1754
Distributed by **GlaxoSmithKline**
Research Triangle Park, NC 27709

©2009, GlaxoSmithKline. All rights reserved.

CEFTIN® Tablets ℞

[*sĕf´tin*]

(cefuroxime axetil tablets)

CEFTIN® for Oral Suspension ℞

(cefuroxime axetil powder for oral suspension)

To reduce the development of drug-resistant bacteria and maintain the effectiveness of CEFTIN and other antibacterial drugs, CEFTIN should be used only to treat or prevent infections that are proven or strongly suspected to be caused by bacteria.

DESCRIPTION

CEFTIN Tablets and CEFTIN for Oral Suspension contain cefuroxime as cefuroxime axetil. CEFTIN is a semisynthetic, broad-spectrum cephalosporin antibiotic for oral administration.

Chemically, cefuroxime axetil, the 1-(acetyloxy) ethyl ester of cefuroxime, is (*RS*)-1-hydroxyethyl (6*R*,7*R*)-7-[2-(2-furyl)glyoxyl-amido]-3-(hydroxymethyl)-8-oxo-5-thia-1-azabicyclo[4.2.0]-oct-2-ene-2-carboxylate, 7^2-(*Z*)-(*O*-methyloxime), 1-acetate 3-carbamate. Its molecular formula is $C_{20}H_{22}N_4O_{10}S$, and it has a molecular weight of 510.48.

Cefuroxime axetil is in the amorphous form.

CEFTIN Tablets are film-coated and contain the equivalent of 250 or 500 mg of cefuroxime as cefuroxime axetil. CEFTIN Tablets contain the inactive ingredients colloidal silicon dioxide, croscarmellose sodium, hydrogenated vegetable oil, hypromellose, methylparaben, microcrystalline cellulose, propylene glycol, propylparaben, sodium benzoate, sodium lauryl sulfate, and titanium dioxide.

CEFTIN for Oral Suspension, when reconstituted with water, provides the equivalent of 125 mg or 250 mg of cefuroxime (as cefuroxime axetil) per 5 mL of suspension. CEFTIN for Oral Suspension contains the inactive ingredients acesulfame potassium, aspartame, povidone K30, stearic acid, sucrose, tutti-frutti flavoring, and xanthan gum.

CLINICAL PHARMACOLOGY

Absorption and Metabolism: After oral administration, cefuroxime axetil is absorbed from the gastrointestinal tract and rapidly hydrolyzed by nonspecific esterases in the intestinal mucosa and blood to cefuroxime. Cefuroxime is subsequently distributed throughout the extracellular fluids. The axetil moiety is metabolized to acetaldehyde and acetic acid.

Pharmacokinetics: Approximately 50% of serum cefuroxime is bound to protein. Serum pharmacokinetic parameters for CEFTIN Tablets and CEFTIN for Oral Suspension are shown in Tables 1 and 2.

[See table 1 at top of next page]
[See table 2 on next page]

Comparative Pharmacokinetic Properties: A 250 mg/5 mL-dose of CEFTIN Suspension is bioequivalent to 2 times 125 mg/5 mL-dose of CEFTIN Suspension when administered with food (see Table 3). **CEFTIN for Oral Suspension was not bioequivalent to CEFTIN Tablets when tested in healthy adults. The tablet and powder for oral suspension formulations are NOT substitutable on a milligram-per-milligram basis.** The area under the curve for the suspension averaged 91% of that for the tablet, and the peak plasma concentration for the suspension averaged 71% of the peak plasma concentration of the tablets. Therefore, the safety and effectiveness of both the tablet and oral suspension formulations had to be established in separate clinical trials.

[See table 3 at top of next page]

Food Effect on Pharmacokinetics: Absorption of the tablet is greater when taken after food (absolute bioavailability of CEFTIN Tablets increases from 37% to 52%). Despite this difference in absorption, the clinical and bacteriologic responses of patients were independent of food intake at the time of tablet administration in 2 studies where this was assessed.

All pharmacokinetic and clinical effectiveness and safety studies in pediatric patients using the suspension formulation were conducted in the fed state. No data are available on the absorption kinetics of the suspension formulation when administered to fasted pediatric patients.

Renal Excretion: Cefuroxime is excreted unchanged in the urine; in adults, approximately 50% of the administered dose is recovered in the urine within 12 hours. The pharmacokinetics of cefuroxime in the urine of pediatric patients have not been studied at this time. Until further data are available, the renal pharmacokinetic properties of cefuroxime axetil established in adults should not be extrapolated to pediatric patients.

Because cefuroxime is renally excreted, the serum half-life is prolonged in patients with reduced renal function. In a study of 20 elderly patients (mean age = 83.9 years) having a mean creatinine clearance of 34.9 mL/min, the mean serum elimination half-life was 3.5 hours. Despite the lower elimination of cefuroxime in geriatric patients, dosage adjustment based on age is not necessary (see PRECAUTIONS: Geriatric Use).

Microbiology: The in vivo bactericidal activity of cefuroxime axetil is due to cefuroxime's binding to essential target proteins and the resultant inhibition of cell-wall synthesis.

Cefuroxime has bactericidal activity against a wide range of common pathogens, including many beta-lactamase–producing strains. Cefuroxime is stable to many bacterial beta-lactamases, especially plasmid-mediated enzymes that are commonly found in enterobacteriaceae.

Cefuroxime has been demonstrated to be active against most strains of the following microorganisms both in vitro and in clinical infections as described in the INDICATIONS AND USAGE (see INDICATIONS AND USAGE).

Aerobic Gram-Positive Microorganisms:

Staphylococcus aureus (including beta-lactamase–producing strains)
Streptococcus pneumoniae
Streptococcus pyogenes

Aerobic Gram-Negative Microorganisms:

Escherichia coli
Haemophilus influenzae (including beta-lactamase–producing strains)
Haemophilus parainfluenzae
Klebsiella pneumoniae
Moraxella catarrhalis (including beta-lactamase–producing strains)

Neisseria gonorrhoeae (including beta-lactamase–producing strains)

Spirochetes:

Borrelia burgdorferi

Cefuroxime has been shown to be active in vitro against most strains of the following microorganisms; however, the clinical significance of these findings is unknown.

Cefuroxime exhibits in vitro minimum inhibitory concentrations (MICs) of 4.0 mcg/mL or less (systemic susceptible breakpoint) against most (≥90%) strains of the following microorganisms; however, the safety and effectiveness of cefuroxime in treating clinical infections due to these microorganisms have not been established in adequate and well-controlled trials.

Aerobic Gram-Positive Microorganisms:

Staphylococcus epidermidis
Staphylococcus saprophyticus
Streptococcus agalactiae

NOTE: *Listeria monocytogenes* and certain strains of enterococci, e.g., *Enterococcus faecalis* (formerly *Streptococcus faecalis*), are resistant to cefuroxime. Methicillin-resistant staphylococci are resistant to cefuroxime.

Aerobic Gram-Negative Microorganisms:

Morganella morganii
Proteus inconstans
Proteus mirabilis
Providencia rettgeri

NOTE: *Pseudomonas* spp., *Campylobacter* spp., *Acinetobacter calcoaceticus*, *Legionella* spp., and most strains of *Serratia* spp. and *Proteus vulgaris* are resistant to most first- and second-generation cephalosporins. Some strains of *Morganella morganii*, *Enterobacter cloacae*, and *Citrobacter* spp. have been shown by in vitro tests to be resistant to cefuroxime and other cephalosporins.

Anaerobic Microorganisms:

Peptococcus niger

NOTE: Most strains of *Clostridium difficile* and *Bacteroides fragilis* are resistant to cefuroxime.

Susceptibility Tests: *Dilution Techniques:* Quantitative methods that are used to determine MICs provide reproducible estimates of the susceptibility of bacteria to antimicrobial compounds. One such standardized procedure uses a standardized dilution method[1] (broth, agar, or microdilution) or equivalent with cefuroxime powder. The MIC values obtained should be interpreted according to the following criteria:

MIC (mcg/mL)	Interpretation
≤4	(S) Susceptible
8-16	(I) Intermediate
≥32	(R) Resistant

A report of "Susceptible" indicates that the pathogen, if in the blood, is likely to be inhibited by usually achievable concentrations of the antimicrobial compound in blood. A report of "Intermediate" indicates that inhibitory concentrations of the antibiotic may be achieved if high dosage is used or if the infection is confined to tissues or fluids in which high antibiotic concentrations are attained. This category also provides a buffer zone that prevents small, uncontrolled technical factors from causing major discrepancies in interpretation. A report of "Resistant" indicates that usually achievable concentrations of the antimicrobial compound in the blood are unlikely to be inhibitory and that other therapy should be selected.

Standardized susceptibility test procedures require the use of laboratory control microorganisms. Standard cefuroxime powder should give the following MIC values:

Microorganism	MIC (mcg/mL)
Escherichia coli ATCC 25922	2-8
Staphylococcus aureus ATCC 29213	0.5-2

Diffusion Techniques: Quantitative methods that require measurement of zone diameters provide estimates of the susceptibility of bacteria to antimicrobial compounds. One such standardized procedure[2] that has been recommended (for use with disks) to test the susceptibility of microorganisms to cefuroxime uses the 30-mcg cefuroxime disk. Interpretation involves correlation of the diameter obtained in the disk test with the MIC for cefuroxime.

Reports from the laboratory providing results of the standard single-disk susceptibility test with a 30-mcg cefuroxime disk should be interpreted according to the following criteria:

Zone Diameter (mm)	Interpretation
≥23	(S) Susceptible
15-22	(I) Intermediate
≤14	(R) Resistant

Interpretation should be as stated above for results using dilution techniques.

Table 1. Postprandial Pharmacokinetics of Cefuroxime Administered as CEFTIN Tablets to Adults[a]

Dose[b] (Cefuroxime Equivalent)	Peak Plasma Concentration (mcg/mL)	Time of Peak Plasma Concentration (hr)	Mean Elimination Half-Life (hr)	AUC (mcg-hr/mL)
125 mg	2.1	2.2	1.2	6.7
250 mg	4.1	2.5	1.2	12.9
500 mg	7.0	3.0	1.2	27.4
1,000 mg	13.6	2.5	1.3	50.0

[a]Mean values of 12 healthy adult volunteers.
[b]Drug administered immediately after a meal.

Table 2. Postprandial Pharmacokinetics of Cefuroxime Administered as CEFTIN for Oral Suspension to Pediatric Patients[a]

Dose[b] (Cefuroxime Equivalent)	n	Peak Plasma Concentration (mcg/mL)	Time of Peak Plasma Concentration (hr)	Mean Elimination Half-Life (hr)	AUC (mcg-hr/mL)
10 mg/kg	8	3.3	3.6	1.4	12.4
15 mg/kg	12	5.1	2.7	1.9	22.5
20 mg/kg	8	7.0	3.1	1.9	32.8

[a]Mean age = 23 months.
[b]Drug administered with milk or milk products.

Table 3. Pharmacokinetics of Cefuroxime Administered as 250 mg/5 mL or 2 × 125 mg/5 mL CEFTIN for Oral Suspension to Adults[a] With Food

Dose (Cefuroxime Equivalent)	Peak Plasma Concentration (mcg/mL)	Time of Peak Plasma Concentration (hr)	Mean Elimination Half-Life (hr)	AUC (mcg-hr/mL)
250 mg/5 mL	2.23	3	1.40	8.92
2 × 125 mg/5 mL	2.37	3	1.44	9.75

[b] Mean values of 18 healthy adult volunteers.

As with standard dilution techniques, diffusion methods require the use of laboratory control microorganisms. The 30-mcg cefuroxime disk provides the following zone diameters in these laboratory test quality control strains:

Microorganism	Zone Diameter (mm)
Escherichia coli ATCC 25922	20-26
Staphylococcus aureus ATCC 25923	27-35

INDICATIONS AND USAGE

NOTE: CEFTIN TABLETS AND CEFTIN FOR ORAL SUSPENSION ARE NOT BIOEQUIVALENT AND ARE NOT SUBSTITUTABLE ON A MILLIGRAM-PER-MILLIGRAM BASIS (SEE CLINICAL PHARMACOLOGY).

CEFTIN Tablets: CEFTIN Tablets are indicated for the treatment of patients with mild to moderate infections caused by susceptible strains of the designated microorganisms in the conditions listed below:

1. **Pharyngitis/Tonsillitis** caused by *Streptococcus pyogenes*.
   NOTE: The usual drug of choice in the treatment and prevention of streptococcal infections, including the prophylaxis of rheumatic fever, is penicillin given by the intramuscular route. CEFTIN Tablets are generally effective in the eradication of streptococci from the nasopharynx; however, substantial data establishing the efficacy of cefuroxime in the subsequent prevention of rheumatic fever are not available. Please also note that in all clinical trials, all isolates had to be sensitive to both penicillin and cefuroxime. There are no data from adequate and well-controlled trials to demonstrate the effectiveness of cefuroxime in the treatment of penicillin-resistant strains of *Streptococcus pyogenes*.

2. **Acute Bacterial Otitis Media** caused by *Streptococcus pneumoniae*, *Haemophilus influenzae* (including beta-lactamase–producing strains), *Moraxella catarrhalis* (including beta-lactamase–producing strains), or *Streptococcus pyogenes*.

3. **Acute Bacterial Maxillary Sinusitis** caused by *Streptococcus pneumoniae* or *Haemophilus influenzae* (non-beta-lactamase–producing strains only) (see CLINICAL STUDIES).
   NOTE: In view of the insufficient numbers of isolates of beta-lactamase–producing strains of *Haemophilus influenzae* and *Moraxella catarrhalis* that were obtained from clinical trials with CEFTIN Tablets for patients with acute bacterial maxillary sinusitis, it was not possible to adequately evaluate the effectiveness of CEFTIN Tablets for sinus infections known, suspected, or considered potentially to be caused by beta-lactamase–producing *Haemophilus influenzae* or *Moraxella catarrhalis*.

4. **Acute Bacterial Exacerbations of Chronic Bronchitis and Secondary Bacterial Infections of Acute Bronchitis** caused by *Streptococcus pneumoniae*, *Haemophilus influenzae* (beta-lactamase negative strains), or *Haemophilus parainfluenzae* (beta-lactamase negative strains) (see DOSAGE AND ADMINISTRATION and CLINICAL STUDIES).

5. **Uncomplicated Skin and Skin-Structure Infections** caused by *Staphylococcus aureus* (including beta-lactamase–producing strains) or *Streptococcus pyogenes*.

6. **Uncomplicated Urinary Tract Infections** caused by *Escherichia coli* or *Klebsiella pneumoniae*.

7. **Uncomplicated Gonorrhea**, urethral and endocervical, caused by penicillinase-producing and non-penicillinase–producing strains of *Neisseria gonorrhoeae* and uncomplicated gonorrhea, rectal, in females, caused by non-penicillinase–producing strains of *Neisseria gonorrhoeae*.

8. **Early Lyme Disease (erythema migrans)** caused by *Borrelia burgdorferi*.

CEFTIN for Oral Suspension: CEFTIN for Oral Suspension is indicated for the treatment of pediatric patients 3 months to 12 years of age with mild to moderate infections caused by susceptible strains of the designated microorganisms in the conditions listed below. The safety and effectiveness of CEFTIN for Oral Suspension in the treatment of infections other than those specifically listed below have not been established either by adequate and well-controlled trials or by pharmacokinetic data with which to determine an effective and safe dosing regimen.

1. **Pharyngitis/Tonsillitis** caused by *Streptococcus pyogenes*.
   NOTE: The usual drug of choice in the treatment and prevention of streptococcal infections, including the prophylaxis of rheumatic fever, is penicillin given by the intramuscular route. CEFTIN for Oral Suspension is generally effective in the eradication of streptococci from the nasopharynx; however, substantial data establishing the efficacy of cefuroxime in the subsequent prevention of rheumatic fever are not available. Please also note that in all clinical trials, all isolates had to be sensitive to both penicillin and cefuroxime. There are no data from adequate and well-controlled trials to demonstrate the effectiveness of cefuroxime in the treatment of penicillin-resistant strains of *Streptococcus pyogenes*.

2. **Acute Bacterial Otitis Media** caused by *Streptococcus pneumoniae*, *Haemophilus influenzae* (including beta-lactamase–producing strains), *Moraxella catarrhalis* (including beta-lactamase–producing strains), or *Streptococcus pyogenes*.

3. **Impetigo** caused by *Staphylococcus aureus* (including beta-lactamase–producing strains) or *Streptococcus pyogenes*.

To reduce the development of drug-resistant bacteria and maintain the effectiveness of CEFTIN and other antibacterial drugs, CEFTIN should be used only to treat or prevent infections that are proven or strongly suspected to be caused by susceptible bacteria. When culture and susceptibility information are available, they should be considered in selecting or modifying antibacterial therapy. In the absence of such data, local epidemiology and susceptibility patterns may contribute to the empiric selection of therapy.

CONTRAINDICATIONS

CEFTIN products are contraindicated in patients with known allergy to the cephalosporin group of antibiotics.

WARNINGS

CEFTIN TABLETS AND CEFTIN FOR ORAL SUSPENSION ARE NOT BIOEQUIVALENT AND ARE THEREFORE NOT SUBSTITUTABLE ON A MILLIGRAM-PER-MILLIGRAM BASIS (SEE CLINICAL PHARMACOLOGY).

BEFORE THERAPY WITH CEFTIN PRODUCTS IS INSTITUTED, CAREFUL INQUIRY SHOULD BE MADE TO DETERMINE WHETHER THE PATIENT HAS HAD PREVIOUS HYPERSENSITIVITY REACTIONS TO CEFTIN PRODUCTS, OTHER CEPHALOSPORINS, PENICILLINS, OR OTHER DRUGS. IF THIS PRODUCT IS TO BE GIVEN TO PENICILLIN-SENSITIVE PATIENTS, CAUTION SHOULD BE EXERCISED BECAUSE CROSS-HYPERSENSITIVITY AMONG BETA-LACTAM ANTIBIOTICS HAS BEEN CLEARLY DOCUMENTED AND MAY OCCUR IN UP TO 10% OF PATIENTS WITH A HISTORY OF PENICILLIN ALLERGY. IF A CLINICALLY SIGNIFICANT ALLERGIC REACTION TO CEFTIN PRODUCTS OCCURS, DISCONTINUE THE DRUG AND INSTITUTE APPROPRIATE THERAPY. SERIOUS ACUTE HYPERSENSITIVITY REACTIONS MAY REQUIRE TREATMENT WITH EPINEPHRINE AND OTHER EMERGENCY MEASURES, INCLUDING OXYGEN, INTRAVENOUS FLUIDS, INTRAVENOUS ANTIHISTAMINES, CORTICOSTEROIDS, PRESSOR AMINES, AND AIRWAY MANAGEMENT, AS CLINICALLY INDICATED.

Clostridium difficile associated diarrhea (CDAD) has been reported with use of nearly all antibacterial agents, including CEFTIN, and may range in severity from mild diarrhea to fatal colitis. Treatment with antibacterial agents alters the normal flora of the colon leading to overgrowth of *C. difficile*.

C. difficile produces toxins A and B which contribute to the development of CDAD. Hypertoxin producing strains of *C. difficile* cause increased morbidity and mortality, as these infections can be refractory to antimicrobial therapy and may require colectomy. CDAD must be considered in all patients who present with diarrhea following antibiotic use. Careful medical history is necessary since CDAD has been reported to occur over 2 months after the administration of antibacterial agents.

If CDAD is suspected or confirmed, ongoing antibiotic use not directed against *C. difficile* may need to be discontinued. Appropriate fluid and electrolyte management, protein supplementation, antibiotic treatment of *C. difficile*, and surgical evaluation should be instituted as clinically indicated.

PRECAUTIONS

General: As with other broad-spectrum antibiotics, prolonged administration of cefuroxime axetil may result in overgrowth of nonsusceptible microorganisms. If superinfection occurs during therapy, appropriate measures should be taken.

Cephalosporins, including cefuroxime axetil, should be given with caution to patients receiving concurrent treatment with potent diuretics because these diuretics are suspected of adversely affecting renal function.

Cefuroxime axetil, as with other broad-spectrum antibiotics, should be prescribed with caution in individuals with a history of colitis. The safety and effectiveness of cefuroxime axetil have not been established in patients with gastrointestinal malabsorption. Patients with gastrointestinal malabsorption were excluded from participating in clinical trials of cefuroxime axetil.

Cephalosporins may be associated with a fall in prothrombin activity. Those at risk include patients with renal or hepatic impairment or poor nutritional state, as well as patients receiving a protracted course of antimicrobial therapy, and patients previously stabilized on anticoagulant therapy. Prothrombin time should be monitored in patients at risk and exogenous Vitamin K administered as indicated. Prescribing CEFTIN in the absence of a proven or strongly suspected bacterial infection or a prophylactic indication is unlikely to provide benefit to the patient and increases the risk of the development of drug-resistant bacteria.

Diarrhea is a common problem caused by antibiotics which usually ends when the antibiotic is discontinued. Sometimes after starting treatment with antibiotics, patients can develop watery and bloody stools (with or without stomach cramps and fever) even as late as 2 or more months after having taken the last dose of the antibiotic. If this occurs, patients should contact their physician as soon as possible.

Information for Patients/Caregivers (Pediatric): *Phenylketonurics:* CEFTIN for Oral Suspension 125 mg/5 mL contains phenylalanine 11.8 mg per 5 mL (1 teaspoonful) constituted suspension. CEFTIN for Oral Suspension 250 mg/5 mL contains phenylalanine 25.2 mg per 5 mL (1 teaspoonful) constituted suspension.

1. During clinical trials, the tablet was tolerated by pediatric patients old enough to swallow the cefuroxime axetil tablet whole. The crushed tablet has a strong, persistent, bitter taste and should not be administered to pediatric patients in this manner. Pediatric patients who cannot swallow the tablet whole should receive the oral suspension.
2. Discontinuation of therapy due to taste and/or problems of administering this drug occurred in 1.4% of pediatric patients given the oral suspension. Complaints about taste (which may impair compliance) occurred in 5% of pediatric patients.
3. Patients should be counseled that antibacterial drugs, including CEFTIN, should only be used to treat bacterial infections. They do not treat viral infections (e.g., the common cold). When CEFTIN is prescribed to treat a bacterial infection, patients should be told that although it is common to feel better early in the course of therapy, the medication should be taken exactly as directed. Skipping doses or not completing the full course of therapy may: (1) decrease the effectiveness of the immediate treatment, and (2) increase the likelihood that bacteria will develop resistance and will not be treatable by CEFTIN or other antibacterial drugs in the future.

Drug/Laboratory Test Interactions: A false-positive reaction for glucose in the urine may occur with copper reduction tests (Benedict's or Fehling's solution or with CLINITEST® tablets), but not with enzyme-based tests for glycosuria (e.g., CLINISTIX®). As a false-negative result may occur in the ferricyanide test, it is recommended that either the glucose oxidase or hexokinase method be used to determine blood/plasma glucose levels in patients receiving cefuroxime axetil. The presence of cefuroxime does not interfere with the assay of serum and urine creatinine by the alkaline picrate method.

Drug/Drug Interactions: Concomitant administration of probenecid with cefuroxime axetil tablets increases the area under the serum concentration versus time curve by 50%. The peak serum cefuroxime concentration after a 1.5-g single dose is greater when taken with 1 g of probenecid (mean = 14.8 mcg/mL) than without probenecid (mean = 12.2 mcg/mL).

Drugs that reduce gastric acidity may result in a lower bioavailability of CEFTIN compared with that of fasting state and tend to cancel the effect of postprandial absorption.

In common with other antibiotics, cefuroxime axetil may affect the gut flora, leading to lower estrogen reabsorption and reduced efficacy of combined oral estrogen/progesterone contraceptives.

Carcinogenesis, Mutagenesis, Impairment of Fertility: Although lifetime studies in animals have not been performed to evaluate carcinogenic potential, no mutagenic activity was found for cefuroxime axetil in a battery of bacterial mutation tests. Positive results were obtained in an in vitro chromosome aberration assay; however, negative results were found in an in vivo micronucleus test at doses up to 1.5 g/kg. Reproduction studies in rats at doses up to 1,000 mg/kg/day (9 times the recommended maximum human dose based on mg/m^2) have revealed no impairment of fertility.

Pregnancy: *Teratogenic Effects:* Pregnancy Category B. Reproduction studies have been performed in mice at doses up to 3,200 mg/kg/day (14 times the recommended maximum human dose based on mg/m^2) and in rats at doses up to 1,000 mg/kg/day (9 times the recommended maximum human dose based on mg/m^2) and have revealed no evidence of impaired fertility or harm to the fetus due to cefuroxime axetil. There are, however, no adequate and well-controlled studies in pregnant women. Because animal reproduction studies are not always predictive of human response, this drug should be used during pregnancy only if clearly needed.

Labor and Delivery: Cefuroxime axetil has not been studied for use during labor and delivery.

Nursing Mothers: Because cefuroxime is excreted in human milk, consideration should be given to discontinuing nursing temporarily during treatment with cefuroxime axetil.

Pediatric Use: The safety and effectiveness of CEFTIN have been established for pediatric patients aged 3 months to 12 years for acute bacterial maxillary sinusitis based upon its approval in adults. Use of CEFTIN in pediatric patients is supported by pharmacokinetic and safety data in adults and pediatric patients, and by clinical and microbiological data from adequate and well-controlled studies of the treatment of acute bacterial maxillary sinusitis in adults and of acute otitis media with effusion in pediatric patients. It is also supported by postmarketing adverse events sur-

veillance (see CLINICAL PHARMACOLOGY, INDICATIONS AND USAGE, ADVERSE REACTIONS, DOSAGE AND ADMINISTRATION, and CLINICAL STUDIES).

Geriatric Use: Of the total number of subjects who received cefuroxime axetil in 20 clinical studies of CEFTIN, 375 were 65 and older while 151 were 75 and older. No overall differences in safety or effectiveness were observed between these subjects and younger adult subjects. The geriatric patients reported somewhat fewer gastrointestinal events and less frequent vaginal candidiasis compared with patients aged 12 to 64 years old; however, no clinically significant differences were reported between the elderly and younger adult patients. Other reported clinical experience has not identified differences in responses between the elderly and younger adult patients.

ADVERSE REACTIONS

CEFTIN TABLETS IN CLINICAL TRIALS: Multiple-Dose Dosing Regimens: *7 to 10 Days Dosing:* Using multiple doses of cefuroxime axetil tablets, 912 patients were treated with cefuroxime axetil (125 to 500 mg twice daily). There were no deaths or permanent disabilities thought related to drug toxicity. Twenty (2.2%) patients discontinued medication due to adverse events thought by the investigators to be possibly, probably, or almost certainly related to drug toxicity. Seventeen (85%) of the 20 patients who discontinued therapy did so because of gastrointestinal disturbances, including diarrhea, nausea, vomiting, and abdominal pain. The percentage of cefuroxime axetil tablet-treated patients who discontinued study drug because of adverse events was very similar at daily doses of 1,000, 500, and 250 mg (2.3%, 2.1%, and 2.2%, respectively). However, the incidence of gastrointestinal adverse events increased with the higher recommended doses.

The following adverse events were thought by the investigators to be possibly, probably, or almost certainly related to cefuroxime axetil tablets in multiple-dose clinical trials (n = 912 cefuroxime axetil-treated patients).

Table 4. Adverse Reactions—CEFTIN Tablets Multiple-Dose Dosing Regimens—Clinical Trials

Incidence ≥1%	Diarrhea/loose stools	3.7%
	Nausea/vomiting	3.0%
	Transient elevation in AST	2.0%
	Transient elevation in ALT	1.6%
	Eosinophilia	1.1%
	Transient elevation in LDH	1.0%
Incidence <1% but >0.1%	Abdominal pain	
	Abdominal cramps	
	Flatulence	
	Indigestion	
	Headache	
	Vaginitis	
	Vulvar itch	
	Rash	
	Hives	
	Itch	
	Dysuria	
	Chills	
	Chest pain	
	Shortness of breath	
	Mouth ulcers	
	Swollen tongue	
	Sleepiness	
	Thirst	
	Anorexia	
	Positive Coombs test	

5-Day Experience (see CLINICAL STUDIES): In clinical trials using CEFTIN in a dose of 250 mg twice daily in the treatment of secondary bacterial infections of acute bronchitis, 399 patients were treated for 5 days and 402 patients were treated for 10 days. No difference in the occurrence of adverse events was found between the 2 regimens.

In Clinical Trials for Early Lyme Disease With 20 Days Dosing: Two multicenter trials assessed cefuroxime axetil tablets 500 mg twice a day for 20 days. The most common drug-related adverse experiences were diarrhea (10.6% of patients), Jarisch-Herxheimer reaction (5.6%), and vaginitis (5.4%). Other adverse experiences occurred with frequencies comparable to those reported with 7 to 10 days dosing.

Single-Dose Regimen for Uncomplicated Gonorrhea: In clinical trials using a single dose of cefuroxime axetil tablets, 1,061 patients were treated with the recommended dosage of cefuroxime axetil (1,000 mg) for the treatment of uncomplicated gonorrhea. There were no deaths or permanent disabilities thought related to drug toxicity in these studies.

The following adverse events were thought by the investigators to be possibly, probably, or almost certainly related to cefuroxime axetil in 1,000-mg single-dose clinical trials of cefuroxime axetil tablets in the treatment of uncomplicated gonorrhea conducted in the United States.

Table 5. Adverse Reactions—CEFTIN Tablets 1-g Single-Dose Regimen for Uncomplicated Gonorrhea—Clinical Trials

Incidence ≥1%	Nausea/vomiting	6.8%
	Diarrhea	4.2%

Incidence <1% but >0.1%	Abdominal pain
	Dyspepsia
	Erythema
	Rash
	Pruritus
	Vaginal candidiasis
	Vaginal itch
	Vaginal discharge
	Headache
	Dizziness
	Somnolence
	Muscle cramps
	Muscle stiffness
	Muscle spasm of neck
	Tightness/pain in chest
	Bleeding/pain in urethra
	Kidney pain
	Tachycardia
	Lockjaw-type reaction

CEFTIN FOR ORAL SUSPENSION IN CLINICAL TRIALS

In clinical trials using multiple doses of cefuroxime axetil powder for oral suspension, pediatric patients (96.7% of whom were younger than 12 years of age) were treated with the recommended dosages of cefuroxime axetil (20 to 30 mg/kg/day divided twice a day up to a maximum dose of 500 or 1,000 mg/day, respectively). There were no deaths or permanent disabilities in any of the patients in these studies. Eleven US patients (1.2%) discontinued medication due to adverse events thought by the investigators to be possibly, probably, or almost certainly related to drug toxicity. The discontinuations were primarily for gastrointestinal disturbances, usually diarrhea or vomiting. During clinical trials, discontinuation of therapy due to the taste and/or problems with administering this drug occurred in 13 (1.4%) pediatric patients enrolled at centers in the United States.

The following adverse events were thought by the investigators to be possibly, probably, or almost certainly related to cefuroxime axetil for oral suspension in multiple-dose clinical trials (n = 931 cefuroxime axetil-treated US patients).

Table 6. Adverse Reactions—CEFTIN for Oral Suspension Multiple-Dose Dosing Regimens—Clinical Trials

Incidence ≥1%	Diarrhea/loose stools	8.6%
	Dislike of taste	5.0%
	Diaper rash	3.4%
	Nausea/vomiting	2.6%

Incidence <1% but >0.1%	Abdominal pain
	Flatulence
	Gastrointestinal infection
	Candidiasis
	Vaginal irritation
	Rash
	Hyperactivity
	Irritable behavior
	Eosinophilia
	Positive direct Coombs test
	Elevated liver enzymes
	Viral illness
	Upper respiratory infection
	Sinusitis
	Cough
	Urinary tract infection
	Joint swelling
	Arthralgia
	Fever
	Ptyalism

POSTMARKETING EXPERIENCE WITH CEFTIN

In addition to adverse events reported during clinical trials, the following events have been identified during clinical practice in patients treated with CEFTIN Tablets or with CEFTIN for Oral Suspension and were reported spontaneously. Data are generally insufficient to allow an estimate of incidence or to establish causation.

Table 7. CEFTIN Tablets
(May be administered without regard to meals.)

Population/Infection	Dosage	Duration (days)
Adolescents and Adults (13 years and older)		
Pharyngitis/tonsillitis	250 mg b.i.d.	10
Acute bacterial maxillary sinusitis	250 mg b.i.d.	10
Acute bacterial exacerbations of chronic bronchitis	250 or 500 mg b.i.d.	10[a]
Secondary bacterial infections of acute bronchitis	250 or 500 mg b.i.d.	5-10
Uncomplicated skin and skin-structure infections	250 or 500 mg b.i.d.	10
Uncomplicated urinary tract infections	250 mg b.i.d.	7-10
Uncomplicated gonorrhea	1,000 mg once	single dose
Early Lyme disease	500 mg b.i.d.	20
Pediatric Patients (who can swallow tablets whole)		
Acute otitis media	250 mg b.i.d.	10
Acute bacterial maxillary sinusitis	250 mg b.i.d.	10

[a] The safety and effectiveness of CEFTIN administered for less than 10 days in patients with acute exacerbations of chronic bronchitis have not been established.

Table 8. CEFTIN for Oral Suspension
(Must be administered with food. Shake well each time before using.)

Population/Infection	Dosage	Daily Maximum Dose	Duration (days)
Pediatric Patients (3 months to 12 years)			
Pharyngitis/tonsillitis	20 mg/kg/day divided b.i.d.	500 mg	10
Acute otitis media	30 mg/kg/day divided b.i.d.	1,000 mg	10
Acute bacterial maxillary sinusitis	30 mg/kg/day divided b.i.d.	1,000 mg	10
Impetigo	30 mg/kg/day divided b.i.d.	1,000 mg	10

General: The following hypersensitivity reactions have been reported: Anaphylaxis, angioedema, pruritus, rash, serum sickness-like reaction, urticaria.
Gastrointestinal: Pseudomembranous colitis (see WARNINGS).
Hematologic: Hemolytic anemia, leukopenia, pancytopenia, thrombocytopenia, and increased prothrombin time.
Hepatic: Hepatic impairment including hepatitis and cholestasis, jaundice.
Neurologic: Seizure.
Skin: Erythema multiforme, Stevens-Johnson syndrome, toxic epidermal necrolysis.
Urologic: Renal dysfunction.

CEPHALOSPORIN-CLASS ADVERSE REACTIONS

In addition to the adverse reactions listed above that have been observed in patients treated with cefuroxime axetil, the following adverse reactions and altered laboratory tests have been reported for cephalosporin-class antibiotics: Toxic nephropathy, aplastic anemia, hemorrhage, increased BUN, increased creatinine, false-positive test for urinary glucose, increased alkaline phosphatase, neutropenia, elevated bilirubin, and agranulocytosis.

Several cephalosporins have been implicated in triggering seizures, particularly in patients with renal impairment when the dosage was not reduced (see DOSAGE AND ADMINISTRATION and OVERDOSAGE). If seizures associated with drug therapy occur, the drug should be discontinued. Anticonvulsant therapy can be given if clinically indicated.

OVERDOSAGE

Overdosage of cephalosporins can cause cerebral irritation leading to convulsions. Serum levels of cefuroxime can be reduced by hemodialysis and peritoneal dialysis.

DOSAGE AND ADMINISTRATION

NOTE: CEFTIN TABLETS AND CEFTIN FOR ORAL SUSPENSION ARE NOT BIOEQUIVALENT AND ARE NOT SUBSTITUTABLE ON A MILLIGRAM-PER-MILLIGRAM BASIS (SEE CLINICAL PHARMACOLOGY).
[See table 7 above]
CEFTIN for Oral Suspension: CEFTIN for Oral Suspension may be administered to pediatric patients ranging in age from 3 months to 12 years, according to dosages in Table 8:
[See table 8 above]
Patients With Renal Failure: The safety and efficacy of cefuroxime axetil in patients with renal failure have not been established. Since cefuroxime is renally eliminated, its half-life will be prolonged in patients with renal failure.
Directions for Mixing CEFTIN for Oral Suspension: Prepare a suspension at the time of dispensing as follows:
1. Shake the bottle to loosen the powder.
2. Remove the cap.
3. Add the total amount of water for reconstitution (see Table 9) and replace the cap.

4. Invert the bottle and vigorously rock the bottle from side to side so that water rises through the powder.
5. Once the sound of the powder against the bottle disappears, turn the bottle upright and vigorously shake it in a diagonal direction.
[See table 9 at top of next page]
NOTE: SHAKE THE ORAL SUSPENSION WELL BEFORE EACH USE. Replace cap securely after each opening. Store the reconstituted suspension between 2° and 8°C (36° and 46°F) (in a refrigerator). DISCARD AFTER 10 DAYS.

HOW SUPPLIED

CEFTIN Tablets: CEFTIN Tablets, 250 mg of cefuroxime (as cefuroxime axetil), are white, capsule-shaped, film-coated tablets engraved with "GX ES7" on one side and blank on the other side as follows:
20 Tablets/Bottle   NDC 0173-0387-00
CEFTIN Tablets, 500 mg of cefuroxime (as cefuroxime axetil), are white, capsule-shaped, film-coated tablets engraved with "GX EG2" on one side and blank on the other side as follows:
20 Tablets/Bottle   NDC 0173-0394-00
Store the tablets between 15° and 30°C (59° and 86°F). Replace cap securely after each opening.
CEFTIN for Oral Suspension: CEFTIN for Oral Suspension is provided as dry, white to off-white, tutti-frutti–flavored powder. When reconstituted as directed, CEFTIN for Oral Suspension provides the equivalent of 125 mg or 250 mg of cefuroxime (as cefuroxime axetil) per 5 mL of suspension. It is supplied in amber glass bottles as follows:
125 mg/5 mL:
100-mL Suspension   NDC 0173-0740-00
250 mg/5 mL:
50-mL Suspension   NDC 0173-0741-10
100-mL Suspension   NDC 0173-0741-00
Before reconstitution, store dry powder between 2° and 30°C (36° and 86°F).
After reconstitution, immediately store suspension between 2° and 8°C (36° and 46°F), in a refrigerator. DISCARD AFTER 10 DAYS.

CLINICAL STUDIES

Ceftin Tablets: *Acute Bacterial Maxillary Sinusitis:* One adequate and well-controlled study was performed in patients with acute bacterial maxillary sinusitis. In this study each patient had a maxillary sinus aspirate collected by sinus puncture before treatment was initiated for presumptive acute bacterial sinusitis. All patients had to have radiographic and clinical evidence of acute maxillary sinusitis. As shown in the following summary of the study, the general clinical effectiveness of CEFTIN Tablets was comparable to an oral antimicrobial agent that contained a specific betalactamase inhibitor in treating acute maxillary sinusitis. However, sufficient microbiology data were obtained to demonstrate the effectiveness of CEFTIN Tablets in treating

Table 9. Amount of Water Required for Reconstitution of Labeled Volumes of CEFTIN for Oral Suspension

CEFTIN for Oral Suspension	Labeled Volume After Reconstitution	Amount of Water Required for Reconstitution
125 mg/5 mL	100 mL	37 mL
250 mg/5 mL	50 mL	19 mL
	100 mL	35 mL

Table 10. Clinical Effectiveness of CEFTIN Tablets Compared to Beta-Lactamase Inhibitor-Containing Control Drug in the Treatment of Acute Bacterial Maxillary Sinusitis

	US Patients[a]		South American Patients[b]	
	CEFTIN (n = 49)	Control (n = 43)	CEFTIN (n = 87)	Control (n = 89)
Clinical success (cure + improvement)	65%	53%	77%	74%
Clinical cure	53%	44%	72%	64%
Clinical improvement	12%	9%	5%	10%

[a] 95% Confidence interval around the success difference [-0.08, +0.32].
[b] 95% Confidence interval around the success difference [-0.10, +0.16].

Table 11. Clinical Effectiveness of CEFTIN Tablets Compared to Doxycycline in the Treatment of Early Lyme Disease

	Part I (1 Month Posttreatment)[a]		Part II (1 Year Posttreatment)[b]	
	CEFTIN (n = 125)	Doxycycline (n = 108)	CEFTIN (n = 105[c])	Doxycycline (n = 83[c])
Satisfactory clinical outcome[d]	91%	93%	84%	87%
Clinical cure/success	72%	73%	73%	73%
Clinical improvement	19%	19%	10%	13%

[a] 95% confidence interval around the satisfactory difference for Part I (-0.08, +0.05).
[b] 95% confidence interval around the satisfactory difference for Part II (-0.13, +0.07).
[c] n's include patients assessed as unsatisfactory clinical outcomes (failure + recurrence) in Part I (CEFTIN - 11 [5 failure, 6 recurrence]; doxycycline - 8 [6 failure, 2 recurrence]).
[d] Satisfactory clinical outcome includes cure + improvement (Part I) and success + improvement (Part II).

Table 12. Clinical Effectiveness of CEFTIN Tablets 250 mg Twice Daily in Secondary Bacterial Infections of Acute Bronchitis: Comparison of 5 Versus 10 Days' Treatment Duration

	CAE-516 and CAE-517[a]		CAEA4001 and CAEA4002[b]	
	5 Day (n = 127)	10 Day (n = 139)	5 Day (n = 173)	10 Day (n = 192)
Clinical success (cure + improvement)	80%	87%	84%	82%
Clinical cure	61%	70%	73%	72%
Clinical improvement	19%	17%	11%	10%

[a] 95% Confidence interval around the success difference [-0.164, +0.029].
[b] 95% Confidence interval around the success difference [-0.061, +0.103].

acute bacterial maxillary sinusitis due only to *Streptococcus pneumoniae* or non-beta-lactamase–producing *Haemophilus influenzae*. An insufficient number of beta-lactamase–producing *Haemophilus influenzae* and *Moraxella catarrhalis* isolates were obtained in this trial to adequately evaluate the effectiveness of CEFTIN Tablets in the treatment of acute bacterial maxillary sinusitis due to these 2 organisms. This study enrolled 317 adult patients, 132 patients in the United States and 185 patients in South America. Patients were randomized in a 1:1 ratio to cefuroxime axetil 250 mg twice daily or an oral antimicrobial agent that contained a specific beta-lactamase inhibitor. An intent-to-treat analysis of the submitted clinical data yielded the following results:
[See table 10 above]
In this trial and in a supporting maxillary puncture trial, 15 evaluable patients had non-beta-lactamase–producing *Haemophilus influenzae* as the identified pathogen. Ten (10) of these 15 patients (67%) had their pathogen (non-beta-lactamase–producing *Haemophilus influenzae*) eradicated. Eighteen (18) evaluable patients had *Streptococcus pneumoniae* as the identified pathogen. Fifteen (15) of these 18 patients (83%) had their pathogen (*Streptococcus pneumoniae*) eradicated.

Safety: The incidence of drug-related gastrointestinal adverse events was statistically significantly higher in the control arm (an oral antimicrobial agent that contained a specific beta-lactamase inhibitor) versus the cefuroxime axetil arm (12% versus 1%, respectively; *P* <.001), particularly drug-related diarrhea (8% versus 1%, respectively; *P* = .001).
Early Lyme Disease: Two adequate and well-controlled studies were performed in patients with early Lyme disease. In these studies all patients had to present with physician-documented erythema migrans, with or without systemic manifestations of infection. Patients were randomized in a 1:1 ratio to a 20-day course of treatment with cefuroxime axetil 500 mg twice daily or doxycycline 100 mg 3 times daily. Patients were assessed at 1 month posttreatment for success in treating early Lyme disease (Part I) and at 1 year posttreatment for success in preventing the progression to the sequelae of late Lyme disease (Part II).
A total of 355 adult patients (181 treated with cefuroxime axetil and 174 treated with doxycycline) were enrolled in the 2 studies. In order to objectively validate the clinical diagnosis of early Lyme disease in these patients, 2 approaches were used: 1) blinded expert reading of photo-

graphs, when available, of the pretreatment erythema migrans skin lesion; and 2) serologic confirmation (using enzyme-linked immunosorbent assay [ELISA] and immuno-blot assay ["Western" blot]) of the presence of antibodies specific to *Borrelia burgdorferi*, the etiologic agent of Lyme disease. By these procedures, it was possible to confirm the physician diagnosis of early Lyme disease in 281 (79%) of the 355 study patients. The efficacy data summarized below are specific to this "validated" patient subset, while the safety data summarized below reflect the entire patient population for the 2 studies.
Analysis of the submitted clinical data for evaluable patients in the "validated" patient subset yielded the following results:
[See table 11 at left]
CEFTIN and doxycycline were effective in prevention of the development of sequelae of late Lyme disease.
Safety: Drug-related adverse events affecting the skin were reported significantly more frequently by patients treated with doxycycline than by patients treated with cefuroxime axetil (12% versus 3%, respectively; *P* = .002), primarily reflecting the statistically significantly higher incidence of drug-related photosensitivity reactions in the doxycycline arm versus the cefuroxime axetil arm (9% versus 0%, respectively; *P*<.001). While the incidence of drug-related gastrointestinal adverse events was similar in the 2 treatment groups (cefuroxime axetil - 13%; doxycycline - 11%), the incidence of drug-related diarrhea was statistically significantly higher in the cefuroxime axetil arm versus the doxycycline arm (11% versus 3%, respectively; *P* = .005).
Secondary Bacterial Infections of Acute Bronchitis: Four randomized, controlled clinical studies were performed comparing 5 days versus 10 days of CEFTIN for the treatment of patients with secondary bacterial infections of acute bronchitis. These studies enrolled a total of 1,253 patients (CAE-516 n = 360; CAE-517 n = 177; CAEA4001 n = 362; CAEA4002 n = 354). The protocols for CAE-516 and CAE-517 were identical and compared CEFTIN 250 mg twice daily for 5 days, CEFTIN 250 mg twice daily for 10 days, and AUGMENTIN® 500 mg 3 times daily for 10 days. These 2 studies were conducted simultaneously. CAEA4001 and CAEA4002 compared CEFTIN 250 mg twice daily for 5 days, CEFTIN 250 mg twice daily for 10 days, and CECLOR® 250 mg 3 times daily for 10 days. They were otherwise identical to CAE-516 and CAE-517 and were conducted over the following 2 years. Patients were required to have polymorphonuclear cells present on the Gram stain of their screening sputum specimen, but isolation of a bacterial pathogen from the sputum culture was not required for inclusion. The following table demonstrates the results of the clinical outcome analysis of the pooled studies CAE-516/CAE-517 and CAEA4001/CAEA4002, respectively:
[See table 12 at left]
The response rates for patients who were both clinically and bacteriologically evaluable were consistent with those reported for the clinically evaluable patients.
Safety: In these clinical trials, 399 patients were treated with CEFTIN for 5 days and 402 patients with CEFTIN for 10 days. No difference in the occurrence of adverse events was observed between the 2 regimens.

REFERENCES

1. National Committee for Clinical Laboratory Standards. *Methods for Dilution Antimicrobial Susceptibility Tests for Bacteria that Grow Aerobically*. 3rd ed. Approved Standard NCCLS Document M7-A3, Vol. 13, No. 25. Villanova, Pa: NCCLS; 1993.
2. National Committee for Clinical Laboratory Standards. *Performance Standards for Antimicrobial Disk Susceptibility Tests*. 4th ed. Approved Standard NCCLS Document M2-A4, Vol. 10, No. 7. Villanova, Pa: NCCLS; 1990.
GlaxoSmithKline Research Triangle Park, NC 27709
CEFTIN and AUGMENTIN are registered trademarks of GlaxoSmithKline.
CLINITEST and CLINISTIX are registered trademarks of Ames Division, Miles Laboratories, Inc.
©2010, GlaxoSmithKline. All rights reserved.
January 2010   CFT-1PI

CERVARIX   ℞
[cer-va-rix]
[Human Papillomavirus Bivalent (Types 16 and 18) Vaccine, Recombinant]
Suspension for Intramuscular Injection

HIGHLIGHTS OF PRESCRIBING INFORMATION
These highlights do not include all the information needed to use CERVARIX safely and effectively. See full prescribing information for CERVARIX.
CERVARIX [Human Papillomavirus Bivalent (Types 16 and 18) Vaccine, Recombinant]
Suspension for Intramuscular Injection
Initial U.S. Approval: 2009
———————INDICATIONS AND USAGE———————
CERVARIX is a vaccine indicated for the prevention of the following diseases caused by oncogenic human papillomavirus (HPV) types 16 and 18:

- cervical cancer,
- cervical intraepithelial neoplasia (CIN) grade 2 or worse and adenocarcinoma *in situ*, and
- cervical intraepithelial neoplasia (CIN) grade 1. (1.1)

CERVARIX is approved for use in females 10 through 25 years of age.

Limitations of Use and Effectiveness (1.2)

- CERVARIX does not provide protection against disease due to all HPV types. (14.3)
- CERVARIX has not been demonstrated to provide protection against disease from vaccine and non-vaccine HPV types to which a woman has previously been exposed through sexual activity. (14.2)

———————DOSAGE AND ADMINISTRATION———————

Three doses (0.5-mL each) by intramuscular injection according to the following schedule: 0, 1, and 6 months. (2.2)

———————DOSAGE FORMS AND STRENGTHS———————

0.5-mL suspension for injection as a single-dose vial or pre-filled syringe. (3)

———————CONTRAINDICATIONS———————

Severe allergic reactions (e.g., anaphylaxis) to any component of CERVARIX. (4)

———————WARNINGS AND PRECAUTIONS———————

- Because vaccinees may develop syncope, sometimes resulting in falling with injury, observation for 15 minutes after administration is recommended. Syncope, sometimes associated with tonic-clonic movements and other seizure-like activity, has been reported following vaccination with CERVARIX. When syncope is associated with tonic-clonic movements, the activity is usually transient and typically responds to restoring cerebral perfusion by maintaining a supine or Trendelenburg position. (5.1)
- Do not use the prefilled syringes in latex sensitive individuals. (5.2)

———————ADVERSE REACTIONS———————

- Most common local adverse reactions in ≥20% of subjects were pain, redness, and swelling at the injection site. (6.1)
- Most common general adverse events in ≥20% of subjects were fatigue, headache, myalgia, gastrointestinal symptoms, and arthralgia. (6.1)

To report SUSPECTED ADVERSE REACTIONS, contact GlaxoSmithKline at 1-888-825-5249 or VAERS at 1-800-822-7967 or www.vaers.hhs.gov

———————DRUG INTERACTIONS———————

Do not mix CERVARIX with any other vaccine in the same syringe or vial. (7.1)

———————USE IN SPECIFIC POPULATIONS———————

- Safety has not been established in pregnant women. Register women who receive CERVARIX while pregnant in the pregnancy registry by calling 1-888-452-9622. (8.1)
- Immunocompromised individuals may have a reduced immune response to CERVARIX. (8.6)

See 17 for PATIENT COUNSELING INFORMATION

Revised: 08/2010

FULL PRESCRIBING INFORMATION: CONTENTS*

Table 1. Rates of Solicited Local Adverse Reactions and General Adverse Events in Females 10 Through 25 Years of Age Within 7 Days of Vaccination (Total Vaccinated Cohort[a])

Adverse Reaction/Event	CERVARIX (10-25 yrs) %	HAV 720[b] (15-25 yrs) %	HAV 360[c] (10-14 yrs) %	Al(OH)₃ Control[d] (15-25 yrs) %
Local Adverse Reaction	**N = 6,431**	**N = 3,079**	**N = 1,027**	**N = 549**
Pain	91.8	78.0	64.2	87.2
Redness	48.0	27.6	25.2	24.4
Swelling	44.1	19.8	17.3	21.3
General Adverse Event	**N = 6,432**	**N = 3,079**	**N = 1,027**	**N = 549**
Fatigue	55.0	53.7	42.3	53.6
Headache	53.4	51.3	45.2	61.4
GI[e]	27.8	27.3	24.6	32.8
Fever (≥99.5°F)	12.8	10.9	16.0	13.5
Rash	9.6	8.4	6.7	10.0
	N = 5,881	**N = 3,079**	**N = 1,027**	—
Myalgia[f]	49.1	44.9	33.1	—
Arthralgia[f]	20.8	17.9	19.9	—
Urticaria[f]	7.4	7.9	5.4	—

[a] Total vaccinated cohort included subjects with at least one documented dose (N).
[b] HAV 720 = Hepatitis A Vaccine control group [720 EL.U. of antigen and 500 mcg Al(OH)₃].
[c] HAV 360 = Hepatitis A Vaccine control group [360 EL.U. of antigen and 250 mcg of Al(OH)₃].
[d] Al(OH)₃ Control = control containing 500 mcg Al(OH)₃.
[e] GI = Gastrointestinal symptoms, including nausea, vomiting, diarrhea, and/or abdominal pain.
[f] Adverse events solicited in a subset of subjects.

FULL PRESCRIBING INFORMATION

1 INDICATIONS AND USAGE

1.1 Indications

CERVARIX® is indicated for the prevention of the following diseases caused by oncogenic human papillomavirus (HPV) types 16 and 18 [see Clinical Studies (14)]:

- cervical cancer,
- cervical intraepithelial neoplasia (CIN) grade 2 or worse and adenocarcinoma *in situ*, and
- cervical intraepithelial neoplasia (CIN) grade 1.

CERVARIX is approved for use in females 10 through 25 years of age.

1.2 Limitations of Use and Effectiveness

CERVARIX does not provide protection against disease due to all HPV types [see Clinical Studies (14.3)].

CERVARIX has not been demonstrated to provide protection against disease from vaccine and non-vaccine HPV types to which a woman has previously been exposed through sexual activity [see Clinical Studies (14.2)].

Females should continue to adhere to recommended cervical cancer screening procedures [see Patient Counseling Information (17)].

Vaccination with CERVARIX may not result in protection in all vaccine recipients.

2 DOSAGE AND ADMINISTRATION

2.1 Preparation for Administration

Shake vial or syringe well before withdrawal and use. Parenteral drug products should be inspected visually for particulate matter and discoloration prior to administration, whenever solution and container permit. CERVARIX also should be inspected visually for cracks in the vial or syringe prior to administration. If any of these conditions exist, the vaccine should not be administered. With thorough agitation, CERVARIX is a homogeneous, turbid, white suspension. Do not administer if it appears otherwise.

2.2 Dose and Schedule

Immunization with CERVARIX consists of 3 doses of 0.5-mL each, by intramuscular injection according to the following schedule: 0, 1, and 6 months. The preferred site of administration is the deltoid region of the upper arm.

Do not administer this product intravenously, intradermally, or subcutaneously.

3 DOSAGE FORMS AND STRENGTHS

CERVARIX is a suspension for intramuscular injection available in 0.5-mL single-dose vials and prefilled TIP-LOK® syringes.

4 CONTRAINDICATIONS

Severe allergic reactions (e.g., anaphylaxis) to any component of CERVARIX [see Description (11)].

5 WARNINGS AND PRECAUTIONS

5.1 Syncope

Because vaccinees may develop syncope, sometimes resulting in falling with injury, observation for 15 minutes after administration is recommended. Syncope, sometimes associated with tonic-clonic movements and other seizure-like activity, has been reported following vaccination with CERVARIX. When syncope is associated with tonic-clonic movements, the activity is usually transient and typically responds to restoring cerebral perfusion by maintaining a supine or Trendelenburg position.

5.2 Latex

The tip cap and the rubber plunger of the needleless prefilled syringes contain dry natural latex rubber that may cause allergic reactions in latex sensitive individuals. The vial stopper does not contain latex.

5.3 Preventing and Managing Allergic Vaccine Reactions

Prior to administration, the healthcare provider should review the immunization history for possible vaccine hypersensitivity and previous vaccination-related adverse reactions to allow an assessment of benefits and risks. Appropriate medical treatment and supervision should be readily available in case of anaphylactic reactions following administration of CERVARIX.

6 ADVERSE REACTIONS

The most common local adverse reactions (≥20% of subjects) were pain, redness, and swelling at the injection site. The most common general adverse events (≥20% of subjects) were fatigue, headache, myalgia, gastrointestinal symptoms, and arthralgia.

6.1 Clinical Studies Experience

Because clinical trials are conducted under widely varying conditions, adverse reaction rates observed in the clinical trials of a vaccine cannot be directly compared with rates in the clinical trials of another vaccine, and may not reflect the rates observed in practice. There is the possibility that broad use of CERVARIX could reveal adverse reactions not observed in clinical trials.

Table 2. Rates of Solicited Local Adverse Reactions in Females 10 Through 25 Years of Age by Dose Within 7 Days of Vaccination (Total Vaccinated Cohort[a])

Adverse Reaction	CERVARIX (10-25 yrs) %			HAV 720[b] (15-25 yrs) %			HAV 360[c] (10-14 yrs) %			Al(OH)₃ Control[d] (15-25 yrs) %		
	Post-Dose			Post-Dose			Post-Dose			Post-Dose		
	1	2	3	1	2	3	1	2	3	1	2	3
N	6,415	6,197	5,936	3,070	2,919	2,758	1,027	1,021	1,011	546	521	500
Pain	86.9	76.2	78.7	65.6	54.4	56.1	48.5	38.5	36.9	79.1	66.8	72.4
Pain, Grade 3[e]	7.5	5.7	7.7	2.0	1.4	2.0	0.8	0.2	1.6	9.0	6.0	8.6
Redness	27.8	29.6	35.6	16.6	15.2	16.1	15.6	13.3	12.1	11.5	11.5	15.6
Redness, >50 mm	0.2	0.5	1.0	0.1	0.1	0.0	0.1	0.2	0.1	0.2	0.0	0.0
Swelling	22.7	25.2	32.7	10.5	9.4	10.5	9.4	8.6	7.6	10.3	10.4	12.0
Swelling, >50 mm	1.2	1.0	1.3	0.2	0.2	0.2	0.4	0.3	0.0	0.0	0.0	0.0

[a] Total vaccinated cohort included subjects with at least one documented dose (N).
[b] HAV 720 = Hepatitis A Vaccine control group [720 EL.U. of antigen and 500 mcg Al(OH)₃].
[c] HAV 360 = Hepatitis A Vaccine control group [360 EL.U. of antigen and 250 mcg of Al(OH)₃].
[d] Al(OH)₃ Control = control containing 500 mcg Al(OH)₃.
[e] Defined as spontaneously painful or pain that prevented normal daily activities.

Table 3. Rates of Unsolicited Adverse Events in Females 10 Through 25 Years of Age Within 30 Days of Vaccination (≥1% For CERVARIX and Greater Than HAV 720, HAV 360, or Al(OH)₃ Control) (Total Vaccinated Cohort[a])

Adverse Event	CERVARIX % (N = 6,654)	HAV 720[b] % (N = 3,186)	HAV 360[c] % (N = 1,032)	Al(OH)₃ Control[d] % (N = 581)
Headache	5.3	7.6	3.3	9.3
Nasopharyngitis	3.6	3.4	5.9	3.3
Influenza	3.2	5.6	1.3	1.9
Pharyngolaryngeal pain	2.9	2.7	2.2	2.2
Dizziness	2.2	2.6	1.5	3.1
Upper respiratory infection	2.0	1.3	6.7	1.5
Chlamydia infection	2.0	4.4	0.0	0.0
Dysmenorrhea	2.0	2.3	1.9	4.0
Pharyngitis	1.5	1.8	2.2	0.5
Injection site bruising	1.4	1.8	0.7	1.5
Vaginal infection	1.4	2.2	0.1	0.9
Injection site pruritus	1.3	0.5	0.6	0.2
Back pain	1.1	1.3	0.7	3.1
Urinary tract infection	1.0	1.4	0.3	1.2

[a] Total vaccinated cohort included subjects with at least one dose administered (N).
[b] HAV 720 = Hepatitis A Vaccine control group [720 EL.U. of antigen and 500 mcg Al(OH)₃].
[c] HAV 360 = Hepatitis A Vaccine control group [360 EL.U. of antigen and 250 mcg of Al(OH)₃].
[d] Al(OH)₃ Control = control containing 500 mcg Al(OH)₃.

Studies in Females 10 Through 25 Years of Age: The safety of CERVARIX was evaluated by pooling data from controlled and uncontrolled clinical trials involving 23,713 females 10 through 25 years of age in the pre-licensure clinical development program. In these studies, 12,785 females (10 through 25 years of age) received at least one dose of CERVARIX and 10,928 females received at least one dose of a control [Hepatitis A Vaccine containing 360 EL.U. (10 through 14 years of age), Hepatitis A Vaccine containing 720 EL.U. (15 through 25 years of age), or Al(OH)₃ (500 mcg, 15 through 25 years of age)].

Data on solicited local and general adverse events were collected by subjects or parents using standardized diary cards for 7 consecutive days following each vaccine dose (i.e., day of vaccination and the next 6 days). Unsolicited adverse events were recorded with diary cards for 30 days following each vaccination (day of vaccination and 29 subsequent days). Parents and/or subjects were also asked at each study visit about the occurrence of any adverse events and instructed to immediately report serious adverse events throughout the study period. These studies were conducted in North America, Latin America, Europe, Asia, and Australia. Overall, the majority of subjects were white (59%), followed by Asian (26%), Hispanic (9%), black (3%), and other racial/ethnic groups (3%).

Solicited Adverse Events: The reported frequencies of solicited local injection site reactions (pain, redness, and swelling) and general adverse events (fatigue, fever, gastrointestinal symptoms, headache, arthralgia, myalgia, and urticaria) within 7 days after vaccination in females 10 through 25 years of age are presented in Table 1. An analysis of solicited local injection site reactions by dose is presented in Table 2. Local reactions were reported more frequently with CERVARIX when compared with the control groups; in ≥84% of recipients of CERVARIX, these local reactions were mild to moderate in intensity. Compared with dose 1, pain was reported less frequently after doses 2 and 3 of CERVARIX, in contrast to redness and swelling where there was a small increased incidence. There was no increase in the frequency of general adverse events with successive doses.

[See table 1 at top of previous page]
[See table 2 at left]
The pattern of solicited local adverse reactions and general adverse events following administration of CERVARIX was similar between the age cohorts (10 through 14 years and 15 through 25 years).

Unsolicited Adverse Events: The frequency of unsolicited adverse events that occurred within 30 days of vaccination (≥1% for CERVARIX and greater than any of the control groups) in females 10 through 25 years of age are presented in Table 3.
[See table 3 at left]

New Onset Autoimmune Diseases (NOADs): The pooled safety database, which included controlled and uncontrolled trials which enrolled females 10 through 25 years of age, was searched for new medical conditions indicative of potential new onset autoimmune diseases. Overall, the incidence of potential NOADs, as well as NOADs, in the group receiving CERVARIX was 0.8% (95/12,533) and comparable to the pooled control group (0.8%, 87/10,730) during the 4.3 years of follow-up (mean 3.0 years) (Table 4).

In the largest randomized, controlled trial (Study 2) which enrolled females 15 through 25 years of age and which included active surveillance for potential NOADs, the incidence of potential NOADs and NOADs was 0.8% among subjects who received CERVARIX (78/9,319) and 0.8% among subjects who received Hepatitis A Vaccine [720 EL.U. of antigen and 500 mcg Al(OH)₃] control (77/9,325).
[See table 4 at top of next page]

Serious Adverse Events: In the pooled safety database, inclusive of controlled and uncontrolled studies, which enrolled females 10 through 72 years of age, 5.3% (862/16,142) of subjects who received CERVARIX and 5.9% (814/13,811) of subjects who received control reported at least one serious adverse event, without regard to causality, during the entire follow-up period (up to 7.4 years). Among females 10 through 25 years of age enrolled in these clinical studies, 6.4% of subjects who received CERVARIX and 7.2% of subjects who received the control reported at least one serious adverse event during the entire follow-up period (up to 7.4 years).

Deaths: In completed and ongoing studies which enrolled 57,323 females 9 through 72 years of age, 37 deaths were reported during the 7.4 years of follow-up: 20 in subjects who received CERVARIX (0.06%, 20/33,623) and 17 in subjects who received control (0.07%, 17/23,700). Causes of death among subjects were consistent with those reported in adolescent and adult female populations. The most common causes of death were motor vehicle accident (5 subjects who received CERVARIX; 5 subjects who received control), and suicide (2 subjects who received CERVARIX; 5 subjects who received control), followed by neoplasm (3 subjects who received CERVARIX; 2 subjects who received control), autoimmune disease (3 subjects who received CERVARIX; 1 subject who received control), infectious disease (3 subjects who received CERVARIX; 1 subject who received control), homicide (2 subjects who received CERVARIX; 1 subject who received control), cardiovascular disorders (2 subjects who received CERVARIX), and death of unknown cause (2 subjects who received control). Among females 10 through 25 years of age, 31 deaths were reported (0.05%, 16/29,467 of subjects who received CERVARIX and 0.07%, 15/20,192 of subjects who received control).

6.2   Postmarketing Experience
In addition to reports in clinical trials, worldwide voluntary reports of adverse events received for CERVARIX since market introduction (2007) are listed below. This list includes serious events or events which have suspected causal association to CERVARIX. Because these events are reported voluntarily from a population of uncertain size, it is not always possible to reliably estimate their frequency or establish a causal relationship to vaccination.

Blood and Lymphatic System Disorders: Lymphadenopathy.

Immune System Disorders: Allergic reactions (including anaphylactic and anaphylactoid reactions), angioedema, erythema multiforme.

Nervous System Disorders: Syncope or vasovagal responses to injection (sometimes accompanied by tonic-clonic movements).

7   DRUG INTERACTIONS
7.1   Concomitant Vaccine Administration
There are no data to assess the concomitant use of CERVARIX with other vaccines.
Do not mix CERVARIX with any other vaccine in the same syringe or vial.
7.2   Hormonal Contraceptives
Among 7,693 subjects 15 through 25 years of age in Study 2 (CERVARIX, N = 3,821 or Hepatitis A Vaccine 720 EL.U., N = 3,872) who used hormonal contraceptives for a mean of 2.8 years, the observed efficacy of CERVARIX was similar to that observed among subjects who did not report use of hormonal contraceptives.

7.3 Immunosuppressive Therapies

Immunosuppressive therapies, including irradiation, anti-metabolites, alkylating agents, cytotoxic drugs, and corticosteroids (used in greater than physiologic doses), may reduce the immune response to CERVARIX [see Use in Specific Populations (8.6)].

8 USE IN SPECIFIC POPULATIONS

8.1 Pregnancy

Pregnancy Category B

Reproduction studies have been performed in rats at a dose approximately 47 times the human dose (on a mg/kg basis) and revealed no evidence of impaired fertility or harm to the fetus due to CERVARIX. There are, however, no adequate and well-controlled studies in pregnant women. Because animal reproduction studies are not always predictive of human response, this drug should be used during pregnancy only if clearly needed.

Non-Clinical Studies: An evaluation of the effect of CERVARIX on embryo-fetal, pre- and post-natal development was conducted using rats. One group of rats was administered CERVARIX 30 days prior to gestation and during the period of organogenesis (gestation days 6, 8, 11, and 15). A second group of rats was administered saline at 30 days prior to gestation followed by CERVARIX on days 6, 8, 11, and 15 of gestation. Two additional groups of rats received either saline or adjuvant following the same dosing regimen. CERVARIX was administered at 0.1 mL/rat/occasion (approximately 47-fold excess relative to the projected human dose on a mg/kg basis) by intramuscular injection. No adverse effects on mating, fertility, pregnancy, parturition, lactation, or embryo-fetal, pre- and post-natal development were observed. There were no vaccine-related fetal malformations or other evidence of teratogenesis.

Clinical Studies: Overall Outcomes: In clinical studies, pregnancy testing was performed prior to each vaccine administration and vaccination was discontinued if a subject had a positive pregnancy test. In all clinical trials, subjects were instructed to take precautions to avoid pregnancy until 2 months after the last vaccination. During pre-licensure clinical development, a total of 7,276 pregnancies were reported among 3,696 females receiving CERVARIX and 3,580 females receiving a control (Hepatitis A Vaccine 360 EL.U., Hepatitis A Vaccine 720 EL.U., or 500 mcg Al(OH)$_3$). The overall proportions of pregnancy outcomes were similar between treatment groups. The majority of women gave birth to normal infants (62.2% and 62.6% of recipients of CERVARIX and control, respectively). Other outcomes included spontaneous abortion (11.0% and 10.8% of recipients of CERVARIX and control, respectively), elective termination (5.8% and 6.1% of recipients of CERVARIX and control, respectively), abnormal infant other than congenital anomaly (2.8% and 3.2% of recipients of CERVARIX and control, respectively), and premature birth (2.0% and 1.7% of recipients of CERVARIX and control, respectively). Other outcomes (congenital anomaly, stillbirth, ectopic pregnancy, and therapeutic abortion) were reported less frequently in 0.1% to 0.8% of pregnancies in both groups.

Outcomes Around Time of Vaccination: Sub-analyses were conducted to describe pregnancy outcomes in 761 women [N = 396 for CERVARIX and N = 365 pooled control, HAV 360 EL.U., HAV 720 EL.U., and 500 mcg Al(OH)$_3$] who had their last menstrual period within 30 days prior to, or 45 days after a vaccine dose and for whom pregnancy outcome was known. The majority of women gave birth to normal infants (65.2% and 69.3% of recipients of CERVARIX and control, respectively). Spontaneous abortion was reported in a total of 11.7% of subjects (13.6% of recipients of CERVARIX and 9.6% of control recipients) and elective termination was reported in a total of 9.7% of subjects (9.9% of recipients of CERVARIX and 9.6% of control recipients). Abnormal infant other than congenital anomaly was reported in a total of 4.9% of subjects (5.1% of recipients of CERVARIX and 4.7% of control recipients) and premature birth was reported in a total of 2.5% of subjects (2.5% of both groups). Other outcomes (congenital anomaly, stillbirth, ectopic pregnancy, and therapeutic abortion) were reported in 0.3% to 1.8% of pregnancies among recipients of CERVARIX and in 0.3% to 1.4% of pregnancies among control recipients.

It is not known whether the observed numerical imbalance in spontaneous abortions in pregnancies which occurred around the time of vaccination is due to a vaccine-related effect.

Pregnancy Registry: Healthcare providers are encouraged to register pregnant women who inadvertently receive CERVARIX in the GlaxoSmithKline vaccination pregnancy registry by calling 1-888-452-9622.

8.3 Nursing Mothers

In non-clinical studies in rats, serological data suggest a transfer of anti-HPV-16 and anti-HPV-18 antibodies via milk during lactation in rats. Excretion of vaccine-induced antibodies in human milk has not been studied for CERVARIX. Because many drugs are excreted in human milk, caution should be exercised when CERVARIX is administered to a nursing woman.

8.4 Pediatric Use

Safety and effectiveness in pediatric patients younger than 10 years of age have not been established. The safety and effectiveness of CERVARIX have been evaluated in 1,193 subjects 10 through 14 years of age and 6,316 subjects 15 through 17 years of age. [See Adverse Reactions (6.1) and Clinical Studies (14.5).]

8.5 Geriatric Use

Clinical studies of CERVARIX did not include sufficient numbers of subjects 65 years of age and older to determine whether they respond differently from younger subjects. CERVARIX is not approved for use in subjects 65 years of age and older.

8.6 Immunocompromised Individuals

The immune response to CERVARIX may be diminished in immunocompromised individuals [see Drug Interactions (7.3)].

11 DESCRIPTION

CERVARIX [Human Papillomavirus Bivalent (Types 16 and 18) Vaccine, Recombinant] is a non-infectious recombinant, AS04-adjuvanted vaccine that contains recombinant L1 protein, the major antigenic protein of the capsid, of oncogenic HPV types 16 and 18. The L1 proteins are produced in separate bioreactors using the recombinant Baculovirus expression vector system in a serum-free culture media composed of chemically-defined lipids, vitamins, amino acids, and mineral salts. Following replication of the L1 encoding recombinant Baculovirus in Trichoplusia ni insect cells, the L1 protein accumulates in the cytoplasm of the cells. The L1 proteins are released by cell disruption and purified by a series of chromatographic and filtration methods. Assembly of the L1 proteins into virus-like particles (VLPs) occurs at the end of the purification process. The purified, non-infectious VLPs are then adsorbed on to aluminum (as hydroxide salt). The adjuvant system, AS04, is composed of 3-O-desacyl-4'-monophosphoryl lipid A (MPL) adsorbed on to aluminum (as hydroxide salt).

CERVARIX is prepared by combining the adsorbed VLPs of each HPV type together with the AS04 adjuvant system in sodium chloride, sodium dihydrogen phosphate dihydrate, and Water for Injection.

CERVARIX is a sterile suspension for intramuscular injection. Each 0.5-mL dose is formulated to contain 20 mcg of HPV type 16 L1 protein, 20 mcg of HPV type 18 L1 protein, 50 mcg of the 3-O-desacyl-4'-monophosphoryl lipid A (MPL), and 0.5 mg of aluminum hydroxide. Each dose also contains 4.4 mg of sodium chloride and 0.624 mg of sodium dihydrogen phosphate dihydrate. Each dose may also contain residual amounts of insect cell and viral protein (<40 ng) and bacterial cell protein (<150 ng) from the manufacturing process. CERVARIX does not contain a preservative.

12 CLINICAL PHARMACOLOGY

12.1 Mechanism of Action

Animal studies suggest that the efficacy of L1 VLP vaccines may be mediated by the development of IgG neutralizing antibodies directed against HPV-L1 capsid proteins generated as a result of vaccination.

Table 4. Incidence of New Medical Conditions Indicative of Potential New Onset Autoimmune Disease and New Onset Autoimmune Disease Throughout the Follow-up Period Regardless of Causality in Females 10 Through 25 Years of Age (Total Vaccinated Cohort[a])

	CERVARIX (N = 12,533)	Pooled Control Group[b] (N = 10,730)
	n (%)[c]	n (%)[c]
Total Number of Subjects With at Least One Medical Condition	95 (0.8)	87 (0.8)
Arthritis[d]	9 (0.0)	4 (0.0)
Celiac disease	2 (0.0)	5 (0.0)
Dermatomyositis	0 (0.0)	1 (0.0)
Diabetes mellitus insulin-dependent (Type 1 or unspecified)	5 (0.0)	5 (0.0)
Erythema nodosum	3 (0.0)	0 (0.0)
Hyperthyroidism[e]	14 (0.1)	15 (0.1)
Hypothyroidism[f]	30 (0.2)	28 (0.3)
Inflammatory bowel disease[g]	8 (0.1)	4 (0.0)
Multiple sclerosis	4 (0.0)	1 (0.0)
Myelitis transverse	1 (0.0)	0 (0.0)
Optic neuritis/Optic neuritis retrobulbar	3 (0.0)	1 (0.0)
Psoriasis[h]	8 (0.1)	11 (0.1)
Raynaud's phenomenon	0 (0.0)	1 (0.0)
Rheumatoid arthritis	4 (0.0)	3 (0.0)
Systemic lupus erythematosus[i]	2 (0.0)	3 (0.0)
Thrombocytopenia[j]	1 (0.0)	1 (0.0)
Vasculitis[k]	1 (0.0)	3 (0.0)
Vitiligo	2 (0.0)	2 (0.0)

[a] Total vaccinated cohort included subjects with at least one documented dose (N).
[b] Pooled Control Group = Hepatitis A Vaccine control group [720 EL.U. of antigen and 500 mcg Al(OH)$_3$], Hepatitis A Vaccine control group [360 EL.U. of antigen and 250 mcg of Al(OH)$_3$], and a control containing 500 mcg Al(OH)$_3$.
[c] n (%): number and percentage of subjects with medical condition.
[d] Term includes reactive arthritis and arthritis.
[e] Term includes Basedow's disease, goiter, and hyperthyroidism.
[f] Term includes thyroiditis, autoimmune thyroiditis, and hypothyroidism.
[g] Term includes colitis ulcerative, Crohn's disease, proctitis ulcerative, and inflammatory bowel disease.
[h] Term includes psoriatic arthropathy, nail psoriasis, guttate psoriasis, and psoriasis.
[i] Term includes systemic lupus erythematosus and cutaneous lupus erythematosus.
[j] Term includes idiopathic thrombocytopenic purpura and thrombocytopenia.
[k] Term includes leukocytoclastic vasculitis and vasculitis.

Table 5. Efficacy of CERVARIX Against Histopathological Lesions Associated With HPV-16 or HPV-18 in Females 15 Through 25 Years of Age (According to Protocol Cohort[a]) (Study 2)

	CERVARIX		Control[b]		% Efficacy (96.1% CI)[c]
	N	Number of Cases	N	Number of Cases	
CIN2/3 or AIS	7,344	4	7,312	56	92.9 (79.9, 98.3)
CIN1/2/3 or AIS	7,344	8	7,312	96	91.7 (82.4, 96.7)

CI = Confidence Interval.
[a] Subjects (including women who had normal cytology, ASC-US, or LSIL at baseline) who received 3 doses of vaccine and were HPV DNA negative and seronegative at baseline and HPV DNA negative at month 6 for the corresponding HPV type (N). The mean follow-up was approximately 35 months.
[b] Hepatitis A Vaccine control group [720 EL.U. of antigen and 500 mcg Al(OH)$_3$].
[c] The 96.1% confidence interval reflected in this final analysis results from statistical adjustment for the previously conducted interim analysis.

Table 6. Efficacy of CERVARIX Against Disease Associated With HPV-16 or HPV-18 in Females 15 Through 25 Years of Age, Regardless of Current or Prior Exposure to Vaccine HPV Types (Study 2)

	CERVARIX		Control		% Efficacy (96.1% CI)[b]
	N	Number of Cases[a]	N	Number of Cases[a]	
CIN1/2/3 or AIS					
Prophylactic Efficacy[c]	5,449	3	5,436	85	96.5 (89.0, 99.4)
HPV-16 or HPV-18 DNA Positive at Baseline[d]	641	90	592	92	—
Regardless of Current Infection or Prior Exposure to HPV-16 or HPV-18[e]	8,667	107	8,682	240	55.5[f] (43.2, 65.3)
CIN2/3 or AIS					
Prophylactic Efficacy[c]	5,449	1	5,436	63	98.4 (90.4, 100)
HPV-16 or HPV-18 DNA Positive at Baseline[d]	641	74	592	73	—
Regardless of Current Infection or Prior Exposure to HPV-16 or HPV-18[e]	8,667	82	8,682	174	52.8[f] (37.5, 64.7)
CIN3 or AIS					
Prophylactic Efficacy[c]	5,449	0	5,436	13	100 (64.7, 100)
HPV-16 or HPV-18 DNA Positive at Baseline[d]	641	41	592	38	—
Regardless of Current Infection or Prior Exposure to HPV-16 or HPV-18[e]	8,667	43	8,682	65	33.6[f] (-1.1, 56.9)

CI = Confidence Interval.
Table does not include disease due to non-vaccine HPV types.
[a] Cases = Histopathological cases associated with HPV-16 and/or HPV-18.
[b] The 96.1% confidence interval reflected in this final analysis results from statistical adjustment for the previously conducted interim analysis.
[c] TVC naïve: includes all vaccinated subjects (who received at least one dose of vaccine) who had normal cytology, were HPV DNA negative for 14 oncogenic HPV types, and seronegative for HPV-16 and HPV-18 at baseline (N). Case counting started on day 1 after the first dose.
[d] TVC subset: includes all vaccinated subjects (who received at least one dose of vaccine) who were HPV DNA positive for HPV-16 or HPV-18 irrespective of serostatus at baseline (N). Case counting started on day 1 after the first dose.
[e] TVC: includes all vaccinated subjects (who received at least one dose of vaccine) irrespective of HPV DNA status and serostatus at baseline (N). Case counting started on day 1 after the first dose.
[f] Observed vaccine efficacy includes the prophylactic efficacy of CERVARIX and the impact of CERVARIX on the course of infections present at first vaccination.

13 NONCLINICAL TOXICOLOGY
13.1 Carcinogenesis, Mutagenesis, Impairment of Fertility
CERVARIX has not been evaluated for its carcinogenic or mutagenic potential. Vaccination of female rats with CERVARIX, at doses shown to be significantly immunogenic in the rat, had no effect on fertility.

14 CLINICAL STUDIES
Cervical intraepithelial neoplasia (CIN) grade 2 and 3 lesions or cervical adenocarcinoma *in situ* (AIS) are the immediate and necessary precursors of squamous cell carcinoma and adenocarcinoma of the cervix, respectively. Their detection and removal has been shown to prevent cancer. Therefore, CIN2/3 and AIS (precancerous lesions) serve as surrogate markers for the prevention of cervical cancer. In clinical studies to evaluate the efficacy of CERVARIX, the endpoints were cases of CIN2/3 and AIS associated with HPV-16, HPV-18, and other oncogenic HPV types. Persistent infection with HPV-16 and HPV-18 that lasts for 12 months was also an endpoint.

The efficacy of CERVARIX to prevent histopathologically-confirmed CIN2/3 or AIS was assessed in 2 double-blind, randomized, controlled clinical studies that enrolled a total of 19,778 females 15 through 25 years of age.

Study 1 (HPV 001) enrolled women who were negative for oncogenic HPV DNA (HPV types 16, 18, 31, 33, 35, 39, 45, 51, 52, 56, 58, 59, 66, and 68) in cervical samples, seronegative for HPV-16 and HPV-18 antibodies and had normal cytology. This represents a population presumed "naïve" without current HPV infection at the time of vaccination and without prior exposure to either HPV-16 or HPV-18. Subjects were enrolled in an extended follow-up study (Study 1 extension [HPV 007]) to evaluate the long-term efficacy, immunogenicity, and safety. These subjects have been followed for up to 6.4 years.

In Study 2 (HPV 008), women were vaccinated regardless of baseline HPV DNA status, serostatus or cytology. This study reflects a population of women naïve (without current infection and without prior exposure) or non-naïve (with current infection and/or with prior exposure) to HPV. Before vaccination, cervical samples were assessed for oncogenic HPV DNA (HPV types 16, 18, 31, 33, 35, 39, 45, 51, 52, 56, 58, 59, 66, and 68) and serostatus of HPV-16 and HPV-18 antibodies.

In both studies, testing for oncogenic HPV types was conducted using SPF$_{10}$-LiPA$_{25}$ PCR to detect HPV DNA in archived biopsy samples.

14.1 Prophylactic Efficacy Against HPV Types 16 and 18
Study 2: A randomized, double-blind, controlled clinical trial was conducted in which 18,665 healthy females 15 through 25 years of age received CERVARIX or Hepatitis A Vaccine control on a 0-, 1-, and 6-month schedule. Among subjects, 54.8% of subjects were white, 31.5% Asian, 7.1% Hispanic, 3.7% black, and 2.9% were of other racial/ethnic groups.

In this study, women were randomized and vaccinated regardless of baseline HPV DNA status, serostatus or cytology. Women with HPV-16 or HPV-18 DNA present in baseline cervical samples (HPV DNA positive) at study entry were considered currently infected with that specific HPV type. If HPV DNA was not detected by PCR, women were considered HPV DNA negative. Additionally, cervical samples were assessed for cytologic abnormalities and serologic testing was performed for anti-HPV-16 and anti-HPV-18 serum antibodies at baseline. Women with anti-HPV serum antibodies present were considered to have prior exposure to HPV and characterized as seropositive. Women seropositive for HPV-16 or HPV-18 but DNA negative for that specific serotype were considered as having cleared a previous natural infection. Women without antibodies to HPV-16 and HPV-18 were characterized as seronegative. Before vaccination, 73.6% of subjects were naïve (without current infection [DNA negative] and without prior exposure [seronegative]) to HPV-16 and/or HPV-18.

Efficacy endpoints included histological evaluation of precancerous and dysplastic lesions (CIN grade 1, grade 2, or grade 3), and AIS. The mean follow-up after the first dose was approximately 39 months. Virological endpoints (HPV DNA in cervical samples detected by PCR) included 12-month persistent infection (defined as at least 2 positive specimens for the same HPV type over a minimum interval of 10 months).

The according to protocol (ATP) cohort for efficacy analyses for HPV-16 and/or HPV-18 included all subjects who received 3 doses of vaccine, for whom efficacy endpoint measures were available and who were HPV-16 and/or HPV-18 DNA negative and seronegative at baseline and HPV-16 and/or HPV-18 DNA negative at month 6 for the HPV type considered in the analysis. Case counting for the ATP cohort started on day 1 after the third dose of vaccine. This cohort included women who had normal or low-grade cytology (cytological abnormalities including atypical squamous cells of undetermined significance [ASC-US] or low grade squamous intraepithelial lesions [LSIL]) at baseline and excluded women with high-grade cytology.

The total vaccinated cohort (TVC) for each efficacy analysis included all subjects who received at least one dose of the vaccine, for whom efficacy endpoint measures were available, irrespective of their HPV DNA status, cytology, and serostatus at baseline. This cohort included women with or without current HPV infection and/or prior exposure. Case counting for the TVC started on day 1 after the first dose. The TVC naïve is a subset of the TVC that had normal cytology, and were HPV DNA negative for 14 oncogenic HPV types and seronegative for HPV-16 and HPV-18 at baseline. CERVARIX was efficacious in the prevention of precancerous lesions or AIS associated with HPV-16 or HPV-18 (Table 5).

[See table 5 at left]

Since CIN3 or AIS represents a more immediate precursor to cervical cancer, cases of CIN3 or AIS associated with HPV-16 or HPV-18 were evaluated. In the ATP cohort, CERVARIX was efficacious in the prevention of CIN3 or AIS associated with HPV-16 or HPV-18 (vaccine efficacy = 80.0% [96.1% CI: 0.3, 98.1]).

Subjects who were already infected with one vaccine HPV type (16 or 18) prior to vaccination were protected from precancerous lesions or AIS and infection caused by the other vaccine HPV type.

Efficacy of CERVARIX against 12-month persistent infection with HPV-16 or HPV-18 was also evaluated. In the ATP cohort, CERVARIX reduced the incidence of 12-month persistent infection with HPV-16 and/or HPV-18 by 91.2% (96.1% CI: 85.9, 94.8). Immune response following natural infection does not reliably confer protection against future infections. Among subjects who received 3 doses of

CERVARIX and who were seropositive at baseline and DNA negative for HPV-16 or HPV-18 at baseline and month 6, CERVARIX reduced the incidence of 12-month persistent infection by 91.5% (96.1% CI: 64.0, 99.2). However, the number of cases of CIN2/3 or AIS was too few to determine efficacy against histopathological endpoints in this population.
Study 1 and Study 1 Extension: In a second double-blind, randomized, controlled study (Study 1), the efficacy of CERVARIX in the prevention of HPV-16 or HPV-18 incident and persistent infections was compared with aluminum hydroxide control in 1,113 females 15 through 25 years of age. The population was naïve to current oncogenic HPV infection or prior exposure to HPV-16 and HPV-18 at the time of vaccination (total cohort). A total of 776 subjects were enrolled in the extended follow-up study (Study 1 Extension) to evaluate the long-term efficacy, immunogenicity, and safety of CERVARIX. These subjects have been followed for up to 6.4 years. In Study 1 and Study 1 Extension, with up to 6.4 years of follow-up (mean 5.9 years), in naïve females 15 through 25 years of age, efficacy against CIN2/3 or AIS associated with HPV-16 or HPV-18 was 100% (98.67% CI: 28.4, 100). Efficacy against 12-month persistent infection with HPV-16 or HPV-18 was 100% (98.67% CI: 74.4, 100). The confidence interval reflected in this final analysis results from statistical adjustment for analyses previously conducted.

14.2   Efficacy Against HPV Types 16 and 18, Regardless of Current Infection or Prior Exposure to HPV-16 or HPV-18
Study 2: The study included women regardless of HPV DNA status (current infection) and serostatus (prior exposure) to vaccine types, HPV-16 or HPV-18 at baseline. Efficacy analyses included lesions arising among women regardless of baseline DNA status and serostatus, including HPV infections present at first vaccination and those from infections acquired after dose 1. In this population which includes naïve (without current infection and prior exposure) and non-naïve women, CERVARIX was efficacious in the prevention of precancerous lesions or AIS associated with HPV-16 or HPV-18 (Table 6).
However, among women HPV DNA positive regardless of serostatus at baseline, there was no clear evidence of efficacy against precancerous lesions or AIS associated with HPV-16 or HPV-18 (Table 6).
[See table 6 on previous page]

14.3   Efficacy Against Cervical Disease Irrespective of HPV Type, Regardless of Current or Prior Infection with Vaccine or Non-Vaccine HPV Types
Study 2: The impact of CERVARIX against the overall burden of HPV-related cervical disease results from a combination of prophylactic efficacy against, and disease contribution of, HPV-16, HPV-18, and non-vaccine HPV types.
In the population naïve to oncogenic HPV (TVC naïve), CERVARIX reduced the overall incidence of CIN1/2/3 or AIS, CIN2/3 or AIS, and CIN3 or AIS regardless of the HPV DNA type in the lesion (Table 7). In the population of women naïve and non-naïve (TVC), vaccine efficacy against CIN1/2/3 or AIS, CIN2/3 or AIS, and CIN3 or AIS was demonstrated in all women regardless of HPV DNA type in the lesion (Table 7).
[See table 7 at right]
In exploratory analyses, CERVARIX reduced definitive cervical therapy procedures (includes loop electrosurgical excision procedure [LEEP], cold-knife Cone, and laser procedures) by 24.7% (96.1% CI: 7.4, 38.9) in the TVC and by 68.8% (96.1% CI: 50.0, 81.2) in the TVC naïve.
To assess reductions in disease caused by non-vaccine HPV types, two analyses were conducted combining 12 non-vaccine oncogenic HPV types, including and excluding lesions in which HPV-16 or HPV-18 were also detected. In these analyses, among females who received 3 doses of CERVARIX and were DNA negative for the specific HPV type at baseline and month 6, CERVARIX reduced the incidence of CIN2/3 or AIS by 54.0% (96.1% CI: 34.0, 68.4) and 37.4% (96.1% CI: 7.4, 58.2), respectively.
Post-hoc analyses, adjusted for multiplicity, were conducted to assess the impact of CERVARIX on CIN2/3 or AIS due to specific non-vaccine HPV types. The ATP cohort for these analyses included all subjects irrespective of serostatus who received 3 doses of CERVARIX and were DNA negative for the specific HPV type at baseline and month 6. These post-hoc analyses were also conducted in the TVC naïve population. In analyses including lesions in which HPV-16 or HPV-18 were also detected, vaccine efficacy in prevention of CIN2/3 or AIS associated with HPV-31 was 92.0% (99.7% CI: 49.0, 99.8) and 100% (99.7% CI: 62.3, 100), respectively. In analyses excluding lesions in which HPV-16 or HPV-18 were detected, vaccine efficacy in prevention of CIN2/3 or AIS associated with HPV-31 was 89.4% (99.7% CI: 29.0, 99.7) and 100% (99.7% CI: 36.3, 100), respectively.

14.4   Immunogenicity
The minimum anti-HPV titer that confers protective efficacy has not been determined.
The antibody response to HPV-16 and HPV-18 was measured using a type-specific binding ELISA (developed by

GlaxoSmithKline) and a pseudovirion-based neutralization assay (PBNA). In a subset of subjects tested for HPV-16 and HPV-18, the ELISA has been shown to correlate with the PBNA. The scales for these assays are unique to each HPV type and each assay, thus, comparison between HPV types or assays is not appropriate.
Duration of Immune Response: The duration of immunity following a complete schedule of immunization with CERVARIX has not been established. In Study 1 and Study 1 Extension, the immune response against HPV-16 and HPV-18 was evaluated for up to 76 months post-dose 1, in females 15 through 25 years of age. Vaccine-induced geometric mean titers (GMTs) for both HPV-16 and HPV-18 peaked at month 7 and thereafter reached a plateau that was sustained from month 18 up to month 76. At all timepoints, >98% of subjects were seropositive for both HPV-16 (≥8 EL.U./mL, the limit of detection) and HPV-18 (≥7 EL.U./mL, the limit of detection) by ELISA.
In Study 2, GMTs for ELISA and PBNA one month post-dose 3 were measured (Table 8). The ATP cohort for immunogenicity included all evaluable subjects for whom data concerning immunogenicity endpoint measures were available. These included subjects for whom assay results were available for antibodies against at least one vaccine type. Subjects who acquired either HPV-16 or HPV-18 infection during the trial were excluded. Of subjects seronegative at baseline, 99.5% were seropositive for anti-HPV-16 and anti-HPV-18 antibodies at month 7 post-vaccination.
[See table 8 above]

14.5   Bridging of Efficacy from Women to Adolescent Girls
The immunogenicity of CERVARIX was evaluated in 2 clinical studies involving 1,193 girls 10 through 14 years of age who received CERVARIX.
Study 3 (HPV 013) was a double-blind, randomized, controlled study in which 1,035 subjects received CERVARIX and 1,032 subjects received a Hepatitis A Vaccine 360 EL.U. as the control vaccine with a subset of subjects evaluated for immunogenicity. All initially seronegative subjects in the group who received CERVARIX were seropositive after vaccination, i.e., had levels of antibody greater than the limit of detection of the assay to both HPV-16 (≥8 EL.U./mL) and HPV-18 (≥7 EL.U./mL) antigens. The GMTs for anti-HPV-16 and anti-HPV-18 antibodies in initially seronegative subjects are presented in Table 9.
[See table 9 at top of next page]
In Study 4 (HPV 012), the immunogenicity of CERVARIX administered to girls 10 through 14 years of age was compared to that in females 15 through 25 years of age. The immune response in girls 10 through 14 years of age mea-

---

Table 7. Efficacy of CERVARIX in Prevention of CIN or AIS Irrespective of Any HPV Type in Females 15 Through 25 Years of Age, Regardless of Current or Prior Infection with Vaccine or Non-Vaccine Types (Study 2)

	CERVARIX		Control		
	N	Number of Cases	N	Number of Cases	% Efficacy (96.1% CI)[a]
CIN1/2/3 or AIS					
Prophylactic Efficacy[b]	5,449	106	5,436	211	50.1 (35.9, 61.4)
Irrespective of HPV DNA at Baseline[c]	8,667	451	8,682	577	21.7 (10.7, 31.4)
CIN2/3 or AIS					
Prophylactic Efficacy[b]	5,449	33	5,436	110	70.2 (54.7, 80.9)
Irrespective of HPV DNA at Baseline[c]	8,667	224	8,682	322	30.4 (16.4, 42.1)
CIN3 or AIS					
Prophylactic Efficacy[b]	5,449	3	5,436	23	87.0 (54.9, 97.7)
Irrespective of HPV DNA at Baseline[c]	8,667	77	8,682	116	33.4 (9.1, 51.5)

CI = Confidence Interval.
[a] The 96.1% confidence interval reflected in this final analysis results from statistical adjustment for the previously conducted interim analysis.
[b] TVC naïve: includes all vaccinated subjects (who received at least one dose of vaccine) who had normal cytology, were HPV DNA negative for 14 oncogenic HPV types (including HPV-16 and HPV-18), and seronegative for HPV-16 and HPV-18 at baseline (N). Case counting started on day 1 after the first dose.
[c] TVC: includes all vaccinated subjects (who received at least one dose of vaccine) irrespective of HPV DNA status and serostatus at baseline (N). Case counting started on day 1 after the first dose.

Table 8. Summary of Anti-HPV Geometric Mean Titers (GMTs) for HPV-16 and HPV-18 at Month 7 for Initially Seronegative Females 15 Through 25 Years of Age (According to Protocol Cohort for Immunogenicity[a]) (Study 2)

Antibody Assay	N	CERVARIX GMT (95% CI)	N	Control GMT (95% CI)
ELISA[b] (EL.U./mL)				
Anti-HPV-16	861	9,206.4 (8,607.2, 9,847.2)	738	4.4 (4.2, 4.6)
Anti-HPV-18	924	4,744.6 (4,454.1, 5,053.9)	769	3.8 (3.6, 3.9)
PBNA[c] (ED$_{50}$)				
Anti-HPV-16	46	27,364.8 (19,780.1, 37,857.9)	44	20.0 (20.0, 20.0)
Anti-HPV-18	46	9,052 (6,851.8, 11,960.5)	44	20.0 (20.0, 20.0)

[a] Subjects who received 3 doses of vaccine for whom assay results were available for at least one post-vaccination antibody measurement (N). Subjects who acquired either HPV-16 or HPV-18 infection during the study were excluded.
[b] Enzyme linked immunosorbent assay (assay cut-off 8 E.L.U./mL for anti-HPV-16 antibody and 7 EL.U./mL for anti-HPV-18 antibody).
[c] Pseudovirion-based neutralization assay (assay cut-off 40 ED$_{50}$ for both anti-HPV-16 antibody and anti-HPV-18 antibody).

Table 9. Geometric Mean Titers (GMTs) at Months 7 and 18 for Initially Seronegative Females 10 Through 14 Years of Age (According To Protocol Cohort for Immunogenicity[a]) (Study 3)

Age Group	Anti-HPV-16 Antibodies GMT EL.U./mL (95% CI)			Anti-HPV-18 Antibodies GMT EL.U./mL (95% CI)		
	N	Month 7	Month 18	N	Month 7	Month 18
10-14 years of age	556-619	19,882.0 (18,626.7, 21,221.9)	3,888.8 (3,605.0, 4,195.0)	562-628	8,262.0 (7,725.0, 8,836.2)	1,539.4 (1,418.8, 1,670.3)

[a] Subjects who received 3 doses of vaccine for whom assay results were available for at least one post-vaccination antibody measurement (N).

Table 10. Geometric Mean Titers (GMTs) and Seropositivity Rates at Month 7 for Initially Seronegative Females 10 Through 14 Years of Age Compared to 15 Through 25 Years of Age (According To Protocol Cohort for Immunogenicity[a]) (Study 4)

Antibody Assay	10-14 Years of Age			15-25 Years of Age		
	N	GMT[b] EL.U./mL (95% CI)	Seropositivity Rate[c] %	N	GMT[b] EL.U./mL (95% CI)	Seropositivity Rate[c] %
Anti-HPV-16	143	17,272.5 (15,117.9, 19,734.1)	100	118	7,438.9 (6,324.6, 8,749.6)	100
Anti-HPV-18	141	6,863.8 (5,976.3, 7,883.0)	100	116	3,070.1 (2,600.0, 3,625.4)	100

[a] Subjects who received 3 doses of vaccine for whom assay results were available for at least one post-vaccination antibody measurement (N).
[b] Non-inferiority based on the upper limit of the 2-sided 95% CI for the GMT ratio (15-25 year olds/10-14 year olds) was <2.
[c] Non-inferiority based on the upper limit of the 2-sided 95% CI for the difference between the seropositivity rates for 10-14 year olds and 15-25 year olds was <10%.

sured one month post-dose 3 was non-inferior to that seen in females 15 through 25 years of age for both HPV-16 and HPV-18 antigens (Table 10).
[See table 10 above]
Based on these immunogenicity data, the efficacy of CERVARIX is inferred in girls 10 through 14 years of age.

16 HOW SUPPLIED/STORAGE AND HANDLING
CERVARIX is available in 0.5-mL single-dose vials and pre-filled TIP-LOK syringes.
Single-Dose Vials
NDC 58160-830-11 (package of 10)
Single-Dose Prefilled Disposable TIP-LOK Syringes (packaged without needles)
NDC 58160-830-32 (package of 1)
NDC 58160-830-46 (package of 5)
Store refrigerated between 2° and 8°C (36° and 46°F). Do not freeze. Discard if the vaccine has been frozen. Upon storage, a fine, white deposit with a clear, colorless supernatant may be observed. This does not constitute a sign of deterioration.

17 PATIENT COUNSELING INFORMATION
Provide the Vaccine Information Statements prior to immunization. This is required by the National Childhood Vaccine Injury Act of 1986 and are available free of charge at the Centers for Disease Control and Prevention (CDC) website (www.cdc.gov/vaccines).
Inform the patient, parent, or guardian:
• Vaccination does not substitute for routine cervical cancer screening. Women who receive CERVARIX should continue to undergo cervical cancer screening per standard of care.
• CERVARIX does not protect against disease from HPV types to which a woman has previously been exposed through sexual activity.
• Since syncope has been reported following vaccination in young females, sometimes resulting in falling with injury, observation for 15 minutes after administration is recommended.
• Information regarding potential benefits and risks associated with vaccination.
• Report any adverse events to their healthcare provider.
• Safety has not been established in pregnant women. CERVARIX is not recommended for use in pregnant women or women planning to become pregnant during the vaccination course. Register women who receive CERVARIX while pregnant in the pregnancy registry by calling 1-888-452-9622.
CERVARIX and TIP-LOK are registered trademarks of GlaxoSmithKline.
Manufactured by **GlaxoSmithKline Biologicals**
Rixensart, Belgium, US License 1617
Distributed by **GlaxoSmithKline**
Research Triangle Park, NC 27709

©2010, GlaxoSmithKline. All rights reserved.
August 2010
CRX:4PI

COREG®   ℞
[kor' eg]
(carvedilol)
Tablets

HIGHLIGHTS OF PRESCRIBING INFORMATION
These highlights do not include all the information needed to use COREG safely and effectively. See full prescribing information for COREG.
COREG® (carvedilol) tablets
Initial U.S. Approval: 1995
——————INDICATIONS AND USAGE——————
COREG is an alpha/beta-adrenergic blocking agent indicated for the treatment of:
• Mild to severe chronic heart failure (1.1)
• Left ventricular dysfunction following myocardial infarction in clinically stable patients (1.2)
• Hypertension (1.3)
——————DOSAGE AND ADMINISTRATION——————
Take with food. Individualize dosage and monitor during up-titration. (2)
• Heart failure: Start at 3.125 mg twice daily and increase to 6.25, 12.5, and then 25 mg twice daily over intervals of at least 2 weeks. Maintain lower doses if higher doses are not tolerated. (2.1)
• Left ventricular dysfunction following myocardial infarction: Start at 6.25 mg twice daily and increase to 12.5 mg then 25 mg twice daily after intervals of 3 to 10 days. A lower starting dose or slower titration may be used. (2.2)
• Hypertension: Start at 6.25 mg twice daily and increase if needed for blood pressure control to 12.5 mg then 25 mg twice daily over intervals of 1 to 2 weeks. (2.3)
——————DOSAGE FORMS AND STRENGTHS——————
Tablets: 3.125, 6.25, 12.5, 25 mg (3)
——————CONTRAINDICATIONS——————
• Bronchial asthma or related bronchospastic conditions (4)
• Second- or third-degree AV block (4)
• Sick sinus syndrome (4)
• Severe bradycardia (unless permanent pacemaker in place) (4)
• Patients in cardiogenic shock or decompensated heart failure requiring the use of IV inotropic therapy. (4)
• Severe hepatic impairment (2.4, 4)
• History of serious hypersensitivity reaction (e.g., Stevens-Johnson syndrome, anaphylactic reaction, angioedema) to any component of this medication or other medications containing carvedilol. (4)

——————WARNINGS AND PRECAUTIONS——————
• Acute exacerbation of coronary artery disease upon cessation of therapy: Do not abruptly discontinue. (5.1)
• Bradycardia, hypotension, worsening heart failure/fluid retention may occur. Reduce the dose as needed. (5.2, 5.3, 5.4)
• Non-allergic bronchospasm (e.g., chronic bronchitis and emphysema): Avoid β-blockers. (4) However, if deemed necessary, use with caution and at lowest effective dose. (5.5)
• Diabetes: Monitor glucose as β-blockers may mask symptoms of hypoglycemia or worsen hyperglycemia. (5.6)
——————ADVERSE REACTIONS——————
Most common adverse events (6.1):
• Heart failure and left ventricular dysfunction following myocardial infarction (≥10%): Dizziness, fatigue, hypotension, diarrhea, hyperglycemia, asthenia, bradycardia, weight increase
• Hypertension (≥5%): Dizziness
To report SUSPECTED ADVERSE REACTIONS, contact GlaxoSmithKline at 1-888-825-5249 or FDA at 1-800-FDA-1088 or www.fda.gov/medwatch.
——————DRUG INTERACTIONS——————
• CYP P450 2D6 enzyme inhibitors may increase and rifampin may decrease carvedilol levels. (7.1, 7.5)
• Hypotensive agents (e.g., reserpine, MAO inhibitors, clonidine) may increase the risk of hypotension and/or severe bradycardia. (7.2)
• Cyclosporine or digoxin levels may increase. (7.3, 7.4)
• Both digitalis glycosides and β-blockers slow atrioventricular conduction and decrease heart rate. Concomitant use can increase the risk of bradycardia. (7.4)
• Amiodarone may increase carvedilol levels resulting in further slowing of the heart rate or cardiac conduction. (7.6)
• Verapamil- or diltiazem-type calcium channel blockers may affect ECG and/or blood pressure. (7.7)
• Insulin and oral hypoglycemics action may be enhanced. (7.8)
Revised: June 2009
CRG:18PI
See 17 for PATIENT COUNSELING INFORMATION and FDA-approved patient labeling.
Revised: 07/2009

FULL PRESCRIBING INFORMATION: CONTENTS*

*** Sections or subsections omitted from the full prescribing information are not listed**

FULL PRESCRIBING INFORMATION

1 INDICATIONS AND USAGE

1.1 Heart Failure

COREG is indicated for the treatment of mild-to-severe chronic heart failure of ischemic or cardiomyopathic origin, usually in addition to diuretics, ACE inhibitors, and digitalis, to increase survival and, also, to reduce the risk of hospitalization *[see Drug Interactions (7.4) and Clinical Studies (14.1)]*.

1.2 Left Ventricular Dysfunction Following Myocardial Infarction

COREG is indicated to reduce cardiovascular mortality in clinically stable patients who have survived the acute phase of a myocardial infarction and have a left ventricular ejection fraction of ≤40% (with or without symptomatic heart failure) *[see Clinical Studies (14.2)]*.

1.3 Hypertension

COREG is indicated for the management of essential hypertension *[see Clinical Studies (14.3, 14.4)]*. It can be used alone or in combination with other antihypertensive agents, especially thiazide-type diuretics *[see Drug Interactions (7.2)]*.

2 DOSAGE AND ADMINISTRATION

COREG should be taken with food to slow the rate of absorption and reduce the incidence of orthostatic effects.

2.1 Heart Failure

DOSAGE MUST BE INDIVIDUALIZED AND CLOSELY MONITORED BY A PHYSICIAN DURING UP-TITRATION. Prior to initiation of COREG, it is recommended that fluid retention be minimized. The recommended starting dose of COREG is 3.125 mg twice daily for 2 weeks. If tolerated, patients may have their dose increased to 6.25, 12.5, and 25 mg twice daily over successive intervals of at least 2 weeks. Patients should be maintained on lower doses if higher doses are not tolerated. A maximum dose of 50 mg twice daily has been administered to patients with mild-to-moderate heart failure weighing over 85 kg (187 lbs).

Patients should be advised that initiation of treatment and (to a lesser extent) dosage increases may be associated with transient symptoms of dizziness or lightheadedness (and rarely syncope) within the first hour after dosing. During these periods, patients should avoid situations such as driving or hazardous tasks, where symptoms could result in injury. Vasodilatory symptoms often do not require treatment, but it may be useful to separate the time of dosing of COREG from that of the ACE inhibitor or to reduce temporarily the dose of the ACE inhibitor. The dose of COREG should not be increased until symptoms of worsening heart failure or vasodilation have been stabilized.

Fluid retention (with or without transient worsening heart failure symptoms) should be treated by an increase in the dose of diuretics.

The dose of COREG should be reduced if patients experience bradycardia (heart rate <55 beats/minute).

Episodes of dizziness or fluid retention during initiation of COREG can generally be managed without discontinuation of treatment and do not preclude subsequent successful titration of, or a favorable response to, carvedilol.

2.2 Left Ventricular Dysfunction Following Myocardial Infarction

DOSAGE MUST BE INDIVIDUALIZED AND MONITORED DURING UP-TITRATION. Treatment with COREG may be started as an inpatient or outpatient and should be started after the patient is hemodynamically stable and fluid retention has been minimized. It is recommended that COREG be started at 6.25 mg twice daily and increased after 3 to 10 days, based on tolerability, to 12.5 mg twice daily, then again to the target dose of 25 mg twice daily. A lower starting dose may be used (3.125 mg twice daily) and/or the rate of up-titration may be slowed if clinically indicated (e.g., due to low blood pressure or heart rate, or fluid retention). Patients should be maintained on lower doses if higher doses are not tolerated. The recommended dosing regimen need not be altered in patients who received treatment with an IV or oral β-blocker during the acute phase of the myocardial infarction.

2.3 Hypertension

DOSAGE MUST BE INDIVIDUALIZED. The recommended starting dose of COREG is 6.25 mg twice daily. If this dose is tolerated, using standing systolic pressure measured about 1 hour after dosing as a guide, the dose should be maintained for 7 to 14 days, and then increased to 12.5 mg twice daily if needed, based on trough blood pressure, again using standing systolic pressure one hour after dosing as a guide for tolerance. This dose should also be maintained for 7 to 14 days and can then be adjusted upward to 25 mg twice daily if tolerated and needed. The full antihypertensive effect of COREG is seen within 7 to 14 days. Total daily dose should not exceed 50 mg.

Concomitant administration with a diuretic can be expected to produce additive effects and exaggerate the orthostatic component of carvedilol action.

2.4 Hepatic Impairment

COREG should not be given to patients with severe hepatic impairment *[see Contraindications (4)]*.

3 DOSAGE FORMS AND STRENGTHS

The white, oval, film-coated tablets are available in the following strengths: 3.125 mg–engraved with 39 and SB, 6.25 mg–engraved with 4140 and SB, 12.5 mg–engraved with 4141 and SB, and 25 mg–engraved with 4142 and SB.

4 CONTRAINDICATIONS

COREG is contraindicated in the following conditions:

- Bronchial asthma or related bronchospastic conditions. Deaths from status asthmaticus have been reported following single doses of COREG.
- Second- or third-degree AV block
- Sick sinus syndrome
- Severe bradycardia (unless a permanent pacemaker is in place)
- Patients with cardiogenic shock or who have decompensated heart failure requiring the use of intravenous inotropic therapy. Such patients should first be weaned from intravenous therapy before initiating COREG.
- Patients with severe hepatic impairment
- Patients with a history of a serious hypersensitivity reaction (e.g., Stevens-Johnson syndrome, anaphylactic reaction, angioedema) to any component of this medication or other medications containing carvedilol.

5 WARNINGS AND PRECAUTIONS

5.1 Cessation of Therapy

Patients with coronary artery disease, who are being treated with COREG, should be advised against abrupt discontinuation of therapy. Severe exacerbation of angina and the occurrence of myocardial infarction and ventricular arrhythmias have been reported in angina patients following the abrupt discontinuation of therapy with β-blockers. The last 2 complications may occur with or without preceding exacerbation of the angina pectoris. As with other β-blockers, when discontinuation of COREG is planned, the patients should be carefully observed and advised to limit physical activity to a minimum. COREG should be discontinued over 1 to 2 weeks whenever possible. If the angina worsens or acute coronary insufficiency develops, it is recommended that COREG be promptly reinstituted, at least temporarily. Because coronary artery disease is common and may be unrecognized, it may be prudent not to discontinue therapy with COREG abruptly even in patients treated only for hypertension or heart failure.

5.2 Bradycardia

In clinical trials, COREG caused bradycardia in about 2% of hypertensive patients, 9% of heart failure patients, and 6.5% of myocardial infarction patients with left ventricular dysfunction. If pulse rate drops below 55 beats/minute, the dosage should be reduced.

5.3 Hypotension

In clinical trials of primarily mild-to-moderate heart failure, hypotension and postural hypotension occurred in 9.7% and syncope in 3.4% of patients receiving COREG compared to 3.6% and 2.5% of placebo patients, respectively. The risk for these events was highest during the first 30 days of dosing, corresponding to the up-titration period and was a cause for discontinuation of therapy in 0.7% of patients receiving COREG, compared to 0.4% of placebo patients. In a long-term, placebo-controlled trial in severe heart failure (COPERNICUS), hypotension and postural hypotension occurred in 15.1% and syncope in 2.9% of heart failure patients receiving COREG compared to 8.7% and 2.3% of placebo patients, respectively. These events were a cause for discontinuation of therapy in 1.1% of patients receiving COREG, compared to 0.8% of placebo patients.

Postural hypotension occurred in 1.8% and syncope in 0.1% of hypertensive patients, primarily following the initial dose or at the time of dose increase and was a cause for discontinuation of therapy in 1% of patients.

In the CAPRICORN study of survivors of an acute myocardial infarction, hypotension or postural hypotension occurred in 20.2% of patients receiving COREG compared to 12.6% of placebo patients. Syncope was reported in 3.9% and 1.9% of patients, respectively. These events were a cause for discontinuation of therapy in 2.5% of patients receiving COREG, compared to 0.2% of placebo patients.

Starting with a low dose, administration with food, and gradual up-titration should decrease the likelihood of syncope or excessive hypotension *[see Dosage and Administration (2.1, 2.2, 2.3)]*. During initiation of therapy, the patient should be cautioned to avoid situations such as driving or hazardous tasks, where injury could result should syncope occur.

5.4 Heart Failure/Fluid Retention

Worsening heart failure or fluid retention may occur during up-titration of carvedilol. If such symptoms occur, diuretics should be increased and the carvedilol dose should not be advanced until clinical stability resumes *[see Dosage and Administration (2)]*. Occasionally it is necessary to lower the carvedilol dose or temporarily discontinue it. Such episodes do not preclude subsequent successful titration of, or a favorable response to, carvedilol. In a placebo-controlled trial of patients with severe heart failure, worsening heart failure during the first 3 months was reported to a similar degree with carvedilol and with placebo. When treatment was maintained beyond 3 months, worsening heart failure was reported less frequently in patients treated with carvedilol than with placebo. Worsening heart failure observed during long-term therapy is more likely to be related to the patients' underlying disease than to treatment with carvedilol.

5.5 Non-allergic Bronchospasm

Patients with bronchospastic disease (e.g., chronic bronchitis and emphysema) should, in general, not receive β-blockers. COREG may be used with caution, however, in patients who do not respond to, or cannot tolerate, other antihypertensive agents. It is prudent, if COREG is used, to use the smallest effective dose, so that inhibition of endogenous or exogenous β-agonists is minimized.

In clinical trials of patients with heart failure, patients with bronchospastic disease were enrolled if they did not require oral or inhaled medication to treat their bronchospastic disease. In such patients, it is recommended that carvedilol be used with caution. The dosing recommendations should be followed closely and the dose should be lowered if any evidence of bronchospasm is observed during up-titration.

5.6 Glycemic Control in Type 2 Diabetes

In general, β-blockers may mask some of the manifestations of hypoglycemia, particularly tachycardia. Nonselective β-blockers may potentiate insulin-induced hypoglycemia and delay recovery of serum glucose levels. Patients subject to spontaneous hypoglycemia, or diabetic patients receiving insulin or oral hypoglycemic agents, should be cautioned about these possibilities.

In heart failure patients with diabetes, carvedilol therapy may lead to worsening hyperglycemia, which responds to intensification of hypoglycemic therapy. It is recommended that blood glucose be monitored when carvedilol dosing is initiated, adjusted, or discontinued. Studies designed to examine the effects of carvedilol on glycemic control in patients with diabetes and heart failure have not been conducted.

In a study designed to examine the effects of carvedilol on glycemic control in a population with mild-to-moderate hypertension and well-controlled type 2 diabetes mellitus, carvedilol had no adverse effect on glycemic control, based on HbA1c measurements *[see Clinical Studies (14.4)]*.

5.7 Peripheral Vascular Disease

β-blockers can precipitate or aggravate symptoms of arterial insufficiency in patients with peripheral vascular disease. Caution should be exercised in such individuals.

5.8 Deterioration of Renal Function

Rarely, use of carvedilol in patients with heart failure has resulted in deterioration of renal function. Patients at risk appear to be those with low blood pressure (systolic blood pressure <100 mm Hg), ischemic heart disease and diffuse vascular disease, and/or underlying renal insufficiency. Renal function has returned to baseline when carvedilol was stopped. In patients with these risk factors it is recommended that renal function be monitored during up-titration of carvedilol and the drug discontinued or dosage reduced if worsening of renal function occurs.

5.9 Anesthesia and Major Surgery

If treatment with COREG is to be continued perioperatively, particular care should be taken when anesthetic agents which depress myocardial function, such as ether, cyclopropane, and trichloroethylene, are used *[see Overdosage (10) for information on treatment of bradycardia and hypertension]*.

5.10 Thyrotoxicosis

β-adrenergic blockade may mask clinical signs of hyperthyroidism, such as tachycardia. Abrupt withdrawal of β-blockade may be followed by an exacerbation of the symptoms of hyperthyroidism or may precipitate thyroid storm.

5.11 Pheochromocytoma

In patients with pheochromocytoma, an α-blocking agent should be initiated prior to the use of any β-blocking agent. Although carvedilol has both α- and β-blocking pharmacologic activities, there has been no experience with its use in this condition. Therefore, caution should be taken in the administration of carvedilol to patients suspected of having pheochromocytoma.

5.12 Prinzmetal's Variant Angina

Agents with non-selective β-blocking activity may provoke chest pain in patients with Prinzmetal's variant angina. There has been no clinical experience with carvedilol in these patients although the α-blocking activity may prevent such symptoms. However, caution should be taken in the administration of carvedilol to patients suspected of having Prinzmetal's variant angina.

5.13 Risk of Anaphylactic Reaction

While taking β-blockers, patients with a history of severe anaphylactic reaction to a variety of allergens may be more reactive to repeated challenge, either accidental, diagnostic, or therapeutic. Such patients may be unresponsive to the usual doses of epinephrine used to treat allergic reaction.

6   ADVERSE REACTIONS

6.1   Clinical Studies Experience

COREG has been evaluated for safety in patients with heart failure (mild, moderate, and severe), in patients with left ventricular dysfunction following myocardial infarction and in hypertensive patients. The observed adverse event profile was consistent with the pharmacology of the drug and the health status of the patients in the clinical trials. Adverse events reported for each of these patient populations are provided below. Excluded are adverse events considered too general to be informative, and those not reasonably associated with the use of the drug because they were associated with the condition being treated or are very common in the treated population. Rates of adverse events were generally similar across demographic subsets (men and women, elderly and non-elderly, blacks and non-blacks).

Heart Failure

COREG has been evaluated for safety in heart failure in more than 4,500 patients worldwide of whom more than 2,100 participated in placebo-controlled clinical trials. Approximately 60% of the total treated population in placebo-controlled clinical trials received COREG for at least 6 months and 30% received COREG for at least 12 months. In the COMET trial, 1,511 patients with mild-to-moderate heart failure were treated with COREG for up to 5.9 years (mean 4.8 years). Both in US clinical trials in mild-to-moderate heart failure that compared COREG in daily doses up to 100 mg (n = 765) to placebo (n = 437), and in a multinational clinical trial in severe heart failure (COPERNICUS) that compared COREG in daily doses up to 50 mg (n = 1,156) with placebo (n = 1,133), discontinuation rates for adverse experiences were similar in carvedilol and placebo patients. In placebo-controlled clinical trials, the only cause of discontinuation >1%, and occurring more often on carvedilol was dizziness (1.3% on carvedilol, 0.6% on placebo in the COPERNICUS trial).

Table 1 shows adverse events reported in patients with mild-to-moderate heart failure enrolled in US placebo-controlled clinical trials, and with severe heart failure enrolled in the COPERNICUS trial. Shown are adverse events that occurred more frequently in drug-treated patients than placebo-treated patients with an incidence of >3% in patients treated with carvedilol regardless of causality. Median study medication exposure was 6.3 months for both carvedilol and placebo patients in the trials of mild-to-moderate heart failure, and 10.4 months in the trial of severe heart failure patients. The adverse event profile of COREG observed in the long-term COMET study was generally similar to that observed in the US Heart Failure Trials.

[See table 1 at left]

Cardiac failure and dyspnea were also reported in these studies, but the rates were equal or greater in patients who received placebo.

The following adverse events were reported with a frequency of >1% but ≤3% and more frequently with COREG in either the US placebo-controlled trials in patients with mild-to-moderate heart failure, or in patients with severe heart failure in the COPERNICUS trial.

Incidence >1% to ≤3%

Body as a Whole: Allergy, malaise, hypovolemia, fever, leg edema.

Cardiovascular: Fluid overload, postural hypotension, aggravated angina pectoris, AV block, palpitation, hypertension.

Central and Peripheral Nervous System: Hypesthesia, vertigo, paresthesia.

Gastrointestinal: Melena, periodontitis.

Liver and Biliary System: SGPT increased, SGOT increased.

Metabolic and Nutritional: Hyperuricemia, hypoglycemia, hyponatremia, increased alkaline phosphatase, glycosuria, hypervolemia, diabetes mellitus, GGT increased, weight loss, hyperkalemia, creatinine increased.

Musculoskeletal: Muscle cramps.

Platelet, Bleeding and Clotting: Prothrombin decreased, purpura, thrombocytopenia.

Psychiatric: Somnolence.

Reproductive, male: Impotence.

Special Senses: Blurred vision.

Urinary System: Renal insufficiency, albuminuria, hematuria.

Left Ventricular Dysfunction Following Myocardial Infarction

COREG has been evaluated for safety in survivors of an acute myocardial infarction with left ventricular dysfunction in the CAPRICORN trial which involved 969 patients who received COREG and 980 who received placebo. Approximately 75% of the patients received COREG for at least 6 months and 53% received COREG for at least 12 months. Patients were treated for an average of 12.9 months and 12.8 months with COREG and placebo, respectively.

The most common adverse events reported with COREG in the CAPRICORN trial were consistent with the profile of the drug in the US heart failure trials and the COPERNICUS trial. The only additional adverse events reported in CAPRICORN in >3% of the patients and more commonly on carvedilol were dyspnea, anemia, and lung edema. The following adverse events were reported with a frequency of >1% but ≤3% and more frequently with COREG: Flu syndrome, cerebrovascular accident, peripheral vascular disorder, hypotonia, depression, gastrointestinal pain, arthritis, and gout. The overall rates of discontinuations due to adverse events were similar in both groups of patients. In this database, the only cause of discontinuation >1%, and occurring more often on carvedilol was hypotension (1.5% on carvedilol, 0.2% on placebo).

Hypertension

COREG has been evaluated for safety in hypertension in more than 2,193 patients in US clinical trials and in 2,976 patients in international clinical trials. Approximately 36% of the total treated population received COREG for at least 6 months. Most adverse events reported during therapy with COREG were of mild to moderate severity. In US controlled clinical trials directly comparing COREG in doses up

Table 1. Adverse Events (%) Occurring More Frequently With COREG Than With Placebo in Patients With Mild-to-Moderate Heart Failure (HF) Enrolled in US Heart Failure Trials or in Patients With Severe Heart Failure in the COPERNICUS Trial (Incidence >3% in Patients Treated With Carvedilol, Regardless of Causality)

	Mild-to-Moderate HF		Severe HF	
	COREG	Placebo	COREG	Placebo
	(n = 765)	(n = 437)	(n = 1,156)	(n = 1,133)
Body as a Whole				
Asthenia	7	7	11	9
Fatigue	24	22	—	—
Digoxin level increased	5	4	2	1
Edema generalized	5	3	6	5
Edema dependent	4	2		
Cardiovascular				
Bradycardia	9	1	10	3
Hypotension	9	3	14	8
Syncope	3	3	8	5
Angina pectoris	2	3	6	4
Central Nervous System				
Dizziness	32	19	24	17
Headache	8	7	5	3
Gastrointestinal				
Diarrhea	12	6	5	3
Nausea	9	5	4	3
Vomiting	6	4	1	2
Metabolic				
Hyperglycemia	12	8	5	3
Weight increase	10	7	12	11
BUN increased	6	5	—	—
NPN increased	6	5	—	—
Hypercholesterolemia	4	3	1	1
Edema peripheral	2	1	7	6
Musculoskeletal				
Arthralgia	6	5	1	1
Respiratory				
Cough increased	8	9	5	4
Rales	4	4	4	2
Vision				
Vision abnormal	5	2	—	—

to 50 mg (n = 1,142) to placebo (n = 462), 4.9% of patients receiving COREG discontinued for adverse events versus 5.2% of placebo patients. Although there was no overall difference in discontinuation rates, discontinuations were more common in the carvedilol group for postural hypotension (1% versus 0). The overall incidence of adverse events in US placebo-controlled trials increased with increasing dose of COREG. For individual adverse events this could only be distinguished for dizziness, which increased in frequency from 2% to 5% as total daily dose increased from 6.25 mg to 50 mg.

Table 2 shows adverse events in US placebo-controlled clinical trials for hypertension that occurred with an incidence of ≥1% regardless of causality, and that were more frequent in drug-treated patients than placebo-treated patients.

Table 2. Adverse Events (%) Occurring in US Placebo-Controlled Hypertension Trials (Incidence ≥1%, Regardless of Causality)*

	COREG	Placebo
	(n = 1,142)	(n = 462)
Cardiovascular		
Bradycardia	2	—
Postural hypotension	2	—
Peripheral edema	1	—
Central Nervous System		
Dizziness	6	5
Insomnia	2	1
Gastrointestinal		
Diarrhea	2	1
Hematologic		
Thrombocytopenia	1	—
Metabolic		
Hypertriglyceridemia	1	—

*Shown are events with rate >1% rounded to nearest integer.

Dyspnea and fatigue were also reported in these studies, but the rates were equal or greater in patients who received placebo.

The following adverse events not described above were reported as possibly or probably related to COREG in worldwide open or controlled trials with COREG in patients with hypertension or heart failure.

Incidence >0.1% to ≤1%
Cardiovascular: Peripheral ischemia, tachycardia.
Central and Peripheral Nervous System: Hypokinesia.
Gastrointestinal: Bilirubinemia, increased hepatic enzymes (0.2% of hypertension patients and 0.4% of heart failure patients were discontinued from therapy because of increases in hepatic enzymes) [see Adverse Reactions (6.2)].
Psychiatric: Nervousness, sleep disorder, aggravated depression, impaired concentration, abnormal thinking, paroniria, emotional lability.
Respiratory System: Asthma [see Contraindications (4)].
Reproductive, male: Decreased libido.
Skin and Appendages: Pruritus, rash erythematous, rash maculopapular, rash psoriaform, photosensitivity reaction.
Special Senses: Tinnitus.
Urinary System: Micturition frequency increased.
Autonomic Nervous System: Dry mouth, sweating increased.
Metabolic and Nutritional: Hypokalemia, hypertriglyceridemia.
Hematologic: Anemia, leukopenia.

The following events were reported in ≤0.1% of patients and are potentially important: Complete AV block, bundle branch block, myocardial ischemia, cerebrovascular disorder, convulsions, migraine, neuralgia, paresis, anaphylactoid reaction, alopecia, exfoliative dermatitis, amnesia, GI hemorrhage, bronchospasm, pulmonary edema, decreased hearing, respiratory alkalosis, increased BUN, decreased HDL, pancytopenia, and atypical lymphocytes.

6.2   Laboratory Abnormalities
Reversible elevations in serum transaminases (ALT or AST) have been observed during treatment with COREG. Rates of transaminase elevations (2- to 3-times the upper limit of normal) observed during controlled clinical trials have generally been similar between patients treated with COREG

and those treated with placebo. However, transaminase elevations, confirmed by rechallenge, have been observed with COREG. In a long-term, placebo-controlled trial in severe heart failure, patients treated with COREG had lower values for hepatic transaminases than patients treated with placebo, possibly because improvements in cardiac function induced by COREG led to less hepatic congestion and/or improved hepatic blood flow.

COREG has not been associated with clinically significant changes in serum potassium, total triglycerides, total cholesterol, HDL cholesterol, uric acid, blood urea nitrogen, or creatinine. No clinically relevant changes were noted in fasting serum glucose in hypertensive patients; fasting serum glucose was not evaluated in the heart failure clinical trials.

6.3   Postmarketing Experience
The following adverse reactions have been identified during post-approval use of COREG. Because these reactions are reported voluntarily from a population of uncertain size, it is not always possible to reliably estimate their frequency or establish a causal relationship to drug exposure.

Reports of aplastic anemia and severe skin reactions (Stevens-Johnson syndrome, toxic epidermal necrolysis, and erythema multiforme) have been rare and received only when carvedilol was administered concomitantly with other medications associated with such reactions. Rare reports of hypersensitivity reactions (e.g., anaphylactic reaction, angioedema, and urticaria) have been received for COREG and COREG CR®, including cases occurring after the initiation of COREG CR in patients previously treated with COREG. Urinary incontinence in women (which resolved upon discontinuation of the medication) and interstitial pneumonitis have been reported rarely.

7   DRUG INTERACTIONS
7.1   CYP2D6 Inhibitors and Poor Metabolizers
Interactions of carvedilol with potent inhibitors of CYP2D6 isoenzyme (such as quinidine, fluoxetine, paroxetine, and propafenone) have not been studied, but these drugs would be expected to increase blood levels of the R(+) enantiomer of carvedilol [see Clinical Pharmacology (12.3)]. Retrospective analysis of side effects in clinical trials showed that poor 2D6 metabolizers had a higher rate of dizziness during up-titration, presumably resulting from vasodilating effects of the higher concentrations of the α-blocking R(+) enantiomer.

7.2   Hypotensive Agents
Patients taking both agents with β-blocking properties and a drug that can deplete catecholamines (e.g., reserpine and monoamine oxidase inhibitors) should be observed closely for signs of hypotension and/or severe bradycardia.
Concomitant administration of clonidine with agents with β-blocking properties may potentiate blood-pressure- and heart-rate-lowering effects. When concomitant treatment with agents with β-blocking properties and clonidine is to be terminated, the β-blocking agent should be discontinued first. Clonidine therapy can then be discontinued several days later by gradually decreasing the dosage.

7.3   Cyclosporine
Modest increases in mean trough cyclosporine concentrations were observed following initiation of carvedilol treatment in 21 renal transplant patients suffering from chronic vascular rejection. In about 30% of patients, the dose of cyclosporine had to be reduced in order to maintain cyclosporine concentrations within the therapeutic range, while in the remainder no adjustment was needed. On the average for the group, the dose of cyclosporine was reduced about 20% in these patients. Due to wide interindividual variability in the dose adjustment required, it is recommended that cyclosporine concentrations be monitored closely after initiation of carvedilol therapy and that the dose of cyclosporine be adjusted as appropriate.

7.4   Digitalis Glycosides
Both digitalis glycosides and β-blockers slow atrioventricular conduction and decrease heart rate. Concomitant use can increase the risk of bradycardia. Digoxin concentrations are increased by about 15% when digoxin and carvedilol are administered concomitantly. Therefore, increased monitoring of digoxin is recommended when initiating, adjusting, or discontinuing COREG [see Clinical Pharmacology (12.5)].

7.5   Inducers/Inhibitors of Hepatic Metabolism
Rifampin reduced plasma concentrations of carvedilol by about 70% [see Clinical Pharmacology (12.5)]. Cimetidine increased AUC by about 30% but caused no change in C_{max} [see Clinical Pharmacology (12.5)].

7.6   Amiodarone
Amiodarone, and its metabolite desethyl amiodarone, inhibitors of CYP2C9 and P-glycoprotein, increased concentrations of the S(-)-enantiomer of carvedilol by at least 2-fold [see Clinical Pharmacology (12.5)]. The concomitant administration of amiodarone or other CYP2C9 inhibitors such as fluconazole with COREG may enhance the β-blocking properties of carvedilol resulting in further slowing of the heart rate or cardiac conduction. Patients should

be observed for signs of bradycardia or heart block, particularly when one agent is added to pre-existing treatment with the other.

7.7   Calcium Channel Blockers
Conduction disturbance (rarely with hemodynamic compromise) has been observed when COREG is co-administered with diltiazem. As with other agents with β-blocking properties, if COREG is to be administered with calcium channel blockers of the verapamil or diltiazem type, it is recommended that ECG and blood pressure be monitored.

7.8   Insulin or Oral Hypoglycemics
Agents with β-blocking properties may enhance the blood-sugar-reducing effect of insulin and oral hypoglycemics. Therefore, in patients taking insulin or oral hypoglycemics, regular monitoring of blood glucose is recommended [see Warnings and Precautions (5.6)].

8   USE IN SPECIFIC POPULATIONS
8.1   Pregnancy
Pregnancy Category C. Studies performed in pregnant rats and rabbits given carvedilol revealed increased post-implantation loss in rats at doses of 300 mg/kg/day (50 times the maximum recommended human dose [MRHD] as mg/m²) and in rabbits at doses of 75 mg/kg/day (25 times the MRHD as mg/m²). In the rats, there was also a decrease in fetal body weight at the maternally toxic dose of 300 mg/kg/day (50 times the MRHD as mg/m²), which was accompanied by an elevation in the frequency of fetuses with delayed skeletal development (missing or stunted 13th rib). In rats the no-observed-effect level for developmental toxicity was 60 mg/kg/day (10 times the MRHD as mg/m²); in rabbits it was 15 mg/kg/day (5 times the MRHD as mg/m²). There are no adequate and well-controlled studies in pregnant women. COREG should be used during pregnancy only if the potential benefit justifies the potential risk to the fetus.

8.3   Nursing Mothers
It is not known whether this drug is excreted in human milk. Studies in rats have shown that carvedilol and/or its metabolites (as well as other β-blockers) cross the placental barrier and are excreted in breast milk. There was increased mortality at one week post-partum in neonates from rats treated with 60 mg/kg/day (10 times the MRHD as mg/m²) and above during the last trimester through day 22 of lactation. Because many drugs are excreted in human milk and because of the potential for serious adverse reactions in nursing infants from β-blockers, especially bradycardia, a decision should be made whether to discontinue nursing or to discontinue the drug, taking into account the importance of the drug to the mother. The effects of other α- and β-blocking agents have included perinatal and neonatal distress.

8.4   Pediatric Use
Effectiveness of COREG in patients younger than 18 years of age has not been established.

In a double-blind trial, 161 children (mean age 6 years, range 2 months to 17 years; 45% less than 2 years old) with chronic heart failure [NYHA class II-IV, left ventricular ejection fraction <40% for children with a systemic left ventricle (LV), and moderate-severe ventricular dysfunction qualitatively by echo for those with a systemic ventricle that was not an LV] who were receiving standard background treatment were randomized to placebo or to 2 dose levels of carvedilol. These dose levels produced placebo-corrected heart rate reduction of 4-6 heart beats per minute, indicative of β-blockade activity. Exposure appeared to be lower in pediatric subjects than adults. After 8 months of follow-up, there was no significant effect of treatment on clinical outcomes. Adverse reactions in this trial that occurred in greater than 10% of patients treated with COREG and at twice the rate of placebo-treated patients included chest pain (17% versus 6%), dizziness (13% versus 2%), and dyspnea (11% versus 0%).

8.5   Geriatric Use
Of the 765 patients with heart failure randomized to COREG in US clinical trials, 31% (235) were 65 years of age or older, and 7.3% (56) were 75 years of age or older. Of the 1,156 patients randomized to COREG in a long-term, placebo-controlled trial in severe heart failure, 47% (547) were 65 years of age or older, and 15% (174) were 75 years of age or older. Of 3,025 patients receiving COREG in heart failure trials worldwide, 42% were 65 years of age or older. Of the 975 myocardial infarction patients randomized to COREG in the CAPRICORN trial, 48% (468) were 65 years of age or older, and 11% (111) were 75 years of age or older. Of the 2,065 hypertensive patients in US clinical trials of efficacy or safety who were treated with COREG, 21% (436) were 65 years of age or older. Of 3,722 patients receiving COREG in hypertension clinical trials conducted worldwide, 24% were 65 years of age or older.

With the exception of dizziness in hypertensive patients (incidence 8.8% in the elderly versus 6% in younger patients), no overall differences in the safety or effectiveness (see Figures 2 and 4) were observed between the older subjects and younger subjects in each of these populations. Similarly, other reported clinical experience has not identified differences in responses between the elderly and younger subjects, but greater sensitivity of some older individuals cannot be ruled out.

10 OVERDOSAGE

Overdosage may cause severe hypotension, bradycardia, cardiac insufficiency, cardiogenic shock, and cardiac arrest. Respiratory problems, bronchospasms, vomiting, lapses of consciousness, and generalized seizures may also occur.

The patient should be placed in a supine position and, where necessary, kept under observation and treated under intensive-care conditions. Gastric lavage or pharmacologically induced emesis may be used shortly after ingestion.

The following agents may be administered:

for excessive bradycardia: Atropine, 2 mg IV.

to support cardiovascular function: Glucagon, 5 to 10 mg IV rapidly over 30 seconds, followed by a continuous infusion of 5 mg/hour; sympathomimetics (dobutamine, isoprenaline, adrenaline) at doses according to body weight and effect.

If peripheral vasodilation dominates, it may be necessary to administer adrenaline or noradrenaline with continuous monitoring of circulatory conditions. For therapy-resistant bradycardia, pacemaker therapy should be performed. For bronchospasm, β-sympathomimetics (as aerosol or IV) or aminophylline IV should be given. In the event of seizures, slow IV injection of diazepam or clonazepam is recommended.

NOTE: In the event of severe intoxication where there are symptoms of shock, treatment with antidotes must be continued for a sufficiently long period of time consistent with the 7- to 10-hour half-life of carvedilol.

Cases of overdosage with COREG alone or in combination with other drugs have been reported. Quantities ingested in some cases exceeded 1,000 milligrams. Symptoms experienced included low blood pressure and heart rate. Standard supportive treatment was provided and individuals recovered.

11 DESCRIPTION

Carvedilol is a nonselective β-adrenergic blocking agent with α_1-blocking activity. It is (±)-1-(Carbazol-4-yloxy)-3-[[2-(o-methoxyphenoxy)ethyl]amino]-2-propanol. Carvedilol is a racemic mixture with the following structure:

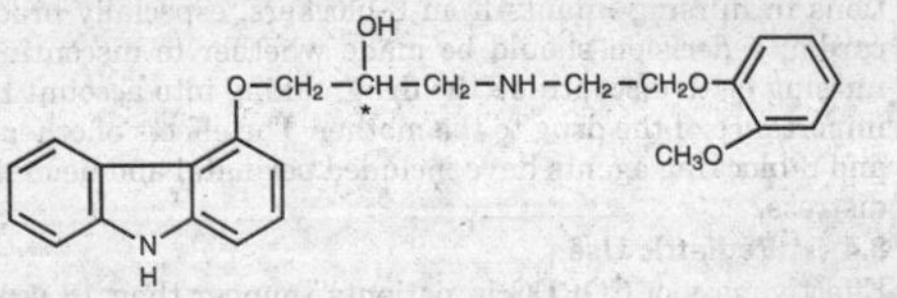

COREG is a white, oval, film-coated tablet containing 3.125 mg, 6.25 mg, 12.5 mg, or 25 mg of carvedilol. The 6.25 mg, 12.5 mg, and 25 mg tablets are TILTAB® tablets. Inactive ingredients consist of colloidal silicon dioxide, crospovidone, hypromellose, lactose, magnesium stearate, polyethylene glycol, polysorbate 80, povidone, sucrose, and titanium dioxide.

Carvedilol is a white to off-white powder with a molecular weight of 406.5 and a molecular formula of $C_{24}H_{26}N_2O_4$. It is freely soluble in dimethylsulfoxide; soluble in methylene chloride and methanol; sparingly soluble in 95% ethanol and isopropanol; slightly soluble in ethyl ether; and practically insoluble in water, gastric fluid (simulated, TS, pH 1.1), and intestinal fluid (simulated, TS without pancreatin, pH 7.5).

12 CLINICAL PHARMACOLOGY

12.1 Mechanism of Action

COREG is a racemic mixture in which nonselective β-adrenoreceptor blocking activity is present in the S(-) enantiomer and α_1-adrenergic blocking activity is present in both R(+) and S(-) enantiomers at equal potency. COREG has no intrinsic sympathomimetic activity.

12.2 Pharmacodynamics

Heart Failure

The basis for the beneficial effects of COREG in heart failure is not established.

Two placebo-controlled studies compared the acute hemodynamic effects of COREG to baseline measurements in 59 and 49 patients with NYHA class II-IV heart failure receiving diuretics, ACE inhibitors, and digitalis. There were significant reductions in systemic blood pressure, pulmonary artery pressure, pulmonary capillary wedge pressure, and heart rate. Initial effects on cardiac output, stroke volume index, and systemic vascular resistance were small and variable.

These studies measured hemodynamic effects again at 12 to 14 weeks. COREG significantly reduced systemic blood pressure, pulmonary artery pressure, right atrial pressure, systemic vascular resistance, and heart rate, while stroke volume index was increased.

Among 839 patients with NYHA class II-III heart failure treated for 26 to 52 weeks in 4 US placebo-controlled trials, average left ventricular ejection fraction (EF) measured by radionuclide ventriculography increased by 9 EF units (%) in patients receiving COREG and by 2 EF units in placebo patients at a target dose of 25-50 mg twice daily. The effects of carvedilol on ejection fraction were related to dose. Doses of 6.25 mg twice daily, 12.5 mg twice daily, and 25 mg twice daily were associated with placebo-corrected increases in EF of 5 EF units, 6 EF units, and 8 EF units, respectively; each of these effects were nominally statistically significant.

Left Ventricular Dysfunction Following Myocardial Infarction

The basis for the beneficial effects of COREG in patients with left ventricular dysfunction following an acute myocardial infarction is not established.

Hypertension

The mechanism by which β-blockade produces an antihypertensive effect has not been established.

β-adrenoreceptor blocking activity has been demonstrated in animal and human studies showing that carvedilol (1) reduces cardiac output in normal subjects; (2) reduces exercise- and/or isoproterenol-induced tachycardia; and (3) reduces reflex orthostatic tachycardia. Significant β-adrenoreceptor blocking effect is usually seen within 1 hour of drug administration.

α_1-adrenoreceptor blocking activity has been demonstrated in human and animal studies, showing that carvedilol (1) attenuates the pressor effects of phenylephrine; (2) causes vasodilation; and (3) reduces peripheral vascular resistance. These effects contribute to the reduction of blood pressure and usually are seen within 30 minutes of drug administration.

Due to the α_1-receptor blocking activity of carvedilol, blood pressure is lowered more in the standing than in the supine position, and symptoms of postural hypotension (1.8%), including rare instances of syncope, can occur. Following oral administration, when postural hypotension has occurred, it has been transient and is uncommon when COREG is administered with food at the recommended starting dose and titration increments are closely followed *[see Dosage and Administration (2)]*.

In hypertensive patients with normal renal function, therapeutic doses of COREG decreased renal vascular resistance with no change in glomerular filtration rate or renal plasma flow. Changes in excretion of sodium, potassium, uric acid, and phosphorus in hypertensive patients with normal renal function were similar after COREG and placebo.

COREG has little effect on plasma catecholamines, plasma aldosterone, or electrolyte levels, but it does significantly reduce plasma renin activity when given for at least 4 weeks. It also increases levels of atrial natriuretic peptide.

12.3 Pharmacokinetics

COREG is rapidly and extensively absorbed following oral administration, with absolute bioavailability of approximately 25% to 35% due to a significant degree of first-pass metabolism. Following oral administration, the apparent mean terminal elimination half-life of carvedilol generally ranges from 7 to 10 hours. Plasma concentrations achieved are proportional to the oral dose administered. When administered with food, the rate of absorption is slowed, as evidenced by a delay in the time to reach peak plasma levels, with no significant difference in extent of bioavailability. Taking COREG with food should minimize the risk of orthostatic hypotension.

Carvedilol is extensively metabolized. Following oral administration of radiolabelled carvedilol to healthy volunteers, carvedilol accounted for only about 7% of the total radioactivity in plasma as measured by area under the curve (AUC). Less than 2% of the dose was excreted unchanged in the urine. Carvedilol is metabolized primarily by aromatic ring oxidation and glucuronidation. The oxidative metabolites are further metabolized by conjugation via glucuronidation and sulfation. The metabolites of carvedilol are excreted primarily via the bile into the feces. Demethylation and hydroxylation at the phenol ring produce 3 active metabolites with β-receptor blocking activity. Based on preclinical studies, the 4′-hydroxyphenyl metabolite is approximately 13 times more potent than carvedilol for β-blockade. Compared to carvedilol, the 3 active metabolites exhibit weak vasodilating activity. Plasma concentrations of the active metabolites are about one-tenth of those observed for carvedilol and have pharmacokinetics similar to the parent.

Carvedilol undergoes stereoselective first-pass metabolism with plasma levels of R(+)-carvedilol approximately 2 to 3 times higher than S(-)-carvedilol following oral administration in healthy subjects. The mean apparent terminal elimination half-lives for R(+)-carvedilol range from 5 to 9 hours compared with 7 to 11 hours for the S(-)-enantiomer.

The primary P450 enzymes responsible for the metabolism of both R(+) and S(-)-carvedilol in human liver microsomes were CYP2D6 and CYP2C9 and to a lesser extent CYP3A4, 2C19, 1A2, and 2E1. CYP2D6 is thought to be the major enzyme in the 4′- and 5′-hydroxylation of carvedilol, with a potential contribution from 3A4. CYP2C9 is thought to be of primary importance in the O-methylation pathway of S(-)-carvedilol.

Carvedilol is subject to the effects of genetic polymorphism with poor metabolizers of debrisoquin (a marker for cytochrome P450 2D6) exhibiting 2- to 3-fold higher plasma concentrations of R(+)-carvedilol compared to extensive metabolizers. In contrast, plasma levels of S(-)-carvedilol are increased only about 20% to 25% in poor metabolizers, indicating this enantiomer is metabolized to a lesser extent by cytochrome P450 2D6 than R(+)-carvedilol. The pharmacokinetics of carvedilol do not appear to be different in poor metabolizers of S-mephenytoin (patients deficient in cytochrome P450 2C19).

Carvedilol is more than 98% bound to plasma proteins, primarily with albumin. The plasma-protein binding is independent of concentration over the therapeutic range. Carvedilol is a basic, lipophilic compound with a steady-state volume of distribution of approximately 115 L, indicating substantial distribution into extravascular tissues. Plasma clearance ranges from 500 to 700 mL/min.

12.4 Specific Populations

Heart Failure

Steady-state plasma concentrations of carvedilol and its enantiomers increased proportionally over the 6.25 to 50 mg dose range in patients with heart failure. Compared to healthy subjects, heart failure patients had increased mean AUC and C_{max} values for carvedilol and its enantiomers, with up to 50% to 100% higher values observed in 6 patients with NYHA class IV heart failure. The mean apparent terminal elimination half-life for carvedilol was similar to that observed in healthy subjects.

Geriatric

Plasma levels of carvedilol average about 50% higher in the elderly compared to young subjects.

Hepatic Impairment

Compared to healthy subjects, patients with severe liver impairment (cirrhosis) exhibit a 4- to 7-fold increase in carvedilol levels. Carvedilol is contraindicated in patients with severe liver impairment.

Renal Impairment

Although carvedilol is metabolized primarily by the liver, plasma concentrations of carvedilol have been reported to be increased in patients with renal impairment. Based on mean AUC data, approximately 40% to 50% higher plasma concentrations of carvedilol were observed in hypertensive patients with moderate to severe renal impairment compared to a control group of hypertensive patients with normal renal function. However, the ranges of AUC values were similar for both groups. Changes in mean peak plasma levels were less pronounced, approximately 12% to 26% higher in patients with impaired renal function.

Consistent with its high degree of plasma protein-binding, carvedilol does not appear to be cleared significantly by hemodialysis.

12.5 Drug-Drug Interactions

Since carvedilol undergoes substantial oxidative metabolism, the metabolism and pharmacokinetics of carvedilol may be affected by induction or inhibition of cytochrome P450 enzymes.

Amiodarone

In a pharmacokinetic study conducted in 106 Japanese patients with heart failure, coadministration of small loading and maintenance doses of amiodarone with carvedilol resulted in at least a 2-fold increase in the steady-state trough concentrations of S(-)-carvedilol *[see Drug Interactions (7.6)]*.

Cimetidine

In a pharmacokinetic study conducted in 10 healthy male subjects, cimetidine (1,000 mg/day) increased the steady-state AUC of carvedilol by 30% with no change in C_{max} *[see Drug Interactions (7.5)]*.

Digoxin

Following concomitant administration of carvedilol (25 mg once daily) and digoxin (0.25 mg once daily) for 14 days, steady-state AUC and trough concentrations of digoxin were increased by 14% and 16%, respectively, in 12 hypertensive patients *[see Drug Interactions (7.4)]*.

Glyburide

In 12 healthy subjects, combined administration of carvedilol (25 mg once daily) and a single dose of glyburide did not result in a clinically relevant pharmacokinetic interaction for either compound.

Hydrochlorothiazide

A single oral dose of carvedilol 25 mg did not alter the pharmacokinetics of a single oral dose of hydrochlorothiazide 25 mg in 12 patients with hypertension. Likewise, hydrochlorothiazide had no effect on the pharmacokinetics of carvedilol.

Rifampin

In a pharmacokinetic study conducted in 8 healthy male subjects, rifampin (600 mg daily for 12 days) decreased the AUC and C_{max} of carvedilol by about 70% *[see Drug Interactions (7.5)]*.

Torsemide

In a study of 12 healthy subjects, combined oral administration of carvedilol 25 mg once daily and torsemide 5 mg once daily for 5 days did not result in any significant differences in their pharmacokinetics compared with administration of the drugs alone.

Warfarin

Carvedilol (12.5 mg twice daily) did not have an effect on the steady-state prothrombin time ratios and did not alter the pharmacokinetics of R(+)- and S(-)-warfarin following concomitant administration with warfarin in 9 healthy volunteers.

13 NONCLINICAL TOXICOLOGY

13.1 Carcinogenesis, Mutagenesis, Impairment of Fertility

In 2-year studies conducted in rats given carvedilol at doses up to 75 mg/kg/day (12 times the MRHD when compared on a mg/m^2 basis) or in mice given up to 200 mg/kg/day (16 times the MRHD on a mg/m^2 basis), carvedilol had no carcinogenic effect.

Carvedilol was negative when tested in a battery of genotoxicity assays, including the Ames and the CHO/HGPRT assays for mutagenicity and the in vitro hamster micronucleus and in vivo human lymphocyte cell tests for clastogenicity.

At doses ≥200 mg/kg/day (≥32 times the MRHD as mg/m^2) carvedilol was toxic to adult rats (sedation, reduced weight gain) and was associated with a reduced number of successful matings, prolonged mating time, significantly fewer corpora lutea and implants per dam, and complete resorption of 18% of the litters. The no-observed-effect dose level for overt toxicity and impairment of fertility was 60 mg/kg/day (10 times the MRHD as mg/m^2).

14 CLINICAL STUDIES

14.1 Heart Failure

A total of 6,975 patients with mild to severe heart failure were evaluated in placebo-controlled studies of carvedilol.

Mild-to-Moderate Heart Failure

Carvedilol was studied in 5 multicenter, placebo-controlled studies, and in 1 active-controlled study (COMET study) involving patients with mild-to-moderate heart failure.

Four US multicenter, double-blind, placebo-controlled studies enrolled 1,094 patients (696 randomized to carvedilol) with NYHA class II-III heart failure and ejection fraction ≤0.35. The vast majority were on digitalis, diuretics, and an ACE inhibitor at study entry. Patients were assigned to the studies based upon exercise ability. An Australia-New Zealand double-blind, placebo-controlled study enrolled 415 patients (half randomized to carvedilol) with less severe heart failure. All protocols excluded patients expected to undergo cardiac transplantation during the 7.5 to 15 months of double-blind follow-up. All randomized patients had tolerated a 2-week course on carvedilol 6.25 mg twice daily.

In each study, there was a primary end point, either progression of heart failure (1 US study) or exercise tolerance (2 US studies meeting enrollment goals and the Australia-New Zealand study). There were many secondary end points specified in these studies, including NYHA classification, patient and physician global assessments, and cardiovascular hospitalization. Other analyses not prospectively planned included the sum of deaths and total cardiovascular hospitalizations. In situations where the primary end points of a trial do not show a significant benefit of treatment, assignment of significance values to the other results is complex, and such values need to be interpreted cautiously.

The results of the US and Australia-New Zealand trials were as follows:

Slowing Progression of Heart Failure: One US multicenter study (366 subjects) had as its primary end point the sum of cardiovascular mortality, cardiovascular hospitalization, and sustained increase in heart failure medications. Heart failure progression was reduced, during an average follow-up of 7 months, by 48% (p = 0.008).

In the Australia-New Zealand study, death and total hospitalizations were reduced by about 25% over 18 to 24 months. In the 3 largest US studies, death and total hospitalizations were reduced by 19%, 39%, and 49%, nominally statistically significant in the last 2 studies. The Australia-New Zealand results were statistically borderline.

Functional Measures: None of the multicenter studies had NYHA classification as a primary end point, but all such studies had it as a secondary end point. There was at least a trend toward improvement in NYHA class in all studies. Exercise tolerance was the primary end point in 3 studies; in none was a statistically significant effect found.

Subjective Measures: Health-related quality of life, as measured with a standard questionnaire (a primary end point in 1 study), was unaffected by carvedilol. However, patients' and investigators' global assessments showed significant improvement in most studies.

Mortality: Death was not a pre-specified end point in any study, but was analyzed in all studies. Overall, in these 4

US trials, mortality was reduced, nominally significantly so in 2 studies.

COMET Trial

In this double-blind trial, 3,029 patients with NYHA class II-IV heart failure (left ventricular ejection fraction ≤35%) were randomized to receive either carvedilol (target dose: 25 mg twice daily) or immediate-release metoprolol tartrate (target dose: 50 mg twice daily). The mean age of the patients was approximately 62 years, 80% were males, and the mean left ventricular ejection fraction at baseline was 26%. Approximately 96% of the patients had NYHA class II or III heart failure. Concomitant treatment included diuretics (99%), ACE inhibitors (91%), digitalis (59%), aldosterone antagonists (11%), and "statin" lipid-lowering agents (21%). The mean duration of follow-up was 4.8 years. The mean dose of carvedilol was 42 mg per day.

The study had 2 primary end points: All-cause mortality and the composite of death plus hospitalization for any reason. The results of COMET are presented in Table 3 below. All-cause mortality carried most of the statistical weight and was the primary determinant of the study size. All-cause mortality was 34% in the patients treated with carvedilol and was 40% in the immediate-release metoprolol group (p = 0.0017; hazard ratio = 0.83, 95%CI 0.74-0.93). The effect on mortality was primarily due to a reduction in cardiovascular death. The difference between the 2 groups with respect to the composite end point was not significant (p = 0.122). The estimated mean survival was 8.0 years with carvedilol and 6.6 years with immediate-release metoprolol.

[See table 3 above]

It is not known whether this formulation of metoprolol at any dose or this low dose of metoprolol in any formulation has any effect on survival or hospitalization in patients with heart failure. Thus, this trial extends the time over which carvedilol manifests benefits on survival in heart failure, but it is not evidence that carvedilol improves outcome over the formulation of metoprolol (TOPROL-XL®) with benefits in heart failure.

Severe Heart Failure (COPERNICUS)

In a double-blind study (COPERNICUS), 2,289 patients with heart failure at rest or with minimal exertion and left ventricular ejection fraction <25% (mean 20%), despite digitalis (66%), diuretics (99%), and ACE inhibitors (89%) were randomized to placebo or carvedilol. Carvedilol was titrated from a starting dose of 3.125 mg twice daily to the maximum tolerated dose or up to 25 mg twice daily over a minimum of 6 weeks. Most subjects achieved the target dose of 25 mg. The study was conducted in Eastern and Western Europe, the United States, Israel, and Canada. Similar numbers of subjects per group (about 100) withdrew during the titration period.

The primary end point of the trial was all-cause mortality, but cause-specific mortality and the risk of death or hospitalization (total, cardiovascular [CV], or heart failure [HF]) were also examined. The developing trial data were followed by a data monitoring committee, and mortality analyses were adjusted for these multiple looks. The trial was stopped after a median follow-up of 10 months because of an observed 35% reduction in mortality (from 19.7% per patient year on placebo to 12.8% on carvedilol, hazard ratio 0.65, 95% CI 0.52–0.81, p = 0.0014, adjusted) (see Figure 1). The results of COPERNICUS are shown in Table 4.

[See table 4 above]

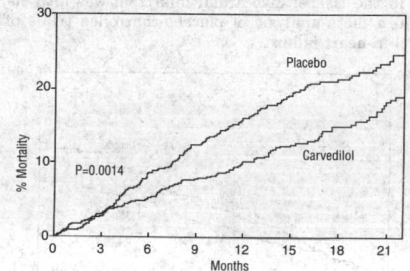

Figure 1. Survival Analysis for COPERNICUS (intent-to-treat)

The effect on mortality was principally the result of a reduction in the rate of sudden death among patients without worsening heart failure.

Patients' global assessments, in which carvedilol-treated patients were compared to placebo, were based on pre-specified, periodic patient self-assessments regarding whether clinical status post-treatment showed improvement, worsening or no change compared to baseline. Patients treated with carvedilol showed significant improvements in global assessments compared with those treated with placebo in COPERNICUS.

The protocol also specified that hospitalizations would be assessed. Fewer patients on COREG than on placebo were hospitalized for any reason (372 versus 432, p = 0.0029), for cardiovascular reasons (246 versus 314, p = 0.0003), or for worsening heart failure (198 versus 268, p = 0.0001).

COREG had a consistent and beneficial effect on all-cause mortality as well as the combined end points of all-cause mortality plus hospitalization (total, CV, or for heart failure) in the overall study population and in all subgroups examined, including men and women, elderly and non-elderly, blacks and non-blacks, and diabetics and non-diabetics (see Figure 2).

[See figure 2 at top of next column]

14.2 Left Ventricular Dysfunction Following Myocardial Infarction

CAPRICORN was a double-blind study comparing carvedilol and placebo in 1,959 patients with a recent myocardial infarction (within 21 days) and left ventricular ejection fraction of ≤40%, with (47%) or without symptoms of heart failure. Patients given carvedilol received 6.25 mg twice daily, titrated as tolerated to 25 mg twice daily. Pa-

Table 3. Results of COMET

End point	Carvedilol N = 1,511	Metoprolol N = 1,518	Hazard ratio	(95% CI)
All-cause mortality	34%	40%	0.83	0.74–0.93
Mortality + all hospitalization	74%	76%	0.94	0.86–1.02
Cardiovascular death	30%	35%	0.80	0.70–0.90
Sudden death	14%	17%	0.81	0.68–0.97
Death due to circulatory failure	11%	13%	0.83	0.67–1.02
Death due to stroke	0.9%	2.5%	0.33	0.18–0.62

Table 4. Results of COPERNICUS Trial in Patients With Severe Heart Failure

End point	Placebo (N = 1,133)	Carvedilol (N = 1,156)	Hazard ratio (95% CI)	% Reduction	Nominal p value
Mortality	190	130	0.65 (0.52–0.81)	35	0.00013
Mortality + all hospitalization	507	425	0.76 (0.67–0.87)	24	0.00004
Mortality + CV hospitalization	395	314	0.73 (0.63–0.84)	27	0.00002
Mortality + HF hospitalization	357	271	0.69 (0.59–0.81)	31	0.000004

Cardiovascular = CV; Heart failure = HF.

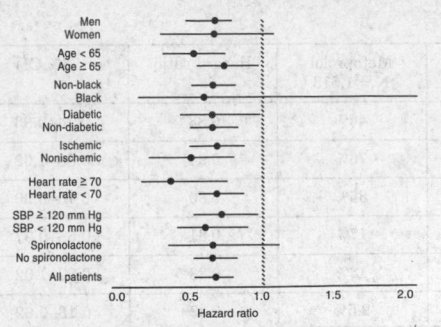

Figure 2. Effects on Mortality for Subgroups in COPERNICUS

tients had to have a systolic blood pressure >90 mm Hg, a sitting heart rate >60 beats/minute, and no contraindication to β-blocker use. Treatment of the index infarction included aspirin (85%), IV or oral β-blockers (37%), nitrates (73%), heparin (64%), thrombolytics (40%), and acute angioplasty (12%). Background treatment included ACE inhibitors or angiotensin receptor blockers (97%), anticoagulants (20%), lipid-lowering agents (23%), and diuretics (34%). Baseline population characteristics included an average age of 63 years, 74% male, 95% Caucasian, mean blood pressure 121/74 mm Hg, 22% with diabetes, and 54% with a history of hypertension. Mean dosage achieved of carvedilol was 20 mg twice daily; mean duration of follow-up was 15 months.

All-cause mortality was 15% in the placebo group and 12% in the carvedilol group, indicating a 23% risk reduction in patients treated with carvedilol (95% CI 2-40%, p = 0.03), as shown in Figure 3. The effects on mortality in various subgroups are shown in Figure 4. Nearly all deaths were cardiovascular (which were reduced by 25% by carvedilol), and most of these deaths were sudden or related to pump failure (both types of death were reduced by carvedilol). Another study end point, total mortality and all-cause hospitalization, did not show a significant improvement.

There was also a significant 40% reduction in fatal or nonfatal myocardial infarction observed in the group treated with carvedilol (95% CI 11% to 60%, p = 0.01). A similar reduction in the risk of myocardial infarction was also observed in a meta-analysis of placebo-controlled trials of carvedilol in heart failure.

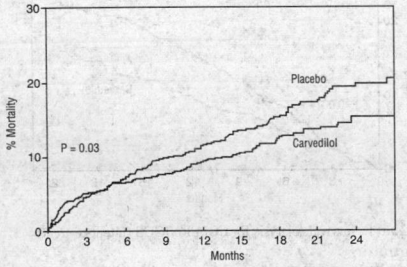

Figure 3. Survival Analysis for CAPRICORN (intent-to-treat)

[See figure 3 below]

14.3 Hypertension

COREG was studied in 2 placebo-controlled trials that utilized twice-daily dosing, at total daily doses of 12.5 to 50 mg. In these and other studies, the starting dose did not exceed 12.5 mg. At 50 mg/day, COREG reduced sitting trough (12-hour) blood pressure by about 9/5.5 mm Hg; at 25 mg/day the effect was about 7.5/3.5 mm Hg. Comparisons of trough to peak blood pressure showed a trough to peak ratio for blood pressure response of about 65%. Heart rate fell by about 7.5 beats/minute at 50 mg/day. In general, as is true for other β-blockers, responses were smaller in black than non-black patients. There were no age- or gender-related differences in response.

The peak antihypertensive effect occurred 1 to 2 hours after a dose. The dose-related blood pressure response was accompanied by a dose-related increase in adverse effects [see Adverse Reactions (6)].

14.4 Hypertension With Type 2 Diabetes Mellitus

In a double-blind study (GEMINI), COREG, added to an ACE inhibitor or angiotensin receptor blocker, was evaluated in a population with mild-to-moderate hypertension and well-controlled type 2 diabetes mellitus. The mean HbA1c at baseline was 7.2%. COREG was titrated to a mean dose of 17.5 mg twice daily and maintained for 5 months. COREG had no adverse effect on glycemic control, based on HbA1c measurements (mean change from baseline of 0.02%, 95% CI -0.06 to 0.10, p = NS) [see Warnings and Precautions (5.6)].

16 HOW SUPPLIED/STORAGE AND HANDLING

The white, oval, film-coated tablets are available in the following strengths: 3.125 mg–engraved with 39 and SB, in bottles of 100; 6.25 mg–engraved with 4140 and SB, in bottles of 100; 12.5 mg–engraved with 4141 and SB, in bottles of 100; 25 mg–engraved with 4142 and SB, in bottles of 100. The 6.25 mg, 12.5 mg, and 25 mg tablets are TILTAB tablets.

- 3.125 mg 100's: NDC 0007-4139-20
- 6.25 mg 100's: NDC 0007-4140-20
- 12.5 mg 100's: NDC 0007-4141-20
- 25 mg 100's: NDC 0007-4142-20

Store below 30°C (86°F). Protect from moisture. Dispense in a tight, light-resistant container.

17 PATIENT COUNSELING INFORMATION

See FDA-Approved Patient Labeling.

17.1 Patient Advice

Patients taking COREG should be advised of the following:
- Patients should take COREG with food.
- Patients should not interrupt or discontinue using COREG without a physician's advice.
- Patients with heart failure should consult their physician if they experience signs or symptoms of worsening heart failure such as weight gain or increasing shortness of breath.
- Patients may experience a drop in blood pressure when standing, resulting in dizziness and, rarely, fainting. Patients should sit or lie down when these symptoms of lowered blood pressure occur.
- If experiencing dizziness or fatigue, patients should avoid driving or hazardous tasks.
- Patients should consult a physician if they experience dizziness or faintness, in case the dosage should be adjusted.

- Diabetic patients should report any changes in blood sugar levels to their physician.
- Contact lens wearers may experience decreased lacrimation.

COREG, COREG CR, and TILTAB are registered trademarks of GlaxoSmithKline.
TOPROL-XL is a registered trademark of the AstraZeneca group of companies.
Manufactured for
GlaxoSmithKline
Research Triangle Park, NC 27709
Manufactured by
Patheon Puerto Rico, Inc.
Manati, PR 00674 USA
©2009, GlaxoSmithKline. All rights reserved.
PHARMACIST-DETACH HERE AND GIVE INSTRUCTIONS TO PATIENT

PATIENT INFORMATION

COREG® (Co-REG)
Carvedilol Tablets
Read the Patient Information that comes with COREG before you start taking it and each time you get a refill. There may be new information. This information does not take the place of talking with your doctor about your medical condition or your treatment. If you have any questions about COREG, ask your doctor or pharmacist.

What is COREG?
COREG is a prescription medicine that belongs to a group of medicines called "beta-blockers". COREG is used, often with other medicines, for the following conditions:
- To treat patients with high blood pressure (hypertension)
- To treat patients who had a heart attack that worsened how well the heart pumps
- To treat patients with certain types of heart failure

COREG is not approved for use in children under 18 years of age.

Who should not take COREG?
Do not take COREG if you:
- Have severe heart failure and are hospitalized in the intensive care unit or require certain intravenous medications that help support circulation (inotropic medications)
- Are prone to asthma or other breathing problems
- Have a slow heartbeat or a heart that skips a beat (irregular heartbeat)
- Have liver problems
- Are allergic to any of the ingredients in COREG. The active ingredient is carvedilol. See the end of this leaflet for a list of all the ingredients in COREG.

What should I tell my doctor before taking COREG?
Tell your doctor about all of your medical conditions, including if you:
- Have asthma or other lung problems (such as bronchitis or emphysema)
- Have problems with blood flow in your feet and legs (peripheral vascular disease) COREG can make some of your symptoms worse.
- Have diabetes
- Have thyroid problems
- Have a condition called pheochromocytoma
- Have had severe allergic reactions
- Are pregnant or trying to become pregnant. It is not known if COREG is safe for your unborn baby. You and your doctor should talk about the best way to control your high blood pressure during pregnancy.
- Are breastfeeding. It is not known if COREG passes into your breast milk. You should not breastfeed while using COREG.
- Are scheduled for surgery and will be given anesthetic agents
- Are taking prescription or non-prescription medicines, vitamins, and herbal supplements. COREG and certain other medicines can affect each other and cause serious side effects. COREG may affect the way other medicines work. Also, other medicines may affect how well COREG works.

Keep a list of all the medicines you take. Show this list to your doctor and pharmacist before you start a new medicine.

How should I take COREG?
It is important for you to take your medicine every day as directed by your doctor. If you stop taking COREG suddenly, you could have chest pain and/or a heart attack. If your doctor decides that you should stop taking COREG, your doctor may slowly lower your dose over a period of time before stopping it completely.
- Take COREG exactly as prescribed. Your doctor will tell you how many tablets to take and how often. In order to minimize possible side effects, your doctor might begin with a low dose and then slowly increase the dose.
- **Do not stop taking COREG and do not change the amount of COREG you take without talking to your doctor.**
- Tell your doctor if you gain weight or have trouble breathing while taking COREG.
- Take COREG with food.
- If you miss a dose of COREG, take your dose as soon as you remember, unless it is time to take your next dose. Take your next dose at the usual time. Do not take 2 doses at the same time.

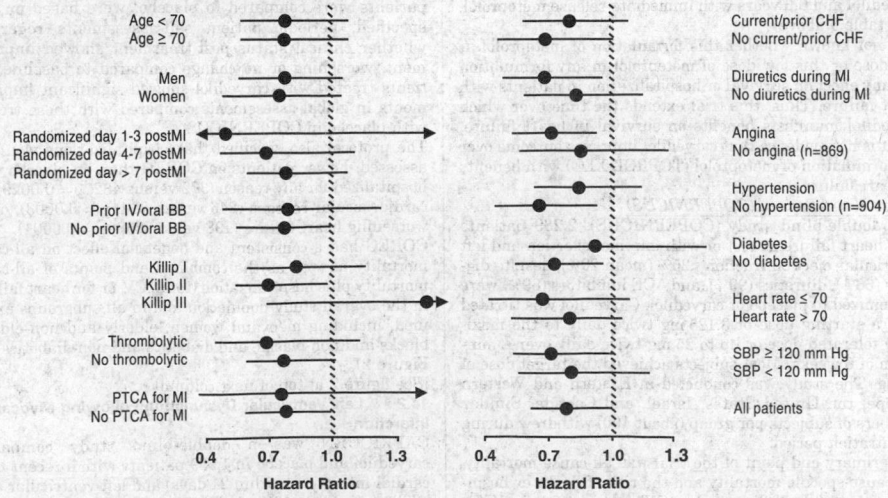

Figure 4. Effects on Mortality for Subgroups in CAPRICORN

- If you take too much COREG, call your doctor or poison control center right away.

What should I avoid while taking COREG?
- COREG can cause you to feel dizzy, tired, or faint. Do not drive a car, use machinery, or do anything that needs you to be alert if you have these symptoms.

What are possible side effects of COREG?
- Low blood pressure (which may cause dizziness or fainting when you stand up). If these happen, sit or lie down right away and tell your doctor.
- **Tiredness.** If you feel tired or dizzy you should not drive, use machinery, or do anything that needs you to be alert.
- Slow heartbeat.
- Changes in your blood sugar. If you have diabetes, tell your doctor if you have any changes in your blood sugar levels.
- COREG may hide some of the symptoms of low blood sugar, especially a fast heartbeat.
- COREG may mask the symptoms of hyperthyroidism (overactive thyroid).
- Worsening of severe allergic reactions.
- Rare but serious allergic reactions (including hives or swelling of the face, lips, tongue, and/or throat that may cause difficulty in breathing or swallowing) have happened in patients who were on COREG. These reactions can be life-threatening.

Other side effects of COREG include shortness of breath, weight gain, diarrhea, and fewer tears or dry eyes that become bothersome if you wear contact lenses.

Call your doctor if you have any side effects that bother you or don't go away.

How should I store COREG?
- Store COREG at less than 86°F (30°C). Keep the tablets dry.
- Safely, throw away COREG that is out of date or no longer needed.
- Keep COREG and all medicines out of the reach of children.

General Information about COREG
Medicines are sometimes prescribed for conditions other than those described in patient information leaflets. Do not use COREG for a condition for which it was not prescribed. Do not give COREG to other people, even if they have the same symptoms you have. It may harm them.

This leaflet summarizes the most important information about COREG. If you would like more information, talk with your doctor. You can ask your doctor or pharmacist for information about COREG that is written for healthcare professionals. You can also find out more about COREG by visiting the website www.COREG.com or calling 1-888-825-5249. This call is free.

What are the ingredients in COREG?
Active Ingredient: Carvedilol.
Inactive Ingredients: Colloidal silicon dioxide, crospovidone, hypromellose, lactose, magnesium stearate, polyethylene glycol, polysorbate 80, povidone, sucrose, and titanium dioxide.
Carvedilol tablets come in the following strengths: 3.125 mg, 6.25 mg, 12.5 mg, 25 mg.
COREG is a registered trademark of GlaxoSmithKline.
Manufactured for
GlaxoSmithKline
Research Triangle Park, NC 27709
Manufactured by
Patheon Puerto Rico, Inc.
Manati, PR 00674 USA
©2009, GlaxoSmithKline. All rights reserved.
Revised: June 2009
CRG:3PIL

COREG CR® ℞
[kor' eg]
(carvedilol phosphate)
Extended-release Capsules

HIGHLIGHTS OF PRESCRIBING INFORMATION
These highlights do not include all the information needed to use COREG CR safely and effectively. See full prescribing information for COREG CR.
COREG CR® (carvedilol phosphate) Extended-release Capsules
Initial U.S. Approval: 1995

———————RECENT MAJOR CHANGES———————
Dosage and Administration, Geriatric Use
(2.5)   December 2008
Warnings and Precautions, Hypotension
(5.3)   December 2008

———————INDICATIONS AND USAGE———————
COREG CR is an alpha/beta-adrenergic blocking agent indicated for the treatment of:
- Mild to severe chronic heart failure (1.1)
- Left ventricular dysfunction following myocardial infarction in clinically stable patients (1.2)

- Hypertension (1.3)

———————DOSAGE AND ADMINISTRATION———————
Take with food. Do not crush or chew capsules. Individualize dosage and monitor during up-titration. (2)
- Heart failure: Start at 10 mg once daily and increase to 20, 40, and then 80 mg once daily over intervals of at least 2 weeks. Maintain lower doses if higher doses are not tolerated. (2.1)
- Left ventricular dysfunction following myocardial infarction: Start at 20 mg once daily and increase to 40 mg then 80 mg once daily after intervals of 3 to 10 days. A lower starting dose or slower titration may be used. (2.2)
- Hypertension: Start at 20 mg once daily and increase if needed for blood pressure control to 40 mg then 80 mg once daily over intervals of 1 to 2 weeks. (2.3)
- Elderly patients (> 65 years of age): When switching from higher doses of immediate-release carvedilol to COREG CR, a lower starting dose should be considered to reduce the risk of hypotension and syncope. (2.5)

———————DOSAGE FORMS AND STRENGTHS———————
Capsules: 10, 20, 40, 80 mg (3)

———————CONTRAINDICATIONS———————
- Bronchial asthma or related bronchospastic conditions (4)
- Second- or third-degree AV block (4)
- Sick sinus syndrome (4)
- Severe bradycardia (unless permanent pacemaker in place) (4)
- Patients in cardiogenic shock or decompensated heart failure requiring the use of IV inotropic therapy. (4)
- Severe hepatic impairment (2.4, 4)
- History of serious hypersensitivity reaction (e.g., Stevens-Johnson syndrome, anaphylactic reaction, angioedema) to carvedilol or any of the components of COREG CR. (4)

———————WARNINGS AND PRECAUTIONS———————
- Acute exacerbation of coronary artery disease upon cessation of therapy: Do not abruptly discontinue. (5.1)
- Bradycardia, hypotension, worsening heart failure/fluid retention may occur. Reduce the dose as needed. (5.2, 5.3, 5.4)
- Non-allergic bronchospasm (e.g., chronic bronchitis and emphysema): Avoid β-blockers. (4) However, if deemed necessary, use with caution and at lowest effective dose. (5.5)
- Diabetes: Monitor glucose as β-blockers may mask symptoms of hypoglycemia or worsen hyperglycemia. (5.6)

———————ADVERSE REACTIONS———————
The safety profile of COREG CR was similar to that observed for immediate-release carvedilol. Most common adverse events seen with immediate-release carvedilol. (6.1):
- Heart failure and left ventricular dysfunction following myocardial infarction (≥10%): Dizziness, fatigue, hypotension, diarrhea, hyperglycemia, asthenia, bradycardia, weight increase
- Hypertension (≥5%): Dizziness

To report SUSPECTED ADVERSE REACTIONS, contact GlaxoSmithKline at 1-888-825-5249 or FDA at 1-800-FDA-1088 or www.fda.gov/medwatch.

———————DRUG INTERACTIONS———————
- CYP P450 2D6 enzyme inhibitors may increase and rifampin may decrease carvedilol levels. (7.1, 7.5)
- Hypotensive agents (e.g., reserpine, MAO inhibitors, clonidine) may increase the risk of hypotension and/or severe bradycardia. (7.2)
- Cyclosporine or digoxin levels may increase. (7.3, 7.4)
- Both digitalis glycosides and β-blockers slow atrioventricular conduction and decrease heart rate. Concomitant use can increase the risk of bradycardia. (7.4)
- Amiodarone may increase carvedilol levels resulting in further slowing of the heart rate or cardiac conduction. (7.6)
- Verapamil- or diltiazem-type calcium channel blockers may affect ECG and/or blood pressure. (7.7)
- Insulin and oral hypoglycemics action may be enhanced. (7.8)

See 17 for PATIENT COUNSELING INFORMATION and FDA-approved patient labeling.

Revised: June 2009
CCR:11PI

FULL PRESCRIBING INFORMATION: CONTENTS*
*Sections or subsections omitted from the full prescribing information are not listed.

FULL PRESCRIBING INFORMATION

1 INDICATIONS AND USAGE

1.1 Heart Failure
COREG CR is indicated for the treatment of mild-to-severe chronic heart failure of ischemic or cardiomyopathic origin, usually in addition to diuretics, ACE inhibitors, and digitalis, to increase survival and, also, to reduce the risk of hospitalization [see Clinical Studies (14.1)].

1.2 Left Ventricular Dysfunction Following Myocardial Infarction
COREG CR is indicated to reduce cardiovascular mortality in clinically stable patients who have survived the acute phase of a myocardial infarction and have a left ventricular ejection fraction of ≤40% (with or without symptomatic heart failure) [see Clinical Studies (14.2)].

1.3 Hypertension
COREG CR is indicated for the management of essential hypertension [see Clinical Studies (14.3, 14.4)]. It can be used alone or in combination with other antihypertensive agents, especially thiazide-type diuretics [see Drug Interactions (7.2)].

2 DOSAGE AND ADMINISTRATION
COREG CR is an extended-release capsule intended for once-daily administration. Patients controlled with immediate-release carvedilol tablets alone or in combination with other medications may be switched to COREG CR extended-release capsules based on the total daily doses shown in Table 1.

Table 1. Dosing Conversion

Daily Dose of Immediate-Release Carvedilol Tablets	Daily Dose of COREG CR Capsules*
6.25 mg (3.125 mg twice daily)	10 mg once daily
12.5 mg (6.25 mg twice daily)	20 mg once daily
25 mg (12.5 mg twice daily)	40 mg once daily
50 mg (25 mg twice daily)	80 mg once daily

* When switching from carvedilol 12.5 mg or 25 mg twice daily, a starting dose of COREG CR 20 mg or 40 mg once daily, respectively, may be warranted for elderly patients or those at increased risk of hypotension, dizziness, or syncope. Subsequent titration to higher doses should, as appropriate, be made after an interval of at least 2 weeks.

COREG CR should be taken once daily in the morning with food. COREG CR should be swallowed as a whole capsule. COREG CR and/or its contents should not be crushed, chewed, or taken in divided doses.

Alternative Administration: The capsules may be carefully opened and the beads sprinkled over a spoonful of applesauce. The applesauce should not be warm because it could affect the modified-release properties of this formulation. The mixture of drug and applesauce should be consumed immediately in its entirety. The drug and applesauce mixture should not be stored for future use. Absorption of the beads sprinkled on other foods has not been tested.

2.1 Heart Failure

DOSAGE MUST BE INDIVIDUALIZED AND CLOSELY MONITORED BY A PHYSICIAN DURING UP-TITRATION. Prior to initiation of COREG CR, it is recommended that fluid retention be minimized. The recommended starting dose of COREG CR is 10 mg once daily for 2 weeks. Patients who tolerate a dose of 10 mg once daily may have their dose increased to 20, 40, and 80 mg over successive intervals of at least 2 weeks. Patients should be maintained on lower doses if higher doses are not tolerated.

Patients should be advised that initiation of treatment and (to a lesser extent) dosage increases may be associated with transient symptoms of dizziness or lightheadedness (and rarely syncope) within the first hour after dosing. Thus during these periods they should avoid situations such as driving or hazardous tasks, where symptoms could result in injury. Vasodilatory symptoms often do not require treatment, but it may be useful to separate the time of dosing of COREG CR from that of the ACE inhibitor or to reduce temporarily the dose of the ACE inhibitor. The dose of COREG CR should not be increased until symptoms of worsening heart failure or vasodilation have been stabilized.

Fluid retention (with or without transient worsening heart failure symptoms) should be treated by an increase in the dose of diuretics.

The dose of COREG CR should be reduced if patients experience bradycardia (heart rate <55 beats/minute).

Episodes of dizziness or fluid retention during initiation of COREG CR can generally be managed without discontinuation of treatment and do not preclude subsequent successful titration of, or a favorable response to, COREG CR.

2.2 Left Ventricular Dysfunction Following Myocardial Infarction

DOSAGE MUST BE INDIVIDUALIZED AND MONITORED DURING UP-TITRATION. Treatment with COREG CR may be started as an inpatient or outpatient and should be started after the patient is hemodynamically stable and fluid retention has been minimized. It is recommended that COREG CR be started at 20 mg once daily and increased after 3 to 10 days, based on tolerability, to 40 mg once daily, then again to the target dose of 80 mg once daily. A lower starting dose may be used (10 mg once daily) and/or the rate of up-titration may be slowed if clinically indicated (e.g., due to low blood pressure or heart rate, or fluid retention). Patients should be maintained on lower doses if higher doses are not tolerated. The recommended dosing regimen need not be altered in patients who received treatment with an IV or oral β-blocker during the acute phase of the myocardial infarction.

2.3 Hypertension

DOSAGE MUST BE INDIVIDUALIZED. The recommended starting dose of COREG CR is 20 mg once daily. If this dose is tolerated, using standing systolic pressure measured about one hour after dosing as a guide, the dose should be maintained for 7 to 14 days, and then increased to 40 mg once daily if needed, based on trough blood pressure, again using standing systolic pressure one hour after dosing as a guide for tolerance. This dose should also be maintained for 7 to 14 days and can then be adjusted upward to 80 mg once daily if tolerated and needed. Although not specifically studied, it is anticipated the full antihypertensive effect of COREG CR would be seen within 7 to 14 days as had been demonstrated with immediate-release carvedilol. Total daily dose should not exceed 80 mg.

Concomitant administration with a diuretic can be expected to produce additive effects and exaggerate the orthostatic component of COREG CR action.

2.4 Hepatic Impairment

COREG CR should not be given to patients with severe hepatic impairment *[see Contraindications (4)]*.

2.5 Geriatric Use

When switching elderly patients (65 years of age or older) who are taking the higher doses of immediate-release carvedilol tablets (25 mg twice daily) to COREG CR, a lower starting dose (40 mg) of COREG CR is recommended to minimize the potential for dizziness, syncope, or hypotension *[see Dosage and Administration (2)]*. Patients who have switched and who tolerate COREG CR should, as appropriate, have their dose increased after an interval of at least 2 weeks *[see Use in Specific Populations (8.5)]*.

3 DOSAGE FORMS AND STRENGTHS

The hard gelatin capsules are filled with white to off-white microparticles and are available in the following strengths:

- 10 mg – white and green capsule shell printed with GSK COREG CR and 10 mg
- 20 mg – white and yellow capsule shell printed with GSK COREG CR and 20 mg
- 40 mg – yellow and green capsule shell printed with GSK COREG CR and 40 mg
- 80 mg – white capsule shell printed with GSK COREG CR and 80 mg

4 CONTRAINDICATIONS

COREG CR is contraindicated in the following conditions:

- Bronchial asthma or related bronchospastic conditions. Deaths from status asthmaticus have been reported following single doses of immediate-release carvedilol.
- Second- or third-degree AV block
- Sick sinus syndrome
- Severe bradycardia (unless a permanent pacemaker is in place)
- Patients with cardiogenic shock or who have decompensated heart failure requiring the use of intravenous inotropic therapy. Such patients should first be weaned from intravenous therapy before initiating COREG CR.
- Patients with severe hepatic impairment
- Patients with a history of a serious hypersensitivity reaction (e.g., Stevens-Johnson syndrome, anaphylactic reaction, angioedema) to carvedilol or any of the components of COREG CR.

5 WARNINGS AND PRECAUTIONS

In clinical trials of COREG CR in patients with hypertension (338 subjects) and in patients with left ventricular dysfunction following a myocardial infarction or heart failure (187 subjects), the profile of adverse events observed with carvedilol phosphate was generally similar to that observed with the administration of immediate-release carvedilol. Therefore, the information included within this section is based on data from controlled clinical trials with COREG CR as well as immediate-release carvedilol.

5.1 Cessation of Therapy

Patients with coronary artery disease, who are being treated with COREG CR, should be advised against abrupt discontinuation of therapy. Severe exacerbation of angina and the occurrence of myocardial infarction and ventricular arrhythmias have been reported in angina patients following the abrupt discontinuation of therapy with β-blockers. The last 2 complications may occur with or without preceding exacerbation of the angina pectoris. As with other β-blockers, when discontinuation of COREG CR is planned, the patients should be carefully observed and advised to limit physical activity to a minimum. COREG CR should be discontinued over 1 to 2 weeks whenever possible. If the angina worsens or acute coronary insufficiency develops, it is recommended that COREG CR be promptly reinstituted, at least temporarily. Because coronary artery disease is common and may be unrecognized, it may be prudent not to discontinue therapy with COREG CR abruptly even in patients treated only for hypertension or heart failure.

5.2 Bradycardia

In clinical trials with immediate-release carvedilol, bradycardia was reported in about 2% of hypertensive patients, 9% of heart failure patients, and 6.5% of myocardial infarction patients with left ventricular dysfunction. Bradycardia was reported in 0.5% of patients receiving COREG CR in a study of heart failure patients and myocardial infarction patients with left ventricular dysfunction. There were no reports of bradycardia in the clinical trial of COREG CR in hypertension. However, if pulse rate drops below 55 beats/minute, the dosage of COREG CR should be reduced.

5.3 Hypotension

In clinical trials of primarily mild-to-moderate heart failure with immediate-release carvedilol, hypotension and postural hypotension occurred in 9.7% and syncope in 3.4% of patients receiving carvedilol compared to 3.6% and 2.5% of placebo patients, respectively. The risk for these events was highest during the first 30 days of dosing, corresponding to the up-titration period and was a cause for discontinuation of therapy in 0.7% of carvedilol patients, compared to 0.4% of placebo patients. In a long-term, placebo-controlled trial in severe heart failure (COPERNICUS), hypotension and postural hypotension occurred in 15.1% and syncope in 2.9% of heart failure patients receiving carvedilol compared to 8.7% and 2.3% of placebo patients, respectively. These events were a cause for discontinuation of therapy in 1.1% of carvedilol patients, compared to 0.8% of placebo patients. In a trial comparing heart failure patients switched to COREG CR or maintained on immediate-release carvedilol, there was a 2-fold increase in the combined incidence of hypotension, syncope or dizziness in elderly patients (> 65 years) switched from the highest dose of carvedilol (25 mg twice daily) to COREG CR 80 mg once daily *[see Dosage and Administration (2), Use in Specific Populations (8.5)]*.

In the clinical trial of COREG CR in hypertensive patients, syncope was reported in 0.3% of patients receiving COREG CR compared to 0% of patients receiving placebo. There were no reports of postural hypotension in this trial. Postural hypotension occurred in 1.8% and syncope in 0.1% of hypertensive patients receiving immediate-release carvedilol, primarily following the initial dose or at the time of dose increase and was a cause for discontinuation of therapy in 1% of patients.

In the CAPRICORN study of survivors of an acute myocardial infarction with left ventricular dysfunction, hypotension or postural hypotension occurred in 20.2% of patients receiving carvedilol compared to 12.6% of placebo patients. Syncope was reported in 3.9% and 1.9% of patients, respectively. These events were a cause for discontinuation of therapy in 2.5% of patients receiving carvedilol, compared to 0.2% of placebo patients.

Starting with a low dose, administration with food, and gradual up-titration should decrease the likelihood of syncope or excessive hypotension *[see Dosage and Administration (2.1, 2.2, 2.3)]*. During initiation of therapy, the patient should be cautioned to avoid situations such as driving or hazardous tasks, where injury could result should syncope occur.

5.4 Heart Failure/Fluid Retention

Worsening heart failure or fluid retention may occur during up-titration of carvedilol. If such symptoms occur, diuretics should be increased and the dose of COREG CR should not be advanced until clinical stability resumes *[see Dosage and Administration (2)]*. Occasionally it is necessary to lower the dose of COREG CR or temporarily discontinue it. Such episodes do not preclude subsequent successful titration of, or a favorable response to, COREG CR. In a placebo-controlled trial of patients with severe heart failure, worsening heart failure during the first 3 months was reported to a similar degree with immediate-release carvedilol and with placebo. When treatment was maintained beyond 3 months, worsening heart failure was reported less frequently in patients treated with carvedilol than with placebo. Worsening heart failure observed during long-term therapy is more likely to be related to the patients' underlying disease than to treatment with carvedilol.

5.5 Nonallergic Bronchospasm

Patients with bronchospastic disease (e.g., chronic bronchitis and emphysema) should, in general, not receive β-blockers. COREG CR may be used with caution, however, in patients who do not respond to, or cannot tolerate, other antihypertensive agents. It is prudent, if COREG CR is used, to use the smallest effective dose, so that inhibition of endogenous or exogenous β-agonists is minimized.

In clinical trials of patients with heart failure, patients with bronchospastic disease were enrolled if they did not require oral or inhaled medication to treat their bronchospastic disease. In such patients, it is recommended that COREG CR be used with caution. The dosing recommendations should be followed closely and the dose should be lowered if any evidence of bronchospasm is observed during up-titration.

5.6 Glycemic Control in Type 2 Diabetes

In general, β-blockers may mask some of the manifestations of hypoglycemia, particularly tachycardia. Nonselective β-blockers may potentiate insulin-induced hypoglycemia and delay recovery of serum glucose levels. Patients subject to spontaneous hypoglycemia, or diabetic patients receiving insulin or oral hypoglycemic agents, should be cautioned about these possibilities.

In heart failure patients with diabetes, carvedilol therapy may lead to worsening hyperglycemia, which responds to intensification of hypoglycemic therapy. It is recommended that blood glucose be monitored when dosing with COREG CR is initiated, adjusted, or discontinued. Studies designed to examine the effects of carvedilol on glycemic control in patients with diabetes and heart failure have not been conducted.

In a study designed to examine the effects of immediate-release carvedilol on glycemic control in a population with mild-to-moderate hypertension and well-controlled type 2 diabetes mellitus, carvedilol had no adverse effect on glycemic control, based on HbA1c measurements [see Clinical Studies (14.4)].

5.7 Peripheral Vascular Disease
β-blockers can precipitate or aggravate symptoms of arterial insufficiency in patients with peripheral vascular disease. Caution should be exercised in such individuals.

5.8 Deterioration of Renal Function
Rarely, use of carvedilol in patients with heart failure has resulted in deterioration of renal function. Patients at risk appear to be those with low blood pressure (systolic blood pressure <100 mm Hg), ischemic heart disease and diffuse vascular disease, and/or underlying renal insufficiency. Renal function has returned to baseline when carvedilol was stopped. In patients with these risk factors it is recommended that renal function be monitored during up-titration of COREG CR and the drug discontinued or dosage reduced if worsening of renal function occurs.

5.9 Anesthesia and Major Surgery
If treatment with COREG CR is to be continued perioperatively, particular care should be taken when anesthetic agents which depress myocardial function, such as ether, cyclopropane, and trichloroethylene, are used [see Overdosage (10) for information on treatment of bradycardia and hypertension].

5.10 Thyrotoxicosis
β-adrenergic blockade may mask clinical signs of hyperthyroidism, such as tachycardia. Abrupt withdrawal of β-blockade may be followed by an exacerbation of the symptoms of hyperthyroidism or may precipitate thyroid storm.

5.11 Pheochromocytoma
In patients with pheochromocytoma, an α-blocking agent should be initiated prior to the use of any β-blocking agent. Although carvedilol has both α- and β-blocking pharmacologic activities, there has been no experience with its use in this condition. Therefore, caution should be taken in the administration of carvedilol to patients suspected of having pheochromocytoma.

5.12 Prinzmetal's Variant Angina
Agents with non-selective β-blocking activity may provoke chest pain in patients with Prinzmetal's variant angina. There has been no clinical experience with carvedilol in these patients although the α-blocking activity may prevent such symptoms. However, caution should be taken in the administration of COREG CR to patients suspected of having Prinzmetal's variant angina.

5.13 Risk of Anaphylactic Reaction
While taking β-blockers, patients with a history of severe anaphylactic reaction to a variety of allergens may be more reactive to repeated challenge, either accidental, diagnostic, or therapeutic. Such patients may be unresponsive to the usual doses of epinephrine used to treat allergic reaction.

6 ADVERSE REACTIONS
6.1 Clinical Trials Experience
Carvedilol has been evaluated for safety in patients with heart failure (mild, moderate, and severe), in patients with left ventricular dysfunction following myocardial infarction, and in hypertensive patients. The observed adverse event profile was consistent with the pharmacology of the drug and the health status of the patients in the clinical trials. Adverse events reported for each of these patient populations reflecting the use of either COREG CR or immediate-release carvedilol are provided below. Excluded are adverse events considered too general to be informative, and those not reasonably associated with the use of the drug because they were associated with the condition being treated or are very common in the treated population. Rates of adverse events were generally similar across demographic subsets (men and women, elderly and non-elderly, blacks and non-blacks). COREG CR has been evaluated for safety in a 4-week (2 weeks of immediate-release carvedilol and 2 weeks of COREG CR) clinical study (n = 187) which included 157 patients with stable mild, moderate, or severe chronic heart failure and 30 patients with left ventricular dysfunction following acute myocardial infarction. The profile of adverse events observed with COREG CR in this small, short-term study was generally similar to that observed with immediate-release carvedilol. Differences in safety would not be expected based on the similarity in plasma levels for COREG CR and immediate-release carvedilol.

Heart Failure: The following information describes the safety experience in heart failure with immediate-release carvedilol.

Carvedilol has been evaluated for safety in heart failure in more than 4,500 patients worldwide of whom more than 2,100 participated in placebo-controlled clinical trials. Approximately 60% of the total treated population in placebo-controlled clinical trials received carvedilol for at least 6 months and 30% received carvedilol for at least 12 months.

Table 2. Adverse Events (%) Occurring More Frequently With Immediate-Release Carvedilol Than With Placebo in Patients With Mild-to-Moderate Heart Failure (HF) Enrolled in US Heart Failure Trials or in Patients With Severe Heart Failure in the COPERNICUS Trial (Incidence >3% in Patients Treated With Carvedilol, Regardless of Causality)

	Mild-to-Moderate HF		Severe HF	
	Carvedilol	Placebo	Carvedilol	Placebo
	(n = 765)	(n = 437)	(n = 1,156)	(n = 1,133)
Body as a Whole				
Asthenia	7	7	11	9
Fatigue	24	22	—	—
Digoxin level increased	5	4	2	1
Edema generalized	5	3	6	5
Edema dependent	4	2	—	—
Cardiovascular				
Bradycardia	9	1	10	3
Hypotension	9	3	14	8
Syncope	3	3	8	5
Angina pectoris	2	3	6	4
Central Nervous System				
Dizziness	32	19	24	17
Headache	8	7	5	3
Gastrointestinal				
Diarrhea	12	6	5	3
Nausea	9	5	4	3
Vomiting	6	4	1	2
Metabolic				
Hyperglycemia	12	8	5	3
Weight increase	10	7	12	11
BUN increased	6	5	—	—
NPN increased	6	5	—	—
Hypercholesterolemia	4	3	1	1
Edema peripheral	2	1	7	6
Musculoskeletal				
Arthralgia	6	5	1	1
Respiratory				
Cough increased	8	9	5	4
Rales	4	4	4	2
Vision				
Vision abnormal	5	2	—	—

In the COMET trial, 1,511 patients with mild-to-moderate heart failure were treated with carvedilol for up to 5.9 years (mean 4.8 years). Both in US clinical trials in mild-to-moderate heart failure that compared carvedilol in daily doses up to 100 mg (n = 765) to placebo (n = 437), and in a multinational clinical trial in severe heart failure (COPERNICUS) that compared carvedilol in daily doses up to 50 mg (n = 1,156) with placebo (n = 1,133), discontinuation rates for adverse experiences were similar in carvedilol and placebo patients. In placebo-controlled clinical trials, the only cause of discontinuation >1%, and occurring more often on carvedilol was dizziness (1.3% on carvedilol, 0.6% on placebo in the COPERNICUS trial).

Table 2 shows adverse events reported in patients with mild-to-moderate heart failure enrolled in US placebo-controlled clinical trials, and with severe heart failure enrolled in the COPERNICUS trial. Shown are adverse events that occurred more frequently in drug-treated patients than placebo-treated patients with an incidence of >3% in patients treated with carvedilol regardless of causality. Median study medication exposure was 6.3 months for both carvedilol and placebo patients in the trials of mild-to-moderate heart failure, and 10.4 months in the trial of severe heart failure patients. The adverse event profile of carvedilol observed in the long-term COMET study was generally similar to that observed in the US Heart Failure Trials.

[See table 2 above]

Cardiac failure and dyspnea were also reported in these studies, but the rates were equal or greater in patients who received placebo.

The following adverse events were reported with a frequency of >1% but ≤3% and more frequently with carvedilol in either the US placebo-controlled trials in patients with mild-to-moderate heart failure, or in patients with severe heart failure in the COPERNICUS trial.

Incidence >1% to ≤3%

Body as a Whole: Allergy, malaise, hypovolemia, fever, leg edema.

Cardiovascular: Fluid overload, postural hypotension, aggravated angina pectoris, AV block, palpitation, hypertension.

Central and Peripheral Nervous System: Hypesthesia, vertigo, paresthesia.
Gastrointestinal: Melena, periodontitis.
Liver and Biliary System: SGPT increased, SGOT increased.
Metabolic and Nutritional: Hyperuricemia, hypoglycemia, hyponatremia, increased alkaline phosphatase, glycosuria, hypervolemia, diabetes mellitus, GGT increased, weight loss, hyperkalemia, creatinine increased.
Musculoskeletal: Muscle cramps.
Platelet, Bleeding and Clotting: Prothrombin decreased, purpura, thrombocytopenia.
Psychiatric: Somnolence.
Reproductive, male: Impotence.
Special Senses: Blurred vision.
Urinary System: Renal insufficiency, albuminuria, hematuria.

Left Ventricular Dysfunction Following Myocardial Infarction: The following information describes the safety experience in left ventricular dysfunction following acute myocardial infarction with immediate-release carvedilol.

Carvedilol has been evaluated for safety in survivors of an acute myocardial infarction with left ventricular dysfunction in the CAPRICORN trial which involved 969 patients who received carvedilol and 980 who received placebo. Approximately 75% of the patients received carvedilol for at least 6 months and 53% received carvedilol for at least 12 months. Patients were treated for an average of 12.9 months and 12.8 months with carvedilol and placebo, respectively.

The most common adverse events reported with carvedilol in the CAPRICORN trial were consistent with the profile of the drug in the US heart failure trials and the COPERNICUS trial. The only additional adverse events reported in CAPRICORN in >3% of the patients and more commonly on carvedilol were dyspnea, anemia, and lung edema. The following adverse events were reported with a frequency of >1% but ≤3% and more frequently with carvedilol: Flu syndrome, cerebrovascular accident, peripheral vascular disorder, hypotonia, depression, gastrointestinal pain, arthritis, and gout. The overall rates of discontinuations due to adverse events were similar in both groups of patients. In this database, the only cause of discontinuation >1%, and occurring more often on carvedilol was hypotension (1.5% on carvedilol, 0.2% on placebo).

Hypertension: COREG CR was evaluated for safety in an 8-week double-blind trial in 337 subjects with essential hypertension. The profile of adverse events observed with COREG CR was generally similar to that observed with immediate-release carvedilol. The overall rates of discontinuations due to adverse events were similar between COREG CR and placebo.

Table 3. Adverse Events (%) Occurring More Frequently With COREG CR Than With Placebo in Patients With Hypertension (Incidence ≥1% in Patients Treated With Carvedilol, Regardless of Causality)

	COREG CR (n = 253)	Placebo (n = 84)
Nasopharyngitis	4	0
Dizziness	2	1
Nausea	2	0
Edema peripheral	2	1
Nasal congestion	1	0
Paresthesia	1	0
Sinus congestion	1	0
Diarrhea	1	0
Insomnia	1	0

The following information describes the safety experience in hypertension with immediate-release carvedilol.

Carvedilol has been evaluated for safety in hypertension in more than 2,193 patients in US clinical trials and in 2,976 patients in international clinical trials. Approximately 36% of the total treated population received carvedilol for at least 6 months. In general, carvedilol was well tolerated at doses up to 50 mg daily. Most adverse events reported during carvedilol therapy were of mild to moderate severity. In US controlled clinical trials directly comparing carvedilol monotherapy in doses up to 50 mg (n = 1,142) to placebo (n = 462), 4.9% of carvedilol patients discontinued for adverse events versus 5.2% of placebo patients. Although there was no overall difference in discontinuation rates, discontinuations were more common in the carvedilol group for postural hypotension (1% versus 0). The overall incidence of adverse events in US placebo-controlled trials was found to increase with increasing dose of carvedilol. For individual adverse events this could only be distinguished for dizziness, which increased in frequency from 2% to 5% as total daily dose increased from 6.25 mg to 50 mg as single or divided doses.

Table 4 shows adverse events in US placebo-controlled clinical trials for hypertension that occurred with an incidence of ≥1% regardless of causality, and that were more frequent in drug-treated patients than placebo-treated patients.

Table 4. Adverse Events (% Occurrence) in US Placebo-Controlled Hypertension Trials With Immediate-Release Carvedilol (Incidence ≥1% in Patients Treated With Carvedilol, Regardless of Causality)*

	Carvedilol (n = 1,142)	Placebo (n = 462)
Cardiovascular		
Bradycardia	2	—
Postural hypotension	2	—
Peripheral edema	1	—
Central Nervous System		
Dizziness	6	5
Insomnia	2	1
Gastrointestinal		
Diarrhea	2	1
Hematologic		
Thrombocytopenia	1	—
Metabolic		
Hypertriglyceridemia	1	—

*Shown are events with rate >1% rounded to nearest integer.

Dyspnea and fatigue were also reported in these studies, but the rates were equal or greater in patients who received placebo.

The following adverse events not described above were reported as possibly or probably related to carvedilol in worldwide open or controlled trials with carvedilol in patients with hypertension or heart failure.

Incidence >0.1% to ≤1%

Cardiovascular: Peripheral ischemia, tachycardia.
Central and Peripheral Nervous System: Hypokinesia.
Gastrointestinal: Bilirubinemia, increased hepatic enzymes (0.2% of hypertension patients and 0.4% of heart failure patients were discontinued from therapy because of increases in hepatic enzymes) *[see Adverse Reactions (6.2)]*.
Psychiatric: Nervousness, sleep disorder, aggravated depression, impaired concentration, abnormal thinking, paroniria, emotional lability.
Respiratory System: Asthma *[see Contraindications (4)]*.
Reproductive, male: Decreased libido.
Skin and Appendages: Pruritus, rash erythematous, rash maculopapular, rash psoriaform, photosensitivity reaction.
Special Senses: Tinnitus.
Urinary System: Micturition frequency increased.
Autonomic Nervous System: Dry mouth, sweating increased.
Metabolic and Nutritional: Hypokalemia, hypertriglyceridemia.
Hematologic: Anemia, leukopenia.

The following events were reported in ≤0.1% of patients and are potentially important: Complete AV block, bundle branch block, myocardial ischemia, cerebrovascular disorder, convulsions, migraine, neuralgia, paresis, anaphylactoid reaction, alopecia, exfoliative dermatitis, amnesia, GI hemorrhage, bronchospasm, pulmonary edema, decreased hearing, respiratory alkalosis, increased BUN, decreased HDL, pancytopenia, and atypical lymphocytes.

6.2 Laboratory Abnormalities

Reversible elevations in serum transaminases (ALT or AST) have been observed during treatment with carvedilol. Rates of transaminase elevations (2- to 3-times the upper limit of normal) observed during controlled clinical trials have generally been similar between patients treated with carvedilol and those treated with placebo. However, transaminase elevations, confirmed by rechallenge, have been observed with carvedilol. In a long-term, placebo-controlled trial in severe heart failure, patients treated with carvedilol had lower values for hepatic transaminases than patients treated with placebo, possibly because carvedilol-induced improvements in cardiac function led to less hepatic congestion and/or improved hepatic blood flow.

Carvedilol therapy has not been associated with clinically significant changes in serum potassium, total triglycerides, total cholesterol, HDL cholesterol, uric acid, blood urea nitrogen, or creatinine. No clinically relevant changes were noted in fasting serum glucose in hypertensive patients; fasting serum glucose was not evaluated in the heart failure clinical trials.

6.3 Postmarketing Experience

The following adverse reactions have been identified during post-approval use of COREG® or COREG CR. Because these reactions are reported voluntarily from a population of uncertain size, it is not always possible to reliably estimate their frequency or establish a causal relationship to drug exposure.

Reports of aplastic anemia and severe skin reactions (Stevens-Johnson syndrome, toxic epidermal necrolysis, and erythema multiforme) have been rare and received only when carvedilol was administered concomitantly with other medications associated with such reactions. Rare reports of hypersensitivity reactions (e.g., anaphylactic reaction, angioedema, and urticaria) have been received for COREG and COREG CR, including cases occurring after the initiation of COREG CR in patients previously treated with COREG. Urinary incontinence in women (which resolved upon discontinuation of the medication) and interstitial pneumonitis have been reported rarely.

7 DRUG INTERACTIONS

7.1 CYP2D6 Inhibitors and Poor Metabolizers

Interactions of carvedilol with potent inhibitors of CYP2D6 isoenzyme (such as quinidine, fluoxetine, paroxetine, and propafenone) have not been studied, but these drugs would be expected to increase blood levels of the R(+) enantiomer of carvedilol *[see Clinical Pharmacology (12.3)]*. Retrospective analysis of side effects in clinical trials showed that poor 2D6 metabolizers had a higher rate of dizziness during up-titration, presumably resulting from vasodilating effects of the higher concentrations of the α-blocking R(+) enantiomer.

7.2 Hypotensive Agents

Patients taking both agents with β-blocking properties and a drug that can deplete catecholamines (e.g., reserpine and monoamine oxidase inhibitors) should be observed closely for signs of hypotension and/or severe bradycardia.

Concomitant administration of clonidine with agents with β-blocking properties may potentiate blood-pressure- and heart-rate-lowering effects. When concomitant treatment with agents with β-blocking properties and clonidine is to be terminated, the β-blocking agent should be discontinued first. Clonidine therapy can then be discontinued several days later by gradually decreasing the dosage.

7.3 Cyclosporine

Modest increases in mean trough cyclosporine concentrations were observed following initiation of carvedilol treatment in 21 renal transplant patients suffering from chronic vascular rejection. In about 30% of patients, the dose of cyclosporine had to be reduced in order to maintain cyclosporine concentrations within the therapeutic range, while in the remainder no adjustment was needed. On the average for the group, the dose of cyclosporine was reduced about 20% in these patients. Due to wide interindividual variability in the dose adjustment required, it is recommended that cyclosporine concentrations be monitored closely after initiation of carvedilol therapy and that the dose of cyclosporine be adjusted as appropriate.

7.4 Digitalis Glycosides

Both digitalis glycosides and β-blockers slow atrioventricular conduction and decrease heart rate. Concomitant use can increase the risk of bradycardia. Digoxin concentrations are increased by about 15% when digoxin and carvedilol are administered concomitantly. Therefore, increased monitoring of digoxin is recommended when initiating, adjusting, or discontinuing COREG CR *[see Clinical Pharmacology (12.5)]*.

7.5 Inducers/Inhibitors of Hepatic Metabolism

Rifampin reduced plasma concentrations of carvedilol by about 70% *[see Clinical Pharmacology (12.5)]*. Cimetidine increased area under the curve (AUC) by about 30% but caused no change in C_{max} *[see Clinical Pharmacology (12.5)]*.

7.6 Amiodarone

Amiodarone, and its metabolite desethyl amiodarone, inhibitors of CYP2C9 and P-glycoprotein, increased concentrations of the S(-) enantiomer of carvedilol by at least 2-fold *[see Clinical Pharmacology (12.5)]*. The concomitant administration of amiodarone or other CYP2C9 inhibitors such as fluconazole with COREG CR may enhance the β-blocking properties of carvedilol resulting in further slowing of the heart rate or cardiac conduction. Patients should be observed for signs of bradycardia or heart block, particularly when one agent is added to pre-existing treatment with the other.

7.7 Calcium Channel Blockers

Conduction disturbance (rarely with hemodynamic compromise) has been observed when carvedilol is co-administered with diltiazem. As with other agents with β-blocking properties, if COREG CR is to be administered orally with calcium channel blockers of the verapamil or diltiazem type, it is recommended that ECG and blood pressure be monitored.

7.8 Insulin or Oral Hypoglycemics

Agents with β-blocking properties may enhance the blood-sugar-reducing effect of insulin and oral hypoglycemics. Therefore, in patients taking insulin or oral hypoglycemics, regular monitoring of blood glucose is recommended *[see Warnings and Precautions (5.6)]*.

7.9 Proton Pump Inhibitors

There is no clinically meaningful increase in AUC and C_{max} with concomitant administration of carvedilol extended-release capsules with pantoprazole.

8 USE IN SPECIFIC POPULATIONS

8.1 Pregnancy

Pregnancy Category C. Studies performed in pregnant rats and rabbits given carvedilol revealed increased post-implantation loss in rats at doses of 300 mg/kg/day (50 times the maximum recommended human dose [MRHD] as mg/m^2) and in rabbits at doses of 75 mg/kg/day (25 times the MRHD as mg/m^2). In the rats, there was also a decrease in fetal body weight at the maternally toxic dose of 300 mg/kg/day (50 times the MRHD as mg/m^2), which was accompanied by an elevation in the frequency of fetuses with delayed skeletal development (missing or stunted 13th rib). In rats the no-observed-effect level for developmental toxicity was 60 mg/kg/day (10 times the MRHD as mg/m^2); in rabbits it was 15 mg/kg/day (5 times the MRHD as mg/m^2). There are no adequate and well-controlled studies in pregnant women. COREG CR should be used during pregnancy only if the potential benefit justifies the potential risk to the fetus.

8.3 Nursing Mothers

It is not known whether this drug is excreted in human milk. Studies in rats have shown that carvedilol and/or its metabolites (as well as other β-blockers) cross the placental barrier and are excreted in breast milk. There was increased mortality at one week post partum in neonates from rats treated with 60 mg/kg/day (10 times the MRHD as mg/m^2) and above during the last trimester through day 22 of lactation. Because many drugs are excreted in human milk and because of the potential for serious adverse reactions in nursing infants from β-blockers, especially bradycardia, a decision should be made whether to discontinue nursing or to discontinue the drug, taking into account the importance of the drug to the mother. The effects of other α- and β-blocking agents have included perinatal and neonatal distress.

8.4 Pediatric Use

Effectiveness of carvedilol in patients younger than 18 years of age has not been established.

In a double-blind trial, 161 children (mean age 6 years, range 2 months to 17 years; 45% younger than 2 years old) with chronic heart failure [NYHA class II-IV, left ventricular ejection fraction <40% for children with a systemic left ventricle (LV), and moderate-severe ventricular dysfunction qualitatively by echo for those with a systemic ventricle that was not an LV] who were receiving standard background treatment were randomized to placebo or to 2 dose levels of carvedilol. These dose levels produced placebo-corrected heart rate reduction of 4-6 heart beats per minute, indicative of β-blockade activity. Exposure appeared to be lower in pediatric subjects than adults. After 8 months of follow-up, there was no significant effect of treatment on clinical outcomes. Adverse reactions in this trial that occurred in greater than 10% of patients treated with immediate-release carvedilol and at twice the rate of placebo-treated patients included chest pain (17% versus 6%), dizziness (13% versus 2%), and dyspnea (11% versus 0%).

8.5 Geriatric Use

The initial clinical studies of COREG CR in patients with hypertension, heart failure, and left ventricular dysfunction following myocardial infarction did not include sufficient numbers of subjects 65 years of age or older to determine whether they respond differently from younger patients.

A randomized study (n = 405) comparing mild to severe heart failure patients switched to COREG CR or maintained on immediate-release carvedilol included 220 patients who were 65 years of age or older. In this elderly subgroup, the combined incidence of dizziness, hypotension, or syncope was 24% (18/75) in patients switched from the highest dose of immediate-release carvedilol (25 mg twice daily) to the highest dose of COREG CR (80 mg once daily) compared to 11% (4/36) in patients maintained on immediate-release carvedilol (25 mg twice daily). When switching from the higher doses of immediate-release carvedilol to COREG CR, a lower starting dose is recommended for elderly patients *[see Dosage and Administration (2.5)]*.

The following information is available for trials with immediate release carvedilol. Of the 765 patients with heart failure randomized to carvedilol in US clinical trials, 31% (235) were 65 years of age or older, and 7.3% (56) were 75 years of age or older. Of the 1,156 patients randomized to carvedilol in a long-term, placebo-controlled trial in severe heart failure, 47% (547) were 65 years of age or older, and 15% (174) were 75 years of age or older. Of 3,025 patients receiving carvedilol in heart failure trials worldwide, 42% were 65 years of age or older. Of the 975 myocardial infarction patients randomized to carvedilol in the CAPRICORN trial, 48% (468) were 65 years of age or older, and 11% (111) were 75 years of age or older. Of the 2,065 hypertensive patients in US clinical trials of efficacy or safety who were treated with carvedilol, 21% (436) were 65 years of age or older. Of 3,722 patients receiving immediate- release carvedilol in hypertension clinical trials conducted worldwide, 24% were 65 years of age or older.

With the exception of dizziness in hypertensive patients (incidence 8.8% in the elderly versus 6% in younger patients), no overall differences in the safety or effectiveness (see Figures 2 and 4) were observed between the older subjects and younger subjects in each of these populations. Similarly, other reported clinical experience has not identified differences in responses between the elderly and younger subjects, but greater sensitivity of some older individuals cannot be ruled out.

10 OVERDOSAGE

Overdosage may cause severe hypotension, bradycardia, cardiac insufficiency, cardiogenic shock, and cardiac arrest. Respiratory problems, bronchospasms, vomiting, lapses of consciousness, and generalized seizures may also occur.

The patient should be placed in a supine position and, where necessary, kept under observation and treated under intensive-care conditions. Gastric lavage or pharmacologically induced emesis may be used shortly after ingestion.

The following agents may be administered:

for excessive bradycardia: atropine, 2 mg IV.

to support cardiovascular function: glucagon, 5 to 10 mg IV rapidly over 30 seconds, followed by a continuous infusion of 5 mg/hour; sympathomimetics (dobutamine, isoprenaline, adrenaline) at doses according to body weight and effect.

If peripheral vasodilation dominates, it may be necessary to administer adrenaline or noradrenaline with continuous monitoring of circulatory conditions. For therapy-resistant bradycardia, pacemaker therapy should be performed. For bronchospasm, β-sympathomimetics (as aerosol or IV) or aminophylline IV should be given. In the event of seizures, slow IV injection of diazepam or clonazepam is recommended.

NOTE: In the event of severe intoxication where there are symptoms of shock, treatment with antidotes must be continued for a sufficiently long period of time consistent with the 7- to 10-hour half-life of carvedilol.

There is no experience of overdosage with COREG CR. Cases of overdosage with carvedilol alone or in combination with other drugs have been reported. Quantities ingested in some cases exceeded 1,000 milligrams. Symptoms experienced included low blood pressure and heart rate. Standard supportive treatment was provided and individuals recovered.

11 DESCRIPTION

Carvedilol phosphate is a nonselective β-adrenergic blocking agent with α_1-blocking activity. It is (2*RS*)-1-(9*H*-Carbazol-4-yloxy)-3-[[2-(2-methoxyphenoxy)ethyl]amino]propan-2-ol phosphate salt (1:1) hemihydrate. It is a racemic mixture with the following structure:

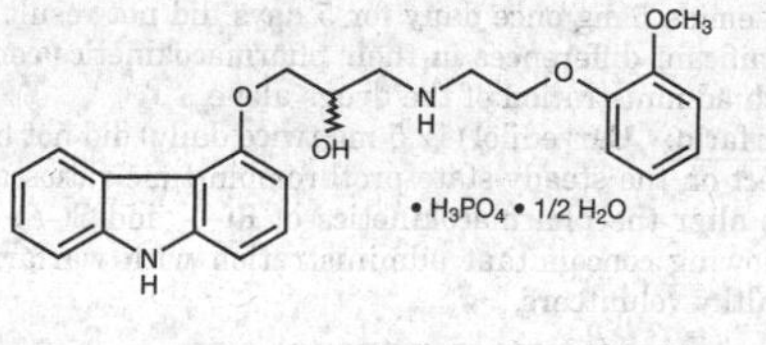

Carvedilol phosphate is a white to almost-white solid with a molecular weight of 513.5 (406.5 carvedilol free base) and a molecular formula of $C_{24}H_{26}N_2O_4 \bullet H_3PO_4 \bullet 1/2\ H_2O$.

COREG CR is available for once-a-day administration as controlled-release oral capsules containing 10, 20, 40, or 80 mg carvedilol phosphate. COREG CR hard gelatin capsules are filled with carvedilol phosphate immediate-release and controlled-release microparticles that are drug-layered and then coated with methacrylic acid copolymers. Inactive ingredients include crospovidone, hydrogenated castor oil, hydrogenated vegetable oil, magnesium stearate, methacrylic acid copolymers, microcrystalline cellulose, and povidone.

12 CLINICAL PHARMACOLOGY

12.1 Mechanism of Action

Carvedilol is a racemic mixture in which nonselective β-adrenoreceptor blocking activity is present in the S(-) enantiomer and α_1-adrenergic blocking activity is present in both R(+) and S(-) enantiomers at equal potency. Carvedilol has no intrinsic sympathomimetic activity.

12.2 Pharmacodynamics

Heart Failure and Left Ventricular Dysfunction Following Myocardial Infarction: The basis for the beneficial effects of carvedilol in patients with heart failure and in patients with left ventricular dysfunction following an acute myocardial infarction is not known. The concentration-response relationship for β_1-blockade following administration of COREG CR is equivalent (±20%) to immediate-release carvedilol tablets.

Hypertension: The mechanism by which β-blockade produces an antihypertensive effect has not been established. β-adrenoreceptor blocking activity has been demonstrated in animal and human studies showing that carvedilol (1) reduces cardiac output in normal subjects; (2) reduces exercise- and/or isoproterenol-induced tachycardia; and (3) reduces reflex orthostatic tachycardia. Significant β-adrenoreceptor blocking effect is usually seen within 1 hour of drug administration.

α_1-adrenoreceptor blocking activity has been demonstrated in human and animal studies, showing that carvedilol (1) attenuates the pressor effects of phenylephrine; (2) causes vasodilation; and (3) reduces peripheral vascular resistance. These effects contribute to the reduction of blood pressure and usually are seen within 30 minutes of drug administration.

Due to the α_1-receptor blocking activity of carvedilol, blood pressure is lowered more in the standing than in the supine position, and symptoms of postural hypotension (1.8%), including rare instances of syncope, can occur. Following oral administration, when postural hypotension has occurred, it has been transient and is uncommon when immediate-release carvedilol is administered with food at the recommended starting dose and titration increments are closely followed *[see Dosage and Administration (2)]*.

In a randomized, double-blind, placebo-controlled trial, the β_1-blocking effect of COREG CR, as measured by heart rate response to submaximal bicycle ergometry, was shown to be equivalent to that observed with immediate-release carvedilol at steady state in adult patients with essential hypertension.

In hypertensive patients with normal renal function, therapeutic doses of carvedilol decreased renal vascular resistance with no change in glomerular filtration rate or renal plasma flow. Changes in excretion of sodium, potassium, uric acid, and phosphorus in hypertensive patients with normal renal function were similar after carvedilol and placebo.

Carvedilol has little effect on plasma catecholamines, plasma aldosterone, or electrolyte levels, but it does significantly reduce plasma renin activity when given for at least 4 weeks. It also increases levels of atrial natriuretic peptide.

12.3 Pharmacokinetics

Absorption: Carvedilol is rapidly and extensively absorbed following oral administration of immediate-release carvedilol tablets, with an absolute bioavailability of approximately 25% to 35% due to a significant degree of first-pass metabolism. COREG CR extended-release capsules have approximately 85% of the bioavailability of immediate-release carvedilol tablets. For corresponding dosages *[see Dosage and Administration (2)]*, the exposure (AUC, C_{max}, trough concentration) of carvedilol as COREG CR extended-release capsules is equivalent to those of immediate-release carvedilol tablets when both are administered with food. The absorption of carvedilol from COREG CR is slower and more prolonged compared to the immediate-release carvedilol tablet with peak concentrations achieved approximately 5 hours after administration. Plasma concentrations of carvedilol increase in a dose-proportional manner over the dosage range of COREG CR 10 to 80 mg. Within-subject and between-subject variability for AUC and C_{max} is similar for COREG CR and immediate-release carvedilol.

Effect of Food: Administration of COREG CR with a high-fat meal resulted in increases (~20%) in AUC and C_{max} compared to COREG CR administered with a standard meal. Decreases in AUC (27%) and C_{max} (43%) were observed when COREG CR was administered in the fasted state compared to administration after a standard meal. COREG CR should be taken with food.

In a study with adult subjects, sprinkling the contents of the COREG CR capsule on applesauce did not appear to have a significant effect on overall exposure (AUC) compared to administration of the intact capsule following a standard meal but did result in a decrease in C_{max} (18%).

Distribution: Carvedilol is more than 98% bound to plasma proteins, primarily with albumin. The plasma-protein binding is independent of concentration over the therapeutic range. Carvedilol is a basic, lipophilic compound with a steady-state volume of distribution of approximately 115 L, indicating substantial distribution into extravascular tissues.

Metabolism and Excretion: Carvedilol is extensively metabolized. Following oral administration of radiolabelled carvedilol to healthy volunteers, carvedilol accounted for only about 7% of the total radioactivity in plasma as mea-

Table 5. Results of COMET

Endpoint	Carvedilol N = 1,511	Metoprolol N = 1,518	Hazard ratio	(95% CI)
All cause mortality	34%	40%	0.83	0.74–0.93
Mortality + all hospitalization	74%	76%	0.94	0.86–1.02
Cardiovascular death	30%	35%	0.80	0.70–0.90
Sudden death	14%	17%	0.81	0.68–0.97
Death due to circulatory failure	11%	13%	0.83	0.67–1.02
Death due to stroke	0.9%	2.5%	0.33	0.18–0.62

sured by AUC. Less than 2% of the dose was excreted unchanged in the urine. Carvedilol is metabolized primarily by aromatic ring oxidation and glucuronidation. The oxidative metabolites are further metabolized by conjugation via glucuronidation and sulfation. The metabolites of carvedilol are excreted primarily via the bile into the feces. Demethylation and hydroxylation at the phenol ring produce 3 active metabolites with β-receptor blocking activity. Based on preclinical studies, the 4′-hydroxyphenyl metabolite is approximately 13 times more potent than carvedilol for β-blockade. Compared to carvedilol, the 3 active metabolites exhibit weak vasodilating activity. Plasma concentrations of the active metabolites are about one-tenth of those observed for carvedilol and have pharmacokinetics similar to the parent.
Carvedilol undergoes stereoselective first-pass metabolism with plasma levels of R(+)-carvedilol approximately 2 to 3 times higher than S(-)-carvedilol following oral administration of COREG CR in healthy subjects. Apparent clearance is 90 L/h and 213 L/h for R(+)- and S(-)-carvedilol, respectively.
The primary P450 enzymes responsible for the metabolism of both R(+) and S(-)-carvedilol in human liver microsomes were CYP2D6 and CYP2C9 and to a lesser extent CYP3A4, 2C19, 1A2, and 2E1. CYP2D6 is thought to be the major enzyme in the 4′- and 5′-hydroxylation of carvedilol, with a potential contribution from 3A4. CYP2C9 is thought to be of primary importance in the O-methylation pathway of S(-)-carvedilol.
Carvedilol is subject to the effects of genetic polymorphism with poor metabolizers of debrisoquin (a marker for cytochrome P450 2D6) exhibiting 2- to 3-fold higher plasma concentrations of R(+)-carvedilol compared to extensive metabolizers. In contrast, plasma levels of S(-)-carvedilol are increased only about 20% to 25% in poor metabolizers, indicating this enantiomer is metabolized to a lesser extent by cytochrome P450 2D6 than R(+)-carvedilol. The pharmacokinetics of carvedilol do not appear to be different in poor metabolizers of S-mephenytoin (patients deficient in cytochrome P450 2C19).

12.4 Specific Populations

Heart Failure: Following administration of immediate-release carvedilol tablets, steady-state plasma concentrations of carvedilol and its enantiomers increased proportionally over the dose range in patients with heart failure. Compared to healthy subjects, heart failure patients had increased mean AUC and C_{max} values for carvedilol and its enantiomers, with up to 50% to 100% higher values observed in 6 patients with NYHA class IV heart failure. The mean apparent terminal elimination half-life for carvedilol was similar to that observed in healthy subjects.
For corresponding dose levels *[see Dosage and Administration (2)]*, the steady-state pharmacokinetics of carvedilol (AUC, C_{max}, trough concentrations) observed after administration of COREG CR to chronic heart failure patients (mild, moderate, and severe) were similar to those observed after administration of immediate-release carvedilol tablets.
Hypertension: For corresponding dose levels *[see Dosage and Administration (2)]*, the pharmacokinetics (AUC, C_{max}, and trough concentrations) observed with administration of COREG CR were equivalent (±20%) to those observed with immediate-release carvedilol tablets following repeat dosing in patients with essential hypertension.
Geriatric: Plasma levels of carvedilol average about 50% higher in the elderly compared to young subjects after administration of immediate-release carvedilol.
Hepatic Impairment: No studies have been performed with COREG CR in patients with hepatic impairment. Compared to healthy subjects, patients with severe liver impairment (cirrhosis) exhibit a 4- to 7-fold increase in carvedilol levels. Carvedilol is contraindicated in patients with severe liver impairment.
Renal Impairment: No studies have been performed with COREG CR in patients with renal impairment. Although carvedilol is metabolized primarily by the liver, plasma concentrations of carvedilol have been reported to be increased in patients with renal impairment after dosing with immediate-release carvedilol. Based on mean AUC data, approximately 40% to 50% higher plasma concentrations of carvedilol were observed in hypertensive patients with moderate to severe renal impairment compared to a control group of hypertensive patients with normal renal function. However, the ranges of AUC values were similar for both groups. Changes in mean peak plasma levels were less pronounced, approximately 12% to 26% higher in patients with impaired renal function.
Consistent with its high degree of plasma protein binding, carvedilol does not appear to be cleared significantly by hemodialysis.

12.5 Drug-Drug Interactions

Since carvedilol undergoes substantial oxidative metabolism, the metabolism and pharmacokinetics of carvedilol may be affected by induction or inhibition of cytochrome P450 enzymes.
The following drug interaction studies were performed with immediate-release carvedilol tablets.
Amiodarone: In a pharmacokinetic study conducted in 106 Japanese patients with heart failure, coadministration of small loading and maintenance doses of amiodarone with carvedilol resulted in at least a 2-fold increase in the steady-state trough concentrations of S(-)-carvedilol *[see Drug Interactions (7.6)]*.
Cimetidine: In a pharmacokinetic study conducted in 10 healthy male subjects, cimetidine (1,000 mg/day) increased the steady-state AUC of carvedilol by 30% with no change in C_{max} *[see Drug Interactions (7.5)]*.
Digoxin: Following concomitant administration of carvedilol (25 mg once daily) and digoxin (0.25 mg once daily) for 14 days, steady-state AUC and trough concentrations of digoxin were increased by 14% and 16%, respectively, in 12 hypertensive patients *[see Drug Interactions (7.4)]*.
Glyburide: In 12 healthy subjects, combined administration of carvedilol (25 mg once daily) and a single dose of glyburide did not result in a clinically relevant pharmacokinetic interaction for either compound.
Hydrochlorothiazide: A single oral dose of carvedilol 25 mg did not alter the pharmacokinetics of a single oral dose of hydrochlorothiazide 25 mg in 12 patients with hypertension. Likewise, hydrochlorothiazide had no effect on the pharmacokinetics of carvedilol.
Rifampin: In a pharmacokinetic study conducted in 8 healthy male subjects, rifampin (600 mg daily for 12 days) decreased the AUC and C_{max} of carvedilol by about 70% *[see Drug Interactions (7.5)]*.
Torsemide: In a study of 12 healthy subjects, combined oral administration of carvedilol 25 mg once daily and torsemide 5 mg once daily for 5 days did not result in any significant differences in their pharmacokinetics compared with administration of the drugs alone.
Warfarin: Carvedilol (12.5 mg twice daily) did not have an effect on the steady-state prothrombin time ratios and did not alter the pharmacokinetics of R(+)- and S(-)-warfarin following concomitant administration with warfarin in 9 healthy volunteers.

13 NONCLINICAL TOXICOLOGY

13.1 Carcinogenesis, Mutagenesis, Impairment of Fertility

In 2-year studies conducted in rats given carvedilol at doses up to 75 mg/kg/day (12 times the MRHD when compared on a mg/m^2 basis) or in mice given up to 200 mg/kg/day (16 times the MRHD on a mg/m^2 basis), carvedilol had no carcinogenic effect.
Carvedilol was negative when tested in a battery of genotoxicity assays, including the Ames and the CHO/HGPRT assays for mutagenicity and the in vitro hamster micronucleus and in vivo human lymphocyte cell tests for clastogenicity.
At doses ≥200 mg/kg/day (≥32 times the MRHD as mg/m^2) carvedilol was toxic to adult rats (sedation, reduced weight gain) and was associated with a reduced number of successful matings, prolonged mating time, significantly fewer corpora lutea and implants per dam, and complete resorption of 18% of the litters. The no-observed-effect dose level for overt toxicity and impairment of fertility was 60 mg/kg/day (10 times the MRHD as mg/m^2).

14 CLINICAL STUDIES

Support for the use of COREG CR extended-release capsules for the treatment of mild- to-severe heart failure and for patients with left ventricular dysfunction following myocardial infarction is based on the equivalence of pharmacokinetic and pharmacodynamic (β_1-blockade) parameters between COREG CR and immediate-release carvedilol *[see Clinical Pharmacology (12.2, 12.3)]*.
The clinical trials performed with immediate-release carvedilol in heart failure and left ventricular dysfunction following myocardial infarction are presented below.

14.1 Heart Failure

A total of 6,975 patients with mild-to-severe heart failure were evaluated in placebo-controlled and active-controlled studies of immediate-release carvedilol.
Mild-to-Moderate Heart Failure: Carvedilol was studied in 5 multicenter, placebo-controlled studies, and in 1 active-controlled study (COMET study) involving patients with mild-to-moderate heart failure.
Four US multicenter, double-blind, placebo-controlled studies enrolled 1,094 patients (696 randomized to carvedilol) with NYHA class II-III heart failure and ejection fraction ≤0.35. The vast majority were on digitalis, diuretics, and an ACE inhibitor at study entry. Patients were assigned to the studies based upon exercise ability. An Australia-New Zealand double-blind, placebo-controlled study enrolled 415 patients (half randomized to immediate-release carvedilol) with less severe heart failure. All protocols excluded patients expected to undergo cardiac transplantation during the 7.5 to 15 months of double-blind follow-up. All randomized patients had tolerated a 2-week course on immediate-release carvedilol 6.25 mg twice daily.
In each study, there was a primary end point, either progression of heart failure (1 US study) or exercise tolerance (2 US studies meeting enrollment goals and the Australia-New Zealand study). There were many secondary end points specified in these studies, including NYHA classification, patient and physician global assessments, and cardiovascular hospitalization. Other analyses not prospectively planned included the sum of deaths and total cardiovascular hospitalizations. In situations where the primary end points of a trial do not show a significant benefit of treatment, assignment of significance values to the other results is complex, and such values need to be interpreted cautiously.
The results of the US and Australia-New Zealand trials were as follows:
Slowing Progression of Heart Failure: One US multicenter study (366 subjects) had as its primary end point the sum of cardiovascular mortality, cardiovascular hospitalization, and sustained increase in heart failure medications. Heart failure progression was reduced, during an average follow-up of 7 months, by 48% (p = 0.008).
In the Australia-New Zealand study, death and total hospitalizations were reduced by about 25% over 18 to 24 months. In the 3 largest US studies, death and total hospitalizations were reduced by 19%, 39%, and 49%, nominally statistically significant in the last 2 studies. The Australia-New Zealand results were statistically borderline.
Functional Measures: None of the multicenter studies had NYHA classification as a primary end point, but all such studies had it as a secondary end point. There was at least a trend toward improvement in NYHA class in all studies. Exercise tolerance was the primary end point in 3 studies; in none was a statistically significant effect found.
Subjective Measures: Health-related quality of life, as measured with a standard questionnaire (a primary end point in 1 study), was unaffected by carvedilol. However, patients' and investigators' global assessments showed significant improvement in most studies.
Mortality: Death was not a pre-specified end point in any study, but was analyzed in all studies. Overall, in these 4 US trials, mortality was reduced, nominally significantly so in 2 studies.
The COMET Trial: In this double-blind trial, 3,029 patients with NYHA class II-IV heart failure (left ventricular ejection fraction ≤35%) were randomized to receive either carvedilol (target dose: 25 mg twice daily) or immediate-release metoprolol tartrate (target dose: 50 mg twice daily). The mean age of the patients was approximately 62 years, 80% were males, and the mean left ventricular ejection fraction at baseline was 26%. Approximately 96% of the patients had NYHA class II or III heart failure. Concomitant treatment included diuretics (99%), ACE inhibitors (91%), digitalis (59%), aldosterone antagonists (11%), and "statin" lipid-lowering agents (21%). The mean duration of follow-up was 4.8 years. The mean dose of carvedilol was 42 mg per day.
The study had 2 primary end points: all-cause mortality and the composite of death plus hospitalization for any reason. The results of COMET are presented in Table 5 below. All-cause mortality carried most of the statistical weight and was the primary determinant of the study size. All-cause

Table 6. Results of COPERNICUS Trial in Patients With Severe Heart Failure

End point	Placebo (N = 1,133)	Carvedilol (N = 1,156)	Hazard ratio (95% CI)	% Reduction	Nominal p value
Mortality	190	130	0.65 (0.52–0.81)	35	0.00013
Mortality + all hospitalization	507	425	0.76 (0.67–0.87)	24	0.00004
Mortality + CV hospitalization	395	314	0.73 (0.63–0.84)	27	0.00002
Mortality + HF hospitalization	357	271	0.69 (0.59–0.81)	31	0.000004

Cardiovascular = CV; Heart failure = HF

mortality was 34% in the patients treated with carvedilol and was 40% in the immediate-release metoprolol group (p = 0.0017; hazard ratio = 0.83, 95% CI 0.74–0.93). The effect on mortality was primarily due to a reduction in cardiovascular death. The difference between the 2 groups with respect to the composite end point was not significant (p = 0.122). The estimated mean survival was 8.0 years with carvedilol and 6.6 years with immediate-release metoprolol. [See table at top of previous page]

It is not known whether this formulation of metoprolol at any dose or this low dose of metoprolol in any formulation has any effect on survival or hospitalization in patients with heart failure. Thus, this trial extends the time over which carvedilol manifests benefits on survival in heart failure, but it is not evidence that carvedilol improves outcome over the formulation of metoprolol (TOPROL-XL®) with benefits in heart failure.

Severe Heart Failure (COPERNICUS): In a double-blind study, 2,289 patients with heart failure at rest or with minimal exertion and left ventricular ejection fraction <25% (mean 20%), despite digitalis (66%), diuretics (99%), and ACE inhibitors (89%) were randomized to placebo or carvedilol. Carvedilol was titrated from a starting dose of 3.125 mg twice daily to the maximum tolerated dose or up to 25 mg twice daily over a minimum of 6 weeks. Most subjects achieved the target dose of 25 mg. The study was conducted in Eastern and Western Europe, the United States, Israel, and Canada. Similar numbers of subjects per group (about 100) withdrew during the titration period.

The primary end point of the trial was all-cause mortality, but cause-specific mortality and the risk of death or hospitalization (total, cardiovascular [CV], or heart failure [HF]) were also examined. The developing trial data were followed by a data monitoring committee, and mortality analyses were adjusted for these multiple looks. The trial was stopped after a median follow-up of 10 months because of an observed 35% reduction in mortality (from 19.7% per patient year on placebo to 12.8% on carvedilol, hazard ratio 0.65, 95% CI 0.52–0.81, p = 0.0014, adjusted) (see Figure 1). The results of COPERNICUS are shown in Table 6. [See table above]

Figure 1. Survival Analysis for COPERNICUS (intent-to-treat)

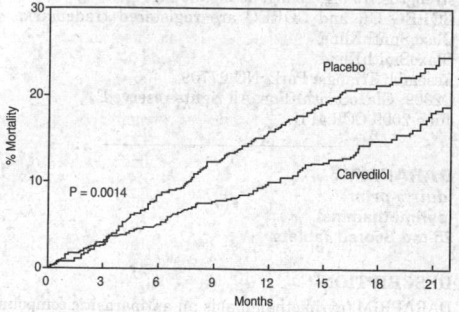

The effect on mortality was principally the result of a reduction in the rate of sudden death among patients without worsening heart failure.

Patients' global assessments, in which carvedilol-treated patients were compared to placebo, were based on prespecified, periodic patient self-assessments regarding whether clinical status post-treatment showed improvement, worsening, or no change compared to baseline. Patients treated with carvedilol showed significant improvements in global assessments compared with those treated with placebo in COPERNICUS.

The protocol also specified that hospitalizations would be assessed. Fewer patients on immediate-release carvedilol than on placebo were hospitalized for any reason (372 ver-

sus 432, p = 0.0029), for cardiovascular reasons (246 versus 314, p = 0.0003), or for worsening heart failure (198 versus 268, p = 0.0001).

Immediate-release carvedilol had a consistent and beneficial effect on all-cause mortality as well as the combined end points of all-cause mortality plus hospitalization (total, CV, or for heart failure) in the overall study population and in all subgroups examined, including men and women, elderly and non-elderly, blacks and non-blacks, and diabetics and non-diabetics (see Figure 2).

Figure 2. Effects on Mortality for Subgroups in COPERNICUS

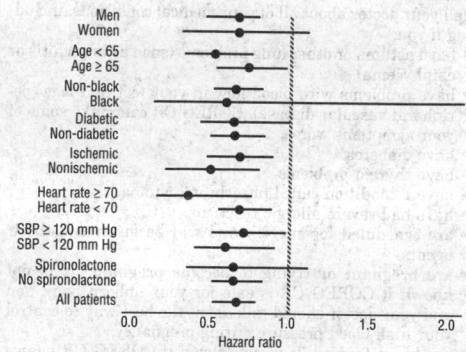

Although the clinical trials used twice-daily dosing, clinical pharmacologic and pharmacokinetic data provide a reasonable basis for concluding that once-daily dosing with COREG CR should be adequate in the treatment of heart failure.

14.2 Left Ventricular Dysfunction Following Myocardial Infarction

CAPRICORN was a double-blind study comparing carvedilol and placebo in 1,959 patients with a recent myocardial infarction (within 21 days) and left ventricular ejection fraction of ≤40%, with (47%) or without symptoms of heart failure. Patients given carvedilol received 6.25 mg twice daily, titrated as tolerated to 25 mg twice daily. Patients had to have a systolic blood pressure >90 mm Hg, a sitting heart rate >60 beats/minute, and no contraindication to β-blocker use. Treatment of the index infarction included aspirin (85%), IV or oral β-blockers (37%), nitrates (73%), heparin (64%), thrombolytics (40%), and acute angioplasty (12%). Background treatment included ACE inhibitors or angiotensin receptor blockers (97%), anticoagulants (20%), lipid-lowering agents (23%), and diuretics (34%). Baseline population characteristics included an average age of 63 years, 74% male, 95% Caucasian, mean blood pressure 121/74 mm Hg, 22% with diabetes, and 54% with a history of hypertension. Mean dosage achieved of carvedilol was 20 mg twice daily; mean duration of follow-up was 15 months.

All-cause mortality was 15% in the placebo group and 12% in the carvedilol group, indicating a 23% risk reduction in patients treated with carvedilol (95% CI 2% to 40%, p = 0.03), as shown in Figure 3. The effects on mortality in various subgroups are shown in Figure 4. Nearly all deaths were cardiovascular (which were reduced by 25% by carvedilol), and most of these deaths were sudden or related to pump failure (both types of death were reduced by carvedilol). Another study end point, total mortality and all-cause hospitalization, did not show a significant improvement.

There was also a significant 40% reduction in fatal or non-fatal myocardial infarction observed in the group treated with carvedilol (95% CI 11% to 60%, p = 0.01). A similar reduction in the risk of myocardial infarction was also ob-

served in a meta-analysis of placebo-controlled trials of carvedilol in heart failure.

Figure 3. Survival Analysis for CAPRICORN (intent-to-treat)

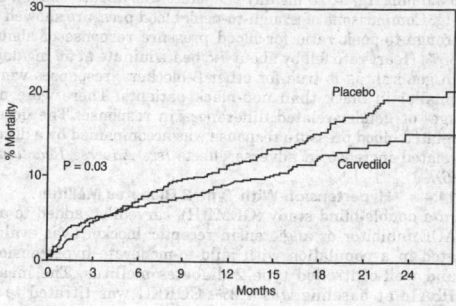

Figure 4. Effects on Mortality for Subgroups in CAPRICORN

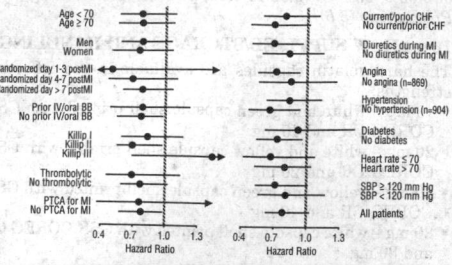

Although the clinical trials used twice-daily dosing, clinical pharmacologic and pharmacokinetic data provide a reasonable basis for concluding that once-daily dosing with COREG CR should be adequate in the treatment of left ventricular dysfunction following myocardial infarction.

14.3 Hypertension

A double-blind, randomized, placebo-controlled, 8-week trial evaluated the blood pressure lowering effects of COREG CR 20 mg, 40 mg, and 80 mg once daily in 338 patients with essential hypertension (sitting diastolic blood pressure [DBP] ≥90 and ≤109 mm Hg). Of 337 evaluable patients, a total of 273 patients (81%) completed the study. Of the 64 (19%) patients withdrawn from the study, 10 (3%) were due to adverse events, 10 (3%) were due to lack of efficacy; the remaining 44 (13%) withdrew for other reasons. The mean age of the patients was approximately 53 years, 66% were male, and the mean sitting systolic blood pressure (SBP) and DBP at baseline were 150 mm Hg and 99 mm Hg, respectively. Dose titration occurred at 2-week intervals. Statistically significant reductions in blood pressure as measured by 24-hour ambulatory blood pressure monitoring (ABPM) were observed with each dose of COREG CR compared to placebo. Placebo-subtracted mean changes from baseline in mean SBP/DBP were -6.1/-4.0 mm Hg, -9.4/-7.6 mm Hg, and -11.8/-9.2 mm Hg for COREG CR 20 mg, 40 mg, and 80 mg, respectively. Placebo-subtracted mean changes from baseline in mean trough (average of hours 20-24) SBP/DBP were -3.3/-2.8 mm Hg, -4.9/-5.2 mm Hg, and -8.4/-7.4 mm Hg for COREG CR 20 mg, 40 mg, and 80 mg, respectively. The placebo-corrected trough to peak (3-7 hr) ratio was approximately 0.6 for COREG CR 80 mg. In this study, assessments of 24-hour ABPM monitoring demonstrated statistically significant blood pressure reductions with COREG CR throughout the dosing period (Figure 5).

Figure 5. Changes from Baseline in Systolic Blood Pressure and Diastolic Blood Pressure Measured by 24-Hour ABPM

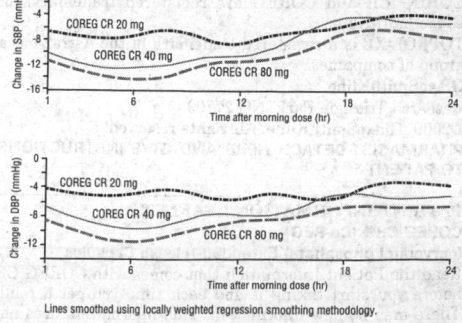

Lines smoothed using locally weighted regression smoothing methodology.

Immediate-release carvedilol was studied in 2 placebo-controlled trials that utilized twice-daily dosing, at total daily doses of 12.5 to 50 mg. In these and other studies, the starting dose did not exceed 12.5 mg. At 50 mg/day, COREG reduced sitting trough (12-hour) blood pressure by about 9/5.5 mm Hg; at 25 mg/day the effect was about 7.5/3.5 mm Hg. Comparisons of trough-to-peak blood pressure showed a trough-to-peak ratio for blood pressure response of about 65%. Heart rate fell by about 7.5 beats/minute at 50 mg/day. In general, as is true for other β-blockers, responses were smaller in black than non-black patients. There were no age- or gender-related differences in response. The dose-related blood pressure response was accompanied by a dose-related increase in adverse effects *[see Adverse Reactions (6)]*.

14.4 Hypertension With Type 2 Diabetes Mellitus

In a double-blind study (GEMINI), carvedilol, added to an ACE inhibitor or angiotensin receptor blocker, was evaluated in a population with mild-to-moderate hypertension and well-controlled type 2 diabetes mellitus. The mean HbA1c at baseline was 7.2%. COREG was titrated to a mean dose of 17.5 mg twice daily and maintained for 5 months. COREG had no adverse effect on glycemic control, based on HbA1c measurements (mean change from baseline of 0.02%, 95% CI -0.06 to 0.10, p = NS) *[see Warnings and Precautions (5.6)]*.

16 HOW SUPPLIED/STORAGE AND HANDLING

The hard gelatin capsules are available in the following strengths:

- 10 mg – white and green capsule shell printed with GSK COREG CR and 10 mg
- 20 mg – white and yellow capsule shell printed with GSK COREG CR and 20 mg
- 40 mg – yellow and green capsule shell printed with GSK COREG CR and 40 mg
- 80 mg – white capsule shell printed with GSK COREG CR and 80 mg
- 10 mg 30's: NDC 0007-3370-13
- 10 mg 90's: NDC 0007-3370-59
- 20 mg 30's: NDC 0007-3371-13
- 20 mg 90's: NDC 0007-3371-59
- 40 mg 30's: NDC 0007-3372-13
- 40 mg 90's: NDC 0007-3372-59
- 80 mg 30's: NDC 0007-3373-13
- 80 mg 90's: NDC 0007-3373-59

Store at 25°C (77°F); excursions 15° to 30°C (59° to 86°F). Dispense in a tight, light-resistant container.

17 PATIENT COUNSELING INFORMATION

See FDA-Approved Patient Labeling (17.2).

17.1 Patient Advice

Patients taking COREG CR should be advised of the following:

- Patients should not interrupt or discontinue using COREG CR without a physician's advice.
- Patients with heart failure should consult their physician if they experience signs or symptoms of worsening heart failure such as weight gain or increasing shortness of breath.
- Patients may experience a drop in blood pressure when standing, resulting in dizziness and, rarely, fainting. Patients should sit or lie down when these symptoms of lowered blood pressure occur.
- If experiencing dizziness or fatigue, patients should avoid driving or hazardous tasks.
- Patients should consult a physician if they experience dizziness or faintness, in case the dosage should be adjusted.
- Patients should not crush or chew COREG CR capsules.
- Patients should take COREG CR with food.
- Diabetic patients should report any changes in blood sugar levels to their physician.
- Contact lens wearers may experience decreased lacrimation.

17.2 FDA-Approved Patient Labeling

Patient labeling is provided as a tear-off leaflet at the end of this full prescribing information.

COREG CR and COREG are registered trademarks of GlaxoSmithKline.

TOPROL-XL is a registered trademark of the AstraZeneca group of companies.

GlaxoSmithKline

Research Triangle Park, NC 27709

©2009, GlaxoSmithKline. All rights reserved.

PHARMACIST-DETACH HERE AND GIVE INSTRUCTIONS TO PATIENT

PATIENT INFORMATION LEAFLET

COREG CR® (Co-REG)

(carvedilol phosphate) Extended-release Capsules

Read the Patient Information that comes with COREG CR before you start taking it and each time you get a refill. There may be new information. This information does not take the place of talking with your doctor about your medical condition or your treatment. If you have any questions about COREG CR, ask your doctor or pharmacist.

What is the most important information I should know about COREG CR?

It is important for you to take your medicine every day as directed by your doctor. If you stop taking COREG CR suddenly, you could have chest pain and a heart attack. If your doctor decides that you should stop taking COREG CR, your doctor may slowly lower your dose over time before stopping it completely.

What is COREG CR?

COREG CR is a prescription medicine that belongs to a group of medicines called "beta-blockers". COREG CR is used, often with other medicines, for the following conditions:

- to treat patients with high blood pressure (hypertension)
- to treat patients who had a heart attack that worsened how well the heart pumps
- to treat patients with certain types of heart failure

COREG CR is not approved for use in children under 18 years of age.

Who should not take COREG CR?

Do not take COREG CR if you:

- have severe heart failure and require certain intravenous medicines that help support circulation.
- have asthma or other breathing problems.
- have a slow heartbeat or certain conditions that cause your heart to skip a beat (irregular heartbeat).
- have liver problems.
- are allergic to any of the ingredients in COREG CR. *See "What are the ingredients in COREG CR?"*

What should I tell my doctor before taking COREG CR?

Tell your doctor about all of your medical conditions, including if you:

- have asthma or other lung problems (such as bronchitis or emphysema).
- have problems with blood flow in your feet and legs (peripheral vascular disease). COREG CR can make some of your symptoms worse.
- have diabetes.
- have thyroid problems.
- have a condition called pheochromocytoma.
- have had severe allergic reactions.
- are scheduled for surgery and will be given anesthetic agents.
- are pregnant or trying to become pregnant. It is not known if COREG CR is safe for your unborn baby. You and your doctor should talk about the best way to control your high blood pressure during pregnancy.
- are breastfeeding. It is not known if COREG CR passes into your breast milk. You should not breastfeed while using COREG CR.

Tell your doctor about all of the medicines you take including prescription and non-prescription medicines, vitamins, and herbal supplements. COREG CR and certain other medicines can affect each other and cause serious side effects. COREG CR may affect the way other medicines work. Also, other medicines may affect how well COREG CR works.

Know the medicines you take. Keep a list of your medicines and show it to your doctor and pharmacist before you start a new medicine.

How should I take COREG CR?

- Take COREG CR exactly as prescribed. Take COREG CR **one** time each day with food. **It is important that you take COREG CR only one time each day.** To lessen possible side effects, your doctor might begin with a low dose and then slowly increase the dose.
- Swallow COREG CR capsules whole. Do not chew or crush COREG CR capsules.
- If you have trouble swallowing COREG CR whole:
  - The capsule may be carefully opened and the beads sprinkled over a spoonful of applesauce which should be eaten right away. The applesauce should not be warm.
  - Do not sprinkle beads on foods other than applesauce.
- **Do not stop taking COREG CR and do not change the amount of COREG CR you take without talking to your doctor.**
- If you miss a dose of COREG CR, take your dose as soon as you remember, unless it is time to take your next dose. Take your next dose at the usual time. Do not take 2 doses at the same time.
- If you take too much COREG CR, call your doctor or poison control center right away.

What should I avoid while taking COREG CR?

COREG CR can cause you to feel dizzy, tired, or faint. Do not drive a car, use machinery, or do anything that needs you to be alert if you have these symptoms.

What are possible side effects of COREG CR?

Serious side effects of COREG CR include:

- **chest pain and heart attack if you suddenly stop taking COREG CR.** *See "What is the most important information I should know about COREG CR?"*
- **slow heart beat.**
- **low blood pressure (which may cause dizziness or fainting when you stand up).** If these happen, sit or lie down, and tell your doctor right away.
- **worsening heart failure.** Tell your doctor right away if you have signs and symptoms that your heart failure may be worse, such as weight gain or increased shortness of breath.
- **changes in your blood sugar. If you have diabetes, tell your doctor if you have any changes in your blood sugar levels.**
- masking (hiding) the symptoms of low blood sugar, especially a fast heartbeat.
- **new or worsening symptoms of peripheral vascular disease.**
  - leg pain that happens when you walk, but goes away when you rest
  - no feeling (numbness) in your legs or feet while you are resting
  - cold legs or feet
- masking the symptoms of hyperthyroidism (overactive thyroid), such as a fast heartbeat.
- **worsening of severe allergic reactions.** Medicines to treat a severe allergic reaction may not work as well while you are taking COREG CR.
- **rare but serious allergic reactions** (including hives or swelling of the face, lips, tongue, and/or throat that may cause difficulty in breathing or swallowing) have happened in patients who were on COREG or COREG CR. These reactions can be life-threatening. In some cases, these reactions happened in patients who had been on COREG before taking COREG CR.

Common side effects of COREG CR include shortness of breath, weight gain, diarrhea, and tiredness. If you wear contact lenses, you may have fewer tears or dry eyes that can become bothersome.

Call your doctor if you have any side effects that bother you or don't go away.

How should I store COREG CR?

Store COREG CR at less than 86°F (30°C).

Safely throw away COREG CR that is out of date or no longer needed.

Keep COREG CR and all medicines out of the reach of children.

General information about COREG CR

Medicines are sometimes prescribed for conditions other than those described in patient information leaflets. Do not use COREG CR for a condition for which it was not prescribed. Do not give COREG CR to other people, even if they have the same symptoms you have. It may harm them.

This leaflet summarizes the most important information about COREG CR. If you would like more information, talk with your doctor. You can ask your doctor or pharmacist for information about COREG CR that is written for healthcare professionals. You can also find out more about COREG CR by visiting the website www.COREGCR.com or calling 1-888-825-5249. This call is free.

What are the ingredients in COREG CR?

Active ingredient: carvedilol phosphate

Inactive ingredients: crospovidone, hydrogenated castor oil, hydrogenated vegetable oil, magnesium stearate, methacrylic acid copolymers, microcrystalline cellulose, and povidone COREG CR capsules come in the following strengths: 10 mg, 20 mg, 40 mg, 80 mg.

COREG CR and COREG are registered trademarks of GlaxoSmithKline.

GlaxoSmithKline

Research Triangle Park, NC 27709

©2009, GlaxoSmithKline. All rights reserved.

June 2009 CCR:4PIL

DARAPRIM® ℞

[dair' ə-prĭm]

(pyrimethamine)

25-mg Scored Tablets

DESCRIPTION

DARAPRIM (pyrimethamine) is an antiparasitic compound available in tablet form for oral administration. Each scored tablet contains 25 mg pyrimethamine and the inactive ingredients corn and potato starch, lactose, and magnesium stearate.

Pyrimethamine, known chemically as 5-(4-chlorophenyl)-6-ethyl-2,4-pyrimidinediamine.

CLINICAL PHARMACOLOGY

Pyrimethamine is well absorbed with peak levels occurring between 2 to 6 hours following administration. It is eliminated slowly and has a plasma half-life of approximately 96 hours. Pyrimethamine is 87% bound to human plasma proteins.

Microbiology: Pyrimethamine is a folic acid antagonist and the rationale for its therapeutic action is based on the

differential requirement between host and parasite for nucleic acid precursors involved in growth. This activity is highly selective against plasmodia and *Toxoplasma gondii*.
Pyrimethamine possesses blood schizonticidal and some tissue schizonticidal activity against malaria parasites of humans. However, the 4-amino-quinoline compounds are more effective against the erythrocytic schizonts. It does not destroy gametocytes, but arrests sporogony in the mosquito.
The action of pyrimethamine against *Toxoplasma gondii* is greatly enhanced when used in conjunction with sulfonamides. This was demonstrated by Eyles and Coleman[1] in the treatment of experimental toxoplasmosis in the mouse. Jacobs et al[2] demonstrated that combination of the 2 drugs effectively prevented the development of severe uveitis in most rabbits following the inoculation of the anterior chamber of the eye with toxoplasma.

INDICATIONS AND USAGE

Treatment of Toxoplasmosis: DARAPRIM is indicated for the treatment of toxoplasmosis when used conjointly with a sulfonamide, since synergism exists with this combination.
Treatment of Acute Malaria: DARAPRIM is also indicated for the treatment of acute malaria. It should not be used alone to treat acute malaria. Fast-acting schizonticides such as chloroquine or quinine are indicated and preferable for the treatment of acute malaria. However, conjoint use of DARAPRIM with a sulfonamide (e.g., sulfadoxine) will initiate transmission control and suppression of susceptible strains of plasmodia.
Chemoprophylaxis of Malaria: DARAPRIM is indicated for the chemoprophylaxis of malaria due to susceptible strains of plasmodia. However, resistance to pyrimethamine is prevalent worldwide. It is not suitable as a prophylactic agent for travelers to most areas.

CONTRAINDICATIONS

Use of DARAPRIM is contraindicated in patients with known hypersensitivity to pyrimethamine or to any component of the formulation. Use of the drug is also contraindicated in patients with documented megaloblastic anemia due to folate deficiency.

WARNINGS

The dosage of pyrimethamine required for the treatment of toxoplasmosis is 10 to 20 times the recommended antimalaria dosage and approaches the toxic level. If signs of folate deficiency develop (see ADVERSE REACTIONS), reduce the dosage or discontinue the drug according to the response of the patient. Folinic acid (leucovorin) should be administered in a dosage of 5 to 15 mg daily (orally, IV, or IM) until normal hematopoiesis is restored.
Data in 2 humans indicate that pyrimethamine may be carcinogenic: a 51-year-old female who developed chronic granulocytic leukemia after taking pyrimethamine for 2 years for toxoplasmosis,[3] and a 56-year-old patient who developed reticulum cell sarcoma after 14 months of pyrimethamine for toxoplasmosis.[4]
Pyrimethamine has been reported to produce a significant increase in the number of lung tumors in mice when given intraperitoneally at doses of 25 mg/kg.[5]
DARAPRIM should be kept out of the reach of infants and children as they are extremely susceptible to adverse effects from an overdose. Deaths in pediatric patients have been reported after accidental ingestion.

PRECAUTIONS

General: The recommended dosage for chemoprophylaxis of malaria should not be exceeded. A small "starting" dose for toxoplasmosis is recommended in patients with convulsive disorders to avoid the potential nervous system toxicity of pyrimethamine. DARAPRIM should be used with caution in patients with impaired renal or hepatic function or in patients with possible folate deficiency, such as individuals with malabsorption syndrome, alcoholism, or pregnancy, and those receiving therapy, such as phenytoin, affecting folate levels (see Pregnancy subsection).
Information for Patients: Patients should be warned that at the first appearance of a skin rash they should stop use of DARAPRIM and seek medical attention immediately. Patients should also be warned that the appearance of sore throat, pallor, purpura, or glossitis may be early indications of serious disorders which require treatment with DARAPRIM to be stopped and medical treatment to be sought.
Women of childbearing potential who are taking DARAPRIM should be warned against becoming pregnant. Patients should be warned to keep DARAPRIM out of the reach of children. Patients should be advised not to exceed recommended doses. Patients should be warned that if anorexia and vomiting occur, they may be minimized by taking the drug with meals.
Concurrent administration of folinic acid is strongly recommended when used for the treatment of toxoplasmosis in all patients.
Laboratory Tests: In patients receiving high dosage, as for the treatment of toxoplasmosis, semiweekly blood counts, including platelet counts, should be performed.
Drug Interactions: Pyrimethamine may be used with sulfonamides, quinine and other antimalarials, and with other antibiotics. However, the concomitant use of other antifolic drugs or agents associated with myelosuppression including sulfonamides or trimethoprim-sulfamethoxazole combinations, proguanil, zidovudine, or cytostatic agents (e.g., methotrexate), while the patient is receiving pyrimethamine, may increase the risk of bone marrow suppression. If signs of folate deficiency develop, pyrimethamine should be discontinued. Folinic acid (leucovorin) should be administered until normal hematopoiesis is restored (see WARNINGS). Mild hepatotoxicity has been reported in some patients when lorazepam and pyrimethamine were administered concomitantly.
Carcinogenesis, Mutagenesis, Impairment of Fertility: See WARNINGS section for information on carcinogenesis.
Mutagenesis: Pyrimethamine has been shown to be nonmutagenic in the following in vitro assays: the Ames point mutation assay, the Rec assay, and the *E. coli* WP2 assay. It was positive in the L5178Y/TK +/- mouse lymphoma assay in the absence of exogenous metabolic activation.[6] Human blood lymphocytes cultured in vitro had structural chromosome aberrations induced by pyrimethamine.
In vivo, chromosomes analyzed from the bone marrow of rats dosed with pyrimethamine showed an increased number of structural and numerical aberrations.
Pregnancy: ***Teratogenic Effects:*** Pregnancy Category C. Pyrimethamine has been shown to be teratogenic in rats when given in oral doses 7 times the human dose for chemoprophylaxis of malaria or 2.5 times the human dose for treatment of toxoplasmosis. At these doses in rats, there was a significant increase in abnormalities such as cleft palate, brachygnathia, oligodactyly, and microphthalmia. Pyrimethamine has also been shown to produce terata such as meningocele in hamsters and cleft palate in miniature pigs when given in oral doses 170 and 5 times the human dose, respectively, for chemoprophylaxis of malaria or for treatment of toxoplasmosis.
There are no adequate and well-controlled studies in pregnant women. DARAPRIM should be used during pregnancy only if the potential benefit justifies the potential risk to the fetus.
Concurrent administration of folinic acid is strongly recommended when used for the treatment of toxoplasmosis during pregnancy.
Nursing Mothers: Pyrimethamine is excreted in human milk. Because of the potential for serious adverse reactions in nursing infants from pyrimethamine and from concurrent use of a sulfonamide with DARAPRIM for treatment of some patients with toxoplasmosis, a decision should be made whether to discontinue nursing or to discontinue the drug, taking into account the importance of the drug to the mother (see WARNINGS and PRECAUTIONS: Pregnancy).
Pediatric Use: See DOSAGE AND ADMINISTRATION section.
Geriatric Use: Clinical studies of DARAPRIM did not include sufficient numbers of subjects aged 65 and over to determine whether they respond differently from younger subjects. Other reported clinical experience has not identified differences in responses between the elderly and younger patients. In general, dose selection for an elderly patient should be cautious, usually starting at the low end of the dosing range, reflecting the greater frequency of decreased hepatic, renal, or cardiac function, and of concomitant disease or other drug therapy.

ADVERSE REACTIONS

Hypersensitivity reactions, occasionally severe (such as Stevens-Johnson syndrome, toxic epidermal necrolysis, erythema multiforme, and anaphylaxis), and hyperphenylalaninemia, can occur particularly when pyrimethamine is administered concomitantly with a sulfonamide. Consult the complete prescribing information for the relevant sulfonamide for sulfonamide-associated adverse events. With doses of pyrimethamine used for the treatment of toxoplasmosis, anorexia and vomiting may occur. Vomiting may be minimized by giving the medication with meals; it usually disappears promptly upon reduction of dosage. Doses used in toxoplasmosis may produce megaloblastic anemia, leukopenia, thrombocytopenia, pancytopenia, atrophic glossitis, hematuria, and disorders of cardiac rhythm. Hematologic effects, however, may also occur at low doses in certain individuals (see PRECAUTIONS: General).
Pulmonary eosinophilia has been reported rarely.

OVERDOSAGE

Following the ingestion of 300 mg or more of pyrimethamine, gastrointestinal and/or central nervous system signs may be present, including convulsions. The initial symptoms are usually gastrointestinal and may include abdominal pain, nausea, severe and repeated vomiting, possibly including hematemesis. Central nervous system toxicity may be manifest by initial excitability, generalized and prolonged convulsions which may be followed by respiratory depression, circulatory collapse, and death within a few hours. Neurological symptoms appear rapidly (30 minutes to 2 hours after drug ingestion), suggesting that in gross overdosage pyrimethamine has a direct toxic effect on the central nervous system.
The fatal dose is variable, with the smallest reported fatal single dose being 375 mg. There are, however, reports of pediatric patients who have recovered after taking 375 to 625 mg.
There is no specific antidote to acute pyrimethamine poisoning. In the event of overdosage, symptomatic and supportive measures should be employed. Gastric lavage is recommended and is effective if carried out very soon after drug ingestion. Parenteral diazepam may be used to control convulsions. Folinic acid should also be administered within 2 hours of drug ingestion to be most effective in counteracting the effects on the hematopoietic system (see WARNINGS). Due to the long half-life of pyrimethamine, daily monitoring of peripheral blood counts is recommended for up to several weeks after the overdose until normal hematologic values are restored.

DOSAGE AND ADMINISTRATION

For Treatment of Toxoplasmosis: The dosage of DARAPRIM for the treatment of toxoplasmosis must be carefully adjusted so as to provide maximum therapeutic effect and a minimum of side effects. At the dosage required, there is a marked variation in the tolerance to the drug. Young patients may tolerate higher doses than older individuals. Concurrent administration of folinic acid is strongly recommended in all patients.
The adult *starting* dose is 50 to 75 mg of the drug daily, together with 1 to 4 g daily of a sulfonamide of the sulfapyrimidine type, e.g., sulfadoxine. This dosage is ordinarily continued for 1 to 3 weeks, depending on the response of the patient and tolerance to therapy. The dosage may then be reduced to about one-half that previously given for each drug and continued for an additional 4 to 5 weeks.
The pediatric dosage of DARAPRIM is 1 mg/kg/day divided into 2 equal daily doses; after 2 to 4 days this dose may be reduced to one half and continued for approximately 1 month. The usual pediatric sulfonamide dosage is used in conjunction with DARAPRIM.
For Treatment of Acute Malaria: DARAPRIM is NOT recommended alone in the treatment of acute malaria. Fast-acting schizonticides, such as chloroquine or quinine, are indicated for treatment of acute malaria. However, DARAPRIM at a dosage of 25 mg daily for 2 days with a sulfonamide will initiate transmission control and suppression of non-falciparum malaria. DARAPRIM is only recommended for patients infected in areas where susceptible plasmodia exist. Should circumstances arise wherein DARAPRIM must be used alone in semi-immune persons, the adult dosage for acute malaria is 50 mg for 2 days; children 4 through 10 years old may be given 25 mg daily for 2 days. In any event, clinical cure should be followed by the once-weekly regimen described below for chemoprophylaxis. Regimens which include suppression should be extended through any characteristic periods of early recrudescence and late relapse, i.e., for at least 10 weeks in each case.
For Chemoprophylaxis of Malaria:
Adults and pediatric patients over 10 years — 25 mg (1 tablet) once weekly
Children 4 through 10 years — 12.5 mg (½ tablet) once weekly
Infants and children under 4 years — 6.25 mg (¼ tablet) once weekly

HOW SUPPLIED

White, scored tablets containing 25 mg pyrimethamine, imprinted with "DARAPRIM" and "A3A" in bottles of 100 (NDC 0173-0201-55).
Store at 15° to 25°C (59° to 77°F) in a dry place and protect from light.

REFERENCES

1. Eyles DE, Coleman N. Synergistic effect of sulfadiazine and Daraprim against experimental toxoplasmosis in the mouse. *Antibiot Chemother.* 1953;3:483-490.
2. Jacobs L, Melton ML, Kaufman HE. Treatment of experimental ocular toxoplasmosis. *Arch Ophthalmol.* 1964;71:111-118.
3. Jim RTS, Elizaga FV. Development of chronic granulocytic leukemia in a patient treated with pyrimethamine. *Hawaii Med J.* 1977;36:173-176.
4. Sadoff L. Antimalarial drugs and Burkitt's lymphoma. *Lancet.* 1973;2:1262-1263.
5. Bahna L. Pyrimethamine. *LARC Monogr Eval Carcinog Risk Chem.* 1977;13:233-242.
6. Clive D, Johnson KO, Spector JKS, et al. Validation and characterization of the L5178Y/TK +/- mouse lymphoma mutagen assay system. *Mut Res.* 1979;59:61-108.

Manufactured by DSM Pharmaceuticals, Inc.
Greenville, NC 27834 for
GlaxoSmithKline, Research Triangle Park, NC 27709
©2003, GlaxoSmithKline. All rights reserved.
March 2003/RL-1179

DEXEDRINE® Ⓒ℞
[*dex' ə-drēn*]
(dextroamphetamine sulfate)
SPANSULE® sustained-release capsules

WARNING

AMPHETAMINES HAVE A HIGH POTENTIAL FOR ABUSE. ADMINISTRATION OF AMPHETAMINES FOR PROLONGED PERIODS OF TIME MAY LEAD TO DRUG DEPENDENCE AND MUST BE AVOIDED. PARTICULAR ATTENTION SHOULD BE PAID TO THE POSSIBILITY OF SUBJECTS OBTAINING AMPHETAMINES FOR NON-THERAPEUTIC USE OR DISTRIBUTION TO OTHERS, AND THE DRUGS SHOULD BE PRESCRIBED OR DISPENSED SPARINGLY.
MISUSE OF AMPHETAMINES MAY CAUSE SUDDEN DEATH AND SERIOUS CARDIOVASCULAR ADVERSE EVENTS.

DESCRIPTION

DEXEDRINE (dextroamphetamine sulfate) is the dextro isomer of the compound *d,l*-amphetamine sulfate, a sympathomimetic amine of the amphetamine group. Chemically, dextroamphetamine is *d*-alpha-methylphenethylamine, and is present in all forms of DEXEDRINE as the neutral sulfate.
Structural formula:

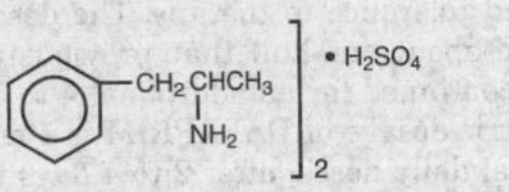

SPANSULE capsules: Each SPANSULE sustained-release capsule is so prepared that an initial dose is released promptly and the remaining medication is released gradually over a prolonged period.
Each capsule, with brown cap and clear body, contains dextroamphetamine sulfate. The 5-mg capsule is imprinted 5 mg and 3512 on the brown cap and is imprinted 5 mg and SB on the clear body. The 10-mg capsule is imprinted 10 mg—3513—on the brown cap and is imprinted 10 mg—SB—on the clear body. The 15-mg capsule is imprinted 15 mg and 3514 on the brown cap and is imprinted 15 mg and SB on the clear body. A narrow bar appears above and below 15 mg and 3514. Product reformulation in 1996 has caused a minor change in the color of the time-released pellets within each capsule. Inactive ingredients now consist of cetyl alcohol, D&C Yellow No. 10, dibutyl sebacate, ethylcellulose, FD&C Blue No. 1, FD&C Blue No. 1 aluminum lake, FD&C Red No. 40, FD&C Yellow No. 6, gelatin, hypromellose, propylene glycol, povidone, silicon dioxide, sodium lauryl sulfate, sugar spheres, and trace amounts of other inactive ingredients.

CLINICAL PHARMACOLOGY

Amphetamines are noncatecholamine, sympathomimetic amines with CNS stimulant activity. Peripheral actions include elevations of systolic and diastolic blood pressures and weak bronchodilator and respiratory stimulant action.
There is neither specific evidence that clearly establishes the mechanism whereby amphetamines produce mental and behavioral effects in children, nor conclusive evidence regarding how these effects relate to the condition of the central nervous system.
DEXEDRINE SPANSULE capsules are formulated to release the active drug substance in vivo in a more gradual fashion than the standard formulation, as demonstrated by blood levels. The formulation has not been shown superior in effectiveness over the same dosage of the standard, noncontrolled-release formulations given in divided doses.
Pharmacokinetics: The pharmacokinetics of the tablet and sustained-release capsule were compared in 12 healthy subjects. The extent of bioavailability of the sustained-release capsule was similar compared to the immediate-release tablet. Following administration of three 5-mg tablets, average maximal dextroamphetamine plasma concentrations (C_{max}) of 36.6 ng/mL were achieved at approximately 3 hours. Following administration of one 15-mg sustained-release capsule, maximal dextroamphetamine plasma concentrations were obtained approximately 8 hours after dosing. The average C_{max} was 23.5 ng/mL. The average plasma $T_{1/2}$ was similar for both the tablet and sustained-release capsule and was approximately 12 hours.
In 12 healthy subjects, the rate and extent of dextroamphetamine absorption were similar following administration of the sustained-release capsule formulation in the fed (58 to 75 gm fat) and fasted state.

INDICATIONS AND USAGE

DEXEDRINE is indicated in:
Narcolepsy
Attention Deficit Disorder with Hyperactivity: As an integral part of a total treatment program that typically includes other measures (psychological, educational, social) for patients (ages 6 years to 16 years) with this syndrome. A diagnosis of Attention Deficit Hyperactivity Disorder (ADHD; DSM-IV) implies the presence of hyperactive-impulsive or inattentive symptoms that caused impairment and were present before age 7 years. The symptoms must cause clinically significant impairment, e.g., in social, academic, or occupational functioning, and be present in 2 or more settings, e.g., school (or work) and at home. The symptoms must not be better accounted for by another mental disorder. For the Inattentive Type, at least 6 of the following symptoms must have persisted for at least 6 months: lack of attention to details/careless mistakes; lack of sustained attention; poor listener; failure to follow through on tasks; poor organization; avoid tasks requiring sustained mental effort; loses things; easily distracted; forgetful. For the Hyperactive-Impulsive Type, at least 6 of the following symptoms must have persisted for at least 6 months: fidgeting/squirming; leaving seat; inappropriate running/climbing; difficulty with quiet activities; "on the go"; excessive talking; blurting answers; can't wait turn; intrusive. The Combined Type requires both inattentive and hyperactive-impulsive criteria to be met.
Special Diagnostic Considerations: Specific etiology of this syndrome is unknown, and there is no single diagnostic test. Adequate diagnosis requires the use of medical and special psychological, educational, and social resources. Learning may or may not be impaired. The diagnosis must be based upon a complete history and evaluation of the patient and not solely on the presences of the required number of DSM-IV characteristics.
Need for Comprehensive Treatment Program: DEXEDRINE is indicated as an integral part of a total treatment program for ADHD that may include other measures (psychological, educational, social) for patients with this syndrome. Drug treatment may not be indicated for all patients with this syndrome. Stimulants are not intended for use in patients who exhibit symptoms secondary to environmental factors and/or other primary psychiatric disorders, including psychosis. Appropriate educational placement is essential and psychosocial intervention is often helpful. When remedial measures alone are insufficient, the decision to prescribe stimulant medication will depend upon the physician's assessment of the chronicity and severity of the patient's symptoms.

CONTRAINDICATIONS

Advanced arteriosclerosis, symptomatic cardiovascular disease, moderate to severe hypertension, hyperthyroidism, known hypersensitivity or idiosyncrasy to the sympathomimetic amines, glaucoma.
Agitated states.
Patients with a history of drug abuse.
During or within 14 days following the administration of monoamine oxidase inhibitors (hypertensive crises may result).

WARNINGS

Serious Cardiovascular Events
Sudden Death in Patients With Pre-existing Structural Cardiac Abnormalities or Other Serious Heart Problems: ***Children and Adolescents:*** Sudden death has been reported in association with CNS stimulant treatment at usual doses in children and adolescents with structural cardiac abnormalities or other serious heart problems. Although some serious heart problems alone carry an increased risk of sudden death, stimulant products generally should not be used in children or adolescents with known serious structural cardiac abnormalities, cardiomyopathy, serious heart rhythm abnormalities, or other serious cardiac problems that may place them at increased vulnerability to the sympathomimetic effects of a stimulant drug.
Adults: Sudden deaths, stroke, and myocardial infarction have been reported in adults taking stimulant drugs at usual doses for ADHD. Although the role of stimulants in these adult cases is also unknown, adults have a greater likelihood than children of having serious structural cardiac abnormalities, cardiomyopathy, serious heart rhythm abnormalities, coronary artery disease, or other serious cardiac problems. Adults with such abnormalities should also generally not be treated with stimulant drugs (see CONTRAINDICATIONS).
Hypertension and Other Cardiovascular Conditions: Stimulant medications cause a modest increase in average blood pressure (about 2–4 mmHg) and average heart rate (about 3–6 bpm), and individuals may have larger increases. While the mean changes alone would not be expected to have short-term consequences, all patients should be monitored for larger changes in heart rate and blood pressure. Caution is indicated in treating patients whose underlying medical conditions might be compromised by increases in blood pressure or heart rate, e.g., those with pre-existing hypertension, heart failure, recent myocardial infarction, or ventricular arrhythmia (see CONTRAINDICATIONS).
Assessing Cardiovascular Status in Patients Being Treated With Stimulant Medications: Children, adolescents, or adults who are being considered for treatment with stimulant medications should have a careful history (including assessment for a family history of sudden death or ventricular arrhythmia) and physical exam to assess for the presence of cardiac disease, and should receive further cardiac evaluation if findings suggest such disease (e.g., electrocardiogram and echocardiogram). Patients who develop symptoms such as exertional chest pain, unexplained syncope, or other symptoms suggestive of cardiac disease during stimulant treatment should undergo a prompt cardiac evaluation.
Psychiatric Adverse Events
Pre-Existing Psychosis: Administration of stimulants may exacerbate symptoms of behavior disturbance and thought disorder in patients with a pre-existing psychotic disorder.
Bipolar Illness: Particular care should be taken in using stimulants to treat ADHD in patients with comorbid bipolar disorder because of concern for possible induction of a mixed/manic episode in such patients. Prior to initiating treatment with a stimulant, patients with comorbid depressive symptoms should be adequately screened to determine if they are at risk for bipolar disorder; such screening should include a detailed psychiatric history, including a family history of suicide, bipolar disorder, and depression.
Emergence of New Psychotic or Manic Symptoms: Treatment emergent psychotic or manic symptoms, e.g., hallucinations, delusional thinking, or mania in children and adolescents without a prior history of psychotic illness or mania can be caused by stimulants at usual doses. If such symptoms occur, consideration should be given to a possible causal role of the stimulant, and discontinuation of treatment may be appropriate. In a pooled analysis of multiple short-term, placebo-controlled studies, such symptoms occurred in about 0.1% (4 patients with events out of 3,482 exposed to methylphenidate or amphetamine for several weeks at usual doses) of stimulant-treated patients compared to 0 in placebo-treated patients.
Aggression: Aggressive behavior or hostility is often observed in children and adolescents with ADHD, and has been reported in clinical trials and the postmarketing experience of some medications indicated for the treatment of ADHD. Although there is no systematic evidence that stimulants cause aggressive behavior or hostility, patients beginning treatment for ADHD should be monitored for the appearance of, or worsening of, aggressive behavior or hostility.
Long-Term Suppression of Growth: Careful follow-up of weight and height in children ages 7 to 10 years who were randomized to either methylphenidate or non-medication treatment groups over 14 months, as well as in naturalistic subgroups of newly methylphenidate-treated and non-medication treated children older than 36 months (to the ages of 10 to 13 years), suggests that consistently medicated children (i.e., treatment for 7 days per week throughout the year) have a temporary slowing in growth rate (on average, a total of about 2 cm less growth in height and 2.7 kg less growth in weight over 3 years), without evidence of growth rebound during this period of development. Published data are inadequate to determine whether chronic use of amphetamines may cause a similar suppression of growth, however, it is anticipated that they likely have this effect as well. Therefore, growth should be monitored during treatment with stimulants, and patients who are not growing or gaining height or weight as expected may need to have their treatment interrupted.
Seizures: There is some clinical evidence that stimulants may lower the convulsive threshold in patients with prior history of seizures, in patients with prior EEG abnormalities in absence of seizures, and, very rarely, in patients without a history of seizures and no prior EEG evidence of seizures. In the presence of seizures, the drug should be discontinued.
Visual Disturbance: Difficulties with accommodation and blurring of vision have been reported with stimulant treatment.

PRECAUTIONS

General: The least amount feasible should be prescribed or dispensed at 1 time in order to minimize the possibility of overdosage.
Information for Patients: Amphetamines may impair the ability of the patient to engage in potentially hazardous ac-

tivities such as operating machinery or vehicles; the patient should therefore be cautioned accordingly.

Prescribers or other health professionals should inform patients, their families, and their caregivers about the benefits and risks associated with treatment with dextroamphetamine and should counsel them in its appropriate use. A patient Medication Guide is available for DEXEDRINE. The prescriber or health professional should instruct patients, their families, and their caregivers to read the Medication Guide and should assist them in understanding its contents. Patients should be given the opportunity to discuss the contents of the Medication Guide and to obtain answers to any questions they may have. The complete text of the Medication Guide is reprinted at the end of this document.

Drug Interactions: ***Acidifying Agents:*** Gastrointestinal acidifying agents (guanethidine, reserpine, glutamic acid HCl, ascorbic acid, fruit juices, etc.) lower absorption of amphetamines. Urinary acidifying agents (ammonium chloride, sodium acid phosphate, etc.) increase the concentration of the ionized species of the amphetamine molecule, thereby increasing urinary excretion. Both groups of agents lower blood levels and efficacy of amphetamines.

Adrenergic Blockers: Adrenergic blockers are inhibited by amphetamines.

Alkalinizing Agents: Gastrointestinal alkalinizing agents (sodium bicarbonate, etc.) increase absorption of amphetamines. Urinary alkalinizing agents (acetazolamide, some thiazides) increase the concentration of the non-ionized species of the amphetamine molecule, thereby decreasing urinary excretion. Both groups of agents increase blood levels and therefore potentiate the actions of amphetamines.

Antidepressants, Tricyclic: Amphetamines may enhance the activity of tricyclic or sympathomimetic agents; d-amphetamine with desipramine or protriptyline and possibly other tricyclics cause striking and sustained increases in the concentration of d-amphetamine in the brain; cardiovascular effects can be potentiated.

MAO Inhibitors: MAOI antidepressants, as well as a metabolite of furazolidone, slow amphetamine metabolism. This slowing potentiates amphetamines, increasing their effect on the release of norepinephrine and other monoamines from adrenergic nerve endings; this can cause headaches and other signs of hypertensive crisis. A variety of neurological toxic effects and malignant hyperpyrexia can occur, sometimes with fatal results.

Antihistamines: Amphetamines may counteract the sedative effect of antihistamines.

Antihypertensives: Amphetamines may antagonize the hypotensive effects of antihypertensives.

Chlorpromazine: Chlorpromazine blocks dopamine and norepinephrine reuptake, thus inhibiting the central stimulant effects of amphetamines, and can be used to treat amphetamine poisoning.

Ethosuximide: Amphetamines may delay intestinal absorption of ethosuximide.

Haloperidol: Haloperidol blocks dopamine and norepinephrine reuptake, thus inhibiting the central stimulant effects of amphetamines.

Lithium Carbonate: The stimulatory effects of amphetamines may be inhibited by lithium carbonate.

Meperidine: Amphetamines potentiate the analgesic effect of meperidine.

Methenamine Therapy: Urinary excretion of amphetamines is increased, and efficacy is reduced, by acidifying agents used in methenamine therapy.

Norepinephrine: Amphetamines enhance the adrenergic effect of norepinephrine.

Phenobarbital: Amphetamines may delay intestinal absorption of phenobarbital; co-administration of phenobarbital may produce a synergistic anticonvulsant action.

Phenytoin: Amphetamines may delay intestinal absorption of phenytoin; co-administration of phenytoin may produce a synergistic anticonvulsant action.

Propoxyphene: In cases of propoxyphene overdosage, amphetamine CNS stimulation is potentiated and fatal convulsions can occur.

Veratrum Alkaloids: Amphetamines inhibit the hypotensive effect of veratrum alkaloids.

Drug/Laboratory Test Interactions: Amphetamines can cause a significant elevation in plasma corticosteroid levels. This increase is greatest in the evening.

Amphetamines may interfere with urinary steroid determinations.

Carcinogenesis/Mutagenesis: Mutagenicity studies and long-term studies in animals to determine the carcinogenic potential of DEXEDRINE have not been performed.

Pregnancy: ***Teratogenic Effects:*** Pregnancy Category C. DEXEDRINE has been shown to have embryotoxic and teratogenic effects when administered to A/Jax mice and C57BL mice in doses approximately 41 times the maximum human dose. Embryotoxic effects were not seen in New Zealand white rabbits given the drug in doses 7 times the human dose nor in rats given 12.5 times the maximum human dose. While there are no adequate and well-controlled studies in pregnant women, there has been 1 report of severe congenital bony deformity, tracheoesophageal fistula, and anal atresia (VATER association) in a baby born to a woman who took dextroamphetamine sulfate with lovastatin during the first trimester of pregnancy. DEXEDRINE should be used during pregnancy only if the potential benefit justifies the potential risk to the fetus.

Nonteratogenic Effects: Infants born to mothers dependent on amphetamines have an increased risk of premature delivery and low birth weight. Also, these infants may experience symptoms of withdrawal as demonstrated by dysphoria, including agitation, and significant lassitude.

Nursing Mothers: Amphetamines are excreted in human milk. Mothers taking amphetamines should be advised to refrain from nursing.

Pediatric Use: Long-term effects of amphetamines in pediatric patients have not been well established.

DEXEDRINE is not recommended for use in pediatric patients younger than 6 years of age with Attention Deficit Disorder with Hyperactivity described under INDICATIONS AND USAGE.

Clinical experience suggests that in psychotic children, administration of amphetamines may exacerbate symptoms of behavior disturbance and thought disorder.

Amphetamines have been reported to exacerbate motor and phonic tics and Tourette's syndrome. Therefore, clinical evaluation for tics and Tourette's syndrome in children and their families should precede use of stimulant medications.

Data are inadequate to determine whether chronic administration of amphetamines may be associated with growth inhibition; therefore, growth should be monitored during treatment.

Drug treatment is not indicated in all cases of Attention Deficit Disorder with Hyperactivity and should be considered only in light of the complete history and evaluation of the child. The decision to prescribe amphetamines should depend on the physician's assessment of the chronicity and severity of the child's symptoms and their appropriateness for his or her age. Prescription should not depend solely on the presence of one or more of the behavioral characteristics.

When these symptoms are associated with acute stress reactions, treatment with amphetamines is usually not indicated.

ADVERSE REACTIONS

Cardiovascular: Palpitations, tachycardia, elevation of blood pressure. There have been isolated reports of cardiomyopathy associated with chronic amphetamine use.

Central Nervous System: Psychotic episodes at recommended doses (rare), overstimulation, restlessness, dizziness, insomnia, euphoria, dyskinesia, dysphoria, tremor, headache, exacerbation of motor and phonic tics, and Tourette's syndrome.

Gastrointestinal: Dryness of the mouth, unpleasant taste, diarrhea, constipation, other gastrointestinal disturbances. Anorexia and weight loss may occur as undesirable effects.

Allergic: Urticaria.

Endocrine: Impotence, changes in libido.

DRUG ABUSE AND DEPENDENCE

Dextroamphetamine sulfate is a Schedule II controlled substance.

Amphetamines have been extensively abused. Tolerance, extreme psychological dependence and severe social disability have occurred. There are reports of patients who have increased the dosage to many times that recommended. Abrupt cessation following prolonged high dosage administration results in extreme fatigue and mental depression; changes are also noted on the sleep EEG.

Manifestations of chronic intoxication with amphetamines include severe dermatoses, marked insomnia, irritability, hyperactivity, and personality changes. The most severe manifestation of chronic intoxication is psychosis, often clinically indistinguishable from schizophrenia. This is rare with oral amphetamines.

OVERDOSAGE

Individual patient response to amphetamines varies widely. While toxic symptoms occasionally occur as an idiosyncrasy at doses as low as 2 mg, they are rare with doses of less than 15 mg; 30 mg can produce severe reactions, yet doses of 400 to 500 mg are not necessarily fatal.

In rats, the oral LD_{50} of dextroamphetamine sulfate is 96.8 mg/kg.

Manifestations of acute overdosage with amphetamines include restlessness, tremor, hyperreflexia, rhabdomyolysis, rapid respiration, hyperpyrexia, confusion, assaultiveness, hallucinations, panic states.

Fatigue and depression usually follow the central stimulation.

Cardiovascular effects include arrhythmias, hypertension or hypotension, and circulatory collapse. Gastrointestinal symptoms include nausea, vomiting, diarrhea, and abdominal cramps. Fatal poisoning is usually preceded by convulsions and coma.

TREATMENT

Consult with a Certified Poison Control Center for up-to-date guidance and advice. Management of acute amphetamine intoxication is largely symptomatic and includes gastric lavage, administration of activated charcoal, administration of a cathartic, and sedation. Experience with hemodialysis or peritoneal dialysis is inadequate to permit recommendation in this regard. Acidification of the urine increases amphetamine excretion, but is believed to increase risk of acute renal failure if myoglobinuria is present. If acute, severe hypertension complicates amphetamine overdosage, administration of intravenous phentolamine (Bedford Laboratories) has been suggested. However, a gradual drop in blood pressure will usually result when sufficient sedation has been achieved.

Chlorpromazine antagonizes the central stimulant effects of amphetamines and can be used to treat amphetamine intoxication.

Since much of the SPANSULE capsule medication is coated for gradual release, therapy directed at reversing the effects of the ingested drug and at supporting the patient should be continued for as long as overdosage symptoms remain. Saline cathartics are useful for hastening the evacuation of pellets that have not already released medication.

DOSAGE AND ADMINISTRATION

Amphetamines should be administered at the lowest effective dosage and dosage should be individually adjusted. Late evening doses should be avoided because of the resulting insomnia.

Narcolepsy: Usual dose is 5 to 60 mg per day in divided doses, depending on the individual patient response.

Narcolepsy seldom occurs in children under 12 years of age; however, when it does, DEXEDRINE may be used. The suggested initial dose for patients aged 6 to 12 is 5 mg daily; daily dose may be raised in increments of 5 mg at weekly intervals until an optimal response is obtained. In patients 12 years of age and older, start with 10 mg daily; daily dosage may be raised in increments of 10 mg at weekly intervals until an optimal response is obtained. If bothersome adverse reactions appear (e.g., insomnia or anorexia), dosage should be reduced. SPANSULE capsules may be used for once-a-day dosage wherever appropriate.

Attention Deficit Disorder with Hyperactivity: The SPANSULE capsule formulation is not recommended for pediatric patients younger than 6 years of age.

In pediatric patients 6 years of age and older, start with 5 mg once or twice daily; daily dosage may be raised in increments of 5 mg at weekly intervals until optimal response is obtained. Only in rare cases will it be necessary to exceed a total of 40 mg per day.

SPANSULE capsules may be used for once-a-day dosage wherever appropriate.

Where possible, drug administration should be interrupted occasionally to determine if there is a recurrence of behavioral symptoms sufficient to require continued therapy.

HOW SUPPLIED

DEXEDRINE SPANSULE capsules: Each capsule, with brown cap and clear body, contains dextroamphetamine sulfate. The 5-mg capsule is imprinted 5 mg and 3512 on the brown cap and is imprinted 5 mg and SB on the clear body. The 10-mg capsule is imprinted 10 mg—3513—on the brown cap and is imprinted 10 mg—SB—on the clear body. The 15-mg capsule is imprinted 15 mg and 3514 on the brown cap and is imprinted 15 mg and SB on the clear body. A narrow bar appears above and below 15 mg and 3514.

5 mg 90s: NDC 0007-3512-59
10 mg 90s: NDC 0007-3513-59
15 mg 90s NDC 0007-3514-59

Store at controlled room temperature between 20° and 25°C (68° and 77°F) [see USP].

Dispense in a tight, light-resistant container.

Medication Guide

DEXEDRINE®

(dextroamphetamine sulfate) SPANSULE® sustained-release capsules CII

Read the Medication Guide that comes with DEXEDRINE before you or your child starts taking it and each time you get a refill. There may be new information. This Medication Guide does not take the place of talking to your doctor about your or your child's treatment with DEXEDRINE.

What is the most important information I should know about DEXEDRINE?

The following have been reported with use of DEXEDRINE and other stimulant medicines.

1. Heart-related problems:

- **Sudden death in patients who have heart problems or heart defects**
- **Stroke and heart attack in adults**
- **Increased blood pressure and heart rate**

Tell your doctor if you or your child have any heart problems, heart defects, high blood pressure, or a family history of these problems.
Your doctor should check you or your child carefully for heart problems before starting DEXEDRINE.
Your doctor should check your or your child's blood pressure and heart rate regularly during treatment with DEXEDRINE.
Call your doctor right away if you or your child has any signs of heart problems such as chest pain, shortness of breath, or fainting while taking DEXEDRINE.

2. Mental (Psychiatric) problems:

All Patients
- **new or worse behavior and thought problems**
- **new or worse bipolar illness**
- **new or worse aggressive behavior or hostility**

Children and Teenagers
- **new psychotic symptoms (such as hearing voices, believing things that are not true, are suspicious) or new manic symptoms**

Tell your doctor about any mental problems you or your child have, or about a family history of suicide, bipolar illness, or depression.
Call your doctor right away if you or your child have any new or worsening mental symptoms or problems while taking DEXEDRINE, especially seeing or hearing things that are not real, believing things that are not real, or are suspicious.

What Is DEXEDRINE?
DEXEDRINE is a central nervous system stimulant prescription medicine. **It is used for the treatment of Attention-Deficit Hyperactivity Disorder (ADHD).**
DEXEDRINE may help increase attention and decrease impulsiveness and hyperactivity in patients with ADHD.
DEXEDRINE should be used as a part of a total treatment program for ADHD that may include counseling or other therapies.
DEXEDRINE is also used in the treatment of a sleep disorder called narcolepsy.

DEXEDRINE is a federally controlled substance (CII) because it can be abused or lead to dependence. Keep DEXEDRINE in a safe place to prevent misuse and abuse. Selling or giving away DEXEDRINE may harm others, and is against the law.
Tell your doctor if you or your child have (or have a family history of) ever abused or been dependent on alcohol, prescription medicines or street drugs.

Who should not take DEXEDRINE?
DEXEDRINE should not be taken if you or your child:
- Have heart disease or hardening of the arteries
- Have moderate to severe high blood pressure
- Have hyperthyroidism
- Have an eye problem called glaucoma
- Are very anxious, tense, or agitated
- Have a history of drug abuse
- Are taking or have taken within the past 14 days an antidepression medicine called a monoamine oxidase inhibitor or MAOI
- Is sensitive to, allergic to, or had a reaction to other stimulant medicines

DEXEDRINE is not recommended for use in children younger than 6 years old.
DEXEDRINE may not be right for you or your child. Before starting DEXEDRINE tell your or your child's doctor about all health conditions (or a family history of) including:
- Heart problems, heart defects, high blood pressure
- Mental problems including psychosis, mania, bipolar illness, or depression
- Tics or Tourette's syndrome
- Thyroid problems
- Seizures or have had an abnormal brain wave test (EEG)

Tell your doctor if you or your child is pregnant, planning to become pregnant, or breastfeeding.
Can DEXEDRINE be taken with other medicines?
Tell your doctor about all of the medicines that you or your child take including prescription and nonprescription medicines, vitamins, and herbal supplements. DEXEDRINE and some medicines may interact with each other and cause serious side effects. Sometimes the doses of other medicines will need to be adjusted while taking DEXEDRINE.
Your doctor will decide whether DEXEDRINE can be taken with other medicines.
Especially tell your doctor if you or your child takes:
- Anti-depression medicines including MAOIs
- Blood pressure medicines
- Antacids
- Seizure medicines

Know the medicines that you or your child takes. Keep a list of your medicines with you to show your doctor and pharmacist.
Do not start any new medicine while taking DEXEDRINE without talking to your doctor first.
How should DEXEDRINE be taken?
- **Take DEXEDRINE exactly as prescribed.** Your doctor may adjust the dose until it is right for you or your child.
- **DEXEDRINE comes as a capsule.**
  - DEXEDRINE SPANSULE capsules are usually taken once a day in the morning. DEXEDRINE SPANSULE is an extended release capsule. It releases medicine into your body throughout the day.
- From time to time, your doctor may stop treatment with DEXEDRINE for a while to check ADHD symptoms.
- Your doctor may do regular checks of the blood, heart, and blood pressure while taking DEXEDRINE. Children should have their height and weight checked often while taking DEXEDRINE. Treatment with DEXEDRINE may be stopped if a problem is found during these check-ups.
- **If you or your child takes too much DEXEDRINE or overdoses, call your doctor or poison control center right away, or get emergency treatment.**

What are possible side effects of DEXEDRINE?
See **"What is the most important information I should know about DEXEDRINE?"** for information on reported heart and mental problems.
Other serious side effects include:
- Slowing of growth (height and weight) in children
- Seizures, mainly in patients with a history of seizures
- Eyesight changes or blurred vision

Common side effects include:
- Fast heartbeat
- Tremors
- Trouble sleeping
- Stomach upset
- Dry mouth
- Decreased appetite
- Headache
- Dizziness
- Weight loss

DEXEDRINE may affect your or your child's ability to drive or do other dangerous activities.
Talk to your doctor if you or your child has side effects that are bothersome or do not go away.
This is not a complete list of possible side effects. Ask your doctor or pharmacist for more information. You may report side effects to FDA at 1-800-FDA-1088.
How should I store DEXEDRINE?
- Store DEXEDRINE SPANSULE capsules in a safe place at room temperature, 68° to 77°F (20° to 25°C). Protect from light.
- **Keep DEXEDRINE and all medicines out of the reach of children.**

General information about DEXEDRINE
Medicines are sometimes prescribed for purposes other than those listed in a Medication Guide. Do not use DEXEDRINE for a condition for which it was not prescribed. Do not give DEXEDRINE to other people, even if they have the same condition. It may harm them and it is against the law.
This Medication Guide summarizes the most important information about DEXEDRINE. If you would like more information, talk with your doctor. You can ask your doctor or pharmacist for information about DEXEDRINE that was written for healthcare professionals. For more information about DEXEDRINE, please contact GlaxoSmithKline (makers of DEXEDRINE) at 1-888-825-5249 or visit www.gsk.com.
What are the ingredients in DEXEDRINE?
Active Ingredient: Dextroamphetamine sulfate
Inactive Ingredients:
SPANSULE Capsules: Cetyl alcohol, D&C Yellow No. 10, dibutyl sebacate, ethylcellulose, FD&C Blue No. 1, FD&C Blue No. 1 aluminum lake, FD&C Red No. 40, FD&C Yellow No. 6, gelatin, hypromellose, propylene glycol, povidone, silicon dioxide, sodium laurate sulfate, and sugar spheres
This Medication Guide has been approved by the U.S. Food and Drug Administration.
July 2008 DXD:3MG
Manufactured by Catalent Pharma Solutions
Winchester, KY 40391 for
GlaxoSmithKline
Research Triangle Park, NC 27709
©2009, GlaxoSmithKline. All rights reserved.
September 2009 DXD:61PI

DYAZIDE® ℞
[dī' ə-zīd]
(hydrochlorothiazide/triamterene)
Capsules

DESCRIPTION
Each capsule of DYAZIDE (hydrochlorothiazide and triamterene) for oral use, with opaque red cap and opaque white body, contains hydrochlorothiazide 25 mg and triamterene 37.5 mg, and is imprinted with the product name DYAZIDE and SB. Hydrochlorothiazide is a diuretic/antihypertensive agent and triamterene is an antikaliuretic agent.
Hydrochlorothiazide is slightly soluble in water. It is soluble in dilute ammonia, dilute aqueous sodium hydroxide, and dimethylformamide. It is sparingly soluble in methanol.
Hydrochlorothiazide is 6-chloro-3,4-dihydro-2H-1, 2, 4-benzothiadiazine-7-sulfonamide 1,1-dioxide, and its structural formula is:

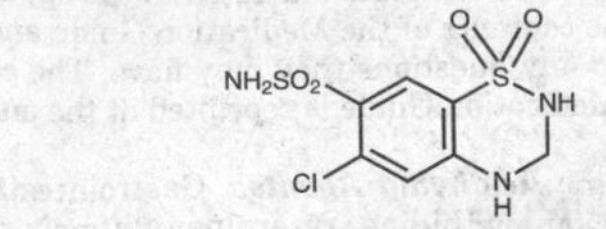

At 50°C, triamterene is practically insoluble in water (less than 0.1%). It is soluble in formic acid, sparingly soluble in methoxyethanol, and very slightly soluble in alcohol.
Triamterene is 2, 4, 7-triamino-6-phenylpteridine and its structural formula is:

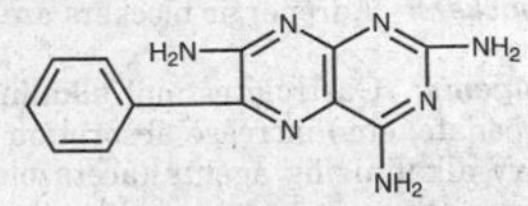

Inactive ingredients consist of benzyl alcohol, cetylpyridinium chloride, D&C Red No. 33, FD&C Yellow No. 6, gelatin, glycine, lactose, magnesium stearate, microcrystalline cellulose, povidone, polysorbate 80, sodium starch glycolate, titanium dioxide, and trace amounts of other inactive ingredients.
Capsules of DYAZIDE meet Drug Release Test 3 as published in the current USP monograph for Triamterene and Hydrochlorothiazide Capsules.

CLINICAL PHARMACOLOGY
DYAZIDE is a diuretic/antihypertensive drug product that combines natriuretic and antikaliuretic effects. Each component complements the action of the other. The hydrochlorothiazide component blocks the reabsorption of sodium and chloride ions, and thereby increases the quantity of sodium traversing the distal tubule and the volume of water excreted. A portion of the additional sodium presented to the distal tubule is exchanged there for potassium and hydrogen ions. With continued use of hydrochlorothiazide and depletion of sodium, compensatory mechanisms tend to increase this exchange and may produce excessive loss of potassium, hydrogen, and chloride ions. Hydrochlorothiazide also decreases the excretion of calcium and uric acid, may increase the excretion of iodide, and may reduce glomerular filtration rate. The exact mechanism of the antihypertensive effect of hydrochlorothiazide is not known.
The triamterene component of DYAZIDE exerts its diuretic effect on the distal renal tubule to inhibit the reabsorption of sodium in exchange for potassium and hydrogen ions. Its natriuretic activity is limited by the amount of sodium reaching its site of action. Although it blocks the increase in this exchange that is stimulated by mineralocorticoids (chiefly aldosterone), it is not a competitive antagonist of aldosterone and its activity can be demonstrated in adrenalectomized rats and patients with Addison's disease. As a result, the dose of triamterene required is not proportionally related to the level of mineralocorticoid activity, but is dictated by the response of the individual patients, and the kaliuretic effect of concomitantly administered drugs. By inhibiting the distal tubular exchange mechanism, triamterene maintains or increases the sodium excretion and reduces the excess loss of potassium, hydrogen and chloride ions induced by hydrochlorothiazide. As with hydrochlorothiazide, triamterene may reduce glomerular filtration and renal plasma flow. Via this mechanism it may reduce uric acid excretion although it has no tubular effect on uric acid reabsorption or secretion. Triamterene does not affect calcium excretion. No predictable antihypertensive effect has been demonstrated for triamterene.
Duration of diuretic activity and effective dosage range of the hydrochlorothiazide and triamterene components of DYAZIDE are similar. Onset of diuresis with DYAZIDE takes place within 1 hour, peaks at 2 to 3 hours and tapers off during the subsequent 7 to 9 hours.
DYAZIDE is well absorbed.
Upon administration of a single oral dose to fasted normal male volunteers, the following mean pharmacokinetic parameters were determined:
[See table at top of next page]
where $AUC_{(0-48)}$, C_{max}, T_{max} and Ae represent area under the plasma concentration versus time plot, maximum plasma concentration, time to reach C_{max}, and amount excreted in urine over 48 hours.

A capsule of DYAZIDE is bioequivalent to a single-entity 25 mg hydrochlorothiazide tablet and 37.5 mg triamterene capsule used in the double-blind clinical trial below (see Clinical Trials).

In a limited study involving 12 subjects, coadministration of DYAZIDE with a high-fat meal resulted in: (1) an increase in the mean bioavailability of triamterene by about 67% (90% confidence interval = 0.99, 1.90), p-hydroxytriamterene sulfate by about 50% (90% confidence interval = 1.06, 1.77), hydrochlorothiazide by about 17% (90% confidence interval = 0.90, 1.34); (2) increases in the peak concentrations of triamterene and p-hydroxytriamterene; and (3) a delay of up to 2 hours in the absorption of the active constituents.

CLINICAL TRIALS

A placebo-controlled, double-blind trial was conducted to evaluate the efficacy of DYAZIDE. This trial demonstrated that DYAZIDE (25 mg hydrochlorothiazide/37.5 mg triamterene) was effective in controlling blood pressure while reducing the incidence of hydrochlorothiazide-induced hypokalemia. This trial involved 636 patients with mild to moderate hypertension controlled by hydrochlorothiazide 25 mg daily and who had hypokalemia (serum potassium <3.5 mEq/L) secondary to the hydrochlorothiazide. Patients were randomly assigned to 4 weeks' treatment with once-daily regimens of 25 mg hydrochlorothiazide plus placebo, or 25 mg hydrochlorothiazide combined with one of the following doses of triamterene: 25 mg, 37.5 mg, 50 mg, or 75 mg.

Blood pressure and serum potassium were monitored at baseline and throughout the trial. All five treatment groups had similar mean blood pressure and serum potassium concentrations at baseline (mean systolic blood pressure range: 137 ± 14 mmHg to 140 ± 16 mmHg; mean diastolic blood pressure range: 86 ± 9 mmHg to 88 ± 8 mmHg; mean serum potassium range: 2.3 to 3.4 mEq/L with the majority of patients having values between 3.1 and 3.4 mEq/L).

While all triamterene regimens reversed hypokalemia, at week 4 the 37.5 mg regimen proved optimal compared with the other tested regimens. On this regimen, 81% of the patients had a significant ($p<0.05$) reversal of hypokalemia vs. 59% of patients on the placebo/hydrochlorothiazide regimen. The mean serum potassium concentration on 37.5 mg triamterene went from 3.2 ± 0.2 mEq/L at baseline to 3.7 ± 0.3 mEq/L at week 4, a significantly greater ($p<0.05$) improvement than that achieved with placebo/hydrochlorothiazide (i.e., 3.2 ± 0.2 mEq/L at baseline and 3.5 ± 0.4 mEq/L at week 4). Also, 51% of patients in the 37.5 mg triamterene group had an increase in serum potassium of ≥ 0.5 mEq/L at week 4 vs. 33% in the placebo group. The 37.5 mg triamterene/25 mg hydrochlorothiazide regimen also maintained control of blood pressure; mean supine systolic blood pressure at week 4 was 138 ± 21 mmHg while mean supine diastolic blood pressure was 87 ± 13 mmHg.

INDICATIONS AND USAGE

This fixed combination drug is not indicated for the initial therapy of edema or hypertension except in individuals in whom the development of hypokalemia cannot be risked.

DYAZIDE is indicated for the treatment of hypertension or edema in patients who develop hypokalemia on hydrochlorothiazide alone.

DYAZIDE is also indicated for those patients who require a thiazide diuretic and in whom the development of hypokalemia cannot be risked.

DYAZIDE may be used alone or as an adjunct to other antihypertensive drugs, such as beta-blockers. Since DYAZIDE may enhance the action of these agents, dosage adjustments may be necessary.

Usage in Pregnancy

The routine use of diuretics in an otherwise healthy woman is inappropriate and exposes mother and fetus to unnecessary hazard. Diuretics do not prevent development of toxemia of pregnancy, and there is no satisfactory evidence that they are useful in the treatment of developed toxemia.

Edema during pregnancy may arise from pathological causes or from the physiologic and mechanical consequences of pregnancy. Diuretics are indicated in pregnancy when edema is due to pathologic causes, just as they are in the absence of pregnancy. Dependent edema in pregnancy resulting from restriction of venous return by the expanded uterus is properly treated through elevation of the lower extremities and use of support hose; use of diuretics to lower intravascular volume in this case is illogical and unnecessary. There is hypervolemia during normal pregnancy which is harmful to neither the fetus nor the mother (in the absence of cardiovascular disease), but which is associated with edema, including generalized edema in the majority of pregnant women. If this edema produces discomfort, increased recumbency will often provide relief. In rare instances this edema may cause extreme discomfort which is not relieved by rest. In these cases a short course of diuretics may provide relief and may be appropriate.

	$AUC_{(0-48)}$ ng*hrs/mL (± SD)	C_{max} ng/mL (± SD)	Median T_{max} Hrs	Ae Mg (± SD)
Triamterene	148.7 (87.9)	46.4 (29.4)	1.1	2.7 (1.4)
hydroxytriamterene sulfate	1,865 (471)	720 (364)	1.3	19.7 (6.1)
hydrochlorothiazide	834 (177)	135.1 (35.7)	2.0	14.3 (3.8)

CONTRAINDICATIONS

Antikaliuretic Therapy and Potassium Supplementation

DYAZIDE should not be given to patients receiving other potassium-sparing agents such as spironolactone, amiloride, or other formulations containing triamterene. Concomitant potassium-containing salt substitutes should also not be used.

Potassium supplementation should not be used with DYAZIDE except in severe cases of hypokalemia. Such concomitant therapy can be associated with rapid increases in serum potassium levels. If potassium supplementation is used, careful monitoring of the serum potassium level is necessary.

Impaired Renal Function

DYAZIDE is contraindicated in patients with anuria, acute and chronic renal insufficiency or significant renal impairment.

Hypersensitivity

Hypersensitivity to either drug in the preparation or to other sulfonamide-derived drugs is a contraindication.

Hyperkalemia

DYAZIDE should not be used in patients with preexisting elevated serum potassium.

WARNINGS

Hyperkalemia: Abnormal elevation of serum potassium levels (greater than or equal to 5.5 mEq/liter) can occur with all potassium-sparing diuretic combinations, including DYAZIDE. Hyperkalemia is more likely to occur in patients with renal impairment and diabetes (even without evidence of renal impairment), and in the elderly or severely ill. Since uncorrected hyperkalemia may be fatal, serum potassium levels must be monitored at frequent intervals especially in patients first receiving DYAZIDE, when dosages are changed or with any illness that may influence renal function.

If hyperkalemia is suspected (warning signs include paresthesias, muscular weakness, fatigue, flaccid paralysis of the extremities, bradycardia, and shock), an electrocardiogram (ECG) should be obtained. However, it is important to monitor serum potassium levels because hyperkalemia may not be associated with ECG changes.

If hyperkalemia is present, DYAZIDE should be discontinued immediately and a thiazide alone should be substituted. If the serum potassium exceeds 6.5 mEq/liter more vigorous therapy is required. The clinical situation dictates the procedures to be employed. These include the intravenous administration of calcium chloride solution, sodium bicarbonate solution, and/or the oral or parenteral administration of glucose with a rapid-acting insulin preparation. Cationic exchange resins such as sodium polystyrene sulfonate may be orally or rectally administered. Persistent hyperkalemia may require dialysis.

The development of hyperkalemia associated with potassium-sparing diuretics is accentuated in the presence of renal impairment (see CONTRAINDICATIONS section). Patients with mild renal functional impairment should not receive this drug without frequent and continuing monitoring of serum electrolytes. Cumulative drug effects may be observed in patients with impaired renal function. The renal clearances of hydrochlorothiazide and the pharmacologically active metabolite of triamterene, the sulfate ester of hydroxytriamterene, have been shown to be reduced and the plasma levels increased following administration of DYAZIDE to elderly patients and patients with impaired renal function.

Hyperkalemia has been reported in diabetic patients with the use of potassium-sparing agents even in the absence of apparent renal impairment. Accordingly, serum electrolytes must be frequently monitored if DYAZIDE is used in diabetic patients.

Metabolic or Respiratory Acidosis

Potassium-sparing therapy should also be avoided in severely ill patients in whom respiratory or metabolic acidosis may occur. Acidosis may be associated with rapid elevations in serum potassium levels. If DYAZIDE is employed, frequent evaluations of acid/base balance and serum electrolytes are necessary.

PRECAUTIONS

Diabetes

Caution should be exercised when administering DYAZIDE to patients with diabetes, since thiazides may cause hyperglycemia, glycosuria, and alter insulin requirements in diabetes. Also, diabetes mellitus may become manifest during thiazide administration.

Impaired Hepatic Function

Thiazides should be used with caution in patients with impaired hepatic function. They can precipitate hepatic coma in patients with severe liver disease. Potassium depletion induced by the thiazide may be important in this connection. Administer DYAZIDE cautiously and be alert for such early signs of impending coma as confusion, drowsiness, and tremor; if mental confusion increases discontinue DYAZIDE for a few days. Attention must be given to other factors that may precipitate hepatic coma, such as blood in the gastrointestinal tract or preexisting potassium depletion.

Hypokalemia

Hypokalemia is uncommon with DYAZIDE; but, should it develop, corrective measures should be taken such as potassium supplementation or increased intake of potassium-rich foods. Institute such measures cautiously with frequent determinations of serum potassium levels, especially in patients receiving digitalis or with a history of cardiac arrhythmias. If serious hypokalemia (serum potassium less than 3.0 mEq/L) is demonstrated by repeat serum potassium determinations, DYAZIDE should be discontinued and potassium chloride supplementation initiated. Less serious hypokalemia should be evaluated with regard to other coexisting conditions and treated accordingly.

Electrolyte Imbalance

Electrolyte imbalance, often encountered in such conditions as heart failure, renal disease or cirrhosis of the liver, may also be aggravated by diuretics and should be considered during therapy with DYAZIDE when using high doses for prolonged periods or in patients on a salt-restricted diet.

Serum determinations of electrolytes should be performed, and are particularly important if the patient is vomiting excessively or receiving fluids parenterally. Possible fluid and electrolyte imbalance may be indicated by such warning signs as: dry mouth, thirst, weakness, lethargy, drowsiness, restlessness, muscle pain or cramps, muscular fatigue, hypotension, oliguria, tachycardia, and gastrointestinal symptoms.

Hypochloremia

Although any chloride deficit is generally mild and usually does not require specific treatment except under extraordinary circumstances (as in liver disease or renal disease), chloride replacement may be required in the treatment of metabolic alkalosis. Dilutional hyponatremia may occur in edematous patients in hot weather; appropriate therapy is water restriction, rather than administration of salt, except in rare instances when the hyponatremia is life threatening. In actual salt depletion, appropriate replacement is the therapy of choice.

Renal Stones

Triamterene has been found in renal stones in association with the other usual calculus components. DYAZIDE should be used with caution in patients with a history of renal stones.

Laboratory Tests

Serum Potassium

The normal adult range of serum potassium is 3.5 to 5.0 mEq per liter with 4.5 mEq often being used for a reference point. If hypokalemia should develop, corrective measures should be taken such as potassium supplementation or increased dietary intake of potassium-rich foods.

Institute such measures cautiously with frequent determinations of serum potassium levels. Potassium levels persistently above 6 mEq per liter require careful observation and treatment. Serum potassium levels do not necessarily indicate true body potassium concentration. A rise in plasma pH may cause a decrease in plasma potassium concentration and an increase in the intracellular potassium concentration. Discontinue corrective measures for hypokalemia immediately if laboratory determinations reveal an abnormal elevation of serum potassium.

Discontinue DYAZIDE and substitute a thiazide diuretic alone until potassium levels return to normal.

Serum Creatinine and BUN

DYAZIDE may produce an elevated blood urea nitrogen level, creatinine level or both. This apparently is secondary to a reversible reduction of glomerular filtration rate or a depletion of intravascular fluid volume (prerenal azotemia) rather than renal toxicity; levels usually return to normal when DYAZIDE is discontinued. If azotemia increases, discontinue DYAZIDE. Periodic BUN or serum creatinine determinations should be made, especially in elderly patients and in patients with suspected or confirmed renal insufficiency.

Serum PBI
Thiazide may decrease serum PBI levels without sign of thyroid disturbance.

Parathyroid Function
Thiazides should be discontinued before carrying out tests for parathyroid function. Calcium excretion is decreased by thiazides. Pathologic changes in the parathyroid glands with hypercalcemia and hypophosphatemia have been observed in a few patients on prolonged thiazide therapy. The common complications of hyperparathyroidism such as bone resorption and peptic ulceration have not been seen.

Drug Interactions

Angiotensin-converting Enzyme Inhibitors
Potassium-sparing agents should be used with caution in conjunction with angiotensin-converting enzyme (ACE) inhibitors due to an increased risk of hyperkalemia.

Oral Hypoglycemic Drugs
Concurrent use with chlorpropamide may increase the risk of severe hyponatremia.

Nonsteroidal Anti-inflammatory Drugs
A possible interaction resulting in acute renal failure has been reported in a few patients on DYAZIDE when treated with indomethacin, a nonsteroidal anti-inflammatory agent. Caution is advised in administering nonsteroidal anti-inflammatory agents with DYAZIDE.

Lithium
Lithium generally should not be given with diuretics because they reduce its renal clearance and increase the risk of lithium toxicity. Read circulars for lithium preparations before use of such concomitant therapy with DYAZIDE.

Surgical Considerations
Thiazides have been shown to decrease arterial responsiveness to norepinephrine (an effect attributed to loss of sodium). This diminution is not sufficient to preclude effectiveness of the pressor agent for therapeutic use. Thiazides have also been shown to increase the paralyzing effect of nondepolarizing muscle relaxants such as tubocurarine (an effect attributed to potassium loss); consequently caution should be observed in patients undergoing surgery.

Other Considerations
Concurrent use of hydrochlorothiazide with amphotericin B or corticosteroids or corticotropin (ACTH) may intensify electrolyte imbalance, particularly hypokalemia, although the presence of triamterene minimizes the hypokalemic effect.

Thiazides may add to or potentiate the action of other antihypertensive drugs. See INDICATIONS AND USAGE for concomitant use with other antihypertensive drugs.

The effect of oral anticoagulants may be decreased when used concurrently with hydrochlorothiazide; dosage adjustments may be necessary.

DYAZIDE may raise the level of blood uric acid; dosage adjustments of antigout medication may be necessary to control hyperuricemia and gout.

The following agents given together with triamterene may promote serum potassium accumulation and possibly result in hyperkalemia because of the potassium-sparing nature of triamterene, especially in patients with renal insufficiency: blood from blood bank (may contain up to 30 mEq of potassium per liter of plasma or up to 65 mEq per liter of whole blood when stored for more than 10 days); low-salt milk (may contain up to 60 mEq of potassium per liter); potassium-containing medications (such as parenteral penicillin G potassium); salt substitutes (most contain substantial amounts of potassium).

Exchange resins, such as sodium polystyrene sulfonate, whether administered orally or rectally, reduce serum potassium levels by sodium replacement of the potassium; fluid retention may occur in some patients because of the increased sodium intake.

Chronic or overuse of laxatives may reduce serum potassium levels by promoting excessive potassium loss from the intestinal tract; laxatives may interfere with the potassium-retaining effects of triamterene.

The effectiveness of methenamine may be decreased when used concurrently with hydrochlorothiazide because of alkalinization of the urine.

Drug/Laboratory Test Interactions
Triamterene and quinidine have similar fluorescence spectra; thus, DYAZIDE will interfere with the fluorescent measurement of quinidine.

Carcinogenesis, Mutagenesis, Impairment of Fertility

Carcinogenesis
Long-term studies have not been conducted with DYAZIDE (the triamterene/hydrochlorothiazide combination), or with triamterene alone.

Hydrochlorothiazide
Two-year feeding studies in mice and rats, conducted under the auspices of the National Toxicology Program (NTP), treated mice and rats with doses of hydrochlorothiazide up to 600 and 100 mg/kg/day, respectively. On a body-weight basis, these doses are 600 times (in mice) and 100 times (in rats) the Maximum Recommended Human Dose (MRHD) for the hydrochlorothiazide component of DYAZIDE at 50 mg/day (or 1.0 mg/kg/day based on 50 kg individuals). On the basis of body-surface area, these doses are 56 times (in mice) and 21 times (in rats) the MRHD. These studies uncovered no evidence of carcinogenic potential of hydrochlorothiazide in rats or female mice, but there was equivocal evidence of hepatocarcinogenicity in male mice.

Mutagenesis
Studies of the mutagenic potential of DYAZIDE (the triamterene/hydrochlorothiazide combination), or of triamterene alone have not been performed.

Hydrochlorothiazide
Hydrochlorothiazide was not genotoxic in in vitro assays using strains TA 98, TA 100, TA 1535, TA 1537 and TA 1538 of *Salmonella typhimurium* (the Ames test); in the Chinese Hamster Ovary (CHO) test for chromosomal aberrations; or in in vivo assays using mouse germinal cell chromosomes, Chinese hamster bone marrow chromosomes, and the *Drosophila* sex-linked recessive lethal trait gene. Positive test results were obtained in the in vitro CHO Sister Chromatid Exchange (clastogenicity) test, and in the mouse Lymphoma Cell (mutagenicity) assays, using concentrations of hydrochlorothiazide of 43 to 1300 mcg/mL. Positive test results were also obtained in the *Aspergillus nidulans* nondisjunction assay, using an unspecified concentration of hydrochlorothiazide.

Impairment of Fertility
Studies of the effects of DYAZIDE (the triamterene/hydrochlorothiazide combination), or of triamterene alone on animal reproductive function have not been conducted.

Hydrochlorothiazide
Hydrochlorothiazide had no adverse effects on the fertility of mice and rats of either sex in studies wherein these species were exposed, via their diet, to doses of up to 100 and 4 mg/kg/day, respectively, prior to mating and throughout gestation. Corresponding multiples of the MRHD are 100 (mice) and 4 (rats) on the basis of body-weight and 9.4 (mice) and 0.8 (rats) on the basis of body-surface area.

Pregnancy: Category C

Teratogenic Effects

DYAZIDE
Animal reproduction studies to determine the potential for fetal harm by DYAZIDE have not been conducted. However, a One Generation Study in the rat approximated composition of DYAZIDE by using a 1:1 ratio of triamterene to hydrochlorothiazide (30:30 mg/kg/day); there was no evidence of teratogenicity at those doses which were, on a body-weight basis, 15 and 30 times, respectively, the MRHD, and on the basis of body-surface area, 3.1 and 6.2 times, respectively, the MRHD.

The safe use of DYAZIDE in pregnancy has not been established since there are no adequate and well-controlled studies with DYAZIDE in pregnant women. DYAZIDE should be used during pregnancy only if the potential benefit justifies the risk to the fetus.

Triamterene
Reproduction studies have been performed in rats at doses as high as 20 times the MRHD on the basis of body-weight, and 6 times the human dose on the basis of body-surface area without evidence of harm to the fetus due to triamterene.

Because animal reproduction studies are not always predictive of human response, this drug should be used during pregnancy only if clearly needed.

Hydrochlorothiazide
Hydrochlorothiazide was orally administered to pregnant mice and rats during respective periods of major organogenesis at doses up to 3,000 and 1,000 mg/kg/day, respectively. At these doses, which are multiples of the MRHD equal to 3,000 for mice and 1,000 for rats, based on body-weight, and equal to 282 for mice and 206 for rats, based on body-surface area, there was no evidence of harm to the fetus.

There are, however, no adequate and well-controlled studies in pregnant women. Because animal reproduction studies are not always predictive of human response, this drug should be used during pregnancy only if clearly needed.

Nonteratogenic Effects
Thiazides and triamterene have been shown to cross the placental barrier and appear in cord blood. The use of thiazides and triamterene in pregnant women requires that the anticipated benefit be weighed against possible hazards to the fetus. These hazards include fetal or neonatal jaundice, pancreatitis, thrombocytopenia, and possible other adverse reactions which have occurred in the adult.

Nursing Mothers
Thiazides and triamterene in combination have not been studied in nursing mothers. Triamterene appears in animal milk; this may occur in humans. Thiazides are excreted in human breast milk. If use of the combination drug product is deemed essential, the patient should stop nursing.

Pediatric Use
Safety and effectiveness in pediatric patients have not been established.

ADVERSE REACTIONS
Adverse effects are listed in decreasing order of severity.

Hypersensitivity
Anaphylaxis, rash, urticaria, subacute cutaneous lupus erythematosus-like reactions, photosensitivity.

Cardiovascular
Arrhythmia, postural hypotension.

Metabolic
Diabetes mellitus, hyperkalemia, hypokalemia, hyponatremia, acidosis, hypercalcemia, hyperglycemia, glycosuria, hyperuricemia, hypochloremia.

Gastrointestinal
Jaundice and/or liver enzyme abnormalities, pancreatitis, nausea and vomiting, diarrhea, constipation, abdominal pain.

Renal
Acute renal failure (one case of irreversible renal failure has been reported), interstitial nephritis, renal stones composed primarily of triamterene, elevated BUN, and serum creatinine, abnormal urinary sediment.

Hematologic
Leukopenia, thrombocytopenia and purpura, megaloblastic anemia.

Musculoskeletal
Muscle cramps.

Central Nervous System
Weakness, fatigue, dizziness, headache, dry mouth.

Miscellaneous
Impotence, sialadenitis.

Thiazides alone have been shown to cause the following additional adverse reactions:

Central Nervous System
Paresthesias, vertigo.

Ophthalmic
Xanthopsia, transient blurred vision.

Respiratory
Allergic pneumonitis, pulmonary edema, respiratory distress.

Other
Necrotizing vasculitis, exacerbation of lupus.

Hematologic
Aplastic anemia, agranulocytosis, hemolytic anemia.

Neonate and infancy
Thrombocytopenia and pancreatitis—rarely, in newborns whose mothers have received thiazides during pregnancy.

Skin
Erythema multiforme including Stevens-Johnson syndrome, exfoliative dermatitis including toxic epidermal necrolysis.

DOSAGE AND ADMINISTRATION
The usual dose of DYAZIDE is one or two capsules given once daily, with appropriate monitoring of serum potassium and of the clinical effect (see WARNINGS, Hyperkalemia).

OVERDOSAGE
Electrolyte imbalance is the major concern (see WARNINGS section). Symptoms reported include: polyuria, nausea, vomiting, weakness, lassitude, fever, flushed face, and hyperactive deep tendon reflexes. If hypotension occurs, it may be treated with pressor agents such as levarterenol to maintain blood pressure. Carefully evaluate the electrolyte pattern and fluid balance. Induce immediate evacuation of the stomach through emesis or gastric lavage. There is no specific antidote.

Reversible acute renal failure following ingestion of 50 tablets of a product containing a combination of 50 mg triamterene and 25 mg hydrochlorothiazide has been reported. Although triamterene is largely protein-bound (approximately 67%), there may be some benefit to dialysis in cases of overdosage.

HOW SUPPLIED
Capsules containing 25 mg hydrochlorothiazide and 37.5 mg triamterene, in bottles of 1,000 capsules; in Patient-Pak™ unit-of-use bottles of 100.

They are supplied as follows:

NDC 0007-3650-22–in Patient-Pak™ unit-of-use bottles of 100.

NDC 0007-3650-30–bottles of 1,000.

Store at controlled room temperature 20° to 25°C (68° to 77°F); excursions permitted to 15° to 30°C (59° to 86°F). Protect from light. Dispense in a tight, light-resistant container.

GlaxoSmithKline
Research Triangle Park, NC 27709
DYAZIDE is a registered trademark of GlaxoSmithKline.
©2009, GlaxoSmithKline. All rights reserved.
October 2009   DYZ:73PI

DYNACIRC CR® ℞

[*di' na-circ*]
(isradipine)
Controlled Release Tablets

DESCRIPTION

DYNACIRC CR contains isradipine, a calcium antagonist. It is available for once-daily oral administration as a controlled-release 5-mg and 10-mg tablet. DYNACIRC CR is a registered trademark for isradipine GITS (Gastrointestinal Therapeutic System) tablets.
The structural formula of isradipine is:

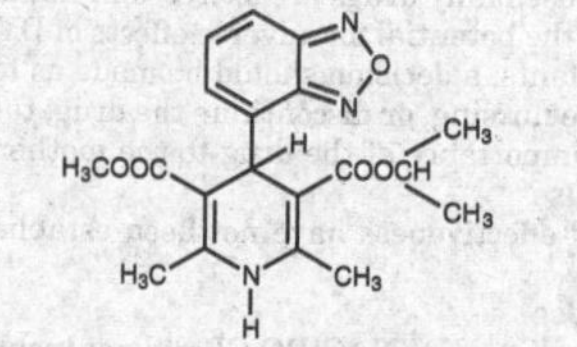

Chemically, isradipine is 3,5-Pyridinedicarboxylic acid, 4-(4-benzofurazanyl)-1,4-dihydro-2,6-dimethyl-, methyl 1-methylethyl ester, with a molecular weight of 371.39. The molecular formula is $C_{19}H_{21}N_3O_5$. Isradipine is a yellow, fine crystalline powder which is odorless or has a faint characteristic odor. Isradipine is practically insoluble in water (<10 mg/L at 37°C), but is soluble in ethanol and freely soluble in acetone, chloroform, and methylene chloride.

Active Ingredient
Isradipine

Inactive Ingredients
Butylated hydroxytoluene, cellulose acetate, hypromellose, magnesium stearate, polyethylene glycol, polyethylene oxide, polysorbate 80, propylene glycol, red ferric oxide, silicon dioxide, sodium chloride, titanium dioxide, yellow ferric oxide.

System Components and Performance
Isradipine is delivered from the DYNACIRC CR Controlled Release Tablet as follows: a semipermeable membrane surrounds an osmotically active drug core. The core is composed of 2 layers: an "active" layer containing the drug, and a pharmacologically inert but osmotically active "push" layer. After ingestion, the tablet overcoating is quickly dissipated in the gastrointestinal tract, allowing water to enter the tablet through the semipermeable membrane. The polyethylene oxide polymer swells in the osmotic ("push") layer and exerts pressure against the "active" drug layer, releasing isradipine as a fine suspension through the laser-drilled tablet orifice which has been positioned on the "active" drug layer side. Drug delivery is essentially constant as long as the osmotic gradient remains constant and, after either 5 mg or 10 mg of isradipine is released, gradually falls to a negligible amount. The controlled rate of drug delivery into the gastrointestinal lumen is independent of pH or gastrointestinal motility. The delivery of isradipine in DYNACIRC CR depends on the existence of an osmotic gradient between the contents of the bilayer core and the fluid in the GI tract. The biologically inert core of the tablet remains intact and, unless it becomes trapped, is eliminated in the feces.

CLINICAL PHARMACOLOGY

Mechanism of Action
Isradipine is a dihydropyridine calcium channel blocker. It binds to calcium channels with high affinity and specificity and inhibits calcium flux into cardiac and smooth muscle. The effects observed in mechanistic experiments in vitro and studied in intact animals and man are compatible with this mechanism of action and are typical of the class.
Except for diuretic activity, the mechanism of which is not clearly understood, the pharmacodynamic effects of isradipine observed in whole animals can also be explained by calcium channel blocking activity, especially dilating effects in arterioles which reduce systemic resistance and lower blood pressure, with a small increase in resting heart rate. Although like other dihydropyridine calcium channel blockers, isradipine has negative inotropic effects in vitro, studies conducted in intact anesthetized animals have shown that the vasodilating effect occurs at doses lower than those which affect contractility. In patients with normal ventricular function, isradipine's afterload-reducing properties lead to some increase in cardiac output.
Effects in patients with impaired ventricular function have not been fully studied.

Clinical Effects
In randomized, placebo-controlled, double-blind, clinical trials, DYNACIRC CR has been shown to have antihypertensive effects proportional to doses between 5 and 20 mg, administered once daily. DYNACIRC CR produced statistically significant reductions in supine and standing blood pressure, compared with placebo, 24 hours postdose. The endpoint results of one parallel-group, dose-ranging trial showed mean responses 24 hours after ingestion of DYNACIRC CR (systolic/diastolic) -5.2/-2.8, -13.4/-9.7, -15.6/-10.2, and -15.5/-11.8 mmHg, for 5-, 10-, 15-, and 20-mg doses, respectively, change from baseline greater than concurrent placebo. The antihypertensive effect of any one dose begins in about 2 hours and reaches a peak at about 8 to 10 hours postdose. At the recommended starting dose (5 mg) the trough response (24 hours after dosing) was about 76% that of the peak. At doses of 10, 15, and 20 mg, the trough blood pressure response was about equal to that at peak effect. In association with the fall in blood pressure, resting heart rate is slightly increased, on average from 1 to 3 beats/minute. The antihypertensive response to DYNACIRC CR has not been detected to be influenced by gender or age.

Hemodynamics
In man, peripheral vasodilation produced by immediate-release DYNACIRC is reflected by decreased systemic vascular resistance and increased cardiac output. Hemodynamic studies conducted in patients with normal left ventricular function produced, following intravenous isradipine administration, increases in cardiac index, stroke volume index, coronary sinus blood flow, heart rate, and peak positive left ventricular dP/dt. Systemic, coronary, and pulmonary vascular resistance was decreased. These studies were conducted with doses of isradipine which produced clinically significant decreases in blood pressure. The clinical consequences of these hemodynamic effects, if any, have not been evaluated.
Effects on heart rate are variable, dependent upon rate of administration and presence of underlying cardiac condition. While increases in both peak positive dP/dt and LV ejection fraction are seen when intravenous isradipine is given, it is impossible to conclude that these represent a positive inotropic effect due to simultaneous changes in preload and afterload. In patients with coronary artery disease undergoing atrial pacing during cardiac catheterization, intravenous isradipine diminished abnormalities of systolic performance. In patients with moderate left ventricular dysfunction, oral and intravenous isradipine in doses which reduce blood pressure by 12% to 30%, resulted in improvement in cardiac index without increase in heart rate, and with no change or reduction in pulmonary capillary wedge pressure. Combination of isradipine and propranolol did not significantly affect left ventricular dP/dt max. The clinical consequences of these effects have not been evaluated.

Electrophysiologic Effects
In general, no detrimental effects on the cardiac conduction system were seen with the use of immediate-release DYNACIRC. Electrophysiologic studies were conducted on patients with normal sinus and atrioventricular node function. Intravenous isradipine in doses which reduce systolic blood pressure did not affect PR, QRS, AH* or HV* intervals.
No changes were seen in Wenckebach cycle length, atrial, and ventricular refractory periods. Slight prolongation of QT_c interval of 3% was seen in one study. Effects on sinus node recovery time (CSNRT) were mild or not seen.
In patients with sick sinus syndrome, at doses which significantly reduced blood pressure, intravenous isradipine resulted in no depressant effect on sinus and atrioventricular node function.
* AH = conduction time from low right atrium to His bundle deflection, or AV nodal conduction time
* HV = conduction time through His bundle and the bundle branch-Purkinje system.

Pharmacokinetics and Metabolism
With the immediate-release formulation DYNACIRC, 90% to 95% of the orally administered dose is absorbed. Because of the biotransformation of isradipine during its first-pass through the portal circulation, the bioavailability of DYNACIRC CR ranges from 15% to 24%. Isradipine is 95% bound to plasma proteins.
Peak concentrations of approximately 1 ng/mL/mg dosed occur about 1.5 hours after administration of immediate-release DYNACIRC. The elimination of isradipine is biphasic with an early half-life of 1½ to 2 hours, and a terminal half-life of about 8 hours, resulting in trough concentrations of about 0.1 ng/mL/mg dosed of immediate-release DYNACIRC.
In single-dose studies of DYNACIRC CR, after a 2 to 3 hour lag time, concentrations of isradipine plateau between 7 and 18 hours post-dosing (reaching a C_{max} of 3 to 4 ng/mL with an AUC of 62 to 73 ng•h/mL for a 10-mg dose) and then a concentration >50% of the peak exists for 17 to 20 hours.
There is no evidence of dose dumping either in the presence or absence of food. Food has been shown to decrease the extent of bioavailability of DYNACIRC CR by up to 25%.
The pharmacokinetics of DYNACIRC CR are linear over the dose range of 5 to 20 mg, in that the plasma drug concentrations are proportional to the dose administered.
Isradipine is completely metabolized prior to excretion, and no unchanged drug is detected in the urine. The major routes of isradipine metabolism are ring oxidation of the dihydropyridine moiety to give the corresponding pyridine, and ester cleavage, with or without concomitant oxidation of the dihydropyridine moiety, giving the corresponding carboxylic acids. The cytochrome P450 3A4 system is implicated in the formation of these metabolites, which are hemodynamically inactive. Approximately 60% to 65% of an administered dose is excreted in the urine and 25% to 30% in the feces. With immediate-release DYNACIRC, mild renal impairment (creatinine clearance 30 to 80 mL/min) increases the AUC of isradipine by 45%. Progressive deterioration reverses this trend, and patients with severe renal failure (creatinine clearance <10 mL/min) who have been on hemodialysis show a 20% to 50% lower AUC than healthy volunteers. In elderly patients administered immediate-release DYNACIRC, C_{max} and AUC are increased by 13% and 40%, respectively; in patients with hepatic impairment, C_{max} and AUC are increased by 32% and 52%, respectively (see DOSAGE AND ADMINISTRATION).

INDICATIONS AND USAGE

Hypertension
DYNACIRC CR is indicated in the management of hypertension. It may be used alone or concurrently with thiazide-type diuretics.

CONTRAINDICATIONS

DYNACIRC CR is contraindicated in individuals who have shown hypersensitivity to any of the ingredients in the formulation.

WARNINGS

None

PRECAUTIONS

General

Blood Pressure
Because DYNACIRC CR decreases peripheral resistance, like other calcium blockers, DYNACIRC CR may occasionally produce symptomatic hypotension. However, symptoms like syncope and severe dizziness have rarely been reported in hypertensive patients administered DYNACIRC CR, particularly at the initial recommended doses (see DOSAGE AND ADMINISTRATION).

Use in Patients with Congestive Heart Failure
Although acute hemodynamic studies in patients with congestive heart failure have shown that immediate-release DYNACIRC reduced afterload without impairing myocardial contractility, it has a negative inotropic effect at high doses in vitro and possibly in some patients. Caution should be exercised when using DYNACIRC CR in congestive heart failure patients, particularly in combination with a beta-blocker.

Peripheral Edema:
Peripheral edema, when it occurs, is usually mild to moderate in severity. It is a localized phenomenon thought to be associated with vasodilation of arterioles and other small blood vessels, and not due to left ventricular dysfunction or generalized fluid retention. Peripheral edema is dose-related with an incidence ranging from approximately 9% at 5 mg, 13% at 10 mg, 16% at 15 mg, and 36% at the highest dose studied (20 mg once-daily). With patients whose hypertension is complicated by congestive heart failure, care should be taken to differentiate this edema from the effects of decreasing left ventricular function. Although the frequency of edema is correlated with dose, no patients treated with DYNACIRC CR discontinued the short-term (6 weeks or less), placebo-controlled hypertension studies as a result of edema. Less than 5% of patients treated with DYNACIRC CR in long-term studies discontinued due to edema.

Other
As with any other non-deformable material, caution should be used when administering DYNACIRC CR in patients with pre-existing severe gastrointestinal narrowing (pathologic or iatrogenic). There have been reports of obstructive symptoms in patients with known strictures associated with ingestion of other GITS products.

Information for Patients
DYNACIRC CR Controlled Release Tablets should be swallowed whole. Do not chew, divide, or crush tablets. Do not be concerned if you occasionally notice in your stool something resembling a tablet. In DYNACIRC CR, the medication is contained within a nonabsorbable shell that has been specially designed to slowly release the drug for your body to absorb. When this process is completed, the empty tablet shell is eliminated in the stool.

Drug Interactions

Nitroglycerin
Immediate-release DYNACIRC has been safely coadministered with nitroglycerin.

Hydrochlorothiazide
A study in normal healthy volunteers has shown that concomitant administration of immediate-release DYNACIRC

Most Frequently Reported Newly-Occurring Adverse Reactions in Dose-Response Study

Adverse Reactions (Excluding Non-Drug Related)	DYNACIRC CR				Placebo Group
	5 mg (N=79)	10 mg (N=79)	15 mg (N=82)	20 mg (N=78)	(N=83)
Headache	13.9%	12.7%	18.3%	10.3%	15.7%
Edema	8.9%	12.7%	15.9%	35.9%	3.6%
Dizziness	5.1%	6.3%	3.7%	6.4%	2.4%
Constipation	3.8%	1.3%	1.2%	2.6%	0.0%
Fatigue	2.5%	7.6%	3.7%	3.8%	2.4%
Flushing	2.5%	3.8%	1.2%	1.3%	1.2%
Abdominal discomfort	1.3%	5.1%	3.7%	5.1%	1.2%
Rash	1.3%	1.3%	0.0%	2.6%	0.0%

Adverse Experience		DYNACIRC			Placebo	Active Controls*
	All Doses	2.5 mg twice-daily	5 mg twice-daily†	10 mg twice-daily††	(N=297) %	(N=414) %
Headache	13.7	12.6	10.7	22.0	14.1	9.4
Dizziness	7.3	8.0	5.3	3.4	4.4	8.2
Edema	7.2	3.5	8.7	8.5	3.0	2.9
Palpitations	4.0	1.0	4.7	5.1	1.4	1.5
Fatigue	3.9	2.5	2.0	8.5	0.3	6.3
Flushing	2.6	3.0	2.0	5.1	0.0	1.2
Chest pain	2.4	2.5	2.7	1.7	2.4	2.9
Nausea	1.8	1.0	2.7	5.1	1.7	3.1
Dyspnea	1.8	0.5	2.7	3.4	1.0	2.2
Abdominal discomfort	1.7	0.0	3.3	1.7	1.7	3.9
Tachycardia	1.5	1.0	1.3	3.4	0.3	0.5
Rash	1.5	1.5	2.0	1.7	0.3	0.7
Pollakiuria	1.5	2.0	1.3	3.4	0.0	<1.0
Weakness	1.2	0.0	0.7	0.0	0.0	1.2
Vomiting	1.1	1.0	1.3	0.0	0.3	0.2
Diarrhea	1.1	0.0	2.7	3.4	2.0	1.9

* Propranolol, prazosin, hydrochlorothiazide, enalapril, and captopril.

† Initial dose of 2.5 mg twice-daily followed by maintenance dose of 5.0 mg twice-daily.

†† Initial dose of 2.5 mg twice-daily followed by sequential titration to 5.0 mg twice-daily, 7.5 mg twice-daily, and maintenance dose of 10.0 mg twice-daily.

and hydrochlorothiazide does not result in altered pharmacokinetics of either drug. In a study in hypertensive patients, addition of isradipine to existing hydrochlorothiazide therapy did not result in any unexpected adverse effects, and isradipine had an additional antihypertensive effect.

Propranolol

In a single-dose study in normal volunteers using immediate-release DYNACIRC, co-administration of propranolol had a small effect on the rate but no effect on the extent of isradipine bioavailability. Significant increases in AUC (27%) and C_{max} (58%) and decreases in T_{max} (23%) of propranolol were noted in this study.

Digoxin

The concomitant administration of immediate-release DYNACIRC and digoxin in a single-dose pharmacokinetic study did not affect renal, non-renal, and total body clearance of digoxin.

Fentanyl Anesthesia

Severe hypotension has been reported during fentanyl anesthesia with concomitant use of a beta blocker and a calcium channel blocker. An increased volume of circulating fluids might be required if such an interaction were to occur.

Carcinogenesis, Mutagenesis, Impairment of Fertility

Treatment of male rats for 2 years with 2.5, 12.5, or 62.5 mg/kg/day isradipine admixed with the diet (approximately 6, 31, and 156 times the maximum recommended daily dose based on a 50 kg man) resulted in dose-dependent increases in the incidence of benign Leydig cell tumors and testicular hyperplasia relative to untreated control animals. These findings, which were replicated in a subsequent experiment, may have been indirectly related to an effect of isradipine on circulating gonadotropin levels in the rats; a comparable endocrine effect was not evident in male patients receiving therapeutic doses of the drug on a chronic basis. Treatment of mice for 2 years with 2.5, 15, or 80 mg/kg/day isradipine in the diet (approximately 6, 38, and 200 times the maximum recommended dose based on a 50 kg man) showed no evidence of oncogenicity. There was no evidence of mutagenic potential based on the results of a battery of mutagenic tests. No effect on fertility was observed in male and female rats treated with up to 60 mg/kg/day isradipine.

Pregnancy

Pregnancy Category C

Isradipine was administered orally to rats and rabbits during organogenesis. Treatment of pregnant rats with doses of 6, 20, or 60 mg/kg/day produced a significant reduction in maternal weight gain during treatment with the highest dose (150 times the maximum recommended human daily dose) but with no lasting effect on the mother or the offspring. Treatment of pregnant rabbits with doses of 1, 3, or 10 mg/kg/day (2.5, 7.5, and 25 times the maximum recommended human daily dose) produced decrements in maternal body weight gain and increased fetal resorption at the 2

higher doses. There was no evidence of embryotoxicity at doses which were not maternotoxic and no evidence of teratogenicity at any dose tested. In a peri/postnatal administration study in rats, reduced maternal body weight gain during late pregnancy at oral doses of 20 and 60 mg/kg/day isradipine was associated with reduced birth weights and decreased peri and postnatal pup survival.

There are no adequate and well controlled studies in pregnant women. The use of DYNACIRC CR during pregnancy should only be considered if the potential benefit outweighs potential risks.

Nursing Mothers

It is not known whether DYNACIRC is excreted in human milk. Because many drugs are excreted in human milk, and because of the potential for adverse effects of DYNACIRC on nursing infants, a decision should be made as to whether to discontinue nursing, or discontinue the drug, taking into account the importance of the drug to the mother.

Pediatric Use

Safety and effectiveness have not been established in children.

Geriatric Use

Clinical studies of DYNACIRC CR did not include sufficient numbers of subjects aged 65 and older to determine whether they respond differently from younger subjects. Other reported clinical experience has not identified differences in responses between the elderly and younger patients. Elderly patients have decreased clearance of DYNACIRC with a higher average AUC and C_{max} (see Pharmacokinetics and Metabolism). The larger extent of bioavailability may be a result of a reduced clearance and/or reduced first-pass metabolism of the drug. In general, dose selection for an elderly patient should be cautious, reflecting the greater frequency of decreased hepatic, renal, or cardiac function, and of concomitant disease or other drug therapy (see DOSAGE AND ADMINISTRATION).

ADVERSE REACTIONS

In a controlled clinical trial with DYNACIRC CR, dose-related edema occurred at an incidence of approximately 9% at 5 mg, 13% at 10 mg, 16% at 15 mg, and 36% at the highest dose studied (20 mg); was mild to moderate in severity; and was not related to age or gender.

The incidences of elicited or volunteered adverse reactions (excluding non-drug related) in the following tables are based on 6-week multicenter, placebo-controlled, double-blind hypertension studies. Less than 1% of patients treated with DYNACIRC CR or placebo discontinued from these studies due to adverse reactions.

The most common adverse experiences (≥1.0%) reported with DYNACIRC CR in a dose-response study are shown in the following table. There were no discontinuations of patients treated with DYNACIRC CR in this study due to these common side effects.

[See first table above]

The table below shows elicited or volunteered adverse experiences for patients treated with DYNACIRC CR in two 6-week, placebo-controlled, multicenter studies, at doses from 5 to 20 mg, and considered by the investigator to be at least possibly drug related. The results for patients treated with DYNACIRC CR are presented for all doses pooled together (reported by at least 1.0% of active drug-treated patients). The incidence of adverse reactions is listed below:

Adverse Reactions (Excluding Non-Drug Related)	Treatment Group	
	DYNACIRC CR (N=422)	Placebo (N=186)
Edema	15.2%	2.2%
Headache	13.0%	12.4%
Dizziness	4.7%	2.7%
Fatigue	4.3%	2.2%
Abdominal discomfort	2.8%	0.5%
Flushing	1.9%	0.5%
Constipation	1.7%	0.0%
Palpitations	1.2%	0.0%
Nausea	1.2%	1.6%
Abdominal distention	1.2%	0.0%

The following adverse experiences were reported in 0.5% to 1.0% or less of patients treated with DYNACIRC CR or immediate-release DYNACIRC in hypertensive studies, or were noted in postmarketing experience with immediate-release DYNACIRC. More serious events are shown in italics. The relationship of these adverse experiences to isradipine administration is uncertain.

Skin
Pruritus, *urticaria, angioedema.*

Musculoskeletal
Backache/pain, joint pain, neck pain/sore/stiff, legs ache/pain, cramps of legs/feet.

Respiratory
Dyspnea, nasal congestion, cough.

Cardiovascular
Epistaxis, tachycardia, chest pain, shortness of breath, hypotension, *syncope, atrial or ventricular fibrillation, myocardial infarction, heart failure.*

Gastrointestinal
Diarrhea, vomiting, appetite increased or decreased.

Urogenital
Pollakiuria, impotence, dysuria, nocturia.

Central Nervous
Drowsiness, insomnia, lethargy, nervousness, libido decrease/frigidity, impotence, depression, *paresthesia* (which includes numbness and tingling), *transient ischemic attack, stroke.*

Autonomic
Dry mouth, hyperhidrosis, visual disturbance.

Miscellaneous
Weight gain, throat discomfort, *drug fever, leukopenia, elevated liver function tests.*

No gastrointestinal bleeding has been reported in clinical trials with DYNACIRC CR Controlled Release Tablets.

In a long-term (one-year) open-label, hypertension trial with DYNACIRC CR, the adverse events reported were generally the same as those seen in the short-term placebo-controlled studies. About 6% of patients treated with DYNACIRC CR discontinued the long-term trial due to adverse reactions.

With immediate-release DYNACIRC, most of the adverse experiences were transient, mild, and related to vasodilatory effects. The following table shows the most common adverse events reported in US clinical trials for immediate-release DYNACIRC, volunteered or elicited, and considered by the investigator to be at least possibly drug related.
[See second table on previous page]

In open-label, long-term studies of up to 2 years in duration with immediate-release DYNACIRC, the adverse experiences reported were generally the same as those reported in the short-term controlled trials. The overall frequencies of these adverse events were slightly higher in the long-term than in the controlled studies, but in the controlled studies most adverse reactions were mild and transient.

OVERDOSAGE

Although there is no well documented experience with DYNACIRC overdosage, available data suggest that, as with other dihydropyridines, gross overdosage would result in excessive peripheral vasodilation with subsequent marked and probably prolonged systemic hypotension. Clinically significant hypotension overdosage calls for active cardiovascular support including monitoring of cardiac and respiratory function, elevation of lower extremities and attention to circulating fluid volume and urine output. A vasoconstrictor (such as epinephrine, norepinephrine, or levarterenol) may be helpful in restoring vascular tone and blood pressure, provided that there is no contraindication to its use. Since isradipine is highly protein bound, dialysis is not likely to be of benefit.

Significant lethality was observed in mice given oral doses of more than 200 mg/kg and rabbits given about 50 mg/kg of isradipine. Rats tolerated doses of more than 2,000 mg/kg without effects on survival.

DOSAGE AND ADMINISTRATION

The dosage of DYNACIRC CR Controlled Release Tablets should be individualized. The recommended initial dose of DYNACIRC CR is 5 mg once-daily as monotherapy or in combination with a thiazide diuretic. An antihypertensive response usually occurs within 2 hours, with the peak antihypertensive response occurring 8 to 10 hours post-dose; blood pressure reduction is maintained for at least 24 hours following drug administration. If necessary, the dose may be adjusted in increments of 5 mg at 2 to 4 week intervals up to a maximum dose of 20 mg/day. Adverse experiences are increased in frequency above 10 mg/day.

DYNACIRC CR Controlled Release Tablets should be swallowed whole and should not be bitten or divided.

The bioavailability (increased AUC) of immediate-release DYNACIRC is increased in elderly patients (older than 65 years of age), patients with hepatic functional impairment, and patients with mild renal impairment. Ordinarily, a starting dose of DYNACIRC CR 5 mg once-daily should be used in these patients.

HOW SUPPLIED

DYNACIRC CR Controlled Release Tablets

5 mg

A light pink, round, standard, biconvex and film coated tablet. Printing is in red with "DynaCirc CR" in a semicircle with "5" centered below the semicircle.

Bottles of 30 controlled-release tablets (NDC 0173-0784-01)

10 mg

A beige, round, standard biconvex and film coated tablet. Printing is in red with "DynaCirc CR" in a semicircle with "10" centered below the semicircle.

Bottles of 30 controlled-release tablets (NDC 0173-0785-01)

Store and Dispense

Below 86°F (30°C) in a tight container, protected from moisture and humidity.

Jointly manufactured for:

GlaxoSmithKline
Research Triangle Park, NC 27709
By: **Novartis Consumer Health, Inc.**
Lincoln, NE 68517 *and*
Patheon Pharmaceuticals Inc.
Cinncinnati, OH 45237
©2009, GlaxoSmithKline. All rights reserved.
February 2009   DCR:2PI

ENGERIX-B®   ℞

[*in' jə-rix*]

[Hepatitis B Vaccine (Recombinant)]

DESCRIPTION

ENGERIX-B [Hepatitis B Vaccine (Recombinant)] is a noninfectious recombinant DNA hepatitis B vaccine developed and manufactured by GlaxoSmithKline Biologicals. It contains purified surface antigen of the virus obtained by culturing genetically engineered *Saccharomyces cerevisiae* cells, which carry the surface antigen gene of the hepatitis B virus. The surface antigen expressed in *Saccharomyces cerevisiae* cells is purified by several physicochemical steps and formulated as a suspension of the antigen adsorbed on aluminum hydroxide. The procedures used to manufacture ENGERIX-B result in a product that contains no more than 5% yeast protein. No substances of human origin are used in its manufacture.

ENGERIX-B is supplied as a sterile suspension for intramuscular administration. The vaccine is ready for use without reconstitution; it must be shaken before administration since a fine white deposit with a clear colorless supernatant may form on storage.

ENGERIX-B is formulated without preservatives.

ENGERIX-B is available in vials and 2 types of prefilled syringes. One type of prefilled syringe has a tip cap which may contain natural rubber latex. The other type has a tip cap and a rubber plunger which contain dry natural latex rubber. The vial stopper does not contain latex. (See HOW SUPPLIED.)

Pediatric/Adolescent:

Each 0.5-mL dose contains 10 mcg of hepatitis B surface antigen adsorbed on 0.25 mg aluminum as aluminum hydroxide. The pediatric formulation contains sodium chloride (9 mg/mL) and phosphate buffers (disodium phosphate dihydrate, 0.98 mg/mL; sodium dihydrogen phosphate dihydrate, 0.71 mg/mL).

Adult:

Each 1-mL adult dose contains 20 mcg of hepatitis B surface antigen adsorbed on 0.5 mg aluminum as aluminum hydroxide. The adult formulation contains sodium chloride (9 mg/mL) and phosphate buffers (disodium phosphate dihydrate, 0.98 mg/mL; sodium dihydrogen phosphate dihydrate, 0.71 mg/mL).

CLINICAL PHARMACOLOGY

Several hepatitis viruses are known to cause a systemic infection resulting in major pathologic changes in the liver (e.g., A, B, C, D, E, and G). The estimated lifetime risk of HBV infection in the United States varies from almost 100% for the highest-risk groups to less than 20% for the population as a whole.[1] Hepatitis B infection can have serious consequences including acute massive hepatic necrosis, chronic active hepatitis, and cirrhosis of the liver. Up to 90% of neonates and 6% to 10% of adults who are infected in the United States will become hepatitis B virus carriers.[1] It has been estimated that 200 to 300 million people in the world today are persistently infected with hepatitis B virus.[1] The Centers for Disease Control and Prevention (CDC) estimates that there are approximately 1 to 1.25 million chronic carriers of hepatitis B virus in the United States.[1] Those patients who become chronic carriers can infect others and are at increased risk of developing primary hepatocellular carcinoma. Among other factors, infection with hepatitis B may be the single most important factor for development of this carcinoma.[1,2]

Reduced Risk of Hepatocellular Carcinoma:

According to the CDC, the hepatitis B vaccine is recognized as the first anti-cancer vaccine because it can prevent primary liver cancer.[3]

A clear link has been demonstrated between chronic hepatitis B infection and the occurrence of hepatocellular carcinoma. In a Taiwanese study, the institution of universal childhood immunization against hepatitis B virus has been shown to decrease the incidence of hepatocellular carcinoma among children.[4] In a Korean study in adult males, vaccination against hepatitis B virus has been shown to decrease the incidence of, and risk of, developing hepatocellular carcinoma in adults.[5]

Considering the serious consequences of infection, immunization should be considered for all persons at potential risk of exposure to the hepatitis B virus. Mothers infected with hepatitis B virus can infect their infants at, or shortly after, birth if they are carriers of the hepatitis B surface antigen (HBsAg) or develop an active infection during the third trimester of pregnancy. Infected infants usually become chronic carriers. Therefore, screening of pregnant women for hepatitis B is recommended.[1] Because a vaccination strategy limited to high-risk individuals has failed to substantially lower the overall incidence of hepatitis B infection, the Advisory Committee on Immunization Practices (ACIP) recommends vaccination of all persons from birth to age 18.[6] The Committee on Infectious Diseases of the American Academy of Pediatrics (AAP) has also endorsed universal infant immunization as part of a comprehensive strategy for the control of hepatitis B infection.[7] The AAP, American Academy of Family Physicians (AAFP), and American Medical Association (AMA) also recommend routine vaccination of adolescents 11 to 12 years of age who have not been vaccinated previously.[8] The AAP further recommends that providers administer hepatitis B vaccine to all previously unvaccinated adolescents.[9] (See INDICATIONS AND USAGE.) There is no specific treatment for acute hepatitis B infection. However, those who develop anti-HBs antibodies after active infection are usually protected against subsequent infection. Antibody titers ≥10 mIU/mL against HBsAg are recognized as conferring protection against hepatitis B.[1] Seroconversion is defined as antibody titers ≥1 mIU/mL.

Protective Efficacy:

Protective efficacy with ENGERIX-B has been demonstrated in a clinical trial in neonates at high risk of hepatitis B infection.[10,11] Fifty-eight neonates born of mothers who were both HBsAg and HBeAg positive were given ENGERIX-B (10 mcg at 0, 1, and 2 months) without concomitant hepatitis B immune globulin. Two infants became chronic carriers in the 12-month follow-up period after initial inoculation. Assuming an expected carrier rate of 70%, the protective efficacy rate against the chronic carrier state during the first 12 months of life was 95%.

Immunogenicity in Neonates:

Immunization with 10 mcg at 0, 1, and 6 months of age produced seroconversion in 100% of infants by month 7, with a geometric mean antibody titer (GMT) of 713 mIU/mL (N = 52), and the seroprotection rate was 97%.

Clinical trials indicate that administration of hepatitis B immune globulin at birth does not alter the response to ENGERIX-B.

Immunization with 10 mcg at 0, 1, and 2 months of age produced a seroprotection rate of 96% in infants by month 4, with a GMT among seroconverters of 210 mIU/mL (N = 311); an additional dose at month 12 produced a GMT among seroconverters of 2,941 mIU/mL at month 13 (N = 126).

Immunogenicity in Pediatric Patients:

In clinical trials with 242 children aged 6 months to, and including, 10 years given 10 mcg at months 0, 1, and 6, the seroprotection rate was 98% 1 to 2 months after the third dose; the GMT of seroconverters was 4,023 mIU/mL.

In a separate clinical trial including both children and adolescents aged 5 to 16 years, 10 mcg of ENGERIX-B was administered at 0, 1, and 6 months (N = 181) or 0, 12, and 24 months (N = 161). Immediately before the third dose of vaccine, seroprotection was achieved in 92.3% of subjects vaccinated on the 0-, 1-, and 6-month schedule and 88.8% of subjects on the 0-, 12-, and 24-month schedule (117.9 mIU/mL versus 162.1 mIU/mL, respectively, *P* = 0.18). One month following the third dose, seroprotection was achieved in 99.5% of children vaccinated on the 0-, 1-, and 6-month schedule compared to 98.1% of those on the 0-, 12-, and 24-month schedule. GMTs were higher (*P* = 0.02) for children receiving vaccine on the 0-, 1-, and 6-month schedule compared to those on the 0-, 12-, and 24-month schedule (5,687.4 mIU/mL versus 3,158.7 mIU/mL, respectively). The clinical relevance of this finding is unknown.

Immunogenicity in Adolescents:

In clinical trials with healthy adolescent subjects 11 through 19 years of age, immunization with 10 mcg using a 0-, 1-, and 6-month schedule produced a seroprotection rate of 97% at month 8 (N = 119) with a GMT of 1,989 mIU/mL (N = 118, 95% confidence intervals = 1,318-3,020). Immunization with 20 mcg using a 0-, 1-, and 6-month schedule produced a seroprotection rate of 99% at month 8 (N = 122) with a GMT of 7,672 mIU/mL (N = 122, 95% confidence intervals = 5,248-10,965).

Immunogenicity in Healthy Adults and Adolescents:

Clinical trials in healthy adult and adolescent subjects have shown that following a course of 3 doses of 20 mcg

ENGERIX-B given according to the ACIP-recommended schedule of injections at months 0, 1, and 6, the seroprotection (antibody titers ≥10 mIU/mL) rate for all individuals was 79% at month 6 and 96% at month 7; the GMT for seroconverters at month 7 was 2,204 mIU/mL. On an alternate schedule (injections at months 0, 1, and 2) designed for certain populations (e.g., neonates born of hepatitis B–infected mothers, individuals who have or might have been recently exposed to the virus, and certain travelers to high-risk areas. See INDICATIONS AND USAGE), 99% of all individuals were seroprotected at month 3 and remained protected through month 12. On the alternate schedule, an additional dose at 12 months produced a GMT for seroconverters at month 13 of 9,163 mIU/mL.

Immunogenicity in Older Subjects:
Among older subjects given 20 mcg at months 0, 1, and 6, the seroprotection rate 1 month after the third dose was 88%. However, as with other hepatitis B vaccines, in adults over 40 years of age, ENGERIX-B vaccine produced anti-HBs titers that were lower than those in younger adults (GMT among seroconverters 1 month after the third 20-mcg dose with a 0-, 1-, and 6-month schedule: 610 mIU/mL for individuals over 40 years of age, N = 50).

Immunogenicity in Subjects With Chronic Hepatitis C:
In a clinical trial of subjects with chronic hepatitis C, 31 subjects received ENGERIX-B on the usual 0-, 1-, and 6-month schedule. All subjects responded with seroprotective titers. The GMT of anti-HBs was 1,260 mIU/mL (95% CI: 709-2,237).

Immunogenicity in Hemodialysis Patients:
Hemodialysis patients given hepatitis B vaccines respond with lower titers,[12] which remain at protective levels for shorter durations than in normal subjects. In a study in which patients on chronic hemodialysis (mean time on dialysis was 24 months; N = 562) received 40 mcg of the plasma-derived vaccine at months 0, 1, and 6, approximately 50% of patients achieved antibody titers ≥10 mIU/mL.[12] Since a fourth dose of ENGERIX-B given to healthy adults at month 12 following the 0-, 1-, and 2-month schedule resulted in a substantial increase in the GMT (see above), a 4-dose regimen was studied in hemodialysis patients. In a clinical trial of adults who had been on hemodialysis for a mean of 56 months (N = 43), 67% of patients were seroprotected 2 months after the last dose of 40 mcg of ENGERIX-B (2 × 20 mcg) given on a 0-, 1-, 2-, and 6-month schedule; the GMT among seroconverters was 93 mIU/mL.

Thimerosal Free Formulation:
In 3 comparative clinical trials with 1,339 adults and 587 children, the thimerosal free formulation performed as well as the preservative free formulation that contained trace amounts of thimerosal.

Interchangeability With Other Hepatitis B Vaccines:
Recombinant DNA vaccines are produced in yeast by expression of a hepatitis B virus gene sequence that codes for the hepatitis B surface antigen. Like plasma-derived vaccine, the yeast-derived vaccines are protein particles visible by electron microscopy and have hepatitis B surface antigen epitopes as determined by monoclonal antibody analyses. Yeast-derived vaccines have been shown by in vitro analyses to induce antibodies (anti-HBs) which are immunologically comparable by epitope specificity and binding affinity to antibodies induced by plasma-derived vaccine.[13] In cross-absorption studies, no differences were detected in the spectra of antibodies induced in man to plasma-derived or to yeast-derived hepatitis B vaccines.[13]
Additionally, patients immunized approximately 3 years previously with plasma-derived vaccine and whose antibody titers were <100 mIU/mL (GMT: 35 mIU/mL; range: 9-94) were given a 20-mcg dose of ENGERIX-B. All patients, including 2 who had not responded to the plasma-derived vaccine, showed a response to ENGERIX-B (GMT: 5,069 mIU/mL; range: 624-15,019). There have been no clinical studies in which a 3-dose vaccine series was initiated with a plasma-derived hepatitis B vaccine and completed with ENGERIX-B, or vice versa. However, because the in vitro and in vivo studies described above indicate the comparability of the antibody produced in response to plasma-derived vaccine and ENGERIX-B, it should be possible to interchange the use of ENGERIX-B and plasma-derived vaccines (but see CONTRAINDICATIONS).
A controlled study (N = 48) demonstrated that completion of a course of immunization with 1 dose of ENGERIX-B (20 mcg, month 6) following 2 doses of RECOMBIVAX HB®* (10 mcg, months 0 and 1) produced a similar GMT (4,077 mIU/mL) to immunization with 3 doses of RECOMBIVAX HB (10 mcg, months 0, 1, and 6; 2,654 mIU/mL). Thus, ENGERIX-B can be used to complete a vaccination course initiated with RECOMBIVAX HB.[14]

Other Clinical Studies:
In 1 study, 4 of 244 (1.6%) adults (homosexual men) at high risk of contracting hepatitis B virus became infected during the period prior to completion of 3 doses of ENGERIX-B (20 mcg at 0, 1, and 6 months).[15] No additional patients became infected during the 18-month follow-up period after completion of the immunization course.

INDICATIONS AND USAGE
ENGERIX-B is indicated for immunization against infection caused by all known subtypes of hepatitis B virus. As hepatitis D (caused by the delta virus) does not occur in the absence of hepatitis B infection, it can be expected that hepatitis D will also be prevented by ENGERIX-B vaccination.
ENGERIX-B will not prevent hepatitis caused by other agents, such as hepatitis A, C, and E viruses, or other pathogens known to infect the liver.
Immunization is recommended in persons of all ages, especially those who are, or will be, at increased risk of exposure to hepatitis B virus,[1] for example:

- Infants, Including Those Born of HBsAg-Positive Mothers *(See DOSAGE AND ADMINISTRATION.)*
- Adolescents *(See CLINICAL PHARMACOLOGY.)*
- Healthcare Personnel: *Dentists and oral surgeons. Dental, medical, and nursing students. Physicians, surgeons, and podiatrists. Nurses. Paramedical and ambulance personnel and custodial staff who may be exposed to the virus via blood or other patient specimens. Dental hygienists and dental nurses. Laboratory and blood bank personnel handling blood, blood products, and other patient specimens. Hospital cleaning staff who handle waste.*
- Selected Patients and Patient Contacts: *Patients and staff in hemodialysis units and hematology/oncology units. Patients requiring frequent and/or large volume blood transfusions or clotting factor concentrates (e.g., persons with hemophilia, thalassemia, sickle cell anemia, cirrhosis). Clients (residents) and staff of institutions for the mentally handicapped. Classroom contacts of deinstitutionalized mentally handicapped persons who have persistent hepatitis B surface antigenemia and who show aggressive behavior. Household and other intimate contacts of persons with persistent hepatitis B surface antigenemia.*
- Subpopulations With a Known High Incidence of the Disease, such as: *Alaskan Eskimos. Pacific Islanders. Indochinese immigrants. Haitian immigrants. Refugees from other HBV-endemic areas. All infants of women born in areas where the infection is highly endemic.*
- Individuals With Chronic Hepatitis C: *Risk factors for hepatitis C are similar to those for hepatitis B. Consequently, immunization with hepatitis B vaccine is recommended for individuals with chronic hepatitis C.*
- Persons Who May Be Exposed to the Hepatitis B Virus by Travel to High-Risk Areas *(See ACIP Guidelines, 1990.)*
- Military Personnel Identified as Being at Increased Risk
- Morticians and Embalmers
- Persons at Increased Risk of the Disease Due to Their Sexual Practices,[1,16] such as: *Persons with more than 1 sexual partner in a 6-month period. Persons who have contracted a sexually transmitted disease. Homosexually active males. Female prostitutes.*
- Prisoners
- Users of Illicit Injectable Drugs
- Others: *Police and fire department personnel who render first aid or medical assistance, and any others who, through their work or personal life-style, may be exposed to the hepatitis B virus. Adoptees from countries of high HBV endemicity.*

Use With Other Vaccines:
The ACIP states that, in general, simultaneous administration of certain live and inactivated pediatric vaccines has not resulted in impaired antibody responses or increased rates of adverse reactions.[17] Separate sites and syringes should be used for simultaneous administration of injectable vaccines.

CONTRAINDICATIONS
Hypersensitivity to any component of the vaccine, including yeast, is a contraindication (see DESCRIPTION). This vaccine is contraindicated in patients with previous hypersensitivity to any hepatitis B-containing vaccine.

WARNINGS
ENGERIX-B is available in vials and 2 types of prefilled syringes. One type of prefilled syringe has a tip cap which may contain natural rubber latex. The other type has a tip cap and a rubber plunger which contain dry natural latex rubber. Use of these syringes may cause allergic reactions in latex sensitive individuals. The vial stopper does not contain latex. (See HOW SUPPLIED.)
Apnea following intramuscular vaccination has been observed in some infants born prematurely. Decisions about when to administer an intramuscular vaccine, including ENGERIX-B, to infants born prematurely should be based on consideration of the individual infant's medical status, and the potential benefits and possible risks of vaccination. For ENGERIX-B, this assessment should include consideration of the mother's hepatitis B antigen status and the high probability of maternal transmission of hepatitis B virus to infants born of mothers who are HBsAg positive if vaccination is delayed.
Hepatitis B has a long incubation period. Hepatitis B vaccination may not prevent hepatitis B infection in individuals who had an unrecognized hepatitis B infection at the time of vaccine administration. Additionally, it may not prevent infection in individuals who do not achieve protective antibody titers.

PRECAUTIONS
General:
As with other vaccines, although a moderate or severe febrile illness is sufficient reason to postpone vaccination, minor illnesses such as mild upper respiratory infections with or without low-grade fever are not contraindications.[17]
Prior to immunization, the patient's medical history should be reviewed. The physician should review the patient's immunization history for possible vaccine sensitivity, previous vaccination-related adverse reactions, and occurrence of any adverse event–related symptoms and/or signs in order to determine the existence of any contraindication to immunization with ENGERIX-B and to allow an assessment of benefits and risks. Epinephrine injection (1:1,000) and other appropriate agents used for the control of immediate allergic reactions must be immediately available should an acute anaphylactic reaction occur.
A separate sterile syringe and needle or a sterile disposable unit should be used for each individual patient to prevent transmission of hepatitis or other infectious agents from one person to another. Needles should be disposed of properly and should not be recapped.
Special care should be taken to prevent injection into a blood vessel.
As with any vaccine administered to immunosuppressed persons or persons receiving immunosuppressive therapy, the expected immune response may not be obtained. For individuals receiving immunosuppressive therapy, deferral of vaccination for at least 3 months after therapy may be considered.[17]
Multiple Sclerosis: Although no causal relationship has been established, rare instances of exacerbation of multiple sclerosis have been reported following administration of hepatitis B vaccines and other vaccines. In persons with multiple sclerosis, the benefit of immunization for prevention of hepatitis B infection and sequelae must be weighed against the risk of exacerbation of the disease.

Information for the Patient:
Patients, parents, or guardians should be informed of the potential benefits and risks of the vaccine, and of the importance of completing the immunization series. As with any vaccine, it is important when a subject returns for the next dose in a series that he or she be questioned concerning occurrence of any symptoms and/or signs of an adverse reaction after a previous dose of the same vaccine. Patients, parents, or guardians should be told to report severe or unusual adverse reactions to their healthcare provider.
The parent or guardian should be given the Vaccine Information Materials, which are required by the National Childhood Vaccine Injury Act of 1986 to be given prior to immunization.

Drug Interactions:
For information regarding simultaneous administration with other vaccines, refer to INDICATIONS AND USAGE.

Carcinogenesis, Mutagenesis, Impairment of Fertility:
ENGERIX-B has not been evaluated for carcinogenic or mutagenic potential, or for impairment of fertility.

Pregnancy:
Pregnancy Category C. Animal reproduction studies have not been conducted with ENGERIX-B. It is also not known whether ENGERIX-B can cause fetal harm when administered to a pregnant woman or can affect reproduction capacity. ENGERIX-B should be given to a pregnant woman only if clearly needed.

Nursing Mothers:
It is not known whether ENGERIX-B is excreted in human milk. Because many drugs are excreted in human milk, caution should be exercised when ENGERIX-B is administered to a nursing woman.

Pediatric Use:
ENGERIX-B has been shown to be well tolerated and highly immunogenic in infants and children of all ages. Newborns also respond well; maternally transferred antibodies do not interfere with the active immune response to the vaccine. (See CLINICAL PHARMACOLOGY for seroconversion rates and titers in neonates and children. See DOSAGE AND ADMINISTRATION for recommended pediatric dosage and for recommended dosage for infants born of HBsAg-positive mothers.)

Geriatric Use:
Clinical studies of ENGERIX-B did not include sufficient numbers of subjects 65 years of age and older to determine whether they respond differently from younger subjects. Other reports from the clinical literature indicate that hepatitis B vaccines are less immunogenic in adults 65 years of age and older than in younger individuals. Other

reported clinical experience has not identified differences in overall safety between these subjects and younger adult subjects.

ADVERSE REACTIONS

ENGERIX-B is generally well tolerated. As with any vaccine, however, it is possible that expanded commercial use of the vaccine could reveal rare adverse reactions.

Ten double-blind studies involving 2,252 subjects showed no significant difference in the frequency or severity of adverse experiences between ENGERIX-B and plasma-derived vaccines. In 36 clinical studies, a total of 13,495 doses of ENGERIX-B were administered to 5,071 healthy adults and children who were initially seronegative for hepatitis B markers, and healthy neonates. All subjects were monitored for 4 days post-administration. Frequency of adverse experiences tended to decrease with successive doses of ENGERIX-B. Using a symptom checklist,[†] the most frequently reported adverse reactions were injection site soreness (22%) and fatigue[†] (14%). Other reactions are listed below.

Incidence 1% to 10% of Injections:
Nervous System Disorders: Dizziness[†], headache.[†]
General Disorders and Administration Site Conditions: Fever (>37.5°C), injection site erythema, injection site induration, injection site swelling.
[†]Parent or guardian completed forms for children and neonates. Neonatal checklist did not include headache, fatigue, or dizziness.

Incidence <1% of Injections:
Infections and Infestations: Upper respiratory tract illnesses.
Blood and Lymphatic System Disorders: Lymphadenopathy.
Metabolism and Nutrition Disorders: Anorexia.
Psychiatric Disorders: Agitation, insomnia.
Nervous System Disorders: Somnolence, tingling.
Vascular Disorders: Flushing, hypotension.
Gastrointestinal Disorders: Abdominal pain/cramps, constipation, diarrhea, nausea, vomiting.
Skin and Subcutaneous Tissue Disorders: Erythema, petechiae, pruritus, rash, sweating, urticaria.
Musculoskeletal and Connective Tissue Disorders: Arthralgia, back pain, myalgia, pain/stiffness in arm, shoulder, or neck.
General Disorders and Administration Site Conditions: Chills, influenza-like symptoms, injection site ecchymosis, injection site pain, injection site pruritus, irritability, malaise, weakness.

Postmarketing Reports:
Additional adverse experiences have been reported with the commercial use of ENGERIX-B. Those listed below are to serve as alerting information to physicians.
Infections and Infestations: Herpes zoster, meningitis.
Blood and Lymphatic System Disorders: Thrombocytopenia.
Immune System Disorders: Allergic reaction, anaphylactoid reaction, anaphylaxis. An apparent hypersensitivity syndrome (serum sickness-like) of delayed onset has been reported days to weeks after vaccination, including: arthralgia/arthritis (usually transient), fever, and dermatologic reactions such as urticaria, erythema multiforme, ecchymoses, and erythema nodosum (see CONTRAINDICATIONS).
Nervous System Disorders: Encephalitis, encephalopathy, migraine, multiple sclerosis, neuritis, neuropathy including hypoesthesia, paresthesia, Guillain-Barré syndrome and Bell's palsy, optic neuritis, paralysis, paresis, seizures, syncope, transverse myelitis.
Eye Disorders: Conjunctivitis, keratitis, visual disturbances.
Ear and Labyrinth Disorders: Earache, tinnitus, vertigo.
Cardiac Disorders: Palpitations, tachycardia.
Vascular Disorders: Vasculitis.
Respiratory, Thoracic and Mediastinal Disorders: Apnea, bronchospasm including asthma-like symptoms.
Gastrointestinal Disorders: Dyspepsia.
Skin and Subcutaneous Tissue Disorders: Alopecia, angioedema, eczema, erythema multiforme including Stevens-Johnson syndrome, erythema nodosum, lichen planus, purpura.
Musculoskeletal and Connective Tissue Disorders: Arthritis, muscular weakness.
General Disorders and Administration Site Conditions: Injection site reaction.
Investigations: Abnormal liver function tests.

Reporting Adverse Events:
The National Childhood Vaccine Injury Act requires that the manufacturer and lot number of the vaccine administered be recorded by the healthcare provider in the vaccine recipient's permanent medical record, along with the date of administration of the vaccine and the name, address, and title of the person administering the vaccine.[18] The Act further requires the healthcare provider to report to the US

Table 1. Recommended Dosage and Administration Schedules

Group	Dose	Schedules
Infants born of:		
HBsAg-negative mothers	10 mcg/0.5 mL	0, 1, 6 months
HBsAg-positive mothers	10 mcg/0.5 mL	0, 1, 6 months
Children:		
Birth through 10 years of age	10 mcg/0.5 mL	0, 1, 6 months
Adolescents:		
11 through 19 years of age	10 mcg/0.5 mL	0, 1, 6 months
Adults (>19 years)	20 mcg/1.0 mL	0, 1, 6 months
Adult hemodialysis	40 mcg/2.0 mL[a]	0, 1, 2, 6 months

[a] Two × 20 mcg in 1 or 2 injections.

Table 2. Alternate Dosage and Administration Schedules

Group	Dose	Schedules
Infants born of:		
HBsAg-positive mothers	10 mcg/0.5 mL	0, 1, 2, 12 months[a]
Children:		
Birth through 10 years of age	10 mcg/0.5 mL	0, 1, 2, 12 months[a]
5 through 10 years of age	10 mcg/0.5 mL	0, 12, 24 months[b]
Adolescents:		
11 through 16 years of age	10 mcg/0.5 mL	0, 12, 24 months[b]
11 through 19 years of age	20 mcg/1.0 mL	0, 1, 6 months
11 through 19 years of age	20 mcg/1.0 mL	0, 1, 2, 12 months[a]
Adults (>19 years)	20 mcg/1.0 mL	0, 1, 2, 12 months[a]

[a] This schedule is designed for certain populations (e.g., neonates born of hepatitis B–infected mothers, others who have or might have been recently exposed to the virus, certain travelers to high-risk areas. See INDICATIONS AND USAGE). On this alternate schedule, an additional dose at 12 months is recommended for prolonged maintenance of protective titers.
[b] For children and adolescents for whom an extended administration schedule is acceptable based on risk of exposure.

Department of Health and Human Services via VAERS the occurrence following immunization of any event set forth in the Vaccine Injury Table including: Anaphylaxis or anaphylactic shock within 4 hours, encephalopathy or encephalitis within 72 hours, or any sequelae thereof (including death).[18,19] In addition, any event considered a contraindication to further doses should be reported. The VAERS toll-free number is 1-800-822-7967.

DOSAGE AND ADMINISTRATION
Injection:
ENGERIX-B should be administered by intramuscular injection. *Do not inject intravenously or intradermally.* In adults, the injection should be given in the deltoid region but it may be preferable to inject in the anterolateral thigh in neonates and infants, who have smaller deltoid muscles. ENGERIX-B should not be administered in the gluteal region; such injections may result in suboptimal response. The attending physician should determine final selection of the injection site and needle size, depending upon the patient's age and the size of the target muscle. A 1-inch, 23-gauge needle is sufficient to penetrate the anterolateral thigh in infants younger than 12 months of age. A 5/8-inch, 25-gauge needle may be used to administer the vaccine in the deltoid region of toddlers and children up to, and including, 10 years of age. The 1-inch, 23-gauge needle is appropriate for use in older children and adults.[17]
ENGERIX-B may be administered subcutaneously to persons at risk of hemorrhage (e.g., hemophiliacs). However, hepatitis B vaccines administered subcutaneously are known to result in lower GMTs. Additionally, when other aluminum-adsorbed vaccines have been administered subcutaneously, an increased incidence of local reactions including subcutaneous nodules has been observed. Therefore, subcutaneous administration should be used only in persons who are at risk of hemorrhage with intramuscular injections.

Preparation for Administration:
Shake well before withdrawal and use. Parenteral drug products should be inspected visually for particulate matter and discoloration prior to administration, whenever solution and container permit. If either of these conditions exists, the vaccine should not be administered. With thorough agitation, ENGERIX-B is a slightly turbid white suspension. Do not administer if it appears otherwise. The vaccine should be used as supplied; no dilution is necessary. The full recommended dose of the vaccine should be used. Any vaccine remaining in a single-dose vial should be discarded.

Dosing Schedules:
The usual immunization regimen (see Table 1) consists of 3 doses of vaccine given according to the following schedule: first dose: at elected date; second dose: 1 month later; third dose: 6 months after first dose.
[See table above]
For hemodialysis patients, in whom vaccine-induced protection is less complete and may persist only as long as antibody levels remain above 10 mIU/mL, the need for booster doses should be assessed by annual antibody testing. 40 mcg (2 × 20 mcg) booster doses with ENGERIX-B should be given when antibody levels decline below 10 mIU/mL.[1] Data show individuals given a booster with ENGERIX-B achieve high antibody titers. (See CLINICAL PHARMACOLOGY.)
There are alternate dosing and administration schedules which may be used for specific populations (see Table 2 and accompanying explanations).
[See table above]
Booster Vaccinations: Whenever administration of a booster dose is appropriate, the dose of ENGERIX-B is 10 mcg for children 10 years of age and younger, 20 mcg for adolescents 11 through 19 years of age, and 20 mcg for adults. Studies have demonstrated a substantial increase in antibody titers after ENGERIX-B booster vaccination fol-

lowing an initial course with both plasma- and yeast-derived vaccines. (See CLINICAL PHARMACOLOGY.)

See previous section for discussion on booster vaccination for adult hemodialysis patients.

Known or Presumed Exposure to Hepatitis B Virus:
Unprotected individuals with known or presumed exposure to the hepatitis B virus (e.g., neonates born of infected mothers, others experiencing percutaneous or permucosal exposure) should be given hepatitis B immune globulin (HBIG) in addition to ENGERIX-B in accordance with ACIP recommendations[1] and with the package insert for HBIG. ENGERIX-B can be given on either dosing schedule (see above).

STORAGE
Store refrigerated between 2° and 8°C (36° and 46°F). *Do not freeze*; discard if product has been frozen. Do not dilute to administer.

HOW SUPPLIED

ENGERIX-B is available in single-dose vials (contain no latex) and prefilled disposable TIP-LOK® syringes (may contain latex) (packaged without needles) (Preservative Free Formulation):

10 mcg/0.5 mL Pediatric/Adolescent Dose
NDC 58160-820-01 Vial (contains no latex) in Package of 10: NDC 58160-820-11
NDC 58160-820-43 Syringe (tip cap may contain latex) in Package of 10: NDC 58160-820-52
NDC 58160-820-32 Syringe (tip cap and plunger contain latex) in Package of 5: NDC 58160-820-46
NDC 58160-820-32 Syringe (tip cap and plunger contain latex) in Package of 10: NDC 58160-820-51

20 mcg/mL Adult Dose
NDC 58160-821-01 Vial (contains no latex) in Package of 10: NDC 58160-821-11
NDC 58160-821-43 Syringe (tip cap may contain latex) in Package of 5: NDC 58160-821-48
NDC 58160-821-32 Syringe (tip cap and plunger contain latex) in Package of 1: NDC 58160-821-32
NDC 58160-821-31 Syringe (tip cap and plunger contain latex) in Package of 5: NDC 58160-821-46

REFERENCES

1. Centers for Disease Control and Prevention. Hepatitis B. In: Atkinson W, Wolfe C, Humiston S, Nelson R, eds. *Epidemiology and Prevention of Vaccine-Preventable Diseases.* 6th ed. Atlanta, GA: Public Health Foundation; 2000:207-229. **2.** Beasley RP, Hwang L-Y, Stevens CE, et al. Efficacy of hepatitis B immune globulin for prevention of perinatal transmission of hepatitis B virus carrier state: final report of a randomized double-blind, placebo-controlled trial. *Hepatology.* 1983;3(2):135-141. **3.** Centers for Disease Control and Prevention. New vaccine information materials for hepatitis B, haemophilus influenzae type B (Hib), and varicella (chickenpox) vaccines, and revised vaccine information materials for measles, mumps, rubella (MMR) vaccines. *Federal Register.* February 23, 1999;64(35):9044-9045. **4.** Chang M-H, Chen C-J, Lai M-S, et al. Universal hepatitis B vaccination in Taiwan and the incidence of hepatocellular carcinoma in children. *N Engl J Med.* 1997;336(26):1855-1859. **5.** Lee M-S, Kim D-H, Kim H, et al. Hepatitis B vaccination and reduced risk of primary liver cancer among male adults: a cohort study in Korea. *Int J Epidemiol.* 1998;27(2):316-319. **6.** Centers for Disease Control and Prevention. Effectiveness of a seventh grade school entry vaccination requirement — statewide and Orange County, Florida, 1997-1998. *MMWR.* 1998;47(34):711-715. **7.** American Academy of Pediatrics. Universal hepatitis B immunization. *Pediatrics.* 1992;89(4):795-800. **8.** Centers for Disease Control and Prevention. Immunization of adolescents: recommendations of the Advisory Committee on Immunization Practices, the American Academy of Pediatrics, the American Academy of Family Physicians, and the American Medical Association. *MMWR.* 1996;45(RR-13):1-16. **9.** American Academy of Pediatrics. Immunization of adolescents: recommendations of the Advisory Committee on Immunization Practices, the American Academy of Pediatrics, the American Academy of Family Physicians, and the American Medical Association. *Pediatrics.* 1997;99(3):479-488. **10.** André FE and Safary A. Clinical experience with a yeast-derived hepatitis B vaccine. In: Zuckerman AJ, ed. *Viral Hepatitis and Liver Disease.* New York, NY: Alan R Liss, Inc.; 1988:1025-1030. **11.** Poovorawan Y, Sanpavat S, Pongpunlert W, et al. Protective efficacy of a recombinant DNA hepatitis B vaccine in neonates of HBe antigen-positive mothers. *JAMA.* 1989;261(22):3278-3281. **12.** Stevens CE, Alter HJ, Taylor PE, et al. Hepatitis B vaccine in patients receiving hemodialysis. *N Engl J Med.* 1984;311(8):496-501. **13.** Hauser P, Voet P, Simoen E, et al. Immunological properties of recombinant HBsAg produced in yeast. *Postgrad Med J.* 1987;63(suppl 2):83-91. **14.** Bush LM, Moonsammy GI, Boscia JA. Evaluation of initiating a hepatitis B vaccination schedule with one vaccine and completing it with another. *Vaccine.* 1991;9(11):807-809. **15.** Goilav C, Prinsen H, Safary A, et al. Immunization of homosexual men with a recombinant DNA vaccine against hepatitis B: immunogenicity and protection. In: Zuckerman AJ, ed. *Viral Hepatitis and Liver Disease.* New York, NY: Alan R Liss, Inc.; 1988:1057-1058. **16.** Centers for Disease Control and Prevention. 1998 Guidelines for treatment of sexually transmitted diseases. *MMWR.* 1998;47(RR-1):102. **17.** Centers for Disease Control and Prevention. General recommendations on immunization: recommendations of the Advisory Committee on Immunization Practices (ACIP). *MMWR.* 1994;43(RR-1):1-38. **18.** Centers for Disease Control. National Childhood Vaccine Injury Act: requirements for permanent vaccination records and for reporting of selected events after vaccination. *MMWR.* 1988;37(13):197-200. **19.** Public Health Service. National Vaccine Injury Compensation Program: revision of the vaccine injury table. *Federal Register.* February 8, 1995;60(26):7694.

*Yeast-derived, Hepatitis B Vaccine, MSD.
ENGERIX-B and TIP-LOK are registered trademarks of GlaxoSmithKline.
RECOMBIVAX HB is a registered trademark of Merck & Co.

Manufactured by **GlaxoSmithKline Biologicals**
Rixensart, Belgium, US License No. 1617
Distributed by **GlaxoSmithKline**
Research Triangle Park, NC 27709
©2010, GlaxoSmithKline. All rights reserved.
July 2010
ENG:45PI

EPIVIR-HBV® ℞
[*ĕp′ə-vir*]
(lamivudine)
Tablets

EPIVIR-HBV® ℞
(lamivudine)
Oral Solution

WARNING
LACTIC ACIDOSIS AND SEVERE HEPATOMEGALY WITH STEATOSIS, INCLUDING FATAL CASES, HAVE BEEN REPORTED WITH THE USE OF NUCLEOSIDE ANALOGUES ALONE OR IN COMBINATION, INCLUDING LAMIVUDINE AND OTHER ANTIRETROVIRALS (SEE WARNINGS).
HUMAN IMMUNODEFICIENCY VIRUS (HIV) COUNSELING AND TESTING SHOULD BE OFFERED TO ALL PATIENTS BEFORE BEGINNING EPIVIR-HBV AND PERIODICALLY DURING TREATMENT (SEE WARNINGS), BECAUSE EPIVIR-HBV TABLETS AND ORAL SOLUTION CONTAIN A LOWER DOSE OF THE SAME ACTIVE INGREDIENT (LAMIVUDINE) AS EPIVIR® TABLETS AND ORAL SOLUTION USED TO TREAT HIV INFECTION. IF TREATMENT WITH EPIVIR-HBV IS PRESCRIBED FOR CHRONIC HEPATITIS B FOR A PATIENT WITH UNRECOGNIZED OR UNTREATED HIV INFECTION, RAPID EMERGENCE OF HIV RESISTANCE IS LIKELY BECAUSE OF SUBTHERAPEUTIC DOSE AND INAPPROPRIATE MONOTHERAPY.
SEVERE ACUTE EXACERBATIONS OF HEPATITIS B HAVE BEEN REPORTED IN PATIENTS WHO HAVE DISCONTINUED ANTI-HEPATITIS B THERAPY (INCLUDING EPIVIR-HBV). HEPATIC FUNCTION SHOULD BE MONITORED CLOSELY WITH BOTH CLINICAL AND LABORATORY FOLLOW-UP FOR AT LEAST SEVERAL MONTHS IN PATIENTS WHO DISCONTINUE ANTI-HEPATITIS B THERAPY. IF APPROPRIATE, INITIATION OF ANTI-HEPATITIS B THERAPY MAY BE WARRANTED (SEE WARNINGS).

DESCRIPTION

EPIVIR-HBV is a brand name for lamivudine, a synthetic nucleoside analogue with activity against hepatitis B virus (HBV) and HIV. Lamivudine was initially developed for the treatment of HIV infection as EPIVIR. Please see the complete prescribing information for EPIVIR Tablets and Oral Solution for additional information. The chemical name of lamivudine is (2R,cis)-4-amino-1-(2-hydroxymethyl-1,3-oxathiolan-5-yl)-(1H)-pyrimidin-2-one. Lamivudine is the (-)enantiomer of a dideoxy analogue of cytidine. Lamivudine has also been referred to as (-)2′,3′-dideoxy, 3′-thiacytidine. It has a molecular formula of $C_8H_{11}N_3O_3S$ and a molecular weight of 229.3. It has the following structural formula:

[See chemical structure at top of next column]

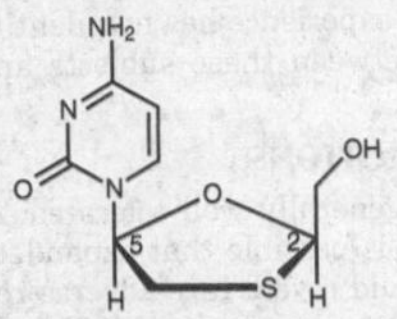

Lamivudine is a white to off-white crystalline solid with a solubility of approximately 70 mg/mL in water at 20°C.

EPIVIR-HBV Tablets are for oral administration. Each tablet contains 100 mg of lamivudine and the inactive ingredients hypromellose, macrogol 400, magnesium stearate, microcrystalline cellulose, polysorbate 80, red iron oxide, sodium starch glycolate, titanium dioxide, and yellow iron oxide.

EPIVIR-HBV Oral Solution is for oral administration. One milliliter (1 mL) of EPIVIR-HBV Oral Solution contains 5 mg of lamivudine (5 mg/mL) in an aqueous solution and the inactive ingredients artificial strawberry and banana flavors, citric acid (anhydrous), methylparaben, propylene glycol, propylparaben, sodium citrate (dihydrate), and sucrose (200 mg).

MICROBIOLOGY
Mechanism of Action
Lamivudine is a synthetic nucleoside analogue. Intracellularly, lamivudine is phosphorylated to its active 5′-triphosphate metabolite, lamivudine triphosphate, 3TC-TP. Incorporation of the monophosphate form into viral DNA by HBV reverse transcriptase results in DNA chain termination. 3TC-TP also inhibits the RNA- and DNA-dependent DNA polymerase activities of HIV-1 reverse transcriptase (RT). 3TC-TP is a weak inhibitor of mammalian α, β, and γ-DNA polymerases.

Antiviral Activity
Activity of lamivudine against HBV in cell culture was assessed in HBV DNA-transfected 2.2.15 cells, HB611 cells, and infected human primary hepatocytes. EC_{50} values (the concentration of drug needed to reduce the level of extracellular HBV DNA by 50%) varied from 0.01 μM (2.3 ng/mL) to 5.6 μM (1.3 mcg/mL) depending upon the duration of exposure of cells to lamivudine, the cell model system, and the protocol used. See the EPIVIR package insert for information regarding activity of lamivudine against HIV.

Resistance
Lamivudine-resistant isolates were identified in patients with virologic breakthrough, defined when using solution hybridization assay as the detection of HBV DNA in serum on 2 or more occasions after failing to detect HBV DNA on 2 or more occasions and defined when using PCR assay as a >1 log_{10} (10-fold) increase in serum HBV DNA from nadir during treatment in a patient who had an initial virologic response.

Lamivudine-resistant HBV isolates develop M204V/I substitutions in the YMDD motif of the catalytic domain of the viral reverse transcriptase. M204V/I substitutions are frequently accompanied by other substitutions (V173L, L180M) which enhance the level of lamivudine resistance or act as compensatory mutations improving replication efficiency. Other substitutions detected in lamivudine-resistant HBV isolates include L80I and A181T.

In 4 controlled clinical trials in adults with HBeAg-positive chronic hepatitis B virus infection (CHB), YMDD-mutant HBV was detected in 81 of 335 patients receiving lamivudine 100 mg once daily for 52 weeks. The prevalence of YMDD substitutions was less than 10% in each of these trials for patients studied at 24 weeks and increased to an average of 24% (range in 4 studies: 16% to 32%) at 52 weeks. In limited data from a long-term follow-up trial in patients who continued 100 mg/day lamivudine after one of these studies, YMDD substitutions further increased from 18% (10 of 57) at 1 year to 41% (20 of 49), 53% (27 of 51), and 69% (31 of 45) after 2, 3, and 4 years of treatment, respectively. Over the 5-year treatment period, the proportion of patients who developed YMDD-mutant HBV at any time was 69% (40 of 58).

In a controlled trial in pediatric patients, YMDD-mutant HBV was detected in 31 of 166 (19%) patients receiving lamivudine for 52 weeks. For a subgroup who remained on lamivudine therapy in a follow-up study, YMDD mutations increased from 24% (29 of 121) at 12 months to 59% (68 of 115) at 24 months and 64% (66 of 103) at 36 months of lamivudine treatment.

In a controlled study, treatment-naive patients with HBeAg-positive CHB were treated with lamivudine or lamivudine plus adefovir dipivoxil combination therapy. Following 104 weeks of therapy, YMDD-mutant HBV was detected in 7 of 40 (18%) patients receiving combination therapy compared with 15 of 35 (43%) patients receiving lamivudine-only therapy. In another controlled study, combination therapy was evaluated in adult patients with HBeAg-positive CHB who had YMDD-mutant HBV and diminished clinical and virologic response to lamivudine. Following 52 weeks of lamivudine plus adefovir dipivoxil combination therapy (n = 46) or lamivudine-only therapy (n = 49), YMDD-mutant HBV was detected less frequently in patients receiving combination therapy, 62% vs 96%.

A published study suggested that the rates of lamivudine resistance in patients treated for HBeAg-negative CHB appear to be more variable (0% to 27% at 1 year and 10% to 56% at 2 years).

Cross-Resistance
HBV
HBV containing lamivudine resistance-associated substitutions (rtL180M, rtM204I, rtM204V, rtL180M + rtM204V, rtV173L + rtL180M + rtM204V) retain susceptibility to adefovir dipivoxil but have reduced susceptibility to entecavir (30 fold) and telbivudine (>100 fold). The lamivudine

resistance-associated substitution rtA181T results in diminished response to adefovir and telbivudine. Similarly, HBV with entecavir resistance-associated substitutions (I169T/M250V and T184G/S202I) have >1,000-fold reductions in susceptibility to lamivudine.

HIV
In studies of HIV-1-infected patients who received lamivudine monotherapy or combination therapy with lamivudine plus zidovudine for at least 12 weeks, HIV-1 isolates with reduced susceptibility in cell culture to lamivudine were detected in most patients (see WARNINGS).

CLINICAL PHARMACOLOGY
Pharmacokinetics in Adults
The pharmacokinetic properties of lamivudine have been studied as single and multiple oral doses ranging from 5 to 600 mg per day administered to HBV-infected patients.
The pharmacokinetic properties of lamivudine have also been studied in asymptomatic, HIV-infected adult patients after administration of single intravenous (IV) doses ranging from 0.25 to 8 mg/kg, as well as single and multiple (twice-daily regimen) oral doses ranging from 0.25 to 10 mg/kg.

Absorption and Bioavailability
Lamivudine was rapidly absorbed after oral administration in HBV-infected patients and in healthy subjects. Following single oral doses of 100 mg, the peak serum lamivudine concentration (C_{max}) in HBV-infected patients (steady state) and healthy subjects (single dose) was 1.28 ± 0.56 mcg/mL and 1.05 ± 0.32 mcg/mL (mean $\pm$ SD), respectively, which occurred between 0.5 and 2 hours after administration. The area under the plasma concentration versus time curve ($AUC_{[0-24 \text{ hr}]}$) following 100 mg lamivudine oral single and repeated daily doses to steady state was 4.3 ± 1.4 (mean $\pm$ SD) and 4.7 ± 1.7 mcg•hr/mL, respectively. The relative bioavailability of the tablet and solution were then demonstrated in healthy subjects. Although the solution demonstrated a slightly higher peak serum concentration (C_{max}), there was no significant difference in systemic exposure (AUC_∞) between the solution and the tablet. Therefore, the solution and the tablet may be used interchangeably. After oral administration of lamivudine once daily to HBV-infected adults, the AUC and C_{max} increased in proportion to dose over the range from 5 mg to 600 mg once daily. The 100-mg tablet was administered orally to 24 healthy subjects on 2 occasions, once in the fasted state and once with food (standard meal: 967 kcal; 67 grams fat, 33 grams protein, 58 grams carbohydrate). There was no significant difference in systemic exposure (AUC_∞) in the fed and fasted states; therefore, EPIVIR-HBV Tablets and Oral Solution may be administered with or without food. Lamivudine was rapidly absorbed after oral administration in HIV-infected patients. Absolute bioavailability in 12 adult patients was $86\% \pm 16\%$ (mean $\pm$ SD) for the 150-mg tablet and $87\% \pm 13\%$ for the 10-mg/mL oral solution.

Distribution
The apparent volume of distribution after IV administration of lamivudine to 20 asymptomatic HIV-infected patients was 1.3 ± 0.4 L/kg, suggesting that lamivudine distributes into extravascular spaces. Volume of distribution was independent of dose and did not correlate with body weight.
Binding of lamivudine to human plasma proteins is low (<36%) and independent of dose. In vitro studies showed that over the concentration range of 0.1 to 100 mcg/mL, the amount of lamivudine associated with erythrocytes ranged from 53% to 57% and was independent of concentration.

Metabolism
Metabolism of lamivudine is a minor route of elimination. In man, the only known metabolite of lamivudine is the trans-sulfoxide metabolite. In 9 healthy subjects receiving 300 mg of lamivudine as single oral doses, a total of 4.2% (range 1.5% to 7.5%) of the dose was excreted as the trans-sulfoxide metabolite in the urine, the majority of which was excreted in the first 12 hours. Serum concentrations of the trans-sulfoxide metabolite have not been determined.

Elimination
The majority of lamivudine is eliminated unchanged in urine by active organic cationic secretion. In 9 healthy subjects given a single 300-mg oral dose of lamivudine, renal clearance was 199.7 ± 56.9 mL/min (mean $\pm$ SD). In 20 HIV-infected patients given a single IV dose, renal clearance was 280.4 ± 75.2 mL/min (mean $\pm$ SD), representing $71\% \pm 16\%$ (mean $\pm$ SD) of total clearance of lamivudine. In most single-dose studies in HIV- or HBV-infected patients or healthy subjects with serum sampling for 24 hours after dosing, the observed mean elimination half-life ($t_{1/2}$) ranged from 5 to 7 hours. In HIV-infected patients, total clearance was 398.5 ± 69.1 mL/min (mean $\pm$ SD). Oral clearance and elimination half-life were independent of dose and body weight over an oral dosing range from 0.25 to 10 mg/kg.

Table 1. Pharmacokinetic Parameters (Mean ± SD) Dose-Normalized to a Single 100-mg Oral Dose of Lamivudine in Patients With Varying Degrees of Renal Function

Parameter	Creatinine Clearance Criterion (Number of Subjects)		
	≥80 mL/min (n = 9)	20-59 mL/min (n = 8)	<20 mL/min (n = 6)
Creatinine clearance (mL/min)	97 (range 82-117)	39 (range 25-49)	15 (range 13-19)
C_{max} (mcg/mL)	1.31 ± 0.35	1.85 ± 0.40	1.55 ± 0.31
AUC_∞ (mcg•hr/mL)	5.28 ± 1.01	14.67 ± 3.74	27.33 ± 6.56
Cl/F (mL/min)	326.4 ± 63.8	120.1 ± 29.5	64.5 ± 18.3

Table 2. Pharmacokinetic Parameters (Mean ± SD) Dose-Normalized to a Single 100-mg Dose of Lamivudine in 3 Groups of Subjects With Normal or Impaired Hepatic Function

Parameter	Normal (n = 8)	Impairment*	
		Moderate (n = 8)	Severe (n = 8)
C_{max} (mcg/mL)	0.92 ± 0.31	1.06 ± 0.58	1.08 ± 0.27
AUC_∞ (mcg•hr/mL)	3.96 ± 0.58	3.97 ± 1.36	4.30 ± 0.63
T_{max} (hr)	1.3 ± 0.8	1.4 ± 0.8	1.4 ± 1.2
Cl/F (mL/min)	424.7 ± 61.9	456.9 ± 129.8	395.2 ± 51.8
Clr (mL/min)	279.2 ± 79.2	323.5 ± 100.9	216.1 ± 58.0

*Hepatic impairment assessed by aminopyrine breath test.

Special Populations
Adults With Impaired Renal Function
The pharmacokinetic properties of lamivudine have been determined in healthy subjects and in subjects with impaired renal function, with and without hemodialysis (Table 1).
[See table 1 above]
Exposure (AUC_∞), C_{max}, and half-life increased with diminishing renal function (as expressed by creatinine clearance). Apparent total oral clearance (Cl/F) of lamivudine decreased as creatinine clearance decreased. T_{max} was not significantly affected by renal function. Based on these observations, it is recommended that the dosage of lamivudine be modified in patients with renal impairment (see DOSAGE AND ADMINISTRATION).
Hemodialysis increases lamivudine clearance from a mean of 64 to 88 mL/min; however, the length of time of hemodialysis (4 hours) was insufficient to significantly alter mean lamivudine exposure after a single-dose administration. Continuous ambulatory peritoneal dialysis and automated peritoneal dialysis have negligible effects on lamivudine clearance. Therefore, it is recommended, following correction of dose for creatinine clearance, that no additional dose modification be made after routine hemodialysis or peritoneal dialysis.
It is not known whether lamivudine can be removed by continuous (24-hour) hemodialysis.
The effect of renal impairment on lamivudine pharmacokinetics in pediatric patients with chronic hepatitis B is not known.

Adults With Impaired Hepatic Function
The pharmacokinetic properties of lamivudine have been determined in adults with impaired hepatic function (Table 2). Patients were stratified by severity of hepatic functional impairment.
[See table 2 above]
Pharmacokinetic parameters were not altered by diminishing hepatic function. Therefore, no dose adjustment for lamivudine is required for patients with impaired hepatic function. Safety and efficacy of EPIVIR-HBV have not been established in the presence of decompensated liver disease (see PRECAUTIONS).

Post-Hepatic Transplant
Fourteen HBV-infected patients received liver transplant following lamivudine therapy and completed pharmacokinetic assessments at enrollment, 2 weeks after 100-mg once-daily dosing (pre-transplant), and 3 months following transplant; there were no significant differences in pharmacokinetic parameters. The overall exposure of lamivudine is primarily affected by renal dysfunction; consequently, transplant patients with reduced renal function had generally higher exposure than patients with normal renal function. Safety and efficacy of EPIVIR-HBV have not been established in this population (see PRECAUTIONS).

Pediatric Patients
Lamivudine pharmacokinetics were evaluated in a 28-day dose-ranging study in 53 pediatric patients with chronic hepatitis B. Patients aged 2 to 12 years were randomized to receive lamivudine 0.35 mg/kg twice daily, 3 mg/kg once daily, 1.5 mg/kg twice daily, or 4 mg/kg twice daily. Patients aged 13 to 17 years received lamivudine 100 mg once daily. Lamivudine was rapidly absorbed (T_{max} 0.5 to 1 hour). In general, both C_{max} and exposure (AUC) showed dose proportionality in the dosing range studied. Weight-corrected oral clearance was highest at age 2 and declined from 2 to 12 years, where values were then similar to those seen in adults. A dose of 3 mg/kg given once daily produced a steady-state lamivudine AUC (mean 5,953 ng•hr/mL ± 1,562 SD) similar to that associated with a dose of 100 mg/day in adults.

Gender
There are no significant gender differences in lamivudine pharmacokinetics.

Race
There are no significant racial differences in lamivudine pharmacokinetics.

Drug Interactions
Multiple doses of lamivudine and a single dose of interferon were coadministered to 19 healthy male subjects in a pharmacokinetics study. Results indicated a small (10%) reduction in lamivudine AUC, but no change in interferon pharmacokinetic parameters when the 2 drugs were given in combination. All other pharmacokinetic parameters (C_{max}, T_{max}, and $t_{1/2}$) were unchanged. There was no significant pharmacokinetic interaction between lamivudine and interferon alfa in this study.
Lamivudine and zidovudine were coadministered to 12 asymptomatic HIV-positive adult patients in a single-center, open-label, randomized, crossover study. No significant differences were observed in AUC_∞ or total clearance for lamivudine or zidovudine when the 2 drugs were administered together. Coadministration of lamivudine with zidovudine resulted in an increase of $39\% \pm 62\%$ (mean $\pm$ SD) in C_{max} of zidovudine.
Lamivudine and trimethoprim/sulfamethoxazole (TMP/SMX) were coadministered to 14 HIV-positive patients in a single-center, open-label, randomized, crossover study. Each patient received treatment with a single 300-mg dose of lamivudine and TMP 160 mg/SMX 800 mg once a day for 5 days with concomitant administration of lamivudine 300 mg with the fifth dose in a crossover design. Coadministration of TMP/SMX with lamivudine resulted in an increase of $44\% \pm 23\%$ (mean $\pm$ SD) in lamivudine AUC_∞, a decrease of $29\% + 13\%$ in lamivudine oral clearance, and a decrease of $30\% \pm 36\%$ in lamivudine renal clearance. The pharmacokinetic properties of TMP and SMX were not altered by coadministration with lamivudine (see PRECAUTIONS: Drug Interactions).

Table 3. Histologic Response at Week 52 Among Adult Patients Receiving EPIVIR-HBV 100 mg Once Daily or Placebo

Assessment	Study 1		Study 2		Study 3	
	EPIVIR-HBV (n = 62)	Placebo (n = 63)	EPIVIR-HBV (n = 131)	Placebo (n = 68)	EPIVIR-HBV (n = 110)	Placebo) (n = 54)
Improvement*	55%	25%	56%	26%	56%	26%
No Improvement	27%	59%	36%	62%	25%	54%
Missing Data	18%	16%	8%	12%	19%	20%

* Improvement was defined as a ≥2-point decrease in the Knodell Histologic Activity Index (HAI)[1] at Week 52 compared with pretreatment HAI. Patients with missing data at baseline were excluded.

Table 4. HBeAg Seroconversion* at Week 52 Among Adult Patients Receiving EPIVIR-HBV 100 mg Once Daily or Placebo

Seroconversion	Study 1		Study 2		Study 3	
	EPIVIR-HBV (n = 63)	Placebo (n = 69)	EPIVIR-HBV (n = 140)	Placebo (n = 70)	EPIVIR-HBV (n = 108)	Placebo (n = 53)
Responder	17%	6%	16%	4%	15%	13%
Nonresponder	67%	78%	80%	91%	69%	68%
Missing Data	16%	16%	4%	4%	17%	19%

* Three-component seroconversion was defined as Week 52 values showing loss of HBeAg, gain of HBeAb, and reduction of HBV DNA to below the solution-hybridization assay limit. Subjects with negative baseline HBeAg or HBV DNA assay were excluded from the analysis.

Lamivudine and zalcitabine may inhibit the intracellular phosphorylation of one another. Therefore, use of lamivudine in combination with zalcitabine is not recommended.

INDICATIONS AND USAGE

EPIVIR-HBV is indicated for the treatment of chronic hepatitis B associated with evidence of hepatitis B viral replication and active liver inflammation. This indication is based on 1-year histologic and serologic responses in adult patients with compensated chronic hepatitis B, and more limited information from a study in pediatric patients ages 2 to 17 years (see Description of Clinical Studies below).

Description of Clinical Studies

Adults

The safety and efficacy of EPIVIR-HBV were evaluated in 4 controlled studies in 967 patients with compensated chronic hepatitis B. All patients were 16 years of age or older and had chronic hepatitis B virus infection (serum HBsAg positive for at least 6 months) accompanied by evidence of HBV replication (serum HBeAg positive and positive for serum HBV DNA, as measured by a research solution-hybridization assay) and persistently elevated ALT levels and/or chronic inflammation on liver biopsy compatible with a diagnosis of chronic viral hepatitis. Three of these studies provided comparisons of EPIVIR-HBV 100 mg once daily versus placebo, and results of these comparisons are summarized below.

- Study 1 was a randomized, double-blind study of EPIVIR-HBV 100 mg once daily versus placebo for 52 weeks followed by a 16-week no-treatment period in treatment-naive US patients.
- Study 2 was a randomized, double-blind, 3-arm study that compared EPIVIR-HBV 25 mg once daily versus EPIVIR-HBV 100 mg once daily versus placebo for 52 weeks in Asian patients.
- Study 3 was a randomized, partially-blind, 3-arm study conducted primarily in North America and Europe in patients who had ongoing evidence of active chronic hepatitis B despite previous treatment with interferon alfa. The study compared EPIVIR-HBV 100 mg once daily for 52 weeks, followed by either EPIVIR-HBV 100 mg or matching placebo once daily for 16 weeks (Arm 1), versus placebo once daily for 68 weeks (Arm 2). (A third arm using a combination of interferon and lamivudine is not presented here because there was not sufficient information to evaluate this regimen.)

Principal endpoint comparisons for the histologic and serologic outcomes in lamivudine (100 mg daily) and placebo recipients in placebo-controlled studies are shown in the following tables.

[See table 3 above]

[See table 4 above]

Normalization of serum ALT levels was more frequent with lamivudine treatment compared with placebo in Studies 1-3.

The majority of lamivudine-treated patients showed a decrease of HBV DNA to below the assay limit early in the course of therapy. However, reappearance of assay-detectable HBV DNA during lamivudine treatment was observed in approximately one third of patients after this initial response.

Pediatrics

The safety and efficacy of EPIVIR-HBV were evaluated in a double-blind clinical trial in 286 patients ranging from 2 to 17 years of age, who were randomized (2:1) to receive 52 weeks of lamivudine (3 mg/kg once daily to a maximum of 100 mg once daily) or placebo. All patients had compensated chronic hepatitis B accompanied by evidence of hepatitis B virus replication (positive serum HBeAg and positive for serum HBV DNA by a research branched-chain DNA assay) and persistently elevated serum ALT levels. The combination of loss of HBeAg and reduction of HBV DNA to below the assay limit of the research assay, evaluated at Week 52, was observed in 23% of lamivudine subjects and 13% of placebo subjects. Normalization of serum ALT was achieved and maintained to Week 52 more frequently in patients treated with EPIVIR-HBV compared with placebo (55% versus 13%). As in the adult controlled trials, most lamivudine-treated subjects had decreases in HBV DNA below the assay limit early in treatment, but about one third of subjects with this initial response had reappearance of assay-detectable HBV DNA during treatment. Adolescents (ages 13 to 17 years) showed less evidence of treatment effect than younger children.

CONTRAINDICATIONS

EPIVIR-HBV Tablets and EPIVIR-HBV Oral Solution are contraindicated in patients with previously demonstrated clinically significant hypersensitivity to any of the components of the products.

WARNINGS

Lactic Acidosis/Severe Hepatomegaly With Steatosis

Lactic acidosis and severe hepatomegaly with steatosis, including fatal cases, have been reported with the use of nucleoside analogues alone or in combination, including lamivudine and other antiretrovirals. A majority of these cases have been in women. Obesity and prolonged nucleoside exposure may be risk factors. Most of these reports have described patients receiving nucleoside analogues for treatment of HIV infection, but there have been reports of lactic acidosis in patients receiving lamivudine for hepatitis B. Particular caution should be exercised when administering EPIVIR or EPIVIR-HBV to any patient with known risk factors for liver disease; however, cases have also been reported in patients with no known risk factors. Treatment with EPIVIR or EPIVIR-HBV should be suspended in any patient who develops clinical or laboratory findings suggestive of lactic acidosis or pronounced hepatotoxicity (which may include hepatomegaly and steatosis even in the absence of marked transaminase elevations).

Important Differences Between Lamivudine-Containing Products, HIV Testing, and Risk of Emergence of Resistant HIV

EPIVIR-HBV Tablets and Oral Solution contain a lower dose of the same active ingredient (lamivudine) as EPIVIR Tablets and Oral Solution, COMBIVIR® (lamivudine/zidovudine) Tablets, EPZICOM® (abacavir sulfate and lamivudine) Tablets, and TRIZIVIR® (abacavir, lamivudine, and zidovudine) Tablets used to treat HIV infection. The formulation and dosage of lamivudine in EPIVIR-HBV are not appropriate for patients dually infected with HBV and HIV. If a decision is made to administer lamivudine to such patients, the higher dosage indicated for HIV therapy should be used as part of an appropriate combination regimen, and the prescribing information for EPIVIR, COMBIVIR, EPZICOM, or TRIZIVIR as well as for EPIVIR-HBV should be consulted. HIV counseling and testing should be offered to all patients before beginning EPIVIR-HBV and periodically during treatment because of the risk of rapid emergence of resistant HIV and limitation of treatment options if EPIVIR-HBV is prescribed to treat chronic hepatitis B in a patient who has unrecognized or untreated HIV infection or acquires HIV infection during treatment.

Posttreatment Exacerbations of Hepatitis

Clinical and laboratory evidence of exacerbations of hepatitis have occurred after discontinuation of EPIVIR-HBV (these have been primarily detected by serum ALT elevations, in addition to the re-emergence of HBV DNA commonly observed after stopping treatment; see Table 7 for more information regarding frequency of posttreatment ALT elevations. Although most events appear to have been self-limited, fatalities have been reported in some cases. The causal relationship to discontinuation of lamivudine treatment is unknown. Patients should be closely monitored with both clinical and laboratory follow-up for at least several months after stopping treatment. There is insufficient evidence to determine whether re-initiation of therapy alters the course of posttreatment exacerbations of hepatitis.

Pancreatitis

Pancreatitis has been reported in patients receiving lamivudine, particularly in HIV-infected pediatric patients with prior nucleoside exposure.

PRECAUTIONS

General

Patients should be assessed before beginning treatment with EPIVIR-HBV by a physician experienced in the management of chronic hepatitis B.

Emergence of Resistance-Associated HBV Mutations

In controlled clinical trials, YMDD-mutant HBV were detected in patients with on-lamivudine re-appearance of HBV DNA after an initial decline below the solution-hybridization assay limit (see MICROBIOLOGY: Drug Resistance). These mutations can be detected by a research assay and have been associated with reduced susceptibility to lamivudine in vitro. Lamivudine-treated patients (adult and pediatric) with YMDD-mutant HBV at 52 weeks showed diminished treatment responses in comparison to lamivudine-treated patients without evidence of YMDD mutations, including lower rates of HBeAg seroconversion and HBeAg loss (no greater than placebo recipients), more frequent return of positive HBV DNA by solution-hybridization or branched-chain DNA assay, and more frequent ALT elevations. In the controlled trials, when patients developed YMDD-mutant HBV, they had a rise in HBV DNA and ALT from their own previous on-treatment levels. Progression of hepatitis B, including death, has been reported in some patients with YMDD-mutant HBV, including patients from the liver transplant setting and from other clinical trials. In clinical practice, monitoring of ALT and HBV DNA levels during lamivudine treatment may aid in treatment decisions if emergence of viral mutants is suspected.

Limitations of Populations Studied

Safety and efficacy of EPIVIR-HBV have not been established in patients with decompensated liver disease or organ transplants; pediatric patients <2 years of age; patients dually infected with HBV and HCV, hepatitis delta, or HIV; or other populations not included in the principal phase III controlled studies. There are no studies in pregnant women and no data regarding effect on vertical transmission, and appropriate infant immunizations should be used to prevent neonatal acquisition of HBV.

Assessing Patients During Treatment

Patients should be monitored regularly during treatment by a physician experienced in the management of chronic hepatitis B. The safety and effectiveness of treatment with EPIVIR-HBV beyond 1 year have not been established. During treatment, combinations of such events such as return of persistently elevated ALT, increasing levels of HBV DNA over time after an initial decline below assay limit, progression of clinical signs or symptoms of hepatic disease, and/or worsening of hepatic necroinflammatory findings may be considered as potentially reflecting loss of therapeutic response. Such observations should be taken into consideration when determining the advisability of continuing therapy with EPIVIR-HBV.

The optimal duration of treatment, the durability of HBeAg seroconversions occurring during treatment, and the relationship between treatment response and long-term outcomes such as hepatocellular carcinoma or decompensated cirrhosis are not known.

Patients With Impaired Renal Function

Reduction of the dosage of EPIVIR-HBV is recommended for patients with impaired renal function (see CLINICAL PHARMACOLOGY and DOSAGE AND ADMINISTRATION).

Information for Patients

A Patient Package Insert (PPI) for EPIVIR-HBV is available for patient information.

Patients should remain under the care of a physician while taking EPIVIR-HBV. They should discuss any new symptoms or concurrent medications with their physician.

Patients should be advised that EPIVIR-HBV is not a cure for hepatitis B, that the long-term treatment benefits of EPIVIR-HBV are unknown at this time, and, in particular, that the relationship of initial treatment response to outcomes such as hepatocellular carcinoma and decompensated cirrhosis is unknown. Patients should be informed that deterioration of liver disease has occurred in some cases when treatment was discontinued. Patients should be advised to discuss any changes in regimen with their physician.

Patients should be informed that emergence of resistant hepatitis B virus and worsening of disease can occur during treatment, and they should promptly report any new symptoms to their physician.

Patients should be counseled on the importance of testing for HIV to avoid inappropriate therapy and development of resistant HIV, and HIV counseling and testing should be offered before starting EPIVIR-HBV and periodically during therapy. Patients should be advised that EPIVIR-HBV Tablets and EPIVIR-HBV Oral Solution contain a lower dose of the same active ingredient (lamivudine) as EPIVIR Tablets, EPIVIR Oral Solution, COMBIVIR Tablets, EPZICOM Tablets, and TRIZIVIR Tablets. EPIVIR-HBV should not be taken concurrently with EPIVIR, COMBIVIR, EPZICOM, or TRIZIVIR (see WARNINGS). Patients infected with both HBV and HIV who are planning to change their HIV treatment regimen to a regimen that does not include EPIVIR, COMBIVIR, EPZICOM, or TRIZIVIR should discuss continued therapy for hepatitis B with their physician.

Patients should be advised that treatment with EPIVIR-HBV has not been shown to reduce the risk of transmission of HBV to others through sexual contact or blood contamination (see Pregnancy section).

Diabetic patients should be advised that each 20-mL dose of EPIVIR-HBV Oral Solution contains 4 grams of sucrose.

Drug Interactions

Lamivudine is predominantly eliminated in the urine by active organic cationic secretion. The possibility of interactions with other drugs administered concurrently should be considered, particularly when their main route of elimination is active renal secretion via the organic cationic transport system (e.g., trimethoprim).

TMP 160 mg/SMX 800 mg once daily has been shown to increase lamivudine exposure (AUC) by 44% (see CLINICAL PHARMACOLOGY). No change in dose of either drug is recommended. There is no information regarding the effect on lamivudine pharmacokinetics of higher doses of TMP/ SMX such as those used in vivo to treat *Pneumocystis carinii* pneumonia. No data are available regarding interactions with other drugs that have renal clearance mechanisms similar to that of lamivudine.

Lamivudine and zalcitabine may inhibit the intracellular phosphorylation of one another. Therefore, use of lamivudine in combination with zalcitabine is not recommended.

Carcinogenesis, Mutagenesis, and Impairment of Fertility

Lamivudine long-term carcinogenicity studies in mice and rats showed no evidence of carcinogenic potential at exposures up to 34 times (mice) and 200 times (rats) those observed in humans at the recommended therapeutic dose for chronic hepatitis B. Lamivudine was not active in a microbial mutagenicity screen or an in vitro cell transformation assay, but showed weak in vitro mutagenic activity in a cytogenetic assay using cultured human lymphocytes and in the mouse lymphoma assay. However, lamivudine showed no evidence of in vivo genotoxic activity in the rat at oral doses of up to 2,000 mg/kg producing plasma levels of 60 to 70 times those in humans at the recommended dose for chronic hepatitis B. In a study of reproductive performance, lamivudine administered to rats at doses up to 4,000 mg/kg/ day, producing plasma levels 80 to 120 times those in humans, revealed no evidence of impaired fertility and no effect on the survival, growth, and development to weaning of the offspring.

Pregnancy

Pregnancy Category C. Reproduction studies have been performed in rats and rabbits at orally administered doses up to 4,000 mg/kg/day and 1,000 mg/kg/day, respectively, producing plasma levels up to approximately 60 times that for the adult HBV dose. No evidence of teratogenicity due to lamivudine was observed. Evidence of early embryolethality was seen in the rabbit at exposure levels similar to those observed in humans, but there was no indication of this ef-

fect in the rat at exposures up to 60 times that in humans. Studies in pregnant rats and rabbits showed that lamivudine is transferred to the fetus through the placenta. There are no adequate and well-controlled studies in pregnant women. Because animal reproductive toxicity studies are not always predictive of human response, lamivudine should be used during pregnancy only if the potential benefits outweigh the risks.

Lamivudine has not been shown to affect the transmission of HBV from mother to infant, and appropriate infant immunizations should be used to prevent neonatal acquisition of HBV.

Pregnancy Registry

To monitor maternal-fetal outcomes of pregnant women exposed to lamivudine, a Pregnancy Registry has been established. Physicians are encouraged to register patients by calling 1-800-258-4263.

Nursing Mothers

A study in lactating rats administered 45 mg/kg of lamivudine showed that lamivudine concentrations in milk were slightly greater than those in plasma. Lamivudine is also excreted in human milk. Samples of breast milk obtained from 20 mothers receiving lamivudine monotherapy (300 mg twice daily) or combination therapy (150 mg lamivudine twice daily and 300 mg zidovudine twice daily) had measurable concentrations of lamivudine.

Because of the potential for serious adverse reactions in nursing infants, **mothers should be instructed not to breastfeed if they are receiving lamivudine.**

Pediatric Use

HBV

Safety and efficacy of lamivudine for treatment of chronic hepatitis B in children have been studied in pediatric patients from 2 to 17 years of age in a controlled clinical trial (see CLINICAL PHARMACOLOGY, INDICATIONS AND USAGE, and DOSAGE AND ADMINISTRATION).

Safety and efficacy in pediatric patients <2 years of age have not been established.

HIV

See the complete prescribing information for EPIVIR Tablets and Oral Solution for additional information on pharmacokinetics of lamivudine in HIV-infected children.

Geriatric Use

Clinical studies of EPIVIR-HBV did not include sufficient numbers of subjects aged 65 and over to determine whether they respond differently from younger subjects. In general, dose selection for an elderly patient should be cautious, reflecting the greater frequency of decreased hepatic, renal, or cardiac function, and of concomitant disease or other drug therapy. In particular, because lamivudine is substantially excreted by the kidney and elderly patients are more likely to have decreased renal function, renal function should be monitored and dosage adjustments should be made accordingly (see PRECAUTIONS: Patients with Impaired Renal Function and DOSAGE AND ADMINISTRATION).

ADVERSE REACTIONS

Several serious adverse events reported with lamivudine (lactic acidosis and severe hepatomegaly with steatosis, posttreatment exacerbations of hepatitis B, pancreatitis, and emergence of viral mutants associated with reduced drug susceptibility and diminished treatment response) are also described in WARNINGS and PRECAUTIONS.

Clinical Trials In Chronic Hepatitis B

Adults

Selected clinical adverse events observed with a ≥5% frequency during therapy with EPIVIR-HBV compared with

Table 6. Frequencies of Specified Laboratory Abnormalities in 3 Placebo-Controlled Trials in Adults During Treatment* (Studies 1-3)

Test (Abnormal Level)	Patients With Abnormality/Patients With Observations	
	EPIVIR-HBV	Placebo
ALT >3 × baseline[†]	37/331 (11%)	26/199 (13%)
Albumin <2.5 g/dL	0/331 (0%)	2/199 (1%)
Amylase >3 × baseline	2/259 (<1%)	4/167 (2%)
Serum Lipase ≥2.5 × ULN[‡]	19/189 (10%)	9/127 (7%)
CPK ≥7 × baseline	31/329 (9%)	9/198 (5%)
Neutrophils <750/mm^3	0/331 (0%)	1/199 (<1%)
Platelets <50,000/mm^3	10/272 (4%)	5/168 (3%)

* Includes patients treated for 52 to 68 weeks.
[†] See Table 7 for posttreatment ALT values.
[‡] Includes observations during and after treatment in the 2 placebo-controlled trials that collected this information.
ULN = Upper limit of normal.

placebo are listed in Table 5. Frequencies of specified laboratory abnormalities during therapy with EPIVIR-HBV compared with placebo are listed in Table 6.

Table 5. Selected Clinical Adverse Events (≥5% Frequency) in 3 Placebo-Controlled Clinical Trials in Adults During Treatment* (Studies 1-3)

Adverse Event	EPIVIR-HBV (n = 332)	Placebo (n = 200)
Non-site Specific		
Malaise and fatigue	24%	28%
Fever or chills	7%	9%
Ear, Nose, and Throat		
Ear, nose, and throat infections	25%	21%
Sore throat	13%	8%
Gastrointestinal		
Nausea and vomiting	15%	17%
Abdominal discomfort and pain	16%	17%
Diarrhea	14%	12%
Musculoskeletal		
Myalgia	14%	17%
Arthralgia	7%	5%
Neurological		
Headache	21%	21%
Skin		
Skin rashes	5%	5%

*Includes patients treated for 52 to 68 weeks.

[See table 6 above]

In patients followed for up to 16 weeks after discontinuation of treatment, posttreatment ALT elevations were observed more frequently in patients who had received EPIVIR-HBV than in patients who had received placebo. A comparison of ALT elevations between Weeks 52 and 68 in patients who discontinued EPIVIR-HBV at Week 52 and patients in the same studies who received placebo throughout the treatment course is shown in Table 7.

[See table 7 at top of next page]

Lamivudine in Patients With HIV

In HIV-infected patients, safety information reflects a higher dose of lamivudine (150 mg b.i.d.) than the dose used to treat chronic hepatitis B in HIV-negative patients. In clinical trials using lamivudine as part of a combination regimen for treatment of HIV infection, several clinical adverse events occurred more often in lamivudine-containing treatment arms than in comparator arms. These included nasal signs and symptoms (20% vs. 11%), dizziness (10% vs. 4%), and depressive disorders (9% vs. 4%). Pancreatitis was observed in 9 of the 2,613 adult patients (<0.5%) who received EPIVIR in controlled clinical trials. Laboratory abnormalities reported more often in lamivudine-containing arms included neutropenia and elevations of liver function tests (also more frequent in lamivudine-containing arms for a retrospective analysis of HIV/HBV dually infected patients in one study), and amylase elevations. Please see the complete prescribing information for EPIVIR Tablets and Oral Solution for more information.

Pediatric Patients With Hepatitis B

Most commonly observed adverse events in the pediatric trials were similar to those in adult trials; in addition, respiratory symptoms (cough, bronchitis, and viral respiratory infections) were reported in both lamivudine and placebo

Table 7. Posttreatment ALT Elevations in 2 Placebo-Controlled Studies in Adults With No-Active-Treatment Follow-up (Studies 1 and 3)

Abnormal Value	Patients With ALT Elevation/ Patients With Observations*	
	EPIVIR-HBV	Placebo
ALT ≥2 × baseline value	37/137 (27%)	22/116 (19%)
ALT ≥3 × baseline value†	29/137 (21%)	9/116 (8%)
ALT ≥2 × baseline value and absolute ALT >500 IU/L	21/137 (15%)	8/116 (7%)
ALT ≥2 × baseline value; and bilirubin >2 × ULN and ≥2 × baseline value	1/137 (0.7%)	1/116 (0.9%)

* Each patient may be represented in one or more category.
† Comparable to a Grade 3 toxicity in accordance with modified WHO criteria.
ULN = Upper limit of normal.

recipients. Posttreatment transaminase elevations were observed in some patients followed after cessation of lamivudine.

Pediatric Patients With HIV Infection
In early open-label studies of lamivudine in children with HIV, peripheral neuropathy and neutropenia were reported, and pancreatitis was observed in 14% to 15% of patients.

Observed During Clinical Practice
The following events have been identified during post-approval use of lamivudine in clinical practice. Because they are reported voluntarily from a population of unknown size, estimates of frequency cannot be made. These events have been chosen for inclusion due to either their seriousness, frequency of reporting, potential causal connection to lamivudine, or a combination of these factors. Post-marketing experience with lamivudine at this time is largely limited to use in HIV-infected patients.

Digestive
Stomatitis.
Endocrine and Metabolic
Hyperglycemia.
General
Weakness.
Hemic and Lymphatic
Anemia (including pure red cell aplasia and severe anemias progressing on therapy), lymphadenopathy, splenomegaly.
Hepatic and Pancreatic
Lactic acidosis and steatosis, pancreatitis, posttreatment exacerbation of hepatitis (see WARNINGS and PRECAUTIONS).
Hypersensitivity
Anaphylaxis, urticaria.
Musculoskeletal
Rhabdomyolysis.
Nervous
Paresthesia, peripheral neuropathy.
Respiratory
Abnormal breath sounds/wheezing.
Skin
Alopecia, pruritus, rash.

OVERDOSAGE
There is no known antidote for EPIVIR-HBV. One case of an adult ingesting 6 g of EPIVIR was reported; there were no clinical signs or symptoms noted and hematologic tests remained normal. Because a negligible amount of lamivudine was removed via (4-hour) hemodialysis, continuous ambulatory peritoneal dialysis, and automated peritoneal dialysis, it is not known if continuous hemodialysis would provide clinical benefit in a lamivudine overdose event. If overdose occurs, the patient should be monitored, and standard supportive treatment applied as required.

DOSAGE AND ADMINISTRATION
Adults
The recommended oral dose of EPIVIR-HBV for treatment of chronic hepatitis B in adults is 100 mg once daily (see paragraph below and WARNINGS). Safety and effectiveness of treatment beyond 1 year have not been established and the optimum duration of treatment is not known (see PRECAUTIONS).
The formulation and dosage of lamivudine in EPIVIR-HBV are not appropriate for patients dually infected with HBV and HIV. If lamivudine is administered to such patients, the higher dosage indicated for HIV therapy should be used as part of an appropriate combination regimen, and the prescribing information for EPIVIR as well as EPIVIR-HBV should be consulted.
Pediatric Patients
The recommended oral dose of EPIVIR-HBV for pediatric patients 2 to 17 years of age with chronic hepatitis B is 3 mg/kg once daily up to a maximum daily dose of 100 mg. Safety and effectiveness of treatment beyond 1 year have not been established and the optimum duration of treatment is not known (see PRECAUTIONS).

EPIVIR-HBV is available in a 5-mg/mL oral solution when a liquid formulation is needed. (Please see information above regarding distinctions between different lamivudine-containing products.)

Dose Adjustment
It is recommended that doses of EPIVIR-HBV be adjusted in accordance with renal function (Table 8) (see CLINICAL PHARMACOLOGY: Special Populations).

Table 8. Adjustment of Adult Dosage of EPIVIR-HBV in Accordance With Creatinine Clearance

Creatinine Clearance (mL/min)	Recommended Dosage of EPIVIR-HBV
≥50	100 mg once daily
30-49	100 mg first dose, then 50 mg once daily
15-29	100 mg first dose, then 25 mg once daily
5-14	35 mg first dose, then 15 mg once daily
<5	35 mg first dose, then 10 mg once daily

No additional dosing of EPIVIR-HBV is required after routine (4-hour) hemodialysis or peritoneal dialysis.
Although there are insufficient data to recommend a specific dose adjustment of EPIVIR-HBV in pediatric patients with renal impairment, a dose reduction should be considered.

HOW SUPPLIED
EPIVIR-HBV Tablets, 100 mg, are butterscotch-colored, film-coated, biconvex, capsule-shaped tablets imprinted with "GX CG5" on one side.
Bottles of 60 tablets (NDC 0173-0662-00) with child-resistant closures.
Store at 25°C (77°F), excursions permitted to 15° to 30°C (59° to 86°F) [see USP Controlled Room Temperature].
EPIVIR-HBV Oral Solution, a clear, colorless to pale yellow, strawberry-banana-flavored liquid, contains 5 mg of lamivudine in each 1 mL in plastic bottles of 240 mL.
Bottles of 240 mL (NDC 0173-0663-00) with child-resistant closures. This product does not require reconstitution.
Store at controlled room temperature of 20° to 25°C (68° to 77°F) (see USP) in tightly closed bottles.

REFERENCES
1. Knodell RG, Ishak KG, Black WC, et al. Formulation and application of a numerical scoring system for assessing histological activity in asymptomatic chronic active hepatitis. *Hepatology*. 1982;1:431-435.
COMBIVIR, EPIVIR, EPIVIR-HBV, EPZICOM, and TRIZIVIR are registered trademarks of GlaxoSmithKline.
GlaxoSmithKline
Research Triangle Park, NC 27709
Manufactured under agreement from
Shire Pharmaceuticals Group plc
Basingstoke, UK
©2007, GlaxoSmithKline. All rights reserved.
October 2007 EPH:1PI
PHARMACIST-DETACH HERE AND GIVE INSTRUCTIONS TO PATIENT

PATIENT INFORMATION
EPIVIR-HBV® (lamivudine) Tablets
EPIVIR-HBV® (lamivudine) Oral Solution
Please read this information before you start taking EPIVIR-HBV (pronounced EP-i-veer h-b-v). Re-read it each time you get your prescription, in case some information has changed. **This information does not take the place of careful discussions with your doctor when you start this** medication and at checkups. Stay under a doctor's care when you take EPIVIR-HBV and do not change or stop treatment without first talking with your doctor.

What is EPIVIR-HBV?
EPIVIR-HBV is the brand name of a product that contains lamivudine, a drug used to treat chronic hepatitis B in patients with actively growing virus and liver inflammation. Hepatitis B can cause damage to cells in the liver. Eventually, this can scar the liver.
The lamivudine in EPIVIR-HBV can reduce the ability of the hepatitis B virus to multiply and infect new liver cells. It may help to lower the amount of hepatitis B virus in your body. EPIVIR-HBV contains a lower dose of lamivudine than the dose in EPIVIR®, COMBIVIR®, EPZICOM®, and TRIZIVIR®.

Why should I consider HIV testing before starting treatment with EPIVIR-HBV?
Your doctor or healthcare provider should offer you counseling and testing for HIV infection (sometimes called the AIDS virus) before treatment for hepatitis B is started with EPIVIR-HBV, and periodically during treatment. EPIVIR-HBV Tablets and EPIVIR-HBV Oral Solution contain a lower dose of the medicine than other lamivudine-containing drugs, such as EPIVIR, COMBIVIR, EPZICOM, and TRIZIVIR which are used to treat HIV. Treatment with EPIVIR-HBV in HIV-infected patients may cause the HIV virus to be less treatable with lamivudine and some other drugs.

If I am HIV-positive, can I take EPIVIR-HBV?
People who have both chronic hepatitis B and HIV should not take EPIVIR-HBV. EPIVIR-HBV Tablets and EPIVIR-HBV Oral Solution contain a lower dose of the same drug (lamivudine) as EPIVIR Tablets, EPIVIR Oral Solution, COMBIVIR Tablets, EPZICOM Tablets, and TRIZIVIR Tablets. If you have both hepatitis B and HIV, make sure that your doctor or healthcare provider is aware that you have both infections. If you are prescribed lamivudine as part of your combination treatment for HIV, you should use only the products and doses that are intended for treatment of HIV infection, because the lower dose of lamivudine in EPIVIR-HBV could cause the HIV virus to be less responsive to treatment. If you are planning to change your HIV treatment to a regimen that does not include EPIVIR, COMBIVIR, EPZICOM, or TRIZIVIR, you should first discuss this change with your doctor or healthcare provider.

Does EPIVIR-HBV cure hepatitis B infection?
EPIVIR-HBV is not a cure for hepatitis B. In studies comparing EPIVIR-HBV with placebo (an inactive sugar pill) for 1 year, more people treated with EPIVIR-HBV had reductions in liver inflammation. It is not known whether EPIVIR-HBV will reduce the risk of getting liver cancer or cirrhosis that may be caused by the hepatitis B virus.
In studies, some patients developed hepatitis B viruses that are resistant to EPIVIR-HBV. These patients generally had less benefit from treatment with EPIVIR-HBV. Some patients have had worsening of hepatitis after resistant virus appears. The long-term importance of a resistant virus is not known.

What happens if I stop taking EPIVIR-HBV?
After stopping treatment with EPIVIR-HBV, some patients have had symptoms or blood tests showing that their hepatitis has gotten worse. Therefore, your doctor should check your health, which may include blood tests, for at least several months after stopping treatment with EPIVIR-HBV. Tell your doctor right away about any new or unusual symptoms that you notice after stopping treatment.

Who should not take EPIVIR-HBV?
You should not take EPIVIR-HBV if you have or may have HIV infection (sometimes called the AIDS virus). EPIVIR-HBV does not contain an appropriate dose of lamivudine for treatment of HIV infection, and using EPIVIR-HBV could cause the HIV virus to become less treatable with lamivudine and some other drugs.
You should not take EPIVIR-HBV if you are also taking EPIVIR, COMBIVIR, EPZICOM, or TRIZIVIR. These drugs all contain lamivudine.
You should not take EPIVIR-HBV if you have had an allergic reaction to lamivudine.
EPIVIR-HBV has not been studied in children less than 2 years old.

Can pregnant women and nursing mothers take EPIVIR-HBV?
There are no studies of EPIVIR-HBV in pregnant women. If you are pregnant or if you become pregnant while taking EPIVIR-HBV, notify your doctor or healthcare provider immediately.
EPIVIR-HBV has not been shown to prevent the spread of the hepatitis B virus from mother to infant.
It is not known whether lamivudine is passed to the infant in breast milk. If there is lamivudine in the breast milk, this could cause side effects in nursing infants. Mothers should not breastfeed while taking EPIVIR-HBV or other forms of lamivudine.

How should I take EPIVIR-HBV?

Your doctor will tell you how much EPIVIR-HBV to take. The usual dose is 1 EPIVIR-HBV Tablet orally (by mouth) once a day. Your doctor may prescribe a lower dose if you have problems with your kidneys. EPIVIR-HBV may be taken with food or on an empty stomach. To help you remember to take your EPIVIR-HBV as prescribed, you should try to take EPIVIR-HBV at the same time each day. You must not skip doses or stop treatment without first talking with your doctor or healthcare provider. A strawberry-banana-flavored liquid of EPIVIR-HBV is available for patients who need a liquid.

If you miss your regular time for taking your dose, but then remember it during that same day, take your missed dose immediately. Then, take your next dose at the regularly scheduled time the following day. Do **not** take 2 doses of EPIVIR-HBV at once to make up for missing a dose. If you are not sure what to do if you miss taking your medication, check with your doctor or healthcare provider for further instructions.

EPIVIR-HBV can usually be taken with many other medications; however, be sure to tell your doctor or healthcare provider about all medications (including over-the-counter and prescription drugs) that you are taking. EPIVIR-HBV Tablets and EPIVIR-HBV Oral Solution contain a lower dose of the same drug (lamivudine) as EPIVIR Tablets, EPIVIR Oral Solution, COMBIVIR Tablets, EPZICOM Tablets, and TRIZIVIR Tablets; therefore, EPIVIR-HBV should not be taken together with EPIVIR, COMBIVIR, EPZICOM, or TRIZIVIR.

You should talk to your doctor about any changes in your treatment.

What are the possible side effects of EPIVIR-HBV?

You should stay under the care of a doctor during treatment so you can be checked for possible serious side effects. Serious side effects such as inflammation of the pancreas can occur with EPIVIR-HBV. Lactic acid buildup in the body and an enlarged liver have been reported with EPIVIR-HBV; this is not common but can result in death.

Hepatitis B virus sometimes becomes resistant to EPIVIR-HBV during treatment, and some people have had tests showing that their hepatitis is getting worse around the time the virus became resistant. Some people also have worsening of hepatitis after stopping EPIVIR-HBV. You should discuss any change in treatment with your doctor.

In studies, the most common side effects seen during treatment with EPIVIR-HBV were ear, nose, and throat infections; malaise and fatigue (feeling tired and run down); headache; abdominal discomfort and pain; nausea and vomiting; diarrhea; muscle pain; sore throat; joint pain; fever or chills; and skin rash.

This list of possible side effects is not complete. Your doctor or pharmacist can discuss with you a more complete list of possible side effects with EPIVIR-HBV. Talk to your doctor right away about any side effects or other unusual symptoms that occur when taking EPIVIR-HBV.

Does EPIVIR-HBV reduce the risk of passing hepatitis B to others?

No, EPIVIR-HBV has not been shown to reduce the risk of passing hepatitis B to others through sexual contact or exposure to infected blood. EPIVIR-HBV also has not been shown to reduce the risk of a mother passing hepatitis B to her baby.

What previous or current medical problems or conditions should I discuss with my doctor or healthcare provider?

Talk to your doctor or healthcare provider if:
• You have HIV infection.
• You are pregnant or if you become pregnant while taking EPIVIR-HBV.
• You are breastfeeding.
• You have diabetes. Each 20-mL dose (100 mg) of EPIVIR-HBV Oral Solution contains 4 grams of sucrose.

Also talk to your doctor or healthcare provider about:
• Problems with your blood counts.
• Problems with your muscles.
• Problems with your kidneys.
• Problems with your pancreas.
• Any side effects or unusual symptoms during treatment.

How should I store EPIVIR-HBV Tablets and Oral Solution?

EPIVIR-HBV Tablets and Oral Solution should be stored at room temperature. They do not require refrigeration. **Keep EPIVIR-HBV and all medicines out of the reach of children.**

Other Information

This medication is prescribed for a particular condition. Do not use it for any other condition or give it to anybody else. For more complete information about EPIVIR-HBV ask your doctor or pharmacist. You can also ask to read the longer information leaflet that is written for health professionals.

Keep EPIVIR-HBV and all medicines out of the reach of children. In case of overdose, get medical help or contact a Poison Control Center right away.

COMBIVIR, EPIVIR, EPIVIR-HBV, EPZICOM, and TRIZIVIR are registered trademarks of GlaxoSmithKline.

GlaxoSmithKline
Research Triangle Park, NC 27709
Manufactured under agreement from
Shire Pharmaceuticals Group plc
Basingstoke, UK
©2007, GlaxoSmithKline.All rights reserved.
October 2007 EPH:1PIL

FLOLAN®
[flō'lan]
(epoprostenol sodium)
for Injection

R

DESCRIPTION

FLOLAN (epoprostenol sodium) for Injection is a sterile sodium salt formulated for intravenous (IV) administration. Each vial of FLOLAN contains epoprostenol sodium equivalent to either 0.5 mg (500,000 ng) or 1.5 mg (1,500,000 ng) epoprostenol, 3.76 mg glycine, 2.93 mg sodium chloride, and 50 mg mannitol. Sodium hydroxide may have been added to adjust pH.

Epoprostenol (PGI_2, PGX, prostacyclin), a metabolite of arachidonic acid, is a naturally occurring prostaglandin with potent vasodilatory activity and inhibitory activity of platelet aggregation.

Epoprostenol is (5Z,9α,11α,13E,15S)-6,9-epoxy-11,15-dihydroxyprosta-5,13-dien-1-oic acid.

Epoprostenol sodium has a molecular weight of 374.45 and a molecular formula of $C_{20}H_{31}NaO_5$. The structural formula is:

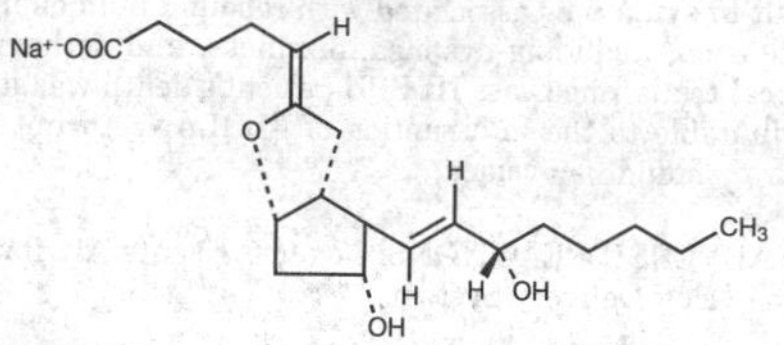

FLOLAN is a white to off-white powder that must be reconstituted with STERILE DILUENT for FLOLAN. STERILE DILUENT for FLOLAN is supplied in glass vials containing 50 mL of 94 mg glycine, 73.3 mg sodium chloride, sodium hydroxide (added to adjust pH), and Water for Injection, USP.

The reconstituted solution of FLOLAN has a pH of 10.2 to 10.8 and is increasingly unstable at a lower pH.

CLINICAL PHARMACOLOGY

General

Epoprostenol has 2 major pharmacological actions: (1) direct vasodilation of pulmonary and systemic arterial vascular beds, and (2) inhibition of platelet aggregation. In animals, the vasodilatory effects reduce right- and left-ventricular afterload and increase cardiac output and stroke volume. The effect of epoprostenol on heart rate in animals varies with dose. At low doses, there is vagally mediated bradycardia, but at higher doses, epoprostenol causes reflex tachycardia in response to direct vasodilation and hypotension. No major effects on cardiac conduction have been observed. Additional pharmacologic effects of epoprostenol in animals include bronchodilation, inhibition of gastric acid secretion, and decreased gastric emptying.

Pharmacokinetics

Epoprostenol is rapidly hydrolyzed at neutral pH in blood and is also subject to enzymatic degradation. Animal studies using tritium-labeled epoprostenol have indicated a high clearance (93 mL/kg/min), small volume of distribution (357 mL/kg), and a short half-life (2.7 minutes). During infusions in animals, steady-state plasma concentrations of tritium-labeled epoprostenol were reached within 15 minutes and were proportional to infusion rates.

No available chemical assay is sufficiently sensitive and specific to assess the in vivo human pharmacokinetics of epoprostenol. The in vitro half-life of epoprostenol in human blood at 37°C and pH 7.4 is approximately 6 minutes; therefore, the in vivo half-life of epoprostenol in humans is expected to be no greater than 6 minutes. The in vitro pharmacologic half-life of epoprostenol in human plasma, based on inhibition of platelet aggregation, was similar for males (n = 954) and females (n = 1,024).

Tritium-labeled epoprostenol has been administered to humans in order to identify the metabolic products of epoprostenol. Epoprostenol is metabolized to 2 primary metabolites: $6\text{-keto-PGF}_{1\alpha}$ (formed by spontaneous degradation) and $6,15\text{-diketo-}13,14\text{-dihydro-PGF}_{1\alpha}$ (enzymatically formed), both of which have pharmacological activity orders of magnitude less than epoprostenol in animal test systems. The recovery of radioactivity in urine and feces over a 1-week period was 82% and 4% of the administered dose, respectively. Fourteen additional minor metabolites have been isolated from urine, indicating that epoprostenol is extensively metabolized in humans.

CLINICAL TRIALS IN PULMONARY HYPERTENSION

Acute Hemodynamic Effects

Acute intravenous infusions of FLOLAN for up to 15 minutes in patients with secondary and primary pulmonary hypertension produce dose-related increases in cardiac index (CI) and stroke volume (SV) and dose-related decreases in pulmonary vascular resistance (PVR), total pulmonary resistance (TPR), and mean systemic arterial pressure (SAPm). The effects of FLOLAN on mean pulmonary artery pressure (PAPm) were variable and minor.

Chronic Infusion in Primary Pulmonary Hypertension (PPH): Hemodynamic Effects

Chronic continuous infusions of FLOLAN in patients with PPH were studied in 2 prospective, open, randomized trials of 8 and 12 weeks' duration comparing FLOLAN plus conventional therapy to conventional therapy alone. Dosage of FLOLAN was determined as described in DOSAGE AND ADMINISTRATION and averaged 9.2 ng/kg/min at study's end. Conventional therapy varied among patients and included some or all of the following: anticoagulants in essentially all patients; oral vasodilators, diuretics, and digoxin in one half to two thirds of patients; and supplemental oxygen in about half the patients. Except for 2 New York Heart Association (NYHA) functional Class II patients, all patients were either functional Class III or Class IV. As results were similar in the 2 studies, the pooled results are described. Chronic hemodynamic effects were generally similar to acute effects. Increases in CI, SV, and arterial oxygen saturation and decreases in PAPm, mean right atrial pressure (RAPm), TPR, and systemic vascular resistance (SVR) were observed in patients who received FLOLAN chronically compared to those who did not. Table 1 illustrates the treatment-related hemodynamic changes in these patients after 8 or 12 weeks of treatment.

[See table 1 below]

These hemodynamic improvements appeared to persist when FLOLAN was administered for at least 36 months in an open, nonrandomized study.

Clinical Effects

Statistically significant improvement was observed in exercise capacity, as measured by the 6-minute walk test in patients receiving continuous intravenous FLOLAN plus conventional therapy (N = 52) for 8 or 12 weeks compared to those receiving conventional therapy alone (N = 54). Improvements were apparent as early as the first week of therapy. Increases in exercise capacity were accompanied by statistically significant improvement in dyspnea and fatigue, as measured by the Chronic Heart Failure Questionnaire and the Dyspnea Fatigue Index.

Survival was improved in NYHA functional Class III and Class IV PPH patients treated with FLOLAN for 12 weeks

Table 1. Hemodynamics During Chronic Administration of FLOLAN in Patients With PPH

Hemodynamic Parameter	Baseline FLOLAN (N = 52)	Baseline Standard Therapy (N = 54)	Mean Change from Baseline at End of Treatment Period* FLOLAN (N = 48)	Mean Change from Baseline at End of Treatment Period* Standard Therapy (N = 41)
CI (L/min/m²)	2.0	2.0	0.3†	-0.1
PAPm (mm Hg)	60	60	-5†	1
PVR (Wood U)	16	17	-4†	1
SAPm (mm Hg)	89	91	-4	-3
SV (mL/beat)	44	43	6†	-1
TPR (Wood U)	20	21	-5†	1

* At 8 weeks: FLOLAN N = 10, conventional therapy N = 11 (N is the number of patients with hemodynamic data).
At 12 weeks: FLOLAN N = 38, conventional therapy N = 30 (N is the number of patients with hemodynamic data).
† Denotes statistically significant difference between FLOLAN and conventional therapy groups.
CI = cardiac index, PAPm = mean pulmonary arterial pressure, PVR = pulmonary vascular resistance, SAPm = mean systemic arterial pressure, SV = stroke volume, TPR = total pulmonary resistance.

Table 2. Hemodynamics During Chronic Administration of FLOLAN in Patients With PH/SSD

Hemodynamic Parameter	Baseline		Mean Change from Baseline at 12 Weeks	
	FLOLAN (N = 56)	Conventional Therapy (N = 55)	FLOLAN (N = 50)	Conventional Therapy (N = 48)
CI (L/min/m^2)	1.9	2.2	0.5*	-0.1
PAPm (mm Hg)	51	49	-5*	1
RAPm (mm Hg)	13	11	-1*	1
PVR (Wood U)	14	11	-5*	1
SAPm (mm Hg)	93	89	-8*	-1

* Denotes statistically significant difference between FLOLAN and conventional therapy groups (N is the number of patients with hemodynamic data).
CI = cardiac index, PAPm = mean pulmonary arterial pressure, RAPm = mean right arterial pressure, PVR = pulmonary vascular resistance, SAPm = mean systemic arterial pressure.

in a multicenter, open, randomized, parallel study. At the end of the treatment period, 8 of 40 (20%) patients receiving conventional therapy alone died, whereas none of the 41 patients receiving FLOLAN died (p = 0.003).

Chronic Infusion in Pulmonary Hypertension Associated with the Scleroderma Spectrum of Diseases (PH/SSD)

Hemodynamic Effects

Chronic continuous infusions of FLOLAN in patients with PH/SSD were studied in a prospective, open, randomized trial of 12 weeks' duration comparing FLOLAN plus conventional therapy (N = 56) to conventional therapy alone (N = 55). Except for 5 NYHA functional Class II patients, all patients were either functional Class III or Class IV. Dosage of FLOLAN was determined as described in DOSAGE AND ADMINISTRATION and averaged 11.2 ng/kg/min at study's end. Conventional therapy varied among patients and included some or all of the following: anticoagulants in essentially all patients, supplemental oxygen and diuretics in two thirds of the patients, oral vasodilators in 40% of the patients, and digoxin in a third of the patients. A statistically significant increase in CI, and statistically significant decreases in PAPm, RAPm, PVR, and SAPm after 12 weeks of treatment were observed in patients who received FLOLAN chronically compared to those who did not. Table 2 illustrates the treatment-related hemodynamic changes in these patients after 12 weeks of treatment.

[See table 2 above]

Clinical Effects

Statistically significant improvement was observed in exercise capacity, as measured by the 6-minute walk, in patients receiving continuous intravenous FLOLAN plus conventional therapy for 12 weeks compared to those receiving conventional therapy alone. Improvements were apparent in some patients at the end of the first week of therapy. Increases in exercise capacity were accompanied by statistically significant improvements in dyspnea and fatigue, as measured by the Borg Dyspnea Index and Dyspnea Fatigue Index. At week 12, NYHA functional class improved in 21 of 51 (41%) patients treated with FLOLAN compared to none of the 48 patients treated with conventional therapy alone. However, more patients in both treatment groups (28/51 [55%] with FLOLAN and 35/48 [73%] with conventional therapy alone) showed no change in functional class, and 2/51 (4%) with FLOLAN and 13/48 (27%) with conventional therapy alone worsened. Of the patients randomized, NYHA functional class data at 12 weeks were not available for 5 patients treated with FLOLAN and 7 patients treated with conventional therapy alone.

No statistical difference in survival over 12 weeks was observed in PH/SSD patients treated with FLOLAN as compared to those receiving conventional therapy alone. At the end of the treatment period, 4 of 56 (7%) patients receiving FLOLAN died, whereas 5 of 55 (9%) patients receiving conventional therapy alone died.

No controlled clinical trials with FLOLAN have been performed in patients with pulmonary hypertension associated with other diseases.

INDICATIONS AND USAGE

FLOLAN is indicated for the long-term intravenous treatment of primary pulmonary hypertension and pulmonary hypertension associated with the scleroderma spectrum of disease in NYHA Class III and Class IV patients who do not respond adequately to conventional therapy (see CLINICAL TRIALS IN PULMONARY HYPERTENSION).

CONTRAINDICATIONS

A large study evaluating the effect of FLOLAN on survival in NYHA Class III and IV patients with congestive heart failure due to severe left ventricular systolic dysfunction was terminated after an interim analysis of 471 patients revealed a higher mortality in patients receiving FLOLAN plus conventional therapy than in those receiving conventional therapy alone. The chronic use of FLOLAN in patients with congestive heart failure due to severe left ventricular systolic dysfunction is therefore contraindicated.

Some patients with pulmonary hypertension have developed pulmonary edema during dose initiation, which may be associated with pulmonary veno-occlusive disease. FLOLAN should not be used chronically in patients who develop pulmonary edema during dose initiation.

FLOLAN is also contraindicated in patients with known hypersensitivity to the drug or to structurally related compounds.

WARNINGS

FLOLAN must be reconstituted only as directed using STERILE DILUENT for FLOLAN. FLOLAN must not be reconstituted or mixed with any other parenteral medications or solutions prior to or during administration.

Abrupt Withdrawal

Abrupt withdrawal (including interruptions in drug delivery) or sudden large reductions in dosage of FLOLAN may result in symptoms associated with rebound pulmonary hypertension, including dyspnea, dizziness, and asthenia. In clinical trials, one Class III PPH patient's death was judged attributable to the interruption of FLOLAN. Abrupt withdrawal should be avoided.

Sepsis

See ADVERSE REACTIONS: Adverse Events Attributable to the Drug Delivery System.

PRECAUTIONS

General

FLOLAN should be used only by clinicians experienced in the diagnosis and treatment of pulmonary hypertension. The diagnosis of PPH or PH/SSD should be carefully established.

FLOLAN is a potent pulmonary and systemic vasodilator. Dose initiation with FLOLAN must be performed in a setting with adequate personnel and equipment for physiologic monitoring and emergency care. Dose initiation in controlled PPH clinical trials was performed during right heart catheterization. In uncontrolled PPH and controlled PH/SSD clinical trials, dose initiation was performed without cardiac catheterization. The risk of cardiac catheterization in patients with pulmonary hypertension should be carefully weighed against the potential benefits. During dose initiation, asymptomatic increases in pulmonary artery pressure coincident with increases in cardiac output occurred rarely. In such cases, dose reduction should be considered, but such an increase does not imply that chronic treatment is contraindicated.

FLOLAN is a potent inhibitor of platelet aggregation. Therefore, an increased risk for hemorrhagic complications should be considered, particularly for patients with other risk factors for bleeding (see PRECAUTIONS: Drug Interactions).

During chronic use, FLOLAN is delivered continuously on an ambulatory basis through a permanent indwelling central venous catheter. Unless contraindicated, anticoagulant therapy should be administered to PPH and PH/SSD patients receiving FLOLAN to reduce the risk of pulmonary thromboembolism or systemic embolism through a patent foramen ovale. In order to reduce the risk of infection, aseptic technique must be used in the reconstitution and administration of FLOLAN as well as in routine catheter care. Because FLOLAN is metabolized rapidly, even brief interruptions in the delivery of FLOLAN may result in symptoms associated with rebound pulmonary hypertension including dyspnea, dizziness, and asthenia. The decision to initiate therapy with FLOLAN should be based upon the understanding that there is a high likelihood that intravenous therapy with FLOLAN will be needed for prolonged periods, possibly years, and the patient's ability to accept and care for a permanent intravenous catheter and infusion pump should be carefully considered.

Based on clinical trials, the acute hemodynamic response to FLOLAN did not correlate well with improvement in exercise tolerance or survival during chronic use of FLOLAN. Dosage of FLOLAN during chronic use should be adjusted at the first sign of recurrence or worsening of symptoms attributable to pulmonary hypertension or the occurrence of adverse events associated with FLOLAN (see DOSAGE AND ADMINISTRATION). Following dosage adjustments, standing and supine blood pressure and heart rate should be monitored closely for several hours.

Information for Patients

Patients receiving FLOLAN should receive the following information. **FLOLAN must be reconstituted only with STERILE DILUENT for FLOLAN.** FLOLAN is infused continuously through a permanent indwelling central venous catheter via a small, portable infusion pump. Thus, therapy with FLOLAN requires commitment by the patient to drug reconstitution, drug administration, and care of the permanent central venous catheter. Sterile technique must be adhered to in preparing the drug and in the care of the catheter, and even brief interruptions in the delivery of FLOLAN may result in rapid symptomatic deterioration. A patient's decision to receive FLOLAN should be based upon the understanding that there is a high likelihood that therapy with FLOLAN will be needed for prolonged periods, possibly years. The patient's ability to accept and care for a permanent intravenous catheter and infusion pump should also be carefully considered.

Drug Interactions

Additional reductions in blood pressure may occur when FLOLAN is administered with diuretics, antihypertensive agents, or other vasodilators. When other antiplatelet agents or anticoagulants are used concomitantly, there is the potential for FLOLAN to increase the risk of bleeding. However, patients receiving infusions of FLOLAN in clinical trials were maintained on anticoagulants without evidence of increased bleeding. In clinical trials, FLOLAN was used with digoxin, diuretics, anticoagulants, oral vasodilators, and supplemental oxygen.

In a pharmacokinetic substudy in patients with congestive heart failure receiving furosemide or digoxin in whom therapy with FLOLAN was initiated, apparent oral clearance values for furosemide (n = 23) and digoxin (n = 30) were decreased by 13% and 15%, respectively, on the second day of therapy and had returned to baseline values by day 87. The change in furosemide clearance value is not likely to be clinically significant. However, patients on digoxin may show elevations of digoxin concentrations after initiation of therapy with FLOLAN, which may be clinically significant in patients prone to digoxin toxicity.

Carcinogenesis, Mutagenesis, Impairment of Fertility

Long-term studies in animals have not been performed to evaluate carcinogenic potential. A micronucleus test in rats revealed no evidence of mutagenicity. The Ames test and DNA elution tests were also negative, although the instability of epoprostenol makes the significance of these tests uncertain. Fertility was not impaired in rats given FLOLAN by subcutaneous injection at doses up to 100 mcg/kg/day (600 mcg/m^2/day, 2.5 times the recommended human dose [4.6 ng/kg/min or 245.1 mcg/m^2/day, IV] based on body surface area).

Pregnancy

Pregnancy Category B. Reproductive studies have been performed in pregnant rats and rabbits at doses up to 100 mcg/kg/day (600 mcg/m^2/day in rats, 2.5 times the recommended human dose, and 1,180 mcg/m^2/day in rabbits, 4.8 times the recommended human dose based on body surface area) and have revealed no evidence of impaired fertility or harm to the fetus due to FLOLAN. There are, however, no adequate and well-controlled studies in pregnant women. Because animal reproduction studies are not always predictive of human response, this drug should be used during pregnancy only if clearly needed.

Labor and Delivery

The use of FLOLAN during labor, vaginal delivery, or cesarean section has not been adequately studied in humans.

Nursing Mothers

It is not known whether this drug is excreted in human milk. Because many drugs are excreted in human milk, caution should be exercised when FLOLAN is administered to a nursing woman.

Pediatric Use

Safety and effectiveness in pediatric patients have not been established.

Geriatric Use

Clinical studies of FLOLAN in pulmonary hypertension did not include sufficient numbers of subjects aged 65 and over to determine whether they respond differently from younger patients. Other reported clinical experience has not identified differences in responses between the elderly and younger patients. In general, dose selection for an elderly patient should be cautious, usually starting at the low end of the dosing range, reflecting the greater frequency of decreased hepatic, renal, or cardiac function and of concomitant disease or other drug therapy.

ADVERSE REACTIONS

During clinical trials, adverse events were classified as follows: (1) adverse events during dose initiation and escalation, (2) adverse events during chronic dosing, and (3) adverse events associated with the drug delivery system.

Adverse Events During Dose Initiation and Escalation

During early clinical trials, FLOLAN was increased in 2-ng/kg/min increments until the patients developed symptomatic intolerance. The most common adverse events and the adverse events that limited further increases in dose were generally related to vasodilation, the major pharmacologic effect of FLOLAN. The most common dose-limiting adverse events (occurring in ≥1% of patients) were nausea, vomiting, headache, hypotension, and flushing, but also include chest pain, anxiety, dizziness, bradycardia, dyspnea, abdominal pain, musculoskeletal pain, and tachycardia. Table 3 lists the adverse events reported during dose initiation and escalation in decreasing order of frequency.

Table 3. Adverse Events During Dose Initiation and Escalation

Adverse Events Occurring in ≥1% of Patients	FLOLAN (n = 391)
Flushing	58%
Headache	49%
Nausea/vomiting	32%
Hypotension	16%
Anxiety, nervousness, agitation	11%
Chest pain	11%
Dizziness	8%
Bradycardia	5%
Abdominal pain	5%
Musculoskeletal pain	3%
Dyspnea	2%
Back pain	2%
Sweating	1%
Dyspepsia	1%
Hypesthesia/paresthesia	1%
Tachycardia	1%

Adverse Events During Chronic Administration

Interpretation of adverse events is complicated by the clinical features of PPH and PH/SSD, which are similar to some of the pharmacologic effects of FLOLAN (e.g., dizziness, syncope). Adverse events probably related to the underlying disease include dyspnea, fatigue, chest pain, edema, hypoxia, right ventricular failure, and pallor. Several adverse events, on the other hand, can clearly be attributed to FLOLAN. These include headache, jaw pain, flushing, diarrhea, nausea and vomiting, flu-like symptoms, and anxiety/nervousness.

Adverse Events During Chronic Administration for PPH

In an effort to separate the adverse effects of the drug from the adverse effects of the underlying disease, Table 4 lists adverse events that occurred at a rate at least 10% different in the 2 groups in controlled trials for PPH.

Table 4. Adverse Events Regardless of Attribution Occurring in Patients With PPH With ≥10% Difference Between FLOLAN and Conventional Therapy Alone

Adverse Event	FLOLAN (n = 52)	Conventional Therapy (n = 54)
Occurrence More Common With FLOLAN		
General		
Chills/fever/sepsis/flu-like symptoms	25%	11%
Cardiovascular		
Tachycardia	35%	24%
Flushing	42%	2%
Gastrointestinal		
Diarrhea	37%	6%
Nausea/vomiting	67%	48%
Musculoskeletal		
Jaw pain	54%	0%
Myalgia	44%	31%
Nonspecific musculoskeletal pain	35%	15%
Neurological		
Anxiety/nervousness/tremor	21%	9%
Dizziness	83%	70%
Headache	83%	33%
Hypesthesia, hyperesthesia, paresthesia	12%	2%
Occurrence More Common With Standard Therapy		
Cardiovascular		
Heart failure	31%	52%
Syncope	13%	24%
Shock	0%	13%
Respiratory		
Hypoxia	25%	37%

Thrombocytopenia has been reported during uncontrolled clinical trials in patients receiving FLOLAN.

Table 5 lists additional adverse events reported in PPH patients receiving FLOLAN plus conventional therapy or conventional therapy alone during controlled clinical trials.

Table 5. Adverse Events Regardless of Attribution Occurring in Patients With PPH With <10% Difference Between FLOLAN and Conventional Therapy Alone

Adverse Event	FLOLAN (n = 52)	Conventional Therapy (n = 54)
General		
Asthenia	87%	81%
Cardiovascular		
Angina pectoris	19%	20%
Arrhythmia	27%	20%
Bradycardia	15%	9%
Supraventricular tachycardia	8%	0%
Pallor	21%	30%
Cyanosis	31%	39%
Palpitation	63%	61%
Cerebrovascular accident	4%	0%
Hemorrhage	19%	11%
Hypotension	27%	31%
Myocardial ischemia	2%	6%
Gastrointestinal		
Abdominal pain	27%	31%
Anorexia	25%	30%
Ascites	12%	17%
Constipation	6%	2%
Metabolic		
Edema	60%	63%
Hypokalemia	6%	4%
Weight reduction	27%	24%
Weight gain	6%	4%
Musculoskeletal		
Arthralgia	6%	0%
Bone pain	0%	4%
Chest pain	67%	65%
Neurological		
Confusion	6%	11%
Convulsion	4%	0%
Depression	37%	44%
Insomnia	4%	4%
Respiratory		
Cough increase	38%	46%
Dyspnea	90%	85%
Epistaxis	4%	2%
Pleural effusion	4%	2%
Skin and Appendages		
Pruritus	4%	0%
Rash	10%	13%
Sweating	15%	20%
Special Senses		
Amblyopia	8%	4%
Vision abnormality	4%	0%

Adverse Events During Chronic Administration for PH/SSD

In an effort to separate the adverse effects of the drug from the adverse effects of the underlying disease, Table 6 lists adverse events that occurred at a rate at least 10% different in the 2 groups in the controlled trial for patients with PH/SSD.

Table 6. Adverse Events Regardless of Attribution Occurring in Patients With PH/SSD With ≥10% Difference Between FLOLAN and Conventional Therapy Alone

Adverse Event	FLOLAN (n = 56)	Conventional Therapy (n = 55)
Occurrence More Common With FLOLAN		
Cardiovascular		
Flushing	23%	0%
Hypotension	13%	0%
Gastrointestinal		
Anorexia	66%	47%
Nausea/vomiting	41%	16%
Diarrhea	50%	5%
Musculoskeletal		
Jaw pain	75%	0%
Pain/neck pain/arthralgia	84%	65%
Neurological		
Headache	46%	5%
Skin and Appendages		
Skin ulcer	39%	24%
Eczema/rash/urticaria	25%	4%
Occurrence More Common With Conventional Therapy		
Cardiovascular		
Cyanosis	54%	80%

	FLOLAN	Conventional
Pallor	32%	53%
Syncope	7%	20%
Gastrointestinal		
Ascites	23%	33%
Esophageal reflux/gastritis	61%	73%
Metabolic		
Weight decrease	45%	56%
Neurological		
Dizziness	59%	76%
Respiratory		
Hypoxia	55%	65%

Table 7 lists additional adverse events reported in PH/SSD patients receiving FLOLAN plus conventional therapy or conventional therapy alone during controlled clinical trials.

Table 7. Adverse Events Regardless of Attribution Occurring in Patients With PH/SSD With <10% Difference Between FLOLAN and Conventional Therapy Alone

Adverse Event*	FLOLAN (n = 56)	Conventional Therapy (n = 55)
General		
Asthenia	100%	98%
Hemorrhage/hemorrhage injection site/hemorrhage rectal	11%	2%
Infection/rhinitis	21%	20%
Chills/fever/sepsis/flu-like symptoms	13%	11%
Blood and Lymphatic		
Thrombocytopenia	4%	0%
Cardiovascular		
Heart failure/heart failure right	11%	13%
Myocardial Infarction	4%	0%
Palpitation	63%	71%
Shock	5%	5%
Tachycardia	43%	42%
Vascular disorder peripheral	96%	100%
Vascular disorder	95%	89%
Gastrointestinal		
Abdominal enlargement	4%	0%
Abdominal pain	14%	7%
Constipation	4%	2%
Flatulence	5%	4%
Metabolic		
Edema/edema peripheral/edema genital	79%	87%
Hypercalcemia	48%	51%
Hyperkalemia	4%	0%
Thirst	0%	4%
Musculoskeletal		
Arthritis	52%	45%
Back pain	13%	5%
Chest pain	52%	45%
Cramps leg	5%	7%
Respiratory		
Cough increase	82%	82%
Dyspnea	100%	100%
Epistaxis	9%	7%
Pharyngitis	5%	2%
Pleural effusion	7%	0%
Pneumonia	5%	0%
Pneumothorax	4%	0%
Pulmonary edema	4%	2%
Respiratory disorder	7%	4%
Sinusitis	4%	4%
Neurological		
Anxiety/hyperkinesia/nervousness/tremor	7%	5%
Depression/depression psychotic	13%	4%
Hyperesthesia/hypesthesia/paresthesia	5%	0%
Insomnia	9%	0%
Somnolence	4%	2%
Skin and Appendages		
Collagen disease	82%	84%
Pruritus	4%	2%
Sweat	41%	36%
Urogenital		
Hematuria	5%	0%
Urinary tract infection	7%	0%

* Adverse events that occurred in at least 2 patients in either treatment group.

$$\text{Infusion Rate (mL/hr)} = \frac{[\text{Dose (ng/kg/min)} \times \text{Weight (kg)} \times 60 \text{ min/hr}]}{\text{Final Concentration (ng/mL)}}$$

Table 9. Infusion Rates for FLOLAN at a Concentration of 3,000 ng/mL

Patient Weight (kg)	Dose or Drug Delivery Rate (ng/kg/min) 2	4	6	8	10	12	14	16
	Infusion Delivery Rate (mL/h)							
10	—	—	1.2	1.6	2.0	2.4	2.8	3.2
20	—	1.6	2.4	3.2	4.0	4.8	5.6	6.4
30	1.2	2.4	3.6	4.8	6.0	7.2	8.4	9.6
40	1.6	3.2	4.8	6.4	8.0	9.6	11.2	12.8
50	2.0	4.0	6.0	8.0	10.0	12.0	14.0	16.0
60	2.4	4.8	7.2	9.6	12.0	14.4	16.8	19.2
70	2.8	5.6	8.4	11.2	14.0	16.8	19.6	22.4
80	3.2	6.4	9.6	12.8	16.0	19.2	22.4	25.6
90	3.6	7.2	10.8	14.4	18.0	21.6	25.2	28.8
100	4.0	8.0	12.0	16.0	20.0	24.0	28.0	32.0

Although the relationship to FLOLAN administration has not been established, pulmonary embolism has been reported in several patients taking FLOLAN and there have been reports of hepatic failure.

Adverse Events Attributable to the Drug Delivery System

Chronic infusions of FLOLAN are delivered using a small, portable infusion pump through an indwelling central venous catheter. During controlled PPH trials of up to 12 weeks' duration, up to 21% of patients reported a local infection and up to 13% of patients reported pain at the injection site. During a controlled PH/SSD trial of 12 weeks' duration, 14% of patients reported a local infection and 9% of patients reported pain at the injection site. During long-term follow-up in the clinical trial of PPH, sepsis was reported at least once in 14% of patients and occurred at a rate of 0.32 infections/patient per year in patients treated with FLOLAN. This rate was higher than reported in patients using chronic indwelling central venous catheters to administer parenteral nutrition, but lower than reported in oncology patients using these catheters. Malfunctions in the delivery system resulting in an inadvertent bolus of or a reduction in FLOLAN were associated with symptoms related to excess or insufficient FLOLAN, respectively (see ADVERSE REACTIONS: Adverse Events During Chronic Administration).

Observed During Clinical Practice

In addition to adverse reactions reported from clinical trials, the following events have been identified during post-approval use of FLOLAN. Because they are reported voluntarily from a population of unknown size, estimates of frequency cannot be made. These events have been chosen for inclusion due to a combination of their seriousness, frequency of reporting, or potential causal connection to FLOLAN.

Blood and Lymphatic

Anemia, hypersplenism, pancytopenia, splenomegaly.

Endocrine and Metabolic

Hyperthyroidism.

OVERDOSAGE

Signs and symptoms of excessive doses of FLOLAN during clinical trials are the expected dose-limiting pharmacologic effects of FLOLAN, including flushing, headache, hypotension, tachycardia, nausea, vomiting, and diarrhea. Treatment will ordinarily require dose reduction of FLOLAN.

One patient with secondary pulmonary hypertension accidentally received 50 mL of an unspecified concentration of FLOLAN. The patient vomited and became unconscious with an initially unrecordable blood pressure. FLOLAN was discontinued and the patient regained consciousness within seconds. In clinical practice, fatal occurrences of hypoxemia, hypotension, and respiratory arrest have been reported following overdosage of FLOLAN.

Single intravenous doses of FLOLAN at 10 and 50 mg/kg (2,703 and 27,027 times the recommended acute phase human dose based on body surface area) were lethal to mice and rats, respectively. Symptoms of acute toxicity were hypoactivity, ataxia, loss of righting reflex, deep slow breathing, and hypothermia.

DOSAGE AND ADMINISTRATION

Important Note

FLOLAN must be reconstituted only with STERILE DILUENT for FLOLAN. Reconstituted solutions of FLOLAN must not be diluted or administered with other parenteral solutions or medications (see WARNINGS).

Dosage

Continuous chronic infusion of FLOLAN should be administered through a central venous catheter. Temporary peripheral intravenous infusion may be used until central access is established. Chronic infusion of FLOLAN should be initiated at 2 ng/kg/min and increased in increments of 2 ng/kg/min every 15 minutes or longer until dose-limiting pharmacologic effects are elicited or until a tolerance limit to the drug is established and further increases in the infusion rate are not clinically warranted (see Dosage Adjustments). If dose-limiting pharmacologic effects occur, then the infusion rate should be decreased to an appropriate chronic infusion rate whereby the pharmacologic effects of FLOLAN are tolerated. In clinical trials, the most common dose-limiting adverse events were nausea, vomiting, hypotension, sepsis, headache, abdominal pain, or respiratory disorder (most treatment-limiting adverse events were not serious). If the initial infusion rate of 2 ng/kg/min is not tolerated, a lower dose that is tolerated by the patient should be identified.

In the controlled 12-week trial in PH/SSD, for example, the dose increased from a mean starting dose of 2.2 ng/kg/min. During the first 7 days of treatment, the dose was increased daily to a mean dose of 4.1 ng/kg/min on day 7 of treatment. At the end of week 12, the mean dose was 11.2 ng/kg/min. The mean incremental increase was 2 to 3 ng/kg/min every 3 weeks.

Dosage Adjustments

Changes in the chronic infusion rate should be based on persistence, recurrence, or worsening of the patient's symptoms of pulmonary hypertension and the occurrence of adverse events due to excessive doses of FLOLAN. In general, increases in dose from the initial chronic dose should be expected.

Increments in dose should be considered if symptoms of pulmonary hypertension persist or recur after improving. The infusion should be increased by 1- to 2-ng/kg/min increments at intervals sufficient to allow assessment of clinical response; these intervals should be at least 15 minutes. In clinical trials, incremental increases in dose occurred at intervals of 24 to 48 hours or longer. Following establishment of a new chronic infusion rate, the patient should be observed, and standing and supine blood pressure and heart rate monitored for several hours to ensure that the new dose is tolerated.

During chronic infusion, the occurrence of dose-limiting pharmacological events may necessitate a decrease in infusion rate, but the adverse event may occasionally resolve without dosage adjustment. Dosage decreases should be made gradually in 2-ng/kg/min decrements every 15 minutes or longer until the dose-limiting effects resolve. Abrupt withdrawal of FLOLAN or sudden large reductions in infusion rates should be avoided. Except in life-threatening situations (e.g., unconsciousness, collapse, etc.), infusion rates of FLOLAN should be adjusted only under the direction of a physician.

In patients receiving lung transplants, doses of FLOLAN were tapered after the initiation of cardiopulmonary bypass.

Administration

FLOLAN is administered by continuous intravenous infusion via a central venous catheter using an ambulatory infusion pump. During initiation of treatment, FLOLAN may be administered peripherally.

The ambulatory infusion pump used to administer FLOLAN should: (1) be small and lightweight, (2) be able to adjust infusion rates in 2-ng/kg/min increments, (3) have occlusion, end-of-infusion, and low-battery alarms, (4) be accurate to ±6% of the programmed rate, and (5) be positive pressure-driven (continuous or pulsatile) with intervals between pulses not exceeding 3 minutes at infusion rates used to deliver FLOLAN. The reservoir should be made of polyvinyl chloride, polypropylene, or glass. The infusion pump used in the most recent clinical trials was the CADD-1 HFX 5100 (SIMS Deltec). A 60-inch microbore non-DEHP extension set with proximal antisyphon valve, low priming volume (0.9 mL), and in-line 0.22 micron filter was used during clinical trials.

To avoid potential interruptions in drug delivery, the patient should have access to a backup infusion pump and intravenous infusion sets. A multi-lumen catheter should be considered if other intravenous therapies are routinely administered.

To facilitate extended use at ambient temperatures exceeding 25°C (77°F), a cold pouch with frozen gel packs was used in clinical trials (see DOSAGE AND ADMINISTRATION: Storage and Stability). The cold pouches and gel packs used in clinical trials were obtained from Palco Labs, Palo Alto, California. Any cold pouch used must be capable of maintaining the temperature of reconstituted FLOLAN between 2° and 8°C for 12 hours.

Reconstitution

FLOLAN is stable only when reconstituted with STERILE DILUENT for FLOLAN. FLOLAN must not be reconstituted or mixed with any other parenteral medications or solutions prior to or during administration.

A concentration for the solution of FLOLAN should be selected that is compatible with the infusion pump being used with respect to minimum and maximum flow rates, reservoir capacity, and the infusion pump criteria listed above. FLOLAN, when administered chronically, should be prepared in a drug delivery reservoir appropriate for the infusion pump with a total reservoir volume of at least 100 mL. FLOLAN should be prepared using 2 vials of STERILE DILUENT for FLOLAN for use during a 24-hour period. Table 8 gives directions for preparing several different concentrations of FLOLAN.

Table 8. Reconstitution and Dilution Instructions

To make 100 mL of solution with Final Concentration (ng/mL) of:	Directions:
3,000 ng/mL	Dissolve contents of one 0.5-mg vial with 5 mL of STERILE DILUENT for FLOLAN. Withdraw 3 mL and add to sufficient STERILE DILUENT for FLOLAN to make a total of 100 mL.
5,000 ng/mL	Dissolve contents of one 0.5-mg vial with 5 mL of STERILE DILUENT for FLOLAN. Withdraw entire vial contents and add sufficient STERILE DILUENT for FLOLAN to make a total of 100 mL.
10,000 ng/mL	Dissolve contents of two 0.5-mg vials each with 5 mL of STERILE DILUENT for FLOLAN. Withdraw entire vial contents and add sufficient STERILE DILUENT for FLOLAN to make a total of 100 mL.
15,000 ng/mL*	Dissolve contents of one 1.5-mg vial with 5 mL of STERILE DILUENT for FLOLAN. Withdraw entire vial contents and add sufficient STERILE DILUENT for FLOLAN to make a total of 100 mL.

* Higher concentrations may be required for patients who receive FLOLAN long-term.

Generally, 3,000 ng/mL and 10,000 ng/mL are satisfactory concentrations to deliver between 2 to 16 ng/kg/min in adults. Infusion rates may be calculated using the following formula:

[See first table above]

Tables 9 through 12 provide infusion delivery rates for doses up to 16 ng/kg/min based upon patient weight, drug delivery rate, and concentration of the solution of FLOLAN to be used. These tables may be used to select the most appropriate concentration of FLOLAN that will result in an infusion rate between the minimum and maximum flow rates of the infusion pump and that will allow the desired duration of infusion from a given reservoir volume. Higher infusion rates, and therefore, more concentrated solutions may be necessary with long-term administration of FLOLAN.

[See table 9 above]
[See table 10 at top of next page]
[See table 11 on next page]
[See table 12 on next page]

Storage and Stability

Unopened vials of FLOLAN are stable until the date indicated on the package when stored at 15° to 25°C (59° to 77°F) and protected from light in the carton. Unopened vials of STERILE DILUENT for FLOLAN are stable until the date indicated on the package when stored at 15° to 25°C (59° to 77°F).

Prior to use, reconstituted solutions of FLOLAN must be protected from light and must be refrigerated at 2° to 8°C (36° to 46°F) if not used immediately. **Do not freeze recon-**

Table 10. Infusion Rates for FLOLAN at a Concentration of 5,000 ng/mL

Patient Weight (kg)	Dose or Drug Delivery Rate (ng/kg/min)							
	2	4	6	8	10	12	14	16
	Infusion Delivery Rate (mL/h)							
10	—	—	—	1.0	1.2	1.4	1.7	1.9
20	—	1.0	1.4	1.9	2.4	2.9	3.4	3.8
30	—	1.4	2.2	2.9	3.6	4.3	5.0	5.8
40	1.0	1.9	2.9	3.8	4.8	5.8	6.7	7.7
50	1.2	2.4	3.6	4.8	6.0	7.2	8.4	9.6
60	1.4	2.9	4.3	5.8	7.2	8.6	10.1	11.5
70	1.7	3.4	5.0	6.7	8.4	10.1	11.8	13.4
80	1.9	3.8	5.8	7.7	9.6	11.5	13.4	15.4
90	2.2	4.3	6.5	8.6	10.8	13.0	15.1	17.3
100	2.4	4.8	7.2	9.6	12.0	14.4	16.8	19.2

Table 11. Infusion Rates for FLOLAN at a Concentration of 10,000 ng/mL

Patient Weight (kg)	Dose or Drug Delivery Rate (ng/kg/min)						
	4	6	8	10	12	14	16
	Infusion Delivery Rate (mL/h)						
20	—	—	1.0	1.2	1.4	1.7	1.9
30	—	1.1	1.4	1.8	2.2	2.5	2.9
40	1.0	1.4	1.9	2.4	2.9	3.4	3.8
50	1.2	1.8	2.4	3.0	3.6	4.2	4.8
60	1.4	2.2	2.9	3.6	4.3	5.0	5.8
70	1.7	2.5	3.4	4.2	5.0	5.9	6.7
80	1.9	2.9	3.8	4.8	5.8	6.7	7.7
90	2.2	3.2	4.3	5.4	6.5	7.6	8.6
100	2.4	3.6	4.8	6.0	7.2	8.4	9.6

Table 12. Infusion Rates for FLOLAN at a Concentration of 15,000 ng/mL

Patient Weight (kg)	Dose or Drug Delivery Rate (ng/kg/min)						
	4	6	8	10	12	14	16
	Infusion Delivery Rate (mL/h)						
30	—	—	1.0	1.2	1.4	1.7	1.9
40	—	1.0	1.3	1.6	1.9	2.2	2.6
50	—	1.2	1.6	2.0	2.4	2.8	3.2
60	1.0	1.4	1.9	2.4	2.9	3.4	3.8
70	1.1	1.7	2.2	2.8	3.4	3.9	4.5
80	1.3	1.9	2.6	3.2	3.8	4.5	5.1
90	1.4	2.2	2.9	3.6	4.3	5.0	5.8
100	1.6	2.4	3.2	4.0	4.8	5.6	6.4

stituted solutions of FLOLAN. Discard any reconstituted solution that has been frozen. Discard any reconstituted solution if it has been refrigerated for more than 48 hours. During use, a single reservoir of reconstituted solution of FLOLAN can be administered at room temperature for a total duration of 8 hours, or it can be used with a cold pouch and administered up to 24 hours with the use of 2 frozen 6-oz gel packs in a cold pouch. When stored or in use, reconstituted FLOLAN must be insulated from temperatures greater than 25°C (77°F) and less than 0°C (32°F), and must not be exposed to direct sunlight.

Use at Room Temperature

Prior to use at room temperature, 15° to 25°C (59° to 77°F), reconstituted solutions of FLOLAN may be stored refrigerated at 2° to 8°C (36° to 46°F) for no longer than 40 hours. When administered at room temperature, reconstituted solutions may be used for no longer than 8 hours. This 48-hour period allows the patient to reconstitute a 2-day supply (200 mL) of FLOLAN. Each 100-mL daily supply may be divided into 3 equal portions. Two of the portions are stored refrigerated at 2° to 8°C (36° to 46°F) until they are used.

Use with a Cold Pouch

Prior to infusion with the use of a cold pouch, solutions may be stored refrigerated at 2° to 8°C (36° to 46°F) for up to 24 hours. When a cold pouch is employed during the infusion, reconstituted solutions of FLOLAN may be used for no longer than 24 hours. The gel packs should be changed every 12 hours. Reconstituted solutions may be kept at 2° to 8°C (36° to 46°F), either in refrigerated storage or in a cold pouch or a combination of the two, for no more than 48 hours.

Parenteral drug products should be inspected visually for particulate matter and discoloration prior to administration whenever solution and container permit. If either occurs, FLOLAN should not be administered.

HOW SUPPLIED

FLOLAN for Injection is supplied as a sterile freeze-dried powder in 17-mL flint glass vials with gray butyl rubber closures, individually packaged in a carton.

17-mL vial containing epoprostenol sodium equivalent to 0.5 mg (500,000 ng), carton of 1 (NDC 0173-0517-00).

17-mL vial containing epoprostenol sodium equivalent to 1.5 mg (1,500,000 ng), carton of 1 (NDC 0173-0519-00).

Store the vials of FLOLAN at 15° to 25°C (59° to 77°F). Protect from light.

The STERILE DILUENT for FLOLAN is supplied in flint glass vials containing 50-mL diluent with fluororesin-faced butyl rubber closures.

50-mL of STERILE DILUENT for FLOLAN, tray of 2 vials (NDC 0173-0518-01).

Store the vials of STERILE DILUENT for FLOLAN at 15° to 25°C (59° to 77°F). DO NOT FREEZE.

GlaxoSmithKline
Research Triangle Park, NC 27709
©2008, GlaxoSmithKline. All rights reserved.
January 2008 FLL:1PI

FLONASE®   ℞

[flō'nāz]
(fluticasone propionate)
Nasal Spray, 50 mcg
For Intranasal Use Only. SHAKE GENTLY BEFORE USE.

DESCRIPTION

Fluticasone propionate, the active component of FLONASE Nasal Spray, is a synthetic corticosteroid having the chemical name S-(fluoromethyl)6α,9-difluoro-11β-17-dihydroxy-16α-methyl-3-oxoandrosta-1,4-diene-17β-carbothioate, 17-propionate and the following chemical structure:

Fluticasone propionate is a white powder with a molecular weight of 500.6, and the empirical formula is $C_{25}H_{31}F_3O_5S$. It is practically insoluble in water, freely soluble in dimethyl sulfoxide and dimethylformamide, and slightly soluble in methanol and 95% ethanol.

FLONASE Nasal Spray, 50 mcg is an aqueous suspension of microfine fluticasone propionate for topical administration to the nasal mucosa by means of a metering, atomizing spray pump. FLONASE Nasal Spray also contains microcrystalline cellulose and carboxymethylcellulose sodium,

dextrose, 0.02% w/w benzalkonium chloride, polysorbate 80, and 0.25% w/w phenylethyl alcohol, and has a pH between 5 and 7.

It is necessary to prime the pump before first use or after a period of non-use (1 week or more). After initial priming (6 actuations), each actuation delivers 50 mcg of fluticasone propionate in 100 mg of formulation through the nasal adapter. Each 16-g bottle of FLONASE Nasal Spray provides 120 metered sprays. After 120 metered sprays, the amount of fluticasone propionate delivered per actuation may not be consistent and the unit should be discarded.

CLINICAL PHARMACOLOGY

Mechanism of Action

Fluticasone propionate is a synthetic trifluorinated corticosteroid with anti-inflammatory activity. In vitro dose response studies on a cloned human glucocorticoid receptor system involving binding and gene expression afforded 50% responses at 1.25 and 0.17 nM concentrations, respectively. Fluticasone propionate was 3-fold to 5-fold more potent than dexamethasone in these assays. Data from the McKenzie vasoconstrictor assay in man also support its potent glucocorticoid activity.

In preclinical studies, fluticasone propionate revealed progesterone-like activity similar to the natural hormone. However, the clinical significance of these findings in relation to the low plasma levels (see Pharmacokinetics) is not known.

The precise mechanism through which fluticasone propionate affects allergic rhinitis symptoms is not known. Corticosteroids have been shown to have a wide range of effects on multiple cell types (e.g., mast cells, eosinophils, neutrophils, macrophages, and lymphocytes) and mediators (e.g., histamine, eicosanoids, leukotrienes, and cytokines) involved in inflammation. In 7 trials in adults, FLONASE Nasal Spray has decreased nasal mucosal eosinophils in 66% (35% for placebo) of patients and basophils in 39% (28% for placebo) of patients. The direct relationship of these findings to long-term symptom relief is not known.

FLONASE Nasal Spray, like other corticosteroids, is an agent that does not have an immediate effect on allergic symptoms. A decrease in nasal symptoms has been noted in some patients 12 hours after initial treatment with FLONASE Nasal Spray. Maximum benefit may not be reached for several days. Similarly, when corticosteroids are discontinued, symptoms may not return for several days.

Pharmacokinetics

Absorption

The activity of FLONASE Nasal Spray is due to the parent drug, fluticasone propionate. Indirect calculations indicate that fluticasone propionate delivered by the intranasal route has an absolute bioavailability averaging less than 2%. After intranasal treatment of patients with allergic rhinitis for 3 weeks, fluticasone propionate plasma concentrations were above the level of detection (50 pg/mL) only when recommended doses were exceeded and then only in occasional samples at low plasma levels. Due to the low bioavailability by the intranasal route, the majority of the pharmacokinetic data was obtained via other routes of administration. Studies using oral dosing of radiolabeled drug have demonstrated that fluticasone propionate is highly extracted from plasma and absorption is low. Oral bioavailability is negligible, and the majority of the circulating radioactivity is due to an inactive metabolite.

Distribution

Following intravenous administration, the initial disposition phase for fluticasone propionate was rapid and consistent with its high lipid solubility and tissue binding. The volume of distribution averaged 4.2 L/kg.

The percentage of fluticasone propionate bound to human plasma proteins averaged 91% with no obvious concentration relationship. Fluticasone propionate is weakly and reversibly bound to erythrocytes and freely equilibrates between erythrocytes and plasma. Fluticasone propionate is not significantly bound to human transcortin.

Metabolism

The total blood clearance of fluticasone propionate is high (average, 1,093 mL/min), with renal clearance accounting for less than 0.02% of the total. The only circulating metabolite detected in man is the 17β-carboxylic acid derivative of fluticasone propionate, which is formed through the cytochrome P450 3A4 pathway. This inactive metabolite had less affinity (approximately 1/2,000) than the parent drug for the glucocorticoid receptor of human lung cytosol in vitro and negligible pharmacological activity in animal studies. Other metabolites detected in vitro using cultured human hepatoma cells have not been detected in man.

Elimination

Following intravenous dosing, fluticasone propionate showed polyexponential kinetics and had a terminal elimination half-life of approximately 7.8 hours. Less than 5% of a radiolabeled oral dose was excreted in the urine as metabolites, with the remainder excreted in the feces as parent drug and metabolites.

Special Populations

Fluticasone propionate nasal spray was not studied in any special populations, and no gender-specific pharmacokinetic data have been obtained.

Drug Interactions

Fluticasone propionate is a substrate of cytochrome P450 3A4. Coadministration of fluticasone propionate and the highly potent cytochrome P450 3A4 inhibitor ritonavir is not recommended based upon a multiple-dose, crossover drug interaction study in 18 healthy subjects. Fluticasone propionate aqueous nasal spray (200 mcg once daily) was coadministered for 7 days with ritonavir (100 mg twice daily). Plasma fluticasone propionate concentrations following fluticasone propionate aqueous nasal spray alone were undetectable (<10 pg/mL) in most subjects, and when concentrations were detectable, peak levels (C_{max}) averaged 11.9 pg/mL (range, 10.8 to 14.1 pg/mL) and $AUC_{(0-\tau)}$ averaged 8.43 pg•hr/mL (range, 4.2 to 18.8 pg•hr/mL). Fluticasone propionate C_{max} and $AUC_{(0-\tau)}$ increased to 318 pg/mL (range, 110 to 648 pg/mL) and 3,102.6 pg•hr/mL (range, 1,207.1 to 5,662.0 pg•hr/mL), respectively, after coadministration of ritonavir with fluticasone propionate aqueous nasal spray. This significant increase in plasma fluticasone propionate exposure resulted in a significant decrease (86%) in plasma cortisol area under the plasma concentration versus time curve (AUC).

Caution should be exercised when other potent cytochrome P450 3A4 inhibitors are coadministered with fluticasone propionate. In a drug interaction study, coadministration of orally inhaled fluticasone propionate (1,000 mcg) and ketoconazole (200 mg once daily) resulted in increased fluticasone propionate exposure and reduced plasma cortisol AUC, but had no effect on urinary excretion of cortisol.

In another multiple-dose drug interaction study, coadministration of orally inhaled fluticasone propionate (500 mcg twice daily) and erythromycin (333 mg 3 times daily) did not affect fluticasone propionate pharmacokinetics.

Pharmacodynamics

In a trial to evaluate the potential systemic and topical effects of FLONASE Nasal Spray on allergic rhinitis symptoms, the benefits of comparable drug blood levels produced by FLONASE Nasal Spray and oral fluticasone propionate were compared. The dosages used were 200 mcg of FLONASE Nasal Spray, the nasal spray vehicle (plus oral placebo), and 5 and 10 mg of oral fluticasone propionate (plus nasal spray vehicle) per day for 14 days. Plasma levels were undetectable in the majority of patients after intranasal dosing, but present at low levels in the majority after oral dosing. FLONASE Nasal Spray was significantly more effective in reducing symptoms of allergic rhinitis than either the oral fluticasone propionate or the nasal vehicle. This trial demonstrated that the therapeutic effect of FLONASE Nasal Spray can be attributed to the topical effects of fluticasone propionate.

In another trial, the potential systemic effects of FLONASE Nasal Spray on the hypothalamic-pituitary-adrenal (HPA) axis were also studied in allergic patients. FLONASE Nasal Spray given as 200 mcg once daily or 400 mcg twice daily was compared with placebo or oral prednisone 7.5 or 15 mg given in the morning. FLONASE Nasal Spray at either dosage for 4 weeks did not affect the adrenal response to 6-hour cosyntropin stimulation, while both dosages of oral prednisone significantly reduced the response to cosyntropin.

CLINICAL TRIALS

A total of 13 randomized, double-blind, parallel-group, multicenter, vehicle placebo-controlled clinical trials were conducted in the United States in adults and pediatric patients (4 years of age and older) to investigate regular use of FLONASE Nasal Spray in patients with seasonal or perennial allergic rhinitis. The trials included 2,633 adults (1,439 men and 1,194 women) with a mean age of 37 (range, 18 to 79 years). A total of 440 adolescents (405 boys and 35 girls), mean age of 14 (range, 12 to 17 years), and 500 children (325 boys and 175 girls), mean age of 9 (range, 4 to 11 years) were also studied. The overall racial distribution was 89% white, 4% black, and 7% other. These trials evaluated the total nasal symptom scores (TNSS) that included rhinorrhea, nasal obstruction, sneezing, and nasal itching in known allergic patients who were treated for 2 to 24 weeks. Subjects treated with FLONASE Nasal Spray exhibited significantly greater decreases in TNSS than vehicle placebo-treated patients. Nasal mucosal basophils and eosinophils were also reduced at the end of treatment in adult studies; however, the clinical significance of this decrease is not known.

There were no significant differences between fluticasone propionate regimens whether administered as a single daily dose of 200 mcg (two 50-mcg sprays in each nostril) or as 100 mcg (one 50-mcg spray in each nostril) twice daily in 6 clinical trials. A clear dose response could not be identified in clinical trials. In 1 trial, 200 mcg/day was slightly more effective than 50 mcg/day during the first few days of treatment; thereafter, no difference was seen.

Two randomized, double-blind, parallel-group, multicenter, vehicle placebo-controlled 28-day trials were conducted in the United States in 732 patients (243 given FLONASE) 12 years of age and older to investigate "as-needed" use of FLONASE Nasal Spray (200 mcg) in patients with seasonal allergic rhinitis. Patients were instructed to take the study medication only on days when they thought they needed the medication for symptom control, not to exceed 2 sprays per nostril on any day, and not more than once daily. "As-needed" use was prospectively defined as average use of study medication no more than 75% of study days. Average use of study medications was 57% to 70% of days for all treatment arms. The studies demonstrated significantly greater reduction in TNSS (sum of nasal congestion, rhinorrhea, sneezing, and nasal itching) with FLONASE Nasal Spray 200 mcg compared to placebo. The relative difference in efficacy with as-needed use as compared to regularly administered doses was not studied.

Three randomized, double-blind, parallel-group, vehicle placebo-controlled trials were conducted in 1,191 patients to investigate regular use of FLONASE Nasal Spray in patients with perennial nonallergic rhinitis. These trials evaluated the patient-rated TNSS (nasal obstruction, postnasal drip, rhinorrhea) in patients treated for 28 days of double-blind therapy and in 1 of the 3 trials for 6 months of open-label treatment. Two of these trials demonstrated that patients treated with FLONASE Nasal Spray at a dosage of 100 mcg twice daily exhibited statistically significant decreases in TNSS compared with patients treated with vehicle.

Individualization of Dosage

Patients should use FLONASE Nasal Spray at regular intervals for optimal effect.

Adult patients may be started on a 200-mcg once-daily regimen (two 50-mcg sprays in each nostril once daily). An alternative 200-mcg/day dosage regimen can be given as 100 mcg twice daily (one 50-mcg spray in each nostril twice daily).

Individual patients will experience a variable time to onset and different degree of symptom relief. In 4 randomized, double-blind, vehicle placebo-controlled, parallel-group allergic rhinitis studies and 2 studies of patients in an outdoor "park" setting (park studies), a decrease in nasal symptoms in treated subjects compared to placebo was shown to occur as soon as 12 hours after treatment with a 200-mcg dose of FLONASE Nasal Spray. Maximum effect may take several days. Regular-use patients who have responded may be able to be maintained (after 4 to 7 days) on 100 mcg/day (1 spray in each nostril once daily).

Some patients (12 years of age and older) with seasonal allergic rhinitis may find as-needed use of FLONASE Nasal Spray (not to exceed 200 mcg daily) effective for symptom control (see CLINICAL TRIALS). Greater symptom control may be achieved with scheduled regular use. Efficacy of as-needed use of FLONASE Nasal Spray has not been studied in pediatric patients under 12 years of age with seasonal allergic rhinitis, or patients with perennial allergic or non-allergic rhinitis.

Pediatric patients (4 years of age and older) should be started with 100 mcg (1 spray in each nostril once daily). Treatment with 200 mcg (2 sprays in each nostril once daily or 1 spray in each nostril twice daily) should be reserved for pediatric patients not adequately responding to 100 mcg daily. Once adequate control is achieved, the dosage should be decreased to 100 mcg (1 spray in each nostril) daily.

Maximum total daily doses should not exceed 2 sprays in each nostril (total dose, 200 mcg/day). There is no evidence that exceeding the recommended dose is more effective.

INDICATIONS AND USAGE

FLONASE Nasal Spray is indicated for the management of the nasal symptoms of seasonal and perennial allergic and nonallergic rhinitis in adults and pediatric patients 4 years of age and older.

Safety and effectiveness of FLONASE Nasal Spray in children below 4 years of age have not been adequately established.

CONTRAINDICATIONS

FLONASE Nasal Spray is contraindicated in patients with a hypersensitivity to any of its ingredients.

WARNINGS

The replacement of a systemic corticosteroid with a topical corticosteroid can be accompanied by signs of adrenal insufficiency, and in addition some patients may experience symptoms of withdrawal, e.g., joint and/or muscular pain, lassitude, and depression. Patients previously treated for prolonged periods with systemic corticosteroids and transferred to topical corticosteroids should be carefully monitored for acute adrenal insufficiency in response to stress. In those patients who have asthma or other clinical conditions requiring long-term systemic corticosteroid treatment, too rapid a decrease in systemic corticosteroids may cause a severe exacerbation of their symptoms.

The concomitant use of intranasal corticosteroids with other inhaled corticosteroids could increase the risk of signs or symptoms of hypercorticism and/or suppression of the HPA axis.

A drug interaction study in healthy subjects has shown that ritonavir (a highly potent cytochrome P450 3A4 inhibitor) can significantly increase plasma fluticasone propionate exposure, resulting in significantly reduced serum cortisol concentrations (see CLINICAL PHARMACOLOGY: Drug Interactions and PRECAUTIONS: Drug Interactions). During postmarketing use, there have been reports of clinically significant drug interactions in patients receiving fluticasone propionate and ritonavir, resulting in systemic corticosteroid effects including Cushing syndrome and adrenal suppression. Therefore, coadministration of fluticasone propionate and ritonavir is not recommended unless the potential benefit to the patient outweighs the risk of systemic corticosteroid side effects.

Persons who are using drugs that suppress the immune system are more susceptible to infections than healthy individuals. Chickenpox and measles, for example, can have a more serious or even fatal course in susceptible children or adults using corticosteroids. In children or adults who have not had these diseases or been properly immunized, particular care should be taken to avoid exposure. How the dose, route, and duration of corticosteroid administration affect the risk of developing a disseminated infection is not known. The contribution of the underlying disease and/or prior corticosteroid treatment to the risk is also not known. If exposed to chickenpox, prophylaxis with varicella zoster immune globulin (VZIG) may be indicated. If exposed to measles, prophylaxis with pooled intramuscular immunoglobulin (IG) may be indicated. (See the respective package inserts for complete VZIG and IG prescribing information.) If chickenpox develops, treatment with antiviral agents may be considered.

Avoid spraying in eyes.

PRECAUTIONS

General

Intranasal corticosteroids may cause a reduction in growth velocity when administered to pediatric patients (see PRECAUTIONS: Pediatric Use).

Rarely, immediate hypersensitivity reactions or contact dermatitis may occur after the administration of FLONASE Nasal Spray. Rare instances of wheezing, nasal septum perforation, cataracts, glaucoma, and increased intraocular pressure have been reported following the intranasal application of corticosteroids, including fluticasone propionate.

Use of excessive doses of corticosteroids may lead to signs or symptoms of hypercorticism and/or suppression of HPA function.

Although systemic effects have been minimal with recommended doses of FLONASE Nasal Spray, potential risk increases with larger doses. Therefore, larger than recommended doses of FLONASE Nasal Spray should be avoided.

When used at higher than recommended doses or in rare individuals at recommended doses, systemic corticosteroid effects such as hypercorticism and adrenal suppression may appear. If such changes occur, the dosage of FLONASE Nasal Spray should be discontinued slowly consistent with accepted procedures for discontinuing oral corticosteroid therapy.

In clinical studies with fluticasone propionate administered intranasally, the development of localized infections of the nose and pharynx with *Candida albicans* has occurred only rarely. When such an infection develops, it may require treatment with appropriate local therapy and discontinuation of treatment with FLONASE Nasal Spray. Patients using FLONASE Nasal Spray over several months or longer should be examined periodically for evidence of *Candida* infection or other signs of adverse effects on the nasal mucosa.

Intranasal corticosteroids should be used with caution, if at all, in patients with active or quiescent tuberculous infections of the respiratory tract; untreated local or systemic fungal or bacterial infections; systemic viral or parasitic infections; or ocular herpes simplex.

Because of the inhibitory effect of corticosteroids on wound healing, patients who have experienced recent nasal septal ulcers, nasal surgery, or nasal trauma should not use a nasal corticosteroid until healing has occurred.

Information for Patients

Patients being treated with FLONASE Nasal Spray should receive the following information and instructions. This information is intended to aid them in the safe and effective use of this medication. It is not a disclosure of all possible adverse or intended effects.

Patients should be warned to avoid exposure to chickenpox or measles and, if exposed, to consult their physician without delay.

Patients should use FLONASE Nasal Spray at regular intervals for optimal effect. Some patients (12 years of age and older) with seasonal allergic rhinitis may find as-needed use of 200 mcg once daily effective for symptom control (see CLINICAL TRIALS).

A decrease in nasal symptoms may occur as soon as 12 hours after starting therapy with FLONASE Nasal Spray. Results in several clinical trials indicate statistically significant improvement within the first day or two of treatment; however, the full benefit of FLONASE Nasal Spray may not be achieved until treatment has been administered for several days. The patient should not increase the prescribed dosage but should contact the physician if symptoms do not improve or if the condition worsens.

For the proper use of FLONASE Nasal Spray and to attain maximum improvement, the patient should read and follow carefully the patient's instructions accompanying the product.

Drug Interactions

Fluticasone propionate is a substrate of cytochrome P450 3A4. A drug interaction study with fluticasone propionate aqueous nasal spray in healthy subjects has shown that ritonavir (a highly potent cytochrome P450 3A4 inhibitor) can significantly increase plasma fluticasone propionate exposure, resulting in significantly reduced serum cortisol concentrations (see CLINICAL PHARMACOLOGY: Drug Interactions). During postmarketing use, there have been reports of clinically significant drug interactions in patients receiving fluticasone propionate and ritonavir, resulting in systemic corticosteroid effects including Cushing syndrome and adrenal suppression. Therefore, coadministration of fluticasone propionate and ritonavir is not recommended unless the potential benefit to the patient outweighs the risk of systemic corticosteroid side effects.

In a placebo-controlled crossover study in 8 healthy volunteers, coadministration of a single dose of orally inhaled fluticasone propionate (1,000 mcg; 5 times the maximum daily intranasal dose) with multiple doses of ketoconazole (200 mg) to steady state resulted in increased plasma fluticasone propionate exposure, a reduction in plasma cortisol AUC, and no effect on urinary excretion of cortisol. Caution should be exercised when FLONASE Nasal Spray is coadministered with ketoconazole and other known potent cytochrome P450 3A4 inhibitors.

Carcinogenesis, Mutagenesis, Impairment of Fertility

Fluticasone propionate demonstrated no tumorigenic potential in mice at oral doses up to 1,000 mcg/kg (approximately 20 times the maximum recommended daily intranasal dose in adults and approximately 10 times the maximum recommended daily intranasal dose in children on a mcg/m^2 basis) for 78 weeks or in rats at inhalation doses up to 57 mcg/kg (approximately 2 times the maximum recommended daily intranasal dose in adults and approximately equivalent to the maximum recommended daily intranasal dose in children on a mcg/m^2 basis) for 104 weeks.

Fluticasone propionate did not induce gene mutation in prokaryotic or eukaryotic cells in vitro. No significant clastogenic effect was seen in cultured human peripheral lymphocytes in vitro or in the mouse micronucleus test.

No evidence of impairment of fertility was observed in reproductive studies conducted in male and female rats at subcutaneous doses up to 50 mcg/kg (approximately 2 times the maximum recommended daily intranasal dose in adults on a mcg/m^2 basis). Prostate weight was significantly reduced at a subcutaneous dose of 50 mcg/kg.

Pregnancy

Teratogenic Effects

Pregnancy Category C. Subcutaneous studies in the mouse and rat at 45 and 100 mcg/kg, respectively (approximately equivalent to and 4 times, respectively, the maximum recommended daily intranasal dose in adults on a mcg/m^2 basis), revealed fetal toxicity characteristic of potent corticosteroid compounds, including embryonic growth retardation, omphalocele, cleft palate, and retarded cranial ossification.

In the rabbit, fetal weight reduction and cleft palate were observed at a subcutaneous dose of 4 mcg/kg (less than the maximum recommended daily intranasal dose in adults on a mcg/m^2 basis). However, no teratogenic effects were reported at oral doses up to 300 mcg/kg (approximately 25 times the maximum recommended daily intranasal dose in adults on a mcg/m^2 basis) of fluticasone propionate to the rabbit. No fluticasone propionate was detected in the plasma in this study, consistent with the established low bioavailability following oral administration (see CLINICAL PHARMACOLOGY).

Fluticasone propionate crossed the placenta following oral administration of 100 mcg/kg to rats and 300 mcg/kg to rabbits (approximately 4 and 25 times, respectively, the maximum recommended daily intranasal dose in adults on a mcg/m^2 basis).

There are no adequate and well-controlled studies in pregnant women. Fluticasone propionate should be used during pregnancy only if the potential benefit justifies the potential risk to the fetus.

Experience with oral corticosteroids since their introduction in pharmacologic, as opposed to physiologic, doses suggests that rodents are more prone to teratogenic effects from corticosteroids than humans. In addition, because there is a natural increase in corticosteroid production during pregnancy, most women will require a lower exogenous corticosteroid dose and many will not need corticosteroid treatment during pregnancy.

Overall Adverse Experiences With >3% Incidence on Fluticasone Propionate in Controlled Clinical Trials With FLONASE Nasal Spray in Patients ≥4 Years With Seasonal or Perennial Allergic Rhinitis

Adverse Experience	Vehicle Placebo (n = 758) %	FLONASE 100 mcg Once Daily (n = 167) %	FLONASE 200 mcg Once Daily (n = 782) %
Headache	14.6	6.6	16.1
Pharyngitis	7.2	6.0	7.8
Epistaxis	5.4	6.0	6.9
Nasal burning/nasal irritation	2.6	2.4	3.2
Nausea/vomiting	2.0	4.8	2.6
Asthma symptoms	2.9	7.2	3.3
Cough	2.8	3.6	3.8

Nursing Mothers

It is not known whether fluticasone propionate is excreted in human breast milk. However, other corticosteroids have been detected in human milk. Subcutaneous administration to lactating rats of 10 mcg/kg of tritiated fluticasone propionate (less than the maximum recommended daily intranasal dose in adults on a mcg/m^2 basis) resulted in measurable radioactivity in the milk. Since there are no data from controlled trials on the use of intranasal fluticasone propionate by nursing mothers, caution should be exercised when FLONASE Nasal Spray is administered to a nursing woman.

Pediatric Use

Six hundred fifty (650) patients aged 4 to 11 years and 440 patients aged 12 to 17 years were studied in US clinical trials with fluticasone propionate nasal spray. The safety and effectiveness of FLONASE Nasal Spray in children below 4 years of age have not been established.

Controlled clinical studies have shown that intranasal corticosteroids may cause a reduction in growth velocity in pediatric patients. This effect has been observed in the absence of laboratory evidence of HPA axis suppression, suggesting that growth velocity is a more sensitive indicator of systemic corticosteroid exposure in pediatric patients than some commonly used tests of HPA axis function. The long-term effects of this reduction in growth velocity associated with intranasal corticosteroids, including the impact on final adult height, are unknown. The potential for "catch-up" growth following discontinuation of treatment with intranasal corticosteroids has not been adequately studied. The growth of pediatric patients receiving intranasal corticosteroids, including FLONASE Nasal Spray, should be monitored routinely (e.g., via stadiometry). The potential growth effects of prolonged treatment should be weighed against the clinical benefits obtained and the risks/benefits of treatment alternatives. To minimize the systemic effects of intranasal corticosteroids, including FLONASE Nasal Spray, each patient should be titrated to the lowest dose that effectively controls his/her symptoms.

A 1-year placebo-controlled clinical growth study was conducted in 150 pediatric patients (ages 3 to 9 years) to assess the effect of FLONASE Nasal Spray (single daily dose of 200 mcg, the maximum approved dose) on growth velocity. From the primary population of 56 patients receiving FLONASE Nasal Spray and 52 receiving placebo, the point estimate for growth velocity with FLONASE Nasal Spray was 0.14 cm/year lower than that noted with placebo (95% confidence interval ranging from 0.54 cm/year lower than placebo to 0.27 cm/year higher than placebo). Thus, no statistically significant effect on growth was noted compared to placebo. No evidence of clinically relevant changes in HPA axis function or bone mineral density was observed as assessed by 12-hour urinary cortisol excretion and dual-energy x-ray absorptiometry, respectively.

The potential for FLONASE Nasal Spray to cause growth suppression in susceptible patients or when given at higher doses cannot be ruled out.

Geriatric Use

A limited number of patients 65 years of age and older (n = 129) or 75 years of age and older (n = 11) have been treated with FLONASE Nasal Spray in US and non-US clinical trials. While the number of patients is too small to permit separate analysis of efficacy and safety, the adverse reactions reported in this population were similar to those reported by younger patients.

ADVERSE REACTIONS

In controlled US studies, more than 3,300 patients with seasonal allergic, perennial allergic, or perennial nonallergic rhinitis received treatment with intranasal fluticasone propionate. In general, adverse reactions in clinical studies have been primarily associated with irritation of the nasal mucous membranes, and the adverse reactions were reported with approximately the same frequency by patients treated with the vehicle itself. The complaints did not usually interfere with treatment. Less than 2% of patients in clinical trials discontinued because of adverse events; this rate was similar for vehicle placebo and active comparators.

Systemic corticosteroid side effects were not reported during controlled clinical studies up to 6 months' duration with FLONASE Nasal Spray. If recommended doses are exceeded, however, or if individuals are particularly sensitive or taking FLONASE Nasal Spray in conjunction with administration of other corticosteroids, symptoms of hypercorticism, e.g., Cushing syndrome, could occur.

The following incidence of common adverse reactions (>3%, where incidence in fluticasone propionate-treated subjects exceeded placebo) is based upon 7 controlled clinical trials in which 536 patients (57 girls and 108 boys aged 4 to 11 years, 137 female and 234 male adolescents and adults) were treated with FLONASE Nasal Spray 200 mcg once daily over 2 to 4 weeks and 2 controlled clinical trials in which 246 patients (119 female and 127 male adolescents and adults) were treated with FLONASE Nasal Spray 200 mcg once daily over 6 months. Also included in the table are adverse events from 2 studies in which 167 children (45 girls and 122 boys aged 4 to 11 years) were treated with FLONASE Nasal Spray 100 mcg once daily for 2 to 4 weeks. [See table above]

Other adverse events that occurred in ≤3% but ≥1% of patients and that were more common with fluticasone propionate (with uncertain relationship to treatment) included: blood in nasal mucus, runny nose, abdominal pain, diarrhea, fever, flu-like symptoms, aches and pains, dizziness, bronchitis.

Observed During Clinical Practice

In addition to adverse events reported from clinical trials, the following events have been identified during postapproval use of intranasal fluticasone propionate in clinical practice. Because they are reported voluntarily from a population of unknown size, estimates of frequency cannot be made. These events have been chosen for inclusion due to either their seriousness, frequency of reporting, or causal connection to fluticasone propionate or a combination of these factors.

General

Hypersensitivity reactions, including angioedema, skin rash, edema of the face and tongue, pruritus, urticaria, bronchospasm, wheezing, dyspnea, and anaphylaxis/anaphylactoid reactions, which in rare instances were severe.

Ear, Nose, and Throat

Alteration or loss of sense of taste and/or smell and, rarely, nasal septal perforation, nasal ulcer, sore throat, throat irritation and dryness, cough, hoarseness, and voice changes.

Eye

Dryness and irritation, conjunctivitis, blurred vision, glaucoma, increased intraocular pressure, and cataracts.

Cases of growth suppression have been reported for intranasal corticosteroids, including FLONASE (see PRECAUTIONS: Pediatric Use).

OVERDOSAGE

Chronic overdosage may result in signs/symptoms of hypercorticism (see PRECAUTIONS). Intranasal administration of 2 mg (10 times the recommended dose) of fluticasone propionate twice daily for 7 days to healthy human volunteers was well tolerated. Single oral doses up to 16 mg have been studied in human volunteers with no acute toxic effects reported. Repeat oral doses up to 80 mg daily for 10 days in volunteers and repeat oral doses up to 10 mg daily for 14 days in patients were well tolerated. Adverse reactions were of mild or moderate severity, and incidences were similar in active and placebo treatment groups. Acute overdosage with this dosage form is unlikely since 1 bottle of FLONASE Nasal Spray contains approximately 8 mg of fluticasone propionate.

The oral and subcutaneous median lethal doses in mice and rats were >1,000 mg/kg (>20,000 and >41,000 times, respectively, the maximum recommended daily intranasal dose in adults and >10,000 and >20,000 times, respectively, the maximum recommended daily intranasal dose in children on a mg/m² basis).

DOSAGE AND ADMINISTRATION

Patients should use FLONASE Nasal Spray at regular intervals for optimal effect.

Adults

The recommended starting dosage in **adults** is 2 sprays (50 mcg of fluticasone propionate each) in each nostril once daily (total daily dose, 200 mcg). The same dosage divided into 100 mcg given twice daily (e.g., 8 a.m. and 8 p.m.) is also effective. After the first few days, patients may be able to reduce their dosage to 100 mcg (1 spray in each nostril) once daily for maintenance therapy. Some patients (12 years of age and older) with seasonal allergic rhinitis may find as-needed use of 200 mcg once daily effective for symptom control (see CLINICAL TRIALS). Greater symptom control may be achieved with scheduled regular use.

Adolescents and Children (4 Years of Age and Older)

Patients should be started with 100 mcg (1 spray in each nostril once daily). Patients not adequately responding to 100 mcg may use 200 mcg (2 sprays in each nostril). Once adequate control is achieved, the dosage should be decreased to 100 mcg (1 spray in each nostril) daily.

The maximum total daily dosage should not exceed 2 sprays in each nostril (200 mcg/day) (see CLINICAL TRIALS: Individualization of Dosage).

FLONASE Nasal Spray is not recommended for children under 4 years of age.

Directions for Use

Illustrated patient's instructions for proper use accompany each package of FLONASE Nasal Spray.

HOW SUPPLIED

FLONASE Nasal Spray, 50 mcg is supplied in an amber glass bottle fitted with a white metering atomizing pump, white nasal adapter, and green dust cover in a box of 1 (NDC 0173-0453-01) with patient's instructions for use. Each bottle contains a net fill weight of 16 g and will provide 120 actuations. Each actuation delivers 50 mcg of fluticasone propionate in 100 mg of formulation through the nasal adapter. The correct amount of medication in each spray cannot be assured after 120 sprays even though the bottle is not completely empty. The bottle should be discarded when the labeled number of actuations has been used.

Store between 4° and 30°C (39° and 86°F).

GlaxoSmithKline
Research Triangle Park, NC 27709
©2007, GlaxoSmithKline. All rights reserved.
August 2007 FLN:1PI

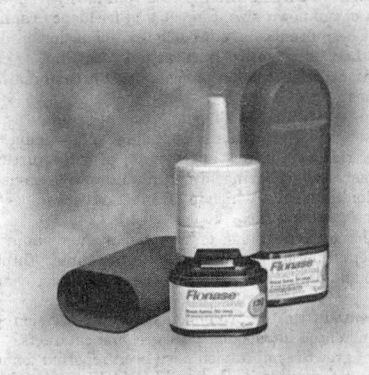

Flonase®
(fluticasone propionate)
Nasal Spray, 50 mcg
Please read this leaflet carefully before you start to take your medicine. It provides a summary of information on your medicine.
For further information ask your doctor or pharmacist.
WHAT YOU SHOULD KNOW ABOUT RHINITIS
Rhinitis is a word that means inflammation of the lining of the nose. If you suffer from rhinitis, your nose becomes stuffy and runny. Rhinitis can also make your nose itchy, and you may sneeze a lot. Rhinitis can be caused by allergies to pollen, animals, molds, or other materials—or it may have a nonallergic cause.

WHAT YOU SHOULD KNOW ABOUT FLONASE NASAL SPRAY

Your doctor has prescribed FLONASE Nasal Spray, a medicine that can help treat your rhinitis. FLONASE Nasal Spray contains fluticasone propionate, which is a synthetic corticosteroid. Corticosteroids are natural substances found in the body that help fight inflammation. When you spray FLONASE into your nose, it helps to reduce the symptoms of allergic reactions and the stuffiness, runniness, itching, and sneezing that can bother you.

THINGS TO REMEMBER ABOUT FLONASE NASAL SPRAY

1. Shake gently before using.
2. Use your nasal spray as directed by your doctor. The directions are on the pharmacy label.
3. Keep your nasal spray **out of the reach of children.**

BEFORE USING YOUR NASAL SPRAY

- If you are pregnant (or intending to become pregnant),
- If you are breastfeeding a baby,
- If you are allergic to FLONASE Nasal Spray or any other nasal corticosteroid,
- If you are taking a medicine containing ritonavir (commonly used to treat HIV infection or AIDS),

TELL YOUR DOCTOR BEFORE STARTING TO TAKE THIS MEDICINE. In some circumstances, this medicine may not be suitable and your doctor may wish to give you a different medicine. Make sure that your doctor knows what other medicines you are taking.

USING YOUR NASAL SPRAY

- Follow the instructions shown in the rest of this leaflet. If you have any problems, tell your doctor or pharmacist.
- It is important that you use it as directed by your doctor. The pharmacist's label will usually tell you what dose to take and how often. If it doesn't, or you are not sure, ask your doctor or pharmacist.

DOSAGE

- For ADULTS, the usual starting dosage is 2 sprays in each nostril once daily. Sometimes your doctor may recommend using 1 spray in each nostril twice a day (morning and evening). You should not use more than a total of 2 sprays in each nostril daily. After you have begun to feel better, 1 spray in each nostril daily may be adequate for you.
- For ADOLESCENTS and CHILDREN (4 years of age and older), the usual starting dosage is 1 spray in each nostril once daily. Sometimes your doctor may recommend using 2 sprays in each nostril daily. Then, after you have begun to feel better, 1 spray in each nostril daily may be adequate for you.
- DO NOT use more of your medicine or take it more often than your doctor advises.
- FLONASE may begin to work within 12 hours of the first dose, but it takes several days of regular use to reach its greatest effect. It is important that you use FLONASE Nasal Spray as prescribed by your doctor. Best results will be obtained by using the spray on a regular basis. If symptoms disappear, contact your doctor for further instructions.
- If you also have itchy, watery eyes, you should tell your doctor. You may be given an additional medicine to treat your eyes. Be careful not to confuse them, particularly if the second medicine is an eye drop.
- If you miss a dose, just take your regularly scheduled next dose when it is due. DO NOT DOUBLE the dose.

HOW TO USE YOUR NASAL SPRAY

Read the complete instructions carefully and use only as directed.

BEFORE USING

1. Shake the bottle gently and then remove the dust cover (Figure 1).
[See figure 1 at top of next column]
2. It is necessary to prime the pump into the air the first time it is used, or when you have not used it for a week or more. To prime the pump, hold the bottle as shown with the nasal applicator pointing away from you and with your forefinger and middle finger on either side of the nasal applicator and your thumb underneath the bottle. When you prime the pump for the first time, press down and release the pump 6 times (Figure 2). The pump is now ready for use. If the pump is not used for 7 days, prime until a fine spray appears.
[See figure 2 in next column]

USING THE SPRAY

3. Blow your nose to clear your nostrils.
4. Close one nostril. Tilt your head forward slightly and, keeping the bottle upright, carefully insert the nasal applicator into the other nostril (Figure 3).
[See figure 3 in next column]
5. Start to breathe in through your nose, and WHILE BREATHING IN press firmly and quickly down once on the applicator to release the spray. To get a full actuation, use your forefinger and middle finger to spray while supporting the base of the bottle with your thumb. Avoid spraying in eyes. Breathe gently inwards through the nostril (Figure 4).
[See figure 4 at top of next page]
6. Breathe out through your mouth.

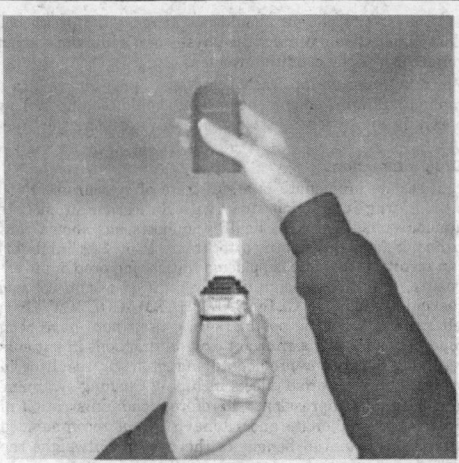

Figure 1

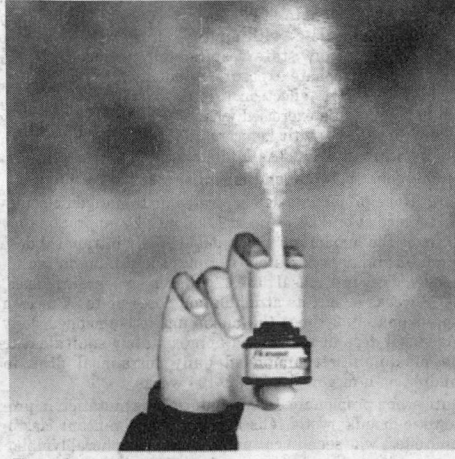

Figure 2

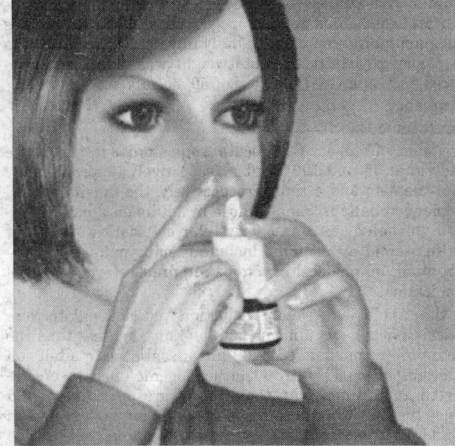

Figure 3

7. If a second spray is required in that nostril, repeat steps 4 through 6.
8. Repeat steps 4 through 7 in the other nostril.
9. Wipe the nasal applicator with a clean tissue and replace the dust cover (Figure 5).
[See figure 5 on next page]
10. Do not use this bottle for more than the labeled number of sprays even though the bottle is not completely empty. Before you throw the bottle away, you should consult your doctor to see if a refill is needed. Do not take extra doses or stop taking FLONASE Nasal Spray without consulting your doctor.

CLEANING

Your nasal spray should be cleaned at least once a week. To do this:
1. Remove the dust cover and then gently pull upwards to free the nasal applicator.
2. Wash the applicator and dust cover under warm tap water. Allow to dry at room temperature, then place the applicator and dust cover back on the bottle.

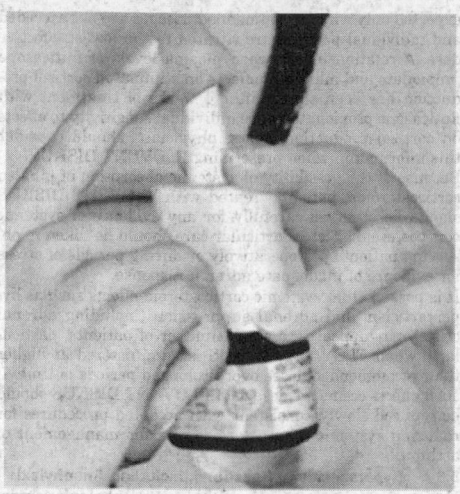

Figure 4

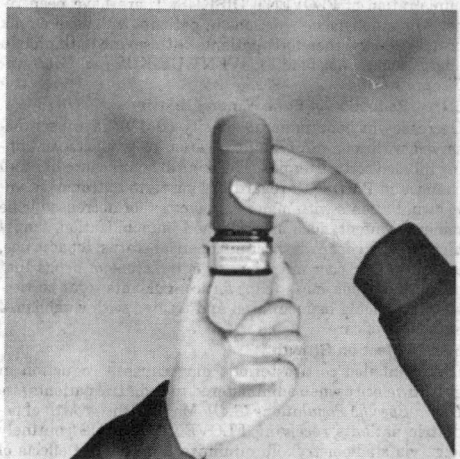

Figure 5

3. If the nasal applicator becomes blocked, it can be removed as above and left to soak in warm water. Rinse with cold tap water, dry, and refit. **Do not try to unblock the nasal applicator by inserting a pin or other sharp object.**

STORING YOUR NASAL SPRAY

• Keep your FLONASE Nasal Spray **out of the reach of children.**
• Avoid spraying in eyes.
• Store between 4° and 30°C (39° and 86°F).
• Do not use your FLONASE Nasal Spray after the date shown as "EXP" on the label or box.

REMEMBER: This medicine has been prescribed for you by your doctor. DO NOT give this medicine to anyone else.

FURTHER INFORMATION

This leaflet does not contain the complete information about your medicine. *If you have any questions, or are not sure about something, then you should ask your doctor or pharmacist.*

You may want to read this leaflet again. Please DO NOT THROW IT AWAY until you have finished your medicine.

GlaxoSmithKline
Research Triangle Park, NC 27709
©2003, GlaxoSmithKline. All rights reserved.
July 2003 RL-2019

FLOVENT® DISKUS® 50 mcg ℞
[flō'vent]
(fluticasone propionate inhalation powder, 50 mcg)
FLOVENT® DISKUS® 100 mcg ℞
(fluticasone propionate inhalation powder, 100 mcg)
FLOVENT® DISKUS® 250 mcg ℞
(fluticasone propionate inhalation powder, 250 mcg)
FOR ORAL INHALATION

HIGHLIGHTS OF PRESCRIBING INFORMATION
These highlights do not include all the information needed to use FLOVENT DISKUS safely and effectively. See full prescribing information for FLOVENT DISKUS.

FLOVENT DISKUS 50 mcg
(fluticasone propionate inhalation powder, 50 mcg)
FLOVENT DISKUS 100 mcg
(fluticasone propionate inhalation powder, 100 mcg)
FLOVENT DISKUS 250 mcg
(fluticasone propionate inhalation powder, 250 mcg)
FOR ORAL INHALATION
Initial U.S. Approval: 1994

———————RECENT MAJOR CHANGES———————

Warnings and Precautions, Hypersensitivity Reactions, Including Anaphylaxis (5.6), Reduction in Bone Mineral Density (5.7), Drug Interaction With Strong Cytochrome P450 3A4 Inhibitors (5.11)	May 2010

———————INDICATIONS AND USAGE———————
FLOVENT DISKUS is an inhaled corticosteroid indicated for:
• Maintenance treatment of asthma as prophylactic therapy in patients 4 years and older. (1)
• Treatment of asthma for patients requiring oral corticosteroid therapy. (1)
FLOVENT DISKUS is NOT indicated for the relief of acute bronchospasm. (1)

———————DOSAGE AND ADMINISTRATION———————
For oral inhalation only. Dosing is based on prior asthma therapy. (2)

Previous Therapy	Recommended Starting Dosage	Highest Recommended Dosage
Patients aged ≥12 years		
Bronchodilators alone	100 mcg twice daily	500 mcg twice daily
Inhaled corticosteroids	100-250 mcg twice daily	500 mcg twice daily
Oral corticosteroids	500-1,000 mcg twice daily	1,000 mcg twice daily
Patients aged 4-11 years	50 mcg twice daily	100 mcg twice daily

———————DOSAGE FORMS AND STRENGTHS———————
Inhalation powder with 50, 100, or 250 mcg per actuation. (3)

———————CONTRAINDICATIONS———————
• Primary treatment of status asthmaticus or acute episodes of asthma requiring intensive measures. (4)
• Severe hypersensitivity to milk proteins. (4)

———————WARNINGS AND PRECAUTIONS———————
• Localized infections: *Candida albicans* infection of the mouth and pharynx. Monitor patients periodically for signs of adverse effects on the oral cavity. Advise patients to rinse mouth following inhalation. (5.1)
• Immunosuppression: Potential worsening of existing tuberculosis; fungal, bacterial, viral, or parasitic infection; or ocular herpes simplex. More serious or even fatal course of chickenpox or measles in susceptible patients. Use caution in patients with above because of the potential for worsening of these infections. (5.3)
• Transferring patients from systemic corticosteroids: Risk of impaired adrenal function when transferring from oral steroids. Taper patients slowly from systemic corticosteroids if transferring to FLOVENT DISKUS. (5.4)
• Hypercorticism and adrenal suppression: May occur with very high dosages or at the regular dosage in susceptible individuals. If such changes occur, discontinue FLOVENT DISKUS slowly. (5.5)
• Hypersensitivity reactions, including anaphylaxis, may occur after administration of FLOVENT DISKUS. Discontinue FLOVENT DISKUS if such reactions occur. (4, 5.6)
• Effect on growth: Monitor growth of pediatric patients. (5.8)
• Glaucoma and cataracts: Close monitoring is warranted. (5.9)

———————ADVERSE REACTIONS———————
Most common adverse reactions (incidence >3%) include upper respiratory tract infection or inflammation, throat irritation, sinusitis, rhinitis, oral candidiasis, nausea and vomiting, gastrointestinal discomfort, fever, cough, bronchitis, and headache. (6.1)

To report SUSPECTED ADVERSE REACTIONS, contact GlaxoSmithKline at 1-888-825-5249 or FDA at 1-800-FDA-1088 or www.fda.gov/medwatch

———————DRUG INTERACTIONS———————
Use with strong cytochrome P450 3A4 inhibitors such as ritonavir and ketoconazole is not recommended. Systemic corticosteroid effects may occur. (7.1, 7.2)

———————USE IN SPECIFIC POPULATIONS———————
Hepatic impairment: Monitor patients for signs of increased drug exposure. (8.6)
See 17 for PATIENT COUNSELING INFORMATION and FDA-approved patient labeling

Revised: 05/2010

FULL PRESCRIBING INFORMATION: CONTENTS*
1 INDICATIONS AND USAGE
2 DOSAGE AND ADMINISTRATION
3 DOSAGE FORMS AND STRENGTHS
4 CONTRAINDICATIONS
5 WARNINGS AND PRECAUTIONS
  5.1 Local Effects
  5.2 Acute Asthma Episodes
  5.3 Immunosuppression
  5.4 Transferring Patients From Systemic Corticosteroid Therapy
  5.5 Hypercorticism and Adrenal Suppression
  5.6 Hypersensitivity Reactions, Including Anaphylaxis
  5.7 Reduction in Bone Mineral Density
  5.8 Effect on Growth
  5.9 Glaucoma and Cataracts
  5.10 Paradoxical Bronchospasm
  5.11 Drug Interaction With Strong Cytochrome P450 3A4 Inhibitors
  5.12 Eosinophilic Conditions and Churg-Strauss Syndrome
6 ADVERSE REACTIONS
  6.1 Clinical Trials Experience
  6.2 Postmarketing Experience
7 DRUG INTERACTIONS
  7.1 Strong Cytochrome P450 3A4 Inhibitors
8 USE IN SPECIFIC POPULATIONS
  8.1 Pregnancy
  8.3 Nursing Mothers
  8.4 Pediatric Use
  8.5 Geriatric Use
  8.6 Hepatic Impairment
  8.7 Renal Impairment
10 OVERDOSAGE
11 DESCRIPTION
12 CLINICAL PHARMACOLOGY
  12.1 Mechanism of Action
  12.2 Pharmacodynamics
  12.3 Pharmacokinetics
13 NONCLINICAL TOXICOLOGY
  13.1 Carcinogenesis, Mutagenesis, Impairment of Fertility
  13.2 Animal Toxicology and/or Pharmacology
14 CLINICAL STUDIES
  14.1 Adult and Adolescent Patients 12 Years and Older
  14.2 Pediatric Patients Aged 4 to 11 Years
16 HOW SUPPLIED/STORAGE AND HANDLING
17 PATIENT COUNSELING INFORMATION
  17.1 Oral Candidiasis
  17.2 Status Asthmaticus and Acute Asthma Symptoms
  17.3 Immunosuppression
  17.4 Hypercorticism and Adrenal Suppression
  17.5 Hypersensitivity Reactions, Including Anaphylaxis
  17.6 Reduction in Bone Mineral Density
  17.7 Reduced Growth Velocity
  17.8 Ocular Effects
  17.9 Use Daily for Best Effect
* Sections or subsections omitted from the full prescribing information are not listed

---

FULL PRESCRIBING INFORMATION

1   INDICATIONS AND USAGE

FLOVENT® DISKUS® is indicated for the maintenance treatment of asthma as prophylactic therapy in patients 4 years and older. It is also indicated for patients requiring oral corticosteroid therapy for asthma. Many of these patients may be able to reduce or eliminate their requirement for oral corticosteroids over time.
FLOVENT DISKUS is NOT indicated for the relief of acute bronchospasm.

2   DOSAGE AND ADMINISTRATION

FLOVENT DISKUS should be administered by the orally inhaled route only in patients 4 years and older. Individual patients will experience a variable time to onset and degree of symptom relief. Maximum benefit may not be achieved for 1 to 2 weeks or longer after starting treatment.
After asthma stability has been achieved, it is always desirable to titrate to the lowest effective dosage to reduce the possibility of side effects. For patients who do not respond

adequately to the starting dosage after 2 weeks of therapy, higher dosages may provide additional asthma control. The safety and efficacy of FLOVENT DISKUS when administered in excess of recommended dosages have not been established.

The recommended starting dosage and the highest recommended dosage of FLOVENT DISKUS, based on prior asthma therapy, are listed in Table 1.

Table 1. Recommended Dosages of FLOVENT DISKUS

NOTE: In all patients, it is desirable to titrate to the lowest effective dosage once asthma stability is achieved.

Previous Therapy	Recommended Starting Dosage	Highest Recommended Dosage
Adult and adolescent patients (aged ≥12 years)		
Bronchodilators alone	100 mcg twice daily	500 mcg twice daily
Inhaled corticosteroids	100-250 mcg twice daily[a]	500 mcg twice daily
Oral corticosteroids[b]	500-1,000 mcg twice daily[c]	1,000 mcg twice daily
Pediatric patients (aged 4-11 years)[d]	50 mcg twice daily[a]	100 mcg twice daily

[a]Starting dosages above 100 mcg twice daily for adult and adolescent patients and 50 mcg twice daily for pediatric patients aged 4 to 11 years may be considered for patients with poorer asthma control or those who have previously required doses of inhaled corticosteroids that are in the higher range for the specific agent.
[b]For patients currently receiving chronic oral corticosteroid therapy, prednisone should be reduced no faster than 2.5 to 5 mg/day on a weekly basis beginning after at least 1 week of therapy with FLOVENT DISKUS. Patients should be carefully monitored for signs of asthma instability, including serial objective measures of airflow, and for signs of adrenal insufficiency [see Warnings and Precautions (5.4)]. Once prednisone reduction is complete, the dosage of FLOVENT DISKUS should be reduced to the lowest effective dosage.
[c]The choice of starting dosage should be made on the basis of individual patient assessment. A controlled clinical study of 111 oral corticosteroid-dependent patients with asthma showed few significant differences between the 2 doses of FLOVENT DISKUS on safety and efficacy endpoints. However, inability to decrease the dose of oral corticosteroids further during corticosteroid reduction may be indicative of the need to increase the dose of fluticasone propionate up to the maximum of 1,000 mcg twice daily.
[d]Because individual responses may vary, pediatric patients previously maintained on other inhaled corticosteroids may require dosage adjustments upon transfer to FLOVENT DISKUS.

3 DOSAGE FORMS AND STRENGTHS

FLOVENT DISKUS is an inhalation powder. Each actuation delivers 46, 94, or 229 mcg of fluticasone propionate from the DISKUS® inhalation unit. FLOVENT DISKUS is supplied as a disposable orange inhalation unit containing 60 blisters of powder formulation packaged in a plastic-coated, moisture-protective foil pouch.

4 CONTRAINDICATIONS

The use of FLOVENT DISKUS is contraindicated in the following conditions:
• Primary treatment of status asthmaticus or other acute episodes of asthma where intensive measures are required [see Warnings and Precautions (5.2)].
• Severe hypersensitivity to milk proteins [see Warnings and Precautions (5.6), Adverse Reactions (6.2), Description (11)].

5 WARNINGS AND PRECAUTIONS

5.1 Local Effects
In clinical studies, the development of localized infections of the mouth and pharynx with Candida albicans has occurred in patients treated with FLOVENT DISKUS. When such an infection develops, it should be treated with appropriate local or systemic (i.e., oral antifungal) therapy while treatment with FLOVENT DISKUS continues, but at times therapy with FLOVENT DISKUS may need to be interrupted. Patients should rinse the mouth after inhalation of FLOVENT DISKUS [see Adverse Reactions (6.1)].

5.2 Acute Asthma Episodes
FLOVENT DISKUS is not to be regarded as a bronchodilator and is not indicated for rapid relief of bronchospasm. Pa-

tients should be instructed to contact their physicians immediately when episodes of asthma that are not responsive to bronchodilators occur during the course of treatment with FLOVENT DISKUS. During such episodes, patients may require therapy with oral corticosteroids.

5.3 Immunosuppression
Persons who are using drugs that suppress the immune system are more susceptible to infections than healthy individuals. Chickenpox and measles, for example, can have a more serious or even fatal course in susceptible children or adults using corticosteroids. In such children or adults who have not had these diseases or been properly immunized, particular care should be taken to avoid exposure. How the dose, route, and duration of corticosteroid administration affect the risk of developing a disseminated infection is not known. The contribution of the underlying disease and/or prior corticosteroid treatment to the risk is also not known. If exposed to chickenpox, prophylaxis with varicella zoster immune globulin (VZIG) may be indicated. If exposed to measles, prophylaxis with pooled intramuscular immunoglobulin (IG) may be indicated. (See the respective package inserts for complete VZIG and IG prescribing information.) If chickenpox develops, treatment with antiviral agents may be considered.
Because of the potential for worsening infections, inhaled corticosteroids should be used with caution, if at all, in patients with active or quiescent tuberculosis infection of the respiratory tract; untreated systemic fungal, bacterial, viral or parasitic infections; or ocular herpes simplex.

5.4 Transferring Patients From Systemic Corticosteroid Therapy
Particular care is needed for patients who have been transferred from systemically active corticosteroids to inhaled corticosteroids because deaths due to adrenal insufficiency have occurred in patients with asthma during and after transfer from systemic corticosteroids to less systemically available inhaled corticosteroids. After withdrawal from systemic corticosteroids, a number of months are required for recovery of hypothalamic-pituitary-adrenal (HPA) function.
Patients requiring oral corticosteroids should be weaned slowly from systemic corticosteroid use after transferring to FLOVENT DISKUS. In a clinical trial of 111 patients, prednisone reduction was accomplished by reducing the daily prednisone dose by 2.5 mg on a weekly basis during transfer to FLOVENT DISKUS. Successive reduction of prednisone dose was allowed only when lung function; symptoms; and as-needed, short-acting beta-agonist use were better than or comparable to that seen before initiation of prednisone dose reduction. Lung function (forced expiratory volume in 1 second [FEV$_1$] or morning peak expiratory flow [AM PEF]), beta-agonist use, and asthma symptoms should be carefully monitored during withdrawal of oral corticosteroids. In addition to monitoring asthma signs and symptoms, patients should be observed for signs and symptoms of adrenal insufficiency such as fatigue, lassitude, weakness, nausea and vomiting, and hypotension.
Patients who have been previously maintained on 20 mg or more per day of prednisone (or its equivalent) may be most susceptible, particularly when their systemic corticosteroids have been almost completely withdrawn. During this period of HPA suppression, patients may exhibit signs and symptoms of adrenal insufficiency when exposed to trauma, surgery, or infection (particularly gastroenteritis) or other conditions associated with severe electrolyte loss. Although inhaled corticosteroids may provide control of asthma symptoms during these episodes, in recommended doses they supply less than normal physiological amounts of glucocorticoid (cortisol) systemically and do NOT provide the mineralocorticoid activity that is necessary for coping with these emergencies.
During periods of stress or a severe asthma attack, patients who have been withdrawn from systemic corticosteroids should be instructed to resume oral corticosteroids immediately and to contact their physicians for further instruction. These patients should also be instructed to carry a warning card indicating that they may need supplementary systemic corticosteroids during periods of stress or a severe asthma attack.
Transfer of patients from systemic corticosteroid therapy to FLOVENT DISKUS may unmask conditions previously suppressed by the systemic corticosteroid therapy, e.g., rhinitis, conjunctivitis, eczema, arthritis, and eosinophilic conditions. Some patients may experience symptoms of systemically active corticosteroid withdrawal, e.g., joint and/or muscular pain, lassitude, and depression, despite maintenance or even improvement of respiratory function.

5.5 Hypercorticism and Adrenal Suppression
Fluticasone propionate will often help control asthma symptoms with less suppression of HPA function than therapeutically equivalent oral doses of prednisone. Since fluticasone propionate is absorbed into the circulation and can be systemically active at higher doses, the beneficial effects of FLOVENT DISKUS in minimizing HPA dysfunction may be

expected only when recommended dosages are not exceeded and individual patients are titrated to the lowest effective dose. A relationship between plasma levels of fluticasone propionate and inhibitory effects on stimulated cortisol production has been shown after 4 weeks of treatment with fluticasone propionate. Since individual sensitivity to effects on cortisol production exists, physicians should consider this information when prescribing FLOVENT DISKUS.
Because of the possibility of systemic absorption of inhaled corticosteroids, patients treated with FLOVENT DISKUS should be observed carefully for any evidence of systemic corticosteroid effects. Particular care should be taken in observing patients postoperatively or during periods of stress for evidence of inadequate adrenal response.
It is possible that systemic corticosteroid effects such as hypercorticism and adrenal suppression (including adrenal crisis) may appear in a small number of patients, particularly when FLOVENT DISKUS is administered at higher than recommended doses over prolonged periods of time. If such effects occur, the dosage of FLOVENT DISKUS should be reduced slowly, consistent with accepted procedures for reducing systemic corticosteroids and for management of asthma.

5.6 Hypersensitivity Reactions, Including Anaphylaxis
Hypersensitivity reactions, including anaphylaxis, angioedema, urticaria, and bronchospasm, may occur after administration of FLOVENT DISKUS. There have been reports of anaphylactic reactions in patients with severe milk protein allergy; therefore, patients with severe milk protein allergy should not take FLOVENT DISKUS [see Contraindications (4)].

5.7 Reduction in Bone Mineral Density
Decreases in bone mineral density (BMD) have been observed with long-term administration of products containing inhaled corticosteroids. The clinical significance of small changes in BMD with regard to long-term outcomes is unknown. Patients with major risk factors for decreased bone mineral content, such as prolonged immobilization, family history of osteoporosis, postmenopausal status, tobacco use, advanced age, poor nutrition, or chronic use of drugs that can reduce bone mass (e.g., anticonvulsants, oral corticosteroids) should be monitored and treated with established standards of care.

5.8 Effect on Growth
Orally inhaled corticosteroids may cause a reduction in growth velocity when administered to pediatric patients [see Use in Specific Populations (8.4)]. Monitor the growth of pediatric patients receiving FLOVENT DISKUS routinely (e.g., via stadiometry). To minimize the systemic effects of orally inhaled corticosteroids, including FLOVENT DISKUS, titrate each patient's dose to the lowest dosage that effectively controls his/her symptoms.

5.9 Glaucoma and Cataracts
Glaucoma, increased intraocular pressure, and cataracts have been reported in patients following the long-term administration of inhaled corticosteroids, including fluticasone propionate. Therefore, close monitoring is warranted in patients with a change in vision or with a history of increased intraocular pressure, glaucoma, and/or cataracts.

5.10 Paradoxical Bronchospasm
As with other inhaled medications, bronchospasm may occur with an immediate increase in wheezing after dosing. If bronchospasm occurs following dosing with FLOVENT DISKUS, it should be treated immediately with a fast-acting inhaled bronchodilator. Treatment with FLOVENT DISKUS should be discontinued immediately and alternative therapy instituted.

5.11 Drug Interaction With Strong Cytochrome P450 3A4 Inhibitors
The use of strong cytochrome P450 [CYP] 3A4 inhibitors (e.g., ritonavir, atazanavir, clarithromycin, indinavir, itraconazole, nefazodone, nelfinavir, saquinavir, ketoconazole, telithromycin) with FLOVENT DISKUS is not recommended because increased systemic corticosteroid adverse effects may occur [see Drug Interactions (7.1), Clinical Pharmacology (12.3)].

5.12 Eosinophilic Conditions and Churg-Strauss Syndrome
In rare cases, patients on inhaled fluticasone propionate may present with systemic eosinophilic conditions. Some of these patients have clinical features of vasculitis consistent with Churg-Strauss syndrome, a condition that is often treated with systemic corticosteroid therapy. These events usually, but not always, have been associated with the reduction and/or withdrawal of oral corticosteroid therapy following the introduction of fluticasone propionate. Cases of serious eosinophilic conditions have also been reported with other inhaled corticosteroids in this clinical setting. Physicians should be alert to eosinophilia, vasculitic rash, worsening pulmonary symptoms, cardiac complications, and/or neuropathy presenting in their patients. A causal relationship between fluticasone propionate and these underlying conditions has not been established.

6 ADVERSE REACTIONS

Systemic and local corticosteroid use may result in the following:

- *Candida albicans* infection *[see Warnings and Precautions (5.1)]*
- Immunosuppression *[see Warnings and Precautions (5.3)]*
- Hypercorticism and adrenal suppression *[see Warnings and Precautions (5.5)]*
- Reduction in bone mineral density *[see Warnings and Precautions (5.7)]*
- Growth effects *[see Warnings and Precautions (5.8)]*
- Glaucoma and cataracts *[see Warnings and Precautions (5.9)]*

6.1 Clinical Trials Experience

Because clinical trials are conducted under widely varying conditions, adverse reaction rates observed in the clinical trials of a drug cannot be directly compared with rates in the clinical trials of another drug and may not reflect the rates observed in practice. The incidence of common adverse reactions in Table 2 is based upon 7 placebo-controlled US clinical trials in which 1,176 pediatric, adolescent, and adult patients (466 females and 710 males) previously treated with as-needed bronchodilators and/or inhaled corticosteroids were treated twice daily for up to 12 weeks with FLOVENT DISKUS (doses of 50 to 500 mcg) or placebo.

[See table 2 at right]

Table 2 includes all events (whether considered drug-related or nondrug-related by the investigator) that occurred at a rate of over 3% in any of the groups treated with FLOVENT DISKUS and were more common than in the placebo group. Less than 2% of patients discontinued from the studies because of adverse reactions. The average duration of exposure was 73 to 79 days in the active treatment groups compared with 56 days in the placebo group.

Additional Adverse Reactions: Other adverse reactions not previously listed, whether considered drug-related or not by the investigators, that were reported more frequently by patients with asthma treated with FLOVENT DISKUS compared with patients treated with placebo include the following: palpitations; soft tissue injuries; contusions and hematomas; wounds and lacerations; burns; poisoning and toxicity; pressure-induced disorders; hoarseness/dysphonia; epistaxis; ear, nose, throat, and tonsil signs and symptoms; ear, nose, and throat polyps; allergic ear, nose, and throat disorders; throat constriction; fluid disturbances; weight gain; appetite disturbances; keratitis and conjunctivitis; blepharoconjunctivitis; gastrointestinal signs and symptoms; oral ulcerations; dental discomfort and pain; oral erythema and rashes; mouth and tongue disorders; oral discomfort and pain; tooth decay; cholecystitis; arthralgia and articular rheumatism; muscle cramps and spasms; musculoskeletal inflammation; dizziness; sleep disorders; migraines; paralysis of cranial nerves; edema and swelling; bacterial infections; fungal infections; mobility disorders; mood disorders; bacterial reproductive infections; photodermatitis; dermatitis and dermatosis; viral skin infections; eczema; pruritus; acne and folliculitis; urinary infections.

Three (3) of the 7 placebo-controlled US clinical trials were pediatric studies. A total of 592 patients 4 to 11 years were treated with FLOVENT DISKUS (dosages of 50 or 100 mcg twice daily) or placebo; an additional 174 patients 4 to 11 years received FLOVENT® ROTADISK® (fluticasone propionate inhalation powder) at the same doses. There were no clinically relevant differences in the pattern or severity of adverse events in children compared with those reported in adults.

In the first 16 weeks of a 52-week clinical trial in adult patients with asthma who previously required oral corticosteroids (daily doses of 5 to 40 mg oral prednisone), the effects of FLOVENT DISKUS 500 mcg twice daily (n = 41) and 1,000 mcg twice daily (n = 36) were compared with placebo (n = 34) for the frequency of reported adverse events. The average duration of exposure for patients taking FLOVENT DISKUS was 105 days compared with 75 days for placebo. Adverse events, whether or not considered drug related by the investigators, reported in more than 5 patients in the group taking FLOVENT DISKUS and that occurred more frequently with FLOVENT DISKUS than with placebo are shown below (percent FLOVENT DISKUS and percent placebo).

Ear, Nose, and Throat: Hoarseness/dysphonia (9% and 0%), nasal congestion/blockage (16% and 0%), oral candidiasis (31% and 21%), rhinitis (13% and 9%), sinusitis/sinus infection (33% and 12%), throat irritation (10% and 9%), and upper respiratory tract infection (31% and 24%).

Gastrointestinal: Nausea and vomiting (9% and 0%).

Lower Respiratory: Cough (9% and 3%) and viral respiratory infections (9% and 6%).

Musculoskeletal: Arthralgia and articular rheumatism (17% and 3%) and muscle pain (12% and 0%).

Non-Site Specific: Malaise and fatigue (16% and 9%) and pain (10% and 3%).

Skin: Pruritus (6% and 0%) and skin rashes (8% and 3%).

Table 2. Adverse Reactions With >3% Incidence in US Controlled Clinical Trials With FLOVENT DISKUS in Patients With Asthma Previously Receiving Bronchodilators and/or Inhaled Corticosteroids

Adverse Event	FLOVENT DISKUS 50 mcg Twice Daily (n = 178) %	FLOVENT DISKUS 100 mcg Twice Daily (n = 305) %	FLOVENT DISKUS 250 mcg Twice Daily (n = 86) %	FLOVENT DISKUS 500 mcg Twice Daily (n = 64) %	Placebo (n = 543) %
Ear, nose, and throat					
Upper respiratory tract infection	20	18	21	14	16
Throat irritation	13	13	3	22	8
Sinusitis/sinus infection	9	10	6	6	6
Upper respiratory inflammation	5	5	0	5	3
Rhinitis	4	3	1	2	2
Oral candidiasis	<1	9	6	5	7
Gastrointestinal					
Nausea and vomiting	8	4	1	2	4
Gastrointestinal discomfort and pain	4	3	2	2	3
Viral gastrointestinal infection	4	3	3	5	1
Non-site specific					
Fever	7	7	1	2	4
Viral infection	2	2	0	5	2
Lower respiratory					
Viral respiratory infection	4	5	1	2	4
Cough	3	5	1	5	4
Bronchitis	2	3	0	8	1
Neurological					
Headache	12	12	2	14	7
Musculoskeletal and trauma					
Muscle injury	2	0	1	5	1
Musculoskeletal pain	4	3	2	5	2
Injury	2	<1	0	5	<1

6.2 Postmarketing Experience

In addition to adverse reactions reported from clinical trials, the following adverse reactions have been identified during postmarketing use of fluticasone propionate. Because these reactions are reported voluntarily from a population of uncertain size, it is not always possible to reliably estimate their frequency or establish a causal relationship to drug exposure. These events have been chosen for inclusion due to either their seriousness, frequency of reporting, or causal connection to fluticasone propionate or a combination of these factors.

Ear, Nose, and Throat: Aphonia, facial and oropharyngeal edema, and throat soreness.

Endocrine and Metabolic: Cushingoid features, growth velocity reduction in children/adolescents, hyperglycemia, and osteoporosis.

Eye: Cataracts.

Immune System Disorders: Immediate and delayed hypersensitivity reactions, including anaphylaxis, rash, angioedema, and bronchospasm, have been reported. Anaphylactic reactions in patients with severe milk protein allergy have been reported.

Psychiatry: Agitation, aggression, anxiety, depression, and restlessness. Behavioral changes, including hyperactivity and irritability, have been reported very rarely and primarily in children.

Respiratory: Asthma exacerbation, bronchospasm, chest tightness, dyspnea, immediate bronchospasm, pneumonia, and wheeze.

Skin: Contusions and ecchymoses.

Eosinophilic Conditions: In rare cases, patients on inhaled fluticasone propionate may present with systemic eosinophilic conditions, with some patients presenting with clinical features of vasculitis consistent with Churg-Strauss syndrome, a condition that is often treated with systemic corticosteroid therapy. These events usually, but not always, have been associated with the reduction and/or withdrawal of oral corticosteroid therapy following the introduction of fluticasone propionate *[see Warnings and Precautions (5.12)]*.

7 DRUG INTERACTIONS

7.1 Strong Cytochrome P450 3A4 Inhibitors

Fluticasone propionate is a substrate of CYP 3A4. The use of strong CYP 3A4 inhibitors (e.g., ritonavir, atazanavir, clarithromycin, indinavir, itraconazole, nefazodone, nelfinavir, saquinavir, ketoconazole, telithromycin) with FLOVENT DISKUS is not recommended because increased systemic corticosteroid adverse effects may occur.

A drug interaction study with fluticasone propionate aqueous nasal spray in healthy subjects has shown that ritonavir (a strong CYP 3A4 inhibitor) can significantly increase plasma fluticasone propionate concentration, resulting in significantly reduced serum cortisol concentrations *[see Clinical Pharmacology (12.3)]*. During postmarketing use, there have been reports of clinically significant drug interactions in patients receiving fluticasone propionate and ritonavir, resulting in systemic corticosteroid effects including Cushing syndrome and adrenal suppression. Therefore, coadministration of fluticasone propionate and ritonavir is not recommended unless the potential benefit to the patient outweighs the risk of systemic corticosteroid side effects. Coadministration of orally inhaled fluticasone propionate (1,000 mcg) and ketoconazole (200 mg once daily) resulted in a 1.9-fold increase in plasma fluticasone propionate exposure and a 45% decrease in plasma cortisol area under the curve (AUC), but had no effect on urinary excretion of cortisol. Coadministration of fluticasone propionate and ketoconazole is not recommended unless the potential benefit to the patient outweighs the risk of systemic corticosteroid side effects.

8 USE IN SPECIFIC POPULATIONS

8.1 Pregnancy

Pregnancy Category C: There are no adequate and well-controlled studies with FLOVENT DISKUS in pregnant women. FLOVENT DISKUS should be used during pregnancy only if the potential benefit justifies the potential risk to the fetus.

Teratogenic Effects: Subcutaneous studies in the mouse and rat at doses approximately 0.1 and 0.4, respectively, times the maximum recommended human daily inhalation dose (MRHD) in adults on a mg/m^2 basis revealed fetal toxicity characteristic of potent corticosteroid compounds, including embryonic growth retardation, omphalocele, cleft palate, and retarded cranial ossification.

In the rabbit, fetal weight reduction and cleft palate were observed at a subcutaneous dose approximately 0.03 times the MRHD in adults on a mg/m^2 basis. However, no teratogenic effects were reported at oral doses up to approximately 2 times the MRHD in adults on a mg/m^2 basis. No fluticasone propionate was detected in the plasma in this study, consistent with the established low bioavailability following oral administration *[see Clinical Pharmacology (12.3)]*.

Experience with oral corticosteroids since their introduction in pharmacologic, as opposed to physiologic, doses suggests that rodents are more prone to teratogenic effects from corticosteroids than humans. In addition, because there is a natural increase in corticosteroid production during pregnancy, most women will require a lower exogenous corticosteroid dose and many will not need corticosteroid treatment during pregnancy.

8.3 Nursing Mothers

It is not known whether fluticasone propionate is excreted in human breast milk. However, other corticosteroids have been detected in human milk. Subcutaneous administration to lactating rats of tritiated fluticasone propionate at a dose approximately 0.04 times the MRHD in adults on a mg/m^2 basis resulted in measurable radioactivity in milk.

Since there are no data from controlled trials on the use of FLOVENT DISKUS by nursing mothers, caution should be exercised when FLOVENT DISKUS is administered to a nursing woman.

8.4 Pediatric Use

The safety and effectiveness of FLOVENT DISKUS in children 4 years and older have been established *[see Adverse Reactions (6.1), Clinical Pharmacology (12.3), Clinical Studies (14.2)]*. The safety and effectiveness of FLOVENT DISKUS in children younger than 4 years have not been established.

Effects on Growth: Orally inhaled corticosteroids may cause a reduction in growth velocity when administered to pediatric patients. A reduction of growth velocity in children or teenagers may occur as a result of poorly controlled asthma or from use of corticosteroids including inhaled corticosteroids. The effects of long-term treatment of children and adolescents with inhaled corticosteroids, including fluticasone propionate, on final adult height are not known. Controlled clinical studies have shown that inhaled corticosteroids may cause a reduction in growth in pediatric patients. In these studies, the mean reduction in growth velocity was approximately 1 cm/year (range: 0.3 to 1.8 cm/year) and appears to depend upon dose and duration of exposure. This effect was observed in the absence of laboratory evidence of HPA axis suppression, suggesting that growth velocity is a more sensitive indicator of systemic corticosteroid exposure in pediatric patients than some commonly used tests of HPA axis function. The long-term effects of this reduction in growth velocity associated with orally inhaled corticosteroids, including the impact on final adult height, are unknown. The potential for "catch-up" growth following discontinuation of treatment with orally inhaled corticosteroids has not been adequately studied. The effects on growth velocity of treatment with orally inhaled corticosteroids for over 1 year, including the impact on final adult height, are unknown. The growth of children and adolescents receiving orally inhaled corticosteroids, including FLOVENT DISKUS, should be monitored routinely (e.g., via stadiometry). The potential growth effects of prolonged treatment should be weighed against the clinical benefits obtained and the risks associated with alternative therapies. To minimize the systemic effects of orally inhaled corticosteroids, including FLOVENT DISKUS, each patient should be titrated to the lowest dose that effectively controls his/her symptoms.

A 52-week placebo-controlled study to assess the potential growth effects of fluticasone propionate inhalation powder (FLOVENT ROTADISK) at 50 and 100 mcg twice daily was conducted in the US in 325 prepubescent children (244 males and 81 females) aged 4 to 11 years. The mean growth velocities at 52 weeks observed in the intent-to-treat population were 6.32 cm/year in the placebo group (n = 76), 6.07 cm/year in the 50-mcg group (n = 98), and 5.66 cm/year in the 100-mcg group (n = 89). An imbalance in the proportion of children entering puberty between groups and a higher dropout rate in the placebo group due to poorly controlled asthma may be confounding factors in interpreting these data. A separate subset analysis of children who remained prepubertal during the study revealed growth rates at 52 weeks of 6.10 cm/year in the placebo group (n = 57), 5.91 cm/year in the 50-mcg group (n = 74), and 5.67 cm/year in the 100-mcg group (n = 79). In children aged 8.5 years, the mean age of children in this study, the range for expected growth velocity is: boys – 3rd percentile = 3.8 cm/year, 50th percentile = 5.4 cm/year, and 97th percentile = 7.0 cm/year; girls – 3rd percentile = 4.2 cm/year, 50th percentile = 5.7 cm/year, and 97th percentile = 7.3 cm/year. The clinical significance of these growth data is not certain.

8.5 Geriatric Use

Safety data have been collected on 280 patients (FLOVENT DISKUS n = 83, FLOVENT ROTADISK n = 197) 65 years or older and 33 patients (FLOVENT DISKUS n = 14, FLOVENT ROTADISK n = 19) 75 years or older who have been treated with fluticasone propionate inhalation powder in US and non-US clinical trials. No overall differences in safety or effectiveness were observed between these patients and younger patients, and other reported clinical experience has not identified differences in responses between the elderly and younger patients, but greater sensitivity of some older individuals cannot be ruled out.

8.6 Hepatic Impairment

Formal pharmacokinetic studies using FLOVENT DISKUS have not been conducted in patients with hepatic impairment. Since fluticasone propionate is predominantly cleared by hepatic metabolism, impairment of liver function may lead to accumulation of fluticasone propionate in plasma. Therefore, patients with hepatic disease should be closely monitored.

8.7 Renal Impairment

Formal pharmacokinetic studies using FLOVENT DISKUS have not been conducted in patients with renal impairment.

10 OVERDOSAGE

Chronic overdosage may result in signs/symptoms of hypercorticism *[see Warnings and Precautions (5.5)]*. Inhalation by healthy volunteers of a single dose of 4,000 mcg of fluticasone propionate inhalation powder or single doses of 1,760 or 3,520 mcg of fluticasone propionate CFC inhalation aerosol was well tolerated. Doses of 1,320 mcg administered to healthy human volunteers twice daily for 7 to 15 days were also well tolerated. Repeat oral doses up to 80 mg daily for 10 days in healthy volunteers and repeat oral doses up to 20 mg daily for 42 days in patients were well tolerated. Adverse reactions were of mild or moderate severity, and incidences were similar in active and placebo treatment groups.

No deaths were seen in mice given an oral dose of 1,000 mg/kg (approximately 2,000 and 9,600 times the MRHD in adults and children aged 4 to 11 years, respectively, on a mg/m^2 basis). No deaths were seen in rats given an oral dose of 1,000 mg/kg (approximately 4,100 and 19,000 times the MRHD in adults and children aged 4 to 11 years, respectively, on a mg/m^2 basis).

11 DESCRIPTION

The active component of FLOVENT DISKUS 50 mcg, FLOVENT DISKUS 100 mcg, and FLOVENT DISKUS 250 mcg is fluticasone propionate, a corticosteroid having the chemical name *S*-(fluoromethyl) 6α,9-difluoro-11β,17-dihydroxy-16α-methyl-3-oxoandrosta-1,4-diene-17β-carbothioate, 17-propionate and the following chemical structure:

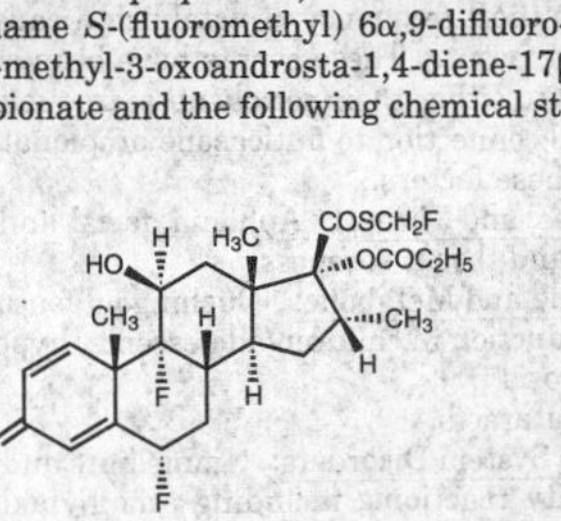

Fluticasone propionate is a white powder with a molecular weight of 500.6, and the empirical formula is $C_{25}H_{31}F_3O_5S$. It is practically insoluble in water, freely soluble in dimethyl sulfoxide and dimethylformamide, and slightly soluble in methanol and 95% ethanol.

FLOVENT DISKUS 50 mcg, FLOVENT DISKUS 100 mcg, and FLOVENT DISKUS 250 mcg are specially designed plastic inhalation delivery systems containing a double-foil blister strip of a powder formulation of fluticasone propionate intended for oral inhalation only. The DISKUS inhalation unit, which is the delivery component, is an integral part of the drug product. Each blister on the double-foil strip within the unit contains 50, 100, or 250 mcg of microfine fluticasone propionate in 12.5 mg of formulation containing lactose (which contains milk proteins). After a blister containing medication is opened by activating the DISKUS, the medication is dispersed into the airstream created by the patient inhaling through the mouthpiece.

Under standardized in vitro test conditions, FLOVENT DISKUS delivers 46, 94, or 229 mcg of fluticasone propionate from FLOVENT DISKUS 50 mcg, FLOVENT DISKUS 100 mcg, or FLOVENT DISKUS 250 mcg, respectively, when tested at a flow rate of 60 L/min for 2 seconds.

In adult patients with obstructive lung disease and severely compromised lung function (FEV_1 20% to 30% of predicted), mean peak inspiratory flow (PIF) through a DISKUS was 82.4 L/min (range: 46.1 to 115.3 L/min). In children with asthma 4 and 8 years old, mean PIF through FLOVENT DISKUS was 70 and 104 L/min, respectively (range: 48 to 123 L/min). The actual amount of drug delivered to the lung may depend on patient factors, such as inspiratory flow profile.

12 CLINICAL PHARMACOLOGY

12.1 Mechanism of Action

Fluticasone propionate is a synthetic trifluorinated corticosteroid with potent anti-inflammatory activity. In vitro assays using human lung cytosol preparations have established fluticasone propionate as a human glucocorticoid receptor agonist with an affinity 18 times greater than dexamethasone, almost twice that of beclomethasone17monopropionate (BMP), the active metabolite of beclomethasone dipropionate, and over 3 times that of budesonide. Data from the McKenzie vasoconstrictor assay in man are consistent with these results. The clinical significance of these findings is unknown.

Inflammation is an important component in the pathogenesis of asthma. Corticosteroids have been shown to inhibit multiple cell types (e.g., mast cells, eosinophils, basophils, lymphocytes, macrophages, neutrophils) and mediator production or secretion (e.g., histamine, eicosanoids, leukotrienes, cytokines) involved in the asthmatic response. These anti-inflammatory actions of corticosteroids contribute to their efficacy in asthma.

Though effective for the treatment of asthma, corticosteroids do not affect asthma symptoms immediately. Individual patients will experience a variable time to onset and degree of symptom relief. Maximum benefit may not be achieved for 1 to 2 weeks or longer after starting treatment. When corticosteroids are discontinued, asthma stability may persist for several days or longer.

Studies in patients with asthma have shown a favorable ratio between topical anti-inflammatory activity and systemic corticosteroid effects with recommended doses of orally inhaled fluticasone propionate. This is explained by a combination of a relatively high local anti-inflammatory effect, negligible oral systemic bioavailability (<1%), and the minimal pharmacological activity of the only metabolite detected in man.

12.2 Pharmacodynamics

In clinical trials with fluticasone propionate inhalation powder using dosages up to and including 250 mcg twice daily, occasional abnormal short cosyntropin tests (peak serum cortisol <18 mcg/dL assessed by radioimmunoassay) were noted both in patients receiving fluticasone propionate and in patients receiving placebo. The incidence of abnormal tests at 500 mcg twice daily was greater than placebo. In a 2-year study carried out with the DISKHALER® inhalation device in 64 patients with mild, persistent asthma (mean FEV_1 91% of predicted) randomized to fluticasone propionate 500 mcg twice daily or placebo, no patient receiving fluticasone propionate had an abnormal response to 6-hour cosyntropin infusion (peak serum cortisol <18 mcg/dL). With a peak cortisol threshold <35 mcg/dL, 1 patient receiving fluticasone propionate (4%) had an abnormal response at 1 year; repeat testing at 18 months and 2 years was normal. Another patient receiving fluticasone propionate (5%) had an abnormal response at 2 years. No patient on placebo had an abnormal response at 1 or 2 years.

In a placebo-controlled clinical study conducted in patients aged 4 to 11 years, a 30-minute cosyntropin stimulation test was performed in 41 patients after 12 weeks of dosing with 50 or 100 mcg twice daily of fluticasone propionate via the DISKUS device. One patient receiving fluticasone propionate via DISKUS had a prestimulation plasma cortisol concentration <5 mcg/dL, and 2 patients had a rise in cortisol of <7 mcg/dL. However, all poststimulation values were >18 mcg/dL.

The potential systemic effects of inhaled fluticasone propionate on the HPA axis were also studied in patients with asthma. Fluticasone propionate given by inhalation aerosol at dosages of 220, 440, 660, or 880 mcg twice daily was compared with placebo or oral prednisone 10 mg given once daily for 4 weeks. For most patients, the ability to increase cortisol production in response to stress, as assessed by 6-hour cosyntropin stimulation, remained intact with inhaled fluticasone propionate treatment. No patient had an abnormal response (peak serum cortisol <18 mcg/dL) after dosing with placebo or fluticasone propionate 220 mcg twice daily. For patients treated with 440, 660, and 880 mcg twice daily, 10%, 16%, and 12%, respectively, had an abnormal response as compared with 29% of patients treated with prednisone.

12.3 Pharmacokinetics

Absorption: Fluticasone propionate acts locally in the lung; therefore, plasma levels do not predict therapeutic effect. Studies using oral dosing of labeled and unlabeled drug have demonstrated that the oral systemic bioavailability of fluticasone propionate is negligible (<1%), primarily due to incomplete absorption and presystemic metabolism in the gut and liver. In contrast, the majority of the fluticasone propionate delivered to the lung is systemically absorbed. The absolute bioavailability of fluticasone propionate from the DISKUS device in healthy volunteers averages 7.8%. Peak steady-state fluticasone propionate plasma concentrations in adult patients with asthma (N = 11) ranged from undetectable to 266 pg/mL after a 500-mcg twice-daily dosage of fluticasone propionate inhalation powder using the DISKUS device. The mean fluticasone propionate plasma concentration was 110 pg/mL.

Distribution: Following intravenous administration, the initial disposition phase for fluticasone propionate was rapid and consistent with its high lipid solubility and tissue binding. The volume of distribution averaged 4.2 L/kg.

The percentage of fluticasone propionate bound to human plasma proteins averages 99%. Fluticasone propionate is weakly and reversibly bound to erythrocytes and is not significantly bound to human transcortin.

Metabolism: The total clearance of fluticasone propionate is high (average, 1,093 mL/min), with renal clearance accounting for less than 0.02% of the total. The only circulating metabolite detected in man is the 17β-carboxylic acid derivative of fluticasone propionate, which is formed through the CYP 3A4 pathway. This metabolite had less affinity (approximately 1/2,000) than the parent drug for the corticosteroid receptor of human lung cytosol in vitro and negligible pharmacological activity in animal studies. Other metabolites detected in vitro using cultured human hepatoma cells have not been detected in man.

Elimination: Following intravenous dosing, fluticasone propionate showed polyexponential kinetics and had a terminal elimination half-life of approximately 7.8 hours. Less than 5% of a radiolabeled oral dose was excreted in the urine as metabolites, with the remainder excreted in the feces as parent drug and metabolites.

Specific Populations: *Gender:* Full pharmacokinetic profiles were obtained from 9 female and 16 male patients given 500 mcg twice daily. No overall differences in fluticasone propionate pharmacokinetics were observed.

Pediatrics: In a clinical study conducted in patients aged 4 to 11 years with mild to moderate asthma, fluticasone propionate concentrations were obtained in 61 patients at 20 and 40 minutes after dosing with 50 and 100 mcg twice daily of fluticasone propionate inhalation powder using the DISKUS. Plasma concentrations were low and ranged from undetectable (about 80% of the plasma samples) to 88 pg/mL. Mean peak fluticasone propionate plasma concentrations at the 50- and 100-mcg dose levels were 5 and 8 pg/mL, respectively.

Hepatic and Renal Impairment: Formal pharmacokinetic studies using FLOVENT DISKUS have not been conducted in patients with hepatic or renal impairment. However, since fluticasone propionate is predominantly cleared by hepatic metabolism, impairment of liver function may lead to accumulation of fluticasone propionate in plasma. Therefore, patients with hepatic disease should be closely monitored.

Drug Interactions: *Ritonavir:* Fluticasone propionate is a substrate of CYP 3A4. Coadministration of fluticasone propionate and the strong CYP 3A4 inhibitor ritonavir is not recommended based upon a multiple-dose, crossover drug interaction study in 18 healthy subjects. Fluticasone propionate aqueous nasal spray (200 mcg once daily) was coadministered for 7 days with ritonavir (100 mg twice daily). Plasma fluticasone propionate concentrations following fluticasone propionate aqueous nasal spray alone were undetectable (<10 pg/mL) in most subjects, and when concentrations were detectable, peak levels (C_{max}) averaged 11.9 pg/mL (range: 10.8 to 14.1 pg/mL) and $AUC_{(0-\tau)}$ averaged 8.43 pg•hr/mL (range: 4.2 to 18.8 pg•hr/mL). Fluticasone propionate C_{max} and $AUC_{(0-\tau)}$ increased to 318 pg/mL (range: 110 to 648 pg/mL) and 3,102.6 pg•hr/mL (range: 1,207.1 to 5,662.0 pg•hr/mL), respectively, after coadministration of ritonavir with fluticasone propionate aqueous nasal spray. This significant increase in plasma fluticasone propionate concentration resulted in a significant decrease (86%) in serum cortisol AUC.

Ketoconazole: In a placebo-controlled, crossover study in 8 healthy adult volunteers, coadministration of a single dose of orally inhaled fluticasone propionate (1,000 mcg) with multiple doses of ketoconazole (200 mg) to steady state resulted in increased plasma fluticasone propionate exposure, a reduction in plasma cortisol AUC, and no effect on urinary excretion of cortisol. Following orally inhaled fluticasone propionate alone, $AUC_{(2-last)}$ averaged 1.559 ng•hr/mL (range: 0.555 to 2.906 ng•hr/mL) and $AUC_{(2-\infty)}$ averaged 2.269 ng•hr/mL (range: 0.836 to 3.707 ng•hr/mL). Fluticasone propionate $AUC_{(2-last)}$ and $AUC_{(2-\infty)}$ increased to 2.781 ng•hr/mL (range: 2.489 to 8.486 ng•hr/mL) and 4.317 ng•hr/mL (range: 3.256 to 9.408 ng•hr/mL), respectively, after coadministration of ketoconazole with orally inhaled fluticasone propionate. This increase in plasma fluticasone propionate concentration resulted in a decrease (45%) in serum cortisol AUC.

Erythromycin: In a multiple-dose drug interaction study, coadministration of orally inhaled fluticasone propionate (500 mcg twice daily) and erythromycin (333 mg 3 times daily) did not affect fluticasone propionate pharmacokinetics.

13 NONCLINICAL TOXICOLOGY

13.1 Carcinogenesis, Mutagenesis, Impairment of Fertility

Fluticasone propionate demonstrated no tumorigenic potential in mice at oral doses up to 1,000 mcg/kg (approximately 2 and 10 times the MRHD in adults and children aged 4 to 11 years, respectively, on a mg/m² basis) for 78 weeks or in rats at inhalation doses up to 57 mcg/kg (approximately 0.2 times and approximately equivalent to the MRHD in adults and children aged 4 to 11 years, respectively, on a mg/m² basis) for 104 weeks.

Fluticasone propionate did not induce gene mutation in prokaryotic or eukaryotic cells in vitro. No significant clastogenic effect was seen in cultured human peripheral lymphocytes in vitro or in the in vivo mouse micronucleus test.

No evidence of impairment of fertility was observed in reproductive studies conducted in male and female rats at subcutaneous doses up to 50 mcg/kg (approximately 0.2 times the MRHD in adults on a mg/m² basis). Prostate weight was significantly reduced at a subcutaneous dose of 50 mcg/kg.

13.2 Animal Toxicology and/or Pharmacology

Reproductive Toxicology: Subcutaneous studies in the mouse and rat at 45 and 100 mcg/kg (approximately 0.1 and 0.4 times the MRHD in adults on a mg/m² basis, respectively) revealed fetal toxicity characteristic of potent corticosteroid compounds, including embryonic growth retardation, omphalocele, cleft palate, and retarded cranial ossification.

In the rabbit, fetal weight reduction and cleft palate were observed at a subcutaneous dose of 4 mcg/kg (approximately 0.03 times the MRHD in adults on a mg/m² basis). However, no teratogenic effects were reported at oral doses up to 300 mcg/kg (approximately 2 times the MRHD in adults on a mg/m² basis) of fluticasone propionate. No fluticasone propionate was detected in the plasma in this study, consistent with the established low bioavailability following oral administration [see Clinical Pharmacology (12.3)].

Fluticasone propionate crossed the placenta following subcutaneous administration to mice and rats and oral administration to rabbits.

14 CLINICAL STUDIES

14.1 Adult and Adolescent Patients 12 Years and Older

Four randomized, double-blind, parallel-group, placebo-controlled, US clinical trials were conducted in 1,036 adult and adolescent patients (aged ≥12 years) with asthma to assess the efficacy and safety of FLOVENT DISKUS in the treatment of asthma. Fixed dosages of 100, 250, and 500 mcg twice daily were compared with placebo to provide information about appropriate dosing to cover a range of asthma severity. Patients in these studies included those inadequately controlled with bronchodilators alone and those already maintained on daily inhaled corticosteroids. All doses were delivered by inhalation of the contents of 1 or 2 blisters from FLOVENT DISKUS twice daily.

Figures 1 through 4 display results of pulmonary function tests (mean percent change from baseline in FEV_1 prior to AM dose) for 3 recommended dosages of FLOVENT DISKUS (100, 250, and 500 mcg twice daily) and placebo from the four 12-week trials in adolescents and adults. These trials used predetermined criteria for lack of efficacy (indicators of worsening asthma), resulting in withdrawal of more patients in the placebo group. Therefore, pulmonary function results at Endpoint (the last evaluable FEV_1 result, including most patients' lung function data) are also displayed. Pulmonary function, as determined by percent change from baseline in FEV_1 at recommended dosages of FLOVENT DISKUS improved significantly compared with placebo by the first week of treatment, and improvement was maintained for up to 1 year or more.

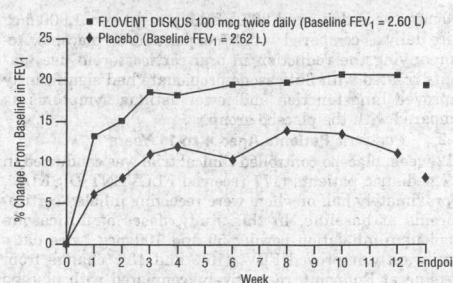

Figure 1. A 12-Week Clinical Trial Evaluating FLOVENT DISKUS 100 mcg Twice Daily in Adolescents and Adults Receiving Bronchodilators Alone

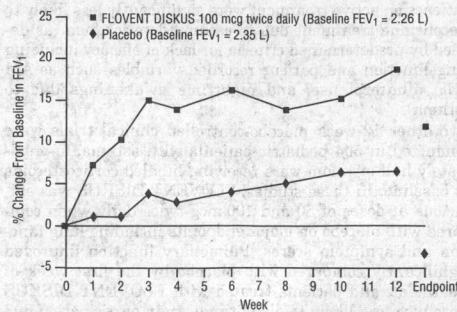

Figure 2. A 12-Week Clinical Trial Evaluating FLOVENT DISKUS 100 mcg Twice Daily in Adolescents and Adults Receiving Inhaled Corticosteroids

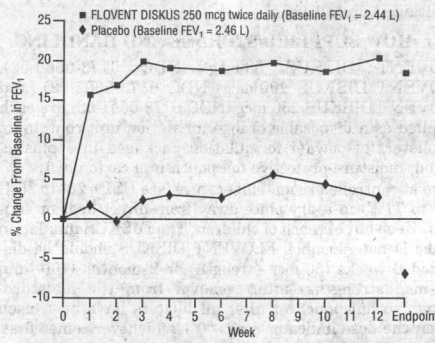

Figure 3. A 12-Week Clinical Trial Evaluating FLOVENT DISKUS 250 mcg Twice Daily in Adolescents and Adults Receiving Inhaled Corticosteroids or Bronchodilators Alone

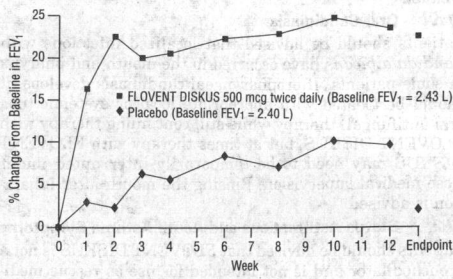

Figure 4. A 12-Week Clinical Trial Evaluating FLOVENT DISKUS 500 mcg Twice Daily in Adolescents and Adults Receiving Inhaled Corticosteroids or Bronchodilators Alone

In all 4 efficacy trials, measures of pulmonary function (FEV_1) were statistically significantly improved as compared with placebo at all twice-daily doses. Patients on all dosages of FLOVENT DISKUS were also less likely to discontinue study participation due to asthma deterioration (as defined by predetermined criteria for lack of efficacy including lung function and patient-recorded variables such as AM PEF, albuterol use, and nighttime awakenings due to asthma) compared with placebo.

In a clinical trial of 111 patients with severe asthma requiring chronic oral prednisone therapy (average baseline daily prednisone dose was 14 mg), fluticasone propionate given by inhalation powder at doses of 500 and 1,000 mcg twice daily was evaluated. Both doses enabled a statistically significantly larger percentage of patients to wean from oral prednisone as compared with placebo (75% of the patients on

500 mcg twice daily and 89% of the patients on 1,000 mcg twice daily as compared with 9% of patients on placebo). Accompanying the reduction in oral corticosteroid use, patients treated with fluticasone propionate had significantly improved lung function and fewer asthma symptoms as compared with the placebo group.

14.2 Pediatric Patients Aged 4 to 11 Years

A 12-week, placebo-controlled clinical trial was conducted in 437 pediatric patients (177 received FLOVENT DISKUS), approximately half of whom were receiving inhaled corticosteroids at baseline. In this study, doses of fluticasone propionate inhalation powder 50 and 100 mcg twice daily significantly improved FEV_1 (15% and 18% change from baseline at Endpoint, respectively) compared with placebo (7% change). AM PEF was also significantly improved with doses of fluticasone propionate 50 and 100 mcg twice daily (26% and 27% change from baseline at Endpoint, respectively) compared with placebo (14% change). In this study, patients on active treatment were significantly less likely to discontinue treatment due to asthma deterioration (as defined by predetermined criteria for lack of efficacy including lung function and patient recorded variables such as AM PEF, albuterol use, and nighttime awakenings due to asthma).

Two other 12-week placebo-controlled clinical trials were conducted in 504 pediatric patients with asthma, approximately half of whom were receiving inhaled corticosteroids at baseline. In these studies, FLOVENT DISKUS was efficacious at doses of 50 and 100 mcg twice daily when compared with placebo on major endpoints including lung function and symptom scores. Pulmonary function improved significantly compared with placebo by the first week of treatment, and patients treated with FLOVENT DISKUS were also less likely to discontinue study participation due to asthma deterioration. One hundred ninety-two (192) patients received FLOVENT DISKUS for up to 1 year during an open-label extension. Data from this open-label extension suggested that lung function improvements could be maintained up to 1 year.

16 HOW SUPPLIED/STORAGE AND HANDLING

FLOVENT DISKUS 50 mcg (NDC 0173-0600-02), FLOVENT DISKUS 100 mcg (NDC 0173-0602-02), and FLOVENT DISKUS 250 mcg (NDC 0173-0601-02) are each supplied as a disposable orange inhalation unit containing 60 blisters of powder formulation packaged in a plastic-coated, moisture-protective foil pouch in a carton of 1.

Store at controlled room temperature (see USP), 20° to 25°C (68° to 77°F) in a dry place away from direct heat or sunlight. Keep out of reach of children. The DISKUS inhalation device is not reusable. FLOVENT DISKUS should be discarded 6 weeks (50-mcg strength) or 2 months (100- and 250-mcg strengths) after removal from the moisture-protective foil pouch or after all blisters have been used (when the dose indicator reads "0"), whichever comes first. Do not attempt to take the device apart.

17 PATIENT COUNSELING INFORMATION

See FDA-Approved Patient Labeling accompanying the product.

17.1 Oral Candidiasis

Patients should be advised that localized infections with *Candida albicans* have occurred in the mouth and pharynx in some patients. If oropharyngeal candidiasis develops, it should be treated with appropriate local or systemic (i.e., oral antifungal) therapy while still continuing therapy with FLOVENT DISKUS, but at times therapy with FLOVENT DISKUS may need to be temporarily interrupted under close medical supervision. Rinsing the mouth after inhalation is advised.

17.2 Status Asthmaticus and Acute Asthma Symptoms

Patients should be advised that FLOVENT DISKUS is not a bronchodilator and is not intended for use as rescue medication for acute asthma exacerbations. Acute asthma symptoms should be treated with an inhaled, short-acting $beta_2$ agonist such as albuterol. Patients should be instructed to contact their physicians immediately if there is deterioration of their asthma.

17.3 Immunosuppression

Patients who are on immunosuppressant doses of corticosteroids should be warned to avoid exposure to chickenpox or measles and if they are exposed to consult their physicians without delay. Patients should be informed of potential worsening of existing tuberculosis, fungal, bacterial, viral, or parasitic infections, or ocular herpes simplex.

17.4 Hypercorticism and Adrenal Suppression

Patients should be advised that FLOVENT DISKUS may cause systemic corticosteroid effects of hypercorticism and adrenal suppression. Additionally, patients should be instructed that deaths due to adrenal insufficiency have occurred during and after transfer from systemic corticosteroids. Patients should taper slowly from systemic corticosteroids if transferring to FLOVENT DISKUS.

17.5 Hypersensitivity Reactions, Including Anaphylaxis

Patients should be advised that hypersensitivity reactions, including anaphylaxis, angioedema, urticaria, and bronchospasm, may occur after administration of FLOVENT DISKUS. Patients should discontinue FLOVENT DISKUS if such reactions occur. There have been reports of anaphylactic reactions in patients with severe milk protein allergy; therefore, patients with severe milk protein allergy should not take FLOVENT DISKUS.

17.6 Reduction in Bone Mineral Density

Patients who are at an increased risk for decreased BMD should be advised that the use of corticosteroids may pose an additional risk.

17.7 Reduced Growth Velocity

Patients should be informed that orally inhaled corticosteroids, including FLOVENT DISKUS, may cause a reduction in growth velocity when administered to pediatric patients. Physicians should closely follow the growth of children and adolescents taking corticosteroids by any route.

17.8 Ocular Effects

Long-term use of inhaled corticosteroids may increase the risk of some eye problems (cataracts or glaucoma); regular eye examinations should be considered.

17.9 Use Daily for Best Effect

Patients should use FLOVENT DISKUS at regular intervals as directed. Individual patients will experience a variable time to onset and degree of symptom relief and the full benefit may not be achieved until treatment has been administered for 1 to 2 weeks or longer. Patients should not increase the prescribed dosage but should contact their physicians if symptoms do not improve or if the condition worsens. Patients should be instructed not to stop use of FLOVENT DISKUS abruptly. Patients should contact their physicians immediately if they discontinue use of FLOVENT DISKUS.

GlaxoSmithKline
Research Triangle Park, NC 27709
©2010, GlaxoSmithKline. All rights reserved.
May 2010
FLD:4PI

Patient Information

FLOVENT® *[flō' vent]* DISKUS® 50 mcg
(fluticasone propionate inhalation powder, 50 mcg)
FLOVENT® DISKUS® 100 mcg
(fluticasone propionate inhalation powder, 100 mcg)
FLOVENT® DISKUS® 250 mcg
(fluticasone propionate inhalation powder, 250 mcg)
FOR ORAL INHALATION ONLY

Read this Patient Information before you start to use FLOVENT DISKUS and each time you get a refill. There may be new information. This information does not take the place of talking with your doctor about your medical condition or your treatment.

What is FLOVENT DISKUS?

FLOVENT DISKUS is an inhaled prescription corticosteroid medicine for the long-term treatment of asthma in people aged 4 and older.

- FLOVENT DISKUS helps to prevent symptoms of asthma
- FLOVENT DISKUS does not treat the sudden symptoms of an asthma attack, such as wheezing, cough, shortness of breath, and chest pain or tightness. **Always have a fast-acting bronchodilator medicine (rescue inhaler) with you to treat sudden symptoms.**

It is not known if FLOVENT DISKUS is safe and effective in children younger than 4 years of age.

Who should not use FLOVENT DISKUS?

Do not use FLOVENT DISKUS

- to treat sudden symptoms of asthma. **FLOVENT DISKUS is not a rescue inhaler and should not be used to give you fast relief from your asthma attack.** Always use a rescue inhaler such as albuterol, during a sudden asthma attack.
- if you have severe allergy to milk proteins or fluticasone propionate. Ask your doctor if you are not sure.

What should I tell my doctor before taking FLOVENT DISKUS?

Before you use FLOVENT DISKUS, tell your doctor if you:

- have liver problems.
- have been exposed to chickenpox or measles.
- have any other medical conditions.
- are pregnant or planning to become pregnant. It is not known if FLOVENT DISKUS will harm your unborn baby. Talk to your doctor if you are pregnant or plan to become pregnant.
- are breast-feeding or plan to breast-feed. It is not known if FLOVENT DISKUS passes into your breast milk. You and your doctor should decide if you should use FLOVENT DISKUS while you breast-feed.

Tell your doctor about all the medicines you take including prescription and non-prescription medicines, vitamins, and herbal supplements. FLOVENT DISKUS may affect the way other medicines work, and other medicines may affect how FLOVENT DISKUS works. Especially, tell your doctor if you take:

- anti-viral medicines, including medicines that contain ritonavir (commonly used to treat HIV infection or AIDS).
- any other corticosteroid medicines.
- ketoconazole (NIZORAL®), an antifungal medicine.

This is not a complete list of medicines that can affect FLOVENT DISKUS. Ask your doctor if you are not sure if any of your medicines are the kinds listed above.

Know the medicines you take. Keep a list of them and show it to your doctor and pharmacist when you get a new medicine.

How should I use FLOVENT DISKUS?

- Read the detailed Instructions for Use at the end of this leaflet.
- An adult should always watch a child use FLOVENT DISKUS to make sure that it is used correctly, as instructed by your doctor.
- FLOVENT DISKUS comes in 3 strengths. Your doctor has prescribed the one that is best for your condition.
- Use FLOVENT DISKUS exactly as your doctor tells you to use it. Do not change the dose yourself. Your doctor will tell you how many times to inhale your FLOVENT DISKUS and when to use your FLOVENT DISKUS. **Do not** inhale more doses or use your FLOVENT DISKUS more often than your doctor has prescribed.
- FLOVENT DISKUS delivers your dose of medicine as a very fine powder **that most people, but not all, can taste or feel.** Whether or not you can taste or feel your dose of medicine, you should not take more than the prescribed dose. If you are not sure you are getting your dose of FLOVENT DISKUS, contact your doctor or pharmacist.
- It may take 1 to 2 weeks or longer after you start FLOVENT DISKUS for your asthma symptoms to get better. You must use FLOVENT DISKUS regularly. **Do not stop using FLOVENT DISKUS, even if you are feeling better, unless your doctor tells you to.**
- If you miss a dose, just take your next dose at your regular time. **Do not take 2 doses at the same time unless your doctor tells you to. If you are not sure about your dosing, call your doctor.**
- Your doctor may prescribe a rescue inhaler for emergency relief of sudden asthma attacks. Contact your doctor right away if:
  - an asthma attack does not respond to your rescue inhaler or
  - you need more of your rescue inhaler than usual.
- If you also use another medicine by inhalation, you should ask your doctor for instructions on when to use it while you are also using FLOVENT DISKUS.
- Do not use FLOVENT DISKUS with a spacer device.

What should I avoid while taking FLOVENT DISKUS?

If you have not had or have not been vaccinated against chickenpox, measles, or active tuberculosis, you should stay away from people who are infected.

What are the possible side effects of FLOVENT DISKUS?

FLOVENT DISKUS can cause serious side effects, including:

- **fungal infection (thrush) in your mouth and throat.** Tell your doctor if you have any redness or white-colored coating in your mouth.
- **decreased ability to fight infections.** Symptoms of infection may include: fever, pain, aches, chills, feeling tired, nausea and vomiting. Tell your doctor about any signs of infection while you use FLOVENT DISKUS.
- **decreased adrenal function (adrenal insufficiency).** Symptoms of decreased adrenal function include tiredness, weakness, nausea and vomiting, and low blood pressure. Decreased adrenal function can lead to death.
- **allergic reaction (anaphylaxis).** Call your doctor and stop FLOVENT DISKUS right away if you have any symptoms of an allergic reaction:

• swelling of the face, throat, and tongue	• rash
• hives	• breathing problems

- **lower bone mineral density.** This may be a problem for people who already have a higher chance of low bone density (osteoporosis).
- **slow growth in children.** The growth of children using FLOVENT DISKUS should be checked regularly.
- **eye problems including glaucoma and cataracts.** Tell your doctor about any vision changes while using FLOVENT DISKUS. Your doctor may tell you to have your eyes checked.
- **increased wheezing (bronchospasm).** Increased wheezing can happen right away after using FLOVENT DISKUS. Always have a rescue inhaler with you to treat sudden wheezing.

Call your doctor right away if you have any of the serious side effects listed above or if you have worsening lung symptoms.

The most common side effects of FLOVENT DISKUS include:

- a cold or upper respiratory tract infection
- throat irritation
- nausea and vomiting
- fever
- headache

Tell your doctor if you have any side effects that bother you or that do not go away. These are not all the possible side effects of FLOVENT DISKUS. For more information ask your doctor or pharmacist.

Call your doctor for medical advice about side effects. You may report side effects to FDA at 1-800-FDA-1088 or 1-800-332-1088.

How should I store FLOVENT DISKUS?

Store FLOVENT DISKUS at room temperature between 68°F to 77°F (20°C to 25°C). Store FLOVENT DISKUS in a dry place away from heat and sunlight.

FLOVENT DISKUS is not reusable. Safely throw away medicine that is out of date or no longer needed.

Do not try to take FLOVENT DISKUS apart.

Keep FLOVENT DISKUS and all medicines out of the reach of children.

General information about the safe and effective use of FLOVENT DISKUS.

Medicines are sometimes prescribed for purposes other than those listed in a Patient Information leaflet. Do not use FLOVENT DISKUS for a condition for which it was not prescribed. Do not give FLOVENT DISKUS to other people, even if they have the same symptoms that you have. It may harm them.

This Patient Information leaflet summarizes the most important information about FLOVENT DISKUS. If you would like more information, talk with your healthcare provider. You can ask your pharmacist or doctor for information about FLOVENT DISKUS that is written for health professionals.

For more information go to www.floventdiskus.com or call 1-888-825-5249.

What are the ingredients in FLOVENT DISKUS?

Active ingredient: fluticasone propionate (microfine)

Inactive ingredient: lactose (which contains milk proteins)

Instructions for Using FLOVENT DISKUS

The parts of your FLOVENT DISKUS

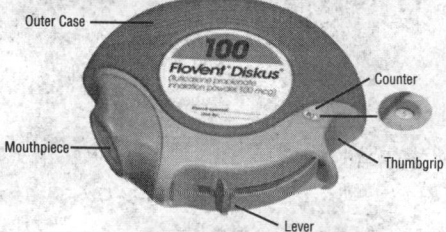

Figure 1

The counter shows you how many doses are left. The counter number will count down each time you use FLOVENT DISKUS. After you have used 55 doses (23 doses from the sample pack), the numbers 5 to 0 will show in **red** to warn you that there are only a few doses left (see Figure 1).

Using your FLOVENT DISKUS

- Take FLOVENT DISKUS out of the moisture-protective foil pouch just before you use it for the first time. Safely throw away the foil pouch.
- FLOVENT DISKUS will be in the closed position. Write the "Pouch opened" and "Use by" dates in the blank lines on the label (see Figure 1). The "Use by" date for FLOVENT DISKUS 50 mcg is 6 weeks from the date you opened the pouch. The "Use by" date for FLOVENT DISKUS 100 mcg and FLOVENT DISKUS 250 mcg is 2 months from the date you opened the pouch.

Read the following steps before using FLOVENT DISKUS and follow them at each use. If you have any questions, ask your doctor or pharmacist.

[See figure 2 at top of next column]

[See figure 3 in next column]

1. Open

Hold FLOVENT DISKUS in one hand and put the thumb of your other hand on the thumbgrip. Push your thumb away from you as far as it will go until the mouthpiece shows and snaps into place (see Figure 2).

2. Click

Hold FLOVENT DISKUS in a level, flat position with the mouthpiece towards you. Slide the lever away from you as

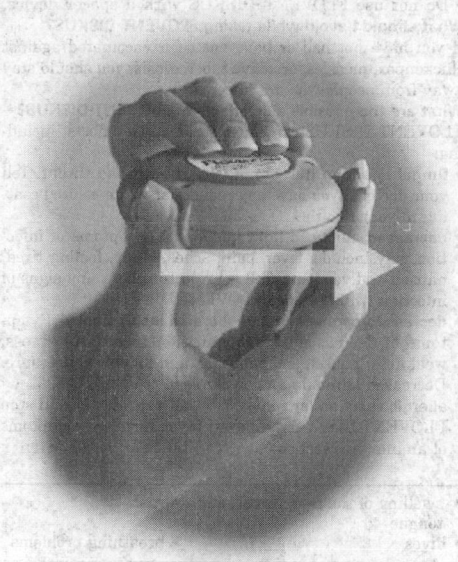

Figure 2

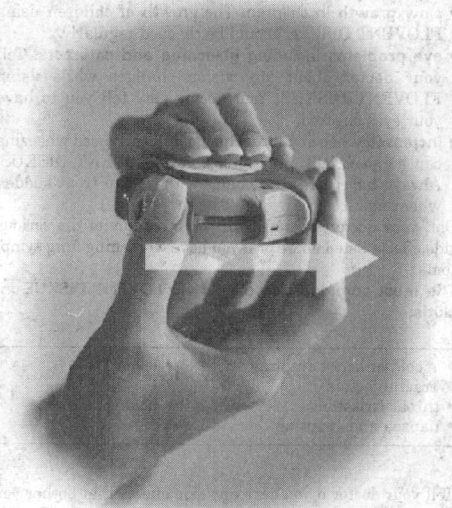

Figure 3

far as it will go until it clicks (see Figure 3). The number on the dose counter will count down by 1. FLOVENT DISKUS is now ready to use.

To avoid releasing a dose by mistake before you are ready to inhale:

- **Do not close FLOVENT DISKUS.**
- **Do not tilt FLOVENT DISKUS.**
- **Do not play with the lever.**
- **Do not slide the lever more than once.**

[See figure 4 at top of next column]

[See figure 5 in next column]

3. Inhale

Before you inhale your dose of FLOVENT DISKUS, breathe out as far as you can while you hold FLOVENT DISKUS level and away from your mouth (see Figure 4). **Never breathe out into the FLOVENT DISKUS mouthpiece.**

Put the mouthpiece to your lips (see Figure 5). Breathe in quickly and deeply through FLOVENT DISKUS. Do not breathe in through your nose.

Remove FLOVENT DISKUS from your mouth. Hold your breath for about 10 seconds, or for as long as is comfortable. Breathe out slowly.

Rinse your mouth with water after inhaling the medicine. Spit out the water. Do not swallow it.

[See figure 6 in next column]

4. Close FLOVENT DISKUS when you are finished taking a dose. Put your thumb on the thumbgrip and slide it back towards you as far as it will go (see Figure 6). FLOVENT DISKUS will click shut. The lever will automatically return to its original position. FLOVENT DISKUS is now ready for you to take your next scheduled dose in about 12 hours. When you are ready for your next dose, you will repeat steps 1 through 4.

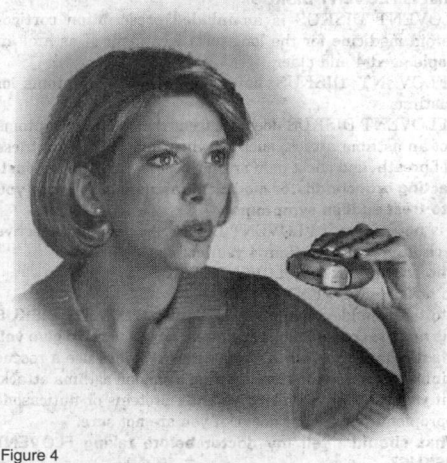

Figure 4

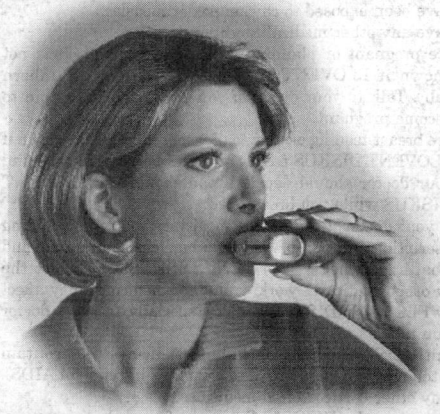

Figure 5

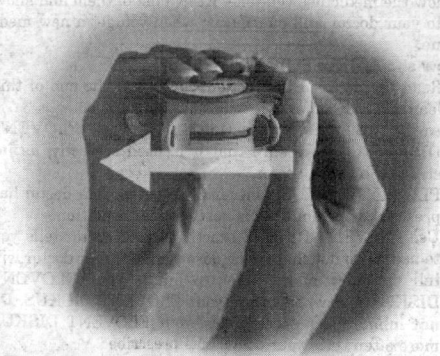

Figure 6

FLOVENT and DISKUS are registered trademarks of GlaxoSmithKline.

NIZORAL is a registered trademark of Janssen Pharmaceutica.

GlaxoSmithKline
Research Triangle Park, NC 27709
©2010, GlaxoSmithKline. All rights reserved.
May 2010 FLD:4PIL

Patient Information

FLOVENT® *[flō′vent]* **DISKUS® 50 mcg**

(fluticasone propionate inhalation powder, 50 mcg)

FLOVENT® DISKUS® 100 mcg

(fluticasone propionate inhalation powder, 100 mcg)

FLOVENT® DISKUS® 250 mcg

(fluticasone propionate inhalation powder, 250 mcg)

FOR ORAL INHALATION

Read this Patient Information before you start to use FLOVENT DISKUS and each time you get a refill. There may be new information. This information does not take the place of talking with your doctor about your medical condition or your treatment.

What is FLOVENT DISKUS?

FLOVENT DISKUS is an inhaled prescription corticosteroid medicine for the long-term treatment of asthma in people aged 4 and older.

- FLOVENT DISKUS helps to prevent symptoms of asthma
- FLOVENT DISKUS does not treat the sudden symptoms of an asthma attack, such as wheezing, cough, shortness of breath, and chest pain or tightness. **Always have a fast-acting bronchodilator medicine (rescue inhaler) with you to treat sudden symptoms.**

It is not known if FLOVENT DISKUS is safe and effective in children younger than 4 years of age.

Who should not use FLOVENT DISKUS?

Do not use FLOVENT DISKUS

- to treat sudden symptoms of asthma. **FLOVENT DISKUS is not a rescue inhaler and should not be used to give you fast relief from your asthma attack.** Always use a rescue inhaler such as albuterol, during a sudden asthma attack.
- if you have severe allergy to milk proteins or fluticasone propionate Ask your doctor if you are not sure.

What should I tell my doctor before taking FLOVENT DISKUS?

Before you use FLOVENT DISKUS, tell your doctor if you:
- have liver problems.
- have been exposed to chickenpox or measles.
- have any other medical conditions.
- are pregnant or planning to become pregnant. It is not known if FLOVENT DISKUS will harm your unborn baby. Talk to your doctor if you are pregnant or plan to become pregnant.
- are breast-feeding or plan to breast-feed. It is not known if FLOVENT DISKUS passes into your breast milk. You and your doctor should decide if you should use FLOVENT DISKUS while you breast-feed.

Tell your doctor about all the medicines you take including prescription and non-prescription medicines, vitamins, and herbal supplements. FLOVENT DISKUS may affect the way other medicines work, and other medicines may affect how FLOVENT DISKUS works. Especially, tell your doctor if you take:
- anti-viral medicines, including medicines that contain ritonavir (commonly used to treat HIV infection or AIDS).
- any other corticosteroid medicines.
- ketoconazole (NIZORAL®), an antifungal medicine.

This is not a complete list of medicines that can affect FLOVENT DISKUS. Ask your doctor if you are not sure if any of your medicines are the kinds listed above.

Know the medicines you take. Keep a list of them and show it to your doctor and pharmacist when you get a new medicine.

How should I use FLOVENT DISKUS?

- Read the detailed Instructions for Use at the end of this leaflet.
- An adult should always watch a child use FLOVENT DISKUS to make sure that it is used correctly, as instructed by your doctor.
- FLOVENT DISKUS comes in 3 strengths. Your doctor has prescribed the one that is best for your condition.
- Use FLOVENT DISKUS exactly as your doctor tells you to use it. Do not change the dose yourself. Your doctor will tell you how many times to inhale your FLOVENT DISKUS and when to use your FLOVENT DISKUS. **Do not inhale more doses or use your FLOVENT DISKUS more often than your doctor has prescribed.**
- FLOVENT DISKUS delivers your dose of medicine as a very fine powder **that most people, but not all, can taste or feel.** Whether or not you can taste or feel your dose of medicine, you should not take more than the prescribed dose. If you are not sure you are getting your dose of FLOVENT DISKUS, contact your doctor or pharmacist.
- It may take 1 to 2 weeks or longer after you start FLOVENT DISKUS for your asthma symptoms to get better. You must use FLOVENT DISKUS regularly. **Do not stop using FLOVENT DISKUS, even if you are feeling better, unless your doctor tells you to.**
- If you miss a dose, just take your next dose at your regular time. **Do not take 2 doses at the same time unless your doctor tells you to. If you are not sure about your dosing, call your doctor.**
- Your doctor may prescribe a rescue inhaler for emergency relief of sudden asthma attacks. Contact your doctor right away if:
  - an asthma attack does not respond to your rescue inhaler or
  - you need more of your rescue inhaler than usual.
- If you also use another medicine by inhalation, you should ask your doctor for instructions on when to use it while you are also using FLOVENT DISKUS.

- Do not use FLOVENT DISKUS with a spacer device.

What should I avoid while taking FLOVENT DISKUS?

If you have not had or have not been vaccinated against chickenpox, measles, or active tuberculosis, you should stay away from people who are infected.

What are the possible side effects of FLOVENT DISKUS?

FLOVENT DISKUS can cause serious side effects, including:
- **fungal infection (thrush) in your mouth and throat.** Tell your doctor if you have any redness or white-colored coating in your mouth.
- **decreased ability to fight infections.** Symptoms of infection may include: fever, pain, aches, chills, feeling tired, nausea and vomiting. Tell your doctor about any signs of infection while you use FLOVENT DISKUS.
- **decreased adrenal function (adrenal insufficiency).** Symptoms of decreased adrenal function include tiredness, weakness, nausea and vomiting, and low blood pressure. Decreased adrenal function can lead to death.
- **allergic reaction (anaphylaxis).** Call your doctor and stop FLOVENT DISKUS right away if you have any symptoms of an allergic reaction:

• swelling of the face, throat, and tongue	• rash
• hives	• breathing problems

- **lower bone mineral density.** This may be a problem for people who already have a higher chance of low bone density (osteoporosis).
- **slow growth in children.** The growth of children using FLOVENT DISKUS should be checked regularly.
- **eye problems including glaucoma and cataracts.** Tell your doctor about any vision changes while using FLOVENT DISKUS. Your doctor may tell you to have your eyes checked.
- **increased wheezing (bronchospasm).** Increased wheezing can happen right away after using FLOVENT DISKUS. Always have a rescue inhaler with you to treat sudden wheezing.

Call your doctor right away if you have any of the serious side effects listed above or if you have worsening lung symptoms.

The most common side effects of FLOVENT DISKUS include:

• a cold or upper respiratory tract infection	• fever
• throat irritation	• headache
• nausea and vomiting	

Tell your doctor if you have any side effects that bother you or that do not go away. These are not all the possible side effects of FLOVENT DISKUS. For more information ask your doctor or pharmacist.

Call your doctor for medical advice about side effects. You may report side effects to FDA at 1-800-FDA-1088 or 1-800-332-1088.

How should I store FLOVENT DISKUS?

Store FLOVENT DISKUS at room temperature between 68°F to 77°F (20°C to 25°C). Store FLOVENT DISKUS in a dry place away from heat and sunlight.

FLOVENT DISKUS is not reusable. Safely throw away medicine that is out of date or no longer needed.

Do not try to take FLOVENT DISKUS apart.

Keep FLOVENT DISKUS and all medicines out of the reach of children.

General information about the safe and effective use of FLOVENT DISKUS.

Medicines are sometimes prescribed for purposes other than those listed in a Patient Information leaflet. Do not use FLOVENT DISKUS for a condition for which it was not prescribed. Do not give FLOVENT DISKUS to other people, even if they have the same symptoms that you have. It may harm them.

This Patient Information leaflet summarizes the most important information about FLOVENT DISKUS. If you would like more information, talk with your healthcare provider. You can ask your pharmacist or doctor for information about FLOVENT DISKUS that is written for health professionals.

For more information go to www.floventdiskus.com or call 1-888-825-5249.

What are the ingredients in FLOVENT DISKUS?

Active ingredient: fluticasone propionate (microfine)
Inactive ingredient: lactose (which contains milk proteins)

Instructions for Using FLOVENT DISKUS
The parts of your FLOVENT DISKUS

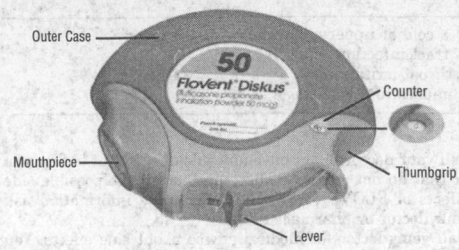

Outer Case
Counter
Mouthpiece
Thumbgrip
Lever

Figure 1

The counter shows you how many doses are left. The counter number will count down each time you use FLOVENT DISKUS. After you have used 55 doses (23 doses from the sample pack), the numbers 5 to 0 will show in **red** to warn you that there are only a few doses left (see Figure 1).

Using your FLOVENT DISKUS

- Take FLOVENT DISKUS out of the moisture-protective foil pouch just before you use it for the first time. Safely throw away the foil pouch.
- FLOVENT DISKUS will be in the closed position. Write the "Pouch opened" and "Use by" dates in the blank lines on the label (see Figure 1). The "Use by" date for FLOVENT DISKUS 50 mcg is 6 weeks from the date you opened the pouch. The "Use by" date for FLOVENT DISKUS 100 mcg and FLOVENT DISKUS 250 mcg is 2 months from the date you opened the pouch.

Read the following steps before using FLOVENT DISKUS and follow them at each use. If you have any questions, ask your doctor or pharmacist.

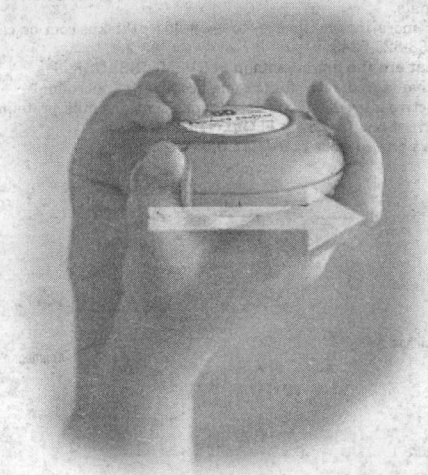

Figure 2

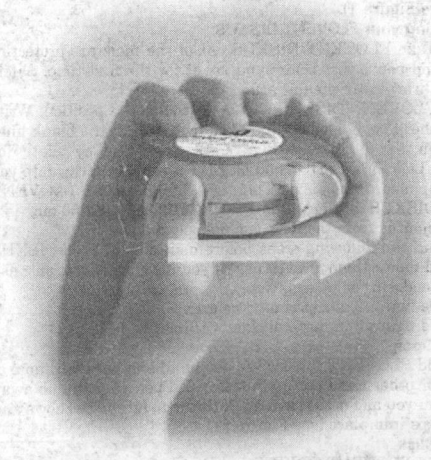

Figure 3

IMPORTANT NOTICE: Updated drug information is sent bi-monthly via the PDR® Update Insert. For _monthly_ email updates, register at PDR.net.

1. Open
Hold FLOVENT DISKUS in one hand and put the thumb of your other hand on the thumbgrip. Push your thumb away from you as far as it will go until the mouthpiece shows and snaps into place (see Figure 2).

2. Click
Hold FLOVENT DISKUS in a level, flat position with the mouthpiece towards you. Slide the lever away from you as far as it will go until it clicks (see Figure 3). The number on the dose counter will count down by 1. FLOVENT DISKUS is now ready to use.

To avoid releasing a dose by mistake before you are ready to inhale:
- **Do not close FLOVENT DISKUS.**
- **Do not tilt FLOVENT DISKUS.**
- **Do not play with the lever.**
- **Do not slide the lever more than once.**

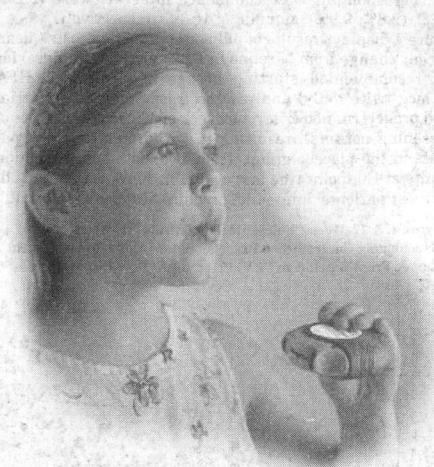

Figure 4

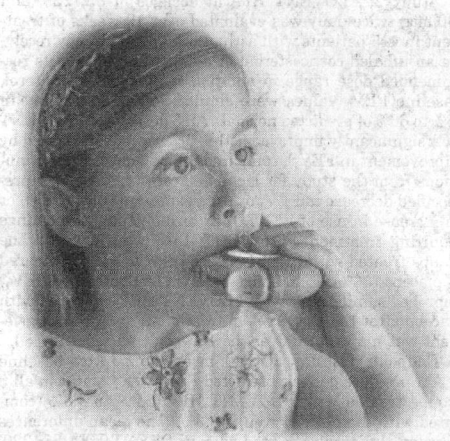

Figure 5

3. Inhale
Before you inhale your dose of FLOVENT DISKUS, breathe out as far as you can while you hold FLOVENT DISKUS level and away from your mouth (see Figure 4). **Never breathe out into the FLOVENT DISKUS mouthpiece.**
Put the mouthpiece to your lips (see Figure 5). Breathe in quickly and deeply through FLOVENT DISKUS. Do not breathe in through your nose.
Remove FLOVENT DISKUS from your mouth. Hold your breath for about 10 seconds, or for as long as is comfortable. Breathe out slowly.
Rinse your mouth with water after inhaling the medicine. Spit out the water. Do not swallow it.
[See figure 6 at top of next column]

4. Close FLOVENT DISKUS when you are finished taking a dose.
Put your thumb on the thumbgrip and slide it back towards you as far as it will go (see Figure 6). FLOVENT DISKUS will click shut. The lever will automatically return to its original position. FLOVENT DISKUS is now ready for you to take your next scheduled dose in about 12 hours. When you are ready for your next dose, you will repeat steps 1 through 4.

FLOVENT and DISKUS are registered trademarks of GlaxoSmithKline.

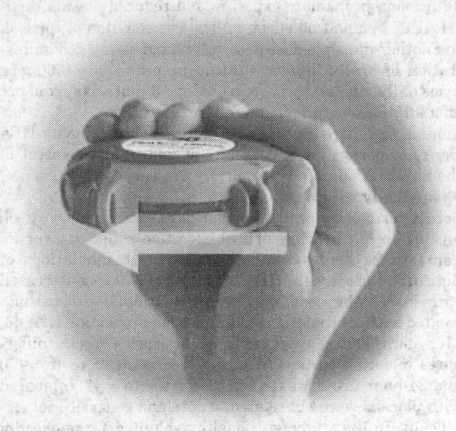

Figure 6

NIZORAL is a registered trademark of Janssen Pharmaceutica.
GlaxoSmithKline
Research Triangle Park, NC 27709
©2010, GlaxoSmithKline. All rights reserved.
May 2010 FLD:4PIL

FLOVENT® HFA 44 mcg ℞
[flō′ vent]
(fluticasone propionate 44 mcg)
Inhalation Aerosol

FLOVENT® HFA 110 mcg ℞
(fluticasone propionate 110 mcg)
Inhalation Aerosol

FLOVENT® HFA 220 mcg ℞
(fluticasone propionate 220 mcg)
Inhalation Aerosol
For Oral Inhalation Only

DESCRIPTION
The active component of FLOVENT HFA 44 mcg Inhalation Aerosol, FLOVENT HFA 110 mcg Inhalation Aerosol, and FLOVENT HFA 220 mcg Inhalation Aerosol is fluticasone propionate, a corticosteroid having the chemical name S-(fluoromethyl) $6\alpha,9$-difluoro-$11\beta,17$-dihydroxy-16α-methyl-3-oxoandrosta-1,4-diene-17β-carbothioate, 17-propionate and the following chemical structure:

$$\text{chemical structure}$$

Fluticasone propionate is a white powder with a molecular weight of 500.6, and the empirical formula is $C_{25}H_{31}F_3O_5S$. It is practically insoluble in water, freely soluble in dimethyl sulfoxide and dimethylformamide, and slightly soluble in methanol and 95% ethanol.
FLOVENT HFA 44 mcg Inhalation Aerosol, FLOVENT HFA 110 mcg Inhalation Aerosol, and FLOVENT HFA 220 mcg Inhalation Aerosol are pressurized metered-dose aerosol units fitted with a counter. FLOVENT HFA is intended for oral inhalation only. Each unit contains a microcrystalline suspension of fluticasone propionate (micronized) in propellant HFA-134a (1,1,1,2-tetrafluoroethane). It contains no other excipients.
After priming, each actuation of the inhaler delivers 50, 125, or 250 mcg of fluticasone propionate in 60 mg of suspension (for the 44-mcg product) or in 75 mg of suspension (for the 110- and 220-mcg products) from the valve. Each actuation delivers 44, 110, or 220 mcg of fluticasone propionate from the actuator. The actual amount of drug delivered to the lung may depend on patient factors, such as the coordination between the actuation of the device and inspiration through the delivery system.
Each 10.6-g canister (44 mcg) and each 12-g canister (110 and 220 mcg) provides 120 inhalations.
FLOVENT HFA should be primed before using for the first time by releasing 4 test sprays into the air away from the face, shaking well for 5 seconds before each spray. In cases where the inhaler has not been used for more than 7 days or when it has been dropped, prime the inhaler again by shaking well for 5 seconds and releasing 1 test spray into the air away from the face.

This product does not contain any chlorofluorocarbon (CFC) as the propellant.

CLINICAL PHARMACOLOGY
Mechanism of Action
Fluticasone propionate is a synthetic trifluorinated corticosteroid with potent anti-inflammatory activity. In vitro assays using human lung cytosol preparations have established fluticasone propionate as a human glucocorticoid receptor agonist with an affinity 18 times greater than dexamethasone, almost twice that of beclomethasone-17-monopropionate (BMP), the active metabolite of beclomethasone dipropionate, and over 3 times that of budesonide. Data from the McKenzie vasoconstrictor assay in man are consistent with these results. The clinical significance of these findings is unknown.
Inflammation is an important component in the pathogenesis of asthma. Corticosteroids have been shown to inhibit multiple cell types (e.g., mast cells, eosinophils, basophils, lymphocytes, macrophages, and neutrophils) and mediator production or secretion (e.g., histamine, eicosanoids, leukotrienes, and cytokines) involved in the asthmatic response. These anti-inflammatory actions of corticosteroids contribute to their efficacy in asthma.
Though effective for the treatment of asthma, corticosteroids do not affect asthma symptoms immediately. Individual patients will experience a variable time to onset and degree of symptom relief. Maximum benefit may not be achieved for 1 to 2 weeks or longer after starting treatment. When corticosteroids are discontinued, asthma stability may persist for several days or longer.
Studies in patients with asthma have shown a favorable ratio between topical anti-inflammatory activity and systemic corticosteroid effects with recommended doses of orally inhaled fluticasone propionate. This is explained by a combination of a relatively high local anti-inflammatory effect, negligible oral systemic bioavailability (<1%), and the minimal pharmacological activity of the only metabolite detected in man.

Preclinical
In animals and humans, propellant HFA-134a was found to be rapidly absorbed and rapidly eliminated, with an elimination half-life of 3 to 27 minutes in animals and 5 to 7 minutes in humans. Time to maximum plasma concentration (T_{max}) and mean residence time are both extremely short, leading to a transient appearance of HFA-134a in the blood with no evidence of accumulation.
Propellant HFA-134a is devoid of pharmacological activity except at very high doses in animals (i.e., 380 to 1,300 times the maximum human exposure based on comparisons of area under the plasma concentration versus time curve [AUC] values), primarily producing ataxia, tremors, dyspnea, or salivation. These events are similar to effects produced by the structurally related CFCs, which have been used extensively in metered-dose inhalers.

Pharmacokinetics
Absorption
Fluticasone propionate acts locally in the lung; therefore, plasma levels do not predict therapeutic effect. Studies using oral dosing of labeled and unlabeled drug have demonstrated that the oral systemic bioavailability of fluticasone propionate is negligible (<1%), primarily due to incomplete absorption and presystemic metabolism in the gut and liver. In contrast, the majority of the fluticasone propionate delivered to the lung is systemically absorbed. Systemic exposure as measured by AUC in healthy subjects (N = 24) who received 8 inhalations, as a single dose, of fluticasone propionate HFA using the 44-, 110-, and 220-mcg strengths increased proportionally with dose. The geometric means (95% CI) of $AUC_{0-24\ hr}$ for the 44-, 110-, and 220-mcg strengths were 488 (362, 657); 1,284 (904; 1,822); and 2,495 (1,945; 3,200) pg•hr/mL, respectively, and the geometric means of C_{max} were 126 (108, 148), 254 (202, 319), and 421 (338, 524) pg/mL, respectively. Systemic exposure from fluticasone propionate HFA 220 mcg was 30% lower than that from the fluticasone propionate CFC inhaler. Systemic exposure was measured in patients with asthma who received 2 inhalations of fluticasone propionate HFA 44 mcg (n = 20), 110 mcg (n = 15), or 220 mcg (n = 17) twice daily for at least 4 weeks. The geometric means (95% CI) of $AUC_{0-12\ hr}$ for the 44-, 110-, and 220-mcg strengths were 76 (33, 175), 298 (191, 464), and 601 (431, 838) pg•hr/mL, respectively. C_{max} occurred in about 1 hour, and the geometric means were 25 (18, 36), 61 (46, 81), and 103 (73, 145) pg/mL, respectively.

Distribution
Following intravenous administration, the initial disposition phase for fluticasone propionate was rapid and consistent with its high lipid solubility and tissue binding. The volume of distribution averaged 4.2 L/kg.
The percentage of fluticasone propionate bound to human plasma proteins averages 99%. Fluticasone propionate is weakly and reversibly bound to erythrocytes and is not significantly bound to human transcortin.

Metabolism

The total clearance of fluticasone propionate is high (average, 1,093 mL/min), with renal clearance accounting for less than 0.02% of the total. The only circulating metabolite detected in man is the 17β-carboxylic acid derivative of fluticasone propionate, which is formed through the cytochrome P450 3A4 pathway. This metabolite had less affinity (approximately 1/2,000) than the parent drug for the corticosteroid receptor of human lung cytosol in vitro and negligible pharmacological activity in animal studies. Other metabolites detected in vitro using cultured human hepatoma cells have not been detected in man.

Elimination

Following intravenous dosing, fluticasone propionate showed polyexponential kinetics and had a terminal elimination half-life of approximately 7.8 hours. Less than 5% of a radiolabeled oral dose was excreted in the urine as metabolites, with the remainder excreted in the feces as parent drug and metabolites.

Special Populations

Hepatic Impairment

Since fluticasone propionate is predominantly cleared by hepatic metabolism, impairment of liver function may lead to accumulation of fluticasone propionate in plasma. Therefore, patients with hepatic disease should be closely monitored.

Pediatric

Two pharmacokinetic studies evaluated the systemic exposure to fluticasone propionate at steady state in children with asthma aged 4 to 11 years following inhalation of fluticasone propionate HFA. In an open-label, multiple-dose, 2-period crossover study, 13 children aged 4 to 11 years received 88 mcg of fluticasone propionate HFA twice daily for 7.5 days in one period and 88 mcg of fluticasone propionate CFC twice daily for 7.5 days in the other period. The geometric means (95% CI) of $AUC_{(last)}$ were 28 pg•hr/mL (10, 80) following fluticasone propionate HFA and 65 pg•hr/mL (27, 153) following fluticasone propionate CFC, indicating that systemic exposure was 55% lower using fluticasone propionate HFA. The geometric means (95% CI) of C_{max} were 15.1 pg/mL (8.5, 27) following fluticasone propionate HFA and 20.4 pg/mL (13, 32) following fluticasone propionate CFC, indicating that C_{max} was 26% lower using fluticasone propionate HFA. T_{max} was similar for both treatments. AUC_{last} and C_{max} in this pediatric population were 37% and 60%, respectively, of those in adult patients receiving the same dose.

In a second open-label, single-dose, 2-period crossover study, 21 children with asthma aged 5 to 11 years received 264 mcg of fluticasone propionate HFA administered with and without an AeroChamber Plus® Valved Holding Chamber (VHC). The geometric means (95% CI) of AUC_{last} were 261 pg•hr/mL (252, 444) with the use of the VHC and 40 pg•hr/mL (16, 208) without the VHC. The geometric means (95% CI) of C_{max} were 52 pg/mL (46, 70) with the VHC and 19 pg/mL (17, 41) without the VHC. The median T_{max} was 1 hour with or without the VHC. Therefore, systemic exposure was higher with the VHC in these pediatric patients with asthma. (See PRECAUTIONS: Pediatric Use for population pharmacokinetics information on children aged 6 months to <4 years.)

Gender

In 19 male and 33 female patients with asthma, systemic exposure was similar from 2 inhalations of fluticasone propionate CFC 44, 110, and 220 mcg twice daily. (See PRECAUTIONS: Pediatric Use for population pharmacokinetics information on children aged 1 to <4 years.)

Drug Interactions

Fluticasone propionate is a substrate of cytochrome P450 3A4. Coadministration of fluticasone propionate and the highly potent cytochrome P450 3A4 inhibitor ritonavir is not recommended based upon a multiple-dose, crossover drug interaction study in 18 healthy subjects. Fluticasone propionate aqueous nasal spray (200 mcg once daily) was coadministered for 7 days with ritonavir (100 mg twice daily). Plasma fluticasone propionate concentrations following fluticasone propionate aqueous nasal spray alone were undetectable (<10 pg/mL) in most subjects, and when concentrations were detectable, peak levels (C_{max}) averaged 11.9 pg/mL (range, 10.8 to 14.1 pg/mL) and $AUC_{(0-\tau)}$ averaged 8.43 pg•hr/mL (range, 4.2 to 18.8 pg•hr/mL). Fluticasone propionate C_{max} and $AUC_{(0-\tau)}$ increased to 318 pg/mL (range, 110 to 648 pg/mL) and 3,102.6 pg•hr/mL (range, 1,207.1 to 5,662.0 pg•hr/mL), respectively, after coadministration of ritonavir with fluticasone propionate aqueous nasal spray. This significant increase in plasma fluticasone propionate exposure resulted in a significant decrease (86%) in serum cortisol AUC.

Caution should be exercised when other potent cytochrome P450 3A4 inhibitors are coadministered with fluticasone propionate. In a drug interaction study, coadministration of orally inhaled fluticasone propionate (1,000 mcg) and ketoconazole (200 mg once daily) resulted in increased systemic fluticasone propionate exposure and reduced plasma cortisol AUC, but had no effect on urinary excretion of cortisol.

In another multiple-dose drug interaction study, coadministration of orally inhaled fluticasone propionate (500 mcg twice daily) and erythromycin (333 mg 3 times daily) did not affect fluticasone propionate pharmacokinetics.

Similar definitive studies with fluticasone propionate HFA were not performed, but results should be independent of the formulation and drug delivery device.

Pharmacodynamics

Serum cortisol concentrations, urinary excretion of cortisol, and urine 6-β-hydroxycortisol excretion collected over 24 hours in 24 healthy subjects following 8 inhalations of fluticasone propionate HFA 44, 110, and 220 mcg decreased with increasing dose. However, in patients with asthma treated with 2 inhalations of fluticasone propionate HFA 44, 110, and 220 mcg twice daily for at least 4 weeks, differences in serum cortisol $AUC_{(0-12\ hr)}$ concentrations (n = 65) and 24-hour urinary excretion of cortisol (n = 47) compared with placebo were not related to dose and generally not significant. In the study with healthy volunteers, the effect of propellant was also evaluated by comparing results following the 220-mcg strength inhaler containing HFA 134a propellant with the same strength of inhaler containing CFC 11/12 propellant. A lesser effect on the hypothalamic-pituitary-adrenal (HPA) axis with the HFA formulation was observed for serum cortisol, but not urine cortisol and 6-betahydroxy cortisol excretion. In addition, in a crossover study of children with asthma aged 4 to 11 years (N = 40), 24-hour urinary excretion of cortisol was not affected after a 4-week treatment period with 88 mcg of fluticasone propionate HFA twice daily compared with urinary excretion after the 2-week placebo period. The ratio (95% CI) of urinary excretion of cortisol over 24 hours following fluticasone propionate HFA versus placebo was 0.987 (0.796, 1.223). (See PRECAUTIONS: Pediatric Use for pharmacodynamic information on children aged 6 months to <4 years.)

The potential systemic effects of fluticasone propionate HFA on the HPA axis were also studied in patients with asthma. Fluticasone propionate given by inhalation aerosol at dosages of 440 or 880 mcg twice daily was compared with placebo in oral corticosteroid-dependent patients with asthma (range of mean dose of prednisone at baseline, 13 to 14 mg/day) in a 16-week study. Consistent with maintenance treatment with oral corticosteroids, abnormal plasma cortisol responses to short cosyntropin stimulation (peak plasma cortisol <18 mcg/dL) were present at baseline in the majority of patients participating in this study (69% of patients later randomized to placebo and 72% to 78% of patients later randomized to fluticasone propionate HFA). At week 16, 8 patients (73%) on placebo compared to 14 (54%) and 13 (68%) patients receiving fluticasone propionate HFA (440 and 880 mcg b.i.d., respectively) had post-stimulation cortisol levels of <18 mcg/dL.

To confirm that systemic absorption does not play a role in the clinical response to inhaled fluticasone propionate, a double-blind clinical study comparing inhaled fluticasone propionate powder and oral fluticasone propionate was conducted. Fluticasone propionate inhalation powder in dosages of 100 and 500 mcg twice daily was compared to oral fluticasone propionate 20,000 mcg once daily and placebo for 6 weeks. Plasma levels of fluticasone propionate were detectable in all 3 active groups, but the mean values were highest in the oral group. Both dosages of inhaled fluticasone propionate were effective in maintaining asthma stability and improving lung function, while oral fluticasone propionate and placebo were ineffective. This demonstrates that the clinical effectiveness of inhaled fluticasone propionate is due to its direct local effect and not to an indirect effect through systemic absorption.

CLINICAL TRIALS

Adolescent and Adult Patients

Three randomized, double-blind, parallel-group, placebo-controlled clinical trials were conducted in the US in 980 adolescent and adult patients (≥12 years of age) with asthma to assess the efficacy and safety of FLOVENT HFA in the treatment of asthma. Fixed dosages of 88, 220, and 440 mcg twice daily (each dose administered as 2 inhalations of the 44-, 110-, and 220-mcg strengths, respectively) and 880 mcg twice daily (administered as 4 inhalations of the 220-mcg strength) were compared with placebo to provide information about appropriate dosing to cover a range of asthma severity. Patients in these studies included those inadequately controlled with bronchodilators alone (Study 1), those already receiving inhaled corticosteroids (Study 2), and those requiring oral corticosteroid therapy (Study 3). In all 3 studies, patients (including placebo-treated patients) were allowed to use VENTOLIN® (albuterol, USP) Inhalation Aerosol as needed for relief of acute asthma symptoms. In Studies 1 and 2, other maintenance asthma therapies were discontinued.

Study 1 enrolled 397 patients with asthma inadequately controlled on bronchodilators alone. FLOVENT HFA was evaluated at dosages of 88, 220, and 440 mcg twice daily for 12 weeks. Baseline FEV_1 values were similar across groups (mean 67% of predicted normal). All 3 dosages of FLOVENT HFA significantly improved asthma control as measured by improvement in AM pre-dose FEV_1 compared with placebo. Pulmonary function (AM pre-dose FEV_1) improved significantly with FLOVENT HFA compared with placebo after the first week of treatment, and this improvement was maintained over the 12-week treatment period.

At Endpoint (last observation), mean change from baseline in AM pre-dose percent predicted FEV_1 was greater in all 3 groups treated with FLOVENT HFA (9.0% to 11.2%) compared with the placebo group (3.4%). The mean differences between the groups treated with FLOVENT HFA 88, 220, and 440 mcg and the placebo group were significant, and the corresponding 95% confidence intervals were (2.2%, 9.2%), (2.8%, 9.9%), and (4.3%, 11.3%), respectively.

Figure 1 displays results of pulmonary function tests (mean percent change from baseline in FEV_1 prior to AM dose) for the recommended starting dosage of FLOVENT HFA (88 mcg twice daily) and placebo from Study 1. This trial used predetermined criteria for lack of efficacy (indicators of worsening asthma), resulting in withdrawal of more patients in the placebo group. Therefore, pulmonary function results at Endpoint (the last evaluable FEV_1 result, including most patients' lung function data) are also displayed.

Figure 1. A 12-Week Clinical Trial in Patients ≥12 Years of Age Inadequately Controlled on Bronchodilators Alone: Mean Percent Change From Baseline in FEV_1 Prior to AM Dose (Study 1)

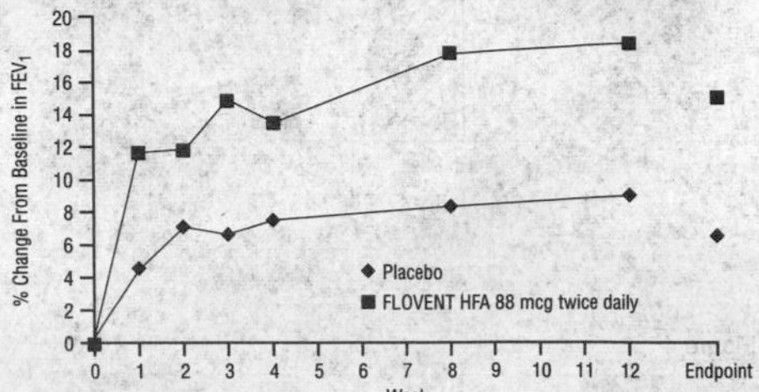

In Study 2, FLOVENT HFA at dosages of 88, 220, and 440 mcg twice daily was evaluated over 12 weeks of treatment in 415 patients with asthma who were already receiving an inhaled corticosteroid at a daily dose within its recommended dose range in addition to as-needed albuterol. Baseline FEV_1 values were similar across groups (mean 65% to 66% of predicted normal). All 3 dosages of FLOVENT HFA significantly improved asthma control (as measured by improvement in FEV_1), compared with placebo. Discontinuations from the study for lack of efficacy (defined by a pre-specified decrease in FEV_1 or peak expiratory flow [PEF], or an increase in use of VENTOLIN or nighttime awakenings requiring treatment with VENTOLIN) were lower in the groups treated with FLOVENT HFA (6% to 11%) compared to placebo (50%). Pulmonary function (AM pre-dose FEV_1) improved significantly with FLOVENT HFA compared with placebo after the first week of treatment, and the improvement was maintained over the 12-week treatment period.

At Endpoint (last observation), mean change from baseline in AM pre-dose percent predicted FEV_1 was greater in all 3 groups treated with FLOVENT HFA (2.2% to 4.6%) compared with the placebo group (-8.3%). The mean differences between the groups treated with FLOVENT HFA 88, 220, and 440 mcg and the placebo group were significant, and the corresponding 95% confidence intervals were (7.1%, 13.8%), (8.2%, 14.9%), and (9.6%, 16.4%), respectively.

Figure 2 displays the mean percent change from baseline in FEV_1 from Week 1 through Week 12. This study also used predetermined criteria for lack of efficacy, resulting in withdrawal of more patients in the placebo group; therefore, pulmonary function results at Endpoint are displayed.

Figure 2. A 12-Week Clinical Trial in Patients ≥12 Years of Age Already Receiving Daily Inhaled Corticosteroids: Mean Percent Change From Baseline in FEV_1 Prior to AM Dose (Study 2)

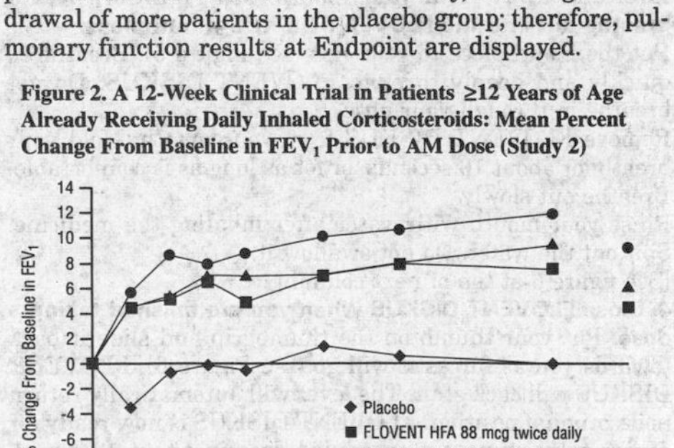

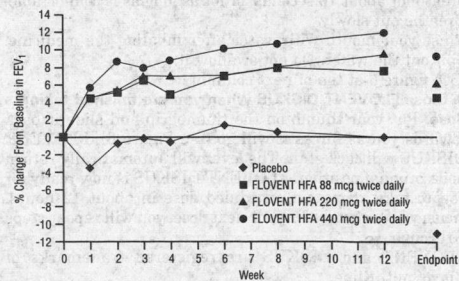

In both studies, use of VENTOLIN, AM and PM PEF, and asthma symptom scores showed numerical improvement with FLOVENT HFA compared to placebo.

Study 3 enrolled 168 patients with asthma requiring oral prednisone therapy (average baseline daily prednisone dose ranged from 13 to 14 mg). FLOVENT HFA at dosages of 440 and 880 mcg twice daily was evaluated over a 16-week treatment period. Baseline FEV_1 values were similar across groups (mean 59% to 62% of predicted normal). Over the course of the study, patients treated with either dosage of FLOVENT HFA required a significantly lower mean daily oral prednisone dose (6 mg) compared with placebo-treated patients (15 mg). Both dosages of FLOVENT HFA enabled a larger percentage of patients (59% and 56% in the groups treated with FLOVENT HFA 440 and 880 mcg, respectively, twice daily) to eliminate oral prednisone as compared with placebo (13%) (see Figure 3). There was no efficacy advantage of FLOVENT HFA 880 mcg twice daily compared to 440 mcg twice daily. Accompanying the reduction in oral corticosteroid use, patients treated with either dosage of FLOVENT HFA had significantly improved lung function, fewer asthma symptoms, and less use of VENTOLIN Inhalation Aerosol compared with the placebo-treated patients.

Figure 3. A 16-Week Clinical Trial in Patients ≥12 Years of Age Requiring Chronic Oral Prednisone Therapy: Change in Maintenance Prednisone Dose

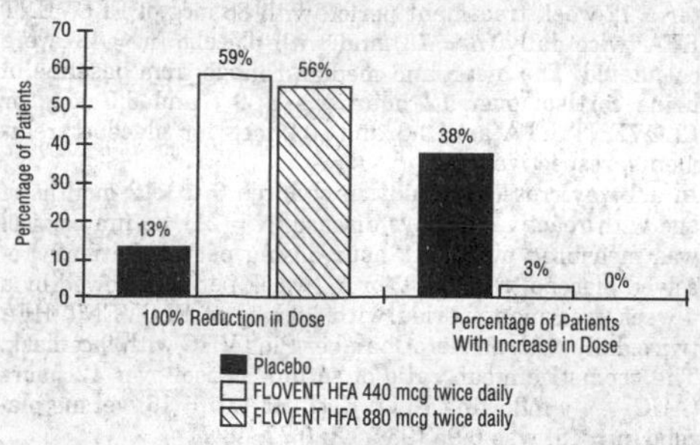

Two long-term safety studies (Study 4 and Study 5) of ≥6 months' duration were conducted in 507 adolescent and adult patients with asthma. Study 4 was designed to monitor the safety of 2 doses of FLOVENT HFA, while Study 5 compared fluticasone propionate HFA and fluticasone propionate CFC. Study 4 enrolled 182 patients who were treated daily with low to high doses of inhaled corticosteroids, beta-agonists (short-acting [as needed or regularly scheduled] or long-acting), theophylline, inhaled cromolyn or nedocromil sodium, leukotriene receptor antagonists, or 5-lipoxygenase inhibitors at baseline. FLOVENT HFA at dosages of 220 and 440 mcg twice daily was evaluated over a 26-week treatment period in 89 and 93 patients, respectively. Study 5 enrolled 325 patients who were treated daily with moderate to high doses of inhaled corticosteroids, with or without concurrent use of salmeterol or albuterol, at baseline. Fluticasone propionate HFA at a dosage of 440 mcg twice daily and fluticasone propionate CFC at a dosage of 440 mcg twice daily were evaluated over a 52-week treatment period in 163 and 162 patients, respectively. Baseline FEV_1 values were similar across groups (mean 81% to 84% of predicted normal). Throughout the 52-week treatment period, asthma control was maintained with both formulations of fluticasone propionate compared to baseline. In both studies, none of the patients were withdrawn due to lack of efficacy.

Pediatric Patients

A 12-week clinical trial conducted in 241 patients aged 4 to 11 years with asthma was supportive of efficacy but inconclusive due to measurable levels of fluticasone propionate in 6/48 (13%) of the plasma samples from patients randomized to placebo. Efficacy in patients 4 to 11 years of age is extrapolated from adult data with FLOVENT HFA and other supporting data (see PRECAUTIONS: Pediatric Use).

INDICATIONS AND USAGE

FLOVENT HFA Inhalation Aerosol is indicated for the maintenance treatment of asthma as prophylactic therapy in patients 4 years of age and older. It is also indicated for patients requiring oral corticosteroid therapy for asthma. Many of these patients may be able to reduce or eliminate their requirement for oral corticosteroids over time.

FLOVENT HFA Inhalation Aerosol is NOT indicated for the relief of acute bronchospasm.

CONTRAINDICATIONS

FLOVENT HFA Inhalation Aerosol is contraindicated in the primary treatment of status asthmaticus or other acute episodes of asthma where intensive measures are required.

Hypersensitivity to any of the ingredients of these preparations contraindicates their use (see DESCRIPTION).

WARNINGS

1. Transferring patients from systemic corticosteroid therapy. Particular care is needed for patients who have been transferred from systemically active corticosteroids to inhaled corticosteroids because deaths due to adrenal insufficiency have occurred in patients with asthma during and after transfer from systemic corticosteroids to less systemically available inhaled corticosteroids. After withdrawal from systemic corticosteroids, a number of months are required for recovery of HPA function.

Patients requiring oral corticosteroids should be weaned slowly from systemic corticosteroid use after transferring to FLOVENT HFA. In a clinical trial of 168 patients, prednisone reduction was successfully accomplished by reducing the daily prednisone dose on a weekly basis following initiation of treatment with FLOVENT HFA. Successive reduction of prednisone dose was allowed only when lung function; symptoms; and as-needed, short-acting beta-agonist use were better than or comparable to that seen before initiation of prednisone dose reduction. Lung function (FEV_1 or AM PEF), beta-agonist use, and asthma symptoms should be carefully monitored during withdrawal of oral corticosteroids. In addition to monitoring asthma signs and symptoms, patients should be observed for signs and symptoms of adrenal insufficiency such as fatigue, lassitude, weakness, nausea and vomiting, and hypotension.

Patients who have been previously maintained on 20 mg or more per day of prednisone (or its equivalent) may be most susceptible, particularly when their systemic corticosteroids have been almost completely withdrawn. During this period of HPA suppression, patients may exhibit signs and symptoms of adrenal insufficiency when exposed to trauma, surgery, or infection (particularly gastroenteritis) or other conditions associated with severe electrolyte loss. Although inhaled corticosteroids may provide control of asthma symptoms during these episodes, in recommended doses they supply less than normal physiological amounts of glucocorticoid (cortisol) systemically and do NOT provide the mineralocorticoid activity that is necessary for coping with these emergencies.

During periods of stress or a severe asthma attack, patients who have been withdrawn from systemic corticosteroids should be instructed to resume oral corticosteroids (in large doses) immediately and to contact their physicians for further instruction. These patients should also be instructed to carry a warning card indicating that they may need supplementary systemic corticosteroids during periods of stress or a severe asthma attack.

Transfer of patients from systemic corticosteroid therapy to FLOVENT HFA may unmask conditions previously suppressed by the systemic corticosteroid therapy, e.g., rhinitis, conjunctivitis, eczema, arthritis, and eosinophilic conditions. Some patients may experience symptoms of systemically active corticosteroid withdrawal, e.g., joint and/or muscular pain, lassitude, and depression, despite maintenance or even improvement of respiratory function.

2. Bronchospasm. As with other inhaled medications, bronchospasm may occur with an immediate increase in wheezing after dosing. If bronchospasm occurs following dosing with FLOVENT HFA, it should be treated immediately with a fast-acting inhaled bronchodilator. Treatment with FLOVENT HFA should be discontinued and alternative therapy instituted.

Patients should be instructed to contact their physicians immediately when episodes of asthma that are not responsive to bronchodilators occur during the course of treatment with FLOVENT HFA. During such episodes, patients may require therapy with oral corticosteroids.

3. Immunosuppression. Persons who are using drugs that suppress the immune system are more susceptible to infections than healthy individuals. Chickenpox and measles, for example, can have a more serious or even fatal course in susceptible children or adults using corticosteroids. In such children or adults who have not had these diseases or been properly immunized, particular care should be taken to avoid exposure. How the dose, route, and duration of corticosteroid administration affect the risk of developing a disseminated infection is not known. The contribution of the underlying disease and/or prior corticosteroid treatment to the risk is also not known. If exposed to chickenpox, prophylaxis with varicella zoster immune globulin (VZIG) may be indicated. If exposed to measles, prophylaxis with pooled intramuscular immunoglobulin (IG) may be indicated. (See the respective package inserts for complete VZIG and IG prescribing information.) If chickenpox develops, treatment with antiviral agents may be considered.

4. Drug interaction with ritonavir. A drug interaction study in healthy subjects has shown that ritonavir (a highly potent cytochrome P450 3A4 inhibitor) can significantly increase systemic fluticasone propionate exposure (AUC), resulting in significantly reduced serum cortisol concentrations (see CLINICAL PHARMACOLOGY: Pharmacokinetics: *Drug Interactions* and PRECAUTIONS: Drug Interactions: *Inhibitors of Cytochrome P450*). During postmarketing use, there have been reports of clinically significant drug interactions in patients receiving fluticasone propionate and ritonavir, resulting in systemic corticosteroid effects including Cushing syndrome and adrenal suppression. Therefore, coadministration of fluticasone propionate and ritonavir is not recommended unless the potential benefit to the patient outweighs the risk of systemic corticosteroid side effects.

5. FLOVENT HFA should not be used to treat acute symptoms. FLOVENT HFA is not to be regarded as a bronchodilator and is not indicated for rapid relief of bronchospasm.

PRECAUTIONS

General

Orally inhaled corticosteroids may cause a reduction in growth velocity when administered to pediatric patients (see PRECAUTIONS: Pediatric Use).

Fluticasone propionate will often help control asthma symptoms with less suppression of HPA function than therapeutically equivalent oral doses of prednisone. Since fluticasone propionate is absorbed into the circulation and can be systemically active at higher doses, the beneficial effects of FLOVENT HFA in minimizing HPA dysfunction may be expected only when recommended dosages are not exceeded and individual patients are titrated to the lowest effective dose. A relationship between plasma levels of fluticasone propionate and inhibitory effects on stimulated cortisol production has been shown after 4 weeks of treatment with fluticasone propionate inhalation aerosol. Since individual sensitivity to effects on cortisol production exists, physicians should consider this information when prescribing FLOVENT HFA.

Because of the possibility of systemic absorption of inhaled corticosteroids, patients treated with FLOVENT HFA should be observed carefully for any evidence of systemic corticosteroid effects. Particular care should be taken in observing patients postoperatively or during periods of stress for evidence of inadequate adrenal response.

It is possible that systemic corticosteroid effects such as hypercorticism and adrenal suppression (including adrenal crisis) may appear in a small number of patients, particularly when FLOVENT HFA is administered at higher than recommended doses over prolonged periods of time. If such effects occur, the dosage of FLOVENT HFA should be reduced slowly, consistent with accepted procedures for reducing systemic corticosteroids and for management of asthma.

The long-term effects of FLOVENT HFA in human subjects are not fully known. In particular, the effects resulting from chronic use of fluticasone propionate on developmental or immunologic processes in the mouth, pharynx, trachea, and lung are unknown. Some patients have received inhaled fluticasone propionate on a continuous basis in a clinical study for up to 4 years. In clinical studies with patients treated for 2 years with inhaled fluticasone propionate, no apparent differences in the type or severity of adverse reactions were observed after long- versus short-term treatment.

Glaucoma, increased intraocular pressure, and cataracts have been reported in patients following the long-term administration of inhaled corticosteroids, including fluticasone propionate.

In clinical studies with inhaled fluticasone propionate, the development of localized infections of the pharynx with *Candida albicans* has occurred. When such an infection develops, it should be treated with appropriate local or systemic (i.e., oral antifungal) therapy while remaining on treatment with FLOVENT HFA, but at times therapy with FLOVENT HFA may need to be interrupted.

Inhaled corticosteroids should be used with caution, if at all, in patients with active or quiescent tuberculosis infection of the respiratory tract; untreated systemic fungal, bacterial, viral or parasitic infections; or ocular herpes simplex.

Eosinophilic Conditions

In rare cases, patients on inhaled fluticasone propionate may present with systemic eosinophilic conditions, with some patients presenting with clinical features of vasculitis consistent with Churg-Strauss syndrome, a condition that is often treated with systemic corticosteroid therapy. These events usually, but not always, have been associated with the reduction and/or withdrawal of oral corticosteroid therapy following the introduction of fluticasone propionate. Cases of serious eosinophilic conditions have also been reported with other inhaled corticosteroids in this clinical setting. Physicians should be alert to eosinophilia, vasculitic rash, worsening pulmonary symptoms, cardiac complications, and/or neuropathy presenting in their patients. A causal relationship between fluticasone propionate and these underlying conditions has not been established (see ADVERSE REACTIONS: Observed During Clinical Practice: *Eosinophilic Conditions*).

Information for Patients

Patients being treated with FLOVENT HFA should receive the following information and instructions. This information is intended to aid them in the safe and effective use of this medication. It is not a disclosure of all possible adverse or intended effects. It is important that patients understand how to use FLOVENT HFA in relation to other asthma medications they are taking.

1. Patients should use FLOVENT HFA at regular intervals as directed. Individual patients will experience a variable time to onset and degree of symptom relief and the full benefit may not be achieved until treatment has been administered for 1 to 2 weeks or longer. The patient should not increase the prescribed dosage but should contact the physician if symptoms do not improve or if the condition worsens.

2. Patients who are pregnant or nursing should contact their physicians about the use of FLOVENT HFA.

3. Patients should be warned to avoid exposure to chickenpox or measles and if they are exposed to consult their physicians without delay.

4. In general, the technique for administering FLOVENT HFA to children is similar to that for adults. Children should use FLOVENT HFA under adult supervision, as instructed by the patient's physician. (See the Information for the Patient leaflet accompanying the product.)

5. Prime the inhaler before using for the first time by releasing 4 test sprays into the air away from the face, shaking well for 5 seconds before each spray. In cases where the inhaler has not been used for more than 7 days or when it has been dropped, prime the inhaler again by shaking well for 5 seconds and releasing 1 test spray into the air away from the face.

6. After inhalation, rinse the mouth with water and spit out. Do not swallow.

7. Clean the inhaler at least once a week after the evening dose. Keeping the canister and plastic actuator clean is important to prevent medicine buildup. (See the cleaning instructions in the Information for the Patient leaflet accompanying the product.)

8. Use FLOVENT HFA only with the actuator supplied with the product. When the counter reads 020, contact the pharmacist for a refill of medication or consult the physician to determine whether a prescription refill is needed. Discard the inhaler when the counter reads 000. Never try to alter the numbers or remove the counter from the metal canister.

9. For important summary information and instructions for the proper use of FLOVENT HFA, the patient should carefully read and follow the Information for the Patient leaflet accompanying the product.

Drug Interactions
Inhibitors of Cytochrome P450
Fluticasone propionate is a substrate of cytochrome P450 3A4. A drug interaction study with fluticasone propionate aqueous nasal spray in healthy subjects has shown that ritonavir (a highly potent cytochrome P450 3A4 inhibitor) can significantly increase plasma fluticasone propionate exposure, resulting in significantly reduced serum cortisol concentrations (see CLINICAL PHARMACOLOGY: Pharmacokinetics: *Drug Interactions*). During postmarketing use, there have been reports of clinically significant drug interactions in patients receiving fluticasone propionate and ritonavir, resulting in systemic corticosteroid effects including Cushing syndrome and adrenal suppression. Therefore, coadministration of fluticasone propionate and ritonavir is not recommended unless the potential benefit to the patient outweighs the risk of systemic corticosteroid side effects.
In a placebo-controlled crossover study in 8 healthy adult volunteers, coadministration of a single dose of orally inhaled fluticasone propionate (1,000 mcg) with multiple doses of ketoconazole (200 mg) to steady state resulted in increased systemic fluticasone propionate exposure, a reduction in plasma cortisol AUC, and no effect on urinary excretion of cortisol. Caution should be exercised when FLOVENT HFA is coadministered with ketoconazole and other known potent cytochrome P450 3A4 inhibitors.
Carcinogenesis, Mutagenesis, Impairment of Fertility
Fluticasone propionate demonstrated no tumorigenic potential in mice at oral doses up to 1,000 mcg/kg (approximately 2 and 10 times the maximum recommended human daily inhalation dose in adults and children, respectively, on a mcg/m^2 basis) for 78 weeks or in rats at inhalation doses up to 57 mcg/kg (less than and equivalent to the maximum recommended human daily inhalation dose in adults and children, respectively, on a mcg/m^2 basis) for 104 weeks.
Fluticasone propionate did not induce gene mutation in prokaryotic or eukaryotic cells in vitro. No significant clastogenic effect was seen in cultured human peripheral lymphocytes in vitro or in the mouse micronucleus test.
No evidence of impairment of fertility was observed in reproductive studies conducted in male and female rats at subcutaneous doses up to 50 mcg/kg (less than the maximum recommended human daily inhalation dose on a mcg/m^2 basis). Prostate weight was significantly reduced at a subcutaneous dose of 50 mcg/kg.
Pregnancy
Teratogenic Effects
Pregnancy Category C. Subcutaneous studies in the mouse and rat at 45 and 100 mcg/kg, respectively (less than the maximum recommended human daily inhalation dose on a mcg/m^2 basis), revealed fetal toxicity characteristic of po-

tent corticosteroid compounds, including embryonic growth retardation, omphalocele, cleft palate, and retarded cranial ossification. No teratogenicity was seen in the rat at inhalation doses up to 68.7 mcg/kg (less than the maximum recommended human daily inhalation dose on a mcg/m^2 basis). In the rabbit, fetal weight reduction and cleft palate were observed at a subcutaneous dose of 4 mcg/kg (less than the maximum recommended human daily inhalation dose on a mcg/m^2 basis). However, no teratogenic effects were reported at oral doses up to 300 mcg/kg (approximately 3 times the maximum recommended human daily inhalation dose on a mcg/m^2 basis) of fluticasone propionate. No fluticasone propionate was detected in the plasma in this study, consistent with the established low bioavailability following oral administration (see CLINICAL PHARMACOLOGY: Pharmacokinetics: *Absorption*).
Fluticasone propionate crossed the placenta following administration of a subcutaneous dose of 100 mcg/kg to mice (less than the maximum recommended human daily inhalation dose on a mcg/m^2 basis), a subcutaneous or an oral dose of 100 mcg/kg to rats (less than the maximum recommended daily inhalation dose on a mcg/m^2 basis), and an oral dose of 300 mcg/kg to rabbits (approximately 3 times the maximum recommended human daily inhalation dose on a mcg/m^2 basis).
There are no adequate and well-controlled studies in pregnant women. FLOVENT HFA should be used during pregnancy only if the potential benefit justifies the potential risk to the fetus.
Experience with oral corticosteroids since their introduction in pharmacologic, as opposed to physiologic, doses suggests that rodents are more prone to teratogenic effects from corticosteroids than humans. In addition, because there is a natural increase in corticosteroid production during pregnancy, most women will require a lower exogenous corticosteroid dose and many will not need corticosteroid treatment during pregnancy.
Nursing Mothers
It is not known whether fluticasone propionate is excreted in human breast milk. However, other corticosteroids have been detected in human milk. Subcutaneous administration to lactating rats of 10 mcg/kg tritiated fluticasone propionate (less than the maximum recommended human daily inhalation dose on a mcg/m^2 basis) resulted in measurable radioactivity in milk.
Since there are no data from controlled trials on the use of FLOVENT HFA by nursing mothers, a decision should be made whether to discontinue nursing or to discontinue FLOVENT HFA, taking into account the importance of FLOVENT HFA to the mother.
Caution should be exercised when FLOVENT HFA is administered to a nursing woman.
Pediatric Use
The safety and effectiveness of FLOVENT HFA in children 12 years of age and older have been established (see CLINICAL PHARMACOLOGY: Pharmacokinetics: *Special Populations: Pediatric* , CLINICAL TRIALS: Pediatric Patients, ADVERSE REACTIONS: Pediatric Patients). Use of FLOVENT HFA in patients 4 to 11 years of age is supported by evidence from adequate and well-controlled studies in adults and adolescents 12 years of age and older, pharmacokinetic studies in patients 4 to 11 years of age, established efficacy of fluticasone propionate formulated as FLOVENT® DISKUS® (fluticasone propionate inhalation powder) and FLOVENT® ROTADISK® (fluticasone propionate inhalation powder) in patients 4 to 11 years of age, and supportive findings with FLOVENT HFA in a study conducted in patients 4 to 11 years of age. Types of adverse events in pediatric patients 4 to 11 years of age were generally similar to those observed in adults and adolescents.
Children Less Than 4 Years of Age
Pharmacokinetics
A 12-week, double-blind, placebo-controlled, parallel-group study was conducted in children with asthma aged 1 to <4 years. Population pharmacokinetics analyses were conducted in 164 children treated with 88 mcg of FLOVENT HFA administered twice daily with the AeroChamber Plus VHC with facemask. The predicted AUC$_{(0-\tau)}$ and C$_{max}$ ranged from 58.30 to 923.90 pg•hr/mL with a median of 129.05 pg•hr/mL and from 15.71 to 85.13 pg/mL with a median of 20.30 pg/mL, respectively. Predicted geometric means for AUC$_{(0-\tau)}$ and C$_{max}$ were 141 pg•hr/mL (95% CI: 127, 156) and 22 pg/mL (95% CI: 21, 23), respectively, indicating higher levels of exposure in children aged 1 to <4 years compared to those in children aged 4 to 11 years (see CLINICAL PHARMACOLOGY: Pharmacokinetics: *Special Populations: Pediatric*). Non-compartmental pharmacokinetic analyses in children aged 4 to 11 years showed AUC$_{(0-\tau)}$ and C$_{max}$ ranged from not calculable to 322 pg•hr/mL with a median of 30.20 pg•hr/mL and from below the limit of quantitation (BLQ) to 87.4 pg/mL with median of 18.8 pg/mL, respectively when the same dosage of FLOVENT HFA was administered without the VHC and facemask.

In a study in children 6 to <12 months of age with reactive airways disease, plasma fluticasone propionate was measured over a 12-hour dosing period after 4 weeks of treatment with 88 mcg of FLOVENT HFA twice daily with an AeroChamber Plus VHC with facemask. The AUC$_{(0-\tau)}$ and C$_{max}$ ranged from not calculable to 671.74 pg•hr/mL with a median of 104.2 pg•hr/mL and from BLQ to 106 pg/mL with a median of 32.0 pg/mL, respectively. The geometric means for AUC$_{(0-\tau)}$ and C$_{max}$ were 75 pg•hr/mL (95% CI: 34, 166; N = 16) and 25 pg/mL (95% CI: 13, 45; N = 17), respectively. The geometric mean AUC$_{(0-\tau)}$ and C$_{max}$ values in children 6 to <12 months of age were higher than those in children aged 4 to 11 years taking the same dosage of FLOVENT HFA without the VHC and facemask (see CLINICAL PHARMACOLOGY: Pharmacokinetics: *Special Populations: Pediatric*).
Population pharmacokinetic analysis of 102 male and 62 female subjects with asthma aged 1 to <4 years indicated that systemic exposure was not influenced by patient demographics, including gender. No overall differences in fluticasone propionate pharmacokinetics were observed between male and female patients with asthma.
Pharmacodynamics
A 12-week, double-blind, placebo-controlled, parallel-group study was conducted in children with asthma aged 1 to <4 years. Twelve-hour overnight urinary cortisol excretion after a 12-week treatment period with 88 mcg of FLOVENT HFA twice daily (n = 73) and with placebo (n = 42) were calculated. The mean and median change from baseline in urine cortisol over 12 hours were -0.7 and 0.0 mcg for FLOVENT HFA and 0.3 and -0.2 mcg for placebo treatments, respectively.
In a 1-way crossover study in children 6 to <12 months of age with reactive airways disease (N = 21), serum cortisol was measured over a 12-hour dosing period. Patients received placebo treatment for a 2-week period followed by a 4-week treatment period with 88 mcg of FLOVENT HFA twice daily with an AeroChamber Plus VHC with facemask. The geometric mean ratio of serum cortisol over 12 hours (AUC$_{0-12\ hr}$) following FLOVENT HFA (n = 16) versus placebo (n = 18) was 0.95 (95% CI: 0.72, 1.27).
Safety
FLOVENT HFA administered as 88 mcg twice daily has been evaluated for safety in 239 pediatric patients 1 to <4 years of age in a 12-week, double-blind, placebo-controlled study. Treatments were administered with an AeroChamber Plus VHC with facemask. In pediatric patients 1 to <4 years of age receiving FLOVENT HFA, the following events occurred with a frequency >3% and more frequently than in pediatric patients who received placebo, regardless of causality assessment: pyrexia, nasopharyngitis, upper respiratory tract infection, vomiting, otitis media, diarrhea, bronchitis, pharyngitis, and viral infection.
FLOVENT HFA administered as 88 mcg twice daily has also been evaluated for safety in 23 pediatric patients 6 to 12 months of age in an open-label placebo-controlled study. Treatments were administered with an AeroChamber Plus VHC with facemask for 2 weeks with placebo followed by 4 weeks with active drug. Adverse events after placebo and active drug were similar in kind and frequency.
In Vitro Testing of Dose Delivery With Holding Chambers
In vitro dose characterization studies were performed to evaluate the delivery of FLOVENT HFA via holding chambers with attached facemasks. The studies were conducted with 2 different holding chambers (AeroChamber Plus VHC and AeroChamber Z-STAT Plus™ VHC) and facemasks (small and medium size) at inspiratory flow rates of 4.9, 8.0, and 12.0 L/min in combination with holding times of 0, 2, 5, and 10 seconds. The flow rates were selected to be representative of inspiratory flow rates of children aged 6 to 12 months, 2 to 5 years, and over 5 years, respectively. The mean delivered dose of fluticasone propionate through the holding chambers with facemasks was lower than the 44 mcg of fluticasone propionate delivered directly from the actuator mouthpiece. The results were similar through both holding chambers (see Table 1 for data for the AeroChamber Plus VHC). The fine particle fraction (approximately 1 to 5 µm) across the flow rates used in these studies was 70% to 84% of the delivered dose, consistent with the removal of the coarser fraction by the holding chamber. In contrast, the fine particle fraction for FLOVENT HFA delivered without a holding chamber typically represents 42% to 55% of the delivered dose measured at the standard flow rate of 28.3 L/min. These data suggest that even at low flow rates and extended holding times potentially experienced in realistic situations with young children, an adequate amount of fluticasone propionate can be delivered to pediatric patients via a holding chamber and facemask at the recommended doses.
[See table 1 at top of next page]
Orally inhaled corticosteroids may cause a reduction in growth velocity when administered to pediatric patients. A reduction of growth velocity in children or teenagers may occur as a result of poorly controlled asthma or from use of

corticosteroids including inhaled corticosteroids. The effects of long-term treatment of children and adolescents with inhaled corticosteroids, including fluticasone propionate, on final adult height are not known.

Controlled clinical studies have shown that inhaled corticosteroids may cause a reduction in growth in pediatric patients. In these studies, the mean reduction in growth velocity was approximately 1 cm/year (range, 0.3 to 1.8 cm/year) and appears to depend upon dose and duration of exposure. This effect was observed in the absence of laboratory evidence of HPA axis suppression, suggesting that growth velocity is a more sensitive indicator of systemic corticosteroid exposure in pediatric patients than some commonly used tests of HPA axis function. The long-term effects of this reduction in growth velocity associated with orally inhaled corticosteroids, including the impact on final adult height, are unknown. The potential for "catch-up" growth following discontinuation of treatment with orally inhaled corticosteroids has not been adequately studied. The effects on growth velocity of treatment with orally inhaled corticosteroids for over 1 year, including the impact on final adult height, are unknown. The growth of children and adolescents receiving orally inhaled corticosteroids, including FLOVENT HFA, should be monitored routinely (e.g., via stadiometry). The potential growth effects of prolonged treatment should be weighed against the clinical benefits obtained and the risks associated with alternative therapies. To minimize the systemic effects of orally inhaled corticosteroids, including FLOVENT HFA, each patient should be titrated to the lowest dose that effectively controls his/her symptoms.

Since a cross study comparison in adolescent and adult patients (≥12 years of age) indicated that systemic exposure of inhaled fluticasone propionate from FLOVENT HFA would be higher than exposure from FLOVENT ROTADISK, results from a study to assess the potential growth effects of FLOVENT ROTADISK in pediatric patients (4 to 11 years of age) are provided.

A 52-week placebo-controlled study to assess the potential growth effects of fluticasone propionate inhalation powder (FLOVENT ROTADISK) at 50 and 100 mcg twice daily was conducted in the US in 325 prepubescent children (244 males and 81 females) aged 4 to 11 years. The mean growth velocities at 52 weeks observed in the intent-to-treat population were 6.32 cm/year in the placebo group (n = 76), 6.07 cm/year in the 50-mcg group (n = 98), and 5.66 cm/year in the 100-mcg group (n = 89). An imbalance in the proportion of children entering puberty between groups and a higher dropout rate in the placebo group due to poorly controlled asthma may be confounding factors in interpreting these data. A separate subset analysis of children who remained prepubertal during the study revealed growth rates at 52 weeks of 6.10 cm/year in the placebo group (n = 57), 5.91 cm/year in the 50-mcg group (n = 74), and 5.67 cm/year in the 100-mcg group (n = 79). In children 8.5 years of age, the mean age of children in this study, the range for expected growth velocity is: boys – 3rd percentile = 3.8 cm/year, 50th percentile = 5.4 cm/year, and 97th percentile = 7.0 cm/year; girls – 3rd percentile = 4.2 cm/year, 50th percentile = 5.7 cm/year, and 97th percentile = 7.3 cm/year.

The clinical significance of these growth data is not certain. Physicians should closely follow the growth of children and adolescents taking corticosteroids by any route, and weigh the benefits of corticosteroid therapy against the possibility of growth suppression if growth appears slowed. Patients should be maintained on the lowest dose of inhaled corticosteroid that effectively controls their asthma.

Geriatric Use
Of the total number of patients treated with FLOVENT HFA in US and non-US clinical trials, 173 were 65 years of age or older, 19 of which were 75 years of age or older. No apparent differences in safety or efficacy were observed between these patients and younger patients. No overall differences in safety were observed between these patients and younger patients, and other reported clinical experience has not identified differences in responses between the elderly and younger patients, but greater sensitivity of some older individuals cannot be ruled out. In general, dose selection for an elderly patient should be cautious, reflecting the greater frequency of decreased hepatic function and of concomitant disease or other drug therapy.

ADVERSE REACTIONS
Adolescent and Adult Patients
The incidence of common adverse events in Table 2 is based upon 2 placebo-controlled US clinical trials in which 812 adolescent and adult patients (457 females and 355 males) previously treated with as-needed bronchodilators and/or inhaled corticosteroids were treated twice daily for up to 12 weeks with 2 inhalations of FLOVENT HFA 44 mcg Inhalation Aerosol, FLOVENT HFA 110 mcg Inhalation Aerosol, FLOVENT HFA 220 mcg Inhalation Aerosol (dosages of 88, 220, or 440 mcg twice daily) or placebo.
[See table 2 above]

Table 1: In Vitro Medication Delivery Through AeroChamber Plus® Valved Holding Chamber With a Facemask

Age	Facemask	Flow Rate (L/min)	Holding Time (seconds)	Mean Medication Delivery Through AeroChamber Plus VHC (mcg/actuation)	Body Weight 50th Percentile (kg)*	Medication Delivered per Actuation (mcg/kg)[†]
6 to 12 Months	Small	4.9	0	8.3	7.5-9.9	0.8-1.1
			2	6.7		0.7-0.9
			5	7.5		0.8-1.0
			10	7.5		0.8-1.0
2 to 5 Years	Small	8.0	0	7.3	12.3-18.0	0.4-0.6
			2	6.8		0.4-0.6
			5	6.7		0.4-0.5
			10	7.7		0.4-0.6
2 to 5 Years	Medium	8.0	0	7.8	12.3-18.0	0.4-0.6
			2	7.7		0.4-0.6
			5	8.1		0.5-0.7
			10	9.0		0.5-0.7
>5 Years	Medium	12.0	0	12.3	18.0	0.7
			2	11.8		0.7
			5	12.0		0.7
			10	10.1		0.6

* Centers for Disease Control growth charts, developed by the National Center for Health Statistics in collaboration with the National Center for Chronic Disease Prevention and Health Promotion (2000). Ranges correspond to the average of the 50th percentile weight for boys and girls at the ages indicated.
[†] A single inhalation of FLOVENT HFA in a 70-kg adult without use of a valved holding chamber and facemask delivers approximately 44 mcg, or 0.6 mcg/kg.

Table 2. Overall Adverse Events With >3% Incidence in US Controlled Clinical Trials With FLOVENT HFA in Patients ≥12 Years of Age With Asthma Previously Receiving Bronchodilators and/or Inhaled Corticosteroids

Adverse Event	FLOVENT HFA 88 mcg Twice Daily (n = 203) %	FLOVENT HFA 220 mcg Twice Daily (n = 204) %	FLOVENT HFA 440 mcg Twice Daily (n = 202) %	Placebo (n = 203) %
Ear, nose, and throat				
Upper respiratory tract infection	18	16	16	14
Throat irritation	8	8	10	5
Upper respiratory inflammation	2	5	5	1
Sinusitis/sinus infection	6	7	4	3
Hoarseness/dysphonia	2	3	6	<1
Gastrointestinal				
Candidiasis mouth/throat & non-site specific	4	2	5	<1
Lower respiratory				
Cough	4	6	4	5
Bronchitis	2	2	6	5
Neurological				
Headache	11	7	5	6
Average duration of exposure (days)	73	74	76	60

Table 2 includes all events (whether considered drug-related or nondrug-related by the investigator) that occurred at a rate of over 3% in any of the groups treated with FLOVENT HFA and were more common than in the placebo group. In considering these data, differences in average duration of exposure should be taken into account. These adverse events were mostly mild to moderate in severity. Rare cases of immediate and delayed hypersensitivity reactions, including urticaria and rash, have been reported.

Other adverse events that occurred in the groups receiving FLOVENT HFA in these studies with an incidence of 1% to 3% and that occurred at a greater incidence than with placebo were:
Ear, Nose, and Throat
Sinusitis/sinus infection, rhinitis, pharyngitis/throat infection, rhinorrhea/post-nasal drip, nasal sinus disorders, laryngitis.
Gastrointestinal
Diarrhea, viral gastrointestinal infections, gastrointestinal signs and symptoms, dyspeptic symptoms, gastrointestinal discomfort and pain, hyposalivation.

Musculoskeletal
Musculoskeletal pain, muscle pain, muscle stiffness/tightness/rigidity.
Neurological
Dizziness, migraines.
Non-Site Specific
Fever, viral infections, pain, chest symptoms.
Skin
Viral skin infections.
Trauma
Muscle injuries, soft tissue injuries, injuries.
Urogenital
Urinary infections.
Fluticasone propionate inhalation aerosol (440 or 880 mcg twice daily) was administered for 16 weeks to patients with asthma requiring oral corticosteroids (Study 3). Adverse events not included in Table 2, but reported by >3 patients in either group treated with FLOVENT HFA and more commonly than in the placebo group included rhinitis, nausea

Table 3. Recommended Dosages of FLOVENT HFA
NOTE: In all patients, it is desirable to titrate to the lowest effective dosage once asthma stability is achieved.

Previous Therapy	Recommended Starting Dosage	Highest Recommended Dosage
Adolescent and adult patients (≥12 years)		
Bronchodilators alone	88 mcg twice daily	440 mcg twice daily
Inhaled corticosteroids	88-220 mcg twice daily[*]	440 mcg twice daily
Oral corticosteroids[†]	440 mcg twice daily	880 mcg twice daily
Pediatric patients (4 to 11 years)[‡]	88 mcg twice daily	88 mcg twice daily

[*]**For Patients Currently Receiving Inhaled Corticosteroid Therapy:** Starting dosages above 88 mcg twice daily may be considered for patients with poorer asthma control or those who have previously required doses of inhaled corticosteroids that are in the higher range for that specific agent.
[†]**For Patients Currently Receiving Chronic Oral Corticosteroid Therapy:** Prednisone should be reduced no faster than 2.5 to 5 mg/day on a weekly basis, beginning after at least 1 week of therapy with FLOVENT HFA. Patients should be carefully monitored for signs of asthma instability, including serial objective measures of airflow, and for signs of adrenal insufficiency (see WARNINGS). Once prednisone reduction is complete, the dosage of fluticasone propionate HFA should be reduced to the lowest effective dosage.
[‡]Recommended pediatric dosage is 88 mcg twice daily regardless of prior therapy.

and vomiting, arthralgia and articular rheumatism, musculoskeletal pain, muscle pain, malaise and fatigue, and sleep disorders.
In 2 long-term studies (26 and 52 weeks), treatment with FLOVENT HFA at dosages up to 440 mcg twice daily was well tolerated. The pattern of adverse events was similar to that observed in the 12-week studies. There were no new and/or unexpected adverse events with long-term treatment.

Pediatric Patients
FLOVENT HFA has been evaluated for safety in 56 pediatric patients aged 4 to 11 years who received 88 mcg twice daily for 4 weeks. Types of adverse events in these pediatric patients were generally similar to those observed in adults and adolescents.

Observed During Clinical Practice
In addition to adverse events reported from clinical trials, the following events have been identified during postmarketing use of fluticasone propionate. Because they are reported voluntarily from a population of unknown size, estimates of frequency cannot be made. These events have been chosen for inclusion due to a combination of their seriousness, frequency of reporting, or potential causal connection to fluticasone propionate.
Ear, Nose, and Throat
Aphonia, facial and oropharyngeal edema, including angioedema, and throat soreness and irritation.
Endocrine and Metabolic
Cushingoid features, growth velocity reduction in children/adolescents, hyperglycemia, osteoporosis, and weight gain.
Eye
Cataracts.
Non-Site Specific
Very rare anaphylactic reaction.
Psychiatry
Agitation, aggression, anxiety, depression, and restlessness. Behavioral changes, including hyperactivity and irritability, have been reported very rarely and primarily in children.
Respiratory
Asthma exacerbation, chest tightness, cough, dyspnea, immediate and delayed bronchospasm, paradoxical bronchospasm, pneumonia, and wheeze.
Skin
Contusions, cutaneous hypersensitivity reactions, ecchymoses, and pruritus.
Eosinophilic Conditions
In rare cases, patients on inhaled fluticasone propionate may present with systemic eosinophilic conditions, with some patients presenting with clinical features of vasculitis consistent with Churg-Strauss syndrome, a condition that is often treated with systemic corticosteroid therapy. These events usually, but not always, have been associated with the reduction and/or withdrawal of oral corticosteroid therapy following the introduction of fluticasone propionate (see PRECAUTIONS: Eosinophilic Conditions).

OVERDOSAGE
Chronic overdosage may result in signs/symptoms of hypercorticism (see PRECAUTIONS: General). Inhalation by healthy volunteers of a single dose of 1,760 or 3,520 mcg of fluticasone propionate CFC inhalation aerosol was well tolerated. Doses of 1,320 mcg administered to healthy human volunteers twice daily for 7 to 15 days were also well tolerated. Repeat oral doses up to 80 mg daily for 10 days in healthy volunteers and repeat oral doses up to 20 mg daily for 42 days in patients were well tolerated. Adverse reactions were of mild or moderate severity, and incidences were similar in active and placebo treatment groups. The oral median lethal dose in mice was >1,000 mg/kg (approximately ≥2,300 and >11,000 times the maximum human daily inhalation dose in adults and children on a mg/m^2 basis, respectively), and the subcutaneous median lethal dose in rats was >1,000 mg/kg (approximately >4,600 and >22,000 times the maximum human daily inhalation dose in adults and children on a mg/m^2 basis, respectively).

DOSAGE AND ADMINISTRATION
FLOVENT HFA should be administered by the orally inhaled route only in patients 4 years of age and older. Individual patients will experience a variable time to onset and degree of symptom relief. Maximum benefit may not be achieved for 1 to 2 weeks or longer after starting treatment. After asthma stability has been achieved, it is always desirable to titrate to the lowest effective dosage to reduce the possibility of side effects. For patients who do not respond adequately to the starting dosage after 2 weeks of therapy, higher dosages may provide additional asthma control. The safety and efficacy of FLOVENT HFA when administered in excess of recommended dosages have not been established. The recommended starting dosage and the highest recommended dosage of FLOVENT HFA, based on prior asthma therapy, are listed in Table 3.
[See table 3 above]
FLOVENT HFA should be primed before using for the first time by releasing 4 test sprays into the air away from the face, shaking well for 5 seconds before each spray. In cases where the inhaler has not been used for more than 7 days or when it has been dropped, prime the inhaler again by shaking well for 5 seconds and releasing 1 test spray into the air away from the face.

Geriatric Use
In studies where geriatric patients (65 years of age or older, see PRECAUTIONS: Geriatric Use) have been treated with fluticasone propionate inhalation aerosol, efficacy and safety did not differ from that in younger patients. Based on available data for FLOVENT HFA, no dosage adjustment is recommended.

Directions for Use
An Information for the Patient leaflet containing illustrated instructions for use accompany each package of FLOVENT HFA.

HOW SUPPLIED
FLOVENT HFA 44 mcg Inhalation Aerosol is supplied in 10.6-g pressurized aluminum canisters containing 120 metered actuations in boxes of 1 (NDC 0173-0718-20).
FLOVENT HFA 110 mcg Inhalation Aerosol is supplied in 12-g pressurized aluminum canisters containing 120 metered actuations in boxes of 1 (NDC 0173-0719-20).
FLOVENT HFA 220 mcg Inhalation Aerosol is supplied in 12-g pressurized aluminum canisters containing 120 metered actuations in boxes of 1 (NDC 0173-0720-20).
Each canister is fitted with a dose counter, supplied with a dark orange oral actuator with a peach strapcap, and sealed in a plastic coated, moisture protective foil pouch with a desiccant that should be discarded when the pouch is opened. Each canister is packaged with an Information for the Patient leaflet.
The dark orange actuator supplied with FLOVENT HFA should not be used with any other product canisters, and actuators from other products should not be used with a FLOVENT HFA canister.
The correct amount of medication in each actuation cannot be assured after the counter reads 000, even though the canister is not completely empty and will continue to operate. The inhaler should be discarded when the counter reads 000.
Keep out of reach of children. Avoid spraying in eyes.

Contents Under Pressure: Do not puncture. Do not use or store near heat or open flame. Exposure to temperatures above 120°F may cause bursting. Never throw into fire or incinerator.
Store at 25°C (77°F); excursions permitted to 15°-30°C (59°-86°F). Store the inhaler with the mouthpiece down. For best results, the inhaler should be at room temperature before use. SHAKE WELL FOR 5 SECONDS BEFORE USING.
FLOVENT HFA does not contain chlorofluorocarbons (CFCs) as the propellant.
DISKUS, FLOVENT, ROTADISK, and VENTOLIN are registered trademarks of GlaxoSmithKline.
AeroChamber Plus is a registered trademark and Aero-Chamber Z-STAT Plus is a trademark of Monaghan Medical Corp. or an affiliate of Monaghan Medical Corp.
GlaxoSmithKline
Research Triangle Park, NC 27709
©2008, GlaxoSmithKline. All rights reserved.
July 2008 FLH:1PI
PHARMACIST—DETACH HERE AND GIVE LEAFLET TO PATIENT

Information for the Patient
FLOVENT® [flō' vent] HFA 44 mcg
(fluticasone propionate 44 mcg)
Inhalation Aerosol
FLOVENT® HFA 110 mcg
(fluticasone propionate 110 mcg)
Inhalation Aerosol
FLOVENT® HFA 220 mcg
(fluticasone propionate 220 mcg)
Inhalation Aerosol
FOR ORAL INHALATION ONLY
Read this leaflet carefully before you start to use FLOVENT HFA Inhalation Aerosol.
Keep this leaflet because it has important summary information about FLOVENT HFA. This leaflet does not contain all the information about your medicine. If you have any questions or are not sure about something, you should ask your doctor or pharmacist.
Read the new leaflet that comes with each refill of your prescription because there may be new information.
What is FLOVENT HFA?
FLOVENT HFA contains a medicine called fluticasone propionate, which is a synthetic corticosteroid. Corticosteroids are natural substances found in the body that help fight inflammation. Corticosteroids are used to treat asthma because they reduce airway inflammation.
FLOVENT HFA is used to treat asthma in patients 4 years of age and older. When inhaled regularly, FLOVENT HFA also helps to prevent symptoms of asthma.
FLOVENT HFA comes in 3 strengths. Your doctor has prescribed the one that is best for your condition.
Who should not use FLOVENT HFA?
Do not use FLOVENT HFA if you:
- are allergic to any of the ingredients in FLOVENT HFA or other inhaled corticosteroids. See "What are the ingredients in FLOVENT HFA?" below.
- have an acute asthma attack or status asthmaticus. **FLOVENT HFA is not a bronchodilator and should not be used to give you fast relief from your breathing problems during an asthma attack.** Always use a short-acting bronchodilator (rescue medicine), such as albuterol inhaler, during a sudden asthma attack. You must take FLOVENT HFA at regular times as recommended by your doctor, and not as an emergency medicine.
What should I tell my doctor before taking FLOVENT HFA?
Tell your doctor if you are:
- pregnant or planning to become pregnant. It is not known if FLOVENT HFA will harm your unborn baby.
- breastfeeding a baby. It is not known if FLOVENT HFA passes into your breast milk.
- exposed to chickenpox or measles.
Tell your doctor about all the medicines you take including prescription and non-prescription medicines, vitamins, and herbal supplements. FLOVENT HFA may affect the way other medicines work, and other medicines may affect how FLOVENT HFA works. Especially, tell your doctor if you take:
- a medicine containing ritonavir (commonly used to treat HIV infection or AIDS). The anti-HIV medicines NORVIR® (ritonavir capsules) Soft Gelatin, NORVIR (ritonavir oral solution), and KALETRA® (lopinavir/ritonavir) Tablets contain ritonavir.
- any other corticosteroids.
How should I use FLOVENT HFA?
1. It is important that you inhale each dose as your doctor has prescribed. The prescription label provided by your pharmacist will usually tell you what dose to take and how often. If it doesn't, or if you are not sure, ask your doctor or pharmacist. DO NOT inhale more doses or use your FLOVENT HFA more often than your doctor has prescribed.
2. It may take 1 to 2 weeks or longer for this medicine to work, and it is very important that you use it regularly.

Do not stop taking FLOVENT HFA, even if you are feeling better, unless your doctor tells you to.

3. If you miss a dose, just take your next scheduled dose when it is due. **Do not double the dose.**

4. Your doctor may prescribe additional medicine (such as fast-acting bronchodilators) for emergency relief if a sudden asthma attack occurs. Contact your doctor if:
   • an asthma attack does not respond to the additional medicine or
   • you need more of the additional medicine than usual.

5. If you also use another medicine by inhalation, you should ask your doctor for instructions on when to use it while you are also using FLOVENT HFA.

What are the possible side effects of FLOVENT HFA?
Common side effects in adults and children using FLOVENT HFA include:
• a cold or upper respiratory tract infection
• throat irritation
• headache
• thrush (fungal infection) in the mouth and throat
Other common side effects in children include:
• fever
• diarrhea
• ear infection
• vomiting
• bronchitis
• inflammation of the nose and throat
• viral infection
Tell your doctor if you have any side effect that bothers you or that does not go away. These are not all the possible side effects of FLOVENT HFA. For more information ask your doctor or pharmacist.
Call your doctor for medical advice about side effects. You may report side effects to FDA at 1-800-FDA-1088.

What are the ingredients in FLOVENT HFA?
Active ingredient: fluticasone propionate (micronized)
Inactive ingredient: propellant HFA-134a

Instructions for Using FLOVENT HFA
The parts of your FLOVENT HFA
There are 2 main parts to your FLOVENT HFA inhaler—the metal canister that holds the medicine and the dark orange plastic actuator that sprays the medicine from the canister (see Figure 1).

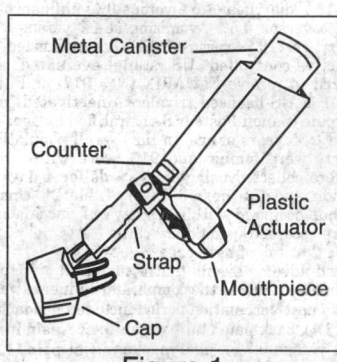

Figure 1

The canister has a counter to show how many sprays of medicine you have left. The number shows through a window in the back of the actuator. The counter starts at 124. The number will count down by 1 each time you spray the inhaler. The counter will stop counting at 000.
Never try to change the numbers or take the counter off the metal canister. The counter cannot be reset, and it is permanently attached to the canister.
The mouthpiece of the actuator is covered by a cap. A strap on this cap keeps it attached to the actuator.
Do not use the actuator with a canister of medicine from any other inhaler. And do not use a FLOVENT HFA canister with an actuator from any other inhaler.
Using your FLOVENT HFA
• The inhaler should be at room temperature before you use it.
• Take your FLOVENT HFA inhaler out of the moisture-protective foil pouch just before you use it for the first time. Safely throw away the foil pouch and the drying packet that comes inside the pouch.
• Priming the inhaler:
Before you use FLOVENT HFA for the first time, you must prime the inhaler so that you will get the right amount of medicine when you use it. To prime the inhaler, take the cap off the mouthpiece and shake the inhaler well for 5 seconds. Then spray the inhaler into the air away from your face. **Avoid spraying in eyes.** Shake and spray the inhaler like this 3 more times to finish priming it. The counter should now read 120.

You must prime the inhaler again if you have not used it in more than 7 days or if you drop it. Take the cap off the mouthpiece and shake the inhaler well for 5 seconds. Then spray it 1 time into the air away from your face.
• An adult should watch a child use the inhaler to be sure it is used correctly. If a child needs help using the inhaler, an adult should help the child use the inhaler with or without a holding chamber attached to a facemask. The adult should follow the instructions that came with the holding chamber.
Read the following 7 steps before using FLOVENT HFA and follow them at each use. If you have any questions, ask your doctor or pharmacist.

1. **Take the cap off the mouthpiece of the actuator** (see Figure 2).
   Look inside the mouthpiece for foreign objects, and take out any you see.
   Make sure the canister fits firmly in the actuator.
   Shake the inhaler well for 5 seconds.

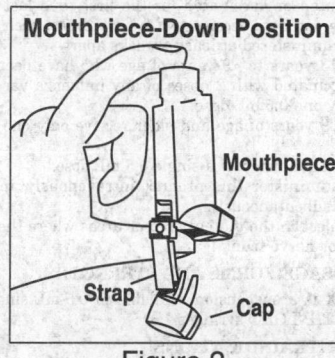

Mouthpiece-Down Position

Mouthpiece

Strap

Cap

Figure 2

2. Hold the inhaler with the mouthpiece down (see Figure 2). **Breathe out through your mouth** and push as much air from your lungs as you can. Put the mouthpiece in your mouth and close your lips around it.

3. Push the top of the canister all the way down while you breathe in deeply and slowly through your mouth (see Figure 3).
   Right after the spray comes out, take your finger off the canister. After you have breathed in all the way, take the inhaler out of your mouth and close your mouth.

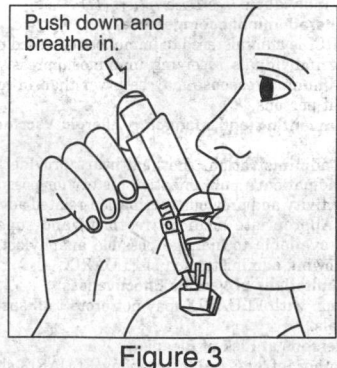

Push down and breathe in.

Figure 3

4. **Hold your breath as long as you can,** up to 10 seconds. Then breathe normally.

5. **Wait about 30 seconds and shake the inhaler well** for 5 seconds. Repeat steps 2 through 4.

6. After you finish taking this medicine, rinse your mouth with water. Spit out the water. Do not swallow it.

7. Put the cap back on the mouthpiece after each time you use the inhaler. Make sure it snaps firmly into place.

Cleaning your FLOVENT HFA
Clean the inhaler at least once a week after your evening dose. It is important to keep the canister and plastic actuator clean so the medicine will not build-up and block the spray.

1. Take the cap off the mouthpiece. The strap on the cap will stay attached to the actuator. Do not take the canister out of the plastic actuator.

2. Use a clean cotton swab dampened with water to clean the small circular opening where the medicine sprays out of the canister. Gently twist the swab in a circular motion to take off any medicine (see Figure 4). Repeat with a new swab dampened with water to take off any medicine still at the opening.

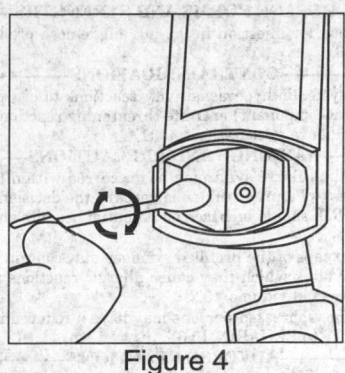

Figure 4

3. Wipe the inside of the mouthpiece with a clean tissue dampened with water. Let the actuator air-dry overnight.

4. Put the cap back on the mouthpiece after the actuator has dried.

Storing your FLOVENT HFA
Store at room temperature with the mouthpiece down. Keep out of reach of children.

Contents Under Pressure: Do not puncture. Do not use or store near heat or open flame. Exposure to temperatures above 120°F may cause bursting. Never throw into fire or incinerator.

Replacing your FLOVENT HFA
• **When the counter reads 020,** you should refill your prescription or ask your doctor if you need a refill of your prescription.
• **When the counter reads 000,** throw the inhaler away. You should not keep using the inhaler because you will not receive the right amount of medicine.
• **Do not use the inhaler** after the expiration date, which is on the packaging it comes in.
For more information go to www.floventdiskus.com or call 1-888-825-5249.
FLOVENT is a registered trademark of GlaxoSmithKline. NORVIR and KALETRA are registered trademarks of Abbott Laboratories.
GlaxoSmithKline
Research Triangle Park, NC 27709
©2008, GlaxoSmithKline. All rights reserved.
July 2008 FLH:1PIL

FLUARIX®   ℞
[flū' a-rix]
(Influenza Virus Vaccine)
Suspension for Intramuscular Injection
2010-2011 Formula

HIGHLIGHTS OF PRESCRIBING INFORMATION
These highlights do not include all the information needed to use FLUARIX safely and effectively. See full prescribing information for FLUARIX.
FLUARIX (Influenza Virus Vaccine)
Suspension for Intramuscular Injection
2010-2011 Formula
Initial U.S. Approval: 2005

———RECENT MAJOR CHANGES———

Indications and Usage (1)	10/2009
Dosage and Administration, Recommended Dose and Schedule (2.2)	10/2009
Warnings and Precautions, Latex (5.2)	07/2010

———INDICATIONS AND USAGE———
FLUARIX is a vaccine indicated for active immunization for the prevention of disease caused by influenza virus subtypes A and type B contained in the vaccine. FLUARIX is approved for use in persons 3 years of age and older. (1)

———DOSAGE AND ADMINISTRATION———
Children: 0.5 mL dose by intramuscular injection (2.2)
• Children 3 years to <9 years of age previously unvaccinated or vaccinated for the first time last season with only one dose receive two 0.5 mL doses; each 0.5 mL dose is administered at least 4 weeks apart.
• Children 3 years to <9 years of age previously vaccinated with 2 doses of any influenza vaccine receive only one 0.5 mL dose.
• Children 9 years of age and older receive only one 0.5 mL dose.
Adults: a single 0.5-mL dose by intramuscular injection. (2.2)

DOSAGE FORMS AND STRENGTHS

Suspension for injection in 0.5-mL single-dose prefilled syringes. (3)

CONTRAINDICATIONS

Known systemic hypersensitivity reactions to egg proteins (a vaccine component) or a life-threatening reaction to previous influenza vaccination. (4, 11)

WARNINGS AND PRECAUTIONS

- If Guillain-Barré syndrome has occurred within 6 weeks of receipt of a prior influenza vaccine, the decision to give FLUARIX should be based on potential benefits and risks. (5.1)
- The tip caps of the prefilled syringes may contain natural rubber latex which may cause allergic reactions in latex sensitive individuals. (5.2)
- Immunosuppressed persons may have a reduced immune response to FLUARIX. (5.3)

ADVERSE REACTIONS

- In adults, the most common (≥10%) local and general adverse events were pain and redness at the injection site, muscle aches, fatigue, and headache. (6.1)
- In children 5 years to <18 years of age, the most common (≥10%) local and general adverse events were similar to those in adults but also included swelling at the injection site. (6.1)
- In children 3 years to <5 years of age, the most common (≥10%) local and general adverse events included pain, redness, and swelling at the injection site, irritability, loss of appetite, and drowsiness. (6.1)

To report SUSPECTED ADVERSE REACTIONS, contact GlaxoSmithKline at 1-888-825-5249 or VAERS at 1-800-822-7967 or www.vaers.hhs.gov.

DRUG INTERACTIONS

Do not mix with any other vaccine in the same syringe or vial. (7.1)

USE IN SPECIFIC POPULATIONS

- Safety and effectiveness have not been established in pregnant women or nursing mothers. (8.1, 8.3)
- In a clinical study of children <3 years of age, antibody titers were lower after FLUARIX than after an active comparator. (8.4)
- Geriatric Use: Antibody responses were lower in geriatric subjects than in younger subjects. (8.5)

See 17 for PATIENT COUNSELING INFORMATION

Revised: 08/2010

FULL PRESCRIBING INFORMATION

1 INDICATIONS AND USAGE

FLUARIX® is indicated for active immunization for the prevention of disease caused by influenza virus subtypes A and type B contained in the vaccine. FLUARIX is approved for use in persons 3 years of age and older.

2 DOSAGE AND ADMINISTRATION

2.1 Preparation for Administration

Shake well before administration. Parenteral drug products should be inspected visually for particulate matter and discoloration prior to administration, whenever solution and container permit. If either of these conditions exists, the vaccine should not be administered.

2.2 Recommended Dose and Schedule

FLUARIX should be administered as an intramuscular injection preferably in the region of the deltoid muscle of the upper arm.

Children: Children 3 years to <9 years of age previously unvaccinated or vaccinated for the first time last season with only one dose receive two 0.5 mL doses; each 0.5 mL dose is administered at least 4 weeks apart.

Children 3 years to <9 years of age who have been previously vaccinated with 2 doses of any influenza vaccine receive only one 0.5 mL dose.

Children 9 years of age and older receive only one 0.5 mL dose.

Adults: Administer as a single 0.5 mL dose.

Do not administer this product intravenously, intradermally, or subcutaneously.

Do not inject in the gluteal area or areas where there may be a major nerve trunk.

3 DOSAGE FORMS AND STRENGTHS

FLUARIX is a suspension available in 0.5-mL single-dose prefilled TIP-LOK® syringes.

4 CONTRAINDICATIONS

Do not administer FLUARIX to anyone with known systemic hypersensitivity reactions to egg proteins (a vaccine component) or a life-threatening reaction to previous administration of any influenza vaccine [see Description (11)].

5 WARNINGS AND PRECAUTIONS

5.1 Guillain-Barré Syndrome

If Guillain-Barré syndrome has occurred within 6 weeks of receipt of a prior influenza vaccine, the decision to give FLUARIX should be based on careful consideration of the potential benefits and risks.

5.2 Latex

The tip caps of the prefilled syringes may contain natural rubber latex which may cause allergic reactions in latex sensitive individuals [see Description (11)].

5.3 Altered Immunocompetence

If FLUARIX is administered to immunosuppressed persons, including those receiving immunosuppressive therapy, the immune response may be lower than in immunocompetent persons.

5.4 Preventing and Managing Allergic Vaccine Reactions

Prior to administration, the healthcare provider should review the patient's immunization history for possible vaccine sensitivity and previous vaccination-related adverse reactions. Appropriate medical treatment and supervision must be available to manage possible anaphylactic reactions following administration of FLUARIX.

5.5 Limitations of Vaccine Effectiveness

Vaccination with FLUARIX may not protect all susceptible individuals.

5.6 Persons at Risk of Bleeding

As with other intramuscular injections, FLUARIX should be given with caution in individuals with bleeding disorders such as hemophilia or on anticoagulant therapy, to avoid the risk of hematoma following the injection.

6 ADVERSE REACTIONS

6.1 Clinical Trials Experience

Because clinical trials are conducted under widely varying conditions, adverse reaction rates observed in the clinical trials of a vaccine cannot be directly compared to rates in the clinical trials of another vaccine, and may not reflect the rates observed in practice. There is the possibility that broad use of FLUARIX could reveal adverse reactions not observed in clinical trials.

Adults: In adults, the most common local adverse reactions and general adverse events observed with FLUARIX were pain and redness at the injection site, muscle aches, fatigue, and headache.

FLUARIX has been administered to 10,317 adults 18 to 64 years of age and 606 subjects ≥65 years of age in 4 clinical trials. One of the 4 clinical trials was a randomized, double-blind, placebo-controlled study that evaluated a total of 952 subjects: FLUARIX (N = 760) and placebo (N = 192). The population was 18 to 64 years of age (mean 39.1), 54% were female and 80% were white. Solicited events were collected

for 4 days (day of vaccination and the next 3 days) (Table 1). Unsolicited events that occurred within 21 days of vaccination (day 0-20) were recorded using diary cards supplemented by spontaneous reports and a medical history as reported by subjects.

Table 1. Percentage of Subjects With Solicited Local Adverse Reactions or General Adverse Events Within 4 Days[a] of Vaccination (Total Vaccinated Cohort)

	FLUARIX N = 760 %	Placebo N = 192 %
Local Adverse Reactions		
Pain	55	12
Redness	18	10
Swelling	9	6
General Adverse Events		
Muscle aches	23	12
Fatigue	20	18
Headache	19	21
Arthralgia	6	6
Shivering	3	3
Fever (≥100.4°F)	2	2

Total vaccinated cohort for safety included all vaccinated subjects for whom safety data were available.

[a] 4 days included day of vaccination and the subsequent 3 days.

Unsolicited adverse events that occurred in ≥1% of recipients of FLUARIX and at a rate greater than placebo included upper respiratory tract infection (3.9% versus 2.6%), nasopharyngitis (2.5% versus 1.6%), nasal congestion (2.2% versus 2.1%), diarrhea (1.6% versus 0%), influenza-like illness (1.6% versus 0.5%), vomiting (1.4% versus 0%), and dysmenorrhea (1.3% versus 1.0%). A randomized, single-blind, active-controlled US study evaluated subjects randomized to receive FLUARIX (N = 917) or FLUZONE (N = 910), a US-licensed trivalent, inactivated influenza virus vaccine (Sanofi Pasteur SA) stratified by age: 18 to 64 years and ≥65 years of age. In the overall population, 59% of subjects were female and 91% were white. Solicited events were collected using diary cards for 4 days (day of vaccination and the next 3 days) (Table 2). Unsolicited events that occurred within 21 days of vaccination (day 0-20) were recorded using diary cards.

[See table 2 at top of next page]

Unsolicited adverse events that occurred in ≥1% of all recipients of FLUARIX or the comparator influenza vaccine in the 21-day post-vaccination period included headache (2.8% versus 2.3%), back pain (1.5% versus 0.4%), pain in extremity (1.2% versus 0.7%), pharyngolaryngeal pain (1.2% versus 0.9%), cough (1.1% versus 0.9%), fatigue (1.1% versus 0.7%), nasopharyngitis (1.0% versus 1.3%), nausea (0.4% versus 1.0%), arthralgia (0.3% versus 1.0%), and injection site pruritus (0.2% versus 1.0%).

A double-blind, placebo-controlled study in subjects 18 to 64 years of age randomized (2:1) to receive FLUARIX (N = 5,103) or placebo (N = 2,549) was conducted to evaluate the efficacy of FLUARIX. In the total population, 60% were female and 99.9% were white. In a subset (FLUARIX [N = 305] and placebo [N = 155]), unsolicited events that occurred within 21 days of vaccination (day 0-20) were recorded on diary cards. The percentage of subjects reporting at least one unsolicited event was similar among the groups (24.3% for FLUARIX and 22.6% for placebo). Unsolicited adverse events that occurred in ≥1% of recipients of FLUARIX and at a rate greater than placebo included injection site pain (5.2% versus 1.3%), dysmenorrhea (1.3% versus 0.6%), and migraine (1.0% versus 0.0%).

Incidence of Adverse Events Reported in ≥1% of Subjects in Non-US Clinical Trials: The following additional adverse events have been observed in adults in non-US clinical trials with FLUARIX. No adverse events were observed at an incidence of >10%.

General Disorders and Administration Site Conditions: Injection site ecchymosis, injection site induration, malaise.

Infections and Infestations: Rhinitis.

Musculoskeletal and Connective Tissue Disorders: Musculoskeletal pain, neck pain.

Skin and Subcutaneous Tissue Disorders: Sweating.

Serious Adverse Events: In the 4 clinical trials in adults (N = 10,923), there was a single case of anaphylaxis reported with FLUARIX (<0.01%).

Children: In children 5 years to <18 years of age, the most common (≥10%) local and general adverse events were similar to those in adults but also included swelling at the injection site. In children 3 years to <5 years of age, the most common (≥10%) local and general adverse events included pain, redness, and swelling at the injection site, irritability, loss of appetite, and drowsiness.

A single-blind, active-controlled US study evaluated subjects 6 months to <18 years of age who received FLUARIX (N = 2,081) or FLUZONE (N = 1,173), a US-licensed trivalent, inactivated influenza virus vaccine (Sanofi Pasteur SA) (Study 005). Children 6 months to <9 years of age with no history of influenza vaccination received 2 doses approximately 28 days apart. Children 6 months to <9 years of age with a history of influenza vaccination and children 9 years of age and older received 1 dose. Children 6 months to <3 years of age received 0.25 mL of FLUARIX or comparator influenza vaccine, and children 3 years of age and older received 0.5 mL of FLUARIX or comparator influenza vaccine. Study subjects were 6 months to <18 years of age and 49% were female; 68% were white, 18% were black, 3% were Asian, and 11% were of other racial/ethnic groups.

Solicited local and general adverse events were collected using diary cards for 4 days (day of vaccination and the next 3 days). Unsolicited adverse events that occurred within 28 days of vaccination (day 0-27) after the first vaccination in all subjects and 21 days (day 0-20) after the second vaccination in unprimed subjects were recorded using diary cards. The frequencies of solicited adverse events for children 3 years to <5 years of age and for children 5 years to <18 years of age were similar for FLUARIX and the comparator vaccine (Table 3).

[See table 3 at right]

In children who received a second dose of FLUARIX or the comparator vaccine, the incidences of adverse events following the second dose were similar to those observed after the first dose.

Unsolicited adverse events that occurred in ≥1% of recipients of FLUARIX 6 months to <18 years of age included upper respiratory tract infection (5.5%), pyrexia (4.8%), cough (4.7%), vomiting (3.2%), headache (2.8%), rhinorrhea (2.7%), diarrhea (2.5%), pharyngolaryngeal pain (2.4%), nasopharyngitis (2.3%), otitis media (2.0%), nasal congestion (1.8%), upper abdominal pain (1.4%), and upper respiratory tract congestion (1.0%). The incidences of these events were similar in recipients of the comparator vaccine.

6.2 Postmarketing Experience

Worldwide voluntary reports of adverse events received for FLUARIX since market introduction of this vaccine are listed below. This list includes serious events or events which have causal connection to FLUARIX. Because these events are reported voluntarily from a population of uncertain size, it is not always possible to reliably estimate their frequency or establish a causal relationship to the vaccine.

Blood and Lymphatic System Disorders: Lymphadenopathy.

Cardiac Disorders: Tachycardia.

Ear and Labyrinth Disorders: Vertigo.

Eye Disorders: Conjunctivitis, eye irritation, eye pain, eye redness, eye swelling, eyelid swelling.

Gastrointestinal Disorders: Abdominal pain or discomfort, nausea, swelling of the mouth, throat, and/or tongue.

General Disorders and Administration Site Conditions: Asthenia, chest pain, chills, feeling hot, injection site mass, injection site reaction, injection site warmth, body aches.

Immune System Disorders: Anaphylactic reaction including shock, anaphylactoid reaction, hypersensitivity, serum sickness.

Infections and Infestations: Injection site abscess, injection site cellulitis, pharyngitis, rhinitis, tonsillitis.

Musculoskeletal and Connective Tissue Disorders: Pain in extremity.

Nervous System Disorders: Convulsion, dizziness, encephalomyelitis, facial palsy, facial paresis, Guillain-Barré syndrome, hypoesthesia, myelitis, neuritis, neuropathy, paresthesia.

Respiratory, Thoracic, and Mediastinal Disorders: Asthma, bronchospasm, cough, dyspnea, respiratory distress, stridor.

Skin and Subcutaneous Tissue Disorders: Angioedema, erythema, erythema multiforme, facial swelling, pruritus, rash, Stevens-Johnson syndrome, urticaria.

Vascular Disorders: Henoch-Schönlein purpura, vasculitis.

6.3 Adverse Events Associated With Influenza Vaccines

Immediate and presumably allergic reactions (e.g., hives, angioedema, allergic asthma, and systemic anaphylaxis) rarely occur after influenza vaccination. These reactions probably result from hypersensitivity to certain vaccine components, such as residual egg protein. Although FLUARIX contains only a limited quantity of egg protein, this protein can induce immediate hypersensitivity reactions among persons who have severe egg allergy [see Contraindications (4)].

Table 2. Percentage of Subjects With Solicited Local Adverse Reactions or General Adverse Events Within 4 Days[a] of Vaccination With FLUARIX or Comparator Influenza Vaccine by Age Group (Total Vaccinated Cohort)

	18-64 Years of Age		≥65 Years of Age	
	FLUARIX N = 315 %	Comparator Influenza Vaccine N = 314 %	FLUARIX N = 601-602 %	Comparator Influenza Vaccine N = 596 %
Local Adverse Reactions				
Pain	48	53	19	18
Redness	13	16	11	13
Swelling	9	11	6	9
General Adverse Events				
Fatigue	21	18	9	10
Headache	20	21	8	8
Muscle aches	16	13	7	7
Arthralgia	9	9	6	5
Shivering	3	5	2	2
Fever (≥99.5°F)	3	1	2	1

Total vaccinated cohort for safety included all vaccinated subjects for whom safety data were available.
[a] 4 days included day of vaccination and the subsequent 3 days.

Table 3. Percentage of Subjects With Solicited Local Adverse Reactions or General Adverse Events Within 4 Days[a] of First Vaccination With FLUARIX or Comparator Influenza Vaccine by Age Group in Children 3 Years to <18 Years of Age

	Age Group: 3 Years to <5 Years		Age Group: 5 Years to <18 Years	
	FLUARIX N = 350 %	Comparator Influenza Vaccine N = 341 %	FLUARIX N = 1,348 %	Comparator Influenza Vaccine N = 451 %
Local Adverse Reactions				
Pain	35	38	56	56
Redness	23	20	18	16
Swelling	14	13	14	13
General Adverse Events				
Irritability	21	22	–	–
Loss of appetite	13	15	–	–
Drowsiness	13	20	–	–
Fever	7	8	4	3
Muscle aches	–	–	29	29
Fatigue	–	–	20	19
Headache	–	–	15	16
Arthralgia	–	–	6	6
Shivering	–	–	3	4

[a] 4 days included day of vaccination and the subsequent 3 days.

The 1976 swine influenza vaccine was associated with an increased frequency of Guillain-Barré syndrome (GBS). Evidence for a causal relation of GBS with subsequent vaccines prepared from other influenza viruses is unclear. If influenza vaccine does pose a risk, it is probably slightly more than 1 additional case/1 million persons vaccinated.

Neurological disorders temporally associated with influenza vaccination such as encephalopathy, optic neuritis/neuropathy, partial facial paralysis, and brachial plexus neuropathy have been reported.

Microscopic polyangitis (vasculitis) has been reported temporally associated with influenza vaccination.

7 DRUG INTERACTIONS

7.1 Concomitant Vaccine Administration

FLUARIX should not be mixed with any other vaccine in the same syringe or vial.

There are insufficient data to assess the concurrent administration of FLUARIX with other vaccines.

7.2 Immunosuppressive Therapies

Immunosuppressive therapies, including irradiation, antimetabolites, alkylating agents, cytotoxic drugs, and corticosteroids (used in greater than physiologic doses), may reduce the immune response to FLUARIX.

8 USE IN SPECIFIC POPULATIONS

8.1 Pregnancy

Pregnancy Category B

A reproductive and developmental toxicity study has been performed in female rats at a dose approximately 56 times the human dose (on a mg/kg basis) and revealed no evidence of impaired female fertility or harm to the fetus due to FLUARIX. There are, however, no adequate and well-controlled studies in pregnant women. Because animal reproduction studies are not always predictive of human response, FLUARIX should be given to a pregnant woman only if clearly needed.

Table 4. Attack Rates and Vaccine Efficacy Against Culture-Confirmed Influenza A and/or B in Adults 18 to 64 Years of Age (Total Vaccinated Cohort)

	N	n	Attack Rates (n/N) %	Vaccine Efficacy %	LL	UL
Antigenically Matched Strains[a]						
FLUARIX	5,103	49	1.0	66.9[b]	51.9	77.4
Placebo	2,549	74	2.9	–	–	–
All Culture-Confirmed Influenza (Matched, Unmatched, and Untyped)[c]						
FLUARIX	5,103	63	1.2	61.6[b]	46.0	72.8
Placebo	2,549	82	3.2	–	–	–

[a] There were no vaccine matched culture-confirmed cases of A/New Caledonia/20/1999 (H1N1) or B/Malaysia/2506/2004 influenza strains with FLUARIX or placebo.
[b] Vaccine efficacy for FLUARIX exceeded a pre-defined threshold of 35% for the lower limit of the 2-sided 95% CI.
[c] Of the 22 additional cases, 18 were unmatched and 4 were untyped; 15 of the 22 cases were A (H3N2) (11 cases with FLUARIX and 4 cases with placebo).

Table 5. Rates With HI Titers ≥1:40 and Rates of Seroconversion to Each Antigen Following FLUARIX or Placebo (21 Days After Vaccination) in Adults 18 to 64 Years of Age (ATP Cohort)

	FLUARIX[a] N = 745 % (95% CI)		Placebo N = 190 % (95% CI)	
% With HI Titers ≥1:40	Pre-vaccination	Post-vaccination	Pre-vaccination	Post-vaccination
A/New Caledonia/20/99 (H1N1)	54.8 (51.1, 58.4)	96.6 (95.1, 97.8)	52.1 (44.8, 59.4)	51.1 (43.7, 58.4)
A/Wyoming/3/2003 (H3N2)	68.7 (65.3, 72)	99.1 (98.1, 99.6)	65.3 (58, 72)	65.3 (58, 72)
B/Jiangsu/10/2003	49.5 (45.9, 53.2)	98.8 (97.7, 99.4)	48.9 (41.6, 56.3)	51.1 (43.7, 58.4)
Seroconversion[b]	Post-vaccination		Post-vaccination	
A/New Caledonia/20/99 (H1N1)	59.6 (56, 63.1)		0 (0, 1.9)	
A/Wyoming/3/2003 (H3N2)	61.9 (58.3, 65.4)		1.1 (0.1, 3.8)	
B/Jiangsu/10/2003	77.6 (74.4, 80.5)		1.1 (0.1, 3.8)	

HI = hemagglutination-inhibition; ATP = according-to-protocol; CI = Confidence Interval.
ATP cohort for immunogenicity included subjects for whom assay results were available after vaccination for at least one study vaccine antigen.
[a] Results obtained following vaccination with FLUARIX manufactured for the 2004-2005 season.
[b] Seroconversion defined as at least a 4-fold increase in serum titers of HI antibodies to ≥1:40.

In a reproductive and developmental toxicity study, the effect of FLUARIX on embryo-fetal and pre-weaning development was evaluated in pregnant rats. Animals were administered FLUARIX by intramuscular injection once prior to gestation, and during the period of organogenesis (gestation days 6, 8, 11, and 15), 0.1 mL/rat/occasion (approximately 56-fold excess relative to the projected human dose on a body weight basis). No adverse effects on mating, female fertility, pregnancy, parturition, lactation parameters, and embryo-fetal or pre-weaning development were observed. There were no vaccine-related fetal malformations or other evidence of teratogenesis.

8.3 Nursing Mothers
It is not known whether FLUARIX is excreted in human milk. Because many drugs are excreted in human milk, caution should be exercised when FLUARIX is administered to a nursing woman.

8.4 Pediatric Use
The immune response of FLUARIX has been evaluated in children 6 months to <5 years of age. In a randomized, controlled study, serum hemagglutination-inhibition (HI) antibody titers were lower in children 6 months to <3 years of age compared to a US-licensed vaccine. Immune responses in children 3 years to <5 years of age receiving FLUARIX or a US-licensed vaccine have been evaluated [see Clinical Studies (14.2)]. Safety has been evaluated in children 6 months to <18 years of age. The frequencies of solicited adverse events for children 3 years to <5 years of age and for children 5 years to <18 years of age were similar for FLUARIX and the comparator vaccine [see Adverse Reactions (6.1)].

8.5 Geriatric Use
A randomized, single-blind, active-controlled study evaluated immunological non-inferiority in a cohort of subjects ≥65 years of age who received FLUARIX (N = 606) or another US-licensed trivalent, inactivated influenza virus vaccine (N = 604) (Sanofi Pasteur SA). In subjects receiving FLUARIX or the comparator vaccine, geometric mean antibody titers post-vaccination were lower in geriatric subjects than in younger subjects (18 to 64 years of age). FLUARIX was non-inferior to the comparator vaccine for each of the 3 influenza strains based on mean antibody titers and seroconversion rates. [See Clinical Studies (14.2).] Solicited local and general adverse events were similar for FLUARIX and the comparator vaccine among geriatric subjects (Table 2). For both vaccines, the frequency of solicited events in subjects ≥65 years of age was lower than in younger subjects (Table 2). [See Adverse Reactions (6.1).]

11 DESCRIPTION
FLUARIX, Influenza Virus Vaccine, for intramuscular injection, is a sterile colorless to slightly opalescent suspension. FLUARIX is a vaccine prepared from influenza viruses propagated in embryonated chicken eggs. Each of the influenza viruses is produced and purified separately. After harvesting the virus-containing fluids, each influenza virus is concentrated and purified by zonal centrifugation using a linear sucrose density gradient solution containing detergent to disrupt the viruses. Following dilution, the vaccine is further purified by diafiltration. Each influenza virus solution is inactivated by the consecutive effects of sodium deoxycholate and formaldehyde leading to the production of a "split virus." Each split inactivated virus is then suspended in sodium phosphate-buffered isotonic sodium chloride solution. The vaccine is formulated from the 3 split inactivated virus solutions. FLUARIX has been standardized according to USPHS requirements for the 2010-2011 influenza season and is formulated to contain 45 micrograms (mcg) hemagglutinin (HA) per 0.5-mL dose, in the recommended ratio of 15 mcg HA of each of the following 3 strains: A/California/7/2009 NYMC X-181 (H1N1), A/Victoria/210/2009 NYMC X-187 (H3N2) (an A/Perth/16/2009-like virus), and B/Brisbane/60/2008.

FLUARIX is formulated without preservatives. FLUARIX does not contain thimerosal. Each 0.5-mL dose also contains octoxynol-10 (TRITON® X-100) ≤0.085 mg, α-tocopheryl hydrogen succinate ≤0.1 mg, and polysorbate 80 (Tween 80) ≤0.415 mg. Each dose may also contain residual amounts of hydrocortisone ≤0.0016 mcg, gentamicin sulfate ≤0.15 mcg, ovalbumin ≤0.05 mcg, formaldehyde ≤5 mcg, and sodium deoxycholate ≤50 mcg from the manufacturing process.

The tip caps of the prefilled syringes may contain natural rubber latex. The rubber plungers do not contain latex.

12 CLINICAL PHARMACOLOGY
12.1 Mechanism of Action
Influenza illness and its complications follow infection with influenza viruses. Global surveillance of influenza identifies yearly antigenic variants. For example, since 1977, antigenic variants of influenza A (H1N1 and H3N2) viruses and influenza B viruses have been in global circulation. Specific levels of hemagglutination-inhibition (HI) antibody titer post-vaccination with inactivated influenza virus vaccines have not been correlated with protection from influenza illness but the HI antibody titers have been used as a measure of vaccine activity. In some human challenge studies, HI antibody titers of ≥1:40 have been associated with protection from influenza illness in up to 50% of subjects.[1,2] Antibody against one influenza virus type or subtype confers little or no protection against another virus. Furthermore, antibody to one antigenic variant of influenza virus might not protect against a new antigenic variant of the same type or subtype. Frequent development of antigenic variants through antigenic drift is the virological basis for seasonal epidemics and the reason for the usual incorporation of one or more new strains in each year's influenza vaccine. Therefore, inactivated influenza vaccines are standardized to contain the hemagglutinins of strains (i.e., typically 2 type A and 1 type B), representing the influenza viruses likely to circulate in the United States in the upcoming winter. Annual revaccination with the current vaccine is recommended because immunity declines during the year after vaccination, and because circulating strains of influenza virus change from year to year.[3]

13 NONCLINICAL TOXICOLOGY
13.1 Carcinogenesis, Mutagenesis, Impairment of Fertility
FLUARIX has not been evaluated for carcinogenic or mutagenic potential, or for impairment of fertility.

14 CLINICAL STUDIES
14.1 Efficacy Against Culture-Confirmed Influenza
The efficacy of FLUARIX was evaluated in a randomized, double-blind, placebo-controlled study conducted in 2 European countries during the 2006-2007 influenza season. Efficacy of FLUARIX, containing A/New Caledonia/20/1999 (H1N1), A/Wisconsin/67/2005 (H3N2), and B/Malaysia/2506/2004 influenza strains, was defined as the prevention of culture-confirmed influenza A and/or B cases, for vaccine antigenically matched strains, compared with placebo. Healthy subjects 18 to 64 years of age (mean 39.9 years) were randomized (2:1) to receive FLUARIX (N = 5,103) or placebo (N = 2,549) and monitored for influenza-like illnesses (ILI) starting 2 weeks post vaccination and lasting for approximately 7 months. In the overall population, 60% of subjects were female and 99.9% were white. Culture-confirmed influenza was assessed by active and passive surveillance of ILI. Influenza-like illness was defined as at least one general symptom (fever ≥100°F and/or myalgia) and at least one respiratory symptom (cough and/or sore throat). After an episode of ILI, nose and throat swab samples were collected for analysis; attack rates and vaccine efficacy were calculated (Table 4).
[See table 4 above]

In a post-hoc, exploratory analysis by age, vaccine efficacy (against culture-confirmed influenza A and/or B cases, for vaccine antigenically matched strains) in subjects 18 to 49 years of age was 73.4% (95% CI: 59.3, 82.8) [number of influenza cases: FLUARIX (n = 35/3,602) and placebo (n = 66/1,810)]. In subjects 50 to 64 years of age, vaccine efficacy was 13.8% (95% CI: -137.0, 66.3) [number of influenza cases: FLUARIX (n = 14/1,501) and placebo (n = 8/739)]. As the study lacked statistical power to evaluate efficacy within age subgroups, the clinical significance of these results is unknown.

14.2 Immunological Evaluation
Adults: In a randomized, double-blind, placebo-controlled study conducted in healthy subjects 18 to 64 years of age (mean 39.1 years) in the United States, the immune responses to each of the antigens contained in FLUARIX were evaluated in sera obtained 21 days after administration of FLUARIX (N = 745) and were compared to those following administration of a placebo vaccine (N = 190). In the overall population, 54% of subjects were female and 80% were

white. For each of the influenza antigens, the percentage of subjects who achieved seroconversion, defined as at least a 4-fold increase in serum hemagglutination-inhibition (HI) titer over baseline to ≥1:40 following vaccination, and the percentage of subjects who achieved HI titers of ≥1:40 are presented in Table 5. The lower limit of the 2-sided 95% CI for the percentage of subjects who achieved seroconversion or an HI titer of ≥1:40 exceeded the pre-defined lower limits of 40% and 70%, respectively.
[See table 5 on previous page]
Non-Inferiority Study: In a randomized, single-blind, active-controlled US study, immunological non-inferiority of FLUARIX (N = 923) was compared with FLUZONE (N = 922), a US-licensed trivalent, inactivated influenza virus vaccine (Sanofi Pasteur SA). Subjects 18 to 64 years and ≥65 years of age were evaluated for immune responses to each of the vaccine antigens 21 days following vaccination *[see Use in Specific Populations (8.5)]*. In the overall population, 59% of subjects were female and 91% were white. The co-primary immunogenicity endpoints were geometric mean titers (GMTs) of serum HI antibodies and the percentage of subjects who achieved seroconversion, defined as at least a 4-fold increase in serum HI titer over baseline to ≥1:40, following vaccination. The primary immunogenicity analyses were performed on the According-to-Protocol (ATP) cohort which included all eligible and evaluable subjects with results of at least one serological assay. For each of the influenza antigens, the GMTs and the percentage of subjects who achieved seroconversion are presented in Table 6. FLUARIX was non-inferior to the comparator influenza vaccine based on antibody GMTs (upper limit of the 2-sided 95% CI for the GMT ratio [comparator influenza vaccine/FLUARIX] ≤1.5) and seroconversion rates (upper limit of the 2-sided 95% CI on difference of the comparator influenza vaccine minus FLUARIX ≤10%).
[See table 6 at right]

<u>Children:</u> The immune response of FLUARIX was compared to FLUZONE, a US-licensed trivalent, inactivated influenza virus vaccine (Sanofi Pasteur SA), in a single-blind, randomized study in a subset of children 6 months to <5 years of age (Study 005). The immune responses to each of the antigens contained in FLUARIX formulated for the 2006-2007 season were evaluated in sera obtained after 1 or 2 doses of FLUARIX (N = 426) and were compared to those following administration of the comparator influenza vaccine (N = 445). Further details on the clinical study design and demographic information have been previously described *[see Adverse Reactions (6.1)]*.
Non-inferiority of the immune response for FLUARIX to comparator influenza vaccine for subjects 6 months to <5 years of age was not demonstrated mainly due to lower antibody response to FLUARIX compared to the comparator influenza vaccine in subjects 6 months to <3 years of age. In subjects 3 years to <5 years of age, FLUARIX met at least one of the pre-specified criteria for demonstration of non-inferiority (GMT and seroconversion rate) for the influenza A strains but not for the influenza B strain. Seroconversion rates and the percentage of subjects with HI titers ≥1:40 were analyzed as secondary endpoints. In subjects 3 years to <5 years of age, the lower limit of the 95% Confidence Interval of the seroconversion rate for FLUARIX or the comparator influenza vaccine exceeded 40% for all 3 strains; also in this age group, the lower limit of the 95% Confidence Interval of the rate with HI titer ≥1:40 for FLUARIX or the comparator influenza vaccine exceeded 70% for both A strains (Table 7).
[See table 7 at right]

15 REFERENCES

1. Hannoun C, Megas F, Piercy J. Immunogenicity and protective efficacy of influenza vaccination. *Virus Res.* 2004;103:133-138.
2. Hobson D, Curry RL, Beare AS, et al. The role of serum haemagglutination-inhibiting antibody in protection against challenge infection with influenza A2 and B viruses. *J Hyg Camb.* 1972;70:767-777.
3. Centers for Disease Control and Prevention. Prevention and control of influenza: Recommendations of the Advisory Committee on Immunization Practices (ACIP). *MMWR* 2006;55(RR-10):1-42.

16 HOW SUPPLIED/STORAGE AND HANDLING

FLUARIX is supplied in 0.5-mL single-dose prefilled TIP-LOK syringes. The tip caps of the needleless prefilled syringes may contain natural rubber latex.
NDC 58160-877-46 (package of 5)
Store refrigerated between 2° and 8°C (36° and 46°F). Do not freeze. Discard if the vaccine has been frozen. Store in the original package to protect from light.

17 PATIENT COUNSELING INFORMATION

The vaccine recipient or guardian should be:
• conformed of the potential benefits and risks of immunization with FLUARIX.
• educated regarding potential side effects, emphasizing that: (1) FLUARIX contains non-infectious killed viruses

Table 6. Immune Responses 21 Days After Vaccination With FLUARIX Compared With Comparator Influenza Vaccine in Adults ≥18 Years of Age (ATP Cohort)

	FLUARIX N = 858-866		Comparator Influenza Vaccine N = 846-854	
GMT (95% CI)	**Pre-vaccination**	**Post-vaccination**	**Pre-vaccination**	**Post-vaccination**
Anti-H1	27.9 (25.6, 30.5)	138.0 (125.2, 152.1)	29.1 (26.6, 31.7)	92.0 (84.5, 100.3)
Anti-H3	16.3 (15.1, 17.6)	121.6 (110.5, 133.7)	16.5 (15.4, 17.6)	114.0 (104.4, 124.5)
Anti-B	47.7 (44.1, 51.6)	231.9 (215.4, 249.6)	54.1 (49.9, 58.6)	273.7 (253.4, 295.7)
Seroconversion[a] (95% CI)	**Post-vaccination**		**Post-vaccination**	
A/New Caledonia/20/99 (H1N1)	45.7 (42.3, 49.1)		33.8 (30.6, 37.1)	
A/New York/55/2004 (H3N2)	67.1 (63.9, 70.3)		65.5 (62.2, 68.7)	
B/Jiangsu/10/2003	52.7 (49.3, 56.1)		53.8 (50.4, 57.2)	

Comparator influenza vaccine manufactured by Sanofi Pasteur SA.
ATP = according-to-protocol; GMT = geometric mean antibody titer; CI = Confidence Interval; H1 = A/New Caledonia/20/99 (H1N1); H3 = A/New York/55/2004 (H3N2) for FLUARIX and A/California/7/2004 (H3N2) for comparator influenza vaccine; B = B/Jiangsu/10/2003.
ATP cohort included all eligible and evaluable subjects with results of at least one serological assay.
[a] Seroconversion defined as at least a 4-fold increase in serum titers of HI antibodies to ≥1:40.

Table 7. Rates With HI Titers ≥1:40 and Rates of Seroconversion to Each Antigen Following FLUARIX or Comparator Influenza Vaccine in Children 3 Years to <5 Years of Age (ATP Cohort)

	FLUARIX[a] % (95% CI)		Comparator Influenza Vaccine[b] % (95% CI)	
% with HI titers ≥1:40	**Pre-vaccination N = 220**	**Post-vaccination N = 220**	**Pre-vaccination N = 220**	**Post-vaccination N = 221**
A/New Caledonia	17.3 (12.5, 22.9)	81.8 (76.1, 86.7)	20.5 (15.3, 26.4)	85.5 (80.2, 89.9)
A/Wisconsin	59.5 (52.7, 66.1)	88.2 (83.2, 92.1)	55.5 (48.6, 62.1)	93.7 (89.6, 96.5)
B/Malaysia	13.6 (9.4, 18.9)	55.0 (48.2, 61.7)	11.8 (7.9, 16.8)	58.4 (51.6, 64.9)
Seroconversion[c]	**Post-vaccination**		**Post-vaccination**	
A/New Caledonia	72.7 (66.3, 78.5)		72.3 (65.9, 78.1)	
A/Wisconsin	70.9 (64.4, 76.8)		70.5 (64.0, 76.4)	
B/Malaysia	53.2 (46.4, 59.9)		55.5 (48.6, 62.1)	

HI = hemagglutination inhibition; ATP = according to protocol; CI = Confidence Interval.
[a] Results obtained following vaccination with FLUARIX manufactured for the 2006-2007 season.
[b] US-licensed trivalent, inactivated influenza virus vaccine (Sanofi Pasteur SA) without preservative manufactured for the 2006-2007 season.
[c] Seroconversion defined as at least a 4-fold increase in serum titers of HI antibodies to ≥1:40.

and cannot cause influenza and (2) FLUARIX is intended to provide protection against illness due to influenza viruses only, and cannot provide protection against all respiratory illness.
• instructed to report any adverse events to their healthcare provider.
• given the Vaccine Information Statements, which are required by the National Childhood Vaccine Injury Act of 1986 to be given prior to immunization. These materials are available free of charge at the Centers for Disease Control and Prevention (CDC) website (www.cdc.gov/vaccines).
• instructed that annual revaccination is recommended.
FLUARIX and TIP-LOK are registered trademarks of GlaxoSmithKline. FLUZONE is a registered trademark of Sanofi Pasteur Limited. TRITON is a registered trademark of Union Carbide Chemicals & Plastics Technology Corp.
Manufactured by **GlaxoSmithKline Biologicals**, Dresden, Germany, a branch of **SmithKline Beecham Pharma GmbH & Co. KG**, Munich, Germany
Licensed by **GlaxoSmithKline Biologicals**, Rixensart, Belgium, US License 1617
Distributed by **GlaxoSmithKline**, Research Triangle Park, NC 27709

FLULAVAL®   ℞
[flū′ la-val]
(Influenza Virus Vaccine)
Suspension for Intramuscular Injection

HIGHLIGHTS OF PRESCRIBING INFORMATION

These highlights do not include all the information needed to use FLULAVAL safely and effectively. See full prescribing information for FLULAVAL.
FLULAVAL (Influenza Virus Vaccine)
Suspension for Intramuscular Injection
2010-2011 Formula
Initial U.S. Approval: 2006

———INDICATIONS AND USAGE———

• FLULAVAL is an inactivated influenza virus vaccine indicated for active immunization of adults 18 years of age and older against influenza disease caused by influenza virus subtypes A and type B contained in the vaccine. (1)

- This indication is based on immune response elicited by FLULAVAL, and there have been no controlled trials demonstrating a decrease in influenza disease after vaccination with FLULAVAL. (1, 14)

———DOSAGE AND ADMINISTRATION———
- A single 0.5-mL intramuscular injection. (2.2)

———DOSAGE FORMS AND STRENGTHS———
- FLULAVAL is a suspension in 5-mL multi-dose vials containing 10 doses (each dose is 0.5 mL). (3)

———CONTRAINDICATIONS———
- Known systemic hypersensitivity reactions to egg proteins (a vaccine component) or a life-threatening reaction to previous influenza vaccination. (4)

———WARNINGS AND PRECAUTIONS———
- If Guillain-Barré syndrome has occurred within 6 weeks of receipt of a prior influenza vaccine, the decision to give FLULAVAL should be based on careful consideration of the potential benefits and risks. (5.1)
- Immunosuppressed persons may have a reduced immune response to FLULAVAL. (5.2)

———ADVERSE REACTIONS———
- Most common (≥10%) local adverse events were pain, redness, and/or swelling at the injection site. (6.1)
- Most common (≥10%) systemic adverse events were headache, fatigue, myalgia, low grade fever, and malaise. (6.1)

To report SUSPECTED ADVERSE REACTIONS, contact GlaxoSmithKline at 1-888-825-5249 or VAERS at 1-800-822-7967 and www.vaers.hhs.gov.

———DRUG INTERACTIONS———
- Do not mix with any other vaccine in the same syringe or vial. (7.1)
- Immunosuppressive therapies may reduce immune responses to FLULAVAL. (7.2)

———USE IN SPECIFIC POPULATIONS———
- Safety and effectiveness of FLULAVAL have not been established in pregnant women, nursing mothers, and children. (8.1, 8.3, 8.4)
- Geriatric Use: Antibody responses were lower in geriatric subjects than in younger subjects. (8.5)

Revised: May 2010
See 17 for PATIENT COUNSELING INFORMATION
Revised: 07/2010

FULL PRESCRIBING INFORMATION: CONTENTS*

FULL PRESCRIBING INFORMATION

1 INDICATIONS AND USAGE

FLULAVAL® is indicated for active immunization of adults (18 years of age and older) against influenza disease caused by influenza virus subtypes A and type B contained in the vaccine.

Table 1. Solicited Adverse Events in the First 4 Days After Administration of FLULAVAL or Comparator Influenza Vaccine

Adverse Events	US Trial Adults 18 to 64 years of age (80% <50 years of age)		Canadian Trial Adults 50 years of age and older
	FLULAVAL N = 721 %	Comparator Influenza Vaccine[a] N = 279 %	FLULAVAL[b] N = 328 %
Local			
Pain	24	31	21
Redness	11	10	14
Swelling	10	10	6
Systemic			
Headache	18	17	10
Fatigue	17	15	10
Myalgia	13	16	11
Fever[c]	11	10	1
Malaise	10	10	4
Sore throat	9	9	5
Reddened eyes	6	5	3
Cough	6	7	3
Chills	5	2	3
Chest tightness	3	1	2
Facial swelling	1	1	1

Results >1% reported to nearest whole percent; results >0 but ≤1 reported as 1%.

[a] US-licensed trivalent, inactivated influenza virus vaccine (FLUZONE).
[b] Includes subjects who received FLULAVAL and a similar investigational formulation of FLULAVAL with reduced thimerosal.
[c] Fever defined as ≥37.5°C in the US study, and ≥38.0°C in the Canadian study.

This indication is based on immune response elicited by FLULAVAL, and there have been no controlled trials demonstrating a decrease in influenza disease after vaccination with FLULAVAL [see Clinical Studies (14)].

2 DOSAGE AND ADMINISTRATION
2.1 Preparation for Administration
Shake the multi-dose vial vigorously each time before withdrawing a dose of vaccine. Parenteral drug products should be inspected visually for particulate matter and discoloration prior to administration, whenever solution and container permit. If either of these conditions exists, the vaccine should not be administered.
Between uses, return the multi-dose vial to the recommended storage conditions, between 2° and 8°C (36° and 46°F). Do not freeze. Discard if the vaccine has been frozen. Once entered, a multi-dose vial, and any residual contents, should be discarded after 28 days.
It is recommended that small syringes (0.5-mL or 1-mL) be used to minimize any product loss.
2.2 Recommended Dose and Schedule
FLULAVAL should be administered as a single 0.5-mL injection by the intramuscular route preferably in the region of the deltoid muscle of the upper arm.
The vaccine should not be injected in the gluteal area or areas where there may be a major nerve trunk. A needle length of ≥1 inch is preferred because needles <1 inch might be of insufficient length to penetrate muscle tissue in certain adults.
Do not administer this product intravenously, intradermally or subcutaneously.

3 DOSAGE FORMS AND STRENGTHS
FLULAVAL is a suspension available in 5-mL multi-dose vials containing 10 doses.

4 CONTRAINDICATIONS
Do not administer FLULAVAL to anyone with known systemic hypersensitivity reactions to egg proteins (a vaccine component) or a life-threatening reaction to previous administration of any influenza vaccination [see Description (11)].

5 WARNINGS AND PRECAUTIONS
5.1 Guillain-Barré Syndrome
If Guillain-Barré syndrome has occurred within 6 weeks of receipt of a prior influenza vaccine, the decision to give FLULAVAL should be based on careful consideration of the potential benefits and risks.

5.2 Altered Immunocompetence
If FLULAVAL is administered to immunosuppressed persons, including individuals receiving immunosuppressive therapy, the immune response may be lower than in immunocompetent persons.
5.3 Persons at Risk of Bleeding
As with other intramuscular injections, FLULAVAL should be given with caution in individuals with bleeding disorders such as hemophilia or on anticoagulant therapy to avoid the risk of hematoma following the injection.
5.4 Preventing and Managing Allergic Vaccine Reactions
Prior to administration, the healthcare provider should review the patient's immunization history for possible vaccine sensitivity and previous vaccination-related adverse reactions. Appropriate medical treatment, including epinephrine, and supervision must be available to manage possible anaphylactic reactions following administration of the vaccine.
5.5 Limitations of Vaccine Effectiveness
Vaccination with FLULAVAL may not protect all susceptible individuals.

6 ADVERSE REACTIONS
6.1 Clinical Trials Experience
Because clinical trials are conducted under widely varying conditions, adverse event rates observed in the clinical trials of a vaccine cannot be directly compared to rates in the clinical trials of another vaccine, and may not reflect the rates observed in practice. As with any vaccine, there is the possibility that broad use of FLULAVAL could reveal adverse events not observed in clinical trials.
In clinical trials, the most common (≥10%) local and systemic adverse events were pain, redness, and/or swelling at the injection site, headache, fatigue, myalgia, low grade fever, and malaise.
Safety information for FLULAVAL was collected in 2 randomized, controlled clinical trials, one in the United States (IDB707-105) and the second in Canada (SPD707-104). The safety population from these trials includes 1,049 adults 18 years of age and older vaccinated with products representative of the licensed formulation of FLULAVAL. The US study included subjects 18 to 64 years of age who were randomized to receive FLULAVAL (N = 721) or a US-licensed trivalent, inactivated influenza virus vaccine (FLUZONE)

(N = 279). The Canadian study compared 4 vaccine groups: FLULAVAL, a similar investigational formulation of FLULAVAL with reduced thimerosal, and 2 Canadian-licensed trivalent influenza vaccines.

Among recipients of FLULAVAL, 56.6% were women; 92.4% of subjects were white, 6.5% black, 2.7% Native American, and 1.0% Asian. In the US study, 74.8% of the recipients of FLULAVAL were Hispanic/Latino. The mean age of subjects in the US study was 38 years (range 18-64 years) and 19% of subjects were 50 to 64 years of age. In the Canadian study, the mean age was 63 years (range 50-92 years), and 46.6% were 65 years of age and older.

A series of symptoms and/or findings were specifically solicited by a diary/memory aid used by subjects for at least the day of vaccination and 3 days post-treatment (Table 1). Subjects were actively queried about changes in their health status through 42 days post-vaccination in the US trial, and six months post-vaccination in the Canadian study. In addition, spontaneous reports of adverse events were also collected (Table 2).

[See table 1 at top of previous page]

Local adverse events occurred with similar frequency in the 2 trials. In the US study, the only significant difference between FLULAVAL and a US-licensed trivalent, inactivated influenza virus vaccine was an increased frequency of chills in subjects receiving FLULAVAL.

Table 2 summarizes the most common adverse events in the 2 clinical trials; adverse events were reported, either spontaneously or in response to queries about changes in health status. The most common events were headache and cough in both studies. These, as well as throat pain, were the only adverse events reported by >1% of subjects in the US trial. The Canadian trial featured a longer safety follow-up (6 months vs. 42 days) and enrolled a population exclusively 50 years of age and older. Therefore, spontaneous adverse event reports were more frequent in this trial. As indicated in Table 2, upper respiratory infection, arthralgia, myalgia, nasopharyngitis, back pain, injection site erythema, diarrhea, fatigue, nausea, and nasal congestion were each reported by ≥5% of the recipients of FLULAVAL in the Canadian study.

[See table 2 at right]

6.2 Postmarketing Experience

The following adverse events have been identified during postapproval use of FLULAVAL. Because these events are reported voluntarily from a population of uncertain size, it is not always possible to reliably estimate their incidence rate or establish a causal relationship to the vaccine. Adverse events described here are included because: a) they represent reactions which are known to occur following immunizations generally or influenza immunizations specifically; b) they are potentially serious; or c) the frequency of reporting.

Blood and Lymphatic System Disorders: Lymphadenopathy.

Eye Disorders: Conjunctivitis, eye pain, photophobia.

Gastrointestinal Disorders: Dysphagia, vomiting.

General Disorders and Administration Site Conditions: Chest pain, injection site inflammation, rigors, asthenia, injection site rash, influenza-like symptoms, abnormal gait, injection site bruising, injection site sterile abscess.

Immune System Disorders: Allergic edema of the face, allergic edema of the mouth, anaphylaxis, allergic edema of the throat.

Infections and Infestations: Pharyngitis, rhinitis, laryngitis, cellulitis.

Musculoskeletal and Connective Tissue Disorders: Muscle weakness, back pain, arthritis.

Nervous System Disorders: Dizziness, paresthesia, hypoesthesia, hypokinesia, tremor, somnolence, syncope, Guillain-Barré syndrome, convulsions/seizures, facial or cranial nerve paralysis, encephalopathy, limb paralysis.

Psychiatric Disorders: Insomnia.

Respiratory, Thoracic, and Mediastinal Disorders: Dyspnea, dysphonia, bronchospasm, throat tightness.

Skin and Subcutaneous Tissue Disorders: Urticaria, localized or generalized rash, pruritus, periorbital edema, sweating.

Vascular Disorders: Flushing, pallor.

6.3 Adverse Events Associated With Influenza Vaccines

Anaphylaxis has been reported after administration of FLULAVAL. Although FLULAVAL contains only a limited quantity of egg protein, this protein can induce immediate hypersensitivity reactions among persons who have severe egg allergy. Allergic reactions include hives, angioedema, allergic asthma, and systemic anaphylaxis [see Contraindications (4)].

The 1976 swine influenza vaccine was associated with an increased frequency of Guillain-Barré syndrome (GBS). Evidence for a causal relation of GBS with subsequent vaccines prepared from other influenza viruses is unclear. If influenza vaccine does pose a risk, it is probably slightly more than 1 additional case/1 million persons vaccinated.

Table 2. Adverse Events Reported Spontaneously[a] by ≥5% of Subjects in Either Clinical Trial of FLULAVAL

Adverse Events	US Trial (safety follow-up 42 days) Adults 18 to 64 years of age (80% <50 years of age)		Canadian Trial (safety follow-up 6 months) Adults 50 years of age and older
	FLULAVAL N = 721 %	Comparator Influenza Vaccine[b] N = 279 %	FLULAVAL[c] N = 328 %
Headache	7	7	19
Cough	2	2	15
Pharyngolaryngeal pain	2	3	12
Upper respiratory infection	1	1	9
Arthralgia	1	1	8
Myalgia	1	1	7
Nasopharyngitis	1	1	7
Back pain	1	1	6
Injection site erythema	1	1	5
Diarrhea	1	0	5
Fatigue	1	1	5
Nausea	1	1	5
Nasal congestion	1	1	5

Results >1% reported to nearest whole percent; results >0 but ≤1 reported as 1%.

[a] Adverse events in this table were reported spontaneously or in response to queries about changes in health status.
[b] US-licensed trivalent, inactivated influenza virus vaccine (FLUZONE).
[c] Includes subjects who received FLULAVAL and a similar investigational formulation of FLULAVAL with reduced thimerosal.

Neurological disorders temporally associated with influenza vaccination such as encephalopathy, optic neuritis/neuropathy, partial facial paralysis, and brachial plexus neuropathy have been reported.

Microscopic polyangitis (vasculitis) has been reported temporally associated with influenza vaccination.

7 DRUG INTERACTIONS

7.1 Concomitant Administration With Other Vaccines

There are no data to assess the concomitant administration of FLULAVAL with other vaccines. If FLULAVAL is to be given at the same time as another injectable vaccine(s), the vaccines should always be administered at different injection sites. FLULAVAL should not be mixed with any other vaccine in the same syringe or vial.

7.2 Immunosuppressive Therapies

Immunosuppressive therapies, including irradiation, antimetabolites, alkylating agents, cytotoxic drugs, and corticosteroids (used in greater than physiologic doses), may reduce the immune response to FLULAVAL.

7.3 Warfarin, Theophylline, and Phenytoin

Although it has been reported that influenza vaccination may inhibit the clearance of warfarin, theophylline, and phenytoin, controlled studies have yielded inconsistent results regarding pharmacokinetic interactions between influenza vaccine and these medications. Nevertheless, clinicians should consider the potential for an interaction when FLULAVAL is administered to persons receiving these drugs.

8 USE IN SPECIFIC POPULATIONS

8.1 Pregnancy

Pregnancy Category B

A reproductive and developmental toxicity study has been performed in female rats at a dose approximately 56 times the human dose (on a mg/kg basis) and revealed no evidence of impaired female fertility or harm to the fetus due to FLULAVAL. There are, however, no adequate and well-controlled studies in pregnant women. Because animal reproduction studies are not always predictive of human response, FLULAVAL should be given to a pregnant woman only if clearly needed.

In a reproductive and developmental toxicity study, the effect of FLULAVAL on embryo-fetal and pre-weaning development was evaluated in pregnant rats. Animals were administered FLULAVAL by intramuscular injection once prior to gestation, and during the period of organogenesis (gestation days 6, 8, 11, and 15), 0.1 mL/rat/occasion (approximately 56-fold excess relative to the projected human dose on a body weight basis). No adverse effects on mating, female fertility, pregnancy, parturition, lactation param-

eters, and embryo-fetal or pre-weaning development were observed. There were no vaccine-related fetal malformations or other evidence of teratogenesis.

8.3 Nursing Mothers

It is not known whether FLULAVAL is excreted in human milk. Because many drugs are excreted in human milk, caution should be exercised when FLULAVAL is administered to a nursing woman.

8.4 Pediatric Use

Safety and effectiveness of FLULAVAL in pediatric patients have not been established.

8.5 Geriatric Use

In the 2 clinical trials, there were 157 subjects who were ≥65 years of age and received FLULAVAL; 21 of these subjects were ≥75 years of age. Hemagglutination-inhibiting (HI) antibody responses were lower in geriatric subjects than younger subjects after administration of FLULAVAL. Solicited adverse events were similar in frequency to those reported in younger subjects [see Adverse Reactions (6.1)].

11 DESCRIPTION

FLULAVAL, Influenza Virus Vaccine, for intramuscular injection, is a trivalent, split-virion, inactivated influenza virus vaccine prepared from virus propagated in the allantoic cavity of embryonated hens' eggs. Each of the influenza virus strains is produced and purified separately. The virus is inactivated with ultraviolet light treatment followed by formaldehyde treatment, purified by centrifugation, and disrupted with sodium deoxycholate.

FLULAVAL is a sterile, translucent to whitish opalescent suspension in a phosphate-buffered saline solution that may sediment slightly. The sediment resuspends upon shaking to form a homogeneous suspension. FLULAVAL has been standardized according to USPHS requirements for the 2010-2011 influenza season and is formulated to contain 45 mcg hemagglutinin per 0.5-mL dose in the recommended ratio of 15 mcg HA of each of the following 3 strains: A/California/7/2009 NYMC X-179A (H1N1), A/Victoria/210/2009 NYMC X-187 (H3N2) (an A/Perth/16/2009-like virus), and B/Brisbane/60/2008. Thimerosal, a mercury derivative, is added as a preservative. Each dose contains 25 mcg mercury. Each dose may also contain residual amounts of egg proteins (≤1 mcg ovalbumin), formaldehyde (≤25 mcg), and sodium deoxycholate (≤50 mcg). Antibiotics are not used in the manufacture of this vaccine.

The vial stopper does not contain latex.

12 CLINICAL PHARMACOLOGY

12.1 Mechanism of Action

Influenza illness and its complications follow infection with influenza viruses. Global surveillance of influenza identifies

Table 3. Serum Hemagglutination-Inhibiting (HI) Antibody Responses to FLULAVAL in 2 Clinical Trials[a] (Per Protocol Cohort)[b]

US Trial in Adults 18 to 64 years of age	% of Subjects (lower bound of 2-sided 95% confidence interval)[c]		
	FLULAVAL N = 692		Primary endpoint met post-vaccination
HI titers ≥1:40 against:	Pre-vaccination	Post-vaccination	
A/New Caledonia/20/99 (H1N1)	24.6	96.5 (94.9)	Yes
A/Wyoming/03/03 (H3N2)	58.7	98.7 (97.6)	Yes
B/Jiangsu/10/03	5.4	62.9 (59.1)	No
Seroconversion[d] to:			
A/New Caledonia/20/99 (H1N1)	85.6 (82.7)		Yes
A/Wyoming/03/03 (H3N2)	79.3 (76.1)		Yes
B/Jiangsu/10/03	58.4 (54.6)		Yes

Canadian Trial in Adults ≥50 years of age	% of Subjects (lower bound of 2-sided 95% confidence interval)[c]		
	FLULAVAL[e] N = 324		Primary endpoint met post-vaccination
HI titers ≥1:40 against:	Pre-vaccination	Post-vaccination	
A/New Caledonia/20/99 (H1N1)	39.5	86.4 (82.2)	Yes
A/Wyoming/03/03 (H3N2)	67.9	99.1 (97.3)	Yes
B/Jiangsu/10/03	10.2	57.1 (51.5)	No
Seroconversion[d] to:			
A/New Caledonia/20/99 (H1N1)	44.8 (39.3)		Yes
A/Wyoming/03/03 (H3N2)	69.1 (63.8)		Yes
B/Jiangsu/10/03	49.1 (43.5)		Yes

[a] Results obtained following vaccination with FLULAVAL manufactured for the 2004–2005 season.

[b] Per Protocol cohort for immunogenicity included subjects with complete pre- and post-dose HI titer data and no major protocol deviations.

[c] Lower bounds were calculated using Clopper-Pearson method.

[d] Seroconversion = a 4-fold increase post-vaccination in HI antibody titer from pre-vaccination titer ≥1:10, or an increase in titer from <1:10 to ≥1:40.

[e] Includes subjects who received FLULAVAL and a similar investigational formulation of FLULAVAL with reduced thimerosal.

yearly antigenic variants. For example, since 1977, antigenic variants of influenza A (H1N1 and H3N2) viruses and influenza B viruses have been in global circulation. Specific levels of HI antibody titer post-vaccination with inactivated influenza virus vaccines have not been correlated with protection from influenza illness but the antibody titers have been used as a measure of vaccine activity. In some human challenge studies, antibody titers of ≥1:40 have been associated with protection from influenza illness in up to 50% of subjects.[1,2] Antibody against one influenza virus type or subtype confers little or no protection against another virus. Furthermore, antibody to one antigenic variant of influenza virus might not protect against a new antigenic variant of the same type or subtype. Frequent development of antigenic variants through antigenic drift is the virological basis for seasonal epidemics and the reason for the usual change of one or more new strains in each year's influenza vaccine. Therefore, inactivated influenza vaccines are standardized to contain the hemagglutinins of strains (i.e., typically 2 type A and 1 type B), representing the influenza viruses likely to circulate in the United States in the upcoming winter.

Annual revaccination with the current vaccine is recommended because immunity declines during the year after vaccination, and because circulating strains of influenza virus change from year to year.[3]

13 NONCLINICAL TOXICOLOGY

13.1 Carcinogenesis, Mutagenesis, Impairment of Fertility

FLULAVAL has not been evaluated for carcinogenic or mutagenic potential, or for impairment of fertility.

14 CLINICAL STUDIES

In 2 randomized, active-controlled trials of FLULAVAL, the immune responses, specifically HI antibody titers to each virus strain in the vaccine, were evaluated in sera obtained 21 days after administration of FLULAVAL. No controlled trials demonstrating a decrease in influenza disease after vaccination with FLULAVAL have been performed.

A 1,000-subject randomized, blinded, and controlled study was performed in the United States in 18- to 64-year-old healthy adults. A total of 721 subjects received FLULAVAL, and 279 received a US-licensed trivalent, inactivated influenza virus vaccine (FLUZONE); 959 subjects had complete serological data and no major protocol deviations. Among recipients of FLULAVAL, 57.4% were women. The mean age of recipients of FLULAVAL was 37.9 years; 80.4% were 18 to 49 years of age and 19.6% were 50 to 64 years of age.

A second, randomized, blinded, and controlled study which enrolled 658 subjects 50 years of age and older (stratified by age <65 and ≥65 years) was conducted in Canada. This study included elderly persons with medically controlled chronic high-risk diagnoses who were clinically stable. This study compared 4 vaccine groups: FLULAVAL, a similar investigational formulation of FLULAVAL with reduced thimerosal, and 2 Canadian-licensed trivalent influenza vaccines. Results from the 2 groups that received FLULAVAL were submitted in support of the US licensure of FLULAVAL. Among these 2 groups, 54.9% of subjects were women. The mean age of recipients of FLULAVAL was 63 years; 53.4% were 50 to 64 years of age and 46.6% were 65 years of age and older.

For both studies, analysis of the following co-primary endpoints (Table 3) were performed for each HA antigen contained in the vaccine: 1) assessment of the lower bounds of 2-sided 95% confidence intervals for the proportion of subjects with HI antibody titers of ≥1:40 after vaccination, and 2) assessment of the lower bounds of 2-sided 95% confidence intervals for rates of seroconversion (defined as a 4-fold increase in post-vaccination HI antibody titer from pre-vaccination titer ≥1:10, or an increase in titer from <1:10 to

≥1:40). The pre-specified targets for the 2 endpoints varied by study because of age of subjects enrolled. The pre-specified target for endpoint 1) was 70% in the US study and 60% in the Canadian study. For endpoint 2) the pre-specified target was 40% in the US study and 30% in the Canadian study. For the Canadian study, the primary endpoints, as originally designed, were descriptive comparisons of immune response; therefore, a post-hoc analysis of the endpoints, as described above, was performed.

[See table 3 at left]

Across both studies, serum HI antibody responses to FLULAVAL met the pre-specified seroconversion criteria for all 3 virus strains, and also the pre-specified criterion for the proportion of subjects with HI titers ≥1:40 for both influenza A viruses. In both trials, both FLULAVAL and the comparator vaccine did not meet the pre-specified criterion for the proportion of subjects with HI titers ≥1:40 for the influenza B virus. The clinical relevance of this finding on vaccine-induced protection against illness caused by influenza type B strains is unknown.

15 REFERENCES

1. Hannoun C, Megas F, Piercy J. Immunogenicity and protective efficacy of influenza vaccination. *Virus Res* 2004;103:133-138.

2. Hobson D, Curry RL, Beare AS, et al. The role of serum haemagglutination-inhibiting antibody in protection against challenge infection with influenza A2 and B viruses. *J Hyg Camb* 1972;70:767-777.

3. Centers for Disease Control and Prevention. Prevention and control of influenza: Recommendations of the Advisory Committee on Immunization Practices (ACIP). *MMWR* 2006;55(RR-10):1-42.

16 HOW SUPPLIED/STORAGE AND HANDLING

FLULAVAL is supplied in a 5-mL multi-dose vial containing ten 0.5-mL doses. Once entered, the multi-dose vial should be discarded after 28 days.

Store refrigerated between 2° and 8°C (36° and 46°F). Do not freeze. Discard if the vaccine has been frozen. Store in the original package to protect from light.

NDC 19515-887-07 (package of 1 vial containing 10 doses)

17 PATIENT COUNSELING INFORMATION

The vaccine recipient or guardian should be:

- informed of the potential benefits and risks of immunization with FLULAVAL.
- educated regarding potential side effects, emphasizing that (1) FLULAVAL contains non-infectious killed viruses and cannot cause influenza and (2) FLULAVAL is intended to provide protection against illness due to influenza viruses only, and cannot provide protection against all respiratory illness.
- instructed to report any adverse events to their healthcare provider.
- given the Vaccine Information Statements, which are required by the National Childhood Vaccine Injury Act of 1986 to be given prior to immunization. These materials are available free of charge at the Centers for Disease Control and Prevention (CDC) website (www.cdc.gov/vaccines).
- instructed that annual revaccination is recommended.

FLULAVAL is a registered trademark of ID Biomedical Corporation of Quebec. FLUZONE is a trademark of Sanofi Pasteur Limited.

Manufactured by **ID Biomedical Corporation of Quebec**
Quebec City, QC, Canada, US License 1739

Distributed by **GlaxoSmithKline**
Research Triangle Park, NC 27709

©2010, GlaxoSmithKline. All rights reserved.

May 2010

FLV:6PI

FORTAZ® ℞

[for' taz]

(ceftazidime for injection)

FORTAZ® ℞

(ceftazidime injection)

To reduce the development of drug-resistant bacteria and maintain the effectiveness of FORTAZ and other antibacterial drugs, FORTAZ should be used only to treat or prevent infections that are proven or strongly suspected to be caused by bacteria.

DESCRIPTION

Ceftazidime is a semisynthetic, broad-spectrum, beta-lactam antibiotic for parenteral administration. It is the pentahydrate of pyridinium, 1-[[7-[[(2-amino-4-thiazolyl)[(1-carboxy-1-methylethoxy)imino]acetyl]amino]-2-carboxy-8-oxo-5-thia-1-azabicyclo[4.2.0]oct-2-en-3-yl]methyl]-, hydroxide, inner salt, [6R-[6α,7β(Z)]]. It has the following structure:

The empirical formula is $C_{22}H_{32}N_6O_{12}S_2$, representing a molecular weight of 636.6.

FORTAZ is a sterile, dry-powdered mixture of ceftazidime pentahydrate and sodium carbonate. The sodium carbonate at a concentration of 118 mg/g of ceftazidime activity has been admixed to facilitate dissolution. The total sodium content of the mixture is approximately 54 mg (2.3 mEq)/g of ceftazidime activity.

FORTAZ in sterile crystalline form is supplied in vials equivalent to 500 mg, 1 g, 2 g, or 6 g of anhydrous ceftazidime and in ADD-Vantage® vials equivalent to 1 or 2 g of anhydrous ceftazidime. Solutions of FORTAZ range in color from light yellow to amber, depending on the diluent and volume used. The pH of freshly constituted solutions usually ranges from 5 to 8.

FORTAZ is available as a frozen, iso-osmotic, sterile, non-pyrogenic solution with 1 or 2 g of ceftazidime as ceftazidime sodium premixed with approximately 2.2 or 1.6 g, respectively, of Dextrose Hydrous, USP. Dextrose has been added to adjust the osmolality. Sodium hydroxide is used to adjust pH and neutralize ceftazidime pentahydrate free acid to the sodium salt. The pH may have been adjusted with hydrochloric acid. Solutions of premixed FORTAZ range in color from light yellow to amber. The solution is intended for intravenous (IV) use after thawing to room temperature. The osmolality of the solution is approximately 300 mOsmol/kg, and the pH of thawed solutions ranges from 5 to 7.5.

The plastic container for the frozen solution is fabricated from a specially designed multilayer plastic, PL 2040. Solutions are in contact with the polyethylene layer of this container and can leach out certain chemical components of the plastic in very small amounts within the expiration period. The suitability of the plastic has been confirmed in tests in animals according to USP biological tests for plastic containers as well as by tissue culture toxicity studies.

CLINICAL PHARMACOLOGY

After IV administration of 500-mg and 1-g doses of ceftazidime over 5 minutes to normal adult male volunteers, mean peak serum concentrations of 45 and 90 mcg/mL, respectively, were achieved. After IV infusion of 500-mg, 1-g, and 2-g doses of ceftazidime over 20 to 30 minutes to normal adult male volunteers, mean peak serum concentrations of 42, 69, and 170 mcg/mL, respectively, were achieved. The average serum concentrations following IV infusion of 500-mg, 1-g, and 2-g doses to these volunteers over an 8-hour interval are given in Table 1.

Table 1. Average Serum Concentrations of Ceftazidime

Ceftazidime	Serum Concentrations (mcg/mL)				
IV Dose	0.5 hr	1 hr	2 hr	4 hr	8 hr
500 mg	42	25	12	6	2
1 g	60	39	23	11	3
2 g	129	75	42	13	5

The absorption and elimination of ceftazidime were directly proportional to the size of the dose. The half-life following IV administration was approximately 1.9 hours. Less than 10% of ceftazidime was protein bound. The degree of protein binding was independent of concentration. There was no evidence of accumulation of ceftazidime in the serum in individuals with normal renal function following multiple IV doses of 1 and 2 g every 8 hours for 10 days.

Following intramuscular (IM) administration of 500-mg and 1-g doses of ceftazidime to normal adult volunteers, the mean peak serum concentrations were 17 and 39 mcg/mL, respectively, at approximately 1 hour. Serum concentrations remained above 4 mcg/mL for 6 and 8 hours after the IM administration of 500-mg and 1-g doses, respectively. The half-life of ceftazidime in these volunteers was approximately 2 hours.

The presence of hepatic dysfunction had no effect on the pharmacokinetics of ceftazidime in individuals administered 2 g intravenously every 8 hours for 5 days. Therefore, a dosage adjustment from the normal recommended dosage is not required for patients with hepatic dysfunction, provided renal function is not impaired.

Approximately 80% to 90% of an IM or IV dose of ceftazidime is excreted unchanged by the kidneys over a 24-

Table 2. Ceftazidime Concentrations in Body Tissues and Fluids

Tissue or Fluid	Dose/Route	No. of Patients	Time of Sample Postdose	Average Tissue or Fluid Level (mcg/mL or mcg/g)
Urine	500 mg IM	6	0-2 hr	2,100.0
	2 g IV	6	0-2 hr	12,000.0
Bile	2 g IV	3	90 min	36.4
Synovial fluid	2 g IV	13	2 hr	25.6
Peritoneal fluid	2 g IV	8	2 hr	48.6
Sputum	1 g IV	8	1 hr	9.0
Cerebrospinal fluid	2 g q8hr IV	5	120 min	9.8
(inflamed meninges)	2 g q8hr IV	6	180 min	9.4
Aqueous humor	2 g IV	13	1-3 hr	11.0
Blister fluid	1 g IV	7	2-3 hr	19.7
Lymphatic fluid	1 g IV	7	2-3 hr	23.4
Bone	2 g IV	8	0.67 hr	31.1
Heart muscle	2 g IV	35	30-280 min	12.7
Skin	2 g IV	22	30-180 min	6.6
Skeletal muscle	2 g IV	35	30-280 min	9.4
Myometrium	2 g IV	31	1-2 hr	18.7

hour period. After the IV administration of single 500-mg or 1-g doses, approximately 50% of the dose appeared in the urine in the first 2 hours. An additional 20% was excreted between 2 and 4 hours after dosing, and approximately another 12% of the dose appeared in the urine between 4 and 8 hours later. The elimination of ceftazidime by the kidneys resulted in high therapeutic concentrations in the urine. The mean renal clearance of ceftazidime was approximately 100 mL/min. The calculated plasma clearance of approximately 115 mL/min indicated nearly complete elimination of ceftazidime by the renal route. Administration of probenecid before dosing had no effect on the elimination kinetics of ceftazidime. This suggested that ceftazidime is eliminated by glomerular filtration and is not actively secreted by renal tubular mechanisms.

Since ceftazidime is eliminated almost solely by the kidneys, its serum half-life is significantly prolonged in patients with impaired renal function. Consequently, dosage adjustments in such patients as described in the DOSAGE AND ADMINISTRATION section are suggested.

Therapeutic concentrations of ceftazidime are achieved in the following body tissues and fluids.

[See table 2 above]

Microbiology

Ceftazidime is bactericidal in action, exerting its effect by inhibition of enzymes responsible for cell-wall synthesis. A wide range of gram-negative organisms is susceptible to ceftazidime in vitro, including strains resistant to gentamicin and other aminoglycosides. In addition, ceftazidime has been shown to be active against gram-positive organisms. It is highly stable to most clinically important beta-lactamases, plasmid or chromosomal, which are produced by both gram-negative and gram-positive organisms and, consequently, is active against many strains resistant to ampicillin and other cephalosporins.

Ceftazidime has been shown to be active against the following organisms both in vitro and in clinical infections (see INDICATIONS AND USAGE).

Aerobes, Gram-negative

Citrobacter spp., including *Citrobacter freundii* and *Citrobacter diversus*; *Enterobacter* spp., including *Enterobacter cloacae* and *Enterobacter aerogenes*; *Escherichia coli*; *Haemophilus influenzae*, including ampicillin-resistant strains; *Klebsiella* spp. (including *Klebsiella pneumoniae*); *Neisseria meningitidis*; *Proteus mirabilis*; *Proteus vulgaris*; *Pseudomonas* spp. (including *Pseudomonas aeruginosa*); and *Serratia* spp.

Aerobes, Gram-positive

Staphylococcus aureus, including penicillinase- and non-penicillinase-producing strains; *Streptococcus agalactiae* (group B streptococci); *Streptococcus pneumoniae*; and *Streptococcus pyogenes* (group A beta-hemolytic streptococci).

Anaerobes

Bacteroides spp. (NOTE: many strains of *Bacteroides fragilis* are resistant).

Ceftazidime has been shown to be active in vitro against most strains of the following organisms; however, the clinical significance of these data is unknown: *Acinetobacter* spp., *Clostridium* spp. (not including *Clostridium difficile*), *Haemophilus parainfluenzae*, *Morganella morganii* (formerly *Proteus morganii*), *Neisseria gonorrhoeae*, *Peptococcus* spp., *Peptostreptococcus* spp., *Providencia* spp. (including *Providencia rettgeri*, formerly *Proteus rettgeri*), *Salmonella* spp., *Shigella* spp., *Staphylococcus epidermidis*, and *Yersinia enterocolitica*.

Ceftazidime and the aminoglycosides have been shown to be synergistic in vitro against *Pseudomonas aeruginosa* and the enterobacteriaceae. Ceftazidime and carbenicillin have also been shown to be synergistic in vitro against *Pseudomonas aeruginosa*.

Ceftazidime is not active in vitro against methicillin-resistant staphylococci, *Streptococcus faecalis* and many other enterococci, *Listeria monocytogenes*, *Campylobacter* spp., or *Clostridium difficile*.

Susceptibility Tests

Diffusion Techniques

Quantitative methods that require measurement of zone diameters give an estimate of antibiotic susceptibility. One such procedure[1-3] has been recommended for use with disks to test susceptibility to ceftazidime.

Reports from the laboratory giving results of the standard single-disk susceptibility test with a 30-mcg ceftazidime disk should be interpreted according to the following criteria:

Susceptible organisms produce zones of 18 mm or greater, indicating that the test organism is likely to respond to therapy.

Organisms that produce zones of 15 to 17 mm are expected to be susceptible if high dosage is used or if the infection is confined to tissues and fluids (e.g., urine) in which high antibiotic levels are attained.

Resistant organisms produce zones of 14 mm or less, indicating that other therapy should be selected.

Organisms should be tested with the ceftazidime disk since ceftazidime has been shown by in vitro tests to be active against certain strains found resistant when other beta-lactam disks are used.

Standardized procedures require the use of laboratory control organisms. The 30-mcg ceftazidime disk should give zone diameters between 25 and 32 mm for *Escherichia coli* ATCC 25922. For *Pseudomonas aeruginosa* ATCC 27853, the zone diameters should be between 22 and 29 mm. For *Staphylococcus aureus* ATCC 25923, the zone diameters should be between 16 and 20 mm.

Dilution Techniques

In other susceptibility testing procedures, e.g., ICS agar dilution or the equivalent, a bacterial isolate may be considered susceptible if the minimum inhibitory concentration (MIC) value for ceftazidime is not more than 16 mcg/mL. Organisms are considered resistant to ceftazidime if the MIC is ≥64 mcg/mL. Organisms having an MIC value of

<64 mcg/mL but >16 mcg/mL are expected to be susceptible if high dosage is used or if the infection is confined to tissues and fluids (e.g., urine) in which high antibiotic levels are attained.

As with standard diffusion methods, dilution procedures require the use of laboratory control organisms. Standard ceftazidime powder should give MIC values in the range of 4 to 16 mcg/mL for *Staphylococcus aureus* ATCC 25923. For *Escherichia coli* ATCC 25922, the MIC range should be between 0.125 and 0.5 mcg/mL. For *Pseudomonas aeruginosa* ATCC 27853, the MIC range should be between 0.5 and 2 mcg/mL.

INDICATIONS AND USAGE

FORTAZ is indicated for the treatment of patients with infections caused by susceptible strains of the designated organisms in the following diseases:

1. **Lower Respiratory Tract Infections,** including pneumonia, caused by *Pseudomonas aeruginosa* and other *Pseudomonas* spp.; *Haemophilus influenzae,* including ampicillin-resistant strains; *Klebsiella* spp.; *Enterobacter* spp.; *Proteus mirabilis; Escherichia coli; Serratia* spp.; *Citrobacter* spp.; *Streptococcus pneumoniae*; and *Staphylococcus aureus* (methicillin-susceptible strains).
2. **Skin and Skin-Structure Infections** caused by *Pseudomonas aeruginosa; Klebsiella* spp.; *Escherichia coli; Proteus* spp., including *Proteus mirabilis* and indole-positive *Proteus; Enterobacter* spp.; *Serratia* spp.; *Staphylococcus aureus* (methicillin-susceptible strains); and *Streptococcus pyogenes* (group A beta-hemolytic streptococci).
3. **Urinary Tract Infections,** both complicated and uncomplicated, caused by *Pseudomonas aeruginosa; Enterobacter* spp.; *Proteus* spp., including *Proteus mirabilis* and indole-positive *Proteus; Klebsiella* spp.; and *Escherichia coli.*
4. **Bacterial Septicemia** caused by *Pseudomonas aeruginosa, Klebsiella* spp., *Haemophilus influenzae, Escherichia coli, Serratia* spp., *Streptococcus pneumoniae,* and *Staphylococcus aureus* (methicillin-susceptible strains).
5. **Bone and Joint Infections** caused by *Pseudomonas aeruginosa, Klebsiella* spp., *Enterobacter* spp., and *Staphylococcus aureus* (methicillin-susceptible strains).
6. **Gynecologic Infections,** including endometritis, pelvic cellulitis, and other infections of the female genital tract caused by *Escherichia coli.*
7. **Intra-abdominal Infections,** including peritonitis caused by *Escherichia coli, Klebsiella* spp., and *Staphylococcus aureus* (methicillin-susceptible strains) and polymicrobial infections caused by aerobic and anaerobic organisms and *Bacteroides* spp. (many strains of *Bacteroides fragilis* are resistant).
8. **Central Nervous System Infections,** including meningitis, caused by *Haemophilus influenzae* and *Neisseria meningitidis*. Ceftazidime has also been used successfully in a limited number of cases of meningitis due to *Pseudomonas aeruginosa* and *Streptococcus pneumoniae.*

FORTAZ may be used alone in cases of confirmed or suspected sepsis. Ceftazidime has been used successfully in clinical trials as empiric therapy in cases where various concomitant therapies with other antibiotics have been used.

FORTAZ may also be used concomitantly with other antibiotics, such as aminoglycosides, vancomycin, and clindamycin; in severe and life-threatening infections; and in the immunocompromised patient. When such concomitant treatment is appropriate, prescribing information in the labeling for the other antibiotics should be followed. The dose depends on the severity of the infection and the patient's condition.

To reduce the development of drug-resistant bacteria and maintain the effectiveness of FORTAZ and other antibacterial drugs, FORTAZ should be used only to treat or prevent infections that are proven or strongly suspected to be caused by susceptible bacteria. When culture and susceptibility information are available, they should be considered in selecting or modifying antibacterial therapy. In the absence of such data, local epidemiology and susceptibility patterns may contribute to the empiric selection of therapy.

CONTRAINDICATIONS

FORTAZ is contraindicated in patients who have shown hypersensitivity to ceftazidime or the cephalosporin group of antibiotics.

WARNINGS

BEFORE THERAPY WITH FORTAZ IS INSTITUTED, CAREFUL INQUIRY SHOULD BE MADE TO DETERMINE WHETHER THE PATIENT HAS HAD PREVIOUS HYPERSENSITIVITY REACTIONS TO CEFTAZIDIME, CEPHALOSPORINS, PENICILLINS, OR OTHER DRUGS. IF THIS PRODUCT IS TO BE GIVEN TO PENICILLIN-SENSITIVE PATIENTS, CAUTION SHOULD BE EXERCISED BECAUSE CROSS-HYPERSENSITIVITY AMONG BETA-LACTAM ANTIBIOTICS HAS BEEN CLEARLY DOCUMENTED AND MAY OCCUR IN UP TO 10% OF PATIENTS WITH A HISTORY OF PENICILLIN ALLERGY. IF AN ALLERGIC REACTION TO FORTAZ OCCURS, DISCONTINUE THE DRUG. SERIOUS ACUTE HYPERSENSITIVITY REACTIONS MAY REQUIRE TREATMENT WITH EPINEPHRINE AND OTHER EMERGENCY MEASURES, INCLUDING OXYGEN, IV FLUIDS, IV ANTIHISTAMINES, CORTICOSTEROIDS, PRESSOR AMINES, AND AIRWAY MANAGEMENT, AS CLINICALLY INDICATED.

Clostridium difficile associated diarrhea (CDAD) has been reported with use of nearly all antibacterial agents, including FORTAZ, and may range in severity from mild diarrhea to fatal colitis. Treatment with antibacterial agents alters the normal flora of the colon leading to overgrowth of *C. difficile.*

C. difficile produces toxins A and B which contribute to the development of CDAD. Hypertoxin producing strains of *C. difficile* cause increased morbidity and mortality, as these infections can be refractory to antimicrobial therapy and may require colectomy. CDAD must be considered in all patients who present with diarrhea following antibiotic use. Careful medical history is necessary since CDAD has been reported to occur over two months after the administration of antibacterial agents.

If CDAD is suspected or confirmed, ongoing antibiotic use not directed against *C. difficile* may need to be discontinued. Appropriate fluid and electrolyte management, protein supplementation, antibiotic treatment of *C. difficile*, and surgical evaluation should be instituted as clinically indicated.

Elevated levels of ceftazidime in patients with renal insufficiency can lead to seizures, encephalopathy, coma, asterixis, neuromuscular excitability, and myoclonia (see PRECAUTIONS).

PRECAUTIONS

General

High and prolonged serum ceftazidime concentrations can occur from usual dosages in patients with transient or persistent reduction of urinary output because of renal insufficiency. The total daily dosage should be reduced when ceftazidime is administered to patients with renal insufficiency (see DOSAGE AND ADMINISTRATION). Elevated levels of ceftazidime in these patients can lead to seizures, encephalopathy, coma, asterixis, neuromuscular excitability, and myoclonia. Continued dosage should be determined by degree of renal impairment, severity of infection, and susceptibility of the causative organisms.

As with other antibiotics, prolonged use of FORTAZ may result in overgrowth of nonsusceptible organisms. Repeated evaluation of the patient's condition is essential. If superinfection occurs during therapy, appropriate measures should be taken.

Inducible type I beta-lactamase resistance has been noted with some organisms (e.g., *Enterobacter* spp., *Pseudomonas* spp., and *Serratia* spp.). As with other extended-spectrum beta-lactam antibiotics, resistance can develop during therapy, leading to clinical failure in some cases. When treating infections caused by these organisms, periodic susceptibility testing should be performed when clinically appropriate. If patients fail to respond to monotherapy, an aminoglycoside or similar agent should be considered.

Cephalosporins may be associated with a fall in prothrombin activity. Those at risk include patients with renal and hepatic impairment, or poor nutritional state, as well as patients receiving a protracted course of antimicrobial therapy. Prothrombin time should be monitored in patients at risk and exogenous vitamin K administered as indicated.

FORTAZ should be prescribed with caution in individuals with a history of gastrointestinal disease, particularly colitis.

Distal necrosis can occur after inadvertent intra-arterial administration of ceftazidime.

Prescribing FORTAZ in the absence of a proven or strongly suspected bacterial infection or a prophylactic indication is unlikely to provide benefit to the patient and increases the risk of the development of drug-resistant bacteria.

Information for Patients

Patients should be counseled that antibacterial drugs, including FORTAZ, should only be used to treat bacterial infections. They do not treat viral infections (e.g., the common cold). When FORTAZ is prescribed to treat a bacterial infection, patients should be told that although it is common to feel better early in the course of therapy, the medication should be taken exactly as directed. Skipping doses or not completing the full course of therapy may: (1) decrease the effectiveness of the immediate treatment, and (2) increase the likelihood that bacteria will develop resistance and will not be treatable by FORTAZ or other antibacterial drugs in the future.

Diarrhea is a common problem caused by antibiotics which usually ends when the antibiotic is discontinued. Sometimes after starting treatment with antibiotics, patients can develop watery and bloody stools (with or without stomach cramps and fever) even as late as 2 or more months after having taken the last dose of the antibiotic. If this occurs, patients should contact their physician as soon as possible.

Drug Interactions

Nephrotoxicity has been reported following concomitant administration of cephalosporins with aminoglycoside antibiotics or potent diuretics such as furosemide. Renal function should be carefully monitored, especially if higher dosages of the aminoglycosides are to be administered or if therapy is prolonged, because of the potential nephrotoxicity and ototoxicity of aminoglycosidic antibiotics. Nephrotoxicity and ototoxicity were not noted when ceftazidime was given alone in clinical trials.

Chloramphenicol has been shown to be antagonistic to beta-lactam antibiotics, including ceftazidime, based on in vitro studies and time kill curves with enteric gram-negative bacilli. Due to the possibility of antagonism in vivo, particularly when bactericidal activity is desired, this drug combination should be avoided.

In common with other antibiotics, ceftazidime may affect the gut flora, leading to lower estrogen reabsorption and reduced efficacy of combined oral estrogen/progesterone contraceptives.

Drug/Laboratory Test Interactions

The administration of ceftazidime may result in a false-positive reaction for glucose in the urine when using CLINITEST® tablets, Benedict's solution, or Fehling's solution. It is recommended that glucose tests based on enzymatic glucose oxidase reactions (such as CLINISTIX®) be used.

Carcinogenesis, Mutagenesis, Impairment of Fertility

Long-term studies in animals have not been performed to evaluate carcinogenic potential. However, a mouse micronucleus test and an Ames test were both negative for mutagenic effects.

Pregnancy

Teratogenic Effects

Pregnancy Category B. Reproduction studies have been performed in mice and rats at doses up to 40 times the human dose and have revealed no evidence of impaired fertility or harm to the fetus due to FORTAZ. There are, however, no adequate and well-controlled studies in pregnant women. Because animal reproduction studies are not always predictive of human response, this drug should be used during pregnancy only if clearly needed.

Nursing Mothers

Ceftazidime is excreted in human milk in low concentrations. Caution should be exercised when FORTAZ is administered to a nursing woman.

Pediatric Use

(see DOSAGE AND ADMINISTRATION).

Geriatric Use

Of the 2,221 subjects who received ceftazidime in 11 clinical studies, 824 (37%) were 65 and older while 391 (18%) were 75 and older. No overall differences in safety or effectiveness were observed between these subjects and younger subjects, and other reported clinical experience has not identified differences in responses between the elderly and younger patients, but greater susceptibility of some older individuals to drug effects cannot be ruled out. This drug is known to be substantially excreted by the kidney, and the risk of toxic reactions to this drug may be greater in patients with impaired renal function. Because elderly patients are more likely to have decreased renal function, care should be taken in dose selection, and it may be useful to monitor renal function (see DOSAGE AND ADMINISTRATION).

ADVERSE REACTIONS

Ceftazidime is generally well tolerated. The incidence of adverse reactions associated with the administration of ceftazidime was low in clinical trials. The most common were local reactions following IV injection and allergic and gastrointestinal reactions. Other adverse reactions were encountered infrequently. No disulfiram-like reactions were reported.

The following adverse effects from clinical trials were considered to be either related to ceftazidime therapy or were of uncertain etiology:

Local Effects, reported in fewer than 2% of patients, were phlebitis and inflammation at the site of injection (1 in 69 patients).

Hypersensitivity Reactions, reported in 2% of patients, were pruritus, rash, and fever. Immediate reactions, generally manifested by rash and/or pruritus, occurred in 1 in 285 patients. Toxic epidermal necrolysis, Stevens-Johnson syndrome, and erythema multiforme have also been reported with cephalosporin antibiotics, including ceftazidime. Angioedema and anaphylaxis (bronchospasm and/or hypotension) have been reported very rarely.

Gastrointestinal Symptoms, reported in fewer than 2% of patients, were diarrhea (1 in 78), nausea (1 in 156), vomiting (1 in 500), and abdominal pain (1 in 416). The onset of pseudomembranous colitis symptoms may occur during or after treatment (see WARNINGS).

Central Nervous System Reactions (fewer than 1%) included headache, dizziness, and paresthesia. Seizures have been reported with several cephalosporins, including ceftazidime. In addition, encephalopathy, coma, asterixis, neuromuscular excitability, and myoclonia have been re-

Table 3. Recommended Dosage Schedule

	Dose	Frequency
Adults		
Usual recommended dosage	**1 gram IV or IM**	**q8-12hr**
Uncomplicated urinary tract infections	250 mg IV or IM	q12hr
Bone and joint infections	2 grams IV	q12hr
Complicated urinary tract infections	500 mg IV or IM	q8-12hr
Uncomplicated pneumonia; mild skin and skin-structure infections	500 mg-1 gram IV or IM	q8hr
Serious gynecologic and intra-abdominal infections	2 grams IV	q8hr
Meningitis	2 grams IV	q8hr
Very severe life-threatening infections, especially in immunocompromised patients	2 grams IV	q8hr
Lung infections caused by *Pseudomonas* spp. in patients with cystic fibrosis with normal renal function*	30-50 mg/kg IV to a maximum of 6 grams per day	q8hr
Neonates (0-4 weeks)	30 mg/kg IV	q12hr
Infants and children (1 month-12 years)	30-50 mg/kg IV to a maximum of 6 grams per day†	q8hr

* Although clinical improvement has been shown, bacteriologic cures cannot be expected in patients with chronic respiratory disease and cystic fibrosis.
† The higher dose should be reserved for immunocompromised pediatric patients or pediatric patients with cystic fibrosis or meningitis.

Males: Creatinine clearance (mL/min) = $\dfrac{\text{Weight (kg)} \times (40 - \text{age})}{72 \times \text{serum creatinine (mg/dL)}}$

Females: $0.85 \times$ male value

ported in renally impaired patients treated with unadjusted dosing regimens of ceftazidime (see PRECAUTIONS: General).

Less Frequent Adverse Events (fewer than 1%) were candidiasis (including oral thrush) and vaginitis.

Hematologic: Rare cases of hemolytic anemia have been reported.

Laboratory Test Changes noted during clinical trials with FORTAZ were transient and included: eosinophilia (1 in 13), positive Coombs test without hemolysis (1 in 23), thrombocytosis (1 in 45), and slight elevations in one or more of the hepatic enzymes, aspartate aminotransferase (AST, SGOT) (1 in 16), alanine aminotransferase (ALT, SGPT) (1 in 15), LDH (1 in 18), GGT (1 in 19), and alkaline phosphatase (1 in 23). As with some other cephalosporins, transient elevations of blood urea, blood urea nitrogen, and/or serum creatinine were observed occasionally. Transient leukopenia, neutropenia, agranulocytosis, thrombocytopenia, and lymphocytosis were seen very rarely.

POSTMARKETING EXPERIENCE WITH FORTAZ PRODUCTS
In addition to the adverse events reported during clinical trials, the following events have been observed during clinical practice in patients treated with FORTAZ and were reported spontaneously. For some of these events, data are insufficient to allow an estimate of incidence or to establish causation.

General
Anaphylaxis; allergic reactions, which, in rare instances, were severe (e.g., cardiopulmonary arrest); urticaria; pain at injection site.

Hepatobiliary Tract
Hyperbilirubinemia, jaundice.

Renal and Genitourinary
Renal impairment.

Cephalosporin-Class Adverse Reactions
In addition to the adverse reactions listed above that have been observed in patients treated with ceftazidime, the following adverse reactions and altered laboratory tests have been reported for cephalosporin-class antibiotics:

Adverse Reactions
Colitis, toxic nephropathy, hepatic dysfunction including cholestasis, aplastic anemia, hemorrhage.

Altered Laboratory Tests
Prolonged prothrombin time, false-positive test for urinary glucose, pancytopenia.

OVERDOSAGE
Ceftazidime overdosage has occurred in patients with renal failure. Reactions have included seizure activity, encephalopathy, asterixis, neuromuscular excitability, and coma. Patients who receive an acute overdosage should be carefully observed and given supportive treatment. In the pres-

ence of renal insufficiency, hemodialysis or peritoneal dialysis may aid in the removal of ceftazidime from the body.

DOSAGE AND ADMINISTRATION
Dosage
The usual adult dosage is 1 gram administered intravenously or intramuscularly every 8 to 12 hours. The dosage and route should be determined by the susceptibility of the causative organisms, the severity of infection, and the condition and renal function of the patient.
The guidelines for dosage of FORTAZ are listed in Table 3. The following dosage schedule is recommended.
[See table 3 above]

Impaired Hepatic Function
No adjustment in dosage is required for patients with hepatic dysfunction.

Impaired Renal Function
Ceftazidime is excreted by the kidneys, almost exclusively by glomerular filtration. Therefore, in patients with impaired renal function (glomerular filtration rate [GFR] <50 mL/min), it is recommended that the dosage of ceftazidime be reduced to compensate for its slower excretion. In patients with suspected renal insufficiency, an initial loading dose of 1 gram of FORTAZ may be given. An estimate of GFR should be made to determine the appropriate maintenance dosage. The recommended dosage is presented in Table 4.

Table 4. Recommended Maintenance Dosages of FORTAZ in Renal Insufficiency

NOTE: IF THE DOSE RECOMMENDED IN TABLE 3 ABOVE IS LOWER THAN THAT RECOMMENDED FOR PATIENTS WITH RENAL INSUFFICIENCY AS OUTLINED IN TABLE 4, THE LOWER DOSE SHOULD BE USED.

Creatinine Clearance (mL/min)	Recommended Unit Dose of FORTAZ	Frequency of Dosing
50-31	1 gram	q12hr
30-16	1 gram	q24hr
15-6	500 mg	q24hr
<5	500 mg	q48hr

When only serum creatinine is available, the following formula (Cockcroft's equation)[4] may be used to estimate creatinine clearance. The serum creatinine should represent a steady state of renal function:

[See table below]
In patients with severe infections who would normally receive 6 grams of FORTAZ daily were it not for renal insufficiency, the unit dose given in the table above may be increased by 50% or the dosing frequency may be increased appropriately. Further dosing should be determined by therapeutic monitoring, severity of the infection, and susceptibility of the causative organism.
In pediatric patients as for adults, the creatinine clearance should be adjusted for body surface area or lean body mass, and the dosing frequency should be reduced in cases of renal insufficiency.
In patients undergoing hemodialysis, a loading dose of 1 gram is recommended, followed by 1 gram after each hemodialysis period.
FORTAZ can also be used in patients undergoing intraperitoneal dialysis and continuous ambulatory peritoneal dialysis. In such patients, a loading dose of 1 gram of FORTAZ may be given, followed by 500 mg every 24 hours. In addition to IV use, FORTAZ can be incorporated in the dialysis fluid at a concentration of 250 mg for 2 L of dialysis fluid.
Note: Generally FORTAZ should be continued for 2 days after the signs and symptoms of infection have disappeared, but in complicated infections longer therapy may be required.

Administration
FORTAZ may be given intravenously or by deep IM injection into a large muscle mass such as the upper outer quadrant of the gluteus maximus or lateral part of the thigh. Intra-arterial administration should be avoided (see PRECAUTIONS).

Intramuscular Administration
For IM administration, FORTAZ should be constituted with one of the following diluents: Sterile Water for Injection, Bacteriostatic Water for Injection, or 0.5% or 1% Lidocaine Hydrochloride Injection. Refer to Table 5.

Intravenous Administration
The IV route is preferable for patients with bacterial septicemia, bacterial meningitis, peritonitis, or other severe or life-threatening infections, or for patients who may be poor risks because of lowered resistance resulting from such debilitating conditions as malnutrition, trauma, surgery, diabetes, heart failure, or malignancy, particularly if shock is present or pending.

For direct intermittent IV administration, constitute FORTAZ as directed in Table 5 with Sterile Water for Injection. Slowly inject directly into the vein over a period of 3 to 5 minutes or give through the tubing of an administration set while the patient is also receiving one of the compatible IV fluids (see COMPATIBILITY AND STABILITY).
For IV infusion, constitute the 500-mg, 1-gram, or 2-gram vial and add an appropriate quantity of the resulting solution to an IV container with one of the compatible IV fluids listed under the COMPATIBILITY AND STABILITY section.

Intermittent IV infusion with a Y-type administration set can be accomplished with compatible solutions. However, during infusion of a solution containing ceftazidime, it is desirable to discontinue the other solution.
ADD-Vantage vials are to be constituted only with 50 or 100 mL of 5% Dextrose Injection, 0.9% Sodium Chloride Injection, or 0.45% Sodium Chloride Injection in Abbott ADD-Vantage flexible diluent containers (see Instructions for Constitution). ADD-Vantage vials that have been joined to Abbott ADD-Vantage diluent containers and activated to dissolve the drug are stable for 12 hours at room temperature or for 3 days under refrigeration. Joined vials that have not been activated may be used within a 14-day period; this period corresponds to that for use of Abbott ADD-Vantage containers following removal of the outer packaging (overwrap).
Freezing solutions of FORTAZ in the ADD-Vantage system is not recommended.
[See table 5 at top of next page]
All vials of FORTAZ as supplied are under reduced pressure. When FORTAZ is dissolved, carbon dioxide is released and a positive pressure develops. For ease of use please follow the recommended techniques of constitution described on the detachable Instructions for Constitution section of this insert.
Solutions of FORTAZ, like those of most beta-lactam antibiotics, should not be added to solutions of aminoglycoside antibiotics because of potential interaction.
However, if concurrent therapy with FORTAZ and an aminoglycoside is indicated, each of these antibiotics can be administered separately to the same patient.
Directions for Use of FORTAZ Frozen in Galaxy® Plastic Containers
FORTAZ supplied as a frozen, sterile, iso-osmotic, nonpyrogenic solution in plastic containers is to be administered after thawing either as a continuous or intermittent IV

Table 5. Preparation of Solutions of FORTAZ

Size	Amount of Diluent to be Added (mL)	Approximate Available Volume (mL)	Approximate Ceftazidime Concentration (mg/mL)
Intramuscular			
500-mg vial	1.5	1.8	280
1-gram vial	3.0	3.6	280
Intravenous			
500-mg vial	5.3	5.7*	100
1-gram vial	10.0	10.8†	100
2-gram vial	10.0	11.5‡	170
Pharmacy bulk package			
6-gram vial	26	30	200

* To obtain a dose of 500 mg, withdraw 5.0 mL from the vial following reconstitution.
† To obtain a dose of 1 g, withdraw 10.0 mL from the vial following reconstitution.
‡ To obtain a dose of 2 g, withdraw 11.5 mL from the vial following reconstitution.

infusion. The thawed solution is stable for 8 hours at room temperature or for 3 days if stored under refrigeration. **Do not refreeze.**

Thaw container at room temperature (25°C) or under refrigeration (5°C). Do not force thaw by immersion in water baths or by microwave irradiation. Components of the solution may precipitate in the frozen state and will dissolve upon reaching room temperature with little or no agitation. Potency is not affected. Mix after solution has reached room temperature. Check for minute leaks by squeezing bag firmly. Discard bag if leaks are found as sterility may be impaired. Do not add supplementary medication. Do not use unless solution is clear and seal is intact.
Use sterile equipment.

Caution: Do not use plastic containers in series connections. Such use could result in air embolism due to residual air being drawn from the primary container before administration of the fluid from the secondary container is complete.

Preparation for Administration
1. Suspend container from eyelet support.
2. Remove protector from outlet port at bottom of container.
3. Attach administration set. Refer to complete directions accompanying set.

COMPATIBILITY AND STABILITY
Intramuscular
FORTAZ, when constituted as directed with Sterile Water for Injection, Bacteriostatic Water for Injection, or 0.5% or 1% Lidocaine Hydrochloride Injection, maintains satisfactory potency for 12 hours at room temperature or for 3 days under refrigeration. Solutions in Sterile Water for Injection that are frozen immediately after constitution in the original container are stable for 3 months when stored at -20°C. Once thawed, solutions should not be refrozen. Thawed solutions may be stored for up to 3 hours at room temperature or for 3 days in a refrigerator.
Intravenous
FORTAZ, when constituted as directed with Sterile Water for Injection, maintains satisfactory potency for 12 hours at room temperature or for 3 days under refrigeration. Solutions in 0.9% Sodium Chloride Injection in VIAFLEX® small-volume containers that are frozen immediately after constitution are stable for 3 months when stored at -20°C. Do not force thaw by immersion in water baths or by microwave irradiation. Once thawed, solutions should not be refrozen. Thawed solutions may be stored for up to 12 hours at room temperature or for 3 days in a refrigerator. More concentrated solutions in Sterile Water for Injection in the original container that are frozen immediately after constitution are stable for 3 months when stored at -20°C. Once thawed, solutions should not be refrozen. Thawed solutions may be stored for up to 8 hours at room temperature or for 3 days in a refrigerator.
FORTAZ is compatible with the more commonly used IV infusion fluids. Solutions at concentrations between 1 and 40 mg/mL in 0.9% Sodium Chloride Injection; 1/6 M Sodium Lactate Injection; 5% Dextrose Injection; 5% Dextrose and 0.225% Sodium Chloride Injection; 5% Dextrose and 0.45% Sodium Chloride Injection; 5% Dextrose and 0.9% Residual Sodium Chloride Injection; 10% Dextrose Injection; Ringer's Injection, USP; Lactated Ringer's Injection, USP; 10% Invert Sugar in Water for Injection; and NORMOSOL®-M in 5% Dextrose Injection may be stored for up to 12 hours at room temperature or for 3 days if refrigerated.

The 1- and 2-g FORTAZ ADD-Vantage vials, when diluted in 50 or 100 mL of 5% Dextrose Injection, 0.9% Sodium Chloride Injection, or 0.45% Sodium Chloride Injection, may be stored for up to 12 hours at room temperature or for 3 days under refrigeration.
FORTAZ is less stable in Sodium Bicarbonate Injection than in other IV fluids. It is not recommended as a diluent. Solutions of FORTAZ in 5% Dextrose Injection and 0.9% Sodium Chloride Injection are stable for at least 6 hours at room temperature in plastic tubing, drip chambers, and volume control devices of common IV infusion sets.
Ceftazidime at a concentration of 4 mg/mL has been found compatible for 12 hours at room temperature or for 3 days under refrigeration in 0.9% Sodium Chloride Injection or 5% Dextrose Injection when admixed with: cefuroxime sodium (ZINACEF®) 3 mg/mL, heparin 10 or 50 U/mL, or potassium chloride 10 or 40 mEq/L.
Vancomycin solution exhibits a physical incompatibility when mixed with a number of drugs, including ceftazidime. The likelihood of precipitation with ceftazidime is dependent on the concentrations of vancomycin and ceftazidime present. It is therefore recommended, when both drugs are to be administered by intermittent IV infusion, that they be given separately, flushing the IV lines (with 1 of the compatible IV fluids) between the administration of these 2 agents.
Note: Parenteral drug products should be inspected visually for particulate matter before administration whenever solution and container permit.
As with other cephalosporins, FORTAZ powder, as well as solutions, tend to darken depending on storage conditions; within the stated recommendations, however, product potency is not adversely affected.

HOW SUPPLIED
FORTAZ in the dry state should be stored between 15° and 30°C (59° and 86°F) and protected from light. FORTAZ is a dry, white to off-white powder supplied in vials as follows:
NDC 0173-0377-10 500-mg* Vial (Tray of 10)
NDC 0173-0378-10 1-g* Vial (Tray of 10)
NDC 0173-0379-34 2-g* Vial (Tray of 10)
NDC 0173-0382-37 6-g* Pharmacy Bulk Package (Tray of 6)
NDC 0173-0434-00 1-g ADD-Vantage® Vial (Tray of 25)
NDC 0173-0435-00 2-g ADD-Vantage® Vial (Tray of 10)
(The above ADD-Vantage vials are to be used only with Abbott ADD-Vantage diluent containers.)
FORTAZ frozen as a premixed solution of ceftazidime sodium should not be stored above -20°C. FORTAZ is supplied frozen in 50-mL, single-dose, plastic containers as follows:
NDC 0173-0412-00 1-g* Plastic Container (Carton of 24)
NDC 0173-0413-00 2-g* Plastic Container (Carton of 24)
*Equivalent to anhydrous ceftazidime.

REFERENCES
1. Bauer AW, Kirby WMM, Sherris JC, Turck M. Antibiotic susceptibility testing by a standardized single disk method. *Am J Clin Pathol.* 1966;45:493-496.
2. National Committee for Clinical Laboratory Standards. Approved Standard: Performance Standards for Antimicrobial Disc Susceptibility Tests. (M2-A3). December 1984.
3. Certification procedure for antibiotic sensitivity discs (21 CFR 460.1). *Federal Register.* May 30, 1974;39: 19182-19184.
4. Cockroft DW, Gault MH. Prediction of creatinine clearance from serum creatinine. *Nephron.* 1976;16:31-41.

GlaxoSmithKline
FORTAZ® (ceftazidime for injection):
GlaxoSmithKline
Research Triangle Park, NC 27709
FORTAZ® (ceftazidime injection):
Manufactured for GlaxoSmithKline
Research Triangle Park, NC 27709
by Baxter Healthcare Corporation
Deerfield, IL 60015
FORTAZ and ZINACEF are registered trademarks of GlaxoSmithKline.
ADD-Vantage is a registered trademark of Abbott Laboratories.
CLINITEST and CLINISTIX are registered trademarks of Ames Division, Miles Laboratories, Inc.
GALAXY and VIAFLEX are registered trademarks of Baxter International Inc.
February 2007   RL-2357

TEAR AWAY

FORTAZ®
(ceftazidime for injection)
Instructions for Constitution
Vials: 500 mg IM/IV, 1 g IM/IV, 2 g IV
1. Insert the syringe needle through the vial closure and inject the recommended volume of diluent. The vacuum may assist entry of the diluent. Remove the syringe needle.
2. Shake to dissolve; a clear solution will be obtained in 1 to 2 minutes.
3. Invert the vial. Ensuring that the syringe plunger is fully depressed, insert the needle through the vial closure and withdraw the total volume of solution into the syringe (the pressure in the vial may aid withdrawal). Ensure that the needle remains within the solution and does not enter the headspace. The withdrawn solution may contain some bubbles of carbon dioxide.
Note: As with the administration of all parenteral products, accumulated gases should be expressed from the syringe immediately before injection of FORTAZ.
ADD-Vantage® Vials: 1 g, 2 g
To Open Diluent Container:
Peel the corner of the ADD-Vantage diluent overwrap and remove flexible diluent container. Some opacity of the plastic flexible container due to moisture absorption during the sterilization process may be observed. This is normal and does not affect the solution quality or safety. The opacity will diminish gradually.
To Assemble Vial and Flexible Diluent Container (Use Aseptic Technique):
1. Remove the protective covers from the top of the vial and the vial port on the diluent container as follows:
a. To remove the breakaway vial cap, swing the pull ring over the top of the vial and pull down far enough to start the opening (see Figure 1), then pull straight up to remove the cap (see Figure 2).

Figure 1

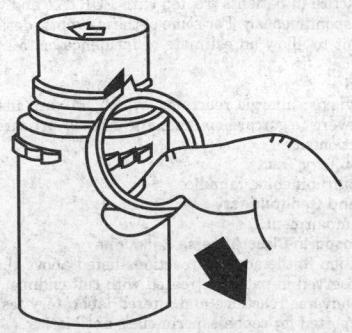

[See figure 2 at top of next page]
Note: Once the breakaway cap has been removed, do not access vial with syringe. b. To remove the vial port cover, grasp the tab on the pull ring, pull up to break the three tie strings, then pull back to remove the cover (see Figure 3). [See figure 3 on next page]
2. Screw the vial into the vial port until it will go no further. THE VIAL MUST BE SCREWED IN TIGHTLY TO ASSURE A SEAL. This occurs approximately one-half turn (180°) after the first audible click (see Figure 4). The clicking sound does not assure a seal; the vial must be turned as far as it will go.

Figure 2

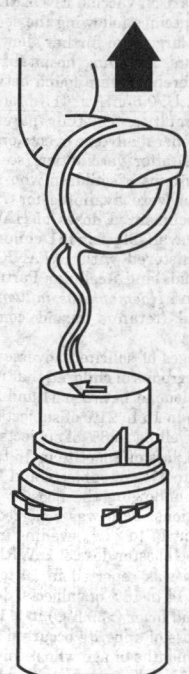

Figure 3

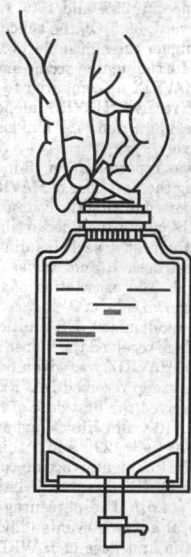

Note: Once vial is seated, do not attempt to remove (see Figure 4).

[See figure 4 at top of next column]

3. Recheck the vial to assure that it is tight by trying to turn it further in the direction of assembly.

4. Label appropriately.

To Prepare Admixture:

1. Squeeze the bottom of the diluent container gently to inflate the portion of the container surrounding the end of the drug vial.

2. With the other hand, push the drug vial down into the container, telescoping the walls of the container. Grasp the inner cap of the vial through the walls of the container (see Figure 5).

[See figure 5 in next column]

3. Pull the inner cap from the drug vial (see Figure 6). Verify that the rubber stopper has been pulled out, allowing the drug and diluent to mix.

[See figure 6 in next column]

4. Mix container contents thoroughly and use within the specified time.

Preparation for Administration (Use Aseptic Technique):

1. Confirm the activation and admixture of vial contents.

2. Check for leaks by squeezing container firmly. If leaks are found, discard unit as sterility may be impaired.

3. Close flow control clamp of administration set.

4. Remove cover from outlet port at bottom of container.

Figure 4

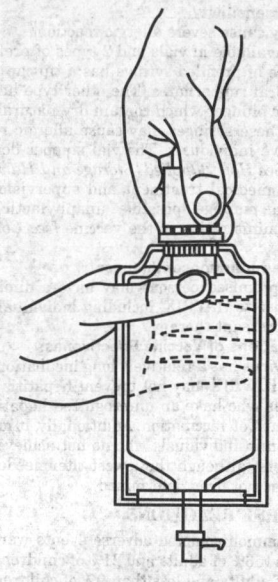

Figure 5

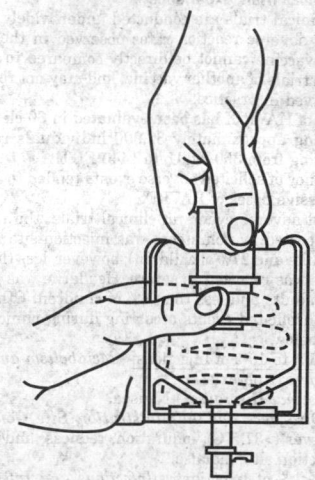

Figure 6

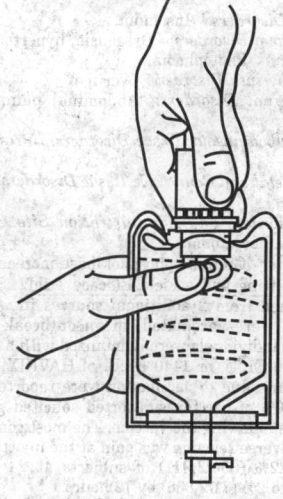

5. Insert piercing pin of administration set into port with a twisting motion until the pin is firmly seated.

Note: See full directions on administration set carton.

6. Lift the free end of the hanger loop on the bottom of the vial, breaking the two tie strings. Bend the loop outward to lock it in the upright position, then suspend container from hanger.

7. Squeeze and release drip chamber to establish proper fluid level in chamber.

8. Open flow control clamp and clear air from set. Close clamp.

9. Attach set to venipuncture device. If device is not indwelling, prime and make venipuncture.

10. Regulate rate of administration with flow control clamp.

WARNING: Do not use flexible container in series connections.

Pharmacy Bulk Package: 6 g

1. Insert the syringe needle through the vial closure and inject 26 mL of diluent. The vacuum may assist entry of the diluent. Remove the syringe needle.

2. Shake to dissolve; a clear solution containing approximately 1 g of ceftazidime activity per 5 mL will be obtained in 1 to 2 minutes.

3. Insert a gas-relief needle through the vial closure to relieve the internal pressure. Remove the gas-relief needle before extracting any solution.

Note: To preserve product sterility, it is important that a gasrelief needle is *not* inserted through the vial closure before the product has dissolved.

GlaxoSmithKline
Research Triangle Park, NC 27709
February 2007   RL-2357

HAVRIX®   ℞
[hav' rix]
(Hepatitis A Vaccine)
Suspension for Intramuscular Injection

HIGHLIGHTS OF PRESCRIBING INFORMATION
These highlights do not include all the information needed to use HAVRIX safely and effectively. See full prescribing information for HAVRIX.
HAVRIX (Hepatitis A Vaccine)
Suspension for Intramuscular Injection
Initial U.S. Approval: 1995

────────RECENT MAJOR CHANGES────────
Warnings and Precautions, Hypersensitivity (5.1) 07/2010

────────INDICATIONS AND USAGE────────
HAVRIX is a vaccine indicated for active immunization against disease caused by hepatitis A virus (HAV) for persons ≥12 months of age. Primary immunization should be administered at least 2 weeks prior to expected exposure to HAV. (1)

────────DOSAGE AND ADMINISTRATION────────
• Children and adolescents: A single 0.5-mL dose and a 0.5-mL booster dose administered between 6 to 12 months later. (2.2)
• Adults: A single 1-mL dose and a 1-mL booster dose administered between 6 to 12 months later. (2.2)
• For intramuscular use only. (2.2)

────────DOSAGE FORMS AND STRENGTHS────────
• HAVRIX is a sterile suspension available in the following presentations:
• 0.5-mL single-dose vials and prefilled syringes. (3, 11, 16)
• 1.0 mL single-dose vials and prefilled syringes. (3, 11, 16)

────────CONTRAINDICATIONS────────
Severe allergic reaction (e.g., anaphylaxis) after a previous dose of any hepatitis A-containing vaccine, or to any component of HAVRIX, including neomycin. (4)

────────WARNINGS AND PRECAUTIONS────────
• HAVRIX is available in vials and 2 types of prefilled syringes. One type of prefilled syringe has a tip cap which may contain natural rubber latex. The other type has a tip cap and a rubber plunger which contain dry natural latex rubber. Use of these syringes may cause allergic reactions in latex sensitive individuals (5.1, 16)
• Immunocompromised persons may have a diminished immune response to HAVRIX. (5.2)
• HAVRIX may not prevent hepatitis A infection in individuals with unrecognized hepatitis A infection at the time of vaccination. (5.3)

────────ADVERSE REACTIONS────────
The most common solicited adverse events were injection-site soreness (56% of adults and 21% of children) and headache (14% of adults and less than 9% of children). (6.1)

To report SUSPECTED ADVERSE REACTIONS, contact GlaxoSmithKline at 1-888-825-5249 or VAERS at 1-800-822-7967 or www.vaers.hhs.gov.

────────DRUG INTERACTIONS────────
• Do not mix HAVRIX with any other vaccine or product in the same syringe or vial. (7.1)
• HAVRIX may be given concurrently at different injection sites with (7.1):
  • INFANRIX® (Diphtheria and Tetanus Toxoids and Acellular Pertussis Vaccine Adsorbed (DTaP).
  • *Haemophilus influenzae* type b (Hib) conjugate vaccine (PRP-T).
  • pneumococcal 7-valent conjugate vaccine.
  • immune globulin.

────────USE IN SPECIFIC POPULATIONS────────
Safety and effectiveness of HAVRIX have not been established in pregnant women and nursing mothers. HAVRIX should only be given to a pregnant woman if clearly needed. (8.1)

See 17 for PATIENT COUNSELING INFORMATION
Revised 08/2010

FULL PRESCRIBING INFORMATION: CONTENTS*

*** Sections or subsections omitted from the full prescribing information are not listed**

FULL PRESCRIBING INFORMATION

1 INDICATIONS AND USAGE

HAVRIX® is indicated for active immunization against disease caused by hepatitis A virus (HAV) for persons equal to or older than 12 months of age. Primary immunization should be administered at least 2 weeks prior to expected exposure to HAV.

2 DOSAGE AND ADMINISTRATION

2.1 Preparation for Administration

Shake vial or syringe well before withdrawal and use. Parenteral drug products should be inspected visually for particulate matter and discoloration prior to administration, whenever solution and container permit. If either of these conditions exists, the vaccine should not be administered. With thorough agitation, HAVRIX is a homogeneous, turbid, white suspension. Do not administer if it appears otherwise.

2.2 Recommended Dose and Schedule

HAVRIX should be administered by intramuscular injection only. HAVRIX should not be administered in the gluteal region; such injections may result in suboptimal response.

Children and Adolescents: Primary immunization for children and adolescents (12 months through 18 years of age) consists of a single 0.5-mL dose and a 0.5-mL booster dose administered anytime between 6 and 12 months later in order to ensure the highest antibody titers. The preferred sites for intramuscular injections are the anterolateral aspect of the thigh in infants and young children or the deltoid muscle of the upper arm in older children.

Adults: Primary immunization for adults consists of a single 1-mL dose and a 1-mL booster dose administered anytime between 6 and 12 months later in order to ensure the highest antibody titers. In adults, the injection should be given in the deltoid region.

3 DOSAGE FORMS AND STRENGTHS

HAVRIX is a sterile suspension available in the following presentations:

- 0.5 mL single-dose vials and prefilled TIP-LOK® syringes.
- 1.0 mL single-dose vials and prefilled TIP-LOK® syringes.

[See Description (11) and How Supplied (16) for a listing of vaccine components.]

4 CONTRAINDICATIONS

Severe allergic reaction (e.g., anaphylaxis) after a previous dose of any hepatitis A-containing vaccine, or to any component of HAVRIX, including neomycin, is a contraindication to administration of HAVRIX *[see Description (11)]*.

5 WARNINGS AND PRECAUTIONS

5.1 Hypersensitivity

HAVRIX may cause severe allergic reaction.

HAVRIX is available in vials and 2 types of prefilled syringes. One type of prefilled syringe has a tip cap which may contain natural rubber latex. The other type has a tip cap and a rubber plunger which contain dry natural latex rubber. Use of these syringes may cause allergic reactions in latex sensitive individuals. The vial stopper does not contain latex. *[See How Supplied/Storage and Handling (16).]*

Appropriate medical treatment and supervision must be available to manage possible anaphylactic reactions following administration of the vaccine *[see Contraindications (4)]*.

5.2 Altered Immunocompetence

Immunocompromised persons may have a diminished immune response to HAVRIX, including individuals receiving immunosuppressant therapy.

5.3 Limitations of Vaccine Effectiveness

Hepatitis A virus has a relatively long incubation period (15 to 50 days). HAVRIX may not prevent hepatitis A infection in individuals who have an unrecognized hepatitis A infection at the time of vaccination. Additionally, it may not prevent infection in individuals who do not achieve protective antibody titers (although the lowest titer needed to confer protection has not been determined).

6 ADVERSE REACTIONS

The most common solicited adverse events were injection-site soreness (56% of adults and 21% of children) and headache (14% of adults and less than 9% of children).

6.1 Clinical Trials Experience

Because clinical trials are conducted under widely varying conditions, adverse reaction rates observed in the clinical trials of a vaccine cannot be directly compared to rates in the clinical trials of another vaccine, and may not reflect the rates observed in practice.

The safety of HAVRIX has been evaluated in 60 clinical trials involving approximately 32,900 individuals receiving doses ranging from 360 EL.U. to 1440 EL.U.

The frequency of solicited adverse events tended to decrease with successive doses of HAVRIX.

Of solicited adverse events in clinical trials, the most frequently reported by volunteers was injection-site soreness (56% of adults and 21% of children); however, less than 0.5% of soreness was reported as severe. Headache was reported by 14% of adults and less than 9% of children. Other solicited and unsolicited events occurring during clinical trials are listed below.

Incidence 1% to 10% of Injections: *Metabolism and Nutrition Disorders:* Anorexia.

Gastrointestinal Disorders: Nausea.

General Disorders and Administration Site Conditions: Fatigue, fever (>37.5°C), induration, redness, and swelling of the injection site; malaise.

Incidence <1% of Injections: *Infections and Infestations:* Pharyngitis, upper respiratory tract infections.

Blood and Lymphatic System Disorders: Lymphadenopathy.

Psychiatric Disorders: Insomnia.

Nervous System Disorders: Dysgeusia, hypertonia.

Eye Disorders: Photophobia.

Ear and Labyrinth Disorders: Vertigo.

Gastrointestinal Disorders: Abdominal pain, diarrhea, vomiting.

Skin and Subcutaneous Tissue Disorders: Pruritus, rash, urticaria.

Musculoskeletal and Connective Tissue Disorders: Arthralgia, myalgia.

General Disorders and Administration Site Conditions: Injection site hematoma.

Investigations: Creatine phosphokinase increased.

Outbreak Setting and a Field Efficacy Trial: Safety data were obtained from 2 additional sources in which large populations were vaccinated. In an outbreak setting in which 4,930 individuals were immunized with a single dose of either 720 EL.U. or 1440 EL.U. of HAVRIX, no serious adverse events due to vaccination were reported. Overall, less than 10% of vaccinees reported solicited general adverse events following the vaccine. The most common solicited local adverse reaction was pain at the injection site, reported in 22% (650/2,911) of subjects at 24 hours and decreasing to 2% (71/2,838) by 72 hours.

In a field efficacy trial, 19,037 children received the 360 EL.U. dose of HAVRIX. The most commonly reported adverse events by children from 2 selected schools following administration of HAVRIX were injection-site pain (10%, 68/719) and tenderness (8%, 58/719), following first doses of HAVRIX. Pain was slightly higher following the first dose of HAVRIX (10%) compared to the group who received the comparison vaccine ENGERIX-B® (6%) but was similar between vaccines following the second dose (6% for both groups). Likewise, tenderness was slightly higher following the first dose of HAVRIX (8%) compared to the group who received the comparison vaccine ENGERIX-B (5%) but was similar between vaccines following the second dose (4% for both groups). The large trial further allowed for analysis of rare adverse events, including hospitalization and death. No significant differences were found between the cohorts.

HAVRIX 720 EL.U./0.5 mL at 11 Months of Age and Older: In a US multicenter study, parents/guardians recorded local and general adverse events on diary cards for 4 days (Days 0 to 3) after vaccination *[see Clinical Studies (14.2)]*. In the 3 groups of children who received HAVRIX alone, safety data were available for 723 children who received 1,396 documented doses of HAVRIX. Additional safety data were available for 181 children who received HAVRIX coadministered with INFANRIX® (Diphtheria and Tetanus Toxoids and Acellular Pertussis Vaccine Adsorbed) (DTaP) and *Haemophilus influenzae* type b (Hib) conjugate vaccine (tetanus toxoid conjugate) (PRP-T) (Sanofi Pasteur SA).

The following ranges of solicited adverse event rates were observed among 3 groups of children that received their first dose of HAVRIX alone at between 11 and 25 months of age: Injection site pain in 15 to 21% of subjects, redness in 16 to 21% of subjects, swelling in 8% of subjects, irritability in 24 to 36% of subjects, loss of appetite in 16 to 19% of subjects, drowsiness in 15 to 17% of subjects and fever (>39.5°C) in ≤2% of subjects. Following the booster dose of HAVRIX, among local reactions: Pain was reported in 16 to 21% of subjects, redness in 17 to 22%, swelling in 8 to 10% of subjects. Following the booster dose of HAVRIX, among general events, irritability was reported in 19 to 29% of subjects, loss of appetite in 14 to 18% of subjects, drowsiness in 13 to 16% of subjects and fever (>39.5°C) in ≤1% of subjects.

Drowsiness and loss of appetite occurred at higher rates in subjects 15 to 18 months of age who received Hib conjugate vaccine and INFANRIX concomitantly with HAVRIX as compared to subjects 15 to 18 months of age who received Hib conjugate vaccine and INFANRIX (drowsiness 34% and 22% and loss of appetite 29% and 19%, respectively). With the exception of fever (>39.5°C), the solicited general symptoms occurred at higher rates in subjects 15 to 18 months of age who received Hib conjugate vaccine and INFANRIX concomitantly with HAVRIX as compared to subjects 15 to 18 months of age who received HAVRIX alone (irritability 46% and 30%, drowsiness 34% and 17%, and loss of appetite 29% and 17%, respectively).

A febrile seizure was reported in an 18-month-old subject 2 days after receiving the first dose of HAVRIX. Other serious adverse events reported during the course of this study with the use of HAVRIX alone included a single case each of hepatitis ~5 months post dose 1, insulin-dependent diabetes ~4 months post dose 1, and Kawasaki's disease ~3½ months post dose 1. The association of these events with vaccination is unknown.

In an open-label, randomized, US multicenter study, children 15 months of age received the 2-dose series of HAVRIX. The second dose of HAVRIX was given 6 to 9 months after the first dose. One group received HAVRIX alone (n = 122); a second group received the first dose of HAVRIX coadministered with INFANRIX and Hib conjugate vaccine (PRP-T) (Sanofi Pasteur SA) (n = 129); and a third group received INFANRIX and Hib conjugate vaccine coadministered and the first dose of HAVRIX one month later (n = 115). *[See Clinical Studies (14.5)]*. The percentages of subjects for whom solicited local adverse events (days 0 to 3) were reported following the first dose of HAVRIX alone, HAVRIX coadministered with INFANRIX and Hib conjugate, and coadministration of INFANRIX and Hib conjugate were as follows: Pain (21%, 45%, 40%), redness (15%, 42%, 42%) and swelling (8%, 30%, 30%). The percentages of subjects for whom solicited local symptoms at the HAVRIX injection site were reported after the first dose of HAVRIX in the HAVRIX alone group compared to subjects who received HAVRIX coadministered with INFANRIX and Hib conjugate vaccine were as follows: Pain (21% versus 35%), redness (15% versus 30%), and swelling (8% versus 16%).

Solicited general adverse events (days 0 to 3) reported among children following the first dose of HAVRIX alone, HAVRIX coadministered with INFANRIX and Hib conjugate vaccine, and coadministration of INFANRIX and Hib conjugate vaccine were as follows: Irritability (33%, 43%, 34%), drowsiness (25%, 34%, 24%), loss of appetite (16%, 24%, 17%), and fever [>38.0°C] (8%, 16%, 19%).

In this trial, 14 subjects reported 24 serious adverse events, including 6 subjects in the HAVRIX group (status asthmaticus, asthma [2 events], failure to thrive, gastroenteritis, arthritis bacterial, developmental delay, expressive language disorder, dehydration [3 events]), 3 subjects in the group who received HAVRIX coadministered with INFANRIX and Hib conjugate vaccine (dehydration, gastroenteritis rotavirus, gastroenteritis, pyrexia, tachycardia), and 5 subjects in the group that received the INFANRIX and Hib conjugate vaccine followed by HAVRIX (bronchial hyperreactivity, respiratory distress, developmental delay, expressive language disorder, dehydration [2 events], gastroenteritis rotavirus, tonsillar hypertrophy). All events were reported as recovered or recovering by the end of the study. No fatalities occurred.

In another US multicenter study, children 15 months of age (range 14 to 16 months) received either HAVRIX coadministered with a US-licensed pneumococcal 7-valent conjugate vaccine (Wyeth Pharmaceuticals Inc.) followed by a second dose of HAVRIX 6 to 9 months later; HAVRIX administered alone followed by a second dose of HAVRIX 6 to 9 months later; or pneumococcal 7-valent conjugate vaccine administered alone followed by a first dose of HAVRIX one month later and a second dose of HAVRIX 6 to 9 months after the first [see Clinical Studies (14.5)]. Parents/guardians recorded local and general symptoms on diary cards for 4 days (Days 0 to 3) after vaccination.

Solicited local adverse events were reported as follows among children who received the first dose of HAVRIX coadministered with pneumococcal 7-valent conjugate vaccine: Pain was reported in 36% of subjects, redness in 41% of subjects, and swelling in 29% of subjects. Reported rates of these local adverse events were similar to those in children who received the first dose of pneumococcal 7-valent conjugate vaccine alone (44%, 46%, and 27%, respectively). Among children who received the first dose of HAVRIX alone, pain was reported in 28% of subjects, redness in 22% of subjects, and swelling in 7% of subjects.

Solicited general adverse events were reported as follows among children who received the first dose of HAVRIX coadministered with pneumococcal 7-valent conjugate vaccine: Irritability was reported in 35% of subjects, drowsiness in 26% of subjects, loss of appetite in 25% of subjects, and fever in 14% of subjects. Reported rates of these general adverse events were similar to those in children who received the first dose of pneumococcal 7-valent conjugate vaccine alone (41%, 32%, 25%, and 16%, respectively). Among children who received the first dose of HAVRIX alone, irritability was reported in 35% of subjects, drowsiness in 29% of subjects, loss of appetite in 26% of subjects, and fever in 9% of subjects.

6.2 Postmarketing Experience

In addition to reports in clinical trials, worldwide voluntary reports of adverse events received for HAVRIX since market introduction of this vaccine are listed below. This list includes serious adverse events or events which have a suspected causal connection to components of HAVRIX or other vaccines or drugs. Because these events are reported voluntarily from a population of uncertain size, it is not always possible to reliably estimate their frequency or establish a causal relationship to the vaccine.

Infections and Infestations: Rhinitis.

Blood and Lymphatic System Disorders: Thrombocytopenia.

Immune System Disorders: Anaphylactic reaction, anaphylactoid reaction, serum sickness–like syndrome.

Nervous System Disorders: Convulsion, dizziness, encephalopathy, Guillain-Barré syndrome, hypoesthesia, multiple sclerosis, myelitis, neuropathy, paresthesia, somnolence, syncope.

Vascular Disorders: Vasculitis.

Respiratory, Thoracic, and Mediastinal Disorders: Dyspnea.

Hepatobiliary Disorders: Hepatitis, jaundice.

Skin and Subcutaneous Tissue Disorders: Angioedema, erythema multiforme, hyperhidrosis.

Congenital, Familial, and Genetic Disorders: Congenital anomaly.

Musculoskeletal and Connective Tissue Disorders: Musculoskeletal stiffness.

General Disorders and Administration Site Conditions: Chills, influenza-like symptoms, injection site reaction, local swelling.

7   DRUG INTERACTIONS

7.1   Concomitant Administration With Vaccines and Immune Globulin

HAVRIX may be given concurrently with INFANRIX (DTaP) and Hib conjugate vaccine (PRP-T) (Sanofi Pasteur SA) [see Adverse Reactions (6.1) and Clinical Studies (14.5)]. HAVRIX may be given concurrently with pneumococcal 7-valent conjugate vaccine (Wyeth Pharmaceuticals Inc.) [see Adverse Reactions (6.1) and Clinical Studies (14.5)]. HAVRIX may be administered concomitantly with immune globulin.

When concomitant administration of other vaccines or immune globulin is required, they should be given with different syringes and at different injection sites. Do not mix HAVRIX with any other vaccine or product in the same syringe or vial.

7.2   Immunosuppressive Therapies

Immunosuppressive therapies, including irradiation, antimetabolites, alkylating agents, cytotoxic drugs, and corticosteroids (used in greater than physiologic doses), may reduce the immune response to HAVRIX.

8   USE IN SPECIFIC POPULATIONS

8.1   Pregnancy

Pregnancy Category C

Animal reproduction studies have not been conducted with HAVRIX. It is also not known whether HAVRIX can cause fetal harm when administered to a pregnant woman or can affect reproduction capacity. HAVRIX should be given to a pregnant woman only if clearly needed.

8.3   Nursing Mothers

It is not known whether HAVRIX is excreted in human milk. Because many drugs are excreted in human milk, caution should be exercised when HAVRIX is administered to a nursing woman.

8.4   Pediatric Use

The safety and effectiveness of HAVRIX have been evaluated in 20,869 subjects 1 year to 18 years of age.

The safety and effectiveness of HAVRIX have not been established in subjects younger than 12 months of age.

8.5   Geriatric Use

Clinical studies of HAVRIX did not include sufficient numbers of subjects 65 years of age and older to determine whether they respond differently from younger subjects. Other reported clinical experience has not identified differences in overall safety between these subjects and younger adult subjects.

8.6   Hepatic Impairment

Subjects with chronic liver disease had a lower antibody response to HAVRIX than healthy subjects [see Clinical Studies (14.3)].

11   DESCRIPTION

HAVRIX (Hepatitis A Vaccine) is a sterile suspension of inactivated virus for intramuscular administration. The virus (strain HM175) is propagated in MRC-5 human diploid cells. After removal of the cell culture medium, the cells are lysed to form a suspension. This suspension is purified through ultrafiltration and gel permeation chromatography procedures. Treatment of this lysate with formalin ensures viral inactivation. Viral antigen activity is referenced to a standard using an enzyme linked immunosorbent assay (ELISA), and is therefore expressed in terms of ELISA Units (EL.U.).

Each 1-mL adult dose of vaccine contains 1440 EL.U. of viral antigen, adsorbed on 0.5 mg of aluminum as aluminum hydroxide.

Each 0.5-mL pediatric dose of vaccine contains 720 EL.U. of viral antigen, adsorbed onto 0.25 mg of aluminum as aluminum hydroxide.

HAVRIX contains the following excipients: Amino acid supplement (0.3% w/v) in a phosphate-buffered saline solution and polysorbate 20 (0.05 mg/mL). From the manufacturing process, HAVRIX also contains residual MRC-5 cellular proteins (not more than 5 mcg/mL), formalin (not more than 0.1 mg/mL), and neomycin sulfate (not more than 40 ng/mL), an aminoglycoside antibiotic included in the cell growth media.

HAVRIX is formulated without preservatives.

HAVRIX is available in vials and 2 types of prefilled syringes. One type of prefilled syringe has a tip cap which may contain natural rubber latex. The other type has a tip cap and a rubber plunger which contain dry natural latex rubber. The vial stopper does not contain latex. [See How Supplied/Storage and Handling (16).]

12   CLINICAL PHARMACOLOGY

12.1   Mechanism of Action

The hepatitis A virus belongs to the picornavirus family. It is one of several hepatitis viruses that cause systemic disease with pathology in the liver.

The incubation period for hepatitis A averages 28 days (range: 15 to 50 days).[1] The course of hepatitis A infection is extremely variable, ranging from asymptomatic infection to icteric hepatitis and death.

The presence of antibodies to HAV confers protection against hepatitis A infection. However, the lowest titer needed to confer protection has not been determined.

13   NONCLINICAL TOXICOLOGY

13.1   Carcinogenesis, Mutagenesis, Impairment of Fertility

HAVRIX has not been evaluated for its carcinogenic potential, mutagenic potential, or potential for impairment of fertility.

14   CLINICAL STUDIES

14.1   Pediatric Effectiveness Studies

Protective efficacy with HAVRIX has been demonstrated in a double-blind, randomized controlled study in school children (age 1 to 16 years) in Thailand who were at high risk of HAV infection. A total of 40,119 children were randomized to be vaccinated with either HAVRIX 360 EL.U. or ENGERIX-B at 0, 1, and 12 months. 19,037 children received a primary course (doses at 0 and 1 months) of HAVRIX and 19,120 children received a primary course (doses at 0 and 1 months) of ENGERIX-B. 38,157 children entered surveillance at day 138 and were observed for an

additional 8 months. Using the protocol-defined endpoint (≥2 days absence from school, ALT level >45 U/mL, and a positive result in the HAVAB-M test), 32 cases of clinical hepatitis A occurred in the control group. In the HAVRIX group, 2 cases were identified. These 2 cases were mild in terms of both biochemical and clinical indices of hepatitis A disease. Thus the calculated efficacy rate for prevention of clinical hepatitis A was 94% (95% Confidence Interval [CI]: 74, 98).

In outbreak investigations occurring in the trial, 26 clinical cases of hepatitis A (of a total of 34 occurring in the trial) occurred. No cases occurred in vaccinees who received HAVRIX.

Using additional virological and serological analyses post hoc, the efficacy of HAVRIX was confirmed. Up to 3 additional cases of mild clinical illness may have occurred in vaccinees. Using available testing, these illnesses could neither be proven nor disproven to have been caused by HAV. By including these as cases, the calculated efficacy rate for prevention of clinical hepatitis A would be 84% (95% CI: 60, 94).

In a study designed to interrupt an epidemic of hepatitis A among Native Americans in Alaska, vaccination with a single dose of HAVRIX (1440 EL.U./mL in adults, 720 EL.U./0.5 mL in children and adolescents) appeared to be efficacious.

14.2   Immunogenicity in Children and Adolescents

Immune Response to HAVRIX 720 EL.U./0.5 mL at 11 Months of Age and Older: In a prospective, open-label, multicenter study, 1,085 children were enrolled into one of 5 groups:

(1) Children 11 to 13 months of age who received HAVRIX on a 0- and 6-month schedule;
(2) Children 15 to 18 months of age who received HAVRIX on a 0- and 6-month schedule;
(3) Children 15 to 18 months of age who received HAVRIX coadministered with INFANRIX and Hib conjugate vaccine (PRP-T) (Sanofi Pasteur SA) at month 0 and HAVRIX at month 6;
(4) Children 15 to 18 months of age who received INFANRIX coadministered with Hib conjugate vaccine (PRP-T) (Sanofi Pasteur SA) at month 0 and HAVRIX at months 1 and 7;
(5) Children 23 to 25 months of age who received HAVRIX on a 0- and 6-month schedule.

Among subjects in all groups, 52% were male; 61% of subjects were white, 9% black, 3% Asian, and 27% were of other racial groups. The anti-hepatitis A antibody vaccine responses and GMTs, calculated on responders for groups 1, 2, and 5 are presented in Table 1. Vaccine response rates were similar among the 3 age groups that received HAVRIX. One month after the second dose of HAVRIX, the GMT in each of the younger age groups (11 to 13 and 15 to 18 months of age) was shown to be similar to that achieved in the 23 to 25 months of age group.

[See table 1 at top of next page]

Immune Response to HAVRIX 360 EL.U. at 2 Years of Age and Older: In 6 clinical studies of subjects 2 to 18 years of age (n = 762) who received 2 doses of HAVRIX (360 EL.U.) given 1 month apart, the GMT ranged from 197 to 660 mIU/mL. Ninety-nine percent of subjects seroconverted following 2 doses. When a booster (third) dose of HAVRIX 360 EL.U. was administered 6 months following the initial dose, all subjects were seropositive 1 month following the booster dose, with GMTs rising to a range of 3,388 to 4,643 mIU/mL. In 1 study in which children were followed for an additional 6 months, all subjects remained seropositive.

Immune Response to HAVRIX 720 EL.U./0.5 mL at 2 Years of Age and Older: In 4 clinical studies, children and adolescents (n = 314), ranging from 2 to 19 years of age, were immunized with 2 doses of HAVRIX 720 EL.U./0.5 mL given 6 months apart. One month after the first dose, seroconversion (anti-HAV ≥20 mIU/mL [lower limit of antibody measurement by assay]) ranged from 96.8% to 100%, with GMTs of 194 mIU/mL to 305 mIU/mL. In studies in which sera were obtained 2 weeks following the initial dose, seroconversion ranged from 91.6% to 96.1%. One month following a booster dose at month 6, all subjects were seropositive, with GMTs ranging from 2,495 mIU/mL to 3,644 mIU/mL. In an additional study in which the booster dose was delayed until 1 year following the initial dose, 95.2% of the subjects were seropositive just prior to administration of the booster dose. One month later, all subjects were seropositive, with a GMT of 2,657 mIU/mL.

Also, HAVRIX has been found to be efficacious in a clinical study of children at high risk of HAV infection [see Clinical Studies (14.1)].

14.3   Immunogenicity in Adults

Over 400 healthy adults 18 to 50 years of age in 3 clinical studies were given a single 1440 EL.U. dose of HAVRIX. All subjects were seronegative for hepatitis A antibodies at baseline. Specific humoral antibodies against HAV were elicited in more than 96% of subjects when measured 1 month after vaccination. By day 15, 80% to 98% of vaccinees had already seroconverted (anti-HAV ≥20 mIU/mL [lower limit of antibody measurement by assay]). GMTs of serocon-

Table 1. Anti-Hepatitis A Immune Response Following 2 Doses of HAVRIX 720 EL.U./0.5 mL Administered 6 Months Apart in Children Given the First Dose of HAVRIX at 11 to 13 Months of Age, 15 to 18 Months of Age, or 23 to 25 Months of Age

| Age group | N | Vaccine Response | | GMT (mIU/mL) |
		%	95% CI	
11-13 months (Group 1)	218	99	97, 100	1,461[a]
15-18 months (Group 2)	200	100	98, 100	1,635[a]
23-25 months (Group 5)	211	100	98, 100	1,911

Vaccine response = Seroconversion (anti-HAV ≥15 mIU/mL [lower limit of antibody measurement by assay]) in children initially seronegative or at least the maintenance of the pre-vaccination anti-HAV concentration in initially seropositive children.

CI = Confidence Interval; GMT = Geometric mean antibody titer.

[a] Calculated on vaccine responders one month post-dose 2. GMTs in children 11 to 13 months of age and 15 to 18 months of age were non-inferior (similar) to the GMT in children 23 to 25 months of age (i.e., the lower limit of the two-sided 95% CI on the GMT ratio for Group 1/Group 5 and for Group 2/Group 5 were both ≥0.5).

verters ranged from 264 to 339 mIU/mL at day 15 and increased to a range of 335 to 637 mIU/mL by 1 month following vaccination.

The GMTs obtained following a single dose of HAVRIX are at least several times higher than that expected following receipt of immune globulin.

In a clinical study using 2.5 to 5 times the standard dose of immune globulin (standard dose = 0.02 to 0.06 mL/kg), the GMT in recipients was 146 mIU/mL at 5 days post-administration, 77 mIU/mL at month 1, and 63 mIU/mL at month 2.

In 2 clinical trials in which a booster dose of 1440 EL.U. was given 6 months following the initial dose, 100% of vaccinees (n = 269) were seropositive 1 month after the booster dose, with GMTs ranging from 3,318 mIU/mL to 5,925 mIU/mL. The titers obtained from this additional dose approximate those observed several years after natural infection.

In a subset of vaccinees (n = 89), a single dose of HAVRIX 1440 EL.U. elicited specific anti-HAV neutralizing antibodies in more than 94% of vaccinees when measured 1 month after vaccination. These neutralizing antibodies persisted until month 6. One hundred percent of vaccinees had neutralizing antibodies when measured 1 month after a booster dose given at month 6.

Immunogenicity of HAVRIX was studied in subjects with chronic liver disease of various etiologies. 189 healthy adults and 220 adults with either chronic hepatitis B (n = 46), chronic hepatitis C (n = 104), or moderate chronic liver disease of other etiology (n = 70) were vaccinated with HAVRIX 1440 EL.U. on a 0- and 6-month schedule. The last group consisted of alcoholic cirrhosis (n = 17), autoimmune hepatitis (n = 10), chronic hepatitis/cryptogenic cirrhosis (n = 9), hemochromatosis (n = 2), primary biliary cirrhosis (n = 15), primary sclerosing cholangitis (n = 4), and unspecified (n = 13). At each time point, geometric mean antibody titers (GMTs) were lower for subjects with chronic liver disease than for healthy subjects. At month 7, the GMTs ranged from 478 mIU/mL (chronic hepatitis C) to 1,245 mIU/mL (healthy). One month after the first dose, seroconversion rates in adults with chronic liver disease were lower than in healthy adults. However, 1 month after the booster dose at month 6, seroconversion rates were similar in all groups; rates ranged from 94.7% to 98.1%. The relevance of these data to the duration of protection afforded by HAVRIX is unknown.

In subjects with chronic liver disease, local injection site reactions with HAVRIX were similar among all 4 groups, and no serious adverse events attributed to the vaccine were reported in subjects with chronic liver disease.

14.4 Duration of Immunity
The duration of immunity following a complete schedule of immunization with HAVRIX has not been established.

14.5 Immune Response to Concomitantly Administered Vaccines
Concomitant Administration With INFANRIX (DTaP) and Hib Conjugate Vaccine (PRP-T): In a US multicenter randomized study, 468 subjects, children 15 months of age (range 14 to 16 months) received either HAVRIX coadministered with INFANRIX (DTaP) and Hib conjugate vaccine (PRP-T) (Sanofi Pasteur SA) followed by a second dose of HAVRIX 6 to 9 months later (n = 127); INFANRIX and Hib conjugate vaccine alone followed by a first dose of HAVRIX one month later and a second dose of HAVRIX 6 to 9 months after the first (n = 132); or HAVRIX administered alone followed by a second dose of HAVRIX 6 to 9 months later (n = 135). Children had completed a primary series of diphtheria, tetanus, acellular pertussis, and Hib conjugate vaccines.

Seropositivity to HAV was defined as anti-HAV ≥15 mIU/mL [lower limit of antibody measurement by assay]. Results of analyses of the co-primary immunogenicity endpoints are as follows: One month after the second dose of HAVRIX, the seropositivity rate (100%, 84/84) in those receiving the first dose of HAVRIX coadministered with INFANRIX and Hib conjugate vaccine was shown to be non-inferior to that achieved (100%, 88/88) in children who received HAVRIX alone (lower limit of 95% CI on the difference of HAVRIX + INFANRIX + Hib conjugate vaccine minus HAVRIX >-5%). One month after the second dose of HAVRIX, anti-HAV GMTs were 1,904 mIU/mL for HAVRIX coadministered with INFANRIX and Hib conjugate vaccine and 1,700 mIU/mL for HAVRIX alone (non-inferior based on the lower limit of 95% CI for the adjusted GMT ratio [HAVRIX + INFANRIX + Hib conjugate vaccine: HAVRIX] ≥0.5).

One month after the first dose of HAVRIX coadministered with INFANRIX and Hib conjugate vaccine, seroprotection rates (≥0.1 mIU/mL) for diphtheria and tetanus were non-inferior to those achieved following INFANRIX and Hib conjugate vaccine alone (lower limit of 95% CI on the difference of HAVRIX + INFANRIX + Hib conjugate vaccine minus INFANRIX + Hib conjugate vaccine >-10%). For each of the pertussis antigens, vaccine response rates were non-inferior to those achieved following INFANRIX and Hib conjugate vaccine alone (antibody concentrations ≥5 EL.U./mL in subjects initially seronegative or post-vaccination antibody concentration ≥2 times the pre-vaccination antibody concentration in subjects initially seropositive; lower limit of 95% CI on the difference of HAVRIX + INFANRIX + Hib conjugate vaccine minus INFANRIX + Hib conjugate vaccine >-10%). GMTs for antibodies against each of the pertussis antigens following HAVRIX coadministered with INFANRIX and Hib conjugate vaccine were non-inferior to those following INFANRIX and Hib conjugate vaccine alone (lower limit of 95% CI for the adjusted GMT ratio [HAVRIX + INFANRIX + Hib conjugate vaccine:INFANRIX + Hib conjugate vaccine] ≥0.66). One month after vaccination, the anti-PRP seroprotection rate (≥1 mcg/mL) following HAVRIX coadministered with INFANRIX and Hib conjugate vaccine (100%, 90/90) was non-inferior to that achieved following INFANRIX and Hib conjugate vaccine alone (97.5%, 79/81) (lower limit of 95% CI on the difference of HAVRIX + INFANRIX + Hib conjugate vaccine minus INFANRIX + Hib conjugate vaccine >-10%).

Concomitant Administration With Pneumococcal 7-Valent Conjugate Vaccine: In a US multicenter study, children 15 months of age (range 14 to 16 months) received one of 3 regimens: (Group 1) HAVRIX coadministered with pneumococcal 7-valent conjugate vaccine (Wyeth Pharmaceuticals Inc.) followed by a second dose of HAVRIX 6 to 9 months later; (Group 2) HAVRIX administered alone followed by a second dose of HAVRIX 6 to 9 months later; or (Group 3) pneumococcal 7-valent conjugate vaccine administered alone followed by a first dose of HAVRIX one month later and a second dose of HAVRIX 6 to 9 months after the first. One month after the second dose, the anti-hepatitis A GMT of HAVRIX coadministered with pneumococcal 7-valent conjugate vaccine was non-inferior to HAVRIX given alone (Group 1 GMT = 1,518 mIU/mL; Group 2 GMT = 1,666 mIU/mL). The difference in anti-hepatitis A seropositivity rates between groups (HAVRIX coadministered with pneumococcal 7-valent conjugate vaccine minus HAVRIX alone) was marginally lower than the pre-defined non-inferiority limit of -5% (lower limit of the two-sided 95% CI -5.78%). However, in all 3 groups, the seropositivity rate ranged between 98% and 100% one month after the second dose of HAVRIX (Group 1, 93/94; Group 2, 106/106; Group 3, 113/115).

One month after vaccination, non-inferiority was demonstrated with respect to GMTs for anti-pneumococcal antibodies to all 7 serotypes after the coadministration of pneumococcal 7-valent conjugate vaccine with HAVRIX compared to pneumococcal 7-valent conjugate vaccine alone.

At least 98% of subjects who received pneumococcal 7-valent conjugate vaccine coadministered with HAVRIX and those who received pneumococcal 7-valent conjugate vaccine alone were seropositive for all 7 pneumococcal serotypes.

There are limited data on the coadministration of HAVRIX with other vaccines.

15 REFERENCES
1. Centers for Disease Control and Prevention. Prevention of hepatitis A through active or passive immunization: Recommendations of the Immunization Practices Advisory Committee (ACIP). MMWR 2006;55(RR-7):1-23.
2. Centers for Disease Control and Prevention. Update: Prevention of hepatitis A after exposure to hepatitis A virus and in international travelers. Updated Recommendations of the Advisory Committee on Immunization Practices (ACIP). MMWR 2007;56(41):1080-1084.

16 HOW SUPPLIED/STORAGE AND HANDLING
HAVRIX is available in single-dose vials (contain no latex) and prefilled TIP-LOK syringes (may contain latex) (packaged without needles) (Preservative Free Formulation):
720 EL.U./0.5 mL
NDC 58160-825-01 Vial (contains no latex) in Package of 10: NDC 58160-825-11
NDC 58160-825-43 Syringe (tip cap may contain latex) in Package of 10: NDC 58160-825-52
NDC 58160-825-41 Syringe (tip cap and plunger contain latex) in Package of 5: NDC 58160-825-46
NDC 58160-825-41 Syringe (tip cap and plunger contain latex) in Package of 10: NDC 58160-825-51
1440 EL.U./mL
NDC 58160-826-01 Vial (contains no latex) in Package of 10: NDC 58160-826-11
NDC 58160-826-43 Syringe (tip cap may contain latex) in Package of 5: NDC 58160-826-48
NDC 58160-826-32 Syringe (tip cap and plunger contain latex) in Package of 1: NDC 58160-826-32
NDC 58160-826-41 Syringe (tip cap and plunger contain latex) in Package of 5: NDC 58160-826-46
Store refrigerated between 2° and 8°C (36° and 46°F). Do not freeze. Discard if the vaccine has been frozen. Do not dilute to administer.

17 PATIENT COUNSELING INFORMATION
- Inform vaccine recipients and parents or guardians of the potential benefits and risks of immunization with HAVRIX.
- Emphasize, when educating vaccine recipients and parents or guardians regarding potential side effects, that HAVRIX contains non-infectious killed viruses and cannot cause hepatitis A infection.
- Instruct vaccine recipients and parents or guardians to report any adverse events to their healthcare provider.
- Give vaccine recipients and parents or guardians the Vaccine Information Statements, which are required by the National Childhood Vaccine Injury Act of 1986 to be given prior to immunization. These materials are available free of charge at the Centers for Disease Control and Prevention (CDC) website (www.cdc.gov/vaccines).

HAVRIX, ENGERIX-B, INFANRIX, and TIP-LOK are registered trademarks of GlaxoSmithKline.
Manufactured by **GlaxoSmithKline Biologicals**
Rixensart, Belgium, US License No. 1617
Distributed by **GlaxoSmithKline**
Research Triangle Park, NC 27709
©2010, GlaxoSmithKline. All rights reserved.
July 2010
HVX:33PI

HYCAMTIN® ℞
[hī-kam′ tin]
(topotecan)
Capsules

HIGHLIGHTS OF PRESCRIBING INFORMATION
These highlights do not include all the information needed to use HYCAMTIN capsules safely and effectively. See full prescribing information for HYCAMTIN capsules.
HYCAMTIN® (topotecan) Capsules
Initial U.S. Approval: 1996

> **WARNING: BONE MARROW SUPPRESSION**
> *See full prescribing information for complete boxed warning*
> HYCAMTIN should be administered only to patients with baseline neutrophil counts of ≥1,500 cells/mm³ and a platelet count ≥100,000 cells/mm³. In order to monitor the occurrence of bone marrow suppression, blood cell counts should be monitored (5.1).

---RECENT MAJOR CHANGES---

Warnings and Precautions, Interstitial Lung Disease (5.3)	06/2010

---INDICATIONS AND USAGE---

HYCAMTIN is a topoisomerase I inhibitor indicated for treatment of patients with relapsed small cell lung cancer. (1)

---DOSAGE AND ADMINISTRATION---

• 2.3 mg/m^2/day orally once daily for 5 consecutive days repeated every 21 days. (2)
• See dose modification guidelines for patients with bone marrow toxicity or Grade 3 or 4 diarrhea. (2.3)

---DOSAGE FORMS AND STRENGTHS---

0.25 mg and 1 mg capsules. (3)

---CONTRAINDICATIONS---

• History of severe hypersensitivity reactions (e.g., anaphylactoid reactions) to topotecan or to any of its ingredients. (4)
• Pregnancy or breastfeeding. (4)
• Severe bone marrow depression. (4)

---WARNINGS AND PRECAUTIONS---

• Bone marrow suppression. HYCAMTIN should be administered only to patients with adequate bone marrow reserves. Peripheral blood counts should be monitored. (5.1) Dose may need to be adjusted. (2.3)
• Topotecan-induced neutropenia can lead to neutropenic colitis. (5.1)
• Diarrhea, including severe diarrhea requiring hospitalization, has been reported during treatment with HYCAMTIN capsules. (5.2) Dose may need to be adjusted. (2.3)
• HYCAMTIN has been associated with reports of interstitial lung disease, some of which have been fatal. (5.3)
• Fetal harm may occur when administered to a pregnant woman. HYCAMTIN should not be used by pregnant women. (5.4)

---ADVERSE REACTIONS---

The most common Grade 3 or 4 hematologic adverse reactions with HYCAMTIN capsules were neutropenia (61%), anemia (25%), and thrombocytopenia (37%). The most common (≥10%) non-hematologic adverse reactions (all grades) were nausea (27%), diarrhea (14%), vomiting (19%), fatigue (11%), and alopecia (10%).

To report SUSPECTED ADVERSE REACTIONS, contact GlaxoSmithKline at 1-888-825-5249 or FDA at 1-800-FDA-1088 or www.fda.gov/medwatch.

---DRUG INTERACTIONS---

• Patients should be carefully monitored for adverse reactions when HYCAMTIN capsules are administered with a drug known to inhibit ABCG2 (BCRP) or ABCB1 (P-glycoprotein). (7.1)

---USE IN SPECIFIC POPULATIONS---

Geriatric use: Among patients who received HYCAMTIN capsules in 4 thoracic cancer studies, drug-related diarrhea was more frequent in patients ≥65 years of age (28%) compared to those <65 years of age (19%). (5.2) (6.1)

See 17 for PATIENT COUNSELING INFORMATION and FDA-approved patient labeling

Revised: June 2010

FULL PRESCRIBING INFORMATION: CONTENTS*
WARNING: BONE MARROW SUPPRESSION

FULL PRESCRIBING INFORMATION

> **WARNING: BONE MARROW SUPPRESSION**
> HYCAMTIN should be administered only to patients with baseline neutrophil counts of ≥1,500 cells/mm^3 and a platelet count ≥100,000 cells/mm^3. In order to assess the occurrence of bone marrow suppression, blood cell counts should be monitored.

1   INDICATIONS AND USAGE

HYCAMTIN capsules are indicated for the treatment of relapsed small cell lung cancer in patients with a prior complete or partial response and who are at least 45 days from the end of first-line chemotherapy.

2   DOSAGE AND ADMINISTRATION

2.1   Recommended Dosing

The recommended dose of HYCAMTIN capsules is 2.3 mg/m^2/day once daily for 5 consecutive days repeated every 21 days. Round the calculated oral daily dose to the nearest 0.25 mg, and prescribe the minimum number of 1 mg and 0.25 mg capsules. The same number of capsules should be prescribed for each of the 5 dosing days.

HYCAMTIN capsules may be taken with or without food. The capsules must be swallowed whole and must not be chewed, crushed, or divided. If your patient vomits after taking the dose of HYCAMTIN, the patient should not take a replacement dose.

2.2   Adjustment of Dose in Special Populations

Renal Function Impairment

No dosage adjustment of HYCAMTIN capsules appears to be required for treating patients with mild renal impairment (CLcr = 50-80 mL/min). A dose adjustment of HYCAMTIN capsules to 1.8 mg/m^2/day is predicted to adjust the area under the curve (AUC) to the normal range for patients with moderate renal impairment (CLcr = 30-49 mL/min). Insufficient data are available in patients with severe renal impairment (CLcr <30 mL/min) to provide a dosage recommendation for HYCAMTIN capsules [see Use in Specific Populations (8.6)].

2.3   Dose Modification Guidelines

Patients should not be treated with subsequent courses of HYCAMTIN until neutrophils recover to >1,000 cells/mm^3, platelets recover to >100,000 cells/mm^3, and hemoglobin levels recover to ≥9.0 g/dL (with transfusion if necessary). For patients who experience severe neutropenia (neutrophils <500 cells/mm^3 associated with fever or infection or lasting for 7 days or more) or neutropenia (neutrophils 500 to 1,000 cells/mm^3 lasting beyond day 21 of the treatment course), the HYCAMTIN capsules dose should be reduced by 0.4 mg/m^2/day for subsequent courses. Doses should be similarly reduced if the platelet count falls below 25,000 cells/mm^3.

For patients who experience Grade 3 or 4 diarrhea, the HYCAMTIN capsules dose should be reduced by 0.4 mg/m^2/day for subsequent courses [see Warnings and Precautions (5.2)]. Patients with Grade 2 diarrhea may need to follow the same dose modification guidelines.

3   DOSAGE FORMS AND STRENGTHS

HYCAMTIN capsules contain topotecan hydrochloride expressed as topotecan free base. The 0.25 mg capsules are opaque white to yellowish-white and imprinted with HYCAMTIN and 0.25 mg. The 1 mg capsules are opaque pink and imprinted with HYCAMTIN and 1 mg.

4   CONTRAINDICATIONS

HYCAMTIN is contraindicated in patients who have a history of severe hypersensitivity reactions (e.g., anaphylactoid reactions) to topotecan or to any of its ingredients.

HYCAMTIN should not be used in patients who are pregnant or breastfeeding, or in patients with severe bone marrow depression.

5   WARNINGS AND PRECAUTIONS

5.1   Bone Marrow Suppression

Bone marrow suppression (primarily neutropenia) is a dose-limiting toxicity of HYCAMTIN. Neutropenia is not cumulative over time. The following data on myelosuppression are based on an integrated safety database from 4 thoracic malignancy studies (N = 682) using HYCAMTIN capsules at 2.3 mg/m^2/day for 5 consecutive days. The median day for neutrophil, red blood cell, and platelet nadirs occurred on day 15.

Neutropenia

Grade 4 neutropenia (<500 cells/mm^3) occurred in 32% of patients with a median duration of 7 days and was most common during course 1 of treatment (20% of patients). Infection, sepsis, and febrile neutropenia occurred in 17%, 2%, and 4% of patients, respectively. Death due to sepsis occurred in 1% of patients. Pancytopenia has been reported. Topotecan-induced neutropenia can lead to neutropenic colitis. Fatalities due to neutropenic colitis have been reported. In patients presenting with fever, neutropenia, and a compatible pattern of abdominal pain, the possibility of neutropenic colitis should be considered. [See Dosage and Administration (2.3).]

Thrombocytopenia

Grade 4 thrombocytopenia (<10,000 cells/mm^3) occurred in 6% of patients, with a median duration of 3 days.

Anemia

Grade 3 or 4 anemia (<8 g/dL) occurred in 25% of patients.

Monitoring of Bone Marrow Function

HYCAMTIN should be administered only in patients with adequate bone marrow reserves, including a baseline neutrophil count of ≥1,500 cells/mm^3 and a platelet count ≥100,000 cells/mm^3. Frequent monitoring of peripheral blood cell counts should be instituted during treatment with HYCAMTIN.

5.2   Diarrhea

Diarrhea, including severe diarrhea requiring hospitalization, has been reported during treatment with HYCAMTIN capsules. Diarrhea related to HYCAMTIN capsules can occur at the same time as drug-related neutropenia and its sequelae. Communication with patients prior to drug administration regarding these side effects and proactive management of early and all signs and symptoms of diarrhea is important. Treatment-related diarrhea is associated with significant morbidity and may be life-threatening. Should diarrhea occur during treatment with HYCAMTIN capsules, physicians are advised to aggressively manage diarrhea. Clinical guidelines describing the aggressive management of diarrhea include specific recommendations on patient communication and awareness, recognition of early warning signs, use of anti-diarrheals and antibiotics, changes in fluid intake and diet, and need for hospitalization.

Of the 682 patients who received HYCAMTIN capsules in the 4 thoracic cancer studies, the overall incidence of drug-related diarrhea was 22%, including 4% with Grade 3 and 0.4% with Grade 4. Drug-related diarrhea was more frequent in patients ≥65 years of age (28%) compared to those <65 years of age (19%). [See Adverse Reactions (6.1) and Use in Specific Populations (8.5).]

5.3   Interstitial Lung Disease

HYCAMTIN has been associated with reports of interstitial lung disease (ILD), some of which have been fatal [see Adverse Reactions (6.2)]. Underlying risk factors include history of ILD, pulmonary fibrosis, lung cancer, thoracic exposure to radiation, and use of pneumotoxic drugs and/or colony stimulating factors. Patients should be monitored for pulmonary symptoms indicative of interstitial lung disease (e.g., cough, fever, dyspnea, and/or hypoxia), and HYCAMTIN should be discontinued if a new diagnosis of ILD is confirmed.

5.4   Pregnancy

Pregnancy Category D

HYCAMTIN may cause fetal harm when administered to a pregnant woman. The effects of topotecan on pregnant women have not been studied. Women should be warned to avoid becoming pregnant. [See Contraindications (4).] In rabbits, an IV dose of 0.10 mg/kg/day (about equal to the clinical IV dose on a mg/m^2 basis) given on days 6 through 20 of gestation caused maternal toxicity, embryolethality, and reduced fetal body weight. In the rat, an IV dose of 0.23 mg/kg/day (about equal to the clinical IV dose on a mg/m^2 basis) given for 14 days before mating through gestation day 6 caused fetal resorption, microphthalmia, preimplant loss, and mild maternal toxicity. An IV dose of 0.10 mg/kg/day (about half the clinical IV dose on a mg/m^2 basis) given to rats on days 6 through 17 of gestation caused an increase in post-implantation mortality. This dose also caused an increase in total fetal malformations. The most frequent malformations were of the eye (microphthalmia, anophthalmia, rosette formation of the retina, coloboma of the retina, ectopic orbit), brain (dilated lateral and third ventricles), skull, and vertebrae. If this drug is used during

Table 1. Incidence (≥5%) of Adverse Reactions in Small Cell Lung Cancer Patients Treated With HYCAMTIN Capsules Plus BSC and in 4 Thoracic Cancer Studies

Adverse Reaction	HYCAMTIN Capsules + BSC (N = 70)			HYCAMTIN Capsules Thoracic Cancer Population (N = 682)		
	All Grades (%)	Grade 3 (%)	Grade 4 (%)	All Grades (%)	Grade 3 (%)	Grade 4 (%)
Hematologic						
Anemia	94	15	10	98	18	7
Leukopenia	90	25	16	86	29	15
Neutropenia	91	28	33	83	24	32
Thrombocytopenia	81	30	7	81	29	6
Non-hematologic						
Nausea	27	1	0	33	3	0
Diarrhea	14	4	1	22	4	0.4
Vomiting	19	1	0	21	3	0.4
Alopecia	10	0	0	20	0.1	0
Fatigue	11	0	0	19	4	0.1
Anorexia	7	0	0	14	2	0
Asthenia	3	0	0	7	2	0
Pyrexia	7	1	0	5	1	1

BSC = Best Supportive Care.
N = total number of patients treated.
Adverse reactions were graded using NCI Common Toxicity Criteria.

pregnancy, or if a patient becomes pregnant while taking this drug, the patient should be apprised of the potential hazard to the fetus.

5.5 Drug Interactions
P-glycoprotein inhibitors (e.g., cyclosporine A, elacridar, ketoconazole, ritonavir, and saquinavir) can cause significant increases in topotecan exposure. The concomitant use of P-glycoprotein inhibitors with HYCAMTIN capsules should be avoided. *[See Drug Interactions (7.1).]*

6 ADVERSE REACTIONS
6.1 Clinical Trials Experience
The safety of HYCAMTIN capsules has been evaluated in 682 patients with thoracic cancer (3 recurrent small cell lung cancer [SCLC] studies and 1 recurrent non-small cell lung cancer [NSCLC] study) who received at least one dose of HYCAMTIN capsules. Because clinical trials are conducted under widely varying conditions, adverse reaction rates observed in the clinical trials of a drug cannot be directly compared to rates in the clinical trials of another drug and may not reflect the rates observed in practice.
Table 1 describes the hematologic and non-hematologic adverse reactions in recurrent SCLC patients treated with HYCAMTIN capsules plus best supportive care (BSC) and in the overall thoracic cancer patient population.
[See table 1 above]
Diarrhea Adverse Reactions
Of the 70 patients who received HYCAMTIN capsules plus BSC, the incidence of drug-related diarrhea was 14%, with 4% Grade 3 and 1% Grade 4.
In the 682 patients who received HYCAMTIN capsules in the 4 thoracic cancer studies, the incidence of drug-related diarrhea was 22%, with 4% Grade 3 and 0.4% Grade 4. The overall incidence of drug-related diarrhea was more frequent in patients ≥65 years of age (28%, n = 225) with 10% Grade 1, 9% Grade 2, 7% Grade 3, and 1% Grade 4 compared to those <65 years of age (19%, n = 457) with 7% Grade 1, 9% Grade 2, 3% Grade 3, and 0% Grade 4. The incidence of Grade 3 or 4 diarrhea proximate (within 5 days) to Grade 3 or 4 neutropenia events in the HYCAMTIN capsules treatment group was 5%. The median time to onset of Grade 2 or worse diarrhea was 9 days in the HYCAMTIN capsules group.
Deaths Occurring Within 30 Days Following the Last Dose of Study Medication
In the 682 patients who received HYCAMTIN capsules in the 4 thoracic cancer studies, 39 deaths occurred within 30 days after the last dose of study medication for a reason other than progressive disease; 13 of these deaths were attributed to hematologic toxicity, 5 were attributed to non-hematologic toxicity, and 21 were attributed to other causes.

One patient death (68 years of age) was attributed to treatment-related diarrhea and one death (68 years of age) attributed diarrhea as a contributory event; both patients received HYCAMTIN capsules.
In addition to the adverse reactions listed previously, the following adverse reactions have been reported with HYCAMTIN for Injection:
• Incidence >10%: Febrile neutropenia, abdominal pain, stomatitis, constipation.
• Incidence 1 to 10%: Sepsis, hypersensitivity (including rash), hyperbilirubinemia, malaise.

6.2 Postmarketing Experience
There is no postmarketing experience with HYCAMTIN capsules. The following adverse reactions have been identified during post-approval use of HYCAMTIN for Injection. Because these reactions are reported voluntarily from a population of uncertain size, it is not always possible to reliably estimate their frequency or establish a causal relationship to drug exposure.
Blood and lymphatic system disorders: Severe bleeding (in association with thrombocytopenia).
Immune system disorders: Allergic manifestations, anaphylactoid reactions.
Respiratory, thoracic, and mediastinal disorders: Interstitial lung disease.
Gastrointestinal disorders: Abdominal pain potentially associated with neutropenic colitis *[see Warnings and Precautions (5.1)].*
Skin and subcutaneous tissue disorders: Angioedema, severe dermatitis, severe pruritus.

7 DRUG INTERACTIONS
7.1 Drugs That Inhibit Drug Efflux Transporters
Topotecan is a substrate for both ABCB1 [P-glycoprotein (P-gp)] and ABCG2 (BCRP). Elacridar (inhibitor of ABCB1 and ABCG2) administered with HYCAMTIN capsules increased topotecan exposure to approximately 2.5-fold of control. Cyclosporine A (inhibitor of ABCB1, ABCC1 [MRP-1], and CYP3A4) with HYCAMTIN capsules increased topotecan exposure to 2- to 3-fold of control. Patients should be carefully monitored for adverse reactions when HYCAMTIN capsules are administered with a drug known to inhibit these transporters. *[See Clinical Pharmacology (12.3).]*

7.2 Effects of Topotecan on Drug Metabolizing Enzymes
In vitro inhibition studies using marker substrates known to be metabolized by human cytochromes P450 (CYP1A2, CYP2A6, CYP2C8/9, CYP2C19, CYP2D6, CYP2E, CYP3A, or CYP4A) or dihydropyrimidine dehydrogenase indicate that the activities of these enzymes were not altered by topotecan. Enzyme inhibition by topotecan has not been evaluated in vivo.

7.3 Effects of Other Drugs on Topotecan Pharmacokinetics
The pharmacokinetics of topotecan were generally unchanged when coadministered with ranitidine.

8 USE IN SPECIFIC POPULATIONS
8.1 Pregnancy
Pregnancy Category D. *[See Contraindications (4) and Warnings and Precautions (5.4).]*
8.3 Nursing Mothers
HYCAMTIN is contraindicated during breastfeeding *[see Contraindications (4)].*
Rats excrete high concentrations of topotecan into milk. Lactating female rats given 4.72 mg/m² IV (about twice the clinical dose on a mg/m² basis) excreted topotecan into milk at concentrations up to 48-fold higher than those in plasma. It is not known whether the drug is excreted in human milk. Breastfeeding should be discontinued when women are receiving HYCAMTIN.
8.4 Pediatric Use
Safety and effectiveness in pediatric patients have not been established.
8.5 Geriatric Use
Of the 682 patients with thoracic cancer in 4 clinical studies who received HYCAMTIN capsules, 33% (n = 225) were 65 years of age and older, while 4.8% (n = 33) were 75 years of age and older. Treatment-related diarrhea was more frequent in patients ≥65 years of age (28%) compared to those <65 years of age (19%). *[See Warnings and Precautions (5.2) and Adverse Reactions (6.1).]* Among patients ≥65 years of age, those receiving HYCAMTIN capsules plus BSC showed a survival benefit compared to those receiving BSC alone. There were no apparent differences in the pharmacokinetics of topotecan in elderly patients with creatinine clearance of ≥60 mL/minute *[see Clinical Pharmacology (12.3)].*
This drug is known to be excreted by the kidney, and the risk of toxic reactions to this drug may be greater in patients with impaired renal function *[see Dosage and Administration (2.2)].*
8.6 Renal Impairment
A cross-study analysis of data collected from 217 patients with advanced solid tumors indicated that exposure (AUC$_{0-\infty}$) to topotecan lactone, the pharmacologically active moiety, was 10% and 20% higher in patients with mild renal (CLcr = 50-80 mL/min) and moderate renal (CLcr = 30-49 mL/min) impairment, respectively, than in patients with normal renal function (CLcr >80 mL/min) *[see Dosage and Administration (2.2)].*
8.7 Hepatic Impairment
In a population pharmacokinetic analysis involving oral topotecan administered at doses of 0.15-2.7 mg/m²/day to 118 cancer patients, the pharmacokinetics of total topotecan did not differ significantly based on patient serum bilirubin, ALT, or AST. No dosage adjustment appeared to be required for patients with impaired hepatic function (serum bilirubin of >1.5 mg/dL).

10 OVERDOSAGE
There is no known antidote for overdosage with HYCAMTIN capsules. The primary anticipated complication of overdosage would consist of hematological toxicity. The patient should be observed closely for bone marrow suppression, and supportive measures (such as the prophylactic use of G-CSF and/or antibiotic therapy) should be considered.

11 DESCRIPTION
Topotecan hydrochloride is a semi-synthetic derivative of camptothecin and is an anti-tumor drug with topoisomerase I-inhibitory activity.
The chemical name for topotecan hydrochloride is (S)-10-[(dimethylamino)methyl]-4-ethyl-4,9-dihydroxy-1H-pyrano[3',4':6,7] indolizino [1,2-b]quinoline-3,14-(4H,12H)-dione monohydrochloride. It has the molecular formula $C_{23}H_{23}N_3O_5 \bullet HCl$ and a molecular weight of 457.9. It is soluble in water and melts with decomposition at 213° to 218°C.
Topotecan hydrochloride has the following structural formula:

HYCAMTIN capsules contain topotecan hydrochloride, the content of which is expressed as topotecan free base. The major excipients are hydrogenated vegetable oil, glyceryl monostearate, gelatin, and titanium dioxide. The capsules are imprinted with edible black ink. The 1 mg capsules also contain red iron oxide.

12 CLINICAL PHARMACOLOGY

12.1 Mechanism of Action

Topoisomerase I relieves torsional strain in DNA by inducing reversible single strand breaks. Topotecan binds to the topoisomerase I-DNA complex and prevents religation of these single strand breaks. The cytotoxicity of topotecan is thought to be due to double strand DNA damage produced during DNA synthesis, when replication enzymes interact with the ternary complex formed by topotecan, topoisomerase I, and DNA. Mammalian cells cannot efficiently repair these double strand breaks.

12.2 Pharmacodynamics

The dose-limiting toxicity of topotecan is leukopenia. White blood cell count decreases with increasing topotecan dose or topotecan AUC. There is a correlation between topotecan lactone AUC day 1 and percent decrease of leukocytes.

12.3 Pharmacokinetics

The pharmacokinetics of HYCAMTIN capsules after oral administration have been evaluated in cancer patients following doses of 1.2 to 3.1 mg/m^2 administered daily for 5 days. Topotecan exhibits biexponential pharmacokinetics with a mean terminal half-life of 3 to 6 hours. Total exposure (AUC) increases approximately proportionally with dose. Plasma protein binding of topotecan is about 35%.

Absorption

Topotecan is rapidly absorbed with peak plasma concentrations occurring between 1 to 2 hours following oral administration. The oral bioavailability of topotecan was about 40%. Following a high-fat meal, the extent of exposure was similar in the fed and fasted states, while t_{max} was delayed from 1.5 to 3 hours (topotecan lactone) and from 3 to 4 hours (total topotecan), respectively. HYCAMTIN capsules can be given without regard to food.

Following coadministration of the ABCG2 (BCRP) and ABCB1 (P-gp) inhibitor elacridar (GF120918) at 100 to 1,000 mg doses with oral topotecan, the $AUC_{0-\infty}$ of topotecan lactone and total topotecan increased approximately 2.5-fold.

Administration of oral cyclosporine A (15 mg/kg), an inhibitor of transporters ABCB1 (P-gp) and ABCC1 (MRP-1) as well as the metabolizing enzyme CYP3A4, within 4 hours of oral topotecan increased the dose-normalized AUC_{0-24} oftopotecan lactone and total topotecan to 2.0- to 3-fold of control. *[See Drug Interactions (7.1).]*

Metabolism and Elimination

Topotecan undergoes a reversible pH-dependent hydrolysis of its lactone moiety; it is the lactone form that is pharmacologically active. At pH ≤4, the lactone is exclusively present, whereas the ring-opened hydroxy-acid form predominates at physiologic pH. The mean metabolite:parent AUC ratio was <10% for total topotecan and topotecan lactone.

In a mass balance study in 4 patients with advanced solid tumors, the overall recovery of drug-related material following 5 daily doses of topotecan was 57% of the administered oral dose. In the urine, 20% of the oral administered dose was excreted as total topotecan and 2% was excreted as N-desmethyl topotecan *[see Use in Specific Populations (8.6)]*. Fecal elimination of total topotecan accounted for 33% while fecal elimination of N-desmethyl topotecan was 1.5%. Overall, the N-desmethyl metabolite contributed a mean of <6% (range 4 to 8%) of the total drug-related material accounted for in the urine and feces. O-glucuronides of both topotecan and N-desmethyl topotecan have been identified in the urine.

Age, Gender, and Race

A cross-study analysis in 217 patients with advanced solid tumors indicated that age and gender did not significantly affect the pharmacokinetics of oral topotecan. There are insufficient data to determine an effect of race on pharmacokinetics of oral topotecan.

13 NONCLINICAL TOXICOLOGY

13.1 Carcinogenesis, Mutagenesis, Impairment of Fertility

Carcinogenicity testing of topotecan has not been done. Nevertheless, topotecan is known to be genotoxic to mammalian cells and is a probable carcinogen. Topotecan was mutagenic to L5178Y mouse lymphoma cells and clastogenic to cultured human lymphocytes with and without metabolic activation. It was also clastogenic to mouse bone marrow. Topotecan did not cause mutations in bacterial cells.

Topotecan given to female rats prior to mating at a dose of 1.4 mg/m^2 IV (about 3/5th of the oral clinical dose on a mg/m^2 basis) caused superovulation possibly related to inhibition of follicular atresia. This dose given to pregnant female rats also caused increased pre-implantation loss. Studies in dogs given 0.4 mg/m^2 IV (about 1/6th the oral clinical dose on a mg/m^2 basis) of topotecan daily for a month suggest that treatment may cause an increase in the incidence of multinucleated spermatogonial giant cells in the testes. Topotecan may impair fertility in women and men.

14 CLINICAL STUDIES

14.1 Small Cell Lung Cancer

HYCAMTIN capsules were studied in patients with relapsed SCLC in a randomized, comparative, open label trial. The patients were prior responders (complete or partial) to first-line chemotherapy, were not considered candidates for standard intravenous chemotherapy, and had relapsed at least 45 days from the end of first-line chemotherapy. Seventy-one patients were randomized to HYCAMTIN capsules (2.3 mg/m^2/day administered for 5 consecutive days repeated every 21 days) and Best Supportive Care (BSC) and 70 patients were randomized to BSC alone. The primary objective was to compare the overall survival between the 2 treatment arms. Patients in the HYCAMTIN capsules plus BSC group received a median of 4 courses (range 1 to 10) and maintained a median dose intensity of HYCAMTIN capsules, 3.77 mg/m^2/week. The median patient age in the HYCAMTIN capsules plus BSC arm and the BSC alone treatment arm was 60 years and 58 years while the percentage of patients ≥65 years of age was 34% and 29%, respectively. All but 1 patient were Caucasian. The HYCAMTIN capsules plus BSC treatment arm included 68% of patients with extensive disease and 28% with liver metastasis. In the BSC alone arm, 61% of patients had extensive disease and 20% had liver metastases. Both treatment arms recruited 73% males. In the HYCAMTIN capsules plus BSC arm, 18% of patients had prior carboplatin and 62% had prior cisplatin. In the BSC alone arm, 26% of patients had prior carboplatin and 51% had prior cisplatin.

The HYCAMTIN capsules plus BSC arm showed a statistically significant improvement in overall survival compared with the BSC alone arm (Log-rank p = 0.0104). Survival results are shown in Table 2 and Figure 1.

Table 2. Overall Survival in Small Cell Lung Cancer Patients With HYCAMTIN Capsules Plus BSC Compared With BSC Alone

	Treatment Group	
	HYCAMTIN Capsules + BSC	BSC
	(N = 71)	(N = 70)
Median (weeks) (95% CI)	25.9 (18.3, 31.6)	13.9 (11.1, 18.6)
Hazard ratio (95% CI)	0.64 (0.45, 0.90)	
Log-rank p-value	0.0104	

BSC = Best Supportive Care.
N = total number of patients randomized.
CI = Confidence Interval.

Figure 1. Kaplan-Meier Estimates for Survival

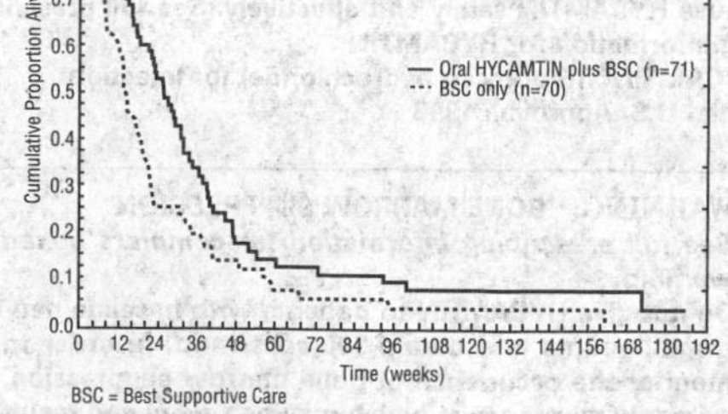

BSC = Best Supportive Care

15 REFERENCES

1. The National Institute for Occupational Safety and Health. NIOSH Alert. Preventing Occupational Exposures to Antineoplastic and Other Hazardous Drugs in Health Care Settings. Available at: www.cdc.gov/niosh/docs/2004-165/ Accessed October 2, 2007.
2. Occupational Safety and Health Administration. Controlling Occupational Exposure to Hazardous Drugs. OSHA Technical Manual, TED 1-0.15A. Section VI: Chapter 2. Available at: www.osha.gov/dts/osta/otm/otm_vi/otm_vi_2.html Accessed October 2, 2007.
3. American Society of Health-System Pharmacists. ASHP Guidelines on Handling Hazardous Drugs. *Am J Health-Syst Pharm.* 2006;63:1172-1193.
4. Polovich, M., White, J.M., Kelleher, L.O., eds. *Chemotherapy and Biotherapy Guidelines and Recommendations for Practice.* 2nd ed. Pittsburgh, PA: Oncology Nursing Society: 2005.

16 HOW SUPPLIED/STORAGE AND HANDLING

The 0.25 mg HYCAMTIN capsules are opaque white to yellowish-white imprinted with HYCAMTIN and 0.25 mg and are available in bottles of 10: NDC 0007-4205-11.

The 1 mg HYCAMTIN capsules are opaque pink imprinted with HYCAMTIN and 1 mg and are available in bottles of 10: NDC 0007-4207-11.

Store refrigerated 2° to 8°C (36° to 46°F). Store the bottles protected from light in the original outer cartons.

Procedures for proper handling and disposal of anticancer drugs should be used. Several guidelines on this subject have been published.[1-4]

HYCAMTIN capsules should not be opened or crushed. Direct contact of the capsule contents with the skin or mucous membranes should be avoided. If such contacts occur, wash thoroughly with soap and water or wash the eyes immediately with gently flowing water for at least 15 minutes. Consult the healthcare provider in case of a skin reaction or if the drug gets in the eyes.

17 PATIENT COUNSELING INFORMATION

See FDA-approved patient labeling (17.4).

17.1 Bone Marrow Suppression

Patients should be informed that HYCAMTIN decreases blood cell counts such as white blood cells, platelets, and red blood cells. Patients who develop fever or other signs of infection such as chills, cough, or burning pain on urination while on therapy should notify their physician promptly. Patients should be told that frequent blood tests will be performed while taking HYCAMTIN to monitor for the occurrence of bone marrow suppression.

17.2 Pregnancy

Patients should be advised to use effective contraceptive measures to prevent pregnancy and to avoid breastfeeding during treatment with HYCAMTIN.

17.3 Diarrhea

Patients should be informed that HYCAMTIN capsules cause diarrhea which may be severe in some cases. Patients should be told how to manage and/or prevent diarrhea and to inform their physician if severe diarrhea occurs during treatment with HYCAMTIN capsules.

17.4 FDA-Approved Patient Labeling

See separate leaflet.

HYCAMTIN is a registered trademark of GlaxoSmithKline.

GlaxoSmithKline
Research Triangle Park, NC 27709

©2010, GlaxoSmithKline. All rights reserved.

June 2010
HYC:4PI

PATIENT INFORMATION

HYCAMTIN® (hi-CAM-tin)
(topotecan) Capsules

Read the Patient Information that comes with HYCAMTIN capsules before you start taking it and each time you get a refill. There may be new information. This information does not take the place of talking with your healthcare provider about your medical condition or treatment.

What is the most important information I should know about taking HYCAMTIN capsules?

HYCAMTIN capsules can cause serious side effects:

Decreased blood counts. Taking HYCAMTIN affects your bone marrow and can cause a severe decrease in your blood cell counts (bone marrow suppression) - neutrophils (a type of white blood cell important in fighting bacterial infections), red blood cells (blood cells that carry oxygen to the tissues), and platelets (important for clotting and control of bleeding).

- You should have blood tests regularly to check your blood counts. A decrease in neutrophils (neutropenia) may affect how your body fights infection.
- Your healthcare provider will tell you if your blood counts are too low before you begin treatment with HYCAMTIN.
- Your dose of HYCAMTIN may need to be changed or stopped until your blood counts recover enough after each cycle of treatment.
- Call your healthcare provider right away if you get any of the following signs of infection:
  - fever (temperature of 100.5°F or greater)
  - chills
  - cough
  - burning or pain on urination
- Tell your healthcare provider about any abnormal bleeding or bruising.

Diarrhea. Diarrhea may occur from taking HYCAMTIN capsules, and may be serious enough that you must be treated in the hospital. Tell your healthcare provider right away if you have:

- diarrhea with fever
- diarrhea 3 or more times a day

- diarrhea with stomach-area pain or cramps

See "What are the possible side effects of HYCAMTIN capsules?"

What are HYCAMTIN capsules?

HYCAMTIN capsules are prescription medicines you take by mouth. HYCAMTIN capsules are used to treat a certain type of lung cancer called small cell lung cancer.

HYCAMTIN capsules may be right for you if:

- your cancer responded to your first chemotherapy
- your cancer came back at least 45 days after you finished your last dose of chemotherapy

HYCAMTIN capsules have not been studied in children.

Who should NOT take HYCAMTIN capsules?

Do not take HYCAMTIN capsules if:

- you are allergic to anything in HYCAMTIN capsules. See the end of this leaflet for a complete list of ingredients in HYCAMTIN capsules.
- the results of your last blood test show blood counts that are too low. Your healthcare provider will tell you.
- you are pregnant or think that you may be pregnant. Taking HYCAMTIN during pregnancy may harm your unborn baby. If you are able to become pregnant, talk with your healthcare provider about how to prevent pregnancy while taking HYCAMTIN.
- you are breastfeeding. Do not breastfeed while you are taking HYCAMTIN.

What else should I tell my healthcare provider before taking HYCAMTIN capsules?

Tell your healthcare provider about all the medicines you take, including prescription and non-prescription medicines, vitamins, and herbal supplements. HYCAMTIN capsules and other medicines may affect each other causing side effects. Especially tell your healthcare provider if you are taking cyclosporine (SANDIMMUNE, GENGRAF, NEORAL).

Know your medicines. Keep a list of your medicines and show it to your healthcare provider and pharmacist when you get a new medicine.

How should I take HYCAMTIN capsules?

- **Take HYCAMTIN capsules exactly as your doctor prescribes them.**
- Your healthcare provider may want you to take both 1 mg and 0.25 mg capsules together to make up your complete dose. You must be able to tell the difference between the capsules. The 1 mg capsule is a pink color and the 0.25 mg capsule is a white to yellowish-white color.
- Take HYCAMTIN capsules once a day for 5 days in a row. This treatment will normally be repeated every 3 weeks (a treatment cycle). Your healthcare provider will decide how long you will take HYCAMTIN capsules.
- Swallow HYCAMTIN capsules whole with water. Do not open, chew, or crush HYCAMTIN capsules. HYCAMTIN capsules may be taken with or without food.
- If any of the HYCAMTIN capsules are broken or leaking, do not touch them with your bare hands. Carefully dispose of the capsules, and then wash your hands well with soap and water.
- If you get any of the contents of HYCAMTIN capsules on your skin or in your eyes, do the following:
  - Wash the area of skin well with soap and water right away,
  - Wash your eyes right away with gently flowing water for at least 15 minutes.
  - Call your healthcare provider if you get a skin reaction or if you get the medicine in your eyes.
- If you take too much HYCAMTIN, contact your healthcare provider right away.
- If you forget to take HYCAMTIN at any time, do not double the dose to make up for a forgotten dose. Wait and take the next scheduled dose. Let your healthcare provider know that you missed a dose.
- If you vomit after taking your HYCAMTIN, do not take another dose on the same day. Let your healthcare provider know right away that you have vomited.

What should I avoid while taking HYCAMTIN capsules?

HYCAMTIN may make you feel drowsy or sleepy both during and for several days after treatment. If you feel tired or weak, do not drive and do not use heavy tools or operate machinery.

What are the possible side effects of HYCAMTIN capsules?

HYCAMTIN can cause serious side effects including decreased blood counts and diarrhea. See "What is the most important information I should know about HYCAMTIN capsules?"

The following side effects have been reported in patients taking HYCAMTIN capsules:

- stomach problems such as nausea (feeling sick) and vomiting
- tiredness
- hair loss
- weakness
- lung problems (may include being short of breath)

Tell your healthcare provider if you have any side effect that bothers you or does not go away. Your healthcare provider may change your dose of HYCAMTIN to a dose that is better for you or may stop your treatment with HYCAMTIN for a while. This can help reduce the side effects and may keep them from getting worse. Let your healthcare provider know if this helps or does not help your side effects.

How should I store HYCAMTIN capsules?

- Store HYCAMTIN capsules in a refrigerator. Protect from light and heat.
- Dispose of HYCAMTIN capsules that are out of date or no longer needed.
- **Keep HYCAMTIN capsules and all other medicines out of the reach of children.**

What are the ingredients in HYCAMTIN capsules?

Active Ingredient: Topotecan

Inactive Ingredients: Hydrogenated vegetable oil, glyceryl monostearate, gelatin, and titanium dioxide. The 1 mg capsules also contain red iron oxide. The capsules are imprinted with edible black ink.

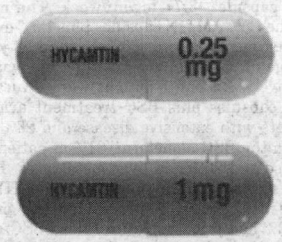

(capsules shown larger than actual size)

General information about HYCAMTIN capsules

Medicines are sometimes prescribed for conditions that are not mentioned in Patient Information leaflets. Only your doctor knows what treatment is best for you. Do not use HYCAMTIN capsules for a condition for which it was not prescribed by your healthcare provider. Do not give HYCAMTIN capsules to other people, even if they have the same condition that you have. It may harm them.

This leaflet summarizes the most important information about HYCAMTIN capsules. If you would like more information, talk with your healthcare provider. You can ask your pharmacist or healthcare provider for information about HYCAMTIN capsules that is written for health professionals. For more information you can call toll-free 1-888-825-5249 or visit www.gsk.com.

HYCAMTIN is a registered trademark of GlaxoSmithKline. The following are registered trademarks of their respective owners: GENGRAF/Abbott Laboratories; NEORAL and SANDIMMUNE/Novartis Pharmaceuticals Corporation.

GlaxoSmithKline

Research Triangle Park, NC 27709

©2010, GlaxoSmithKline. All rights reserved.

June 2010

HYC:4PIL

HYCAMTIN®   ℞

[hī-kam′tin]

(topotecan hydrochloride)
for Injection

HIGHLIGHTS OF PRESCRIBING INFORMATION

These highlights do not include all the information needed to use HYCAMTIN safely and effectively. See full prescribing information for HYCAMTIN.

HYCAMTIN® (topotecan hydrochloride) for Injection
Initial U.S. Approval: 1996

WARNING: BONE MARROW SUPPRESSION

See full prescribing information for complete boxed warning

Do not give HYCAMTIN to patients with baseline neutrophil counts less than 1,500 cells/mm³. In order to monitor the occurrence of bone marrow suppression, primarily neutropenia, which may be severe and result in infection and death, monitor peripheral blood cell counts frequently on all patients receiving HYCAMTIN. (5.1)

———INDICATIONS AND USAGE———

HYCAMTIN for Injection is a topoisomerase inhibitor indicated for:

- metastatic carcinoma of the ovary after failure of initial or subsequent chemotherapy. (1)
- small cell lung cancer sensitive disease after failure of first-line chemotherapy. (1)
- combination therapy with cisplatin for stage IV-B, recurrent, or persistent carcinoma of the cervix which is not amenable to curative treatment with surgery and/or radiation therapy. (1)

———DOSAGE AND ADMINISTRATION———

- Ovarian cancer and small cell lung cancer: 1.5mg/m² by intravenous infusion over 30 minutes daily for 5 consecutive days, starting on day one of a 21-day course. (2.1)
- Cervical cancer: 0.75mg/m² by intravenous infusion over 30 minutes on days 1, 2, and 3 followed by cisplatin 50mg/m² by intravenous infusion on day 1 repeated every 21 days. (2.2)

See Dosage Modification Guidelines for patients with neutropenia or reduced platelets. (2.1, 2.2)

See Dosage Adjustment in Renal Impairment. (2.3)

———DOSAGE FORMS AND STRENGTHS———

4-mg (free base) single-dose vial. (3)

———CONTRAINDICATIONS———

- History of severe hypersensitivity reactions (e.g., anaphylactoid reactions) to topotecan or any of its ingredients (4)
- Severe bone marrow depression (4)

———WARNINGS AND PRECAUTIONS———

- Bone marrow suppression: Administer HYCAMTIN only to patients with adequate bone marrow reserves. Monitor peripheral blood counts and adjust the dose if needed. (5.1)
- Topotecan-induced neutropenia can lead to neutropenic colitis. (5.2)
- Interstitial lung disease: HYCAMTIN has been associated with reports of interstitial lung disease. Monitor patients for symptoms and discontinue HYCAMTIN if the diagnosis is confirmed. (5.3)
- Pregnancy: Can cause fetal harm. Advise women of potential risk to the fetus. (5.4, 8.1)

———ADVERSE REACTIONS———

Ovarian and small cell lung cancer:

- The most common hematologic adverse reactions were: neutropenia (97%), leukopenia (97%), anemia (89%), and thrombocytopenia (69%). (6.1)
- The most common (>25%) non-hematologic adverse reactions (all grades) were: nausea, alopecia, vomiting, sepsis or pyrexia/infection with neutropenia, diarrhea, constipation, fatigue, and pyrexia. (6.1)

Cervical cancer (HYCAMTIN plus cisplatin):

- The most common hematologic adverse reactions (all grades) were: anemia (94%), leukopenia (91%), neutropenia (89%), and thrombocytopenia (74%). (6.1)
- The most common (>25%) non-hematologic adverse reactions (all grades) were: pain, nausea, vomiting, and infection/febrile neutropenia. (6.1)

To report SUSPECTED ADVERSE REACTIONS, contact GlaxoSmithKline at 1-888-825-5249 or FDA at 1-800-FDA-1088 or www.fda.gov/medwatch.

———DRUG INTERACTIONS———

- Do not initiate G-CSF until 24 hours after completion of treatment with HYCAMTIN. Concomitant administration can prolong duration of neutropenia. (7)
- Greater myelosuppression is likely to be seen when used in combination with other cytotoxic agents. (7)

———USE IN SPECIFIC POPULATIONS———

- Nursing Mothers: Discontinue nursing when receiving HYCAMTIN. (8.3)

See 17 for PATIENT COUNSELING INFORMATION

Revised: 04/2010

FULL PRESCRIBING INFORMATION: CONTENTS*

WARNING: BONE MARROW SUPPRESSION

FULL PRESCRIBING INFORMATION

> **WARNING: BONE MARROW SUPPRESSION**
> Do not give HYCAMTIN to patients with baseline neutrophil counts less than 1,500 cells/mm^3. In order to monitor the occurrence of bone marrow suppression, primarily neutropenia, which may be severe and result in infection and death, monitor peripheral blood counts frequently on all patients receiving HYCAMTIN [see Warnings and Precautions (5.1)].

1 INDICATIONS AND USAGE

HYCAMTIN is indicated for the treatment of:
• metastatic carcinoma of the ovary after failure of initial or subsequent chemotherapy.
• small cell lung cancer sensitive disease after failure of first-line chemotherapy. In clinical studies submitted to support approval, sensitive disease was defined as disease responding to chemotherapy but subsequently progressing at least 60 days (in the Phase 3 study) or at least 90 days (in the Phase 2 studies) after chemotherapy [see Clinical Studies (14)].

HYCAMTIN in combination with cisplatin is indicated for the treatment of:
• stage IV-B, recurrent, or persistent carcinoma of the cervix which is not amenable to curative treatment with surgery and/or radiation therapy.

2 DOSAGE AND ADMINISTRATION

Prior to administration of the first course of HYCAMTIN, patients must have a baseline neutrophil count of >1,500 cells/mm^3 and a platelet count of >100,000 cells/mm^3.

2.1 Ovarian Cancer and Small Cell Lung Cancer

Recommended Dosage:
• The recommended dose of HYCAMTIN is 1.5 mg/m^2 by intravenous infusion over 30 minutes daily for 5 consecutive days, starting on day 1 of a 21-day course.
• In the absence of tumor progression, a minimum of 4 courses is recommended because tumor response may be delayed. The median time to response in 3 ovarian clinical trials was 9 to 12 weeks, and median time to response in 4 small cell lung cancer trials was 5 to 7 weeks.

Dosage Modification Guidelines:
• In the event of severe neutropenia (defined as <500 cells/mm^3) during any course, reduce the dose by 0.25 mg/m^2 (to 1.25 mg/m^2) for subsequent courses.
• Alternatively, in the event of severe neutropenia, administer G-CSF (granulocyte-colony stimulating factor) following the subsequent course (before resorting to dose reduction) starting from day 6 of the course (24 hours after completion of topotecan administration).
• In the event the platelet count falls below 25,000 cells/mm^3, reduce doses by 0.25 mg/m^2 (to 1.25 mg/m^2) for subsequent courses.

2.2 Cervical Cancer

Recommended Dosage:
The recommended dose of HYCAMTIN is 0.75 mg/m^2 by intravenous infusion over 30 minutes daily on days 1, 2, and 3; followed by cisplatin 50 mg/m^2 by intravenous infusion on day 1 repeated every 21 days (a 21-day course).

Dosage Modification Guidelines:
Dosage adjustments for subsequent courses of HYCAMTIN in combination with cisplatin are specific for each drug. See manufacturer's prescribing information for cisplatin administration and hydration guidelines and for cisplatin dosage adjustment in the event of hematologic toxicity.
• In the event of severe febrile neutropenia (defined as <1,000 cells/mm^3 with temperature of 38.0°C or 100.4°F), reduce the dose of HYCAMTIN to 0.60 mg/m^2 for subsequent courses.
• Alternatively, in the event of severe febrile neutropenia, administer G-CSF following the subsequent course (before resorting to dose reduction) starting from day 4 of the course (24 hours after completion of administration of HYCAMTIN).
• If febrile neutropenia occurs despite the use of G-CSF, reduce the dose of HYCAMTIN to 0.45 mg/m^2 for subsequent courses.
• In the event the platelet count falls below 25,000 cells/mm^3, reduce doses to 0.60 mg/m^2 for subsequent courses.

2.3 Dosage Adjustment in Specific Populations

Renal Impairment:
No dosage adjustment of HYCAMTIN appears to be required for patients with mild renal impairment (Cl$_{cr}$ 40 to 60 mL/min.). Dosage adjustment of HYCAMTIN to 0.75 mg/m^2 is recommended for patients with moderate renal impairment (20 to 39 mL/min.). Insufficient data are available in patients with severe renal impairment to provide a dosage recommendation for HYCAMTIN [see Use in Specific Populations (8.6) and Clinical Pharmacology (12.3)].
HYCAMTIN in combination with cisplatin for the treatment of cervical cancer should only be initiated in patients with serum creatinine ≤1.5 mg/dL. In the clinical trial, cisplatin was discontinued for a serum creatinine >1.5 mg/dL. Insufficient data are available regarding continuing monotherapy with HYCAMTIN after cisplatin discontinuation in patients with cervical cancer.

2.4 Instructions for Handling, Preparation and Intravenous Administration

Handling:
HYCAMTIN is a cytotoxic anticancer drug. Prepare HYCAMTIN under a vertical laminar flow hood while wearing gloves and protective clothing. If HYCAMTIN solution contacts the skin, wash the skin immediately and thoroughly with soap and water. If HYCAMTIN contacts mucous membranes, flush thoroughly with water.
Use procedures for proper handling and disposal of anticancer drugs. Several guidelines on this subject have been published.[1-4]

Preparation and Administration:
Each 4-mg vial of HYCAMTIN is reconstituted with 4 mL Sterile Water for Injection. Then the appropriate volume of the reconstituted solution is diluted in either 0.9% Sodium Chloride Intravenous Infusion or 5% Dextrose Intravenous Infusion prior to administration.

Stability:
Unopened vials of HYCAMTIN are stable until the date indicated on the package when stored between 20° and 25°C (68° and 77°F) [see USP] and protected from light in the original package. Because the vials contain no preservative, contents should be used immediately after reconstitution. Reconstituted vials of HYCAMTIN diluted for infusion are stable at approximately 20° to 25°C (68° to 77°F) and ambient lighting conditions for 24 hours.

3 DOSAGE FORMS AND STRENGTHS

4-mg (free base) single-dose vial, light yellow to greenish powder.

4 CONTRAINDICATIONS

HYCAMTIN is contraindicated in patients who have a history of severe hypersensitivity reactions (e.g., anaphylactoid reactions) to topotecan or to any of its ingredients. HYCAMTIN should not be used in patients with severe bone marrow depression.

5 WARNINGS AND PRECAUTIONS

5.1 Bone Marrow Suppression

Bone marrow suppression (primarily neutropenia) is the dose-limiting toxicity of HYCAMTIN. Neutropenia is not cumulative over time. In the comparative study in small cell lung cancer, however, the treatment-related death rate was 1%. In the comparative study in small cell lung cancer, however, the treatment-related death rates were 5% for HYCAMTIN and 4% for CAV (cyclophosphamide-doxorubicin-vincristine).

Neutropenia:
• Ovarian and small cell lung cancer experience: Grade 4 neutropenia (<500 cells/mm^3) was most common during course 1 of treatment (60% of patients) and occurred in 39% of all courses, with a median duration of 7 days. The nadir neutrophil count occurred at a median of 12 days. Therapy-related sepsis or febrile neutropenia occurred in 23% of patients, and sepsis was fatal in 1%. Pancytopenia has been reported.
• Cervical cancer experience: Grade 3 and grade 4 neutropenia affected 26% and 48% of patients, respectively.

Thrombocytopenia:
• Ovarian and small cell lung cancer experience: Grade 4 thrombocytopenia (<25,000/mm^3) occurred in 27% of patients and in 9% of courses, with a median duration of 5 days and platelet nadir at a median of 15 days. Platelet transfusions were given to 15% of patients in 4% of courses.
• Cervical cancer experience: Grade 3 and grade 4 thrombocytopenia affected 26% and 7% of patients, respectively.

Anemia:
• Ovarian and small cell lung cancer experience: Grade 3/4 anemia (<8 g/dL) occurred in 37% of patients and in 14% of courses. Median nadir was at day 15. Transfusions were needed in 52% of patients in 22% of courses.
• Cervical cancer experience: Grade 3 and grade 4 anemia affected 34% and 6% of patients, respectively.

Monitoring of Bone Marrow Function:
Administer HYCAMTIN only in patients with adequate bone marrow reserves, including baseline neutrophil count of at least 1,500 cells/mm^3 and platelet count at least 100,000/mm^3. Monitor peripheral blood counts frequently during treatment with HYCAMTIN. Do not treat patients with subsequent courses of HYCAMTIN until neutrophils recover to >1,000 cells/mm^3, platelets recover to >100,000 cells/mm^3, and hemoglobin levels recover to 9.0 g/dL (with transfusion if necessary). Severe myelotoxicity has been reported when HYCAMTIN is used in combination with cisplatin [see Drug Interactions (7.1)].

5.2 Neutropenic Colitis

Topotecan-induced neutropenia can lead to neutropenic colitis. Fatalities due to neutropenic colitis have been reported in clinical trials with HYCAMTIN. In patients presenting with fever, neutropenia, and a compatible pattern of abdominal pain, consider the possibility of neutropenic colitis.

5.3 Interstitial Lung Disease

HYCAMTIN has been associated with reports of interstitial lung disease (ILD), some of which have been fatal [see Adverse Reactions (6.2)]. Underlying risk factors include history of ILD, pulmonary fibrosis, lung cancer, thoracic exposure to radiation, and use of pneumotoxic drugs and/or colony stimulating factors. Monitor patients for pulmonary symptoms indicative of interstitial lung disease (e.g., cough, fever, dyspnea, and/or hypoxia), and discontinue HYCAMTIN if a new diagnosis of ILD is confirmed.

5.4 Pregnancy

Pregnancy Category D
HYCAMTIN can cause fetal harm when administered to a pregnant woman.
Topotecan caused embryolethality, fetotoxicity, and teratogenicity in rats and rabbits when administered during organogenesis. There are no adequate and well controlled studies of HYCAMTIN in pregnant women. If this drug is used during pregnancy, or if a patient becomes pregnant while receiving HYCAMTIN, the patient should be apprised of the potential hazard to the fetus. [see Use in Specific Populations, Pregnancy (8.1)].

5.5 Inadvertent Extravasation

Inadvertent extravasation with HYCAMTIN has been observed, most reactions have been mild but severe cases have been reported.

6 ADVERSE REACTIONS

6.1 Clinical Trials Experience

Because clinical trials are conducted under widely varying conditions, adverse reaction rates observed in the clinical trials of a drug cannot be directly compared to rates in the clinical trials of another drug and may not reflect the rates observed in practice.

Ovarian Cancer and Small Cell Lung Cancer:
Data in the following section are based on the combined experience of 453 patients with metastatic ovarian carcinoma, and 426 patients with small cell lung cancer treated with HYCAMTIN. Table 1 lists the principal hematologic adverse reactions and Table 2 lists non-hematologic adverse reactions occurring in at least 15% of patients.

Table 1. Hematologic Adverse Reactions Experienced in ≥15% Ovarian Cancer and Small Cell Lung Cancer Patients Receiving HYCAMTIN

Hematologic Adverse Reaction	Patients (n = 879) % Incidence
Neutropenia	
<1,500 cells/mm^3	97
<500 cells/mm^3	78
Leukopenia	
<3,000 cells/mm^3	97
<1,000 cells/mm^3	32
Thrombocytopenia	
<75,000/mm^3	69
<25,000/mm^3	27

Anemia	
<10 g/dL	89
<8 g/dL	37

Table 2. Non-hematologic Adverse Reactions Experienced by ≥15% of Ovarian Cancer and Small Cell Lung Cancer Patients Receiving HYCAMTIN

Non-hematologic Adverse Reaction	Percentage of Patients with Adverse Reaction (879 Patients)		
	All Grades	Grade 3	Grade 4
Infections and infestations			
Sepsis or pyrexia/ infection with neutropenia[a]	43	NR	23
Metabolism and nutrition disorders			
Anorexia	19	2	<1
Nervous system disorders			
Headache	18	1	<1
Respiratory, thoracic, and mediastinal disorders			
Dyspnea	22	5	3
Coughing	15	1	0
Gastrointestinal disorders			
Nausea	64	7	1
Vomiting	45	4	1
Diarrhea	32	3	1
Constipation	29	2	1
Abdominal pain	22	2	2
Stomatitis	18	1	<1
Skin and subcutaneous tissue disorders			
Alopecia	49	NA	NA
Rash[b]	16	1	0
General disorders and administrative site conditions			
Fatigue	29	5	0
Pyrexia	28	1	<1
Pain[c]	23	2	1
Asthenia	25	4	2

NA = Not applicable
NR = Not reported separately
[a] Does not include Grade 1 sepsis or pyrexia.
[b] Rash also includes pruritus, rash erythematous, urticaria, dermatitis, bullous eruption, and maculopapular rash.
[c] Pain includes body pain, back pain, and skeletal pain.

Nervous System Disorders:
Paresthesia occurred in 7% of patients but was generally grade 1.
Hepatobiliary Disorders:
Grade 1 transient elevations in hepatic enzymes occurred in 8% of patients. Greater elevations, grade 3/4, occurred in 4%. Grade 3/4 elevated bilirubin occurred in <2% of patients.

Table 3 shows the grade 3/4 hematologic and major non-hematologic adverse reactions in the topotecan/paclitaxel comparator trial in ovarian cancer.

Table 3. Adverse Reactions Experienced by ≥5% of Ovarian Cancer Patients Randomized to Receive HYCAMTIN or Paclitaxel

Adverse Reaction	HYCAMTIN (n = 112)	Paclitaxel (n = 114)
Hematologic Grade 3/4	%	%
Grade 4 neutropenia (<500 cells/mm[3])	80	21
Grade 3/4 anemia (Hgb <8 g/dL)	41	6
Grade 4 thrombocytopenia (<25,000 plts/mm[3])	27	3
Pyrexia/Grade 4 neutropenia	23	4
Non-hematologic Grade 3/4	%	%
Infections and infestations		
Documented sepsis[a]	5	2
Respiratory, thoracic, and mediastinal disorders		
Dyspnea	6	5
Gastrointestinal disorders		
Abdominal pain	5	4
Constipation	5	0
Diarrhea	6	1
Intestinal obstruction	5	4
Nausea	10	2
Vomiting	10	3
General disorders and administrative site conditions		
Fatigue	7	6
Asthenia	5	3
Pain[b]	5	7

[a] Death related to sepsis occurred in 2% of patients receiving HYCAMTIN, and 0% of patients receiving paclitaxel.
[b] Pain includes body pain, skeletal pain, and back pain.

Table 4 shows the grade 3/4 hematologic and major non-hematologic adverse reactions in the topotecan/CAV comparator trial in small cell lung cancer.

Table 4. Adverse Reactions Experienced by ≥5% of Small Cell Lung Cancer Patients Randomized to Receive HYCAMTIN or CAV

Adverse Reaction	HYCAMTIN (n = 107)	CAV (n = 104)
Hematologic Grade 3/4	%	%
Grade 4 neutropenia (<500 cells/mm[3])	70	72
Grade 3/4 anemia (Hgb <8 g/dL)	42	20
Grade 4 thrombocytopenia (<25,000 plts/mm[3])	29	5
Pyrexia/Grade 4 neutropenia	28	26
Non-hematologic Grade 3/4	%	%
Infections and infestations		
Documented sepsis[a]	5	5
Respiratory, thoracic, and mediastinal disorders		
Dyspnea	9	14
Pneumonia	8	6
Gastrointestinal disorders		
Abdominal pain	6	4
Nausea	8	6
General disorders and administrative site conditions		
Fatigue	6	10
Asthenia	9	7
Pain[b]	5	7

[a] Death related to sepsis occurred in 3% of patients receiving HYCAMTIN, and 1% of patients receiving CAV.
[b] Pain includes body pain, skeletal pain, and back pain.

Cervical Cancer:
In the comparative trial with HYCAMTIN plus cisplatin versus cisplatin in patients with cervical cancer, the most common dose-limiting adverse reaction was myelosuppression. Table 5 shows the hematologic adverse reactions and Table 6 shows the non-hematologic adverse reactions in patients with cervical cancer.

Table 5. Hematologic Adverse Reactions in Patients with Cervical Cancer Treated with HYCAMTIN Plus Cisplatin or Cisplatin Monotherapy[a]

Hematologic Adverse Reaction	HYCAMTIN Plus Cisplatin (n = 140)	Cisplatin (n = 144)
Anemia		
All grades (Hgb <12 g/dL)	131 (94%)	130 (90%)
Grade 3 (Hgb <8-6.5 g/dL)	47 (34%)	28 (19%)
Grade 4 (Hgb <6.5 g/dL)	9 (6%)	5 (3%)
Leukopenia		
All grades (<3,800 cells/mm3)	128 (91%)	43 (30%)
Grade 3 (<2,000-1,000 cells/mm3)	58 (41%)	1 (1%)
Grade 4 (<1,000 cells/mm3)	35 (25%)	0 (0%)
Neutropenia		
All grades (<2,000 cells/mm3)	125 (89%)	28 (19%)
Grade 3 (<1,000-500 cells/mm3)	36 (26%)	1 (1%)
Grade 4 (<500 cells/mm3)	67 (48%)	1 (1%)
Thrombocytopenia		
All grades (<130,000 cells/mm3)	104 (74%)	21 (15%)
Grade 3 (<50,000-10,000 cells/mm3)	36 (26%)	5 (3%)
Grade 4 (<10,000 cells/mm3)	10 (7%)	0 (0%)

[a] Includes patients who were eligible and treated.

[See table 6 at top of next page]
6.2   Postmarketing Experience
In addition to adverse reactions reported from clinical trials or listed in other sections of the prescribing information, the following reactions have been identified during postmarketing use of HYCAMTIN. Because they are reported voluntarily from a population of unknown size, estimates of frequency cannot be made. These reactions have been chosen for inclusion due to a combination of their seriousness, frequency of reporting, or potential causal connection to HYCAMTIN.

Blood and Lymphatic System Disorders:
Severe bleeding (in association with thrombocytopenia) [see Warnings and Precautions (5.1)].
Immune System Disorders:
Allergic manifestations; Anaphylactoid reactions.
Gastrointestinal Disorders:
Abdominal pain potentially associated with neutropenic colitis [see Warnings and Precautions (5.2)].
Pulmonary Disorders:
Interstitial lung disease [see Warnings and Precautions (5.3)].
Skin and Subcutaneous Tissue Disorders:
Angioedema, severe dermatitis, severe pruritus.
General Disorders and Administrative Site Conditions:
Inadvertant extravastation [see Warnings and Precautions (5.5)].

7 DRUG INTERACTIONS

G-CSF: Concomitant administration of G-CSF can prolong the duration of neutropenia, so if G-CSF is to be used, do not initiat it until day 6 of the course of therapy, 24 hours after completion of treatment with HYCAMTIN.

Platinum and Other Cytotoxic Agents: Myelosuppression was more severe when HYCAMTIN, at a dose of 1.25 mg/m^2/day for 5 days, was given in combination with cisplatin at a dose of 50 mg/m^2 in Phase 1 studies. In one study, 1 of 3 patients had severe neutropenia for 12 days and a second patient died with neutropenic sepsis.

Greater myelosuppression is also likely to be seen when HYCAMTIN is used in combination with other cytotoxic agents, thereby necessitating a dose reduction. However, when combining HYCAMTIN with platinum agents (e.g., cisplatin or carboplatin), a distinct sequence-dependent interaction on myelosuppression has been reported. Coadministration of a platinum agent on day 1 of dosing with HYCAMTIN required lower doses of each agent compared to coadministration on day 5 of the dosing schedule for HYCAMTIN.

For information on the pharmacokinetics, efficacy, safety, and dosing of HYCAMTIN at a dose of 0.75 mg/m^2/day on days 1, 2, and 3 in combination with cisplatin 50 mg/m^2 on day 1 for cervical cancer, see Dosage and Administration (2), Adverse Reactions (6), Clinical Pharmacology (12.3), and Clinical Studies (14).

8 USE IN SPECIFIC POPULATIONS

8.1 Pregnancy

Pregnancy Category D [see Warnings and Precautions (5.4)]. HYCAMTIN can cause fetal harm when administered to a pregnant woman. In rabbits, a dose of 0.10 mg/kg/day (about equal to the clinical dose on a mg/m^2 basis) given on days 6 through 20 of gestation caused maternal toxicity, embryolethality, and reduced fetal body weight. In the rat, a dose of 0.23 mg/kg/day (about equal to the clinical dose on a mg/m^2 basis) given for 14 days before mating through gestation day 6 caused fetal resorption, microphthalmia, pre-implant loss, and mild maternal toxicity. A dose of 0.10 mg/kg/day (about half the clinical dose on a mg/m^2 basis) given to rats on days 6 through 17 of gestation caused an increase in post-implantation mortality. This dose also caused an increase in total fetal malformations. The most frequent malformations were of the eye (microphthalmia, anophthalmia, rosette formation of the retina, coloboma of the retina, ectopic orbit), brain (dilated lateral and third ventricles), skull, and vertebrae.

There are no adequate and well controlled studies of HYCAMTIN in pregnant women. If this drug is used during pregnancy, or if a patient becomes pregnant while receiving HYCAMTIN, the patient should be apprised of the potential hazard to the fetus. [see Warnings and Precautions (5.4)]

8.3 Nursing Mothers

Rats excrete high concentrations of topotecan into milk. Lactating female rats given 4.72 mg/m^2 IV (about twice the clinical dose on a mg/m^2 basis) excreted topotecan into milk at concentrations up to 48-fold higher than those in plasma. It is not known whether the drug is excreted in human milk. Because many drugs are excreted in human milk and because of the potential for serious adverse reactions in nursing infants from HYCAMTIN, discontinue breastfeeding when women are receiving HYCAMTIN.

8.4 Pediatric Use

Safety and effectiveness in pediatric patients have not been established.

8.5 Geriatric Use

Of the 879 patients with metastatic ovarian cancer or small cell lung cancer in clinical studies of HYCAMTIN, 32% (n = 281) were 65 years of age and older, while 3.8% (n = 33) were 75 years of age and older. Of the 140 patients with stage IV-B, relapsed, or refractory cervical cancer in clinical studies of HYCAMTIN who received HYCAMTIN plus cisplatin in the randomized clinical trial, 6% (n = 9) were 65 years of age and older, while 3% (n = 4) were 75 years of age and older. No overall differences in effectiveness or safety were observed between these patients and younger adult patients, and other reported clinical experience has not

Table 6. Non-hematologic Adverse Reactions Experienced by ≥5% of Patients with Cervical Cancer Treated with HYCAMTIN Plus Cisplatin or Cisplatin Monotherapy[a]

Adverse Event	HYCAMTIN Plus Cisplatin (n = 140)			Cisplatin (n = 144)		
	All Grades[b]	Grade 3	Grade 4	All Grades[b]	Grade 3	Grade 4
General disorders and administrative site conditions						
Constitutional[c]	96 (69%)	11 (8%)	0	89 (62%)	17 (12%)	0
Pain[d]	82 (59%)	28 (20%)	3 (2%)	72 (50%)	18 (13%)	5 (3%)
Gastrointestinal disorders						
Vomiting	56 (40%)	20 (14%)	2 (1%)	53 (37%)	13 (9%)	0
Nausea	77 (55%)	18 (13%)	2 (1%)	79 (55%)	13 (9%)	0
Stomatitis-pharyngitis	8 (6%)	1 (<1%)	0	0	0	0
Other	88 (63%)	16 (11%)	4 (3%)	80 (56%)	12 (8%)	3 (2%)
Dermatology	67 (48%)	1 (<1%)	0	29 (20%)	0	0
Metabolic-Laboratory	55 (39%)	13 (9%)	7 (5%)	44 (31%)	14 (10%)	1 (<1%)
Genitourinary	51 (36%)	9 (6%)	9 (6%)	49 (34%)	7 (5%)	7 (5%)
Nervous system disorders						
Neuropathy	4 (3%)	1 (<1%)	0	3 (2%)	1 (<1%)	0
Other	49 (35%)	3 (2%)	1 (<1%)	43 (30%)	7 (5%)	2 (1%)
Infection-febrile neutropenia	39 (28%)	21 (15%)	5 (4%)	26 (18%)	11 (8%)	0
Cardiovascular	35 (25%)	7 (5%)	6 (4%)	22 (15%)	8 (6%)	3 (2%)
Hepatic	34 (24%)	5 (4%)	2 (1%)	23 (16%)	2 (1%)	0
Pulmonary	24 (17%)	4 (3%)	0	23 (16%)	5 (3%)	3 (2%)
Vascular disorders						
Hemorrhage	21 (15%)	8 (6%)	1 (<1%)	20 (14%)	3 (2%)	1 (<1%)
Coagulation	8 (6%)	4 (3%)	3 (2%)	10 (7%)	7 (5%)	0
Musculoskeletal	19 (14%)	3 (2%)	0	7 (5%)	1 (<1%)	1 (<1%)
Allergy-Immunology	8 (6%)	2 (1%)	1 (<1%)	4 (3%)	0	1 (<1%)
Endocrine	8 (6%)	0	0	4 (3%)	2 (1%)	0
Sexual reproduction function	7 (5%)	0	0	10 (7%)	1 (<1%)	0
Ocular-visual	7 (5%)	0	0	7 (5%)	1 (<1%)	0

Data were collected using NCI Common Toxicity Criteria, v. 2.0.
[a] Includes patients who were eligible and treated.
[b] Grades 1 through 4 only. There were 3 patients who experienced grade 5 deaths with investigator-designated attribution. One was a grade 5 hemorrhage in which the drug-related thrombocytopenia aggravated the event. A second patient experienced bowel obstruction, cardiac arrest, pleural effusion and respiratory failure which were not treatment related but probably aggravated by treatment. A third patient experienced a pulmonary embolism and adult respiratory distress syndrome, the latter was indirectly treatment-related.
[c] Constitutional includes fatigue (lethargy, malaise, asthenia), fever (in the absence of neutropenia), rigors, chills, sweating, and weight gain or loss.
[d] Pain includes abdominal pain or cramping, arthralgia, bone pain, chest pain (non-cardiac and non-pleuritic), dysmenorrhea, dyspareunia, earache, headache, hepatic pain, myalgia, neuropathic pain, pain due to radiation, pelvic pain, pleuritic pain, rectal or perirectal pain, and tumor pain.

identified differences in responses between the elderly and younger adult patients, but greater sensitivity of some older individuals cannot be ruled out.

There were no apparent differences in the pharmacokinetics of topotecan in elderly patients, once the age-related decrease in renal function was considered [see Clinical Pharmacology (12.3)].

This drug is known to be substantially excreted by the kidney, and the risk of toxic reactions to this drug may be greater in patients with impaired renal function. Because elderly patients are more likely to have decreased renal function, care should be taken in dose selection, and it may be useful to monitor renal function [see Dosage and Administration (2.3)].

8.6 Renal Impairment

No dosage adjustment of HYCAMTIN appears to be required for patients with mild renal impairment (Cl$_{cr}$ 40 to 60 mL/min.). Dosage reduction is recommended for patients with moderate renal impairment (Cl$_{cr}$ 20 to 39 mL/min.). Insufficient data are available in patients with severe renal

impairment to provide a dosage recommendation for HYCAMTIN. [see Dosage and Administration (2.3) and Clinical Pharmacology (12.3)].

10 OVERDOSAGE

There is no known antidote for overdosage with HYCAMTIN. The primary anticipated complication of overdosage would consist of bone marrow suppression.

One patient on a single-dose regimen of 17.5 mg/m^2 given on day 1 of a 21-day cycle had received a single dose of 35 mg/m^2. This patient experienced severe neutropenia (nadir of 320/mm^3) 14 days later but recovered without incident.

Observe patients closely for bone marrow suppression, and supportive measures (such as the prophylactic use of G-CSF and/or antibiotic therapy).

11 DESCRIPTION

HYCAMTIN (topotecan hydrochloride) is a semi-synthetic derivative of camptothecin and is an anti-tumor drug with topoisomerase I-inhibitory activity.

HYCAMTIN for Injection is supplied as a sterile lyophilized, buffered, light yellow to greenish powder available in single-dose vials. Each vial contains topotecan hydrochloride equivalent to 4 mg of topotecan as free base. The reconstituted solution ranges in color from yellow to yellow-green and is intended for administration by intravenous infusion. Inactive ingredients are mannitol, 48 mg, and tartaric acid, 20 mg. Hydrochloric acid and sodium hydroxide may be used to adjust the pH. The solution pH ranges from 2.5 to 3.5.

The chemical name for topotecan hydrochloride is (S)-10-[(dimethylamino)methyl]-4-ethyl-4,9-dihydroxy-1H-pyrano[3′,4′:6,7] indolizino [1,2-b]quinoline-3,14-(4H,12H)-dione monohydrochloride. It has the molecular formula $C_{23}H_{23}N_3O_5 \cdot HCl$ and a molecular weight of 457.9.

Topotecan hydrochloride has the following structural formula:

It is soluble in water and melts with decomposition at 213° to 218°C.

12   CLINICAL PHARMACOLOGY

12.1   Mechanism of Action

Topoisomerase I relieves torsional strain in DNA by inducing reversible single strand breaks. Topotecan binds to the topoisomerase I-DNA complex and prevents religation of these single strand breaks. The cytotoxicity of topotecan is thought to be due to double strand DNA damage produced during DNA synthesis, when replication enzymes interact with the ternary complex formed by topotecan, topoisomerase I, and DNA. Mammalian cells cannot efficiently repair these double strand breaks.

12.2   Pharmacodynamics

The dose-limiting toxicity of topotecan is leukopenia. White blood cell count decreases with increasing topotecan dose or topotecan AUC. When topotecan is administered at a dose of 1.5 mg/m²/day for 5 days, an 80% to 90% decrease in white blood cell count at nadir is typically observed after the first cycle of therapy.

12.3   Pharmacokinetics

The pharmacokinetics of topotecan have been evaluated in cancer patients following doses of 0.5 to 1.5 mg/m² administered as a 30-minute infusion. Topotecan exhibits multiexponential pharmacokinetics with a terminal half-life of 2 to 3 hours. Total exposure (AUC) is approximately dose-proportional.

Distribution:
Binding of topotecan to plasma proteins is about 35%.

Metabolism:
Topotecan undergoes a reversible pH dependent hydrolysis of its lactone moiety; it is the lactone form that is pharmacologically active. At pH ≤ 4, the lactone is exclusively present, whereas the ring-opened hydroxy-acid form predominates at physiologic pH. In vitro studies in human liver microsomes indicate topotecan is metabolized to an N-demethylated metabolite. The mean metabolite:parent AUC ratio was about 3% for total topotecan and topotecan lactone following IV administration.

Excretion:
Renal clearance is an important determinant of topotecan elimination.

In a mass balance/excretion study in 4 patients with solid tumors, the overall recovery of total topotecan and its N-desmethyl metabolite in urine and feces over 9 days averaged 73.4 ± 2.3% of the administered IV dose. Mean values of 50.8 ± 2.9% as total topotecan and 3.1 ± 1.0% as N-desmethyl topotecan were excreted in the urine following IV administration. Fecal elimination of total topotecan accounted for 17.9 ± 3.6% while fecal elimination of N-desmethyl topotecan was 1.7 ± 0.6%. An O-glucuronidation metabolite of topotecan and N-desmethyl topotecan has been identified in the urine. These metabolites, topotecan-O-glucuronide and N-desmethyl topotecan-O-glucuronide, were less than 2% of the administered dose.

Effect of Gender:
The overall mean topotecan plasma clearance in male patients was approximately 24% higher than that in female patients, largely reflecting difference in body size.

Effect of Age:
Topotecan pharmacokinetics have not been specifically studied in an elderly population, but population pharmacokinetic analysis in female patients did not identify age as a significant factor. Decreased renal clearance, which is common in the elderly, is a more important determinant of topotecan clearance [see Dosage and Administration (2.3) and Use in Specific Populations (8.5)].

Effect of Race:
The effect of race on topotecan pharmacokinetics has not been studied.

Effect of Renal Impairment:
In patients with mild renal impairment (creatinine clearance of 40 to 60 mL/min.), topotecan plasma clearance was decreased to about 67% of the value in patients with normal renal function. In patients with moderate renal impairment (Cl_{cr} of 20 to 39 mL/min.), topotecan plasma clearance was reduced to about 34% of the value in control patients, with an increase in half-life. Mean half-life, estimated in 3 renally impaired patients, was about 5.0 hours. Dosage adjustment is recommended for these patients [see Dosage and Administration (2.3)].

Effect of Hepatic Impairment:
Plasma clearance in patients with hepatic impairment (serum bilirubin levels between 1.7 and 15.0 mg/dL) was decreased to about 67% of the value in patients without hepatic impairment. Topotecan half-life increased slightly, from 2.0 hours to 2.5 hours, but these hepatically impaired patients tolerated the usual recommended topotecan dosage regimen.

Drug Interactions:
Pharmacokinetic studies of the interaction of topotecan with concomitantly administered medications have not been formally investigated.

In vitro inhibition studies using marker substrates known to be metabolized by human P450 CYP1A2, CYP2A6, CYP2C8/9, CYP2C19, CYP2D6, CYP2E, CYP3A, or CYP4A or dihydropyrimidine dehydrogenase indicate that the activities of these enzymes were not altered by topotecan. Enzyme inhibition by topotecan has not been evaluated in vivo.

Cisplatin:
Administration of cisplatin (60 or 75 mg/m² on day 1) before topotecan (0.75 mg/m²/day on days 1 to 5) in 9 patients with ovarian cancer had no significant effect on the C_{max} and AUC of total topotecan.

Topotecan had no effect on the pharmacokinetics of free platinum in 15 patients with ovarian cancer who were administered cisplatin 50 mg/m² (n = 9) or 75 mg/m² (n = 6) on day 2 after paclitaxel 110 mg/m² on day 1 before topotecan 0.3 mg/m² IV daily on days 2-6. Topotecan had no effect on dose-normalized (60 mg/m²) C_{max} values of free platinum in 13 patients with ovarian cancer who were administered 60 mg/m² (n = 10) or 75 mg/m² (n = 3) cisplatin on day 1 before topotecan 0.75 mg/m² IV daily on days 1 to 5.

No pharmacokinetic data are available following topotecan (0.75 mg/m²/day for 3 consecutive days) and cisplatin (50 mg/m²/day on day 1) in patients with cervical cancer. Myelosuppression was more severe when HYCAMTIN was given in combination with cisplatin. [see Drug Interactions (7)].

13   NONCLINICAL TOXICOLOGY

13.1   Carcinogenesis, Mutagenesis, Impairment of Fertility

Carcinogenicity testing of topotecan has not been performed. Topotecan is known to be genotoxic to mammalian cells and is a probable carcinogen. Topotecan was mutagenic to L5178Y mouse lymphoma cells and clastogenic to cultured human lymphocytes with and without metabolic activation. It was also clastogenic to mouse bone marrow. Topotecan did not cause mutations in bacterial cells.

Topotecan given to female rats prior to mating at a dose of 1.4 mg/m² IV (about equal to the clinical dose on a mg/m² basis) caused superovulation possibly related to inhibition of follicular atresia. This dose given to pregnant female rats also caused increased pre-implantation loss. Studies in dogs given 0.4 mg/m² IV (about 1/4th the clinical dose on a mg/m² basis) of topotecan daily for a month suggest that treatment may cause an increase in the incidence of multinucleated spermatogonial giant cells in the testes. Topotecan may impair fertility in women and men.

14   CLINICAL STUDIES

14.1   Ovarian Cancer

HYCAMTIN was studied in 2 clinical trials of 223 patients given topotecan with metastatic ovarian carcinoma. All patients had disease that had recurred on, or was unresponsive to, a platinum-containing regimen. Patients in these 2 studies received an initial dose of 1.5 mg/m² given by intravenous infusion over 30 minutes for 5 consecutive days, starting on day 1 of a 21-day course.

One study was a randomized trial of 112 patients treated with HYCAMTIN (1.5 mg/m²/day × 5 days starting on day 1 of a 21-day course) and 114 patients treated with paclitaxel (175 mg/m² over 3 hours on day 1 of a 21-day course). All patients had recurrent ovarian cancer after a platinum-containing regimen or had not responded to at least 1 prior platinum-containing regimen. Patients who did not respond to the study therapy, or who progressed, could be given the alternative treatment.

Response rates, response duration, and time to progression are shown in Table 7.

Table 7. Efficacy of HYCAMTIN Versus Paclitaxel in Ovarian Cancer

Parameter	HYCAMTIN (n = 112)	Paclitaxel (n = 114)
Complete response rate	5%	3%
Partial response rate	16%	11%
Overall response rate	21%	14%
95% Confidence interval	13 to 28%	8 to 20%
(P-value)	(0.20)	
Response duration[a] (weeks)	n = 23	n = 16
Median	25.9	21.6
95% Confidence interval	22.1 to 32.9	16.0 to 34.0
hazard-ratio		
(HYCAMTIN:paclitaxel)	0.78	
(P-value)	(0.48)	
Time to progression (weeks)		
Median	18.9	14.7
95% Confidence interval	12.1 to 23.6	11.9 to 18.3
hazard-ratio		
(HYCAMTIN:paclitaxel)	0.76	
(P-value)	(0.07)	
Survival (weeks)		
Median	63.0	53.0
95% Confidence interval	46.6 to 71.9	42.3 to 68.7
hazard-ratio		
(HYCAMTIN:paclitaxel)	0.97	
(P-value)	(0.87)	

[a] The calculation for duration of response was based on the interval between first response and time to progression.

The median time to response was 7.6 weeks (range 3.1 to 21.7) with HYCAMTIN compared to 6.0 weeks (range 2.4 to 18.1) with paclitaxel. Consequently, the efficacy of HYCAMTIN may not be achieved if patients are withdrawn from treatment prematurely.

In the crossover phase, 8 of 61 (13%) patients who received HYCAMTIN after paclitaxel had a partial response and 5 of 49 (10%) patients who received paclitaxel after HYCAMTIN had a response (2 complete responses).

HYCAMTIN was active in ovarian cancer patients who had developed resistance to platinum-containing therapy, defined as tumor progression while on, or tumor relapse within 6 months after completion of, a platinum-containing regimen. One complete and 6 partial responses were seen in 60 patients, for a response rate of 12%. In the same study, there were no complete responders and 4 partial responders on the paclitaxel arm, for a response rate of 7%.

HYCAMTIN was also studied in an open-label, noncomparative trial in 111 patients with recurrent ovarian cancer after treatment with a platinum-containing regimen, or who had not responded to 1 prior platinum-containing regimen. The response rate was 14% (95% CI = 7% to 20%). The median duration of response was 22 weeks (range 4.6 to 41.9 weeks). The time to progression was 11.3 weeks (range 0.7 to 72.1 weeks). The median survival was 67.9 weeks (range 1.4 to 112.9 weeks).

14.2   Small Cell Lung Cancer

HYCAMTIN was studied in 426 patients with recurrent or progressive small cell lung cancer in 1 randomized, comparative study and in 3 single-arm studies.

Randomized Comparative Study:
In a randomized, comparative, Phase 3 trial, 107 patients were treated with HYCAMTIN (1.5 mg/m²/day × 5 days starting on day 1 of a 21-day course) and 104 patients were treated with CAV (1,000 mg/m² cyclophosphamide, 45 mg/m² doxorubicin, 2 mg vincristine administered sequentially on day 1 of a 21-day course). All patients were

considered sensitive to first-line chemotherapy (responders who then subsequently progressed ≥60 days after completion of first-line therapy). A total of 77% of patients treated with HYCAMTIN and 79% of patients treated with CAV received platinum/etoposide with or without other agents as first-line chemotherapy.

Response rates, response duration, time to progression, and survival are shown in Table 8.

Table 8. Efficacy of HYCAMTIN Versus CAV (cyclophosphamide-doxorubicin-vincristine) in Small Cell Lung Cancer Patients Sensitive to First-Line Chemotherapy

Parameter	HYCAMTIN (n = 107)	CAV (n = 104)
Complete response rate	0%	1%
Partial response rate	24%	17%
Overall response rate	24%	18%
Difference in overall response rates	6%	
95% Confidence interval of the difference	(−6 to 18%)	
Response duration[a] (weeks)	n = 26	n = 19
Median	14.4	15.3
95% Confidence interval	13.1 to 18.0	13.1 to 23.1
hazard-ratio		
(HYCAMTIN:CAV) (95% CI)	1.42 (0.73 to 2.76)	
(P-value)	(0.30)	
Time to progression (weeks)		
Median	13.3	12.3
95% Confidence interval	11.4 to 16.4	11.0 to 14.1
hazard-ratio		
(HYCAMTIN:CAV) (95% CI)	0.92 (0.69 to 1.22)	
(P-value)	(0.55)	
Survival (weeks)		
Median	25.0	24.7
95% Confidence interval	20.6 to 29.6	21.7 to 30.3
hazard-ratio		
(HYCAMTIN:CAV) (95% CI)	1.04 (0.78 to 1.39)	
(P-value)	(0.80)	

[a] The calculation for duration of response was based on the interval between first response and time to progression.

The time to response was similar in both arms: HYCAMTIN median of 6 weeks (range 2.4 to 15.7) versus CAV median 6 weeks (range 5.1 to 18.1).

Changes on a disease-related symptom scale in patients who received HYCAMTIN or who received CAV are presented in Table 9. It should be noted that not all patients had all symptoms, nor did all patients respond to all questions. Each symptom was rated on a 4-category scale with an improvement defined as a change in 1 category from baseline sustained over 2 courses. Limitations in interpretation of the rating scale and responses preclude formal statistical analysis.

[See table 9 above]

Single-Arm Studies:

HYCAMTIN was also studied in 3 open-label, noncomparative trials in a total of 319 patients with recurrent or progressive small cell lung cancer after treatment with first-line chemotherapy. In all 3 studies, patients were stratified as either sensitive (responders who then subsequently progressed ≥90 days after completion of first-line therapy) or refractory (no response to first-line chemotherapy or who

Table 9. Percentage of Patients With Symptom Improvement[a]: HYCAMTIN Versus CAV in Patients With Small Cell Lung Cancer

Symptom	HYCAMTIN (n = 107)		CAV (n = 104)	
	n[b]	(%)	n[b]	(%)
Shortness of breath	68	(28)	61	(7)
Interference with daily activity	67	(27)	63	(11)
Fatigue	70	(23)	65	(9)
Hoarseness	40	(33)	38	(13)
Cough	69	(25)	61	(15)
Insomnia	57	(33)	53	(19)
Anorexia	56	(32)	57	(16)
Chest pain	44	(25)	41	(17)
Hemoptysis	15	(27)	12	(33)

[a] Defined as improvement sustained over at least 2 courses compared to baseline.
[b] Number of patients with baseline and at least 1 post-baseline assessment.

responded to first-line therapy and then progressed within 90 days of completing first-line therapy). Response rates ranged from 11% to 31% for sensitive patients and 2% to 7% for refractory patients. Median time to progression and median survival were similar in all 3 studies and the comparative study.

14.3 Cervical Cancer

In a comparative trial, 147 eligible women were randomized to HYCAMTIN (0.75 mg/m²/day IV over 30 minutes × 3 consecutive days starting on day 1 of a 21-day course) plus cisplatin (50 mg/m² on day 1) and 146 eligible women were randomized to cisplatin (50 mg/m² IV on day 1 of a 21-day course). All patients had histologically confirmed Stage IV-B, recurrent, or persistent carcinoma of the cervix considered not amenable to curative treatment with surgery and/or radiation. Fifty-six percent (56%) of patients treated with HYCAMTIN plus cisplatin and 56% of patients treated with cisplatin had received prior cisplatin with or without other agents as first-line chemotherapy.

Median survival of eligible patients receiving HYCAMTIN plus cisplatin was 9.4 months (95% CI: 7.9 to 11.9) compared to 6.5 months (95% CI: 5.8 to 8.8) among patients randomized to cisplatin alone with a log rank P-value of 0.033 (significance level was 0.044 after adjusting for the interim analysis). The unadjusted hazard ratio for overall survival was 0.76 (95% CI: 0.59 to 0.98).

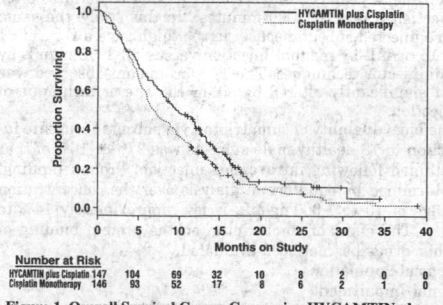

Number at Risk

HYCAMTIN plus Cisplatin	147	104	69	32	10	4	2	0	0
Cisplatin Monotherapy	146	93	52	14	8	2	1	0	0

Figure 1. Overall Survival Curves Comparing HYCAMTIN plus Cisplatin versus Cisplatin Monotherapy in Cervical Cancer Patients

15 REFERENCES

1. Preventing Occupational Exposures to Antineoplastic and Other Hazardous Drugs in Health Care Settings. NIOSH Alert 2004-165.
2. OSHA Technical Manual, TED 1-0.15A, Section VI: Chapter 2. Controlling Occupational Exposure to Hazardous Drugs. OSHA, 1999. http://www.osha.gov/dts/osta/otm/otm_vi/otm_vi_2.html
3. American Society of Health-System Pharmacists. ASHP Guidelines on Handling Hazardous Drugs. Am J Health-Syst Pharm. 2006;63:1172-1193.
4. Polovich M, White JM, Kelleher LO (eds.) 2005. Chemotherapy and Biotherapy Guidelines and Recommendations for Practice. (2nd ed) Pittsburgh, PA: Oncology Nursing Society.

16 HOW SUPPLIED/STORAGE AND HANDLING

HYCAMTIN for Injection is supplied in 4-mg (free base) single-dose vials.
NDC 0007-4201-01 (package of 1)
NDC 0007-4201-05 (package of 5)

Storage: Store the vials protected from light in the original cartons at controlled room temperature between 20° and 25°C (68° and 77°F) [see USP].

17 PATIENT COUNSELING INFORMATION

17.1 Bone Marrow Suppression

Inform patients that HYCAMTIN decreases blood cell counts such as white blood cells, platelets, and red blood cells. Patients who develop fever or other signs of infection (e.g., chills, cough, or burning pain on urination), while on therapy should notify their physician promptly. Inform patients that frequent blood tests will be performed while taking HYCAMTIN to monitor for the occurrence of bone marrow suppression.

17.2 Pregnancy and Breastfeeding

Advise patients to use effective contraceptive measures to prevent pregnancy and to avoid breastfeeding during treatment with HYCAMTIN.

17.3 Asthenia and Fatigue

Inform patients that HYCAMTIN may cause asthenia or fatigue. If these symptoms occur, caution should be observed when driving or operating machinery.

HYCAMTIN is a registered trademark of GlaxoSmithKline.

GlaxoSmithKline
Research Triangle Park, NC 27709
©2010, GlaxoSmithKline. All rights reserved.
April 2010
HYJ:20PI

IMITREX®

[ĭm' ĭ-trĕx]
(sumatriptan succinate)
Injection
For Subcutaneous Use Only.

DESCRIPTION

IMITREX (sumatriptan succinate) Injection is a selective 5-hydroxytryptamine₁ receptor subtype agonist. Sumatriptan succinate is chemically designated as 3-[2-(dimethylamino)ethyl]-N-methyl-indole-5-methanesulfonamide succinate (1:1), and it has the following structure:

$CH_3NHSO_2CH_2$ — ... — $CH_2CH_2N(CH_3)_2$ ... COOH CH₂ • CH₂ COOH

The empirical formula is $C_{14}H_{21}N_3O_2S•C_4H_6O_4$, representing a molecular weight of 413.5.

Sumatriptan succinate is a white to off-white powder that is readily soluble in water and in saline.

IMITREX Injection is a clear, colorless to pale yellow, sterile, nonpyrogenic solution for subcutaneous injection. Each 0.5 mL of IMITREX Injection 8 mg/mL solution contains 4 mg of sumatriptan (base) as the succinate salt and 3.8 mg of sodium chloride, USP in Water for Injection, USP. Each 0.5 mL of IMITREX Injection 12 mg/mL solution contains 6 mg of sumatriptan (base) as the succinate salt and 3.5 mg of sodium chloride, USP in Water for Injection, USP. The pH range of both solutions is approximately 4.2 to 5.3. The osmolality of both injections is 291 mOsmol.

Table 1. Dose Response Relationship for Efficacy

IMITREX Dose (mg)	% Patients With Relief[a] at 10 Minutes	% Patients With Relief[a] at 30 Minutes	% Patients With Relief[a] at 1 Hour	% Patients With Relief[a] at 2 Hours	Adverse Events Incidence (%)
Placebo	5	15	24	21	55
1	10	40	43	40	63
2	7	23	57	43	63
3	17	47	57	60	77
4	13	37	50	57	80
6	10	63	73	70	83
8	23	57	80	83	93

[a] Relief is defined as the reduction of moderate or severe pain to no or mild pain after dosing without use of rescue medication.

Table 2. Efficacy Data From US Phase III Trials

1-Hour Data	Study 1		Study 2	
	Placebo (n = 190)	IMITREX 6 mg (n = 384)	Placebo (n = 180)	IMITREX 6 mg (n = 350)
Patients with pain relief (grade 0/1)	18%	70%[a]	26%	70%[a]
Patients with no pain	5%	48%[a]	13%	49%
Patients without nausea	48%	73%[a]	50%	73%[a]
Patients without photophobia	23%	56%[a]	25%	58%*
Patients with little or no clinical disability[b]	34%	76%[a]	34%	76%[a]

2-Hour Data	Study 1		Study 2	
	Placebo[c]	IMITREX 6 mg[d]	Placebo[c]	IMITREX 6 mg[d]
Patients with pain relief (grade 0/1)	31%	81%[a]	39%	82%[a]
Patients with no pain	11%	63%[a]	19%	65%[a]
Patients without nausea	56%	82%[a]	63%	81%[a]
Patients without photophobia	31%	72%[a]	35%	71%[a]
Patients with little or no clinical disability[b]	42%	85%[a]	49%	84%[a]

[a] $p<0.05$ versus placebo.
[b] A successful outcome in terms of clinical disability was defined prospectively as ability to work mildly impaired or ability to work and function normally.
[c] Includes patients that may have received an additional placebo injection 1 hour after the initial injection.
[d] Includes patients that may have received an additional 6 mg of IMITREX Injection 1 hour after the initial injection.

CLINICAL PHARMACOLOGY

Mechanism of Action
Sumatriptan is a selective agonist for a vascular 5-hydroxytryptamine$_1$ receptor subtype (probably a member of the 5-HT$_{1D}$ family) with no significant affinity (as measured using standard radioligand binding assays) or pharmacological activity at 5-HT$_2$, 5-HT$_3$ receptor subtypes or at alpha$_1$-, alpha$_2$-, or beta-adrenergic; dopamine$_1$; dopamine$_2$; muscarinic; or benzodiazepine receptors.

The vascular 5-HT$_1$ receptor subtype to which sumatriptan binds selectively, and through which it presumably exerts its antimigrainous effect, is present on cranial arteries in both dog and primate, on the human basilar artery, and in the vasculature of the isolated dura mater of humans. In these tissues, sumatriptan activates this receptor to cause vasoconstriction, an action in humans correlating with the relief of migraine and cluster headache. In the anesthetized dog, sumatriptan selectively reduces the carotid arterial blood flow with little or no effect on arterial blood pressure or total peripheral resistance. In the cat, sumatriptan selectively constricts the carotid arteriovenous anastomoses while having little effect on blood flow or resistance in cerebral or extracerebral tissues.

Corneal Opacities
Dogs receiving oral sumatriptan developed corneal opacities and defects in the corneal epithelium. Corneal opacities were seen at the lowest dosage tested, 2 mg/kg/day, and were present after 1 month of treatment. Defects in the corneal epithelium were noted in a 60-week study. Earlier examinations for these toxicities were not conducted and no-effect doses were not established; however, the relative exposure at the lowest dose tested was approximately 5 times the human exposure after a 100-mg oral dose or 3 times the human exposure after a 6-mg subcutaneous dose.

Melanin Binding
In rats with a single subcutaneous dose (0.5 mg/kg) of radiolabeled sumatriptan, the elimination half-life of radioactivity from the eye was 15 days, suggesting that sumatriptan and its metabolites bind to the melanin of the eye. The clinical significance of this binding is unknown.

Pharmacokinetics
Pharmacokinetic parameters following a 6-mg subcutaneous injection into the deltoid area of the arm in 9 males (mean age: 33 years, mean weight: 77 kg) were systemic clearance: $1,194 \pm 149$ mL/min (mean $\pm$ S.D.), distribution half-life: 15 ± 2 minutes, terminal half-life: 115 ± 19 min-

utes, and volume of distribution central compartment: 50 ± 8 liters. Of this dose, $22\% \pm 4\%$ was excreted in the urine as unchanged sumatriptan and $38\% \pm 7\%$ as the indole acetic acid metabolite.

After a single 6-mg subcutaneous manual injection into the deltoid area of the arm in 18 healthy males (age: 24 ± 6 years, weight: 70 kg), the maximum serum concentration (C_{max}) was (mean $\pm$ standard deviation) 74 ± 15 ng/mL and the time to peak concentration (T_{max}) was 12 minutes after injection (range: 5 to 20 minutes). In this study, the same dose injected subcutaneously in the thigh gave a C_{max} of 61 ± 15 ng/mL by manual injection versus 52 ± 15 ng/mL by autoinjector techniques. The T_{max} or amount absorbed was not significantly altered by either the site or technique of injection.

The bioavailability of sumatriptan via subcutaneous site injection to 18 healthy male subjects was $97\% \pm 16\%$ of that obtained following intravenous injection. Protein binding, determined by equilibrium dialysis over the concentration range of 10 to 1,000 ng/mL, is low, approximately 14% to 21%. The effect of sumatriptan on the protein binding of other drugs has not been evaluated.

Special Populations

Renal Impairment
The effect of renal impairment on the pharmacokinetics of sumatriptan has not been examined, but little clinical effect would be expected as sumatriptan is largely metabolized to an inactive substance.

Hepatic Impairment
The effect of hepatic disease on the pharmacokinetics of subcutaneously and orally administered sumatriptan has been evaluated. There were no statistically significant differences in the pharmacokinetics of subcutaneously administered sumatriptan in hepatically impaired patients compared with healthy controls. However, the liver plays an important role in the presystemic clearance of orally administered sumatriptan. Accordingly, the bioavailability of sumatriptan following oral administration may be markedly increased in patients with liver disease. In 1 small study of hepatically impaired patients (N = 8) matched for sex, age, and weight with healthy subjects, the hepatically impaired patients had an approximately 70% increase in AUC and C_{max} and a T_{max} 40 minutes earlier compared with the healthy subjects.

Age
The pharmacokinetics of sumatriptan in the elderly (mean age: 72 years, 2 males and 4 females) and in patients with

migraine (mean age: 38 years, 25 males and 155 females) were similar to that in healthy male subjects (mean age: 30 years) (see PRECAUTIONS: Geriatric Use).

Race
The systemic clearance and C_{max} of sumatriptan were similar in black (n = 34) and Caucasian (n = 38) healthy male subjects.

Drug Interactions

Monoamine Oxidase Inhibitors
In vitro studies with human microsomes suggest that sumatriptan is metabolized by monoamine oxidase (MAO), predominantly the A isoenzyme. In a study of 14 healthy females, pretreatment with MAO-A inhibitor decreased the clearance of sumatriptan. Under the conditions of this experiment, the result was a 2-fold increase in the area under the sumatriptan plasma concentration × time curve (AUC), corresponding to a 40% increase in elimination half-life. No significant effect was seen with an MAO-B inhibitor.

Pharmacodynamics

Typical Physiologic Responses

Blood Pressure
See WARNINGS: Increase in Blood Pressure.

Peripheral (Small) Arteries
In healthy volunteers (N = 18), a study evaluating the effects of sumatriptan on peripheral (small vessel) arterial reactivity failed to detect a clinically significant increase in peripheral resistance.

Heart Rate
Transient increases in blood pressure observed in some patients in clinical studies carried out during sumatriptan's development as a treatment for migraine were not accompanied by any clinically significant changes in heart rate.

Respiratory Rate
Experience gained during the clinical development of sumatriptan as a treatment for migraine failed to detect an effect of the drug on respiratory rate.

CLINICAL TRIALS

Migraine
In US controlled clinical trials enrolling more than 1,000 patients during migraine attacks who were experiencing moderate or severe pain and 1 or more of the symptoms enumerated in Table 2, onset of relief began as early as 10 minutes following a 6-mg IMITREX Injection. Smaller doses of sumatriptan may also prove effective, although the proportion of patients obtaining adequate relief is decreased and the latency to that relief is greater.

In 1 well-controlled study where placebo (n = 62) was compared with 6 different doses of IMITREX Injection (n = 30 each group) in a single-attack, parallel-group design, the dose response relationship was found to be as shown in Table 1.

[See table 1 above]

In 2 US well-controlled clinical trials in 1,104 migraine patients with moderate or severe migraine pain, the onset of relief was rapid (less than 10 minutes) with IMITREX Injection 6 mg. Headache relief, as evidenced by a reduction in pain from severe or moderately severe to mild or no headache, was achieved in 70% of the patients within 1 hour of a single 6-mg subcutaneous dose of IMITREX Injection. Headache relief was achieved in approximately 82% of patients within 2 hours, and 65% of all patients were pain free within 2 hours.

Table 2 shows the 1- and 2-hour efficacy results for IMITREX Injection 6 mg.

[See table 2 above]

IMITREX Injection also relieved photophobia, phonophobia (sound sensitivity), nausea, and vomiting associated with migraine attacks. Similar efficacy was seen when patients self-administered IMITREX Injection using an autoinjector. The efficacy of IMITREX Injection is unaffected by whether or not migraine is associated with aura, duration of attack, gender or age of the patient, or concomitant use of common migraine prophylactic drugs (e.g., beta-blockers).

Cluster Headache
The efficacy of IMITREX Injection in the acute treatment of cluster headache was demonstrated in 2 randomized, double-blind, placebo-controlled, 2-period crossover trials. Patients age 21 to 65 were enrolled and were instructed to treat a moderate to very severe headache within 10 minutes of onset. Headache relief was defined as a reduction in headache severity to mild or no pain. In both trials, the proportion of individuals gaining relief at 10 or 15 minutes was significantly greater among patients receiving 6 mg of IMITREX Injection compared with those who received placebo (see Table 3). One study evaluated a 12-mg dose; there was no statistically significant difference in outcome between patients randomized to the 6- and 12-mg doses.

[See table 3 at top of next page]

The Kaplan-Meier (product limit) Survivorship Plot (Figure 1) provides an estimate of the cumulative probability of a patient with a cluster headache obtaining relief after being treated with either sumatriptan or placebo.

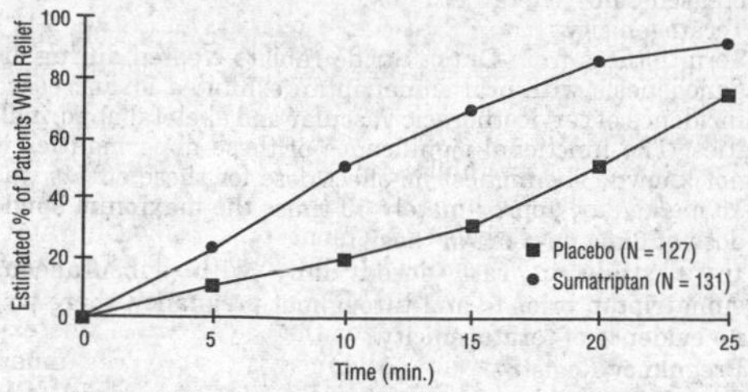

Figure 1. Time to Relief From Time of Injection[a]

[a]Patients taking rescue medication were censored at 15 minutes.

The plot was constructed with data from patients who either experienced relief or did not require (request) rescue medication within a period of 2 hours following treatment. As a consequence, the data in the plot are derived from only a subset of the 258 headaches treated (rescue medication was required in 52 of the 127 placebo-treated headaches and 18 of the 131 sumatriptan-treated headaches).

Other data suggest that treatment with sumatriptan is not associated with an increase in early recurrence of headache and has little effect on the incidence of latter-occurring headaches (i.e., those occurring after 2, but before 18 or 24 hours).

INDICATIONS AND USAGE

IMITREX Injection is indicated for 1) the acute treatment of migraine attacks with or without aura and 2) the acute treatment of cluster headache episodes.

IMITREX Injection is not for use in the management of hemiplegic or basilar migraine (see CONTRAINDICATIONS).

CONTRAINDICATIONS

IMITREX Injection should not be given intravenously because of its potential to cause coronary vasospasm.

IMITREX Injection should not be given to patients with history, symptoms, or signs of ischemic cardiac, cerebrovascular, or peripheral vascular syndromes. In addition, patients with other significant underlying cardiovascular diseases should not receive IMITREX Injection. Ischemic cardiac syndromes include, but are not limited to, angina pectoris of any type (e.g., stable angina of effort, vasospastic forms of angina such as the Prinzmetal variant), all forms of myocardial infarction, and silent myocardial ischemia. Cerebrovascular syndromes include, but are not limited to, strokes of any type as well as transient ischemic attacks. Peripheral vascular disease includes, but is not limited to, ischemic bowel disease (see WARNINGS: Other Vasospasm-Related Events and WARNINGS: Risk of Myocardial Ischemia and/or Infarction and Other Adverse Cardiac Events).

Because IMITREX Injection may increase blood pressure, it should not be given to patients with uncontrolled hypertension.

IMITREX Injection and any ergotamine-containing or ergot-type medication (like dihydroergotamine or methysergide) should not be used within 24 hours of each other, nor should IMITREX Injection and another 5-HT_1 agonist.

IMITREX Injection should not be administered to patients with hemiplegic or basilar migraine.

IMITREX Injection is contraindicated in patients with hypersensitivity to sumatriptan or any of its components.

IMITREX Injection is contraindicated in patients with severe hepatic impairment.

WARNINGS

IMITREX Injection should only be used where a clear diagnosis of migraine or cluster headache has been established. The prescriber should be aware that cluster headache patients often possess one or more predictive risk factors for coronary artery disease (CAD).

Risk of Myocardial Ischemia and/or Infarction and Other Adverse Cardiac Events

Sumatriptan should not be given to patients with documented ischemic or vasospastic CAD (see CONTRAINDICATIONS). It is strongly recommended that sumatriptan not be given to patients in whom unrecognized CAD is predicted by the presence of risk factors (e.g., hypertension, hypercholesterolemia, smoker, obesity, diabetes, strong family history of CAD, female with surgical or physiological menopause, male over 40 years of age) unless a cardiovascular evaluation provides satisfactory clinical evidence that the patient is reasonably free of coronary artery and ischemic myocardial disease or other significant underlying cardiovascular disease. The sensitivity of cardiac diagnostic procedures to detect cardiovascular disease or predisposition to coronary artery vasospasm is modest, at best. If, during the cardiovascular evaluation, the patient's medical history or electrocardiographic investigations reveal findings indicative of or consistent with coronary artery vasospasm or myocardial ischemia, sumatriptan should not be administered (see CONTRAINDICATIONS).

For patients with risk factors predictive of CAD who are determined to have a satisfactory cardiovascular evaluation, it is strongly recommended that administration of the first dose of sumatriptan injection take place in the setting of a physician's office or similar medically staffed and equipped facility. Because cardiac ischemia can occur in the absence of clinical symptoms, consideration should be given to obtaining an electrocardiogram (ECG) during the interval immediately following the first dose in these patients with risk factors.

It is recommended that patients who are intermittent long-term users of sumatriptan and who have or acquire risk factors predictive of CAD, as described above, undergo periodic interval cardiovascular evaluation as they continue to use sumatriptan. In considering this recommendation for periodic cardiovascular evaluation, it is noted that patients with cluster headache are predominantly male and over 40 years of age, which are risk factors for CAD.

The systematic approach described above is intended to reduce the likelihood that patients with unrecognized cardiovascular disease will be inadvertently exposed to sumatriptan.

Drug-Associated Cardiac Events and Fatalities

Serious adverse cardiac events, including acute myocardial infarction, life-threatening disturbances of cardiac rhythm, and death have been reported within a few hours following the administration of IMITREX Injection or IMITREX® (sumatriptan succinate) Tablets. Considering the extent of use of sumatriptan in patients with migraine, the incidence of these events is extremely low.

The fact that sumatriptan can cause coronary vasospasm, that some of these events have occurred in patients with no prior cardiac disease history and with documented absence of CAD, and the close proximity of the events to sumatriptan use support the conclusion that some of these cases were caused by the drug. In many cases, however, where there has been known underlying CAD, the relationship is uncertain.

Premarketing Experience With Sumatriptan

Among the more than 1,900 patients with migraine who participated in premarketing controlled clinical trials of subcutaneous sumatriptan, there were 8 patients who sustained clinical events during or shortly after receiving sumatriptan that may have reflected coronary artery vasospasm. Six of these 8 patients had ECG changes consistent with transient ischemia, but without accompanying clinical symptoms or signs. Of these 8 patients, 4 had either findings suggestive of CAD or risk factors predictive of CAD prior to study enrollment.

Of 6,348 patients with migraine who participated in premarketing controlled and uncontrolled clinical trials of oral sumatriptan, 2 experienced clinical adverse events shortly after receiving oral sumatriptan that may have reflected coronary vasospasm. Neither of these adverse events was associated with a serious clinical outcome.

Among approximately 4,000 patients with migraine who participated in premarketing controlled and uncontrolled clinical trials of sumatriptan nasal spray, 1 patient experienced an asymptomatic subendocardial infarction possibly subsequent to a coronary vasospastic event.

Postmarketing Experience With Sumatriptan

Serious cardiovascular events, some resulting in death, have been reported in association with the use of IMITREX Injection or IMITREX Tablets. The uncontrolled nature of postmarketing surveillance, however, makes it impossible to determine definitively the proportion of the reported cases that were actually caused by sumatriptan or to reliably assess causation in individual cases. On clinical grounds, the longer the latency between the administration of IMITREX and the onset of the clinical event, the less likely the association is to be causative. Accordingly, interest has focused on events beginning within 1 hour of the administration of IMITREX.

Cardiac events that have been observed to have onset within 1 hour of sumatriptan administration include: coronary artery vasospasm, transient ischemia, myocardial infarction, ventricular tachycardia and ventricular fibrillation, cardiac arrest, and death.

Some of these events occurred in patients who had no findings of CAD and appear to represent consequences of coronary artery vasospasm. However, among domestic reports of serious cardiac events within 1 hour of sumatriptan administration, the majority had risk factors predictive of CAD and the presence of significant underlying CAD was established in most cases (see CONTRAINDICATIONS).

Drug-Associated Cerebrovascular Events and Fatalities

Cerebral hemorrhage, subarachnoid hemorrhage, stroke, and other cerebrovascular events have been reported in patients treated with oral or subcutaneous sumatriptan, and some have resulted in fatalities. The relationship of sumatriptan to these events is uncertain. In a number of cases, it appears possible that the cerebrovascular events were primary, sumatriptan having been administered in the incorrect belief the symptoms experienced were a consequence of migraine when they were not. As with other acute migraine therapies, before treating headaches in patients not previously diagnosed as migraineurs, and in migraineurs who present with atypical symptoms, care should be taken to exclude other potentially serious neurological conditions. It should also be noted that patients with migraine may be at increased risk of certain cerebrovascular events (e.g., cerebrovascular accident, transient ischemic attack).

Other Vasospasm-Related Events

Sumatriptan may cause vasospastic reactions other than coronary artery vasospasm. Both peripheral vascular ischemia and colonic ischemia with abdominal pain and bloody diarrhea have been reported. Very rare reports of transient and permanent blindness and significant partial vision loss have been reported with the use of sumatriptan. Visual disorders may also be part of a migraine attack.

Serotonin Syndrome

The development of a potentially life-threatening serotonin syndrome may occur with triptans, including treatment with IMITREX, particularly during combined use with selective serotonin reuptake inhibitors (SSRIs) or serotonin norepinephrine reuptake inhibitors (SNRIs). If concomitant treatment with sumatriptan and an SSRI (e.g., fluoxetine, paroxetine, sertraline, fluvoxamine, citalopram, escitalopram) or SNRI (e.g., venlafaxine, duloxetine) is clinically warranted, careful observation of the patient is advised, particularly during treatment initiation and dose increases. Serotonin syndrome symptoms may include mental status changes (e.g., agitation, hallucinations, coma), autonomic instability (e.g., tachycardia, labile blood pressure, hyperthermia), neuromuscular aberrations (e.g., hyperreflexia, incoordination), and/or gastrointestinal symptoms (e.g., nausea, vomiting, diarrhea).

Increase in Blood Pressure

Significant elevation in blood pressure, including hypertensive crisis, has been reported on rare occasions in patients with and without a history of hypertension. Sumatriptan is contraindicated in patients with uncontrolled hypertension (see CONTRAINDICATIONS). Sumatriptan should be administered with caution to patients with controlled hypertension as transient increases in blood pressure and peripheral vascular resistance have been observed in a small proportion of patients.

Concomitant Drug Use

In patients taking MAO-A inhibitors, sumatriptan plasma levels attained after treatment with recommended doses are nearly double those obtained under other conditions. Accordingly, the coadministration of sumatriptan and an MAO-A inhibitor is not generally recommended. If such

Table 3. Efficacy Data From the Pivotal Cluster Headache Studies

	Study 1		Study 2	
	Placebo (n = 39)	IMITREX 6 mg (n = 39)	Placebo (n = 88)	IMITREX 6 mg (n = 92)
Patients with pain relief (no/mild)				
5 minutes postinjection	8%	21%	7%	23%[a]
10 minutes postinjection	10%	49%[a]	25%	49%
15 minutes postinjection	26%	74%[a]	35%	75%[a]

[a] $p<0.05$.

(n = Number of headaches treated.)

therapy is clinically warranted, however, suitable dose adjustment and appropriate observation of the patient is advised (see CLINICAL PHARMACOLOGY: Drug Interactions: *Monoamine Oxidase Inhibitors*).

Use in Women of Childbearing Potential
See PRECAUTIONS: Pregnancy.

Hypersensitivity
Hypersensitivity (anaphylaxis/anaphylactoid) reactions have occurred on rare occasions in patients receiving sumatriptan. Such reactions can be life threatening or fatal. In general, hypersensitivity reactions to drugs are more likely to occur in individuals with a history of sensitivity to multiple allergens (see CONTRAINDICATIONS).

PRECAUTIONS
General
Chest, jaw, or neck tightness is relatively common after administration of IMITREX Injection. Chest discomfort and jaw or neck tightness have been reported following use of IMITREX Tablets and have also been reported infrequently following the administration of IMITREX® (sumatriptan) Nasal Spray. Only rarely have these symptoms been associated with ischemic ECG changes. However, because sumatriptan may cause coronary artery vasospasm, patients who experience signs or symptoms suggestive of angina following sumatriptan should be evaluated for the presence of CAD or a predisposition to Prinzmetal variant angina before receiving additional doses of sumatriptan and should be monitored electrocardiographically if dosing is resumed and similar symptoms recur. Similarly, patients who experience other symptoms or signs suggestive of decreased arterial flow, such as ischemic bowel syndrome or Raynaud syndrome, following sumatriptan should be evaluated for atherosclerosis or predisposition to vasospasm (see WARNINGS: Risk of Myocardial Ischemia and/or Infarction and Other Adverse Cardiac Events and WARNINGS: Other Vasospasm-Related Events).

IMITREX should also be administered with caution to patients with diseases that may alter the absorption, metabolism, or excretion of drugs, such as impaired hepatic or renal function.

There have been rare reports of seizure following administration of sumatriptan. Sumatriptan should be used with caution in patients with a history of epilepsy or conditions associated with a lowered seizure threshold.

Care should be taken to exclude other potentially serious neurologic conditions before treating headache in patients not previously diagnosed with migraine or cluster headache or who experience a headache that is atypical for them. There have been rare reports where patients received sumatriptan for severe headaches that were subsequently shown to have been secondary to an evolving neurologic lesion (see WARNINGS: Drug-Associated Cerebrovascular Events and Fatalities). For a given attack, if a patient does not respond to the first dose of sumatriptan, the diagnosis of migraine or cluster headache should be reconsidered before administration of a second dose.

Overuse of acute migraine treatments has been associated with the exacerbation of headache (medication overuse headache) in susceptible patients. Withdrawal of the treatment may be necessary.

Binding to Melanin-Containing Tissues
Because sumatriptan binds to melanin, it could accumulate in melanin-rich tissues (such as the eye) over time. This raises the possibility that sumatriptan could cause toxicity in these tissues after extended use. However, no effects on the retina related to treatment with sumatriptan were noted in any of the toxicity studies. Although no systematic monitoring of ophthalmologic function was undertaken in clinical trials, and no specific recommendations for ophthalmologic monitoring are offered, prescribers should be aware of the possibility of long-term ophthalmologic effects (see CLINICAL PHARMACOLOGY: Melanin Binding).

Corneal Opacities
Sumatriptan causes corneal opacities and defects in the corneal epithelium in dogs; this raises the possibility that these changes may occur in humans. While patients were not systematically evaluated for these changes in clinical trials, and no specific recommendations for monitoring are being offered, prescribers should be aware of the possibility of these changes (see CLINICAL PHARMACOLOGY: Corneal Opacities).

Patients who are advised to self-administer IMITREX Injection in medically unsupervised situations should receive instruction on the proper use of the product from the physician or other suitably qualified health care professional prior to doing so for the first time.

Information for Patients
With the autoinjector, the needle penetrates approximately 1/4 of an inch (5 to 6 mm). Since the injection is intended to be given subcutaneously, intramuscular or intravascular delivery should be avoided. Patients should be directed to use injection sites with an adequate skin and subcutaneous thickness to accommodate the length of the needle. See PATIENT INFORMATION at the end of this labeling for the text of the separate leaflet provided for patients.

Patients should be cautioned about the risk of serotonin syndrome with the use of sumatriptan or other triptans, especially during combined use with SSRIs or SNRIs.

Laboratory Tests
No specific laboratory tests are recommended for monitoring patients prior to and/or after treatment with sumatriptan.

Drug Interactions
Selective Serotonin Reuptake Inhibitors/Serotonin Norepinephrine Reuptake Inhibitors and Serotonin Syndrome
Cases of life-threatening serotonin syndrome have been reported during combined use of SSRIs or SNRIs and triptans (see WARNINGS).

Migraine Prophylactic Medications
There is no evidence that concomitant use of migraine prophylactic medications has any effect on the efficacy of sumatriptan. In 2 Phase III trials in the US, a retrospective analysis of 282 patients who had been using prophylactic drugs (verapamil n = 63, amitriptyline n = 57, propranolol n = 94, for 45 other drugs n = 123) were compared with those who had not used prophylaxis (N = 452). There were no differences in relief rates at 60 minutes postdose for IMITREX Injection, whether or not prophylactic medications were used.

Ergot-Containing Drugs
Ergot-containing drugs have been reported to cause prolonged vasospastic reactions. Because there is a theoretical basis that these effects may be additive, use of ergotamine-containing or ergot-type medications (like dihydroergotamine or methysergide) and sumatriptan within 24 hours of each other should be avoided (see CONTRAINDICATIONS).

Monoamine Oxidase-A Inhibitors
MAO-A inhibitors reduce sumatriptan clearance, significantly increasing systemic exposure. Therefore, the use of sumatriptan in patients receiving MAO-A inhibitors is not ordinarily recommended. If the clinical situation warrants the combined use of sumatriptan and an MAOI, the dose of sumatriptan employed should be reduced (see CLINICAL PHARMACOLOGY: Drug Interactions: *Monoamine Oxidase Inhibitors* and WARNINGS: Concomitant Drug Use).

Drug/Laboratory Test Interactions
IMITREX is not known to interfere with commonly employed clinical laboratory tests.

Carcinogenesis, Mutagenesis, Impairment of Fertility
In carcinogenicity studies, rats and mice were given sumatriptan by oral gavage (rats: 104 weeks) or drinking water (mice: 78 weeks). Average exposures achieved in mice receiving the highest dose were approximately 110 times the exposure attained in humans after the maximum recommended single dose of 6 mg. The highest dose to rats was approximately 260 times the maximum single dose of 6 mg on a mg/m² basis. There was no evidence of an increase in tumors in either species related to sumatriptan administration.

Sumatriptan was not mutagenic in the presence or absence of metabolic activation when tested in 2 gene mutation assays (the Ames test and the in vitro mammalian Chinese hamster V79/HGPRT assay). In 2 cytogenetics assays (the in vitro human lymphocyte assay and the in vivo rat micronucleus assay) sumatriptan was not associated with clastogenic activity.

A fertility study (Segment I) by the subcutaneous route, during which male and female rats were dosed daily with sumatriptan prior to and throughout the mating period, has shown no evidence of impaired fertility at doses equivalent to approximately 100 times the maximum recommended single human dose of 6 mg on a mg/m² basis. However, following oral administration, a treatment-related decrease in fertility, secondary to a decrease in mating, was seen for rats treated with 50 and 500 mg/kg/day. The no-effect dose for this finding was approximately 8 times the maximum recommended single human dose of 6 mg on a mg/m² basis. It is not clear whether the problem is associated with the treatment of males or females or both.

Pregnancy
Pregnancy Category C. Sumatriptan has been shown to be embryolethal in rabbits when given daily at a dose approximately equivalent to the maximum recommended single human subcutaneous dose of 6 mg on a mg/m² basis. There is no evidence that establishes that sumatriptan is a human teratogen; however, there are no adequate and well-controlled studies in pregnant women. IMITREX Injection should be used during pregnancy only if the potential benefit justifies the potential risk to the fetus.

In assessing this information, the following additional findings should be considered.

Embryolethality
When given intravenously to pregnant rabbits daily throughout the period of organogenesis, sumatriptan caused embryolethality at doses at or close to those producing maternal toxicity. The mechanism of the embryolethality is not known. These doses were approximately equivalent to the maximum single human dose of 6 mg on a mg/m² basis.

The intravenous administration of sumatriptan to pregnant rats throughout organogenesis at doses that are approximately 20 times a human dose of 6 mg on a mg/m² basis, did

not cause embryolethality. Additionally, in a study of pregnant rats given subcutaneous sumatriptan daily prior to and throughout pregnancy, there was no evidence of increased embryo/fetal lethality.

Teratogenicity
Term fetuses from Dutch Stride rabbits treated during organogenesis with oral sumatriptan exhibited an increased incidence of cervicothoracic vascular and skeletal abnormalities. The functional significance of these abnormalities is not known. The highest no-effect dose for these effects was 15 mg/kg/day, approximately 50 times the maximum single dose of 6 mg on a mg/m² basis.

In a study in rats dosed daily with subcutaneous sumatriptan prior to and throughout pregnancy, there was no evidence of teratogenicity.

Pregnancy Registry
To monitor fetal outcomes of pregnant women exposed to IMITREX, GlaxoSmithKline maintains a Sumatriptan Pregnancy Registry. Physicians are encouraged to register patients by calling (800) 336-2176.

Nursing Mothers
Sumatriptan is excreted in human breast milk following subcutaneous administration. Infant exposure to sumatriptan can be minimized by avoiding breastfeeding for 12 hours after treatment with IMITREX Injection.

Pediatric Use
Safety and effectiveness of IMITREX Injection in pediatric patients under 18 years of age have not been established; therefore, IMITREX Injection is not recommended for use in patients under 18 years of age.

Two controlled clinical trials evaluated sumatriptan nasal spray (5 to 20 mg) in 1,248 adolescent migraineurs aged 12 to 17 years who treated a single attack. The studies did not establish the efficacy of sumatriptan nasal spray compared with placebo in the treatment of migraine in adolescents. Adverse events observed in these clinical trials were similar in nature to those reported in clinical trials in adults.

Five controlled clinical trials (2 single-attack studies, 3 multiple-attack studies) evaluating oral sumatriptan (25 to 100 mg) in pediatric patients aged 12 to 17 years enrolled a total of 701 adolescent migraineurs. These studies did not establish the efficacy of oral sumatriptan compared with placebo in the treatment of migraine in adolescents. Adverse events observed in these clinical trials were similar in nature to those reported in clinical trials in adults. The frequency of all adverse events in these patients appeared to be both dose- and age-dependent, with younger patients reporting events more commonly than older adolescents.

Postmarketing experience documents that serious adverse events have occurred in the pediatric population after use of subcutaneous, oral, and/or intranasal sumatriptan. These reports include events similar in nature to those reported rarely in adults, including stroke, visual loss, and death. A myocardial infarction has been reported in a 14-year-old male following the use of oral sumatriptan; clinical signs occurred within 1 day of drug administration. Since clinical data to determine the frequency of serious adverse events in pediatric patients who might receive injectable, oral, or intranasal sumatriptan are not presently available, the use of sumatriptan in patients aged younger than 18 years is not recommended.

Geriatric Use
The use of sumatriptan in elderly patients is not recommended because elderly patients are more likely to have decreased hepatic function, they are at higher risk for CAD, and blood pressure increases may be more pronounced in the elderly (see WARNINGS: Risk of Myocardial Ischemia and/or Infarction and Other Adverse Cardiac Events).

ADVERSE REACTIONS

Serious cardiac events, including some that have been fatal, have occurred following the use of IMITREX Injection or Tablets. These events are extremely rare and most have been reported in patients with risk factors predictive of CAD. Events reported have included coronary artery vasospasm, transient myocardial ischemia, myocardial infarction, ventricular tachycardia, and ventricular fibrillation (see CONTRAINDICATIONS, WARNINGS: Risk of Myocardial Ischemia and/or Infarction and Other Adverse Cardiac Events, and PRECAUTIONS: General).

Significant hypertensive episodes, including hypertensive crises, have been reported on rare occasions in patients with or without a history of hypertension (see WARNINGS: Increase in Blood Pressure).

Among patients in clinical trials of subcutaneous IMITREX Injection (N = 6,218), up to 3.5% of patients withdrew for reasons related to adverse events.

Incidence in Controlled Clinical Trials of Migraine Headache
Table 4 lists adverse events that occurred in 2 large US, Phase III, placebo-controlled clinical trials in migraine patients following either a single 6-mg dose of IMITREX Injection or placebo. Only events that occurred at a frequency of 2% or more in groups treated with IMITREX Injection 6 mg and occurred at a frequency greater than the placebo group are included in Table 4.

Table 4. Treatment Emergent Adverse Experience Incidence in 2 Large Placebo-Controlled Migraine Clinical Trials: Events Reported by at Least 2% of Patients Treated With IMITREX Injection 6 mg[a]

Adverse Event	Percent of Patients Reporting	
	IMITREX Injection 6 mg Subcutaneous (n = 547)	Placebo (n = 370)
Atypical sensations	42	9
Tingling	14	3
Warm/hot sensation	11	4
Burning sensation	7	<1
Feeling of heaviness	7	1
Pressure sensation	7	2
Feeling of tightness	5	<1
Numbness	5	2
Feeling strange	2	<1
Tight feeling in head	2	<1
Cardiovascular		
Flushing	7	2
Chest discomfort	5	1
Tightness in chest	3	<1
Pressure in chest	2	<1
Ear, nose, and throat		
Throat discomfort	3	<1
Discomfort: nasal cavity/sinuses	2	<1
Injection site reaction	59	24
Miscellaneous		
Jaw discomfort	2	0
Musculoskeletal		
Weakness	5	<1
Neck pain/stiffness	5	<1
Myalgia	2	<1
Neurological		
Dizziness/vertigo	12	4
Drowsiness/sedation	3	2
Headache	2	<1
Skin		
Sweating	2	1

[a]The sum of the percentages cited is greater than 100% because patients may experience more than 1 type of adverse event. Only events that occurred at a frequency of 2% or more in groups treated with IMITREX Injection and occurred at a frequency greater than the placebo groups are included.

The incidence of adverse events in controlled clinical trials was not affected by gender or age of the patients. There were insufficient data to assess the impact of race on the incidence of adverse events.

Incidence in Controlled Trials of Cluster Headache
In the controlled clinical trials assessing sumatriptan's efficacy as a treatment for cluster headache, no new significant adverse events associated with the use of sumatriptan were detected that had not already been identified in association with the drug's use in migraine.

Overall, the frequency of adverse events reported in the studies of cluster headache were generally lower. Exceptions include reports of paresthesia (5% IMITREX, 0% placebo), nausea and vomiting (4% IMITREX, 0% placebo), and bronchospasm (1% IMITREX, 0% placebo).

Other Events Observed in Association With the Administration of IMITREX Injection
In the paragraphs that follow, the frequencies of less commonly reported adverse clinical events are presented. Because the reports include events observed in open and uncontrolled studies, the role of IMITREX Injection in their causation cannot be reliably determined. Furthermore, variability associated with adverse event reporting, the terminology used to describe adverse events, etc., limit the value of the quantitative frequency estimates provided.

Event frequencies are calculated as the number of patients reporting an event divided by the total number of patients (N = 6,218) exposed to subcutaneous IMITREX Injection. All reported events are included except those already listed in the previous table, those too general to be informative, and those not reasonably associated with the use of the drug. Events are further classified within body system categories and enumerated in order of decreasing frequency using the following definitions: frequent adverse events are defined as those occurring in at least 1/100 patients, infrequent adverse events are those occurring in 1/100 to 1/1,000 patients, and rare adverse events are those occurring in fewer than 1/1,000 patients.

Cardiovascular
Infrequent were hypertension, hypotension, bradycardia, tachycardia, palpitations, pulsating sensations, various transient ECG changes (nonspecific ST or T wave changes,

prolongation of PR or QTc intervals, sinus arrhythmia, non-sustained ventricular premature beats, isolated junctional ectopic beats, atrial ectopic beats, delayed activation of the right ventricle), and syncope. Rare were pallor, arrhythmia, abnormal pulse, vasodilatation, and Raynaud syndrome.

Endocrine and Metabolic
Infrequent was thirst. Rare were polydipsia and dehydration.

Eye
Frequent was vision alterations. Infrequent was irritation of the eye.

Gastrointestinal
Frequent were abdominal discomfort and dysphagia. Infrequent were gastroesophageal reflux and diarrhea. Rare were peptic ulcer, retching, flatulence/eructation, and gallstones.

Musculoskeletal
Frequent were muscle cramps. Infrequent were various joint disturbances (pain, stiffness, swelling, ache). Rare were muscle stiffness, need to flex calf muscles, backache, muscle tiredness, and swelling of the extremities.

Neurological
Frequent was anxiety. Infrequent were mental confusion, euphoria, agitation, relaxation, chills, sensation of lightness, tremor, shivering, disturbances of taste, prickling sensations, paresthesia, stinging sensations, facial pain, photophobia, and lacrimation. Rare were transient hemiplegia, hysteria, globus hystericus, intoxication, depression, myoclonia, monoplegia/diplegia, sleep disturbance, difficulties in concentration, disturbances of smell, hyperesthesia, dysesthesia, simultaneous hot and cold sensations, tickling sensations, dysarthria, yawning, reduced appetite, hunger, and dystonia.

Respiratory
Infrequent was dyspnea. Rare were influenza, diseases of the lower respiratory tract, and hiccoughs.

Skin
Infrequent were erythema, pruritus, and skin rashes and eruptions. Rare was skin tenderness.

Urogenital
Rare were dysuria, frequency, dysmenorrhea, and renal calculus.

Miscellaneous
Infrequent were miscellaneous laboratory abnormalities, including minor disturbances in liver function tests, "serotonin agonist effect," and hypersensitivity to various agents. Rare was fever.

Other Events Observed in the Clinical Development of IMITREX
The following adverse events occurred in clinical trials with IMITREX Tablets and IMITREX Nasal Spray. Because the reports include events observed in open and uncontrolled studies, the role of IMITREX in their causation cannot be reliably determined. All reported events are included except those already listed, those too general to be informative, and those not reasonably associated with the use of the drug.

Breasts
Breast swelling, cysts, disorder of breasts, lumps, masses of breasts, nipple discharge, primary malignant breast neoplasm, and tenderness.

Cardiovascular
Abdominal aortic aneurysm, angina, atherosclerosis, cerebral ischemia, cerebrovascular lesion, heart block, peripheral cyanosis, phlebitis, thrombosis, and transient myocardial ischemia.

Ear, Nose, and Throat
Allergic rhinitis; disorder of nasal cavity/sinuses; ear, nose, and throat hemorrhage; ear infection; external otitis; feeling of fullness in the ear(s); hearing disturbances; hearing loss; Meniere disease; nasal inflammation; otalgia; sensitivity to noise; sinusitis; tinnitus; and upper respiratory inflammation.

Endocrine and Metabolic
Elevated thyrotropin stimulating hormone (TSH) levels; endocrine cysts, lumps, and masses; fluid disturbances; galactorrhea; hyperglycemia; hypoglycemia; hypothyroidism; weight gain; and weight loss.

Eye
Accommodation disorders, blindness and low vision, conjunctivitis, disorders of sclera, external ocular muscle disorders, eye edema and swelling, eye hemorrhage, eye itching, eye pain, keratitis, mydriasis, and visual disturbances.

Gastrointestinal
Abdominal distention, colitis, constipation, dental pain, dyspeptic symptoms, feelings of gastrointestinal pressure, gastric symptoms, gastritis, gastroenteritis, gastrointestinal bleeding, gastrointestinal pain, hematemesis, hypersalivation, hyposalivation, intestinal obstruction, melena, nausea and/or vomiting, oral itching and irritation, pancreatitis, salivary gland swelling, and swallowing disorders.

Hematological Disorders
Anemia.

Mouth and Teeth
Disorder of mouth and tongue (e.g., burning of tongue, numbness of tongue, dry mouth).

Musculoskeletal
Acquired musculoskeletal deformity, arthralgia and articular rheumatitis, arthritis, intervertebral disc disorder, muscle atrophy, muscle tightness and rigidity, musculoskeletal inflammation, and tetany.

Neurological
Apathy, aggressiveness, bad/unusual taste, bradylogia, cluster headache, convulsions, depressive disorders, detachment, disturbance of emotions, drug abuse, facial paralysis, hallucinations, heat sensitivity, incoordination, increased alertness, memory disturbance, migraine, motor dysfunction, neoplasm of pituitary, neuralgia, neurotic disorders, paralysis, personality change, phobia, phonophobia, psychomotor disorders, radiculopathy, raised intracranial pressure, rigidity, stress, syncope, suicide, and twitching.

Respiratory
Asthma, breathing disorders, bronchitis, cough, and lower respiratory tract infection.

Skin
Dry/scaly skin, eczema, herpes, seborrheic dermatitis, skin nodules, tightness of skin, and wrinkling of skin.

Urogenital
Abnormal menstrual cycle, abortion, bladder inflammation, endometriosis, hematuria, increased urination, inflammation of fallopian tubes, intermenstrual bleeding, menstruation symptoms, micturition disorders, urethritis, and urinary infections.

Miscellaneous
Contusions, difficulty in walking, edema, hematoma, hypersensitivity, fever, fluid retention, lymphadenopathy, overdose, speech disturbance, swelling of extremities, swelling of face, and voice disturbances.

Pain and Other Pressure Sensations
Chest pain and/or heaviness, neck/throat/jaw pain/tightness/pressure, and pain (location specified).

Postmarketing Experience (Reports for Subcutaneous or Oral Sumatriptan)
The following section enumerates potentially important adverse events that have occurred in clinical practice and that have been reported spontaneously to various surveillance systems. The events enumerated represent reports arising from both domestic and nondomestic use of oral or subcutaneous dosage forms of sumatriptan. The events enumerated include all except those already listed in the ADVERSE REACTIONS section above or those too general to be informative. Because the reports cite events reported spontaneously from worldwide postmarketing experience, frequency of events and the role of IMITREX Injection in their causation cannot be reliably determined. It is assumed, however, that systemic reactions following sumatriptan use are likely to be similar regardless of route of administration.

Blood
Hemolytic anemia, pancytopenia, thrombocytopenia.

Cardiovascular
Atrial fibrillation, cardiomyopathy, colonic ischemia (see WARNINGS), Prinzmetal variant angina, pulmonary embolism, shock, thrombophlebitis.

Ear, Nose, and Throat
Deafness.

Eye
Ischemic optic neuropathy, retinal artery occlusion, retinal vein thrombosis, loss of vision.

Gastrointestinal
Ischemic colitis with rectal bleeding (see WARNINGS), xerostomia.

Hepatic
Elevated liver function tests.

Neurological
Central nervous system vasculitis, cerebrovascular accident, dysphasia, serotonin syndrome, subarachnoid hemorrhage.

Non-Site Specific
Angioneurotic edema, cyanosis, death (see WARNINGS), temporal arteritis.

Psychiatry
Panic disorder.

Respiratory
Bronchospasm in patients with and without a history of asthma.

Skin
Exacerbation of sunburn, hypersensitivity reactions (allergic vasculitis, erythema, pruritus, rash, shortness of breath, urticaria; in addition, severe anaphylaxis/anaphylactoid reactions have been reported [see WARNINGS: Hypersensitivity]), photosensitivity. Following subcutaneous administration of sumatriptan, pain, redness, stinging, induration, swelling, contusion, subcutaneous bleeding, and, on rare occasions, lipoatrophy (depression in the skin) or lipohypertrophy (enlargement or thickening of tissue) have been reported.

Urogenital
Acute renal failure.

DRUG ABUSE AND DEPENDENCE

The abuse potential of IMITREX Injection cannot be fully delineated in advance of extensive marketing experience. One clinical study enrolling 12 patients with a history of substance abuse failed to induce subjective behavior and/or physiologic response ordinarily associated with drugs that have an established potential for abuse.

OVERDOSAGE

Patients (N = 269) have received single injections of 8 to 12 mg without significant adverse effects. Volunteers (N = 47) have received single subcutaneous doses of up to 16 mg without serious adverse events.

No gross overdoses in clinical practice have been reported. Coronary vasospasm was observed after intravenous administration of IMITREX Injection (see CONTRAINDICATIONS). Overdoses would be expected from animal data (dogs at 0.1 g/kg, rats at 2 g/kg) to possibly cause convulsions, tremor, inactivity, erythema of the extremities, reduced respiratory rate, cyanosis, ataxia, mydriasis, injection site reactions (desquamation, hair loss, and scab formation), and paralysis. The half-life of elimination of sumatriptan is about 2 hours (see CLINICAL PHARMACOLOGY: Pharmacokinetics), and therefore monitoring of patients after overdose with IMITREX Injection should continue while symptoms or signs persist, and for at least 10 hours.

It is unknown what effect hemodialysis or peritoneal dialysis has on the serum concentrations of sumatriptan.

DOSAGE AND ADMINISTRATION

The maximum single recommended adult dose of IMITREX Injection is 6 mg injected subcutaneously. If side effects are dose limiting, then lower doses may be used (see Table 1). The maximum recommended dose that may be given in 24 hours is two 6-mg injections separated by at least 1 hour. Controlled clinical trials have failed to show that clear benefit is associated with the administration of a second 6-mg dose in patients who have failed to respond to a first injection.

In patients receiving MAO inhibitors, decreased doses of sumatriptan should be considered (see WARNINGS: Concomitant Drug Use and CLINICAL PHARMACOLOGY: Drug Interactions: *Monoamine Oxidase Inhibitors*).

An autoinjection device is available for use with the 4- and 6-mg prefilled syringe cartridges to facilitate self-administration in patients using the 4- or 6-mg dose. With this device, the needle penetrates approximately 1/4 inch (5 to 6 mm). Since the injection is intended to be given subcutaneously, intramuscular or intravascular delivery should be avoided. Patients should be directed to use injection sites with an adequate skin and subcutaneous thickness to accommodate the length of the needle.

In patients receiving doses other than 4 or 6 mg, only the 6-mg single-dose vial dosage form should be used. Parenteral drug products should be inspected visually for particulate matter and discoloration before administration whenever solution and container permit.

HOW SUPPLIED

IMITREX Injection contains sumatriptan (base) as the succinate salt and is supplied as a clear, colorless to pale yellow, sterile, nonpyrogenic solution as follows:

(NDC 0173-0739-00) IMITREX STATdose System®, 4 mg, containing 2 prefilled single-dose syringe cartridges, 1 IMITREX STATdose Pen®, 1 carrying case, and a patient information leaflet with instructions for use.

(NDC 0173-0739-02) Two 4-mg single-dose prefilled syringe cartridges for use with IMITREX STATdose System with a patient information leaflet with instructions for use.

(NDC 0173-0479-00) IMITREX STATdose System, 6 mg, containing 2 prefilled single-dose syringe cartridges, 1 IMITREX STATdose Pen, 1 carrying case, and a patient information leaflet with instructions for use.

(NDC 0173-0478-00) Two 6-mg single-dose prefilled syringe cartridges for use with IMITREX STATdose System with a patient information leaflet with instructions for use.

(NDC 0173-0449-02) IMITREX Injection single-dose vial (6 mg/0.5 mL) in cartons containing 5 vials.

Store between 2° and 30°C (36° and 86°F). Protect from light.

IMITREX, IMITREX STATdose System, and IMITREX STATdose Pen are registered trademarks of GlaxoSmithKline.

This product's prescribing information may have been updated. Please refer to ww.gsk.com for the most current version.

GlaxoSmithKline
Research Triangle Park, NC 27709
©2010, GlaxoSmithKline. All rights reserved.

February 2010
IMJ:3PI

PATIENT INFORMATION

The following wording is contained in a separate leaflet provided for patients.

How to Use the IMITREX STATdose System®
Read this leaflet carefully several times before you start to use the IMITREX STATdose System. If you have any questions, ask your healthcare provider.
Keep the IMITREX STATdose System out of the reach of children.

Before you use the IMITREX STATdose System
When you first open the IMITREX STATdose System box, the Cartridge Pack and the IMITREX STATdose Pen® are already in the Carrying Case for your convenience.

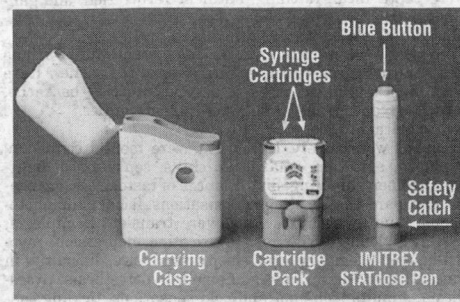

The grey and blue **Carrying Case** is used for storing the unloaded Pen and the Cartridge Pack when they are not being used.

The **Cartridge Pack** holds 2 individually sealed **Syringe Cartridges**. Each Syringe Cartridge holds 1 dose of IMITREX® (sumatriptan succinate) Injection. The Cartridge Pack for the 4-mg strength of this medicine is yellow, and the Cartridge Pack for the 6-mg strength is blue (as shown). Refill Cartridge Packs are available.

The grey and blue **Pen** is used to automatically inject 1 dose of medicine from a Syringe Cartridge. Do not touch the **Blue Button** until you have pressed the Pen against your skin to give a dose. If you press it at any other time, you might lose a dose. The **Safety Catch** keeps the Pen from accidentally firing until you are ready. The Pen will only work when you slide the grey part of the barrel down to the blue part. Always check to make sure that the white Priming Rod is <u>not</u> sticking out from the end of the Pen (as shown in Figure 2) before you load a new Syringe Cartridge. If it is sticking out, you will lose that dose.

How to load the IMITREX STATdose Pen
Do not load the Pen until you are ready to give yourself an injection. Do not touch the Blue Button on top of the Pen (see Figure 1) while you are loading the Pen.

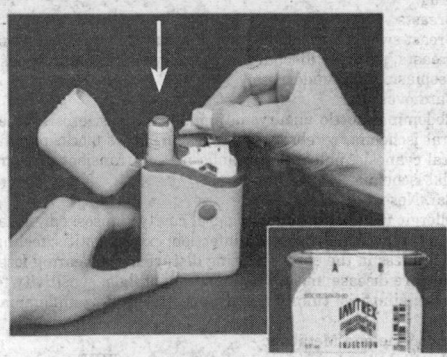

Figure 1

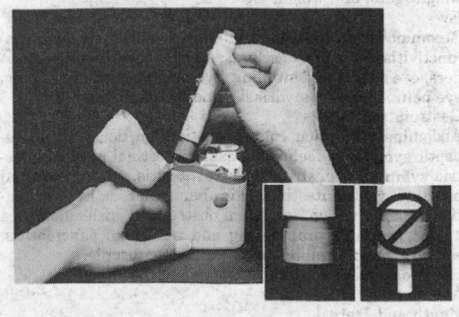

Figure 2

1. Open the lid of the Carrying Case.

The tamper-evident seals over the 2 Syringe Cartridges are labeled "A" and "B" (see Figure 1 inset). Always use the Syringe Cartridge marked "A" before the one marked "B" to help you keep track of your doses. **Do not use if either seal is broken or missing when you first open the Carrying Case.**

2. Tear off one of the tamper-evident seals (see Figure 1). Throw away the seal. Open the lid over the Syringe Cartridge.

3. Hold the Pen by the ridges at the top. Take it out of the Carrying Case (see Figure 2).
Check to make sure the white Priming Rod is <u>not</u> sticking out from the lower end of the Pen (see Figure 2 inset). If it is sticking out, put the Pen back into the Carrying Case and press down firmly until you feel it click. Then take the Pen out of the Carrying Case.

4. Put the Pen in the Cartridge Pack. Turn it to the right (clockwise) until it will not turn any more (about half a turn) (see Figure 3).

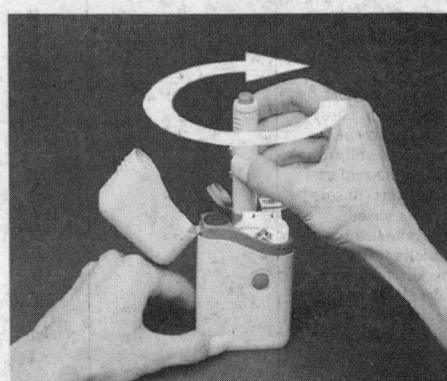

Figure 3

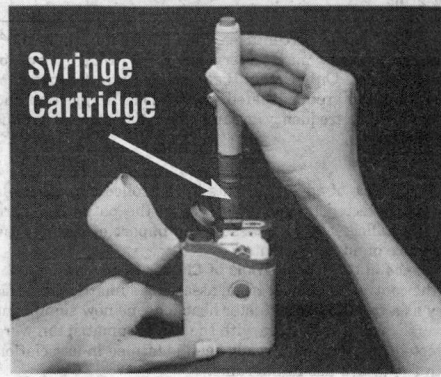

Figure 4

5. Hold the loaded Pen by the ridges and pull it **straight out** (see Figure 4). You may need to pull hard on the Pen, but this is normal.
Do not press the Blue Button yet.
The Pen is now ready to use. Do not put the <u>loaded</u> Pen back into the Carrying Case because that will damage the needle.
How to use the IMITREX STATdose Pen to take your medicine
Before injecting your medicine, choose an area with a fatty tissue layer (see Figure 5a **or** Figure 5b). Ask your healthcare provider if you have a question about where to inject. Clean the skin around this area.
[See figure 5a at top of next page]
or
[See figure 5b on next page]
[See figures 6, 7, 8 and 9 on next page]
1. Without pushing the Blue Button, press the loaded Pen firmly against the skin so that the grey barrel slides down toward the blue section that holds the Syringe Cartridge (see Figure 4). (This releases the Safety Catch that keeps the Pen from firing by mistake until you are ready.)
2. Push the Blue Button. Hold the Pen still for **at least 5 seconds.** If the Pen is taken away from the skin too soon, not all the medicine will come out.
3. **After 5 seconds,** carefully take the Pen away from your skin. The needle will be showing (see Figure 6). **Do not touch the needle.**
How to unload the IMITREX STATdose Pen after taking your medicine
Right after you take a dose with the Pen, you need to return the used Syringe Cartridge to the Cartridge Pack.

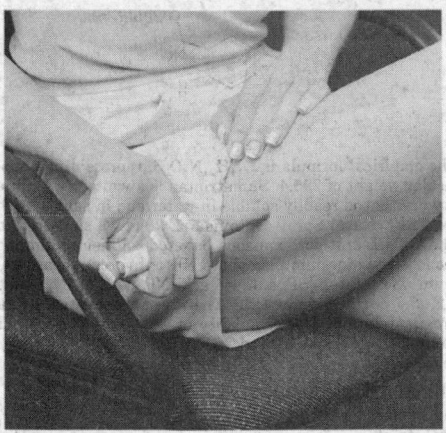

Figure 5a

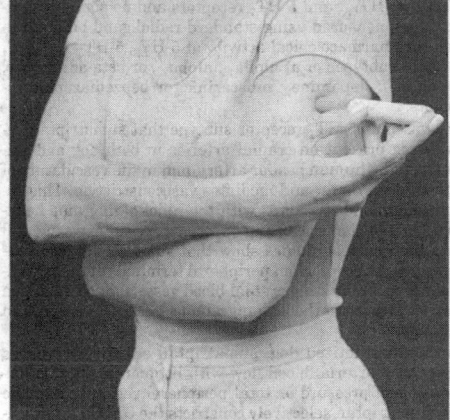

Figure 5b

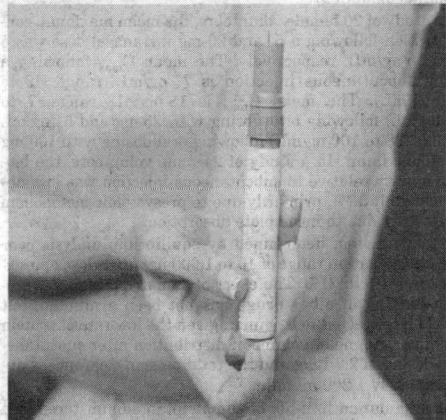

Figure 6

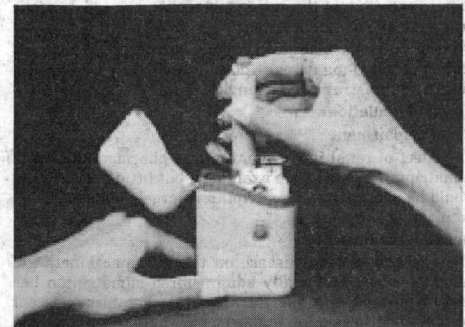

Figure 7

1. Push the Pen down into the empty side of the Cartridge Pack as far as it will go (see Figure 7).

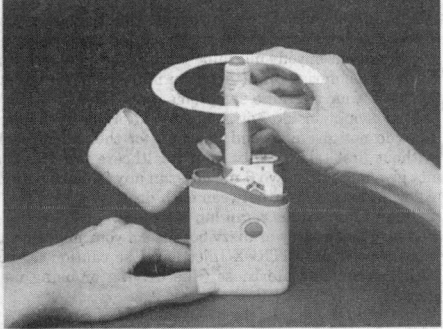

Figure 8

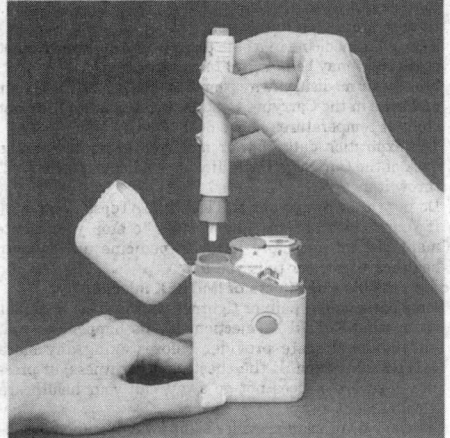

Figure 9

2. Turn the Pen to the left (counterclockwise) about half a turn until it is released from the Syringe Cartridge (see Figure 8).

3. Pull the empty Pen out of the Cartridge Pack (see Figure 9).
Because the Pen has now been used, the white Priming Rod will stick out from the lower end of the Pen.

4. Close the Cartridge Pack lid over the used Syringe Cartridge. When the used Syringe Cartridges are inserted correctly, the Cartridge Pack is a disposable, protective case to help you avoid needle sticks and use the syringes correctly.

5. Put the Pen back into the Carrying Case and press it down firmly until you feel it click. Close the Carrying Case lid. This gets the Pen ready for the next use.
If the lid will not close, push the Pen down until you feel it click. Then close the lid.

How to take out a used Cartridge Pack
After both Syringe Cartridges have been used, take the Cartridge Pack out of the Carrying Case and throw it away. **Never reuse a Syringe Cartridge.**

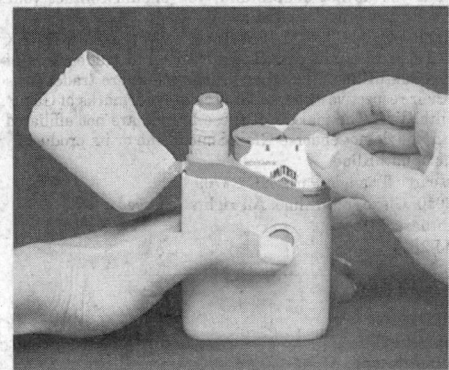

Figure 10

[See figure 11 at top of next column]
1. Open the Carrying Case lid.
2. Hold the Carrying Case with one hand and press the 2 buttons on either side of the Carrying Case (see Figure 10).
3. Gently pull out the Cartridge Pack with the other hand (see Figure 11).

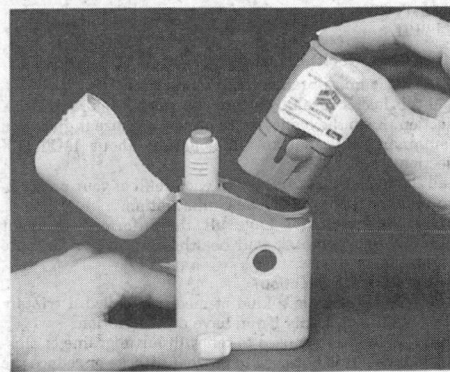

Figure 11
How to insert a new Cartridge Pack

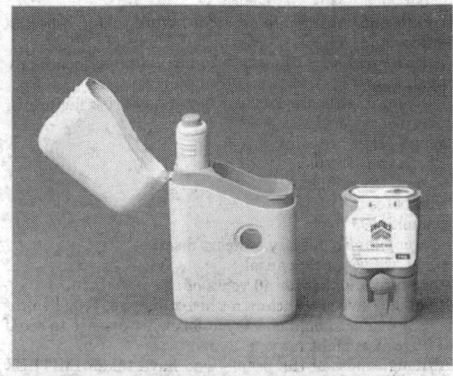

Figure 12

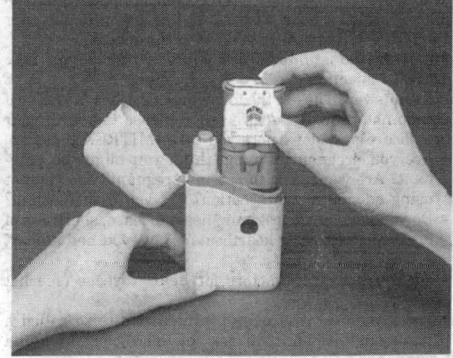

Figure 13

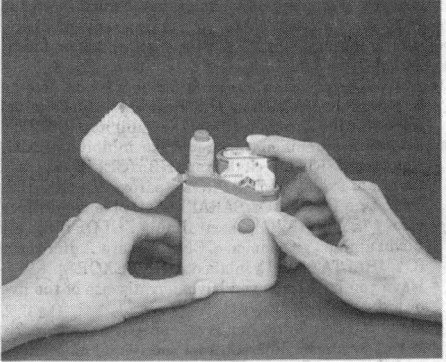

Figure 14

1. Take the new Cartridge Pack out of its box. **Do not take off the tamper-evident seals** (see Figure 12).
2. Put the Cartridge Pack in the Carrying Case. Slide it down smoothly (see Figure 13).
3. The Cartridge Pack will click into place when the 2 buttons show through the holes in the Carrying Case (see Figure 14). Close the lid.

February 2008
IMJ:2PIL

Information for the Patient

IMITREX® (sumatriptan succinate) Injection

Read this leaflet carefully before you start to take IMITREX Injection. Keep the leaflet for reference because it gives you a summary of important information about IMITREX Injection.

Read the leaflet that comes with each refill of your prescription because there may be new information.

This leaflet does not have all the information about IMITREX Injection. Ask your healthcare provider for more information or advice.

What is IMITREX Injection?

IMITREX Injection is a kind of medicine called a triptan. You should take it only if you have a prescription.

IMITREX Injection is used to relieve your migraine or cluster headache. It is **not** used to prevent attacks or reduce the number of attacks you have. Use IMITREX Injection only to treat an actual migraine or cluster headache attack.

The decision to use IMITREX Injection is one that you and your healthcare provider should make together, based on your personal needs and health.

Talk with your healthcare provider before taking IMITREX Injection

1. **Risk factors for heart disease to tell your healthcare provider:**

   Tell your healthcare provider if you have risk factors for heat disease such as:
   - high blood pressure
   - high cholesterol
   - being overweight
   - diabetes
   - smoking
   - strong family history of heart disease
   - you are postmenopausal
   - you are a male over 40 years of age

   If you do have risk factors for heart disease, your healthcare provider should check you for heart disease to see if IMITREX is right for you.

   Although most of the people who have taken IMITREX have not had any serious side effects, some have had serious heart problems. Deaths have been reported, but these were rare considering the extensive worldwide use of IMITREX. Usually, serious problems happened in people with known heart disease. It was not clear whether IMITREX had anything to do with these deaths.

2. **Important questions to ask yourself before you take IMITREX Injection:**

   If the answer to any of the following questions is **YES** or if you do not know the answer, then please talk with your healthcare provider before you take IMITREX Injection.
   - Are you pregnant? Do you think you might be pregnant? Are you trying to become pregnant? Are you not using adequate contraception? Are you breastfeeding?
   - Do you have any chest pain, heart disease, shortness of breath, or irregular heartbeats? Have you had a heart attack?
   - Do you have risk factors for heart disease (see list above)?
   - Have you had a stroke, a mini-stroke (also called a transient ischemic attack or TIA), or Raynaud syndrome?
   - Do you have high blood pressure?
   - Have you ever had to stop taking this or any other medicine because of an allergy or other problems?
   - Are you taking any other migraine medicines, including other triptans? Are you taking any medicines containing ergotamine, dihydroergotamine, or methysergide?
   - Are you taking any medicine for depression or other health problems such as a monoamine oxidase inhibitor, selective serotonin reuptake inhibitor (SSRI), or serotonin norepinephrine reuptake inhibitor (SNRI)? Common SSRIs are citalopram HBr (CELEXA®), escitalopram oxalate (LEXAPRO®), paroxetine (PAXIL®), fluoxetine (PROZAC®/SARAFEM®), olanzapine/fluoxetine (SYMBYAX®), sertraline (ZOLOFT®), and fluvoxamine. Common SNRIs are duloxetine (CYMBALTA®) and venlafaxine (EFFEXOR®).
   - Have you had, or do you have, any disease of the liver or kidney?
   - Have you had, or do you have, epilepsy or seizures?
   - Is this headache different from your usual migraine attacks?

   Remember, if you answered **YES** to any of the above questions, then talk with your healthcare provider about it.

Important points about IMITREX Injection

1. **The use of IMITREX Injection during pregnancy:**

   Do not take IMITREX Injection if you are pregnant, think you might be pregnant, are trying to become pregnant, or are not using adequate contraception unless you have talked with your healthcare provider about this.

2. **How to take IMITREX Injection:**

   For adults, the usual dose is a single injection given just below the skin. You should give an injection as soon as the symptoms of your migraine start, but it may be given at any time during an attack. You may give a second injection if your migraine symptoms come back.

   If your symptoms do not get better after the first injection, do not give a second injection for the same attack without first talking with your healthcare provider. Do not give more than two 6-mg doses in any 24-hour period. Allow at least 1 hour between each dose.

3. **Caution for activities requiring alertness:**

   You may feel drowsy or dizzy because of your migraine or treatment with IMITREX Injection. Use caution for activities requiring alertness (like driving or using machines).

4. **What to do if you take an overdose:**

   If you have taken more medicine than has been prescribed for you, contact either your healthcare provider, hospital emergency department, or nearest poison control center right away.

5. **How to store your medicine:**

   Keep your medicine in a safe place where children cannot reach it. It may be harmful to children.

   Store your medicine away from heat and light. Keep your medicine in the Carrying Case that comes with it. Do not store at temperatures above 86°F (30°C).

   The expiration date of your medicine is printed on the back of the Cartridge Pack. If your medicine has expired, throw it away.

   Do not throw away your IMITREX STATdose Pen®.

   If your healthcare provider decides to stop your treatment, do not keep any leftover medicine unless your healthcare provider tells you to.

Some possible side effects of IMITREX Injection

- Some patients feel pain or tightness in the chest or throat when using IMITREX Injection. If this happens to you, tell your healthcare provider before taking any more IMITREX Injection. If the chest pain, tightness, or pressure is severe or does not go away, call your healthcare provider right away.
- Call your healthcare provider right away if you have sudden and/or severe abdominal pain after you take IMITREX Injection.
- Some people may have a reaction called serotonin syndrome when they take certain kinds of medicines for depression called SSRIs or SNRIs while they are taking IMITREX Injection. Symptoms may include confusion, hallucinations, fast heartbeat, feeling faint, fever, sweating, muscle spasm, difficulty walking, and/or diarrhea. Call your healthcare provider right away if you have any of these symptoms after taking IMITREX Injection.
- Shortness of breath; wheeziness; heart throbbing; swelling of eyelids, face, or lips; or a skin rash, skin lumps, or hives happens rarely. If it happens to you, then tell your healthcare provider right away. Do not take any more IMITREX Injection unless your healthcare provider tells you to.
- Some people may feel tingling, heat, flushing (redness of face lasting a short time), heaviness, or pressure after taking IMITREX Injection. A few people may feel drowsy, dizzy, tired, or sick. If you have any of these symptoms, tell your healthcare provider at your next visit.
- You may have pain or redness at the site of injection, but this usually lasts less than an hour.
- If you feel unwell in any other way or have any symptoms that you do not understand, you should contact your healthcare provider right away.

IMITREX, IMITREX STATdose System, IMITREX STATdose Pen, and PAXIL are registered trademarks of GlaxoSmithKline. The other brands listed are trademarks of their respective owners and are not trademarks of GlaxoSmithKline. The makers of these brands are not affiliated with and do not endorse GlaxoSmithKline or its products.

GlaxoSmithKline
Research Triangle Park, NC 27709
©2010, GlaxoSmithKline. All rights reserved.
February 2010
IMJ:2PPI

IMITREX®
[im' ĭ-trĕx]
(sumatriptan)
Nasal Spray
℞

DESCRIPTION

IMITREX (sumatriptan) Nasal Spray contains sumatriptan, a selective 5-hydroxytryptamine₁ receptor subtype agonist. Sumatriptan is chemically designated as 3-[2-(dimethylamino)ethyl]-N-methyl-1H-indole-5-methanesulfonamide, and it has the following structure:

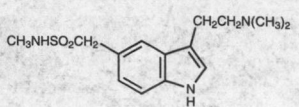

The empirical formula is $C_{14}H_{21}N_3O_2S$, representing a molecular weight of 295.4. Sumatriptan is a white to off-white powder that is readily soluble in water and in saline. Each IMITREX Nasal Spray contains 5 or 20 mg of sumatriptan in a 100-μL unit dose aqueous buffered solution containing monobasic potassium phosphate NF, anhydrous dibasic sodium phosphate USP, sulfuric acid NF, sodium hydroxide NF, and purified water USP. The pH of the solution is approximately 5.5. The osmolality of the solution is 372 or 742 mOsmol for the 5- and 20-mg IMITREX Nasal Spray, respectively.

CLINICAL PHARMACOLOGY

Mechanism of Action

Sumatriptan is an agonist for a vascular 5-hydroxytryptamine₁ receptor subtype (probably a member of the 5-HT₁D family) having only a weak affinity for 5-HT₁A, 5-HT₅A, and 5-HT₇ receptors and no significant affinity (as measured using standard radioligand binding assays) or pharmacological activity at 5-HT₂, 5-HT₃, or 5-HT₄ receptor subtypes or at alpha₁-, alpha₂-, or beta-adrenergic; dopamine₁; dopamine₂; muscarinic; or benzodiazepine receptors.

The vascular 5-HT₁ receptor subtype that sumatriptan activates is present on cranial arteries in both dog and primate, on the human basilar artery, and in the vasculature of human dura mater and mediates vasoconstriction. This action in humans correlates with the relief of migraine headache. In addition to causing vasoconstriction, experimental data from animal studies show that sumatriptan also activates 5-HT₁ receptors on peripheral terminals of the trigeminal nerve innervating cranial blood vessels. Such an action may contribute to the antimigrainous effect of sumatriptan in humans.

In the anesthetized dog, sumatriptan selectively reduces the carotid arterial blood flow with little or no effect on arterial blood pressure or total peripheral resistance. In the cat, sumatriptan selectively constricts the carotid arteriovenous anastomoses while having little effect on blood flow or resistance in cerebral or extracerebral tissues.

Pharmacokinetics

In a study of 20 female volunteers, the mean maximum concentration following a 5- and 20-mg intranasal dose was 5 and 16 ng/mL, respectively. The mean C_{max} following a 6-mg subcutaneous injection is 71 ng/mL (range: 49 to 110 ng/mL). The mean C_{max} is 18 ng/mL (range: 7 to 47 ng/mL) following oral dosing with 25 mg and 51 ng/mL (range: 28 to 100 ng/mL) following oral dosing with 100 mg of sumatriptan. In a study of 24 male volunteers, the bioavailability relative to subcutaneous dosing was low, approximately 17%, primarily due to presystemic metabolism and partly due to incomplete absorption.

Protein binding, determined by equilibrium dialysis over the concentration range of 10 to 1,000 ng/mL, is low, approximately 14% to 21%. The effect of sumatriptan on the protein binding of other drugs has not been evaluated, but would be expected to be minor, given the low rate of protein binding. The mean volume of distribution after subcutaneous dosing is 2.7 L/kg and the total plasma clearance is approximately 1,200 mL/min.

The elimination half-life of sumatriptan administered as a nasal spray is approximately 2 hours, similar to the half-life seen after subcutaneous injection. Only 3% of the dose is excreted in the urine as unchanged sumatriptan; 42% of the dose is excreted as the major metabolite, the indole acetic acid analogue of sumatriptan.

Clinical and pharmacokinetic data indicate that administration of two 5-mg doses, 1 dose in each nostril, is equivalent to administration of a single 10-mg dose in 1 nostril.

Special Populations

Renal Impairment

The effect of renal impairment on the pharmacokinetics of sumatriptan has not been examined, but little clinical effect would be expected as sumatriptan is largely metabolized to an inactive substance.

Hepatic Impairment

The effect of hepatic disease on the pharmacokinetics of subcutaneously and orally administered sumatriptan has been evaluated, but the intranasal dosage form has not been studied in hepatic impairment. There were no statistically significant differences in the pharmacokinetics of subcutaneously administered sumatriptan in hepatically impaired patients compared to healthy controls. However, the liver plays an important role in the presystemic clearance of orally administered sumatriptan. In 1 small study involving oral sumatriptan in hepatically impaired patients (N = 8) matched for sex, age, and weight with healthy subjects, the hepatically impaired patients had an approximately 70% increase in AUC and C_{max} and a T_{max} 40 minutes earlier compared to the healthy subjects. The bioavailability of nasally absorbed sumatriptan following intranasal administration, which would not undergo first-pass metabolism, should not be altered in hepatically impaired patients. The bioavailability of the swallowed portion of the intranasal sumatriptan dose has not been determined, but would be increased in these patients. The swallowed intranasal dose is small, however, compared to the usual oral dose, so that its impact should be minimal.

Age

The pharmacokinetics of oral sumatriptan in the elderly (mean age: 72 years, 2 males and 4 females) and in patients with migraine (mean age: 38 years, 25 males and 155 females) were similar to that in healthy male subjects (mean age: 30 years). Intranasal sumatriptan has not been evaluated for age differences (see PRECAUTIONS: Geriatric Use).

Race

The systemic clearance and C_{max} of sumatriptan were similar in black (n = 34) and Caucasian (n = 38) healthy male subjects. Intranasal sumatriptan has not been evaluated for race differences.

Drug Interactions

Monoamine Oxidase Inhibitors

Treatment with monoamine oxidase inhibitors (MAOIs) generally leads to an increase of sumatriptan plasma levels (see CONTRAINDICATIONS and PRECAUTIONS).

MAOI interaction studies have not been performed with intranasal sumatriptan. Due to gut and hepatic metabolic first-pass effects, the increase of systemic exposure after coadministration of an MAO-A inhibitor with oral sumatriptan is greater than after coadministration of the MAOI with subcutaneous sumatriptan. The effects of an MAOI on systemic exposure after intranasal sumatriptan would be expected to be greater than the effect after subcutaneous sumatriptan but smaller than the effect after oral sumatriptan because only swallowed drug would be subject to first-pass effects.

In a study of 14 healthy females, pretreatment with an MAO-A inhibitor decreased the clearance of subcutaneous sumatriptan. Under the conditions of this experiment, the result was a 2-fold increase in the area under the sumatriptan plasma concentration x time curve (AUC), corresponding to a 40% increase in elimination half-life. This interaction was not evident with an MAO-B inhibitor.

A small study evaluating the effect of pretreatment with an MAO-A inhibitor on the bioavailability from a 25-mg oral sumatriptan tablet resulted in an approximately 7-fold increase in systemic exposure.

Xylometazoline

An in vivo drug interaction study indicated that 3 drops of xylometazoline (0.1% w/v), a decongestant, administered 15 minutes prior to a 20-mg nasal dose of sumatriptan did not alter the pharmacokinetics of sumatriptan.

CLINICAL TRIALS

The efficacy of IMITREX Nasal Spray in the acute treatment of migraine headaches was demonstrated in 8, randomized, double-blind, placebo-controlled studies, of which 5 used the recommended dosing regimen and used the marketed formulation. Patients enrolled in these 5 studies were predominately female (86%) and Caucasian (95%), with a mean age of 41 (range of 18 to 65). Patients were instructed to treat a moderate to severe headache. Headache response, defined as a reduction in headache severity from moderate or severe pain to mild or no pain, was assessed up to 2 hours after dosing. Associated symptoms such as nausea, photophobia, and phonophobia were also assessed. Maintenance of response was assessed for up to 24 hours postdose. A second dose of IMITREX Nasal Spray or other medication was allowed 2 to 24 hours after the initial treatment for recurrent headache. The frequency and time to use of these additional treatments were also determined. In all studies, doses of 10 and 20 mg were compared to placebo in the treatment of 1 to 3 migraine attacks. Patients received doses as a single spray into 1 nostril. In 2 studies, a 5-mg dose was also evaluated.

In all 5 trials utilizing the market formulation and recommended dosage regimen, the percentage of patients achieving headache response 2 hours after treatment was significantly greater among patients receiving IMITREX Nasal Spray at all doses (with one exception) compared to those who received placebo. In 4 of the 5 studies, there was a statistically significant greater percentage of patients with headache response at 2 hours in the 20-mg group when compared to the lower dose groups (5 and 10 mg). There were no statistically significant differences between the 5- and 10-mg dose groups in any study. The results from the 5 controlled clinical trials are summarized in Table 1. Note that, in general, comparisons of results obtained in studies conducted under different conditions by different investigators with different samples of patients are ordinarily unreliable for purposes of quantitative comparison.

[See table 1 above]

The estimated probability of achieving an initial headache response over the 2 hours following treatment is depicted in Figure 1.

Table 1. Percentage of Patients With Headache Response (No or Mild Pain) 2 Hours Following Treatment				
	Placebo	IMITREX Nasal Spray 5 mg	IMITREX Nasal Spray 10 mg	IMITREX Nasal Spray 20 mg
Study 1	25% (n = 63)	49%[a] (n = 121)	46%[a] (n = 112)	64%[abc] (n = 118)
Study 2	25% (n = 138)	Not applicable	44%[a] (n = 273)	55%[ab] (n = 277)
Study 3	35% (n = 100)	Not applicable	54%[a] (n = 106)	63%[a] (n = 202)
Study 4	29% (n = 112)	Not applicable	43% (n = 106)	62%[ab] (n = 215)
Study 5[d]	36% (n = 198)	45%[a] (n = 296)	53%[a] (n = 291)	60%[ac] (n = 286)

[a] p<0.05 in comparison with placebo.
[b] p<0.05 in comparison with 10 mg.
[c] p<0.05 in comparison with 5 mg.
[d] Data are for attack 1 only of multiattack study for comparison.

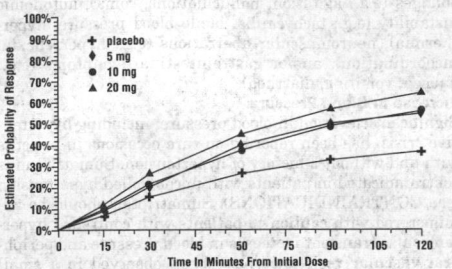

Figure 1. Estimated Probability of Achieving Initial Headache Response Within 120 Minutes[a]

[a] The figure shows the probability over time of obtaining headache response (no or mild pain) following treatment with intranasal sumatriptan. The averages displayed are based on pooled data from the 5 clinical controlled trials providing evidence of efficacy. Kaplan-Meier plot with patients not achieving response within 120 minutes censored to 120 minutes.

For patients with migraine-associated nausea, photophobia, and phonophobia at baseline, there was a lower incidence of these symptoms at 2 hours following administration of IMITREX Nasal Spray compared to placebo.

Two to 24 hours following the initial dose of study treatment, patients were allowed to use additional treatment for pain relief in the form of a second dose of study treatment or other medication. The estimated probability of patients taking a second dose or other medication for migraine over the 24 hours following the initial dose of study treatment is summarized in Figure 2.

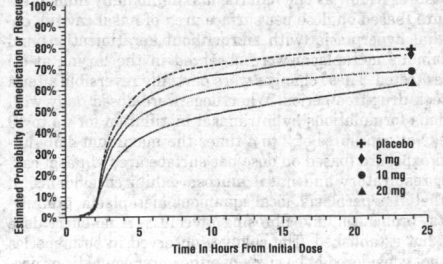

Figure 2. The Estimated Probability of Patients Taking a Second Dose or Other Medication for Migraine Over the 24 Hours Following the Initial Dose of Study Treatment[a]

[a] Kaplan-Meier plot based on data obtained in the 3 clinical controlled trials providing evidence of efficacy with patients not using additional treatments censored to 24 hours. Plot also includes patients who had no response to the initial dose. No remediation was allowed within 2 hours postdose.

There is evidence that doses above 20 mg do not provide a greater effect than 20 mg. There was no evidence to suggest that treatment with sumatriptan was associated with an increase in the severity of recurrent headaches. The efficacy of IMITREX Nasal Spray was unaffected by presence of aura; duration of headache prior to treatment; gender, age, or weight of the patient; or concomitant use of common migraine prophylactic drugs (e.g., beta-blockers, calcium channel blockers, tricyclic antidepressants). There were insufficient data to assess the impact of race on efficacy.

INDICATIONS AND USAGE

IMITREX Nasal Spray is indicated for the acute treatment of migraine attacks with or without aura in adults.

IMITREX Nasal Spray is not intended for the prophylactic therapy of migraine or for use in the management of hemiplegic or basilar migraine (see CONTRAINDICATIONS). Safety and effectiveness of IMITREX Nasal Spray have not been established for cluster headache, which is present in an older, predominantly male population.

CONTRAINDICATIONS

IMITREX Nasal Spray should not be given to patients with history, symptoms, or signs of ischemic cardiac, cerebrovascular, or peripheral vascular syndromes. In addition, patients with other significant underlying cardiovascular diseases should not receive IMITREX Nasal Spray. Ischemic cardiac syndromes include, but are not limited to, angina pectoris of any type (e.g., stable angina of effort, vasospastic forms of angina such as the Prinzmetal variant), all forms of myocardial infarction, and silent myocardial ischemia. Cerebrovascular syndromes include, but are not limited to, strokes of any type as well as transient ischemic attacks. Peripheral vascular disease includes, but is not limited to, ischemic bowel disease (see WARNINGS).

Because IMITREX Nasal Spray may increase blood pressure, it should not be given to patients with uncontrolled hypertension.

Concurrent administration of MAO-A inhibitors or use within 2 weeks of discontinuation of MAO-A inhibitor therapy is contraindicated (see CLINICAL PHARMACOLOGY: Drug Interactions and PRECAUTIONS: Drug Interactions).

IMITREX Nasal Spray and any ergotamine-containing or ergot-type medication (like dihydroergotamine or methysergide) should not be used within 24 hours of each other, nor should IMITREX Nasal Spray and another 5-HT$_1$ agonist.

IMITREX Nasal Spray should not be administered to patients with hemiplegic or basilar migraine.

IMITREX Nasal Spray is contraindicated in patients with hypersensitivity to sumatriptan or any of its components.

IMITREX Nasal Spray is contraindicated in patients with severe hepatic impairment.

WARNINGS

IMITREX Nasal Spray should only be used where a clear diagnosis of migraine headache has been established.

Risk of Myocardial Ischemia and/or Infarction and Other Adverse Cardiac Events

Sumatriptan should not be given to patients with documented ischemic or vasospastic coronary artery disease (CAD) (see CONTRAINDICATIONS). It is strongly recommended that sumatriptan not be given to patients in whom unrecognized CAD is predicted by the presence of risk factors (e.g., hypertension, hypercholesterolemia, smoker, obesity, diabetes, strong family history of CAD, female with surgical or physiological menopause, male over 40 years of age) unless a cardiovascular evaluation provides satisfactory clinical evidence that the patient is reasonably free of coronary artery and ischemic myocardial disease or other significant underlying cardiovascular disease. The sensitivity of cardiac diagnostic procedures to detect cardiovascular disease or predisposition to coronary artery vasospasm is modest, at best. If, during the cardiovascular evaluation, the patient's medical history or electrocardiographic investigations reveal findings indicative of, or consistent with, coronary artery vasospasm or myocardial ischemia, sumatriptan should not be administered (see CONTRAINDICATIONS).

For patients with risk factors predictive of CAD, who are determined to have a satisfactory cardiovascular evaluation, it is strongly recommended that administration of the first dose of sumatriptan nasal spray take place in the setting of a physician's office or similar medically staffed and equipped facility unless the patient has previously received sumatriptan. Because cardiac ischemia can occur in the absence of clinical symptoms, consideration should be given to obtaining on the first occasion of use an electrocardiogram (ECG) during the interval immediately following IMITREX Nasal Spray in these patients with risk factors.

It is recommended that patients who are intermittent long-term users of sumatriptan and who have or acquire risk factors predictive of CAD, as described above, undergo periodic interval cardiovascular evaluation as they continue to use sumatriptan.

The systematic approach described above is intended to reduce the likelihood that patients with unrecognized cardiovascular disease will be inadvertently exposed to sumatriptan.

Drug-Associated Cardiac Events and Fatalities
Serious adverse cardiac events, including acute myocardial infarction, life-threatening disturbances of cardiac rhythm, and death have been reported within a few hours following the administration of IMITREX® (sumatriptan succinate) Injection or IMITREX® (sumatriptan succinate) Tablets. Considering the extent of use of sumatriptan in patients with migraine, the incidence of these events is extremely low.

The fact that sumatriptan can cause coronary vasospasm, that some of these events have occurred in patients with no prior cardiac disease history and with documented absence of CAD, and the close proximity of the events to sumatriptan use support the conclusion that some of these cases were caused by the drug. In many cases, however, where there has been known underlying coronary artery disease, the relationship is uncertain.

Premarketing Experience With Sumatriptan
Among approximately 4,000 patients with migraine who participated in premarketing controlled and uncontrolled clinical trials of sumatriptan nasal spray, 1 patient experienced an asymptomatic subendocardial infarction possibly subsequent to a coronary vasospastic event.

Of 6,348 patients with migraine who participated in premarketing controlled and uncontrolled clinical trials of oral sumatriptan, 2 experienced clinical adverse events shortly after receiving oral sumatriptan that may have reflected coronary vasospasm. Neither of these adverse events was associated with a serious clinical outcome.

Among the more than 1,900 patients with migraine who participated in premarketing controlled clinical trials of subcutaneous sumatriptan, there were 8 patients who sustained clinical events during or shortly after receiving sumatriptan that may have reflected coronary artery vasospasm. Six of these 8 patients had ECG changes consistent with transient ischemia, but without accompanying clinical symptoms or signs. Of these 8 patients, 4 had either findings suggestive of CAD or risk factors predictive of CAD prior to study enrollment.

Postmarketing Experience With Sumatriptan
Serious cardiovascular events, some resulting in death, have been reported in association with the use of IMITREX Injection or IMITREX Tablets. The uncontrolled nature of postmarketing surveillance, however, makes it impossible to determine definitively the proportion of the reported cases that were actually caused by sumatriptan or to reliably assess causation in individual cases. On clinical grounds, the longer the latency between the administration of IMITREX and the onset of the clinical event, the less likely the association is to be causative. Accordingly, interest has focused on events beginning within 1 hour of the administration of IMITREX.

Cardiac events that have been observed to have onset within 1 hour of sumatriptan administration include: coronary artery vasospasm, transient ischemia, myocardial infarction, ventricular tachycardia and ventricular fibrillation, cardiac arrest, and death.

Some of these events occurred in patients who had no findings of CAD and appear to represent consequences of coronary artery vasospasm. However, among domestic reports of serious cardiac events within 1 hour of sumatriptan administration, almost all of the patients had risk factors predictive of CAD and the presence of significant underlying CAD was established in most cases (see CONTRAINDICATIONS).

Drug-Associated Cerebrovascular Events and Fatalities
Cerebral hemorrhage, subarachnoid hemorrhage, stroke, and other cerebrovascular events have been reported in pa-

tients treated with oral or subcutaneous sumatriptan, and some have resulted in fatalities. The relationship of sumatriptan to these events is uncertain. In a number of cases, it appears possible that the cerebrovascular events were primary, sumatriptan having been administered in the incorrect belief that the symptoms experienced were a consequence of migraine when they were not. As with other acute migraine therapies, before treating headaches in patients not previously diagnosed as migraineurs, and in migraineurs who present with atypical symptoms, care should be taken to exclude other potentially serious neurological conditions. It should also be noted that patients with migraine may be at increased risk of certain cerebrovascular events (e.g., cerebrovascular accident, transient ischemic attack).

Other Vasospasm-Related Events
Sumatriptan may cause vasospastic reactions other than coronary artery vasospasm. Both peripheral vascular ischemia and colonic ischemia with abdominal pain and bloody diarrhea have been reported. Very rare reports of transient and permanent blindness and significant partial vision loss have been reported with the use of sumatriptan. Visual disorders may also be part of a migraine attack.

Serotonin Syndrome
The development of a potentially life-threatening serotonin syndrome may occur with triptans, including treatment with IMITREX, particularly during combined use with selective serotonin reuptake inhibitors (SSRIs) or serotonin norepinephrine reuptake inhibitors (SNRIs). If concomitant treatment with sumatriptan and an SSRI (e.g., fluoxetine, paroxetine, sertraline, fluvoxamine, citalopram, escitalopram) or SNRI (e.g., venlafaxine, duloxetine) is clinically warranted, careful observation of the patient is advised, particularly during treatment initiation and dose increases. Serotonin syndrome symptoms may include mental status changes (e.g., agitation, hallucinations, coma), autonomic instability (e.g., tachycardia, labile blood pressure, hyperthermia), neuromuscular aberrations (e.g., hyperreflexia, incoordination), and/or gastrointestinal symptoms (e.g., nausea, vomiting, diarrhea).

Increase in Blood Pressure
Significant elevation in blood pressure, including hypertensive crisis, has been reported on rare occasions in patients with and without a history of hypertension. Sumatriptan is contraindicated in patients with uncontrolled hypertension (see CONTRAINDICATIONS). Sumatriptan should be administered with caution to patients with controlled hypertension as transient increases in blood pressure and peripheral vascular resistance have been observed in a small proportion of patients.

Local Irritation
Of the 3,378 patients using the nasal spray (5-, 10-, or 20-mg doses) on 1 or 2 occasions in controlled clinical studies, approximately 5% noted irritation in the nose and throat. Irritative symptoms such as burning, numbness, paresthesia, discharge, and pain or soreness were noted to be severe in about 1% of patients treated. The symptoms were transient and in approximately 60% of the cases, the symptoms resolved in less than 2 hours. Limited examinations of the nose and throat did not reveal any clinically noticeable injury in these patients.

The consequences of extended and repeated use of IMITREX Nasal Spray on the nasal and/or respiratory mucosa have not been systematically evaluated in patients. No increase in the incidence of local irritation was observed in patients using IMITREX Nasal Spray repeatedly for up to 1 year.

In inhalation studies in rats dosed daily for up to 1 month at exposures as low as one half the maximum daily human exposure (based on dose per surface area of nasal cavity), epithelial hyperplasia (with and without keratinization) and squamous metaplasia were observed in the larynx at all doses tested. These changes were partially reversible after a 2-week drug-free period. When dogs were dosed daily with various formulations by intranasal instillation for up to 13 weeks at exposures of 2 to 4 times the maximum daily human exposure (based on dose per surface area of nasal cavity), respiratory and nasal mucosa exhibited evidence of epithelial hyperplasia, focal squamous metaplasia, granulomata, bronchitis, and fibrosing alveolitis. A no-effect dose was not established. The changes observed in both species are not considered to be signs of either preneoplastic or neoplastic transformation.

Local effects on nasal and respiratory tissues after chronic intranasal dosing in animals have not been studied.

Concomitant Drug Use
In patients taking MAO-A inhibitors, sumatriptan plasma levels attained after treatment with recommended doses are 2-fold (following subcutaneous administration) to 7-fold (following oral administration) higher than those obtained under other conditions. Accordingly, the coadministration of IMITREX Nasal Spray and an MAO-A inhibitor is contraindicated (see CLINICAL PHARMACOLOGY and CONTRAINDICATIONS).

Hypersensitivity
Hypersensitivity (anaphylaxis/anaphylactoid) reactions have occurred on rare occasions in patients receiving sumatriptan. Such reactions can be life threatening or fatal. In general, hypersensitivity reactions to drugs are more likely to occur in individuals with a history of sensitivity to multiple allergens (see CONTRAINDICATIONS).

PRECAUTIONS
General
Chest discomfort and jaw or neck tightness have been reported infrequently following the administration of IMITREX Nasal Spray and have also been reported following use of IMITREX Tablets. Chest, jaw, or neck tightness is relatively common after administration of IMITREX Injection. Only rarely have these symptoms been associated with ischemic ECG changes. However, because sumatriptan may cause coronary artery vasospasm, patients who experience signs or symptoms suggestive of angina following sumatriptan should be evaluated for the presence of CAD or a predisposition to Prinzmetal variant angina before receiving additional doses of sumatriptan, and should be monitored electrocardiographically if dosing is resumed and similar symptoms recur. Similarly, patients who experience other symptoms or signs suggestive of decreased arterial flow, such as ischemic bowel syndrome or Raynaud syndrome following sumatriptan should be evaluated for atherosclerosis or predisposition to vasospasm (see WARNINGS).

IMITREX Nasal Spray should also be administered with caution to patients with diseases that may alter the absorption, metabolism, or excretion of drugs, such as impaired hepatic or renal function.

There have been rare reports of seizure following administration of sumatriptan. Sumatriptan should be used with caution in patients with a history of epilepsy or conditions associated with a lowered seizure threshold.

Care should be taken to exclude other potentially serious neurologic conditions before treating headache in patients not previously diagnosed with migraine headache or who experience a headache that is atypical for them. There have been rare reports where patients received sumatriptan for severe headaches that were subsequently shown to have been secondary to an evolving neurologic lesion (see WARNINGS).

For a given attack, if a patient does not respond to the first dose of sumatriptan, the diagnosis of migraine headache should be reconsidered before administration of a second dose.

Overuse of acute migraine treatments has been associated with the exacerbation of headache (medication overuse headache) in susceptible patients. Withdrawal of the treatment may be necessary.

Binding to Melanin-Containing Tissues
In rats treated with a single subcutaneous dose (0.5 mg/kg) or oral dose (2 mg/kg) of radiolabeled sumatriptan, the elimination half-life of radioactivity from the eye was 15 and 23 days, respectively, suggesting that sumatriptan and/or its metabolites bind to the melanin of the eye. Comparable studies were not performed by the intranasal route. Because there could be an accumulation in melanin-rich tissues over time, this raises the possibility that sumatriptan could cause toxicity in these tissues after extended use. However, no effects on the retina related to treatment with sumatriptan were noted in any of the oral or subcutaneous toxicity studies. Although no systematic monitoring of ophthalmologic function was undertaken in clinical trials, and no specific recommendations for ophthalmologic monitoring are offered, prescribers should be aware of the possibility of long-term ophthalmologic effects.

Corneal Opacities
Sumatriptan causes corneal opacities and defects in the corneal epithelium in dogs; this raises the possibility that these changes may occur in humans. While patients were not systematically evaluated for these changes in clinical trials, and no specific recommendations for monitoring are being offered, prescribers should be aware of the possibility of these changes (see ANIMAL TOXICOLOGY).

Information for Patients
See PATIENT INFORMATION at the end of this labeling for the text of the separate leaflet provided for patients.

Patients should be cautioned about the risk of serotonin syndrome with the use of sumatriptan or other triptans, especially during combined use with SSRIs or SNRIs.

Laboratory Tests
No specific laboratory tests are recommended for monitoring patients prior to and/or after treatment with sumatriptan.

Drug Interactions
Selective Serotonin Reuptake Inhibitors/Serotonin Norepinephrine Reuptake Inhibitors and Serotonin Syndrome
Cases of life-threatening serotonin syndrome have been reported during combined use of SSRIs or SNRIs and triptans (see WARNINGS).

Ergot-Containing Drugs
Ergot-containing drugs have been reported to cause prolonged vasospastic reactions. Because there is a theoretical basis that these effects may be additive, use of ergotamine-containing or ergot-type medications (like dihydroergotamine or methysergide) and sumatriptan within 24 hours of each other should be avoided (see CONTRAINDICATIONS).
Monoamine Oxidase-A Inhibitors
MAO-A inhibitors reduce sumatriptan clearance, significantly increasing systemic exposure. Therefore, the use of IMITREX Nasal Spray in patients receiving MAO-A inhibitors is contraindicated (see CLINICAL PHARMACOLOGY and CONTRAINDICATIONS).

Drug/Laboratory Test Interactions
IMITREX Nasal Spray is not known to interfere with commonly employed clinical laboratory tests.

Carcinogenesis, Mutagenesis, Impairment of Fertility
Carcinogenesis
In carcinogenicity studies, rats and mice were given sumatriptan by oral gavage (rats: 104 weeks) or drinking water (mice: 78 weeks). Average exposures achieved in mice receiving the highest dose (target dose of 160 mg/kg/day) were approximately 184 times the exposure attained in humans after the maximum recommended single intranasal dose of 20 mg. The highest dose administered to rats (160 mg/kg/day, reduced from 360 mg/kg/day during week 21) was approximately 78 times the maximum recommended single intranasal dose of 20 mg on a mg/m^2 basis. There was no evidence of an increase in tumors in either species related to sumatriptan administration. Local effects on nasal and respiratory tissue after chronic intranasal dosing in animals have not been evaluated (see WARNINGS).
Mutagenesis
Sumatriptan was not mutagenic in the presence or absence of metabolic activation when tested in 2 gene mutation assays (the Ames test and the in vitro mammalian Chinese hamster V79/HGPRT assay). In 2 cytogenetics assays (the in vitro human lymphocyte assay and the in vivo rat micronucleus assay) sumatriptan was not associated with clastogenic activity.
Impairment of Fertility
In a study in which male and female rats were dosed daily with oral sumatriptan prior to and throughout the mating period, there was a treatment-related decrease in fertility secondary to a decrease in mating in animals treated with 50 and 500 mg/kg/day. The highest no-effect dose for this finding was 5 mg/kg/day, or approximately twice the maximum recommended single human intranasal dose of 20 mg on a mg/m^2 basis. It is not clear whether the problem is associated with treatment of the males or females or both combined. In a similar study by the subcutaneous route there was no evidence of impaired fertility at 60 mg/kg/day, the maximum dose tested, which is equivalent to approximately 29 times the maximum recommended single human intranasal dose of 20 mg on a mg/m^2 basis. Fertility studies, in which sumatriptan was administered by the intranasal route, were not conducted.

Pregnancy
Pregnancy Category C. In reproductive toxicity studies in rats and rabbits, oral treatment with sumatriptan was associated with embryolethality, fetal abnormalities, and pup mortality. When administered by the intravenous route to rabbits, sumatriptan has been shown to be embryolethal. Reproductive toxicity studies for sumatriptan by the intranasal route have not been conducted.
There are no adequate and well-controlled studies in pregnant women. Therefore, IMITREX Nasal Spray should be used during pregnancy only if the potential benefit justifies the potential risk to the fetus. In assessing this information, the following findings should be considered.
Embryolethality
When given orally or intravenously to pregnant rabbits daily throughout the period of organogenesis, sumatriptan caused embryolethality at doses at or close to those producing maternal toxicity. In the oral studies this dose was 100 mg/kg/day, and in the intravenous studies this dose was 2.0 mg/kg/day. The mechanism of the embryolethality is not known. The highest no-effect dose for embryolethality by the oral route was 50 mg/kg/day, which is approximately 48 times the maximum single recommended human intranasal dose of 20 mg on a mg/m^2 basis. By the intravenous route, the highest no-effect dose was 0.75 mg/kg/day, or approximately 0.7 times the maximum single recommended human intranasal dose of 20 mg on a mg/m^2 basis.
The intravenous administration of sumatriptan to pregnant rats throughout organogenesis at 12.5 mg/kg/day, the maximum dose tested, did not cause embryolethality. This dose is approximately 6 times the maximum single recommended human intranasal dose of 20 mg on a mg/m^2 basis. Additionally, in a study in rats given subcutaneous sumatriptan daily, prior to and throughout pregnancy, at 60 mg/kg/day, the maximum dose tested, there was no evidence of increased embryo/fetal lethality. This dose is equivalent to approximately 29 times the maximum recommended single human intranasal dose of 20 mg on a mg/m^2 basis.
Teratogenicity
Oral treatment of pregnant rats with sumatriptan during the period of organogenesis resulted in an increased incidence of blood vessel abnormalities (cervicothoracic and umbilical) at doses of approximately 250 mg/kg/day or higher. The highest no-effect dose was approximately 60 mg/kg/day, which is approximately 29 times the maximum single recommended human intranasal dose of 20 mg on a mg/m^2 basis. Oral treatment of pregnant rabbits with sumatriptan during the period of organogenesis resulted in an increased incidence of cervicothoracic vascular and skeletal abnormalities. The highest no-effect dose for these effects was 15 mg/kg/day, or approximately 14 times the maximum single recommended human intranasal dose of 20 mg on a mg/m^2 basis.
A study in which rats were dosed daily with oral sumatriptan prior to and throughout gestation demonstrated embryo/fetal toxicity (decreased body weight, decreased ossification, increased incidence of rib variations) and an increased incidence of a syndrome of malformations (short tail/short body and vertebral disorganization) at 500 mg/kg/day. The highest no-effect dose was 50 mg/kg/day, or approximately 24 times the maximum single recommended human intranasal dose of 20 mg on a mg/m^2 basis. In a study in rats dosed daily with subcutaneous sumatriptan prior to and throughout pregnancy, at a dose of 60 mg/kg/day, the maximum dose tested, there was no evidence of teratogenicity. This dose is equivalent to approximately 29 times the maximum recommended single human intranasal dose of 20 mg on a mg/m^2 basis.
Pup Deaths
Oral treatment of pregnant rats with sumatriptan during the period of organogenesis resulted in a decrease in pup survival between birth and postnatal day 4 at doses of approximately 250 mg/kg/day or higher. The highest no-effect dose for this effect was approximately 60 mg/kg/day, or 29 times the maximum single recommended human intranasal dose of 20 mg on a mg/m^2 basis.
Oral treatment of pregnant rats with sumatriptan from gestational day 17 through postnatal day 21 demonstrated a decrease in pup survival measured at postnatal days 2, 4, and 20 at the dose of 1,000 mg/kg/day. The highest no-effect dose for this finding was 100 mg/kg/day, approximately 49 times the maximum single recommended human intranasal dose of 20 mg on a mg/m^2 basis. In a similar study in rats by the subcutaneous route there was no increase in pup death at 81 mg/kg/day, the highest dose tested, which is equivalent to 40 times the maximum single recommended human intranasal dose of 20 mg on a mg/m^2 basis.
Pregnancy Registry
To monitor fetal outcomes of pregnant women exposed to IMITREX, GlaxoSmithKline maintains a Sumatriptan Pregnancy Registry. Physicians are encouraged to register patients by calling (800) 336-2176.

Nursing Mothers
Sumatriptan is excreted in human breast milk following subcutaneous administration. Infant exposure to sumatriptan can be minimized by avoiding breastfeeding for 12 hours after treatment with IMITREX Nasal Spray.

Pediatric Use
Safety and effectiveness of IMITREX Nasal Spray in pediatric patients under 18 years of age have not been established; therefore, IMITREX Nasal Spray is not recommended for use in patients under 18 years of age.
Two controlled clinical trials evaluating sumatriptan nasal spray (5 to 20 mg) in pediatric patients aged 12 to 17 years enrolled a total of 1,248 adolescent migraineurs who treated a single attack. The studies did not establish the efficacy of sumatriptan nasal spray compared to placebo in the treatment of migraine in adolescents. Adverse events observed in these clinical trials were similar in nature to those reported in clinical trials in adults.
Five controlled clinical trials (2 single attack studies, 3 multiple attack studies) evaluating oral sumatriptan (25 to 100 mg) in pediatric patients aged 12 to 17 years enrolled a total of 701 adolescent migraineurs. These studies did not establish the efficacy of oral sumatriptan compared to placebo in the treatment of migraine in adolescents. Adverse events observed in these clinical trials were similar in nature to those reported in clinical trials in adults. The frequency of all adverse events in these patients appeared to be both dose- and age-dependent, with younger patients reporting events more commonly than older adolescents.
Postmarketing experience documents that serious adverse events have occurred in the pediatric population after use of subcutaneous, oral, and/or intranasal sumatriptan. These reports include events similar in nature to those reported rarely in adults, including stroke, visual loss, and death. A myocardial infarction has been reported in a 14-year-old male following the use of oral sumatriptan; clinical signs occurred within 1 day of drug administration. Since clinical data to determine the frequency of serious adverse events in pediatric patients who might receive injectable, oral, or intranasal sumatriptan are not presently available, the use of sumatriptan in patients aged younger than 18 years is not recommended.

Geriatric Use
The use of sumatriptan in elderly patients is not recommended because elderly patients are more likely to have decreased hepatic function, they are at higher risk for CAD, and blood pressure increases may be more pronounced in the elderly (see WARNINGS).

ADVERSE REACTIONS

Serious cardiac events, including some that have been fatal, have occurred following the use of IMITREX Injection or Tablets. These events are extremely rare and most have been reported in patients with risk factors predictive of CAD. Events reported have included coronary artery vasospasm, transient myocardial ischemia, myocardial infarction, ventricular tachycardia, and ventricular fibrillation (see CONTRAINDICATIONS, WARNINGS, and PRECAUTIONS).
Significant hypertensive episodes, including hypertensive crises, have been reported on rare occasions in patients with or without a history of hypertension (see WARNINGS).

Incidence in Controlled Clinical Trials
Among 3,653 patients treated with IMITREX Nasal Spray in active- and placebo-controlled clinical trials, less than 0.4% of patients withdrew for reasons related to adverse events. Table 2 lists adverse events that occurred in worldwide placebo-controlled clinical trials in 3,419 migraineurs. The events cited reflect experience gained under closely monitored conditions of clinical trials in a highly selected patient population. In actual clinical practice or in other clinical trials, these frequency estimates may not apply, as the conditions of use, reporting behavior, and the kinds of patients treated may differ.
Only events that occurred at a frequency of 1% or more in the IMITREX Nasal Spray 20-mg treatment group and were more frequent in that group than in the placebo group are included in Table 2.
[See table 2 above]
Phonophobia also occurred in more than 1% of patients but was more frequent on placebo.
IMITREX Nasal Spray is generally well tolerated. Across all doses, most adverse reactions were mild and transient and did not lead to long-lasting effects. The incidence of adverse events in controlled clinical trials was not affected by gen-

Table 2. Treatment-Emergent Adverse Events Reported by at Least 1% of Patients in Controlled Migraine Trials

Adverse Event Type	Percent of Patients Reporting			
	Placebo (n = 704)	IMITREX 5 mg (n = 496)	IMITREX 10 mg (n = 1,007)	IMITREX 20 mg (n = 1,212)
Atypical sensations				
Burning sensation	0.1%	0.4%	0.6%	1.4%
Ear, nose, and throat				
Disorder/discomfort of nasal cavity/sinuses	2.4%	2.8%	2.5%	3.8%
Throat discomfort	0.9%	0.8%	1.8%	2.4%
Gastrointestinal				
Nausea and/or vomiting	11.3%	12.2%	11.0%	13.5%
Neurological				
Bad/unusual taste	1.7%	13.5%	19.3%	24.5%
Dizziness/vertigo	0.9%	1.0%	1.7%	1.4%

der, weight, or age of the patients; use of prophylactic medications; or presence of aura. There were insufficient data to assess the impact of race on the incidence of adverse events.

Other Events Observed in Association With the Administration of IMITREX Nasal Spray

In the paragraphs that follow, the frequencies of less commonly reported adverse clinical events are presented. Because the reports include events observed in open and uncontrolled studies, the role of IMITREX Nasal Spray in their causation cannot be reliably determined. Furthermore, variability associated with adverse event reporting, the terminology used to describe adverse events, etc., limit the value of the quantitative frequency estimates provided. Event frequencies are calculated as the number of patients who used IMITREX Nasal Spray (5, 10, or 20 mg in controlled and uncontrolled trials) and reported an event divided by the total number of patients (N = 3,711) exposed to IMITREX Nasal Spray. All reported events are included except those already listed in the previous table, those too general to be informative, and those not reasonably associated with the use of the drug. Events are further classified within body system categories and enumerated in order of decreasing frequency using the following definitions: infrequent adverse events are those occurring in 1/100 to 1/1,000 patients and rare adverse events are those occurring in fewer than 1/1,000 patients.

Atypical Sensations
Infrequent were tingling, warm/hot sensation, numbness, pressure sensation, feeling strange, feeling of heaviness, feeling of tightness, paresthesia, cold sensation, and tight feeling in head. Rare were dysesthesia and prickling sensation.

Cardiovascular
Infrequent were flushing and hypertension (see WARNINGS), palpitations, tachycardia, changes in ECG, and arrhythmia (see WARNINGS and PRECAUTIONS). Rare were abdominal aortic aneurysm, hypotension, bradycardia, pallor, and phlebitis.

Chest Symptoms
Infrequent were chest tightness, chest discomfort, and chest pressure/heaviness (see PRECAUTIONS: General).

Ear, Nose, and Throat
Infrequent were disturbance of hearing and ear infection. Rare were otalgia and Meniere disease.

Endocrine and Metabolic
Infrequent was thirst. Rare were galactorrhea, hypothyroidism, and weight loss.

Eye
Infrequent were irritation of eyes and visual disturbance.

Gastrointestinal
Infrequent were abdominal discomfort, diarrhea, dysphagia, and gastroesophageal reflux. Rare were constipation, flatulence/eructation, hematemesis, intestinal obstruction, melena, gastroenteritis, colitis, hemorrhage of gastrointestinal tract, and pancreatitis.

Mouth and Teeth
Infrequent was disorder of mouth and tongue (e.g., burning of tongue, numbness of tongue, dry mouth).

Musculoskeletal
Infrequent were neck pain/stiffness, backache, weakness, joint symptoms, arthritis, and myalgia. Rare were muscle cramps, tetany, intervertebral disc disorder, and muscle stiffness.

Neurological
Infrequent were drowsiness/sedation, anxiety, sleep disturbances, tremors, syncope, shivers, chills, depression, agitation, sensation of lightness, and mental confusion. Rare were difficulty concentrating, hunger, lacrimation, memory disturbances, monoplegia/diplegia, apathy, disturbance of smell, disturbance of emotions, dysarthria, facial pain, intoxication, stress, decreased appetite, difficulty coordinating, euphoria, and neoplasm of pituitary.

Respiratory
Infrequent were dyspnea and lower respiratory tract infection. Rare was asthma.

Skin
Infrequent were rash/skin eruption, pruritus, and erythema. Rare were herpes, swelling of face, sweating, and peeling of skin.

Urogenital
Infrequent were dysuria, disorder of breasts, and dysmenorrhea. Rare were endometriosis and increased urination.

Miscellaneous
Infrequent were cough, edema, and fever. Rare were hypersensitivity, swelling of extremities, voice disturbances, difficulty in walking, and lymphadenopathy.

Other Events Observed in the Clinical Development of IMITREX

The following adverse events occurred in clinical trials with IMITREX Injection and IMITREX Tablets. Because the reports include events observed in open and uncontrolled studies, the role of IMITREX in their causation cannot be reliably determined. All reported events are included except

those already listed, those too general to be informative, and those not reasonably associated with the use of the drug.

Breasts
Breast swelling; cysts, lumps, and masses of breasts; nipple discharge; primary malignant breast neoplasm; and tenderness.

Cardiovascular
Abnormal pulse, angina, atherosclerosis, cerebral ischemia, cerebrovascular lesion, heart block, peripheral cyanosis, pulsating sensations, Raynaud syndrome, thrombosis, transient myocardial ischemia, various transient ECG changes (nonspecific ST or T wave changes, prolongation of PR or QTc intervals, sinus arrhythmia, nonsustained ventricular premature beats, isolated junctional ectopic beats, atrial ectopic beats, delayed activation of the right ventricle), and vasodilation.

Ear, Nose, and Throat
Allergic rhinitis; ear, nose, and throat hemorrhage; external otitis; feeling of fullness in the ear(s); hearing disturbances; hearing loss; nasal inflammation; sensitivity to noise; sinusitis; tinnitus; and upper respiratory inflammation.

Endocrine and Metabolic
Dehydration; endocrine cysts, lumps, and masses; elevated thyrotropin stimulating hormone (TSH) levels; fluid disturbances; hyperglycemia; hypoglycemia; polydipsia; and weight gain.

Eye
Accommodation disorders, blindness and low vision, conjunctivitis, disorders of sclera, external ocular muscle disorders, eye edema and swelling, eye itching, eye hemorrhage, eye pain, keratitis, mydriasis, and vision alterations.

Gastrointestinal
Abdominal distention, dental pain, disturbances of liver function tests, dyspeptic symptoms, feelings of gastrointestinal pressure, gallstones, gastric symptoms, gastritis, gastrointestinal pain, hypersalivation, hyposalivation, oral itching and irritation, peptic ulcer, retching, salivary gland swelling, and swallowing disorders.

Hematological Disorders
Anemia.

Injection Site Reaction

Miscellaneous
Contusions, fluid retention, hematoma, hypersensitivity to various agents, jaw discomfort, miscellaneous laboratory abnormalities, overdose, "serotonin agonist effect," and speech disturbance.

Musculoskeletal
Acquired musculoskeletal deformity, arthralgia and articular rheumatitis, muscle atrophy, muscle tiredness, musculoskeletal inflammation, need to flex calf muscles, rigidity, tightness, and various joint disturbances (pain, stiffness, swelling, ache).

Neurological
Aggressiveness, bradylogia, cluster headache, convulsions, detachment, disturbances of taste, drug abuse, dystonia, facial paralysis, globus hystericus, hallucinations, headache, heat sensitivity, hyperesthesia, hysteria, increased alertness, malaise/fatigue, migraine, motor dysfunction, myoclonia, neuralgia, neurotic disorders, paralysis, personality change, phobia, photophobia, psychomotor disorders, radiculopathy, raised intracranial pressure, relaxation, stinging sensations, transient hemiplegia, simultaneous hot and cold sensations, suicide, tickling sensations, twitching, and yawning.

Pain and Other Pressure Sensations
Chest pain, neck tightness/pressure, throat/jaw pain/tightness/pressure, and pain (location specified).

Respiratory
Breathing disorders, bronchitis, diseases of the lower respiratory tract, hiccoughs, and influenza.

Skin
Dry/scaly skin, eczema, seborrheic dermatitis, skin nodules, skin tenderness, tightness of skin, and wrinkling of skin.

Urogenital
Abortion, abnormal menstrual cycle, bladder inflammation, hematuria, inflammation of fallopian tubes, intermenstrual bleeding, menstruation symptoms, micturition disorders, renal calculus, urethritis, urinary frequency, and urinary infections.

Postmarketing Experience (Reports for Subcutaneous or Oral Sumatriptan)

The following section enumerates potentially important adverse events that have occurred in clinical practice and that have been reported spontaneously to various surveillance systems. The events enumerated represent reports arising from both domestic and nondomestic use of oral or subcutaneous dosage forms of sumatriptan. The events enumerated include all except those already listed in the ADVERSE REACTIONS section above or those too general to be informative. Because the reports cite events reported spontaneously from worldwide postmarketing experience, frequency of events and the role of sumatriptan in their causation cannot

be reliably determined. It is assumed, however, that systemic reactions following sumatriptan use are likely to be similar regardless of route of administration.

Blood
Hemolytic anemia, pancytopenia, thrombocytopenia.

Cardiovascular
Atrial fibrillation, cardiomyopathy, colonic ischemia (see WARNINGS), Prinzmetal variant angina, pulmonary embolism, shock, thrombophlebitis.

Ear, Nose, and Throat
Deafness.

Eye
Ischemic optic neuropathy, retinal artery occlusion, retinal vein thrombosis, loss of vision.

Gastrointestinal
Ischemic colitis with rectal bleeding (see WARNINGS), xerostomia.

Hepatic
Elevated liver function tests.

Neurological
Central nervous system vasculitis, cerebrovascular accident, dysphasia, serotonin syndrome, subarachnoid hemorrhage.

Non-Site Specific
Angioneurotic edema, cyanosis, death (see WARNINGS), temporal arteritis.

Psychiatry
Panic disorder.

Respiratory
Bronchospasm in patients with and without a history of asthma.

Skin
Exacerbation of sunburn, hypersensitivity reactions (allergic vasculitis, erythema, pruritus, rash, shortness of breath, urticaria; in addition, severe anaphylaxis/anaphylactoid reactions have been reported [see WARNINGS]), photosensitivity.

Urogenital
Acute renal failure.

DRUG ABUSE AND DEPENDENCE

One clinical study with IMITREX (sumatriptan succinate) Injection enrolling 12 patients with a history of substance abuse failed to induce subjective behavior and/or physiologic response ordinarily associated with drugs that have an established potential for abuse.

OVERDOSAGE

In clinical trials, the highest single doses of IMITREX Nasal Spray administered without significant adverse effects were 40 mg to 12 volunteers and 40 mg to 85 migraine patients, which is twice the highest single recommended dose. In addition, 12 volunteers were administered a total daily dose of 60 mg (20 mg 3 times daily) for 3.5 days without significant adverse events.

Overdose in animals has been fatal and has been heralded by convulsions, tremor, paralysis, inactivity, ptosis, erythema of the extremities, abnormal respiration, cyanosis, ataxia, mydriasis, salivation, and lacrimation. The elimination half-life of sumatriptan is about 2 hours (see CLINICAL PHARMACOLOGY), and therefore monitoring of patients after overdose with IMITREX Nasal Spray should continue for at least 10 hours or while symptoms or signs persist. It is unknown what effect hemodialysis or peritoneal dialysis has on the serum concentrations of sumatriptan.

DOSAGE AND ADMINISTRATION

In controlled clinical trials, single doses of 5, 10, or 20 mg of IMITREX Nasal Spray administered into 1 nostril were effective for the acute treatment of migraine in adults. A greater proportion of patients had headache response following a 20-mg dose than following a 5- or 10-mg dose (see CLINICAL TRIALS). Individuals may vary in response to doses of IMITREX Nasal Spray. The choice of dose should therefore be made on an individual basis, weighing the possible benefit of the 20-mg dose with the potential for a greater risk of adverse events. A 10-mg dose may be achieved by the administration of a single 5-mg dose in each nostril. There is evidence that doses above 20 mg do not provide a greater effect than 20 mg.

If the headache returns, the dose may be repeated once after 2 hours, not to exceed a total daily dose of 40 mg. The safety of treating an average of more than 4 headaches in a 30-day period has not been established.

HOW SUPPLIED

IMITREX Nasal Spray 5 mg (NDC 0173-0524-00) and 20 mg (NDC 0173-0523-00) are each supplied in boxes of 6 nasal spray devices. Each unit dose spray supplies 5 and 20 mg, respectively, of sumatriptan.

Store between 36° and 86°F (2° and 30°C). Protect from light.

ANIMAL TOXICOLOGY

Corneal Opacities

Dogs receiving oral sumatriptan developed corneal opacities and defects in the corneal epithelium. Corneal opacities were seen at the lowest dosage tested, 2 mg/kg/day, and were present after 1 month of treatment. Defects in the corneal epithelium were noted in a 60-week study. Earlier examinations for these toxicities were not conducted and no-effect doses were not established; however, the relative exposure at the lowest dose tested was approximately 5 times the human exposure after a 100-mg oral dose or 3 times the human exposure after a 6-mg subcutaneous dose or 22 times the human exposure after a single 20-mg intranasal dose. There is evidence of alterations in corneal appearance on the first day of intranasal dosing to dogs. Changes were noted at the lowest dose tested, which was approximately 2 times the maximum single human intranasal dose of 20 mg on a mg/m^2 basis.

This product's prescribing information may have been updated. Please refer to www.gsk.com for the most current version.

GlaxoSmithKline
Research Triangle Park, NC 27709
©2010, GlaxoSmithKline. All rights reserved.
February 2010
IMN:2PI

PATIENT INFORMATION

The following wording is contained in a separate leaflet provided for patients.

Information for the Patient

IMITREX® (sumatriptan) Nasal Spray

Read this leaflet carefully before you start to take IMITREX Nasal Spray. Keep the leaflet for reference because it gives you a summary of important information about IMITREX Nasal Spray.

Read the leaflet that comes with each refill of your prescription because there may be new information.

This leaflet does not have all the information about IMITREX Nasal Spray. Ask your healthcare provider for more information or advice.

What is IMITREX Nasal Spray?

IMITREX Nasal Spray is a kind of medicine called a triptan. You should take it only if you have a prescription.

IMITREX Nasal Spray is used to relieve your migraine. It is **not** used to prevent attacks or reduce the number of attacks you have. Use IMITREX Nasal Spray only to treat an actual migraine attack.

The decision to use IMITREX Nasal Spray is one that you and your healthcare provider should make together, based on your personal needs and health.

Talk with your healthcare provider before taking IMITREX Nasal Spray

1. **Risk factors for heart disease to tell your healthcare provider:**

   Tell your healthcare provider if you have risk factors for heart disease such as:
   - high blood pressure
   - high cholesterol
   - being overweight
   - diabetes
   - smoking
   - strong family history of heart disease
   - you are postmenopausal
   - you are a male over 40 years of age

   If you do have risk factors for heart disease, your healthcare provider should check you for heart disease to see if IMITREX is right for you.

   Although most of the people who have taken IMITREX have not had any serious side effects, some have had serious heart problems. Deaths have been reported, but these were rare considering the extensive worldwide use of IMITREX. Usually, serious problems happened in people with known heart disease. It was not clear whether IMITREX had anything to do with these deaths.

2. **Important questions to ask yourself before you take IMITREX Nasal Spray:**

   If the answer to any of the following questions is **YES** or if you do not know the answer, then please talk with your healthcare provider before you take IMITREX Nasal Spray.
   - Are you pregnant? Do you think you might be pregnant? Are you trying to become pregnant? Are you not using adequate contraception? Are you breastfeeding?
   - Do you have any chest pain, heart disease, shortness of breath, or irregular heartbeats? Have you had a heart attack?
   - Do you have risk factors for heart disease (see list above)?
   - Have you had a stroke, a mini-stroke (also called a transient ischemic attack or TIA), or Raynaud syndrome?
   - Do you have high blood pressure?
   - Have you ever had to stop taking this or any other medicine because of an allergy or other problems?
   - Are you taking any other migraine medicines, including other triptans? Are you taking any medicines containing ergotamine, dihydroergotamine, or methysergide?
   - Are you taking any medicine for depression or other health problems such as a monoamine oxidase inhibitor, selective serotonin reuptake inhibitor (SSRI), or serotonin norepinephrine reuptake inhibitor (SNRI)? Common SSRIs are citalopram HBr (CELEXA®), escitalopram oxalate (LEXAPRO®), paroxetine (PAXIL®), fluoxetine (PROZAC®/SARAFEM®), olanzapine/fluoxetine (SYMBYAX®), sertraline (ZOLOFT®), and fluvoxamine. Common SNRIs are duloxetine (CYMBALTA®) and venlafaxine (EFFEXOR®).
   - Have you had, or do you have, any disease of the liver or kidney?
   - Have you had, or do you have, epilepsy or seizures?
   - Is this headache different from your usual migraine attacks?

Remember, if you answered **YES** to any of the above questions, then talk with your healthcare provider about it.

Important points about IMITREX Nasal Spray

1. The use of IMITREX Nasal Spray during pregnancy:

Do not take IMITREX Nasal Spray if you are pregnant, think you might be pregnant, are trying to become pregnant, or are not using adequate contraception unless you have talked with your healthcare provider about this.

2. How to take IMITREX Nasal Spray:

Before taking IMITREX Nasal Spray, see the enclosed instructions leaflet.

For adults, the usual dose is a single nasal spray in 1 nostril. If your headache comes back, you can take a second nasal spray anytime after 2 hours after you took the first spray.

For any attack where you have no response to the first nasal spray, do not take a second nasal spray without first talking with your healthcare provider. Do not take more than a total of 40 mg of IMITREX Nasal Spray in any 24-hour period.

The safety of treating an average of more than 4 headaches in a 30-day period has not been established.

The effects of long-term repeated use of IMITREX Nasal Spray on the surfaces of the nose and throat have not been specifically studied.

3. Caution for activities requiring alertness:

You may feel drowsy or dizzy because of your migraine or treatment with IMITREX Nasal Spray. Use caution for activities requiring alertness (like driving or using machines).

4. What to do if you take an overdose:

If you have taken more medicine than has been prescribed for you, contact either your healthcare provider, hospital emergency department, or nearest poison control center right away.

5. How to store your medicine:

Keep your medicine in a safe place where children cannot reach it. It may be harmful to children.

Store your medicine away from heat and light. Do not store at temperatures above 86°F (30°C) or below 36°F (2°C).

The expiration date of your medicine is printed on the packaging. If your medicine has expired, throw it away.

If your healthcare provider decides to stop your treatment, do not keep any leftover medicine unless your healthcare provider tells you to.

Some possible side effects of IMITREX Nasal Spray

- Some patients feel pain or tightness in the chest or throat when using IMITREX Nasal Spray. If this happens to you, tell your healthcare provider before taking any more IMITREX Nasal Spray. If the chest pain, tightness, or pressure is severe or does not go away, call your healthcare provider right away.
- Call your healthcare provider right away if you have sudden and/or severe abdominal pain after you take IMITREX Nasal Spray.
- Some people may have a reaction called serotonin syndrome when they take certain kinds of medicines for depression called SSRIs or SNRIs while they are taking IMITREX Nasal Spray. Symptoms may include confusion, hallucinations, fast heartbeat, feeling faint, fever, sweating, muscle spasm, difficulty walking, and/or diarrhea. Call your healthcare provider right away if you have any of these symptoms after taking IMITREX Nasal Spray.
- Shortness of breath; wheeziness; heart throbbing; swelling of eyelids, face, or lips; or a skin rash, skin lumps, or hives happens rarely. If it happens to you, then tell your healthcare provider right away. Do not take any more IMITREX Nasal Spray unless your healthcare provider tells you to.
- Some people may feel tingling, heat, flushing (redness of face lasting a short time), heaviness, or pressure after taking IMITREX Nasal Spray. A few people may feel drowsy, dizzy, tired, sick, or may experience nasal irritation. If you have any of these symptoms, tell your healthcare provider at your next visit.
- If you feel unwell in any other way or have any symptoms that you do not understand, you should contact your healthcare provider right away.

IMITREX and PAXIL are registered trademarks of GlaxoSmithKline. The other brands listed are trademarks of their respective owners and are not trademarks of GlaxoSmithKline. The makers of these brands are not affiliated with and do not endorse GlaxoSmithKline or its products.

GlaxoSmithKline
Research Triangle Park, NC 27709
©2010, GlaxoSmithKline. All rights reserved.
February 2010
IMN:2PIL

IMITREX® ℞

[ĭm' ĭ-trĕx]

(sumatriptan succinate)

Tablets

DESCRIPTION

IMITREX Tablets contain sumatriptan (as the succinate), a selective 5-hydroxytryptamine$_1$ receptor subtype agonist. Sumatriptan succinate is chemically designated as 3-[2-(dimethylamino)ethyl]-N-methyl-indole-5-methanesulfonamide succinate (1:1), and it has the following structure:

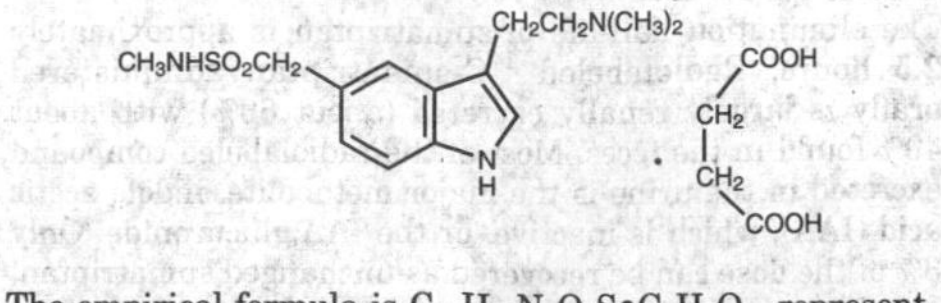

The empirical formula is $C_{14}H_{21}N_3O_2S \cdot C_4H_6O_4$, representing a molecular weight of 413.5. Sumatriptan succinate is a white to off-white powder that is readily soluble in water and in saline. Each IMITREX Tablet for oral administration contains 35, 70, or 140 mg of sumatriptan succinate equivalent to 25, 50, or 100 mg of sumatriptan, respectively. Each tablet also contains the inactive ingredients croscarmellose sodium, dibasic calcium phosphate, magnesium stearate, microcrystalline cellulose, and sodium bicarbonate. Each 100-mg tablet also contains hypromellose, iron oxide, titanium dioxide, and triacetin.

CLINICAL PHARMACOLOGY

Mechanism of Action

Sumatriptan is an agonist for a vascular 5-hydroxytryptamine$_1$ receptor subtype (probably a member of the 5-HT$_{1D}$ family) having only a weak affinity for 5-HT$_{1A}$, 5-HT$_{5A}$, and 5-HT$_7$ receptors and no significant affinity (as measured using standard radioligand binding assays) or pharmacological activity at 5-HT$_2$, 5-HT$_3$, or 5-HT$_4$ receptor subtypes or at alpha$_1$-, alpha$_2$-, or beta-adrenergic; dopamine$_1$; dopamine$_2$; muscarinic; or benzodiazepine receptors.

The vascular 5-HT$_1$ receptor subtype that sumatriptan activates is present on cranial arteries in both dog and primate, on the human basilar artery, and in the vasculature of human dura mater and mediates vasoconstriction. This action in humans correlates with the relief of migraine headache. In addition to causing vasoconstriction, experimental data from animal studies show that sumatriptan also activates 5-HT$_1$ receptors on peripheral terminals of the trigeminal nerve innervating cranial blood vessels. Such an action may also contribute to the antimigrainous effect of sumatriptan in humans.

In the anesthetized dog, sumatriptan selectively reduces the carotid arterial blood flow with little or no effect on arterial blood pressure or total peripheral resistance. In the cat, sumatriptan selectively constricts the carotid arteriovenous anastomoses while having little effect on blood flow or resistance in cerebral or extracerebral tissues.

Pharmacokinetics

The mean maximum concentration following oral dosing with 25 mg is 18 ng/mL (range: 7 to 47 ng/mL) and 51 ng/mL (range: 28 to 100 ng/mL) following oral dosing with 100 mg of sumatriptan. This compares with a C_{max} of 5 and 16 ng/mL following dosing with a 5- and 20-mg intranasal dose, respectively. The mean C_{max} following a 6-mg subcutaneous injection is 71 ng/mL (range: 49 to 110 ng/mL). The bioavailability is approximately 15%, primarily due to presystemic metabolism and partly due to incomplete absorption. The C_{max} is similar during a migraine attack and during a migraine-free period, but the T_{max} is slightly later during the attack, approximately 2.5 hours compared to 2.0 hours. When given as a single dose, sumatriptan displays dose proportionality in its extent of absorption (area under the curve [AUC]) over the dose range of 25 to 200 mg, but the C_{max} after 100 mg is approximately 25% less than expected (based on the 25-mg dose). A food effect study involving administration of IMITREX Tablets 100 mg to healthy volunteers under fasting condi-

Table 1. Percentage of Patients With Headache Response (No or Mild Pain) 2 and 4 Hours Following Treatment

	Placebo 2 hr 4 hr	IMITREX Tablets 25 mg 2 hr 4 hr	IMITREX Tablets 50 mg 2 hr 4 hr	IMITREX Tablets 100 mg 2 hr 4 hr
Study 1	27% 38% (N = 94)	52%[a] 67%[a] (N = 298)	61%[ab] 78%[ab] (N = 296)	62%[ab] 79%[ab] (N = 296)
Study 2	26% 38% (N = 65)	52%[a] 70%[a] (N = 66)	50%[a] 68%[a] (N = 62)	56%[a] 71%[a] (N = 66)
Study 3	17% 19% (N = 47)	52%[a] 65%[a] (N = 48)	54%[a] 72%[a] (N = 46)	57%[a] 78%[a] (N = 46)

[a] $p < 0.05$ in comparison with placebo.
[b] $p < 0.05$ in comparison with 25 mg.

tions and with a high-fat meal indicated that the C_{max} and AUC were increased by 15% and 12%, respectively, when administered in the fed state.

Plasma protein binding is low (14% to 21%). The effect of sumatriptan on the protein binding of other drugs has not been evaluated, but would be expected to be minor, given the low rate of protein binding. The apparent volume of distribution is 2.4 L/kg.

The elimination half-life of sumatriptan is approximately 2.5 hours. Radiolabeled ^{14}C-sumatriptan administered orally is largely renally excreted (about 60%) with about 40% found in the feces. Most of the radiolabeled compound excreted in the urine is the major metabolite, indole acetic acid (IAA), which is inactive, or the IAA glucuronide. Only 3% of the dose can be recovered as unchanged sumatriptan. In vitro studies with human microsomes suggest that sumatriptan is metabolized by monoamine oxidase (MAO), predominantly the A isoenzyme, and inhibitors of that enzyme may alter sumatriptan pharmacokinetics to increase systemic exposure. No significant effect was seen with an MAO-B inhibitor (see CONTRAINDICATIONS, WARNINGS, and PRECAUTIONS: Drug Interactions).

Special Populations
Renal Impairment
The effect of renal impairment on the pharmacokinetics of sumatriptan has not been examined, but little clinical effect would be expected as sumatriptan is largely metabolized to an inactive substance.

Hepatic Impairment
The liver plays an important role in the presystemic clearance of orally administered sumatriptan. Accordingly, the bioavailability of sumatriptan following oral administration may be markedly increased in patients with liver disease. In 1 small study of hepatically impaired patients (N = 8) matched for sex, age, and weight with healthy subjects, the hepatically impaired patients had an approximately 70% increase in AUC and C_{max} and a T_{max} 40 minutes earlier compared to the healthy subjects (see DOSAGE AND ADMINISTRATION).

Age
The pharmacokinetics of oral sumatriptan in the elderly (mean age: 72 years, 2 males and 4 females) and in patients with migraine (mean age: 38 years, 25 males and 155 females) were similar to that in healthy male subjects (mean age: 30 years) (see PRECAUTIONS: Geriatric Use).

Gender
In a study comparing females to males, no pharmacokinetic differences were observed between genders for AUC, C_{max}, T_{max}, and half-life.

Race
The systemic clearance and C_{max} of sumatriptan were similar in black (N = 34) and Caucasian (N = 38) healthy male subjects.

Drug Interactions
Monoamine Oxidase Inhibitors
Treatment with MAO-A inhibitors generally leads to an increase of sumatriptan plasma levels (see CONTRAINDICATIONS and PRECAUTIONS).

Due to gut and hepatic metabolic first-pass effects, the increase of systemic exposure after coadministration of an MAO-A inhibitor with oral sumatriptan is greater than after coadministration of the monoamine oxidase inhibitors (MAOI) with subcutaneous sumatriptan. In a study of 14 healthy females, pretreatment with an MAO-A inhibitor decreased the clearance of subcutaneous sumatriptan. Under the conditions of this experiment, the result was a 2-fold increase in the area under the sumatriptan plasma concentration x time curve (AUC), corresponding to a 40% increase in elimination half-life. This interaction was not evident with an MAO-A inhibitor.

A small study evaluating the effect of pretreatment with an MAO-A inhibitor on the bioavailability from a 25-mg oral sumatriptan tablet resulted in an approximately 7-fold increase in systemic exposure.

Alcohol
Alcohol consumed 30 minutes prior to sumatriptan ingestion had no effect on the pharmacokinetics of sumatriptan.

CLINICAL STUDIES
The efficacy of IMITREX Tablets in the acute treatment of migraine headaches was demonstrated in 3, randomized, double-blind, placebo-controlled studies. Patients enrolled in these 3 studies were predominantly female (87%) and Caucasian (97%), with a mean age of 40 years (range, 18 to 65 years). Patients were instructed to treat a moderate to severe headache. Headache response, defined as a reduction in headache severity from moderate or severe pain to mild or no pain, was assessed up to 4 hours after dosing. Associated symptoms such as nausea, photophobia, and phonophobia were also assessed. Maintenance of response was assessed for up to 24 hours postdose. A second dose of IMITREX Tablets or other medication was allowed 4 to 24 hours after the initial treatment for recurrent headache. Acetaminophen was offered to patients in Studies 2 and 3 beginning at 2 hours after initial treatment if the migraine pain had not improved or worsened. Additional medications were allowed 4 to 24 hours after the initial treatment for recurrent headache or as rescue in all 3 studies. The frequency and time to use of these additional treatments were also determined. In all studies, doses of 25, 50, and 100 mg were compared to placebo in the treatment of migraine attacks. In 1 study, doses of 25, 50, and 100 mg were also compared to each other.

In all 3 trials, the percentage of patients achieving headache response 2 and 4 hours after treatment was significantly greater among patients receiving IMITREX Tablets at all doses compared to those who received placebo. In 1 of the 3 studies, there was a statistically significant greater percentage of patients with headache response at 2 and 4 hours in the 50- or 100-mg group when compared to the 25-mg dose groups. There were no statistically significant differences between the 50- and 100-mg dose groups in any study. The results from the 3 controlled clinical trials are summarized in Table 1.

Comparisons of drug performance based upon results obtained in different clinical trials are never reliable. Because studies are conducted at different times, with different samples of patients, by different investigators, employing different criteria and/or different interpretations of the same criteria, under different conditions (dose, dosing regimen, etc.), quantitative estimates of treatment response and the timing of response may be expected to vary considerably from study to study.

[See table 1 above]

The estimated probability of achieving an initial headache response over the 4 hours following treatment is depicted in Figure 1.

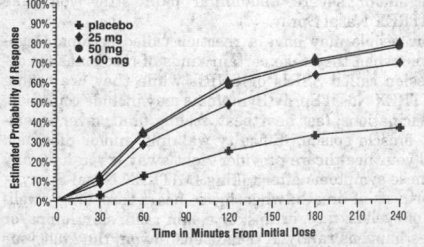

Figure 1. Estimated Probability of Achieving Initial Headache Response Within 240 Minutes[a]

[a]The figure shows the probability over time of obtaining headache response (no or mild pain) following treatment with sumatriptan. The averages displayed are based on pooled data from the 3 clinical controlled trials providing evidence of efficacy. Kaplan-Meier plot with patients not achieving response and/or taking rescue within 240 minutes censored to 240 minutes.

For patients with migraine-associated nausea, photophobia, and/or phonophobia at baseline, there was a lower incidence

of these symptoms at 2 hours (Study 1) and at 4 hours (Studies 1, 2, and 3) following administration of IMITREX Tablets compared to placebo.

As early as 2 hours in Studies 2 and 3 or 4 hours in Study 1, through 24 hours following the initial dose of study treatment, patients were allowed to use additional treatment for pain relief in the form of a second dose of study treatment or other medication. The estimated probability of patients taking a second dose or other medication for migraine over the 24 hours following the initial dose of study treatment is summarized in Figure 2.

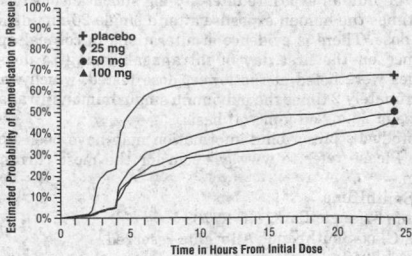

Figure 2. The Estimated Probability of Patients Taking a Second Dose or Other Medication for Migraine Over the 24 Hours Following the Initial Dose of Study Treatment[a]

[a] Kaplan-Meier plot based on data obtained in the 3 clinical controlled trials providing evidence of efficacy with patients not using additional treatments censored to 24 hours. Plot also includes patients who had no response to the initial dose. No remediation was allowed within 2 hours postdose.

There is evidence that doses above 50 mg do not provide a greater effect than 50 mg. There was no evidence to suggest that treatment with sumatriptan was associated with an increase in the severity of recurrent headaches. The efficacy of IMITREX Tablets was unaffected by presence of aura; duration of headache prior to treatment; gender, age, or weight of the patient; relationship to menses; or concomitant use of common migraine prophylactic drugs (e.g., beta-blockers, calcium channel blockers, tricyclic antidepressants). There were insufficient data to assess the impact of race on efficacy.

INDICATIONS AND USAGE
IMITREX Tablets are indicated for the acute treatment of migraine attacks with or without aura in adults.

IMITREX Tablets are not intended for the prophylactic therapy of migraine or for use in the management of hemiplegic or basilar migraine (see CONTRAINDICATIONS). Safety and effectiveness of IMITREX Tablets have not been established for cluster headache, which is present in an older, predominantly male population.

CONTRAINDICATIONS
IMITREX Tablets should not be given to patients with history, symptoms, or signs of ischemic cardiac, cerebrovascular, or peripheral vascular syndromes. In addition, patients with other significant underlying cardiovascular diseases should not receive IMITREX Tablets. Ischemic cardiac syndromes include, but are not limited to, angina pectoris of any type (e.g., stable angina of effort, vasospastic forms of angina such as the Prinzmetal variant), all forms of myocardial infarction, and silent myocardial ischemia. Cerebrovascular syndromes include, but are not limited to, strokes of any type as well as transient ischemic attacks. Peripheral vascular disease includes, but is not limited to, ischemic bowel disease (see WARNINGS).

Because IMITREX Tablets may increase blood pressure, they should not be given to patients with uncontrolled hypertension.

Concurrent administration of MAO-A inhibitors or use within 2 weeks of discontinuation of MAO-A inhibitor therapy is contraindicated (see CLINICAL PHARMACOLOGY: Drug Interactions and PRECAUTIONS: Drug Interactions).

IMITREX Tablets should not be administered to patients with hemiplegic or basilar migraine.

IMITREX Tablets and any ergotamine-containing or ergot-type medication (like dihydroergotamine or methysergide) should not be used within 24 hours of each other, nor should IMITREX and another 5-HT$_1$ agonist.

IMITREX Tablets are contraindicated in patients with hypersensitivity to sumatriptan or any of their components.

IMITREX Tablets are contraindicated in patients with severe hepatic impairment.

WARNINGS
IMITREX Tablets should only be used where a clear diagnosis of migraine headache has been established.

Risk of Myocardial Ischemia and/or Infarction and Other Adverse Cardiac Events

Sumatriptan should not be given to patients with documented ischemic or vasospastic coronary artery disease

(CAD) (see CONTRAINDICATIONS). It is strongly recommended that sumatriptan not be given to patients in whom unrecognized CAD is predicted by the presence of risk factors (e.g., hypertension, hypercholesterolemia, smoker, obesity, diabetes, strong family history of CAD, female with surgical or physiological menopause, male over 40 years of age) unless a cardiovascular evaluation provides satisfactory clinical evidence that the patient is reasonably free of coronary artery and ischemic myocardial disease or other significant underlying cardiovascular disease. The sensitivity of cardiac diagnostic procedures to detect cardiovascular disease or predisposition to coronary artery vasospasm is modest, at best. If, during the cardiovascular evaluation, the patient's medical history or electrocardiographic investigations reveal findings indicative of, or consistent with, coronary artery vasospasm or myocardial ischemia, sumatriptan should not be administered (see CONTRAINDICATIONS).

For patients with risk factors predictive of CAD, who are determined to have a satisfactory cardiovascular evaluation, it is strongly recommended that administration of the first dose of sumatriptan tablets take place in the setting of a physician's office or similar medically staffed and equipped facility unless the patient has previously received sumatriptan. Because cardiac ischemia can occur in the absence of clinical symptoms, consideration should be given to obtaining on the first occasion of use an electrocardiogram (ECG) during the interval immediately following IMITREX Tablets in these patients with risk factors.

It is recommended that patients who are intermittent long-term users of sumatriptan and who have or acquire risk factors predictive of CAD, as described above, undergo periodic interval cardiovascular evaluation as they continue to use sumatriptan.

The systematic approach described above is intended to reduce the likelihood that patients with unrecognized cardiovascular disease will be inadvertently exposed to sumatriptan.

Drug-Associated Cardiac Events and Fatalities

Serious adverse cardiac events, including acute myocardial infarction, life-threatening disturbances of cardiac rhythm, and death have been reported within a few hours following the administration of IMITREX® (sumatriptan succinate) Injection or IMITREX Tablets. Considering the extent of use of sumatriptan in patients with migraine, the incidence of these events is extremely low.

The fact that sumatriptan can cause coronary vasospasm, that some of these events have occurred in patients with no prior cardiac disease history and with documented absence of CAD, and the close proximity of the events to sumatriptan use support the conclusion that some of these cases were caused by the drug. In many cases, however, where there has been known underlying coronary artery disease, the relationship is uncertain.

Premarketing Experience With Sumatriptan

Of 6,348 patients with migraine who participated in premarketing controlled and uncontrolled clinical trials of oral sumatriptan, 2 experienced clinical adverse events shortly after receiving oral sumatriptan that may have reflected coronary vasospasm. Neither of these adverse events was associated with a serious clinical outcome.

Among the more than 1,900 patients with migraine who participated in premarketing controlled clinical trials of subcutaneous sumatriptan, there were 8 patients who sustained clinical events during or shortly after receiving sumatriptan that may have reflected coronary artery vasospasm. Six of these 8 patients had ECG changes consistent with transient ischemia, but without accompanying clinical symptoms or signs. Of these 8 patients, 4 had either findings suggestive of CAD or risk factors predictive of CAD prior to study enrollment.

Among approximately 4,000 patients with migraine who participated in premarketing controlled and uncontrolled clinical trials of sumatriptan nasal spray, 1 patient experienced an asymptomatic subendocardial infarction possibly subsequent to a coronary vasospastic event.

Postmarketing Experience With Sumatriptan

Serious cardiovascular events, some resulting in death, have been reported in association with the use of IMITREX Injection or IMITREX Tablets. The uncontrolled nature of postmarketing surveillance, however, makes it impossible to determine definitively the proportion of the reported cases that were actually caused by sumatriptan or to reliably assess causation in individual cases. On clinical grounds, the longer the latency between the administration of IMITREX and the onset of the clinical event, the less likely the association is to be causative. Accordingly, interest has focused on events beginning within 1 hour of the administration of IMITREX.

Cardiac events that have been observed to have onset within 1 hour of sumatriptan administration include: coronary artery vasospasm, transient ischemia, myocardial infarction, ventricular tachycardia and ventricular fibrillation, cardiac arrest, and death.

Some of these events occurred in patients who had no findings of CAD and appear to represent consequences of coronary artery vasospasm. However, among domestic reports of serious cardiac events within 1 hour of sumatriptan administration, almost all of the patients had risk factors predictive of CAD and the presence of significant underlying CAD was established in most cases (see CONTRAINDICATIONS).

Drug-Associated Cerebrovascular Events and Fatalities

Cerebral hemorrhage, subarachnoid hemorrhage, stroke, and other cerebrovascular events have been reported in patients treated with oral or subcutaneous sumatriptan, and some have resulted in fatalities. The relationship of sumatriptan to these events is uncertain. In a number of cases, it appears possible that the cerebrovascular events were primary, sumatriptan having been administered in the incorrect belief that the symptoms experienced were a consequence of migraine when they were not. As with other acute migraine therapies, before treating headaches in patients not previously diagnosed as migraineurs, and in migraineurs who present with atypical symptoms, care should be taken to exclude other potentially serious neurological conditions. It should also be noted that patients with migraine may be at increased risk of certain cerebrovascular events (e.g., cerebrovascular accident, transient ischemic attack).

Other Vasospasm-Related Events

Sumatriptan may cause vasospastic reactions other than coronary artery vasospasm. Both peripheral vascular ischemia and colonic ischemia with abdominal pain and bloody diarrhea have been reported. Very rare reports of transient and permanent blindness and significant partial vision loss have been reported with the use of sumatriptan. Visual disorders may also be part of a migraine attack.

Serotonin Syndrome

The development of a potentially life-threatening serotonin syndrome may occur with triptans, including treatment with IMITREX, particularly during combined use with selective serotonin reuptake inhibitors (SSRIs) or serotonin norepinephrine reuptake inhibitors (SNRIs). If concomitant treatment with sumatriptan and an SSRI (e.g., fluoxetine, paroxetine, sertraline, fluvoxamine, citalopram, escitalopram) or SNRI (e.g., venlafaxine, duloxetine) is clinically warranted, careful observation of the patient is advised, particularly during treatment initiation and dose increases. Serotonin syndrome symptoms may include mental status changes (e.g., agitation, hallucinations, coma), autonomic instability (e.g., tachycardia, labile blood pressure, hyperthermia), neuromuscular aberrations (e.g., hyperreflexia, incoordination), and/or gastrointestinal symptoms (e.g., nausea, vomiting, diarrhea).

Increase in Blood Pressure

Significant elevation in blood pressure, including hypertensive crisis, has been reported on rare occasions in patients with and without a history of hypertension. Sumatriptan is contraindicated in patients with uncontrolled hypertension (see CONTRAINDICATIONS). Sumatriptan should be administered with caution to patients with controlled hypertension as transient increases in blood pressure and peripheral vascular resistance have been observed in a small proportion of patients.

Concomitant Drug Use

In patients taking MAO-A inhibitors, sumatriptan plasma levels attained after treatment with recommended doses are 7-fold higher following oral administration than those obtained under other conditions. Accordingly, the coadministration of IMITREX Tablets and an MAO-A inhibitor is contraindicated (see CLINICAL PHARMACOLOGY and CONTRAINDICATIONS).

Hypersensitivity

Hypersensitivity (anaphylaxis/anaphylactoid) reactions have occurred on rare occasions in patients receiving sumatriptan. Such reactions can be life threatening or fatal. In general, hypersensitivity reactions to drugs are more likely to occur in individuals with a history of sensitivity to multiple allergens (see CONTRAINDICATIONS).

PRECAUTIONS

General

Chest discomfort and jaw or neck tightness have been reported following use of IMITREX Tablets and have also been reported infrequently following administration of IMITREX® (sumatriptan) Nasal Spray. Chest, jaw, or neck tightness is relatively common after administration of IMITREX Injection. Only rarely have these symptoms been associated with ischemic ECG changes. However, because sumatriptan may cause coronary artery vasospasm, patients who experience signs or symptoms suggestive of angina following sumatriptan should be evaluated for the presence of CAD or a predisposition to Prinzmetal variant angina before receiving additional doses of sumatriptan, and should be monitored electrocardiographically if dosing is resumed and similar symptoms recur. Similarly, patients who experience other symptoms or signs suggestive of de-

creased arterial flow, such as ischemic bowel syndrome or Raynaud syndrome following sumatriptan should be evaluated for atherosclerosis or predisposition to vasospasm (see WARNINGS).

IMITREX should also be administered with caution to patients with diseases that may alter the absorption, metabolism, or excretion of drugs, such as impaired hepatic or renal function.

There have been rare reports of seizure following administration of sumatriptan. Sumatriptan should be used with caution in patients with a history of epilepsy or conditions associated with a lowered seizure threshold.

Care should be taken to exclude other potentially serious neurologic conditions before treating headache in patients not previously diagnosed with migraine headache or who experience a headache that is atypical for them. There have been rare reports where patients received sumatriptan for severe headaches that were subsequently shown to have been secondary to an evolving neurologic lesion (see WARNINGS).

For a given attack, if a patient does not respond to the first dose of sumatriptan, the diagnosis of migraine should be reconsidered before administration of a second dose.

Overuse of acute migraine treatments has been associated with the exacerbation of headache (medication overuse headache) in susceptible patients. Withdrawal of the treatment may be necessary.

Binding to Melanin-Containing Tissues

In rats treated with a single subcutaneous dose (0.5 mg/kg) or oral dose (2 mg/kg) of radiolabeled sumatriptan, the elimination half-life of radioactivity from the eye was 15 and 23 days, respectively, suggesting that sumatriptan and/or its metabolites bind to the melanin of the eye. Because there could be an accumulation in melanin-rich tissues over time, this raises the possibility that sumatriptan could cause toxicity in these tissues after extended use. However, no effects on the retina related to treatment with sumatriptan were noted in any of the oral or subcutaneous toxicity studies. Although no systematic monitoring of ophthalmologic function was undertaken in clinical trials, and no specific recommendations for ophthalmologic monitoring are offered, prescribers should be aware of the possibility of long-term ophthalmologic effects.

Corneal Opacities

Sumatriptan causes corneal opacities and defects in the corneal epithelium in dogs; this raises the possibility that these changes may occur in humans. While patients were not systematically evaluated for these changes in clinical trials, and no specific recommendations for monitoring are being offered, prescribers should be aware of the possibility of these changes (see ANIMAL TOXICOLOGY).

Information for Patients

See PATIENT INFORMATION at the end of this labeling for the text of the separate leaflet provided for patients.

Patients should be cautioned about the risk of serotonin syndrome with the use of sumatriptan or other triptans, especially during combined use with SSRIs or SNRIs.

Laboratory Tests

No specific laboratory tests are recommended for monitoring patients prior to and/or after treatment with sumatriptan.

Drug Interactions

Selective Serotonin Reuptake Inhibitors/Serotonin Norepinephrine Reuptake Inhibitors and Serotonin Syndrome

Cases of life-threatening serotonin syndrome have been reported during combined use of SSRIs or SNRIs and triptans (see WARNINGS).

Ergot-Containing Drugs

Ergot-containing drugs have been reported to cause prolonged vasospastic reactions. Because there is a theoretical basis that these effects may be additive, use of ergotamine-containing or ergot-type medications (like dihydroergotamine or methysergide) and sumatriptan within 24 hours of each other should be avoided (see CONTRAINDICATIONS).

Monoamine Oxidase-A Inhibitors

MAO-A inhibitors reduce sumatriptan clearance, significantly increasing systemic exposure. Therefore, the use of IMITREX Tablets in patients receiving MAO-A inhibitors is contraindicated (see CLINICAL PHARMACOLOGY and CONTRAINDICATIONS).

Drug/Laboratory Test Interactions

IMITREX Tablets are not known to interfere with commonly employed clinical laboratory tests.

Carcinogenesis, Mutagenesis, Impairment of Fertility

Carcinogenesis

In carcinogenicity studies, rats and mice were given sumatriptan by oral gavage (rats: 104 weeks) or drinking water (mice: 78 weeks). Average exposures achieved in mice receiving the highest dose (target dose of 160 mg/kg/day) were approximately 40 times the exposure attained in humans after the maximum recommended single oral dose of 100 mg. The highest dose administered to rats (160 mg/kg/day, reduced from 360 mg/kg/day during week

21) was approximately 15 times the maximum recommended single human oral dose of 100 mg on a mg/m^2 basis. There was no evidence of an increase in tumors in either species related to sumatriptan administration.

Mutagenesis

Sumatriptan was not mutagenic in the presence or absence of metabolic activation when tested in 2 gene mutation assays (the Ames test and the in vitro mammalian Chinese hamster V79/HGPRT assay). In 2 cytogenetics assays (the in vitro human lymphocyte assay and the in vivo rat micronucleus assay) sumatriptan was not associated with clastogenic activity.

Impairment of Fertility

In a study in which male and female rats were dosed daily with oral sumatriptan prior to and throughout the mating period, there was a treatment-related decrease in fertility secondary to a decrease in mating in animals treated with 50 and 500 mg/kg/day. The highest no-effect dose for this finding was 5 mg/kg/day, or approximately one half of the maximum recommended single human oral dose of 100 mg on a mg/m^2 basis. It is not clear whether the problem is associated with treatment of the males or females or both combined. In a similar study by the subcutaneous route there was no evidence of impaired fertility at 60 mg/kg/day, the maximum dose tested, which is equivalent to approximately 6 times the maximum recommended single human oral dose of 100 mg on a mg/m^2 basis.

Pregnancy

Pregnancy Category C. In reproductive toxicity studies in rats and rabbits, oral treatment with sumatriptan was associated with embryolethality, fetal abnormalities, and pup mortality. When administered by the intravenous route to rabbits, sumatriptan has been shown to be embryolethal. There are no adequate and well-controlled studies in pregnant women. Therefore, IMITREX should be used during pregnancy only if the potential benefit justifies the potential risk to the fetus. In assessing this information, the following findings should be considered.

Embryolethality

When given orally or intravenously to pregnant rabbits daily throughout the period of organogenesis, sumatriptan caused embryolethality at doses at or close to those producing maternal toxicity. In the oral studies this dose was 100 mg/kg/day, and in the intravenous studies this dose was 2.0 mg/kg/day. The mechanism of the embryolethality is not known. The highest no-effect dose for embryolethality by the oral route was 50 mg/kg/day, which is approximately 9 times the maximum single recommended human oral dose of 100 mg on a mg/m^2 basis. By the intravenous route, the highest no-effect dose was 0.75 mg/kg/day, or approximately one tenth of the maximum single recommended human oral dose of 100 mg on a mg/m^2 basis.

The intravenous administration of sumatriptan to pregnant rats throughout organogenesis at 12.5 mg/kg/day, the maximum dose tested, did not cause embryolethality. This dose is equivalent to the maximum single recommended human oral dose of 100 mg on a mg/m^2 basis. Additionally, in a study in rats given subcutaneous sumatriptan daily prior to and throughout pregnancy at 60 mg/kg/day, the maximum dose tested, there was no evidence of increased embryo/fetal lethality. This dose is equivalent to approximately 6 times the maximum recommended single human oral dose of 100 mg on a mg/m^2 basis.

Teratogenicity

Oral treatment of pregnant rats with sumatriptan during the period of organogenesis resulted in an increased incidence of blood vessel abnormalities (cervicothoracic and umbilical) at doses of approximately 250 mg/kg/day or higher. The highest no-effect dose was approximately 60 mg/kg/day, which is approximately 6 times the maximum single recommended human oral dose of 100 mg on a mg/m^2 basis. Oral treatment of pregnant rabbits with sumatriptan during the period of organogenesis resulted in an increased incidence of cervicothoracic vascular and skeletal abnormalities. The highest no-effect dose for these effects was 15 mg/kg/day, or approximately 3 times the maximum single recommended human oral dose of 100 mg on a mg/m^2 basis.

A study in which rats were dosed daily with oral sumatriptan prior to and throughout gestation demonstrated embryo/fetal toxicity (decreased body weight, decreased ossification, increased incidence of rib variations) and an increased incidence of a syndrome of malformations (short tail/short body and vertebral disorganization) at 500 mg/kg/day. The highest no-effect dose was 50 mg/kg/day, or approximately 5 times the maximum single recommended human oral dose of 100 mg on a mg/m^2 basis. In a study in rats dosed daily with subcutaneous sumatriptan prior to and throughout pregnancy, at a dose of 60 mg/kg/day, the maximum dose tested, there was no evidence of teratogenicity. This dose is equivalent to approximately 6 times the maximum recommended single human oral dose of 100 mg on a mg/m^2 basis.

Pup Deaths

Oral treatment of pregnant rats with sumatriptan during the period of organogenesis resulted in a decrease in pup survival between birth and postnatal day 4 at doses of approximately 250 mg/kg/day or higher. The highest no-effect dose for this effect was approximately 60 mg/kg/day, or 6 times the maximum single recommended human oral dose of 100 mg on a mg/m^2 basis.

Oral treatment of pregnant rats with sumatriptan from gestational day 17 through postnatal day 21 demonstrated a decrease in pup survival measured at postnatal days 2, 4, and 20 at the dose of 1,000 mg/kg/day. The highest no-effect dose for this finding was 100 mg/kg/day, approximately 10 times the maximum single recommended human oral dose of 100 mg on a mg/m^2 basis. In a similar study in rats by the subcutaneous route there was no increase in pup death at 81 mg/kg/day, the highest dose tested, which is equivalent to 8 times the maximum single recommended human oral dose of 100 mg on a mg/m^2 basis.

Pregnancy Registry

To monitor fetal outcomes of pregnant women exposed to IMITREX, GlaxoSmithKline maintains a Sumatriptan Pregnancy Registry. Physicians are encouraged to register patients by calling (800) 336-2176.

Nursing Mothers

Sumatriptan is excreted in human breast milk following subcutaneous administration. Infant exposure to sumatriptan can be minimized by avoiding breastfeeding for 12 hours after treatment with IMITREX Tablets.

Pediatric Use

Safety and effectiveness of IMITREX Tablets in pediatric patients under 18 years of age have not been established; therefore, IMITREX Tablets are not recommended for use in patients under 18 years of age.

Two controlled clinical trials evaluating sumatriptan nasal spray (5 to 20 mg) in pediatric patients aged 12 to 17 years enrolled a total of 1,248 adolescent migraineurs who treated a single attack. The studies did not establish the efficacy of sumatriptan nasal spray compared to placebo in the treatment of migraine in adolescents. Adverse events observed in these clinical trials were similar in nature to those reported in clinical trials in adults.

Five controlled clinical trials (2 single attack studies, 3 multiple attack studies) evaluating oral sumatriptan (25 to 100 mg) in pediatric patients aged 12 to 17 years enrolled a total of 701 adolescent migraineurs. These studies did not establish the efficacy of oral sumatriptan compared to placebo in the treatment of migraine in adolescents. Adverse events observed in these clinical trials were similar in nature to those reported in clinical trials in adults. The frequency of all adverse events in these patients appeared to be both dose- and age-dependent, with younger patients reporting events more commonly than older adolescents.

Postmarketing experience documents that serious adverse events have occurred in the pediatric population after use of subcutaneous, oral, and/or intranasal sumatriptan. These reports include events similar in nature to those reported rarely in adults, including stroke, visual loss, and death. A myocardial infarction has been reported in a 14-year-old male following the use of oral sumatriptan; clinical signs occurred within 1 day of drug administration. Since clinical data to determine the frequency of serious adverse events in pediatric patients who might receive injectable, oral, or intranasal sumatriptan are not presently available, the use of sumatriptan in patients aged younger than 18 years is not recommended.

Geriatric Use

The use of sumatriptan in elderly patients is not recommended because elderly patients are more likely to have decreased hepatic function, they are at higher risk for CAD, and blood pressure increases may be more pronounced in the elderly (see WARNINGS).

ADVERSE REACTIONS

Serious cardiac events, including some that have been fatal, have occurred following the use of IMITREX Injection or Tablets. These events are extremely rare and most have been reported in patients with risk factors predictive of CAD. Events reported have included coronary artery vasospasm, transient myocardial ischemia, myocardial infarction, ventricular tachycardia, and ventricular fibrillation (see CONTRAINDICATIONS, WARNINGS, and PRECAUTIONS).

Significant hypertensive episodes, including hypertensive crises, have been reported on rare occasions in patients with or without a history of hypertension (see WARNINGS).

Incidence in Controlled Clinical Trials

Table 2 lists adverse events that occurred in placebo-controlled clinical trials in patients who took at least 1 dose of study drug. Only events that occurred at a frequency of 2% or more in any group treated with IMITREX Tablets and were more frequent in that group than in the placebo group are included in Table 2. The events cited reflect experience gained under closely monitored conditions of clinical trials in a highly selected patient population. In actual clinical practice or in other clinical trials, these frequency estimates may not apply, as the conditions of use, reporting behavior, and the kinds of patients treated may differ.

[See table 2 at left]

Table 2. Treatment Emergent Adverse Events Reported by at Least 2% of Patients in Controlled Migraine Trials[a]

Adverse Event Type	Percent of Patients Reporting			
	Placebo (N = 309)	IMITREX 25 mg (N = 417)	IMITREX 50 mg (N = 771)	IMITREX 100 mg (N = 437)
Atypical sensations	4%	5%	6%	6%
Paresthesia (all types)	2%	3%	5%	3%
Sensation warm/cold	2%	3%	2%	3%
Pain and other pressure sensations	4%	6%	6%	8%
Chest - pain/tightness/pressure and/or heaviness	1%	1%	2%	2%
Neck/throat/jaw - pain/tightness/pressure	<1%	<1%	2%	3%
Pain - location specified	1%	2%	1%	1%
Other - pressure/tightness/heaviness	2%	1%	1%	3%
Neurological				
Vertigo	<1%	<1%	<1%	2%
Other				
Malaise/fatigue	<1%	2%	2%	3%

[a] Events that occurred at a frequency of 2% or more in the group treated with IMITREX Tablets and that occurred more frequently in that group than the placebo group.

Other events that occurred in more than 1% of patients receiving IMITREX Tablets and at least as often on placebo included nausea and/or vomiting, migraine, headache, hyposalivation, dizziness, and drowsiness/sleepiness.

IMITREX Tablets are generally well tolerated. Across all doses, most adverse reactions were mild and transient and did not lead to long-lasting effects. The incidence of adverse events in controlled clinical trials was not affected by gender or age of the patients. There were insufficient data to assess the impact of race on the incidence of adverse events.

Other Events Observed in Association With the Administration of IMITREX Tablets

In the paragraphs that follow, the frequencies of less commonly reported adverse clinical events are presented. Because the reports include events observed in open and uncontrolled studies, the role of IMITREX Tablets in their causation cannot be reliably determined. Furthermore, variability associated with adverse event reporting, the terminology used to describe adverse events, etc., limit the value of quantitative frequency estimates provided. Event frequencies are calculated as the number of patients who used IMITREX Tablets (25, 50, or 100 mg) and reported an event divided by the total number of patients (N = 6,348) exposed to IMITREX Tablets. All reported events are included except those already listed in the previous table, those too general to be informative, and those not reasonably associated with the use of the drug. Events are further classified within body system categories and enumerated in order of decreasing frequency using the following definitions: frequent adverse events are defined as those occurring in at least 1/100 patients, infrequent adverse events are those occurring in 1/100 to 1/1,000 patients, and rare adverse events are those occurring in fewer than 1/1,000 patients.

Atypical Sensations

Frequent were burning sensation and numbness. Infrequent was tight feeling in head. Rare were dysesthesia.

Cardiovascular

Frequent were palpitations, syncope, decreased blood pressure, and increased blood pressure. Infrequent were arrhythmia, changes in ECG, hypertension, hypotension, pallor, pulsating sensations, and tachycardia. Rare were angina, atherosclerosis, bradycardia, cerebral ischemia, cerebrovascular lesion, heart block, peripheral cyanosis, thrombosis, transient myocardial ischemia, and vasodilation.

Ear, Nose, and Throat

Frequent were sinusitis, tinnitus; allergic rhinitis; upper respiratory inflammation; ear, nose, and throat hemorrhage; external otitis; hearing loss; nasal inflammation; and sensitivity to noise. Infrequent were hearing disturbances and otalgia. Rare was feeling of fullness in the ear(s).

Endocrine and Metabolic

Infrequent was thirst. Rare were elevated thyrotropin stimulating hormone (TSH) levels; galactorrhea; hyperglycemia; hypoglycemia; hypothyroidism; polydipsia; weight gain; weight loss; endocrine cysts, lumps, and masses; and fluid disturbances.

Eye

Rare were disorders of sclera, mydriasis, blindness and low vision, visual disturbances, eye edema and swelling, eye irritation and itching, accommodation disorders, external ocular muscle disorders, eye hemorrhage, eye pain, and keratitis and conjunctivitis.

Gastrointestinal

Frequent were diarrhea and gastric symptoms. Infrequent were constipation, dysphagia, and gastroesophageal reflux. Rare were gastrointestinal bleeding, hematemesis, melena, peptic ulcer, gastrointestinal pain, dyspeptic symptoms, dental pain, feelings of gastrointestinal pressure, gastritis, gastroenteritis, hypersalivation, abdominal distention, oral itching and irritation, salivary gland swelling, and swallowing disorders.

Hematological Disorders

Rare was anemia.

Musculoskeletal

Frequent was myalgia. Infrequent was muscle cramps. Rare were tetany; muscle atrophy, weakness, and tiredness; arthralgia and articular rheumatitis; acquired musculoskeletal deformity; muscle stiffness, tightness, and rigidity; and musculoskeletal inflammation.

Neurological

Frequent were phonophobia and photophobia. Infrequent were confusion, depression, difficulty concentrating, disturbance of smell, dysarthria, euphoria, facial pain, heat sensitivity, incoordination, lacrimation, monoplegia, sleep disturbance, shivering, syncope, and tremor. Rare were aggressiveness, apathy, bradylogia, cluster headache, convulsions, decreased appetite, drug abuse, dystonic reaction, facial paralysis, hallucinations, hunger, hyperesthesia, hysteria, increased alertness, memory disturbance, neuralgia, paralysis, personality change, phobia, radiculopathy, rigidity, suicide, twitching, agitation, anxiety, depressive disorders, detachment, motor dysfunction, neurotic disorders, psychomotor disorders, taste disturbances, and raised intracranial pressure.

Respiratory

Frequent was dyspnea. Infrequent was asthma. Rare were hiccoughs, breathing disorders, cough, and bronchitis.

Skin

Frequent was sweating. Infrequent were erythema, pruritus, rash, and skin tenderness. Rare were dry/scaly skin, tightness of skin, wrinkling of skin, eczema, seborrheic dermatitis, and skin nodules.

Breasts

Infrequent was tenderness. Rare were nipple discharge; breast swelling; cysts, lumps, and masses of breasts; and primary malignant breast neoplasm.

Urogenital

Infrequent were dysmenorrhea, increased urination, and intermenstrual bleeding. Rare were abortion and hematuria, urinary frequency, bladder inflammation, micturition disorders, urethritis, urinary infections, menstruation symptoms, abnormal menstrual cycle, inflammation of fallopian tubes, and menstrual cycle symptoms.

Miscellaneous

Frequent was hypersensitivity. Infrequent were fever, fluid retention, and overdose. Rare were edema, hematoma, lymphadenopathy, speech disturbance, voice disturbances, contusions.

Other Events Observed in the Clinical Development of IMITREX

The following adverse events occurred in clinical trials with IMITREX Injection and IMITREX Nasal Spray. Because the reports include events observed in open and uncontrolled studies, the role of IMITREX in their causation cannot be reliably determined. All reported events are included except those already listed, those too general to be informative, and those not reasonably associated with the use of the drug.

Atypical Sensations

Feeling strange, prickling sensation, tingling, and hot sensation.

Cardiovascular

Abdominal aortic aneurysm, abnormal pulse, flushing, phlebitis, Raynaud syndrome, and various transient ECG changes (nonspecific ST or T wave changes, prolongation of PR or QTc intervals, sinus arrhythmia, nonsustained ventricular premature beats, isolated junctional ectopic beats, atrial ectopic beats, delayed activation of the right ventricle).

Chest Symptoms

Chest discomfort.

Endocrine and Metabolic

Dehydration.

Ear, Nose, and Throat

Disorder/discomfort nasal cavity and sinuses, ear infection, Meniere disease, and throat discomfort.

Eye

Vision alterations.

Gastrointestinal

Abdominal discomfort, colitis, disturbance of liver function tests, flatulence/eructation, gallstones, intestinal obstruction, pancreatitis, and retching.

Injection Site Reaction

Miscellaneous

Difficulty in walking, hypersensitivity to various agents, jaw discomfort, miscellaneous laboratory abnormalities, "serotonin agonist effect," swelling of the extremities, and swelling of the face.

Mouth and Teeth

Disorder of mouth and tongue (e.g., burning of tongue, numbness of tongue, dry mouth).

Musculoskeletal

Arthritis, backache, intervertebral disc disorder, neck pain/stiffness, need to flex calf muscles, and various joint disturbances (pain, stiffness, swelling, ache).

Neurological

Bad/unusual taste, chills, diplegia, disturbance of emotions, sedation, globus hystericus, intoxication, myoclonia, neoplasm of pituitary, relaxation, sensation of lightness, simultaneous hot and cold sensations, stinging sensations, stress, tickling sensations, transient hemiplegia, and yawning.

Respiratory

Influenza and diseases of the lower respiratory tract and lower respiratory tract infection.

Skin

Skin eruption, herpes, and peeling of the skin.

Urogenital

Disorder of breasts, endometriosis, and renal calculus.

Postmarketing Experience (Reports for Subcutaneous or Oral Sumatriptan)

The following section enumerates potentially important adverse events that have occurred in clinical practice and that have been reported spontaneously to various surveillance systems. The events enumerated represent reports arising from both domestic and nondomestic use of oral or subcutaneous dosage forms of sumatriptan. The events enumerated include all except those already listed in the ADVERSE REACTIONS section above or those too general to be informative. Because the reports cite events reported spontaneously from worldwide postmarketing experience, frequency of events and the role of sumatriptan in their causation cannot be reliably determined. It is assumed, however, that systemic reactions following sumatriptan use are likely to be similar regardless of route of administration.

Blood

Hemolytic anemia, pancytopenia, thrombocytopenia.

Cardiovascular

Atrial fibrillation, cardiomyopathy, colonic ischemia (see WARNINGS), Prinzmetal variant angina, pulmonary embolism, shock, thrombophlebitis.

Ear, Nose, and Throat

Deafness.

Eye

Ischemic optic neuropathy, retinal artery occlusion, retinal vein thrombosis, loss of vision.

Gastrointestinal

Ischemic colitis with rectal bleeding (see WARNINGS), xerostomia.

Hepatic

Elevated liver function tests.

Neurological

Central nervous system vasculitis, cerebrovascular accident, dysphasia, serotonin syndrome, subarachnoid hemorrhage.

Non-Site Specific

Angioneurotic edema, cyanosis, death (see WARNINGS), temporal arteritis.

Psychiatry

Panic disorder.

Respiratory

Bronchospasm in patients with and without a history of asthma.

Skin

Exacerbation of sunburn, hypersensitivity reactions (allergic vasculitis, erythema, pruritus, rash, shortness of breath, urticaria; in addition, severe anaphylaxis/anaphylactoid reactions have been reported [see WARNINGS]), photosensitivity.

Urogenital

Acute renal failure.

DRUG ABUSE AND DEPENDENCE

One clinical study with IMITREX Injection enrolling 12 patients with a history of substance abuse failed to induce subjective behavior and/or physiologic response ordinarily associated with drugs that have an established potential for abuse.

OVERDOSAGE

Patients (N = 670) have received single oral doses of 140 to 300 mg without significant adverse effects. Volunteers (N = 174) have received single oral doses of 140 to 400 mg without serious adverse events.

Overdose in animals has been fatal and has been heralded by convulsions, tremor, paralysis, inactivity, ptosis, erythema of the extremities, abnormal respiration, cyanosis, ataxia, mydriasis, salivation, and lacrimation. The elimination half-life of sumatriptan is approximately 2.5 hours (see CLINICAL PHARMACOLOGY), and therefore monitoring of patients after overdose with IMITREX Tablets should continue for at least 12 hours or while symptoms or signs persist.

It is unknown what effect hemodialysis or peritoneal dialysis has on the serum concentrations of sumatriptan.

DOSAGE AND ADMINISTRATION

In controlled clinical trials, single doses of 25, 50, or 100 mg of IMITREX Tablets were effective for the acute treatment of migraine in adults. There is evidence that doses of 50 and 100 mg may provide a greater effect than 25 mg (see CLINICAL TRIALS). There is also evidence that doses of 100 mg do not provide a greater effect than 50 mg. Individuals may vary in response to doses of IMITREX Tablets. The choice of dose should therefore be made on an individual basis, weighing the possible benefit of a higher dose with the potential for a greater risk of adverse events.

If the headache returns or the patient has a partial response to the initial dose, the dose may be repeated after 2 hours, not to exceed a total daily dose of 200 mg. If a headache returns following an initial treatment with IMITREX Injection, additional single IMITREX Tablets (up to 100 mg/day) may be given with an interval of at least 2 hours between tablet doses. The safety of treating an average of more than 4 headaches in a 30-day period has not been established.

Because of the potential of MAO-A inhibitors to cause unpredictable elevations in the bioavailability of oral sumatriptan, their combined use is contraindicated (see CONTRAINDICATIONS).

Hepatic disease/functional impairment may also cause unpredictable elevations in the bioavailability of orally administered sumatriptan. Consequently, if treatment is deemed advisable in the presence of liver disease, the maximum single dose should in general not exceed 50 mg (see CLINICAL PHARMACOLOGY for the basis of this recommendation).

HOW SUPPLIED

IMITREX Tablets, 25, 50, and 100 mg of sumatriptan (base) as the succinate.

IMITREX Tablets, 25 mg are white, triangular-shaped, film-coated tablets debossed with "I" on one side and "25" on the other in blister packs of 9 tablets (NDC 0173-0735-00).

IMITREX Tablets, 50 mg are white, triangular-shaped, film-coated tablets debossed with "IMITREX 50" on one side and a chevron shape (^) on the other in blister packs of 9 tablets (NDC 0173-0736-01).

IMITREX Tablets, 100 mg, are pink, triangular-shaped, film-coated tablets debossed with "IMITREX 100" on one side and a chevron shape (^) on the other in blister packs of 9 tablets (NDC 0173-0737-01).

Store between 36° and 86°F (2° and 30°C).

ANIMAL TOXICOLOGY

Corneal Opacities

Dogs receiving oral sumatriptan developed corneal opacities and defects in the corneal epithelium. Corneal opacities were seen at the lowest dosage tested, 2 mg/kg/day, and were present after 1 month of treatment. Defects in the corneal epithelium were noted in a 60-week study. Earlier examinations for these toxicities were not conducted and no-effect doses were not established; however, the relative exposure at the lowest dose tested was approximately 5 times the human exposure after a 100-mg oral dose. There is evidence of alterations in corneal appearance on the first day of intranasal dosing to dogs. Changes were noted at the lowest dose tested, which was approximately one half the maximum single human oral dose of 100 mg on a mg/m² basis.

This product's prescribing information may have been updated. Please refer to www.gsk.com for the most current version.

GlaxoSmithKline
Research Triangle Park, NC 27709
©2010, GlaxoSmithKline. All rights reserved.
February 2010
IMT:2PI

PATIENT INFORMATION

The following wording is contained in a separate leaflet provided for patients.

Information for the Patient
IMITREX® (sumatriptan succinate) Tablets

Read this leaflet carefully before you start to take IMITREX Tablets. Keep the leaflet for reference because it gives you a summary of important information about IMITREX Tablets.

Read the leaflet that comes with each refill of your prescription because there may be new information.

This leaflet does not have all the information about IMITREX Tablets. Ask your healthcare provider for more information or advice.

What are IMITREX Tablets?

IMITREX Tablets are a kind of medicine called a triptan. You should take it only if you have a prescription.

IMITREX Tablets are used to relieve your migraine. They are **not** used to prevent attacks or reduce the number of attacks you have. Use IMITREX Tablets only to treat an actual migraine attack.

The decision to use IMITREX Tablets is one that you and your healthcare provider should make together, based on your personal needs and health.

Talk with your healthcare provider before taking IMITREX Tablets

1. **Risk factors for heart disease to tell your healthcare provider:**

Tell your healthcare provider if you have risk factors for heart disease such as:
- high blood pressure
- high cholesterol
- being overweight
- diabetes
- smoking
- strong family history of heart disease
- you are postmenopausal
- you are a male over 40 years of age

If you do have risk factors for heart disease, your healthcare provider should check you for heart disease to see if IMITREX is right for you.

Although most of the people who have taken IMITREX have not had any serious side effects, some have had serious heart problems. Deaths have been reported, but these were rare considering the extensive worldwide use of IMITREX Tablets. Usually, serious problems happened in people with known heart disease. It was not clear whether IMITREX had anything to do with these deaths.

2. **Important questions to ask yourself before you take IMITREX Tablets:**

If the answer to any of the following questions is **YES** or if you do not know the answer, then please talk with your healthcare provider before you take IMITREX Tablets.
- Are you pregnant? Do you think you might be pregnant? Are you trying to become pregnant? Are you not using adequate contraception? Are you breastfeeding?
- Do you have any chest pain, heart disease, shortness of breath, or irregular heartbeats? Have you had a heart attack?
- Do you have risk factors for heart disease (see list above)?
- Have you had a stroke, a mini-stroke (also called a transient ischemic attack or TIA), or Raynaud syndrome?
- Do you have high blood pressure?
- Have you ever had to stop taking this or any other medicine because of an allergy or other problems?
- Are you taking any other migraine medicines, including other triptans? Are you taking any medicines containing ergotamine, dihydroergotamine, or methysergide?
- Are you taking any medicine for depression or other health problems such as a monoamine oxidase inhibitor, selective serotonin reuptake inhibitor (SSRI), or serotonin norepinephrine reuptake inhibitor (SNRI)? Common SSRIs are citalopram HBr (CELEXA®), escitalopram oxalate (LEXAPRO®), paroxetine (PAXIL®), fluoxetine (PROZAC®/SARAFEM®), olanzapine/fluoxetine (SYMBYAX®), sertraline (ZOLOFT®), and fluvoxamine (SYMBYAX®). Common SNRIs are duloxetine (CYMBALTA®) and venlafaxine (EFFEXOR®).

- Have you had, or do you have, any disease of the liver or kidney?
- Have you had, or do you have, epilepsy or seizures?
- Is this headache different from your usual migraine attacks?

Remember, if you answered **YES** to any of the above questions, then talk with your healthcare provider about it.

Important points about IMITREX Tablets

1. **The use of IMITREX Tablets during pregnancy:**

Do not take IMITREX Tablets if you are pregnant, think you might be pregnant, are trying to become pregnant, or are not using adequate contraception unless you have talked with your healthcare provider about this.

2. **How to take IMITREX Tablets:**

For adults, the usual dose is a single tablet swallowed whole with water or other liquids. Do not split tablets. If your symptoms of migraine come back or if you have a partial response to the first dose, you can take a second tablet 2 hours after the first tablet, but not sooner.

For any attack where you have no response to the first tablet, do not take a second tablet without first talking to your healthcare provider. Do not take more than a total of 200 mg of IMITREX Tablets in any 24-hour period. The safety of treating an average of more than 4 headaches in a 30 day period has not been established.

3. **Caution for activities requiring alertness:**

You may feel drowsy or dizzy because of your migraine or treatment with IMITREX Tablets. Use caution for activities requiring alertness (like driving or using machines).

4. **What to do if you take an overdose:**

If you have taken more medicine than has been prescribed for you, contact either your healthcare provider, hospital emergency department, or nearest poison control center right away.

5. **How to store your medicine:**

Keep your medicine in a safe place where children cannot reach it. It may be harmful to children.

Do not take tablets out of the packaging until you are ready to take them. Do not store the tablets in any other container.

Store your medicine away from heat and light. Do not store at temperatures above 86°F (30°C) or below 36°F (2°C).

The expiration date of your medicine is printed on the packaging. If your medicine has expired, throw it away. If your healthcare provider decides to stop your treatment, do not keep any leftover medicine unless your healthcare provider tells you to.

Some possible side effects of IMITREX Tablets

- Some patients feel pain or tightness in the chest or throat when using IMITREX Tablets. If this happens to you, tell your healthcare provider before taking any more IMITREX Tablets. If the chest pain, tightness, or pressure is severe or does not go away, call your healthcare provider right away.
- Call your healthcare provider right away if you have sudden and/or severe abdominal pain after you take IMITREX Tablets.
- Some people may have a reaction called serotonin syndrome when they take certain kinds of medicines for depression called SSRIs or SNRIs while they are taking IMITREX Tablets. Symptoms may include confusion, hallucinations, fast heartbeat, feeling faint, fever, sweating, muscle spasm, difficulty walking, and/or diarrhea. Call your healthcare provider right away if you have any of these symptoms after taking IMITREX Tablets.
- Shortness of breath; wheeziness; heart throbbing; swelling of eyelids, face, or lips; or a skin rash, skin lumps, or hives happens rarely. If it happens to you, then tell your healthcare provider right away. Do not take any more IMITREX Tablets unless your healthcare provider tells you to.
- Some people may feel tingling, heat, flushing (redness of face lasting a short time), heaviness, or pressure after taking IMITREX Tablets. A few people may feel drowsy, dizzy, tired, or sick. If you have any of these symptoms, tell your healthcare provider at your next visit.
- If you feel unwell in any other way or have any symptoms that you do not understand, you should contact your healthcare provider right away.

IMITREX and PAXIL are registered trademarks of GlaxoSmithKline. The other brands listed are trademarks of their respective owners and are not trademarks of GlaxoSmithKline. The makers of these brands are not affiliated with and do not endorse GlaxoSmithKline or its products.

GlaxoSmithKline
Research Triangle Park, NC 27709
©2010, GlaxoSmithKline. All rights reserved.
February 2010
IMT:2PIL

INFANRIX® ℞
[in' fan-rix]
(Diphtheria and Tetanus Toxoids
and Acellular Pertussis Vaccine Adsorbed)

HIGHLIGHTS OF PRESCRIBING INFORMATION

These highlights do not include all the information needed to use INFANRIX safely and effectively. See full prescribing information for INFANRIX.

INFANRIX (Diphtheria and Tetanus Toxoids and Acellular Pertussis Vaccine Adsorbed)
Initial U.S. Approval: 1997

——————RECENT MAJOR CHANGES——————

Warnings and Precautions, Apnea in Premature Infants (5.5)	02/2010

—————— INDICATIONS AND USAGE ——————

INFANRIX is a vaccine indicated for active immunization against diphtheria, tetanus, and pertussis as a 5-dose series in infants and children 6 weeks to 7 years of age. (1)

——————DOSAGE AND ADMINISTRATION——————

A 0.5-mL intramuscular injection given as a 5-dose series: (2.2)
- One dose each at 2, 4, and 6 months of age.
- One booster dose at 15 to 20 months of age and another booster dose at 4 to 6 years of age.

——————DOSAGE FORMS AND STRENGTHS——————

Suspension for intramuscular injection supplied in single-dose (0.5-mL) vials and prefilled syringes. (3)

——————CONTRAINDICATIONS——————

- Severe allergic reaction (e.g., anaphylaxis) after a previous dose of any diphtheria toxoid, tetanus toxoid, or pertussis-containing vaccine, or to any component of INFANRIX. (4.1)
- Encephalopathy within 7 days of administration of a previous pertussis-containing vaccine. (4.2)
- Progressive neurologic disorders. (4.3)

——————WARNINGS AND PRECAUTIONS——————

- If Guillain-Barré syndrome occurs within 6 weeks of receipt of a prior vaccine containing tetanus toxoid, the decision to give INFANRIX should be based on potential benefits and risks. (5.1)
- The needleless prefilled syringes contain dry natural latex rubber and may cause allergic reactions. (5.2)
- If temperature ≥105°F, collapse or shock-like state, or persistent, inconsolable crying lasting ≥3 hours have occurred within 48 hours after receipt of a pertussis-containing vaccine, or if seizures have occurred within 3 days after receipt of a pertussis-containing vaccine, the decision to give INFANRIX should be based on potential benefits and risks. (5.3)
- For children at higher risk for seizures, an antipyretic may be administered at the time of vaccination with INFANRIX. (5.4)
- Apnea following intramuscular vaccination has been observed in some infants born prematurely. Decisions about when to administer an intramuscular vaccine, including INFANRIX, to infants born prematurely should be based on consideration of the individual infant's medical status, and the potential benefits and possible risks of vaccination. (5.5)

——————ADVERSE REACTIONS——————

Rates of injection site reactions (pain, redness, swelling) ranged from 10% to 53%, depending on reaction and dose number, and were highest following doses 4 and 5. Fever was common (20% to 30%) following doses 1-3. Other common solicited adverse events were drowsiness, irritability/fussiness, and loss of appetite, reported in approximately 15% to 60% of subjects, depending on event and dose number. (6.1)

To report SUSPECTED ADVERSE REACTIONS, contact GlaxoSmithKline at 1-888-825-5249 or VAERS at 1-800-822-7967 or www.vaers.hhs.gov.

——————DRUG INTERACTIONS——————

Do not mix INFANRIX with any other vaccine in the same syringe or vial. (7.1)

Revised: 02/2010
See 17 for PATIENT COUNSELING INFORMATION
Revised: 02/2010

FULL PRESCRIBING INFORMATION: CONTENTS*

FULL PRESCRIBING INFORMATION

1 INDICATIONS AND USAGE

INFANRIX® is indicated for active immunization against diphtheria, tetanus, and pertussis as a 5-dose series in infants and children 6 weeks to 7 years of age (prior to seventh birthday).

2 DOSAGE AND ADMINISTRATION

2.1 Preparation for Administration

Shake vigorously to obtain a homogeneous, turbid, white suspension. Do not use if resuspension does not occur with vigorous shaking. Parenteral drug products should be inspected visually for particulate matter and discoloration prior to administration, whenever solution and container permit. INFANRIX also should be inspected visually for cracks in the vial or syringe prior to administration. If any of these conditions exist, the vaccine should not be administered.

2.2 Dose and Schedule

A 0.5-mL dose of INFANRIX is approved for intramuscular administration in infants and children 6 weeks to 7 years of age (prior to the seventh birthday) as a 5-dose series. The series consists of a primary immunization course of 3 doses administered at 2, 4, and 6 months of age (at intervals of 4 to 8 weeks), followed by 2 booster doses, administered at 15 to 20 months of age and at 4 to 6 years of age. The first dose may be given as early as 6 weeks of age.

The preferred administration site is the anterolateral aspect of the thigh for most infants younger than 12 months of age and the deltoid muscle of the upper arm for most children 12 months of age to 7 years of age.

Do not administer this product intravenously, intradermally, or subcutaneously.

2.3 Use of INFANRIX With Other DTaP Vaccines

Sufficient data are not available on the safety and effectiveness of interchanging INFANRIX and Diphtheria and Tetanus Toxoids and Acellular Pertussis (DTaP) vaccines from different manufacturers for successive doses of the DTaP vaccination series. Because the pertussis antigen components of INFANRIX and PEDIARIX® [Diphtheria and Tetanus Toxoids and Acellular Pertussis Adsorbed, Hepatitis B (Recombinant) and Inactivated Poliovirus Vaccine Combined] are the same, INFANRIX may be used to complete a DTaP vaccination series initiated with PEDIARIX.

2.4 Additional Dosing Information

If any recommended dose of pertussis vaccine cannot be given [see Contraindications (4.2, 4.3) and Warnings and Precautions (5.3)], Diphtheria and Tetanus Toxoids Adsorbed (DT) For Pediatric Use should be given according to its prescribing information.

3 DOSAGE FORMS AND STRENGTHS

INFANRIX is a suspension for intramuscular injection available in 0.5-mL single-dose vials and prefilled TIP-LOK® syringes.

Table 1. Solicited Local Reactions and General Adverse Events (%) Occurring Within 4 Days of Vaccination[a] With Separate Concomitant Administration of INFANRIX, ENGERIX-B, IPV, Haemophilus b (Hib) Conjugate Vaccine, and Pneumococcal Conjugate Vaccine (PCV7) (Modified Intent To Treat Cohort)

	INFANRIX, ENGERIX-B, IPV, Hib Vaccine, & PCV7		
	Dose 1	Dose 2	Dose 3
Local[b]			
N	335	323	315
Pain, any	31.9	30.0	29.8
Pain, grade 2 or 3	9.0	8.7	8.9
Pain, grade 3	2.7	1.5	1.3
Redness, any	18.2	32.8	39.0
Redness, >20 mm	0.3	0.0	1.9
Swelling, any	9.6	20.4	24.8
Swelling, >20 mm	0.6	0.0	1.3
General			
N	333	321	311
Fever[c] (≥100.4°F)	19.8	30.2	23.8
Fever[c] (>101.3°F)	4.5	9.7	5.8
Fever[c] (>102.2°F)	0.3	3.1	2.3
Fever[c] (>103.1°F)	0.0	0.3	0.3
N	335	323	315
Drowsiness, any	54.0	48.3	38.4
Drowsiness, grade 2 or 3	17.6	12.4	11.1
Drowsiness, grade 3	3.6	0.6	1.9
Irritability/Fussiness, any	61.5	61.6	56.5
Irritability/Fussiness, grade 2 or 3	19.4	21.1	19.4
Irritability/Fussiness, grade 3	3.9	3.4	3.2
Loss of appetite, any	27.8	26.6	23.8
Loss of appetite, grade 2 or 3	5.1	3.4	5.4
Loss of appetite, grade 3	0.6	0.3	0.0

Hib conjugate vaccine and PCV7 manufactured by Wyeth Pharmaceuticals Inc. IPV manufactured by Sanofi Pasteur SA. Modified intent to treat cohort = all vaccinated subjects for whom safety data were available.

N = number of infants for whom at least one symptom sheet was completed; for fever, numbers exclude missing temperature recordings or tympanic measurements.

Grade 2: pain defined as cried/protested on touch; drowsiness defined as interfered with normal daily activities; irritability/fussiness defined as crying more than usual/interfered with normal daily activities; loss of appetite defined as eating less than usual/interfered with normal daily activities.

Grade 3: pain defined as cried when limb was moved/spontaneously painful; drowsiness defined as prevented normal daily activities; irritability/fussiness defined as crying that could not be comforted/prevented normal daily activities; loss of appetite defined as no eating at all.

[a] Within 4 days of vaccination defined as day of vaccination and the next 3 days.
[b] Local reactions at the injection site for INFANRIX.
[c] Axillary temperatures increased by 1°C and oral temperatures increased by 0.5°C to derive equivalent rectal temperature.

4 CONTRAINDICATIONS

4.1 Hypersensitivity

Severe allergic reaction (e.g., anaphylaxis) after a previous dose of any diphtheria toxoid, tetanus toxoid, or pertussis-containing vaccine, or to any component of INFANRIX is a contraindication [see Description (11)]. Because of the uncertainty as to which component of the vaccine might be responsible, no further vaccination with any of these components should be given. Alternatively, such individuals may be referred to an allergist for evaluation if immunization with any of these components is being considered.

4.2 Encephalopathy

Encephalopathy (e.g., coma, decreased level of consciousness, prolonged seizures) within 7 days of administration of a previous dose of a pertussis-containing vaccine that is not attributable to another identifiable cause is a contraindication to administration of any pertussis-containing vaccine, including INFANRIX.

4.3 Progressive Neurologic Disorder

Progressive neurologic disorder, including infantile spasms, uncontrolled epilepsy, or progressive encephalopathy is a contraindication to administration of any pertussis-

containing vaccine, including INFANRIX. Pertussis vaccine should not be administered to individuals with these conditions until a treatment regimen has been established and the condition has stabilized.

5 WARNINGS AND PRECAUTIONS

5.1 Guillain-Barré Syndrome

If Guillain-Barré syndrome occurs within 6 weeks of receipt of a prior vaccine containing tetanus toxoid, the decision to give any tetanus toxoid-containing vaccine, including INFANRIX, should be based on careful consideration of the potential benefits and possible risks. When a decision is made to withhold tetanus toxoid, other available vaccines should be given, as indicated.

5.2 Latex

The tip cap and the rubber plunger of the needleless prefilled syringes contain dry natural latex rubber that may cause allergic reactions in latex sensitive individuals. The vial stopper does not contain latex.

5.3 Adverse Events Following Prior Pertussis Vaccination

If any of the following events occur in temporal relation to receipt of a pertussis-containing vaccine, the decision to give

Table 2. Solicited Local Reactions and General Adverse Events (%) Occurring Within 4 Days of Vaccination[a] With INFANRIX Administered as the Fourth Dose Following 3 Previous Doses of INFANRIX or PEDIARIX (Total Vaccinated Cohort)

	Group Primed With INFANRIX[b] N = 247	Group Primed With PEDIARIX[c] N = 553
Local[d]		
Pain, any	44.5	48.3
Pain, grade 2 or 3	19.0	18.6
Pain, grade 3	3.6	3.4
Redness, any	48.2	49.9
Redness, >20 mm	6.1	6.0
Swelling, any	32.8	32.7
Swelling, >20 mm	3.6	5.2
Increase in mid-thigh circumference, any	33.2	26.2
Increase in mid-thigh circumference, >40 mm	0.0	1.3
General		
Fever[e] (>99.5°F)	8.9	15.4
Fever[e] (>100.4°F)	4.5	6.7
Fever[e] (>101.3°F)	2.0	2.0
Drowsiness, any	35.6	31.3
Drowsiness, grade 2 or 3	9.3	6.7
Drowsiness, grade 3	2.4	1.3
Irritability, any	52.2	53.9
Irritability, grade 2 or 3	18.2	19.7
Irritability, grade 3	3.2	1.4
Loss of appetite, any	24.7	23.3
Loss of appetite, grade 2 or 3	5.3	4.9
Loss of appetite, grade 3	2.4	0.5

Total Vaccinated Cohort = all subjects who received a dose of study vaccine.
N = number of subjects for whom at least one symptom sheet was completed.
Grade 2: pain defined as cried/protested on touch; drowsiness defined as interfered with normal daily activities; irritability defined as crying more than usual/interfered with normal daily activities; loss of appetite defined as eating less than usual/no effect on normal daily activities.
Grade 3: pain defined as cried when limb was moved/spontaneously painful; drowsiness defined as prevented normal daily activities; irritability defined as crying that could not be comforted/prevented normal daily activities; loss of appetite defined as eating less than usual/interfered with normal daily activities.
[a] Within 4 days of vaccination defined as day of vaccination and the next 3 days.
[b] Received INFANRIX, ENGERIX-B, IPV (Sanofi Pasteur SA), PCV7 vaccine (Wyeth Pharmaceuticals Inc.), and Hib conjugate vaccine (Wyeth Pharmaceuticals Inc.) at 2, 4, and 6 months of age.
[c] Received PEDIARIX, PCV7 vaccine (Wyeth Pharmaceuticals Inc.), and Hib conjugate vaccine (Wyeth Pharmaceuticals Inc.) at 2, 4, and 6 months of age or PCV7 vaccine 2 weeks later.
[d] Local reactions at the injection site for INFANRIX.
[e] Axillary temperatures.

any pertussis-containing vaccine, including INFANRIX, should be based on careful consideration of the potential benefits and possible risks:

- Temperature of ≥40.5°C (105°F) within 48 hours not due to another identifiable cause;
- Collapse or shock-like state (hypotonic-hyporesponsive episode) within 48 hours;
- Persistent, inconsolable crying lasting ≥3 hours, occurring within 48 hours;
- Seizures with or without fever occurring within 3 days.

5.4   Children at Risk for Seizures
For children at higher risk for seizures than the general population, an appropriate antipyretic may be administered at the time of vaccination with a pertussis-containing vaccine, including INFANRIX, and for the ensuing 24 hours to reduce the possibility of post-vaccination fever.

5.5   Apnea in Premature Infants
Apnea following intramuscular vaccination has been observed in some infants born prematurely. Decisions about when to administer an intramuscular vaccine, including INFANRIX, to infants born prematurely should be based on

consideration of the individual infant's medical status, and the potential benefits and possible risks of vaccination.
5.6   Preventing and Managing Allergic Vaccine Reactions
Prior to administration, the healthcare provider should review the patient's immunization history for possible vaccine hypersensitivity. Epinephrine and other appropriate agents used for the control of immediate allergic reactions must be immediately available should an acute anaphylactic reaction occur.

6   ADVERSE REACTIONS
6.1   Clinical Trials Experience
Because clinical trials are conducted under widely varying conditions, adverse reaction rates observed in the clinical trials of a vaccine cannot be directly compared to rates in the clinical trials of another vaccine and may not reflect the rates observed in practice. There is the possibility that broad use of INFANRIX could reveal adverse reactions not observed in clinical trials.
Approximately 95,000 doses of INFANRIX have been administered in clinical studies. In these studies, 29,243 in-

fants have received INFANRIX in primary series studies, 6,081 children have received a fourth consecutive dose of INFANRIX, 1,764 children have received a fifth consecutive dose of INFANRIX, and 559 children have received a dose of INFANRIX following 3 doses of PEDIARIX.
Solicited Adverse Events: In a US study, 335 infants received INFANRIX, ENGERIX-B® [Hepatitis B Vaccine (Recombinant)], inactivated poliovirus vaccine (IPV, Sanofi Pasteur SA), Haemophilus b (Hib) conjugate vaccine (Wyeth Pharmaceuticals Inc.), and pneumococcal 7-valent conjugate (PCV7) vaccine (Wyeth Pharmaceuticals Inc.) concomitantly at separate sites. All vaccines were administered at 2, 4, and 6 months of age. Data on solicited local reactions and general adverse events were collected by parents using standardized diary cards for 4 consecutive days following each vaccine dose (i.e., day of vaccination and the next 3 days) (Table 1). Among subjects, 69% were White, 16% were Hispanic, 8% were Black, 4% were Asian, and 2% were of other racial/ethnic groups.
[See table 1 at top of previous page]
In a US study, the safety of a booster dose of INFANRIX was evaluated in children 15 to 18 months of age whose previous 3 DTaP doses were with INFANRIX (N = 251) or PEDIARIX (N = 559). Vaccines administered concurrently with the fourth dose of INFANRIX included measles, mumps, and rubella (MMR) vaccine (Merck & Co., Inc.), varicella vaccine (Merck & Co., Inc.), pneumococcal 7-valent conjugate (PCV7) vaccine (Wyeth Pharmaceuticals Inc.), and any US-licensed Hib conjugate vaccine; these were given concomitantly in 13.2%, 6.3%, 37.4%, and 41.2% of subjects, respectively. Data on solicited adverse events were collected by parents using standardized diary cards for 4 consecutive days following each vaccine dose (i.e., day of vaccination and the next 3 days) (Table 2). Among subjects, 85% were White, 6% were Hispanic, 6% were Black, 1% were Asian, and 2% were of other racial/ethnic groups.
[See table 2 at left]
In a US study, the safety of a fifth consecutive dose of INFANRIX coadministered at separate sites with a fourth dose of IPV (Sanofi Pasteur SA) and a second dose of MMR vaccine (Merck & Co., Inc.) was evaluated in 1,053 children 4 to 6 years of age. Data on solicited adverse events were collected by parents using standardized diary cards for 4 consecutive days following each vaccine dose (i.e., day of vaccination and the next 3 days) (Table 3). Among subjects, 43% were White, 18% Hispanic, 15% Asian, 7% Black, and 17% were of other racial/ethnic groups.

Table 3. Solicited Local Reactions and General Adverse Events (%) Occurring Within 4 Days of Vaccination[a] With a Fifth Consecutive Dose of INFANRIX When Coadministered With IPV and MMR Vaccine (Total Vaccinated Cohort)

Local[b]	N = 1,039-1,043
Pain, any	53.3
Pain, grade 2 or 3[c]	12.0
Pain, grade 3[c]	0.6
Redness, any	36.6
Redness, ≥50 mm	20.0
Redness, ≥110 mm	4.1
Arm circumference increase, any	37.8
Arm circumference increase, >20 mm	7.4
Arm circumference increase, >30 mm	3.2
Swelling, any	27.0
Swelling, ≥50 mm	11.5
Swelling, ≥110 mm	1.8
General	N = 993-1,036
Drowsiness, any	17.5
Drowsiness, grade 3[d]	0.8
Fever, ≥99.5°F	14.8
Fever, >100.4°F	4.4
Fever, >102.2°F	1.1
Fever, >104°F	0.0

Loss of appetite, any	16.0
Loss of appetite, grade 3[e]	0.6

IPV manufactured by Sanofi Pasteur SA. MMR vaccine manufactured by Merck & Co., Inc.

Total Vaccinated Cohort = all vaccinated subjects for whom safety data were available.

N = number of children with evaluable data for the events listed.

[a] Within 4 days of vaccination defined as day of vaccination and the next 3 days.

[b] Local reactions at the injection site for INFANRIX.

[c] Grade 2 defined as painful when the limb was moved; Grade 3 defined as preventing normal daily activities.

[d] Grade 3 defined as preventing normal daily activities.

[e] Grade 3 defined as not eating at all.

In the US booster immunization studies in which INFANRIX was administered as the fourth or fifth dose in the DTaP series following previous doses with INFANRIX or PEDIARIX, large swelling reactions of the limb injected with INFANRIX were assessed.

In the fourth dose study, a large swelling reaction was defined as injection site swelling with a diameter of >50 mm, a >50 mm increase in the mid-thigh circumference compared to the pre-vaccination measurement, and/or any diffuse swelling that interfered with or prevented daily activities. The overall incidence of large swelling reactions occurring within 4 days (Day 0-Day 3) following INFANRIX was 2.3%.

In the fifth dose study, a large swelling reaction was defined as swelling that involved >50% of the injected upper arm length and that was associated with a >30 mm increase in mid-upper arm circumference within 4 days following vaccination. The incidence of large swelling reactions following the fifth consecutive dose of INFANRIX was 1.0%.

Less Common and Serious General Adverse Events: Selected adverse events reported from a double-blind, randomized Italian clinical efficacy trial involving 4,696 children administered INFANRIX or 4,678 children administered whole-cell DTP vaccine (DTwP) (manufactured by Connaught Laboratories, Inc.) as a 3-dose primary series are shown in Table 4. The incidence of rectal temperature ≥104°F, hypotonic-hyporesponsive episodes and persistent crying ≥3 hours following administration of INFANRIX was significantly less than that following administration of whole-cell DTP vaccine.

[See table 4 above]

In a German safety study that enrolled 22,505 infants (66,867 doses of INFANRIX administered as a 3-dose primary series at 3, 4, and 5 months of age), all subjects were monitored for unsolicited adverse events that occurred within 28 days following vaccination using report cards. In a subset of subjects (N = 2,457), these cards were standardized diaries which solicited specific adverse events that occurred within 8 days of each vaccination in addition to unsolicited adverse events which occurred from enrollment until approximately 30 days following the third vaccination. Cards from the whole cohort were returned at subsequent visits and were supplemented by spontaneous reporting by parents and a medical history after the first and second doses of vaccine. In the subset of 2,457, adverse events following the third dose of vaccine were reported via standardized diaries and spontaneous reporting at a follow-up visit. Adverse events in the remainder of the cohort were reported via report cards which were returned by mail approximately 28 days after the third dose of vaccine. Adverse events (rates per 1,000 doses) occurring within 7 days following any of the first 3 doses included: unusual crying (0.09), febrile seizure (0.0), afebrile seizure (0.13), and hypotonic-hyporesponsive episodes (0.01).

6.2 Postmarketing Experience

In addition to reports in clinical trials, worldwide voluntary reports of adverse events received for INFANRIX since market introduction are listed below. This list includes serious events and events which have a plausible causal connection to INFANRIX. These adverse events were reported voluntarily from a population of uncertain size; therefore, it is not always possible to reliably estimate their frequency or establish a causal relationship to vaccination.

Infections and Infestations: Bronchitis, cellulitis, respiratory tract infection.

Blood and Lymphatic System Disorders: Lymphadenopathy, thrombocytopenia.

Immune System Disorders: Anaphylactic reaction, hypersensitivity.

Nervous System Disorders: Encephalopathy, headache, hypotonia.

Ear and Labyrinth Disorders: Ear pain.

Cardiac Disorders: Cyanosis.

Respiratory, Thoracic, and Mediastinal Disorders: Apnea, cough.

Skin and Subcutaneous Tissue Disorders: Angioedema, erythema, pruritus, rash, urticaria.

General Disorders and Administration Site Conditions: Fatigue, injection site induration, injection site reaction, Sudden Infant Death Syndrome.

7 DRUG INTERACTIONS

7.1 Concomitant Vaccine Administration

In clinical trials, INFANRIX was given concomitantly with Hib conjugate vaccine, pneumococcal 7-valent conjugate vaccine, hepatitis B vaccine, IPV, and the second dose of MMR vaccine [see Adverse Reactions (6.1) and Clinical Studies (14.3)].

When INFANRIX is administered concomitantly with other injectable vaccines, they should be given with separate syringes. INFANRIX should not be mixed with any other vaccine in the same syringe or vial.

7.2 Immunosuppressive Therapies

Immunosuppressive therapies, including irradiation, antimetabolites, alkylating agents, cytotoxic drugs, and corticosteroids (used in greater than physiologic doses), may reduce the immune response to INFANRIX.

8 USE IN SPECIFIC POPULATIONS

8.1 Pregnancy

Pregnancy Category C

Animal reproduction studies have not been conducted with INFANRIX. It is also not known whether INFANRIX can cause fetal harm when administered to a pregnant woman or can affect reproduction capacity.

8.4 Pediatric Use

Safety and effectiveness of INFANRIX in infants younger than 6 weeks of age and children 7 to 16 years of age have not been established. INFANRIX is not approved for use in these age groups.

11 DESCRIPTION

INFANRIX (Diphtheria and Tetanus Toxoids and Acellular Pertussis Vaccine Adsorbed) is a noninfectious, sterile vaccine for intramuscular administration. Each 0.5-mL dose is formulated to contain 25 Lf of diphtheria toxoid, 10 Lf of tetanus toxoid, 25 mcg of inactivated pertussis toxin (PT), 25 mcg of filamentous hemagglutinin (FHA), and 8 mcg of pertactin (69 kiloDalton outer membrane protein).

The diphtheria toxin is produced by growing *Corynebacterium diphtheriae* in Fenton medium containing a bovine extract. Tetanus toxin is produced by growing *Clostridium tetani* in a modified Latham medium derived from bovine casein. The bovine materials used in these extracts are sourced from countries which the United States Department of Agriculture (USDA) has determined neither have nor present an undue risk for bovine spongiform encephalopathy (BSE). Both toxins are detoxified with formaldehyde, concentrated by ultrafiltration, and purified by precipitation, dialysis, and sterile filtration.

The acellular pertussis antigens (PT, FHA, and pertactin) are isolated from *Bordetella pertussis* culture grown in modified Stainer-Scholte liquid medium. PT and FHA are isolated from the fermentation broth; pertactin is extracted from the cells by heat treatment and flocculation. The antigens are purified in successive chromatographic and precipitation steps. PT is detoxified using glutaraldehyde and formaldehyde. FHA and pertactin are treated with formaldehyde.

Diphtheria and tetanus toxoids and pertussis antigens (PT, FHA, and pertactin) are individually adsorbed onto aluminum hydroxide.

Diphtheria and tetanus toxoid potency is determined by measuring the amount of neutralizing antitoxin in previously immunized guinea pigs. The potency of the acellular pertussis components (PT, FHA, and pertactin) is determined by enzyme-linked immunosorbent assay (ELISA) on sera from previously immunized mice.

Each 0.5-mL dose contains aluminum hydroxide as adjuvant (not more than 0.625 mg aluminum by assay) and 4.5 mg of sodium chloride. Each dose also contains ≤100 mcg of residual formaldehyde and ≤100 mcg of polysorbate 80 (Tween 80).

The tip cap and the rubber plunger of the needleless prefilled syringes contain dry natural latex rubber. The vial stopper does not contain latex.

INFANRIX is formulated without preservatives.

12 CLINICAL PHARMACOLOGY

12.1 Mechanism of Action

Diphtheria: Diphtheria is an acute toxin-mediated infectious disease caused by toxigenic strains of *C. diphtheriae*. Protection against disease is due to the development of neutralizing antibodies to the diphtheria toxin. A serum diphtheria antitoxin level of 0.01 IU/mL is the lowest level giving some degree of protection; a level of 0.1 IU/mL is regarded as protective.[1]

Tetanus: Tetanus is an acute toxin-mediated infectious disease caused by a potent exotoxin released by *C. tetani*. Protection against disease is due to the development of neutralizing antibodies to the tetanus toxin. A serum tetanus antitoxin level of at least 0.01 IU/mL, measured by neutralization assays, is considered the minimum protective level.[2,3] A level of 0.1 IU/mL is considered protective.[4]

Pertussis: Pertussis (whooping cough) is a disease of the respiratory tract caused by *B. pertussis*. The role of the different components produced by *B. pertussis* in either the pathogenesis of, or the immunity to, pertussis is not well understood. There is no well established serological correlate of protection for pertussis.

13 NONCLINICAL TOXICOLOGY

13.1 Carcinogenesis, Mutagenesis, Impairment of Fertility

INFANRIX has not been evaluated for carcinogenic or mutagenic potential, or for impairment of fertility.

14 CLINICAL STUDIES

14.1 Diphtheria and Tetanus

Efficacy of diphtheria toxoid used in INFANRIX was determined on the basis of immunogenicity studies. A VERO cell toxin neutralizing test confirmed the ability of infant sera (N = 45), obtained one month after a 3-dose primary series, to neutralize diphtheria toxin. Levels of diphtheria antitoxin ≥0.01 IU/mL were achieved in 100% of the sera tested.

Efficacy of tetanus toxoid used in INFANRIX was determined on the basis of immunogenicity studies. An in vivo mouse neutralization assay confirmed the ability of infant sera (N = 45), obtained one month after a 3-dose primary series, to neutralize tetanus toxin. Levels of tetanus antitoxin ≥0.01 IU/mL were achieved in 100% of the sera tested.

14.2 Pertussis

Efficacy of a 3-dose primary series of INFANRIX has been assessed in 2 clinical studies.

A double-blind, randomized, active Diphtheria and Tetanus Toxoids (DT)-controlled trial conducted in Italy assessed the absolute protective efficacy of INFANRIX when administered at 2, 4, and 6 months of age. The population used in the primary analysis of the efficacy of INFANRIX included 4,481 infants vaccinated with INFANRIX and 1,470 DT vaccinees. The mean length of follow-up was 17 months, beginning 30 days after the third dose of vaccine. After 3 doses, the absolute protective efficacy of INFANRIX against WHO-

Table 4. Selected Adverse Events Occurring Within 48 Hours Following Vaccination With INFANRIX or Whole-Cell DTP in Italian Infants at 2, 4, or 6 Months of Age

Event	INFANRIX (N = 13,761 Doses)		Whole-Cell DTP Vaccine (N = 13,520 Doses)	
	Number	Rate/1,000 Doses	Number	Rate/1,000 Doses
Fever (≥104°F)[ab]	5	0.36	32	2.4
Hypotonic-hyporesponsive episode[c]	0	0	9	0.67
Persistent crying ≥3 hours[a]	6	0.44	54	4.0
Seizures[d]	1[e]	0.07	3[f]	0.22

[a] P <0.001.
[b] Rectal temperatures.
[c] P = 0.002.
[d] Not statistically significant at P <0.05.
[e] Maximum rectal temperature within 72 hours of vaccination = 103.1°F.
[f] Maximum rectal temperature within 72 hours of vaccination = 99.5°F, 101.3°F, and 102.2°F.

defined typical pertussis (21 days or more of paroxysmal cough with infection confirmed by culture and/or serologic testing) was 84% (95% CI: 76, 89). When the definition of pertussis was expanded to include clinically milder disease with respect to type and duration of cough, with infection confirmed by culture and/or serologic testing, the efficacy of INFANRIX was calculated to be 71% (95% CI: 60, 78) against >7 days of any cough and 73% (95% CI: 63, 80) against ≥14 days of any cough. Vaccine efficacy after 3 doses and with no booster dose in the second year of life was assessed in 2 subsequent follow-up periods. A follow-up period from 24 months to a mean age of 33 months was conducted in a partially unblinded cohort (children who received DT were offered pertussis vaccine and those who declined were retained in the study cohort). During this period, the efficacy of INFANRIX against WHO-defined pertussis was 78% (95% CI: 62, 87). During the third follow-up period which was conducted in an unblinded manner among children from 3 to 6 years of age, the efficacy of INFANRIX against WHO-defined pertussis was 86% (95% CI: 79, 91). Thus, protection against pertussis in children administered 3 doses of INFANRIX in infancy was sustained to 6 years of age.

A prospective efficacy trial was also conducted in Germany employing a household contact study design. In preparation for this study, 3 doses of INFANRIX were administered at 3, 4, and 5 months of age to more than 22,000 children living in 6 areas of Germany in a safety and immunogenicity study. Infants who did not participate in the safety and immunogenicity study could have received a DTwP vaccine or DT vaccine. Index cases were identified by spontaneous presentation to a physician. Households with at least one other member (i.e., besides index case) aged 6 through 47 months were enrolled. Household contacts of index cases were monitored for incidence of pertussis by a physician who was blinded to the vaccination status of the household. Calculation of vaccine efficacy was based on attack rates of pertussis in household contacts classified by vaccination status. Of the 173 household contacts who had not received a pertussis vaccine, 96 developed WHO-defined pertussis, as compared with 7 of 112 contacts vaccinated with INFANRIX. The protective efficacy of INFANRIX was calculated to be 89% (95% CI: 77, 95), with no indication of waning of protection up until the time of the booster vaccination. The average age of infants vaccinated with INFANRIX at the end of follow-up in this trial was 13 months (range 6 to 25 months). When the definition of pertussis was expanded to include clinically milder disease, with infection confirmed by culture and/or serologic testing, the efficacy of INFANRIX against ≥7 days of any cough was 67% (95% CI: 52, 78) and against ≥7 days of paroxysmal cough was 81% (95% CI: 68, 89). The corresponding efficacy of INFANRIX against ≥14 days of any cough or paroxysmal cough were 73% (95% CI: 59, 82) and 84% (95% CI: 71, 91), respectively.

Pertussis Immune Response to INFANRIX Administered as a 3-Dose Primary Series: The immune responses to each of the 3 pertussis antigens contained in INFANRIX were evaluated in sera obtained 1 month after the third dose of vaccine in each of 3 studies (schedule of administration: 2, 4, and 6 months of age in the Italian efficacy study and one US study; 3, 4, and 5 months of age in the German efficacy study). One month after the third dose of INFANRIX, the response rates to each pertussis antigen were similar in all 3 studies. Thus, although a serologic correlate of protection for pertussis has not been established, the antibody responses to these 3 pertussis antigens (PT, FHA, and pertactin) in a US population were similar to those achieved in 2 populations in which efficacy of INFANRIX was demonstrated.

14.3 Immune Response to Concomitantly Administered Vaccines

In a US study, INFANRIX was given concomitantly, at separate sites, with Hib conjugate vaccine (Sanofi Pasteur SA) at 2, 4, and 6 months of age. Subjects also received ENGERIX-B and oral poliovirus vaccine (OPV). One month after the third dose of Hib conjugate vaccine, 90% of 72 infants had anti-PRP (polyribosyl-ribitol-phosphate) ≥1.0 mcg/mL.

In a US study, INFANRIX was given concomitantly, at separate sites, with ENGERIX-B, IPV (Sanofi Pasteur SA), pneumococcal 7-valent conjugate (PCV7), and Hib conjugate vaccines (Wyeth Pharmaceuticals Inc.) at 2, 4, and 6 months of age. Immune responses were measured in sera obtained approximately one month after the third dose of vaccines. Among 121 subjects who had not received a birth dose of hepatitis B vaccine, 99.2% had anti-HBsAg (hepatitis B surface antigen) ≥10 mIU/mL following the third dose of ENGERIX-B. Among 153 subjects, 100% had anti-poliovirus 1, 2, and 3, ≥1:8 following the third dose of IPV. Although serological correlates for protection have not been established for the pneumococcal serotypes, a threshold level of ≥0.3 mcg/mL was evaluated. Following the third dose of PCV7 vaccine, 91.8% to 99.4% of subjects (N = 146-156) had anti-pneumococcal polysaccharide ≥0.3 mcg/mL for serotypes 4, 9V, 14, 18C, 19F, and 23F, and 73.0% had a level ≥0.3 mcg/mL for serotype 6B.

15 REFERENCES

1. Vitek CR and Wharton M. Diphtheria Toxoid. In: Plotkin SA, Orenstein WA, and Offit PA, eds. *Vaccines*. 5th ed. Saunders; 2008:139-156.
2. Wassilak SGF, Roper MH, Kretsinger K, and Orenstein WA. Tetanus Toxoid. In: Plotkin SA, Orenstein WA, and Offit PA, eds. *Vaccines*. 5th ed. Saunders; 2008:805-839.
3. Department of Health and Human Services, Food and Drug Administration. Biological products; Bacterial vaccines and toxoids; Implementation of efficacy review; Proposed rule. *Federal Register* December 13, 1985;50(240):51002-51117.
4. Centers for Disease Control and Prevention. General Recommendations on Immunization. Recommendations of the Advisory Committee on Immunization Practices (ACIP). *MMWR* 2006;55(RR-15):1-48.

16 HOW SUPPLIED/STORAGE AND HANDLING

INFANRIX is available in 0.5-mL single-dose vials and disposable prefilled TIP-LOK syringes.

Single-Dose Vials and Prefilled Syringes
NDC 58160-810-11 Package of 10 Single-Dose Vials
NDC 58160-810-46 Package of 5 Single-Dose Prefilled Disposable TIP-LOK Syringes (packaged without needles)
NDC 58160-810-51 Package of 10 Single-Dose Prefilled Disposable TIP-LOK Syringes (packaged without needles)

Store refrigerated between 2° and 8°C (36° and 46°F). Do not freeze. Discard if the vaccine has been frozen.

17 PATIENT COUNSELING INFORMATION

The parent or guardian should be:

- informed of the potential benefits and risks of immunization with INFANRIX, and of the importance of completing the immunization series.
- informed about the potential for adverse reactions that have been temporally associated with administration of INFANRIX or other vaccines containing similar components.
- instructed to report any adverse events to their health-care provider.
- given the Vaccine Information Statements, which are required by the National Childhood Vaccine Injury Act of 1986 to be given prior to immunization. These materials are available free of charge at the Centers for Disease Control and Prevention (CDC) website (www.cdc.gov/vaccines).

ENGERIX-B, INFANRIX, PEDIARIX, and TIP-LOK are registered trademarks of GlaxoSmithKline.

Manufactured by **GlaxoSmithKline Biologicals**
Rixensart, Belgium, US License 1617
Novartis Vaccines and Diagnostics GmbH & Co. KG
Marburg, Germany, US License 1754
Distributed by **GlaxoSmithKline**
Research Triangle Park, NC 27709
©2010, GlaxoSmithKline. All rights reserved.
February 2010
INF:18PI

INNOPRAN XL® ℞

[*in' ō-pran*]
(propranolol hydrochloride)
Extended Release Capsules

DESCRIPTION

INNOPRAN XL (propranolol hydrochloride) is a nonselective, beta-adrenergic receptor-blocking agent for oral administration, available as an extended release product. INNOPRAN XL is available as 80-mg and 120-mg capsules which contain sustained-release beads. Each of the beads contains propranolol hydrochloride and is coated with dual membranes. These membranes are designed to retard release of propranolol hydrochloride for several hours after ingestion followed by the sustained release of propranolol.

The active ingredient in INNOPRAN XL is a synthetic beta-adrenergic receptor-blocking agent chemically described as 1-(Isopropylamino)-3-(1-naphthyloxy)-2-propanol hydrochloride. Its structural formula is:

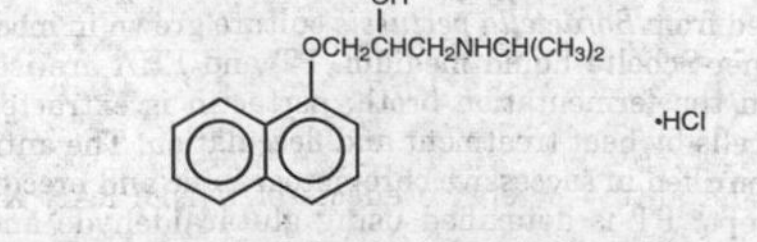

Propranolol hydrochloride is a stable, white, crystalline solid, which is readily soluble in water and ethanol. Its molecular weight is 295.81. Each capsule for oral administration contains sugar spheres, ethylcellulose, povidone, hypromellose phthalate, diethyl phthalate, hypromellose, polyethylene glycol, gelatin, titanium dioxide, and black iron oxide. In addition, INNOPRAN XL 120 mg capsules contain yellow iron oxide.

CLINICAL PHARMACOLOGY

General

Propranolol is a nonselective, beta-adrenergic receptor-blocking agent possessing no other autonomic nervous system activity. It specifically competes with beta-adrenergic receptor-stimulating agents for available receptor sites. When access to beta-receptor sites is blocked by propranolol, chronotropic, inotropic, and vasodilator responses to beta-adrenergic stimulation are decreased proportionately. At dosages greater than required for beta blockade, propranolol also exerts a quinidine-like or anesthetic-like membrane action, which affects the cardiac action potential. The significance of the membrane action in the treatment of arrhythmias is uncertain.

Mechanism of Action

The mechanism of the antihypertensive effect of propranolol has not been established. Among factors that contribute to the antihypertensive action are: (1) decreased cardiac output, (2) inhibition of renin release by the kidneys, and (3) diminution of tonic sympathetic nerve outflow from vasomotor centers in the brain. Although total peripheral resistance may increase initially, it readjusts to or below the pretreatment level with chronic use of propranolol. Effects of propranolol on plasma volume appear to be minor and somewhat variable.

Pharmacokinetics and Drug Metabolism

Absorption

Propranolol is highly lipophilic and is almost completely absorbed after oral administration. However, it undergoes high first-pass metabolism by the liver and on average, only about 25% of propranolol reaches the systemic circulation.

A single-dose, food-effect study in 36 healthy subjects showed that a high fat meal administered with INNOPRAN XL at 10 p.m., increased the lag time from 3 to 5 hours and the time to reach the maximum concentration from 11.5 to 15.4 hours, under fed conditions, with no effect on the AUC (see DOSAGE AND ADMINISTRATION).

Following multiple-dose administration of INNOPRAN XL at 10 p.m. under fasting conditions, the steady state lag time was between 4 and 5 hours and propranolol peak plasma concentrations were reached approximately 12 to 14 hours after dosing. Propranolol trough levels were achieved 24 to 27 hours after dosing, and persisted for 3 to 5 hours after the next dose. The elimination half-life of propranolol was approximately 8 hours.

The plasma levels of propranolol showed dose-proportional increases after single and multiple administration of 80-, 120-, and 160-mg of INNOPRAN XL.

At steady state, the bioavailability of a 160-mg dose of INNOPRAN XL and propranolol hydrochloride long-acting capsules did not differ significantly.

Distribution

Approximately 90% of circulating propranolol is bound to plasma proteins (albumin and alpha$_1$ acid glycoprotein). The binding is enantiomer-selective. The S-isomer is preferentially bound to alpha$_1$ glycoprotein and the R-isomer preferentially bound to albumin. The volume of distribution of propranolol is approximately 4 liters.

Metabolism and Elimination

Propranolol is extensively metabolized with most metabolites appearing in the urine. Propranolol is metabolized through 3 primary routes: Aromatic hydroxylation (mainly 4-hydroxylation), N-dealkylation followed by further side-chain oxidation, and direct glucuronidation. It has been estimated that the percentage contributions of these routes to total metabolism are 42%, 41%, and 17%, respectively, but with considerable variability between individuals. The 4 major metabolites are propranolol glucuronide, naphthyloxylactic acid, and glucuronic acid and sulfate conjugates of 4-hydroxy propranolol.

In vitro studies have indicated that the aromatic hydroxylation of propranolol is catalyzed mainly by polymorphic CYP2D6. Side-chain oxidation is mediated mainly by CYP1A2 and to some extent by CYP2D6. 4-hydroxy propranolol is a weak inhibitor of CYP2D6.

Propranolol is also a substrate for CYP2C19 and a substrate for the intestinal efflux transporter, p-glycoprotein (p-gp). Studies suggest however that p-gp is not dose-limiting for intestinal absorption of propranolol in the usual therapeutic dose range.

In healthy subjects, no difference was observed between CYP2D6 extensive metabolizers (EMs) and poor metabolizers (PMs) with respect to oral clearance or elimination half-life. Partial clearance to 4-hydroxy propranolol was significantly higher and to naphthyloxylactic acid was significantly lower in EMs than PMs.

Enantiomers

Of the 2 enantiomers of propranolol, the S-enantiomer blocks beta adrenergic receptors. In normal subjects receiving oral doses of racemic propranolol, S-enantiomer concentrations exceeded those of the R-enantiomer by 40 to 90% as a result of stereoselective hepatic metabolism.

Special Populations

Pediatric

The pharmacokinetics of INNOPRAN XL have not been investigated in patients younger than 18 years of age.

Geriatric

The pharmacokinetics of INNOPRAN XL have not been investigated in patients older than 65 years of age. In a study of 12 elderly (62 to 79 years old) and 12 young (25 to 33 years old) healthy subjects, the clearance of the S-enantiomer of propranolol was decreased in the elderly. Additionally, the half-lives of both R- and S-propranolol were prolonged in the elderly compared with the young (11 hours versus 5 hours).

Gender

In a dose-proportionality study, the pharmacokinetics of INNOPRAN XL were evaluated in 22 male and 14 female healthy volunteers. Following single doses under fasting conditions, the mean AUC and C_{max} were about 49% and 16% higher for females across the dosage range. The mean elimination half-life was longer in females than in males (11 hours versus 7.5 hours).

Race

A study conducted in 12 white and 13 African-American male subjects taking propranolol showed, that at steady state, the clearance of R- and S-propranolol were about 76% and 53% higher in African-Americans than in whites, respectively.

Renal Insufficiency

The pharmacokinetics of INNOPRAN XL have not been evaluated in patients with renal insufficiency. In a study conducted in 5 patients with chronic renal failure, 6 patients on regular dialysis, and 5 healthy subjects, who received a single oral dose of 40 mg of propranolol, the peak plasma concentrations (C_{max}) of propranolol in the chronic renal failure group were 2- to 3-fold higher (161±41 ng/mL) than those observed in the dialysis patients (47±9 ng/mL) and in the healthy subjects (26±1 ng/mL). Propranolol plasma clearance was also reduced in the patients with chronic renal failure.

Chronic renal failure has been associated with a decrease in drug metabolism via down regulation of hepatic cytochrome P450 activity.

Hepatic Insufficiency

The pharmacokinetics of INNOPRAN XL have not been evaluated in patients with hepatic impairment. However, propranolol is extensively metabolized by the liver. In a study conducted in 7 patients with cirrhosis and 9 healthy subjects receiving 80-mg oral propranolol every 8 hours for 7 doses, the steady-state unbound propranolol concentration in patients with cirrhosis was increased 3-fold in comparison to controls. In cirrhosis, the half-life increased to 11 hours compared to 4 hours (see PRECAUTIONS).

Drug Interactions

Interactions with Substrates, Inhibitors or Inducers of Cytochrome P-450 Enzymes

Because propranolol's metabolism involves multiple pathways in the cytochrome P-450 system (CYP2D6, 1A2, 2C19), administration of INNOPRAN XL with drugs that are metabolized by, or affect the activity (induction or inhibition) of one or more of these pathways may lead to clinically relevant drug interactions (see PRECAUTIONS, Drug Interactions).

Substrates or Inhibitors of CYP2D6

Blood levels and/or toxicity of propranolol may be increased by administration of INNOPRAN XL with substrates or inhibitors of CYP2D6, such as amiodarone, cimetidine, delavudin, fluoxetine, paroxetine, quinidine, and ritonavir. No interactions were observed with either ranitidine or lansoprazole.

Substrates or Inhibitors of CYP1A2

Blood levels and/or toxicity of propranolol may be increased by administration of INNOPRAN XL with substrates or inhibitors of CYP1A2, such as imipramine, cimetidine, ciprofloxacin, fluvoxamine, isoniazid, ritonavir, theophylline, zileuton, zolmitriptan, and rizatriptan.

Substrates or Inhibitors of CYP2C19

Blood levels and/or toxicity of propranolol may be increased by administration of INNOPRAN XL with substrates or inhibitors of CYP2C19, such as fluconazole, cimetidine, fluoxetine, fluvoxamine, teniposide, and tolbutamide. No interaction was observed with omeprazole.

Inducers of Hepatic Drug Metabolism

Blood levels of propranolol may be decreased by administration of INNOPRAN XL with inducers such as rifampin and ethanol. Cigarette smoking also induces hepatic metabolism and has been shown to increase up to 100% the clearance of propranolol, resulting in decreased plasma concentrations.

Cardiovascular Drugs

Antiarrhythmics

The concomitant administration of propranolol and propafenone increased propranolol average steady-state plasma concentrations (213%), AUC (113%), C_{max} (83%), T_{max} (55%), and $T_{1/2}$ (30%), and significantly decreased plasma levels of 4-hydroxy-propranolol. Co-administration of propranolol and propafenone did not produce any significant change in propafenone pharmacokinetics. While the therapeutic range for propranolol is wide, a reduction in dosage may be necessary during concomitant administration with propafenone.

The metabolism of propranolol is reduced by co-administration of quinidine, leading to a 2-to 3-fold increase in blood concentrations and greater degrees of clinical beta-blockade.

Concomitant administration of propranolol with lidocaine, bupivacaine or mepivacaine has been reported to decrease the clearance of these amide anesthetics significantly, resulting in higher serum concentrations of the anesthetic.

Calcium channel blockers

The mean C_{max} and AUC of propranolol are increased respectively, by 50% and 30% by co-administration of nisoldipine and by 80% and 47%, by co-administration of nicardipine.

The mean C_{max} and AUC of nifedipine are increased by 64% and 79%, respectively, by co-administration of propranolol. Propranolol does not affect the pharmacokinetics of verapamil and norverapamil. Verapamil does not affect the pharmacokinetics of propranolol.

Non-Cardiovascular Drugs

Anti-Ulcer Drugs

Co-administration of propranolol with cimetidine, a non-specific CYP450 inhibitor, increased propranolol concentrations by about 40%. Co-administration with aluminum hydroxide gel (1,200 mg) resulted in a 50% decrease in propranolol concentrations.

Co-administration of metoclopramide with propranolol did not have a significant effect on propranolol's pharmacokinetics.

Benzodiazepines

Propranolol can inhibit the metabolism of diazepam, resulting in increased concentrations of diazepam and its metabolites. Diazepam does not alter the pharmacokinetics of propranolol.

The pharmacokinetics of oxazepam, triazolam, lorazepam, and alprazolam are not affected by co-administration of propranolol.

Lipid Lowering Drugs

Co-administration of cholesteramine or colestipol with propranolol resulted in up to a 50% decrease in propranolol concentrations.

Co-administration of propranolol with lovastatin or pravastatin decreased 20% to 25% the AUC of both, but did not alter their pharmacodynamics. Propranolol did not have an effect on the pharmacokinetics of fluvastatin.

Migraine Drugs

Administration of zolmitriptan or rizatriptan with propranolol resulted in increased concentrations of zolmitriptan (AUC increased by 56% and C_{max} by 37%) or rizatriptan (the AUC and C_{max} were increased by 67% and 75%, respectively).

Neuroleptic Drugs

Co-administration of propranolol at doses greater than or equal to 160 mg/day resulted in increased thioridazine plasma concentrations ranging from 50% to 370% and increased thioridazine metabolites concentrations ranging from 33% to 210%.

Co-administration of chlorpromazine with propranolol resulted in increased plasma levels of both drugs (70% increase in propranolol concentrations).

Theophylline

Co-administration of theophylline with propranolol decreases theophylline oral clearance by 33% to 52%.

Warfarin

Concomitant administration of propranolol and warfarin has been shown to increase warfarin bioavailability and increase prothrombin time.

Pharmacodynamics and Clinical Effects

Hypertension

In a double-blind, parallel dose-response study in patients with mild-to-moderate hypertension (n=434), doses of INNOPRAN XL from 80 to 640 mg were taken once daily at approximately 10 p.m. INNOPRAN XL significantly lowered sitting systolic and diastolic blood pressure when measurements were taken approximately 16 hours later. The placebo-subtracted diastolic blood pressure effect for the 80- and 120-mg doses was -3.0 and -4.0 mm Hg, respectively. Higher doses of INNOPRAN XL (160, 640 mg) had no additional blood pressure lowering effect when compared with 120 mg. The antihypertensive effects of INNOPRAN XL were seen in the elderly (≥65 years old) and men and women. There were too few non-white patients to assess the efficacy of INNOPRAN XL in these patients.

INDICATIONS AND USAGE

Hypertension

INNOPRAN XL is indicated in the management of hypertension; it may be used alone or in combination with other antihypertensive agents.

CONTRAINDICATIONS

Propranolol is contraindicated in 1) cardiogenic shock; 2) sinus bradycardia, sick sinus syndrome, and greater than first-degree block unless a permanent pacemaker is in place; 3) bronchial asthma; and 4) in patients with known hypersensitivity to propranolol hydrochloride.

WARNINGS

Cardiac Failure

Sympathetic stimulation may be a vital component supporting circulatory function in patients with congestive heart failure, and its inhibition by beta-blockade may precipitate more severe failure. Although beta-blockers should be avoided in overt congestive heart failure, some have been shown to be highly beneficial when used with close follow-up in patients with a history of failure who are well compensated and are receiving additional therapies, including diuretics as needed. Beta-adrenergic blocking agents do not abolish the inotropic action of digitalis on heart muscle.

Angina Pectoris: There have been reports of exacerbation of angina and, in some cases, myocardial infarction, following abrupt discontinuance of propranolol therapy. Therefore, when discontinuance of propranolol is planned, the dosage should be gradually reduced over at least a few weeks, and the patient should be cautioned against interruption or cessation of therapy without a physician's advice. If propranolol therapy is interrupted and exacerbation of angina occurs, it is usually advisable to reinstitute propranolol therapy and take other measures appropriate for the management of angina pectoris. Since coronary artery disease may be unrecognized, it may be prudent to follow the above advice in patients considered at risk of having occult atherosclerotic heart disease who are given propranolol for other indications.

Nonallergic Bronchospasm (e.g., Chronic Bronchitis, Emphysema)

In general, patients with bronchospastic lung disease should not receive beta-blockers. Propranolol should be administered with caution in this setting since it may block bronchodilation produced by endogenous and exogenous catecholamine stimulation of beta-receptors.

Major Surgery

The necessity or desirability of withdrawal of beta-blocking therapy prior to major surgery is controversial. It should be noted, however, that the impaired ability of the heart to respond to reflex adrenergic stimuli in propranolol-treated patients may augment the risks of general anesthesia and surgical procedures.

Propranolol is a competitive inhibitor of beta-receptor agonists, and its effects can be reversed by administration of such agents, e.g., dobutamine or isoproterenol. However, such patients may be subject to protracted severe hypotension.

Diabetes and Hypoglycemia

Beta-adrenergic blockade may prevent the appearance of certain premonitory signs and symptoms (pulse rate and blood pressure changes) of acute hypoglycemia, especially in labile insulin-dependent diabetics. In these patients, it may be more difficult to adjust the dosage of insulin.

Propranolol therapy, particularly in infants and children, diabetic or not, has been associated with hypoglycemia especially during fasting, as in preparation for surgery. Hypoglycemia has been reported with propranolol use after prolonged physical exertion and in patients with renal insufficiency.

Thyrotoxicosis

Beta-adrenergic blockade may mask certain clinical signs of hyperthyroidism. Therefore, abrupt withdrawal of propranolol may be followed by an exacerbation of symptoms of hyperthyroidism, including thyroid storm. Propranolol may change thyroid-function tests, increasing T_4 and reversing T_3, and decreasing T_3.

Wolff-Parkinson-White Syndrome

Beta-adrenergic blockade in patients with Wolff-Parkinson-White syndrome and tachycardia has been associated with severe bradycardia requiring treatment with a pacemaker. In one case, this resulted after an initial dose of 5-mg propranolol.

PRECAUTIONS

General

Propranolol should be used with caution in patients with impaired hepatic or renal function. INNOPRAN XL is not indicated for the treatment of hypertensive emergencies.

Beta-adrenergic receptor blockade can cause reduction of intraocular pressure. Patients should be told that

INNOPRAN XL may interfere with the glaucoma screening test. Withdrawal may lead to a return of intraocular pressure.

Myopathy

Caution should be exercised when administering propranolol to patients with underlying skeletal muscle disease. Isolated cases of exacerbation of myopathy and myotonia have been reported.

Risk of Anaphylactic Reaction

While taking beta-blockers, patients with a history of severe anaphylactic reaction to a variety of allergens may be more reactive to repeated challenge, either accidental, diagnostic, or therapeutic. Such patients may be unresponsive to the usual doses of epinephrine used to treat allergic reaction.

Clinical Laboratory Tests

In patients with hypertension, use of propranolol has been associated with elevated levels of serum potassium, and serum transaminases and alkaline phosphatase. In severe heart failure, the use of propranolol has been associated with increases in blood urea nitrogen.

Drug Interactions

Caution should be exercised when INNOPRAN XL is administered with drugs that have an effect on CYP2D6, 1A2, or 2C19 metabolic pathways. Co-administration of such drugs with propranolol may lead to clinically relevant drug interactions and changes on its efficacy and/or toxicity (see CLINICAL PHARMACOLOGY, Drug Interactions).

Cardiovascular Drugs

ACE Inhibitors

When combined with beta-blockers, ACE inhibitors can cause hypotension, particularly in the setting of acute myocardial infraction.

Certain ACE inhibitors have been reported to increase bronchial hyperreactivity when administered with propranolol.

The antihypertensive effects of clonidine may be antagonized by beta-blockers. INNOPRAN XL should be administered cautiously to patients withdrawing from clonidine.

Alpha Blockers

Prazosin has been associated with prolongation of first dose hypotension in the presence of beta-blockers.

Postural hypotension has been reported in patients taking both beta-blockers and terazosin or doxazosin.

Antiarrhythmics

Propafenone has negative inotropic and beta-blocking properties that can be additive to those of propranolol.

Quinidine increases the concentration of propranolol and produces greater degrees of clinical beta-blockade and may cause postural hypotension.

Disopyramide is a Type I antiarrhythmic drug with potent negative inotropic and chronotropic effects and has been associated with severe bradycardia, asystole, and heart failure when administered with propranolol.

Amiodarone is an antiarrhythmic agent with negative chronotropic properties that may be additive to those seen with propranolol.

The clearance of lidocaine and bupivacaine are significantly reduced with administration of propranolol. Lidocaine and bupivacaine toxicity has been reported following coadministration with propranolol. (see also PRECAUTIONS, Drug Interactions, Non-Cardiovascular Drugs, Anesthetic Agents)

Caution should be exercised when administering INNOPRAN XL with drugs that slow A-V nodal conduction, e.g. digitalis, lidocaine, and calcium channel blockers.

Calcium Channel Blockers

Caution should be exercised when patients receiving a beta-blocker are administered a calcium-channel-blocking drug with negative inotropic and/or chronotropic effects. Both agents may depress myocardial contractility or atrioventricular conduction.

There have been reports of significant bradycardia, heart failure, and cardiovascular collapse with concurrent use of verapamil and beta-blockers.

Co-administration of propranolol and diltiazem in patients with cardiac disease has been associated with bradycardia, hypotension, high degree heart block, and heart failure.

Digitalis Glycosides

Both digitalis glycosides and beta-blockers slow atrioventricular conduction and decrease heart rate. Concomitant use can increase the risk of bradycardia.

Inotropic Agents

Patients on long-term therapy with propranolol may experience uncontrolled hypertension if administered epinephrine as a consequence of unopposed alpha-receptor stimulation. Epinephrine is therefore not indicated in the treatment of propranolol overdose (see OVERDOSAGE).

Isoproterenol and Dobutamine

Propranolol is a competitive inhibitor of beta-receptor agonists, and its effects can be reversed by administration of such agents, e.g., dobutamine or isoproterenol. Also, propranolol may reduce sensitivity to dobutamine stress echocardiography in patients undergoing evaluation for myocardial ischemia.

Reserpine

Patients receiving catecholamine-depleting drugs, such as reserpine and INNOPRAN XL, should be closely observed for excessive reduction of resting sympathetic nervous activity, which may result in hypotension, marked bradycardia, vertigo, syncopal attacks, or orthostatic hypotension. Administration of reserpine with propranolol may also potentiate depression.

Non-Cardiovascular Drugs

Anesthetic Agents

Methoxyflurane and trichloroethylene may depress myocardial contractility when administered with propranolol.

The clearance of local amide anesthetics (e.g., lidocaine, bupivacaine, mepivacaine) is reduced with administration of propranolol.

Lidocaine and bupivacaine toxicity has been reported following coadministration with propranolol. Caution should be exercised when amide anesthetic agents are administered concomitantly with propanolol.

Antidepressants

The hypotensive effects of MAO inhibitors or tricyclic antidepressants may be exacerbated when administered with beta-blockers by interfering with the beta-blocking activity of propranolol.

Neuroleptic Drugs

Hypotension and cardiac arrest have been reported with the concomitant use of propranolol and haloperidol.

Non-Steroidal Anti-Inflammatory Drugs

Nonsteroidal anti-inflammatory drugs (NSAIDS) have been reported to blunt the antihypertensive effect of beta-adrenoreceptor blocking agents.

Administration of indomethacin with propranolol may reduce the efficacy of propranolol in reducing blood pressure and heart rate.

Thyroxine

Thyroxine may result in a lower than expected T_3 concentration when used concomitantly with propranolol.

Warfarin

Propranolol when administered with warfarin increases the concentration of warfarin. Prothrombin time, therefore, should be monitored.

Carcinogenesis, Mutagenesis, Impairment of Fertility

In dietary administration studies in which mice and rats were treated with propranolol HCl for up to 18 months at doses of up to 150 mg/kg/day, there was no evidence of drug-related tumorigenesis. On a body surface area basis, this dose in the mouse and rat is, respectively, about equal to and about twice the maximum recommended human oral daily dose (MRHD) of 640 mg propranolol HCl. In a study in which both male and female rats were exposed to propranolol HCl in their diets at concentrations of up to 0.05% (about 50 mg/kg body weight and less than the MRHD), from 60 days prior to mating and throughout pregnancy and lactation for 2 generations, there were no effects on fertility. Based on differing results from Ames tests performed by different laboratories, there is equivocal evidence for a genotoxic effect of propranolol HCl in bacteria (S. typhimurium strain TA 1538).

Pregnancy

Pregnancy Category C

In a series of reproductive and developmental toxicology studies, propranolol was given to rats by gavage or in the diet throughout pregnancy and lactation. At doses of 150 mg/kg/day, but not at doses of 80 mg/kg/day (equivalent to the MRHD on a body surface area basis), treatment was associated with embryotoxicity (reduced litter size and increased resorption rates) as well as neonatal toxicity (deaths). Propranolol HCl also was administered (in the feed) to rabbits (throughout pregnancy and lactation) at doses as high as 150 mg/kg/day (about 5 times the maximum recommended human oral daily dose). No evidence of embryo or neonatal toxicity was noted.

There are no adequate and well-controlled studies in pregnant women. Intrauterine growth retardation has been reported for neonates whose mothers received propranolol HCl during pregnancy. Neonates whose mothers received propranolol HCl at parturition have exhibited bradycardia, hypoglycemia, and respiratory depression. Adequate facilities for monitoring such infants at birth should be available. INNOPRAN XL should be used during pregnancy only if the potential benefit justifies the potential risk to the fetus.

Nursing Mothers

Propranolol is excreted in human milk. Caution should be exercised when INNOPRAN XL is administered to a nursing woman.

Pediatric Use

Safety and effectiveness of propranolol in pediatric patients have not been established.

Geriatric Use

Clinical studies of INNOPRAN XL did not include sufficient numbers of subjects aged 65 and over to determine whether they respond differently from younger subjects. Other reported clinical experience has not identified differences in responses between the elderly and younger patients. In general, dose selection for an elderly patient should be cautious, usually starting at the low end of the dosing range, reflecting the greater frequency of decreased hepatic, renal, or cardiac function, and of concomitant disease or other drug therapy.

ADVERSE REACTIONS

Adverse events occurring at a rate of ≥3%, excluding those reported more commonly in placebo, encountered in the INNOPRAN XL placebo-controlled hypertension trials and plausibly related to treatment are shown in Table 1.

Table 1. Treatment Emergent Adverse Events Reported In ≥3% of Subjects

		INNOPRAN XL	
	Placebo	80 mg	120 mg
Body System	(N=88)	(N=89)	(N=85)
Fatigue	3 (3.0%)	4 (5.0%)	6 (7.0%)
Dizziness (except vertigo)	2 (2.0%)	6 (7.0%)	3 (4.0%)
Constipation	0	3 (3.0%)	1 (1.0%)

The following adverse events were observed and have been reported with use of formulations of sustained- or immediate-release propranolol.

Cardiovascular

Bradycardia; congestive heart failure; intensification of AV block; hypotension; paresthesia of hands; thrombocytopenic purpura; arterial insufficiency, usually of the Raynaud type.

Central Nervous System

Light-headedness, mental depression manifested by insomnia, lassitude, weakness, fatigue; reversible mental depression progressing to catatonia; visual disturbances; hallucinations; vivid dreams; an acute reversible syndrome characterized by disorientation for time and place, short-term memory loss, emotional lability, slightly clouded sensorium, and decreased performance on neuropsychometrics. For immediate-release formulations, fatigue, lethargy, and vivid dreams appear dose related.

Gastrointestinal

Nausea, vomiting, epigastric distress, abdominal cramping, diarrhea, constipation, mesenteric arterial thrombosis, ischemic colitis.

Allergic

Pharyngitis and agranulocytosis; erythematous rash, fever combined with aching and sore throat, laryngospasm, and respiratory distress.

Respiratory

Bronchospasm.

Hematologic

Agranulocytosis, nonthrombocytopenic purpura, thrombocytopenic purpura.

Musculoskeletal

Myopathy, myotonia (see PRECAUTIONS).

Autoimmune

In extremely rare instances, systemic lupus erythematosus has been reported.

Miscellaneous

Alopecia, LE-like reactions, psoriasiform rashes, dry eyes, male impotence, and Peyronie's disease have been reported rarely. Oculomucocutaneous reactions involving the skin, serous membranes, and conjunctivae reported for a beta blocker (practolol) have not been associated with propranolol.

DOSAGE AND ADMINISTRATION

INNOPRAN XL should be administered once daily at bedtime (approximately 10 p.m.) and should be taken consistently either on an empty stomach or with food. The starting dose is 80 mg but dosage should be individualized and titration may be needed to a dose of 120 mg. In the clinical trial, doses of INNOPRAN XL above 120 mg had no additional effects on blood pressure (see CLINICAL PHARMACOLOGY, Pharmacodynamics and Clinical Effects). The time needed for full antihypertensive response is variable, but is usually achieved within 2 to 3 weeks.

OVERDOSAGE

Most overdoses of propranolol are mild and respond to supportive care.

Propranolol is not significantly dialyzable. In the event of overdose or exaggerated response, the following measures should be employed.

Hypotension and bradycardia have been reported following propranolol overdose and should be treated appropriately. Glucagon can exert potent inotropic and chronotropic effects and may be particularly useful for the treatment of hypotension or depressed myocardial function after a propranolol overdose.

Glucagon should be administered as 50-150 mcg/kg intravenously followed by continuous drip of 1-5 mg/hour for positive chronotropic effect. Isoproterenol, dopamine or phosphodiesterase inhibitors may also be useful. Epinephrine, however, may provoke uncontrolled hypertension. Bradycardia can be treated with atropine or isoproterenol. Serious bradycardia may require temporary cardiac pacing.

The electrocardiogram, pulse, blood pressure, neurobehavioral status and intake and output balance must be monitored. Isoproterenol and aminophylline may be used for bronchospasm.

HOW SUPPLIED

INNOPRAN XL (propranolol hydrochloride) Extended Release Capsules

Each gray/white capsule, imprinted with "80", 2 segmented bands, "InnoPran XL", and the Reliant logo, contains 80 mg of propranolol hydrochloride in bottles of 30 (NDC 0173-0790-01), bottles of 100 (NDC 0173-0790-02).

Each gray/off-white capsule, imprinted with "120", 3 segmented bands, "InnoPran XL", and the Reliant logo, contains 120 mg of propranolol hydrochloride in bottles of 30 (NDC 0173-0791-01), bottles of 100 (NDC 0173-0791-02).

Store at 25°C (77°F); excursions permitted to 15 and 30°C (59 and 86°F) [see USP Controlled Room Temperature] in a tightly closed container.

Manufactured for:
GlaxoSmithKline
Research Triangle Park, NC 27709
By: Eurand America, Inc.
Vandalia, OH 45377
©2010 GlaxoSmithKline. All rights reserved.
May 2010   INN:5PI

JALYN™ ℞
[*JAY-LIN*]
(dutasteride and tamsulosin hydrochloride)
Capsules

HIGHLIGHTS OF PRESCRIBING INFORMATION
These highlights do not include all the information needed to use JALYN safely and effectively. See full prescribing information for JALYN.

JALYN (dutasteride and tamsulosin hydrochloride) Capsules
Initial U.S. Approval: 2010

————INDICATIONS AND USAGE————
JALYN, a combination of dutasteride, a 5α-reductase inhibitor, and tamsulosin, an alpha-adrenergic antagonist, is indicated for the treatment of symptomatic benign prostatic hyperplasia (BPH) in men with an enlarged prostate. (1)

————DOSAGE AND ADMINISTRATION————
• Take one capsule daily approximately 30 minutes after the same meal each day. (2)
• Swallow capsule whole. (2)

————DOSAGE FORMS AND STRENGTHS————
Each capsule contains 0.5 mg dutasteride and 0.4 mg tamsulosin hydrochloride. (3)

————CONTRAINDICATIONS————
• Pregnancy and women of childbearing potential. (4, 5.1, 8.1)
• Pediatric patients. (4)
• Patients with previously demonstrated, clinically significant hypersensitivity (e.g., serious skin reactions, angioedema) to dutasteride, tamsulosin, other 5α-reductase inhibitors, or any component of the formulation. (4)

————WARNINGS AND PRECAUTIONS————
• Orthostatic hypotension and/or syncope can occur. Advise patients of symptoms related to postural hypotension and to avoid situations where injury could result if syncope occurs. (5.1)
• JALYN should not be combined with strong inhibitors of cytochrome P450 (CYP) 3A4. Exercise caution in combination of JALYN with moderate CYP3A4 inhibitors, with strong or moderate CYP2D6 inhibitors, or in patients known to be poor metabolizers of CYP2D6. (5.2, 7.1, 12.3)
• JALYN should not be used with other alpha-adrenergic antagonists, as this may increase the risk of hypotension. (5.2)
• Women who are pregnant or may become pregnant should not handle JALYN Capsules. (5.3, 8.1)
• Assess patients to rule out other urological diseases, including prostate cancer, prior to treatment with JALYN. (5.4)
• JALYN reduces total serum prostate-specific antigen (PSA) concentration by approximately 50%. Evaluate any confirmed increases in PSA levels from nadir while on JALYN, even if those values are within normal range, for the presence of prostate cancer. (5.5)
• Exercise caution with concomitant administration of warfarin. (5.2, 7.1, 12.3)

• Advise patients about the possibility and seriousness of priapism. (5.6)
• Advise patients to not donate blood until 6 months after their last dose. (5.7)
• Intraoperative Floppy Iris Syndrome has been observed during cataract surgery after alpha-adrenergic antagonist exposure. Advise patients considering cataract surgery to tell their ophthalmologist that they take or have taken JALYN Capsules. (5.8)

————ADVERSE REACTIONS————
The most common adverse reactions, reported in ≥1% of patients treated with coadministered dutasteride and tamsulosin are ejaculation disorders, impotence, decreased libido, dizziness, and breast disorders. (6.1)

To report SUSPECTED ADVERSE REACTIONS, contact GlaxoSmithKline at 1-888-825-5249 or FDA at 1-800-FDA-1088 or www.fda.gov/medwatch.

————DRUG INTERACTIONS————
• CYP Inhibitors: JALYN is metabolized by both CYP3A4 and CYP2D6. Concomitant use with known inhibitors can cause a marked increase in plasma levels resulting in an increased rate of side effects. Use of JALYN with ketoconazole and paroxetine is not recommended. Caution should be exercised when used with less potent inhibitors, such as, but not limited to terbinafine and erythromycin. (5.2, 7.1, 12.3)
• PDE-5 inhibitors: Use caution as this can increase risk of hypotension. (5.2, 7.3, 12.3)

————USE IN SPECIFIC POPULATIONS————
• Renal Impairment: Has not been studied in patients with end-stage renal disease. (8.6, 12.3)
• Hepatic Impairment: Has not been studied in patients with severe hepatic impairment. (8.7, 12.3)

See 17 for PATIENT COUNSELING INFORMATION and FDA-approved patient labeling

Revised: 06/2010

————————————————————————

————————————————————————

FULL PRESCRIBING INFORMATION

1   INDICATIONS AND USAGE

JALYN™ (dutasteride and tamsulosin hydrochloride) Capsules are indicated for the treatment of symptomatic benign prostatic hyperplasia (BPH) in men with an enlarged prostate.

2   DOSAGE AND ADMINISTRATION

The recommended dosage of JALYN is 1 capsule (0.5 mg dutasteride and 0.4 mg tamsulosin hydrochloride) taken once daily approximately 30 minutes after the same meal each day.

The capsules should be swallowed whole and not chewed or opened. Contact with the contents of the JALYN capsule may result in irritation of the oropharyngeal mucosa.

JALYN should not be used in combination with strong inhibitors of CYP3A4 (e.g., ketoconazole) [see Warnings and Precautions (5.2), Drug Interactions (7.1), Clinical Pharmacology (12.3)].

2.1   Dosage Adjustment in Specific Populations

Renal Impairment: No dosage adjustment is necessary for patients with moderate to severe renal impairment ($10 \leq CL_{cr} < 30$ mL/min/1.73 m²). However, there are no data of JALYN or its individual components in patients with end-stage renal disease [see Use in Specific Populations (8.6), Clinical Pharmacology (12.3)].

Hepatic Impairment: No dosage recommendation can be made due to the absence of data in patients with hepatic impairment [see Use in Specific Populations (8.7), Clinical Pharmacology (12.3)].

Elderly: No dosage adjustment is necessary [see Use in Specific Populations (8.6), Clinical Pharmacology (12.3)].

3   DOSAGE FORMS AND STRENGTHS

JALYN Capsules, containing 0.5 mg dutasteride and 0.4 mg tamsulosin hydrochloride, are oblong, hard-shell capsules with a brown body and an orange cap imprinted with "GS 7CZ" in black ink.

4   CONTRAINDICATIONS

JALYN is contraindicated for use in:
• Pregnancy. Dutasteride inhibits the activity of 5α-reductase and prevents conversion of testosterone to dihydrotestosterone, a hormone necessary for normal development of male genitalia. In animal reproduction and developmental toxicity studies, dutasteride inhibited development of male fetus external genitalia. Therefore, JALYN may cause fetal harm when administered to a pregnant woman. If JALYN is used during pregnancy, or if the patient becomes pregnant while taking JALYN, the patient should be apprised of the potential hazard to the fetus [see Warnings and Precautions (5.3), Use in Specific Populations (8.1)].
• Women of childbearing potential [see Warnings and Precautions (5.3), Use in Specific Populations (8.1)].
• Pediatric patients [see Use in Specific Populations (8.4)].
• Patients with previously demonstrated, clinically significant hypersensitivity (e.g., serious skin reactions, angioedema) to dutasteride, other 5α-reductase inhibitors, tamsulosin, or any other component of the formulation.

5   WARNINGS AND PRECAUTIONS

5.1   Orthostatic Hypotension

As with other alpha-adrenergic antagonists, orthostatic hypotension (postural hypotension, dizziness, and vertigo) may occur in patients treated with tamsulosin-containing products, including JALYN, and can result in syncope. Patients starting treatment with JALYN should be cautioned to avoid situations where syncope could result in an injury [see Adverse Reactions (6.1)].

5.2   Drug-Drug Interactions

Strong Inhibitors of CYP3A4: Tamsulosin-containing products, including JALYN, should not be coadministered with strong CYP3A4 inhibitors (e.g., ketoconazole) as this can significantly decrease tamsulosin metabolism and increase tamsulosin exposure [see Drug Interactions (7.1), Clinical Pharmacology (12.3)].

Inhibitors of CYP2D6 and Moderate Inhibitors of CYP3A4: Tamsulosin-containing products, including JALYN, should be used with caution when coadministered with moderate inhibitors of CYP3A4 (e.g., erythromycin), when coadministered with strong (e.g., paroxetine) or moderate (e.g., terbinafine) inhibitors of CYP2D6, or in patients known to be poor metabolizers of CYP2D6 as there is a potential for significant increase in tamsulosin exposure [see Drug Interactions (7.1), Clinical Pharmacology (12.3)].

Cimetidine: Caution is advised when tamsulosin-containing products, including JALYN, are coadministered with cimetidine [see Drug Interactions (7.1), Clinical Pharmacology (12.3)].

Other Alpha-adrenergic Antagonists: Tamsulosin-containing products, including JALYN, should not be coadministered with other alpha-adrenergic antagonists because of the increased risk of symptomatic hypotension *[see Drug Interactions (7.2), Clinical Pharmacology (12.3)]*.
Phosphodiesterase-5 Inhibitors (PDE-5 Inhibitors): Caution is advised when alpha-adrenergic antagonist-containing products, including JALYN, are coadministered with PDE-5 inhibitors. Alpha-adrenergic blockers and PDE-5 inhibitors are both vasodilators that can lower blood pressure. Concomitant use of these 2 drug classes can potentially cause symptomatic hypotension *[see Drug Interactions (7.3), Clinical Pharmacology (12.3)]*.
Warfarin: Caution should be exercised with concomitant administration of warfarin and tamsulosin-containing products, including JALYN *[see Drug Interactions (7.4), Clinical Pharmacology (12.3)]*.

5.3 Exposure of Women—Risk to Male Fetus
JALYN Capsules should not be handled by a woman who is pregnant or who may become pregnant. Dutasteride is absorbed through the skin and could result in unintended fetal exposure. If a woman who is pregnant or may become pregnant comes in contact with a leaking capsule, the contact area should be washed immediately with soap and water *[see Use in Specific Populations (8.1)]*.

5.4 Evaluation for Other Urological Diseases
Lower urinary tract symptoms of BPH can be indicative of other urological diseases, including prostate cancer. Patients should be assessed to rule out prostate cancer and other urological diseases prior to treatment with JALYN and periodically thereafter. Patients with a large residual urinary volume and/or severely diminished urinary flow may not be good candidates for 5α-reductase inhibitor therapy and should be carefully monitored for obstructive uropathy.

5.5 Effects on Prostate-Specific Antigen and the Use of Prostate-Specific Antigen in Prostate Cancer Detection
Coadministration of dutasteride with tamsulosin resulted in similar changes to total prostate-specific antigen (PSA) as with dutasteride monotherapy.
Dutasteride: Dutasteride reduces total serum PSA concentration by approximately 40% following 3 months of treatment and by approximately 50% following 6, 12, and 24 months of treatment. This decrease is predictable over the entire range of PSA values, although it may vary in individual patients. Therefore, for interpretation of serial PSAs in a man taking a dutasteride-containing product, including JALYN, a new baseline PSA concentration should be established after 3 to 6 months of treatment, and this new value should be used to assess potentially cancer-related changes in PSA. To interpret an isolated PSA value in a man treated with a dutasteride-containing product, including JALYN, for 6 months or more, the PSA value should be doubled for comparison with normal values in untreated men. Any confirmed increases in PSA levels from nadir while on dutasteride-containing products, including JALYN, may signal the presence of prostate cancer and should be carefully evaluated, even if those values are still within the normal range for men not taking a 5α-reductase inhibitor.
The free-to-total PSA ratio (percent free PSA) remains constant at Month 12, even under the influence of dutasteride. If clinicians elect to use percent free PSA as an aid in the detection of prostate cancer in men receiving JALYN, no adjustment to its value appears necessary.
Tamsulosin: Treatment with tamsulosin for up to 24 months had no significant effect on PSA.

5.6 Priapism
Priapism (persistent painful penile erection unrelated to sexual activity) has been associated (probably less than 1 in 50,000) with the use of alpha-adrenergic antagonists, including tamsulosin, which is a component of JALYN. Because this condition can lead to permanent impotence if not properly treated, patients must be advised about the seriousness of the condition.

5.7 Blood Donation
Men being treated with any dutasteride-containing products, including JALYN, should not donate blood until at least 6 months have passed following their last dose. The purpose of this deferred period is to prevent administration of dutasteride to a pregnant female transfusion recipient.

5.8 Intraoperative Floppy Iris Syndrome
Intraoperative Floppy Iris Syndrome (IFIS) has been observed during cataract surgery in some patients treated with alpha-adrenergic antagonists, including tamsulosin, which is a component of JALYN. Most reports were in patients taking the alpha-adrenergic antagonist when IFIS occurred, but in some cases, the alpha-adrenergic antagonist had been stopped prior to surgery. In most of these cases, the alpha-adrenergic antagonist had been stopped recently prior to surgery (2 to 14 days), but in a few cases IFIS was reported after the patient had been taken off the alpha-adrenergic antagonist for a longer period (5 weeks to 9 months). IFIS is a variant of small pupil syndrome and is characterized by the combination of a flaccid iris that billows in response to intraoperative irrigation currents, progressive intraoperative miosis despite preoperative dilation with standard mydriatic drugs, and potential prolapse of the iris toward the phacoemulsification incisions. The patient's ophthalmologist should be prepared for possible modification to their surgical technique, such as the utilization of iris hooks, iris dilator rings, or visoelastic substances. The benefit of stopping alpha-adrenergic antagonist therapy prior to cataract surgery has not been established.

5.9 Sulfa Allergy
In patients with sulfa allergy, allergic reaction to tamsulosin has been rarely reported. If a patient reports a serious or life-threatening sulfa allergy, caution is warranted when administering tamsulosin-containing products, including JALYN.

5.10 Effect on Semen Characteristics
Dutasteride: The effects of dutasteride 0.5 mg/day on semen characteristics were evaluated in normal volunteers aged 18 to 52 years (n = 27 dutasteride, n = 23 placebo) throughout 52 weeks of treatment and 24 weeks of post-treatment follow-up. At 52 weeks, the mean percent reductions from baseline in total sperm count, semen volume, and sperm motility were 23%, 26%, and 18%, respectively, in the dutasteride group when adjusted for changes from baseline in the placebo group. Sperm concentration and sperm morphology were unaffected. After 24 weeks of follow-up, the mean percent change in total sperm count in the dutasteride group remained 23% lower than baseline. While mean values for all semen parameters at all time-points remained within the normal ranges and did not meet predefined criteria for a clinically significant change (30%), 2 subjects in the dutasteride group had decreases in sperm count of greater than 90% from baseline at 52 weeks, with partial recovery at the 24-week follow-up. The clinical significance of dutasteride's effect on semen characteristics for an individual patient's fertility is not known.
Tamsulosin: The effects of tamsulosin hydrochloride on sperm counts or sperm function have not been evaluated.

6 ADVERSE REACTIONS

6.1 Clinical Trials Experience
There have been no clinical trials conducted with JALYN; however, the clinical efficacy and safety of coadministered dutasteride and tamsulosin, which are individual components of JALYN, have been evaluated in a multicenter, randomized, double-blind, parallel group study (the Combination with Alpha-Blocker Therapy, or CombAT, study).
Because clinical trials are conducted under widely varying conditions, adverse reaction rates observed in the clinical trials of a drug cannot be directly compared to rates in the clinical trial of another drug and may not reflect the rates observed in practice.

- The most common adverse reactions reported in subjects receiving coadministered dutasteride and tamsulosin were impotence, decreased libido, breast disorders (including breast enlargement and tenderness), ejaculation disorders, and dizziness. Over 2 years of treatment, drug-related ejaculation disorders occurred more frequently in subjects receiving coadministration therapy (9%) compared to dutasteride (2%) or tamsulosin (3%) as monotherapy.
- Study withdrawal due to adverse reactions occurred in 5% of subjects receiving coadministered dutasteride and tamsulosin and 3% of subjects receiving dutasteride or tamsulosin as monotherapy. The most common adverse reaction leading to study withdrawal in subjects receiving coadministration therapy was impotence (1%).

In the CombAT study, over 4,800 male subjects with BPH were randomly assigned to receive either 0.5 mg dutasteride, 0.4 mg tamsulosin hydrochloride, or coadministration therapy (0.5 mg dutasteride and 0.4 mg tamsulosin hydrochloride) administered once daily in a 4-year double-blind study. Adverse reaction information over the first 2 years of treatment is presented below; information for years 2 to 4 is not yet available. During the first 2 years, 1,623 subjects received monotherapy with dutasteride; 1,611 subjects received monotherapy with tamsulosin; and 1,610 subjects received coadministration therapy. The population was aged 49 to 88 years (mean age: 66 years) and 88% Caucasian. Table 1 presents clinical adverse reactions considered by the investigator to be possibly drug-related for which the incidence was ≥1% in any treatment group.
[See table 1 at left]

Table 1. Adverse Reactions Reported Over a 24-Month Period in ≥1% of Subjects in Any Treatment Group (CombAT) by Time of Onset

	Adverse Reaction Time of Onset			
Adverse Reactions	Months 0-6	Months 7-12	Months 13-18	Months 19-24
Coadministration (n)[a]	(n = 1,610)	(n = 1,524)	(n = 1,424)	(n = 1,345)
Dutasteride (n)	(n = 1,623)	(n = 1,547)	(n = 1,457)	(n = 1,378)
Tamsulosin (n)	(n = 1,611)	(n = 1,542)	(n = 1,468)	(n = 1,363)
Ejaculation disorders				
Combination	7.6%	1.6%	0.4%	<0.1%
Dutasteride	1.1%	0.6%	0.1%	0.1%
Tamsulosin	2.2%	0.5%	0.4%	0.1%
Impotence				
Combination	5.5%	1.2%	0.8%	0.3%
Dutasteride	3.9%	1.2%	0.6%	0.7%
Tamsulosin	2.7%	0.8%	0.4%	0.4%
Decreased libido				
Combination	4.5%	0.9%	0.4%	<0.1%
Dutasteride	3.3%	0.6%	0.7%	0.2%
Tamsulosin	1.9%	0.6%	0.4%	0.2%
Dizziness				
Combination	1.1%	0.4%	0.2%	0.0%
Dutasteride	0.4%	0.2%	<0.1%	<0.1%
Tamsulosin	0.9%	0.5%	0.3%	0.1%
Breast disorders[b]				
Combination	1.0%	1.1%	0.7%	0.3%
Dutasteride	0.9%	1.0%	0.8%	0.5%
Tamsulosin	0.4%	0.4%	0.2%	0.1%

[a] Coadministration = Dutasteride 0.5 mg once daily plus tamsulosin hydrochloride 0.4 mg once daily.
[b] Includes breast tenderness and breast enlargement.

Cardiac Failure: In CombAT, after 4 years of treatment, the incidence of the composite term cardiac failure in the co-administration group (12/1,610; 0.7%) was higher than in either monotherapy group: AVODART, 2/1,623 (0.1%) and tamsulosin, 9/1,611 (0.6%). Composite cardiac failure was also examined in a separate 4-year placebo-controlled trial evaluating AVODART in men at risk for development of prostate cancer. The incidence of cardiac failure in subjects taking AVODART was 0.6% (26/4,105) compared to 0.4% (15/4,126) in subjects on placebo. A majority of subjects with cardiac failure in both studies had co-morbidities associated with an increased risk of cardiac failure. Therefore, the clinical significance of the numerical imbalances in cardiac failure is unknown. No causal relationship between AVODART, alone or co-administered with tamsulosin, and cardiac failure has been established. No imbalance was observed in the incidence of overall cardiovascular adverse events in either study.
Additional information regarding adverse reactions in controlled trials with dutasteride and tamsulosin monotherapy follows:
Dutasteride: There is no evidence of increased sexual adverse reactions (impotence, decreased libido, and ejaculation disorders) or breast disorders with increased duration of dutasteride monotherapy (up to 4 years). The relationship between long-term use of dutasteride and male breast neoplasia is currently unknown.
Tamsulosin: According to the tamsulosin prescribing information, in two 13-week treatment trials with tamsulosin

monotherapy, treatment-emergent adverse reactions occurring in ≥2% of subjects receiving 0.4 mg tamsulosin hydrochloride and at an incidence higher than in subjects receiving placebo were: infection, asthenia, back pain, chest pain, somnolence, insomnia, rhinitis, pharyngitis, cough increased, sinusitis, and diarrhea.

Signs and Symptoms of Orthostasis: According to the tamsulosin prescribing information, in clinical studies with tamsulosin monotherapy, a positive orthostatic test result was observed in 16% (81/502) of subjects receiving 0.4 mg tamsulosin hydrochloride vs. 11% (54/493) of subjects receiving placebo. Because orthostasis was detected more frequently in the tamsulosin-treated subjects than in placebo recipients, there is a potential risk of syncope *[see Warnings and Precaution (5.1)]*.

6.2 Postmarketing Experience

The following adverse reactions have been identified during post-approval use of the individual components of JALYN. Because these reactions are reported voluntarily from a population of uncertain size, it is not always possible to reliably estimate their frequency or establish a causal relationship to drug exposure. These reactions have been chosen for inclusion due to a combination of their seriousness, frequency of reporting, or potential causal connection to drug exposure.

Dutasteride:

Immune System Disorders: Hypersensitivity reactions, including rash, pruritus, urticaria, localized edema, serious skin reactions, and angioedema.

Tamsulosin:

Immune System Disorders: Hypersensitivity reactions, including rash, urticaria, pruritus, angioedema, and respiratory problems.

Cardiac Disorders: Palpitations.

Skin Disorders: Skin desquamation.

Gastrointestinal Disorders: Constipation, vomiting.

Reproductive System and Breast Disorders: Priapism.

Vascular Disorders: Hypotension.

Ophthalmologic Disorders: During cataract surgery, a variant of small pupil syndrome known as Intraoperative floppy iris syndrome (IFIS) associated with alpha-adrenergic antagonist therapy *[see Warnings and Precautions (5.8)]*.

7 DRUG INTERACTIONS

There have been no drug interaction studies using JALYN. The following sections reflect information available for the individual components.

7.1 Cytochrome P450 Inhibitors

Dutasteride: Dutasteride is extensively metabolized in humans by the CYP3A4 and CYP3A5 isoenzymes. The effect of strong CYP3A4 inhibitors on dutasteride has not been studied *[see Clinical Pharmacology (12.3)]*.

Tamsulosin: *Strong and Moderate Inhibitors of CYP3A4 or CYP2D6:* Tamsulosin is extensively metabolized, mainly by CYP3A4 or CYP2D6.

Concomitant treatment with ketoconazole (a strong inhibitor of CYP3A4) resulted in increases in the C_{max} and AUC of tamsulosin by factors of 2.2 and 2.8, respectively *[see Warnings and Precautions (5.2), Clinical Pharmacology (12.3)]*. The effects of concomitant administration of a moderate CYP3A4 inhibitor (e.g., erythromycin) on the pharmacokinetics of tamsulosin have not been evaluated *[see Warnings and Precautions (5.2), Clinical Pharmacology (12.3)]*. Concomitant treatment with paroxetine (a strong inhibitor of CYP2D6) resulted in increases in the C_{max} and AUC of tamsulosin by factors of 1.3 and 1.6, respectively *[see Warnings and Precautions (5.2), Clinical Pharmacology (12.3)]*. A similar increase in exposure is expected in poor metabolizers (PM) of CYP2D6 as compared to extensive metabolizers (EM). Since CYP2D6 PMs cannot be readily identified and the potential for significant increase in tamsulosin exposure exists when tamsulosin 0.4 mg is coadministered with strong CYP3A4 inhibitors in CYP2D6 PMs, tamsulosin 0.4 mg capsules should not be used in combination with strong inhibitors of CYP3A4 (e.g., ketoconazole) *[see Warnings and Precautions (5.2), Clinical Pharmacology (12.3)]*. The effects of concomitant administration of a moderate CYP2D6 inhibitor (e.g., terbinafine) on the pharmacokinetics of tamsulosin have not been evaluated *[see Warnings and Precautions (5.2), Clinical Pharmacology (12.3)]*. The effects of coadministration of both a CYP3A4 and a CYP2D6 inhibitor with tamsulosin have not been evaluated. However, there is a potential for significant increase in tamsulosin exposure when tamsulosin 0.4 mg is coadministered with a combination of both CYP3A4 and CYP2D6 inhibitors *[see Warnings and Precautions (5.2), Clinical Pharmacology (12.3)]*.

Cimetidine: Treatment with cimetidine resulted in a significant decrease (26%) in the clearance of tamsulosin hydrochloride, which resulted in a moderate increase in tamsulosin hydrochloride AUC (44%) *[see Warnings and Precautions (5.2), Clinical Pharmacology (12.3)]*.

7.2 Alpha-Adrenergic Antagonists

Tamsulosin-containing products, including JALYN, should not be used in combination with other alpha-adrenergic antagonists. The pharmacokinetic and pharmacodynamic interactions between tamsulosin and other alpha-adrenergic antagonists have not been determined. However, interactions may be expected *[see Warnings and Precautions (5.2), Clinical Pharmacology (12.3)]*.

7.3 PDE-5 Inhibitors

Caution is advised when alpha-adrenergic antagonists, including tamsulosin-containing products such as JALYN, are coadministered with PDE-5 inhibitors. Alpha-adrenergic antagonists and PDE-5 inhibitors are both vasodilators that can lower blood pressure. Concomitant use of these 2 drug classes can potentially cause symptomatic hypotension *[see Warnings and Precautions (5.2), Clinical Pharmacology (12.3)]*.

7.4 Warfarin

Dutasteride: Concomitant administration of dutasteride 0.5 mg/day for 3 weeks with warfarin does not alter the steady-state pharmacokinetics of the S- or R-warfarin isomers or alter the effect of warfarin on prothrombin time *[see Clinical Pharmacology (12.3)]*.

Tamsulosin: A definitive drug-drug interaction study between tamsulosin hydrochloride and warfarin was not conducted. Results from limited in vitro and in vivo studies are inconclusive. Caution should be exercised with concomitant administration of warfarin and tamsulosin-containing products, including JALYN *[see Warnings and Precautions (5.2), Clinical Pharmacology (12.3)]*.

7.5 Nifedipine, Atenolol, Enalapril

Tamsulosin: Dosage adjustments are not necessary when tamsulosin is administered concomitantly with nifedipine, atenolol, or enalapril *[see Clinical Pharmacology (12.3)]*.

7.6 Digoxin and Theophylline

Dutasteride: Dutasteride does not alter the steady-state pharmacokinetics of digoxin when administered concomitantly at a dose of 0.5 mg/day for 3 weeks *[see Clinical Pharmacology (12.3)]*.

Tamsulosin: Dosage adjustments are not necessary when tamsulosin is administered concomitantly with digoxin or theophylline *[see Clinical Pharmacology (12.3)]*.

7.7 Furosemide

Tamsulosin: Tamsulosin had no effect on the pharmacodynamics (excretion of electrolytes) of furosemide. While furosemide produced an 11% to 12% reduction in tamsulosin hydrochloride C_{max} and AUC, these changes are expected to be clinically insignificant and do not require adjustment of the dose of tamsulosin *[see Clinical Pharmacology (12.3)]*.

7.8 Calcium Channel Blockers

Dutasteride: Coadministration of verapamil or diltiazem decreases dutasteride clearance and leads to increased exposure to dutasteride. However, the change in dutasteride exposure is not considered to be clinically significant. No dosage adjustment of dutasteride is recommended *[see Clinical Pharmacology (12.3)]*.

7.9 Cholestyramine

Dutasteride: Administration of a single 5-mg dose of dutasteride followed 1 hour later by a 12-g dose of cholestyramine does not affect the relative bioavailability of dutasteride *[see Clinical Pharmacology (12.3)]*.

8 USE IN SPECIFIC POPULATIONS

8.1 Pregnancy

Pregnancy Category X *[see Contraindications (4)]*. There are no adequate and well-controlled studies in pregnant women with JALYN or its individual components.

Dutasteride: Dutasteride is contraindicated for use in women of childbearing potential and during pregnancy. Dutasteride is a 5α-reductase inhibitor that prevents conversion of testosterone to dihydrotestosterone (DHT), a hormone necessary for normal development of male genitalia. In animal reproduction and developmental toxicity studies, dutasteride inhibited normal development of external genitalia in male fetuses. Therefore, dutasteride may cause fetal harm when administered to a pregnant woman. If dutasteride is used during pregnancy or if the patient becomes pregnant while taking dutasteride, the patient should be apprised of the potential hazard to the fetus.

Abnormalities in the genitalia of male fetuses is an expected physiological consequence of inhibition of the conversion of testosterone to DHT by 5α-reductase inhibitors. These results are similar to observations in male infants with genetic 5α-reductase deficiency. Dutasteride is absorbed through the skin. To avoid potential fetal exposure, women who are pregnant or may become pregnant should not handle dutasteride-containing capsules. If contact is made with leaking capsules, the contact area should be washed immediately with soap and water. Dutasteride is secreted into male semen. The highest measured semen concentration of dutasteride in treated men was 14 ng/mL. Assuming exposure of a 50-kg woman to 5 mL of semen and 100% absorption, the woman's dutasteride concentration would be about 0.175 ng/mL. This concentration is more than 100 times less than concentrations producing abnormalities of male genitalia in animal studies. Dutasteride is highly protein bound in human semen (greater than 96%), which may reduce the amount of dutasteride available for vaginal absorption *[see Warnings and Precautions (5.3)]*.

In an embryo-fetal development study in female rats, oral administration of dutasteride at doses 10 times less than the maximum recommended human dose (MRHD) of 0.5 mg daily resulted in abnormalities of male genitalia in the fetus (decreased anogenital distance at 0.05 mg/kg/day), and nipple development, hypospadias, and distended preputial glands in male offspring (at all doses of 0.05, 2.5, 12.5, and 30 mg/kg/day). An increase in stillborn pups was observed at 111 times the MRHD, and reduced fetal body weight was observed at doses of about 15 times the MRHD (animal dose of 2.5 mg/kg/day). Increased incidences of skeletal variations considered to be delays in ossification associated with reduced body weight were observed at doses at about 56 times the MRHD (animal dose of 12.5 mg/kg/day).

In a rabbit embryo-fetal study, doses 28- to 93-fold the MRHD (animal doses of 30, 100, and 200 mg/kg/day) were administered orally during the period of major organogenesis (gestation days 7 to 29) to encompass the late period of external genitalia development. Histological evaluation of the genital papilla of fetuses revealed evidence of feminization of the male fetus at all doses. A second embryo-fetal study in rabbits at 0.3- to 53-fold the expected clinical exposure (animal doses of 0.05, 0.4, 3.0, and 30 mg/kg/day) also produced evidence of feminization of the genitalia in male fetuses at all doses.

In an oral pre- and post-natal development study in rats, dutasteride doses of 0.05, 2.5, 12.5, or 30 mg/kg/day were administered. Unequivocal evidence of feminization of the genitalia (i.e., decreased anogenital distance, increased incidence of hypospadias, nipple development) of male offspring occurred at 14- to 90-fold the MRHD (animal doses of 2.5 mg/kg/day or greater). At 0.05-fold the expected clinical exposure (animal dose of 0.05 mg/kg/day), evidence of feminization was limited to a small, but statistically significant, decrease in anogenital distance. Animal doses of 2.5 to 30 mg/kg/day resulted in prolonged gestation in the parental females and a decrease in time to vaginal patency for female offspring and a decrease in prostate and seminal vesicle weights in male offspring. Effects on newborn startle response were noted at doses greater than or equal to 12.5 mg/kg/day. Increased stillbirths were noted at 30 mg/kg/day.

In an embryo-fetal development study, pregnant rhesus monkeys were exposed intravenously to a dutasteride blood level comparable to the dutasteride concentration found in human semen. Dutasteride was administered on gestation days 20 to 100 at doses of 400, 780, 1,325, or 2,010 ng/day (12 monkeys/group). The development of male external genitalia of monkey offspring was not adversely affected. Reduction of fetal adrenal weights, reduction in fetal prostate weights, and increases in fetal ovarian and testis weights were observed at the highest dose tested in monkeys. Based on the highest measured semen concentration of dutasteride in treated men (14 ng/mL), these doses represent 0.8 to 16 times based on blood levels of parent drug (32 to 186 times based on a ng/kg daily dose) the potential maximum exposure of a 50-kg human female to 5 mL semen daily from a dutasteride-treated man, assuming 100% absorption. Dutasteride is highly bound to proteins in human semen (greater than 96%), potentially reducing the amount of dutasteride available for vaginal absorption. It is not known whether rabbits or rhesus monkeys produce any of the major human metabolites.

Estimates of exposure multiples comparing animal studies to the MRHD for dutasteride are based on clinical serum concentration at steady state.

Tamsulosin: Administration of tamsulosin to pregnant female rats at dose levels up to approximately 50 times the human therapeutic AUC exposure (animal dose of 300 mg/kg/day) revealed no evidence of harm to the fetus. Administration of tamsulosin hydrochloride to pregnant rabbits at dose levels up to 50 mg/kg/day produced no evidence of fetal harm. However, because of the effect of dutasteride on the fetus, JALYN is contraindicated for use in pregnant women. Estimates of exposure multiples comparing animal studies to the MRHD for tamsulosin are based on AUC.

8.3 Nursing Mothers

JALYN is contraindicated for use in women of childbearing potential, including nursing women. It is not known whether dutasteride or tamsulosin is excreted in human milk.

8.4 Pediatric Use

JALYN is contraindicated for use in pediatric patients. Safety and effectiveness of JALYN in pediatric patients have not been established.

8.5 Geriatric Use

Of 1,610 male subjects treated with coadministered dutasteride and tamsulosin in the CombAT trial, 58% of enrolled subjects were 65 years of age and over and 13% of enrolled subjects were 75 years of age and over. No overall differences in safety or efficacy were observed between these subjects and younger subjects *[see Clinical Pharmacology (12.3)]*.

8.6 Renal Impairment

The effect of renal impairment on dutasteride and tamsulosin pharmacokinetics has not been studied using JALYN. Because no dosage adjustment is necessary for dutasteride or tamsulosin in patients with moderate-to-severe renal impairment ($10 \le CL_{cr} < 30$ mL/min/1.73 m^2), no dosage adjustment is necessary for JALYN in patients with moderate-to-severe renal impairment. However, patients with end-stage renal disease ($CL_{cr} < 10$ mL/min/1.73 m^2) have not been studied *[see Clinical Pharmacology (12.3)]*.

8.7 Hepatic Impairment

The effect of hepatic impairment on dutasteride and tamsulosin pharmacokinetics has not been studied using JALYN. The following text reflects information available for the individual components.

Dutasteride: The effect of hepatic impairment on dutasteride pharmacokinetics has not been studied. Because dutasteride is extensively metabolized, exposure could be higher in hepatically impaired patients. However, in a clinical study where 60 subjects received 5 mg (10 times the therapeutic dose) daily for 24 weeks, no additional adverse events were observed compared with those observed at the therapeutic dose of 0.5 mg *[see Clinical Pharmacology (12.3)]*.

Tamsulosin: Patients with moderate hepatic impairment do not require an adjustment in tamsulosin dosage. Tamsulosin has not been studied in patients with severe hepatic impairment *[see Clinical Pharmacology (12.3)]*.

10 OVERDOSAGE

No data are available with regard to overdosage with JALYN. The following text reflects information available for the individual components.

Dutasteride: In volunteer studies, single doses of dutasteride up to 40 mg (80 times the therapeutic dose) for 7 days have been administered without significant safety concerns. In a clinical study, daily doses of 5 mg (10 times the therapeutic dose) were administered to 60 subjects for 6 months with no additional adverse effects to those seen at therapeutic doses of 0.5 mg. There is no specific antidote for dutasteride. Therefore, in cases of suspected overdosage symptomatic and supportive treatment should be given as appropriate, taking the long half-life of dutasteride into consideration.

Tamsulosin: Should overdosage of tamsulosin lead to hypotension *[see Warnings and Precautions (5.1), Adverse Reactions (6.1)]*, support of the cardiovascular system is of first importance. Restoration of blood pressure and normalization of heart rate may be accomplished by keeping the patient in the supine position. If this measure is inadequate, then administration of intravenous fluids should be considered. If necessary, vasopressors should then be used and renal function should be monitored and supported as needed. Laboratory data indicate that tamsulosin is 94% to 99% protein bound; therefore, dialysis is unlikely to be of benefit.

11 DESCRIPTION

JALYN (dutasteride and tamsulosin hydrochloride) Capsules contain dutasteride (a selective inhibitor of both the type 1 and type 2 isoforms of steroid 5α-reductase, an intracellular enzyme that converts testosterone to dihydrotestosterone (DHT) and tamsulosin (an antagonist of alpha$_{1A}$-adrenoceptors in the prostate). Each JALYN Capsule contains the following:

- One dutasteride oblong, opaque, dull-yellow soft gelatin capsule, containing 0.5 mg of dutasteride dissolved in a mixture of butylated hydroxytoluene and mono-diglycerides of caprylic/capric acid. The inactive ingredients in the soft-gelatin capsule shell are ferric oxide (yellow), gelatin (from certified BSE-free bovine sources), glycerin, and titanium dioxide.
- Tamsulosin hydrochloride white to off-white pellets, containing 0.4 mg tamsulosin hydrochloride and the inactive ingredients: methacrylic acid copolymer dispersion, microcrystalline cellulose, talc, and triethyl citrate.

The above components are encapsulated in a hard-shell capsule made with the inactive ingredients of carrageenan, FD&C yellow 6, hypromellose, iron oxide red, potassium chloride, titanium dioxide, and imprinted with "GS 7CZ" in black ink.

Dutasteride: Dutasteride is a synthetic 4-azasteroid compound chemically designated as (5α,17β)-N-{2,5 bis(trifluoromethyl)phenyl}-3-oxo-4-azaandrost-1-ene-17-carboxamide. The empirical formula of dutasteride is $C_{27}H_{30}F_6N_2O_2$, representing a molecular weight of 528.5 with the following structural formula:

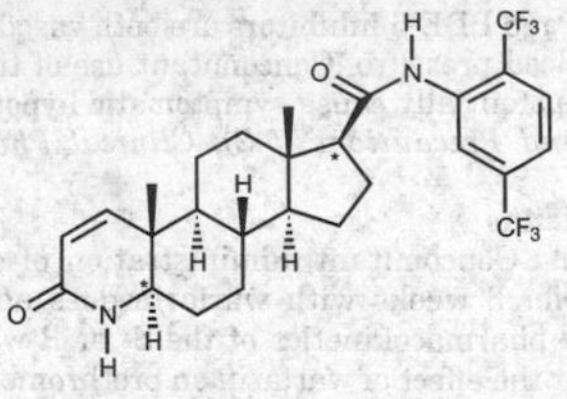

Dutasteride is a white to pale yellow powder with a melting point of 242° to 250°C. It is soluble in ethanol (44 mg/mL), methanol (64 mg/mL), and polyethylene glycol 400 (3 mg/mL), but it is insoluble in water.

Tamsulosin: Tamsulosin hydrochloride is a synthetic compound chemically designated as (-)-(*R*)-5-[2-[[2-(o-Ethoxyphenoxy) ethyl]amino]propyl]-2-methoxybenzenesulfonamide, monohydrochloride.

The empirical formula of tamsulosin hydrochloride is $C_{20}H_{28}N_2O_5S \cdot HCl$. The molecular weight of tamsulosin hydrochloride is 444.97. Its structural formula is:

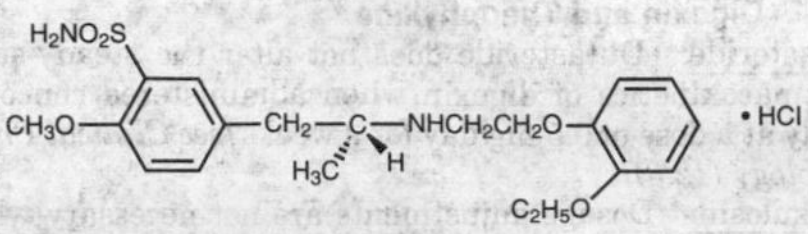

Tamsulosin hydrochloride is a white or almost white crystalline powder that melts with decomposition at approximately 234°C. It is sparingly soluble in water and slightly soluble in methanol, ethanol, acetone, and ethyl acetate.

12 CLINICAL PHARMACOLOGY

12.1 Mechanism of Action

JALYN is a combination of 2 drugs with different mechanisms of action to improve symptoms in patients with BPH: dutasteride, a 5α-reductase inhibitor (5 ARI), and tamsulosin, an antagonist of alpha$_{1A}$-adrenoreceptors.

Dutasteride: Dutasteride inhibits the conversion of testosterone to dihydrotestosterone (DHT). DHT is the androgen primarily responsible for the initial development and subsequent enlargement of the prostate gland. Testosterone is converted to DHT by the enzyme 5α-reductase, which exists as 2 isoforms, type 1 and type 2. The type 2 isoenzyme is primarily active in the reproductive tissues, while the type 1 isoenzyme is also responsible for testosterone conversion in the skin and liver.

Dutasteride is a competitive and specific inhibitor of both type 1 and type 2 5α-reductase isoenzymes, with which it forms a stable enzyme complex. Dissociation from this complex has been evaluated under in vitro and in vivo conditions and is extremely slow. Dutasteride does not bind to the human androgen receptor.

Tamsulosin: Smooth muscle tone is mediated by the sympathetic nervous stimulation of alpha1-adrenoceptors, which are abundant in the prostate, prostatic capsule, prostatic urethra, and bladder neck. Blockade of these adrenoceptors can cause smooth muscles in the bladder neck and prostate to relax, resulting in an improvement in urine flow rate and a reduction in symptoms of BPH.

Tamsulosin, an alpha$_1$-adrenoceptor blocking agent, exhibits selectivity for alpha$_1$-receptors in the human prostate. At least 3 discrete alpha$_1$-adrenoceptor subtypes have been identified: alpha$_{1A}$, alpha$_{1B}$, and alpha$_{1D}$; their distribution differs between human organs and tissue. Approximately 70% of the alpha$_1$-receptors in human prostate are of the alpha$_{1A}$ subtype. Tamsulosin is not intended for use as an antihypertensive.

12.2 Pharmacodynamics

Dutasteride: *Effect on 5α-Dihydrotestosterone and Testosterone:* The maximum effect of daily doses of dutasteride on the reduction of DHT is dose-dependent and is observed within 1 to 2 weeks. After 1 and 2 weeks of daily dosing with dutasteride 0.5 mg, median serum DHT concentrations were reduced by 85% and 90%, respectively. In patients with BPH treated with dutasteride 0.5 mg/day for 4 years, the median decrease in serum DHT was 94% at 1 year, 93% at 2 years, and 95% at both 3 and 4 years. The median increase in serum testosterone was 19% at both 1 and 2 years, 26% at 3 years, and 22% at 4 years, but the mean and median levels remained within the physiologic range.

In patients with BPH treated with 5 mg/day of dutasteride or placebo for up to 12 weeks prior to transurethral resection of the prostate, mean DHT concentrations in prostatic tissue were significantly lower in the dutasteride group compared with placebo (784 and 5,793 pg/g, respectively, $P<0.001$). Mean prostatic tissue concentrations of testosterone were significantly higher in the dutasteride group compared with placebo (2,073 and 93 pg/g, respectively, $P<0.001$).

Adult males with genetically inherited type 2 5α-reductase deficiency also have decreased DHT levels. These 5α-reductase deficient males have a small prostate gland throughout life and do not develop BPH. Except for the associated urogenital defects present at birth, no other clinical abnormalities related to 5α-reductase deficiency have been observed in these individuals.

Effects on Other Hormones: In healthy volunteers, 52 weeks of treatment with dutasteride 0.5 mg/day (n = 26) resulted in no clinically significant change compared with placebo (n = 23) in sex hormone-binding globulin, estradiol, luteinizing hormone, follicle-stimulating hormone, thyroxine (free T4), and dehydroepiandrosterone. Statistically significant, baseline-adjusted mean increases compared with placebo were observed for total testosterone at 8 weeks (97.1 ng/dL, $P<0.003$) and thyroid-stimulating hormone at 52 weeks (0.4 mcIU/mL, $P<0.05$). The median percentage changes from baseline within the dutasteride group were 17.9% for testosterone at 8 weeks and 12.4% for thyroid-stimulating hormone at 52 weeks. After stopping dutasteride for 24 weeks, the mean levels of testosterone and thyroid-stimulating hormone had returned to baseline in the group of subjects with available data at the visit. In patients with BPH treated with dutasteride in a large randomized, double-blind, placebo-controlled study, there was a median percent increase in luteinizing hormone of 12% at 6 months and 19% at both 12 and 24 months.

Other Effects: Plasma lipid panel and bone mineral density were evaluated following 52 weeks of dutasteride 0.5 mg once daily in healthy volunteers. There was no change in bone mineral density as measured by dual energy x-ray absorptiometry compared with either placebo or baseline. In addition, the plasma lipid profile (i.e., total cholesterol, low density lipoproteins, high density lipoproteins, and triglycerides) was unaffected by dutasteride. No clinically significant changes in adrenal hormone responses to ACTH stimulation were observed in a subset population (n = 13) of the 1-year healthy volunteer study.

12.3 Pharmacokinetics

The pharmacokinetics of dutasteride and tamsulosin from JALYN are comparable to the pharmacokinetics of dutasteride and tamsulosin when administered separately.

Absorption: The pharmacokinetic parameters of dutasteride and tamsulosin observed after administration of JALYN in a single dose, randomized, 3-period partial cross-over study are summarized in Table 2 below.

[See table 2 at left]

Dutasteride: Following administration of a single 0.5-mg dose of a soft gelatin capsule, time to peak absolute bioavailability in 5 healthy subjects is approximately 60% (range: 40% to 94%).

Tamsulosin: Absorption of tamsulosin is essentially complete (>90%) following oral administration of 0.4-mg tamsulosin hydrochloride capsules under fasting conditions. Tamsulosin exhibits linear kinetics following single and multiple dosing, with achievement of steady-state concentrations by the fifth day of once-daily dosing.

Effect of Food: Food does not affect the pharmacokinetics of dutasteride following administration of JALYN. However, a mean 30% decrease in tamsulosin C_{max} was observed when JALYN was administered with food, similar to that seen when tamsulosin monotherapy was administered under fed versus fasting conditions.

Distribution: *Dutasteride:* Pharmacokinetic data following single and repeat oral doses show that dutasteride has a large volume of distribution (300 to 500 L). Dutasteride is highly bound to plasma albumin (99.0%) and alpha-1 acid glycoprotein (96.6%).

In a study of healthy subjects (n = 26) receiving dutasteride 0.5 mg/day for 12 months, semen dutasteride concentrations averaged 3.4 ng/mL (range: 0.4 to 14 ng/mL) at 12

Table 2. Arithmetic Means (SD) of Serum Dutasteride and Tamsulosin in Single-dose Pharmacokinetic Parameters Under Fed Conditions

Component	N	$AUC_{(0\text{-}t)}$ (ng hr/mL)	C_{max} (ng/mL)	T_{max} (hr)[a]	$t_{1/2}$ (hr)
Dutasteride	92	39.6 (23.1)	2.14 (0.77)	3.00 (1.00-10.00)	
Tamsulosin	92	187.2 (95.7)	11.3 (4.44)	6.00 (2.00-24.00)	13.5 (3.92)[b]

[a] Median (range).
[b] N = 91.

months and, similar to serum, achieved steady-state concentrations at 6 months. On average, at 12 months 11.5% of serum dutasteride concentrations partitioned into semen.

Tamsulosin: The mean steady-state apparent volume of distribution of tamsulosin after intravenous administration to 10 healthy male adults was 16 L, which is suggestive of distribution into extracellular fluids in the body.

Tamsulosin is extensively bound to human plasma proteins (94% to 99%), primarily alpha-1 acid glycoprotein (AAG), with linear binding over a wide concentration range (20 to 600 ng/mL). The results of 2-way in vitro studies indicate that the binding of tamsulosin to human plasma proteins is not affected by amitriptyline, diclofenac, glyburide, simvastatin plus simvastatin-hydroxy acid metabolite, warfarin, diazepam, or propranolol. Likewise, tamsulosin had no effect on the extent of binding of these drugs.

Metabolism: *Dutasteride:* Dutasteride is extensively metabolized in humans. In vitro studies showed that dutasteride is metabolized by the CYP3A4 and CYP3A5 isoenzymes. Both of these isoenzymes produced the 4′-hydroxydutasteride, 6-hydroxydutasteride, and the 6,4′-dihydroxydutasteride metabolites. In addition, the 15-hydroxydutasteride metabolite was formed by CYP3A4. Dutasteride is not metabolized in vitro by human cytochrome P450 isoenzymes CYP1A2, CYP2A6, CYP2B6, CYP2C8, CYP2C9, CYP2C19, CYP2D6, and CYP2E1. In human serum following dosing to steady state, unchanged dutasteride, 3 major metabolites (4′-hydroxydutasteride, 1,2-dihydrodutasteride, and 6-hydroxydutasteride), and 2 minor metabolites (6,4′-dihydroxydutasteride and 15-hydroxydutasteride), as assessed by mass spectrometric response, have been detected. The absolute stereochemistry of the hydroxyl additions in the 6 and 15 positions is not known. In vitro, the 4′-hydroxydutasteride and 1,2-dihydrodutasteride metabolites are much less potent than dutasteride against both isoforms of human 5α-reductase. The activity of 6β-hydroxydutasteride is comparable to that of dutasteride.

Tamsulosin: There is no enantiomeric bioconversion from tamsulosin [R(-) isomer] to the S(+) isomer in humans. Tamsulosin is extensively metabolized by cytochrome P450 enzymes in the liver and less than 10% of the dose is excreted in urine unchanged. However, the pharmacokinetic profile of the metabolites in humans has not been established. In vitro studies indicate that CYP3A4 and CYP2D6 are involved in metabolism of tamsulosin as well as some minor participation of other CYP isoenzymes. Inhibition of hepatic drug metabolizing enzymes may lead to increased exposure to tamsulosin *[see Drug Interactions (7.2)]*. The metabolites of tamsulosin undergo extensive conjugation to glucuronide or sulfate prior to renal excretion.

Incubations with human liver microsomes showed no evidence of clinically significant metabolic interactions between tamsulosin and amitriptyline, albuterol, glyburide, and finasteride. However, results of the in vitro testing of the tamsulosin interaction with diclofenac and warfarin were equivocal.

Excretion: *Dutasteride:* Dutasteride and its metabolites were excreted mainly in feces. As a percent of dose, there was approximately 5% unchanged dutasteride (approximately 1% to approximately 15%) and 40% as dutasteride-related metabolites (~2% to ~90%). Only trace amounts of unchanged dutasteride were found in urine (<1%). Therefore, on average, the dose unaccounted for approximated 55% (range: 5% to 97%). The terminal elimination half-life of dutasteride is approximately 5 weeks at steady state. The average steady-state serum dutasteride concentration was 40 ng/mL following 0.5 mg/day for 1 year. Following daily dosing, dutasteride serum concentrations achieve 65% of steady-state concentration after 1 month and approximately 90% after 3 months. Due to the long half-life of dutasteride, serum concentrations remain detectable (greater than 0.1 ng/mL) for up to 4 to 6 months after discontinuation of treatment.

Tamsulosin: On administration of the radiolabeled dose of tamsulosin to 4 healthy volunteers, 97% of the administered radioactivity was recovered, with urine (76%) representing the primary route of excretion compared to feces (21%) over 168 hours.

Following intravenous or oral administration of an immediate-release formulation, the elimination half-life of tamsulosin in plasma ranges from 5 to 7 hours. Because of absorption rate-controlled pharmacokinetics with tamsulosin hydrochloride capsules, the apparent half-life of tamsulosin is approximately 9 to 13 hours in healthy volunteers and 14 to 15 hours in the target population.

Tamsulosin undergoes restrictive clearance in humans, with a relatively low systemic clearance (2.88 L/hr).

Specific Populations: *Pediatric Patients:* The pharmacokinetics of dutasteride and tamsulosin administered together have not been investigated in subjects younger than 18 years.

Geriatric Patients: Dutasteride and tamsulosin pharmacokinetics using JALYN have not been studied in geriatric patients. The following text reflects information for the individual components.

Dutasteride: No dosage adjustment is necessary in the elderly. The pharmacokinetics and pharmacodynamics of dutasteride were evaluated in 36 healthy male subjects aged between 24 and 87 years following administration of a single 5-mg dose of dutasteride. In this single-dose study, dutasteride half-life increased with age (approximately 170 hours in men aged 20 to 49 years, approximately 260 hours in men aged 50 to 69 years, and approximately 300 hours in men older than 70 years).

Tamsulosin: Cross-study comparison of tamsulosin overall exposure (AUC) and half-life indicate that the pharmacokinetic disposition of tamsulosin may be slightly prolonged in geriatric males compared to young, healthy male volunteers. Intrinsic clearance is independent of tamsulosin binding to AAG, but diminishes with age, resulting in a 40% overall higher exposure (AUC) in subjects aged 55 to 75 years compared to subjects aged 20 to 32 years.

Gender: Dutasteride: Dutasteride is contraindicated in pregnancy and women of childbearing potential and is not indicated for use in other women *[see Contraindications (4), Warnings and Precautions (5.3)]*. The pharmacokinetics of dutasteride in women have not been studied.

Tamsulosin: Tamsulosin is not indicated for use in women. No information is available on the pharmacokinetics of tamsulosin in women.

Race: The effect of race on pharmacokinetics of dutasteride and tamsulosin administered together or separately has not been studied.

Renal Impairment: The effect of renal impairment on dutasteride and tamsulosin pharmacokinetics has not been studied using JALYN. The following text reflects information for the individual components.

Dutasteride: The effect of renal impairment on dutasteride pharmacokinetics has not been studied. However, less than 0.1% of a steady-state 0.5-mg dose of dutasteride is recovered in human urine, so no adjustment in dosage is anticipated for patients with renal impairment.

Tamsulosin: The pharmacokinetics of tamsulosin have been compared in 6 subjects with mild-moderate (30≤ CL_{cr} <70 mL/min/1.73 m^2) or moderate-severe (10≤ CL_{cr} <30 mL/min/1.73 m^2) renal impairment and 6 normal subjects (CL_{cr} >90 mL/min/1.73 m^2). While a change in the overall plasma concentration of tamsulosin was observed as the result of altered binding to AAG, the unbound (active) concentration of tamsulosin, as well as the intrinsic clearance, remained relatively constant. Therefore, patients with renal impairment do not require an adjustment in tamsulosin dosing. However, patients with end-stage renal disease (CL_{cr} <10 mL/min/1.73 m^2) have not been studied.

Hepatic Impairment: The effect of hepatic impairment on dutasteride and tamsulosin pharmacokinetics has not been studied using JALYN. The following text reflects information available for the individual components.

Dutasteride: The effect of hepatic impairment on dutasteride pharmacokinetics has not been studied. Because dutasteride is extensively metabolized, exposure could be higher in hepatically impaired patients.

Tamsulosin: The pharmacokinetics of tamsulosin have been compared in 8 subjects with moderate hepatic impairment (Child-Pugh classification: Grades A and B) and 8 normal subjects. While a change in the overall plasma concentration of tamsulosin was observed as the result of altered binding to AAG, the unbound (active) concentration of tamsulosin does not change significantly with only a modest (32%) change in intrinsic clearance of unbound tamsulosin. Therefore, patients with moderate hepatic impairment do not require an adjustment in tamsulosin dosage. Tamsulosin has not been studied in patients with severe hepatic impairment.

Drug Interactions: There have been no drug interaction studies using JALYN. The following text reflects information available for the individual components.

Cytochrome P450 Inhibitors: Dutasteride: No clinical drug interaction studies have been performed to evaluate the impact of CYP3A enzyme inhibitors on dutasteride pharmacokinetics. However, based on in vitro data, blood concentrations of dutasteride may increase in the presence of inhibitors of CYP3A4/5 such as ritonavir, ketoconazole, verapamil, diltiazem, cimetidine, troleandomycin, and ciprofloxacin.

Dutasteride does not inhibit the in vitro metabolism of model substrates for the major human cytochrome P450 isoenzymes (CYP1A2, CYP2C9, CYP2C19, CYP2D6, and CYP3A4) at a concentration of 1,000 ng/mL, 25 times greater than steady-state serum concentrations in humans.

Tamsulosin: Strong and Moderate Inhibitors of CYP3A4 or CYP2D6: The effects of ketoconazole (a strong inhibitor of CYP3A4) at 400 mg once daily for 5 days on the pharmacokinetics of a single tamsulosin hydrochloride capsule 0.4 mg dose was investigated in 24 healthy volunteers (age range: 23 to 47 years). Concomitant treatment with ketoconazole resulted in increases in the C_{max} and AUC of tamsulosin by factors of 2.2 and 2.8, respectively. The effects of concomitant administration of a moderate CYP3A4 inhibitor (e.g., erythromycin) on the pharmacokinetics of tamsulosin have not been evaluated.

The effects of paroxetine (a strong inhibitor of CYP2D6) at 20 mg once daily for 9 days on the pharmacokinetics of a single tamsulosin capsule 0.4 mg dose was investigated in 24 healthy volunteers (age range: 23 to 47 years). Concomitant treatment with paroxetine resulted in increases in the C_{max} and AUC of tamsulosin by factors of 1.3 and 1.6, respectively. A similar increase in exposure is expected in poor metabolizers (PM) of CYP2D6 as compared to extensive metabolizers (EM). A fraction of the population (about 7% of Caucasians and 2% of African-Americans) are CYP2D6 PMs. Since CYP2D6 PMs cannot be readily identified and the potential for significant increase in tamsulosin exposure exists when tamsulosin 0.4 mg is coadministered with strong CYP3A4 inhibitors in CYP2D6 PMs, tamsulosin 0.4 mg capsules should not be used in combination with strong inhibitors of CYP3A4 (e.g., ketoconazole).

The effects of concomitant administration of a moderate CYP2D6 inhibitor (e.g., terbinafine) on the pharmacokinetics of tamsulosin have not been evaluated.

The effects of co-administration of both a CYP3A4 and a CYP2D6 inhibitor with tamsulosin capsules have not been evaluated. However, there is a potential for significant increase in tamsulosin exposure when tamsulosin 0.4 mg is coadministered with a combination of both CYP3A4 and CYP2D6 inhibitors.

Cimetidine: The effects of cimetidine at the highest recommended dose (400 mg every 6 hours for 6 days) on the pharmacokinetics of a single tamsulosin capsule 0.4 mg dose was investigated in 10 healthy volunteers (age range: 21 to 38 years). Treatment with cimetidine resulted in a significant decrease (26%) in the clearance of tamsulosin hydrochloride, which resulted in a moderate increase in tamsulosin hydrochloride AUC (44%).

Alpha-Adrenergic Antagonists: Dutasteride: In a single-sequence, crossover study in healthy volunteers, the administration of tamsulosin or terazosin in combination with dutasteride had no effect on the steady-state pharmacokinetics of either alpha-adrenergic antagonist. Although the effect of administration of tamsulosin or terazosin on dutasteride pharmacokinetic parameters was not evaluated, the percent change in DHT concentrations was similar for dutasteride, alone or in combination with tamsulosin or terazosin.

Tamsulosin: Tamsulosin-containing products, including JALYN, should not be used in combination with other alpha-adrenergic antagonists. The pharmacokinetic and pharmacodynamic interactions between tamsulosin and other alpha-adrenergic antagonists have not been determined. However, interactions may be expected *[see Warnings and Precautions (5.2), Drug Interactions (7.2)]*.

PDE-5 Inhibitors: Caution is advised when alpha-adrenergic antagonists, including tamsulosin-containing products such as JALYN, are co-administered with PDE-5 inhibitors. Alpha-adrenergic antagonists and PDE-5 inhibitors are both vasodilators that can lower blood pressure. Concomitant use of these 2 drug classes can potentially cause symptomatic hypotension.

Warfarin: Dutasteride: In a study of 23 healthy volunteers, 3 weeks of treatment with dutasteride 0.5 mg/day did not alter the steady-state pharmacokinetics of the S- or R-warfarin isomers or alter the effect of warfarin on prothrombin time when administered with warfarin.

Tamsulosin: A definitive drug-drug interaction study between tamsulosin and warfarin was not conducted. Results from limited in vitro and in vivo studies are inconclusive. Therefore, caution should be exercised with concomitant administration of warfarin and tamsulosin.

Nifedipine, Atenolol, Enalapril: Tamsulosin: In 3 studies in hypertensive subjects (age range: 47 to 79 years) whose blood pressure was controlled with stable doses of nifedipine extended-release, atenolol, or enalapril for at least 3 months, tamsulosin hydrochloride capsules 0.4 mg for 7 days followed by tamsulosin hydrochloride capsules 0.8 mg for another 7 days (n = 8 per study) resulted in no clinically significant effects on blood pressure and pulse rate compared with placebo (n = 4 per study). Therefore, dosage adjustments are not necessary when tamsulosin is administered concomitantly with nifedipine extended-release, atenolol, or enalapril.

Digoxin and Theophylline: Dutasteride: In a study of 20 healthy volunteers, dutasteride did not alter the steady-state pharmacokinetics of digoxin when administered concomitantly at a dose of 0.5 mg/day for 3 weeks.

Tamsulosin: In 2 studies in healthy volunteers (n = 10 per study; age range: 19 to 39 years) receiving tamsulosin capsules 0.4 mg/day for 2 days, followed by tamsulosin capsules 0.8 mg/day for 5 to 8 days, single intravenous doses of digoxin 0.5 mg or theophylline 5 mg/kg resulted in no change in the pharmacokinetics of digoxin or theophylline. Therefore, dosage adjustments are not necessary when a tamsulosin capsule is administered concomitantly with digoxin or theophylline.

Furosemide: Tamsulosin: The pharmacokinetic and pharmacodynamic interaction between tamsulosin hydrochloride capsules 0.8 mg/day (steady-state) and furosemide 20 mg intravenously (single dose) was evaluated in 10 healthy volunteers (age range: 21 to 40 years). Tamsulosin had no effect on the pharmacodynamics (excretion of electrolytes) of furosemide. While furosemide produced an 11% to 12% reduction in tamsulosin C_{max} and AUC, these changes are expected to be clinically insignificant and do not require dose adjustment for tamsulosin.

Calcium Channel Blockers: Dutasteride: In a population pharmacokinetics analysis, a decrease in clearance of dutasteride was noted when coadministered with the CYP3A4 inhibitors verapamil (-37%, n = 6) and diltiazem (-44%, n = 5). In contrast, no decrease in clearance was seen when amlodipine, another calcium channel antagonist that is not a CYP3A4 inhibitor, was coadministered with dutasteride (+7%, n = 4). The decrease in clearance and subsequent increase in exposure to dutasteride in the presence of verapamil and diltiazem is not considered to be clinically significant. No dosage adjustment is recommended.

Cholestyramine: Dutasteride: Administration of a single 5-mg dose of dutasteride followed 1 hour later by 12 g cholestyramine did not affect the relative bioavailability of dutasteride in 12 normal volunteers.

13 NONCLINICAL TOXICOLOGY

13.1 Carcinogenesis, Mutagenesis, Impairment of Fertility

No non-clinical studies have been conducted with JALYN. The following information is based on studies performed with dutasteride or tamsulosin.

Carcinogenesis: *Dutasteride:* A 2-year carcinogenicity study was conducted in B6C3F1 mice at doses of 3, 35, 250, and 500 mg/kg/day for males and 3, 35, and 250 mg/kg/day for females; an increased incidence of benign hepatocellular adenomas was noted at 250 mg/kg/day (290-fold the maximum recommended human dose (MRHD) of 0.5-mg daily) in female mice only dosed at 250 mg/kg/day. Two of the 3 major human metabolites have been detected in mice. The exposure to these metabolites in mice is either lower than in humans or is not known.

In a 2-year carcinogenicity study in Han Wistar rats, at doses of 1.5, 7.5, and 53 mg/kg/day for males and 0.8, 6.3, and 15 mg/kg/day for females, there was an increase in Leydig cell adenomas in the testes at 135-fold the MRHD (53 mg/kg/day). An increased incidence of Leydig cell hyperplasia was present at 52-fold the MRHD (male rate doses of 7.5 mg/kg/day and greater). A positive correlation between proliferative changes in the Leydig cells and an increase in circulating luteinizing hormone levels has been demonstrated with 5α-reductase inhibitors and is consistent with an effect on the hypothalamic-pituitary-testicular axis following 5α-reductase inhibition. At tumorigenic doses in rats, luteinizing hormone levels in rats were increased by 167%. In this study, the major human metabolites were tested for carcinogenicity at approximately 1 to 3 times the expected clinical exposure.

Tamsulosin: In a rat carcinogenicity assay, no increases in tumor incidence was observed in rats administered up to 3 times the MRHD of 0.8 mg/day (based on AUC of animal doses up to 43 mg/kg/day in males and up to 52 mg/kg/day in females), with the exception of a modest increase in the frequency of mammary gland fibroadenomas in female rats receiving doses of 5.4 mg/kg or greater.

In a carcinogenicity assay, mice were administered up to 8 times the MRHD of tamsulosin (oral doses up to 127 mg/kg/day in males and 158 mg/kg/day in females). There were no significant tumor findings in male mice. Female mice treated for 2 years with the 2 highest doses of 45 and 158 mg/kg/day had statistically significant increases in the incidence of mammary gland fibroadenomas (P<0.0001) and adenocarcinomas.

The increased incidences of mammary gland neoplasms in female rats and mice were considered secondary to tamsulosin-induced hyperprolactinemia. It is not known if tamsulosin elevates prolactin in humans. The relevance for human risk of the findings of prolactin-mediated endocrine tumors in rodents is not known.

Mutagenesis: *Dutasteride:* Dutasteride was tested for genotoxicity in a bacterial mutagenesis assay (Ames test), a chromosomal aberration assay in CHO cells, and a micronucleus assay in rats. The results did not indicate any genotoxic potential of the parent drug. Two major human metabolites were also negative in either the Ames test or an abbreviated Ames test.

Tamsulosin: Tamsulosin produced no evidence of mutagenic potential in vitro in the Ames reverse mutation test, mouse lymphoma thymidine kinase assay, unscheduled DNA repair synthesis assay, and chromosomal aberration assays in CHO cells or human lymphocytes. There were no mutagenic effects in the in vivo sister chromatid exchange and mouse micronucleus assay.

Impairment of Fertility: *Dutasteride:* Treatment of sexually mature male rats with dutasteride at 0.1- to 110-fold the MRHD (animal doses of 0.05, 10, 50, and 500 mg/kg/day) for up to 31 weeks resulted in dose- and time-dependent decreases in fertility; reduced cauda epididymal (absolute) sperm counts but not sperm concentration (at 50 and 500 mg/kg/day); reduced weights of the epididymis, prostate, and seminal vesicles; and microscopic changes in the male reproductive organs. The fertility effects were reversed by recovery week 6 at all doses, and sperm counts were normal at the end of a 14-week recovery period. The 5α-reductase–related changes consisted of cytoplasmic vacuolation of tubular epithelium in the epididymides and decreased cytoplasmic content of epithelium, consistent with decreased secretory activity in the prostate and seminal vesicles. The microscopic changes were no longer present at recovery week 14 in the low-dose group and were partly recovered in the remaining treatment groups. Low levels of dutasteride (0.6 to 17 ng/mL) were detected in the serum of untreated female rats mated to males dosed at 10, 50, or 500 mg/kg/day for 29 to 30 weeks.

In a fertility study in female rats, oral administration of dutasteride at doses of 0.05, 2.5, 12.5, and 30 mg/kg/day resulted in reduced litter size, increased embryo resorption and feminization of male fetuses (decreased anogenital distance) at 2- to 10-fold the MRHD (animal doses of 2.5 mg/kg/day or greater). Fetal body weights were also reduced at less than 0.02-fold the MRHD in rats (0.5 mg/kg/day).

Tamsulosin: Studies in rats revealed significantly reduced fertility in males at approximately 50 times the MRHD based on AUC (single or multiple daily doses of 300 mg/kg/day of tamsulosin hydrochloride). The mechanism of decreased fertility in male rats is considered to be an effect of the compound on the vaginal plug formation possibly due to changes of semen content or impairment of ejaculation. The effects on fertility were reversible showing improvement by 3 days after a single dose and 4 weeks after multiple dosing. Effects on fertility in males were completely reversed within nine weeks of discontinuation of multiple dosing. Multiple doses of 0.2 and 16 times the MRHD (animal doses of 10 and 100 mg/kg/day tamsulosin hydrochloride) did not significantly alter fertility in male rats. Effects of tamsulosin on sperm counts or sperm function have not been evaluated.

Studies in female rats revealed significant reductions in fertility after single or multiple dosing with 300 mg/kg/day of the R-isomer or racemic mixture of tamsulosin hydrochloride, respectively. In female rats, the reductions in fertility after single doses were considered to be associated with impairments in fertilization. Multiple dosing with 10 or 100 mg/kg/day of the racemic mixture did not significantly alter fertility in female rats.

Estimates of exposure multiples comparing animal studies to the MRHD for dutasteride are based on clinical serum concentration at steady state.

Estimates of exposure multiples comparing animal studies to the MRHD for tamsulosin are based on AUC.

13.2 Animal Toxicology and/or Pharmacology

Central Nervous System Toxicology Studies: *Dutasteride:* In rats and dogs, repeated oral administration of dutasteride resulted in some animals showing signs of non-specific, reversible, centrally-mediated toxicity without associated histopathological changes at exposures 425- and 315-fold the expected clinical exposure (of parent drug), respectively.

14 CLINICAL STUDIES

The trial supporting the efficacy of JALYN was a 4-year multicenter, randomized, double-blind, parallel group study (CombAT study) investigating the efficacy of the coadministration of dutasteride 0.5 mg/day and tamsulosin hydrochloride 0.4 mg/day (n = 1,610) compared with dutasteride alone (n = 1,623) or tamsulosin alone (n = 1,611). Subjects were at least 50 years of age with a serum PSA ≥1.5 ng/mL and <10 ng/mL and BPH diagnosed by medical history and physical examination, including enlarged prostate (≥30 cc) and BPH symptoms that were moderate to severe according to the International Prostate Symptom Score (IPSS). The results presented below are from data collected following the first 2 years of treatment in the 4-year study. Eighty-eight percent (88%) of the enrolled study population was Caucasian. Approximately 52% of subjects had previous exposure to 5α-reductase inhibitor or alpha-blocker treatment. The primary efficacy endpoint evaluated during the first 2 years of treatment was change in IPSS. Most of the 4,844 subjects randomly assigned to receive coadministration therapy, dutasteride, or tamsulosin completed 2 years of double-blind treatment (79%, 80%, and 78%, respectively).

Effect on Symptom Score: Symptoms were quantified using the first 7 questions of the IPSS. The baseline score was approximately 16.4 units for each treatment group. Coadministration therapy was statistically superior to each of the monotherapy treatments in decreasing symptom score at Month 24. This difference was seen by Month 9 and continued through Month 24. At Month 24, the mean changes from baseline (±SD) in IPSS symptom scores were -6.2 (±7.14) for the coadministration group, -4.9 (±6.81) for dutasteride, and -4.3 (±7.01) for tamsulosin, with a mean difference between combination and dutasteride of -1.3 units (P<0.001; [95% CI: -1.69, -0.86]), and between coadministration and tamsulosin of -1.8 units (P<0.001; [95% CI: -2.23, -1.40]). See Figure 1.

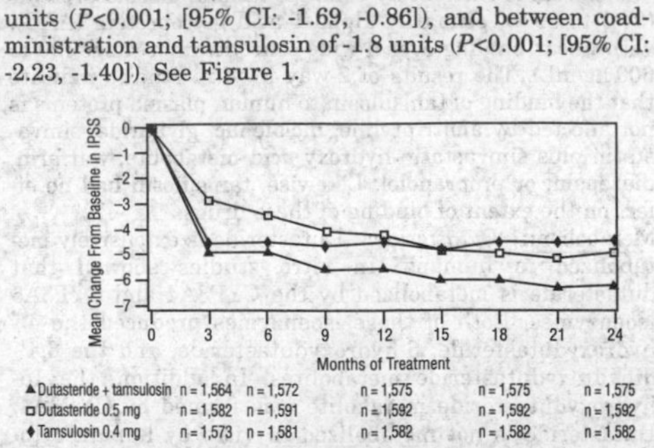

Figure 1. International Prostate Symptom Score Changes from Baseline (CombAT study)

Effect on Maximum Urine Flow Rate: The baseline Q_{max} was approximately 10.7 mL/sec for each treatment group. Coadministration therapy was statistically superior to each of the monotherapy treatments in increasing Q_{max} at Month 24. This difference was seen by Month 6 and continued through Month 24. At Month 24, the mean increases from baseline (±SD) in Q_{max} were 2.4 (±1;5.26) mL/sec for coadministration group, 1.9 (±5.10) mL/sec for dutasteride, and 0.9 (±4.57) mL/sec for tamsulosin, with a mean difference between coadministration and dutasteride of 0.5 mL/sec (P = 0.003; [95% CI: 0.17, 0.84]), and between coadministration and tamsulosin of 1.5 mL/sec (P<0.001; [95% CI: 1.19, 1.86]). See Figure 2.

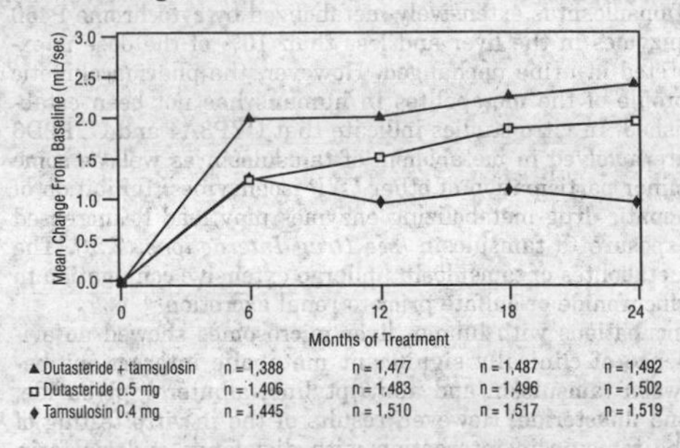

Figure 2. Q_{max} Change from Baseline (CombAT study)

Effect on Prostate Volume: The mean prostate volume at study entry was approximately 55 cc. At Month 24, the mean percent changes from baseline (±SD) in prostate volume were -26.9% (±22.57) for coadministration therapy, -28.0% (±24.88) for dutasteride, and 0% (±31.14) for tamsulosin, with a mean difference between coadministration and dutasteride of 1.1% (P = NS; [95% CI: -0.6, 2.8]), and between coadministration and tamsulosin of -26.9% (P<0.001; [95% CI: -28.9, -24.9]).

16 HOW SUPPLIED/STORAGE AND HANDLING

JALYN Capsules, containing 0.5 mg dutasteride and 0.4 mg tamsulosin hydrochloride, are oblong hard-shell capsules with a brown body and an orange cap imprinted with "GS 7CZ" in black ink. They are available in bottles with child-resistant closures as follows:

Bottle of 30 (NDC 0173-0809-13).

Bottle of 90 (NDC 0173-0809-59).

Store at 25°C (77°F); excursions permitted 15° to 30°C (59° to 86°F). [see USP Controlled Room Temperature]. Capsules may become deformed and/or discolored if kept at high temperatures.

Dutasteride is absorbed through the skin. JALYN Capsules should not be handled by women who are pregnant or who may become pregnant because of the potential for absorption of dutasteride and the subsequent potential risk to a developing male fetus *[see Warnings and Precautions (5.3)]*.

17 PATIENT COUNSELING INFORMATION

See FDA-approved patient labeling.

17.1 Orthostatic Hypotension

Patients should be informed about the possible occurrence of symptoms related to orthostatic hypotension, such as dizziness and vertigo, and the potential risk of syncope when taking JALYN. Patients starting treatment with JALYN should be cautioned to avoid situations where injury could result should syncope occur (e.g., driving, operating machinery, performing hazardous tasks). Patients should sit or lie down at the first signs of orthostatic hypotension [see Warnings and Precautions (5.1)].

17.2 Exposure of Women—Risk to Male Fetus

JALYN Capsules should not be handled by a woman who is pregnant or who may become pregnant because of the potential for absorption of dutasteride and the subsequent potential risk to a developing male fetus. Dutasteride is absorbed through the skin and could result in unintended fetal exposure. If a pregnant woman or woman of childbearing potential comes in contact with leaking JALYN Capsules, the contact area should be washed immediately with soap and water [see Warnings and Precautions (5.3), Use in Specific Populations (8.1)].

17.3 Instructions for Use

JALYN Capsules should be swallowed whole and not chewed, crushed, or opened. JALYN Capsules may become deformed and/or discolored if kept at high temperatures. If this occurs, capsules should not be used.

17.4 Priapism

Patients should be informed about the possibility of priapism as a result of treatment with JALYN or other alpha-adrenergic antagonist-containing medications. Patients should be informed that this reaction is extremely rare, but can lead to permanent erectile dysfunction if not brought to immediate medical attention [see Warnings and Precautions (5.6)].

17.5 Blood Donation

Patients treated with JALYN should not donate blood until at least 6 months following their last dose to prevent pregnant women from receiving dutasteride through blood transfusion [see Warnings and Precautions (5.7)]. Serum levels of dutasteride are detectable for 4 to 6 months after treatment ends [see Clinical Pharmacology (12.3)].

17.6 Intraoperative Floppy Iris Syndrome (IFIS)

Advise patients considering cataract surgery to tell their ophthalmologist that they take or have taken JALYN, an alpha-adrenergic antagonist-containing product [see Warnings and Precautions (5.8)].

JALYN and AVODART are trademarks of GlaxoSmithKline. The other brands listed are trademarks of their respective owners and are not trademarks of GlaxoSmithKline. The makers of these brands are not affiliated with and do not endorse GlaxoSmithKline or its products.

Jointly Manufactured by
Catalent Pharma Solutions
F-67930 Beinheim, France
D-73614 Schorndorf, Germany
and
Rottendorf Pharma GmbH
D-59320 Ennigerloh, Germany
Distributed by
GlaxoSmithKline
Research Triangle Park, NC 27709
©2010, GlaxoSmithKline. All rights reserved.
June 2010
JLN:1PI

PHARMACIST—DETACH HERE AND GIVE INSTRUCTIONS TO PATIENT

PATIENT INFORMATION
JALYN™ [JAY-LIN]
(dutasteride and tamsulosin hydrochloride)
Capsules
JALYN is for use by men only.

Read this patient information before you start taking JALYN and each time you get a refill. There may be new information. This information does not take the place of talking with your doctor about your medical condition or your treatment.

What is JALYN?

JALYN is a prescription medicine that contains 2 medicines: dutasteride and tamsulosin. JALYN is used to treat the symptoms of benign prostatic hyperplasia (BPH) in men with an enlarged prostate.

Who should not take JALYN?

Do Not Take JALYN if you are:

- pregnant or may become pregnant. JALYN may harm your unborn baby. Pregnant women should not touch JALYN Capsules. If a woman who is pregnant with a male baby gets enough JALYN in her body by swallowing or touching JALYN, the male baby may be born with sex organs that are not normal.
- a child or teenager.
- allergic to dutasteride, tamsulosin, or any of the ingredients in JALYN. See the end of this leaflet for a complete list of ingredients in JALYN.
- taking another medicine that contains an alpha-blocker.

What should I tell my doctor before taking JALYN?

Before you take JALYN, tell your doctor if you:

- have a history of low blood pressure
- take medicines to treat high blood pressure
- plan to have cataract surgery
- have liver problems

- are allergic to sulfa medications
- have any other medical conditions

Tell your doctor about all the medicines you take, including prescription and non-prescription medicines, vitamins, and herbal supplements. JALYN and other medicines may affect each other, causing side effects. JALYN may affect the way other medicines work, and other medicines may affect how JALYN works.

Know the medicines you take. Keep a list of them to show your doctor and pharmacist when you get a new medicine.

How should I take JALYN?

- Take JALYN exactly as your doctor tells you to take it.
- Swallow JALYN Capsules whole. Do not crush, chew, or open JALYN Capsules.
- Take your JALYN 1 time each day, about 30 minutes after the same meal every day. For example, you may take JALYN 30 minutes after dinner every day.
- If you miss a dose, you can take it later that same day, 30 minutes after a meal. Do not take 2 JALYN capsules in the same day. If you stop or forget to take JALYN for several days, talk with your doctor before starting again.
- If you take too much JALYN, call your doctor or go to the nearest hospital emergency room right away.
- Your doctor may check you for other prostate problems, including prostate cancer before you start and while you take JALYN. A blood test called PSA (prostate-specific antigen) is sometimes used to see if you might have prostate cancer. JALYN will reduce the amount of PSA measured in your blood. Your doctor is aware of this effect and can still use PSA to see if you might have prostate cancer. Increases in your PSA levels from their lowest point while on JALYN (even if the PSA levels are in the normal range) should be evaluated by your doctor.

What should I avoid while taking JALYN?

- Avoid driving, operating machinery, or other dangerous activities when starting treatment with JALYN until you know how JALYN affects you. JALYN can cause a sudden drop in your blood pressure, especially at the start of treatment. A sudden drop in blood pressure may cause you to faint, feel dizzy or lightheaded.
- You should not donate blood while taking JALYN or for 6 months after you have stopped JALYN. This is important to prevent pregnant women from receiving JALYN through blood transfusions.

What are the possible side effects of JALYN?
JALYN may cause serious side effects, including:

- **Decreased blood pressure.** JALYN may cause a sudden drop in your blood pressure upon standing from a sitting or lying position, especially at the start of treatment. Symptoms of low blood pressure may include:
  - fainting
  - dizziness
  - feeling lightheaded
- **Eye problems during cataract surgery.** During cataract surgery, a condition called intraoperative floppy iris syndrome (IFIS) can happen if you take or have taken JALYN in the past. If you need to have cataract surgery, tell your surgeon if you take or have taken JALYN.
- **A painful erection that will not go away.** Rarely, JALYN can cause a painful erection (priapism), which cannot be relieved by having sex. If this happens, get medical help right away. If priapism is not treated, there could be lasting damage to your penis, including not being able to have an erection.
- **Allergic reactions.** Call your doctor if you get any signs of an allergic reaction while taking JALYN, including:
  - itching
  - hives
  - rash

Rare and more serious allergic reactions may include:
- swelling of your face, tongue, or throat
- difficulty breathing

Get medical help right away if you have swelling of the face, tongue, or throat or difficulty breathing.

The most common side effects of JALYN include:
- ejaculation problems
- trouble getting or keeping an erection (impotence)
- a decrease in sex drive (libido)
- decreased amount of semen released during sex
- dizziness
- enlarged or painful breast
- runny nose

Tell your doctor if you have any side effect that bothers you or that does not go away.

These are not all the possible side effects with JALYN. For more information, ask your doctor or pharmacist.

Call your doctor for medical advice about side effects. You may report side effects to FDA at 1-800-FDA-1088.

How should I store JALYN?

- Store JALYN Capsules at room temperature (59° to 86°F or 15° to 30°C).
- JALYN Capsules may become deformed and/or discolored if kept at high temperatures.

- Do not use or touch JALYN if your capsules are deformed, discolored, or leaking.
- Safely throw away medicine that is no longer needed.

Keep JALYN and all medicines out of the reach of children.

Medicines are sometimes prescribed for purposes other than those listed in a patient leaflet. Do not use JALYN for a condition for which it was not prescribed. Do not give JALYN to other people, even if they have the same symptoms that you have. It may harm them.

This patient information leaflet summarizes the most important information about JALYN. If you like more information, talk with your doctor. You can ask your pharmacist or doctor for information about JALYN that is written for health professionals.

For more information, go to www.gsk.com or call 1-888-825-5249.

What are the ingredients in JALYN?

Active ingredients: dutasteride and tamsulosin hydrochloride

Inactive ingredients: black ink, butylated hydroxytoluene, carrageenan, FD&C yellow 6, ferric oxide (yellow), gelatin (from certified BSE-free bovine sources), glycerin, hypromellose, iron oxide red, methacrylic acid copolymer dispersion, microcrystalline cellulose, mono-di-glycerides of caprylic/capric acid, potassium chloride, talc, titanium dioxide, and triethyl citrate.

How does JALYN work?

JALYN contains 2 medications, dutasteride and tamsulosin. These 2 medications work in different ways to improve symptoms of BPH. Dutasteride shrinks the enlarged prostate and tamsulosin relaxes muscles in the prostate and neck of the bladder. These 2 medications, when used together, can improve symptoms of BPH better than either medication when used alone.

Jointly Manufactured by
Catalent Pharma Solutions
F-67930 Beinheim, France
D-73614 Schorndorf, Germany
and
Rottendorf Pharma GmbH
D-59320 Ennigerloh, Germany
Distributed by
GlaxoSmithKline
Research Triangle Park, NC 27709
©2010, GlaxoSmithKline. All rights reserved.
June 2010
JLN:1PIL

KINRIX®
[kin' rix]   ℞
(Diphtheria and Tetanus Toxoids and Acellular Pertussis Adsorbed and Inactivated Poliovirus Vaccine) Suspension for Intramuscular Injection

HIGHLIGHTS OF PRESCRIBING INFORMATION

These highlights do not include all the information needed to use KINRIX safely and effectively. See full prescribing information for KINRIX.

KINRIX (Diphtheria and Tetanus Toxoids and Acellular Pertussis Adsorbed and Inactivated Poliovirus Vaccine) Suspension for Intramuscular Injection
Initial U.S. Approval: 2008

---INDICATIONS AND USAGE---
A single dose of KINRIX is indicated for active immunization against diphtheria, tetanus, pertussis, and poliomyelitis as the fifth dose in the diphtheria, tetanus, and acellular pertussis (DTaP) vaccine series and the fourth dose in the inactivated poliovirus vaccine (IPV) series in children 4 through 6 years of age whose previous DTaP vaccine doses have been with INFANRIX and/or PEDIARIX for the first three doses and INFANRIX for the fourth dose. (1)

---DOSAGE AND ADMINISTRATION---
A single intramuscular injection (0.5 mL). (2.2)

---DOSAGE FORMS AND STRENGTHS---
Single-dose vial and prefilled syringe containing a 0.5-mL suspension for injection of diphtheria and tetanus toxoids, acellular pertussis antigens, and inactivated poliovirus types 1, 2, and 3. (3)

---CONTRAINDICATIONS---
- Severe allergic reaction (e.g., anaphylaxis) after a previous dose of any diphtheria toxoid, tetanus toxoid, pertussis- or poliovirus-containing vaccine, or to any component of KINRIX, including neomycin and polymyxin B. (4.1)
- Encephalopathy within 7 days of administration of a previous pertussis-containing vaccine. (4.2)
- Progressive neurologic disorders. (4.3)

---WARNINGS AND PRECAUTIONS---
- If Guillain-Barré syndrome occurs within 6 weeks of receipt of a prior vaccine containing tetanus toxoid, the decision to give KINRIX should be based on potential benefits and risks. (5.1)

- The needleless prefilled syringes contain dry natural latex rubber and may cause allergic reactions. (5.2)
- If adverse events (i.e., temperature ≥105°F, collapse or shock-like state, persistent, inconsolable crying lasting ≥3 hours, occurring within 48 hours of vaccination; seizures within 3 days of vaccination) have occurred in temporal relation to receipt of a pertussis-containing vaccine, the decision to give KINRIX should be based on potential benefits and risks. (5.3)
- For children at higher risk for seizures, an antipyretic may be administered at the time of vaccination with KINRIX. (5.4)

-------------------ADVERSE REACTIONS-------------------
- The most frequently reported solicited local reaction (>50%) was injection site pain. Other common solicited local reactions (≥25%) were redness, increase in arm circumference, and swelling. (6.1)
- Common solicited general adverse events (≥15%) were drowsiness, fever (≥99.5°F), and loss of appetite. (6.1)

To report SUSPECTED ADVERSE REACTIONS, contact GlaxoSmithKline at 1-888-825-5249 or VAERS at 1-800-822-7967 or www.vaers.hhs.gov.

-------------------DRUG INTERACTIONS-------------------
Do not mix KINRIX with any other vaccine in the same syringe or vial. (7.1)
Revised: January 2010
KNX:4PI
See 17 for PATIENT COUNSELING INFORMATION
Revised: 06/2010

FULL PRESCRIBING INFORMATION: CONTENTS*

FULL PRESCRIBING INFORMATION

1 INDICATIONS AND USAGE
A single dose of KINRIX® is indicated for active immunization against diphtheria, tetanus, pertussis, and poliomyelitis as the fifth dose in the diphtheria, tetanus, and acellular pertussis (DTaP) vaccine series and the fourth dose in the inactivated poliovirus vaccine (IPV) series in children 4 through 6 years of age whose previous DTaP vaccine doses have been with INFANRIX® (Diphtheria and Tetanus Toxoids and Acellular Pertussis Vaccine Adsorbed) and/or PEDIARIX® [Diphtheria and Tetanus Toxoids and Acellular Pertussis Adsorbed, Hepatitis B (Recombinant) and Inactivated Poliovirus Vaccine Combined] for the first three doses and INFANRIX for the fourth dose.

2 DOSAGE AND ADMINISTRATION
2.1 Preparation for Administration
Shake vigorously to obtain a homogeneous, turbid, white suspension. Do not use if resuspension does not occur with vigorous shaking. Parenteral drug products should be in-

spected visually for particulate matter and discoloration prior to administration, whenever solution and container permit. KINRIX also should be inspected visually for cracks in the vial or syringe prior to administration. If any of these conditions exist, the vaccine should not be administered. After removal of the dose, any vaccine remaining in the vial should be discarded.

2.2 Recommended Dose and Schedule
KINRIX is to be administered as a 0.5-mL dose by intramuscular injection. The preferred site of administration is the deltoid muscle of the upper arm. Do not administer this product intravenously, intradermally, or subcutaneously. KINRIX may be used for the fifth dose in the DTaP immunization series and the fourth dose in the IPV immunization series in children 4 through 6 years of age (prior to the seventh birthday) whose previous DTaP vaccine doses have been with INFANRIX and/or PEDIARIX for the first three doses and INFANRIX for the fourth dose [see Indications and Usage (1)].

3 DOSAGE FORMS AND STRENGTHS
KINRIX is available in 0.5-mL single-dose vials and prefilled TIP-LOK® syringes.
Each 0.5-mL dose contains a suspension for injection of diphtheria and tetanus toxoids, acellular pertussis antigens, and inactivated poliovirus types 1, 2, and 3. See Description (11) for the complete listing of ingredients.

4 CONTRAINDICATIONS
4.1 Hypersensitivity
Severe allergic reaction (e.g., anaphylaxis) after a previous dose of any diphtheria toxoid, tetanus toxoid, pertussis- or poliovirus-containing vaccine, or to any component of KINRIX, including neomycin and polymyxin B, is a contraindication to administration of KINRIX [see Description (11)]. Because of the uncertainty as to which component of the vaccine might be responsible, no further vaccination with any of these components should be given. Alternatively, such individuals may be referred to an allergist for evaluation if immunization with any of these components is considered.

4.2 Encephalopathy
Encephalopathy (e.g., coma, decreased level of consciousness, prolonged seizures) within 7 days of administration of a previous dose of a pertussis-containing vaccine that is not attributable to another identifiable cause is a contraindication to administration of any pertussis-containing vaccine, including KINRIX.

4.3 Progressive Neurologic Disorder
Progressive neurologic disorder, including infantile spasms, uncontrolled epilepsy, or progressive encephalopathy is a contraindication to administration of any pertussis-containing vaccine, including KINRIX. Pertussis vaccine should not be administered to individuals with such conditions until a treatment regimen has been established and the condition has stabilized.

5 WARNINGS AND PRECAUTIONS
5.1 Guillain-Barré Syndrome
If Guillain-Barré syndrome occurs within 6 weeks of receipt of a prior vaccine containing tetanus toxoid, the decision to give any tetanus toxoid-containing vaccine, including KINRIX, should be based on careful consideration of the potential benefits and possible risks. When a decision is made to withhold tetanus toxoid, other available vaccines should be given, as indicated.

5.2 Latex
The tip cap and the rubber plunger of the needleless prefilled syringes contain dry natural latex rubber that may cause allergic reactions in latex sensitive individuals. The vial stopper is latex-free.

5.3 Adverse Events Following Prior Pertussis Vaccination
If any of the following events occur in temporal relation to receipt of a pertussis-containing vaccine, the decision to give any pertussis-containing vaccine, including KINRIX, should be based on careful consideration of the potential benefits and possible risks:
- Temperature of ≥40.5°C (105°F) within 48 hours not due to another identifiable cause;
- Collapse or shock-like state (hypotonic-hyporesponsive episode) within 48 hours;
- Persistent, inconsolable crying lasting ≥3 hours, occurring within 48 hours;
- Seizures with or without fever occurring within 3 days.
When a decision is made to withhold pertussis vaccination, other available vaccines should be given, as indicated.

5.4 Children at Risk for Seizures
For children at higher risk for seizures than the general population, an appropriate antipyretic may be administered at the time of vaccination with a pertussis-containing vaccine, including KINRIX, and for the ensuing 24 hours to reduce the possibility of post-vaccination fever.

5.5 Preventing and Managing Allergic Vaccine Reactions
Prior to administration, the healthcare provider should review the patient's immunization history for possible vaccine sensitivity and previous vaccination-related adverse reactions to allow an assessment of benefits and risks. Epinephrine and other appropriate agents used for the control of immediate allergic reactions must be immediately available should an acute anaphylactic reaction occur.

6 ADVERSE REACTIONS
6.1 Clinical Trials Experience
Because clinical trials are conducted under widely varying conditions, adverse reaction rates observed in the clinical trials of a vaccine cannot be directly compared with rates in the clinical trials of another vaccine, and may not reflect the rates observed in practice.
A total of 3,537 children were vaccinated with a single dose of KINRIX in 3 clinical trials. Of these, 381 children received a non-US formulation of KINRIX (containing ≤2.5 mg 2-phenoxyethanol per dose as preservative). The primary study (Study 048), conducted in the United States, was a randomized, controlled clinical trial in which children 4 to 6 years of age were vaccinated with KINRIX (N = 3,156) or control vaccines (INFANRIX and IPOL® vaccine [IPV, Sanofi Pasteur SA]; N = 1,053) as a fifth DTaP vaccine dose following 4 doses of INFANRIX and as a fourth IPV dose following 3 doses of IPOL. Subjects also received the second dose of US-licensed measles, mumps, and rubella (MMR) vaccine (Merck & Co., Inc.) administered concomitantly, at separate sites.
Data on adverse events were collected by parents/guardians using standardized forms for 4 consecutive days following vaccination with KINRIX or control vaccines (i.e., day of vaccination and the next 3 days). The reported frequencies of solicited local reactions and general adverse events in Study 048 are presented in Table 1.
In 3 studies (Study 046, 047, and 048), children were monitored for unsolicited adverse events, that occurred in the 31-day period following vaccination and in 2 studies (Study 047 and 048), parents/guardians were actively queried about changes in the child's health status, including the occurrence of serious adverse events, through 6 months post-vaccination.

Table 1. Percentage of Children 4 to 6 Years of Age Reporting Solicited Local Reactions or General Adverse Events Within 4 Days of Vaccination[a] With KINRIX or Separate Concomitant Administration of INFANRIX and IPV When Coadministered With MMR Vaccine (Study 048) (Total Vaccinated Cohort)

	KINRIX	INFANRIX + IPV
Local[b]	N = 3,121-3,128	N = 1,039-1,043
Pain, any	57.0[c]	53.3
Pain, grade 2 or 3[d]	13.7	12.0
Pain, grade 3[d]	1.6[c]	0.6
Redness, any	36.6	36.6
Redness, ≥50 mm	17.6	20.0
Redness, ≥110 mm	2.9	4.1
Arm circumference increase, any	36.0	38.1
Arm circumference increase, >20 mm	6.9	7.4
Arm circumference increase, >30 mm	2.4	3.2
Swelling, any	26.0	27.0
Swelling, ≥50 mm	10.2	11.5
Swelling, ≥110 mm	1.4	1.8
General	N = 3,037-3,120	N = 993-1,036
Drowsiness, any	19.1	17.5
Drowsiness, grade 3[e]	0.8	0.8
Fever, ≥99.5°F	16.0	14.8
Fever, >100.4°F	6.5[c]	4.4
Fever, >102.2°F	1.1	1.1

Fever, >104°F	0.1	0.0
Loss of appetite, any	15.5	16.0
Loss of appetite, grade 3[f]	0.8	0.6

IPV manufactured by Sanofi Pasteur SA. MMR vaccine manufactured by Merck & Co., Inc.
Total Vaccinated Cohort = all vaccinated subjects for whom safety data were available.
N = number of children with evaluable data for the events listed.
[a] Within 4 days of vaccination defined as day of vaccination and the next 3 days.
[b] Local reactions at the injection site for KINRIX or INFANRIX.
[c] Statistically higher than comparator group (P <0.05).
[d] Grade 2 defined as painful when the limb was moved; Grade 3 defined as preventing normal daily activities.
[e] Grade 3 defined as preventing normal daily activities.
[f] Grade 3 defined as not eating at all.

In Study 048, KINRIX was non-inferior to INFANRIX with regard to swelling that involved >50% of the injected upper arm length and that was associated with a >30 mm increase in mid-upper arm circumference within 4 days following vaccination (upper limit of two-sided 95% Confidence Interval for difference in percentage of KINRIX [0.6%, n = 20] minus INFANRIX [1.0%, n = 11] ≤2%).
Serious Adverse Events: Within the 31-day period following study vaccination in 3 studies (Study 046, 047, and 048), in which all subjects received concomitant MMR vaccine (US-licensed MMR vaccine [Merck & Co., Inc.] in Study 047 and 048; non-US-licensed MMR vaccine in Study 046), 3 subjects (0.1% [3/3,537]) who received KINRIX reported serious adverse events (dehydration and hypernatremia; cerebrovascular accident; dehydration and gastroenteritis) and 4 subjects (0.3% [4/1,434]) who received INFANRIX and IPV (Sanofi Pasteur SA) reported serious adverse events (cellulitis; constipation; foreign body trauma; fever without identified etiology).

6.2   Postmarketing Experience
In addition to reports in clinical trials, the following adverse events, for which a causal relationship to components of KINRIX is plausible, have been reported since market introduction of DTaP-IPV manufactured by GlaxoSmithKline outside the U.S. Because these events are reported voluntarily from a population of uncertain size, it is not always possible to reliably estimate their frequency or establish a causal relationship to vaccination.
General Disorders and Administration Site Conditions: Injection site vesicles.
Skin and Subcutaneous Tissue Disorders: Pruritus.
Additional adverse events reported following postmarketing use of INFANRIX, for which a causal relationship to vaccination is plausible, are: Allergic reactions, including anaphylactoid reactions, anaphylaxis, angioedema, and urticaria, apnea, collapse or shock-like state (hypotonic-hyporesponsive episode), convulsions (with or without fever), lymphadenopathy, and thrombocytopenia.

7   DRUG INTERACTIONS
7.1   Concomitant Vaccine Administration
In clinical trials, KINRIX was administered concomitantly with the second dose of MMR vaccine [see Clinical Studies (14)].
Data are not available on concomitant use of KINRIX and varicella vaccine.
When KINRIX is administered concomitantly with other injectable vaccines, they should be given with separate syringes. KINRIX should not be mixed with any other vaccine in the same syringe or vial.
7.2   Immunosuppressive Therapies
Immunosuppressive therapies, including irradiation, antimetabolites, alkylating agents, cytotoxic drugs, and corticosteroids (used in greater than physiologic doses), may reduce the immune response to KINRIX.

8   USE IN SPECIFIC POPULATIONS
8.1   Pregnancy
Pregnancy Category C
Animal reproduction studies have not been conducted with KINRIX. It is also not known whether KINRIX can cause fetal harm when administered to a pregnant woman or can affect reproduction capacity.
8.4   Pediatric Use
Safety and effectiveness of KINRIX in children younger than 4 years of age and children 7 to 16 years of age have not been evaluated. KINRIX is not approved for use in persons in these age groups.

11   DESCRIPTION
KINRIX (Diphtheria and Tetanus Toxoids and Acellular Pertussis Adsorbed and Inactivated Poliovirus Vaccine) is a noninfectious, sterile vaccine for intramuscular administration. Each 0.5-mL dose is formulated to contain 25 Lf of diphtheria toxoid, 10 Lf of tetanus toxoid, 25 mcg of inactivated pertussin toxin (PT), 25 mcg of filamentous

Table 2. Pre-Vaccination Antibody Levels and Post-Vaccination[a] Antibody Responses Following KINRIX Compared With Separate Concomitant Administration of INFANRIX and IPV in Children 4 to 6 Years of Age When Coadministered With MMR Vaccine (Study 048) (ATP Cohort for Immunogenicity)

	KINRIX N = 787-851	INFANRIX + IPV N = 237-262
Anti-Diphtheria Toxoid		
Pre-vaccination % ≥0.1 IU/mL (95% CI)[b]	87.7 (85.3, 89.9)	85.5 (80.6, 89.5)
Post-vaccination % ≥0.1 IU/mL (95% CI)[b]	100 (99.6, 100)	100 (98.6, 100)
% Booster Response (95% CI)[c]	99.5 (98.8, 99.9)[d]	100 (98.6, 100)
Anti-Tetanus Toxoid		
Pre-vaccination % ≥0.1 IU/mL (95% CI)[b]	87.8 (85.4, 90.0)	88.2 (83.6, 91.8)
Post-vaccination % ≥0.1 IU/mL (95% CI)[b]	100 (99.6, 100)	100 (98.6, 100)
% Booster Response (95% CI)[c]	96.7 (95.2, 97.8)[d]	93.9 (90.2, 96.5)
Anti-PT		
% Booster Response (95% CI)[e]	92.2 (90.2, 94.0)[d]	92.6 (88.7, 95.5)
Anti-FHA		
% Booster Response (95% CI)[e]	95.4 (93.7, 96.7)[d]	96.2 (93.1, 98.1)
Anti-Pertactin		
% Booster Response (95% CI)[e]	97.8 (96.5, 98.6)[d]	96.9 (94.1, 98.7)
Anti-Poliovirus 1		
Pre-vaccination % ≥1:8 (95% CI)[b]	88.3 (85.9, 90.4)	85.1 (80.1, 89.2)
Post-vaccination % ≥1:8 (95% CI)[b]	99.9 (99.3, 100)	100 (98.5, 100)
Post-vaccination GMT (95% CI)	2,127 (1,976, 2,290)[f]	1,685 (1,475, 1,925)
Anti-Poliovirus 2		
Pre-vaccination % ≥1:8 (95% CI)[b]	91.8 (89.7, 93.6)	87.0 (82.3, 90.8)
Post-vaccination % ≥1:8 (95% CI)[b]	100 (99.6, 100)	100 (98.5, 100)
Post-vaccination GMT (95% CI)	2,265 (2,114, 2,427)[f]	1,818 (1,606, 2,057)
Anti-Poliovirus 3		
Pre-vaccination % ≥1:8 (95% CI)[b]	84.7 (82.0, 87.0)	85.0 (80.1, 89.1)
Post-vaccination % ≥1:8 (95% CI)[b]	100 (99.5, 100)	100 (98.5, 100)
Post-vaccination GMT (95% CI)	3,588 (3,345, 3,849)[f]	3,365 (2,961, 3,824)

IPV manufactured by Sanofi Pasteur SA. MMR vaccine manufactured by Merck & Co., Inc.
ATP = according-to-protocol; CI = Confidence Interval; GMT = geometric mean antibody titer
N = number of subjects with available results.
[a] One month blood sampling, range 31 to 48 days.
[b] Seroprotection defined as anti-diphtheria toxoid and anti-tetanus toxoid antibody concentrations ≥0.1 IU/mL by ELISA and as anti-poliovirus Type 1, Type 2, and Type 3 antibody titer ≥1:8 by micro-neutralization assay for poliovirus.
[c] Booster response: In subjects with pre-vaccination <0.1 IU/mL, post-vaccination concentration ≥0.4 IU/mL. In subjects with pre-vaccination concentration ≥0.1 IU/mL, an increase of at least 4 times the pre-vaccination concentration.
[d] KINRIX was non-inferior to INFANRIX + IPV based on booster response rates (upper limit of two-sided 95% CI on the difference of INFANRIX + IPV minus KINRIX ≤10%).
[e] Booster response: In subjects with pre-vaccination <5 EL.U./mL, post-vaccination concentration ≥20 EL.U./mL. In subjects with pre-vaccination ≥5 EL.U./mL and <20 EL.U./mL, an increase of at least 4 times the pre-vaccination concentration. In subjects with pre-vaccination ≥20 EL.U./mL, an increase of at least 2 times the pre-vaccination concentration.
[f] KINRIX was non-inferior to INFANRIX + IPV based on post-vaccination anti-poliovirus antibody GMTs adjusted for baseline titer (upper limit of two-sided 95% CI for the GMT ratio [INFANRIX + IPV:KINRIX] ≤1.5).

hemagglutinin (FHA), 8 mcg of pertactin (69 kiloDalton outer membrane protein), 40 D-antigen Units (DU) of Type 1 poliovirus (Mahoney), 8 DU of Type 2 poliovirus (MEF-1), and 32 DU of Type 3 poliovirus (Saukett). The diphtheria, tetanus, and pertussis components of KINRIX are the same as those in INFANRIX and PEDIARIX and the poliovirus component is the same as that in PEDIARIX.
The diphtheria toxin is produced by growing Corynebacterium diphtheriae in Fenton medium containing a bovine extract. Tetanus toxin is produced by growing Clostridium tetani in a modified Latham medium derived from bovine casein. The bovine materials used in these extracts are sourced from countries which the United States Department of Agriculture (USDA) has determined neither have nor are at risk of bovine spongiform encephalopathy (BSE). Both toxins are detoxified with formaldehyde, concentrated by ultrafiltration, and purified by precipitation, dialysis, and sterile filtration.

The acellular pertussis antigens (PT, FHA, and pertactin) are isolated from Bordetella pertussis culture grown in modified Stainer-Scholte liquid medium. PT and FHA are isolated from the fermentation broth; pertactin is extracted from the cells by heat treatment and flocculation. The antigens are purified in successive chromatographic and precipitation steps. PT is detoxified using glutaraldehyde and formaldehyde. FHA and pertactin are treated with formaldehyde.
Diphtheria and tetanus toxoids and pertussis antigens (inactivated PT, FHA, and pertactin) are individually adsorbed onto aluminum hydroxide.
The inactivated poliovirus component of KINRIX is an enhanced potency component. Each of the 3 strains of poliovirus is individually grown in VERO cells, a continuous line of monkey kidney cells, cultivated on microcarriers. Calf serum and lactalbumin hydrolysate are used during VERO cell culture and/or virus culture. Calf serum is sourced from

countries the USDA has determined neither have nor are at risk of BSE. After clarification, each viral suspension is purified by ultrafiltration, diafiltration, and successive chromatographic steps, and inactivated with formaldehyde. The 3 purified viral strains are then pooled to form a trivalent concentrate.

Diphtheria and tetanus toxoid potency is determined by measuring the amount of neutralizing antitoxin in previously immunized guinea pigs. The potency of the acellular pertussis components (inactivated PT, FHA, and pertactin) is determined by enzyme-linked immunosorbent assay (ELISA) on sera from previously immunized mice. The potency of the inactivated poliovirus component is determined by using the D-antigen ELISA and by a poliovirus neutralizing cell culture assay on sera from previously immunized rats.

Each 0.5-mL dose contains 4.5 mg of NaCl and aluminum adjuvant (not more than 0.6 mg aluminum by assay). Each dose also contains ≤100 mcg of residual formaldehyde and ≤100 mcg of polysorbate 80 (Tween 80). Neomycin sulfate and polymyxin B are used in the poliovirus vaccine manufacturing process and may be present in the final vaccine at ≤0.05 ng neomycin and ≤0.01 ng polymyxin B per dose. KINRIX does not contain a preservative.

12   CLINICAL PHARMACOLOGY

12.1   Mechanism of Action

Diphtheria: Diphtheria is an acute toxin-mediated infectious disease caused by toxigenic strains of *C. diphtheriae*. Protection against disease is due to the development of neutralizing antibodies to the diphtheria toxin. A serum diphtheria antitoxin level of 0.01 IU/mL is the lowest level giving some degree of protection; a level of 0.1 IU/mL is regarded as protective.[1]

Tetanus: Tetanus is an acute toxin-mediated disease caused by a potent exotoxin released by *C. tetani*. Protection against disease is due to the development of neutralizing antibodies to the tetanus toxin. A serum tetanus antitoxin level of at least 0.01 IU/mL, measured by neutralization assays, is considered the minimum protective level.[2,3] A level of ≥0.1 IU/mL is considered protective.[4]

Pertussis: Pertussis (whooping cough) is a disease of the respiratory tract caused by *B. pertussis*. The role of the different components produced by *B. pertussis* in either the pathogenesis of, or the immunity to, pertussis is not well understood. There is no well established serological correlate of protection for pertussis. The efficacy of the pertussis component of KINRIX was determined in clinical trials of INFANRIX administered as a 3-dose series in infants (see INFANRIX prescribing information).

Poliomyelitis: Poliovirus is an enterovirus that belongs to the picornavirus family. Three serotypes of poliovirus have been identified (Types 1, 2, and 3). Neutralizing antibodies against the 3 poliovirus serotypes are recognized as conferring protection against poliomyelitis disease.[5]

13   NONCLINICAL TOXICOLOGY

13.1   Carcinogenesis, Mutagenesis, Impairment of Fertility

KINRIX has not been evaluated for carcinogenic or mutagenic potential, or for impairment of fertility.

14   CLINICAL STUDIES

14.1   Immunological Evaluation

In a US multicenter study (Study 048), 4,209 children were randomized in a 3:1 ratio to receive either KINRIX or INFANRIX and IPV (Sanofi Pasteur SA) administered concomitantly at separate sites. Subjects also received MMR vaccine (Merck & Co., Inc.) administered concomitantly at a separate site. Subjects were children 4 through 6 years of age who previously received 4 doses of INFANRIX, 3 doses of IPV, and 1 dose of MMR vaccine. Among subjects in both vaccine groups combined, 49.6% were female; 45.6% of subjects were White, 18.8% Hispanic, 13.6% Asian, 7.0% Black, and 15.0% were of other racial/ethnic groups.

Levels of antibodies to the diphtheria, tetanus, pertussis (PT, FHA, and pertactin), and poliovirus antigens were measured in sera obtained immediately prior to vaccination and 1 month (range 31 to 48 days) after vaccination (Table 2). The co-primary immunogenicity endpoints were anti-diphtheria toxoid, anti-tetanus toxoid, anti-PT, anti-FHA, and anti-pertactin booster responses, and anti-poliovirus Type 1, Type 2, and Type 3 geometric mean antibody titers (GMTs) 1 month after vaccination. KINRIX was shown to be non-inferior to INFANRIX and IPV administered separately, in terms of booster responses to DTaP antigens and post-vaccination GMTs for anti-poliovirus antibodies (Table 2).

[See table 2 at top of previous page]

14.2   Concomitant Vaccine Administration

In a US study (Study 047), among recipients of DTaP-IPV (same formulation as KINRIX but also containing 2-phenoxyethanol) and the second dose of MMR vaccine (Merck & Co., Inc.) who had pre-vaccination sera tested for antibodies to measles, mumps, and rubella (N = 175-181), 99% of subjects were seropositive for antibodies to measles, mumps, and rubella prior to vaccination.

15   REFERENCES

1. Vitek CR and Wharton M. Diphtheria Toxoid. In: Plotkin SA, Orenstein WA, and Offit PA, eds. *Vaccines*. 5th ed. Saunders; 2008:139-156.
2. Wassilak SGF, Roper MH, Kretsinger K, and Orenstein WA. Tetanus Toxoid. In: Plotkin SA, Orenstein WA, and Offit PA, eds. *Vaccines*. 5th ed. Saunders; 2008:805-839.
3. Department of Health and Human Services, Food and Drug Administration. Biological products; Bacterial vaccines and toxoids; Implementation of efficacy review; Proposed rule. *Federal Register* December 13, 1985; 50(240):51002-51117.
4. Centers for Disease Control and Prevention. General Recommendations on Immunization. Recommendations of the Advisory Committee on Immunization Practices (ACIP). *MMWR* 2006;55(RR-15):1-48.
5. Sutter RW, Pallansch MA, Sawyer LA, et al. Defining surrogate serologic tests with respect to predicting protective vaccine efficacy: Poliovirus vaccination. In: Williams JC, Goldenthal KL, Burns DL, Lewis Jr BP, eds. Combined vaccines and simultaneous administration. Current issues and perspectives. New York, NY: The New York Academy of Sciences; 1995:289-299.

16   HOW SUPPLIED/STORAGE AND HANDLING

KINRIX is available in 0.5-mL single-dose vials and disposable prefilled TIP-LOK syringes.

Single-Dose Vials
NDC 58160-812-11 (package of 10)
Single-Dose Prefilled Disposable TIP-LOK Syringes (packaged without needles)
NDC 58160-812-46 (package of 5)
NDC 58160-812-51 (package of 10)
Store refrigerated between 2° and 8°C (36° and 46°F). Do not freeze. Discard if the vaccine has been frozen.

17   PATIENT COUNSELING INFORMATION

Parents or guardians should be:
• informed of the potential benefits and risks of immunization with KINRIX.
• informed about the potential for adverse reactions that have been temporally associated with administration of KINRIX or other vaccines containing similar components.
• instructed to report any adverse events to their healthcare provider where the vaccine was administered.
• given the Vaccine Information Statements, which are required by the National Childhood Vaccine Injury Act of 1986 to be given prior to immunization. These materials are available free of charge at the Centers for Disease Control and Prevention (CDC) website (www.cdc.gov/vaccines).

INFANRIX, KINRIX, PEDIARIX, and TIP-LOK are registered trademarks of GlaxoSmithKline. IPOL is a registered trademark of Sanofi Pasteur Limited.

Manufactured by **GlaxoSmithKline Biologicals**
Rixensart, Belgium, US License 1617, and
Novartis Vaccines and Diagnostics GmbH & Co. KG
Marburg, Germany, US License 1754
Distributed by **GlaxoSmithKline**
Research Triangle Park, NC 27709
©2010, GlaxoSmithKline. All rights reserved.

LAMICTAL®   ℞
[la-mĭk' tal]
(lamotrigine)
Tablets

LAMICTAL   ℞
(lamotrigine)
Chewable Dispersible Tablets

LAMICTAL ODT   ℞
(lamotrigine)
Orally Disintegrating Tablets

HIGHLIGHTS OF PRESCRIBING INFORMATION

These highlights do not include all the information needed to use LAMICTAL safely and effectively. See full prescribing information for LAMICTAL.

LAMICTAL (lamotrigine) Tablets
LAMICTAL (lamotrigine) Chewable Dispersible Tablets
LAMICTAL ODT (lamotrigine) Orally Disintegrating Tablets
Initial U.S. Approval: 1994

WARNING: SERIOUS SKIN RASHES
See full prescribing information for complete boxed warning
Cases of life-threatening serious rashes, including Stevens-Johnson syndrome, toxic epidermal necrolysis, and/or rash-related death, have been caused by LAMICTAL. The rate of serious rash is greater in pedi-

---

atric patients than in adults. Additional factors that may increase the risk of rash include (5.1):
• coadministration with valproate
• exceeding recommended initial dose of LAMICTAL
• exceeding recommended dose escalation of LAMICTAL
Benign rashes are also caused by LAMICTAL; however, it is not possible to predict which rashes will prove to be serious or life-threatening. LAMICTAL should be discontinued at the first sign of rash, unless the rash is clearly not drug-related. (5.1)

—RECENT MAJOR CHANGES—

Dosage and Administration, LAMICTAL ODT (2.6)	May/2009
Warnings and Precautions, Suicidal Behavior and Ideation (5.5)	April/2009

—INDICATIONS AND USAGE—

LAMICTAL is an antiepileptic drug (AED) indicated for:
Epilepsy—adjunctive therapy in patients ≥2 years of age: (1.1)
• partial seizures.
• primary generalized tonic-clonic seizures.
• generalized seizures of Lennox-Gastaut syndrome.
Epilepsy—monotherapy in patients ≥16 years of age: conversion to monotherapy in patients with partial seizures who are receiving treatment with carbamazepine, phenobarbital, phenytoin, primidone, or valproate as the single AED. (1.1)
Bipolar Disorder in patients ≥18 years of age: maintenance treatment of Bipolar I Disorder to delay the time to occurrence of mood episodes in patients treated for acute mood episodes with standard therapy. (1.2)

—DOSAGE AND ADMINISTRATION—

• Dosing is based on concomitant medications, indication, and patient age. (2.2, 2.4)
• To avoid an increased risk of rash, the recommended initial dose and subsequent dose escalations should not be exceeded. LAMICTAL Starter Kits and LAMICTAL ODT Patient Titration Kits are available for the first 5 weeks of treatment. (2.1, 16)
• Do not restart LAMICTAL in patients who discontinued due to rash unless the potential benefits clearly outweigh the risks. (2.1)
• Adjustments to maintenance doses will in most cases be required in patients starting or stopping estrogen-containing oral contraceptives. (2.1, 5.8)
• LAMICTAL should be discontinued over a period of at least 2 weeks (approximately 50% reduction per week). (2.1, 5.9)
Epilepsy
• Adjunctive therapy—See Table 1 for patients >12 years of age and Tables 2 and 3 for patients 2 to 12 years. (2.2)
• Conversion to monotherapy—See Table 4. (2.3)
Bipolar Disorder: See Tables 5 and 6. (2.4)

—DOSAGE FORMS AND STRENGTHS—

Tablets: 25 mg, 100 mg, 150 mg, and 200 mg scored. (3.1, 16)
Chewable Dispersible Tablets: 2 mg, 5 mg, and 25 mg. (3.2, 16)
Orally Disintegrating Tablets: 25 mg, 50 mg, 100 mg, and 200 mg. (3.3, 16)

—CONTRAINDICATIONS—

Hypersensitivity to the drug or its ingredients. (Boxed Warning, 4)

—WARNINGS AND PRECAUTIONS—

• Life-threatening serious rash and/or rash-related death may result. (Boxed Warning, 5.1)
• Hypersensitivity reaction may be fatal or life-threatening. Early signs of hypersensitivity (e.g., fever, lymphadenopathy) may present without rash; if signs present, patient should be evaluated immediately. LAMICTAL should be discontinued if alternate etiology for hypersensitivity signs is not found. (5.2)
• Acute multiorgan failure has resulted (some cases fatal). (5.3)
• Blood dyscrasias (e.g., neutropenia, thrombocytopenia, pancytopenia), may result either with or without an associated hypersensitivity syndrome. (5.4)
• Suicidal behavior and ideation. (5.5)
• Clinical worsening, emergence of new symptoms, and suicidal ideation/behaviors may be associated with treatment of bipolar disorder. Patients should be closely monitored, particularly early in treatment or during dosage changes. (5.6)
• Medication errors involving LAMICTAL have occurred. In particular the names LAMICTAL or lamotrigine can be confused with names of other commonly used medications. Medication errors may also occur between the different formulations of LAMICTAL. (3.4, 5.7, 16, 17.9)

—ADVERSE REACTIONS—

• Most common adverse reactions (incidence ≥10%) in adult epilepsy clinical studies were dizziness, headache, diplopia, ataxia, nausea, blurred vision, somnolence, rhinitis, and rash. Additional adverse reactions (incidence ≥10%) reported in children in epilepsy clinical studies included vomiting, infection, fever, accidental injury, pharyngitis, abdominal pain, and tremor. (6.1)

- Most common adverse reactions (incidence >5%) in adult bipolar clinical studies were nausea, insomnia, somnolence, back pain, fatigue, rash, rhinitis, abdominal pain, and xerostomia. (6.1)

To report SUSPECTED ADVERSE REACTIONS, contact GlaxoSmithKline at 1-888-825-5249 or FDA at 1-800-FDA-1088 or www.fda.gov/medwatch.

—————————DRUG INTERACTIONS—————————

- Valproate increases lamotrigine concentrations more than 2-fold. (7, 12.3)
- Carbamazepine, phenytoin, phenobarbital, and primidone decrease lamotrigine concentrations by approximately 40%. (7, 12.3)
- Oral estrogen-containing contraceptives and rifampin also decrease lamotrigine concentrations by approximately 50%. (7, 12.3)

—————————USE IN SPECIFIC POPULATIONS—————————

- Hepatic impairment: Dosage adjustments required. (2.1)
- Healthcare professionals can enroll patients in the Lamotrigine Pregnancy Registry (1-800-336-2176). Patients can enroll themselves in the North American Antiepileptic Drug Pregnancy Registry (1-888-233-2334). (8.1)
- Efficacy of LAMICTAL, used as adjunctive treatment for partial seizures, was not demonstrated in a small randomized, double-blind, placebo-controlled study in very young pediatric patients (1 to 24 months). (8.4)

Revised: September 2009
LMT:3PI

See 17 for PATIENT COUNSELING INFORMATION and Medication Guide

Revised: 10/2009

FULL PRESCRIBING INFORMATION: CONTENTS*
WARNING: SERIOUS SKIN RASHES

FULL PRESCRIBING INFORMATION

> **WARNING: SERIOUS SKIN RASHES**
> LAMICTAL® can cause serious rashes requiring hospitalization and discontinuation of treatment. The incidence of these rashes, which have included Stevens-Johnson syndrome, is approximately 0.8% (8 per 1,000) in pediatric patients (2 to 16 years of age) receiving LAMICTAL as adjunctive therapy for epilepsy and 0.3% (3 per 1,000) in adults on adjunctive therapy for epilepsy. In clinical trials of bipolar and other mood disorders, the rate of serious rash was 0.08% (0.8 per 1,000) in adult patients receiving LAMICTAL as initial monotherapy and 0.13% (1.3 per 1,000) in adult patients receiving LAMICTAL as adjunctive therapy. In a prospectively followed cohort of 1,983 pediatric patients (2 to 16 years of age) with epilepsy taking adjunctive LAMICTAL, there was 1 rash-related death. In worldwide postmarketing experience, rare cases of toxic epidermal necrolysis and/or rash-related death have been reported in adult and pediatric patients, but their numbers are too few to permit a precise estimate of the rate.
>
> Other than age, there are as yet no factors identified that are known to predict the risk of occurrence or the severity of rash caused by LAMICTAL. There are suggestions, yet to be proven, that the risk of rash may also be increased by (1) coadministration of LAMICTAL with valproate (includes valproic acid and divalproex sodium), (2) exceeding the recommended initial dose of LAMICTAL, or (3) exceeding the recommended dose escalation for LAMICTAL. However, cases have occurred in the absence of these factors.
>
> Nearly all cases of life-threatening rashes caused by LAMICTAL have occurred within 2 to 8 weeks of treatment initiation. However, isolated cases have occurred after prolonged treatment (e.g., 6 months). Accordingly, duration of therapy cannot be relied upon as means to predict the potential risk heralded by the first appearance of a rash.
>
> Although benign rashes are also caused by LAMICTAL, it is not possible to predict reliably which rashes will prove to be serious or life-threatening. Accordingly, LAMICTAL should ordinarily be discontinued at the first sign of rash, unless the rash is clearly not drug-related. Discontinuation of treatment may not prevent a rash from becoming life-threatening or permanently disabling or disfiguring [(see Warnings and Precautions (5.1)].

1 INDICATIONS AND USAGE

1.1 Epilepsy

Adjunctive Therapy: LAMICTAL is indicated as adjunctive therapy for the following seizure types in patients ≥2 years of age:

- partial seizures.
- primary generalized tonic-clonic seizures.
- generalized seizures of Lennox-Gastaut syndrome.

Monotherapy: LAMICTAL is indicated for conversion to monotherapy in adults (≥16 years of age) with partial seizures who are receiving treatment with carbamazepine, phenytoin, phenobarbital, primidone, or valproate as the single antiepileptic drug (AED).

Safety and effectiveness of LAMICTAL have not been established (1) as initial monotherapy; (2) for conversion to monotherapy from AEDs other than carbamazepine, phenytoin, phenobarbital, primidone, or valproate; or (3) for simultaneous conversion to monotherapy from 2 or more concomitant AEDs.

1.2 Bipolar Disorder

LAMICTAL is indicated for the maintenance treatment of Bipolar I Disorder to delay the time to occurrence of mood episodes (depression, mania, hypomania, mixed episodes) in adults (≥18 years of age) treated for acute mood episodes with standard therapy. The effectiveness of LAMICTAL in the acute treatment of mood episodes has not been established.

The effectiveness of LAMICTAL as maintenance treatment was established in 2 placebo-controlled trials in patients with Bipolar I Disorder as defined by DSM-IV [see Clinical Studies (14.2)]. The physician who elects to prescribe LAMICTAL for periods extending beyond 16 weeks should periodically re-evaluate the long-term usefulness of the drug for the individual patient.

2 DOSAGE AND ADMINISTRATION

2.1 General Dosing Considerations

Rash: There are suggestions, yet to be proven, that the risk of severe, potentially life-threatening rash may be increased by (1) coadministration of LAMICTAL with valproate, (2) exceeding the recommended initial dose of LAMICTAL, or (3) exceeding the recommended dose escalation for LAMICTAL. However, cases have occurred in the absence of these factors [see Boxed Warning]. Therefore, it is important that the dosing recommendations be followed closely.

The risk of nonserious rash may be increased when the recommended initial dose and/or the rate of dose escalation of LAMICTAL is exceeded and in patients with a history of allergy or rash to other AEDs.

LAMICTAL Starter Kits and LAMICTAL® ODT™ Patient Titration Kits provide LAMICTAL at doses consistent with the recommended titration schedule for the first 5 weeks of treatment, based upon concomitant medications, for patients with epilepsy (>12 years of age) and Bipolar I Disorder (≥18 years of age) and are intended to help reduce the potential for rash. The use of LAMICTAL Starter Kits and LAMICTAL ODT Patient Titration Kits is recommended for appropriate patients who are starting or restarting LAMICTAL [see How Supplied/Storage and Handling (16)]. It is recommended that LAMICTAL not be restarted in patients who discontinued due to rash associated with prior treatment with lamotrigine, unless the potential benefits clearly outweigh the risks. If the decision is made to restart a patient who has discontinued lamotrigine, the need to restart with the initial dosing recommendations should be assessed. The greater the interval of time since the previous dose, the greater consideration should be given to restarting with the initial dosing recommendations. If a patient has discontinued lamotrigine for a period of more than 5 half-lives, it is recommended that initial dosing recommendations and guidelines be followed. The half-life of lamotrigine is affected by other concomitant medications [see Clinical Pharmacology (12.3)].

LAMICTAL Added to Drugs Known to Induce or Inhibit Glucuronidation: Drugs other than those listed in the Clinical Pharmacology section [see Clinical Pharmacology (12.3)] have not been systematically evaluated in combination with lamotrigine. Because lamotrigine is metabolized predominantly by glucuronic acid conjugation, drugs that are known to induce or inhibit glucuronidation may affect the apparent clearance of lamotrigine and doses of LAMICTAL may require adjustment based on clinical response.

Target Plasma Levels for Patients With Epilepsy or Bipolar Disorder: A therapeutic plasma concentration range has not been established for lamotrigine. Dosing of LAMICTAL should be based on therapeutic response [see Clinical Pharmacology (12.3)].

Women Taking Estrogen-Containing Oral Contraceptives:
Starting LAMICTAL in Women Taking Estrogen-Containing Oral Contraceptives: Although estrogen-containing oral contraceptives have been shown to increase the clearance of lamotrigine [see Clinical Pharmacology (12.3)], no adjustments to the recommended dose-escalation guidelines for LAMICTAL should be necessary solely based on the use of estrogen-containing oral contraceptives. Therefore, dose escalation should follow the recommended guidelines for initiating adjunctive therapy with LAMICTAL based on the concomitant AED or other concomitant medications (see Table 1 or Table 5). See below for adjustments to maintenance doses of LAMICTAL in women taking estrogen-containing oral contraceptives.

Adjustments to the Maintenance Dose of LAMICTAL In Women Taking Estrogen-Containing Oral Contraceptives:
(1) Taking Estrogen-Containing Oral Contraceptives: For women not taking carbamazepine, phenytoin, phenobarbital, primidone, or other drugs such as rifampin that induce lamotrigine glucuronidation [see Drug Interactions (7), Clinical Pharmacology (12.3)], the maintenance dose of LAMICTAL will in most cases need to be increased, by as much as 2-fold over the recommended target maintenance dose, in order to maintain a consistent lamotrigine plasma level [see Clinical Pharmacology (12.3)].
(2) Starting Estrogen-Containing Oral Contraceptives: In women taking a stable dose of LAMICTAL and not taking carbamazepine, phenytoin, phenobarbital, primidone, or

Table 1. Escalation Regimen for LAMICTAL in Patients Over 12 Years of Age With Epilepsy

	For Patients TAKING Valproate[a]	For Patients NOT TAKING Carbamazepine, Phenytoin, Phenobarbital, Primidone,[b] or Valproate[a]	For Patients TAKING Carbamazepine, Phenytoin, Phenobarbital, or Primidone,[b] and NOT TAKING Valproate[a]
Weeks 1 and 2	25 mg every *other* day	25 mg every day	50 mg/day
Weeks 3 and 4	25 mg every day	50 mg/day	100 mg/day (in 2 divided doses)
Weeks 5 onwards to maintenance	Increase by 25 to 50 mg/day every 1 to 2 weeks	Increase by 50 mg/day every 1 to 2 weeks	Increase by 100 mg/day every 1 to 2 weeks.
Usual Maintenance Dose	100 to 200 mg/day with valproate alone 100 to 400 mg/day with valproate and other drugs that induce glucuronidation in 1 or 2 divided doses	225 to 375 mg/day (in 2 divided doses)	300 to 500 mg/day (in 2 divided doses)

[a] Valproate has been shown to inhibit glucuronidation and decrease the apparent clearance of lamotrigine *[see Drug Interactions (7), Clinical Pharmacology (12.3)].*
[b] These drugs induce lamotrigine glucuronidation and increase clearance *[see Drug Interactions (7), Clinical Pharmacology (12.3)].* Other drugs which have similar effects include estrogen-containing oral contraceptives *[see Drug Interactions (7), Clinical Pharmacology (12.3)].* Dosing recommendations for oral contraceptives can be found in General Dosing Considerations *[see Dosage and Administration (2.1)].* Patients on rifampin, or other drugs that induce lamotrigine glucuronidation and increase clearance, should follow the same dosing titration/maintenance regimen as that used with anticonvulsants that have this effect.

other drugs such as rifampin that induce lamotrigine glucuronidation *[see Drug Interactions (7), Clinical Pharmacology (12.3)],* the maintenance dose will in most cases need to be increased by as much as 2-fold in order to maintain a consistent lamotrigine plasma level. The dose increases should begin at the same time that the oral contraceptive is introduced and continue, based on clinical response, no more rapidly than 50 to 100 mg/day every week. Dose increases should not exceed the recommended rate (see Table 1 or Table 5) unless lamotrigine plasma levels or clinical response support larger increases. Gradual transient increases in lamotrigine plasma levels may occur during the week of inactive hormonal preparation ("pill-free" week), and these increases will be greater if dose increases are made in the days before or during the week of inactive hormonal preparation. Increased lamotrigine plasma levels could result in additional adverse reactions, such as dizziness, ataxia, and diplopia. If adverse reactions attributable to LAMICTAL consistently occur during the "pill-free" week, dose adjustments to the overall maintenance dose may be necessary. Dose adjustments limited to the "pill-free" week are not recommended. For women taking LAMICTAL in addition to carbamazepine, phenytoin, phenobarbital, primidone, or other drugs such as rifampin that induce lamotrigine glucuronidation *[see Drug Interactions (7), Clinical Pharmacology (12.3)],* no adjustment to the dose of LAMICTAL should be necessary.
(3) Stopping Estrogen-Containing Oral Contraceptives: For women not taking carbamazepine, phenytoin, phenobarbital, primidone, or other drugs such as rifampin that induce lamotrigine glucuronidation *[see Drug Interactions (7), Clinical Pharmacology (12.3)],* the maintenance dose of LAMICTAL will in most cases need to be decreased by as much as 50% in order to maintain a consistent lamotrigine plasma level. The decrease in dose of LAMICTAL should not exceed 25% of the total daily dose per week over a 2-week period, unless clinical response or lamotrigine plasma levels indicate otherwise *[see Clinical Pharmacology (12.3)].* For women taking LAMICTAL in addition to carbamazepine, phenytoin, phenobarbital, primidone, or other drugs such as rifampin that induce lamotrigine glucuronidation *[see Drug Interactions (7), Clinical Pharmacology (12.3)],* no adjustment to the dose of LAMICTAL should be necessary.
Women and Other Hormonal Contraceptive Preparations or Hormone Replacement Therapy: The effect of other hormonal contraceptive preparations or hormone replacement therapy on the pharmacokinetics of lamotrigine has not been systematically evaluated. It has been reported that ethinylestradiol, not progestogens, increased the clearance of lamotrigine up to 2-fold, and the progestin-only pills had no effect on lamotrigine plasma levels. Therefore, adjustments to the dosage of LAMICTAL in the presence of progestogens alone will likely not be needed.
Patients With Hepatic Impairment: Experience in patients with hepatic impairment is limited. Based on a clinical pharmacology study in 24 patients with mild, moderate, and severe liver impairment *[see Use in Specific Populations*

(8.6), Clinical Pharmacology (12.3)], the following general recommendations can be made. No dosage adjustment is needed in patients with mild liver impairment. Initial, escalation, and maintenance doses should generally be reduced by approximately 25% in patients with moderate and severe liver impairment without ascites and 50% in patients with severe liver impairment with ascites. Escalation and maintenance doses may be adjusted according to clinical response.
Patients With Renal Impairment: Initial doses of LAMICTAL should be based on patients' concomitant medications (see Tables 1-3 or Table 5); reduced maintenance doses may be effective for patients with significant renal impairment *[see Use in Specific Populations (8.7), Clinical Pharmacology (12.3)].* Few patients with severe renal impairment have been evaluated during chronic treatment with LAMICTAL. Because there is inadequate experience in this population, LAMICTAL should be used with caution in these patients.
Discontinuation Strategy: *Epilepsy:* For patients receiving LAMICTAL in combination with other AEDs, a re-evaluation of all AEDs in the regimen should be considered if a change in seizure control or an appearance or worsening of adverse experiences is observed.
If a decision is made to discontinue therapy with LAMICTAL, a step-wise reduction of dose over at least 2 weeks (approximately 50% per week) is recommended unless safety concerns require a more rapid withdrawal *[see Warnings and Precautions (5.9)].*
Discontinuing carbamazepine, phenytoin, phenobarbital, primidone, or other drugs such as rifampin that induce lamotrigine glucuronidation, should prolong the half-life of lamotrigine; discontinuing valproate should shorten the half-life of lamotrigine.
Bipolar Disorder: In the controlled clinical trials, there was no increase in the incidence, type, or severity of adverse reactions following abrupt termination of LAMICTAL. In clinical trials in patients with Bipolar Disorder, 2 patients experienced seizures shortly after abrupt withdrawal of LAMICTAL. However, there were confounding factors that may have contributed to the occurrence of seizures in these bipolar patients. Discontinuation of LAMICTAL should involve a step-wise reduction of dose over at least 2 weeks (approximately 50% per week) unless safety concerns require a more rapid withdrawal *[see Warnings and Precautions (5.9)].*
2.2   Epilepsy – Adjunctive Therapy
This section provides specific dosing recommendations for patients greater than 12 years of age and patients 2 to 12 years of age. Within each of these age-groups, specific dosing recommendations are provided depending upon concomitant AED or other concomitant medications (Table 1 for patients greater than 12 years of age and Table 2 for patients 2 to 12 years of age). A weight-based dosing guide for patients 2 to 12 years of age on concomitant valproate is provided in Table 3.
Patients Over 12 Years of Age: Recommended dosing guidelines are summarized in Table 1.

[See table 1 at left]
Patients 2 to 12 Years of Age: Recommended dosing guidelines are summarized in Table 2.
Smaller starting doses and slower dose escalations than those used in clinical trials are recommended because of the suggestion that the risk of rash may be decreased by smaller starting doses and slower dose escalations. Therefore, maintenance doses will take longer to reach in clinical practice than in clinical trials. It may take several weeks to months to achieve an individualized maintenance dose. Maintenance doses in patients weighing less than 30 kg, regardless of age or concomitant AED, may need to be increased as much as 50%, based on clinical response.
The smallest available strength of LAMICTAL Chewable Dispersible Tablets is 2 mg, and only whole tablets should be administered. If the calculated dose cannot be achieved using whole tablets, the dose should be rounded down to the nearest whole tablet *[see How Supplied/Storage and Handling (16) and Medication Guide].*
[See table 2 at top of next page]
[See table 3 on next page]
Usual Adjunctive Maintenance Dose for Epilepsy: The usual maintenance doses identified in Tables 1 and 2 are derived from dosing regimens employed in the placebo-controlled adjunctive studies in which the efficacy of LAMICTAL was established. In patients receiving multidrug regimens employing carbamazepine, phenytoin, phenobarbital, or primidone **without valproate**, maintenance doses of adjunctive LAMICTAL as high as 700 mg/day have been used. In patients receiving **valproate alone**, maintenance doses of adjunctive LAMICTAL as high as 200 mg/day have been used. The advantage of using doses above those recommended in Tables 1 through 4 has not been established in controlled trials.
2.3   Epilepsy – Conversion From Adjunctive Therapy to Monotherapy
The goal of the transition regimen is to effect the conversion to monotherapy with LAMICTAL under conditions that ensure adequate seizure control while mitigating the risk of serious rash associated with the rapid titration of LAMICTAL.
The recommended maintenance dose of LAMICTAL as monotherapy is 500 mg/day given in 2 divided doses.
To avoid an increased risk of rash, the recommended initial dose and subsequent dose escalations of LAMICTAL should not be exceeded *[see Boxed Warning].*
Conversion From Adjunctive Therapy With Carbamazepine, Phenytoin, Phenobarbital, or Primidone to Monotherapy With LAMICTAL: After achieving a dose of 500 mg/day of LAMICTAL according to the guidelines in Table 1, the concomitant AED should be withdrawn by 20% decrements each week over a 4-week period. The regimen for the withdrawal of the concomitant AED is based on experience gained in the controlled monotherapy clinical trial.
Conversion From Adjunctive Therapy With Valproate to Monotherapy With LAMICTAL: The conversion regimen involves 4 steps outlined in Table 4.
[See table 4 at top of page 1440]
Conversion From Adjunctive Therapy With AEDs Other Than Carbamazepine, Phenytoin, Phenobarbital, Primidone, or Valproate to Monotherapy With LAMICTAL: No specific dosing guidelines can be provided for conversion to monotherapy with LAMICTAL with AEDs other than carbamazepine, phenobarbital, phenytoin, primidone, or valproate.
2.4   Bipolar Disorder
The goal of maintenance treatment with LAMICTAL is to delay the time to occurrence of mood episodes (depression, mania, hypomania, mixed episodes) in patients treated for acute mood episodes with standard therapy. The target dose of LAMICTAL is 200 mg/day (100 mg/day in patients taking valproate, which decreases the apparent clearance of lamotrigine, and 400 mg/day in patients not taking valproate and taking either carbamazepine, phenytoin, phenobarbital, primidone, or other drugs such as rifampin that increase the apparent clearance of lamotrigine). In the clinical trials, doses up to 400 mg/day as monotherapy were evaluated; however, no additional benefit was seen at 400 mg/day compared with 200 mg/day *[see Clinical Studies (14.2)].* Accordingly, doses above 200 mg/day are not recommended. Treatment with LAMICTAL is introduced, based on concurrent medications, according to the regimen outlined in Table 5. If other psychotropic medications are withdrawn following stabilization, the dose of LAMICTAL should be adjusted. For patients discontinuing valproate, the dose of LAMICTAL should be doubled over a 2-week period in equal weekly increments (see Table 6). For patients discontinuing carbamazepine, phenytoin, phenobarbital, primidone, or other drugs such as rifampin that induce lamotrigine glucuronidation, the dose of LAMICTAL should remain constant for the first week and then should be decreased by half over a 2-week period in equal weekly decre-

ments (see Table 6). The dose of LAMICTAL may then be further adjusted to the target dose (200 mg) as clinically indicated.

If other drugs are subsequently introduced, the dose of LAMICTAL may need to be adjusted. In particular, the introduction of valproate requires reduction in the dose of LAMICTAL [see Drug Interactions (7), Clinical Pharmacology (12.3)].

To avoid an increased risk of rash, the recommended initial dose and subsequent dose escalations of LAMICTAL should not be exceeded [see Boxed Warning].

[See table 5 on next page]
[See table 6 on next page]

The benefit of continuing treatment in patients who had been stabilized in an 8- to 16-week open-label phase with LAMICTAL was established in 2 randomized, placebo-controlled clinical maintenance trials [see Clinical Studies (14.2)]. However, the optimal duration of treatment with LAMICTAL has not been established. Thus, patients should be periodically reassessed to determine the need for maintenance treatment.

2.5 Administration of LAMICTAL Chewable Dispersible Tablets

LAMICTAL Chewable Dispersible Tablets may be swallowed whole, chewed, or dispersed in water or diluted fruit juice. If the tablets are chewed, consume a small amount of water or diluted fruit juice to aid in swallowing.

To disperse LAMICTAL Chewable Dispersible Tablets, add the tablets to a small amount of liquid (1 teaspoon, or enough to cover the medication). Approximately 1 minute later, when the tablets are completely dispersed, swirl the solution and consume the entire quantity immediately. *No attempt should be made to administer partial quantities of the dispersed tablets.*

2.6 Administration of LAMICTAL ODT Orally Disintegrating Tablets

LAMICTAL ODT Orally Disintegrating Tablets should be placed onto the tongue and moved around in the mouth. The tablet will disintegrate rapidly, can be swallowed with or without water, and can be taken with or without food.

3 DOSAGE FORMS AND STRENGTHS

3.1 Tablets

25 mg, white, scored, shield-shaped tablets debossed with "LAMICTAL" and "25"

100 mg, peach, scored, shield-shaped tablets debossed with "LAMICTAL" and "100"

150 mg, cream, scored, shield-shaped tablets debossed with "LAMICTAL" and "150"

200 mg, blue, scored, shield-shaped tablets debossed with "LAMICTAL" and "200"

3.2 Chewable Dispersible Tablets

2 mg, white to off-white, round tablets debossed with "LTG" over "2"

5 mg, white to off-white, caplet-shaped tablets debossed with "GX CL2"

25 mg, white, super elliptical-shaped tablets debossed with "GX CL5"

3.3 Orally Disintegrating Tablets

25 mg, white to off-white, round, flat-faced, radius edge, tablets debossed with "LMT" on one side and "25" on the other side.

50 mg, white to off-white, round, flat-faced, radius edge, tablets debossed with "LMT" on one side and "50" on the other side.

100 mg, white to off-white, round, flat-faced, radius edge, tablets debossed with "LAMICTAL" on one side and "100" on the other side.

200 mg, white to off-white, round, flat-faced, radius edge, tablets debossed with "LAMICTAL" on one side and "200" on the other side.

3.4 Potential Medication Errors

Patients should be strongly advised to visually inspect their tablets to verify that they are receiving LAMICTAL as well as the correct formulation of LAMICTAL each time they fill their prescription. Depictions of the LAMICTAL Tablets, Chewable Dispersible Tablets, and Orally Disintegrating Tablets can be found in the Medication Guide that accompanies the product.

4 CONTRAINDICATIONS

LAMICTAL is contraindicated in patients who have demonstrated hypersensitivity to the drug or its ingredients [see Boxed Warning, Warnings and Precautions (5.1), (5.2)].

5 WARNINGS AND PRECAUTIONS

5.1 Serious Skin Rashes [see Boxed Warning]

Pediatric Population: The incidence of serious rash associated with hospitalization and discontinuation of LAMICTAL in a prospectively followed cohort of pediatric patients (2 to 16 years of age) with epilepsy receiving adjunctive therapy was approximately 0.8% (16 of 1,983). When 14 of these cases were reviewed by 3 expert dermatologists, there was considerable disagreement as to their proper classification. To illustrate, one dermatologist consid-

Table 2. Escalation Regimen for LAMICTAL in Patients 2 to 12 Years of Age With Epilepsy

	For Patients TAKING Valproate[a]	For Patients NOT TAKING Carbamazepine, Phenytoin, Phenobarbital, Primidone[b], or Valproate[a]	For Patients TAKING Carbamazepine, Phenytoin, Phenobarbital, or Primidone[b] and NOT TAKING Valproate[a]
Weeks 1 and 2	**0.15 mg/kg/day** in 1 or 2 divided doses, rounded down to the nearest whole tablet (see Table 3 for weight based dosing guide)	**0.3 mg/kg/day** in 1 or 2 divided doses, rounded down to the nearest whole tablet	**0.6 mg/kg/day** in 2 divided doses, rounded down to the nearest whole tablet
Weeks 3 and 4	**0.3 mg/kg/day** in 1 or 2 divided doses, rounded down to the nearest whole tablet (see Table 3 for weight based dosing guide)	**0.6 mg/kg/day** in 2 divided doses, rounded down to the nearest whole tablet	**1.2 mg/kg/day** in 2 divided doses, rounded down to the nearest whole tablet
Weeks 5 onwards to maintenance	The dose should be increased every 1 to 2 weeks as follows: calculate 0.3 mg/kg/day, round this amount down to the nearest whole tablet, and add this amount to the previously administered daily dose	The dose should be increased every 1 to 2 weeks as follows: calculate 0.6 mg/kg/day, round this amount down to the nearest whole tablet, and add this amount to the previously administered daily dose	The dose should be increased every 1 to 2 weeks as follows: calculate 1.2 mg/kg/day, round this amount down to the nearest whole tablet, and add this amount to the previously administered daily dose
Usual Maintenance Dose	**1 to 5 mg/kg/day** (maximum 200 mg/day in 1 or 2 divided doses). **1 to 3 mg/kg/day** with valproate alone	**4.5 to 7.5 mg/kg/day** (maximum 300 mg/day in 2 divided doses)	**5 to 15 mg/kg/day** (maximum 400 mg/day in 2 divided doses)
Maintenance dose in patients less than 30 kg	May need to be increased by as much as 50%, based on clinical response	May need to be increased by as much as 50%, based on clinical response	May need to be increased by as much as 50%, based on clinical response

Note: Only whole tablets should be used for dosing.

[a] Valproate has been shown to inhibit glucuronidation and decrease the apparent clearance of lamotrigine [see Drug Interactions (7), Clinical Pharmacology (12.3)].

[b] These drugs induce lamotrigine glucuronidation and increase clearance [see Drug Interactions (7), Clinical Pharmacology (12.3)]. Other drugs which have similar effects include estrogen-containing oral contraceptives [see Drug Interactions (7), Clinical Pharmacology (12.3)]. Dosing recommendations for oral contraceptives can be found in General Dosing Considerations [see Dosage and Administration (2.1)]. Patients on rifampin, or other drugs that induce lamotrigine glucuronidation and increase clearance, should follow the same dosing titration/maintenance regimen as that used with anticonvulsants that have this effect.

Table 3. The Initial Weight-Based Dosing Guide for Patients 2 to 12 Years Taking Valproate (Weeks 1 to 4) With Epilepsy

If the patient's weight is		Give this daily dose, using the most appropriate combination of LAMICTAL 2-mg and 5-mg tablets	
Greater than	And less than	Weeks 1 and 2	Weeks 3 and 4
6.7 kg	14 kg	2 mg every *other* day	2 mg every day
14.1 kg	27 kg	2 mg every day	4 mg every day
27.1 kg	34 kg	4 mg every day	8 mg every day
34.1 kg	40 kg	5 mg every day	10 mg every day

ered none of the cases to be Stevens-Johnson syndrome; another assigned 7 of the 14 to this diagnosis. There was 1 rash-related death in this 1,983-patient cohort. Additionally, there have been rare cases of toxic epidermal necrolysis with and without permanent sequelae and/or death in US and foreign postmarketing experience.

There is evidence that the inclusion of valproate in a multidrug regimen increases the risk of serious, potentially life-threatening rash in pediatric patients. In pediatric patients who used valproate concomitantly, 1.2% (6 of 482) experienced a serious rash compared with 0.6% (6 of 952) patients not taking valproate.

Adult Population: Serious rash associated with hospitalization and discontinuation of LAMICTAL occurred in 0.3% (11 of 3,348) of adult patients who received LAMICTAL in premarketing clinical trials of epilepsy. In the bipolar and other mood disorders clinical trials, the rate of serious rash was 0.08% (1 of 1,233) of adult patients who received LAMICTAL as initial monotherapy and 0.13% (2 of 1,538) of adult patients who received LAMICTAL as adjunctive ther-

apy. No fatalities occurred among these individuals. However, in worldwide postmarketing experience, rare cases of rash-related death have been reported, but their numbers are too few to permit a precise estimate of the rate.

Among the rashes leading to hospitalization were Stevens-Johnson syndrome, toxic epidermal necrolysis, angioedema, and a rash associated with a variable number of the following systemic manifestations: fever, lymphadenopathy, facial swelling, and hematologic and hepatologic abnormalities. There is evidence that the inclusion of valproate in a multidrug regimen increases the risk of serious, potentially life-threatening rash in adults. Specifically, of 584 patients administered LAMICTAL with valproate in epilepsy clinical trials, 6 (1%) were hospitalized in association with rash; in contrast, 4 (0.16%) of 2,398 clinical trial patients and volunteers administered LAMICTAL in the absence of valproate were hospitalized.

Patients With History of Allergy or Rash to Other AEDs: The risk of nonserious rash may be increased when the recommended initial dose and/or the rate of dose escalation of

Table 4. Conversion From Adjunctive Therapy With Valproate to Monotherapy With LAMICTAL in Patients ≥16 Years of Age with Epilepsy

	LAMICTAL	Valproate
Step 1	Achieve a dose of 200 mg/day according to guidelines in Table 1 (if not already on 200 mg/day).	Maintain previous stable dose.
Step 2	Maintain at 200 mg/day.	Decrease to 500 mg/day by decrements no greater than 500 mg/day/week and then maintain the dose of 500 mg/day for 1 week.
Step 3	Increase to 300 mg/day and maintain for 1 week.	Simultaneously decrease to 250 mg/day and maintain for 1 week.
Step 4	Increase by 100 mg/day every week to achieve maintenance dose of 500 mg/day.	Discontinue.

Table 5. Escalation Regimen for LAMICTAL for Patients With Bipolar Disorder

	For Patients TAKING Valproate[a]	For Patients NOT TAKING Carbamazepine, Phenytoin, Phenobarbital, Primidone,[b] or Valproate[a]	For Patients TAKING Carbamazepine, Phenytoin, Phenobarbital, or Primidone[b] and NOT TAKING Valproate[a]
Weeks 1 and 2	25 mg every *other* day	25 mg daily	50 mg daily
Weeks 3 and 4	25 mg daily	50 mg daily	100 mg daily, in divided doses
Week 5	50 mg daily	100 mg daily	200 mg daily, in divided doses
Week 6	100 mg daily	200 mg daily	300 mg daily, in divided doses
Week 7	100 mg daily	200 mg daily	up to 400 mg daily, in divided doses

[a] Valproate has been shown to inhibit glucuronidation and decrease the apparent clearance of lamotrigine *[see Drug Interactions (7), Clinical Pharmacology (12.3)]*.
[b] These drugs induce lamotrigine glucuronidation and increase clearance *[see Drug Interactions (7), Clinical Pharmacology (12.3)]*. Other drugs which have similar effects include estrogen-containing oral contraceptives *[see Drug Interactions (7), Clinical Pharmacology (12.3)]*. Dosing recommendations for oral contraceptives can be found in General Dosing Considerations *[see Dosage and Administration (2.1)]*. Patients on rifampin, or other drugs that induce lamotrigine glucuronidation and increase clearance, should follow the same dosing titration/maintenance regimen as that used with anticonvulsants that have this effect.

Table 6. Dosage Adjustments to LAMICTAL for Patients With Bipolar Disorder Following Discontinuation of Psychotropic Medications

	Discontinuation of Psychotropic Drugs (excluding Carbamazepine, Phenytoin, Phenobarbital, Primidone,[b] or Valproate[a])	After Discontinuation of Valproate[a]	After Discontinuation of Carbamazepine, Phenytoin, Phenobarbital, or Primidone[b]
		Current dose of LAMICTAL (mg/day) 100	Current dose of LAMICTAL (mg/day) 400
Week 1	Maintain current dose of LAMICTAL	150	400
Week 2	Maintain current dose of LAMICTAL	200	300
Week 3 onward	Maintain current dose of LAMICTAL	200	200

[a] Valproate has been shown to inhibit glucuronidation and decrease the apparent clearance of lamotrigine *[see Drug Interactions (7), Clinical Pharmacology (12.3)]*.
[b] These drugs induce lamotrigine glucuronidation and increase clearance *[see Drug Interactions (7), Clinical Pharmacology (12.3)]*. Other drugs which have similar effects include estrogen-containing oral contraceptives *[see Drug Interactions (7), Clinical Pharmacology (12.3)]*. Dosing recommendations for oral contraceptives can be found in General Dosing Considerations *[see Dosage and Administration (2.1)]*. Patients on rifampin, or other drugs that induce lamotrigine glucuronidation and increase clearance, should follow the same dosing titration/maintenance regimen as that used with anticonvulsants that have this effect.

LAMICTAL is exceeded and in patients with a history of allergy or rash to other AEDs.

5.2 Hypersensitivity Reactions
Hypersensitivity reactions, some fatal or life-threatening, have also occurred. Some of these reactions have included clinical features of multiorgan failure/dysfunction, including hepatic abnormalities and evidence of disseminated intravascular coagulation. It is important to note that early manifestations of hypersensitivity (e.g., fever, lymphadenopathy) may be present even though a rash is not evident. If such signs or symptoms are present, the patient should be evaluated immediately. LAMICTAL should be discontinued if an alternative etiology for the signs or symptoms cannot be established.

Prior to initiation of treatment with LAMICTAL, the patient should be instructed that a rash or other signs or symptoms of hypersensitivity (e.g., fever, lymphadenopathy) may herald a serious medical event and that the patient should report any such occurrence to a physician immediately.

5.3 Acute Multiorgan Failure
Multiorgan failure, which in some cases has been fatal or irreversible, has been observed in patients receiving LAMICTAL. Fatalities associated with multiorgan failure and various degrees of hepatic failure have been reported in 2 of 3,796 adult patients and 4 of 2,435 pediatric patients who received LAMICTAL in epilepsy clinical trials. No such fatalities have been reported in bipolar patients in clinical trials. Rare fatalities from multiorgan failure have also been reported in compassionate plea and postmarketing use. The majority of these deaths occurred in association with other serious medical events, including status epilepticus and overwhelming sepsis, and hantavirus, making it difficult to identify the initial cause.

Additionally, 3 patients (a 45-year-old woman, a 3.5-year-old boy, and an 11-year-old girl) developed multiorgan dysfunction and disseminated intravascular coagulation 9 to 14 days after LAMICTAL was added to their AED regimens. Rash and elevated transaminases were also present in all patients and rhabdomyolysis was noted in 2 patients. Both pediatric patients were receiving concomitant therapy with valproate, while the adult patient was being treated with carbamazepine and clonazepam. All patients subsequently recovered with supportive care after treatment with LAMICTAL was discontinued.

5.4 Blood Dyscrasias
There have been reports of blood dyscrasias that may or may not be associated with the hypersensitivity syndrome. These have included neutropenia, leukopenia, anemia, thrombocytopenia, pancytopenia, and, rarely, aplastic anemia and pure red cell aplasia.

5.5 Suicidal Behavior and Ideation
Antiepileptic drugs (AEDs), including LAMICTAL, increase the risk of suicidal thoughts or behavior in patients taking these drugs for any indication. Patients treated with any AED for any indication should be monitored for the emergence or worsening of depression, suicidal thoughts or behavior, and/or any unusual changes in mood or behavior.

Pooled analyses of 199 placebo-controlled clinical trials (mono- and adjunctive therapy) of 11 different AEDs showed that patients randomized to one of the AEDs had approximately twice the risk (adjusted Relative Risk 1.8, 95% CI: 1.2, 2.7) of suicidal thinking or behavior compared to patients randomized to placebo. In these trials, which had a median treatment duration of 12 weeks, the estimated incidence of suicidal behavior or ideation among 27,863 AED-treated patients was 0.43%, compared to 0.24% among 16,029 placebo-treated patients, representing an increase of approximately 1 case of suicidal thinking or behavior for every 530 patients treated. There were 4 suicides in drug-treated patients in the trials and none in placebo-treated patients, but the number of events is too small to allow any conclusion about drug effect on suicide.

The increased risk of suicidal thoughts or behavior with AEDs was observed as early as 1 week after starting treatment with AEDs and persisted for the duration of treatment assessed. Because most trials included in the analysis did not extend beyond 24 weeks, the risk of suicidal thoughts or behavior beyond 24 weeks could not be assessed.

The risk of suicidal thoughts or behavior was generally consistent among drugs in the data analyzed. The finding of increased risk with AEDs of varying mechanism of action and across a range of indications suggests that the risk applies to all AEDs used for any indication. The risk did not vary substantially by age (5 to 100 years) in the clinical trials analyzed.

Table 7 shows absolute and relative risk by indication for all evaluated AEDs.

[See table 7 at top of next page]

The relative risk for suicidal thoughts or behavior was higher in clinical trials for epilepsy than in clinical trials for psychiatric or other conditions, but the absolute risk differences were similar for the epilepsy and psychiatric indications.

Anyone considering prescribing LAMICTAL or any other AED must balance the risk of suicidal thoughts or behavior with the risk of untreated illness. Epilepsy and many other illnesses for which AEDs are prescribed are themselves associated with morbidity and mortality and an increased risk of suicidal thoughts and behavior. Should suicidal thoughts and behavior emerge during treatment, the prescriber needs to consider whether the emergence of these symptoms in any given patient may be related to the illness being treated.

Patients, their caregivers, and families should be informed that AEDs increase the risk of suicidal thoughts and behavior and should be advised of the need to be alert for the emergence or worsening of the signs and symptoms of depression, any unusual changes in mood or behavior, or the emergence of suicidal thoughts, behavior, or thoughts about self-harm. Behaviors of concern should be reported immediately to healthcare providers.

5.6 Use in Patients With Bipolar Disorder

Acute Treatment of Mood Episodes: Safety and effectiveness of LAMICTAL in the acute treatment of mood episodes have not been established.

Children and Adolescents (less than 18 years of age): Safety and effectiveness of LAMICTAL in patients below the age of 18 years with mood disorders have not been established [see Suicidal Behavior and Ideation (5.5)].

Clinical Worsening and Suicide Risk Associated With Bipolar Disorder: Patients with bipolar disorder may experience worsening of their depressive symptoms and/or the emergence of suicidal ideation and behaviors (suicidality) whether or not they are taking medications for bipolar disorder. Patients should be closely monitored for clinical worsening (including development of new symptoms) and suicidality, especially at the beginning of a course of treatment or at the time of dose changes.

In addition, patients with a history of suicidal behavior or thoughts, those patients exhibiting a significant degree of suicidal ideation prior to commencement of treatment, and young adults are at an increased risk of suicidal thoughts or suicide attempts, and should receive careful monitoring during treatment [see Suicidal Behavior and Ideation (5.5)]. Consideration should be given to changing the therapeutic regimen, including possibly discontinuing the medication, in patients who experience clinical worsening (including development of new symptoms) and/or the emergence of suicidal ideation/behavior especially if these symptoms are severe, abrupt in onset, or were not part of the patient's presenting symptoms.

Prescriptions for LAMICTAL should be written for the smallest quantity of tablets consistent with good patient management in order to reduce the risk of overdose. Overdoses have been reported for LAMICTAL, some of which have been fatal [see Overdosage (10.1)].

5.7 Potential Medication Errors

Medication errors involving LAMICTAL have occurred. In particular, the names LAMICTAL or lamotrigine can be confused with the names of other commonly used medications. Medication errors may also occur between the different formulations of LAMICTAL. To reduce the potential of medication errors, write and say LAMICTAL clearly. Depictions of the LAMICTAL Tablets, Chewable Dispersible Tablets, and Orally Disintegrating Tablets can be found in the Medication Guide that accompanies the product to highlight the distinctive markings, colors, and shapes that serve to identify the different presentations of the drug and thus may help reduce the risk of medication errors. To avoid the medication error of using the wrong drug or formulation, patients should be strongly advised to visually inspect their tablets to verify that they are LAMICTAL, as well as the correct formulation of LAMICTAL, each time they fill their prescription.

5.8 Concomitant Use With Oral Contraceptives

Some estrogen-containing oral contraceptives have been shown to decrease serum concentrations of lamotrigine [see Clinical Pharmacology (12.3)]. Dosage adjustments will be necessary in most patients who start or stop estrogen-containing oral contraceptives while taking LAMICTAL [see Dosage and Administration (2.1)]. During the week of inactive hormone preparation ("pill-free" week) of oral contraceptive therapy, plasma lamotrigine levels are expected to rise, as much as doubling at the end of the week. Adverse reactions consistent with elevated levels of lamotrigine, such as dizziness, ataxia, and diplopia, could occur.

5.9 Withdrawal Seizures

As with other AEDs, LAMICTAL should not be abruptly discontinued. In patients with epilepsy there is a possibility of increasing seizure frequency. In clinical trials in patients with Bipolar Disorder, 2 patients experienced seizures shortly after abrupt withdrawal of LAMICTAL; however, there were confounding factors that may have contributed to the occurrence of seizures in these bipolar patients. Unless safety concerns require a more rapid withdrawal, the dose of LAMICTAL should be tapered over a period of at least 2 weeks (approximately 50% reduction per week) [see Dosage and Administration (2.1)].

5.10 Status Epilepticus

Valid estimates of the incidence of treatment-emergent status epilepticus among patients treated with LAMICTAL are difficult to obtain because reporters participating in clinical trials did not all employ identical rules for identifying cases. At a minimum, 7 of 2,343 adult patients had episodes that could unequivocally be described as status epilepticus. In addition, a number of reports of variably defined episodes of seizure exacerbation (e.g., seizure clusters, seizure flurries, etc.) were made.

5.11 Sudden Unexplained Death in Epilepsy (SUDEP)

During the premarketing development of LAMICTAL, 20 sudden and unexplained deaths were recorded among a cohort of 4,700 patients with epilepsy (5,747 patient-years of exposure).

Table 7. Risk by Indication for Antiepileptic Drugs in the Pooled Analysis

Indication	Placebo Patients With Events Per 1,000 Patients	Drug Patients With Events Per 1,000 Patients	Relative Risk: Incidence of Events in Drug Patients/ Incidence in Placebo Patients	Risk Difference: Additional Drug Patients With Events Per 1,000 Patients
Epilepsy	1.0	3.4	3.5	2.4
Psychiatric	5.7	8.5	1.5	2.9
Other	1.0	1.8	1.9	0.9
Total	2.4	4.3	1.8	1.9

Some of these could represent seizure-related deaths in which the seizure was not observed, e.g., at night. This represents an incidence of 0.0035 deaths per patient-year. Although this rate exceeds that expected in a healthy population matched for age and sex, it is within the range of estimates for the incidence of sudden unexplained deaths in patients with epilepsy not receiving LAMICTAL (ranging from 0.0005 for the general population of patients with epilepsy, to 0.004 for a recently studied clinical trial population similar to that in the clinical development program for LAMICTAL, to 0.005 for patients with refractory epilepsy). Consequently, whether these figures are reassuring or suggest concern depends on the comparability of the populations reported upon to the cohort receiving LAMICTAL and the accuracy of the estimates provided. Probably most reassuring is the similarity of estimated SUDEP rates in patients receiving LAMICTAL and those receiving other AEDs, chemically unrelated to each other, that underwent clinical testing in similar populations. Importantly, that drug is chemically unrelated to LAMICTAL. This evidence suggests, although it certainly does not prove, that the high SUDEP rates reflect population rates, not a drug effect.

5.12 Addition of LAMICTAL to a Multidrug Regimen That Includes Valproate

Because valproate reduces the clearance of lamotrigine, the dosage of lamotrigine in the presence of valproate is less than half of that required in its absence.

5.13 Binding in the Eye and Other Melanin-Containing Tissues

Because lamotrigine binds to melanin, it could accumulate in melanin-rich tissues over time. This raises the possibility that lamotrigine may cause toxicity in these tissues after extended use. Although ophthalmological testing was performed in one controlled clinical trial, the testing was inadequate to exclude subtle effects or injury occurring after long-term exposure. Moreover, the capacity of available tests to detect potentially adverse consequences, if any, of lamotrigine's binding to melanin is unknown [see Clinical Pharmacology (12.2)].

Accordingly, although there are no specific recommendations for periodic ophthalmological monitoring, prescribers should be aware of the possibility of long-term ophthalmologic effects.

5.14 Laboratory Tests

The value of monitoring plasma concentrations of lamotrigine in patients treated with LAMICTAL has not been established. Because of the possible pharmacokinetic interactions between lamotrigine and other drugs including AEDs (see Table 15), monitoring of the plasma levels of lamotrigine and concomitant drugs may be indicated, particularly during dosage adjustments. In general, clinical judgment should be exercised regarding monitoring of plasma levels of lamotrigine and other drugs and whether or not dosage adjustments are necessary.

6 ADVERSE REACTIONS

The following adverse reactions are described in more detail in the Warnings and Precautions section of the label:

• Serious skin rashes [see Warnings and Precautions (5.1)]
• Hypersensitivity reactions [see Warnings and Precautions (5.2)]
• Acute multiorgan failure [see Warnings and Precautions (5.3)]
• Blood dyscrasias [see Warnings and Precautions (5.4)]
• Suicidal behavior and ideation [see Warnings and Precautions (5.5)]
• Withdrawal seizures [see Warnings and Precautions (5.9)]
• Status epilepticus [see Warnings and Precautions (5.10)]
• Sudden unexplained death in epilepsy [see Warnings and Precautions (5.11)]

6.1 Clinical Trials

Because clinical trials are conducted under widely varying conditions, adverse reaction rates observed in the clinical trials of a drug cannot be directly compared with rates in the clinical trials of another drug and may not reflect the rates observed in practice.

LAMICTAL has been evaluated for safety in patients with epilepsy and in patients with Bipolar I Disorder. Adverse

reactions reported for each of these patient populations are provided below. Excluded are adverse reactions considered too general to be informative and those not reasonably attributable to the use of the drug.

Epilepsy: Most Common Adverse Reactions in All Clinical Studies: Adjunctive Therapy in Adults With Epilepsy: The most commonly observed (≥5% for LAMICTAL and more common on drug than placebo) adverse reactions seen in association with LAMICTAL during adjunctive therapy in adults and not seen at an equivalent frequency among placebo-treated patients were: dizziness, ataxia, somnolence, headache, diplopia, blurred vision, nausea, vomiting, and rash. Dizziness, diplopia, ataxia, blurred vision, nausea, and vomiting were dose-related. Dizziness, diplopia, ataxia, and blurred vision occurred more commonly in patients receiving carbamazepine with LAMICTAL than in patients receiving other AEDs with LAMICTAL. Clinical data suggest a higher incidence of rash, including serious rash, in patients receiving concomitant valproate than in patients not receiving valproate [see Warnings and Precautions (5.1)].

Approximately 11% of the 3,378 adult patients who received LAMICTAL as adjunctive therapy in premarketing clinical trials discontinued treatment because of an adverse reaction. The adverse reactions most commonly associated with discontinuation were rash (3.0%), dizziness (2.8%), and headache (2.5%).

In a dose-response study in adults, the rate of discontinuation of LAMICTAL for dizziness, ataxia, diplopia, blurred vision, nausea, and vomiting was dose-related.

Monotherapy in Adults With Epilepsy: The most commonly observed (≥5% for LAMICTAL and more common on drug than placebo) adverse reactions seen in association with the use of LAMICTAL during the monotherapy phase of the controlled trial in adults not seen at an equivalent rate in the control group were vomiting, coordination abnormality, dyspepsia, nausea, dizziness, rhinitis, anxiety, insomnia, infection, pain, weight decrease, chest pain, and dysmenorrhea. The most commonly observed (≥5% for LAMICTAL and more common on drug than placebo) adverse reactions associated with the use of LAMICTAL during the conversion to monotherapy (add-on) period, not seen at an equivalent frequency among low-dose valproate-treated patients, were dizziness, headache, nausea, asthenia, coordination abnormality, vomiting, rash, somnolence, diplopia, ataxia, accidental injury, tremor, blurred vision, insomnia, nystagmus, diarrhea, lymphadenopathy, pruritus, and sinusitis.

Approximately 10% of the 420 adult patients who received LAMICTAL as monotherapy in premarketing clinical trials discontinued treatment because of an adverse reaction. The adverse reactions most commonly associated with discontinuation were rash (4.5%), headache (3.1%), and asthenia (2.4%).

Adjunctive Therapy in Pediatric Patients With Epilepsy: The most commonly observed (≥5% for LAMICTAL and more common on drug than placebo) adverse reactions seen in association with the use of LAMICTAL as adjunctive treatment in pediatric patients 2 to 16 years of age and not seen at an equivalent rate in the control group were infection, vomiting, rash, fever, somnolence, accidental injury, dizziness, diarrhea, abdominal pain, nausea, ataxia, tremor, asthenia, bronchitis, flu syndrome, and diplopia.

In 339 patients 2 to 16 years of age with partial seizures or generalized seizures of Lennox-Gastaut syndrome, 4.2% of patients on LAMICTAL and 2.9% of patients on placebo discontinued due to adverse reactions. The most commonly reported adverse reaction that led to discontinuation of LAMICTAL was rash.

Approximately 11.5% of the 1,081 pediatric patients 2 to 16 years of age who received LAMICTAL as adjunctive therapy in premarketing clinical trials discontinued treatment because of an adverse reaction. The adverse reactions most commonly associated with discontinuation were rash (4.4%), reaction aggravated (1.7%), and ataxia (0.6%).

Controlled Adjunctive Clinical Studies in Adults With Epilepsy: Table 8 lists treatment-emergent adverse reactions that occurred in at least 2% of adult patients with epilepsy treated with LAMICTAL in placebo-controlled trials and were numerically more common in the patients treated with LAMICTAL. In these studies, either LAMICTAL or placebo was added to the patient's current AED therapy. Adverse reactions were usually mild to moderate in intensity.

Table 8. Treatment-Emergent Adverse Reaction Incidence in Placebo-Controlled Adjunctive Trials in Adult Patients With Epilepsy[a] (Adverse reactions in at least 2% of patients treated with LAMICTAL and numerically more frequent than in the placebo group.)

Body System/ Adverse Reaction	Percent of Patients Receiving Adjunctive LAMICTAL (n = 711)	Percent of Patients Receiving Adjunctive Placebo (n = 419)
Body as a whole		
Headache	29	19
Flu syndrome	7	6
Fever	6	4
Abdominal pain	5	4
Neck pain	2	1
Reaction aggravated (seizure exacerbation)	2	1
Digestive		
Nausea	19	10
Vomiting	9	4
Diarrhea	6	4
Dyspepsia	5	2
Constipation	4	3
Anorexia	2	1
Musculoskeletal		
Arthralgia	2	0
Nervous		
Dizziness	38	13
Ataxia	22	6
Somnolence	14	7
Incoordination	6	2
Insomnia	6	2
Tremor	4	1
Depression	4	3
Anxiety	4	3
Convulsion	3	1
Irritability	3	2
Speech disorder	3	0
Concentration disturbance	2	1
Respiratory		
Rhinitis	14	9
Pharyngitis	10	9
Cough increased	8	6
Skin and appendages		
Rash	10	5
Pruritus	3	2
Special senses		
Diplopia	28	7
Blurred vision	16	5
Vision abnormality	3	1
Urogenital		
Female patients only	(n = 365)	(n = 207)
Dysmenorrhea	7	6
Vaginitis	4	1
Amenorrhea	2	1

[a] Patients in these adjunctive studies were receiving 1 to 3 of the following concomitant AEDs (carbamazepine, phenytoin, phenobarbital, or primidone) in addition to LAMICTAL or placebo. Patients may have reported multiple adverse reactions during the study or at discontinuation; thus, patients may be included in more than one category.

In a randomized, parallel study comparing placebo and 300 and 500 mg/day of LAMICTAL, some of the more common drug-related adverse reactions were dose-related (see Table 9).

Table 9. Dose-Related Adverse Reactions From a Randomized, Placebo-Controlled Adjunctive Trial in Adults With Epilepsy

Adverse Reaction	Percent of Patients Experiencing Adverse Reactions		
	Placebo (n = 73)	LAMICTAL 300 mg (n = 71)	LAMICTAL 500 mg (n = 72)
Ataxia	10	10	28[ab]
Blurred vision	10	11	25[ab]
Diplopia	8	24[a]	49[ab]
Dizziness	27	31	54[ab]
Nausea	11	18	25[a]
Vomiting	4	11	18[a]

[a] Significantly greater than placebo group ($p<0.05$).
[b] Significantly greater than group receiving LAMICTAL 300 mg ($p<0.05$).

The overall adverse reaction profile for LAMICTAL was similar between females and males, and was independent of age. Because the largest non-Caucasian racial subgroup was only 6% of patients exposed to LAMICTAL in placebo-controlled trials, there are insufficient data to support a statement regarding the distribution of adverse reaction reports by race. Generally, females receiving either LAMICTAL as adjunctive therapy or placebo were more likely to report adverse reactions than males. The only adverse reaction for which the reports on LAMICTAL were greater than 10% more frequent in females than males (without a corresponding difference by gender on placebo) was dizziness (difference = 16.5%). There was little difference between females and males in the rates of discontinuation of LAMICTAL for individual adverse reactions.

Controlled Monotherapy Trial in Adults With Partial Seizures: Table 10 lists treatment-emergent adverse reactions that occurred in at least 5% of patients with epilepsy treated with monotherapy with LAMICTAL in a double-blind trial following discontinuation of either concomitant carbamazepine or phenytoin not seen at an equivalent frequency in the control group.

Table 10. Treatment-Emergent Adverse Reaction Incidence in Adults With Partial Seizures in a Controlled Monotherapy Trial[a] (Adverse reactions in at least 5% of patients treated with LAMICTAL and numerically more frequent than in the valproate group.)

Body System/ Adverse Reaction	Percent of Patients Receiving LAMICTAL as Monotherapy[b] (n = 43)	Percent of Patients Receiving Low-Dose Valproate[c] Monotherapy (n = 44)
Body as a whole		
Pain	5	0
Infection	5	2
Chest pain	5	2
Digestive		
Vomiting	9	0
Dyspepsia	7	2
Nausea	7	2
Metabolic and nutritional		
Weight decrease	5	2
Nervous		
Coordination abnormality	7	0
Dizziness	7	0
Anxiety	5	0
Insomnia	5	2
Respiratory		
Rhinitis	7	2
Urogenital (female patients only)	(n = 21)	(n = 28)
Dysmenorrhea	5	0

[a] Patients in these studies were converted to LAMICTAL or valproate monotherapy from adjunctive therapy with carbamazepine or phenytoin. Patients may have reported multiple adverse reactions during the study; thus, patients may be included in more than one category.
[b] Up to 500 mg/day.
[c] 1,000 mg/day.

Adverse reactions that occurred with a frequency of less than 5% and greater than 2% of patients receiving LAMICTAL and numerically more frequent than placebo were:
Body as a Whole: Asthenia, fever.
Digestive: Anorexia, dry mouth, rectal hemorrhage, peptic ulcer.
Metabolic and Nutritional: Peripheral edema.
Nervous System: Amnesia, ataxia, depression, hypesthesia, libido increase, decreased reflexes, increased reflexes, nystagmus, irritability, suicidal ideation.
Respiratory: Epistaxis, bronchitis, dyspnea.
Skin and Appendages: Contact dermatitis, dry skin, sweating.
Special Senses: Vision abnormality.
Incidence in Controlled Adjunctive Trials in Pediatric Patients With Epilepsy: Table 11 lists adverse reactions that occurred in at least 2% of 339 pediatric patients with partial seizures or generalized seizures of Lennox-Gastaut syndrome, who received LAMICTAL up to 15 mg/kg/day or a maximum of 750 mg/day. Reported adverse reactions were classified using COSTART terminology.

Table 11. Treatment-Emergent Adverse Reaction Incidence in Placebo-Controlled Adjunctive Trials in Pediatric Patients With Epilepsy (Adverse reactions in at least 2% of patients treated with LAMICTAL and numerically more frequent than in the placebo group.)

Body System/ Adverse Reaction	Percent of Patients Receiving LAMICTAL (n = 168)	Percent of Patients Receiving Placebo (n = 171)
Body as a whole		
Infection	20	17
Fever	15	14
Accidental injury	14	12
Abdominal pain	10	5
Asthenia	8	4
Flu syndrome	7	6
Pain	5	4

Facial edema	2	1
Photosensitivity	2	0
Cardiovascular		
Hemorrhage	2	1
Digestive		
Vomiting	20	16
Diarrhea	11	9
Nausea	10	2
Constipation	4	2
Dyspepsia	2	1
Hemic and lymphatic		
Lymphadenopathy	2	1
Metabolic and nutritional		
Edema	2	0
Nervous system		
Somnolence	17	15
Dizziness	14	4
Ataxia	11	3
Tremor	10	1
Emotional lability	4	2
Gait abnormality	4	2
Thinking abnormality	3	2
Convulsions	2	1
Nervousness	2	1
Vertigo	2	1
Respiratory		
Pharyngitis	14	11
Bronchitis	7	5
Increased cough	7	6
Sinusitis	2	1
Bronchospasm	2	1
Skin		
Rash	14	12
Eczema	2	1
Pruritus	2	1
Special senses		
Diplopia	5	1
Blurred vision	4	1
Visual abnormality	2	0
Urogenital		
Male and female patients		
Urinary tract infection	3	0

Bipolar Disorder: The most commonly observed (≥5%) treatment-emergent adverse reactions seen in association with the use of LAMICTAL as monotherapy (100 to 400 mg/day) in adult patients (≥18 years of age) with Bipolar Disorder in the 2 double-blind, placebo-controlled trials of 18 months' duration, and numerically more frequent than in placebo-treated patients are included in Table 12. Adverse reactions that occurred in at least 5% of patients and were numerically more common during the dose-escalation phase of LAMICTAL in these trials (when patients may have been receiving concomitant medications) compared with the monotherapy phase were: headache (25%), rash (11%), dizziness (10%), diarrhea (8%), dream abnormality (6%), and pruritus (6%).

During the monotherapy phase of the double-blind, placebo-controlled trials of 18 months' duration, 13% of 227 patients who received LAMICTAL (100 to 400 mg/day), 16% of 190 patients who received placebo, and 23% of 166 patients who received lithium discontinued therapy because of an adverse reaction. The adverse reactions which most commonly led to discontinuation of LAMICTAL were rash (3%) and mania/hypomania/mixed mood adverse reactions (2%). Approximately 16% of 2,401 patients who received LAMICTAL (50 to 500 mg/day) for Bipolar Disorder in premarketing trials discontinued therapy because of an adverse reaction; most commonly due to rash (5%) and mania/hypomania/mixed mood adverse reactions (2%).

The overall adverse reaction profile for LAMICTAL was similar between females and males, between elderly and nonelderly patients, and among racial groups.

Table 12. Treatment-Emergent Adverse Reaction Incidence in 2 Placebo-Controlled Trials in Adults With Bipolar I Disorder[a] (Adverse reactions in at least 5% of patients treated with LAMICTAL as monotherapy and numerically more frequent than in the placebo group.)

Body System/ Adverse Reaction	Percent of Patients Receiving LAMICTAL (n = 227)	Percent of Patients Receiving Placebo (n = 190)
General		
Back pain	8	6
Fatigue	8	5
Abdominal pain	6	3
Digestive		
Nausea	14	11
Constipation	5	2
Vomiting	5	2
Nervous System		
Insomnia	10	6
Somnolence	9	7
Xerostomia (dry mouth)	6	4
Respiratory		
Rhinitis	7	4
Exacerbation of cough	5	3
Pharyngitis	5	4
Skin		
Rash (nonserious)[b]	7	5

[a] Patients in these studies were converted to LAMICTAL (100 to 400 mg/day) or placebo monotherapy from add-on therapy with other psychotropic medications. Patients may have reported multiple adverse reactions during the study; thus, patients may be included in more than one category.
[b] In the overall bipolar and other mood disorders clinical trials, the rate of serious rash was 0.08% (1 of 1,233) of adult patients who received LAMICTAL as initial monotherapy and 0.13% (2 of 1,538) of adult patients who received LAMICTAL as adjunctive therapy [see Warnings and Precautions (5.1)].

These adverse reactions were usually mild to moderate in intensity. Other reactions that occurred in 5% or more patients but equally or more frequently in the placebo group included: dizziness, mania, headache, infection, influenza, pain, accidental injury, diarrhea, and dyspepsia.

Adverse reactions that occurred with a frequency of less than 5% and greater than 1% of patients receiving LAMICTAL and numerically more frequent than placebo were:
General: Fever, neck pain.
Cardiovascular: Migraine.
Digestive: Flatulence
Metabolic and Nutritional: Weight gain, edema.

Musculoskeletal: Arthralgia, myalgia.
Nervous System: Amnesia, depression, agitation, emotional lability, dyspraxia, abnormal thoughts, dream abnormality, hypoesthesia.
Respiratory: Sinusitis.
Urogenital: Urinary frequency.
Adverse Reactions Following Abrupt Discontinuation: In the 2 maintenance trials, there was no increase in the incidence, severity or type of adverse reactions in Bipolar Disorder patients after abruptly terminating therapy with LAMICTAL. In clinical trials in patients with Bipolar Disorder, 2 patients experienced seizures shortly after abrupt withdrawal of LAMICTAL. However, there were confounding factors that may have contributed to the occurrence of seizures in these bipolar patients [see Warnings and Precautions (5.9)].
Mania/Hypomania/Mixed Episodes: During the double-blind, placebo-controlled clinical trials in Bipolar I Disorder in which patients were converted to monotherapy with LAMICTAL (100 to 400 mg/day) from other psychotropic medications and followed for up to 18 months, the rates of manic or hypomanic or mixed mood episodes reported as adverse reactions were 5% for patients treated with LAMICTAL (n = 227), 4% for patients treated with lithium (n = 166), and 7% for patients treated with placebo (n = 190). In all bipolar controlled trials combined, adverse reactions of mania (including hypomania and mixed mood episodes) were reported in 5% of patients treated with LAMICTAL (n = 956), 3% of patients treated with lithium (n = 280), and 4% of patients treated with placebo (n = 803).
6.2 Other Adverse Reactions Observed in All Clinical Trials
LAMICTAL has been administered to 6,694 individuals for whom complete adverse reaction data was captured during all clinical trials, only some of which were placebo controlled. During these trials, all adverse reactions were recorded by the clinical investigators using terminology of their own choosing. To provide a meaningful estimate of the proportion of individuals having adverse reactions, similar types of adverse reactions were grouped into a smaller number of standardized categories using modified COSTART dictionary terminology. The frequencies presented represent the proportion of the 6,694 individuals exposed to LAMICTAL who experienced an event of the type cited on at least one occasion while receiving LAMICTAL. All reported adverse reactions are included except those already listed in the previous tables or elsewhere in the labeling, those too general to be informative, and those not reasonably associated with the use of the drug.
Adverse reactions are further classified within body system categories and enumerated in order of decreasing frequency using the following definitions: *frequent* adverse reactions are defined as those occurring in at least 1/100 patients; *infrequent* adverse reactions are those occurring in 1/100 to 1/1,000 patients; *rare* adverse reactions are those occurring in fewer than 1/1,000 patients.
Body as a Whole: *Infrequent:* Allergic reaction, chills, and malaise.
Cardiovascular System: *Infrequent:* Flushing, hot flashes, hypertension, palpitations, postural hypotension, syncope, tachycardia, and vasodilation.
Dermatological: *Infrequent:* Acne, alopecia, hirsutism, maculopapular rash, skin discoloration, and urticaria. *Rare:* Angioedema, erythema, exfoliative dermatitis, fungal dermatitis, herpes zoster, leukoderma, multiforme erythema, petechial rash, pustular rash, Stevens-Johnson syndrome, and vesiculobullous rash.
Digestive System: *Infrequent:* Dysphagia, eructation, gastritis, gingivitis, increased appetite, increased salivation, liver function tests abnormal, and mouth ulceration. *Rare:* Gastrointestinal hemorrhage, glossitis, gum hemorrhage, gum hyperplasia, hematemesis, hemorrhagic colitis, hepatitis, melena, stomach ulcer, stomatitis, and tongue edema.
Endocrine System: *Rare:* Goiter and hypothyroidism.
Hematologic and Lymphatic System: *Infrequent:* Ecchymosis and leukopenia. *Rare:* Anemia, eosinophilia, fibrin decrease, fibrinogen decrease, iron deficiency anemia, leukocytosis, lymphocytosis, macrocytic anemia, petechia, and thrombocytopenia.
Metabolic and Nutritional Disorders: *Infrequent:* Aspartate transaminase increased. *Rare:* Alcohol intolerance, alkaline phosphatase increase, alanine transaminase increase, bilirubinemia, general edema, gamma glutamyl transpeptidase increase, and hyperglycemia.
Musculoskeletal System: *Infrequent:* Arthritis, leg cramps, myasthenia, and twitching. *Rare:* Bursitis, muscle atrophy, pathological fracture, and tendinous contracture.
Nervous System: *Frequent:* Confusion and paresthesia. *Infrequent:* Akathisia, apathy, aphasia, CNS depression, depersonalization, dysarthria, dyskinesia, euphoria, hallucinations, hostility, hyperkinesia, hypertonia, libido decreased, memory decrease, mind racing, movement disorder, myoclonus, panic attack, paranoid reaction, personality disorder, psychosis, sleep disorder, stupor, and suicidal ide-

ation. *Rare:* Choreoathetosis, delirium, delusions, dysphoria, dystonia, extrapyramidal syndrome, faintness, grand mal convulsions, hemiplegia, hyperalgesia, hyperesthesia, hypokinesia, hypotonia, manic depression reaction, muscle spasm, neuralgia, neurosis, paralysis, and peripheral neuritis.

Respiratory System: *Infrequent:* Yawn. *Rare:* Hiccup and hyperventilation.

Special Senses: *Frequent:* Amblyopia. *Infrequent:* Abnormality of accommodation, conjunctivitis, dry eyes, ear pain, photophobia, taste perversion, and tinnitus. *Rare:* Deafness, lacrimation disorder, oscillopsia, parosmia, ptosis, strabismus, taste loss, uveitis, and visual field defect.

Urogenital System: *Infrequent:* Abnormal ejaculation, hematuria, impotence, menorrhagia, polyuria, and urinary incontinence. *Rare:* Acute kidney failure, anorgasmia, breast abscess, breast neoplasm, creatinine increase, cystitis, dysuria, epididymitis, female lactation, kidney failure, kidney pain, nocturia, urinary retention, and urinary urgency.

6.3 Postmarketing Experience
The following adverse events (not listed above in clinical trials or other sections of the prescribing information) have been identified during postapproval use of LAMICTAL. Because these events are reported voluntarily from a population of uncertain size, it is not always possible to reliably estimate their frequency or establish a causal relationship to drug exposure.

Blood and Lymphatic: Agranulocytosis, hemolytic anemia, lymphadenopathy not associated with hypersensitivity disorder.

Gastrointestinal: Esophagitis.

Hepatobiliary Tract and Pancreas: Pancreatitis.

Immunologic: Lupus-like reaction, vasculitis.

Lower Respiratory: Apnea.

Musculoskeletal: Rhabdomyolysis has been observed in patients experiencing hypersensitivity reactions.

Nervous System: Aseptic meningitis.

Neurology: Exacerbation of Parkinsonian symptoms in patients with pre-existing Parkinson's disease, tics.

Non-site Specific: Progressive immunosuppression.

7 DRUG INTERACTIONS
Significant drug interactions with lamotrigine are summarized in Table 13. Additional details of these drug interaction studies are provided in the Clinical Pharmacology section [*see Clinical Pharmacology (12.3)*].

Table 13. Established and Other Potentially Significant Drug Interactions

Concomitant Drug	Effect on Concentration of Lamotrigine or Concomitant Drug	Clinical Comment
Estrogen-containing oral contraceptive preparations containing 30 mcg ethinylestradiol and 150 mcg levonorgestrel	↓ lamotrigine	Decreased lamotrigine levels approximately 50%.
	↓ levonorgestrel	Decrease in levonorgestrel component by 19%.
Carbamazepine (CBZ) and CBZ epoxide	↓ lamotrigine	Addition of carbamazepine decreases lamotrigine concentration approximately 40%.
	? CBZ epoxide	May increase CBZ epoxide levels.
Phenobarbital/Primidone	↓ lamotrigine	Decreased lamotrigine concentration approximately 40%.
Phenytoin (PHT)	↓ lamotrigine	Decreased lamotrigine concentration approximately 40%.
Rifampin	↓ lamotrigine	Decreased lamotrigine AUC approximately 40%.
Valproate	↑ lamotrigine	Increased lamotrigine concentrations slightly more than 2-fold.
	? valproate	Decreased valproate concentrations an average of 25% over a 3-week period then stabilized in healthy volunteers; no change in controlled clinical trials in epilepsy patients.

↓ = Decreased (induces lamotrigine glucuronidation).
↑ = Increased (inhibits lamotrigine glucuronidation).
? = Conflicting data.

8 USE IN SPECIFIC POPULATIONS
8.1 Pregnancy
Teratogenic Effects: Pregnancy Category C. No evidence of teratogenicity was found in mice, rats, or rabbits when lamotrigine was orally administered to pregnant animals during the period of organogenesis at doses up to 1.2, 0.5, and 1.1 times, respectively, on a mg/m² basis, the highest usual human maintenance dose (i.e., 500 mg/day). However, maternal toxicity and secondary fetal toxicity producing reduced fetal weight and/or delayed ossification were seen in mice and rats, but not in rabbits at these doses. Teratology studies were also conducted using bolus intravenous administration of the isethionate salt of lamotrigine in rats and rabbits. In rat dams administered an intravenous dose at 0.6 times the highest usual human maintenance dose, the incidence of intrauterine death without signs of teratogenicity was increased.

A behavioral teratology study was conducted in rats dosed during the period of organogenesis. At day 21 postpartum, offspring of dams receiving 5 mg/kg/day or higher displayed a significantly longer latent period for open field exploration and a lower frequency of rearing. In a swimming maze test performed on days 39 to 44 postpartum, time to completion was increased in offspring of dams receiving 25 mg/kg/day. These doses represent 0.1 and 0.5 times the clinical dose on a mg/m² basis, respectively.

Lamotrigine did not affect fertility, teratogenesis, or postnatal development when rats were dosed prior to and during mating, and throughout gestation and lactation at doses equivalent to 0.4 times the highest usual human maintenance dose on a mg/m² basis.

When pregnant rats were orally dosed at 0.1, 0.14, or 0.3 times the highest human maintenance dose (on a mg/m² basis) during the latter part of gestation (days 15 to 20), maternal toxicity and fetal death were seen. In dams, food consumption and weight gain were reduced, and the gestation period was slightly prolonged (22.6 vs. 22.0 days in the control group). Stillborn pups were found in all 3 drug-treated groups with the highest number in the high-dose group. Postnatal death was also seen, but only in the 2 highest doses, and occurred between days 1 and 20. Some of these deaths appear to be drug-related and not secondary to the maternal toxicity. A no-observed-effect level (NOEL) could not be determined for this study.

Although lamotrigine was not found to be teratogenic in the above studies, lamotrigine decreases fetal folate concentrations in rats, an effect known to be associated with teratogenesis in animals and humans. There are no adequate and well-controlled studies in pregnant women. Because animal reproduction studies are not always predictive of human response, this drug should be used during pregnancy only if the potential benefit justifies the potential risk to the fetus.

Non-Teratogenic Effects: As with other AEDs, physiological changes during pregnancy may affect lamotrigine concentrations and/or therapeutic effect. There have been reports of decreased lamotrigine concentrations during pregnancy and restoration of pre-partum concentrations after delivery. Dosage adjustments may be necessary to maintain clinical response.

Pregnancy Exposure Registry: To provide information regarding the effects of in utero exposure to LAMICTAL, physicians are advised to recommend that pregnant patients taking LAMICTAL enroll in the North American Antiepileptic Drug (NAAED) Pregnancy Registry. This can be done by calling the toll-free number 1-888-233-2334, and must be done by patients themselves. Information on the registry can also be found at the website http://www.aedpregnancyregistry.org/.

Physicians are also encouraged to register patients in the Lamotrigine Pregnancy Registry; enrollment in this registry must be done prior to any prenatal diagnostic tests and **before fetal outcome is known. Physicians** can obtain information by calling the Lamotrigine Pregnancy Registry at 1-800-336-2176 (toll-free).

8.2 Labor and Delivery
The effect of LAMICTAL on labor and delivery in humans is unknown.

8.3 Nursing Mothers
Preliminary data indicate that lamotrigine passes into human milk. Because the effects on the infant exposed to lamotrigine by this route are unknown, breastfeeding while taking LAMICTAL is not recommended.

8.4 Pediatric Use
LAMICTAL is indicated for adjunctive therapy in patients ≥2 years of age for partial seizures, the generalized seizures of Lennox-Gastaut syndrome, and primary generalized tonic-clonic seizures.

Safety and efficacy of LAMICTAL, used as adjunctive treatment for partial seizures, were not demonstrated in a small randomized, double-blind, placebo-controlled, withdrawal study in very young pediatric patients (1 to 24 months). LAMICTAL was associated with an increased risk for infectious adverse reactions (LAMICTAL 37%, Placebo 5%), and respiratory adverse reactions (LAMICTAL 26%, Placebo 5%). Infectious adverse reactions included bronchiolitis, bronchitis, ear infection, eye infection, otitis externa, pharyngitis, urinary tract infection, and viral infection. Respiratory adverse reactions included nasal congestion, cough, and apnea.

Safety and effectiveness in patients below the age of 18 years with Bipolar Disorder have not been established.

8.5 Geriatric Use
Clinical studies of LAMICTAL for epilepsy and in Bipolar Disorder did not include sufficient numbers of subjects 65 years of age and over to determine whether they respond differently from younger subjects or exhibit a different safety profile than that of younger patients. In general, dose selection for an elderly patient should be cautious, usually starting at the low end of the dosing range, reflecting the greater frequency of decreased hepatic, renal, or cardiac function, and of concomitant disease or other drug therapy.

8.6 Patients With Hepatic Impairment
Experience in patients with hepatic impairment is limited. Based on a clinical pharmacology study in 24 patients with mild, moderate, and severe liver impairment [*see Clinical Pharmacology (12.3)*], the following general recommendations can be made. No dosage adjustment is needed in patients with mild liver impairment. Initial, escalation, and maintenance doses should generally be reduced by approximately 25% in patients with moderate and severe liver impairment without ascites and 50% in patients with severe liver impairment with ascites. Escalation and maintenance doses may be adjusted according to clinical response [*see Dosage and Administration (2.1)*].

8.7 Patients With Renal Impairment
Lamotrigine is metabolized mainly by glucuronic acid conjugation, with the majority of the metabolites being recovered in the urine. In a small study comparing a single dose of lamotrigine in patients with varying degrees of renal impairment with healthy volunteers, the plasma half-life of lamotrigine was significantly longer in the patients with renal impairment [*see Clinical Pharmacology (12.3)*].

Initial doses of LAMICTAL should be based on patients' AED regimens; reduced maintenance doses may be effective for patients with significant renal impairment. Few patients with severe renal impairment have been evaluated during chronic treatment with LAMICTAL. Because there is inadequate experience in this population, LAMICTAL should be used with caution in these patients [*see Dosage and Administration (2.1)*].

10 OVERDOSAGE
10.1 Human Overdose Experience
Overdoses involving quantities up to 15 g have been reported for LAMICTAL, some of which have been fatal. Overdose has resulted in ataxia, nystagmus, increased seizures, decreased level of consciousness, coma, and intraventricular conduction delay.

10.2 Management of Overdose
There are no specific antidotes for lamotrigine. Following a suspected overdose, hospitalization of the patient is advised. General supportive care is indicated, including frequent monitoring of vital signs and close observation of the patient. If indicated, emesis should be induced; usual precautions should be taken to protect the airway. It should be kept in mind that lamotrigine is rapidly absorbed [*see Clinical Pharmacology (12.3)*]. It is uncertain whether hemodialysis is an effective means of removing lamotrigine from the blood. In 6 renal failure patients, about 20% of the amount of lamotrigine in the body was removed by hemodialysis during a 4-hour session. A Poison Control Center should be contacted for information on the management of overdosage of LAMICTAL.

11 DESCRIPTION
LAMICTAL (lamotrigine), an AED of the phenyltriazine class, is chemically unrelated to existing AEDs. Its chemical name is 3,5-diamino-6-(2,3-dichlorophenyl)-*as*-triazine, its molecular formula is $C_9H_7N_5Cl_2$, and its molecular weight is

256.09. Lamotrigine is a white to pale cream-colored powder and has a pK_a of 5.7. Lamotrigine is very slightly soluble in water (0.17 mg/mL at 25°C) and slightly soluble in 0.1 M HCl (4.1 mg/mL at 25°C). The structural formula is:

LAMICTAL Tablets are supplied for oral administration as 25 mg (white), 100 mg (peach), 150 mg (cream), and 200 mg (blue) tablets. Each tablet contains the labeled amount of lamotrigine and the following inactive ingredients: lactose; magnesium stearate; microcrystalline cellulose; povidone; sodium starch glycolate; FD&C Yellow No. 6 Lake (100 mg tablet only); ferric oxide, yellow (150 mg tablet only); and FD&C Blue No. 2 Lake (200 mg tablet only).

LAMICTAL Chewable Dispersible Tablets are supplied for oral administration. The tablets contain 2 mg (white), 5 mg (white), or 25 mg (white) of lamotrigine and the following inactive ingredients: blackcurrant flavor, calcium carbonate, low-substituted hydroxypropylcellulose, magnesium aluminum silicate, magnesium stearate, povidone, saccharin sodium, and sodium starch glycolate.

LAMICTAL ODT Orally Disintegrating Tablets are supplied for oral administration. The tablets contain 25 mg (white to off-white), 50 mg (white to off-white), 100 mg (white to off-white), or 200 mg (white to off-white) of lamotrigine and the following inactive ingredients: artificial cherry flavor, crospovidone, ethylcellulose, magnesium stearate, mannitol, polyethylene, and sucralose.

LAMICTAL ODT Orally Disintegrating Tablets are formulated using technologies (Microcaps® and AdvaTab®) designed to mask the bitter taste of lamotrigine and achieve a rapid dissolution profile. Tablet characteristics including flavor, mouth-feel, after-taste, and ease of use were rated as favorable in a study of 108 healthy volunteers.

12 CLINICAL PHARMACOLOGY

12.1 Mechanism of Action

The precise mechanism(s) by which lamotrigine exerts its anticonvulsant action are unknown. In animal models designed to detect anticonvulsant activity, lamotrigine was effective in preventing seizure spread in the maximum electroshock (MES) and pentylenetetrazol (scMet) tests, and prevented seizures in the visually and electrically evoked after-discharge (EEAD) tests for antiepileptic activity. Lamotrigine also displayed inhibitory properties in the kindling model in rats both during kindling development and in the fully kindled state. The relevance of these models to human epilepsy, however, is not known.

One proposed mechanism of action of lamotrigine, the relevance of which remains to be established in humans, involves an effect on sodium channels. In vitro pharmacological studies suggest that lamotrigine inhibits voltage-sensitive sodium channels, thereby stabilizing neuronal membranes and consequently modulating presynaptic transmitter release of excitatory amino acids (e.g., glutamate and aspartate).

Although the relevance for human use is unknown, the following data characterize the performance of lamotrigine in receptor binding assays. Lamotrigine had a weak inhibitory effect on the serotonin 5-HT$_3$ receptor (IC_{50} = 18 μM). It does not exhibit high affinity binding (IC_{50}>100 μM) to the following neurotransmitter receptors: adenosine A$_1$ and A$_2$; adrenergic α$_1$, α$_2$, and β; dopamine D$_1$ and D$_2$; γ-aminobutyric acid (GABA) A and B; histamine H$_1$; kappa opioid; muscarinic acetylcholine; and serotonin 5-HT$_2$. Studies have failed to detect an effect of lamotrigine on dihydropyridine-sensitive calcium channels. It had weak effects at sigma opioid receptors (IC_{50} = 145 μM). Lamotrigine did not inhibit the uptake of norepinephrine, dopamine, or serotonin (IC_{50}>200 μM) when tested in rat synaptosomes and/or human platelets in vitro.

Effect of Lamotrigine on N-Methyl d-Aspartate-Receptor Mediated Activity: Lamotrigine did not inhibit N-methyl d-aspartate (NMDA)-induced depolarizations in rat cortical slices or NMDA-induced cyclic GMP formation in immature rat cerebellum, nor did lamotrigine displace compounds that are either competitive or noncompetitive ligands at this glutamate receptor complex (CNQX, CGS, TCHP). The IC_{50} for lamotrigine action on NMDA-induced currents (in the presence of 3 μM of glycine) in cultured hippocampal neurons exceeded 100 μM.

The mechanisms by which lamotrigine exerts its therapeutic action in Bipolar Disorder have not been established.

12.2 Pharmacodynamics

Folate Metabolism: In vitro, lamotrigine inhibited dihydrofolate reductase, the enzyme that catalyzes the reduction of dihydrofolate to tetrahydrofolate. Inhibition of this enzyme may interfere with the biosynthesis of nucleic acids and proteins. When oral daily doses of lamotrigine were given to pregnant rats during organogenesis, fetal, placental, and maternal folate concentrations were reduced. Significantly reduced concentrations of folate are associated with teratogenesis [see Use in Specific Populations (8.1)]. Folate concentrations were also reduced in male rats given repeated oral doses of lamotrigine. Reduced concentrations were partially returned to normal when supplemented with folinic acid.

Accumulation in Kidneys: Lamotrigine accumulated in the kidney of the male rat, causing chronic progressive nephrosis, necrosis, and mineralization. These findings are attributed to α-2 microglobulin, a species- and sex-specific protein that has not been detected in humans or other animal species.

Melanin Binding: Lamotrigine binds to melanin-containing tissues, e.g., in the eye and pigmented skin. It has been found in the uveal tract up to 52 weeks after a single dose in rodents.

Cardiovascular: In dogs, lamotrigine is extensively metabolized to a 2-N-methyl metabolite. This metabolite causes dose-dependent prolongations of the PR interval, widening of the QRS complex, and, at higher doses, complete AV conduction block. Similar cardiovascular effects are not anticipated in humans because only trace amounts of the 2-N-methyl metabolite (<0.6% of lamotrigine dose) have been found in human urine [see Clinical Pharmacology (12.3)]. However, it is conceivable that plasma concentrations of this metabolite could be increased in patients with a reduced capacity to glucuronidate lamotrigine (e.g., in patients with liver disease).

12.3 Pharmacokinetics

The pharmacokinetics of lamotrigine have been studied in patients with epilepsy, healthy young and elderly volunteers, and volunteers with chronic renal failure. Lamotrigine pharmacokinetic parameters for adult and pediatric patients and healthy normal volunteers are summarized in Tables 14 and 16.

[See table 14 above]

Absorption: Lamotrigine is rapidly and completely absorbed after oral administration with negligible first-pass metabolism (absolute bioavailability is 98%). The bioavailability is not affected by food. Peak plasma concentrations occur anywhere from 1.4 to 4.8 hours following drug administration. The lamotrigine chewable/dispersible tablets were found to be equivalent, whether they were administered as dispersed in water, chewed and swallowed, or swallowed as whole, to the lamotrigine compressed tablets in terms of rate and extent of absorption. In terms of rate and extent of absorption, lamotrigine orally disintegrating tablets whether disintegrated in the mouth or swallowed whole with water were equivalent to the lamotrigine compressed tablets swallowed with water.

Dose Proportionality: In healthy volunteers not receiving any other medications and given single doses, the plasma concentrations of lamotrigine increased in direct proportion to the dose administered over the range of 50 to 400 mg. In 2 small studies (n = 7 and 8) of patients with epilepsy who were maintained on other AEDs, there also was a linear relationship between dose and lamotrigine plasma concentrations at steady state following doses of 50 to 350 mg twice daily.

Distribution: Estimates of the mean apparent volume of distribution (Vd/F) of lamotrigine following oral administration ranged from 0.9 to 1.3 L/kg. Vd/F is independent of dose and is similar following single and multiple doses in both patients with epilepsy and healthy volunteers.

Protein Binding: Data from in vitro studies indicate that lamotrigine is approximately 55% bound to human plasma proteins at plasma lamotrigine concentrations from 1 to 10 mcg/mL (10 mcg/mL is 4 to 6 times the trough plasma concentration observed in the controlled efficacy trials). Because lamotrigine is not highly bound to plasma proteins, clinically significant interactions with other drugs through competition for protein binding sites are unlikely. The binding of lamotrigine to plasma proteins did not change in the

Table 14. Mean[a] Pharmacokinetic Parameters in Healthy Volunteers and Adult Patients With Epilepsy

Adult Study Population	Number of Subjects	T$_{max}$: Time of Maximum Plasma Concentration (h)	t$_{1/2}$: Elimination Half-life (h)	Cl/F: Apparent Plasma Clearance (mL/min/kg)
Healthy volunteers taking no other medications:				
Single-dose LAMICTAL	179	2.2 (0.25-12.0)	32.8 (14.0-103.0)	0.44 (0.12-1.10)
Multiple-dose LAMICTAL	36	1.7 (0.5-4.0)	25.4 (11.6-61.6)	0.58 (0.24-1.15)
Healthy volunteers taking valproate:				
Single-dose LAMICTAL	6	1.8 (1.0-4.0)	48.3 (31.5-88.6)	0.30 (0.14-0.42)
Multiple-dose LAMICTAL	18	1.9 (0.5-3.5)	70.3 (41.9-113.5)	0.18 (0.12-0.33)
Patients with epilepsy taking valproate only:				
Single-dose LAMICTAL	4	4.8 (1.8-8.4)	58.8 (30.5-88.8)	0.28 (0.16-0.40)
Patients with epilepsy taking carbamazepine, phenytoin, phenobarbital, or primidone[b] plus valproate:				
Single-dose LAMICTAL	25	3.8 (1.0-10.0)	27.2 (11.2-51.6)	0.53 (0.27-1.04)
Patients with epilepsy taking carbamazepine, phenytoin, phenobarbital, or primidone:[b]				
Single-dose LAMICTAL	24	2.3 (0.5-5.0)	14.4 (6.4-30.4)	1.10 (0.51-2.22)
Multiple-dose LAMICTAL	17	2.0 (0.75-5.93)	12.6 (7.5-23.1)	1.21 (0.66-1.82)

[a] The majority of parameter means determined in each study had coefficients of variation between 20% and 40% for half-life and Cl/F and between 30% and 70% for T$_{max}$. The overall mean values were calculated from individual study means that were weighted based on the number of volunteers/patients in each study. The numbers in parentheses below each parameter mean represent the range of individual volunteer/patient values across studies.
[b] Carbamazepine, phenobarbital, phenytoin, and primidone have been shown to increase the apparent clearance of lamotrigine. Estrogen-containing oral contraceptives and other drugs such as rifampin that induce lamotrigine glucuronidation have also been shown to increase the apparent clearance of lamotrigine [see Drug Interactions (7)].

Table 15. Summary of Drug Interactions With LAMICTAL

Drug	Drug Plasma Concentration With Adjunctive LAMICTAL[a]	Lamotrigine Plasma Concentration With Adjunctive Drugs[b]
Oral contraceptives (e.g., ethinylestradiol/levonorgestrel)[c]	↔[d]	↓
Bupropion	Not assessed	↔
Carbamazepine (CBZ)	↔	↓
CBZ epoxide[e]	?	
Felbamate	Not assessed	↔
Gabapentin	Not assessed	↔
Levetiracetam	↔	↔
Lithium	↔	Not assessed
Olanzapine	↔	↔[f]
Oxcarbazepine	↔	↔
10-monohydroxy oxcarbazepine metabolite[g]	↔	
Phenobarbital/primidone	↔	↓
Phenytoin (PHT)	↔	↓
Pregabalin	↔	
Rifampin	Not assessed	↓
Topiramate	↔[h]	↔
Valproate	↓	↑
Valproate + PHT and/or CBZ	Not assessed	↔
Zonisamide	Not assessed	↔

[a] From adjunctive clinical trials and volunteer studies.
[b] Net effects were estimated by comparing the mean clearance values obtained in adjunctive clinical trials and volunteers studies.
[c] The effect of other hormonal contraceptive preparations or hormone replacement therapy on the pharmacokinetics of lamotrigine has not been systematically evaluated in clinical trials, although the effect may be similar to that seen with the ethinylestradiol/levonorgestrel combinations.
[d] Modest decrease in levonorgestrel.
[e] Not administered, but an active metabolite of carbamazepine.
[f] Slight decrease, not expected to be clinically relevant.
[g] Not administered, but an active metabolite of oxcarbazepine.
[h] Slight increase, not expected to be clinically relevant.
↔ = No significant effect.
? = Conflicting data.

presence of therapeutic concentrations of phenytoin, phenobarbital, or valproate. Lamotrigine did not displace other AEDs (carbamazepine, phenytoin, phenobarbital) from protein-binding sites.
Metabolism: Lamotrigine is metabolized predominantly by glucuronic acid conjugation; the major metabolite is an inactive 2-N-glucuronide conjugate. After oral administration of 240 mg of ^{14}C-lamotrigine (15 μCi) to 6 healthy volunteers, 94% was recovered in the urine and 2% was recovered in the feces. The radioactivity in the urine consisted of unchanged lamotrigine (10%), the 2-N-glucuronide (76%), a 5-N-glucuronide (10%), a 2-N-methyl metabolite (0.14%), and other unidentified minor metabolites (4%).
Enzyme Induction: The effects of lamotrigine on the induction of specific families of mixed-function oxidase isozymes have not been systematically evaluated.
Following multiple administrations (150 mg twice daily) to normal volunteers taking no other medications, lamotrigine induced its own metabolism, resulting in a 25% decrease in $t_{1/2}$ and a 37% increase in Cl/F at steady state compared with values obtained in the same volunteers following a single dose. Evidence gathered from other sources suggests that self-induction by lamotrigine may not occur when lamotrigine is given as adjunctive therapy in patients receiving enzyme-inducing drugs such as carbamazepine, phenytoin, phenobarbital, primidone, or drugs such as rifampin that induce lamotrigine glucuronidation [see Drug Interactions (7)].
Elimination: The elimination half-life and apparent clearance of lamotrigine following administration of LAMICTAL to adult patients with epilepsy and healthy volunteers is summarized in Table 14. Half-life and apparent oral clearance vary depending on concomitant AEDs.
Drug Interactions: The apparent clearance of lamotrigine is affected by the coadministration of certain medications

[see Warnings and Precautions (5.8, 5.12), Drug Interactions (7)].
The net effects of drug interactions with LAMICTAL are summarized in Tables 13 and 15, followed by details of the drug interaction studies below.
[See table 15 above]
Estrogen-Containing Oral Contraceptives: In 16 female volunteers, an oral contraceptive preparation containing 30 mcg ethinylestradiol and 150 mcg levonorgestrel increased the apparent clearance of lamotrigine (300 mg/day) by approximately 2-fold with mean decreases in AUC of 52% and in C_{max} of 39%. In this study, trough serum lamotrigine concentrations gradually increased and were approximately 2-fold higher on average at the end of the week of the inactive hormone preparation compared with trough lamotrigine concentrations at the end of the active hormone cycle.
Gradual transient increases in lamotrigine plasma levels (approximate 2-fold increase) occurred during the week of inactive hormone preparation ("pill-free" week) for women not also taking a drug that increased the clearance of lamotrigine (carbamazepine, phenytoin, phenobarbital, primidone, or other drugs such as rifampin that induce lamotrigine glucuronidation [see Drug Interactions (7)]). The increase in lamotrigine plasma levels will be greater if the dose of LAMICTAL is increased in the few days before or during the "pill-free" week. Increases in lamotrigine plasma levels could result in dose-dependent adverse reactions.
In the same study, coadministration of LAMICTAL (300 mg/day) in 16 female volunteers did not affect the pharmacokinetics of the ethinylestradiol component of the oral contraceptive preparation. There were mean decreases in the AUC and C_{max} of the levonorgestrel component of 19% and 12%, respectively. Measurement of serum progesterone indicated that there was no hormonal evidence of ovulation

in any of the 16 volunteers, although measurement of serum FSH, LH, and estradiol indicated that there was some loss of suppression of the hypothalamic-pituitary-ovarian axis.
The effects of doses of LAMICTAL other than 300 mg/day have not been systematically evaluated in controlled clinical trials.
The clinical significance of the observed hormonal changes on ovulatory activity is unknown. However, the possibility of decreased contraceptive efficacy in some patients cannot be excluded. Therefore, patients should be instructed to promptly report changes in their menstrual pattern (e.g., break-through bleeding).
Dosage adjustments may be necessary for women receiving estrogen-containing oral contraceptive preparations [see Dosage and Administration (2.1)].
Other Hormonal Contraceptives or Hormone Replacement Therapy: The effect of other hormonal contraceptive preparations or hormone replacement therapy on the pharmacokinetics of lamotrigine has not been systematically evaluated. It has been reported that ethinylestradiol, not progestogens, increased the clearance of lamotrigine up to 2-fold, and the progestin-only pills had no effect on lamotrigine plasma levels. Therefore, adjustments to the dosage of LAMICTAL in the presence of progestogens alone will likely not be needed.
Bupropion: The pharmacokinetics of a 100-mg single dose of LAMICTAL in healthy volunteers (n = 12) were not changed by coadministration of bupropion sustained-release formulation (150 mg twice daily) starting 11 days before LAMICTAL.
Carbamazepine: LAMICTAL has no appreciable effect on steady-state carbamazepine plasma concentration. Limited clinical data suggest there is a higher incidence of dizziness, diplopia, ataxia, and blurred vision in patients receiving carbamazepine with lamotrigine than in patients receiving other AEDs with lamotrigine [see Adverse Reactions (6.1)]. The mechanism of this interaction is unclear. The effect of lamotrigine on plasma concentrations of carbamazepine-epoxide is unclear. In a small subset of patients (n = 7) studied in a placebo-controlled trial, lamotrigine had no effect on carbamazepine-epoxide plasma concentrations, but in a small, uncontrolled study (n = 9), carbamazepine-epoxide levels increased.
The addition of carbamazepine decreases lamotrigine steady-state concentrations by approximately 40%.
Felbamate: In a study of 21 healthy volunteers, coadministration of felbamate (1,200 mg twice daily) with lamotrigine (100 mg twice daily for 10 days) appeared to have no clinically relevant effects on the pharmacokinetics of lamotrigine.
Folate Inhibitors: Lamotrigine is a weak inhibitor of dihydrofolate reductase. Prescribers should be aware of this action when prescribing other medications that inhibit folate metabolism.
Gabapentin: Based on a retrospective analysis of plasma levels in 34 patients who received lamotrigine both with and without gabapentin, gabapentin does not appear to change the apparent clearance of lamotrigine.
Levetiracetam: Potential drug interactions between levetiracetam and lamotrigine were assessed by evaluating serum concentrations of both agents during placebo-controlled clinical trials. These data indicate that lamotrigine does not influence the pharmacokinetics of levetiracetam and that levetiracetam does not influence the pharmacokinetics of lamotrigine.
Lithium: The pharmacokinetics of lithium were not altered in healthy subjects (n = 20) by coadministration of lamotrigine (100 mg/day) for 6 days.
Olanzapine: The AUC and C_{max} of olanzapine were similar following the addition of olanzapine (15 mg once daily) to lamotrigine (200 mg once daily) in healthy male volunteers (n = 16) compared with the AUC and C_{max} in healthy male volunteers receiving olanzapine alone (n = 16).
In the same study, the AUC and C_{max} of lamotrigine were reduced on average by 24% and 20%, respectively, following the addition of olanzapine to lamotrigine in healthy male volunteers compared with those receiving lamotrigine alone. This reduction in lamotrigine plasma concentrations is not expected to be clinically relevant.
Oxcarbazepine: The AUC and C_{max} of oxcarbazepine and its active 10-monohydroxy oxcarbazepine metabolite were not significantly different following the addition of oxcarbazepine (600 mg twice daily) to lamotrigine (200 mg once daily) in healthy male volunteers (n = 13) compared with healthy male volunteers receiving oxcarbazepine alone (n = 13).
In the same study, the AUC and C_{max} of lamotrigine were similar following the addition of oxcarbazepine (600 mg twice daily) to LAMICTAL in healthy male volunteers compared with those receiving LAMICTAL alone. Limited clinical data suggest a higher incidence of headache, dizzi-

ness, nausea, and somnolence with coadministration of lamotrigine and oxcarbazepine compared with lamotrigine alone or oxcarbazepine alone.

Phenobarbital, Primidone: The addition of phenobarbital or primidone decreases lamotrigine steady-state concentrations by approximately 40%.

Phenytoin: Lamotrigine has no appreciable effect on steady-state phenytoin plasma concentrations in patients with epilepsy. The addition of phenytoin decreases lamotrigine steady-state concentrations by approximately 40%.

Pregabalin: Steady-state trough plasma concentrations of lamotrigine were not affected by concomitant pregabalin (200 mg 3 times daily) administration. There are no pharmacokinetic interactions between lamotrigine and pregabalin.

Rifampin: In 10 male volunteers, rifampin (600 mg/day for 5 days) significantly increased the apparent clearance of a single 25-mg dose of lamotrigine by approximately 2-fold (AUC decreased by approximately 40%).

Topiramate: Topiramate resulted in no change in plasma concentrations of lamotrigine. Administration of lamotrigine resulted in a 15% increase in topiramate concentrations.

Valproate: When lamotrigine was administered to healthy volunteers (n = 18) receiving valproate, the trough steady-state valproate plasma concentrations decreased by an average of 25% over a 3-week period, and then stabilized. However, adding lamotrigine to the existing therapy did not cause a change in valproate plasma concentrations in either adult or pediatric patients in controlled clinical trials.

The addition of valproate increased lamotrigine steady-state concentrations in normal volunteers by slightly more than 2-fold. In one study, maximal inhibition of lamotrigine clearance was reached at valproate doses between 250 and 500 mg/day and did not increase as the valproate dose was further increased.

Zonisamide: In a study of 18 patients with epilepsy, coadministration of zonisamide (200 to 400 mg/day) with lamotrigine (150 to 500 mg/day for 35 days) had no significant effect on the pharmacokinetics of lamotrigine.

Known Inducers or Inhibitors of Glucuronidation: Drugs other than those listed above have not been systematically evaluated in combination with lamotrigine. Since lamotrigine is metabolized predominantly by glucuronic acid conjugation, drugs that are known to induce or inhibit glucuronidation may affect the apparent clearance of lamotrigine and doses of lamotrigine may require adjustment based on clinical response.

Other: Results of in vitro experiments suggest that clearance of lamotrigine is unlikely to be reduced by concomitant administration of amitriptyline, clonazepam, clozapine, fluoxetine, haloperidol, lorazepam, phenelzine, risperidone, sertraline, or trazodone.

Results of in vitro experiments suggest that lamotrigine does not reduce the clearance of drugs eliminated predominantly by CYP2D6.

Special Populations: *Patients With Renal Impairment:* Twelve volunteers with chronic renal failure (mean creatinine clearance: 13 mL/min; range: 6 to 33) and another 6 individuals undergoing hemodialysis were each given a single 100-mg dose of lamotrigine. The mean plasma half-lives determined in the study were 42.9 hours (chronic renal failure), 13.0 hours (during hemodialysis), and 57.4 hours (between hemodialysis) compared with 26.2 hours in healthy volunteers. On average, approximately 20% (range: 5.6 to 35.1) of the amount of lamotrigine present in the body was eliminated by hemodialysis during a 4-hour session *[see Dosage and Administration (2.1)]*.

Hepatic Disease: The pharmacokinetics of lamotrigine following a single 100-mg dose of lamotrigine were evaluated in 24 subjects with mild, moderate, and severe hepatic impairment (Child-Pugh Classification system) and compared with 12 subjects without hepatic impairment. The patients with severe hepatic impairment were without ascites (n = 2) or with ascites (n = 5). The mean apparent clearances of lamotrigine in patients with mild (n = 12), moderate (n = 5), severe without ascites (n = 2), and severe with ascites (n = 5) liver impairment were 0.30 ± 0.09, 0.24 ± 0.1, 0.21 ± 0.04, and 0.15 ± 0.09 mL/min/kg, respectively, as compared with 0.37 ± 0.1 mL/min/kg in the healthy controls. Mean half-lives of lamotrigine in patients with mild, moderate, severe without ascites, and severe with ascites hepatic impairment were 46 ± 20, 72 ± 44, 67 ± 11, and 100 ± 48 hours, respectively, as compared with 33 ± 7 hours in healthy controls *[see Dosage and Administration (2.1)]*.

Age: Pediatric Patients: The pharmacokinetics of lamotrigine following a single 2-mg/kg dose were evaluated in 2 studies of pediatric patients (n = 29 for patients 10 months to 5.9 years of age and n = 26 for patients 5 to 11 years of age). Forty-three patients received concomitant therapy with other AEDs and 12 patients received lamotrigine as monotherapy. Lamotrigine pharmacokinetic

Table 16. Mean Pharmacokinetic Parameters in Pediatric Patients With Epilepsy

Pediatric Study Population	Number of Subjects	T_{max} (h)	$t_{1/2}$ (h)	Cl/F (mL/min/kg)
Ages 10 months-5.3 years				
Patients taking carbamazepine, phenytoin, phenobarbital, or primidone[a]	10	3.0 (1.0-5.9)	7.7 (5.7-11.4)	3.62 (2.44-5.28)
Patients taking AEDs with no known effect on the apparent clearance of lamotrigine	7	5.2 (2.9-6.1)	19.0 (12.9-27.1)	1.2 (0.75-2.42)
Patients taking valproate only	8	2.9 (1.0-6.0)	44.9 (29.5-52.5)	0.47 (0.23-0.77)
Ages 5-11 years				
Patients taking carbamazepine, phenytoin, phenobarbital, or primidone[a]	7	1.6 (1.0-3.0)	7.0 (3.8-9.8)	2.54 (1.35-5.58)
Patients taking carbamazepine, phenytoin, phenobarbital, or primidone[a] plus valproate	8	3.3 (1.0-6.4)	19.1 (7.0-31.2)	0.89 (0.39-1.93)
Patients taking valproate only[b]	3	4.5 (3.0-6.0)	65.8 (50.7-73.7)	0.24 (0.21-0.26)
Ages 13-18 years				
Patients taking carbamazepine, phenytoin, phenobarbital, or primidone[a]	11	c	c	1.3
Patients taking carbamazepine, phenytoin, phenobarbital, or primidone[a] plus valproate	8	c	c	0.5
Patients taking valproate only	4	c	c	0.3

[a] Carbamazepine, phenobarbital, phenytoin, and primidone have been shown to increase the apparent clearance of lamotrigine. Estrogen-containing oral contraceptives and rifampin have also been shown to increase the apparent clearance of lamotrigine *[see Drug Interactions (7)]*.
[b] Two subjects were included in the calculation for mean T_{max}.
[c] Parameter not estimated.

parameters for pediatric patients are summarized in Table 16.

Population pharmacokinetic analyses involving patients 2 to 18 years of age demonstrated that lamotrigine clearance was influenced predominantly by total body weight and concurrent AED therapy. The oral clearance of lamotrigine was higher, on a body weight basis, in pediatric patients than in adults. Weight-normalized lamotrigine clearance was higher in those subjects weighing less than 30 kg, compared with those weighing greater than 30 kg. Accordingly, patients weighing less than 30 kg may need an increase of as much as 50% in maintenance doses, based on clinical response, as compared with subjects weighing more than 30 kg being administered the same AEDs *[see Dosage and Administration (2.2)]*. These analyses also revealed that, after accounting for body weight, lamotrigine clearance was not significantly influenced by age. Thus, the same weight-adjusted doses should be administered to children irrespective of differences in age. Concomitant AEDs which influence lamotrigine clearance in adults were found to have similar effects in children.

[See table 16 above]

Elderly: The pharmacokinetics of lamotrigine following a single 150-mg dose of LAMICTAL were evaluated in 12 elderly volunteers between the ages of 65 and 76 years (mean creatinine clearance = 61 mL/min, range: 33 to 108 mL/min). The mean half-life of lamotrigine in these subjects was 31.2 hours (range: 24.5 to 43.4 hours), and the mean clearance was 0.40 mL/min/kg (range: 0.26 to 0.48 mL/min/kg).

Gender: The clearance of lamotrigine is not affected by gender. However, during dose escalation of LAMICTAL in one clinical trial in patients with epilepsy on a stable dose of valproate (n = 77), mean trough lamotrigine concentrations, unadjusted for weight, were 24% to 45% higher (0.3 to 1.7 mcg/mL) in females than in males.

Race: The apparent oral clearance of lamotrigine was 25% lower in non-Caucasians than Caucasians.

13 NONCLINICAL TOXICOLOGY

13.1 Carcinogenesis, Mutagenesis, Impairment of Fertility

No evidence of carcinogenicity was seen in 1 mouse study or 2 rat studies following oral administration of lamotrigine for up to 2 years at maximum tolerated doses (30 mg/kg/day for mice and 10 to 15 mg/kg/day for rats, doses that are equivalent to 90 mg/m² and 60 to 90 mg/m², respectively). Steady-state plasma concentrations ranged from 1 to 4 mcg/mL in the mouse study and 1 to 10 mcg/mL in the rat study. Plasma concentrations associated with the recom-

mended human doses of 300 to 500 mg/day are generally in the range of 2 to 5 mcg/mL, but concentrations as high as 19 mcg/mL have been recorded.

Lamotrigine was not mutagenic in the presence or absence of metabolic activation when tested in 2 gene mutation assays (the Ames test and the in vitro mammalian mouse lymphoma assay). In 2 cytogenetic assays (the in vitro human lymphocyte assay and the in vivo rat bone marrow assay), lamotrigine did not increase the incidence of structural or numerical chromosomal abnormalities.

No evidence of impairment of fertility was detected in rats given oral doses of lamotrigine up to 2.4 times the highest usual human maintenance dose of 8.33 mg/kg/day or 0.4 times the human dose on a mg/m² basis. The effect of lamotrigine on human fertility is unknown.

14 CLINICAL STUDIES

14.1 Epilepsy

Monotherapy With LAMICTAL in Adults With Partial Seizures Already Receiving Treatment With Carbamazepine, Phenytoin, Phenobarbital, or Primidone as the Single AED

The effectiveness of monotherapy with LAMICTAL was established in a multicenter, double-blind clinical trial enrolling 156 adult outpatients with partial seizures. The patients experienced at least 4 simple partial, complex partial, and/or secondarily generalized seizures during each of 2 consecutive 4-week periods while receiving carbamazepine or phenytoin monotherapy during baseline. LAMICTAL (target dose of 500 mg/day) or valproate (1,000 mg/day) was added to either carbamazepine or phenytoin monotherapy over a 4-week period. Patients were then converted to monotherapy with LAMICTAL or valproate during the next 4 weeks, then continued on monotherapy for an additional 12-week period.

Study endpoints were completion of all weeks of study treatment or meeting an escape criterion. Criteria for escape relative to baseline were: (1) doubling of average monthly seizure count, (2) doubling of highest consecutive 2-day seizure frequency, (3) emergence of a new seizure type (defined as a seizure that did not occur during the 8-week baseline) that is more severe than seizure types that occur during study treatment, or (4) clinically significant prolongation of generalized tonic-clonic (GTC) seizures. The primary efficacy variable was the proportion of patients in each treatment group who met escape criteria.

The percentages of patients who met escape criteria were 42% (32/76) in the group receiving LAMICTAL and 69% (55/80) in the valproate group. The difference in the percentage of patients meeting escape criteria was statistically significant (p = 0.0012) in favor of LAMICTAL. No differences in efficacy based on age, sex, or race were detected.

Patients in the control group were intentionally treated with a relatively low dose of valproate; as such, the sole objective of this study was to demonstrate the effectiveness and safety of monotherapy with LAMICTAL, and cannot be interpreted to imply the superiority of LAMICTAL to an adequate dose of valproate.

Adjunctive Therapy With LAMICTAL in Adults With Partial Seizures

The effectiveness of LAMICTAL as adjunctive therapy (added to other AEDs) was established in 3 multicenter, placebo-controlled, double-blind clinical trials in 355 adults with refractory partial seizures. The patients had a history of at least 4 partial seizures per month in spite of receiving one or more AEDs at therapeutic concentrations and, in 2 of the studies, were observed on their established AED regimen during baselines that varied between 8 to 12 weeks. In the third, patients were not observed in a prospective baseline. In patients continuing to have at least 4 seizures per month during the baseline, LAMICTAL or placebo was then added to the existing therapy. In all 3 studies, change from baseline in seizure frequency was the primary measure of effectiveness. The results given below are for all partial seizures in the intent-to-treat population (all patients who received at least one dose of treatment) in each study, unless otherwise indicated. The median seizure frequency at baseline was 3 per week while the mean at baseline was 6.6 per week for all patients enrolled in efficacy studies.

One study (n = 216) was a double-blind, placebo-controlled, parallel trial consisting of a 24-week treatment period. Patients could not be on more than 2 other anticonvulsants and valproate was not allowed. Patients were randomized to receive placebo, a target dose of 300 mg/day of LAMICTAL, or a target dose of 500 mg/day of LAMICTAL. The median reductions in the frequency of all partial seizures relative to baseline were 8% in patients receiving placebo, 20% in patients receiving 300 mg/day of LAMICTAL, and 36% in patients receiving 500 mg/day of LAMICTAL. The seizure frequency reduction was statistically significant in the 500-mg/day group compared with the placebo group, but not in the 300-mg/day group.

A second study (n = 98) was a double-blind, placebo-controlled, randomized, crossover trial consisting of two 14-week treatment periods (the last 2 weeks of which consisted of dose tapering) separated by a 4-week washout period. Patients could not be on more than 2 other anticonvulsants and valproate was not allowed. The target dose of LAMICTAL was 400 mg/day. When the first 12 weeks of the treatment periods were analyzed, the median change in seizure frequency was a 25% reduction on LAMICTAL compared with placebo (p<0.001).

The third study (n = 41) was a double-blind, placebo-controlled, crossover trial consisting of two 12-week treatment periods separated by a 4-week washout period. Patients could not be on more than 2 other anticonvulsants. Thirteen patients were on concomitant valproate; these patients received 150 mg/day of LAMICTAL. The 28 other patients had a target dose of 300 mg/day of LAMICTAL. The median change in seizure frequency was a 26% reduction on LAMICTAL compared with placebo (p<0.01).

No differences in efficacy based on age, sex, or race, as measured by change in seizure frequency, were detected.

Adjunctive Therapy With LAMICTAL in Pediatric Patients With Partial Seizures

The effectiveness of LAMICTAL as adjunctive therapy in pediatric patients with partial seizures was established in a multicenter, double-blind, placebo-controlled trial in 199 patients 2 to 16 years of age (n = 98 on LAMICTAL, n = 101 on placebo). Following an 8-week baseline phase, patients were randomized to 18 weeks of treatment with LAMICTAL or placebo added to their current AED regimen of up to 2 drugs. Patients were dosed based on body weight and valproate use. Target doses were designed to approximate 5 mg/kg/day for patients taking valproate (maximum dose: 250 mg/day) and 15 mg/kg/day for the patients not taking valproate (maximum dose: 750 mg/day). The primary efficacy endpoint was percentage change from baseline in all partial seizures. For the intent-to-treat population, the median reduction of all partial seizures was 36% in patients treated with LAMICTAL and 7% on placebo, a difference that was statistically significant (p<0.01).

Adjunctive Therapy With LAMICTAL in Pediatric and Adult Patients With Lennox-Gastaut Syndrome

The effectiveness of LAMICTAL as adjunctive therapy in patients with Lennox-Gastaut syndrome was established in a multicenter, double-blind, placebo-controlled trial in 169 patients 3 to 25 years of age (n = 79 on LAMICTAL, n = 90 on placebo). Following a 4-week single-blind, placebo phase, patients were randomized to 16 weeks of treatment with LAMICTAL or placebo added to their current AED regimen of up to 3 drugs. Patients were dosed on a fixed-dose regimen based on body weight and valproate use. Target doses were designed to approximate 5 mg/kg/day for patients taking valproate (maximum dose: 200 mg/day) and 15 mg/kg/day for patients not taking valproate (maximum dose: 400 mg/day). The primary efficacy endpoint was percentage change from baseline in major motor seizures (atonic, tonic, major myoclonic, and tonic-clonic seizures). For the intent-to-treat population, the median reduction of major motor seizures was 32% in patients treated with LAMICTAL and 9% on placebo, a difference that was statistically significant (p<0.05). Drop attacks were significantly reduced by LAMICTAL (34%) compared with placebo (9%), as were tonic-clonic seizures (36% reduction versus 10% increase for LAMICTAL and placebo, respectively).

Adjunctive Therapy With LAMICTAL in Pediatric and Adult Patients With Primary Generalized Tonic-Clonic Seizures

The effectiveness of LAMICTAL as adjunctive therapy in patients with primary generalized tonic-clonic seizures was established in a multicenter, double-blind, placebo-controlled trial in 117 pediatric and adult patients ≥2 years (n = 58 on LAMICTAL, n = 59 on placebo). Patients with at least 3 primary generalized tonic-clonic seizures during an 8-week baseline phase were randomized to 19 to 24 weeks of treatment with LAMICTAL or placebo added to their current AED regimen of up to 2 drugs. Patients were dosed on a fixed-dose regimen, with target doses ranging from 3 mg/kg/day to 12 mg/kg/day for pediatric patients and from 200 mg/day to 400 mg/day for adult patients based on concomitant AED.

The primary efficacy endpoint was percentage change from baseline in primary generalized tonic-clonic seizures. For the intent-to-treat population, the median percent reduction of primary generalized tonic-clonic seizures was 66% in patients treated with LAMICTAL and 34% on placebo, a difference that was statistically significant (p = 0.006).

14.2 Bipolar Disorder

The effectiveness of LAMICTAL in the maintenance treatment of Bipolar I Disorder was established in 2 multicenter, double-blind, placebo-controlled studies in adult patients who met DSM-IV criteria for Bipolar I Disorder. Study 1 enrolled patients with a current or recent (within 60 days) depressive episode as defined by DSM-IV and Study 2 included patients with a current or recent (within 60 days) episode of mania or hypomania as defined by DSM-IV. Both studies included a cohort of patients (30% of 404 patients in Study 1 and 28% of 171 patients in Study 2) with rapid cycling Bipolar Disorder (4 to 6 episodes per year).

In both studies, patients were titrated to a target dose of 200 mg of LAMICTAL, as add-on therapy or as monotherapy, with gradual withdrawal of any psychotropic medications during an 8- to 16-week open-label period. Overall 81% of 1,305 patients participating in the open-label period were receiving 1 or more other psychotropic medications, including benzodiazepines, selective serotonin reuptake inhibitors (SSRIs), atypical antipsychotics (including olanzapine), valproate, or lithium, during titration of LAMICTAL. Patients with a CGI-severity score of 3 or less maintained for at least 4 continuous weeks, including at least the final week on monotherapy with LAMICTAL, were randomized to a placebo-controlled, double-blind treatment period for up to 18 months. The primary endpoint was TIME (time to intervention for a mood episode or one that was emerging, time to discontinuation for either an adverse event that was judged to be related to Bipolar Disorder, or for lack of efficacy). The mood episode could be depression, mania, hypomania, or a mixed episode.

In Study 1, patients received double-blind monotherapy with LAMICTAL 50 mg/day (n = 50), LAMICTAL 200 mg/day (n = 124), LAMICTAL 400 mg/day (n = 47), or placebo (n = 121). LAMICTAL (200- and 400-mg/day treatment groups combined) was superior to placebo in delaying the time to occurrence of a mood episode. Separate analyses of the 200- and 400-mg/day dose groups revealed no added benefit from the higher dose.

In Study 2, patients received double-blind monotherapy with LAMICTAL (100 to 400 mg/day, n = 59), or placebo (n = 70). LAMICTAL was superior to placebo in delaying time to occurrence of a mood episode. The mean dose of LAMICTAL was about 211 mg/day.

Although these studies were not designed to separately evaluate time to the occurrence of depression or mania, a combined analysis for the 2 studies revealed a statistically significant benefit for LAMICTAL over placebo in delaying the time to occurrence of both depression and mania, although the finding was more robust for depression.

16 HOW SUPPLIED/STORAGE AND HANDLING

LAMICTAL (lamotrigine) Tablets

25 mg, white, scored, shield-shaped tablets debossed with "LAMICTAL" and "25", bottles of 100 (NDC 0173-0633-02).

Store at 25°C (77°F); excursions permitted to 15-30°C (59-86°F) [see USP Controlled Room Temperature] in a dry place.

100 mg, peach, scored, shield-shaped tablets debossed with "LAMICTAL" and "100", bottles of 100 (NDC 0173-0642-55).

150 mg, cream, scored, shield-shaped tablets debossed with "LAMICTAL" and "150", bottles of 60 (NDC 0173-0643-60).

200 mg, blue, scored, shield-shaped tablets debossed with "LAMICTAL" and "200", bottles of 60 (NDC 0173-0644-60).

Store at 25°C (77°F); excursions permitted to 15-30°C (59-86°F) [see USP Controlled Room Temperature] in a dry place and protect from light.

LAMICTAL (lamotrigine) Starter Kit for Patients Taking Valproate (Blue Kit)

25 mg, white, scored, shield-shaped tablets debossed with "LAMICTAL" and "25", blisterpack of 35 tablets (NDC 0173-0633-10).

Store at 25°C (77°F); excursions permitted to 15-30°C (59-86°F) [see USP Controlled Room Temperature] in a dry place.

LAMICTAL (lamotrigine) Starter Kit for Patients Taking Carbamazepine, Phenytoin, Phenobarbital, or Primidone and Not Taking Valproate (Green Kit)

25 mg, white, scored, shield-shaped tablets debossed with "LAMICTAL" and "25" and 100 mg, peach, scored, shield-shaped tablets debossed with "LAMICTAL" and "100", blisterpack of 98 tablets (84/25-mg tablets and 14/100-mg tablets) (NDC 0173-0817-28).

Store at 25°C (77°F); excursions permitted to 15-30°C (59-86°F) [see USP Controlled Room Temperature] in a dry place and protect from light.

LAMICTAL (lamotrigine) Starter Kit for Patients Not Taking Carbamazepine, Phenytoin, Phenobarbital, Primidone, or Valproate (Orange Kit)

25 mg, white, scored, shield-shaped tablets debossed with "LAMICTAL" and "25" and 100 mg, peach, scored, shield-shaped tablets debossed with "LAMICTAL" and "100", blisterpack of 49 tablets (42/25-mg tablets and 7/100-mg tablets) (NDC 0173-0594-02).

Store at 25°C (77°F); excursions permitted to 15-30°C (59-86°F) [see USP Controlled Room Temperature] in a dry place and protect from light.

LAMICTAL (lamotrigine) Chewable Dispersible Tablets

2 mg, white to off-white, round tablets debossed with "LTG" over "2", bottles of 30 (NDC 0173-0699-00). ORDER DIRECTLY FROM GlaxoSmithKline 1-800-334-4153.

5 mg, white to off-white, caplet-shaped tablets debossed with "GX CL2", bottles of 100 (NDC 0173-0526-00).

25 mg, white, super elliptical-shaped tablets debossed with "GX CL5", bottles of 100 (NDC 0173-0527-00).

Store at 25°C (77°F); excursions permitted to 15-30°C (59-86°F) [see USP Controlled Room Temperature] in a dry place.

LAMICTAL ODT (lamotrigine) Orally Disintegrating Tablets

25 mg, white to off-white, round, flat-faced, radius edge, tablets debossed with "LMT" on one side and "25" on the other, Maintenance Packs of 30 (NDC 0173-0772-02).

50 mg, white to off-white, round, flat-faced, radius edge, tablets debossed with "LMT" on one side and "50" on the other, Maintenance Packs of 30 (NDC 0173-0774-02).

100 mg, white to off-white, round, flat-faced, radius edge, tablets debossed with "LAMICTAL" on one side and "100" on the other, Maintenance Packs of 30 (NDC 0173-0776-02).

200 mg, white to off-white, round, flat-faced, radius edge, tablets debossed with "LAMICTAL" on one side and "200" on the other, Maintenance Packs of 30 (NDC 0173-0777-02).

Store between 20°C to 25°C (68°F to 77°F); with excursions permitted between 15°C and 30°C (59°F and 86°F).

LAMICTAL ODT (lamotrigine) Patient Titration Kit for Patients Taking Valproate (Blue ODT Kit)

25 mg, white to off-white, round, flat-faced, radius edge, tablets debossed with "LMT" on one side and "25" on the other, and 50 mg, white to off-white, round, flat-faced, radius edge, tablets debossed with "LMT" on one side and "50" on the other, blisterpack of 28 tablets (21/25-mg tablets and 7/50-mg tablets) (NDC 0173-0779-00).

LAMICTAL ODT (lamotrigine) Patient Titration Kit for Patients Taking Carbamazepine, Phenytoin, Phenobarbital, or Primidone and Not Taking Valproate (Green ODT Kit)

50 mg, white to off-white, round, flat-faced, radius edge, tablets debossed with "LMT" on one side and "50" on the other, and 100 mg, white to off-white, round, flat-faced, radius edge, tablets debossed with "LAMICTAL" on one side and "100"; on the other, blisterpack of 56 tablets (42/50-mg tablets and 14/100-mg tablets) (NDC 0173-0780-00).

LAMICTAL ODT (lamotrigine) Patient Titration Kit for Patients Not Taking Carbamazepine, Phenytoin, Phenobarbital, Primidone, or Valproate (Orange ODT Kit)

25 mg, white to off-white, round, flat-faced, radius edge, tablets debossed with "LMT" on one side and "25" on the other, 50 mg, white to off-white, round, flat-faced, radius edge, tablets debossed with "LMT" on one side and "50" on the other, and 100 mg, white to off-white, round, flat-faced, radius edge, tablets debossed with "LAMICTAL" on one side and "100" on the other, blisterpack of 35 (14/25-mg tablets, 14/50-mg tablets, and 7/100-mg tablets) (NDC 0173-0778-00).

Store between 20°C to 25°C (68°F to 77°F); with excursions permitted between 15°C and 30°C (59°F and 86°F).

Blisterpacks: If the product is dispensed in a blisterpack, the patient should be advised to examine the blisterpack before use and not use if blisters are torn, broken, or missing.

17   PATIENT COUNSELING INFORMATION

See Medication Guide that accompanies the product.

17.1   Rash

Prior to initiation of treatment with LAMICTAL, the patient should be instructed that a rash or other signs or symptoms of hypersensitivity (e.g., fever, lymphadenopathy) may herald a serious medical event and that the patient should report any such occurrence to a physician immediately.

17.2   Suicidal Thinking and Behavior

Patients, their caregivers, and families should be counseled that AEDs, including LAMICTAL, may increase the risk of suicidal thoughts and behavior and should be advised of the need to be alert for the emergence or worsening of symptoms of depression, any unusual changes in mood or behavior, or the emergence of suicidal thoughts, behavior, or thoughts about self-harm. Behaviors of concern should be reported immediately to healthcare providers.

17.3   Worsening of Seizures

Patients should be advised to notify their physician if worsening of seizure control occurs.

17.4   CNS Adverse Effects

Patients should be advised that LAMICTAL may cause dizziness, somnolence, and other symptoms and signs of central nervous system (CNS) depression. Accordingly, they should be advised neither to drive a car nor to operate other complex machinery until they have gained sufficient experience on LAMICTAL to gauge whether or not it adversely affects their mental and/or motor performance.

17.5   Blood Dyscrasias and/or Acute Multiorgan Failure

Patients should be advised of the possibility of blood dyscrasias and/or acute multiorgan failure and to contact their physician immediately if they experience any signs or symptoms of these conditions [see Warnings and Precautions (5.3, 5.4)].

17.6   Pregnancy

Patients should be advised to notify their physicians if they become pregnant or intend to become pregnant during therapy. Patients should be advised to notify their physicians if they intend to breastfeed or are breastfeeding an infant. Patients should also be encouraged to enroll in the NAAED Pregnancy Registry if they become pregnant. This registry is collecting information about the safety of antiepileptic drugs during pregnancy. To enroll, patients can call the toll-free number 1-888-233-2334 [see Use in Specific Populations (8.1)].

17.7   Oral Contraceptive Use

Women should be advised to notify their physician if they plan to start or stop use of oral contraceptives or other female hormonal preparations. Starting estrogen-containing oral contraceptives may significantly decrease lamotrigine plasma levels and stopping estrogen-containing oral contraceptives (including the "pill-free" week) may significantly increase lamotrigine plasma levels [see Warnings and Precautions (5.8), Clinical Pharmacology (12.3)]. Women should also be advised to promptly notify their physician if they experience adverse reactions or changes in menstrual pattern (e.g., break-through bleeding) while receiving LAMICTAL in combination with these medications.

17.8   Discontinuing LAMICTAL

Patients should be advised to notify their physician if they stop taking LAMICTAL for any reason and not to resume LAMICTAL without consulting their physician.

17.9   Potential Medication Errors

Medication errors involving LAMICTAL have occurred. In particular the names LAMICTAL or lamotrigine can be confused with the names of other commonly used medications. Medication errors may also occur between the different formulations of LAMICTAL. To reduce the potential of medication errors, write and say LAMICTAL clearly. Depictions of the LAMICTAL Tablets, Chewable Dispersible Tablets, and Orally Disintegrating Tablets can be found in the Medication Guide that accompanies the product to highlight the distinctive markings, colors, and shapes that serve to identify the different presentations of the drug and thus may help reduce the risk of medication errors. **To avoid a medication error of using the wrong drug or formulation, patients should be strongly advised to visually inspect their tablets to verify that they are LAMICTAL, as well as the correct formulation of LAMICTAL, each time they fill their prescription** [see Dosage Forms and Strengths (3.1, 3.2, 3.3), How Supplied/Storage and Handling (16)].

GlaxoSmithKline
Research Triangle Park, NC 27709
LAMICTAL Tablets and Chewable Dispersible Tablets are manufactured by
DSM Pharmaceuticals, Inc., Greenville, NC 27834 or GlaxoSmithKline, Research Triangle Park, NC 27709
LAMICTAL Orally Disintegrating Tablets are manufactured by
Eurand, Inc., Vandalia, OH 45377

LAMICTAL (lamotrigine) Tablets

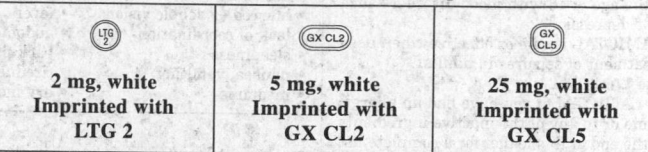

25 mg, white Imprinted with LAMICTAL 25	100 mg, peach Imprinted with LAMICTAL 100	150 mg, cream Imprinted with LAMICTAL 150	200 mg, blue Imprinted with LAMICTAL 200

LAMICTAL (lamotrigine) Chewable Dispersible Tablets

2 mg, white Imprinted with LTG 2	5 mg, white Imprinted with GX CL2	25 mg, white Imprinted with GX CL5

LAMICTAL ODT (lamotrigine) Orally Disintegrating Tablets

25 mg, white to off-white Imprinted with LMT on one side 25 on the other	50 mg, white to off-white Imprinted with LMT on one side 50 on the other	100 mg, white to off-white Imprinted with LAMICTAL on one side 100 on the other	200 mg, white to off-white Imprinted with LAMICTAL on one side 200 on the other

LAMICTAL is a registered trademark of GlaxoSmithKline Microcaps and AdvaTab are registered trademarks of Eurand, Inc.
©2009, GlaxoSmithKline. All rights reserved.

MEDICATION GUIDE

LAMICTAL® (la-MIK-tal) (lamotrigine) Tablets and Chewable Dispersible Tablets
LAMICTAL® ODT™ (lamotrigine) Orally Disintegrating Tablets

Read this Medication Guide before you start taking LAMICTAL and each time you get a refill. There may be new information. This information does not take the place of talking with your healthcare provider about your medical condition or treatment. If you have questions about LAMICTAL, ask your healthcare provider or pharmacist.

What is the most important information I should know about LAMICTAL?

1. LAMICTAL may cause a serious skin rash that may cause you to be hospitalized or to stop LAMICTAL; it may rarely cause death.

There is no way to tell if a mild rash will develop into a more serious reaction. These serious skin reactions are more likely to happen when you begin taking LAMICTAL, within the first 2 to 8 weeks of treatment. But it can happen in people who have taken LAMICTAL for any period of time. Children between 2 to 16 years of age have a higher chance of getting this serious skin reaction while taking LAMICTAL.

The risk of getting a rash is higher if you:
• take LAMICTAL while taking valproate (DEPAKENE (valproic acid) or DEPAKOTE (divalproex sodium))
• take a higher starting dose of LAMICTAL than your healthcare provider prescribed
• increase your dose of LAMICTAL faster than prescribed

LAMICTAL can also cause other types of allergic reactions or serious problems which may affect organs and other parts of your body like the liver or blood cells. You may or may not have a rash with these types of reactions.

Call your healthcare provider right away if you have any of the following:
• a skin rash
• hives
• fever
• swollen lymph glands
• painful sores in the mouth or around your eyes
• swelling of your lips or tongue
• yellowing of your skin or eyes
• unusual bruising or bleeding
• severe fatigue or weakness
• severe muscle pain
• frequent infections

These symptoms may be the first signs of a serious reaction. A healthcare provider should examine you to decide if you should continue taking LAMICTAL.

2. Like other antiepileptic drugs, LAMICTAL may cause suicidal thoughts or actions in a very small number of people, about 1 in 500.

Call a healthcare provider right away if you have any of these symptoms, especially if they are new, worse, or worry you:
• thoughts about suicide or dying
• attempt to commit suicide
• new or worse depression
• new or worse anxiety
• feeling agitated or restless
• panic attacks
• trouble sleeping (insomnia)
• new or worse irritability
• acting aggressive, being angry, or violent
• acting on dangerous impulses
• an extreme increase in activity and talking (mania)
• other unusual changes in behavior or mood

Do not stop LAMICTAL without first talking to a healthcare provider.
• Stopping LAMICTAL suddenly can cause serious problems.
• Suicidal thoughts or actions can be caused by things other than medicines. If you have suicidal thoughts or actions, your healthcare provider may check for other causes.

How can I watch for early symptoms of suicidal thoughts and actions?
• Pay attention to any changes, especially sudden changes, in mood, behaviors, thoughts, or feelings.
• Keep all follow-up visits with your healthcare provider as scheduled.
• Call your healthcare provider between visits as needed, especially if you are worried about symptoms.

LAMICTAL can have other serious side effects. For more information ask your healthcare provider or pharmacist. Tell your healthcare provider if you have any side effect that bothers you. Be sure to read the section below entitled "What are the possible side effects of LAMICTAL?"

3. Patients prescribed LAMICTAL have sometimes been given the wrong medicine because many medicines have names similar to LAMICTAL, so always check that you receive LAMICTAL.

Taking the wrong medication can cause serious health problems. When your healthcare provider gives you a prescription for LAMICTAL:
• Make sure you can read it clearly.
• Talk to your pharmacist to check that you are given the correct medicine.
• Each time you fill your prescription, check the tablets you receive against the pictures of the tablets below.

These pictures show the distinct wording, colors, and shapes of the tablets that help to identify the right strength of LAMICTAL Tablets, Chewable Dispersible Tablets, and Orally Disintegrating Tablets. Immediately call your pharmacist if you receive a LAMICTAL tablet that does not look like one of the tablets shown below, as you may have received the wrong medication.

[See figure above]

What is LAMICTAL?

LAMICTAL is a prescription medicine used:

1. together with other medicines to treat certain types of seizures (partial seizures, primary generalized tonic-clonic seizures, generalized seizures of Lennox-Gastaut syndrome) in people 2 years or older.
2. alone when changing from other medicines used to treat partial seizures in people 16 years or older.
3. for the long-term treatment of Bipolar I Disorder to lengthen the time between mood episodes in people 18 years or older who have been treated for mood episodes with other medicine.

It is not known if LAMICTAL is safe or effective in children or teenagers under the age of 18 with mood disorders such as bipolar disorder or depression.

It is not known if LAMICTAL is safe or effective when used alone as the first treatment of seizures in adults.

Who should not take LAMICTAL?

You should not take LAMICTAL if you have had an allergic reaction to lamotrigine or to any of the inactive ingredients in LAMICTAL. See the end of this leaflet for a complete list of ingredients in LAMICTAL.

What should I tell my healthcare provider before taking LAMICTAL?

Before taking LAMICTAL, tell your healthcare provider about all of your medical conditions, including if you:

- have had a rash or allergic reaction to another antiseizure medicine.
- have or have had depression, mood problems or suicidal thoughts or behavior.
- are taking oral contraceptives (birth control pills) or other female hormonal medicines. Do not start or stop taking birth control pills or other female hormonal medicine until you have talked with your healthcare provider. Tell your healthcare provider if you have any changes in your menstrual pattern such as breakthrough bleeding. Stopping or starting these medicines may cause side effects (such as dizziness, lack of coordination, or double vision) or lessen how well LAMICTAL works.
- are pregnant or plan to become pregnant. It is not known if LAMICTAL will harm your unborn baby. If you become pregnant while taking LAMICTAL, talk to your healthcare provider about registering with the North American Antiepileptic Drug Pregnancy Registry. You can enroll in this registry by calling 1-888-233-2334. The purpose of this registry is to collect information about the safety of antiepileptic drugs during pregnancy.
- are breastfeeding. LAMICTAL can pass into your breast milk. You and your healthcare provider should decide if you should take LAMICTAL or breastfeed. Breastfeeding while taking LAMICTAL is not recommended.

Tell your healthcare provider about all the medicines you take or if you are planning to take a new medicine, including prescription and non-prescription medicines, vitamins, and herbal supplements. Using LAMICTAL with certain other medicines can affect each other, causing side effects.

How should I take LAMICTAL?

- Take LAMICTAL exactly as prescribed.
- Your healthcare provider may change your dose. Do not change your dose without talking to your healthcare provider.
- Do not stop taking LAMICTAL without talking to your healthcare provider. Stopping LAMICTAL suddenly may cause serious problems. For example, if you have epilepsy and you stop taking LAMICTAL suddenly, you may get seizures that do not stop. Talk with your healthcare provider about how to stop LAMICTAL slowly.
- If you miss a dose of LAMICTAL, take it as soon as you remember. If it is almost time for your next dose, just skip the missed dose. Take the next dose at your regular time. **Do not take two doses at the same time.**
- You may not feel the full effect of LAMICTAL for several weeks.
- If you have epilepsy, tell your healthcare provider if your seizures get worse or if you have any new types of seizures.
- Swallow LAMICTAL tablets whole.
- If you have trouble swallowing LAMICTAL Tablets, there may be another form of LAMICTAL you can take.
- LAMICTAL ODT should be placed on the tongue and moved around the mouth. The tablet will rapidly disintegrate, can be swallowed with or without water, and can be taken with or without food.
- LAMICTAL Chewable Dispersible tablets may be swallowed whole, chewed, or mixed in water or diluted fruit juice. If the tablets are chewed, drink a small amount of water or diluted fruit juice to help in swallowing. To break up LAMICTAL Chewable Dispersible tablets, add the tablets to a small amount of liquid (1 teaspoon, or enough to cover the medicine) in a glass or spoon. Wait at least 1 minute or until the tablets are completely broken up, mix the solution together and take the whole amount right away.
- If you receive LAMICTAL in a blisterpack, examine the blisterpack before use. Do not use if blisters are torn, broken, or missing.

What should I avoid while taking LAMICTAL?

- Do not drive a car or operate complex, hazardous machinery until you know how LAMICTAL affects you.

What are possible side effects of LAMICTAL?

- See "What is the most important information I should know about LAMICTAL?"

Common side effects of LAMICTAL include:

• dizziness	• tremor
• headache	• rash
• blurred or double vision	• fever
• lack of coordination	• abdominal pain
• sleepiness	• back pain
• nausea, vomiting	• tiredness
• insomnia	• dry mouth

Tell your healthcare provider about any side effect that bothers you or that does not go away.

These are not all the possible side effects of LAMICTAL. For more information, ask your healthcare provider or pharmacist.

Call your doctor for medical advice about side effects. You may report side effects to FDA at 1-800-FDA-1088.

How should I store LAMICTAL?

- Store LAMICTAL at room temperature between 68°F to 77°F (20°C to 25°C).
- **Keep LAMICTAL and all medicines out of the reach of children.**

General information about LAMICTAL

Medicines are sometimes prescribed for purposes other than those listed in a Medication Guide. Do not use LAMICTAL for a condition for which it was not prescribed. Do not give LAMICTAL to other people, even if they have the same symptoms you have. It may harm them.

This Medication Guide summarizes the most important information about LAMICTAL. If you would like more information, talk with your healthcare provider. You can ask your healthcare provider or pharmacist for information about LAMICTAL that is written for healthcare professionals.

For more information, go to www.lamictal.com or call 1-888-825-5249.

What are the ingredients in LAMICTAL?

LAMICTAL Tablets

Active ingredient: lamotrigine.

Inactive ingredients: lactose; magnesium stearate, microcrystalline cellulose, povidone, sodium starch glycolate, FD&C Yellow No. 6 Lake (100-mg tablet only), ferric oxide, yellow (150-mg tablet only), and FD&C Blue No. 2 Lake (200-mg tablet only).

LAMICTAL Chewable Dispersible Tablets

Active ingredient: lamotrigine.

Inactive ingredients: blackcurrant flavor, calcium carbonate, low-substituted hydroxypropylcellulose, magnesium aluminum silicate, magnesium stearate, povidone, saccharin sodium, and sodium starch glycolate.

LAMICTAL ODT Orally Disintegrating Tablets

Active ingredient: lamotrigine.

Inactive ingredients: artificial cherry flavor, crospovidone, ethylcellulose, magnesium stearate, mannitol, polyethylene, and sucralose.

This Medication Guide has been approved by the U.S. Food and Drug Administration.

GlaxoSmithKline
Research Triangle Park, NC 27709
LAMICTAL Tablets and Chewable Dispersible Tablets are manufactured by
DSM Pharmaceuticals, Inc., Greenville, NC 27834 or
GlaxoSmithKline, Research Triangle Park, NC 27709
LAMICTAL Orally Disintegrating Tablets are manufactured by
Eurand, Inc., Vandalia, OH 45377
LAMICTAL is a registered trademark of GlaxoSmithKline.
DEPAKENE and DEPAKOTE are registered trademarks of Abbott Laboratories.
©2009, GlaxoSmithKline. All rights reserved.
May 2009
LMT:2MG

LAMICTAL® XR™ ℞

[la-mĭk' tal]
(lamotrigine)
Extended-Release Tablets

HIGHLIGHTS OF PRESCRIBING INFORMATION

These highlights do not include all the information needed to use LAMICTAL XR safely and effectively. See full prescribing information for LAMICTAL XR.

LAMICTAL XR (lamotrigine) Extended-Release Tablets
Initial U.S. Approval: 1994

> **WARNING: SERIOUS SKIN RASHES**
> ***See full prescribing information for complete boxed warning.***
> **Cases of life-threatening serious rashes, including Stevens-Johnson syndrome, toxic-epidermal necrolysis, and/or rash-related death, have been caused by lamotrigine. The rate of serious rash is greater in pediatric patients than in adults. Additional factors that may increase the risk of rash include (5.1):**
> - **coadministration with valproate**
> - **exceeding recommended initial dose of LAMICTAL XR**
> - **exceeding recommended dose escalation of LAMICTAL XR**
>
> **Benign rashes are also caused by lamotrigine; however, it is not possible to predict which rashes will prove to be serious or life-threatening. LAMICTAL XR should be discontinued at the first sign of rash unless the rash is clearly not drug-related. (5.1)**

RECENT MAJOR CHANGES

Indications and Usage (1) January/2010
Dosage and Administration (2.2) January/2010

INDICATIONS AND USAGE

LAMICTAL XR is an antiepileptic drug (AED) indicated as adjunctive therapy for primary generalized tonic-clonic (PGTC) seizures and partial onset seizures with or without secondary generalization in patients ≥13 years of age. (1.1)

DOSAGE AND ADMINISTRATION

- Doses are administered once daily. Dose escalation and maintenance doses are based on concomitant medications. (2.1, 2.2)
- To avoid an increased risk of rash, the recommended initial dose and subsequent dose escalations should not be exceeded. LAMICTAL XR Patient Titration Kits are available for the first 5 weeks of treatment. (2.1, 16)
- For patients being converted from immediate-release lamotrigine to LAMICTAL XR, the initial dose of LAMICTAL XR should match the total daily dose of the immediate-release lamotrigine. Patients should be closely monitored for seizure control after conversion to LAMICTAL XR. (2.3)
- Do not restart LAMICTAL XR in patients who discontinued due to rash unless the potential benefits clearly outweigh the risks. (2.1, 5.1)
- Adjustments to maintenance doses will in most cases be required in patients starting or stopping estrogen-containing oral contraceptives. (2.1, 5.7)
- LAMICTAL XR should be discontinued over a period of at least 2 weeks (approximately 50% reduction per week). (2.1, 5.8)

DOSAGE FORMS AND STRENGTHS

Extended-Release Tablets: 25 mg, 50 mg, 100 mg, and 200 mg. (3.1, 16)

CONTRAINDICATIONS

Hypersensitivity to the drug or its ingredients. (Boxed Warning, 4)

WARNINGS AND PRECAUTIONS

- Life-threatening serious rash, and/or rash-related death, may result. (Boxed Warning, 5.1)
- Hypersensitivity reaction may be fatal or life-threatening. Early signs of hypersensitivity (e.g., fever, lymphadenopathy) may present without rash; if signs present, patient should be evaluated immediately.
- LAMICTAL XR should be discontinued if alternate etiology for hypersensitivity signs is not found. (5.2)
- Acute multiorgan failure has resulted (some cases fatal). (5.3)
- Blood dyscrasias (e.g., neutropenia, thrombocytopenia, pancytopenia) may result, either with or without an associated hypersensitivity syndrome. (5.4)
- Suicidal behavior and ideation. (5.5)
- Medication errors involving LAMICTAL have occurred. In particular, the names LAMICTAL or lamotrigine can be confused with the names of other commonly used medications. Medication errors may also occur between the different formulations of LAMICTAL. (3.2, 5.6, 16, 17.9)

ADVERSE REACTIONS

- Most common adverse reactions (treatment difference ≥4%, LAMICTAL XR - Placebo) are dizziness, tremor/intention tremor, vomiting, and diplopia. (6.1)

To report SUSPECTED ADVERSE REACTIONS, contact GlaxoSmithKline at 1-888-825-5249 or FDA at 1-800-FDA-1088 or www.fda.gov/medwatch.

DRUG INTERACTIONS

- Valproate increases lamotrigine concentrations more than 2-fold. (7, 12.3)
- Carbamazepine, phenytoin, phenobarbital, and primidone decrease lamotrigine concentrations by approximately 40%. (7, 12.3)
- Oral estrogen-containing contraceptives and rifampin also decrease lamotrigine concentrations by approximately 50%. (7, 12.3)

USE IN SPECIFIC POPULATIONS

- Pediatric use: Safety and effectiveness in patients below the age of 13 have not been established. (8.4)

- Effectiveness of lamotrigine, used as adjunctive treatment for partial seizures, was not demonstrated in a small randomized, double-blind, placebo-controlled, withdrawal study in very young pediatric patients (1 to 24 months). (8.4)
- Hepatic impairment: Dosage adjustments required. (2.1)
- Healthcare professionals can enroll patients in the Lamotrigine Pregnancy Registry (1-800-336-2176). Patients can enroll themselves in the North American Antiepileptic Drug Pregnancy Registry (1 888 233 2334). (8.1)

See 17 for PATIENT COUNSELING INFORMATION and Medication Guide

Revised: 01/2010

FULL PRESCRIBING INFORMATION

> **WARNING: SERIOUS SKIN RASHES**
>
> LAMICTAL® XR™ can cause serious rashes requiring hospitalization and discontinuation of treatment. The incidence of these rashes, which have included Stevens-Johnson syndrome, is approximately 0.8% (8 per 1,000) in pediatric patients (2 to 16 years of age) receiving the immediate-release formulation of LAMICTAL as adjunctive therapy for epilepsy and 0.3% (3 per 1,000) in adults on adjunctive therapy for epilepsy. In a prospectively followed cohort of 1,983 pediatric patients (2 to 16 years of age) with epilepsy taking the adjunctive immediate-release formulation of LAMICTAL, there was 1 rash-related death. LAMICTAL XR is not approved for patients under the age of 13 years. In worldwide postmarketing experience, rare cases of toxic epidermal necrolysis and/or rash-related death have been reported in adult and pediatric patients, but their numbers are too few to permit a precise estimate of the rate.
>
> The risk of serious rash caused by treatment with LAMICTAL XR is not expected to differ from that with the immediate-release formulation of LAMICTAL. However, the relatively limited treatment experience with LAMICTAL XR makes it difficult to characterize the frequency and risk of serious rashes caused by treatment with LAMICTAL XR.
>
> Other than age, there are as yet no factors identified that are known to predict the risk of occurrence or the severity of rash caused by LAMICTAL XR. There are suggestions, yet to be proven, that the risk of rash may also be increased by (1) coadministration of LAMICTAL XR with valproate (includes valproic acid and divalproex sodium), (2) exceeding the recommended initial dose of LAMICTAL XR, or (3) exceeding the recommended dose escalation for LAMICTAL XR. However, cases have occurred in the absence of these factors.
>
> Nearly all cases of life-threatening rashes caused by the immediate-release formulation of LAMICTAL have occurred within 2 to 8 weeks of treatment initiation. However, isolated cases have occurred after prolonged treatment (e.g., 6 months). Accordingly, duration of therapy cannot be relied upon as means to predict the potential risk heralded by the first appearance of a rash. Although benign rashes are also caused by LAMICTAL XR, it is not possible to predict reliably which rashes will prove to be serious or life-threatening. Accordingly, LAMICTAL XR should ordinarily be discontinued at the first sign of rash, unless the rash is clearly not drug-related. Discontinuation of treatment may not prevent a rash from becoming life-threatening or permanently disabling or disfiguring *[see Warnings and Precautions (5.1)]*.

---

1   INDICATIONS AND USAGE

LAMICTAL XR is indicated as adjunctive therapy for primary generalized tonic-clonic (PGTC) seizures and partial onset seizures with or without secondary generalization in patients ≥13 years of age.

Safety and effectiveness of LAMICTAL XR for use in patients below the age of 13 have not been established.

2   DOSAGE AND ADMINISTRATION

LAMICTAL XR Extended-Release Tablets are taken once daily, with or without food. Tablets must be swallowed whole and must not be chewed, crushed, or divided.

2.1   General Dosing Considerations

Rash: There are suggestions, yet to be proven, that the risk of severe, potentially life-threatening rash may be increased by (1) coadministration of LAMICTAL XR with valproate, (2) exceeding the recommended initial dose of LAMICTAL XR, or (3) exceeding the recommended dose escalation for LAMICTAL XR. However, cases have occurred in the absence of these factors *[see Boxed Warning]*. Therefore, it is important that the dosing recommendations be followed closely.

The risk of nonserious rash may be increased when the recommended initial dose and/or the rate of dose escalation of LAMICTAL XR is exceeded and in patients with a history of allergy or rash to other AEDs.

LAMICTAL XR Patient Titration Kits provide LAMICTAL XR at doses consistent with the recommended titration schedule for the first 5 weeks of treatment, based upon concomitant medications for patients with partial onset seizures and are intended to help reduce the potential for rash. The use of LAMICTAL XR Patient Titration Kits is recommended for appropriate patients who are starting or restarting LAMICTAL XR *[see How Supplied/Storage and Handling (16)]*.

It is recommended that LAMICTAL XR not be restarted in patients who discontinued due to rash associated with prior treatment with lamotrigine, unless the potential benefits clearly outweigh the risks. If the decision is made to restart a patient who has discontinued LAMICTAL XR, the need to restart with the initial dosing recommendations should be assessed. The greater the interval of time since the previous dose, the greater consideration should be given to restarting with the initial dosing recommendations. If a patient has discontinued lamotrigine for a period of more than 5 half-lives, it is recommended that initial dosing recommendations and guidelines be followed. The half-life of lamotrigine is affected by other concomitant medications *[see Clinical Pharmacology (12.3)]*.

LAMICTAL XR Added to Drugs Known to Induce or Inhibit Glucuronidation: Drugs other than those listed in the Clinical Pharmacology section *[see Clinical Pharmacology (12.3)]* have not been systematically evaluated in combination with lamotrigine. Because lamotrigine is metabolized predominantly by glucuronic acid conjugation, drugs that are known to induce or inhibit glucuronidation may affect the apparent clearance of lamotrigine and doses of LAMICTAL XR may require adjustment based on clinical response.

Target Plasma Levels: A therapeutic plasma concentration range has not been established for lamotrigine. Dosing of LAMICTAL XR should be based on therapeutic response *[see Clinical Pharmacology (12.3)]*.

Women Taking Estrogen-Containing Oral Contraceptives: *Starting LAMICTAL XR in Women Taking Estrogen-Containing Oral Contraceptives:* Although estrogen-containing oral contraceptives have been shown to increase the clearance of lamotrigine *[see Clinical Pharmacology (12.3)]*, no adjustments to the recommended dose-escalation guidelines for LAMICTAL XR should be necessary solely based on the use of estrogen-containing oral contraceptives. Therefore, dose escalation should follow the recommended guidelines for initiating adjunctive therapy with LAMICTAL XR based on the concomitant AED or other concomitant medications (see Table 1). See below for adjustments to maintenance doses of LAMICTAL XR in women taking estrogen-containing oral contraceptives.

Adjustments to the Maintenance Dose of LAMICTAL XR In Women Taking Estrogen-Containing Oral Contraceptives: (1) *Taking Estrogen-Containing Oral Contraceptives:*   For women not taking carbamazepine, phenytoin, phenobarbital, primidone, or other drugs such as rifampin that induce lamotrigine glucuronidation *[see Drug Interactions (7), Clinical Pharmacology (12.3)]*, the maintenance dose of LAMICTAL XR will in most cases need to be increased, by as much as 2-fold over the recommended target maintenance dose, in order to maintain a consistent lamotrigine plasma level *[see Clinical Pharmacology (12.3)]*.

(2) *Starting Estrogen-Containing Oral Contraceptives:*   In women taking a stable dose of LAMICTAL XR and not taking carbamazepine, phenytoin, phenobarbital, primidone, or other drugs such as rifampin that induce lamotrigine glucuronidation *[see Drug Interactions (7), Clinical Pharmacology (12.3)]*, the maintenance dose will in most cases need to be increased by as much as 2-fold in order to maintain a consistent lamotrigine plasma level. The dose increases should begin at the same time that the oral contraceptive is introduced and continue, based on clinical response, no more rapidly than 50 to 100 mg/day every week. Dose increases should not exceed the recommended rate (see Table 1) unless lamotrigine plasma levels or clinical response support larger increases. Gradual transient increases in lamotrigine plasma levels may occur during the week of inactive hormonal preparation ("pill-free" week), and these increases will be greater if dose increases are made in the days before or during the week of inactive hormonal preparation. Increased lamotrigine plasma levels could result in additional adverse reactions, such as dizziness, ataxia, and diplopia. If adverse reactions attributable to LAMICTAL XR consistently occur during the "pill-free" week, dose adjustments to the overall maintenance dose may be necessary. Dose adjustments limited to the "pill-free" week are not recommended. For women taking LAMICTAL XR in addition to carbamazepine, phenytoin, phenobarbital, primidone, or other drugs such as rifampin that induce lamotrigine glucuronidation *[see Drug Interactions (7), Clinical Pharmacology (12.3)]*, no adjustment to the dose of LAMICTAL XR should be necessary.

(3) *Stopping Estrogen-Containing Oral Contraceptives:* For women not taking carbamazepine, phenytoin, phenobarbital, primidone, or other drugs such as rifampin that induce lamotrigine glucuronidation *[see Drug Interactions (7), Clinical Pharmacology (12.3)]*, the maintenance dose of LAMICTAL XR will in most cases need to be decreased by as much as 50% in order to maintain a consistent lamotrigine plasma level. The decrease in dose of LAMICTAL XR should not exceed 25% of the total daily dose per week over a 2-week period, unless clinical response or lamotrigine plasma levels indicate otherwise *[see Clinical Pharmacology (12.3)]*. For women taking LAMICTAL XR in addition to carbamazepine, phenytoin, phenobarbital, primidone, or other drugs such as rifampin that induce lamotrigine glucuronidation *[see Drug Interactions (7), Clin-*

Table 1. Escalation Regimen for LAMICTAL XR in Patients ≥13 Years of Age

	For Patients TAKING Valproate[a]	For Patients NOT TAKING Carbamazepine, Phenytoin, Phenobarbital, Primidone,[b] or Valproate[a]	For Patients TAKING Carbamazepine, Phenytoin, Phenobarbital, or Primidone[b] and NOT TAKING Valproate[a]
Weeks 1 and 2	25 mg every *other* day	25 mg every day	50 mg every day
Weeks 3 and 4	25 mg every day	50 mg every day	100 mg every day
Week 5	50 mg every day	100 mg every day	200 mg every day
Week 6	100 mg every day	150 mg every day	300 mg every day
Week 7	150 mg every day	200 mg every day	400 mg every day
Maintenance Range (Week 8 and onward)	200 to 250 mg every day[c]	300 to 400 mg every day[c]	400 to 600 mg every day[c]

[a] Valproate has been shown to inhibit glucuronidation and decrease the apparent clearance of lamotrigine *[see Drug Interactions (7), Clinical Pharmacology (12.3)].*

[b] These drugs induce lamotrigine glucuronidation and increase clearance *[see Drug Interactions (7), Clinical Pharmacology (12.3)].* Other drugs which have similar effects include estrogen-containing oral contraceptives *[see Drug Interactions (7), Clinical Pharmacology (12.3)].* Dosing recommendations for oral contraceptives can be found in General Dosing Considerations *[see Dosage and Administration (2.1)].* Patients on rifampin, or other drugs that induce lamotrigine glucuronidation and increase clearance, should follow the same dosing titration/maintenance regimen as that used with anticonvulsants that have this effect.

[c] Dose increases at week 8 or later should not exceed 100 mg daily at weekly intervals.

ical Pharmacology (12.3)], no adjustment to the dose of LAMICTAL XR should be necessary.

Women and Other Hormonal Contraceptive Preparations or Hormone Replacement Therapy: The effect of other hormonal contraceptive preparations or hormone replacement therapy on the pharmacokinetics of lamotrigine has not been systematically evaluated. It has been reported that ethinylestradiol, not progestogens, increased the clearance of lamotrigine up to 2-fold, and the progestin-only pills had no effect on lamotrigine plasma levels. Therefore, adjustments to the dosage of LAMICTAL XR in the presence of progestogens alone will likely not be needed.

Patients With Hepatic Impairment: Experience in patients with hepatic impairment is limited. Based on a clinical pharmacology study in 24 patients with mild, moderate, and severe liver impairment *[see Use in Specific Populations (8.6), Clinical Pharmacology (12.3)],* the following general recommendations can be made. No dosage adjustment is needed in patients with mild liver impairment. Initial, escalation, and maintenance doses should generally be reduced by approximately 25% in patients with moderate and severe liver impairment without ascites and 50% in patients with severe liver impairment with ascites. Escalation and maintenance doses may be adjusted according to clinical response.

Patients With Renal Impairment: Initial doses of LAMICTAL XR should be based on patients' concomitant medications (see Table 1); reduced maintenance doses may be effective for patients with significant renal impairment *[see Use in Specific Populations (8.7), Clinical Pharmacology (12.3)].* Few patients with severe renal impairment have been evaluated during chronic treatment with immediate-release lamotrigine. Because there is inadequate experience in this population, LAMICTAL XR should be used with caution in these patients.

Discontinuation Strategy: For patients receiving LAMICTAL XR in combination with other AEDs, a re-evaluation of all AEDs in the regimen should be considered if a change in seizure control or an appearance or worsening of adverse reactions is observed. If a decision is made to discontinue therapy with LAMICTAL XR, a step-wise reduction of dose over at least 2 weeks (approximately 50% per week) is recommended unless safety concerns require a more rapid withdrawal *[see Warnings and Precautions (5.8)].* Discontinuing carbamazepine, phenytoin, phenobarbital, primidone, or other drugs such as rifampin that induce lamotrigine glucuronidation should prolong the half-life of lamotrigine; discontinuing valproate should shorten the half-life of lamotrigine.

2.2 Primary Generalized Tonic-Clonic and Partial Onset Seizures

This section provides specific dosing recommendations for patients ≥13 years of age. Specific dosing recommendations are provided depending upon concomitant AED or other concomitant medications.

[See table 1 above]

2.3 Conversion From Immediate-Release Lamotrigine Tablets to LAMICTAL XR

Patients may be converted directly from immediate-release lamotrigine to LAMICTAL XR Extended-Release Tablets. The initial dose of LAMICTAL XR should match the total daily dose of immediate-release lamotrigine. However, some subjects on concomitant enzyme-inducing agents may have lower plasma levels of lamotrigine on conversion and should be monitored *[see Clinical Pharmacology (12.3)].*

Following conversion to LAMICTAL XR, all patients (but especially those on drugs that induce lamotrigine glucuronidation) should be closely monitored for seizure control *[see Drug Interactions (7)].* Depending on the therapeutic response after conversion, the total daily dose may need to be adjusted within the recommended dosing instructions (Table 1).

3 DOSAGE FORMS AND STRENGTHS

3.1 Extended-Release Tablets

25 mg, yellow with white center, round, biconvex, film-coated tablets printed with "LAMICTAL" and "XR 25."

50 mg, green with white center, round, biconvex, film-coated tablets printed with "LAMICTAL" and "XR 50."

100 mg, orange with white center, round, biconvex, film-coated tablets printed with "LAMICTAL" and "XR 100."

200 mg, blue with white center, round, biconvex, film-coated tablets printed with "LAMICTAL" and "XR 200."

3.2 Potential Medication Errors

Patients should be strongly advised to visually inspect their tablets to verify that they are receiving LAMICTAL XR, as opposed to other medications, and that they are receiving the correct formulation of LAMICTAL each time they fill their prescription. Depictions of the LAMICTAL XR tablets can be found in the Medication Guide,

4 CONTRAINDICATIONS

LAMICTAL XR is contraindicated in patients who have demonstrated hypersensitivity to the drug or its ingredients *[see Boxed Warning, Warnings and Precautions (5.1), (5.2)].*

5 WARNINGS AND PRECAUTIONS

5.1 Serious Skin Rashes

[see Boxed Warning]

The risk of serious rash caused by treatment with LAMICTAL XR is not expected to differ from that with the immediate-release formulation of LAMICTAL *[see Boxed Warning].* However, the relatively limited treatment experience with LAMICTAL XR makes it difficult to characterize the frequency and risk of serious rashes caused by treatment with LAMICTAL XR.

Pediatric Population: The incidence of serious rash associated with hospitalization and discontinuation of the immediate-release formulation of LAMICTAL in a prospectively followed cohort of pediatric patients (2 to 16 years of age) with epilepsy receiving adjunctive therapy with immediate-release lamotrigine was approximately 0.8% (16 of 1,983). When 14 of these cases were reviewed by 3 expert dermatologists, there was considerable disagreement as to their proper classification. To illustrate, one dermatologist considered none of the cases to be Stevens-Johnson syndrome; another assigned 7 of the 14 to this diagnosis. There was 1 rash-related death in this 1,983-patient cohort. Additionally, there have been rare cases of toxic epidermal necrolysis with and without permanent sequelae and/or death in US and foreign postmarketing experience.

There is evidence that the inclusion of valproate in a multidrug regimen increases the risk of serious, potentially life-threatening rash in pediatric patients. In pediatric patients who used valproate concomitantly, 1.2% (6 of 482) experienced a serious rash compared with 0.6% (6 of 952) patients not taking valproate.

LAMICTAL XR is not approved in patients under the age of 13 years.

Adult Population: Serious rash associated with hospitalization and discontinuation of the immediate-release formulation of LAMICTAL occurred in 0.3% (11 of 3,348) of adult patients who received the immediate-release formulation of LAMICTAL in premarketing clinical trials of epilepsy. In worldwide postmarketing experience, rare cases of rash-related death have been reported, but their numbers are too few to permit a precise estimate of the rate.

Among the rashes leading to hospitalization were Stevens-Johnson syndrome, toxic epidermal necrolysis, angioedema, and a rash associated with a variable number of the following systemic manifestations: fever, lymphadenopathy, facial swelling, and hematologic and hepatologic abnormalities. There is evidence that the inclusion of valproate in a multidrug regimen increases the risk of serious, potentially life-threatening rash in adults. Specifically, of 584 patients administered the immediate-release formulation of LAMICTAL with valproate in epilepsy clinical trials, 6 (1%) were hospitalized in association with rash; in contrast, 4 (0.16%) of 2,398 clinical trial patients and volunteers administered the immediate-release formulation of LAMICTAL in the absence of valproate were hospitalized.

Patients With History of Allergy or Rash to Other AEDs: The risk of nonserious rash may be increased when the recommended initial dose and/or the rate of dose escalation of LAMICTAL is exceeded and in patients with a history of allergy or rash to other AEDs.

5.2 Hypersensitivity Reactions

Hypersensitivity reactions, some fatal or life-threatening, have also occurred. Some of these reactions have included clinical features of multiorgan failure/dysfunction, including hepatic abnormalities and evidence of disseminated intravascular coagulation. It is important to note that early manifestations of hypersensitivity (e.g., fever, lymphadenopathy) may be present even though a rash is not evident. If such signs or symptoms are present, the patient should be evaluated immediately. LAMICTAL XR should be discontinued if an alternative etiology for the signs or symptoms cannot be established.

Prior to initiation of treatment with LAMICTAL XR, the patient should be instructed that a rash or other signs or symptoms of hypersensitivity (e.g., fever, lymphadenopathy) may herald a serious medical event and that the patient should report any such occurrence to a physician immediately.

5.3 Acute Multiorgan Failure

Multiorgan failure, which in some cases has been fatal or irreversible, has been observed in patients receiving the immediate-release formulation of LAMICTAL. Fatalities associated with multiorgan failure and various degrees of hepatic failure have been reported in 2 of 3,796 adult patients and 4 of 2,435 pediatric patients who received the immediate-release formulation of LAMICTAL in epilepsy clinical trials. Rare fatalities from multiorgan failure have been reported in compassionate plea and postmarketing use. The majority of these deaths occurred in association with other serious medical events, including status epilepticus and overwhelming sepsis, and hantavirus, making it difficult to identify the initial cause.

Additionally, 3 patients (a 45-year-old woman, a 3.5-year-old boy, and an 11-year-old girl) developed multiorgan dysfunction and disseminated intravascular coagulation 9 to 14 days after the immediate-release formulation of LAMICTAL was added to their AED regimens. Rash and elevated transaminases were also present in all patients and rhabdomyolysis was noted in 2 patients. Both pediatric patients were receiving concomitant therapy with valproate, while the adult patient was being treated with carbamazepine and clonazepam. All patients subsequently recovered with supportive care after treatment with the immediate-release formulation of LAMICTAL was discontinued.

5.4 Blood Dyscrasias

There have been reports of blood dyscrasias with the immediate-release formulation of LAMICTAL that may or may not be associated with the hypersensitivity syndrome. These have included neutropenia, leukopenia, anemia, thrombocytopenia, pancytopenia, and, rarely, aplastic anemia and pure red cell aplasia.

5.5 Suicidal Behavior and Ideation

Antiepileptic drugs (AEDs), including LAMICTAL XR, increase the risk of suicidal thoughts or behavior in patients taking these drugs for any indication. Patients treated with any AED for any indication should be monitored for the emergence or worsening of depression, suicidal thoughts or behavior, and/or any unusual changes in mood or behavior. Pooled analyses of 199 placebo-controlled clinical trials (mono- and adjunctive therapy) of 11 different AEDs showed that patients randomized to one of the AEDs had approximately twice the risk (adjusted Relative Risk 1.8, 95%

CI: 1.2, 2.7) of suicidal thinking or behavior compared to patients randomized to placebo. In these trials, which had a median treatment duration of 12 weeks, the estimated incidence of suicidal behavior or ideation among 27,863 AED-treated patients was 0.43%, compared to 0.24% among 16,029 placebo-treated patients, representing an increase of approximately 1 case of suicidal thinking or behavior for every 530 patients treated. There were 4 suicides in drug-treated patients in the trials and none in placebo-treated patients, but the number of events is too small to allow any conclusion about drug effect on suicide.

The increased risk of suicidal thoughts or behavior with AEDs was observed as early as 1 week after starting treatment with AEDs and persisted for the duration of treatment assessed. Because most trials included in the analysis did not extend beyond 24 weeks, the risk of suicidal thoughts or behavior beyond 24 weeks could not be assessed.

The risk of suicidal thoughts or behavior was generally consistent among drugs in the data analyzed. The finding of increased risk with AEDs of varying mechanism of action and across a range of indications suggests that the risk applies to all AEDs used for any indication. The risk did not vary substantially by age (5 to 100 years) in the clinical trials analyzed.

Table 2 shows absolute and relative risk by indication for all evaluated AEDs.

[See table 2 above]

Table 2. Risk by Indication for Antiepileptic Drugs in the Pooled Analysis

Indication	Placebo Patients With Events Per 1,000 Patients	Drug Patients With Events Per 1,000 Patients	Relative Risk: Incidence of Events in Drug Patients/Incidence in Placebo Patients	Risk Difference: Additional Drug Patients With Events Per 1,000 Patients
Epilepsy	1.0	3.4	3.5	2.4
Psychiatric	5.7	8.5	1.5	2.9
Other	1.0	1.8	1.9	0.9
Total	2.4	4.3	1.8	1.9

The relative risk for suicidal thoughts or behavior was higher in clinical trials for epilepsy than in clinical trials for psychiatric or other conditions, but the absolute risk differences were similar for the epilepsy and psychiatric indications.

Anyone considering prescribing LAMICTAL XR or any other AED must balance the risk of suicidal thoughts or behavior with the risk of untreated illness. Epilepsy and many other illnesses for which AEDs are prescribed are themselves associated with morbidity and mortality and an increased risk of suicidal thoughts and behavior. Should suicidal thoughts and behavior emerge during treatment, the prescriber needs to consider whether the emergence of these symptoms in any given patient may be related to the illness being treated.

Patients, their caregivers, and families should be informed that AEDs increase the risk of suicidal thoughts and behavior and should be advised of the need to be alert for the emergence or worsening of the signs and symptoms of depression, any unusual changes in mood or behavior, or the emergence of suicidal thoughts, behavior, or thoughts about self-harm. Behaviors of concern should be reported immediately to healthcare providers.

5.6 Potential Medication Errors

Medication errors involving LAMICTAL have occurred. In particular, the names LAMICTAL or lamotrigine can be confused with the names of other commonly used medications. Medication errors may also occur between the different formulations of LAMICTAL. To reduce the potential of medication errors, write and say LAMICTAL XR clearly. Depictions of the LAMICTAL XR Extended-Release Tablets can be found in the Medication Guide. Each LAMICTAL XR tablet has a distinct color and white center, and is printed with "LAMICTAL XR" and the tablet strength. These distinctive features serve to identify the different presentations of the drug and thus may help reduce the risk of medication errors. LAMICTAL XR is supplied in round, unit-of-use bottles with orange caps containing 30 tablets. The label on the bottle includes a depiction of the tablets which further communicates to patients and pharmacists that the medication is LAMICTAL XR and the specific tablet strength included in the bottle. The unit-of-use bottle with a distinctive orange cap and distinctive bottle label features serves to identify the different presentations of the drug and thus may help to reduce the risk of medication errors. To avoid the medication error of using the wrong drug or formulation, patients should be strongly advised to visually inspect their tablets to verify that they are LAMICTAL XR each time they fill their prescription.

5.7 Concomitant Use With Oral Contraceptives

Some estrogen-containing oral contraceptives have been shown to decrease serum concentrations of lamotrigine *[see Clinical Pharmacology (12.3)]*. **Dosage adjustments will be necessary in most patients who start or stop estrogen-containing oral contraceptives while taking LAMICTAL XR** *[see Dosage and Administration (2.1)]*. During the week of inactive hormone preparation ("pill-free" week) of oral contraceptive therapy, plasma lamotrigine levels are expected to rise, as much as doubling at the end of the week. Adverse reactions consistent with elevated levels of lamotrigine, such as dizziness, ataxia, and diplopia, could occur.

5.8 Withdrawal Seizures

As with other AEDs, LAMICTAL XR should not be abruptly discontinued. In patients with epilepsy there is a possibility of increasing seizure frequency. Unless safety concerns require a more rapid withdrawal, the dose of LAMICTAL XR should be tapered over a period of at least 2 weeks (approximately 50% reduction per week) *[see Dosage and Administration (2.1)]*.

5.9 Status Epilepticus

Valid estimates of the incidence of treatment-emergent status epilepticus among patients treated with immediate-release lamotrigine are difficult to obtain because reporters participating in clinical trials did not all employ identical rules for identifying cases. At a minimum, 7 of 2,343 adult patients had episodes that could unequivocally be described as status epilepticus. In addition, a number of reports of variably defined episodes of seizure exacerbation (e.g., seizure clusters, seizure flurries, etc.) were made.

5.10 Sudden Unexplained Death in Epilepsy (SUDEP)

During the premarketing development of the immediate-release formulation of LAMICTAL, 20 sudden and unexplained deaths were recorded among a cohort of 4,700 patients with epilepsy (5,747 patient-years of exposure).

Some of these could represent seizure-related deaths in which the seizure was not observed, e.g., at night. This represents an incidence of 0.0035 deaths per patient-year. Although this rate exceeds that expected in a healthy population matched for age and sex, it is within the range of estimates for the incidence of sudden unexplained deaths in patients with epilepsy not receiving lamotrigine (ranging from 0.0005 for the general population of patients with epilepsy, to 0.004 for a recently studied clinical trial population similar to that in the clinical development program for immediate-release lamotrigine, to 0.005 for patients with refractory epilepsy). Consequently, whether these figures are reassuring or suggest concern depends on the comparability of the populations reported upon to the cohort receiving immediate-release lamotrigine and the accuracy of the estimates provided. Probably most reassuring is the similarity of estimated SUDEP rates in patients receiving immediate-release lamotrigine and those receiving other AEDs, chemically unrelated to each other, that underwent clinical testing in similar populations. Importantly, that drug is chemically unrelated to lamotrigine. This evidence suggests, although it certainly does not prove, that the high SUDEP rates reflect population rates, not a drug effect.

5.11 Addition of LAMICTAL XR to a Multidrug Regimen That Includes Valproate

Because valproate reduces the clearance of lamotrigine, the dosage of lamotrigine in the presence of valproate is less than half of that required in its absence.

5.12 Binding in the Eye and Other Melanin-Containing Tissues

Because lamotrigine binds to melanin, it could accumulate in melanin-rich tissues over time. This raises the possibility that lamotrigine may cause toxicity in these tissues after extended use. Although ophthalmological testing was performed in one controlled clinical trial, the testing was inadequate to exclude subtle effects or injury occurring after long-term exposure. Moreover, the capacity of available tests to detect potentially adverse consequences, if any, of lamotrigine binding to melanin is unknown *[see Clinical Pharmacology (12.2)]*.

Accordingly, although there are no specific recommendations for periodic ophthalmological monitoring, prescribers should be aware of the possibility of long-term ophthalmologic effects.

5.13 Laboratory Tests

The value of monitoring plasma concentrations of lamotrigine in patients treated with LAMICTAL XR has not been established. Because of the possible pharmacokinetic interactions between lamotrigine and other drugs including AEDs (see Table 4), monitoring of the plasma levels of lamotrigine and concomitant drugs may be indicated, particularly during dosage adjustments. In general, clinical judgment should be exercised regarding monitoring of plasma levels of lamotrigine and other drugs and whether or not dosage adjustments are necessary.

Treatment with LAMICTAL XR caused an increased incidence of subnormal (below the reference range) values in some hematology analytes (e.g., total white blood cells, monocytes). The treatment effect (LAMICTAL XR % - Placebo %) incidence of subnormal counts was 3% for total white blood cells and 4% for monocytes.

6 ADVERSE REACTIONS

The following adverse reactions are described in more detail in the *Warnings and Precautions* section of the label:

- Serious skin rashes *[see Warnings and Precautions (5.1)]*
- Hypersensitivity reactions *[see Warnings and Precautions (5.2)]*
- Acute multiorgan failure *[see Warnings and Precautions (5.3)]*
- Blood dyscrasias *[see Warnings and Precautions (5.4)]*
- Suicidal behavior and ideation *[see Warnings and Precautions (5.5)]*
- Withdrawal seizures *[see Warnings and Precautions (5.8)]*
- Status epilepticus *[see Warnings and Precautions (5.9)]*
- Sudden unexplained death in epilepsy *[see Warnings and Precautions (5.10)]*

6.1 Clinical Trial Experience With LAMICTAL XR for Treatment of PGTC and Partial Onset Seizures

Because clinical trials are conducted under widely varying conditions, adverse reaction rates observed in the clinical trials of a drug cannot be directly compared with rates in the clinical trials of another drug and may not reflect the rates observed in practice.

LAMICTAL XR has been evaluated for safety in patients ≥13 years of age with PGTC and partial onset seizures. The most commonly observed adverse reactions (≥4% for LAMICTAL XR and more common on drug than placebo) in these 2 double-blind, placebo-controlled trials of adjunctive therapy with LAMICTAL XR were, in order of decreasing treatment difference (LAMICTAL XR % - Placebo %) incidence: dizziness, tremor/intention tremor, vomiting, and diplopia.

In these 2 trials, adverse reactions led to withdrawal of 4 (2%) patients in the group receiving placebo and 10 (5%) patients in the group receiving LAMICTAL XR. Dizziness was the most common reason for withdrawal in the group receiving LAMICTAL XR (5 patients [3%]). The next most common adverse reactions leading to withdrawal in 2 patients each (1%) were rash, headache, nausea, and nystagmus.

Table 3 displays the incidence of adverse reactions in these two 19-week, double-blind, placebo-controlled studies of patients with PGTC and partial onset seizures.

[See table 3 at top of next page]

Note: In these trials the incidence of nonserious rash was 2% for LAMICTAL XR and 3% for placebo. In clinical trials evaluating the immediate-release formulation of LAMICTAL, the rate of serious rash was 0.3% in adults on adjunctive therapy for epilepsy *[see Boxed Warning]*.

Adverse reactions were also analyzed to assess the incidence of the onset of an event in the titration period, and in the maintenance period, and if adverse reactions occurring in the titration phase persisted in the maintenance phase.

The incidence for many adverse reactions caused by LAMICTAL XR treatment was increased relative to placebo (i.e., LAMICTAL XR % - Placebo % = treatment difference ≥2%) in either the titration or maintenance phases of the study. During the titration phase, an increased incidence (shown in descending order of % treatment difference) was observed for diarrhea, nausea, vomiting, somnolence, vertigo, myalgia, hot flush, and anxiety. During the maintenance phase, an increased incidence was observed for dizziness, tremor, and diplopia. Some adverse reactions developing in the titration phase were notable for persisting (>7 days) into the maintenance phase. These "persistent" adverse reactions included somnolence and dizziness.

There were inadequate data to evaluate the effect of dose and/or concentration on the incidence of adverse reactions because although patients were randomized to different target doses based upon concomitant AED, the plasma exposure was expected to be generally similar among all patients receiving different doses. However, in a randomized, parallel study comparing placebo and 300 and 500 mg/day of immediate-release formulation of LAMICTAL, the inci-

Table 3. Treatment-Emergent Adverse Reaction Incidence in Double-Blind, Placebo-Controlled Adjunctive Trials of Patients With Epilepsy (Adverse Reactions ≥2% of Patients Treated With LAMICTAL XR and Numerically More Frequent Than in the Placebo Group)

Body System/Adverse Reaction	LAMICTAL XR (n = 190) %	Placebo (n = 195) %
Ear and Labyrinth Disorders		
Vertigo	3	<1
Eye Disorders		
Diplopia	5	<1
Vision blurred	3	2
Gastrointestinal Disorders		
Nausea	7	4
Vomiting	6	3
Diarrhea	5	3
Constipation	2	<1
Dry mouth	2	1
General Disorders and Administration Site Conditions		
Asthenia and fatigue	6	4
Infections and Infestations		
Sinusitis	2	1
Metabolic and Nutritional Disorders		
Anorexia	3	2
Musculoskeletal and Connective Tissue Disorder		
Myalgia	2	0
Nervous System		
Dizziness	14	6
Tremor and intention tremor	6	1
Somnolence	5	3
Cerebellar coordination and balance disorder	3	0
Nystagmus	2	<1
Psychiatric Disorders		
Depression	3	<1
Anxiety	3	0
Respiratory, Thoracic, and Mediastinal Disorders		
Pharnygolaryngeal pain	3	2
Vascular disorder		
Hot flush	2	0

dence of the most common adverse reactions (≥5%) such as ataxia, blurred vision, diplopia, and dizziness were dose-related. Less common adverse reactions (<5%) were not assessed for dose-response relationships.

There were insufficient data to evaluate the effect of gender, age, and race on the adverse reaction profile for LAMICTAL XR.

6.2   Other Adverse Reactions Observed During the Clinical Development of the Immediate-Release Formulation of LAMICTAL

All reported reactions are included except those already listed in the previous tables or elsewhere in the labeling, those too general to be informative, and those not reasonably associated with the use of the drug.

Adjunctive Therapy in Adults With Epilepsy: In addition to the adverse reactions reported above from the development of LAMICTAL XR, the following adverse reactions with an uncertain relationship to lamotrigine were reported during the clinical development of the immediate-release formulation of LAMICTAL for treatment of epilepsy in adults. These reactions occurred in ≥2% of patients receiving the immediate-release formulation of LAMICTAL and more frequently than in the placebo group.

Body as a Whole: Flu syndrome, fever, abdominal pain, neck pain.
Musculoskeletal: Arthralgia.
Nervous: Insomnia, convulsion, irritability, speech disorder, concentration disturbance.
Respiratory: Rhinitis, pharyngitis, cough increased.
Skin and Appendages: Rash, pruritus.
Urogenital: (female patients only) Vaginitis, amenorrhea, dysmenorrhea.
Other Clinical Trial Experience: The immediate-release formulation of LAMICTAL has been administered to 6,694 individuals for whom complete adverse reaction data was captured during all clinical trials, only some of which were placebo controlled. During these trials, all adverse reactions were recorded by the clinical investigators using terminology of their own choosing. To provide a meaningful estimate of the proportion of individuals having adverse reactions, similar types of reactions were grouped into a smaller number of standardized categories using modified COSTART dictionary terminology. The frequencies presented represent the proportion of the 6,694 individuals exposed to LAMICTAL who experienced an event of the type cited on at least one occasion while receiving LAMICTAL.

Adverse reactions are further classified within body system categories and enumerated in order of decreasing frequency using the following definitions: frequent adverse reactions are defined as those occurring in at least 1/100 patients; infrequent adverse reactions are those occurring in 1/100 to 1/1,000 patients; rare adverse reactions are those occurring in fewer than 1/1,000 patients.

Body as a Whole: Infrequent: Allergic reaction, chills, and malaise.
Cardiovascular System: Infrequent: Flushing, hypertension, palpitations, postural hypotension, syncope, tachycardia, and vasodilation.
Dermatological: Infrequent: Acne, hirsutism, maculopapular rash, skin discoloration, and urticaria. Rare: Angioedema, erythema, exfoliative dermatitis, fungal dermatitis, herpes zoster, leukoderma, multiforme erythema, petechial rash, pustular rash, Stevens-Johnson syndrome, and vesiculobullous rash.
Digestive System: Infrequent: Dysphagia, eructation, gastritis, gingivitis, increased appetite, increased salivation, liver function tests abnormal, and mouth ulceration. Rare: Gastrointestinal hemorrhage, glossitis, gum hemorrhage, gum hyperplasia, hematemesis, hemorrhagic colitis, hepatitis, melena, stomach ulcer, stomatitis, and tongue edema.
Endocrine System: Rare: Goiter and hypothyroidism.
Hematologic and Lymphatic System: Infrequent: Ecchymosis and leukopenia. Rare: Anemia, eosinophilia, fibrin decrease, fibrinogen decrease, iron deficiency anemia, leukocytosis, lymphocytosis, macrocytic anemia, petechia, and thrombocytopenia.
Metabolic and Nutritional Disorders: Infrequent: Aspartate transaminase increased. Rare: Alcohol intolerance, alkaline phosphatase increase, alanine transaminase increase, bilirubinemia, general edema, gamma glutamyl transpeptidase increase, and hyperglycemia.
Musculoskeletal System: Infrequent: Arthritis, leg cramps, myasthenia, and twitching. Rare: Bursitis, muscle atrophy, pathological fracture, and tendinous contracture.
Nervous System: Frequent: Confusion and paresthesia. Infrequent: Akathisia, apathy, aphasia, CNS depression, depersonalization, dysarthria, dyskinesia, euphoria, hallucinations, hostility, hyperkinesia, hypertonia, libido decreased, memory decrease, mind racing, movement disorder, myoclonus, panic attack, paranoid reaction, personality disorder, psychosis, stupor, and suicidal ideation. Rare: Choreoathetosis, delirium, delusions, dysphoria, dystonia, extrapyramidal syndrome, faintness, grand mal convulsions, hemiplegia, hyperalgesia, hyperesthesia, hypokinesia, hypotonia, manic depression reaction, muscle spasm, neuralgia, neurosis, paralysis, and peripheral neuritis.
Respiratory System: Infrequent: Yawn. Rare: Hiccup and hyperventilation.
Special Senses: Frequent: Amblyopia. Infrequent: Abnormality of accommodation, conjunctivitis, dry eyes, ear pain, photophobia, taste perversion, and tinnitus. Rare: Deafness, lacrimation disorder, oscillopsia, parosmia, ptosis, strabismus, taste loss, uveitis, and visual field defect.
Urogenital System: Infrequent: Abnormal ejaculation, hematuria, impotence, menorrhagia, polyuria, and urinary incontinence. Rare: Acute kidney failure, anorgasmia, breast abscess, breast neoplasm, creatinine increase, cystitis, dysuria, epididymitis, female lactation, kidney failure, kidney pain, nocturia, urinary retention, and urinary urgency.

6.3   Postmarketing Experience with the Immediate-Release Formulation of LAMICTAL

The following adverse events (not listed above in clinical trials or other sections of the prescribing information) have been identified during postapproval use of the immediate-release formulation of LAMICTAL. Because these events are reported voluntarily from a population of uncertain size, it is not always possible to reliably estimate their frequency or establish a causal relationship to drug exposure.

Blood and Lymphatic: Agranulocytosis, hemolytic anemia, lymphadenopathy not associated with hypersensitivity disorder.
Gastrointestinal: Esophagitis.
Hepatobiliary Tract and Pancreas: Pancreatitis.
Immunologic: Lupus-like reaction, vasculitis.
Lower Respiratory: Apnea.
Musculoskeletal: Rhabdomyolysis has been observed in patients experiencing hypersensitivity reactions.
Nervous System: Aseptic meningitis.
Neurology: Exacerbation of Parkinsonian symptoms in patients with pre-existing Parkinson's disease, tics.
Non-site Specific: Progressive immunosuppression.

7   DRUG INTERACTIONS

Significant drug interactions with lamotrigine are summarized in Table 4. Additional details of these drug interaction studies, which were conducted using the immediate-release formulation of LAMICTAL, are provided in the Clinical Pharmacology section [see Clinical Pharmacology (12.3)].

[See table 4 at right]

8 USE IN SPECIFIC POPULATIONS

8.1 Pregnancy

Teratogenic Effects: Pregnancy Category C. No evidence of teratogenicity was found in mice, rats, or rabbits when lamotrigine was orally administered to pregnant animals during the period of organogenesis at doses up to 1.2, 0.5, and 1.1 times, respectively, on a mg/m^2 basis, the highest usual human maintenance dose (i.e., 500 mg/day). However, maternal toxicity and secondary fetal toxicity producing reduced fetal weight and/or delayed ossification were seen in mice and rats, but not in rabbits at these doses. Teratology studies were also conducted using bolus intravenous administration of the isethionate salt of lamotrigine in rats and rabbits. In rat dams administered an intravenous dose at 0.6 times the highest usual human maintenance dose, the incidence of intrauterine death without signs of teratogenicity was increased.

A behavioral teratology study was conducted in rats dosed during the period of organogenesis. At day 21 postpartum, offspring of dams receiving 5 mg/kg/day or higher displayed a significantly longer latent period for open field exploration and a lower frequency of rearing. In a swimming maze test performed on days 39 to 44 postpartum, time to completion was increased in offspring of dams receiving 25 mg/kg/day. These doses represent 0.1 and 0.5 times the clinical dose on a mg/m^2 basis, respectively.

Lamotrigine did not affect fertility, teratogenesis, or postnatal development when rats were dosed prior to and during mating, and throughout gestation and lactation at doses equivalent to 0.4 times the highest usual human maintenance dose on a mg/m^2 basis.

When pregnant rats were orally dosed at 0.1, 0.14, or 0.3 times the highest human maintenance dose (on a mg/m^2 basis) during the latter part of gestation (days 15 to 20), maternal toxicity and fetal death were seen. In dams, food consumption and weight gain were reduced, and the gestation period was slightly prolonged (22.6 vs. 22.0 days in the control group). Stillborn pups were found in all 3 drug-treated groups with the highest number in the high-dose group. Postnatal death was also seen, but only in the 2 highest doses, and occurred between days 1 and 20. Some of these deaths appear to be drug-related and not secondary to the maternal toxicity. A no-observed-effect level (NOEL) could not be determined for this study.

Although lamotrigine was not found to be teratogenic in the above studies, lamotrigine decreases fetal folate concentrations in rats, an effect known to be associated with teratogenesis in animals and humans. There are no adequate and well-controlled studies in pregnant women. Because animal reproduction studies are not always predictive of human response, this drug should be used during pregnancy only if the potential benefit justifies the potential risk to the fetus.

Non-Teratogenic Effects: As with other AEDs, physiological changes during pregnancy may affect lamotrigine concentrations and/or therapeutic effect. There have been reports of decreased lamotrigine concentrations during pregnancy and restoration of pre-partum concentrations after delivery. Dosage adjustments may be necessary to maintain clinical response.

Pregnancy Exposure Registry: To provide information regarding the effects of in utero exposure to LAMICTAL XR, physicians are advised to recommend that pregnant patients taking LAMICTAL XR enroll in the North American Antiepileptic Drug (NAAED) Pregnancy Registry. This can be done by calling the toll-free number 1-888-233-2334, and must be done by patients themselves. Information on the registry can also be found at the website http://www.aedpregnancyregistry.org/.

Physicians are also encouraged to register patients in the Lamotrigine Pregnancy Registry; enrollment in this registry must be done prior to any prenatal diagnostic tests and **before fetal outcome is known. Physicians** can obtain information by calling the Lamotrigine Pregnancy Registry at 1-800-336-2176 (toll-free).

8.2 Labor and Delivery

The effect of LAMICTAL XR on labor and delivery in humans is unknown.

8.3 Nursing Mothers

Preliminary data indicate that lamotrigine passes into human milk. Because the effects on the infant exposed to lamotrigine by this route are unknown, breastfeeding while taking LAMICTAL XR is not recommended.

8.4 Pediatric Use

LAMICTAL XR is indicated as adjunctive therapy for PGTC and partial onset seizures with or without secondary generalization in patients ≥13 years of age. Safety and effectiveness of LAMICTAL XR for any use in patients below the age of 13 have not been established.

The immediate-release formulation of LAMICTAL is indicated for adjunctive therapy in patients ≥2 years of age for partial seizures, the generalized seizures of Lennox-Gastaut syndrome, and primary generalized tonic-clonic seizures.

Table 4. Established and Other Potentially Significant Drug Interactions

Concomitant Drug	Effect on Concentration of Lamotrigine or Concomitant Drug	Clinical Comment
Estrogen-containing oral contraceptive preparations containing 30 mcg ethinylestradiol and 150 mcg levonorgestrel	↓ lamotrigine ↓ levonorgestrel	Decreased lamotrigine levels approximately 50%. Decrease in levonorgestrel component by 19%.
Carbamazepine (CBZ) and CBZ epoxide	↓ lamotrigine ? CBZ epoxide	Addition of carbamazepine decreases lamotrigine concentration approximately 40%. May increase CBZ epoxide levels.
Phenobarbital/Primidone	↓ lamotrigine	Decreased lamotrigine concentration approximately 40%.
Phenytoin (PHT)	↓ lamotrigine	Decreased lamotrigine concentration approximately 40%.
Rifampin	↓ lamotrigine	Decreased lamotrigine AUC approximately 40%.
Valproate	↑ lamotrigine ? valproate	Increased lamotrigine concentrations slightly more than 2-fold. Decreased valproate concentrations an average of 25% over a 3-week period then stabilized in healthy volunteers; no change in controlled clinical trials in epilepsy patients.

↓ = Decreased (induces lamotrigine glucuronidation).
↑ = Increased (inhibits lamotrigine glucuronidation).
? = Conflicting data.

Safety and efficacy of the immediate-release formulation of LAMICTAL, used as adjunctive treatment for partial seizures, were not demonstrated in a small randomized, double-blind, placebo-controlled, withdrawal study in very young pediatric patients (1 to 24 months). The immediate-release formulation of LAMICTAL was associated with an increased risk for infectious adverse reactions (LAMICTAL 37%, Placebo 5%), and respiratory adverse reactions (LAMICTAL 26%, Placebo 5%). Infectious adverse reactions included bronchiolitis, bronchitis, ear infection, eye infection, otitis externa, pharyngitis, urinary tract infection, and viral infection. Respiratory adverse reactions included nasal congestion, cough, and apnea.

8.5 Geriatric Use

Clinical studies of LAMICTAL XR for epilepsy did not include sufficient numbers of subjects 65 years of age and over to determine whether they respond differently from younger subjects or exhibit a different safety profile than that of younger patients. In general, dose selection for an elderly patient should be cautious, usually starting at the low end of the dosing range, reflecting the greater frequency of decreased hepatic, renal, or cardiac function, and of concomitant disease or other drug therapy.

8.6 Patients With Hepatic Impairment

Experience in patients with hepatic impairment is limited. Based on a clinical pharmacology study with the immediate-release formulation of LAMICTAL in 24 patients with mild, moderate, and severe liver impairment *[see Clinical Pharmacology (12.3)]*, the following general recommendations can be made. No dosage adjustment is needed in patients with mild liver impairment. Initial, escalation, and maintenance doses should generally be reduced by approximately 25% in patients with moderate and severe liver impairment without ascites and 50% in patients with severe liver impairment with ascites. Escalation and maintenance doses may be adjusted according to clinical response *[see Dosage and Administration (2.1)]*.

8.7 Patients With Renal Impairment

Lamotrigine is metabolized mainly by glucuronic acid conjugation, with the majority of the metabolites being recovered in the urine. In a small study comparing a single dose of immediate-release lamotrigine in patients with varying degrees of renal impairment with healthy volunteers, the plasma half-life of lamotrigine was significantly longer in the patients with renal impairment *[see Clinical Pharmacology (12.3)]*.

Initial doses of LAMICTAL XR should be based on patients' AED regimens; reduced maintenance doses may be effective for patients with significant renal impairment. Few patients with severe renal impairment have been evaluated during chronic treatment with lamotrigine. Because there is inadequate experience in this population, LAMICTAL XR should be used with caution in these patients *[see Dosage and Administration (2.1)]*.

10 OVERDOSAGE

10.1 Human Overdose Experience

Overdoses involving quantities up to 15 g have been reported for the immediate-release formulation of LAMICTAL, some of which have been fatal. Overdose has resulted in ataxia, nystagmus, increased seizures, decreased level of consciousness, coma, and intraventricular conduction delay.

10.2 Management of Overdose

There are no specific antidotes for lamotrigine. Following a suspected overdose, hospitalization of the patient is advised. General supportive care is indicated, including frequent monitoring of vital signs and close observation of the patient. If indicated, emesis should be induced; usual precautions should be taken to protect the airway. It is uncertain whether hemodialysis is an effective means of removing lamotrigine from the blood. In 6 renal failure patients, about 20% of the amount of lamotrigine in the body was removed by hemodialysis during a 4-hour session. A Poison Control Center should be contacted for information on the management of overdosage of LAMICTAL XR.

11 DESCRIPTION

LAMICTAL XR (lamotrigine), an AED of the phenyltriazine class, is chemically unrelated to existing AEDs. Its chemical name is 3,5-diamino-6-(2,3-dichlorophenyl)-*as*-triazine, its molecular formula is $C_9H_7N_5Cl_2$, and its molecular weight is 256.09. Lamotrigine is a white to pale cream-colored powder and has a pK_a of 5.7. Lamotrigine is very slightly soluble in water (0.17 mg/mL at 25°C) and slightly soluble in 0.1 M HCl (4.1 mg/mL at 25°C). The structural formula is:

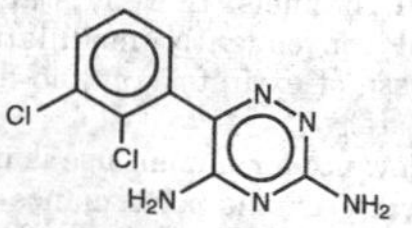

LAMICTAL XR Extended-Release Tablets are supplied for oral administration as 25-mg (yellow with white center), 50-mg (green with white center), 100-mg (orange with white center), and 200-mg (blue with white center) tablets. Each tablet contains the labeled amount of lamotrigine and the following inactive ingredients: glycerol monostearate, hypromellose, lactose monohydrate; magnesium stearate; methacrylic acid copolymer dispersion, polyethylene glycol 400, polysorbate 80, silicon dioxide (25-mg and 50-mg tablets only), titanium dioxide, triethyl citrate, iron oxide black (50-mg tablet only), iron oxide yellow (25-mg, 50-mg, 100-mg tablets only), iron oxide red (100-mg tablet only), FD&C Blue No. 2 Aluminum Lake (200-mg tablet only). Tablets are printed with edible black ink.

LAMICTAL XR Extended-Release Tablets contain a modified-release eroding formulation as the core. The tablets are coated with a clear enteric coat and have an aperture drilled through the coats on both faces of the tablet (DiffCORE™) to enable a controlled release of drug in the acidic environment of the stomach. The combination of this and the modified-release core are designed to control the dissolution rate of lamotrigine over a period of approximately 12 to 15 hours, leading to a gradual increase in serum lamotrigine levels.

Table 6. Mean[a] Pharmacokinetic Parameters of Immediate-Release Lamotrigine in Healthy Volunteers and Adult Patients With Epilepsy

Adult Study Population	Number of Subjects	$t_{1/2}$: Elimination Half-life (hr)	Cl/F: Apparent Plasma Clearance (mL/min/kg)
Healthy volunteers taking no other medications:			
Single-dose lamotrigine	179	32.8 (14.0-103.0)	0.44 (0.12-1.10)
Multiple-dose lamotrigine	36	25.4 (11.6-61.6)	0.58 (0.24-1.15)
Healthy volunteers taking valproate:			
Single-dose lamotrigine	6	48.3 (31.5-88.6)	0.30 (0.14-0.42)
Multiple-dose lamotrigine	18	70.3 (41.9-113.5)	0.18 (0.12-0.33)
Patients with epilepsy taking valproate only:			
Single-dose lamotrigine	4	58.8 (30.5-88.8)	0.28 (0.16-0.40)
Patients with epilepsy taking carbamazepine, phenytoin, phenobarbital, or primidone[b] plus valproate:			
Single-dose lamotrigine	25	27.2 (11.2-51.6)	0.53 (0.27-1.04)
Patients with epilepsy taking carbamazepine, phenytoin, phenobarbital, or primidone:[b]			
Single-dose lamotrigine	24	14.4 (6.4-30.4)	1.10 (0.51-2.22)
Multiple-dose lamotrigine	17	12.6 (7.5-23.1)	1.21 (0.66-1.82)

[a] The majority of parameter means determined in each study had coefficients of variation between 20% and 40% for half-life and Cl/F and between 30% and 70% for T_{max}. The overall mean values were calculated from individual study means that were weighted based on the number of volunteers/patients in each study. The numbers in parentheses below each parameter mean represent the range of individual volunteer/patient values across studies.
[b] Carbamazepine, phenobarbital, phenytoin, and primidone have been shown to increase the apparent clearance of lamotrigine. Estrogen-containing oral contraceptives and other drugs such as rifampin that induce lamotrigine glucuronidation have also been shown to increase the apparent clearance of lamotrigine [see Drug Interactions (7)].

12   CLINICAL PHARMACOLOGY

12.1   Mechanism of Action

The precise mechanism(s) by which lamotrigine exerts its anticonvulsant action are unknown. In animal models designed to detect anticonvulsant activity, lamotrigine was effective in preventing seizure spread in the maximum electroshock (MES) and pentylenetetrazol (scMet) tests, and prevented seizures in the visually and electrically evoked after-discharge (EEAD) tests for antiepileptic activity. Lamotrigine also displayed inhibitory properties in the kindling model in rats both during kindling development and in the fully kindled state. The relevance of these models to human epilepsy, however, is not known.

One proposed mechanism of action of lamotrigine, the relevance of which remains to be established in humans, involves an effect on sodium channels. In vitro pharmacological studies suggest that lamotrigine inhibits voltage-sensitive sodium channels, thereby stabilizing neuronal membranes and consequently modulating presynaptic transmitter release of excitatory amino acids (e.g., glutamate and aspartate).

Although the relevance for human use is unknown, the following data characterize the performance of lamotrigine in receptor binding assays. Lamotrigine had a weak inhibitory effect on the serotonin 5-HT_3 receptor (IC_{50} = 18 μM). It does not exhibit high affinity binding (IC_{50}>100 μM) to the following neurotransmitter receptors: adenosine A_1 and A_2; adrenergic α_1, α_2, and β; dopamine D_1 and D_2; γ-aminobutyric acid (GABA) A and B; histamine H_1; kappa opioid; muscarinic acetylcholine; and serotonin 5-HT_2. Studies have failed to detect an effect of lamotrigine on dihydropyridine-sensitive calcium channels. It had weak effects at sigma opioid receptors (IC_{50} = 145 μM). Lamotrigine did not inhibit the uptake of norepinephrine, dopamine, or serotonin, (IC_{50}>200 μM) when tested in rat synaptosomes and/or human platelets in vitro.

Effect of Lamotrigine on N-Methyl d-Aspartate-Receptor Mediated Activity: Lamotrigine did not inhibit N-methyl d-aspartate (NMDA)-induced depolarizations in rat cortical slices or NMDA-induced cyclic GMP formation in immature rat cerebellum, nor did lamotrigine displace compounds that are either competitive or noncompetitive ligands at this glutamate receptor complex (CNQX, CGS, TCHP). The IC_{50} for lamotrigine effects on NMDA-induced currents (in the presence of 3 μM of glycine) in cultured hippocampal neurons exceeded 100 μM.

12.2   Pharmacodynamics

Folate Metabolism: In vitro, lamotrigine inhibited dihydrofolate reductase, the enzyme that catalyzes the reduc-

tion of dihydrofolate to tetrahydrofolate. Inhibition of this enzyme may interfere with the biosynthesis of nucleic acids and proteins. When oral daily doses of lamotrigine were given to pregnant rats during organogenesis, fetal, placental, and maternal folate concentrations were reduced. Significantly reduced concentrations of folate are associated with teratogenesis [see Use in Specific Populations (8.1)]. Folate concentrations were also reduced in male rats given repeated oral doses of lamotrigine. Reduced concentrations were partially returned to normal when supplemented with folinic acid.

Accumulation in Kidneys: Lamotrigine accumulated in the kidney of the male rat, causing chronic progressive nephrosis, necrosis, and mineralization. These findings are attributed to α-2 microglobulin, a species- and sex-specific protein that has not been detected in humans or other animal species.

Melanin Binding: Lamotrigine binds to melanin-containing tissues, e.g., in the eye and pigmented skin. It has been found in the uveal tract up to 52 weeks after a single dose in rodents.

Cardiovascular: In dogs, lamotrigine is extensively metabolized to a 2-N-methyl metabolite. This metabolite causes dose-dependent prolongations of the PR interval, widening of the QRS complex, and, at higher doses, complete AV conduction block. Similar cardiovascular effects are not anticipated in humans because only trace amounts of the 2-N-methyl metabolite (<0.6% of lamotrigine dose) have been found in human urine [see Clinical Pharmacology (12.3)]. However, it is conceivable that plasma concentrations of this metabolite could be increased in patients with a reduced capacity to glucuronidate lamotrigine (e.g., in patients with liver disease).

12.3   Pharmacokinetics

In comparison to immediate-release lamotrigine, the plasma lamotrigine levels following administration of LAMICTAL XR are not associated with any significant changes in trough plasma concentrations, and are characterized by lower peaks, longer time to peaks, and lower peak-to-trough fluctuation, as described in detail below.

Absorption: Lamotrigine is absorbed after oral administration with negligible first-pass metabolism. The bioavailability of lamotrigine is not affected by food.

In an open-label, crossover study of 44 subjects with epilepsy receiving concomitant AEDs, the steady-state pharmacokinetics of lamotrigine were compared following administration of equivalent total doses of LAMICTAL XR given once daily with those of lamotrigine immediate-release given twice daily. In this study, the median time to

peak concentration (T_{max}) following administration of LAMICTAL XR were 4 to 6 hours in patients taking carbamazepine, phenytoin, phenobarbital, or primidone; 9 to 11 hours in patients taking VPA; and 6 to 10 hours in patients taking AEDs other than carbamazepine, phenytoin, phenobarbital, primidone, or VPA. In comparison, the median T_{max} following administration of immediate-release lamotrigine was between 1 and 1.5 hours.

The steady-state trough concentrations for extended-release lamotrigine were similar to or higher than those of immediate-release lamotrigine depending on concomitant AED (Table 5). A mean reduction in the lamotrigine C_{max} by 11% to 29% was observed for LAMICTAL XR compared to immediate-release lamotrigine resulting in a decrease in the peak-to-trough fluctuation in serum lamotrigine concentrations. However, in some subjects receiving enzyme-inducing AEDs, a reduction in C_{max} of 44% to 77% was observed. The degree of fluctuation was reduced by 17% in patients taking enzyme-inducing AEDs, 34% in patients taking VPA, and 37% in patients taking AEDs other than carbamazepine, phenytoin, phenobarbital, primidone, or VPA. LAMICTAL XR and immediate-release lamotrigine regimens were similar with respect to area under the curve (AUC, a measure of the extent of bioavailability) for patients receiving AEDs other than those known to induce the metabolism of lamotrigine. The relative bioavailability of extended-release lamotrigine was approximately 21% lower than immediate-release lamotrigine in subjects receiving enzyme-inducing AEDs. However, in some subjects in this group a reduction in exposure of up to 70% was observed when switched to LAMICTAL XR. Therefore, doses may need to be adjusted in some subjects based on therapeutic response.

Table 5. Steady-State Bioavailability of LAMICTAL XR Relative to Immediate-Release Lamotrigine at Equivalent Daily Doses (Ratio of XR to IR 90% CI)

Concomitant AED	AUC $_{(0-24ss)}$	C_{max}	C_{min}
EIAEDs[a]	0.79 (0.69, 0.90)	0.71 (0.61, 0.82)	0.99 (0.89, 1.09)
VPA	0.94 (0.81, 1.08)	0.88 (0.75, 1.03)	0.99 (0.88, 1.10)
AEDs other than EIAEDs[a] or VPA	1.00 (0.88, 1.14)	0.89 (0.78, 1.03)	1.14 (1.03, 1.25)

[a] EIAEDs include carbamazepine, phenytoin, phenobarbital, and primidone.

Dose Proportionality: In healthy volunteers not receiving any other medications and given LAMICTAL XR once daily, the systemic exposure to lamotrigine increased in direct proportion to the dose administered over the range of 50 to 200 mg. At doses between 25 and 50 mg, the increase was less than dose proportional, with a 2-fold increase in dose resulting in an approximately 1.6-fold increase in systemic exposure.

Distribution: Estimates of the mean apparent volume of distribution (Vd/F) of lamotrigine following oral administration ranged from 0.9 to 1.3 L/kg. Vd/F is independent of dose and is similar following single and multiple doses in both patients with epilepsy and in healthy volunteers.

Protein Binding: Data from in vitro studies indicate that lamotrigine is approximately 55% bound to human plasma proteins at plasma lamotrigine concentrations from 1 to 10 mcg/mL (10 mcg/mL is 4 to 6 times the trough plasma concentration observed in the controlled efficacy trials). Because lamotrigine is not highly bound to plasma proteins, clinically significant interactions with other drugs through competition for protein binding sites are unlikely. The binding of lamotrigine to plasma proteins did not change in the presence of therapeutic concentrations of phenytoin, phenobarbital, or valproate. Lamotrigine did not displace other AEDs (carbamazepine, phenytoin, phenobarbital) from protein-binding sites.

Metabolism: Lamotrigine is metabolized predominantly by glucuronic acid conjugation; the major metabolite is an inactive 2-N-glucuronide conjugate. After oral administration of 240 mg of ^{14}C-lamotrigine (15 μCi) to 6 healthy volunteers, 94% was recovered in the urine and 2% was recovered in the feces. The radioactivity in the urine consisted of unchanged lamotrigine (10%), the 2-N-glucuronide (76%), a 5-N-glucuronide (10%), a 2-N-methyl metabolite (0.14%), and other unidentified minor metabolites (4%).

Enzyme Induction: The effects of lamotrigine on the induction of specific families of mixed-function oxidase isozymes have not been systematically evaluated.

Following multiple administrations (150 mg twice daily) to normal volunteers taking no other medications, lamotrigine induced its own metabolism, resulting in a 25% decrease in $t_{1/2}$ and a 37% increase in Cl/F at steady state compared with values obtained in the same volunteers following a single dose. Evidence gathered from other sources suggests that self-induction by lamotrigine may not occur when lamotrigine is given as adjunctive therapy in patients receiving enzyme-inducing drugs such as carbamazepine, phenytoin, phenobarbital, primidone, or other drugs such as rifampin that induce lamotrigine glucuronidation [see Drug Interactions (7)].

Elimination: The elimination half-life and apparent clearance of lamotrigine following administration of immediate-release lamotrigine to adult patients with epilepsy and healthy volunteers is summarized in Table 6. Half-life and apparent oral clearance vary depending on concomitant AEDs.

Since the half-life of lamotrigine following administration of single doses of immediate-release lamotrigine is comparable to that observed following administration of LAMICTAL XR, similar changes in the half-life of lamotrigine would be expected for LAMICTAL XR.

[See table 6 at top of previous page]

Drug Interactions: The apparent clearance of lamotrigine is affected by the coadministration of certain medications [see Warnings and Precautions (5.7, 5.11), Drug Interactions (7)].

The net effects of drug interactions with lamotrigine are summarized in Table 7. Details of the drug interaction studies, which were done using immediate-release lamotrigine, are provided following Table 7.

[See table 7 at right]

Estrogen-Containing Oral Contraceptives: In 16 female volunteers, an oral contraceptive preparation containing 30 mcg ethinylestradiol and 150 mcg levonorgestrel increased the apparent clearance of lamotrigine (300 mg/day) by approximately 2-fold with mean decreases in AUC of 52% and in C_{max} of 39%. In this study, trough serum lamotrigine concentrations gradually increased and were approximately 2-fold higher on average at the end of the week of the inactive hormone preparation compared with trough lamotrigine concentrations at the end of the active hormone cycle.

Gradual transient increases in lamotrigine plasma levels (approximate 2-fold increase) occurred during the week of inactive hormone preparation ("pill-free" week) for women not also taking a drug that increased the clearance of lamotrigine (carbamazepine, phenytoin, phenobarbital, primidone, or other drugs such as rifampin that induce lamotrigine glucuronidation [see Drug Interactions (7)]. The increase in lamotrigine plasma levels will be greater if the dose of LAMICTAL XR is increased in the few days before or during the "pill-free" week. Increases in lamotrigine plasma levels could result in dose-dependent adverse reactions.

In the same study, coadministration of lamotrigine (300 mg/day) in 16 female volunteers did not affect the pharmacokinetics of the ethinylestradiol component of the oral contraceptive preparation. There were mean decreases in the AUC and C_{max} of the levonorgestrel component of 19% and 12%, respectively. Measurement of serum progesterone indicated that there was no hormonal evidence of ovulation in any of the 16 volunteers, although measurement of serum FSH, LH, and estradiol indicated that there was some loss of suppression of the hypothalamic-pituitary-ovarian axis.

The effects of doses of lamotrigine other than 300 mg/day have not been systematically evaluated in controlled clinical trials.

The clinical significance of the observed hormonal changes on ovulatory activity is unknown. However, the possibility of decreased contraceptive efficacy in some patients cannot be excluded. Therefore, patients should be instructed to promptly report changes in their menstrual pattern (e.g., break-through bleeding).

Dosage adjustments may be necessary for women receiving estrogen-containing oral contraceptive preparations [see Dosage and Administration (2.1)].

Other Hormonal Contraceptives or Hormone Replacement Therapy: The effect of other hormonal contraceptive preparations or hormone replacement therapy on the pharmacokinetics of lamotrigine has not been systematically evaluated. It has been reported that ethinylestradiol, not progestogens, increased the clearance of lamotrigine up to 2-fold, and the progestin-only pills had no effect on lamotrigine plasma levels. Therefore, adjustments to the dosage of LAMICTAL XR in the presence of progestogens alone will likely not be needed.

Bupropion: The pharmacokinetics of a 100-mg single dose of lamotrigine in healthy volunteers (n = 12) were not changed by coadministration of bupropion sustained-release formulation (150 mg twice daily) starting 11 days before lamotrigine.

Carbamazepine: Lamotrigine has no appreciable effect on steady-state carbamazepine plasma concentration. Limited clinical data suggest there is a higher incidence of dizziness,

diplopia, ataxia, and blurred vision in patients receiving carbamazepine with lamotrigine than in patients receiving other AEDs with lamotrigine [see Adverse Reactions (6.1)]. The mechanism of this interaction is unclear. The effect of lamotrigine on plasma concentrations of carbamazepine-epoxide is unclear. In a small subset of patients (n = 7) studied in a placebo-controlled trial, lamotrigine had no effect on carbamazepine-epoxide plasma concentrations, but in a small, uncontrolled study (n = 9), carbamazepine-epoxide levels increased.

The addition of carbamazepine decreases lamotrigine steady-state concentrations by approximately 40%.

Esomeprazole: In a study of 30 subjects, coadministration of LAMICTAL XR with esomeprazole resulted in no significant change in lamotrigine levels and a small decrease in T_{max}. The levels of gastric pH were not altered compared with pre-lamotrigine dosing.

Felbamate: In a study of 21 healthy volunteers, coadministration of felbamate (1,200 mg twice daily) with lamotrigine (100 mg twice daily for 10 days) appeared to have no clinically relevant effects on the pharmacokinetics of lamotrigine.

Folate Inhibitors: Lamotrigine is a weak inhibitor of dihydrofolate reductase. Prescribers should be aware of this action when prescribing other medications that inhibit folate metabolism.

Gabapentin: Based on a retrospective analysis of plasma levels in 34 patients who received lamotrigine both with and without gabapentin, gabapentin does not appear to change the apparent clearance of lamotrigine.

Levetiracetam: Potential drug interactions between levetiracetam and lamotrigine were assessed by evaluating serum concentrations of both agents during placebo-controlled clinical trials. These data indicate that lamotrigine does not influence the pharmacokinetics of le-

vetiracetam and that levetiracetam does not influence the pharmacokinetics of lamotrigine.

Lithium: The pharmacokinetics of lithium were not altered in healthy subjects (n = 20) by coadministration of lamotrigine (100 mg/day) for 6 days.

Olanzapine: The AUC and C_{max} of olanzapine were similar following the addition of olanzapine (15 mg once daily) to lamotrigine (200 mg once daily) in healthy male volunteers (n = 16) compared with the AUC and C_{max} in healthy male volunteers receiving olanzapine alone (n = 16).

In the same study, the AUC and C_{max} of lamotrigine were reduced on average by 24% and 20%, respectively, following the addition of olanzapine to lamotrigine in healthy male volunteers compared with those receiving lamotrigine alone. This reduction in lamotrigine plasma concentrations is not expected to be clinically relevant.

Oxcarbazepine: The AUC and C_{max} of oxcarbazepine and its active 10-monohydroxy oxcarbazepine metabolite were not significantly different following the addition of oxcarbazepine (600 mg twice daily) to lamotrigine (200 mg once daily) in healthy male volunteers (n = 13) compared with healthy male volunteers receiving oxcarbazepine alone (n = 13).

In the same study, the AUC and C_{max} of lamotrigine were similar following the addition of oxcarbazepine (600 mg twice daily) to lamotrigine in healthy male volunteers compared with those receiving lamotrigine alone. Limited clinical data suggest a higher incidence of headache, dizziness, nausea, and somnolence with coadministration of lamotrigine and oxcarbazepine compared with lamotrigine alone or oxcarbazepine alone.

Phenobarbital, Primidone: The addition of phenobarbital or primidone decreases lamotrigine steady-state concentrations by approximately 40%.

Table 7. Summary of Drug Interactions With Lamotrigine

Drug	Drug Plasma Concentration With Adjunctive Lamotrigine[a]	Lamotrigine Plasma Concentration With Adjunctive Drugs[b]
Oral contraceptives (e.g., ethinylestradiol/levonorgestrel[c])	↔[d]	↓
Bupropion	Not assessed	↔
Carbamazepine (CBZ)	↔	↓
CBZ epoxide[e]	?	
Felbamate	Not assessed	↔
Gabapentin	Not assessed	↔
Levetiracetam	↔	↔
Lithium	↔	Not assessed
Olanzapine	↔	↔[f]
Oxcarbazepine	↔	↔
10-monohydroxy oxcarbazepine metabolite[g]	↔	
Phenobarbital/primidone	↔	↓
Phenytoin (PHT)	↔	↓
Pregabalin	↔	↔
Rifampin	Not assessed	↓
Topiramate	↔[h]	↔
Valproate	↓	↑
Valproate + PHT and/or CBZ	Not assessed	↔
Zonisamide	Not assessed	↔

[a] From adjunctive clinical trials and volunteer studies.
[b] Net effects were estimated by comparing the mean clearance values obtained in adjunctive clinical trials and volunteer studies.
[c] The effect of other hormonal contraceptive preparations or hormone replacement therapy on the pharmacokinetics of lamotrigine has not been systematically evaluated in clinical trials, although the effect may be similar to that seen with the ethinylestradiol/levonorgestrel combinations.
[d] Modest decrease in levonorgestrel.
[e] Not administered, but an active metabolite of carbamazepine.
[f] Slight decrease, not expected to be clinically relevant.
[g] Not administered, but an active metabolite of oxcarbazepine.
[h] Slight increase not expected to be clinically relevant.
↔ = No significant effect.
? = Conflicting data.

Phenytoin: Lamotrigine has no appreciable effect on steady-state phenytoin plasma concentrations in patients with epilepsy. The addition of phenytoin decreases lamotrigine steady-state concentrations by approximately 40%.

Pregabalin: Steady-state trough plasma concentrations of lamotrigine were not affected by concomitant pregabalin (200 mg 3 times daily) administration. There are no pharmacokinetic interactions between lamotrigine and pregabalin.

Rifampin: In 10 male volunteers, rifampin (600 mg/day for 5 days) significantly increased the apparent clearance of a single 25-mg dose of lamotrigine by approximately 2-fold (AUC decreased by approximately 40%).

Topiramate: Topiramate resulted in no change in plasma concentrations of lamotrigine. Administration of lamotrigine resulted in a 15% increase in topiramate concentrations.

Valproate: When lamotrigine was administered to healthy volunteers (n = 18) receiving valproate, the trough steady-state valproate plasma concentrations decreased by an average of 25% over a 3-week period, and then stabilized. However, adding lamotrigine to the existing therapy did not cause a change in valproate plasma concentrations in either adult or pediatric patients in controlled clinical trials.

The addition of valproate increased lamotrigine steady-state concentrations in normal volunteers by slightly more than 2-fold. In one study, maximal inhibition of lamotrigine clearance was reached at valproate doses between 250 and 500 mg/day and did not increase as the valproate dose was further increased.

Zonisamide: In a study of 18 patients with epilepsy, coadministration of zonisamide (200 to 400 mg/day) with lamotrigine (150 to 500 mg/day for 35 days) had no significant effect on the pharmacokinetics of lamotrigine.

Known Inducers or Inhibitors of Glucuronidation: Drugs other than those listed above have not been systematically evaluated in combination with lamotrigine. Since lamotrigine is metabolized predominately by glucuronic acid conjugation, drugs that are known to induce or inhibit glucuronidation may affect the apparent clearance of lamotrigine, and doses of LAMICTAL XR may require adjustment based on clinical response.

Other: Results of in vitro experiments suggest that clearance of lamotrigine is unlikely to be reduced by concomitant administration of amitriptyline, clonazepam, clozapine, fluoxetine, haloperidol, lorazepam, phenelzine, risperidone, sertraline, or trazodone.

Results of in vitro experiments suggest that lamotrigine does not reduce the clearance of drugs eliminated predominantly by CYP2D6.

Special Populations: *Patients With Renal Impairment:* Twelve volunteers with chronic renal failure (mean creatinine clearance: 13 mL/min; range: 6 to 23) and another 6 individuals undergoing hemodialysis were each given a single 100 mg dose of immediate-release lamotrigine. The mean plasma half-lives determined in the study were 42.9 hours (chronic renal failure), 13.0 hours (during hemodialysis), and 57.4 hours (between hemodialysis) compared with 26.2 hours in healthy volunteers. On average, approximately 20% (range: 5.6 to 35.1) of the amount of lamotrigine present in the body was eliminated by hemodialysis during a 4-hour session *[see Dosage and Administration (2.1)]*.

Hepatic Disease: The pharmacokinetics of lamotrigine following a single 100-mg dose of immediate-release lamotrigine were evaluated in 24 subjects with mild, moderate, and severe hepatic impairment (Child-Pugh Classification system) and compared with 12 subjects without hepatic impairment. The patients with severe hepatic impairment were without ascites (n = 2) or with ascites (n = 5). The mean apparent clearances of lamotrigine in patients with mild (n = 12), moderate (n = 5), severe without ascites (n = 2), and severe with ascites (n = 5) liver impairment were 0.30 ± 0.09, 0.24 ± 0.1, 0.21 ± 0.04, and 0.15 ± 0.09 mL/min/kg, respectively, as compared with 0.37 ± 0.1 mL/min/kg in the healthy controls. Mean half-lives of lamotrigine in patients with mild, moderate, severe without ascites, and severe with ascites hepatic impairment were 46 ± 20, 72 ± 44, 67 ± 11, and 100 ± 48 hours, respectively, as compared with 33 ± 7 hours in healthy controls *[see Dosage and Administration (2.1)]*.

Elderly: The pharmacokinetics of lamotrigine following a single 150 mg dose of immediate-release lamotrigine were evaluated in 12 elderly volunteers between the ages of 65 and 76 years (mean creatinine clearance: 61 mL/min, range: 33 to 108 mL/min). The mean half-life of lamotrigine in these subjects was 31.2 hours (range: 24.5 to 43.4 hours), and the mean clearance was 0.40 mL/min/kg (range: 0.26 to 0.48 mL/min/kg).

Gender: The clearance of lamotrigine is not affected by gender. However, during dose escalation of immediate-release lamotrigine in one clinical trial in patients with epilepsy on a stable dose of valproate (n = 77), mean trough lamotrigine concentrations, unadjusted for weight, were 24% to 45% higher (0.3 to 1.7 mcg/mL) in females than in males.

Race: The apparent oral clearance of lamotrigine was 25% lower in non-Caucasians than Caucasians.

Pediatric Patients: Safety and effectiveness of LAMICTAL XR for use in patients below the age of 13 have not been established.

13 NONCLINICAL TOXICOLOGY

13.1 Carcinogenesis, Mutagenesis, Impairment of Fertility

No evidence of carcinogenicity was seen in 1 mouse study or 2 rat studies following oral administration of lamotrigine for up to 2 years at maximum tolerated doses (30 mg/kg/day for mice and 10 to 15 mg/kg/day for rats, doses that are equivalent to 90 mg/m^2 and 60 to 90 mg/m^2, respectively). Steady-state plasma concentrations ranged from 1 to 4 mcg/mL in the mouse study and 1 to 10 mcg/mL in the rat study. Plasma concentrations associated with the recommended human doses of 300 to 500 mg/day are generally in the range of 2 to 5 mcg/mL, but concentrations as high as 19 mcg/mL have been recorded.

Lamotrigine was not mutagenic in the presence or absence of metabolic activation when tested in 2 gene mutation assays (the Ames test and the in vitro mammalian mouse lymphoma assay). In 2 cytogenetic assays (the in vitro human lymphocyte assay and the in vivo rat bone marrow assay), lamotrigine did not increase the incidence of structural or numerical chromosomal abnormalities.

No evidence of impairment of fertility was detected in rats given oral doses of lamotrigine up to 2.4 times the highest usual human maintenance dose of 8.33 mg/kg/day or 0.4 times the human dose on a mg/m^2 basis. The effect of lamotrigine on human fertility is unknown.

14 CLINICAL STUDIES

14.1 PGTC Seizures

The effectiveness of LAMICTAL XR as adjunctive therapy was established in PGTC seizures in a 19-week, international, multicenter, double-blind, randomized, placebo-controlled study in 143 patients 13 years of age and older (n = 70 on LAMICTAL XR and n = 73 on placebo). Patients with at least 3 PGTC seizures during an 8-week baseline phase were randomized to 19 weeks of treatment with LAMICTAL XR or placebo added to their current AED regimen of up to 2 drugs. Patients were dosed on a fixed-dose regimen, with target doses ranging from 200 mg/day to 500 mg/day of LAMICTAL XR based on concomitant AED(s) (target dose = 200 mg for valproate, 300 mg for AEDs not altering plasma lamotrigine levels, and 500 mg for enzyme-inducing AEDs).

The primary efficacy endpoint was percent change from baseline in PGTC seizure frequency during the double-blind treatment phase. For the intent-to-treat population, the median percent reduction in PGTC seizure frequency was 75% in patients treated with LAMICTAL XR and 32% in patients treated with placebo, a difference that was statistically significant, defined as a 2-sided p value ≤0.05.

Figure 1 presents the percentage of patients (X-axis) with a percent reduction in PGTC seizure frequency (responder rate) from baseline through the entire treatment period at least as great as that represented on the Y-axis. A positive value on the Y-axis indicates an improvement from baseline (i.e., a decrease in seizure frequency), while a negative value indicates a worsening from baseline (i.e., an increase in seizure frequency). Thus, in a display of this type, a curve for an effective treatment is shifted to the left of the curve for placebo. The proportion of patients achieving any particular level of reduction in PGTC seizure frequency was consistently higher for the group treated with LAMICTAL XR compared with the placebo group. For example, 70% of patients randomized to LAMICTAL XR experienced a 50% or greater reduction in PGTC seizure frequency, compared with 32% of patients randomized to placebo. Patients with an increase in seizure frequency >100% are represented on the Y-axis as equal to or greater than -100%.

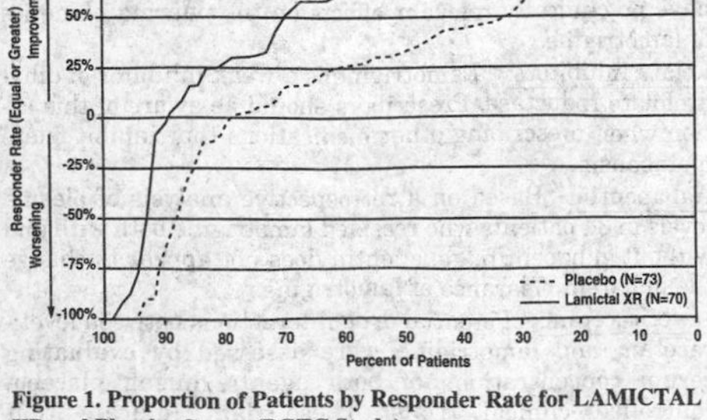

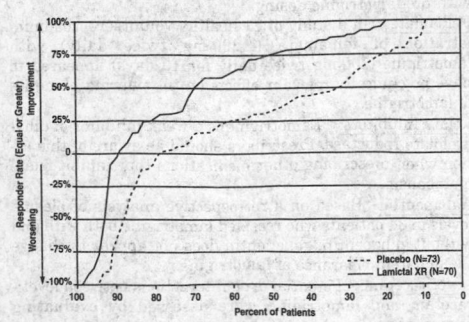

Figure 1. Proportion of Patients by Responder Rate for LAMICTAL XR and Placebo Group (PGTC Study)

14.2 Partial Onset Seizures

The effectiveness of immediate-release lamotrigine as adjunctive therapy was initially established in 3 pivotal multicenter, placebo-controlled, double-blind clinical trials in 355 adults with refractory partial onset seizures.

The effectiveness of LAMICTAL XR as adjunctive therapy in partial onset seizures, with or without secondary generalization, was established in a 19-week, multicenter, double-blind, placebo-controlled trial in 236 patients, 13 years of age and older (approximately 93% of patients were 16 to 65 years old). Approximately 36% were from the U.S. and approximately 64% were from other countries including Argentina, Brazil, Chile, Germany, India, Korea, Russian Federation, and Ukraine. Patients with at least 8 partial onset seizures during an 8-week prospective baseline phase (or 4-week prospective baseline coupled with a 4-week historical baseline documented with seizure diary data) were randomized to treatment with LAMICTAL XR (n = 116) or placebo (n = 120) added to their current regimen of 1 or 2 AEDs. Approximately half of the patients were taking 2 concomitant AEDs at baseline. Target doses ranged from 200 to 500 mg/day of LAMICTAL XR based on concomitant AED (target dose = 200 mg for valproate, 300 mg for AEDs not altering plasma lamotrigine, and 500 mg for enzyme-inducing AEDs). The median partial seizure frequency per week at baseline was 2.3 for LAMICTAL XR and 2.1 for placebo.

The primary endpoint was the median percent change from baseline in partial onset seizure frequency during the entire double-blind treatment phase. The median percent reductions in weekly partial onset seizures were 47% in patients treated with LAMICTAL XR and 25% on placebo, a difference that was statistically significant, defined as a 2-sided p value ≤0.05.

Figure 2 presents the percentage of patients (X-axis) with a percent reduction in partial seizure frequency (responder rate) from baseline through the entire treatment period at least as great as that represented on the Y-axis. The proportion of patients achieving any particular level of reduction in partial seizure frequency was consistently higher for the group treated with LAMICTAL XR compared with the placebo group. For example, 44% of patients randomized to LAMICTAL XR experienced a 50% or greater reduction in partial seizure frequency, compared with 21% of patients randomized to placebo.

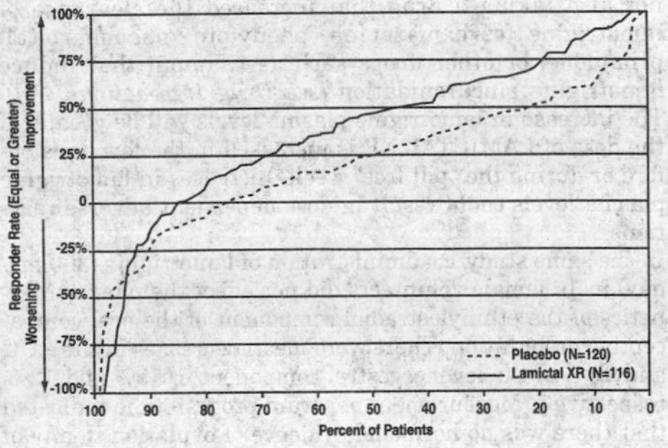

Figure 2. Proportion of Patients by Responder Rate for LAMICTAL XR and Placebo Group (Partial Onset Seizure Study)

16 HOW SUPPLIED/STORAGE AND HANDLING

LAMICTAL XR (lamotrigine) Extended-Release Tablets

25 mg, yellow with a white center, round, biconvex, film-coated tablets printed on one face in black ink with "LAMICTAL" and "XR 25", unit-of-use bottles of 30 with orange caps (NDC 0173-0754-00).

50 mg, green with a white center, round, biconvex, film-coated tablets printed on one face in black ink with "LAMICTAL" and "XR 50", unit-of-use bottles of 30 with orange caps (NDC 0173-0755-00).

100 mg, orange with a white center, round, biconvex, film-coated tablets printed on one face in black ink with "LAMICTAL" and "XR 100", unit-of-use bottles of 30 with orange caps (NDC 0173-0756-00).

200 mg, blue with a white center, round, biconvex, film-coated tablets printed on one face in black ink with "LAMICTAL" and "XR 200", unit-of-use bottles of 30 with orange caps (NDC 0173-0757-00).

LAMICTAL XR (lamotrigine) Patient Titration Kit for Patients Taking Valproate (Blue XR Kit)

25 mg, yellow with a white center, round, biconvex, film-coated tablets printed on one face in black ink with "LAMICTAL" and "XR 25" and 50 mg, green with a white center, round, biconvex, film-coated tablets printed on one face in black ink with "LAMICTAL" and "XR 50"; blisterpack of 21/25-mg tablets and 7/50-mg tablets (NDC 0173-0758-00).

LAMICTAL XR (lamotrigine) Patient Titration Kit for Patients Taking Carbamazepine, Phenytoin, Phenobarbital, or Primidone, and Not Taking Valproate (Green XR Kit)

50 mg, green with a white center, round, biconvex, film-coated tablets printed on one face in black ink with "LAMICTAL" and "XR 50"; 100 mg, orange with a white center, round, biconvex, film-coated tablets printed on one face in black ink with "LAMICTAL" and "XR 100"; and 200 mg, blue with a white center, round, biconvex, film-coated tablets printed on one face in black ink with "LAMICTAL" and "XR 200"; blisterpack of 14/50-mg tablets, 14/100-mg tablets, and 7/200-mg tablets (NDC 0173-0759-00).

LAMICTAL XR (lamotrigine) Patient Titration Kit for Patients Not Taking Carbamazepine, Phenytoin, Phenobarbital, Primidone, or Valproate (Orange XR Kit) 25 mg, yellow with a white center, round, biconvex, film-coated tablets printed on one face in black ink with "LAMICTAL" and "XR 25"; 50 mg, green with a white center, round, biconvex, film-coated tablets printed on one face in black ink with "LAMICTAL" and "XR 50"; and 100 mg, orange with a white center, round, biconvex, film-coated tablets printed on one face in black ink with "LAMICTAL" and "XR 100"; blisterpack of 14/25-mg tablets, 14/50-mg tablets, and 7/100-mg tablets (NDC 0173-0760-00).

Storage: Store at 25°C (77°F); excursions permitted to 15-30°C (59-86°F) [see USP Controlled Room Temperature].

17 PATIENT COUNSELING INFORMATION

See Medication Guide.

17.1 Rash

Prior to initiation of treatment with LAMICTAL XR, the patient should be instructed that a rash or other signs or symptoms of hypersensitivity (e.g., fow supplieedever, lymphadenopathy) may herald a serious medical event and that the patient should report any such occurrence to a physician immediately.

17.2 Suicidal Thinking and Behavior

Patients, their caregivers, and families should be counseled that AEDs, including LAMICTAL XR, may increase the risk of suicidal thoughts and behavior and should be advised of the need to be alert for the emergence or worsening of symptoms of depression, any unusual changes in mood or behavior, or the emergence of suicidal thoughts, behavior, or thoughts about self-harm. Behaviors of concern should be reported immediately to healthcare providers.

17.3 Worsening of Seizures

Patients should be advised to notify their physician if worsening of seizure control occurs.

17.4 CNS Adverse Effects

Patients should be advised that LAMICTAL XR may cause dizziness, somnolence, and other symptoms and signs of central nervous system (CNS) depression. Accordingly, they should be advised neither to drive a car nor to operate other complex machinery until they have gained sufficient experience on LAMICTAL XR to gauge whether or not it adversely affects their mental and/or motor performance.

17.5 Blood Dyscrasias and/or Acute Multiorgan Failure

Patients should be advised of the possibility of blood dyscrasias and/or acute multiorgan failure and to contact their physician immediately if they experience any signs or symptoms of these conditions [see Warnings and Precautions (5.3, 5.4)].

17.6 Pregnancy

Patients should be advised to notify their physicians if they become pregnant or intend to become pregnant during therapy. Patients should be advised to notify their physicians if they intend to breastfeed or are breastfeeding an infant. Patients should also be encouraged to enroll in the NAAED Pregnancy Registry if they become pregnant. This registry is collecting information about the safety of antiepileptic drugs during pregnancy. To enroll, patients can call the toll-free number 1-888-233-2334 [see Use in Specific Populations (8.1)].

17.7 Oral Contraceptive Use

Women should be advised to notify their physician if they plan to start or stop use of oral contraceptives or other female hormonal preparations. Starting estrogen-containing oral contraceptives may significantly decrease lamotrigine plasma levels and stopping estrogen-containing oral contraceptives (including the "pill-free" week) may significantly increase lamotrigine plasma levels [see Warnings and Precautions (5.7), Clinical Pharmacology (12.3)]. Women should also be advised to promptly notify their physician if they experience adverse reactions or changes in menstrual pattern (e.g., break-through bleeding) while receiving LAMICTAL XR in combination with these medications.

17.8 Discontinuing LAMICTAL XR

Patients should be advised to notify their physician if they stop taking LAMICTAL XR for any reason and not to resume LAMICTAL XR without consulting their physician.

17.9 Potential Medication Errors

Medication errors involving LAMICTAL have occurred. In particular the names LAMICTAL or lamotrigine can be confused with the names of other commonly used medications. Medication errors may also occur between the different formulations of LAMICTAL. To reduce the potential of medi-

cation errors, write and say LAMICTAL XR clearly. Depictions of the LAMICTAL XR Extended-Release Tablets can be found in the Medication Guide. Each LAMICTAL XR tablet has a distinct color and white center, and is printed with "LAMICTAL XR" and the tablet strength. These distinctive features serve to identify the different presentations of the drug and thus may help reduce the risk of medication errors. LAMICTAL XR is supplied in round, unit-of-use bottles with orange caps containing 30 tablets. The label on the bottle includes a depiction of the tablets which further communicates to patients and pharmacists that the medication is LAMICTAL XR and the specific tablet strength included in the bottle. The unit-of-use bottle with a distinctive orange cap and distinctive bottle label features serves to identify the different presentations of the drug and thus may help to reduce the risk of medication errors. **To avoid a medication error of using the wrong drug or formulation, patients should be strongly advised to visually inspect their tablets to verify that they are LAMICTAL XR each time they fill their prescription and to immediately talk to their doctor/pharmacist if they receive a LAMICTAL XR tablet without a white center and without "LAMICTAL XR" and the strength printed on the tablet as they may have received the wrong medication** [see Dosage Forms and Strengths (3), How Supplied/Storage and Handling (16)].

LAMICTAL XR and DiffCORE are trademarks of GlaxoSmithKline.

GlaxoSmithKline
Research Triangle Park, NC 27709
©2010, GlaxoSmithKline. All rights reserved.
January 2010
LXR:3PI

MEDICATION GUIDE

LAMICTAL® (la-MIK-tal) XR™ (lamotrigine) Extended-Release Tablets

Read this Medication Guide before you start taking LAMICTAL XR and each time you get a refill. There may be new information. This information does not take the place of talking with your healthcare provider about your medical condition or treatment. If you have questions about LAMICTAL XR, ask your healthcare provider or pharmacist.

What is the most important information I should know about LAMICTAL XR?

1. LAMICTAL XR may cause a serious skin rash that may cause you to be hospitalized or to stop LAMICTAL XR; it may rarely cause death.

There is no way to tell if a mild rash will develop into a more serious reaction. These serious skin reactions are more likely to happen when you begin taking LAMICTAL XR, within the first 2 to 8 weeks of treatment. But it can happen in people who have taken LAMICTAL XR for any period of time. Children between 2 to 16 years of age have a higher chance of getting this serious skin reaction while taking lamotrigine. LAMICTAL XR is not approved for use in children less than 13 years old.

The risk of getting a rash is higher if you:

• take LAMICTAL XR while taking valproate (DEPAKENE (valproic acid) or DEPAKOTE (divalproex sodium)).

• take a higher starting dose of LAMICTAL XR than your healthcare provider prescribed.

• increase your dose of LAMICTAL XR faster than prescribed.

LAMICTAL XR can also cause other types of allergic reactions or serious problems which may affect organs and other parts of your body like the liver or blood cells. You may or may not have a rash with these types of reactions. Call your healthcare provider right away if you have any of the following:

• a skin rash
• hives
• fever
• swollen lymph glands
• painful sores in the mouth or around your eyes
• swelling of your lips or tongue
• yellowing of your skin or eyes
• unusual bruising or bleeding
• severe fatigue or weakness
• severe muscle pain
• frequent infections

These symptoms may be the first signs of a serious reaction. A healthcare provider should examine you to decide if you should continue taking LAMICTAL XR.

2. Like other antiepileptic drugs, LAMICTAL XR may cause suicidal thoughts or actions in a very small number of people, about 1 in 500.

Call a healthcare provider right away if you have any of these symptoms, especially if they are new, worse, or worry you:

• thoughts about suicide or dying
• attempt to commit suicide
• new or worse depression
• new or worse anxiety
• feeling agitated or restless

• panic attacks
• trouble sleeping (insomnia)
• new or worse irritability
• acting aggressive, being angry, or violent
• acting on dangerous impulses
• an extreme increase in activity and talking (mania)
• other unusual changes in behavior or mood

Do not stop LAMICTAL XR without first talking to a healthcare provider.

• Stopping LAMICTAL XR suddenly can cause serious problems.
• Suicidal thoughts or actions can be caused by things other than medicines. If you have suicidal thoughts or actions, your healthcare provider may check for other causes.

How can I watch for early symptoms of suicidal thoughts and actions?

• Pay attention to any changes, especially sudden changes, in mood, behaviors, thoughts, or feelings.
• Keep all follow-up visits with your healthcare provider as scheduled.
• Call your healthcare provider between visits as needed, especially if you are worried about symptoms.

LAMICTAL XR can have other serious side effects. For more information ask your healthcare provider or pharmacist. Tell your healthcare provider if you have any side effect that bothers you. Be sure to read the section below entitled "What are the possible side effects of LAMICTAL XR?"

3. Patients prescribed LAMICTAL have sometimes been given the wrong medicine because many medicines have names similar to LAMICTAL, so always check that you receive LAMICTAL XR.

Taking the wrong medication can cause serious health problems. When your healthcare provider gives you a prescription for LAMICTAL XR:

• Make sure you can read it clearly.
• Talk to your pharmacist to check that you are given the correct medicine.
• Each time you fill your prescription, check the tablets you receive against the pictures of the tablets below.

These pictures show the distinct wording, colors, and shapes of the tablets that help to identify the right strength of LAMICTAL XR. Immediately call your pharmacist if you receive a LAMICTAL XR tablet that does not look like one of the tablets shown below, as you may have received the wrong medication.

LAMICTAL XR (lamotrigine)
Extended-Release Tablets

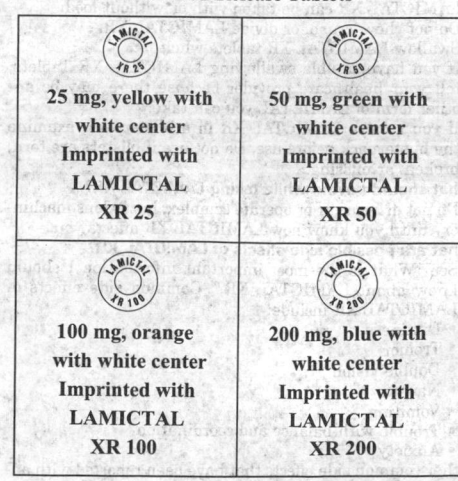

25 mg, yellow with white center Imprinted with LAMICTAL XR 25	50 mg, green with white center Imprinted with LAMICTAL XR 50
100 mg, orange with white center Imprinted with LAMICTAL XR 100	200 mg, blue with white center Imprinted with LAMICTAL XR 200

What is LAMICTAL XR?

LAMICTAL XR is a prescription medicine used together with other medicines to treat primary generalized tonic-clonic seizures and partial onset seizures in people 13 years or older.

It is not known if LAMICTAL XR is safe or effective in children under the age of 13. Other forms of LAMICTAL can be used in children 2 to 12 years.

Who should not take LAMICTAL XR?

You should not take LAMICTAL XR if you have had an allergic reaction to lamotrigine or to any of the inactive ingredients in LAMICTAL XR. See the end of this leaflet for a complete list of ingredients in LAMICTAL XR.

What should I tell my healthcare provider before taking LAMICTAL XR?

Before taking LAMICTAL XR, tell your healthcare provider about all of your medical conditions, including if you:

• have had a rash or allergic reaction to another antiseizure medicine.
• have or have had depression, mood problems or suicidal thoughts or behavior.

- are taking oral contraceptives (birth control pills) or other female hormonal medicines. Do not start or stop taking birth control pills or other female hormonal medicine until you have talked with your healthcare provider. Tell your healthcare provider if you have any changes in your menstrual pattern such as breakthrough bleeding. Stopping these medicines may cause side effects (such as dizziness, lack of coordination, or double vision). Starting these medicines may lessen how well LAMICTAL XR works.
- are pregnant or plan to become pregnant. It is not known if LAMICTAL XR will harm your unborn baby. If you become pregnant while taking LAMICTAL XR, talk to your healthcare provider about registering with the North American Antiepileptic Drug Pregnancy Registry. You can enroll in this registry by calling 1-888-233-2334. The purpose of this registry is to collect information about the safety of antiepileptic drugs during pregnancy.
- are breastfeeding. LAMICTAL XR can pass into your breast milk. You and your healthcare provider should decide if you should take LAMICTAL XR or breastfeed. Breastfeeding while taking LAMICTAL XR is not recommended.

Tell your healthcare provider about all the medicines you take or if you are planning to take a new medicine, including prescription and non-prescription medicines, vitamins, and herbal supplements. Using LAMICTAL XR with certain other medicines can affect each other, causing side effects.

How should I take LAMICTAL XR?

- Take LAMICTAL XR exactly as prescribed.
- Your healthcare provider may change your dose. Do not change your dose without talking to your healthcare provider.
- Do not stop taking LAMICTAL XR without talking to your healthcare provider. Stopping LAMICTAL XR suddenly may cause serious problems. For example, if you have epilepsy and you stop taking LAMICTAL XR suddenly, you may get seizures that do not stop. Talk with your healthcare provider about how to stop LAMICTAL XR slowly.
- If you miss a dose of LAMICTAL XR, take it as soon as you remember. If it is almost time for your next dose, just skip the missed dose. Take the next dose at your regular time. **Do not take two doses at the same time.**
- You may not feel the full effect of LAMICTAL XR for several weeks.
- If you have epilepsy, tell your healthcare provider if your seizures get worse or if you have any new types of seizures.
- LAMICTAL XR can be taken with or without food.
- Do not chew, crush, or divide LAMICTAL XR.
- Swallow LAMICTAL XR tablets whole.
- If you have trouble swallowing LAMICTAL XR Tablets, tell your healthcare provider because there may be another form of LAMICTAL you can take.
- If you receive LAMICTAL XR in a blisterpack, examine the blisterpack before use. Do not use if blisters are torn, broken, or missing.

What should I avoid while taking LAMICTAL XR?

- Do not drive a car or operate complex, hazardous machinery until you know how LAMICTAL XR affects you.

What are possible side effects of LAMICTAL XR?

- See "What is the most important information I should know about LAMICTAL XR?" Common side effects of LAMICTAL XR include:
  - Dizziness
  - Tremor
  - Double vision
  - Nausea
  - Vomiting
  - Trouble with balance and coordination
  - Anxiety

Other common side effects that have been reported with another form of LAMICTAL include headache, sleepiness, blurred vision, runny nose, and rash.

Tell your healthcare provider about any side effect that bothers you or that does not go away.

These are not all the possible side effects of LAMICTAL XR. For more information, ask your healthcare provider or pharmacist.

Call your doctor for medical advice about side effects. You may report side effects to FDA at 1-800-FDA-1088.

How should I store LAMICTAL XR?

- Store LAMICTAL XR at room temperature between 59°F to 86°F (15°C to 30°C).
- **Keep LAMICTAL XR and all medicines out of the reach of children.**

General information about LAMICTAL XR

Medicines are sometimes prescribed for purposes other than those listed in a Medication Guide. Do not use LAMICTAL XR for a condition for which it was not prescribed. Do not give LAMICTAL XR to other people, even if they have the same symptoms you have. It may harm them.

This Medication Guide summarizes the most important information about LAMICTAL XR. If you would like more information, talk with your healthcare provider. You can ask your healthcare provider or pharmacist for information about LAMICTAL XR that is written for healthcare professionals.

For more information, go to www.lamictalxr.com or call 1-888-825-5249.

What are the ingredients in LAMICTAL XR?

Active ingredient: Lamotrigine.

Inactive ingredients: glycero monostearate, hypromellose, lactose monohydrate, magnesium stearate, methacrylic acid copolymer dispersion, polyethylene glycol 400, polysorbate 80, silicon dioxide (25-mg and 50-mg tablets only), titanium dioxide, triethyl citrate, iron oxide black (50-mg tablet only), iron oxide yellow (25-mg, 50-mg, 100-mg tablets only), iron oxide red (100-mg tablet only), FD&C Blue No. 2 Aluminum Lake (200-mg tablet only). Tablets are printed with edible black ink.

This Medication Guide has been approved by the U.S. Food and Drug Administration.

LAMICTAL XR is a trademark of GlaxoSmithKline.
DEPAKENE and DEPAKOTE are registered trademarks of Abbott Laboratories.
GlaxoSmithKline
Research Triangle Park, NC 27709
©2010, GlaxoSmithKline. All rights reserved.
January 2010
LXR:2MG

LANOXIN® ℞
[lă-nŏx′ĭn]
(digoxin)
Injection
500 mcg (0.5 mg) in 2 mL (250 mcg [0.25 mg] per mL)

DESCRIPTION

LANOXIN (digoxin) is one of the cardiac (or digitalis) glycosides, a closely related group of drugs having in common specific effects on the myocardium. These drugs are found in a number of plants. Digoxin is extracted from the leaves of *Digitalis lanata*. The term "digitalis" is used to designate the whole group of glycosides. The glycosides are composed of 2 portions: a sugar and a cardenolide (hence "glycosides"). Digoxin is described chemically as (3β,5β,12β)-3-[(O-2, 6-dideoxy-β-D-ribo-hexopyranosyl-(1→4)-O-2,6-dideoxy-β-D-ribo-hexopyranosyl-(1→4)-2,6-dideoxy-β-D-ribo-hexopyranosyl)oxy]-12,14-dihydroxy-card-20(22)-enolide. Its molecular formula is $C_{41}H_{64}O_{14}$, its molecular weight is 780.95, and its structural formula is:

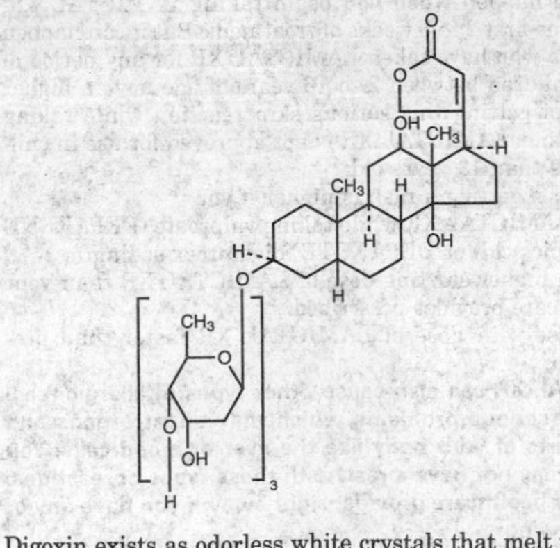

Digoxin exists as odorless white crystals that melt with decomposition above 230°C. The drug is practically insoluble in water and in alcohol; slightly soluble in diluted (50%) alcohol and in chloroform; and freely soluble in pyridine.

LANOXIN Injection is a sterile solution of digoxin for intravenous or intramuscular injection. The vehicle contains 40% propylene glycol and 10% alcohol. The injection is buffered to a pH of 6.8 to 7.2 with 0.17% dibasic sodium phosphate and 0.08% anhydrous citric acid. Each 2-mL ampul contains 500 mcg (0.5 mg) digoxin (250 mcg [0.25 mg] per mL). Dilution is not required.

CLINICAL PHARMACOLOGY

Mechanism of Action

Digoxin inhibits sodium-potassium ATPase, an enzyme that regulates the quantity of sodium and potassium inside cells. Inhibition of the enzyme leads to an increase in the intracellular concentration of sodium and thus (by stimulation of sodium-calcium exchange) an increase in the intracellular concentration of calcium. The beneficial effects of digoxin result from direct actions on cardiac muscle, as well as indirect actions on the cardiovascular system mediated by effects on the autonomic nervous system. The autonomic effects include: (1) a vagomimetic action, which is responsible for the effects of digoxin on the sinoatrial and atrioventricular (AV) nodes; and (2) baroreceptor sensitization,

which results in increased afferent inhibitory activity and reduced activity of the sympathetic nervous system and renin-angiotensin system for any given increment in mean arterial pressure. The pharmacologic consequences of these direct and indirect effects are: (1) an increase in the force and velocity of myocardial systolic contraction (positive inotropic action); (2) a decrease in the degree of activation of the sympathetic nervous system and renin-angiotensin system (neurohormonal deactivating effect); and (3) slowing of the heart rate and decreased conduction velocity through the AV node (vagomimetic effect). The effects of digoxin in heart failure are mediated by its positive inotropic and neurohormonal deactivating effects, whereas the effects of the drug in atrial arrhythmias are related to its vagomimetic actions. In high doses, digoxin increases sympathetic outflow from the central nervous system (CNS). This increase in sympathetic activity may be an important factor in digitalis toxicity.

Pharmacokinetics

Note: the following data are from studies performed in adults, unless otherwise stated.

Absorption

Comparisons of the systemic availability and equivalent doses for preparations of LANOXIN are shown in Table 1.
[See table 1 at top of next page]

Distribution

Following drug administration, a 6- to 8-hour tissue distribution phase is observed. This is followed by a much more gradual decline in the serum concentration of the drug, which is dependent on the elimination of digoxin from the body. The peak height and slope of the early portion (absorption/distribution phases) of the serum concentration-time curve are dependent upon the route of administration and the absorption characteristics of the formulation. Clinical evidence indicates that the early high serum concentrations do not reflect the concentration of digoxin at its site of action, but that with chronic use, the steady-state post-distribution serum concentrations are in equilibrium with tissue concentrations and correlate with pharmacologic effects. In individual patients, these post-distribution serum concentrations may be useful in evaluating therapeutic and toxic effects (see DOSAGE AND ADMINISTRATION: Serum Digoxin Concentrations).

Digoxin is concentrated in tissues and therefore has a large apparent volume of distribution. Digoxin crosses both the blood-brain barrier and the placenta. At delivery, the serum digoxin concentration in the newborn is similar to the serum concentration in the mother. Approximately 25% of digoxin in the plasma is bound to protein. Serum digoxin concentrations are not significantly altered by large changes in fat tissue weight, so that its distribution space correlates best with lean (i.e., ideal) body weight, not total body weight.

Metabolism

Only a small percentage (16%) of a dose of digoxin is metabolized. The end metabolites, which include 3 β-digoxigenin, 3-keto-digoxigenin, and their glucuronide and sulfate conjugates, are polar in nature and are postulated to be formed via hydrolysis, oxidation, and conjugation. The metabolism of digoxin is not dependent upon the cytochrome P-450 system, and digoxin is not known to induce or inhibit the cytochrome P-450 system.

Excretion

Elimination of digoxin follows first-order kinetics (that is, the quantity of digoxin eliminated at any time is proportional to the total body content). Following intravenous administration to healthy volunteers, 50% to 70% of a digoxin dose is excreted unchanged in the urine. Renal excretion of digoxin is proportional to glomerular filtration rate and is largely independent of urine flow. In healthy volunteers with normal renal function, digoxin has a half-life of 1.5 to 2.0 hours. The half-life in anuric patients is prolonged to 3.5 to 5 days. Digoxin is not effectively removed from the body by dialysis, exchange transfusion, or during cardiopulmonary bypass because most of the drug is bound to tissue and does not circulate in the blood.

Special Populations

Race differences in digoxin pharmacokinetics have not been formally studied. Because digoxin is primarily eliminated as unchanged drug via the kidney and because there are no important differences in creatinine clearance among races, pharmacokinetic differences due to race are not expected. The clearance of digoxin can be primarily correlated with renal function as indicated by creatinine clearance. The Cockcroft and Gault formula for estimation of creatinine clearance includes age, body weight, and gender. Table 5 that provides the usual daily maintenance dose requirements of LANOXIN Tablets based on creatinine clearance (per 70 kg) is presented in the DOSAGE AND ADMINISTRATION section.

Plasma digoxin concentration profiles in patients with acute hepatitis generally fell within the range of profiles in a group of healthy subjects.

Pharmacodynamic and Clinical Effects

The times to onset of pharmacologic effect and to peak effect of preparations of LANOXIN are shown in Table 2.

[See table 2 at right]

Hemodynamic Effects

Digoxin produces hemodynamic improvement in patients with heart failure. Short- and long-term therapy with the drug increases cardiac output and lowers pulmonary artery pressure, pulmonary capillary wedge pressure, and systemic vascular resistance. These hemodynamic effects are accompanied by an increase in the left ventricular ejection fraction and a decrease in end-systolic and end-diastolic dimensions.

Chronic Heart Failure

Two 12-week, double-blind, placebo-controlled studies enrolled 178 (RADIANCE trial) and 88 (PROVED trial) patients with NYHA class II or III heart failure previously treated with oral digoxin, a diuretic, and an ACE inhibitor (RADIANCE only) and randomized them to placebo or treatment with LANOXIN Tablets. Both trials demonstrated better preservation of exercise capacity in patients randomized to LANOXIN. Continued treatment with LANOXIN reduced the risk of developing worsening heart failure, as evidenced by heart failure-related hospitalizations and emergency care and the need for concomitant heart failure therapy. The larger study also showed treatment-related benefits in NYHA class and patients' global assessment. In the smaller trial, these trended in favor of a treatment benefit.

The Digitalis Investigation Group (DIG) main trial was a multicenter, randomized, double-blind, placebo-controlled mortality study of 6,801 patients with heart failure and left ventricular ejection fraction ≤0.45. At randomization, 67% were NYHA class I or II, 71% had heart failure of ischemic etiology, 44% had been receiving digoxin, and most were receiving concomitant ACE inhibitor (94%) and diuretic (82%). Patients were randomized to placebo or LANOXIN Tablets, the dose of which was adjusted for the patient's age, sex, lean body weight, and serum creatinine (see DOSAGE AND ADMINISTRATION), and followed for up to 58 months (median 37 months). The median daily dose prescribed was 0.25 mg. Overall all-cause mortality was 35% with no difference between groups (95% confidence limits for relative risk of 0.91 to 1.07). LANOXIN was associated with a 25% reduction in the number of hospitalizations for heart failure, a 28% reduction in the risk of a patient having at least 1 hospitalization for heart failure, and a 6.5% reduction in total hospitalizations (for any cause).

Use of LANOXIN was associated with a trend to increase time to all-cause death or hospitalization. The trend was evident in subgroups of patients with mild heart failure as well as more severe disease, as shown in Table 3. Although the effect on all-cause death or hospitalization was not statistically significant, much of the apparent benefit derived from effects on mortality and hospitalization attributed to heart failure.

[See table 3 at right]

In situations where there is no statistically significant benefit of treatment evident from a trial's primary endpoint, results pertaining to a secondary endpoint should be interpreted cautiously.

Chronic Atrial Fibrillation

In patients with chronic atrial fibrillation, digoxin slows rapid ventricular response rate in a linear dose-response fashion from 0.25 to 0.75 mg/day. Digoxin should not be used for the treatment of multifocal atrial tachycardia.

INDICATIONS AND USAGE

Heart Failure

LANOXIN is indicated for the treatment of mild to moderate heart failure. LANOXIN increases left ventricular ejection fraction and improves heart failure symptoms as evidenced by exercise capacity and heart failure-related hospitalizations and emergency care, while having no effect on mortality. Where possible, LANOXIN should be used with a diuretic and an angiotensin-converting enzyme inhibitor, but an optimal order for starting these 3 drugs cannot be specified.

Atrial Fibrillation

LANOXIN is indicated for the control of ventricular response rate in patients with chronic atrial fibrillation.

CONTRAINDICATIONS

Digitalis glycosides are contraindicated in patients with ventricular fibrillation or in patients with a known hypersensitivity to digoxin. A hypersensitivity reaction to other digitalis preparations usually constitutes a contraindication to digoxin.

WARNINGS

Sinus Node Disease and AV Block

Because digoxin slows sinoatrial and AV conduction, the drug commonly prolongs the PR interval. The drug may cause severe sinus bradycardia or sinoatrial block in patients with pre-existing sinus node disease and may cause

Table 1. Comparisons of the Systemic Availability and Equivalent Doses for Preparations of LANOXIN

Product	Absolute Bioavailability	Equivalent Doses (mcg)[a] Among Dosage Forms			
LANOXIN Tablets	60-80%	62.5	125	250	500
LANOXIN Injection/IV	100%	50	100	200	400

[a] For example, 125 mcg LANOXIN Tablets equivalent to 100 mcg LANOXIN Injection/IV.

Table 2. Times to Onset of Pharmacologic Effect and to Peak Effect of Preparations of LANOXIN

Product	Time to Onset of Effect[a]	Time to Peak Effect[a]
LANOXIN Tablets	0.5-2 hours	2-6 hours
LANOXIN Injection/IV	5-30 minutes[b]	1-4 hours

[a] Documented for ventricular response rate in atrial fibrillation, inotropic effects and electrocardiographic changes.
[b] Depending upon rate of infusion.

Table 3. Subgroup Analyses of Mortality and Hospitalization During the First 2 Years Following Randomization

	n	Risk of All-Cause Mortality or All-Cause Hospitalization[a]			Risk of HF-Related Mortality or HF-Related Hospitalization[a]		
		Placebo	LANOXIN	Relative risk[b]	Placebo	LANOXIN	Relative risk[b]
All patients (EF ≤0.45)	6,801	604	593	0.94 (0.88-1.00)	294	217	0.69 (0.63-0.76)
NYHA I/II	4,571	549	541	0.96 (0.89-1.04)	242	178	0.70 (0.62-0.80)
EF 0.25-0.45	4,543	568	571	0.99 (0.91-1.07)	244	190	0.74 (0.66-0.84)
CTR ≤0.55	4,455	561	563	0.98 (0.91-1.06)	239	180	0.71 (0.63-0.81)
NYHA III/IV	2,224	719	696	0.88 (0.80-0.97)	402	295	0.65 (0.57-0.75)
EF <0.25	2,258	677	637	0.84 (0.76-0.93)	394	270	0.61 (0.53-0.71)
CTR >0.55	2,346	687	650	0.85 (0.77-0.94)	398	287	0.65 (0.57-0.75)
EF >0.45[c]	987	571	585	1.04 (0.88-1.23)	179	136	0.72 (0.53-0.99)

[a] Number of patients with an event during the first 2 years per 1,000 randomized patients.
[b] Relative risk (95% confidence interval).
[c] DIG Ancillary Study.

advanced or complete heart block in patients with pre-existing incomplete AV block. In such patients consideration should be given to the insertion of a pacemaker before treatment with digoxin.

Accessory AV Pathway (Wolff-Parkinson-White Syndrome)

After intravenous digoxin therapy, some patients with paroxysmal atrial fibrillation or flutter and a coexisting accessory AV pathway have developed increased antegrade conduction across the accessory pathway bypassing the AV node, leading to a very rapid ventricular response or ventricular fibrillation. Unless conduction down the accessory pathway has been blocked (either pharmacologically or by surgery), digoxin should not be used in such patients. The treatment of paroxysmal supraventricular tachycardia in such patients is usually direct-current cardioversion.

Use in Patients With Preserved Left Ventricular Systolic Function

Patients with certain disorders involving heart failure associated with preserved left ventricular ejection fraction may be particularly susceptible to toxicity of the drug. Such disorders include restrictive cardiomyopathy, constrictive pericarditis, amyloid heart disease, and acute cor pulmonale. Patients with idiopathic hypertrophic subaortic stenosis may have worsening of the outflow obstruction due to the inotropic effects of digoxin. Digoxin should generally be avoided in these patients, although it has been used for ventricular rate control in the subgroup of patients with atrial fibrillation.

PRECAUTIONS

Use in Patients With Impaired Renal Function

Digoxin is primarily excreted by the kidneys; therefore, patients with impaired renal function require smaller than usual maintenance doses of digoxin (see DOSAGE AND ADMINISTRATION). Because of the prolonged elimination half-life, a longer period of time is required to achieve an initial or new steady-state serum concentration in patients with renal impairment than in patients with normal renal function. If appropriate care is not taken to reduce the dose of digoxin, such patients are at high risk for toxicity, and toxic effects will last longer in such patients than in patients with normal renal function.

Use in Patients With Electrolyte Disorders

In patients with hypokalemia or hypomagnesemia, toxicity may occur despite serum digoxin concentrations below 2.0 ng/mL, because potassium or magnesium depletion sensitizes the myocardium to digoxin. Therefore, it is desirable to maintain normal serum potassium and magnesium concentrations in patients being treated with digoxin. Deficiencies of these electrolytes may result from malnutrition, diarrhea, or prolonged vomiting, as well as the use of the following drugs or procedures: diuretics, amphotericin B, corticosteroids, antacids, dialysis, and mechanical suction of gastrointestinal secretions.

Hypercalcemia from any cause predisposes the patient to digitalis toxicity. Calcium, particularly when administered rapidly by the intravenous route, may produce serious arrhythmias in digitalized patients. On the other hand, hypocalcemia can nullify the effects of digoxin in humans; thus, digoxin may be ineffective until serum calcium is restored to normal. These interactions are related to the fact that digoxin affects contractility and excitability of the heart in a manner similar to that of calcium.

Use in Thyroid Disorders and Hypermetabolic States

Hypothyroidism may reduce the requirements for digoxin. Heart failure and/or atrial arrhythmias resulting from hypermetabolic or hyperdynamic states (e.g., hyperthyroidism, hypoxia, or arteriovenous shunt) are best treated by addressing the underlying condition. Atrial arrhythmias associated with hypermetabolic states are particularly resistant to digoxin treatment. Care must be taken to avoid toxicity if digoxin is used.

Use in Patients With Acute Myocardial Infarction

Digoxin should be used with caution in patients with acute myocardial infarction. The use of inotropic drugs in some patients in this setting may result in undesirable increases in myocardial oxygen demand and ischemia.

Use During Electrical Cardioversion
It may be desirable to reduce the dose of digoxin for 1 to 2 days prior to electrical cardioversion of atrial fibrillation to avoid the induction of ventricular arrhythmias, but physicians must consider the consequences of increasing the ventricular response if digoxin is withdrawn. If digitalis toxicity is suspected, elective cardioversion should be delayed. If it is not prudent to delay cardioversion, the lowest possible energy level should be selected to avoid provoking ventricular arrhythmias.

Use in Patients With Myocarditis
Digoxin can rarely precipitate vasoconstriction and therefore should be avoided in patients with myocarditis.

Use in Patients With Beri Beri Heart Disease
Patients with beri beri heart disease may fail to respond adequately to digoxin if the underlying thiamine deficiency is not treated concomitantly.

Laboratory Test Monitoring
Patients receiving digoxin should have their serum electrolytes and renal function (serum creatinine concentrations) assessed periodically; the frequency of assessments will depend on the clinical setting. For discussion of serum digoxin concentrations, see DOSAGE AND ADMINISTRATION.

Drug Interactions
Potassium-depleting *diuretics* are a major contributing factor to digitalis toxicity. *Calcium*, particularly if administered rapidly by the intravenous route, may produce serious arrhythmias in digitalized patients. *Quinidine, verapamil, amiodarone, propafenone, indomethacin, itraconazole, alprazolam,* and *spironolactone* raise the serum digoxin concentration due to a reduction in clearance and/or in volume of distribution of the drug, with the implication that digitalis intoxication may result. *Erythromycin* and *clarithromycin* (and possibly other *macrolide antibiotics*) and *tetracycline* may increase digoxin absorption in patients who inactivate digoxin by bacterial metabolism in the lower intestine, so that digitalis intoxication may result. *Propantheline* and *diphenoxylate*, by decreasing gut motility, may increase digoxin absorption. *Antacids, kaolin-pectin, sulfasalazine, neomycin, cholestyramine,* certain *anticancer drugs*, and *metoclopramide* may interfere with intestinal digoxin absorption, resulting in unexpectedly low serum concentrations. *Rifampin* may decrease serum digoxin concentration, especially in patients with renal dysfunction, by increasing the non-renal clearance of digoxin. There have been inconsistent reports regarding the effects of other drugs (e.g., *quinine, penicillamine*) on serum digoxin concentration. *Thyroid* administration to a digitalized, hypothyroid patient may increase the dose requirement of digoxin. Concomitant use of digoxin and *sympathomimetics* increases the risk of cardiac arrhythmias. *Succinylcholine* may cause a sudden extrusion of potassium from muscle cells, and may thereby cause arrhythmias in digitalized patients. Although calcium channel blockers and digoxin may be useful in combination to control atrial fibrillation, their additive effects on AV node conduction can result in advanced or complete heart block. Both digitalis glycosides and beta-blockers slow atrioventricular conduction and decrease heart rate. Concomitant use can increase the risk of bradycardia. Digoxin concentrations are increased by about 15% when digoxin and carvedilol are administered concomitantly. Therefore, increased monitoring of digoxin is recommended when initiating, adjusting, or discontinuing carvedilol.
Due to the considerable variability of these interactions, the dosage of digoxin should be individualized when patients receive these medications concurrently. Furthermore, caution should be exercised when combining digoxin with any drug that may cause a significant deterioration in renal function, since a decline in glomerular filtration or tubular secretion may impair the excretion of digoxin.

Drug/Laboratory Test Interactions
The use of therapeutic doses of digoxin may cause prolongation of the PR interval and depression of the ST segment on the electrocardiogram. Digoxin may produce false positive ST-T changes on the electrocardiogram during exercise testing. These electrophysiologic effects reflect an expected effect of the drug and are not indicative of toxicity.

Carcinogenesis, Mutagenesis, Impairment of Fertility
There have been no long-term studies performed in animals to evaluate carcinogenic potential, nor have studies been conducted to assess the mutagenic potential of digoxin or its potential to affect fertility.

Pregnancy
Teratogenic Effects
Pregnancy Category C. Animal reproduction studies have not been conducted with digoxin. It is also not known whether digoxin can cause fetal harm when administered to a pregnant woman or can affect reproductive capacity. Digoxin should be given to a pregnant woman only if clearly needed.

Nursing Mothers
Studies have shown that digoxin concentrations in the mother's serum and milk are similar. However, the estimated exposure of a nursing infant to digoxin via breastfeeding will be far below the usual infant maintenance dose. Therefore, this amount should have no pharmacologic effect upon the infant. Nevertheless, caution should be exercised when digoxin is administered to a nursing woman.

Pediatric Use
Newborn infants display considerable variability in their tolerance to digoxin. Premature and immature infants are particularly sensitive to the effects of digoxin, and the dosage of the drug must not only be reduced but must be individualized according to their degree of maturity. Digitalis glycosides can cause poisoning in children due to accidental ingestion.

Geriatric Use
The majority of clinical experience gained with digoxin has been in the elderly population. This experience has not identified differences in response or adverse effects between the elderly and younger patients. However, this drug is known to be substantially excreted by the kidney, and the risk of toxic reactions to this drug may be greater in patients with impaired renal function. Because elderly patients are more likely to have decreased renal function, care should be taken in dose selection, which should be based on renal function, and it may be useful to monitor renal function (see DOSAGE AND ADMINISTRATION).

ADVERSE REACTIONS

In general, the adverse reactions of digoxin are dose-dependent and occur at doses higher than those needed to achieve a therapeutic effect. Hence, adverse reactions are less common when digoxin is used within the recommended dose range or therapeutic serum concentration range and when there is careful attention to concurrent medications and conditions.
Because some patients may be particularly susceptible to side effects with digoxin, the dosage of the drug should always be selected carefully and adjusted as the clinical condition of the patient warrants. In the past, when high doses of digoxin were used and little attention was paid to clinical status or concurrent medications, adverse reactions to digoxin were more frequent and severe. Cardiac adverse reactions accounted for about one-half, gastrointestinal disturbances for about one-fourth, and CNS and other toxicity for about one-fourth of these adverse reactions. However, available evidence suggests that the incidence and severity of digoxin toxicity has decreased substantially in recent years. In recent controlled clinical trials, in patients with predominantly mild to moderate heart failure, the incidence of adverse experiences was comparable in patients taking digoxin and in those taking placebo. In a large mortality trial, the incidence of hospitalization for suspected digoxin toxicity was 2% in patients taking LANOXIN Tablets compared to 0.9% in patients taking placebo. In this trial, the most common manifestations of digoxin toxicity included gastrointestinal and cardiac disturbances; CNS manifestations were less common.

Adults:
Cardiac
Therapeutic doses of digoxin may cause heart block in patients with pre-existing sinoatrial or AV conduction disorders; heart block can be avoided by adjusting the dose of digoxin. Prophylactic use of a cardiac pacemaker may be considered if the risk of heart block is considered unacceptable. High doses of digoxin may produce a variety of rhythm disturbances, such as first-degree, second-degree (Wenckebach), or third-degree heart block (including asystole); atrial tachycardia with block; AV dissociation; accelerated junctional (nodal) rhythm; unifocal or multiform ventricular premature contractions (especially bigeminy or trigeminy); ventricular tachycardia; and ventricular fibrillation. Digoxin produces PR prolongation and ST segment depression which should not by themselves be considered digoxin toxicity. Cardiac toxicity can also occur at therapeutic doses in patients who have conditions which may alter their sensitivity to digoxin (see WARNINGS and PRECAUTIONS).
Gastrointestinal
Digoxin may cause anorexia, nausea, vomiting, and diarrhea. Rarely, the use of digoxin has been associated with abdominal pain, intestinal ischemia, and hemorrhagic necrosis of the intestines.
CNS
Digoxin can produce visual disturbances (blurred or yellow vision), headache, weakness, dizziness, apathy, confusion, and mental disturbances (such as anxiety, depression, delirium, and hallucination).
Other
Gynecomastia has been occasionally observed following the prolonged use of digoxin. Thrombocytopenia and maculopapular rash and other skin reactions have been rarely observed.
Table 4 summarizes the incidence of those adverse experiences listed above for patients treated with LANOXIN Tablets or placebo from 2 randomized, double-blind, placebo-controlled withdrawal trials. Patients in these trials were also receiving diuretics with or without angiotensin-converting enzyme inhibitors. These patients had been stable on digoxin, and were randomized to digoxin or placebo. The results shown in Table 4 reflect the experience in patients following dosage titration with the use of serum digoxin concentrations and careful follow-up. These adverse experiences are consistent with results from a large, placebo-controlled mortality trial (DIG trial) wherein over half the patients were not receiving digoxin prior to enrollment.

Table 4. Adverse Experiences In 2 Parallel, Double-Blind, Placebo-Controlled Withdrawal Trials (Number of Patients Reporting)

Adverse Experience	Digoxin Patients (n = 123)	Placebo Patients (n = 125)
Cardiac		
Palpitation	1	4
Ventricular extrasystole	1	1
Tachycardia	2	1
Heart arrest	1	1
Gastrointestinal		
Anorexia	1	4
Nausea	4	2
Vomiting	2	1
Diarrhea	4	1
Abdominal pain	0	6
CNS		
Headache	4	4
Dizziness	6	5
Mental disturbances	5	1
Other		
Rash	2	1
Death	4	3

Infants and Children
The side effects of digoxin in infants and children differ from those seen in adults in several respects. Although digoxin may produce anorexia, nausea, vomiting, diarrhea, and CNS disturbances in young patients, these are rarely the initial symptoms of overdosage. Rather, the earliest and most frequent manifestation of excessive dosing with digoxin in infants and children is the appearance of cardiac arrhythmias, including sinus bradycardia. In children, the use of digoxin may produce any arrhythmia. The most common are conduction disturbances or supraventricular tachyarrhythmias, such as atrial tachycardia (with or without block) and junctional (nodal) tachycardia. Ventricular arrhythmias are less common. Sinus bradycardia may be a sign of impending digoxin intoxication, especially in infants, even in the absence of first-degree heart block. Any arrhythmia or alteration in cardiac conduction that develops in a child taking digoxin should be assumed to be caused by digoxin, until further evaluation proves otherwise.

OVERDOSAGE

Signs and Symptoms
The signs and symptoms of toxicity are generally similar to those described in the ADVERSE REACTIONS section but may be more frequent and can be more severe. Signs and symptoms of digoxin toxicity become more frequent with levels above 2 ng/mL. However, in deciding whether a patient's symptoms are due to digoxin, the clinical state together with serum electrolyte levels and thyroid function are important factors (see DOSAGE AND ADMINISTRATION).
Adults
In adults without heart disease, clinical observation suggests that an overdose of digoxin of 10 to 15 mg was the dose resulting in death of half of the patients. If more than 25 mg of digoxin was ingested by an adult without heart disease, death or progressive toxicity responsive only to digoxin-binding Fab antibody fragments resulted. Cardiac manifestations are the most frequent and serious sign of both acute and chronic toxicity. Peak cardiac effects generally occur 3 to 6 hours following overdosage and may persist for the ensuing 24 hours or longer. Digoxin toxicity may result in almost any type of arrhythmia (see ADVERSE REACTIONS). Multiple rhythm disturbances in the same patient are common. Cardiac arrest from asystole or ventricular fibrillation due to digoxin toxicity is usually fatal.
Among the extra-cardiac manifestations, gastrointestinal symptoms (e.g. nausea, vomiting, anorexia) are very common (up to 80% incidence) and precede cardiac manifestations in approximately half of the patients in most literature reports. Neurologic manifestations (e.g. dizziness, various CNS disturbances), fatigue, and malaise are very common. Visual manifestations may also occur with aberration in color vision (predominance of yellow green) the most

frequent. Neurological and visual symptoms may persist after other signs of toxicity have resolved. In chronic toxicity, non-specific extra-cardiac symptoms, such as malaise and weakness, may predominate.

Children

In children aged 1 to 3 years without heart disease, clinical observation suggests that an overdose of digoxin of 6 to 10 mg was the dose resulting in death in half of the patients. If more than 10 mg of digoxin was ingested by a child aged 1 to 3 years without heart disease, the outcome was uniformly fatal when Fab fragment treatment was not given. Most manifestations of toxicity in children occur during or shortly after the loading phase with digoxin. The same arrhythmias or combination of arrhythmias that occur in adults can occur in pediatrics. Sinus tachycardia, supraventricular tachycardia, and rapid atrial fibrillation are seen less frequently in the pediatric population. Pediatric patients are more likely to present with an AV conduction disturbance or a sinus bradycardia. Any arrhythmia or alteration in cardiac conduction that develops in a child taking digoxin should be assumed to be caused by digoxin, until further evaluation proves otherwise.

The frequent extracardiac manifestations similar to those seen in adults are gastrointestinal, CNS, and visual. However, nausea and vomiting are not frequent in infants and small children.

In addition to the undesirable effects seen with recommended doses, weight loss in older age groups and failure to thrive in infants, abdominal pain due to mesenteric artery ischemia, drowsiness, and behavioral disturbances including psychotic manifestations have been reported in overdose.

Treatment

In addition to cardiac monitoring, digoxin should be temporarily discontinued until the adverse reaction resolves and may be all that is required to treat the adverse reaction such as in asymptomatic bradycardia or digoxin-related heart block. Every effort should also be made to correct factors that may contribute to the adverse reaction (such as electrolyte disturbances, thyroid function, or concurrent medications) (see WARNINGS and PRECAUTIONS: Drug Interactions). Once the adverse reaction has resolved, therapy with digoxin may be reinstituted, following a careful reassessment of dose.

When the primary manifestation of digoxin overdosage is a cardiac arrhythmia, additional therapy may be needed.

If the rhythm disturbance is a symptomatic bradyarrhythmia or heart block, consideration should be given to the reversal of toxicity with Digoxin Immune Fab (Ovine) [DIGIBIND® or DIGIFAB®] (see Massive Digitalis Overdosage subsection), the use of atropine, or the insertion of a temporary cardiac pacemaker. Digoxin Immune Fab (Ovine) is a specific antidote for digoxin and may be used to reverse potentially life-threatening ventricular arrhythmias due to digoxin overdosage.

If the rhythm disturbance is a ventricular arrhythmia, consideration should be given to the correction of electrolyte disorders, particularly if hypokalemia (see Administration of Potassium subsection) or hypomagnesemia is present. Ventricular arrhythmias may respond to lidocaine or phenytoin.

Administration of Potassium

Before administering potassium in digoxin overdose for hypokalemia, the serum potassium must be known and every effort should be made to maintain the serum potassium concentration between 4 and 5.5 mmol/L. Potassium salts should be avoided as they may be dangerous in patients who manifest bradycardia or heart block due to digoxin (unless primarily related to supraventricular tachycardia) and in the setting of massive digitalis overdosage. Potassium is usually administered orally, but when correction of the arrhythmia is urgent and the serum potassium concentration is low, potassium may be administered cautiously by the intravenous route. The electrocardiogram should be monitored for any evidence of potassium toxicity (e.g., peaking of T waves) and to observe the effect on the arrhythmia.

Massive Digitalis Overdosage

Manifestations of life-threatening toxicity include ventricular tachycardia or ventricular fibrillation, or progressive bradyarrhythmias, or heart block.

Digoxin Immune Fab (Ovine) should be used to reverse the toxic effects of ingestion of a massive overdose. The decision to administer Digoxin Immune Fab (Ovine) to a patient who has ingested a massive dose of digoxin but who has not yet manifested life-threatening toxicity should depend on the likelihood that life-threatening toxicity will occur (see above).

Digoxin is not effectively removed from the body by dialysis due to its large extravascular volume of distribution. Patients with massive digitalis ingestion should receive large doses of activated charcoal to prevent absorption and bind digoxin in the gut during enteroenteric recirculation. Emesis may be indicated especially if ingestion has occurred within 30 minutes of the patient's presentation at the hospital. Emesis should not be induced in patients who are obtunded. If a patient presents more than 2 hours after ingestion or already has toxic manifestations, it may be unsafe to induce vomiting because such maneuvers may induce an acute vagal episode that can worsen digitalis-related arrhythmias.

In cases where a large amount of digoxin has been ingested, hyperkalemia may be present due to release of potassium from skeletal muscle. Hyperkalemia caused by massive digitalis toxicity is best treated with Digoxin Immune Fab (Ovine); initial treatment with glucose and insulin may also be required if hyperkalemia itself is acutely life-threatening.

DOSAGE AND ADMINISTRATION

General

Recommended dosages of digoxin may require considerable modification because of individual sensitivity of the patient to the drug, the presence of associated conditions, or the use of concurrent medications.

Parenteral administration of digoxin should be used only when the need for rapid digitalization is urgent or when the drug cannot be taken orally. Intramuscular injection can lead to severe pain at the injection site, thus intravenous administration is preferred. If the drug must be administered by the intramuscular route, it should be injected deep into the muscle followed by massage. No more than 500 mcg (2 mL) should be injected into a single site.

LANOXIN Injection can be administered undiluted or diluted with a 4-fold or greater volume of Sterile Water for Injection, 0.9% Sodium Chloride Injection, or 5% Dextrose Injection. The use of less than a 4-fold volume of diluent could lead to precipitation of the digoxin. Immediate use of the diluted product is recommended.

If tuberculin syringes are used to measure very small doses, one must be aware of the problem of inadvertent overadministration of digoxin. The syringe should *not* be flushed with the parenteral solution after its contents are expelled into an indwelling vascular catheter.

Slow infusion of LANOXIN Injection is preferable to bolus administration. Rapid infusion of digitalis glycosides has been shown to cause systemic and coronary arteriolar constriction, which may be clinically undesirable. Caution is thus advised and LANOXIN Injection should probably be administered over a period of 5 minutes or longer. Mixing of LANOXIN Injection with other drugs in the same container or simultaneous administration in the same intravenous line is not recommended.

In selecting a dose of digoxin, the following factors must be considered:

1. The body weight of the patient. Doses should be calculated based upon lean (i.e., ideal) body weight.
2. The patient's renal function, preferably evaluated on the basis of estimated creatinine clearance.
3. The patient's age. Infants and children require different doses of digoxin than adults. Also, advanced age may be indicative of diminished renal function even in patients with normal serum creatinine concentration (i.e., below 1.5 mg/dL).
4. Concomitant disease states, concurrent medications, or other factors likely to alter the pharmacokinetic or pharmacodynamic profile of digoxin (see PRECAUTIONS).

Serum Digoxin Concentrations

In general, the dose of digoxin used should be determined on clinical grounds. However, measurement of serum digoxin concentrations can be helpful to the clinician in determining the adequacy of digoxin therapy and in assigning certain probabilities to the likelihood of digoxin intoxication. About two-thirds of adults considered adequately digitalized (without evidence of toxicity) have serum digoxin concentrations ranging from 0.8 to 2.0 ng/mL (lower serum trough concentrations of 0.5 to 1 ng/mL may be appropriate in some adult patients, see Maintenance Dosing). However, digoxin may produce clinical benefits even at serum concentrations below this range. About two-thirds of adult patients with clinical toxicity have serum digoxin concentrations greater than 2.0 ng/mL. However, since one-third of patients with clinical toxicity have concentrations less than 2.0 ng/mL, values below 2.0 ng/mL do not rule out the possibility that a certain sign or symptom is related to digoxin therapy. Rarely, there are patients who are unable to tolerate digoxin at serum concentrations below 0.8 ng/mL. Consequently, the serum concentration of digoxin should always be interpreted in the overall clinical context, and an isolated measurement should not be used alone as the basis for increasing or decreasing the dose of the drug.

To allow adequate time for equilibration of digoxin between serum and tissue, sampling of serum concentrations should be done just before the next scheduled dose of the drug. If this is not possible, sampling should be done at least 6 to 8 hours after the last dose, regardless of the route of administration or the formulation used. On a once-daily dosing schedule, the concentration of digoxin will be 10% to 25% lower when sampled at 24 versus 8 hours, depending upon the patient's renal function. On a twice-daily dosing schedule, there will be only minor differences in serum digoxin concentrations whether sampling is done at 8 or 12 hours after a dose.

If a discrepancy exists between the reported serum concentration and the observed clinical response, the clinician should consider the following possibilities:

1. Analytical problems in the assay procedure.
2. Inappropriate serum sampling time.
3. Administration of a digitalis glycoside other than digoxin.
4. Conditions (described in WARNINGS and PRECAUTIONS) causing an alteration in the sensitivity of the patient to digoxin.
5. Serum digoxin concentration may decrease acutely during periods of exercise without any associated change in clinical efficacy due to increased binding of digoxin to skeletal muscle.

Heart Failure

Adults

Digitalization may be accomplished by either of 2 general approaches that vary in dosage and frequency of administration, but reach the same endpoint in terms of total amount of digoxin accumulated in the body.

1. If rapid digitalization is considered medically appropriate, it may be achieved by administering a loading dose based upon projected peak digoxin body stores. Maintenance dose can be calculated as a percentage of the loading dose.
2. More gradual digitalization may be obtained by beginning an appropriate maintenance dose, thus allowing digoxin body stores to accumulate slowly. Steady-state serum digoxin concentrations will be achieved in approximately 5 half-lives of the drug for the individual patient. Depending upon the patient's renal function, this will take between 1 and 3 weeks.

Rapid Digitalization With a Loading Dose

LANOXIN Injection is frequently used to achieve rapid digitalization, with conversion to LANOXIN Tablets for maintenance therapy. If patients are switched from intravenous to oral digoxin formulations, allowances must be made for differences in bioavailability when calculating maintenance dosages (see Table 1, CLINICAL PHARMACOLOGY: Pharmacokinetics and dosing Table 5).

Intramuscular injection of digoxin is extremely painful and offers no advantages unless other routes of administration are contraindicated.

Peak digoxin body stores of 8 to 12 mcg/kg should provide therapeutic effect with minimum risk of toxicity in most patients with heart failure and normal sinus rhythm. Because of altered digoxin distribution and elimination, projected peak body stores for patients with renal insufficiency should be conservative (i.e., 6 to 10 mcg/kg) (see PRECAUTIONS).

The loading dose should be administered in several portions, with roughly half the total given as the first dose. Additional fractions of this planned total dose may be given at 6- to 8-hour intervals, **with careful assessment of clinical response before each additional dose.** If the patient's clinical response necessitates a change from the calculated loading dose of digoxin, then calculation of the maintenance dose should be based upon the amount actually given.

A single initial intravenous dose of 400 to 600 mcg (0.4 to 0.6 mg) of LANOXIN Injection usually produces a detectable effect in 5 to 30 minutes that becomes maximal in 1 to 4 hours. Additional doses of 100 to 300 mcg (0.1 to 0.3 mg) may be given cautiously at 6- to 8-hour intervals until clinical evidence of an adequate effect is noted. The usual amount of LANOXIN Injection that a 70-kg patient requires to achieve 8- to 12-mcg/kg peak body stores is 600 to 1,000 mcg (0.6 to 1.0 mg).

Maintenance Dosing

The doses of oral digoxin used in controlled trials in patients with heart failure have ranged from 125 to 500 mcg (0.125 to 0.5 mg) once daily. In these studies, the digoxin dose has been generally titrated according to the patient's age, lean body weight, and renal function. Therapy is generally initiated at a dose of 250 mcg (0.25 mg) once daily in patients under age 70 with good renal function, at a dose of 125 mcg (0.125 mg) once daily in patients over age 70 or with impaired renal function, and at a dose of 62.5 mcg (0.0625 mg) in patients with marked renal impairment. Doses may be increased every 2 weeks according to clinical response.

In a subset of approximately 1,800 patients enrolled in the DIG trial (wherein dosing was based on an algorithm similar to that in Table 5) the mean (± SD) serum digoxin concentrations at 1 month and 12 months were 1.01 ± 0.47 ng/mL and 0.97 ± 0.43 ng/mL, respectively. There are no rigid guidelines as to the range of serum concentrations that are most efficacious. Several post hoc analyses of heart failure patients in the DIG trial suggest that the optimal trough digoxin serum level may be 0.5 ng/mL to 1 ng/mL.

The maintenance dose should be based upon the percentage of the peak body stores lost each day through elimination. The following formula has had wide clinical use:

Table 5. Usual Daily Maintenance Dose Requirements (mcg) of LANOXIN Injection for Estimated Peak Body Stores of 10 mcg/kg[a]

Corrected Ccr (mL/min per 70 kg)[b]	Lean Body Weight							Number of Days Before Steady State Achieved[c]
	kg	50	60	70	80	90	100	
	lb	110	132	154	176	198	220	
0		75[d]	75	100	100	125	150	22
10		75	100	100	125	150	150	19
20		100	100	125	150	150	175	16
30		100	125	150	150	175	200	14
40		100	125	150	175	200	225	13
50		125	150	175	200	225	250	12
60		125	150	175	200	225	250	11
70		150	175	200	225	250	275	10
80		150	175	200	250	275	300	9
90		150	200	225	250	300	325	8
100		175	200	250	275	300	350	7

[a] Daily maintenance doses have been rounded to the nearest 25-mcg increment.
[b] Ccr is creatinine clearance, corrected to 70-kg body weight or 1.73 m² body surface area. *For adults,* if only serum creatinine concentrations (Scr) are available, a Ccr (corrected to 70 kg body weight) may be estimated in men as (140 - Age)/Scr. For women, this result should be multiplied by 0.85. *Note: This equation cannot be used for estimating creatinine clearance in infants or children.*
[c] If no loading dose administered.
[d] 75mcg = 0.075 mg.

Maintenance Dose = Peak Body Stores (i.e., Loading Dose) × % Daily Loss/100
Where: % Daily Loss = 14 + Ccr/5
(Ccr is creatinine clearance, corrected to 70 kg body weight or 1.73 m² body surface area.)
Table 5 provides average daily maintenance dose requirements of LANOXIN Injection for patients with heart failure based upon lean body weight and renal function:
[See table 5 above]
Example: Based on the above table, a patient in heart failure with an estimated lean body weight of 70 kg and a Ccr of 60 mL/min should be given a dose of 175 mcg (0.175 mg) daily of LANOXIN Injection. If no loading dose is administered, steady-state serum concentrations in this patient should be anticipated at approximately 11 days.
Infants and Children
See the full prescribing information for LANOXIN Injection Pediatric for specific recommendations.
It cannot be overemphasized that dosage guidelines provided are based upon average patient response and substantial individual variation can be expected. Accordingly, ultimate dosage selection must be based upon clinical assessment of the patient.
Atrial Fibrillation
Peak digoxin body stores larger than the 8 to 12 mcg/kg required for most patients with heart failure and normal sinus rhythm have been used for control of ventricular rate in patients with atrial fibrillation. Doses of digoxin used for the treatment of chronic atrial fibrillation should be titrated to the minimum dose that achieves the desired ventricular rate control without causing undesirable side effects. Data are not available to establish the appropriate resting or exercise target rates that should be achieved.
Dosage Adjustment When Changing Preparations
The difference in bioavailability between LANOXIN Injection or LANOXIN Tablets must be considered when changing patients from one dosage form to the other.

HOW SUPPLIED
LANOXIN (digoxin) Injection, 500 mcg (0.5 mg) in 2 mL (250 mcg [0.25 mg] per mL); Boxes of 10 (NDC 0173-0260-10) and 50 ampuls (NDC 0173-0260-35).
Store at 25°C (77°F); excursions permitted to 15 to 30°C (59 to 86°F) [see USP Controlled Room Temperature] and protect from light.
LANOXIN and DIGIBIND are registered trademarks of GlaxoSmithKline
DIGIFAB is a registered trademark of Prostherics Inc.
Manufactured by
Draxis Pharma Inc.
Kirkland, Canada H9H 4J4 for
GlaxoSmithKline
Research Triangle Park, NC 27709
©2009, GlaxoSmithKline. All rights reserved.
August 2009
LNJ:1PI

LANOXIN®
[lă-nŏx'ĭn]
(digoxin)
Injection Pediatric
100 mcg (0.1 mg) in 1 mL

DESCRIPTION
LANOXIN (digoxin) is one of the cardiac (or digitalis) glycosides, a closely related group of drugs having in common specific effects on the myocardium. These drugs are found in a number of plants. Digoxin is extracted from the leaves of *Digitalis lanata*. The term "digitalis" is used to designate the whole group of glycosides. The glycosides are composed of 2 portions: a sugar and a cardenolide (hence "glycosides"). Digoxin is described chemically as (3β,5β,12β)-3-[(O-2,6-dideoxy-β-D-ribo-hexopyranosyl-(1→4)-O-2,6-dideoxy-β-D-ribo-hexopyranosyl-(1→4)-2,6-dideoxy-β-D-ribo-hexopyranosyl]oxy]-12,14-dihydroxy-card-20(22)-enolide. Its molecular formula is $C_{41}H_{64}O_{14}$, its molecular weight is 780.95, and its structural formula is:

Digoxin exists as odorless white crystals that melt with decomposition above 230°C. The drug is practically insoluble in water and in ether; slightly soluble in diluted (50%) alcohol and in chloroform; and freely soluble in pyridine.
LANOXIN Injection Pediatric is a sterile solution of digoxin for intravenous or intramuscular injection. The vehicle contains 40% propylene glycol and 10% alcohol. The injection is buffered to a pH of 6.8 to 7.2 with 0.17% sodium phosphate and 0.08% anhydrous citric acid. Each 1-mL ampul contains 100 mcg (0.1 mg) digoxin. Dilution is not required.

CLINICAL PHARMACOLOGY
Mechanism of Action
Digoxin inhibits sodium-potassium ATPase, an enzyme that regulates the quantity of sodium and potassium inside cells. Inhibition of the enzyme leads to an increase in the intracellular concentration of sodium and thus (by stimulation of sodium-calcium exchange) an increase in the intracellular concentration of calcium. The beneficial effects of digoxin result from direct actions on cardiac muscle, as well as indirect actions on the cardiovascular system mediated by effects on the autonomic nervous system. The autonomic effects include: (1) a vagomimetic action, which is responsible for the effects of digoxin on the sinoatrial and atrioventricular (AV) nodes; and (2) baroreceptor sensitization, which results in increased afferent inhibitory activity and reduced activity of the sympathetic nervous system and renin-angiotensin system for any given increment in mean arterial pressure. The pharmacologic consequences of these direct and indirect effects are: (1) an increase in the force and velocity of myocardial systolic contraction (positive inotropic action); (2) a decrease in the degree of activation of the sympathetic nervous system and renin-angiotensin system (neurohormonal deactivating effect); and (3) slowing of the heart rate and decreased conduction velocity through the AV node (vagomimetic effect). The effects of digoxin in heart failure are mediated by its positive inotropic and neurohormonal deactivating effects, whereas the effects of the drug in atrial arrhythmias are related to its vagomimetic actions. In high doses, digoxin increases sympathetic outflow from the central nervous system (CNS). This increase in sympathetic activity may be an important factor in digitalis toxicity.
Pharmacokinetics
Note: The following data are from studies performed in adults, unless otherwise stated.
Absorption
Comparisons of the systemic availability and equivalent doses for preparations of digoxin are shown in Table 1.
[See table 1 at top of next page]
Distribution
Following drug administration, a 6- to 8-hour tissue distribution phase is observed. This is followed by a much more gradual decline in the serum concentration of the drug, which is dependent on the elimination of digoxin from the body. The peak height and slope of the early portion (absorption/distribution phases) of the serum concentration-time curve are dependent upon the route of administration and the absorption characteristics of the formulation. Clinical evidence indicates that the early high serum concentrations do not reflect the concentration of digoxin at its site of action, but that with chronic use, the steady-state post-distribution serum concentrations are in equilibrium with tissue concentrations and correlate with pharmacologic effects. In individual patients, these post-distribution serum concentrations may be useful in evaluating therapeutic and toxic effects (see DOSAGE AND ADMINISTRATION: Serum Digoxin Concentrations).
Digoxin is concentrated in tissues and therefore has a large apparent volume of distribution. Digoxin crosses both the blood-brain barrier and the placenta. At delivery, the serum digoxin concentration in the newborn is similar to the serum concentration in the mother. Approximately 25% of digoxin in the plasma is bound to protein. Serum digoxin concentrations are not significantly altered by large changes in fat tissue weight, so that its distribution space correlates best with lean (i.e., ideal) body weight, not total body weight.
Metabolism
Only a small percentage (16%) of a dose of digoxin is metabolized. The end metabolites, which include 3 β-digoxigenin, 3-keto-digoxigenin, and their glucuronide and sulfate conjugates, are polar in nature and are postulated to be formed via hydrolysis, oxidation, and conjugation. The metabolism of digoxin is not dependent upon the cytochrome P-450 system, and digoxin is not known to induce or inhibit the cytochrome P-450 system.
Excretion
Elimination of digoxin follows first-order kinetics (that is, the quantity of digoxin eliminated at any time is proportional to the total body content). Following intravenous administration to healthy volunteers, 50% to 70% of a digoxin dose is excreted unchanged in the urine. Renal excretion of digoxin is proportional to glomerular filtration rate and is largely independent of urine flow. In healthy volunteers with normal renal function, digoxin has a half-life of 1.5 to 2.0 days. The half-life in anuric patients is prolonged to 3.5 to 5 days. Digoxin is not effectively removed from the body by dialysis, exchange transfusion, or during cardiopulmonary bypass because most of the drug is bound to tissue and does not circulate in the blood.
Special Populations
Race differences in digoxin pharmacokinetics have not been formally studied. Because digoxin is primarily eliminated as unchanged drug via the kidney and because there are no important differences in creatinine clearance among races, pharmacokinetic differences due to race are not expected.
The clearance of digoxin can be primarily correlated with renal function as indicated by creatinine clearance. In children with renal disease, digoxin must be carefully titrated based upon clinical response.
Plasma digoxin concentration profiles in patients with acute hepatitis generally fell within the range of profiles in a group of healthy subjects.
Pharmacodynamic and Clinical Effects
The times to onset of pharmacologic effect and to peak effect of preparations of LANOXIN are shown in Table 2.
[See table 2 on next page]
Hemodynamic Effects
Digoxin produces hemodynamic improvement in patients with heart failure. Short- and long-term therapy with the drug increases cardiac output and lowers pulmonary artery pressure, pulmonary capillary wedge pressure, and systemic vascular resistance. These hemodynamic effects are

accompanied by an increase in the left ventricular ejection fraction and a decrease in end-systolic and end-diastolic dimensions.

Chronic Heart Failure

Two 12-week, double-blind, placebo-controlled studies enrolled 178 (RADIANCE trial) and 88 (PROVED trial) adult patients with NYHA class II or III heart failure previously treated with oral digoxin, a diuretic, and an ACE inhibitor (RADIANCE only) and randomized them to placebo or treatment with LANOXIN Tablets. Both trials demonstrated better preservation of exercise capacity in patients randomized to LANOXIN. Continued treatment with LANOXIN reduced the risk of developing worsening heart failure, as evidenced by heart failure-related hospitalizations and emergency care and the need for concomitant heart failure therapy. The larger study also showed treatment-related benefits in NYHA class and patients' global assessment. In the smaller trial, these trended in favor of a treatment benefit.

The Digitalis Investigation Group (DIG) main trial was a multicenter, randomized, double-blind, placebo-controlled mortality study of 6,801 adult patients with heart failure and left ventricular ejection fraction ≤0.45. At randomization, 67% were NYHA class I or II, 71% had heart failure of ischemic etiology, 44% had been receiving digoxin, and most were receiving concomitant ACE inhibitor (94%) and diuretic (82%). Patients were randomized to placebo or LANOXIN Tablets, the dose of which was adjusted for the patient's age, sex, lean body weight, and serum creatinine (see DOSAGE AND ADMINISTRATION), and followed for up to 58 months (median 37 months). The median daily dose prescribed was 0.25 mg. Overall all-cause mortality was 35% with no difference between groups (95% confidence limits for relative risk of 0.91 to 1.07). LANOXIN was associated with a 25% reduction in the number of hospitalizations for heart failure, a 28% reduction in the risk of a patient having at least 1 hospitalization for heart failure, and a 6.5% reduction in total hospitalizations (for any cause).

Use of LANOXIN was associated with a trend to increase time to all-cause death or hospitalization. The trend was evident in subgroups of patients with mild heart failure as well as more severe disease, as shown in Table 3. Although the effect on all-cause death or hospitalization was not statistically significant, much of the apparent benefit derived from effects on mortality and hospitalization attributed to heart failure.

[See table 3 at right]

In situations where there is no statistically significant benefit of treatment evident from a trial's primary endpoint, results pertaining to a secondary endpoint should be interpreted cautiously.

Chronic Atrial Fibrillation

In adult patients with chronic atrial fibrillation, digoxin slows rapid ventricular response rate in a linear dose-response fashion from 0.25 to 0.75 mg/day. Digoxin should not be used for the treatment of multifocal atrial tachycardia.

INDICATIONS AND USAGE

Heart Failure

LANOXIN is indicated for the treatment of mild to moderate heart failure. LANOXIN increases left ventricular ejection fraction and improves heart failure symptoms as evidenced by exercise capacity and heart failure-related hospitalizations and emergency care, while having no effect on mortality. Where possible, LANOXIN should be used with a diuretic and an angiotensin-converting enzyme inhibitor, but an optimal order for starting these 3 drugs cannot be specified.

Atrial Fibrillation

LANOXIN is indicated for the control of ventricular response rate in patients with chronic atrial fibrillation.

CONTRAINDICATIONS

Digitalis glycosides are contraindicated in patients with ventricular fibrillation or in patients with a known hypersensitivity to digoxin. A hypersensitivity reaction to other digitalis preparations usually constitutes a contraindication to digoxin.

WARNINGS

Sinus Node Disease and AV Block

Because digoxin slows sinoatrial and AV conduction, the drug commonly prolongs the PR interval. The drug may cause severe sinus bradycardia or sinoatrial block in patients with pre-existing sinus node disease and may cause advanced or complete heart block in patients with pre-existing incomplete AV block. In such patients consideration should be given to the insertion of a pacemaker before treatment with digoxin.

Accessory AV Pathway (Wolff-Parkinson-White Syndrome)

After intravenous digoxin therapy, some patients with paroxysmal atrial fibrillation or flutter and a coexisting accessory AV pathway have developed increased antegrade conduction across the accessory pathway bypassing the AV

Table 1. Comparisons of the Systemic Availability and Equivalent Doses for Preparations of LANOXIN

Product	Absolute Bioavailability	Equivalent Doses (mcg)[a] Among Dosage Forms			
LANOXIN Tablets	60-80%	62.5	125	250	500
LANOXIN Injection/IV	100%	50	100	200	400

[a] For example, 125 mcg LANOXIN Tablets equivalent to 100 mcg LANOXIN Injection/IV.

Table 2. Times to Onset of Pharmacologic Effect and to Peak Effect of Preparations of LANOXIN

Product	Time to Onset of Effect[a]	Time to Peak Effect[a]
LANOXIN Tablets	0.5-2 hours	2-6 hours
LANOXIN Injection/IV	5-30 minutes[b]	1-4 hours

[a] Documented for ventricular response rate in atrial fibrillation, inotropic effects and electrocardiographic changes.
[b] Depending upon rate of infusion.

Table 3. Subgroup Analyses of Mortality and Hospitalization During the First 2 Years Following Randomization

	n	Risk of All-Cause Mortality or All-Cause Hospitalization[a]			Risk of HF-Related Mortality or HF-Related Hospitalization[a]		
		Placebo	LANOXIN	Relative risk[b]	Placebo	LANOXIN	Relative risk[b]
All patients (EF ≤0.45)	6,801	604	593	0.94 (0.88-1.00)	294	217	0.69 (0.63-0.76)
NYHA I/II	4,571	549	541	0.96 (0.89-1.04)	242	178	0.70 (0.62-0.80)
EF 0.25-0.45	4,543	568	571	0.99 (0.91-1.07)	244	190	0.74 (0.66-0.84)
CTR ≤0.55	4,455	561	563	0.98 (0.91-1.06)	239	180	0.71 (0.63-0.81)
NYHA III/IV	2,224	719	696	0.88 (0.80-0.97)	402	295	0.65 (0.57-0.75)
EF <0.25	2,258	677	637	0.84 (0.76-0.93)	394	270	0.61 (0.53-0.71)
CTR >0.55	2,346	687	650	0.85 (0.77-0.94)	398	287	0.65 (0.57-0.75)
EF >0.45[c]	987	571	585	1.04 (0.88-1.23)	179	136	0.72 (0.53-0.99)

[a] Number of patients with an event during the first 2 years per 1,000 randomized patients.
[b] Relative risk (95% confidence interval).
[c] DIG Ancillary Study.

node, leading to a very rapid ventricular response or ventricular fibrillation. Unless conduction down the accessory pathway has been blocked (either pharmacologically or by surgery), digoxin should not be used in such patients. The treatment of paroxysmal supraventricular tachycardia in such patients is usually direct-current cardioversion.

Use in Patients With Preserved Left Ventricular Systolic Function

Patients with certain disorders involving heart failure associated with preserved left ventricular ejection fraction may be particularly susceptible to toxicity of the drug. Such disorders include restrictive cardiomyopathy, constrictive pericarditis, amyloid heart disease, and acute cor pulmonale. Patients with idiopathic hypertrophic subaortic stenosis may have worsening of the outflow obstruction due to the inotropic effects of digoxin. Digoxin should generally be avoided in these patients, although it has been used for ventricular rate control in the subgroup of patients with atrial fibrillation.

PRECAUTIONS

Use in Patients With Impaired Renal Function

Digoxin is primarily excreted by the kidneys; therefore, patients with impaired renal function require smaller than usual maintenance doses of digoxin (see DOSAGE AND ADMINISTRATION). Because of the prolonged elimination half-life, a longer period of time is required to achieve an initial or new steady-state serum concentration in patients with renal impairment than in patients with normal renal function. If appropriate care is not taken to reduce the dose of digoxin, such patients are at high risk for toxicity, and toxic effects will last longer in such patients than in patients with normal renal function.

Use in Patients With Electrolyte Disorders

In patients with hypokalemia or hypomagnesemia, toxicity may occur despite serum digoxin concentrations below 2.0 ng/mL, because potassium or magnesium depletion sensitizes the myocardium to digoxin. It is desirable to maintain normal serum potassium and magnesium concentrations in patients being treated with digoxin. Deficiencies of these electrolytes may result from malnutrition, di-

arrhea, or prolonged vomiting, as well as the use of the following drugs or procedures: diuretics, amphotericin B, corticosteroids, antacids, dialysis, and mechanical suction of gastrointestinal secretions.

Hypercalcemia from any cause predisposes the patient to digitalis toxicity. Calcium, particularly when administered rapidly by the intravenous route, may produce serious arrhythmias in digitalized patients. On the other hand, hypocalcemia can nullify the effects of digoxin in humans; thus, digoxin may be ineffective until serum calcium is restored to normal. These interactions are related to the fact that digoxin affects contractility and excitability of the heart in a manner similar to that of calcium.

Use in Thyroid Disorders and Hypermetabolic States

Hypothyroidism may reduce the requirements for digoxin. Heart failure and/or atrial arrhythmias resulting from hypermetabolic or hyperdynamic states (e.g., hyperthyroidism, hypoxia, or arteriovenous shunt) are best treated by addressing the underlying condition. Atrial arrhythmias associated with hypermetabolic states are particularly resistant to digoxin treatment. Care must be taken to avoid toxicity if digoxin is used.

Use in Patients With Acute Myocardial Infarction

Digoxin should be used with caution in patients with acute myocardial infarction. The use of inotropic drugs in some patients in this setting may result in undesirable increases in myocardial oxygen demand and ischemia.

Use During Electrical Cardioversion

It may be desirable to reduce the dose of digoxin for 1 to 2 days prior to electrical cardioversion of atrial fibrillation to avoid the induction of ventricular arrhythmias, but physicians must consider the consequences of increasing the ventricular response if digoxin is withdrawn. If digitalis toxicity is suspected, elective cardioversion should be delayed. If it is not prudent to delay cardioversion, the lowest possible energy level should be selected to avoid provoking ventricular arrhythmias.

Use in Patients With Myocarditis

Digoxin can rarely precipitate vasoconstriction and therefore should be avoided in patients with myocarditis.

Use in Patients With Beri Beri Heart Disease
Patients with beri beri heart disease may fail to respond adequately to digoxin if the underlying thiamine deficiency is not treated concomitantly.

Laboratory Test Monitoring
Patients receiving digoxin should have their serum electrolytes and renal function (serum creatinine concentrations) assessed periodically; the frequency of assessments will depend on the clinical setting. For discussion of serum digoxin concentrations, see DOSAGE AND ADMINISTRATION.

Drug Interactions
Potassium-depleting *diuretics* are a major contributing factor to digitalis toxicity. *Calcium*, particularly if administered rapidly by the intravenous route, may produce serious arrhythmias in digitalized patients. *Quinidine, verapamil, amiodarone, propafenone, indomethacin, itraconazole, alprazolam*, and *spironolactone* raise the serum digoxin concentration due to a reduction in clearance and/or volume of distribution of the drug, with the implication that digitalis intoxication may result. *Erythromycin* and *clarithromycin* (and possibly other *macrolide antibiotics*) and *tetracycline* may increase digoxin absorption in patients who inactivate digoxin by bacterial metabolism in the lower intestine, so that digitalis intoxication may result. *Propantheline* and *diphenoxylate*, by decreasing gut motility, may increase digoxin absorption. *Antacids, kaolin-pectin, sulfasalazine, neomycin, cholestyramine*, certain *anticancer drugs*, and *metoclopramide* may interfere with intestinal digoxin absorption, resulting in unexpectedly low serum concentrations. *Rifampin* may decrease serum digoxin concentration, especially in patients with renal dysfunction, by increasing the non-renal clearance of digoxin. There have been inconsistent reports regarding the effects of other drugs (e.g., *quinine, penicillamine*) on serum digoxin concentration. *Thyroid* administration to a digitalized, hypothyroid patient may increase the dose requirement of digoxin. Concomitant use of digoxin and *sympathomimetics* increases the risk of cardiac arrhythmias. *Succinylcholine* may cause a sudden extrusion of potassium from muscle cells, and may thereby cause arrhythmias in digitalized patients. Although calcium channel blockers and digoxin may be useful in combination to control atrial fibrillation, their additive effects on AV node conduction can result in advanced or complete heart block. Both digitalis glycosides and beta-blockers slow atrioventricular conduction and decrease heart rate. Concomitant use can increase the risk of bradycardia. Digoxin concentrations are increased by about 15% when digoxin and carvedilol are administered concomitantly. Therefore, increased monitoring of digoxin is recommended when initiating, adjusting, or discontinuing carvedilol.

Due to the considerable variability of these interactions, dosage of digoxin should be individualized when patients receive these medications concurrently. Furthermore, caution should be exercised when combining digoxin with any drug that may cause a significant deterioration in renal function, since a decline in glomerular filtration or tubular secretion may impair the excretion of digoxin.

Drug/Laboratory Test Interactions
The use of therapeutic doses of digoxin may cause prolongation of the PR interval and depression of the ST segment on the electrocardiogram. Digoxin may produce false positive ST-T changes on the electrocardiogram during exercise testing. These electrophysiologic effects reflect an expected effect of the drug and are not indicative of toxicity.

Carcinogenesis, Mutagenesis, Impairment of Fertility
There have been no long-term studies performed in animals to evaluate carcinogenic potential, nor have studies been conducted to assess the mutagenic potential of digoxin or its potential to affect fertility.

Pregnancy
Teratogenic Effects
Pregnancy Category C. Animal reproduction studies have not been conducted with digoxin. It is also not known whether digoxin can cause fetal harm when administered to a pregnant woman or can affect reproductive capacity. Digoxin should be given to a pregnant woman only if clearly needed.

Nursing Mothers
Studies have shown that digoxin concentrations in the mother's serum and milk are similar. However, the estimated exposure of a nursing infant to digoxin via breastfeeding will be far below the usual infant maintenance dose. Therefore, this amount should have no pharmacologic effect upon the infant. Nevertheless, caution should be exercised when digoxin is administered to a nursing woman.

Pediatric Use
Newborn infants display considerable variability in their tolerance to digoxin. Premature and immature infants are particularly sensitive to the effects of digoxin, and the dosage of the drug must not only be reduced but must be individualized according to their degree of maturity. Digitalis glycosides can cause poisoning in children due to accidental ingestion.

Geriatric Use
The majority of clinical experience gained with digoxin has been in the elderly population. This experience has not identified differences in response or adverse effects between the elderly and younger patients. However, this drug is known to be substantially excreted by the kidney, and the risk of toxic reactions to this drug may be greater in patients with impaired renal function. Because elderly patients are more likely to have decreased renal function, care should be taken in dose selection, which should be based on renal function, and it may be useful to monitor renal function.

ADVERSE REACTIONS
In general, the adverse reactions of digoxin are dose-dependent and occur at doses higher than those needed to achieve a therapeutic effect. Hence, adverse reactions are less common when digoxin is used within the recommended dose range or therapeutic serum concentration range and when there is careful attention to concurrent medications and conditions.

Because some patients may be particularly susceptible to side effects with digoxin, the dosage of the drug should always be selected carefully and adjusted as the clinical condition of the patient warrants. In the past, when high doses of digoxin were used and little attention was paid to clinical status or concurrent medications, adverse reactions to digoxin were more frequent and severe. Cardiac adverse reactions accounted for about one-half, gastrointestinal disturbances for about one-fourth, and CNS and other toxicity for about one-fourth of these adverse reactions. However, available evidence suggests that the incidence and severity of digoxin toxicity has decreased substantially in recent years. In recent controlled clinical trials, in patients with predominantly mild to moderate heart failure, the incidence of adverse experiences was comparable in patients taking digoxin and in those taking placebo. In a large mortality trial, the incidence of hospitalization for suspected digoxin toxicity was 2% in patients taking LANOXIN Tablets compared to 0.9% in patients taking placebo. In this trial, the most common manifestations of digoxin toxicity included gastrointestinal and cardiac disturbances; CNS manifestations were less common.

Adults
Cardiac
Therapeutic doses of digoxin may cause heart block in patients with pre-existing sinoatrial or AV conduction disorders; heart block can be avoided by adjusting the dose of digoxin. Prophylactic use of a cardiac pacemaker may be considered if the risk of heart block is considered unacceptable. High doses of digoxin may produce a variety of rhythm disturbances, such as first-degree, second-degree (Wenckebach), or third-degree heart block (including asystole); atrial tachycardia with block; AV dissociation; accelerated junctional (nodal) rhythm; unifocal or multiform ventricular premature contractions (especially bigeminy or trigeminy); ventricular tachycardia; and ventricular fibrillation. Digoxin produces PR prolongation and ST segment depression which should not by themselves be considered digoxin toxicity. Cardiac toxicity can also occur at therapeutic doses in patients who have conditions which may alter their sensitivity to digoxin (see WARNINGS and PRECAUTIONS).

Gastrointestinal
Digoxin may cause anorexia, nausea, vomiting, and diarrhea. Rarely, the use of digoxin has been associated with abdominal pain, intestinal ischemia, and hemorrhagic necrosis of the intestines.

CNS
Digoxin can produce visual disturbances (blurred or yellow vision), headache, weakness, dizziness, apathy, confusion, and mental disturbances (such as anxiety, depression, delirium, and hallucination).

Other
Gynecomastia has been occasionally observed following the prolonged use of digoxin. Thrombocytopenia and maculopapular rash and other skin reactions have been rarely observed.

Table 4 summarizes the incidence of those adverse experiences listed above for patients treated with LANOXIN Tablets or placebo from 2 randomized, double-blind, placebo-controlled withdrawal trials. Patients in these trials were also receiving diuretics with or without angiotensin-converting enzyme inhibitors. These patients had been stable on digoxin, and were randomized to digoxin or placebo. The results shown in Table 4 reflect the experience in patients following dosage titration with the use of serum digoxin concentrations and careful follow-up. These adverse experiences are consistent with results from a large, placebo-controlled mortality trial (DIG trial) wherein over half the patients were not receiving digoxin prior to enrollment.

Table 4. Adverse Experiences in 2 Parallel, Double-Blind, Placebo-Controlled Withdrawal Trials (Number of Patients Reporting)

Adverse Experience	Digoxin Patients (n = 123)	Placebo Patients (n = 125)
Cardiac		
Palpitation	1	4
Ventricular extrasystole	1	1
Tachycardia	2	1
Heart arrest	1	1
Gastrointestinal		
Anorexia	1	4
Nausea	4	2
Vomiting	2	1
Diarrhea	4	1
Abdominal pain	0	6
CNS		
Headache	4	4
Dizziness	6	5
Mental disturbances	5	1
Other		
Rash	2	1
Death	4	3

Infants and Children
The side effects of digoxin in infants and children differ from those seen in adults in several respects. Although digoxin may produce anorexia, nausea, vomiting, diarrhea, and CNS disturbances in young patients, these are rarely the initial symptoms of overdosage. Rather, the earliest and most frequent manifestation of excessive dosing with digoxin in infants and children is the appearance of cardiac arrhythmias, including sinus bradycardia. In children, the use of digoxin may produce any arrhythmia. The most common are conduction disturbances or supraventricular tachyarrhythmias, such as atrial tachycardia (with or without block) and junctional (nodal) tachycardia. Ventricular arrhythmias are less common. Sinus bradycardia may be a sign of impending digoxin intoxication, especially in infants, even in the absence of first-degree heart block. Any arrhythmia or alteration in cardiac conduction that develops in a child taking digoxin should be assumed to be caused by digoxin, until further evaluation proves otherwise.

OVERDOSAGE
Signs and Symptoms
The signs and symptoms of toxicity are generally similar to those described in the ADVERSE REACTIONS section but may be more frequent and can be more severe. Signs and symptoms of digoxin toxicity become more frequent with levels above 2 ng/mL. However, in deciding whether a patient's symptoms are due to digoxin, the clinical state together with serum electrolyte levels and thyroid function are important factors (see DOSAGE AND ADMINISTRATION).

Adults
In adults without heart disease, clinical observation suggests that an overdose of digoxin of 10 to 15 mg was the dose resulting in death of half of the patients. If more than 25 mg of digoxin was ingested by an adult without heart disease, death or progressive toxicity responsive only to digoxin-binding Fab antibody fragments resulted. Cardiac manifestations are the most frequent and serious sign of both acute and chronic toxicity. Peak cardiac effects generally occur 3 to 6 hours following overdosage and may persist for the ensuing 24 hours or longer. Digoxin toxicity may result in almost any type of arrhythmia (see ADVERSE REACTIONS). Multiple rhythm disturbances in the same patient are common. Cardiac arrest from asystole or ventricular fibrillation due to digoxin toxicity is usually fatal.

Among the extra-cardiac manifestations, gastrointestinal symptoms (e.g. nausea, vomiting, anorexia) are very common (up to 80% incidence) and precede cardiac manifestations in approximately half of the patients in most literature reports. Neurologic manifestations (e.g. dizziness, various CNS disturbances), fatigue, and malaise are very common. Visual manifestations may also occur with aberration in color vision (predominance of yellow green) the most frequent. Neurological and visual symptoms may persist after other signs of toxicity have resolved. In chronic toxicity, non-specific extra-cardiac symptoms, such as malaise and weakness, may predominate.

Children
In children aged 1 to 3 years without heart disease, clinical observation suggests that an overdose of digoxin of 6 to 10 mg was the dose resulting in death in half of the patients. If more than 10 mg of digoxin was ingested by a child

aged 1 to 3 years without heart disease, the outcome was uniformly fatal when Fab fragment treatment was not given. Most manifestations of toxicity in children occur during or shortly after the loading phase with digoxin. The same arrhythmias or combination of arrhythmias that occur in adults can occur in pediatrics. Sinus tachycardia, supraventricular tachycardia, and rapid atrial fibrillation are seen less frequently in the pediatric population. Pediatric patients are more likely to present with an AV conduction disturbance or a sinus bradycardia. Any arrhythmia or alteration in cardiac conduction that develops in a child taking digoxin should be assumed to be caused by digoxin, until further evaluation proves otherwise.

The frequent extracardiac manifestations similar to those seen in adults are gastrointestinal, CNS, and visual. However, nausea and vomiting are not frequent in infants and small children.

In addition to the undesirable effects seen with recommended doses, weight loss in older age groups and failure to thrive in infants, abdominal pain due to mesenteric artery ischemia, drowsiness, and behavioral disturbances including psychotic manifestations have been reported in overdose.

Treatment

In addition to cardiac monitoring, digoxin should be temporarily discontinued until the adverse reaction resolves and may be all that is required to treat the adverse reaction such as in asymptomatic bradycardia or digoxin-related heart block. Every effort should also be made to correct factors that may contribute to the adverse reaction (such as electrolyte disturbances, thyroid function, or concurrent medications) (see WARNINGS and PRECAUTIONS: Drug Interactions). Once the adverse reaction has resolved, therapy with digoxin may be reinstituted, following a careful reassessment of dose.

When the primary manifestation of digoxin overdosage is a cardiac arrhythmia, additional therapy may be needed.

If the rhythm disturbance is a symptomatic bradyarrhythmia or heart block, consideration should be given to the reversal of toxicity with Digoxin Immune Fab (Ovine) [DIGIBIND® or DIGIFAB®] (see Massive Digitalis Overdosage subsection), the use of atropine, or the insertion of a temporary cardiac pacemaker. Digoxin Immune Fab (Ovine) is a specific antidote for digoxin and may be used to reverse potentially life-threatening ventricular arrhythmias due to digoxin overdosage.

If the rhythm disturbance is a ventricular arrhythmia, consideration should be given to the correction of electrolyte disorders, particularly if hypokalemia (see Administration of Potassium subsection) or hypomagnesemia is present. Ventricular arrhythmias may respond to lidocaine or phenytoin.

Administration of Potassium

Before administering potassium in digoxin overdose for hypokalemia, the serum potassium must be known and every effort should be made to maintain the serum potassium concentration between 4 and 5.5 mmol/L. Potassium salts should be avoided as they may be dangerous in patients who manifest bradycardia or heart block due to digoxin (unless primarily related to supraventricular tachycardia) and in the setting of massive digitalis overdosage. Potassium is usually administered orally, but when correction of the arrhythmia is urgent and the serum potassium concentration is low, potassium may be administered cautiously by the intravenous route. The electrocardiogram should be monitored for any evidence of potassium toxicity (e.g., peaking of T waves) and to observe the effect on the arrhythmia.

Massive Digitalis Overdosage

Manifestations of life-threatening toxicity include ventricular tachycardia or ventricular fibrillation, or progressive bradyarrhythmias, or heart block.

Digoxin Immune Fab (Ovine) should be used to reverse the toxic effects of ingestion of a massive overdose. The decision to administer Digoxin Immune Fab (Ovine) to a patient who has ingested a massive dose of digoxin but who has not yet manifested life-threatening toxicity should depend on the likelihood that life-threatening toxicity will occur (see above).

Digoxin is not effectively removed from the body by dialysis due to its large extravascular volume of distribution. Patients with massive digitalis ingestion should receive large doses of activated charcoal to prevent absorption and bind digoxin in the gut during enteroenteric recirculation. Emesis may be indicated especially if ingestion has occurred within 30 minutes of the patient's presentation at the hospital. Emesis should not be induced in patients who are obtunded. If a patient presents more than 2 hours after ingestion or already has toxic manifestations, it may be unsafe to induce vomiting because such maneuvers may induce an acute vagal episode that can worsen digitalis-related arrhythmias.

In cases where a large amount of digoxin has been ingested, hyperkalemia may be present due to release of potassium from skeletal muscle. Hyperkalemia caused by massive digitalis toxicity is best treated with Digoxin Immune Fab (Ovine); initial treatment with glucose and insulin may also be required if hyperkalemia itself is acutely life-threatening.

Table 5. Usual Digitalizing and Maintenance Dosages for LANOXIN® Injection Pediatric in Children with Normal Renal Function Based on Lean Body Weight

Age	IV Digitalizing[a] Dose (mcg/kg)	Daily IV Maintenance Dose[b] (mcg/kg)
Premature	15 to 25	20% to 30% of the IV digitalizing dose[c]
Full-Term	20 to 30	
1 to 24 Months	30 to 50	
2 to 5 Years	25 to 35	25% to 35% of the IV digitalizing dose[c]
5 to 10 Years	15 to 30	
Over 10 Years	8 to 12	

[a] IV digitalizing doses are 80% of oral digitalizing doses.
[b] Divided daily dosing is recommended for children under 10 years of age.
[c] Projected or actual digitalizing dose providing clinical response.

DOSAGE AND ADMINISTRATION

General

Recommended dosages of digoxin may require considerable modification because of individual sensitivity of the patient to the drug, the presence of associated conditions, or the use of concurrent medications.

Parenteral administration of digoxin should be used only when the need for rapid digitalization is urgent or when the drug cannot be taken orally. Intramuscular injection can lead to severe pain at the injection site, thus intravenous administration is preferred. If the drug must be administered by the intramuscular route, it should be injected deep into the muscle followed by massage. No more than 200 mcg (2 mL) should be injected into a single site.

LANOXIN Injection Pediatric can be administered undiluted or diluted with a 4-fold or greater volume of Sterile Water for Injection, 0.9% Sodium Chloride Injection, or 5% Dextrose Injection. The use of less than a 4-fold volume of diluent could lead to precipitation of the digoxin. Immediate use of the diluted product is recommended.

If tuberculin syringes are used to measure very small doses, one must be aware of the problem of inadvertent overadministration of digoxin. The syringe should *not* be flushed with the parenteral solution after its contents are expelled into an indwelling vascular catheter.

Slow infusion of LANOXIN Injection Pediatric is preferable to bolus administration. Rapid infusion of digitalis glycosides has been shown to cause systemic and coronary arteriolar constriction, which may be clinically undesirable. Caution is thus advised and LANOXIN Injection Pediatric should probably be administered over a period of 5 minutes or longer. Mixing of LANOXIN Injection Pediatric with other drugs in the same container or simultaneous administration in the same intravenous line is not recommended.

In selecting a dose of digoxin, the following factors must be considered:

1. The body weight of the patient. Doses should be calculated based upon lean (i.e., ideal) body weight.
2. The patient's renal function, preferably evaluated on the basis of estimated creatinine clearance.
3. The patient's age. Infants and children require different doses of digoxin than adults. Also, advanced age may be indicative of diminished renal function even in patients with normal serum creatinine concentration (i.e., below 1.5 mg/dL).
4. Concomitant disease states, concurrent medications, or other factors likely to alter the pharmacokinetic or pharmacodynamic profile of digoxin (see PRECAUTIONS).

Serum Digoxin Concentrations

In general, the dose of digoxin used should be determined on clinical grounds. However, measurement of serum digoxin concentrations can be helpful to the clinician in determining the adequacy of digoxin therapy and in assigning certain probabilities to the likelihood of digoxin intoxication. About two-thirds of adults considered adequately digitalized (without evidence of toxicity) have serum digoxin concentrations ranging from 0.8 to 2.0 ng/mL. However, digoxin may produce clinical benefits even at serum concentrations below this range. About two-thirds of adult patients with clinical toxicity have serum digoxin concentrations greater than 2.0 ng/mL. However, since one-third of patients with clinical toxicity have concentrations less than 2.0 ng/mL, values below 2.0 ng/mL do not rule out the possibility that a certain sign or symptom is related to digoxin therapy. Rarely, there are patients who are unable to tolerate digoxin at serum concentrations below 0.8 ng/mL. Consequently, the serum concentration of digoxin should always be interpreted in the overall clinical context, and an isolated measurement should not be used alone as the basis for increasing or decreasing the dose of the drug.

To allow adequate time for equilibration of digoxin between serum and tissue, sampling of serum concentrations should be done just before the next scheduled dose of the drug. If this is not possible, sampling should be done at least 6 to 8 hours after the last dose, regardless of the route of administration or the formulation used. On a once-daily dosing schedule, the concentration of digoxin will be 10% to 25% lower when sampled at 24 versus 8 hours, depending upon the patient's renal function. On a twice-daily dosing schedule, there will be only minor differences in serum digoxin concentrations whether sampling is done at 8 or 12 hours after a dose.

If a discrepancy exists between the reported serum concentration and the observed clinical response, the clinician should consider the following possibilities:

1. Analytical problems in the assay procedure.
2. Inappropriate serum sampling time.
3. Administration of a digitalis glycoside other than digoxin.
4. Conditions (described in WARNINGS and PRECAUTIONS) causing an alteration in the sensitivity of the patient to digoxin.
5. Serum digoxin concentration may decrease acutely during periods of exercise without any associated change in clinical efficacy due to increased binding of digoxin to skeletal muscle.

Heart Failure

Adults

See the full prescribing information for LANOXIN Injection for specific recommendations.

Infants and Children

In general, divided daily dosing is recommended for infants and young children (under age 10). In the newborn period, renal clearance of digoxin is diminished and suitable dosage adjustments must be observed. This is especially pronounced in the premature infant. Beyond the immediate newborn period, children generally require proportionally larger doses than adults on the basis of body weight or body surface area. Children over 10 years of age require adult dosages in proportion to their body weight. Some researchers have suggested that infants and young children tolerate slightly higher serum concentrations than do adults.

Digitalization may be accomplished by either of two general approaches that vary in dosage and frequency of administration, but reach the same endpoint in terms of total amount of digoxin accumulated in the body.

1. If rapid digitalization is considered medically appropriate, it may be achieved by administering a loading dose based upon projected peak digoxin body stores. Maintenance dose can be calculated as a percentage of the loading dose.
2. More gradual digitalization may be obtained by beginning an appropriate maintenance dose, thus allowing digoxin body stores to accumulate slowly. Steady-state serum digoxin concentrations will be achieved in approximately five half-lives of the drug for the individual patient. Depending upon the patient's renal function, this will take between 1 and 3 weeks.

Rapid Digitalization With a Loading Dose

LANOXIN Injection Pediatric can be used to achieve rapid digitalization, with conversion to an oral formulation of LANOXIN for maintenance therapy. If patients are switched from intravenous to oral digoxin formulations, allowances must be made for differences in bioavailability when calculating maintenance dosages (see Table 1 in CLINICAL PHARMACOLOGY: Pharmacokinetics and dosing Table 5).

Intramuscular injection of digoxin is extremely painful and offers no advantages unless other routes of administration are contraindicated.

Peak digoxin body stores of 8 to 12 mcg/kg should provide therapeutic effect with minimum risk of toxicity in most patients with heart failure and normal sinus rhythm. Because of altered digoxin distribution and elimination, projected peak body stores for patients with renal insufficiency should be conservative (i.e., 6 to 10 mcg/kg) (see PRECAUTIONS). Digitalizing and daily maintenance doses for each age group are given in Table 5 and should provide therapeutic effect with minimum risk of toxicity in most patients with heart failure and normal sinus rhythm. These recommendations assume the presence of normal renal function.

The loading dose should be administered in several portions, with roughly half the total given as the first dose. Additional fractions of this planned total dose may be given at 4- to 8-hour intervals, **with careful assessment of clinical response before each additional dose.** If the patient's clinical response necessitates a change from the calculated loading dose of digoxin, then calculation of the maintenance dose should be based upon the amount actually given.

[See table 5 at top of previous page]

In children with renal disease, digoxin dosing must be carefully titrated based on clinical response.

Gradual Digitalization With A Maintenance Dose

More gradual digitalization can also be accomplished by beginning an appropriate maintenance dose. The range of percentages provided in Table 5 can be used in calculating this dose for patients with normal renal function.

It cannot be overemphasized that these pediatric dosage guidelines are based upon average patient response and substantial individual variation can be expected. Accordingly, ultimate dosage selection must be based upon clinical assessment of the patient.

Atrial Fibrillation

Peak digoxin body stores larger than the 8 to 12 mcg/kg required for most patients with heart failure and normal sinus rhythm have been used for control of ventricular rate in patients with atrial fibrillation. Doses of digoxin used for the treatment of chronic atrial fibrillation should be titrated to the minimum dose that achieves the desired ventricular rate control without causing undesirable side effects. Data are not available to establish the appropriate resting or exercise target rates that should be achieved.

Dosage Adjustment When Changing Preparations

The differences in bioavailability between injectable LANOXIN or LANOXIN Tablets must be considered when changing patients from one dosage form to another.

HOW SUPPLIED

LANOXIN (digoxin) Injection Pediatric, 100 mcg (0.1 mg) in 1 mL; box of 10 ampuls (NDC 0173-0262-10).

Store at 25°C (77°F); excursions permitted to 15 to 30°C (59 to 86°F) [see USP Controlled Room Temperature] and protect from light.

LANOXIN and DIGIBIND are registered trademarks of GlaxoSmithKline

DIGIFAB is a registered trademark of Prostherics Inc.

Manufactured by
DSM Pharmaceuticals, Inc.
Greenville, NC 27834 for
GlaxoSmithKline
Research Triangle Park, NC 27709
©2009, GlaxoSmithKline. All rights reserved.

August 2009
LNP:1PI

LANOXIN®

[lă-nŏx' ĭn]
(digoxin)
Tablets, USP
125 mcg (0.125 mg) Scored I.D. Imprint Y3B (yellow)
250 mcg (0.25 mg) Scored I.D. Imprint X3A (white)

Rx

DESCRIPTION

LANOXIN (digoxin) is one of the cardiac (or digitalis) glycosides, a closely related group of drugs having in common specific effects on the myocardium. These drugs are found in a number of plants. Digoxin is extracted from the leaves of *Digitalis lanata*. The term "digitalis" is used to designate the whole group of glycosides. The glycosides are composed of 2 portions: a sugar and a cardenolide (hence "glycosides"). Digoxin is described chemically as $(3\beta,5\beta,12\beta)$-3-$[(O$-2,6-dideoxy-β-D-$ribo$-hexopyranosyl-$(1{\rightarrow}4)$-O-2,6-dideoxy-β-D-$ribo$-hexopyranosyl-$(1{\rightarrow}4)$-2,6-dideoxy-β-D-$ribo$-hexopyranosyl)oxy]-12,14-dihydroxy-card-20(22)-enolide. Its molecular formula is $C_{41}H_{64}O_{14}$, its molecular weight is 780.95, and its structural formula is:

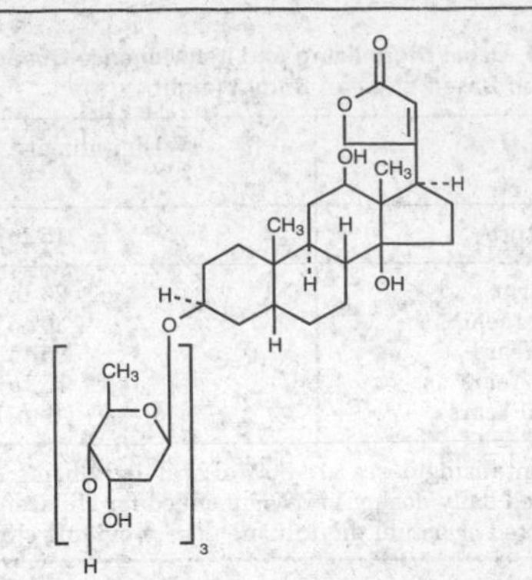

Digoxin exists as odorless white crystals that melt with decomposition above 230°C. The drug is practically insoluble in water and in ether; slightly soluble in diluted (50%) alcohol and in chloroform; and freely soluble in pyridine.

LANOXIN is supplied as 125-mcg (0.125-mg) or 250-mcg (0.25-mg) tablets for oral administration. Each tablet contains the labeled amount of digoxin USP and the following inactive ingredients: corn and potato starches, lactose, and magnesium stearate. In addition, the dyes used in the 125-mcg (0.125-mg) tablets are D&C Yellow No. 10 and FD&C Yellow No. 6.

CLINICAL PHARMACOLOGY

Mechanism of Action

Digoxin inhibits sodium-potassium ATPase, an enzyme that regulates the quantity of sodium and potassium inside cells. Inhibition of the enzyme leads to an increase in the intracellular concentration of sodium and thus (by stimulation of sodium-calcium exchange) an increase in the intracellular concentration of calcium. The beneficial effects of digoxin result from direct actions on cardiac muscle, as well as indirect actions on the cardiovascular system mediated by effects on the autonomic nervous system. The autonomic effects include: (1) a vagomimetic action, which is responsible for the effects of digoxin on the sinoatrial and atrioventricular (AV) nodes; and (2) baroreceptor sensitization, which results in increased afferent inhibitory activity and reduced activity of the sympathetic nervous system and renin-angiotensin system for any given increment in mean arterial pressure. The pharmacologic consequences of these direct and indirect effects are: (1) an increase in the force and velocity of myocardial systolic contraction (positive inotropic action); (2) a decrease in the degree of activation of the sympathetic nervous system and renin-angiotensin system (neurohormonal deactivating effect); and (3) slowing of the heart rate and decreased conduction velocity through the AV node (vagomimetic effect). The effects of digoxin in heart failure are mediated by its positive inotropic and neurohormonal deactivating effects, whereas the effects of the drug in atrial arrhythmias are related to its vagomimetic actions. In high doses, digoxin increases sympathetic outflow from the central nervous system (CNS). This increase in sympathetic activity may be an important factor in digitalis toxicity.

Pharmacokinetics

Absorption

Following oral administration, peak serum concentrations of digoxin occur at 1 to 3 hours. Absorption of digoxin from LANOXIN Tablets has been demonstrated to be 60% to 80% complete compared to an identical intravenous dose of digoxin (absolute bioavailability). When LANOXIN Tablets are taken after meals, the rate of absorption is slowed, but the total amount of digoxin absorbed is usually unchanged. When taken with meals high in bran fiber, however, the amount absorbed from an oral dose may be reduced. Comparisons of the systemic availability and equivalent doses for oral preparations of LANOXIN are shown in Table 1.

[See table 1 below]

In some patients, orally administered digoxin is converted to inactive reduction products (e.g., dihydrodigoxin) by colonic bacteria in the gut. Data suggest that 1 in 10 patients treated with digoxin tablets will degrade 40% or more of the ingested dose. As a result, certain antibiotics may increase the absorption of digoxin in such patients. Although inactivation of these bacteria by antibiotics is rapid, the serum

digoxin concentration will rise at a rate consistent with the elimination half-life of digoxin. The magnitude of rise in serum digoxin concentration relates to the extent of bacterial inactivation, and may be as much as 2-fold in some cases.

Distribution

Following drug administration, a 6- to 8-hour tissue distribution phase is observed. This is followed by a much more gradual decline in the serum concentration of the drug, which is dependent on the elimination of digoxin from the body. The peak height and slope of the early portion (absorption/distribution phases) of the serum concentration-time curve are dependent upon the route of administration and the absorption characteristics of the formulation. Clinical evidence indicates that the early high serum concentrations do not reflect the concentration of digoxin at its site of action, but that with chronic use, the steady-state post-distribution serum concentrations are in equilibrium with tissue concentrations and correlate with pharmacologic effects. In individual patients, these post-distribution serum concentrations may be useful in evaluating therapeutic and toxic effects (see DOSAGE AND ADMINISTRATION: Serum Digoxin Concentrations).

Digoxin is concentrated in tissues and therefore has a large apparent volume of distribution. Digoxin crosses both the blood-brain barrier and the placenta. At delivery, the serum digoxin concentration in the newborn is similar to the serum concentration in the mother. Approximately 25% of digoxin in the plasma is bound to protein. Serum digoxin concentrations are not significantly altered by large changes in fat tissue weight, so that its distribution space correlates best with lean (i.e., ideal) body weight, not total body weight.

Metabolism

Only a small percentage (16%) of a dose of digoxin is metabolized. The end metabolites, which include 3 β-digoxigenin, 3-keto-digoxigenin, and their glucuronide and sulfate conjugates, are polar in nature and are postulated to be formed via hydrolysis, oxidation, and conjugation. The metabolism of digoxin is not dependent upon the cytochrome P-450 system, and digoxin is not known to induce or inhibit the cytochrome P-450 system.

Excretion

Elimination of digoxin follows first-order kinetics (that is, the quantity of digoxin eliminated at any time is proportional to the total body content). Following intravenous administration to healthy volunteers, 50% to 70% of a digoxin dose is excreted unchanged in the urine. Renal excretion of digoxin is proportional to glomerular filtration rate and is largely independent of urine flow. In healthy volunteers with normal renal function, digoxin has a half-life of 1.5 to 2.0 days. The half-life in anuric patients is prolonged to 3.5 to 5 days. Digoxin is not effectively removed from the body by dialysis, exchange transfusion, or during cardiopulmonary bypass because most of the drug is bound to tissue and does not circulate in the blood.

Special Populations

Race differences in digoxin pharmacokinetics have not been formally studied. Because digoxin is primarily eliminated as unchanged drug via the kidney and because there are no important differences in creatinine clearance among races, pharmacokinetic differences due to race are not expected.

The clearance of digoxin can be primarily correlated with renal function as indicated by creatinine clearance. The Cockcroft and Gault formula for estimation of creatinine clearance includes age, body weight, and gender. Table 5 that provides the usual daily maintenance dose requirements of LANOXIN Tablets based on creatinine clearance (per 70 kg) is presented in the DOSAGE AND ADMINISTRATION section.

Plasma digoxin concentration profiles in patients with acute hepatitis generally fell within the range of profiles in a group of healthy subjects.

Pharmacodynamic and Clinical Effects

The times to onset of pharmacologic effect and to peak effect of preparations of LANOXIN are shown in Table 2.

[See table 2 at top of next page]

Hemodynamic Effects

Digoxin produces hemodynamic improvement in patients with heart failure. Short- and long-term therapy with the drug increases cardiac output and lowers pulmonary artery pressure, pulmonary capillary wedge pressure, and systemic vascular resistance. These hemodynamic effects are accompanied by an increase in the left ventricular ejection fraction and a decrease in end-systolic and end-diastolic dimensions.

Chronic Heart Failure

Two 12-week, double-blind, placebo-controlled studies enrolled 178 (RADIANCE trial) and 88 (PROVED trial) patients with NYHA class II or III heart failure previously treated with digoxin, a diuretic, and an ACE inhibitor (RADIANCE only) and randomized them to placebo or treatment with LANOXIN. Both trials demonstrated better preservation of exercise capacity in patients randomized to

Table 1. Comparisons of the Systemic Availability and Equivalent Doses for Oral Preparations of LANOXIN

Product	Absolute Bioavailability	Equivalent Doses (mcg)[a] Among Dosage Forms			
LANOXIN Tablets	60-80%	62.5	125	250	500
LANOXIN Injection/IV	100%	50	100	200	400

[a] For example, 125-mcg LANOXIN Tablets equivalent to 100-mcg LANOXIN Injection/IV.

LANOXIN. Continued treatment with LANOXIN reduced the risk of developing worsening heart failure, as evidenced by heart failure-related hospitalizations and emergency care and the need for concomitant heart failure therapy. The larger study also showed treatment-related benefits in NYHA class and patients' global assessment. In the smaller trial, these trended in favor of a treatment benefit.

The Digitalis Investigation Group (DIG) main trial was a multicenter, randomized, double-blind, placebo-controlled mortality study of 6,801 patients with heart failure and left ventricular ejection fraction ≤0.45. At randomization, 67% were NYHA class I or II, 71% had heart failure of ischemic etiology, 44% had been receiving digoxin, and most were receiving concomitant ACE inhibitor (94%) and diuretic (82%). Patients were randomized to placebo or LANOXIN, the dose of which was adjusted for the patient's age, sex, lean body weight, and serum creatinine (see DOSAGE AND ADMINISTRATION), and followed for up to 58 months (median 37 months). The median daily dose prescribed was 0.25 mg. Overall all-cause mortality was 35% with no difference between groups (95% confidence limits for relative risk of 0.91 to 1.07). LANOXIN was associated with a 25% reduction in the number of hospitalizations for heart failure, a 28% reduction in the risk of a patient having at least 1 hospitalization for heart failure, and a 6.5% reduction in total hospitalizations (for any cause).

Use of LANOXIN was associated with a trend to increase time to all-cause death or hospitalization. The trend was evident in subgroups of patients with mild heart failure as well as more severe disease, as shown in Table 3. Although the effect on all-cause death or hospitalization was not statistically significant, much of the apparent benefit derived from effects on mortality and hospitalization attributed to heart failure.

[See table 3 at right]

In situations where there is no statistically significant benefit of treatment evident from a trial's primary endpoint, results pertaining to a secondary endpoint should be interpreted cautiously.

Chronic Atrial Fibrillation

In patients with chronic atrial fibrillation, digoxin slows rapid ventricular response rate in a linear dose-response fashion from 0.25 to 0.75 mg/day. Digoxin should not be used for the treatment of multifocal atrial tachycardia.

INDICATIONS AND USAGE

Heart Failure

LANOXIN is indicated for the treatment of mild to moderate heart failure. LANOXIN increases left ventricular ejection fraction and improves heart failure symptoms as evidenced by exercise capacity and heart failure-related hospitalizations and emergency care, while having no effect on mortality. Where possible, LANOXIN should be used with a diuretic and an angiotensin-converting enzyme inhibitor, but an optimal order for starting these 3 drugs cannot be specified.

Atrial Fibrillation

LANOXIN is indicated for the control of ventricular response rate in patients with chronic atrial fibrillation.

CONTRAINDICATIONS

Digitalis glycosides are contraindicated in patients with ventricular fibrillation or in patients with a known hypersensitivity to digoxin. A hypersensitivity reaction to other digitalis preparations usually constitutes a contraindication to digoxin.

WARNINGS

Sinus Node Disease and AV Block

Because digoxin slows sinoatrial and AV conduction, the drug commonly prolongs the PR interval. The drug may cause severe sinus bradycardia or sinoatrial block in patients with pre-existing sinus node disease and may cause advanced or complete heart block in patients with pre-existing incomplete AV block. In such patients consideration should be given to the insertion of a pacemaker before treatment with digoxin.

Accessory AV Pathway (Wolff-Parkinson-White Syndrome)

After intravenous digoxin therapy, some patients with paroxysmal atrial fibrillation or flutter and a coexisting accessory AV pathway have developed increased antegrade conduction across the accessory pathway bypassing the AV node, leading to a very rapid ventricular response or ventricular fibrillation. Unless conduction down the accessory pathway has been blocked (either pharmacologically or by surgery), digoxin should not be used in such patients. The treatment of paroxysmal supraventricular tachycardia in such patients is usually direct-current cardioversion.

Use in Patients With Preserved Left Ventricular Systolic Function

Patients with certain disorders involving heart failure associated with preserved left ventricular ejection fraction may be particularly susceptible to toxicity of the drug. Such disorders include restrictive cardiomyopathy, constrictive pericarditis, amyloid heart disease, and acute cor pulmonale.

Table 2. Times to Onset of Pharmacologic Effect and to Peak Effect of Preparations of LANOXIN

Product	Time to Onset of Effect[a]	Time to Peak Effect[a]
LANOXIN Tablets	0.5-2 hours	2-6 hours
LANOXIN Injection/IV	5-30 minutes[b]	1-4 hours

[a] Documented for ventricular response rate in atrial fibrillation, inotropic effects and electrocardiographic changes.
[b] Depending upon rate of infusion.

Table 3. Subgroup Analyses of Mortality and Hospitalization During the First 2 Years Following Randomization

	n	Risk of All-Cause Mortality or All-Cause Hospitalization[a]			Risk of HF-Related Mortality or HF-Related Hospitalization[a]		
		Placebo	LANOXIN	Relative risk[b]	Placebo	LANOXIN	Relative risk[b]
All patients (EF≤0.45)	6,801	604	593	0.94 (0.88-1.00)	294	217	0.69 (0.63-0.76)
NYHA I/II	4,571	549	541	0.96 (0.89-1.04)	242	178	0.70 (0.62-0.80)
EF 0.25-0.45	4,543	568	571	0.99 (0.91-1.07)	244	190	0.74 (0.66-0.84)
CTR ≤0.55	4,455	561	563	0.98 (0.91-1.06)	239	180	0.71 (0.63-0.81)
NYHA III/IV	2,224	719	696	0.88 (0.80-0.97)	402	295	0.65 (0.57-0.75)
EF <0.25	2,258	677	637	0.84 (0.76-0.93)	394	270	0.61 (0.53-0.71)
CTR >0.55	2,346	687	650	0.85 (0.77-0.94)	398	287	0.65 (0.57-0.75)
EF >0.45[c]	987	571	585	1.04 (0.88-1.23)	179	136	0.72 (0.53-0.99)

[a] Number of patients with an event during the first 2 years per 1,000 randomized patients.
[b] Relative risk (95% confidence interval).
[c] DIG Ancillary Study.

Patients with idiopathic hypertrophic subaortic stenosis may have worsening of the outflow obstruction due to the inotropic effects of digoxin. Digoxin should generally be avoided in these patients, although it has been used for ventricular rate control in the subgroup of patients with atrial fibrillation.

PRECAUTIONS

Use in Patients With Impaired Renal Function

Digoxin is primarily excreted by the kidneys; therefore, patients with impaired renal function require smaller than usual maintenance doses of digoxin (see DOSAGE AND ADMINISTRATION). Because of the prolonged elimination half-life, a longer period of time is required to achieve an initial or new steady-state serum concentration in patients with renal impairment than in patients with normal renal function. If appropriate care is not taken to reduce the dose of digoxin, such patients are at high risk for toxicity, and toxic effects will last longer in such patients than in patients with normal renal function.

Use in Patients With Electrolyte Disorders

In patients with hypokalemia or hypomagnesemia, toxicity may occur despite serum digoxin concentrations below 2.0 ng/mL, because potassium or magnesium depletion sensitizes the myocardium to digoxin. Therefore, it is desirable to maintain normal serum potassium and magnesium concentrations in patients being treated with digoxin. Deficiencies of these electrolytes may result from malnutrition, diarrhea, or prolonged vomiting, as well as the use of the following drugs or procedures: diuretics, amphotericin B, corticosteroids, antacids, dialysis, and mechanical suction of gastrointestinal secretions.

Hypercalcemia from any cause predisposes the patient to digitalis toxicity. Calcium, particularly when administered rapidly by the intravenous route, may produce serious arrhythmias in digitalized patients. On the other hand, hypocalcemia can nullify the effects of digoxin in humans; thus, digoxin may be ineffective until serum calcium is restored to normal. These interactions are related to the fact that digoxin affects contractility and excitability of the heart in a manner similar to that of calcium.

Use in Thyroid Disorders and Hypermetabolic States

Hypothyroidism may reduce the requirements for digoxin. Heart failure and/or atrial arrhythmias resulting from hypermetabolic or hyperdynamic states (e.g., hyperthyroidism, hypoxia, or arteriovenous shunt) are best treated by addressing the underlying condition. Atrial arrhythmias associated with hypermetabolic states are particularly resistant to digoxin treatment. Care must be taken to avoid toxicity if digoxin is used.

Use in Patients With Acute Myocardial Infarction

Digoxin should be used with caution in patients with acute myocardial infarction. The use of inotropic drugs in some patients in this setting may result in undesirable increases in myocardial oxygen demand and ischemia.

Use During Electrical Cardioversion

It may be desirable to reduce the dose of digoxin for 1 to 2 days prior to electrical cardioversion of atrial fibrillation to avoid the induction of ventricular arrhythmias, but physicians must consider the consequences of increasing the ventricular response if digoxin is withdrawn. If digitalis toxicity is suspected, elective cardioversion should be delayed. If it is not prudent to delay cardioversion, the lowest possible energy level should be selected to avoid provoking ventricular arrhythmias.

Use in Patients With Myocarditis

Digoxin can rarely precipitate vasoconstriction and therefore should be avoided in patients with myocarditis.

Use in Patients With Beri Beri Heart Disease

Patients with beri beri heart disease may fail to respond adequately to digoxin if the underlying thiamine deficiency is not treated concomitantly.

Laboratory Test Monitoring

Patients receiving digoxin should have their serum electrolytes and renal function (serum creatinine concentrations) assessed periodically; the frequency of assessments will depend on the clinical setting. For discussion of serum digoxin concentrations, see DOSAGE AND ADMINISTRATION section.

Drug Interactions

Potassium-depleting *diuretics* are a major contributing factor to digitalis toxicity. *Calcium*, particularly if administered rapidly by the intravenous route, may produce serious arrhythmias in digitalized patients. *Quinidine, verapamil, amiodarone, propafenone, indomethacin, itraconazole, alprazolam*, and *spironolactone* raise the serum digoxin concentration due to a reduction in clearance and/or in volume of distribution of the drug, with the implication that digitalis intoxication may result. *Erythromycin* and *clarithromycin* (and possibly other *macrolide antibiotics*) and *tetracycline* may increase digoxin absorption in patients who inactivate digoxin by bacterial metabolism in the lower intestine, so that digitalis intoxication may result (see CLINICAL PHARMACOLOGY: Absorption). *Propantheline* and *diphenoxylate*, by decreasing gut motility, may increase digoxin absorption. *Antacids, kaolin-pectin, sulfasalazine, neomycin, cholestyramine*, certain *anticancer drugs*, and *metoclopramide* may interfere with intestinal digoxin absorption, resulting in unexpectedly low serum digoxin concentrations. *Rifampin* may reduce serum digoxin concentration, especially in patients with renal dysfunction, by increasing the non-renal clearance of digoxin. There have been inconsistent reports regarding the effects of other drugs (e.g., *quinine, penicillamine*) on serum digoxin concentration. *Thyroid* administration to a digitalized, hypothyroid patient may increase the dose requirement of digoxin. Concomitant use of digoxin and *sympathomimetics* increases the risk of cardiac arrhythmias. *Succinylcholine* may cause a sudden extrusion of potassium from muscle cells, and may thereby cause arrhythmias in digitalized patients. Although calcium channel blockers and digoxin may be useful in combination to control atrial fibrillation, their additive effects on AV node conduction can result in advanced or complete heart block. Both digitalis glycosides and beta-blockers slow atrioventricular conduction and decrease heart rate. Concomitant use can increase the risk of bradycardia.

Digoxin concentrations are increased by about 15% when digoxin and carvedilol are administered concomitantly. Therefore, increased monitoring of digoxin is recommended when initiating, adjusting, or discontinuing carvedilol.

Due to the considerable variability of these interactions, the dosage of digoxin should be individualized when patients receive these medications concurrently. Furthermore, caution should be exercised when combining digoxin with any drug that may cause a significant deterioration in renal function, since a decline in glomerular filtration or tubular secretion may impair the excretion of digoxin.

Drug/Laboratory Test Interactions

The use of therapeutic doses of digoxin may cause prolongation of the PR interval and depression of the ST segment on the electrocardiogram. Digoxin may produce false positive ST-T changes on the electrocardiogram during exercise testing. These electrophysiologic effects reflect an expected effect of the drug and are not indicative of toxicity.

Carcinogenesis, Mutagenesis, Impairment of Fertility

There have been no long-term studies performed in animals to evaluate carcinogenic potential, nor have studies been conducted to assess the mutagenic potential of digoxin or its potential to affect fertility.

Pregnancy

Teratogenic Effects

Pregnancy Category C. Animal reproduction studies have not been conducted with digoxin. It is also not known whether digoxin can cause fetal harm when administered to a pregnant woman or can affect reproductive capacity. Digoxin should be given to a pregnant woman only if clearly needed.

Nursing Mothers

Studies have shown that digoxin concentrations in the mother's serum and milk are similar. However, the estimated exposure of a nursing infant to digoxin via breast-feeding will be far below the usual infant maintenance dose. Therefore, this amount should have no pharmacologic effect upon the infant. Nevertheless, caution should be exercised when digoxin is administered to a nursing woman.

Pediatric Use

Newborn infants display considerable variability in their tolerance to digoxin. Premature and immature infants are particularly sensitive to the effects of digoxin, and the dosage of the drug must not only be reduced but must be individualized according to their degree of maturity. Digitalis glycosides can cause poisoning in children due to accidental ingestion.

Geriatric Use

The majority of clinical experience gained with digoxin has been in the elderly population. This experience has not identified differences in response or adverse effects between the elderly and younger patients. However, this drug is known to be substantially excreted by the kidney, and the risk of toxic reactions to this drug may be greater in patients with impaired renal function. Because elderly patients are more likely to have decreased renal function, care should be taken in dose selection, which should be based on renal function, and it may be useful to monitor renal function (see DOSAGE AND ADMINISTRATION).

ADVERSE REACTIONS

In general, the adverse reactions of digoxin are dose-dependent and occur at doses higher than those needed to achieve a therapeutic effect. Hence, adverse reactions are less common when digoxin is used within the recommended dose range or therapeutic serum concentration range and when there is careful attention to concurrent medications and conditions.

Because some patients may be particularly susceptible to side effects with digoxin, the dosage of the drug should always be selected carefully and adjusted as the clinical condition of the patient warrants. In the past, when high doses of digoxin were used and little attention was paid to clinical status or concurrent medications, adverse reactions to digoxin were more frequent and severe. Cardiac adverse reactions accounted for about one-half, gastrointestinal disturbances for about one-fourth, and CNS and other toxicity for about one-fourth of these adverse reactions. However, available evidence suggests that the incidence and severity of digoxin toxicity has decreased substantially in recent

years. In recent controlled clinical trials, in patients with predominantly mild to moderate heart failure, the incidence of adverse experiences was comparable in patients taking digoxin and in those taking placebo. In a large mortality trial, the incidence of hospitalization for suspected digoxin toxicity was 2% in patients taking LANOXIN compared to 0.9% in patients taking placebo. In this trial, the most common manifestations of digoxin toxicity included gastrointestinal and cardiac disturbances; CNS manifestations were less common.

Adults

Cardiac

Therapeutic doses of digoxin may cause heart block in patients with pre-existing sinoatrial or AV conduction disorders; heart block can be avoided by adjusting the dose of digoxin. Prophylactic use of a cardiac pacemaker may be considered if the risk of heart block is considered unacceptable. High doses of digoxin may produce a variety of rhythm disturbances, such as first-degree, second-degree (Wenckebach), or third-degree heart block (including asystole); atrial tachycardia with block; AV dissociation; accelerated junctional (nodal) rhythm; unifocal or multiform ventricular premature contractions (especially bigeminy or trigeminy); ventricular tachycardia; and ventricular fibrillation. Digoxin produces PR prolongation and ST segment depression which should not by themselves be considered digoxin toxicity. Cardiac toxicity can also occur at therapeutic doses in patients who have conditions which may alter their sensitivity to digoxin (see WARNINGS and PRECAUTIONS).

Gastrointestinal

Digoxin may cause anorexia, nausea, vomiting, and diarrhea. Rarely, the use of digoxin has been associated with abdominal pain, intestinal ischemia, and hemorrhagic necrosis of the intestines.

CNS

Digoxin can produce visual disturbances (blurred or yellow vision), headache, weakness, dizziness, apathy, confusion, and mental disturbances (such as anxiety, depression, delirium, and hallucination).

Other

Gynecomastia has been occasionally observed following the prolonged use of digoxin. Thrombocytopenia and maculopapular rash and other skin reactions have been rarely observed.

Table 4 summarizes the incidence of those adverse experiences listed above for patients treated with LANOXIN Tablets or placebo from 2 randomized, double-blind, placebo-controlled withdrawal trials. Patients in these trials were also receiving diuretics with or without angiotensin-converting enzyme inhibitors. These patients had been stable on digoxin, and were randomized to digoxin or placebo. The results shown in Table 4 reflect the experience in patients following dosage titration with the use of serum digoxin concentrations and careful follow-up. These adverse experiences are consistent with results from a large, placebo-controlled mortality trial (DIG trial) wherein over half the patients were not receiving digoxin prior to enrollment.

Table 4. Adverse Experiences In 2 Parallel, Double-Blind, Placebo-Controlled Withdrawal Trials (Number of Patients Reporting)

Adverse Experience	Digoxin Patients (n = 123)	Placebo Patients (n = 125)
Cardiac		
Palpitation	1	4
Ventricular extrasystole	1	1
Tachycardia	2	1
Heart arrest	1	1
Gastrointestinal		
Anorexia	1	4
Nausea	4	2
Vomiting	2	1
Diarrhea	4	1
Abdominal pain	0	6
CNS		
Headache	4	4
Dizziness	6	5
Mental disturbances	5	1
Other		
Rash	2	1
Death	4	3

Infants and Children

The side effects of digoxin in infants and children differ from those seen in adults in several respects. Although digoxin may produce anorexia, nausea, vomiting, diarrhea, and CNS disturbances in young patients, these are rarely the initial symptoms of overdosage. Rather, the earliest and most frequent manifestation of excessive dosing with

digoxin in infants and children is the appearance of cardiac arrhythmias, including sinus bradycardia. In children, the use of digoxin may produce any arrhythmia. The most common are conduction disturbances or supraventricular tachyarrhythmias, such as atrial tachycardia (with or without block) and junctional (nodal) tachycardia. Ventricular arrhythmias are less common. Sinus bradycardia may be a sign of impending digoxin intoxication, especially in infants, even in the absence of first-degree heart block. Any arrhythmia or alteration in cardiac conduction that develops in a child taking digoxin should be assumed to be caused by digoxin, until further evaluation proves otherwise.

OVERDOSAGE

Signs and Symptoms

The signs and symptoms of toxicity are generally similar to those described in the ADVERSE REACTIONS section but may be more frequent and can be more severe. Signs and symptoms of digoxin toxicity become more frequent with levels above 2 ng/mL. However, in deciding whether a patient's symptoms are due to digoxin, the clinical state together with serum electrolyte levels and thyroid function are important factors (see DOSAGE AND ADMINISTRATION).

Adults

In adults without heart disease, clinical observation suggests that an overdose of digoxin of 10 to 15 mg was the dose resulting in death of half of the patients. If more than 25 mg of digoxin was ingested by an adult without heart disease, death or progressive toxicity responsive only to digoxin-binding Fab antibody fragments resulted. Cardiac manifestations are the most frequent and serious sign of both acute and chronic toxicity. Peak cardiac effects generally occur 3 to 6 hours following overdosage and may persist for the ensuing 24 hours or longer. Digoxin toxicity may result in almost any type of arrhythmia (see ADVERSE REACTIONS). Multiple rhythm disturbances in the same patient are common. Cardiac arrest from asystole or ventricular fibrillation due to digoxin toxicity is usually fatal.

Among the extra-cardiac manifestations, gastrointestinal symptoms (e.g. nausea, vomiting, anorexia) are very common (up to 80% incidence) and precede cardiac manifestations in approximately half of the patients in most literature reports. Neurologic manifestations (e.g. dizziness, various CNS disturbances), fatigue, and malaise are very common. Visual manifestations may also occur with aberration in color vision (predominance of yellow green) the most frequent. Neurological and visual symptoms may persist after other signs of toxicity have resolved. In chronic toxicity, non-specific extra-cardiac symptoms, such as malaise and weakness, may predominate.

Children

In children aged 1 to 3 years without heart disease, clinical observation suggests that an overdose of digoxin of 6 to 10 mg was the dose resulting in death in half of the patients. If more than 10 mg of digoxin was ingested by a child aged 1 to 3 years without heart disease, the outcome was uniformly fatal when Fab fragment treatment was not given. Most manifestations of toxicity in children occur during or shortly after the loading phase with digoxin. The same arrhythmias or combination of arrhythmias that occur in adults can occur in pediatrics. Sinus tachycardia, supraventricular tachycardia, and rapid atrial fibrillation are seen less frequently in the pediatric population. Pediatric patients are more likely to present with an AV conduction disturbance or a sinus bradycardia. Any arrhythmia or alteration in cardiac conduction that develops in a child taking digoxin should be assumed to be caused by digoxin, until further evaluation proves otherwise.

The frequent extracardiac manifestations similar to those seen in adults are gastrointestinal, CNS, and visual. However, nausea and vomiting are not frequent in infants and small children.

In addition to the undesirable effects seen with recommended doses, weight loss in older age groups and failure to thrive in infants, abdominal pain due to mesenteric artery ischemia, drowsiness, and behavioral disturbances including psychotic manifestations have been reported in overdose.

Treatment

In addition to cardiac monitoring, digoxin should be temporarily discontinued until the adverse reaction resolves and may be all that is required to treat the adverse reaction such as in asymptomatic bradycardia or digoxin-related heart block. Every effort should also be made to correct factors that may contribute to the adverse reaction (such as electrolyte disturbances, thyroid function, or concurrent medications) (see WARNINGS and PRECAUTIONS: Drug Interactions). Once the adverse reaction has resolved, therapy with digoxin may be reinstituted, following a careful reassessment of dose.

When the primary manifestation of digoxin overdosage is a cardiac arrhythmia, additional therapy may be needed.

Table 5. Usual Daily Maintenance Dose Requirements (mcg) of LANOXIN for Estimated Peak Body Stores of 10 mcg/kg

Corrected Ccr		Lean Body Weight						
Corrected Ccr (mL/min per 70 kg)[a]	kg / lb	50 / 110	60 / 132	70 / 154	80 / 176	90 / 198	100 / 220	Number of Days Before Steady State Achieved[b]
0		62.5[c]	125	125	125	187.5	187.5	22
10		125	125	125	187.5	187.5	187.5	19
20		125	125	187.5	187.5	187.5	250	16
30		125	187.5	187.5	187.5	250	250	14
40		125	187.5	187.5	250	250	250	13
50		187.5	187.5	250	250	250	250	12
60		187.5	187.5	250	250	250	375	11
70		187.5	250	250	250	250	375	10
80		187.5	250	250	250	375	375	9
90		187.5	250	250	250	375	500	8
100		250	250	250	375	375	500	7

[a] Ccr is creatinine clearance, corrected to 70 kg body weight or 1.73 m^2 body surface area. *For adults*, if only serum creatinine concentrations (Scr) are available, a Ccr (corrected to 70 kg body weight) may be estimated in men as (140 - Age)/Scr. For women, this result should be multiplied by 0.85. *Note:* This equation cannot be used for estimating creatinine clearance in infants or children.
[b] If no loading dose administered.
[c] 62.5 mcg = 0.0625 mg.

If the rhythm disturbance is a symptomatic bradyarrhythmia or heart block, consideration should be given to the reversal of toxicity with Digoxin Immune Fab (Ovine) [DIGIBIND® or DIGIFAB®] (see Massive Digitalis Overdosage subsection), the use of atropine, or the insertion of a temporary cardiac pacemaker. Digoxin Immune Fab (Ovine) is a specific antidote for digoxin and may be used to reverse potentially life-threatening ventricular arrhythmias due to digoxin overdosage.

If the rhythm disturbance is a ventricular arrhythmia, consideration should be given to the correction of electrolyte disorders, particularly if hypokalemia (see Administration of Potassium subsection) or hypomagnesemia is present. Ventricular arrhythmias may respond to lidocaine or phenytoin.

Administration of Potassium

Before administering potassium in digoxin overdose for hypokalemia, the serum potassium must be known and every effort should be made to maintain the serum potassium concentration between 4 and 5.5 mmol/L. Potassium salts should be avoided as they may be dangerous in patients who manifest bradycardia or heart block due to digoxin (unless primarily related to supraventricular tachycardia) and in the setting of massive digitalis overdosage. Potassium is usually administered orally, but when correction of the arrhythmia is urgent and the serum potassium concentration is low, potassium may be administered cautiously by the intravenous route. The electrocardiogram should be monitored for any evidence of potassium toxicity (e.g., peaking of T waves) and to observe the effect on the arrhythmia.

Massive Digitalis Overdosage

Manifestations of life-threatening toxicity include ventricular tachycardia or ventricular fibrillation, or progressive bradyarrhythmias, or heart block.

Digoxin Immune Fab (Ovine) should be used to reverse the toxic effects of ingestion of a massive overdose. The decision to administer Digoxin Immune Fab (Ovine) to a patient who has ingested a massive dose of digoxin but who has not yet manifested life-threatening toxicity should depend on the likelihood that life-threatening toxicity will occur (see above).

Digoxin is not effectively removed from the body by dialysis due to its large extravascular volume of distribution. Patients with massive digitalis ingestion should receive large doses of activated charcoal to prevent absorption and bind digoxin in the gut during enteroenteric recirculation. Emesis may be indicated especially if ingestion has occurred within 30 minutes of the patient's presentation at the hospital. Emesis should not be induced in patients who are obtunded. If a patient presents more than 2 hours after ingestion or already has toxic manifestations, it may be unsafe to induce vomiting because such maneuvers may induce an acute vagal episode that can worsen digitalis-related arrhythmias.

In cases where a large amount of digoxin has been ingested, hyperkalemia may be present due to release of potassium from skeletal muscle. Hyperkalemia caused by massive digitalis toxicity is best treated with Digoxin Immune Fab (Ovine); initial treatment with glucose and insulin may also be required if hyperkalemia itself is acutely life-threatening.

DOSAGE AND ADMINISTRATION

General

Recommended dosages of digoxin may require considerable modification because of individual sensitivity of the patient to the drug, the presence of associated conditions, or the use of concurrent medications. In selecting a dose of digoxin, the following factors must be considered:

1. The body weight of the patient. Doses should be calculated based upon lean (i.e., ideal) body weight.
2. The patient's renal function, preferably evaluated on the basis of estimated creatinine clearance.
3. The patient's age. Infants and children require different doses of digoxin than adults. Also, advanced age may be indicative of diminished renal function even in patients with normal serum creatinine concentration (i.e., below 1.5 mg/dL).
4. Concomitant disease states, concurrent medications, or other factors likely to alter the pharmacokinetic or pharmacodynamic profile of digoxin (see PRECAUTIONS).

Serum Digoxin Concentrations

In general, the dose of digoxin used should be determined on clinical grounds. However, measurement of serum digoxin concentrations can be helpful to the clinician in determining the adequacy of digoxin therapy and in assigning certain probabilities to the likelihood of digoxin intoxication. About two-thirds of adults considered adequately digitalized (without evidence of toxicity) have serum digoxin concentrations ranging from 0.8 to 2.0 ng/mL (lower serum trough concentrations of 0.5 to 1 ng/mL may be appropriate in some adult patients, see Maintenance Dosing). However, digoxin may produce clinical benefits even at serum concentrations below this range. About two-thirds of adult patients with clinical toxicity have serum digoxin concentrations greater than 2.0 ng/mL. However, since one-third of patients with clinical toxicity have concentrations less than 2.0 ng/mL, values below 2.0 ng/mL do not rule out the possibility that a certain sign or symptom is related to digoxin therapy. Rarely, there are patients who are unable to tolerate digoxin at serum concentrations below 0.8 ng/mL. Consequently, the serum concentration of digoxin should always be interpreted in the overall clinical context, and an isolated measurement should not be used alone as the basis for increasing or decreasing the dose of the drug.

To allow adequate time for equilibration of digoxin between serum and tissue, sampling of serum concentrations should be done just before the next scheduled dose of the drug. If this is not possible, sampling should be done at least 6 to 8 hours after the last dose, regardless of the route of administration or the formulation used. On a once-daily dosing schedule, the concentration of digoxin will be 10% to 25% lower when sampled at 24 versus 8 hours, depending upon the patient's renal function. On a twice-daily dosing schedule, there will be only minor differences in serum digoxin concentrations whether sampling is done at 8 or 12 hours after a dose.

If a discrepancy exists between the reported serum concentration and the observed clinical response, the clinician should consider the following possibilities:

1. Analytical problems in the assay procedure.
2. Inappropriate serum sampling time.
3. Administration of a digitalis glycoside other than digoxin.
4. Conditions (described in WARNINGS and PRECAUTIONS) causing an alteration in the sensitivity of the patient to digoxin.
5. Serum digoxin concentration may decrease acutely during periods of exercise without any associated change in clinical efficacy due to increased binding of digoxin to skeletal muscle.

Heart Failure

Adults

Digitalization may be accomplished by either of 2 general approaches that vary in dosage and frequency of administration, but reach the same endpoint in terms of total amount of digoxin accumulated in the body.

1. If rapid digitalization is considered medically appropriate, it may be achieved by administering a loading dose based upon projected peak digoxin body stores. Maintenance dose can be calculated as a percentage of the loading dose.
2. More gradual digitalization may be obtained by beginning an appropriate maintenance dose, thus allowing digoxin body stores to accumulate slowly. Steady-state serum digoxin concentrations will be achieved in approximately 5 half-lives of the drug for the individual patient. Depending upon the patient's renal function, this will take between 1 and 3 weeks.

Rapid Digitalization With a Loading Dose

Peak digoxin body stores of 8 to 12 mcg/kg should provide therapeutic effect with minimum risk of toxicity in most patients with heart failure and normal sinus rhythm. Because of altered digoxin distribution and elimination, projected peak body stores for patients with renal insufficiency should be conservative (i.e., 6 to 10 mcg/kg) (see PRECAUTIONS).

The loading dose should be administered in several portions, with roughly half the total given as the first dose. Additional fractions of this planned total dose may be given at 6- to 8-hour intervals, **with careful assessment of clinical response before each additional dose.**

If the patient's clinical response necessitates a change from the calculated loading dose of digoxin, then calculation of the maintenance dose should be based upon the amount actually given.

A single initial dose of 500 to 750 mcg (0.5 to 0.75 mg) of LANOXIN Tablets usually produces a detectable effect in 0.5 to 2 hours that becomes maximal in 2 to 6 hours. Additional doses of 125 to 375 mcg (0.125 to 0.375 mg) may be given cautiously at 6- to 8-hour intervals until clinical evidence of an adequate effect is noted. The usual amount of LANOXIN Tablets that a 70-kg patient requires to achieve 8 to 12 mcg/kg peak body stores is 750 to 1,250 mcg (0.75 to 1.25 mg).

LANOXIN Injection is frequently used to achieve rapid digitalization, with conversion to LANOXIN Tablets for maintenance therapy. If patients are switched from intravenous to oral digoxin formulations, allowances must be made for differences in bioavailability when calculating maintenance dosages (see Table 1, CLINICAL PHARMACOLOGY).

Maintenance Dosing

The doses of digoxin used in controlled trials in patients with heart failure have ranged from 125 to 500 mcg (0.125 to 0.5 mg) once daily. In these studies, the digoxin dose has been generally titrated according to the patient's age, lean body weight, and renal function. Therapy is generally initiated at a dose of 250 mcg (0.25 mg) once daily in patients under age 70 with good renal function, at a dose of 125 mcg (0.125 mg) once daily in patients over age 70 or with impaired renal function, and at a dose of 62.5 mcg (0.0625 mg) in patients with marked renal impairment. Doses may be increased every 2 weeks according to clinical response.

In a subset of approximately 1,800 patients enrolled in the DIG trial (wherein dosing was based on an algorithm similar to that in Table 5) the mean (± SD) serum digoxin concentrations at 1 month and 12 months were 1.01 ± 0.47 ng/mL and 0.97 ± 0.43 ng/mL, respectively.

There are no rigid guidelines as to the range of serum concentrations that are most efficacious. Several post hoc analyses of heart failure patients in the DIG trial suggest that the optimal trough digoxin serum level may be 0.5 ng/mL to 1 ng/mL.

The maintenance dose should be based upon the percentage of the peak body stores lost each day through elimination. The following formula has had wide clinical use:

Maintenance Dose = Peak Body Stores (i.e., Loading Dose) × % Daily Loss/100

Where: % Daily Loss = 14 + Ccr/5

(Ccr is creatinine clearance, corrected to 70 kg body weight or 1.73 m^2 body surface area.)

Table 5 provides average daily maintenance dose requirements of LANOXIN Tablets for patients with heart failure based upon lean body weight and renal function:

[See table 5 above]

Example: Based on Table 5, a patient in heart failure with an estimated lean body weight of 70 kg and a Ccr of 60 mL/min should be given a dose of 250 mcg (0.25 mg) daily of LANOXIN Tablets, usually taken after the morning meal. If no loading dose is administered, steady-state serum concentrations in this patient should be anticipated at approximately 11 days.

Infants and Children

In general, divided daily dosing is recommended for infants and young children (under age 10). In the newborn period, renal clearance of digoxin is diminished and suitable dosage adjustments must be observed. This is especially pronounced in the premature infant. Beyond the immediate newborn period, children generally require proportionally larger doses than adults on the basis of body weight or body surface area. Children over 10 years of age require adult dosages in proportion to their body weight. Some researchers have suggested that infants and young children tolerate slightly higher serum concentrations than do adults.

Daily maintenance doses for each age group are given in Table 6 and should provide therapeutic effects with minimum risk of toxicity in most patients with heart failure and normal sinus rhythm. These recommendations assume the presence of normal renal function:

Table 6. Daily Maintenance Doses in Children With Normal Renal Function

Age	Daily Maintenance Dose (mcg/kg)
2 to 5 Years	10 to 15
5 to 10 Years	7 to 10
Over 10 Years	3 to 5

In children with renal disease, digoxin must be carefully titrated based upon clinical response.

It cannot be overemphasized that both the adult and pediatric dosage guidelines provided are based upon average patient response and substantial individual variation can be expected. Accordingly, ultimate dosage selection must be based upon clinical assessment of the patient.

Atrial Fibrillation
Peak digoxin body stores larger than the 8 to 12 mcg/kg required for most patients with heart failure and normal sinus rhythm have been used for control of ventricular rate in patients with atrial fibrillation. Doses of digoxin used for the treatment of chronic atrial fibrillation should be titrated to the minimum dose that achieves the desired ventricular rate control without causing undesirable side effects. Data are not available to establish the appropriate resting or exercise target rates that should be achieved.

Dosage Adjustment When Changing Preparations
The difference in bioavailability between LANOXIN Injection or LANOXIN Tablets must be considered when changing patients from one dosage form to the other.

HOW SUPPLIED
LANOXIN (digoxin) Tablets, Scored 125 mcg (0.125 mg): Bottles of 100 with child-resistant cap (NDC 0173-0242-55) and 1,000 (NDC 0173-0242-75); unit dose pack of 100 (NDC 0173-0242-56). Imprinted with LANOXIN and Y3B (yellow).

Store at 25°C (77°F); excursions permitted to 15 to 30°C (59 to 86°F) [see USP Controlled Room Temperature] in a dry place and protect from light.
LANOXIN (digoxin) Tablets, Scored 250 mcg (0.25 mg): Bottles of 100 with child-resistant cap (NDC 0173-0249-55), 1,000 (NDC 0173-0249-75), and 5,000 (NDC 0173-0249-80); unit dose pack of 100 (NDC 0173-0249-56). Imprinted with LANOXIN and X3A (white).

Store at 25°C (77°F); excursions permitted to 15 to 30°C (59 to 86°F) [see USP Controlled Room Temperature] in a dry place.
LANOXIN and DIGIBIND are registered trademarks of GlaxoSmithKline
DIGIFAB is a registered trademark of Prostherics Inc.
Manufactured for
GlaxoSmithKline
Research Triangle Park, NC 27709
by DSM Pharmaceuticals, Inc.
Greenville, NC 27834 or
GlaxoSmithKline
Research Triangle Park, NC 27709
©2009, GlaxoSmithKline. All rights reserved.
August 2009
LNT:1PI

LEUKERAN®
[lū´kŭh-răn]
(chlorambucil)
Tablets

℞

DESCRIPTION
LEUKERAN (chlorambucil) was first synthesized by Everett et al. It is a bifunctional alkylating agent of the nitrogen mustard type that has been found active against selected human neoplastic diseases. Chlorambucil is known chemically as 4-[bis(2-chlorethyl)amino]benzenebutanoic acid. Chlorambucil hydrolyzes in water and has a pKa of 5.8.

LEUKERAN (chlorambucil) is available in tablet form for oral administration. Each film-coated tablet contains 2 mg chlorambucil and the inactive ingredients colloidal silicon dioxide, hypromellose, lactose (anhydrous), macrogol/PEG 400, microcrystalline cellulose, red iron oxide, stearic acid, titanium dioxide, and yellow iron oxide.

CLINICAL PHARMACOLOGY
Chlorambucil is rapidly and completely absorbed from the gastrointestinal tract. After single oral doses of 0.6 to 1.2 mg/kg, peak plasma chlorambucil levels (C_{max}) are reached within 1 hour and the terminal elimination half-life ($t_{1/2}$) of the parent drug is estimated at 1.5 hours. Chlorambucil undergoes rapid metabolism to phenylacetic acid mustard, the major metabolite, and the combined chlorambucil and phenylacetic acid mustard urinary excretion is extremely low — less than 1% in 24 hours. In a study of 12 patients given single oral doses of 0.2 mg/kg of LEUKERAN, the mean dose (12 mg) adjusted (± SD) plasma chlorambucil C_{max} was 492 ± 160 ng/mL, the AUC was 883 ± 329 ng•h/mL, $t_{1/2}$ was 1.3 ± 0.5 hours, and the t_{max} was 0.83 ± 0.53 hours. For the major metabolite, phenylacetic acid mustard, the mean dose (12 mg) adjusted (± SD) plasma C_{max} was 306 ± 73 ng/mL, the AUC was 1204 ± 285 ng•h/mL, the $t_{1/2}$ was 1.8 ± 0.4 hours, and the t_{max} was 1.9 ± 0.7 hours.

Chlorambucil and its metabolites are extensively bound to plasma and tissue proteins. In vitro, chlorambucil is 99% bound to plasma proteins, specifically albumin. Cerebrospinal fluid levels of chlorambucil have not been determined. Evidence of human teratogenicity suggests that the drug crosses the placenta.

Chlorambucil is extensively metabolized in the liver primarily to phenylacetic acid mustard, which has antineoplastic activity. Chlorambucil and its major metabolite spontaneously degrade in vivo forming monohydroxy and dihydroxy derivatives. After a single dose of radiolabeled chlorambucil (¹⁴C), approximately 15% to 60% of the radioactivity appears in the urine after 24 hours. Again, less than 1% of the urinary radioactivity is in the form of chlorambucil or phenylacetic acid mustard. In summary, the pharmacokinetic data suggest that oral chlorambucil undergoes rapid gastrointestinal absorption and plasma clearance and that it is almost completely metabolized, having extremely low urinary excretion.

INDICATIONS AND USAGE
LEUKERAN (chlorambucil) is indicated in the treatment of chronic lymphatic (lymphocytic) leukemia, malignant lymphomas including lymphosarcoma, giant follicular lymphoma, and Hodgkin's disease. It is not curative in any of these disorders but may produce clinically useful palliation.

CONTRAINDICATIONS
Chlorambucil should not be used in patients whose disease has demonstrated a prior resistance to the agent. Patients who have demonstrated hypersensitivity to chlorambucil should not be given the drug. There may be cross-hypersensitivity (skin rash) between chlorambucil and other alkylating agents.

WARNINGS
Because of its carcinogenic properties, chlorambucil should not be given to patients with conditions other than chronic lymphatic leukemia or malignant lymphomas. Convulsions, infertility, leukemia, and secondary malignancies have been observed when chlorambucil was employed in the therapy of malignant and non-malignant diseases.

There are many reports of acute leukemia arising in patients with both malignant and non-malignant diseases following chlorambucil treatment. In many instances, these patients also received other chemotherapeutic agents or some form of radiation therapy. The quantitation of the risk of chlorambucil-induction of leukemia or carcinoma in humans is not possible. Evaluation of published reports of leukemia developing in patients who have received chlorambucil (and other alkylating agents) suggests that the risk of leukemogenesis increases with both chronicity of treatment and large cumulative doses. However, it has proved impossible to define a cumulative dose below which there is no risk of the induction of secondary malignancy. The potential benefits from chlorambucil therapy must be weighed on an individual basis against the possible risk of the induction of a secondary malignancy.

Chlorambucil has been shown to cause chromatid or chromosome damage in humans. Both reversible and permanent sterility have been observed in both sexes receiving chlorambucil.

A high incidence of sterility has been documented when chlorambucil is administered to prepubertal and pubertal males. Prolonged or permanent azoospermia has also been observed in adult males. While most reports of gonadal dysfunction secondary to chlorambucil have related to males, the induction of amenorrhea in females with alkylating agents is well documented and chlorambucil is capable of producing amenorrhea. Autopsy studies of the ovaries from women with malignant lymphoma treated with combination chemotherapy including chlorambucil have shown varying degrees of fibrosis, vasculitis, and depletion of primordial follicles.

Rare instances of skin rash progressing to erythema multiforme, toxic epidermal necrolysis, or Stevens-Johnson syndrome have been reported. Chlorambucil should be discontinued promptly in patients who develop skin reactions.

Pregnancy: Pregnancy Category D. Chlorambucil can cause fetal harm when administered to a pregnant woman. Unilateral renal agenesis has been observed in 2 offspring whose mothers received chlorambucil during the first trimester. Urogenital malformations, including absence of a kidney, were found in fetuses of rats given chlorambucil. There are no adequate and well-controlled studies in pregnant women. If this drug is used during pregnancy, or if the patient becomes pregnant while taking this drug, the patient should be apprised of the potential hazard to the fetus. Women of childbearing potential should be advised to avoid becoming pregnant.

PRECAUTIONS
General: Many patients develop a slowly progressive lymphopenia during treatment. The lymphocyte count usually rapidly returns to normal levels upon completion of drug therapy. Most patients have some neutropenia after the third week of treatment and this may continue for up to 10 days after the last dose. Subsequently, the neutrophil count usually rapidly returns to normal. Severe neutropenia appears to be related to dosage and usually occurs only in patients who have received a total dosage of 6.5 mg/kg or more in one course of therapy with continuous dosing. About one quarter of all patients receiving the continuous-dose schedule, and one third of those receiving this dosage in 8 weeks or less may be expected to develop severe neutropenia.

While it is not necessary to discontinue chlorambucil at the first evidence of a fall in neutrophil count, it must be remembered that the fall may continue for 10 days after the last dose, and that as the total dose approaches 6.5 mg/kg, there is a risk of causing irreversible bone marrow damage. The dose of chlorambucil should be decreased if leukocyte or platelet counts fall below normal values and should be discontinued for more severe depression.

Chlorambucil should not be given at full dosages before 4 weeks after a full course of radiation therapy or chemotherapy because of the vulnerability of the bone marrow to damage under these conditions. If the pretherapy leukocyte or platelet counts are depressed from bone marrow disease process prior to institution of therapy, the treatment should be instituted at a reduced dosage.

Persistently low neutrophil and platelet counts or peripheral lymphocytosis suggest bone marrow infiltration. If confirmed by bone marrow examination, the daily dosage of chlorambucil should not exceed 0.1 mg/kg. Chlorambucil appears to be relatively free from gastrointestinal side effects or other evidence of toxicity apart from the bone marrow depressant action. In humans, single oral doses of 20 mg or more may produce nausea and vomiting.

Children with nephrotic syndrome and patients receiving high pulse doses of chlorambucil may have an increased risk of seizures. As with any potentially epileptogenic drug, caution should be exercised when administering chlorambucil to patients with a history of seizure disorder or head trauma, or who are receiving other potentially epileptogenic drugs.

Administration of live vaccines to immunocompromised patients should be avoided.

Information for Patients: Patients should be informed that the major toxicities of chlorambucil are related to hypersensitivity, drug fever, myelosuppression, hepatotoxicity, infertility, seizures, gastrointestinal toxicity, and secondary malignancies. Patients should never be allowed to take the drug without medical supervision and should consult their physician if they experience skin rash, bleeding, fever, jaundice, persistent cough, seizures, nausea, vomiting, amenorrhea, or unusual lumps/masses. Women of childbearing potential should be advised to avoid becoming pregnant.

Laboratory Tests: Patients must be followed carefully to avoid life-endangering damage to the bone marrow during treatment. Weekly examination of the blood should be made to determine hemoglobin levels, total and differential leukocyte counts, and quantitative platelet counts. Also, during the first 3 to 6 weeks of therapy, it is recommended that white blood cell counts be made 3 or 4 days after each of the weekly complete blood counts. Galton et al have suggested that in following patients it is helpful to plot the blood counts on a chart at the same time that body weight, temperature, spleen size, etc., are recorded. It is considered dangerous to allow a patient to go more than 2 weeks without hematological and clinical examination during treatment.

Drug Interactions: There are no known drug/drug interactions with chlorambucil.

Carcinogenesis, Mutagenesis, Impairment of Fertility: See WARNINGS section for information on carcinogenesis, mutagenesis, and impairment of fertility.

Pregnancy: *Teratogenic Effects:* Pregnancy Category D: See WARNINGS section.

Nursing Mothers: It is not known whether this drug is excreted in human milk. Because many drugs are excreted in human milk and because of the potential for serious adverse reactions in nursing infants from chlorambucil, a decision should be made whether to discontinue nursing or to discontinue the drug, taking into account the importance of the drug to the mother.

Pediatric Use: The safety and effectiveness in pediatric patients have not been established.

Geriatric Use: Clinical studies of chlorambucil did not include sufficient numbers of subjects aged 65 and over to determine whether they respond differently from younger subjects. Other reported clinical experience has not identified differences in responses between the elderly and younger patients. In general, dose selection for an elderly patient should be cautious, usually starting at the low end of the dosing range, reflecting the greater frequency of decreased hepatic, renal, or cardiac function, and of concomitant disease or other drug therapy.

ADVERSE REACTIONS

Hematologic: The most common side effect is bone marrow suppression, anemia, leukopenia, neutropenia, thrombocytopenia, or pancytopenia. Although bone marrow suppression frequently occurs, it is usually reversible if the chlorambucil is withdrawn early enough. However, irreversible bone marrow failure has been reported.

Gastrointestinal: Gastrointestinal disturbances such as nausea and vomiting, diarrhea, and oral ulceration occur infrequently.

CNS: Tremors, muscular twitching, myoclonia, confusion, agitation, ataxia, flaccid paresis, and hallucinations have been reported as rare adverse experiences to chlorambucil which resolve upon discontinuation of drug. Rare, focal and/or generalized seizures have been reported to occur in both children and adults at both therapeutic daily doses and pulse-dosing regimens, and in acute overdose (see PRECAUTIONS: General).

Dermatologic: Allergic reactions such as urticaria and angioneurotic edema have been reported following initial or subsequent dosing. Skin hypersensitivity (including rare reports of skin rash progressing to erythema multiforme, toxic epidermal necrolysis, and Stevens-Johnson syndrome) has been reported (see WARNINGS).

Miscellaneous: Other reported adverse reactions include: pulmonary fibrosis, hepatotoxicity and jaundice, drug fever, peripheral neuropathy, interstitial pneumonia, sterile cystitis, infertility, leukemia, and secondary malignancies (see WARNINGS).

OVERDOSAGE

Reversible pancytopenia was the main finding of inadvertent overdoses of chlorambucil. Neurological toxicity ranging from agitated behavior and ataxia to multiple grand mal seizures has also occurred. As there is no known antidote, the blood picture should be closely monitored and general supportive measures should be instituted, together with appropriate blood transfusions, if necessary. Chlorambucil is not dialyzable.

Oral LD_{50} single doses in mice are 123 mg/kg. In rats, a single intraperitoneal dose of 12.5 mg/kg of chlorambucil produces typical nitrogen-mustard effects; these include atrophy of the intestinal mucous membrane and lymphoid tissues, severe lymphopenia becoming maximal in 4 days, anemia, and thrombocytopenia. After this dose, the animals begin to recover within 3 days and appear normal in about a week, although the bone marrow may not become completely normal for about 3 weeks. An intraperitoneal dose of 18.5 mg/kg kills about 50% of the rats with development of convulsions. As much as 50 mg/kg has been given orally to rats as a single dose, with recovery. Such a dose causes bradycardia, excessive salivation, hematuria, convulsions, and respiratory dysfunction.

DOSAGE AND ADMINISTRATION

The usual oral dosage is 0.1 to 0.2 mg/kg body weight daily for 3 to 6 weeks as required. This usually amounts to 4 to 10 mg per day for the average patient. The entire daily dose may be given at one time. These dosages are for initiation of therapy or for short courses of treatment. The dosage must be carefully adjusted according to the response of the patient and must be reduced as soon as there is an abrupt fall in the white blood cell count. Patients with Hodgkin's disease usually require 0.2 mg/kg daily, whereas patients with other lymphomas or chronic lymphocytic leukemia usually require only 0.1 mg/kg daily. When lymphocytic infiltration of the bone marrow is present, or when the bone marrow is hypoplastic, the daily dose should not exceed 0.1 mg/kg (about 6 mg for the average patient).

Alternate schedules for the treatment of chronic lymphocytic leukemia employing intermittent, biweekly, or once-monthly pulse doses of chlorambucil have been reported. Intermittent schedules of chlorambucil begin with an initial single dose of 0.4 mg/kg. Doses are generally increased by 0.1 mg/kg until control of lymphocytosis or toxicity is observed. Subsequent doses are modified to produce mild hematologic toxicity. It is felt that the response rate of chronic lymphocytic leukemia to the biweekly or once-monthly schedule of chlorambucil administration is similar or better to that previously reported with daily administration and that hematologic toxicity was less than or equal to that encountered in studies using daily chlorambucil.

Radiation and cytotoxic drugs render the bone marrow more vulnerable to damage, and chlorambucil should be used with particular caution within 4 weeks of a full course of radiation therapy or chemotherapy. However, small doses of palliative radiation over isolated foci remote from the bone marrow will not usually depress the neutrophil and platelet count. In these cases chlorambucil may be given in the customary dosage.

It is presently felt that short courses of treatment are safer than continuous maintenance therapy, although both methods have been effective. It must be recognized that continuous therapy may give the appearance of "maintenance" in patients who are actually in remission and have no immediate need for further drug. If maintenance dosage is used, it should not exceed 0.1 mg/kg daily and may well be as low as 0.03 mg/kg daily. A typical maintenance dose is 2 mg to 4 mg daily, or less, depending on the status of the blood counts. It may, therefore, be desirable to withdraw the drug after maximal control has been achieved, since intermittent therapy reinstituted at time of relapse may be as effective as continuous treatment.

Procedures for proper handling and disposal of anticancer drugs should be used. Several guidelines on this subject have been published.[1-8] There is no general agreement that all of the procedures recommended in the guidelines are necessary or appropriate.

HOW SUPPLIED

Leukeran is supplied as brown, film-coated, round, biconvex tablets containing 2 mg chlorambucil in amber glass bottles with child-resistant closures. One side is engraved with "GX EG3" and the other side is engraved with an "L."

Bottle of 50 (NDC 0173-0635-35).

Store in a refrigerator, 2° to 8°C (36° to 46°F).

REFERENCES

1. ONS Clinical Practice Committee. Cancer Chemotherapy Guidelines and Recommendations for Practice. Pittsburgh, PA: Oncology Nursing Society; 1999:32-41.
2. Recommendations for the safe handling of parenteral antineoplastic drugs. Washington, DC: Division of Safety, Clinical Center Pharmacy Department and Cancer Nursing Services, National Institutes of Health and Human Services, 1992, US Dept of Health and Human Services, Public Health Service publication NIH 92-2621.
3. AMA Council on Scientific Affairs. Guidelines for handling parenteral antineoplastics. *JAMA.* 1985;253:1590-1591.
4. National Study Commission on Cytotoxic Exposure. Recommendations for handling cytotoxic agents. 1987. Available from Louis P. Jeffrey, Chairman, National Study Commission on Cytotoxic Exposure. Massachusetts College of Pharmacy and Allied Health Sciences, 179 Longwood Avenue, Boston, MA 02115.
5. Clinical Oncological Society of Australia. Guidelines and recommendations for safe handling of antineoplastic agents. *Med J Australia.* 1983;1:426-428.
6. Jones RB, Frank R, Mass T. Safe handling of chemotherapeutic agents: a report from the Mount Sinai Medical Center. *CA-A Cancer J for Clin.* 1983;33:258-263.
7. American Society of Hospital Pharmacists. ASHP technical assistance bulletin on handling cytotoxic and hazardous drugs. *Am J Hosp Pharm.* 1990;47:1033-1049.
8. Controlling Occupational Exposure to Hazardous Drugs. (OSHA Work-Practice Guidelines.) *Am J Health-Syst Pharm.* 1996;53:1669-1685.

GlaxoSmithKline, Research Triangle Park, NC 27709
©2006, GlaxoSmithKline. All rights reserved.
November 2006   RL-2328

LOVAZA® ℞

[lō-vā' ză]
(omega-3-acid ethyl esters)
Capsules

HIGHLIGHTS OF PRESCRIBING INFORMATION

These highlights do not include all the information needed to use LOVAZA safely and effectively. See full prescribing information for LOVAZA.

LOVAZA® (omega-3-acid ethyl esters) Capsules
Initial U.S. Approval: 2004

───────INDICATIONS AND USAGE───────
LOVAZA is a combination of ethyl esters of omega 3 fatty acids, principally EPA and DHA, indicated as an adjunct to diet to reduce triglyceride (TG) levels in adult patients with severe (≥500 mg/dL) hypertriglyceridemia. (1)

Limitations of Use: The effect of LOVAZA on cardiovascular mortality and morbidity in patients with elevated triglycerides has not been determined. (1)

──────DOSAGE AND ADMINISTRATION──────
• The daily dose of LOVAZA is 4 grams per day taken as a single 4-gram dose (4 capsules) or as two 2-gram doses (2 capsules given twice daily). (2)
• Patients should be advised to swallow LOVAZA capsules whole. Do not break open, crush, dissolve or chew LOVAZA. (2)

─────DOSAGE FORMS AND STRENGTHS─────
1-gram transparent soft-gelatin capsules. (3)

────────CONTRAINDICATIONS────────
LOVAZA is contraindicated in patients with known hypersensitivity (e.g., anaphylactic reaction) to LOVAZA or any of its components. (4)

─────WARNINGS AND PRECAUTIONS─────
• In patients with hepatic impairment, monitor ALT and AST levels periodically during therapy. (5.1)
• LOVAZA may increase levels of LDL. Monitor LDL levels periodically during therapy. (5.1)
• Use with caution in patients with known hypersensitivity to fish and/or shellfish. (5.2)

────────ADVERSE REACTIONS────────
The most common adverse events (incidence >3% and greater than placebo) were eructation, infection, flu syndrome, and dyspepsia. (6)

To report SUSPECTED ADVERSE REACTIONS, contact GlaxoSmithKline at 1-888-825-5249 or FDA at 1-800-FDA-1088 or www.fda.gov/medwatch

────────DRUG INTERACTIONS────────
Omega-3-acids may prolong bleeding time. Patients taking LOVAZA and an anticoagulant or other drug affecting coagulation should be monitored periodically. (7.1)

─────USE IN SPECIFIC POPULATIONS─────
• Pregnancy: Use during pregnancy only if the potential benefit justifies the potential risk to the fetus. (8.1)
• Pediatric Use: The safety and effectiveness in pediatric patients have not been established. (8.4)

See 17 for PATIENT COUNSELING INFORMATION and FDA-approved patient labeling

Revised: 12/2009

───────────────────────────────

FULL PRESCRIBING INFORMATION: CONTENTS*

───────────────────────────────

FULL PRESCRIBING INFORMATION

1   INDICATIONS AND USAGE

LOVAZA® (omega-3-acid ethyl esters) is indicated as an adjunct to diet to reduce triglyceride (TG) levels in adult patients with severe (≥500 mg/dL) hypertriglyceridemia.

Usage Considerations: Patients should be placed on an appropriate lipid-lowering diet before receiving LOVAZA and should continue this diet during treatment with LOVAZA.

Table 1. Adverse Events in Randomized, Placebo-Controlled, Double-Blind, Parallel-Group Studies for Very High TG Levels (≥500 mg/dL) that used LOVAZA

BODY SYSTEM	LOVAZA 4 grams/day (N = 226)		Placebo (N = 228)	
Adverse Event*	n	%	n	%
Subjects with at least 1 adverse event	80	35.4	63	27.6
Body as a whole				
Infection	10	4.4	5	2.2
Flu syndrome	8	3.5	3	1.3
Back pain	5	2.2	3	1.3
Pain	4	1.8	3	1.3
Cardiovascular				
Angina pectoris	3	1.3	2	0.9
Digestive				
Eructation	11	4.9	5	2.2
Dyspepsia	7	3.1	6	2.6
Skin				
Rash	4	1.8	1	0.4
Special senses				
Taste perversion	6	2.7	0	0.0

* Adverse events were coded using COSTART, version 5.0. Subjects were counted only once for each body system and for each preferred term.

Laboratory studies should be done to ascertain that the lipid levels are consistently abnormal before instituting LOVAZA therapy. Every attempt should be made to control serum lipids with appropriate diet, exercise, weight loss in obese patients, and control of any medical problems such as diabetes mellitus and hypothyroidism that are contributing to the lipid abnormalities. Medications known to exacerbate hypertriglyceridemia (such as beta blockers, thiazides, estrogens) should be discontinued or changed if possible prior to consideration of triglyceride-lowering drug therapy.

Limitations of Use: The effect of LOVAZA on cardiovascular mortality and morbidity in patients with elevated triglycerides has not been determined.

2 DOSAGE AND ADMINISTRATION

- Assess triglyceride levels carefully before initiating therapy. Identify other causes (e.g., diabetes mellitus, hypothyroidism, or medications) of high triglyceride levels and manage as appropriate. *[see Indications and Usage (1)].*
- Patients should be placed on an appropriate lipid-lowering diet before receiving LOVAZA, and should continue this diet during treatment with LOVAZA. In clinical studies, LOVAZA was administered with meals.

The daily dose of LOVAZA is 4 grams per day. The daily dose may be taken as a single 4-gram dose (4 capsules) or as two 2-gram doses (2 capsules given twice daily).

Patients should be advised to swallow LOVAZA capsules whole. Do not break open, crush, dissolve or chew LOVAZA.

3 DOSAGE FORMS AND STRENGTHS

LOVAZA (omega-3-acid ethyl esters) capsules are supplied as 1-gram transparent soft-gelatin capsules filled with light-yellow oil and bearing the designation LOVAZA.

4 CONTRAINDICATIONS

LOVAZA is contraindicated in patients with known hypersensitivity (e.g., anaphylactic reaction) to LOVAZA or any of its components.

5 WARNINGS AND PRECAUTIONS

5.1 Monitoring: Laboratory Tests

In patients with hepatic impairment, alanine aminotransferase (ALT) and aspartate aminotransferase (AST) levels should be monitored periodically during therapy with LOVAZA. In some patients, increases in ALT levels without a concurrent increase in AST levels were observed.

In some patients, LOVAZA increases LDL-C levels. LDL-C levels should be monitored periodically during therapy with LOVAZA.

Laboratory studies should be performed periodically to measure the patient's TG levels during therapy with LOVAZA.

5.2 Fish Allergy

LOVAZA contains ethyl esters of omega-3 fatty acids (EPA and DHA) obtained from the oil of several fish sources. It is not known whether patients with allergies to fish and/or shellfish, are at increased risk of an allergic reaction to LOVAZA. LOVAZA should be used with caution in patients with known hypersensitivity to fish and/or shellfish.

6 ADVERSE REACTIONS

6.1 Clinical Trials Experience

Because clinical trials are conducted under widely varying conditions, adverse reaction rates observed in the clinical trials of a drug cannot be directly compared to rates in the clinical trials of another drug and may not reflect the rates observed in practice.

Adverse events reported in at least 1% of patients treated with LOVAZA 4 grams per day or placebo during 8 randomized, placebo-controlled, double-blind, parallel-group studies for HTG are listed in Table 1. Adverse events led to discontinuation of treatment in 3.5% of patients treated with LOVAZA and 2.6% of patients treated with placebo.

[See table 1 above]

Additional adverse events reported by 1 or more patients from clinical studies for HTG are listed below:

Body as a Whole: Enlarged abdomen, asthenia, body odor, chest pain, chills, suicide, fever, generalized edema, fungal infection, malaise, neck pain, neoplasm, rheumatoid arthritis, and sudden death.

Cardiovascular System: Arrhythmia, bypass surgery, cardiac arrest, hyperlipemia, hypertension, migraine, myocardial infarct, myocardial ischemia, occlusion, peripheral vascular disorder, syncope, and tachycardia.

Digestive System: Anorexia, constipation, dry mouth, dysphagia, colitis, fecal incontinence, gastritis, gastroenteritis, gastrointestinal disorder, increased appetite, intestinal obstruction, melena, pancreatitis, tenesmus, and vomiting.

Hematologic-Lymphatic System: Lymphadenopathy.

Infections and Infestations: Viral infection.

Metabolic and Nutritional Disorders: Edema, hyperglycemia, increased ALT, and increased AST.

Musculoskeletal System: Arthralgia, arthritis, myalgia, pathological fracture, and tendon disorder.

Nervous System: Central nervous system neoplasia, depression, dizziness, emotional lability, facial paralysis, insomnia, vasodilatation, and vertigo.

Respiratory System: Asthma, bronchitis, increased cough, dyspnea, epistaxis, laryngitis, pharyngitis, pneumonia, rhinitis, and sinusitis.

Skin: Alopecia, eczema, pruritus, and sweating.

Special Senses: Cataract.

Urogenital System: Cervix disorder, endometrial carcinoma, epididymitis, and impotence.

6.2 Postmarketing Experience

In addition to adverse reactions reported from clinical trials, the events described below have been identified during post-approval use of LOVAZA. Because these events are reported voluntarily from a population of unknown size, it is not possible to reliably estimate their frequency or to always establish a causal relationship to drug exposure. The following events have been reported: anaphylactic reaction, hemorrhagic diathesis.

7 DRUG INTERACTIONS

7.1 Anticoagulants or Other Drugs Affecting Coagulation

Some studies with omega-3-acids demonstrated prolongation of bleeding time. The prolongation of bleeding time reported in these studies has not exceeded normal limits and did not produce clinically significant bleeding episodes. Clinical studies have not been done to thoroughly examine the effect of LOVAZA and concomitant anticoagulants. Patients receiving treatment with LOVAZA and an anticoagulant or other drug affecting coagulation should be monitored periodically (e.g., aspirin, NSAIDS, warfarin, coumarin).

8 USE IN SPECIFIC POPULATIONS

8.1 Pregnancy

Pregnancy Category C: There are no adequate and well-controlled studies in pregnant women. It is unknown whether LOVAZA can cause fetal harm when administered to a pregnant woman or can affect reproductive capacity. LOVAZA should be used during pregnancy only if the potential benefit to the patient justifies the potential risk to the fetus.

Animal Data

Omega-3-acid ethyl esters have been shown to have an embryocidal effect in pregnant rats when given in doses resulting in exposures 7 times the recommended human dose of 4 grams/day based on a body surface area comparison.

In female rats given oral gavage doses of 100, 600, and 2,000 mg/kg/day beginning 2 weeks prior to mating and continuing through gestation and lactation, no adverse effects were observed in the high dose group (5 times human systemic exposure following an oral dose of 4 grams/day based on body surface area comparison).

In pregnant rats given oral gavage doses of 1,000, 3,000, and 6,000 mg/kg/day from gestation day 6 through 15, no adverse effects were observed (14 times human systemic exposure following an oral dose of 4 grams/day based on a body surface area comparison).

In pregnant rats given oral gavage doses of 100, 600, and 2,000 mg/kg/day from gestation day 14 through lactation day 21, no adverse effects were seen at 2,000 mg/kg/day (5 times the human systemic exposure following an oral dose of 4 grams/day based on a body surface area comparison). However, decreased live births (20% reduction) and decreased survival to postnatal day 4 (40% reduction) were observed in a dose-ranging study using higher doses of 3,000 mg/kg/day (7 times the human systemic exposure following an oral dose of 4 grams/day based on a body surface area comparison).

In pregnant rabbits given oral gavage doses of 375, 750, and 1,500 mg/kg/day from gestation day 7 through 19, no findings were observed in the fetuses in groups given 375 mg/kg/day (2 times human systemic exposure following an oral dose of 4 grams/day based on a body surface area comparison). However, at higher doses, evidence of maternal toxicity was observed (4 times human systemic exposure following an oral dose of 4 grams/day based on a body surface area comparison).

8.3 Nursing Mothers

It is not known whether omega-3-acid ethyl esters are excreted in human milk. Because many drugs are excreted in human milk, caution should be exercised when LOVAZA is administered to a nursing woman.

8.4 Pediatric Use

Safety and effectiveness in pediatric patients have not been established.

8.5 Geriatric Use

A limited number of patients older than 65 years were enrolled in the clinical studies of LOVAZA. Safety and efficacy findings in subjects older than 60 years did not appear to differ from those of subjects younger than 60 years.

9 DRUG ABUSE AND DEPENDENCE

LOVAZA does not have any known drug abuse or withdrawal effects.

10 OVERDOSAGE

In the event of an overdose, the patient should be treated symptomatically, and general supportive care measures instituted, as required.

11 DESCRIPTION

LOVAZA, a lipid-regulating agent, is supplied as a liquid-filled gel capsule for oral administration. Each 1-gram capsule of LOVAZA contains at least 900 mg of the ethyl esters of omega-3 fatty acids sourced from fish oils. These are predominantly a combination of ethyl esters of eicosapentaenoic acid (EPA - approximately 465 mg) and docosahexaenoic acid (DHA - approximately 375 mg).

IMPORTANT NOTICE: Updated drug information is sent bi-monthly via the PDR® Update Insert. For *monthly* email updates, register at PDR.net.

The empirical formula of EPA ethyl ester is $C_{22}H_{34}O_2$, and the molecular weight of EPA ethyl ester is 330.51. The structural formula of EPA ethyl ester is:

The empirical formula of DHA ethyl ester is $C_{24}H_{36}O_2$, and the molecular weight of DHA ethyl ester is 356.55. The structural formula of DHA ethyl ester is:

LOVAZA capsules also contain the following inactive ingredients: 4 mg α-tocopherol (in a carrier of soybean oil), and gelatin, glycerol, and purified water (components of the capsule shell).

12 CLINICAL PHARMACOLOGY

12.1 Mechanism of Action

The mechanism of action of LOVAZA is not completely understood. Potential mechanisms of action include inhibition of acyl-CoA:1,2-diacylglycerol acyltransferase, increased mitochondrial and peroxisomal β-oxidation in the liver, decreased lipogenesis in the liver, and increased plasma lipoprotein lipase activity. LOVAZA may reduce the synthesis of triglycerides in the liver because EPA and DHA are poor substrates for the enzymes responsible for TG synthesis, and EPA and DHA inhibit esterification of other fatty acids.

12.3 Pharmacokinetics

In healthy volunteers and in patients with hypertriglyceridemia, EPA and DHA were absorbed when administered as ethyl esters orally. Omega-3-acids administered as ethyl esters (LOVAZA) induced significant, dose-dependent increases in serum phospholipid EPA content, though increases in DHA content were less marked and not dose-dependent when administered as ethyl esters.

Specific Populations

Age

Uptake of EPA and DHA into serum phospholipids in subjects treated with LOVAZA was independent of age (<49 years versus ≥49 years).

Gender

Females tended to have more uptake of EPA into serum phospholipids than males. The clinical significance of this is unknown.

Pediatric

Pharmacokinetics of LOVAZA in pediatric patients have not been established [see Use in Specific Populations (8.4)].

Renal or Hepatic Impairment

LOVAZA has not been studied in patients with renal or hepatic impairment.

Drug-Drug Interactions

Simvastatin

In a 14-day study of 24 healthy adult subjects, daily co-administration of simvastatin 80 mg with LOVAZA 4 grams did not affect the extent (AUC) or rate (C_{max}) of exposure to simvastatin or the major active metabolite, beta-hydroxy simvastatin at steady state.

Atorvastatin

In a 14-day study of 50 healthy adult subjects, daily co-administration of atorvastatin 80 mg with LOVAZA 4 grams did not affect AUC or C_{max} of exposure to atorvastatin, 2-hydroxyatorvastatin, or 4-hydroxyatorvastatin at steady state.

Rosuvastatin

In a 14-day study of 48 healthy adult subjects, daily co-administration of rosuvastatin 40 mg with LOVAZA 4 grams did not affect AUC or C_{max} of exposure to rosuvastatin at steady state.

In vitro studies using human liver microsomes indicated that clinically significant cytochrome P450 mediated inhibition by EPA/DHA combinations are not expected in humans.

13 NONCLINICAL TOXICOLOGY

13.1 Carcinogenesis, Mutagenesis, Impairment of Fertility

In a rat carcinogenicity study with oral gavage doses of 100, 600, and 2,000 mg/kg/day, males were treated with omega-3-acid ethyl esters for 101 weeks and females for 89 weeks without an increased incidence of tumors (up to 5 times human systemic exposures following an oral dose of 4 grams/day based on a body surface area comparison). Standard lifetime carcinogenicity bioassays were not conducted in mice.

Omega-3-acid ethyl esters were not mutagenic or clastogenic with or without metabolic activation in the bacterial mutagenesis (Ames) test with *Salmonella typhimurium* and *Escherichia coli* or in the chromosomal aberration assay in Chinese hamster V79 lung cells or human lymphocytes. Omega-3-acid ethyl esters were negative in the in vivo mouse micronucleus assay.

In a rat fertility study with oral gavage doses of 100, 600, and 2,000 mg/kg/day, males were treated for 10 weeks prior to mating and females were treated for 2 weeks prior to and throughout mating, gestation, and lactation. No adverse effect on fertility was observed at 2,000 mg/kg/day (5 times human systemic exposure following an oral dose of 4 grams/day based on a body surface area comparison).

14 CLINICAL STUDIES

14.1 Severe Hypertriglyceridemia

The effects of LOVAZA 4 grams per day were assessed in 2 randomized, placebo-controlled, double-blind, parallel-group studies of 84 adult patients (42 on LOVAZA, 42 on placebo) with very high triglyceride levels. Patients whose baseline triglyceride levels were between 500 and 2,000 mg/dL were enrolled in these 2 studies of 6 and 16 weeks duration. The median triglyceride and LDL-C levels in these patients were 792 mg/dL and 100 mg/dL, respectively. Median HDL-C level was 23.0 mg/dL.

The changes in the major lipoprotein lipid parameters for the groups receiving LOVAZA or placebo are shown in Table 2.

Table 2. Median Baseline and Percent Change From Baseline in Lipid Parameters in Patients with Very High TG Levels (≥500 mg/dL)

Parameter	LOVAZA N = 42		Placebo N = 42		Difference
	BL	% Change	BL	% Change	
TG	816	-44.9	788	+6.7	-51.6
Non-HDL-C	271	-13.8	292	-3.6	-10.2
TC	296	-9.7	314	-1.7	-8.0
VLDL-C	175	-41.7	175	-0.9	-40.8
HDL-C	22	+9.1	24	0.0	+9.1
LDL-C	89	+44.5	108	-4.8	+49.3

BL = Baseline (mg/dL); % Change = Median Percent Change from Baseline; Difference = LOVAZA Median % Change – Placebo Median % Change

LOVAZA 4 grams per day reduced median TG, VLDL-C, and non-HDL-C levels and increased median HDL-C from baseline relative to placebo. Treatment with LOVAZA to reduce very high TG levels may result in elevations in LDL-C and non-HDL-C in some individuals. Patients should be monitored to ensure that the LDL-C level does not increase excessively.

The effect of LOVAZA on the risk of pancreatitis in patients with very high TG levels has not been evaluated.

The effect of LOVAZA on cardiovascular mortality and morbidity in patients with elevated TG levels has not been determined.

14.2 Other Clinical Experience

The effects of LOVAZA 4 grams per day as add-on therapy to treatment with simvastatin were evaluated in a randomized, placebo-controlled, double-blind, parallel-group study of 254 adult patients (122 on LOVAZA and 132 on placebo) with persistent high triglycerides (200 to 499 mg/dL) despite simvastatin therapy. Patients were treated with open-

Table 3. Response to the Addition of LOVAZA 4 grams per day to Ongoing Simvastatin 40 mg per day Therapy in Patients with High Triglycerides (200 to 499 mg/dL)

Parameter	LOVAZA + Simvastatin N = 122			Placebo + Simvastatin N = 132			Difference	P-Value
	BL	EOT	Median % Change	BL	EOT	Median % Change		
Non-HDL-C	137	123	-9.0	141	134	-2.2	-6.8	<0.0001
TG	268	182	-29.5	271	260	-6.3	-23.2	<0.0001
TC	184	172	-4.8	184	178	-1.7	-3.1	<0.05
VLDL-C	52	37	-27.5	52	49	-7.2	-20.3	<0.05
Apo-B	86	80	-4.2	87	85	-1.9	-2.3	<0.05
HDL-C	46	48	+3.4	43	44	-1.2	+4.6	<0.05
LDL-C	91	88	+0.7	88	85	-2.8	+3.5	=0.05

BL = Baseline (mg/dL); EOT = End of Treatment (mg/dL); Median % Change = Median Percent Change from Baseline; Difference = LOVAZA Median % Change – Placebo Median % Change

label simvastatin 40 mg per day for 8 weeks prior to randomization to control their LDL-C to no greater than 10% above NCEP ATP III goal and remained on this dose throughout the study. Following 8 weeks of open-label treatment with simvastatin, patients were randomized to either LOVAZA 4 grams per day or placebo for an additional 8 weeks with simvastatin co-therapy. The median baseline triglyceride and LDL-C levels in these patients were 268 mg/dL and 89 mg/dL, respectively. Median baseline non-HDL-C and HDL-C levels were 138 mg/dL and 45 mg/dL, respectively.

The changes in the major lipoprotein lipid parameters for the groups receiving LOVAZA plus simvastatin or placebo plus simvastatin are shown in Table 3.

[See table 3 above]

LOVAZA 4 grams per day significantly reduced non-HDL-C, TG, TC, VLDL-C, and Apo-B levels and increased HDL-C and LDL-C from baseline relative to placebo.

16 HOW SUPPLIED/STORAGE AND HANDLING

LOVAZA (omega-3-acid ethyl esters) capsules are supplied as 1-gram transparent soft-gelatin capsules filled with light-yellow oil and bearing the designation LOVAZA.

Bottles of 60: NDC 0173-0783-01

Bottles of 120: NDC 0173-0783-02

Store at 25°C (77°F); excursions permitted to 15° to 30°C (59° to 86°F) [see USP Controlled Room Temperature]. Do not freeze. Keep out of reach of children.

17 PATIENT COUNSELING INFORMATION

See FDA-approved patient labeling

- LOVAZA should be used with caution in patients with known sensitivity or allergy to fish and/or shellfish [see Warnings and Precautions (5.3)].
- Patients should be advised that use of lipid-regulating agents does not reduce the importance of adhering to diet [see Dosage and Administration (2)].
- Patients should be advised not to alter LOVAZA capsules in any way and to ingest intact capsules only [see Dosage and Administration (2)].

Manufactured for GlaxoSmithKline by:

Catalent Pharma Solutions

2725 Scherer Drive

St. Petersburg, FL 33716-1016

Accucaps Industries Limited

2125 Ambassador Drive

Windsor, Ontario, Canada N9B 3R5

Banner Pharmaceuticals Inc.

4125 Premier Drive

High Point, NC 27265

Distributed by:

GlaxoSmithKline

Research Triangle Park, NC 27709

LOVAZA is a registered trademark of the GlaxoSmithKline group of companies.

©2009 GlaxoSmithKline. All rights reserved.

September 2009   LVZ:5PI

PHARMACIST-DETACH HERE AND GIVE INSTRUCTIONS TO PATIENT

PATIENT INFORMATION

LOVAZA® (lō-vā-ză)

(omega-3-acid ethyl esters) Capsules

Read the Patient Information that comes with LOVAZA before you start taking it, and each time you get a refill. There may be new information. This leaflet does not take the place of talking with your doctor about your condition or treatment.

What is LOVAZA?

LOVAZA is a prescription medicine, called a lipid-regulating medicine, for adults. LOVAZA is made of omega-3 fatty acids from oils of fish, such as salmon and mackerel. Omega-3 fatty acids are substances that your body needs but cannot produce itself.

LOVAZA is used along with a low-fat and low-cholesterol diet to lower very high triglycerides (fats) in your blood. Before taking LOVAZA, talk to your healthcare provider about how you can lower high blood fats by:

- losing weight, if you are overweight
- increasing physical exercise
- lowering alcohol use
- treating diseases such as diabetes and low thyroid (hypothyroidism)
- adjusting the dose or changing other medicines that raise triglyceride levels such as certain blood pressure medicines and estrogens

Treatment with LOVAZA has not been shown to prevent heart attacks or strokes.

LOVAZA has not been studied in children under the age of 18 years.

Who should not take LOVAZA?

Do not take LOVAZA if you:

- **are allergic to LOVAZA or any of its ingredients.** See the end of this leaflet for a complete list of ingredients in LOVAZA.

What should I tell my doctor before taking LOVAZA?

Tell your doctor about all of your medical conditions, including if you:

- drink more than 2 glasses of alcohol daily.
- have diabetes.
- have a thyroid problem called hypothyroidism.
- have a liver problem.
- have a pancreas problem.
- are allergic to fish and/or shellfish. LOVAZA may not be right for you.
- are pregnant, or planning to become pregnant. It is not known if LOVAZA can harm your unborn baby.
- are breastfeeding. It is not known if LOVAZA passes into your milk and if it can harm your baby.

Tell your doctor about all the medicines you take, including prescription and non-prescription medicine, vitamins, and herbal supplements. LOVAZA and certain other medicines can interact. Especially tell your doctor if you take medicines that affect clotting such as anticoagulants or blood thinners. Examples of these medicines include aspirin, nonsteroidal anti-inflammatory agents (NSAIDS), warfarin, coumarin, and clopidogrel (PLAVIX®).

Know all the medicines you take. Keep a list of them with you to show your doctor and pharmacist.

How should I take LOVAZA?

- Take LOVAZA exactly as prescribed. Do not change your dose or stop LOVAZA without talking to your doctor.
- The usual dose of LOVAZA is 4 capsules:
  - Take all 4 capsules at the same time, or
  - Take 2 capsules two times a day
- Take LOVAZA at the same time or times each day.
- Take LOVAZA with or without food. You may find it easier to take LOVAZA with food.
- Do not take more than 4 capsules a day. Taking more than 4 capsules per day may increase the chance of side effects.
- Take LOVAZA capsules whole. Do not break, crush, dissolve, or chew LOVAZA capsules before swallowing. If you cannot swallow LOVAZA capsules whole, tell your doctor. You may need a different medicine.
- Your doctor should start you on a low-fat and low-cholesterol diet before giving you LOVAZA. Stay on this low-fat and low-cholesterol diet while taking LOVAZA.
- Your doctor should do blood tests to check your triglyceride and cholesterol levels during treatment with LOVAZA.
- If you have liver disease, your doctor should do blood tests to check your liver function during treatment with LOVAZA.
- If you miss a dose of LOVAZA, take it as soon as you remember. However, if you miss one day of LOVAZA, do not double your dose when you next take it.
- If you take too much LOVAZA or overdose, call your doctor or Poison Control Center right away.

What are the possible side effects of LOVAZA?

The most common side effects with LOVAZA are burping, infection, flu symptoms, upset stomach, a change in your sense of taste, back pain, and skin rash.

LOVAZA may affect certain blood tests. It may change:

- one of the tests to check liver function (ALT)
- one of the tests to measure cholesterol levels (LDL-C)

Talk to your doctor if you have side effects that bother you or that will not go away. You may report side effects to FDA at 1-800-FDA-1088.

These are not all the side effects with LOVAZA. For more information, ask your doctor or pharmacist.

How should I store LOVAZA?

- Store LOVAZA at room temperature, 59° to 86° F (15° to 30° C). Do not freeze.

- Do not keep medicine that is out of date or that you no longer need.
- **Keep LOVAZA out of the reach of children.** Be sure that if you throw medicines away, it is out of the reach of children.

General information about LOVAZA

Medicines are sometimes prescribed for conditions that are not mentioned in patient information leaflets. Do not use LOVAZA for a condition for which it was not prescribed. Do not give LOVAZA to other people, even if they have the same problem you have. It may harm them.

This leaflet summarizes the most important information about LOVAZA. If you would like more information, talk with your doctor. You can ask your doctor or pharmacist for information about LOVAZA that is written for health professionals or go to www.LOVAZA.com.

What are the ingredients in LOVAZA?

Active Ingredient: Omega-3-acid ethyl esters
Inactive Ingredients: Gelatin, glycerol, purified water, alpha-tocopherol (in soybean oil)

LOVAZA is a registered trademark of the GlaxoSmithKline group of companies.
PLAVIX is a registered trademark of Sanofi-Synthelabo.

Manufactured for GlaxoSmithKline by:
Catalent Pharma Solutions
2725 Scherer Drive
St. Petersburg, FL 33716-1016
Accucaps Industries Limited
2125 Ambassador Drive
Windsor, Ontario, Canada N9B 3R5
Banner Pharmaceuticals Inc.
4125 Premier Drive
High Point, NC 27265
Distributed by:
GlaxoSmithKline
Research Triangle Park, NC 27709
©2009 GlaxoSmithKline. All rights reserved.
September 2009   LVZ:2PIL

MALARONE®   ℞
[mal' ə-rōn]
(atovaquone and proguanil hydrochloride)
Tablets

MALARONE®   ℞
(atovaquone and proguanil hydrochloride)
Pediatric Tablets

DESCRIPTION

MALARONE (atovaquone and proguanil hydrochloride) is a fixed-dose combination of the antimalarial agents atovaquone and proguanil hydrochloride. The chemical name of atovaquone is trans-2-[4-(4-chlorophenyl)-cyclohexyl]-3-hydroxy-1,4-naphthalenedione. Atovaquone is a yellow crystalline solid that is practically insoluble in water. It has a molecular weight of 366.84 and the molecular formula $C_{22}H_{19}ClO_3$. The compound has the following structural formula:

The chemical name of proguanil hydrochloride is 1-(4-chlorophenyl)-5-isopropyl-biguanide hydrochloride. Proguanil hydrochloride is a white crystalline solid that is sparingly soluble in water. It has a molecular weight of 290.22 and the molecular formula $C_{11}H_{16}ClN_5$•HCl. The compound has the following structural formula:

MALARONE Tablets and MALARONE Pediatric Tablets are for oral administration. Each MALARONE Tablet contains 250 mg of atovaquone and 100 mg of proguanil hydrochloride and each MALARONE Pediatric Tablet contains 62.5 mg of atovaquone and 25 mg of proguanil hydrochloride. The inactive ingredients in both tablets are low-substituted hydroxypropyl cellulose, magnesium stearate, microcrystalline cellulose, poloxamer 188, povidone K30, and sodium starch glycolate. The tablet coating contains hypromellose, polyethylene glycol 400, polyethylene glycol 8000, red iron oxide, and titanium dioxide.

CLINICAL PHARMACOLOGY

Microbiology

Mechanism of Action

The constituents of MALARONE, atovaquone and proguanil hydrochloride, interfere with 2 different pathways involved in the biosynthesis of pyrimidines required for nucleic acid replication. Atovaquone is a selective inhibitor of parasite mitochondrial electron transport. Proguanil hydrochloride primarily exerts its effect by means of the metabolite cycloguanil, a dihydrofolate reductase inhibitor. Inhibition of dihydrofolate reductase in the malaria parasite disrupts deoxythymidylate synthesis.

Activity In Vitro and In Vivo

Atovaquone and cycloguanil (an active metabolite of proguanil) are active against the erythrocytic and exoerythrocytic stages of Plasmodium spp. Enhanced efficacy of the combination compared to either atovaquone or proguanil hydrochloride alone was demonstrated in clinical studies in both immune and non-immune patients (see CLINICAL STUDIES).

Drug Resistance

Strains of P. falciparum with decreased susceptibility to atovaquone or proguanil/cycloguanil alone can be selected in vitro or in vivo. The combination of atovaquone and proguanil hydrochloride may not be effective for treatment of recrudescent malaria that develops after prior therapy with the combination.

Pharmacokinetics

Absorption

Atovaquone is a highly lipophilic compound with low aqueous solubility. The bioavailability of atovaquone shows considerable inter-individual variability.

Dietary fat taken with atovaquone increases the rate and extent of absorption, increasing AUC 2 to 3 times and C_{max} 5 times over fasting. The absolute bioavailability of the tablet formulation of atovaquone when taken with food is 23%. MALARONE Tablets should be taken with food or a milky drink.

Proguanil hydrochloride is extensively absorbed regardless of food intake.

Distribution

Atovaquone is highly protein bound (>99%) over the concentration range of 1 to 90 mcg/mL. A population pharmacokinetic analysis demonstrated that the apparent volume of distribution of atovaquone (V/F) in adult and pediatric patients after oral administration is approximately 8.8 L/kg. Proguanil is 75% protein bound. A population pharmacokinetic analysis demonstrated that the apparent V/F of proguanil in adult and pediatric patients >15 years of age with body weights from 31 to 110 kg ranged from 1,617 to 2,502 L. In pediatric patients ≤15 years of age with body weights from 11 to 56 kg, the V/F of proguanil ranged from 462 to 966 L.

In human plasma, the binding of atovaquone and proguanil was unaffected by the presence of the other.

Metabolism

In a study where ^{14}C-labeled atovaquone was administered to healthy volunteers, greater than 94% of the dose was recovered as unchanged atovaquone in the feces over 21 days. There was little or no excretion of atovaquone in the urine (less than 0.6%). There is indirect evidence that atovaquone may undergo limited metabolism; however, a specific metabolite has not been identified. Between 40% to 60% of proguanil is excreted by the kidneys. Proguanil is metabolized to cycloguanil (primarily via CYP2C19) and 4-chlorophenylbiguanide. The main routes of elimination are hepatic biotransformation and renal excretion.

Elimination

The elimination half-life of atovaquone is about 2 to 3 days in adult patients.

The elimination half-life of proguanil is 12 to 21 hours in both adult patients and pediatric patients, but may be longer in individuals who are slow metabolizers.

A population pharmacokinetic analysis in adult and pediatric patients showed that the apparent clearance (CL/F) of both atovaquone and proguanil are related to the body weight. The values CL/F for both atovaquone and proguanil in subjects with body weight ≥11 kg are shown in Table 1.
[See table 1 at top of next page]

The pharmacokinetics of atovaquone and proguanil in patients with body weight below 11 kg have not been adequately characterized.

Special Populations

Pediatrics

The pharmacokinetics of proguanil and cycloguanil are similar in adult patients and pediatric patients. However, the elimination half-life of atovaquone is shorter in pediatric patients (1 to 2 days) than in adult patients (2 to 3 days). In clinical trials, plasma trough levels of atovaquone and proguanil in pediatric patients weighing 5 to 40 kg were within the range observed in adults after dosing by body weight.

Geriatrics

In a single-dose study, the pharmacokinetics of atovaquone, proguanil, and cycloguanil were compared in 13 elderly subjects (age 65 to 79 years) to 13 younger subjects (age 30 to 45 years). In the elderly subjects, the extent of systemic exposure (AUC) of cycloguanil was increased (point estimate = 2.36, CI = 1.70, 3.28). T_{max} was longer in elderly subjects (median 8 hours) compared with younger subjects (median 4 hours) and average elimination half-life was longer in elderly subjects (mean 14.9 hours) compared with younger subjects (mean 8.3 hours).

Hepatic Impairment

In a single-dose study, the pharmacokinetics of atovaquone, proguanil, and cycloguanil were compared in 13 subjects with hepatic impairment (9 mild, 4 moderate, as indicated by the Child-Pugh method) to 13 subjects with normal hepatic function. In subjects with mild or moderate hepatic impairment as compared to healthy subjects, there were no marked differences (<50%) in the rate or extent of systemic exposure of atovaquone. However, in subjects with moderate hepatic impairment, the elimination half-life of atovaquone was increased (point estimate = 1.28, 90% CI = 1.00 to 1.63). Proguanil AUC, C_{max}, and its $t_{1/2}$ increased in subjects with mild hepatic impairment when compared to healthy subjects (Table 2). Also, the proguanil AUC and its $t_{1/2}$ increased in subjects with moderate hepatic impairment when compared to healthy subjects. Consistent with the increase in proguanil AUC, there were marked decreases in the systemic exposure of cycloguanil (C_{max} and AUC) and an increase in its elimination half-life in subjects with mild hepatic impairment when compared to healthy volunteers (Table 2). There were few measurable cycloguanil concentrations in subjects with moderate hepatic impairment (see DOSAGE AND ADMINISTRATION). The pharmacokinetics of atovaquone, proguanil, and cycloguanil after administration of MALARONE have not been studied in patients with severe hepatic impairment.
[See table 2 at right]

Renal Impairment

In patients with mild renal impairment (creatinine clearance 50 to 80 mL/min), oral clearance and/or AUC data for atovaquone, proguanil, and cycloguanil are within the range of values observed in patients with normal renal function (creatinine clearance >80 mL/min). In patients with moderate renal impairment (creatinine clearance 30 to 50 mL/min), mean oral clearance for proguanil was reduced by approximately 35% compared with patients with normal renal function (creatinine clearance >80 mL/min) and the oral clearance of atovaquone was comparable between patients with normal renal function and mild renal impairment. No data exist on the use of MALARONE for long-term prophylaxis (over 2 months) in individuals with moderate renal failure. In patients with severe renal impairment (creatinine clearance <30 mL/min), atovaquone C_{max} and AUC are reduced but the elimination half-lives for proguanil and cycloguanil are prolonged, with corresponding increases in AUC, resulting in the potential of drug accumulation and toxicity with repeated dosing (see CONTRAINDICATIONS).

Drug Interactions

There are no pharmacokinetic interactions between atovaquone and proguanil at the recommended dose.
Concomitant treatment with **tetracycline** has been associated with approximately a 40% reduction in plasma concentrations of atovaquone.
Concomitant treatment with **metoclopramide** has also been associated with decreased bioavailability of atovaquone.
Concomitant administration of **rifampin** or **rifabutin** is known to reduce atovaquone levels by approximately 50% and 34%, respectively (see PRECAUTIONS: Drug Interactions). The mechanisms of these interactions are unknown.
Concomitant administration of atovaquone (750 mg BID with food for 14 days) and indinavir (800 mg TID without food for 14 days) did not result in any change in the steady-state AUC and C_{max} of indinavir but resulted in a decrease in the C_{trough} of indinavir (23% decrease [90% CI 8%, 35%]). Caution should be exercised when prescribing atovaquone with indinavir due to the decrease in trough levels of indinavir.
Atovaquone is highly protein bound (>99%) but does not displace other highly protein-bound drugs in vitro, indicating significant drug interactions arising from displacement are unlikely (see PRECAUTIONS: Drug Interactions). Proguanil is metabolized primarily by CYP2C19. Potential pharmacokinetic interactions with other substrates or inhibitors of this pathway are unknown.

INDICATIONS AND USAGE

Prevention of Malaria

MALARONE is indicated for the prophylaxis of *P. falciparum* malaria, including in areas where chloroquine resistance has been reported (see CLINICAL STUDIES).

Treatment of Malaria

MALARONE is indicated for the treatment of acute, uncomplicated *P. falciparum* malaria. MALARONE has been

Table 1. Apparent Clearance for Atovaquone and Proguanil in Patients as a Function of Body Weight

Body Weight	Atovaquone		Proguanil	
	N	CL/F (L/hr) Mean ± SD* (range)	N	CL/F (L/hr) Mean ± SD* (range)
11-20 kg	159	1.34 ± 0.63 (0.52-4.26)	146	29.5 ± 6.5 (10.3-48.3)
21-30 kg	117	1.87 ± 0.81 (0.52-5.38)	113	40.0 ± 7.5 (15.9-62.7)
31-40 kg	95	2.76 ± 2.07 (0.97-12.5)	91	49.5 ± 8.30 (25.8-71.5)
>40 kg	368	6.61 ± 3.92 (1.32-20.3)	282	67.9 ± 19.9 (14.0-145)

* SD = standard deviation.

Table 2. Point Estimates (90% CI) for Proguanil and Cycloguanil Parameters in Subjects With Mild and Moderate Hepatic Impairment Compared to Healthy Volunteers

Parameter	Comparison	Proguanil	Cycloguanil
$AUC_{(0-inf)}$*	mild:healthy	1.96 (1.51, 2.54)	0.32 (0.22, 0.45)
C_{max}*	mild:healthy	1.41 (1.16, 1.71)	0.35 (0.24, 0.50)
$t_{1/2}$†	mild:healthy	1.21 (0.92, 1.60)	0.86 (0.49, 1.48)
$AUC_{(0-inf)}$*	moderate:healthy	1.64 (1.14, 2.34)	ND
C_{max}*	moderate:healthy	0.97 (0.69, 1.36)	ND
$t_{1/2}$†	moderate:healthy	1.46 (1.05, 2.05)	ND

ND = not determined due to lack of quantifiable data.
* Ratio of geometric means.
† Mean difference.

shown to be effective in regions where the drugs chloroquine, halofantrine, mefloquine, and amodiaquine may have unacceptable failure rates, presumably due to drug resistance.

CONTRAINDICATIONS

MALARONE is contraindicated in individuals with known hypersensitivity to atovaquone or proguanil hydrochloride or any component of the formulation. Rare cases of anaphylaxis following treatment with atovaquone/proguanil have been reported.
MALARONE is contraindicated for prophylaxis of *P. falciparum* malaria in patients with severe renal impairment (creatinine clearance <30 mL/min) (see CLINICAL PHARMACOLOGY: Special Populations: Renal Impairment).

PRECAUTIONS

General

MALARONE has not been evaluated for the treatment of cerebral malaria or other severe manifestations of complicated malaria, including hyperparasitemia, pulmonary edema, or renal failure. Patients with severe malaria are not candidates for oral therapy.
Elevated liver function tests and rare cases of hepatitis have been reported with prophylactic use of MALARONE. A single case of hepatic failure requiring liver transplantation has also been reported with prophylactic use.
Absorption of atovaquone may be reduced in patients with diarrhea or vomiting. If MALARONE is used in patients who are vomiting (see DOSAGE AND ADMINISTRATION), parasitemia should be closely monitored and the use of an antiemetic considered. Vomiting occurred in up to 19% of pediatric patients given treatment doses of MALARONE. In the controlled clinical trials of MALARONE, 15.3% of adults who were treated with atovaquone/proguanil received an antiemetic drug during that part of the trial when they received atovaquone/proguanil. Of these patients, 98.3% were successfully treated. In patients with severe or persistent diarrhea or vomiting, alternative antimalarial therapy may be required.
Parasite relapse occurred commonly when *P. vivax* malaria was treated with MALARONE alone.
In the event of recrudescent *P. falciparum* infections after treatment with MALARONE or failure of chemoprophylaxis with MALARONE, patients should be treated with a different blood schizonticide.

Information for Patients

Patients should be instructed:
• to take MALARONE tablets at the same time each day with food or a milky drink.
• to take a repeat dose of MALARONE if vomiting occurs within 1 hour after dosing.

• to take a dose as soon as possible if a dose is missed, then return to their normal dosing schedule. However, if a dose is skipped, the patient should not double the next dose.
• that rare serious adverse events such as hepatitis, severe skin reactions, neurological, and hematological events have been reported when MALARONE was used for the prophylaxis or treatment of malaria.
• to consult a healthcare professional regarding alternative forms of prophylaxis if prophylaxis with MALARONE is prematurely discontinued for any reason.
• that protective clothing, insect repellents, and bednets are important components of malaria prophylaxis.
• that no chemoprophylactic regimen is 100% effective; therefore, patients should seek medical attention for any febrile illness that occurs during or after return from a malaria-endemic area and inform their healthcare professional that they may have been exposed to malaria.
• that falciparum malaria carries a higher risk of death and serious complications in pregnant women than in the general population. Pregnant women anticipating travel to malarious areas should discuss the risks and benefits of such travel with their physicians (see Pregnancy section).

Drug Interactions

Concomitant treatment with **tetracycline** has been associated with approximately a 40% reduction in plasma concentrations of atovaquone. Parasitemia should be closely monitored in patients receiving tetracycline. While antiemetics may be indicated for patients receiving MALARONE, **metoclopramide** may reduce the bioavailability of atovaquone and should be used only if other antiemetics are not available.
Concomitant administration of **rifampin** or **rifabutin** is known to reduce atovaquone levels by approximately 50% and 34%, respectively. The concomitant administration of MALARONE and rifampin or rifabutin is not recommended. Proguanil may potentiate the anticoagulant effect of warfarin and other coumarin-based anticoagulants. The mechanism of this potential drug interaction has not been established. Caution is advised when initiating or withdrawing malaria prophylaxis or treatment with MALARONE in patients on continuous treatment with coumarin-based anticoagulants. When these products are administered concomitantly, suitable coagulation tests should be closely monitored.
Atovaquone is highly protein bound (>99%) but does not displace other highly protein-bound drugs in vitro, indicating significant drug interactions arising from displacement are unlikely.
Potential interactions between proguanil or cycloguanil and other drugs that are CYP2C19 substrates or inhibitors are unknown.

Carcinogenesis, Mutagenesis, Impairment of Fertility

Atovaquone

Carcinogenicity studies in rats were negative; 24-month studies in mice showed treatment-related increases in incidence of hepatocellular adenoma and hepatocellular carcinoma at all doses tested which ranged from approximately 5 to 8 times the average steady-state plasma concentrations in humans during prophylaxis of malaria. Atovaquone was negative with or without metabolic activation in the Ames *Salmonella* mutagenicity assay, the Mouse Lymphoma mutagenesis assay, and the Cultured Human Lymphocyte cytogenetic assay. No evidence of genotoxicity was observed in the in vivo Mouse Micronucleus assay.

Proguanil

No evidence of a carcinogenic effect was observed in 24-month studies conducted in CD-1 mice (doses up to 1.5 times the average systemic human exposure based on AUC) and in Wistar Hannover rats (doses up to 1.1 times the average systemic human exposure).

Proguanil was negative with or without metabolic activation in the Ames *Salmonella* mutagenicity assay and the Mouse Lymphoma mutagenesis assay. No evidence of genotoxicity was observed in the in vivo Mouse Micronucleus assay.

Cycloguanil, the active metabolite of proguanil, was also negative in the Ames test, but was positive in the Mouse Lymphoma assay and the Mouse Micronucleus assay. These positive effects with cycloguanil, a dihydrofolate reductase inhibitor, were significantly reduced or abolished with folinic acid supplementation.

A fertility study in Sprague-Dawley rats revealed no adverse effects at doses up to 16 mg/kg/day of proguanil hydrochloride (up to 0.2-times the average human exposure based on AUC comparisons.) Fertility studies of proguanil in animals at exposures similar to or greater than those observed in humans have not been conducted.

Genotoxicity studies have not been performed with atovaquone in combination with proguanil. Effects of MALARONE on male and female reproductive performance are unknown.

Pregnancy

Pregnancy Category C. Falciparum malaria carries a higher risk of morbidity and mortality in pregnant women than in the general population. Maternal death and fetal loss are both known complications of falciparum malaria in pregnancy. In pregnant women who must travel to malaria-endemic areas, personal protection against mosquito bites should always be employed (see Information for Patients) in addition to antimalarials.

Atovaquone was not teratogenic and did not cause reproductive toxicity in rats at maternal plasma concentrations up to 5 to 6.5 times the estimated human exposure during treatment of malaria. Following single-dose administration of ^{14}C-labeled atovaquone to pregnant rats, concentrations of radiolabel in rat fetuses were 18% (mid-gestation) and 60% (late gestation) of concurrent maternal plasma concentrations. In rabbits, atovaquone caused maternal toxicity at plasma concentrations that were approximately 0.6 to 1.3 times the estimated human exposure during treatment of malaria. Adverse fetal effects in rabbits, including decreased fetal body lengths and increased early resorptions and post-implantation losses, were observed only in the presence of maternal toxicity. Concentrations of atovaquone in rabbit fetuses averaged 30% of the concurrent maternal plasma concentrations.

A pre- and post-natal study in Sprague-Dawley rats revealed no adverse effects at doses up to 16 mg/kg/day of proguanil hydrochloride (up to 0.2-times the average human exposure based on AUC comparisons). Pre- and post-natal studies of proguanil in animals at exposures similar to or greater than those observed in humans have not been conducted.

The combination of atovaquone and proguanil hydrochloride was not teratogenic in rats at plasma concentrations up to 1.7 and 0.10 times, respectively, the estimated human exposure during treatment of malaria. In rabbits, the combination of atovaquone and proguanil hydrochloride was not teratogenic or embryotoxic to rabbit fetuses at plasma concentrations up to 0.34 and 0.82 times, respectively, the estimated human exposure during treatment of malaria.

While there are no adequate and well-controlled studies of atovaquone and/or proguanil hydrochloride in pregnant women, MALARONE may be used if the potential benefit justifies the potential risk to the fetus. The proguanil component of MALARONE acts by inhibiting the parasitic dihydrofolate reductase (see CLINICAL PHARMACOLOGY: Microbiology: Mechanism of Action). However, there are no clinical data indicating that folate supplementation diminishes drug efficacy, and for women of childbearing age receiving folate supplements to prevent neural tube birth defects, such supplements may be continued while taking MALARONE.

Nursing Mothers

It is not known whether atovaquone is excreted into human milk. In a rat study, atovaquone concentrations in the milk were 30% of the concurrent atovaquone concentrations in the maternal plasma.

Proguanil is excreted into human milk in small quantities. Caution should be exercised when MALARONE is administered to a nursing woman.

Pediatric Use

Treatment of Malaria

The efficacy and safety of MALARONE for the treatment of malaria have been established in controlled studies involving pediatric patients weighing 5 kg or more (see CLINICAL STUDIES). Safety and effectiveness have not been established in pediatric patients who weigh less than 5 kg.

Prophylaxis of Malaria

The efficacy and safety of MALARONE have been established for the prophylaxis of malaria in controlled studies involving pediatric patients weighing 11 kg or more (see CLINICAL STUDIES). Safety and effectiveness have not been established in pediatric patients who weigh less than 11 kg.

Geriatric Use

Clinical studies of MALARONE did not include sufficient numbers of subjects aged 65 and over to determine whether they respond differently from younger subjects. In general, dose selection for an elderly patient should be cautious, reflecting the greater frequency of decreased hepatic, renal, or cardiac function, the higher systemic exposure to cycloguanil (see CLINICAL PHARMACOLOGY: Special Populations: Geriatrics), and the greater frequency of concomitant disease or other drug therapy.

ADVERSE REACTIONS

Because MALARONE contains atovaquone and proguanil hydrochloride, the type and severity of adverse reactions associated with each of the compounds may be expected. The higher treatment doses of MALARONE were less well tolerated than the lower prophylactic doses.

Among adults who received MALARONE for treatment of malaria, attributable adverse experiences that occurred in ≥5% of patients were abdominal pain (17%), nausea (12%), vomiting (12%), headache (10%), diarrhea (8%), asthenia (8%), anorexia (5%), and dizziness (5%). Treatment was discontinued prematurely due to an adverse experience in 4 of 436 adults treated with MALARONE.

Among pediatric patients (weighing 11 to 40 kg) who received MALARONE for the treatment of malaria, attributable adverse experiences that occurred in ≥5% of patients were vomiting (10%) and pruritus (6%). Vomiting occurred in 43 of 319 (13%) pediatric patients who did not have symptomatic malaria but were given treatment doses of MALARONE for 3 days in a clinical trial. The design of this clinical trial required that any patient who vomited be withdrawn from the trial. Among pediatric patients with symptomatic malaria treated with MALARONE, treatment was discontinued prematurely due to an adverse experience in 1 of 116 (0.9%).

In a study of 100 pediatric patients (5 to <11 kg body weight) who received MALARONE for the treatment of uncomplicated *P. falciparum* malaria, only diarrhea (6%) occurred in ≥5% of patients as an adverse experience attributable to MALARONE. In 3 patients (3%), treatment was discontinued prematurely due to an adverse experience.

Abnormalities in laboratory tests reported in clinical trials were limited to elevations of transaminases in malaria patients being treated with MALARONE. The frequency of these abnormalities varied substantially across studies of treatment and were not observed in the randomized portions of the prophylaxis trials.

In one phase III trial of malaria treatment in Thai adults, early elevations of ALT and AST were observed to occur more frequently in patients treated with MALARONE compared to patients treated with an active control drug. Rates for patients who had normal baseline levels of these clinical laboratory parameters were: Day 7: ALT 26.7% vs. 15.6%; AST 16.9% vs. 8.6%. By day 14 of this 28-day study, the frequency of transaminase elevations equalized across the 2 groups.

In this and other studies in which transaminase elevations occurred, they were noted to persist for up to 4 weeks following treatment with MALARONE for malaria. None were associated with untoward clinical events.

Among subjects who received MALARONE for prophylaxis of malaria in placebo-controlled trials, adverse experiences occurred in similar proportions of subjects receiving MALARONE or placebo (Table 3). The most commonly reported adverse experiences possibly attributable to MALARONE or placebo were headache and abdominal pain. Prophylaxis with MALARONE was discontinued prematurely due to a treatment-related adverse experience in 3 of 381 adults and 0 of 125 pediatric patients.

[See table 3 at left]

Table 3. Adverse Experiences in Placebo-Controlled Clinical Trials of MALARONE for Prophylaxis of Malaria

Adverse Experience	Percent of Subjects With Adverse Experiences (Percent of Subjects With Adverse Experiences Attributable to Therapy)									
	Adults						Children and Adolescents			
	Placebo n = 206		MALARONE* n = 206		MALARONE† n = 381		Placebo n = 140		MALARONE n = 125	
Headache	27	(7)	22	(3)	17	(5)	21	(14)	19	(14)
Fever	13	(1)	5	(0)	3	(0)	11	(<1)	6	(0)
Myalgia	11	(0)	12	(0)	7	(0)	0	(0)	0	(0)
Abdominal pain	10	(5)	9	(4)	6	(3)	29	(29)	33	(31)
Cough	8	(<1)	6	(<1)	4	(1)	9	(0)	9	(0)
Diarrhea	8	(3)	6	(2)	4	(1)	3	(1)	2	(0)
Upper respiratory infection	7	(0)	8	(0)	5	(0)	0	(0)	<1	(0)
Dyspepsia	5	(4)	3	(2)	2	(1)	0	(0)	0	(0)
Back pain	4	(0)	8	(0)	4	(0)	0	(0)	0	(0)
Gastritis	3	(2)	3	(3)	2	(2)	0	(0)	0	(0)
Vomiting	2	(<1)	1	(<1)	<1	(<1)	6	(6)	7	(7)
Flu syndrome	1	(0)	2	(0)	4	(0)	6	(0)	9	(0)
Any adverse experience	65	(32)	54	(17)	49	(17)	62	(41)	60	(42)

* Subjects receiving the recommended dose of atovaquone and proguanil hydrochloride in placebo-controlled trials.
† Subjects receiving the recommended dose of atovaquone and proguanil hydrochloride in any trial.

In an additional placebo-controlled study of malaria prophylaxis with MALARONE involving 330 pediatric patients in a malaria-endemic area (see CLINICAL STUDIES), the safety profile of MALARONE was consistent with that described above. The most common treatment-emergent adverse events with MALARONE were abdominal pain (13%), headache (13%), and cough (10%). Abdominal pain (13% vs. 8%) and vomiting (5% vs. 3%) were reported more often with MALARONE than with placebo, while fever (5% vs. 12%) and diarrhea (1% vs. 5%) were more common with placebo. No patient withdrew from the study due to an adverse experience with MALARONE. No routine laboratory data were obtained during this study.

Among subjects who received MALARONE for prophylaxis of malaria in clinical trials with an active comparator, adverse experiences occurred in a similar or lower proportion of subjects receiving MALARONE than an active comparator (Table 4). The mean durations of dosing and the periods for which the adverse experiences are summarized in Table

Table 4. Adverse Experiences in Active-Controlled Clinical Trials of MALARONE for Prophylaxis of Malaria

	Percent of Subjects With Adverse Experiences* (Percent of Subjects With Adverse Experiences Attributable to Therapy)							
	Study 1				Study 2			
Adverse Experience	MALARONE n = 493		Mefloquine n = 483		MALARONE n = 511		Chloroquine plus Proguanil n = 511	
Diarrhea	38	(8)	36	(7)	34	(5)	39	(7)
Nausea	14	(3)	20	(8)	11	(2)	18	(7)
Abdominal pain	17	(5)	16	(5)	14	(3)	22	(6)
Headache	12	(4)	17	(7)	12	(4)	14	(4)
Dreams	7	(7)	16	(14)	6	(4)	7	(3)
Insomnia	5	(3)	16	(13)	4	(2)	5	(2)
Fever	9	(<1)	11	(1)	8	(<1)	8	(<1)
Dizziness	5	(2)	14	(9)	7	(3)	8	(4)
Vomiting	8	(1)	10	(2)	8	(0)	14	(2)
Oral ulcers	9	(6)	6	(4)	5	(4)	7	(5)
Pruritus	4	(2)	5	(2)	3	(1)	2	(<1)
Visual difficulties	2	(2)	5	(3)	3	(2)	3	(2)
Depression	<1	(<1)	5	(4)	<1	(<1)	1	(<1)
Anxiety	1	(<1)	5	(4)	<1	(<1)	1	(<1)
Any adverse experience	64	(30)	69	(42)	58	(22)	66	(28)
Any neuropsychiatric event	20	(14)	37	(29)	16	(10)	20	(10)
Any GI event	49	(16)	50	(19)	43	(12)	54	(20)

*Adverse experiences that started while receiving active study drug.

4, were 28 days (Study 1) and 26 days (Study 2) for MALARONE, 53 days for mefloquine, and 49 days for chloroquine plus proguanil (reflecting the different recommended dosing regimens). Fewer neuropsychiatric adverse experiences occurred in subjects who received MALARONE than mefloquine. Fewer gastrointestinal adverse experiences occurred in subjects receiving MALARONE than chloroquine/proguanil. Compared with active comparator drugs, subjects receiving MALARONE had fewer adverse experiences overall that were attributed to prophylactic therapy (Table 4). Prophylaxis with MALARONE was discontinued prematurely due to a treatment-related adverse experience in 7 of 1,004 travelers.

[See table 4 above]

In a third active-controlled study, MALARONE (n = 110) was compared with chloroquine/proguanil (n = 111) for the prophylaxis of malaria in 221 non-immune pediatric patients (see CLINICAL STUDIES). The mean duration of exposure was 23 days for MALARONE, 46 days for chloroquine, and 43 days for proguanil, reflecting the different recommended dosage regimens for these products. Fewer patients treated with MALARONE reported abdominal pain (2% vs. 7%) or nausea (<1% vs. 7%) than children who received chloroquine/proguanil. Oral ulceration (2% vs. 2%), vivid dreams (2% vs. <1%), and blurred vision (0% vs. 2%) occurred in similar proportions of patients receiving either MALARONE or chloroquine/proguanil, respectively. Two patients discontinued prophylaxis with chloroquine/proguanil due to adverse events, while none of those receiving MALARONE discontinued due to adverse events.

Post-Marketing Adverse Reactions

In addition to adverse events reported from clinical trials, the following events have been identified during world-wide post-approval use of MALARONE. Because they are reported voluntarily from a population of unknown size, estimates of frequency cannot be made. These events have been chosen for inclusion due to a combination of their seriousness, frequency of reporting, or potential causal connection to MALARONE.

Blood and Lymphatic System Disorders

Neutropenia and rarely anemia. Pancytopenia in patients with severe renal impairment treated with proguanil.

Immune System Disorders

Allergic reactions including angioedema, urticaria, and rare cases of anaphylaxis and vasculitis.

Nervous System Disorders

Rare cases of seizures and psychotic events (such as hallucinations); however, a causal relationship has not been established.

Gastrointestinal Disorders

Stomatitis.

Hepatobiliary Disorders

Elevated liver function tests and rare cases of hepatitis, cholestasis; a single case of hepatic failure requiring transplant has been reported.

Skin and Subcutaneous Tissue Disorders

Photosensitivity, rash, and rare cases of erythema multiforme and Stevens-Johnson syndrome.

OVERDOSAGE

There is no information on overdoses of MALARONE substantially higher than the doses recommended for treatment.

There is no known antidote for atovaquone, and it is currently unknown if atovaquone is dialyzable. The median lethal dose is higher than the maximum oral dose tested in mice and rats (1,825 mg/kg/day). Overdoses up to 31,500 mg of atovaquone have been reported. In one such patient who also took an unspecified dose of dapsone, methemoglobinemia occurred. Rash has also been reported after overdose. Overdoses of proguanil hydrochloride as large as 1,500 mg have been followed by complete recovery, and doses as high as 700 mg twice daily have been taken for over 2 weeks without serious toxicity. Adverse experiences occasionally associated with proguanil hydrochloride doses of 100 to 200 mg/day, such as epigastric discomfort and vomiting, would be likely to occur with overdose. There are also reports of reversible hair loss and scaling of the skin on the palms and/or soles, reversible aphthous ulceration, and hematologic side effects.

DOSAGE AND ADMINISTRATION

The daily dose should be taken at the same time each day with food or a milky drink. In the event of vomiting within 1 hour after dosing, a repeat dose should be taken.

Prevention of Malaria

Prophylactic treatment with MALARONE should be started 1 or 2 days before entering a malaria-endemic area and continued daily during the stay and for 7 days after return.

Adults

One MALARONE Tablet (adult strength = 250 mg atovaquone/100 mg proguanil hydrochloride) per day.

Pediatric Patients

The dosage for prevention of malaria in pediatric patients is based upon body weight (Table 5).

Table 5. Dosage for Prevention of Malaria in Pediatric Patients

Weight (kg)	Atovaquone/ Proguanil HCl Total Daily Dose	Dosage Regimen
11-20	62.5 mg/25 mg	1 MALARONE Pediatric Tablet daily
21-30	125 mg/50 mg	2 MALARONE Pediatric Tablets as a single dose daily
31-40	187.5 mg/75 mg	3 MALARONE Pediatric Tablets as a single dose daily
>40	250 mg/100 mg	1 MALARONE Tablet (adult strength) as a single dose daily

Treatment of Acute Malaria

Adults

Four MALARONE Tablets (adult strength; total daily dose 1 g atovaquone/400 mg proguanil hydrochloride) as a single dose for 3 consecutive days.

Pediatric Patients

The dosage for treatment of acute malaria in pediatric patients is based upon body weight (Table 6).

Table 6. Dosage for Treatment of Acute Malaria in Pediatric Patients

Weight (kg)	Atovaquone/ Proguanil HCl Total Daily Dose	Dosage Regimen
5-8	125 mg/50 mg	2 MALARONE Pediatric Tablets daily for 3 consecutive days
9-10	187.5 mg/75 mg	3 MALARONE Pediatric Tablets daily for 3 consecutive days
11-20	250 mg/100 mg	1 MALARONE Tablet (adult strength) daily for 3 consecutive days
21-30	500 mg/200 mg	2 MALARONE Tablets (adult strength) as a single dose daily for 3 consecutive days
31-40	750 mg/300 mg	3 MALARONE Tablets (adult strength) as a single dose daily for 3 consecutive days
>40	1 g/400 mg	4 MALARONE Tablets (adult strength) as a single dose daily for 3 consecutive days

MALARONE Tablets may be crushed and mixed with condensed milk just prior to administration for children who may have difficulty swallowing tablets.

Patients With Renal Impairment

MALARONE should not be used for malaria prophylaxis in patients with severe renal impairment (creatinine clearance <30 mL/min). MALARONE may be used with caution for the treatment of malaria in patients with severe renal impairment (creatinine clearance <30 mL/min), only if the benefits of the 3-day treatment regimen outweigh the potential risks associated with increased drug exposure (see CLINICAL PHARMACOLOGY: Special Populations: Renal Impairment). No dosage adjustments are needed in patients with mild (creatinine clearance 50 to 80 mL/min) and moderate (creatinine clearance 30 to 50 mL/min) renal impairment (see CLINICAL PHARMACOLOGY: Special Populations).

Patients With Hepatic Impairment

No dosage adjustments are needed in patients with mild to moderate hepatic impairment. No studies have been conducted in patients with severe hepatic impairment (see CLINICAL PHARMACOLOGY: Special Populations: Hepatic Impairment).

Table 7. Parasitological Response in Clinical Trials of MALARONE for Treatment of P. falciparum Malaria

Study Site	MALARONE*		Comparator			
	Evaluable Patients (n)	% Sensitive Response[†]	Drug(s)	Evaluable Patients (n)	% Sensitive Response[†]	
Brazil	74	98.6%	Quinine and tetracycline	76	100.0%	
Thailand	79	100.0%	Mefloquine	79	86.1%	
France[‡]	21	100.0%	Halofantrine	18	100.0%	
Kenya[‡,§]	81	93.8%	Halofantrine	83	90.4%	
Zambia	80	100.0%	Pyrimethamine/sulfadoxine (P/S)	80	98.8%	
Gabon[‡]	63	98.4%	Amodiaquine	63	81.0%	
Philippines	54	100.0%	Chloroquine (Cq) Cq and P/S	23 32	30.4% 87.5%	
Peru	19	100.0%	Chloroquine P/S	13 7	7.7% 100.0%	

* MALARONE = 1,000 mg atovaquone and 400 mg proguanil hydrochloride (or equivalent based on body weight for patients weighing ≤40 kg) once daily for 3 days.
[†] Elimination of parasitemia with no recurrent parasitemia during follow-up for 28 days.
[‡] Patients hospitalized only for acute care. Follow-up conducted in outpatients.
[§] Study in pediatric patients 3 to 12 years of age.

Table 9. Prevention of Parasitemia in Active-Controlled Clinical Trials of MALARONE for Prophylaxis of P. falciparum Malaria in Non-Immune Travelers

Total number of randomized patients who received study drug	MALARONE	Mefloquine	Chloroquine plus Proguanil
	1,004	483	511
Failed to complete study	14	6	4
Developed parasitemia (P. falciparum)	0	0	3

HOW SUPPLIED

MALARONE Tablets, containing 250 mg atovaquone and 100 mg proguanil hydrochloride, are pink, film-coated, round, biconvex tablets engraved with "GX CM3" on one side.
Bottle of 100 tablets with child-resistant closure (NDC 0173-0675-01).
Unit Dose Pack of 24 (NDC 0173-0675-02).
MALARONE Pediatric Tablets, containing 62.5 mg atovaquone and 25 mg proguanil hydrochloride, are pink, film-coated, round, biconvex tablets engraved with "GX CG7" on one side.
Bottle of 100 tablets with child-resistant closure (NDC 0173-0676-01).
Store at 25°C (77°F); excursions permitted to 15° to 30°C (59° to 86°F) (see USP Controlled Room Temperature).

ANIMAL TOXICOLOGY

Fibrovascular proliferation in the right atrium, pyelonephritis, bone marrow hypocellularity, lymphoid atrophy, and gastritis/enteritis were observed in dogs treated with proguanil hydrochloride for 6 months at a dose of 12 mg/kg/day (approximately 3.9 times the recommended daily human dose for malaria prophylaxis on a mg/m² basis). Bile duct hyperplasia, gall bladder mucosal atrophy, and interstitial pneumonia were observed in dogs treated with proguanil hydrochloride for 6 months at a dose of 4 mg/kg/day (approximately 1.3 times the recommended daily human dose for malaria prophylaxis on a mg/m² basis). Mucosal hyperplasia of the cecum and renal tubular basophilia were observed in rats treated with proguanil hydrochloride for 6 months at a dose of 20 mg/kg/day (approximately 1.6 times the recommended daily human dose for malaria prophylaxis on a mg/m² basis). Adverse heart, lung, liver, and gall bladder effects observed in dogs and kidney effects observed in rats were not shown to be reversible.

CLINICAL STUDIES
Treatment of Acute Malarial Infections

In 3 phase II clinical trials, atovaquone alone, proguanil hydrochloride alone, and the combination of atovaquone and proguanil hydrochloride were evaluated for the treatment of acute, uncomplicated malaria caused by P. falciparum. Among 156 evaluable patients, the parasitological cure rate was 59/89 (66%) with atovaquone alone, 1/17 (6%) with proguanil hydrochloride alone, and 50/50 (100%) with the combination of atovaquone and proguanil hydrochloride.

MALARONE was evaluated for treatment of acute, uncomplicated malaria caused by P. falciparum in 8 phase III controlled clinical trials. Among 471 evaluable patients treated with the equivalent of 4 MALARONE Tablets once daily for 3 days, 464 had a sensitive response (elimination of parasitemia with no recurrent parasitemia during follow-up for 28 days) (see Table 7). Seven patients had a response of RI resistance (elimination of parasitemia but with recurrent parasitemia between 7 and 28 days after starting treatment). In these trials, the response to treatment with MALARONE was similar to treatment with the comparator drug in 4 trials, and better than the response to treatment with the comparator drug in the other 4 trials.
The overall efficacy in 521 evaluable patients was 98.7% (Table 7).
[See table 7 above]
Eighteen of 521 (3.5%) evaluable patients with acute falciparum malaria presented with a pretreatment serum creatinine greater than 2.0 mg/dL (range 2.1 to 4.3 mg/dL). All were successfully treated with MALARONE and 17 of 18 (94.4%) had normal serum creatinine levels by day 7.
Data from a phase II trial of atovaquone conducted in Zambia suggested that approximately 40% of the study population in this country were HIV-infected patients. The enrollment criteria were similar for the phase III trial of MALARONE conducted in Zambia and the results are presented in Table 7. Efficacy rates for MALARONE in this study population were high and comparable to other populations studied.
The efficacy of MALARONE in the treatment of the erythrocytic phase of nonfalciparum malaria was assessed in a small number of patients. Of the 23 patients in Thailand infected with P. vivax and treated with atovaquone/proguanil hydrochloride 1,000 mg/400 mg daily for 3 days, parasitemia cleared in 21 (91.3%) at 7 days. Parasite relapse occurred commonly when P. vivax malaria was treated with MALARONE alone. Seven patients in Gabon with malaria due to P. ovale or P. malariae were treated with atovaquone/proguanil hydrochloride 1,000 mg/400 mg daily for 3 days. All 6 evaluable patients (3 with P. malariae, 2 with P. ovale, and 1 with mixed P. falciparum and P. ovale) were cured at 28 days. Relapsing malarias including P. vivax and P. ovale require additional treatment to prevent relapse.
The efficacy of MALARONE in treating acute uncomplicated P. falciparum malaria in children weighing ≥5 and <11 kg was examined in an open-label, randomized trial conducted in Gabon. Patients received either MALARONE

(2 or 3 MALARONE Pediatric Tablets once daily depending upon body weight) for 3 days (n = 100) or amodiaquine (10 mg/kg/day) for 3 days (n = 100). In this study, the MALARONE Tablets were crushed and mixed with condensed milk just prior to administration. In the per-protocol population, adequate clinical response was obtained in 95% (87/92) of the pediatric patients who received MALARONE and in 53% (41/78) of those who received amodiaquine. A response of RI resistance (elimination of parasitemia but with recurrent parasitemia between 7 and 28 days after starting treatment) was noted in 3% and 40% of the patients, respectively. Two cases of RIII resistance (rising parasite count despite therapy) were reported in the patients receiving MALARONE. There were 4 cases of RIII in the amodiaquine arm.

Prevention of Malaria

MALARONE was evaluated for prophylaxis of malaria in 5 clinical trials in malaria-endemic areas and in 3 active-controlled trials in non-immune travelers to malaria-endemic areas.
Three placebo-controlled studies of 10 to 12 weeks' duration were conducted among residents of malaria-endemic areas in Kenya, Zambia, and Gabon. Of a total of 669 randomized patients (including 264 pediatric patients 5 to 16 years of age), 103 were withdrawn for reasons other than falciparum malaria or drug-related adverse events. (Fifty-five percent of these were lost to follow-up and 45% were withdrawn for protocol violations.) The results are listed in Table 8.

Table 8. Prevention of Parasitemia in Placebo-Controlled Clinical Trials of MALARONE for Prophylaxis of P. falciparum Malaria in Residents of Malaria-Endemic Areas

Total number of patients randomized	MALARONE	Placebo
	326	341
Failed to complete study	57	44
Developed parasitemia (P. falciparum)	2	92

In another study, 330 Gabonese pediatric patients (weighing 13 to 40 kg, and aged 4 to 14 years) who had received successful open-label radical cure treatment with artesunate, were randomized to receive either MALARONE (dosage based on body weight) or placebo in a double-blind fashion for 12 weeks. Blood smears were obtained weekly and any time malaria was suspected. Nineteen of the 165 children given MALARONE and 18 of 165 patients given placebo withdrew from the study for reasons other than parasitemia (primary reason was lost to follow-up). In the per-protocol population, 1 out of 150 patients (<1%) who received MALARONE developed P. falciparum parasitemia while receiving prophylaxis with MALARONE compared with 31 (22%) of the 144 placebo recipients.
In a 10-week study in 175 South African subjects who moved into malaria-endemic areas and were given prophylaxis with 1 MALARONE Tablet daily, parasitemia developed in 1 subject who missed several doses of medication. Since no placebo control was included, the incidence of malaria in this study was not known.
Two active-controlled studies were conducted in non-immune travelers who visited a malaria-endemic area. The mean duration of travel was 18 days (range 2 to 38 days). Of a total of 1,998 randomized patients who received MALARONE or controlled drug, 24 discontinued from the study before follow-up evaluation 60 days after leaving the endemic area. Nine of these were lost to follow-up, 2 withdrew because of an adverse experience, and 13 were discontinued for other reasons. These studies were not large enough to allow for statements of comparative efficacy. In addition, the true exposure rate to P. falciparum malaria in both studies is unknown. The results are listed in Table 9.
[See table 9 above]
A third randomized, open-label study was conducted which included 221 otherwise healthy pediatric patients (weighing ≥11 kg and 2 to 17 years of age) who were at risk of contracting malaria by traveling to an endemic area. The mean duration of travel was 15 days (range 1 to 30 days). Prophylaxis with MALARONE (n = 110, dosage based on body weight) began 1 or 2 days before entering the endemic area and lasted until 7 days after leaving the area. A control group (n = 111) received prophylaxis with chloroquine/proguanil dosed according to WHO guidelines. No cases of malaria occurred in either group of children. However, the study was not large enough to allow for statements of comparative efficacy. In addition, the true exposure rate to P. falciparum malaria in this study is unknown.
In a malaria challenge study conducted in healthy US volunteers, atovaquone alone prevented malaria in 6 of 6 individuals, whereas 4 of 4 placebo-treated volunteers developed malaria.

Causal Prophylaxis

In separate studies with small numbers of volunteers, atovaquone and proguanil hydrochloride were independently shown to have causal prophylactic activity directed against liver-stage parasites of *P. falciparum*. Six patients given a single dose of atovaquone 250 mg 24 hours prior to malaria challenge were protected from developing malaria, whereas all 4 placebo-treated patients developed malaria. During the 4 weeks following cessation of prophylaxis in clinical trial participants who remained in malaria-endemic areas and were available for evaluation, malaria developed in 24 of 211 (11.4%) subjects who took placebo and 9 of 328 (2.7%) who took MALARONE. While new infections could not be distinguished from recrudescent infections, all but 1 of the infections in patients treated with MALARONE occurred more than 15 days after stopping therapy, probably representing new infections. The single case occurring on day 8 following cessation of therapy with MALARONE probably represents a failure of prophylaxis with MALARONE.

The possibility that delayed cases of *P. falciparum* malaria may occur some time after stopping prophylaxis with MALARONE cannot be ruled out. Hence, returning travelers developing febrile illnesses should be investigated for malaria.

GlaxoSmithKline
Research Triangle Park, NC 27709
©2009, GlaxoSmithKline. All rights reserved.
September 2009   MLR:4PI

MEPRON®
[mĕ′prŏn]
(atovaquone)
Suspension

℞

DESCRIPTION

MEPRON (atovaquone) is an antiprotozoal agent. The chemical name of atovaquone is *trans*-2-[4-(4-chlorophenyl) cyclohexyl]-3-hydroxy-1,4-naphthalenedione. Atovaquone is a yellow crystalline solid that is practically insoluble in water. It has a molecular weight of 366.84 and the molecular formula $C_{22}H_{19}ClO_3$. The compound has the following structural formula:

MEPRON Suspension is a formulation of micro-fine particles of atovaquone. The atovaquone particles, reduced in size to facilitate absorption, are significantly smaller than those in the previously marketed tablet formulation. MEPRON Suspension is for oral administration and is bright yellow with a citrus flavor. Each teaspoonful (5 mL) contains 750 mg of atovaquone and the inactive ingredients benzyl alcohol, flavor, poloxamer 188, purified water, saccharin sodium, and xanthan gum.

MICROBIOLOGY
Mechanism of Action

Atovaquone is a hydroxy-1,4-naphthoquinone, an analog of ubiquinone, with antipneumocystis activity. The mechanism of action against *Pneumocystis carinii* has not been fully elucidated. In *Plasmodium* species, the site of action appears to be the cytochrome bc_1 complex (Complex III). Several metabolic enzymes are linked to the mitochondrial electron transport chain via ubiquinone. Inhibition of electron transport by atovaquone will result in indirect inhibition of these enzymes. The ultimate metabolic effects of such blockade may include inhibition of nucleic acid and ATP synthesis.

Activity In Vitro

Several laboratories, using different in vitro methodologies, have shown the IC_{50} (50% inhibitory concentration) of atovaquone against rat *P. carinii* to be in the range of 0.1 to 3.0 mcg/mL.

Drug Resistance

Phenotypic resistance to atovaquone in vitro has not been demonstrated for *P. carinii*. However, in 2 patients who developed *P. carinii* pneumonia (PCP) after prophylaxis with atovaquone, DNA sequence analysis identified mutations in the predicted amino acid sequence of *P. carinii* cytochrome b (a likely target site for atovaquone). The clinical significance of this is unknown.

CLINICAL PHARMACOLOGY
Pharmacokinetics
Absorption

Atovaquone is a highly lipophilic compound with low aqueous solubility. The bioavailability of atovaquone is highly dependent on formulation and diet. The suspension formulation provides an approximately 2-fold increase in atovaquone bioavailability in the fasting or fed state compared to the previously marketed tablet formulation. The absolute bioavailability of a 750-mg dose of MEPRON Suspension administered under fed conditions in 9 HIV-infected (CD4 >100 cells/mm³) volunteers was 47% ± 15%. In the same study, the bioavailability of a 750-mg dose of the previously marketed tablet formulation was 23% ± 11%. Administering atovaquone with food enhances its absorption by approximately 2 fold. In one study, 16 healthy volunteers received a single dose of 750 mg MEPRON Suspension after an overnight fast and following a standard breakfast (23 g fat: 610 kCal). The mean (±SD) area under the concentration-time curve (AUC) values were 324 ± 115 and 801 ± 320 hr•mcg/mL under fasting and fed conditions, respectively, representing a 2.6 ± 1.0-fold increase. The effect of food (23 g fat: 400 kCal) on plasma atovaquone concentrations was also evaluated in a multiple-dose, randomized, crossover study in 19 HIV-infected volunteers (CD4 <200 cells/mm³) receiving daily doses of 500 mg MEPRON Suspension. AUC was 280 ± 114 hr•mcg/mL when atovaquone was administered with food as compared to 169 ± 77 hr•mcg/mL under fasting conditions. Maximum plasma atovaquone concentration (C_{max}) was 15.1 ± 6.1 and 8.8 ± 3.7 mcg/mL when atovaquone was administered with food and under fasting conditions, respectively.

Dose Proportionality

Plasma atovaquone concentrations do not increase proportionally with dose. When MEPRON Suspension was administered with food at dosage regimens of 500 mg once daily, 750 mg once daily, and 1,000 mg once daily, average steady-state plasma atovaquone concentrations were 11.7 ± 4.8, 12.5 ± 5.8, and 13.5 ± 5.1 mcg/mL, respectively. The corresponding C_{max} concentrations were 15.1 ± 6.1, 15.3 ± 7.6, and 16.8 ± 6.4 mcg/mL. When MEPRON Suspension was administered to 5 HIV-infected volunteers at a dose of 750 mg twice daily, the average steady-state plasma atovaquone concentration was 21.0 ± 4.9 mcg/mL and C_{max} was 24.0 ± 5.7 mcg/mL. The minimum plasma atovaquone concentration (C_{min}) associated with the 750-mg twice-daily regimen was 16.7 ± 4.6 mcg/mL.

Distribution

Following the intravenous administration of atovaquone, the volume of distribution at steady state (Vd_{ss}) was 0.60 ± 0.17 L/kg (n = 9). Atovaquone is extensively bound to plasma proteins (99.9%) over the concentration range of 1 to 90 mcg/mL. In 3 HIV-infected children who received 750 mg atovaquone as the tablet formulation 4 times daily for 2 weeks, the cerebrospinal fluid concentrations of atovaquone were 0.04, 0.14, and 0.26 mcg/mL, representing less than 1% of the plasma concentration.

Elimination

The plasma clearance of atovaquone following intravenous (IV) administration in 9 HIV-infected volunteers was 10.4 ± 5.5 mL/min (0.15 ± 0.09 mL/min/kg). The half-life of atovaquone was 62.5 ± 35.3 hours after IV administration and ranged from 67.0 ± 33.4 to 77.6 ± 23.1 hours across studies following administration of MEPRON Suspension. The half-life of atovaquone is long due to presumed enterohepatic cycling and eventual fecal elimination. In a study where ¹⁴C-labelled atovaquone was administered to healthy volunteers, greater than 94% of the dose was recovered as unchanged atovaquone in the feces over 21 days. There was little or no excretion of atovaquone in the urine (less than 0.6%). There is indirect evidence that atovaquone may undergo limited metabolism; however, a specific metabolite has not been identified.

Special Populations
Pediatrics

In a study of MEPRON Suspension in 27 HIV-infected, asymptomatic infants and children between 1 month and 13 years of age, the pharmacokinetics of atovaquone were age dependent. These patients were dosed once daily with food for 12 days. The average steady-state plasma atovaquone concentrations in the 24 patients with available concentration data are shown in Table 1.
[See table 1 above]

Hepatic/Renal Impairment

The pharmacokinetics of atovaquone have not been studied in patients with hepatic or renal impairment.

Drug Interactions
Rifampin

In a study with 13 HIV-infected volunteers, the oral administration of rifampin 600 mg every 24 hours with MEPRON Suspension 750 mg every 12 hours resulted in a 52% ± 13% decrease in the average steady-state plasma atovaquone concentration and a 37% ± 42% increase in the average steady-state plasma rifampin concentration. The half-life of atovaquone decreased from 82 ± 36 hours when administered without rifampin to 50 ± 16 hours with rifampin. Rifabutin, another rifamycin, is structurally similar to rifampin and may possibly have some of the same drug interactions as rifampin. No interaction trials have been conducted with MEPRON and rifabutin.

Trimethoprim/Sulfamethoxazole (TMP-SMX)

The possible interaction between atovaquone and TMP-SMX was evaluated in 6 HIV-infected adult volunteers as part of a larger multiple-dose, dose-escalation, and chronic dosing study of MEPRON Suspension. In this crossover study, MEPRON Suspension 500 mg once daily, or TMP-SMX tablets (160 mg trimethoprim and 800 mg sulfamethoxazole) twice daily, or the combination were administered with food to achieve steady state. No difference was observed in the average steady-state plasma atovaquone concentration after coadministration with TMP-SMX. Coadministration of MEPRON with TMP-SMX resulted in a 17% and 8% decrease in average steady-state concentrations of trimethoprim and sulfamethoxazole in plasma, respectively. This effect is minor and would not be expected to produce clinically significant events.

Zidovudine

Data from 14 HIV-infected volunteers who were given atovaquone tablets 750 mg every 12 hours with zidovudine 200 mg every 8 hours showed a 24% ± 12% decrease in zidovudine apparent oral clearance, leading to a 35% ± 23% increase in plasma zidovudine AUC. The glucuronide metabolite:parent ratio decreased from a mean of 4.5 when zidovudine was administered alone to 3.1 when zidovudine was administered with atovaquone tablets. This effect is minor and would not be expected to produce clinically significant events. Zidovudine had no effect on atovaquone pharmacokinetics.

Relationship Between Plasma Atovaquone Concentration and Clinical Outcome

In a comparative study of atovaquone tablets with TMP-SMX for oral treatment of mild-to-moderate *Pneumocystis carinii* pneumonia (PCP) (see INDICATIONS AND USAGE), where AIDS patients received 750 mg atovaquone tablets 3 times daily for 21 days, the mean steady-state atovaquone concentration was 13.9 ± 6.9 mcg/mL (n = 133). Analysis of these data established a relationship between plasma atovaquone concentration and successful treatment. This is shown in Table 2.
[See table 2 at top of next page]

A dosing regimen of MEPRON Suspension for the treatment of mild-to-moderate PCP has been selected to achieve average plasma atovaquone concentrations of approximately 20 mcg/mL, because this plasma concentration was previously shown to be well tolerated and associated with the highest treatment success rates (Table 2). In an open-label PCP treatment study with MEPRON Suspension, dosing regimens of 1,000 mg once daily, 750 mg twice daily, 1,500 mg once daily, and 1,000 mg twice daily were explored. The average steady-state plasma atovaquone concentration achieved at the 750-mg twice-daily dose given with meals was 22.0 ± 10.1 mcg/mL (n = 18).

Table 1. Average Steady-State Plasma Atovaquone Concentrations in Pediatric Patients

| | Dose of MEPRON Suspension | | |
| | 10 mg/kg | 30 mg/kg | 45 mg/kg |
Age	Average C_{ss} in mcg/mL (mean ± SD)		
1-3 months	5.9 (n = 1)	27.8 ± 5.8 (n = 4)	—
>3-24 months	5.7 ± 5.1 (n = 4)	9.8 ± 3.2 (n = 4)	15.4 ± 6.6 (n = 4)
>2-13 years	16.8 ± 6.4 (n = 4)	37.1 ± 10.9 (n = 3)	—

Table 2. Relationship Between Plasma Atovaquone Concentration and Successful Treatment

Steady-State Plasma Atovaquone Concentrations (mcg/mL)	Successful Treatment* (No. Successes/No. in Group) (%)			
	Observed		Predicted[†]	
0 to <5	0/6	(0%)	1.5/6	(25%)
5 to <10	18/26	(69%)	14.7/26	(57%)
10 to <15	30/38	(79%)	31.9/38	(84%)
15 to <20	18/19	(95%)	18.1/19	(95%)
20 to <25	18/18	(100%)	17.8/18	(99%)
25+	6/6	(100%)	6/6	(100%)

*Successful treatment was defined as improvement in clinical and respiratory measures persisting at least 4 weeks after cessation of therapy. This was based on data from patients for which both outcome and steady-state plasma atovaquone concentration data are available.
[†] Based on logistic regression analysis.

Table 3. Confirmed or Presumed/Probable PCP Events (As-Treated Analysis)*

Assessment	Study 115-211		Study 115-213		
	Atovaquone 1,500 mg/day (n = 527)	Dapsone 100 mg/day (n = 510)	Atovaquone 750 mg/day (n = 188)	Atovaquone 1,500 mg/day (n = 172)	Aerosolized Pentamidine 300 mg/month (n = 169)
%	15%	19%	23%	18%	17%
Relative Risk[†] (CI)[‡]	0.77 (0.57, 1.04)		1.47 (0.86, 2.50)	1.14 (0.63, 2.06)	

*Those events occurring during or within 30 days of stopping assigned treatment.
[†] Relative risk <1 favors atovaquone and values >1 favor comparator. These trials were designed to show superiority of atovaquone to the comparator. This was not shown.
[‡] The confidence level of the interval for the dapsone comparative study was 95% and for the pentamidine comparative study was 97.5%.

Table 4. Outcome of Treatment for PCP-Positive Patients Enrolled in the TMP-SMX Comparative Study

Outcome of Therapy*	Number of Patients (% of Total)				
	MEPRON (n = 160)		TMP-SMX (n = 162)		P Value
Therapy success	99	(62%)	103	(64%)	0.75
Therapy failure					
- Lack of response	28	(17%)	10	(6%)	<0.01
- Adverse experience	11	(7%)	33	(20%)	<0.01
- Unevaluable	22	(14%)	16	(10%)	0.28
Required alternate PCP therapy during study	55	(34%)	55	(34%)	0.95

*As defined by the protocol and described in study description above.

Table 5. Outcome of Treatment for PCP-Positive Patients Enrolled in the Pentamidine Comparative Study

Outcome of Therapy	Primary Treatment				Salvage Treatment				
	MEPRON (n = 56)		Pentamidine (n = 53)		P Value	MEPRON (n = 14)		Pentamidine (n = 11)		P Value
Therapy success	32	(57%)	21	(40%)	0.09	13	(93%)	7	(64%)	0.14
Therapy failure										
- Lack of response	16	(29%)	9	(17%)	0.18	0		0		—
- Adverse experience	2	(3.6%)	19	(36%)	<0.01	0		3	(27%)	0.07
- Unevaluable	6	(11%)	4	(8%)	0.75	1	(7%)	1	(9%)	1.00
Required alternate PCP therapy during study	19	(34%)	29	(55%)	0.04			4	(36%)	0.03

INDICATIONS AND USAGE

MEPRON Suspension is indicated for the prevention of *Pneumocystis carinii* pneumonia in patients who are intolerant to trimethoprim-sulfamethoxazole (TMP-SMX).
MEPRON Suspension is also indicated for the acute oral treatment of mild-to-moderate PCP in patients who are intolerant to TMP-SMX.

Prevention of PCP

The indication for prevention of PCP is based on the results of 2 clinical trials comparing MEPRON Suspension to dapsone or aerosolized pentamidine in HIV-infected adult and adolescent patients at risk of PCP (CD4 count <200 cells/mm[3] or a prior episode of PCP) and intolerant to TMP-SMX.

Dapsone Comparative Study

This randomized, open-label trial enrolled a total of 1,057 patients at 48 study centers. Patients were randomized to receive 1,500 mg MEPRON Suspension once daily (n = 536) or 100 mg dapsone once daily (n = 521). Median follow-up was 24 months. Patients randomized to the dapsone arm who were seropositive for *Toxoplasma gondii* and had a CD4 count <100 cells/mm[3] also received pyrimethamine and folinic acid. PCP event rates are shown in Table 3. There was no significant difference in mortality rates between the groups.

Aerosolized Pentamidine Comparative Study

This randomized, open-label trial enrolled a total of 549 patients at 35 study centers. Patients were randomized to receive 1,500 mg MEPRON Suspension once daily (n = 175), 750 mg MEPRON Suspension once daily (n = 188), or 300 mg aerosolized pentamidine once monthly (n = 186). Median follow-up was 11.3 months. The results of the PCP event rates appear in Table 3. There were no significant differences in mortality rates among the groups.
[See table 3 at left]
An analysis of all PCP events (intent-to-treat analysis) showed results similar to those above.

Treatment of PCP

The indication for treatment of mild-to-moderate PCP is based on the results of comparative pharmacokinetic studies of the suspension and tablet formulations (see CLINICAL PHARMACOLOGY) and clinical efficacy studies of the tablet formulation which established a relationship between plasma atovaquone concentration and successful treatment. The results of a randomized, double-blind trial comparing MEPRON to TMP-SMX in AIDS patients with mild-to-moderate PCP (defined in the study protocol as an alveolar-arterial oxygen diffusion gradient $[(A-a)DO_2]^1 \leq 45$ mm Hg and $PaO_2 \geq 60$ mm Hg on room air) and a randomized trial comparing MEPRON to IV pentamidine isethionate in patients with mild-to-moderate PCP intolerant to trimethoprim or sulfa-antimicrobials are summarized below:

TMP-SMX Comparative Study

This double-blind, randomized trial initiated in 1990 was designed to compare the safety and efficacy of MEPRON to that of TMP-SMX for the treatment of AIDS patients with histologically confirmed PCP. Only patients with mild-to-moderate PCP were eligible for enrollment.
A total of 408 patients were enrolled into the trial at 37 study centers. Eighty-six patients without histologic confirmation of PCP were excluded from the efficacy analyses. Of the 322 patients with histologically confirmed PCP, 160 were randomized to receive MEPRON and 162 to TMP-SMX.
Study participants randomized to treatment with MEPRON were to receive 750 mg MEPRON (three 250-mg tablets) 3 times daily for 21 days and those randomized to TMP-SMX were to receive 320 mg TMP plus 1,600 mg SMX 3 times daily for 21 days.
Therapy success was defined as improvement in clinical and respiratory measures persisting at least 4 weeks after cessation of therapy. Therapy failures included lack of response, treatment discontinuation due to an adverse experience, and unevaluable.
There was a significant difference (P = 0.03) in mortality rates between the treatment groups. Among the 322 patients with confirmed PCP, 13 of 160 (8%) patients treated with MEPRON and 4 of 162 (2.5%) patients receiving TMP-SMX died during the 21-day treatment course or 8-week follow-up period. In the intent-to-treat analysis for all 408 randomized patients, there were 16 (8%) deaths in the arm treated with MEPRON and 7 (3.4%) deaths in the TMP-SMX arm (P = 0.051). Of the 13 patients treated with MEPRON who died, 4 died of PCP and 5 died with a combination of bacterial infections and PCP; bacterial infections did not appear to be a factor in any of the 4 deaths among TMP-SMX-treated patients.
A correlation between plasma atovaquone concentrations and death was demonstrated; in general, patients with lower plasma concentrations were more likely to die. For those patients for whom day 4 plasma atovaquone concentration data are available, 5 (63%) of the 8 patients with concentrations <5 mcg/mL died during participation in the study. However, only 1 (2.0%) of the 49 patients with day 4 plasma atovaquone concentrations ≥5 mcg/mL died.
Sixty-two percent of patients on MEPRON and 64% of patients on TMP-SMX were classified as protocol-defined therapy successes (Table 4).
[See table 4 above]
The failure rate due to lack of response was significantly larger for patients receiving MEPRON while the failure rate due to adverse experiences was significantly larger for patients receiving TMP-SMX.
There were no significant differences in the effect of either treatment on additional indicators of response (i.e., arterial blood gas measurements, vital signs, serum LDH levels, clinical symptoms, and chest radiographs).

Pentamidine Comparative Study

This unblinded, randomized trial initiated in 1991 was designed to compare the safety and efficacy of MEPRON to that of pentamidine for the treatment of histologically confirmed mild or moderate PCP in AIDS patients. Approximately 80% of the patients either had a history of intolerance to trimethoprim or sulfa-antimicrobials (the primary therapy group) or were experiencing intolerance to TMP-SMX with treatment of an episode of PCP at the time of enrollment in the study (the salvage treatment group). Patients randomized to MEPRON were to receive 750 mg atovaquone (three 250-mg tablets) 3 times daily for 21 days and those randomized to pentamidine isethionate were to receive a 3- to 4-mg/kg single IV infusion daily for 21 days. A total of 174 patients were enrolled into the trial at 22 study centers. Thirty-nine patients without histologic confirmation of PCP were excluded from the efficacy analyses. Of the 135 patients with histologically confirmed PCP, 70 were randomized to receive MEPRON and 65 to pentamidine. One hundred and ten (110) of these were in the primary therapy group and 25 were in the salvage therapy group. One patient in the primary therapy group randomized to receive pentamidine did not receive study medication.

There was no difference in mortality rates between the treatment groups. Among the 135 patients with confirmed PCP, 10 of 70 (14%) randomized to MEPRON and 9 of 65 (14%) patients randomized to pentamidine died during the 21-day treatment course or 8-week follow-up period. In the intent-to-treat analysis for all randomized patients, there were 11 (12.5%) deaths in the arm treated with MEPRON and 12 (14%) deaths in the pentamidine arm. For those patients for whom day 4 plasma atovaquone concentrations are available, 3 of 5 (60%) patients with concentrations <5 mcg/mL died during participation in the study. However, only 2 of 21 (9%) patients with day 4 plasma concentrations ≥5 mcg/mL died.

The therapeutic outcomes for the 134 patients who received study medication in this trial are presented in Table 5. [See table 5 on previous page]

CONTRAINDICATIONS

MEPRON Suspension is contraindicated for patients who develop or have a history of potentially life-threatening allergic reactions to any of the components of the formulation.

WARNINGS

Clinical experience with MEPRON for the treatment of PCP has been limited to patients with mild-to-moderate PCP [(A-a)DO$_2$≤45 mm Hg]. Treatment of more severe episodes of PCP has not been systematically studied with this agent. Also, the efficacy of MEPRON in patients who are failing therapy with TMP-SMX has not been systematically studied.

PRECAUTIONS
General
Absorption of orally administered MEPRON is limited but can be significantly increased when the drug is taken with food. Plasma atovaquone concentrations have been shown to correlate with the likelihood of successful treatment and survival. Therefore, parenteral therapy with other agents should be considered for patients who have difficulty taking MEPRON with food (see CLINICAL PHARMACOLOGY). Gastrointestinal disorders may limit absorption of orally administered drugs. Patients with these disorders also may not achieve plasma concentrations of atovaquone associated with response to therapy in controlled trials.

Based upon the spectrum of in vitro antimicrobial activity, atovaquone is not effective therapy for concurrent pulmonary conditions such as bacterial, viral, or fungal pneumonia or mycobacterial diseases. Clinical deterioration in patients may be due to infections with other pathogens, as well as progressive PCP. All patients with acute PCP should be carefully evaluated for other possible causes of pulmonary disease and treated with additional agents as appropriate.

Rare cases of hepatitis, elevated liver function tests, and one case of fatal liver failure have been reported in patients treated with atovaquone. A causal relationship between atovaquone use and these events could not be established because of numerous confounding medical conditions and concomitant drug therapies. (See ADVERSE REACTIONS.) If it is necessary to treat patients with severe hepatic impairment, caution is advised and administration should be closely monitored.

Information for Patients
The importance of taking the prescribed dose of MEPRON should be stressed. Patients should be instructed to take their daily doses of MEPRON with meals, as the presence of food will significantly improve the absorption of the drug.

Drug Interactions
Atovaquone is highly bound to plasma protein (>99.9%). Therefore, caution should be used when administering MEPRON concurrently with other highly plasma protein-bound drugs with narrow therapeutic indices, as competition for binding sites may occur. The extent of plasma protein binding of atovaquone in human plasma is not affected by the presence of therapeutic concentrations of phenytoin (15 mcg/mL), nor is the binding of phenytoin affected by the presence of atovaquone.

Rifampin: Coadministration of rifampin and MEPRON Suspension results in a significant decrease in average steady-state plasma atovaquone concentrations (see CLINICAL PHARMACOLOGY: Drug Interactions). Alternatives to rifampin should be considered during the course of PCP treatment with MEPRON.

Rifabutin, another rifamycin, is structurally similar to rifampin and may possibly have some of the same drug interactions as rifampin. No interaction trials have been conducted with MEPRON and rifabutin.

Drug/Laboratory Test Interactions
It is not known if MEPRON interferes with clinical laboratory test or assay results.

Carcinogenesis, Mutagenesis, Impairment of Fertility
Carcinogenicity studies in rats were negative; 24-month studies in mice showed treatment-related increases in incidence of hepatocellular adenoma and hepatocellular carcinoma at all doses tested which ranged from 1.4 to 3.6 times the average steady-state plasma concentrations in humans during acute treatment of *Pneumocystis carinii* pneumonia. Atovaquone was negative with or without metabolic activation in the Ames *Salmonella* mutagenicity assay, the Mouse Lymphoma mutagenesis assay, and the Cultured Human Lymphocyte cytogenetic assay. No evidence of genotoxicity was observed in the in vivo Mouse Micronucleus assay.

Pregnancy
Pregnancy Category C. Atovaquone was not teratogenic and did not cause reproductive toxicity in rats at plasma concentrations up to 2 to 3 times the estimated human exposure. Atovaquone caused maternal toxicity in rabbits at plasma concentrations that were approximately one half the estimated human exposure. Mean fetal body lengths and weights were decreased and there were higher numbers of early resorption and post-implantation loss per dam. It is not clear whether these effects were caused by atovaquone directly or were secondary to maternal toxicity. Concentrations of atovaquone in rabbit fetuses averaged 30% of the concurrent maternal plasma concentrations. In a separate study in rats given a single ^{14}C-radiolabelled dose, concentrations of radiocarbon in rat fetuses were 18% (middle gestation) and 60% (late gestation) of concurrent maternal plasma concentrations. There are no adequate and well-controlled studies in pregnant women. MEPRON should be used during pregnancy only if the potential benefit justifies the potential risk to the fetus.

Nursing Mothers
It is not known whether atovaquone is excreted into human milk. Because many drugs are excreted into human milk, caution should be exercised when MEPRON is administered to a nursing woman. In a rat study, atovaquone concentrations in the milk were 30% of the concurrent atovaquone concentrations in the maternal plasma.

Table 6. Treatment-Limiting Adverse Experiences in the Dapsone Comparative PCP Prevention Study

	Percentage of Patients with Treatment-Limiting Adverse Experience			
	All Patients		Patients Not Taking Either Drug at Enrollment	
Treatment-Limiting Adverse Experience	MEPRON 1,500 mg/day (n = 536)	Dapsone 100 mg/day (n = 521)	MEPRON 1,500 mg/day (n = 238)	Dapsone 100 mg/day (n = 249)
Any event	24.4%	25.9%	20.2%	43.4%
Rash	6.3%	8.8%	7.6%	16.1%
Nausea	4.1%	0.6%	2.5%	0.8%
Diarrhea	3.2%	0.2%	2.1%	0.4%
Vomiting	2.2%	0.6%	1.3%	0.8%
Allergic reaction	1.1%	2.9%	0.8%	4.8%
Fever	0.6%	2.9%	0%	5.6%
Anemia	0%	1.5%	0%	2.0%

Table 7. Treatment-Emergent Adverse Experiences in the Aerosolized Pentamidine Comparative PCP Prevention Study

	Percentage of Patients with Treatment-Emergent Adverse Experience		
Treatment-Emergent Adverse Experience	MEPRON 1,500 mg/day (n = 175)	MEPRON 750 mg/day (n = 188)	Aerosolized Pentamidine (n = 186)
Diarrhea	42%	42%	35%
Rash	39%	46%	28%
Headache	28%	31%	22%
Nausea	26%	32%	23%
Cough increased	25%	25%	31%
Fever	25%	31%	18%
Rhinitis	24%	18%	17%
Asthenia	22%	31%	31%
Infection	22%	18%	19%
Abdominal pain	20%	21%	20%
Dyspnea	15%	21%	16%
Vomiting	15%	22%	11%
Patients discontinuing therapy due to an adverse experience	25%	16%	7%
Patients reporting at least 1 adverse experience	98%	96%	89%

Table 8. Treatment-Emergent Adverse Experiences in the TMP-SMX Comparative PCP Treatment Study

Treatment-Emergent Adverse Experience	Percentage of Patients with Treatment-Emergent Adverse Experience	
	MEPRON (n = 203)	TMP-SMX (n = 205)
Rash (including maculopapular)	23%	34%
Nausea	21%	44%
Diarrhea	19%	7%
Headache	16%	22%
Vomiting	14%	35%
Fever	14%	25%
Insomnia	10%	9%
Asthenia	8%	8%
Pruritus	5%	9%
Monilia, oral	5%	10%
Abdominal pain	4%	7%
Constipation	3%	17%
Dizziness	3%	8%
Patients discontinuing therapy due to an adverse experience	9%	24%
Patients reporting at least 1 adverse experience	63%	65%

Table 9. Treatment-Emergent Laboratory Test Abnormalities in the TMP-SMX Comparative PCP Treatment Study

Laboratory Test Abnormality	Percentage of Patients Developing a Laboratory Test Abnormality	
	MEPRON	TMP-SMX
Anemia (Hgb<8.0 g/dL)	6%	7%
Neutropenia (ANC<750 cells/mm^3)	3%	9%
Elevated ALT (>5 × ULN)	6%	16%
Elevated AST (>5 × ULN)	4%	14%
Elevated alkaline phosphatase (>2.5 × ULN)	8%	6%
Elevated amylase (>1.5 × ULN)	7%	12%
Hyponatremia (<0.96 × LLN)	7%	26%

ULN = upper limit of normal range.
LLN = lower limit of normal range.

Pediatric Use

Evidence of safety and effectiveness in pediatric patients has not been established. A relationship between plasma atovaquone concentrations and successful treatment of PCP has been established in adults (see Table 2). In a study of MEPRON Suspension in 27 HIV-infected, asymptomatic infants and children between 1 month and 13 years of age, the pharmacokinetics of atovaquone were age-dependent (see CLINICAL PHARMACOLOGY: Special Populations). No drug-related treatment-limiting adverse events were observed in the pharmacokinetic study.

Geriatric Use

Clinical studies of MEPRON did not include sufficient numbers of subjects aged 65 and over to determine whether they respond differently from younger subjects. Other reported clinical experience has not identified differences in responses between the elderly and younger patients. In general, dose selection for an elderly patient should be cautious, reflecting the greater frequency of decreased hepatic, renal, or cardiac function, and of concomitant disease or other drug therapy.

ADVERSE REACTIONS

Because many patients who participated in clinical trials with MEPRON had complications of advanced HIV disease, it was often difficult to distinguish adverse events caused by MEPRON from those caused by underlying medical conditions. There were no life-threatening or fatal adverse experiences caused by MEPRON.

PCP Prevention Studies

In the dapsone comparative study of MEPRON Suspension, adverse experience data were collected only for treatment-limiting events. Among the entire population (n = 1,057), treatment-limiting events occurred at similar frequencies in patients treated with MEPRON Suspension or dapsone (Table 6). Among patients who were taking neither dapsone nor atovaquone at enrollment (n = 487), treatment-limiting events occurred in 43% of patients treated with dapsone and 20% of patients treated with MEPRON Suspension (P <0.001). In both populations, the type of treatment-limiting events differed between the 2 treatment arms. Hypersensitivity reactions (rash, fever, allergic reaction) and anemia were more common in patients treated with dapsone, while gastrointestinal events (nausea, diarrhea, and vomiting) were more common in patients treated with MEPRON Suspension.
[See table 6 at top of previous page]

Table 7 summarizes the clinical adverse experiences reported by ≥20% of patients in any group in the aerosolized pentamidine comparative study of MEPRON Suspension (n = 549), regardless of attribution. The incidence of adverse experiences at the recommended dose was similar to that seen with aerosolized pentamidine. Rash was the only individual adverse experience that occurred significantly more commonly in patients treated with both dosages of MEPRON Suspension (39% to 46%) than in patients treated with aerosolized pentamidine (28%). Among patients treated with MEPRON Suspension, there was no evidence of a dose-related increase in the incidence of adverse experiences. Treatment-limiting adverse experiences occurred less often in patients treated with aerosolized pentamidine (7%) than in patients treated with 1,500 mg MEPRON Suspension once daily (25%, P≤0.001) or 750 mg MEPRON Suspension once daily (16%, P = 0.004). The most common

adverse experiences requiring discontinuation of dosing in the group receiving 1,500 mg MEPRON Suspension once daily were rash (6%), diarrhea (4%), and nausea (3%). The most common adverse experience requiring discontinuation of dosing in the group receiving aerosolized pentamidine was bronchospasm (2%).
[See table 7 on previous page]

Other events occurring in ≥10% of the patients receiving the recommended dose of MEPRON included sweating, flu syndrome, pain, sinusitis, pruritus, insomnia, depression, and myalgia. Bronchospasm occurred more frequently in patients receiving aerosolized pentamidine (11%) than in patients receiving MEPRON 1,500 mg/day (4%) and MEPRON 750 mg/day (2%).

Neither MEPRON nor aerosolized pentamidine was associated with a substantial change from baseline values in any measured laboratory parameter, nor were there any significant differences in any measured laboratory parameter between MEPRON and aerosolized pentamidine. Some patients had laboratory abnormalities considered serious by the investigator or that contributed to discontinuation of therapy.

PCP Treatment Studies

Table 8 summarizes all the clinical adverse experiences reported by ≥5% of the study population during the TMP-SMX comparative study of MEPRON (n = 408), regardless of attribution. The incidence of adverse experiences with MEPRON Suspension at the recommended dose was similar to that seen with the tablet formulation of atovaquone.
[See table 8 at left]

Although an equal percentage of patients receiving MEPRON and TMP-SMX reported at least 1 adverse experience, more patients receiving TMP-SMX required discontinuation of therapy due to an adverse event. Twenty-four percent of patients receiving TMP-SMX were prematurely discontinued from therapy due to an adverse experience versus 9% of patients receiving MEPRON. Four percent of patients receiving MEPRON had therapy discontinued due to development of rash. The majority of cases of rash among patients receiving MEPRON were mild and did not require the discontinuation of dosing. The only other clinical adverse experience that led to premature discontinuation of dosing of MEPRON by more than 1 patient was vomiting (<1%). The most common adverse experience requiring discontinuation of dosing in the TMP-SMX group was rash (8%).

Laboratory test abnormalities reported for ≥5% of the study population during the treatment period are summarized in Table 9. Two percent of patients treated with MEPRON and 7% of patients treated with TMP-SMX had therapy prematurely discontinued due to elevations in ALT/AST. In general, patients treated with MEPRON developed fewer abnormalities in measures of hepatocellular function (ALT, AST, alkaline phosphatase) or amylase values than patients treated with TMP-SMX.
[See table 9 at left]

Table 10 summarizes the clinical adverse experiences reported by ≥5% of the primary therapy study population (n = 144) during the comparative trial of MEPRON and intravenous pentamidine, regardless of attribution. A slightly lower percentage of patients who received MEPRON reported occurrence of adverse events than did those who received pentamidine (63% vs 72%). However, only 7% of patients discontinued treatment with MEPRON due to adverse events, while 41% of patients who received pentamidine discontinued treatment for this reason (P<0.001). Of the 5 patients who discontinued therapy with MEPRON, 3 reported rash (4%). Rash was not severe in any patient. No other reason for discontinuation of MEPRON was cited more than once. The most frequently cited reasons for discontinuation of pentamidine therapy were hypoglycemia (11%) and vomiting (9%).
[See table 10 at top of next page]

Laboratory test abnormalities reported in ≥5% of patients in the pentamidine comparative study are presented in Table 11. Laboratory abnormality was reported as the reason for discontinuation of treatment in 2 of 73 patients who received MEPRON. One patient (1%) had elevated creatinine and BUN levels and 1 patient (1%) had elevated amylase levels. Laboratory abnormalities were the sole or contributing factor in 14 patients who prematurely discontinued pentamidine therapy. In the 71 patients who received pentamidine, laboratory parameters most frequently reported as reasons for discontinuation were hypoglycemia (11%), elevated creatinine levels (6%), and leukopenia (4%).
[See table 11 on next page]

Postmarketing Experience

In addition to adverse events reported from clinical trials, the following events have been identified during post-approval use of MEPRON. Because they are reported voluntarily from a population of unknown size, estimates of frequency cannot be made. These events have been chosen

Table 10. Treatment-Emergent Adverse Experiences in the Pentamidine Comparative PCP Treatment Study (Primary Therapy Group)

Treatment-Emergent Adverse Experience	Percentage of Patients with Treatment-Emergent Adverse Experience	
	MEPRON (n = 73)	Pentamidine (n = 71)
Fever	40%	25%
Nausea	22%	37%
Rash	22%	13%
Diarrhea	21%	31%
Insomnia	19%	14%
Headache	18%	28%
Vomiting	14%	17%
Cough	14%	1%
Abdominal pain	10%	11%
Pain	10%	10%
Sweat	10%	3%
Monilia, oral	10%	3%
Asthenia	8%	14%
Dizziness	8%	14%
Anxiety	7%	10%
Anorexia	7%	10%
Sinusitis	7%	6%
Dyspepsia	5%	10%
Rhinitis	5%	7%
Taste perversion	3%	13%
Hypoglycemia	1%	15%
Hypotension	1%	10%
Patients discontinuing therapy due to an adverse experience	7%	41%
Patients reporting at least 1 adverse experience	63%	72%

Table 11. Treatment-Emergent Laboratory Test Abnormalities in the Pentamidine Comparative PCP Treatment Study

Laboratory Test Abnormality	Percentage of Patients Developing a Laboratory Test Abnormality	
	MEPRON	Pentamidine
Anemia (Hgb<8.0 g/dL)	4%	9%
Neutropenia (ANC<750 cells/mm^3)	5%	9%
Hyponatremia (<0.96 × LLN)	10%	10%
Hyperkalemia (>1.18 × ULN)	0%	5%
Alkaline phosphatase (>2.5 × ULN)	5%	2%
Hyperglycemia (>1.8 × ULN)	9%	13%
Elevated AST (>5 × ULN)	0%	5%
Elevated amylase (>1.5 × ULN)	8%	4%
Elevated creatinine (>1.5 × ULN)	0%	7%

ULN = upper limit of normal range.
LLN = lower limit of normal range.

for inclusion due to a combination of their seriousness, frequency of reporting, or potential causal connection to MEPRON.
Blood and Lymphatic System Disorders
Methemoglobinemia, thrombocytopenia.
Immune System Disorders
Hypersensitivity reactions including angioedema, bronchospasm, throat tightness, and urticaria.

Eye Disorders
Vortex keratopathy.
Gastrointestinal Disorders: Pancreatitis
Hepatobiliary Disorders: Rare cases of hepatitis, and one case of fatal liver failure have been reported with atovaquone usage.
Skin and Subcutaneous Tissue Disorders: Erythema multiforme, Stevens-Johnson syndrome, and skin desquama-

tion have been reported in patients receiving multiple drug therapy including atovaquone.
Renal and Urinary Disorders: Acute renal impairment.

OVERDOSAGE

There is no known antidote for atovaquone, and it is currently unknown if atovaquone is dialyzable. The median lethal dose is higher than the maximum oral dose tested in mice and rats (1,825 mg/kg/day). Overdoses up to 31,500 mg of atovaquone have been reported. In 1 such patient who also took an unspecified dose of dapsone, methemoglobinemia occurred. Rash has also been reported after overdose.

DOSAGE AND ADMINISTRATION
Dosage
Prevention of PCP: Adults and Adolescents (13 to 16 Years):
The recommended oral dose is 1,500 mg (10 mL) once daily administered with a meal.
Treatment of Mild-to-Moderate PCP: Adults and Adolescents (13 to 16 Years):
The recommended oral dose is 750 mg (5 mL) administered with meals twice daily for 21 days (total daily dose 1,500 mg).
Note: Failure to administer MEPRON Suspension with meals may result in lower plasma atovaquone concentrations and may limit response to therapy (see CLINICAL PHARMACOLOGY and PRECAUTIONS).
Administration
Foil Pouch
Open pouch by removing tab at perforation and tear at notch. Take entire contents by mouth. Can be discharged into a dosing spoon or cup or directly into the mouth.
Bottle
SHAKE BOTTLE GENTLY BEFORE USING.

HOW SUPPLIED
MEPRON Suspension (bright yellow, citrus flavored) containing 750 mg atovaquone in each teaspoonful 5 mL).
Bottle of 210 mL with child-resistant cap (NDC 0173-0665-18).
Store at 15° to 25°C (59° to 77°F). DO NOT FREEZE. Dispense in tight container as defined in USP.
5-mL child-resistant foil pouch - unit dose pack of 42 (NDC 0173-0547-00).
Store at 15° to 25°C (59° to 77°F). DO NOT FREEZE.
[1](A-a)DO$_2$ = [(713 × FiO$_2$) − (PaCO$_2$/0.8)] − PaO$_2$ (mm Hg)
GlaxoSmithKline
Research Triangle Park, NC 27709
©2008, GlaxoSmithKline. All rights reserved.
May 2008 MPR:1PI

MYLERAN®
[mī 'lə-răn]
(busulfan)
Tablets

℞

WARNING

MYLERAN is a potent drug. It should not be used unless a diagnosis of chronic myelogenous leukemia has been adequately established and the responsible physician is knowledgeable in assessing response to chemotherapy. MYLERAN can induce severe bone marrow hypoplasia. Reduce or discontinue the dosage immediately at the first sign of any unusual depression of bone marrow function as reflected by an abnormal decrease in any of the formed elements of the blood. A bone marrow examination should be performed if the bone marrow status is uncertain.
SEE WARNINGS FOR INFORMATION REGARDING BUSULFAN-INDUCED LEUKEMOGENESIS IN HUMANS.

DESCRIPTION
MYLERAN (busulfan) is a bifunctional alkylating agent. Busulfan is known chemically as 1,4-butanediol dimethanesulfonate and has the following structural formula:
$$CH_3SO_2O(CH_2)_4OSO_2CH_3$$
Busulfan is *not* a structural analog of the nitrogen mustards. MYLERAN is available in tablet form for oral administration. Each film-coated tablet contains 2 mg busulfan and the inactive ingredients hypromellose, lactose (anhydrous), magnesium stearate, pregelatinized starch, triacetin, and titanium dioxide.
The activity of busulfan in chronic myelogenous leukemia was first reported by D.A.G. Galton in 1953.

CLINICAL PHARMACOLOGY
Busulfan is a small, highly lipophilic molecule that easily crosses the blood brain barrier. Following absorption, 32% and 47% of busulfan are bound to plasma proteins and red blood cells, respectively.
Busulfan absorption from the gastrointestinal tract is essentially complete. This has been demonstrated in radioac-

tive studies after both intravenous and oral administration of ^{35}S-busulfan, ^{14}C-busulfan, and ^{3}H-busulfan. Following intravenous administration of a single therapeutic dose of ^{35}S-busulfan, there was rapid disappearance of radioactivity from the blood and 90% to 95% of the ^{35}S-label disappeared within 3 to 5 minutes after injection. After either oral or intravenous administration of ^{35}S-busulfan, 45% to 60% of the radioactivity was recovered in the urine in the 48 hours after administration; the majority of the total urinary excretion occurring in the first 24 hours. Over 95% of the urinary ^{35}S-label occurs as ^{35}S-methanesulfonic acid. Oral and intravenous administration of 1,4-^{14}C-busulfan showed the same rapid initial disappearance of plasma radioactivity as observed following the administration of ^{35}S-labeled drug. Cumulative radioactivity in the urine after 48 hours was 25% to 30% of the administered dose (contrasting with 45% to 60% for ^{35}S-busulfan), and suggests a slower excretion of the alkylating portion of the molecule and its metabolites than for the sulfonoxymethyl moieties. Regardless of the route of administration, 1,4-^{14}C-busulfan yielded a complex mixture of at least 12 radiolabeled metabolites in urine; the main metabolite being 3-hydroxytetrahydrothiophene-1,1-dioxide. Pharmacokinetic studies employing ^{3}H-busulfan labeled on the tetramethylene chain confirmed a rapid initial clearance of the radioactivity from plasma, irrespective of whether the drug was given orally or intravenously.

A study compared a 2-mg single IV bolus injection to a single oral dose of a 2-mg tablet of nonradioactive busulfan in 8 adult patients 13 to 60 years of age. The study demonstrated that the mean ± SD absolute bioavailability was 80% ± 20% in adults. However, the absolute bioavailability for 8 children 1.5 to 6 years of age was 68% ± 31%.

In another study of 2, 4, and 6 mg of busulfan, given as a single oral dose on consecutive days (starting with the lowest dose) in 5 adult patients, the mean dose-normalized (to 2 mg dose) area under the plasma concentration-time curve (AUC) was about 130 ng•hr/mL, while the mean intra- and inter-patient variability was about 16% and 21%, respectively. Busulfan was eliminated with a plasma terminal elimination half-life ($t_{1/2}$) of about 2.6 hours, and demonstrated linear kinetics within the range of 2 to 6 mg for both the maximum plasma concentration (C_{max}) and AUC. The mean C_{max} for the 2-, 4-, and 6-mg doses (after dose normalization to 2 mg) was about 30 ng/mL. A recent study of 4 to 8 mg as single oral doses in 12 patients showed that the mean ± SD C_{max} (after dose normalization to 4 mg) was 68.2 ± 24.4 ng/mL, occurring at about 0.9 hours and the mean ± SD AUC (after dose normalization to 4 mg) was 269 ± 62 ng•hr/mL. These results are consistent with previous results. In addition, the mean ± SD elimination half-life was 2.69 ± 0.49 hours.

The elimination of busulfan appears to be independent of renal function. This probably reflects the extensive metabolism of the drug in the liver, since less than 2% of the administered dose is excreted in the urine unchanged within 24 hours. The drug is metabolized by enzymatic activity to at least 12 metabolites, among which tetrahydrothiophene, tetrahydrothiophene 12-oxide, sulfolane, and 3-hydroxysulfolane were identified. These metabolites do not have cytotoxic activity.

There is no experience with the use of dialysis in an attempt to modify the clinical toxicity of busulfan. One technical difficulty would derive from the extremely poor water solubility of busulfan. Additionally, all studies of the metabolism of busulfan employing radiolabeled materials indicate rapid chemical reactivity of the parent compound with prolonged retention of some of the metabolites (particularly the metabolites arising from the "alkylating" portion of the molecule). The effectiveness of dialysis at removing significant quantities of unreacted drug would be expected to be minimal in such a situation.

Currently, there are no available data on the effect of food on busulfan bioavailability.

Pharmacokinetics in Hemodialysis Patients: The impact of hemodialysis on the clearance of busulfan was determined in a patient with chronic renal failure undergoing autologous stem cell transplantation. The apparent oral clearance of busulfan during a 4-hour hemodialysis session was increased by 65%, but the 24-hour oral clearance of busulfan was increased by only 11%.

The incidence of veno-occlusive disease was higher (33.3% versus 3.0%) in patients with busulfan AUC_{0-6hr} >1,500 µM.min (C_{ss} >900 mcg/L) compared to patients with busulfan AUC_{0-6hr} <1,500 µM.min (C_{ss} <900 mcg/L) (see WARNINGS).

Drug Interactions: Itraconazole reduced busulfan clearance by up to 25% in patients receiving itraconazole compared to patients who did not receive itraconazole. Higher busulfan exposure due to concomitant itraconazole could lead to toxic plasma levels in some patients. Fluconazole had no effect on the clearance of busulfan. Patients treated with concomitant cyclophosphamide and busulfan with phenytoin pretreatment have increased cyclophosphamide and busulfan clearance, which may lead to decreased concentrations of both cyclophosphamide and busulfan. However, busulfan clearance may be reduced in the presence of cyclophosphamide alone, presumably due to competition for glutathione.

Diazepam had no effect on the clearance of busulfan.

No information is available regarding the penetration of busulfan into brain or cerebrospinal fluid.

Biochemical Pharmacology: In aqueous media, busulfan undergoes a wide range of nucleophilic substitution reactions. While this chemical reactivity is relatively nonspecific, alkylation of the DNA is felt to be an important biological mechanism for its cytotoxic effect. Coliphage T7 exposed to busulfan was found to have the DNA crosslinked by intrastrand crosslinkages, but no interstrand linkages were found.

The metabolic fate of busulfan has been studied in rats and humans using [14]C- and ^{35}S-labeled materials. In humans, as in the rat, almost all of the radioactivity in ^{35}S-labeled busulfan is excreted in the urine in the form of ^{35}S-methanesulfonic acid. Roberts and Warwick demonstrated that the formation of methanesulfonic acid in vivo in the rat is not due to a simple hydrolysis of busulfan to 1,4-butanediol, since only about 4% of 2,3-^{14}C-busulfan was excreted as carbon dioxide, whereas 2,3-^{14}C-1,4-butanediol was converted almost exclusively to carbon dioxide. The predominant reaction of busulfan in the rat is the alkylation of sulfhydryl groups (particularly cysteine and cysteine-containing compounds) to produce a cyclic sulfonium compound which is the precursor of the major urinary metabolite of the 4-carbon portion of the molecule, 3-hydroxytetrahydrothiophene-1,1-dioxide. This has been termed a "sulfur-stripping" action of busulfan and it may modify the function of certain sulfur-containing amino acids, polypeptides, and proteins; whether this action makes an important contribution to the cytotoxicity of busulfan is unknown.

The biochemical basis for acquired resistance to busulfan is largely a matter of speculation. Although altered transport of busulfan into the cell is one possibility, increased intracellular inactivation of the drug before it reaches the DNA is also possible. Experiments with other alkylating agents have shown that resistance to this class of compounds may reflect an acquired ability of the resistant cell to repair alkylation damage more effectively.

Clinical Studies: Although not curative, busulfan reduces the total granulocyte mass, relieves symptoms of the disease, and improves the clinical state of the patient. Approximately 90% of adults with previously untreated chronic myelogenous leukemia will obtain hematologic remission with regression or stabilization of organomegaly following the use of busulfan. It has been shown to be superior to splenic irradiation with respect to survival times and maintenance of hemoglobin levels, and to be equivalent to irradiation at controlling splenomegaly.

It is not clear whether busulfan unequivocally prolongs the survival of responding patients beyond the 31 months experienced by an untreated group of historical controls. Median survival figures of 31 to 42 months have been reported for several groups of patients treated with busulfan, but concurrent control groups of comparable, untreated patients are not available. The median survival figures reported from different studies will be influenced by the percentage of "poor risk" patients initially entered into the particular study. Patients who are alive 2 years following the diagnosis of chronic myelogenous leukemia, and who have been treated during that period with busulfan, are estimated to have a mean annual mortality rate during the second to fifth year which is approximately two thirds that of patients who received either no treatment, conventional x-ray or ^{32}P-irradiation, or chemotherapy with minimally active drugs. Busulfan is clearly less effective in patients with chronic myelogenous leukemia who lack the Philadelphia (Ph^1) chromosome. Also, the so-called "juvenile" type of chronic myelogenous leukemia, typically occurring in young children and associated with the absence of a Philadelphia chromosome, responds poorly to busulfan. The drug is of no benefit in patients whose chronic myelogenous leukemia has entered a "blastic" phase.

MYLERAN should not be used in patients whose chronic myelogenous leukemia has demonstrated prior resistance to this drug.

MYLERAN is of no value in chronic lymphocytic leukemia, acute leukemia, or in the "blastic crisis" of chronic myelogenous leukemia.

INDICATIONS AND USAGE

MYLERAN (busulfan) is indicated for the palliative treatment of chronic myelogenous (myeloid, myelocytic, granulocytic) leukemia.

CONTRAINDICATIONS

MYLERAN is contraindicated in patients in whom a definitive diagnosis of chronic myelogenous leukemia has not been firmly established.

MYLERAN is contraindicated in patients who have previously suffered a hypersensitivity reaction to busulfan or any other component of the preparation.

WARNINGS

The most frequent, serious side effect of treatment with busulfan is the induction of bone marrow failure (which may or may not be anatomically hypoplastic) resulting in severe pancytopenia. The pancytopenia caused by busulfan may be more prolonged than that induced with other alkylating agents. It is generally felt that the usual cause of busulfan-induced pancytopenia is the failure to stop administration of the drug soon enough; individual idiosyncrasy to the drug does not seem to be an important factor. *MYLERAN should be used with extreme caution and exceptional vigilance in patients whose bone marrow reserve may have been compromised by prior irradiation or chemotherapy, or whose marrow function is recovering from previous cytotoxic therapy.* Although recovery from busulfan-induced pancytopenia may take from 1 month to 2 years, this complication is potentially reversible, and the patient should be vigorously supported through any period of severe pancytopenia.

A rare, important complication of busulfan therapy is the development of bronchopulmonary dysplasia with pulmonary fibrosis. Symptoms have been reported to occur within 8 months to 10 years after initiation of therapy—the average duration of therapy being 4 years. The histologic findings associated with "busulfan lung" mimic those seen following pulmonary irradiation. Clinically, patients have reported the insidious onset of cough, dyspnea, and low-grade fever. In some cases, however, onset of symptoms may be acute. Pulmonary function studies have revealed diminished diffusion capacity and decreased pulmonary compliance. It is important to exclude more common conditions (such as opportunistic infections or leukemic infiltration of the lungs) with appropriate diagnostic techniques. If measures such as sputum cultures, virologic studies, and exfoliative cytology fail to establish an etiology for the pulmonary infiltrates, lung biopsy may be necessary to establish the diagnosis. Treatment of established busulfan-induced pulmonary fibrosis is unsatisfactory; in most cases the patients have died within 6 months after the diagnosis was established. There is no specific therapy for this complication. MYLERAN should be discontinued if this lung toxicity develops. The administration of corticosteroids has been suggested, but the results have not been impressive or uniformly successful.

Busulfan may cause cellular dysplasia in many organs in addition to the lung. Cytologic abnormalities characterized by giant, hyperchromatic nuclei have been reported in lymph nodes, pancreas, thyroid, adrenal glands, liver, and bone marrow. This cytologic dysplasia may be severe enough to cause difficulty in interpretation of exfoliative cytologic examinations from the lung, bladder, breast, and the uterine cervix.

In addition to the widespread epithelial dysplasia that has been observed during busulfan therapy, chromosome aberrations have been reported in cells from patients receiving busulfan.

Busulfan is mutagenic in mice and, possibly, in humans. Malignant tumors and acute leukemias have been reported in patients who have received busulfan therapy, and this drug may be a human carcinogen. The World Health Organization has concluded that there is a causal relationship between busulfan exposure and the development of secondary malignancies. Four cases of acute leukemia occurred among 243 patients treated with busulfan as adjuvant chemotherapy following surgical resection of bronchogenic carcinoma. All 4 cases were from a subgroup of 19 of these 243 patients who developed pancytopenia while taking busulfan 5 to 8 years before leukemia became clinically apparent. These findings suggest that busulfan is leukemogenic, although its mode of action is uncertain.

Ovarian suppression and amenorrhea with menopausal symptoms commonly occur during busulfan therapy in premenopausal patients. Busulfan has been associated with ovarian failure including failure to achieve puberty in females. Busulfan interferes with spermatogenesis in experimental animals, and there have been clinical reports of sterility, azoospermia, and testicular atrophy in male patients. Hepatic veno-occlusive disease, which may be life threatening, has been reported in patients receiving busulfan, usually in combination with cyclophosphamide or other chemotherapeutic agents prior to bone marrow transplantation. Possible risk factors for the development of hepatic veno-occlusive disease include: total busulfan dose exceeding 16 mg/kg based on ideal body weight, and concurrent use of multiple alkylating agents (see CLINICAL PHARMACOLOGY and Drug Interactions).

A clear cause-and-effect relationship with busulfan has not been demonstrated. Periodic measurement of serum transaminases, alkaline phosphatase, and bilirubin is indicated for early detection of hepatotoxicity. A reduced incidence of hepatic veno-occlusive disease and other regimen-related toxicities have been observed in patients treated with high-dose MYLERAN and cyclophosphamide when the first dose of cyclophosphamide has been delayed for >24 hours after the last dose of busulfan (see CLINICAL PHARMACOLOGY and Drug Interactions).

Cardiac tamponade has been reported in a small number of patients with thalassemia (2% in one series) who received busulfan and cyclophosphamide as the preparatory regimen for bone marrow transplantation. In this series, the cardiac tamponade was often fatal. Abdominal pain and vomiting preceded the tamponade in most patients.

Pregnancy: Pregnancy Category D. Busulfan may cause fetal harm when administered to a pregnant woman. Although there have been a number of cases reported where apparently normal children have been born after busulfan treatment during pregnancy, one case has been cited where a malformed baby was delivered by a mother treated with busulfan. During the pregnancy that resulted in the malformed infant, the mother received x-ray therapy early in the first trimester, mercaptopurine until the third month, then busulfan until delivery. In pregnant rats, busulfan produces sterility in both male and female offspring due to the absence of germinal cells in testes and ovaries. Germinal cell aplasia or sterility in offspring of mothers receiving busulfan during pregnancy has not been reported in humans. There are no adequate and well-controlled studies in pregnant women. If this drug is used during pregnancy, or if the patient becomes pregnant while taking this drug, the patient should be apprised of the potential hazard to the fetus. Women of childbearing potential should be advised to avoid becoming pregnant.

PRECAUTIONS

General: The most consistent, dose-related toxicity is bone marrow suppression. This may be manifest by anemia, leukopenia, thrombocytopenia, or any combination of these. It is imperative that patients be instructed to report promptly the development of fever, sore throat, signs of local infection, bleeding from any site, or symptoms suggestive of anemia. Any one of these findings may indicate busulfan toxicity; however, they may also indicate transformation of the disease to an acute "blastic" form. Since busulfan may have a delayed effect, it is important to withdraw the medication temporarily at the first sign of an abnormally large or exceptionally rapid fall in any of the formed elements of the blood. *Patients should never be allowed to take the drug without close medical supervision.*

Seizures have been reported in patients receiving busulfan. As with any potentially epileptogenic drug, caution should be exercised when administering busulfan to patients with a history of seizure disorder, head trauma, or receiving other potentially epileptogenic drugs. Some investigators have used prophylactic anticonvulsant therapy in this setting.

Information for Patients: Patients beginning therapy with busulfan should be informed of the importance of having periodic blood counts and to immediately report any unusual fever or bleeding. Aside from the major toxicity of myelosuppression, patients should be instructed to report any difficulty in breathing, persistent cough, or congestion. They should be told that diffuse pulmonary fibrosis is an infrequent, but serious and potentially life-threatening complication of long-term busulfan therapy. Patients should be alerted to report any signs of abrupt weakness, unusual fatigue, anorexia, weight loss, nausea and vomiting, and melanoderma that could be associated with a syndrome resembling adrenal insufficiency. Patients should never be allowed to take the drug without medical supervision and they should be informed that other encountered toxicities to busulfan include infertility, amenorrhea, skin hyperpigmentation, drug hypersensitivity, dryness of the mucous membranes, and rarely, cataract formation. Women of childbearing potential should be advised to avoid becoming pregnant. The increased risk of a second malignancy should be explained to the patient.

Laboratory Tests: It is recommended that evaluation of the hemoglobin or hematocrit, total white blood cell count and differential count, and quantitative platelet count be obtained weekly while the patient is on busulfan therapy. In cases where the cause of fluctuation in the formed elements of the peripheral blood is obscure, bone marrow examination may be useful for evaluation of marrow status. A decision to increase, decrease, continue, or discontinue a given dose of busulfan must be based not only on the absolute hematologic values, but also on the rapidity with which changes are occurring. The dosage of busulfan may need to be reduced if this agent is combined with other drugs whose primary toxicity is myelosuppression. Occasional patients may be unusually sensitive to busulfan administered at standard dosage and suffer neutropenia or thrombocytopenia after a relatively short exposure to the drug. Busulfan should not be used where facilities for complete blood counts, including quantitative platelet counts, are not available at weekly (or more frequent) intervals.

Drug Interactions: Busulfan may cause additive myelosuppression when used with other myelosuppressive drugs.

In one study, 12 of approximately 330 patients receiving continuous busulfan and thioguanine therapy for treatment of chronic myelogenous leukemia were found to have portal hypertension and esophageal varices associated with abnormal liver function tests. Subsequent liver biopsies were performed in 4 of these patients, all of which showed evidence of nodular regenerative hyperplasia. Duration of combination therapy prior to the appearance of esophageal varices ranged from 6 to 45 months. With the present analysis of the data, no cases of hepatotoxicity have appeared in the busulfan-alone arm of the study. Long-term continuous therapy with thioguanine and busulfan should be used with caution.

Busulfan-induced pulmonary toxicity may be additive to the effects produced by other cytotoxic agents.

The concomitant systemic administration of itraconazole to patients receiving high-dose MYLERAN may result in reduced busulfan clearance (see CLINICAL PHARMACOLOGY). Patients should be monitored for signs of busulfan toxicity when itraconazole is used concomitantly with MYLERAN.

Carcinogenesis, Mutagenesis, Impairment of Fertility: See WARNINGS section. The World Health Organization has concluded that there is a causal relationship between busulfan exposure and the development of secondary malignancies.

Pregnancy: ***Teratogenic Effects:*** Pregnancy Category D. See WARNINGS section.

Nonteratogenic Effects: There have been reports in the literature of small infants being born after the mothers received busulfan during pregnancy, in particular, during the third trimester. One case was reported where an infant had mild anemia and neutropenia at birth after busulfan was administered to the mother from the eighth week of pregnancy to term.

Nursing Mothers: It is not known whether this drug is excreted in human milk. Because of the potential for tumorigenicity shown for busulfan in animal and human studies, a decision should be made whether to discontinue nursing or to discontinue the drug, taking into account the importance of the drug to the mother.

Pediatric Use: See INDICATIONS AND USAGE and DOSAGE AND ADMINISTRATION sections.

Geriatric Use: Clinical studies of busulfan did not include sufficient numbers of subjects aged 65 and over to determine whether they respond differently from younger subjects. Other reported clinical experience has not identified differences in responses between the elderly and younger patients. In general, dose selection for an elderly patient should be cautious, usually starting at the low end of the dosing range, reflecting the greater frequency of decreased hepatic, renal, or cardiac function, and of concomitant disease or other drug therapy.

ADVERSE REACTIONS

Hematological Effects: The most frequent, serious, toxic effect of busulfan is dose-related myelosuppression resulting in leukopenia, thrombocytopenia, and anemia. Myelosuppression is most frequently the result of a failure to discontinue dosage in the face of an undetected decrease in leukocyte or platelet counts.

Aplastic anemia (sometimes irreversible) has been reported rarely, often following long-term conventional doses and also high doses of MYLERAN.

Pulmonary: Interstitial pulmonary fibrosis has been reported rarely, but it is a clinically significant adverse effect when observed and calls for immediate discontinuation of further administration of the drug. The role of corticosteroids in arresting or reversing the fibrosis has been reported to be beneficial in some cases and without effect in others.

Cardiac: Cardiac tamponade has been reported in a small number of patients with thalassemia who received busulfan and cyclophosphamide as the preparatory regimen for bone marrow transplantation (see WARNINGS).

One case of endocardial fibrosis has been reported in a 79-year-old woman who received a total dose of 7,200 mg of busulfan over a period of 9 years for the management of chronic myelogenous leukemia. At autopsy, she was found to have endocardial fibrosis of the left ventricle in addition to interstitial pulmonary fibrosis.

Ocular: Busulfan is capable of inducing cataracts in rats and there have been several reports indicating that this is a rare complication in humans.

Dermatologic: Hyperpigmentation is the most common adverse skin reaction and occurs in 5% to 10% of patients, particularly those with a dark complexion.

Metabolic: In a few cases, a clinical syndrome closely resembling adrenal insufficiency and characterized by weakness, severe fatigue, anorexia, weight loss, nausea and vomiting, and melanoderma has developed after prolonged busulfan therapy. The symptoms have sometimes been reversible when busulfan was withdrawn. Adrenal responsiveness to exogenously administered ACTH has usually been normal. However, pituitary function testing with metyrapone revealed a blunted urinary 17-hydroxycorticosteroid excretion in 2 patients. Following the discontinuation of busulfan (which was associated with clinical improvement), rechallenge with metyrapone revealed normal pituitary-adrenal function.

Hyperuricemia and/or hyperuricosuria are not uncommon in patients with chronic myelogenous leukemia. Additional rapid destruction of granulocytes may accompany the initiation of chemotherapy and increase the urate pool. Adverse effects can be minimized by increased hydration, urine alkalinization, and the prophylactic administration of a xanthine oxidase inhibitor such as allopurinol.

Hepatic Effects: Esophageal varices have been reported in patients receiving continuous busulfan and thioguanine therapy for treatment of chronic myelogenous leukemia (see PRECAUTIONS: Drug Interactions). Hepatic veno-occlusive disease has been observed in patients receiving busulfan (see WARNINGS).

Miscellaneous: Other reported adverse reactions include: urticaria, erythema multiforme, erythema nodosum, alopecia, porphyria cutanea tarda, excessive dryness and fragility of the skin with anhidrosis, dryness of the oral mucous membranes and cheilosis, gynecomastia, cholestatic jaundice, and myasthenia gravis. Most of these are single case reports, and in many, a clear cause-and-effect relationship with busulfan has not been demonstrated.

Seizures (see PRECAUTIONS: General) have been observed in patients receiving higher than recommended doses of busulfan.

Observed During Clinical Practice: The following events have been identified during post-approval use of busulfan. Because they are reported voluntarily from a population of unknown size, estimates of frequency cannot be made. These events have been chosen for inclusion due to a combination of their seriousness, frequency of reporting, or potential causal connection to busulfan.

Blood and Lymphatic: Aplastic anemia.

Eye: Cataracts, corneal thinning, lens changes.

Hepatobiliary Tract and Pancreas: Centrilobular sinusoidal fibrosis, hepatic veno- occlusive disease, hepatocellular atrophy, hepatocellular necrosis, hyperbilirubinemia (see WARNINGS).

Non-site Specific: Infection, mucositis, sepsis.

Respiratory: Pneumonia.

Skin: Rash. An increased local cutaneous reaction has been observed in patients receiving radiotherapy soon after busulfan.

OVERDOSAGE

There is no known antidote to busulfan. The principal toxic effects are bone marrow depression and pancytopenia. The hematologic status should be closely monitored and vigorous supportive measures instituted if necessary. Induction of vomiting or gastric lavage followed by administration of charcoal would be indicated if ingestion were recent. Dialysis may be considered in the management of overdose as there is 1 report of successful dialysis of busulfan (see CLINICAL PHARMACOLOGY).

Gastrointestinal toxicity with mucositis, nausea, vomiting, and diarrhea has been observed when MYLERAN was used in association with bone marrow transplantation.

Oral LD_{50} single doses in mice are 120 mg/kg. Two distinct types of toxic response are seen at median lethal doses given intraperitoneally. Within a matter of hours there are signs of stimulation of the central nervous system with convulsions and death on the first day. Mice are more sensitive to this effect than are rats. With doses at the LD_{50} there is also delayed death due to damage to the bone marrow. At 3 times the LD_{50}, atrophy of the mucosa of the large intestine is found after a week, whereas that of the small intestine is little affected. After doses in the order of 10 times those used therapeutically were added to the diet of rats, irreversible cataracts were produced after several weeks. Small doses had no such effect.

DOSAGE AND ADMINISTRATION

Busulfan is administered orally. The usual adult dose range for *remission induction* is 4 to 8 mg, total dose, daily. Dosing on a weight basis is the same for both pediatric patients and adults, approximately 60 mcg/kg of body weight or 1.8 mg/m^2 of body surface, daily. Since the rate of fall of the leukocyte count is dose related, daily doses exceeding 4 mg per day should be reserved for patients with the most compelling symptoms; the greater the total daily dose, the greater is the possibility of inducing bone marrow aplasia.

A decrease in the leukocyte count is not usually seen during the first 10 to 15 days of treatment; the leukocyte count may actually increase during this period and it should not be interpreted as resistance to the drug, nor should the dose be increased. Since the leukocyte count may continue to fall for more than 1 month after discontinuing the drug, it is important that busulfan be discontinued *prior* to the total leukocyte count falling into the normal range. When the total leukocyte count has declined to approximately 15,000/mcL, the drug should be withheld.

With a constant dose of busulfan, the total leukocyte count declines exponentially; a weekly plot of the leukocyte count on semi-logarithmic graph paper aids in predicting the time when therapy should be discontinued. With the recommended dose of busulfan, a normal leukocyte count is usually achieved in 12 to 20 weeks.

During remission, the patient is examined at monthly intervals and treatment resumed with the induction dosage when the total leukocyte count reaches approximately 50,000/mcL. When remission is shorter than 3 months, maintenance therapy of 1 to 3 mg daily may be advisable in order to keep the hematological status under control and prevent rapid relapse.

Procedures for proper handling and disposal of anticancer drugs should be considered. Several guidelines on this subject have been published.[1-8]

There is no general agreement that all of the procedures recommended in the guidelines are necessary or appropriate.

HOW SUPPLIED

MYLERAN is supplied as white, film-coated, round, biconvex tablets containing 2 mg busulfan in amber glass bottles with child-resistant closures. One side is imprinted with "GX EF3" and the other side is imprinted with an "M."
Bottle of 25 (NDC 0173-0713-25).

Store at 25°C (77°F); excursions permitted to 15° to 30°C (59° to 86°F) (see USP Controlled Room Temperature).

REFERENCES

1. ONS Clinical Practice Committee. Cancer Chemotherapy Guidelines and Recommendations for Practice. Pittsburgh, PA. Oncology Nursing Society; 1999:32-41.
2. Recommendations for the safe handling of parenteral antineoplastic drugs. Washington, DC: Division of Safety, Clinical Center Pharmacy Department and Cancer Nursing Services, National Institutes of Health and Human Services; 1992. US Dept of Health and Human Services, Public Health Service publication NIH 92-2621.
3. AMA Council on Scientific Affairs. Guidelines for handling parenteral antineoplastics. *JAMA.* 1985;253:1590-1591.
4. National Study Commission on Cytotoxic Exposure. Recommendations for handling cytotoxic agents. 1987. Available from Louis P. Jeffrey, Chairman, National Study Commission on Cytotoxic Exposure. Massachusetts College of Pharmacy and Allied Health Sciences, 179 Longwood Avenue, Boston, MA 02115.
5. Clinical Oncological Society of Australia. Guidelines and recommendations for safe handling of antineoplastic agents. *Med J Australia.* 1983;1:426-428.
6. Jones RB, Frank R, Mass T. Safe handling of chemotherapeutic agents: a report from the Mount Sinai Medical Center. *CA-A Cancer J for Clin.* 1983;33:258-263.
7. American Society of Hospital Pharmacists. ASHP technical assistance bulletin on handling cytotoxic and hazardous drugs. *Am J Hosp Pharm.* 1990;47:1033-1049.
8. Controlling Occupational Exposure to Hazardous Drugs. (OSHA Work-Practice Guidelines.) *Am J. Health-Syst Pharm.* 1996:53:1669-1685.

Manufactured by
Heumann Pharma GmbH
90537 Feucht, Germany
for GlaxoSmithKline
Research Triangle Park, NC 27709
©2004, GlaxoSmithKline. All rights reserved.
January 2004/RL-2065

PARNATE®   ℞

[par'nāt]
(tranylcypromine sulfate)
tablets 10 mg

Suicidality and Antidepressant Drugs
Antidepressants increased the risk compared to placebo of suicidal thinking and behavior (suicidality) in children, adolescents, and young adults in short-term studies of major depressive disorder (MDD) and other psychiatric disorders. Anyone considering the use of PARNATE or any other antidepressant in a child, adolescent, or young adult must balance this risk with the clinical need. Short-term studies did not show an increase in the risk of suicidality with antidepressants compared to placebo in adults beyond age 24; there was a reduction in risk with antidepressants compared to placebo in adults aged 65 and older. Depression and certain other psychiatric disorders are themselves associated with increases in the risk of suicide. Patients of all ages who are started on antidepressant therapy should be monitored appropriately and observed

---

closely for clinical worsening, suicidality, or unusual changes in behavior. Families and caregivers should be advised of the need for close observation and communication with the prescriber. PARNATE is not approved for use in pediatric patients. (See WARNINGS TO PHYSICIANS: Clinical Worsening and Suicide Risk, PRECAUTIONS: Information for Patients, and PRECAUTIONS: Pediatric Use.)

DESCRIPTION

Chemically, tranylcypromine sulfate is (±)-*trans*-2-phenylcyclopropylamine sulfate (2:1). Each round, rose-red, film-coated tablet is debossed with the product name PARNATE and SB and contains tranylcypromine sulfate equivalent to 10 mg of tranylcypromine. Inactive ingredients consist of cellulose, citric acid, croscarmellose sodium, D&C Red No. 7, FD&C Blue No. 2, FD&C Red No. 40, FD&C Yellow No. 6, gelatin, lactose, magnesium stearate, talc, titanium dioxide, and trace amounts of other inactive ingredients.

ACTION

Tranylcypromine is a non-hydrazine monoamine oxidase inhibitor with a rapid onset of activity. It increases the concentration of epinephrine, norepinephrine, and serotonin in storage sites throughout the nervous system and, in theory, this increased concentration of monoamines in the brain stem is the basis for its antidepressant activity. When tranylcypromine is withdrawn, monoamine oxidase activity is recovered in 3 to 5 days, although the drug is excreted in 24 hours.

INDICATIONS

For the treatment of Major Depressive Episode Without Melancholia.
PARNATE should be used in adult patients who can be closely supervised. It should rarely be the first antidepressant drug given. Rather, the drug is suited for patients who have failed to respond to the drugs more commonly administered for depression.
The effectiveness of PARNATE has been established in adult outpatients, most of whom had a depressive illness which would correspond to a diagnosis of Major Depressive Episode Without Melancholia. As described in the American Psychiatric Association's Diagnostic and Statistical Manual, third edition (DSM III), Major Depressive Episode implies a prominent and relatively persistent (nearly every day for at least 2 weeks) depressed or dysphoric mood that usually interferes with daily functioning and includes at least 4 of the following 8 symptoms: change in appetite, change in sleep, psychomotor agitation or retardation, loss of interest in usual activities or decrease in sexual drive, increased fatigability, feelings of guilt or worthlessness, slowed thinking or impaired concentration, and suicidal ideation or attempts.
The effectiveness of PARNATE in patients who meet the criteria for Major Depressive Episode with Melancholia (endogenous features) has not been established.

SUMMARY OF CONTRAINDICATIONS

PARNATE should not be administered in combination with any of the following: MAO inhibitors or dibenzazepine derivatives; sympathomimetics (including amphetamines); some central nervous system depressants (including narcotics and alcohol); antihypertensive, diuretic, antihistaminic, sedative, or anesthetic drugs; bupropion HCl; buspirone HCl; dextromethorphan; cheese or other foods with a high tyramine content; or excessive quantities of caffeine.
PARNATE should not be administered to any patient with a confirmed or suspected cerebrovascular defect or to any patient with cardiovascular disease, hypertension, or history of headache.
(For complete discussion of contraindications and warnings, see below.)

CONTRAINDICATIONS

PARNATE is contraindicated:
1. In patients with cerebrovascular defects or cardiovascular disorders
PARNATE should not be administered to any patient with a confirmed or suspected cerebrovascular defect or to any patient with cardiovascular disease or hypertension.
2. In the presence of pheochromocytoma
PARNATE should not be used in the presence of pheochromocytoma since such tumors secrete pressor substances.
3. In combination with MAO inhibitors or with dibenzazepine-related entities
PARNATE should not be administered together or in rapid succession with other MAO inhibitors or with dibenzazepine-related entities. Hypertensive crises or severe convulsive seizures may occur in patients receiving such combinations.
In patients being transferred to PARNATE from another MAO inhibitor or from a dibenzazepine-related entity, allow a medication-free interval of at least a week, then initiate

---

PARNATE using half the normal starting dosage for at least the first week of therapy. Similarly, at least a week should elapse between the discontinuance of PARNATE and the administration of another MAO inhibitor or a dibenzazepine-related entity, or the readministration of PARNATE.
The following list includes some other MAO inhibitors, dibenzazepine-related entities and tricyclic antidepressants, and the companies which market them.

Other MAO Inhibitors

Generic Name	Source
Furazolidone	
Isocarboxazid	Marplan® (Oxford Pharm Services)
Pargyline HCl	
Pargyline HCl and methyclothiazide	
Phenelzine sulfate	Nardil® (Pfizer)
Procarbazine HCl	Matulane® (Sigma Tau)

Dibenzazepine-Related and Other Tricyclics

Generic Name	Source
Amitriptyline HCl	(Sandoz)
Perphenazine and amitriptyline HCl	(Sandoz)
Clomipramine hydrochloride	Anafranil® (Mallinckrodt)
Desipramine HCl	(Sandoz)
Imipramine HCl	(Sandoz)
	Tofranil® (Mallinckrodt)
Nortriptyline HCl	(Mylan)
	Pamelor® (Mallinckrodt)
Protriptyline HCl	Vivactil® (Odyssey Pharmaceuticals, Inc.)
Doxepin HCl	Sinequan® (Pfizer)
Carbamazepine	Tegretol® (Novartis)
Cyclobenzaprine HCl	(Mylan)
	Flexeril® (McNeil)
Amoxapine	(Watson)
Maprotiline HCl	(Mylan)
Trimipramine maleate	Surmontil® (Odyssey Pharmaceuticals, Inc.)

4. In combination with bupropion
The concurrent administration of an MAO inhibitor and bupropion hydrochloride (Wellbutrin®, Wellbutrin SR®, Wellbutrin XL®, Zyban®, GlaxoSmithKline) is contraindicated. At least 14 days should elapse between discontinuation of an MAO inhibitor and initiation of treatment with bupropion hydrochloride.
5. In combination with selective serotonin reuptake inhibitors (SSRIs) or selective norepinephrine reuptake inhibitors (SNRIs)
As a general rule, PARNATE should not be administered in combination with any SSRI or SNRI. There have been reports of serious, sometimes fatal, reactions (including hyperthermia, rigidity, myoclonus, autonomic instability with possible rapid fluctuations of vital signs, and mental status changes that include extreme agitation progressing to delirium and coma) in patients receiving a SSRI (e.g., fluoxetine, Prozac®, Eli Lilly and Company) or a SNRI (e.g., venlafaxine, Effexor®, Effexor XR®, Wyeth) in combination with a monoamine oxidase inhibitor (MAOI), and in patients who have recently discontinued a SSRI or SNRI and are then started on an MAOI. Some cases presented with features resembling neuroleptic malignant syndrome. Therefore SSRIs and SNRIs should not be used in combination with an MAOI, or within 14 days of discontinuing therapy with an MAOI.
Since fluoxetine and its major metabolite have very long elimination half-lives, at least 5 weeks should be allowed after stopping fluoxetine before starting an MAOI.
At least 2 weeks should be allowed after stopping sertraline (Zoloft®, Pfizer) or paroxetine (Paxil®, Paxil CR®, GlaxoSmithKline) before starting an MAOI.
At least one week should be allowed after stopping a SNRI (e.g., venlafaxine) before starting a MAOI.
6. In combination with buspirone
PARNATE should not be used in combination with buspirone HCl, since several cases of elevated blood pressure have been reported in patients taking MAO inhibitors who were then given buspirone HCl. At least 10 days should elapse between the discontinuation of PARNATE and the institution of buspirone HCl.
7. In combination with sympathomimetics
PARNATE should not be administered in combination with sympathomimetics, including amphetamines which may be found in many herbal preparations as well as over-the-counter drugs such as cold, hay fever or weight-reducing preparations that contain vasoconstrictors.

During therapy with PARNATE, it appears that certain patients are particularly vulnerable to the effects of sympathomimetics when the activity of certain enzymes is inhibited. Use of sympathomimetics and compounds such as guanethidine, methyldopa, reserpine, dopamine, levodopa, and tryptophan with PARNATE may precipitate hypertension, headache, and related symptoms. Cerebral hemorrhage may also occur. The combination of MAOIs and tryptophan has been reported to cause behavioral and neurologic syndromes including disorientation, confusion, amnesia, delirium, agitation, hypomanic signs, ataxia, myoclonus, hyperreflexia, shivering, ocular oscillations, and Babinski's signs.

8. In combination with meperidine

Do not use meperidine concomitantly with MAO inhibitors or within 2 or 3 weeks following MAOI therapy. Serious reactions have been precipitated with concomitant use, including coma, severe hypertension or hypotension, severe respiratory depression, convulsions, malignant hyperpyrexia, excitation, peripheral vascular collapse, and death. It is thought that these reactions may be mediated by accumulation of 5-HT (serotonin) consequent to MAO inhibition.

9. In combination with dextromethorphan

The combination of MAO inhibitors and dextromethorphan has been reported to cause brief episodes of psychosis or bizarre behavior.

10. In combination with cheese or other foods with a high tyramine content

When excessive amounts of tyramine are consumed in conjunction with tranylcypromine, or within 2 weeks of stopping treatment, a serious and sometimes fatal hypertensive reaction may occur.

Tyramine occurs naturally in some foods or may occur from the bacterial breakdown of protein in foods which are fermented, aged, or spoiled. Foods that have reliably been shown to contain a high tyramine content and may also have been reported to induce a serious hypertensive reaction when consumed with tranylcypromine are:

- all matured or aged cheeses (note: all cheeses are considered matured or aged except fresh cottage cheese, cream cheese, ricotta, and processed cheese. All non-cheese dairy products can be consumed providing they are fresh)
- all aged, cured or fermented meat, fish, or poultry (note: meat, fish, or poultry that has not undergone aging, curing or fermenting and that is bought fresh, stored correctly and eaten fresh is not contraindicated)
- all fermented soybean products (e.g., soy sauce, miso, fermented tofu)
- sauerkraut
- fava or broad bean pods
- banana peel (but not the pulp)
- concentrated yeast extracts (e.g., Marmite or Vegemite spread)
- all tap/draught beers (note: some bottled beers, including non-alcoholic beer, may also pose a risk).

Patients should be advised to minimize or avoid use of all alcoholic beverages while taking PARNATE. Patients should be advised to adhere to the following dietary guidance about eating fresh foods:

Foods may be deliberately aged as part of their processing and these are contraindicated (*see list above*). Foods may also naturally age over time, even if they are refrigerated. It is therefore extremely important that patients are instructed to buy and eat only fresh foods or those which have been properly frozen. They should avoid eating foods if they are unsure of their storage conditions or freshness and they should be cautious of foods of unknown age or composition even if refrigerated.

The longer food is left to deteriorate and the larger the quantity of food eaten, the greater the potential quantity of tyramine ingested. Where there is any doubt, patients should be advised to either avoid the food or consume it in strict moderation if it is not otherwise contraindicated.

Patients should also be warned that tyramine levels may vary by brand or even batch and a person may absorb different amounts of tyramine from a particular food at different times. Therefore, if they have accidentally consumed a prohibited food on one occasion and not had a reaction, this does not mean that they will not have a serious hypertensive reaction if they consume the same food on a different occasion.

11. In patients undergoing elective surgery

Patients taking PARNATE should not undergo elective surgery requiring general anesthesia. Also, they should not be given cocaine or local anesthesia containing sympathomimetic vasoconstrictors. The possible combined hypotensive effects of PARNATE and spinal anesthesia should be kept in mind. PARNATE should be discontinued at least 10 days prior to elective surgery.

ADDITIONAL CONTRAINDICATIONS

In general, the physician should bear in mind the possibility of a lowered margin of safety when PARNATE is administered in combination with potent drugs.

1. PARNATE should not be used in combination with some central nervous system depressants such as narcotics and alcohol, or with hypotensive agents. A marked potentiating effect on these classes of drugs has been reported.

2. Anti-parkinsonism drugs should be used with caution in patients receiving PARNATE since severe reactions have been reported.

3. PARNATE should not be used in patients with a history of liver disease or in those with abnormal liver function tests.

4. Excessive use of caffeine in any form should be avoided in patients receiving PARNATE.

WARNINGS TO PHYSICIANS

Clinical Worsening and Suicide Risk

Patients with major depressive disorder (MDD), both adult and pediatric, may experience worsening of their depression and/or the emergence of suicidal ideation and behavior (suicidality) or unusual changes in behavior, whether or not they are taking antidepressant medications, and this risk may persist until significant remission occurs. Suicide is a known risk of depression and certain other psychiatric disorders, and these disorders themselves are the strongest predictors of suicide. There has been a long-standing concern, however, that antidepressants may have a role in inducing worsening of depression and the emergence of suicidality in certain patients during the early phases of treatment. Pooled analyses of short-term placebo-controlled trials of antidepressant drugs (SSRIs and others) showed that these drugs increase the risk of suicidal thinking and behavior (suicidality) in children, adolescents, and young adults (ages 18-24) with major depressive disorder (MDD) and other psychiatric disorders. Short-term studies did not show an increase in the risk of suicidality with antidepressants compared to placebo in adults beyond age 24; there was a reduction with antidepressants compared to placebo in adults aged 65 and older.

The pooled analyses of placebo-controlled trials in children and adolescents with MDD, obsessive compulsive disorder (OCD), or other psychiatric disorders included a total of 24 short-term trials of 9 antidepressant drugs in over 4,400 patients. The pooled analyses of placebo-controlled trials in adults with MDD or other psychiatric disorders included a total of 295 short-term trials (median duration of 2 months) of 11 antidepressant drugs in over 77,000 patients. There was considerable variation in risk of suicidality among drugs, but a tendency toward an increase in the younger patients for almost all drugs studied. There were differences in absolute risk of suicidality across the different indications, with the highest incidence in MDD. The risk differences (drug vs placebo), however, were relatively stable within age strata and across indications. These risk differences (drug-placebo difference in the number of cases of suicidality per 1,000 patients treated) are provided in Table 1.

Table 1.

Age Range	Drug-Placebo Difference in Number of Cases of Suicidality per 1,000 Patients Treated
Increases Compared to Placebo	
<18	14 additional cases
18-24	5 additional cases
Decreases Compared to Placebo	
25-64	1 fewer case
≥65	6 fewer cases

No suicides occurred in any of the pediatric trials. There were suicides in the adult trials, but the number was not sufficient to reach any conclusion about drug effect on suicide.

It is unknown whether the suicidality risk extends to longer-term use, i.e., beyond several months. However, there is substantial evidence from placebo-controlled maintenance trials in adults with depression that the use of antidepressants can delay the recurrence of depression.

All patients being treated with antidepressants for any indication should be monitored appropriately and observed closely for clinical worsening, suicidality, and unusual changes in behavior, especially during the initial few months of a course of drug therapy, or at times of dose changes, either increases or decreases.

The following symptoms, anxiety, agitation, panic attacks, insomnia, irritability, hostility, aggressiveness, impulsivity, akathisia (psychomotor restlessness), hypomania, and mania, have been reported in adult and pediatric patients being treated with antidepressants for major depressive disorder as well as for other indications, both psychiatric and nonpsychiatric. Although a causal link between the emergence of such symptoms and either the worsening of depression and/or the emergence of suicidal impulses has not been established, there is concern that such symptoms may represent precursors to emerging suicidality.

Consideration should be given to changing the therapeutic regimen, including possibly discontinuing the medication, in patients whose depression is persistently worse, or who are experiencing emergent suicidality or symptoms that might be precursors to worsening depression or suicidality, especially if these symptoms are severe, abrupt in onset, or were not part of the patient's presenting symptoms.

Families and caregivers of patients being treated with antidepressants for major depressive disorder or other indications, both psychiatric and nonpsychiatric, should be alerted about the need to monitor patients for the emergence of agitation, irritability, unusual changes in behavior, and the other symptoms described above, as well as the emergence of suicidality, and to report such symptoms immediately to healthcare providers. Such monitoring should include daily observation by families and caregivers. Prescriptions for PARNATE should be written for the smallest quantity of tablets consistent with good patient management, in order to reduce the risk of overdose.

Screening Patients for Bipolar Disorder

A major depressive episode may be the initial presentation of bipolar disorder. It is generally believed (though not established in controlled trials) that treating such an episode with an antidepressant alone may increase the likelihood of precipitation of a mixed/manic episode in patients at risk for bipolar disorder. Whether any of the symptoms described above represent such a conversion is unknown. However, prior to initiating treatment with an antidepressant, patients with depressive symptoms should be adequately screened to determine if they are at risk for bipolar disorder; such screening should include a detailed psychiatric history, including a family history of suicide, bipolar disorder, and depression. It should be noted that PARNATE is not approved for use in treating bipolar depression.

PARNATE is a potent agent with the capability of producing serious side effects. PARNATE is not recommended in those depressive reactions where other antidepressant drugs may be effective. **It should be reserved for patients who can be closely supervised and who have not responded satisfactorily to the drugs more commonly administered for depression.**

Before prescribing, the physician should be completely familiar with the full material on dosage, side effects, and contraindications on these pages, with the principles of MAO inhibitor therapy and the side effects of this class of drugs. Also, the physician should be familiar with the symptomatology of mental depressions and alternate methods of treatment to aid in the careful selection of patients for therapy with PARNATE.

Pregnancy Warning

Use of any drug in pregnancy, during lactation or in women of childbearing age requires that the potential benefits of the drug be weighed against its possible hazards to mother and child.

Animal reproductive studies show that PARNATE passes through the placental barrier into the fetus of the rat, and into the milk of the lactating dog. The absence of a harmful action of PARNATE on fertility or on postnatal development by either prenatal treatment or from the milk of treated animals has not been demonstrated. Tranylcypromine is excreted in human milk.

WARNING TO THE PATIENT

Patients should be instructed to report promptly the occurrence of headache or other unusual symptoms, i.e., palpitation and/or tachycardia, a sense of constriction in the throat or chest, sweating, dizziness, neck stiffness, nausea, or vomiting.

Patients should be warned against eating the foods listed in Section 11 under Contraindications while on therapy with PARNATE. Also, they should be told not to drink alcoholic beverages. The patient should also be warned about the possibility of hypotension and faintness, as well as drowsiness sufficient to impair performance of potentially hazardous tasks such as driving a car or operating machinery.

Patients should also be cautioned not to take concomitant medications, whether prescription or over-the-counter drugs such as cold, hay fever, or weight-reducing preparations, without the advice of a physician. They should be advised not to consume excessive amounts of caffeine in any form. Likewise, they should inform other physicians, and their dentist, about their use of PARNATE.

See PRECAUTIONS—Information for Patients for information regarding clinical worsening and suicide risk.

WARNINGS

Hypertensive Crisis

The most important reaction associated with PARNATE is the occurrence of hypertensive crises which have sometimes been fatal.

These crises are characterized by some or all of the following symptoms: occipital headache which may radiate frontally, palpitation, neck stiffness or soreness, nausea or vomiting, sweating (sometimes with fever and sometimes with cold, clammy skin), and photophobia. Either tachycardia or bradycardia may be present, and associated constricting chest pain and dilated pupils may occur. **Intracranial bleeding, sometimes fatal in outcome, has been reported in association with the paradoxical increase in blood pressure.**

In all patients taking PARNATE, blood pressure should be followed closely to detect evidence of any pressor response. It is emphasized that full reliance should not be placed on blood pressure readings, but that the patient should also be observed frequently.

Therapy should be discontinued immediately upon the occurrence of palpitation or frequent headaches during therapy with PARNATE. These signs may be prodromal of a hypertensive crisis.

Important:

Recommended treatment in hypertensive crises

If a hypertensive crisis occurs, PARNATE should be discontinued and therapy to lower blood pressure should be instituted immediately. Headache tends to abate as blood pressure is lowered. On the basis of present evidence, phentolamine is recommended. (The dosage reported for phentolamine is 5 mg I.V.) Care should be taken to administer this drug slowly in order to avoid producing an excessive hypotensive effect. Fever should be managed by means of external cooling. Other symptomatic and supportive measures may be desirable in particular cases. Do not use parenteral reserpine.

PRECAUTIONS

Hypotension

Hypotension has been observed during therapy with PARNATE. Symptoms of postural hypotension are seen most commonly but not exclusively in patients with pre-existent hypertension; blood pressure usually returns rapidly to pretreatment levels upon discontinuation of the drug. At doses above 30 mg daily, postural hypotension is a major side effect and may result in syncope. Dosage increases should be made more gradually in patients showing a tendency toward hypotension at the beginning of therapy. Postural hypotension may be relieved by having the patient lie down until blood pressure returns to normal.

Also, when PARNATE is combined with those phenothiazine derivatives or other compounds known to cause hypotension, the possibility of additive hypotensive effects should be considered.

There have been reports of drug dependency in patients using doses of tranylcypromine significantly in excess of the therapeutic range. Some of these patients had a history of previous substance abuse. The following withdrawal symptoms have been reported: restlessness, anxiety, depression, confusion, hallucinations, headache, weakness, and diarrhea.

Drugs which lower the seizure threshold, including MAO inhibitors, should not be used with Amipaque®*. As with other MAO inhibitors, PARNATE should be discontinued at least 48 hours before myelography and should not be resumed for at least 24 hours postprocedure.

MAO inhibitors may have the capacity to suppress anginal pain that would otherwise serve as a warning of myocardial ischemia.

The usual precautions should be observed in patients with impaired renal function since there is a possibility of cumulative effects in such patients.

Older patients may suffer more morbidity than younger patients during and following an episode of hypertension or malignant hyperthermia. Older patients have less compensatory reserve to cope with any serious adverse reaction. Therefore, PARNATE should be used with caution in the elderly population.

Although excretion of PARNATE is rapid, inhibition of MAO may persist up to 10 days following discontinuation.

Because the influence of PARNATE on the convulsive threshold is variable in animal experiments, suitable precautions should be taken if epileptic patients are treated.

Some MAO inhibitors have contributed to hypoglycemic episodes in diabetic patients receiving insulin or oral hypoglycemic agents. Therefore, PARNATE should be used with caution in diabetics using these drugs.

PARNATE may aggravate coexisting symptoms in depression, such as anxiety and agitation.

Use PARNATE with caution in hyperthyroid patients because of their increased sensitivity to pressor amines.

PARNATE should be administered with caution to patients receiving Antabuse®†. In a single study, rats given high intraperitoneal doses of *d* or *l* isomers of tranylcypromine sulfate plus disulfiram experienced severe toxicity including convulsions and death. Additional studies in rats given high oral doses of racemic tranylcypromine sulfate (PARNATE) and disulfiram produced no adverse interaction.

Information for Patients

Prescribers or other health professionals should inform patients, their families, and their caregivers about the benefits and risks associated with treatment with PARNATE and should counsel them in its appropriate use. A patient Medication Guide about "Antidepressant Medicines, Depression and Other Serious Mental Illnesses, and Suicidal Thoughts or Actions" is available for PARNATE. The prescriber or health professional should instruct patients, their families, and their caregivers to read the Medication Guide and should assist them in understanding its contents. Patients should be given the opportunity to discuss the contents of the Medication Guide and to obtain answers to any questions they may have. The complete text of the Medication Guide is reprinted at the end of this document.

Patients should be advised of the following issues and asked to alert their prescriber if these occur while taking PARNATE.

Clinical Worsening and Suicide Risk

Patients, their families, and their caregivers should be encouraged to be alert to the emergence of anxiety, agitation, panic attacks, insomnia, irritability, hostility, aggressiveness, impulsivity, akathisia (psychomotor restlessness), hypomania, mania, other unusual changes in behavior, worsening of depression, and suicidal ideation, especially early during antidepressant treatment and when the dose is adjusted up or down. Families and caregivers of patients should be advised to look for the emergence of such symptoms on a day-to-day basis, since changes may be abrupt. Such symptoms should be reported to the patient's prescriber or health professional, especially if they are severe, abrupt in onset, or were not part of the patient's presenting symptoms. Symptoms such as these may be associated with an increased risk for suicidal thinking and behavior and indicate a need for very close monitoring and possibly changes in the medication.

Pediatric Use

Safety and effectiveness in the pediatric population have not been established (see BOX WARNING and WARNINGS—Clinical Worsening and Suicide Risk). Anyone considering the use of PARNATE in a child or adolescent must balance the potential risks with the clinical need.

ADVERSE REACTIONS

Overstimulation which may include increased anxiety, agitation, and manic symptoms is usually evidence of excessive therapeutic action. Dosage should be reduced, or a phenothiazine tranquilizer should be administered concomitantly. Patients may experience restlessness or insomnia; may notice some weakness, drowsiness, episodes of dizziness or dry mouth; or may report nausea, diarrhea, abdominal pain, or constipation. Most of these effects can be relieved by lowering the dosage or by giving suitable concomitant medication.

Tachycardia, significant anorexia, edema, palpitation, blurred vision, chills, and impotence have each been reported.

Headaches without blood pressure elevation have occurred. Rare instances of hepatitis, skin rash, and alopecia have been reported.

Impaired water excretion compatible with the syndrome of inappropriate secretion of antidiuretic hormone (SIADH) has been reported.

Tinnitus, muscle spasm, tremors, myoclonic jerks, numbness, paresthesia, urinary retention, and retarded ejaculation have been reported.

Hematologic disorders including anemia, leukopenia, agranulocytosis, and thrombocytopenia have been reported.

Post-Introduction Reports

The following are spontaneously reported adverse events temporally associated with use of PARNATE. No clear relationship between PARNATE and these events has been established. Localized scleroderma, flare-up of cystic acne, ataxia, confusion, disorientation, memory loss, urinary frequency, urinary incontinence, urticaria, fissuring in corner of mouth, akinesia.

DOSAGE AND ADMINISTRATION

Dosage should be adjusted to the requirements of the individual patient. Improvement should be seen within 48 hours to 3 weeks after starting therapy.

The usual effective dosage is 30 mg per day, usually given in divided doses. If there are no signs of improvement after a reasonable period (up to 2 weeks), then the dosage may be increased in 10 mg per day increments at intervals of 1 to 3 weeks; the dosage range may be extended to a maximum of 60 mg per day from the usual 30 mg per day.

OVERDOSAGE

Symptoms

The characteristic symptoms that may be caused by overdosage are usually those described above.

However, an intensification of these symptoms and sometimes severe additional manifestations may be seen, depending on the degree of overdosage and on individual

susceptibility. Some patients exhibit insomnia, restlessness and anxiety, progressing in severe cases to agitation, mental confusion, and incoherence. Hypotension, dizziness, weakness, and drowsiness may occur, progressing in severe cases to extreme dizziness and shock. A few patients have displayed hypertension with severe headache and other symptoms. Rare instances have been reported in which hypertension was accompanied by twitching or myoclonic fibrillation of skeletal muscles with hyperpyrexia, sometimes progressing to generalized rigidity and coma.

Treatment

Because strategies for the management of overdose are continually evolving, it is advisable to contact a Poison Control Center to determine the latest recommendations for the management of an overdose of any drug. Telephone numbers for the certified Poison Control Centers are listed in the *Physicians' Desk Reference* (PDR).

Treatment should normally consist of general supportive measures, close observation of vital signs and steps to counteract specific symptoms as they occur, since MAO inhibition may persist. The management of hypertensive crises is described under WARNINGS in the HYPERTENSIVE CRISES section.

External cooling is recommended if hyperpyrexia occurs. Barbiturates have been reported to help relieve myoclonic reactions, but frequency of administration should be controlled carefully because PARNATE may prolong barbiturate activity. When hypotension requires treatment, the standard measures for managing circulatory shock should be initiated. If pressor agents are used, the rate of infusion should be regulated by careful observation of the patient because an exaggerated pressor response sometimes occurs in the presence of MAO inhibition. Remember that the toxic effect of PARNATE may be delayed or prolonged following the last dose of the drug. Therefore, the patient should be closely observed for at least a week. It is not known if tranylcypromine is dialyzable.

HOW SUPPLIED

PARNATE is supplied as round, rose-red, film-coated tablets debossed with the product name PARNATE and SB and contains tranylcypromine sulfate equivalent to 10 mg of tranylcypromine, in bottles of 100 with a desiccant.

10 mg 100's: NDC 0007-4471-20

Store between 15° and 30°C (59° and 86°F).

*metrizamide, The Sanofi-Aventis Group.

†disulfiram, Odyssey Pharmaceuticals, Inc.

Medication Guide

Antidepressant Medicines, Depression and Other Serious Mental Illnesses, and Suicidal Thoughts or Actions

PARNATE® (PAR-nate) (tranylcypromine sulfate) Tablets

Read the Medication Guide that comes with you or your family member's antidepressant medicine. This Medication Guide is only about the risk of suicidal thoughts and actions with antidepressant medicines. **Talk to your, or your family member's, healthcare provider about:**

• All risks and benefits of treatment with antidepressant medicines

• All treatment choices for depression or other serious mental illness

What is the most important information I should know about antidepressant medicines, depression and other serious mental illnesses, and suicidal thoughts or actions?

1. Antidepressant medicines may increase suicidal thoughts or actions in some children, teenagers, and young adults within the first few months of treatment.

2. Depression and other serious mental illnesses are the most important causes of suicidal thoughts and actions. Some people may have a particularly high risk of having suicidal thoughts or actions. These include people who have (or have a family history of) bipolar illness (also called manic-depressive illness) or suicidal thoughts or actions.

3. How can I watch for and try to prevent suicidal thoughts and actions in myself or a family member?

• Pay close attention to any changes, especially sudden changes, in mood, behaviors, thoughts, or feelings. This is very important when an antidepressant medicine is started or when the dose is changed.

• Call the healthcare provider right away to report new or sudden changes in mood, behavior, thoughts, or feelings.

• Keep all follow-up visits with the healthcare provider as scheduled. Call the healthcare provider between visits as needed, especially if you have concerns about symptoms.

Call a healthcare provider right away if you or your family member has any of the following symptoms, especially if they are new, worse, or worry you:

• Thoughts about suicide or dying

• Attempts to commit suicide

• New or worse depression

• New or worse anxiety

• Feeling very agitated or restless

• Panic attacks

• Trouble sleeping (insomnia)

• New or worse irritability

- Acting aggressive, being angry, or violent
- Acting on dangerous impulses
- An extreme increase in activity and talking (mania)
- Other unusual changes in behavior or mood

What else do I need to know about antidepressant medicines?

- **Never stop an antidepressant medicine without first talking to a healthcare provider.** Stopping an antidepressant medicine suddenly can cause other symptoms.
- **Antidepressants are medicines used to treat depression and other illnesses.** It is important to discuss all the risks of treating depression and also the risks of not treating it. Patients and their families or other caregivers should discuss all treatment choices with the healthcare provider, not just the use of antidepressants.
- **Antidepressant medicines have other side effects.** Call your doctor for medical advice about side effects. You may report side effects to FDA at 1-800-FDA-1088.
- **Antidepressant medicines can interact with other medicines.** Know all of the medicines that you or your family member takes. Keep a list of all medicines to show the healthcare provider. Do not start new medicines without first checking with your healthcare provider.
- **Not all antidepressant medicines prescribed for children are FDA approved for use in children.** Talk to your child's healthcare provider for more information.

This Medication Guide has been approved by the U.S. Food and Drug Administration for all antidepressants.

July 2008 PRT:4MG
GlaxoSmithKline
Research Triangle Park, NC 27709
©2010, GlaxoSmithKline. All rights reserved.
May 2010 PRT:75PI

PAXIL® ℞
[pax'il]
(paroxetine hydrochloride)
Tablets and Oral Suspension

SUICIDALITY AND ANTIDEPRESSANT DRUGS
Antidepressants increased the risk compared to placebo of suicidal thinking and behavior (suicidality) in children, adolescents, and young adults in short-term studies of major depressive disorder (MDD) and other psychiatric disorders. Anyone considering the use of PAXIL or any other antidepressant in a child, adolescent, or young adult must balance this risk with the clinical need. Short-term studies did not show an increase in the risk of suicidality with antidepressants compared to placebo in adults beyond age 24; there was a reduction in risk with antidepressants compared to placebo in adults aged 65 and older. Depression and certain other psychiatric disorders are themselves associated with increases in the risk of suicide. Patients of all ages who are started on antidepressant therapy should be monitored appropriately and observed closely for clinical worsening, suicidality, or unusual changes in behavior. Families and caregivers should be advised of the need for close observation and communication with the prescriber. PAXIL is not approved for use in pediatric patients. (See WARNINGS: Clinical Worsening and Suicide Risk, PRECAUTIONS: Information for Patients, and PRECAUTIONS: Pediatric Use.)

DESCRIPTION
PAXIL (paroxetine hydrochloride) is an orally administered psychotropic drug. It is the hydrochloride salt of a phenylpiperidine compound identified chemically as (-)-*trans*-4R-(4'-fluorophenyl)-3S-[(3',4'-methylenedioxyphenoxy) methyl] piperidine hydrochloride hemihydrate and has the empirical formula of $C_{19}H_{20}FNO_3 \cdot HCl \cdot 1/2H_2O$. The molecular weight is 374.8 (329.4 as free base). The structural formula of paroxetine hydrochloride is:

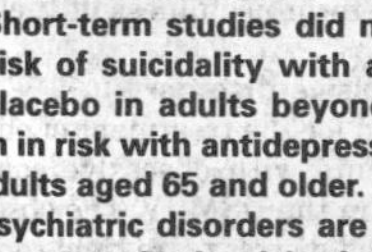

Paroxetine hydrochloride is an odorless, off-white powder, having a melting point range of 120° to 138°C and a solubility of 5.4 mg/mL in water.

Tablets
Each film-coated tablet contains paroxetine hydrochloride equivalent to paroxetine as follows: 10 mg—yellow (scored);

20 mg—pink (scored); 30 mg—blue, 40 mg—green. Inactive ingredients consist of dibasic calcium phosphate dihydrate, hypromellose, magnesium stearate, polyethylene glycols, polysorbate 80, sodium starch glycolate, titanium dioxide, and 1 or more of the following: D&C Red No. 30 aluminum lake, D&C Yellow No. 10 aluminum lake, FD&C Blue No. 2 aluminum lake, FD&C Yellow No. 6 aluminum lake.

Suspension for Oral Administration
Each 5 mL of orange-colored, orange-flavored liquid contains paroxetine hydrochloride equivalent to paroxetine, 10 mg. Inactive ingredients consist of polacrilin potassium, microcrystalline cellulose, propylene glycol, glycerin, sorbitol, methylparaben, propylparaben, sodium citrate dihydrate, citric acid anhydrous, sodium saccharin, flavorings, FD&C Yellow No. 6 aluminum lake, and simethicone emulsion, USP.

CLINICAL PHARMACOLOGY
Pharmacodynamics
The efficacy of paroxetine in the treatment of major depressive disorder, social anxiety disorder, obsessive compulsive disorder (OCD), panic disorder (PD), generalized anxiety disorder (GAD), and posttraumatic stress disorder (PTSD) is presumed to be linked to potentiation of serotonergic activity in the central nervous system resulting from inhibition of neuronal reuptake of serotonin (5-hydroxytryptamine, 5-HT). Studies at clinically relevant doses in humans have demonstrated that paroxetine blocks the uptake of serotonin into human platelets. In vitro studies in animals also suggest that paroxetine is a potent and highly selective inhibitor of neuronal serotonin reuptake and has only very weak effects on norepinephrine and dopamine neuronal reuptake. In vitro radioligand binding studies indicate that paroxetine has little affinity for muscarinic, alpha$_1$-, alpha$_2$-, beta-adrenergic-, dopamine (D$_2$)-, 5-HT$_1$-, 5-HT$_2$-, and histamine (H$_1$)-receptors; antagonism of muscarinic, histaminergic, and alpha$_1$-adrenergic receptors has been associated with various anticholinergic, sedative, and cardiovascular effects for other psychotropic drugs.
Because the relative potencies of paroxetine's major metabolites are at most 1/50 of the parent compound, they are essentially inactive.

Pharmacokinetics
Paroxetine hydrochloride is completely absorbed after oral dosing of a solution of the hydrochloride salt. The mean elimination half-life is approximately 21 hours (CV 32%) after oral dosing of 30 mg tablets of PAXIL daily for 30 days. Paroxetine is extensively metabolized and the metabolites are considered to be inactive. Nonlinearity in pharmacokinetics is observed with increasing doses. Paroxetine metabolism is mediated in part by CYP2D6, and the metabolites are primarily excreted in the urine and to some extent in the feces. Pharmacokinetic behavior of paroxetine has not been evaluated in subjects who are deficient in CYP2D6 (poor metabolizers).

Absorption and Distribution
Paroxetine is equally bioavailable from the oral suspension and tablet.
Paroxetine hydrochloride is completely absorbed after oral dosing of a solution of the hydrochloride salt. In a study in which normal male subjects (n = 15) received 30 mg tablets daily for 30 days, steady-state paroxetine concentrations were achieved by approximately 10 days for most subjects, although it may take substantially longer in an occasional patient. At steady state, mean values of C$_{max}$, T$_{max}$, C$_{min}$, and T$_{1/2}$ were 61.7 ng/mL (CV 45%), 5.2 hr. (CV 10%), 30.7 ng/mL (CV 67%), and 21.0 hours (CV 32%), respectively. The steady-state C$_{max}$ and C$_{min}$ values were about 6 and 14 times what would be predicted from single-dose studies. Steady-state drug exposure based on AUC$_{0-24}$ was about 8 times greater than would have been predicted from single-dose data in these subjects. The excess accumulation is a consequence of the fact that 1 of the enzymes that metabolizes paroxetine is readily saturable.
The effects of food on the bioavailability of paroxetine were studied in subjects administered a single dose with and without food. AUC was only slightly increased (6%) when drug was administered with food but the C$_{max}$ was 29% greater, while the time to reach peak plasma concentration decreased from 6.4 hours post-dosing to 4.9 hours.
Paroxetine distributes throughout the body, including the CNS, with only 1% remaining in the plasma.
Approximately 95% and 93% of paroxetine is bound to plasma protein at 100 ng/mL and 400 ng/mL, respectively. Under clinical conditions, paroxetine concentrations would normally be less than 400 ng/mL. Paroxetine does not alter the in vitro protein binding of phenytoin or warfarin.

Metabolism and Excretion
The mean elimination half-life is approximately 21 hours (CV 32%) after oral dosing of 30 mg tablets daily for 30 days of PAXIL. In steady-state dose proportionality studies involving elderly and nonelderly patients, at doses of 20 mg to 40 mg daily for the elderly and 20 mg to 50 mg daily for the nonelderly, some nonlinearity was observed in both popula-

tions, again reflecting a saturable metabolic pathway. In comparison to C$_{min}$ values after 20 mg daily, values after 40 mg daily were only about 2 to 3 times greater than doubled.
Paroxetine is extensively metabolized after oral administration. The principal metabolites are polar and conjugated products of oxidation and methylation, which are readily cleared. Conjugates with glucuronic acid and sulfate predominate, and major metabolites have been isolated and identified. Data indicate that the metabolites have no more than 1/50 the potency of the parent compound at inhibiting serotonin uptake. The metabolism of paroxetine is accomplished in part by CYP2D6. Saturation of this enzyme at clinical doses appears to account for the nonlinearity of paroxetine kinetics with increasing dose and increasing duration of treatment. The role of this enzyme in paroxetine metabolism also suggests potential drug-drug interactions (see PRECAUTIONS).
Approximately 64% of a 30-mg oral solution dose of paroxetine was excreted in the urine with 2% as the parent compound and 62% as metabolites over a 10-day post-dosing period. About 36% was excreted in the feces (probably via the bile), mostly as metabolites and less than 1% as the parent compound over the 10-day post-dosing period.

Other Clinical Pharmacology Information
Specific Populations
Renal and Liver Disease
Increased plasma concentrations of paroxetine occur in subjects with renal and hepatic impairment. The mean plasma concentrations in patients with creatinine clearance below 30 mL/min. were approximately 4 times greater than seen in normal volunteers. Patients with creatinine clearance of 30 to 60 mL/min. and patients with hepatic functional impairment had about a 2-fold increase in plasma concentrations (AUC, C$_{max}$).
The initial dosage should therefore be reduced in patients with severe renal or hepatic impairment, and upward titration, if necessary, should be at increased intervals (see DOSAGE AND ADMINISTRATION).

Elderly Patients
In a multiple-dose study in the elderly at daily paroxetine doses of 20, 30, and 40 mg, C$_{min}$ concentrations were about 70% to 80% greater than the respective C$_{min}$ concentrations in nonelderly subjects. Therefore the initial dosage in the elderly should be reduced (see DOSAGE AND ADMINISTRATION).

Drug-Drug Interactions
In vitro drug interaction studies reveal that paroxetine inhibits CYP2D6. Clinical drug interaction studies have been performed with substrates of CYP2D6 and show that paroxetine can inhibit the metabolism of drugs metabolized by CYP2D6 including desipramine, risperidone, and atomoxetine (see PRECAUTIONS—Drug Interactions).

Clinical Trials
Major Depressive Disorder
The efficacy of PAXIL as a treatment for major depressive disorder has been established in 6 placebo-controlled studies of patients with major depressive disorder (aged 18 to 73). In these studies, PAXIL was shown to be significantly more effective than placebo in treating major depressive disorder by at least 2 of the following measures: Hamilton Depression Rating Scale (HDRS), the Hamilton depressed mood item, and the Clinical Global Impression (CGI)-Severity of Illness. PAXIL was significantly better than placebo in improvement of the HDRS sub-factor scores, including the depressed mood item, sleep disturbance factor, and anxiety factor.
A study of outpatients with major depressive disorder who had responded to PAXIL (HDRS total score <8) during an initial 8-week open-treatment phase and were then randomized to continuation on PAXIL or placebo for 1 year demonstrated a significantly lower relapse rate for patients taking PAXIL (15%) compared to those on placebo (39%). Effectiveness was similar for male and female patients.

Obsessive Compulsive Disorder
The effectiveness of PAXIL in the treatment of obsessive compulsive disorder (OCD) was demonstrated in two 12-week multicenter placebo-controlled studies of adult outpatients (Studies 1 and 2). Patients in all studies had moderate to severe OCD (DSM-IIIR) with mean baseline ratings on the Yale Brown Obsessive Compulsive Scale (YBOCS) total score ranging from 23 to 26. Study 1, a dose-range finding study where patients were treated with fixed doses of 20, 40, or 60 mg of paroxetine/day demonstrated that daily doses of paroxetine 40 and 60 mg are effective in the treatment of OCD. Patients receiving doses of 40 and 60 mg paroxetine experienced a mean reduction of approximately 6 and 7 points, respectively, on the YBOCS total score which was significantly greater than the approximate 4-point reduction at 20 mg and a 3-point reduction in the placebo-treated patients. Study 2 was a flexible-dose study comparing paroxetine (20 to 60 mg daily) with clomipramine (25 to 250 mg daily). In this study, patients receiving paroxetine experienced a mean reduction of approximately 7 points on

Outcome Classification (%) on CGI-Global Improvement Item for Completers in Study 1

Outcome Classification	Placebo (n = 74)	PAXIL 20 mg (n = 75)	PAXIL 40 mg (n = 66)	PAXIL 60 mg (n = 66)
Worse	14%	7%	7%	3%
No Change	44%	35%	22%	19%
Minimally Improved	24%	33%	29%	34%
Much Improved	11%	18%	22%	24%
Very Much Improved	7%	7%	20%	20%

the YBOCS total score, which was significantly greater than the mean reduction of approximately 4 points in placebo-treated patients.

The following table provides the outcome classification by treatment group on Global Improvement items of the Clinical Global Impression (CGI) scale for Study 1.

[See table above]

Subgroup analyses did not indicate that there were any differences in treatment outcomes as a function of age or gender.

The long-term maintenance effects of PAXIL in OCD were demonstrated in a long-term extension to Study 1. Patients who were responders on paroxetine during the 3-month double-blind phase and a 6-month extension on open-label paroxetine (20 to 60 mg/day) were randomized to either paroxetine or placebo in a 6-month double-blind relapse prevention phase. Patients randomized to paroxetine were significantly less likely to relapse than comparably treated patients who were randomized to placebo.

Panic Disorder

The effectiveness of PAXIL in the treatment of panic disorder was demonstrated in three 10- to 12-week multicenter, placebo-controlled studies of adult outpatients (Studies 1-3). Patients in all studies had panic disorder (DSM-IIIR), with or without agoraphobia. In these studies, PAXIL was shown to be significantly more effective than placebo in treating panic disorder by at least 2 out of 3 measures of panic attack frequency and on the Clinical Global Impression Severity of Illness score.

Study 1 was a 10-week dose-range finding study; patients were treated with fixed paroxetine doses of 10, 20, or 40 mg/day or placebo. A significant difference from placebo was observed only for the 40 mg/day group. At endpoint, 76% of patients receiving paroxetine 40 mg/day were free of panic attacks, compared to 44% of placebo-treated patients.

Study 2 was a 12-week flexible-dose study comparing paroxetine (10 to 60 mg daily) and placebo. At endpoint, 51% of paroxetine patients were free of panic attacks compared to 32% of placebo-treated patients.

Study 3 was a 12-week flexible-dose study comparing paroxetine (10 to 60 mg daily) to placebo in patients concurrently receiving standardized cognitive behavioral therapy. At endpoint, 33% of the paroxetine-treated patients showed a reduction to 0 or 1 panic attacks compared to 14% of placebo patients.

In both Studies 2 and 3, the mean paroxetine dose for completers at endpoint was approximately 40 mg/day of paroxetine.

Long-term maintenance effects of PAXIL in panic disorder were demonstrated in an extension to Study 1. Patients who were responders during the 10-week double-blind phase and during a 3-month double-blind extension phase were randomized to either paroxetine (10, 20, or 40 mg/day) or placebo in a 3-month double-blind relapse prevention phase. Patients randomized to paroxetine were significantly less likely to relapse than comparably treated patients who were randomized to placebo.

Subgroup analyses did not indicate that there were any differences in treatment outcomes as a function of age or gender.

Social Anxiety Disorder

The effectiveness of PAXIL in the treatment of social anxiety disorder was demonstrated in three 12-week, multicenter, placebo-controlled studies (Studies 1, 2, and 3) of adult outpatients with social anxiety disorder (DSM-IV). In these studies, the effectiveness of PAXIL compared to placebo was evaluated on the basis of (1) the proportion of responders, as defined by a Clinical Global Impression (CGI) Improvement score of 1 (very much improved) or 2 (much improved), and (2) change from baseline in the Liebowitz Social Anxiety Scale (LSAS).

Studies 1 and 2 were flexible-dose studies comparing paroxetine (20 to 50 mg daily) and placebo. Paroxetine demonstrated statistically significant superiority over placebo on both the CGI Improvement responder criterion and the Liebowitz Social Anxiety Scale (LSAS). In Study 1, for patients who completed to week 12, 69% of paroxetine-treated

patients compared to 29% of placebo-treated patients were CGI Improvement responders. In Study 2, CGI Improvement responders were 77% and 42% for the paroxetine- and placebo-treated patients, respectively.

Study 3 was a 12-week study comparing fixed paroxetine doses of 20, 40, or 60 mg/day with placebo. Paroxetine 20 mg was demonstrated to be significantly superior to placebo on both the LSAS Total Score and the CGI Improvement responder criterion; there were trends for superiority over placebo for the 40 mg and 60 mg/day dose groups. There was no indication in this study of any additional benefit for doses higher than 20 mg/day.

Subgroup analyses generally did not indicate differences in treatment outcomes as a function of age, race, or gender.

Generalized Anxiety Disorder

The effectiveness of PAXIL in the treatment of Generalized Anxiety Disorder (GAD) was demonstrated in two 8-week, multicenter, placebo-controlled studies (Studies 1 and 2) of adult outpatients with Generalized Anxiety Disorder (DSM-IV).

Study 1 was an 8-week study comparing fixed paroxetine doses of 20 mg or 40 mg/day with placebo. Doses of 20 mg or 40 mg of PAXIL were both demonstrated to be significantly superior to placebo on the Hamilton Rating Scale for Anxiety (HAM-A) total score. There was not sufficient evidence in this study to suggest a greater benefit for the 40 mg/day dose compared to the 20 mg/day dose.

Study 2 was a flexible-dose study comparing paroxetine (20 mg to 50 mg daily) and placebo. PAXIL demonstrated statistically significant superiority over placebo on the Hamilton Rating Scale for Anxiety (HAM-A) total score. A third study, also flexible-dose comparing paroxetine (20 mg to 50 mg daily), did not demonstrate statistically significant superiority of PAXIL over placebo on the Hamilton Rating Scale for Anxiety (HAM-A) total score, the primary outcome.

Subgroup analyses did not indicate differences in treatment outcomes as a function of race or gender. There were insufficient elderly patients to conduct subgroup analyses on the basis of age.

In a longer-term trial, 566 patients meeting DSM-IV criteria for Generalized Anxiety Disorder, who had responded during a single-blind, 8-week acute treatment phase with 20 to 50 mg/day of PAXIL, were randomized to continuation of PAXIL at their same dose, or to placebo, for up to 24 weeks of observation for relapse. Response during the single-blind phase was defined by having a decrease of ≥2 points compared to baseline on the CGI-Severity of Illness scale, to a score of ≤3. Relapse during the double-blind phase was defined as an increase of ≥2 points compared to baseline on the CGI-Severity of Illness scale to a score of ≥4, or withdrawal due to lack of efficacy. Patients receiving continued PAXIL experienced a significantly lower relapse rate over the subsequent 24 weeks compared to those receiving placebo.

Posttraumatic Stress Disorder

The effectiveness of PAXIL in the treatment of Posttraumatic Stress Disorder (PTSD) was demonstrated in two 12-week, multicenter, placebo-controlled studies (Studies 1 and 2) of adult outpatients who met DSM-IV criteria for PTSD. The mean duration of PTSD symptoms for the 2 studies combined was 13 years (ranging from .1 year to 57 years). The percentage of patients with secondary major depressive disorder or non-PTSD anxiety disorders in the combined 2 studies was 41% (356 out of 858 patients) and 40% (345 out of 858 patients), respectively. Study outcome was assessed by (i) the Clinician-Administered PTSD Scale Part 2 (CAPS-2) score and (ii) the Clinical Global Impression-Global Improvement Scale (CGI-I). The CAPS-2 is a multi-item instrument that measures 3 aspects of PTSD with the following symptom clusters: Reexperiencing/intrusion, avoidance/numbing and hyperarousal. The 2 primary outcomes for each trial were (i) change from baseline to endpoint on the CAPS-2 total score (17 items), and (ii) proportion of responders on the CGI-I, where responders were defined as patients having a score of 1 (very much improved) or 2 (much improved).

Study 1 was a 12-week study comparing fixed paroxetine doses of 20 mg or 40 mg/day to placebo. Doses of 20 mg and 40 mg of PAXIL were demonstrated to be significantly superior to placebo on change from baseline for the CAPS-2 total score and on proportion of responders on the CGI-I. There was not sufficient evidence in this study to suggest a greater benefit for the 40 mg/day dose compared to the 20 mg/day dose.

Study 2 was a 12-week flexible-dose study comparing paroxetine (20 to 50 mg daily) to placebo. PAXIL was demonstrated to be significantly superior to placebo on change from baseline for the CAPS-2 total score and on proportion of responders on the CGI-I.

A third study, also a flexible-dose study comparing paroxetine (20 to 50 mg daily) to placebo, demonstrated PAXIL to be significantly superior to placebo on change from baseline for CAPS-2 total score, but not on proportion of responders on the CGI-I.

The majority of patients in these trials were women (68% women: 377 out of 551 subjects in Study 1 and 66% women: 202 out of 303 subjects in Study 2). Subgroup analyses did not indicate differences in treatment outcomes as a function of gender. There were an insufficient number of patients who were 65 years and older or were non-Caucasian to conduct subgroup analyses on the basis of age or race, respectively.

INDICATIONS AND USAGE

Major Depressive Disorder

PAXIL is indicated for the treatment of major depressive disorder.

The efficacy of PAXIL in the treatment of a major depressive episode was established in 6-week controlled trials of outpatients whose diagnoses corresponded most closely to the DSM-III category of major depressive disorder (see CLINICAL PHARMACOLOGY—Clinical Trials). A major depressive episode implies a prominent and relatively persistent depressed or dysphoric mood that usually interferes with daily functioning (nearly every day for at least 2 weeks); it should include at least 4 of the following 8 symptoms: Change in appetite, change in sleep, psychomotor agitation or retardation, loss of interest in usual activities or decrease in sexual drive, increased fatigue, feelings of guilt or worthlessness, slowed thinking or impaired concentration, and a suicide attempt or suicidal ideation.

The effects of PAXIL in hospitalized depressed patients have not been adequately studied.

The efficacy of PAXIL in maintaining a response in major depressive disorder for up to 1 year was demonstrated in a placebo-controlled trial (see CLINICAL PHARMACOLOGY—Clinical Trials). Nevertheless, the physician who elects to use PAXIL for extended periods should periodically re-evaluate the long-term usefulness of the drug for the individual patient.

Obsessive Compulsive Disorder

PAXIL is indicated for the treatment of obsessions and compulsions in patients with obsessive compulsive disorder (OCD) as defined in the DSM-IV. The obsessions or compulsions cause marked distress, are time-consuming, or significantly interfere with social or occupational functioning.

The efficacy of PAXIL was established in two 12-week trials with obsessive compulsive outpatients whose diagnoses corresponded most closely to the DSM-IIIR category of obsessive compulsive disorder (see CLINICAL PHARMACOLOGY—Clinical Trials).

Obsessive compulsive disorder is characterized by recurrent and persistent ideas, thoughts, impulses, or images (obsessions) that are ego-dystonic and/or repetitive, purposeful, and intentional behaviors (compulsions) that are recognized by the person as excessive or unreasonable.

Long-term maintenance of efficacy was demonstrated in a 6-month relapse prevention trial. In this trial, patients assigned to paroxetine showed a lower relapse rate compared to patients on placebo (see CLINICAL PHARMACOLOGY—Clinical Trials). Nevertheless, the physician who elects to use PAXIL for extended periods should periodically re-evaluate the long-term usefulness of the drug for the individual patient (see DOSAGE AND ADMINISTRATION).

Panic Disorder

PAXIL is indicated for the treatment of panic disorder, with or without agoraphobia, as defined in DSM-IV. Panic disorder is characterized by the occurrence of unexpected panic attacks and associated concern about having additional attacks, worry about the implications or consequences of the attacks, and/or a significant change in behavior related to the attacks.

The efficacy of PAXIL was established in three 10- to 12-week trials in panic disorder patients whose diagnoses corresponded to the DSM-IIIR category of panic disorder (see CLINICAL PHARMACOLOGY—Clinical Trials).

Panic disorder (DSM-IV) is characterized by recurrent unexpected panic attacks, i.e., a discrete period of intense fear or discomfort in which 4 (or more) of the following symptoms develop abruptly and reach a peak within 10 minutes: (1) palpitations, pounding heart, or accelerated heart rate; (2) sweating; (3) trembling or shaking; (4) sensations of shortness of breath or smothering; (5) feeling of choking;

(6) chest pain or discomfort; (7) nausea or abdominal distress; (8) feeling dizzy, unsteady, lightheaded, or faint; (9) derealization (feelings of unreality) or depersonalization (being detached from oneself); (10) fear of losing control; (11) fear of dying; (12) paresthesias (numbness or tingling sensations); (13) chills or hot flushes.

Long-term maintenance of efficacy was demonstrated in a 3-month relapse prevention trial. In this trial, patients with panic disorder assigned to paroxetine demonstrated a lower relapse rate compared to patients on placebo (see CLINICAL PHARMACOLOGY—Clinical Trials). Nevertheless, the physician who prescribes PAXIL for extended periods should periodically re-evaluate the long-term usefulness of the drug for the individual patient.

Social Anxiety Disorder

PAXIL is indicated for the treatment of social anxiety disorder, also known as social phobia, as defined in DSM-IV (300.23). Social anxiety disorder is characterized by a marked and persistent fear of 1 or more social or performance situations in which the person is exposed to unfamiliar people or to possible scrutiny by others. Exposure to the feared situation almost invariably provokes anxiety, which may approach the intensity of a panic attack. The feared situations are avoided or endured with intense anxiety or distress. The avoidance, anxious anticipation, or distress in the feared situation(s) interferes significantly with the person's normal routine, occupational or academic functioning, or social activities or relationships, or there is marked distress about having the phobias. Lesser degrees of performance anxiety or shyness generally do not require psychopharmacological treatment.

The efficacy of PAXIL was established in three 12-week trials in adult patients with social anxiety disorder (DSM-IV). PAXIL has not been studied in children or adolescents with social phobia (see CLINICAL PHARMACOLOGY—Clinical Trials).

The effectiveness of PAXIL in long-term treatment of social anxiety disorder, i.e., for more than 12 weeks, has not been systematically evaluated in adequate and well-controlled trials. Therefore, the physician who elects to prescribe PAXIL for extended periods should periodically re-evaluate the long-term usefulness of the drug for the individual patient (see DOSAGE AND ADMINISTRATION).

Generalized Anxiety Disorder

PAXIL is indicated for the treatment of Generalized Anxiety Disorder (GAD), as defined in DSM-IV. Anxiety or tension associated with the stress of everyday life usually does not require treatment with an anxiolytic.

The efficacy of PAXIL in the treatment of GAD was established in two 8-week placebo-controlled trials in adults with GAD. PAXIL has not been studied in children or adolescents with Generalized Anxiety Disorder (see CLINICAL PHARMACOLOGY—Clinical Trials).

Generalized Anxiety Disorder (DSM-IV) is characterized by excessive anxiety and worry (apprehensive expectation) that is persistent for at least 6 months and which the person finds difficult to control. It must be associated with at least 3 of the following 6 symptoms: Restlessness or feeling keyed up or on edge, being easily fatigued, difficulty concentrating or mind going blank, irritability, muscle tension, sleep disturbance.

The efficacy of PAXIL in maintaining a response in patients with Generalized Anxiety Disorder, who responded during an 8-week acute treatment phase while taking PAXIL and were then observed for relapse during a period of up to 24 weeks, was demonstrated in a placebo-controlled trial (see CLINICAL PHARMACOLOGY—Clinical Trials). Nevertheless, the physician who elects to use PAXIL for extended periods should periodically re-evaluate the long-term usefulness of the drug for the individual patient (see DOSAGE AND ADMINISTRATION).

Posttraumatic Stress Disorder

PAXIL is indicated for the treatment of Posttraumatic Stress Disorder (PTSD).

The efficacy of PAXIL in the treatment of PTSD was established in two 12-week placebo-controlled trials in adults with PTSD (DSM-IV) (see CLINICAL PHARMACOLOGY—Clinical Trials).

PTSD, as defined by DSM-IV, requires exposure to a traumatic event that involved actual or threatened death or serious injury, or threat to the physical integrity of self or others, and a response that involves intense fear, helplessness, or horror. Symptoms that occur as a result of exposure to the traumatic event include reexperiencing of the event in the form of intrusive thoughts, flashbacks, or dreams, and intense psychological distress and physiological reactivity on exposure to cues to the event; avoidance of situations reminiscent of the traumatic event, inability to recall details of the event, and/or numbing of general responsiveness manifested as diminished interest in significant activities, estrangement from others, restricted range of affect, or sense of foreshortened future; and symptoms of autonomic arousal including hypervigilance, exaggerated startle response, sleep disturbance, impaired concentration, and irri-

tability or outbursts of anger. A PTSD diagnosis requires that the symptoms are present for at least a month and that they cause clinically significant distress or impairment in social, occupational, or other important areas of functioning. The efficacy of PAXIL in longer-term treatment of PTSD, i.e., for more than 12 weeks, has not been systematically evaluated in placebo-controlled trials. Therefore, the physician who elects to prescribe PAXIL for extended periods should periodically re-evaluate the long-term usefulness of the drug for the individual patient (see DOSAGE AND ADMINISTRATION).

CONTRAINDICATIONS

Concomitant use in patients taking either monoamine oxidase inhibitors (MAOIs), including linezolid, an antibiotic which is a reversible non-selective MAOI, or thioridazine is contraindicated (see WARNINGS and PRECAUTIONS). Concomitant use in patients taking pimozide is contraindicated (see PRECAUTIONS).

PAXIL is contraindicated in patients with a hypersensitivity to paroxetine or any of the inactive ingredients in PAXIL.

WARNINGS

Clinical Worsening and Suicide Risk

Patients with major depressive disorder (MDD), both adult and pediatric, may experience worsening of their depression and/or the emergence of suicidal ideation and behavior (suicidality) or unusual changes in behavior, whether or not they are taking antidepressant medications, and this risk may persist until significant remission occurs. Suicide is a known risk of depression and certain other psychiatric disorders, and these disorders themselves are the strongest predictors of suicide. There has been a long-standing concern, however, that antidepressants may have a role in inducing worsening of depression and the emergence of suicidality in certain patients during the early phases of treatment. Pooled analyses of short-term placebo-controlled trials of antidepressant drugs (SSRIs and others) showed that these drugs increase the risk of suicidal thinking and behavior (suicidality) in children, adolescents, and young adults (ages 18-24) with major depressive disorder (MDD) and other psychiatric disorders. Short-term studies did not show an increase in the risk of suicidality with antidepressants compared to placebo in adults beyond age 24; there was a reduction with antidepressants compared to placebo in adults aged 65 and older.

The pooled analyses of placebo-controlled trials in children and adolescents with MDD, obsessive compulsive disorder (OCD), or other psychiatric disorders included a total of 24 short-term trials of 9 antidepressant drugs in over 4,400 patients. The pooled analyses of placebo-controlled trials in adults with MDD or other psychiatric disorders included a total of 295 short-term trials (median duration of 2 months) of 11 antidepressant drugs in over 77,000 patients. There was considerable variation in risk of suicidality among drugs, but a tendency toward an increase in the younger patients for almost all drugs studied. There were differences in absolute risk of suicidality across the different indications, with the highest incidence in MDD. The risk differences (drug vs placebo), however, were relatively stable within age strata and across indications. These risk differences (drug-placebo difference in the number of cases of suicidality per 1,000 patients treated) are provided in Table 1.

Table 1.

Age Range	Drug-Placebo Difference in Number of Cases of Suicidality per 1,000 Patients Treated
Increases Compared to Placebo	
<18	14 additional cases
18-24	5 additional cases
Decreases Compared to Placebo	
25-64	1 fewer case
≥65	6 fewer cases

No suicides occurred in any of the pediatric trials. There were suicides in the adult trials, but the number was not sufficient to reach any conclusion about drug effect on suicide.

It is unknown whether the suicidality risk extends to longer-term use, i.e., beyond several months. However, there is substantial evidence from placebo-controlled maintenance trials in adults with depression that the use of antidepressants can delay the recurrence of depression.

All patients being treated with antidepressants for any indication should be monitored appropriately and observed closely for clinical worsening, suicidality, and unusual

changes in behavior, especially during the initial few months of a course of drug therapy, or at times of dose changes, either increases or decreases.

The following symptoms, anxiety, agitation, panic attacks, insomnia, irritability, hostility, aggressiveness, impulsivity, akathisia (psychomotor restlessness), hypomania, and mania, have been reported in adult and pediatric patients being treated with antidepressants for major depressive disorder as well as for other indications, both psychiatric and nonpsychiatric. Although a causal link between the emergence of such symptoms and either the worsening of depression and/or the emergence of suicidal impulses has not been established, there is concern that such symptoms may represent precursors to emerging suicidality.

Consideration should be given to changing the therapeutic regimen, including possibly discontinuing the medication, in patients whose depression is persistently worse, or who are experiencing emergent suicidality or symptoms that might be precursors to worsening depression or suicidality, especially if these symptoms are severe, abrupt in onset, or were not part of the patient's presenting symptoms.

If the decision has been made to discontinue treatment, medication should be tapered, as rapidly as is feasible, but with recognition that abrupt discontinuation can be associated with certain symptoms (see PRECAUTIONS and DOSAGE AND ADMINISTRATION—Discontinuation of Treatment With PAXIL, for a description of the risks of discontinuation of PAXIL).

Families and caregivers of patients being treated with antidepressants for major depressive disorder or other indications, both psychiatric and nonpsychiatric, should be alerted about the need to monitor patients for the emergence of agitation, irritability, unusual changes in behavior, and the other symptoms described above, as well as the emergence of suicidality, and to report such symptoms immediately to healthcare providers. Such monitoring should include daily observation by families and caregivers. Prescriptions for PAXIL should be written for the smallest quantity of tablets consistent with good patient management, in order to reduce the risk of overdose.

Screening Patients for Bipolar Disorder

A major depressive episode may be the initial presentation of bipolar disorder. It is generally believed (though not established in controlled trials) that treating such an episode with an antidepressant alone may increase the likelihood of precipitation of a mixed/manic episode in patients at risk for bipolar disorder. Whether any of the symptoms described above represent such a conversion is unknown. However, prior to initiating treatment with an antidepressant, patients with depressive symptoms should be adequately screened to determine if they are at risk for bipolar disorder; such screening should include a detailed psychiatric history, including a family history of suicide, bipolar disorder, and depression. It should be noted that PAXIL is not approved for use in treating bipolar depression.

Potential for Interaction With Monoamine Oxidase Inhibitors

In patients receiving another serotonin reuptake inhibitor drug in combination with a monoamine oxidase inhibitor (MAOI), there have been reports of serious, sometimes fatal, reactions including hyperthermia, rigidity, myoclonus, autonomic instability with possible rapid fluctuations of vital signs, and mental status changes that include extreme agitation progressing to delirium and coma. These reactions have also been reported in patients who have recently discontinued that drug and have been started on an MAOI. Some cases presented with features resembling neuroleptic malignant syndrome. While there are no human data showing such an interaction with PAXIL, limited animal data on the effects of combined use of paroxetine and MAOIs suggest that these drugs may act synergistically to elevate blood pressure and evoke behavioral excitation. Therefore, it is recommended that PAXIL not be used in combination with an MAOI (including linezolid, an antibiotic which is a reversible non-selective MAOI), or within 14 days of discontinuing treatment with an MAOI (see CONTRAINDICATIONS). At least 2 weeks should be allowed after stopping PAXIL before starting an MAOI.

Serotonin Syndrome or Neuroleptic Malignant Syndrome (NMS)-like Reactions

The development of a potentially life-threatening serotonin syndrome or Neuroleptic Malignant Syndrome (NMS)-like reactions have been reported with SNRIs and SSRIs alone, including treatment with PAXIL, but particularly with concomitant use of serotonergic drugs (including triptans) with drugs which impair metabolism of serotonin (including MAOIs), or with antipsychotics or other dopamine antagonists. Serotonin syndrome symptoms may include mental status changes (e.g., agitation, hallucinations, coma), autonomic instability (e.g., tachycardia, labile blood pressure, hyperthermia), neuromuscular aberrations (e.g., hyperreflexia, incoordination) and/or gastrointestinal symptoms (e.g., nausea, vomiting, diarrhea). Serotonin syndrome, in its most severe form can resemble neurolep-

	Major Depressive Disorder		OCD		Panic Disorder		Social Anxiety Disorder		Generalized Anxiety Disorder		PTSD	
	PAXIL	Placebo	PAXIL	Placebo	PAXIL	Placebo	PAXIL	Placebo	PAXIL	Placebo	PAXIL	Placebo
CNS												
Somnolence	2.3%	0.7%	—		1.9%	0.3%	3.4%	0.3%	2.0%	0.2%	2.8%	0.6%
Insomnia	—	—	1.7%	0%	1.3%	0.3%	3.1%	0%			—	—
Agitation	1.1%	0.5%	—								—	—
Tremor	1.1%	0.3%	—				1.7%	0%			1.0%	0.2%
Anxiety	—	—	—				1.1%	0%			—	—
Dizziness	—	—	1.5%	0%			1.9%	0%	1.0%	0.2%	—	—
Gastrointestinal												
Constipation	—		1.1%	0%							—	—
Nausea	3.2%	1.1%	1.9%	0%	3.2%	1.2%	4.0%	0.3%	2.0%	0.2%	2.2%	0.6%
Diarrhea	1.0%	0.3%	—									
Dry mouth	1.0%	0.3%	—								—	—
Vomiting	1.0%	0.3%	—				1.0%	0%			—	—
Flatulence							1.0%	0.3%			—	—
Other												
Asthenia	1.6%	0.4%	1.9%	0.4%			2.5%	0.6%	1.8%	0.2%	1.6%	0.2%
Abnormal ejaculation[1]	1.6%	0%	2.1%	0%			4.9%	0.6%	2.5%	0.5%	—	—
Sweating	1.0%	0.3%	—				1.1%	0%	1.1%	0.2%	—	—
Impotence[1]	—		1.5%	0%							—	—
Libido Decreased							1.0%	0%			—	—

Where numbers are not provided the incidence of the adverse events in patients treated with PAXIL was not >1% or was not greater than or equal to 2 times the incidence of placebo.
[1] Incidence corrected for gender.

tic malignant syndrome, which includes hyperthermia, muscle rigidity, autonomic instability with possible rapid fluctuation of vital signs, and mental status changes.
Patients should be monitored for the emergence of serotonin syndrome or NMS-like signs and symptoms.
The concomitant use of PAXIL with MAOIs intended to treat depression is contraindicated.
If concomitant treatment of PAXIL with a 5-hydroxytryptamine receptor agonist (triptan) is clinically warranted, careful observation of the patient is advised, particularly during treatment initiation and dose increases.
The concomitant use of PAXIL with serotonin precursors (such as tryptophan) is not recommended.
Treatment with PAXIL and any concomitant serotonergic or antidopaminergic agents, including antipsychotics, should be discontinued immediately if the above events occur and supportive symptomatic treatment should be initiated.

Potential Interaction With Thioridazine
Thioridazine administration alone produces prolongation of the QTc interval, which is associated with serious ventricular arrhythmias, such as torsade de pointes–type arrhythmias, and sudden death. This effect appears to be dose related.
An in vivo study suggests that drugs which inhibit CYP2D6, such as paroxetine, will elevate plasma levels of thioridazine. Therefore, it is recommended that paroxetine not be used in combination with thioridazine (see CONTRAINDICATIONS and PRECAUTIONS).

Usage in Pregnancy
Teratogenic Effects
Epidemiological studies have shown that infants exposed to paroxetine in the first trimester of pregnancy have an increased risk of congenital malformations, particularly cardiovascular malformations. The findings from these studies are summarized below:

- A study based on Swedish national registry data demonstrated that infants exposed to paroxetine during pregnancy (n = 815) had an increased risk of cardiovascular malformations (2% risk in paroxetine-exposed infants) compared to the entire registry population (1% risk), for an odds ratio (OR) of 1.8 (95% confidence interval 1.1 to 2.8). No increase in the risk of overall congenital malformations was seen in the paroxetine-exposed infants. The cardiac malformations in the paroxetine-exposed infants were primarily ventricular septal defects (VSDs) and atrial septal defects (ASDs). Septal defects range in severity from those that resolve spontaneously to those which require surgery.
- A separate retrospective cohort study from the United States (United Healthcare data) evaluated 5,956 infants of mothers dispensed antidepressants during the first trimester (n = 815 for paroxetine). This study showed a trend towards an increased risk for cardiovascular malformations for paroxetine (risk of 1.5%) compared to other antidepressants (risk of 1%), for an OR of 1.5 (95% confidence interval 0.8 to 2.9). Of the 12 paroxetine-exposed infants with cardiovascular malformations, 9 had VSDs. This study also suggested an increased risk of overall major congenital malformations including cardiovascular defects for paroxetine (4% risk) compared to other (2% risk) antidepressants (OR 1.8; 95% confidence interval 1.2 to 2.8).
- Two large case-control studies using separate databases, each with >9,000 birth defect cases and >4,000 controls, found that maternal use of paroxetine during the first trimester of pregnancy was associated with a 2- to 3-fold increased risk of right ventricular outflow tract obstructions. In one study the odds ratio was 2.5 (95% confidence interval, 1.0 to 6.0, 7 exposed infants) and in the other study the odds ratio was 3.3 (95% confidence interval, 1.3 to 8.8, 6 exposed infants).

Other studies have found varying results as to whether there was an increased risk of overall, cardiovascular, or specific congenital malformations. A meta-analysis of epidemiological data over a 16-year period (1992 to 2008) on first trimester paroxetine use in pregnancy and congenital malformations included the above-noted studies in addition to others (n = 17 studies that included overall malformations and n = 14 studies that included cardiovascular malformations; n = 20 distinct studies). While subject to limitations, this meta-analysis suggested an increased occurrence of cardiovascular malformations (prevalence odds ratio [POR] 1.5; 95% confidence interval 1.2 to 1.9) and overall malformations (POR 1.2; 95% confidence interval 1.1 to 1.4) with paroxetine use during the first trimester. It was not possible in this meta-analysis to determine the extent to which the observed prevalence of cardiovascular malformations might have contributed to that of overall malformations, nor was it possible to determine whether any specific types of cardiovascular malformations might have contributed to the observed prevalence of all cardiovascular malformations.
If a patient becomes pregnant while taking paroxetine, she should be advised of the potential harm to the fetus. Unless the benefits of paroxetine to the mother justify continuing treatment, consideration should be given to either discontinuing paroxetine therapy or switching to another antidepressant (see PRECAUTIONS—Discontinuation of Treatment With PAXIL). For women who intend to become pregnant or are in their first trimester of pregnancy, paroxetine should only be initiated after consideration of the other available treatment options.

Animal Findings
Reproduction studies were performed at doses up to 50 mg/kg/day in rats and 6 mg/kg/day in rabbits administered during organogenesis. These doses are approximately 8 (rat) and 2 (rabbit) times the maximum recommended human dose (MRHD) on an mg/m^2 basis. These studies have revealed no evidence of teratogenic effects. However, in rats, there was an increase in pup deaths during the first 4 days of lactation when dosing occurred during the last trimester of gestation and continued throughout lactation. This effect occurred at a dose of 1 mg/kg/day or approximately one-sixth of the MRHD on an mg/m^2 basis. The no-effect dose for rat pup mortality was not determined. The cause of these deaths is not known.

Nonteratogenic Effects
Neonates exposed to PAXIL and other SSRIs or serotonin and norepinephrine reuptake inhibitors (SNRIs), late in the third trimester have developed complications requiring prolonged hospitalization, respiratory support, and tube feeding. Such complications can arise immediately upon delivery. Reported clinical findings have included respiratory distress, cyanosis, apnea, seizures, temperature instability, feeding difficulty, vomiting, hypoglycemia, hypotonia, hypertonia, hyperreflexia, tremor, jitteriness, irritability, and constant crying. These features are consistent with either a direct toxic effect of SSRIs and SNRIs or, possibly, a drug discontinuation syndrome. It should be noted that, in some cases, the clinical picture is consistent with serotonin syndrome (see WARNINGS—Potential for Interaction With Monoamine Oxidase Inhibitors).
Infants exposed to SSRIs in late pregnancy may have an increased risk for persistent pulmonary hypertension of the newborn (PPHN). PPHN occurs in 1–2 per 1,000 live births in the general population and is associated with substantial neonatal morbidity and mortality. In a retrospective case-control study of 377 women whose infants were born with PPHN and 836 women whose infants were born healthy, the risk for developing PPHN was approximately six-fold higher for infants exposed to SSRIs after the 20th week of gestation compared to infants who had not been exposed to antidepressants during pregnancy. There is currently no corroborative evidence regarding the risk for PPHN following exposure to SSRIs in pregnancy; this is the first study that has investigated the potential risk. The study did not include enough cases with exposure to individual SSRIs to determine if all SSRIs posed similar levels of PPHN risk.
There have also been postmarketing reports of premature births in pregnant women exposed to paroxetine or other SSRIs.
When treating a pregnant woman with paroxetine during the third trimester, the physician should carefully consider both the potential risks and benefits of treatment (see DOSAGE AND ADMINISTRATION). Physicians should note that in a prospective longitudinal study of 201 women with a history of major depression who were euthymic at the beginning of pregnancy, women who discontinued antidepressant medication during pregnancy were more likely to experience a relapse of major depression than women who continued antidepressant medication.

PRECAUTIONS
General
Activation of Mania/Hypomania
During premarketing testing, hypomania or mania occurred in approximately 1.0% of unipolar patients treated with PAXIL compared to 1.1% of active-control and 0.3% of placebo-treated unipolar patients. In a subset of patients classified as bipolar, the rate of manic episodes was 2.2% for PAXIL and 11.6% for the combined active-control groups. As with all drugs effective in the treatment of major depressive disorder, PAXIL should be used cautiously in patients with a history of mania.

Seizures
During premarketing testing, seizures occurred in 0.1% of patients treated with PAXIL, a rate similar to that associated with other drugs effective in the treatment of major depressive disorder. PAXIL should be used cautiously in patients with a history of seizures. It should be discontinued in any patient who develops seizures.

Discontinuation of Treatment With PAXIL
Recent clinical trials supporting the various approved indications for PAXIL employed a taper-phase regimen, rather than an abrupt discontinuation of treatment. The taper-phase regimen used in GAD and PTSD clinical trials involved an incremental decrease in the daily dose by 10 mg/day at weekly intervals. When a daily dose of 20 mg/day was reached, patients were continued on this dose for 1 week before treatment was stopped.
With this regimen in those studies, the following adverse events were reported at an incidence of 2% or greater for PAXIL and were at least twice that reported for placebo: Abnormal dreams, paresthesia, and dizziness. In the majority of patients, these events were mild to moderate and were self-limiting and did not require medical intervention.
During marketing of PAXIL and other SSRIs and SNRIs, there have been spontaneous reports of adverse events occurring upon the discontinuation of these drugs (particularly when abrupt), including the following: Dysphoric mood, irritability, agitation, dizziness, sensory disturbances (e.g., paresthesias such as electric shock sensations and tinnitus), anxiety, confusion, headache, lethargy, emotional lability, insomnia, and hypomania. While these events are generally self-limiting, there have been reports of serious discontinuation symptoms.
Patients should be monitored for these symptoms when discontinuing treatment with PAXIL. A gradual reduction in the dose rather than abrupt cessation is recommended whenever possible. If intolerable symptoms occur following

a decrease in the dose or upon discontinuation of treatment, then resuming the previously prescribed dose may be considered. Subsequently, the physician may continue decreasing the dose but at a more gradual rate (see DOSAGE AND ADMINISTRATION).

See also PRECAUTIONS—Pediatric Use, for adverse events reported upon discontinuation of treatment with PAXIL in pediatric patients.

Tamoxifen

Some studies have shown that the efficacy of tamoxifen, as measured by the risk of breast cancer relapse/mortality, may be reduced when co-prescribed with paroxetine as a result of paroxetine's irreversible inhibition of CYP2D6 (see Drug Interactions). This risk may increase with longer duration of coadministration. When tamoxifen is used for the treatment or prevention of breast cancer, prescribers should consider using an alternative antidepressant with little or no CYP2D6 inhibition.

Akathisia

The use of paroxetine or other SSRIs has been associated with the development of akathisia, which is characterized by an inner sense of restlessness and psychomotor agitation such as an inability to sit or stand still usually associated with subjective distress. This is most likely to occur within the first few weeks of treatment.

Hyponatremia

Hyponatremia may occur as a result of treatment with SSRIs and SNRIs, including PAXIL. In many cases, this hyponatremia appears to be the result of the syndrome of inappropriate antidiuretic hormone secretion (SIADH). Cases with serum sodium lower than 110 mmol/L have been reported. Elderly patients may be at greater risk of developing hyponatremia with SSRIs and SNRIs. Also, patients taking diuretics or who are otherwise volume depleted may be at greater risk (see Geriatric Use). Discontinuation of PAXIL should be considered in patients with symptomatic hyponatremia and appropriate medical intervention should be instituted.

Signs and symptoms of hyponatremia include headache, difficulty concentrating, memory impairment, confusion, weakness, and unsteadiness, which may lead to falls. Signs and symptoms associated with more severe and/or acute cases have included hallucination, syncope, seizure, coma, respiratory arrest, and death.

Abnormal Bleeding

SSRIs and SNRIs, including paroxetine, may increase the risk of bleeding events. Concomitant use of aspirin, nonsteroidal anti-inflammatory drugs, warfarin, and other anticoagulants may add to this risk. Case reports and epidemiological studies (case-control and cohort design) have demonstrated an association between use of drugs that interfere with serotonin reuptake and the occurrence of gastrointestinal bleeding. Bleeding events related to SSRIs and SNRIs use have ranged from ecchymoses, hematomas, epistaxis, and petechiae to life-threatening hemorrhages. Patients should be cautioned about the risk of bleeding associated with the concomitant use of paroxetine and NSAIDs, aspirin, or other drugs that affect coagulation.

Use in Patients With Concomitant Illness

Clinical experience with PAXIL in patients with certain concomitant systemic illness is limited. Caution is advisable in using PAXIL in patients with diseases or conditions that could affect metabolism or hemodynamic responses.

As with other SSRIs, mydriasis has been infrequently reported in premarketing studies with PAXIL. A few cases of acute angle closure glaucoma associated with paroxetine therapy have been reported in the literature. As mydriasis can cause acute angle closure in patients with narrow angle glaucoma, caution should be used when PAXIL is prescribed for patients with narrow angle glaucoma.

PAXIL has not been evaluated or used to any appreciable extent in patients with a recent history of myocardial infarction or unstable heart disease. Patients with these diagnoses were excluded from clinical studies during the product's premarket testing. Evaluation of electrocardiograms of 682 patients who received PAXIL in double-blind, placebo-controlled trials, however, did not indicate that PAXIL is associated with the development of significant ECG abnormalities. Similarly, PAXIL does not cause any clinically important changes in heart rate or blood pressure.

Increased plasma concentrations of paroxetine occur in patients with severe renal impairment (creatinine clearance <30 mL/min.) or severe hepatic impairment. A lower starting dose should be used in such patients (see DOSAGE AND ADMINISTRATION).

Information for Patients

PAXIL should not be chewed or crushed, and should be swallowed whole.

Patients should be cautioned about the risk of serotonin syndrome with the concomitant use of PAXIL and triptans, tramadol, or other serotonergic agents.

Table 2. Treatment-Emergent Adverse Experience Incidence in Placebo-Controlled Clinical Trials for Major Depressive Disorder[1]

Body System	Preferred Term	PAXIL (n = 421)	Placebo (n = 421)
Body as a Whole	Headache	18%	17%
	Asthenia	15%	6%
Cardiovascular	Palpitation	3%	1%
	Vasodilation	3%	1%
Dermatologic	Sweating	11%	2%
	Rash	2%	1%
Gastrointestinal	Nausea	26%	9%
	Dry Mouth	18%	12%
	Constipation	14%	9%
	Diarrhea	12%	8%
	Decreased Appetite	6%	2%
	Flatulence	4%	2%
	Oropharynx Disorder[2]	2%	0%
	Dyspepsia	2%	1%
Musculoskeletal	Myopathy	2%	1%
	Myalgia	2%	1%
	Myasthenia	1%	0%
Nervous System	Somnolence	23%	9%
	Dizziness	13%	6%
	Insomnia	13%	6%
	Tremor	8%	2%
	Nervousness	5%	3%
	Anxiety	5%	3%
	Paresthesia	4%	2%
	Libido Decreased	3%	0%
	Drugged Feeling	2%	1%
	Confusion	1%	0%
Respiration	Yawn	4%	0%
Special Senses	Blurred Vision	4%	1%
	Taste Perversion	2%	0%
Urogenital System	Ejaculatory Disturbance[3,4]	13%	0%
	Other Male Genital Disorders[3,5]	10%	0%
	Urinary Frequency	3%	1%
	Urination Disorder[6]	3%	0%
	Female Genital Disorders[3,7]	2%	0%

[1] Events reported by at least 1% of patients treated with PAXIL are included, except the following events which had an incidence on placebo ≥ PAXIL: Abdominal pain, agitation, back pain, chest pain, CNS stimulation, fever, increased appetite, myoclonus, pharyngitis, postural hypotension, respiratory disorder (includes mostly "cold symptoms" or "URI"), trauma, and vomiting.
[2] Includes mostly "lump in throat" and "tightness in throat."
[3] Percentage corrected for gender.
[4] Mostly "ejaculatory delay."
[5] Includes "anorgasmia," "erectile difficulties," "delayed ejaculation/orgasm," and "sexual dysfunction," and "impotence."
[6] Includes mostly "difficulty with micturition" and "urinary hesitancy."
[7] Includes mostly "anorgasmia" and "difficulty reaching climax/orgasm."

Prescribers or other health professionals should inform patients, their families, and their caregivers about the benefits and risks associated with treatment with PAXIL and should counsel them in its appropriate use. A patient Medication Guide about "Antidepressant Medicines, Depression and Other Serious Mental Illnesses, and Suicidal Thoughts or Actions" is available for PAXIL. The prescriber or health professional should instruct patients, their families, and their caregivers to read the Medication Guide and should assist them in understanding its contents. Patients should be given the opportunity to discuss the contents of the Medication Guide and to obtain answers to any questions they may have. The complete text of the Medication Guide is reprinted at the end of this document.

Patients should be advised of the following issues and asked to alert their prescriber if these occur while taking PAXIL.

Table 3. Treatment-Emergent Adverse Experience Incidence in Placebo-Controlled Clinical Trials for Obsessive Compulsive Disorder, Panic Disorder, and Social Anxiety Disorder[1]

Body System	Preferred Term	Obsessive Compulsive Disorder		Panic Disorder		Social Anxiety Disorder	
		PAXIL (n = 542)	Placebo (n = 265)	PAXIL (n = 469)	Placebo (n = 324)	PAXIL (n = 425)	Placebo (n = 339)
Body as a Whole	Asthenia	22%	14%	14%	5%	22%	14%
	Abdominal Pain	—	—	4%	3%	—	—
	Chest Pain	3%	2%	—	—	—	—
	Back Pain	—	—	3%	2%	—	—
	Chills	2%	1%	2%	1%	—	—
	Trauma	—	—	—	—	3%	1%
Cardiovascular	Vasodilation	4%	1%	—	—	—	—
	Palpitation	2%	0%	—	—	—	—
Dermatologic	Sweating	9%	3%	14%	6%	9%	2%
	Rash	3%	2%	—	—	—	—
Gastrointestinal	Nausea	23%	10%	23%	17%	25%	7%
	Dry Mouth	18%	9%	18%	11%	9%	3%
	Constipation	16%	6%	8%	5%	5%	2%
	Diarrhea	10%	10%	12%	7%	9%	6%
	Decreased Appetite	9%	3%	7%	3%	8%	2%
	Dyspepsia	—	—	—	—	4%	2%
	Flatulence	—	—	—	—	4%	2%
	Increased Appetite	4%	3%	2%	1%	—	—
	Vomiting	—	—	—	—	2%	1%
Musculoskeletal	Myalgia	—	—	—	—	4%	3%
Nervous System	Insomnia	24%	13%	18%	10%	21%	16%
	Somnolence	24%	7%	19%	11%	22%	5%
	Dizziness	12%	6%	14%	10%	11%	7%
	Tremor	11%	1%	9%	1%	9%	1%
	Nervousness	9%	8%	—	—	8%	7%
	Libido Decreased	7%	4%	9%	1%	12%	1%
	Agitation	—	—	5%	4%	3%	1%
	Anxiety	—	—	5%	4%	5%	4%
	Abnormal Dreams	4%	1%	—	—	—	—
	Concentration Impaired	3%	2%	—	—	4%	1%
	Depersonalization	3%	0%	—	—	—	—
	Myoclonus	3%	0%	3%	2%	2%	1%
	Amnesia	2%	1%	—	—	—	—

(Table continued on next page)

Clinical Worsening and Suicide Risk

Patients, their families, and their caregivers should be encouraged to be alert to the emergence of anxiety, agitation, panic attacks, insomnia, irritability, hostility, aggressiveness, impulsivity, akathisia (psychomotor restlessness), hypomania, mania, other unusual changes in behavior, worsening of depression, and suicidal ideation, especially early during antidepressant treatment and when the dose is adjusted up or down. Families and caregivers of patients should be advised to look for the emergence of such symptoms on a day-to-day basis, since changes may be abrupt. Such symptoms should be reported to the patient's prescriber or health professional, especially if they are severe, abrupt in onset, or were not part of the patient's presenting symptoms. Symptoms such as these may be associated with an increased risk for suicidal thinking and behavior and indicate a need for very close monitoring and possibly changes in the medication.

Drugs That Interfere With Hemostasis (e.g., NSAIDs, Aspirin, and Warfarin)

Patients should be cautioned about the concomitant use of paroxetine and NSAIDs, aspirin, warfarin, or other drugs that affect coagulation since the combined use of psychotropic drugs that interfere with serotonin reuptake and these agents has been associated with an increased risk of bleeding.

Interference With Cognitive and Motor Performance

Any psychoactive drug may impair judgment, thinking, or motor skills. Although in controlled studies PAXIL has not been shown to impair psychomotor performance, patients should be cautioned about operating hazardous machinery, including automobiles, until they are reasonably certain that therapy with PAXIL does not affect their ability to engage in such activities.

Completing Course of Therapy

While patients may notice improvement with treatment with PAXIL in 1 to 4 weeks, they should be advised to continue therapy as directed.

Concomitant Medication

Patients should be advised to inform their physician if they are taking, or plan to take, any prescription or over-the-counter drugs, since there is a potential for interactions.

Alcohol

Although PAXIL has not been shown to increase the impairment of mental and motor skills caused by alcohol, patients should be advised to avoid alcohol while taking PAXIL.

Pregnancy

Patients should be advised to notify their physician if they become pregnant or intend to become pregnant during therapy (see WARNINGS—Usage in Pregnancy: *Teratogenic and Nonteratogenic Effects*).

Nursing

Patients should be advised to notify their physician if they are breastfeeding an infant (see PRECAUTIONS—Nursing Mothers).

Laboratory Tests

There are no specific laboratory tests recommended.

Drug Interactions

Tryptophan

As with other serotonin reuptake inhibitors, an interaction between paroxetine and tryptophan may occur when they are coadministered. Adverse experiences, consisting primarily of headache, nausea, sweating, and dizziness, have been reported when tryptophan was administered to patients taking PAXIL. Consequently, concomitant use of PAXIL with tryptophan is not recommended (see WARNINGS—Serotonin Syndrome).

Monoamine Oxidase Inhibitors

See CONTRAINDICATIONS and WARNINGS.

Pimozide

In a controlled study of healthy volunteers, after PAXIL was titrated to 60 mg daily, co-administration of a single dose of 2 mg pimozide was associated with mean increases in pimozide AUC of 151% and C_{max} of 62%, compared to pimozide administered alone. The increase in pimozide AUC and C_{max} is due to the CYP2D6 inhibitory properties of paroxetine. Due to the narrow therapeutic index of pimozide and its known ability to prolong the QT interval, concomitant use of pimozide and PAXIL is contraindicated (see CONTRAINDICATIONS).

Serotonergic Drugs

Based on the mechanism of action of SNRIs and SSRIs, including paroxetine hydrochloride, and the potential for serotonin syndrome, caution is advised when PAXIL is co-administered with other drugs that may affect the serotonergic neurotransmitter systems, such as triptans, linezolid (an antibiotic which is a reversible non-selective MAOI), lithium, tramadol, or St. John's Wort (see WARNINGS—Serotonin Syndrome). The concomitant use of PAXIL with MAOIs (including linezolid) is contraindicated (see CONTRAINDICATIONS). The concomitant use of PAXIL with other SSRIs, SNRIs or tryptophan is not recommended (see PRECAUTIONS—Drug Interactions, *Tryptophan*).

Thioridazine

See CONTRAINDICATIONS and WARNINGS.

Warfarin

Preliminary data suggest that there may be a pharmacodynamic interaction (that causes an increased bleeding diathesis in the face of unaltered prothrombin time) between paroxetine and warfarin. Since there is little clinical experience, the concomitant administration of PAXIL and warfarin should be undertaken with caution (see *Drugs That Interfere With Hemostasis*).

Triptans

There have been rare postmarketing reports of serotonin syndrome with the use of an SSRI and a triptan. If concomitant use of PAXIL with a triptan is clinically warranted, careful observation of the patient is advised, particularly during treatment initiation and dose increases (see WARNINGS—Serotonin Syndrome).

Drugs Affecting Hepatic Metabolism

The metabolism and pharmacokinetics of paroxetine may be affected by the induction or inhibition of drug-metabolizing enzymes.

Cimetidine

Cimetidine inhibits many cytochrome P_{450} (oxidative) enzymes. In a study where PAXIL (30 mg once daily) was dosed orally for 4 weeks, steady-state plasma concentrations of paroxetine were increased by approximately 50% during coadministration with oral cimetidine (300 mg three times daily) for the final week. Therefore, when these drugs are administered concurrently, dosage adjustment of PAXIL after the 20-mg starting dose should be guided by clinical effect. The effect of paroxetine on cimetidine's pharmacokinetics was not studied.

Phenobarbital

Phenobarbital induces many cytochrome P_{450} (oxidative) enzymes. When a single oral 30-mg dose of PAXIL was administered at phenobarbital steady state (100 mg once daily for 14 days), paroxetine AUC and $T_{1/2}$ were reduced (by an average of 25% and 38%, respectively) compared to paroxetine administered alone. The effect of paroxetine on phenobarbital pharmacokinetics was not studied. Since PAXIL exhibits nonlinear pharmacokinetics, the results of this study may not address the case where the 2 drugs are both being chronically dosed. No initial dosage adjustment of PAXIL is considered necessary when coadministered with phenobarbital; any subsequent adjustment should be guided by clinical effect.

Phenytoin

When a single oral 30-mg dose of PAXIL was administered at phenytoin steady state (300 mg once daily for 14 days), paroxetine AUC and $T_{1/2}$ were reduced (by an average of 50% and 35%, respectively) compared to PAXIL administered alone. In a separate study, when a single oral 300-mg dose of phenytoin was administered at paroxetine steady state (30 mg once daily for 14 days), phenytoin AUC was slightly reduced (12% on average) compared to phenytoin administered alone. Since both drugs exhibit nonlinear pharmacokinetics, the above studies may not address the case where the 2 drugs are both being chronically dosed. No initial dosage adjustments are considered necessary when these drugs are coadministered; any subsequent adjustments should be guided by clinical effect (see ADVERSE REACTIONS—Postmarketing Reports).

Drugs Metabolized by CYP2D6

Many drugs, including most drugs effective in the treatment of major depressive disorder (paroxetine, other SSRIs and many tricyclics), are metabolized by the cytochrome P_{450} isozyme CYP2D6. Like other agents that are metabolized by CYP2D6, paroxetine may significantly inhibit the activity of this isozyme. In most patients (>90%), this CYP2D6 isozyme is saturated early during dosing with PAXIL. In 1 study, daily dosing of PAXIL (20 mg once daily) under steady-state conditions increased single dose desipramine (100 mg) C_{max}, AUC, and $T_{1/2}$ by an average of approximately 2-, 5-, and 3-fold, respectively. Concomitant use of paroxetine with risperidone, a CYP2D6 substrate has also been evaluated. In 1 study, daily dosing of paroxetine 20 mg in patients stabilized on risperidone (4 to 8 mg/day) increased mean plasma concentrations of risperidone approximately 4-fold, decreased 9-hydroxyrisperidone concentrations approximately 10%, and increased concentrations of the active moiety (the sum of risperidone plus 9-hydroxyrisperidone) approximately 1.4-fold. The effect of paroxetine on the pharmacokinetics of atomoxetine has been evaluated when both drugs were at steady state. In healthy volunteers who were extensive metabolizers of CYP2D6, paroxetine 20 mg daily was given in combination with 20 mg atomoxetine every 12 hours. This resulted in increases in steady state atomoxetine AUC values that were 6- to 8-fold greater and in atomoxetine C_{max} values that were 3- to 4-fold greater than when atomoxetine was given alone.

Dosage adjustment of atomoxetine may be necessary and it is recommended that atomoxetine be initiated at a reduced dose when it is given with paroxetine.

Concomitant use of PAXIL with other drugs metabolized by cytochrome CYP2D6 has not been formally studied but may require lower doses than usually prescribed for either PAXIL or the other drug.

Therefore, coadministration of PAXIL with other drugs that are metabolized by this isozyme, including certain drugs effective in the treatment of major depressive disorder (e.g., nortriptyline, amitriptyline, imipramine, desipramine, and fluoxetine), phenothiazines, risperidone, and Type 1C antiarrhythmics (e.g., propafenone, flecainide, and encainide), or that inhibit this enzyme (e.g., quinidine), should be approached with caution.

However, due to the risk of serious ventricular arrhythmias and sudden death potentially associated with elevated plasma levels of thioridazine, paroxetine and thioridazine should not be coadministered (see CONTRAINDICATIONS and WARNINGS).

Tamoxifen is a pro-drug requiring metabolic activation by CYP2D6. Inhibition of CYP2D6 by paroxetine may lead to reduced plasma concentrations of an active metabolite (endoxifen) and hence reduced efficacy of tamoxifen (see PRECAUTIONS).

At steady state, when the CYP2D6 pathway is essentially saturated, paroxetine clearance is governed by alternative P_{450} isozymes that, unlike CYP2D6, show no evidence of saturation (see PRECAUTIONS—Tricyclic Antidepressants).

Table 3 (cont.). Treatment-Emergent Adverse Experience Incidence in Placebo-Controlled Clinical Trials for Obsessive Compulsive Disorder, Panic Disorder, and Social Anxiety Disorder[1]

Body System	Preferred Term	Obsessive Compulsive Disorder PAXIL (n = 542)	Obsessive Compulsive Disorder Placebo (n = 265)	Panic Disorder PAXIL (n = 469)	Panic Disorder Placebo (n = 324)	Social Anxiety Disorder PAXIL (n = 425)	Social Anxiety Disorder Placebo (n = 339)
Respiratory System	Rhinitis	—	—	3%	0%	—	—
	Pharyngitis	—	—	—	—	4%	2%
	Yawn	—	—	—	—	5%	1%
Special Senses	Abnormal Vision	4%	2%	—	—	4%	1%
	Taste Perversion	2%	0%	—	—	—	—
Urogenital System	Abnormal Ejaculation[2]	23%	1%	21%	1%	28%	1%
	Dysmenorrhea	—	—	—	—	5%	4%
	Female Genital Disorder[2]	3%	0%	9%	1%	9%	1%
	Impotence[2]	8%	1%	5%	0%	5%	1%
	Urinary Frequency	3%	1%	2%	0%	—	—
	Urination Impaired	3%	0%	—	—	—	—
	Urinary Tract Infection	2%	1%	2%	1%	—	—

[1] Events reported by at least 2% of OCD, panic disorder, and social anxiety disorder in patients treated with PAXIL are included, except the following events which had an incidence on placebo ≥PAXIL: [OCD]: Abdominal pain, agitation, anxiety, back pain, cough increased, depression, headache, hyperkinesia, infection, paresthesia, pharyngitis, respiratory disorder, rhinitis, and sinusitis. [panic disorder]: Abnormal dreams, abnormal vision, chest pain, cough increased, depersonalization, depression, dysmenorrhea, dyspepsia, flu syndrome, headache, infection, myalgia, nervousness, palpitation, paresthesia, pharyngitis, rash, respiratory disorder, sinusitis, taste perversion, trauma, urination impaired, and vasodilation. [social anxiety disorder]: Abdominal pain, depression, headache, infection, respiratory disorder, and sinusitis.

[2] Percentage corrected for gender.

Drugs Metabolized by Cytochrome CYP3A4

An in vivo interaction study involving the coadministration under steady-state conditions of paroxetine and terfenadine, a substrate for cytochrome CYP3A4, revealed no effect of paroxetine on terfenadine pharmacokinetics. In addition, in vitro studies have shown ketoconazole, a potent inhibitor of CYP3A4 activity, to be at least 100 times more potent than paroxetine as an inhibitor of the metabolism of several substrates for this enzyme, including terfenadine, astemizole, cisapride, triazolam, and cyclosporine. Based on the assumption that the relationship between paroxetine's in vitro K_i and its lack of effect on terfenadine's in vivo clearance predicts its effect on other CYP3A4 substrates, paroxetine's extent of inhibition of CYP3A4 activity is not likely to be of clinical significance.

Tricyclic Antidepressants (TCAs)

Caution is indicated in the coadministration of tricyclic antidepressants (TCAs) with PAXIL, because paroxetine may inhibit TCA metabolism. Plasma TCA concentrations may need to be monitored, and the dose of TCA may need to be reduced, if a TCA is coadministered with PAXIL (see PRECAUTIONS—Drugs Metabolized by Cytochrome CYP2D6).

Drugs Highly Bound to Plasma Protein

Because paroxetine is highly bound to plasma protein, administration of PAXIL to a patient taking another drug that is highly protein bound may cause increased free concentrations of the other drug, potentially resulting in adverse events. Conversely, adverse effects could result from displacement of paroxetine by other highly bound drugs.

Drugs That Interfere With Hemostasis (e.g., NSAIDs, Aspirin, and Warfarin)

Serotonin release by platelets plays an important role in hemostasis. Epidemiological studies of the case-control and cohort design that have demonstrated an association between use of psychotropic drugs that interfere with serotonin reuptake and the occurrence of upper gastrointestinal bleeding have also shown that concurrent use of an NSAID or aspirin may potentiate this risk of bleeding. Altered anticoagulant effects, including increased bleeding, have been reported when SSRIs or SNRIs are coadministered with warfarin. Patients receiving warfarin therapy should be carefully monitored when paroxetine is initiated or discontinued.

Alcohol

Although PAXIL does not increase the impairment of mental and motor skills caused by alcohol, patients should be advised to avoid alcohol while taking PAXIL.

Lithium

A multiple-dose study has shown that there is no pharmacokinetic interaction between PAXIL and lithium carbonate. However, due to the potential for serotonin syndrome, caution is advised when PAXIL is coadministered with lithium.

Digoxin

The steady-state pharmacokinetics of paroxetine was not altered when administered with digoxin at steady state. Mean digoxin AUC at steady state decreased by 15% in the presence of paroxetine. Since there is little clinical experience, the concurrent administration of paroxetine and digoxin should be undertaken with caution.

Diazepam

Under steady-state conditions, diazepam does not appear to affect paroxetine kinetics. The effects of paroxetine on diazepam were not evaluated.

Procyclidine

Daily dosing of PAXIL (30 mg once daily) increased steady-state AUC_{0-24}, C_{max}, and C_{min} values of procyclidine (5 mg oral once daily) by 35%, 37%, and 67%, respectively, compared to procyclidine alone at steady state. If anticholinergic effects are seen, the dose of procyclidine should be reduced.

Beta-Blockers

In a study where propranolol (80 mg twice daily) was dosed orally for 18 days, the established steady-state plasma concentrations of propranolol were unaltered during coadministration with PAXIL (30 mg once daily) for the final 10 days. The effects of propranolol on paroxetine have not been evaluated (see ADVERSE REACTIONS—Postmarketing Reports).

Theophylline

Reports of elevated theophylline levels associated with treatment with PAXIL have been reported. While this interaction has not been formally studied, it is recommended that theophylline levels be monitored when these drugs are concurrently administered.

Fosamprenavir/Ritonavir

Co-administration of fosamprenavir/ritonavir with paroxetine significantly decreased plasma levels of paroxetine. Any dose adjustment should be guided by clinical effect (tolerability and efficacy).

Electroconvulsive Therapy (ECT)

There are no clinical studies of the combined use of ECT and PAXIL.

Carcinogenesis, Mutagenesis, Impairment of Fertility

Carcinogenesis

Two-year carcinogenicity studies were conducted in rodents given paroxetine in the diet at 1, 5, and 25 mg/kg/day (mice) and 1, 5, and 20 mg/kg/day (rats). These doses are up to 2.4 (mouse) and 3.9 (rat) times the MRHD for major depressive disorder, social anxiety disorder, GAD, and PTSD on a mg/m[2] basis. Because the MRHD for major depressive

Table 4. Treatment-Emergent Adverse Experience Incidence in Placebo-Controlled Clinical Trials for Generalized Anxiety Disorder and Posttraumatic Stress Disorder[1]

Body System	Preferred Term	Generalized Anxiety Disorder		Posttraumatic Stress Disorder	
		PAXIL (n = 735)	Placebo (n = 529)	PAXIL (n = 676)	Placebo (n = 504)
Body as a Whole	Asthenia	14%	6%	12%	4%
	Headache	17%	14%	—	—
	Infection	6%	3%	5%	4%
	Abdominal Pain			4%	3%
	Trauma			6%	5%
Cardiovascular	Vasodilation	3%	1%	2%	1%
Dermatologic	Sweating	6%	2%	5%	1%
Gastrointestinal	Nausea	20%	5%	19%	8%
	Dry Mouth	11%	5%	10%	5%
	Constipation	10%	2%	5%	3%
	Diarrhea	9%	7%	11%	5%
	Decreased Appetite	5%	1%	6%	3%
	Vomiting	3%	2%	3%	2%
	Dyspepsia	—	—	5%	3%
Nervous System	Insomnia	11%	8%	12%	11%
	Somnolence	15%	5%	16%	5%
	Dizziness	6%	5%	6%	5%
	Tremor	5%	1%	4%	1%
	Nervousness	4%	3%	—	—
	Libido Decreased	9%	2%	5%	2%
	Abnormal Dreams			3%	2%
Respiratory System	Respiratory Disorder	7%	5%	—	—
	Sinusitis	4%	3%	—	—
	Yawn	4%	—	2%	<1%
Special Senses	Abnormal Vision	2%	1%	3%	1%
Urogenital System	Abnormal Ejaculation[2]	25%	2%	13%	2%
	Female Genital Disorder[2]	4%	1%	5%	1%
	Impotence[2]	4%	3%	9%	1%

[1] Events reported by at least 2% of GAD and PTSD in patients treated with PAXIL are included, except the following events which had an incidence on placebo ≥PAXIL [GAD]: Abdominal pain, back pain, trauma, dyspepsia, myalgia, and pharyngitis. [PTSD]: Back pain, headache, anxiety, depression, nervousness, respiratory disorder, pharyngitis, and sinusitis.
[2] Percentage corrected for gender.

disorder is slightly less than that for OCD (50 mg versus 60 mg), the doses used in these carcinogenicity studies were only 2.0 (mouse) and 3.2 (rat) times the MRHD for OCD. There was a significantly greater number of male rats in the high-dose group with reticulum cell sarcomas (1/100, 0/50, 0/50, and 4/50 for control, low-, middle-, and high-dose groups, respectively) and a significantly increased linear trend across dose groups for the occurrence of lymphoreticular tumors in male rats. Female rats were not affected. Although there was a dose-related increase in the number of tumors in mice, there was no drug-related increase in the number of mice with tumors. The relevance of these findings to humans is unknown.

Mutagenesis
Paroxetine produced no genotoxic effects in a battery of 5 in vitro and 2 in vivo assays that included the following: Bacterial mutation assay, mouse lymphoma mutation assay, unscheduled DNA synthesis assay, and tests for cytogenetic aberrations in vivo in mouse bone marrow and in vitro in human lymphocytes and in a dominant lethal test in rats.

Impairment of Fertility
A reduced pregnancy rate was found in reproduction studies in rats at a dose of paroxetine of 15 mg/kg/day, which is 2.9 times the MRHD for major depressive disorder, social anxiety disorder, GAD, and PTSD or 2.4 times the MRHD for OCD on a mg/m[2] basis. Irreversible lesions occurred in the reproductive tract of male rats after dosing in toxicity studies for 2 to 52 weeks. These lesions consisted of vacuolation of epididymal tubular epithelium at 50 mg/kg/day and atrophic changes in the seminiferous tubules of the testes with arrested spermatogenesis at 25 mg/kg/day (9.8 and 4.9 times the MRHD for major depressive disorder, social anxiety disorder, and GAD; 8.2 and 4.1 times the MRHD for OCD and PD on a mg/m[2] basis).

Pregnancy
Pregnancy Category D. See WARNINGS— Usage in Pregnancy: Teratogenic and Nonteratogenic Effects.

Labor and Delivery
The effect of paroxetine on labor and delivery in humans is unknown.

Nursing Mothers
Like many other drugs, paroxetine is secreted in human milk, and caution should be exercised when PAXIL is administered to a nursing woman.

Pediatric Use
Safety and effectiveness in the pediatric population have not been established (see BOX WARNING and WARNINGS—Clinical Worsening and Suicide Risk). Three placebo-controlled trials in 752 pediatric patients with MDD have been conducted with PAXIL, and the data were not sufficient to support a claim for use in pediatric patients. Anyone considering the use of PAXIL in a child or adolescent must balance the potential risks with the clinical need.

In placebo-controlled clinical trials conducted with pediatric patients, the following adverse events were reported in at least 2% of pediatric patients treated with PAXIL and occurred at a rate at least twice that for pediatric patients receiving placebo: emotional lability (including self-harm, suicidal thoughts, attempted suicide, crying, and mood fluctuations), hostility, decreased appetite, tremor, sweating, hyperkinesia, and agitation.

Events reported upon discontinuation of treatment with PAXIL in the pediatric clinical trials that included a taper phase regimen, which occurred in at least 2% of patients who received PAXIL and which occurred at a rate at least twice that of placebo, were: emotional lability (including suicidal ideation, suicide attempt, mood changes, and tearfulness), nervousness, dizziness, nausea, and abdominal pain (see Discontinuation of Treatment With PAXIL).

Geriatric Use
SSRIs and SNRIs, including PAXIL, have been associated with cases of clinically significant hyponatremia in elderly patients, who may be at greater risk for this adverse event (see PRECAUTIONS, Hyponatremia).

In worldwide premarketing clinical trials with PAXIL, 17% of patients treated with PAXIL (approximately 700) were 65 years of age or older. Pharmacokinetic studies revealed a decreased clearance in the elderly, and a lower starting dose is recommended; there were, however, no overall differences in the adverse event profile between elderly and younger patients, and effectiveness was similar in younger and older patients (see CLINICAL PHARMACOLOGY and DOSAGE AND ADMINISTRATION).

ADVERSE REACTIONS
Associated With Discontinuation of Treatment
Twenty percent (1,199/6,145) of patients treated with PAXIL in worldwide clinical trials in major depressive disorder and 16.1% (84/522), 11.8% (64/542), 9.4% (44/469), 10.7% (79/735), and 11.7% (79/676) of patients treated with PAXIL in worldwide trials in social anxiety disorder, OCD, panic disorder, GAD, and PTSD, respectively, discontinued treatment due to an adverse event. The most common events (≥1%) associated with discontinuation and considered to be drug related (i.e., those events associated with dropout at a rate approximately twice or greater for PAXIL compared to placebo) included the following:
[See table at top of page 1494]

Commonly Observed Adverse Events
Major Depressive Disorder
The most commonly observed adverse events associated with the use of paroxetine (incidence of 5% or greater and incidence for PAXIL at least twice that for placebo, derived from Table 2) were: Asthenia, sweating, nausea, decreased appetite, somnolence, dizziness, insomnia, tremor, nervousness, ejaculatory disturbance, and other male genital disorders.

Obsessive Compulsive Disorder
The most commonly observed adverse events associated with the use of paroxetine (incidence of 5% or greater and incidence for PAXIL at least twice that for placebo, derived from Table 3) were: Nausea, dry mouth, decreased appetite, constipation, dizziness, somnolence, tremor, sweating, impotence, and abnormal ejaculation.

Panic Disorder
The most commonly observed adverse events associated with the use of paroxetine (incidence of 5% or greater and incidence for PAXIL at least twice that for placebo, derived from Table 3) were: Asthenia, sweating, decreased appetite, libido decreased, tremor, abnormal ejaculation, female genital disorders, and impotence.

Social Anxiety Disorder
The most commonly observed adverse events associated with the use of paroxetine (incidence of 5% or greater and incidence for PAXIL at least twice that for placebo, derived from Table 3) were: Sweating, nausea, dry mouth, constipation, decreased appetite, somnolence, tremor, libido decreased, yawn, abnormal ejaculation, female genital disorders, and impotence.

Generalized Anxiety Disorder
The most commonly observed adverse events associated with the use of paroxetine (incidence of 5% or greater and incidence for PAXIL at least twice that for placebo, derived from Table 4) were: Asthenia, infection, constipation, decreased appetite, dry mouth, nausea, libido decreased, somnolence, tremor, sweating, and abnormal ejaculation.

Posttraumatic Stress Disorder
The most commonly observed adverse events associated with the use of paroxetine (incidence of 5% or greater and incidence for PAXIL at least twice that for placebo, derived from Table 4) were: Asthenia, sweating, nausea, dry mouth,

Table 5. Treatment-Emergent Adverse Experience Incidence in a Dose-Comparison Trial in the Treatment of Major Depressive Disorder*

Body System/Preferred Term	Placebo n = 51	PAXIL			
		10 mg n = 102	20 mg n = 104	30 mg n = 101	40 mg n = 102
Body as a Whole					
Asthenia	0.0%	2.9%	10.6%	13.9%	12.7%
Dermatology					
Sweating	2.0%	1.0%	6.7%	8.9%	11.8%
Gastrointestinal					
Constipation	5.9%	4.9%	7.7%	9.9%	12.7%
Decreased Appetite	2.0%	2.0%	5.8%	4.0%	4.9%
Diarrhea	7.8%	9.8%	19.2%	7.9%	14.7%
Dry Mouth	2.0%	10.8%	18.3%	15.8%	20.6%
Nausea	13.7%	14.7%	26.9%	34.7%	36.3%
Nervous System					
Anxiety	0.0%	2.0%	5.8%	5.9%	5.9%
Dizziness	3.9%	6.9%	6.7%	8.9%	12.7%
Nervousness	0.0%	5.9%	5.8%	4.0%	2.9%
Paresthesia	0.0%	2.9%	1.0%	5.0%	5.9%
Somnolence	7.8%	12.7%	18.3%	20.8%	21.6%
Tremor	0.0%	0.0%	7.7%	7.9%	14.7%
Special Senses					
Blurred Vision	2.0%	2.9%	2.9%	2.0%	7.8%
Urogenital System					
Abnormal Ejaculation	0.0%	5.8%	6.5%	10.6%	13.0%
Impotence	0.0%	1.9%	4.3%	6.4%	1.9%
Male Genital Disorders	0.0%	3.8%	8.7%	6.4%	3.7%

* Rule for including adverse events in table: Incidence at least 5% for 1 of paroxetine groups and ≥ twice the placebo incidence for at least 1 paroxetine group.

diarrhea, decreased appetite, somnolence, libido decreased, abnormal ejaculation, female genital disorders, and impotence.

Incidence in Controlled Clinical Trials
The prescriber should be aware that the figures in the tables following cannot be used to predict the incidence of side effects in the course of usual medical practice where patient characteristics and other factors differ from those that prevailed in the clinical trials. Similarly, the cited frequencies cannot be compared with figures obtained from other clinical investigations involving different treatments, uses, and investigators. The cited figures, however, do provide the prescribing physician with some basis for estimating the relative contribution of drug and nondrug factors to the side effect incidence rate in the populations studied.

Major Depressive Disorder
Table 2 enumerates adverse events that occurred at an incidence of 1% or more among paroxetine-treated patients who participated in short-term (6-week) placebo-controlled trials in which patients were dosed in a range of 20 mg to 50 mg/day. Reported adverse events were classified using a standard COSTART-based Dictionary terminology.
[See table 2 at top of page 1495]

Obsessive Compulsive Disorder, Panic Disorder, and Social Anxiety Disorder
Table 3 enumerates adverse events that occurred at a frequency of 2% or more among OCD patients on PAXIL who participated in placebo-controlled trials of 12-weeks duration in which patients were dosed in a range of 20 mg to 60 mg/day or among patients with panic disorder on PAXIL who participated in placebo-controlled trials of 10- to 12-weeks duration in which patients were dosed in a range of 10 mg to 60 mg/day or among patients with social anxiety disorder on PAXIL who participated in placebo-controlled trials of 12-weeks duration in which patients were dosed in a range of 20 mg to 50 mg/day.
[See table 3 on pages 1496 and 1497]

Generalized Anxiety Disorder and Posttraumatic Stress Disorder
Table 4 enumerates adverse events that occurred at a frequency of 2% or more among GAD patients on PAXIL who participated in placebo-controlled trials of 8-weeks duration in which patients were dosed in a range of 10 mg/day to 50 mg/day or among PTSD patients on PAXIL who participated in placebo-controlled trials of 12-weeks duration in which patients were dosed in a range of 20 mg/day to 50 mg/day.
[See table 4 at top of previous page]

Dose Dependency of Adverse Events
A comparison of adverse event rates in a fixed-dose study comparing 10, 20, 30, and 40 mg/day of PAXIL with placebo in the treatment of major depressive disorder revealed a clear dose dependency for some of the more common adverse events associated with use of PAXIL, as shown in the following table:
[See table 5 above]

In a fixed-dose study comparing placebo and 20, 40, and 60 mg/day of PAXIL in the treatment of OCD, there was no clear relationship between adverse events and the dose of PAXIL to which patients were assigned. No new adverse events were observed in the group treated with 60 mg of PAXIL compared to any of the other treatment groups.

In a fixed-dose study comparing placebo and 10, 20, and 40 mg/day of PAXIL in the treatment of panic disorder, there was no clear relationship between adverse events and the dose of PAXIL to which patients were assigned, except for asthenia, dry mouth, anxiety, libido decreased, tremor, and abnormal ejaculation. In flexible-dose studies, no new adverse events were observed in patients receiving 60 mg of PAXIL compared to any of the other treatment groups.

In a fixed-dose study comparing placebo and 20, 40, and 60 mg of PAXIL in the treatment of social anxiety disorder, for most of the adverse events, there was no clear relationship between adverse events and the dose of PAXIL to which patients were assigned.

In a fixed-dose study comparing placebo and 20 and 40 mg of PAXIL in the treatment of generalized anxiety disorder, for most of the adverse events, there was no clear relationship between adverse events and the dose of PAXIL to which patients were assigned, except for the following adverse events: Asthenia, constipation, and abnormal ejaculation.

In a fixed-dose study comparing placebo and 20 and 40 mg of PAXIL in the treatment of posttraumatic stress disorder, for most of the adverse events, there was no clear relationship between adverse events and the dose of PAXIL to which patients were assigned, except for impotence and abnormal ejaculation.

Adaptation to Certain Adverse Events
Over a 4- to 6-week period, there was evidence of adaptation to some adverse events with continued therapy (e.g., nausea and dizziness), but less to other effects (e.g., dry mouth, somnolence, and asthenia).

Male and Female Sexual Dysfunction With SSRIs
Although changes in sexual desire, sexual performance, and sexual satisfaction often occur as manifestations of a psychiatric disorder, they may also be a consequence of pharmacologic treatment. In particular, some evidence suggests that selective serotonin reuptake inhibitors (SSRIs) can cause such untoward sexual experiences.

Reliable estimates of the incidence and severity of untoward experiences involving sexual desire, performance, and satisfaction are difficult to obtain, however, in part because patients and physicians may be reluctant to discuss them. Accordingly, estimates of the incidence of untoward sexual experience and performance cited in product labeling, are likely to underestimate their actual incidence.

In placebo-controlled clinical trials involving more than 3,200 patients, the ranges for the reported incidence of sexual side effects in males and females with major depressive disorder, OCD, panic disorder, social anxiety disorder, GAD, and PTSD are displayed in Table 6.

Table 6. Incidence of Sexual Adverse Events in Controlled Clinical Trials

	PAXIL	Placebo
n (males)	1446	1042
Decreased Libido	6-15%	0-5%
Ejaculatory Disturbance	13-28%	0-2%
Impotence	2-9%	0-3%
n (females)	1822	1340
Decreased Libido	0-9%	0-2%
Orgasmic Disturbance	2-9%	0-1%

There are no adequate and well-controlled studies examining sexual dysfunction with paroxetine treatment.

Paroxetine treatment has been associated with several cases of priapism. In those cases with a known outcome, patients recovered without sequelae.

While it is difficult to know the precise risk of sexual dysfunction associated with the use of SSRIs, physicians should routinely inquire about such possible side effects.

Weight and Vital Sign Changes
Significant weight loss may be an undesirable result of treatment with PAXIL for some patients but, on average, patients in controlled trials had minimal (about 1 pound) weight loss versus smaller changes on placebo and active control. No significant changes in vital signs (systolic and diastolic blood pressure, pulse and temperature) were observed in patients treated with PAXIL in controlled clinical trials.

ECG Changes
In an analysis of ECGs obtained in 682 patients treated with PAXIL and 415 patients treated with placebo in controlled clinical trials, no clinically significant changes were seen in the ECGs of either group.

Liver Function Tests
In placebo-controlled clinical trials, patients treated with PAXIL exhibited abnormal values on liver function tests at no greater rate than that seen in placebo-treated patients. In particular, the PAXIL-versus-placebo comparisons for alkaline phosphatase, SGOT, SGPT, and bilirubin revealed no differences in the percentage of patients with marked abnormalities.

Hallucinations
In pooled clinical trials of immediate-release paroxetine hydrochloride, hallucinations were observed in 22 of 9089 patients receiving drug and 4 of 3187 patients receiving placebo.

Other Events Observed During the Premarketing Evaluation of PAXIL

During its premarketing assessment in major depressive disorder, multiple doses of PAXIL were administered to 6,145 patients in phase 2 and 3 studies. The conditions and duration of exposure to PAXIL varied greatly and included (in overlapping categories) open and double-blind studies, uncontrolled and controlled studies, inpatient and outpatient studies, and fixed-dose, and titration studies. During premarketing clinical trials in OCD, panic disorder, social anxiety disorder, generalized anxiety disorder, and posttraumatic stress disorder, 542, 469, 522, 735, and 676 patients, respectively, received multiple doses of PAXIL. Untoward events associated with this exposure were recorded by clinical investigators using terminology of their own choosing. Consequently, it is not possible to provide a meaningful estimate of the proportion of individuals experiencing adverse events without first grouping similar types of untoward events into a smaller number of standardized event categories.

In the tabulations that follow, reported adverse events were classified using a standard COSTART-based Dictionary terminology. The frequencies presented, therefore, represent the proportion of the 9,089 patients exposed to multiple doses of PAXIL who experienced an event of the type cited on at least 1 occasion while receiving PAXIL. All reported events are included except those already listed in Tables 2 to 4, those reported in terms so general as to be uninformative and those events where a drug cause was remote. It is important to emphasize that although the events reported occurred during treatment with paroxetine, they were not necessarily caused by it.

Events are further categorized by body system and listed in order of decreasing frequency according to the following definitions: Frequent adverse events are those occurring on 1 or more occasions in at least 1/100 patients (only those not already listed in the tabulated results from placebo-controlled trials appear in this listing); infrequent adverse events are those occurring in 1/100 to 1/1,000 patients; rare events are those occurring in fewer than 1/1,000 patients. Events of major clinical importance are also described in the PRECAUTIONS section.

Body as a Whole

Infrequent: Allergic reaction, chills, face edema, malaise, neck pain; *rare:* Adrenergic syndrome, cellulitis, moniliasis, neck rigidity, pelvic pain, peritonitis, sepsis, ulcer.

Cardiovascular System

Frequent: Hypertension, tachycardia; *infrequent:* Bradycardia, hematoma, hypotension, migraine, postural hypotension, syncope; *rare:* Angina pectoris, arrhythmia nodal, atrial fibrillation, bundle branch block, cerebral ischemia, cerebrovascular accident, congestive heart failure, heart block, low cardiac output, myocardial infarct, myocardial ischemia, pallor, phlebitis, pulmonary embolus, supraventricular extrasystoles, thrombophlebitis, thrombosis, varicose vein, vascular headache, ventricular extrasystoles.

Digestive System

Infrequent: Bruxism, colitis, dysphagia, eructation, gastritis, gastroenteritis, gingivitis, glossitis, increased salivation, liver function tests abnormal, rectal hemorrhage, ulcerative stomatitis; *rare:* Aphthous stomatitis, bloody diarrhea, bulimia, cardiospasm, cholelithiasis, duodenitis, enteritis, esophagitis, fecal impactions, fecal incontinence, gum hemorrhage, hematemesis, hepatitis, ileitis, ileus, intestinal obstruction, jaundice, melena, mouth ulceration, peptic ulcer, salivary gland enlargement, sialadenitis, stomach ulcer, stomatitis, tongue discoloration, tongue edema, tooth caries.

Endocrine System

Rare: Diabetes mellitus, goiter, hyperthyroidism, hypothyroidism, thyroiditis.

Hemic and Lymphatic Systems

Infrequent: Anemia, leukopenia, lymphadenopathy, purpura; *rare:* Abnormal erythrocytes, basophilia, bleeding time increased, eosinophilia, hypochromic anemia, iron deficiency anemia, leukocytosis, lymphedema, abnormal lymphocytes, lymphocytosis, microcytic anemia, monocytosis, normocytic anemia, thrombocythemia, thrombocytopenia.

Metabolic and Nutritional

Frequent: Weight gain; *infrequent:* Edema, peripheral edema, SGOT increased, SGPT increased, thirst, weight loss; *rare:* Alkaline phosphatase increased, bilirubinemia, BUN increased, creatinine phosphokinase increased, dehydration, gamma globulins increased, gout, hypercalcemia, hypercholesteremia, hyperglycemia, hyperkalemia, hyperphosphatemia, hypocalcemia, hypoglycemia, hypokalemia, hyponatremia, ketosis, lactic dehydrogenase increased, nonprotein nitrogen (NPN) increased.

Musculoskeletal System

Frequent: Arthralgia; *infrequent:* Arthritis, arthrosis; *rare:* Bursitis, myositis, osteoporosis, generalized spasm, tenosynovitis, tetany.

Nervous System

Frequent: Emotional lability, vertigo; *infrequent:* Abnormal thinking, alcohol abuse, ataxia, dystonia, dyskinesia, euphoria, hallucinations, hostility, hypertonia, hypesthesia, hypokinesia, incoordination, lack of emotion, libido increased, manic reaction, neurosis, paralysis, paranoid reaction; *rare:* Abnormal gait, akinesia, antisocial reaction, aphasia, choreoathetosis, circumoral paresthesias, convulsion, delirium, delusions, diplopia, drug dependence, dysarthria, extrapyramidal syndrome, fasciculations, grand mal convulsion, hyperalgesia, hysteria, manic-depressive reaction, meningitis, myelitis, neuralgia, neuropathy, nystagmus, peripheral neuritis, psychotic depression, psychosis, reflexes decreased, reflexes increased, stupor, torticollis, trismus, withdrawal syndrome.

Respiratory System

Infrequent: Asthma, bronchitis, dyspnea, epistaxis, hyperventilation, pneumonia, respiratory flu; *rare:* Emphysema, hemoptysis, hiccups, lung fibrosis, pulmonary edema, sputum increased, stridor, voice alteration.

Skin and Appendages

Frequent: Pruritus; *infrequent:* Acne, alopecia, contact dermatitis, dry skin, ecchymosis, eczema, herpes simplex, photosensitivity, urticaria; *rare:* Angioedema, erythema nodosum, erythema multiforme, exfoliative dermatitis, fungal dermatitis, furunculosis; herpes zoster, hirsutism, maculopapular rash, seborrhea, skin discoloration, skin hypertrophy, skin ulcer, sweating decreased, vesiculobullous rash.

Special Senses

Frequent: Tinnitus; *infrequent:* Abnormality of accommodation, conjunctivitis, ear pain, eye pain, keratoconjunctivitis, mydriasis, otitis media; *rare:* Amblyopia, anisocoria, blepharitis, cataract, conjunctival edema, corneal ulcer, deafness, exophthalmos, eye hemorrhage, glaucoma, hyperacusis, night blindness, otitis externa, parosmia, photophobia, ptosis, retinal hemorrhage, taste loss, visual field defect.

Urogenital System

Infrequent: Amenorrhea, breast pain, cystitis, dysuria, hematuria, menorrhagia, nocturia, polyuria, pyuria, urinary incontinence, urinary retention, urinary urgency, vaginitis; *rare:* Abortion, breast atrophy, breast enlargement, endometrial disorder, epididymitis, female lactation, fibrocystic breast, kidney calculus, kidney pain, leukorrhea, mastitis, metrorrhagia, nephritis, oliguria, salpingitis, urethritis, urinary casts, uterine spasm, urolith, vaginal hemorrhage, vaginal moniliasis.

Postmarketing Reports

Voluntary reports of adverse events in patients taking PAXIL that have been received since market introduction and not listed above that may have no causal relationship with the drug include acute pancreatitis, elevated liver function tests (the most severe cases were deaths due to liver necrosis, and grossly elevated transaminases associated with severe liver dysfunction), Guillain-Barré syndrome, toxic epidermal necrolysis, priapism, syndrome of inappropriate ADH secretion, symptoms suggestive of prolactinemia and galactorrhea; extrapyramidal symptoms which have included akathisia, bradykinesia, cogwheel rigidity, dystonia, hypertonia, oculogyric crisis which has been associated with concomitant use of pimozide; tremor and trismus; status epilepticus, acute renal failure, pulmonary hypertension, allergic alveolitis, anaphylaxis, eclampsia, laryngismus, optic neuritis, porphyria, ventricular fibrillation, ventricular tachycardia (including torsade de pointes), thrombocytopenia, hemolytic anemia, events related to impaired hematopoiesis (including aplastic anemia, pancytopenia, bone marrow aplasia, and agranulocytosis), and vasculitic syndromes (such as Henoch-Schönlein purpura). There has been a case report of an elevated phenytoin level after 4 weeks of PAXIL and phenytoin coadministration. There has been a case report of severe hypotension when PAXIL was added to chronic metoprolol treatment.

DRUG ABUSE AND DEPENDENCE

Controlled Substance Class

PAXIL is not a controlled substance.

Physical and Psychologic Dependence

PAXIL has not been systematically studied in animals or humans for its potential for abuse, tolerance or physical dependence. While the clinical trials did not reveal any tendency for any drug-seeking behavior, these observations were not systematic and it is not possible to predict on the basis of this limited experience the extent to which a CNS-active drug will be misused, diverted, and/or abused once marketed. Consequently, patients should be evaluated carefully for history of drug abuse, and such patients should be observed closely for signs of misuse or abuse of PAXIL (e.g., development of tolerance, incrementations of dose, drug-seeking behavior).

OVERDOSAGE

Human Experience

Since the introduction of PAXIL in the United States, 342 spontaneous cases of deliberate or accidental overdosage during paroxetine treatment have been reported worldwide (circa 1999). These include overdoses with paroxetine alone and in combination with other substances. Of these, 48 cases were fatal and of the fatalities, 17 appeared to involve paroxetine alone. Eight fatal cases that documented the amount of paroxetine ingested were generally confounded by the ingestion of other drugs or alcohol or the presence of significant comorbid conditions. Of 145 non-fatal cases with known outcome, most recovered without sequelae. The largest known ingestion involved 2,000 mg of paroxetine (33 times the maximum recommended daily dose) in a patient who recovered.

Commonly reported adverse events associated with paroxetine overdosage include somnolence, coma, nausea, tremor, tachycardia, confusion, vomiting, and dizziness. Other notable signs and symptoms observed with overdoses involving paroxetine (alone or with other substances) include mydriasis, convulsions (including status epilepticus), ventricular dysrhythmias (including torsade de pointes), hypertension, aggressive reactions, syncope, hypotension, stupor, bradycardia, dystonia, rhabdomyolysis, symptoms of hepatic dysfunction (including hepatic failure, hepatic necrosis, jaundice, hepatitis, and hepatic steatosis), serotonin syndrome, manic reactions, myoclonus, acute renal failure, and urinary retention.

Overdosage Management

Treatment should consist of those general measures employed in the management of overdosage with any drugs effective in the treatment of major depressive disorder.

Ensure an adequate airway, oxygenation, and ventilation. Monitor cardiac rhythm and vital signs. General supportive and symptomatic measures are also recommended. Induction of emesis is not recommended. Gastric lavage with a large-bore orogastric tube with appropriate airway protection, if needed, may be indicated if performed soon after ingestion, or in symptomatic patients.

Activated charcoal should be administered. Due to the large volume of distribution of this drug, forced diuresis, dialysis, hemoperfusion, and exchange transfusion are unlikely to be of benefit. No specific antidotes for paroxetine are known.

A specific caution involves patients who are taking or have recently taken paroxetine who might ingest excessive quantities of a tricyclic antidepressant. In such a case, accumulation of the parent tricyclic and/or an active metabolite may increase the possibility of clinically significant sequelae and extend the time needed for close medical observation (see PRECAUTIONS—*Drugs Metabolized by Cytochrome CYP2D6*).

In managing overdosage, consider the possibility of multiple drug involvement. The physician should consider contacting a poison control center for additional information on the treatment of any overdose. Telephone numbers for certified poison control centers are listed in the *Physicians' Desk Reference* (PDR).

DOSAGE AND ADMINISTRATION

Major Depressive Disorder

Usual Initial Dosage

PAXIL should be administered as a single daily dose with or without food, usually in the morning. The recommended initial dose is 20 mg/day. Patients were dosed in a range of 20 to 50 mg/day in the clinical trials demonstrating the effectiveness of PAXIL in the treatment of major depressive disorder. As with all drugs effective in the treatment of major depressive disorder, the full effect may be delayed. Some patients not responding to a 20-mg dose may benefit from dose increases, in 10-mg/day increments, up to a maximum of 50 mg/day. Dose changes should occur at intervals of at least 1 week.

Maintenance Therapy

There is no body of evidence available to answer the question of how long the patient treated with PAXIL should remain on it. It is generally agreed that acute episodes of major depressive disorder require several months or longer of sustained pharmacologic therapy. Whether the dose needed to induce remission is identical to the dose needed to maintain and/or sustain euthymia is unknown.

Systematic evaluation of the efficacy of PAXIL has shown that efficacy is maintained for periods of up to 1 year with doses that averaged about 30 mg.

Obsessive Compulsive Disorder

Usual Initial Dosage

PAXIL should be administered as a single daily dose with or without food, usually in the morning. The recommended dose of PAXIL in the treatment of OCD is 40 mg daily. Patients should be started on 20 mg/day and the dose can be increased in 10-mg/day increments. Dose changes should occur at intervals of at least 1 week. Patients were dosed in a range of 20 to 60 mg/day in the clinical trials demonstrating the effectiveness of PAXIL in the treatment of OCD. The maximum dosage should not exceed 60 mg/day.

Maintenance Therapy

Long-term maintenance of efficacy was demonstrated in a 6-month relapse prevention trial. In this trial, patients with OCD assigned to paroxetine demonstrated a lower relapse rate compared to patients on placebo (see CLINICAL PHARMACOLOGY—Clinical Trials). OCD is a chronic condition, and it is reasonable to consider continuation for a responding patient. Dosage adjustments should be made to maintain the patient on the lowest effective dosage, and patients should be periodically reassessed to determine the need for continued treatment.

Panic Disorder
Usual Initial Dosage
PAXIL should be administered as a single daily dose with or without food, usually in the morning. The target dose of PAXIL in the treatment of panic disorder is 40 mg/day. Patients should be started on 10 mg/day. Dose changes should occur in 10-mg/day increments and at intervals of at least 1 week. Patients were dosed in a range of 10 to 60 mg/day in the clinical trials demonstrating the effectiveness of PAXIL. The maximum dosage should not exceed 60 mg/day.
Maintenance Therapy
Long-term maintenance of efficacy was demonstrated in a 3-month relapse prevention trial. In this trial, patients with panic disorder assigned to paroxetine demonstrated a lower relapse rate compared to patients on placebo (see CLINICAL PHARMACOLOGY—Clinical Trials). Panic disorder is a chronic condition, and it is reasonable to consider continuation for a responding patient. Dosage adjustments should be made to maintain the patient on the lowest effective dosage, and patients should be periodically reassessed to determine the need for continued treatment.

Social Anxiety Disorder
Usual Initial Dosage
PAXIL should be administered as a single daily dose with or without food, usually in the morning. The recommended and initial dosage is 20 mg/day. In clinical trials the effectiveness of PAXIL was demonstrated in patients dosed in a range of 20 to 60 mg/day. While the safety of PAXIL has been evaluated in patients with social anxiety disorder at doses up to 60 mg/day, available information does not suggest any additional benefit for doses above 20 mg/day (see CLINICAL PHARMACOLOGY—Clinical Trials).
Maintenance Therapy
There is no body of evidence available to answer the question of how long the patient treated with PAXIL should remain on it. Although the efficacy of PAXIL beyond 12 weeks of dosing has not been demonstrated in controlled clinical trials, social anxiety disorder is recognized as a chronic condition, and it is reasonable to consider continuation of treatment for a responding patient. Dosage adjustments should be made to maintain the patient on the lowest effective dosage, and patients should be periodically reassessed to determine the need for continued treatment.

Generalized Anxiety Disorder
Usual Initial Dosage
PAXIL should be administered as a single daily dose with or without food, usually in the morning. In clinical trials the effectiveness of PAXIL was demonstrated in patients dosed in a range of 20 to 50 mg/day. The recommended starting dosage and the established effective dosage is 20 mg/day. There is not sufficient evidence to suggest a greater benefit to doses higher than 20 mg/day. Dose changes should occur in 10 mg/day increments and at intervals of at least 1 week.
Maintenance Therapy
Systematic evaluation of continuing PAXIL for periods of up to 24 weeks in patients with Generalized Anxiety Disorder who had responded while taking PAXIL during an 8-week acute treatment phase has demonstrated a benefit of such maintenance (see CLINICAL PHARMACOLOGY—Clinical Trials). Nevertheless, patients should be periodically reassessed to determine the need for maintenance treatment.

Posttraumatic Stress Disorder
Usual Initial Dosage
PAXIL should be administered as a single daily dose with or without food, usually in the morning. The recommended starting dosage and the established effective dosage is 20 mg/day. In 1 clinical trial, the effectiveness of PAXIL was demonstrated in patients dosed in a range of 20 to 50 mg/day. However, in a fixed dose study, there was not sufficient evidence to suggest a greater benefit for a dose of 40 mg/day compared to 20 mg/day. Dose changes, if indicated, should occur in 10 mg/day increments and at intervals of at least 1 week.
Maintenance Therapy
There is no body of evidence available to answer the question of how long the patient treated with PAXIL should remain on it. Although the efficacy of PAXIL beyond 12 weeks of dosing has not been demonstrated in controlled clinical trials, PTSD is recognized as a chronic condition, and it is reasonable to consider continuation of treatment for a responding patient. Dosage adjustments should be made to maintain the patient on the lowest effective dosage, and patients should be periodically reassessed to determine the need for continued treatment.

Special Populations
Treatment of Pregnant Women During the Third Trimester
Neonates exposed to PAXIL and other SSRIs or SNRIs, late in the third trimester have developed complications requiring prolonged hospitalization, respiratory support, and tube feeding (see WARNINGS). When treating pregnant women with paroxetine during the third trimester, the physician should carefully consider the potential risks and benefits of treatment. The physician may consider tapering paroxetine in the third trimester.

Dosage for Elderly or Debilitated Patients, and Patients With Severe Renal or Hepatic Impairment
The recommended initial dose is 10 mg/day for elderly patients, debilitated patients, and/or patients with severe renal or hepatic impairment. Increases may be made if indicated. Dosage should not exceed 40 mg/day.
Switching Patients to or From a Monoamine Oxidase Inhibitor
At least 14 days should elapse between discontinuation of an MAOI and initiation of therapy with PAXIL. Similarly, at least 14 days should be allowed after stopping PAXIL before starting an MAOI.
Discontinuation of Treatment With PAXIL
Symptoms associated with discontinuation of PAXIL have been reported (see PRECAUTIONS). Patients should be monitored for these symptoms when discontinuing treatment, regardless of the indication for which PAXIL is being prescribed. A gradual reduction in the dose rather than abrupt cessation is recommended whenever possible. If intolerable symptoms occur following a decrease in the dose or upon discontinuation of treatment, then resuming the previously prescribed dose may be considered. Subsequently, the physician may continue decreasing the dose but at a more gradual rate.
NOTE: SHAKE SUSPENSION WELL BEFORE USING.

HOW SUPPLIED
Tablets
Film-coated, modified-oval as follows:
10-mg yellow, scored tablets engraved on the front with PAXIL and on the back with 10.
NDC 0029-3210-13 Bottles of 30
20-mg pink, scored tablets engraved on the front with PAXIL and on the back with 20.
NDC 0029-3211-13 Bottles of 30
NDC 0029-3211-59 Bottles of 90
NDC 0029-3211-21 SUP 100s (intended for institutional use only)
30-mg blue tablets engraved on the front with PAXIL and on the back with 30.
NDC 0029-3212-13 Bottles of 30
40-mg green tablets engraved on the front with PAXIL and on the back with 40.
NDC 0029-3213-13 Bottles of 30
Store tablets between 15° and 30°C (59° and 86°F).
Oral Suspension
Orange-colored, orange-flavored, 10 mg/5 mL, in 250 mL white bottles.
NDC 0029-3215-48
Store suspension at or below 25°C (77°F).
PAXIL is a registered trademark of GlaxoSmithKline.

MEDICATION GUIDE
Antidepressant Medicines, Depression and Other Serious Mental Illnesses, and Suicidal Thoughts or Actions
PAXIL® (PAX-il) (paroxetine hydrochloride) Tablets and Oral Suspension
Read the Medication Guide that comes with your or your family member's antidepressant medicine. This Medication Guide is only about the risk of suicidal thoughts and actions with antidepressant medicines. **Talk to your, or your family member's, healthcare provider about:**
• All risks and benefits of treatment with antidepressant medicines
• All treatment choices for depression or other serious mental illness
What is the most important information I should know about antidepressant medicines, depression and other serious mental illnesses, and suicidal thoughts or action?
1. Antidepressant medicines may increase suicidal thoughts or actions in some children, teenagers, and young adults within the first few months of treatment.
2. Depression and other serious mental illnesses are the most important causes of suicidal thoughts and actions. Some people may have a particularly high risk of having suicidal thoughts or actions. These include people who have (or have a family history of) bipolar illness (also called manic-depressive illness) or suicidal thoughts or actions.
3. How can I watch for and try to prevent suicidal thoughts and actions in myself or a family member?
• Pay close attention to any changes, especially sudden changes, in mood, behaviors, thoughts, or feelings. This is very important when an antidepressant medicine is started or when the dose is changed.
• Call the healthcare provider right away to report new or sudden changes in mood, behavior, thoughts, or feelings.
• Keep all follow-up visits with the healthcare provider as scheduled. Call the healthcare provider between visits as needed, especially if you have concerns about symptoms.
Call a healthcare provider right away if you or your family member has any of the following symptoms, especially if they are new, worse, or worry you:
• Thoughts about suicide or dying
• Attempts to commit suicide
• New or worse depression

• New or worse anxiety
• Feeling very agitated or restless
• Panic attacks
• Trouble sleeping (insomnia)
• New or worse irritability
• Acting aggressive, being angry, or violent
• Acting on dangerous impulses
• An extreme increase in activity and talking (mania)
• Other unusual changes in behavior or mood
What else do I need to know about antidepressant medicines?
• **Never stop an antidepressant medicine without first talking to a healthcare provider.** Stopping an antidepressant medicine suddenly can cause other symptoms.
• **Antidepressants are medicines used to treat depression and other illnesses.** It is important to discuss all the risks of treating depression and also the risks of not treating it. Patients and their families or other caregivers should discuss all treatment choices with the healthcare provider, not just the use of antidepressants.
• **Antidepressant medicines have other side effects.** Call your doctor for medical advice about side effects. You may report side effects to FDA at 1–800–FDA-1088.
• **Antidepressant medicines can interact with other medicines.** Know all of the medicines that you or your family member takes. Keep a list of all medicines to show the healthcare provider. Do not start new medicines without first checking with your healthcare provider.
• **Not all antidepressant medicines prescribed for children are FDA approved for use in children.** Talk to your child's healthcare provider for more information.
This Medication Guide has been approved by the U.S. Food and Drug Administration for all antidepressants.
January 2008   PXL:4MG
GlaxoSmithKline
Research Triangle Park, NC 27709
©2010, GlaxoSmithKline. All rights reserved.
June 2010   PXL:53PI

PAXIL CR®   ℞
[*pax' il*]
(paroxetine hydrochloride)
Controlled-Release Tablets

SUICIDALITY AND ANTIDEPRESSANT DRUGS
Antidepressants increased the risk compared to placebo of suicidal thinking and behavior (suicidality) in children, adolescents, and young adults in short-term studies of major depressive disorder (MDD) and other psychiatric disorders. Anyone considering the use of PAXIL CR or any other antidepressant in a child, adolescent, or young adult must balance this risk with the clinical need. Short-term studies did not show an increase in the risk of suicidality with antidepressants compared to placebo in adults beyond age 24; there was a reduction in risk with antidepressants compared to placebo in adults aged 65 and older. Depression and certain other psychiatric disorders are themselves associated with increases in the risk of suicide. Patients of all ages who are started on antidepressant therapy should be monitored appropriately and observed closely for clinical worsening, suicidality, or unusual changes in behavior. Families and caregivers should be advised of the need for close observation and communication with the prescriber. PAXIL CR is not approved for use in pediatric patients. (See WARNINGS: Clinical Worsening and Suicide Risk, PRECAUTIONS: Information for Patients, and PRECAUTIONS: Pediatric Use.)

DESCRIPTION
PAXIL CR (paroxetine hydrochloride) is an orally administered psychotropic drug with a chemical structure unrelated to other selective serotonin reuptake inhibitors or to tricyclic, tetracyclic, or other available antidepressant or antipanic agents. It is the hydrochloride salt of a phenylpiperidine compound identified chemically as (-)-*trans*-4R-(4'-fluorophenyl)-3S-[(3',4'-methylenedioxyphenoxy) methyl] piperidine hydrochloride hemihydrate and has the empirical formula of $C_{19}H_{20}FNO_3 \cdot HCl \cdot 1/2H_2O$. The molecular weight is 374.8 (329.4 as free base). The structural formula of paroxetine hydrochloride is:
[See chemical structure at top of next page]
Paroxetine hydrochloride is an odorless, off-white powder, having a melting point range of 120° to 138°C and a solubility of 5.4 mg/mL in water.
Each enteric, film-coated, controlled-release tablet contains paroxetine hydrochloride equivalent to paroxetine as follows: 12.5 mg–yellow, 25 mg–pink, 37.5 mg–blue. One layer of the tablet consists of a degradable barrier layer and the other contains the active material in a hydrophilic matrix.

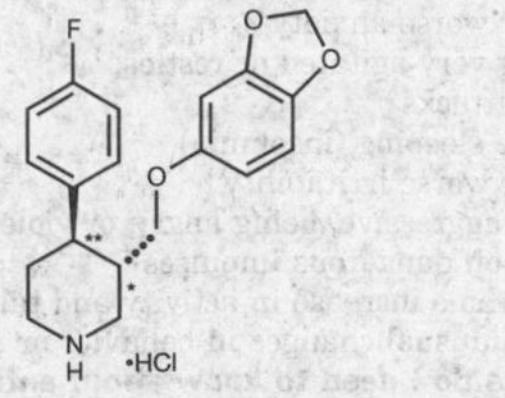

Inactive ingredients consist of hypromellose, polyvinylpyrrolidone, lactose monohydrate, magnesium stearate, silicon dioxide, glyceryl behenate, methacrylic acid copolymer type C, sodium lauryl sulfate, polysorbate 80, talc, triethyl citrate, titanium dioxide, polyethylene glycols, and 1 or more of the following colorants: Yellow ferric oxide, red ferric oxide, D&C Red No. 30 aluminum lake, FD&C Yellow No. 6 aluminum lake, D&C Yellow No. 10 aluminum lake, FD&C Blue No. 2 aluminum lake.

CLINICAL PHARMACOLOGY

Pharmacodynamics

The efficacy of paroxetine in the treatment of major depressive disorder, panic disorder, social anxiety disorder, and premenstrual dysphoric disorder (PMDD) is presumed to be linked to potentiation of serotonergic activity in the central nervous system resulting from inhibition of neuronal reuptake of serotonin (5-hydroxy-tryptamine, 5-HT). Studies at clinically relevant doses in humans have demonstrated that paroxetine blocks the uptake of serotonin into human platelets. In vitro studies in animals also suggest that paroxetine is a potent and highly selective inhibitor of neuronal serotonin reuptake and has only very weak effects on norepinephrine and dopamine neuronal reuptake. In vitro radioligand binding studies indicate that paroxetine has little affinity for muscarinic, alpha$_1$-, alpha$_2$-, beta-adrenergic-, dopamine (D_2)-, 5-HT_1-, 5-HT_2-, and histamine (H_1)-receptors; antagonism of muscarinic, histaminergic, and alpha$_1$-adrenergic receptors has been associated with various anticholinergic, sedative, and cardiovascular effects for other psychotropic drugs.

Because the relative potencies of paroxetine's major metabolites are at most 1/50 of the parent compound, they are essentially inactive.

Pharmacokinetics

Paroxetine hydrochloride is completely absorbed after oral dosing of a solution of the hydrochloride salt. The elimination half-life is approximately 15 to 20 hours after a single dose of PAXIL CR. Paroxetine is extensively metabolized and the metabolites are considered to be inactive. Nonlinearity in pharmacokinetics is observed with increasing doses. Paroxetine metabolism is mediated in part by CYP2D6, and the metabolites are primarily excreted in the urine and to some extent in the feces. Pharmacokinetic behavior of paroxetine has not been evaluated in subjects who are deficient in CYP2D6 (poor metabolizers).

Absorption and Distribution

Tablets of PAXIL CR contain a degradable polymeric matrix (GEOMATRIX™) designed to control the dissolution rate of paroxetine over a period of approximately 4 to 5 hours. In addition to controlling the rate of drug release in vivo, an enteric coat delays the start of drug release until tablets of PAXIL CR have left the stomach.

Paroxetine hydrochloride is completely absorbed after oral dosing of a solution of the hydrochloride salt. In a study in which normal male and female subjects (n = 23) received single oral doses of PAXIL CR at 4 dosage strengths (12.5 mg, 25 mg, 37.5 mg, and 50 mg), paroxetine C_{max} and $AUC_{0\text{-}inf}$ increased disproportionately with dose (as seen also with immediate-release formulations). Mean C_{max} and $AUC_{0\text{-}inf}$ values at these doses were 2.0, 5.5, 9.0, and 12.5 ng/mL, and 121, 261, 338, and 540 ng•hr./mL, respectively. T_{max} was observed typically between 6 and 10 hours post-dose, reflecting a reduction in absorption rate compared with immediate-release formulations. The bioavailability of 25 mg PAXIL CR is not affected by food.

Paroxetine distributes throughout the body, including the CNS, with only 1% remaining in the plasma.

Approximately 95% and 93% of paroxetine is bound to plasma protein at 100 ng/mL and 400 ng/mL, respectively. Under clinical conditions, paroxetine concentrations would normally be less than 400 ng/mL. Paroxetine does not alter the in vitro protein binding of phenytoin or warfarin.

Metabolism and Excretion

The mean elimination half-life of paroxetine was 15 to 20 hours throughout a range of single doses of PAXIL CR (12.5 mg, 25 mg, 37.5 mg, and 50 mg). During repeated administration of PAXIL CR (25 mg once daily), steady state was reached within 2 weeks (i.e., comparable to immediate-release formulations). In a repeat-dose study in which normal male and female subjects (n = 23) received PAXIL CR (25 mg daily), mean steady state C_{max}, C_{min}, and $AUC_{0\text{-}24}$ values were 30 ng/mL, 20 ng/mL, and 550 ng•hr./mL, respectively.

Based on studies using immediate-release formulations, steady-state drug exposure based on $AUC_{0\text{-}24}$ was several-fold greater than would have been predicted from single-dose data. The excess accumulation is a consequence of the fact that 1 of the enzymes that metabolizes paroxetine is readily saturable.

In steady-state dose proportionality studies involving elderly and nonelderly patients, at doses of the immediate-release formulation of 20 mg to 40 mg daily for the elderly and 20 mg to 50 mg daily for the nonelderly, some nonlinearity was observed in both populations, again reflecting a saturable metabolic pathway. In comparison to C_{min} values after 20 mg daily, values after 40 mg daily were only about 2 to 3 times greater than doubled.

Paroxetine is extensively metabolized after oral administration. The principal metabolites are polar and conjugated products of oxidation and methylation, which are readily cleared. Conjugates with glucuronic acid and sulfate predominate, and major metabolites have been isolated and identified. Data indicate that the metabolites have no more than 1/50 the potency of the parent compound at inhibiting serotonin uptake. The metabolism of paroxetine is accomplished in part by CYP2D6. Saturation of this enzyme at clinical doses appears to account for the nonlinearity of paroxetine kinetics with increasing dose and increasing duration of treatment. The role of this enzyme in paroxetine metabolism also suggests potential drug-drug interactions (see PRECAUTIONS).

Approximately 64% of a 30-mg oral solution dose of paroxetine was excreted in the urine with 2% as the parent compound and 62% as metabolites over a 10-day post-dosing period. About 36% was excreted in the feces (probably via the bile), mostly as metabolites and less than 1% as the parent compound over the 10-day post-dosing period.

Other Clinical Pharmacology Information

Specific Populations

Renal and Liver Disease

Increased plasma concentrations of paroxetine occur in subjects with renal and hepatic impairment. The mean plasma concentrations in patients with creatinine clearance below 30 mL/min. were approximately 4 times greater than seen in normal volunteers. Patients with creatinine clearance of 30 to 60 mL/min. and patients with hepatic functional impairment had about a 2-fold increase in plasma concentrations (AUC, C_{max}).

The initial dosage should therefore be reduced in patients with severe renal or hepatic impairment, and upward titration, if necessary, should be at increased intervals (see DOSAGE AND ADMINISTRATION).

Elderly Patients

In a multiple-dose study in the elderly at daily doses of 20, 30, and 40 mg of the immediate-release formulation, C_{min} concentrations were about 70% to 80% greater than the respective C_{min} concentrations in nonelderly subjects. Therefore the initial dosage in the elderly should be reduced (see DOSAGE AND ADMINISTRATION).

Drug-Drug Interactions

In vitro drug interaction studies reveal that paroxetine inhibits CYP2D6. Clinical drug interaction studies have been performed with substrates of CYP2D6 and show that paroxetine can inhibit the metabolism of drugs metabolized by CYP2D6 including desipramine, risperidone, and atomoxetine (see PRECAUTIONS—Drug Interactions).

Clinical Trials

Major Depressive Disorder

The efficacy of PAXIL CR controlled-release tablets as a treatment for major depressive disorder has been established in two 12-week, flexible-dose, placebo-controlled studies of patients with DSM-IV Major Depressive Disorder. One study included patients in the age range 18 to 65 years, and a second study included elderly patients, ranging in age from 60 to 88. In both studies, PAXIL CR was shown to be significantly more effective than placebo in treating major depressive disorder as measured by the following: Hamilton Depression Rating Scale (HDRS), the Hamilton depressed mood item, and the Clinical Global Impression (CGI)–Severity of Illness score.

A study of outpatients with major depressive disorder who had responded to immediate-release paroxetine tablets (HDRS total score <8) during an initial 8-week open-treatment phase and were then randomized to continuation on immediate-release paroxetine tablets or placebo for 1 year demonstrated a significantly lower relapse rate for patients taking immediate-release paroxetine tablets (15%) compared to those on placebo (39%). Effectiveness was similar for male and female patients.

Panic Disorder

The effectiveness of PAXIL CR in the treatment of panic disorder was evaluated in three 10-week, multicenter, flexible-dose studies (Studies 1, 2, and 3) comparing paroxetine controlled-release (12.5 to 75 mg daily) to placebo in adult outpatients who had panic disorder (DSM-IV), with or without agoraphobia. These trials were assessed on the basis of their outcomes on 3 variables: (1) the proportions of patients free of full panic attacks at endpoint; (2) change from baseline to endpoint in the median number of full panic attacks; and (3) change from baseline to endpoint in the median Clinical Global Impression Severity score. For Studies 1 and 2, PAXIL CR was consistently superior to placebo on 2 of these 3 variables. Study 3 failed to consistently demonstrate a significant difference between PAXIL CR and placebo on any of these variables.

For all 3 studies, the mean dose of PAXIL CR for completers at endpoint was approximately 50 mg/day. Subgroup analyses did not indicate that there were any differences in treatment outcomes as a function of age or gender.

Long-term maintenance effects of the immediate-release formulation of paroxetine in panic disorder were demonstrated in an extension study. Patients who were responders during a 10-week double-blind phase with immediate-release paroxetine and during a 3-month double-blind extension phase were randomized to either immediate-release paroxetine or placebo in a 3-month double-blind relapse prevention phase. Patients randomized to paroxetine were significantly less likely to relapse than comparably treated patients who were randomized to placebo.

Social Anxiety Disorder

The efficacy of PAXIL CR as a treatment for social anxiety disorder has been established, in part, on the basis of extrapolation from the established effectiveness of the immediate-release formulation of paroxetine. In addition, the effectiveness of PAXIL CR in the treatment of social anxiety disorder was demonstrated in a 12-week, multicenter, double-blind, flexible-dose, placebo-controlled study of adult outpatients with a primary diagnosis of social anxiety disorder (DSM-IV). In the study, the effectiveness of PAXIL CR (12.5 to 37.5 mg daily) compared to placebo was evaluated on the basis of (1) change from baseline in the Liebowitz Social Anxiety Scale (LSAS) total score and (2) the proportion of responders who scored 1 or 2 (very much improved or much improved) on the Clinical Global Impression (CGI) Global Improvement score.

PAXIL CR demonstrated statistically significant superiority over placebo on both the LSAS total score and the CGI Improvement responder criterion. For patients who completed the trial, 64% of patients treated with PAXIL CR compared to 34.7% of patients treated with placebo were CGI Improvement responders.

Subgroup analyses did not indicate that there were any differences in treatment outcomes as a function of gender. Subgroup analyses of studies utilizing the immediate-release formulation of paroxetine generally did not indicate differences in treatment outcomes as a function of age, race, or gender.

Premenstrual Dysphoric Disorder

The effectiveness of PAXIL CR for the treatment of PMDD utilizing a continuous dosing regimen has been established in 2 placebo-controlled trials. Patients in these trials met DSM-IV criteria for PMDD. In a pool of 1,030 patients, treated with daily doses of PAXIL CR 12.5 or 25 mg/day, or placebo the mean duration of the PMDD symptoms was approximately 11 ± 7 years. Patients on systemic hormonal contraceptives were excluded from these trials. Therefore, the efficacy of PAXIL CR in combination with systemic (including oral) hormonal contraceptives for the continuous daily treatment of PMDD is unknown. In both positive studies, patients (N = 672) were treated with 12.5 mg/day or 25 mg/day of PAXIL CR or placebo continuously throughout the menstrual cycle for a period of 3 menstrual cycles. The VAS-Total score is a patient-rated instrument that mirrors the diagnostic criteria of PMDD as identified in the DSM-IV, and includes assessments for mood, physical symptoms, and other symptoms. 12.5 mg/day and 25 mg/day of PAXIL CR were significantly more effective than placebo as measured by change from baseline to the endpoint on the luteal phase VAS-Total score.

In a third study employing intermittent dosing, patients (N = 366) were treated for the 2 weeks prior to the onset of menses (luteal phase dosing, also known as intermittent dosing) with 12.5 mg/day or 25 mg/day of PAXIL CR or placebo for a period of 3 months. 12.5 mg/day and 25 mg/day of PAXIL CR, as luteal phase dosing, was significantly more effective than placebo as measured by change from baseline luteal phase VAS total score.

There is insufficient information to determine the effect of race or age on outcome in these studies.

INDICATIONS AND USAGE

Major Depressive Disorder

PAXIL CR is indicated for the treatment of major depressive disorder.

The efficacy of PAXIL CR in the treatment of a major depressive episode was established in two 12-week controlled trials of outpatients whose diagnoses corresponded to the DSM-IV category of major depressive disorder (see CLINICAL PHARMACOLOGY—Clinical Trials).

A major depressive episode (DSM-IV) implies a prominent and relatively persistent (nearly every day for at least 2 weeks) depressed mood or loss of interest or pleasure in nearly all activities, representing a change from previous functioning, and includes the presence of at least 5 of the following 9 symptoms during the same 2-week period: Depressed mood, markedly diminished interest or pleasure in usual activities, significant change in weight and/or appetite, insomnia or hypersomnia, psychomotor agitation or retardation, increased fatigue, feelings of guilt or worthlessness, slowed thinking or impaired concentration, a suicide attempt, or suicidal ideation.

The antidepressant action of paroxetine in hospitalized depressed patients has not been adequately studied.

PAXIL CR has not been systematically evaluated beyond 12 weeks in controlled clinical trials; however, the effectiveness of immediate-release paroxetine hydrochloride in maintaining a response in major depressive disorder for up to 1 year has been demonstrated in a placebo-controlled trial (see CLINICAL PHARMACOLOGY—Clinical Trials). The physician who elects to use PAXIL CR for extended periods should periodically re-evaluate the long-term usefulness of the drug for the individual patient.

Panic Disorder

PAXIL CR is indicated for the treatment of panic disorder, with or without agoraphobia, as defined in DSM-IV. Panic disorder is characterized by the occurrence of unexpected panic attacks and associated concern about having additional attacks, worry about the implications or consequences of the attacks, and/or a significant change in behavior related to the attacks.

The efficacy of PAXIL CR controlled-release tablets was established in two 10-week trials in panic disorder patients whose diagnoses corresponded to the DSM-IV category of panic disorder (see CLINICAL PHARMACOLOGY—Clinical Trials).

Panic disorder (DSM-IV) is characterized by recurrent unexpected panic attacks, i.e., a discrete period of intense fear or discomfort in which 4 (or more) of the following symptoms develop abruptly and reach a peak within 10 minutes: (1) palpitations, pounding heart, or accelerated heart rate; (2) sweating; (3) trembling or shaking; (4) sensations of shortness of breath or smothering; (5) feeling of choking; (6) chest pain or discomfort; (7) nausea or abdominal distress; (8) feeling dizzy, unsteady, lightheaded, or faint; (9) derealization (feelings of unreality) or depersonalization (being detached from oneself); (10) fear of losing control; (11) fear of dying; (12) paresthesias (numbness or tingling sensations); (13) chills or hot flushes.

Long-term maintenance of efficacy with the immediate-release formulation of paroxetine was demonstrated in a 3-month relapse prevention trial. In this trial, patients with panic disorder assigned to immediate-release paroxetine demonstrated a lower relapse rate compared to patients on placebo (see CLINICAL PHARMACOLOGY—Clinical Trials). Nevertheless, the physician who prescribes PAXIL CR for extended periods should periodically re-evaluate the long-term usefulness of the drug for the individual patient.

Social Anxiety Disorder

PAXIL CR is indicated for the treatment of social anxiety disorder, also known as social phobia, as defined in DSM-IV (300.23). Social anxiety disorder is characterized by a marked and persistent fear of 1 or more social or performance situations in which the person is exposed to unfamiliar people or to possible scrutiny by others. Exposure to the feared situation almost invariably provokes anxiety, which may approach the intensity of a panic attack. The feared situations are avoided or endured with intense anxiety or distress. The avoidance, anxious anticipation, or distress in the feared situation(s) interferes significantly with the person's normal routine, occupational or academic functioning, or social activities or relationships, or there is marked distress about having the phobias. Lesser degrees of performance anxiety or shyness generally do not require psychopharmacological treatment.

The efficacy of PAXIL CR as a treatment for social anxiety disorder has been established, in part, on the basis of extrapolation from the established effectiveness of the immediate-release formulation of paroxetine. In addition, the efficacy of PAXIL CR was established in a 12-week trial, in adult outpatients with social anxiety disorder (DSM-IV). PAXIL CR has not been studied in children or adolescents with social phobia (see CLINICAL PHARMACOLOGY—Clinical Trials).

The effectiveness of PAXIL CR in long-term treatment of social anxiety disorder, i.e., for more than 12 weeks, has not been systematically evaluated in adequate and well-controlled trials. Therefore, the physician who elects to prescribe PAXIL CR for extended periods should periodically re-evaluate the long-term usefulness of the drug for the individual patient (see DOSAGE AND ADMINISTRATION).

Premenstrual Dysphoric Disorder

PAXIL CR is indicated for the treatment of PMDD.

The efficacy of PAXIL CR in the treatment of PMDD has been established in 3 placebo-controlled trials (see CLINICAL PHARMACOLOGY—Clinical Trials).

The essential features of PMDD, according to DSM-IV, include markedly depressed mood, anxiety or tension, affective lability, and persistent anger or irritability. Other features include decreased interest in usual activities, difficulty concentrating, lack of energy, change in appetite or sleep, and feeling out of control. Physical symptoms associated with PMDD include breast tenderness, headache, joint and muscle pain, bloating, and weight gain. These symptoms occur regularly during the luteal phase and remit within a few days following the onset of menses; the disturbance markedly interferes with work or school or with usual social activities and relationships with others. In making the diagnosis, care should be taken to rule out other cyclical mood disorders that may be exacerbated by treatment with an antidepressant.

The effectiveness of PAXIL CR in long-term use, that is, for more than 3 menstrual cycles, has not been systematically evaluated in controlled trials. Therefore, the physician who elects to use PAXIL CR for extended periods should periodically re-evaluate the long-term usefulness of the drug for the individual patient.

CONTRAINDICATIONS

Concomitant use in patients taking either monoamine oxidase inhibitors (MAOIs), including linezolid, an antibiotic which is a reversible non-selective MAOI, or thioridazine is contraindicated (see WARNINGS and PRECAUTIONS). Concomitant use in patients taking pimozide is contraindicated (see PRECAUTIONS).

PAXIL CR is contraindicated in patients with a hypersensitivity to paroxetine or to any of the inactive ingredients in PAXIL CR.

WARNINGS

Clinical Worsening and Suicide Risk

Patients with major depressive disorder (MDD), both adult and pediatric, may experience worsening of their depression and/or the emergence of suicidal ideation and behavior (suicidality) or unusual changes in behavior, whether or not they are taking antidepressant medications, and this risk may persist until significant remission occurs. Suicide is a known risk of depression and certain other psychiatric disorders, and these disorders themselves are the strongest predictors of suicide. There has been a long-standing concern, however, that antidepressants may have a role in inducing worsening of depression and the emergence of suicidality in certain patients during the early phases of treatment. Pooled analyses of short-term placebo-controlled trials of antidepressant drugs (SSRIs and others) showed that these drugs increase the risk of suicidal thinking and behavior (suicidality) in children, adolescents, and young adults (ages 18-24) with major depressive disorder (MDD) and other psychiatric disorders. Short-term studies did not show an increase in the risk of suicidality with antidepressants compared to placebo in adults beyond age 24; there was a reduction with antidepressants compared to placebo in adults aged 65 and older.

The pooled analyses of placebo-controlled trials in children and adolescents with MDD, obsessive compulsive disorder (OCD), or other psychiatric disorders included a total of 24 short-term trials of 9 antidepressant drugs in over 4,400 patients. The pooled analyses of placebo-controlled trials in adults with MDD or other psychiatric disorders included a total of 295 short-term trials (median duration of 2 months) of 11 antidepressant drugs in over 77,000 patients. There was considerable variation in risk of suicidality among drugs, but a tendency toward an increase in the younger patients for almost all drugs studied. There were differences in absolute risk of suicidality across the different indications, with the highest incidence in MDD. The risk differences (drug vs placebo), however, were relatively stable within age strata and across indications. These risk differences (drug-placebo difference in the number of cases of suicidality per 1,000 patients treated) are provided in Table 1.

Table 1

Age Range	Drug-Placebo Difference in Number of Cases of Suicidality per 1,000 Patients Treated
Increases Compared to Placebo	
<18	14 additional cases
18-24	5 additional cases
Decreases Compared to Placebo	
25-64	1 fewer case
≥65	6 fewer cases

No suicides occurred in any of the pediatric trials. There were suicides in the adult trials, but the number was not sufficient to reach any conclusion about drug effect on suicide.

It is unknown whether the suicidality risk extends to longer-term use, i.e., beyond several months. However, there is substantial evidence from placebo-controlled maintenance trials in adults with depression that the use of antidepressants can delay the recurrence of depression.

All patients being treated with antidepressants for any indication should be monitored appropriately and observed closely for clinical worsening, suicidality, and unusual changes in behavior, especially during the initial few months of a course of drug therapy, or at times of dose changes, either increases or decreases.

The following symptoms, anxiety, agitation, panic attacks, insomnia, irritability, hostility, aggressiveness, impulsivity, akathisia (psychomotor restlessness), hypomania, and mania, have been reported in adult and pediatric patients being treated with antidepressants for major depressive disorder as well as for other indications, both psychiatric and nonpsychiatric. Although a causal link between the emergence of such symptoms and either the worsening of depression and/or the emergence of suicidal impulses has not been established, there is concern that such symptoms may represent precursors to emerging suicidality.

Consideration should be given to changing the therapeutic regimen, including possibly discontinuing the medication, in patients whose depression is persistently worse, or who are experiencing emergent suicidality or symptoms that might be precursors to worsening depression or suicidality, especially if these symptoms are severe, abrupt in onset, or were not part of the patient's presenting symptoms.

If the decision has been made to discontinue treatment, medication should be tapered, as rapidly as is feasible, but with recognition that abrupt discontinuation can be associated with certain symptoms (see PRECAUTIONS and DOSAGE AND ADMINISTRATION—Discontinuation of Treatment With PAXIL CR, for a description of the risks of discontinuation of PAXIL CR).

Families and caregivers of patients being treated with antidepressants for major depressive disorder or other indications, both psychiatric and nonpsychiatric, should be alerted about the need to monitor patients for the emergence of agitation, irritability, unusual changes in behavior, and the other symptoms described above, as well as the emergence of suicidality, and to report such symptoms immediately to healthcare providers. Such monitoring should include daily observation by families and caregivers. Prescriptions for PAXIL CR should be written for the smallest quantity of tablets consistent with good patient management, in order to reduce the risk of overdose.

Screening Patients for Bipolar Disorder

A major depressive episode may be the initial presentation of bipolar disorder. It is generally believed (though not established in controlled trials) that treating such an episode with an antidepressant alone may increase the likelihood of precipitation of a mixed/manic episode in patients at risk for bipolar disorder. Whether any of the symptoms described above represent such a conversion is unknown. However, prior to initiating treatment with an antidepressant, patients with depressive symptoms should be adequately screened to determine if they are at risk for bipolar disorder; such screening should include a detailed psychiatric history, including a family history of suicide, bipolar disorder, and depression. It should be noted that PAXIL CR is not approved for use in treating bipolar depression.

Potential for Interaction With Monoamine Oxidase Inhibitors

In patients receiving another serotonin reuptake inhibitor drug in combination with an MAOI, there have been reports of serious, sometimes fatal, reactions including hyperthermia, rigidity, myoclonus, autonomic instability with possible rapid fluctuations of vital signs, and mental status changes that include extreme agitation progressing to delirium and coma. These reactions have also been reported in patients who have recently discontinued that drug and have been started on an MAOI. Some cases presented with features resembling neuroleptic malignant syndrome. While there are no human data showing such an interaction with paroxetine hydrochloride, limited animal data on the effects of combined use of paroxetine and MAOIs suggest that these drugs may act synergistically to elevate blood pressure and evoke behavioral excitation. Therefore, it is recommended that PAXIL CR not be used in combination with an MAOI (including linezolid, an antibiotic which is a reversible non-selective MAOI), or within 14 days of discontinuing treatment with an MAOI (see CONTRAINDICATIONS). At least 2 weeks should be allowed after stopping PAXIL CR before starting an MAOI.

Serotonin Syndrome or Neuroleptic Malignant Syndrome (NMS)-like Reactions

The development of a potentially life-threatening serotonin syndrome or Neuroleptic Malignant Syndrome (NMS)-like reactions have been reported with SNRIs and SSRIs alone, including treatment with PAXIL CR, but particularly with concomitant use of serotonergic drugs (including triptans) with drugs which impair metabolism of serotonin (includ-

ing MAOIs), or with antipsychotics or other dopamine antagonists. Serotonin syndrome symptoms may include mental status changes (e.g., agitation, hallucinations, coma), autonomic instability (e.g., tachycardia, labile blood pressure, hyperthermia), neuromuscular aberrations (e.g., hyperreflexia, incoordination) and/or gastrointestinal symptoms (e.g., nausea, vomiting, diarrhea). Serotonin syndrome, in its most severe form can resemble neuroleptic malignant syndrome, which includes hyperthermia, muscle rigidity, autonomic instability with possible rapid fluctuation of vital signs, and mental status changes. Patients should be monitored for the emergence of serotonin syndrome or NMS-like signs and symptoms.

The concomitant use of PAXIL CR with MAOIs intended to treat depression is contraindicated.

If concomitant treatment of PAXIL CR with a 5-hydroxytryptamine receptor agonist (triptan) is clinically warranted, careful observation of the patient is advised, particularly during treatment initiation and dose increases. The concomitant use of PAXIL CR with serotonin precursors (such as tryptophan) is not recommended.

Treatment with PAXIL CR and any concomitant serotonergic or antidopaminergic agents, including antipsychotics, should be discontinued immediately if the above events occur and supportive symptomatic treatment should be initiated.

Potential Interaction With Thioridazine

Thioridazine administration alone produces prolongation of the QTc interval, which is associated with serious ventricular arrhythmias, such as torsade de pointes–type arrhythmias, and sudden death. This effect appears to be dose related.

An in vivo study suggests that drugs which inhibit CYP2D6, such as paroxetine, will elevate plasma levels of thioridazine. Therefore, it is recommended that paroxetine not be used in combination with thioridazine (see CONTRAINDICATIONS and PRECAUTIONS).

Usage in Pregnancy

Teratogenic Effects

Epidemiological studies have shown that infants exposed to paroxetine in the first trimester of pregnancy have an increased risk of congenital malformations, particularly cardiovascular malformations. The findings from these studies are summarized below:

- A study based on Swedish national registry data demonstrated that infants exposed to paroxetine during pregnancy (n = 815) had an increased risk of cardiovascular malformations (2% risk in paroxetine-exposed infants) compared to the entire registry population (1% risk), for an odds ratio (OR) of 1.8 (95% confidence interval 1.1 to 2.8). No increase in the risk of overall congenital malformations was seen in the paroxetine-exposed infants. The cardiac malformations in the paroxetine-exposed infants were primarily ventricular septal defects (VSDs) and atrial septal defects (ASDs). Septal defects range in severity from those that resolve spontaneously to those which require surgery.
- A separate retrospective cohort study from the United States (United Healthcare data) evaluated 5,956 infants of mothers dispensed antidepressants during the first trimester (n = 815 for paroxetine). This study showed a trend towards an increased risk for cardiovascular malformations for paroxetine (risk of 1.5%) compared to other antidepressants (risk of 1%), for an OR of 1.5 (95% confidence interval 0.8 to 2.9). Of the 12 paroxetine-exposed infants with cardiovascular malformations, 9 had VSDs. This study also suggested an increased risk of overall major congenital malformations including cardiovascular defects for paroxetine (4% risk) compared to other (2% risk) antidepressants (OR 1.8; 95% confidence interval 1.2 to 2.8).
- Two large case-control studies using separate databases, each with >9,000 birth defect cases and >4,000 controls, found that maternal use of paroxetine during the first trimester of pregnancy was associated with a 2- to 3-fold increased risk of right ventricular outflow tract obstructions. In one study the OR was 2.5 (95% confidence interval, 1.0 to 6.0, 7 exposed infants) and in the other study the OR was 3.3 (95% confidence interval, 1.3 to 8.8, 6 exposed infants).

Other studies have found varying results as to whether there was an increased risk of overall, cardiovascular, or specific congenital malformations. A meta-analysis of epidemiological data over a 16-year period (1992 to 2008) on first trimester paroxetine use in pregnancy and congenital malformations included the above-noted studies in addition to others (n = 17 studies that included overall malformations and n = 14 studies that included cardiovascular malformations; n = 20 distinct studies). While subject to limitations, this meta-analysis suggested an increased occurrence of cardiovascular malformations (prevalence odds ratio [POR] 1.5; 95% confidence interval 1.2 to 1.9) and overall malformations (POR 1.2; 95% confidence interval 1.1 to 1.4) with paroxetine use during the first trimester. It was not possible in this meta-analysis to determine the extent to which the observed prevalence of cardiovascular malformations might have contributed to that of overall malformations, nor was it possible to determine whether any specific types of cardiovascular malformations might have contributed to the observed prevalence of all cardiovascular malformations.

If a patient becomes pregnant while taking paroxetine, she should be advised of the potential harm to the fetus. Unless the benefits of paroxetine to the mother justify continuing treatment, consideration should be given to either discontinuing paroxetine therapy or switching to another antidepressant (see PRECAUTIONS—Discontinuation of Treatment With PAXIL CR). For women who intend to become pregnant or are in their first trimester of pregnancy, paroxetine should only be initiated after consideration of the other available treatment options.

Animal Findings

Reproduction studies were performed at doses up to 50 mg/kg/day in rats and 6 mg/kg/day in rabbits administered during organogenesis. These doses are approximately 8 (rat) and 2 (rabbit) times the maximum recommended human dose (MRHD) on an mg/m^2 basis. These studies have revealed no evidence of teratogenic effects. However, in rats, there was an increase in pup deaths during the first 4 days of lactation when dosing occurred during the last trimester of gestation and continued throughout lactation. This effect occurred at a dose of 1 mg/kg/day or approximately one-sixth of the MRHD on an mg/m^2 basis. The no-effect dose for rat pup mortality was not determined. The cause of these deaths is not known.

Nonteratogenic Effects

Neonates exposed to PAXIL CR and other SSRIs or serotonin and norepinephrine reuptake inhibitors (SNRIs), late in the third trimester have developed complications requiring prolonged hospitalization, respiratory support, and tube feeding. Such complications can arise immediately upon delivery. Reported clinical findings have included respiratory distress, cyanosis, apnea, seizures, temperature instability, feeding difficulty, vomiting, hypoglycemia, hypotonia, hypertonia, hyperreflexia, tremor, jitteriness, irritability, and constant crying. These features are consistent with either a direct toxic effect of SSRIs and SNRIs or, possibly, a drug discontinuation syndrome. It should be noted that, in some cases, the clinical picture is consistent with serotonin syndrome (see WARNINGS—Potential for Interaction With Monoamine Oxidase Inhibitors).

Infants exposed to SSRIs in late pregnancy may have an increased risk for persistent pulmonary hypertension of the newborn (PPHN). PPHN occurs in 1–2 per 1,000 live births in the general population and is associated with substantial neonatal morbidity and mortality. In a retrospective case-control study of 377 women whose infants were born with PPHN and 836 women whose infants were born healthy, the risk for developing PPHN was approximately six-fold higher for infants exposed to SSRIs after the 20th week of gestation compared to infants who had not been exposed to antidepressants during pregnancy. There is currently no corroborative evidence regarding the risk for PPHN following exposure to SSRIs in pregnancy; this is the first study that has investigated the potential risk. The study did not include enough cases with exposure to individual SSRIs to determine if all SSRIs posed similar levels of PPHN risk.

There have also been postmarketing reports of premature births in pregnant women exposed to paroxetine or other SSRIs.

When treating a pregnant woman with paroxetine during the third trimester, the physician should carefully consider both the potential risks and benefits of treatment (see DOSAGE AND ADMINISTRATION). Physicians should note that in a prospective longitudinal study of 201 women with a history of major depression who were euthymic at the beginning of pregnancy, women who discontinued antidepressant medication during pregnancy were more likely to experience a relapse of major depression than women who continued antidepressant medication.

PRECAUTIONS

General

Activation of Mania/Hypomania

During premarketing testing of immediate-release paroxetine hydrochloride, hypomania or mania occurred in approximately 1.0% of paroxetine-treated unipolar patients compared to 1.1% of active-control and 0.3% of placebo-treated unipolar patients. In a subset of patients classified as bipolar, the rate of manic episodes was 2.2% for immediate-release paroxetine and 11.6% for the combined active-control groups. Among 1,627 patients with major depressive disorder, panic disorder, social anxiety disorder, or PMDD treated with PAXIL CR in controlled clinical studies, there were no reports of mania or hypomania. As with all drugs effective in the treatment of major depressive disorder, PAXIL CR should be used cautiously in patients with a history of mania.

Seizures

During premarketing testing of immediate-release paroxetine hydrochloride, seizures occurred in 0.1% of paroxetine-treated patients, a rate similar to that associated with other drugs effective in the treatment of major depressive disorder. Among 1,627 patients who received PAXIL CR in controlled clinical trials in major depressive disorder, panic disorder, social anxiety disorder, or PMDD, 1 patient (0.1%) experienced a seizure. PAXIL CR should be used cautiously in patients with a history of seizures. It should be discontinued in any patient who develops seizures.

Discontinuation of Treatment With PAXIL CR

Adverse events while discontinuing therapy with PAXIL CR were not systematically evaluated in most clinical trials; however, in recent placebo-controlled clinical trials utilizing daily doses of PAXIL CR up to 37.5 mg/day, spontaneously reported adverse events while discontinuing therapy with PAXIL CR were evaluated. Patients receiving 37.5 mg/day underwent an incremental decrease in the daily dose by 12.5 mg/day to a dose of 25 mg/day for 1 week before treatment was stopped. For patients receiving 25 mg/day or 12.5 mg/day, treatment was stopped without an incremental decrease in dose. With this regimen in those studies, the following adverse events were reported for PAXIL CR, at an incidence of 2% or greater for PAXIL CR and were at least twice that reported for placebo: Dizziness, nausea, nervousness, and additional symptoms described by the investigator as associated with tapering or discontinuing PAXIL CR (e.g., emotional lability, headache, agitation, electric shock sensations, fatigue, and sleep disturbances). These events were reported as serious in 0.3% of patients who discontinued therapy with PAXIL CR.

During marketing of PAXIL CR and other SSRIs and SNRIs, there have been spontaneous reports of adverse events occurring upon discontinuation of these drugs, (particularly when abrupt), including the following: Dysphoric mood, irritability, agitation, dizziness, sensory disturbances (e.g., paresthesias such as electric shock sensations and tinnitus), anxiety, confusion, headache, lethargy, emotional lability, insomnia, and hypomania. While these events are generally self-limiting, there have been reports of serious discontinuation symptoms.

Patients should be monitored for these symptoms when discontinuing treatment with PAXIL CR. A gradual reduction in the dose rather than abrupt cessation is recommended whenever possible. If intolerable symptoms occur following a decrease in the dose or upon discontinuation of treatment, then resuming the previously prescribed dose may be considered. Subsequently, the physician may continue decreasing the dose but at a more gradual rate (see DOSAGE AND ADMINISTRATION).

See also PRECAUTIONS—Pediatric Use, for adverse events reported upon discontinuation of treatment with paroxetine in pediatric patients.

Tamoxifen

Some studies have shown that the efficacy of tamoxifen, as measured by the risk of breast cancer relapse/mortality, may be reduced when co-prescribed with paroxetine as a result of paroxetine's irreversible inhibition of CYP2D6 (see Drug Interactions). This risk may increase with longer duration of coadministration. When tamoxifen is used for the treatment or prevention of breast cancer, prescribers should consider using an alternative antidepressant with little or no CYP2D6 inhibition.

Akathisia

The use of paroxetine or other SSRIs has been associated with the development of akathisia, which is characterized by an inner sense of restlessness and psychomotor agitation such as an inability to sit or stand still usually associated with subjective distress. This is most likely to occur within the first few weeks of treatment.

Hyponatremia

Hyponatremia may occur as a result of treatment with SSRIs and SNRIs, including PAXIL CR. In many cases, this hyponatremia appears to be the result of the syndrome of inappropriate antidiuretic hormone secretion (SIADH). Cases with serum sodium lower than 110 mmol/L have been reported. Elderly patients may be at greater risk of developing hyponatremia with SSRIs and SNRIs. Also, patients taking diuretics or who are otherwise volume depleted may be at greater risk (see Geriatric Use). Discontinuation of PAXIL CR should be considered in patients with symptomatic hyponatremia and appropriate medical intervention should be instituted.

Signs and symptoms of hyponatremia include headache, difficulty concentrating, memory impairment, confusion, weakness, and unsteadiness, which may lead to falls. Signs and symptoms associated with more severe and/or acute cases have included hallucination, syncope, seizure, coma, respiratory arrest, and death.

Abnormal Bleeding

SSRIs and SNRIs, including paroxetine, may increase the risk of bleeding events. Concomitant use of aspirin, nonsteroidal anti-inflammatory drugs, warfarin, and other anticoagulants may add to this risk. Case reports and epidemiological studies (case-control and cohort design) have demonstrated an association between use of drugs that interfere with serotonin reuptake and the occurrence of gastrointestinal bleeding. Bleeding events related to SSRIs and SNRIs use have ranged from ecchymoses, hematomas, epistaxis, and petechiae to life-threatening hemorrhages. Patients should be cautioned about the risk of bleeding associated with the concomitant use of paroxetine and NSAIDs, aspirin, or other drugs that affect coagulation.

Use in Patients With Concomitant Illness
Clinical experience with immediate-release paroxetine hydrochloride in patients with certain concomitant systemic illness is limited. Caution is advisable in using PAXIL CR in patients with diseases or conditions that could affect metabolism or hemodynamic responses.

As with other SSRIs, mydriasis has been infrequently reported in premarketing studies with paroxetine hydrochloride. A few cases of acute angle closure glaucoma associated with therapy with immediate-release paroxetine have been reported in the literature. As mydriasis can cause acute angle closure in patients with narrow angle glaucoma, caution should be used when PAXIL CR is prescribed for patients with narrow angle glaucoma.

PAXIL CR or the immediate-release formulation has not been evaluated or used to any appreciable extent in patients with a recent history of myocardial infarction or unstable heart disease. Patients with these diagnoses were excluded from clinical studies during premarket testing. Evaluation of electrocardiograms of 682 patients who received immediate-release paroxetine hydrochloride in double-blind, placebo-controlled trials, however, did not indicate that paroxetine is associated with the development of significant ECG abnormalities. Similarly, paroxetine hydrochloride does not cause any clinically important changes in heart rate or blood pressure.

Increased plasma concentrations of paroxetine occur in patients with severe renal impairment (creatinine clearance <30 mL/min.) or severe hepatic impairment. A lower starting dose should be used in such patients (see DOSAGE AND ADMINISTRATION).

Information for Patients
PAXIL CR should not be chewed or crushed, and should be swallowed whole.

Patients should be cautioned about the risk of serotonin syndrome with the concomitant use of PAXIL CR and triptans, tramadol, or other serotonergic agents.

Prescribers or other health professionals should inform patients, their families, and their caregivers about the benefits and risks associated with treatment with PAXIL CR and should counsel them in its appropriate use. A patient Medication Guide about "Antidepressant Medicines, Depression and Other Serious Mental Illnesses, and Suicidal Thoughts or Actions" is available for PAXIL CR. The prescriber or health professional should instruct patients, their families, and their caregivers to read the Medication Guide and should assist them in understanding its contents. Patients should be given the opportunity to discuss the contents of the Medication Guide and to obtain answers to any questions they may have. The complete text of the Medication Guide is reprinted at the end of this document.

Patients should be advised of the following issues and asked to alert their prescriber if these occur while taking PAXIL CR.

Clinical Worsening and Suicide Risk
Patients, their families, and their caregivers should be encouraged to be alert to the emergence of anxiety, agitation, panic attacks, insomnia, irritability, hostility, aggressiveness, impulsivity, akathisia (psychomotor restlessness), hypomania, mania, other unusual changes in behavior, worsening of depression, and suicidal ideation, especially early during antidepressant treatment and when the dose is adjusted up or down. Families and caregivers of patients should be advised to look for the emergence of such symptoms on a day-to-day basis, since changes may be abrupt. Such symptoms should be reported to the patient's prescriber or health professional, especially if they are severe, abrupt in onset, or were not part of the patient's presenting symptoms. Symptoms such as these may be associated with an increased risk for suicidal thinking and behavior and indicate a need for very close monitoring and possibly changes in the medication.

Drugs That Interfere With Hemostasis (e.g., NSAIDs, Aspirin, and Warfarin)
Patients should be cautioned about the concomitant use of paroxetine and NSAIDs, aspirin, warfarin, or other drugs that affect coagulation since combined use of psychotropic drugs that interfere with serotonin reuptake and these agents has been associated with an increased risk of bleeding.

Interference With Cognitive and Motor Performance
Any psychoactive drug may impair judgment, thinking, or motor skills. Although in controlled studies immediate-release paroxetine hydrochloride has not been shown to impair psychomotor performance, patients should be cautioned about operating hazardous machinery, including automobiles, until they are reasonably certain that therapy with PAXIL CR does not affect their ability to engage in such activities.

Completing Course of Therapy
While patients may notice improvement with use of PAXIL CR in 1 to 4 weeks, they should be advised to continue therapy as directed.

Concomitant Medications
Patients should be advised to inform their physician if they are taking, or plan to take, any prescription or over-the-counter drugs, since there is a potential for interactions.

Alcohol
Although immediate-release paroxetine hydrochloride has not been shown to increase the impairment of mental and motor skills caused by alcohol, patients should be advised to avoid alcohol while taking PAXIL CR.

Pregnancy
Patients should be advised to notify their physician if they become pregnant or intend to become pregnant during therapy (see WARNINGS—Usage in Pregnancy: *Teratogenic and Nonteratogenic Effects*).

Nursing
Patients should be advised to notify their physician if they are breastfeeding an infant (see PRECAUTIONS—Nursing Mothers).

Laboratory Tests
There are no specific laboratory tests recommended.

Drug Interactions

Tryptophan
As with other serotonin reuptake inhibitors, an interaction between paroxetine and tryptophan may occur when they are coadministered. Adverse experiences, consisting primarily of headache, nausea, sweating, and dizziness, have been reported when tryptophan was administered to patients taking immediate-release paroxetine. Consequently, concomitant use of PAXIL CR with tryptophan is not recommended (see WARNINGS—Serotonin Syndrome).

Monoamine Oxidase Inhibitors
See CONTRAINDICATIONS and WARNINGS.

Pimozide
In a controlled study of healthy volunteers, after immediate-release paroxetine hydrochloride was titrated to 60 mg daily, co-administration of a single dose of 2 mg pimozide was associated with mean increases in pimozide AUC of 151% and C_{max} of 62%, compared to pimozide administered alone. The increase in pimozide AUC and C_{max} is due to the CYP2D6 inhibitory properties of paroxetine. Due to the narrow therapeutic index of pimozide and its known ability to prolong the QT interval, concomitant use of pimozide and PAXIL CR is contraindicated (see CONTRAINDICATIONS).

Serotonergic Drugs
Based on the mechanism of action of SNRIs and SSRIs, including paroxetine hydrochloride, and the potential for serotonin syndrome, caution is advised when PAXIL CR is coadministered with other drugs that may affect the serotonergic neurotransmitter systems, such as triptans, linezolid (an antibiotic which is a reversible non-selective MAOI), lithium, tramadol, or St. John's Wort (see WARNINGS—Serotonin Syndrome). The concomitant use of PAXIL CR with MAOIs (including linezolid) is contraindicated (see CONTRAINDICATIONS). The concomitant use of PAXIL CR with other SSRIs, SNRIs or tryptophan is not recommended (see PRECAUTIONS—Drug Interactions, *Tryptophan*).

Thioridazine
See CONTRAINDICATIONS and WARNINGS.

Warfarin
Preliminary data suggest that there may be a pharmacodynamic interaction (that causes an increased bleeding diathesis in the face of unaltered prothrombin time) between paroxetine and warfarin. Since there is little clinical experience, the concomitant administration of PAXIL CR and warfarin should be undertaken with caution (see Drugs That Interfere With Hemostasis).

Triptans
There have been rare postmarketing reports of serotonin syndrome with the use of an SSRI and a triptan. If concomitant use of PAXIL CR with a triptan is clinically warranted, careful observation of the patient is advised, particularly during treatment initiation and dose increases (see WARNINGS—Serotonin Syndrome).

Drugs Affecting Hepatic Metabolism
The metabolism and pharmacokinetics of paroxetine may be affected by the induction or inhibition of drug-metabolizing enzymes.

Cimetidine
Cimetidine inhibits many cytochrome P_{450} (oxidative) enzymes. In a study where immediate-release paroxetine (30 mg once daily) was dosed orally for 4 weeks, steady-state plasma concentrations of paroxetine were increased by approximately 50% during coadministration with oral cimetidine (300 mg three times daily) for the final week. Therefore, when these drugs are administered concurrently, dosage adjustment of PAXIL CR after the starting dose should be guided by clinical effect. The effect of paroxetine on cimetidine's pharmacokinetics was not studied.

Phenobarbital
Phenobarbital induces many cytochrome P_{450} (oxidative) enzymes. When a single oral 30-mg dose of immediate-release paroxetine was administered at phenobarbital steady state (100 mg once daily for 14 days), paroxetine AUC and $T_{1/2}$ were reduced (by an average of 25% and 38%, respectively) compared to paroxetine administered alone. The effect of paroxetine on phenobarbital pharmacokinetics was not studied. Since paroxetine exhibits nonlinear pharmacokinetics, the results of this study may not address the case where the 2 drugs are both being chronically dosed. No initial dosage adjustment with PAXIL CR is considered necessary when coadministered with phenobarbital; any subsequent adjustment should be guided by clinical effect.

Phenytoin
When a single oral 30-mg dose of immediate-release paroxetine was administered at phenytoin steady state (300 mg once daily for 14 days), paroxetine AUC and $T_{1/2}$ were reduced (by an average of 50% and 35%, respectively) compared to immediate-release paroxetine administered alone. In a separate study, when a single oral 300-mg dose of phenytoin was administered at paroxetine steady state (30 mg once daily for 14 days), phenytoin AUC was slightly reduced (12% on average) compared to phenytoin administered alone. Since both drugs exhibit nonlinear pharmacokinetics, the above studies may not address the case where the 2 drugs are both being chronically dosed. No initial dosage adjustments are considered necessary when PAXIL CR is coadministered with phenytoin; any subsequent adjustments should be guided by clinical effect (see ADVERSE REACTIONS—Postmarketing Reports).

Drugs Metabolized by CYP2D6
Many drugs, including most drugs effective in the treatment of major depressive disorder (paroxetine, other SSRIs, and many tricyclics), are metabolized by the cytochrome P_{450} isozyme CYP2D6. Like other agents that are metabolized by CYP2D6, paroxetine may significantly inhibit the activity of this isozyme. In most patients (>90%), this CYP2D6 isozyme is saturated early during paroxetine dosing. In 1 study, daily dosing of immediate-release paroxetine (20 mg once daily) under steady-state conditions increased single-dose desipramine (100 mg) C_{max}, AUC, and $T_{1/2}$ by an average of approximately 2-, 5-, and 3-fold, respectively. Concomitant use of paroxetine with risperidone, a CYP2D6 substrate has also been evaluated. In 1 study, daily dosing of paroxetine 20 mg in patients stabilized on risperidone (4 to 8 mg/day) increased mean plasma concentrations of risperidone approximately 4-fold, decreased 9-hydroxyrisperidone concentrations approximately 10%, and increased concentrations of the active moiety (the sum of risperidone plus 9-hydroxyrisperidone) approximately 1.4-fold. The effect of paroxetine on the pharmacokinetics of atomoxetine has been evaluated when both drugs were at steady state. In healthy volunteers who were extensive metabolizers of CYP2D6, paroxetine 20 mg daily was given in combination with 20 mg atomoxetine every 12 hours. This resulted in increases in steady state atomoxetine AUC values that were 6- to 8-fold greater and in atomoxetine C_{max} values that were 3- to 4-fold greater than when atomoxetine was given alone. Dosage adjustment of atomoxetine may be necessary and it is recommended that atomoxetine be initiated at a reduced dose when given with paroxetine.

Concomitant use of PAXIL CR with other drugs metabolized by cytochrome CYP2D6 has not been formally studied but may require lower doses than usually prescribed for either PAXIL CR or the other drug.

Therefore, coadministration of PAXIL CR with other drugs that are metabolized by this isozyme, including certain drugs effective in the treatment of major depressive disorder (e.g., nortriptyline, amitriptyline, imipramine, desipramine, and fluoxetine), phenothiazines, risperidone, and Type 1C antiarrhythmics (e.g., propafenone, flecainide, and encainide), or that inhibit this enzyme (e.g., quinidine), should be approached with caution.

However, due to the risk of serious ventricular arrhythmias and sudden death potentially associated with elevated plasma levels of thioridazine, paroxetine and thioridazine should not be coadministered (see CONTRAINDICATIONS and WARNINGS).

Tamoxifen is a pro-drug requiring metabolic activation by CYP2D6. Inhibition of CYP2D6 by paroxetine may lead to reduced plasma concentrations of an active metabolite (endoxifen) and hence reduced efficacy of tamoxifen (see PRECAUTIONS).

At steady state, when the CYP2D6 pathway is essentially saturated, paroxetine clearance is governed by alternative P_{450} isozymes that, unlike CYP2D6, show no evidence of saturation (see PRECAUTIONS—Tricyclic Antidepressants).

Drugs Metabolized by Cytochrome CYP3A4
An in vivo interaction study involving the coadministration under steady-state conditions of paroxetine and terfenadine, a substrate for CYP3A4, revealed no effect of paroxetine on terfenadine pharmacokinetics. In addition, in vitro studies have shown ketoconazole, a potent inhibitor of CYP3A4 activity, to be at least 100 times more potent than paroxetine as an inhibitor of the metabolism of several

substrates for this enzyme, including terfenadine, astemizole, cisapride, triazolam, and cyclosporine. Based on the assumption that the relationship between paroxetine's in vitro K_i and its lack of effect on terfenadine's in vivo clearance predicts its effect on other CYP3A4 substrates, paroxetine's extent of inhibition of CYP3A4 activity is not likely to be of clinical significance.

Tricyclic Antidepressants (TCAs)
Caution is indicated in the coadministration of TCAs with PAXIL CR, because paroxetine may inhibit TCA metabolism. Plasma TCA concentrations may need to be monitored, and the dose of TCA may need to be reduced, if a TCA is coadministered with PAXIL CR (see PRECAUTIONS—Drugs Metabolized by Cytochrome CYP2D6).

Drugs Highly Bound to Plasma Protein
Because paroxetine is highly bound to plasma protein, administration of PAXIL CR to a patient taking another drug that is highly protein bound may cause increased free concentrations of the other drug, potentially resulting in adverse events. Conversely, adverse effects could result from displacement of paroxetine by other highly bound drugs.

Drugs That Interfere With Hemostasis (e.g., NSAIDs, Aspirin, and Warfarin)
Serotonin release by platelets plays an important role in hemostasis. Epidemiological studies of the case-control and cohort design that have demonstrated an association between use of psychotropic drugs that interfere with serotonin reuptake and the occurrence of upper gastrointestinal bleeding have also shown that concurrent use of an NSAID or aspirin may potentiate this risk of bleeding. Altered anticoagulant effects, including increased bleeding, have been reported when SSRIs or SNRIs are coadministered with warfarin. Patients receiving warfarin therapy should be carefully monitored when paroxetine is initiated or discontinued.

Alcohol
Although paroxetine does not increase the impairment of mental and motor skills caused by alcohol, patients should be advised to avoid alcohol while taking PAXIL CR.

Lithium
A multiple-dose study with immediate-release paroxetine hydrochloride has shown that there is no pharmacokinetic interaction between paroxetine and lithium carbonate. However, due to the potential for serotonin syndrome, caution is advised when immediate-release paroxetine hydrochloride is coadministered with lithium.

Digoxin
The steady-state pharmacokinetics of paroxetine was not altered when administered with digoxin at steady state. Mean digoxin AUC at steady state decreased by 15% in the presence of paroxetine. Since there is little clinical experience, the concurrent administration of PAXIL CR and digoxin should be undertaken with caution.

Diazepam
Under steady-state conditions, diazepam does not appear to affect paroxetine kinetics. The effects of paroxetine on diazepam were not evaluated.

Procyclidine
Daily oral dosing of immediate-release paroxetine (30 mg once daily) increased steady-state AUC_{0-24}, C_{max}, and C_{min} values of procyclidine (5 mg oral once daily) by 35%, 37%, and 67%, respectively, compared to procyclidine alone at steady state. If anticholinergic effects are seen, the dose of procyclidine should be reduced.

Beta-Blockers
In a study where propranolol (80 mg twice daily) was dosed orally for 18 days, the established steady-state plasma concentrations of propranolol were unaltered during coadministration with immediate-release paroxetine (30 mg once daily) for the final 10 days. The effects of propranolol on paroxetine have not been evaluated (see ADVERSE REACTIONS—Postmarketing Reports).

Theophylline
Reports of elevated theophylline levels associated with immediate-release paroxetine treatment have been reported. While this interaction has not been formally studied, it is recommended that theophylline levels be monitored when these drugs are concurrently administered.

Fosamprenavir/Ritonavir
Co-administration of fosamprenavir/ritonavir with paroxetine significantly decreased plasma levels of paroxetine. Any dose adjustment should be guided by clinical effect (tolerability and efficacy).

Electroconvulsive Therapy (ECT)
There are no clinical studies of the combined use of ECT and PAXIL CR.

Carcinogenesis, Mutagenesis, Impairment of Fertility
Carcinogenesis
Two-year carcinogenicity studies were conducted in rodents given paroxetine in the diet at 1, 5, and 25 mg/kg/day (mice) and 1, 5, and 20 mg/kg/day (rats). These doses are up to approximately 2 (mouse) and 3 (rat) times the MRHD on a mg/m² basis. There was a significantly greater number of male rats in the high-dose group with reticulum cell sarcomas (1/100, 0/50, 0/50, and 4/50 for control, low-, middle-, and high-dose groups, respectively) and a significantly increased linear trend across dose groups for the occurrence of lymphoreticular tumors in male rats. Female rats were not affected. Although there was a dose-related increase in the number of tumors in mice, there was no drug-related increase in the number of mice with tumors. The relevance of these findings to humans is unknown.

Mutagenesis
Paroxetine produced no genotoxic effects in a battery of 5 in vitro and 2 in vivo assays that included the following: Bacterial mutation assay, mouse lymphoma mutation assay, unscheduled DNA synthesis assay, and tests for cytogenetic aberrations in vivo in mouse bone marrow and in vitro in human lymphocytes and in a dominant lethal test in rats.

Impairment of Fertility
A reduced pregnancy rate was found in reproduction studies in rats at a dose of paroxetine of 15 mg/kg/day, which is approximately twice the MRHD on a mg/m² basis. Irreversible lesions occurred in the reproductive tract of male rats after dosing in toxicity studies for 2 to 52 weeks. These lesions consisted of vacuolation of epididymal tubular epithelium at 50 mg/kg/day and atrophic changes in the seminiferous tubules of the testes with arrested spermatogenesis at 25 mg/kg/day (approximately 8 and 4 times the MRHD on a mg/m² basis)

Pregnancy
Pregnancy Category D. See WARNINGS—Usage in Pregnancy: Teratogenic and Nonteratogenic Effects.

Labor and Delivery
The effect of paroxetine on labor and delivery in humans is unknown.

Nursing Mothers
Like many other drugs, paroxetine is secreted in human milk, and caution should be exercised when PAXIL CR is administered to a nursing woman.

Pediatric Use
Safety and effectiveness in the pediatric population have not been established (see BOX WARNING and WARNINGS—Clinical Worsening and Suicide Risk). Three placebo-controlled trials in 752 pediatric patients with MDD have been conducted with PAXIL, and the data were not sufficient to support a claim for use in pediatric patients. Anyone considering the use of PAXIL CR in a child or adolescent must balance the potential risks with the clinical need.

In placebo-controlled clinical trials conducted with pediatric patients, the following adverse events were reported in at least 2% of pediatric patients treated with immediate-release paroxetine hydrochloride and occurred at a rate at least twice that for pediatric patients receiving placebo: emotional lability (including self-harm, suicidal thoughts, attempted suicide, crying, and mood fluctuations), hostility, decreased appetite, tremor, sweating, hyperkinesia, and agitation.

Events reported upon discontinuation of treatment with immediate-release paroxetine hydrochloride in the pediatric clinical trials that included a taper phase regimen, which occurred in at least 2% of patients who received immediate-release paroxetine hydrochloride and which occurred at a rate at least twice that of placebo, were: emotional lability (including suicidal ideation, suicide attempt, mood changes, and tearfulness), nervousness, dizziness, nausea, and abdominal pain (see Discontinuation of Treatment With PAXIL CR).

Geriatric Use
SSRIs and SNRIs, including PAXIL CR, have been associated with cases of clinically significant hyponatremia in elderly patients, who may be at greater risk for this adverse event (see PRECAUTIONS, Hyponatremia).

In worldwide premarketing clinical trials with immediate-release paroxetine hydrochloride, 17% of paroxetine-treated patients (approximately 700) were 65 years or older. Pharmacokinetic studies revealed a decreased clearance in the elderly, and a lower starting dose is recommended; there were, however, no overall differences in the adverse event profile between elderly and younger patients, and effectiveness was similar in younger and older patients (see CLINICAL PHARMACOLOGY and DOSAGE AND ADMINISTRATION).

In a controlled study focusing specifically on elderly patients with major depressive disorder, PAXIL CR was demonstrated to be safe and effective in the treatment of elderly patients (>60 years) with major depressive disorder. (See CLINICAL PHARMACOLOGY—Clinical Trials and ADVERSE REACTIONS—Table 2.)

ADVERSE REACTIONS
The information included under the "Adverse Findings Observed in Short-Term, Placebo-Controlled Trials With PAXIL CR" subsection of ADVERSE REACTIONS is based on data from 11 placebo-controlled clinical trials. Three of these studies were conducted in patients with major depressive disorder, 3 studies were done in patients with panic disorder, 1 study was conducted in patients with social anxiety disorder, and 4 studies were done in female patients with PMDD. Two of the studies in major depressive disorder, which enrolled patients in the age range 18 to 65 years, are pooled. Information from a third study of major depressive disorder, which focused on elderly patients (60 to 88 years), is presented separately as is the information from the panic disorder studies and the information from the PMDD studies. Information on additional adverse events associated with PAXIL CR and the immediate-release formulation of paroxetine hydrochloride is included in a separate subsection (see Other Events).

Adverse Findings Observed in Short-Term, Placebo-Controlled Trials With PAXIL CR:
Adverse Events Associated With Discontinuation of Treatment
Major Depressive Disorder
Ten percent (21/212) of patients treated with PAXIL CR discontinued treatment due to an adverse event in a pool of 2 studies of patients with major depressive disorder. The most common events (≥1%) associated with discontinuation and considered to be drug related (i.e., those events associated with dropout at a rate approximately twice or greater for PAXIL CR compared to placebo) included the following:

	PAXIL CR 25 mg (n = 348)	PAXIL CR 12.5 mg (n = 333)	Placebo (n = 349)
TOTAL	15%	9.9%	6.3%
Nausea*	6.0%	2.4%	0.9%
Asthenia	4.9%	3.0%	1.4%
Somnolence*	4.3%	1.8%	0.3%
Insomnia	2.3%	1.5%	0.0%
Concentration Impaired*	2.0%	0.6%	0.3%
Dry mouth*	2.0%	0.6%	0.3%
Dizziness*	1.7%	0.6%	0.6%
Decreased Appetite*	1.4%	0.6%	0.0%
Sweating*	1.4%	0.0%	0.3%
Tremor*	1.4%	0.3%	0.0%
Yawn*	1.1%	0.0%	0.0%
Diarrhea	0.9%	1.2%	0.0%

* Events considered to be dose dependent are defined as events having an incidence rate with 25 mg of PAXIL CR that was at least twice that with 12.5 mg of PAXIL CR (as well as the placebo group).

	PAXIL CR (n = 212)	Placebo (n = 211)
Nausea	3.7%	0.5%
Asthenia	1.9%	0.5%
Dizziness	1.4%	0.0%
Somnolence	1.4%	0.0%

In a placebo-controlled study of elderly patients with major depressive disorder, 13% (13/104) of patients treated with PAXIL CR discontinued due to an adverse event. Events meeting the above criteria included the following:

	PAXIL CR (n = 104)	Placebo (n = 109)
Nausea	2.9%	0.0%
Headache	1.9%	0.9%
Depression	1.9%	0.0%
LFT's abnormal	1.9%	0.0%

Panic Disorder
Eleven percent (50/444) of patients treated with PAXIL CR in panic disorder studies discontinued treatment due to an adverse event. Events meeting the above criteria included the following:

	PAXIL CR (n = 444)	Placebo (n = 445)
Nausea	2.9%	0.4%
Insomnia	1.8%	0.0%
Headache	1.4%	0.2%
Asthenia	1.1%	0.0%

Social Anxiety Disorder
Three percent (5/186) of patients treated with PAXIL CR in the social anxiety disorder study discontinued treatment due to an adverse event. Events meeting the above criteria included the following:

	PAXIL CR (n = 186)	Placebo (n = 184)
Nausea	2.2%	0.5%
Headache	1.6%	0.5%
Diarrhea	1.1%	0.5%

Premenstrual Dysphoric Disorder
Spontaneously reported adverse events were monitored in studies of both continuous and intermittent dosing of PAXIL CR in the treatment of PMDD. Generally, there were few differences in the adverse event profiles of the 2 dosing regimens. Thirteen percent (88/681) of patients treated with PAXIL CR in PMDD studies of continuous dosing discontinued treatment due to an adverse event.

The most common events (≥1%) associated with discontinuation in either group treated with PAXIL CR with an incidence rate that is at least twice that of placebo in PMDD trials that employed a continuous dosing regimen are shown in the following table. This table also shows those events that were dose dependent (indicated with an asterisk) as defined as events having an incidence rate with 25 mg of PAXIL CR that was at least twice that with 12.5 mg of PAXIL CR (as well as the placebo group). [See table at top of previous page]

Commonly Observed Adverse Events
Major Depressive Disorder
The most commonly observed adverse events associated with the use of PAXIL CR in a pool of 2 trials (incidence of 5.0% or greater and incidence for PAXIL CR at least twice that for placebo, derived from Table 2) were: Abnormal ejaculation, abnormal vision, constipation, decreased libido, diarrhea, dizziness, female genital disorders, nausea, somnolence, sweating, trauma, tremor, and yawning.

Using the same criteria, the adverse events associated with the use of PAXIL CR in a study of elderly patients with major depressive disorder were: Abnormal ejaculation, constipation, decreased appetite, dry mouth, impotence, infection, libido decreased, sweating, and tremor.
Panic Disorder
In the pool of panic disorder studies, the adverse events meeting these criteria were: Abnormal ejaculation, somnolence, impotence, libido decreased, tremor, sweating, and female genital disorders (generally anorgasmia or difficulty achieving orgasm).
Social Anxiety Disorder
In the social anxiety disorder study, the adverse events meeting these criteria were: Nausea, asthenia, abnormal ejaculation, sweating, somnolence, impotence, insomnia, and libido decreased.
Premenstrual Dysphoric Disorder
The most commonly observed adverse events associated with the use of PAXIL CR either during continuous dosing or luteal phase dosing (incidence of 5% or greater and incidence for PAXIL CR at least twice that for placebo, derived from Table 6) were: Nausea, asthenia, libido decreased, somnolence, insomnia, female genital disorders, sweating, dizziness, diarrhea, and constipation.
In the luteal phase dosing PMDD trial, which employed dosing of 12.5 mg/day or 25 mg/day of PAXIL CR limited to the 2 weeks prior to the onset of menses over 3 consecutive menstrual cycles, adverse events were evaluated during the first 14 days of each off-drug phase. When the 3 off-drug phases were combined, the following adverse events were reported at an incidence of 2% or greater for PAXIL CR and were at least twice the rate of that reported for placebo: Infection (5.3% versus 2.5%), depression (2.8% versus 0.8%), insomnia (2.4% versus 0.8%), sinusitis (2.4% versus 0%), and asthenia (2.0% versus 0.8%).

Incidence in Controlled Clinical Trials
Table 2 enumerates adverse events that occurred at an incidence of 1% or more among patients treated with PAXIL CR, aged 18 to 65, who participated in 2 short-term (12-week) placebo-controlled trials in major depressive disorder in which patients were dosed in a range of 25 mg to 62.5 mg/day. Table 3 enumerates adverse events reported at an incidence of 5% or greater among elderly patients (ages 60 to 88) treated with PAXIL CR who participated in a short-term (12-week) placebo-controlled trial in major depressive disorder in which patients were dosed in a range of 12.5 mg to 50 mg/day. Table 4 enumerates adverse events reported at an incidence of 1% or greater among patients (19 to 72 years) treated with PAXIL CR who participated in short-term (10-week) placebo-controlled trials in panic disorder in which patients were dosed in a range of 12.5 mg to 75 mg/day. Table 5 enumerates adverse events reported at an incidence of 1% or greater among adult patients treated with PAXIL CR who participated in a short-term (12-week), double-blind, placebo-controlled trial in social anxiety disorder in which patients were dosed in a range of 12.5 to 37.5 mg/day. Table 6 enumerates adverse events that occurred at an incidence of 1% or more among patients treated with PAXIL CR who participated in three, 12-week, placebo-controlled trials in PMDD in which patients were dosed at 12.5 mg/day or 25 mg/day and in one 12-week placebo-controlled trial in which patients were dosed for 2 weeks prior to the onset of menses (luteal phase dosing) at 12.5 mg/day or 25 mg/day. Reported adverse events were classified using a standard COSTART-based Dictionary terminology.

The prescriber should be aware that these figures cannot be used to predict the incidence of side effects in the course of usual medical practice where patient characteristics and other factors differ from those that prevailed in the clinical trials. Similarly, the cited frequencies cannot be compared with figures obtained from other clinical investigations involving different treatments, uses, and investigators. The cited figures, however, do provide the prescribing physician with some basis for estimating the relative contribution of drug and nondrug factors to the side effect incidence rate in the population studied.

Table 2. Treatment-Emergent Adverse Events Occurring in ≥1% of Patients Treated With PAXIL CR in a Pool of 2 Studies in Major Depressive Disorder[1,2]

Body System/Adverse Event	% Reporting Event	
	PAXIL CR (n = 212)	Placebo (n = 211)
Body as a Whole		
Headache	27%	20%
Asthenia	14%	9%
Infection[3]	8%	5%
Abdominal Pain	7%	4%
Back Pain	5%	3%
Trauma[4]	5%	1%
Pain[5]	3%	1%
Allergic Reaction[6]	2%	1%
Cardiovascular System		
Tachycardia	1%	0%
Vasodilatation[7]	2%	0%
Digestive System		
Nausea	22%	10%
Diarrhea	18%	7%
Dry Mouth	15%	8%
Constipation	10%	4%
Flatulence	6%	4%
Decreased Appetite	4%	2%
Vomiting	2%	1%
Nervous System		
Somnolence	22%	8%
Insomnia	17%	9%
Dizziness	14%	4%
Libido Decreased	7%	3%
Tremor	7%	1%
Hypertonia	3%	1%
Paresthesia	3%	1%
Agitation	2%	1%
Confusion	1%	0%
Respiratory System		
Yawn	5%	0%
Rhinitis	4%	1%
Cough Increased	2%	1%
Bronchitis	1%	0%
Skin and Appendages		
Sweating	6%	2%
Photosensitivity	2%	0%
Special Senses		
Abnormal Vision[8]	5%	1%
Taste Perversion	2%	0%
Urogenital System		
Abnormal Ejaculation[9,10]	26%	1%
Female Genital Disorder[9,11]	10%	<1%
Impotence[9]	5%	3%
Urinary Tract Infection	3%	1%
Menstrual Disorder[9]	2%	<1%
Vaginitis[9]	2%	0%

[1] Adverse events for which the PAXIL CR reporting incidence was less than or equal to the placebo incidence are not included. These events are: Abnormal dreams, anxiety, arthralgia, depersonalization, dysmenorrhea, dyspepsia, hyperkinesia, increased appetite, myalgia, nervousness, pharyngitis, purpura, rash, respiratory disorder, sinusitis, urinary frequency, and weight gain.

[2] <1% means greater than zero and less than 1%.
[3] Mostly flu.
[4] A wide variety of injuries with no obvious pattern.
[5] Pain in a variety of locations with no obvious pattern.
[6] Most frequently seasonal allergic symptoms.
[7] Usually flushing.
[8] Mostly blurred vision.
[9] Based on the number of males or females.
[10] Mostly anorgasmia or delayed ejaculation.
[11] Mostly anorgasmia or delayed orgasm.

Table 3. Treatment-Emergent Adverse Events Occurring in ≥5% of Patients Treated With PAXIL CR in a Study of Elderly Patients With Major Depressive Disorder[1,2]

Body System/Adverse Event	% Reporting Event	
	PAXIL CR (n = 104)	Placebo (n = 109)
Body as a Whole		
Headache	17%	13%
Asthenia	15%	14%
Trauma	8%	5%
Infection	6%	2%
Digestive System		
Dry Mouth	18%	7%
Diarrhea	15%	9%
Constipation	13%	5%
Dyspepsia	13%	10%
Decreased Appetite	12%	5%
Flatulence	8%	7%
Nervous System		
Somnolence	21%	12%
Insomnia	10%	8%
Dizziness	9%	5%
Libido Decreased	8%	<1%
Tremor	7%	0%
Skin and Appendages		
Sweating	10%	<1%
Urogenital System		
Abnormal Ejaculation[3,4]	17%	3%
Impotence[3]	9%	3%

[1] Adverse events for which the PAXIL CR reporting incidence was less than or equal to the placebo incidence are not included. These events are nausea and respiratory disorder.
[2] <1% means greater than zero and less than 1%.
[3] Based on the number of males.
[4] Mostly anorgasmia or delayed ejaculation.

Table 4. Treatment-Emergent Adverse Events Occurring in ≥1% of Patients Treated With PAXIL CR in a Pool of 3 Panic Disorder Studies[1,2]

Body System/Adverse Event	% Reporting Event	
	PAXIL CR (n = 444)	Placebo (n = 445)
Body as a Whole		
Asthenia	15%	10%
Abdominal Pain	6%	4%
Trauma[3]	5%	4%

Cardiovascular System

Vasodilation[4]	3%	2%
Digestive System		
Nausea	23%	17%
Dry Mouth	13%	9%
Diarrhea	12%	9%
Constipation	9%	6%
Decreased Appetite	8%	6%
Metabolic/Nutritional Disorders		
Weight Loss	1%	0%
Musculoskeletal System		
Myalgia	5%	3%
Nervous System		
Insomnia	20%	11%
Somnolence	20%	9%
Libido Decreased	9%	4%
Nervousness	8%	7%
Tremor	8%	2%
Anxiety	5%	4%
Agitation	3%	2%
Hypertonia[5]	2%	<1%
Myoclonus	2%	<1%
Respiratory System		
Sinusitis	8%	5%
Yawn	3%	0%
Skin and Appendages		
Sweating	7%	2%
Special Senses		
Abnormal Vision[6]	3%	<1%
Urogenital System		
Abnormal Ejaculation[7,8]	27%	3%
Impotence[7]	10%	1%
Female Genital Disorders[9,10]	7%	1%
Urinary Frequency	2%	<1%
Urination Impaired	2%	<1%
Vaginitis[9]	1%	<1%

[1] Adverse events for which the reporting rate for PAXIL CR was less than or equal to the placebo rate are not included. These events are: Abnormal dreams, allergic reaction, back pain, bronchitis, chest pain, concentration impaired, confusion, cough increased, depression, dizziness, dysmenorrhea, dyspepsia, fever, flatulence, headache, increased appetite, infection, menstrual disorder, migraine, pain, paresthesia, pharyngitis, respiratory disorder, rhinitis, tachycardia, taste perversion, thinking abnormal, urinary tract infection, and vomiting.
[2] <1% means greater than zero and less than 1%.
[3] Various physical injuries.
[4] Mostly flushing.
[5] Mostly muscle tightness or stiffness.
[6] Mostly blurred vision.
[7] Based on the number of male patients.
[8] Mostly anorgasmia or delayed ejaculation.
[9] Based on the number of female patients.
[10] Mostly anorgasmia or difficulty achieving orgasm.

Table 5. Treatment-Emergent Adverse Effects Occurring in ≥1% of Patients Treated With PAXIL CR in a Social Anxiety Disorder Study[1,2]

Body System/Adverse Event	% Reporting Event	
	PAXIL CR (n = 186)	Placebo (n = 184)
Body as a Whole		
Headache	23%	17%
Asthenia	18%	7%
Abdominal Pain	5%	4%
Back Pain	4%	1%
Trauma[3]	3%	<1%
Allergic Reaction[4]	2%	<1%
Chest Pain	1%	<1%
Cardiovascular System		
Hypertension	2%	0%
Migraine	2%	1%
Tachycardia	2%	1%
Digestive System		
Nausea	22%	6%
Diarrhea	9%	8%
Constipation	5%	2%
Dry Mouth	3%	2%
Dyspepsia	2%	<1%
Decreased Appetite	1%	<1%
Tooth Disorder	1%	0%
Metabolic/Nutritional Disorders		
Weight Gain	3%	1%
Weight Loss	1%	0%
Nervous System		
Insomnia	9%	4%
Somnolence	9%	4%
Libido Decreased	8%	1%
Dizziness	7%	4%
Tremor	4%	2%
Anxiety	2%	1%
Concentration Impaired	2%	0%
Depression	2%	1%
Myoclonus	1%	<1%
Paresthesia	1%	<1%
Respiratory System		
Yawn	2%	0%
Skin and Appendages		
Sweating	14%	3%
Eczema	1%	0%
Special Senses		
Abnormal Vision[5]	2%	0%
Abnormality of Accommodation	2%	0%

Urogenital System

Abnormal Ejaculation[6,7]	15%	1%
Impotence[6]	9%	0%
Female Genital Disorders[8,9]	3%	0%

[1] Adverse events for which the reporting rate for PAXIL CR was less than or equal to the placebo rate are not included. These events are: Dysmenorrhea, flatulence, gastroenteritis, hypertonia, infection, pain, pharyngitis, rash, respiratory disorder, rhinitis, and vomiting.
[2] <1% means greater than zero and less than 1%.
[3] Various physical injuries.
[4] Most frequently seasonal allergic symptoms.
[5] Mostly blurred vision.
[6] Based on the number of male patients.
[7] Mostly anorgasmia or delayed ejaculation.
[8] Based on the number of female patients.
[9] Mostly anorgasmia or difficulty achieving orgasm.

[See table 6 at right and on next page]

Dose Dependency of Adverse Events

The following table shows results in PMDD trials of common adverse events, defined as events with an incidence of ≥1% with 25 mg of PAXIL CR that was at least twice that with 12.5 mg of PAXIL CR and with placebo.

Incidence of Common Adverse Events in Placebo, 12.5 mg and 25 mg of PAXIL CR in a Pool of 3 Fixed-Dose PMDD Trials

	PAXIL CR 25 mg (n = 348)	PAXIL CR 12.5 mg (n = 333)	Placebo (n = 349)
Common Adverse Event			
Sweating	8.9%	4.2%	0.9%
Tremor	6.0%	1.5%	0.3%
Concentration Impaired	4.3%	1.5%	0.6%
Yawn	3.2%	0.9%	0.3%
Paresthesia	1.4%	0.3%	0.3%
Hyperkinesia	1.1%	0.3%	0.0%
Vaginitis	1.1%	0.3%	0.3%

A comparison of adverse event rates in a fixed-dose study comparing immediate-release paroxetine with placebo in the treatment of major depressive disorder revealed a clear dose dependency for some of the more common adverse events associated with the use of immediate-release paroxetine.

Male and Female Sexual Dysfunction With SSRIs

Although changes in sexual desire, sexual performance, and sexual satisfaction often occur as manifestations of a psychiatric disorder, they may also be a consequence of pharmacologic treatment. In particular, some evidence suggests that SSRIs can cause such untoward sexual experiences.

Reliable estimates of the incidence and severity of untoward experiences involving sexual desire, performance, and satisfaction are difficult to obtain; however, in part because patients and physicians may be reluctant to discuss them. Accordingly, estimates of the incidence of untoward sexual experience and performance cited in product labeling, are likely to underestimate their actual incidence.

The percentage of patients reporting symptoms of sexual dysfunction in the pool of 2 placebo-controlled trials in nonelderly patients with major depressive disorder, in the pool of 3 placebo-controlled trials in patients with panic disorder, in the placebo-controlled trial in patients with social anxiety disorder, and in the intermittent dosing and the pool of 3 placebo-controlled continuous dosing trials in female patients with PMDD are as follows:

[See table on next page]

There are no adequate, controlled studies examining sexual dysfunction with paroxetine treatment.

Paroxetine treatment has been associated with several cases of priapism. In those cases with a known outcome, patients recovered without sequelae.

While it is difficult to know the precise risk of sexual dysfunction associated with the use of SSRIs, physicians should routinely inquire about such possible side effects.

Table 6. Treatment-Emergent Adverse Events Occurring in ≥1% of Patients Treated With PAXIL CR in a Pool of 3 Premenstrual Dysphoric Disorder Studies With Continuous Dosing or in 1 Premenstrual Dysphoric Disorder Study With Luteal Phase Dosing[1,2,3]

Body System/Adverse Event	% Reporting Event			
	Continuous Dosing		Luteal Phase Dosing	
	PAXIL CR (n = 681)	Placebo (n = 349)	PAXIL CR (n = 246)	Placebo (n = 120)
Body as a Whole				
Asthenia	17%	6%	15%	4%
Headache	15%	12%	-	-
Infection	6%	4%	-	-
Abdominal pain	-	-	3%	0%
Cardiovascular System				
Migraine	1%	<1%	-	-
Digestive System				
Nausea	17%	7%	18%	2%
Diarrhea	6%	2%	6%	0%
Constipation	5%	1%	2%	<1%
Dry Mouth	4%	2%	2%	<1%
Increased Appetite	3%	<1%	-	-
Decreased Appetite	2%	<1%	2%	0%
Dyspepsia	2%	1%	2%	2%
Gingivitis	-	-	1%	0%
Metabolic and Nutritional Disorders				
Generalized Edema	-	-	1%	<1%
Weight Gain	-	-	1%	<1%
Musculoskeletal System				
Arthralgia	2%	1%	-	-
Nervous System				
Libido Decreased	12%	5%	9%	6%
Somnolence	9%	2%	3%	<1%
Insomnia	8%	2%	7%	3%
Dizziness	7%	3%	6%	3%
Tremor	4%	<1%	5%	0%
Concentration Impaired	3%	<1%	1%	0%
Nervousness	2%	<1%	3%	2%
Anxiety	2%	1%	-	-
Lack of Emotion	2%	<1%	-	-
Depression	-	-	2%	<1%
Vertigo	-	-	2%	<1%
Abnormal Dreams	1%	<1%	-	-
Amnesia	-	-	1%	0%

(Table continued on next page)

Weight and Vital Sign Changes

Significant weight loss may be an undesirable result of treatment with paroxetine for some patients but, on average, patients in controlled trials with PAXIL CR or the immediate-release formulation, had minimal weight loss (about 1 pound). No significant changes in vital signs (systolic and diastolic blood pressure, pulse, and temperature) were observed in patients treated with PAXIL CR, or immediate-release paroxetine hydrochloride, in controlled clinical trials.

ECG Changes

In an analysis of ECGs obtained in 682 patients treated with immediate-release paroxetine and 415 patients treated with placebo in controlled clinical trials, no clinically significant changes were seen in the ECGs of either group.

Liver Function Tests

In a pool of 2 placebo-controlled clinical trials, patients treated with PAXIL CR or placebo exhibited abnormal values on liver function tests at comparable rates. In particular, the controlled-release paroxetine-versus-placebo com-

Table 6 (cont.). Treatment-Emergent Adverse Events Occurring in ≥1% of Patients Treated With PAXIL CR in a Pool of 3 Premenstrual Dysphoric Disorder Studies With Continuous Dosing or in 1 Premenstrual Dysphoric Disorder Study With Luteal Phase Dosing[1,2,3]

Body System/Adverse Event	% Reporting Event			
	Continuous Dosing		Luteal Phase Dosing	
	PAXIL CR (n = 681)	Placebo (n = 349)	PAXIL CR (n = 246)	Placebo (n = 120)
Respiratory System				
Sinusitis	-	-	4%	2%
Yawn	2%	<1%	-	-
Bronchitis	-	-	2%	0%
Cough Increased	1%	<1%	-	-
Skin and Appendages				
Sweating	7%	<1%	6%	<1%
Special Senses				
Abnormal Vision	-	-	1%	0%
Urogenital System				
Female Genital Disorders[4]	8%	1%	2%	0%
Menorrhagia	1%	<1%	-	-
Vaginal Moniliasis	1%	<1%	-	-
Menstrual Disorder	-	-	1%	0%

[1] Adverse events for which the reporting rate of PAXIL CR was less than or equal to the placebo rate are not included. These events for continuous dosing are: Abdominal pain, back pain, pain, trauma, weight gain, myalgia, pharyngitis, respiratory disorder, rhinitis, sinusitis, pruritis, dysmenorrhea, menstrual disorder, urinary tract infection, and vomiting. The events for luteal phase dosing are: Allergic reaction, back pain, headache, infection, pain, trauma, myalgia, anxiety, pharyngitis, respiratory disorder, cystitis, and dysmenorrhea.
[2] <1% means greater than zero and less than 1%.
[3] The luteal phase and continuous dosing PMDD trials were not designed for making direct comparisons between the 2 dosing regimens. Therefore, a comparison between the 2 dosing regimens of the PMDD trials of incidence rates shown in Table 5 should be avoided.
[4] Mostly anorgasmia or difficulty achieving orgasm.

	Major Depressive Disorder		Panic Disorder		Social Anxiety Disorder		PMDD Continuous Dosing		PMDD Luteal Phase Dosing	
	PAXIL CR	Placebo	PAXIL CR	Placebo	PAXIL CR	Placebo	PAXIL CR	Placebo	PAXIL CR	Placebo
n (males)	78	78	162	194	88	97	n/a	n/a	n/a	n/a
Decreased Libido	10%	5%	9%	6%	13%	1%	n/a	n/a	n/a	n/a
Ejaculatory Disturbance	26%	1%	27%	3%	15%	1%	n/a	n/a	n/a	n/a
Impotence	5%	3%	10%	1%	9%	0%	n/a	n/a	n/a	n/a
n (females)	134	133	282	251	98	87	681	349	246	120
Decreased Libido	4%	2%	8%	2%	4%	1%	12%	5%	9%	6%
Orgasmic Disturbance	10%	<1%	7%	1%	3%	0%	8%	1%	2%	0%

parisons for alkaline phosphatase, SGOT, SGPT, and bilirubin revealed no differences in the percentage of patients with marked abnormalities.

In a study of elderly patients with major depressive disorder, 3 of 104 patients treated with PAXIL CR and none of 109 placebo patients experienced liver transaminase elevations of potential clinical concern.

Two of the patients treated with PAXIL CR dropped out of the study due to abnormal liver function tests; the third patient experienced normalization of transaminase levels with continued treatment. Also, in the pool of 3 studies of patients with panic disorder, 4 of 444 patients treated with PAXIL CR and none of 445 placebo patients experienced liver transaminase elevations of potential clinical concern. Elevations in all 4 patients decreased substantially after discontinuation of PAXIL CR. The clinical significance of these findings is unknown.

In placebo-controlled clinical trials with the immediate-release formulation of paroxetine, patients exhibited abnormal values on liver function tests at no greater rate than that seen in placebo-treated patients.

Hallucinations
In pooled clinical trials of immediate-release paroxetine hydrochloride, hallucinations were observed in 22 of 9,089 patients receiving drug and in 4 of 3,187 patients receiving placebo.

Other Events Observed During the Clinical Development of Paroxetine
The following adverse events were reported during the clinical development of PAXIL CR and/or the clinical development of the immediate-release formulation of paroxetine.

Adverse events for which frequencies are provided below occurred in clinical trials with the controlled-release formulation of paroxetine. During its premarketing assessment in major depressive disorder, panic disorder, social anxiety disorder, and PMDD, multiple doses of PAXIL CR were administered to 1,627 patients in phase 3 double-blind, controlled, outpatient studies. Untoward events associated with this exposure were recorded by clinical investigators using terminology of their own choosing. Consequently, it is not possible to provide a meaningful estimate of the proportion of individuals experiencing adverse events without first grouping similar types of untoward events into a smaller number of standardized event categories.

In the tabulations that follow, reported adverse events were classified using a COSTART-based dictionary. The frequencies presented, therefore, represent the proportion of the 1,627 patients exposed to PAXIL CR who experienced an event of the type cited on at least 1 occasion while receiving PAXIL CR. All reported events are included except those already listed in Tables 2 through 6 and those events where a drug cause was remote. If the COSTART term for an event was so general as to be uninformative, it was deleted or, when possible, replaced with a more informative term. It is important to emphasize that although the events reported occurred during treatment with paroxetine, they were not necessarily caused by it.

Events are further categorized by body system and listed in order of decreasing frequency according to the following definitions: Frequent adverse events are those occurring on 1 or more occasions in at least 1/100 patients (only those not already listed in the tabulated results from placebo-controlled trials appear in this listing); infrequent adverse events are those occurring in 1/100 to 1/1,000 patients; rare events are those occurring in fewer than 1/1,000 patients.

Adverse events for which frequencies are not provided occurred during the premarketing assessment of immediate-release paroxetine in phase 2 and 3 studies of major depressive disorder, obsessive compulsive disorder, panic disorder, social anxiety disorder, generalized anxiety disorder, and posttraumatic stress disorder. The conditions and duration of exposure to immediate-release paroxetine varied greatly and included (in overlapping categories) open and double-blind studies, uncontrolled and controlled studies, inpatient and outpatient studies, and fixed-dose and titration studies. Only those events not previously listed for controlled-release paroxetine are included. The extent to which these events may be associated with PAXIL CR is unknown.

Events are listed alphabetically within the respective body system. Events of major clinical importance are also described in the PRECAUTIONS section.

Body as a Whole
Infrequent were chills, face edema, fever, flu syndrome, malaise; rare were abscess, anaphylactoid reaction, anticholinergic syndrome, hypothermia; also observed were adrenergic syndrome, neck rigidity, sepsis.

Cardiovascular System
Infrequent were angina pectoris, bradycardia, hematoma, hypertension, hypotension, palpitation, postural hypotension, supraventricular tachycardia, syncope; rare were bundle branch block; also observed were arrhythmia nodal, atrial fibrillation, cerebrovascular accident, congestive heart failure, low cardiac output, myocardial infarct, myocardial ischemia, pallor, phlebitis, pulmonary embolus, supraventricular extrasystoles, thrombophlebitis, thrombosis, vascular headache, ventricular extrasystoles.

Digestive System
Infrequent were bruxism, dysphagia, eructation, gastritis, gastroenteritis, gastroesophageal reflux, gingivitis, hemorrhoids, liver function test abnormal, melena, pancreatitis, rectal hemorrhage, toothache, ulcerative stomatitis; rare were colitis, glossitis, gum hyperplasia, hepatosplenomegaly, increased salivation, intestinal obstruction, peptic ulcer, stomach ulcer, throat tightness; also observed were aphthous stomatitis, bloody diarrhea, bulimia, cardiospasm, cholelithiasis, duodenitis, enteritis, esophagitis, fecal impactions, fecal incontinence, gum hemorrhage, hematemesis, hepatitis, ileitis, ileus, jaundice, mouth ulceration, salivary gland enlargement, sialadenitis, stomatitis, tongue discoloration, tongue edema.

Endocrine System
Infrequent were ovarian cyst, testes pain; rare were diabetes mellitus, hyperthyroidism; also observed were goiter, hypothyroidism, thyroiditis.

Hemic and Lymphatic System
Infrequent were anemia, eosinophilia, hypochromic anemia, leukocytosis, leukopenia, lymphadenopathy, purpura; rare were thrombocytopenia; also observed were anisocytosis, basophilia, bleeding time increased, lymphedema, lymphocytosis, lymphopenia, microcytic anemia, monocytosis, normocytic anemia, thrombocythemia.

Metabolic and Nutritional Disorders
Infrequent were generalized edema, hyperglycemia, hypokalemia, peripheral edema, SGOT increased, SGPT increased, thirst; rare were bilirubinemia, dehydration, hyperkalemia, obesity; also observed were alkaline phosphatase increased, BUN increased, creatinine phosphokinase

increased, gamma globulins increased, gout, hypercalcemia, hypercholesteremia, hyperphosphatemia, hypocalcemia, hypoglycemia, hyponatremia, ketosis, lactic dehydrogenase increased, non-protein nitrogen (NPN) increased.

Musculoskeletal System

Infrequent were arthritis, bursitis, tendonitis; rare were myasthenia, myopathy, myositis; also observed were generalized spasm, osteoporosis, tenosynovitis, tetany.

Nervous System

Frequent were depression; infrequent were amnesia, convulsion, depersonalization, dystonia, emotional lability, hallucinations, hyperkinesia, hypesthesia, hypokinesia, incoordination, libido increased, neuralgia, neuropathy, nystagmus, paralysis, vertigo; rare were ataxia, coma, diplopia, dyskinesia, hostility, paranoid reaction, torticollis, withdrawal syndrome; also observed were abnormal gait, akathisia, akinesia, aphasia, choreoathetosis, circumoral paresthesia, delirium, delusions, dysarthria, euphoria, extrapyramidal syndrome, fasciculations, grand mal convulsion, hyperalgesia, irritability, manic reaction, manic-depressive reaction, meningitis, myelitis, peripheral neuritis, psychosis, psychotic depression, reflexes decreased, reflexes increased, stupor, trismus.

Respiratory System

Frequent were pharyngitis; infrequent were asthma, dyspnea, epistaxis, laryngitis, pneumonia; rare were stridor; also observed were dysphonia, emphysema, hemoptysis, hiccups, hyperventilation, lung fibrosis, pulmonary edema, respiratory flu, sputum increased.

Skin and Appendages

Frequent were rash; infrequent were acne, alopecia, dry skin, eczema, pruritus, urticaria; rare were exfoliative dermatitis, furunculosis, pustular rash, seborrhea; also observed were angioedema, ecchymosis, erythema multiforme, erythema nodosum, hirsutism, maculopapular rash, skin discoloration, skin hypertrophy, skin ulcer, sweating decreased, vesiculobullous rash.

Special Senses

Infrequent were conjunctivitis, earache, keratoconjunctivitis, mydriasis, photophobia, retinal hemorrhage, tinnitus; rare were blepharitis, visual field defect; also observed were amblyopia, anisocoria, blurred vision, cataract, conjunctival edema, corneal ulcer, deafness, exophthalmos, glaucoma, hyperacusis, night blindness, parosmia, ptosis, taste loss.

Urogenital System

Frequent were dysmenorrhea*; infrequent were albuminuria, amenorrhea*, breast pain*, cystitis, dysuria, prostatitis*, urinary retention; rare were breast enlargement*, breast neoplasm*, female lactation, hematuria, kidney calculus, metrorrhagia*, nephritis, nocturia, pregnancy and puerperal disorders*, salpingitis, urinary incontinence, uterine fibroids enlarged*; also observed were breast atrophy, ejaculatory disturbance, endometrial disorder, epididymitis, fibrocystic breast, leukorrhea, mastitis, oliguria, polyuria, pyuria, urethritis, urinary casts, urinary urgency, urolith, uterine spasm, vaginal hemorrhage.

*Based on the number of men and women as appropriate.

Postmarketing Reports

Voluntary reports of adverse events in patients taking immediate-release paroxetine hydrochloride that have been received since market introduction and not listed above that may have no causal relationship with the drug include acute pancreatitis, elevated liver function tests (the most severe cases were deaths due to liver necrosis, and grossly elevated transaminases associated with severe liver dysfunction), Guillain-Barré syndrome, toxic epidermal necrolysis, priapism, syndrome of inappropriate ADH secretion, symptoms suggestive of prolactinemia and galactorrhea; extrapyramidal symptoms which have included akathisia, bradykinesia, cogwheel rigidity, dystonia, hypertonia, oculogyric crisis which has been associated with concomitant use of pimozide; tremor and trismus; status epilepticus, acute renal failure, pulmonary hypertension, allergic alveolitis, anaphylaxis, eclampsia, laryngismus, optic neuritis, porphyria, ventricular fibrillation, ventricular tachycardia (including torsade de pointes), thrombocytopenia, hemolytic anemia, events related to impaired hematopoiesis (including aplastic anemia, pancytopenia, bone marrow aplasia, and agranulocytosis), and vasculitic syndromes (such as Henoch-Schönlein purpura). There has been a case report of an elevated phenytoin level after 4 weeks of immediate-release paroxetine and phenytoin coadministration. There has been a case report of severe hypotension when immediate-release paroxetine was added to chronic metoprolol treatment.

DRUG ABUSE AND DEPENDENCE

Controlled Substance Class

PAXIL CR is not a controlled substance.

Physical and Psychologic Dependence

PAXIL CR has not been systematically studied in animals or humans for its potential for abuse, tolerance or physical dependence. While the clinical trials did not reveal any tendency for any drug-seeking behavior, these observations were not systematic and it is not possible to predict on the basis of this limited experience the extent to which a CNS-active drug will be misused, diverted, and/or abused once marketed. Consequently, patients should be evaluated carefully for history of drug abuse, and such patients should be observed closely for signs of misuse or abuse of PAXIL CR (e.g., development of tolerance, incrementations of dose, drug-seeking behavior).

OVERDOSAGE

Human Experience

Since the introduction of immediate-release paroxetine hydrochloride in the United States, 342 spontaneous cases of deliberate or accidental overdosage during paroxetine treatment have been reported worldwide (circa 1999). These include overdoses with paroxetine alone and in combination with other substances. Of these, 48 cases were fatal and of the fatalities, 17 appeared to involve paroxetine alone. Eight fatal cases that documented the amount of paroxetine ingested were generally confounded by the ingestion of other drugs or alcohol or the presence of significant comorbid conditions. Of 145 non-fatal cases with known outcome, most recovered without sequelae. The largest known ingestion involved 2,000 mg of paroxetine (33 times the maximum recommended daily dose) in a patient who recovered.

Commonly reported adverse events associated with paroxetine overdosage include somnolence, coma, nausea, tremor, tachycardia, confusion, vomiting, and dizziness. Other notable signs and symptoms observed with overdoses involving paroxetine (alone or with other substances) include mydriasis, convulsions (including status epilepticus), ventricular dysrhythmias (including torsade de pointes), hypertension, aggressive reactions, syncope, hypotension, stupor, bradycardia, dystonia, rhabdomyolysis, symptoms of hepatic dysfunction (including hepatic failure, hepatic necrosis, jaundice, hepatitis, and hepatic steatosis), serotonin syndrome, manic reactions, myoclonus, acute renal failure, and urinary retention.

Overdosage Management

Treatment should consist of those general measures employed in the management of overdosage with any drugs effective in the treatment of major depressive disorder.

Ensure an adequate airway, oxygenation, and ventilation. Monitor cardiac rhythm and vital signs. General supportive and symptomatic measures are also recommended. Induction of emesis is not recommended. Gastric lavage with a large-bore orogastric tube with appropriate airway protection, if needed, may be indicated if performed soon after ingestion, or in symptomatic patients.

Activated charcoal should be administered. Due to the large volume of distribution of this drug, forced diuresis, dialysis, hemoperfusion, and exchange transfusion are unlikely to be of benefit. No specific antidotes for paroxetine are known.

A specific caution involves patients taking or recently having taken paroxetine who might ingest excessive quantities of a tricyclic antidepressant. In such a case, accumulation of the parent tricyclic and an active metabolite may increase the possibility of clinically significant sequelae and extend the time needed for close medical observation (see PRECAUTIONS—*Drugs Metabolized by Cytochrome CYP2D6*).

In managing overdosage, consider the possibility of multiple-drug involvement. The physician should consider contacting a poison control center for additional information on the treatment of any overdose. Telephone numbers for certified poison control centers are listed in the *Physicians' Desk Reference* (PDR).

DOSAGE AND ADMINISTRATION

Major Depressive Disorder

Usual Initial Dosage

PAXIL CR should be administered as a single daily dose, usually in the morning, with or without food. The recommended initial dose is 25 mg/day. Patients were dosed in a range of 25 mg to 62.5 mg/day in the clinical trials demonstrating the effectiveness of PAXIL CR in the treatment of major depressive disorder. As with all drugs effective in the treatment of major depressive disorder, the full effect may be delayed. Some patients not responding to a 25-mg dose may benefit from dose increases, in 12.5-mg/day increments, up to a maximum of 62.5 mg/day. Dose changes should occur at intervals of at least 1 week.

Patients should be cautioned that PAXIL CR should not be chewed or crushed, and should be swallowed whole.

Maintenance Therapy

There is no body of evidence available to answer the question of how long the patient treated with PAXIL CR should remain on it. It is generally agreed that acute episodes of major depressive disorder require several months or longer of sustained pharmacologic therapy. Whether the dose of an antidepressant needed to induce remission is identical to the dose needed to maintain and/or sustain euthymia is unknown.

Systematic evaluation of the efficacy of immediate-release paroxetine hydrochloride has shown that efficacy is maintained for periods of up to 1 year with doses that averaged about 30 mg, which corresponds to a 37.5-mg dose of PAXIL CR, based on relative bioavailability considerations (see CLINICAL PHARMACOLOGY—Pharmacokinetics).

Panic Disorder

Usual Initial Dosage

PAXIL CR should be administered as a single daily dose, usually in the morning. Patients should be started on 12.5 mg/day. Dose changes should occur in 12.5-mg/day increments and at intervals of at least 1 week. Patients were dosed in a range of 12.5 to 75 mg/day in the clinical trials demonstrating the effectiveness of PAXIL CR. The maximum dosage should not exceed 75 mg/day.

Patients should be cautioned that PAXIL CR should not be chewed or crushed, and should be swallowed whole.

Maintenance Therapy

Long-term maintenance of efficacy with the immediate-release formulation of paroxetine was demonstrated in a 3-month relapse prevention trial. In this trial, patients with panic disorder assigned to immediate-release paroxetine demonstrated a lower relapse rate compared to patients on placebo. Panic disorder is a chronic condition, and it is reasonable to consider continuation for a responding patient. Dosage adjustments should be made to maintain the patient on the lowest effective dosage, and patients should be periodically reassessed to determine the need for continued treatment.

Social Anxiety Disorder

Usual Initial Dosage

PAXIL CR should be administered as a single daily dose, usually in the morning, with or without food. The recommended initial dose is 12.5 mg/day. Patients were dosed in a range of 12.5 mg to 37.5 mg/day in the clinical trial demonstrating the effectiveness of PAXIL CR in the treatment of social anxiety disorder. If the dose is increased, this should occur at intervals of at least 1 week, in increments of 12.5 mg/day, up to a maximum of 37.5 mg/day.

Patients should be cautioned that PAXIL CR should not be chewed or crushed, and should be swallowed whole.

Maintenance Therapy

There is no body of evidence available to answer the question of how long the patient treated with PAXIL CR should remain on it. Although the efficacy of PAXIL CR beyond 12 weeks of dosing has not been demonstrated in controlled clinical trials, social anxiety disorder is recognized as a chronic condition, and it is reasonable to consider continuation of treatment for a responding patient. Dosage adjustments should be made to maintain the patient on the lowest effective dosage, and patients should be periodically reassessed to determine the need for continued treatment.

Premenstrual Dysphoric Disorder

Usual Initial Dosage

PAXIL CR should be administered as a single daily dose, usually in the morning, with or without food. PAXIL CR may be administered either daily throughout the menstrual cycle or limited to the luteal phase of the menstrual cycle, depending on physician assessment. The recommended initial dose is 12.5 mg/day. In clinical trials, both 12.5 mg/day and 25 mg/day were shown to be effective. Dose changes should occur at intervals of at least 1 week.

Patients should be cautioned that PAXIL CR should not be chewed or crushed, and should be swallowed whole.

Maintenance/Continuation Therapy

The effectiveness of PAXIL CR for a period exceeding 3 menstrual cycles has not been systematically evaluated in controlled trials. However, women commonly report that symptoms worsen with age until relieved by the onset of menopause. Therefore, it is reasonable to consider continuation of a responding patient. Patients should be periodically reassessed to determine the need for continued treatment.

Special Populations

Treatment of Pregnant Women During the Third Trimester

Neonates exposed to PAXIL CR and other SSRIs or SNRIs, late in the third trimester have developed complications requiring prolonged hospitalization, respiratory support, and tube feeding (see WARNINGS). When treating pregnant women with paroxetine during the third trimester, the physician should carefully consider the potential risks and benefits of treatment. The physician may consider tapering paroxetine in the third trimester.

Dosage for Elderly or Debilitated Patients, and Patients With Severe Renal or Hepatic Impairment

The recommended initial dose of PAXIL CR is 12.5 mg/day for elderly patients, debilitated patients, and/or patients with severe renal or hepatic impairment. Increases may be made if indicated. Dosage should not exceed 50 mg/day.

Switching Patients to or From a Monoamine Oxidase Inhibitor

At least 14 days should elapse between discontinuation of an MAOI and initiation of therapy with PAXIL CR. Similarly, at least 14 days should be allowed after stopping PAXIL CR before starting an MAOI.

Discontinuation of Treatment With PAXIL CR

Symptoms associated with discontinuation of immediate-release paroxetine hydrochloride or PAXIL CR have been reported (see PRECAUTIONS). Patients should be monitored for these symptoms when discontinuing treatment, regardless of the indication for which PAXIL CR is being prescribed. A gradual reduction in the dose rather than abrupt cessation is recommended whenever possible. If intolerable symptoms occur following a decrease in the dose or upon discontinuation of treatment, then resuming the previously prescribed dose may be considered. Subsequently, the physician may continue decreasing the dose but at a more gradual rate.

HOW SUPPLIED

PAXIL CR is supplied as an enteric film-coated, controlled-release, round tablet, as follows:

12.5-mg yellow tablets

NDC 0029-3206-13	Bottles of 30 (engraved with PAXIL CR and 12.5)
NDC 0029-4606-13	Bottles of 30 (engraved with GSK and 12.5)

25-mg pink tablets

NDC 0029-3207-13	Bottles of 30 (engraved with PAXIL CR and 25)
NDC 0029-4607-13	Bottles of 30 (engraved with GSK and 25)

37.5 mg blue tablets

NDC 0029-3208-13	Bottles of 30 (engraved with PAXIL CR and 37.5)
NDC 0029-4608-13	Bottles of 30 (engraved with GSK and 37.5)

Store at or below 25°C (77°F) [see USP].

PAXIL CR is a registered trademark of GlaxoSmithKline.
GEOMATRIX is a trademark of Jago Pharma, Muttenz, Switzerland.

MEDICATION GUIDE

Antidepressant Medicines, Depression and Other Serious Mental Illnesses, and Suicidal Thoughts or Actions

PAXIL CR® (PAX-il) (paroxetine hydrochloride) Controlled-Release Tablets

Read the Medication Guide that comes with your or your family member's antidepressant medicine. This Medication Guide is only about the risk of suicidal thoughts and actions with antidepressant medicines. **Talk to your, or your family member's, healthcare provider about:**

- All risks and benefits of treatment with antidepressant medicines
- All treatment choices for depression or other serious mental illness

What is the most important information I should know about antidepressant medicines, depression and other serious mental illnesses, and suicidal thoughts or action?

1. Antidepressant medicines may increase suicidal thoughts or actions in some children, teenagers, and young adults within the first few months of treatment.

2. Depression and other serious mental illnesses are the most important causes of suicidal thoughts and actions. Some people may have a particularly high risk of having suicidal thoughts or actions. These include people who have (or have a family history of) bipolar illness (also called manic-depressive illness) or suicidal thoughts or actions.

3. How can I watch for and try to prevent suicidal thoughts and actions in myself or a family member?

- Pay close attention to any changes, especially sudden changes, in mood, behaviors, thoughts, or feelings. This is very important when an antidepressant medicine is started or when the dose is changed.
- Call the healthcare provider right away to report new or sudden changes in mood, behavior, thoughts, or feelings.
- Keep all follow-up visits with the healthcare provider as scheduled. Call the healthcare provider between visits as needed, especially if you have concerns about symptoms.

Call a healthcare provider right away if you or your family member has any of the following symptoms, especially if they are new, worse, or worry you:

- Thoughts about suicide or dying
- Attempts to commit suicide
- New or worse depression
- New or worse anxiety
- Feeling very agitated or restless
- Panic attacks
- Trouble sleeping (insomnia)
- New or worse irritability
- Acting aggressive, being angry, or violent
- Acting on dangerous impulses
- An extreme increase in activity and talking (mania)
- Other unusual changes in behavior or mood

What else do I need to know about antidepressant medicines?

- **Never stop an antidepressant medicine without first talking to a healthcare provider.** Stopping an antidepressant medicine suddenly can cause other symptoms.
- **Antidepressants are medicines used to treat depression and other illnesses.** It is important to discuss all the risks of treating depression and also the risks of not treating it. Patients and their families or other caregivers should discuss all treatment choices with the healthcare provider, not just the use of antidepressants.

- **Antidepressant medicines have other side effects.** Call your doctor for medical advice about side effects. You may report side effects to FDA at 1–800–FDA–1088.
- **Antidepressant medicines can interact with other medicines.** Know all of the medicines that you or your family member takes. Keep a list of all medicines to show the healthcare provider. Do not start new medicines without first checking with your healthcare provider.
- **Not all antidepressant medicines prescribed for children are FDA approved for use in children.** Talk to your child's healthcare provider for more information.

This Medication Guide has been approved by the U.S. Food and Drug Administration for all antidepressants.

January 2008   PCR:3MG

GlaxoSmithKline
Research Triangle Park, NC 27709
©2010, GlaxoSmithKline. All rights reserved.

June 2010   PCR:34PI

PEDIARIX®   ℞

[pĕd'ē-ə-rix]

[Diphtheria and Tetanus Toxoids and Acellular Pertussis Adsorbed, Hepatitis B (Recombinant) and Inactivated Poliovirus Vaccine]

Suspension for Intramuscular Injection

HIGHLIGHTS OF PRESCRIBING INFORMATION

These highlights do not include all the information needed to use PEDIARIX safely and effectively. See full prescribing information for PEDIARIX.

PEDIARIX [Diphtheria and Tetanus Toxoids and Acellular Pertussis Adsorbed, Hepatitis B (Recombinant) and Inactivated Poliovirus Vaccine]
Suspension for Intramuscular Injection
Initial U.S. Approval: 2002

RECENT MAJOR CHANGES

Warnings and Precautions, Apnea in Premature Infants (5.6) 02/2010

INDICATIONS AND USAGE

PEDIARIX is a vaccine indicated for active immunization against diphtheria, tetanus, pertussis, infection caused by all known subtypes of hepatitis B virus, and poliomyelitis. PEDIARIX is approved for use as a three-dose series in infants born of hepatitis B surface antigen (HBsAg)-negative mothers. PEDIARIX may be given as early as 6 weeks of age through 6 years of age (prior to the 7th birthday). (1)

DOSAGE AND ADMINISTRATION

Three doses (0.5 mL each) by intramuscular injection at 2, 4, and 6 months of age. (2.2)

DOSAGE FORMS AND STRENGTHS

Suspension for injection in 0.5 mL single-dose vials or syringes. (3)

CONTRAINDICATIONS

- Severe allergic reaction (e.g., anaphylaxis) after a previous dose of any diphtheria toxoid, tetanus toxoid, pertussis, hepatitis B, or poliovirus-containing vaccine, or to any component of PEDIARIX. (4.1)
- Encephalopathy within 7 days of administration of a previous pertussis-containing vaccine. (4.2)
- Progressive neurologic disorders. (4.3)

WARNINGS AND PRECAUTIONS

- In clinical trials, PEDIARIX was associated with higher rates of fever, relative to separately administered vaccines. (5.1)
- If Guillain-Barré syndrome occurs within 6 weeks of receipt of a prior vaccine containing tetanus toxoid, the decision to give PEDIARIX should be based on potential benefits and risks. (5.2)
- The needleless prefilled syringes contain dry natural latex rubber and may cause allergic reactions. (5.3)
- If specified adverse events (i.e., temperature ≥105°F, collapse or shock-like state, or inconsolable crying lasting ≥3 hours, within 48 hours after vaccination; seizures within 3 days after vaccination) have occurred following a pertussis-containing vaccine, the decision to give PEDIARIX should be based on potential benefits and risks. (5.4)
- For children at higher risk for seizures, an antipyretic may be administered at the time of vaccination with PEDIARIX. (5.5)
- Apnea following intramuscular vaccination has been observed in some infants born prematurely. Decisions about when to administer an intramuscular vaccine, including PEDIARIX, to infants born prematurely should be based on consideration of the individual infant's medical status, and the potential benefits and possible risks of vaccination. (5.6)

ADVERSE REACTIONS

Common solicited adverse events following any dose (≥25%) included local injection site reactions (pain, redness, and swelling), fever (≥100.4°F), drowsiness, irritability/fussiness and loss of appetite. (6.1)

To report SUSPECTED ADVERSE REACTIONS, contact GlaxoSmithKline at 1-888-825-5249 or VAERS at 1-800-822-7967 or www.vaers.hhs.gov

DRUG INTERACTIONS

Do not mix PEDIARIX with any other vaccine in the same syringe or vial. (7.1)

See 17 for PATIENT COUNSELING INFORMATION

Revised: 04/2010

FULL PRESCRIBING INFORMATION

1   INDICATIONS AND USAGE

PEDIARIX® is indicated for active immunization against diphtheria, tetanus, pertussis, infection caused by all known subtypes of hepatitis B virus, and poliomyelitis. PEDIARIX is approved for use as a three-dose series in infants born of hepatitis B surface antigen (HBsAg)-negative mothers. PEDIARIX may be given as early as 6 weeks of age through 6 years of age (prior to the 7th birthday).

2   DOSAGE AND ADMINISTRATION

2.1   Preparation for Administration

Shake vigorously to obtain a homogeneous, turbid, white suspension. Do not use if resuspension does not occur with vigorous shaking. Parenteral drug products should be inspected visually for particulate matter and discoloration prior to administration, whenever solution and container permit. PEDIARIX also should be inspected visually for cracks in the vial or syringe prior to administration. If any of these conditions exist, the vaccine should not be administered.

The preferred administration site is the anterolateral aspect of the thigh for children younger than 1 year. In older children, the deltoid muscle is usually large enough for an intramuscular injection. The vaccine should not be injected in the gluteal area or areas where there may be a major nerve trunk. Gluteal injections may result in suboptimal hepatitis B immune response.

Do not administer PEDIARIX intravenously, intradermally, or subcutaneously.

2.2 Recommended Dose and Schedule

Immunization with PEDIARIX consists of 3 doses of 0.5 mL each, by intramuscular injection, at 2, 4, and 6 months of age (at intervals of 6 to 8 weeks, preferably 8 weeks). The first dose may be given as early as 6 weeks of age. Three doses of PEDIARIX constitute a primary immunization course for diphtheria, tetanus, pertussis, and poliomyelitis and the complete vaccination course for hepatitis B.

2.3 Modified Schedules in Previously Vaccinated Children

Children Previously Vaccinated With Diphtheria and Tetanus Toxoids and Acellular Pertussis Vaccine Adsorbed (DTaP): PEDIARIX may be used to complete the first 3 doses of the DTaP series in children who have received 1 or 2 doses of INFANRIX® (Diphtheria and Tetanus Toxoids and Acellular Pertussis Vaccine Adsorbed), manufactured by GlaxoSmithKline, identical to the DTaP component of PEDIARIX *[see Description (11)]* and are also scheduled to receive the other vaccine components of PEDIARIX. Data are not available on the safety and effectiveness of using PEDIARIX following one or more doses of a DTaP vaccine from a different manufacturer.

Children Previously Vaccinated With Hepatitis B Vaccine: PEDIARIX may be used to complete the hepatitis B vaccination series following 1 or 2 doses of another hepatitis B vaccine (monovalent or as part of a combination vaccine), including vaccines from other manufacturers, in children born of HBsAg-negative mothers who are also scheduled to receive the other vaccine components of PEDIARIX.

A 3-dose series of PEDIARIX may be administered to infants born of HBsAg-negative mothers and who received a dose of hepatitis B vaccine at or shortly after birth. However, data are limited regarding the safety of PEDIARIX in such infants *[see Adverse Reactions (6.1)]*. There are no data to support the use of a 3-dose series of PEDIARIX in infants who have previously received more than one dose of hepatitis B vaccine.

Children Previously Vaccinated With Inactivated Poliovirus Vaccine (IPV): PEDIARIX may be used to complete the first 3 doses of the IPV series in children who have received 1 or 2 doses of IPV from a different manufacturer and are also scheduled to receive the other vaccine components of PEDIARIX.

2.4 Booster Immunization Following PEDIARIX

Children who have received a 3-dose series with PEDIARIX should complete the DTaP and IPV series according to the recommended schedule.[1] Because the pertussis antigens contained in INFANRIX and KINRIX® (Diphtheria and Tetanus Toxoids and Acellular Pertussis Adsorbed and Inactivated Poliovirus Vaccine), manufactured by GlaxoSmithKline, are the same as those in PEDIARIX, these children should receive INFANRIX as their fourth dose of DTaP and either INFANRIX or KINRIX as their fifth dose of DTaP, according to the respective prescribing information for these vaccines. KINRIX or another manufacturer's IPV may be used to complete the 4-dose IPV series according to the respective prescribing information.

3 DOSAGE FORMS AND STRENGTHS

PEDIARIX is a suspension for injection available in 0.5-mL single-dose vials and prefilled TIP-LOK® syringes.

4 CONTRAINDICATIONS

4.1 Hypersensitivity

A severe allergic reaction (e.g., anaphylaxis) after a previous dose of any diphtheria toxoid-, tetanus toxoid-, pertussis antigen-, hepatitis B-, or poliovirus-containing vaccine or any component of this vaccine, including yeast, neomycin, and polymyxin B, is a contraindication to administration of PEDIARIX *[see Description (11)]*.

4.2 Encephalopathy

Encephalopathy (e.g., coma, decreased level of consciousness, prolonged seizures) within 7 days of administration of a previous dose of a pertussis-containing vaccine that is not attributable to another identifiable cause is a contraindication to administration of any pertussis-containing vaccine, including PEDIARIX.

4.3 Progressive Neurologic Disorder

Progressive neurologic disorder, including infantile spasms, uncontrolled epilepsy, or progressive encephalopathy is a contraindication to administration of any pertussis-containing vaccine, including PEDIARIX. PEDIARIX should not be administered to individuals with such conditions until the neurologic status is clarified and stabilized.

5 WARNINGS AND PRECAUTIONS

5.1 Fever

In clinical trials, administration of PEDIARIX in infants was associated with higher rates of fever, relative to separately administered vaccines *[see Adverse Reactions (6.1)]*.

5.2 Guillain-Barré Syndrome

If Guillain-Barré syndrome occurs within 6 weeks of receipt of a prior vaccine containing tetanus toxoid, the decision to give PEDIARIX or any vaccine containing tetanus toxoid should be based on careful consideration of the potential benefits and possible risks.

5.3 Latex

The tip cap and the rubber plunger of the needleless prefilled syringes contain dry natural latex rubber that may cause allergic reactions in latex sensitive individuals. The vial stopper does not contain latex.

5.4 Adverse Events Following Prior Pertussis Vaccination

If any of the following events occur in temporal relation to receipt of a vaccine containing a pertussis component, the decision to give any pertussis-containing vaccine, including PEDIARIX, should be based on careful consideration of the potential benefits and possible risks:

- Temperature of ≥40.5°C (105°F) within 48 hours not due to another identifiable cause;
- Collapse or shock-like state (hypotonic-hyporesponsive episode) within 48 hours;
- Persistent, inconsolable crying lasting ≥3 hours, occurring within 48 hours;
- Seizures with or without fever occurring within 3 days.

5.5 Children at Risk for Seizures

For children at higher risk for seizures than the general population, an appropriate antipyretic may be administered at the time of vaccination with a vaccine containing a pertussis component, including PEDIARIX, and for the ensuing 24 hours to reduce the possibility of post-vaccination fever.

5.6 Apnea in Premature Infants

Apnea following intramuscular vaccination has been observed in some infants born prematurely. Decisions about when to administer an intramuscular vaccine, including PEDIARIX, to infants born prematurely should be based on consideration of the individual infant's medical status, and the potential benefits and possible risks of vaccination.

5.7 Preventing and Managing Allergic Vaccine Reactions

Prior to administration, the healthcare provider should review the immunization history for possible vaccine sensitivity and previous vaccination-related adverse reactions to allow an assessment of benefits and risks. Epinephrine and other appropriate agents used for the control of immediate allergic reactions must be immediately available should an acute anaphylactic reaction occur.

6 ADVERSE REACTIONS

6.1 Clinical Trials Experience

Because clinical trials are conducted under widely varying conditions, adverse event rates observed in the clinical trials of a vaccine cannot be directly compared to rates in the clinical trials of another vaccine, and may not reflect the rates observed in practice.

A total of 23,849 doses of PEDIARIX have been administered to 8,088 infants who received one or more doses as part of the 3-dose series during 14 clinical studies. Common adverse events that occurred in ≥25% of subjects following any dose of PEDIARIX included local injection site reactions (pain, redness, and swelling), fever, drowsiness, irritability/fussiness, and loss of appetite. In comparative studies (including the German and US studies described below), administration of PEDIARIX was associated with higher rates of fever relative to separately administered vaccines *[see Warnings and Precautions (5.1)]*. The prevalence of fever was highest on the day of vaccination and the day following vaccination. More than 96% of episodes of fever resolved within the 4-day period following vaccination (i.e., the period including the day of vaccination and the next 3 days).

In the largest of the 14 studies, conducted in Germany, safety data were available for 4,666 infants who received PEDIARIX administered concomitantly at separate sites with 1 of 4 *Haemophilus influenzae* type b (Hib) conjugate vaccines (GlaxoSmithKline [licensed in the US only for booster immunization], Wyeth Pharmaceuticals Inc. [no longer licensed in the US], Sanofi Pasteur SA [US-licensed], or Merck & Co, Inc. [US-licensed]) at 3, 4, and 5 months of age and for 768 infants in the control group that received separate US-licensed vaccines (INFANRIX, Hib conjugate vaccine [Sanofi Pasteur SA], and oral poliovirus vaccine [OPV] [Wyeth Pharmaceuticals, Inc.; no longer licensed in the US]). In this study, information on adverse events that occurred within 30 days following vaccination was collected. More than 95% of study participants were white.

In a US study, the safety of PEDIARIX administered to 673 infants was compared to the safety of separately administered INFANRIX, ENGERIX-B® [Hepatitis B Vaccine (Recombinant)], and IPV (Sanofi Pasteur SA) in 335 infants. In both groups, infants received Hib conjugate vaccine (Wyeth Pharmaceuticals Inc.; no longer licensed in the US) and 7-valent pneumococcal conjugate vaccine (Wyeth Pharmaceuticals Inc.) concomitantly at separate sites. All vaccines were administered at 2, 4, and 6 months of age. Data on solicited local reactions and general adverse events were collected by parents using standardized diary cards for 4 consecutive days following each vaccine dose (i.e., day of vaccination and the next 3 days). Telephone follow-up was conducted 1 month and 6 months after the third vaccination to inquire about serious adverse events. At the 6-month follow-up, information also was collected on new onset of chronic illnesses. A total of 638 subjects who received PEDIARIX and 313 subjects who received INFANRIX, ENGERIX-B, and IPV completed the 6-month follow-up. Among subjects in both study groups combined, 69% were white, 18% were Hispanic, 7% were black, 3% were Oriental, and 3% were of other racial/ethnic groups.

Solicited Adverse Events: Data on solicited local reactions and general adverse events from the US safety study are presented in Table 1. This study was powered to evaluate fever >101.3°F following dose 1. The rate of fever ≥100.4°F following each dose was significantly higher in the group that received PEDIARIX compared to separately administered vaccines. Other statistically significant differences between groups in rates of fever, as well as other solicited adverse events, are noted in Table 1. Medical attention (a visit to or from medical personnel) for fever within 4 days following vaccination was sought in the group who received PEDIARIX for 8 infants after the first dose (1.2%), 1 infant following the second dose (0.2%), and 5 infants following the third dose (0.8%) (Table 1). Following dose 2, medical attention for fever was sought for 2 infants (0.6%) who received separately administered vaccines (Table 1). Among infants who had a medical visit for fever within 4 days following vaccination, 9 of 14 who received PEDIARIX and 1 of 2 who received separately administered vaccines, had one or more diagnostic studies performed to evaluate the cause of fever.

[See table 1 at top of next page]

Serious Adverse Events: Within 30 days following any dose of vaccine in the US study in which all subjects received concomitant Hib and pneumococcal conjugate vaccines, 7 serious adverse events were reported in 7 subjects (1% [7/673]) who received PEDIARIX (1 case each of pyrexia, gastroenteritis, and culture negative clinical sepsis and 4 cases of bronchiolitis) and 5 serious adverse events were reported in 4 subjects (1% [4/335]) who received INFANRIX, ENGERIX-B, and IPV (uteropelvic junction obstruction and testicular atrophy in one subject and 3 cases of bronchiolitis).

Deaths: In 14 clinical trials, 5 deaths were reported among 8,088 (0.06%) recipients of PEDIARIX and 1 death was reported among 2,287 (0.04%) recipients of comparator vaccines. Causes of death in the group that received PEDIARIX included 2 cases of Sudden Infant Death Syndrome (SIDS) and one case of each of the following: convulsive disorder, congenital immunodeficiency with sepsis, and neuroblastoma. One case of SIDS was reported in the comparator group. The rate of SIDS among all recipients of PEDIARIX across the 14 trials was 0.25/1,000. The rate of SIDS observed for recipients of PEDIARIX in the German safety study was 0.2/1,000 infants (reported rate of SIDS in Germany in the latter part of the 1990s was 0.7/1,000 newborns). The reported rate of SIDS in the United States from 1990 to 1994 was 1.2/1,000 live births. By chance alone, some cases of SIDS can be expected to follow receipt of pertussis-containing vaccines.

Onset of Chronic Illnesses: In the US safety study in which all subjects received concomitant Hib and pneumococcal conjugate vaccines, 21 subjects (3%) who received PEDIARIX and 14 subjects (4%) who received INFANRIX, ENGERIX-B, and IPV reported new onset of a chronic illness during the period from 1 to 6 months following the last dose of study vaccines. Among the chronic illnesses reported in the subjects who received PEDIARIX, there were 4 cases of asthma and 1 case each of diabetes mellitus and chronic neutropenia. There were 4 cases of asthma in subjects who received INFANRIX, ENGERIX-B, and IPV.

Seizures: In the German safety study over the entire study period, 6 subjects in the group that received PEDIARIX (N = 4,666) reported seizures. Two of these subjects had a febrile seizure, 1 of whom also developed afebrile seizures. The remaining 4 subjects had afebrile seizures, including 2 with infantile spasms. Two subjects reported seizures within 7 days following vaccination (1 subject had both febrile and afebrile seizures, and 1 subject had afebrile seizures), corresponding to a rate of 0.22 seizures per 1,000 doses (febrile seizures 0.07 per 1,000 doses, afebrile seizures 0.14 per 1,000 doses). No subject who received concomitant INFANRIX, Hib vaccine, and OPV (N = 768) reported seizures. In a separate German study that evaluated the safety of INFANRIX in 22,505 infants who received 66,867 doses of INFANRIX administered as a 3-dose primary series, the rate of seizures within 7 days of vaccination with INFANRIX was 0.13 per 1,000 doses (febrile seizures 0.0 per 1,000 doses, afebrile seizures 0.13 per 1,000 doses).

Over the entire study period in the US safety study in which all subjects received concomitant Hib and pneumococcal conjugate vaccines, 4 subjects in the group that received PEDIARIX (N = 673) reported seizures. Three of these subjects had a febrile seizure and 1 had an afebrile seizure.

Over the entire study period, 2 subjects in the group that received INFANRIX, ENGERIX-B, and IPV (N = 335) reported febrile seizures. There were no afebrile seizures in this group. No subject in either study group had seizures within 7 days following vaccination.

Other Neurological Events of Interest: No cases of hypotonic-hyporesponsiveness or encephalopathy were reported in either the German or US safety studies.

Safety of PEDIARIX After a Previous Dose of Hepatitis B Vaccine: Limited data are available on the safety of administering PEDIARIX after a previous dose of hepatitis B vaccine. In 2 separate studies, 160 Moldovan infants and 96 US infants, respectively, received 3 doses of PEDIARIX following 1 previous dose of hepatitis B vaccine. Neither study was designed to detect significant differences in rates of adverse events associated with PEDIARIX administered after a previous dose of hepatitis B vaccine compared to PEDIARIX administered without a previous dose of hepatitis B vaccine.

6.2 Postmarketing Safety Surveillance Study
In a safety surveillance study conducted at a health maintenance organization in the US, infants who received one or more doses of PEDIARIX from approximately mid-2003 through mid-2005 were compared to age-, gender-, and area-matched historical controls who received one or more doses of separately administered US-licensed DTaP vaccine from 2002 through approximately mid-2003. Only infants who received 7-valent pneumococcal conjugate vaccine (Wyeth Pharmaceuticals Inc.) concomitantly with PEDIARIX or DTaP vaccine were included in the cohorts. Other US-licensed vaccines were administered according to routine practices at the study sites, but concomitant administration with PEDIARIX or DTaP was not a criterion for inclusion in the cohorts. A birth dose of hepatitis B vaccine had been administered routinely to infants in the historical DTaP control cohort, but not to infants who received PEDIARIX. For each of Doses 1-3, a random sample of 40,000 infants who received PEDIARIX was compared to the historical DTaP control cohort for the incidence of seizures (with or without fever) during the 8-day period following vaccination. For each dose, random samples of 7,500 infants in each cohort were also compared for the incidence of medically-attended fever (fever ≥100.4°F that resulted in hospitalization, an emergency department visit, or an outpatient visit) during the 4-day period following vaccination. Possible seizures and medical visits plausibly related to fever were identified by searching automated inpatient and outpatient data files. Medical record reviews of identified events were conducted to verify the occurrence of seizures or medically-attended fever. The incidence of verified seizures and medically-attended fever from this study are presented in Table 2.

[See table 2 at top of next page]

6.3 Postmarketing Spontaneous Reports for PEDIARIX
In addition to reports in clinical trials, worldwide voluntary reports of adverse events received for PEDIARIX since market introduction of this vaccine are listed below. This list includes serious adverse events or events which have a suspected causal connection to components of PEDIARIX. Because these events are reported voluntarily from a population of uncertain size, it is not possible to reliably estimate their frequency or establish a causal relationship to vaccine exposure.

Cardiac Disorders: Cyanosis.
Gastrointestinal Disorders: Diarrhea, vomiting.
General Disorders and Administration Site Conditions: Fatigue, injection site cellulitis, injection site induration, injection site itching, injection site nodule/lump, injection site reaction, injection site vesicles, injection site warmth, limb pain, limb swelling.
Immune System Disorders: Anaphylactic reaction, anaphylactoid reaction, hypersensitivity.
Infections and Infestations: Upper respiratory tract infection.
Investigations: Abnormal liver function tests.
Nervous System Disorders: Bulging fontanelle, depressed level of consciousness, encephalitis, hypotonia, hypotonic-hyporesponsive episode, lethargy, somnolence.
Psychiatric Disorders: Crying, insomnia, nervousness, restlessness, screaming, unusual crying.
Respiratory, Thoracic, and Mediastinal Disorders: Apnea, cough, dyspnea.
Skin and Subcutaneous Tissue Disorders: Angioedema, erythema, rash, urticaria.
Vascular Disorders: Pallor, petechiae.

6.4 Postmarketing Spontaneous Reports for INFANRIX and/or ENGERIX-B
Worldwide voluntary reports of adverse events received for INFANRIX and/or ENGERIX-B in children younger than 7 years of age but not already reported for PEDIARIX are listed below. This list includes serious adverse events or events which have a suspected causal connection to components of INFANRIX and/or ENGERIX-B. Because these events are reported voluntarily from a population of uncertain size, it is not possible to reliably estimate their frequency or establish a causal relationship to vaccine exposure.
Blood and Lymphatic System Disorders: Idiopathic thrombocytopenic purpura[a,b], lymphadenopathy[a], thrombocytopenia[a,b].
Gastrointestinal Disorders: Abdominal pain[b], intussusception[a,b], nausea[b].
General Disorders and Administration Site Conditions: Asthenia[b], malaise[b].
Hepatobiliary Disorders: Jaundice[b].
Immune System Disorders: Anaphylactic shock[a], serum sickness-like disease[b].
Musculoskeletal and Connective Tissue Disorders: Arthralgia[b], arthritis[b], muscular weakness[b], myalgia[b].
Nervous System Disorders: Encephalopathy[a], headache[a], meningitis[b], neuritis[b], neuropathy[b], paralysis[b].
Skin and Subcutaneous Tissue Disorders: Alopecia[b], erythema multiforme[b], lichen planus[b], pruritus[a,b], Stevens Johnson syndrome[a].
Vascular Disorders: Vasculitis[b].
[a] Following INFANRIX (licensed in the United States in 1997).

Table 1. Percentage of Infants With Solicited Local Reactions or General Adverse Events Within 4 Days of Vaccination[a] at 2, 4, and 6 Months of Age With PEDIARIX Administered Concomitantly With Hib Conjugate Vaccine and 7-valent Pneumococcal Conjugate Vaccine (PCV7) or With Separate Concomitant Administration of INFANRIX, ENGERIX-B, IPV, Hib Conjugate Vaccine, and PCV7 (Modified Intent To Treat Cohort)

	PEDIARIX, Hib Vaccine, & PCV7			INFANRIX, ENGERIX-B, IPV, Hib Vaccine, & PCV7		
	Dose 1	Dose 2	Dose 3	Dose 1	Dose 2	Dose 3
Local[b]						
N	671	653	648	335	323	315
Pain, any	36.1	36.1	31.2	31.9	30.0	29.8
Pain, grade 2 or 3	11.5	10.9	10.6	9.0	8.7	8.9
Pain, grade 3	2.4	2.5	1.7	2.7	1.5	1.3
Redness, any	24.9[c]	37.2	40.1	18.2	32.8	39.0
Redness, >5 mm	6.0[c]	9.6[c]	12.7[c]	1.8	5.9	7.3
Redness, >20 mm	0.9	1.2[c]	2.8	0.3	0.0	1.9
Swelling, any	17.3[c]	26.5[c]	28.7	9.6	20.4	24.8
Swelling, >5 mm	5.8[c]	9.6[c]	9.3[c]	1.8	5.0	4.1
Swelling, >20 mm	1.9	2.5[c]	3.1	0.6	0.0	1.3
General						
N	667	644	645	333	321	311
Fever[d], ≥100.4°F	27.9[c]	38.8[c]	33.5[c]	19.8	30.2	23.8
Fever[d], >101.3°F	7.0	14.1[c]	8.8	4.5	9.7	5.8
Fever[d], >102.2°F	2.2[c]	3.6	3.4	0.3	3.1	2.3
Fever[d], >103.1°F	0.4	1.4	1.1	0.0	0.3	0.3
Fever[d], M.A.	1.2[c]	0.2	0.8	0.0	0.6	0.0
N	671	653	648	335	323	315
Drowsiness, any	57.2	51.6	40.9	54.0	48.3	38.4
Drowsiness, grade 2 or 3	15.8	13.8	11.4	17.6	12.4	11.1
Drowsiness, grade 3	2.5	1.2	0.9	3.6	0.6	1.9
Irritability/Fussiness, any	60.5	64.9	61.1	61.5	61.6	56.5
Irritability/Fussiness, grade 2 or 3	19.8	27.9[c]	25.2[c]	19.4	21.1	19.4
Irritability/Fussiness, grade 3	3.4	4.4	3.5	3.9	3.4	3.2
Loss of appetite, any	30.4	30.6	26.2	27.8	26.6	23.8
Loss of appetite, grade 2 or 3	6.6	7.8[c]	5.9	5.1	3.4	5.4
Loss of appetite, grade 3	0.7	0.3	0.2	0.6	0.3	0.0

Hib conjugate vaccine (Wyeth Pharmaceuticals Inc.; no longer licensed in the US); PCV7 (Wyeth Pharmaceuticals Inc.); IPV (Sanofi Pasteur SA).
Modified intent to treat cohort = all vaccinated subjects for whom safety data were available.
N = number of infants for whom at least one symptom sheet was completed; for fever, numbers exclude missing temperature recordings or tympanic measurements.
M.A. = medically attended (a visit to or from medical personnel).
Grade 2 defined as sufficiently discomforting to interfere with daily activities.
Grade 3 defined as preventing normal daily activities.
[a] Within 4 days of vaccination defined as day of vaccination and the next 3 days.
[b] Local reactions at the injection site for PEDIARIX or INFANRIX.
[c] Rate significantly higher in the group that received PEDIARIX compared to separately administered vaccines [P value <0.05 (2-sided Fisher Exact test) or the 95% CI on the difference between groups (Separate minus PEDIARIX) does not include 0].
[d] Axillary temperatures increased by 1°C and oral temperatures increased by 0.5°C to derive equivalent rectal temperature.

[b] Following ENGERIX-B (licensed in the United States in 1989).

7 DRUG INTERACTIONS

7.1 Concomitant Vaccine Administration

Immune responses following concomitant administration of PEDIARIX, Hib conjugate vaccine (Wyeth Pharmaceuticals Inc.; no longer licensed in the US), and 7-valent pneumococcal conjugate vaccine (Wyeth Pharmaceuticals Inc.) were evaluated in a clinical trial *[see Clinical Studies (14.3)]*. When PEDIARIX is administered concomitantly with other injectable vaccines, they should be given with separate syringes and at different injection sites. PEDIARIX should not be mixed with any other vaccine in the same syringe or vial.

7.2 Immunosuppressive Therapies

Immunosuppressive therapies, including irradiation, antimetabolites, alkylating agents, cytotoxic drugs, and corticosteroids (used in greater than physiologic doses), may reduce the immune response to PEDIARIX.

8 USE IN SPECIFIC POPULATIONS

8.1 Pregnancy

Pregnancy Category C

Animal reproduction studies have not been conducted with PEDIARIX. It is not known whether PEDIARIX can cause fetal harm when administered to a pregnant woman or if PEDIARIX can affect reproduction capacity.

8.4 Pediatric Use

Safety and effectiveness of PEDIARIX were established in the age group 6 weeks through 6 months on the basis of clinical studies *[see Adverse Reactions (6.1) and Clinical Studies (14.1, 14.2)]*. Safety and effectiveness of PEDIARIX in the age group 7 months through 6 years are supported by evidence in infants 6 weeks through 6 months of age. Safety and effectiveness of PEDIARIX in infants younger than 6 weeks of age and children 7 to 16 years of age have not been evaluated.

11 DESCRIPTION

PEDIARIX [Diphtheria and Tetanus Toxoids and Acellular Pertussis Adsorbed, Hepatitis B (Recombinant) and Inactivated Poliovirus Vaccine] is a noninfectious, sterile vaccine for intramuscular administration. Each 0.5-mL dose is formulated to contain 25 Lf of diphtheria toxoid, 10 Lf of tetanus toxoid, 25 mcg of inactivated pertussis toxin (PT), 25 mcg of filamentous hemagglutinin (FHA), 8 mcg of pertactin (69 kiloDalton outer membrane protein), 10 mcg of HBsAg, 40 D-antigen Units (DU) of Type 1 poliovirus (Mahoney), 8 DU of Type 2 poliovirus (MEF-1), and 32 DU of Type 3 poliovirus (Saukett). The diphtheria, tetanus, and pertussis components are the same as those in INFANRIX and KINRIX. The hepatitis B surface antigen is the same as that in ENGERIX-B.

The diphtheria toxin is produced by growing *Corynebacterium diphtheriae* in Fenton medium containing a bovine extract. Tetanus toxin is produced by growing *Clostridium tetani* in a modified Latham medium derived from bovine casein. The bovine materials used in these extracts are sourced from countries which the United States Department of Agriculture (USDA) has determined neither have nor present an undue risk for bovine spongiform encephalopathy (BSE). Both toxins are detoxified with formaldehyde, concentrated by ultrafiltration, and purified by precipitation, dialysis, and sterile filtration.

The acellular pertussis antigens (PT, FHA, and pertactin) are isolated from *Bordetella pertussis* culture grown in modified Stainer-Scholte liquid medium. PT and FHA are isolated from the fermentation broth; pertactin is extracted from the cells by heat treatment and flocculation. The antigens are purified in successive chromatographic and precipitation steps. PT is detoxified using glutaraldehyde and formaldehyde. FHA and pertactin are treated with formaldehyde.

The hepatitis B surface antigen is obtained by culturing genetically engineered *Saccharomyces cerevisiae* cells, which carry the surface antigen gene of the hepatitis B virus, in synthetic medium. The surface antigen expressed in the *S. cerevisiae* cells is purified by several physiochemical steps, which include precipitation, ion exchange chromatography, and ultrafiltration.

The inactivated poliovirus component is an enhanced potency component. Each of the 3 strains of poliovirus is individually grown in VERO cells, a continuous line of monkey kidney cells, cultivated on microcarriers. Calf serum and lactalbumin hydrolysate are used during VERO cell culture and/or virus culture. Calf serum is sourced from countries the USDA has determined neither have nor present an undue risk for BSE. After clarification, each viral suspension is purified by ultrafiltration, diafiltration, and successive chromatographic steps, and inactivated with formaldehyde. The 3 purified viral strains are then pooled to form a trivalent concentrate. Diphtheria and tetanus toxoids and pertussis antigens (inactivated PT, FHA, and pertactin) are individually adsorbed onto aluminum hydroxide. The hepatitis B component is adsorbed onto aluminum phosphate.

Table 2. Percentage of Infants With Seizures (With or Without Fever) Within 8 Days of Vaccination and Medically-Attended Fever Within 4 Days of Vaccination With PEDIARIX Compared With Historical Controls

	PEDIARIX			Historical DTaP Controls			Difference (PEDIARIX– DTaP Controls)
	N	n	% (95% CI)	N	n	% (95% CI)	% (95% CI)
All seizures (with or without fever)							
Dose 1, Days 0-7	40,000	7	0.02 (0.01, 0.04)	39,232	6	0.02 (0.01, 0.03)	0.00 (-0.02, 0.02)
Dose 2, Days 0-7	40,000	3	0.01 (0.00, 0.02)	37,405	4	0.01 (0.00, 0.03)	0.00 (-0.02, 0.01)
Dose 3, Days 0-7	40,000	6	0.02 (0.01, 0.03)	40,000	5	0.01 (0.00, 0.03)	0.00 (-0.01, 0.02)
Total doses	120,000	16	0.01 (0.01, 0.02)	116,637	15	0.01 (0.01, 0.02)	0.00 (-0.01, 0.01)
Medically-attended fever[a]							
Dose 1, Days 0-3	7,500	14	0.19 (0.11, 0.30)	7,500	14	0.19 (0.11, 0.30)	0.00 (-0.14, 0.14)
Dose 2, Days 0-3	7,500	25	0.33 (0.22, 0.48)	7,500	15	0.20 (0.11, 0.33)	0.13 (-0.03, 0.30)
Dose 3, Days 0-3	7,500	21	0.28 (0.17, 0.43)	7,500	19	0.25 (0.15, 0.34)	0.03 (-0.14, 0.19)
Total doses	22,500	60	0.27 (0.20, 0.34)	22,500	48	0.21 (0.16, 0.28)	0.05 (-0.01, 0.14)

DTaP – any US-licensed DTaP vaccine. Infants received 7-valent pneumococcal conjugate vaccine (Wyeth Pharmaceuticals Inc.) concomitantly with each dose of PEDIARIX or DTaP. Other US-licensed vaccines were administered according to routine practices at the study sites.
N = number of subjects in the given cohort.
n = number of subjects with events reported in the given cohort.
[a] Medically-attended fever defined as fever ≥100.4°F that resulted in hospitalization, an emergency department visit, or an outpatient visit.

12 CLINICAL PHARMACOLOGY

12.1 Mechanism of Action

Diphtheria: Diphtheria is an acute toxin-mediated infectious disease caused by toxigenic strains of *C. diphtheriae*. Protection against disease is due to the development of neutralizing antibodies to the diphtheria toxin. A serum diphtheria antitoxin level of 0.01 IU/mL is the lowest level giving some degree of protection; a level of 0.1 IU/mL is regarded as protective.[2]

Tetanus: Tetanus is an acute toxin-mediated disease caused by a potent exotoxin released by *C. tetani*. Protection against disease is due to the development of neutralizing antibodies to the tetanus toxin. A serum tetanus antitoxin level of at least 0.01 IU/mL, measured by neutralization assays, is considered the minimum protective level.[3,4] A level ≥0.1 IU/mL is considered protective.[5]

Pertussis: Pertussis (whooping cough) is a disease of the respiratory tract caused by *B. pertussis*. The role of the different components produced by *B. pertussis* in either the pathogenesis of, or the immunity to, pertussis is not well understood. There is no established serological correlate of protection for pertussis.

Hepatitis B: Infection with hepatitis B virus can have serious consequences including acute massive hepatic necrosis and chronic active hepatitis. Chronically infected persons are at increased risk for cirrhosis and hepatocellular carcinoma.

Antibody concentrations ≥10 mIU/mL against HBsAg are recognized as conferring protection against hepatitis B virus infection.[6]

Poliomyelitis: Poliovirus is an enterovirus that belongs to the picornavirus family. Three serotypes of poliovirus have been identified (Types 1, 2, and 3). Poliovirus neutralizing antibodies confer protection against poliomyelitis disease.[7]

13 NONCLINICAL TOXICOLOGY

13.1 Carcinogenesis, Mutagenesis, Impairment of Fertility

PEDIARIX has not been evaluated for carcinogenic or mutagenic potential, or for impairment of fertility.

14 CLINICAL STUDIES

The efficacy of PEDIARIX is based on the immunogenicity of the individual antigens compared to licensed vaccines. Serological correlates of protection exist for the diphtheria, tetanus, hepatitis B, and poliovirus components. The efficacy of the pertussis component, which does not have a well established correlate of protection, was determined in clinical trials of INFANRIX.

14.1 Efficacy of INFANRIX

Efficacy of a 3-dose primary series of INFANRIX has been assessed in 2 clinical studies.

A double-blind, randomized, active Diphtheria and Tetanus Toxoids (DT)-controlled trial conducted in Italy, sponsored by the National Institutes of Health (NIH), assessed the absolute protective efficacy of INFANRIX when administered at 2, 4, and 6 months of age. The population used in the primary analysis of the efficacy of INFANRIX included 4,481 infants vaccinated with INFANRIX and 1,470 DT vaccinees. After 3 doses, the absolute protective efficacy of INFANRIX against WHO-defined typical pertussis (21 days or more of paroxysmal cough with infection confirmed by culture and/or serologic testing) was 84% (95% CI: 76%, 89%). When the definition of pertussis was expanded to include clinically milder disease, with infection confirmed by culture and/or serologic testing, the efficacy of INFANRIX was 71% (95% CI: 60%, 78%) against >7 days of any cough and 73% (95% CI: 63%, 80%) against ≥14 days of any cough. A longer unblinded follow-up period showed that after 3 doses and with no booster dose in the second year of life, the efficacy of INFANRIX against WHO-defined pertussis was 86% (95% CI: 79%, 91%) among children followed to 6 years of age. For details see INFANRIX prescribing information.

Diphtheria and tetanus toxoid potency is determined by measuring the amount of neutralizing antitoxin in previously immunized guinea pigs. The potency of the acellular pertussis component (inactivated PT, FHA, and pertactin) is determined by enzyme-linked immunosorbent assay (ELISA) on sera from previously immunized mice. Potency of the hepatitis B component is established by HBsAg ELISA. The potency of the inactivated poliovirus component is determined by using the D-antigen ELISA and by a poliovirus neutralizing cell culture assay on sera from previously immunized rats.

Each 0.5-mL dose contains aluminum salts as adjuvant (not more than 0.85 mg aluminum by assay) and 4.5 mg of sodium chloride. Each dose also contains ≤100 mcg of residual formaldehyde and ≤100 mcg of polysorbate 80 (Tween 80). Neomycin sulfate and polymyxin B are used in the poliovirus vaccine manufacturing process and may be present in the final vaccine at ≤0.05 ng neomycin and ≤0.01 ng polymyxin B per dose. The procedures used to manufacture the HBsAg antigen result in a product that contains ≤5% yeast protein.

PEDIARIX is formulated without preservatives.

A prospective efficacy trial was also conducted in Germany employing a household contact study design. In this study, the protective efficacy of INFANRIX administered to infants at 3, 4, and 5 months of age, against WHO-defined pertussis was 89% (95% CI: 77%, 95%). When the definition of pertussis was expanded to include clinically milder disease, with infection confirmed by culture and/or serologic testing, the efficacy of INFANRIX against ≥7 days of any cough was 67% (95% CI: 52%, 78%) and against ≥7 days of paroxysmal cough was 81% (95% CI: 68%, 89%). For details see INFANRIX prescribing information.

14.2 Immunological Evaluation of PEDIARIX

In a US multicenter study, infants were randomized to 1 of 3 groups: (1) a combination vaccine group that received PEDIARIX concomitantly with Hib conjugate vaccine (Wyeth Pharmaceuticals Inc.; no longer licensed in the US) and US-licensed 7-valent pneumococcal conjugate vaccine (Wyeth Pharmaceuticals Inc.); (2) a separate vaccine group that received US-licensed INFANRIX, ENGERIX-B, and IPV (Sanofi Pasteur SA) concomitantly with the same Hib and pneumococcal conjugate vaccines; and (3) a staggered vaccine group that received PEDIARIX concomitantly with the same Hib conjugate vaccine but with the same pneumococcal conjugate vaccine administered 2 weeks later. The schedule of administration was 2, 4, and 6 months of age. Infants either did not receive a dose of hepatitis B vaccine prior to enrollment or were permitted to receive one dose of hepatitis B vaccine administered at least 30 days prior to enrollment. For the separate vaccine group, ENGERIX-B was not administered at 4 months of age to subjects who received a dose of hepatitis B vaccine prior to enrollment. Among subjects in all 3 vaccine groups combined, 84% were white, 7% were Hispanic, 6% were black, 0.7% were Oriental, and 2.4% were of other racial/ethnic groups.

The immune responses to the pertussis (PT, FHA, and pertactin), diphtheria, tetanus, poliovirus, and hepatitis B antigens were evaluated in sera obtained one month (range 20 to 60 days) after the third dose of PEDIARIX or INFANRIX. Geometric mean antibody concentrations (GMCs) adjusted for pre-vaccination values for PT, FHA, and pertactin and the seroprotection rates for diphtheria, tetanus, and the polioviruses among subjects who received PEDIARIX in the combination vaccine group were shown to be non-inferior to those achieved following separately administered vaccines (Table 3).

Because of differences in the hepatitis B vaccination schedule among subjects in the study, no clinical limit for non-inferiority was pre-defined for the hepatitis B immune response. However, in a previous US study, non-inferiority of PEDIARIX relative to separately administered INFANRIX, ENGERIX-B, and an oral poliovirus vaccine, with respect to the hepatitis B immune response was demonstrated.

Table 3. Antibody Responses Following PEDIARIX as Compared to Separate Concomitant Administration of INFANRIX, ENGERIX-B, and IPV (One Month[a] After Administration of Dose 3) in Infants Vaccinated at 2, 4, and 6 Months of Age When Administered Concomitantly With Hib Conjugate Vaccine and Pneumococcal Conjugate Vaccine (PCV7)

	PEDIARIX, Hib Vaccine, & PCV7	INFANRIX, ENGERIX-B, IPV, Hib Vaccine, & PCV7
	(N = 154-168)	(N = 141-155)
Anti-Diphtheria Toxoid		
% ≥0.1 IU/mL[b]	99.4	98.7
Anti-Tetanus Toxoid		
% ≥0.1 IU/mL[b]	100	98.1
Anti-PT		
% VR[c]	98.7	95.1
GMC[b]	48.1	28.6
Anti-FHA		
% VR[c]	98.7	96.5
GMC[b]	111.9	97.6
Anti-Pertactin		
% VR[c]	91.7	95.1
GMC[b]	95.3	80.6

Anti-Polio 1		
% ≥1:8[bd]	100	100
Anti-Polio 2		
% ≥1:8[bd]	100	100
Anti-Polio 3		
% ≥1:8[bd]	100	100
	(N = 114-128)	(N = 111-121)
Anti-HBsAg[e]		
% ≥10 mIU/mL[f]	97.7	99.2
GMC (mIU/mL)[f]	1032.1	614.5

Hib conjugate vaccine (Wyeth Pharmaceuticals Inc.; no longer licensed in the US); PCV7 (Wyeth Pharmaceuticals Inc.); IPV (Sanofi Pasteur SA).

Assay methods used: ELISA for anti-diphtheria, anti-tetanus, anti-PT, anti-FHA, anti-pertactin, and anti-HBsAg; micro-neutralization for anti-polio (1, 2, and 3).

VR = vaccine response: In initially seronegative infants, appearance of antibodies (concentration ≥5 EL.U./mL); in initially seropositive infants, at least maintenance of pre-vaccination concentration.

GMC = geometric mean antibody concentration. GMCs are adjusted for pre-vaccination levels.

[a] One month blood sampling, range 20 to 60 days.

[b] Seroprotection rate or GMC for PEDIARIX not inferior to separately administered vaccines [upper limit of 90% CI on GMC ratio (separate vaccine group/combination vaccine group) <1.5 for anti-PT, anti-FHA, and anti-pertactin, and upper limit of 95% CI for the difference in seroprotection rates (separate vaccine group minus combination vaccine group) <10% for diphtheria and tetanus and <5% for the 3 polioviruses]. GMCs are adjusted for pre-vaccination levels.

[c] The upper limit of 95% CI for differences in vaccine response rates (separate vaccine group minus combination group) was 0.31, 1.52, and 9.46 for PT, FHA, and pertactin, respectively. No clinical limit defined for non-inferiority.

[d] Poliovirus neutralizing antibody titer.

[e] Subjects who received a previous dose of hepatitis B vaccine were excluded from the analysis of hepatitis B seroprotection rates and GMCs presented in the table.

[f] No clinical limit defined for non-inferiority.

14.3 Concomitant Vaccine Administration

In a US multicenter study [see Clinical Studies (14.2)], there was no evidence for interference with the immune responses to PEDIARIX when administered concomitantly with 7-valent pneumococcal conjugate vaccine (Wyeth Pharmaceuticals Inc.) relative to 2 weeks prior.

Anti-PRP (Hib polyribosyl-ribitol-phosphate) seroprotection rates and GMCs of pnemococcal antibodies one month (range 20 to 60 days) after the third dose of vaccines for the combination vaccine group and the separate vaccine group from the US multicenter study [see Clinical Studies (14.2)], are presented in Table 4.

Table 4. Anti-PRP Seroprotection Rates and GMCs (mcg/mL) of Pneumococcal Antibodies One Month[a] Following the Third Dose of Hib Conjugate Vaccine and Pneumococcal Conjugate Vaccine (PCV7) Administered Concomitantly With PEDIARIX or With INFANRIX, ENGERIX-B, and IPV

	PEDIARIX, Hib Vaccine, & PCV7	INFANRIX, ENGERIX-B, IPV, Hib Vaccine, & PCV7
	(N = 161-168)	(N = 146-156)
	% (95% CI)	% (95% CI)
Anti-PRP		
≥0.15 mcg/mL	100 (97.8, 100)	99.4 (96.5, 100)
Anti-PRP		
≥1.0 mcg/mL	95.8 (91.6, 98.3)	91.0 (85.3, 95.0)
	GMC (95% CI)	GMC (95% CI)

Pneumococcal Serotype		
4	1.7 (1.5, 2.0)	2.1 (1.8, 2.4)
6B	0.8 (0.7, 1.0)	0.7 (0.5, 0.9)
9V	1.6 (1.4, 1.8)	1.6 (1.4, 1.9)
14	4.7 (4.0, 5.4)	6.3 (5.4, 7.4)
18C	2.6 (2.3, 3.0)	3.0 (2.5, 3.5)
19F	1.1 (1.0, 1.3)	1.1 (0.9, 1.2)
23F	1.5 (1.2, 1.8)	1.8 (1.5, 2.3)

Hib conjugate vaccine (Wyeth Pharmaceuticals Inc.; no longer licensed in the US); PCV7 (Wyeth Pharmaceuticals Inc.); IPV (Sanofi Pasteur SA).

Assay method used: ELISA for anti-PRP and 7 pneumococcal serotypes.

GMC = geometric mean antibody concentration.

[a] One month blood sampling, range 20 to 60 days.

15 REFERENCES

1. Centers for Disease and Control and Prevention. Recommended immunization schedules for persons aged 0-18 years—United States, 2010. MMWR 2010;58(51&52).
2. Vitek CR and Wharton M. Diphtheria Toxoid. In: Plotkin SA, Orenstein WA, and Offit PA, eds. Vaccines. 5th ed. Saunders;2008:139-156.
3. Wassilak SGF, Roper MH, Kretsinger K, and Orenstein WA. Tetanus Toxoid. In: Plotkin SA, Orenstein WA, and Offit PA, eds. Vaccines. 5th ed. Saunders;2008:805-839.
4. Department of Health and Human Services, Food and Drug Administration. Biological products; Bacterial vaccines and toxoids; Implementation of efficacy review; Proposed rule. Federal Register December 13, 1985;50(240):51002-51117.
5. Centers for Disease Control and Prevention. General Recommendations on Immunization. Recommendations of the Advisory Committee on Immunization Practices (ACIP). MMWR 2006;55(RR-15):1-48.
6. Ambrosch F, Frisch-Niggemeyer W, Kremsner P, et al. Persistence of vaccine-induced antibodies to hepatitis B surface antigen and the need for booster vaccination in adult subjects. Postgrad Med J 1987;63(Suppl. 2):129-135.
7. Sutter RW, Pallansch MA, Sawyer LA, et al. Defining surrogate serologic tests with respect to predicting protective vaccine efficacy: Poliovirus vaccination. In: Williams JC, Goldenthal KL, Burns DL, Lewis Jr BP, eds. Combined vaccines and simultaneous administration. Current issues and perspectives. New York, NY: The New York Academy of Sciences; 1995:289-299.

16 HOW SUPPLIED/STORAGE AND HANDLING

PEDIARIX is available in 0.5 mL single-dose vials and disposable prefilled TIP-LOK syringes.

Single-Dose Vials and Prefilled Syringes

NDC 58160-811-11 Package of 10 Single-Dose Vials

NDC 58160-811-46 Package of 5 Single-Dose Prefilled Disposable TIP-LOK Syringes (packaged without needles)

NDC 58160-811-51 Package of 10 Single-Dose Prefilled Disposable TIP-LOK Syringes (packaged without needles)

Store refrigerated between 2° and 8°C (36° and 46°F). Do not freeze. Discard if the vaccine has been frozen.

17 PATIENT COUNSELING INFORMATION

The parent or guardian should be:

- informed of the potential benefits and risks of immunization with PEDIARIX, and of the importance of completing the immunization series.
- informed about the potential for adverse reactions that have been temporally associated with administration of PEDIARIX or other vaccines containing similar components.
- instructed to report any adverse events to their healthcare provider.
- given the Vaccine Information Statements, which are required by the National Childhood Vaccine Injury Act of 1986 to be given prior to immunization. These materials are available free of charge at the Centers for Disease Control and Prevention (CDC) website (www.cdc.gov/nip).

PEDIARIX, INFANRIX, KINRIX, TIP-LOK, and ENGERIX-B are registered trademarks of GlaxoSmithKline.

Manufactured by **GlaxoSmithKline Biologicals**

Rixensart, Belgium, US License 1617, and

Novartis Vaccines and Diagnostics GmbH & Co. KG

Marburg, Germany, US License 1754

Distributed by **GlaxoSmithKline**

Research Triangle Park, NC 27709

PROMACTA®
(eltrombopag)
Tablets

HIGHLIGHTS OF PRESCRIBING INFORMATION
These highlights do not include all the information needed to use PROMACTA safely and effectively. See full prescribing information for PROMACTA.
PROMACTA® (eltrombopag) Tablets
For oral use
Initial U.S. Approval: 2008

WARNING: RISK FOR HEPATOTOXICITY
See full prescribing information for complete boxed warning
PROMACTA may cause hepatotoxicity:
• **Measure serum alanine aminotransferase (ALT), aspartate aminotransferase (AST), and bilirubin prior to initiation of PROMACTA, every 2 weeks during the dose adjustment phase and monthly following establishment of a stable dose. If bilirubin is elevated, perform fractionation.**
• **Evaluate abnormal serum liver tests with repeat testing within 3 to 5 days. If the abnormalities are confirmed, monitor serum liver tests weekly until the abnormality(ies) resolve, stabilize, or return to baseline levels.**
• **Discontinue PROMACTA if ALT levels increase to ≥3× upper limit of normal (ULN) and are:**
  • **progressive, or**
  • **persistent for ≥4 weeks, or**
  • **accompanied by increased direct bilirubin, or**
  • **accompanied by clinical symptoms of liver injury or evidence for hepatic decompensation.**

———INDICATIONS AND USAGE———
PROMACTA is a thrombopoietin receptor agonist indicated for the treatment of thrombocytopenia in patients with chronic immune (idiopathic) thrombocytopenic purpura who have had an insufficient response to corticosteroids, immunoglobulins, or splenectomy.
PROMACTA should be used only in patients with ITP whose degree of thrombocytopenia and clinical condition increase the risk for bleeding. PROMACTA should not be used in an attempt to normalize platelet counts. (1)
———DOSAGE AND ADMINISTRATION———
• The starting dose of PROMACTA is 50 mg once daily for most patients; for patients of East Asian ancestry or patients with moderate or severe hepatic insufficiency, the starting dose is 25 mg once daily. (2)
• Give on an empty stomach (1 hour before or 2 hours after a meal). (2)
• Allow a 4-hour interval between PROMACTA and other medications, foods, or supplements containing polyvalent cations (e.g., iron, calcium, aluminum, magnesium, selenium, and zinc). (2, 7.4)
• Adjust the daily dose to achieve and maintain a platelet count ≥50 × 10⁹/L in order to reduce the risk for bleeding. (2)
• Do not exceed a daily dose of 75 mg. (2)
• Discontinue PROMACTA if the platelet count does not increase after 4 weeks at the maximum dose; also discontinue PROMACTA for important liver test abnormalities or excessive platelet count responses. (2)
———DOSAGE FORMS AND STRENGTHS———
25 mg, 50 mg, and 75 mg tablets. Each tablet, for oral administration, contains eltrombopag olamine, equivalent to 25 mg, 50 mg, or 75 mg of eltrombopag free acid. (3)
———CONTRAINDICATIONS———
None. (4)
———WARNINGS AND PRECAUTIONS———
• PROMACTA may cause hepatotoxicity. Increases in serum aminotransferase levels and bilirubin were observed. Liver chemistries must be measured before the initiation of treatment and regularly during treatment. (5.1)
• Exercise caution when administering to patients with hepatic impairment. (5.1, 8.6)
• PROMACTA is a thrombopoietin receptor agonist and TPO-receptor agonists increase the risk for development or progression of reticulin fiber deposition within the bone marrow. Monitor peripheral blood for signs of marrow fibrosis. (5.2)
• Discontinuation may result in worsened thrombocytopenia than was present prior to therapy. Monitor weekly complete blood counts (CBCs), including platelet counts for at least 4 weeks after discontinuation. (5.3)

• Excessive doses of PROMACTA may increase platelet counts to a level that produces thrombotic/thromboembolic complications. (5.4)
• PROMACTA may increase the risk for hematological malignancies, especially in patients with myelodysplastic syndrome. (5.5)
• Monitor CBCs, including platelet counts and peripheral blood smears, weekly during the dose adjustment phase of therapy with PROMACTA and then monthly following establishment of a stable dose of PROMACTA. (5.6)
• Because of the risk for hepatotoxicity and other risks, PROMACTA is available only through a restricted distribution program. To enroll in the restricted distribution program, PROMACTA *CARES*, call 1-877-9-PROMACTA. (5.8)
———ADVERSE REACTIONS———
The most common adverse reactions (occurring in more than 1 patient receiving PROMACTA and at a higher rate in PROMACTA versus placebo) were: nausea, vomiting, menorrhagia, myalgia, paresthesia, cataract, dyspepsia, ecchymosis, thrombocytopenia, increased ALT/AST and conjunctival hemorrhage. (6.1)
To report SUSPECTED ADVERSE REACTIONS, contact GlaxoSmithKline at 1-888-825-5249 or FDA at 1-800-FDA-1088 or www.fda.gov/medwatch.
———DRUG INTERACTIONS———
• Eltrombopag is an inhibitor of OATP1B1 transporter. Monitor patients closely for signs and symptoms of excessive exposure to the drugs that are substrates of OATP1B1 (e.g., rosuvastatin) and consider reduction of the dose of these drugs. (7.2)
• Polyvalent cations (e.g., iron, calcium, aluminum, magnesium, selenium, and zinc) significantly reduce the absorption of eltrombopag; PROMACTA must not be taken within 4 hours of any medications or products containing polyvalent cations such as antacids, dairy products, and mineral supplements. (7.3)
———USE IN SPECIFIC POPULATIONS———
• Pregnancy: May cause fetal harm. Enroll pregnant patients in the PROMACTA pregnancy registry by calling 1-888-825-5249. (8.1)
• Nursing Mothers: A decision should be made to discontinue PROMACTA or nursing, taking into account the importance of PROMACTA to the mother. (8.3)
Revised: October 2009
PRM:2PI
See 17 for PATIENT COUNSELING INFORMATION and Medication Guide

Revised: 03/2010

FULL PRESCRIBING INFORMATION

WARNING: RISK FOR HEPATOTOXICITY
PROMACTA may cause hepatotoxicity:
• **Measure serum alanine aminotransferase (ALT), aspartate aminotransferase (AST), and bilirubin prior to initiation of PROMACTA, every 2 weeks during the dose adjustment phase and monthly following establishment of a stable dose. If bilirubin is elevated, perform fractionation.**
• **Evaluate abnormal serum liver tests with repeat testing within 3 to 5 days. If the abnormalities are confirmed, monitor serum liver tests weekly until the abnormality(ies) resolve, stabilize, or return to baseline levels.**
• **Discontinue PROMACTA if ALT levels increase to ≥3× the upper limit of normal (ULN) and are:**
  • **progressive, or**
  • **persistent for ≥4 weeks, or**
  • **accompanied by increased direct bilirubin, or**
  • **accompanied by clinical symptoms of liver injury or evidence for hepatic decompensation.**
Because of the risk for hepatotoxicity and other risks *[see Warnings and Precautions (5.1-5.6)]*, PROMACTA is available only through a restricted distribution program called PROMACTA *CARES*. Under PROMACTA *CARES*, only prescribers, pharmacies, and patients registered with the program are able to prescribe, dispense, and receive PROMACTA. To enroll in PROMACTA *CARES*, call 1-877-9-PROMACTA *[see Warnings and Precautions (5.8)]*.

---

1   INDICATIONS AND USAGE

PROMACTA is indicated for the treatment of thrombocytopenia in patients with chronic immune (idiopathic) thrombocytopenic purpura (ITP) who have had an insufficient response to corticosteroids, immunoglobulins, or splenectomy. PROMACTA should be used only in patients with ITP whose degree of thrombocytopenia and clinical condition increases the risk for bleeding. PROMACTA should not be used in an attempt to normalize platelet counts.

2   DOSAGE AND ADMINISTRATION

Only prescribers enrolled in PROMACTA *CARES* may prescribe PROMACTA *[see Warnings and Precautions (5.8)]*.
Monitor liver tests (ALT, AST, and bilirubin) and complete blood counts (CBCs), including platelet counts and peripheral blood smears, prior to initiation of PROMACTA and throughout therapy with PROMACTA. If bilirubin is elevated, perform fractionation. Monitor CBCs, including platelet counts, for at least 4 weeks following discontinuation of PROMACTA *[see Warnings and Precautions (5.3)]*. In clinical studies, platelet counts generally increased within 1 to 2 weeks after starting PROMACTA and decreased within 1 to 2 weeks after discontinuing PROMACTA *[see Clinical Studies (14)]*.
Use the lowest dose of PROMACTA to achieve and maintain a platelet count ≥50 × 10⁹/L as necessary to reduce the risk for bleeding. Dose adjustments are based upon the platelet count response. Do not use PROMACTA in an attempt to normalize platelet counts *[see Warnings and Precautions (5.4)]*.
Take PROMACTA on an empty stomach (1 hour before or 2 hours after a meal) *[see Clinical Pharmacology (12.3)]*. Allow at least a 4-hour interval between PROMACTA and other medications (e.g., antacids), calcium-rich foods (e.g., dairy products and calcium fortified juices), or supplements containing polyvalent cations such as iron, calcium, aluminum, magnesium, selenium, and zinc *[see Drug Interactions (7.4) and Clinical Pharmacology (12.3)]*.

2.1   Initial Dose Regimen
Initiate PROMACTA at a dose of 50 mg once daily except in patients who are of East Asian ancestry or who have moderate to severe hepatic impairment.
For patients of East Asian ancestry (such as Chinese, Japanese, Taiwanese, or Korean), initiate PROMACTA at a reduced dose of 25 mg once daily *[see Clinical Pharmacology (12.3)]*.
For patients with moderate or severe hepatic impairment, initiate PROMACTA at a reduced dose of 25 mg once daily *[see Use in Specific Populations (8.6)]*.

2.2 Monitoring and Dose Adjustment
After initiating PROMACTA, adjust the dose to achieve and maintain a platelet count $\geq 50 \times 10^9$/L as necessary to reduce the risk for bleeding. Do not exceed a dose of 75 mg daily. Monitor clinical hematology and liver tests regularly throughout therapy with PROMACTA and modify the dosage regimen of PROMACTA based on platelet counts as outlined in Table 1. During therapy with PROMACTA, assess CBCs, including platelet count and peripheral blood smears, weekly until a stable platelet count has been achieved. Obtain CBCs including platelet counts and peripheral blood smears, monthly thereafter.

Table 1. Dose Adjustments of PROMACTA

Platelet Count Result	Dose Adjustment or Response
$<50 \times 10^9$/L following at least 2 weeks of PROMACTA	Increase daily dose by 25 mg to a maximum of 75 mg/day.
$\geq 200 \times 10^9$/L to $\leq 400 \times 10^9$/L at any time	Decrease the daily dose by 25 mg. Wait 2 weeks to assess the effects of this and any subsequent dose adjustments.
$>400 \times 10^9$/L	Stop PROMACTA; increase the frequency of platelet monitoring to twice weekly. Once the platelet count is $<150 \times 10^9$/L, reinitiate therapy at a daily dose reduced by 25 mg.
$>400 \times 10^9$/L after 2 weeks of therapy at lowest dose of PROMACTA	Permanently discontinue PROMACTA.

Modify the dosage regimen of concomitant ITP medications, as medically appropriate, to avoid excessive increases in platelet counts during therapy with PROMACTA. Do not administer more than one dose of PROMACTA within any 24-hour period.

2.3 Discontinuation
Discontinue PROMACTA if the platelet count does not increase to a level sufficient to avoid clinically important bleeding after 4 weeks of therapy with PROMACTA at the maximum daily dose of 75 mg. Excessive platelet count responses, as outlined in Table 1, or important liver test abnormalities also necessitate discontinuation of PROMACTA *[see Warnings and Precautions (5.1)]*.

3 DOSAGE FORMS AND STRENGTHS

25 mg tablets—round, biconvex, orange, film-coated tablets debossed with GS NX3 and 25 on one side. Each tablet, for oral administration, contains eltrombopag olamine, equivalent to 25 mg of eltrombopag free acid.
50 mg tablets—round, biconvex, blue, film-coated tablets debossed with GS UFU and 50 on one side. Each tablet, for oral administration, contains eltrombopag olamine, equivalent to 50 mg of eltrombopag free acid.
75 mg tablets—round, biconvex, pink, film-coated tablets debossed with GS FSS and 75 on one side. Each tablet, for oral administration, contains eltrombopag olamine, equivalent to 75 mg of eltrombopag free acid.

4 CONTRAINDICATIONS

None.

5 WARNINGS AND PRECAUTIONS

5.1 Risk for Hepatotoxicity
PROMACTA administration may cause hepatotoxicity. In the controlled clinical studies, one patient experienced Grade 4 (NCI Common Terminology Criteria for Adverse Events [NCI CTCAE] toxicity scale) elevations in serum liver test values during therapy with PROMACTA, worsening of underlying cardiopulmonary disease, and death. No patients in the placebo group experienced Grade 4 liver test abnormalities. Overall, serum liver test abnormalities (predominantly Grade 2 or less in severity) were reported in 10% and 8% of the PROMACTA and placebo groups, respectively. In the controlled studies, two patients (1%) treated with PROMACTA and two patients in the placebo group (3%) discontinued treatment due to hepatobiliary laboratory abnormalities. Seven of the patients treated with PROMACTA in the controlled studies with hepatobiliary laboratory abnormalities were re-exposed to PROMACTA in the extension study. Six of these patients again experienced liver test abnormalities (predominantly Grade 1) resulting in discontinuation of PROMACTA in one patient. In the extension study, one additional patient had PROMACTA discontinued due to liver test abnormalities ($\leq$Grade 3).

Measure serum ALT, AST, and bilirubin prior to initiation of PROMACTA, every 2 weeks during the dose adjustment phase and monthly following establishment of a stable dose. If bilirubin is elevated, perform fractionation. Evaluate abnormal serum liver tests with repeat testing within 3 to 5 days. If the abnormalities are confirmed, monitor serum liver tests weekly until the abnormality(ies) resolve, stabilize, or return to baseline levels. Discontinue PROMACTA if ALT levels increase to $\geq 3\times$ the upper limit of normal (ULN) and are:

- progressive, or
- persistent for $\geq$4 weeks, or
- accompanied by increased direct bilirubin, or
- accompanied by clinical symptoms of liver injury or evidence for hepatic decompensation.

Reinitiating treatment with PROMACTA is not recommended. If the potential benefit for reinitiating PROMACTA treatment is considered to outweigh the risk for hepatotoxicity, then cautiously reintroduce PROMACTA and measure serum liver tests weekly during the dose adjustment phase. If liver tests abnormalities persist, worsen or recur, then permanently discontinue PROMACTA.
Exercise caution when administering PROMACTA to patients with hepatic disease. Use a lower starting dose of PROMACTA in patients with moderate to severe hepatic disease and monitor closely *[see Dosage and Administration (2.1)]*.

5.2 Bone Marrow Reticulin Formation and Risk for Bone Marrow Fibrosis
PROMACTA is a thrombopoietin (TPO) receptor agonist and TPO-receptor agonists increase the risk for development or progression of reticulin fiber deposition within the bone marrow.
In the extension study, seven patients had reticulin fiber deposition reported in bone marrow biopsies, including two patients who also had collagen fiber deposition. The fiber deposition was not associated with cytopenias and did not necessitate discontinuation of PROMACTA. However, clinical studies have not excluded a risk of bone marrow fibrosis with cytopenias.
Prior to initiation of PROMACTA, examine the peripheral blood smear closely to establish a baseline level of cellular morphologic abnormalities. Following identification of a stable dose of PROMACTA, examine peripheral blood smears and CBCs monthly for new or worsening morphological abnormalities (e.g., teardrop and nucleated red blood cells, immature white blood cells) or cytopenia(s). If the patient develops new or worsening morphological abnormalities or cytopenia(s), discontinue treatment with PROMACTA and consider a bone marrow biopsy, including staining for fibrosis.

5.3 Worsened Thrombocytopenia and Hemorrhage Risk After Cessation of PROMACTA
Discontinuation of PROMACTA may result in thrombocytopenia of greater severity than was present prior to therapy with PROMACTA. This worsened thrombocytopenia may increase the patient's risk of bleeding, particularly if PROMACTA is discontinued while the patient is on anticoagulants or antiplatelet agents. In the controlled clinical studies, transient decreases in platelet counts to levels lower than baseline were observed following discontinuation of treatment in 10% and 6% of the PROMACTA and placebo groups, respectively. Serious hemorrhagic events requiring the use of supportive ITP medications occurred in 3 severely thrombocytopenic patients within one month following the discontinuation of PROMACTA; none were reported among the placebo group.
Following discontinuation of PROMACTA, obtain weekly CBCs, including platelet counts for at least 4 weeks and consider alternative treatments for worsening thrombocytopenia, according to current treatment guidelines *[see Adverse Reactions (6.1)]*.

5.4 Thrombotic/Thromboembolic Complications
Thrombotic/thromboembolic complications may result from excessive increases in platelet counts. Excessive doses of PROMACTA or medication errors that result in excessive doses of PROMACTA may increase platelet counts to a level that produces thrombotic/thromboembolic complications. In the controlled clinical studies, one thrombotic/thromboembolic complication was reported within the groups that received PROMACTA and none within the placebo groups. Seven patients experienced thrombotic/thromboembolic complications in the extension study. Use caution when administering PROMACTA to patients with known risk factors for thromboembolism (e.g., Factor V Leiden, ATIII deficiency, antiphospholipid syndrome, etc). To minimize the risk for thrombotic/thromboembolic complications, do not use PROMACTA in an attempt to normalize platelet counts. Follow the dose adjustment guidelines to achieve and maintain a platelet count of $\geq 50 \times 10^9$/L *[see Dosage and Administration (2.2)]*.

5.5 Malignancies and Progression of Malignancies
PROMACTA stimulation of the TPO receptor on the surface of hematopoietic cells may increase the risk for hematologic malignancies. In the controlled clinical studies, patients were treated with PROMACTA for a maximum of 6 weeks and during this period no hematologic malignancies were reported. One hematologic malignancy (non-Hodgkin's lymphoma) was reported in the extension study. PROMACTA is not indicated for the treatment of thrombocytopenia due to causes of thrombocytopenia (e.g., myelodysplasia or chemotherapy) other than chronic ITP.

5.6 Laboratory Monitoring
Complete Blood Counts (CBCs): Monitor CBCs, including platelet counts and peripheral blood smears, prior to initiation, throughout, and following discontinuation of therapy with PROMACTA. Prior to the initiation of PROMACTA, examine the peripheral blood differential to establish the extent of red and white blood cell abnormalities. Obtain CBCs, including platelet counts and peripheral blood smears, weekly during the dose adjustment phase of therapy with PROMACTA and then monthly following establishment of a stable dose of PROMACTA. Obtain CBCs, including platelet counts, weekly for at least 4 weeks following discontinuation of PROMACTA *[see Dosage and Administration (2) and Warnings and Precautions (5.2, 5.3)]*.
Liver Tests: Monitor serum liver tests (ALT, AST, and bilirubin) prior to initiation of PROMACTA, every 2 weeks during the dose adjustment phase and monthly following establishment of a stable dose. If bilirubin is elevated, perform fractionation. If abnormal levels are detected, repeat the tests within 3 to 5 days. If the abnormalities are confirmed, monitor serum liver tests weekly until the abnormality(ies) resolve, stabilize, or return to baseline levels. Discontinue PROMACTA for the development of important liver test abnormalities *[see Warnings and Precautions (5.1)]*.

5.7 Cataracts
In the controlled clinical studies, cataracts developed or worsened in five (5%) patients who received 50 mg PROMACTA daily and two (3%) placebo-group patients. In the extension study, cataracts developed or worsened in 4% of patients who underwent ocular examination prior to therapy with PROMACTA. Cataracts were observed in toxicology studies of eltrombopag in rodents *[see Nonclinical Toxicology (13.2)]*. Perform a baseline ocular examination prior to administration of PROMACTA and, during therapy with PROMACTA, regularly monitor patients for signs and symptoms of cataracts.

5.8 PROMACTA Distribution Program
PROMACTA is available only through a restricted distribution program called PROMACTA *CARES*. Under PROMACTA *CARES*, only prescribers, pharmacies, and patients registered with the program are able to prescribe, dispense, and receive PROMACTA. This program provides educational materials and a mechanism for the proper use of PROMACTA. To enroll in PROMACTA *CARES*, call 1-877-9-PROMACTA. Prescribers and patients are required to understand the risks of therapy with PROMACTA. Prescribers are required to understand the information in the prescribing information and be able to:

- Educate patients on the benefits and risks of treatment with PROMACTA, ensure that the patient receives the Medication Guide, instruct them to read it, and encourage them to ask questions when considering PROMACTA. Patients may be educated by the enrolled prescriber or a healthcare provider under that prescriber's direction.
- Review the PROMACTA *CARES* Prescriber Enrollment Forms, sign the form, and return the form according to PROMACTA *CARES* Program instructions.
- As part of the initial prescription process for PROMACTA, obtain the patient's signature on the Patient Enrollment and Consent form, sign it, place the original signed form in the patient's medical record, send a copy to PROMACTA *CARES*, and give a copy to the patient.
- Report any serious adverse events associated with the use of PROMACTA to PROMACTA *CARES* Call Center at 1-877-9-PROMACTA or to the FDA's MedWatch Program at 1-800-FDA-1088.
- Report serious adverse events observed in patients receiving PROMACTA, including events actively solicited at 6-month intervals.

6 ADVERSE REACTIONS

6.1 Clinical Trials Experience
In clinical studies, hemorrhage was the most common serious adverse reaction and most hemorrhagic reactions followed discontinuation of PROMACTA. Other serious adverse reactions included liver test abnormalities and thrombotic/thromboembolic complications *[see Warnings and Precautions (5.1, 5.2)]*.
The data described below reflect PROMACTA exposure to 313 patients with chronic ITP aged 18 to 85, of whom 65% were female. PROMACTA was studied in 2 randomized, placebo-controlled studies in which patients received the drug for no more than 6 weeks. PROMACTA was also studied in an open-label, single-arm study in which patients

received the drug over an extended period of time. Overall, PROMACTA was administered to 81 patients for at least 6 months and 39 patients for at least 1 year.

Because clinical trials are conducted under widely varying conditions, adverse reaction rates observed in the clinical trials of a drug cannot be directly compared to rates in the clinical trials of another drug and may not reflect the rates observed in practice.

Table 2 presents the most common adverse drug reactions (experienced by more than 1 patient receiving PROMACTA) from the placebo-controlled studies, with a higher incidence in PROMACTA versus placebo.

Table 2. Adverse Reactions Identified in Two Placebo-Controlled Studies

Preferred Term	PROMACTA 50mg n = 106 (%)	Placebo n = 67 (%)
Nausea	6	4
Vomiting	4	3
Menorrhagia	4	1
Myalgia	3	1
Paresthesia	3	1
Cataract	3	1
Dyspepsia	2	0
Ecchymosis	2	1
Thrombocytopenia	2	0
Increased ALT	2	0
Increased AST	2	0
Conjunctival hemorrhage	2	1

Among 207 patients with chronic ITP who received PROMACTA in the single-arm extended study, the adverse reactions occurred in a pattern similar to those reported in the placebo-controlled studies.

7 DRUG INTERACTIONS

7.1 Cytochrome P450

In vitro studies demonstrate that CYP1A2 and CYP2C8 are involved in the oxidative metabolism of eltrombopag. The significance of coadministration of PROMACTA with 1) moderate or strong inhibitors of CYP 1A2 (e.g., ciprofloxacin, fluvoxamine) and CYP 2C8 (e.g., gemfibrozil, trimethoprim); 2) inducers of CYP 1A2 (e.g., tobacco, omeprazole) and CYP 2C8 (e.g., rifampin); or 3) other substrates of these CYP enzymes on the systemic exposure of PROMACTA has not been established in clinical studies. Monitor patients for signs and symptoms of excessive eltrombopag exposure when PROMACTA is administered concomitantly with these moderate or strong inhibitors of CYP1A2 or CYP2C8.

7.2 Transporters

In vitro studies demonstrate that eltrombopag is an inhibitor of the organic anion transporting polypeptide OATP1B1 and can increase the systemic exposure of other drugs that are substrates of this transporter (e.g., benzylpenicillin, atorvastatin, fluvastatin, pravastatin, rosuvastatin, methotrexate, nateglinide, repaglinide, rifampin). In a clinical study of healthy adult subjects, administration of a single dose of rosuvastatin following repeated daily PROMACTA dosing increased plasma rosuvastatin $AUC_{0-\infty}$ by 55% and C_{max} by 103% [see Clinical Pharmacology (12.3)].

Use caution when concomitantly administering PROMACTA and drugs that are substrates of OATP1B1. Monitor patients closely for signs and symptoms of excessive exposure to the drugs that are substrates of OATP1B1 and consider reduction of the dose of these drugs. In clinical trials with eltrombopag, a dose reduction of rosuvastatin by 50% was recommended for coadministration with eltrombopag.

7.3 UDP-glucuronosyltransferases (UGTs)

In vitro studies demonstrate that eltrombopag is an inhibitor of UGT1A1, UGT1A3, UGT1A4, UGT1A6, UGT1A9, UGT2B7, and UGT2B15, enzymes involved in the metabolism of multiple drugs, such as acetaminophen, narcotics, and nonsteroidal anti-inflammatory drugs (NSAIDs). The significance of this inhibition on the potential for increased systemic exposure of drugs that are substrates of these UGTs following coadministration with PROMACTA has not

been evaluated in clinical studies. Monitor patients closely for signs or symptoms of excessive exposure to these drugs when concomitantly administered with PROMACTA.

In vitro studies demonstrate that UGT1A1 and UGT1A3 are responsible for the glucuronidation of PROMACTA. The significance of coadministration of PROMACTA with moderate or strong inhibitors or inducers on the systemic exposure of PROMACTA has not been evaluated in clinical studies. Monitor patients closely for signs or symptoms of excessive exposure to PROMACTA when concomitantly administered with these moderate or strong inhibitors of UGT1A1 or UGT1A3.

7.4 Polyvalent Cations (Chelation)

Eltrombopag chelates polyvalent cations (such as iron, calcium, aluminum, magnesium, selenium, and zinc) in foods, mineral supplements, and antacids. In a clinical study, administration of PROMACTA with a polyvalent cation-containing antacid (1,524 mg aluminum hydroxide, 1,425 mg magnesium carbonate, and sodium alginate) decreased plasma eltrombopag systemic exposure by approximately 70% [see Clinical Pharmacology (12.3)]. PROMACTA must not be taken within 4 hours of any medications or products containing polyvalent cations such as antacids, dairy products, and mineral supplements to avoid significant reduction in PROMACTA absorption due to chelation [see Dosage and Administration (2)].

8 USE IN SPECIFIC POPULATIONS

8.1 Pregnancy

Pregnancy Category C

There are no adequate and well-controlled studies of eltrombopag use in pregnancy. In animal reproduction and developmental toxicity studies, there was evidence of embryolethality and reduced fetal weights at maternally toxic doses. PROMACTA should be used in pregnancy only if the potential benefit to the mother justifies the potential risk to the fetus.

Pregnancy Registry: A pregnancy registry has been established to collect information about the effects of PROMACTA during pregnancy. Physicians are encouraged to register pregnant patients, or pregnant women may enroll themselves in the PROMACTA pregnancy registry by calling 1-888-825-5249.

In an early embryonic development study, female rats received eltrombopag at doses of 0.8, 2, and 7 times the human clinical exposure (based on AUC). Increased pre- and post-implantation loss and reduced fetal weight were observed at the highest dose which also caused maternal toxicity.

In an embryofetal development study, pregnant rats received eltrombopag at doses of 0.8, 2, and 7 times the human clinical exposure (based on AUC). Decreased fetal weights and a slight increase in the presence of cervical ribs were observed at the highest dose which also caused maternal toxicity. However, no evidence of major structural malformations was observed.

In an embryofetal development study in pregnant rabbits treated with oral eltrombopag doses of 0.1, 0.3, and 0.6 times the human clinical exposure (based on AUC) no evidence of fetotoxicity, embryolethality, or teratogenicity was observed.

In a pre- and post-natal developmental toxicity study in pregnant rats (F0), no adverse effects on maternal reproductive function or on the development of the offspring (F1) were observed at doses up to 2 times the human clinical exposure (based on AUC). Eltrombopag was detected in the plasma of offspring (F1). The plasma concentrations in pups increased with dose (0.8 and 2 times the human clinical exposure based on AUC) following administration of drug to the F0 dams.

8.3 Nursing Mothers

It is not known whether eltrombopag is excreted in human milk. Because many drugs are excreted in human milk and because of the potential for serious adverse reactions in nursing infants from PROMACTA, a decision should be made whether to discontinue nursing or to discontinue PROMACTA taking into account the importance of PROMACTA to the mother and the known benefits of nursing.

8.4 Pediatric Use

The safety and efficacy of PROMACTA in pediatric patients have not been established.

8.5 Geriatric Use

Of the 106 patients in 2 randomized clinical studies of PROMACTA 50-mg dose, 22% were 65 years of age and older, and 9% were 75 years of age and older. No overall differences in safety or efficacy have been observed between older and younger patients in the placebo-controlled studies, but greater sensitivity of some older individuals cannot be ruled out. In general, dose adjustment for an elderly patient should be cautious, reflecting the greater frequency of decreased hepatic, renal, or cardiac function, and of concomitant disease or other drug therapy.

8.6 Hepatic Impairment

The disposition of PROMACTA was compared in patients with hepatic impairment to subjects with normal hepatic function. Apparent clearance of PROMACTA was reduced by approximately 50% in patients with moderate and severe (as indicated by the Child-Pugh method) hepatic impairment. In this clinical study that did not evaluate protein binding effects, the half-life of PROMACTA was prolonged 2-fold in patients with moderate and severe hepatic impairment.

For patients with moderate and severe hepatic impairment, initiate PROMACTA at a reduced dose of 25 mg once daily [see Dosage and Administration (2.1) and Warnings and Precautions (5.1)].

8.7 Renal Impairment

The safety and efficacy of PROMACTA in patients with varying degrees of renal function have not been established. Closely monitor patients with impaired renal function when administering PROMACTA.

10 OVERDOSAGE

In the event of overdose, platelet counts may increase excessively and result in thrombotic/thromboembolic complications. In case of an overdose, consider oral administration of a metal cation-containing preparation, such as calcium, aluminum, or magnesium preparations to chelate eltrombopag and thus limit absorption. Closely monitor platelet counts. Reinitiate treatment with PROMACTA in accordance with dosing and administration recommendations [see Dosage and Administration (2.2)].

In one report, a subject ingested 5,000 mg of PROMACTA and was treated with gastric lavage, oral lactulose, intravenous fluids, omeprazole, atropine, furosemide, calcium, dexamethasone, and plasmapheresis. The patient's platelet count increased to a maximum of $929 \times 10^9/L$ at 13 days following the ingestion. The patient also experienced rash, bradycardia, ALT/AST elevations, and fatigue. The abnormal platelet count and liver test abnormalities persisted for 3 weeks. After 2 months follow-up, all events had resolved without sequelae.

Hemodialysis is not expected to enhance the elimination of PROMACTA because eltrombopag is not significantly renally excreted and is highly bound to plasma proteins.

11 DESCRIPTION

PROMACTA (eltrombopag) Tablets contain eltrombopag olamine, a small molecule thrombopoietin (TPO) receptor agonist for oral administration. Eltrombopag interacts with the transmembrane domain of the TPO receptor (also known as cMpl) leading to increased platelet production. Each tablet contains eltrombopag olamine in the amount equivalent to 25 mg or 50 mg of eltrombopag free acid.

Eltrombopag olamine is a biphenyl hydrazone. The chemical name for eltrombopag olamine is 3'-[(2Z)-2-[1-(3,4-dimethylphenyl)-3-methyl-5-oxo-1,5-dihydro-4H-pyrazol-4-ylidene]hydrazino]-3-methyl-5-oxo-1,5-dihydro-4H-pyrazol-4-ylidene]hydrazino]-2'-hydroxy-3-biphenylcarboxylic acid - 2-aminoethanol (1:2). It has the molecular formula $C_{25}H_{22}N_4O_4 \cdot 2(C_2H_7NO)$. The molecular weight is 564.65 for eltrombopag olamine and 442.5 for eltrombopag free acid. Eltrombopag olamine has the following structural formula:

Eltrombopag olamine is practically insoluble in aqueous buffer across a pH range of 1 to 7.4, and is sparingly soluble in water.

The inactive ingredients of PROMACTA are: **Tablet Core:** magnesium stearate, mannitol, microcrystalline cellulose, povidone, and sodium starch glycolate. **Coating:** hypromellose, polyethylene glycol 400, titanium dioxide, and FD&C Yellow No. 6 aluminum lake (25 mg tablet), FD&C Blue No. 2 aluminum lake (50 mg tablet), or Iron Oxide Red and Iron Oxide Black (75 mg tablet).

12 CLINICAL PHARMACOLOGY

12.1 Mechanism of Action

Eltrombopag is an orally bioavailable, small-molecule TPO-receptor agonist that interacts with the transmembrane domain of the human TPO-receptor and initiates signaling cascades that induce proliferation and differentiation of megakaryocytes from bone marrow progenitor cells.

12.2 Pharmacodynamics
ECG Effects: There is no indication of a QT/QTc prolonging effect of PROMACTA in doses up to 150 mg daily for 5 days. The effects of PROMACTA at doses up to 150 mg daily for 5 days (supratherapeutic doses) on the QT/QTc interval was evaluated in a double-blind, randomized, placebo- and positive-controlled (moxifloxacin 400 mg, single oral dose) crossover trial in healthy adult subjects. Assay sensitivity was confirmed by significant QTc prolongation by moxifloxacin.

12.3 Pharmacokinetics
A population pharmacokinetic model analysis suggests that the pharmacokinetic profile for eltrombopag following oral administration is best described by a 2-compartment model. Based on this model, the estimated exposures of eltrombopag after administration to patients with ITP are shown in Table 3.

Table 3. Geometric Mean (95% Confidence Intervals) of Steady-State Plasma Eltrombopag Pharmacokinetic Parameters in Adults With Idiopathic Thrombocytopenic Purpura

Regimen of PROMACTA	$AUC_{(0-T)}$ (mcg.hr/mL)
50 mg once daily (N = 34)	91.9 (73.6, 115)
75 mg once daily (N = 26)	146 (122, 176)

Absorption: Eltrombopag is absorbed with a peak concentration occurring 2 to 6 hours after oral administration. Based on urinary excretion and biotransformation products eliminated in feces, the oral absorption of drug-related material following administration of a single 75 mg solution dose was estimated to be at least 52%.
In a clinical study, administration of a single 75 mg-dose of PROMACTA with a polyvalent cation-containing antacid (1,524 mg aluminum hydroxide, 1,425 mg magnesium carbonate, and sodium alginate) decreased plasma eltrombopag $AUC_{0-\infty}$ and C_{max} by 70%. The contribution of sodium alginate to this interaction is not known [see Drug Interactions (7.4)].
An open-label, randomized, crossover study was conducted to assess the effect of food on the bioavailability of eltrombopag. A standard high-fat breakfast significantly decreased plasma eltrombopag $AUC_{0-\infty}$ by approximately 59% and C_{max} by 65% and delayed t_{max} by 1 hour. The calcium content of this meal may have also contributed to this decrease in exposure.
Distribution: The concentration of eltrombopag in blood cells is approximately 50 to 79% of plasma concentrations based on a radiolabel study. In vitro studies suggest that eltrombopag is highly bound to human plasma proteins (>99%). Eltrombopag is not a substrate for p-glycoprotein (Pgp) or OATP1B1.
Metabolism: Absorbed eltrombopag is extensively metabolized, predominantly through pathways including cleavage, oxidation, and conjugation with glucuronic acid, glutathione, or cysteine. In a human radiolabel study, eltrombopag accounted for approximately 64% of plasma radiocarbon $AUC_{0-\infty}$. Metabolites due to glucuronidation and oxidation were also detected. In vitro studies suggest that CYP 1A2 and 2C8 are responsible for the oxidative metabolism of eltrombopag. UGT1A1 and UGT1A3 are responsible for the glucuronidation of eltrombopag.
Elimination: The predominant route of eltrombopag excretion is via feces (59%), and 31% of the dose is found in the urine. Unchanged eltrombopag in feces accounts for approximately 20% of the dose; unchanged eltrombopag is not detectable in urine. The plasma elimination half-life of eltrombopag is approximately 21 to 32 hours in healthy subjects and 26 to 35 hours in ITP patients.
Race: Based on both non-compartment analysis and population pharmacokinetic analysis, plasma eltrombopag exposure was approximately 70% higher in some Asian subjects of Japanese, Chinese, Taiwanese, and Korean ancestry (i.e., East Asian) with ITP as compared to non-Asian subjects who were predominantly Caucasian [see Dosage and Administration (2.1)]. In addition, the pharmacodynamic (PD) response to eltrombopag was qualitatively similar in the Asian subjects, but the absolute PD response was somewhat greater.
An approximately 40% higher systemic eltrombopag exposure in healthy African-American subjects was noted in at least one clinical pharmacology study. The effect of African-American ethnicity on exposure and related safety and efficacy of eltrombopag has not been established.

Gender: Results from a population pharmacokinetic model suggest that males have a 27% greater apparent eltrombopag clearance than females, after adjustment for the body weight difference.
Hepatic Impairment: Plasma eltrombopag pharmacokinetics in subjects with mild, moderate, and severe hepatic impairment compared to healthy subjects was investigated following administration of a single 50-mg dose of eltrombopag. The degree of hepatic impairment was based on Child-Pugh score. Plasma eltrombopag $AUC_{0-\infty}$ was 41% higher in subjects with mild hepatic impairment, and 80% to 93% higher in subjects with moderate to severe hepatic impairment compared with healthy subjects. A corresponding reduction in apparent clearance was also reported. The impact of hepatic impairment was highly variable between subjects. Unbound eltrombopag (active) concentrations for this highly protein bound drug was not measured [see Dosage and Administration (2.1) and Use in Specific Populations (8.6)].
Renal Impairment: The pharmacokinetics of eltrombopag have not been established in patients with renal impairment [see Use in Specific Populations (8.7)].
Drug Interactions: Cytochrome P450: In vitro studies report that eltrombopag is an inhibitor of CYP2C8 and CYP2C9 as measured using paclitaxel and diclofenac as the probe substrates. A clinical study where PROMACTA 75 mg once daily was administered for 7 days to 24 healthy male subjects did not show inhibition or induction of the metabolism of a combination of probe substrates for CYP 1A2 (caffeine), CYP2C19 (omeprazole), CYP2C9 (flurbiprofen), or CYP3A4 (midazolam) in humans. Probe substrates for CYP2C8 were not evaluated in this study.
In vitro studies suggest that CYP 1A2 and 2C8 are responsible for oxidative metabolism of eltrombopag. Clinical studies evaluating the effect of strong inducers or inhibitors of these CYP enzymes responsible for the metabolism of eltrombopag have not been conducted.
Transporters: In vitro studies demonstrated that eltrombopag is an inhibitor of the OATP1B1. Administration of 75 mg of PROMACTA once daily for 5 days with a single 10 mg-dose of the OATP1B1 substrate, rosuvastatin, to 39 healthy adult subjects increased plasma rosuvastatin $AUC_{0-\infty}$ by 55% and C_{max} by 103% [see Drug Interactions (7.2)].
UDP-glucuronosyltransferases (UGTs): See Drug Interactions (7.3).

13 NONCLINICAL TOXICOLOGY
13.1 Carcinogenesis, Mutagenesis, Impairment of Fertility
Eltrombopag does not stimulate platelet production in rats, mice, or dogs because of unique TPO receptor specificity. Data from these animals do not fully model effects in humans.
Eltrombopag was not carcinogenic in mice at doses up to 75 mg/kg/day or in rats at doses up to 40 mg/kg/day (exposures up to 4 and 5 times the human clinical exposure based on AUC, respectively).
Eltrombopag was not mutagenic or clastogenic in a bacterial mutation assay or in 2 in vivo assays in rats (micronucleus and unscheduled DNA synthesis, 11 times the human clinical exposure based on C_{max}). In the in vitro mouse lymphoma assay, eltrombopag was marginally positive (<3-fold increase in mutation frequency).
Eltrombopag did not affect female fertility in rats at doses up to 20 mg/kg/day (2 times the human clinical exposure based on AUC). Eltrombopag did not affect male fertility in rats at doses up to 40 mg/kg/day, the highest dose tested (5 times the human clinical exposure based on AUC).

13.2 Animal Pharmacology/Toxicology
Eltrombopag is phototoxic and photoclastogenic in vitro. In vitro photoclastogenic effects were observed only at cytotoxic drug concentrations (≥15 mcg/mL) and at UV light exposure intensity (30 MED, minimal erythematous dose). No evidence of in vitro photoclastogenicity was observed at higher drug concentrations (up to 58.4 mcg/mL) and UV light exposure of 15 MED. There was no evidence of in vivo cutaneous phototoxicity in mice, photo-ocular toxicity in rats or photo-ocular toxicity in mice at exposures up to 11, 6, and 7 times the human clinical exposure based on AUC, respectively.
Treatment-related cataracts were detected in rodents in a dose- and time-dependent manner. At ≥7 times the human clinical exposure based on AUC, cataracts were observed in mice after 6 weeks and in rats after 28 weeks of dosing. At ≥5 times the human clinical exposure based on AUC, cataracts were observed in mice after 13 weeks and in rats after 39 weeks of dosing. Cataracts were not observed in dogs after 52 weeks of dosing (3 times the human clinical exposure based on AUC). The clinical relevance of these findings is unknown [see Warnings and Precautions (5.7)].
Renal tubular toxicity was observed in studies up to 14 days in duration in mice and rats at exposures that were generally associated with morbidity and mortality. Tubular toxic-

ity was also observed in a 2-year oral carcinogenicity study in mice at doses of 25, 75, and 150 mg/kg/day. The exposure at the lowest dose was 1.4 times the human clinical exposure based on AUC. No similar effects were observed after 13 weeks at exposures greater than those associated with renal changes in the 2-year study, suggesting that this effect is both dose- and time-dependent. Renal tubular toxicity was not observed in rats in a 2-year carcinogenicity study or in dogs after 52 weeks at exposures 5 and 3 times the human clinical exposure based on AUC, respectively.
Eltrombopag produced hepatocellular hypertrophy in mice (7 times the human clinical exposure based on AUC), rats (5 times the human clinical exposure based on AUC), rabbits (1.4 times the human clinical exposure based on AUC), and dogs (4 times the human clinical exposure based on AUC) and hepatocellular vacuolation in rats (2 times the human clinical exposure based on AUC).

13.3 Reproductive and Developmental Toxicology
Eltrombopag was administered orally to pregnant rats in an embryofetal development study at 10, 20, or 60 mg/kg/day (0.8, 2, and 7 times the human clinical exposure, respectively, based on AUC). Decreases in maternal body weight gain and food consumption occurred in the 60 mg/kg/day dose group. At this maternally toxic dose, male and female fetal weights were significantly reduced (6% to 7%) and there was a slight increase in the presence of cervical ribs, a fetal variation.
In an embryofetal development study in mated female rabbits, eltrombopag was administered orally at 30, 80, or 150 mg/kg/day (0.1, 0.3, and 0.6 times the human clinical exposure, respectively, based on AUC). There was no evidence of fetotoxicity, embryolethality, or teratogenicity at any dose.
In a pre- and post-natal developmental toxicity study in pregnant rats (F0), no adverse effects on maternal reproductive function or on the development of the offspring (F1) were observed at doses up to 2 times the human clinical exposure (based on AUC). Eltrombopag was detected in the plasma of offspring (F1). The plasma concentrations in pups increased with dose (0.8 and 2 times the human clinical exposure based on AUC) following administration of drug to the F0 dams.

14 CLINICAL STUDIES
The efficacy and safety of PROMACTA in adult patients with chronic ITP were evaluated in 2 randomized double-blind, placebo-controlled studies and in an open-label extension study.
14.1 Studies 1 and 2
In studies 1 and 2, patients who had completed at least one prior ITP therapy and who had a platelet count <30 × 10^9/L were randomized to either daily placebo or PROMACTA administered over a maximum treatment period of 6 weeks, followed by 6 weeks off therapy. During the studies, PROMACTA or placebo were discontinued if the platelet count exceeded 200 × 10^9/L. The primary efficacy endpoint was response rate, defined as a shift from a baseline platelet count of <30 × 10^9/L to ≥50 × 10^9/L at any time during the treatment period.
The median age of the patients was 50 years and 60% were female. Approximately 70% of the patients had received at least 2 prior ITP therapies (predominantly corticosteroids, immunoglobulins, rituximab, cytotoxic therapies, danazol, and azathioprine) and 40% of the patients had undergone splenectomy. The median baseline platelet counts (approximately 18 × 10^9/L) were similar among all treatment groups.
Study 1 randomized 114 patients (2:1) to PROMACTA 50 mg or placebo. Study 2 randomized 117 patients (1:1:1:1) among placebo or one of three dose regimens of PROMACTA, 30 mg, 50 mg, or 75 mg each administered daily.
Table 4 shows the outcomes for the placebo groups and the groups of patients who received the 50 mg daily regimen of PROMACTA.

Table 4. Studies 1 and 2 Platelet Count Response (≥50 × 10^9/L) Rates

Study	PROMACTA 50 mg Daily	Placebo
1	43/73 (59%)[a]	6/37 (16%)
2	19/27 (70%)[a]	3/27 (11%)

[a] p <0.001 for PROMACTA versus placebo.

The platelet count response to PROMACTA was similar among patients who had or had not undergone splenectomy. In general, increases in platelet counts were detected 1 week following initiation of PROMACTA and the maximum response observed after 2 weeks of therapy. Within the placebo and 50 mg-dose group of PROMACTA, the study drug was discontinued due to an increase in platelet counts to

>200 × 10⁹/L in 3% and 27% of the patients, respectively. The median duration of treatment with the 50 mg-dose of PROMACTA in Study 1 was 42 days and Study 2 was 43 days.

Of seven patients (three in the placebo group and four in the group that received PROMACTA) who underwent hemostatic challenges, additional ITP medications were required in all placebo group patients and none of the patients treated with PROMACTA. Surgical procedures accounted for most of the hemostatic challenges. Hemorrhage requiring transfusion occurred in one placebo group patient and no patients treated with PROMACTA.

14.2 Extension Study

Patients who completed any prior clinical study with PROMACTA were enrolled in an open-label, single-arm study in which attempts were made to decrease the dose or eliminate the need for any concomitant ITP medications. PROMACTA was administered to 109 patients; 74 completed 3 months of treatment, 53 completed 6 months and three patients completed 1 year of therapy. The median baseline platelet count was 18 × 10⁹/L prior to administration of PROMACTA. Median platelet counts at 3, 6, and 9 months on study were 74 × 10⁹/L, 67 × 10⁹/L, and 95 × 10⁹/L, respectively. The median daily dose of PROMACTA following 6 months of therapy was 50 mg (n = 53); the median daily dose was also 50 mg among patients with no change in the dose regimen of PROMACTA over 2 months or more of therapy (n = 45).

16 HOW SUPPLIED/STORAGE AND HANDLING

The 25 mg tablets are round, biconvex, orange, film-coated tablets debossed with GS NX3 and 25 on one side and are available in bottles of 30: NDC 0007-4640-13.

The 50 mg tablets are round, biconvex, blue, film-coated tablets debossed with GS UFU and 50 on one side and are available in bottles of 30: NDC 0007-4641-13.

The 75 mg tablets are round, biconvex, pink, film-coated tablets debossed with GS FFS and 75 on one side and are available in bottles of 30: NDC 0007-4642-13.

Store at 25°C (77°F); excursions permitted to 15° to 30°C (59° to 86°F) [see USP Controlled Room Temperature].

17 PATIENT COUNSELING INFORMATION

See FDA-Approved Medication Guide.

17.1 Information for Patients

Prior to treatment, patients should fully understand the risks and benefits of PROMACTA. Inform patients that the risks associated with long-term administration of PROMACTA are unknown and that they must enroll in PROMACTA *CARES*, which provides for the proper use of PROMACTA in ITP patients.

Inform patients of the following risks and considerations for PROMACTA:

- Therapy with PROMACTA is administered to achieve and maintain a platelet count ≥50 × 10⁹/L as necessary to reduce the risk for bleeding; PROMACTA is not used to normalize platelet counts.
- Therapy with PROMACTA may be associated with hepatobiliary laboratory abnormalities. Monitor serum liver tests (ALT, AST, and bilirubin) prior to initiation of PROMACTA, every 2 weeks during the dose adjustment phase and monthly following establishment of a stable dose. If bilirubin is elevated, perform fractionation.
- Inform patients that they should report any of the following signs and symptoms of liver problems to their healthcare provider right away.
  ○ yellowing of the skin or the whites of the eyes (jaundice),
  ○ unusual darkening of the urine,
  ○ unusual tiredness,
  ○ right upper stomach area pain.
- Following discontinuation of PROMACTA, thrombocytopenia and risk of bleeding may develop that is worse than that experienced prior to therapy with PROMACTA, particularly if PROMACTA is discontinued while the patient is on anticoagulants or antiplatelet agents.
- Therapy with PROMACTA increases the risk of reticulin fiber formation within the bone marrow, and further fiber formation may progress to marrow fibrosis. Detection of peripheral blood cell abnormalities may necessitate a bone marrow examination.
- Too much PROMACTA may result in excessive platelet counts and a risk for thrombotic/thromboembolic complications.
- PROMACTA stimulates certain bone marrow cells to make platelets and may increase the risk for progression of underlying MDS or hematological malignancies.
- Platelet counts and CBCs, including peripheral blood smears, must be performed weekly until a stable dose of PROMACTA has been achieved; thereafter, platelet counts and CBCs, including peripheral blood smears, must be performed monthly while taking PROMACTA.

- Patients must be closely monitored with weekly platelet counts and CBCs for at least 4 weeks following discontinuation of PROMACTA.
- Even during therapy with PROMACTA, patients should continue to avoid situations or medications that may increase the risk for bleeding.
- Patients must be advised to keep at least a 4-hour interval between PROMACTA and foods, mineral supplements, and antacids which contain polyvalent cations such as iron, calcium, aluminum, magnesium, selenium, and zinc.

PROMACTA is a registered trademark of GlaxoSmithKline.

GlaxoSmithKline
Research Triangle Park, NC 27709
©2009, GlaxoSmithKline. All rights reserved.

MEDICATION GUIDE
PROMACTA® (pro-MAC-ta)
(eltrombopag)
Tablets

Read the Medication Guide that comes with PROMACTA before you start taking it and each time you get a refill. There may be new information. This Medication Guide does not take the place of talking with your healthcare provider about your medical condition or treatment.

What is the most important information I should know about PROMACTA?

PROMACTA can cause uncommon but serious side effects:

- **Liver problems.** PROMACTA may damage your liver and cause serious illness and death. You must have blood tests to check your liver before you start taking PROMACTA and during treatment with PROMACTA. Your healthcare provider will order these blood tests. In some cases PROMACTA treatment may need to be stopped. Tell your healthcare provider right away if you have any of these signs and symptoms of liver problems:
  ○ yellowing of the skin or the whites of the eyes (jaundice),
  ○ unusual darkening of the urine,
  ○ unusual tiredness,
  ○ right upper stomach area pain.
- **Bone marrow changes (increased reticulin and possible bone marrow fibrosis).** Long-term use of PROMACTA may cause changes in your bone marrow. These changes may lead to abnormal blood cells or your body making less blood cells. The mild form of these bone marrow changes is called "increased reticulin." It is not known if this may progress to a more severe form called "fibrosis." The mild form may cause no problems while the severe form may cause life-threatening blood problems. Signs of bone marrow changes may show up as abnormal results in your blood tests. Your healthcare provider will decide if abnormal blood test results mean that you should have bone marrow tests or if you should stop PROMACTA.
- **Worsening low blood platelet count (thrombocytopenia) and risk of bleeding shortly after stopping PROMACTA.** When you stop taking PROMACTA, your low blood platelet count (thrombocytopenia) may become worse than before you started taking PROMACTA. These effects are most likely to happen within 4 weeks after you stop taking PROMACTA. The lower platelet counts during this time period may increase your risk of bleeding, especially if you take a blood thinner or other medicines that affects platelets. Your healthcare provider will check your blood platelet counts for at least 4 weeks after you stop taking PROMACTA. Call your healthcare provider right away to report any bruising or bleeding.
- **High platelet counts and higher chance for blood clots.** You may have a higher chance of getting a blood clot if your platelet count is too high during treatment with PROMACTA but blood clots can occur with normal or even low platelet counts. You may have severe complications or die from some forms of blood clots, such as clots that travel to the lungs or that cause heart attacks or strokes. Your healthcare provider will check your blood platelet counts, and change your dose or stop PROMACTA if your platelet counts get too high. Tell your healthcare provider right away if you have signs and symptoms of a blood clot in the leg, such as swelling, pain, or tenderness in your leg.
- **Worsening of blood cancers.** PROMACTA is not for use in patients with blood cancer or a precancerous condition called myelodysplastic syndrome (MDS). If you have one of these conditions, PROMACTA may worsen your cancer or condition and may cause you to die sooner.

When you are being treated with PROMACTA, your healthcare provider will closely monitor your dose of PROMACTA and blood tests, including platelet counts and liver tests. PROMACTA is available only through a program called "PROMACTA *CARES*". To receive PROMACTA, you must talk to your healthcare provider, understand the benefits and risks of PROMACTA and agree to enroll into PROMACTA *CARES*.

- During therapy with PROMACTA, your healthcare provider may change your dose of PROMACTA, depending

upon the change in your blood platelet count. You must have blood platelet count tests done before, during and after your therapy with PROMACTA.

- PROMACTA is used to try to keep your platelet count about 50,000 per microliter in order to lower your risk for bleeding. PROMACTA is not used to make your platelet count normal.

See "What are the possible side effects of PROMACTA?" for other side effects of PROMACTA.

What is PROMACTA?

PROMACTA is a prescription medicine used to treat low blood platelet counts in adults with chronic immune (idiopathic) thrombocytopenic purpura (ITP), when other medicines to treat your ITP or surgery to remove the spleen have not worked well enough.

PROMACTA is only:

- prescribed by healthcare providers who are enrolled in PROMACTA *CARES*.
- given to people who are enrolled in PROMACTA *CARES*.

It is not known if PROMACTA works or if it is safe in people under the age of 18 years.

PROMACTA is for treatment of certain people with low platelet counts caused by chronic ITP, not low platelet counts caused by other conditions or diseases.

What should I tell my healthcare provider before taking PROMACTA?

Tell your healthcare provider if you:

- have liver problems
- have or had a blood clot
- have a history of cataracts
- have had surgery to remove your spleen (splenectomy)
- have a bone marrow problem, including a blood cancer or Myelodysplastic Syndrome (MDS)
- have bleeding problems
- are Asian and you are of Chinese, Japanese, Taiwanese, or Korean ancestry, you may need a lower dose of PROMACTA.
- have any other medical conditions
- are pregnant, think you may be pregnant, or plan to get pregnant. It is not known if PROMACTA will harm an unborn baby.

Pregnancy Registry: There is a registry for women who become pregnant during treatment with PROMACTA. If you become pregnant, consider this registry. The purpose of the registry is to collect safety information about the health of you and your baby. Contact the registry as soon as you become aware of the pregnancy, or ask your healthcare provider to contact the registry for you. You and your healthcare provider can get information and enroll in the registry by calling 1-888-825-5249.

- are breast-feeding or plan to breast-feed. It is not known if PROMACTA passes into your breast milk. You and your healthcare provider should decide whether you will take PROMACTA or breast-feed. You should not do both.

Tell your healthcare provider about all the medicines you take, including prescription and non-prescription medicines, vitamins, and herbal products. PROMACTA may affect the way certain medicines work. Certain other medicines may affect the way PROMACTA works.

Especially tell your healthcare provider if you take:

- certain medicines used to treat high cholesterol, called "statins".
- a blood thinner medicine.

Certain medicines may keep PROMACTA from working correctly. Take PROMACTA either 4 hours before or 4 hours after taking these products:

- antacids used to treat stomach ulcers or heartburn.
- multivitamins or products that contain iron, calcium, aluminum, magnesium, selenium, and zinc which may be found in mineral supplements.

Ask your healthcare provider if you are not sure if your medicine is one that is listed above.

Know the medicines you take. Keep a list of them and show it to your healthcare provider and pharmacist when you get a new medicine.

How should I take PROMACTA?

To receive PROMACTA, you must first talk with your healthcare provider and understand the benefits and risks of PROMACTA. You must agree to and follow all of the instructions in PROMACTA *CARES*.

- Before you can begin to receive PROMACTA, your healthcare provider will:
  ○ explain PROMACTA *CARES* to you.
  ○ answer all of your questions about PROMACTA and PROMACTA *CARES*.
  ○ make sure you read this PROMACTA Medication Guide.
  ○ have you sign the PROMACTA *CARES* Patient Enrollment Form.
- Take PROMACTA exactly as your healthcare provider tells you. Do not stop using PROMACTA without talking with your healthcare provider first. Do not change your

dose or schedule for taking PROMACTA unless your healthcare provider tells you to change it.
- Take PROMACTA on an empty stomach, either 1 hour before or 2 hours after eating food.
- Take PROMACTA at least 4 hours before or 4 hours after eating dairy products and calcium fortified juices.
- If you miss a dose of PROMACTA, wait and take your next scheduled dose. Do not take more than one dose of PROMACTA in one day.
- If you take too much PROMACTA, you may have a higher chance of serious side effects. Call your healthcare provider right away.
- Your healthcare provider will check your platelet count every week and change your dose of PROMACTA as needed. This will happen every week until your healthcare provider decides that your dose of PROMACTA can stay the same. After that, you will need to have blood tests every month. When you stop taking PROMACTA, you will need to have blood tests for at least 4 weeks to check if your platelet count drops too low.
- Tell your healthcare provider about any bruising or bleeding that happens while you take and after you stop taking PROMACTA.

What should I avoid while taking PROMACTA?
Avoid situations and medicines that may increase your risk of bleeding.

What are the possible side effects of PROMACTA?
Promacta may cause serious side effects.
- **See "What is the most important information I should know about PROMACTA?".**
- **New or worsened cataracts (a clouding of the lens in the eye).** New or worsened cataracts have happened in people taking PROMACTA. Your healthcare provider will check your eyes before and during your treatment with PROMACTA. Tell your healthcare provider about any changes in your eyesight while taking PROMACTA.

The most common side effects of PROMACTA are:
- nausea
- vomiting
- heavy or longer than normal menstrual periods
- muscle aches
- abnormal skin sensations such as tingling, itching, or burning
- indigestion
- bruising
- bleeding into the tissue that covers the eye and under side of the eyelid (conjunctiva).

These are not all the possible side effects of PROMACTA. Tell your healthcare provider if you have any side effect that bothers you or that does not go away. For more information, ask your healthcare provider or pharmacist.

Call your doctor for medical advice about side effects. You may report side effects to FDA at 1-800-FDA-1088.

How should I store PROMACTA Tablets?
- Store at room temperature, 59°F to 86°F (15°C to 30°C).
- **Keep PROMACTA and all medicines out of the reach of children.**

What are the ingredients in PROMACTA?
Active Ingredient: eltrombopag olamine.
Inactive Ingredients:
- Tablet Core: Magnesium stearate, mannitol, microcrystalline cellulose, povidone, and sodium starch glycolate.
- Coating: Hypromellose, polyethylene glycol 400, titanium dioxide, and FD&C Yellow No. 6 aluminum lake (25 mg tablet), FD&C Blue No. 2 aluminum lake (50 mg tablet), or Iron Oxide Red and Iron Oxide Black (75 mg tablet).

General information about the safe and effective use of PROMACTA
Medicines are sometimes prescribed for purposes other than those listed in a Medication Guide. Do not use PROMACTA for a condition for which it was not prescribed. Do not give PROMACTA to other people even if they have the same symptoms that you have. It may harm them.
This Medication Guide summarizes the most important information about PROMACTA. If you would like more information, talk with your healthcare provider. You can ask your healthcare provider or pharmacist for information about PROMACTA that is written for healthcare professionals. For more information you can call toll-free 1-888-825-5249.
PROMACTA is a registered trademark of GlaxoSmithKline.
This Medication Guide has been approved by the U.S. Food and Drug Administration.
GlaxoSmithKline
Research Triangle Park, NC 27709
©2010, GlaxoSmithKline. All rights reserved.
Revised: March 2010
PRM:3MG

RELENZA®   ℞
[rə-lin'zə]
(zanamivir)
Inhalation Powder, for oral inhalation

HIGHLIGHTS OF PRESCRIBING INFORMATION
These highlights do not include all the information needed to use RELENZA safely and effectively. See full prescribing information for RELENZA.
RELENZA (zanamivir) Inhalation Powder, for oral inhalation
Initial U.S. Approval: 1999
————————INDICATIONS AND USAGE————————
RELENZA, an influenza neuraminidase inhibitor, is indicated for:
Treatment of influenza in patients 7 years of age and older who have been symptomatic for no more than 2 days. (1.1)
Prophylaxis of influenza in patients 5 years of age and older. (1.2)
Important Limitations on Use of RELENZA:
Not recommended for treatment or prophylaxis of influenza in:
- Individuals with underlying airways disease. (5.1)

Not proven effective for:
- Treatment in individuals with underlying airways disease. (1.3)
- Prophylaxis in nursing home residents. (1.3)

Not a substitute for annual influenza vaccination. (1.3)
Consider available information on influenza drug susceptibility patterns and treatment effects when deciding whether to use RELENZA. (1.3)
————————DOSAGE AND ADMINISTRATION————————

Indication	Dose
Treatment of Influenza (2.2)	10 mg twice daily for 5 days
Prophylaxis: (2.3) Household Setting	10 mg once daily for 10 days
Community Outbreaks	10 mg once daily for 28 days

Note: The 10 mg dose is provided by 2 inhalations (one 5 mg blister per inhalation). (2.1)
————————DOSAGE FORMS AND STRENGTHS————————
Blister for oral inhalation: 5 mg. Four 5 mg blisters of powder on a ROTADISK® for oral inhalation via DISKHALER®. Packaged in carton containing 5 ROTADISKs (total of 10 doses) and 1 DISKHALER inhalation device. (3)
————————CONTRAINDICATIONS————————
Do not use in patients with history of allergic reaction to any ingredient of RELENZA, including lactose (which contains milk proteins). (4)
————————WARNINGS AND PRECAUTIONS————————
- **Bronchospasm:** Serious, sometimes fatal, cases have occurred. Not recommended in individuals with underlying airways disease. Discontinue RELENZA if bronchospasm or decline in respiratory function develops. (5.1)
- **Allergic Reactions:** Discontinue RELENZA and initiate appropriate treatment if an allergic reaction occurs or is suspected. (5.2)
- **Neuropsychiatric Events:** Patients with influenza, particularly pediatric patients, may be at an increased risk of seizures, confusion, or abnormal behavior early in their illness. Monitor for signs of abnormal behavior. (5.3)
- **High-risk Underlying Medical Conditions:** Safety and effectiveness have not been demonstrated in these patients. (5.4)

————————ADVERSE REACTIONS————————
The most common adverse events reported in >1.5% of patients treated with RELENZA and more commonly than in patients treated with placebo are:
- Treatment Studies – sinusitis, dizziness.
- Prophylaxis Studies – fever and/or chills, arthralgia and articular rheumatism. (6.1)

To report SUSPECTED ADVERSE REACTIONS, contact GlaxoSmithKline at 1-888-825-5249 or FDA at 1-800-FDA-1088 or www.fda.gov/medwatch.
————————DRUG INTERACTIONS————————
Live attenuated influenza vaccine, intranasal (7):
- Do not administer until 48 hours following cessation of RELENZA.
- Do not administer RELENZA until 2 weeks following administration of the live attenuated influenza vaccine, unless medically indicated.

Revised: March 2010
See 17 for PATIENT COUNSELING INFORMATION and FDA-approved patient labeling
Revised: 03/2010

FULL PRESCRIBING INFORMATION: CONTENTS*
1   INDICATIONS AND USAGE
  1.1   Treatment of Influenza

* Sections or subsections omitted from the full prescribing information are not listed

FULL PRESCRIBING INFORMATION

1   INDICATIONS AND USAGE
1.1   Treatment of Influenza
RELENZA® (zanamivir) Inhalation Powder is indicated for treatment of uncomplicated acute illness due to influenza A and B virus in adults and pediatric patients 7 years of age and older who have been symptomatic for no more than 2 days.
1.2   Prophylaxis of Influenza
RELENZA is indicated for prophylaxis of influenza in adults and pediatric patients 5 years of age and older.
1.3   Important Limitations on Use of RELENZA
- RELENZA is not recommended for treatment or prophylaxis of influenza in individuals with underlying airways disease (such as asthma or chronic obstructive pulmonary disease) due to risk of serious bronchospasm [see Warnings and Precautions (5.1)].
- RELENZA has not been proven effective for treatment of influenza in individuals with underlying airways disease.
- RELENZA has not been proven effective for prophylaxis of influenza in the nursing home setting.
- RELENZA is not a substitute for early influenza vaccination on an annual basis as recommended by the Centers for Disease Control's Immunization Practices Advisory Committee.
- Influenza viruses change over time. Emergence of resistance mutations could decrease drug effectiveness. Other factors (for example, changes in viral virulence) might also diminish clinical benefit of antiviral drugs. Prescribers should consider available information on influenza drug susceptibility patterns and treatment effects when deciding whether to use RELENZA.
- There is no evidence for efficacy of zanamivir in any illness caused by agents other than influenza virus A and B.
- Patients should be advised that the use of RELENZA for treatment of influenza has not been shown to reduce the risk of transmission of influenza to others.

2   DOSAGE AND ADMINISTRATION
2.1   Dosing Considerations
- RELENZA is for administration to the respiratory tract by oral inhalation only, using the DISKHALER device provided.
- The 10 mg dose is provided by 2 inhalations (one 5 mg blister per inhalation).
- Patients should be instructed in the use of the delivery system. Instructions should include a demonstration whenever possible. If RELENZA is prescribed for

children, it should be used only under adult supervision and instruction, and the supervising adult should first be instructed by a healthcare professional [see Patient Counseling Information (17.4)].

- Patients scheduled to use an inhaled bronchodilator at the same time as RELENZA should use their bronchodilator before taking RELENZA [see Patient Counseling Information (17.2)].

2.2 Treatment of Influenza

- The recommended dose of RELENZA for treatment of influenza in adults and pediatric patients 7 years of age and older is 10 mg twice daily (approximately 12 hours apart) for 5 days.
- Two doses should be taken on the first day of treatment whenever possible provided there is at least 2 hours between doses.
- On subsequent days, doses should be about 12 hours apart (e.g., morning and evening) at approximately the same time each day.
- The safety and efficacy of repeated treatment courses have not been studied.

2.3 Prophylaxis of Influenza

Household Setting:

- The recommended dose of RELENZA for prophylaxis of influenza in adults and pediatric patients 5 years of age and older in a household setting is 10 mg once daily for 10 days.
- The dose should be administered at approximately the same time each day.
- There are no data on the effectiveness of prophylaxis with RELENZA in a household setting when initiated more than 1.5 days after the onset of signs or symptoms in the index case.

Community Outbreaks:

- The recommended dose of RELENZA for prophylaxis of influenza in adults and adolescents in a community setting is 10 mg once daily for 28 days.
- The dose should be administered at approximately the same time each day.
- There are no data on the effectiveness of prophylaxis with RELENZA in a community outbreak when initiated more than 5 days after the outbreak was identified in the community.
- The safety and effectiveness of prophylaxis with RELENZA have not been evaluated for longer than 28 days' duration.

3 DOSAGE FORMS AND STRENGTHS

Blister for oral inhalation: 5 mg. Four 5 mg blisters of powder on a ROTADISK for oral inhalation via DISKHALER. Packaged in carton containing 5 ROTADISKs (total of 10 doses) and 1 DISKHALER inhalation device [see How Supplied/Storage and Handling (16)].

4 CONTRAINDICATIONS

Do not use in patients with history of allergic reaction to any ingredient of RELENZA including lactose (which contains milk proteins) [see Warnings and Precautions (5.2), Description (11)].

5 WARNINGS AND PRECAUTIONS

5.1 Bronchospasm

RELENZA is not recommended for treatment or prophylaxis of influenza in individuals with underlying airways disease (such as asthma or chronic obstructive pulmonary disease).

Serious cases of bronchospasm, including fatalities, have been reported during treatment with RELENZA in patients with and without underlying airways disease. Many of these cases were reported during postmarketing and causality was difficult to assess.

RELENZA should be discontinued in any patient who develops bronchospasm or decline in respiratory function; immediate treatment and hospitalization may be required.

Some patients without prior pulmonary disease may also have respiratory abnormalities from acute respiratory infection that could resemble adverse drug reactions or increase patient vulnerability to adverse drug reactions.

Bronchospasm was documented following administration of zanamivir in 1 of 13 patients with mild or moderate asthma (but without acute influenza-like illness) in a Phase I study. In a Phase III study in patients with acute influenza-like illness superimposed on underlying asthma or chronic obstructive pulmonary disease, 10% (24 of 244) of patients on zanamivir and 9% (22 of 237) on placebo experienced a greater than 20% decline in FEV$_1$ following treatment for 5 days.

If use of RELENZA is considered for a patient with underlying airways disease, the potential risks and benefits should be carefully weighed. If a decision is made to prescribe RELENZA for such a patient, this should be done only under conditions of careful monitoring of respiratory

function, close observation, and appropriate supportive care including availability of fast-acting bronchodilators.

5.2 Allergic Reactions

Allergic-like reactions, including oropharyngeal edema, serious skin rashes, and anaphylaxis have been reported in postmarketing experience with RELENZA. RELENZA should be stopped and appropriate treatment instituted if an allergic reaction occurs or is suspected.

5.3 Neuropsychiatric Events

Influenza can be associated with a variety of neurologic and behavioral symptoms which can include events such as seizures, hallucinations, delirium, and abnormal behavior, in some cases resulting in fatal outcomes. These events may occur in the setting of encephalitis or encephalopathy but can occur without obvious severe disease.

There have been postmarketing reports (mostly from Japan) of delirium and abnormal behavior leading to injury in patients with influenza who were receiving neuraminidase inhibitors, including RELENZA. Because these events were reported voluntarily during clinical practice, estimates of frequency cannot be made, but they appear to be uncommon based on usage data for RELENZA. These events were reported primarily among pediatric patients and often had an abrupt onset and rapid resolution. The contribution of RELENZA to these events has not been established. Patients with influenza should be closely monitored for signs of abnormal behavior. If neuropsychiatric symptoms occur, the risks and benefits of continuing treatment should be evaluated for each patient.

5.4 Limitations of Populations Studied

Safety and efficacy have not been demonstrated in patients with high-risk underlying medical conditions. No information is available regarding treatment of influenza in patients with any medical condition sufficiently severe or unstable to be considered at imminent risk of requiring inpatient management.

5.5 Bacterial Infections

Serious bacterial infections may begin with influenza-like symptoms or may coexist with or occur as complications during the course of influenza. RELENZA has not been shown to prevent such complications.

5.6 Importance of Proper Use of DISKHALER

Effective and safe use of RELENZA requires proper use of the DISKHALER to inhale the drug. Prescribers should carefully evaluate the ability of young children to use the delivery system if use of RELENZA is considered [see Use in Specific Populations (8.4)].

6 ADVERSE REACTIONS

See Warnings and Precautions for information about risk of serious adverse events such as bronchospasm (5.1) and allergic-like reactions (5.2), and for safety information in patients with underlying airways disease (5.1).

6.1 Clinical Trials Experience

Because clinical trials are conducted under widely varying conditions, adverse reaction rates observed in the clinical trials of a drug cannot be directly compared with rates in the clinical trials of another drug and may not reflect the rates observed in practice.

The placebo used in clinical studies consisted of inhaled lactose powder, which is also the vehicle for the active drug; therefore, some adverse events occurring at similar frequencies in different treatment groups could be related to lactose vehicle inhalation.

Treatment of Influenza: Clinical Trials in Adults and Adolescents: Adverse events that occurred with an incidence ≥1.5% in treatment studies are listed in Table 1. This table shows adverse events occurring in patients ≥12 years of age receiving RELENZA 10 mg inhaled twice daily, RELENZA in all inhalation regimens, and placebo inhaled twice daily (where placebo consisted of the same lactose vehicle used in RELENZA).

Table 1. Summary of Adverse Events ≥1.5% Incidence During Treatment in Adults and Adolescents

Adverse Event	RELENZA 10 mg b.i.d. Inhaled (n = 1,132)	RELENZA All Dosing Regimens[a] (n = 2,289)	Placebo (Lactose Vehicle) (n = 1,520)
Body as a whole			
Headaches	2%	2%	3%
Digestive			
Diarrhea	3%	3%	4%
Nausea	3%	3%	3%
Vomiting	1%	1%	2%
Respiratory			
Nasal signs and symptoms	2%	3%	3%
Bronchitis	2%	2%	3%
Cough	2%	2%	3%
Sinusitis	3%	2%	2%
Ear, nose, and throat infections	2%	1%	2%
Nervous system			
Dizziness	2%	1%	<1%

[a] Includes studies where RELENZA was administered intranasally (6.4 mg 2 to 4 times per day in addition to inhaled preparation) and/or inhaled more frequently (q.i.d.) than the currently recommended dose.

Additional adverse reactions occurring in less than 1.5% of patients receiving RELENZA included malaise, fatigue, fever, abdominal pain, myalgia, arthralgia, and urticaria. The most frequent laboratory abnormalities in Phase III treatment studies included elevations of liver enzymes and CPK, lymphopenia, and neutropenia. These were reported in similar proportions of zanamivir and lactose vehicle placebo recipients with acute influenza-like illness.

Clinical Trials in Pediatric Patients: Adverse events that occurred with an incidence ≥1.5% in children receiving treatment doses of RELENZA in 2 Phase III studies are listed in Table 2. This table shows adverse events occurring in pediatric patients 5 to 12 years old receiving RELENZA 10 mg inhaled twice daily and placebo inhaled twice daily (where placebo consisted of the same lactose vehicle used in RELENZA).

Table 2. Summary of Adverse Events ≥1.5% Incidence During Treatment in Pediatric Patients[a]

Adverse Event	RELENZA 10 mg b.i.d. Inhaled (n = 291)	Placebo (Lactose Vehicle) (n = 318)
Respiratory		
Ear, nose, and throat infections	5%	5%
Ear, nose, and throat hemorrhage	<1%	2%
Asthma	<1%	2%
Cough	<1%	2%
Digestive		
Vomiting	2%	3%
Diarrhea	2%	2%
Nausea	<1%	2%

[a] Includes a subset of patients receiving RELENZA for treatment of influenza in a prophylaxis study.

In 1 of the 2 studies described in Table 2, some additional information is available from children (5 to 12 years old) without acute influenza-like illness who received an investigational prophylaxis regimen of RELENZA; 132 children received RELENZA and 145 children received placebo. Among these children, nasal signs and symptoms (zanamivir 20%, placebo 9%), cough (zanamivir 16%, placebo 8%), and throat/tonsil discomfort and pain (zanamivir 11%, placebo 6%) were reported more frequently with RELENZA than placebo. In a subset with chronic pulmonary disease, lower respiratory adverse events (described as asthma, cough, or viral respiratory infections which could include influenza-like symptoms) were reported in 7 of 7 zanamivir recipients and 5 of 12 placebo recipients.

Prophylaxis of Influenza: Family/Household Prophylaxis Studies: Adverse events that occurred with an incidence of ≥1.5% in the 2 prophylaxis studies are listed in Table 3. This table shows adverse events occurring in patients ≥5 years of age receiving RELENZA 10 mg inhaled once daily for 10 days.

Table 3. Summary of Adverse Events ≥1.5% Incidence During 10-Day Prophylaxis Studies in Adults, Adolescents, and Children[a]

Adverse Event	Contact Cases	
	RELENZA (n = 1,068)	Placebo (n = 1,059)
Lower respiratory		
Viral respiratory infections	13%	19%
Cough	7%	9%
Neurologic		
Headaches	13%	14%
Ear, nose, and throat		
Nasal signs and symptoms	12%	12%
Throat and tonsil discomfort and pain	8%	9%

Nasal inflammation	1%	2%
Musculoskeletal		
Muscle pain	3%	3%
Endocrine and metabolic		
Feeding problems (decreased or increased appetite and anorexia)	2%	2%
Gastrointestinal		
Nausea and vomiting	1%	2%
Non-site specific		
Malaise and fatigue	5%	5%
Temperature regulation disturbances (fever and/or chills)	5%	4%

[a] In prophylaxis studies, symptoms associated with influenza-like illness were captured as adverse events; subjects were enrolled during a winter respiratory season during which time any symptoms that occurred were captured as adverse events.

Community Prophylaxis Studies: Adverse events that occurred with an incidence of ≥1.5% in 2 prophylaxis studies are listed in Table 4. This table shows adverse events occurring in patients ≥5 years of age receiving RELENZA 10 mg inhaled once daily for 28 days.

Table 4. Summary of Adverse Events ≥1.5% Incidence During 28-Day Prophylaxis Studies in Adults, Adolescents, and Children[a]

Adverse Event	RELENZA (n = 2,231)	Placebo (n = 2,239)
Neurologic		
Headaches	24%	26%
Ear, nose, and throat		
Throat and tonsil discomfort and pain	19%	20%
Nasal signs and symptoms	12%	13%
Ear, nose, and throat infections	2%	2%
Lower respiratory		
Cough	17%	18%
Viral respiratory infections	3%	4%
Musculoskeletal		
Muscle pain	8%	8%
Musculoskeletal pain	6%	6%
Arthralgia and articular rheumatism	2%	<1%
Endocrine and metabolic		
Feeding problems (decreased or increased appetite and anorexia)	4%	4%
Gastrointestinal		
Nausea and vomiting	2%	3%
Diarrhea	2%	2%
Non-site specific		
Temperature regulation disturbances (fever and/or chills)	9%	10%
Malaise and fatigue	8%	8%

[a] In prophylaxis studies, symptoms associated with influenza-like illness were captured as adverse events; subjects were enrolled during a winter respiratory season during which time any symptoms that occurred were captured as adverse events.

6.2 Postmarketing Experience

In addition to adverse events reported from clinical trials, the following events have been identified during post-marketing use of zanamivir (RELENZA). Because they are reported voluntarily from a population of unknown size, estimates of frequency cannot be made. These events have been chosen for inclusion due to a combination of their seriousness, frequency of reporting, or potential causal connection to zanamivir (RELENZA).

Allergic Reactions: Allergic or allergic-like reaction, including oropharyngeal edema *[see Warnings and Precautions (5.2)]*.

Psychiatric: Delirium, including symptoms such as altered level of consciousness, confusion, abnormal behavior, delusions, hallucinations, agitation, anxiety, nightmares *[see Warnings and Precautions (5.3)]*.

Cardiac: Arrhythmias, syncope.

Neurologic: Seizures.

Respiratory: Bronchospasm, dyspnea *[see Warnings and Precautions (5.1)]*.

Skin: Facial edema; rash, including serious cutaneous reactions (e.g., erythema multiforme, Stevens-Johnson syndrome, toxic epidermal necrolysis); urticaria *[see Warnings and Precautions (5.2)]*.

7 DRUG INTERACTIONS

Zanamivir is not a substrate nor does it affect cytochrome P450 (CYP) isoenzymes (CYP1A1/2, 2A6, 2C9, 2C18, 2D6, 2E1, and 3A4) in human liver microsomes. No clinically significant pharmacokinetic drug interactions are predicted based on data from in vitro studies.

The concurrent use of RELENZA with live attenuated influenza vaccine (LAIV) intranasal has not been evaluated. However, because of potential interference between these products, LAIV should not be administered within 2 weeks before or 48 hours after administration of RELENZA, unless medically indicated. The concern about possible interference arises from the potential for antiviral drugs to inhibit replication of live vaccine virus.

Trivalent inactivated influenza vaccine can be administered at any time relative to use of RELENZA *[see Clinical Pharmacology (12.4)]*.

8 USE IN SPECIFIC POPULATIONS

8.1 Pregnancy

Pregnancy Category C. There are no adequate and well-controlled studies of zanamivir in pregnant women. Zanamivir should be used during pregnancy only if the potential benefit justifies the potential risk to the fetus.

Embryo/fetal development studies were conducted in rats (dosed from days 6 to 15 of pregnancy) and rabbits (dosed from days 7 to 19 of pregnancy) using the same IV doses (1, 9, and 90 mg/kg/day). Pre- and post-natal developmental studies were performed in rats (dosed from day 16 of pregnancy until litter day 21 to 23). No malformations, maternal toxicity, or embryotoxicity were observed in pregnant rats or rabbits and their fetuses. Because of insufficient blood sampling timepoints in rat and rabbit reproductive toxicity studies, AUC values were not available. In a subchronic study in rats at the 90 mg/kg/day IV dose, the AUC values were greater than 300 times the human exposure at the proposed clinical dose.

An additional embryo/fetal study, in a different strain of rat, was conducted using subcutaneous administration of zanamivir, 3 times daily, at doses of 1, 9, or 80 mg/kg during days 7 to 17 of pregnancy. There was an increase in the incidence rates of a variety of minor skeleton alterations and variants in the exposed offspring in this study. Based on AUC measurements, the 80 mg/kg dose produced an exposure greater than 1,000 times the human exposure at the proposed clinical dose. However, in most instances, the individual incidence rate of each skeletal alteration or variant remained within the background rates of the historical occurrence in the strain studied.

Zanamivir has been shown to cross the placenta in rats and rabbits. In these animals, fetal blood concentrations of zanamivir were significantly lower than zanamivir concentrations in the maternal blood.

8.3 Nursing Mothers

Studies in rats have demonstrated that zanamivir is excreted in milk. However, nursing mothers should be instructed that it is not known whether zanamivir is excreted in human milk. Because many drugs are excreted in human milk, caution should be exercised when RELENZA is administered to a nursing mother.

8.4 Pediatric Use

Treatment of Influenza: Safety and effectiveness of RELENZA for treatment of influenza have not been assessed in pediatric patients less than 7 years of age, but were studied in a Phase III treatment study in pediatric patients, where 471 children 5 to 12 years of age received zanamivir or placebo *[see Clinical Studies (14.1)]*. Adolescents were included in the 3 principal Phase III adult treatment studies. In these studies, 67 patients were 12 to 16 years of age. No definite differences in safety and efficacy were observed between these adolescent patients and young adults.

In a Phase I study of 16 children ages 6 to 12 years with signs and symptoms of respiratory disease, 4 did not produce a measurable peak inspiratory flow rate (PIFR) through the DISKHALER (3 with no adequate inhalation on request, 1 with missing data), 9 had measurable PIFR on each of 2 inhalations, and 3 achieved measurable PIFR on only 1 of 2 inhalations. Neither of two 6-year-olds and one of two 7-year-olds produced measurable PIFR. Overall, 8 of the 16 children (including all those under 8 years old) either did not produce measurable inspiratory flow through the DISKHALER or produced peak inspiratory flow rates below the 60 L/min considered optimal for the device under standardized in vitro testing; lack of measurable flow rate was related to low or undetectable serum concentrations *[see Clinical Pharmacology (12.3), Clinical Studies (14.1)]*. Prescribers should carefully evaluate the ability of young children to use the delivery system if prescription of RELENZA is considered.

Prophylaxis of Influenza: The safety and effectiveness of RELENZA for prophylaxis of influenza have been studied in 4 Phase III studies where 273 children 5 to 11 years of age and 239 adolescents 12 to 16 years of age received RELENZA. No differences in safety and effectiveness were observed between pediatric and adult subjects *[see Clinical Studies (14.2)]*.

8.5 Geriatric Use

Of the total number of patients in 6 clinical studies of RELENZA for treatment of influenza, 59 patients were 65 years of age and older, while 24 patients were 75 years of age and older. Of the total number of patients in 4 clinical studies of RELENZA for prophylaxis of influenza in households and community settings, 954 patients were 65 years of age and older, while 347 patients were 75 years of age and older. No overall differences in safety or effectiveness were observed between these patients and younger patients, and other reported clinical experience has not identified differences in responses between the elderly and younger patients, but greater sensitivity of some older individuals cannot be ruled out. Elderly patients may need assistance with use of the device.

In 2 additional studies of RELENZA for prophylaxis of influenza in the nursing home setting, efficacy was not demonstrated *[see Indications and Usage (1.3)]*.

10 OVERDOSAGE

There have been no reports of overdosage from administration of RELENZA.

11 DESCRIPTION

The active component of RELENZA is zanamivir. The chemical name of zanamivir is 5-(acetylamino)-4-[(aminoiminomethyl)-amino]-2,6-anhydro-3,4,5-trideoxy-D-glycero-D-galacto-non-2-enonic acid. It has a molecular formula of $C_{12}H_{20}N_4O_7$ and a molecular weight of 332.3. It has the following structural formula:

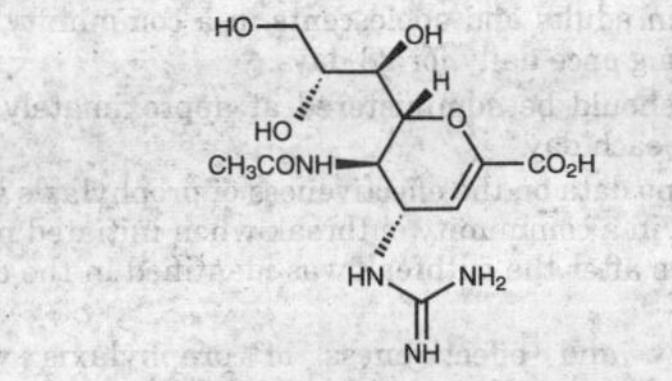

Zanamivir is a white to off-white powder for oral inhalation with a solubility of approximately 18 mg/mL in water at 20°C.

RELENZA is for administration to the respiratory tract by oral inhalation only. Each RELENZA ROTADISK contains 4 regularly spaced double-foil blisters with each blister containing a powder mixture of 5 mg of zanamivir and 20 mg of lactose (which contains milk proteins). The contents of each blister are inhaled using a specially designed breath-activated plastic device for inhaling powder called the DISKHALER. After a RELENZA ROTADISK is loaded into the DISKHALER, a blister that contains medication is pierced and the zanamivir is dispersed into the air stream created when the patient inhales through the mouthpiece. The amount of drug delivered to the respiratory tract will depend on patient factors such as inspiratory flow. Under standardized in vitro testing, RELENZA ROTADISK delivers 4 mg of zanamivir from the DISKHALER device when tested at a pressure drop of 3 kPa (corresponding to a flow rate of about 62 to 65 L/min) for 3 seconds.

12 CLINICAL PHARMACOLOGY

12.1 Mechanism of Action

Zanamivir is an antiviral drug *[see Clinical Pharmacology (12.4)]*.

12.3 Pharmacokinetics

Absorption and Bioavailability: Pharmacokinetic studies of orally inhaled zanamivir indicate that approximately 4% to 17% of the inhaled dose is systemically absorbed. The peak serum concentrations ranged from 17 to 142 ng/mL within 1 to 2 hours following a 10 mg dose. The area under the serum concentration versus time curve (AUC_∞) ranged from 111 to 1,364 ng•hr/mL.

Distribution: Zanamivir has limited plasma protein binding (<10%).

Metabolism: Zanamivir is renally excreted as unchanged drug. No metabolites have been detected in humans.

Elimination: The serum half-life of zanamivir following administration by oral inhalation ranges from 2.5 to 5.1 hours. It is excreted unchanged in the urine with excretion of a single dose completed within 24 hours. Total clearance ranges from 2.5 to 10.9 L/hr. Unabsorbed drug is excreted in the feces.

Impaired Hepatic Function: The pharmacokinetics of zanamivir have not been studied in patients with impaired hepatic function.

Impaired Renal Function: After a single intravenous dose of 4 mg or 2 mg of zanamivir in volunteers with mild/moderate or severe renal impairment, respectively, significant decreases in renal clearance (and hence total clearance: normals 5.3 L/hr, mild/moderate 2.7 L/hr, and severe 0.8 L/hr; median values) and significant increases in half-life (normals 3.1 hr, mild/moderate 4.7 hr, and severe 18.5 hr; median values) and systemic exposure were observed. Safety and efficacy have not been documented in the presence of severe renal insufficiency. Due to the low systemic bioavailability of zanamivir following oral inhalation, no dosage adjustments are necessary in patients with renal impairment. However, the potential for drug accumulation should be considered.

Pediatric Patients: The pharmacokinetics of zanamivir were evaluated in pediatric patients with signs and symptoms of respiratory illness. Sixteen patients, 6 to 12 years of age, received a single dose of 10 mg zanamivir dry powder via DISKHALER. Five patients had either undetectable zanamivir serum concentrations or had low drug concentrations (8.32 to 10.38 ng/mL) that were not detectable after 1.5 hours. Eleven patients had C_{max} median values of 43 ng/mL (range 15 to 74) and AUC_{∞} median values of 167 ng•hr/mL (range 58 to 279). Low or undetectable serum concentrations were related to lack of measurable PIFR in individual patients *[see Use in Specific Populations (8.4), Clinical Studies (14.1)]*.

Geriatric Patients: The pharmacokinetics of zanamivir have not been studied in patients over 65 years of age *[see Use in Specific Populations (8.5)]*.

Gender, Race, and Weight: In a population pharmacokinetic analysis in patient studies, no clinically significant differences in serum concentrations and/or pharmacokinetic parameters (V/F, CL/F, ka, AUC_{0-3}, C_{max}, T_{max}, CLr, and % excreted in urine) were observed when demographic variables (gender, age, race, and weight) and indices of infection (laboratory evidence of infection, overall symptoms, symptoms of upper respiratory illness, and viral titers) were considered. There were no significant correlations between measures of systemic exposure and safety parameters.

12.4 Microbiology

Mechanism of Action: Zanamivir is an inhibitor of influenza virus neuraminidase affecting release of viral particles.

Antiviral Activity: The antiviral activity of zanamivir against laboratory and clinical isolates of influenza virus was determined in cell culture assays. The concentrations of zanamivir required for inhibition of influenza virus were highly variable depending on the assay method used and virus isolate tested. The 50% and 90% effective concentrations (EC_{50} and EC_{90}) of zanamivir were in the range of 0.005 to 16.0 µM and 0.05 to >100 µM, respectively (1 µM = 0.33 mcg/mL). The relationship between the cell culture inhibition of influenza virus by zanamivir and the inhibition of influenza virus replication in humans has not been established.

Resistance: Influenza viruses with reduced susceptibility to zanamivir have been selected in cell culture by multiple passages of the virus in the presence of increasing concentrations of the drug. Genetic analysis of these viruses showed that the reduced susceptibility in cell culture to zanamivir is associated with mutations that result in amino acid changes in the viral neuraminidase or viral hemagglutinin or both. Resistance mutations selected in cell culture which result in neuraminidase amino acid substitutions include E119G/A/D and R292K. Mutations selected in cell culture in hemagglutinin include: K68R, G75E, E114K, N145S, S165N, S186F, N199S, and K222T.

In an immunocompromised patient infected with influenza B virus, a variant virus emerged after treatment with an investigational nebulized solution of zanamivir for 2 weeks. Analysis of this variant showed a hemagglutinin substitution (T198I) which resulted in a reduced affinity for human cell receptors, and a substitution in the neuraminidase active site (R152K) which reduced the enzyme's activity to zanamivir by 1,000-fold. Insufficient information is available to characterize the risk of emergence of zanamivir resistance in clinical use.

Cross-Resistance: Cross-resistance has been observed between some zanamivir-resistant and some oseltamivir-resistant influenza virus mutants generated in cell culture. However, some of the in cell culture zanamivir-induced resistance mutations, E119G/A/D and R292K, occurred at the same neuraminidase amino acid positions as in the clinical isolates resistant to oseltamivir, E119V and R292K. No studies have been performed to assess risk of emergence of cross-resistance during clinical use.

Influenza Vaccine Interaction Study: An interaction study (n = 138) was conducted to evaluate the effects of zanamivir (10 mg once daily) on the serological response to a single dose of trivalent inactivated influenza vaccine, as measured by hemagglutination inhibition titers. There was no difference in hemagglutination inhibition antibody titers at 2 weeks and 4 weeks after vaccine administration between zanamivir and placebo recipients.

Influenza Challenge Studies: Antiviral activity of zanamivir was supported for infection with influenza A virus, and to a more limited extent for infection with influenza B virus, by Phase I studies in volunteers who received intranasal inoculations of challenge strains of influenza virus, and received an intranasal formulation of zanamivir or placebo starting before or shortly after viral inoculation.

13 NONCLINICAL TOXICOLOGY

13.1 Carcinogenesis, Mutagenesis, Impairment of Fertility

Carcinogenesis: In 2-year carcinogenicity studies conducted in rats and mice using a powder formulation administered through inhalation, zanamivir induced no statistically significant increases in tumors over controls. The maximum daily exposures in rats and mice were approximately 23 to 25 and 20 to 22 times, respectively, greater than those in humans at the proposed clinical dose based on AUC comparisons.

Mutagenesis: Zanamivir was not mutagenic in in vitro and in vivo genotoxicity assays which included bacterial mutation assays in *S. typhimurium* and *E. coli*, mammalian mutation assays in mouse lymphoma, chromosomal aberration assays in human peripheral blood lymphocytes, and the in vivo mouse bone marrow micronucleus assay.

Impairment of Fertility: The effects of zanamivir on fertility and general reproductive performance were investigated in male (dosed for 10 weeks prior to mating, and throughout mating, gestation/lactation, and shortly after weaning) and female rats (dosed for 3 weeks prior to mating through Day 19 of pregnancy, or Day 21 post partum) at IV doses 1, 9, and 90 mg/kg/day. Zanamivir did not impair mating or fertility of male or female rats, and did not affect the sperm of treated male rats. The reproductive performance of the F1 generation born to female rats given zanamivir was not affected. Based on a subchronic study in rats at a 90 mg/kg/day IV dose, AUC values ranged between 142 and 199 mcg•hr/mL (>300 times the human exposure at the proposed clinical dose).

14 CLINICAL STUDIES

14.1 Treatment of Influenza

Adults and Adolescents: The efficacy of RELENZA 10 mg inhaled twice daily for 5 days in the treatment of influenza has been evaluated in placebo-controlled studies conducted in North America, the Southern Hemisphere, and Europe during their respective influenza seasons. The magnitude of treatment effect varied between studies, with possible relationships to population-related factors including amount of symptomatic relief medication used.

Populations Studied: The principal Phase III studies enrolled 1,588 patients ages 12 years and older (median age 34 years, 49% male, 91% Caucasian), with uncomplicated influenza-like illness within 2 days of symptom onset. Influenza was confirmed by culture, hemagglutination inhibition antibodies, or investigational direct tests. Of 1,164 patients with confirmed influenza, 89% had influenza A and 11% had influenza B. These studies served as the principal basis for efficacy evaluation, with more limited Phase II studies providing supporting information where necessary. Following randomization to either zanamivir or placebo (inhaled lactose vehicle), all patients received instruction and supervision by a healthcare professional for the initial dose.

Principal Results: The definition of time to improvement in major symptoms of influenza included no fever and self-assessment of "none" or "mild" for headache, myalgia, cough, and sore throat. A Phase II and a Phase III study conducted in North America (total of over 600 influenza-positive patients) suggested up to 1 day of shortening of median time to this defined improvement in symptoms in patients receiving zanamivir compared with placebo, although statistical significance was not reached in either of these studies. In a study conducted in the Southern Hemisphere (321 influenza-positive patients), a 1.5-day difference in median time to symptom improvement was observed. Additional evidence of efficacy was provided by the European study.

Other Findings: There was no consistent difference in treatment effect in patients with influenza A compared with influenza B; however, these trials enrolled smaller numbers of patients with influenza B and thus provided less evidence in support of efficacy in influenza B.

In general, patients with lower temperature (e.g., 38.2°C or less) or investigator-rated as having less severe symptoms at entry derived less benefit from therapy.

No consistent treatment effect was demonstrated in patients with underlying chronic medical conditions, including respiratory or cardiovascular disease *[see Warnings and Precautions (5.4)]*.

No consistent differences in rate of development of complications were observed between treatment groups.

Some fluctuation of symptoms was observed after the primary study endpoint in both treatment groups.

Pediatric Patients: The efficacy of RELENZA 10 mg inhaled twice daily for 5 days in the treatment of influenza in pediatric patients has been evaluated in a placebo-controlled study conducted in North America and Europe, enrolling 471 patients, ages 5 to 12 years (55% male, 90% Caucasian), within 36 hours of symptom onset. Of 346 patients with confirmed influenza, 65% had influenza A and 35% had influenza B. The definition of time to improvement included no fever and parental assessment of no or mild cough and absent/minimal muscle and joint aches or pains, sore throat, chills/feverishness, and headache. Median time to symptom improvement was 1 day shorter in patients receiving zanamivir compared with placebo. No consistent differences in rate of development of complications were observed between treatment groups. Some fluctuation of symptoms was observed after the primary study endpoint in both treatment groups.

Although this study was designed to enroll children ages 5 to 12 years, the product is indicated only for children 7 years of age and older. This evaluation is based on the combination of lower estimates of treatment effect in 5- and 6-year-olds compared with the overall study population, and evidence of inadequate inhalation through the DISKHALER in a pharmacokinetic study *[see Use in Specific Populations (8.4), Clinical Pharmacology (12.3)]*.

14.2 Prophylaxis of Influenza

The efficacy of RELENZA in preventing naturally occurring influenza illness has been demonstrated in 2 post-exposure prophylaxis studies in households and 2 seasonal prophylaxis studies during community outbreaks of influenza. The primary efficacy endpoint in these studies was the incidence of symptomatic, laboratory-confirmed influenza, defined as the presence of 2 or more of the following symptoms: oral temperature ≥100°F/37.8°C or feverishness, cough, headache, sore throat, and myalgia; and laboratory confirmation of influenza A or B by culture, PCR, or seroconversion (defined as a 4-fold increase in convalescent antibody titer from baseline).

Household Prophylaxis Studies: Two studies assessed post-exposure prophylaxis in household contacts of an index case. Within 1.5 days of onset of symptoms in an index case, each household (including all family members ≥5 years of age) was randomized to RELENZA 10 mg inhaled once daily or placebo inhaled once daily for 10 days. In the first study only, each index case was randomized to RELENZA 10 mg inhaled twice daily for 5 days or inhaled placebo twice daily for 5 days. In this study, the proportion of households with at least 1 new case of symptomatic laboratory-confirmed influenza was reduced from 19.0% (32 of 168 households) for the placebo group to 4.1% (7 of 169 households) for the group receiving RELENZA.

In the second study, index cases were not treated. The incidence of symptomatic laboratory-confirmed influenza was reduced from 19.0% (46 of 242 households) for the placebo group to 4.1% (10 of 245 households) for the group receiving RELENZA.

Seasonal Prophylaxis Studies: Two seasonal prophylaxis studies assessed RELENZA 10 mg inhaled once daily versus placebo inhaled once daily for 28 days during community outbreaks. The first study enrolled subjects 18 years of age or greater (mean age 29 years) from 2 university communities. The majority of subjects were unvaccinated (86%). In this study, the incidence of symptomatic laboratory-confirmed influenza was reduced from 6.1% (34 of 554) for the placebo group to 2.0% (11 of 553) for the group receiving RELENZA.

The second seasonal prophylaxis study enrolled subjects 12 to 94 years of age (mean age 60 years) with 56% of them older than 65 years of age. Sixty-seven percent of the subjects were vaccinated. In this study, the incidence of symptomatic laboratory-confirmed influenza was reduced from 1.4% (23 of 1,685) for the placebo group to 0.2% (4 of 1,678) for the group receiving RELENZA.

16 HOW SUPPLIED/STORAGE AND HANDLING

RELENZA is supplied in a circular double-foil pack (a ROTADISK) containing 4 blisters of the drug. Five ROTADISKs are packaged in a white polypropylene tube. The tube is packaged in a carton with 1 blue and gray DISKHALER inhalation device (NDC 0173-0681-01).

Store at 25°C (77°F); excursions permitted to 15° to 30°C (59° to 86°F) (see USP Controlled Room Temperature). Keep out of reach of children. Do not puncture any RELENZA ROTADISK blister until taking a dose using the DISKHALER.

17 PATIENT COUNSELING INFORMATION

See FDA-Approved Patient Labeling.

17.1 Bronchospasm

Patients should be advised of the risk of bronchospasm, especially in the setting of underlying airways disease, and should stop RELENZA and contact their physician if they experience increased respiratory symptoms during treatment such as worsening wheezing, shortness of breath, or other signs or symptoms of bronchospasm *[see Warnings and Precautions (5.1)]*. If a decision is made to prescribe RELENZA for a patient with asthma or chronic obstructive

pulmonary disease, the patient should be made aware of the risks and should have a fast-acting bronchodilator available.

17.2 Concomitant Bronchodilator Use
Patients scheduled to take inhaled bronchodilators at the same time as RELENZA should be advised to use their bronchodilators before taking RELENZA.

17.3 Neuropsychiatric Events
Patients with influenza (the flu), particularly children and adolescents, may be at an increased risk of seizures, confusion, or abnormal behavior early in their illness. These events may occur after beginning RELENZA or may occur when flu is not treated. These events are uncommon but may result in accidental injury to the patient. Therefore, patients should be observed for signs of unusual behavior and a healthcare professional should be contacted immediately if the patient shows any signs of unusual behavior *[see Warnings and Precautions (5.3)]*.

17.4 Instructions for Use
Patients should be instructed in use of the delivery system. Instructions should include a demonstration whenever possible. For the proper use of RELENZA, the patient should read and follow carefully the accompanying Patient Instructions for Use.

If RELENZA is prescribed for children, it should be used only under adult supervision and instruction, and the supervising adult should first be instructed by a healthcare professional *[see Dosage and Administration (2.1)]*.

17.5 Risk of Influenza Transmission to Others
Patients should be advised that the use of RELENZA for treatment of influenza has not been shown to reduce the risk of transmission of influenza to others.

RELENZA, DISKHALER, and ROTADISK are registered trademarks of GlaxoSmithKline.

This product's prescribing information may have been updated. Please refer to www.gsk.com for the most current version.

GlaxoSmithKline
Research Triangle Park, NC 27709
©2010, GlaxoSmithKline. All rights reserved.
March 2010
RLZ:7PI

PATIENT LABELING
RELENZA® (zanamivir) Inhalation Powder
This leaflet contains important patient information about RELENZA (zanamivir) Inhalation Powder, and should be read completely before beginning treatment. It does not, however, take the place of discussions with your healthcare provider about your medical condition or your treatment. This summary does not list all benefits and risks of RELENZA. The medication described here can only be prescribed and dispensed by a licensed healthcare provider, who has information about your medical condition and more information about the drug, including how to take it, what to expect, and potential side effects. If you have any questions about RELENZA, talk with your healthcare provider.

What is RELENZA?
RELENZA (ruh-LENS-uh) is a medicine for the treatment of influenza (flu, infection caused by influenza virus) and for reducing the chance of getting the flu in community and household settings. It belongs to a group of medicines called neuraminidase inhibitors. These medications attack the influenza virus and prevent it from spreading inside your body. RELENZA treats the cause of influenza at its source, rather than simply masking the symptoms.

Important Safety Information About RELENZA
Some patients have had bronchospasm (wheezing) or serious breathing problems when they used RELENZA. Many but not all of these patients had previous asthma or chronic obstructive pulmonary disease. RELENZA has not been shown to shorten the duration of influenza in people with these diseases. Because of the risk of side effects and because it has not been shown to help them, RELENZA is not recommended for people with chronic respiratory disease such as asthma or chronic obstructive pulmonary disease.

If you develop worsening respiratory symptoms such as wheezing or shortness of breath, stop using RELENZA and contact your healthcare provider right away.

If you have chronic respiratory disease such as asthma and chronic obstructive pulmonary disease and your healthcare provider has prescribed RELENZA, you should have a fast-acting, inhaled bronchodilator available for your use. If you are scheduled to use an inhaled bronchodilator at the same time as RELENZA, use the inhaled bronchodilator **before** using RELENZA.

Read the rest of this leaflet for more information about side effects and risks.

Other kinds of infections can appear like influenza or occur along with influenza, and need different kinds of treatment. Contact your healthcare provider if you feel worse or develop new symptoms during or after treatment, or if your influenza symptoms do not start to get better.

Who should not take RELENZA?
RELENZA is not recommended for people who have chronic lung disease such as asthma or chronic obstructive pulmonary disease. RELENZA has not been shown to shorten the duration of influenza in people with these diseases, and some people have had serious side effects of bronchospasm and worsening lung function. (See the section of this Patient Information entitled "**Important Safety Information About RELENZA**.")

You should not take RELENZA if you are allergic to zanamivir or any other ingredient of RELENZA. Also tell your healthcare provider if you have any type of chronic condition including lung or heart disease, if you are allergic to any other medicines or food products, or if you are pregnant.

RELENZA was not effective in reducing the chance of getting the flu in 2 studies in nursing home patients.

RELENZA does not treat flu-like illness that is not caused by influenza virus.

Who should consider taking RELENZA?
Adult and pediatric patients at least 7 years of age who have influenza symptoms that appeared within the previous day or two. Typical symptoms of influenza include sudden onset of fever, cough, headache, fatigue, muscular weakness, and sore throat.

RELENZA can also help reduce the chance of getting the flu in adults and children at least 5 years of age who have a higher chance of getting the flu because they spend time with someone who has the flu. RELENZA can also reduce the chance of getting the flu if there is a flu outbreak in the community.

The use of RELENZA for the treatment of flu has not been shown to reduce the risk of spreading the virus to others.

Can I take other medications with RELENZA?
RELENZA has been shown to have an acceptable safety profile when used as labeled, with minimal risk of drug interactions. Your healthcare provider may recommend taking other medications, including over-the-counter medications, to reduce fever or other symptoms while you are taking RELENZA. Before starting treatment, make sure that your healthcare provider knows if you are taking other medicines. If you are scheduled to use an inhaled bronchodilator at the same time as RELENZA, you should use the inhaled bronchodilator **before** using RELENZA.

Before taking RELENZA, please let your healthcare provider know if you received live attenuated influenza vaccine (FLUMIST®) intranasal in the past 2 weeks.

How and when should I take RELENZA?
RELENZA is packaged in medicine disks called ROTADISKS® and is inhaled by mouth using a delivery device called a DISKHALER®. Each ROTADISK contains 4 blisters. Each blister contains 5 mg of active drug and 20 mg of lactose powder (which contains milk proteins).

You should receive a demonstration on how to use RELENZA in the DISKHALER from a healthcare provider. Before taking RELENZA, read the "Patient Instructions for Use." Make sure that you understand these instructions and talk to your healthcare provider if you have any questions. Children who use RELENZA should always be supervised by an adult who understands how to use RELENZA. Proper use of the DISKHALER to inhale the drug is necessary for safe and effective use of RELENZA.

If you have the flu the usual dose for treatment is 2 inhalations of RELENZA (1 blister per inhalation) twice daily (in the morning and evening) for 5 days. It is important that you begin your treatment with RELENZA as soon as possible from the first appearance of your flu symptoms. Take 2 doses on the first day of treatment whenever possible if there are at least 2 hours between doses.

To reduce the chance of getting the flu, the usual dose is 2 inhalations of RELENZA (1 blister per inhalation) once daily for 10 or 28 days as prescribed by your healthcare provider.

Never share RELENZA with anyone, even if they have the same symptoms. If you feel worse or develop new symptoms during treatment with RELENZA, or if your flu symptoms do not start to get better, stop using the medicine and contact your healthcare provider.

What if I miss a dose?
If you forget to take your medicine at any time, take the missed dose as soon as you remember, except if it is near the next dose (within 2 hours). Then continue to take RELENZA at the usual times. You do not need to take a double dose. If you have missed several doses, inform your healthcare provider and follow the advice given to you.

What are important or common possible side effects of taking RELENZA?
Some patients have had breathing problems while taking RELENZA. This can be very serious and need treatment right away. Most of the patients who had this problem had asthma or chronic obstructive pulmonary disease, but some did not. If you have trouble breathing or have wheezing after your dose of RELENZA, stop taking RELENZA and get medical attention.

In studies, the most common side effects with RELENZA have been headaches; diarrhea; nausea; vomiting; nasal irritation; bronchitis; cough; sinusitis; ear, nose, and throat infections; and dizziness. Other side effects that have been reported, but were not as common, include rashes and allergic reactions, some of which were severe.

People with influenza (the flu), particularly children and adolescents, may be at an increased risk of seizures, confusion, or abnormal behavior early in their illness. These events may occur after beginning RELENZA or may occur when flu is not treated. These events are uncommon but may result in accidental injury to the patient. Therefore, patients should be observed for signs of unusual behavior and a healthcare professional should be contacted immediately if the patient shows any signs of unusual behavior.

This list of side effects is not complete. Your healthcare provider or pharmacist can discuss with you a more complete list of possible side effects with RELENZA. Talk to your healthcare provider promptly about any side effects you have.

Please refer to the section entitled "**Important Safety Information About RELENZA**" for additional information.

Should I get a flu shot?
RELENZA is not a substitute for a flu shot. You should receive an annual flu shot according to guidelines on immunization practices that your healthcare provider can share with you.

What if I am pregnant or nursing?
If you are pregnant or planning to become pregnant while taking RELENZA, talk to your healthcare provider before taking this medication. RELENZA is normally not recommended for use during pregnancy or nursing, as the effects on the unborn child or nursing infant are unknown.

How and where should I store RELENZA?
RELENZA should be stored at room temperature below 77°F (25°C). RELENZA is not in a childproof container. Keep RELENZA out of the reach of children. Discard the DISKHALER after finishing your treatment.

PATIENT INSTRUCTIONS FOR USE

RELENZA®
(ZANAMIVIR) INHALATION POWDER

IMPORTANT: Read Step-by-Step Instructions before using the DISKHALER®.
Be sure to take the dose your healthcare provider has prescribed.

BEFORE YOU START:
Please read the entire Patient Labeling for important information about the effects of RELENZA including the section "Important Safety Information About RELENZA" for information about the risk of breathing difficulties.
If RELENZA is prescribed for a child, dosing should be supervised by an adult who understands how to use RELENZA and has been instructed in its use by a healthcare provider.

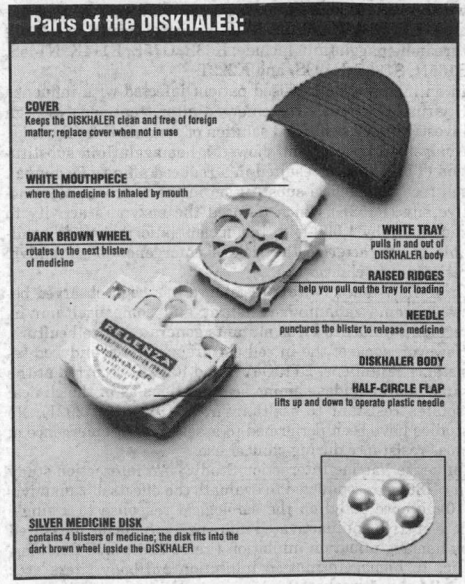

Parts of the DISKHALER:

COVER
Keeps the DISKHALER clean and free of foreign matter; replace cover when not in use

WHITE MOUTHPIECE
where the medicine is inhaled by mouth

DARK BROWN WHEEL
rotates to the next blister of medicine

WHITE TRAY
pulls in and out of DISKHALER body

RAISED RIDGES
help you pull out the tray for loading

NEEDLE
punctures the blister to release medicine

DISKHALER BODY

HALF-CIRCLE FLAP
lifts up and down to operate plastic needle

SILVER MEDICINE DISK
contains 4 blisters of medicine; the disk fits into the dark brown wheel inside the DISKHALER

Step-by-step instructions for using the DISKHALER®
Step A: Load the medicine into the DISKHALER
1. Start by pulling off the blue cover.

2. **Always check inside the mouthpiece to make sure it is clear before each use. If foreign objects are in the mouthpiece, they could be inhaled and cause serious harm.**

3. Pull the white mouthpiece by the edges to extend the white tray all the way.

4. Once the white tray is extended all the way, find the raised ridges on each side of it. Press in these ridges, both sides at the same time, and **pull the whole white tray out of the DISKHALER body.**

5. Place one silver medicine disk onto the dark brown wheel, flat side up. The four silver blisters on the underside of the medicine disk will drop neatly into the four holes in the wheel.

6. Push in the white tray as far as it will go. Now the DISKHALER is loaded with medicine.

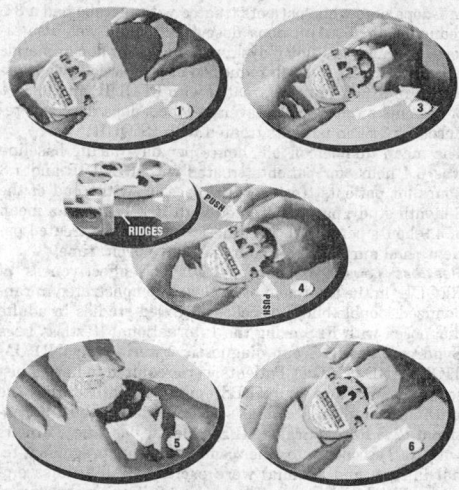

Step B: Puncture the blister
Be sure to keep the DISKHALER level.

The DISKHALER punctures one blister of medicine at a time so you can inhale the right amount. It does not matter which blister you start with. Check to make sure that the silver foil is unbroken.

1. Be sure to keep the DISKHALER level so the medicine does not spill out.

2. Locate the half-circle flap with the name "RELENZA" on top of the DISKHALER.

3. Lift this flap from the outer edge until it cannot go any farther. Flap must be **straight up** for the plastic needle to puncture both the **top** and **bottom** of the silver medicine disk inside.

4. Keeping the DISKHALER level, click the flap down into place.

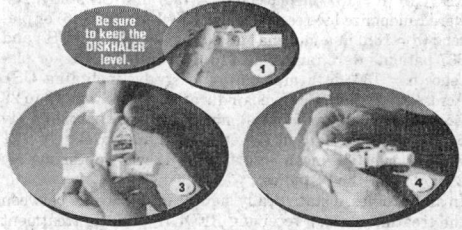

Step C: Inhale
1. Before putting the white mouthpiece into your mouth, breathe all the way out (exhale).

Then put the white mouthpiece into your mouth. Be sure to keep the DISKHALER level so the medicine does not spill out.

2. Close your lips firmly around the mouthpiece. Be sure not to cover the small holes on either side of it.

3. Breathe in through your mouth steadily and as deeply as you can. Your breath pulls the medicine into your airways and lungs.

4. Hold your breath for a few seconds to help RELENZA stay in your lungs where it can work.

To take another inhalation, move to the next blister by following Step D below.

Once you've inhaled the number of blisters prescribed by your healthcare provider, replace the cover until your next dose.

[See figure at top of next column]

Step D: Move the medicine disk to the next blister
1. **Pull** the mouthpiece to extend the white tray, without removing it.

2. Then **push** it back until it clicks. This pull-push motion rotates the medicine disk to the next blister.

3. To take your next inhalation, repeat Steps B and C.

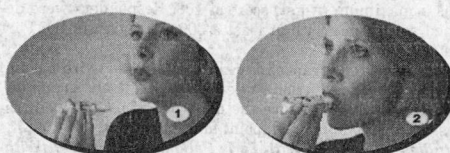

If all four blisters in the medicine disk have been used, you are ready to start a new medicine disk (see Step A). Check to make sure that the silver foil is unbroken each time you are ready to puncture the next blister.

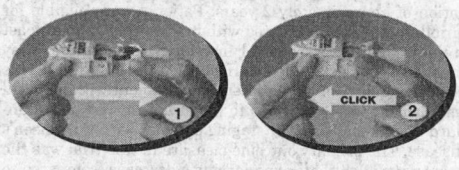

IMPORTANT INSTRUCTIONS

Read this entire leaflet before using RELENZA. Even if you have had a previous prescription for RELENZA, read this leaflet to see if any information has changed.

If you have the flu, the usual dose is 2 inhalations twice daily. To reduce the chance of getting the flu, the usual dose is 2 inhalations once daily. However, you must take the number of inhalations your healthcare provider has prescribed.

If you feel worse or develop new symptoms during or after treatment, or if your flu symptoms do not start to improve, stop using the medicine and contact your healthcare provider.

Keep out of reach of children.

Always check inside the mouthpiece to make sure it is clear before each use. If foreign objects are in the mouthpiece, they could be inhaled and cause serious harm.

Always replace the cover after each use.

Throw away the DISKHALER after treatment is completed. This DISKHALER is for use only with RELENZA. Do not use the RELENZA DISKHALER device with FLOVENT® (fluticasone propionate) and do not use RELENZA with the FLOVENT DISKHALER device.

Store at 25°C (77°F); excursions permitted to 15° to 30°C (59° to 86°F) (see USP Controlled Room Temperature).

REMEMBER: This medicine has been prescribed for you by your healthcare provider. DO NOT give this medicine to anyone else.

RELENZA, FLOVENT, ROTADISK, and DISKHALER are registered trademarks of GlaxoSmithKline.
FLUMIST is a registered trademark of MedImmune, Inc.
GlaxoSmithKline
Research Triangle Park, NC 27709
©2008, GlaxoSmithKline. All rights reserved.
February 2008
RLZ:3PIL

REQUIP®   ℞
[rē′kwip]
(ropinirole tablets)
Patient Information Included

DESCRIPTION
REQUIP (ropinirole) is an orally administered non-ergoline dopamine agonist. It is the hydrochloride salt of 4-[2-(dipropylamino)ethyl]-1,3-dihydro-2H-indol-2-one monohydrochloride and has an empirical formula of $C_{16}H_{24}N_2O \cdot HCl$. The molecular weight is 296.84 (260.38 as the free base).
The structural formula is:

$$N(CH_2CH_2CH_3)_2 \cdot HCl$$

Ropinirole hydrochloride is a white to yellow solid with a melting range of 243° to 250°C and a solubility of 133 mg/mL in water.

Each pentagonal film-coated TILTAB® tablet with beveled edges contains 0.29 mg, 0.57 mg, 1.14 mg, 2.28 mg, 3.42 mg, 4.56 mg, or 5.70 mg ropinirole hydrochloride equivalent to ropinirole, 0.25 mg, 0.5 mg, 1 mg, 2 mg, 3 mg, 4 mg, or 5 mg. Inactive ingredients consist of: croscarmellose sodium, hydrous lactose, magnesium stearate, microcrystalline cellulose, and one or more of the following: carmine,

FD&C Blue No. 2 aluminum lake, FD&C Yellow No. 6 aluminum lake, hypromellose, iron oxides, polyethylene glycol, polysorbate 80, titanium dioxide.

CLINICAL PHARMACOLOGY
Mechanism of Action: REQUIP is a non-ergoline dopamine agonist with high relative in vitro specificity and full intrinsic activity at the D_2 and D_3 dopamine receptor subtypes, binding with higher affinity to D_3 than to D_2 or D_4 receptor subtypes.

Ropinirole has moderate in vitro affinity for opioid receptors. Ropinirole and its metabolites have negligible in vitro affinity for dopamine D_1, 5-HT_1, 5-HT_2, benzodiazepine, GABA, muscarinic, alpha$_1$-, alpha$_2$-, and beta-adrenoreceptors.

Parkinson's Disease: The precise mechanism of action of REQUIP as a treatment for Parkinson's disease is unknown, although it is believed to be due to stimulation of postsynaptic dopamine D_2-type receptors within the caudate-putamen in the brain. This conclusion is supported by studies that show that ropinirole improves motor function in various animal models of Parkinson's disease. In particular, ropinirole attenuates the motor deficits induced by lesioning the ascending nigrostriatal dopaminergic pathway with the neurotoxin 1-methyl-4-phenyl-1,2,3,6-tetrahydropyridine (MPTP) in primates. The relevance of D_3 receptor binding in Parkinson's disease is unknown.

Restless Legs Syndrome (RLS): The precise mechanism of action of REQUIP as a treatment for Restless Legs Syndrome (also known as Ekbom Syndrome) is unknown. Although the pathophysiology of RLS is largely unknown, neuropharmacological evidence suggests primary dopaminergic system involvement. Positron emission tomographic (PET) studies suggest that a mild striatal presynaptic dopaminergic dysfunction may be involved in the pathogenesis of RLS.

Clinical Pharmacology Studies: In healthy normotensive subjects, single oral doses of REQUIP in the range 0.01 to 2.5 mg had little or no effect on supine blood pressure and pulse rates. Upon standing, REQUIP caused decreases in systolic and diastolic blood pressure at doses above 0.25 mg. In some subjects, these changes were associated with the emergence of orthostatic symptoms, bradycardia, and, in one case, transient sinus arrest with syncope. With repeat dosing and slow titration up to 4 mg once daily in healthy volunteers, postural hypotension or hypotension-related adverse events were noted in 13% of subjects on REQUIP and none of the subjects on placebo.

The mechanism of postural hypotension induced by REQUIP is presumed to be due to a D_2-mediated blunting of the noradrenergic response to standing and subsequent decrease in peripheral vascular resistance. Nausea is a common concomitant symptom of orthostatic signs and symptoms.

At oral doses as low as 0.2 mg, REQUIP suppressed serum prolactin concentrations in healthy male volunteers.

REQUIP had no dose-related effect on ECG wave form and rhythm in young, healthy, male volunteers in the range of 0.01 to 2.5 mg.

REQUIP had no dose- or exposure-related effect on mean QT intervals in healthy male and female volunteers titrated to doses up to 4 mg/day. The effect of REQUIP on QT intervals at higher exposures achieved either due to drug interactions or at doses used in Parkinson's disease has not been systematically evaluated.

Pharmacokinetics: ***Absorption, Distribution, Metabolism, and Elimination:*** The pharmacokinetics of ropinirole are similar in Parkinson's disease patients and patients with Restless Legs Syndrome. Ropinirole is rapidly absorbed after oral administration, reaching peak concentration in approximately 1-2 hours. In clinical studies, over 88% of a radiolabeled dose was recovered in urine and the absolute bioavailability was 55%, indicating a first-pass effect. Relative bioavailability from a tablet compared to an oral solution is 85%. Food does not affect the extent of absorption of ropinirole, although its T_{max} is increased by 2.5 hours and its C_{max} is decreased by approximately 25% when the drug is taken with a high-fat meal. The clearance of ropinirole after oral administration to patients is 47 L/hr (cv = 45%) and its elimination half-life is approximately 6 hours. Ropinirole is extensively metabolized by the liver to inactive metabolites and displays linear kinetics over the therapeutic dosing range of 1 to 8 mg 3 times daily. Steady-state concentrations are expected to be achieved within 2 days of dosing. Accumulation upon multiple dosing is predictive from single dosing.

Ropinirole is widely distributed throughout the body, with an apparent volume of distribution of 7.5 L/kg (cv = 32%). It is up to 40% bound to plasma proteins and has a blood-to-plasma ratio of 1:1.

The major metabolic pathways are N-despropylation and hydroxylation to form the inactive N-despropyl and hydroxy metabolites. In vitro studies indicate that the major cytochrome P_{450} isozyme involved in the metabolism of ropinirole is CYP1A2, an enzyme known to be stimulated by smoking and omeprazole, and inhibited by, for example, fluvoxamine, mexiletine, and the older fluoroquinolones such as ciprofloxacin and norfloxacin. The N-despropyl metabolite is converted to carbamyl glucuronide, carboxylic acid, and N-despropyl hydroxy metabolites. The hydroxy metabolite of ropinirole is rapidly glucuronidated. Less than 10% of the administered dose is excreted as unchanged drug in urine. N-despropyl ropinirole is the predominant metabolite found in urine (40%), followed by the carboxylic acid metabolite (10%), and the glucuronide of the hydroxy metabolite (10%).

P_{450} Interaction: In vitro metabolism studies showed that CYP1A2 was the major enzyme responsible for the metabolism of ropinirole. Inhibitors or inducers of this enzyme have been shown to alter its clearance when coadministered with ropinirole. Therefore, if therapy with a drug known to be a potent inhibitor of CYP1A2 is stopped or started during treatment with REQUIP, adjustment of the dose of REQUIP may be required.

Population Subgroups: Because therapy with REQUIP is initiated at a low dose and gradually titrated upward according to clinical tolerability to obtain the optimum therapeutic effect, adjustment of the initial dose based on gender, weight, or age is not necessary.

Age: Oral clearance of ropinirole is reduced by 15% in patients above 65 years of age compared to younger patients. Dosage adjustment is not necessary in the elderly (above 65 years), as the dose of ropinirole is to be individually titrated to clinical response.

Gender: Female and male patients showed similar oral clearance.

Race: The influence of race on the pharmacokinetics of ropinirole has not been evaluated.

Cigarette Smoking: Smoking is expected to increase the clearance of ropinirole since CYP1A2 is known to be induced by smoking. In a study in patients with RLS, smokers (n = 7) had an approximate 30% lower C_{max} and a 38% lower AUC than did nonsmokers (n = 11), when those parameters were normalized for dose.

Renal Impairment: Based on population pharmacokinetic analysis, no difference was observed in the pharmacokinetics of ropinirole in patients with moderate renal impairment (creatinine clearance between 30 to 50 mL/min.) compared to an age-matched population with creatinine clearance above 50 mL/min. Therefore, no dosage adjustment is necessary in moderately renally impaired patients. The use of REQUIP in patients with severe renal impairment has not been studied.

The effect of hemodialysis on drug removal is not known, but because of the relatively high apparent volume of distribution of ropinirole (525 L), the removal of the drug by hemodialysis is unlikely.

Hepatic Impairment: The pharmacokinetics of ropinirole have not been studied in hepatically impaired patients. These patients may have higher plasma levels and lower clearance of the drug than patients with normal hepatic function. The drug should be titrated with caution in this population.

Other Diseases: Population pharmacokinetic analysis revealed no change in the oral clearance of ropinirole in patients with concomitant diseases such as hypertension, depression, osteoporosis/arthritis, and insomnia compared to patients with Parkinson's disease only.

Clinical Trials: Parkinson's Disease: The effectiveness of REQUIP in the treatment of Parkinson's disease was evaluated in a multinational drug development program consisting of 11 randomized, controlled trials. Four were conducted in patients with early Parkinson's disease and no concomitant levodopa (L-dopa), and 7 were conducted in patients with advanced Parkinson's disease with concomitant L-dopa.

Among these 11 studies, 3 placebo-controlled studies provide the most persuasive evidence of ropinirole's effectiveness in the management of patients with Parkinson's disease who were and were not receiving concomitant L-dopa. Two of these 3 trials enrolled patients with early Parkinson's disease (without L-dopa) and 1 enrolled patients receiving L-dopa.

In these studies a variety of measures were used to assess the effects of treatment (e.g., the Unified Parkinson's Disease Rating Scale [UPDRS], Clinical Global Impression [CGI] scores, patient diaries recording time "on" and "off," and tolerability of L-dopa dose reductions).

In both studies of early Parkinson's disease (without L-dopa) patients, the motor component (Part III) of the UPDRS was the primary outcome assessment. The UPDRS is a 4-part multi-item rating scale intended to evaluate mentation (Part I), activities of daily living (Part II), motor performance (Part III), and complications of therapy (Part IV). Part III of the UPDRS contains 14 items designed to assess the severity of the cardinal motor findings in patients with Parkinson's disease (e.g., tremor, rigidity, bradykinesia, postural instability, etc.) scored for different body regions and

has a maximum (worst) score of 108. Responders were defined as patients with at least a 30% reduction in the Part III score.

In the study of advanced Parkinson's disease (with L-dopa) patients, both reduction in percent awake time spent "off" and the ability to reduce the daily use of L-dopa were assessed as a combined endpoint and individually.

Studies in Patients With Early Parkinson's Disease (Without L-dopa): One early therapy study was a 12-week multicenter study in which 63 patients (41 on REQUIP) with idiopathic Parkinson's disease receiving concomitant anti-Parkinson medication (but not L-dopa) were randomized to either REQUIP or placebo. Patients had a mean disease duration of approximately 2 years. Patients were eligible for enrollment if they presented with bradykinesia and at least tremor, rigidity, or postural instability. In addition, they must have been classified as Hoehn & Yahr Stage I-IV. This scale, ranging from I = unilateral involvement with minimal impairment to V = confined to wheelchair or bed, is a standard instrument used for staging patients with Parkinson's disease. The primary outcome measure in this trial was the proportion of patients experiencing a decrease (compared to baseline) of at least 30% in the UPDRS motor score. Patients were titrated for up to 10 weeks, starting at 0.5 mg twice daily, with weekly increments of 0.5 mg twice daily to a maximum of 5 mg twice daily. Once patients reached their maximally tolerated dose (or 5 mg twice daily), they were maintained on that dose through 12 weeks. The mean dose achieved by patients at study endpoint was 7.4 mg/day. At the end of 12 weeks, 71% of patients treated with REQUIP were responders, compared with 41% of patients in the placebo group (p = 0.021).

Statistically significant differences between the percentage of responders on REQUIP compared to placebo were seen after 8 weeks of treatment.

In addition, the mean percentage improvement from baseline in the Total Motor Score was 43% in patients treated with REQUIP compared with 21% in patients treated with placebo (p = 0.018).

Statistically significant differences in UPDRS motor score between REQUIP and placebo were seen after 2 weeks of treatment.

The median daily dose at which a 30% reduction in UPDRS motor score was sustained was 4 mg.

The second trial in early Parkinson's disease (without L-dopa) patients was a double-blind, randomized, placebo-controlled, 6-month study. Patients were essentially similar to those in the study described above; concomitant use of selegiline was allowed, but patients were not permitted to use anticholinergics or amantadine during the study. Patients had a mean disease duration of 2 years and limited (not more than a 6-week period) or no prior exposure to L-dopa. The starting dose of REQUIP in this trial was 0.25 mg 3 times daily. The dose was titrated at weekly intervals by increments of 0.25 mg 3 times daily to a dose of 1 mg 3 times daily. Further titrations at weekly intervals were at increments of 0.5 mg 3 times daily up to a dose of 3 mg 3 times daily, and then weekly at increments of 1 mg 3 times daily. Patients were to be titrated to a dose of at least 1.5 mg 3 times daily and then to their maximally tolerated dose, up to a maximum of 8 mg 3 times daily. The mean dose attained in patients at study endpoint was 15.7 mg/day.

The primary measure of effectiveness was the mean percent reduction (improvement) from baseline in the UPDRS Motor Score. In this study 241 patients were enrolled. At the end of the 6-month study, patients treated with REQUIP had 22% improvement in motor score, compared with a 4% worsening in the placebo group (p<0.001).

Statistically significant differences in UPDRS motor score improvement between REQUIP and placebo were seen after 12 weeks of treatment.

Study in Patients With Advanced Parkinson's Disease (With L-dopa): This double-blind, randomized, placebo-controlled, 6-month trial evaluated 148 patients (Hoehn & Yahr II-IV) who were not adequately controlled on L-dopa. Patients in this study had a mean disease duration of approximately 9 years, had been exposed to L-dopa for approximately 7 years, and had experienced "on-off" periods with L-dopa therapy. Patients previously receiving stable doses of selegiline, amantadine, and/or anticholinergic agents could continue on these agents during the study. Patients were started at a dose of 0.25 mg 3 times daily of REQUIP and titrated upward by weekly intervals until an optimal therapeutic response was achieved. The maximum dose of study medication was 8 mg 3 times daily. All patients had to be titrated to at least a dose of 2.5 mg 3 times daily. Patients could then be maintained on this dose level or higher for the remainder of the study. Once a dose of 2.5 mg 3 times daily was achieved, patients underwent a mandatory reduction in their L-dopa dose, to be followed by additional mandatory reductions with continued escalation of the dose of REQUIP. Reductions in the dosage of L-dopa were also allowed if patients experienced adverse events that the investigator con-

sidered related to dopaminergic therapy. The mean dose attained at study endpoint was 16.3 mg/day. The primary outcome was the proportion of responders, defined as patients who were able both to achieve a decrease (compared to baseline) of at least 20% in their L-dopa dose and a decrease of at least 20% in the proportion of the time awake in the "off" condition (a period of time during the day when patients are particularly immobile), as determined by patient diary. In addition, the mean percent change from baseline in daily L-dopa dose was examined.

At the end of 6 months, 28% of patients treated with REQUIP were classified as responders (based on combined endpoint) while 11% of patients treated with placebo were responders (p = 0.02). Based on the protocol-mandated reductions in L-dopa dosage with escalating doses of REQUIP, patients treated with REQUIP had a 19.4% mean reduction in L-dopa dose while patients treated with placebo had a 3% reduction (p<0.001). L-dopa dosage reduction was also allowed during the study if dyskinesias or other dopaminergic effects occurred. Overall, reduction of L-dopa dose was sustained in 87% of patients treated with REQUIP and in 57% of patients on placebo. On average, the L-dopa dose was reduced by 31% in patients treated with REQUIP.

The mean number of "off" hours per day during baseline was 6.4 hours for patients treated with REQUIP and 7.3 hours for patients treated with placebo. At the end of the 6-month study, patients treated with REQUIP had a mean of 4.9 hours per day of "off" time, while placebo-treated patients had a mean of 6.4 hours per day of "off" time.

Restless Legs Syndrome (RLS): The effectiveness of REQUIP in the treatment of RLS was demonstrated in randomized, double-blind, placebo-controlled studies in adults diagnosed with RLS using the International Restless Legs Syndrome Study Group diagnostic criteria (see INDICATIONS AND USAGE). Patients were required to have a history of a minimum of 15 RLS episodes/month during the previous month and a total score of ≥15 on the International RLS Rating Scale (IRLS scale) at baseline. Patients with RLS secondary to other conditions (e.g., pregnancy, renal failure, and anemia) were excluded. All studies employed flexible dosing, with patients initiating therapy at 0.25 mg REQUIP once daily. Patients were titrated based on clinical response and tolerability over 7 weeks to a maximum of 4 mg once daily. All doses were taken between 1 and 3 hours before bedtime.

A variety of measures were used to assess the effects of treatment, including the IRLS Scale and Clinical Global Impression-Global Improvement (CGI-I) scores. The IRLS Scale contains 10 items designed to assess the severity of sensory and motor symptoms, sleep disturbance, daytime somnolence, and impact on activities of daily living and mood associated with RLS. The range of scores is 0 to 40, with 0 being absence of RLS symptoms and 40 the most severe symptoms. Three of the controlled studies utilized the change from baseline in the IRLS Scale at the week 12 endpoint as the primary efficacy outcome.

Three hundred eighty patients were randomized to receive REQUIP (n = 187) or placebo (n = 193) in a US study; 284 were randomized to receive either REQUIP (n = 146) or placebo (n = 138) in a multinational study (excluding US); and 267 patients were randomized to REQUIP (n = 131) or placebo (n = 136) in a multinational study (including US). Across the 3 studies, the mean duration of RLS was 16 to 22 years (range of 0 to 65 years), mean age was approximately 54 years (range of 18 to 79 years), and approximately 61% were women. The mean dose at week 12 was approximately 2 mg/day for the 3 studies.

In all 3 studies, a statistically significant difference between the treatment group receiving REQUIP and the treatment group receiving placebo was observed at week 12 for both the mean change from baseline in the IRLS Scale total score and the percentage of patients rated as responders (much improved or very much improved) on the CGI-I (see Table 1).

[See table 1 at top of next page]

Long-term maintenance of efficacy in the treatment of RLS was demonstrated in a 36-week study. Following a 24-week single-blind treatment phase (flexible doses of REQUIP of 0.25 to 4 mg once daily), patients who were responders (defined as a decrease of >6 points on the IRLS Scale total score relative to baseline) were randomized in double-blind fashion to placebo or continuation of REQUIP for an additional 12 weeks. Relapse was defined as an increase of at least 6 points on the IRLS Scale total score to a total score of at least 15, or withdrawal due to lack of efficacy. For patients who were responders at week 24, the mean dose of ropinirole was 2 mg (range 0.25 to 4 mg). Patients continued on REQUIP demonstrated a significantly lower relapse rate compared with patients randomized to placebo (32.6% vs 57.8%, p = 0.0156).

INDICATIONS AND USAGE
Parkinson's Disease: REQUIP is indicated for the treatment of the signs and symptoms of idiopathic Parkinson's disease.

The effectiveness of REQUIP was demonstrated in randomized, controlled trials in patients with early Parkinson's disease who were not receiving concomitant L-dopa therapy as well as in patients with advanced disease on concomitant L-dopa (see CLINICAL PHARMACOLOGY: Clinical Trials).

Restless Legs Syndrome: REQUIP is indicated for the treatment of moderate-to-severe primary Restless Legs Syndrome (RLS).

Key diagnostic criteria for RLS are: an urge to move the legs usually accompanied or caused by uncomfortable and unpleasant leg sensations; symptoms begin or worsen during periods of rest or inactivity such as lying or sitting; symptoms are partially or totally relieved by movement such as walking or stretching at least as long as the activity continues; and symptoms are worse or occur only in the evening or night. Difficulty falling asleep may frequently be associated with moderate-to-severe RLS.

CONTRAINDICATIONS

REQUIP is contraindicated for patients known to have hypersensitivity reaction (including urticaria, angioedema, rash, pruritus) to ropinirole or to any of the excipients.

WARNINGS

Falling Asleep During Activities of Daily Living: Patients treated with REQUIP have reported falling asleep while engaged in activities of daily living, including the operation of motor vehicles, which sometimes resulted in accidents. Although many of these patients reported somnolence while on REQUIP, some perceived that they had no warning signs such as excessive drowsiness, and believed that they were alert immediately prior to the event. Some of these events have been reported as late as 1 year after initiation of treatment.

In controlled clinical trials, somnolence was a common occurrence in patients receiving REQUIP and is more frequent in Parkinson's disease (up to 40% REQUIP, 6% placebo) than in Restless Legs Syndrome (12% REQUIP, 6% placebo). Many clinical experts believe that falling asleep while engaged in activities of daily living always occurs in a setting of preexisting somnolence, although patients may not give such a history. For this reason, prescribers should continually reassess patients for drowsiness or sleepiness, especially since some of the events occur well after the start of treatment. Prescribers should also be aware that patients may not acknowledge drowsiness or sleepiness until directly questioned about drowsiness or sleepiness during specific activities.

Before initiating treatment with REQUIP, patients should be advised of the potential to develop drowsiness and specifically asked about factors that may increase the risk with REQUIP such as concomitant sedating medications, the presence of sleep disorders (other than Restless Legs Syndrome), and concomitant medications that increase ropinirole plasma levels (e.g., ciprofloxacin—see PRECAUTIONS: Drug Interactions). If a patient develops significant daytime sleepiness or episodes of falling asleep during activities that require active participation (e.g., conversations, eating, etc.), REQUIP should ordinarily be discontinued. (See DOSAGE AND ADMINISTRATION for guidance in discontinuing REQUIP.) If a decision is made to continue REQUIP, patients should be advised to not drive and to avoid other potentially dangerous activities. There is insufficient information to establish that dose reduction will eliminate episodes of falling asleep while engaged in activities of daily living.

Syncope: Syncope, sometimes associated with bradycardia, was observed in association with ropinirole in both Parkinson's disease patients and RLS patients. In the 2 double-blind, placebo-controlled studies of REQUIP in patients with Parkinson's disease who were not being treated with L-dopa, 11.5% (18 of 157) of patients on REQUIP had syncope compared to 1.4% (2 of 147) of patients on placebo. Most of these cases occurred more than 4 weeks after initiation of therapy with REQUIP, and were usually associated with a recent increase in dose.

Of 208 patients being treated with both L-dopa and REQUIP in placebo-controlled advanced Parkinson's disease trials, there were reports of syncope in 6 (2.9%) compared to 2 of 120 (1.7%) of placebo/L-dopa patients.

In patients with RLS, of 496 patients treated with REQUIP in 12-week placebo-controlled trials, there were reports of syncope in 5 (1.0%) compared with 1 of 500 (0.2%) patients treated with placebo.

Because the studies of REQUIP excluded patients with significant cardiovascular disease, it is not known to what extent the estimated incidence figures apply to either Parkinson's disease or RLS patients in clinical practice. Therefore, patients with severe cardiovascular disease should be treated with caution.

Two of 47 Parkinson's disease patient volunteers enrolled in phase 1 studies had syncope following a 1-mg dose. In 2 studies in RLS patients that used a forced titration regimen and orthostatic challenge with intensive blood pressure monitoring, 1 of 55 RLS patients treated with REQUIP compared with 0 of 27 patients receiving placebo reported syncope. In phase 1 studies including 110 healthy volunteers, 1 patient developed hypotension, bradycardia, and sinus arrest of 26 seconds accompanied by syncope; the patient recovered spontaneously without intervention. One other healthy volunteer reported syncope.

Table 1. Mean Change in IRLS Score and Percent Responders on CGI-I

	REQUIP	Placebo	p-value
Mean Change in IRLS score at Week 12			
US study	-13.5	-9.8	p<0.0001
Multinational study (excluding US)	-11.0	-8.0	p=0.0036
Multinational study (including US)	-11.2	-8.7	p=0.0197
Percent responders on CGI-I at Week 12			
US study	73.3%	56.5%	p=0.0006
Multinational study (excluding US)	53.4%	40.9%	p=0.0416
Multinational study (including US)	59.5%	39.6%	p=0.0010

Symptomatic Hypotension: Dopamine agonists, in clinical studies and clinical experience, appear to impair the systemic regulation of blood pressure, with resulting postural hypotension, especially during dose escalation. Parkinson's disease patients, in addition, appear to have an impaired capacity to respond to a postural challenge. For these reasons, Parkinson's patients being treated with dopaminergic agonists ordinarily (1) require careful monitoring for signs and symptoms of postural hypotension, especially during dose escalation, and (2) should be informed of this risk (see PRECAUTIONS: Information for Patients).

Although the clinical trials were not designed to systematically monitor blood pressure, there were individual reported cases of postural hypotension in early Parkinson's disease (without L-dopa) in patients treated with REQUIP. Most of these cases occurred more than 4 weeks after initiation of therapy with REQUIP and were usually associated with a recent increase in dose.

In 12-week placebo-controlled trials of patients with RLS, the adverse event orthostatic hypotension was reported by 4 of 496 patients (0.8%) treated with REQUIP compared with 2 of 500 patients (0.4%) receiving placebo.

In two phase 2 studies in patients with RLS that used a forced-titration regimen and orthostatic challenges with intensive blood pressure monitoring, 14 of 55 patients (25%) receiving REQUIP experienced an adverse event of hypotension or postural hypotension. As described above, one additional patient was noted to have an episode of vasovagal syncope (although no blood pressure recording was documented). None of the 27 patients receiving placebo had a similar adverse event. In these studies, 11 of the 55 patients (20%) receiving REQUIP and 3 of the 26 patients (12%) who had post-dose blood pressure assessments following placebo, experienced an orthostatic blood pressure decrease of at least 40 mm Hg systolic and/or at least 20 mm Hg diastolic; not all of these changes were associated with clinical symptoms. Except for its forced nature these studies used a similar titration schedule as those in the phase 3 efficacy trials.

In phase 1 studies of REQUIP that included 110 healthy volunteers, 9 subjects had documented symptomatic postural hypotension. These episodes appeared mainly at doses above 0.8 mg and these doses are higher than the starting doses recommended for either Parkinson's disease patients or RLS patients. In 8 of these 9 individuals, the hypotension was accompanied by bradycardia, but did not develop into syncope (see Syncope subsection). None of these events resulted in death or hospitalization.

One of 47 Parkinson's disease patient volunteers enrolled in phase 1 studies had documented hypotension following a 2-mg dose on 2 occasions.

Hallucinations: In double-blind, placebo-controlled, early-therapy studies in patients with Parkinson's disease who were not treated with L-dopa, 5.2% (8 of 157) of patients treated with REQUIP reported hallucinations, compared to 1.4% of patients on placebo (2 of 147). Among those patients receiving both REQUIP and L-dopa in advanced Parkinson's disease (with L-dopa) studies, 10.1% (21 of 208) were reported to experience hallucinations, compared to 4.2% (5 of 120) of patients treated with placebo and L-dopa.

Hallucinations were of sufficient severity to cause discontinuation of treatment in 1.3% of the early Parkinson's disease (without L-dopa) patients and 1.9% of the advanced Parkinson's disease (with L-dopa) patients, compared to 0% and 1.7% of placebo patients, respectively.

In patients with RLS, hallucinations were reported by 0% of patients treated with REQUIP (0 of 496) compared with 0.2% of patients who received placebo (1 of 500) in the 12-week placebo-controlled trials; in premarketing long-term open-label studies, 0.5% of patients reported hallucinations during therapy with REQUIP (2 of 390) but did not discontinue treatment and symptoms resolved.

PRECAUTIONS

General: ***Dyskinesia:*** REQUIP may potentiate the dopaminergic side effects of L-dopa and may cause and/or exacerbate preexisting dyskinesia in patients treated with L-dopa for Parkinson's disease. Decreasing the dose of L-dopa may ameliorate this side effect.

Renal Impairment: No dosage adjustment is needed in patients with mild to moderate renal impairment (creatinine clearance of 30 to 50 mL/min). The use of REQUIP in patients with severe renal impairment has not been studied.

Hepatic Impairment: The pharmacokinetics of ropinirole have not been studied in patients with hepatic impairment. Since patients with hepatic impairment may have higher plasma levels and lower clearance, REQUIP should be titrated with caution in these patients.

Events Reported With Dopaminergic Therapy: Withdrawal-Emergent Hyperpyrexia and Confusion: Although not reported with REQUIP, a symptom complex resembling the neuroleptic malignant syndrome (characterized by elevated temperature, muscular rigidity, altered consciousness, and autonomic instability), with no other obvious etiology, has been reported in association with rapid dose reduction, withdrawal of, or changes in anti-Parkinsonian therapy.

Fibrotic Complications: Cases of retroperitoneal fibrosis, pulmonary infiltrates, pleural effusion, pleural thickening, pericarditis, and cardiac valvulopathy have been reported in some patients treated with ergot-derived dopaminergic agents. While these complications may resolve when the drug is discontinued, complete resolution does not always occur.

Although these adverse events are believed to be related to the ergoline structure of these compounds, whether other, nonergot-derived dopamine agonists can cause them is unknown.

A small number of reports have been received of possible fibrotic complications, including pleural effusion, pleural fibrosis, interstitial lung disease, and cardiac valvulopathy, in the development program and postmarketing experience for REQUIP. While the evidence is not sufficient to establish a causal relationship between REQUIP and these fibrotic complications, a contribution of REQUIP cannot be completely ruled out in rare cases.

Melanoma: Epidemiologic studies have shown that patients with Parkinson's disease have a higher risk (2- to approximately 6-fold higher) of developing melanoma than the general population. Whether the increased risk observed was due to Parkinson's disease or other factors, such as drugs used to treat Parkinson's disease, is unclear.

For the reasons stated above, patients and providers are advised to monitor for melanomas frequently and on a regular basis when using REQUIP for *any* indication. Ideally, periodic skin examinations should be performed by appropriately qualified individuals (e.g., dermatologists).

Augmentation and Rebound in RLS: Reports in the literature indicate treatment of RLS with dopaminergic medications can result in a worsening of symptoms in the early morning hours, referred to as rebound. Augmentation has also been described during therapy for RLS. Augmentation refers to the earlier onset of symptoms in the evening (or even the afternoon), increase in symptoms, and spread of symptoms to involve other extremities. The controlled trials of REQUIP in patients with RLS excluded patients with augmentation and rebound and were generally not of sufficient duration to capture these phenomena. The frequency of augmentation and/or rebound after longer use of REQUIP and the appropriate management of these events, have not been evaluated in controlled clinical trials.

Retinal Pathology: Albino Rats: Retinal degeneration was observed in albino rats in the 2-year carcinogenicity study at all doses tested (equivalent to 0.6 to 20 times the maximum recommended human dose on a mg/m^2 basis), but was statistically significant at the highest dose (50 mg/kg/day). Additional studies to further evaluate the specific pathology (e.g., loss of photoreceptor cells) have not been performed. Similar changes were not observed in a 2-year carcinogenicity study in albino mice or in rats or monkeys treated for 1 year. The potential significance of this effect in humans has not been established, but cannot be disregarded because disruption of a mechanism that is universally present in vertebrates (e.g., disk shedding) may be involved.

Human: In order to evaluate the effect of REQUIP in humans, ocular electroretinogram (ERG) assessments were conducted during a 2-year, double-blind, multicenter, flexible dose, L-dopa controlled clinical study of REQUIP in patients with Parkinson's disease. A total of 156 patients (78 on ropinirole, mean dose 11.9 mg/day and 78 on L-dopa, mean dose 555.2 mg/day) were evaluated for evidence of retinal dysfunction through electroretinograms. There was no clinically meaningful difference between the treatment groups in retinal function over the duration of the study.

Binding to Melanin: REQUIP binds to melanin-containing tissues (i.e., eyes, skin) in pigmented rats. After a single dose, long-term retention of drug was demonstrated, with a half-life in the eye of 20 days. It is not known if REQUIP accumulates in these tissues over time.

Information for Patients: Physicians should instruct their patients to read the Patient Information leaflet before starting therapy with REQUIP and to reread it upon prescription renewal for new information regarding the use of REQUIP.

Patients should be instructed to take REQUIP only as prescribed. If a dose is missed, patients should be advised not to double their next dose.

REQUIP can be taken with or without food. Patients may be advised that taking REQUIP with food may reduce the occurrence of nausea. However, this has not been established in controlled clinical trials.

Patients should be advised that they may develop postural (orthostatic) hypotension with or without symptoms such as dizziness, nausea, syncope, and sometimes sweating. Hypotension and/or orthostatic symptoms may occur more frequently during initial therapy or with an increase in dose at any time (cases have been seen after weeks of treatment). Accordingly, patients should be cautioned against rising rapidly after sitting or lying down, especially if they have been doing so for prolonged periods, and especially at the initiation of treatment with REQUIP.

Patients should be alerted to the potential sedating effects associated with REQUIP, including somnolence and the possibility of falling asleep while engaged in activities of daily living. Since somnolence is a frequent adverse event with potentially serious consequences, patients should neither drive a car nor engage in other potentially dangerous activities until they have gained sufficient experience with REQUIP to gauge whether or not it affects their mental and/or motor performance adversely. Patients should be advised that if increased somnolence or episodes of falling asleep during activities of daily living (e.g., watching television, passenger in a car, etc.) are experienced at any time during treatment, they should not drive or participate in potentially dangerous activities until they have contacted their physician.

Because of possible additive effects, caution should be advised when patients are taking other sedating medications or alcohol in combination with REQUIP and when taking concomitant medications that increase plasma levels of ropinirole (e.g., ciprofloxacin).

Because of the possible additive sedative effects, caution should also be used when patients are taking alcohol or other CNS depressants (e.g., benzodiazepines, antipsychotics, antidepressants, etc.) in combination with REQUIP.

Patients should be informed they may experience hallucinations (unreal visions, sounds, or sensations) while taking REQUIP. These were uncommon in patients taking REQUIP for Restless Legs Syndrome. The risk is greater in patients with Parkinson's disease; the elderly are at greater risk than younger patients with Parkinson's disease; and the risk is greater in patients who are taking REQUIP with L-dopa, or taking higher doses of REQUIP.

Impulse Control Symptoms Including Compulsive Behaviors: There have been reports of patients experiencing intense urges to gamble, increased sexual urges, and other intense urges and the inability to control these urges while taking one or more of the medications that increase central dopaminergic tone, that are generally used for the treatment of Parkinson's disease or Restless Legs Syndrome, including REQUIP. Although it is not proven that the medications caused these events, these urges were reported to have stopped in some cases when the dose was reduced or the medication was stopped. Prescribers should ask patients about the development of new or increased gambling urges, sexual urges or other urges while being treated with REQUIP. Patients should inform their physician if they experience new or increased gambling urges, increased sexual urges or other intense urges while taking REQUIP. Physicians should consider dose reduction or stopping the medication if a patient develops such urges while taking REQUIP.

Because of the possibility that ropinirole may be excreted in breast milk, patients should be advised to notify their physicians if they intend to breastfeed or are breastfeeding an infant.

Because ropinirole has been shown to have adverse effects on embryo-fetal development, including teratogenic effects, in animals, and because experience in humans is limited, patients should be advised to notify their physician if they become pregnant or intend to become pregnant during therapy (see PRECAUTIONS: Pregnancy).

Drug Interactions: ***P_{450} Interaction:*** In vitro metabolism studies showed that CYP1A2 was the major enzyme responsible for the metabolism of ropinirole. There is thus the potential for substrates or inhibitors of this enzyme when coadministered with ropinirole to alter its clearance. Therefore, if therapy with a drug known to be a potent inhibitor of CYP1A2 is stopped or started during treatment with REQUIP, adjustment of the dose of REQUIP may be required.

L-dopa: Coadministration of carbidopa + L-dopa (SINEMET® 10/100 mg twice daily) with ropinirole (2 mg 3 times daily) had no effect on the steady-state pharmacokinetics of ropinirole (n = 28 patients). Oral administration of REQUIP 2 mg 3 times daily increased mean steady state C_{max} of L-dopa by 20%, but its AUC was unaffected (n = 23 patients).

Digoxin: Coadministration of REQUIP (2 mg 3 times daily) with digoxin (0.125 to 0.25 mg once daily) did not alter the steady-state pharmacokinetics of digoxin in 10 patients.

Theophylline: Administration of theophylline (300 mg twice daily, a substrate of CYP1A2) did not alter the steady-state pharmacokinetics of ropinirole (2 mg 3 times daily) in 12 patients with Parkinson's disease. Ropinirole (2 mg 3 times daily) did not alter the pharmacokinetics of theophylline (5 mg/kg IV) in 12 patients with Parkinson's disease.

Ciprofloxacin: Coadministration of ciprofloxacin (500 mg twice daily), an inhibitor of CYP1A2, with ropinirole (2 mg 3 times daily) increased ropinirole AUC by 84% on average and C_{max} by 60% (n = 12 patients).

Estrogens: Population pharmacokinetic analysis revealed that estrogens (mainly ethinylestradiol: intake 0.6 to 3 mg over 4-month to 23-year period) reduced the oral clearance of ropinirole by 36% in 16 patients. Dosage adjustment may not be needed for REQUIP in patients on estrogen therapy because patients must be carefully titrated with ropinirole to tolerance or adequate effect. However, if estrogen therapy is stopped or started during treatment with REQUIP, then adjustment of the dose of REQUIP may be required.

Dopamine Antagonists: Since ropinirole is a dopamine agonist, it is possible that dopamine antagonists such as neuroleptics (phenothiazines, butyrophenones, thioxanthenes) or metoclopramide may diminish the effectiveness of REQUIP. Patients with major psychotic disorders treated with neuroleptics should only be treated with dopamine agonists if the potential benefits outweigh the risks.

Population analysis showed that commonly administered drugs, e.g., selegiline, amantadine, tricyclic antidepressants, benzodiazepines, ibuprofen, thiazides, antihistamines, and anticholinergics, did not affect the oral clearance of ropinirole.

Carcinogenesis, Mutagenesis, Impairment of Fertility: Two-year carcinogenicity studies were conducted in Charles River CD-1 mice at doses of 5, 15, and 50 mg/kg/day and in Sprague-Dawley rats at doses of 1.5, 15, and 50 mg/kg/day (top doses equivalent to 10 and 20 times, respectively, the maximum recommended human dose (MRHD) of 24 mg/day on a mg/m^2 basis). In the male rat, there was a significant increase in testicular Leydig cell adenomas at all doses tested, i.e., ≥1.5 mg/kg (0.6 times the MRHD on a mg/m^2 basis). This finding is of questionable significance because the endocrine mechanisms believed to be involved in the production of Leydig cell hyperplasia and adenomas in rats are not relevant to humans. In the female mouse, there was an increase in benign uterine endometrial polyps at a dose of 50 mg/kg/day (10 times the MRHD on a mg/m^2 basis).

Ropinirole was not mutagenic or clastogenic in the in vitro Ames test, the in vitro chromosome aberration test in human lymphocytes, the in vitro mouse lymphoma (L1578Y cells) assay, and the in vivo mouse micronucleus test.

When administered to female rats prior to and during mating and throughout pregnancy, ropinirole caused disruption of implantation at doses of 20 mg/kg/day (8 times the MRHD on a mg/m^2 basis) or greater. This effect is thought to be due to the prolactin-lowering effect of ropinirole. In humans, chorionic gonadotropin, not prolactin, is essential for implantation. In rat studies using low doses (5 mg/kg) during the prolactin-dependent phase of early pregnancy (gestation days 0 to 8), ropinirole did not affect female fertility at dosages up to 100 mg/kg/day (40 times the MRHD on a mg/m^2 basis). No effect on male fertility was observed in rats at dosages up to 125 mg/kg/day (50 times the MRHD on a mg/m^2 basis).

Pregnancy: Pregnancy Category C. In animal reproduction studies, ropinirole has been shown to have adverse effects on embryo-fetal development, including teratogenic effects. Ropinirole given to pregnant rats during organogenesis (20 mg/kg on gestation days 6 and 7 followed by 20, 60, 90, 120, or 150 mg/kg on gestation days 8 through 15) resulted in decreased fetal body weight at 60 mg/kg/day, increased fetal death at 90 mg/kg/day, and digital malformations at 150 mg/kg/day (24, 36, and 60 times the MRHD on a mg/m^2 basis, respectively). The combined administration of ropinirole (10 mg/kg/day, 8 times the MRHD on a mg/m^2 basis) and L-dopa (250 mg/kg/day) to pregnant rabbits during organogenesis produced a greater incidence and severity of fetal malformations (primarily digit defects) than were seen in the offspring of rabbits treated with L-dopa alone. No indication of an effect on development of the conceptus was observed in rabbits when a maternally toxic dose of ropinirole was administered alone (20 mg/kg/day, 16 times the MRHD on a mg/m^2 basis). In a perinatal-postnatal study in rats, 10 mg/kg/day (4 times the MRHD on a mg/m^2 basis) of ropinirole impaired growth and development of nursing offspring and altered neurological development of female offspring.

There are no adequate and well-controlled studies using REQUIP in pregnant women. REQUIP should be used during pregnancy only if the potential benefit outweighs the potential risk to the fetus.

Nursing Mothers: REQUIP inhibits prolactin secretion in humans and could potentially inhibit lactation.

Studies in rats have shown that REQUIP and/or its metabolite(s) is excreted in breast milk. It is not known whether this drug is excreted in human milk. Because many drugs are excreted in human milk and because of the potential for serious adverse reactions in nursing infants from REQUIP, a decision should be made whether to discontinue nursing or to discontinue the drug, taking into account the importance of the drug to the mother.

Pediatric Use: Safety and effectiveness in the pediatric population have not been established.

ADVERSE REACTIONS

Parkinson's Disease: During the premarketing development of REQUIP, patients received REQUIP either without L-dopa (early Parkinson's disease studies) or as concomitant therapy with L-dopa (advanced Parkinson's disease studies). Because these 2 populations may have differential risks for various adverse events, this section will, in general, present adverse event data for these 2 populations separately.

Early Parkinson's Disease (Without L-dopa): The most commonly observed adverse events (>5%) in the double-blind, placebo-controlled early Parkinson's disease trials associated with the use of REQUIP (n = 157) not seen at an equivalent frequency among the placebo-treated patients (n = 147) were, in order of decreasing incidence: nausea, dizziness, somnolence, headache, vomiting, syncope, fatigue, dyspepsia, viral infection, constipation, pain, increased sweating, asthenia, dependent/leg edema, orthostatic symptoms, abdominal pain, pharyngitis, confusion, hallucinations, urinary tract infections, and abnormal vision.

Approximately 24% of 157 patients treated with REQUIP who participated in the double-blind, placebo-controlled early Parkinson's disease (without L-dopa) trials discontinued treatment due to adverse events compared to 13% of 147 patients who received placebo. The adverse events most commonly causing discontinuation of treatment by patients treated with REQUIP were: nausea (6.4%), dizziness (3.8%), aggravated Parkinson's disease (1.3%), hallucinations (1.3%), somnolence (1.3%), vomiting (1.3%), and headache (1.3%). Of these, hallucinations appear to be dose-related. While other adverse events leading to discontinuation may be dose-related, the titration design utilized in these trials precluded an adequate assessment of the dose response. For example, in the larger of the 2 trials described in CLINICAL PHARMACOLOGY: Clinical Trials, the difference in the rate of discontinuations emerged only after 10 weeks of treatment, suggesting, although not proving, that the effect could be related to dose.

Adverse Event Incidence in Controlled Clinical Studies: Table 2 lists treatment-emergent adverse events that occurred in ≥2% of patients with early Parkinson's disease (without L-dopa) treated with REQUIP participating in the double-blind, placebo-controlled studies and were numerically more common in the group treated with REQUIP. In these studies, either REQUIP or placebo was used as early therapy (i.e., without L-dopa).

The prescriber should be aware that these figures cannot be used to predict the incidence of adverse events in the course of usual medical practice where patient characteristics and other factors differ from those that prevailed in the clinical studies. Similarly, the cited frequencies cannot be compared with figures obtained from other clinical investigations involving different treatments, uses, and investigators. However, the cited figures do provide the prescribing physician with some basis for estimating the relative contribution of drug and non-drug factors to the adverse-events incidence rate in the population studied.

Table 2. Treatment-Emergent Adverse Event* Incidence in Double-Blind, Placebo-Controlled Early Parkinson's Disease (Without L-dopa) Trials (Events ≥2% of Patients Treated With REQUIP and Numerically More Frequent Than the Placebo Group)

Adverse Experience	REQUIP (n = 157) (%)	Placebo (n = 147) (%)
Autonomic nervous system		
Flushing	3	1
Dry mouth	5	3
Increased sweating	6	4
Body as a whole		
Asthenia	6	1
Chest pain	4	2
Dependent edema	6	3
Leg edema	7	1
Fatigue	11	4
Malaise	3	1
Pain	8	4
Cardiovascular general		
Hypertension	5	3
Hypotension	2	0
Orthostatic symptoms	6	5
Syncope	12	1
Central/peripheral nervous system		
Dizziness	40	22
Hyperkinesia	2	1
Hypesthesia	4	2
Vertigo	2	0
Gastrointestinal system		
Abdominal pain	6	3
Anorexia	4	1
Dyspepsia	10	5
Flatulence	3	1
Nausea	60	22
Vomiting	12	7
Heart rate/rhythm		
Extrasystoles	2	1
Atrial fibrillation	2	0
Palpitation	3	2
Tachycardia	2	0
Metabolic/nutritional		
Increased alkaline phosphatase	3	1
Psychiatric		
Amnesia	3	1
Impaired concentration	2	0
Confusion	5	1
Hallucination	5	1
Somnolence	40	6
Yawning	3	0
Reproductive male		
Impotence	3	1
Resistance mechanism		
Viral infection	11	3
Respiratory system		
Bronchitis	3	1
Dyspnea	3	0
Pharyngitis	6	4
Rhinitis	4	3
Sinusitis	4	3
Urinary system		
Urinary tract infection	5	4
Vascular extracardiac		
Peripheral ischemia	3	0
Vision		
Eye abnormality	3	1
Abnormal vision	6	3
Xerophthalmia	2	0

*Patients may have reported multiple adverse experiences during the study or at discontinuation; thus, patients may be included in more than one category.

Other events reported by 1% or more of early Parkinson's disease (without L-dopa) patients treated with REQUIP, but that were equally or more frequent in the placebo group, were: headache, upper respiratory infection, insomnia, arthralgia, tremor, back pain, anxiety, dyskinesias, aggravated Parkinsonism, depression, falls, myalgia, leg cramps, paresthesias, nervousness, diarrhea, arthritis, hot flushes, weight loss, rash, cough, hyperglycemia, muscle spasm, arthrosis, abnormal dreams, dystonia, increased salivation, bradycardia, gout, basal cell carcinoma, gingivitis, hematuria, and rigors.

Among the treatment-emergent adverse events in patients treated with REQUIP, hallucinations appear to be dose-related.

The incidence of adverse events was not materially different between women and men.

Advanced Parkinson's Disease (With L-dopa): The most commonly observed adverse events (>5%), in the double-blind, placebo-controlled advanced Parkinson's disease (with L-dopa) trials associated with the use of REQUIP (n = 208) as an adjunct to L-dopa not seen at an equivalent frequency among the placebo-treated patients (n = 120) were, in order of decreasing incidence: dyskinesias, nausea, dizziness, aggravated Parkinsonism, somnolence, headache, insomnia, injury, hallucinations, falls, abdominal pain, upper respiratory infection, confusion, increased sweating, vomiting, viral infection, increased drug level, arthralgia, tremor, anxiety, urinary tract infection, constipation, dry mouth, pain, hypokinesia, and paresthesia.

Approximately 24% of 208 patients who received REQUIP in the double-blind, placebo-controlled advanced Parkinson's disease (with L-dopa) trials discontinued treatment due to adverse events compared to 18% of 120 patients who received placebo. The events most commonly (≥1%) causing discontinuation of treatment by patients treated with REQUIP were: dizziness (2.9%), dyskinesias (2.4%), vomiting (2.4%), confusion (2.4%), nausea (1.9%), hallucinations (1.9%), anxiety (1.9%), and increased sweating (1.4%). Of these, hallucinations and dyskinesias appear to be dose-related.

Adverse Event Incidence in Controlled Clinical Studies: Table 3 lists treatment-emergent adverse events that occurred in ≥2% of patients with advanced Parkinson's disease (with L-dopa) treated with REQUIP who participated in the double-blind, placebo-controlled studies and were numerically more common in the group treated with REQUIP. In these studies, either REQUIP or placebo was used as an adjunct to L-dopa. Adverse events were usually mild or moderate in intensity.

The prescriber should be aware that these figures cannot be used to predict the incidence of adverse events in the course of usual medical practice where patient characteristics and other factors differ from those that prevailed in the clinical studies. Similarly, the cited frequencies cannot be compared with figures obtained from other clinical investigations involving different treatments, uses, and investigators. However, the cited figures do provide the prescribing physician with some basis for estimating the relative contribution of drug and non-drug factors to the adverse events incidence rate in the population studied.

Table 3. Treatment-Emergent Adverse Event* Incidence in Double-Blind, Placebo-Controlled Advanced Parkinson's Disease (With L-dopa) Trials (Events ≥2% of Patients Treated With REQUIP and Numerically More Frequent Than the Placebo Group)

Adverse Experience	REQUIP (n = 208) (%)	Placebo (n = 120) (%)
Autonomic nervous system		
Dry mouth	5	1
Increased sweating	7	2
Body as a whole		
Increased drug level	7	3
Pain	5	3
Cardiovascular general		
Hypotension	2	1
Syncope	3	2
Central/peripheral nervous system		
Dizziness	26	16
Dyskinesia	34	13
Falls	10	7
Headache	17	12
Hypokinesia	5	4
Paresis	3	0
Paresthesia	5	3
Tremor	6	3
Gastrointestinal system		
Abdominal pain	9	8
Constipation	6	3
Diarrhea	5	3
Dysphagia	2	1
Flatulence	2	1
Nausea	30	18
Increased saliva	2	1
Vomiting	7	4
Metabolic/nutritional		
Weight decrease	2	1
Musculoskeletal system		
Arthralgia	7	5
Arthritis	3	1
Psychiatric		
Amnesia	5	1
Anxiety	6	3
Confusion	9	2
Abnormal dreaming	3	2
Hallucinations	10	4
Nervousness	5	3
Somnolence	20	8
Red blood cell		
Anemia	2	0
Resistance mechanism		
Upper respiratory tract infection	9	8
Respiratory system		
Dyspnea	3	2
Urinary system		
Pyuria	2	1
Urinary incontinence	2	1
Urinary tract infection	6	3
Vision		
Diplopia	2	1

*Patients may have reported multiple adverse experiences during the study or at discontinuation; thus, patients may be included in more than one category.

Other events reported by 1% or more of patients treated with both REQUIP and L-dopa, but equally or more frequent in the placebo/L-dopa group, were: myocardial infarction, orthostatic symptoms, virus infections, asthenia, dyspepsia, myalgia, back pain, depression, leg cramps, fatigue, rhinitis, chest pain, hematuria, vertigo, tinnitus, leg edema, hot flushes, abnormal gait, hyperkinesia, and pharyngitis.

Among the treatment-emergent adverse events in patients treated with REQUIP, hallucinations and dyskinesias appear to be dose-related.

Restless Legs Syndrome: The most commonly observed adverse events (>5%) in the 12-week double-blind, placebo-controlled trials in the treatment of Restless Legs Syndrome with REQUIP (n = 496) and at least twice the rate for placebo-treated patients (n = 500) were, in order of decreasing incidence: nausea, somnolence, vomiting, dizziness, and fatigue (see Table 4). Occurrences of nausea in clinical trials were generally mild to moderate in intensity (see also DOSAGE AND ADMINISTRATION: General Dosing Considerations).

Approximately 5% of 496 patients treated with REQUIP who participated in the double-blind, placebo-controlled trials in the treatment of RLS discontinued treatment due to adverse events compared to 4% of 500 patients who received placebo. The adverse events most commonly causing discontinuation of treatment by patients treated with REQUIP were: nausea (1.6%), dizziness (0.8 %), and headache (0.8%).

Adverse Event Incidence in Controlled Clinical Studies: Table 4 lists treatment-emergent adverse events that occurred in ≥2% of patients with RLS treated with REQUIP participating in the 12-week double-blind, placebo-controlled studies and were numerically more common in the group treated with REQUIP.

The prescriber should be aware that these figures cannot be used to predict the incidence of adverse events in the course of usual medical practice where patient characteristics and other factors differ from those that prevailed in the clinical studies. Similarly, the cited frequencies cannot be compared with figures obtained from other clinical investigations involving different treatments, uses, and investigators. However, the cited figures do provide the prescribing physician with some basis for estimating the relative contribution of drug and non-drug factors to the adverse-events incidence rate in the population studied.

Table 4. Treatment-Emergent Adverse Event Incidence in Double-Blind, Placebo-Controlled RLS Trials (Events ≥2% of Patients Treated With REQUIP and Numerically More Frequent Than the Placebo Group)

Adverse Experience	REQUIP (n = 496) (%)	Placebo (n = 500) (%)
Ear and labyrinth disorders		
Vertigo	2	1
Gastrointestinal disorders		
Nausea	40	8
Vomiting	11	2
Diarrhea	5	3
Dyspepsia	4	3
Dry mouth	3	2
Abdominal pain upper	3	1
General disorders and administration site conditions		
Fatigue	8	4
Edema peripheral	2	1
Infections and infestations		
Nasopharyngitis	9	8
Influenza	3	2
Musculoskeletal and connective tissue disorders		
Arthralgia	4	3
Muscle cramps	3	2
Pain in extremity	3	2
Nervous system disorders		
Somnolence	12	6
Dizziness	11	5
Paresthesia	3	1
Respiratory, thoracic, and mediastinal disorders		
Cough	3	2
Nasal congestion	2	1
Skin and subcutaneous tissue disorders		
Hyperhidrosis	3	1

Other events reported by 2% or more of patients treated with REQUIP, but equally or more frequent in the placebo group, were headache, insomnia, restless legs syndrome, upper respiratory tract infection, back pain, and sinusitis.

Other Adverse Events Observed During All Phase 2/3 Clinical Trials for Parkinson's Disease: REQUIP has been administered to 1,599 individuals in clinical trials. During these trials, all adverse events were recorded by the clinical investigators using terminology of their own choosing. To provide a meaningful estimate of the proportion of individuals having adverse events, similar types of events were grouped into a smaller number of standardized categories using modified WHOART dictionary terminology. These categories are used in the listing below. The frequencies presented represent the proportion of the 1,599 individuals exposed to REQUIP who experienced events of the type cited on at least 1 occasion while receiving REQUIP. All reported events that occurred at least twice (or once for serious or potentially serious events), except those already listed above, trivial events, and terms too vague to be meaningful, are included without regard to determination of a causal relationship to REQUIP, except that events very unlikely to be drug-related have been deleted.

Events are further classified within body system categories and enumerated in order of decreasing frequency using the following definitions: frequent adverse events are defined as those occurring in at least 1/100 patients and infrequent adverse events are those occurring in 1/100 to 1/1,000 patients and rare events are those occurring in fewer than 1/1,000 patients.

Body as a Whole: Infrequent: Cellulitis, peripheral edema, fever, influenza-like symptoms, enlarged abdomen, precordial chest pain, and generalized edema. *Rare:* Ascites.

Cardiovascular: Infrequent: Cardiac failure, bradycardia, tachycardia, supraventricular tachycardia, angina pectoris, bundle branch block, cardiac arrest, cardiomegaly, aneurysm, mitral insufficiency. *Rare:* Ventricular tachycardia.

Central/Peripheral Nervous System: Frequent: Neuralgia. *Infrequent:* Involuntary muscle contractions, hypertonia, dysphonia, abnormal coordination, extrapyramidal disorder, migraine, choreoathetosis, coma, stupor, aphasia, convulsions, hypotonia, peripheral neuropathy, paralysis. *Rare:* Grand mal convulsions, hemiparesis, hemiplegia.

Endocrine: Infrequent: Hypothyroidism, gynecomastia, hyperthyroidism. *Rare:* Goiter, SIADH.

Gastrointestinal: Infrequent: Increased hepatic enzymes, bilirubinemia, cholecystitis, cholelithiasis colitis, dysphagia, periodontitis, fecal incontinence, gastroesophageal reflux, hemorrhoids, toothache, eructation, gastritis, esophagitis, hiccups, diverticulitis, duodenal ulcer, gastric ulcer, melena, duodenitis, gastrointestinal hemorrhage, glossitis, rectal hemorrhage, pancreatitis, stomatitis and ulcerative stomatitis, tongue edema. *Rare:* Biliary pain, hemorrhagic gastritis, hematemesis, salivary duct obstruction.

Hematologic: Infrequent: Purpura, thrombocytopenia, hematoma, Vitamin B12 deficiency, hypochromic anemia, eosinophilia, leukocytosis, leukopenia, lymphocytosis, lymphopenia, lymphedema.

Metabolic/Nutritional: Frequent: Increased BUN. *Infrequent:* Hypoglycemia, increased alkaline phosphatase, increased LDH, weight increase, hyperphosphatemia, hyperuricemia, diabetes mellitus, glycosuria, hypokalemia, hypercholesterolemia, hyperkalemia, acidosis, hyponatremia, thirst, increased CPK, dehydration. *Rare:* Hypochloremia.

Musculoskeletal: Infrequent: Aggravated arthritis, tendonitis, osteoporosis, bursitis, polymyalgia rheumatica, muscle weakness, skeletal pain, torticollis. *Rare:* Dupuytren's contracture requiring surgery.

Neoplasm: Infrequent: Malignant breast neoplasm. *Rare:* Bladder carcinoma, benign brain neoplasm, esophageal carcinoma, malignant laryngeal neoplasm, lipoma, rectal carcinoma, uterine neoplasm.

Psychiatric: Infrequent: Increased libido, agitation, apathy, impaired concentration, depersonalization, paranoid reaction, personality disorder, euphoria, delirium, dementia, delusion, emotional lability, decreased libido, manic reaction, somnambulism, aggressive reaction, neurosis. *Rare:* Suicide attempt.

Genitourinary: Infrequent: Amenorrhea, vaginal hemorrhage, penile disorder, prostatic disorder, balanoposthitis, epididymitis, perineal pain, dysuria, micturition frequency, albuminuria, nocturia, polyuria, renal calculus. *Rare:* Breast enlargement, mastitis, uterine hemorrhage, ejaculation disorder, Peyronie's disease, pyelonephritis, acute renal failure, uremia.

Resistance Mechanism: Infrequent: Herpes zoster, otitis media, sepsis, abscess, herpes simplex, fungal infection, genital moniliasis.

Respiratory: Infrequent: Asthma, epistaxis, laryngitis, pleurisy, pulmonary edema.

Skin/Appendage: Infrequent: Pruritus, dermatitis, eczema, skin ulceration, alopecia, skin hypertrophy, skin discoloration, urticaria, fungal dermatitis, furunculosis, hyperkeratosis, photosensitivity reaction, psoriasis, maculopapular rash, psoriaform rash, seborrhea.

Special Senses: Infrequent: Tinnitus, earache, decreased hearing, abnormal lacrimation, conjunctivitis, blepharitis, glaucoma, abnormal accommodation, blepharospasm, eye pain, photophobia. *Rare:* Scotoma.

Vascular Extracardiac: Infrequent: Varicose veins, phlebitis, peripheral gangrene. *Rare:* Limb embolism, pulmonary embolism, gangrene, subarachnoid hemorrhage, deep thrombophlebitis, leg thrombophlebitis, thrombosis.

Falling Asleep During Activities of Daily Living: Patients treated with REQUIP have reported falling asleep while engaged in activities of daily living, including operation of a motor vehicle which sometimes resulted in accidents (see bolded WARNING).

Other Adverse Events Observed During Phase 2/3 Clinical Trials for RLS: REQUIP has been administered to 911 individuals in clinical trials. During these trials, all adverse events were recorded by the clinical investigators using terminology of their own choosing. To provide a meaningful estimate of the proportion of individuals having adverse events, similar types of events were grouped into a smaller number of standardized categories using MedDRA dictionary terminology. These categories are used in the listing below. The frequencies presented represent the proportion of the 911 individuals exposed to REQUIP who experienced events of the type cited on at least one occasion while receiving REQUIP. All reported events that occurred at least twice (or once for serious or potentially serious events), except those already listed, trivial events, and terms too vague to be meaningful, are included without regard to determination of a causal relationship to REQUIP, except that events very unlikely to be drug-related have been deleted. Events are further classified within body system categories and enumerated in order of decreasing frequency using the following definitions: frequent adverse events are defined as those occurring in at least 1/100 patients and infrequent adverse events are those occurring in 1/100 to 1/1,000 patients.

Blood and Lymphatic System Disorders: Infrequent: Anemia, lymphadenopathy.

Cardiac Disorders: Frequent: Palpitations. *Infrequent:* Acute coronary syndrome, angina pectoris, angina unstable, bradycardia, cardiac failure, cardiovascular disorder, coronary artery disease, myocardial infarction, sick sinus syndrome, tachycardia.

Congenital, Familial, and Genetic Disorders: Infrequent: Pigmented nevus.

Ear and Labyrinth Disorders: Infrequent: Ear pain, middle ear effusion, tinnitus.

Endocrine Disorders: Infrequent: Goiter, hypothyroidism.

Eye Disorders: Infrequent: Blepharitis, conjunctival hemorrhage, conjunctivitis, eye irritation, eye pain, keratoconjunctivitis sicca, vision blurred, visual acuity reduced, visual disturbance.

Gastrointestinal Disorders: Frequent: Abdominal pain, constipation, gastroesophageal reflux disease, stomach discomfort, toothache. *Infrequent:* Abdominal adhesions, abdominal discomfort, abdominal distension, abdominal pain lower, duodenal ulcer, dysphagia, eructation, flatulence, gastric disorder, gastric hemorrhage, gastric polyps, gastric ulcer, gastritis, gastrointestinal pain, hematemesis, hemorrhoids, hiatus hernia, intestinal obstruction, irritable bowel syndrome, loose stools, mouth ulceration, pancreatitis acute, peptic ulcer, rectal hemorrhage, reflux esophagitis.

General Disorders and Administration Site Conditions: Frequent: Asthenia, chest pain, influenza-like illness, rigors. *Infrequent:* Chest discomfort, feeling cold, feeling hot, hunger, lethargy, malaise, edema, pain, pyrexia.

Hepatobiliary Disorders: Infrequent: Cholecystitis, cholelithiasis, ischemic hepatitis.

Immune System Disorders: Infrequent: Hypersensitivity.

Infections and Infestations: Frequent: Bronchitis, gastroenteritis, gastroenteritis viral, lower respiratory tract infection, rhinitis, tooth abscess, urinary tract infection. *Infrequent:* Appendicitis, bacterial infection, bladder infection, bronchitis acute, candidiasis, cellulitis, cystitis, diarrhea infectious, diverticulitis, ear infection, folliculitis, fungal infection, gastrointestinal infection, herpes simplex, infected cyst, laryngitis, localized infection, mastitis, otitis externa, otitis media, pharyngitis, pneumonia, postoperative infection, respiratory tract infection, tonsillitis, tooth infection, vaginal candidiasis, vaginal infection, vaginal mycosis, viral infection, viral upper respiratory tract infection, wound infection.

Injury, Poisoning, and Procedural Complications: Infrequent: Concussion, lower limb fracture, post procedural hemorrhage, road traffic accident.

Investigations: Infrequent: Blood cholesterol increased, blood iron decreased, blood pressure increased, blood urine present, hemoglobin decreased, heart rate increased, protein urine present, weight decreased, weight increased.

Metabolism and Nutrition Disorders: Infrequent: Anorexia, decreased appetite, diabetes mellitus non-insulin-dependent, fluid retention, gout, hypercholesterolemia.

Musculoskeletal and Connective Tissue Disorders: Frequent: Muscle spasms, musculoskeletal stiffness, myalgia, neck pain, osteoarthritis, tendonitis. *Infrequent:* Arthritis, aseptic necrosis bone, bone pain, bone spur, bursitis, groin pain, intervertebral disc degeneration, intervertebral disc protrusion, joint stiffness, joint swelling, localized osteoarthritis, monoarthritis, muscle contracture, muscle tightness, muscle twitching, osteoporosis, rotator cuff syndrome, sacroiliitis, synovitis.

Neoplasms Benign, Malignant, and Unspecified: Infrequent: Anaplastic thyroid cancer, angiomyolipoma, basal cell carcinoma, breast cancer, gastric cancer, gastrointestinal stromal tumor, malignant melanoma, prostate cancer, skin papilloma, squamous cell carcinoma, uterine leiomyoma.

Nervous System Disorders: Frequent: Hypoesthesia, migraine. *Infrequent:* Amnesia, aphasia, ataxia, balance disorder, benign intracranial hypertension, burning sensation, carpal tunnel syndrome, disturbance in attention, dizziness postural, dysgeusia, dyskinesia, head discomfort, hyperesthesia, hypersomnia, lethargy, loss of consciousness, memory impairment, migraine with aura, migraine without aura, neuralgia, sciatica, sedation, sinus headache, sleep apnea syndrome, syncope vasovagal, tension headache, transient ischemic attack, tremor.

Psychiatric Disorders: Frequent: Anxiety, depression, irritability, sleep disorder. *Infrequent:* Abnormal dreams, agitation, bruxism, confusional state, depressed mood, disorientation, early morning awakening, libido decreased, loss of libido, mood swings, nervousness, nightmare, panic attack, stress symptoms, tension.

Renal and Urinary Disorders: Infrequent: Dysuria, hematuria, hypertonic bladder, micturition disorder, nephrolithiasis, nocturia, pollakiuria, proteinuria, urinary retention.

Reproductive System and Breast Disorders: Frequent: Erectile dysfunction. ***Infrequent:*** Breast cyst, dysmenorrhea, menorrhagia, pelvic peritoneal adhesions, postmenopausal hemorrhage, premenstrual syndrome, prostatitis.
Respiratory, Thoracic and Mediastinal Disorders: Frequent: Asthma, pharyngolaryngeal pain. ***Infrequent:*** Dry throat, dyspnea, epistaxis, hemoptysis, hoarseness, interstitial lung disease, nasal mucosal disorder, nasal polyps, respiratory tract congestion, rhinorrhea, sinus congestion, sneezing, wheezing, yawning.
Skin and Subcutaneous Tissue Disorders: Frequent: Night sweats, rash. ***Infrequent:*** Acne, actinic keratosis, alopecia, cold sweat, dermatitis, dermatitis allergic, dermatitis contact, eczema, exanthem, face edema, photosensitivity reaction, pruritus, psoriasis, rash pruritic, skin lesion, urticaria.
Vascular Disorders: Frequent: Hot flush, hypertension, hypotension. ***Infrequent:*** Atherosclerosis, circulatory collapse, flushing, hematoma, thrombosis, varicose vein.
Postmarketing Reports: The following adverse events (not listed above in clinical trials or other sections of the prescribing information) have been identified during postapproval use of ropinirole. Because these events are reported voluntarily from a population of uncertain size, it is not always possible to reliably estimate their frequency or establish a causal relationship to drug exposure.
Immune Systems Disorders: Hypersensitivity reactions (including urticaria, angioedema, rash, and pruritus).
Psychiatric Disorders: Impulse control symptoms, pathological gambling, increased libido including hypersexuality.

DRUG ABUSE AND DEPENDENCE

Controlled Substance Class: REQUIP is not a controlled substance.
Physical and Psychological Dependence: Animal studies and human clinical trials with REQUIP did not reveal any potential for drug-seeking behavior or physical dependence.

OVERDOSAGE

In the Parkinson's disease program, there have been patients who accidentally or intentionally took more than their prescribed dose of ropinirole. The largest overdose reported in the Parkinson's disease clinical trials was 435 mg taken over a 7-day period (62.1 mg/day). Of patients who received a dose greater than 24 mg/day, reported symptoms included adverse events commonly reported during dopaminergic therapy (nausea, dizziness), as well as visual hallucinations, hyperhidrosis, claustrophobia, chorea, palpitations, asthenia, and nightmares. Additional symptoms reported for doses of 24 mg or less or for overdoses of unknown amount included vomiting, increased coughing, fatigue, syncope, vasovagal syncope, dyskinesia, agitation, chest pain, orthostatic hypotension, somnolence, and confusional state.
Overdose Management: It is anticipated that the symptoms of overdose with REQUIP will be related to its dopaminergic activity. General supportive measures are recommended. Vital signs should be maintained, if necessary. Removal of any unabsorbed material (e.g., by gastric lavage) should be considered.

DOSAGE AND ADMINISTRATION

General Dosing Considerations for Parkinson's Disease and RLS: REQUIP can be taken with or without food. Patients may be advised that taking REQUIP with food may reduce the occurrence of nausea. However, this has not been established in controlled clinical trials.
If a significant interruption in therapy with REQUIP has occurred, retitration of therapy may be warranted.
Geriatric Use: Pharmacokinetic studies demonstrated a reduced clearance of ropinirole in the elderly (see CLINICAL PHARMACOLOGY). Dose adjustment is not necessary since the dose is individually titrated to clinical response.
Renal Impairment: The pharmacokinetics of ropinirole were not altered in patients with moderate renal impairment (see CLINICAL PHARMACOLOGY). Therefore, no dosage adjustment is necessary in patients with moderate renal impairment. The use of REQUIP in patients with severe renal impairment has not been studied.
Hepatic Impairment: The pharmacokinetics of ropinirole have not been studied in patients with hepatic impairment. Since patients with hepatic impairment may have higher plasma levels and lower clearance, REQUIP should be titrated with caution in these patients.
Dosing for Parkinson's Disease: In all clinical studies, dosage was initiated at a subtherapeutic level and gradually titrated to therapeutic response. The dosage should be increased to achieve a maximum therapeutic effect, balanced against the principal side effects of nausea, dizziness, somnolence, and dyskinesia.
The recommended starting dose for Parkinson's disease is 0.25 mg 3 times daily. Based on individual patient response, dosage should then be titrated with weekly increments as described in Table 5. After week 4, if necessary, daily dosage may be increased by 1.5 mg/day on a weekly basis up to a dose of 9 mg/day, and then by up to 3 mg/day weekly to a total dose of 24 mg/day. Doses greater than 24 mg/day have not been tested in clinical trials.

Table 5. Ascending-Dose Schedule of REQUIP for Parkinson's Disease

Week	Dosage	Total Daily Dose
1	0.25 mg 3 times daily	0.75 mg
2	0.5 mg 3 times daily	1.5 mg
3	0.75 mg 3 times daily	2.25 mg
4	1 mg 3 times daily	3 mg

When REQUIP is administered as adjunct therapy to L-dopa, the concurrent dose of L-dopa may be decreased gradually as tolerated. L-dopa dosage reduction was allowed during the advanced Parkinson's disease (with L-dopa) study if dyskinesias or other dopaminergic effects occurred. Overall, reduction of L-dopa dose was sustained in 87% of patients treated with REQUIP and in 57% of patients on placebo. On average the L-dopa dose was reduced by 31% in patients treated with REQUIP.
REQUIP for Parkinson's disease patients should be discontinued gradually over a 7-day period. The frequency of administration should be reduced from 3 times daily to twice daily for 4 days. For the remaining 3 days, the frequency should be reduced to once daily prior to complete withdrawal of REQUIP.
Dosing for Restless Legs Syndrome: In all clinical trials, the dose for REQUIP was initiated at 0.25 mg once daily, 1 to 3 hours before bedtime. Patients were titrated based on clinical response and tolerability.
The recommended adult starting dosage for RLS is 0.25 mg once daily, 1 to 3 hours before bedtime. After 2 days, the dosage can be increased to 0.5 mg once daily and to 1 mg once daily at the end of the first week of dosing, then as shown in Table 6 as needed to achieve efficacy. For RLS, the safety and effectiveness of doses greater than 4 mg once daily have not been established.

Table 6. Dose Titration Schedule for RLS

Day/Week	Dosage to be taken once daily, 1 to 3 hours before bedtime
Days 1 and 2	0.25 mg
Days 3-7	0.5 mg
Week 2	1 mg
Week 3	1.5 mg
Week 4	2 mg
Week 5	2.5 mg
Week 6	3 mg
Week 7	4 mg

In clinical trials of patients being treated for RLS with doses up to 4 mg once daily, REQUIP was discontinued without a taper.

HOW SUPPLIED

Tablets: Each pentagonal film-coated TILTAB® tablet with beveled edges contains ropinirole hydrochloride equivalent to the labeled amount of ropinirole as follows:
0.25 mg: white tablets imprinted with "SB" and "4890" in bottles of 100 (NDC 0007-4890-20).
0.5 mg: yellow tablets imprinted with "SB" and "4891" in bottles of 100 (NDC 0007-4891-20).
1 mg: green tablets imprinted with "SB" and "4892" in bottles of 100 (NDC 0007-4892-20).
2 mg: pale yellowish-pink tablets imprinted with "SB" and "4893" in bottles of 100 (NDC 0007-4893-20).
3 mg: pale to moderate reddish-purple tablets, imprinted with "SB" and "4895" in bottles of 100 (NDC 0007-4895-20).
4 mg: pale brown tablets imprinted with "SB" and "4896" in bottles of 100 (NDC 0007-4896-20).
5 mg: blue tablets imprinted with "SB" and "4894" in bottles of 100 (NDC 0007-4894-20).
STORAGE: Protect from light and moisture. Close container tightly after each use. Store at controlled room temperature 20°-25°C (68°-77°F) [see USP].

GlaxoSmithKline
Research Triangle Park, NC 27709
REQUIP and TILTAB are registered trademarks of GlaxoSmithKline.
SINEMET is a registered trademark of Merck & Co., Inc.
©2009, GlaxoSmithKline. All rights reserved.
May 2009 REP: 3PI

PHARMACIST--DETACH HERE AND GIVE INSTRUCTIONS TO PATIENT

PATIENT INFORMATION

REQUIP® (ropinirole tablets)
If you have Restless Legs Syndrome (RLS, also known as Ekbom Syndrome), read this side
Read this information completely before you start taking REQUIP. Read the information each time you get more medicine. There may be new information. This leaflet provides a summary about REQUIP. It does not include everything there is to know about your medicine. This information should not take the place of discussions with your doctor about your medical condition or REQUIP.
What is REQUIP?
REQUIP is a prescription medicine to treat moderate-to-severe primary Restless Legs Syndrome. It is sometimes used to treat Parkinson's disease. Having one of these conditions does not mean you have or will develop the other.
What is the most important information I should know about REQUIP?
- Patients with RLS should take REQUIP differently than patients with Parkinson's disease (see **How should I take REQUIP for RLS?** for the recommended dosing for RLS). A lower dose of REQUIP is generally needed for patients with RLS, and is taken once daily before bedtime.
- There are known side effects of REQUIP. If you fall asleep or feel very sleepy while doing normal activities such as driving, faint, feel dizzy, nauseated, or sweaty when you stand up from sitting or lying down, you should talk with your doctor (see **What are the possible side effects of REQUIP?**).
- Before starting REQUIP, be sure to tell your doctor if you are taking any medicines that make you drowsy.

Unusual urges: Some patients taking REQUIP or REQUIP XL get urges to behave in a way unusual for them. Examples of this are an unusual urge to gamble or increased sexual urges and behaviors. If you notice or your family notices that you are developing any unusual behaviors, talk to your healthcare provider.
Who should not take REQUIP?
You should not take REQUIP if you are allergic to the active ingredient ropinirole or to any of the inactive ingredients. Your doctor and pharmacist have a list of the inactive ingredients.
What should I tell my doctor?
Be sure to tell your doctor if:
- you are pregnant or plan to become pregnant.
- you are breastfeeding.
- you have daytime sleepiness from a sleep disorder other than RLS or have unexpected sleepiness or periods of sleep while taking REQUIP.
- you are taking any other prescription or over-the-counter medicines. Some of these medicines may increase your chances of getting side effects while taking REQUIP.
- you start or stop taking other medicines while you are taking REQUIP. This may increase your chances of getting side effects.
- you start or stop smoking while you are taking REQUIP. Smoking may decrease the treatment effect of REQUIP.
- you feel dizzy, nauseated, sweaty, or faint when you stand up from sitting or lying down.
- you drink alcoholic beverages. This may increase your chances of becoming drowsy or sleepy while taking REQUIP.

How should I take REQUIP for RLS?
- Be sure to take REQUIP exactly as directed by your doctor or healthcare provider.
- The usual way to take REQUIP is once in the evening, 1 to 3 hours before bedtime.
- Your doctor will start you on a low dose of REQUIP. Your doctor may change the dose until you are taking the amount of medicine that is right for you to control your symptoms.
- **If you miss your dose, do not double your next dose.** Take only your usual dose 1 to 3 hours before your next bedtime.
- Contact your doctor, if you stop taking REQUIP for any reason. Do not restart without consulting your doctor.
- You can take REQUIP with or without food. Taking REQUIP with food may decrease the chances of feeling nauseated.

What are the possible side effects of REQUIP?
- Most people who take REQUIP tolerate it well. The most commonly reported side effects in people taking REQUIP for RLS are nausea, vomiting, dizziness, and drowsiness or sleepiness. You should be careful until you know if REQUIP affects your ability to remain alert while doing normal daily activities, and you should watch for the development of significant daytime sleepiness or episodes of falling asleep. It is possible that you could fall asleep

while doing normal activities such as driving a car, doing physical tasks, or using hazardous machinery while taking REQUIP. Your chances of falling asleep while doing normal activities while taking REQUIP are greater if you are taking other medicines that cause drowsiness.

- When you start taking REQUIP or when you increase your dose, you may feel dizzy, nauseated, sweaty or faint, when first standing up from sitting or lying down. Therefore, do not stand up quickly after sitting or lying down, particularly if you have been sitting or lying down for a long period of time. Take a minute sitting on the edge of the bed or chair before you get up.
- Hallucinations (unreal sounds, visions, or sensations) have been reported in patients taking REQUIP. These were uncommon in patients taking REQUIP for RLS. The risk is greater in patients with Parkinson's disease who are elderly, taking REQUIP with L-dopa, or taking higher doses of REQUIP than recommended for RLS.

Some patients taking REQUIP get urges to behave in a way unusual for them. Examples of this are an unusual urge to gamble or increased sexual urges and behaviors. If you notice or your family notices that you are developing any unusual behaviors, talk to your healthcare provider.

This is not a complete list of side effects and should not take the place of discussions with your healthcare providers. Your doctor or pharmacist can give you a more complete list of possible side effects.

Call your healthcare provider for medical advice about side effects. You may report side effects to FDA at 1-800-FDA-1088.

Other Information about REQUIP

- Studies of people with Parkinson's disease show that they may be at an increased risk of developing melanoma, a form of skin cancer, when compared to people without Parkinson's disease. It is not known if this problem is associated with Parkinson's disease or the medicines used to treat Parkinson's disease. REQUIP is one of the medicines used to treat Parkinson's disease, therefore, patients being treated with REQUIP should have periodic skin examinations.
- Take REQUIP exactly as your doctor prescribes it.
- Do not share REQUIP with other people, even if they have the same symptoms you have.
- Keep REQUIP out of the reach of children.
- Store REQUIP at room temperature out of direct sunlight.
- Keep REQUIP in a tightly closed container.

This leaflet summarizes important information about REQUIP. Medicines are sometimes prescribed for purposes other than those listed in this leaflet. Do not take REQUIP for a condition for which it was not prescribed. For more information, talk with your doctor or pharmacist. They can give you information about REQUIP that is written for healthcare professionals.

PATIENT INFORMATION

REQUIP® (ropinirole tablets)

If you have Parkinson's disease, read this side

Read this information completely before you start taking REQUIP. Read the information each time you get more medicine. There may be new information. This leaflet provides a summary about REQUIP. It does not include everything there is to know about your medicine. This information should not take the place of discussions with your doctor about your medical condition or REQUIP.

What is REQUIP?

REQUIP is a prescription medicine used to treat Parkinson's disease. It is also used to treat moderate-to-severe primary Restless Legs Syndrome. Having one of these conditions does not mean you have or will develop the other.

What is the most important information I should know about REQUIP?

- Patients with Parkinson's disease should take REQUIP differently than patients with Restless Legs Syndrome (see **How should I take REQUIP for Parkinson's disease?**). For Parkinson's disease, a higher dose of REQUIP is generally needed, and is taken more frequently throughout the day.
- There are known side effects of REQUIP (see **What are the possible side effects of REQUIP?**).
- If you fall asleep or feel very sleepy while doing normal activities such as driving, faint, feel dizzy, nauseated, or sweaty when you stand up from sitting or lying down, you should talk with your doctor.
- Hallucinations (unreal visions, sounds, or sensations) have been reported in patients taking REQUIP. The risk is greater in patients with Parkinson's disease who are elderly, taking REQUIP with L-dopa or taking higher doses of REQUIP. If these occur, you should discuss them with your doctor.
- REQUIP may make some of the side effects of L-dopa worse. REQUIP may cause uncontrolled sudden movements or make such movements you already have worse or more frequent. You should notify your doctor in such a case as dosage adjustments to your anti-Parkinson's medications may be necessary.
- Before starting REQUIP, be sure to tell your doctor if you are taking any medicines that make you drowsy.

Unusual urges: Some patients taking REQUIP or REQUIP XL get urges to behave in a way unusual for them. Examples of this are an unusual urge to gamble or increased sexual urges and behaviors. If you notice or your family notices that you are developing any unusual behaviors, talk to your healthcare provider.

Who should not take REQUIP?

You should not take REQUIP if you are allergic to the active ingredient ropinirole or to any of the inactive ingredients. Your doctor and pharmacist have a list of the inactive ingredients.

What should I tell my doctor?

Be sure to tell your doctor if:

- you are pregnant or plan to become pregnant.
- you are breastfeeding.
- you have daytime sleepiness from a sleep disorder or have unexpected sleepiness or periods of sleep while taking REQUIP.
- you are taking any other prescription or over-the-counter medicines. Some of these medicines may increase your chances of getting side effects while taking REQUIP.
- you start or stop taking other medicines while you are taking REQUIP. This may increase your chances of getting side effects.
- you start or stop smoking while you are taking REQUIP. Smoking may decrease the treatment effect of REQUIP.
- you feel dizzy, nauseated, sweaty, or faint when you first stand up from sitting or lying down.
- you drink alcoholic beverages. This may increase your chances of becoming drowsy or sleepy while taking REQUIP.

How should I take REQUIP for Parkinson's disease?

- Be sure to take your REQUIP exactly as directed by your doctor or healthcare provider.
- Three times a day is the usual way to take REQUIP for Parkinson's disease.
- Your doctor will start you on a low dose of REQUIP. Your doctor will change the dose until you are taking the right amount of medicine to control your symptoms. It may take several weeks before you reach a dose that controls your symptoms.
- **If you miss a dose, do not double your next dose.**
- Contact your doctor, if you stop taking REQUIP for any reason. Do not restart without consulting your doctor.
- Your doctor may prescribe REQUIP alone or add REQUIP to medicine that you are already taking for Parkinson's disease.
- You can take REQUIP with or without food. Taking REQUIP with food may decrease the chances of feeling nauseated.

What are the possible side effects of REQUIP?

- Most people who take REQUIP tolerate it well. The most commonly reported side effects in people taking REQUIP are nausea, headache, dizziness, drowsiness or sleepiness.
- You should be careful until you know if REQUIP affects your ability to remain alert while doing normal daily activities, and you should watch for the development of significant daytime sleepiness or episodes of falling asleep. It is possible that you could fall asleep while doing normal activities such as driving a car, doing physical tasks, or using hazardous machinery while taking REQUIP. Your chances of falling asleep while doing normal activities while taking REQUIP are greater if you are taking other medicines that cause drowsiness.
- When you start taking REQUIP or when you increase your dose, you may feel dizzy, nauseated, sweaty or faint, when first standing up from sitting or lying down. Therefore, do not stand up quickly after sitting or lying down, particularly if you have been sitting or lying down for a long period of time. Take a minute sitting on the edge of the bed or chair before you get up.
- Hallucinations (unreal visions, sounds, or sensations) have been reported in patients taking REQUIP. The risk is greater in patients with Parkinson's disease who are elderly, taking REQUIP with L-dopa, or taking higher amounts of REQUIP.
- If you are taking L-dopa for Parkinson's disease, REQUIP may make some of the side effects of L-dopa worse. REQUIP may cause uncontrolled sudden movements or make such movements you already have worse or more frequent.

Some patients taking REQUIP get urges to behave in a way unusual for them. Examples of this are an unusual urge to gamble or increased sexual urges and behaviors. If you notice or your family notices that you are developing any unusual behaviors, talk to your healthcare provider.

This is not a complete list of side effects and should not take the place of discussions with your healthcare providers. Your doctor or pharmacist can give you a more complete list of possible side effects.

Call your healthcare provider for medical advice about side effects. You may report side effects to FDA at 1-800-FDA-1088.

Other Information about REQUIP

- Studies of people with Parkinson's disease show that they may be at an increased risk of developing melanoma, a form of skin cancer, when compared to people without Parkinson's disease. It is not known if this problem is associated with Parkinson's disease or the medicines used to treat Parkinson's disease, therefore, patients being treated with REQUIP should have periodic skin examinations.
- Take REQUIP exactly as your doctor prescribes it.
- Do not share REQUIP with other people, even if they have the same symptoms you have.
- Keep REQUIP out of the reach of children.
- Store REQUIP at room temperature out of direct sunlight.
- Keep REQUIP in a tightly closed container.

This leaflet summarizes important information about REQUIP. Medicines are sometimes prescribed for purposes other than those listed in this leaflet. Do not take REQUIP for a condition for which it was not prescribed. For more information, talk with your doctor or pharmacist. They can give you information about REQUIP that is written for healthcare professionals.

GlaxoSmithKline
Research Triangle Park, NC 27709
©2009, GlaxoSmithKline. All rights reserved.
April 2009 REP:2PIL

REQUIP® XL™ ℞

[rē′ kwip]

(ropinirole extended-release tablets)

HIGHLIGHTS OF PRESCRIBING INFORMATION

These highlights do not include all the information needed to use REQUIP XL safely and effectively. See full prescribing information for REQUIP XL.

REQUIP® XL™ (ropinirole extended-release tablets)

Initial U.S. Approval: 1997

INDICATIONS AND USAGE

REQUIP XL is an orally administered, non-ergoline dopamine agonist indicated for the treatment of signs and symptoms of idiopathic Parkinson's disease. (1.1)

DOSAGE AND ADMINISTRATION

- REQUIP XL Tablets are taken once daily, with or without food. Tablets must be swallowed whole and must not be chewed, crushed, or divided. (2.1)
- The starting dose is 2 mg taken once daily for 1 to 2 weeks, followed by increases of 2 mg/day at 1 week or longer intervals as appropriate, depending on therapeutic response and tolerability, up to a maximally recommended dose of 24 mg/day. Patients should be assessed for therapeutic response and tolerability at a minimal interval of 1 week or longer after each dose increment. Caution should be exercised during dose titration because too rapid a rate of titration can lead to dose selection that does not provide additional benefit, but that increases the risk of adverse reactions. (2.2, 14.2)
- Patients may be switched directly from immediate-release ropinirole to REQUIP XL. The initial switching dose of REQUIP XL should most closely match the total daily dose of immediate-release ropinirole, see Table 1. (2.3)
- If REQUIP XL must be discontinued, it should be tapered gradually over a 7-day period. (2.2)

DOSAGE FORMS AND STRENGTHS

Tablets: 2 mg, 4 mg, 6 mg, 8 mg, and 12 mg (3)

CONTRAINDICATIONS

None

WARNINGS AND PRECAUTIONS

- Falling asleep during activities of daily living may occur, including the operation of motor vehicles, which sometimes resulted in accidents. Sudden onset of sleep may occur without apparent warning or daytime drowsiness. Sedating medications (such as alcohol or CNS depressants), the presence of sleeping disorders, or other medications that increase plasma levels of ropinirole, may increase the risk of somnolence or falling asleep while engaged in activities of daily living. Before initiating treatment, patients should be advised of the potential of sudden onset of sleep or to develop drowsiness and asked about risk factors they may have. If a patient develops sudden onset of sleep during activities that require active participation (e.g., conversations, eating, etc.) and/or cannot avoid high-risk activities in the future, REQUIP XL should ordinarily be discontinued. (5.1)
- Syncope, sometimes associated with bradycardia, may occur. (5.2)
- Symptomatic hypotension (including postural/orthostatic hypotension) may occur, especially during dose escalation. (5.3)

- Elevation of blood pressure and changes in heart rate may occur. (5.4)
- Hallucination may occur. (5.5)
- Dyskinesia may be caused or exacerbated. Decreasing the L-dopa dose may lessen or eliminate this side effect. (5.6)

———————ADVERSE REACTIONS———————

- Most common adverse reactions (incidence ≥5% and greater than placebo) in advanced Parkinson's disease with concomitant L-dopa were dyskinesia, nausea, dizziness, hallucination, somnolence, abdominal pain/discomfort, and orthostatic hypotension. (6.1)
- Most common adverse reactions (incidence ≥5%) in early Parkinson's disease without L-dopa were nausea, somnolence, abdominal pain/discomfort, dizziness, headache, and constipation. (6.1)

To report SUSPECTED ADVERSE REACTIONS, contact GlaxoSmithKline at 1-888-825-5249 or FDA at 1-800-FDA-1088 or www.fda.gov/medwatch.

———————DRUG INTERACTIONS———————

- CYP1A2 is the major enzyme responsible for the metabolism of ropinirole. Thus inhibitors (e.g., ciprofloxacin, fluvoxamine) or inducers (e.g., omeprazole or smoking) of CYP1A2 may alter the clearance of ropinirole. Adjustment of dosage of REQUIP XL may be required. (7.1)
- Higher doses of estrogens, usually associated with hormone replacement therapy (HRT), reduced oral clearance of ropinirole. Starting or stopping HRT treatment may require adjustment of dosage of REQUIP XL. (7.3)
- Dopamine antagonists, such as neuroleptics (e.g., phenothiazines, butyrophenones, thioxanthenes) or metoclopramide, may diminish effectiveness of ropinirole. (7.4)

———————USE IN SPECIFIC POPULATIONS———————

Pregnancy: REQUIP XL should be used during pregnancy only if the potential benefit outweighs the potential risk to the fetus. (8.1)

See 17 for PATIENT COUNSELING INFORMATION and FDA-approved patient labeling.

**Revised: April 2009
RXL:4PI**

FULL PRESCRIBING INFORMATION

1 INDICATIONS AND USAGE

1.1 Parkinson's Disease

REQUIP XL (ropinirole extended-release tablets) is indicated for the treatment of the signs and symptoms of idiopathic Parkinson's disease.

2 DOSAGE AND ADMINISTRATION

2.1 General Dosing Considerations

- REQUIP XL Extended-Release Tablets are taken once daily, with or without food. Taking REQUIP XL with food may reduce the occurrence of nausea; this has not been established in controlled clinical trials [see Clinical Pharmacology (12.3)].
- Tablets must be swallowed whole and must not be chewed, crushed, or divided.
- If a significant interruption in therapy with REQUIP XL has occurred, retitration of therapy may be warranted.

2.2 Dosing for Parkinson's Disease

The starting dose is 2 mg taken once daily for 1 to 2 weeks, followed by increases of 2 mg/day at 1-week or longer intervals as appropriate, depending on therapeutic response and tolerability, up to a maximally recommended dose of 24 mg/day.

In clinical trials, dosage was initiated at 2 mg/day and gradually titrated based on individual therapeutic response and tolerability. Doses greater than 24 mg/day have not been studied in clinical trials. Patients should be assessed for therapeutic response and tolerability at a minimal interval of 1 week or longer after each dose increment. Caution should be exercised during dose titration because too rapid a rate of titration may lead to dose selection that may not provide additional benefit, but that may increase the risk of adverse reactions [see Clinical Studies (14.2)]. Due to the flexible dosing design used in clinical studies, specific dose response information could not be determined.

When REQUIP XL is administered as adjunct therapy to L-dopa, the concurrent dose of L-dopa may be decreased gradually as tolerated. In the placebo-controlled advanced Parkinson's disease study, the L-dopa dose was reduced once patients reached a dose of REQUIP XL of 8 mg/day. Overall, L-dopa dose reduction was sustained in 93% of patients treated with REQUIP XL and in 72% of patients on placebo. On average the L-dopa dose was reduced by 34% in patients treated with REQUIP XL [see Clinical Studies (14)]. REQUIP XL should be discontinued gradually over a 7-day period.

2.3 Switching From Immediate-Release Ropinirole Tablets to REQUIP XL

Patients may be switched directly from immediate-release ropinirole to REQUIP XL Tablets. The initial dose of REQUIP XL should most closely match the total daily dose of the immediate-release formulation of REQUIP, as shown in Table 1.

Table 1. Conversion from Immediate-Release REQUIP to REQUIP XL

Immediate-Release Ropinirole Tablets Total Daily Dose (mg)	REQUIP XL Tablets Total Daily Dose (mg)
0.75 to 2.25	2
3 to 4.5	4
6	6
7.5 to 9	8
12	12
15 to 18	16
21	20
24	24

Following conversion to REQUIP XL, the dose may be adjusted depending on therapeutic response and tolerability [see Dosage and Administration (2.2)].

3 DOSAGE FORMS AND STRENGTHS

- 2 mg, pink, biconvex, capsule-shaped, film-coated, tablets debossed with "GS" and "3V2"
- 4 mg, light brown, biconvex, capsule-shaped, film-coated, tablets debossed with "GS" and "WXG"
- 6 mg, white, biconvex, capsule-shaped, film-coated, tablets debossed with "GS" and "11F"
- 8 mg, red, biconvex, capsule-shaped, film-coated, tablets debossed with "GS" and "5CC"
- 12 mg, green, biconvex, capsule-shaped, film-coated, tablets debossed with "GS" and "YX7"

4 CONTRAINDICATIONS

None.

5 WARNINGS AND PRECAUTIONS

5.1 Falling Asleep During Activities of Daily Living

Patients treated with ropinirole have reported falling asleep while engaged in activities of daily living, including the operation of motor vehicles, which sometimes resulted in accidents. Although many of these patients reported somnolence while on ropinirole, some perceived that they had no warning signs such as excessive drowsiness, and believed that they were alert immediately prior to the event. Some of these events have been reported more than 1 year after initiation of treatment.

Among the 613 patients who received REQUIP XL in clinical trials, there were 5 cases of sudden onset of sleep and 2 cases of motor vehicle accident in which it is not known if falling asleep was a contributing factor.

During the 6-month trial in advanced Parkinson's disease, somnolence was reported in 7% (14 of 202) of patients receiving REQUIP XL compared with 4% (7 of 191) of patients receiving placebo. During the 36-week trial in early Parkinson's disease, somnolence was reported in 11% (16 of 140) of patients receiving REQUIP XL compared with 15% (22 of 149) of patients receiving the immediate-release formulation of REQUIP [see Adverse Reactions (6)]. However, because dose-response was not systematically studied with REQUIP XL, the occurrence of somnolence at the highest recommended doses may be higher than these reported frequencies [see Adverse Reactions (6)].

Many clinical experts believe that falling asleep while engaged in activities of daily living always occurs in a setting of preexisting somnolence, although patients may not give such a history. For this reason, prescribers should continually reassess patients for drowsiness or sleepiness, especially since some of the events occur well after the start of treatment. Prescribers should also be aware that patients may not acknowledge drowsiness or sleepiness until directly questioned about drowsiness or sleepiness during specific activities.

Before initiating treatment with REQUIP XL, patients should be advised of the potential to develop drowsiness and specifically asked about factors that may increase the risk with REQUIP XL such as concomitant sedating medications, the presence of sleep disorders, and concomitant medications that increase ropinirole plasma levels (e.g., ciprofloxacin) [see Drug Interactions (7.1)]. If a patient develops significant daytime sleepiness or episodes of falling asleep during activities that require active participation (e.g., driving a motor vehicle, conversations, eating, etc.), REQUIP XL should ordinarily be discontinued [see Dosage and Administration for guidance in discontinuing REQUIP XL (2.2)]. If a decision is made to continue REQUIP XL, patients should be advised to not drive and to avoid other potentially dangerous activities. There is insufficient information to establish that dose reduction will eliminate episodes of falling asleep while engaged in activities of daily living.

5.2 Syncope

Syncope, sometimes associated with bradycardia, was observed during treatment with ropinirole in Parkinson's disease patients.

In a placebo-controlled study involving patients with advanced Parkinson's disease, syncope occurred in 2 of the 202 patients (1%) who received REQUIP XL, and in none of the 191 patients who received placebo.

Because the study of REQUIP XL excluded patients with significant cardiovascular disease, it is not known to what extent the estimated incidence figure applies to patients with Parkinson's disease in clinical practice. Therefore, patients with significant cardiovascular disease should be treated with caution.

5.3 Hypotension

Dopamine agonists, in clinical studies and clinical experience, appear to impair the systemic regulation of blood pressure, with resulting postural hypotension, especially during dose escalation. In addition, patients with Parkinson's disease appear to have an impaired capacity to respond to a postural challenge. For these reasons, patients being treated with dopaminergic agonists ordinarily (1) require careful monitoring for signs and symptoms of postural hypotension, especially during dose escalation, and (2) should be informed of this risk *[see Patient Counseling Information (17.2)]*.

In a placebo-controlled trial involving patients with advanced Parkinson's disease, hypotension was reported as an adverse event in 5 of 202 patients (2%) receiving REQUIP XL and in none of the 191 patients receiving placebo. Orthostatic hypotension was reported as an adverse event in 5% of patients receiving REQUIP XL, and in 1% of placebo recipients.

An analysis of the randomized, double-blinded, placebo-controlled study in advanced Parkinson's disease was conducted using a variety of adverse event terms possibly suggestive of hypotension, including hypotension, orthostatic hypotension, dizziness, vertigo, and blood pressure decreased. This analysis showed a higher incidence of these events with REQUIP XL (7%, 15 of 202) vs. placebo (3%, 6 of 191). This increased incidence was observed in a setting in which patients were very carefully titrated, and patients with clinically relevant cardiovascular disease or symptomatic orthostatic hypotension at baseline had been excluded from this study.

Orthostatic vital signs (semi-supine to standing) were monitored throughout the study in the advanced Parkinson's disease study and changes related to REQUIP XL (compared with placebo) from baseline were assessed.

The frequency of any orthostatic hypotension at any time during the study was 38% for REQUIP XL vs. 31% for placebo for mild to moderate systolic blood pressure decrements (≥20 mm Hg), 63% for REQUIP XL vs. 58% for placebo for mild to moderate diastolic blood pressure decrements (≥10 mm Hg), 10% for REQUIP XL vs. 7% for placebo for severe diastolic blood pressure decrements (≥20 mm Hg), and 23% for REQUIP XL vs. 19% for placebo for mild to moderate combined systolic and diastolic blood pressure decrements.

Significant decrements in blood pressure unrelated to standing were also reported in some patients taking REQUIP XL. In the semi-supine position, the frequency was 10% for REQUIP XL vs. 8% for placebo for severe systolic blood pressure decrease (≥40 mm Hg), and was 25% for REQUIP XL vs. 21% for placebo for severe diastolic blood pressure decrease (≥20 mm Hg).

The increased incidence for hypotension and/or orthostatic hypotension was observed in both the titration and maintenance phases and in some cases persisted into the maintenance period after developing in the titration phase.

5.4 Elevation of Blood Pressure and Changes in Heart Rate

In the placebo-controlled study in advanced Parkinson's disease, there were no clear effects of REQUIP XL on average changes in blood pressure or heart rate compared with placebo. However, there was an increased incidence of patients treated with REQUIP XL who met various outlier criteria, as described below.

In the semi-supine position, the frequency was 8% for REQUIP XL vs. 5% for placebo for severe systolic blood pressure increase (≥40 mm Hg). In the standing position, the frequency was 9% for REQUIP XL vs. 6% for placebo for severe systolic blood pressure increase (≥40 mm Hg).

In the semi-supine position, the frequency was 23% for REQUIP XL vs. 18% for placebo for moderate pulse increase (≥15 beats/minute), and 19% for REQUIP XL vs. 17% for placebo for moderate pulse decrease (≥15 beats/minute). In the standing position, the frequency was 2% for REQUIP XL vs. <1% for placebo for severe pulse increase (≥30 beats/minute), and 24% for REQUIP XL vs. 19% for placebo for moderate pulse decrease (≥15 beats/minute).

The increased incidence for various elevations of systolic and/or diastolic blood pressure and/or changes in pulse was observed in both the titration and maintenance phases as well as persisting into the maintenance period after developing in the titration phase.

Elevation of blood pressure and/or changes in heart rate in patients taking REQUIP XL should be considered when treating patients with cardiovascular disease.

5.5 Hallucination

In the double-blind, placebo-controlled, advanced Parkinson's disease trial 8% (17 of 202) of patients receiving REQUIP XL reported hallucination compared with 2% (4 of 191) patients receiving placebo. Hallucination led to discontinuation of treatment in 2% (4 of 202) of patients on REQUIP XL and 1% (2 of 191) of patients on placebo.

The incidence of hallucination is increased in patients over age 65. Coadministration of entacapone and L-dopa with ropinirole may also increase the risk of hallucination. In a placebo-controlled clinical trial, hallucination occurred in 0 of 43 patients taking entacapone plus L-dopa, in 9 of 155 patients taking REQUIP XL plus L-dopa (6%), and in 7 of 47 patients taking entacapone with REQUIP XL plus L-dopa (15%).

5.6 Dyskinesia

REQUIP XL may potentiate the dopaminergic side effects of L-dopa and may cause and/or exacerbate preexisting dyskinesia in patients treated with L-dopa for Parkinson's disease. Decreasing the dose of a dopaminergic drug may ameliorate this side effect.

5.7 Major Psychotic Disorders

Patients with a major psychotic disorder should ordinarily not be treated with REQUIP XL because of the risk of exacerbating the psychosis. In addition, many treatments for psychosis may decrease the effectiveness of REQUIP XL *[see Drug Interactions (7.4)]*.

5.8 Events Reported With Dopaminergic Therapy

Withdrawal-Emergent Hyperpyrexia and Confusion: Although not reported during the clinical development of ropinirole, a symptom complex resembling the neuroleptic malignant syndrome (characterized by elevated temperature, muscular rigidity, altered consciousness, and autonomic instability), with no other obvious etiology, has been reported in association with rapid dose reduction, withdrawal of, or changes in dopaminergic therapy. Therefore, it is recommended that the dose be tapered at the end of treatment with REQUIP XL as a prophylactic measure *[see Dosage and Administration (2.2)]*.

Fibrotic Complications: Cases of retroperitoneal fibrosis, pulmonary infiltrates, pleural effusion, pleural thickening, pericarditis, and cardiac valvulopathy have been reported in some patients treated with ergot-derived dopaminergic agents. While these complications may resolve when the drug is discontinued, complete resolution does not always occur.

Although these adverse reactions are believed to be related to the ergoline structure of these compounds, whether other, nonergot-derived dopamine agonists, such as REQUIP or REQUIP XL, can cause them is unknown.

A small number of reports have been received of possible fibrotic complications, including pleural effusion, pleural fibrosis, interstitial lung disease, and cardiac valvulopathy, in the development program and postmarketing experience for ropinirole. In the clinical development program (N = 613), 2 patients treated with REQUIP XL had pleural effusion. While the evidence is not sufficient to establish a causal relationship between ropinirole and these fibrotic complications, a contribution of ropinirole cannot be completely ruled out in rare cases.

Melanoma: Some epidemiologic studies have shown that patients with Parkinson's disease have a higher risk (perhaps 2- to 4-fold higher) of developing melanoma than the general population. Whether the observed increased risk was due to Parkinson's disease or other factors, such as drugs used to treat Parkinson's disease, was unclear. Ropinirole is one of the dopamine agonists used to treat Parkinson's disease. Although ropinirole has not been associated with an increased risk of melanoma specifically, its potential role as a risk factor has not been systematically studied. In the clinical development program (N = 613), one patient treated with REQUIP XL and also levodopa/carbidopa developed melanoma. Patients using REQUIP XL should be made aware of these results and undergo periodic dermatologic screening.

5.9 Retinal Pathology

Human: Because of observations made in albino rats (see below), ocular electroretinogram (ERG) assessments were conducted during a 2-year, double-blind, multicenter, flexible-dose, L-dopa controlled clinical study of immediate-release ropinirole in patients with Parkinson's disease. A total of 156 patients (78 on immediate-release ropinirole, mean dose 11.9 mg/day and 78 on L-dopa, mean dose 555.2 mg/day) were evaluated for evidence of retinal dysfunction through electroretinograms. There was no clinically meaningful difference between the treatment groups in retinal function over the duration of the study.

Albino Rats: Retinal degeneration was observed in albino rats in the 2-year carcinogenicity study at all doses tested (equivalent to 0.6 to 20 times the maximum recommended human dose (MRHD) of 24 mg/day on a mg/m^2 basis), but was statistically significant at the highest dose (50 mg/kg/day). Retinal degeneration was not observed in pigmented rats after 3 months in a 2-year carcinogenicity study in albino mice, or in 1-year studies in monkeys or albino rats. The potential significance of this effect for humans has not been established, but cannot be disregarded because disruption of a mechanism that is universally present in vertebrates (e.g., disk shedding) may be involved.

5.10 Binding to Melanin

Ropinirole binds to melanin-containing tissues (i.e., eyes, skin) in pigmented rats. After a single dose, long-term retention of drug was demonstrated, with a half-life in the eye of 20 days.

6 ADVERSE REACTIONS

The following adverse reactions are described in more detail in the *Warnings and Precautions* section of the label:

- Falling asleep during activities of daily living (5.1)
- Syncope (5.2)
- Symptomatic hypotension, hypotension, postural/orthostatic hypotension (5.3)
- Elevation of blood pressure and changes in heart rate (5.4)
- Hallucination (5.5)
- Dyskinesia (5.6)
- Major psychotic disorders (5.7)
- Events with dopaminergic therapy (5.8)
- Retinal pathology (5.9)

6.1 Clinical Trial Experience

Because clinical trials are conducted under widely varying conditions, adverse reaction rates observed in the clinical trials of a drug cannot be directly compared with rates in the clinical trials of another drug (or of another development program of a different formulation of the same drug) and may not reflect the rates observed in practice.

During the premarketing development of REQUIP XL, patients with advanced Parkinson's disease received REQUIP XL or placebo as adjunctive therapy in 1 clinical trial. In a second trial, patients with early Parkinson's disease were treated with REQUIP XL or the immediate-release formulation of REQUIP without L-dopa.

Advanced Parkinson's Disease (With L-dopa): The most commonly observed adverse reactions (≥5% and numerically greater than placebo) in the 24-week, double-blind, placebo-controlled trial for the treatment of advanced Parkinson's disease during treatment with REQUIP XL were, in order of decreasing incidence: dyskinesia, nausea, dizziness, hallucination, somnolence, abdominal pain/discomfort, and orthostatic hypotension.

Approximately 6% of 202 patients treated with REQUIP XL discontinued treatment due to adverse event(s) compared with 5% of 191 patients who received placebo. The adverse event most commonly causing discontinuation of treatment with REQUIP XL was hallucination (2%).

Table 2 lists adverse reactions that occurred with a frequency of at least 2% (and were numerically greater than placebo) in patients with advanced Parkinson's disease treated with REQUIP XL who participated in the 26-week, double-blind, placebo-controlled study. In this study, either REQUIP XL or placebo was used as an adjunct to L-dopa. Adverse reactions were generally mild or moderate in intensity.

Table 2. Treatment-Emergent Adverse Reaction Incidence in a Double-Blind, Placebo-Controlled Trial in Advanced Stage Parkinson's Disease (With L-dopa) (Events ≥2% of Patients Treated with REQUIP XL and >% with Placebo)

Body System/Adverse Reaction	REQUIP XL (n = 202) %	Placebo (n = 191) %
Ear and labyrinth disorders		
Vertigo	4	2
Gastrointestinal disorders		
Nausea	11	4
Constipation	4	2
Abdominal pain/discomfort	6	3
Diarrhea	3	2
Dry mouth	2	<1
General disorders		
Edema peripheral	4	1
Injury, poisoning, and procedural complications		
Fall*	2	1
Musculoskeletal and connective tissue disorders		
Back pain	3	2
Nervous system disorders		
Dyskinesia*	13	3
Dizziness	8	3
Somnolence	7	4
Psychiatric disorders		
Hallucination	8	2
Anxiety	2	1
Vascular disorders		
Orthostatic hypotension	5	1
Hypotension	2	0
Hypertension*	3	2

*Dose-related.

Although this study was not designed for optimally characterizing dose-related adverse reactions, there was a suggestion (based upon comparison of incidence of adverse reactions across dose ranges for REQUIP XL and placebo) that the incidence for dyskinesia, hypertension, and fall was dose-related to REQUIP XL.

The incidence for many adverse reactions with REQUIP XL treatment was increased relative to placebo (i.e., REQUIP XL % - Placebo % = treatment difference ≥2%) in either the titration or maintenance phases of the study. During the titration phase, an increased incidence (shown in descending order of % treatment difference) was observed for dyskinesia, nausea, abdominal pain/discomfort, orthostatic hypotension, dizziness, vertigo, hypertension, peripheral edema, and dry mouth. During the maintenance phase, an increased incidence was observed for dyskinesia, nausea, dizziness, hallucination, somnolence, fall, hypertension, abnormal dreams, constipation, chest pain, bronchitis, and nasopharyngitis. Some adverse reactions developing in the titration phase persisted (≥7 days) into the maintenance phase. These "persistent" adverse reactions included dyskinesia, hallucination, orthostatic hypotension, and dry mouth.

The incidence of adverse reactions was not clearly different between women and men.

Early Parkinson's Disease (Without L-dopa): The most commonly observed adverse reactions (≥5%) in the 36-week early Parkinson's disease trial during treatment with REQUIP XL were, in order of decreasing incidence: nausea (19%), somnolence (11%), abdominal pain/discomfort (7%), dizziness (6%), headache (6%), and constipation (5%). The type of adverse reactions and the frequency (i.e. incidence) with which they occurred were generally similar over the whole treatment period in this study of early Parkinson's disease patients who were initially treated with REQUIP XL or the immediate-release formulation of REQUIP and subsequently crossed over to treatment with the other formulation.

During the titration phase, an increased incidence with REQUIP XL compared with the immediate-release formulation of REQUIP (i.e., REQUIP XL % - REQUIP IR % = treatment difference ≥2%), shown in descending order of % treatment difference, was observed for: constipation, hallucination, vertigo, abdominal pain/discomfort, nausea, vomiting, fall, headache, diarrhea, pyrexia, and flatulence. During the maintenance phase, an increased incidence was observed for fall, myalgia, and sleep disorder. Several adverse reactions developing in the titration phase persisted (≥7 days) into the maintenance phase. These "persistent" adverse reactions included: constipation, hallucination, muscle spasms, flatulence, insomnia, sleep disorder, abdominal pain/discomfort, cough, and nasopharyngitis.

6.2 Adverse Reactions Observed During the Clinical Development of the Immediate-Release Formulation of REQUIP for Parkinson's Disease (Advanced and Early)

Because clinical trials are conducted under widely varying conditions, adverse reaction rates observed in the clinical trials of a drug cannot be directly compared to rates in the clinical trials of another drug (or of another development program of a different formulation of the same drug) and may not reflect the rates observed in practice.

In patients with advanced Parkinson's disease who were treated with the immediate-release formulation of REQUIP, the most common adverse reactions (≥5% treatment difference from placebo; presented in order of decreasing treatment difference frequency) were dyskinesia (21%), somnolence (12%), nausea (12%), dizziness (10%), confusion (7%), hallucinations (6%), headache (5%), and increased sweating (5%). In patients with early Parkinson's disease who were treated with the immediate-release formulation of REQUIP, the most common adverse reactions (≥5% treatment difference from placebo; presented in order of decreasing treatment difference frequency) were nausea (38%), somnolence (34%), dizziness (18%), syncope (11%), viral infection (8%), fatigue (7%), leg edema (6%), asthenia (5%), and dyspepsia (5%).

7 DRUG INTERACTIONS

7.1 P450 Interaction

In vitro metabolism studies showed that CYP1A2 is the major enzyme responsible for the metabolism of ropinirole. There is thus the potential for inducers or inhibitors of this enzyme to alter the clearance of ropinirole. Therefore, if therapy with a drug known to be a potent inducer or inhibitor of CYP1A2 is stopped or started during treatment with ropinirole, adjustment of the dose of ropinirole may be required.

Coadministration of ciprofloxacin, an inhibitor of CYP1A2, with immediate-release ropinirole increased the AUC of ropinirole by 84% on average and C_{max} by 60% *[see Clinical Pharmacology (12.3)]*.

Cigarette smoking is expected to increase the clearance of ropinirole since CYP1A2 is known to be induced by smoking. In one study in patients with Restless Legs Syndrome, cigarette smokers had an approximate 30% lower C_{max} and a 38% lower AUC than did nonsmokers, when those parameters were normalized for dose.

There is no evidence of interaction between ropinirole and other CYP1A2 substrates (e.g., theophylline).

Ropinirole and its circulating metabolites do not inhibit or induce P450 enzymes therefore ropinirole is unlikely to affect the pharmacokinetics of other drugs by a P450 mechanism *[see Clinical Pharmacology (12.3)]*.

7.2 L-dopa

Coadministration of carbidopa + L-dopa (SINEMET®*) with immediate-release ropinirole had no effect on the steady-state pharmacokinetics of ropinirole. Oral administration of immediate-release ropinirole increased mean steady-state C_{max} of L-dopa by 20%, but its AUC was unaffected *[see Clinical Pharmacology (12.3)]*.

7.3 Estrogens

Population pharmacokinetic analysis revealed that higher doses of estrogens (usually associated with hormone replacement therapy [HRT]) reduced the oral clearance of ropinirole by approximately 35%. Dosage adjustment is not needed for initiating REQUIP XL in patients on estrogen therapy because patients are individually titrated with REQUIP XL to tolerance or adequate effect. If estrogen therapy is stopped or started during treatment with REQUIP XL, then adjustment of the dose of REQUIP XL may be required.

7.4 Dopamine Antagonists

Since ropinirole is a dopamine agonist, it is possible that dopamine antagonists such as neuroleptics (e.g., phenothiazines, butyrophenones, thioxanthenes) or metoclopramide may diminish the effectiveness of REQUIP XL. Patients with a history or presence of major psychotic disorders should be treated with dopamine agonists only if the potential benefits outweigh the risks.

8 USE IN SPECIFIC POPULATIONS

8.1 Pregnancy

Pregnancy Category C. There are no adequate and well-controlled studies using ropinirole in pregnant women. REQUIP XL should be used during pregnancy only if the potential benefit outweighs the potential risk to the fetus.

In animal reproduction studies, ropinirole has been shown to have adverse effects on embryo-fetal development, including teratogenic effects. Treatment of pregnant rats with ropinirole during organogenesis resulted in decreased fetal body weight, increased fetal death, and digital malformations at 24, 36, and 60 times the MRHD, respectively. The combined administration of ropinirole at 8 times the MRHD and a clinically relevant dose of L-dopa to pregnant rabbits during organogenesis produced a greater incidence and severity of fetal malformations (primarily digit defects) than were seen in the offspring of rabbits treated with L-dopa alone. In a perinatal-postnatal study in rats, impaired growth and development of nursing offspring and altered neurological development of female offspring were observed when dams were treated with 4 times the MRHD.

8.3 Nursing Mothers

Ropinirole inhibits prolactin secretion in humans and could potentially inhibit lactation.

Ropinirole has been detected in the milk of lactating rats. Although many drugs are excreted in human milk, transfer of ropinirole into human milk has not been demonstrated. Due to the potential for serious adverse reactions in nursing infants, a decision should be made whether to discontinue nursing or to discontinue the drug, taking into account the importance of ropinirole to the mother.

8.4 Pediatric Use

Safety and effectiveness in the pediatric population have not been established.

8.5 Geriatric Use

Dosage adjustment is not necessary in the elderly (above 65 years), as the dose of REQUIP XL is to be individually titrated to clinical response *[see Clinical Pharmacology (12.3)]*. Pharmacokinetic studies conducted in patients demonstrated that oral clearance of ropinirole is reduced by 15% in patients above 65 years of age compared to younger patients.

Of the total number of patients who participated in clinical trials of REQUIP XL for Parkinson's disease, 387 patients were 65 and over and 107 patients were 75 and over. Among patients receiving REQUIP XL, hallucination was more common in elderly subjects (10%) compared with non-elderly subjects (2%). The incidence of overall adverse events increased with increasing age for both patients receiving REQUIP XL and placebo.

8.6 Renal Impairment

No dosage adjustment of ropinirole is needed in patients with moderate renal impairment (creatinine clearance of 30 to 50 mL/min). The use of ropinirole in patients with severe renal impairment has not been studied.

8.7 Hepatic Impairment

The pharmacokinetics of ropinirole have not been studied in patients with hepatic impairment. Since patients with hepatic impairment may have higher plasma levels and lower clearance, ropinirole should be titrated with caution in these patients.

9 DRUG ABUSE AND DEPENDENCE

9.1 Controlled Substance

Ropinirole is not a controlled substance.

9.3 Dependence

Animal studies and human clinical trials with ropinirole did not reveal any potential for drug-seeking behavior or physical dependence.

10 OVERDOSAGE

10.1 Human Overdose Experience

In the Parkinson's disease program, there have been patients who accidentally or intentionally took more than their prescribed dose of ropinirole. The largest overdose reported with immediate-release ropinirole in clinical trials was 435 mg taken over a 7-day period (62.1 mg/day). Of patients who received a dose greater than 24 mg/day, reported symptoms included adverse events commonly reported during dopaminergic therapy (nausea, dizziness), as well as visual hallucination, hyperhidrosis, claustrophobia, chorea, palpitations, asthenia, and nightmares. Additional symptoms reported for doses of 24 mg or less or for overdoses of unknown amount included vomiting, increased coughing, fatigue, syncope, vasovagal syncope, dyskinesia, agitation, chest pain, orthostatic hypotension, somnolence, and confusional state.

10.2 Overdose Management

The symptoms of overdose with ropinirole are generally related to its dopaminergic activity; these symptoms may be alleviated by appropriate treatment with dopamine antagonists such as neuroleptics or metoclopramide. General supportive measures are recommended. Vital signs should be maintained, if necessary. Removal of any unabsorbed material (e.g., by gastric lavage) may be considered.

11 DESCRIPTION

REQUIP (ropinirole) is an orally administered non-ergoline dopamine agonist. It is supplied as the hydrochloride salt of ropinirole 4-[2-(dipropylamino)ethyl]-1,3-dihydro-2H-indol-2-one and has an empirical formula of $C_{16}H_{24}N_2O \bullet HCl$. The molecular weight is 296.84 (260.38 as the free base).

The structural formula is:

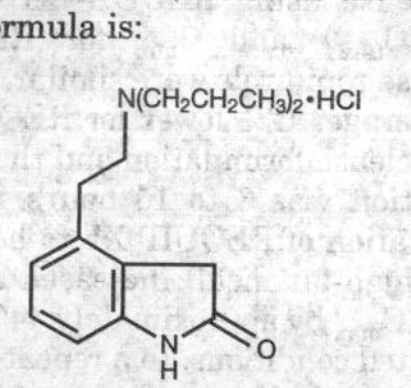

Ropinirole hydrochloride is a white to yellow solid with a melting range of 243° to 250°C and a solubility of 133 mg/mL in water.

REQUIP XL Extended-Release Tablets are formulated as a three-layered tablet with a central, active-containing, slow-release layer, and 2 placebo outer layers acting as barrier layers which control the surface area available for drug release. Each biconvex, capsule-shaped tablet contains 2.28 mg, 4.56 mg, 6.84 mg, 9.12 mg, or 13.68 mg ropinirole hydrochloride equivalent to ropinirole 2 mg, 4 mg, 6 mg, 8 mg, or 12 mg, respectively. Inactive ingredients consist of carboxymethylcellulose sodium, colloidal silicon dioxide, glyceryl behenate, hydrogenated castor oil, hypromellose, lactose monohydrate, magnesium stearate, maltodextrin, mannitol, povidone, and one or more of the following: FD&C Yellow No. 6 aluminum lake, FD&C Blue No. 2 aluminum lake, ferric oxides (black, red, yellow), polyethylene glycol 400, titanium dioxide.

12 CLINICAL PHARMACOLOGY

12.1 Mechanism of Action

Ropinirole is a non-ergoline dopamine agonist with high relative in vitro specificity and full intrinsic activity at the D_2 and D_3 dopamine receptor subtypes, binding with higher affinity to D_3 than to D_2 or D_4 receptor subtypes.

Ropinirole has moderate in vitro affinity for opioid receptors. Ropinirole and its metabolites have negligible in vitro affinity for dopamine D_1, 5-HT_1, 5-HT_2, benzodiazepine, GABA, muscarinic, alpha$_1$-, alpha$_2$-, and beta-adrenoreceptors.

The precise mechanism of action of ropinirole as a treatment for Parkinson's disease is unknown, although it is believed to be due to stimulation of postsynaptic dopamine D_2-type receptors within the caudate-putamen in the brain. This conclusion is supported by studies that show that ropinirole improves motor function in various animal models of Parkinson's disease. In particular, ropinirole attenuates the motor deficits induced by lesioning the ascending nigrostriatal dopaminergic pathway with the neurotoxin 1-methyl-4-phenyl-1,2,3,6-tetrahydropyridine (MPTP) in primates. The relevance of D_3 receptor binding in Parkinson's disease is unknown.

12.2 Pharmacodynamics

Clinical experience with dopamine agonists, including ropinirole, suggests an association with impaired ability to regulate blood pressure with resulting postural hypotension, especially during dose escalation. In some subjects in clinical trials, blood pressure changes were associated with the emergence of orthostatic symptoms, bradycardia, and, in one case in a healthy volunteer, transient sinus arrest with syncope.

The mechanism of postural hypotension induced by ropinirole is presumed to be due to a D_2-mediated blunting of the noradrenergic response to standing and subsequent decrease in peripheral vascular resistance. Nausea is a common concomitant symptom of orthostatic signs and symptoms.

At oral doses as low as 0.2 mg, ropinirole suppressed serum prolactin concentrations in healthy male volunteers.

Immediate-release ropinirole had no dose-related effect on ECG wave form and rhythm in young, healthy, male volunteers in the range of 0.01 to 2.5 mg. Immediate-release ropinirole had no dose- or exposure-related effect on mean QT intervals in healthy male and female volunteers titrated to doses up to 4 mg/day. The effect of ropinirole on QTc intervals at higher exposures achieved either due to drug interactions, hepatic impairment, or at higher doses has not been systematically evaluated.

12.3 Pharmacokinetics

Absorption: In clinical studies with immediate-release ropinirole, over 88% of a radiolabeled dose was recovered in urine, and the absolute bioavailability was 45% to 55%, indicating approximately 50% first-pass effect.

Ropinirole displayed linear kinetics up to doses of 24 mg/day (8 mg immediate-release, 3 times a day). Increase in systemic exposure of ropinirole following oral administration of 2 to 12 mg of REQUIP XL was approximately dose-proportional. For REQUIP XL, steady-state concentrations of ropinirole are expected to be achieved within 4 days of dosing.

Relative bioavailability of REQUIP XL Extended-Release Tablets compared with immediate-release tablets was approximately 100%. In a repeat-dose study in patients with Parkinson's disease using REQUIP XL 8 mg, the dose-normalized $AUC_{(0-24)}$ and C_{min} for REQUIP XL and immediate-release ropinirole were similar. Dose-normalized C_{max} was, on average, 12% lower for REQUIP XL than for the immediate-release formulation and the median time-to-peak concentration was 6 to 10 hours. In a single-dose study, administration of REQUIP XL to healthy volunteers with food (i.e., high-fat meal) increased AUC by approximately 30% and C_{max} by approximately 44%, compared with dosing under fasted conditions. In a repeat-dose study in patients with Parkinson's disease, food (i.e., high-fat meal) increased AUC by approximately 20% and C_{max} by approximately 44%; T_{max} was prolonged by 3 hours (median prolongation) compared with dosing under fasted conditions *[see Dosage and Administration (2.1)]*.

Distribution: Ropinirole is widely distributed throughout the body, with an apparent volume of distribution of 7.5 L/kg (cv = 32%). It is up to 40% bound to plasma proteins and has a blood-to-plasma ratio of 1:1.

Metabolism: Ropinirole is extensively metabolized by the liver. The major metabolic pathways are N-despropylation and hydroxylation to form the inactive N-despropyl metabolite and hydroxy metabolites. The N-despropyl metabolite is converted to carbamyl glucuronide, carboxylic acid, and N-despropyl hydroxy metabolites. The hydroxy metabolite of ropinirole is rapidly glucuronidated.

In vitro studies indicate that the major cytochrome P450 isozyme involved in the metabolism of ropinirole is CYP1A2, an enzyme known to be induced by smoking and omeprazole, and inhibited by, for example, fluvoxamine, mexiletine, and the older fluoroquinolones such as ciprofloxacin and norfloxacin.

Elimination: The clearance of ropinirole after oral administration to patients is 47 L/hr (cv = 45%) and its elimination half-life is approximately 6 hours. Less than 10% of the administered dose is excreted as unchanged drug in urine. N-despropyl ropinirole is the predominant metabolite found in urine (40%), followed by the carboxylic acid metabolite (10%), and the glucuronide of the hydroxy metabolite (10%).

Drug Interactions: *Ciprofloxacin:* Coadministration of ciprofloxacin (500 mg twice daily), an inhibitor of CYP1A2, with immediate-release ropinirole (2 mg 3 times daily) increased ropinirole AUC by 84% on average and C_{max} by 60% (n = 12 patients).

Digoxin: Coadministration of immediate-release ropinirole (2 mg 3 times daily) with digoxin (0.125 to 0.25 mg once daily) did not alter the steady-state pharmacokinetics of digoxin in 10 patients.

Theophylline: Administration of theophylline (300 mg twice daily, a substrate of CYP1A2) did not alter the steady-state pharmacokinetics of immediate-release ropinirole (2 mg 3 times daily) in 12 patients with Parkinson's disease. Immediate-release ropinirole (2 mg 3 times daily) did not alter the pharmacokinetics of theophylline (5 mg/kg IV) in 12 patients with Parkinson's disease.

L-dopa: Coadministration of carbidopa + L-dopa (SINEMET 10/100 mg twice daily) with immediate-release ropinirole (2 mg 3 times daily) had no effect on the steady-state pharmacokinetics of ropinirole (n = 28 patients). Oral administration of immediate-release ropinirole 2 mg 3 times daily increased mean steady-state C_{max} of L-dopa by 20%, but its AUC was unaffected (n = 23 patients).

Estrogens: Population pharmacokinetic analysis revealed that higher doses of estrogens (usually associated with hormone replacement therapy [HRT]) reduced the oral clearance of ropinirole by approximately 35%.

Commonly Administered Drugs: Population analysis showed that commonly administered drugs, e.g., selegiline, amantadine, tricyclic antidepressants, benzodiazepines, ibuprofen, thiazides, antihistamines, and anticholinergics, did not affect the oral clearance of ropinirole.

Population Subgroups: Because therapy with REQUIP XL is initiated at a low dose and gradually titrated upward according to clinical tolerability to obtain the optimum therapeutic effect, adjustment of the initial dose based on gender, weight, or age is not necessary.

Age: Oral clearance of ropinirole is reduced by approximately 15% in patients above 65 years of age compared with younger patients. Dosage adjustment is not necessary in the elderly (above 65 years), as the dose of ropinirole is individually titrated to clinical response.

Gender: Female and male patients showed similar oral clearance.

Race: The influence of race on the pharmacokinetics of ropinirole has not been evaluated.

Renal Impairment: Based on population pharmacokinetic analysis, no difference was observed in the pharmacokinetics of ropinirole in patients with moderate renal impairment (creatinine clearance between 30 to 50 mL/min) compared with an age-matched population with creatinine clearance above 50 mL/min. Therefore, no dosage adjustment is necessary in patients with moderate renal impairment. The use of ropinirole in patients with severe renal impairment has not been studied.

The effect of hemodialysis on ropinirole clearance is not known, but because of the relatively high apparent volume of distribution of ropinirole (7.5 L/kg), significant removal of ropinirole by hemodialysis is unlikely.

Hepatic Impairment: The pharmacokinetics of ropinirole have not been studied in patients with hepatic impairment. These patients may have higher plasma levels and lower clearance of ropinirole than patients with normal hepatic function. REQUIP XL should be titrated with caution in this population.

Other Diseases: Population pharmacokinetic analysis revealed no change in the oral clearance of ropinirole in patients with concomitant diseases such as hypertension, depression, osteoporosis/arthritis, and insomnia compared with patients who had Parkinson's disease only.

13 NONCLINICAL TOXICOLOGY

13.1 Carcinogenesis, Mutagenesis, Impairment of Fertility

Two-year carcinogenicity studies were conducted in Charles River CD-1 mice at doses of 5, 15, and 50 mg/kg/day and in Sprague-Dawley rats at doses of 1.5, 15, and 50 mg/kg/day (top doses which, based on mg/m^2, are equivalent to 10 and 20 times, respectively, the MRHD of 24 mg/day). In the male rat, there was a significant increase in testicular Leydig cell adenomas at all doses tested, i.e., ≥1.5 mg/kg (0.6 times the MRHD on a mg/m^2 basis). This finding is of questionable significance because the endocrine mechanisms believed to be involved in the production of Leydig cell hyperplasia and adenomas in rats are not relevant to humans. In the female mouse, there was an increase in benign uterine endometrial polyps at a dose of 50 mg/kg/day (10 times the MRHD on a mg/m^2 basis).

Ropinirole was not mutagenic or clastogenic in the in vitro Ames test, the in vitro chromosome aberration test in human lymphocytes, the in vitro mouse lymphoma (L1578Y cells) assay, and the in vivo mouse micronucleus test.

When administered to female rats prior to and during mating and throughout pregnancy, ropinirole caused disruption of implantation at doses of 20 mg/kg/day (8 times the MRHD on a mg/m^2 basis) or greater. This effect is thought to be due to the prolactin-lowering effect of ropinirole. In humans, chorionic gonadotropin, not prolactin, is essential for implantation. In rat studies using low doses (5 mg/kg) during the prolactin-dependent phase of early pregnancy (gestation days 0 to 8), ropinirole did not affect female fertility at dosages up to 100 mg/kg/day (40 times the MRHD on a mg/m^2 basis). No effect on male fertility was observed in rats at dosages up to 125 mg/kg/day (50 times the MRHD on a mg/m^2 basis).

14 CLINICAL STUDIES

The effectiveness of the immediate-release formulation of ropinirole (REQUIP Tablets) in the treatment of early and advanced Parkinson's disease was initially established in 3 randomized, double-blind, placebo-controlled trials.

The effectiveness of REQUIP XL in the treatment of Parkinson's disease was supported by 2 randomized, double-blind, multicenter clinical trials and clinical pharmacokinetic considerations. One trial conducted in advanced Parkinson's disease patients compared REQUIP XL with placebo as adjunctive therapy to L-dopa. A second trial compared REQUIP XL with REQUIP Tablets in early phase Parkinson's disease patients not receiving L-dopa.

In these studies a variety of measures were used to assess the effects of treatment (e.g., patient diaries recording time "on" and "off," tolerability of L-dopa dose reductions, and the Unified Parkinson's Disease Rating Scale [UPDRS] scores). The UPDRS is a multi-item rating scale evaluating mentation (Part I), activities of daily living (Part II), motor performance (Part III), and complications of therapy (Part IV). Part III of the UPDRS contains 14 items designed to assess the severity of the cardinal motor findings in patients with Parkinson's disease (e.g., tremor, rigidity, bradykinesia, postural instability, etc.) scored for different body regions and has a maximum (worst) score of 108.

14.1 Study in Patients With Advanced Parkinson's Disease (With L-dopa)

The effectiveness of REQUIP XL as adjunctive therapy to L-dopa in patients with Parkinson's disease was established in a randomized, double-blind, placebo-controlled, parallel group, 24-week clinical trial in 393 patients (Hoehn & Yahr criteria Stages II-IV) who were not adequately controlled by L-dopa therapy. Patients were allowed to be on concomitant selegiline, amantadine, anticholinergics, and catechol-O-methyltransferase (COMT) inhibitors provided the doses were stable for at least 4 weeks prior to screening and throughout the trial. The primary efficacy endpoint evaluated was the mean change from baseline in total awake time spent "off".

Patients in this study had a mean disease duration of 8.6 years, a mean duration of exposure to L-dopa of 6.5 years, had experienced a minimum of 3 hours awake time "off" with a baseline average of approximately 7 hours awake time "off", and had a mean baseline UPDRS motor score of approximately 30 points with similar mean data in each treatment group. The mean baseline dose of L-dopa in the group receiving REQUIP XL was 824 mg/day and 776 mg/day for the placebo group. Patients initiated treatment at 2 mg/day for 1 week followed by increases of 2 mg/day at weekly intervals to a minimum dose of 6 mg/day. The following week, the REQUIP XL total daily dose could be further increased (based upon therapeutic response and tolerability) to 8 mg/day. Once a daily dose of 8 mg/day was reached, the background L-dopa dosage was reduced. Thereafter, the daily dose could be increased by up to 4 mg/day approximately every 2 weeks until an optimal dose was achieved (based upon therapeutic response and tolerability). The mean dose of REQUIP XL at the end of Week 24 was 18.8 mg/day. Dose titrations were based upon the degree of symptom control, planned L-dopa dosage reduction, and/or tolerability. The maximal allowed daily dosage for REQUIP XL was 24 mg/day.

The primary efficacy endpoint was mean change from baseline in total awake time spent "off" at Week 24. At baseline the mean total awake time spent "off" was approximately 7 hours in each treatment group. At Week 24, the total awake time spent "off", on average, had decreased by approximately 2 hours in the group receiving REQUIP XL and by approximately half an hour in the placebo group. The adjusted mean difference in total awake time spent "off" between REQUIP XL and placebo was -1.7 hours, which was statistically significant (ANCOVA, p< 0.0001). Results for this endpoint showing the statistical superiority of REQUIP XL over Placebo are presented in Table 3.

Table 3. Change from Baseline in Total Awake Time Spent "Off" at Week 24

	REQUIP XL (n = 201)	Placebo (n = 190)
Mean "Off" time at Baseline (hours)	7.0	7.0
Mean Change from Baseline in "Off" time (hours)	-2.1	-0.4

The difference between groups in favor of REQUIP XL, with regard to a decrease in total "off" hours, was primarily related to an increase in total "on" hours without troublesome dyskinesia. Patients treated with REQUIP XL had a mean reduction in L-dopa dose of 278 mg/day (34%) while patients treated with placebo had a mean reduction of 164 mg/day (21%). In patients who reduced their L-dopa dose, reduction was sustained in 93% of patients treated with REQUIP XL and in 72% of patients treated with placebo (p<0.001).

14.2 Study in Patients With Early Parkinson's Disease (Without L-dopa)

A 36-week multicenter, double-blind, titration/3-period maintenance, cross-over study compared the efficacy of

REQUIP XL with the immediate-release formulation of REQUIP (IR) in 161 patients with early phase Parkinson's disease (Hoehn & Yahr Stages I-III) with limited prior exposure to L-dopa or dopamine agonists. Eligible subjects were randomized (1:1:1:1) to 4 treatment sequences (2 were titrated on REQUIP IR and 2 on REQUIP XL). The REQUIP IR titration was slower in rate than that of the REQUIP XL. Patients were titrated, during the 12-week titration period, to their optimal dosage, based upon tolerance and therapeutic response. This was followed by 3 consecutive 8-week maintenance periods, during which patients were either maintained on the prior formulation or switched to the alternative formulation. All switches were performed overnight by using the approximately equivalent doses of ropinirole. The primary efficacy endpoint was the change of UPDRS motor score within each maintenance period.

Patients in all 4 groups started out with similar UPDRS motor scores (about 21) at baseline. All 4 groups exhibited similar improvement in UPDRS total motor scores from baseline until the completion of the titration phase, with a change in score of about -9 observed for the groups started on REQUIP IR and of about -10 for the groups started on REQUIP XL. No difference was observed between groups when switches were made between identical formulations or between different formulations. This suggests therapeutic dosage equivalence between REQUIP IR and REQUIP XL formulations.

The optimal daily dose at the end of the titration period for patients on REQUIP IR was substantially lower (mean 7 mg) compared to the dose at the end of the titration period for patients on REQUIP XL (mean 18 mg). In this study, the marked difference in the final optimal dosages suggests that the higher doses afforded no additional benefit when compared to the lower doses [see Dosage and Administration (2)].

16 HOW SUPPLIED/STORAGE AND HANDLING

Each biconvex, capsule-shaped, film-coated tablet contains ropinirole hydrochloride equivalent to the labeled amount of ropinirole as follows:

- 2 mg: pink tablets debossed with "GS" and "3V2", in bottles of 30 (NDC 0007-4885-13) and 90 (NDC 0007-4885-59).
- 4 mg: light brown tablets debossed with "GS" and "WXG", in bottles of 30 (NDC 0007-4887-13) and 90 (NDC 0007-4887-59).
- 6 mg: white tablets debossed with "GS" and "11F", in bottles of 30 (NDC 0007-4883-13).
- 8 mg: red tablets debossed with "GS" and "5CC", in bottles of 30 (NDC 0007-4888-13) and 90 (NDC 0007-4888-59).
- 12 mg: green tablets debossed with "GS" and "YX7", in bottles of 30 (NDC 0007-4882-13).

Storage: Store at 25°C (77°F); excursions permitted to 15-30°C (59-86°F) [see USP Controlled Room Temperature]. Dispense in a tight, light-resistant container as defined in the USP.

17 PATIENT COUNSELING INFORMATION

See FDA-Approved Patient Labeling (17.9)
Physicians should instruct their patients to read the Patient Information leaflet before starting therapy with REQUIP XL and to reread it upon prescription renewal for new information regarding the use of REQUIP XL.

17.1 Dosing Instructions
- Patients should be instructed to take REQUIP XL only as prescribed. If a dose is missed, patients should be advised not to double their next dose.
- REQUIP XL can be taken with or without food. Taking REQUIP XL with food may reduce the occurrence of nausea [see Dosage and Administration (2.1)].
- REQUIP XL Tablets should be swallowed whole. They should not be chewed, crushed, or divided [see Dosage and Administration (2.1)].
- Ropinirole is the active ingredient that is in both REQUIP XL and REQUIP Tablets (the immediate-release formulation). Ask your patient if they are taking another medication containing ropinirole.

17.2 Postural (Orthostatic) Hypotension
Patients should be advised that they may develop postural (orthostatic) hypotension with or without symptoms such as dizziness, nausea, syncope, and sometimes sweating. Hypotension and/or orthostatic symptoms may occur more frequently during initial therapy or with an increase in dose at any time (cases have been seen after weeks of treatment). Accordingly, patients should be cautioned against standing up rapidly after sitting or lying down, especially if they have been doing so for prolonged periods, and especially at the initiation of treatment with REQUIP XL [see Warnings and Precautions (5.2, 5.3)].

17.3 Elevation of Blood Pressure and Changes in Heart Rate
Patients should be alerted to the possibility of increases in blood pressure during treatment with REQUIP XL.

Exacerbation of hypertension may occur. Medication dose adjustment may be necessary if elevation of blood pressure is sustained over multiple evaluations. Patients with cardiovascular disease, who may not tolerate marked changes in heart rate, should also be alerted to the possibility that they may experience significant increases or decreases in heart rate during treatment with REQUIP XL [see Warnings and Precautions (5.4)].

17.4 Sedating Effects
Patients should be alerted to the potential sedating effects caused by REQUIP XL, including somnolence and the possibility of falling asleep while engaged in activities of daily living. Since somnolence is a frequent adverse reaction with potentially serious consequences, patients should neither drive a car nor engage in other potentially dangerous activities until they have gained sufficient experience with REQUIP XL to gauge whether or not it affects their mental and/or motor performance adversely. Patients should be advised that if increased somnolence or episodes of falling asleep during activities of daily living (e.g., conversations, eating, driving a motor vehicle, etc.) are experienced at any time during treatment, they should not drive or participate in potentially dangerous activities until they have contacted their physician.

Because of possible additive effects, caution should be advised when patients are taking other sedating medications, alcohol, or other CNS depressants (e.g., benzodiazepines, antipsychotics, antidepressants, etc.) in combination with REQUIP XL or when taking concomitant medications that increase plasma levels of ropinirole (e.g., ciprofloxacin) [see Warnings and Precautions (5.1)].

17.5 Hallucinations
Patients should be informed they may experience hallucinations (unreal visions, sounds, or sensations) while taking ropinirole. The elderly are at greater risk than younger patients with Parkinson's disease; and the risk is greater in patients who use taking ropinirole with L-dopa or taking higher doses of ropinirole, and may also be further increased in patients taking any other drugs that increase dopaminergic tone [see Warnings and Precautions (5.5)].

17.6 Impulse Control Symptoms Including Compulsive Behaviors
There have been reports of patients experiencing intense urges to gamble, increased sexual urges, and other intense urges and the inability to control these urges while taking one or more of the medications that increase central dopaminergic tone, that are generally used for the treatment of Parkinson's disease or Restless Legs Syndrome, including ropinirole. In the clinical development program (N = 613), 6 patients treated with REQUIP XL exhibited compulsive behaviors consisting of pathological gambling and/or hypersexuality. Although it is not proven that the medications caused these events, these urges were reported to have stopped in some cases when the dose was reduced or the medication was stopped. Prescribers should ask patients about the development of new or increased gambling urges, sexual urges or other urges while being treated with REQUIP XL. Patients should inform their physician if they experience new or increased gambling urges, increased sexual urges or other intense urges while taking REQUIP XL. Physicians should consider dose reduction or stopping the medication if a patient develops such urges while taking REQUIP XL.

17.7 Nursing Mothers
Because of the possibility that ropinirole may be excreted in breast milk, a decision should be made whether to discontinue nursing or to discontinue the drug, taking into account the importance of the drug to the mother [see Use in Specific Populations (8.3)].
Patients should be advised that ropinirole could inhibit lactation, as ropinirole inhibits prolactin secretion.

17.8 Pregnancy
Because ropinirole has been shown to have adverse effects on embryo-fetal development, including teratogenic effects, in animals, and because experience in humans is limited, patients should be advised to notify their physician if they become pregnant or intend to become pregnant during therapy [see Use in Specific Populations (8.1)].

17.9 FDA-Approved Patient Labeling
Patient labeling is provided as a tear-off leaflet at the end of this full prescribing information.
Physicians should instruct their patients to read the Patient Information leaflet before starting therapy with REQUIP XL and to reread it upon prescription renewal for new information regarding the use of REQUIP XL.
REQUIP XL is a trademark of GlaxoSmithKline.
*SINEMET is a registered trademark of Merck & Co., Inc.
GlaxoSmithKline
Research Triangle Park, NC 27709
©2009, GlaxoSmithKline. All rights reserved.

What should I tell my healthcare provider before taking REQUIP or REQUIP XL?

Be sure to tell your healthcare provider if you:

- have daytime sleepiness from a sleep disorder or have unexpected or unpredictable sleepiness or periods of sleep.
- are taking any other prescription or over-the-counter medicines. Some of these medicines may increase your chances of getting side effects while taking REQUIP or REQUIP XL.
- start or stop taking other medicines while you are taking REQUIP or REQUIP XL. This may increase your chances of getting side effects.
- start or stop smoking while you are taking REQUIP or REQUIP XL. Smoking may decrease the treatment effect of REQUIP or REQUIP XL.
- feel dizzy, nauseated, sweaty, or faint when you first stand up from sitting or lying down.
- drink alcoholic beverages. This may increase your chances of becoming drowsy or sleepy while taking REQUIP or REQUIP XL.
- have high or low blood pressure.
- are pregnant or plan to become pregnant. REQUIP and REQUIP XL should only be used during pregnancy if needed.
- are breastfeeding. It is not known if REQUIP or REQUIP XL passes into your breast milk. Talk to your healthcare provider to decide whether you will breastfeed or take REQUIP or REQUIP XL.
- are allergic to any of the ingredients in REQUIP or REQUIP XL. See the end of this Patient Information leaflet for a complete list of the ingredients in REQUIP and REQUIP XL.

How should I take REQUIP or REQUIP XL for Parkinson's disease?

- Take REQUIP or REQUIP XL exactly as directed by your healthcare provider.
- Do not suddenly stop taking REQUIP or REQUIP XL without talking to your healthcare provider. If you stop this medicine suddenly, you may develop fever, confusion, or severe muscle stiffness.
- Before starting REQUIP or REQUIP XL, you should talk to your healthcare provider about what to do if you miss a dose. If you have missed the previous dose and it is time for your next dose, **do not double the dose.**
- Your healthcare provider will start you on a low dose of REQUIP or REQUIP XL. Your healthcare provider will change the dose until you are taking the right amount of medicine to control your symptoms. **It may take several weeks before you reach a dose that controls your symptoms.**

If you are taking REQUIP:

- REQUIP Tablets are usually taken 3 times each day for Parkinson's disease.

If you are taking REQUIP XL:

- Take REQUIP XL Tablets 1 time each day for Parkinson's disease, preferably at or around the same time of day.
- Swallow REQUIP XL Tablets whole. Do not chew, crush, or split REQUIP XL Tablets.

If you are taking either REQUIP or REQUIP XL:

- Contact your healthcare provider if you stop taking REQUIP or REQUIP XL for any reason. Do not restart without talking with your healthcare provider.
- Your healthcare provider may prescribe REQUIP or REQUIP XL alone, or add REQUIP or REQUIP XL to medicine that you are already taking for Parkinson's disease.
- You should not substitute REQUIP for REQUIP XL or REQUIP XL for REQUIP without talking with your healthcare provider.
- You can take REQUIP or REQUIP XL with or without food. If you experience nausea you may try taking REQUIP or REQUIP XL with food.

What are the possible side effects of REQUIP and REQUIP XL?

Serious side effects in people taking REQUIP and REQUIP XL are described in the section "REQUIP and REQUIP XL can cause serious side effects including" and include:

- Falling asleep during normal activities
- Changes in blood pressure
- Fainting
- Hallucinations
- Uncontrolled sudden movements

Some patients taking REQUIP or REQUIP XL get urges to behave in a way unusual for them. Examples of this are an unusual urge to gamble or increased sexual urges and behaviors. If you notice or your family notices that you are developing any unusual behaviors, talk to your healthcare provider.

You should be careful until you know if REQUIP or REQUIP XL affects your ability to remain alert while doing normal daily activities, driving a car, operating machinery,

or working at heights. You should also watch for the development of significant daytime sleepiness or episodes of falling asleep.

Common side effects in people taking REQUIP and REQUIP XL include:

- Fainting
- Sleepiness
- Hallucinations
- Dizziness
- Nausea or vomiting
- Uncontrolled sudden movements
- Leg swelling
- Fatigue
- Headache
- Upset stomach
- Increased sweating

This is not a complete list of side effects and should not take the place of discussions with your healthcare providers. Your healthcare provider or pharmacist can give you a more complete list of possible side effects.

Call your healthcare provider for medical advice about side effects. You may report side effects to FDA at 1-800-FDA-1088.

How should I store REQUIP and REQUIP XL?

- Store REQUIP Tablets between 68°-77°F (20°-25°C).
- Store REQUIP XL Tablets between 59°-86°F (15°-30°C).
- Store REQUIP or REQUIP XL at room temperature out of direct sunlight.
- Keep REQUIP or REQUIP XL in a tightly closed container.
- Keep REQUIP or REQUIP XL out of the reach of children.

Other Information about REQUIP and REQUIP XL:

- Do not share REQUIP or REQUIP XL with other people, even if they have the same symptoms you have.
- Studies of people with Parkinson's disease show that they may be at an increased risk of developing melanoma, a form of skin cancer, when compared to people without Parkinson's disease. It is not known if this problem is associated with Parkinson's disease or the medicines used to treat Parkinson's disease. REQUIP and REQUIP XL are two of the medicines used to treat Parkinson's disease, therefore, patients being treated with REQUIP or REQUIP XL should have periodic skin examinations.

This patient information leaflet summarizes the most important information about REQUIP and REQUIP XL for Parkinson's disease. Medicines are sometimes prescribed for purposes other than those listed in this leaflet. Do not take REQUIP or REQUIP XL for a condition for which it was not prescribed. For more information, talk with your healthcare provider or pharmacist. They can give you information about REQUIP and REQUIP XL that is written for healthcare professionals. For more information call 1-888-825-5249 (toll-free) or visit www.requipxl.com.

What are the ingredients in REQUIP and REQUIP XL?
The following ingredients are in REQUIP:

Active ingredient: ropinirole (as ropinirole hydrochloride)
Inactive ingredients: croscarmellose sodium, hydrous lactose, magnesium stearate, microcrystalline cellulose, and one or more of the following: carmine, FD&C Blue No. 2 aluminum lake, FD&C Yellow No. 6 aluminum lake, hypromellose, iron oxides, polyethylene glycol, polysorbate 80, titanium dioxide.

The following ingredients are in REQUIP XL:

Active ingredient: ropinirole (as ropinirole hydrochloride)
Inactive ingredients: carboxymethylcellulose sodium, colloidal silicon dioxide, glycerol behenate, hydrogenated castor oil, hypromellose, lactose monohydrate, magnesium stearate, maltodextrin, mannitol, povidone, and one or more of the following: FD&C Yellow No. 6 aluminum lake, FD&C Blue No. 2 aluminum lake, ferric oxides (black, red, yellow), polyethylene glycol 400, titanium dioxide.

PATIENT INFORMATION
REQUIP® (RE-qwip) (ropinirole) Tablets
IF YOU HAVE RESTLESS LEGS SYNDROME (RLS), READ THIS SIDE
IF YOU HAVE PARKINSON'S DISEASE, READ THE OTHER SIDE

Read this information completely before you start taking REQUIP. Read the information each time you get more medicine. There may be new information. This leaflet provides a summary about REQUIP. It does not include everything there is to know about your medicine. This information should not take the place of discussions with your healthcare provider about your medical condition or treatment with REQUIP.

Patients with RLS should take REQUIP differently than patients with Parkinson's disease (see **How should I take REQUIP for RLS?** for the recommended dosing for RLS). A lower dose of REQUIP is generally needed for patients with RLS, and is taken once daily before bedtime.

What is the most important information I should know about REQUIP?
REQUIP can cause serious side effects including:

- **Falling asleep during normal activities.** You may fall asleep while doing normal activities such as driving a car,

doing physical tasks, or using hazardous machinery while taking REQUIP. You may suddenly fall asleep without being drowsy or without warning. This may result in having accidents. Your chances of falling asleep while doing normal activities while taking REQUIP are greater if you take other medicines that cause drowsiness. Tell your healthcare provider right away if this happens. Before starting REQUIP, be sure to tell your healthcare provider if you take any medicines that make you drowsy.

- **Decrease in blood pressure.** REQUIP can decrease your blood pressure. Lowering of your blood pressure is of special concern. If you faint, feel dizzy, nauseated, or sweaty when you stand up from sitting or lying down, this may mean that your blood pressure is decreased. If you notice this, you should contact your healthcare provider. Also, when changing position from lying down or sitting to standing up, you should do it carefully and slowly. Lowering of your blood pressure can happen especially when you start taking REQUIP or when your dose is increased.
- **Fainting.** Fainting can occur, and sometimes your heart rate may be decreased. This can happen especially when you start taking REQUIP or your dose is increased. Tell your healthcare provider if you faint or feel dizzy.
- **Hallucinations** (unreal visions, sounds, or sensations) can occur in patients taking REQUIP. If you have hallucinations, talk with your healthcare provider.

Unusual urges. Some patients taking REQUIP get urges to behave in a way unusual for them. Examples of this are an unusual urge to gamble or increased sexual urges and behaviors. If you notice or your family notices that you are developing any unusual behaviors, talk to your healthcare provider.

See "What are the possible side effects of REQUIP?"
What is REQUIP?

REQUIP is a prescription medicine containing ropinirole used to treat moderate-to-severe primary Restless Legs Syndrome. It is also used to treat Parkinson's disease. Having one of these conditions does not mean you have or will develop the other.

REQUIP has not been studied in children.

What should I tell my healthcare provider before taking REQUIP?

Be sure to tell your healthcare provider if you:

- have daytime sleepiness from a sleep disorder or have unexpected or unpredictable sleepiness or periods of sleep.
- are taking any other prescription or over-the-counter medicines. Some of these medicines may increase your chances of getting side effects while taking REQUIP.
- start or stop taking other medicines while you are taking REQUIP. This may increase your chances of getting side effects.
- start or stop smoking while you are taking REQUIP. Smoking may decrease the treatment effect of REQUIP.
- feel dizzy, nauseated, sweaty, or faint when you first stand up from sitting or lying down.
- drink alcoholic beverages. This may increase your chances of becoming drowsy or sleepy while taking REQUIP.
- have high or low blood pressure.
- are pregnant or plan to become pregnant. REQUIP should only be used during pregnancy if needed.
- are breastfeeding. It is not known if REQUIP passes into your breast milk. Talk to your healthcare provider to decide whether you will breastfeed or take REQUIP.
- are allergic to any of the ingredients in REQUIP. See the end of this Patient Information leaflet for a complete list of the ingredients in REQUIP.

How should I take REQUIP for RLS?

- Take REQUIP exactly as directed by your healthcare provider.
- The usual way to take REQUIP is once in the evening, 1 to 3 hours before bedtime.
- Your healthcare provider will start you on a low dose of REQUIP. Your healthcare provider may change the dose until you are taking the right amount of medicine to control your symptoms.
- **If you miss your dose, do not double your next dose.** Take only your usual dose 1 to 3 hours before your next bedtime.
- Contact your healthcare provider if you stop taking REQUIP for any reason. Do not restart without consulting your healthcare provider.
- You can take REQUIP with or without food. Taking REQUIP with food may decrease the chances of feeling nauseated.

What are the possible side effects of REQUIP?

Serious side effects in people taking REQUIP are described in the section "REQUIP can cause serious side effects including" and include:

- Falling asleep during normal activities
- Decrease in blood pressure
- Fainting
- Hallucinations

Some patients taking REQUIP get urges to behave in a way unusual for them. Examples of this are an unusual urge to gamble or increased sexual urges and behaviors. If you notice or your family notices that you are developing any unusual behaviors, talk to your healthcare provider.

You should be careful until you know if REQUIP affects your ability to remain alert while doing normal daily activities, driving a car, operating machinery, or working at heights. You should also watch for the development of significant daytime sleepiness or episodes of falling asleep. Common side effects in people taking REQUIP include:
- Nausea or vomiting
- Sleepiness or drowsiness
- Dizziness
- Fatigue

This is not a complete list of side effects and should not take the place of discussions with your healthcare providers. Your healthcare provider or pharmacist can give you a more complete list of possible side effects.

Call your healthcare provider for medical advice about side effects. You may report side effects to FDA at 1-800-FDA-1088.

How should I store REQUIP?
- Store REQUIP Tablets between 68°-77°F (20°-25°C).
- Store REQUIP at room temperature out of direct sunlight.
- Keep REQUIP in a tightly closed container.
- Keep REQUIP out of the reach of children.

Other Information about REQUIP
- Do not share REQUIP with other people, even if they have the same symptoms you have.
- Studies of people with Parkinson's disease show that they may be at an increased risk of developing melanoma, a form of skin cancer, when compared to people without Parkinson's disease. It is not known if this problem is associated with Parkinson's disease or the medicines used to treat Parkinson's disease. REQUIP is one of the medicines used to treat Parkinson's disease, therefore, patients being treated with REQUIP should have periodic skin examinations.

This patient information leaflet summarizes important information about REQUIP for Restless Legs Syndrome. Medicines are sometimes prescribed for purposes other than those listed in this leaflet. Do not take REQUIP for a condition for which it was not prescribed. For more information, talk with your healthcare provider or pharmacist. They can give you information about REQUIP that is written for healthcare professionals. For more information call 1-888-825-5249 (toll-free) or visit www.requip.com.

What are the ingredients in REQUIP?
The following ingredients are in REQUIP:
Active ingredient: ropinirole (as ropinirole hydrochloride)
Inactive ingredients: croscarmellose sodium, hydrous lactose, magnesium stearate, microcrystalline cellulose, and one or more of the following: carmine, FD&C Blue No. 2 aluminum lake, FD&C Yellow No. 6 aluminum lake, hypromellose, iron oxides, polyethylene glycol, polysorbate 80, titanium dioxide.

GlaxoSmithKline
Research Triangle Park, NC 27709
©2008, GlaxoSmithKline. All rights reserved.
RXL:2PIL
July 2008

ROTARIX®   ℞
[rōt' ə-rix]
(Rotavirus Vaccine, Live, Oral)
Oral Suspension

HIGHLIGHTS OF PRESCRIBING INFORMATION
These highlights do not include all the information needed to use ROTARIX safely and effectively. See full prescribing information for ROTARIX.
ROTARIX (Rotavirus Vaccine, Live, Oral)
Oral Suspension
Initial U.S. Approval: 2008

———————RECENT MAJOR CHANGES———————
Contraindications (4.1)   01/2010
Contraindications (4.3)   02/2010
———————INDICATIONS AND USAGE———————
ROTARIX is a vaccine indicated for the prevention of rotavirus gastroenteritis caused by G1 and non-G1 types (G3, G4, and G9). ROTARIX is approved for use in infants 6 weeks to 24 weeks of age. (1)
——————DOSAGE AND ADMINISTRATION——————
FOR ORAL USE ONLY. (2.1)
- Each dose is 1-mL administered orally. (2.2)
- Administer first dose to infants beginning at 6 weeks of age. (2.2)
- Administer second dose after an interval of at least 4 weeks and prior to 24 weeks of age. (2.2)
——————DOSAGE FORMS AND STRENGTHS——————
- Vial of lyophilized vaccine to be reconstituted with a liquid diluent in a prefilled oral applicator. (3)
- Each 1-mL dose contains a suspension of at least $10^{6.0}$ median Cell Culture Infective Dose ($CCID_{50}$) of live, attenuated human G1P[8] rotavirus after reconstitution. (3)

———————CONTRAINDICATIONS———————
- A demonstrated history of hypersensitivity to the vaccine or any component of the vaccine including latex rubber (contained in the oral applicator). (4.1, 11)
- History of uncorrected congenital malformation of the gastrointestinal tract that would predispose the infant to intussusception. (4.2)
- History of Severe Combined Immunodeficiency Disease (SCID). (4.3, 6.2)
——————WARNINGS AND PRECAUTIONS——————
- Administration of ROTARIX in infants suffering from acute diarrhea or vomiting should be delayed. Safety and effectiveness of ROTARIX in infants with chronic gastrointestinal disorders have not been evaluated. (5.1)
- Since ROTARIX is a live virus, safety and effectiveness in infants with known primary or secondary immunodeficiencies have not been evaluated. (5.2)
———————ADVERSE REACTIONS———————
Common (≥5%) solicited adverse events included fussiness/irritability, cough/runny nose, fever, loss of appetite, and vomiting. (6.1)
To report SUSPECTED ADVERSE REACTIONS, contact GlaxoSmithKline at 1-888-825-5249 or VAERS at 1-800-822-7967 or www.vaers.hhs.gov.
See 17 for PATIENT COUNSELING INFORMATION and FDA-approved patient labeling

Revised: 02/2010

———————————————————————————————
FULL PRESCRIBING INFORMATION: CONTENTS*
* Sections or subsections omitted from the full prescribing information are not listed

———————————————————————————————
FULL PRESCRIBING INFORMATION

1   INDICATIONS AND USAGE
ROTARIX® is indicated for the prevention of rotavirus gastroenteritis caused by G1 and non-G1 types (G3, G4, and G9) when administered as a 2-dose series *[see Clinical Studies (14.3)]*. ROTARIX is approved for use in infants 6 weeks to 24 weeks of age.

2   DOSAGE AND ADMINISTRATION
2.1   Reconstitution Instructions for Oral Administration
For oral use only. Not for injection.
Reconstitute only with accompanying diluent. Do not mix ROTARIX with other vaccines or solutions. Inspect vials visually for any cracks prior to administration. If any cracks exist, the vaccine should not be administered.

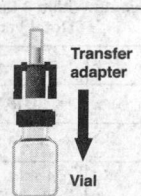

Transfer adapter

Vial

Remove vial cap and push transfer adapter onto vial (lyophilized vaccine).

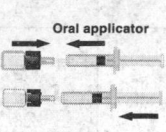

Oral applicator

Shake diluent in oral applicator (white, turbid suspension). Connect oral applicator to transfer adapter.

Push plunger of oral applicator to transfer diluent into vial. Suspension will appear white and turbid.

Withdraw vaccine into oral applicator.

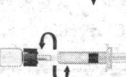

Twist and remove the oral applicator.

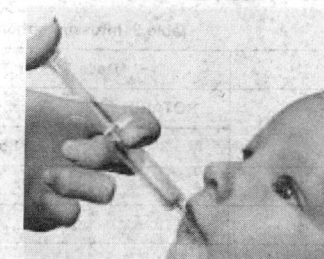

Ready for **oral** administration.

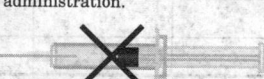

Do not use a needle with ROTARIX. Not for injection.

2.2   Recommended Dose and Schedule
The vaccination series consists of two 1-mL doses administered **orally**. The first dose should be administered to infants beginning at 6 weeks of age. There should be an interval of at least 4 weeks between the first and second dose. The 2-dose series should be completed by 24 weeks of age. Safety and effectiveness have not been evaluated if ROTARIX were administered for the first dose and another rotavirus vaccine were administered for the second dose or vice versa.
In the event that the infant spits out or regurgitates most of the vaccine dose, a single replacement dose may be considered at the same vaccination visit.
2.3   Infant Feeding
Breast-feeding was permitted in clinical studies. There was no evidence to suggest that breast-feeding reduced the protection against rotavirus gastroenteritis afforded by ROTARIX. There are no restrictions on the infant's liquid consumption, including breast-milk, either before or after vaccination with ROTARIX.

3   DOSAGE FORMS AND STRENGTHS
ROTARIX is available as a vial of lyophilized vaccine to be reconstituted with a liquid diluent in a prefilled oral applicator.
Each 1-mL dose contains a suspension of at least $10^{6.0}$ median Cell Culture Infective Dose ($CCID_{50}$) of live, attenuated human G1P[8] rotavirus after reconstitution.

4   CONTRAINDICATIONS
4.1   Hypersensitivity
A demonstrated history of hypersensitivity to any component of the vaccine.
Infants who develop symptoms suggestive of hypersensitivity after receiving a dose of ROTARIX should not receive further doses of ROTARIX.
4.2   Gastrointestinal Tract Congenital Malformation
History of uncorrected congenital malformation of the gastrointestinal tract (such as Meckel's diverticulum) that would predispose the infant for intussusception.
4.3   Severe Combined Immunodeficiency Disease
Infants with Severe Combined Immunodeficiency Disease (SCID) should not receive ROTARIX. Postmarketing reports of gastroenteritis, including severe diarrhea and prolonged

Table 1. Solicited Adverse Events Within 8 Days Following Doses 1 and 2 of ROTARIX or Placebo (Total Vaccinated Cohort)

	Dose 1		Dose 2	
	ROTARIX	Placebo	ROTARIX	Placebo
	N = 3,284	N = 2,013	N = 3,201	N = 1,973
	%	%	%	%
Fussiness/irritability[a]	52	52	42	42
Cough/runny nose[b]	28	30	31	33
Fever[c]	25	33	28	34
Loss of appetite[d]	25	25	21	21
Vomiting	13	11	8	8
Diarrhea	4	3	3	3

Total vaccinated cohort = all vaccinated infants for whom safety data were available.
N = number of infants for whom at least one symptom sheet was completed.
[a]Defined as crying more than usual.
[b]Data not collected in 1 of 7 studies; Dose 1: ROTARIX N = 2,583; placebo N = 1,897; Dose 2: ROTARIX N = 2,522; placebo N = 1,863.
[c]Defined as temperature ≥100.4°F (≥38.0°C) rectally or ≥99.5°F (≥37.5°C) orally.
[d]Defined as eating less than usual.

Table 3. Intussusception Cases by Day Range in Relation to Dose

	Dose 1		Dose 2		Any Dose	
	ROTARIX	Placebo	ROTARIX	Placebo	ROTARIX	Placebo
Day Range	N = 31,673	N = 31,552	N = 29,616	N = 29,465	N = 31,673	N = 31,552
0-7	0	0	2	0	2	0
8-14	0	0	0	2	0	2
15-21	1	1	2	1	3	2
22-30	0	1	1	2	1	3
Total (0-30)	1	2	5	5	6	7

shedding of vaccine virus, have been reported in infants who were administered live, oral rotavirus vaccines and later identified as having SCID [see Adverse Reactions (6.2)].

5 WARNINGS AND PRECAUTIONS

5.1 Gastrointestinal Disorders
Administration of ROTARIX should be delayed in infants suffering from acute diarrhea or vomiting.
Safety and effectiveness of ROTARIX in infants with chronic gastrointestinal disorders have not been evaluated. [See Contraindications (4.2).]

5.2 Altered Immunocompetence
Safety and effectiveness of ROTARIX in infants with known primary or secondary immunodeficiencies, including infants with human immunodeficiency virus (HIV), infants on immunosuppressive therapy, or infants with malignant neoplasms affecting the bone marrow or lymphatic system have not been evaluated.

5.3 Shedding and Transmission
Rotavirus shedding in stool occurs after vaccination with peak excretion occurring around day 7 after dose 1. Live rotavirus shedding was evaluated in 2 studies among a subset of infants at day 7 after dose 1. In these studies, the estimated percentages of recipients of ROTARIX who shed live rotavirus were 25.6% (95% Confidence Interval [CI]: 10.2, 41.1) and 26.5% (95% CI: 15.5, 37.5), respectively. Transmission of virus was not evaluated. There is a possibility that the live vaccine virus can be transmitted to non-vaccinated contacts. The potential for transmission of vaccine virus following vaccination should be weighed against the possibility of acquiring and transmitting natural rotavirus.

5.4 Intussusception
Following administration of a previously licensed oral live rhesus rotavirus-based vaccine, an increased risk of intussusception was observed.[1] The risk of intussusception with ROTARIX was evaluated in a safety study (including 63,225 infants) conducted in Latin America and Finland. No increased risk of intussusception was observed in this clinical trial following administration of ROTARIX when compared with placebo. [See Adverse Reactions (6.1).] In post-marketing experience, cases of intussusception have been reported in temporal association with ROTARIX [see Adverse Reactions (6.2)].

5.5 Post-Exposure Prophylaxis
Safety and effectiveness of ROTARIX when administered after exposure to rotavirus have not been evaluated.

6 ADVERSE REACTIONS

6.1 Clinical Trials Experience
Because clinical trials are conducted under widely varying conditions, adverse reaction rates observed in the clinical trials of a vaccine cannot be directly compared to rates in the clinical trials of another vaccine, and may not reflect the rates observed in practice. As with any vaccine, there is the possibility that broad use of ROTARIX could reveal adverse reactions not observed in clinical trials.
Solicited and unsolicited adverse events, serious adverse events and cases of intussusception were collected in 7 clinical studies. Cases of intussusception and serious adverse events were collected in an additional large safety study. These 8 clinical studies evaluated a total of 71,209 infants who received ROTARIX (N = 36,755) or placebo (N = 34,454). The racial distribution for these studies was as follows: Hispanic 73.4%, white 16.2%, black 1.0%, and other 9.4%; 51% were male.
Solicited Adverse Events: In 7 clinical studies, detailed safety information was collected by parents/guardians for 8 consecutive days following vaccination with ROTARIX (i.e., day of vaccination and the next 7 days). A diary card was completed to record fussiness/irritability, cough/runny nose, the infant's temperature, loss of appetite, vomiting, or diarrhea on a daily basis during the first week following each dose of ROTARIX or placebo. Adverse events among recipients of ROTARIX and placebo occurred at similar rates (Table 1).
[See table 1 above]
Unsolicited Adverse Events: Infants were monitored for unsolicited serious and non-serious adverse events that occurred in the 31-day period following vaccination in 7 clinical studies. The following adverse events occurred at a statistically higher incidence (95% CI of Relative Risk excluding 1) among recipients of ROTARIX (N = 5,082) as compared with placebo recipients (N = 2,902): irritability (ROTARIX 11.4%, placebo 8.7%) and flatulence (ROTARIX 2.2%, placebo 1.3%).
Serious Adverse Events (SAEs): Infants were monitored for serious adverse events that occurred in the 31-day period following vaccination in 8 clinical studies. Serious adverse events occurred in 1.7% of recipients of ROTARIX (N = 36,755) as compared with 1.9% of placebo recipients (N = 34,454). Among placebo recipients, diarrhea (placebo 0.07%, ROTARIX 0.02%), dehydration (placebo 0.06%, ROTARIX 0.02%), and gastroenteritis (placebo 0.3%, ROTARIX 0.2%) occurred at a statistically higher incidence (95% CI of Relative Risk excluding 1) as compared with recipients of ROTARIX.
Deaths: During the entire course of 8 clinical studies, there were 68 (0.19%) deaths following administration of ROTARIX (N = 36,755) and 50 (0.15%) deaths following placebo administration (N = 34,454). The most commonly reported cause of death following vaccination was pneumonia, which was observed in 19 (0.05%) recipients of ROTARIX and 10 (0.03%) placebo recipients (Relative Risk: 1.74, 95% CI: 0.76, 4.23).
Intussusception: In a controlled safety study conducted in Latin America and Finland, the risk of intussusception was evaluated in 63,225 infants (31,673 received ROTARIX and 31,552 received placebo). Infants were monitored by active surveillance including independent, complementary methods (prospective hospital surveillance and parent reporting at scheduled study visits) to identify potential cases of intussusception within 31 days after vaccination and, in a subset of 20,169 infants (10,159 received ROTARIX and 10,010 received placebo), up to one year after the first dose. No increased risk of intussusception following administration of ROTARIX was observed within a 31-day period following any dose, and rates were comparable to the placebo group after a median of 100 days (Table 2). In a subset of 20,169 infants (10,159 received ROTARIX and 10,010 received placebo) followed up to one year after dose 1, there were 4 cases of intussusception with ROTARIX compared with 14 cases of intussusception with placebo [Relative Risk: 0.28 (95% CI: 0.10, 0.81)]. All of the infants who developed intussusception recovered without sequelae.

Table 2. Intussusception and Relative Risk With ROTARIX Compared With Placebo

Confirmed Cases of Intussusception	ROTARIX N = 31,673	Placebo N = 31,552
Within 31 days of diagnosis after any dose	6	7
Relative Risk (95% CI)	0.85 (0.30, 2.42)	
Within 100 days of dose 1[a]	9	16
Relative Risk (95% CI)	0.56 (0.25, 1.24)	

CI = Confidence Interval.
[a]Median duration after dose 1 (follow-up visit at 30 to 90 days after dose 2).

Among vaccine recipients, there were no confirmed cases of intussusception within the 0- to 14-day period after the first dose (Table 3), which was the period of highest risk for the previously licensed oral live rhesus rotavirus-based vaccine.[1]
[See table 3 above]
Kawasaki Disease: Kawasaki disease has been reported in 18 (0.035%) recipients of ROTARIX and 9 (0.021%) placebo recipients from 16 completed or ongoing clinical trials. Of the 27 cases, 5 occurred following ROTARIX in clinical trials that were either not placebo-controlled or 1:1 randomized. In placebo-controlled trials, Kawasaki disease was reported in 17 recipients of ROTARIX and 9 placebo recipients [Relative Risk: 1.71 (95% CI: 0.71, 4.38)]. Three of the 27 cases were reported within 30 days post-vaccination: 2 cases (ROTARIX = 1, placebo = 1) were from placebo-controlled trials [Relative Risk: 1.00 (95% CI: 0.01, 78.35)] and one case following ROTARIX was from a non-placebo-controlled trial. Among recipients of ROTARIX, the time of onset after study dose ranged 3 days to 19 months.

6.2 Postmarketing Experience
The following adverse events have been reported since market introduction of ROTARIX. Because these events are reported voluntarily from a population of uncertain size, it is not always possible to reliably estimate their frequency or establish a causal relationship to vaccination with ROTARIX.
Gastrointestinal Disorders: Intussusception (including death), hematochezia, gastroenteritis with vaccine viral shedding in infants with Severe Combined Immunodeficiency Disease (SCID).

Blood and Lymphatic System Disorders: Idiopathic thrombocytopenic purpura.
Vascular Disorders: Kawasaki disease.
General Disorders and Administration Site Conditions: Maladministration.

7   DRUG INTERACTIONS
7.1   Concomitant Vaccine Administration
In clinical trials, ROTARIX was administered concomitantly with US-licensed and non-US-licensed vaccines. In a US coadministration study in 484 infants, there was no evidence of interference in the immune responses to any of the antigens when PEDIARIX® [Diphtheria and Tetanus Toxoids and Acellular Pertussis Adsorbed, Hepatitis B (Recombinant) and Inactivated Poliovirus Vaccine Combined], a US-licensed 7-valent pneumococcal conjugate vaccine (Wyeth Pharmaceuticals Inc.), and a US-licensed Hib conjugate vaccine (Sanofi Pasteur SA) were coadministered with ROTARIX as compared with separate administration of ROTARIX.
7.2   Immunosuppressive Therapies
Immunosuppressive therapies, including irradiation, antimetabolites, alkylating agents, cytotoxic drugs, and corticosteroids (used in greater than physiologic doses), may reduce the immune response to ROTARIX. [See Warnings and Precautions (5.2).]

8   USE IN SPECIFIC POPULATIONS
8.1   Pregnancy
Pregnancy Category C
Animal reproduction studies have not been conducted with ROTARIX. It is also not known whether ROTARIX can cause fetal harm when administered to a pregnant woman or can affect reproduction capacity.
8.4   Pediatric Use
Safety and effectiveness of ROTARIX in infants younger than 6 weeks or older than 24 weeks of age have not been evaluated.
The effectiveness of ROTARIX in pre-term infants has not been established. Safety data are available in pre-term infants (ROTARIX = 134, placebo = 120) with a reported gestational age ≤36 weeks. These pre-term infants were followed for serious adverse events up to 30 to 90 days after dose 2. Serious adverse events were observed in 5.2% of recipients of ROTARIX as compared with 5.0% of placebo recipients. No deaths or cases of intussusception were reported in this population.

11   DESCRIPTION
ROTARIX (Rotavirus Vaccine, Live, Oral), for oral administration, is a live, attenuated rotavirus vaccine derived from the human 89-12 strain which belongs to G1P[8] type. The rotavirus strain is propagated on Vero cells. After reconstitution, the final formulation (1 mL) contains at least $10^{6.0}$ median Cell Culture Infective Dose ($CCID_{50}$) of live, attenuated rotavirus.
The lyophilized vaccine contains amino acids, dextran, Dulbecco's Modified Eagle Medium (DMEM), sorbitol, and sucrose. DMEM contains the following ingredients: sodium chloride, potassium chloride, magnesium sulfate, ferric (III) nitrate, sodium phosphate, sodium pyruvate, D-glucose, concentrated vitamin solution, L-cystine, L-tyrosine, amino acids solution, L-glutamine, calcium chloride, sodium hydrogenocarbonate, and phenol red. The liquid diluent contains calcium carbonate, sterile water, and xanthan. The diluent includes an antacid component (calcium carbonate) to protect the vaccine during passage through the stomach and prevent its inactivation due to the acidic environment of the stomach.
ROTARIX contains no preservatives.
The tip cap and the rubber plunger of the oral applicator contain dry natural latex rubber. The vial stopper and transfer adapter are latex-free.

12   CLINICAL PHARMACOLOGY
12.1   Mechanism of Action
Prior to rotavirus vaccination programs, rotavirus infected nearly all children by the time they were 5 years of age. Severe, dehydrating rotavirus gastroenteritis occurs primarily among children aged 3 to 35 months.[2] Among children up to 3 years of age, approximately 16% of cases before 6 months of age result in hospitalization.[3]
The exact immunologic mechanism by which ROTARIX protects against rotavirus gastroenteritis is unknown [see Clinical Pharmacology (12.2)]. ROTARIX contains a live, attenuated human rotavirus that replicates in the small intestine and induces immunity.
12.2   Pharmacodynamics
Immunogenicity: A relationship between antibody responses to rotavirus vaccination and protection against rotavirus gastroenteritis has not been established. Seroconversion was defined as the appearance of anti-rotavirus IgA antibodies (concentration ≥20 U/mL) post-vaccination in the serum of infants previously negative for rotavirus. In 2 safety and efficacy studies, one to two months after a 2-dose series, 86.5% of 787 recipients of ROTARIX seroconverted

compared with 6.7% of 420 placebo recipients and 76.8% of 393 recipients of ROTARIX seroconverted compared with 9.7% of 341 placebo recipients, respectively.

13   NONCLINICAL TOXICOLOGY
13.1   Carcinogenesis, Mutagenesis, Impairment of Fertility
ROTARIX has not been evaluated for carcinogenic or mutagenic potential, or for impairment of fertility.

14   CLINICAL STUDIES
14.1   Efficacy Studies
The data demonstrating the efficacy of ROTARIX in preventing rotavirus gastroenteritis come from 24,163 infants randomized in two placebo-controlled studies conducted in 17 countries in Europe and Latin America. In these studies, oral polio vaccine (OPV) was not coadministered; however, other routine childhood vaccines could be concomitantly administered. Breast-feeding was permitted in both studies.
A randomized, double-blind, placebo-controlled study was conducted in 6 European countries. A total of 3,994 infants were enrolled to receive ROTARIX (n = 2,646) or placebo (n = 1,348). Vaccine or placebo was given to healthy infants as a 2-dose series with the first dose administered orally from 6 through 14 weeks of age followed by one additional dose administered at least 4 weeks after the first dose. The

2-dose series was completed by 24 weeks of age. For both vaccination groups, 98.3% of infants were white and 53% were male.
The clinical case definition of rotavirus gastroenteritis was an episode of diarrhea (passage of 3 or more loose or watery stools within a day), with or without vomiting, where rotavirus was identified in a stool sample. Severity of gastroenteritis was determined by a clinical scoring system, the Vesikari scale, assessing the duration and intensity of diarrhea and vomiting, the intensity of fever, use of rehydration therapy or hospitalization for each episode. Scores range from 0 to 20, where higher scores indicate greater severity. An episode of gastroenteritis with a score of 11 or greater was considered severe.[4]
The primary efficacy endpoint was prevention of any grade of severity of rotavirus gastroenteritis caused by naturally occurring rotavirus from 2 weeks after the second dose through one rotavirus season (according to protocol, ATP). Other efficacy evaluations included prevention of severe rotavirus gastroenteritis, as defined by the Vesikari scale, and reductions in hospitalizations due to rotavirus gastroenteritis and all cause gastroenteritis regardless of presumed etiology. Analyses were also done to evaluate the efficacy of ROTARIX against rotavirus gastroenteritis among infants who received at least one vaccination (total vaccinated cohort, TVC).

Table 4. Efficacy Evaluation of ROTARIX Through One Rotavirus Season

	According to Protocol[a]		Total Vaccinated Cohort[b]	
	ROTARIX	Placebo	ROTARIX	Placebo
Infants in Cohort	N = 2,572	N = 1,302	N = 2,646	N = 1,348
Gastroenteritis cases				
Any severity	24	94	26	104
Severe[c]	5	60	5	64
Efficacy estimate against RV GE				
Any severity	87.1%[d]		87.3%[d]	
(95% CI)	(79.6, 92.1)		(80.3, 92.0)	
Severe[c]	95.8%[d]		96.0%[d]	
(95% CI)	(89.6, 98.7)		(90.2, 98.8)	
Cases of hospitalization due to RV GE	0	12	0	12
Efficacy in reducing hospitalizations due to RV GE	100%[d]		100%[d]	
(95% CI)	(81.8, 100)		(81.7, 100)	

RV GE = rotavirus gastroenteritis; CI = Confidence Interval.
[a]ATP analysis includes all infants in the efficacy cohort who received two doses of vaccine according to randomization.
[b]TVC analysis includes all infants in the efficacy cohort who received at least one dose of vaccine or placebo.
[c]Severe gastroenteritis defined as ≥11 on the Vesikari scale.
[d]Statistically significant vs. placebo (P<0.001).

Table 5. Efficacy Evaluation of ROTARIX Through One Year

	According to Protocol[a]		Total Vaccinated Cohort[b]	
	ROTARIX	Placebo	ROTARIX	Placebo
Infants in Cohort	N = 9,009	N = 8,858	N = 10,159	N = 10,010
Gastroenteritis cases				
Severe	12	77	18	94
Efficacy estimate against RV GE				
Severe	84.7%[c]		81.1%[c]	
(95% CI)	(71.7, 92.4)		(68.5, 89.3)	
Cases of hospitalization due to RV GE	9	59	14	72
Efficacy in reducing hospitalizations due to RV GE	85.0%[c]		80.8%[c]	
(95% CI)	(69.6, 93.5)		(65.7, 90.0)	

RV GE = rotavirus gastroenteritis; CI = Confidence Interval.
[a]ATP analysis includes all infants in the efficacy cohort who received two doses of vaccine according to randomization.
[b]TVC analysis includes all infants in the efficacy cohort who received at least one dose of vaccine or placebo.
[c]Statistically significant vs. placebo (P<0.001).

Table 6. Type-Specific Efficacy of ROTARIX Against Any Grade of Severity and Severe Rotavirus Gastroenteritis (According to Protocol)

	Through One Rotavirus Season			Through Two Rotavirus Seasons		
	Number of Cases			Number of Cases		
	ROTARIX	Placebo	% Efficacy	ROTARIX	Placebo	% Efficacy
Type Identified[a]	N = 2,572	N = 1,302	(95% CI)	N = 2,572	N = 1,302	(95% CI)
ANY GRADE OF SEVERITY						
G1P[8]	4	46	95.6%[b] (87.9, 98.8)	18	89[c,d]	89.8%[b] (82.9, 94.2)
G2P[4]	3	4[c]	NS	14	17[c]	58.3%[b] (10.1, 81.0)
G3P[8]	1	5	89.9%[b] (9.5, 99.8)	3	10	84.8%[b] (41.0, 97.3)
G4P[8]	3	13	88.3%[b] (57.5, 97.9)	6	18	83.1%[b] (55.6, 94.5)
G9P[8]	13	27	75.6%[b] (51.1, 88.5)	38	71[d]	72.9%[b] (59.3, 82.2)
Combined non-G1 (G2, G3, G4, G9, G12) types[e]	20	49	79.3%[b] (64.6, 88.4)	62	116	72.9%[b] (62.9, 80.5)
SEVERE						
G1P[8]	2	28	96.4%[b] (85.7, 99.6)	4	57	96.4%[b] (90.4, 99.1)
G2P[4]	1	2[c]	NS	2	7[c]	85.5%[b] (24.0, 98.5)
G3P[8]	0	5	100%[b] (44.8, 100)	1	8	93.7%[b] (52.8, 99.9)
G4P[8]	0	7	100%[b] (64.9, 100)	1	11	95.4%[b] (68.3, 99.9)
G9P[8]	2	19	94.7%[b] (77.9, 99.4)	13	44[d]	85.0%[b] (71.7, 92.6)
Combined non-G1 (G2, G3, G4, G9, G12) types[e]	3	33	95.4%[b] (85.3, 99.1)	17	70	87.7%[b] (78.9, 93.2)

CI = Confidence Interval; NS = Not significant.
[a]Statistical analyses done by G type; if more than one rotavirus type was detected from a rotavirus gastroenteritis episode, the episode was counted in each of the detected rotavirus type categories.
[b]Statistically significant vs. placebo (P<0.05).
[c]The P genotype was not typeable for one episode.
[d]P[8] genotype was not detected in one episode.
[e]Two cases of G12P[8] were isolated in the second season (one in each group).

Efficacy of ROTARIX against any grade of severity of rotavirus gastroenteritis through one rotavirus season was 87.1% (95% CI: 79.6, 92.1); TVC efficacy was 87.3% (95% CI: 80.3, 92.0). Efficacy against severe rotavirus gastroenteritis through one rotavirus season was 95.8% (95% CI: 89.6, 98.7); TVC efficacy was 96.0% (95% CI: 90.2, 98.8) (Table 4). The protective effect of ROTARIX against any grade of severity of rotavirus gastroenteritis observed immediately following dose 1 administration and prior to dose 2 was 89.8% (95% CI: 8.9, 99.8).
Efficacy of ROTARIX in reducing hospitalizations for rotavirus gastroenteritis through one rotavirus season was 100% (95% CI: 81.8, 100); TVC efficacy was 100% (95% CI: 81.7, 100) (Table 4). ROTARIX reduced hospitalizations for all cause gastroenteritis regardless of presumed etiology by 74.7% (95% CI: 45.5, 88.9).
[See table 4 at top of previous page]
A randomized, double-blind, placebo-controlled study was conducted in 11 countries in Latin America and Finland. A total of 63,225 infants received ROTARIX (n = 31,673) or placebo (n = 31,552). An efficacy subset of these infants consisting of 20,169 infants from Latin America received ROTARIX (n = 10,159) or placebo (n = 10,010). Vaccine or placebo was given to healthy infants as a 2-dose series with the first dose administered orally from 6 through 13 weeks of age followed by one additional dose administered at least 4 weeks after the first dose. The 2-dose series was completed by the age of 24 weeks of age. For both vaccination groups, the racial distribution of the efficacy subset was as follows: Hispanic 85.8%, white 7.9%, black 1.1%, and other 5.2%; 51% were male.
The clinical case definition of severe rotavirus gastroenteritis was an episode of diarrhea (passage of 3 or more loose or watery stools within a day), with or without vomiting, where rotavirus was identified in a stool sample, requiring hospitalization and/or rehydration therapy equivalent to World Health Organization (WHO) plan B (oral rehydration therapy) or plan C (intravenous rehydration therapy) in a medical facility.
The primary efficacy endpoint was prevention of severe rotavirus gastroenteritis caused by naturally occurring rotavirus from 2 weeks after the second dose through one year (ATP). Analyses were done to evaluate the efficacy of ROTARIX against severe rotavirus gastroenteritis among infants who received at least one vaccination (TVC). Reduction in hospitalizations due to rotavirus gastroenteritis was also evaluated (ATP).
Efficacy of ROTARIX against severe rotavirus gastroenteritis through one year was 84.7% (95% CI: 71.7, 92.4); TVC efficacy was 81.1% (95% CI: 68.5, 89.3) (Table 5).
Efficacy of ROTARIX in reducing hospitalizations for rotavirus gastroenteritis through one year was 85.0% (95% CI: 69.6, 93.5); TVC efficacy was 80.8% (95% CI: 65.7, 90.0) (Table 5).
[See table 5 on previous page]

14.2 Efficacy Through Two Rotavirus Seasons
The efficacy of ROTARIX persisting through two rotavirus seasons was evaluated in two studies.
In the European study, the efficacy of ROTARIX against any grade of severity of rotavirus gastroenteritis through two rotavirus seasons was 78.9% (95% CI: 72.7, 83.8). Efficacy in preventing any grade of severity of rotavirus gastroenteritis cases occurring only during the second season post-vaccination was 71.9% (95% CI: 61.2, 79.8). The efficacy of ROTARIX against severe rotavirus gastroenteritis through two rotavirus seasons was 90.4% (95% CI: 85.1, 94.1). Efficacy in preventing severe rotavirus gastroenteritis cases occurring only during the second season post-vaccination was 85.6% (95% CI: 75.8, 91.9). The efficacy of ROTARIX in reducing hospitalizations for rotavirus gastroenteritis through two rotavirus seasons was 96.0% (95% CI: 83.8, 99.5).

In the Latin American study, the efficacy of ROTARIX against severe rotavirus gastroenteritis through two years was 80.5% (95% CI: 71.3, 87.1). Efficacy in preventing severe rotavirus gastroenteritis cases occurring only during the second year post-vaccination was 79.0% (95% CI: 66.4, 87.4). The efficacy of ROTARIX in reducing hospitalizations for rotavirus gastroenteritis through two years was 83.0% (95% CI: 73.1, 89.7).
The efficacy of ROTARIX beyond the second season post-vaccination was not evaluated.

14.3 Efficacy Against Specific Rotavirus Types
The type-specific efficacy against any grade of severity and severe rotavirus gastroenteritis caused by G1P[8], G3P[8], G4P[8], G9P[8], and combined non-G1 (G2, G3, G4, G9) types was statistically significant through one year. Additionally, type-specific efficacy against any grade of severity and severe rotavirus gastroenteritis caused by G1P[8], G2P[4], G3P[8], G4P[8], G9P[8], and combined non-G1 (G2, G3, G4, G9) types was statistically significant through two years (Table 6).
[See table 6 at left]

15 REFERENCES
1. Murphy TV, Gargiullo PM, Massoudi MS, et al. Intussusception among infants given an oral rotavirus vaccine. *N Engl J Med* 2001;344:564–572.
2. Centers for Disease Control and Prevention. Prevention of rotavirus gastroenteritis among infants and children. Recommendations of the Advisory Committee on Immunization Practices (ACIP). *MMWR* 2006;55(No. RR-12): 1-13.
3. Parashar UD, Holman RC, Clarke MJ, et al. Hospitalizations associated with rotavirus diarrhea in the United States, 1993 through 1995: surveillance based on the new ICD-9-CM rotavirus-specific diagnostic code. *J Infect Dis* 1998;177:13-17.
4. Ruuska T, Vesikari T. Rotavirus disease in Finnish children: use of numerical scores for severity of diarrheal episodes. *Scand J Infect Dis* 1990;22:259-267.

16 HOW SUPPLIED/STORAGE AND HANDLING
ROTARIX is available as a vial of lyophilized vaccine, a prefilled oral applicator of liquid diluent (1 mL) with a plunger stopper, and a transfer adapter for reconstitution.
Supplied as:
NDC 58160-805-11 (package of 10)
16.1 Storage Before Reconstitution
• Vials: Store the vials of lyophilized ROTARIX refrigerated at 2° to 8°C (36° to 46°F). **Protect vials from light.**
• Diluent: The diluent may be stored at a controlled room temperature 20° to 25°C (68° to 77°F). **Do not freeze. Discard if the diluent has been frozen.**
16.2 Storage After Reconstitution
ROTARIX should be administered within 24 hours of reconstitution. It may be stored refrigerated at 2° to 8°C (36° to 46°F) or at room temperature up to 25°C (77°F), after reconstitution. Discard the reconstituted vaccine if not used within 24 hours in biological waste container. **Do not freeze. Discard if the vaccine has been frozen.**

17 PATIENT COUNSELING INFORMATION
See FDA-approved patient labeling (17.2).
17.1 Patient Advice
• Parents or guardians should be informed by the healthcare provider of the potential benefits and risks of immunization with ROTARIX, and of the importance of completing the immunization series.
• The healthcare provider should inform the parents or guardians about the potential for adverse reactions that have been temporally associated with administration of ROTARIX or other vaccines containing similar components.
• The parent or guardian accompanying the recipient should be instructed to report any adverse events to their healthcare provider.
• The parent or guardian should be given the Vaccine Information Statements, which are required by the National Childhood Vaccine Injury Act of 1986 to be given prior to immunization. These materials are available free of charge at the Centers for Disease Control and Prevention (CDC) website (www.cdc.gov/vaccines).
17.2 FDA-Approved Patient Labeling
Patient labeling is provided as a tear-off leaflet at the end of this full prescribing information.
ROTARIX and PEDIARIX are registered trademarks of GlaxoSmithKline.
Manufactured by **GlaxoSmithKline Biologicals**
Rixensart, Belgium, US License 1617
Distributed by **GlaxoSmithKline**
Research Triangle Park, NC 27709
©2010, GlaxoSmithKline. All rights reserved.
February 2010
RTX:6PI

PATIENT INFORMATION
ROTARIX® (ROW-tah-rix)
Rotavirus Vaccine, Live, Oral

Read this Patient Information carefully before your baby gets ROTARIX and before your baby receives the next dose of ROTARIX. This leaflet is a summary of information about ROTARIX and does not take the place of talking with your baby's doctor.

What is ROTARIX?
ROTARIX is a vaccine that protects your baby from a kind of virus (called a rotavirus) that can cause bad diarrhea and vomiting. Rotavirus can cause diarrhea and vomiting that is so bad that your baby can lose too much body fluid and need to go to the hospital.
Rotavirus vaccine is a liquid that is given to your baby by mouth. It is not a shot.

Who should not take ROTARIX?
Your baby should not get ROTARIX if:
- He or she has had an allergic reaction after getting a dose of ROTARIX.
- He or she is allergic to any of the ingredients of this vaccine. A list of ingredients can be found at the end of this leaflet.
- A doctor has told you that your baby's digestive system has a defect (is not normal).
- He or she has Severe Combined Immunodeficiency Disease (SCID), a severe problem with his/her immune system.

Tell your doctor if your baby:
- Has problems with his/her immune system.
- Has cancer.
- Will be in close contact with someone who has problems with his/her immune system or is getting treated for cancer.

If your baby has been having diarrhea and vomiting, your doctor may want to wait before giving your baby a dose of ROTARIX.

What are possible side effects of ROTARIX?
The most common side effects of ROTARIX are:
- Crying
- Fussiness
- Cough
- Runny nose
- Fever
- Loss of appetite
- Vomiting.

Call your doctor right away or go to the emergency department if your baby has any of these problems after getting ROTARIX even if it has been several weeks since the last vaccine dose because these may be signs of a serious problem called intussusception that happens when a part of the intestine gets blocked or twisted:
- Bad vomiting
- Bad diarrhea
- Bloody bowel movement
- High fever
- Severe stomach pain (if your baby brings his/her knees to his/her chest while crying or screaming).

Since FDA approval, reports of infants with intussusception have been received by Vaccine Adverse Event Reporting System (VAERS). Intussusception occurred days and sometimes weeks after vaccination. Some infants needed hospitalization, surgery on their intestines, or a special enema to treat this problem. Death due to intussusception has occurred.

Other reported side effects include: Kawasaki disease (a serious condition that can affect the heart; symptoms may include fever, rash, red eyes, red mouth, swollen glands, swollen hands, and feet and, if not treated, death can occur). Talk to your baby's doctor if your baby has any problems that concern you.

How is ROTARIX given?
ROTARIX is a liquid that is dropped into your baby's mouth and swallowed.

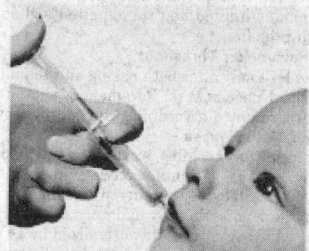

Figure 1. Administration of ROTARIX

Your baby will get the first dose at around 6 weeks old. The second dose will be at least 4 weeks after the first dose (before 6 months old).

Be sure to plan the time for your baby's second dose with the doctor because it is important that your baby gets both doses of ROTARIX before your baby is 6 months old.
The doctor may decide to give your baby shots at the same time as ROTARIX.
Your baby can be fed normally after getting ROTARIX.

What are the ingredients in ROTARIX?
ROTARIX contains weakened human rotavirus.
ROTARIX also contains dextran, sorbitol, xanthan, and Dulbecco's Modified Eagle Medium (DMEM). The ingredients of DMEM are as follows: sodium chloride, potassium chloride, magnesium sulphate, ferric (III) nitrate, sodium phosphate, sodium pyruvate, D-glucose, concentrated vitamin solution, L-cystine, L-tyrosine, amino acids solution, L-glutamine, calcium chloride, sodium hydrogenocarbonate, and phenol red. ROTARIX contains no preservatives.
The dropper used to give your baby ROTARIX contains latex.
ROTARIX is a registered trademark of GlaxoSmithKline.
Manufactured by **GlaxoSmithKline Biologicals**
Rixensart, Belgium, US License 1617
Distributed by **GlaxoSmithKline**
Research Triangle Park, NC 27709
©2010, GlaxoSmithKline. All rights reserved.
February 2010
RTX:4PIL

RYTHMOL® ℞
[rith'-mol]
(propafenone hydrochloride)
Tablets

DESCRIPTION
RYTHMOL (propafenone hydrochloride) is an antiarrhythmic drug supplied in scored, film-coated tablets of 150, 225, and 300 mg for oral administration. Propafenone has some structural similarities to beta-blocking agents.
Chemically, propafenone hydrochloride (HCl) is 2′-[2-Hydroxy-3-(propylamino)-propoxy]-3-phenylpropiophenone hydrochloride, with a molecular weight of 377.92. The molecular formula is $C_{21}H_{27}NO_3 \cdot HCl$. The structural formula of propafenone HCl is given below:

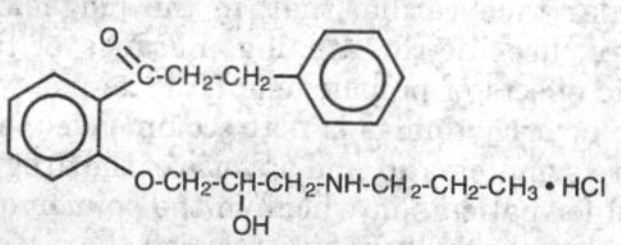

$$\text{C-CH}_2\text{-CH}_2$$
$$\text{O-CH}_2\text{-CH-CH}_2\text{-NH-CH}_2\text{-CH}_2\text{-CH}_3 \cdot \text{HCl}$$
$$\text{OH}$$

Propafenone HCl occurs as colorless crystals or white crystalline powder with a very bitter taste. It is slightly soluble in water (20°C), chloroform and ethanol. The following inactive ingredients are contained in the tablet: corn starch, hypromellose, magnesium stearate, polyethylene glycol, polysorbate, povidone, propylene glycol, sodium starch glycolate, and titanium dioxide.

CLINICAL PHARMACOLOGY
Mechanism of Action
RYTHMOL is a Class 1C antiarrhythmic drug with local anesthetic effects, and a direct stabilizing action on myocardial membranes. The electrophysiological effect of RYTHMOL manifests itself in a reduction of upstroke velocity (Phase 0) of the monophasic action potential. In Purkinje fibers, and to a lesser extent myocardial fibers, RYTHMOL reduces the fast inward current carried by sodium ions. Diastolic excitability threshold is increased and effective refractory period prolonged. Propafenone reduces spontaneous automaticity and depresses triggered activity.
Studies in anesthetized dogs and isolated organ preparations show that RYTHMOL has beta-sympatholytic activity at about 1/50 the potency of propranolol. Clinical studies employing isoproterenol challenge and exercise testing after single doses of propafenone indicate a beta-adrenergic blocking potency (per mg) about 1/40 that of propranolol in man. In clinical trials, resting heart rate decreases of about 8% were noted at the higher end of the therapeutic plasma concentration range. At very high concentrations in vitro, propafenone can inhibit the slow inward current carried by calcium, but this calcium antagonist effect probably does not contribute to antiarrhythmic efficacy. Propafenone has local anesthetic activity approximately equal to procaine.

Electrophysiology
Electrophysiology studies in patients with ventricular tachycardia (VT) have shown that propafenone HCl prolongs atrioventricular (AV) conduction while having little or no effect on sinus node function. Both AV nodal conduction time (AH interval) and His-Purkinje conduction time (HV interval) are prolonged. Propafenone has little or no effect on the atrial functional refractory period, but AV nodal functional and effective refractory periods are prolonged. In patients with Wolff-Parkinson-White (WPW) syndrome, RYTHMOL reduces conduction and increases the effective refractory period of the accessory pathway in both directions. Propafenone slows conduction and consequently produces dose-related changes in the PR interval and QRS duration. QTc interval does not change.
[See table 1 at top of next page]
In any individual patient, the above ECG changes cannot be readily used to predict either efficacy or plasma concentration.
RYTHMOL causes a dose-related and concentration-related decrease in the rate of single and multiple premature ventricular contractions (PVCs) and can suppress recurrence of ventricular tachycardia. Based on the percent of patients attaining substantial (80% to 90%) suppression of ventricular ectopic activity, it appears that trough plasma levels of 0.2 to 1.5 µg/mL can provide good suppression, with higher concentrations giving a greater rate of good response.
When 600 mg/day propafenone was administered to patients with paroxysmal atrial tachyarrhythmias, mean heart rate during arrhythmia decreased 14 beats/min and 37 beats/min for paroxysmal atrial fibrillation/flutter (PAF) patients and paroxysmal supraventricular tachycardia (PSVT) patients, respectively.

Hemodynamics
Sympathetic stimulation may be a vital component supporting circulatory function in patients with congestive heart failure, and its inhibition by the beta blockade produced by propafenone HCl may in itself aggravate congestive heart failure.
Additionally, like other Class 1C antiarrhythmic drugs, studies in humans have shown that propafenone HCl exerts a negative inotropic effect on the myocardium. Cardiac catheterization studies in patients with moderately impaired ventricular function (mean C.I. = 2.61 L/min/m²) utilizing intravenous propafenone infusions (2 mg/kg over 10 min + 2 mg/min for 30 min) that gave mean plasma concentrations of 3.0 µg/mL (well above the therapeutic range of 0.2 to 1.5 µg/mL) showed significant increases in pulmonary capillary wedge pressure, systemic and pulmonary vascular resistances and depression of cardiac output and cardiac index.

Pharmacokinetics and Metabolism
Propafenone HCl is nearly completely absorbed after oral administration with peak plasma levels occurring approximately 3.5 hours after administration in most individuals. Propafenone exhibits extensive saturable presystemic biotransformation (first pass effect) resulting in a dose dependent and dosage form dependent absolute bioavailability; e.g., a 150 mg tablet had absolute bioavailability of 3.4%, while a 300 mg tablet had absolute bioavailability of 10.6%. A 300 mg solution was rapidly absorbed, had absolute bioavailability of 21.4%. At still larger doses, above those recommended, bioavailability increases still further. Decreased liver function also increases bioavailability; bioavailability is inversely related to indocyanine green clearance reaching 60% to 70% at clearances of 7 mL/min and below. The clearance of propafenone is reduced and the elimination half-life increased in patients with significant hepatic dysfunction (see PRECAUTIONS).
Propafenone HCl follows a nonlinear pharmacokinetic disposition presumably due to saturation of first pass hepatic metabolism as the liver is exposed to higher concentrations of propafenone and shows a very high degree of interindividual variability. For example, for a three-fold increase in daily dose from 300 to 900 mg/day there is a tenfold increase in steady-state plasma concentration. The top 25% of patients given 337.5 mg/day, however, had a mean concentration of propafenone larger than the bottom 25%, and about equal to the second 25%, of patients given a dose of 900 mg. Although food increased peak blood level and bioavailability in a single dose study, during multiple dose administration of propafenone to healthy volunteers food did not change bioavailability significantly.
There are two genetically determined patterns of propafenone metabolism. In over 90% of patients, the drug is rapidly and extensively metabolized with an elimination half-life from 2 to 10 hours. These patients metabolize propafenone into two active metabolites: 5-hydroxypropafenone which is formed by CYP2D6 and N-depropylpropafenone which is formed by both CYP3A4 and CYP1A2.
In vitro preparations have shown these two metabolites to have antiarrhythmic activity comparable to propafenone but in man they both are usually present in concentrations less than 20% of propafenone. Nine additional metabolites have been identified, most only in trace amounts. It is the saturable hydroxylation pathway that is responsible for nonlinear pharmacokinetic disposition.
In less than 10% of patients (and in any patient also receiving quinidine, see PRECAUTIONS), metabolism of propafenone is slower because the 5-hydroxy metabolite is not formed or is minimally formed. The estimated propafenone elimination half-life ranges from 10 to 32 hours. Decreased ability to form the 5-hydroxy metabolite of propafenone is associated with a diminished ability to me-

Table 1: Mean Changes in Electrocardiogram Intervals[a]

| | Total Daily Dose (mg) | | | | | | | |
| | 337.5 mg | | 450 mg | | 675 mg | | 900 mg | |
Interval	msec	%	msec	%	msec	%	msec	%
RR	-14.5	-1.8	30.6	3.8	31.5	3.9	41.7	5.1
PR	3.6	2.1	19.1	11.6	28.9	17.8	35.6	21.9
QRS	5.6	6.4	5.5	6.1	7.7	8.4	15.6	17.3
QTc	2.7	0.7	-7.5	-1.8	5.0	1.2	14.7	3.7

[a] Change and percent change based on mean baseline values for each treatment group.

Table 2: Reduction of Arrythmias in Patients with PAF or PSVT

| | Study 1 | | Study 2 | |
	Propafenone	Placebo	Propafenone	Placebo
PAF	n = 30	n = 30	n = 9	n = 9
Percent attack free	53%	13%	67%	22%
Median time to first recurrence	> 98 days	8 days	62 days	5 days
PSVT	n = 45	n = 45	n = 15	N = 15
Percent attack free	47%	16%	38%	7%
Median time to first recurrence	> 98 days	12 days	31 days	8 days

tabolize debrisoquine and a variety of other drugs (encainide, metoprolol, dextromethorphan). In these patients, the N-depropylpropafenone occurs in quantities comparable to the levels occurring in extensive metabolizers (EM). In slow metabolizers (SM) propafenone pharmacokinetics are linear.

There are significant differences in plasma concentrations of propafenone in slow and extensive metabolizers, the former achieving concentrations 1.5 to 2.0 times those of the extensive metabolizers at daily doses of 675 to 900 mg/day. At low doses the differences are greater, with slow metabolizers attaining concentrations more than five times that of extensive metabolizers. Because the difference decreases at high doses and is mitigated by the lack of the active 5-hydroxy metabolite in the slow metabolizers, and because steady-state conditions are achieved after 4 to 5 days of dosing in all patients, the recommended dosing regimen is the same for all patients. The greater variability in blood levels require that the drug be titrated carefully in patients with close attention paid to clinical and ECG evidence of toxicity (See DOSAGE AND ADMINISTRATION).

In vitro and in vivo studies have shown that the R-isomer of propafenone is cleared faster than the S-isomer via the 5-hydroxylation pathway (CYP2D6). This results in a higher ratio of S-propafenone during steady state.

Clinical Trials

In two randomized, crossover, placebo-controlled, double-blind trials of 60 to 90 days duration in patients with paroxysmal supraventricular arrhythmias [paroxysmal atrial fibrillation/flutter (PAF), or paroxysmal supraventricular tachycardia (PSVT)], propafenone reduced the rate of both arrhythmias, as shown in Table 2.
[See table 2 above]
The patient population in the above trials was 50% male with a mean age of 57.3 years. Fifty percent of the patients had a diagnosis of PAF and 50% had PSVT. Eighty percent of the patients received 600 mg/day propafenone. No patient died in the above 2 studies.

In U.S. long-term safety trials, 474 patients (mean age: 57.4 ± 14.5 years) with supraventricular arrhythmias [195 with PAF, 274 with PSVT and 5 with both PAF and PSVT] were treated up to 5 years (mean: 14.4 months) with propafenone. Fourteen of the patients died. When this mortality rate was compared to the rate in a similar patient population (n = 194 patients; mean age: 43.0 ± 16.8 years) studied in an arrhythmia clinic, there was no age-adjusted difference in mortality. This comparison was not, however, a randomized trial and the 95% confidence interval around the comparison was large, such that neither a significant adverse or favorable effect could be ruled out.

INDICATIONS AND USAGE

In patients without structural heart disease, RYTHMOL is indicated to prolong the time to recurrence of:
• paroxysmal atrial fibrillation/flutter (PAF) associated with disabling symptoms.
• paroxysmal supraventricular tachycardia (PSVT) associated with disabling symptoms.
As with other agents, some patients with atrial flutter treated with propafenone have developed 1:1 conduction,

producing an increase in ventricular rate. Concomitant treatment with drugs that increase the functional AV refractory period is recommended.
The use of propafenone HCl in patients with chronic atrial fibrillation has not been evaluated. Propafenone HCl should not be used to control ventricular rate during atrial fibrillation.
Propafenone HCl is also indicated for the treatment of:
• documented ventricular arrhythmias, such as sustained ventricular tachycardia, that, in the judgement of the physician, are life-threatening. Because of the proarrhythmic effects of propafenone HCl, its use with lesser ventricular arrhythmias is not recommended, even if patients are symptomatic, and any use of the drug should be reserved for patients in whom, in the opinion of the physician, the potential benefits outweigh the risks.
Initiation of propafenone HCl treatment, as with other antiarrhythmics used to treat life-threatening ventricular arrhythmias, should be carried out in the hospital.
Propafenone HCl, like other antiarrhythmic drugs, has not been shown to enhance survival in patients with ventricular or atrial arrhythmias.

CONTRAINDICATIONS

Propafenone HCl is contraindicated in the presence of uncontrolled congestive heart failure, cardiogenic shock, sinoatrial, atrioventricular and intraventricular disorders of impulse generation and/or conduction (e.g., sick sinus node syndrome, atrioventricular block) in the absence of an artificial pacemaker, bradycardia, marked hypotension, bronchospastic disorders, manifest electrolyte imbalance, and known hypersensitivity to the drug.

WARNINGS

MORTALITY:
In the National Heart, Lung and Blood Institute's Cardiac Arrhythmia Suppression Trial (CAST), a long-term, multi-center, randomized, double-blind study in patients with asymptomatic non-life-threatening ventricular arrhythmias who had a myocardial infarction more than six days but less than two years previously, an increased rate of death or reversed cardiac arrest rate (7.7%; 56/730) was seen in patients treated with encainide or flecainide (Class 1C antiarrhythmics) compared with that seen in patients assigned to placebo (3.0%; 22/725). The average duration of treatment with encainide or flecainide in this study was ten months. The applicability of the CAST results to other populations (e.g., those without recent myocardial infarction) or other antiarrhythmic drugs is uncertain, but at present it is prudent to consider any 1C antiarrhythmic to have a significant risk in patients with structural heart disease. Given the lack of any evidence that these drugs improve survival, antiarrhythmic agents should generally be avoided in patients with non-life-threatening ventricular arrhythmias, even if the patients are experiencing unpleasant, but not life-threatening, symptoms or signs.

Proarrhythmic Effects

Propafenone HCl, like other antiarrhythmic agents, may cause new or worsened arrhythmias. Such proarrhythmic effects range from an increase in frequency of PVCs to the development of more severe ventricular tachycardia, ventricular fibrillation or torsade de pointes; i.e., tachycardia that is more sustained or more rapid which may lead to fatal consequences. It is therefore essential that each patient given propafenone HCl be evaluated electrocardiographically and clinically prior to, and during therapy to determine whether the response to propafenone HCl supports continued treatment.
Overall in clinical trials with propafenone, 4.7% of all patients had new or worsened ventricular arrhythmia possibly representing a pro-arrhythmic event (0.7% was an increase in PVCs; 4.0% a worsening, or new appearance, of VT or ventricular fibrillation [VF]). Of the patients who had worsening of VT (4%), 92% had a history of VT and/or VT/VF, 71% had coronary artery disease, and 68% had a prior myocardial infarction. The incidence of proarrhythmia in patients with less serious or benign arrhythmias, which include patients with an increase in frequency of PVCs, was 1.6%. Although most proarrhythmic events occurred during the first week of therapy, late events also were seen and the CAST study (see above) suggests that an increased risk is present throughout treatment.
In the 474 patient U.S. multicenter trial in patients with symptomatic supraventricular tachycardia (SVT), 1.9% (9/474) of these patients experienced ventricular tachycardia (VT) or ventricular fibrillation (VF) during the study. However, in 4 of the 9 patients, the ventricular tachycardia was of atrial origin. Six of the nine patients that developed ventricular arrhythmias did so within 14 days of onset of therapy. About 2.3% (11/474) of all patients had a recurrence of SVT during the study which could have been a change in the patients' arrhythmia behavior or could represent a proarrhythmic event. Case reports in patients treated with propafenone HCl for atrial fibrillation/flutter have included increased PVCs, VT, VF, and death.

Nonallergic Bronchospasm (e.g., chronic bronchitis, emphysema)

PATIENTS WITH BRONCHOSPASTIC DISEASE SHOULD, IN GENERAL, NOT RECEIVE PROPAFENONE or other agents with beta-adrenergic-blocking activity.

Congestive Heart Failure

During treatment with oral propafenone in patients with depressed baseline function (mean ejection fraction [EF] = 33.5%), no significant decreases in ejection fraction were seen. In clinical trial experience, new or worsened CHF has been reported in 3.7% of patients with ventricular arrhythmia; of those 0.9% were considered probably or definitely related to propafenone HCl. Of the patients with congestive heart failure probably related to propafenone, 80% had preexisting heart failure and 85% had coronary artery disease. CHF attributable to propafenone HCl developed rarely (< 0.2%) in ventricular arrhythmia patients who had no previous history of CHF. CHF occurred in 1.9% of patients studied with PAF or PSVT.
As propafenone HCl exerts both beta blockade and a (dose-related) negative inotropic effect on cardiac muscle, patients with congestive heart failure should be fully compensated before receiving propafenone HCl. If congestive heart failure worsens, propafenone HCl should be discontinued (unless congestive heart failure is due to the cardiac arrhythmia) and, if indicated, restarted at a lower dosage only after adequate cardiac compensation has been established.

Conduction Disturbances

Propafenone HCl slows atrioventricular conduction and also causes first degree AV block. Average PR interval prolongation and increases in QRS duration are closely correlated with dosage increases and concomitant increases in propafenone plasma concentrations. The incidence of first degree, second degree, and third degree AV block observed in 2,127 ventricular arrhythmia patients was 2.5%, 0.6%, and 0.2%, respectively. Development of second or third degree AV block requires a reduction in dosage or discontinuation of propafenone HCl. Bundle branch block (1.2%) and intraventricular conduction delay (1.1%) have been reported in patients receiving propafenone. Bradycardia has also been reported (1.5%). Experience in patients with sick sinus node syndrome is limited and these patients should not be treated with propafenone.

Effects on Pacemaker Threshold

Propafenone HCl may alter both pacing and sensing thresholds of artificial pacemakers. Pacemakers should be monitored and programmed accordingly during therapy.

Hematologic Disturbances

Agranulocytosis (fever, chills, weakness, and neutropenia) has been reported in patients receiving propafenone. Generally, the agranulocytosis occurred within the first two months of propafenone therapy and upon discontinuation of therapy, the white count usually normalized by 14 days. Unexplained fever and/or decrease in white cell count, particularly during the initial three months of therapy, warrant consideration of possible agranulocytosis/granulocytopenia. Patients should be instructed to promptly report the development of any signs of infection such as fever, sore throat, or chills.

PRECAUTIONS

Hepatic Dysfunction

Propafenone is highly metabolized by the liver and should, therefore, be administered cautiously to patients with impaired hepatic function. Severe liver dysfunction increases the bioavailability of propafenone to approximately 70% compared to 3 to 40% for patients with normal liver function. In eight patients with moderate to severe liver disease, the mean half-life was approximately 9 hours. As a result, the dose of propafenone given to patients with impaired hepatic function should be approximately 20 to 30% of the dose given to patients with normal hepatic function (see DOSAGE AND ADMINISTRATION). Careful monitoring for excessive pharmacological effects (see OVERDOSAGE) should be carried out.

Renal Dysfunction

A considerable percentage of propafenone metabolites (18.5% to 38% of the dose/48 hours) are excreted in the urine.

Until further data are available, propafenone HCl should be administered cautiously to patients with impaired renal function. These patients should be carefully monitored for signs of overdosage (see OVERDOSAGE).

Elevated ANA Titers

Positive ANA titers have been reported in patients receiving propafenone. They have been reversible upon cessation of treatment and may disappear even in the face of continued propafenone therapy. These laboratory findings were usually not associated with clinical symptoms, but there is one published case of drug-induced lupus erythematosis (positive rechallenge); it resolved completely upon discontinuation of therapy. Patients who develop an abnormal ANA test should be carefully evaluated and, if persistent or worsening elevation of ANA titers is detected, consideration should be given to discontinuing therapy.

Impaired Spermatogenesis

Reversible disorders of spermatogenesis have been demonstrated in monkeys, dogs and rabbits after high dose intravenous administration of propafenone HCl. Evaluation of the effects of short-term RYTHMOL administration on spermatogenesis in 11 normal subjects had suggested that propafenone HCl produced a reversible, short-term drop (within normal range) in sperm count. Subsequent evaluations in 11 patients receiving RYTHMOL chronically have suggested no effect of propafenone HCl on sperm count.

Neuromuscular Dysfunction

Exacerbation of myasthenia gravis has been reported during propafenone therapy.

Drug Interactions

Propafenone is metabolized by CYP2D6 (major pathway) and CYP1A2 and CYP3A4. Drugs that inhibit CYP2D6 (such as desipramine, paroxetine, ritonavir, sertraline), CYP1A2 (such as amiodarone), and CYP3A4 (such as ketaconazole, ritonavir, saquinavir, erythromycin, and grapefruit juice) can be expected to cause increased plasma levels of propafenone. Appropriate monitoring is recommended when RYTHMOL SR is used together with such drugs. In addition, propafenone is an inhibitor of CYP2D6. Coadministration of propafenone with drugs metabolized by CYP2D6 (such as desipramine, imipramine, haloperidol, venlafaxine) might lead to increased plasma concentrations of these drugs. The effect of propafenone on the P-Glycoprotein transporter has not been studied.

Quinidine

Small doses of quinidine completely inhibit the CYP2D6 hydroxylation metabolic pathway, making all patients, in effect, slow metabolizers (see CLINICAL PHARMACOLOGY). Concomitant administration of quinidine (50 mg three times daily) with 150 mg immediate release propafenone three times daily decreased the clearance of propafenone by 60% in EM, making them SM. Steady-state plasma concentrations increased by more that 2-fold for propafenone, and decreased 50% for 5-OH-propafenone A 100 mg dose of quinidine increased steady state concentrations of propafenone 3-fold. Concomitant use of propafenone and quinidine is not recommended.

Digoxin

Concomitant use of propafenone and digoxin increased steady-state serum digoxin exposure (AUC) in patients by 60% to 270%, and decreased the clearance of digoxin by 31% to 67%. Plasma digoxin levels of patients receiving propafenone should be monitored and digoxin dosage adjusted as needed.

Lidocaine

No significant effects on the pharmacokinetics of propafenone or lidocaine have been seen following their concomitant use in patients. However, concomitant use of propafenone and lidocaine have been reported to increase the risks of central nervous system side effects of lidocaine.

Beta-Antagonists

Concomitant use of propafenone and propranolol in healthy subjects increased propranolol plasma concentrations at steady state by 113%. In 4 patients, administration of metoprolol with propafenone increased the metoprolol plasma concentrations at steady state by 100% to 400%. The pharmacokinetics of propafenone was not affected by the coadministration of either propranolol or metoprolol. In clinical trials using propafenone immediate release tablets, patients who were receiving beta-blockers concurrently did not experience an increased incidence of side effects.

Warfarin

The concomitant administration of propafenone and warfarin increased warfarin plasma concentrations at steady state by 39% in healthy volunteers and prolonged the prothrombin time in patients taking warfarin. Adjustment of the warfarin dose should be guided by monitoring of the prothrombin time.

Cimetidine

Concomitant administration of propafenone immediate release tablets and cimetidine in 12 healthy subjects resulted in a 20% increase in steady-state plasma concentrations of propafenone.

Rifampin

Concomitant administration of rifampin and propafenone in extensive metabolizers decreased the plasma concentrations of propafenone by 67% with a corresponding decrease of 5OH-propafenone by 65%. The concentrations of norpropafenone increased by 30%. In slow metabolizers, there was a 50% decrease in propafenone plasma concentrations and increased the AUC and C_{max} of norpropafenone by 74% and 20%, respectively. Urinary excretion of propafenone and its metabolites decreased significantly. Similar results were noted in elderly patients: Both the AUC and C_{max} propafenone decreased by 84%, with a corresponding decrease in AUC and C_{max} of 5OH-propafenone by 69% and 57%.

Fluoxetine

Concomitant administration of propafenone and fluoxetine in extensive metabolizers increased the S-propafenone C_{max} and AUC by 39% and 50% and the R propafenone C_{max} and AUC by 71% and 50%.

Amiodarone

Concomitant administration of propafenone and amiodarone can affect conduction and repolarization and is not recommended.

Post Marketing Reports

Orlistat may limit the fraction of propafenone available for absorption. In post marketing reports, abrupt cessation of orlistat in patients stabilized on propafenone has resulted in severe adverse events including convulsions, atrioventricular block and acute circulatory failure.

Renal and Hepatic Toxicity in Animals

Renal changes have been observed in the rat following 6 months of oral administration of propafenone HCl at doses of 180 and 360 mg/kg/day (about 2 and 4 times, respectively, the maximum recommended human daily dose [MRHD] on a mg/m^2 basis). Both inflammatory and non-inflammatory changes in the renal tubules, with accompanying interstitial nephritis, were observed. These changes were reversible, as they were not found in rats allowed to recover for 6 weeks. Fatty degenerative changes of the liver were found in rats following longer durations of administration of propafenone HCl at a dose of 270 mg/kg/day (about 3 times the MRHD on a mg/m^2 basis). There were no renal or hepatic changes at 90 mg/kg/day (equivalent to the MRHD on a mg/m^2 basis).

Carcinogenesis, Mutagenesis, Impairment of Fertility

Lifetime maximally tolerated oral dose studies in mice (up to 360 mg/kg/day, about twice the maximum recommended human oral daily dose [MRHD] on a mg/m^2 basis) and rats (up to 270 mg/kg/day, about 3 times the MRHD on a mg/m^2 basis) provided no evidence of a carcinogenic potential for propafenone HCl.

Propafenone HCl tested negative for mutagenicity in the Ames (salmonella) test and the mouse dominant lethal test, and tested negative for clastogenicity in the Chinese hamster micronucleus test, and other *in vivo* tests for chromosomal aberrations in rat bone marrow and Chinese hamster bone marrow and spermatogonia.

Propafenone HCl, administered intravenously to rabbits, dogs, and monkeys, has been shown to decrease spermatogenesis. These effects were reversible, were not found following oral dosing of propafenone HCl, were seen at lethal or near lethal dose levels and were not seen in rats treated either orally or intravenously (see PRECAUTIONS, Impaired Spermatogenesis). Treatment of male rabbits for 10 weeks prior to mating at an oral dose of 120 mg/kg/day (about 2.4 times the MRHD on a mg/m^2 basis) or an intravenous dose of 3.5 mg/kg/day (a spermatogenesis-impairing dose) did not result in evidence of impaired fertility. Nor was there evidence of impaired fertility when propafenone HCl was administered orally to male and female rats at dose levels up to 270 mg/kg/day (about 3 times the MRHD on mg/m^2 basis).

Pregnancy

Teratogenic Effects

Pregnancy Category C. Propafenone HCl has been shown to be embryotoxic (decreased survival) in rabbits and rats when given in oral maternally toxic doses of 150 mg/kg day (about 3 times the maximum recommended human dose [MRHD] on a mg/m^2 basis) and 600 mg/kg/day (about 6 times the MRHD on a mg/m^2 basis), respectively. Although maternally tolerated doses (up to 270 mg/kg/day, about 3 times the MRHD on a mg/m^2 basis) produced no evidence of embryotoxicity in rats, post-implantation loss was elevated in all rabbit treatment groups (doses as low as 15 mg/kg/day, about 1/3 the MRHD on a mg/m^2 basis). There are no adequate and well-controlled studies in pregnant women. RYTHMOL should be used during pregnancy only if the potential benefit justifies the potential risk to the fetus.

Non-teratogenic Effects

In a study in which female rats received daily oral doses of propafenone HCl from mid-gestation through weaning of their offspring, doses as low as 90 mg/kg/day (equivalent to the MRHD on a mg/m^2 basis) produced increases in maternal deaths. Doses of 360 or more mg/kg/day (4 or more times the MRHD on a mg/m^2 basis) resulted in reductions in neonatal survival, body weight gain and physiological development.

Labor and Delivery

It is not known whether the use of propafenone during labor or delivery has immediate or delayed adverse effects on the fetus, or whether it prolongs the duration of labor or increases the need for forceps delivery or other obstetrical intervention.

Nursing Mothers

It is not known whether this drug is excreted in human milk. Because many drugs are excreted in human milk and because of the potential for serous adverse reactions in nursing infants from propafenone HCl, a decision should be made whether to discontinue nursing or to discontinue the drug, taking into account the importance of the drug to the mother.

Pediatric Use

The safety and effectiveness of propafenone HCl in pediatric patients have not been established.

Geriatric Use

Clinical studies of RYTHMOL did not include sufficient numbers of subjects aged 65 and over to determine whether they respond differently from younger subjects. Other reported clinical experience has not identified differences in responses between the elderly and younger patients. In general, dose selection for an elderly patient should be cautious, usually starting at the low end of the dosing range, reflecting the greater frequency of decreased hepatic, renal, or cardiac function, and of concomitant disease or other drug therapy.

ADVERSE REACTIONS

Adverse reactions associated with propafenone HCl occur most frequently in the gastrointestinal, cardiovascular, and central nervous systems. About 20% of patients treated with propafenone HCl have discontinued treatment because of adverse reactions.

Adverse reactions reported for > 1.5% of 474 SVT patients who received propafenone in U.S. clinical trials are presented in Table 3 by incidence and percent discontinuation, reported to the nearest percent.

Table 3: Adverse Reactions Reported for > 1.5% of SVT Patients

	Incidence (N = 480)	% of Pts. Who Discontinued
Unusual Taste	14%	1.3%
Nausea and/or Vomiting	11%	2.9%
Dizziness	9%	1.7%
Constipation	8%	0.2%
Headache	6%	0.8%
Fatigue	6%	1.5%
Blurred Vision	3%	0.6%
Weakness	3%	1.3%
Dyspnea	2%	1.0%
Wide Complex Tachycardia	2%	1.9%
CHF	2%	0.6%
Bradycardia	2%	0.2%
Palpitations	2%	0.2%
Tremor	2%	0.4%

Anorexia	2%	0.2%
Diarrhea	2%	0.4%
Ataxia	2%	0.0%

Results of controlled trials in ventricular arrhythmia patients comparing adverse reaction rates on propafenone and placebo, and on propafenone and quinidine are shown in Table 4. Adverse reactions reported for ≥ 1% of the patients receiving propafenone as shown, unless they were more frequent on placebo than propafenone. The most common events were unusual taste, dizziness, first degree AV block, intraventricular conduction delay, nausea and/or vomiting, and constipation. Headache was relatively common also, but was not increased compared to placebo.
[See table 4 at right]

Adverse reactions reported for ≥ 1% of 2,127 ventricular arrhythmia patients who received propafenone in U.S. clinical trials are presented in Table 5 by propafenone daily dose. The most common adverse reactions in controlled clinical trials appeared dose-related (but note that most patients spent more time at the larger doses), especially dizziness, nausea and/or vomiting, unusual taste, constipation, and blurred vision. Some less common reactions may also have been dose-related such as first degree AV block, congestive heart failure, dyspepsia, and weakness. The principal causes of discontinuation were the most common events and are shown in the table.
[See table 5 below and on next page]

In addition, the following adverse reactions were reported less frequently than 1% either in clinical trials or in marketing experience (*adverse events for marketing experience are given in italics*). Causality and relationship to propafenone therapy cannot necessarily be judged from these events.

Cardiovascular System
Atrial flutter, AV dissociation, cardiac arrest, flushing, hot flashes, sick sinus syndrome, sinus pause or arrest, supraventricular tachycardia.

Nervous System
Abnormal dreams, abnormal speech, abnormal vision, *apnea, coma,* confusion, depression, memory loss, numbness, paresthesias, psychosis/mania, seizures (0.3%), tinnitus, unusual smell sensation, vertigo.

Gastrointestinal
A number of patients with liver abnormalities associated with propafenone therapy have been reported in postmarketing experience. Some appeared due to hepatocellular injury, some were cholestatic and some showed a mixed picture. Some of these reports were simply discovered through clinical chemistries, others because of clinical symptoms including fulminant hepatitis and death. One case was rechallenged with a positive outcome. Cholestasis (0.1%), elevated liver enzymes (alkaline phosphatase, serum transaminases) (0.2%), gastroenteritis, hepatitis (0.03%).

Hematologic
Agranulocytosis, anemia, bruising, granulocytopenia, *increased bleeding time,* leukopenia, purpura, thrombocytopenia.

Other
Alopecia, eye irritation, *hyponatremia/inappropriate ADH secretion,* impotence, increased glucose, *kidney failure,* positive ANA (0.7%), *lupus erythematosis,* muscle cramps, muscle weakness, nephrotic syndrome, pain, pruritus.

OVERDOSAGE

The symptoms of overdosage, which are usually most severe within 3 hours of ingestion, may include hypotension, somnolence, bradycardia, intra-atrial and intraventricular conduction disturbances, and rarely convulsions and high grade ventricular arrhythmias. Defibrillation as well as infusion of dopamine and isoproterenol have been effective in controlling rhythm and blood pressure. Convulsions have been alleviated with intravenous diazepam. General supportive measures such as mechanical respiratory assistance and external cardiac massage may be necessary.

DOSAGE AND ADMINISTRATION

The dose of RYTHMOL must be individually titrated on the basis of response and tolerance. It is recommended that therapy be initiated with 150 mg propafenone given every eight hours (450 mg/day). Dosage may be increased at a minimum of 3 to 4 day intervals to 225 mg every 8 hours (675 mg/day) and, if necessary, to 300 mg every 8 hours (900 mg/day). The usefulness and safety of dosages exceeding 900 mg per day have not been established. In those patients in whom significant widening of the QRS complex or second or third degree AV block occurs, dose reduction should be considered.

As with other antiarrhythmic agents, in the elderly or in ventricular arrhythmia patients with marked previous myocardial damage, the dose of RYTHMOL should be increased more gradually during the initial phase of treatment.

Table 4: Adverse Reactions Reported for ≥ 1% of Ventricular Arrhythmia Patients

	Prop./Placebo Trials		Prop./Quinidine Trials	
	Prop.	Placebo	Prop.	Quinidine
	(N = 247)	(N = 111)	(N = 53)	(N = 52)
Unusual Taste	7%	1%	23%	0%
Dizziness	7%	5%	15%	10%
First Degree AV Block	5%	1%	2%	0%
Headache(s)	5%	5%	2%	8%
Constipation	4%	0%	6%	2%
Intraventricular Conduction Delay	4%	0%	-	-
Nausea and/or Vomiting	3%	1%	6%	15%
Fatigue	-	-	4%	2%
Palpitations	2%	1%	-	-
Blurred Vision	2%	1%	6%	2%
Dry Mouth	2%	1%	6%	6%
Dyspnea	2%	3%	4%	0%
Abdominal Pain/Cramps	-	-	2%	8%
Dyspepsia	-	-	2%	8%
CHF	-	-	2%	0%
Fever	-	-	2%	10%
Tinnitus	-	-	2%	2%
Vision, Abnormal	-	-	2%	2%
Esophagitis	-	-	2%	0%
Gastroenteritis	-	-	2%	0%
Anxiety	2%	2%	-	-
Anorexia	2%	1%	0%	2%
Proarrhythmia	1%	0%	2%	0%
Flatulence	1%	0%	2%	0%
Angina	1%	0%	2%	4%
Second Degree AV Block	1%	0%	-	-
Bundle Branch Block	1%	0%	2%	2%
Loss of Balance	1%	0%	-	-
Diarrhea	1%	1%	6%	39%

Table 5: Adverse Reactions Reported for ≥ 1% of Ventricular Arrhythmia Patients (N=2127)

	Incidence by Total Daily Dose			Total Incidence	% of Pts. Who Discont.
	450 mg	600 mg	≥ 900 mg		
	(N = 1430)	(N = 1337)	(N = 1333)	(N = 2127)	
Dizziness	4%	7%	11%	13%	2.4%
Nausea and/or Vomiting	2%	6%	9%	11%	3.4%
Unusual Taste	3%	5%	6%	9%	0.7%
Constipation	2%	4%	5%	7%	0.5%

(Table continued on next page)

HOW SUPPLIED
RYTHMOL tablets are supplied as scored, round, film-coated tablets containing either 150 mg, 225 mg, or 300 mg

Table 5 *(cont.):* Adverse Reactions Reported for ≥ 1% of Ventricular Arrhythmia Patients (N=2127)

	Incidence by Total Daily Dose			Total Incidence	% of Pts. Who Discont.
	450 mg	600 mg	≥ 900 mg		
	(N = 1430)	(N = 1337)	(N = 1333)	(N = 2127)	
Fatigue	2%	3%	4%	6%	1.0%
Dyspnea	2%	2%	4%	5%	1.6%
Proarrhythmia	2%	2%	3%	5%	4.7%
Angina	2%	2%	3%	5%	0.5%
Headache(s)	2%	3%	3%	5%	1.0%
Blurred Vision	1%	2%	3%	4%	0.8%
CHF	1%	2%	3%	4%	1.4%
Ventricular Tachycardia	1%	2%	3%	3%	1.2%
Dyspepsia	1%	2%	3%	3%	0.9%
Palpitations	1%	2%	3%	3%	0.5%
Rash	1%	1%	2%	3%	0.8%
AV Block, First Degree	1%	1%	2%	3%	0.3%
Diarrhea	1%	2%	2%	3%	0.6%
Weakness	1%	2%	2%	2%	0.7%
Dry Mouth	1%	1%	1%	2%	0.2%
Syncope/Near Syncope	1%	1%	1%	2%	0.7%
QRS Duration, Increased	1%	1%	2%	2%	0.5%
Chest Pain	1%	1%	1%	2%	0.2%
Anorexia	1%	1%	2%	2%	0.4%
Abdominal Pain, Cramps	1%	1%	1%	2%	0.4%
Ataxia	0%	1%	2%	2%	0.2%
Insomnia	0%	1%	1%	2%	0.3%
Premature Ventricular Contraction(s)	1%	1%	1%	2%	0.1%
Bradycardia	1%	1%	1%	2%	0.5%
Anxiety	1%	1%	1%	2%	0.6%
Edema	1%	0%	1%	1%	0.2%
Tremor(s)	0%	1%	1%	1%	0.3%
Diaphoresis	1%	0%	1%	1%	0.3%
Bundle Branch Block	0%	1%	1%	1%	0.5%
Drowsiness	1%	1%	1%	1%	0.2%
Atrial Fibrillation	1%	1%	1%	1%	0.4%
Flatulence	0%	1%	1%	1%	0.1%
Hypotension	0%	1%	1%	1%	0.4%
Intraventricular Conduction Delay	0%	1%	1%	1%	0.1%
Pain, Joints	0%	0%	1%	1%	0.1%

of propafenone hydrochloride and embossed (on the same side) with GS and TF5 for the 150 mg tablet, GS and F1X for the 225 mg tablet, and GS and 1FY for the 300 mg tablet, in the following package sizes:

150 mg bottles of 100: NDC 0173-0792-20
225 mg bottles of 100: NDC 0173-0794-20
300 mg bottles of 100: NDC 0173-0795-20

Storage
Store at 25°C (77°F); excursions permitted to 15°C to 30°C (59°F to 86°F). Dispense in a tight, light-resistant container.
RYTHMOL is a registered trademark of G. Petrik used under license by Abbott Laboratories.
Manufactured for GlaxoSmithKline by:
Halo Pharmaceutical, Inc.
30 North Jefferson Road
Whippany, NJ 07981

Distributed by:
GlaxoSmithKline
Research Triangle Park, NC 27709
©2009 GlaxoSmithKline. All rights reserved.
October 2009   RML:1PI

RYTHMOL® SR   ℞
[rith' mol]
(propafenone hydrochloride)
Extended Release Capsules

DESCRIPTION
RYTHMOL SR (propafenone hydrochloride) is an antiarrhythmic drug supplied in extended-release capsules of 225, 325 and 425 mg for oral administration.

The structural formula of propafenone HCl is given below:

Chemically, propafenone hydrochloride is 2'-[2-Hydroxy-3-(propylamino)-propoxy]-3-phenylpropiophenone hydrochloride, with a molecular weight of 377.92. The molecular formula is $C_{21}H_{27}NO_3$•HCl. Propafenone HCl has some structural similarities to beta-blocking agents. Propafenone HCl occurs as colorless crystals or white crystalline power with a very bitter taste. It is slightly soluble in water (20°C), chloroform, and ethanol. RYTHMOL SR capsules are filled with cylindrical-shaped 2×2 mm microtablets containing propafenone and the following inactive ingredients: antifoam, gelatin, hypromellose, red iron oxide, magnesium stearate, shellac, sodium lauryl sulfate, sodium dodecyl sulfate, soy lecithin, and titanium dioxide.

CLINICAL PHARMACOLOGY
Mechanism of Action: Propafenone is a Class 1C antiarrhythmic drug with local anesthetic effects, and a direct stabilizing action on myocardial membranes. The electrophysiological effect of propafenone manifests itself in a reduction of upstroke velocity (Phase 0) of the monophasic action potential. In Purkinje fibers, and to a lesser extent myocardial fibers, propafenone reduces the fast inward current carried by sodium ions. Diastolic excitability threshold is increased and effective refractory period prolonged. Propafenone reduces spontaneous automaticity and depresses triggered activity.

Studies in anesthetized dogs and isolated organ preparations show that propafenone has beta-sympatholytic activity at about 1/50 the potency of propranolol. Clinical studies employing isoproterenol challenge and exercise testing after single doses of propafenone indicate a beta-adrenergic blocking potency (per mg) about 1/40 that of propranolol in man. In clinical trials with the immediate-release formulation, resting heart rate decreases of about 8% were noted at the higher end of the therapeutic plasma concentration range. At very high concentrations in vitro, propafenone can inhibit the slow inward current carried by calcium, but this calcium antagonist effect probably does not contribute to antiarrhythmic efficacy. Moreover, propafenone inhibits a variety of cardiac potassium currents in in vitro studies (i.e. the transient outward, the delayed rectifier, and the inward rectifier current). Propafenone has local anesthetic activity approximately equal to procaine. Compared to propafenone, the main metabolite, 5-hydroxypropafenone, has similar sodium and calcium channel activity, but about 10 times less beta-blocking activity (N-depropylpropafenone has weaker sodium channel activity but equivalent affinity for beta-receptors).

Electrophysiology: Electrophysiology studies in patients with ventricular tachycardia (VT) have shown that propafenone prolongs atrioventricular (AV) conduction while having little or no effect on sinus node function. Both atrioventricular (AV) nodal conduction time (AH interval) and His-Purkinje conduction time (HV interval) are prolonged. Propafenone has little or no effect on the atrial functional refractory period, but AV nodal functional and effective refractory periods are prolonged. In patients with Wolff-Parkinson-White (WPW) syndrome, RYTHMOL immediate-release tablets reduce conduction and increase the effective refractory period of the accessory pathway in both directions (see ADVERSE REACTIONS, *Electrocardiograms*).

Hemodynamics: Studies in humans have shown that propafenone exerts a negative inotropic effect on the myocardium. Cardiac catheterization studies in patients with moderately impaired ventricular function (mean C.I.=2.61 L/min/m²), utilizing intravenous propafenone infusions (loading dose of 2 mg/kg over 10 min+ followed by 2 mg/min for 30 min) that gave mean plasma concentrations of 3.0 mcg/mL (a dose that produces plasma levels of propafenone greater than does recommended oral dosing), showed significant increases in pulmonary capillary wedge pressure, systemic and pulmonary vascular resistances, and depression of cardiac output and cardiac index.

Pharmacokinetics and Metabolism: *Absorption/Bioavailability:* Maximal plasma levels of propafenone are reached between 3 to 8 hours following the administration of

Table 1. Analysis of Tachycardia-Free Period (Days) From Day 1 of Randomization

Parameter	RYTHMOL SR Dose 225 mg twice daily (N = 126) n (%)	325 mg twice daily (N = 135) n (%)	425 mg twice daily (N = 136) n (%)	Placebo (N = 126) n (%)
Patients completing with terminating event*	66 (52)	56 (41)	41 (30)	87 (69)
Comparison of tachycardia-free periods				
Kaplan-Meier median	112	291	†	41
Range	0-285	0-293	0-300	0-289
p-Value (Log-rank test)	0.014	<0.0001	<0.0001	—
Hazard ratio compared to placebo	0.67	0.43	0.35	—
95% CI for hazard ratio	(0.49, 0.93)	(0.31, 0.61)	(0.24, 0.51)	—

*Fewer than 50% of the patients had events. The median time is not calculable.
†Terminating events comprised 91% atrial fibrillation, 5% atrial flutter, and 4% PSVT.

RYTHMOL SR. Propafenone is known to undergo extensive and saturable presystemic biotransformation which results in a dose- and dosage form-dependent absolute bioavailability; e.g., a 150-mg immediate-release tablet had an absolute bioavailability of 3.4%, while a 300-mg immediate-release tablet had an absolute bioavailability of 10.6%. Absorption from a 300-mg solution dose was rapid, with an absolute bioavailability of 21.4%. At still larger doses, above those recommended, bioavailability of propafenone from immediate-release tablets increased still further.

Relative bioavailability assessments have been performed between RYTHMOL SR capsules and RYTHMOL immediate-release tablets. In extensive metabolizers, the bioavailability of propafenone from the SR formulation was less than that of the immediate-release formulation as the more gradual release of propafenone from the prolonged-release preparations resulted in an increase of overall first-pass metabolism (see CLINICAL PHARMACOLOGY, *Metabolism*). As a result of the increased first-pass effect, higher daily doses of propafenone were required from the SR formulation relative to the immediate-release formulation, to obtain similar exposure to propafenone. The relative bioavailability of propafenone from the 325 twice-daily regimen of RYTHMOL SR approximates that of RYTHMOL immediate-release 150 mg three times daily regimen. Mean exposure to 5-hydroxypropafenone was about 20 to 25% higher after SR capsule administration than after immediate-release tablet administration.

Food increased the exposure to propafenone 4-fold after single dose administration of 425 mg of RYTHMOL SR. However, in the multiple dose study (425 mg dose twice daily), the difference between the fed and fasted state was not significant.

Distribution: Following intravenous administration of propafenone, plasma levels decline in a bi-phasic manner consistent with a 2-compartment pharmacokinetic model. The average distribution half-life corresponding to the first phase was about 5 minutes. The volume of the central compartment was about 88 liters (1.1 L/kg) and the total volume of distribution about 252 liters.

In serum, propafenone is greater than 95% bound to proteins within the concentration range of 0.5 to 2 mcg/mL. Protein binding decreases to about 88% in patients with severe hepatic dysfunction.

Metabolism: There are 2 genetically determined patterns of propafenone metabolism. In more than 90% of patients, the drug is rapidly and extensively metabolized with an elimination half-life from 2 to 10 hours. These patients metabolize propafenone into 2 active metabolites: 5-hydroxypropafenone which is formed by CYP2D6, and N-depropylpropafenone (norpropafenone) which is formed by both CYP3A4 and CYP1A2. In less than 10% of patients, metabolism of propafenone is slower because the 5-hydroxy metabolite is not formed or is minimally formed. In these patients, the estimated propafenone elimination half-life ranges from 10 to 32 hours. Decreased ability to form the 5-hydroxy metabolite of propafenone is associated with a diminished ability to metabolize debrisoquine and a variety of other drugs such as encainide, metoprolol, and dextromethorphan whose metabolism is mediated by the CYP2D6 isozyme. In these patients, the N-depropylpropafenone metabolite occurs in quantities comparable to the levels occurring in extensive metabolizers.

As a consequence of the observed differences in metabolism, administration of RYTHMOL SR to slow and extensive metabolizers results in significant differences in plasma concentrations of propafenone, with slow metabolizers achieving concentrations about twice those of the extensive metabolizers at daily doses of 850 mg/day. At low doses the differences are greater, with slow metabolizers attaining concentrations about 3 to 4 times higher than extensive metabolizers. In extensive metabolizers, saturation of the hydroxylation pathway (CYP2D6) results in greater-than-linear increases in plasma levels following administration of RYTHMOL SR capsules. In slow metabolizers, propafenone pharmacokinetics are linear. Because the difference decreases at high doses and is mitigated by the lack of the active 5-hydroxy metabolite in the slow metabolizers, and because steady-state conditions are achieved after 4 to 5 days of dosing in all patients, the recommended dosing regimen of RYTHMOL SR is the same for all patients. The larger inter-subject variability in blood levels require that the dose of the drug be titrated carefully in patients with close attention paid to clinical and ECG evidence of toxicity (see DOSAGE AND ADMINISTRATION).

The 5-hydroxypropafenone and norpropafenone metabolites have electrophysiologic properties similar to propafenone in vitro. In man after administration of RYTHMOL SR, the 5-hydroxypropafenone metabolite is usually present in concentrations less than 40% of propafenone. The norpropafenone metabolite is usually present in concentrations less than 10% of propafenone.

Inter-Subject Variability: With propafenone, there is a considerable degree of inter-subject variability in pharmacokinetics which is due in large part to the first-pass hepatic effect and non-linear pharmacokinetics in extensive metabolizers. A higher degree of inter-subject variability in pharmacokinetic parameters of propafenone was observed following both single and multiple dose administration of RYTHMOL SR capsules. Inter-subject variability appears to be substantially less in the poor metabolizer group than in the extensive metabolizer group, suggesting that a large portion of the variability is intrinsic to CYP2D6 polymorphism rather than to the formulation.

The clearance of propafenone is reduced and the elimination half-life increased in patients with significant hepatic dysfunction (see PRECAUTIONS). Decreased liver function also increases the bioavailability of propafenone. Absolute bioavailability assessments have not been determined for the RYTHMOL SR capsule formulation. Absolute bioavailability of RYTHMOL immediate-release tablets has been demonstrated to be inversely related to indocyanine green clearance, reaching 60 to 70% at clearances of 7 mL/min and below.

Stereochemistry: RYTHMOL is a racemic mixture. The R- and S-enantiomers of propafenone display stereoselective disposition characteristics. In vitro and in vivo studies have shown that the R-isomer of propafenone is cleared faster than the S-isomer via the 5-hydroxylation pathway (CYP2D6). This results in a higher ratio of S-propafenone to R-propafenone at steady state. Both enantiomers have equivalent potency to block sodium channels; however, the S-enantiomer is a more potent β-antagonist than the R-enantiomer. Following administration of RYTHMOL immediate-release tablets or RYTHMOL SR capsules, the S/R ratio for the area under the plasma concentration-time curve was about 1.7. The S/R ratios of propafenone obtained after administration of 225, 325, and 425 mg RYTHMOL SR are independent of dose. In addition, no difference in the average values of the S/R ratios is evident between genotypes or over time.

CLINICAL TRIALS

RYTHMOL SR has been evaluated in patients with a history of electrocardiographically documented recurrent episodes of symptomatic atrial fibrillation in 2 randomized, double-blind, placebo-controlled trials.

RAFT: In one US multicenter study (Rythmol SR Atrial Fibrillation Trial, RAFT), 3 doses of RYTHMOL SR (225 mg twice daily, 325 mg twice daily and 425 mg twice daily) and placebo were compared in 523 patients with symptomatic, episodic atrial fibrillation. The patient population in this trial was 59% male with a mean age of 63 years, 91% white and 6% black. The patients had a median history of atrial fibrillation of 13 months, and documented symptomatic atrial fibrillation within 12 months of study entry. More than 90% were NYHA Class I, and 21% had a prior electrical cardioversion. At baseline, 24% were treated with calcium channel blockers, 37% with beta blockers, and 38% with digoxin. Symptomatic arrhythmias after randomization were documented by transtelephonic electrocardiogram and centrally read and adjudicated by a blinded adverse event committee. RYTHMOL SR administered for up to 39 weeks was shown to prolong significantly the time to the first recurrence of symptomatic atrial arrhythmia, predominantly atrial fibrillation, from Day 1 of randomization (primary efficacy variable) compared to placebo, as shown in Table 1.

[See table 1 at left]

There was a dose response for RYTHMOL SR for the tachycardia-free period as shown in the proportional hazard analysis and the Kaplan-Meier curves presented in Figure 1.

Figure 1: RAFT Kaplan-Meier Analysis for the Tachycardia-Free Period From Day 1 of Randomization:

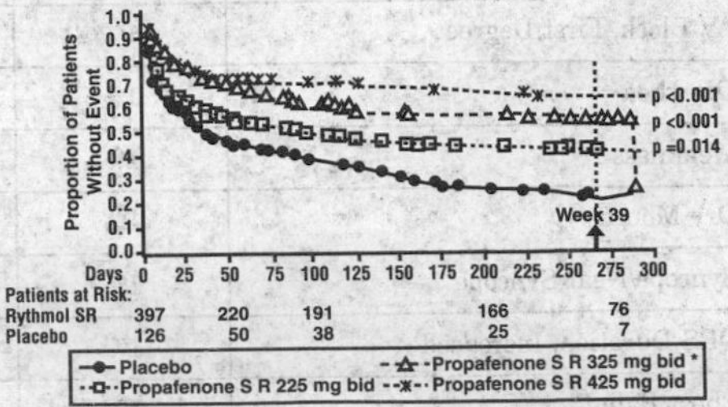
Proportion of Patients Without Event
1.0
0.9
0.8
0.7
0.6
0.5
0.4
0.3
0.2
0.1
0.0
p <0.001
p <0.001
p =0.014
Week 39
Days 0 25 50 75 100 125 150 175 200 225 250 275 300
Patients at Risk:
Rythmol SR 397 220 191 166 76
Placebo 126 50 38 25 7
Placebo
Propafenone S R 225 mg bid
Propafenone S R 325 mg bid *
Propafenone S R 425 mg bid

* Patient closeout started on Day 273 (week 39) and lasted until 300 days. On day 291, of the 2 patients that were left on 325 mg, 1 had an event, causing a 50% decline in the Kaplan-Meier curves

In additional analyses, RYTHMOL SR (225 mg twice daily, 325 mg twice daily, and 425 mg twice daily) was also shown to prolong time to the first recurrence of symptomatic atrial fibrillation from Day 5 (steady-state pharmacokinetics were attained). The antiarrhythmic effect of RYTHMOL SR was not influenced by age, gender, history of cardioversion, duration of atrial fibrillation, frequency of atrial fibrillation, or use of medication that lowers heart rate. Similarly, the antiarrhythmic effect of RYTHMOL SR was not influenced by the individual use of calcium channel blockers, beta-blockers, or digoxin. Too few non-white patients were enrolled to assess the influence of race on effects of RYTHMOL SR.

No difference in the average heart rate during the first recurrence of symptomatic arrhythmia between RYTHMOL SR and placebo was observed.

ERAFT: In a European multicenter trial [European Rythmonorm SR Atrial Fibrillation Trial (ERAFT)], 2 doses of RYTHMOL SR (325 mg twice daily and 425 mg twice daily) and placebo were compared in 293 patients. The patient population in this trial was 61% male, 100% white with a mean age of 61 years. Patients had a median duration of atrial fibrillation of 3.3 years, and 61% were taking medications that lowered heart rate. At baseline, 15% of the patients were treated with calcium channel blockers (verapamil and diltiazem), 42% with beta-blockers and 8% with digoxin. During a qualifying period of up to 28 days, patients had to have one ECG-documented incident of symptomatic atrial fibrillation. The double-blind treatment phase consisted of a 4-day loading period followed by a 91-day efficacy period. Symptomatic arrhythmias were documented by electrocardiogram monitoring.

In ERAFT, RYTHMOL SR was shown to prolong the time to the first recurrence of symptomatic atrial arrhythmia from Day 5 of randomization (primary efficacy analysis). The proportional hazard analysis revealed that both RYTHMOL SR doses were superior to placebo. The antiarrhythmic effect of propafenone SR was not influenced by age, gender, duration of atrial fibrillation, frequency of atrial fibrillation, or use of medication that lowers heart rate. It was also not influenced by the individual use of calcium channel blockers, beta-blockers, or digoxin. Too few non-white patients were enrolled to assess the influence of race on the effects of RYTHMOL SR. There was a slight increase in the incidence of centrally diagnosed asymptomatic atrial fibrillation or atrial flutter in each of the 2 groups treated with RYTHMOL SR compared to placebo.

INDICATIONS AND USAGE

RYTHMOL SR is indicated to prolong the time to recurrence of symptomatic atrial fibrillation in patients without structural heart disease.

The use of RYTHMOL SR in patients with permanent atrial fibrillation or in patients exclusively with atrial flutter or PSVT has not been evaluated. RYTHMOL SR should not be used to control ventricular rate during atrial fibrillation.

The effect of RYTHMOL SR on mortality has not been determined (see black box WARNINGS).

CONTRAINDICATIONS

RYTHMOL SR is contraindicated in the presence of congestive heart failure, cardiogenic shock, sinoatrial, atrioventricular, and intraventricular disorders of impulse generation or conduction (e.g., sick sinus node syndrome, atrioventricular block) in the absence of an artificial pacemaker, bradycardia, marked hypotension, bronchospastic disorders, electrolyte imbalance, or hypersensitivity to the drug.

WARNINGS

Mortality:

In the National Heart, Lung and Blood Institute's Cardiac Arrhythmia Suppression Trial (CAST), a long-term, multi-center, randomized, double-blind study in patients with asymptomatic non-life-threatening ventricular arrhythmias who had a myocardial infarction more than 6 days but less than 2 years previously, an increased rate of death or reversed cardiac arrest rate (7.7%; 56/730) was seen in patients treated with encainide or flecainide (Class 1C antiarrhythmics) compared with that seen in patients assigned to placebo (3.0%; 22/725). The average duration of treatment with encainide or flecainide in this study was 10 months.

The applicability of the CAST results to other populations (e.g., those without recent myocardial infarction) or other antiarrhythmic drugs is uncertain, but at present, it is prudent to consider any 1C antiarrhythmic to have a significant risk in patients with structural heart disease. Given the lack of any evidence that these drugs improve survival, antiarrhythmic agents should generally be avoided in patients with non-life-threatening ventricular arrhythmias, even if the patients are experiencing unpleasant, but not life-threatening, symptoms or signs.

Proarrhythmic Effects: Propafenone has caused new or worsened arrhythmias. Such proarrhythmic effects include sudden death and life-threatening ventricular arrhythmias such as ventricular fibrillation, ventricular tachycardia, asystole and torsade de pointes. It may also worsen premature ventricular contractions or supraventricular arrhythmias, and it may prolong the QT interval. It is therefore essential that each patient given RYTHMOL SR be evaluated electrocardiographically prior to and during therapy, to determine whether the response to RYTHMOL SR supports continued treatment. Because propafenone prolongs the QRS interval in the electrocardiogram, changes in the QT interval are difficult to interpret.

In a 474 patient US uncontrolled, open-label multicenter trial using the immediate-release formulation in patients with symptomatic SVT, 1.9% (9/474) of these patients experienced ventricular tachycardia (VT) or ventricular fibrillation (VF) during the study. However, in 4 of the 9 patients, the ventricular tachycardia was of atrial origin: Six of the 9 patients that developed ventricular arrhythmias did so within 14 days of onset of therapy. About 2.3% (11/474) of all patients had recurrence of SVT during the study which could have been a change in the patients' arrhythmia behavior or could represent a proarrhythmic event. Case reports in patients treated with RYTHMOL for atrial fibrillation/flutter have included increased PVCs, VT, VF, torsade de pointes, asystole, and death.

In the RAFT study, there were 5 deaths, 3 in the pooled RYTHMOL SR group (0.8%) and 2 in the placebo group (1.6%). In the overall RYTHMOL SR and RYTHMOL immediate-release database of 8 studies, the mortality rate was 2.5% per year on RYTHMOL and 4.0% per year on placebo. Concurrent use of propafenone with other antiarrhythmic agents has not been well studied.

Use With Drugs That Prolong the QT Interval and Antiarrhythmic Agents: The use of RYTHMOL SR in conjunction with other drugs that prolong the QT interval has not been extensively studied and is not recommended. Such drugs may include many antiarrhythmics, some phenothiazines, cisapride, bepridil, tricyclic antidepressants, and oral macrolides. Class Ia and III antiarrhythmic agents should be withheld for at least 5 half-lives prior to dosing with RYTHMOL SR. The use of propafenone with Class Ia and III antiarrhythmic agents (including quinidine and amiodarone) is not recommended. There is only limited experience with the concomitant use of Class Ib or Ic antiarrhythmics.

Nonallergic Bronchospasm (e.g., Chronic Bronchitis, Emphysema): Patients with bronchospastic disease should not, in general, receive propafenone or other agents with beta-adrenergic-blocking activity.

Congestive Heart Failure: Propafenone exerts a negative inotropic activity on the myocardium as well as beta-blockade effects and may provoke overt congestive heart failure. In the US trial (RAFT) in patients with symptomatic atrial fibrillation, congestive heart failure was reported in four (1.0%) patients receiving RYTHMOL SR (all doses), compared to one (0.8%) patient receiving placebo. Proarrhythmic effects are more likely to occur when propafenone is administered to patients with congestive heart failure (NYHA III and IV) or severe myocardial ischemia (see CONTRAINDICATIONS).

Conduction Disturbances: Propafenone causes dose-related first-degree AV block. Average PR interval prolongation and increases in QRS duration are also dose-related. Propafenone should not be given to patients with atrioventricular and intraventricular conduction defects in the absence of a pacemaker (see CONTRAINDICATIONS).

In a US trial (RAFT) in 523 patients with a history of symptomatic atrial fibrillation treated with RYTHMOL SR, electrocardiograms obtained in response to symptoms were associated with no patients having sinus rhythm with Mobitz Type I (Wenckebach) second degree AV block, sinus rhythm with Mobitz Type II second degree AV block, or third degree AV block. Sinus bradycardia (rate <50 beats/min) was reported with the same frequency with RYTHMOL SR and placebo.

Effects on Pacemaker Threshold: Propafenone may alter both pacing and sensing thresholds of artificial pacemakers. Pacemakers should be monitored and programmed accordingly during therapy.

Hematologic Disturbances: Agranulocytosis (fever, chills, weakness, and neutropenia) has been reported in patients receiving propafenone. Generally, the agranulocytosis occurred within the first 2 months of propafenone therapy and upon discontinuation of therapy, the white count usually normalized by 14 days. Unexplained fever and/or decrease in white cell count, particularly during the initial 3 months of therapy, warrant consideration of possible agranulocytosis or granulocytopenia. Patients should be instructed to report promptly the development of any signs of infection such as fever, sore throat, or chills.

PRECAUTIONS

Hepatic Dysfunction: Propafenone is highly metabolized by the liver and should, therefore, be administered cautiously to patients with impaired hepatic function. Severe liver dysfunction increases the bioavailability of propafenone to approximately 70% compared to 3 to 40% in patients with normal liver function when given RYTHMOL immediate-release tablets. In 8 patients with moderate to severe liver disease administered RYTHMOL immediate-release tablets, the mean half-life was approximately 9 hours. No studies are currently available comparing bioavailability of propafenone from RYTHMOL SR in patients with normal and impaired hepatic function. Increased bioavailability of propafenone in these patients may result in excessive accumulation. Careful monitoring for excessive pharmacological effects (see OVERDOSAGE) should be performed for patients with impaired hepatic function.

Renal Dysfunction: Approximately 50% of propafenone metabolites are excreted in the urine following administration of RYTHMOL immediate-release tablets. No studies have been performed to assess the percentage of metabolites eliminated in the urine following the administration of RYTHMOL SR capsules.

Until further data are available, RYTHMOL SR should be administered cautiously to patients with impaired renal function. These patients should be carefully monitored for signs of overdosage (see OVERDOSAGE).

Information for Patients: *Medications and Supplements:* Assessment of patients' medication history should include all over-the-counter, prescription, and herbal/natural preparations with emphasis on preparations that may affect the pharmacodynamics or kinetics of RYTHMOL SR (see WARNINGS, Use With Drugs That Prolong QT Interval and Antiarrhythmic Agents). Patients should be instructed to notify their healthcare providers of any change in over-the-counter, prescription, and supplement use. If a patient is hospitalized, or is prescribed new medication for any condition, the patient must inform the healthcare provider of ongoing therapy with RYTHMOL SR. Patients should also check with their healthcare providers prior to taking a new over-the-counter medicine.

Electrolyte Imbalance: If patients experience symptoms that may be associated with altered electrolyte balance, such as excessive or prolonged diarrhea, sweating, vomiting, or loss of appetite or thirst, these conditions should be immediately reported to their healthcare provider.

Dosing Schedule: Patients should be instructed NOT to double the next dose if a dose is missed. The next dose should be taken at the usual time.

Elevated ANA Titers: Positive ANA titers have been reported in patients receiving propafenone. They have been reversible upon cessation of treatment and may disappear even in the face of continued propafenone therapy. These laboratory findings were usually not associated with clinical symptoms, but there is one published case of drug-induced lupus erythematosus (positive rechallenge); it resolved completely upon discontinuation of therapy. Patients who develop an abnormal ANA test should be carefully evaluated and, if persistent or worsening elevation of ANA titers is detected, consideration should be given to discontinuing therapy.

Impaired Spermatogenesis: Reversible disorders of spermatogenesis have been demonstrated in monkeys, dogs, and rabbits after high-dose intravenous administration of propafenone. Evaluation of the effects of short-term administration of propafenone on spermatogenesis in 11 normal subjects suggested that propafenone produced a reversible, short-term drop (within normal range) in sperm count. Subsequent evaluations in 11 patients receiving RYTHMOL chronically have found no effect of propafenone on sperm count.

Neuromuscular Dysfunction: Exacerbation of myasthenia gravis has been reported during therapy with RYTHMOL immediate-release tablets.

Drug Interactions: Propafenone is metabolized by CYP2D6 (major pathway) and CYP1A2 and CYP3A4. Drugs that inhibit CYP2D6 (such as desipramine, paroxetine, ritonavir, sertraline), CYP1A2 (such as amiodarone), and CYP3A4 (such as ketaconazole, ritonavir, saquinavir, erythromycin, and grapefruit juice) can be expected to cause increased plasma levels of propafenone. Appropriate monitoring is recommended when RYTHMOL SR is used together with such drugs. In addition, propafenone is an inhibitor of CYP2D6. Coadministration of propafenone with drugs metabolized by CYP2D6 (such as desipramine, imipramine, haloperidol, venlafaxine) might lead to increased plasma concentrations of these drugs. The effect of propafenone on the P-Glycoprotein transporter has not been studied.

Quinidine: Small doses of quinidine completely inhibit the CYP2D6 hydroxylation metabolic pathway, making all patients, in effect, slow metabolizers (see CLINICAL PHARMACOLOGY). Concomitant administration of quinidine (50 mg three times daily) with 150 mg immediate-release propafenone three times daily decreased the clearance of propafenone by 60% in extensive metabolizers, making them poor metabolizers. Steady-state plasma concentrations increased by more than 2-fold for propafenone, and decreased 50% for 5-OH-propafenone. A 100-mg dose of quinidine increased steady state concentrations of propafenone 3-fold. Concomitant use of propafenone and quinidine is not recommended.

Digoxin: Concomitant use of propafenone and digoxin increased steady-state serum digoxin exposure (AUC) in patients by 60 to 270%, and decreased the clearance of digoxin by 31 to 67%. Plasma digoxin levels of patients receiving propafenone should be monitored and digoxin dosage adjusted as needed.

Lidocaine: No significant effects on the pharmacokinetics of propafenone or lidocaine have been seen following their concomitant use in patients. However, concomitant use of propafenone and lidocaine has been reported to increase the risks of central nervous system side effects of lidocaine.

Beta-Antagonists: Concomitant use of propafenone and propranolol in healthy subjects increased propranolol plasma concentrations at steady state by 113%. In 4 patients, administration of metoprolol with propafenone increased the metoprolol plasma concentrations at steady state by 100 to 400%. The pharmacokinetics of propafenone was not affected by the coadministration of either propranolol or metoprolol. In clinical trials using propafenone immediate-release tablets, patients who were receiving beta-blockers concurrently did not experience an increased incidence of side effects.

Warfarin: The concomitant administration of propafenone and warfarin increased warfarin plasma concentrations at steady state by 39% in healthy volunteers and prolonged the prothrombin time in patients taking warfarin. Adjustment of the warfarin dose should be guided by monitoring of the prothrombin time.

Cimetidine: Concomitant administration of propafenone immediate-release tablets and cimetidine in 12 healthy subjects resulted in a 20% increase in steady-state plasma concentrations of propafenone.

Rifampin: Concomitant administration of rifampin and propafenone in extensive metabolizers decreased the plasma concentrations of propafenone by 67% with a corresponding decrease of 5OH-propafenone by 65%. The concentrations of norpropafenone increased by 30%. In poor metabolizers, there was a 50% decrease in propafenone plasma concentrations and an increase in AUC and C_{max} of norpropafenone by 74 and 20%, respectively. Urinary excretion of propafenone and its metabolites decreased significantly. Similar results were noted in elderly patients: Both

Table 2: Most Common Adverse Events (≥2.0% in any RAFT Propafenone SR Treatment Group and More Common on Propafenone Than on Placebo)

MedDRA Body System/Preferred Term	RYTHMOL SR			
	225 mg twice daily (N = 126) n (%)	325 mg twice daily (N = 135) n (%)	425 mg twice daily (N = 136) n (%)	Placebo (N = 126) n (%)
Mean exposure (days)	124	149	141	91
Cardiac disorders				
Angina pectoris	0 (0)	0 (0)	3 (2)	0 (0)
Atrial flutter	3 (2)	2 (1)	0 (0)	1 (1)
AV block first degree	3 (2)	3 (2)	4 (3)	0 (0)
Bradycardia	4 (3)	4 (3)	6 (4)	1 (1)
Cardiac failure congestive	0 (0)	1 (1)	3 (2)	1 (1)
Cardiac murmur	2 (2)	3 (2)	6 (4)	0 (0)
Edema	6 (5)	18 (13)	10 (7)	8 (6)
Eye disorders				
Vision blurred	1 (1)	1 (1)	5 (4)	0 (0)
Gastrointestinal disorders				
Constipation	10 (8)	19 (14)	16 (12)	3 (2)
Diarrhea	2 (2)	3 (2)	5 (4)	3 (2)
Dry mouth	1 (1)	1 (1)	5 (4)	1 (1)
Flatulence	3 (2)	3 (2)	1 (1)	0 (0)
Nausea	11 (9)	15 (11)	23 (17)	11 (9)
Vomiting	1 (1)	0 (0)	8 (6)	3 (2)
General disorder and administration site				
Fatigue	14 (11)	17 (13)	17 (13)	7 (6)
Weakness	4 (3)	6 (4)	6 (4)	3 (2)
Infections and infestations				
Upper respiratory tract infection	11 (9)	16 (12)	11 (8)	7 (6)
Investigations				
Blood alkaline phosphatase increased	0 (0)	0 (0)	4 (3)	0 (0)
Cardioactive drug level above therapeutic	1 (1)	1 (1)	3 (2)	1 (1)
Hematuria	2 (2)	2 (1)	4 (3)	3 (2)
Musculoskeletal, connective tissue and bone				
Muscle weakness	1 (1)	5 (4)	1 (1)	0 (0)
Nervous system disorders				
Dizziness (excluding vertigo)	29 (23)	28 (21)	29 (21)	18 (14)
Headache	8 (6)	12 (9)	14 (10)	11 (9)
Taste disturbance	7 (6)	18 (13)	30 (22)	1 (1)
Tremor	2 (2)	0 (0)	3 (2)	1 (1)
Somnolence	1 (1)	1 (1)	4 (3)	0 (0)
Psychiatric disorders				
Anxiety	12 (10)	17 (13)	16 (12)	13 (10)
Depression	1 (1)	4 (3)	0 (0)	2 (2)
Respiratory, thoracic and mediastinal disorder				
Dyspnea	16 (13)	23 (17)	17 (13)	9 (7)
Rales	2 (2)	1 (1)	3 (2)	0 (0)
Wheezing	0 (0)	0 (0)	3 (2)	0 (0)
Skin & subcutaneous tissue disorders				
Ecchymosis	2 (2)	3 (2)	5 (4)	0 (0)

the AUC and C_{max} of propafenone decreased by 84%, with a corresponding decrease in AUC and C_{max} of 5OH-propafenone by 69 and 57%.

Fluoxetine: Concomitant administration of propafenone and fluoxetine in extensive metabolizers increased the S-propafenone C_{max} and AUC by 39 and 50% and the R-propafenone C_{max} and AUC by 71 and 50%, respectively.

Amiodarone: Concomitant administration of propafenone and amiodarone can affect conduction and repolarization and is not recommended.

Postmarketing Reports: Orlistat may limit the fraction of propafenone available for absorption. In postmarketing reports, abrupt cessation of orlistat in patients stabilized on propafenone has resulted in severe adverse events including convulsions, atrioventricular block, and acute circulatory failure.

Renal and Hepatic Toxicity in Animals: Renal changes have been observed in the rat following 6 months of oral administration of propafenone HCl at doses of 180 and 360 mg/kg/day (about 2 and 4 times, respectively, the maximum recommended human daily dose [MRHD] on a mg/m² basis). Both inflammatory and non-inflammatory changes in the renal tubules, with accompanying interstitial nephritis, were observed. These changes were reversible, as they were not found in rats allowed to recover for 6 weeks. Fatty degenerative changes of the liver were found in rats following longer durations of administration of propafenone HCl at a dose of 270 mg/kg/day (about 3 times the MRHD on a mg/m² basis). There were no renal or hepatic changes at 90 mg/kg/day (equivalent to the MRHD on a mg/m² basis).

Carcinogenesis, Mutagenesis, Impairment of Fertility: Lifetime maximally tolerated oral dose studies in mice (up to 360 mg/kg/day, about twice the maximum recommended human oral daily dose [MRHD] on a mg/m² basis) and rats (up to 270 mg/kg/day, about 3 times the MRHD on a mg/m² basis) provided no evidence of a carcinogenic potential for propafenone HCl.

Propafenone HCl tested negative for mutagenicity in the Ames (salmonella) test and in the in vivo mouse dominant lethal test. It tested negative for clastogenicity in the human lymphocyte chromosome aberration assay in vitro and in rat and Chinese hamster micronucleus tests, and other *in vivo* tests for chromosomal aberrations in rat bone marrow and Chinese hamster bone marrow and spermatogonia.

Propafenone HCl, administered intravenously to rabbits, dogs, and monkeys, has been shown to decrease spermatogenesis. These effects were reversible, were not found following oral dosing of propafenone HCl, were seen at lethal or near lethal dose levels and were not seen in rats treated either orally or intravenously (see PRECAUTIONS, Impaired Spermatogenesis). Treatment of male rabbits for 10 weeks prior to mating at an oral dose of 120 mg/kg/day (about 2.4 times the MRHD on a mg/m² basis) or an intravenous dose of 3.5 mg/kg/day (a spermatogenesis-impairing dose) did not result in evidence of impaired fertility. Nor was there evidence of impaired fertility when propafenone HCl was administered orally to male and female rats at dose levels up to 270 mg/kg/day (about 3 times the MRHD on a mg/m² basis).

Pregnancy: *Teratogenic Effects:* *Pregnancy Category C.* Propafenone HCl has been shown to be embryotoxic (decreased survival) in rabbits and rats when given in oral maternally toxic doses of 150 mg/kg/day (about 3 times the maximum recommended human dose [MRHD] on a mg/m² basis) and 600 mg/kg/day (about 6 times the MRHD on a mg/m² basis), respectively. Although maternally tolerated doses (up to 270 mg/kg/day, about 3 times the MRHD on a mg/m² basis) produced no evidence of embryotoxicity in rats, post-implantation loss was elevated in all rabbit treatment groups (doses as low as 15 mg/kg/day, about 1/3 the MRHD on a mg/m² basis). There are no adequate and well-controlled studies in pregnant women. RYTHMOL SR should be used during pregnancy only if the potential benefit justifies the potential risk to the fetus.

Non-teratogenic Effects: In a study in which female rats received daily oral doses of propafenone HCl from midgestation through weaning of their offspring, doses as low as 90 mg/kg/day (equivalent to the MRHD on a mg/m² basis) produced increases in maternal deaths. Doses of 360 or more mg/kg/day (4 or more times the MRHD on a mg/m² basis) resulted in reductions in neonatal survival, body weight gain, and physiological development.

Labor and Delivery: It is not known whether the use of propafenone during labor or delivery has immediate or delayed adverse effects on the fetus, or whether it prolongs the duration of labor or increases the need for forceps delivery or other obstetrical intervention.

Nursing Mothers: Propafenone is excreted in human milk. Caution should be exercised when RYTHMOL SR is administered to a nursing mother.

Pediatric Use: The safety and effectiveness of propafenone in pediatric patients have not been established.

Geriatric Use: Of the total number of subjects in Phase III clinical studies of RYTHMOL SR 45.7 percent were 65 and older, while 15.7 percent were 75 and older. No overall differences in safety or effectiveness were observed between these subjects and younger subjects, but greater sensitivity of some older individuals at higher doses cannot be ruled out. The effect of age on the pharmacokinetics and pharmacodynamics of propafenone has not been studied.

ADVERSE REACTIONS

The data described below reflect exposure to RYTHMOL SR 225 mg twice daily in 126 patients, to RYTHMOL SR 325 mg twice daily in 135 patients, to RYTHMOL SR 425 mg twice daily in 136 patients, and to placebo in 126 patients for up to 39 weeks in a placebo-controlled trial (RAFT) conducted in the US. The most commonly reported adverse events in the trial included dizziness, chest pain, palpitations, taste disturbance, dyspnea, nausea, constipation, anxiety, fatigue, upper respiratory tract infection, influenza, first-degree heart block, and vomiting. The frequency of discontinuation due to adverse events was highest during the first 14 days of treatment. The majority of the patients with serious adverse events who withdrew or were discontinued recovered without sequelae.

Adverse events occurring in 2% or more of the patients in any of the RAFT propafenone SR treatment groups and more common with propafenone than with placebo, excluding those that are common in the population and those not plausibly related to drug therapy, are listed in Table 2.

[See table 2 at top of previous page]

No clinically important differences in incidence of adverse reactions were noted by age, or gender. Too few non-white patients were enrolled to assess adverse events according to race. Adverse events occurring in 2% or more of the patients in any of the ERAFT propafenone SR treatment groups and not listed in Table 2 include the following: bundle branch block left, bundle branch block right, conduction disorders, sinus bradycardia, and hypotension.

Other adverse events reported with propafenone clinical trials not already listed in Table 2 include the following adverse events by body and preferred term.

Blood and Lymphatic System Disorders: Anemia, lymphadenopathy, spleen disorder, thrombocytopenia.

Cardiac Disorders: Angina unstable, arrhythmia, atrial hypertrophy, atrioventricular block, bundle branch block, bunch branch block left, bundle branch block right, cardiac arrest, cardiac disorder, conduction disorder, coronary artery disease, extrasystoles, myocardial infarction, nodal arrhythmia, palpitations, pericarditis, sinoatrial block, sinus arrest, sinus arrhythmia, sinus bradycardia, supraventricular extrasystoles, supraventricular tachycardia, ventricular arrhythmia, ventricular extrasystoles, ventricular hypertrophy.

Ear and Labyrinth Disorders: Hearing impaired, tinnitus, vertigo.

Eye Disorders: Eye hemorrhage, eye inflammation, eyelid ptosis, miosis, retinal disorder, visual acuity reduced.

Gastrointestinal Disorders: Abdominal distension, abdominal pain, dry throat, duodenitis, dyspepsia, dysphagia, eructation, gastritis, gastroesophageal reflux disease, gingival bleeding, glossitis, glossodynia, gum pain, halitosis, intestinal obstruction, melena, mouth ulceration, pancreatitis, peptic ulcer, rectal bleeding, sore throat.

General Disorders and Administration Site Conditions: Chest pain, feeling hot, hemorrhage, malaise, pain, pyrexia.

Hepatobiliary Disorders: Hepatomegaly.

Investigations: Abnormal electrocardiogram, abnormal heart sounds, abnormal liver function tests, abnormal pulse, carotid bruit, decreased blood chloride, decreased blood pressure, decreased blood sodium, decreased hemoglobin, decreased neutrophil count, decreased platelet count, decreased prothrombin level, decreased red blood cell count, decreased weight, electrocardiogram QT prolonged, glycosuria present, heart rate irregular, increased alanine aminotransferase, increased aspartate aminotransferase, increased blood bilirubin, increased blood cholesterol, increased blood creatinine, increased blood glucose, increased blood lactate dehydrogenase, increased blood pressure, increased blood prolactin, increased blood triglycerides, increased blood urea, increased blood uric acid, increased eosinophil count, increased gamma-glutamyltransferase, increased monocyte count, increased prostatic specific antigen, increased prothrombin level, increased weight, increased white blood cell count, ketonuria present, proteinuria present.

Metabolism and Nutrition Disorders: Anorexia, dehydration, diabetes mellitus, gout, hypercholesterolemia, hyperglycemia, hyperlipidemia, hypokalemia.

Musculoskeletal, Connective Tissue and Bone Disorders: Arthritis, bursitis, collagen-vascular disease, costochondritis, joint disorder, muscle cramps, muscle spasms, myalgia, neck pain, pain in jaw, sciatica, tendonitis.

Nervous System Disorders: Amnesia, ataxia, balance impaired, brain damage, cerebrovascular accident, dementia,

gait abnormal, hypertonia, hypothesia, insomnia, paralysis, paresthesia, peripheral neuropathy, speech disorder, syncope, tongue hypoesthesia.

Psychiatric Disorders: Decreased libido, emotional disturbance, mental disorder, neurosis, nightmare, sleep disorder.

Renal and Urinary Disorders: Dysuria, nocturia, oliguria, pyuria, renal failure, urinary casts, urinary frequency, urinary incontinence, urinary retention, urine abnormal.

Reproductive System and Breast Disorders: Breast pain, impotence, prostatism.

Respiratory, Thoracic and Mediastinal Disorders Disorders: Atelectasis, breath sounds decreased, chronic obstructive airways disease, cough, epistaxis, hemoptysis, lung disorder, pleural effusion, pulmonary congestion, rales, respiratory failure, rhinitis, throat tightness.

Skin and Subcutaneous Tissue Disorders: Alopecia, dermatitis, dry skin, erythema, nail abnormality, petechiae, pruritis, sweating increased, urticaria.

Vascular Disorders: Arterial embolism limb, deep limb venous thrombosis, flushing, hematoma, hypertension, hypertensive crisis, hypotension, labile blood pressure, pallor, peripheral coldness, peripheral vascular disease, thrombosis.

Laboratory: *Electrocardiograms:* Propafenone prolongs the PR and QRS intervals in patients with atrial and ventricular arrythmias. Prolongation of the QRS interval makes it difficult to interpret the effect of propafenone on the QT interval.

Table 3: Mean Change in 12-Lead Electrocardiogram Results (RAFT)

	RYTHMOL SR twice-daily dosing			
	225 mg	325 mg	425 mg	Placebo
	n = 126	n = 135	n = 136	n = 126
PR (ms)	9±22	12±23	21±24	1±16
QRS (ms)	4±14	6±15	6±15	-2±12
QTc* (ms)	2±30	5±36	6±37	5±35

*Calculated using Bazett's correction factor

In RAFT, the distribution of the maximum changes in QTc compared to baseline over the study in each patient was similar in the RYTHMOL SR 225 mg twice daily, 325 mg twice daily, and 425 mg twice daily and placebo dose groups. Similar results were seen in the ERAFT study.

[See table 4 above]

OVERDOSAGE

The symptoms of overdosage may include hypotension, somnolence, bradycardia, intra-atrial and intraventricular conduction disturbances, and rarely convulsions and high grade ventricular arrhythmias. Defibrillation as well as infusion of dopamine and isoproterenol have been effective in controlling abnormal ventricular rhythm and blood pressure. Convulsions have been alleviated with intravenous diazepam. General supportive measures such as mechanical respiratory assistance and external cardiac massage may be necessary.

The hemodialysis of propafenone in patients with an overdose is expected to be of limited value in the removal of propafenone as a result of both its high protein binding (>95%) and large volume of distribution.

DOSAGE AND ADMINISTRATION

The dose of RYTHMOL SR must be individually titrated on the basis of response and tolerance. Therapy should be initiated with RYTHMOL SR 225 mg given every 12 hours. Dosage may be increased at a minimum of 5-day interval to 325 mg given every 12 hours. If additional therapeutic effect is needed, the dose of RYTHMOL SR may be increased to 425 mg given every 12 hours.

Table 4: Number of Patients According to the Range of Maximum QTc Change Compared to Baseline Over the Study in Each Dose Group (RAFT Study)

Range of maximum QTc change	RYTHMOL SR			Placebo
	225 mg twice daily	325 mg twice daily	425 mg twice daily	
	N = 119	N = 129	N = 123	N = 120
	n (%)	n (%)	n (%)	n (%)
>20%	1 (1%)	6 (5%)	3 (2%)	5 (4%)
10-20%	19 (16%)	28 (22%)	32 (26%)	24 (20%)
≤10%	99 (83%)	95 (74%)	88 (72%)	91 (76%)

In patients with hepatic impairment or having significant widening of the QRS complex or second or third degree AV block, dose reduction should be considered.

RYTHMOL SR can be taken with or without food. Do not crush or further divide the contents of the capsule.

HOW SUPPLIED

RYTHMOL® SR (propafenone HCl) capsules are supplied as white, opaque, hard-gelatin capsules containing either 225 mg, 325 mg, or 425 mg of propafenone HCl and imprinted in red with ⓡReliant and strength. The 325-mg strength is also imprinted with a single red band around ¾ of the circumference of the body; the 425-mg strength is imprinted with three bands around ¾ of the circumference of the body.

Capsule Strength	60 count bottle NDC
225 mg	0173-0786-01
325 mg	0173-0788-01
425 mg	0173-0789-01

Storage: Store at 25°C (77°F); excursions permitted to 15° to 30°C (59° to 86°F) [see USP Controlled Room Temperature]. Dispense in a tight container as defined in the USP. RYTHMOL is a registered trademark of G. Petrik used under license by Abbott Laboratories.

Manufactured for:
GlaxoSmithKline
Research Triangle Park, NC 27709
Manufactured by:
Abbott Laboratories
North Chicago, IL 60064
©2008 GlaxoSmithKline. All rights reserved.
November 2008 RMS:2PI

SEREVENT® DISKUS® ℞
[ser' ə-vent disk' us]
(salmeterol xinafoate inhalation powder)
For Oral Inhalation Only

> **WARNING: ASTHMA-RELATED DEATH**
> Long-acting beta₂-adrenergic agonists (LABAs), such as salmeterol, the active ingredient in SEREVENT DISKUS, increase the risk of asthma-related death. Data from a large placebo-controlled US study that compared the safety of salmeterol (SEREVENT® Inhalation Aerosol) or placebo added to usual asthma therapy showed an increase in asthma-related deaths in patients receiving salmeterol (13 deaths out of 13,176 patients treated for 28 weeks on salmeterol versus 3 deaths out of 13,179 patients on placebo) (see WARNINGS and CLINICAL TRIALS: Asthma: *Salmeterol Multi-center Asthma Research Trial*). Currently available data are inadequate to determine whether concurrent use of inhaled corticosteroids or other long-term asthma control drugs mitigates the increased risk of asthma-related death from LABAs.
> Because of this risk, use of SEREVENT DISKUS for the treatment of asthma without a concomitant long-term asthma control medication, such as an inhaled corticosteroid, is contraindicated. Use SEREVENT DISKUS only as additional therapy for patients with asthma who are currently taking but are inadequately controlled on a long-term asthma control medication, such as an inhaled corticosteroid. Once asthma control is achieved and maintained, assess the patient at regular intervals and step down therapy (e.g., discontinue SEREVENT DISKUS) if possible without loss of asthma control and maintain the patient on a long-term asthma control medication, such as an inhaled cortico-

steroid. Do not use SEREVENT DISKUS for patients whose asthma is adequately controlled on low- or medium-dose inhaled corticosteroids.

Pediatric and Adolescent Patients: Available data from controlled clinical trials suggest that LABAs increase the risk of asthma-related hospitalization in pediatric and adolescent patients. For pediatric and adolescent patients with asthma who require addition of a LABA to an inhaled corticosteroid, a fixed-dose combination product containing both an inhaled corticosteroid and a LABA should ordinarily be used to ensure adherence with both drugs. In cases where use of a separate long-term asthma control medication (e.g., inhaled corticosteroid) and a LABA is clinically indicated, appropriate steps must be taken to ensure adherence with both treatment components. If adherence cannot be assured, a fixed-dose combination product containing both an inhaled corticosteroid and a LABA is recommended.

DESCRIPTION

SEREVENT DISKUS (salmeterol xinafoate inhalation powder) contains salmeterol xinafoate as the racemic form of the 1-hydroxy-2-naphthoic acid salt of salmeterol. The active component of the formulation is salmeterol base, a highly selective beta$_2$-adrenergic bronchodilator. The chemical name of salmeterol xinafoate is 4-hydroxy-α^1-[[[6-(4-phenylbutoxy)hexyl]amino]methyl]-1,3-benzenedimethanol, 1-hydroxy-2-naphthalenecarboxylate. Salmeterol xinafoate has the following chemical structure:

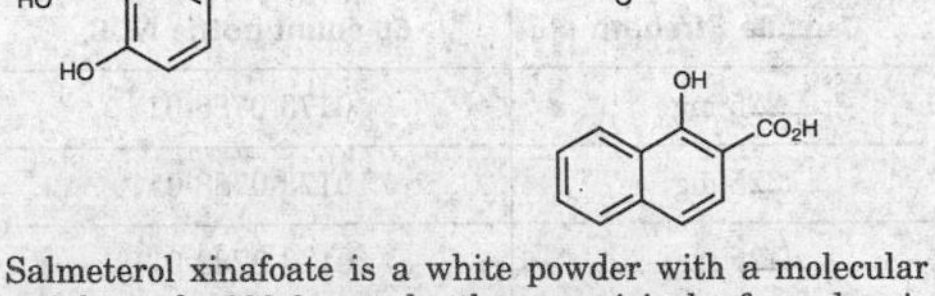

Salmeterol xinafoate is a white powder with a molecular weight of 603.8, and the empirical formula is $C_{25}H_{37}NO_4 \bullet C_{11}H_8O_3$. It is freely soluble in methanol; slightly soluble in ethanol, chloroform, and isopropanol; and sparingly soluble in water.

SEREVENT DISKUS is a specially designed plastic inhalation delivery system containing a double-foil blister strip of a powder formulation of salmeterol xinafoate intended for oral inhalation only. The DISKUS®, which is the delivery component, is an integral part of the drug product. Each blister on the double-foil strip within the unit contains 50 mcg of salmeterol administered as the salmeterol xinafoate salt in 12.5 mg of formulation containing lactose (which contains milk proteins). After a blister containing medication is opened by activating the DISKUS, the medication is dispersed into the airstream created by the patient inhaling through the mouthpiece.

Under standardized in vitro test conditions, SEREVENT DISKUS delivers 47 mcg when tested at a flow rate of 60 L/min for 2 seconds. In adult patients with obstructive lung disease and severely compromised lung function (mean forced expiratory volume in 1 second [FEV$_1$] 20% to 30% of predicted), mean peak inspiratory flow (PIF) through a DISKUS was 82.4 L/min (range, 46.1 to 115.3 L/min).

The actual amount of drug delivered to the lung will depend on patient factors, such as inspiratory flow profile.

CLINICAL PHARMACOLOGY

Mechanism of Action

Salmeterol is a long-acting beta$_2$-adrenergic agonist (LABA). In vitro studies and in vivo pharmacologic studies demonstrate that salmeterol is selective for beta$_2$-adrenoceptors compared with isoproterenol, which has approximately equal agonist activity on beta$_1$- and beta$_2$-adrenoceptors. In vitro studies show salmeterol to be at least 50 times more selective for beta$_2$-adrenoceptors than albuterol. Although beta$_2$-adrenoceptors are the predominant adrenergic receptors in bronchial smooth muscle and beta$_1$-adrenoceptors are the predominant receptors in the heart, there are also beta$_2$-adrenoceptors in the human heart comprising 10% to 50% of the total beta-adrenoceptors. The precise function of these receptors has not been established, but they raise the possibility that even highly selective beta$_2$-agonists may have cardiac effects.

The pharmacologic effects of beta$_2$-adrenoceptor agonist drugs, including salmeterol, are at least in part attributable to stimulation of intracellular adenyl cyclase, the enzyme that catalyzes the conversion of adenosine triphosphate (ATP) to cyclic-3',5'-adenosine monophosphate (cyclic AMP). Increased cyclic AMP levels cause relaxation of bronchial smooth muscle and inhibition of release of mediators of immediate hypersensitivity from cells, especially from mast cells.

In vitro tests show that salmeterol is a potent and long-lasting inhibitor of the release of mast cell mediators, such as histamine, leukotrienes, and prostaglandin D_2, from human lung. Salmeterol inhibits histamine-induced plasma protein extravasation and inhibits platelet-activating factor–induced eosinophil accumulation in the lungs of guinea pigs when administered by the inhaled route. In humans, single doses of salmeterol administered via inhalation aerosol attenuate allergen-induced bronchial hyper-responsiveness.

Pharmacokinetics

Salmeterol xinafoate, an ionic salt, dissociates in solution so that the salmeterol and 1-hydroxy-2-naphthoic acid (xinafoate) moieties are absorbed, distributed, metabolized, and eliminated independently. Salmeterol acts locally in the lung; therefore, plasma levels do not predict therapeutic effect.

Absorption

Because of the small therapeutic dose, systemic levels of salmeterol are low or undetectable after inhalation of recommended doses (50 mcg of salmeterol inhalation powder twice daily). Following chronic administration of an inhaled dose of 50 mcg of salmeterol inhalation powder twice daily, salmeterol was detected in plasma within 5 to 45 minutes in 7 patients with asthma; plasma concentrations were very low, with mean peak concentrations of 167 pg/mL at 20 minutes and no accumulation with repeated doses.

Distribution

The percentage of salmeterol bound to human plasma proteins averages 96% in vitro over the concentration range of 8 to 7,722 ng of salmeterol base per milliliter, much higher concentrations than those achieved following therapeutic doses of salmeterol.

Metabolism

Salmeterol base is extensively metabolized by hydroxylation, with subsequent elimination predominantly in the feces. No significant amount of unchanged salmeterol base has been detected in either urine or feces.

An in vitro study using human liver microsomes showed that salmeterol is extensively metabolized to α-hydroxysalmeterol (aliphatic oxidation) by cytochrome P450 3A4 (CYP3A4). Ketoconazole, a strong inhibitor of CYP3A4, essentially completely inhibited the formation of α-hydroxysalmeterol in vitro.

Elimination

In 2 healthy subjects who received 1 mg of radiolabeled salmeterol (as salmeterol xinafoate) orally, approximately 25% and 60% of the radiolabeled salmeterol was eliminated in urine and feces, respectively, over a period of 7 days. The terminal elimination half-life was about 5.5 hours (1 volunteer only).

The xinafoate moiety has no apparent pharmacologic activity. The xinafoate moiety is highly protein bound (>99%) and has a long elimination half-life of 11 days.

Special Populations

The pharmacokinetics of salmeterol base has not been studied in elderly patients nor in patients with hepatic or renal impairment. Since salmeterol is predominantly cleared by hepatic metabolism, liver function impairment may lead to accumulation of salmeterol in plasma. Therefore, patients with hepatic disease should be closely monitored.

Drug Interactions

Salmeterol is a substrate of CYP3A4.

Inhibitors of Cytochrome P450 3A4

Ketoconazole

In a placebo-controlled, crossover drug interaction study in 20 healthy male and female subjects, coadministration of salmeterol (50 mcg twice daily) and the strong CYP3A4 inhibitor ketoconazole (400 mg once daily) for 7 days resulted in a significant increase in plasma salmeterol exposure as determined by a 16-fold increase in AUC (ratio with and without ketoconazole 15.76; 90% CI: 10.66, 23.31) mainly due to increased bioavailability of the swallowed portion of the dose. Peak plasma salmeterol concentrations were increased by 1.4-fold (90% CI: 1.23, 1.68). Three (3) out of 20 subjects (15%) were withdrawn from salmeterol and ketoconazole coadministration due to beta-agonist–mediated systemic effects (2 with QTc prolongation and 1 with palpitations and sinus tachycardia). Coadministration of salmeterol and ketoconazole did not result in a clinically significant effect on mean heart rate, mean blood potassium, or mean blood glucose. Although there was no statistical effect on the mean QTc, coadministration of salmeterol and ketoconazole was associated with more frequent increases in QTc duration compared with salmeterol and placebo administration. Due to the potential increased risk of cardiovascular adverse events, the concomitant use of salmeterol with strong CYP3A4 inhibitors (e.g., ketoconazole, ritonavir, atazanavir, clarithromycin, indinavir, itraconazole, nefazodone, nelfinavir, saquinavir, telithromycin) is not recommended.

Erythromycin

In a repeat-dose study in 13 healthy subjects, concomitant administration of erythromycin (a moderate CYP3A4 inhibitor) and salmeterol inhalation aerosol resulted in a 40% increase in salmeterol C_{max} at steady state (ratio with and without erythromycin 1.4; 90% CI: 0.96, 2.03; $p = 0.12$), a 3.6-beat/min increase in heart rate (95% CI: 0.19, 7.03; $p<0.04$), a 5.8-msec increase in QTc interval (95% CI: -6.14, 17.77; $p = 0.34$), and no change in plasma potassium.

Pharmacodynamics

Inhaled salmeterol, like other beta-adrenergic agonist drugs, can in some patients produce dose-related cardiovascular effects and effects on blood glucose and/or serum potassium (see PRECAUTIONS: General). The cardiovascular effects (heart rate, blood pressure) associated with salmeterol inhalation aerosol occur with similar frequency, and are of similar type and severity, as those noted following albuterol administration.

The effects of rising doses of salmeterol and standard inhaled doses of albuterol were studied in volunteers and in patients with asthma. Salmeterol doses up to 84 mcg administered as inhalation aerosol resulted in heart rate increases of 3 to 16 beats/min, about the same as albuterol dosed at 180 mcg by inhalation aerosol (4 to 10 beats/min). Adolescent and adult patients receiving 50-mcg doses of salmeterol inhalation powder (N = 60) underwent continuous electrocardiographic monitoring during two 12-hour periods after the first dose and after 1 month of therapy, and no clinically significant dysrhythmias were noted. Also, pediatric patients receiving 50-mcg doses of salmeterol inhalation powder (N = 67) underwent continuous electrocardiographic monitoring during two 12-hour periods after the first dose and after 3 months of therapy, and no clinically significant dysrhythmias were noted.

In 24-week clinical studies in patients with chronic obstructive pulmonary disease (COPD), the incidence of clinically significant abnormalities on the predose electrocardiograms (ECGs) at Weeks 12 and 24 in patients who received salmeterol 50 mcg was not different compared with placebo.

No effect of treatment with salmeterol 50 mcg was observed on pulse rate and systolic and diastolic blood pressure in a subset of patients with COPD who underwent 12-hour serial vital sign measurements after the first dose (N = 91) and after 12 weeks of therapy (N = 74). Median changes from baseline in pulse rate and systolic and diastolic blood pressure were similar for patients receiving either salmeterol or placebo (see ADVERSE REACTIONS).

Studies in laboratory animals (minipigs, rodents, and dogs) have demonstrated the occurrence of cardiac arrhythmias and sudden death (with histologic evidence of myocardial necrosis) when beta-agonists and methylxanthines are administered concurrently. The clinical significance of these findings is unknown.

CLINICAL TRIALS

Asthma

During the initial treatment day in several multiple-dose clinical trials with SEREVENT DISKUS in patients with asthma, the median time to onset of clinically significant bronchodilatation (≥15% improvement in FEV$_1$) ranged from 30 to 48 minutes after a 50-mcg dose.

One hour after a single dose of 50 mcg of SEREVENT DISKUS, the majority of patients had ≥15% improvement in FEV$_1$. Maximum improvement in FEV$_1$ generally occurred within 180 minutes, and clinically significant improvement continued for 12 hours in most patients.

In 2 randomized, double-blind studies, SEREVENT DISKUS was compared with albuterol inhalation aerosol and placebo in adolescent and adult patients with mild-to-moderate asthma (protocol defined as 50% to 80% predicted FEV$_1$, actual mean of 67.7% at baseline), including patients who did and who did not receive concurrent inhaled corticosteroids. The efficacy of SEREVENT DISKUS was demonstrated over the 12-week period with no change in effectiveness over this time period (see Figure 1). There were no gender- or age-related differences in safety or efficacy. No development of tachyphylaxis to the bronchodilator effect was noted in these studies. FEV$_1$ measurements (mean change from baseline) from these two 12-week studies are shown in Figure 1 for both the first and last treatment days.

[See figure 1 at top of next column]

Table 1 shows the treatment effects seen during daily treatment with SEREVENT DISKUS for 12 weeks in adolescent and adult patients with mild-to-moderate asthma.

[See table 1 at top of next page]

Maintenance of efficacy for periods up to 1 year has been documented.

SEREVENT DISKUS and SEREVENT® (salmeterol xinafoate) Inhalation Aerosol were compared to placebo in 2 additional randomized, double-blind clinical trials in adolescent and adult patients with mild-to-moderate asthma. SEREVENT DISKUS 50 mcg and SEREVENT Inhalation Aerosol 42 mcg, both administered twice daily, produced significant improvements in pulmonary function compared with placebo over the 12-week period. While no statistically significant differences were observed between the active treatments for any of the efficacy assessments or safety evaluations performed, there were some efficacy measures on which the metered-dose inhaler appeared to provide bet-

First Treatment Day

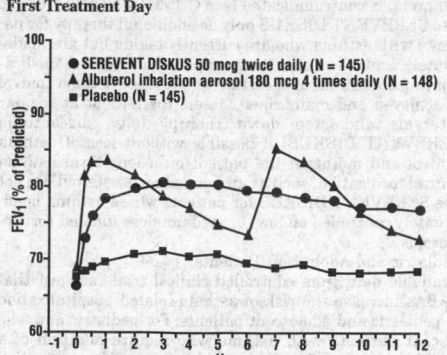

● SEREVENT DISKUS 50 mcg twice daily (N = 145)
▲ Albuterol inhalation aerosol 180 mcg 4 times daily (N = 148)
■ Placebo (N = 145)

Last Treatment Day (Week 12)

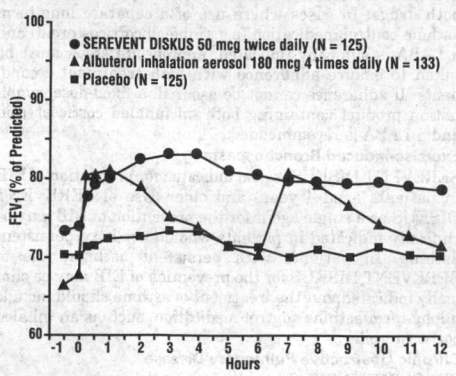

● SEREVENT DISKUS 50 mcg twice daily (N = 125)
▲ Albuterol inhalation aerosol 180 mcg 4 times daily (N = 133)
■ Placebo (N = 125)

Figure 1. Serial 12-Hour FEV_1 From Two 12-Week Clinical Trials in Patients With Asthma

Table 1. Daily Efficacy Measurements in Two 12-Week Clinical Trials (Combined Data)

Parameter	Time	Placebo	SEREVENT DISKUS	Albuterol Inhalation Aerosol
No. of randomized subjects		152	149	148
Mean AM peak expiratory flow (L/min)	baseline 12 weeks	394 396	395 427[a]	394 394
Mean % days with no asthma symptoms	baseline 12 weeks	14 20	13 33	12 21
Mean % nights with no awakenings	baseline 12 weeks	70 73	63 85[a]	68 71
Rescue medications (mean no. of inhalations per day)	baseline 12 weeks	4.2 3.3	4.3 1.6[b]	4.3 2.2
Asthma exacerbations		14%	15%	16%

[a]Statistically superior to placebo and albuterol (p<0.001).
[a]Statistically superior to placebo (p<0.001).

Table 2. Results of 2 Exercise-Induced Bronchospasm Studies in Adolescents and Adults

		Placebo (N = 52)		SEREVENT DISKUS (N = 52)	
		n	% Total	n	% Total
0.5-Hour postdose exercise challenge	% Fall in FEV_1				
	<10%	15	29	31	60
	≥10%, <20%	3	6	11	21
	≥20%	34	65	10	19
Mean maximal % fall in FEV_1 (SE)		-25% (1.8)		-11% (1.9)	
8.5-Hour postdose exercise challenge	% Fall in FEV_1				
	<10%	12	23	26	50
	≥10%, <20%	7	13	12	23
	≥20%	33	63	14	27
Mean maximal % fall in FEV_1 (SE)		-27% (1.5)		-16% (2.0)	

ter results. Similar findings were noted in 2 randomized, single-dose, crossover comparisons of SEREVENT DISKUS and SEREVENT Inhalation Aerosol for the prevention of exercise-induced bronchospasm (EIB). Therefore, while SEREVENT DISKUS was comparable to SEREVENT Inhalation Aerosol in clinical trials in mild-to-moderate patients with asthma, it should not be assumed that they will produce clinically equivalent outcomes in all patients.

In a randomized, double-blind, controlled study (N = 449), 50 mcg of SEREVENT DISKUS was administered twice daily to pediatric patients with asthma who did and who did not receive concurrent inhaled corticosteroids. The efficacy of salmeterol inhalation powder was demonstrated over the 12-week treatment period with respect to periodic serial peak expiratory flow (PEF) (36% to 39% postdose increase from baseline) and FEV_1 (32% to 33% postdose increase from baseline). Salmeterol was effective in demographic subgroup analyses (gender and age) and was effective when coadministered with other inhaled asthma medications such as short-acting bronchodilators and inhaled corticosteroids. A second randomized, double-blind, placebo-controlled study (N = 207) with 50 mcg of salmeterol inhalation powder via an alternate device supported the findings of the trial with the DISKUS.

Effects in Patients With Asthma on Concomitant Inhaled Corticosteroids

In 4 clinical trials in adult and adolescent patients with asthma (N = 1,922), the effect of adding salmeterol to inhaled corticosteroid therapy was evaluated. The studies utilized the inhalation aerosol formulation of salmeterol xinafoate for a treatment period of 6 months. They compared the addition of salmeterol therapy to an increase (at least doubling) of the inhaled corticosteroid dose.

Two randomized, double-blind, controlled, parallel-group clinical trials (N = 997) enrolled patients (aged 18 to 82 years) with persistent asthma who were previously maintained but not adequately controlled on inhaled corticosteroid therapy. During the 2-week run-in period, all patients were switched to beclomethasone dipropionate 168 mcg twice daily. Patients still not adequately controlled were randomized to either the addition of SEREVENT Inhalation Aerosol 42 mcg twice daily or an increase of beclomethasone dipropionate to 336 mcg twice daily. As compared to the doubled dose of beclomethasone dipropionate, the addition of SEREVENT Inhalation Aerosol resulted in statistically significantly greater improvements in pulmonary function and asthma symptoms, and statistically significantly greater reduction in supplemental albuterol use. The percent of patients who experienced asthma exacerbations overall was not different between groups (i.e., 16.2% in the

group receiving SEREVENT Inhalation Aerosol versus 17.9% in the higher-dose beclomethasone dipropionate group).

Two randomized, double-blind, parallel-group clinical trials (N = 925) enrolled patients (aged 12 to 78 years) with persistent asthma who were previously maintained but not adequately controlled on prior therapy. During the 2- to 4-week run-in period, all patients were switched to fluticasone propionate 88 mcg twice daily. Patients still not adequately controlled were randomized to either the addition of SEREVENT Inhalation Aerosol 42 mcg twice daily or an increase of fluticasone propionate to 220 mcg twice daily. As compared to the increased (2.5 times) dose of fluticasone propionate, the addition of SEREVENT Inhalation Aerosol resulted in statistically significantly greater improvements in pulmonary function and asthma symptoms, and statistically significantly greater reductions in supplemental albuterol use. Fewer patients receiving SEREVENT Inhalation Aerosol experienced asthma exacerbations than those receiving the higher dose of fluticasone propionate (8.8% versus 13.8%).

Exercise-Induced Bronchospasm

In 2 randomized, single-dose, crossover studies in adolescents and adults with EIB (N = 53), 50 mcg of SEREVENT DISKUS prevented EIB when dosed 30 minutes prior to exercise. For many patients, this protective effect against EIB was still apparent up to 8.5 hours following a single dose.
[See table 2 above]

In 2 randomized studies in children aged 4 to 11 years with asthma and EIB (N = 50), a single 50-mcg dose of SEREVENT DISKUS prevented EIB when dosed 30 minutes prior to exercise, with protection lasting up to 11.5 hours in repeat testing following this single dose in many patients.

Salmeterol Multi-center Asthma Research Trial

The Salmeterol Multi-center Asthma Research Trial (SMART) was a randomized, double-blind study that enrolled LABA-naive patients with asthma (average age of 39 years; 71% Caucasian, 18% African American, 8% Hispanic) to assess the safety of salmeterol (SEREVENT Inhalation Aerosol) 42 mcg twice daily over 28 weeks compared with placebo when added to usual asthma therapy.

A planned interim analysis was conducted when approximately half of the intended number of patients had been enrolled (N = 26,355), which led to premature termination of the study. The results of the interim analysis showed that patients receiving salmeterol were at increased risk for fa-

tal asthma events (see Table 3 and Figure 2). In the total population, a higher rate of asthma-related death occurred in patients treated with salmeterol than those treated with placebo (0.10% versus 0.02%; relative risk: 4.37 [95% CI: 1.25, 15.34]).

Post-hoc subpopulation analyses were performed. In Caucasians, asthma-related death occurred at a higher rate in patients treated with salmeterol than in patients treated with placebo (0.07% versus 0.01%; relative risk: 5.82 [95% CI: 0.70, 48.37]). In African Americans also, asthma-related death occurred at a higher rate in patients treated with salmeterol than those treated with placebo (0.31% versus 0.04%; relative risk: 7.26 [95% CI: 0.89, 58.94]). Although the relative risks of asthma-related death were similar in Caucasians and African Americans, the estimate of excess deaths in patients treated with salmeterol was greater in African Americans because there was a higher overall rate of asthma-related death in African American patients (see Table 3).

Post-hoc analyses in pediatric patients aged 12 to 18 years were also performed. Pediatric patients accounted for approximately 12% of patients in each treatment arm. Respiratory-related death or life-threatening experience occurred at a similar rate in the salmeterol group (0.12% [2/1,653]) and the placebo group (0.12% [2/1,622]; relative risk: 1.0 [95% CI: 0.1, 7.2]). All-cause hospitalization, however, was increased in the salmeterol group (2% [35/1,653]) versus the placebo group (<1% [16/1,622]; relative risk: 2.1 [95% CI: 1.1, 3.7]).

The data from the SMART study are not adequate to determine whether concurrent use of inhaled corticosteroids or other long-term asthma control therapy mitigates the risk of asthma-related death.
[See table 3 at top of next page]
[See figure 2 in next page]

Chronic Obstructive Pulmonary Disease

In 2 clinical trials evaluating twice-daily treatment with SEREVENT DISKUS 50 mcg (N = 336) compared to placebo (N = 366) in patients with chronic bronchitis with airflow limitation, with or without emphysema, improvements in pulmonary function endpoints were greater with salmeterol 50 mcg than with placebo. Treatment with SEREVENT DISKUS did not result in significant improvements in secondary endpoints assessing COPD symptoms in either clinical trial. Both trials were randomized, double-blind, parallel-group studies of 24 weeks' duration and were identical in design, patient entrance criteria, and overall conduct.

Figure 3 displays the integrated 2-hour postdose FEV_1 results from the 2 clinical trials. The percent change in FEV_1

Table 3: Asthma-Related Deaths in the 28-Week Salmeterol Multi-center Asthma Research Trial (SMART)

	Salmeterol n (%[a])	Placebo n (%[a])	Relative Risk[b] (95% Confidence Interval)	Excess Deaths Expressed per 10,000 Patients[c] (95% Confidence Interval)
Total Population[d]				
Salmeterol: N = 13,176	13 (0.10%)		4.37 (1.25, 15.34)	8 (3, 13)
Placebo: N = 13,179		3 (0.02%)		
Caucasian				
Salmeterol: N = 9,281	6 (0.07%)		5.82 (0.70, 48.37)	6 (1, 10)
Placebo: N = 9,361		1 (0.01%)		
African American				
Salmeterol: N = 2,366	7 (0.31%)		7.26 (0.89, 58.94)	27 (8, 46)
Placebo: N = 2,319		1 (0.04%)		

[a] Life-table 28-week estimate, adjusted according to the patients' actual lengths of exposure to study treatment to account for early withdrawal of patients from the study.

[b] Relative risk is the ratio of the rate of asthma-related death in the salmeterol group and the rate in the placebo group. The relative risk indicates how many more times likely an asthma-related death occurred in the salmeterol group than in the placebo group in a 28-week treatment period.

[c] Estimate of the number of additional asthma-related deaths in patients treated with salmeterol in SMART, assuming 10,000 patients received salmeterol for a 28-week treatment period. Estimate calculated as the difference between the salmeterol and placebo groups in the rates of asthma-related death multiplied by 10,000.

[d] The Total Population includes the following ethnic origins listed on the case report form: Caucasian, African American, Hispanic, Asian, and "Other." In addition, the Total Population includes those patients whose ethnic origin was not reported. The results for Caucasian and African American subpopulations are shown above. No asthma-related deaths occurred in the Hispanic (salmeterol n = 996, placebo n = 999), Asian (salmeterol n = 173, placebo n = 149), or "Other" (salmeterol n = 230, placebo n = 224) subpopulations. One asthma-related death occurred in the placebo group in the subpopulation whose ethnic origin was not reported (salmeterol n = 130, placebo n = 127).

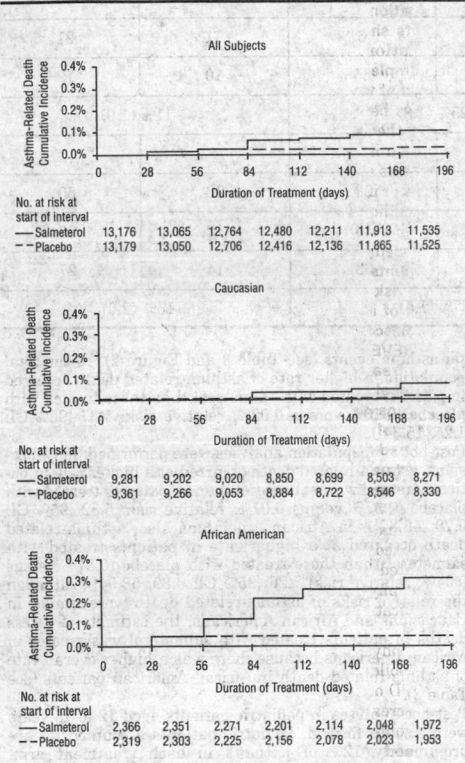

Figure 2. Cumulative Incidence of Asthma-Related Deaths in the 28-Week Salmeterol Multi-center Asthma Research Trial (SMART), by Duration of Treatment

refers to the change from baseline, defined as the predose value on Treatment Day 1. To account for patient withdrawals during the study, Endpoint (last evaluable FEV$_1$) data are provided. Patients receiving SEREVENT DISKUS 50 mcg had significantly greater improvements in 2-hour postdose FEV$_1$ at Endpoint (216 mL, 20%) compared to placebo (43 mL, 5%). Improvement was apparent on the first day of treatment and maintained throughout the 24 weeks of treatment.

[See figure 3 in next column]

Onset of Action and Duration of Effect

The onset of action and duration of effect of SEREVENT DISKUS were evaluated in a subset of patients (n = 87) from 1 of the 2 clinical trials discussed above. Following the first 50-mcg dose, significant improvement in pulmonary function (mean FEV$_1$ increase of 12% or more and at least 200 mL) occurred at 2 hours. The mean time to peak bronchodilator effect was 4.75 hours. As seen in Figure 4, evidence of bronchodilatation was seen throughout the 12-hour period. Figure 4 also demonstrates that the bronchodilating effect after 12 weeks of treatment was similar to that ob-

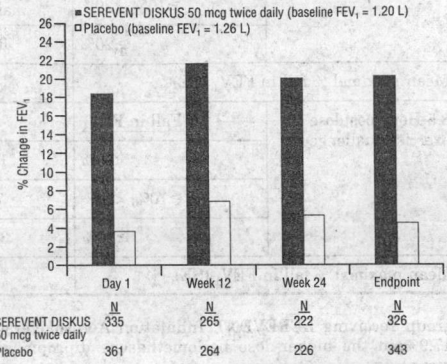

Figure 3. Mean Percent Change From Baseline in Postdose FEV$_1$ Integrated Data From 2 Trials of Patients With Chronic Bronchitis and Airflow Limitation

served after the first dose. The mean time to peak bronchodilator effect after 12 weeks of treatment was 3.27 hours.

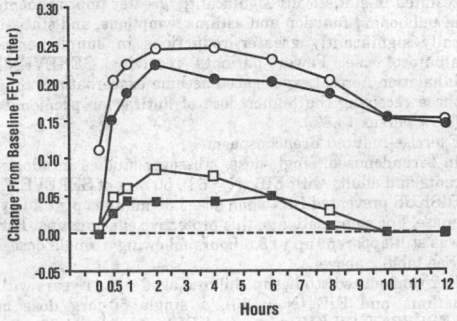

Figure 4. Serial 12-Hour FEV$_1$ on the First Day and at Week 12 of Treatment

INDICATIONS AND USAGE

Asthma

SEREVENT DISKUS is indicated for the treatment of asthma and in the prevention of bronchospasm only as concomitant therapy with a long-term asthma control medication, such as an inhaled corticosteroid, in patients aged 4 years and older with reversible obstructive airway disease, including patients with symptoms of nocturnal asthma. LABAs, such as salmeterol, the active ingredient in SEREVENT DISKUS, increase the risk of asthma-related death (see WARNINGS). Use of SEREVENT DISKUS for the treatment of asthma without concomitant use of a long-term asthma control medication, such as an inhaled corti-

costeroid, is contraindicated (see CONTRAINDICATIONS). Use SEREVENT DISKUS only as additional therapy for patients with asthma who are currently taking but are inadequately controlled on a long-term asthma control medication, such as an inhaled corticosteroid. Once asthma control is achieved and maintained, assess the patient at regular intervals and step down therapy (e.g., discontinue SEREVENT DISKUS) if possible without loss of asthma control and maintain the patient on a long-term asthma control medication, such as an inhaled corticosteroid. Do not use SEREVENT DISKUS for patients whose asthma is adequately controlled on low- or medium-dose inhaled corticosteroids.

Pediatric and Adolescent Patients

Available data from controlled clinical trials suggest that LABAs increase the risk of asthma-related hospitalization in pediatric and adolescent patients. For pediatric and adolescent patients with asthma who require addition of a LABA to an inhaled corticosteroid, a fixed-dose combination product containing both an inhaled corticosteroid and a LABA should ordinarily be used to ensure adherence with both drugs. In cases where use of a separate long-term asthma control medication (e.g., inhaled corticosteroid) and a LABA is clinically indicated, appropriate steps must be taken to ensure adherence with both treatment components. If adherence cannot be assured, a fixed-dose combination product containing both an inhaled corticosteroid and a LABA is recommended.

Exercise-Induced Bronchospasm

SEREVENT DISKUS is also indicated for prevention of EIB in patients aged 4 years and older. Use of SEREVENT DISKUS as a single agent for the prevention of EIB may be clinically indicated in patients who do not have persistent asthma. In patients with persistent asthma, use of SEREVENT DISKUS for the prevention of EIB may be clinically indicated, but the treatment of asthma should include a long-term asthma control medication, such as an inhaled corticosteroid.

Chronic Obstructive Pulmonary Disease

SEREVENT DISKUS is indicated for the long-term, twice-daily (morning and evening) administration in the maintenance treatment of bronchospasm associated with COPD (including emphysema and chronic bronchitis).

CONTRAINDICATIONS

Because of the risk of asthma-related death and hospitalization, use of SEREVENT DISKUS for the treatment of asthma without concomitant use of a long-term asthma control medication, such as an inhaled corticosteroid, is contraindicated (see WARNINGS: Asthma-Related Death). SEREVENT DISKUS is contraindicated in patients with a history of hypersensitivity to salmeterol or any other component of the drug product (see DESCRIPTION and ADVERSE REACTIONS: Observed During Clinical Practice: *Non-Site Specific*).

WARNINGS

Asthma-Related Death

LABAs, such as salmeterol, the active ingredient in SEREVENT DISKUS, increase the risk of asthma-related death. Currently available data are inadequate to determine whether concurrent use of inhaled corticosteroids or other long-term asthma control drugs mitigates the increased risk of asthma-related death from LABAs.

Because of this risk, use of SEREVENT DISKUS for the treatment of asthma without concomitant use of a long-term asthma control medication, such as an inhaled corticosteroid, is contraindicated. Use SEREVENT DISKUS only as additional therapy for patients with asthma who are currently taking but are inadequately controlled on a long-term asthma control medication, such as an inhaled corticosteroid. Once asthma control is achieved and maintained, assess the patient at regular intervals and step down therapy (e.g., discontinue SEREVENT DISKUS) if possible without loss of asthma control and maintain the patient on a long-term asthma control medication, such as an inhaled corticosteroid. Do not use SEREVENT DISKUS for patients whose asthma is adequately controlled on low- or medium-dose inhaled corticosteroids.

Pediatric and Adolescent Patients

Available data from controlled clinical trials suggest that LABAs increase the risk of asthma-related hospitalization in pediatric and adolescent patients. For pediatric and adolescent patients with asthma who require addition of a LABA to an inhaled corticosteroid, a fixed-dose combination product containing both an inhaled corticosteroid and a LABA should ordinarily be used to ensure adherence with both drugs. In cases where use of a separate long-term asthma control medication (e.g., inhaled corticosteroid) and a LABA is clinically indicated, appropriate steps must be taken to ensure adherence with both treatment components. If adherence cannot be assured, a fixed-dose combination product containing both an inhaled corticosteroid and a LABA is recommended.

Salmeterol Multi-center Asthma Research Trial and Salmeterol Nationwide Surveillance Studies

A large 28-week placebo-controlled US study comparing the safety of salmeterol (SEREVENT Inhalation Aerosol) with placebo, each added to usual asthma therapy, showed an increase in asthma-related deaths in patients receiving salmeterol (see CLINICAL TRIALS: Asthma: *Salmeterol Multi-center Asthma Research Trial*). Given the similar basic mechanisms of action of beta$_2$-agonists, the findings seen in the SMART study are considered a class effect.

A 16-week clinical study performed in the United Kingdom, the Salmeterol Nationwide Surveillance (SNS) study, showed results similar to the SMART study. In the SNS study, the rate of asthma-related death was numerically, though not statistically significantly, greater in patients with asthma treated with salmeterol (42 mcg twice daily) than those treated with albuterol (180 mcg 4 times daily) added to usual asthma therapy.

The SNS and SMART studies enrolled patients with asthma. No studies have been conducted that were adequate to determine whether the rate of death in patients with COPD is increased by LABAs.

- **It is important to watch for signs of worsening asthma, such as increasing use of inhaled, short-acting beta$_2$-agonists or a significant decrease in PEF or lung function. Such findings require immediate evaluation. Patients should be advised to seek immediate medical attention should their condition deteriorate.**
- **SEREVENT DISKUS should not be used to treat acute symptoms. It is crucial to inform patients of this and prescribe an inhaled, short-acting beta$_2$-agonist for this purpose and to warn them that increasing inhaled beta$_2$-agonist use is a signal of deteriorating asthma that requires prompt consultation with a physician.**
- **SEREVENT DISKUS should not be initiated in patients with significantly worsening or acutely deteriorating asthma, which may be a life-threatening condition. Serious acute respiratory events, including fatalities, have been reported both in the United States and worldwide when SEREVENT has been initiated in this situation. Although it is not possible from these reports to determine whether SEREVENT contributed to these adverse events or simply failed to relieve the deteriorating asthma, the use of SEREVENT DISKUS in this setting is inappropriate.**
- **SEREVENT DISKUS is not a substitute for inhaled or oral corticosteroids. Corticosteroids should not be stopped or reduced when SEREVENT DISKUS is initiated.**

See PRECAUTIONS: Information for Patients and the Medication Guide accompanying the product.

The following additional WARNINGS about SEREVENT DISKUS should be noted.

1. SEREVENT DISKUS should not be used as a treatment for acutely deteriorating asthma. SEREVENT DISKUS should not be introduced in acutely deteriorating asthma, which is a potentially life-threatening condition. There are no data demonstrating that SEREVENT DISKUS provides greater efficacy than or additional efficacy to inhaled, short-acting beta$_2$-agonists in patients with worsening asthma. Serious acute respiratory events, including fatalities, have been reported both in the United States and worldwide in patients receiving SEREVENT. In most cases, these have occurred in patients with severe asthma (e.g., patients with a history of corticosteroid dependence, low pulmonary function, intubation, mechanical ventilation, frequent hospitalizations, previous life-threatening acute asthma exacerbations) and/or in some patients in whom asthma has been acutely deteriorating (e.g., unresponsive to usual medications; increasing need for inhaled, short-acting beta$_2$-agonists; increasing need for systemic corticosteroids; significant increase in symptoms; recent emergency room visits; sudden or progressive deterioration in pulmonary function). However, they have occurred in a few patients with less severe asthma as well. It was not possible from these reports to determine whether SEREVENT contributed to these events.
2. SEREVENT DISKUS should not be used to treat acute symptoms. An inhaled, short-acting beta$_2$-agonist, not SEREVENT DISKUS, should be used to relieve acute asthma or COPD symptoms. When prescribing SEREVENT DISKUS, the physician must also provide the patient with an inhaled, short-acting beta$_2$-agonist (e.g., albuterol) for treatment of symptoms that occur acutely, despite regular twice-daily (morning and evening) use of SEREVENT DISKUS.

   When beginning treatment with SEREVENT DISKUS, patients who have been taking inhaled, short-acting beta$_2$-agonists on a regular basis (e.g., 4 times a day) should be instructed to discontinue the regular use of these drugs and use them only for symptomatic relief of acute asthma or COPD symptoms (see PRECAUTIONS: Information for Patients).
3. Increasing use of inhaled, short-acting beta$_2$-agonists is a marker of deteriorating asthma or COPD. The physician and patient should be alert to such changes. The patient's condition may deteriorate acutely over a period of hours or chronically over several days or longer. If the patient's inhaled, short-acting beta$_2$-agonist becomes less effective, the patient needs more inhalations than usual, or the patient develops a significant decrease in PEF or lung function, these may be markers of destabilization of their disease. In this setting, the patient requires immediate reevaluation with reassessment of the treatment regimen, giving special consideration to the possible need for corticosteroids. If the patient uses 4 or more inhalations per day of an inhaled, short-acting beta$_2$-agonist for 2 or more consecutive days, or if more than 1 canister (200 inhalations per canister) of inhaled, short-acting beta$_2$-agonist is used in an 8-week period in conjunction with SEREVENT DISKUS, then the patient should consult the physician for reevaluation. **Increasing the daily dosage of SEREVENT DISKUS in this situation is not appropriate. SEREVENT DISKUS should not be used more frequently than twice daily (morning and evening) at the recommended dose of 1 inhalation.**
4. SEREVENT DISKUS should not be used in conjunction with an inhaled LABA. SEREVENT DISKUS should not be used with other medications containing inhaled LABAs.
5. SEREVENT DISKUS is not a substitute for oral or inhaled corticosteroids. There are no data demonstrating that SEREVENT DISKUS has a clinical anti-inflammatory effect and could be expected to take the place of corticosteroids. When initiating SEREVENT DISKUS in patients receiving oral or inhaled corticosteroids for treatment of asthma, patients should be continued on a suitable dose of corticosteroids to maintain clinical stability even if they feel better as a result of initiating SEREVENT DISKUS. Any change in corticosteroid dosage should be made ONLY after clinical evaluation (see PRECAUTIONS: Information for Patients).
6. The recommended dosage should not be exceeded. As with other inhaled beta$_2$-adrenergic drugs, SEREVENT DISKUS should not be used more often or at higher doses than recommended. Fatalities have been reported in association with excessive use of inhaled sympathomimetic drugs. Large doses of inhaled or oral salmeterol (12 to 20 times the recommended dose) have been associated with clinically significant prolongation of the QTc interval, which has the potential for producing ventricular arrhythmias.
7. Paradoxical bronchospasm. As with other inhaled asthma and COPD medications, SEREVENT DISKUS can produce paradoxical bronchospasm, which may be life threatening. If paradoxical bronchospasm occurs following dosing with SEREVENT DISKUS, it should be treated immediately with an inhaled, short-acting bronchodilator; SEREVENT DISKUS should be discontinued immediately; and alternative therapy should be instituted.
8. Immediate hypersensitivity reactions. Immediate hypersensitivity reactions may occur after administration of SEREVENT DISKUS, as demonstrated by cases of urticaria, angioedema, rash, and bronchospasm.
9. Upper airway symptoms. Symptoms of laryngeal spasm, irritation, or swelling, such as stridor and choking, have been reported in patients receiving SEREVENT DISKUS.
10. Cardiovascular disorders. SEREVENT DISKUS, like all sympathomimetic amines, should be used with caution in patients with cardiovascular disorders, especially coronary insufficiency, cardiac arrhythmias, and hypertension. SEREVENT DISKUS, like all other beta-adrenergic agonists, can produce a clinically significant cardiovascular effect in some patients as measured by pulse rate, blood pressure, and/or symptoms. Although such effects are uncommon after administration of SEREVENT DISKUS at recommended doses, if they occur, the drug may need to be discontinued. In addition, beta-agonists have been reported to produce ECG changes, such as flattening of the T wave, prolongation of the QTc interval, and ST segment depression. The clinical significance of these findings is unknown.
11. Potential drug interactions. Because of the potential for drug interactions and the potential for increased risk of cardiovascular adverse events, the concomitant use of SEREVENT DISKUS with strong CYP3A4 inhibitors (e.g., ketoconazole, ritonavir, atazanavir, clarithromycin, indinavir, itraconazole, nefazodone, nelfinavir, saquinavir, telithromycin) is not recommended (see CLINICAL PHARMACOLOGY: Pharmacokinetics: *Drug Interactions*).

PRECAUTIONS

General

Cardiovascular Effects

No effect on the cardiovascular system is usually seen after the administration of inhaled salmeterol at recommended doses, but the cardiovascular and central nervous system effects seen with all sympathomimetic drugs (e.g., increased blood pressure, heart rate, excitement) can occur after use of salmeterol and may require discontinuation of SEREVENT DISKUS. SEREVENT DISKUS, like all sympathomimetic amines, should be used with caution in patients with cardiovascular disorders, especially coronary insufficiency, cardiac arrhythmias, and hypertension; in patients with convulsive disorders or thyrotoxicosis; and in patients who are unusually responsive to sympathomimetic amines.

As has been described with other beta-adrenergic agonist bronchodilators, clinically significant changes in systolic and/or diastolic blood pressure, pulse rate, and ECGs have been seen infrequently in individual patients in controlled clinical studies with salmeterol.

Metabolic Effects

Doses of the related beta$_2$-adrenoceptor agonist albuterol, when administered intravenously, have been reported to aggravate preexisting diabetes mellitus and ketoacidosis. Beta-adrenergic agonist medications may produce significant hypokalemia in some patients, possibly through intracellular shunting, which has the potential to produce adverse cardiovascular effects. The decrease in serum potassium is usually transient, not requiring supplementation.

Clinically significant changes in blood glucose and/or serum potassium were seen rarely during clinical studies with long-term administration of SEREVENT DISKUS at recommended doses.

Information for Patients

Patients should be instructed to read the accompanying Medication Guide with each new prescription and refill. The complete text of the Medication Guide is reprinted at the end of this document.

Patients being treated with SEREVENT DISKUS should receive the following information and instructions. This information is intended to aid them in the safe and effective use of this medication. It is not a disclosure of all possible adverse or intended effects. It is important that patients understand how to use the DISKUS appropriately and how to use SEREVENT DISKUS in relation to other asthma or COPD medications they are taking.

1. **Patients should be informed that salmeterol increases the risk of asthma-related death and may increase the risk of asthma-related hospitalization in pediatric and adolescent patients. Patients should be informed that SEREVENT DISKUS should not be the only therapy for the treatment of asthma and must only be used as additional therapy when long-term asthma control medications (e.g., inhaled corticosteroids) do not adequately control asthma symptoms. Patients should be informed that when SEREVENT DISKUS is added to their treatment regimen they must continue to use their long-term asthma control medication.**
2. SEREVENT DISKUS is not meant to relieve acute asthma or COPD symptoms and extra doses should not be used for that purpose. Acute symptoms should be treated with an inhaled, short-acting bronchodilator. The physician should provide the patient with such medication and instruct the patient in how it should be used.
3. The physician should be notified immediately if any of the following signs of seriously worsening asthma or COPD occur:
   - decreasing effectiveness of inhaled, short-acting beta$_2$-agonists;
   - need for more inhalations than usual of inhaled, short-acting beta$_2$-agonists;
   - significant decrease in PEF or lung function as outlined by the physician;
   - use of 4 or more inhalations per day of a short-acting beta$_2$-agonist for 2 or more days consecutively;
   - use of more than 1 canister (200 inhalations per canister) of an inhaled, short-acting beta$_2$-agonist in an 8-week period.
4. Patients should not stop therapy with SEREVENT DISKUS for asthma or COPD without physician/provider guidance since symptoms may worsen after discontinuation.
5. SEREVENT DISKUS should not be used as a substitute for oral or inhaled corticosteroids. The dosage of these medications should not be changed and they should not be stopped without consulting the physician, even if the patient feels better after initiating treatment with SEREVENT DISKUS.
6. Patients should be cautioned regarding adverse effects associated with beta$_2$-agonists, such as palpitations, chest pain, rapid heart rate, tremor, or nervousness.
7. When patients are prescribed SEREVENT DISKUS, other medications for asthma and COPD should be used only as directed by the physician.
8. SEREVENT DISKUS should not be used with a spacer device.

9. Patients who are pregnant or nursing should contact the physician about the use of SEREVENT DISKUS.

10. The action of SEREVENT DISKUS may last up to 12 hours or longer. The recommended dosage (1 inhalation twice daily, morning and evening) should not be exceeded.

11. When used for the treatment of EIB, 1 inhalation of SEREVENT DISKUS should be taken 30 minutes before exercise.
    - Additional doses of SEREVENT should not be used for 12 hours.
    - Patients who are receiving SEREVENT DISKUS twice daily should not use additional SEREVENT for prevention of EIB.

12. Effective and safe use of SEREVENT DISKUS includes an understanding of the way that it should be used:
    - Never exhale into the DISKUS.
    - Never attempt to take the DISKUS apart.
    - Always activate and use the DISKUS in a level, horizontal position.
    - Never wash the mouthpiece or any part of the DISKUS. KEEP IT DRY.
    - Always keep the DISKUS in a dry place.
    - Discard **6 weeks** after removal from the moisture-protective foil overwrap pouch or after all blisters have been used (when the dose indicator reads "0"), whichever comes first.

13. For the proper use of SEREVENT DISKUS and to attain maximum benefit, the patient should read and follow carefully the Instructions for Using SEREVENT DISKUS in the Medication Guide accompanying the product.

14. Most patients are able to taste or feel a dose delivered from SEREVENT DISKUS. However, whether or not patients are able to sense delivery of a dose, they should not exceed the recommended dose of 1 inhalation twice daily, morning and evening. Patients should contact a physician or pharmacist if they have questions.

Drug Interactions

Inhibitors of Cytochrome P450 3A4

In a drug interaction study in 20 healthy subjects, coadministration of salmeterol (50 mcg twice daily) and ketoconazole (400 mg once daily) for 7 days resulted in greater systemic exposure to salmeterol (AUC increased 16-fold and C_{max} increased 1.4-fold). Three (3) subjects were withdrawn due to beta$_2$-agonist side effects (2 with prolonged QTc and 1 with palpitations and sinus tachycardia). Although there was no statistical effect on the mean QTc, coadministration of salmeterol and ketoconazole was associated with more frequent increases in QTc duration compared with salmeterol and placebo administration. Due to the potential increased risk of cardiovascular adverse events, the concomitant use of salmeterol with strong CYP3A4 inhibitors (e.g., ketoconazole, ritonavir, atazanavir, clarithromycin, indinavir, itraconazole, nefazodone, nelfinavir, saquinavir, telithromycin) is not recommended.

Short-Acting Beta$_2$-Agonists

In two 12-week, repetitive-dose adolescent and adult clinical trials in patients with asthma (N = 149), the mean daily need for additional beta$_2$-agonist in patients using SEREVENT DISKUS was approximately 1½ inhalations/day. Twenty-six percent (26%) of the patients in these trials used between 8 and 24 inhalations of short-acting beta-agonist per day on 1 or more occasions. Nine percent (9%) of the patients in these trials averaged over 4 inhalations/day over the course of the 12-week trials. No increase in frequency of cardiovascular events was observed among the 3 patients who averaged 8 to 11 inhalations/day; however, the safety of concomitant use of more than 8 inhalations/day of short-acting beta$_2$-agonist with SEREVENT DISKUS has not been established. In 29 patients who experienced worsening of asthma while receiving SEREVENT DISKUS during these trials, albuterol therapy administered via either nebulizer or inhalation aerosol (1 dose in most cases) led to improvement in FEV$_1$ and no increase in occurrence of cardiovascular adverse events.

In 2 clinical trials in patients with COPD, the mean daily need for additional beta$_2$-agonist for patients using SEREVENT DISKUS was approximately 4 inhalations/day. Twenty-four percent (24%) of the patients using SEREVENT DISKUS in these trials averaged 6 or more inhalations of albuterol per day over the course of the 24-week trials. No increase in frequency of cardiovascular events was observed among patients who averaged 6 or more inhalations per day.

Monoamine Oxidase Inhibitors and Tricyclic Antidepressants

Salmeterol should be administered with extreme caution to patients being treated with monoamine oxidase inhibitors or tricyclic antidepressants, or within 2 weeks of discontinuation of such agents, because the action of salmeterol on the vascular system may be potentiated by these agents.

Corticosteroids and Cromoglycate

In clinical trials, inhaled corticosteroids and/or inhaled cromolyn sodium did not alter the safety profile of salmeterol when administered concurrently.

Methylxanthines

The concurrent use of intravenously or orally administered methylxanthines (e.g., aminophylline, theophylline) by patients receiving salmeterol has not been completely evaluated. In 1 clinical asthma trial, 87 patients receiving SEREVENT Inhalation Aerosol 42 mcg twice daily concurrently with a theophylline product had adverse event rates similar to those in 71 patients receiving SEREVENT Inhalation Aerosol without theophylline. Resting heart rates were slightly higher in the patients on theophylline but were little affected by therapy with SEREVENT Inhalation Aerosol.

In 2 clinical trials in patients with COPD, 39 subjects receiving SEREVENT DISKUS concurrently with a theophylline product had adverse event rates similar to those in 302 patients receiving SEREVENT DISKUS without theophylline. Based on the available data, the concomitant administration of methylxanthines with SEREVENT DISKUS did not alter the observed adverse event profile.

Beta-Adrenergic Receptor Blocking Agents

Beta-blockers not only block the pulmonary effect of beta-agonists, such as SEREVENT DISKUS, but may also produce severe bronchospasm in patients with asthma or COPD. Therefore, patients with asthma or COPD should not normally be treated with beta-blockers. However, under certain circumstances, e.g., as prophylaxis after myocardial infarction, there may be no acceptable alternatives to the use of beta-adrenergic blocking agents in patients with asthma or COPD. In this setting, cardioselective beta-blockers could be considered, although they should be administered with caution.

Diuretics

The ECG changes and/or hypokalemia that may result from the administration of nonpotassium-sparing diuretics (such as loop or thiazide diuretics) can be acutely worsened by beta-agonists, especially when the recommended dose of the beta-agonist is exceeded. Although the clinical significance of these effects is not known, caution is advised in the coadministration of beta-agonists with nonpotassium-sparing diuretics.

Carcinogenesis, Mutagenesis, Impairment of Fertility

In an 18-month oral carcinogenicity study in CD-mice, salmeterol xinafoate caused a dose-related increase in the incidence of smooth muscle hyperplasia, cystic glandular hyperplasia, leiomyomas of the uterus, and ovarian cysts at doses of 1.4 mg/kg and above (approximately 20 times the maximum recommended daily inhalation dose [MRHD] for adults and children based on comparison of the area under the plasma concentration versus time curves [AUCs]). The incidence of leiomyosarcomas was not statistically significant. No tumors were seen at 0.2 mg/kg (approximately 3 times the MRHD for adults and children based on comparison of the AUCs).

In a 24-month oral and inhalation carcinogenicity study in Sprague Dawley rats, salmeterol caused a dose-related increase in the incidence of mesovarian leiomyomas and ovarian cysts at doses of 0.68 mg/kg and above (approximately 55 and 25 times the MRHD for adults and children, respectively, MRHD on an mg/m^2 basis). No tumors were seen at 0.21 mg/kg (approximately 15 and 8 times the MRHD for adults and children, respectively, on an mg/m^2 basis). These findings in rodents are similar to those reported previously for other beta-adrenergic agonist drugs. The relevance of these findings to human use is unknown.

Salmeterol produced no detectable or reproducible increases in microbial and mammalian gene mutation in vitro. No clastogenic activity occurred in vitro in human lymphocytes or in vivo in a rat micronucleus test. No effects on fertility were identified in male and female rats treated with salmeterol at oral doses up to 2 mg/kg (approximately 160 times the MRHD for adults on an mg/m^2 basis).

Pregnancy

Teratogenic Effects

Pregnancy Category C. No teratogenic effects occurred in rats at oral doses up to 2 mg/kg (approximately 160 times the MRHD for adults on an mg/m^2 basis). In pregnant Dutch rabbits administered oral doses of 1 mg/kg and above (approximately 50 times the MRHD for adults based on comparison of the AUCs), salmeterol exhibited fetal toxic effects characteristically resulting from beta-adrenoceptor stimulation. These included precocious eyelid openings, cleft palate, sternebral fusion, limb and paw flexures, and delayed ossification of the frontal bones. No significant effects occurred at an oral dose of 0.6 mg/kg (approximately 20 times the MRHD for adults based on comparison of the AUCs).

New Zealand White rabbits were less sensitive since only delayed ossification of the frontal cranial bones was seen at an oral dose of 10 mg/kg (approximately 1,600 times the MRHD for adults on an mg/m^2 basis). Extensive use of other

beta-agonists has provided no evidence that these class effects in animals are relevant to their use in humans. There are no adequate and well-controlled studies with SEREVENT DISKUS in pregnant women. SEREVENT DISKUS should be used during pregnancy only if the potential benefit justifies the potential risk to the fetus.

Salmeterol xinafoate crossed the placenta following oral administration of 10 mg/kg to mice and rats (approximately 410 and 810 times, respectively, the MRHD for adults on an mg/m^2 basis).

Use in Labor and Delivery

There are no well-controlled human studies that have investigated effects of salmeterol on preterm labor or labor at term. Because of the potential for beta-agonist interference with uterine contractility, use of SEREVENT DISKUS during labor should be restricted to those patients in whom the benefits clearly outweigh the risks.

Nursing Mothers

Plasma levels of salmeterol after inhaled therapeutic doses are very low. In rats, salmeterol xinafoate is excreted in the milk. However, since there are no data from controlled trials on the use of salmeterol by nursing mothers, a decision should be made whether to discontinue nursing or to discontinue SEREVENT DISKUS, taking into account the importance of SEREVENT DISKUS to the mother. Caution should be exercised when SEREVENT DISKUS is administered to a nursing woman.

Pediatric Use

Available data from controlled clinical trials suggest that LABAs increase the risk of asthma-related hospitalization in pediatric and adolescent patients. For pediatric and adolescent patients with asthma who require addition of a LABA to an inhaled corticosteroid, a fixed-dose combination product containing both an inhaled corticosteroid and a LABA should ordinarily be used to ensure adherence with both drugs (see INDICATIONS AND USAGE and WARNINGS).

The safety and efficacy of SEREVENT DISKUS in adolescents (aged 12 years and older) has been established based on adequate and well-controlled trials conducted in adults and adolescents (see CLINICAL TRIALS). A large 28-week placebo-controlled US study, comparing salmeterol (SEREVENT Inhalation Aerosol) and placebo, each added to usual asthma therapy, showed an increase in asthma-related deaths in patients receiving salmeterol (see CLINICAL TRIALS: Asthma: *Salmeterol Multi-center Asthma Research Trial*). Post-hoc analyses in pediatric patients aged 12 to 18 years were also performed. Pediatric patients accounted for approximately 12% of patients in each treatment arm. Respiratory-related death or life-threatening experience occurred at a similar rate in the salmeterol group (0.12% [2/1,653]) and the placebo group (0.12% [2/1,622]; relative risk: 1.0 [95% CI: 0.1, 7.2]). All-cause hospitalization, however, was increased in the salmeterol group (2% [35/1,653]) versus the placebo group (<1% [16/1,622]; relative risk: 2.1 [95% CI: 1.1, 3.7]).

The safety and efficacy of SEREVENT DISKUS has been evaluated in over 2,500 patients aged 4 to 11 years with asthma, 346 of whom were administered SEREVENT DISKUS for 1 year. Based on available data, no adjustment of dosage of SEREVENT DISKUS in pediatric patients is warranted for either asthma or EIB (see DOSAGE AND ADMINISTRATION).

In 2 randomized, double-blind, controlled clinical trials of 12 weeks' duration, SEREVENT DISKUS 50 mcg was administered to 211 pediatric patients with asthma who did and who did not receive concurrent inhaled corticosteroids. The efficacy of SEREVENT DISKUS was demonstrated over the 12-week treatment period with respect to PEF and FEV$_1$. SEREVENT DISKUS was effective in demographic subgroups (gender and age) of the population.

In 2 randomized studies in children aged 4 to 11 years with asthma and EIB, a single 50-mcg dose of SEREVENT DISKUS prevented EIB when dosed 30 minutes prior to exercise, with protection lasting up to 11.5 hours in repeat testing following this single dose in many patients.

Geriatric Use

Of the total number of adolescent and adult patients with asthma who received SEREVENT DISKUS in chronic dosing clinical trials, 209 were aged 65 years or older. Of the total number of patients with COPD who received SEREVENT DISKUS in chronic dosing clinical trials, 167 were aged 65 years or older and 45 were aged 75 years or older. No apparent differences in the safety of SEREVENT DISKUS were observed when geriatric patients were compared with younger patients in clinical trials. As with other beta$_2$-agonists, however, special caution should be observed when using SEREVENT DISKUS in geriatric patients who have concomitant cardiovascular disease that could be adversely affected by this class of drug. Data from the trials in patients with COPD suggested a greater effect on FEV$_1$ of SEREVENT DISKUS in the <65 years age-group, as compared with the ≥65 years age-group. However, based on available data, no adjustment of dosage of SEREVENT DISKUS in geriatric patients is warranted.

ADVERSE REACTIONS

LABAs, including salmeterol, the active ingredient in SEREVENT DISKUS, increase the risk of asthma-related death. Data from a large 28-week placebo-controlled US study that compared the safety of salmeterol (SEREVENT Inhalation Aerosol) or placebo added to usual asthma therapy showed an increase in asthma-related deaths in patients receiving salmeterol. Available data from controlled clinical trials suggest that LABAs increase the risk of asthma-related hospitalization in pediatric and adolescent patients (see WARNINGS and CLINICAL TRIALS: Asthma: *Salmeterol Multi-center Asthma Research Trial*).

Asthma

Two multicenter 12-week controlled studies have evaluated twice-daily doses of SEREVENT DISKUS in patients aged 12 years and older with asthma. Table 4 reports the incidence of adverse events in these 2 studies.

[See table 4 at right]

Table 4 includes all events (whether considered drug-related or nondrug-related by the investigator) that occurred at a rate of 3% or greater in the group receiving SEREVENT DISKUS and were more common than in the placebo group.

Pharyngitis, sinusitis, upper respiratory tract infection, and cough occurred at ≥3% but were more common in the placebo group. However, throat irritation has been described at rates exceeding that of placebo in other controlled clinical trials.

Other adverse events that occurred in the group receiving SEREVENT DISKUS in these studies with an incidence of 1% to 3% and that occurred at a greater incidence than with placebo were:

Ear, Nose, and Throat
Sinus headache.
Gastrointestinal
Nausea.
Mouth and Teeth
Oral mucosal abnormality.
Musculoskeletal
Pain in joint.
Neurological
Sleep disturbance, paresthesia.
Skin
Contact dermatitis, eczema.
Miscellaneous
Localized aches and pains, pyrexia of unknown origin.

Two multicenter 12-week controlled studies have evaluated twice-daily doses of SEREVENT DISKUS in patients aged 4 to 11 years with asthma. Table 5 includes all events (whether considered drug-related or nondrug-related by the investigator) that occurred at a rate of 3% or greater in the group receiving SEREVENT DISKUS and were more common than in the placebo group.

[See table 5 above]

The following events were reported at an incidence of 1% to 2% (3 to 4 patients) in the salmeterol group and with a higher incidence than in the albuterol and placebo groups: gastrointestinal signs and symptoms, lower respiratory signs and symptoms, photodermatitis, and arthralgia and articular rheumatism.

In clinical trials evaluating concurrent therapy of salmeterol with inhaled corticosteroids, adverse events were consistent with those previously reported for salmeterol, or with events that would be expected with the use of inhaled corticosteroids.

Chronic Obstructive Pulmonary Disease

Two multicenter 24-week controlled studies have evaluated twice-daily doses of SEREVENT DISKUS in patients with COPD. For presentation (Table 6), the placebo data from a third trial, identical in design, patient entrance criteria, and overall conduct but comparing fluticasone propionate with placebo, were integrated with the placebo data from these 2 studies (total N = 341 for salmeterol and 576 for placebo).

[See table 6 above]

Other events occurring in the group receiving SEREVENT DISKUS that occurred at a frequency of 1% to <3% and were more common than in the placebo group were as follows:

Endocrine and Metabolic
Hyperglycemia.
Eye
Keratitis and conjunctivitis.
Gastrointestinal
Candidiasis mouth/throat, dyspeptic symptoms, hyposalivation, dental discomfort and pain, gastrointestinal infections.
Lower Respiratory
Lower respiratory signs and symptoms.

Musculoskeletal
Arthralgia and articular rheumatism; muscle pain; bone and skeletal pain; musculoskeletal inflammation; muscle stiffness, tightness, and rigidity.
Neurology
Migraines.
Non-Site Specific
Pain, edema and swelling.
Psychiatry
Anxiety.
Skin
Skin rashes.
Adverse reactions to salmeterol are similar in nature to those seen with other selective beta$_2$-adrenoceptor agonists, e.g., tachycardia; palpitations; immediate hypersensitivity reactions, including urticaria, angioedema, rash, bronchospasm (see WARNINGS); headache; tremor; nervousness; and paradoxical bronchospasm (see WARNINGS).

Observed During Clinical Practice

In addition to adverse events reported from clinical trials, the following events have been identified during postapproval use of salmeterol. Because they are reported voluntarily from a population of unknown size, estimates of frequency cannot be made. These events have been chosen for inclusion due to either their seriousness, frequency of reporting, or causal connection to salmeterol or a combination of these factors.

In extensive US and worldwide postmarketing experience with salmeterol, serious exacerbations of asthma, including some that have been fatal, have been reported. In most cases, these have occurred in patients with severe asthma and/or in some patients in whom asthma has been acutely deteriorating (see WARNINGS), but they have also occurred in a few patients with less severe asthma. It was not possible from these reports to determine whether salmeterol contributed to these events.

Respiratory
Reports of upper airway symptoms of laryngeal spasm, irritation, or swelling such as stridor or choking; oropharyngeal irritation.
Cardiovascular
Arrhythmias (including atrial fibrillation, supraventricular tachycardia, extrasystoles), and anaphylaxis.
Non-Site Specific
Very rare anaphylactic reaction in patients with severe milk protein allergy.

Table 4. Adverse Event Incidence in Two 12-Week Adolescent and Adult Clinical Trials in Patients With Asthma

Adverse Event	Percent of Patients		
	Placebo (N = 152)	SEREVENT DISKUS 50 mcg Twice Daily (N = 149)	Albuterol Inhalation Aerosol 180 mcg 4 Times Daily (N = 150)
Ear, nose, and throat			
Nasal/sinus congestion, pallor	6	9	8
Rhinitis	4	5	4
Neurological			
Headache	9	13	12
Respiratory			
Asthma	1	3	<1
Tracheitis/bronchitis	4	7	3
Influenza	2	5	5

Table 5. Adverse Event Incidence in Two 12-Week Pediatric Clinical Trials in Patients With Asthma

Adverse Event	Percent of Patients		
	Placebo (N = 215)	SEREVENT DISKUS 50 mcg Twice Daily (N = 211)	Albuterol Inhalation Powder 200 mcg 4 Times Daily (N = 115)
Ear, nose, and throat			
Ear signs and symptoms	3	4	9
Pharyngitis	3	6	3
Neurological			
Headache	14	17	20
Respiratory			
Asthma	2	4	<1
Skin			
Skin rashes	3	4	2
Urticaria	0	3	2

Table 6. Adverse Events With ≥3% Incidence in US Controlled Clinical Trials With SEREVENT DISKUS in Patients With Chronic Obstructive Pulmonary Disease[a]

Adverse Event	Percent of Patients	
	Placebo (N = 576)	SEREVENT DISKUS 50 mcg Twice Daily (N = 341)
Cardiovascular		
Hypertension	2	4
Ear, nose, and throat		
Throat irritation	6	7
Nasal congestion/blockage	3	4
Sinusitis	2	4
Ear signs and symptoms	1	3
Gastrointestinal		
Nausea and vomiting	3	3
Lower respiratory		
Cough	4	5
Rhinitis	2	4
Viral respiratory infection	4	5
Musculoskeletal		
Musculoskeletal pain	10	12
Muscle cramps and spasms	1	3
Neurological		
Headache	11	14
Dizziness	2	4
Average duration of exposure (days)	128.9	138.5

[a] Table 6 includes all events (whether considered drug-related or nondrug-related by the investigator) that occurred at a rate of 3% or greater in the group receiving SEREVENT DISKUS and were more common in the group receiving SEREVENT DISKUS than in the placebo group.

OVERDOSAGE

The expected signs and symptoms with overdosage of SEREVENT DISKUS are those of excessive beta-adrenergic stimulation and/or occurrence or exaggeration of any of the signs and symptoms listed under ADVERSE REACTIONS, e.g., seizures, angina, hypertension or hypotension, tachycardia with rates up to 200 beats/min, arrhythmias, nervousness, headache, tremor, muscle cramps, dry mouth, palpitation, nausea, dizziness, fatigue, malaise, insomnia.

Overdosage with SEREVENT DISKUS may be expected to result in exaggeration of the pharmacologic adverse effects associated with beta-adrenoceptor agonists, including tachycardia and/or arrhythmia, tremor, headache, and muscle cramps. Overdosage with SEREVENT DISKUS can lead to clinically significant prolongation of the QTc interval, which can produce ventricular arrhythmias. Other signs of overdosage may include hypokalemia and hyperglycemia.

As with all sympathomimetic medications, cardiac arrest and even death may be associated with abuse of SEREVENT DISKUS.

Treatment consists of discontinuation of SEREVENT DISKUS together with appropriate symptomatic therapy. The judicious use of a cardioselective beta-receptor blocker may be considered, bearing in mind that such medication can produce bronchospasm. There is insufficient evidence to determine if dialysis is beneficial for overdosage of SEREVENT DISKUS. Cardiac monitoring is recommended in cases of overdosage.

No deaths were seen in rats at an inhalation dose of 2.9 mg/kg (approximately 240 and 110 times the MRHD for adults and children, respectively, on an mg/m^2 basis) and in dogs at an inhalation dose of 0.7 mg/kg (approximately 190 and 90 times the MRHD for adults and children, respectively, on an mg/m^2 basis). By the oral route, no deaths occurred in mice at 150 mg/kg (approximately 6,100 and 2,900 times the MRHD for adults and children, respectively on an mg/m^2 basis) and in rats at 1,000 mg/kg (approximately 81,000 and 38,000 times the MRHD for adults and children, respectively, on an mg/m^2 basis).

DOSAGE AND ADMINISTRATION

SEREVENT DISKUS should be administered by the orally inhaled route only (see Instructions for Using SEREVENT DISKUS in the Medication Guide accompanying the product). The patient must not exhale into the DISKUS and the DISKUS should only be activated and used in a level, horizontal position.

Asthma

LABAs, such as salmeterol, the active ingredient in SEREVENT DISKUS, increase the risk of asthma-related death (see WARNINGS).

Because of this risk, use of SEREVENT DISKUS for the treatment of asthma without concomitant use of a long-term asthma control medication, such as an inhaled corticosteroid is contraindicated. Use SEREVENT DISKUS only as additional therapy for patients with asthma who are currently taking but are inadequately controlled on a long-term asthma control medication, such as an inhaled corticosteroid. Once asthma control is achieved and maintained, assess the patient at regular intervals and step down therapy (e.g., discontinue SEREVENT DISKUS) if possible without loss of asthma control and maintain the patient on a long-term asthma control medication, such as an inhaled corticosteroid. Do not use SEREVENT DISKUS for patients whose asthma is adequately controlled on low- or medium-dose inhaled corticosteroids.

Pediatric and Adolescent Patients

Available data from controlled clinical trials suggest that LABAs increase the risk of asthma-related hospitalization in pediatric and adolescent patients. For patients with asthma less than 18 years of age who require addition of a LABA to an inhaled corticosteroid, a fixed-dose combination product containing both an inhaled corticosteroid and a LABA should ordinarily be used to ensure adherence with both drugs. In cases where use of a separate long-term asthma control medication (e.g., inhaled corticosteroid) and a LABA is clinically indicated, appropriate steps must be taken to ensure adherence with both treatment components. If adherence cannot be assured, a fixed-dose combination product containing both an inhaled corticosteroid and a LABA is recommended.

For bronchodilatation and prevention of symptoms of asthma, including the symptoms of nocturnal asthma, the usual dosage for adults and children aged 4 years and older is 1 inhalation (50 mcg) twice daily (morning and evening, approximately 12 hours apart). If a previously effective dosage regimen fails to provide the usual response, medical advice should be sought immediately as this is often a sign of destabilization of asthma. Under these circumstances, the therapeutic regimen should be reevaluated. If symptoms arise in the period between doses, an inhaled, short-acting beta$_2$-agonist should be taken for immediate relief.

Chronic Obstructive Pulmonary Disease

For maintenance treatment of bronchospasm associated with COPD (including chronic bronchitis and emphysema), the usual dosage for adults is 1 inhalation (50 mcg) twice daily (morning and evening, approximately 12 hours apart). For both asthma and COPD, adverse effects are more likely to occur with higher doses of salmeterol, and more frequent administration or administration of a larger number of inhalations is not recommended.

To gain full therapeutic benefit, SEREVENT DISKUS should be administered twice daily (morning and evening) in the treatment of reversible airway obstruction.

Geriatric Use

Based on available data for SEREVENT DISKUS, no dosage adjustment is recommended.

Prevention of Exercise-Induced Bronchospasm

Use of SEREVENT DISKUS as a single agent for the prevention of EIB may be clinically indicated in patients who do not have persistent asthma. In patients with persistent asthma, use of SEREVENT DISKUS for the prevention of EIB may be clinically indicated, but the treatment of asthma should include a long-term asthma control medication, such as an inhaled corticosteroid. One inhalation of SEREVENT DISKUS at least 30 minutes before exercise has been shown to protect patients against EIB. When used intermittently as needed for prevention of EIB, this protection may last up to 9 hours in adolescents and adults and up to 12 hours in patients aged 4 to 11 years. Additional doses of SEREVENT should not be used for 12 hours after the administration of this drug. Patients who are receiving SEREVENT DISKUS twice daily should not use additional SEREVENT for prevention of EIB.

HOW SUPPLIED

SEREVENT DISKUS is supplied as a disposable teal green unit containing 60 blisters. The drug product is packaged within a plastic-coated, moisture-protective foil pouch (NDC 0173-0521-00).

SEREVENT DISKUS is also supplied in an institutional pack of 1 disposable teal green unit containing 28 blisters. The drug product is packaged within a plastic-coated, moisture-protective foil pouch (NDC 0173-0520-00).

Store at controlled room temperature (see USP), 20° to 25°C (68° to 77°F) in a dry place away from direct heat or sunlight. Keep out of reach of children. SEREVENT DISKUS should be discarded 6 weeks after removal from the moisture-protective foil pouch or after all blisters have been used (when the dose indicator reads "0"), whichever comes first. The DISKUS is not reusable. Do not attempt to take the DISKUS apart.

SEREVENT and DISKUS are registered trademarks of GlaxoSmithKline

GlaxoSmithKline
Research Triangle Park, NC 27709

©2010, GlaxoSmithKline. All rights reserved.

June 2010
SRD:5PI

MEDICATION GUIDE

SEREVENT® [*ser' uh-vent*] DISKUS®

(salmeterol xinafoate inhalation powder)

Read the Medication Guide that comes with SEREVENT DISKUS before you start using it and each time you get a refill. There may be new information. This Medication Guide does not take the place of talking to your healthcare provider about your medical condition or treatment.

What is the most important information I should know about SEREVENT DISKUS?

SEREVENT DISKUS can cause serious side effects, including:

1. **People with asthma who take long-acting beta$_2$-adrenergic agonist (LABA) medicines, such as salmeterol (SEREVENT DISKUS), have an increased risk of death from asthma problems.**
   - **Call your healthcare provider if breathing problems worsen over time while using SEREVENT DISKUS.** You may need different treatment.
   - **Get emergency medical care if:**
     - breathing problems worsen quickly and
     - you use your rescue inhaler medicine, but it does not relieve your breathing problems.
2. **Do not use SEREVENT DISKUS as your only asthma medicine. SEREVENT DISKUS must only be used with a long-term asthma control medicine, such as an inhaled corticosteroid.**
3. When your asthma is well controlled, your healthcare provider may tell you to stop taking SEREVENT DISKUS. Your healthcare provider will decide if you can stop SEREVENT DISKUS without loss of asthma control. You will continue taking your other asthma control medicine, such as an inhaled corticosteroid.
4. Children and adolescents who take LABA medicines may have an increased risk of being hospitalized for asthma problems.

What is SEREVENT DISKUS?

- SEREVENT DISKUS is a LABA medicine. LABA medicines help the muscles around the airways in your lungs stay relaxed to prevent symptoms, such as wheezing and shortness of breath. These symptoms can happen when the muscles around the airways tighten. This makes it hard to breathe. In severe cases, wheezing can stop your breathing and cause death if not treated right away.
- SEREVENT DISKUS is used for asthma, exercise-induced bronchospasm (EIB), and chronic obstructive pulmonary disease (COPD) as follows:

Asthma:

SEREVENT DISKUS is used in adults and children aged 4 years and older, with a long-term asthma control medicines, such as an inhaled corticosteroid:

- to control symptoms of asthma and
- to prevent symptoms such as wheezing.

LABA medicines, such as SEREVENT DISKUS, increase the risk of death from asthma problems. SEREVENT DISKUS is not for adults and children with asthma who are well controlled with a long-term asthma control medicine, such as a low to medium dose of an inhaled corticosteroid medicine.

EIB:

SEREVENT DISKUS is used to prevent wheezing caused by exercise in adults and children aged 4 years and older.

- If you have EIB only, your healthcare provider may prescribe only SEREVENT DISKUS for your condition.
- If you have EIB and asthma, your healthcare provider should also prescribe an asthma control medicine, such as an inhaled corticosteroid.

COPD:

SEREVENT DISKUS is used long term, 2 times each day (morning and evening) to control symptoms of COPD and prevent wheezing in adults with COPD.

Who should not use SEREVENT DISKUS?

Do not use SEREVENT DISKUS:

- to treat your asthma without an asthma medicine known as an inhaled corticosteroid and
- if you are allergic to salmeterol or any of the ingredients in SEREVENT DISKUS. Ask your healthcare provider if you are not sure. See the end of this Medication Guide for a list of ingredients in SEREVENT DISKUS.

What should I tell my healthcare provider before using SEREVENT DISKUS?

Tell your healthcare provider about all of your health conditions, including if you:

- **have heart problems**
- **have high blood pressure**
- **have seizures**
- **have thyroid problems**
- **have diabetes**
- **have liver problems**
- **are pregnant or planning to become pregnant.** It is not known if SEREVENT DISKUS may harm your unborn baby.
- **are breastfeeding.** It is not known if SEREVENT DISKUS passes into your milk and if it can harm your baby.
- **are allergic to SEREVENT DISKUS, any other medicines, or food products.** See the end of this Medication Guide for a complete list of the ingredients in SEREVENT DISKUS.

Tell your healthcare provider about all the medicines you take including prescription and non-prescription medicines, vitamins, and herbal supplements. SEREVENT DISKUS and certain other medicines, especially those used to treat infections, may interact with each other. This may cause serious side effects.

Know the medicines you take. Keep a list and show it to your healthcare provider and pharmacist each time you get a new medicine.

How do I use SEREVENT DISKUS?

See the step-by-step instructions for using SEREVENT DISKUS at the end of this Medication Guide. Do not use SEREVENT DISKUS unless your healthcare provider has taught you and you understand everything. Ask your healthcare provider or pharmacist if you have any questions.

- Children should use SEREVENT DISKUS with an adult's help, as instructed by the child's healthcare provider.
- Use SEREVENT DISKUS exactly as prescribed. **Do not use SEREVENT DISKUS more often than prescribed.**
- For asthma and COPD, the usual dosage is 1 inhalation 2 times each day (morning and evening). The 2 doses should be about 12 hours apart.
- For preventing EIB, take 1 inhalation at least 30 minutes before exercise. Do not use SEREVENT DISKUS more often than every 12 hours. Do not use extra SEREVENT DISKUS before exercise if you already use it 2 times each day.
- If you miss a dose of SEREVENT DISKUS, just skip that dose. Take your next dose at your usual time. Do not take 2 doses at one time.
- Do not use a spacer device with SEREVENT DISKUS.

- Do not breathe into SEREVENT DISKUS.
- **While you are using SEREVENT DISKUS 2 times each day, do not use other medicines that contain a LABA for any reason.** Ask your healthcare provider or pharmacist for a list of these medicines.
- Do not stop using SEREVENT DISKUS or any of your asthma medicines unless told to do so by your healthcare provider because your symptoms might get worse. Your healthcare provider will change your medicines as needed.
- SEREVENT DISKUS does not relieve sudden symptoms. Always have a rescue inhaler medicine with you to treat sudden symptoms. If you do not have an inhaled, short-acting bronchodilator, call your healthcare provider to have one prescribed for you.
- Call your healthcare provider or get medical care right away if:
  - your breathing problems worsen with SEREVENT DISKUS
  - you need to use your rescue inhaler medicine more often than usual
  - your rescue inhaler medicine does not work as well for you at relieving symptoms
  - you need to use 4 or more inhalations of your rescue inhaler medicine for 2 or more days in a row
  - you use 1 whole canister of your rescue inhaler medicine in 8 weeks' time
  - your peak flow meter results decrease. Your healthcare provider will tell you the numbers that are right for you.
  - you have asthma and your symptoms do not improve after using SEREVENT DISKUS regularly for 1 week
  - after a change in your asthma medicines you have any worsening of your asthma symptoms or an increase in the need for your rescue inhaler medicine.

What are the possible side effects with SEREVENT DISKUS?
SEREVENT DISKUS can cause serious side effects, including:
- **See "What is the most important information I should know about SEREVENT DISKUS?"**
- **serious allergic reactions.** Call your healthcare provider or get emergency medical care if you get any of the following symptoms of a serious allergic reaction:
  - rash
  - hives
  - swelling of the face, mouth, and tongue
  - breathing problems
- **sudden breathing problems immediately after inhaling your medicine**
- **effects on heart**
  - increased blood pressure
  - a fast and irregular heartbeat
  - chest pain
- **effects on nervous system**
  - tremor
  - nervousness
- **changes in blood (sugar, potassium)**

Common side effects of SEREVENT DISKUS include:
Asthma in adults and children:
- headache
- nasal congestion
- bronchitis
- throat irritation
- runny nose
- flu

COPD:
- headache
- musculoskeletal pain
- throat irritation
- cough
- respiratory infection

Tell your healthcare provider about any side effect that bothers you or that does not go away.
These are not all the side effects with SEREVENT DISKUS. Ask your healthcare provider or pharmacist for more information.
Call your doctor for medical advice about side effects. You may report side effects to FDA at 1-800-FDA-1088 or 1-800-332-1088.

How do I store SEREVENT DISKUS?
- Store SEREVENT DISKUS at room temperature between 68° to 77° F (20° to 25° C). Keep in a dry place away from heat and sunlight.
- Safely discard SEREVENT DISKUS 6 weeks after you remove it from the foil pouch, or after the dose indicator reads "0", whichever comes first.
- Keep SEREVENT DISKUS and all medicines out of the reach of children.

General Information About SEREVENT DISKUS
Medicines are sometimes prescribed for purposes not mentioned in a Medication Guide. Do not use SEREVENT DISKUS for a condition for which it was not prescribed. Do

not give your SEREVENT DISKUS to other people, even if they have the same condition that you have. It may harm them.
This Medication Guide summarizes the most important information about SEREVENT DISKUS. If you would like more information, talk with your healthcare provider or pharmacist. You can ask your healthcare provider or pharmacist for information about SEREVENT DISKUS that was written for healthcare professionals. You can also contact the company that makes SEREVENT DISKUS (toll free) at 1-888-825-5249 or at www.serevent.com.

What are the ingredients in SEREVENT DISKUS?
Active ingredient: salmeterol xinafoate
Inactive ingredient: lactose (contains milk proteins)

Instructions for Using SEREVENT DISKUS
Follow the instructions below for using your SEREVENT DISKUS. **You will breathe in (inhale) the medicine from the DISKUS.** If you have any questions, ask your healthcare provider or pharmacist.

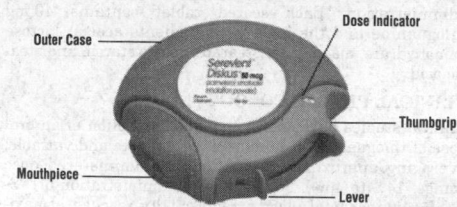

Take the SEREVENT DISKUS out of the box and foil pouch. Write the **"Pouch opened"** and **"Use by"** dates on the label on top of the DISKUS. **The "Use by" date is 6 weeks from date of opening the pouch.**
- The DISKUS will be in the closed position when the pouch is opened.
- The **dose indicator** on the top of the DISKUS tells you how many doses are left. The dose indicator number will decrease each time you use the DISKUS. After you have used 55 doses from the DISKUS, the numbers 5 to 0 will appear in **red** to warn you that there are only a few doses left (*see Figure 1*).

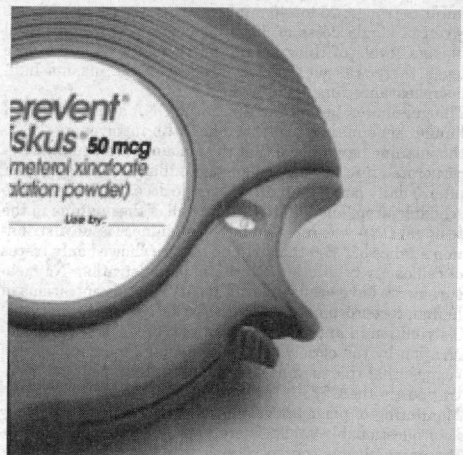

Figure 1

Taking a dose from the DISKUS requires the following 3 simple steps: Open, Click, Inhale.

1. OPEN
Hold the DISKUS in one hand and put the thumb of your other hand on the **thumbgrip**. Push your thumb away from you as far as it will go until the mouthpiece appears and snaps into position (*see Figure 2*).
[See figure 2 at top of next column]

2. CLICK
Hold the DISKUS in a level, flat position with the mouthpiece towards you. Slide the **lever** away from you as far as it will go until it **clicks** (*see Figure 3*). The DISKUS is now ready to use.
[See figure 3 in next column]
Every time the **lever** is pushed back, a dose is ready to be inhaled. This is shown by a decrease in numbers on the dose counter. **To avoid releasing or wasting doses once the DISKUS is ready:**
- **Do not close the DISKUS.**
- **Do not tilt the DISKUS.**
- **Do not play with the lever.**
- **Do not move the lever more than once.**

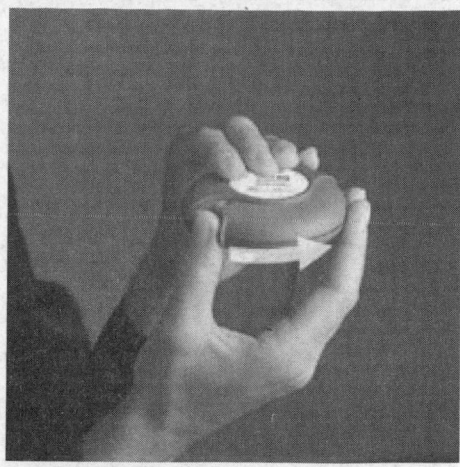

Figure 2

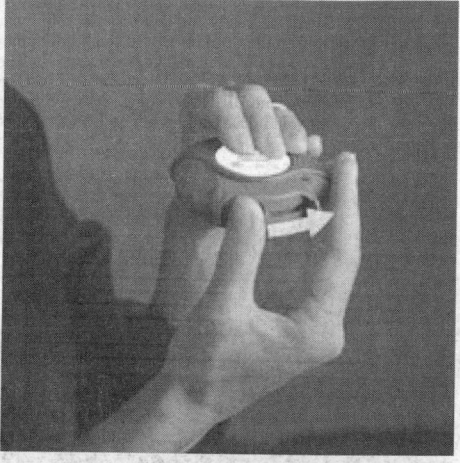

Figure 3

3. INHALE
Before inhaling your dose from the DISKUS, breathe out (exhale) fully while holding the DISKUS level and away from your mouth (*see Figure 4*). **Remember, never breathe out into the DISKUS mouthpiece.**

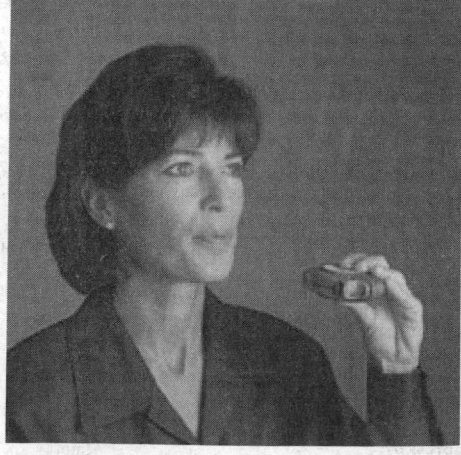

Figure 4

Put the mouthpiece to your lips (*see Figure 5*). Breathe in quickly and deeply through the DISKUS. Do not breathe in through your nose.
[See figure 5 at top of next column]
Remove the DISKUS from your mouth. Hold your breath for about 10 seconds, or for as long as is comfortable. Breathe out slowly.
The DISKUS delivers your dose of medicine as a very fine powder. Most patients can taste or feel the powder. Do not use another dose from the DISKUS if you do not feel or taste the medicine.

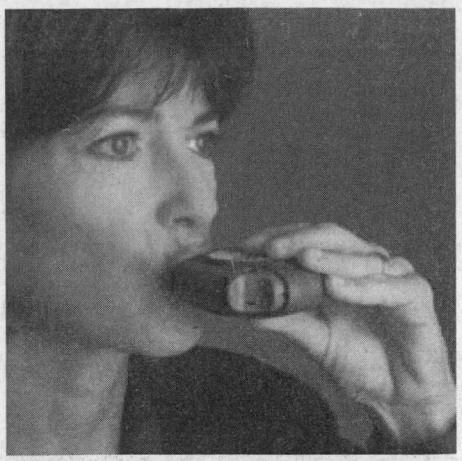

Figure 5

4. Close the DISKUS when you are finished taking a dose so that the DISKUS will be ready for you to take your next dose. Put your thumb on the thumbgrip and slide the thumbgrip back towards you as far as it will go *(see Figure 6)*. The DISKUS will click shut. The lever will automatically return to its original position. The DISKUS is now ready for you to take your next scheduled dose, due in about 12 hours. (Repeat steps 1 to 4.)

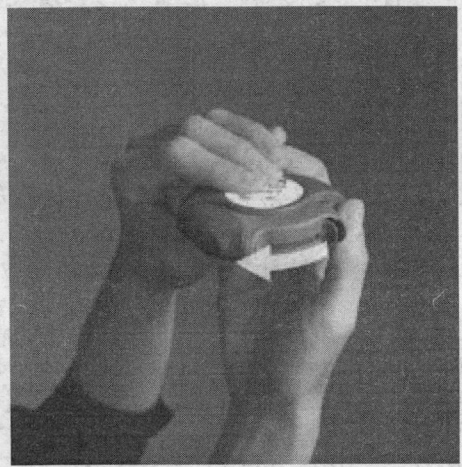

Figure 6

Remember:
• Never breathe into the DISKUS.
• Never take the DISKUS apart.
• Always ready and use the DISKUS in a level, flat position.
• Do not use the DISKUS with a spacer device.
• Never wash the mouthpiece or any part of the DISKUS. **Keep it dry.**
• Always keep the DISKUS in a dry place.
• Never take an extra dose, even if you did not taste or feel the medicine.

This Medication Guide has been approved by the U.S. Food and Drug Administration.

SEREVENT and DISKUS are registered trademarks of GlaxoSmithKline.
GlaxoSmithKline
Research Triangle Park, NC 27709
©2010, GlaxoSmithKline. All rights reserved.
June 2010
SRD:3MG

TABLOID®   ℞
[tab' loid]
brand Thioguanine
40-mg Scored Tablets

CAUTION
TABLOID brand Thioguanine is a potent drug. It should not be used unless a diagnosis of acute nonlymphocytic leukemia has been adequately established and the responsible physician is knowledgeable in assessing response to chemotherapy.

DESCRIPTION

TABLOID brand Thioguanine was synthesized and developed by Hitchings, Elion, and associates at the Wellcome Research Laboratories. It is one of a large series of purine analogues which interfere with nucleic acid biosynthesis, and has been found active against selected human neoplastic diseases.

Thioguanine, known chemically as 2-amino-1,7-dihydro-6*H*-purine-6-thione, is an analogue of the nucleic acid constituent guanine, and is closely related structurally and functionally to PURINETHOL® (mercaptopurine). Its structural formula is:

$$\text{... } \cdot x\,H_2O$$

TABLOID brand Thioguanine is available in tablets for oral administration. Each scored tablet contains 40 mg thioguanine and the inactive ingredients acacia, lactose monohydrate, magnesium stearate, potato starch, and stearic acid.

CLINICAL PHARMACOLOGY

Clinical studies have shown that the absorption of an oral dose of thioguanine in humans is incomplete and variable, averaging approximately 30% of the administered dose (range: 14% to 46%). Following oral administration of ^{35}S-6-thioguanine, total plasma radioactivity reached a maximum at 8 hours and declined slowly thereafter. Parent drug represented only a very small fraction of the total plasma radioactivity at any time, being virtually undetectable throughout the period of measurements.

The oral administration of radiolabeled thioguanine revealed only trace quantities of parent drug in the urine. However, a methylated metabolite, 2-amino-6-methylthiopurine (MTG), appeared very early, rose to a maximum 6 to 8 hours after drug administration, and was still being excreted after 12 to 22 hours. Radiolabeled sulfate appeared somewhat later than MTG but was the principal metabolite after 8 hours. Thiouric acid and some unidentified products were found in the urine in small amounts. Intravenous administration of ^{35}S-6-thioguanine disclosed a median plasma half-disappearance time of 80 minutes (range: 25 to 240 minutes) when the compound was given in single doses of 65 to 300 mg/m^2. Although initial plasma levels of thioguanine did correlate with the dose level, there was no correlation between the plasma half-disappearance time and the dose.

Thioguanine is incorporated into the DNA and the RNA of human bone marrow cells. Studies with intravenous ^{35}S-6-thioguanine have shown that the amount of thioguanine incorporated into nucleic acids is more than 100 times higher after 5 daily doses than after a single dose. With the 5-dose schedule, from one-half to virtually all of the guanine in the residual DNA was replaced by thioguanine. Tissue distribution studies of ^{35}S-6-thioguanine in mice showed only traces of radioactivity in brain after oral administration. No measurements have been made of thioguanine concentrations in human cerebrospinal fluid (CSF), but observations on tissue distribution in animals, together with the lack of CNS penetration by the closely related compound, mercaptopurine, suggest that thioguanine does not reach therapeutic concentrations in the CSF.

Monitoring of plasma levels of thioguanine during therapy is of questionable value. There is technical difficulty in determining plasma concentrations, which are seldom greater than 1 to 2 mcg/mL after a therapeutic oral dose. More significantly, thioguanine enters rapidly into the anabolic and catabolic pathways for purines, and the active intracellular metabolites have appreciably longer half-lives than the parent drug. The biochemical effects of a single dose of thioguanine are evident long after the parent drug has disappeared from plasma. Because of this rapid metabolism of thioguanine to active intracellular derivatives, hemodialysis would not be expected to appreciably reduce toxicity of the drug.

Thioguanine competes with hypoxanthine and guanine for the enzyme hypoxanthine-guanine phosphoribosyltransferase (HGPRTase) and is itself converted to 6-thioguanylic acid (TGMP). This nucleotide reaches high intracellular concentrations at therapeutic doses. TGMP interferes at several points with the synthesis of guanine nucleotides. It inhibits de novo purine biosynthesis by pseudo-feedback inhibition of glutamine-5-phosphoribosylpyrophosphate amidotransferase—the first enzyme unique to the de novo pathway for purine ribonucleotide synthesis. TGMP also inhibits the conversion of inosinic acid (IMP) to xanthylic acid (XMP) by competition for the enzyme IMP dehydrogenase. At one time TGMP was felt to be a significant inhibitor of ATP:GMP phosphotransferase (guanylate kinase), but recent results have shown this not to be so.

Thioguanylic acid is further converted to the di- and triphosphates, thioguanosine diphosphate (TGDP) and thioguanosine triphosphate (TGTP) (as well as their 2'-deoxyribosyl analogues) by the same enzymes which metabolize guanine nucleotides. Thioguanine nucleotides are incorporated into both the RNA and the DNA by phosphodiester linkages and it has been argued that incorporation of such fraudulent bases contributes to the cytotoxicity of thioguanine.

Thus, thioguanine has multiple metabolic effects and at present it is not possible to designate one major site of action. Its tumor inhibitory properties may be due to one or more of its effects on (a) feedback inhibition of de novo purine synthesis; (b) inhibition of purine nucleotide interconversions; or (c) incorporation into the DNA and the RNA. The net consequence of its actions is a sequential blockade of the synthesis and utilization of the purine nucleotides.

The catabolism of thioguanine and its metabolites is complex and shows significant differences between humans and the mouse. In both humans and mice, after oral administration of ^{35}S-6-thioguanine, urine contains virtually no detectable intact thioguanine. While deamination and subsequent oxidation to thiouric acid occurs only to a small extent in humans, it is the main pathway in mice. The product of deamination by guanase, 6-thioxanthine is inactive, having negligible antitumor activity. This pathway of thioguanine inactivation is not dependent on the action of xanthine oxidase, and an inhibitor of that enzyme (such as allopurinol) will not block the detoxification of thioguanine even though the inactive 6-thioxanthine is normally further oxidized by xanthine oxidase to thiouric acid before it is eliminated. In humans, methylation of thioguanine is much more extensive than in the mouse. The product of methylation, 2-amino-6-methylthiopurine, is also substantially less active and less toxic than thioguanine and its formation is likewise unaffected by the presence of allopurinol. Appreciable amounts of inorganic sulfate are also found in both murine and human urine, presumably arising from further metabolism of the methylated derivatives.

In some animal tumors, resistance to the effect of thioguanine correlates with the loss of HGPRTase activity and the resulting inability to convert thioguanine to thioguanylic acid. However, other resistance mechanisms, such as increased catabolism of TGMP by a nonspecific phosphatase, may be operative. Although not invariable, it is usual to find cross-resistance between thioguanine and its close analogue, PURINETHOL (mercaptopurine).

INDICATIONS AND USAGE
a) Acute Nonlymphocytic Leukemias
TABLOID brand Thioguanine is indicated for remission induction and remission consolidation treatment of acute nonlymphocytic leukemias. However, it is not recommended for use during maintenance therapy or similar long-term continuous treatments due to the high risk of liver toxicity (see WARNINGS and ADVERSE REACTIONS).

The response to this agent depends upon the age of the patient (younger patients faring better than older) and whether thioguanine is used in previously treated or previously untreated patients. Reliance upon thioguanine alone is seldom justified for initial remission induction of acute nonlymphocytic leukemias because combination chemotherapy including thioguanine results in more frequent remission induction and longer duration of remission than thioguanine alone.

b) Other Neoplasms
TABLOID brand Thioguanine is not effective in chronic lymphocytic leukemia, Hodgkin's lymphoma, multiple myeloma, or solid tumors. Although thioguanine is one of several agents with activity in the treatment of the chronic phase of chronic myelogenous leukemia, more objective responses are observed with MYLERAN® (busulfan), and therefore busulfan is usually regarded as the preferred drug.

CONTRAINDICATIONS

Thioguanine should not be used in patients whose disease has demonstrated prior resistance to this drug. In animals and humans, there is usually complete cross-resistance between PURINETHOL (mercaptopurine) and TABLOID brand Thioguanine.

WARNINGS

SINCE DRUGS USED IN CANCER CHEMOTHERAPY ARE POTENTIALLY HAZARDOUS, IT IS RECOMMENDED THAT ONLY PHYSICIANS EXPERIENCED WITH THE RISKS OF THIOGUANINE AND KNOWLEDGEABLE IN THE NATURAL HISTORY OF ACUTE NONLYMPHOCYTIC LEUKEMIAS ADMINISTER THIS DRUG.

THIOGUANINE IS NOT RECOMMENDED FOR MAINTENANCE THERAPY OR SIMILAR LONG-TERM CONTINUOUS TREATMENTS DUE TO THE HIGH RISK OF LIVER TOXICITY ASSOCIATED WITH VASCULAR ENDOTHELIAL DAMAGE (see DOSAGE AND ADMINISTRATION and ADVERSE REACTIONS). This liver toxicity has been observed in a high proportion of children receiving thioguanine as part of maintenance therapy for acute lymphoblastic leukemia and in other conditions associated with continuous use of thioguanine. This liver toxicity is particularly prevalent in males. Liver toxicity usually presents as the clinical syndrome of hepatic veno-occlusive disease (hyperbilirubinemia, tender hepatomegaly, weight gain due to fluid retention, and ascites) or with signs of portal hypertension (splenomegaly, thrombocytopenia, and oesophageal varices). Histopathological features associated with this toxicity include hepatoportal sclerosis, nodular regenerative hyperplasia, peliosis hepatitis, and periportal fibrosis.

Thioguanine therapy should be discontinued in patients with evidence of liver toxicity as reversal of signs and symptoms of liver toxicity have been reported upon withdrawal. Patients must be carefully monitored (see PRECAUTIONS, Laboratory Tests). Early indications of liver toxicity are signs associated with portal hypertension such as thrombocytopenia out of proportion with neutropenia and splenomegaly. Elevations of liver enzymes have also been reported in association with liver toxicity but do not always occur.

The most consistent, dose-related toxicity is bone marrow suppression. This may be manifested by anemia, leukopenia, thrombocytopenia, or any combination of these. Any one of these findings may also reflect progression of the underlying disease. Since thioguanine may have a delayed effect, it is important to withdraw the medication temporarily at the first sign of an abnormally large fall in any of the formed elements of the blood.

There are individuals with an inherited deficiency of the enzyme thiopurine methyltransferase (TPMT) who may be unusually sensitive to the myelosuppressive effects of thioguanine and prone to developing rapid bone marrow suppression following the initiation of treatment. Substantial dosage reductions may be required to avoid the development of life-threatening bone marrow suppression in these patients. Prescribers should be aware that some laboratories offer testing for TPMT deficiency. Since bone marrow suppression may be associated with factors other than TPMT deficiency, TPMT testing may not identify all patients at risk for severe toxicity. Therefore, close monitoring of clinical and hematologic parameters is important. Bone marrow suppression could be exacerbated by coadministration with drugs that inhibit TPMT, such as olsalazine, mesalazine, or sulphasalazine.

It is recommended that evaluation of the hemoglobin concentration or hematocrit, total white blood cell count and differential count, and quantitative platelet count be obtained frequently while the patient is on thioguanine therapy. In cases where the cause of fluctuations in the formed elements in the peripheral blood is obscure, bone marrow examination may be useful for the evaluation of marrow status. The decision to increase, decrease, continue, or discontinue a given dosage of thioguanine must be based not only on the absolute hematologic values, but also upon the rapidity with which changes are occurring. In many instances, particularly during the induction phase of acute leukemia, complete blood counts will need to be done more frequently in order to evaluate the effect of the therapy. The dosage of thioguanine may need to be reduced when this agent is combined with other drugs whose primary toxicity is myelosuppression.

Myelosuppression is often unavoidable during the induction phase of adult acute nonlymphocytic leukemias if remission induction is to be successful. Whether or not this demands modification or cessation of dosage depends both upon the response of the underlying disease and a careful consideration of supportive facilities (granulocyte and platelet transfusions) which may be available. Life-threatening infections and bleeding have been observed as consequences of thioguanine-induced granulocytopenia and thrombocytopenia.

The effect of thioguanine on the immunocompetence of patients is unknown.

Pregnancy

Pregnancy Category D. Drugs such as thioguanine are potential mutagens and teratogens. Thioguanine may cause fetal harm when administered to a pregnant woman. Thioguanine has been shown to be teratogenic in rats when given in doses 5 times the human dose. When given to the rat on the 4th and 5th days of gestation, 13% of surviving placentas did not contain fetuses, and 19% of offspring were malformed or stunted. The malformations noted included generalized edema, cranial defects, and general skeletal hypoplasia, hydrocephalus, ventral hernia, situs inversus, and incomplete development of the limbs. There are no adequate and well-controlled studies in pregnant women. If this drug is used during pregnancy, or if the patient becomes pregnant while taking the drug, the patient should be apprised of the potential hazard to the fetus. Women of childbearing potential should be advised to avoid becoming pregnant.

PRECAUTIONS

General

Although the primary toxicity of thioguanine is myelosuppression, other toxicities have occasionally been observed, particularly when thioguanine is used in combination with other cancer chemotherapeutic agents.

A few cases of jaundice have been reported in patients with leukemia receiving thioguanine. Among these were 2 adult male patients and 4 pediatric patients with acute myelogenous leukemia and an adult male with acute lymphocytic leukemia who developed hepatic veno-occlusive disease while receiving chemotherapy for their leukemia. Six patients had received cytarabine prior to treatment with thioguanine, and some were receiving other chemotherapy in addition to thioguanine when they became symptomatic. While hepatic veno-occlusive disease has not been reported in patients treated with thioguanine alone, it is recommended that thioguanine be withheld if there is evidence of toxic hepatitis or biliary stasis, and that appropriate clinical and laboratory investigations be initiated to establish the etiology of the hepatic dysfunction. Deterioration in liver function studies during thioguanine therapy should prompt discontinuation of treatment and a search for an explanation of the hepatotoxicity.

Administration of live vaccines to immunocompromised patients should be avoided.

Information for Patients

Patients should be informed that the major toxicities of thioguanine are related to myelosuppression, hepatotoxicity, and gastrointestinal toxicity. Patients should never be allowed to take the drug without medical supervision and should be advised to consult their physician if they experience fever, sore throat, jaundice, nausea, vomiting, signs of local infection, bleeding from any site, or symptoms suggestive of anemia. Women of childbearing potential should be advised to avoid becoming pregnant.

Laboratory Tests

Prescribers should be aware that some laboratories offer testing for TPMT deficiency (see WARNINGS).

It is advisable to monitor liver function tests (serum transaminases, alkaline phosphatase, bilirubin) at weekly intervals when first beginning therapy and at monthly intervals thereafter. It may be advisable to perform liver function tests more frequently in patients with known pre-existing liver disease or in patients who are receiving thioguanine and other hepatotoxic drugs. Patients should be instructed to discontinue thioguanine immediately if clinical jaundice is detected (see WARNINGS).

Drug Interactions

There is usually complete cross-resistance between PURINETHOL (mercaptopurine) and TABLOID brand Thioguanine.

As there is in vitro evidence that aminosalicylate derivatives (e.g., olsalazine, mesalazine, or sulphasalazine) inhibit the TPMT enzyme, they should be administered with caution to patients receiving concurrent thioguanine therapy (see WARNINGS).

Carcinogenesis, Mutagenesis, Impairment of Fertility

In view of its action on cellular DNA, thioguanine is potentially mutagenic and carcinogenic, and consideration should be given to the theoretical risk of carcinogenesis when thioguanine is administered (see WARNINGS).

Pregnancy

Teratogenic Effects

Pregnancy Category D. See WARNINGS section.

Nursing Mothers

It is not known whether this drug is excreted in human milk. Because of the potential for tumorigenicity shown for thioguanine, a decision should be made whether to discontinue nursing or to discontinue the drug, taking into account the importance of the drug to the mother.

Pediatric Use

See DOSAGE AND ADMINISTRATION section.

Geriatric Use

Clinical studies of thioguanine did not include sufficient numbers of subjects aged 65 and over to determine whether they respond differently from younger subjects. Other reported clinical experience has not identified differences in responses between the elderly and younger patients. In general, dose selection for an elderly patient should be cautious, usually starting at the low end of the dosing range, reflecting the greater frequency of decreased hepatic, renal, or cardiac function, and of concomitant disease or other drug therapy.

ADVERSE REACTIONS

The most frequent adverse reaction to thioguanine is myelosuppression. The induction of complete remission of acute myelogenous leukemia usually requires combination chemotherapy in dosages which produce marrow hypoplasia. Since consolidation and maintenance of remission are also effected by multiple-drug regimens whose component agents cause myelosuppression, pancytopenia is observed in nearly all patients. Dosages and schedules must be adjusted to prevent life-threatening cytopenias whenever these adverse reactions are observed.

Hyperuricemia frequently occurs in patients receiving thioguanine as a consequence of rapid cell lysis accompanying the antineoplastic effect. Adverse effects can be minimized by increased hydration, urine alkalinization, and the prophylactic administration of a xanthine oxidase inhibitor such as ZYLOPRIM® (allopurinol). Unlike PURINETHOL (mercaptopurine) and IMURAN® (azathioprine), thioguanine may be continued in the usual dosage when allopurinol is used conjointly to inhibit uric acid formation.

Less frequent adverse reactions include nausea, vomiting, anorexia, and stomatitis. Intestinal necrosis and perforation have been reported in patients who received multiple-drug chemotherapy including thioguanine.

Hepatic Effects

Liver toxicity associated with vascular endothelial damage has been reported when thioguanine is used in maintenance or similar long-term continuous therapy which is not recommended (see WARNINGS and DOSAGE AND ADMINISTRATION). This usually presents as the clinical syndrome of hepatic veno-occlusive disease (hyperbilirubinemia, tender hepatomegaly, weight gain due to fluid retention, and ascites) or signs and symptoms of portal hypertension (splenomegaly, thrombocytopenia, and esophageal varices). Elevation of liver transaminases, alkaline phosphatase, and gamma glutamyl transferase and jaundice may also occur. Histopathological features associated with this toxicity include hepatoportal sclerosis, nodular regenerative hyperplasia, peliosis hepatitis, and periportal fibrosis.

Liver toxicity during short-term cyclical therapy presents as veno-occlusive disease. Reversal of signs and symptoms of this liver toxicity has been reported upon withdrawal of short-term or long-term continuous therapy.

Centrilobular hepatic necrosis has been reported in a few cases; however, the reports are confounded by the use of high doses of thioguanine, other chemotherapeutic agents, and oral contraceptives and chronic alcohol abuse.

OVERDOSAGE

Signs and symptoms of overdosage may be immediate, such as nausea, vomiting, malaise, hypotension, and diaphoresis; or delayed, such as myelosuppression and azotemia. It is not known whether thioguanine is dialyzable. Hemodialysis is thought to be of marginal use due to the rapid intracellular incorporation of thioguanine into active metabolites with long persistence. The oral LD_{50} of thioguanine was determined to be 823 mg/kg ± 50.73 mg/kg and 740 mg/kg ± 45.24 mg/kg for male and female rats, respectively. Symptoms of overdosage may occur after a single dose of as little as 2.0 to 3.0 mg/kg thioguanine. As much as 35 mg/kg has been given in a single oral dose with reversible myelosuppression observed. There is no known pharmacologic antagonist of thioguanine. The drug should be discontinued immediately if unintended toxicity occurs during treatment. Severe hematologic toxicity may require supportive therapy with platelet transfusions for bleeding, and granulocyte transfusions and antibiotics if sepsis is documented. If a patient is seen immediately following an accidental overdosage of the drug, it may be useful to induce emesis.

DOSAGE AND ADMINISTRATION

TABLOID brand Thioguanine is administered orally. The dosage which will be tolerated and effective varies according to the stage and type of neoplastic process being treated. Because the usual therapies for adult and pediatric acute nonlymphocytic leukemias involve the use of thioguanine with other agents in combination, physicians responsible for administering these therapies should be experienced in the use of cancer chemotherapy and in the chosen protocol.

There are individuals with an inherited deficiency of the enzyme thiopurine methyltransferase (TPMT) who may be unusually sensitive to the myelosuppressive effects of thioguanine and prone to developing rapid bone marrow suppression following the initiation of treatment. Substantial dosage reductions may be required to avoid the development of life-threatening bone marrow suppression in these patients (see WARNINGS). Prescribers should be aware that some laboratories offer testing for TPMT deficiency.

Ninety-six (59%) of 163 pediatric patients with previously untreated acute nonlymphocytic leukemia obtained complete remission with a multiple-drug protocol including thioguanine, prednisone, cytarabine, cyclophosphamide, and vincristine. Remission was maintained with daily thioguanine, 4-day pulses of cytarabine and cyclophosphamide, and a single dose of vincristine every 28 days. The median duration of remission was 11.5 months.

Fifty-three percent of previously untreated adults with acute nonlymphocytic leukemias attained remission following use of the combination of thioguanine and cytarabine according to a protocol developed at The Memorial Sloan-Kettering Cancer Center. A median duration of remission of 8.8 months was achieved with the multiple-drug maintenance regimen which included thioguanine.

On those occasions when single-agent chemotherapy with thioguanine may be appropriate, the usual initial dosage for pediatric patients and adults is approximately 2 mg/kg of body weight per day. If, after 4 weeks on this dosage, there is no clinical improvement and no leukocyte or platelet depression, the dosage may be cautiously increased to 3 mg/kg/day. The total daily dose may be given at one time.

The dosage of thioguanine used does not depend on whether or not the patient is receiving ZYLOPRIM (allopurinol); **this is in contradistinction to the dosage reduction which is mandatory when PURINETHOL (mercaptopurine) or IMURAN (azathioprine) is given simultaneously with allopurinol.**

Procedures for proper handling and disposal of anticancer drugs should be considered. Several guidelines on this subject have been published.[1-8]

There is no general agreement that all of the procedures recommended in the guidelines are necessary or appropriate.

HOW SUPPLIED

Greenish-yellow, scored, round tablets containing 40 mg thioguanine, imprinted with "WELLCOME" and "U3B" on each tablet; in bottles of 25 (NDC 0173-0880-25).

Store at 15° to 25°C (59° to 77°F) in a dry place.

REFERENCES

1. ONS Clinical Practice Committee. Cancer Chemotherapy Guidelines and Recommendations for Practice. Pittsburgh, PA: Oncology Nursing Society; 1999:32-41.
2. Recommendations for the safe handling of parenteral antineoplastic drugs. Washington, DC: Division of Safety, Clinical Center Pharmacy Department and Cancer Nursing Services, National Institutes of Health and Human Services, 1992 US Dept of Health and Human Services, Public Health Service publication NIH 92-2621.
3. AMA Council on Scientific Affairs. Guidelines for handling parenteral antineoplastics. *JAMA.* 1985;253: 1590-1591.
4. National Study Commission on Cytotoxic Exposure. Recommendations for handling cytotoxic agents. 1987. Available from Louis P. Jeffrey, Chairman, National Study Commission on Cytotoxic Exposure. Massachusetts College of Pharmacy and Allied Health Sciences, 179 Longwood Avenue, Boston, MA 02115.
5. Clinical Oncological Society of Australia. Guidelines and recommendations for safe handling of antineoplastic agents. *Med J Australia.* 1983;1:426-428.
6. Jones RB, Frank R, Mass T. Safe handling of chemotherapeutic agents: a report from the Mount Sinai Medical Center. *CA-A Cancer J for Clin.* 1983;33:258-263.
7. American Society of Hospital Pharmacists. ASHP technical assistance bulletin on handling cytotoxic and hazardous drugs. *Am J Hosp Pharm.* 1990;47:1033-1049.
8. Controlling Occupational Exposure to Hazardous Drugs. (OSHA Work-Practice Guidelines.) *Am J Health-Syst Pharm.* 1996;53:1669-1685.

TABLOID and MYLERAN are registered trademarks of GlaxoSmithKline. The following are registered trademarks of their respective owners: PURINETHOL/Teva Pharmaceutical Works; ZYLOPRIM and IMURAN/Promethius Laboratories Inc.

Manufactured by
DSM Pharmaceuticals, Inc.
Greenville, NC 27834
for GlaxoSmithKline
Research Triangle Park, NC 27709
©2009, GlaxoSmithKline. All rights reserved.
June 2009 TBL:1PI

TIMENTIN® ℞

[tī-měn'tin]
**(sterile ticarcillin disodium
and clavulanate potassium)
for Intravenous Administration**

To reduce the development of drug-resistant bacteria and maintain the effectiveness of TIMENTIN (ticarcillin disodium and clavulanate potassium) and other antibacterial drugs, TIMENTIN should be used only to treat or prevent infections that are proven or strongly suspected to be caused by bacteria.

DESCRIPTION

TIMENTIN is a sterile injectable antibacterial combination consisting of the semisynthetic antibiotic ticarcillin disodium and the β-lactamase inhibitor clavulanate potassium (the potassium salt of clavulanic acid) for intravenous administration. Ticarcillin is derived from the basic penicillin nucleus, 6-amino-penicillanic acid.

Chemically, ticarcillin disodium is *N*-(2-Carboxy-3,3-dimethyl-7-oxo-4-thia-1-azabicyclo[3.2.0]hept-6-yl)-3-thiophenemalonamic acid disodium salt and may be represented as:

Clavulanic acid is produced by the fermentation of *Streptomyces clavuligerus*. It is a β-lactam structurally re-

SERUM LEVELS IN ADULTS AFTER A 30-MINUTE IV INFUSION OF TIMENTIN®

TICARCILLIN SERUM LEVELS (mcg/mL)

Dose	0	15 min.	30 min.	1 hr.	1.5 hr.	3.5 hr.	5.5 hr.
3.1 gram	324	223	176	131	90	27	6
	(293 to 388)	(184 to 293)	(135 to 235)	(102 to 195)	(65 to 119)	(19 to 37)	(5 to 7)

CLAVULANIC ACID SERUM LEVELS (mcg/mL)

Dose	0	15 min.	30 min.	1 hr.	1.5 hr.	3.5 hr.	5.5 hr.
3.1 gram	8.0	4.6	2.6	1.8	1.2	0.3	0
	(5.3 to 10.3)	(3.0 to 7.6)	(1.8 to 3.4)	(1.6 to 2.2)	(0.8 to 1.6)	(0.2 to 0.3)	

lated to the penicillins and possesses the ability to inactivate a wide variety of β-lactamases by blocking the active sites of these enzymes. Clavulanic acid is particularly active against the clinically important plasmid-mediated β-lactamases frequently responsible for transferred drug resistance to penicillins and cephalosporins.

Chemically, clavulanate potassium is potassium (*Z*)-(2*R*,5*R*)-3-(2-hydroxyethylidene)-7-oxo-4-oxa-1-azabicyclo [3.2.0]heptane-2-carboxylate and may be represented structurally as:

TIMENTIN is supplied as a white to pale yellow powder for reconstitution. TIMENTIN is very soluble in water, its solubility being greater than 600 mg/mL. The reconstituted solution is clear, colorless or pale yellow, having a pH of 5.5 to 7.5.

For the 3.1-gram dosage of TIMENTIN, the theoretical sodium content is 4.51 mEq (103.6 mg) per gram of TIMENTIN. The theoretical potassium content is 0.15 mEq (6 mg) per gram of TIMENTIN.

CLINICAL PHARMACOLOGY

After an intravenous infusion (30 min.) of 3.1 grams of TIMENTIN, peak serum concentrations of both ticarcillin and clavulanic acid are attained immediately after completion of infusion. Ticarcillin serum levels are similar to those produced by the administration of equivalent amounts of ticarcillin alone with a mean peak serum level of 330 mcg/mL. The corresponding mean peak serum level for clavulanic acid is 8 mcg/mL. (See following table.)

[See table above]

The mean area under the serum concentration curve was 485 mcg•hr/mL for ticarcillin and 8.2 mcg•hr/mL for clavulanic acid.

The mean serum half-lives of ticarcillin and clavulanic acid in healthy volunteers are 1.1 hours and 1.1 hours, respectively.

In pediatric patients receiving approximately 50 mg/kg of TIMENTIN (30:1 ratio ticarcillin to clavulanate), mean ticarcillin serum half-lives were 4.4 hours in neonates (n = 18) and 1.0 hour in infants and children (n = 41). The corresponding clavulanate serum half-lives averaged 1.9 hours in neonates (n = 14) and 0.9 hour in infants and children (n = 40). Area under the serum concentration time curves averaged 339 mcg•hr/mL in infants and children (n = 41), whereas the corresponding mean clavulanate area under the serum concentration time curves was approximately 7 mcg•hr/mL in the same population (n = 40).

Approximately 60% to 70% of ticarcillin and approximately 35% to 45% of clavulanic acid are excreted unchanged in urine during the first 6 hours after administration of a single dose of TIMENTIN to normal volunteers with normal renal function. Two hours after an intravenous injection of 3.1 grams of TIMENTIN, concentrations of ticarcillin in urine generally exceed 1,500 mcg/mL. The corresponding concentrations of clavulanic acid in urine generally exceed 40 mcg/mL. By 4 to 6 hours after injection, the urine concentrations of ticarcillin and clavulanic acid usually decline to approximately 190 mcg/mL and 2 mcg/mL, respectively. Neither component of TIMENTIN is highly protein bound; ticarcillin has been found to be approximately 45% bound to human serum protein and clavulanic acid approximately 25% bound.

Somewhat higher and more prolonged serum levels of ticarcillin can be achieved with the concurrent administration of probenecid; however, probenecid does not enhance the serum levels of clavulanic acid.

Ticarcillin can be detected in tissues and interstitial fluid following parenteral administration.

Penetration of ticarcillin into bile and pleural fluid has been demonstrated. The results of experiments involving the administration of clavulanic acid to animals suggest that this compound, like ticarcillin, is well distributed in body tissues.

An inverse relationship exists between the serum half-life of ticarcillin and creatinine clearance. The dosage of TIMENTIN need only be adjusted in cases of severe renal impairment. (See DOSAGE AND ADMINISTRATION.)

Ticarcillin may be removed from patients undergoing dialysis; the actual amount removed depends on the duration and type of dialysis.

Microbiology: Ticarcillin is a semisynthetic antibiotic with a broad spectrum of bactericidal activity against many gram-positive and gram-negative aerobic and anaerobic bacteria.

Ticarcillin is, however, susceptible to degradation by β-lactamases, and therefore, the spectrum of activity does not normally include organisms which produce these enzymes.

Clavulanic acid is a β-lactam, structurally related to the penicillins, which possesses the ability to inactivate a wide range of β-lactamase enzymes commonly found in microorganisms resistant to penicillins and cephalosporins. In particular, it has good activity against the clinically important plasmid-mediated β-lactamases frequently responsible for transferred drug resistance.

The formulation of ticarcillin with clavulanic acid in TIMENTIN protects ticarcillin from degradation by β-lactamase enzymes and effectively extends the antibiotic spectrum of ticarcillin to include many bacteria normally resistant to ticarcillin and other β-lactam antibiotics. Thus, TIMENTIN possesses the distinctive properties of a broad-spectrum antibiotic and a β-lactamase inhibitor. Ticarcillin/clavulanic acid has been shown to be active against most strains of the following microorganisms, both in vitro and in clinical infections as described in the INDICATIONS AND USAGE section.

Gram-Positive Aerobes:
Staphylococcus aureus (β-lactamase and non–β-lactamase–producing)*
Staphylococcus epidermidis (β-lactamase and non–β-lactamase–producing)*
*Staphylococci that are resistant to methicillin/oxacillin must be considered resistant to ticarcillin/clavulanic acid.

Gram-Negative Aerobes:
Citrobacter species (β-lactamase and non–β-lactamase–producing)
Enterobacter species including *E. cloacae* (β-lactamase and non–β-lactamase–producing)
(Although most strains of *Enterobacter* species are resistant in vitro, clinical efficacy has been demonstrated with TIMENTIN in urinary tract infections and gynecologic infections caused by these organisms.)
Escherichia coli (β-lactamase and non–β-lactamase–producing)
Haemophilus influenzae (β-lactamase and non–β-lactamase–producing)†
Klebsiella species including *K. pneumoniae* (β-lactamase and non–β-lactamase–producing)
Pseudomonas species including *P. aeruginosa* (β-lactamase and non–β-lactamase–producing)
Serratia marcescens (β-lactamase and non–β-lactamase–producing)
† β-lactamase–negative, ampicillin-resistant (BLNAR) strains of *H. influenzae* must be considered resistant to ticarcillin/clavulanic acid.

Anaerobic Bacteria:
Bacteroides fragilis group (β-lactamase and non–β-lactamase–producing)
Prevotella (formerly *Bacteroides*) *melaninogenicus* (β-lactamase and non–β-lactamase–producing)
The following in vitro data are available, **but their clinical significance is unknown.**
The following strains exhibit an in vitro minimum inhibitory concentration (MIC) less than or equal to the susceptible breakpoint for ticarcillin/clavulanic acid. However, with the exception of organisms shown to respond to ticarcillin alone, the safety and effectiveness of ticarcillin/clavulanic acid in treating infections due to these microorganisms have not been established in adequate and well-controlled clinical trials.

Gram-Positive Aerobes:
Staphylococcus saprophyticus (β-lactamase and non–β-lactamase–producing)

Streptococcus agalactiae[‡] (Group B)
Streptococcus bovis[‡]
Streptococcus pneumoniae[‡] (penicillin-susceptible strains only)
Streptococcus pyogenes[‡]
Viridans group streptococci[‡]

Gram-Negative Aerobes:
Acinetobacter baumannii (β-lactamase and non–β-lactamase–producing)
Acinetobacter calcoaceticus (β-lactamase and non–β-lactamase–producing)
Acinetobacter haemolyticus (β-lactamase and non–β-lactamase–producing)
Acinetobacter lwoffi (β-lactamase and non–β-lactamase–producing)
Moraxella catarrhalis (β-lactamase and non–β-lactamase–producing)
Morganella morganii (β-lactamase and non–β-lactamase–producing)
Neisseria gonorrhoeae (β-lactamase and non–β-lactamase–producing)
Pasteurella multocida (β-lactamase and non–β-lactamase–producing)
Proteus mirabilis (β-lactamase and non–β-lactamase–producing)
Proteus penneri (β-lactamase and non–β-lactamase–producing)
Proteus vulgaris (β-lactamase and non–β-lactamase–producing)
Providencia rettgeri (β-lactamase and non–β-lactamase–producing)
Providencia stuartii (β-lactamase and non–β-lactamase–producing)
Stenotrophomonas maltophilia (β-lactamase and non–β-lactamase–producing)

Anaerobic Bacteria:
Clostridium species including *C. perfringens, C. difficile, C. sporogenes, C. ramosum,* and *C. bifermentans* (β-lactamase and non–β-lactamase–producing)
Eubacterium species
Fusobacterium species including *F. nucleatum* and *F. necrophorum* (β-lactamase and non–β-lactamase–producing)
Peptostreptococcus species[‡]
Veillonella species[‡]

[‡]These are non–β-lactamase–producing strains, and therefore, are susceptible to ticarcillin.

In vitro synergism between TIMENTIN and gentamicin, tobramycin, or amikacin against multiresistant strains of *Pseudomonas aeruginosa* has been demonstrated.

Susceptibility Testing: *Dilution Techniques:* Quantitative methods are used to determine antimicrobial MICs. These MICs provide estimates of the susceptibility of bacteria to antimicrobial compounds. The MICs should be determined using a standardized procedure. Standardized procedures are based on a dilution method[1,3] (broth or agar) or equivalent with standardized inoculum concentrations and standardized concentrations of ticarcillin/clavulanate potassium powder.

The recommended dilution pattern utilizes a constant level of 2 mcg/mL clavulanic acid in all tubes with varying amounts of ticarcillin. MICs are expressed in terms of the ticarcillin concentration in the presence of clavulanic acid at a constant 2 mcg/mL. The MIC values should be interpreted according to the following criteria:

RECOMMENDED RANGES FOR TICARCILLIN/ CLAVULANIC ACID SUSCEPTIBILITY TESTING*

For *Pseudomonas aeruginosa:*

MIC (mcg/mL)	Interpretation	
≤64	Susceptible	(S)
≥128	Resistant	(R)

For Enterobacteriaceae:

MIC (mcg/mL)	Interpretation	
≤16	Susceptible	(S)
32-64	Intermediate	(I)
≥128	Resistant	(R)

For Staphylococci[†]:

MIC (mcg/mL)	Interpretation	
≤8	Susceptible	(S)
≥16	Resistant	(R)

* Expressed as concentration of ticarcillin in the presence of clavulanic acid at a constant 2 mcg/mL.
[†] Staphylococci that are susceptible to ticarcillin/ clavulanic acid but resistant to methicillin/oxacillin must be considered as resistant.

A report of "Susceptible" indicates that the pathogen is likely to be inhibited if the antimicrobial compound in the blood reaches the concentrations usually achievable. A report of "Intermediate" indicates that the result should be considered equivocal, and, if the microorganism is not fully susceptible to alternative, clinically feasible drugs, the test should be repeated. This category implies possible clinical applicability in body sites where the drug is physiologically concentrated or in situations where high dosage of drug can be used. This category also provides a buffer zone that prevents small uncontrolled technical factors from causing major discrepancies in interpretation. A report of "Resistant" indicates that the pathogen is not likely to be inhibited if the antimicrobial compound in the blood reaches the concentrations usually achievable; other therapy should be selected.

Standardized susceptibility test procedures require the use of laboratory control microorganisms to control the technical aspects of the laboratory procedures. Standard ticarcillin/clavulanate potassium powder should provide the following MIC values:

Microorganism		MIC (mcg/mL)[‡]
Escherichia coli	ATCC 25922	4-16
Escherichia coli	ATCC 35218	4-16
Pseudomonas aeruginosa	ATCC 27853	8-32
Staphylococcus aureus	ATCC 29213	0.5-2

[‡] Expressed as concentration of ticarcillin in the presence of clavulanic acid at a constant 2 mcg/mL.

Diffusion Techniques: Quantitative methods that require measurement of zone diameters also provide reproducible estimates of the susceptibility of bacteria to antimicrobial compounds. One such standardized procedure[2,3] requires the use of standardized inoculum concentrations. This procedure uses paper disks impregnated with 85 mcg of ticarcillin/clavulanate potassium (75 mcg ticarcillin plus 10 mcg clavulanate potassium) to test the susceptibility of microorganisms to ticarcillin/clavulanic acid.

Reports from the laboratory providing results of the standard single-disk susceptibility test with an 85 mcg of ticarcillin/clavulanate potassium (75 mcg ticarcillin plus 10 mcg clavulanate potassium) disk should be interpreted according to the following criteria:

RECOMMENDED RANGES FOR TICARCILLIN/ CLAVULANIC ACID SUSCEPTIBILITY TESTING

For *Pseudomonas aeruginosa:*

Zone Diameter (mm)	Interpretation	
≥15	Susceptible	(S)
≤14	Resistant	(R)

For Enterobacteriaceae:

Zone Diameter (mm)	Interpretation	
≥20	Susceptible	(S)
15-19	Intermediate	(I)
≤14	Resistant	(R)

For Staphylococci[§]:

Zone Diameter (mm)	Interpretation	
≥23	Susceptible	(S)
≤22	Resistant	(R)

[§] Staphylococci that are resistant to methicillin/oxacillin must be considered as resistant to ticarcillin/clavulanic acid.

Interpretation should be as stated above for results using dilution techniques. Interpretation involves correlation of the diameter obtained in the disk test with the MIC for ticarcillin/clavulanic acid.

As with standardized dilution techniques, diffusion methods require the use of laboratory control microorganisms that are used to control the technical aspects of the laboratory procedures. For the diffusion technique, the 85 mcg of ticarcillin/clavulanate potassium (75 mcg ticarcillin plus 10 mcg clavulanate potassium) disk should provide the following zone diameters in these laboratory test quality control strains:

Microorganism		Zone Diameter (mm)
Escherichia coli	ATCC 25922	24-30
Escherichia coli	ATCC 35218	21-25
Pseudomonas aeruginosa	ATCC 27853	20-28
Staphylococcus aureus	ATCC 25923	29-37

Anaerobic Techniques: For anaerobic bacteria, the susceptibility to ticarcillin/clavulanic acid can be determined by standardized test methods[3,4]. The MIC values obtained should be interpreted according to the following criteria:

Microorganism		Agar dilution MIC Range (mcg/mL)[‖]	Broth microdilution MIC Range (mcg/mL)[‖]
Bacteroides thetaiotaomicron	ATCC 29741	0.5-2	0.5-2
Eubacterium lentum	ATCC 43055	16-64	8-32

[‖] Expressed as concentration of ticarcillin in the presence of clavulanic acid at a constant 2 mcg/mL.

RECOMMENDED RANGES FOR TICARCILLIN/ CLAVULANIC ACID SUSCEPTIBILITY TESTING[‖]

MIC (mcg/mL)	Interpretation	
≤32	Susceptible	(S)
64	Intermediate	(I)
≥128	Resistant	(R)

[‖] Expressed as concentration of ticarcillin in the presence of clavulanic acid at a constant 2 mcg/mL.

Interpretation is identical to that stated above for results using dilution techniques.

As with other susceptibility techniques, the use of laboratory control microorganisms is required to control the technical aspects of the laboratory standardized procedures. Standardized ticarcillin/clavulanate potassium powder should provide the following MIC values:

[See table above]

INDICATIONS AND USAGE

TIMENTIN is indicated in the treatment of infections caused by susceptible strains of the designated microorganisms in the conditions listed below:

Septicemia (including bacteremia) caused by β-lactamase–producing strains of *Klebsiella* spp.*, *E. coli**, *S. aureus**, or *P. aeruginosa** (or other *Pseudomonas* species*)

Lower Respiratory Infections caused by β-lactamase–producing strains of *S. aureus*, *H. influenzae**, or *Klebsiella* spp.*

Bone and Joint Infections caused by β-lactamase–producing strains of *S. aureus*

Skin and Skin Structure Infections caused by β-lactamase–producing strains of *S. aureus*, *Klebsiella* spp.*, or *E. coli**

Urinary Tract Infections (complicated and uncomplicated) caused by β-lactamase–producing strains of *E. coli*, *Klebsiella* spp., *P. aeruginosa** (or other *Pseudomonas* spp.*), *Citrobacter* spp.*, *Enterobacter cloacae**, *S. marcescens**, or *S. aureus**

Gynecologic Infections endometritis caused by β-lactamase–producing strains of *P. melaninogenicus**, *Enterobacter* spp. (including *E. cloacae**), *E. coli*, *K. pneumoniae**, *S. aureus*, or *S. epidermidis*

Intra-abdominal Infections peritonitis caused by β-lactamase–producing strains of *E. coli*, *K. pneumoniae*, or *B. fragilis** group

*Efficacy for this organism in this organ system was studied in fewer than 10 infections.

NOTE: For information on use in pediatric patients (≥3 months of age) see PRECAUTIONS—Pediatric Use and CLINICAL STUDIES sections. There are insufficient data to support the use of TIMENTIN in pediatric patients under 3 months of age or for the treatment of septicemia and/or infections in the pediatric population where the suspected or proven pathogen is *H. influenzae* type b.

While TIMENTIN is indicated only for the conditions listed above, infections caused by ticarcillin-susceptible organisms are also amenable to treatment with TIMENTIN due to its ticarcillin content. Therefore, mixed infections caused by ticarcillin-susceptible organisms and β-lactamase–producing organisms susceptible to ticarcillin/clavulanic acid should not require the addition of another antibiotic.

Appropriate culture and susceptibility tests should be performed before treatment in order to isolate and identify organisms causing infection and to determine their susceptibility to ticarcillin/clavulanic acid. Because of its broad spectrum of bactericidal activity against gram-positive and gram-negative bacteria, TIMENTIN is particularly useful for the treatment of mixed infections and for presumptive therapy prior to the identification of the causative organisms. TIMENTIN has been shown to be effective as single drug therapy in the treatment of some serious infections where normally combination antibiotic therapy might be employed. Therapy with TIMENTIN may be initiated before results of such tests are known when there is reason to believe the infection may involve any of the β-lactamase–producing organisms listed above.

Based on in vitro synergism between ticarcillin/clavulanic acid and aminoglycosides against certain strains of *P. aeruginosa*, combined therapy has been successful, especially in patients with impaired host defenses. Both drugs should be used in full therapeutic doses.

To reduce the development of drug-resistant bacteria and maintain the effectiveness of TIMENTIN and other antibacterial drugs, TIMENTIN should be used only to treat or prevent infections that are proven or strongly suspected to be caused by susceptible bacteria. When culture and susceptibility information are available, they should be considered in selecting or modifying antibacterial therapy. In the absence of such data, local epidemiology and susceptibility patterns may contribute to the empiric selection of therapy.

CONTRAINDICATIONS

TIMENTIN is contraindicated in patients with a history of hypersensitivity reactions to any of the penicillins.

WARNINGS

SERIOUS AND OCCASIONALLY FATAL HYPERSENSITIVITY (ANAPHYLACTIC) REACTIONS HAVE BEEN REPORTED IN PATIENTS ON PENICILLIN THERAPY. THESE REACTIONS ARE MORE LIKELY TO OCCUR IN INDIVIDUALS WITH A HISTORY OF PENICILLIN HYPERSENSITIVITY AND/OR A HISTORY OF SENSITIVITY TO MULTIPLE ALLERGENS. THERE HAVE BEEN REPORTS OF INDIVIDUALS WITH A HISTORY OF PENICILLIN HYPERSENSITIVITY WHO HAVE EXPERIENCED SEVERE REACTIONS WHEN TREATED WITH CEPHALOSPORINS. BEFORE INITIATING THERAPY WITH TIMENTIN, CAREFUL INQUIRY SHOULD BE MADE CONCERNING PREVIOUS HYPERSENSITIVITY REACTIONS TO PENICILLINS, CEPHALOSPORINS, OR OTHER ALLERGENS. IF AN ALLERGIC REACTION OCCURS, TIMENTIN SHOULD BE DISCONTINUED AND THE APPROPRIATE THERAPY INSTITUTED. SERIOUS ANAPHYLACTIC REACTIONS REQUIRE IMMEDIATE EMERGENCY TREATMENT WITH EPINEPHRINE. OXYGEN, INTRAVENOUS STEROIDS, AND AIRWAY MANAGEMENT, INCLUDING INTUBATION, SHOULD ALSO BE PROVIDED AS INDICATED.

Clostridium difficile associated diarrhea (CDAD) has been reported with use of nearly all antibacterial agents, including TIMENTIN, and may range in severity from mild diarrhea to fatal colitis. Treatment with antibacterial agents alters the normal flora of the colon leading to overgrowth of *C. difficile*.

C. difficile produces toxins A and B which contribute to the development of CDAD. Hypertoxin producing strains of *C. difficile* cause increased morbidity and mortality, as these infections can be refractory to antimicrobial therapy and may require colectomy. CDAD must be considered in all patients who present with diarrhea following antibiotic use. Careful medical history is necessary since CDAD has been reported to occur over two months after the administration of antibacterial agents.

If CDAD is suspected or confirmed, ongoing antibiotic use not directed against *C. difficile* may need to be discontinued. Appropriate fluid and electrolyte management, protein supplementation, antibiotic treatment of *C. difficile*, and surgical evaluation should be instituted as clinically indicated.

When very high doses of TIMENTIN are administered, especially in the presence of impaired renal function, patients may experience convulsions. (See ADVERSE REACTIONS and OVERDOSAGE.)

PRECAUTIONS

General: While TIMENTIN possesses the characteristic low toxicity of the penicillin group of antibiotics, periodic assessment of organ system functions, including renal, hepatic, and hematopoietic function, is advisable during prolonged therapy.

Bleeding manifestations have occurred in some patients receiving β-lactam antibiotics. These reactions have been associated with abnormalities of coagulation tests such as clotting time, platelet aggregation, and prothrombin time and are more likely to occur in patients with renal impairment. If bleeding manifestations appear, treatment with TIMENTIN should be discontinued and appropriate therapy instituted.

TIMENTIN has only rarely been reported to cause hypokalemia; however, the possibility of this occurring should be kept in mind particularly when treating patients with fluid and electrolyte imbalance. Periodic monitoring of serum potassium may be advisable in patients receiving prolonged therapy.

The theoretical sodium content is 4.51 mEq (103.6 mg) per gram of TIMENTIN. This should be considered when treating patients requiring restricted salt intake.

As with any penicillin, an allergic reaction, including anaphylaxis, may occur during administration of TIMENTIN, particularly in a hypersensitive individual.

The possibility of superinfections with mycotic or bacterial pathogens should be kept in mind, particularly during prolonged treatment. If superinfections occur, appropriate measures should be taken.

Prescribing TIMENTIN in the absence of a proven or strongly suspected bacterial infection or a prophylactic indication is unlikely to provide benefit to the patient and increases the risk of the development of drug-resistant bacteria.

Information for Patients: Patients should be counseled that antibacterial drugs, including TIMENTIN, should only be used to treat bacterial infections. They do not treat viral infections (e.g., the common cold). When TIMENTIN is prescribed to treat a bacterial infection, patients should be told that although it is common to feel better early in the course of therapy, the medication should be taken exactly as directed. Skipping doses or not completing the full course of therapy may: (1) decrease the effectiveness of the immediate treatment, and (2) increase the likelihood that bacteria will develop resistance and will not be treatable by TIMENTIN or other antibacterial drugs in the future.

Diarrhea is a common problem caused by antibiotics which usually ends when the antibiotic is discontinued. Sometimes after starting treatment with antibiotics, patients can develop watery and bloody stools (with or without stomach cramps and fever) even as late as 2 or more months after having taken the last dose of the antibiotic. If this occurs, patients should contact their physician as soon as possible.

Drug/Laboratory Test Interactions: As with other penicillins, the mixing of TIMENTIN with an aminoglycoside in solutions for parenteral administration can result in substantial inactivation of the aminoglycoside.

Probenecid interferes with the renal tubular secretion of ticarcillin, thereby increasing serum concentrations and prolonging serum half-life of the antibiotic.

In common with other antibiotics, ticarcillin disodium/clavulanate potassium may affect the gut flora, leading to lower estrogen reabsorption and reduced efficacy of combined oral estrogen/progesterone contraceptives.

High urine concentrations of ticarcillin may produce false-positive protein reactions (pseudoproteinuria) with the following methods: Sulfosalicylic acid and boiling test, acetic acid test, biuret reaction, and nitric acid test. The bromphenol blue (MULTI-STIX®) reagent strip test has been reported to be reliable.

The presence of clavulanic acid in TIMENTIN may cause a nonspecific binding of IgG and albumin by red cell membranes leading to a false-positive Coombs test.

Carcinogenesis, Mutagenesis, Impairment of Fertility: Long-term studies in animals have not been performed to evaluate carcinogenic potential. However, results from assays for gene mutation in vitro using bacteria (Ames tests) and yeast, and for chromosomal effects in vitro in human lymphocytes, and in vivo in mouse bone marrow (micronucleus test) indicate that TIMENTIN is without any mutagenic potential.

Pregnancy (Category B): Reproduction studies have been performed in rats given doses up to 1,050 mg/kg/day and have revealed no evidence of impaired fertility or harm to the fetus due to TIMENTIN. There are, however, no adequate and well-controlled studies in pregnant women. Because animal reproduction studies are not always predictive of human response, this drug should be used during pregnancy only if clearly needed.

Nursing Mothers: It is not known whether this drug is excreted in human milk. Because many drugs are excreted in human milk, caution should be exercised when TIMENTIN is administered to a nursing woman.

Pediatric Use: The safety and effectiveness of TIMENTIN have been established in the age group of 3 months to 16 years. Use of TIMENTIN in these age groups is supported by evidence from adequate and well-controlled studies of TIMENTIN in adults with additional efficacy, safety, and pharmacokinetic data from both comparative and noncomparative studies in pediatric patients. There are insufficient data to support the use of TIMENTIN in pediatric patients under 3 months of age or for the treatment of septicemia and/or infections in the pediatric population where the suspected or proven pathogen is *H. influenzae* type b.

In those patients in whom meningeal seeding from a distant infection site or in whom meningitis is suspected or documented, or in patients who require prophylaxis against central nervous system infection, an alternate agent with demonstrated clinical efficacy in this setting should be used.

Geriatric Use: An analysis of clinical studies of TIMENTIN was conducted to determine whether subjects aged 65 and over respond differently from younger subjects. Of the 1,078 subjects treated with at least one dose of TIMENTIN, 67.5% were <65 years old, and 32.5% were ≥65 years old. No overall differences in safety or efficacy were observed between these subjects and younger subjects, and other reported clinical experience have not identified differences in responses between the elderly and younger patients, but a greater sensitivity of some older individuals cannot be ruled out.

This drug is known to be substantially excreted by the kidney, and the risk of toxic reactions to this drug may be greater in patients with impaired renal function. Because elderly patients are more likely to have decreased renal function, care should be taken in dose selection, and it may be useful to monitor renal function (see DOSAGE and ADMINISTRATION).

TIMENTIN contains 103.6 mg (4.51 mEq) of sodium per gram of TIMENTIN. At the usual recommended doses, patients would receive between 1,285 and 1,927 mg/day (56 and 84 mEq) of sodium. The geriatric population may respond with a blunted natriuresis to salt loading. This may be clinically important with regard to such diseases as congestive heart failure.

ADVERSE REACTIONS

As with other penicillins, the following adverse reactions may occur:

Hypersensitivity Reactions: Skin rash, pruritus, urticaria, arthralgia, myalgia, drug fever, chills, chest discomfort, erythema multiforme, toxic epidermal necrolysis, Stevens-Johnson syndrome, and anaphylactic reactions.

Central Nervous System: Headache, giddiness, neuromuscular hyperirritability, or convulsive seizures.

Gastrointestinal Disturbances: Disturbances of taste and smell, stomatitis, flatulence, nausea, vomiting and diarrhea, epigastric pain, and pseudomembranous colitis have been reported. Onset of pseudomembranous colitis symptoms may occur during or after antibiotic treatment. (See WARNINGS.)

Hemic and Lymphatic Systems: Thrombocytopenia, leukopenia, neutropenia, eosinophilia, reduction of hemoglobin or hematocrit, and prolongation of prothrombin time and bleeding time.

Abnormalities of Hepatic Function Tests: Elevation of serum aspartate aminotransferase (SGOT), serum alanine aminotransferase (SGPT), serum alkaline phosphatase, serum LDH, serum bilirubin. There have been reports of transient hepatitis and cholestatic jaundice—as with some other penicillins and some cephalosporins.

Renal and Urinary Effects: Elevation of serum creatinine and/or BUN, hypernatremia, reduction in serum potassium, and uric acid. Rare reports of hemorrhagic cystitis.

Local Reactions: Pain, burning, swelling, and induration at the injection site and thrombophlebitis with intravenous administration.

Available safety data for pediatric patients treated with TIMENTIN demonstrate a similar adverse event profile to that observed in adult patients.

DRUG ABUSE AND DEPENDENCE

Neither abuse of nor dependence on TIMENTIN has been reported.

OVERDOSAGE

As with other penicillins, neurotoxic reactions may arise when very high doses of TIMENTIN are administered, especially in patients with impaired renal function. (See WARNINGS and ADVERSE REACTIONS — Central Nervous System.)

In case of overdosage, discontinue TIMENTIN, treat symptomatically, and institute supportive measures as required. Ticarcillin may be removed from circulation by hemodialysis. The molecular weight, degree of protein binding, and pharmacokinetic profile of clavulanic acid together with information from a single patient with renal insufficiency all suggest that this compound may also be removed by hemodialysis.

DOSAGE AND ADMINISTRATION

TIMENTIN should be administered by intravenous infusion (30 min.).

Adults: The usual recommended dosage for systemic and urinary tract infections for average (60 kg) adults is 3.1 grams of TIMENTIN (3.1-gram vial containing 3 grams ticarcillin and 100 mg clavulanic acid) given every 4 to 6 hours. For gynecologic infections, TIMENTIN should be administered as follows: Moderate infections, 200 mg/kg/day in divided doses every 6 hours, and for severe infections, 300 mg/kg/day in divided doses every 4 hours. For patients weighing less than 60 kg, the recommended dosage is 200 to 300 mg/kg/day, based on ticarcillin content, given in divided doses every 4 to 6 hours.

Pediatric Patients (≥3 months): *For patients <60 kg:* In patients <60 kg, TIMENTIN is dosed at 50 mg/kg/dose based on the ticarcillin component. TIMENTIN should be administered as follows: Mild to moderate infections, 200 mg/kg/day in divided doses every 6 hours; for severe infections, 300 mg/kg/day in divided doses every 4 hours.

For patients ≥60 kg: For mild to moderate infections, 3.1 grams of TIMENTIN (3 grams of ticarcillin and 100 mg of clavulanic acid) administered every 6 hours; for severe infections, 3.1 grams every 4 hours.

Renal Impairment: For infections complicated by renal insufficiency†, an initial loading dose of 3.1 grams should be followed by doses based on creatinine clearance and type of dialysis as indicated below:

[See first table at top of next page]

†The half-life of ticarcillin in patients with renal failure is approximately 13 hours.

Dosage for any individual patient must take into consideration the site and severity of infection, the susceptibility of the organisms causing infection, and the status of the patient's host defense mechanisms.

The duration of therapy depends upon the severity of infection. Generally, TIMENTIN should be continued for at least 2 days after the signs and symptoms of infection have disappeared. The usual duration is 10 to 14 days; however, in difficult and complicated infections, more prolonged therapy may be required.

Frequent bacteriologic and clinical appraisals are necessary during therapy of chronic urinary tract infection and may be required for several months after therapy has been completed. Persistent infections may require treatment for several weeks, and doses smaller than those indicated above should not be used.

In certain infections, involving abscess formation, appropriate surgical drainage should be performed in conjunction with antimicrobial therapy.

INTRAVENOUS ADMINISTRATION
DIRECTIONS FOR USE
3.1-gram Vials

The 3.1-gram vial should be reconstituted by adding approximately 13 mL of Sterile Water for Injection, USP, or Sodium Chloride Injection, USP, and shaking well. When dissolved, the concentration of ticarcillin will be approximately 200 mg/mL with a corresponding concentration of 6.7 mg/mL for clavulanic acid. Conversely, each 5.0 mL of the 3.1-gram dose reconstituted with approximately 13 mL of diluent will contain approximately 1 gram of ticarcillin and 33 mg of clavulanic acid.

Intravenous Infusion: The dissolved drug should be further diluted to desired volume using the recommended solution listed in the COMPATIBILITY AND STABILITY Section (STABILITY PERIOD) to a concentration between 10 mg/mL to 100 mg/mL. The solution of reconstituted drug may then be administered over a period of 30 minutes by direct infusion or through a Y-type intravenous infusion set. If this method of administration is used, it is advisable to discontinue temporarily the administration of any other solutions during the infusion of TIMENTIN.

Stability: For I.V. solutions, see STABILITY PERIOD below.

When TIMENTIN is given in combination with another antimicrobial, such as an aminoglycoside, each drug should be given separately in accordance with the recommended dosage and routes of administration for each drug.

After reconstitution and prior to administration, TIMENTIN, as with other parenteral drugs, should be inspected visually for particulate matter. If this condition is evident, the solution should be discarded.

The color of reconstituted solutions of TIMENTIN normally ranges from light to dark yellow, depending on concentration, duration, and temperature of storage while maintaining label claim characteristics.

COMPATIBILITY AND STABILITY
3.1-gram Vials
(Dilutions derived from a stock solution of 200 mg/mL)

The concentrated stock solution at 200 mg/mL is stable for up to 6 hours at room temperature 21° to 24°C (70° to 75°F) or up to 72 hours under refrigeration 4°C (40°F).

If the concentrated stock solution (200 mg/mL) is held for up to 6 hours at room temperature 21° to 24°C (70° to 75°F) or up to 72 hours under refrigeration 4°C (40°F) and further diluted to a concentration between 10 mg/mL and 100 mg/mL with any of the diluents listed below, then the following stability periods apply.

[See second table above]

If the concentrated stock solution (200 mg/mL) is stored for up to 6 hours at room temperature and then further diluted to a concentration between 10 mg/mL and 100 mg/mL, solutions of Sodium Chloride Injection, USP, and Lactated Ringer's Injection, USP, may be stored frozen −18°C (0°F) for up to 30 days. Solutions prepared with Dextrose Injection 5%, USP, may be stored frozen −18°C (0°F) for up to 7 days. All thawed solutions should be used within 8 hours or discarded. Once thawed, solutions should not be refrozen.

NOTE: TIMENTIN is incompatible with Sodium Bicarbonate.

Unused solutions must be discarded after the time periods listed above.

HOW SUPPLIED

Each 3.1-gram vial of TIMENTIN contains sterile ticarcillin disodium equivalent to 3 grams ticarcillin and sterile clavulanate potassium equivalent to 0.1 gram clavulanic acid.

NDC 0029-6571-26   3.1-gram Vial
TIMENTIN is also supplied as:
NDC 0029-6571-40   3.1-gram ADD-Vantage® Antibiotic Vial

Creatinine clearance mL/min.	Dosage
over 60	3.1 grams every 4 hrs.
30 to 60	2 grams every 4 hrs.
10 to 30	2 grams every 8 hrs.
less than 10	2 grams every 12 hrs.
less than 10 with hepatic dysfunction	2 grams every 24 hrs.
patients on peritoneal dialysis	3.1 grams every 12 hrs.
patients on hemodialysis	2 grams every 12 hrs. supplemented with 3.1 grams after each dialysis

To calculate creatinine clearance[‡] from a serum creatinine value use the following formula:

$$C_{cr} = \frac{(140 - Age)\ (wt.\ in\ kg)}{72 \times S_{cr}\ (mg/100\ mL)}$$

This is the calculated creatinine clearance for adult males; for females it is 15% less.

[‡] Cockcroft, D.W., et al: Prediction of Creatinine Clearance from Serum Creatinine. Nephron 16:31-41, 1976.

STABILITY PERIOD
(3.1-gram Vials)

Intravenous Solution (ticarcillin concentrations of 10 mg/mL to 100 mg/mL)	Room Temperature 21° to 24°C (70° to 75°F)	Refrigerated 4°C (40°F)
Dextrose Injection 5%, USP	24 hours	3 days
Sodium Chloride Injection, USP	24 hours	7 days
Lactated Ringer's Injection, USP	24 hours	7 days

Each 31 gram Pharmacy Bulk Package contains sterile ticarcillin disodium equivalent to 30 grams ticarcillin and sterile clavulanate potassium equivalent to 1 gram clavulanic acid.
NDC 0029-6579-21   31 gram Pharmacy Bulk Package Vials of TIMENTIN should be stored at or below 24°C (75°F).
NDC 0029-6571-31 TIMENTIN as an iso-osmotic, sterile, nonpyrogenic, frozen solution in GALAXY® (PL 2040) Plastic Containers—supplied in 100 mL single-dose containers equivalent to 3 grams ticarcillin and clavulanate potassium equivalent to 0.1 gram clavulanic acid.

CLINICAL STUDIES

TIMENTIN has been studied in a total of 296 pediatric patients (excluding neonates and infants less than 3 months) in 6 controlled clinical trials. The majority of patients studied had intra-abdominal infections, and the primary comparator was clindamycin and gentamicin with or without ampicillin. At the end-of-therapy visit, comparable efficacy was reported in the trial arms using TIMENTIN and an appropriate comparator.

TIMENTIN was also evaluated in an additional 408 pediatric patients (excluding neonates and infants less than 3 months) in 3 uncontrolled US clinical trials. Patients were treated across a broad range of presenting diagnoses including: Infections in bone and joint, skin and skin structure, lower respiratory tract, urinary tract, as well as intra-abdominal and gynecologic infections. Patients received TIMENTIN either 300 mg/kg/day (based on the ticarcillin component) divided every 4 hours for severe infection or 200 mg/kg/day (based on the ticarcillin component) divided every 6 hours for mild to moderate infections. The efficacy rates were comparable to those obtained in the controlled trials.

The adverse event profile in these 704 pediatric patients treated with TIMENTIN was comparable to that seen in adult patients.

REFERENCES

1. National Committee for Clinical Microbiology Standards. *Methods for Dilution Antimicrobial Susceptibility Tests for Bacteria that Grow Aerobically* - Sixth Edition. Approved Standard. NCCLS Document M7-A6, Vol. 23, No. 2 (ISBN 1-56238-486-4). NCCLS, 940 West Valley Road, Suite 1400, Wayne, PA 19087-1898, January, 2003.
2. National Committee for Clinical Microbiology Standards. *Performance Standards for Antimicrobial Disk Susceptibility Tests* - Eighth Edition. Approved Standard. NCCLS Document M2-A8, Vol. 23, No. 1 (ISBN 1-56238-485-6). NCCLS, 940 West Valley Road, Suite 1400, Wayne, PA 19087-1898, January, 2003.
3. National Committee for Clinical Microbiology Standards. *Performance Standards for Antimicrobial Susceptibility Testing* - Thirteenth Informational Supplement. NCCLS Document M100-S13 (M7), Vol. 23, No. 2. NCCLS, 940 West Valley Road, Suite 1400, Wayne, PA 19087-1898, January, 2003.
4. National Committee for Clinical Laboratory Standards. *Methods for Antimicrobial Susceptibility Testing of Anaerobic Bacteria* - Fifth Edition. Approved Standard. NCCLS Document M11-A5, Vol. 21, No. 2 (ISBN 1-56238-429-5). NCCLS, 940 West Valley Road, Suite 1400, Wayne, PA 19087-1898, January, 2001.

TIMENTIN is a registered trademark of GlaxoSmithKline. The following are registered trademarks of their respective owners: ADD-VANTAGE/Abbott Laboratories; GALAXY/Baxter International Inc.; MULTI-STIX/Bayer Corporation.

GlaxoSmithKline
Research Triangle Park, NC 27709
©2008, GlaxoSmithKline. All rights reserved.
July 2008   TMN:18PI

TIMENTIN®   ℞
[tī-měn' tin]
(sterile ticarcillin disodium and clavulanate potassium) for Intravenous Administration ADD-VANTAGE® ANTIBIOTIC VIAL

To reduce the development of drug-resistant bacteria and maintain the effectiveness of TIMENTIN (ticarcillin disodium and clavulanate potassium) and other antibacterial drugs, TIMENTIN should be used only to treat or prevent infections that are proven or strongly suspected to be caused by bacteria.

DESCRIPTION

TIMENTIN is a sterile injectable antibacterial combination consisting of the semisynthetic antibiotic ticarcillin disodium, and the β-lactamase inhibitor clavulanate potassium (the potassium salt of clavulanic acid) for intravenous administration. Ticarcillin is derived from the basic penicillin nucleus, 6-amino-penicillanic acid.
Chemically, ticarcillin disodium is N-(2-Carboxy-3,3-dimethyl-7-oxo-4-thia-1-azabicyclo[3.2.0]hept-6-yl)-3-thiophenemalonamic acid disodium salt and may be represented as:

Clavulanic acid is produced by the fermentation of *Streptomyces clavuligerus*. It is a β-lactam structurally related to the penicillins and possesses the ability to inactivate a wide variety of β-lactamases by blocking the active sites of these enzymes. Clavulanic acid is particularly active against the clinically important plasmid-mediated β-lactamases frequently responsible for transferred drug resistance to penicillins and cephalosporins.
Chemically, clavulanate potassium is potassium (Z)-(2R,5R)-3-(2-hydroxyethylidene)-7-oxo-4-oxa-1-azabicyclo[3.2.0]heptane-2-carboxylate and may be represented structurally as:

TIMENTIN is supplied as a white to pale yellow powder for reconstitution. TIMENTIN is very soluble in water, its solubility being greater than 600 mg/mL. The reconstituted solution is clear, colorless or pale yellow, having a pH of 5.5 to 7.5.
For the 3.1-gram dosage of TIMENTIN, the theoretical sodium content is 4.51 mEq (103.6 mg) per gram of TIMENTIN. The theoretical potassium content is 0.15 mEq (6 mg) per gram of TIMENTIN.

CLINICAL PHARMACOLOGY

After an intravenous infusion (30 min.) of 3.1 grams of TIMENTIN, peak serum concentrations of both ticarcillin and clavulanic acid are attained immediately after

SERUM LEVELS IN ADULTS
AFTER A 30-MINUTE IV INFUSION OF TIMENTIN®
TICARCILLIN SERUM LEVELS (mcg/mL)

Dose	0	15 min.	30 min.	1 hr.	1.5 hr.	3.5 hr.	5.5 hr.
3.1 gram	324 (293 to 388)	223 (184 to 293)	176 (135 to 235)	131 (102 to 195)	90 (65 to 119)	27 (19 to 37)	6 (5 to 7)

CLAVULANIC ACID SERUM LEVELS (mcg/mL)

Dose	0	15 min.	30 min.	1 hr.	1.5 hr.	3.5 hr.	5.5 hr.
3.1 gram	8.0 (5.3 to 10.3)	4.6 (3.0 to 7.6)	2.6 (1.8 to 3.4)	1.8 (1.6 to 2.2)	1.2 (0.8 to 1.6)	0.3 (0.2 to 0.3)	0

completion of infusion. Ticarcillin serum levels are similar to those produced by the administration of equivalent amounts of ticarcillin alone with a mean peak serum level of 330 mcg/mL. The corresponding mean peak serum level for clavulanic acid was 8 mcg/mL. (See following table.)
[See table above]

The mean area under the serum concentration curve was 485 mcg•hr/mL for ticarcillin and 8.2 mcg•hr/mL for clavulanic acid.

The mean serum half-lives of ticarcillin and clavulanic acid in healthy volunteers are 1.1 hours and 1.1 hours, respectively.

In pediatric patients receiving approximately 50 mg/kg of TIMENTIN (30:1 ratio ticarcillin to clavulanate), mean ticarcillin serum half-lives were 4.4 hours in neonates (n = 18) and 1.0 hour in infants and children (n = 41). The corresponding clavulanate serum half-lives averaged 1.9 hours in neonates (n = 14) and 0.9 hour in infants and children (n = 40). Area under the serum concentration time curves averaged 339 mcg•hr/mL in infants and children (n = 41), whereas the corresponding mean clavulanate area under the serum concentration time curves was approximately 7 mcg•hr/mL in the same population (n = 40).

Approximately 60% to 70% of ticarcillin and approximately 35% to 45% of clavulanic acid are excreted unchanged in urine during the first 6 hours after administration of a single dose of TIMENTIN to normal volunteers with normal renal function. Two hours after an intravenous injection of 3.1 grams of TIMENTIN, concentrations of ticarcillin in urine generally exceed 1,500 mcg/mL. The corresponding concentrations of clavulanic acid in urine generally exceed 40 mcg/mL. By 4 to 6 hours after injection, the urine concentrations of ticarcillin and clavulanic acid usually decline to approximately 190 mcg/mL and 2 mcg/mL, respectively. Neither component of TIMENTIN is highly protein bound; ticarcillin has been found to be approximately 45% bound to human serum protein and clavulanic acid approximately 25% bound.

Somewhat higher and more prolonged serum levels of ticarcillin can be achieved with the concurrent administration of probenecid; however, probenecid does not enhance the serum levels of clavulanic acid.

Ticarcillin can be detected in tissues and interstitial fluid following parenteral administration.

Penetration of ticarcillin into bile and pleural fluid has been demonstrated. The results of experiments involving the administration of clavulanic acid to animals suggest that this compound, like ticarcillin, is well distributed in body tissues.

An inverse relationship exists between the serum half-life of ticarcillin and creatinine clearance. The dosage of TIMENTIN need only be adjusted in cases of severe renal impairment. (See DOSAGE AND ADMINISTRATION.)

Ticarcillin may be removed from patients undergoing dialysis; the actual amount removed depends on the duration and type of dialysis.

Microbiology: Ticarcillin is a semisynthetic antibiotic with a broad spectrum of bactericidal activity against many gram-positive and gram-negative aerobic and anaerobic bacteria.

Ticarcillin is, however, susceptible to degradation by β-lactamases, and therefore, the spectrum of activity does not normally include organisms which produce these enzymes.

Clavulanic acid is a β-lactam, structurally related to the penicillins, which possesses the ability to inactivate a wide range of β-lactamase enzymes commonly found in microorganisms resistant to penicillins and cephalosporins. In particular, it has good activity against the clinically important plasmid-mediated β-lactamases frequently responsible for transferred drug resistance.

The formulation of ticarcillin with clavulanic acid in TIMENTIN protects ticarcillin from degradation by β-lactamase enzymes and effectively extends the antibiotic spectrum of ticarcillin to include many bacteria normally resistant to ticarcillin and other β-lactam antibiotics. Thus, TIMENTIN possesses the distinctive properties of a broad-spectrum antibiotic and a β-lactamase inhibitor. Ticarcillin/clavulanic acid has been shown to be active against most strains of the following microorganisms, both in vitro and in clinical infections as described in the INDICATIONS AND USAGE section.

Gram-Positive Aerobes:
Staphylococcus aureus (β-lactamase and non–β-lactamase–producing)*
Staphylococcus epidermidis (β-lactamase and non–β-lactamase–producing)*
*Staphylococci that are resistant to methicillin/oxacillin must be considered resistant to ticarcillin/clavulanic acid.

Gram-Negative Aerobes:
Citrobacter species (β-lactamase and non–β-lactamase–producing)
Enterobacter species including *E. cloacae* (β-lactamase and non–β-lactamase–producing)
(Although most strains of *Enterobacter* species are resistant in vitro, clinical efficacy has been demonstrated with TIMENTIN in urinary tract infections and gynecologic infections caused by these organisms.)
Escherichia coli (β-lactamase and non–β-lactamase–producing)
Haemophilus influenzae (β-lactamase and non–β-lactamase–producing)†
Klebsiella species including *K. pneumoniae* (β-lactamase and non–β-lactamase–producing)
Pseudomonas species including *P. aeruginosa* (β-lactamase and non–β-lactamase–producing)
Serratia marcescens (β-lactamase and non–β-lactamase–producing)
†β-lactamase–negative, ampicillin-resistant (BLNAR) strains of *H. influenzae* must be considered resistant to ticarcillin/clavulanic acid.

Anaerobic Bacteria:
Bacteroides fragilis group (β-lactamase and non–β-lactamase–producing)
Prevotella (formerly *Bacteroides*) *melaninogenicus* (β-lactamase and non–β-lactamase–producing)

The following in vitro data are available, **but their clinical significance is unknown.**

The following strains exhibit an in vitro minimum inhibitory concentration (MIC) less than or equal to the susceptible breakpoint for ticarcillin/clavulanic acid. However, with the exception of organisms shown to respond to ticarcillin alone, the safety and effectiveness of ticarcillin/clavulanic acid in treating infections due to these microorganisms have not been established in adequate and well-controlled clinical trials.

Gram-Positive Aerobes:
Staphylococcus saprophyticus (β-lactamase and non–β-lactamase–producing)
Streptococcus agalactiae‡ (Group B)
Streptococcus bovis‡
Streptococcus pneumoniae‡ (penicillin-susceptible strains only)
Streptococcus pyogenes‡
Viridans group streptococci‡

Gram-Negative Aerobes:
Acinetobacter baumannii (β-lactamase and non–β-lactamase–producing)
Acinetobacter calcoaceticus (β-lactamase and non–β-lactamase–producing)
Acinetobacter haemolyticus (β-lactamase and non–β-lactamase–producing)
Acinetobacter lwoffi (β-lactamase and non–β-lactamase–producing)
Moraxella catarrhalis (β-lactamase and non–β-lactamase–producing)
Morganella morganii (β-lactamase and non–β-lactamase–producing)
Neisseria gonorrhoeae (β-lactamase and non–β-lactamase–producing)
Pasteurella multocida (β-lactamase and non–β-lactamase–producing)
Proteus mirabilis (β-lactamase and non–β-lactamase–producing)
Proteus penneri (β-lactamase and non–β-lactamase–producing)
Proteus vulgaris (β-lactamase and non–β-lactamase–producing)

Providencia rettgeri (β-lactamase and non–β-lactamase–producing)
Providencia stuartii (β-lactamase and non–β-lactamase–producing)
Stenotrophomonas maltophilia (β-lactamase and non–β-lactamase–producing)
Anaerobic Bacteria:
Clostridium species including *C. perfringens, C. difficile, C. sporogenes, C. ramosum,* and *C. bifermentans* (β-lactamase and non–β-lactamase–producing)
Eubacterium species
Fusobacterium species including *F. nucleatum* and *F. necrophorum* (β-lactamase and non–β-lactamase–producing)
Peptostreptococcus species‡
Veillonella species‡
‡These are non–β-lactamase–producing strains, and therefore, are susceptible to ticarcillin.

In vitro synergism between TIMENTIN and gentamicin, tobramycin, or amikacin against multiresistant strains of *Pseudomonas aeruginosa* has been demonstrated.

Susceptibility Testing: Dilution Techniques: Quantitative methods are used to determine antimicrobial MICs. These MICs provide estimates of the susceptibility of bacteria to antimicrobial compounds. The MICs should be determined using a standardized procedure. Standardized procedures are based on a dilution method[1,3] (broth or agar) or equivalent with standardized inoculum concentrations and standardized concentrations of ticarcillin/clavulanate potassium powder.

The recommended dilution pattern utilizes a constant level of 2 mcg/mL clavulanic acid in all tubes with varying amounts of ticarcillin. MICs are expressed in terms of the ticarcillin concentration in the presence of clavulanic acid at a constant 2 mcg/mL. The MIC values should be interpreted according to the following criteria:

RECOMMENDED RANGES FOR TICARCILLIN/CLAVULANIC ACID SUSCEPTIBILITY TESTING*

For *Pseudomonas aeruginosa:*

MIC (mcg/mL)	Interpretation	
≤64	Susceptible	(S)
≥128	Resistant	(R)

For Enterobacteriaceae:

MIC (mcg/mL)	Interpretation	
≤16	Susceptible	(S)
32–64	Intermediate	(I)
≥128	Resistant	(R)

For Staphylococci†:

MIC (mcg/mL)	Interpretation	
≤8	Susceptible	(S)
≥16	Resistant	(R)

* Expressed as concentration of ticarcillin in the presence of clavulanic acid at a constant 2 mcg/mL.
† Staphylococci that are susceptible to ticarcillin/clavulanic acid but resistant to methicillin/oxacillin must be considered as resistant.

A report of "Susceptible" indicates that the pathogen is likely to be inhibited if the antimicrobial compound in the blood reaches the concentrations usually achievable. A report of "Intermediate" indicates that the result should be considered equivocal, and if the microorganism is not fully susceptible to alternative, clinically feasible drugs, the test should be repeated. This category implies possible clinical applicability in body sites where the drug is physiologically concentrated or in situations where high dosage of drug can be used. This category also provides a buffer zone that prevents small uncontrolled technical factors from causing major discrepancies in interpretation. A report of "Resistant" indicates that the pathogen is not likely to be inhibited if the antimicrobial compound in the blood reaches the concentrations usually achievable; other therapy should be selected.

Standardized susceptibility test procedures require the use of laboratory control microorganisms to control the technical aspects of the laboratory procedures. Standard ticarcillin/clavulanate potassium powder should provide the following MIC values:

Microorganism		MIC (mcg/mL)‡
Escherichia coli	ATCC 25922	4-16
Escherichia coli	ATCC 35218	4-16
Pseudomonas aeruginosa	ATCC 27853	8-32
Staphylococcus aureus	ATCC 29213	0.5-2

‡ Expressed as concentration of ticarcillin in the presence of clavulanic acid at a constant 2 mcg/mL.

Diffusion Techniques: Quantitative methods that require measurement of zone diameters also provide reproducible estimates of the susceptibility of bacteria to antimicrobial compounds. One such standardized procedure[2,3] requires the use of standardized inoculum concentrations. This procedure uses paper disks impregnated with 85 mcg of ticarcillin/clavulanate potassium (75 mcg ticarcillin plus 10 mcg clavulanate potassium) to test the susceptibility of microorganisms to ticarcillin/clavulanic acid.

Reports from the laboratory providing results of the standard single-disk susceptibility test with an 85 mcg of ticarcillin/clavulanate potassium (75 mcg ticarcillin plus 10 mcg clavulanate potassium) disk should be interpreted according to the following criteria:

RECOMMENDED RANGES FOR TICARCILLIN/CLAVULANIC ACID SUSCEPTIBILITY TESTING

For *Pseudomonas aeruginosa*:

Zone Diameter (mm)	Interpretation	
≥15	Susceptible	(S)
≤14	Resistant	(R)

For Enterobacteriaceae:

Zone Diameter (mm)	Interpretation	
≥20	Susceptible	(S)
15-19	Intermediate	(I)
≤14	Resistant	(R)

For Staphylococci§:

Zone Diameter (mm)	Interpretation	
≥23	Susceptible	(S)
≤22	Resistant	(R)

§Staphylococci that are resistant to methicillin/oxacillin must be considered as resistant to ticarcillin/clavulanic acid.

Interpretation should be as stated above for results using dilution techniques. Interpretation involves correlation of the diameter obtained in the disk test with the MIC for ticarcillin/clavulanic acid.

As with standardized dilution techniques, diffusion methods require the use of laboratory control microorganisms that are used to control the technical aspects of the laboratory procedures. For the diffusion technique, the 85 mcg of ticarcillin/clavulanate potassium (75 mcg ticarcillin plus 10 mcg clavulanate potassium) disk should provide the following zone diameters in these laboratory test quality control strains:

Microorganism		Zone Diameter (mm)
Escherichia coli	ATCC 25922	24-30
Escherichia coli	ATCC 35218	21-25
Pseudomonas aeruginosa	ATCC 27853	20-28
Staphylococcus aureus	ATCC 25923	29-37

Anaerobic Techniques: For anaerobic bacteria, the susceptibility to ticarcillin/clavulanic acid can be determined by standardized test methods.[3,4] The MIC values obtained should be interpreted according to the following criteria:

RECOMMENDED RANGES FOR TICARCILLIN/CLAVULANIC ACID SUSCEPTIBILITY TESTING‖

MIC (mcg/mL)	Interpretation	
≤32	Susceptible	(S)
64	Intermediate	(I)
≥128	Resistant	(R)

‖ Expressed as concentration of ticarcillin in the presence of clavulanic acid at a constant 2 mcg/mL.

Interpretation is identical to that stated above for results using dilution techniques.

As with other susceptibility techniques, the use of laboratory control microorganisms is required to control the technical aspects of the laboratory standardized procedures. Standardized ticarcillin/clavulanate potassium powder should provide the following MIC values:

[See table above]

INDICATIONS AND USAGE

TIMENTIN is indicated in the treatment of infections caused by susceptible strains of the designated microorganisms in the conditions listed below:

Septicemia (including bacteremia) caused by β-lactamase–producing strains of *Klebsiella* spp.*, *E. coli**, *S. aureus**, or *P. aeruginosa** (or other *Pseudomonas* species*)

Lower Respiratory Infections caused by β-lactamase–producing strains of *S. aureus, H. influenzae**, or *Klebsiella* spp.*

Bone and Joint Infections caused by β-lactamase–producing strains of *S. aureus*

Skin and Skin Structure Infections caused by β-lactamase–producing strains of *S. aureus*, *Klebsiella* spp.*, or *E. coli**

Urinary Tract Infections (complicated and uncomplicated) caused by β-lactamase–producing strains of *E. coli, Klebsiella* spp., *P. aeruginosa** (or other *Pseudomonas* spp.*), *Citrobacter* spp.*, *Enterobacter cloacae**, *S. marcescens**, or *S. aureus**

Gynecologic Infections endometritis caused by β-lactamase–producing strains of *P. melaninogenicus**, *Enterobacter* spp. (including *E. cloacae**), *E. coli, K. pneumoniae**, *S. aureus*, or *S. epidermidis*

Microorganism		Agar dilution MIC Range (mcg/mL)‖	Broth microdilution MIC Range (mcg/mL)‖
Bacteroides thetaiotaomicron	ATCC 29741	0.5-2	0.5-2
Eubacterium lentum	ATCC 43055	16-64	8-32

‖Expressed as concentration of ticarcillin in the presence of clavulanic acid at a constant 2 mcg/mL.

Intra-abdominal Infections peritonitis caused by β-lactamase–producing strains of *E. coli, K. pneumoniae*, or *B. fragilis** group

*Efficacy for this organism in this organ system was studied in fewer than 10 infections.

NOTE: For information on use in pediatric patients (≥3 months of age) see PRECAUTIONS-Pediatric Use and CLINICAL STUDIES sections. There are insufficient data to support the use of TIMENTIN in pediatric patients under 3 months of age or for the treatment of septicemia and/or infections in the pediatric population where the suspected or proven pathogen is *H. influenzae* type b.

While TIMENTIN is indicated only for the conditions listed above, infections caused by ticarcillin-susceptible organisms are also amenable to treatment with TIMENTIN due to its ticarcillin content. Therefore, mixed infections caused by ticarcillin-susceptible organisms and β-lactamase–producing organisms susceptible to ticarcillin/clavulanic acid should not require the addition of another antibiotic.

Appropriate culture and susceptibility tests should be performed before treatment in order to isolate and identify organisms causing infection and to determine their susceptibility to ticarcillin/clavulanic acid. Because of its broad spectrum of bactericidal activity against gram-positive and gram-negative bacteria, TIMENTIN is particularly useful for the treatment of mixed infections and for presumptive therapy prior to the identification of the causative organisms. TIMENTIN has been shown to be effective as single drug therapy in the treatment of some serious infections where normally combination antibiotic therapy might be employed. Therapy with TIMENTIN may be initiated before results of such tests are known when there is reason to believe the infection may involve any of the β-lactamase–producing organisms listed above.

Based on the in vitro synergism between ticarcillin/clavulanic acid and aminoglycosides against certain strains of *P. aeruginosa*, combined therapy has been successful, especially in patients with impaired host defenses. Both drugs should be used in full therapeutic doses.

To reduce the development of drug-resistant bacteria and maintain the effectiveness of TIMENTIN and other antibacterial drugs, TIMENTIN should be used only to treat or prevent infections that are proven or strongly suspected to be caused by susceptible bacteria. When culture and susceptibility information are available, they should be considered in selecting or modifying antibacterial therapy. In the absence of such data, local epidemiology and susceptibility patterns may contribute to the empiric selection of therapy.

CONTRAINDICATIONS

TIMENTIN is contraindicated in patients with a history of hypersensitivity reactions to any of the penicillins.

WARNINGS

SERIOUS AND OCCASIONALLY FATAL HYPERSENSITIVITY (ANAPHYLACTIC) REACTIONS HAVE BEEN REPORTED IN PATIENTS ON PENICILLIN THERAPY. THESE REACTIONS ARE MORE LIKELY TO OCCUR IN INDIVIDUALS WITH A HISTORY OF PENICILLIN HYPERSENSITIVITY AND/OR A HISTORY OF SENSITIVITY TO MULTIPLE ALLERGENS. THERE HAVE BEEN REPORTS OF INDIVIDUALS WITH A HISTORY OF PENICILLIN HYPERSENSITIVITY WHO HAVE EXPERIENCED SEVERE REACTIONS WHEN TREATED WITH CEPHALOSPORINS. BEFORE INITIATING THERAPY WITH TIMENTIN CAREFUL INQUIRY SHOULD BE MADE CONCERNING PREVIOUS HYPERSENSITIVITY REACTIONS TO PENICILLINS, CEPHALOSPORINS, OR OTHER ALLERGENS. IF AN ALLERGIC REACTION OCCURS, TIMENTIN SHOULD BE DISCONTINUED AND THE APPROPRIATE THERAPY INSTITUTED. **SERIOUS ANAPHYLACTIC REACTIONS REQUIRE IMMEDIATE EMERGENCY TREATMENT WITH EPINEPHRINE. OXYGEN, INTRAVENOUS STEROIDS, AND AIRWAY MANAGEMENT, INCLUDING INTUBATION, SHOULD ALSO BE PROVIDED AS INDICATED.**

Clostridium difficile associated diarrhea (CDAD) has been reported with use of nearly all antibacterial agents, including TIMENTIN, and may range in severity from mild diarrhea to fatal colitis. Treatment with antibacterial agents alters the normal flora of the colon leading to overgrowth of *C. difficile*.

C. difficile produces toxins A and B which contribute to the development of CDAD. Hypertoxin producing strains of *C. difficile* cause increased morbidity and mortality, as these infections can be refractory to antimicrobial therapy and may require colectomy. CDAD must be considered in all patients who present with diarrhea following antibiotic use. Careful medical history is necessary since CDAD has been reported to occur over two months after the administration of antibacterial agents.

If CDAD is suspected or confirmed, ongoing antibiotic use not directed against *C. difficile* may need to be discontinued. Appropriate fluid and electrolyte management, protein supplementation, antibiotic treatment of *C. difficile*, and surgical evaluation should be instituted as clinically indicated.

When very high doses of TIMENTIN are administered, especially in the presence of impaired renal function, patients may experience convulsions. (See ADVERSE REACTIONS and OVERDOSAGE.)

PRECAUTIONS

General: While TIMENTIN possesses the characteristic low toxicity of the penicillin group of antibiotics, periodic assessment of organ system functions, including renal, hepatic, and hematopoietic function, is advisable during prolonged therapy.

Bleeding manifestations have occurred in some patients receiving β-lactam antibiotics. These reactions have been associated with abnormalities of coagulation tests such as clotting time, platelet aggregation, and prothrombin time and are more likely to occur in patients with renal impairment. If bleeding manifestations appear, treatment with TIMENTIN should be discontinued and appropriate therapy instituted.

TIMENTIN has only rarely been reported to cause hypokalemia; however, the possibility of this occurring should be kept in mind particularly when treating patients with fluid and electrolyte imbalance. Periodic monitoring of serum potassium may be advisable in patients receiving prolonged therapy.

The theoretical sodium content is 4.51 mEq (103.6 mg) per gram of TIMENTIN. This should be considered when treating patients requiring restricted salt intake.

As with any penicillin, an allergic reaction, including anaphylaxis, may occur during administration of TIMENTIN, particularly in a hypersensitive individual.

The possibility of superinfections with mycotic or bacterial pathogens should be kept in mind, particularly during prolonged treatment. If superinfections occur, appropriate measures should be taken.

Prescribing TIMENTIN in the absence of a proven or strongly suspected bacterial infection or a prophylactic indication is unlikely to provide benefit to the patient and increases the risk of the development of drug-resistant bacteria.

Information for Patients: Patients should be counseled that antibacterial drugs, including TIMENTIN, should only be used to treat bacterial infections. They do not treat viral infections (e.g., the common cold). When TIMENTIN is prescribed to treat a bacterial infection, patients should be told that although it is common to feel better early in the course of therapy, the medication should be taken exactly as directed. Skipping doses or not completing the full course of therapy may: (1) decrease the effectiveness of the immediate treatment, and (2) increase the likelihood that bacteria will develop resistance and will not be treatable by TIMENTIN or other antibacterial drugs in the future.

Diarrhea is a common problem caused by antibiotics which usually ends when the antibiotic is discontinued. Sometimes after starting treatment with antibiotics, patients can develop watery and bloody stools (with or without stomach cramps and fever) even as late as 2 or more months after having taken the last dose of the antibiotic. If this occurs, patients should contact their physician as soon as possible.

Drug/Laboratory Test Interactions: As with other penicillins, the mixing of TIMENTIN with an aminoglycoside in solutions for parenteral administration can result in substantial inactivation of the aminoglycoside.

Probenecid interferes with the renal tubular secretion of ticarcillin, thereby increasing serum concentrations and prolonging serum half-life of the antibiotic.

In common with other antibiotics, ticarcillin disodium/clavulanate potassium may affect the gut flora, leading to lower estrogen reabsorption and reduced efficacy of combined oral estrogen/progesterone contraceptives.

High urine concentrations of ticarcillin may produce false-positive protein reactions (pseudoproteinuria) with the following methods: Sulfosalicylic acid and boiling test, acetic acid test, biuret reaction and nitric acid test. The bromphenol blue (MULTI-STIX®) reagent strip test has been reported to be reliable.

Creatinine clearance mL/min.	Dosage
over 60	3.1 grams every 4 hrs.
30 to 60	2 grams every 4 hrs.
10 to 30	2 grams every 8 hrs.
less than 10	2 grams every 12 hrs.
less than 10 with hepatic dysfunction	2 grams every 24 hrs.
patients on peritoneal dialysis	3.1 grams every 12 hrs.
patients on hemodialysis	2 grams every 12 hrs. supplemented with 3.1 grams after each dialysis

To calculate creatinine clearance[‡] from a serum creatinine value use the following formula:

$$C_{cr} = \frac{(140 - Age)\ (wt.\ in\ kg)}{72 \times S_{cr}\ (mg/100\ mL)}$$

This is the calculated creatinine clearance for adult males; for females it is 15% less.

[‡] Cockcroft, D.W., et al: Prediction of Creatinine Clearance from Serum Creatinine. Nephron 16:31-41, 1976.

The presence of clavulanic acid in TIMENTIN may cause a nonspecific binding of IgG and albumin by red cell membranes, leading to a false-positive Coombs test.

Carcinogenesis, Mutagenesis, Impairment of Fertility: Long-term studies in animals have not been performed to evaluate carcinogenic potential. However, results from assays for gene mutation in vitro using bacteria (Ames tests) and yeast, and for chromosomal effects in vitro in human lymphocytes, and in vivo in mouse bone marrow (micronucleus test) indicate that TIMENTIN is without any mutagenic potential.

Pregnancy (Category B): Reproduction studies have been performed in rats given doses up to 1,050 mg/kg/day and have revealed no evidence of impaired fertility or harm to the fetus due to TIMENTIN. There are, however, no adequate and well-controlled studies in pregnant women. Because animal reproduction studies are not always predictive of human response, this drug should be used during pregnancy only if clearly needed.

Nursing Mothers: It is not known whether this drug is excreted in human milk. Because many drugs are excreted in human milk, caution should be exercised when TIMENTIN is administered to a nursing woman.

Pediatric Use: The safety and effectiveness of TIMENTIN have been established in the age group of 3 months to 16 years. Use of TIMENTIN in these age groups is supported by evidence from adequate and well-controlled studies of TIMENTIN in adults with additional efficacy, safety, and pharmacokinetic data from both comparative and noncomparative studies in pediatric patients. There are insufficient data to support the use of TIMENTIN in pediatric patients under 3 months of age or for the treatment of septicemia and/or infections in the pediatric population where the suspected or proven pathogen is *H. influenzae* type b.

In those patients in whom meningeal seeding from a distant infection site or in whom meningitis is suspected or documented, or in patients who require prophylaxis against central nervous system infection, an alternate agent with demonstrated clinical efficacy in this setting should be used.

Geriatric Use: An analysis of clinical studies of TIMENTIN was conducted to determine whether subjects aged 65 and over respond differently from younger subjects. Of the 1,078 subjects treated with at least one dose of TIMENTIN, 67.5% were <65 years old, and 32.5% were ≥65 years old. No overall differences in safety or efficacy were observed between these subjects and younger subjects, and other reported clinical experience have not identified differences in responses between the elderly and younger patients, but a greater sensitivity of some older individuals cannot be ruled out.

This drug is known to be substantially excreted by the kidney, and the risk of toxic reactions to this drug may be greater in patients with impaired renal function. Because elderly patients are more likely to have decreased renal function, care should be taken in dose selection, and it may be useful to monitor renal function (see DOSAGE and ADMINISTRATION).

TIMENTIN contains 103.6 mg (4.51 mEq) of sodium per gram of TIMENTIN. At the usual recommended doses, patients would receive between 1,285 and 1,927 mg/day (56 and 84 mEq) of sodium. The geriatric population may respond with a blunted natriuresis to salt loading. This may be clinically important with regard to such diseases as congestive heart failure.

ADVERSE REACTIONS

As with other penicillins, the following adverse reactions may occur:

Hypersensitivity Reactions: Skin rash, pruritus, urticaria, arthralgia, myalgia, drug fever, chills, chest discomfort, erythema multiforme, toxic epidermal necrolysis, Stevens-Johnson syndrome, and anaphylactic reactions.

Central Nervous System: Headache, giddiness, neuromuscular hyperirritability, or convulsive seizures.

Gastrointestinal Disturbances: Disturbances of taste and smell, stomatitis, flatulence, nausea, vomiting and diarrhea, epigastric pain, and pseudomembranous colitis have been reported. Onset of pseudomembranous colitis symptoms may occur during or after antibiotic treatment. (See WARNINGS.)

Hemic and Lymphatic Systems: Thrombocytopenia, leukopenia, neutropenia, eosinophilia, reduction of hemoglobin or hematocrit, and prolongation of prothrombin time and bleeding time.

Abnormalities of Hepatic Function Tests: Elevation of serum aspartate aminotransferase (SGOT), serum alanine aminotransferase (SGPT), serum alkaline phosphatase, serum LDH, serum bilirubin. There have been reports of transient hepatitis and cholestatic jaundice—as with some other penicillins and some cephalosporins.

Renal and Urinary Effects: Elevation of serum creatinine and/or BUN, hypernatremia, reduction in serum potassium and uric acid. Rare reports of hemorrhagic cystitis.

Local Reactions: Pain, burning, swelling, and induration at the injection site and thrombophlebitis with intravenous administration.

Available safety data for pediatric patients treated with TIMENTIN demonstrate a similar adverse event profile to that observed in adult patients.

DRUG ABUSE AND DEPENDENCE

Neither abuse of nor dependence on TIMENTIN has been reported.

OVERDOSAGE

As with other penicillins, neurotoxic reactions may arise when very high doses of TIMENTIN are administered, especially in patients with impaired renal function. (See WARNINGS and ADVERSE REACTIONS-Central Nervous System.)

In case of overdosage, discontinue TIMENTIN, treat symptomatically, and institute supportive measures as required. Ticarcillin may be removed from circulation by hemodialysis. The molecular weight, degree of protein binding, and pharmacokinetic profile of clavulanic acid, together with information from a single patient with renal insufficiency all suggest that this compound may also be removed by hemodialysis.

DOSAGE AND ADMINISTRATION

TIMENTIN should be administered by intravenous infusion (30 min.).

Adults: The usual recommended dosage for systemic and urinary tract infections for average (60 kg) adults is 3.1 grams of TIMENTIN (3.1-gram vial containing 3 grams ticarcillin and 100 mg clavulanic acid) given every 4 to 6 hours. For gynecologic infections, TIMENTIN should be administered as follows: Moderate infections 200 mg/kg/day in divided doses every 6 hours and for severe infections 300 mg/kg/day in divided doses every 4 hours. For patients weighing less than 60 kg, the recommended dosage is 200 to 300 mg/kg/day, based on ticarcillin content, given in divided doses every 4 to 6 hours.

Pediatric Patients (≥3 months): *For patients <60 kg:* In patients <60 kg, TIMENTIN is dosed at 50 mg/kg/dose based on the ticarcillin component. TIMENTIN should be administered as follows: Mild to moderate infections, 200 mg/kg/day in divided doses every 6 hours; for severe infections, 300 mg/kg/day in divided doses every 4 hours.

For patients ≥60 kg: For mild to moderate infections, 3.1 grams of TIMENTIN (3 grams of ticarcillin and 100 mg of clavulanic acid) administered every 6 hours; for severe infections, 3.1 grams every 4 hours.

Renal Impairment: For infections complicated by renal insufficiency[†], an initial loading dose of 3.1 grams should be followed by doses based on creatinine clearance and type of dialysis as indicated below:

[See table above]

NOTE: TIMENTIN in the ADD-VANTAGE® system should only be administered for 3.1-gram dosing.

[†]The half-life of ticarcillin in patients with renal failure is approximately 13 hours.

Dosage for any individual patient must take into consideration the site and severity of infection, the susceptibility of the organisms causing infection, and the status of the patient's host defense mechanisms.

The duration of therapy depends upon the severity of infection. Generally, TIMENTIN should be continued for at least 2 days after the signs and symptoms of infection have disappeared. The usual duration is 10 to 14 days; however, in difficult and complicated infections, more prolonged therapy may be required.

Frequent bacteriologic and clinical appraisals are necessary during therapy of chronic urinary tract infection and may be required for several months after therapy has been completed. Persistent infections may require treatment for several weeks, and doses smaller than those indicated above should not be used.

In certain infections, involving abscess formation, appropriate surgical drainage should be performed in conjunction with antimicrobial therapy.

INSTRUCTIONS FOR USE

To Open Diluent Container:
Peel overwrap at corner and remove solution container. Some opacity of the plastic due to moisture absorption during the sterilization process may be observed.

This is normal and does not affect the solution quality or safety. The opacity will diminish gradually.

To Assemble Vial and Flexible Diluent Container:
(Use Aseptic Technique):

1. Remove the protective covers from the top of the vial and the vial port on the diluent container as follows:

    a. To remove the breakaway vial cap, swing the pull ring over the top of the vial and pull down far enough to start the opening (see Figure 1), then pull straight up to remove the cap (see Figure 2).

    NOTE: Do not access vial with syringe.

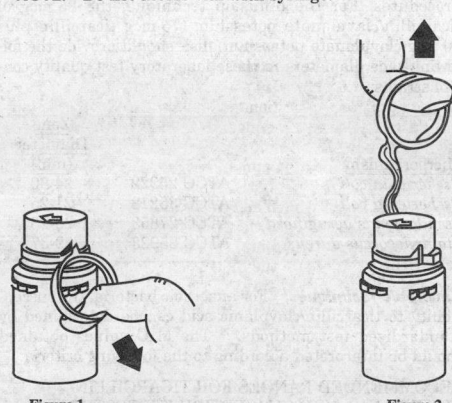

Figure 1   **Figure 2**

    b. To remove the vial port cover, grasp the tab on the pull ring, pull up to break the 3 tie strings, then pull back to remove the cover (see Figure 3).

2. Screw the vial into the vial port until it will go no further. THE VIAL MUST BE SCREWED IN TIGHTLY TO ASSURE A SEAL. This occurs approximately ½ turn (180°) after the first audible click (see Figure 4). The clicking sound does not assure a seal; the vial must be turned as far as it will go.

    NOTE: Once vial is sealed, do not attempt to remove (see Figure 4).

3. Recheck the vial to assure that it is tight by trying to turn it further in the direction of assembly.

4. Label appropriately.

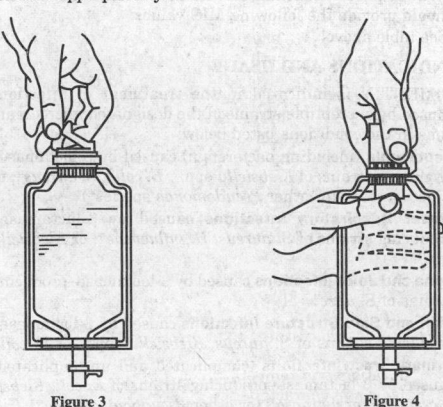

Figure 3   **Figure 4**

To Reconstitute the Drug:
1. Squeeze the bottom of the diluent container gently to inflate the portion of the container surrounding the end of the drug vial.
2. With the other hand, push the drug vial down into the container telescoping the walls of the container. Grasp

STABILITY PERIOD

INTRAVENOUS SOLUTION (ticarcillin concentration of ~ 30 mg/mL or ~ 60 mg/mL)	ROOM TEMPERATURE 21° to 24°C (70° to 75°F)
Sodium Chloride Injection, USP	24 hours
5% Dextrose in Water	12 hours

the inner cap of the vial through the walls of the container (see Figure 5).

3. Pull the inner cap from the drug vial (see Figure 6). Verify that the rubber stopper has been pulled out, allowing the drug and diluent to mix.
4. Mix container contents thoroughly and use within the specified time.

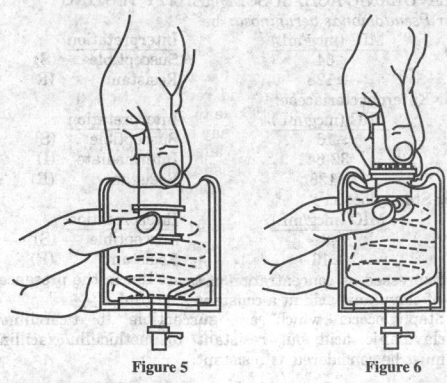

Figure 5   Figure 6

Preparation for Administration:
(Use Aseptic Technique):
1. Confirm the activation and admixture of vial contents.
2. Check for leaks by squeezing container firmly. If leaks are found discard unit as sterility may be impaired.
3. Close flow control clamp of administration set.
4. Remove cover from outlet port at bottom of container.
5. Insert piercing pin of administration set into port with a twisting motion until the pin is firmly seated. **NOTE:** See full directions on administration set carton.
6. Lift the free end of the hanger loop on the bottom of the vial, breaking the 2 tie strings. Bend the loop outward to lock it in the upright position, then suspend container from hanger.
7. Squeeze and release drip chamber to establish proper fluid level in chamber.
8. Open flow control clamp and clear air from set. Close clamp.
9. Attach set to venipuncture device. If device is not indwelling, prime and make venipuncture.
10. Regulate rate of administration with flow control clamp.
WARNING: Do not use flexible container in series connections.

RECONSTITUTION DIRECTIONS
Intravenous Infusion: Use a 50-mL or 100-mL ADD-VANTAGE® DILUENT CONTAINER containing either Sodium Chloride Injection, USP, or 5% Dextrose in Water (refer to INSTRUCTIONS FOR USE section). The resulting concentration of the 3.1-gram dose reconstituted in 50 mL of diluent is approximately 60 mg/mL of ticarcillin and approximately 2 mg/mL of clavulanic acid. The resulting concentration of the 3.1-gram dose reconstituted in 100 mL of diluent is approximately 30 mg/mL of ticarcillin and approximately 1 mg/mL of clavulanic acid.

The solution of reconstituted drug may then be administered over a period of 30 minutes by direct infusion or through a Y-type intravenous infusion set, which may already be in place. If this method of administration is used, it is advisable to discontinue temporarily the administration of any other solutions during the infusion of TIMENTIN. When TIMENTIN is given in combination with another antimicrobial, such as an aminoglycoside, each drug should be given separately in accordance with the recommended dosage and routes of administration for each drug. After reconstitution and prior to administration, TIMENTIN, as with other parenteral drugs, should be inspected visually for particulate matter. If this condition is evident, the solution should be discarded.

The color of reconstituted solutions of TIMENTIN normally ranges from light to dark yellow, depending on concentration, duration, and temperature of storage while maintaining label claim characteristics.
[See table above]
NOTE: TIMENTIN is incompatible with Sodium Bicarbonate.

Unused portions of solutions should be discarded after the time periods listed above.
Avoid excessive heat.
Protect from freezing.

HOW SUPPLIED
Each 3.1-gram vial of TIMENTIN contains sterile ticarcillin disodium equivalent to 3 grams ticarcillin and sterile clavulanate potassium equivalent to 0.1 gram clavulanic acid.
NDC 0029-6571-40   3.1-gram ADD-VANTAGE® Antibiotic Vial
TIMENTIN is also supplied as:
NDC 0029-6571-26   3.1-gram Vial
Each 31-gram Pharmacy Bulk Package contains sterile ticarcillin disodium equivalent to 30 grams ticarcillin and sterile clavulanate potassium equivalent to 1 gram clavulanic acid.
NDC 0029-6579-21   31-gram Pharmacy Bulk Package
TIMENTIN should be stored at or below 24°C (75°F).
NDC 0029-6571-31   TIMENTIN as an iso-osmotic, sterile, nonpyrogenic, frozen solution in GALAXY® (PL 2040) Plastic Containers—supplied in 100-mL single-dose containers equivalent to 3 grams ticarcillin and clavulanate potassium equivalent to 0.1 gram clavulanic acid.

CLINICAL STUDIES
TIMENTIN has been studied in a total of 296 pediatric patients (excluding neonates and infants less than 3 months) in 6 controlled clinical trials. The majority of patients studied had intra-abdominal infections, and the primary comparator was clindamycin and gentamicin with or without ampicillin. At the end-of-therapy visit, comparable efficacy was reported in the trial arms using TIMENTIN and an appropriate comparator.
TIMENTIN was also evaluated in an additional 408 pediatric patients (excluding neonates and infants less than 3 months) in 3 uncontrolled US clinical trials. Patients were treated across a broad range of presenting diagnoses including: Infections in bone and joint, skin and skin structure, lower respiratory tract, urinary tract, as well as intra-abdominal and gynecologic infections. Patients received TIMENTIN either 300 mg/kg/day (based on the ticarcillin component) divided every 4 hours for severe infection or 200 mg/kg/day (based on the ticarcillin component) divided every 6 hours for mild to moderate infections. The efficacy rates were comparable to those obtained in the controlled trials.
The adverse event profile in these 704 pediatric patients treated with TIMENTIN was comparable to that seen in adult patients.

REFERENCES
1. National Committee for Clinical Microbiology Standards. *Methods for Dilution Antimicrobial Susceptibility Tests for Bacteria that Grow Aerobically* - Sixth Edition. Approved Standard. NCCLS Document M7-A6, Vol. 23, No. 2 (ISBN 1-56238-486-4). NCCLS, 940 West Valley Road, Suite 1400, Wayne, PA 19087-1898, January, 2003.
2. National Committee for Clinical Microbiology Standards. *Performance Standards for Antimicrobial Disk Susceptibility Tests* - Eighth Edition. Approved Standard. NCCLS Document M2-A8, Vol. 23, No. 1 (ISBN 1-56238-485-6). NCCLS, 940 West Valley Road, Suite 1400, Wayne, PA 19087-1898, January, 2003.
3. National Committee for Clinical Microbiology Standards. *Performance Standards for Antimicrobial Susceptibility Testing* - Thirteenth Informational Supplement. NCCLS Document M100-S13 (M7), Vol. 23, No. 2. NCCLS, 940 West Valley Road, Suite 1400, Wayne, PA 19087-1898, January, 2003.
4. National Committee for Clinical Laboratory Standards. *Methods for Antimicrobial Susceptibility Testing of Anaerobic Bacteria* - Fifth Edition. Approved Standard. NCCLS Document M11-A5, Vol. 21, No. 2 (ISBN 1–56238-429-5). NCCLS, 940 West Valley Road, Suite 1400, Wayne, PA 19087-1898, January, 2001.
TIMENTIN is a registered trademark of GlaxoSmithKline. The following are registered trademarks of their respective owners: ADD-VANTAGE/Abbott Laboratories; GALAXY/Baxter International Inc.; MULTI-STIX/Bayer Corporation. GlaxoSmithKline
Research Triangle Park, NC 27709
©2009, GlaxoSmithKline. All rights reserved.
February 2009 TMV:17PI

TIMENTIN®
[tī-měn' tin]
(ticarcillin disodium and clavulanate potassium) Injection
GALAXY® (PL 2040) Plastic Container (Product Package)   ℞

To reduce the development of drug-resistant bacteria and maintain the effectiveness of TIMENTIN (ticarcillin disodium and clavulanate potassium) and other antibacterial drugs, TIMENTIN should be used only to treat or prevent infections that are proven or strongly suspected to be caused by bacteria.

DESCRIPTION
TIMENTIN is an injectable antibacterial combination consisting of the semisynthetic antibiotic, ticarcillin disodium, and the β-lactamase inhibitor, clavulanate potassium (the potassium salt of clavulanic acid), for intravenous administration. Ticarcillin is derived from the basic penicillin nucleus, 6-amino-penicillanic acid.
Chemically, ticarcillin disodium is N-(2-Carboxy-3,3-dimethyl-7-oxo-4-thia-1-azabicyclo[3.2.0]hept-6-yl)-3-thiophenemalonamic acid disodium salt and may be represented as:

Clavulanic acid is produced by the fermentation of *Streptomyces clavuligerus*. It is a β-lactam structurally related to the penicillins and possesses the ability to inactivate a wide variety of β-lactamases by blocking the active sites of these enzymes. Clavulanic acid is particularly active against the clinically important plasmid-mediated β-lactamases frequently responsible for transferred drug resistance to penicillins and cephalosporins.
Chemically, clavulanate potassium is potassium (Z)-$(2R,5R)$-3-(2-hydroxyethylidene)-7-oxo-4-oxa-1-azabicyclo[3.2.0]heptane-2-carboxylate and may be represented structurally as:

TIMENTIN is an iso-osmotic, sterile, nonpyrogenic, frozen solution consisting of 3.0 grams ticarcillin as ticarcillin disodium and 0.1 gram clavulanic acid as clavulanate potassium. Approximately 0.3 gram sodium citrate hydrous, USP, is added as a buffer. Sodium hydroxide is used to adjust pH and convert ticarcillin monosodium to ticarcillin disodium. The pH may have been adjusted with hydrochloric acid. The solution is intended for intravenous use after thawing to room temperature. The pH of thawed solution ranges from 5.5 to 7.5.
For the 3.1 gram of TIMENTIN in the GALAXY® (PL 2040) Plastic Container, the theoretical total sodium content of the 100-mL solution is 18.7 mEq (429 mg), of which 15.6 mEq (359 mg) is contributed by the ticarcillin disodium component of TIMENTIN. The total theoretical potassium content of the 100-mL solution is 0.50 mEq (19.63 mg).
This plastic container is fabricated from a specially designed multilayer plastic (PL 2040). Solutions are in contact with the polyethylene layer of this container and can leach out certain chemical components of the plastic in very small amounts within the expiration period. The suitability of the plastic has been confirmed in tests in animals according to USP biological tests for plastic containers, as well as by tissue culture toxicity studies.

CLINICAL PHARMACOLOGY
After an intravenous infusion (30 min.) of 3.1 grams of TIMENTIN, peak serum concentrations of both ticarcillin and clavulanic acid are attained immediately after completion of the infusion. Ticarcillin serum levels are similar to those produced by the administration of equivalent amounts of ticarcillin alone with a mean peak serum level of 324 mcg/mL. The corresponding mean peak serum level for clavulanic acid is 8 mcg/mL. (See following table.)
[See table at top of next page]
The mean area under the serum concentration curve was 485 mcg•hr/mL for ticarcillin and 8.2 mcg•hr/mL for clavulanic acid.
The mean serum half-lives of ticarcillin and clavulanic acid in healthy volunteers are 1.1 hours and 1.1 hours, respectively.
In pediatric patients receiving approximately 50 mg/kg of TIMENTIN (30:1 ratio ticarcillin to clavulanate), mean ticarcillin serum half-lives were 4.4 hours in neonates (n = 18) and 1.0 hour in infants and children (n = 41). The corresponding clavulanate serum half-lives averaged 1.9 hours in neonates (n = 14) and 0.9 hour in infants and children (n = 40). Area under the serum concentration time curves averaged 339 mcg•hr/mL in infants and children (n = 41), whereas the corresponding mean clavulanate area under the serum concentration time curves was approximately 7 mcg•hr/mL in the same population (n = 40).

SERUM LEVELS IN ADULTS
AFTER A 30-MINUTE I.V. INFUSION OF TIMENTIN®
TICARCILLIN SERUM LEVELS (mcg/mL)

Dose	0	15 min.	30 min.	1 hr.	1.5 hr.	3.5 hr.	5.5 hr.
3.1 gram	324 (293-388)	223 (184-293)	176 (135-235)	131 (102-195)	90 (65-119)	27 (19-37)	6 (5-7)

CLAVULANIC ACID SERUM LEVELS (mcg/mL)

Dose	0	15 min.	30 min.	1 hr.	1.5 hr.	3.5 hr.	5.5 hr.
3.1 gram	8.0 (5.3-10.3)	4.6 (3.0-7.6)	2.6 (1.8-3.4)	1.8 (1.6-2.2)	1.2 (0.8-1.6)	0.3 (0.2-0.3)	0

Approximately 60% to 70% of ticarcillin and approximately 35% to 45% of clavulanic acid are excreted unchanged in urine during the first 6 hours after administration of a single dose of TIMENTIN to normal volunteers with normal renal function. Two hours after an intravenous injection of 3.1 grams of TIMENTIN, concentrations of ticarcillin in urine generally exceed 1,500 mcg/mL. The corresponding concentration of clavulanic acid in urine generally exceeds 40 mcg/mL. By 4 to 6 hours after injection, the urine concentrations of ticarcillin and clavulanic acid usually decline to approximately 190 mcg/mL and 2 mcg/mL, respectively. Neither component of TIMENTIN is highly protein bound; ticarcillin has been found to be approximately 45% bound to human serum protein and clavulanic acid approximately 25% bound.

Somewhat higher and more prolonged serum levels of ticarcillin can be achieved with the concurrent administration of probenecid; however, probenecid does not enhance the serum levels of clavulanic acid.

Ticarcillin can be detected in tissues and interstitial fluid following parenteral administration.

Penetration of ticarcillin into bile and pleural fluid has been demonstrated. The results of experiments involving the administration of clavulanic acid to animals suggest that this compound, like ticarcillin, is well distributed in body tissues.

An inverse relationship exists between the serum half-life of ticarcillin and creatinine clearance. The dosage of TIMENTIN need only be adjusted in cases of severe renal impairment. (See DOSAGE AND ADMINISTRATION.)

Ticarcillin may be removed from patients undergoing dialysis; the actual amount removed depends on the duration and type of dialysis.

Microbiology: Ticarcillin is a semisynthetic antibiotic with a broad spectrum of bactericidal activity against many gram-positive and gram-negative aerobic and anaerobic bacteria.

Ticarcillin is, however, susceptible to degradation by β-lactamases, and therefore, the spectrum of activity does not normally include organisms which produce these enzymes.

Clavulanic acid is a β-lactam, structurally related to the penicillins, which possesses the ability to inactivate a wide range of β-lactamase enzymes commonly found in microorganisms resistant to penicillins and cephalosporins. In particular, it has good activity against the clinically important plasmid-mediated β-lactamases frequently responsible for transferred drug resistance.

The formulation of ticarcillin with clavulanic acid in TIMENTIN protects ticarcillin from degradation by β-lactamase enzymes and effectively extends the antibiotic spectrum of ticarcillin to include many bacteria normally resistant to ticarcillin and other β-lactam antibiotics. Thus, TIMENTIN possesses the distinctive properties of a broad-spectrum antibiotic and a β-lactamase inhibitor. Ticarcillin/clavulanic acid has been shown to be active against most strains of the following microorganisms, both in vitro and in clinical infections as described in the INDICATIONS AND USAGE section.

Gram-Positive Aerobes:
Staphylococcus aureus (β-lactamase and non-β-lactamase-producing)*
Staphylococcus epidermidis (β-lactamase and non-β-lactamase-producing)*
*Staphylococci which are resistant to methicillin/oxacillin must be considered resistant to ticarcillin/clavulanic acid.

Gram-Negative Aerobes:
Citrobacter species (β-lactamase and non-β-lactamase-producing)
Enterobacter species including *E. cloacae* (β-lactamase and non-β-lactamase-producing)
(Although most strains of *Enterobacter* species are resistant in vitro, clinical efficacy has been demonstrated with TIMENTIN in urinary tract infections and gynecologic infections caused by these organisms).
Escherichia coli (β-lactamase and non-β-lactamase-producing)
Haemophilus influenzae (β-lactamase and non-β-lactamase-producing)†

Klebsiella species including *K. pneumoniae* (β-lactamase and non-β-lactamase-producing)
Pseudomonas species including *P. aeruginosa* (β-lactamase and non-β-lactamase-producing)
Serratia marcescens (β-lactamase and non-β-lactamase-producing)
† β-lactamase-negative, ampicillin-resistant (BLNAR) strains of *H. influenzae* must be considered resistant to ticarcillin/clavulanic acid.

Anaerobic Bacteria:
Bacteroides fragilis group (β-lactamase and non-β-lactamase-producing)
Prevotella (formerly *Bacteroides*) *melaninogenicus* (β-lactamase and non-β-lactamase-producing)

The following in vitro data are available, **but their clinical significance is unknown.**
The following strains exhibit an in vitro minimum inhibitory concentration (MIC) less than or equal to the susceptible breakpoint for ticarcillin/clavulanic acid. However, with the exception of organisms shown to respond to ticarcillin alone, the safety and effectiveness of ticarcillin/clavulanic acid in treating infections due to these microorganisms have not been established in adequate and well-controlled clinical trials.

Gram-Positive Aerobes:
Staphylococcus saprophyticus (β-lactamase and non-β-lactamase-producing)
Streptococcus agalactiae‡ (Group B)
Streptococcus bovis‡
Streptococcus pneumoniae‡ (penicillin-susceptible strains only)
Streptococcus pyogenes‡
Viridans group streptococci‡

Gram-Negative Aerobes:
Acinetobacter baumannii (β-lactamase and non-β-lactamase-producing)
Acinetobacter calcoaceticus (β-lactamase and non-β-lactamase-producing)
Acinetobacter haemolyticus (β-lactamase and non-β-lactamase-producing)
Acinetobacter lwoffi (β-lactamase and non-β-lactamase-producing)
Moraxella catarrhalis (β-lactamase and non-β-lactamase-producing)
Morganella morganii (β-lactamase and non-β-lactamase-producing)
Neisseria gonorrhoeae (β-lactamase and non-β-lactamase-producing)
Pasteurella multocida (β-lactamase and non-β-lactamase-producing)
Proteus mirabilis (β-lactamase and non-β-lactamase-producing)
Proteus penneri (β-lactamase and non-β-lactamase-producing)
Proteus vulgaris (β-lactamase and non-β-lactamase-producing)
Providencia rettgeri (β-lactamase and non-β-lactamase-producing)
Providencia stuartii (β-lactamase and non-β-lactamase-producing)
Stenotrophomonas maltophilia (β-lactamase and non-β-lactamase-producing)

Anaerobic Bacteria:
Clostridium species including *C. perfringens, C. difficile, C. sporogenes, C. ramosum,* and *C. bifermentans* (β-lactamase and non-β-lactamase-producing)
Eubacterium species
Fusobacterium species including *F. nucleatum* and *F. necrophorum* (β-lactamase and non-β-lactamase-producing)
Peptostreptococcus species‡
Veillonella species‡
‡ These are non-β-lactamase-producing strains, and therefore, are susceptible to ticarcillin. In vitro synergism between TIMENTIN and gentamicin, tobramycin, or amikacin against multiresistant strains of *Pseudomonas aeruginosa* has been demonstrated.

Susceptibility Testing: Dilution Techniques: Quantitative methods are used to determine antimicrobial MICs. These MICs provide estimates of the susceptibility of bacteria to antimicrobial compounds. The MICs should be determined using a standardized procedure. Standardized procedures are based on a dilution method[1,3] (broth or agar) or equivalent with standardized inoculum concentrations and standardized concentrations of ticarcillin/clavulanate potassium powder.

The recommended dilution pattern utilizes a constant level of 2 mcg/mL clavulanic acid in all tubes with varying amounts of ticarcillin. MICs are expressed in terms of the ticarcillin concentration in the presence of clavulanic acid at a constant 2 mcg/mL. The MIC values should be interpreted according to the following criteria:

RECOMMENDED RANGES FOR TICARCILLIN/ CLAVULANIC ACID SUSCEPTIBILITY TESTING*
For *Pseudomonas aeruginosa:*

MIC (mcg/mL)	Interpretation	
≤64	Susceptible	(S)
≥128	Resistant	(R)

For Enterobacteriaceae:

MIC (mcg/mL)	Interpretation	
≤16	Susceptible	(S)
32-64	Intermediate	(I)
≥128	Resistant	(R)

For Staphylococci†:

MIC (mcg/mL)	Interpretation	
≤8	Susceptible	(S)
≥16	Resistant	(R)

* Expressed as concentration of ticarcillin in the presence of clavulanic acid at a constant 2 mcg/mL.
† Staphylococci which are susceptible to ticarcillin/clavulanic acid but resistant to methicillin/oxacillin must be considered as resistant.

A report of "Susceptible" indicates that the pathogen is likely to be inhibited if the antimicrobial compound in the blood reaches the concentrations usually achievable. A report of "Intermediate" indicates that the result should be considered equivocal, and, if the microorganism is not fully susceptible to alternative, clinically feasible drugs, the test should be repeated. This category implies possible clinical applicability in body sites where the drug is physiologically concentrated or in situations where high dosage of drug can be used. This category also provides a buffer zone which prevents small uncontrolled technical factors from causing major discrepancies in interpretation. A report of "Resistant" indicates that the pathogen is not likely to be inhibited if the antimicrobial compound in the blood reaches the concentrations usually achievable; other therapy should be selected.

Standardized susceptibility test procedures require the use of laboratory control microorganisms to control the technical aspects of the laboratory procedures. Standard ticarcillin/clavulanate potassium powder should provide the following MIC values:

Microorganism		MIC (mcg/mL)‡
Escherichia coli	ATCC 25922	4-16
Escherichia coli	ATCC 35218	4-16
Pseudomonas aeruginosa	ATCC 27853	8-32
Staphylococcus aureus	ATCC 29213	0.5-2

‡ Expressed as concentration of ticarcillin in the presence of clavulanic acid at a constant 2 mcg/mL.

Diffusion Techniques: Quantitative methods that require measurement of zone diameters also provide reproducible estimates of the susceptibility of bacteria to antimicrobial compounds. One such standardized procedure[2,3] requires the use of standardized inoculum concentrations. This procedure uses paper disks impregnated with 85 mcg of ticarcillin/clavulanate potassium (75 mcg ticarcillin plus 10 mcg clavulanate potassium) to test the susceptibility of microorganisms to ticarcillin/clavulanic acid.

Reports from the laboratory providing results of the standard single-disk susceptibility test with an 85 mcg of ticarcillin/clavulanate potassium (75 mcg ticarcillin plus 10 mcg clavulanate potassium) disk should be interpreted according to the following criteria:

RECOMMENDED RANGES FOR TICARCILLIN/ CLAVULANIC ACID SUSCEPTIBILITY TESTING
For *Pseudomonas aeruginosa:*

Zone Diameter (mm)	Interpretation	
≥15	Susceptible	(S)
≤14	Resistant	(R)

For Enterobacteriaceae:

Zone Diameter (mm)	Interpretation	
≥20	Susceptible	(S)
15-19	Intermediate	(I)
≤14	Resistant	(R)

For Staphylococci§:

Zone Diameter (mm)	Interpretation	
≥23	Susceptible	(S)
≥22	Resistant	(R)

§ Staphylococci which are resistant to methicillin/oxacillin must be considered as resistant to ticarcillin/clavulanic acid.

Interpretation should be as stated above for results using dilution techniques. Interpretation involves correlation of the diameter obtained in the disk test with the MIC for ticarcillin/clavulanic acid.
As with standardized dilution techniques, diffusion methods require the use of laboratory control microorganisms that are used to control the technical aspects of the laboratory procedures. For the diffusion technique, the 85 mcg of ticarcillin/clavulanate potassium (75 mcg ticarcillin plus 10 mcg clavulanate potassium) disk should provide the following zone diameters in these laboratory test quality control strains:

Microorganism		Zone Diameter (mm)
Escherichia coli	ATCC 25922	24-30
Escherichia coli	ATCC 35218	21-25
Pseudomonas aeruginosa	ATCC 27853	20-28
Staphylococcus aureus	ATCC 25923	29-37

Anaerobic Techniques: For anaerobic bacteria, the susceptibility to ticarcillin/clavulanic acid can be determined by standardized test methods[3,4]. The MIC values obtained should be interpreted according to the following criteria:

RECOMMENDED RANGES FOR TICARCILLIN/ CLAVULANIC ACID SUSCEPTIBILITY TESTING‖

MIC (mcg/mL)	Interpretation	
≤32	Susceptible	(S)
64	Intermediate	(I)
≥128	Resistant	(R)

‖ Expressed as concentration of ticarcillin in the presence of clavulanic acid at a constant 2 mcg/mL.

Interpretation is identical to that stated above for results using dilution techniques.
As with other susceptibility techniques, the use of laboratory control microorganisms is required to control the technical aspects of the laboratory standardized procedures. Standardized ticarcillin/clavulanate potassium powder should provide the following MIC values:
[See table above]

Microorganism		Agar dilution MIC Range (mcg/mL)‖	Broth microdilution MIC Range (mcg/mL)‖
Bacteroides thetaiotaomicron	ATCC 29741	0.5-2	0.5-2
Eubacterium lentum	ATCC 43055	16-64	8-32

‖ Expressed as concentration of ticarcillin in the presence of clavulanic acid at a constant 2 mcg/mL.

INDICATIONS AND USAGE

TIMENTIN is indicated in the treatment of infections caused by susceptible strains of the designated microorganisms in the conditions listed below:
Septicemia (including bacteremia) caused by β-lactamase–producing strains of *Klebsiella* spp.*, *E. coli**, *S. aureus**, or *P. aeruginosa** (or other *Pseudomonas* species*)
Lower Respiratory Infections caused by β-lactamase–producing strains of *S. aureus, H. influenzae**, or *Klebsiella* spp.*
Bone and Joint Infections caused by β-lactamase–producing strains of *S. aureus*
Skin and Skin Structure Infections caused by β-lactamase–producing strains of *S. aureus, Klebsiella* spp.*, or *E. coli**
Urinary Tract Infections (complicated and uncomplicated) caused by β-lactamase–producing strains of *E. coli, Klebsiella* spp., *P. aeruginosa** (or other *Pseudomonas* spp.*), *Citrobacter* spp.*, *Enterobacter cloacae**, *S. marcescens**, or *S. aureus**
Gynecologic Infections endometritis caused by β-lactamase–producing strains of *P. melaninogenicus**, Enterobacter spp. (including *E. cloacae**), *E. coli, Klebsiella pneumoniae**, *S. aureus*, or *S. epidermidis*
Intra-abdominal Infections peritonitis caused by β-lactamase–producing strains of *E. coli, K. pneumoniae*, or *B. fragilis** group
*Efficacy for this organism in this organ system was studied in fewer than 10 infections.
NOTE: For information on use in pediatric patients (≥3 months of age) see PRECAUTIONS—Pediatric Use and CLINICAL STUDIES sections. There are insufficient data to support the use of TIMENTIN in pediatric patients under 3 months of age or for the treatment of septicemia and/or infections in the pediatric population where the suspected or proven pathogen is *H. influenzae* type b.
While TIMENTIN is indicated only for the conditions listed above, infections caused by ticarcillin-susceptible organisms are also amenable to treatment with TIMENTIN due to its ticarcillin content. Therefore, mixed infections caused by ticarcillin-susceptible organisms and β-lactamase–producing organisms susceptible to ticarcillin/clavulanic acid should not require the addition of another antibiotic.
Appropriate culture and susceptibility tests should be performed before treatment in order to isolate and identify organisms causing infection and to determine their susceptibility to ticarcillin/clavulanic acid. Because of its broad spectrum of bactericidal activity against gram-positive and gram-negative bacteria, TIMENTIN is particularly useful for the treatment of mixed infections and for presumptive therapy prior to the identification of the causative organisms. TIMENTIN has been shown to be effective as single drug therapy in the treatment of some serious infections where normally combination antibiotic therapy might be employed. Therapy with TIMENTIN may be initiated before results of such tests are known when there is reason to believe the infection may involve any of the β-lactamase–producing organisms listed above.
Based on the in vitro synergism between ticarcillin/clavulanic acid and aminoglycosides against certain strains of *P. aeruginosa*, combined therapy has been successful, especially in patients with impaired host defenses. Both drugs should be used in full therapeutic doses.
To reduce the development of drug-resistant bacteria and maintain the effectiveness of TIMENTIN and other antibacterial drugs, TIMENTIN should be used only to treat or prevent infections that are proven or strongly suspected to be caused by susceptible bacteria. When culture and susceptibility information are available, they should be considered in selecting or modifying antibacterial therapy. In the absence of such data, local epidemiology and susceptibility patterns may contribute to the empiric selection of therapy.

CONTRAINDICATIONS

TIMENTIN is contraindicated in patients with a history of hypersensitivity reactions to any of the penicillins.

WARNINGS

SERIOUS AND OCCASIONALLY FATAL HYPERSENSITIVITY (ANAPHYLACTIC) REACTIONS HAVE BEEN REPORTED IN PATIENTS ON PENICILLIN THERAPY. THESE REACTIONS ARE MORE LIKELY TO OCCUR IN INDIVIDUALS WITH A HISTORY OF PENICILLIN HYPERSENSITIVITY AND/OR A HISTORY OF SENSITIVITY TO MULTIPLE ALLERGENS. THERE HAVE BEEN REPORTS OF INDIVIDUALS WITH A HISTORY OF PENICILLIN HYPERSENSITIVITY WHO HAVE EXPERIENCED SEVERE REACTIONS WHEN TREATED WITH CEPHALOSPORINS. BEFORE INITIATING THERAPY WITH TIMENTIN, CAREFUL INQUIRY SHOULD BE MADE CONCERNING PREVIOUS HYPERSENSITIVITY REACTIONS TO PENICILLINS, CEPHALOSPORINS, OR OTHER ALLERGENS. IF AN ALLERGIC REACTION OCCURS, TIMENTIN SHOULD BE DISCONTINUED AND THE APPROPRIATE THERAPY INSTITUTED. **SERIOUS ANAPHYLACTIC REACTIONS REQUIRE IMMEDIATE EMERGENCY TREATMENT WITH EPINEPHRINE. OXYGEN, INTRAVENOUS STEROIDS, AND AIRWAY MANAGEMENT, INCLUDING INTUBATION, SHOULD ALSO BE PROVIDED AS INDICATED.**
Clostridium difficile associated diarrhea (CDAD) has been reported with use of nearly all antibacterial agents, including TIMENTIN, and may range in severity from mild diarrhea to fatal colitis. Treatment with antibacterial agents alters the normal flora of the colon leading to overgrowth of *C. difficile*.
C. difficile produces toxins A and B which contribute to the development of CDAD. Hypertoxin producing strains of *C. difficile* cause increased morbidity and mortality, as these infections can be refractory to antimicrobial therapy and may require colectomy. CDAD must be considered in all patients who present with diarrhea following antibiotic use. Careful medical history is necessary since CDAD has been reported to occur over two months after the administration of antibacterial agents.
If CDAD is suspected or confirmed, ongoing antibiotic use not directed against *C. difficile* may need to be discontinued. Appropriate fluid and electrolyte management, protein supplementation, antibiotic treatment of *C. difficile*, and surgical evaluation should be instituted as clinically indicated.
When very high doses of TIMENTIN are administered, especially in the presence of impaired renal function, patients may experience convulsions. (See ADVERSE REACTIONS and OVERDOSAGE.)

PRECAUTIONS

General: While TIMENTIN possesses the characteristic low toxicity of the penicillin group of antibiotics, periodic assessment of organ system functions, including renal, hepatic, and hematopoietic function, is advisable during prolonged therapy.
Bleeding manifestations have occurred in some patients receiving β-lactam antibiotics. These reactions have been associated with abnormalities of coagulation tests such as clotting time, platelet aggregation, and prothrombin time and are more likely to occur in patients with renal impairment. If bleeding manifestations appear, treatment with TIMENTIN should be discontinued and appropriate therapy instituted.
TIMENTIN has only rarely been reported to cause hypokalemia; however, the possibility of this occurring should be kept in mind particularly when treating patients with fluid and electrolyte imbalance. Periodic monitoring of serum potassium may be advisable in patients receiving prolonged therapy.
The theoretical total sodium content of the 100 mL premixed solution is 429 mg (359 mg contributed by the ticarcillin disodium component of TIMENTIN). This should be considered when treating patients requiring restricted salt intake.
As with any penicillin, an allergic reaction, including anaphylaxis, may occur during administration of TIMENTIN, particularly in a hypersensitive individual.
The possibility of superinfections with mycotic or bacterial pathogens should be kept in mind, particularly during prolonged treatment. If superinfections occur, appropriate measures should be taken.
Prescribing TIMENTIN in the absence of a proven or strongly suspected bacterial infection or a prophylactic indication is unlikely to provide benefit to the patient and increases the risk of the development of drug-resistant bacteria.
Information for Patients: Patients should be counseled that antibacterial drugs, including TIMENTIN, should only be used to treat bacterial infections. They do not treat viral infections (e.g., the common cold). When TIMENTIN is prescribed to treat a bacterial infection, patients should be told that although it is common to feel better early in the course of therapy, the medication should be taken exactly as directed. Skipping doses or not completing the full course of therapy may: (1) decrease the effectiveness of the immediate treatment, and (2) increase the likelihood that bacteria will develop resistance and will not be treatable by TIMENTIN or other antibacterial drugs in the future.
Diarrhea is a common problem caused by antibiotics which usually ends when the antibiotic is discontinued. Sometimes after starting treatment with antibiotics, patients can develop watery and bloody stools (with or without stomach cramps and fever) even as late as 2 or more months after having taken the last dose of the antibiotic. If this occurs, patients should contact their physician as soon as possible.
Drug/Laboratory Test Interactions: As with other penicillins, the mixing of TIMENTIN with an aminoglycoside in solutions for parenteral administration can result in substantial inactivation of the aminoglycoside.
Probenecid interferes with the renal tubular secretion of ticarcillin, thereby increasing serum concentrations and prolonging serum half-life of the antibiotic.
In common with other antibiotics, ticarcillin disodium/clavulanate potassium may affect the gut flora, leading to lower estrogen reabsorption and reduced efficacy of combined oral estrogen/progesterone contraceptives.
High urine concentrations of ticarcillin may produce false-positive protein reactions (pseudoproteinuria) with the following methods: Sulfosalicylic acid and boiling test, acetic acid test, biuret reaction, and nitric acid test. The bromphenol blue (MULTI-STIX®) reagent strip test has been reported to be reliable.
The presence of clavulanic acid in TIMENTIN may cause a nonspecific binding of IgG and albumin by red cell membranes leading to a false-positive Coombs test.
Carcinogenesis, Mutagenesis, Impairment of Fertility: Long-term studies in animals have not been performed to evaluate carcinogenic potential. However, results from assays for gene mutation in vitro using bacteria (Ames tests) and yeast, and for chromosomal effects in vitro in human lymphocytes, and in vivo in mouse bone marrow (micronucleus test) indicate that TIMENTIN is without any mutagenic potential.
Pregnancy (Category B): Reproduction studies have been performed in rats given doses up to 1,050 mg/kg/day and have revealed no evidence of impaired fertility or harm to the fetus due to TIMENTIN. There are, however, no adequate and well-controlled studies in pregnant women. Because animal reproduction studies are not always predictive of human response, this drug should be used during pregnancy only if clearly needed.

Creatinine clearance mL/min.	Dosage
over 60	3.1 grams every 4 hrs.
30 to 60	2 grams every 4 hrs.
10 to 30	2 grams every 8 hrs.
less than 10	2 grams every 12 hrs.
less than 10 with hepatic dysfunction	2 grams every 24 hrs.
patients on peritoneal dialysis	3.1 grams every 12 hrs.
patients on hemodialysis	2 grams every 12 hrs. supplemented with 3.1 grams after each dialysis

To calculate creatinine clearance[‡] from a serum creatinine value use the following formula:

$$C_{cr} = \frac{(140-Age) \text{ (wt. in kg)}}{72 \times S_{cr} \text{ (mg/100 mL)}}$$

This is the calculated creatinine clearance for adult males; for females it is 15% less.

[‡] Cockcroft, D.W., et al: Prediction of Creatinine Clearance from Serum Creatinine. Nephron 16:31-41, 1976.

Nursing Mothers: It is not known whether this drug is excreted in human milk. Because many drugs are excreted in human milk, caution should be exercised when TIMENTIN is administered to a nursing woman.

Pediatric Use: The safety and effectiveness of TIMENTIN have been established in the age group of 3 months to 16 years. Use of TIMENTIN in these age groups is supported by evidence from adequate and well-controlled studies of TIMENTIN in adults with additional efficacy, safety, and pharmacokinetic data from both comparative and noncomparative studies in pediatric patients. There are insufficient data to support the use of TIMENTIN in pediatric patients under 3 months of age or for the treatment of septicemia and/or infections in the pediatric population where the suspected or proven pathogen is H. influenzae type b. The potential for toxic effects in children from chemicals that may leach from the single dose premixed intravenous preparation in plastic containers has not been determined. **In those patients in whom meningeal seeding from a distant infection site or in whom meningitis is suspected or documented, or in patients who require prophylaxis against central nervous system infection, an alternate agent with demonstrated clinical efficacy in this setting should be used.**

Geriatric Use: An analysis of clinical studies of TIMENTIN was conducted to determine whether subjects aged 65 and over respond differently from younger subjects. Of the 1,078 subjects treated with at least one dose of TIMENTIN, 67.5% were <65 years old, and 32.5% were ≥65 years old. No overall differences in safety or efficacy were observed between these subjects and younger subjects, and other reported clinical experience have not identified differences in responses between the elderly and younger patients, but a greater sensitivity of some older individuals cannot be ruled out.

This drug is known to be substantially excreted by the kidney, and the risk of toxic reactions to this drug may be greater in patients with impaired renal function. Because elderly patients are more likely to have decreased renal function, care should be taken in dose selection, and it may be useful to monitor renal function (see DOSAGE and ADMINISTRATION).

TIMENTIN contains 103.6 mg (4.51 mEq) of sodium per gram of TIMENTIN. At the usual recommended doses, patients would receive between 1,285 and 1,927 mg/day (56 and 84 mEq) of sodium. The geriatric population may respond with a blunted natriuresis to salt loading. This may be clinically important with regard to such diseases as congestive heart failure.

ADVERSE REACTIONS

As with other penicillins, the following adverse reactions may occur:

Hypersensitivity Reactions: Skin rash, pruritus, urticaria, arthralgia, myalgia, drug fever, chills, chest discomfort, erythema multiforme, toxic epidermal necrolysis, Stevens-Johnson syndrome, and anaphylactic reactions.

Central Nervous System: Headache, giddiness, neuromuscular hyperirritability, or convulsive seizures.

Gastrointestinal Disturbances: Disturbances of taste and smell, stomatitis, flatulence, nausea, vomiting and diarrhea, epigastric pain, and pseudomembranous colitis have been reported. Onset of pseudomembranous colitis symptoms may occur during or after antibiotic treatment. (See WARNINGS.)

Hemic and Lymphatic Systems: Thrombocytopenia, leukopenia, neutropenia, eosinophilia, reduction of hemoglobin or hematocrit, and prolongation of prothrombin time and bleeding time.

Abnormalities of Hepatic Function Tests: Elevation of serum aspartate aminotransferase (SGOT), serum alanine aminotransferase (SGPT), serum alkaline phosphatase, serum LDH, serum bilirubin. There have been reports of transient hepatitis and cholestatic jaundice—as with some other penicillins and some cephalosporins.

Renal and Urinary Effects: Elevation of serum creatinine and/or BUN, hypernatremia, reduction in serum potassium and uric acid. Rare reports of hemorrhagic cystitis.

Local Reactions: Pain, burning, swelling and induration at the infusion site and thrombophlebitis with intravenous administration.

Available safety data for pediatric patients treated with TIMENTIN demonstrate a similar adverse event profile to that observed in adult patients.

DRUG ABUSE AND DEPENDENCE

Neither abuse of nor dependence on TIMENTIN has been reported.

OVERDOSAGE

As with other penicillins, neurotoxic reactions may arise when very high doses of TIMENTIN are administered, especially in patients with impaired renal function. (See WARNINGS and ADVERSE REACTIONS–Central Nervous System.)

In case of overdosage, discontinue TIMENTIN, treat symptomatically, and institute supportive measures as required. Ticarcillin may be removed from circulation by hemodialysis. The molecular weight, degree of protein binding, and pharmacokinetic profile of clavulanic acid together with information from a single patient with renal insufficiency all suggest that this compound may also be removed by hemodialysis.

DOSAGE AND ADMINISTRATION

TIMENTIN should be administered by intravenous infusion (30 min.).

Adults: The usual recommended dosage for systemic and urinary tract infections for average (60 kg) adults is 3.1 grams of TIMENTIN (3.1-gram vial containing 3 grams ticarcillin and 100 mg clavulanic acid) given every 4 to 6 hours. For gynecologic infections, TIMENTIN should be administered as follows: Moderate infections 200 mg/kg/day in divided doses every 6 hours and for severe infections 300 mg/kg/day in divided doses every 4 hours. For patients weighing less than 60 kg, the recommended dosage is 200 to 300 mg/kg/day, based on ticarcillin content, given in divided doses every 4 to 6 hours.

Pediatric Patients (≥3 months): *For patients <60 kg:* In patients <60 kg, TIMENTIN is dosed at 50 mg/kg/dose based on the ticarcillin component. TIMENTIN should be administered as follows: Mild to moderate infections 200 mg/kg/day in divided doses every 6 hours; for severe infections, 300 mg/kg/day in divided doses every 4 hours.

For patients ≥60 kg: For mild to moderate infections, 3.1 grams of TIMENTIN (3 grams of ticarcillin and 100 mg of clavulanic acid) administered every 6 hours; for severe infections, 3.1 grams every 4 hours.

Renal Impairment: For infections complicated by renal insufficiency[†], an initial loading dose of 3.1 grams should be followed by doses based on creatinine clearance and type of dialysis as indicated below:

[See table above]

[†] The half-life of ticarcillin in patients with renal failure is approximately 13 hours.

Dosage for any individual patient must take into consideration the site and severity of infection, the susceptibility of the organisms causing infection, and the status of the patient's host defense mechanisms.

The duration of therapy depends upon the severity of infection. Generally, TIMENTIN should be continued for at least 2 days after the signs and symptoms of infection have disappeared. The usual duration is 10 to 14 days; however, in difficult and complicated infections, more prolonged therapy may be required.

Frequent bacteriologic and clinical appraisals are necessary during therapy of chronic urinary tract infection and may be required for several months after therapy has been completed. Persistent infections may require treatment for several weeks and doses smaller than those indicated above should not be used.

In certain infections, involving abscess formation, appropriate surgical drainage should be performed in conjunction with antimicrobial therapy.

DIRECTIONS FOR USE OF TIMENTIN
Injection
in Plastic Containers
GALAXY® (PL 2040) Plastic Container

TIMENTIN supplied as an iso-osmotic, sterile, nonpyrogenic, frozen solution in GALAXY® (PL 2040) Plastic Containers is for intravenous administration only.

Storage: Avoid unnecessary handling of bags. Store in a freezer capable of maintaining a temperature -20°C (-4°F).

Thawing of Plastic Containers: Thaw frozen bag at room temperature 22°C (72°F) or in a refrigerator 4°C (39°F). [DO NOT FORCE THAW BY IMMERSION IN WATER BATHS OR BY MICROWAVE IRRADIATION.] Check for minute leaks by squeezing bag firmly. If leaks are detected discard solution as sterility may be impaired. Do not add supplementary medication.

The bag should be visually inspected. Thawed solutions should not be used unless clear; solutions will be light to dark yellow in color. Components of the solution may precipitate in the frozen state and will dissolve upon reaching room temperature with little or no agitation. If, after visual inspection, the solution remains cloudy or if an insoluble precipitate is noted or if any seals or outlet ports are not intact, the bag should be discarded.

Use sterile equipment.

The thawed solution is stable for 24 hours at room temperature 22°C (72°F) or for 7 days under refrigeration 4°C (39°F).

DO NOT REFREEZE

Caution: Do not use plastic containers in series connections. Such use could result in an embolism due to residual air being drawn from the primary container before administration of the fluid from the secondary container is complete.

Preparation for Administration:
1. Suspend container from eyelet support.
2. Remove protector from outlet port at bottom of container.
3. Attach administration set. Refer to complete directions accompanying set.

HOW SUPPLIED

TIMENTIN Injection intravenous solution is supplied as a frozen solution in 100-mL single-dose GALAXY® (PL 2040) Plastic Containers.

Each 100-mL single-dose container of TIMENTIN contains ticarcillin disodium equivalent to 3.0 grams ticarcillin and clavulanate potassium equivalent to 0.1 gram clavulanic acid (NDC 0029-6571-31).

Store at or below -20°C (-4°F) [see DIRECTIONS FOR USE OF TIMENTIN Injection in Plastic Containers].

TIMENTIN Injection in GALAXY® (PL 2040) Plastic Containers is manufactured for GlaxoSmithKline by Baxter Healthcare Corporation, Deerfield, Illinois 60015.

TIMENTIN is also supplied as:

NDC 0029-6571-40   3.1-gram ADD-VANTAGE® Antibiotic Vial

Each 31-gram Pharmacy Bulk Package contains sterile ticarcillin disodium equivalent to 30 grams ticarcillin and sterile clavulanate potassium equivalent to 1 gram clavulanic acid.

NDC 0029-6579-21   31-gram Pharmacy Bulk Package

Each 3.1-gram vial contains sterile ticarcillin disodium equivalent to 3 grams ticarcillin and sterile clavulanate potassium equivalent to 0.1 gram clavulanic acid.

NDC 0029-6571-26   3.1-gram Vial

CLINICAL STUDIES

TIMENTIN has been studied in a total of 296 pediatric patients (excluding neonates and infants less than 3 months) in 6 controlled clinical trials. The majority of patients studied had intra-abdominal infections, and the primary comparator was clindamycin and gentamicin with or without ampicillin. At the end-of-therapy visit, comparable efficacy was reported in the trial arms using TIMENTIN and an appropriate comparator.

TIMENTIN was also evaluated in an additional 408 pediatric patients (excluding neonates and infants less than 3 months) in 3 uncontrolled US clinical trials. Patients were treated across a broad range of presenting diagnoses including: Infections in bone and joint, skin and skin structure, lower respiratory tract, urinary tract, as well as intra-abdominal and gynecologic infections. Patients received TIMENTIN either 300 mg/kg/day (based on the ticarcillin component) divided every 4 hours for severe infection or 200 mg/kg/day (based on the ticarcillin component) divided every 6 hours for mild to moderate infections. The efficacy rates were comparable to those obtained in the controlled trials.

The adverse event profile in these 704 pediatric patients treated with TIMENTIN was comparable to that seen in adult patients.

REFERENCES

1. National Committee for Clinical Microbiology Standards. Methods for Dilution Antimicrobial Susceptibility Tests for Bacteria that Grow Aerobically - Sixth Edition. Approved Standard. NCCLS Document M7-A6, Vol. 23,

No. 2 (ISBN 1-56238-486-4). NCCLS, 940 West Valley Road, Suite 1400, Wayne, PA 19087-1898, January, 2003.
2. National Committee for Clinical Microbiology Standards. *Performance Standards for Antimicrobial Disk Suscepti-bility Tests* - Eighth Edition. Approved Standard. NCCLS Document M2-A8, Vol. 23, No. 1 (ISBN 1-56238-485-6). NCCLS, 940 West Valley Road, Suite 1400, Wayne, PA 19087-1898, January, 2003.
3. National Committee for Clinical Microbiology Standards. *Performance Standards for Antimicrobial Susceptibility Testing* - Thirteenth Informational Supplement. NCCLS Document M100-S13 (M7), Vol. 23, No. 2. NCCLS, 940 West Valley Road, Suite 1400, Wayne, PA 19087-1898, January, 2003.
4. National Committee for Clinical Laboratory Standards. *Methods for Antimicrobial Susceptibility Testing of An-aerobic Bacteria* - Fifth Edition. Approved Standard. NCCLS Document M11-A5, Vol. 21, No. 2 (ISBN 1-56238-429-5). NCCLS, 940 West Valley Road, Suite 1400, Wayne, PA 19087-1898, January, 2001.
TIMENTIN is a registered trademark of GlaxoSmithKline. The following are registered trademarks of their respective owners: ADD-VANTAGE/Abbott Laboratories; GALAXY/Baxter International Inc.; MULTI-STIX/Bayer Corporation. GlaxoSmithKline

Research Triangle Park, NC 27709
©2008, GlaxoSmithKline. All rights reserved.
July 2008 TMG:20PI

TIMENTIN®

[tī-měn' tin]
(sterile ticarcillin disodium
and clavulanate potassium)
for Intravenous Administration

Rx

PHARMACY BULK PACKAGE
NOT FOR DIRECT INFUSION

RECONSTITUTED STOCK SOLUTION MUST BE TRANS-FERRED AND FURTHER DILUTED FOR IV INFUSION.

To reduce the development of drug-resistant bacteria and maintain the effectiveness of TIMENTIN (ticarcillin disodium and clavulanate potassium) and other antibacte-rial drugs, TIMENTIN should be used only to treat or pre-vent infections that are proven or strongly suspected to be caused by bacteria.

PACKAGE DESCRIPTION

TIMENTIN is available in a 31-gram Pharmacy Bulk Pack-age. This sterile dosage form contains multiple-single doses for use in a pharmacy admixture program for the prepara-tion of parenteral fluids.

PRODUCT DESCRIPTION

TIMENTIN is a sterile injectable antibacterial combination consisting of the semisynthetic antibiotic ticarcillin disodium and the β-lactamase inhibitor clavulanate potassium (the potassium salt of clavulanic acid) for intra-venous administration. Ticarcillin is derived from the basic penicillin nucleus, 6-amino-penicillanic acid.
Chemically, ticarcillin disodium is N-(2-Carboxy-3,3-dimethyl-7-oxo-4-thia-1-azabicyclo[3.2.0]hept-6-yl)-3-thiophenemalonamic acid disodium salt and may be represented as:

Clavulanic acid is produced by the fermentation of *Strepto-myces clavuligerus*. It is a β-lactam structurally related to the penicillins and possesses the ability to inactivate a wide variety of β-lactamases by blocking the active sites of these enzymes. Clavulanic acid is particularly active against the clinically important plasmid-mediated β-lactamases frequently responsible for transferred drug resistance to penicillins and cephalosporins.
Chemically, clavulanate potassium is potassium (Z)-$(2R,5R)$-3-(2-hydroxyethylidene)-7-oxo-4-oxa-1-azabicyclo [3.2.0]heptane-2-carboxylate and may be represented struc-turally as:

TIMENTIN is supplied as a white to pale yellow powder for reconstitution. TIMENTIN is very soluble in water, its sol-ubility being greater than 600 mg/mL. The reconstituted so-lution is clear, colorless or pale yellow, having a pH of 5.5 to 7.5.

SERUM LEVELS IN ADULTS AFTER A 30-MINUTE IV INFUSION OF TIMENTIN®

TICARCILLIN SERUM LEVELS (mcg/mL)

Dose	0	15 min.	30 min.	1 hr.	1.5 hr.	3.5 hr.	5.5 hr.
3.1 gram	324 (293 to 388)	223 (184 to 293)	176 (135 to 235)	131 (102 to 195)	90 (65 to 119)	27 (19 to 37)	6 (5 to 7)

CLAVULANIC ACID SERUM LEVELS (mcg/mL)

Dose	0	15 min.	30 min.	1 hr.	1.5 hr.	3.5 hr.	5.5 hr.
3.1 gram	8.0 (5.3 to 10.3)	4.6 (3.0 to 7.6)	2.6 (1.8 to 3.4)	1.8 (1.6 to 2.2)	1.2 (0.8 to 1.6)	0.3 (0.2 to 0.3)	0

For the 3.1-gram dosage of TIMENTIN, the theoretical so-dium content is 4.51 mEq (103.6 mg) per gram of TIMENTIN. The theoretical potassium content is 0.15 mEq (6 mg) per gram of TIMENTIN.

CLINICAL PHARMACOLOGY

After an intravenous infusion (30 min.) of 3.1 grams of TIMENTIN, peak serum concentrations of both ticarcillin and clavulanic acid are attained immediately after comple-tion of infusion. Ticarcillin serum levels are similar to those produced by the administration of equivalent amounts of ticarcillin alone with a mean peak serum level of 330 mcg/mL. The corresponding mean peak serum level for clavulanic acid was 8 mcg/mL. (See following table.)
[See table above]
The mean area under the serum concentration curve was 485 mcg•hr/mL for ticarcillin and 8.2 mcg•hr/mL for clavulanic acid.
The mean serum half-lives of ticarcillin and clavulanic acid in healthy volunteers are 1.1 hours and 1.1 hours, respec-tively.
In pediatric patients receiving approximately 50 mg/kg of TIMENTIN (30:1 ratio ticarcillin to clavulanate), mean ticarcillin serum half-lives were 4.4 hours in neonates (n = 18) and 1.0 hour in infants and children (n = 41). The cor-responding clavulanate serum half-lives averaged 1.9 hours in neonates (n = 14) and 0.9 hour in infants and children (n = 40). Area under the serum concentration time curves av-eraged 339 mcg•hr/mL in infants and children (n = 41), whereas the corresponding mean clavulanate area under the serum concentration time curves was approximately 7 mcg•hr/mL in the same population (n = 40).
Approximately 60% to 70% of ticarcillin and approximately 35% to 45% of clavulanic acid are excreted unchanged in urine during the first 6 hours after administration of a sin-gle dose of TIMENTIN to normal volunteers with normal renal function. Two hours after an intravenous injection of 3.1 grams of TIMENTIN, concentrations of ticarcillin in urine generally exceed 1,500 mcg/mL. The corresponding concentrations of clavulanic acid in urine generally exceed 40 mcg/mL. By 4 to 6 hours after injection, the urine con-centrations of ticarcillin and clavulanic acid usually decline to approximately 190 mcg/mL. Neither component of TIMENTIN is highly protein bound; ticarcillin has been found to be approximately 45% bound to human serum pro-tein and clavulanic acid approximately 25% bound.
Somewhat higher and more prolonged serum levels of ticarcillin can be achieved with the concurrent administra-tion of probenecid; however, probenecid does not enhance the serum levels of clavulanic acid.
Ticarcillin can be detected in tissues and interstitial fluid following parenteral administration.
Penetration of ticarcillin into bile and pleural fluid has been demonstrated. The results of experiments involving the ad-ministration of clavulanic acid to animals suggest that this compound, like ticarcillin, is well distributed in body tis-sues.
An inverse relationship exists between the serum half-life of ticarcillin and creatinine clearance. The dosage of TIMENTIN need only be adjusted in cases of severe renal impairment. (See DOSAGE AND ADMINISTRATION.)
Ticarcillin may be removed from patients undergoing dialy-sis; the actual amount removed depends on the duration and type of dialysis.

Microbiology: Ticarcillin is a semisynthetic antibiotic with a broad spectrum of bactericidal activity against many gram-positive and gram-negative aerobic and anaerobic bacteria.
Ticarcillin is, however, susceptible to degradation by β-lactamases, and therefore, the spectrum of activity does not normally include organisms which produce these enzymes.
Clavulanic acid is a β-lactam, structurally related to the penicillins, which possesses the ability to inactivate a wide range of β-lactamase enzymes commonly found in microor-ganisms resistant to penicillins and cephalosporins. In par-ticular, it has good activity against the clinically important plasmid-mediated β-lactamases frequently responsible for transferred drug resistance.

The formulation of ticarcillin with clavulanic acid in TIMENTIN protects ticarcillin from degradation by β-lactamase enzymes and effectively extends the antibiotic spectrum of ticarcillin to include many bacteria normally re-sistant to ticarcillin and other β-lactam antibiotics. Thus, TIMENTIN possesses the distinctive properties of a broad-spectrum antibiotic and a β-lactamase inhibitor. Ticarcillin/clavulanic acid has been shown to be active against most strains of the following microorganisms, both in vitro and in clinical infections as described in the INDICATIONS AND USAGE section.

Gram-Positive Aerobes:
Staphylococcus aureus (β-lactamase and non–β-lactamase–producing)*
Staphylococcus epidermidis (β-lactamase and non–β-lactamase–producing)*
*Staphylococci that are resistant to methicillin/oxacillin must be considered resistant to ticarcillin/clavulanic acid.

Gram-Negative Aerobes:
Citrobacter species (β-lactamase and non–β-lactamase–producing)
Enterobacter species including *E. cloacae* (β-lactamase and non–β-lactamase–producing)
(Although most strains of *Enterobacter* species are resistant in vitro, clinical efficacy has been demonstrated with TIMENTIN in urinary tract infections and gynecologic in-fections caused by these organisms.)
Escherichia coli (β-lactamase and non–β-lactamase–producing)
Haemophilus influenzae (β-lactamase and non–β-lactamase–producing)†
Klebsiella species including *K. pneumoniae* (β-lactamase and non–β-lactamase–producing)
Pseudomonas species including *P. aeruginosa* (β-lactamase and non–β-lactamase–producing)
Serratia marcescens (β-lactamase and non–β-lactamase–producing)
†β-lactamase–negative, ampicillin-resistant (BLNAR) strains of *H. influenzae* must be considered resistant to ticarcillin/clavulanic acid.

Anaerobic Bacteria:
Bacteroides fragilis group (β-lactamase and non–β-lactamase–producing)
Prevotella (formerly *Bacteroides*) *melaninogenicus* (β-lactamase and non–β-lactamase–producing)
The following in vitro data are available, **but their clinical significance is unknown.**
The following strains exhibit an in vitro minimum inhibi-tory concentration (MIC) less than or equal to the suscepti-ble breakpoint for ticarcillin/clavulanic acid. However, with the exception of organisms shown to respond to ticarcillin alone, the safety and effectiveness of ticarcillin/clavulanic acid in treating infections due to these microorganisms have not been established in adequate and well-controlled clini-cal trials.

Gram-Positive Aerobes:
Staphylococcus saprophyticus (β-lactamase and non–β-lactamase–producing)
Streptococcus agalactiae‡ (Group B)
Streptococcus bovis‡
Streptococcus pneumoniae‡ (penicillin-susceptible strains only)
Streptococcus pyogenes‡
Viridans group streptococci‡

Gram-Negative Aerobes:
Acinetobacter baumannii (β-lactamase and non–β-lactamase–producing)
Acinetobacter calcoaceticus (β-lactamase and non–β-lactamase–producing)
Acinetobacter haemolyticus (β-lactamase and non–β-lactamase–producing)
Acinetobacter lwoffi (β-lactamase and non–β-lactamase–producing)
Moraxella catarrhalis (β-lactamase and non–β-lactamase–producing)
Morganella morganii (β-lactamase and non–β-lactamase–producing)
Neisseria gonorrhoeae (β-lactamase and non–β-lactamase–producing)

Pasteurella multocida (β-lactamase and non–β-lactamase–producing)
Proteus mirabilis (β-lactamase and non–β-lactamase–producing)
Proteus penneri (β-lactamase and non–β-lactamase–producing)
Proteus vulgaris (β-lactamase and non–β-lactamase–producing)
Providencia rettgeri (β-lactamase and non–β-lactamase–producing)
Providencia stuartii (β-lactamase and non–β-lactamase–producing)
Stenotrophomonas maltophilia (β-lactamase and non–β-lactamase–producing)

Anaerobic Bacteria:
Clostridium species including *C. perfringens, C. difficile, C. sporogenes, C. ramosum,* and *C. bifermentans* (β-lactamase and non–β-lactamase–producing)
Eubacterium species
Fusobacterium species including *F. nucleatum* and *F. necrophorum* (β-lactamase and non–β-lactamase–producing)
Peptostreptococcus species[‡]
Veillonella species[‡]

[‡]These are non–β-lactamase–producing strains, and therefore, are susceptible to ticarcillin.

In vitro synergism between TIMENTIN and gentamicin, tobramycin, or amikacin against multiresistant strains of *Pseudomonas aeruginosa* has been demonstrated.

Susceptibility Testing: *Dilution Techniques:* Quantitative methods are used to determine antimicrobial MICs. These MICs provide estimates of the susceptibility of bacteria to antimicrobial compounds. The MICs should be determined using a standardized procedure. Standardized procedures are based on a dilution method[1,3] (broth or agar) or equivalent with standardized inoculum concentrations and standardized concentrations of ticarcillin/clavulanate potassium powder.

The recommended dilution pattern utilizes a constant level of 2 mcg/mL clavulanic acid in all tubes with varying amounts of ticarcillin. MICs are expressed in terms of the ticarcillin concentration in the presence of clavulanic acid at a constant 2 mcg/mL. The MIC values should be interpreted according to the following criteria:

RECOMMENDED RANGES FOR TICARCILLIN/ CLAVULANIC ACID SUSCEPTIBILITY TESTING*
For *Pseudomonas aeruginosa:*

MIC (mcg/mL)	Interpretation
≤64	Susceptible (S)
≥128	Resistant (R)

For *Enterobacteriaceae:*

MIC (mcg/mL)	Interpretation
≤16	Susceptible (S)
32-64	Intermediate (I)
≥128	Resistant (R)

For *Staphylococci*[†]:

MIC (mcg/mL)	Interpretation
≤8	Susceptible (S)
≥16	Resistant (R)

* Expressed as concentration of ticarcillin in the presence of clavulanic acid at a constant 2 mcg/mL.
† Staphylococci that are susceptible to ticarcillin/clavulanic acid but resistant to methicillin/oxacillin must be considered as resistant.

A report of "Susceptible" indicates that the pathogen is likely to be inhibited if the antimicrobial compound in the blood reaches the concentrations usually achievable. A report of "Intermediate" indicates that the result should be considered equivocal, and, if the microorganism is not fully susceptible to alternative, clinically feasible drugs, the test should be repeated. This category implies possible clinical applicability in body sites where the drug is physiologically concentrated or in situations where high dosage of drug can be used. This category also provides a buffer zone that prevents small uncontrolled technical factors from causing major discrepancies in interpretation. A report of "Resistant" indicates that the pathogen is not likely to be inhibited if the antimicrobial compound in the blood reaches the concentrations usually achievable; other therapy should be selected.

Standardized susceptibility test procedures require the use of laboratory control microorganisms to control the technical aspects of the laboratory procedures. Standard ticarcillin/clavulanate potassium powder should provide the following MIC values:

Microorganism		MIC (mcg/mL)[‡]
Escherichia coli	ATCC 25922	4-16
Escherichia coli	ATCC 35218	4-16
Pseudomonas aeruginosa	ATCC 27853	8-32
Staphylococcus aureus	ATCC 29213	0.5-2

‡ Expressed as concentration of ticarcillin in the presence of clavulanic acid at a constant 2 mcg/mL.

Diffusion Techniques: Quantitative methods that require measurement of zone diameters also provide reproducible estimates of the susceptibility of bacteria to antimicrobial compounds. One such standardized procedure[2,3] requires the use of standardized inoculum concentrations. This procedure uses paper disks impregnated with 85 mcg of ticarcillin/clavulanate potassium (75 mcg ticarcillin plus 10 mcg clavulanate potassium) to test the susceptibility of microorganisms to ticarcillin/clavulanic acid.

Reports from the laboratory providing results of the standard single-disk susceptibility test with an 85 mcg of ticarcillin/clavulanate potassium (75 mcg ticarcillin plus 10 mcg clavulanate potassium) disk should be interpreted according to the following criteria:

RECOMMENDED RANGES FOR TICARCILLIN/ CLAVULANIC ACID SUSCEPTIBILITY TESTING
For *Pseudomonas aeruginosa:*

Zone Diameter (mm)	Interpretation
≥15	Susceptible (S)
≤14	Resistant (R)

For *Enterobacteriaceae:*

Zone Diameter (mm)	Interpretation
≥20	Susceptible (S)
15-19	Intermediate (I)
≤14	Resistant (R)

For *Staphylococci*[§]:

Zone Diameter (mm)	Interpretation
≥23	Susceptible (S)
≤22	Resistant (R)

§ Staphylococci that are resistant to methicillin/oxacillin must be considered as resistant to ticarcillin/clavulanic acid.

Interpretation should be as stated above for results using dilution techniques. Interpretation involves correlation of the diameter obtained in the disk test with the MIC for ticarcillin/clavulanic acid.

As with standardized dilution techniques, diffusion methods require the use of laboratory control microorganisms that are used to control the technical aspects of the laboratory procedures. For the diffusion technique, the 85 mcg of ticarcillin/clavulanate potassium (75 mcg ticarcillin plus 10 mcg clavulanate potassium) disk should provide the following zone diameters in these laboratory test quality control strains:

Microorganism		Zone Diameter (mm)
Escherichia coli	ATCC 25922	24-30
Escherichia coli	ATCC 35218	21-25
Pseudomonas aeruginosa	ATCC 27853	20-28
Staphylococcus aureus	ATCC 25923	29-37

Anaerobic Techniques: For anaerobic bacteria, the susceptibility to ticarcillin/clavulanic acid can be determined by standardized test methods[3,4]. The MIC values obtained should be interpreted according to the following criteria:

RECOMMENDED RANGES FOR TICARCILLIN/ CLAVULANIC ACID SUSCEPTIBILITY TESTING‖

MIC (mcg/mL)	Interpretation
≤32	Susceptible (S)
64	Intermediate (I)
≥128	Resistant (R)

‖ Expressed as concentration of ticarcillin in the presence of clavulanic acid at a constant 2 mcg/mL.

Interpretation is identical to that stated above for results using dilution techniques.

As with other susceptibility techniques, the use of laboratory control microorganisms is required to control the technical aspects of the laboratory standardized procedures. Standardized ticarcillin/clavulanate potassium powder should provide the following MIC values:
[See table below]

INDICATIONS AND USAGE

TIMENTIN is indicated in the treatment of infections caused by susceptible strains of the designated microorganisms in the conditions listed below:
Septicemia (including bacteremia) caused by β-lactamase–producing strains of *Klebsiella* spp.*, *E. coli**, *S. aureus**, or *P. aeruginosa** (or other *Pseudomonas* species*)
Lower Respiratory Infections caused by β-lactamase–producing strains of *S. aureus, H. influenzae**, or *Klebsiella* spp.*
Bone and Joint Infections caused by β-lactamase–producing strains of *S. aureus*
Skin and Skin Structure Infections caused by β-lactamase–producing strains of *S. aureus, Klebsiella* spp.*, or *E. coli**
Urinary Tract Infections (complicated and uncomplicated) caused by β-lactamase–producing strains of *E. coli, Klebsiella* spp.*, *P. aeruginosa** (or other *Pseudomonas* spp.*), *Citrobacter* spp.*, *Enterobacter cloacae**, *S. marcescens**, or *S. aureus**
Gynecologic Infections endometritis caused by β-lactamase–producing strains of *P. melaninogenicus**, *Enterobacter* spp. (including *E. cloacae**), *E. coli, K. pneumoniae**, *S. aureus*, or *S. epidermidis*
Intra-abdominal Infections peritonitis caused by β-lactamase–producing strains of *E. coli, K. pneumoniae*, or *B. fragilis** group
*Efficacy for this organism in this organ system was studied in fewer than 10 infections.
NOTE: For information on use in pediatric patients (≥3 months of age) see PRECAUTIONS—Pediatric Use and CLINICAL STUDIES sections. There are insufficient data to support the use of TIMENTIN in pediatric patients under 3 months of age or for the treatment of septicemia and/or infections in the pediatric population where the suspected or proven pathogen is *H. influenzae* type b.

While TIMENTIN is indicated only for the conditions listed above, infections caused by ticarcillin-susceptible organisms are also amenable to treatment with TIMENTIN due to its ticarcillin content. Therefore, mixed infections caused by ticarcillin-susceptible organisms and β-lactamase–producing organisms susceptible to ticarcillin/clavulanic acid should not require the addition of another antibiotic. Appropriate culture and susceptibility tests should be performed before treatment in order to isolate and identify organisms causing infection and to determine their susceptibility to ticarcillin/clavulanic acid. Because of its broad spectrum of bactericidal activity against gram-positive and gram-negative bacteria, TIMENTIN is particularly useful for the treatment of mixed infections and for presumptive therapy prior to the identification of the causative organisms. TIMENTIN has been shown to be effective as single drug therapy in the treatment of some serious infections where normally combination antibiotic therapy might be employed. Therapy with TIMENTIN may be initiated before results of such tests are known when there is reason to believe the infection may involve any of the β-lactamase–producing organisms listed above.

Based on the in vitro synergism between ticarcillin/clavulanic acid and aminoglycosides against certain strains of *P. aeruginosa*, combined therapy has been successful, especially in patients with impaired host defenses. Both drugs should be used in full therapeutic doses.

To reduce the development of drug-resistant bacteria and maintain the effectiveness of TIMENTIN and other antibacterial drugs, TIMENTIN should be used only to treat or prevent infections that are proven or strongly suspected to be caused by susceptible bacteria. When culture and susceptibility information are available, they should be considered in selecting or modifying antibacterial therapy. In the absence of such data, local epidemiology and susceptibility patterns may contribute to the empiric selection of therapy.

CONTRAINDICATIONS

TIMENTIN is contraindicated in patients with a history of hypersensitivity reactions to any of the penicillins.

WARNINGS

SERIOUS AND OCCASIONALLY FATAL HYPERSENSITIVITY (ANAPHYLACTIC) REACTIONS HAVE BEEN REPORTED IN PATIENTS ON PENICILLIN THERAPY. THESE REACTIONS ARE MORE LIKELY TO OCCUR IN INDIVIDUALS WITH A HISTORY OF PENICILLIN HYPERSENSITIVITY AND/OR A HISTORY OF SENSITIVITY TO MULTIPLE ALLERGENS. THERE HAVE BEEN REPORTS OF INDIVIDUALS WITH A HISTORY OF PENICILLIN HYPERSENSITIVITY WHO HAVE EXPERIENCED SEVERE REACTIONS WHEN TREATED WITH CEPHALOSPORINS. BEFORE INITIATING THERAPY

Microorganism		Agar dilution MIC Range (mcg/mL)‖	Broth microdilution MIC Range (mcg/mL)‖
Bacteroides thetaiotaomicron	ATCC 29741	0.5-2	0.5-2
Eubacterium lentum	ATCC 43055	16-64	8-32

‖ Expressed as concentration of ticarcillin in the presence of clavulanic acid at a constant 2 mcg/mL.

WITH TIMENTIN, CAREFUL INQUIRY SHOULD BE MADE CONCERNING PREVIOUS HYPERSENSITIVITY REACTIONS TO PENICILLINS, CEPHALOSPORINS, OR OTHER ALLERGENS. IF AN ALLERGIC REACTION OCCURS, TIMENTIN SHOULD BE DISCONTINUED AND THE APPROPRIATE THERAPY INSTITUTED. **SERIOUS ANAPHYLACTIC REACTIONS REQUIRE IMMEDIATE EMERGENCY TREATMENT WITH EPINEPHRINE. OXYGEN, INTRAVENOUS STEROIDS, AND AIRWAY MANAGEMENT, INCLUDING INTUBATION, SHOULD ALSO BE PROVIDED AS INDICATED.**

Clostridium difficile associated diarrhea (CDAD) has been reported with use of nearly all antibacterial agents, including TIMENTIN, and may range in severity from mild diarrhea to fatal colitis. Treatment with antibacterial agents alters the normal flora of the colon leading to overgrowth of *C. difficile.*

C. difficile produces toxins A and B which contribute to the development of CDAD. Hypertoxin producing strains of *C. difficile* cause increased morbidity and mortality, as these infections can be refractory to antimicrobial therapy and may require colectomy. CDAD must be considered in all patients who present with diarrhea following antibiotic use. Careful medical history is necessary since CDAD has been reported to occur over two months after the administration of antibacterial agents.

If CDAD is suspected or confirmed, ongoing antibiotic use not directed against *C. difficile* may need to be discontinued. Appropriate fluid and electrolyte management, protein supplementation, antibiotic treatment of *C. difficile,* and surgical evaluation should be instituted as clinically indicated.

When very high doses of TIMENTIN are administered, especially in the presence of impaired renal function, patients may experience convulsions. (See ADVERSE REACTIONS and OVERDOSAGE.)

PRECAUTIONS
General: While TIMENTIN possesses the characteristic low toxicity of the penicillin group of antibiotics, periodic assessment of organ system functions, including renal, hepatic, and hematopoietic function, is advisable during prolonged therapy.

Bleeding manifestations have occurred in some patients receiving β-lactam antibiotics. These reactions have been associated with abnormalities of coagulation tests such as clotting time, platelet aggregation, and prothrombin time and are more likely to occur in patients with renal impairment. If bleeding manifestations appear, treatment with TIMENTIN should be discontinued and appropriate therapy instituted.

TIMENTIN has only rarely been reported to cause hypokalemia; however, the possibility of this occurring should be kept in mind particularly when treating patients with fluid and electrolyte imbalance. Periodic monitoring of serum potassium may be advisable in patients receiving prolonged therapy.

The theoretical sodium content is 4.51 mEq (103.6 mg) per gram of TIMENTIN. This should be considered when treating patients requiring restricted salt intake.

As with any penicillin, an allergic reaction, including anaphylaxis, may occur during TIMENTIN administration, particularly in a hypersensitive individual.

The possibility of superinfections with mycotic or bacterial pathogens should be kept in mind, particularly during prolonged treatment. If superinfections occur, appropriate measures should be taken.

Prescribing TIMENTIN in the absence of a proven or strongly suspected bacterial infection or a prophylactic indication is unlikely to provide benefit to the patient and increases the risk of the development of drug-resistant bacteria.

Information for Patients: Patients should be counseled that antibacterial drugs, including TIMENTIN, should only be used to treat bacterial infections. They do not treat viral infections (e.g., the common cold). When TIMENTIN is prescribed to treat a bacterial infection, patients should be told that although it is common to feel better early in the course of therapy, the medication should be taken exactly as directed. Skipping doses or not completing the full course of therapy may: (1) decrease the effectiveness of the immediate treatment, and (2) increase the likelihood that bacteria will develop resistance and will not be treatable by TIMENTIN or other antibacterial drugs in the future.

Diarrhea is a common problem caused by antibiotics which usually ends when the antibiotic is discontinued. Sometimes after starting treatment with antibiotics, patients can develop watery and bloody stools (with or without stomach cramps and fever) even as late as 2 or more months after having taken the last dose of the antibiotic. If this occurs, patients should contact their physician as soon as possible.

Drug/Laboratory Test Interactions: As with other penicillins, the mixing of TIMENTIN with an aminoglycoside in solutions for parenteral administration can result in substantial inactivation of the aminoglycoside.

Probenecid interferes with the renal tubular secretion of ticarcillin, thereby increasing serum concentrations and prolonging serum half-life of the antibiotic.

In common with other antibiotics, ticarcillin disodium/clavulanate potassium may affect the gut flora, leading to lower estrogen reabsorption and reduced efficacy of combined oral estrogen/progesterone contraceptives.

High urine concentrations of ticarcillin may produce false-positive protein reactions (pseudoproteinuria) with the following methods: Sulfosalicylic acid and boiling test, acetic acid test, biuret reaction, and nitric acid test. The bromphenol blue (MULTI-STIX®) reagent strip test has been reported to be reliable.

The presence of clavulanic acid in TIMENTIN may cause a nonspecific binding of IgG and albumin by red cell membranes leading to a false-positive Coombs test.

Carcinogenesis, Mutagenesis, Impairment of Fertility: Long-term studies in animals have not been performed to evaluate carcinogenic potential. However, results from assays for gene mutation in vitro using bacteria (Ames tests) and yeast, and for chromosomal effects in vitro in human lymphocytes, and in vivo in mouse bone marrow (micronucleus test) indicate that TIMENTIN is without any mutagenic potential.

Pregnancy (Category B): Reproduction studies have been performed in rats given doses up to 1,050 mg/kg/day and have revealed no evidence of impaired fertility or harm to the fetus due to TIMENTIN. There are, however, no adequate and well-controlled studies in pregnant women. Because animal reproduction studies are not always predictive of human response, this drug should be used during pregnancy only if clearly needed.

Nursing Mothers: It is not known whether this drug is excreted in human milk. Because many drugs are excreted in human milk, caution should be exercised when TIMENTIN is administered to a nursing woman.

Pediatric Use: The safety and effectiveness of TIMENTIN have been established in the age group of 3 months to 16 years. Use of TIMENTIN in these age groups is supported by evidence from adequate and well-controlled studies of TIMENTIN in adults with additional efficacy, safety, and pharmacokinetic data from both comparative and noncomparative studies in pediatric patients. There are insufficient data to support the use of TIMENTIN in pediatric patients under 3 months of age or for the treatment of septicemia and/or infections in the pediatric population where the suspected or proven pathogen is *H. influenzae* type b.

In those patients in whom meningeal seeding from a distant infection site or in whom meningitis is suspected or documented, or in patients who require prophylaxis against central nervous system infection, an alternate agent with demonstrated clinical efficacy in this setting should be used.

Geriatric Use: An analysis of clinical studies of TIMENTIN was conducted to determine whether subjects aged 65 and over respond differently from younger subjects. Of the 1,078 subjects treated with at least one dose of TIMENTIN, 67.5% were <65 years old, and 32.5% were ≥65 years old. No overall differences in safety or efficacy were observed between these subjects and younger subjects, and other reported clinical experience have not identified differences in responses between the elderly and younger patients, but a greater sensitivity of some older individuals cannot be ruled out.

This drug is known to be substantially excreted by the kidney, and the risk of toxic reactions to this drug may be greater in patients with impaired renal function. Because elderly patients are more likely to have decreased renal function, care should be taken in dose selection, and it may be useful to monitor renal function (see DOSAGE and ADMINISTRATION).

TIMENTIN contains 103.6 mg (4.51 mEq) of sodium per gram of TIMENTIN. At the usual recommended doses, patients would receive between 1,285 and 1,927 mg/day (56 and 84 mEq) of sodium. The geriatric population may respond with a blunted natriuresis to salt loading. This may be clinically important with regard to such diseases as congestive heart failure.

ADVERSE REACTIONS

As with other penicillins, the following adverse reactions may occur:

Hypersensitivity Reactions: Skin rash, pruritus, urticaria, arthralgia, myalgia, drug fever, chills, chest discomfort, erythema multiforme, toxic epidermal necrolysis, Stevens-Johnson syndrome, and anaphylactic reactions.

Central Nervous System: Headache, giddiness, neuromuscular hyperirritability, or convulsive seizures.

Gastrointestinal Disturbances: Disturbances of taste and smell, stomatitis, flatulence, nausea, vomiting and diarrhea, epigastric pain, and pseudomembranous colitis have been reported. Onset of pseudomembranous colitis symptoms may occur during or after antibiotic treatment. (See WARNINGS.)

Hemic and Lymphatic Systems: Thrombocytopenia, leukopenia, neutropenia, eosinophilia, reduction of hemoglobin or hematocrit, and prolongation of prothrombin time and bleeding time.

Abnormalities of Hepatic Function Tests: Elevation of serum aspartate aminotransferase (SGOT), serum alanine aminotransferase (SGPT), serum alkaline phosphatase, serum LDH, serum bilirubin. There have been reports of transient hepatitis and cholestatic jaundice—as with some other penicillins and some cephalosporins.

Renal and Urinary Effects: Elevation of serum creatinine and/or BUN, hypernatremia, reduction in serum potassium, and uric acid. Rare reports of hemorrhagic cystitis.

Local Reactions: Pain, burning, swelling, and induration at the injection site and thrombophlebitis with intravenous administration.

Available safety data for pediatric patients treated with TIMENTIN demonstrate a similar adverse event profile to that observed in adult patients.

DRUG ABUSE AND DEPENDENCE

Neither abuse of nor dependence on TIMENTIN has been reported.

OVERDOSAGE

As with other penicillins, neurotoxic reactions may arise when very high doses of TIMENTIN are administered, especially in patients with impaired renal function. (See WARNINGS and ADVERSE REACTIONS—Central Nervous System.)

In case of overdosage, discontinue TIMENTIN, treat symptomatically, and institute supportive measures as required. Ticarcillin may be removed from circulation by hemodialysis. The molecular weight, degree of protein binding, and pharmacokinetic profile of clavulanic acid, together with information from a single patient with renal insufficiency all suggest that this compound may also be removed by hemodialysis.

DOSAGE AND ADMINISTRATION

TIMENTIN should be administered by intravenous infusion (30 min.).

Adults: The usual recommended dosage for systemic and urinary tract infections for average (60 kg) adults is 3.1 grams TIMENTIN (3.1-gram vial containing 3 grams ticarcillin and 100 mg clavulanic acid) given every 4 to 6 hours. For gynecologic infections, TIMENTIN should be administered as follows: Moderate infections, 200 mg/kg/day in divided doses every 6 hours, and for severe infections, 300 mg/kg/day in divided doses every 4 hours. For patients weighing less than 60 kg, the recommended dosage is 200 to 300 mg/kg/day, based on ticarcillin content, given in divided doses every 4 to 6 hours.

Pediatric Patients (≥3 months): *For patients <60 kg:* In patients <60 kg, TIMENTIN is dosed at 50 mg/kg/dose based on the ticarcillin component. TIMENTIN should be administered as follows: Mild to moderate infections 200 mg/kg/day in divided doses every 6 hours; for severe infections, 300 mg/kg/day in divided doses every 4 hours.

For patients ≥60 kg: For mild to moderate infections, 3.1 grams of TIMENTIN (3 grams of ticarcillin and 100 mg of clavulanic acid) administered every 6 hours; for severe infections, 3.1 grams every 4 hours.

Renal Impairment: For infections complicated by renal insufficiency†, an initial loading dose of 3.1 grams should be followed by doses based on creatinine clearance and type of dialysis as indicated below:

[See first table at top of next page]

†The half-life of ticarcillin in patients with renal failure is approximately 13 hours.

Dosage for any individual patient must take into consideration the site and severity of infection, the susceptibility of the organisms causing infection, and the status of the patient's host defense mechanisms.

The duration of therapy depends upon the severity of infection. Generally, TIMENTIN should be continued for at least 2 days after the signs and symptoms of infection have disappeared. The usual duration is 10 to 14 days; however, in difficult and complicated infections, more prolonged therapy may be required.

Frequent bacteriologic and clinical appraisals are necessary during therapy of chronic urinary tract infection and may be required for several months after therapy has been completed. Persistent infections may require treatment for several weeks, and doses smaller than those indicated above should not be used.

In certain infections, involving abscess formation, appropriate surgical drainage should be performed in conjunction with antimicrobial therapy.

INTRAVENOUS ADMINISTRATION
DIRECTIONS FOR PROPER USE OF PHARMACY BULK PACKAGE
RECONSTITUTED STOCK SOLUTION MUST BE TRANSFERRED AND FURTHER DILUTED FOR I.V. INFUSION.

Creatinine clearance mL/min.	Dosage
over 60	3.1 grams every 4 hrs.
30 to 60	2 grams every 4 hrs.
10 to 30	2 grams every 8 hrs.
less than 10	2 grams every 12 hrs.
less than 10 with hepatic dysfunction	2 grams every 24 hrs.
patients on peritoneal dialysis	3.1 grams every 12 hrs.
patients on hemodialysis	2 grams every 12 hrs. supplemented with 3.1 grams after each dialysis

To calculate creatinine clearance[‡] from a serum creatinine value use the following formula:

$$C_{cr} = \frac{(140-Age)\ (wt.\ in\ kg)}{72 \times S_{cr}\ (mg/100\ mL)}$$

This is the calculated creatinine clearance for adult males; for females it is 15% less.

[‡] Cockcroft, D.W., et al: Prediction of Creatinine Clearance from Serum Creatinine. Nephron 16:31-41, 1976.

STABILITY PERIOD
(31-gram Pharmacy Bulk Package)

Intravenous Solution (ticarcillin concentrations of 10 mg/mL to 100 mg/mL)	Room Temperature 21° to 24°C (70° to 75°F)	Refrigerated 4°C (40°F)
Dextrose Injection 5%, USP	24 hours	3 days
Sodium Chloride Injection 0.9%, USP	24 hours	4 days
Lactated Ringer's Injection, USP	24 hours	4 days
Sterile Water for Injection, USP	24 hours	4 days

The container closure may be penetrated only one time utilizing a suitable sterile transfer device or dispensing set that allows measured distribution of the contents. A sterile substance that must be reconstituted prior to use may require a separate closure entry.
Restrict use of Pharmacy Bulk Packages to an aseptic area such as a laminar flow hood.
Reconstituted contents of the vial should be withdrawn immediately. However, if this is not possible, aliquoting operations must be completed within 4 hours of reconstitution.
Discard the reconstituted stock solution 4 hours after initial entry.
Add 76 mL of Sterile Water for Injection, USP, or Sodium Chloride Injection, USP, to the 31-gram Pharmacy Bulk Package and shake well. For ease of reconstitution, the diluent may be added in 2 portions. Each 1.0 mL of the resulting concentrated stock solution contains approximately 300 mg of ticarcillin and 10 mg of clavulanic acid.
Intravenous Infusion: The desired dosage should be withdrawn from the stock solution and further diluted to desired volume using the recommended solution listed in the COMPATIBILITY AND STABILITY section (STABILITY PERIOD) to a concentration between 10 mg/mL to 100 mg/mL. The solution of reconstituted drug may then be administered over a period of 30 minutes by direct infusion, or through a Y-type intravenous infusion set. If this method of administration is used, it is advisable to discontinue temporarily the administration of any other solution during the infusion of TIMENTIN.
Stability: For I.V. solutions, see STABILITY PERIOD below.
When TIMENTIN is given in combination with another antimicrobial, such as an aminoglycoside, each drug should be given separately in accordance with the recommended dosage and routes of administration for each drug.
After reconstitution and prior to administration, TIMENTIN, as with other parenteral drugs, should be inspected visually for particulate matter. If this condition is evident, the solution should be discarded.
The color of reconstituted solutions of TIMENTIN normally ranges from light to dark yellow, depending on concentration, duration, and temperature of storage while maintaining label claim characteristics.
COMPATIBILITY AND STABILITY
31-gram Pharmacy Bulk Package
(Dilutions derived from a stock solution of 300 mg/mL)
Aliquots of the reconstituted stock solution at 300 mg/mL are stable for up to 6 hours between 21° and 24°C (70° and 75°F) or up to 72 hours under refrigeration 4°C (40°F). The reconstituted stock solution should be held under refrigeration 4°C (40°F).
If the aliquots of the reconstituted stock solution (300 mg/mL) are held up to 6 hours between 21° and 24°C (70° and 75°F) or up to 72 hours under refrigeration 4°C (40°F) and further diluted to a concentration between 10 mg/mL and 100 mg/mL with any of the diluents listed below, then the following stability periods apply.
[See second table above]
If an aliquot of concentrated stock solution (300 mg/mL) is stored for up to 6 hours between 21° and 24°C (70° and 75°F) and then further diluted to a concentration between 10 mg/mL and 100 mg/mL, solutions of Sodium Chloride Injection, USP, Lactated Ringer's Injection, USP, and Sterile Water for Injection, USP, may be stored frozen −18°C (0°F) for up to 30 days. Solutions prepared with Dextrose Injection 5%, USP, may be stored frozen −18°C (0°F) for up to 7 days. All thawed solutions should be used within 8 hours or discarded. Once thawed, solutions should not be refrozen.
NOTE: TIMENTIN is incompatible with Sodium Bicarbonate.
Unused solutions must be discarded after the time periods listed above.
HOW SUPPLIED
Each 31-gram vial of TIMENTIN contains sterile ticarcillin disodium equivalent to 30 grams ticarcillin and sterile clavulanate potassium equivalent to 1 gram clavulanic acid.
NDC 0029-6579-21   31-gram Pharmacy Bulk Package
TIMENTIN is also supplied as:
NDC 0029-6571-26   3.1-gram Vial
NDC 0029-6571-40   3.1-gram ADD-VANTAGE® Antibiotic Vial
Vials of TIMENTIN should be stored at or below 24°C (75°F).
NDC 0029-6571-31   TIMENTIN as an iso-osmotic, sterile, nonpyrogenic, frozen solution in GALAXY® (PL 2040) Plastic Containers—supplied in 100 mL single-dose containers equivalent to 3 grams ticarcillin and clavulanate potassium equivalent to 0.1 gram clavulanic acid.
CLINICAL STUDIES
TIMENTIN has been studied in a total of 296 pediatric patients (excluding neonates and infants less than 3 months) in 6 controlled clinical trials. The majority of patients studied had intra-abdominal infections, and the primary comparator was clindamycin and gentamicin with or without ampicillin. At the end-of-therapy visit, comparable efficacy was reported in the trial arms using TIMENTIN and an appropriate comparator.
TIMENTIN was also evaluated in an additional 408 pediatric patients (excluding neonates and infants less than 3 months) in 3 uncontrolled US clinical trials. Patients were treated across a broad range of presenting diagnoses including: Infections in bone and joint, skin and skin structure, lower respiratory tract, urinary tract, as well as intra-abdominal and gynecologic infections. Patients received TIMENTIN either 300 mg/kg/day (based on the ticarcillin component) divided every 4 hours for severe infection or 200 mg/kg/day (based on the ticarcillin component) divided every 6 hours for mild to moderate infections. The efficacy rates were comparable to those obtained in the controlled trials.
The adverse event profile in these 704 pediatric patients treated with TIMENTIN was comparable to that seen in adult patients.

REFERENCES
1. National Committee for Clinical Microbiology Standards. *Methods for Dilution Antimicrobial Susceptibility Tests for Bacteria that Grow Aerobically* - Sixth Edition. Approved Standard. NCCLS Document M7-A6, Vol. 23, No. 2 (ISBN 1-56238-486-4). NCCLS, 940 West Valley Road, Suite 1400, Wayne, PA 19087-1898, January, 2003.
2. National Committee for Clinical Microbiology Standards. *Performance Standards for Antimicrobial Disk Susceptibility Tests* - Eighth Edition. Approved Standard. NCCLS Document M2-A8, Vol. 23, No. 1 (ISBN 1-56238-485-6). NCCLS, 940 West Valley Road, Suite 1400, Wayne, PA 19087-1898, January, 2003.
3. National Committee for Clinical Microbiology Standards. *Performance Standards for Antimicrobial Susceptibility Testing* - Thirteenth Informational Supplement. NCCLS Document M100-S13 (M7), Vol. 23, No. 2. NCCLS, 940 West Valley Road, Suite 1400, Wayne, PA 19087-1898, January, 2003.
4. National Committee for Clinical Laboratory Standards. *Methods for Antimicrobial Susceptibility Testing of Anaerobic Bacteria* - Fifth Edition. Approved Standard. NCCLS Document M11-A5, Vol. 21, No. 2 (ISBN 1–56238-429-5). NCCLS, 940 West Valley Road, Suite 1400, Wayne, PA 19087-1898, January, 2001.
TIMENTIN is a registered trademark of GlaxoSmithKline. The following are registered trademarks of their respective owners: ADD-VANTAGE/Abbott Laboratories; GALAXY/Baxter International Inc.; MULTI-STIX/Bayer Corporation.
GlaxoSmithKline
Research Triangle Park, NC 27709
©2008, GlaxoSmithKline. All rights reserved.
July 2008 TMP:18PI

TREXIMET®   ℞
[trĕx' ə-mĕt]
(sumatriptan and naproxen sodium)
Tablets

> **WARNINGS**
> **Cardiovascular Risk**
> TREXIMET may cause an increased risk of serious cardiovascular thrombotic events, myocardial infarction, and stroke, which can be fatal. This risk may increase with duration of use. Patients with cardiovascular disease or risk factors for cardiovascular disease may be at greater risk (see WARNINGS: Cardiovascular Effects).
> **Gastrointestinal Risk**
> TREXIMET contains a nonsteroidal anti-inflammatory drug (NSAID). NSAID-containing products cause an increased risk of serious gastrointestinal adverse events including bleeding, ulceration, and perforation of the stomach or intestines, which can be fatal. These events can occur at any time during use and without warning symptoms. Elderly patients are at greater risk for serious gastrointestinal events (see WARNINGS: Risk of Gastrointestinal Ulceration, Bleeding, and Perforation With Nonsteroidal Anti-inflammatory Drug Therapy).

DESCRIPTION
TREXIMET contains sumatriptan (as the succinate), a selective 5-hydroxytryptamine$_1$ (5-HT$_1$) receptor subtype agonist, and naproxen sodium, a member of the arylacetic acid group of nonsteroidal anti-inflammatory drugs (NSAIDs).
Sumatriptan succinate is chemically designated as 3-[2-(dimethylamino)ethyl]-N-methyl-indole-5-methanesulfonamide succinate (1:1), and it has the following structure:

The empirical formula is $C_{14}H_{21}N_3O_2S \cdot C_4H_6O_4$, representing a molecular weight of 413.5. Sumatriptan succinate is a white to off-white powder that is readily soluble in water and in saline.
Naproxen sodium is chemically designated as (S)-6-methoxy-α-methyl-2-naphthaleneacetic acid, sodium salt, and it has the following structure:

The empirical formula is $C_{14}H_{13}NaO_3$, representing a molecular weight of 252.23. Naproxen sodium is a white-to-creamy white crystalline solid, freely soluble in water at neutral pH.
Each TREXIMET Tablet for oral administration contains 119 mg of sumatriptan succinate equivalent to 85 mg of sumatriptan and 500 mg of naproxen sodium. Each tablet also contains the inactive ingredients croscarmellose sodium, dextrose monohydrate, dibasic calcium phosphate, FD&C Blue No. 2, lecithin, magnesium stearate, maltodextrin, microcrystalline cellulose, povidone, sodium bicarbonate, sodium carboxymethylcellulose, talc, and titanium dioxide.

CLINICAL PHARMACOLOGY
Mechanism of Action
TREXIMET contains sumatriptan, a 5-HT$_1$ receptor agonist that mediates vasoconstriction of the human basilar artery and vasculature of human dura mater, which correlates with the relief of migraine headache. It also contains

naproxen, an NSAID that inhibits the synthesis of inflammatory mediators. Therefore, sumatriptan and naproxen contribute to the relief of migraine through pharmacologically different mechanisms of action.

Sumatriptan is a 5-HT_1 receptor agonist that binds with high affinity to 5-HT_{1B} and 5-HT_{1D} receptors. Sumatriptan has only a weak affinity for 5-HT_{1A}, 5-HT_{5A}, and 5-HT_7 receptors and no significant affinity (as measured using standard radioligand binding assays) or pharmacological activity at 5-HT_2, 5-HT_3, or 5-HT_4 receptor subtypes or at $alpha_1$-, $alpha_2$-, or beta-adrenergic; $dopamine_1$; $dopamine_2$; muscarinic; or benzodiazepine receptors. In addition to causing vasoconstriction, experimental data from animal studies show that sumatriptan also activates 5-HT_1 receptors on peripheral terminals of the trigeminal nerve innervating cranial blood vessels. Such an action may contribute to the antimigrainous effect of sumatriptan in humans. In the anesthetized dog, sumatriptan selectively reduces carotid arterial blood flow with little or no effect on arterial blood pressure or total peripheral resistance.

Naproxen sodium is an NSAID with analgesic and antipyretic properties. The sodium salt of naproxen has been developed as a more rapidly absorbed formulation of naproxen for use as an analgesic. The mechanism of action of the naproxen anion, like that of other NSAIDs, is not completely understood but may be related to prostaglandin synthetase inhibition.

Pharmacokinetics

TREXIMET is a formulation of 85 mg of sumatriptan (as sumatriptan succinate) and 500 mg of naproxen sodium with a distinct pharmacokinetic profile. C_{max} (median, range) for sumatriptan following administration of TREXIMET occurs at approximately 1 hour (0.3 to 4.0 hours). C_{max} (median, range) for naproxen following administration of TREXIMET occurs at approximately 5 hours (0.3 to 12 hours). The sumatriptan half-life is approximately 2 hours (15% to 43% CV) and the naproxen half-life is approximately 19 hours (13% to 15% CV). The mean C_{max} for sumatriptan when given as TREXIMET is similar to that of sumatriptan when given as IMITREX® (sumatriptan succinate) Tablets 100 mg alone. The median sumatriptan T_{max} is only slightly different (1 hour for TREXIMET and 1.5 hours for IMITREX). The C_{max} for naproxen is approximately 36% lower, and the T_{max} occurs approximately 4 hours later from TREXIMET than from ANAPROX® DS (naproxen sodium tablets) 550 mg. AUC values for sumatriptan and for naproxen are similar for TREXIMET compared to IMITREX or ANAPROX DS, respectively. In a crossover study in 16 patients, the pharmacokinetics of both components administered as TREXIMET were similar during a migraine attack and during a migraine-free period.

Absorption and Bioavailability

Bioavailability of sumatriptan is approximately 15%, primarily due to presystemic (first-pass) metabolism and partly due to incomplete absorption.

Naproxen is rapidly and completely absorbed from the gastrointestinal tract with an in vivo bioavailability of 95%.

Food Effects

Food had no significant effect on the bioavailability of sumatriptan or naproxen administered as TREXIMET, but slightly delayed the T_{max} of sumatriptan by about 0.6 hour. These data indicate that TREXIMET may be administered without regard to food.

Distribution

The volume of distribution of sumatriptan is 2.4 L/kg. Plasma protein binding is 14% to 21%. The effect of sumatriptan on the protein binding of other drugs has not been evaluated, but would be expected to be minor, given the low protein binding.

The volume of distribution of naproxen is 0.16 L/kg. At therapeutic levels naproxen is greater than 99% albumin bound. At doses of naproxen greater than 500 mg/day, there is a less than proportional increase in plasma levels due to an increase in clearance caused by saturation of plasma protein binding at higher doses (average trough C_{ss} = 36.5, 49.2, and 56.4 mg/L with 500, 1,000, and 1,500 mg daily doses of naproxen, respectively). However, the concentration of unbound naproxen continues to increase proportionally to dose.

Metabolism

Most of a radiolabeled dose of sumatriptan excreted in the urine is the major metabolite indole acetic acid (IAA) or the IAA glucuronide, both of which are inactive. Three percent of the dose can be recovered as unchanged sumatriptan. In vitro studies with human microsomes suggest that sumatriptan is metabolized by monoamine oxidase (MAO), predominantly the A isoenzyme, and inhibitors of that enzyme may alter sumatriptan pharmacokinetics to increase systemic exposure (see CONTRAINDICATIONS and PRECAUTIONS: Drug Interactions: *Monoamine Oxidase-A Inhibitors*). No significant effect was seen with an MAO-B inhibitor.

Naproxen is extensively metabolized to 6-0-desmethyl naproxen, and both parent and metabolites do not induce metabolizing enzymes.

Table 1. Percentage of Patients With 2-Hour Pain Relief and Sustained Pain Free Following Treatment[a]

	TREXIMET	Sumatriptan 85 mg	Naproxen Sodium 500 mg	Placebo
2-Hour Pain Relief				
Study 1 (all patients)	65%[b] n = 364	55% n = 361	44% n = 356	28% n = 360
Study 2 (all patients)	57%[b] n = 362	50% n = 362	43% n = 364	29% n = 382
Sustained Pain Free (2-24 Hours)				
Study 1	25%[c] n = 364	16% n = 361	10% n = 356	8% n = 360
Study 2	23%[c] n = 362	14% n = 362	10% n = 364	7% n = 382

[a] p values provided only for prespecified comparisons.
[b] p<0.05 versus placebo and sumatriptan.
[c] p<0.01 versus placebo, sumatriptan, and naproxen sodium.

Elimination

Radiolabeled ^{14}C-sumatriptan administered orally is largely renally excreted (about 60%), with about 40% found in the feces. The elimination half-life of sumatriptan is approximately 2 hours.

The clearance of naproxen is 0.13 mL/min/kg. Approximately 95% of the naproxen from any dose is excreted in the urine, primarily as naproxen (less than 1%), 6-0-desmethyl naproxen (less than 1%), or their conjugates (66% to 92%). The plasma half-life of the naproxen anion in humans is approximately 19 hours. The corresponding half-lives of both metabolites and conjugates of naproxen are shorter than 12 hours, and their rates of excretion have been found to coincide closely with the rate of naproxen disappearance from the plasma. In patients with renal failure, metabolites may accumulate (see PRECAUTIONS: Renal Effects).

Special Populations

Renal Impairment

TREXIMET is not recommended for use in patients with creatinine clearance less than 30 mL/min (see PRECAUTIONS: Renal Effects). The effect of renal impairment on the pharmacokinetics of TREXIMET has not been studied. Minimal change in clinical effect would be expected with regard to sumatriptan as it is largely metabolized to an inactive substance.

Since naproxen and its metabolites and conjugates are primarily excreted by the kidney, the potential exists for naproxen metabolites to accumulate in the presence of renal insufficiency. Elimination of naproxen is decreased in patients with severe renal impairment.

Hepatic Impairment

Because TREXIMET is a fixed-dose combination that cannot be adjusted for this patient population, it is contraindicated in patients with hepatic impairment (see CONTRAINDICATIONS and PRECAUTIONS: Hepatic Effects). The effect of hepatic impairment on the pharmacokinetics of TREXIMET has not been studied. Sumatriptan is contraindicated in patients with severe hepatic impairment and the dose is limited to 50 mg in patients with liver disease.

Age

The effect of age (elderly or pediatric patients) on the pharmacokinetics of TREXIMET has not been studied. Elderly patients are more likely to have decreased hepatic function and decreased renal function (see PRECAUTIONS: Geriatric Use).

The pharmacokinetics of oral sumatriptan in the elderly (mean age: 72 years, 2 males and 4 females) and in patients with migraine (mean age: 38 years, 25 males and 155 females) were similar to that in healthy male subjects (mean age: 30 years).

Gender

In a pooled analysis of 5 pharmacokinetic studies, there was no effect of gender on the systemic exposure of TREXIMET. In a study comparing the pharmacokinetics of sumatriptan in females and males, no differences were observed between genders for AUC, C_{max}, T_{max}, and $T_{1/2}$.

Race

The effect of race on the pharmacokinetics of TREXIMET has not been studied. The systemic clearance and C_{max} of sumatriptan were similar in black (n = 34) and Caucasian (n = 38) healthy male subjects.

Drug Interactions

No formal drug interaction studies have been conducted with TREXIMET.

Monoamine Oxidase Inhibitors

TREXIMET is contraindicated in patients taking MAO-A inhibitors (see CONTRAINDICATIONS and PRECAUTIONS: Drug Interactions). Treatment with MAO-A inhibitors generally leads to an increase of sumatriptan plasma levels. This interaction has not been seen with an MAO-B inhibitor.

Alcohol

The effect of alcohol consumption on the pharmacokinetics of TREXIMET has not been studied. Alcohol consumed 30 minutes prior to sumatriptan ingestion had no effect on the pharmacokinetics of sumatriptan.

CLINICAL TRIALS

The efficacy of TREXIMET in providing relief from migraine was demonstrated in 2 randomized, double-blind, multicenter, parallel-group trials utilizing placebo and each individual active component of TREXIMET (sumatriptan and naproxen sodium) as comparison treatments. Patients enrolled in these 2 trials were predominately female (87%) and Caucasian (88%), with a mean age of 40 years (range 18 to 65 years). Patients were instructed to treat a migraine of moderate to severe pain with 1 tablet. No rescue medication was allowed within 2 hours postdose. Patients evaluated their headache pain 2 hours after taking 1 dose of study medication; headache relief was defined as a reduction in headache severity from moderate or severe pain to mild or no pain. Associated symptoms of nausea, photophobia, and phonophobia were also evaluated. Sustained pain free was defined as a reduction in headache severity from moderate or severe pain to no pain at 2 hours postdose without a return of mild, moderate, or severe pain and no use of rescue medication for 24 hours postdose. The results from the 2 controlled clinical trials are summarized in Table 1. In both trials, the percentage of patients achieving headache pain relief 2 hours after treatment was significantly greater among patients receiving TREXIMET (65% and 57%) compared with those who received placebo (28% and 29%).

Further, the percentage of patients who remained pain free without use of other medications through 24 hours postdose was significantly greater among patients receiving a single dose of TREXIMET (25% and 23%) compared with those who received placebo (8% and 7%) or either sumatriptan (16% and 14%) or naproxen sodium (10%) alone.

[See table 1 above]

Note that comparisons of the performance of different drugs based upon results obtained in different clinical trials are never reliable. Because studies are generally conducted at different times, with different samples of patients, by different investigators, employing different criteria and/or different interpretations of the same criteria, under different conditions (dose, dosing regimen, etc.), quantitative estimates of treatment response and the timing of response may be expected to vary considerably from study to study.

The percentage of patients achieving initial headache pain relief within 2 hours following treatment with TREXIMET is shown in Figure 1.

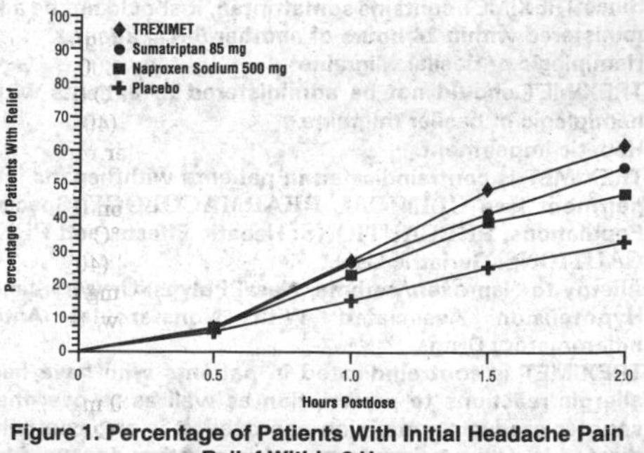

Figure 1. Percentage of Patients With Initial Headache Pain Relief Within 2 Hours

Compared with placebo, there was a decreased incidence of photophobia, phonophobia, and nausea 2 hours after the administration of TREXIMET. The estimated probability of taking a rescue medication over the first 24 hours is shown in Figure 2.

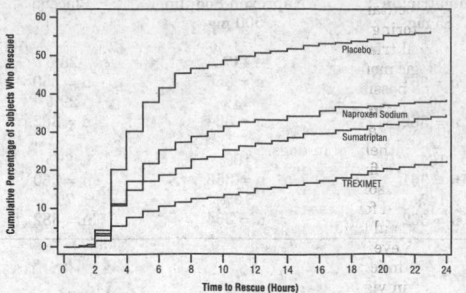

Figure 2. Cumulative Percentage of Subjects Taking a Rescue Medication Over the 24 Hours Following the First Dose[a]

[a]Plot also includes patients who had no response to the initial dose.

TREXIMET was more effective than placebo regardless of the presence of aura; duration of headache prior to treatment; gender, age, or weight of the patient; or concomitant use of oral contraceptives or common migraine prophylactic drugs (e.g., beta-blockers, anti-epileptic drugs, tricyclic antidepressants).

INDICATIONS AND USAGE

TREXIMET is indicated for the acute treatment of migraine attacks with or without aura in adults. Carefully consider the potential benefits and risks of TREXIMET and other treatment options when deciding to use TREXIMET. TREXIMET is not intended for the prophylactic therapy of migraine or for use in the management of hemiplegic or basilar migraine (see CONTRAINDICATIONS). Safety and effectiveness of TREXIMET have not been established for cluster headache.

CONTRAINDICATIONS

Cardiac, Cerebrovascular, or Peripheral Vascular Disease
TREXIMET should not be given to patients with history, symptoms, or signs of ischemic cardiac, cerebrovascular, or peripheral vascular syndromes. In addition, patients with other significant underlying cardiovascular diseases should not receive TREXIMET, nor should patients who have had coronary artery bypass graft (CABG) surgery. Ischemic cardiac syndromes include, but are not limited to, angina pectoris of any type (e.g., stable angina of effort and vasospastic forms of angina, such as the Prinzmetal variant), all forms of myocardial infarction, and silent myocardial ischemia. Cerebrovascular syndromes include, but are not limited to, strokes of any type as well as transient ischemic attacks. Peripheral vascular disease includes, but is not limited to, ischemic bowel disease (see WARNINGS: Cardiovascular Effects).

Uncontrolled Hypertension
TREXIMET should not be given to patients with uncontrolled hypertension because the components have been shown to increase blood pressure.

Monoamine Oxidase-A Inhibitors
Concurrent administration of MAO-A inhibitors or use of TREXIMET within 2 weeks of discontinuation of MAO-A inhibitor therapy is contraindicated (see CLINICAL PHARMACOLOGY: Drug Interactions and PRECAUTIONS: Drug Interactions).

Ergotamine-Containing or Ergot-Type Medications
TREXIMET and any ergotamine-containing or ergot-type medication (like dihydroergotamine or methysergide) should not be used within 24 hours of each other (see PRECAUTIONS: Drug Interactions).

Other 5-HT₁ Agonists
Since TREXIMET contains sumatriptan, it should not be administered within 24 hours of another 5-HT₁ agonist.

Hemiplegic or Basilar Migraine
TREXIMET should not be administered to patients with hemiplegic or basilar migraine.

Hepatic Impairment
TREXIMET is contraindicated in patients with hepatic impairment (see CLINICAL PHARMACOLOGY: Special Populations, PRECAUTIONS: Hepatic Effects, and PRECAUTIONS: Geriatric Use).

Allergy to Naproxen/Asthma, Nasal Polyps, Urticaria, and Hypotension Associated With Nonsteroidal Anti-inflammatory Drugs
TREXIMET is contraindicated in patients who have had allergic reactions to prescription as well as to over-the-counter products containing naproxen. It is also contraindicated in patients in whom aspirin or other nonsteroidal anti-inflammatory/analgesic drugs induce the syndrome of asthma, rhinitis, and nasal polyps. Anaphylactic/anaphylactoid reactions to naproxen, whether of the true allergic type or the pharmacologic idiosyncratic type (e.g., aspirin

hypersensitivity syndrome), usually but not always occur in patients with a known history of such reactions. Both types of reactions have the potential of being fatal. Therefore, careful questioning of patients for medical conditions such as asthma, nasal polyps, urticaria, and hypotension associated with NSAIDs before starting therapy is important. In addition, if such symptoms occur during therapy, treatment should be discontinued (see WARNINGS: Anaphylactic/Anaphylactoid Reactions and PRECAUTIONS: Preexisting Asthma).

Hypersensitivity to Sumatriptan or Naproxen
TREXIMET is contraindicated in patients with hypersensitivity to sumatriptan, naproxen, or any other component of the product.

WARNINGS

TREXIMET should only be used where a clear diagnosis of migraine headache has been established.

Cardiovascular Effects

Risk of Myocardial Ischemia and/or Infarction and Other Adverse Cardiac Events
TREXIMET should not be given to patients with documented ischemic or vasospastic coronary artery disease (CAD) or to patients with a history of CABG surgery (see CONTRAINDICATIONS). It is strongly recommended that sumatriptan-containing products not be given to patients in whom unrecognized CAD is predicted by the presence of risk factors (e.g., hypertension, hypercholesterolemia, smoker, obesity, diabetes, strong family history of CAD, female with surgical or physiological menopause, male over 40 years of age) unless a cardiovascular evaluation provides satisfactory clinical evidence that the patient is reasonably free of CAD and ischemic myocardial disease or other significant underlying cardiovascular disease. The sensitivity of cardiac diagnostic procedures to detect cardiovascular disease or predisposition to coronary artery vasospasm is modest, at best. If, during the cardiovascular evaluation, the patient's medical history or electrocardiographic investigations reveal findings indicative of, or consistent with, coronary artery vasospasm or myocardial ischemia, TREXIMET should not be administered (see CONTRAINDICATIONS).

For patients with risk factors predictive of CAD who are determined to have a satisfactory cardiovascular evaluation, it is strongly recommended that administration of the first dose of TREXIMET take place in the setting of a physician's office or similar medically staffed and equipped facility unless the patient has previously received sumatriptan. Because cardiac ischemia can occur in the absence of clinical symptoms, consideration should be given to obtaining an electrocardiogram (ECG) immediately following first-time use of TREXIMET in patients with risk factors.

It is recommended that patients who are intermittent long-term users of TREXIMET and who have or acquire risk factors predictive of CAD as described above undergo periodic cardiovascular evaluation as they continue to use TREXIMET.

The systematic approach described above is intended to reduce the likelihood that patients with unrecognized cardiovascular disease will be inadvertently exposed to sumatriptan-containing products.

Cardiac Events and Fatalities Associated With 5-HT₁ Agonists
Serious adverse cardiac events, including acute myocardial infarction, life-threatening disturbances of cardiac rhythm, and death have been reported within a few hours following the administration of sumatriptan. Considering the extent of use of 5-HT₁ agonists in patients with migraine, the incidence of these events is extremely low.

The fact that sumatriptan can cause coronary vasospasm, that some of these events have occurred in patients with no prior cardiac disease history and with documented absence of CAD, and the close proximity of the events to sumatriptan use support the conclusion that some of these cases were caused by the drug. In cases, however, where there has been known underlying coronary artery disease, the relationship is uncertain.

Cardiovascular Thrombotic Events and Fatalities Associated With Nonsteroidal Anti-inflammatory Drugs
Clinical trials of several COX-2 selective and nonselective NSAIDs of up to 3 years' duration have shown an increased risk of serious cardiovascular thrombotic events, myocardial infarction, and stroke, which can be fatal. All NSAIDs, both COX-2 selective and nonselective, may have a similar risk. Patients with known cardiovascular disease or risk factors for cardiovascular disease may be at greater risk. To minimize the potential risk for an adverse cardiovascular event in patients treated with an NSAID, the lowest effective dose should be used for the shortest duration possible. Physicians and patients should remain alert for the development of such events, even in the absence of previous cardiovascular symptoms. Patients should be informed about the signs and/or symptoms of serious cardiovascular events and the steps to take if they occur.

There is no consistent evidence that concurrent use of aspirin mitigates the increased risk of serious cardiovascular thrombotic events associated with NSAID use. The concurrent use of aspirin and an NSAID does increase the risk of serious gastrointestinal events (see WARNINGS: Risk of Gastrointestinal Ulceration, Bleeding, and Perforation With Nonsteroidal Anti-inflammatory Drug Therapy).

Premarketing Experience With TREXIMET
Among 3,302 patients with migraine who received TREXIMET in premarketing controlled and uncontrolled clinical trials, a 47-year-old female with cardiac risk factors in an open-label 12-month safety study experienced signs and symptoms of acute coronary syndrome approximately 2 hours after receiving TREXIMET.

Drug-Associated Cerebrovascular Events and Fatalities
Cerebral hemorrhage, subarachnoid hemorrhage, stroke, and other cerebrovascular events have been reported in patients treated with oral or subcutaneous sumatriptan, and some have resulted in fatalities. The relationship of sumatriptan to these events is uncertain. In a number of cases, it appears possible that the cerebrovascular events were primary, sumatriptan having been administered in the incorrect belief that the symptoms experienced were a consequence of migraine when they were not. As with other acute migraine therapies, before treating headaches in patients not previously diagnosed as migraineurs, and in migraineurs who present with atypical symptoms, care should be taken to exclude other potentially serious neurological conditions. It should also be noted that patients with migraine may be at increased risk of certain cerebrovascular events (e.g., cerebrovascular accident, transient ischemic attack).

Other Vasospasm-Related Events
Sumatriptan may cause vasospastic reactions other than coronary artery vasospasm. Both peripheral vascular ischemia and colonic ischemia with abdominal pain and bloody diarrhea have been reported. Transient and permanent blindness and significant partial vision loss have been reported with the use of sumatriptan. Visual disorders may also be part of a migraine attack.

Increase in Blood Pressure
TREXIMET is contraindicated in patients with uncontrolled hypertension (see CONTRAINDICATIONS). TREXIMET should be used with caution in patients with controlled hypertension.

Significant elevation in blood pressure, including hypertensive crisis, has been reported in patients with and without a history of hypertension receiving sumatriptan. Sumatriptan-containing products should be administered with caution to patients with controlled hypertension as transient increases in blood pressure and peripheral vascular resistance have been observed.

NSAID-containing products can lead to onset of new hypertension or worsening of preexisting hypertension, either of which may contribute to the increased incidence of cardiovascular events. Patients taking thiazides or loop diuretics may have impaired response to these therapies when taking NSAIDs. The potential effect on blood pressure associated with long-term use of TREXIMET has not been studied. Blood pressure should be monitored closely during the initiation of NSAID treatment and throughout the course of therapy.

Congestive Heart Failure and Edema
TREXIMET should be used with caution in patients with fluid retention or heart failure. Fluid retention and edema have been observed in some patients taking NSAIDs. Since each TREXIMET tablet contains 61.2 mg of sodium (about 2.7 mEq/500 mg of naproxen sodium), this should be considered in patients whose overall intake of sodium must be severely restricted.

Serotonin Syndrome
The development of a potentially life-threatening serotonin syndrome may occur with triptans, including treatment with TREXIMET, particularly during combined use with selective serotonin reuptake inhibitors (SSRIs) or serotonin norepinephrine reuptake inhibitors (SNRIs). If concomitant treatment with TREXIMET and an SSRI (e.g., fluoxetine, paroxetine, sertraline, fluvoxamine, citalopram, escitalopram) or SNRI (e.g., venlafaxine, duloxetine) is clinically warranted, careful observation of the patient is advised, particularly during treatment initiation and dose increases. Serotonin syndrome symptoms may include mental status changes (e.g., agitation, hallucinations, coma), autonomic instability (e.g., tachycardia, labile blood pressure, hyperthermia), neuromuscular aberrations (e.g., hyperreflexia, incoordination), and/or gastrointestinal symptoms (e.g., nausea, vomiting, diarrhea) (see PRECAUTIONS: Drug Interactions).

Risk of Gastrointestinal Ulceration, Bleeding, and Perforation With Nonsteroidal Anti-inflammatory Drug Therapy
TREXIMET contains an NSAID. NSAID-containing products can cause serious gastrointestinal adverse events

including inflammation, bleeding, ulceration, and perforation of the stomach, small intestine, or large intestine, which can be fatal.

These serious adverse events can occur at any time, with or without warning symptoms, in patients treated with NSAIDs. Only 1 in 5 patients who develop a serious upper gastrointestinal adverse event on NSAID therapy is symptomatic. Upper gastrointestinal ulcers, gross bleeding, or perforation caused by NSAIDs appear to occur in approximately 1% of patients treated daily for 3 to 6 months and in about 2% to 4% of patients treated for 1 year. These trends continue with longer duration of use, increasing the likelihood of developing a serious gastrointestinal event at some time during the course of therapy. However, even short-term therapy is not without risk. Among 3,302 patients with migraine who received TREXIMET in premarketing controlled and uncontrolled clinical trials, 1 patient experienced a recurrence of gastric ulcer after taking 8 doses over 3 weeks, and 1 patient developed a gastric ulcer after treating an average of 8 attacks per month over 7 months.

NSAID-containing products, including TREXIMET, should be prescribed with extreme caution in those with a prior history of ulcer disease or gastrointestinal bleeding. Patients with a prior history of peptic ulcer disease and/or gastrointestinal bleeding who use NSAIDs have a greater than 10-fold increased risk for developing gastrointestinal bleeding compared to patients with neither of these risk factors. Other factors that increase the risk for gastrointestinal bleeding in patients treated with NSAIDs include concomitant use of oral corticosteroids or anticoagulants, longer duration of NSAID therapy, smoking, use of alcohol, older age, and poor general health status. Most spontaneous reports of fatal gastrointestinal events are in elderly or debilitated patients, and therefore special care should be taken in treating this population.

To minimize the potential risk for an adverse gastrointestinal event in patients treated with an NSAID-containing product, the lowest effective dose should be used for the shortest possible duration. Patients and physicians should remain alert for signs and symptoms of gastrointestinal ulceration and bleeding during NSAID therapy and promptly initiate additional evaluation and treatment if a serious gastrointestinal adverse event is suspected. This should include discontinuation of the NSAID until a serious gastrointestinal adverse event is ruled out. For high-risk patients, alternate therapies that do not involve NSAIDs should be considered.

NSAIDs should be given with care to patients with a history of inflammatory bowel disease (ulcerative colitis, Crohn's disease) as their condition may be exacerbated.

Renal Effects

Long-term administration of NSAIDs has resulted in renal papillary necrosis and other renal injury. Renal toxicity has also been seen in patients in whom renal prostaglandins have a compensatory role in the maintenance of renal perfusion. In these patients administration of an NSAID may cause a dose-dependent reduction in prostaglandin formation and, secondarily, in renal blood flow, which may precipitate overt renal decompensation. Patients at greatest risk of this reaction are those with impaired renal function, heart failure, liver dysfunction, those taking diuretics and angiotensin-converting enzyme (ACE) inhibitors, and the elderly. Discontinuation of NSAID therapy is usually followed by recovery to the pretreatment state.

Advanced Renal Disease

Treatment with TREXIMET is not recommended in patients with advanced renal disease. If therapy with TREXIMET must be initiated, close monitoring of the patient's renal function is advisable (see CLINICAL PHARMACOLOGY: Pharmacokinetics and PRECAUTIONS: Renal Effects). No information is available from controlled clinical studies regarding the use of TREXIMET in patients with advanced renal disease.

Anaphylactic/Anaphylactoid Reactions

As with other NSAID-containing products, anaphylactic/anaphylactoid reactions may occur in patients without known prior exposure to naproxen. TREXIMET should not be given to patients with the aspirin triad. This symptom complex typically occurs in patients with asthma who experience rhinitis with or without nasal polyps, or who exhibit severe, potentially fatal bronchospasm after taking aspirin or other NSAIDs (see CONTRAINDICATIONS, PRECAUTIONS: Preexisting Asthma, and PRECAUTIONS: Drug Interactions).

Anaphylactic/anaphylactoid reactions have occurred in patients receiving sumatriptan. Such reactions can be life-threatening or fatal. In general, anaphylactic reactions to drugs are more likely to occur in individuals with a history of sensitivity to multiple allergens (see CONTRAINDICATIONS). Emergency help should be sought in cases where an anaphylactoid reaction occurs. Anaphylactoid reactions, like anaphylaxis, may have a fatal outcome.

Skin Reactions

NSAID-containing products, including TREXIMET, can cause serious adverse events such as exfoliative dermatitis, Stevens-Johnson syndrome, and toxic epidermal necrolysis, which can be fatal. These serious events may occur without warning. Patients should be informed about the signs and symptoms of serious skin manifestations and use of the drug should be discontinued at the first appearance of skin rash or any other sign of hypersensitivity.

Pregnancy

TREXIMET should not be used in late pregnancy because NSAID-containing products have been shown to cause premature closure of the ductus arteriosus. TREXIMET should not be used during early pregnancy unless the potential benefit justifies the potential risk to the fetus (see PRECAUTIONS: Pregnancy).

PRECAUTIONS

Naproxen-Containing Products

TREXIMET and other naproxen-containing products should not be used concomitantly since they all circulate in the plasma as the naproxen anion.

Chest, Jaw, or Neck Pain/Discomfort

Chest discomfort and jaw or neck tightness have been reported following use of sumatriptan. Only rarely have these symptoms been associated with ischemic ECG changes. However, because sumatriptan may cause coronary artery vasospasm, patients who experience signs or symptoms suggestive of angina following TREXIMET should be evaluated for the presence of CAD or a predisposition to Prinzmetal variant angina before receiving additional doses of TREXIMET and should be monitored electrocardiographically if dosing is resumed and similar symptoms recur. Similarly, patients who experience other symptoms or signs suggestive of decreased arterial flow, such as ischemic bowel syndrome or Raynaud syndrome, following TREXIMET should be evaluated for atherosclerosis or predisposition to vasospasm (see WARNINGS: Cardiovascular Effects).

Diseases That May Alter the Absorption, Metabolism, or Excretion of Drugs

TREXIMET should also be administered with caution to patients with diseases that may alter the absorption, metabolism, or excretion of drugs, such as impaired renal function.

Seizures

TREXIMET should be used with caution in patients with a history of epilepsy or conditions associated with a lowered seizure threshold. There have been reports of seizure following administration of sumatriptan.

Other Potentially Serious Neurologic Conditions

Care should be taken to exclude other potentially serious neurologic conditions before treating headache in patients not previously diagnosed with migraine headache or who experience a headache that is atypical for them. There have been reports where patients received sumatriptan for severe headaches that were subsequently shown to have been secondary to an evolving neurologic lesion (see WARNINGS: Drug-Associated Cerebrovascular Events and Fatalities). For a given attack, if a patient does not respond to the first dose of TREXIMET, the diagnosis of migraine should be reconsidered before administration of a second dose.

Hepatic Effects

TREXIMET is contraindicated in patients with hepatic impairment (see CONTRAINDICATIONS and CLINICAL PHARMACOLOGY). A patient with symptoms and/or signs suggesting liver dysfunction or in whom an abnormal liver test has occurred should be evaluated for evidence of the development of a more severe hepatic reaction while on therapy with TREXIMET. Borderline elevations of 1 or more liver tests may occur in up to 15% of patients who take NSAID-containing products. These abnormalities may progress, may remain essentially unchanged, or may be transient with continued therapy. Notable (3 times the upper limit of normal) elevations of SGPT (ALT) or SGOT (AST) have been reported in approximately 1% of patients in clinical trials with NSAIDs. In addition, cases of severe hepatic reactions, including jaundice and fatal fulminant hepatitis, liver necrosis, and hepatic failure, some of them with fatal outcomes, have been reported with NSAIDs. A patient with symptoms and/or signs suggesting liver dysfunction, or in whom an abnormal liver test has occurred, should be evaluated for evidence of the development of a more severe hepatic reaction while on therapy with TREXIMET. If clinical signs and symptoms consistent with liver disease develop, or if systemic manifestations occur (e.g., eosinophilia, rash), TREXIMET should be discontinued.

Overuse

Overuse of acute migraine treatments has been associated with the exacerbation of headache (medication overuse headache) in susceptible patients. Withdrawal of the treatment may be necessary.

Binding to Melanin-Containing Tissues

In rats treated with a single subcutaneous dose (0.5 mg/kg) or oral dose (2 mg/kg) of radiolabeled sumatriptan, the elimination half-life of radioactivity from the eye was 15 and 23 days, respectively, suggesting that sumatriptan and/or its metabolites bind to the melanin of the eye. Because there could be an accumulation in melanin-rich tissues over time, sumatriptan could possibly cause toxicity in these tissues after extended use. However, no effects on the retina related to treatment with sumatriptan were noted in any of the oral or subcutaneous toxicity studies. Although no systematic monitoring of ophthalmologic function was undertaken in clinical trials and no specific recommendations for ophthalmologic monitoring are offered, prescribers should be aware of the possibility of long-term ophthalmologic effects.

Corneal Opacities

Sumatriptan causes corneal opacities and defects in the corneal epithelium in dogs (see ANIMAL TOXICOLOGY). Adverse eye findings have also been observed in animal studies with some NSAIDs. Patients were not systematically evaluated for these changes in clinical trials. However, since the animal findings raise the possibility that adverse effects on the eye may occur in humans, it is recommended that ophthalmic studies be carried out if any change or disturbance in vision occurs.

Renal Effects

Caution is recommended in patients with preexisting kidney disease or dehydration (see WARNINGS: Renal Effects). Naproxen and its metabolites are eliminated primarily by the kidneys; therefore, TREXIMET should be used with caution in patients with significantly impaired renal function, and monitoring of serum creatinine and/or creatinine clearance is advised in these patients. TREXIMET is not recommended for use in patients with creatinine clearance less than 30 mL/min (see CLINICAL PHARMACOLOGY: Special Populations).

Hematological Effects

Patients on long-term treatment with NSAIDs, including TREXIMET, should have their hemoglobin or hematocrit checked if they exhibit any signs or symptoms of anemia. Anemia is sometimes seen in patients receiving NSAIDs. This may be due to fluid retention, occult or gross gastrointestinal blood loss, or an incompletely described effect upon erythropoiesis. Patients receiving TREXIMET who may be adversely affected by alterations in platelet function, such as those with coagulation disorders or patients receiving anticoagulants, should be carefully monitored. NSAID-containing products inhibit platelet aggregation and have been shown to prolong bleeding time in some patients. Unlike aspirin, their effect on platelet function is quantitatively less, of shorter duration, and reversible.

Preexisting Asthma

Patients with asthma may have aspirin-sensitive asthma. The use of aspirin in patients with aspirin-sensitive asthma has been associated with severe bronchospasm that can be fatal. Since cross reactivity, including bronchospasm, between aspirin and other NSAIDs has been reported in such aspirin-sensitive patients, TREXIMET should not be administered to patients with this form of aspirin sensitivity and should be used with caution in patients with preexisting asthma.

Information for Patients

Patients should be informed of the following information before initiating therapy with TREXIMET and periodically during the course of ongoing therapy. Patients should also be encouraged to read the Medication Guide that accompanies each prescription dispensed.

1. TREXIMET may cause serious cardiovascular side effects such as myocardial infarction or stroke, which may result in hospitalization and even death. Although serious cardiovascular events can occur without warning symptoms, patients should be alert for the signs and symptoms of chest pain, shortness of breath, weakness, slurring of speech, and should ask for medical advice when observing any indicative sign or symptoms. Patients should be apprised of the importance of this follow-up (see WARNINGS: Cardiovascular Effects).
2. TREXIMET, like other NSAID-containing products, may cause gastrointestinal discomfort and, rarely, serious gastrointestinal side effects such as ulcers and bleeding, which may result in hospitalization and even death. Although serious gastrointestinal tract ulcerations and bleeding can occur without warning symptoms, patients should be alert for the signs and symptoms of ulcerations and bleeding and should ask for medical advice when observing any indicative sign or symptoms, including epigastric pain, dyspepsia, melena, and hematemesis. Patients should be apprised of the importance of this follow-up (see WARNINGS: Risk of Gastrointestinal Ulceration, Bleeding, and Perforation With Nonsteroidal Anti-inflammatory Drug Therapy).
3. TREXIMET, like other NSAID-containing products, may increase the risk of serious skin side effects such as exfoliative dermatitis, Stevens-Johnson syndrome, and toxic epidermal necrolysis, which may result in hospitalizations and even death. Although serious skin reactions may occur without warning, patients should be alert for the signs and symptoms of skin rash and blisters, fever, or other signs of hypersensitivity such as itching and should ask for medical advice when observing any

indicative signs or symptoms. Patients should be advised to stop the drug immediately if they develop any type of rash and contact their physicians as soon as possible.

4. Patients should promptly report signs or symptoms of unexplained weight gain or edema to their physicians.

5. Patients should be informed of the warning signs and symptoms of hepatotoxicity (e.g., nausea, fatigue, lethargy, pruritus, jaundice, right upper quadrant tenderness, flu-like symptoms). If these occur, patients should be instructed to stop therapy and seek immediate medical therapy.

6. Patients should be informed of the signs of an anaphylactic/anaphylactoid reaction (e.g., difficulty breathing, swelling of the face or throat). If these occur, patients should be instructed to seek immediate emergency help (see WARNINGS: Anaphylactic/Anaphylactoid Reactions).

7. TREXIMET should not be used in late pregnancy because NSAID-containing products have been shown to cause premature closure of the ductus arteriosus. TREXIMET should not be used during early pregnancy unless the potential benefit justifies the potential risk to the fetus.

8. Patients should be cautioned about the risk of serotonin syndrome, particularly during concomitant use with SSRIs or SNRIs.

9. Caution should be exercised by patients whose activities require alertness if they experience drowsiness, dizziness, vertigo, or depression during therapy with TREXIMET.

Laboratory Tests

Because serious gastrointestinal tract ulcerations and bleeding can occur without warning symptoms, physicians should monitor for signs or symptoms of gastrointestinal bleeding. If clinical signs and symptoms consistent with liver or renal disease develop, systemic manifestations occur (e.g., eosinophilia, rash), or abnormal liver tests persist or worsen, TREXIMET should be discontinued.

Drug Interactions

Monoamine Oxidase-A Inhibitors

The use of TREXIMET in patients receiving MAO-A inhibitors is contraindicated (see CLINICAL PHARMACOLOGY: Drug Interactions and CONTRAINDICATIONS). MAO-A inhibitors reduce sumatriptan clearance, significantly increasing systemic exposure. In patients taking MAO-A inhibitors, sumatriptan plasma levels attained after treatment with recommended doses are 7-fold higher following oral administration than those obtained under other conditions.

Ergot-Containing Drugs

Ergot-containing drugs have been reported to cause prolonged vasospastic reactions. Because there is a theoretical basis that these effects may be additive, use of ergotamine-containing or ergot-type medications (e.g., dihydroergotamine, methysergide) and TREXIMET within 24 hours of each other should be avoided (see CONTRAINDICATIONS).

Methotrexate

Caution should be used if TREXIMET is administered concomitantly with methotrexate. Naproxen sodium and other NSAIDs have been reported to reduce the tubular secretion of methotrexate in an animal model, possibly increasing the toxicity of methotrexate. Concomitant administration of some NSAIDs with high-dose methotrexate therapy has been reported to elevate and prolong serum methotrexate levels, resulting in deaths from severe hematologic and gastrointestinal toxicity.

Aspirin

When naproxen is administered with aspirin, its protein binding is reduced, although the clearance of free naproxen is not altered. The clinical significance of this interaction is not known; however, as with other NSAID-containing products, concomitant administration of TREXIMET and aspirin is not generally recommended because of the potential of increased adverse effects.

Selective Serotonin Reuptake Inhibitors/Serotonin Norepinephrine Reuptake Inhibitors and Serotonin Syndrome

Cases of life-threatening serotonin syndrome have been reported during combined use of SSRIs or SNRIs and triptans (see WARNINGS: Serotonin Syndrome).

Angiotensin-Converting Enzyme Inhibitors

Reports suggest that NSAIDs may diminish the antihypertensive effect of ACE inhibitors. The use of TREXIMET in patients who are receiving ACE inhibitors may potentiate renal disease states (see WARNINGS: Renal Effects).

Furosemide

Clinical studies, as well as postmarketing observations, have shown that NSAIDs can reduce the natriuretic effect of furosemide and thiazides in some patients. This response has been attributed to inhibition of renal prostaglandin synthesis. During concomitant therapy with NSAIDs, the patient should be observed closely for signs of renal failure (see WARNINGS: Renal Effects), as well as to assure diuretic efficacy.

Lithium

NSAIDs have produced an elevation of plasma lithium levels and a reduction in renal lithium clearance. The mean minimum lithium concentration increased 15%, and the renal clearance was decreased by approximately 20%. These effects have been attributed to inhibition of renal prostaglandin synthesis by the NSAID. Thus, when TREXIMET and lithium are administered concurrently, patients should be observed carefully for signs of lithium toxicity.

Probenecid

Probenecid given concurrently increases naproxen anion plasma levels and extends its plasma half-life significantly.

Propranolol and Other Beta-Blockers

Propranolol 80 mg given twice daily had no significant effect on sumatriptan pharmacokinetics. Naproxen and other NSAIDs can reduce the antihypertensive effect of propranolol and other beta-blockers.

Warfarin

The effects of warfarin and NSAIDs on gastrointestinal bleeding are synergistic, such that patients taking both drugs have a higher risk of serious gastrointestinal bleeding than patients taking either drug alone.

Drug/Laboratory Test Interactions

The ability of TREXIMET to interfere with commonly employed clinical laboratory tests has not been investigated. Sumatriptan is not known to interfere with commonly employed clinical laboratory tests. Naproxen may decrease platelet aggregation and prolong bleeding time. This effect should be kept in mind when bleeding times are determined.

The administration of naproxen sodium may result in increased urinary values for 17-ketogenic steroids because of an interaction between the drug and/or its metabolites with m-di-nitrobenzene used in this assay. Although 17-hydroxycorticosteroid measurements (Porter-Silber test) do not appear to be artifactually altered, it is suggested that therapy with naproxen be temporarily discontinued 72 hours before adrenal function tests are performed if the Porter-Silber test is to be used.

Naproxen may interfere with some urinary assays of 5-hydroxy indoleacetic acid (5HIAA).

Carcinogenesis, Mutagenesis, Impairment of Fertility

Carcinogenesis

The carcinogenic potential of TREXIMET has not been studied.

The carcinogenic potential of sumatriptan was evaluated in oral carcinogenicity studies in mice (78 weeks) and rats (104 weeks). The highest dose administered to mice and rats (160 mg/kg/day) is approximately 9 and 18 times, respectively, the recommended human oral daily dose of 85 mg sumatriptan on a mg/m² basis. There was no evidence of an increase in tumors in either species related to sumatriptan administration.

The carcinogenic potential of naproxen sodium was evaluated in a 2-year oral carcinogenicity study in rats at doses of 8, 16, and 24 mg/kg/day and in another 2-year oral carcinogenicity study in rats at a dose of 8 mg/kg/day. No evidence of tumorigenicity was found in either study, at doses up to approximately 0.5 times the recommended human oral daily dose of 500 mg/day naproxen sodium on a mg/m² basis.

Mutagenesis

Sumatriptan and naproxen sodium tested alone and in combination were negative in an in vitro bacterial reverse mutation assay, and in an in vivo micronucleus assay in mice. The combination of sumatriptan and naproxen sodium was negative in an in vitro mouse lymphoma tk assay in the presence and absence of metabolic activation. However, in separate in vitro mouse lymphoma tk assays, naproxen sodium alone was reproducibly positive in the presence of metabolic activation.

Naproxen sodium alone and in combination with sumatriptan was positive in an in vitro clastogenicity assay in mammalian cells in the presence and absence of metabolic activation. The clastogenic effect for the combination was reproducible within this assay and was greater than observed with naproxen sodium alone. Sumatriptan alone was negative in these assays.

Chromosomal aberrations were not induced in peripheral blood lymphocytes following 7 days of twice-daily dosing with TREXIMET in human volunteers.

In previous studies, sumatriptan alone was not mutagenic in 2 gene mutation assays (the Ames test and the in vitro Chinese Hamster V79/HGPRT assay) and was not clastogenic in 2 cytogenetics assays (the in vitro human lymphocyte assay and the in vivo rat micronucleus assay).

Impairment of Fertility

The effect of TREXIMET on fertility in animals has not been studied.

In a study in which male and female rats were dosed daily with oral sumatriptan prior to and throughout the mating period, there was a treatment-related decrease in fertility secondary to a decrease in mating in animals treated with 50 and 500 mg/kg/day. The highest no-effect dose for this finding was 5 mg/kg/day, or approximately 0.5 times the recommended human oral daily dose of 85 mg sumatriptan on a mg/m² basis. It is not clear whether the problem is associated with treatment of the males or females or both combined. In a similar study of sumatriptan by the subcutaneous route there was no evidence of impaired fertility at doses up to 60 mg/kg/day.

Pregnancy

Pregnancy Category C. In developmental toxicity studies in rabbits, oral treatment with sumatriptan combined with naproxen sodium (5/9, 25/45, or 50/90 mg/kg/day sumatriptan/naproxen sodium) or each drug alone (50/0 or 0/90 mg/kg/day sumatriptan/naproxen sodium) resulted in decreased fetal body weight in all treated groups and in increased embryofetal death at the highest dose of naproxen, alone and in combination with sumatriptan. Naproxen sodium, alone and in combination with sumatriptan, increased the total incidences of fetal abnormalities at all doses and increased the incidences of specific malformations (cardiac interventricular septal defect in the 50/90-mg/kg/day group, fused caudal vertebrae in the 50/0- and 0/90-mg/kg/day groups) and variations (absent intermediate lobe of the lung, irregular ossification of the skull, incompletely ossified sternal centra) in the 50/0- and 0/90-mg/kg/day groups. A no-effect dose for development toxicity in rabbits was not established. The lowest effect dose was 5/9 mg/kg/day sumatriptan/naproxen sodium, which was associated with plasma exposures (AUC) to sumatriptan and naproxen that were 1.4 and 0.14 times, respectively, those attained at the maximum recommended human oral daily dose of 85 mg sumatriptan and 500 mg naproxen sodium.

In previous developmental toxicity studies in rats and rabbits, oral treatment with sumatriptan was associated with embryolethality, fetal abnormalities, and pup mortality. Oral treatment of pregnant rats with sumatriptan during the period of organogenesis resulted in an increased incidence of fetal blood vessel (cervicothoracic and umbilical) abnormalities and decreased pup survival at doses of 250 mg/kg/day or higher. The highest no-effect dose was approximately 60 mg/kg/day, which is approximately 7 times the recommended human oral daily dose of 85 mg sumatriptan on a mg/m² basis. Oral treatment of pregnant rabbits with sumatriptan during the period of organogenesis resulted in an increased incidence of cervicothoracic vascular and skeletal abnormalities at a dose of 50 mg/kg/day and embryolethality at 100 mg/kg/day. The highest no-effect dose for embryotoxicity in rabbits was 15 mg/kg/day, or approximately 3 times the recommended human oral daily dose of 85 mg sumatriptan on a mg/m² basis.

Inhibitors of prostaglandin synthesis (including naproxen) are known to delay parturition. Because of this and the known effects of drugs of this class on the human fetal cardiovascular system (closure of the ductus arteriosus), use during third trimester should be avoided.

There are no adequate and well-controlled studies in pregnant women.

TREXIMET should not be used during pregnancy unless the potential benefit justifies the potential risk to the fetus.

Pregnancy Registry

To monitor fetal outcomes of pregnant women exposed to TREXIMET, GlaxoSmithKline maintains a TREXIMET Pregnancy Registry. Physicians are encouraged to register patients as soon as possible after they become pregnant and (if possible) before the outcome of the pregnancy is known by calling (800) 336-2176.

Labor and Delivery

In rat studies with NSAIDs, as with other drugs known to inhibit prostaglandin synthesis, an increased incidence of dystocia, delayed parturition, and decreased pup survival occurred. Naproxen-containing products are not recommended in labor and delivery because, through its prostaglandin synthesis inhibitory effect, naproxen may adversely affect fetal circulation and inhibit uterine contractions, thus increasing the risk of uterine hemorrhage.

Nursing Mothers

Both active components of TREXIMET, sumatriptan and naproxen sodium, have been reported to be excreted in human breast milk. Because of the possible adverse effects of these drugs on neonates, use of TREXIMET in nursing mothers should be avoided.

Pediatric Use

Safety and effectiveness of TREXIMET in pediatric patients have not been established.

Geriatric Use

TREXIMET is contraindicated for use in elderly patients who have abnormal hepatic function, and is not recommended for use in elderly patients who have decreased renal function, higher risk for unrecognized CAD, and increases in blood pressure that may be more pronounced in the elderly (see CONTRAINDICATIONS: Hepatic Impairment, WARNINGS: Cardiovascular Effects, and CLINICAL PHARMACOLOGY: Pharmacokinetics).

ADVERSE REACTIONS

The adverse reactions reported below are specific to the clinical trials with TREXIMET. See also the full prescribing information for naproxen and sumatriptan products.

Incidence in Controlled Clinical Trials

Table 2 lists adverse events that occurred in 2 placebo-controlled clinical trials evaluating patients who took at least 1 dose of study drug. Only events that occurred at a frequency of 2% or more with TREXIMET and were more frequent than in the placebo group are included in Table 2. The events cited reflect experience gained under closely monitored conditions of clinical trials in a highly selected patient population. In actual clinical practice or in other clinical trials, these frequency estimates may not apply, as the conditions of use, reporting behavior, and the kinds of patients treated may differ.

[See table 2 at right]

Table 2. Treatment-Emergent Adverse Events Reported by at Least 2% of Patients in 2 Controlled Migraine Trials[a]

Adverse Event	TREXIMET (n = 737)	Placebo (n = 752)	Sumatriptan 85 mg (n = 735)	Naproxen Sodium 500 mg (n = 732)
Nervous system disorders				
Dizziness	4	2	2	2
Somnolence	3	2	2	2
Paresthesia	2	<1	2	<1
Gastrointestinal disorders				
Nausea	3	1	3	<1
Dyspepsia	2	1	2	1
Dry mouth	2	1	2	<1
Pain and other pressure sensations				
Chest discomfort/chest pain	3	<1	2	1
Neck/throat/jaw pain/tightness/pressure	3	1	3	1

[a]Events that occurred at a frequency of 2% or more in the group treated with TREXIMET and that occurred more frequently in the group treated with TREXIMET than in the placebo group.

Other events that occurred in more than 1% of patients receiving TREXIMET and occurred at a frequency greater than the placebo group included asthenia, feeling hot, muscle tightness, and palpitations.

TREXIMET was generally well tolerated. Most adverse reactions were mild and transient. The incidence of adverse events in controlled clinical trials was not affected by gender or age of the patients. There were insufficient data to assess the impact of race on the incidence of adverse events.

Other Events Observed in Migraine Clinical Trials Associated With the Administration of TREXIMET

The occurrence of less commonly reported adverse clinical events is presented in this section. Because the reports include events observed in an open-label, long-term safety study in which TREXIMET was used as needed for up to 12 months, the role of TREXIMET cannot be reliably determined. Furthermore, variability associated with adverse event reporting, the terminology used to describe adverse events, etc., limit the value of quantitative frequency estimates provided. Event frequencies are calculated as the number of patients who used TREXIMET and reported an event divided by the total number of patients (N = 3,302) exposed to TREXIMET. Events listed in the previous table and text are not included below. Those events described too generally to be informative or those unlikely to be associated with the use of TREXIMET are excluded. Events are further classified within body system categories and enumerated in order of decreasing frequency using the following definitions: frequent adverse events are those occurring in at least 1/100 patients, infrequent adverse events are those occurring in 1/100 to 1/1,000 patients, and rare adverse events are those occurring in fewer than 1/1,000 patients.

Blood and Lymphatic Disorders

Infrequent was lymphadenopathy. Rare were anemia, ecchymosis, leukopenia.

Cardiac Disorders

Infrequent was tachycardia. Rare were acute coronary syndrome, cardiac flutter, congestive cardiac failure, right ventricular failure, ventricular extrasystoles.

Ear and Labyrinth Disorders

Infrequent were ear pain, tinnitus. Rare were motion sickness, vertigo.

Endocrine, Metabolic, and Nutrition Disorders

Rare were diabetes mellitus, goiter, hypoglycemia, hypothyroidism.

Eye Disorders

Infrequent was conjunctivitis. Rare were cataract, conjunctival hemorrhage, visual disturbance.

Gastrointestinal Disorders

Frequent was abdominal pain. Infrequent were abdominal distention, constipation, diarrhea, dysgeusia, dysphagia, flatulence, gastritis, gastroesophageal reflux disease, vomiting. Rare were colitis, diverticulitis, gastric ulcer, irritable bowel syndrome, oral mucosal blistering, swollen tongue.

General Disorders

Frequent was fatigue. Infrequent were feeling jittery, lethargy, malaise, peripheral edema, pyrexia, temperature intolerance, thirst. Rare was difficulty in walking.

Hepatobiliary Disorders

Rare was biliary colic.

Infections and Infestations

Rare were kidney infection, pneumonia, sepsis, staphylococcal infection, viral myocarditis.

Musculoskeletal and Connective Tissue

Infrequent were arthralgia, back pain, muscular weakness, myalgia, sensation of heaviness.

Nervous System Disorders

Infrequent were burning sensation, disturbance of attention, insomnia, mental impairment, tremor. Rare were aphasia, facial palsy, impairment of psychomotor skills, sedation.

Psychiatric Disorders

Infrequent were anxiety, depression, irritability, nervousness. Rare were disorientation, panic attack.

Renal and Urinary Disorders

Infrequent was nephrolithiasis. Rare was renal insufficiency.

Respiratory, Thoracic, and Mediastinal

Infrequent were asthma, cough, dyspnea, oropharyngeal swelling. Rare was pleurisy.

Skin and Subcutaneous Disorders

Infrequent were facial swelling, hyperhydrosis, pruritus, rash, urticaria. Rare was systemic lupus erythematosus.

Vascular Disorders

Infrequent were flushing, hot flush, hypertension. Rare were epistaxis, peripheral coldness.

DRUG ABUSE AND DEPENDENCE

The potential for abuse with TREXIMET has not been studied.

One clinical study with sumatriptan succinate injection enrolling 12 patients with a history of substance abuse failed to induce subjective behavior and/or physiologic response ordinarily associated with drugs that have an established potential for abuse.

OVERDOSAGE

Because strategies for the management of overdose are continually evolving, it is advisable to contact a Poison Control Center to determine the latest recommendations for the management of an overdose of any drug.

There have been no reports of overdosage with TREXIMET. Since sumatriptan and naproxen have pharmacologically different actions, it is difficult to predict how an individual will respond to an overdosage with TREXIMET.

Patients (N = 670) have received single oral doses of 140 to 300 mg of sumatriptan without significant adverse effects. Volunteers (N = 174) have received single oral doses of 140 to 400 mg without serious adverse events. Overdose of sumatriptan in animals has been fatal and has been heralded by convulsions, tremor, paralysis, inactivity, ptosis, erythema of the extremities, abnormal respiration, cyanosis, ataxia, mydriasis, salivation, and lacrimation.

Significant naproxen overdosage may be characterized by lethargy, dizziness, drowsiness, epigastric pain, abdominal discomfort, heartburn, indigestion, nausea, transient alterations in liver function, hypoprothrombinemia, renal dysfunction, metabolic acidosis, apnea, disorientation, or vomiting. Gastrointestinal bleeding can occur. Hypertension, acute renal failure, respiratory depression, and coma may occur, but are rare. Anaphylactoid reactions have been reported with therapeutic ingestion of NSAIDs, and may occur following an overdose. Because naproxen sodium may be rapidly absorbed, high and early blood levels should be anticipated. A few patients have experienced seizures, but it is not clear whether or not these were drug related. It is not known what dose of the drug would be life threatening.

In animals 0.5 g/kg of activated charcoal was effective in reducing plasma levels of naproxen. Patients should be managed by symptomatic and supportive care. There are no specific antidotes. Hemodialysis does not decrease the plasma concentration of naproxen because of the high degree of its protein binding. It is unknown what effect hemodialysis or peritoneal dialysis has on the serum concentrations of sumatriptan. Emesis and/or activated charcoal (60 to 100 g in adults, 1 to 2 g/kg in children) and/or osmotic cathartic may be indicated in patients seen within 4 hours of ingestion with symptoms or following a large overdose. Forced diuresis, alkalinization of urine, or hemoperfusion may not be useful due to high protein binding.

DOSAGE AND ADMINISTRATION

TREXIMET is a fixed combination containing doses of sumatriptan (85 mg) and naproxen sodium (500 mg) within the approved dosage ranges of the individual components (25 to 100 mg of sumatriptan and 220 to 825 mg of naproxen sodium). TREXIMET contains a dose of sumatriptan higher than the lowest effective dose. Individuals may vary in response to doses of sumatriptan. The choice of the dose of sumatriptan, and of the use of a fixed combination such as in TREXIMET should therefore be made on an individual basis, weighing the possible benefit of a higher dose of sumatriptan with the potential for a greater risk of adverse events. Carefully consider the potential benefits and risks of TREXIMET and other treatment options when deciding to use TREXIMET.

The recommended dose is 1 tablet. In controlled clinical trials, single doses of TREXIMET were effective for the acute treatment of migraine in adults (see CLINICAL TRIALS). The efficacy of taking a second dose has not been established. Do not take more than 2 TREXIMET tablets in 24 hours. Dosing of tablets should be at least 2 hours apart. The safety of treating an average of more than 5 migraine headaches in a 30-day period has not been established.

TREXIMET may be administered with or without food. Tablets should not be split, crushed, or chewed.

The combined use of TREXIMET with MAO-A inhibitors or use of TREXIMET within 2 weeks of discontinuation of MAO-A inhibitor therapy is contraindicated (see CONTRAINDICATIONS, CLINICAL PHARMACOLOGY: Drug Interactions, PRECAUTIONS: Drug Interactions).

TREXIMET and any ergotamine-containing or ergot-type medication (like dihydroergotamine or methysergide) should not be used within 24 hours of each other. TREXIMET and other 5-HT_1 agonists should not be administered within 24 hours of each other (see CONTRAINDICATIONS and PRECAUTIONS: Drug Interactions).

TREXIMET is contraindicated in patients with hepatic impairment (see CONTRAINDICATIONS and CLINICAL PHARMACOLOGY: Special Populations).

TREXIMET is not recommended for use in patients with creatinine clearance less than 30 mL/min (see CLINICAL PHARMACOLOGY: Special Populations and PRECAUTIONS: Renal Effects).

HOW SUPPLIED

TREXIMET contains 119 mg of sumatriptan succinate equivalent to 85 mg of sumatriptan and 500 mg of naproxen sodium and is supplied as blue film-coated tablets debossed on one side with *TREXIMET* in compact containers of 9 tablets with a specially formulated, non-removable desiccant (NDC 0173-0750-00).

Store at 25°C (77°F); excursions permitted to 15°-30°C (59°-86°F) [see USP Controlled Room Temperature]. Do not repackage; dispense and store in original container.

ANIMAL TOXICOLOGY

Corneal Opacities

Dogs receiving oral sumatriptan developed corneal opacities and defects in the corneal epithelium. Corneal opacities were seen at the lowest dosage tested, 2 mg/kg/day, and were present after 1 month of treatment. Defects in the corneal epithelium were noted in a 60-week study. Earlier examinations for these toxicities were not conducted and no-effect doses were not established; the lowest dose tested is approximately 0.8 times the recommended human oral daily dose of 85 mg sumatriptan on a mg/m^2 basis. There was evidence of alterations in corneal appearance on the first day of intranasal dosing to dogs at all doses tested.

PATIENT INFORMATION

MEDICATION GUIDE

TREXIMET® *[trex' i-met]* Tablets
(sumatriptan and naproxen sodium)

What is the most important information I should know about TREXIMET?

TREXIMET, which contains sumatriptan and naproxen sodium [a nonsteroidal anti-inflammatory drug (NSAID)], may increase the chance of a heart attack or stroke that can lead to death. This chance increases:

Serious side effects include:

- heart attack
- heartbeat problems
- stroke
- high blood pressure
- heart failure from body swelling (fluid retention)
- kidney problems including kidney failure
- bleeding and ulcers in the stomach and intestine
- low red blood cells (anemia)
- life-threatening skin reactions
- life-threatening allergic reactions
- liver problems including liver failure
- asthma attacks in people who have asthma
- loss of blood circulation to areas of your body
- serotonin syndrome (See list of symptoms in "What is the most important information I should know about TREXIMET?")

Other side effects include:

- pain, tightness, or pressure in the chest, neck, and throat
- stomach pain
- constipation
- diarrhea
- gas
- heartburn
- nausea
- vomiting
- dizziness
- drowsiness
- tiredness
- weakness
- tingling and numbness
- unusual body sensations
- redness of face (flushed)

- sudden/severe pain in your belly
- vomit blood
- blood in your bowel movement or it is black and sticky like tar
- itching
- skin rash or blisters with fever
- yellow skin or eyes
- swelling of the arms and legs, hands, feet, face, lips, or tongue
- unusual weight gain
- more tired or weaker than usual
- flu-like symptoms
- serotonin syndrome. See list of symptoms in "What is the most important information I should know about TREXIMET?"

Tell your healthcare provider if you have any side effects that bother you or do not go away. These are not all of the side effects of TREXIMET. For more information ask your healthcare provider.

Call your healthcare provider for medical advice about side effects. You may report side effects at FDA at 1-800-FDA-1088.

How should I store TREXIMET?

- Store TREXIMET at room temperature, 59° to 86°F (15° to 30°C).
- Keep TREXIMET and all medicines out of the reach of children.

General information about TREXIMET

- Medicines are sometimes prescribed for purposes other than those listed in a Medication Guide. Do not use TREXIMET for a condition for which it was not prescribed.
- Do not give TREXIMET to other people, even if they have the same problem you have. It may harm them.
- This Medication Guide contains the most important information about TREXIMET. If you would like more information, talk with your healthcare provider.
- You can ask your healthcare provider for information written for healthcare professionals.
- For more information call 1-888-825-5249 (toll-free), or visit www.TREXIMET.com.

What are the ingredients in TREXIMET?

Active ingredients: sumatriptan succinate and naproxen sodium

Inactive ingredients: croscarmellose sodium, dextrose monohydrate, dibasic calcium phosphate, FD&C Blue No. 2, lecithin, magnesium stearate, maltodextrin, microcrystalline cellulose, povidone, sodium bicarbonate, sodium carboxymethylcellulose, talc, and titanium dioxide.

This Medication Guide has been approved by the U.S. Food and Drug Administration.

June 2009 TRX:3MG

TREXIMET is a trademark of GlaxoSmithKline. IMITREX, PARNATE, and PAXIL are registered trademarks of GlaxoSmithKline.

The other brands listed are trademarks of their respective owners and are not trademarks of GlaxoSmithKline. The makers of these brands are not affiliated with and do not endorse GlaxoSmithKline or its products.

GlaxoSmithKline

Research Triangle Park, NC 27709

©2009, GlaxoSmithKline. All rights reserved.

December 2009 TRX:5PI

- with longer use of NSAID medicines
- in people who have heart disease.

NSAID-containing medicines, such as TREXIMET, should never be used right before or after a heart surgery called a coronary artery bypass graft (CABG).

NSAID-containing medicines, such as TREXIMET, can cause ulcers and bleeding in the stomach and intestines at any time during treatment. Ulcers and bleeding:

- can happen without warning symptoms
- may cause death.

The chance of a person getting an ulcer or bleeding increases with:

- the use of medicines called steroid hormones (corticosteroids) and blood thinners (anticoagulants)
- longer use
- more frequent use
- smoking
- drinking alcohol
- older age
- having poor health.

TREXIMET is not recommended for people with risk factors for heart disease unless a heart exam is done and shows no problems.

The risk factors for heart disease include:

- high blood pressure
- high cholesterol levels
- smoking
- obesity
- diabetes
- family history of heart disease
- female who has gone through menopause
- male over age 40.

"Serotonin syndrome" is a serious and life-threatening problem that may occur with TREXIMET, especially if used with antidepressant medicines called selective serotonin reuptake inhibitors (SSRIs) or selective norepinephrine reuptake inhibitors (SNRIs).

Commonly used SSRIs are:

- CELEXA® (citalopram HBr)
- LEXAPRO® (escitalopram oxalate)
- PAXIL® (paroxetine)
- PROZAC®/SARAFEM® (fluoxetine)
- SYMBYAX® (olanzapine/fluoxetine)
- ZOLOFT® (sertraline)
- LUVOX® (fluvoxamine).

Commonly used SNRIs are:

- CYMBALTA® (duloxetine)
- EFFEXOR® (venlafaxine).

Call your healthcare provider if you have symptoms of serotonin syndrome, which include:

- mental changes (hallucinations, agitation, coma)
- fast heartbeat
- changes in blood pressure
- high body temperature or sweating
- tight muscles
- trouble walking
- nausea, vomiting, diarrhea.

TREXIMET should only be used:

- exactly as prescribed
- at the lowest dose possible for your treatment
- for the shortest time needed.

TREXIMET already contains an NSAID (naproxen). Do not use TREXIMET with other medicines to lessen pain or fever without talking to your healthcare provider first, because they may contain an NSAID also.

What is TREXIMET?

TREXIMET is a prescription medicine used to treat migraine attacks in adults. It does not prevent or lessen the number of migraines you have, and it is not for other types of headaches. TREXIMET contains 2 medicines: sumatriptan and naproxen sodium (an NSAID). This Medication Guide provides important information you need to know before taking TREXIMET. It does not take the place of talking with your healthcare provider about your medical condition or your treatment.

How should I take TREXIMET?

- Take 1 TREXIMET tablet to treat your migraine headache. Do not take more than 2 TREXIMET tablets in 24 hours. Doses should be separated by at least 2 hours.
- TREXIMET can be taken with or without food.
- Do not split, crush, or chew TREXIMET tablets.
- If you take too much TREXIMET, call the Poison Control Center at 1-800-222-1222.

Who should not take TREXIMET?

Do not take TREXIMET right before or after heart bypass surgery.

Do not take TREXIMET if you have or have had:

- uncontrolled high blood pressure
- hemiplegic or basilar migraine. (Ask your doctor if you are not sure what type of migraine you have.)
- liver problems
- an asthma attack, hives, or other allergic reaction with aspirin or any other NSAID medicine
- a heart attack or a history or symptoms of heart disease (such as chest pain or angina)
- a stroke, mini-stroke (transient ischemic attack or TIA), or other stroke-like syndrome
- problems with blood circulation to parts of your body, such as less blood flow to your intestines (ischemic bowel disease)
- allergic reactions to sumatriptan, naproxen, or other ingredients in TREXIMET.

Do not take TREXIMET if you take or have taken an antidepressant medicine called a monoamine oxidase (MAO) inhibitor within the last 2 weeks. Common MAO inhibitors are isocarboxazid (MARPLAN®), phenelzine (NARDIL®), tranylcypromine (PARNATE®), and selegiline (ELDEPRYL®, EMSAM®). Ask your healthcare provider if you are not sure if your medicine is an MAO inhibitor.

Do not take TREXIMET if you have taken other migraine medicines in the last 24 hours such as:

- ergotamine-containing medicine or
- another triptan medicine.

Before starting TREXIMET, tell your healthcare provider about:

- all of your medical conditions including kidney or liver problems
- all allergies to any medicines
- chest pain, shortness of breath, irregular heartbeats
- medicines you may take for migraines, depression, or other health problems such as MAO inhibitors, SSRIs, or SNRIs
- all the prescription and non-prescription medicines you take, including vitamins and herbal supplements. Some medicines can interact with TREXIMET and cause serious side effects.

Keep a list of your medicines to show to your healthcare provider.

Before starting TREXIMET, tell your healthcare provider if you:

- are pregnant, think you might be pregnant, or are trying to become pregnant. **TREXIMET should not be used by pregnant women late in their pregnancy.**
- are breastfeeding
- have a headache that is different from your usual migraine
- have or have had epilepsy or seizures.

What are the possible side effects of TREXIMET?

[See table above]

Get emergency help right away if you have any of the following symptoms:

- shortness of breath or trouble breathing
- chest pain
- swelling of the face or throat
- weakness in one part or on one side of your body
- slurred speech.

Stop TREXIMET and call your healthcare provider right away if you have any of the following symptoms:

- nausea that seems out of proportion to your migraine
- stomach pain

TWINRIX® ℞

[twin'rix]

Hepatitis A Inactivated
& Hepatitis B (Recombinant) Vaccine

DESCRIPTION

TWINRIX® [Hepatitis A Inactivated & Hepatitis B (Recombinant) Vaccine] is a sterile bivalent vaccine containing the antigenic components used in producing HAVRIX® (Hepatitis A Vaccine, Inactivated) and ENGERIX-B® [Hepatitis B Vaccine (Recombinant)]. TWINRIX is a sterile suspension of inactivated hepatitis A virus (strain HM175) propagated in MRC-5 cells, and combined with purified surface antigen of the hepatitis B virus. The purified hepatitis B surface antigen (HBsAg) is obtained by culturing genetically engineered *Saccharomyces cerevisiae* cells, which carry the surface antigen gene of the hepatitis B virus, in synthetic media containing inorganic salts, amino acids, dextrose, and vitamins. Bulk preparations of each antigen are adsorbed separately onto aluminum salts and then pooled during formulation.

A 1.0-mL dose of vaccine contains 720 ELISA Units of inactivated hepatitis A virus and 20 mcg of recombinant HBsAg protein. One dose of vaccine also contains 0.45 mg of aluminum in the form of aluminum phosphate and aluminum hydroxide as adjuvants, amino acids, sodium chloride, phosphate buffer, polysorbate 20, Water for Injection, traces of formalin (not more than 0.1 mg), and residual MRC-5 cellular proteins (not more than 2.5 mcg). Neomycin sulfate, an aminoglycoside antibiotic, is included in the cell growth media; only trace amounts (not more than 20 ng) remain following purification. The manufacturing procedures used to manufacture TWINRIX result in a product that contains no more than 5% yeast protein.

TWINRIX is formulated without preservatives.

TWINRIX is supplied as a sterile suspension for intramuscular administration. The vaccine is ready for use without reconstitution; it must be well shaken before administration to obtain a homogeneous, turbid, white suspension.

CLINICAL PHARMACOLOGY

Several hepatitis viruses (A, B, C, D, and E) are known to cause a systemic infection resulting in major pathologic changes in the liver. Features of hepatitis A and hepatitis B are described below.

Hepatitis A:

The hepatitis A virus (HAV) belongs to the picornavirus family.

Hepatitis A is a highly contagious disease with the predominant mode of transmission being person-to-person via the fecal-oral route. Infection has been shown to be spread (1) by contaminated water or food; (2) by infected food handlers[1]; (3) after breakdown in usual sanitary conditions or after floods or natural disasters; (4) by ingestion of raw or undercooked shellfish (oysters, clams, mussels) from contaminated waters[2]; (5) during travel to areas of the world with poor hygienic conditions[3]; (6) among institutionalized children and adults[4]; (7) in day-care centers[5]; (8) by parenteral transmission, either blood transfusions or sharing needles with infected people[6]; and (9) sexually, especially among men who have sex with men.[7]

The incubation period for hepatitis A averages 28 days (range: 15 to 50 days).[7] The course of hepatitis A infection is extremely variable, ranging from asymptomatic infection to icteric hepatitis and death.[8]

Chronic shedding of HAV in feces has not been demonstrated, but relapses of hepatitis A can occur in as many as 20% of patients[9,10] and fecal shedding of HAV may recur at this time.[9] Approximately 70% of pediatric patients less than 6 years of age infected with hepatitis A are asymptomatic, and serve as a reservoir for infection among adults.[7] The presence of antibodies to HAV (anti-HAV) confers protection against hepatitis A disease. However, the lowest titer needed to confer protection has not been determined. Natural infection provides lifelong immunity even when antibodies to hepatitis A are undetectable. At present, studies show the duration of protection afforded by TWINRIX against hepatitis A lasts at least 4 years.[11]

Hepatitis B:

The hepatitis B virus (HBV) belongs to a family of genetically related DNA-containing animal viruses, which are hepatotropic. The incubation period of hepatitis B ranges between 30 and 180 days.[12]

HBV infection occurs throughout the world with highly variable prevalences. A human reservoir of persistently infected persons is present in nearly all communities of the world. In the United States, parenteral drug abuse, unprotected sexual activity, occupationally acquired infection, or travelers returning from high prevalence countries may be the principal mechanisms of HBV transmission.

Modes of transmission of hepatitis B virus include sexual contact with an infected person, percutaneous or mucosal exposure to infectious blood, and perinatal exposure to an infected mother. Antibody concentrations ≥10 mIU/mL against HBsAg are recognized as conferring protection against hepatitis B.[13]

Clinical infection with hepatitis B may occur in 2 major forms: Asymptomatic or symptomatic hepatitis. Asymptomatic HBV infection can be subclinical or inapparent. In subclinical infection, patients have abnormal liver enzymes without jaundice, while inapparent asymptomatic infection is identified only by serological testing. One in 4 adults who has symptomatic disease has jaundice (anicteric/icteric hepatitis).

HBV infection can have serious consequences including acute massive hepatic necrosis, chronic active hepatitis, and cirrhosis of the liver. As many as 90% of infants and approximately 5% of adults who are infected with HBV will become HBV carriers.[7] More than 350 million people are chronic carriers of HBV worldwide.[7] The Centers for Disease Control and Prevention (CDC) estimates that there are approximately 1 million to 1.25 million chronic carriers of HBV in the United States.[7] The annual number of unreported infections may be 10 times greater than the number of reported cases.[7] Close contact (sexual contact or household contact) or exposure to blood from infected individuals is associated with increased risk of infection.[7] Those patients who become chronic carriers can infect others and are at increased risk of developing primary hepatocellular carcinoma. Among other factors, infection with HBV may be the single most important factor for development of this carcinoma.[7,14]

Reduced Risk of Hepatocellular Carcinoma:

According to the Centers for Disease Control and Prevention (CDC), hepatitis B vaccine is recognized as an anti-

cancer vaccine because it can prevent primary liver cancer.[15] In a Taiwanese study, the institution of universal childhood immunization against hepatitis B virus has been shown to decrease the incidence of hepatocellular carcinoma among children.[16] In a Korean study in adult males, vaccination against the hepatitis B virus has been shown to decrease the incidence and risk of developing hepatocellular carcinoma in adults.[17]

Clinical Trials:

Immunogenicity in Adults: Sera from 1,551 healthy adult volunteers ages 17 to 70, including 555 male subjects and 996 female subjects, in 11 clinical trials were analyzed following administration of 3 doses of TWINRIX on a 0-, 1-, and 6-month schedule. Seroconversion for antibodies against HAV was elicited in 99.9% of vaccinees, and protective antibodies against HBV were detected in 98.5%, 1 month after completion of the 3-dose series.

[See table 1 above]

One of the 11 trials was a comparative trial conducted in a US population given either TWINRIX (on a 0-, 1-, 6-month schedule) or HAVRIX (0- and 6-month schedule) and ENGERIX-B (0-, 1-, and 6-month schedule). The monovalent vaccines were given concurrently in opposite arms. Of a total of 773 adults (ages 18 to 70 years) enrolled in this trial, an immunogenicity analysis was performed in 533 subjects who completed the study according to protocol. Of these, 264 subjects received TWINRIX and 269 subjects received HAVRIX and ENGERIX-B. Seroconversion against HAV and seroprotection against HBV are shown in Table 2.

[See table 2 above]

Since the immune responses to hepatitis A and hepatitis B induced by TWINRIX were non-inferior to the monovalent vaccines, efficacy is expected to be similar to the efficacy for each of the monovalent vaccines (Table 3).

[See table 3 above]

It was noted that the antibody titers achieved 1 month after the final dose of TWINRIX were higher than titers achieved 1 month after the final dose of HAVRIX in these clinical trials. This may have been due to a difference in the recommended dosage regimens for these 2 vaccines, whereby TWINRIX vaccinees received 3 doses of 720 EL.U. of hepatitis A antigen at 0, 1, and 6 months, whereas HAVRIX vaccinees received 2 doses of 1440 EL.U. of the same antigen (at 0 and 6 months). However, these differences in peak titer have not been shown to be clinically significant.

Two clinical trials involving a total of 129 subjects demonstrated that antibodies to both HAV and HBV persisted for at least 4 years after the first vaccine dose in a 3-dose series

of TWINRIX, given on a 0-, 1-, and 6-month schedule. For comparison, after the recommended immunization regimens for HAVRIX and ENGERIX-B, respectively, similar studies involving a total of 114 subjects have shown that seropositivity to HAV and HBV also persists for at least 4 years.

The effect of age on immune response to TWINRIX was studied in 2 trials comparing subjects over 40 years of age (n = 183, mean age = 48 in one trial and n = 72, mean age = 50 in the other) with those ≤40 (n = 191; mean age 32.5). The response to the hepatitis A component of TWINRIX declined slightly with age, but >99% of subjects achieved protective antibody levels in both age groups, and antibody titers were comparable to 2 doses of hepatitis A vaccine alone in age matched controls.

The response to hepatitis B immunization is known to decline in vaccinees over 40 years of age. TWINRIX elicited a seroprotective response to hepatitis B in 97% of younger subjects and 93% to 94% of the older subjects, as compared to 92% of older subjects given hepatitis B vaccine alone. Geometric mean titers elicited by TWINRIX were 2,285 in the younger subjects and 1,890 or 1,038 for the older subjects in the 2 trials. Hepatitis B vaccine alone gave titers of 2,896 in younger subjects and 1,157 in those over 40 years of age.

It has been shown in open randomized clinical trials that combining the hepatitis A antigen with the hepatitis B surface antigen in TWINRIX resulted in comparable anti-HAV or anti-HBsAg titers, relative to vaccination with the individual monovalent vaccines or the concomitant administration of each vaccine in opposite arms.

Accelerated Dosing Schedule: In 496 healthy adults, the safety and immunogenicity of TWINRIX given on a 0-, 7-, and 21- to 30-day schedule followed by a booster dose at 12 months (N = 250), was compared to separate vaccinations with monovalent hepatitis A vaccine (HAVRIX at 0 and 12 months) and hepatitis B vaccine (ENGERIX-B at 0, 1, 2, and 12 months) as a control group (N = 246).

Following a booster dose at month 12, the seroprotection rate for hepatitis B and seroconversion rate for hepatitis A at month 13 (the coprimary endpoints) following TWINRIX were non-inferior as compared to the control group. The immune responses for the According to Protocol (ATP) cohort for immunogenicity are shown in Table 4 and Figure 1.

At day 37, following 3 doses of TWINRIX, the seroprotection rate for hepatitis B was 63.2% and in the control group, who received 2 doses of ENGERIX-B, was 43.5%. This difference of 19.76% [95% CI for the difference is 10.16% to 28.99%] is

Table 1. Immunogenicity in TWINRIX Worldwide Clinical Trials

TWINRIX Dose	N	% Seroconversion for Hepatitis A[a]	% Seroprotection for Hepatitis B[b]
1	1587	93.8	30.8
2	1571	98.8	78.2
3	1551	99.9	98.5

[a]Anti-HAV titer ≥assay cut-off: 20 mIU/mL (HAVAB Test) or 33 mIU/mL (ENZYMUN-TEST®).
[b]Anti-HBsAg titer ≥10 mIU/mL (AUSAB®).

Table 2. Percentage of Seroconversion or Seroprotection Rates in the TWINRIX US Clinical Trial

Vaccine	N	Timepoint	% Seroconversion for Hepatitis A[a] (95% CI)	% Seroprotection for Hepatitis B[b] (95% CI)
TWINRIX	264	Month 1	91.6	17.9
		Month 2	97.7	61.2
		Month 7	99.6 (97.9-100.0)	95.1 (91.7-97.4)
HAVRIX and ENGERIX-B	269	Month 1	98.1	7.5
		Month 2	98.9	50.4
		Month 7	99.3 (97.3-99.9)	92.2 (88.3-95.1)

[a]Anti-HAV titer ≥assay cut-off: 33 mIU/mL (ENZYMUN-TEST®).
[b]Anti-HBsAg titer ≥10 mIU/mL (AUSAB®).

Table 3. Geometric Mean Titers in the TWINRIX US Clinical Trial

Vaccine	N	Timepoint	GMT to Hepatitis A (95% CI)	GMT to Hepatitis B (95% CI)
TWINRIX	263	Month 1	335	8
	259	Month 2	636	23
	264	Month 7	4756 (4152-5448)	2099 (1663-2649)
HAVRIX and ENGERIX-B	268	Month 1	444	6
	269	Month 2	257	18
	269	Month 7	2948 (2638-3294)	1871 (1428-2450)

Table 4. Seroconversion and Seroprotection Rates Up to One Month After the Last Dose of Vaccines (According To Protocol Cohort)

	Timepoint	TWINRIX[a]	HAVRIX and ENGERIX-B[b]
		(N = 194-204)	(N = 197-207)
% Seroconversion for Hepatitis A[c] (95% CI)	Day 37	98.5 (95.8-99.7)	98.6 (95.8-99.7)
	Day 90	100 (98.2-100)	95.6 (91.9-98.0)
	Month 12	96.9 (93.4-98.9)	86.9 (81.4-91.2)
	Month 13	100 (98.1-100)	100 (98.1-100)
% Seroprotection for Hepatitis B[d] (95% CI)	Day 37	63.2 (56.2-69.9)	43.5 (36.6-50.5)
	Day 90	83.2 (77.3-88.1)	76.7 (70.3-82.3)
	Month 12	82.1 (75.9-87.2)	77.8 (71.3-83.4)
	Month 13	96.4 (92.7-98.5)	93.4 (89.0-96.4)

[a]TWINRIX given on a 0-, 7-, and 21- to 30-day schedule followed by a booster at month 12.
[b]HAVRIX 1440 EL.U./1 mL given on a 0- and 12-month schedule and ENGERIX-B 20 mcg/1 mL given on a 0-, 1-, 2-, and 12-month schedule.
[c]Anti-HAV titer ≥assay cut-off: 15 mIU/mL (anti-HAV Behring).
[d]Anti-HBsAg titer ≥10 mIU/mL (AUSAB®).

statistically significant (P <0.001). No statistical significant difference in the hepatitis A seroconversion rates was observed between groups at day 37. At day 90, the hepatitis A seroconversion rate following TWINRIX was 100% compared to 95.6% in the control group (P = 0.004). At month 12 before the booster dose, the hepatitis A seroconversion rates between groups, 96.9% following TWINRIX and 86.9% in the control group, were statistically significantly different (P <0.001).
[See table 4 above]

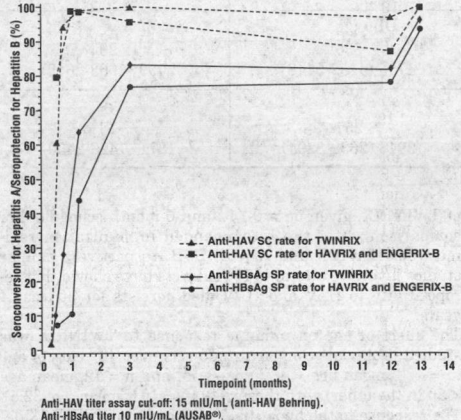

Anti-HAV titer assay cut-off: 15 mIU/mL (anti-HAV Behring).
Anti-HBsAg titer 10 mIU/mL (AUSAB®).

Figure 1. Seroconversion and Seroprotection Rates Up to One Month After the Last Dose of Vaccines (According To Protocol Cohort)

Immune Response to Simultaneously Administered Vaccines: Limited immunogenicity data are available on the concurrent administration of TWINRIX with other vaccines.
Preservative Free, Thimerosal Free Formulation:
In one randomized comparative clinical trial with 446 adults, the preservative free, thimerosal free formulation performed as well as the formulation that contained 2-phenyoxyethanol and trace amounts of thimerosal.

INDICATIONS AND USAGE

TWINRIX is indicated for active immunization of persons 18 years of age or older against disease caused by hepatitis A virus and infection by all known subtypes of hepatitis B virus. As with any vaccine, vaccination with TWINRIX may not protect 100% of recipients. As hepatitis D (caused by the delta virus) does not occur in the absence of HBV infection, it can be expected that hepatitis D will also be prevented by vaccination with TWINRIX.
Immunization is recommended for all susceptible persons 18 years of age or older who are, or will be, at risk of exposure to both hepatitis A and hepatitis B viruses, including but not limited to:

• *Travelers:* Persons traveling to areas of high/intermediate endemicity for *both* HAV and HBV *who are at increased risk of HBV infection due to behavioral or occupational factors.* (See CLINICAL PHARMACOLOGY.) Vaccine recipients should consult with CDC to determine regions of high or intermediate endemicity for hepatitis A and hepatitis B.
• *Patients With Chronic Liver Disease,* including:
– alcoholic cirrhosis
– chronic hepatitis C

– autoimmune hepatitis
– primary biliary cirrhosis
• *Persons at Risk Through Their Work:*
– Laboratory workers who handle live hepatitis A and hepatitis B virus.
– Police and other personnel who render first-aid or medical assistance.
– Workers who come in contact with feces or sewage.
– Healthcare personnel who render first-aid or emergency medical assistance.
– Personnel employed in day-care centers and correctional facilities.
– Staff of hemodialysis units.
– Military recruits and other military personnel at increased risk for HBV.
• *Persons at Increased Risk of Disease due to Their Sexual Practices:*[18,19]
Men who have sex with men.
• *Others:*
– Residents of drug and alcohol treatment centers.
– People living in, or relocating to, areas of high/intermediate endemicity of HAV and who have risk factors for HBV.
– Patients frequently receiving blood products including persons who have clotting factor disorders (hemophiliacs and other recipients of therapeutic blood products).
– Users of injectable illicit drugs.
– Individuals who are at increased risk for HBV infection and who are close household contacts of patients with acute or relapsing hepatitis A and individuals who are at increased risk for HAV infection and who are close household contacts of individuals with acute or chronic hepatitis B infection.

CONTRAINDICATIONS

Hypersensitivity to any component of the vaccine, including yeast and neomycin, is a contraindication (see DESCRIPTION). This vaccine is contraindicated in patients with previous hypersensitivity to TWINRIX or monovalent hepatitis A or hepatitis B vaccines.

WARNINGS

There have been rare reports of anaphylaxis/anaphylactoid reactions following routine clinical use of TWINRIX. (See ADVERSE REACTIONS, Postmarketing Reports.)
The tip cap and the rubber plunger of the needleless prefilled syringes contain dry natural latex rubber that may cause allergic reactions in latex sensitive individuals. The vial stopper is latex-free.
Hepatitis A and hepatitis B have relatively long incubation periods. The vaccine may not prevent hepatitis A or hepatitis B infection in individuals who have an unrecognized hepatitis A or hepatitis B infection at the time of vaccination. Additionally, it may not prevent infection in individuals who do not achieve protective antibody titers.

PRECAUTIONS

General:
Prior to immunization with TWINRIX, the patient's current health status and medical history should be reviewed. The physician should review the patient's immunization history for possible vaccine sensitivity, previous vaccination-related adverse reactions and occurrence of any adverse–event-related symptoms and/or signs, in order to determine the existence of any contraindication to immunization with TWINRIX and to allow an assessment of benefits and risks. Appropriate medical treatment and supervision should be readily available for immediate use in case of a rare anaphylactic reaction following the administration of the vaccine. Epinephrine injection (1:1,000) and other appropriate

agents used for the control of immediate allergic reactions must be immediately available. As with other vaccines, although a moderate or severe acute illness is sufficient reason to postpone vaccination, minor illnesses such as mild upper respiratory infections with or without low-grade fever are not contraindications.[20]
TWINRIX should be given with caution in persons with bleeding disorders such as hemophilia or thrombocytopenia and in persons on anticoagulant therapy, with steps taken to avoid the risk of hematoma following the injection.[20]
A separate, sterile syringe and needle or a sterile disposable unit should be used for each patient to prevent the transmission of other infectious agents from person to person. Needles should be disposed of properly and should not be recapped.
As with any vaccine, if administered to immunosuppressed persons, including individuals receiving immunosuppressive therapy, the expected immune response may not be obtained.
Multiple Sclerosis: Results from 2 clinical studies indicate that there is no association between hepatitis B vaccination and the development of multiple sclerosis,[21] and that vaccination with hepatitis B vaccine does not appear to increase the short-term risk of relapse in multiple sclerosis.[22]
Information for Vaccine Recipients:
Vaccine recipients should be informed by their healthcare provider of the potential benefits and risks of immunization with TWINRIX. When educating vaccine recipients regarding potential side effects, clinicians should emphasize that components of TWINRIX cannot cause hepatitis A or hepatitis B infection.
Vaccine recipients should be instructed to report any severe or unusual adverse reactions to their healthcare provider. The vaccine recipients should be given the Vaccine Information Statements, which are required by the National Childhood Vaccine Injury Act of 1986 to be given prior to immunization. These materials are available free of charge at the CDC website (www.cdc.gov/vaccines). The Vaccine Adverse Events Reporting System (VAERS) toll-free number is 1-800-822-7967. Reporting forms may also be obtained at the VAERS website at www.vaers.hhs.gov.
Carcinogenesis, Mutagenesis, Impairment of Fertility:
TWINRIX has not been evaluated for its carcinogenic potential, mutagenic potential, or potential for impairment of fertility.
Pregnancy:
Pregnancy Category C. Animal reproduction studies have not been conducted with TWINRIX. It is also not known whether TWINRIX can cause fetal harm when administered to a pregnant woman or can affect reproduction capacity. TWINRIX should be given to a pregnant woman only if clearly indicated (see INDICATIONS AND USAGE).
Pregnancy Exposure Registry:
Healthcare providers are encouraged to register pregnant women who receive TWINRIX in the GlaxoSmithKline vaccination pregnancy registry by calling 1-888-452-9622.
Nursing Mothers:
It is not known whether TWINRIX is excreted in human milk. Because many drugs are excreted in human milk, caution should be exercised when TWINRIX is administered to a nursing woman.
Pediatric Use:
Safety and effectiveness in pediatric patients below the age of 18 years have not been established.
Geriatric Use:
Clinical studies of TWINRIX did not include sufficient numbers of subjects aged 65 and over to determine whether they respond differently from younger subjects.

ADVERSE REACTIONS

Because clinical trials are conducted under widely varying conditions, adverse event rates observed in the clinical trials of a vaccine cannot be directly compared to rates in the clinical trials of another vaccine, and may not reflect the rates observed in practice. As with any vaccine, there is the possibility that broad use of TWINRIX could reveal adverse events not observed in clinical trials.
The safety of TWINRIX has been evaluated in clinical trials involving the administration of approximately 7,500 doses to more than 2,500 individuals.
Of 773 volunteers who participated in the comparative trial conducted in the United States, 389 subjects received at least 1 dose of TWINRIX (0-, 1-, and 6-month schedule) and 384 received at least 1 dose each of ENGERIX-B and HAVRIX as separate but simultaneous injections. Solicited adverse events reported following the administration of TWINRIX are shown in Table 5, compared with adverse events reported after administration of ENGERIX-B and HAVRIX.

[See table 5 at right]

Adverse reactions seen with TWINRIX were similar to those observed after vaccination with the monovalent components. The frequency of solicited adverse events did not increase with successive doses of TWINRIX. Most events reported were considered by the subjects as mild and self-limiting and did not last more than 48 hours.

In a clinical trial in which TWINRIX was given on a 0-, 7-, and 21- to 30-day schedule followed by a booster dose at 12 months, solicited local or general adverse events were comparable to those seen in other clinical trials of TWINRIX given on a 0-, 1-, and 6-month schedule.

Among 2,299 subjects in 14 clinical trials, the following adverse experiences were reported to occur within 30 days following vaccination with the frequency shown below. Adverse experiences within 30 days of vaccination in the US clinical trial of TWINRIX given on a 0-, 7-, and 21- to 30-day schedule followed by a booster dose at 12 months were similar to those reported in other clinical trials and postmarketing surveillance.

Incidence 1% to 10% of Injections, Seen in Clinical Trials With TWINRIX:

Infections and Infestations: Upper respiratory tract infections.

General Disorders and Administration Site Conditions: Injection site induration.

Incidence <1% of Injections, Seen in Clinical Trials With TWINRIX:

Infections and Infestations: Respiratory tract illnesses.

Metabolism and Nutrition Disorders: Anorexia.

Psychiatric Disorders: Agitation, insomnia.

Nervous System Disorders: Dizziness, migraine, paresthesia, somnolence, syncope.

Ear and Labyrinth Disorders: Vertigo.

Vascular Disorders: Flushing.

Gastrointestinal System: Abdominal pain, vomiting.

Skin and Subcutaneous Tissue Disorders: Erythema, petechiae, rash, sweating, urticaria.

Musculoskeletal and Connective Tissue Disorders: Arthralgia, back pain, myalgia.

General Disorders and Administration Site Conditions: Injection site ecchymosis, injection site pruritus, influenza-like symptoms, irritability, weakness.

Incidence <1% of Injections, Seen in Clinical Trials With HAVRIX[a] and/or ENGERIX-B[b]:

Blood and Lymphatic System Disorders: Lymphadenopathy.[a+b]

Nervous System: Dysgeusia,[a] hypertonic episode,[a] tingling.[b]

Eye Disorders: Photophobia.[a]

Vascular Disorders: Hypotension.[b]

Gastrointestinal Disorders: Constipation.[b]

Investigations: Elevation of creatine phosphokinase.[a]

Postmarketing Reports:

Worldwide voluntary reports of adverse events received for TWINRIX, HAVRIX, and/or ENGERIX-B since market introduction of these vaccines are listed below. These lists include serious events or events which have suspected causal connections to components of these or other vaccines or drugs. Because these events are reported voluntarily from a population of uncertain size, it is not possible to reliably estimate their frequency or establish a causal relationship to vaccine exposure.

Postmarketing Reports With TWINRIX:

Infections and Infestations: Herpes zoster, meningitis.

Blood and Lymphatic System Disorders: Thrombocytopenia, thrombocytopenic purpura.

Immune System Disorders: Allergic reaction, anaphylactoid reaction, anaphylaxis, serum sickness–like syndrome days to weeks after vaccination including arthralgia/arthritis (usually transient), fever, urticaria, erythema multiforme, ecchymoses, and erythema nodosum.

Nervous System Disorders: Bell's palsy, convulsions, encephalitis, encephalopathy, Guillain-Barré syndrome, hypoesthesia, myelitis, multiple sclerosis, neuritis, neuropathy, optic neuritis, paralysis, paresis, transverse myelitis.

Eye Disorders: Conjunctivitis, visual disturbances.

Ear and Labyrinth Disorders: Earache, tinnitus.

Cardiac Disorders: Palpitations, tachycardia.

Vascular Disorders: Vasculitis.

Respiratory, Thoracic and Mediastinal Disorders: Bronchospasm including asthma-like symptoms, dyspnea.

Gastrointestinal Disorders: Dyspepsia.

Hepatobiliary disorders: Hepatitis, jaundice.

Skin and Subcutaneous Tissue Disorders: Alopecia, angioedema, eczema, erythema multiforme, erythema nodosum, hyperhydrosis, lichen planus.

Musculoskeletal and Connective Tissue Disorders: Arthritis, muscular weakness.

General Disorders and Administration Site Conditions: Chills, injection site reaction, malaise.

Investigations: Abnormal liver function tests.

Postmarketing Reports With HAVRIX and/or ENGERIX-B:

Worldwide voluntary reports of adverse events received for HAVRIX and/or ENGERIX-B but not already reported for TWINRIX are listed below.

Eye Disorders: Keratitis.[b]

Skin and Subcutaneous Tissue Disorders: Stevens-Johnson syndrome.[b]

Congenital, Familial and Genetic Disorders: Congenital abnormality.[a]

[a]Following HAVRIX.

[b]Following ENGERIX-B.

[a+b]Following either HAVRIX or ENGERIX-B.

Table 5. Rate of Adverse Events Reported After Administration of TWINRIX or ENGERIX-B and HAVRIX

Adverse Event	TWINRIX			ENGERIX-B			HAVRIX	
	Dose 1	Dose 2	Dose 3	Dose 1	Dose 2	Dose 3	Dose 1	Dose 2
Local	(N = 385) %	(N = 382) %	(N = 374) %	(N = 382) %	(N = 376) %	(N = 369) %	(N = 382) %	(N = 369) %
Soreness	37	35	41	41	25	30	53	47
Redness	8	9	11	6	7	9	7	9
Swelling	4	4	6	3	5	5	5	5

Adverse Event	TWINRIX			ENGERIX-B and HAVRIX		
	Dose 1	Dose 2	Dose 3	Dose 1	Dose 2	Dose 3
General	(N = 385) %	(N = 382) %	(N = 374) %	(N = 382) %	(N = 376) %	(N = 369) %
Headache	22	15	13	19	12	14
Fatigue	14	13	11	14	9	10
Diarrhea	5	4	6	5	3	3
Nausea	4	3	2	7	3	5
Fever	4	3	2	4	2	4
Vomiting	1	1	0	1	1	1

Reporting of Adverse Events:

The US Department of Health and Human Services has established VAERS to accept reports of suspected adverse events after the administration of any vaccine, including, but not limited to, the reporting of events required by the National Childhood Vaccine Injury Act of 1986. The toll-free number for VAERS forms and information is 1-800-822-7967.[23] Reporting forms may also be obtained at the VAERS website at www.vaers.hhs.gov.

DOSAGE AND ADMINISTRATION

TWINRIX should be administered by intramuscular injection. *Do not inject intravenously or intradermally.* In adults, the injection should be given in the deltoid region. TWINRIX should not be administered in the gluteal region; such injections may result in a suboptimal response.

Primary immunization for adults consists of 3 doses, given on a 0-, 1-, and 6-month schedule. Alternatively, a 4-dose schedule, given on days 0, 7 and 21 to 30 followed by a booster dose at month 12 may be used. Each 1-mL dose contains 720 EL.U. of inactivated hepatitis A virus and 20 mcg of hepatitis B surface antigen.

When concomitant administration of other vaccines or immunoglobulin (IG) is required, they should be given with different syringes and at different injection sites.

Preparation for Administration:

Shake vial or syringe well before withdrawal and use. Inspect TWINRIX visually for particulate matter, discoloration, and cracks in the vial or syringe prior to administration, whenever solution and container permit. If any of these conditions exist, the vaccine should not be administered. With thorough agitation, TWINRIX is a slightly turbid white suspension. Discard if it appears otherwise.

The vaccine should be used as supplied; no dilution or reconstitution is necessary. The full recommended dose of the vaccine should be used. After removal of the appropriate volume from a single-dose vial, any vaccine remaining in the vial should be discarded.

STORAGE

Store TWINRIX refrigerated between 2° and 8° C (36° and 46° F). **Do not freeze.** Discard if the vaccine has been frozen. Do not use after expiration date shown on the label.

HOW SUPPLIED

TWINRIX is supplied as a slightly turbid white suspension in vials and prefilled TIP-LOK® syringes containing a 1.0-mL single dose.

Single-Dose Vials (Preservative Free Formulation)
NDC 58160-815-11 (package of 10)

Single-Dose Prefilled Disposable TIP-LOK Syringes (packaged without needles) (Preservative Free Formulation)
NDC 58160-815-32 (package of 1)
NDC 58160-815-46 (package of 5)

REFERENCES

1. Dienstag JL, Routenberg JA, Purcell RH, et al. Foodhandler-associated outbreak of hepatitis Type A: an immune electron microscopic study. *Ann Intern Med.* 1975;83:647-650. **2.** Mackowiak PA, Caraway CT, Portnoy BL. Oyster-associated hepatitis: lessons from the Louisiana experience. *Am J Epidemiol.* 1976;103(2):181-191. **3.** Woodson RD, Clinton JJ. Hepatitis prophylaxis abroad. Effectiveness of immune serum globulin in protecting Peace Corps volunteers. *JAMA.* 1969;209(7):1053-1058. **4.** Krugman S, Giles JP. Viral hepatitis. New light on an old disease. *JAMA.* 1970;212(6):1019-1029. **5.** Hadler SC, Erben JJ, Francis DP, et al. Risk factors for hepatitis A in day-care centers. *J Infect Dis.* 1982;145(2):255-261. **6.** Hadler SC. Global impact of hepatitis A virus infection changing patterns. In: Hollinger FB, Lemon SM, Margolis H, eds. *Viral Hepatitis and Liver Disease.* Baltimore, MD: Williams & Wilkins; 1991:14-20. **7.** Centers for Disease Control and Prevention. Epidemiology and prevention of vaccine-preventable diseases. Atkinson W, Hamborsky J, McIntyre L, Wolfe S, eds. 10th ed. Washington DC: Public Health Foundation; 2007:197-234. **8.** Lemon SM. Type A viral hepatitis: new developments in an old disease. *N Engl J Med.* 1985;313(17):1059-1067. **9.** Sjogren MH, Tanno H, Fay O, et al. Hepatitis A virus in stool during clinical relapse. *Ann Intern Med.* 1987;106:221-226. **10.** Chiriaco P, Guadalupi C, Armigliato M, et al. Polyphasic course of hepatitis type A in children. *J Infect Dis.* 1986;153(2):378-379. **11.** Data on file (TWR101), GlaxoSmithKline. **12.** Koff RS. Hepatitis B and hepatitis D. In: Gorbach SL, Bartlett JG, Blacklow NR, eds. *Infectious Diseases.* Philadelphia, PA: WB Saunders Company; 1992:709-716. **13.** Frisch-Niggemeyer W, Ambrosch F, Hofmann H. The assessment of immunity against hepatitis B after vaccination. *J Bio Stand.* 1986;14(3):255-258. **14.** Beasley RP, Hwang LY, Stevens CE, et al. Efficacy of hepatitis B immune globulin for prevention of perinatal transmission of the hepatitis B virus carrier state: final report of a randomized double-blind, placebo-controlled trial. *Hepatology.* 1983;3(2):135-141. **15.** Centers for Disease Control and Prevention. Proposed vaccine information materials for hepatitis B, haemophilus influenza type B (Hib), varicella (chickenpox), and measles, mumps, rubella (MMR) vaccines. *Federal Register.* September 3, 1998;63(171):47026-47031. **16.** Chang MH, Chen CJ, Lai MS. Universal hepatitis B vaccination in Taiwan and the incidence of hepatocellular carcinoma in children. *N Engl J Med.* 1997;336(26):1855-1859. **17.** Lee MS, Kim DH, Kim H, et al. Hepatitis B vaccination and reduced risk of primary liver cancer among male adults: A cohort study in Korea. *Int J Epidemiol.* 1998;27:316-319. **18.** Centers for Disease Control and Prevention. 1998 Guidelines for treatment of sexually transmitted diseases. *MMWR.* 1999;47(RR-1):99-104. **19.** Centers for Disease Control and Prevention. Hepatitis surveillance report No. 57. Atlanta, GA: DHHS; 2000:12. **20.** Centers for Disease Control and Prevention. General recommendations on immunization: recommendations of the Advisory Committee on Immunization Practices (ACIP). *MMWR.* 2006;55(RR-15):1-48. **21.** Ascherio A, Zhang SM, Hernán MA, et al. Hepatitis B vaccination and the risk of multiple sclerosis. *N Engl J Med.* 2001;344(5):327-332. **22.** Confavreux C, Suissa S, Saddier P, et al. Vaccination and the risk of relapse in multiple sclerosis. *N Engl J Med.* 2001;344(5):319-326. **23.** Centers for Disease Control and Prevention. Vaccine adverse event reporting system — United States. *MMWR.* 1990;39(41):730-733.

TWINRIX, HAVRIX, ENGERIX-B, and TIP-LOK are registered trademarks of GlaxoSmithKline. ENZYMUN-TEST is a registered trademark of Boehringer Mannheim Immunodiagnostics. AUSAB is a registered trademark of Abbott Laboratories.

Manufactured by **GlaxoSmithKline Biologicals**
Rixensart, Belgium, US License No. 1617

Distributed by **GlaxoSmithKline** Research Triangle Park, NC 27709
©2009, GlaxoSmithKline. All rights reserved.
August 2009
TWR:12PI

TYKERB®   ℞
[ti'kerb]
(lapatinib)
tablets

HIGHLIGHTS OF PRESCRIBING INFORMATION
These highlights do not include all the information needed to use TYKERB safely and effectively. See full prescribing information for TYKERB.
TYKERB (lapatinib) tablets
Initial U.S. Approval: 2007

> **WARNING: HEPATOTOXICITY**
> *See full prescribing information for complete boxed warning.*
> Hepatotoxicity has been observed in clinical trials and postmarketing experience. The hepatotoxicity may be severe and deaths have been reported. Causality of the deaths is uncertain. *[See Warnings and Precautions (5.2).]*

---RECENT MAJOR CHANGES---
Indications and Usage. (1)   January 2010
Dosage and Administration. (2)   January 2010
Contraindications. (4)   January 2010

---INDICATIONS AND USAGE---
TYKERB, a kinase inhibitor, is indicated in combination with: (1)
- capecitabine, for the treatment of patients with advanced or metastatic breast cancer whose tumors overexpress HER2 and who have received prior therapy including an anthracycline, a taxane, and trastuzumab.
- letrozole for the treatment of postmenopausal women with hormone receptor positive metastatic breast cancer that overexpresses the HER2 receptor for whom hormonal therapy is indicated.

TYKERB in combination with an aromatase inhibitor has not been compared to a trastuzumab-containing chemotherapy regimen for the treatment of metastatic breast cancer.

---DOSAGE AND ADMINISTRATION---
The recommended dosage of TYKERB for advanced or metastatic breast cancer is 1,250 mg (5 tablets) given orally once daily on Days 1-21 continuously in combination with capecitabine 2,000 mg/m^2/day (administered orally in 2 doses approximately 12 hours apart) on Days 1-14 in a repeating 21 day cycle. (2.1)
The recommended dose of TYKERB for hormone receptor positive, HER2 positive metastatic breast cancer is 1500 mg (6 tablets) given orally once daily continuously in combination with letrozole. When TYKERB is coadministered with letrozole, the recommended dose of letrozole is 2.5 mg once daily. (2.1)
- TYKERB should be taken at least one hour before or one hour after a meal. However, capecitabine should be taken with food or within 30 minutes after food. (2.1)
- TYKERB should be taken once daily. Do not divide daily doses of TYKERB. (2.1, 12.3)
- Modify dose for cardiac and other toxicities, severe hepatic impairment, and CYP3A4 drug interactions. (2.2)

---DOSAGE FORMS AND STRENGTHS---
250 mg tablets (3)

---CONTRAINDICATIONS---
Known severe hypersensitivity (e.g., anaphylaxis) to this product or any of its components. (4)

---WARNINGS AND PRECAUTIONS---
- Decreases in left ventricular ejection fraction have been reported. Confirm normal LVEF before starting TYKERB and continue evaluations during treatment. (5.1)
- Lapatinib has been associated with hepatotoxicity. Monitor liver function tests before initiation of treatment, every 4 to 6 weeks during treatment, and as clinically indicated. Discontinue and do not restart TYKERB if patients experience severe changes in liver function tests. (5.2)
- Dose reduction in patients with severe hepatic impairment should be considered. (2.2, 5.3, 8.7)
- Diarrhea, including severe diarrhea, has been reported during treatment. Manage with anti-diarrheal agents, and replace fluids and electrolytes if severe. (5.4)
- Lapatinib has been associated with interstitial lung disease and pneumonitis. Discontinue TYKERB if patients experience severe pulmonary symptoms. (5.5)
- Lapatinib may prolong the QT interval in some patients. Consider ECG and electrolyte monitoring. (5.6, 12.4)
- Fetal harm can occur when administered to a pregnant woman. Women should be advised not to become pregnant when taking TYKERB. (5.7)

---ADVERSE REACTIONS---
The most common (>20%) adverse reactions during treatment with TYKERB plus capecitabine were diarrhea, palmar-plantar erythrodysesthesia, nausea, rash, vomiting, and fatigue. The most common ((20%) adverse reactions during treatment with TYKERB plus letrozole were diarrhea, rash, nausea, and fatigue. (6.1)
To report **SUSPECTED ADVERSE REACTIONS**, contact GlaxoSmithKline at 1-888-825-5249 or FDA at 1-800-FDA-1088 or www.fda.gov/medwatch.

---DRUG INTERACTIONS---
- TYKERB is likely to increase exposure to concomitantly administered drugs which are metabolized by CYP3A4 or CYP2C8. (7.1)
- Avoid strong CYP3A4 inhibitors. If unavoidable, consider dose reduction of TYKERB in patients coadministered a strong CYP3A4 inhibitor. (2.2, 7.2)
- Avoid strong CYP3A4 inducers. If unavoidable, consider gradual dose increase of TYKERB in patients coadministered a strong CYP3A4 inducer. (2.2, 7.2)

See 17 for **PATIENT COUNSELING INFORMATION** and FDA-approved patient labeling

Revised: 04/2010

FULL PRESCRIBING INFORMATION: CONTENTS*

FULL PRESCRIBING INFORMATION

> **WARNING: HEPATOTOXICITY**
> Hepatotoxicity has been observed in clinical trials and postmarketing experience. The hepatotoxicity may be severe and deaths have been reported. Causality of the deaths is uncertain. *[See Warnings and Precautions (5.2).]*

1   INDICATIONS AND USAGE

TYKERB® is indicated in combination with:
- capecitabine for the treatment of patients with advanced or metastatic breast cancer whose tumors overexpress HER2 and who have received prior therapy including an anthracycline, a taxane, and trastuzumab.

- letrozole for the treatment of postmenopausal women with hormone receptor positive metastatic breast cancer that overexpresses the HER2 receptor for whom hormonal therapy is indicated.

TYKERB in combination with an aromatase inhibitor has not been compared to a trastuzumab-containing chemotherapy regimen for the treatment of metastatic breast cancer.

2   DOSAGE AND ADMINISTRATION
2.1   Recommended Dosing
Underline: HER2 Positive Metastatic Breast Cancer: The recommended dose of TYKERB is 1,250 mg given orally once daily on Days 1-21 continuously in combination with capecitabine 2,000 mg/m^2/day (administered orally in 2 doses approximately 12 hours apart) on Days 1-14 in a repeating 21 day cycle. TYKERB should be taken at least one hour before or one hour after a meal. The dose of TYKERB should be once daily (5 tablets administered all at once); dividing the daily dose is not recommended *[see Clinical Pharmacology (12.3)].* Capecitabine should be taken with food or within 30 minutes after food. If a day's dose is missed, the patient should not double the dose the next day. Treatment should be continued until disease progression or unacceptable toxicity occurs.

Hormone Receptor Positive, HER2 Positive Metastatic Breast Cancer: The recommended dose of TYKERB is 1,500 mg given orally once daily continuously in combination with letrozole. When coadministered with TYKERB, the recommended dose of letrozole is 2.5 mg once daily. TYKERB should be taken at least one hour before or one hour after a meal. The dose of TYKERB should be once daily (6 tablets administered all at once); dividing the daily dose is not recommended *[see Clinical Pharmacology (12.3)].*

2.2   Dose Modification Guidelines
Cardiac Events: TYKERB should be discontinued in patients with a decreased left ventricular ejection fraction (LVEF) that is Grade 2 or greater by National Cancer Institute Common Terminology Criteria for Adverse Events (NCI CTCAE) and in patients with an LVEF that drops below the institution's lower limit of normal *[see Warnings and Precautions (5.1) and Adverse Reactions (6.1)].* TYKERB in combination with capecitabine may be restarted at a reduced dose (1,000 mg/day) and in combination with letrozole may be restarted at a reduced dose of 1,250 mg/day after a minimum of 2 weeks if the LVEF recovers to normal and the patient is asymptomatic.
Hepatic Impairment: Patients with severe hepatic impairment (Child-Pugh Class C) should have their dose of TYKERB reduced. A dose reduction from 1,250 mg/day to 750 mg/day (HER2 positive metastatic breast cancer indication) or from 1,500 mg/day to 1,000 mg/day (hormone receptor positive, HER2 positive breast cancer indication) in patients with severe hepatic impairment is predicted to adjust the area under the curve (AUC) to the normal range and should be considered. However, there are no clinical data with this dose adjustment in patients with severe hepatic impairment.
Concomitant Strong CYP3A4 Inhibitors: The concomitant use of strong CYP3A4 inhibitors should be avoided (e.g., ketoconazole, itraconazole, clarithromycin, atazanavir, indinavir, nefazodone, nelfinavir, ritonavir, saquinavir, telithromycin, voriconazole). Grapefruit may also increase plasma concentrations of lapatinib and should be avoided. If patients must be coadministered a strong CYP3A4 inhibitor, based on pharmacokinetic studies, a dose reduction to 500 mg/day of lapatinib is predicted to adjust the lapatinib AUC to the range observed without inhibitors and should be considered. However, there are no clinical data with this dose adjustment in patients receiving strong CYP3A4 inhibitors. If the strong inhibitor is discontinued, a washout period of approximately 1 week should be allowed before the lapatinib dose is adjusted upward to the indicated dose. *[See Drug Interactions (7.2).]*
Concomitant Strong CYP3A4 Inducers: The concomitant use of strong CYP3A4 inducers should be avoided (e.g., dexamethasone, phenytoin, carbamazepine, rifampin, rifabutin, rifapentin, phenobarbital, St. John's Wort). If patients must be coadministered a strong CYP3A4 inducer, based on pharmacokinetic studies, the dose of lapatinib should be titrated gradually from 1,250 mg/day up to 4,500 mg/day (HER2 positive metastatic breast cancer indication) or from 1,500 mg/day up to 5,500 mg/day (hormone receptor positive, HER2 positive breast cancer indication) based on tolerability. This dose of lapatinib is predicted to adjust the lapatinib AUC to the range observed without inducers and should be considered. However, there are no clinical data with this dose adjustment in patients receiving strong CYP3A4 inducers. If the strong inducer is discontinued the lapatinib dose should be reduced to the indicated dose. *[See Drug Interactions (7.2).]*
Other Toxicities: Discontinuation or interruption of dosing with TYKERB may be considered when patients develop ≥Grade 2 NCI CTCAE toxicity and can be restarted at 1,250 mg/day when the toxicity improves to Grade 1 or less. If the toxicity recurs, then TYKERB in combination with

capecitabine should be restarted at a lower dose (1,000 mg/day) and in combination with letrozole should be restarted at a lower dose of 1,250 mg/day.

See manufacturer's prescribing information for the coadministered product dosage adjustment guidelines in the event of toxicity and other relevant safety information or contraindications.

3 DOSAGE FORMS AND STRENGTHS

250 mg tablets—oval, biconvex, orange, film-coated with GS XJG debossed on one side.

4 CONTRAINDICATIONS

TYKERB is contraindicated in patients with known severe hypersensitivity (e.g., anaphylaxis) to this product or any of its components.

5 WARNINGS AND PRECAUTIONS

5.1 Decreased Left Ventricular Ejection Fraction

TYKERB has been reported to decrease LVEF *[see Adverse Reactions (6.1)]*. In clinical trials, the majority (>57%) of LVEF decreases occurred within the first 12 weeks of treatment; however, data on long-term exposure are limited. Caution should be taken if TYKERB is to be administered to patients with conditions that could impair left ventricular function. LVEF should be evaluated in all patients prior to initiation of treatment with TYKERB to ensure that the patient has a baseline LVEF that is within the institution's normal limits. LVEF should continue to be evaluated during treatment with TYKERB to ensure that LVEF does not decline below the institution's normal limits *[see Dosage and Administration (2.2)]*.

5.2 Hepatotoxicity

Hepatotoxicity (ALT or AST >3 times the upper limit of normal and total bilirubin >2 times the upper limit of normal) has been observed in clinical trials (<1% of patients) and postmarketing experience. The hepatotoxicity may be severe and deaths have been reported. Causality of the deaths is uncertain. The hepatotoxicity may occur days to several months after initiation of treatment. Liver function tests (transaminases, bilirubin, and alkaline phosphatase) should be monitored before initiation of treatment, every 4 to 6 weeks during treatment, and as clinically indicated. If changes in liver function are severe, therapy with TYKERB should be discontinued and patients should not be retreated with TYKERB *[see Adverse Reactions (6.1)]*.

5.3 Patients with Severe Hepatic Impairment

If TYKERB is to be administered to patients with severe pre-existing hepatic impairment, dose reduction should be considered *[see Dosage and Administration (2.2) and Use in Specific Populations (8.7)]*. In patients who develop severe hepatotoxicity while on therapy, TYKERB should be discontinued and patients should not be retreated with TYKERB *[see Warnings and Precautions (5.2)]*.

5.4 Diarrhea

Diarrhea, including severe diarrhea, has been reported during treatment with TYKERB *[see Adverse Reactions (6.1)]*. Proactive management of diarrhea with anti-diarrheal agents is important. Severe cases of diarrhea may require administration of oral or intravenous electrolytes and fluids, and interruption or discontinuation of therapy with TYKERB.

5.5 Interstitial Lung Disease/Pneumonitis

Lapatinib has been associated with interstitial lung disease and pneumonitis in monotherapy or in combination with other chemotherapies *[see Adverse Reactions (6.1)]*. Patients should be monitored for pulmonary symptoms indicative of interstitial lung disease or pneumonitis. TYKERB should be discontinued in patients who experience pulmonary symptoms which are ≥Grade 3 (NCI CTCAE).

5.6 QT Prolongation

QT prolongation was observed in an uncontrolled, open-label dose escalation study of lapatinib in advanced cancer patients *[see Clinical Pharmacology (12.4)]*. Lapatinib should be administered with caution to patients who have or may develop prolongation of QTc. These conditions include patients with hypokalemia or hypomagnesemia, with congenital long QT syndrome, patients taking antiarrhythmic medicines or other medicinal products that lead to QT prolongation, and cumulative high-dose anthracycline therapy. Hypokalemia or hypomagnesemia should be corrected prior to lapatinib administration.

5.7 Use in Pregnancy

TYKERB can cause fetal harm when administered to a pregnant woman. Based on findings in animals, TYKERB is expected to result in adverse reproductive effects. Lapatinib administered to rats during organogenesis and through lactation led to death of offspring within the first 4 days after birth *[see Use in Specific Populations (8.1)]*.

There are no adequate and well-controlled studies with TYKERB in pregnant women. Women should be advised not to become pregnant when taking TYKERB. If this drug is used during pregnancy, or if the patient becomes pregnant while taking this drug, the patient should be apprised of the potential hazard to the fetus.

6 ADVERSE REACTIONS

6.1 Clinical Trials Experience

Because clinical trials are conducted under widely varying conditions, adverse reaction rates observed in the clinical trials of a drug cannot be directly compared to rates in the clinical trials of another drug and may not reflect the rates observed in practice.

HER2 Positive Metastatic Breast Cancer: The safety of TYKERB has been evaluated in more than 12,000 patients in clinical trials. The efficacy and safety of TYKERB in combination with capecitabine in breast cancer was evaluated in 198 patients in a randomized, Phase 3 trial. *[See Clinical Studies (14.1).]* Adverse reactions which occurred in at least 10% of patients in either treatment arm and were higher in the combination arm are shown in Table 1.

The most common adverse reactions (>20%) during therapy with TYKERB plus capecitabine were gastrointestinal (diarrhea, nausea, and vomiting), dermatologic (palmar-plantar erythrodysesthesia and rash), and fatigue. Diarrhea was the most common adverse reaction resulting in discontinuation of study medication.

The most common Grade 3 and 4 adverse reactions (NCI CTCAE v3) were diarrhea and palmar-plantar erythrodysesthesia. Selected laboratory abnormalities are shown in Table 2.

[See table 1 above]
[See table 2 at top of next page]

Hormone Receptor Positive, Metastatic Breast Cancer: In a randomized clinical trial of patients (N = 1,286) with hormone receptor positive, metastatic breast cancer, who had not received chemotherapy for their metastatic disease, patients received letrozole with or without TYKERB. In this trial, the safety profile of TYKERB was consistent with previously reported results from trials of TYKERB in the advanced or metastatic breast cancer population. Adverse reactions which occurred in at least 10% of patients in either treatment arm and were higher in the combination arm are shown in Table 3. Selected laboratory abnormalities are shown in Table 4.

[See table 3 on next page]
[See table 4 at top of page 1591]

Decreases in Left Ventricular Ejection Fraction

Due to potential cardiac toxicity with HER2 (ErbB2) inhibitors, LVEF was monitored in clinical trials at approximately 8-week intervals. LVEF decreases were defined as signs or symptoms of deterioration in left ventricular cardiac function that are ≥Grade 3 (NCI CTCAE), or a ≥20% decrease in left ventricular cardiac ejection fraction relative to baseline which is below the institution's lower limit of normal. Among 198 patients who received TYKERB/capecitabine combination treatment, 3 experienced Grade 2 and one had Grade 3 LVEF adverse reactions *[See Warnings and Precautions (5.1).]* Among 654 patients who received TYKERB/letrozole combination treatment, 26 patients experienced Grade 1 or 2 and 6 patients had Grade 3 or 4 LVEF adverse reactions.

Hepatotoxicity: TYKERB has been associated with hepatotoxicity *[see Boxed Warning and Warnings and Precautions (5.2)]*.

Interstitial Lung Disease/Pneumonitis: TYKERB has been associated with interstitial lung disease and pneumonitis in monotherapy or in combination with other chemotherapies *[see Warnings and Precautions (5.5)]*.

6.2 Postmarketing Experience

The following adverse reactions have been identified during post-approval use of TYKERB. Because these reactions are reported voluntarily from a population of uncertain size, it is not always possible to reliably estimate their frequency or establish a causal relationship to drug exposure.

Immune System Disorders: Hypersensitivity reactions including anaphylaxis *[see Contraindications (4)]*.

Skin and Subcutaneous Tissue Disorders: Nail disorders including paronychia.

Table 1. Adverse Reactions Occurring in ≥10% of Patients

Reactions	TYKERB 1,250 mg/day + Capecitabine 2,000 mg/m²/day (N = 198)			Capecitabine 2,500 mg/m²/day (N = 191)		
	All Grades[a]	Grade 3	Grade 4	All Grades[a]	Grade 3	Grade 4
	%	%	%	%	%	%
Gastrointestinal disorders						
Diarrhea	65	13	1	40	10	0
Nausea	44	2	0	43	2	0
Vomiting	26	2	0	21	2	0
Stomatitis	14	0	0	11	<1	0
Dyspepsia	11	<1	0	3	0	0
Skin and subcutaneous tissue disorders						
Palmar-plantar erythrodysesthesia	53	12	0	51	14	0
Rash[b]	28	2	0	14	1	0
Dry skin	10	0	0	6	0	0
General disorders and administrative site conditions						
Mucosal inflammation	15	0	0	12	2	0
Musculoskeletal and connective tissue disorders						
Pain in extremity	12	1	0	7	<1	0
Back pain	11	1	0	6	<1	0
Respiratory, thoracic, and mediastinal disorders						
Dyspnea	12	3	0	8	2	0
Psychiatric disorders						
Insomnia	10	<1	0	6	0	0

[a] National Cancer Institute Common Terminology Criteria for Adverse Events, version 3.
[b] Grade 3 dermatitis acneiform was reported in <1% of patients in TYKERB plus capecitabine group.

Table 2. Selected Laboratory Abnormalities

Parameters	TYKERB 1,250 mg/day + Capecitabine 2,000 mg/m²/day			Capecitabine 2,500 mg/m²/day		
	All Grades[a]	Grade 3	Grade 4	All Grades[a]	Grade 3	Grade 4
	%	%	%	%	%	%
Hematologic						
Hemoglobin	56	<1	0	53	1	0
Platelets	18	<1	0	17	<1	<1
Neutrophils	22	3	<1	31	2	1
Hepatic						
Total Bilirubin	45	4	0	30	3	0
AST	49	2	<1	43	2	0
ALT	37	2	0	33	1	0

[a] National Cancer Institute Common Terminology Criteria for Adverse Events, version 3.

Table 3. Adverse Reactions Occurring in ≥10% of Patients

Reactions	TYKERB 1,500 mg/day + Letrozole 2.5 mg/day (N = 654)			Letrozole 2.5 mg/day (N = 624)		
	All Grades[a]	Grade 3	Grade 4	All Grades[a]	Grade 3	Grade 4
	%	%	%	%	%	%
Gastrointestinal disorders						
Diarrhea	64	9	<1	20	<1	0
Nausea	31	<1	0	21	<1	0
Vomiting	17	1	<1	11	<1	<1
Anorexia	11	<1	0	9	<1	0
Skin and subcutaneous tissue disorders						
Rash[b]	44	1	0	13	0	0
Dry skin	13	<1	0	4	0	0
Alopecia	13	<1	0	7	0	0
Pruritus	12	<1	0	9	<1	0
Nail Disorder	11	<1	0	<1	0	0
General disorders and administrative site conditions						
Fatigue	20	2	0	17	<1	0
Asthenia	12	<1	0	11	<1	0
Nervous system disorders						
Headache	14	<1	0	13	<1	0
Respiratory, thoracic, and mediastinal disorders						
Epistaxis	11	<1	0	2	<1	0

[a] National Cancer Institute Common Terminology Criteria for Adverse Events, version 3.
[b] In addition to the rash reported under "Skin and subcutaneous tissue disorders", 3 additional subjects in each treatment arm had rash under "Infections and infestations"; none were Grade 3 or 4.

7 DRUG INTERACTIONS

7.1 Effects of Lapatinib on Drug Metabolizing Enzymes and Drug Transport Systems

Lapatinib inhibits CYP3A4 and CYP2C8 in vitro at clinically relevant concentrations. Caution should be exercised and dose reduction of the concomitant substrate drug should be considered when dosing lapatinib concurrently with medications with narrow therapeutic windows that are substrates of CYP3A4 or CYP2C8. Lapatinib did not significantly inhibit the following enzymes in human liver microsomes: CYP1A2, CYP2C9, CYP2C19, and CYP2D6 or UGT enzymes in vitro, however, the clinical significance is unknown.

Lapatinib inhibits human P-glycoprotein. If TYKERB is administered with drugs that are substrates of P-gp, increased concentrations of the substrate drug are likely, and caution should be exercised.

Paclitaxel: In cancer patients receiving TYKERB and the CYP2C8 substrate paclitaxel, 24-hour systemic exposure (AUC) of paclitaxel was increased 23%. This increase in paclitaxel exposure may have been underestimated from the in vivo evaluation due to study design limitations.

7.2 Drugs that Inhibit or Induce Cytochrome P450 3A4 Enzymes

Lapatinib undergoes extensive metabolism by CYP3A4, and concomitant administration of strong inhibitors or inducers of CYP3A4 alter lapatinib concentrations significantly (see Ketoconazole and Carbamazepine sections, below). Dose adjustment of lapatinib should be considered for patients who must receive concomitant strong inhibitors or concomitant strong inducers of CYP3A4 enzymes [see Dosage and Administration (2.2)].

Ketoconazole: In healthy subjects receiving ketoconazole, a CYP3A4 inhibitor, at 200 mg twice daily for 7 days, systemic exposure (AUC) to lapatinib was increased to approximately 3.6-fold of control and half-life increased to 1.7-fold of control.

Carbamazepine: In healthy subjects receiving the CYP3A4 inducer, carbamazepine, at 100 mg twice daily for 3 days and 200 mg twice daily for 17 days, systemic exposure (AUC) to lapatinib was decreased approximately 72%.

7.3 Drugs that Inhibit Drug Transport Systems

Lapatinib is a substrate of the efflux transporter P-glycoprotein (P-gp, ABCB1). If TYKERB is administered with drugs that inhibit P-gp, increased concentrations of lapatinib are likely, and caution should be exercised.

8 USE IN SPECIFIC POPULATIONS

8.1 Pregnancy

Pregnancy Category D *[see Warnings and Precautions (5.7)].*

Based on findings in animals, TYKERB can cause fetal harm when administered to a pregnant woman. Lapatinib administered to rats during organogenesis and through lactation led to death of offspring within the first 4 days after birth. When administered to pregnant animals during the period of organogenesis, lapatinib caused fetal anomalies (rats) or abortions (rabbits) at maternally toxic doses. There are no adequate and well-controlled studies with TYKERB in pregnant women. Women should be advised not to become pregnant when taking TYKERB. If this drug is used during pregnancy, or if the patient becomes pregnant while taking this drug, the patient should be apprised of the potential hazard to the fetus.

In a study where pregnant rats were dosed with lapatinib during organogenesis and through lactation, at a dose of 120 mg/kg/day (approximately 6.4 times the human clinical exposure based on AUC following 1,250 mg dose of lapatinib plus capecitabine), 91% of the pups had died by the fourth day after birth, while 34% of the 60 mg/kg/day pups were dead. The highest no-effect dose for this study was 20 mg/kg/day (approximately equal to the human clinical exposure based on AUC).

Lapatinib was studied for effects on embryo-fetal development in pregnant rats and rabbits given oral doses of 30, 60, and 120 mg/kg/day. There were no teratogenic effects; however, minor anomalies (left-sided umbilical artery, cervical rib, and precocious ossification) occurred in rats at the maternally toxic dose of 120 mg/kg/day (approximately 6.4 times the human clinical exposure based on AUC following 1,250 mg dose of lapatinib plus capecitabine). In rabbits, lapatinib was associated with maternal toxicity at 60 and 120 mg/kg/day (approximately 0.07 and 0.2 times the human clinical exposure, respectively, based on AUC following 1,250 mg dose of lapatinib plus capecitabine) and abortions at 120 mg/kg/day. Maternal toxicity was associated with decreased fetal body weights and minor skeletal variations.

8.3 Nursing Mothers

It is not known whether lapatinib is excreted in human milk. Because many drugs are excreted in human milk and because of the potential for serious adverse reactions in nursing infants from TYKERB, a decision should be made whether to discontinue nursing or to discontinue the drug, taking into account the importance of the drug to the mother.

8.4 Pediatric Use

The safety and effectiveness of TYKERB in pediatric patients have not been established.

8.5 Geriatric Use

Of the total number of metastatic breast cancer patients in clinical studies of TYKERB in combination with capecitabine (N = 198), 17% were 65 years of age and older, and 1% were 75 years of age and older. Of the total number of hormone receptor positive, HER2 positive metastatic breast cancer patients in clinical studies of TYKERB in combination with letrozole (N = 642), 44% were 65 years of age and older, and 12% were 75 years of age and older. No overall differences in safety or effectiveness were observed between elderly subjects and younger subjects, and other reported clinical experience has not identified differences in responses between the elderly and younger patients, but greater sensitivity of some older individuals cannot be ruled out.

8.6 Renal Impairment

Lapatinib pharmacokinetics have not been specifically studied in patients with renal impairment or in patients undergoing hemodialysis. There is no experience with TYKERB in patients with severe renal impairment. However, renal impairment is unlikely to affect the pharmacokinetics of lapatinib given that less than 2% (lapatinib and metabolites) of an administered dose is eliminated by the kidneys.

8.7 Hepatic Impairment

The pharmacokinetics of lapatinib were examined in subjects with pre-existing moderate (n = 8) or severe (n = 4) hepatic impairment (Child-Pugh Class B/C, respectively) and in 8 healthy control subjects. Systemic exposure (AUC) to lapatinib after a single oral 100-mg dose increased approximately 14% and 63% in subjects with moderate and severe pre-existing hepatic impairment, respectively. Administration of TYKERB in patients with severe hepatic impairment should be undertaken with caution due to increased exposure to the drug. A dose reduction should be considered for patients with severe pre-existing hepatic impairment *[see Dosage and Administration (2.2)]*. In patients who develop severe hepatotoxicity while on therapy, TYKERB should be discontinued and patients should not be retreated with TYKERB *[see Warnings and Precautions (5.2)]*.

10 OVERDOSAGE

There is no known antidote for overdoses of TYKERB. The maximum oral doses of lapatinib that have been administered in clinical trials are 1,800 mg once daily. More frequent ingestion of TYKERB could result in serum concentrations exceeding those observed in clinical trials and could result in increased toxicity. Therefore, missed doses should not be replaced and dosing should resume with the next scheduled daily dose.

Asymptomatic and symptomatic cases of overdose have been reported in patients being treated with lapatinib. Symptoms observed include lapatinib-associated events *[see Adverse Reactions (6.1)]* and in some cases sore scalp, sinus tachycardia (with otherwise normal ECG) and/or mucosal inflammation.

Because lapatinib is not significantly renally excreted and is highly bound to plasma proteins, hemodialysis would not be expected to be an effective method to enhance the elimination of lapatinib.

Treatment of overdose with TYKERB should consist of general supportive measures.

11 DESCRIPTION

Lapatinib is a small molecule and a member of the 4-anilinoquinazoline class of kinase inhibitors. It is present as the monohydrate of the ditosylate salt, with chemical name N-(3-chloro-4-{[(3-fluorophenyl)methyl]oxy}phenyl)-6-[5-({[2-(methylsulfonyl)ethyl]amino}methyl)-2-furanyl]-4-quinazolinamine bis(4-methylbenzenesulfonate) monohydrate. It has the molecular formula $C_{29}H_{26}ClFN_4O_4S$ $(C_7H_8O_3S)_2 \cdot H_2O$ and a molecular weight of 943.5. Lapatinib ditosylate monohydrate has the following chemical structure:

Lapatinib is a yellow solid, and its solubility in water is 0.007 mg/mL and in 0.1N HCl is 0.001 mg/mL at 25°C.

Each 250 mg tablet of TYKERB contains 405 mg of lapatinib ditosylate monohydrate, equivalent to 398 mg of lapatinib ditosylate or 250 mg lapatinib free base.

The inactive ingredients of TYKERB are: **Tablet Core:** Magnesium stearate, microcrystalline cellulose, povidone, sodium starch glycolate. **Coating:** Orange film-coat: FD&C yellow No. 6/sunset yellow FCF aluminum lake, hypromellose, macrogol/PEG 400, polysorbate 80, titanium dioxide.

12 CLINICAL PHARMACOLOGY

12.1 Mechanism of Action

Lapatinib is a 4-anilinoquinazoline kinase inhibitor of the intracellular tyrosine kinase domains of both Epidermal Growth Factor Receptor (EGFR [ErbB1]) and of Human Epidermal Receptor Type 2 (HER2 [ErbB2]) receptors (estimated K_i^{app} values of 3nM and 13nM, respectively) with a dissociation half-life of ≥ 300 minutes. Lapatinib inhibits ErbB-driven tumor cell growth in vitro and in various animal models.

An additive effect was demonstrated in an in vitro study when lapatinib and 5-FU (the active metabolite of capecitabine) were used in combination in the 4 tumor cell lines tested. The growth inhibitory effects of lapatinib were evaluated in trastuzumab-conditioned cell lines. Lapatinib retained significant activity against breast cancer cell lines selected for long-term growth in trastuzumab-containing medium in vitro. These in vitro findings suggest non-cross-resistance between these two agents.

Hormone receptor positive breast cancer cells (with ER [Estrogen Receptor] and/or PgR [Progesterone Receptor]) that coexpress the HER2 tend to be resistant to established endocrine therapies. Similarly, hormone receptor positive breast cancer cells that initially lack EGFR or HER2 upregulate these receptor proteins as the tumor becomes resistant to endocrine therapy.

12.3 Pharmacokinetics

Absorption: Absorption following oral administration of TYKERB is incomplete and variable. Serum concentrations appear after a median lag time of 0.25 hours (range 0 to 1.5 hour). Peak plasma concentrations (C_{max}) of lapatinib are achieved approximately 4 hours after administration. Daily dosing of TYKERB results in achievement of steady state within 6 to 7 days, indicating an effective half-life of 24 hours.

At the dose of 1,250 mg daily, steady state geometric mean (95% confidence interval) values of C_{max} were 2.43 mcg/mL (1.57 to 3.77 mcg/mL) and AUC were 36.2 mcg.hr/mL (23.4 to 56 mcg.hr/mL).

Divided daily doses of TYKERB resulted in approximately 2-fold higher exposure at steady state (steady state AUC) compared to the same total dose administered once daily.

Systemic exposure to lapatinib is increased when administered with food. Lapatinib AUC values were approximately 3- and 4-fold higher (C_{max} approximately 2.5- and 3-fold higher) when administered with a low fat (5% fat-500 calories) or with a high fat (50% fat-1,000 calories) meal, respectively.

Distribution: Lapatinib is highly bound (>99%) to albumin and alpha-1 acid glycoprotein. In vitro studies indicate that lapatinib is a substrate for the transporters breast cancer resistance protein (BCRP, ABCG2) and P-glycoprotein (P-gp, ABCB1). Lapatinib has also been shown in vitro to inhibit these efflux transporters, as well as the hepatic uptake transporter OATP 1B1, at clinically relevant concentrations.

Metabolism: Lapatinib undergoes extensive metabolism, primarily by CYP3A4 and CYP3A5, with minor contributions from CYP2C19 and CYP2C8 to a variety of oxidated metabolites, none of which accounts for more than 14% of the dose recovered in the feces or 10% of lapatinib concentration in plasma.

Elimination: At clinical doses, the terminal phase half-life following a single dose was 14.2 hours; accumulation with repeated dosing indicates an effective half-life of 24 hours. Elimination of lapatinib is predominantly through metabolism by CYP3A4/5 with negligible (<2%) renal excretion. Recovery of parent lapatinib in feces accounts for a median of 27% (range 3 to 67%) of an oral dose.

Effects of Age, Gender, or Race: Studies of the effects of age, gender, or race on the pharmacokinetics of lapatinib have not been performed.

12.4 QT Prolongation

The QT prolongation potential of lapatinib was assessed as part of an uncontrolled, open-label dose escalation study in advanced cancer patients. Eighty-one patients received daily doses of lapatinib ranging from 175 mg/day to 1,800 mg/day. Serial ECGs were collected on Day 1 and Day 14 to evaluate the effect of lapatinib on QT intervals. Analysis of the data suggested a consistent concentration-dependent increase in QTc interval.

13 NONCLINICAL TOXICOLOGY

13.1 Carcinogenesis, Mutagenesis, Impairment of Fertility

Two-year carcinogenicity studies with lapatinib are ongoing.

Lapatinib was not clastogenic or mutagenic in the Chinese hamster ovary chromosome aberration assay, microbial mutagenesis (Ames) assay, human lymphocyte chromosome aberration assay or the in vivo rat bone marrow chromosome aberration assay at single doses up to 2,000 mg/kg. However, an impurity in the drug product (up to 4 ppm or 8 mcg/day) was genotoxic when tested alone in both in vitro and in vivo assays.

There were no effects on male or female rat mating or fertility at doses up to 120 mg/kg/day in females and 180 mg/kg/day in males (approximately 6.4 times and 2.6 times the expected human clinical exposure based on AUC following 1,250 mg dose of lapatinib plus capecitabine, respectively). The effect of lapatinib on human fertility is unknown. However, when female rats were given oral doses of lapatinib during breeding and through the first 6 days of gestation, a significant decrease in the number of live fetuses was seen at 120 mg/kg/day and in the fetal body weights at ≥60 mg/kg/day (approximately 6.4 times and 3.3 times the expected human clinical exposure based on AUC following 1,250 mg dose of lapatinib plus capecitabine, respectively).

14 CLINICAL STUDIES

14.1 HER2 Positive Metastatic Breast Cancer

The efficacy and safety of TYKERB in combination with capecitabine in breast cancer were evaluated in a random-

Table 4. Selected Laboratory Abnormalities

Hepatic Parameters	TYKERB 1,500 mg/day + Letrozole 2.5 mg/day			Letrozole 2.5 mg/day		
	All Grades[a]	Grade 3	Grade 4	All Grades[a]	Grade 3	Grade 4
	%	%	%	%	%	%
AST	53	6	0	36	2	<1
ALT	46	5	<1	35	1	0
Total Bilirubin	22	<1	<1	11	1	<1

[a] National Cancer Institute Common Terminology Criteria for Adverse Events, version 3.

Table 5. Efficacy Results

	Independent Assessment[a]		Investigator Assessment	
	TYKERB 1,250 mg/day + Capecitabine 2,000 mg/m²/day	Capecitabine 2,500 mg/m²/day	TYKERB 1,250 mg/day + Capecitabine 2,000 mg/m²/day	Capecitabine 2,500 mg/m²/day
	(N = 198)	(N = 201)	(N = 198)	(N = 201)
Number of TTP events	82	102	121	126
Median TTP, weeks	27.1	18.6	23.9	18.3
(25th, 75th, Percentile), weeks	(17.4, 49.4)	(9.1, 36.9)	(12.0, 44.0)	(6.9, 35.7)
Hazard Ratio	0.57		0.72	
(95% CI)	(0.43, 0.77)		(0.56, 0.92)	
P value	0.00013		0.00762	
Response Rate (%)	23.7	13.9	31.8	17.4
(95% CI)	(18.0, 30.3)	(9.5, 19.5)	(25.4, 38.8)	(12.4, 23.4)

TTP = Time to progression.

[a] The time from last tumor assessment to the data cut-off date was >100 days in approximately 30% of patients in the independent assessment. The pre-specified assessment interval was 42 or 84 days.

ized, Phase 3 trial. Patients eligible for enrollment had HER2 (ErbB2) overexpressing (IHC 3+ or IHC 2+ confirmed by FISH), locally advanced or metastatic breast cancer, progressing after prior treatment that included anthracyclines, taxanes, and trastuzumab.

Patients were randomized to receive either TYKERB 1,250 mg once daily (continuously) plus capecitabine 2,000 mg/m²/day on Days 1-14 every 21 days, or to receive capecitabine alone at a dose of 2,500 mg/m²/day on Days 1-14 every 21 days. The endpoint was time to progression (TTP). TTP was defined as time from randomization to tumor progression or death related to breast cancer. Based on the results of a pre-specified interim analysis, further enrollment was discontinued. Three hundred and ninety-nine (399) patients were enrolled in this study. The median age was 53 years and 14% were older than 65 years. Ninety-one percent (91%) were Caucasian. Ninety-seven percent (97%) had stage IV breast cancer, 48% were estrogen receptor+ (ER+) or progesterone receptor+ (PR+), and 95% were ErbB2 IHC 3+ or IHC 2+ with FISH confirmation. Approximately 95% of patients had prior treatment with anthracyclines, taxanes, and trastuzumab.

Efficacy analyses 4 months after the interim analysis are presented in Table 5, Figure 1, and Figure 2.
[See table 5 on previous page]

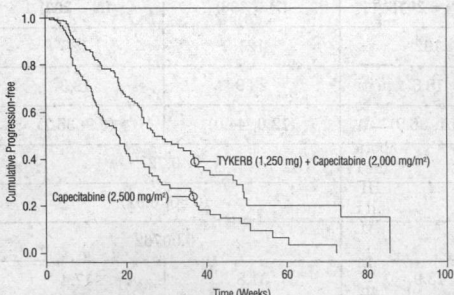

Figure 1. Kaplan-Meier Estimates for Independent Review Panel-evaluated Time to Progression

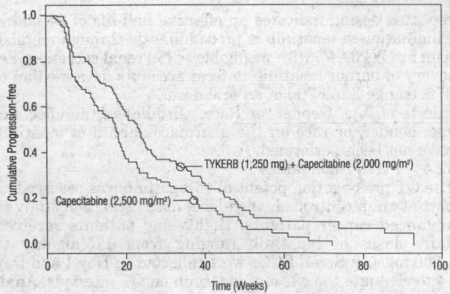

Figure 2. Kaplan-Meier Estimates for Investigator Assessment Time to Progression

At the time of above efficacy analysis, the overall survival data were not mature (32% events). However, based on the TTP results, the study was unblinded and patients receiving capecitabine alone were allowed to cross over to TYKERB plus capecitabine treatment. The survival data

were followed for an additional 2 years to be mature and the analysis is summarized in Table 6.

Table 6: Overall Survival Data

	TYKERB 1,250 mg/day + Capecitabine 2,000 mg/m²/day (N = 207)	Capecitabine 2,500 mg/m²/day (N = 201)
Overall Survival		
Died	76%	82%
Median Overall Survival (weeks)	75.0	65.9
Hazard ratio, 95% CI (P value)	0.89 (0.71, 1.10) 0.276	

CI = confidence interval

14.2 Hormone Receptor Positive, HER2 Positive Metastatic Breast Cancer

The efficacy and safety of TYKERB in combination with letrozole were evaluated in a double-blind, placebo-controlled, multi-center study. A total of 1,286 postmenopausal women with hormone receptor positive (ER positive and/or PgR positive) metastatic breast cancer, who had not received prior therapy for metastatic disease, were randomly assigned to receive either TYKERB (1,500 mg once daily) plus letrozole (2.5 mg once daily) (n = 642) or letrozole (2.5 mg once daily) alone (n = 644). Of all patients randomized to treatment, 219 (17%) patients had tumors overexpressing the HER2 receptor, defined as fluorescence in situ hybridization (FISH) (≥2 or 3+ immunohistochemistry (IHC)). There were 952 (74%) patients who were HER2 negative and 115 (9%) patients did not have their HER2 receptor status confirmed. The primary objective was to evaluate and compare progression-free survival (PFS) in the HER2 positive population. Progression-free survival was defined as the interval of time between date of randomization and the earlier date of first documented sign of disease progression or death due to any cause.

The baseline demographic and disease characteristics were balanced between the two treatment arms. The median age was 63 years and 45% were 65 years of age or older. Eighty-four percent (84%) of the patients were White. Approximately 50% of the HER2 positive population had prior adjuvant/neo-adjuvant chemotherapy and 56% had prior hormonal therapy. Only 2 patients had prior trastuzumab. In the HER2 positive subgroup (n = 219), the addition of TYKERB to letrozole resulted in an improvement in PFS. In the HER2 negative subgroup, there was no improvement in PFS of the TYKERB plus letrozole combination compared to the letrozole plus placebo. Overall response rate (ORR) was also improved with the TYKERB plus letrozole combination therapy. The overall survival (OS) data were not mature. Efficacy analyses for the hormone receptor positive, HER2 positive and HER2 negative subgroups are presented in Table 7 and Figure 3.
[See table 7 below]
[See figure 3 at top of next column]

16 HOW SUPPLIED/STORAGE AND HANDLING

The 250 mg tablets of TYKERB are oval, biconvex, orange, and film-coated with GS XJG debossed on one side and are available in:
Bottles of 150 tablets: NDC 0173-0752-00

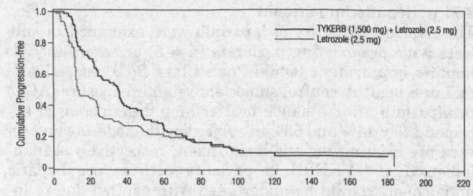

Figure 3. Kaplan-Meier Estimates for Progression-Free Survival for the HER2 Positive Population

Store at 25°C (77°F); excursions permitted to 15° to 30°C (59° to 86°F) [see USP Controlled Room Temperature].

17 PATIENT COUNSELING INFORMATION
See FDA-approved patient labeling (17.2).
17.1 Information for Patients
Patients should be informed of the following:
- TYKERB has been reported to decrease left ventricular ejection fraction which may result in shortness of breath, palpitations, and/or fatigue. Patients should inform their physician if they develop these symptoms while taking TYKERB.
- TYKERB often causes diarrhea which may be severe in some cases. Patients should be told how to manage and/or prevent diarrhea and to inform their physician if severe diarrhea occurs during treatment with TYKERB.
- TYKERB may interact with many drugs; therefore, patients should be advised to report to their healthcare provider the use of any other prescription or nonprescription medication or herbal products.
- TYKERB may interact with grapefruit. Patients should not take TYKERB with grapefruit products.
- TYKERB should be taken at least one hour before or one hour after a meal, in contrast to capecitabine which should be taken with food or within 30 minutes after food.
- The dose of TYKERB should be taken once daily. Dividing the daily dose is not recommended.
17.2 FDA-Approved Patient Labeling
Patient labeling is provided as a tear-off leaflet at the end of this full prescribing information.
TYKERB is a registered trademark of GlaxoSmithKline.
GlaxoSmithKline
Research Triangle Park, NC 27709
©2010, GlaxoSmithKline. All rights reserved.
April 2010
TKB:7PI
PHARMACIST - DETACH HERE AND GIVE INSTRUCTIONS TO PATIENT

PATIENT INFORMATION
TYKERB (TIE-curb)
(lapatinib) tablets
Read this leaflet before you start taking TYKERB® and each time you get a refill. There may be new information. This information does not take the place of talking with your doctor about your medical condition or treatment.
What is TYKERB?
TYKERB is used with the medicine capecitabine for the treatment of patients with advanced or metastatic breast cancer that is HER2 positive (tumors that produce large amounts of a protein called human epidermal growth factor receptor-2), and who have already had certain other breast cancer treatments.
TYKERB is also used with a type of medicine called letrozole for the treatment of postmenopausal women with hormone receptor positive, HER2 positive metastatic breast cancer for whom hormonal therapy is indicated. TYKERB in combination with an aromatase inhibitor has not been compared to a trastuzumab-containing chemotherapy regimen for the treatment of metastatic breast cancer.
Who should not take TYKERB?
Do not take TYKERB if you are allergic to any of its ingredients. See the end of this leaflet for a list of ingredients in TYKERB.
Before you start taking TYKERB, tell your doctor about all of your medical conditions, including if you:
- ever had a severe allergic (hypersensitivity) reaction to TYKERB. Check with your doctor if you think this applies to you. Don't take TYKERB.
- have heart problems.
- have liver problems. You may need a lower dose of TYKERB.
- are pregnant or may become pregnant. TYKERB may harm an unborn baby. If you become pregnant during treatment with TYKERB, tell your doctor as soon as possible.
- are breast-feeding. It is not known if TYKERB passes into your breast milk or if it can harm your baby. If you are a woman who has or will have a baby, talk with your doctor about the best way to feed your baby.

Table 7. Efficacy Results

	HER2(+) Population		HER2(-) Population	
	TYKERB 1500 mg/day + Letrozole 2.5 mg/day	Letrozole 2.5 mg/day	TYKERB 1500 mg/day + Letrozole 2.5 mg/day	Letrozole 2.5 mg/day
	(N = 111)	(N = 108)	(N = 478)	(N = 474)
Median PFS[a], weeks (95% CI)	35.4 (24.1, 39.4)	13.0 (12.0, 23.7)	59.7 (48.6, 69.7)	58.3 (47.9, 62.0)
Hazard Ratio (95% CI) P value	0.71 (0.53, 0.96) 0.019		0.90 (0.77, 1.05) 0.188	
Response Rate (%) (95% CI)	27.9 (19.8, 37.2)	14.8 (8.7, 22.9)	32.6 (28.4, 37.0)	31.6 (27.5, 36.0)

PFS = progression-free survival; CI = confidence interval.
[a] Kaplan-Meier estimate.

Tell your doctor about all the medicines you take, including prescription and nonprescription medicines, vitamins, and herbal and dietary supplements. TYKERB and many other medicines may interact with each other. Your doctor needs to know what medicines you take so he or she can choose the right dose of TYKERB for you.

Especially tell your doctor if you take:

- antibiotics and anti-fungals (drugs used to treat infections)
- HIV (AIDS) treatments
- anticonvulsant drugs (drugs used to treat seizures)
- calcium channel blockers (drugs used to treat certain heart disorders or high blood pressure)
- antidepressants
- drugs used for stomach ulcers
- St. John's Wort or other herbal supplements

Know the medicines you take. Keep a list of your medicines with you to show your doctor. Do not take other medicines during treatment with TYKERB without first checking with your doctor.

Because TYKERB is given with other drugs called capecitabine or letrozole, you should also discuss with your doctor or pharmacist any medicines that should be avoided during treatment.

How should I take TYKERB?

- Take TYKERB exactly as your doctor tells you to take it. Your doctor may change your dose of TYKERB if needed.
  - For patients with advanced or metastatic breast cancer, TYKERB and capecitabine are taken in 21 day cycles. The usual dose of TYKERB is 1,250 mg (5 tablets) taken by mouth all at once, **one time a day on days 1 to 21**. Your doctor will tell you the dose of capecitabine you should take and when you should take it.
  - For patients with hormone receptor positive, HER2 positive breast cancer, TYKERB and letrozole are taken daily. The usual dose of TYKERB is 1,500 mg (6 tablets) taken by mouth all at once, **one time a day**. Your doctor will tell you the dose of letrozole you should take and when you should take it.
- TYKERB should be taken at least one hour before, or at least one hour after food.
- Do not eat or drink grapefruit products while taking TYKERB.
- If you forget to take your dose of TYKERB, do not take two doses at one time. Take your next dose at your scheduled time.
- If you take too much TYKERB, call your doctor or poison control center right away.

What are the possible side effects of TYKERB?

Serious side effects include:

- **heart problems** including, decreased pumping of blood from the heart and an abnormal heartbeat. Signs and symptoms of an abnormal heartbeat include:
  - feeling like your heart is pounding or racing
  - dizziness
  - tiredness
  - feeling lightheaded
  - shortness of breath
    - Your doctor should check your heart function before you start taking TYKERB and during treatment.
- **liver problems.** Signs and symptoms of liver problems include:
  - itching
  - yellow eyes or skin
  - dark urine
  - pain or discomfort in the right upper stomach area
  - death
    - Your doctor should do blood tests to check your liver before you start taking TYKERB and during treatment.
- **diarrhea**, which may cause you to become dehydrated. Follow your doctors instructions for what to do to help prevent or treat diarrhea.
- **lung problems.** Symptoms of a lung problem with TYKERB include a cough that will not go away or shortness of breath.

Call your doctor right away if you have any of the signs or symptoms of the serious side effects listed above.

Common side effects of TYKERB in combination with capecitabine or letrozole include:

- diarrhea
- red, painful hands and feet
- nausea
- rash
- vomiting
- tiredness or weakness
- mouth sores
- loss of appetite
- indigestion
- unusual hair loss or thinning
- nose bleeds
- headache
- dry skin
- itching

- nail disorders such as nail bed changes, nail pain, infection and swelling of the cuticles.

Tell your doctor about any side effect that gets serious or that does not go away.

These are not all the side effects with TYKERB. Ask your doctor or pharmacist for more information.

Call your doctor for medical advice about side effects. You may report side effects to FDA at 1-800-FDA-1088.

You may also get side effects from the other drugs taken with TYKERB. Talk to your doctor about possible side effects you may get during treatment.

How should I store TYKERB tablets?

- Store TYKERB tablets at room temperature at 59° to 86°F (15° to 30°C). Keep the container closed tightly.
- Do not keep medicine that is out of date or that you no longer need. Be sure that if you throw any medicine away, it is out of the reach of children.
- **Keep TYKERB and all medicines out of the reach of children.**

General information about TYKERB

Medicines are sometimes prescribed for conditions that are not mentioned in patient information leaflets. Do not use TYKERB for any other condition for which it was not prescribed. Do not give TYKERB to other people, even if they have the same condition that you have. It may harm them. This leaflet summarizes the most important information about TYKERB. If you would like more information, talk with your doctor. You can ask your doctor or pharmacist for information about TYKERB that is written for health professionals. For more information, you can call toll-free 1-888-825-5249 or by visiting the website www.tykerb.com.

What are the ingredients in TYKERB?

Active Ingredient: Lapatinib.

Inactive Ingredients: Tablet Core: Magnesium stearate, microcrystalline cellulose, povidone, sodium starch glycolate. **Coating:** Orange film-coat: FD&C yellow #6/sunset yellow FCF aluminum lake, hypromellose, macrogol/PEG 400, polysorbate 80, titanium dioxide.

TYKERB tablets are oval, biconvex, orange, film-coated with GS XJG printed on one side.

TYKERB is a registered trademark of GlaxoSmithKline.
GlaxoSmithKline
Research Triangle Park, NC 27709
©2010, GlaxoSmithKline. All rights reserved.
Revised: April 2010
TKB:6PIL

VALTREX®   ℞
[val′trĕx]
(valacyclovir hydrochloride)
Caplets

HIGHLIGHTS OF PRESCRIBING INFORMATION
These highlights do not include all the information needed to use VALTREX safely and effectively. See full prescribing information for VALTREX.
VALTREX (valacyclovir hydrochloride) Caplets
Initial U.S. Approval: 1995

━━━━━━**RECENT MAJOR CHANGES**━━━━━━
Warnings and Precautions, Central Nervous System Effects (5.3) 3/2010

━━━━━━━**INDICATIONS AND USAGE**━━━━━━━
VALTREX is a nucleoside analogue DNA polymerase inhibitor indicated for:
Adult Patients (1.1)
- Cold Sores (Herpes Labialis)
- Genital Herpes
  - Treatment in immunocompetent patients (initial or recurrent episode)
  - Suppression in immunocompetent or HIV-infected patients
  - Reduction of transmission
- Herpes Zoster
Pediatric Patients (1.2)
- Cold Sores (Herpes Labialis)
- Chickenpox
Limitations of Use (1.3)
- The efficacy and safety of VALTREX have not been established in immunocompromised patients other than for the suppression of genital herpes in HIV-infected patients.

━━━━━━**DOSAGE AND ADMINISTRATION**━━━━━━

Adult Dosage (2.1)

Cold Sores	2 grams every 12 hours for 1 day
Genital Herpes	
Initial episode	1 gram twice daily for 10 days
Recurrent episodes	500 mg twice daily for 3 days
Suppressive therapy Immunocompetent patients	1 gram once daily
Alternate dose in patients with ≤ 9 recurrences/yr	500 mg once daily
HIV-infected patients	500 mg twice daily
Reduction of transmission	500 mg once daily
Herpes Zoster	1 gram 3 times daily for 7 days

Pediatric Dosage (2.2)

Cold Sores (≥12 years of age)	2 grams every 12 hours for 1 day
Chickenpox (2 to <18 years of age)	20 mg/kg 3 times daily for 5 days; not to exceed 1 gram 3 times daily

Valacyclovir oral suspension (25 mg/mL or 50 mg/mL) can be prepared from the 500 mg VALTREX Caplets. (2.3)

━━━**DOSAGE FORMS AND STRENGTHS**━━━
Caplets: 500 mg (unscored), 1 gram (partially scored) (3)

━━━━━━━━**CONTRAINDICATIONS**━━━━━━━━
Hypersensitivity to valacyclovir (e.g., anaphylaxis), acyclovir, or any component of the formulation. (4)

━━━━━━**WARNINGS AND PRECAUTIONS**━━━━━━
- Thrombotic thrombocytopenic purpura/hemolytic uremic syndrome (TTP/HUS): Has occurred in patients with advanced HIV disease and in allogenic bone marrow transplant and renal transplant patients receiving 8 grams per day of VALTREX in clinical trials. Discontinue treatment if clinical symptoms and laboratory findings consistent with TTP/HUS occur. (5.1)
- Acute renal failure: May occur in elderly patients (with or without reduced renal function), patients with underlying renal disease who receive higher than recommended doses of VALTREX for their level of renal function, patients who receive concomitant nephrotoxic drugs, or inadequately hydrated patients. Use with caution in elderly patients and reduce dosage in patients with renal impairment. (2.4, 5.2)
- Central nervous system adverse reactions (e.g., agitation, hallucinations, confusion, and encephalopathy): May occur in both adult and pediatric patients (with or without reduced renal function) and in patients with underlying renal disease who receive higher than recommended doses of VALTREX for their level of renal function. Elderly patients are more likely to have central nervous system adverse reactions. Use with caution in elderly patients and reduce dosage in patients with renal impairment. (2.4, 5.3)

━━━━━━━━━**ADVERSE REACTIONS**━━━━━━━━━
- The most common adverse reactions reported in at least one indication by >10% of adult patients treated with VALTREX and more commonly than in patients treated with placebo are headache, nausea, and abdominal pain. (6.1)
- The only adverse reaction occurring in >10% of pediatric patients <18 years of age was headache. (6.2)

To report SUSPECTED ADVERSE REACTIONS, contact GlaxoSmithKline at 1-888-825-5249 or FDA at 1-800-FDA-1088 or www.fda.gov/medwatch.

See 17 for PATIENT COUNSELING INFORMATION and FDA-approved patient labeling

Revised: 03/2010

FULL PRESCRIBING INFORMATION

1 INDICATIONS AND USAGE

1.1 Adult Patients

Cold Sores (Herpes Labialis): VALTREX® (valacyclovir hydrochloride) Caplets are indicated for treatment of cold sores (herpes labialis). The efficacy of VALTREX initiated after the development of clinical signs of a cold sore (e.g., papule, vesicle, or ulcer) has not been established.

Genital Herpes: Initial Episode: VALTREX is indicated for treatment of the initial episode of genital herpes in immunocompetent adults. The efficacy of treatment with VALTREX when initiated more than 72 hours after the onset of signs and symptoms has not been established.

Recurrent Episodes: VALTREX is indicated for treatment of recurrent episodes of genital herpes in immunocompetent adults. The efficacy of treatment with VALTREX when initiated more than 24 hours after the onset of signs and symptoms has not been established.

Suppressive Therapy: VALTREX is indicated for chronic suppressive therapy of recurrent episodes of genital herpes in immunocompetent and in HIV-infected adults. The efficacy and safety of VALTREX for the suppression of genital herpes beyond 1 year in immunocompetent patients and beyond 6 months in HIV-infected patients have not been established.

Reduction of Transmission: VALTREX is indicated for the reduction of transmission of genital herpes in immunocompetent adults. The efficacy of VALTREX for the reduction of transmission of genital herpes beyond 8 months in discordant couples has not been established. The efficacy of VALTREX for the reduction of transmission of genital herpes in individuals with multiple partners and nonheterosexual couples has not been established. Safer sex practices should be used with suppressive therapy (see current Centers for Disease Control and Prevention [CDC] Sexually Transmitted Diseases Treatment Guidelines).

Herpes Zoster: VALTREX is indicated for the treatment of herpes zoster (shingles) in immunocompetent adults. The efficacy of VALTREX when initiated more than 72 hours after the onset of rash and the efficacy and safety of VALTREX for treatment of disseminated herpes zoster have not been established.

1.2 Pediatric Patients

Cold Sores (Herpes Labialis): VALTREX is indicated for the treatment of cold sores (herpes labialis) in pediatric patients ≥12 years of age. The efficacy of VALTREX initiated after the development of clinical signs of a cold sore (e.g., papule, vesicle, or ulcer) has not been established.

Chickenpox: VALTREX is indicated for the treatment of chickenpox in immunocompetent pediatric patients 2 to <18 years of age. Based on efficacy data from clinical studies with oral acyclovir, treatment with VALTREX should be initiated within 24 hours after the onset of rash [see Clinical Studies (14.4)].

1.3 Limitations of Use

The efficacy and safety of VALTREX have not been established in:

- Immunocompromised patients other than for the suppression of genital herpes in HIV-infected patients with a CD4+ cell count ≥100 cells/mm³.
- Patients <12 years of age with cold sores (herpes labialis).
- Patients <2 years of age or ≥18 years of age with chickenpox.
- Patients <18 years of age with genital herpes.
- Patients <18 years of age with herpes zoster.
- Neonates and infants as suppressive therapy following neonatal herpes simplex virus (HSV) infection.

2 DOSAGE AND ADMINISTRATION

- VALTREX may be given without regard to meals.
- Valacyclovir oral suspension (25 mg/mL or 50 mg/mL) may be prepared extemporaneously from 500 mg VALTREX Caplets for use in pediatric patients for whom a solid dosage form is not appropriate [see Dosage and Administration (2.3)].

2.1 Adult Dosing Recommendations

Cold Sores (Herpes Labialis): The recommended dosage of VALTREX for treatment of cold sores is 2 grams twice daily for 1 day taken 12 hours apart. Therapy should be initiated at the earliest symptom of a cold sore (e.g., tingling, itching, or burning).

Genital Herpes: Initial Episode: The recommended dosage of VALTREX for treatment of initial genital herpes is 1 gram twice daily for 10 days. Therapy was most effective when administered within 48 hours of the onset of signs and symptoms.

Recurrent Episodes: The recommended dosage of VALTREX for treatment of recurrent genital herpes is 500 mg twice daily for 3 days. Initiate treatment at the first sign or symptom of an episode.

Suppressive Therapy: The recommended dosage of VALTREX for chronic suppressive therapy of recurrent genital herpes is 1 gram once daily in patients with normal immune function. In patients with a history of 9 or fewer recurrences per year, an alternative dose is 500 mg once daily. In HIV-infected patients with a CD4+ cell count ≥100 cells/mm³, the recommended dosage of VALTREX for chronic suppressive therapy of recurrent genital herpes is 500 mg twice daily.

Reduction of Transmission: The recommended dosage of VALTREX for reduction of transmission of genital herpes in patients with a history of 9 or fewer recurrences per year is 500 mg once daily for the source partner.

Herpes Zoster: The recommended dosage of VALTREX for treatment of herpes zoster is 1 gram 3 times daily for 7 days. Therapy should be initiated at the earliest sign or symptom of herpes zoster and is most effective when started within 48 hours of the onset of rash.

2.2 Pediatric Dosing Recommendations

Cold Sores (Herpes Labialis): The recommended dosage of VALTREX for the treatment of cold sores in pediatric patients ≥12 years of age is 2 grams twice daily for 1 day taken 12 hours apart. Therapy should be initiated at the earliest symptom of a cold sore (e.g., tingling, itching, or burning).

Chickenpox: The recommended dosage of VALTREX for treatment of chickenpox in immunocompetent pediatric patients 2 to <18 years of age is 20 mg/kg administered 3 times daily for 5 days. The total dose should not exceed 1 gram 3 times daily. Therapy should be initiated at the earliest sign or symptom [see Use in Specific Populations (8.4), Clinical Pharmacology (12.3), Clinical Studies (14.4)].

2.3 Extemporaneous Preparation of Oral Suspension

Ingredients and Preparation per USP-NF: VALTREX Caplets 500 mg, cherry flavor, and Suspension Structured Vehicle USP-NF (SSV). Valacyclovir oral suspension (25 mg/mL or 50 mg/mL) should be prepared in lots of 100 mL.

Prepare Suspension at Time of Dispensing as Follows:

- Prepare SSV according to the USP-NF.
- Using a pestle and mortar, grind the required number of VALTREX 500 mg Caplets until a fine powder is produced (5 VALTREX Caplets for 25 mg/mL suspension; 10 VALTREX Caplets for 50 mg/mL suspension).
- Gradually add approximately 5 mL aliquots of SSV to the mortar and triturate the powder until a paste has been produced. Ensure that the powder has been adequately wetted.
- Continue to add approximately 5 mL aliquots of SSV to the mortar, mixing thoroughly between additions, until a concentrated suspension is produced, to a minimum total quantity of 20 mL SSV and a maximum total quantity of 40 mL SSV for both the 25 mg/mL and 50 mg/mL suspensions.
- Transfer the mixture to a suitable 100 mL measuring flask.
- Transfer the cherry flavor* to the mortar and dissolve in approximately 5 mL of SSV. Once dissolved, add to the measuring flask.
- Rinse the mortar at least 3 times with approximately 5 mL aliquots of SSV, transferring the rinsing to the measuring flask between additions.
- Make the suspension to volume (100 mL) with SSV and shake thoroughly to mix.
- Transfer the suspension to an amber glass medicine bottle with a child-resistant closure.
- The prepared suspension should be labeled with the following information "Shake well before using. Store suspension between 2° to 8°C (36° to 46°F) in a refrigerator. Discard after 28 days."

* The amount of cherry flavor added is as instructed by the suppliers of the cherry flavor.

2.4 Patients With Renal Impairment

Dosage recommendations for adult patients with reduced renal function are provided in Table 1 [see Use in Specific Populations (8.5, 8.6), Clinical Pharmacology (12.3)]. Data are not available for the use of VALTREX in pediatric patients with a creatinine clearance <50 mL/min/1.73 m². [See table 1 at left]

Hemodialysis: Patients requiring hemodialysis should receive the recommended dose of VALTREX after hemodialysis. During hemodialysis, the half-life of acyclovir after administration of VALTREX is approximately 4 hours. About one third of acyclovir in the body is removed by dialysis during a 4-hour hemodialysis session.

Peritoneal Dialysis: There is no information specific to administration of VALTREX in patients receiving peritoneal dialysis. The effect of chronic ambulatory peritoneal dialysis (CAPD) and continuous arteriovenous hemofiltration/dialysis (CAVHD) on acyclovir pharmacokinetics has been studied. The removal of acyclovir after CAPD and CAVHD is less pronounced than with hemodialysis, and the pharmacokinetic parameters closely resemble those observed in patients with end-stage renal disease (ESRD) not receiving hemodialysis. Therefore, supplemental doses of VALTREX should not be required following CAPD or CAVHD.

Table 1. VALTREX Dosage Recommendations for Adults With Renal Impairment

Indications	Normal Dosage Regimen (Creatinine Clearance ≥50 mL/min)	Creatinine Clearance (mL/min)		
		30-49	10-29	<10
Cold sores (Herpes labialis) Do not exceed 1 day of treatment.	Two 2 gram doses taken 12 hours apart	Two 1 gram doses taken 12 hours apart	Two 500 mg doses taken 12 hours apart	500 mg single dose
Genital herpes: Initial episode	1 gram every 12 hours	no reduction	1 gram every 24 hours	500 mg every 24 hours
Genital herpes: Recurrent episode	500 mg every 12 hours	no reduction	500 mg every 24 hours	500 mg every 24 hours
Genital herpes: Suppressive therapy Immunocompetent patients	1 gram every 24 hours	no reduction	500 mg every 24 hours	500 mg every 24 hours
Alternate dose for immunocompetent patients with ≤9 recurrences/year	500 mg every 24 hours	no reduction	500 mg every 48 hours	500 mg every 48 hours
HIV-infected patients	500 mg every 12 hours	no reduction	500 mg every 24 hours	500 mg every 24 hours
Herpes zoster	1 gram every 8 hours	1 gram every 12 hours	1 gram every 24 hours	500 mg every 24 hours

3 DOSAGE FORMS AND STRENGTHS

Caplets:
- 500 mg: blue, film-coated, capsule-shaped tablets printed with "VALTREX 500 mg."
- 1 gram: blue, film-coated, capsule-shaped tablets, with a partial scorebar on both sides, printed with "VALTREX 1 gram."

4 CONTRAINDICATIONS

VALTREX is contraindicated in patients who have had a demonstrated clinically significant hypersensitivity reaction (e.g., anaphylaxis) to valacyclovir, acyclovir, or any component of the formulation [see Adverse Reactions (6.3)].

5 WARNINGS AND PRECAUTIONS

5.1 Thrombotic Thrombocytopenic Purpura/Hemolytic Uremic Syndrome (TTP/HUS)

TTP/HUS, in some cases resulting in death, has occurred in patients with advanced HIV disease and also in allogeneic bone marrow transplant and renal transplant recipients participating in clinical trials of VALTREX at doses of 8 grams per day. Treatment with VALTREX should be stopped immediately if clinical signs, symptoms, and laboratory abnormalities consistent with TTP/HUS occur.

5.2 Acute Renal Failure

Cases of acute renal failure have been reported in:
- Elderly patients with or without reduced renal function. Caution should be exercised when administering VALTREX to geriatric patients, and dosage reduction is recommended for those with impaired renal function [see Dosage and Administration (2.4), Use in Specific Populations (8.5)].
- Patients with underlying renal disease who received higher than recommended doses of VALTREX for their level of renal function. Dosage reduction is recommended when administering VALTREX to patients with renal impairment [see Dosage and Administration (2.4), Use in Specific Populations (8.6)].
- Patients receiving other nephrotoxic drugs. Caution should be exercised when administering VALTREX to patients receiving potentially nephrotoxic drugs.
- Patients without adequate hydration. Precipitation of acyclovir in renal tubules may occur when the solubility (2.5 mg/mL) is exceeded in the intratubular fluid. Adequate hydration should be maintained for all patients.

In the event of acute renal failure and anuria, the patient may benefit from hemodialysis until renal function is restored [see Dosage and Administration (2.4), Adverse Reactions (6.3)].

5.3 Central Nervous System Effects

Central nervous system adverse reactions, including agitation, hallucinations, confusion, delirium, seizures, and encephalopathy, have been reported in both adult and pediatric patients with or without reduced renal function and in patients with underlying renal disease who received higher than recommended doses of VALTREX for their level of renal function. Elderly patients are more likely to have central nervous system adverse reactions. VALTREX should be discontinued if central nervous system adverse reactions occur [see Adverse Reactions (6.3), Use in Specific Populations (8.5, 8.6)].

6 ADVERSE REACTIONS

The following serious adverse reactions are discussed in greater detail in other sections of the labeling:
- Thrombotic Thrombocytopenic Purpura/Hemolytic Uremic Syndrome [see Warnings and Precautions (5.1)].
- Acute Renal Failure [see Warnings and Precautions (5.2)].
- Central Nervous System Effects [see Warnings and Precautions (5.3)].

The most common adverse reactions reported in at least 1 indication by >10% of adult patients treated with VALTREX and observed more frequently with VALTREX compared to placebo are headache, nausea, and abdominal pain. The only adverse reaction reported in >10% of pediatric patients <18 years of age was headache.

6.1 Clinical Trials Experience in Adult Patients

Because clinical trials are conducted under widely varying conditions, adverse reaction rates observed in the clinical trials of a drug cannot be directly compared with rates in the clinical trials of another drug and may not reflect the rates observed in practice.

Cold Sores (Herpes Labialis): In clinical studies for the treatment of cold sores, the adverse reactions reported by patients receiving VALTREX 2 grams twice daily (n = 609) or placebo (n = 609) for 1 day, respectively, included headache (14%, 10%) and dizziness (2%, 1%). The frequencies of abnormal ALT (>2 × ULN) were 1.8% for patients receiving VALTREX compared with 0.8% for placebo. Other laboratory abnormalities (hemoglobin, white blood cells, alkaline phosphatase, and serum creatinine) occurred with similar frequencies in the 2 groups.

Genital Herpes: Initial Episode: In a clinical study for the treatment of initial episodes of genital herpes, the adverse reactions reported by ≥5% of patients receiving VALTREX

1 gram twice daily for 10 days (n = 318) or oral acyclovir 200 mg 5 times daily for 10 days (n = 318), respectively, included headache (13%, 10%) and nausea (6%, 6%). For the incidence of laboratory abnormalities see Table 2.

Recurrent Episodes: In 3 clinical studies for the episodic treatment of recurrent genital herpes, the adverse reactions reported by ≥5% of patients receiving VALTREX 500 mg twice daily for 3 days (n = 402), VALTREX 500 mg twice daily for 5 days (n = 1,136) or placebo (n = 259), respectively, included headache (16%, 11%, 14%) and nausea (5%, 4%, 5%). For the incidence of laboratory abnormalities see Table 2.

Suppressive Therapy: Suppression of Recurrent Genital Herpes in Immunocompetent Adults: In a clinical study for the suppression of recurrent genital herpes infections, the adverse reactions reported by patients receiving VALTREX 1 gram once daily (n = 269), VALTREX 500 mg once daily (n = 266), or placebo (n = 134), respectively, included headache (35%, 38%, 34%), nausea (11%, 11%, 8%), abdominal pain (11%, 9%, 6%), dysmenorrhea (8%, 5%, 4%), depression (7%, 5%, 5%), arthralgia (6%, 5%, 4%), vomiting (3%, 3%, 2%), and dizziness (4%, 2%, 1%). For the incidence of laboratory abnormalities see Table 2.

Suppression of Recurrent Genital Herpes in HIV-Infected Patients: In HIV-infected patients, frequently reported adverse reactions for VALTREX (500 mg twice daily; n = 194, median days on therapy = 172) and placebo (n = 99, median days on therapy = 59), respectively, included headache (13%, 8%), fatigue (8%, 5%), and rash (8%, 1%). Postrandomization laboratory abnormalities that were reported more frequently in valacyclovir subjects versus placebo included elevated alkaline phosphatase (4%, 2%), elevated ALT (14%, 10%), elevated AST (16%, 11%), decreased neutrophil counts (18%, 10%), and decreased platelet counts (3%, 0%), respectively.

Reduction of Transmission: In a clinical study for the reduction of transmission of genital herpes, the adverse reactions reported by patients receiving VALTREX 500 mg once daily (n = 743) or placebo once daily (n = 741), respectively, included headache (29%, 26%), nasopharyngitis (16%, 15%), and upper respiratory tract infection (9%, 10%).

Herpes Zoster: In 2 clinical studies for the treatment of herpes zoster, the adverse reactions reported by patients receiving VALTREX 1 gram 3 times daily for 7 to 14 days (n = 967) or placebo (n = 195), respectively, included nausea (15%, 8%), headache (14%, 12%), vomiting (6%, 3%), dizziness (3%, 2%), and abdominal pain (3%, 2%). For the incidence of laboratory abnormalities see Table 2.
[See table 2 above]

6.2 Clinical Trials Experience in Pediatric Patients

The safety profile of VALTREX has been studied in 177 pediatric patients 1 month to <18 years of age. Sixty-five of these pediatric patients, 12 to <18 years of age, received oral caplets for 1 to 2 days for treatment of cold sores. The remaining 112 pediatric patients, 1 month to <12 years of age, participated in 3 pharmacokinetic and safety studies and received valacyclovir oral suspension. Fifty-one of these 112 pediatric patients received oral suspension for 3 to 6

days. The frequency, intensity, and nature of clinical adverse reactions and laboratory abnormalities were similar to those seen in adults.

Pediatric Patients 12 to <18 Years of Age (Cold Sores): In clinical studies for the treatment of cold sores, the adverse reactions reported by adolescent patients receiving VALTREX 2 grams twice daily for 1 day, or VALTREX 2 grams twice daily for 1 day followed by 1 gram twice daily for 1 day (n = 65, across both dosing groups), or placebo (n = 30), respectively, included headache (17%, 3%) and nausea (8%, 0%).

Pediatric Patients 1 Month to <12 Years of Age: Adverse events reported in more than 1 subject across the 3 pharmacokinetic and safety studies in children 1 month to <12 years of age were diarrhea (5%), pyrexia (4%), dehydration (2%), herpes simplex (2%), and rhinorrhea (2%). No clinically meaningful changes in laboratory values were observed.

6.3 Postmarketing Experience

In addition to adverse events reported from clinical trials, the following events have been identified during postmarketing use of VALTREX. Because they are reported voluntarily from a population of unknown size, estimates of frequency cannot be made. These events have been chosen for inclusion due to a combination of their seriousness, frequency of reporting, or potential causal connection to VALTREX.

General: Facial edema, hypertension, tachycardia.
Allergic: Acute hypersensitivity reactions including anaphylaxis, angioedema, dyspnea, pruritus, rash, and urticaria [see Contraindications (4)].
CNS Symptoms: Aggressive behavior; agitation; ataxia; coma; confusion; decreased consciousness; dysarthria; encephalopathy; mania; and psychosis, including auditory and visual hallucinations, seizures, tremors [see Warnings and Precautions (5.3), Use in Specific Populations (8.5), (8.6)].
Eye: Visual abnormalities.
Gastrointestinal: Diarrhea.
Hepatobiliary Tract and Pancreas: Liver enzyme abnormalities, hepatitis.
Renal: Renal failure, renal pain (may be associated with renal failure) [see Warnings and Precautions (5.2), Use in Specific Populations (8.5), (8.6)].
Hematologic: Thrombocytopenia, aplastic anemia, leukocytoclastic vasculitis, TTP/HUS [see Warnings and Precautions (5.1)].
Skin: Erythema multiforme, rashes including photosensitivity, alopecia.

7 DRUG INTERACTIONS

No clinically significant drug-drug or drug-food interactions with VALTREX are known [see Clinical Pharmacology (12.3)].

8 USE IN SPECIFIC POPULATIONS

8.1 Pregnancy

Pregnancy Category B. There are no adequate and well-controlled studies of VALTREX or acyclovir in pregnant women. Based on prospective pregnancy registry data on

Table 2. Incidence (%) of Laboratory Abnormalities in Herpes Zoster and Genital Herpes Study Populations

Laboratory Abnormality	Herpes Zoster		Genital Herpes Treatment			Genital Herpes Suppression		
	VALTREX 1 gram 3 times daily (n = 967)	Placebo (n = 195)	VALTREX 1 gram twice daily (n = 1,194)	VALTREX 500 mg twice daily (n = 1,159)	Placebo (n = 439)	VALTREX 1 mg once daily (n = 269)	VALTREX 500 mg once daily (n = 266)	Placebo (n = 134)
Hemoglobin (<0.8 × LLN)	0.8%	0%	0.3%	0.2%	0%	0%	0.8%	0.8%
White blood cells (<0.75 × LLN)	1.3%	0.6%	0.7%	0.6%	0.2%	0.7%	0.8%	1.5%
Platelet count (<100,000/mm³)	1.0%	1.2%	0.3%	0.1%	0.7%	0.4%	1.1%	1.5%
AST (SGOT) (>2 × ULN)	1.0%	0%	1.0%	a	0.5%	4.1%	3.8%	3.0%
Serum creatinine (>1.5 × ULN)	0.2%	0%	0.7%	0%	0%	0%	0%	0%

a Data were not collected prospectively.
LLN = Lower limit of normal.
ULN = Upper limit of normal.

749 pregnancies, the overall rate of birth defects in infants exposed to acyclovir in-utero appears similar to the rate for infants in the general population. VALTREX should be used during pregnancy only if the potential benefit justifies the potential risk to the fetus.

A prospective epidemiologic registry of acyclovir use during pregnancy was established in 1984 and completed in April 1999. There were 749 pregnancies followed in women exposed to systemic acyclovir during the first trimester of pregnancy resulting in 756 outcomes. The occurrence rate of birth defects approximates that found in the general population. However, the small size of the registry is insufficient to evaluate the risk for less common defects or to permit reliable or definitive conclusions regarding the safety of acyclovir in pregnant women and their developing fetuses.

Animal reproduction studies performed at oral doses that provided up to 10 and 7 times the human plasma levels during the period of major organogenesis in rats and rabbits, respectively, revealed no evidence of teratogenicity.

8.3 Nursing Mothers

Following oral administration of a 500 mg dose of VALTREX to 5 nursing mothers, peak acyclovir concentrations (C_{max}) in breast milk ranged from 0.5 to 2.3 times (median 1.4) the corresponding maternal acyclovir serum concentrations. The acyclovir breast milk AUC ranged from 1.4 to 2.6 times (median 2.2) maternal serum AUC. A 500 mg maternal dosage of VALTREX twice daily would provide a nursing infant with an oral acyclovir dosage of approximately 0.6 mg/kg/day. This would result in less than 2% of the exposure obtained after administration of a standard neonatal dose of 30 mg/kg/day of intravenous acyclovir to the nursing infant. Unchanged valacyclovir was not detected in maternal serum, breast milk, or infant urine. Caution should be exercised when VALTREX is administered to a nursing woman.

8.4 Pediatric Use

VALTREX is indicated for treatment of cold sores in pediatric patients ≥12 years of age and for treatment of chickenpox in pediatric patients 2 to <18 years of age *[see Indications and Usage (1.2), Dosage and Administration (2.2)]*.

The use of VALTREX for treatment of cold sores is based on 2 double-blind, placebo-controlled clinical trials in healthy adults and adolescents (≥12 years of age) with a history of recurrent cold sores *[see Clinical Studies (14.1)]*.

The use of VALTREX for treatment of chickenpox in pediatric patients 2 to <18 years of age is based on single-dose pharmacokinetic and multiple-dose safety data from an open-label trial with valacyclovir and supported by efficacy and safety data from 3 randomized, double-blind, placebo-controlled trials evaluating oral acyclovir in pediatric patients with chickenpox *[see Dosage and Administration (2.2), Adverse Reactions (6.2), Clinical Pharmacology (12.3), Clinical Studies (14.4)]*.

The efficacy and safety of valacyclovir have not been established in pediatric patients:

- <12 years of age with cold sores
- <18 years of age with genital herpes
- <18 years of age with herpes zoster
- <2 years of age with chickenpox
- for suppressive therapy following neonatal HSV infection.

The pharmacokinetic profile and safety of valacyclovir oral suspension in children <12 years of age were studied in 3 open-label studies. No efficacy evaluations were conducted in any of the 3 studies.

Study 1 was a single-dose pharmacokinetic, multiple-dose safety study in 27 pediatric patients 1 to <12 years of age with clinically suspected varicella-zoster virus (VZV) infection *[see Dosage and Administration (2.2), Adverse Reactions (6.2), Clinical Pharmacology (12.3), Clinical Studies (14.4)]*.

Study 2 was a single-dose pharmacokinetic and safety study in pediatric patients 1 month to <6 years of age who had an active herpes virus infection or who were at risk for herpes virus infection. Fifty-seven subjects were enrolled and received a single dose of 25 mg/kg valacyclovir oral suspension. In infants and children 3 months to <6 years of age, this dose provided comparable systemic acyclovir exposures to that from a 1 gram dose of valacyclovir in adults (historical data). In infants 1 month to <3 months of age, mean acyclovir exposures resulting from a 25 mg/kg dose were higher (C_{max}: ↑ 30%, AUC: ↑ 60%) than acyclovir exposures following a 1 gram dose of valacyclovir in adults. Acyclovir is not approved for suppressive therapy in infants and children following neonatal HSV infections; therefore valacyclovir is not recommended for this indication because efficacy cannot be extrapolated from acyclovir.

Study 3 was a single-dose pharmacokinetic, multiple-dose safety study in 28 pediatric patients 1 to <12 years of age with clinically suspected HSV infection. None of the children enrolled in this study had genital herpes. Each subject was dosed with valacyclovir oral suspension, 10 mg/kg twice daily for 3 to 5 days. Acyclovir systemic exposures in pediatric patients following valacyclovir oral suspension were compared with historical acyclovir systemic exposures in immunocompetent adults receiving the solid oral dosage form of valacyclovir or acyclovir for the treatment of recurrent genital herpes. The mean projected daily acyclovir systemic exposures in pediatric patients across all age-groups (1 to <12 years of age) were lower (C_{max}: ↓ 20%, AUC: ↓ 33%) compared with the acyclovir systemic exposures in adults receiving valacyclovir 500 mg twice daily, but were higher (daily AUC: ↑ 16%) than systemic exposures in adults receiving acyclovir 200 mg 5 times daily. Insufficient data are available to support valacyclovir for the treatment of recurrent genital herpes in this age-group because clinical information on recurrent genital herpes in young children is limited; therefore, extrapolating efficacy data from adults to this population is not possible. Moreover, valacyclovir has not been studied in children 1 to <12 years of age with recurrent genital herpes.

8.5 Geriatric Use

Of the total number of subjects in clinical studies of VALTREX, 906 were 65 and over, and 352 were 75 and over. In a clinical study of herpes zoster, the duration of pain after healing (post-herpetic neuralgia) was longer in patients 65 and older compared with younger adults. Elderly patients are more likely to have reduced renal function and require dose reduction. Elderly patients are also more likely to have renal or CNS adverse events *[see Dosage and Administration (2.4), Warnings and Precautions (5.2, 5.3), Clinical Pharmacology (12.3)]*.

8.6 Renal Impairment

Dosage reduction is recommended when administering VALTREX to patients with renal impairment *[see Dosage and Administration (2.4), Warnings and Precautions (5.2, 5.3)]*.

10 OVERDOSAGE

Caution should be exercised to prevent inadvertent overdose *[see Use in Specific Populations (8.5), (8.6)]*. Precipitation of acyclovir in renal tubules may occur when the solubility (2.5 mg/mL) is exceeded in the intratubular fluid. In the event of acute renal failure and anuria, the patient may benefit from hemodialysis until renal function is restored *[see Dosage and Administration (2.4)]*.

11 DESCRIPTION

VALTREX (valacyclovir hydrochloride) is the hydrochloride salt of the *L*-valyl ester of the antiviral drug acyclovir.

VALTREX Caplets are for oral administration. Each caplet contains valacyclovir hydrochloride equivalent to 500 mg or 1 gram valacyclovir and the inactive ingredients carnauba wax, colloidal silicon dioxide, crospovidone, FD&C Blue No. 2 Lake, hypromellose, magnesium stearate, microcrystalline cellulose, polyethylene glycol, polysorbate 80, povidone, and titanium dioxide. The blue, film-coated caplets are printed with edible white ink.

The chemical name of valacyclovir hydrochloride is *L*-valine, 2-[(2-amino-1,6-dihydro-6-oxo-9*H*-purin-9-yl) methoxy]ethyl ester, monohydrochloride. It has the following structural formula:

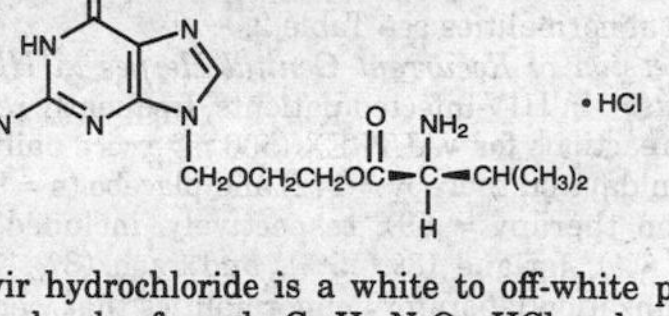

Valacyclovir hydrochloride is a white to off-white powder with the molecular formula $C_{13}H_{20}N_6O_4$•HCl and a molecular weight of 360.80. The maximum solubility in water at 25°C is 174 mg/mL. The pk_as for valacyclovir hydrochloride are 1.90, 7.47, and 9.43.

12 CLINICAL PHARMACOLOGY

12.1 Mechanism of Action

Valacyclovir is an antiviral drug *[see Clinical Pharmacology (12.4)]*.

12.3 Pharmacokinetics

The pharmacokinetics of valacyclovir and acyclovir after oral administration of VALTREX have been investigated in 14 volunteer studies involving 283 adults and in 3 studies involving 112 pediatric subjects from 1 month to <12 years of age.

Pharmacokinetics in Adults: *Absorption and Bioavailability:* After oral administration, valacyclovir hydrochloride is rapidly absorbed from the gastrointestinal tract and nearly completely converted to acyclovir and *L*-valine by first-pass intestinal and/or hepatic metabolism.

The absolute bioavailability of acyclovir after administration of VALTREX is 54.5% ± 9.1% as determined following a 1 gram oral dose of VALTREX and a 350 mg intravenous acyclovir dose to 12 healthy volunteers. Acyclovir bioavailability from the administration of VALTREX is not altered by administration with food (30 minutes after an 873 Kcal breakfast, which included 51 grams of fat).

Acyclovir pharmacokinetic parameter estimates following administration of VALTREX to healthy adult volunteers are presented in Table 3. There was a less than dose-proportional increase in acyclovir maximum concentration (C_{max}) and area under the acyclovir concentration-time curve (AUC) after single-dose and multiple-dose administration (4 times daily) of VALTREX from doses between 250 mg to 1 gram.

There is no accumulation of acyclovir after the administration of valacyclovir at the recommended dosage regimens in adults with normal renal function.

Table 3. Mean (± SD) Plasma Acyclovir Pharmacokinetic Parameters Following Administration of VALTREX to Healthy Adult Volunteers

	Single-Dose Administration (N = 8)		Multiple-Dose Administration[a] (N = 24, 8 per treatment arm)	
Dose	C_{max} (±SD) (mcg/mL)	AUC (±SD) (hr•mcg/mL)	C_{max} (±SD) (mcg/mL)	AUC (±SD) (hr•mcg/mL)
100 mg	0.83 (±0.14)	2.28 (±0.40)	ND	ND
250 mg	2.15 (±0.50)	5.76 (±0.60)	2.11 (±0.33)	5.66 (±1.09)
500 mg	3.28 (±0.83)	11.59 (±1.79)	3.69 (±0.87)	9.88 (±2.01)
750 mg	4.17 (±1.14)	14.11 (±3.54)	ND	ND
1,000 mg	5.65 (±2.37)	19.52 (±6.04)	4.96 (±0.64)	15.70 (±2.27)

[a] Administered 4 times daily for 11 days.
ND = not done.

Distribution: The binding of valacyclovir to human plasma proteins ranges from 13.5% to 17.9%. The binding of acyclovir to human plasma proteins ranges from 9% to 33%.

Metabolism: Valacyclovir is converted to acyclovir and L-valine by first-pass intestinal and/or hepatic metabolism. Acyclovir is converted to a small extent to inactive metabolites by aldehyde oxidase and by alcohol and aldehyde dehydrogenase. Neither valacyclovir nor acyclovir is metabolized by cytochrome P450 enzymes. Plasma concentrations of unconverted valacyclovir are low and transient, generally becoming non- quantifiable by 3 hours after administration. Peak plasma valacyclovir concentrations are generally less than 0.5 mcg/mL at all doses. After single-dose administration of 1 gram of VALTREX, average plasma valacyclovir concentrations observed were 0.5, 0.4, and 0.8 mcg/mL in patients with hepatic dysfunction, renal insufficiency, and in healthy volunteers who received concomitant cimetidine and probenecid, respectively.

Elimination: The pharmacokinetic disposition of acyclovir delivered by valacyclovir is consistent with previous experience from intravenous and oral acyclovir. Following the oral administration of a single 1 gram dose of radiolabeled valacyclovir to 4 healthy subjects, 46% and 47% of administered radioactivity was recovered in urine and feces, respectively, over 96 hours. Acyclovir accounted for 89% of the radioactivity excreted in the urine. Renal clearance of acyclovir following the administration of a single 1 gram dose of VALTREX to 12 healthy volunteers was approximately 255 ± 86 mL/min which represents 42% of total acyclovir apparent plasma clearance.

The plasma elimination half-life of acyclovir typically averaged 2.5 to 3.3 hours in all studies of VALTREX in volunteers with normal renal function.

Specific Populations: *Renal Impairment:* Reduction in dosage is recommended in patients with renal impairment *[see Dosage and Administration (2.4), Use in Specific Populations (8.5), (8.6)]*.

Following administration of VALTREX to volunteers with ESRD, the average acyclovir half-life is approximately 14 hours. During hemodialysis, the acyclovir half-life is approximately 4 hours. Approximately one third of acyclovir in the body is removed by dialysis during a 4-hour hemodialysis session. Apparent plasma clearance of acyclovir in dialysis patients was 86.3 ± 21.3 mL/min/1.73 m^2 compared with 679.16 ± 162.76 mL/min/1.73 m^2 in healthy volunteers.

Hepatic Impairment: Administration of VALTREX to patients with moderate (biopsy-proven cirrhosis) or severe (with and without ascites and biopsy-proven cirrhosis) liver disease indicated that the rate but not the extent of conversion of valacyclovir to acyclovir is reduced, and the acyclovir half-life is not affected. Dosage modification is not recommended for patients with cirrhosis.

HIV Disease: In 9 patients with HIV disease and CD4+ cell counts <150 cells/mm^3 who received VALTREX at a dosage of 1 gram 4 times daily for 30 days, the pharmacokinetics of valacyclovir and acyclovir were not different from that observed in healthy volunteers.

Geriatrics: After single-dose administration of 1 gram of VALTREX in healthy geriatric volunteers, the half-life of acyclovir was 3.11 ± 0.51 hours, compared with 2.91 ± 0.63 hours in healthy younger adult volunteers. The pharmacokinetics of acyclovir following single- and multiple-dose oral administration of VALTREX in geriatric volunteers varied with renal function. Dose reduction may be required in geriatric patients, depending on the underlying renal status of the patient *[see Dosage and Administration (2.4), Use in Specific Populations (8.5), (8.6)]*.

Pediatrics: Acyclovir pharmacokinetics have been evaluated in a total of 98 pediatric patients (1 month to <12 years of age) following administration of the first dose of an extemporaneous oral suspension of valacyclovir *[see Adverse Reactions (6.2), Use in Specific Populations (8.4)]*. Acyclovir pharmacokinetic parameter estimates following a 20 mg/kg dose are provided in Table 4.

Table 4: Mean (±SD) Plasma Acyclovir Pharmacokinetic Parameter Estimates Following First-Dose Administration of 20 mg/kg Valacyclovir Oral Suspension to Pediatric Patients vs. 1 Gram Single Dose of VALTREX to Adults

Parameter	Pediatric Patients (20 mg/kg Oral Suspension) 1-<2 yr (N = 6)	2-<6 yr (N = 12)	6-<12 yr (N = 8)	Adults 1 gram Solid Dose of VALTREX[a] (N = 15)
AUC (mcg•hr/mL)	14.4 (±6.26)	10.1 (±3.35)	13.1 (±3.43)	17.2 (±3.10)
C_{max} (mcg/mL)	4.03 (±1.37)	3.75 (±1.14)	4.71 (±1.20)	4.72 (±1.37)

[a] Historical estimates using pediatric pharmacokinetic sampling schedule.

Drug Interactions: When VALTREX is coadministered with antacids, cimetidine and/or probenecid, digoxin, or thiazide diuretics in patients with normal renal function, the effects are not considered to be of clinical significance (see below). Therefore, when VALTREX is coadministered with these drugs in patients with normal renal function, no dosage adjustment is recommended.

Antacids: The pharmacokinetics of acyclovir after a single dose of VALTREX (1 gram) were unchanged by coadministration of a single dose of antacids (Al^{3+} or Mg^{++}).

Cimetidine: Acyclovir C_{max} and AUC following a single dose of VALTREX (1 gram) increased by 8% and 32%, respectively, after a single dose of cimetidine (800 mg).

Cimetidine Plus Probenecid: Acyclovir C_{max} and AUC following a single dose of VALTREX (1 gram) increased by 30% and 78%, respectively, after a combination of cimetidine and probenecid, primarily due to a reduction in renal clearance of acyclovir.

Digoxin: The pharmacokinetics of digoxin were not affected by coadministration of VALTREX 1 gram 3 times daily, and the pharmacokinetics of acyclovir after a single dose of VALTREX (1 gram) was unchanged by coadministration of digoxin (2 doses of 0.75 mg).

Probenecid: Acyclovir C_{max} and AUC following a single dose of VALTREX (1 gram) increased by 22% and 49%, respectively, after probenecid (1 gram).

Thiazide Diuretics: The pharmacokinetics of acyclovir after a single dose of VALTREX (1 gram) were unchanged by coadministration of multiple doses of thiazide diuretics.

12.4 Microbiology

Mechanism of Action: Valacyclovir is a nucleoside analogue DNA polymerase inhibitor. Valacyclovir hydrochloride is rapidly converted to acyclovir which has demonstrated antiviral activity against HSV types 1 (HSV-1) and 2 (HSV-2) and VZV both in cell culture and in vivo.

The inhibitory activity of acyclovir is highly selective due to its affinity for the enzyme thymidine kinase (TK) encoded by HSV and VZV. This viral enzyme converts acyclovir into acyclovir monophosphate, a nucleotide analogue. The monophosphate is further converted into diphosphate by cellular guanylate kinase and into triphosphate by a number of cellular enzymes. In biochemical assays, acyclovir triphosphate inhibits replication of herpes viral DNA. This is accomplished in 3 ways: 1) competitive inhibition of viral DNA polymerase, 2) incorporation and termination of the growing viral DNA chain, and 3) inactivation of the viral DNA polymerase. The greater antiviral activity of acyclovir against HSV compared with VZV is due to its more efficient phosphorylation by the viral TK.

Antiviral Activities: The quantitative relationship between the cell culture susceptibility of herpesviruses to antivirals and the clinical response to therapy has not been established in humans, and virus sensitivity testing has not been standardized. Sensitivity testing results, expressed as the concentration of drug required to inhibit by 50% the growth of virus in cell culture (EC_{50}), vary greatly depending upon a number of factors. Using plaque-reduction assays, the EC_{50} values against herpes simplex virus isolates range from 0.09 to 60 µM (0.02 to 13.5 mcg/mL) for HSV-1 and from 0.04 to 44 µM (0.01 to 9.9 mcg/mL) for HSV-2. The EC_{50} values for acyclovir against most laboratory strains and clinical isolates of VZV range from 0.53 to 48 µM (0.12 to 10.8 mcg/mL). Acyclovir also demonstrates activity against the Oka vaccine strain of VZV with a mean EC_{50} of 6 µM (1.35 mcg/mL).

Resistance: Resistance of HSV and VZV to acyclovir can result from qualitative and quantitative changes in the viral TK and/or DNA polymerase. Clinical isolates of VZV with reduced susceptibility to acyclovir have been recovered from patients with AIDS. In these cases, TK-deficient mutants of VZV have been recovered.

Resistance of HSV and VZV to acyclovir occurs by the same mechanisms. While most of the acyclovir-resistant mutants isolated thus far from immunocompromised patients have been found to be TK-deficient mutants, other mutants involving the viral TK gene (TK partial and TK altered) and DNA polymerase have also been isolated. TK-negative mutants may cause severe disease in immunocompromised patients. The possibility of viral resistance to valacyclovir (and therefore, to acyclovir) should be considered in patients who show poor clinical response during therapy.

13 NONCLINICAL TOXICOLOGY

13.1 Carcinogenesis, Mutagenesis, Impairment of Fertility

The data presented below include references to the steady-state acyclovir AUC observed in humans treated with 1 gram VALTREX given orally 3 times a day to treat herpes zoster. Plasma drug concentrations in animal studies are expressed as multiples of human exposure to acyclovir *[see Clinical Pharmacology (12.3)]*.

Valacyclovir was noncarcinogenic in lifetime carcinogenicity bioassays at single daily doses (gavage) of valacyclovir giving plasma acyclovir concentrations equivalent to human levels in the mouse bioassay and 1.4 to 2.3 times human levels in the rat bioassay. There was no significant difference in the incidence of tumors between treated and control animals, nor did valacyclovir shorten the latency of tumors.

Valacyclovir was tested in 5 genetic toxicity assays. An Ames assay was negative in the absence or presence of metabolic activation. Also negative were an in vitro cytogenetic study with human lymphocytes and a rat cytogenetic study. In the mouse lymphoma assay, valacyclovir was not mutagenic in the absence of metabolic activation. In the presence of metabolic activation (76% to 88% conversion to acyclovir), valacyclovir was mutagenic.

Valacyclovir was mutagenic in a mouse micronucleus assay.

Valacyclovir did not impair fertility or reproduction in rats at 6 times human plasma levels.

14 CLINICAL STUDIES

14.1 Cold Sores (Herpes Labialis)

Two double-blind, placebo-controlled clinical trials were conducted in 1,856 healthy adults and adolescents (≥12 years old) with a history of recurrent cold sores. Patients self-initiated therapy at the earliest symptoms and prior to any signs of a cold sore. The majority of patients initiated treatment within 2 hours of onset of symptoms. Patients were randomized to VALTREX 2 grams twice daily on Day 1 followed by placebo on Day 2, VALTREX 2 grams twice daily on Day 1 followed by 1 gram twice daily on Day 2, or placebo on Days 1 and 2.

The mean duration of cold sore episodes was about 1 day shorter in treated subjects as compared with placebo. The 2 day regimen did not offer additional benefit over the 1-day regimen.

No significant difference was observed between subjects receiving VALTREX or placebo in the prevention of progression of cold sore lesions beyond the papular stage.

14.2 Genital Herpes Infections

Initial Episode: Six hundred forty-three immunocompetent adults with first-episode genital herpes who presented within 72 hours of symptom onset were randomized in a double-blind trial to receive 10 days of VALTREX 1 gram twice daily (n = 323) or oral acyclovir 200 mg 5 times a day (n = 320). For both treatment groups: the median time to lesion healing was 9 days, the median time to cessation of pain was 5 days, the median time to cessation of viral shedding was 3 days.

Recurrent Episodes: Three double-blind trials (2 of them placebo-controlled) in immunocompetent adults with recurrent genital herpes were conducted. Patients self-initiated therapy within 24 hours of the first sign or symptom of a recurrent genital herpes episode.

In 1 study, patients were randomized to receive 5 days of treatment with either VALTREX 500 mg twice daily (n = 360) or placebo (n = 259). The median time to lesion healing was 4 days in the group receiving VALTREX 500 mg versus 6 days in the placebo group, and the median time to cessation of viral shedding in patients with at least 1 positive culture (42% of the overall study population) was 2 days in the group receiving VALTREX 500 mg versus 4 days in the placebo group. The median time to cessation of pain was 3 days in the group receiving VALTREX 500 mg versus 4 days in the placebo group. Results supporting efficacy were replicated in a second trial.

In a third study, patients were randomized to receive VALTREX 500 mg twice daily for 5 days (n = 398) or VALTREX 500 mg twice daily for 3 days (and matching placebo twice daily for 2 additional days) (n = 402). The median time to lesion healing was about 4½ days in both treatment groups. The median time to cessation of pain was about 3 days in both treatment groups.

Suppressive Therapy: Two clinical studies were conducted, one in immunocompetent adults and one in HIV-infected adults.

A double-blind, 12-month, placebo- and active-controlled study enrolled immunocompetent adults with a history of 6 or more recurrences per year. Outcomes for the overall study population are shown in Table 5.

[See table 5 above]

Table 5. Recurrence Rates in Immunocompetent Adults at 6 and 12 Months

Outcome	6 Months: VALTREX 1 gram once daily (n = 269)	6 Months: Oral acyclovir 400 mg twice daily (n = 267)	6 Months: Placebo (n = 134)	12 Months: VALTREX 1 gram once daily (n = 269)	12 Months: Oral acyclovir 400 mg twice daily (n = 267)	12 Months: Placebo (n = 134)
Recurrence free	55%	54%	7%	34%	34%	4%
Recurrences	35%	36%	83%	46%	46%	85%
Unknown[a]	10%	10%	10%	19%	19%	10%

[a] Includes lost to follow-up, discontinuations due to adverse events, and consent withdrawn.

Subjects with 9 or fewer recurrences per year showed comparable results with VALTREX 500 mg once daily.

In a second study, 293 HIV-infected adults on stable antiretroviral therapy with a history of 4 or more recurrences of ano-genital herpes per year were randomized to receive either VALTREX 500 mg twice daily (n = 194) or matching placebo (n = 99) for 6 months. The median duration of recurrent genital herpes in enrolled subjects was 8 years, and the median number of recurrences in the year prior to enrollment was 5. Overall, the median prestudy HIV-1 RNA was 2.6 $\log_{10}$ copies/mL. Among patients who received VALTREX, the prestudy median CD4+ cell count was 336 cells/mm^3; 11% had <100 cells/mm^3, 16% had 100 to 199 cells/mm^3, 42% had 200 to 499 cells/mm^3, and 31% had ≥500 cells/mm^3. Outcomes for the overall study population are shown in Table 6.

Table 6. Recurrence Rates in HIV-Infected Adults at 6 Months

Outcome	VALTREX 500 mg twice daily (n = 194)	Placebo (n = 99)
Recurrence free	65%	26%
Recurrences	17%	57%
Unknown[a]	18%	17%

[a] Includes lost to follow-up, discontinuations due to adverse events, and consent withdrawn.

Reduction of Transmission of Genital Herpes: A double-blind, placebo-controlled study to assess transmission of genital herpes was conducted in 1,484 monogamous, heterosexual, immunocompetent adult couples. The couples were discordant for HSV-2 infection. The source partner had a history of 9 or fewer genital herpes episodes per year. Both partners were counseled on safer sex practices and were advised to use condoms throughout the study period. Source partners were randomized to treatment with either VALTREX 500 mg once daily or placebo once daily for 8 months. The primary efficacy endpoint was symptomatic acquisition of HSV-2 in susceptible partners. Overall HSV-2 acquisition was defined as symptomatic HSV-2 acquisition and/or HSV-2 seroconversion in susceptible partners. The efficacy results are summarized in Table 7.

Table 7. Percentage of Susceptible Partners Who Acquired HSV-2 Defined by the Primary and Selected Secondary Endpoints

Endpoint	VALTREX[a] (n = 743)	Placebo (n = 741)
Symptomatic HSV-2 acquisition	4 (0.5%)	16 (2.2%)
HSV-2 seroconversion	12 (1.6%)	24 (3.2%)
Overall HSV-2 acquisition	14 (1.9%)	27 (3.6%)

[a] Results show reductions in risk of 75% (symptomatic HSV-2 acquisition), 50% (HSV-2 seroconversion), and 48% (overall HSV-2 acquisition) with VALTREX versus placebo. Individual results may vary based on consistency of safer sex practices.

14.3 Herpes Zoster

Two randomized double-blind clinical trials in immunocompetent adults with localized herpes zoster were conducted. VALTREX was compared with placebo in patients less than 50 years of age, and with oral acyclovir in patients greater than 50 years of age. All patients were treated within 72 hours of appearance of zoster rash. In patients less than 50 years of age, the median time to cessation of new lesion formation was 2 days for those treated with VALTREX compared with 3 days for those treated with placebo. In patients greater than 50 years of age, the median time to cessation of new lesions was 3 days in patients treated with either VALTREX or oral acyclovir. In patients less than 50 years of age, no difference was found with respect to the duration of pain after healing (post-herpetic neuralgia) between the recipients of VALTREX and placebo. In patients greater than 50 years of age, among the 83% who reported pain after healing (post-herpetic neuralgia), the median duration of pain after healing [95% confidence interval] in days was: 40 [31, 51], 43 [36, 55], and 59 [41, 77] for 7-day VALTREX, 14-day VALTREX, and 7-day oral acyclovir, respectively.

14.4 Chickenpox

The use of VALTREX for treatment of chickenpox in pediatric patients 2 to <18 years of age is based on single-dose pharmacokinetic and multiple-dose safety data from an open-label trial with valacyclovir and supported by safety and extrapolated efficacy data from 3 randomized, double-blind, placebo-controlled trials evaluating oral acyclovir in pediatric patients.

The single-dose pharmacokinetic and multiple-dose safety study enrolled 27 pediatric patients 1 to <12 years of age with clinically suspected VZV infection. Each subject was dosed with valacyclovir oral suspension, 20 mg/kg 3 times daily for 5 days. Acyclovir systemic exposures in pediatric patients following valacyclovir oral suspension were compared with historical acyclovir systemic exposures in immunocompetent adults receiving the solid oral dosage form of valacyclovir or acyclovir for the treatment of herpes zoster. The mean projected daily acyclovir exposures in pediatric patients across all age-groups (1 to <12 years of age) were lower (C_{max}: ↓ 13%, AUC: ↓ 30%) than the mean daily historical exposures in adults receiving valacyclovir 1 gram 3 times daily, but were higher (daily AUC: ↑ 50%) than the mean daily historical exposures in adults receiving acyclovir 800 mg 5 times daily. The projected daily exposures in pediatric patients were greater (daily AUC approximately 100% greater) than the exposures seen in immunocompetent pediatric patients receiving acyclovir 20 mg/kg 4 times daily for the treatment of chickenpox. Based on the pharmacokinetic and safety data from this study and the safety and extrapolated efficacy data from the acyclovir studies, oral valacyclovir 20 mg/kg 3 times a day for 5 days (not to exceed 1 gram 3 times daily) is recommended for the treatment of chickenpox in pediatric patients 2 to <18 years of age. Because the efficacy and safety of acyclovir for the treatment of chickenpox in children <2 years of age have not been established, efficacy data cannot be extrapolated to support valacyclovir treatment in children <2 years of age with chickenpox. Valacyclovir is also not recommended for the treatment of herpes zoster in children because safety data up to 7 days' duration are not available *[see Use in Specific Populations (8.4)]*.

16 HOW SUPPLIED/STORAGE AND HANDLING

VALTREX Caplets (blue, film-coated, capsule-shaped tablets) containing valacyclovir hydrochloride equivalent to 500 mg valacyclovir and printed with "VALTREX 500 mg."
Bottle of 30 (NDC 0173-0933-08).
Bottle of 90 (NDC 0173-0933-10).
Unit dose pack of 100 (NDC 0173-0933-56).
VALTREX Caplets (blue, film-coated, capsule-shaped tablets, with a partial scorebar on both sides) containing valacyclovir hydrochloride equivalent to 1 gram valacyclovir and printed with "VALTREX 1 gram."
Bottle of 30 (NDC 0173-0565-04).
Bottle of 90 (NDC 0173-0565-10).

Storage:
Store at 15° to 25°C (59° to 77°F). Dispense in a well-closed container as defined in the USP.

17 PATIENT COUNSELING INFORMATION

See FDA-Approved Patient Labeling.

17.1 Importance of Adequate Hydration

Patients should be advised to maintain adequate hydration.

17.2 Cold Sores (Herpes Labialis)

Patients should be advised to initiate treatment at the earliest symptom of a cold sore (e.g., tingling, itching, or burning). There are no data on the effectiveness of treatment initiated after the development of clinical signs of a cold sore (e.g., papule, vesicle, or ulcer). Patients should be instructed that treatment for cold sores should not exceed 1 day (2 doses) and that their doses should be taken about 12 hours apart. Patients should be informed that VALTREX is not a cure for cold sores.

17.3 Genital Herpes

Patients should be informed that VALTREX is not a cure for genital herpes. Because genital herpes is a sexually transmitted disease, patients should avoid contact with lesions or intercourse when lesions and/or symptoms are present to avoid infecting partners. Genital herpes is frequently transmitted in the absence of symptoms through asymptomatic viral shedding. Therefore, patients should be counseled to use safer sex practices in combination with suppressive therapy with VALTREX. Sex partners of infected persons should be advised that they might be infected even if they have no symptoms. Type-specific serologic testing of asymptomatic partners of persons with genital herpes can determine whether risk for HSV-2 acquisition exists.

VALTREX has not been shown to reduce transmission of sexually transmitted infections other than HSV-2.

If medical management of a genital herpes recurrence is indicated, patients should be advised to initiate therapy at the first sign or symptom of an episode.

There are no data on the effectiveness of treatment initiated more than 72 hours after the onset of signs and symptoms of a first episode of genital herpes or more than 24 hours after the onset of signs and symptoms of a recurrent episode.

There are no data on the safety or effectiveness of chronic suppressive therapy of more than 1 year's duration in otherwise healthy patients. There are no data on the safety or effectiveness of chronic suppressive therapy of more than 6 months' duration in HIV-infected patients.

17.4 Herpes Zoster

There are no data on treatment initiated more than 72 hours after onset of the zoster rash. Patients should be advised to initiate treatment as soon as possible after a diagnosis of herpes zoster.

17.5 Chickenpox

Patients should be advised to initiate treatment at the earliest sign or symptom of chickenpox.

This product's prescribing information may have been updated. Please refer to www.gsk.com for the most current version.

Distributed by:
GlaxoSmithKline
Research Triangle Park, NC 27709
Manufactured by:
GlaxoSmithKline
Research Triangle Park, NC 27709
or
DSM Pharmaceuticals, Inc.
Greenville, NC 27834
©2010, GlaxoSmithKline. All rights reserved.
March 2010
VTX:3PI

PHARMACIST-DETACH HERE AND GIVE INSTRUCTIONS TO PATIENT

Patient Information

VALTREX® (VAL-trex)
(valacyclovir hydrochloride) Caplets

Read the Patient Information that comes with VALTREX before you start using it and each time you get a refill. There may be new information. This information does not take the place of talking to your healthcare provider about your medical condition or treatment. Ask your healthcare provider or pharmacist if you have questions.

What is VALTREX?

VALTREX is a prescription antiviral medicine. VALTREX lowers the ability of herpes viruses to multiply in your body.

VALTREX is used in adults:
- to treat cold sores (also called fever blisters or herpes labialis)
- to treat shingles (also called herpes zoster)
- to treat or control genital herpes outbreaks in adults with normal immune systems
- to control genital herpes outbreaks in adults infected with the human immunodeficiency virus (HIV) with CD4+ cell count greater than 100 cells/mm^3
- with safer sex practices to lower the chances of spreading genital herpes to others. Even with safer sex practices, it is still possible to spread genital herpes.

VALTREX used daily with the following safer sex practices can lower the chances of passing genital herpes to your partner.
- **Do not have sexual contact with your partner when you have any symptom or outbreak of genital herpes.**
- **Use a condom** made of latex or polyurethane whenever you have sexual contact.

VALTREX is used in children:
- to treat cold sores (for children ≥12 years of age)
- to treat chickenpox (for children 2 to <18 years of age).

VALTREX does not cure herpes infections (cold sores, chickenpox, shingles, or genital herpes).

The efficacy of VALTREX has not been studied in children who have not reached puberty.

What are cold sores, chickenpox, shingles, and genital herpes?

Cold sores are caused by a herpes virus that may be spread by kissing or other physical contact with the infected area of the skin. They are small, painful ulcers that you get in or around your mouth. It is not known if VALTREX can stop the spread of cold sores to others.

Chickenpox is caused by a herpes virus. It causes an itchy rash of multiple small, red bumps that look like pimples or insect bites usually appearing first on the abdomen or back and face. It can spread to almost everywhere else on the body and may be accompanied by flu-like symptoms.

Shingles is caused by the same herpes virus that causes chickenpox. It causes small, painful blisters that happen on your skin. Shingles occurs in people who have already had chickenpox. Shingles can be spread to people who have not had chickenpox or the chickenpox vaccine by contact with the infected areas of the skin. It is not known if VALTREX can stop the spread of shingles to others.

Genital herpes is a sexually transmitted disease. It causes small, painful blisters on your genital area. You can spread genital herpes to others, even when you have no symptoms. If you are sexually active, you can still pass herpes to your partner, even if you are taking VALTREX. VALTREX, taken every day as prescribed and used with the following **safer sex practices,** can lower the chances of passing genital herpes to your partner.
- Do not have sexual contact with your partner when you have any symptom or outbreak of genital herpes.
- Use a condom made of latex or polyurethane whenever you have sexual contact.

Ask your healthcare provider for more information about safer sex practices.

Who should not take VALTREX?

Do not take VALTREX if you are allergic to any of its ingredients or to acyclovir. The active ingredient is valacyclovir. See the end of this leaflet for a complete list of ingredients in VALTREX.

Before taking VALTREX, tell your healthcare provider:

About all your medical conditions, including:
- **if you have had a bone marrow transplant or kidney transplant, or if you have advanced HIV disease or "AIDS".** Patients with these conditions may have a higher chance for getting a blood disorder called thrombotic thrombocytopenic purpura/hemolytic uremic syndrome (TTP/HUS). TTP/HUS can result in death.
- **if you have kidney problems.** Patients with kidney problems may have a higher chance for getting side effects or more kidney problems with VALTREX. Your healthcare provider may give you a lower dose of VALTREX.

- **if you are 65 years of age or older.** Elderly patients have a higher chance of certain side effects. Also, elderly patients are more likely to have kidney problems. Your healthcare provider may give you a lower dose of VALTREX.
- **if you are pregnant or planning to become pregnant.** Talk with your healthcare provider about the risks and benefits of taking prescription drugs (including VALTREX) during pregnancy.
- **if you are breastfeeding.** VALTREX may pass into your milk and it may harm your baby. Talk with your healthcare provider about the best way to feed your baby if you are taking VALTREX.
- **about all the medicines you take,** including prescription and non-prescription medicines, vitamins, and herbal supplements. VALTREX may affect other medicines, and other medicines may affect VALTREX. It is a good idea to keep a complete list of all the medicines you take. Show this list to your healthcare provider and pharmacist any time you get a new medicine.

How should I take VALTREX?
Take VALTREX exactly as prescribed by your healthcare provider. Your dose of VALTREX and length of treatment will depend on the type of herpes infection that you have and any other medical problems that you have.

- Do not stop VALTREX or change your treatment without talking to your healthcare provider.
- VALTREX can be taken with or without food.
- If you are taking VALTREX to treat cold sores, chickenpox, shingles, or genital herpes, you should start treatment as soon as possible after your symptoms start. VALTREX may not help you if you start treatment too late.
- If you miss a dose of VALTREX, take it as soon as you remember and then take your next dose at its regular time. However, if it is almost time for your next dose, do not take the missed dose. Wait and take the next dose at the regular time.
- Do not take more than the prescribed number of VALTREX Caplets each day. Call your healthcare provider right away if you take too much VALTREX.

What are the possible side effects of VALTREX?
Kidney failure and nervous system problems are not common, but can be serious in some patients taking VALTREX. Nervous system problems include aggressive behavior, unsteady movement, shaky movements, confusion, speech problems, hallucinations (seeing or hearing things that are really not there), seizures, and coma. Kidney failure and nervous system problems have happened in patients who already have kidney disease and in elderly patients whose kidneys do not work well due to age. **Always tell your healthcare provider if you have kidney problems before taking VALTREX. Call your doctor right away if you get a nervous system problem while you are taking VALTREX.**
Common side effects of VALTREX in adults include headache, nausea, stomach pain, vomiting, and dizziness. Side effects in HIV-infected adults include headache, tiredness, and rash. These side effects usually are mild and do not cause patients to stop taking VALTREX.
Other less common side effects in adults include painful periods in women, joint pain, depression, low blood cell counts, and changes in tests that measure how well the liver and kidneys work.
The most common side effect seen in children <18 years of age was headache.
Talk to your healthcare provider if you develop any side effects that concern you.
These are not all the side effects of VALTREX. For more information ask your healthcare provider or pharmacist.

How should I store VALTREX?
- Store VALTREX Caplets at room temperature, 59° to 77°F (15° to 25°C).
- Store VALTREX suspension between 2° to 8°C (36° to 46°F) in a refrigerator. Discard after 28 days.
- Keep VALTREX in a tightly closed container.
- Do not keep medicine that is out of date or that you no longer need.
- Keep VALTREX and all medicines out of the reach of children.

General information about VALTREX
Medicines are sometimes prescribed for conditions that are not mentioned in patient information leaflets. Do not use VALTREX for a condition for which it was not prescribed. Do not give VALTREX to other people, even if they have the same symptoms you have. It may harm them.
This leaflet summarizes the most important information about VALTREX. If you would like more information, talk with your healthcare provider. You can ask your healthcare provider or pharmacist for information about VALTREX that is written for health professionals. More information is available at www.VALTREX.com.

What are the ingredients in VALTREX?
Active Ingredient: valacyclovir hydrochloride
Inactive Ingredients: carnauba wax, colloidal silicon dioxide, crospovidone, FD&C Blue No. 2 Lake, hypromellose,

magnesium stearate, microcrystalline cellulose, polyethylene glycol, polysorbate 80, povidone, and titanium dioxide.
Distributed by:
GlaxoSmithKline
Research Triangle Park, NC 27709
Manufactured by:
GlaxoSmithKline
Research Triangle Park, NC 27709
or
DSM Pharmaceuticals, Inc.
Greenville, NC 27834
©2008, GlaxoSmithKline. All rights reserved.
September 2008
VTX:2PIL

VENTOLIN® HFA   ℞
[vent' ō-lin]
(albuterol sulfate)
Inhalation Aerosol

HIGHLIGHTS OF PRESCRIBING INFORMATION
These highlights do not include all the information needed to use VENTOLIN HFA Inhalation Aerosol safely and effectively. See full prescribing information for VENTOLIN HFA Inhalation Aerosol.
VENTOLIN® HFA (albuterol sulfate) Inhalation Aerosol
Initial U.S. Approval: 1981

————INDICATIONS AND USAGE————
VENTOLIN HFA is a beta$_2$-adrenergic agonist indicated for:
- Treatment or prevention of bronchospasm in patients 4 years of age and older with reversible obstructive airway disease. (1.1)
- Prevention of exercise-induced bronchospasm in patients 4 years of age and older. (1.2)

————DOSAGE AND ADMINISTRATION————
FOR ORAL INHALATION ONLY.
- Treatment or prevention of bronchospasm in adults and children 4 years of age and older: 2 inhalations every 4 to 6 hours. For some patients, 1 inhalation every 4 hours may be sufficient. (2.1)
- Prevention of exercise-induced bronchospasm in adults and children 4 years of age and older: 2 inhalations 15 to 30 minutes before exercise. (2.2)
- Priming information: Prime VENTOLIN HFA before using for the first time, when the inhaler has not been used for more than 2 weeks, or when the inhaler has been dropped. To prime VENTOLIN HFA, release 4 sprays into the air away from the face, shaking well before each spray. (2.3)
- Cleaning information: At least once a week, wash the actuator with warm water and let it air-dry completely. (2.3)

————DOSAGE FORMS AND STRENGTHS————
Inhalation aerosol: 108 mcg albuterol sulfate (90 mcg albuterol base) from mouthpiece per actuation. Supplied in 18-g canister containing 200 actuations and 8-g canister containing 60 actuations. (3)

————CONTRAINDICATIONS————
Hypersensitivity to albuterol sulfate or any of the ingredients of VENTOLIN HFA. (4)

————WARNINGS AND PRECAUTIONS————
- Paradoxical bronchospasm may occur and should be treated immediately with alternative therapy. (5.1)
- Need for more doses of VENTOLIN HFA than usual may be a sign of deterioration of asthma and requires re-evaluation of treatment. (5.2)
- Cardiovascular effects may occur with beta-adrenergic agonists use. Consider discontinuation of VENTOLIN HFA if these effects occur. Use with caution in patients with underlying cardiovascular disorders. (5.4)
- Immediate hypersensitivity reactions may occur. Discontinue VENTOLIN HFA if immediate hypersensitivity reactions occur. (5.6)

————ADVERSE REACTIONS————
Most common adverse reactions (incidence ≥3%) are throat irritation, viral respiratory infections, upper respiratory inflammation, cough, and musculoskeletal pain. (6)
To report SUSPECTED ADVERSE REACTIONS, contact GlaxoSmithKline at 1-888-825-5249 or FDA at 1-800-FDA-1088 or www.fda.gov/medwatch.

————DRUG INTERACTIONS————
- Beta-blockers: May block bronchodilatory effects of beta-agonists and produce severe bronchospasm. Patients with asthma should not normally be treated with beta-blockers. (7.1)
- Diuretics: Electrocardiographic changes and/or hypokalemia associated with diuretics may worsen with concomitant beta-agonists. Consider monitoring potassium levels. (7.2)
- Monoamine oxidase inhibitors (MAOs) or tricyclic antidepressants: May potentiate effect of albuterol on the vas-

cular system. Consider alternative therapy in patients taking MAOs or tricyclic antidepressants. (7.4)
Revised: June 2009
VNT:6PI
See 17 for PATIENT COUNSELING INFORMATION and FDA-approved patient labeling
Revised: 01/2010

FULL PRESCRIBING INFORMATION

1 INDICATIONS AND USAGE
1.1 Bronchospasm
VENTOLIN HFA is indicated for the treatment or prevention of bronchospasm in patients 4 years of age and older with reversible obstructive airway disease.
1.2 Exercise-Induced Bronchospasm
VENTOLIN HFA is indicated for the prevention of exercise-induced bronchospasm in patients 4 years of age and older.

2 DOSAGE AND ADMINISTRATION
Administer VENTOLIN HFA by oral inhalation only. Shake VENTOLIN HFA well before each spray.
2.1 Bronchospasm
For treatment of acute episodes of bronchospasm or prevention of symptoms associated with bronchospasm, the usual dosage for adults and children is 2 inhalations repeated every 4 to 6 hours; in some patients, 1 inhalation every 4 hours may be sufficient. More frequent administration or a larger number of inhalations is not recommended.
2.2 Exercise-Induced Bronchospasm
The usual dosage for adults and children 4 years of age and older is 2 inhalations 15 to 30 minutes before exercise.
2.3 Administration Information
Priming: Priming VENTOLIN HFA is essential to ensure appropriate albuterol content in each actuation. Prime VENTOLIN HFA before using for the first time, when the inhaler has not been used for more than 2 weeks, or when the inhaler has been dropped. To prime VENTOLIN HFA,

Table 1. Overall Adverse Reactions With ≥3% Incidence in 2 Large 12-Week Clinical Trials in Adolescents and Adults*

	Percent of Patients		
Adverse Reaction	VENTOLIN HFA (n = 202) %	CFC 11/12-Propelled Albuterol Inhaler (n = 207) %	Placebo HFA-134a (n = 201) %
Ear, nose, and throat			
Throat irritation	10	6	7
Upper respiratory inflammation	5	5	2
Lower respiratory			
Viral respiratory infections	7	4	4
Cough	5	2	2
Musculoskeletal			
Musculoskeletal pain	5	5	4

*This table includes all adverse reactions (whether considered by the investigator to be drug-related or unrelated to drug) that occurred at an incidence rate of at least 3.0% in the group treated with VENTOLIN HFA and more frequently in the group treated with VENTOLIN HFA than in the HFA-134a placebo inhaler group.

release 4 sprays into the air away from the face, shaking well before each spray.

Cleaning: To ensure proper dosing and to prevent actuator orifice blockage, wash the actuator with warm water and let it air-dry completely at least once a week.

Dose Counter: VENTOLIN HFA has a dose counter attached to the canister that starts at 204 or 64 and counts down each time a spray is released *[see Dosage Forms and Strengths (3)]*. When the counter reads 020, the patient should contact the pharmacist for a refill of medication or consult the physician to determine whether a prescription refill is needed.

VENTOLIN HFA comes in a moisture-protective foil pouch, which should be removed prior to use. Discard VENTOLIN HFA when the counter reads 000 or 12 months after removal from the moisture-protective foil pouch, whichever comes first *[see Dosage Forms and Strengths (3)]*.

See 17.8 FDA-Approved Patient Labeling for instructions on how to prime and clean the inhaler to ensure proper dosing and to prevent actuator orifice blockage.

3 DOSAGE FORMS AND STRENGTHS

VENTOLIN HFA is an inhalation aerosol. Each actuation contains 108 mcg albuterol sulfate (90 mcg albuterol base) from the mouthpiece. VENTOLIN HFA is supplied as an 18-g pressurized aluminum canister with dose counter fitted with a blue plastic actuator and a blue strapcap; this canister contains 200 actuations. VENTOLIN HFA is also supplied as an 8-g pressurized aluminum canister with dose counter fitted with a blue plastic actuator and a blue strapcap; this canister contains 60 actuations.

4 CONTRAINDICATIONS

VENTOLIN HFA is contraindicated in patients with a history of hypersensitivity to albuterol or any other components of VENTOLIN HFA. Rare cases of hypersensitivity reactions, including urticaria, angioedema, and rash have been reported after the use of albuterol sulfate.

5 WARNINGS AND PRECAUTIONS

5.1 Paradoxical Bronchospasm

Inhaled albuterol sulfate can produce paradoxical bronchospasm, which may be life threatening. If paradoxical bronchospasm occurs, VENTOLIN HFA should be discontinued immediately and alternative therapy instituted. It should be recognized that paradoxical bronchospasm, when associated with inhaled formulations, frequently occurs with the first use of a new canister.

5.2 Deterioration of Asthma

Asthma may deteriorate acutely over a period of hours or chronically over several days or longer. If the patient needs more doses of VENTOLIN HFA than usual, this may be a marker of destabilization of asthma and requires reevaluation of the patient and treatment regimen, giving special consideration to the possible need for anti-inflammatory treatment, e.g., corticosteroids.

5.3 Use of Anti-Inflammatory Agents

The use of beta-adrenergic agonist bronchodilators alone may not be adequate to control asthma in many patients. Early consideration should be given to adding anti-inflammatory agents, e.g., corticosteroids, to the therapeutic regimen.

5.4 Cardiovascular Effects

VENTOLIN HFA, like all other beta$_2$-adrenergic agonists, can produce clinically significant cardiovascular effects in some patients such as changes in pulse rate or blood pressure. If such effects occur, VENTOLIN HFA may need to be discontinued. In addition, beta-agonists have been reported to produce electrocardiogram (ECG) changes, such as flattening of the T wave, prolongation of the QTc interval, and ST segment depression. The clinical relevance of these findings is unknown. Therefore, VENTOLIN HFA, like all other sympathomimetic amines, should be used with caution in patients with underlying cardiovascular disorders, especially coronary insufficiency, cardiac arrhythmias, and hypertension.

5.5 Do Not Exceed Recommended Dose

Fatalities have been reported in association with excessive use of inhaled sympathomimetic drugs in patients with asthma. The exact cause of death is unknown, but cardiac arrest following an unexpected development of a severe acute asthmatic crisis and subsequent hypoxia is suspected.

5.6 Immediate Hypersensitivity Reactions

Immediate hypersensitivity reactions may occur after administration of albuterol sulfate inhalation aerosol, as demonstrated by cases of urticaria, angioedema, rash, bronchospasm, anaphylaxis, and oropharyngeal edema. Discontinue VENTOLIN HFA if immediate hypersensitivity reactions occur.

5.7 Coexisting Conditions

VENTOLIN HFA, like other sympathomimetic amines, should be used with caution in patients with convulsive disorders, hyperthyroidism, or diabetes mellitus and in patients who are unusually responsive to sympathomimetic amines. Large doses of intravenous albuterol have been reported to aggravate preexisting diabetes mellitus and ketoacidosis.

5.8 Hypokalemia

As with other beta-agonists, albuterol may produce significant hypokalemia in some patients, possibly through intracellular shunting, which has the potential to produce adverse cardiovascular effects. The decrease is usually transient, not requiring supplementation.

6 ADVERSE REACTIONS

Use of VENTOLIN HFA may be associated with the following:

- Paradoxical bronchospasm *[see Warnings and Precautions (5.1)]*
- Cardiovascular effects *[see Warnings and Precautions (5.4)]*
- Immediate hypersensitivity reactions *[see Warnings and Precautions (5.6)]*
- Hypokalemia *[see Warnings and Precautions (5.8)]*

6.1 Clinical Trials Experience

The safety data described below reflects exposure to VENTOLIN HFA in 248 patients treated with VENTOLIN HFA in 3 placebo-controlled clinical trials of 2 to 12 weeks' duration. The data from adults and adolescents is based upon 2 clinical trials in which 202 patients with asthma 12 years of age and older were treated with VENTOLIN HFA 2 inhalations 4 times daily for 12 weeks' duration. The adult/adolescent population was 92 female, 110 male and 163 white, 19 black, 18 Hispanic, 2 other. The data from pediatric patients are based upon 1 clinical trial in which 46 patients with asthma 4 to 11 years of age were treated with VENTOLIN HFA 2 inhalations 4 times daily for 2 weeks' duration. The population was 21 female, 25 male and 25 white, 17 black, 3 Hispanic, 1 other.

Because clinical trials are conducted under widely varying conditions, adverse reaction rates observed in the clinical trials of a drug cannot be directly compared to rates in the clinical trials of another drug and may not reflect the rates observed in practice.

Adults and Adolescents 12 Years of Age and Older

The two 12-week, randomized, double-blind studies in 610 adolescent and adult patients with asthma that compared VENTOLIN HFA, a CFC 11/12-propelled albuterol inhaler, and an HFA-134a placebo inhaler. Overall, the incidence and nature of the adverse reactions reported for VENTOLIN HFA and a CFC 11/12-propelled albuterol inhaler were comparable. Table 1 lists the incidence of all adverse reactions (whether considered by the investigator to be related or unrelated to drug) from these studies that occurred at a rate of 3% or greater in the group treated with VENTOLIN HFA and more frequently in the group treated with VENTOLIN HFA than in the HFA-134a placebo inhaler group.

[See table 1 at left]

Adverse reactions reported by less than 3% of the adolescent and adult patients receiving VENTOLIN HFA and by a greater proportion of patients receiving VENTOLIN HFA than receiving HFA-134a placebo inhaler and that have the potential to be related to VENTOLIN HFA include diarrhea, laryngitis, oropharyngeal edema, cough, lung disorders, tachycardia, and extrasystoles. Palpitation and dizziness have also been observed with VENTOLIN HFA.

Pediatric Patients

Results from the 2-week pediatric clinical study in patients with asthma 4 to 11 years of age showed that this pediatric population had an adverse reaction profile similar to that of the adolescent and adult populations.

Three studies have been conducted to evaluate the safety and efficacy of VENTOLIN HFA in patients between birth and 4 years of age. The results of these studies did not establish the efficacy of VENTOLIN HFA in this age-group *[see Pediatric Use (8.4)]*. Since the efficacy of VENTOLIN HFA has not been demonstrated in children between birth and 48 months of age, the safety of VENTOLIN HFA in this age-group cannot be established. However, the safety profile observed in the pediatric population under 4 years of age was comparable to that observed in the older pediatric patients and in adolescents and adults. Where adverse reaction incidence rates were greater in patients under 4 years of age compared with older patients, the higher incidence rates were noted in all treatment arms, including placebo. These adverse reactions included upper respiratory tract infection, nasopharyngitis, pyrexia, and tachycardia.

6.2 Postmarketing Experience

In addition to the adverse reactions listed in section 6.1, the following adverse reactions have been identified during postapproval use of VENTOLIN HFA. Because these reactions are reported voluntarily from a population of uncertain size, it is not always possible to reliably estimate their frequency or establish a causal relationship to drug exposure.

Cases of paradoxical bronchospasm, hoarseness, arrhythmias (including atrial fibrillation, supraventricular tachycardia), and hypersensitivity reactions (including urticaria, angioedema, rash) have been reported after the use of VENTOLIN HFA.

In addition, albuterol, like other sympathomimetic agents, can cause adverse reactions such as hypokalemia, hypertension, peripheral vasodilatation, angina, tremor, central nervous system stimulation, hyperactivity, sleeplessness, headache, muscle cramps, and drying or irritation of the oropharynx.

7 DRUG INTERACTIONS

Other short-acting sympathomimetic aerosol bronchodilators should not be used concomitantly with albuterol. If additional adrenergic drugs are to be administered by any route, they should be used with caution to avoid deleterious cardiovascular effects.

7.1 Beta-Blockers

Beta-adrenergic receptor blocking agents not only block the pulmonary effect of beta-agonists, such as VENTOLIN HFA, but may produce severe bronchospasm in patients with asthma. Therefore, patients with asthma should not normally be treated with beta-blockers. However, under certain circumstances, e.g., as prophylaxis after myocardial infarction, there may be no acceptable alternatives to the use of beta-adrenergic blocking agents in patients with asthma. In this setting, cardioselective beta-blockers should be considered, although they should be administered with caution.

7.2 Diuretics

The ECG changes and/or hypokalemia that may result from the administration of nonpotassium-sparing diuretics (such as loop or thiazide diuretics) can be acutely worsened by beta-agonists, especially when the recommended dose of the beta-agonist is exceeded. Although the clinical relevance of these effects is not known, caution is advised in the coadministration of beta-agonists with nonpotassium-sparing diuretics. Consider monitoring potassium levels.

7.3 Digoxin

Mean decreases of 16% to 22% in serum digoxin levels were demonstrated after single-dose intravenous and oral administration of albuterol, respectively, to normal volunteers who had received digoxin for 10 days. The clinical relevance of these findings for patients with obstructive airway disease who are receiving inhaled albuterol and digoxin on a chronic basis is unclear. Nevertheless, it would be prudent to carefully evaluate the serum digoxin levels in patients who are currently receiving digoxin and albuterol.

IMPORTANT NOTICE: Updated drug information is sent bi-monthly via the PDR® Update Insert. For *monthly* email updates, register at PDR.net.

7.4 Monoamine Oxidase Inhibitors or Tricyclic Antidepressants

VENTOLIN HFA should be administered with extreme caution to patients being treated with monoamine oxidase inhibitors or tricyclic antidepressants, or within 2 weeks of discontinuation of such agents, because the action of albuterol on the vascular system may be potentiated. Consider alternative therapy in patients taking MAOs or tricyclic antidepressants.

8 USE IN SPECIFIC POPULATIONS

8.1 Pregnancy
Teratogenic Effects
Pregnancy Category C.
There are no adequate and well-controlled studies of VENTOLIN HFA or albuterol sulfate in pregnant women. During worldwide marketing experience, various congenital anomalies, including cleft palate and limb defects, have been reported in the offspring of patients being treated with albuterol. Some of the mothers were taking multiple medications during their pregnancies. No consistent pattern of defects can be discerned, and a relationship between albuterol use and congenital anomalies has not been established. Animal reproduction studies in mice and rabbits revealed evidence of teratogenicity. VENTOLIN HFA should be used during pregnancy only if the potential benefit justifies the potential risk to the fetus.

In a mouse reproduction study, subcutaneously administered albuterol sulfate produced cleft palate formation in 5 of 111 (4.5%) fetuses at exposures approximately equal to the maximum recommended human dose (MRHD) for adults on a mg/m² basis and in 10 of 108 (9.3%) fetuses at approximately 8 times the MRHD. Similar effects were not observed at approximately one eleventh of the MRHD. Cleft palate also occurred in 22 of 72 (30.5%) fetuses from females treated subcutaneously with isoproterenol (positive control). In a rabbit reproduction study, orally administered albuterol sulfate produced cranioschisis in 7 of 19 fetuses (37%) at approximately 680 times the MRHD.

In another rabbit study, an albuterol sulfate/HFA-134a formulation administered by inhalation produced enlargement of the frontal portion of the fetal fontanelles at approximately one third of the MRHD [see Animal Toxicology and/or Pharmacology (13.2)].

8.2 Labor and Delivery
Because of the potential for beta-agonist interference with uterine contractility, use of VENTOLIN HFA for relief of bronchospasm during labor should be restricted to those patients in whom the benefits clearly outweigh the risk.

8.3 Nursing Mothers
Plasma levels of albuterol sulfate and HFA-134a after inhaled therapeutic doses are very low in humans, but it is not known whether the components of VENTOLIN HFA are excreted in human milk. Because of the potential for tumorigenicity shown for albuterol in animal studies and lack of experience with the use of VENTOLIN HFA by nursing mothers, a decision should be made whether to discontinue nursing or to discontinue the drug, taking into account the importance of the drug to the mother. Caution should be exercised when VENTOLIN HFA is administered to a nursing woman.

8.4 Pediatric Use
The safety and effectiveness of VENTOLIN HFA in children 4 years of age and older has been established based upon two 12-week clinical trials in patients 12 years of age and older with asthma and one 2-week clinical trial in patients 4 to 11 years of age with asthma [see Clinical Studies (14.1), Adverse Reactions (6.1)]. The safety and effectiveness of VENTOLIN HFA in children under 4 years of age has not been established. Three studies have been conducted to evaluate the safety and efficacy of VENTOLIN HFA in patients under 4 years of age and the findings are described below.

Two 4-week randomized, double-blind, placebo-controlled studies were conducted in 163 pediatric patients from birth to 48 months of age with symptoms of bronchospasm associated with obstructive airway disease (presenting symptoms included: wheeze, cough, dyspnea, or chest tightness). VENTOLIN HFA or placebo HFA was delivered with either an AeroChamber Plus® Valved Holding Chamber or an Optichamber® Valved Holding Chamber with mask 3 times daily. In one study, VENTOLIN HFA 90 mcg (N = 26), VENTOLIN HFA 180 mcg (N = 25), and placebo HFA (N = 26) were administered to children between 24 and 48 months of age. In the second study, VENTOLIN HFA 90 mcg (N = 29), VENTOLIN HFA 180 mcg (N = 29), and placebo HFA (N = 28) were administered to children between birth and 24 months of age. Over the 4-week treatment period, there were no treatment differences in asthma symptom scores between the groups receiving VENTOLIN HFA 90 mcg, VENTOLIN HFA 180 mcg, and placebo in either study.

In a third study, VENTOLIN HFA was evaluated in 87 pediatric patients younger than 24 months of age for the treatment of acute wheezing. VENTOLIN HFA was delivered with an AeroChamber Plus Valved Holding Chamber in this study. There were no significant differences in asthma symptom scores and mean change from baseline in an asthma symptom score between VENTOLIN HFA 180 mcg and VENTOLIN HFA 360 mcg.

In vitro dose characterization studies were performed to evaluate the delivery of VENTOLIN HFA via holding chambers with facemasks. The studies were conducted with 2 different holding chambers with facemasks (small and medium size). The in vitro study data when simulated to patients suggest that the dose of VENTOLIN HFA presented for inhalation via a valved holding chamber with facemask will be comparable to the dose delivered in adults without a spacer and facemask per kilogram of body weight (Table 2). However, clinical studies in children under 4 years of age described above suggest that either the optimal dose of VENTOLIN HFA has not been defined in this age-group or VENTOLIN HFA is not effective in this age-group. The safety and effectiveness of VENTOLIN HFA administered with or without a spacer device in children under 4 years of age has not been demonstrated.
[See table 2 above]

8.5 Geriatric Use
Clinical studies of VENTOLIN HFA did not include sufficient numbers of subjects aged 65 and over to determine whether they respond differently from younger subjects. Other reported clinical experience has not identified differences in responses between the elderly and younger patients. In general, dose selection for an elderly patient should be cautious, usually starting at the low end of the dosing range, reflecting the greater frequency of decreased hepatic, renal, or cardiac function, and of concomitant disease or other drug therapy.

10 OVERDOSAGE
The expected symptoms with overdosage are those of excessive beta-adrenergic stimulation and/or occurrence or exaggeration of any of the symptoms listed under ADVERSE REACTIONS, e.g., seizures, angina, hypertension or hypotension, tachycardia with rates up to 200 beats/min, arrhythmias, nervousness, headache, tremor, dry mouth, palpitation, nausea, dizziness, fatigue, malaise, sleeplessness. Hypokalemia may also occur.

As with all sympathomimetic aerosol medications, cardiac arrest and even death may be associated with abuse of VENTOLIN HFA. Treatment consists of discontinuation of VENTOLIN HFA together with appropriate symptomatic therapy. The judicious use of a cardioselective beta-receptor blocker may be considered, bearing in mind that such medication can produce bronchospasm. There is insufficient evidence to determine if dialysis is beneficial for overdosage of VENTOLIN HFA.

The oral median lethal dose of albuterol sulfate in mice is greater than 2,000 mg/kg (approximately 6,800 times the maximum recommended daily inhalation dose for adults on a mg/m² basis and approximately 3,200 times the maximum recommended daily inhalation dose for children on a mg/m² basis). In mature rats, the subcutaneous median lethal dose of albuterol sulfate is approximately 450 mg/kg (approximately 3,000 times the maximum recommended daily inhalation dose for adults on a mg/m² basis and approximately 1,400 times the maximum recommended daily inhalation dose for children on a mg/m² basis). In young rats, the subcutaneous median lethal dose is approximately 2,000 mg/kg (approximately 14,000 times the maximum recommended daily inhalation dose for adults on a mg/m² basis and approximately 6,400 times the maximum recommended daily inhalation dose for children on a mg/m² basis). The inhalation median lethal dose has not been determined in animals.

11 DESCRIPTION
The active component of VENTOLIN HFA is albuterol sulfate, USP, the racemic form of albuterol and a relatively selective beta₂-adrenergic bronchodilator. Albuterol sulfate has the chemical name α^1-[(*tert*-butylamino)methyl]-4-hydroxy-*m*-xylene-α, α'-diol sulfate (2:1)(salt) and the following chemical structure:

Albuterol sulfate is a white crystalline powder with a molecular weight of 576.7, and the empirical formula is $(C_{13}H_{21}NO_3)_2 \cdot H_2SO_4$. It is soluble in water and slightly soluble in ethanol.

The World Health Organization recommended name for albuterol base is salbutamol.

VENTOLIN HFA is a pressurized metered-dose aerosol unit fitted with a counter. VENTOLIN HFA is intended for oral inhalation only. Each unit contains a microcrystalline suspension of albuterol sulfate in propellant HFA-134a (1,1,1,2-tetrafluoroethane). It contains no other excipients.

Priming VENTOLIN HFA is essential to ensure appropriate albuterol content in each actuation. To prime the inhaler, release 4 sprays into the air away from the face, shaking well before each spray. The inhaler should be primed before using it for the first time, when it has not been used for more than 2 weeks, or when it has been dropped.

After priming, each actuation of the inhaler delivers 120 mcg of albuterol sulfate, USP in 75 mg of suspension from the valve and 108 mcg of albuterol sulfate, USP from the mouthpiece (equivalent to 90 mcg of albuterol base from the mouthpiece).

Each 18-g canister provides 200 inhalations. Each 8-g canister provides 60 inhalations.

This product does not contain chlorofluorocarbons (CFCs) as the propellant.

12 CLINICAL PHARMACOLOGY
12.1 Mechanism of Action
In vitro studies and in vivo pharmacologic studies have demonstrated that albuterol has a preferential effect on beta₂-adrenergic receptors compared with isoproterenol. While it is recognized that beta₂-adrenergic receptors are the predominant receptors in bronchial smooth muscle, data indicate that there is a population of beta₂-receptors in the

---

Table 2: In Vitro Medication Delivery Through AeroChamber Plus® Valved Holding Chamber With a Facemask

Age	Facemask	Flow Rate (L/min)	Holding Time (seconds)	Mean Medication Delivery Through AeroChamber Plus (mcg/actuation)	Body Weight 50th Percentile (kg)*	Medication Delivered per Actuation (mcg/kg)†
6 to 12 Months	Small	4.9	0	18.2	7.5-9.9	1.8-2.4
			2	19.8		2.0-2.6
			5	13.8		1.4-1.8
			10	15.4		1.6-2.1
2 to 5 Years	Small	8.0	0	17.8	12.3-18.0	1.0-1.4
			2	16.0		0.9-1.3
			5	16.3		0.9-1.3
			10	18.3		1.0-1.5
2 to 5 Years	Medium	8.0	0	21.1	12.3-18.0	1.2-1.7
			2	15.3		0.8-1.2
			5	18.3		1.0-1.5
			10	18.2		1.0-1.5
>5 Years	Medium	12.0	0	26.8	18.0	1.5
			2	20.9		1.2
			5	19.6		1.1
			10	20.3		1.1

* Centers for Disease Control growth charts, developed by the National Center for Health Statistics in collaboration with the National Center for Chronic Disease Prevention and Health Promotion (2000). Ranges correspond to the average of the 50th percentile weight for boys and girls at the ages indicated.
† A single inhalation of VENTOLIN HFA in a 70-kg adult without use of a valved holding chamber and facemask delivers approximately 90 mcg, or 1.3 mcg/kg.

human heart existing in a concentration between 10% and 50% of cardiac beta-adrenergic receptors. The precise function of these receptors has not been established *[see Warnings and Precautions (5.4)]*.

Activation of beta$_2$-adrenergic receptors on airway smooth muscle leads to the activation of adenylcyclase and to an increase in the intracellular concentration of cyclic-3′,5′-adenosine monophosphate (cyclic AMP). This increase of cyclic AMP leads to the activation of protein kinase A, which inhibits the phosphorylation of myosin and lowers intracellular ionic calcium concentrations, resulting in relaxation. Albuterol relaxes the smooth muscles of all airways, from the trachea to the terminal bronchioles. Albuterol acts as a functional antagonist to relax the airway irrespective of the spasmogen involved, thus protecting against all bronchoconstrictor challenges. Increased cyclic AMP concentrations are also associated with the inhibition of release of mediators from mast cells in the airway.

Albuterol has been shown in most controlled clinical trials to have more effect on the respiratory tract, in the form of bronchial smooth muscle relaxation, than isoproterenol at comparable doses while producing fewer cardiovascular effects. Controlled clinical studies and other clinical experience have shown that inhaled albuterol, like other beta-adrenergic agonist drugs, can produce a significant cardiovascular effect in some patients, as measured by pulse rate, blood pressure, symptoms, and/or electrocardiographic changes *[see Warnings and Precautions (5.4)]*

12.2 Pharmacokinetics

The systemic levels of albuterol are low after inhalation of recommended doses. A study conducted in 12 healthy male and female subjects using a higher dose (1,080 mcg of albuterol base) showed that mean peak plasma concentrations of approximately 3 ng/mL occurred after dosing when albuterol was delivered using propellant HFA-134a. The mean time to peak concentrations (T_{max}) was delayed after administration of VENTOLIN HFA (T_{max} = 0.42 hours) as compared to CFC-propelled albuterol inhaler (T_{max} = 0.17 hours). Apparent terminal plasma half-life of albuterol is approximately 4.6 hours. No further pharmacokinetic studies for VENTOLIN HFA were conducted in neonates, children, or elderly subjects.

13 NONCLINICAL TOXICOLOGY

13.1 Carcinogenesis, Mutagenesis, Impairment of Fertility

In a 2-year study in Sprague-Dawley rats, albuterol sulfate caused a dose-related increase in the incidence of benign leiomyomas of the mesovarium at and above dietary doses of 2.0 mg/kg (approximately 14 times the maximum recommended daily inhalation dose for adults on a mg/m^2 basis and approximately 6 times the maximum recommended daily inhalation dose for children on a mg/m^2 basis). In another study this effect was blocked by the coadministration of propranolol, a non-selective beta-adrenergic antagonist.

In an 18-month study in CD-1 mice, albuterol sulfate showed no evidence of tumorigenicity at dietary doses of up to 500 mg/kg (approximately 1,700 times the maximum recommended daily inhalation dose for adults on a mg/m^2 basis and approximately 800 times the maximum recommended daily inhalation dose for children on a mg/m^2 basis). In a 22-month study in Golden hamsters, albuterol sulfate showed no evidence of tumorigenicity at dietary doses of up to 50 mg/kg (approximately 225 times the maximum recommended daily inhalation dose for adults on a mg/m^2 basis and approximately 110 times the maximum recommended daily inhalation dose for children on a mg/m^2 basis).

Albuterol sulfate was not mutagenic in the Ames test or a mutation test in yeast. Albuterol sulfate was not clastogenic in a human peripheral lymphocyte assay or in an AH1 strain mouse micronucleus assay.

Reproduction studies in rats demonstrated no evidence of impaired fertility at oral doses of albuterol sulfate up to 50 mg/kg (approximately 340 times the maximum recommended daily inhalation dose for adults on a mg/m^2 basis).

13.2 Animal Toxicology and/or Pharmacology

Preclinical: Intravenous studies in rats with albuterol sulfate have demonstrated that albuterol crosses the blood-brain barrier and reaches brain concentrations amounting to approximately 5.0% of the plasma concentrations. In structures outside the blood-brain barrier (pineal and pituitary glands), albuterol concentrations were found to be 100 times those in the whole brain.

Studies in laboratory animals (minipigs, rodents, and dogs) have demonstrated the occurrence of cardiac arrhythmias and sudden death (with histologic evidence of myocardial necrosis) when beta-agonists and methylxanthines are administered concurrently. The clinical relevance of these findings is unknown.

Propellant HFA-134a is devoid of pharmacological activity except at very high doses in animals (380 to 1,300 times the maximum human exposure based on comparisons of AUC values), primarily producing ataxia, tremors, dyspnea, or salivation. These are similar to effects produced by the structurally related CFCs, which have been used extensively in metered-dose inhalers.

In animals and humans, propellant HFA-134a was found to be rapidly absorbed and rapidly eliminated, with an elimination half-life of 3 to 27 minutes in animals and 5 to 7 minutes in humans. Time to maximum plasma concentration (T_{max}) and mean residence time are both extremely short, leading to a transient appearance of HFA-134a in the blood with no evidence of accumulation.

Reproductive Toxicology Studies: A study in CD-1 mice given albuterol sulfate subcutaneously showed cleft palate formation in 5 of 111 (4.5%) fetuses at 0.25 mg/kg (less than the maximum recommended daily inhalation dose for adults on a mg/m^2 basis) and in 10 of 108 (9.3%) fetuses at 2.5 mg/kg (approximately 8 times the maximum recommended daily inhalation dose for adults on a mg/m^2 basis). The drug did not induce cleft palate formation at a dose of 0.025 mg/kg (less than the maximum recommended daily inhalation dose for adults on a mg/m^2 basis). Cleft palate also occurred in 22 of 72 (30.5%) fetuses from females treated subcutaneously with 2.5 mg/kg of isoproterenol (positive control).

A reproduction study in Stride Dutch rabbits revealed cranioschisis in 7 of 19 fetuses (37%) when albuterol sulfate was administered orally at a 50 mg/kg dose (approximately 680 times the maximum recommended daily inhalation dose for adults on a mg/m^2 basis).

In an inhalation reproduction study in New Zealand white rabbits, albuterol sulfate/HFA-134a formulation exhibited enlargement of the frontal portion of the fetal fontanelles at and above inhalation doses of 0.0193 mg/kg (less than the maximum recommended daily inhalation dose for adults on a mg/m^2 basis).

A study in which pregnant rats were dosed with radiolabeled albuterol sulfate demonstrated that drug-related material is transferred from the maternal circulation to the fetus.

14 CLINICAL STUDIES

14.1 Bronchospasm Associated With Asthma

Adult and Adolescent Patients 12 Years of Age and Older

The efficacy of VENTOLIN HFA was evaluated in two 12-week, randomized, double-blind, placebo controlled trials in patients 12 years of age and older with mild to moderate asthma. These trials included a total of 610 patients (323 males, 287 females). In each trial, patients received 2 inhalations of VENTOLIN HFA, CFC 11/12-propelled albuterol, or HFA-134a placebo 4 times daily for 12 weeks' duration. Patients taking the HFA-134a placebo inhaler also took VENTOLIN HFA for asthma symptom relief on an as-needed basis. Some patients who participated in these clinical trials were using concomitant inhaled steroid therapy. Efficacy was assessed by serial forced expiratory volume in 1 second (FEV$_1$). In each of these trials, 2 inhalations of VENTOLIN HFA produced significantly greater improvement in FEV$_1$ over the pretreatment value than placebo. Results from the 2 clinical trials are described below.

In a 12-week, randomized, double-blind study, VENTOLIN HFA (101 patients) was compared to CFC 11/12-propelled albuterol (99 patients) and an HFA-134a placebo inhaler (97 patients) in adolescent and adult patients 12 to 76 years of age with mild to moderate asthma. Serial FEV$_1$ measurements [shown below as percent change from test-day baseline at Day 1 (n = 297) and at Week 12 (n = 249)] demonstrated that 2 inhalations of VENTOLIN HFA produced significantly greater improvement in FEV$_1$ over the pretreatment value than placebo.

[See first figure at top of next column]

[See second figure in next column]

In the responder population (≥15% increase in FEV$_1$ within 30 minutes postdose) treated with VENTOLIN HFA, the mean time to onset of a 15% increase in FEV$_1$ over the pretreatment value was 5.4 minutes, and the mean time to peak effect was 56 minutes. The mean duration of effect as measured by a 15% increase in FEV$_1$ over the pretreatment value was approximately 4 hours. In some patients, duration of effect was as long as 6 hours.

The second 12-week randomized, double-blind study was conducted to evaluate the efficacy and safety of switching patients from CFC 11/12-propelled albuterol to VENTOLIN HFA. During the 3-week run-in phase of the study, all patients received CFC 11/12-propelled albuterol. During the double-blind treatment phase, VENTOLIN HFA (91 patients) was compared to CFC 11/12-propelled albuterol (100 patients) and an HFA-134a placebo inhaler (95 patients) in adolescent and adult patients with mild to moderate asthma. Serial FEV$_1$ measurements demonstrated that 2 inhalations of VENTOLIN HFA produced significantly greater improvement in pulmonary function than placebo. The switching from CFC 11/12-propelled albuterol inhaler to VENTOLIN HFA did not reveal any clinically significant changes in the efficacy profile.

FEV$_1$ as Percent Change From Predose in a Large, 12-Week Clinical Trial

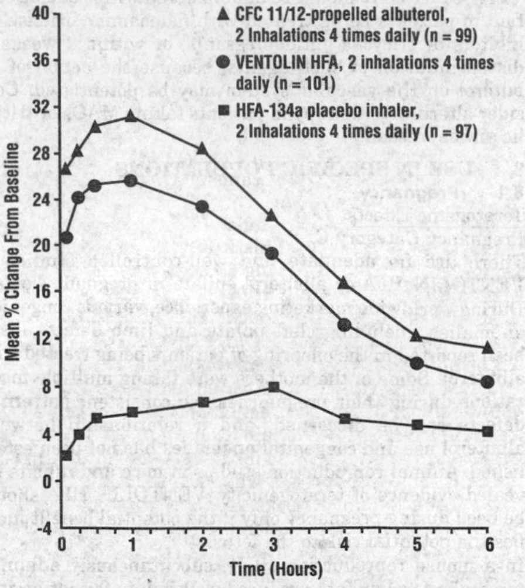

Day 1

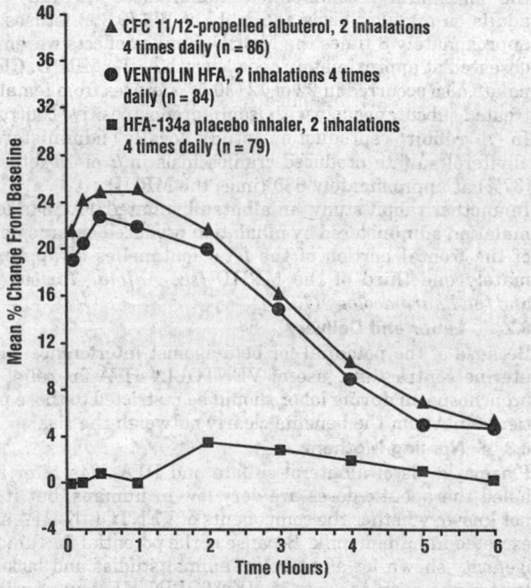

Week 12

In the 2 adult studies, the efficacy results from VENTOLIN HFA were significantly greater than placebo and were clinically comparable to those achieved with CFC 11/12-propelled albuterol, although small numerical differences in mean FEV$_1$ response and other measures were observed. Physicians should recognize that individual responses to beta-adrenergic agonists administered via different propellants may vary and that equivalent responses in individual patients should not be assumed.

Pediatric Patients 4 Years of Age

The efficacy of VENTOLIN HFA was evaluated in one 2-week, randomized, double-blind, placebo-controlled trial in 135 pediatric patients 4 to 11 years of age with mild to moderate asthma. In this trial, patients received VENTOLIN HFA, CFC 11/12-propelled albuterol, or HFA-134a placebo. Serial pulmonary function measurements demonstrated that 2 inhalations of VENTOLIN HFA produced significantly greater improvement in pulmonary function than placebo and that there were no significant differences between the groups treated with VENTOLIN HFA and CFC 11/12-propelled albuterol. In the responder population treated with VENTOLIN HFA, the mean time to onset of a 15% increase in peak expiratory flow rate (PEFR) over the pretreatment value was 7.8 minutes, and the mean time to peak effect was approximately 90 minutes. The mean duration of effect as measured by a 15% increase in PEFR over the pretreatment value was greater than 3 hours. In some patients, duration of effect was as long as 6 hours.

14.2 Exercise-Induced Bronchospasm

One controlled clinical study in adult patients with asthma (N = 24) demonstrated that 2 inhalations of VENTOLIN HFA taken approximately 30 minutes prior to exercise significantly prevented exercise-induced bronchospasm (as measured by maximum percentage fall in FEV$_1$ following exercise) compared to an HFA-134a placebo inhaler. In addition, VENTOLIN HFA was shown to be clinically comparable to a CFC 11/12-propelled albuterol inhaler for this indication.

16   HOW SUPPLIED/STORAGE AND HANDLING

VENTOLIN HFA (albuterol sulfate) Inhalation Aerosol is supplied in the following packs as a pressurized aluminum canister fitted with a counter with a blue plastic actuator and a blue strapcap packaged within a moisture-protective foil pouch that also contains a desiccant:

NDC 0173-0682-20   18-g canister containing 200 actuations

NDC 0173-0682-21   8-g canister containing 60 actuations

NDC 0173-0682-24   8-g institutional pack canister containing 60 actuations

Before using, VENTOLIN HFA should be removed from the moisture-protective foil pouch. The pouch and dessicant should be discarded. VENTOLIN HFA should be discarded 12 months after removal from the pouch.

Priming VENTOLIN HFA is essential to ensure appropriate albuterol content in each actuation. To prime the inhaler, release 4 sprays into the air away from the face, shaking well before each spray. The inhaler should be primed before using it for the first time, when the inhaler has not been used for more than 2 weeks, or when it has been dropped. After priming, each actuation delivers 120 mcg of albuterol sulfate, USP in 75 mg of suspension from the valve and 108 mcg of albuterol sulfate, USP from the mouthpiece (equivalent to 90 mcg of albuterol base from the mouthpiece).

To ensure proper dosing and to prevent actuator orifice blockage, wash the actuator with warm water and let it air-dry completely at least once a week *[see FDA-Approved Patient Labeling (17.8)]*.

The blue actuator supplied with VENTOLIN HFA should not be used with any other product canisters, and actuators from other products should not be used with a VENTOLIN HFA canister.

VENTOLIN HFA has a counter attached to the canister. The counter starts at 204 or 64 and counts down each time a spray is released. The correct amount of medication in each inhalation cannot be assured after the counter reads 000, even though the canister is not completely empty and will continue to operate. VENTOLIN HFA should be discarded when the counter reads 000 or 12 months after removal from the moisture-protective foil pouch, whichever comes first. Never immerse the canister in water to determine the amount of drug remaining in the canister.

Keep out of reach of children. Avoid spraying in eyes.

Contents Under Pressure: Do not puncture. Do not use or store near heat or open flame. Exposure to temperatures above 120°F may cause bursting. Never throw container into fire or incinerator.

Store between 15° and 25°C (59° and 77°F). Store the inhaler with the mouthpiece down. For best results, the inhaler should be at room temperature before use. SHAKE WELL BEFORE EACH SPRAY.

VENTOLIN HFA does not contain chlorofluorocarbons (CFCs) as the propellant.

17   PATIENT COUNSELING INFORMATION

See FDA-Approved Patient Labeling (17.8)

17.1   Frequency of Use

The action of VENTOLIN HFA should last up to 4 to 6 hours. VENTOLIN HFA should not be used more frequently than recommended. Do not increase the dose or frequency of doses of VENTOLIN HFA without consulting the physician. If patients find that treatment with VENTOLIN HFA becomes less effective for symptomatic relief, symptoms become worse, and/or they need to use the product more frequently than usual, they should seek medical attention immediately.

17.2   Priming and Cleaning

Priming: Patients should be instructed that priming VENTOLIN HFA is essential to ensure appropriate albuterol content in each actuation. Patients should prime VENTOLIN HFA before using for the first time, when the inhaler has not been used for more than 2 weeks, or when the inhaler has been dropped. To prime VENTOLIN HFA, patients should release 4 sprays into the air away from the face, shaking well before each spray.

Cleaning: To ensure proper dosing and to prevent actuator orifice blockage, patients should be instructed to wash the actuator and dry thoroughly at least once a week. Patients should be informed that detailed cleaning instructions are included in the Information for the Patient leaflet.

17.3   Dose Counter

Patients should be informed that VENTOLIN HFA has a dose counter that starts at 204 or 64 and counts down each time a spray is released. Patients should be informed to discard VENTOLIN HFA when the counter reads 000 or 12 months after removal from the moisture-protective foil pouch, whichever comes first. When the counter reads 020, the patient should contact the pharmacist for a refill of med-

ication or consult the physician to determine whether a prescription refill is needed. Patients should never try to alter the numbers or remove the counter from the metal canister. Patients should never immerse the canister in water to determine the amount of drug remaining in the canister.

17.4   Paradoxical Bronchospasm

Patients should be informed that VENTOLIN HFA can produce paradoxical bronchospasm. If paradoxical bronchospasm occurs, patients should discontinue VENTOLIN HFA.

17.5   Concomitant Drug Use

While patients are using VENTOLIN HFA, other inhaled drugs and asthma medications should be taken only as directed by the physician.

17.6   Common Adverse Effects

Common adverse effects of treatment with inhaled albuterol include palpitations, chest pain, rapid heart rate, tremor, and nervousness.

17.7   Pregnancy

Patients who are pregnant or nursing should contact their physicians about the use of VENTOLIN HFA.

17.8   FDA-Approved Patient Labeling

See tear-off leaflet below.

VENTOLIN is a registered trademark of GlaxoSmithKline.

AeroChamber Plus is a registered trademark of Monaghan Medical Inc.

OptiChamber is a registered trademark of Respironics Inc.

GlaxoSmithKline

Research Triangle Park, NC 27709

©2009, GlaxoSmithKline. All rights reserved.

PHARMACIST—DETACH HERE AND GIVE LEAFLET TO PATIENT

INFORMATION FOR THE PATIENT

VENTOLIN® HFA Inhalation Aerosol

(albuterol sulfate)

Read this leaflet carefully before you start to use VENTOLIN HFA.

Keep this leaflet because it has important summary information about VENTOLIN HFA. Your healthcare provider has more information or advice.

Read the new leaflet that comes with each refill of your prescription because there may be new information.

What is VENTOLIN HFA?

VENTOLIN HFA is a kind of medicine called a fast-acting bronchodilator. Fast-acting bronchodilators help to quickly open the airways in your lungs so that you can breathe more easily.

Each dose of VENTOLIN HFA should last up to 4 to 6 hours. Take VENTOLIN HFA as directed by your doctor. Do not take extra doses or take more often without asking your doctor.

Get medical help right away if VENTOLIN HFA no longer helps your symptoms. Also get medical help if your symptoms get worse or if you need to use your inhaler more often. While you are using VENTOLIN HFA, use other inhaled medicines and asthma medicines only as directed by your doctor. Tell your doctor if you are pregnant or nursing, and ask about the use of VENTOLIN HFA.

Possible side effects of taking VENTOLIN HFA include fast or irregular heartbeat, chest pain, shakiness, and nervousness. With the first use of a new canister, worsening of wheezing may occur.

The parts of your VENTOLIN HFA inhaler:

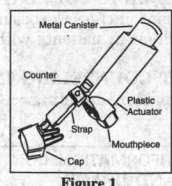

Figure 1

There are 2 main parts to your VENTOLIN HFA inhaler—the metal canister that holds the medicine and the blue plastic actuator that sprays the medicine from the canister (see Figure 1).

The inhaler also has a cap that covers the mouthpiece of the actuator. The strap on the cap will stay attached to the actuator.

Do not use the actuator with a canister of medicine from any other inhaler. And do not use a VENTOLIN HFA canister with an actuator from any other inhaler.

The canister has a counter to show how many sprays of medicine you have left. The number shows through a window in the back of the actuator.

The counter starts at either 204 or at 64, depending on which size inhaler you have. The number will count down by 1 each time you spray the inhaler. The counter will stop counting at 000.

Never try to change the numbers or take the counter off the metal canister. The counter cannot be reset, and it is permanently attached to the canister.

How to Use Your VENTOLIN HFA

Before using your VENTOLIN HFA

Take the inhaler out of the foil pouch. Safely throw away the pouch and the drying packet that comes inside the pouch. The counter should read 204 or 64.

If a child needs help using the inhaler, an adult should help the child use the inhaler with or without a holding chamber attached to a facemask. The adult should follow the instructions that came with the holding chamber. An adult should watch a child use the inhaler to be sure it is used correctly. The inhaler should be at room temperature before you use it.

Check each time to make sure the canister fits firmly in the plastic actuator. Also look into the mouthpiece to make sure there are no foreign objects there, especially if the strap is no longer attached to the actuator or if the cap is not being used to cover the mouthpiece.

Priming your VENTOLIN HFA

You must prime the inhaler to get the right amount of medicine. Prime the inhaler before you use it for the first time, if you have not used it for more than 14 days, or if it has been dropped. To prime the inhaler, take the cap off the mouthpiece of the actuator. Then shake the inhaler well, and spray it into the air away from your face. Shake and spray the inhaler like this 3 more times to finish priming it. The counter should now read 200 or 60.

Instructions for taking a dose from your VENTOLIN HFA:

Read through the 6 steps below before using VENTOLIN HFA. If you have any questions, ask your doctor or pharmacist.

1. Take the cap off the mouthpiece of the actuator. **Shake the inhaler well** before each spray.

2. Hold the inhaler with the mouthpiece down (see Figure 2). **Breathe out through your mouth** and push as much air from your lungs as you can. Put the mouthpiece in your mouth and close your lips around it.

3. **Push the top of the canister all the way down while you breathe in deeply and slowly through your mouth** (see Figure 3). Right after the spray comes out, take your finger off the canister. After you have breathed in all the way, take the inhaler out of your mouth and close your mouth.

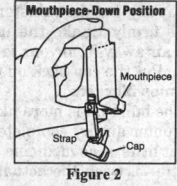

Figure 2

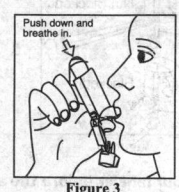

Figure 3

4. **Hold your breath as long as you can,** up to 10 seconds, then breathe normally.

5. If your doctor has prescribed more sprays, wait 1 minute and **shake** the inhaler again. Repeat steps 2 through 4.

6. Put the cap back on the mouthpiece after every time you use the inhaler, and make sure it snaps firmly into place.

When to Replace Your VENTOLIN HFA

• **When the counter reads 020,** you should refill your prescription or ask your doctor if you need another prescription for VENTOLIN HFA.

• **Throw the inhaler away** when the counter reads 000 or 12 months after you have taken the inhaler out of the foil pouch, whichever happens first. You should not keep using the inhaler when the counter reads 000 because you will not receive the right amount of medicine.

• **Do not use the inhaler** after the expiration date, which is on the packaging it comes in.

How to Clean Your VENTOLIN HFA

It is very important to keep the plastic actuator clean so the medicine will not build-up and block the spray. Do not try to clean the metal canister or let it get wet. The inhaler may stop spraying if it is not cleaned correctly.

Wash the actuator at least once a week.

Cleaning instructions:

1. Take the canister out of the actuator, and take the cap off the mouthpiece. The strap on the cap will stay attached to the actuator.

2. Wash the actuator through the top with warm running water for 30 seconds (see Figure 4). Then wash the actuator again through the mouthpiece (see Figure 5).

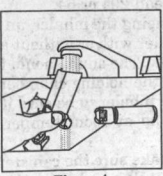

Figure 4

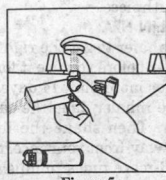

Figure 5

3. Shake off as much water from the actuator as you can. Look into the mouthpiece to make sure any medicine build-up has been completely washed away. If there is any build-up, repeat step 2.

4. Let the actuator air-dry completely, such as overnight (see Figure 6).

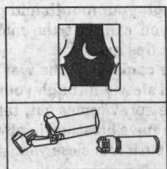

Figure 6

5. When the actuator is dry, put the canister in the actuator and make sure it fits firmly. Shake the inhaler well and spray it once into the air away from your face. (The counter will count down by 1.) Put the cap back on the mouthpiece.

If your actuator becomes blocked:

Blockage from medicine build-up is more likely to happen if you do not let the actuator air-dry completely. If the actuator gets blocked so that little or no medicine comes out of the mouthpiece (see Figure 7), wash the actuator as described in cleaning steps 1-5.

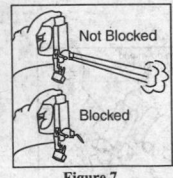

Not Blocked

Blocked

Figure 7

If you need to use your inhaler before the actuator is completely dry, shake as much water off the actuator as you can. Put the canister in the actuator and make sure it fits firmly. Shake the inhaler well and spray it once into the air away from your face. Then take your dose as prescribed. Then clean and air-dry it completely.

Storing Your VENTOLIN HFA

Store at room temperature with the mouthpiece down. Keep out of reach of children.

Contents Under Pressure: Do not puncture. Do not use or store near heat or open flame. Exposure to temperatures above 120°F may cause bursting. Never throw into fire or incinerator.

GlaxoSmithKline
Research Triangle Park, NC 27709
©2009, GlaxoSmithKline. All rights reserved.
June 2009 VNT:6PIL

VERAMYST®   ℞
[ver' ə-mist]
(fluticasone furoate)
Nasal Spray

HIGHLIGHTS OF PRESCRIBING INFORMATION
These highlights do not include all the information needed to use VERAMYST safely and effectively. See full prescribing information for VERAMYST.
VERAMYST (fluticasone furoate) Nasal Spray
Initial U.S. Approval: 2007

---RECENT MAJOR CHANGES---
Contraindications (4)   September 2009
Warnings and Precautions (5.3)   September 2009

---INDICATIONS AND USAGE---
VERAMYST Nasal Spray is a corticosteroid indicated for treatment of symptoms of seasonal and perennial allergic rhinitis in adults and children ≥2 years. (1.1)

---DOSAGE AND ADMINISTRATION---
For intranasal use only. Usual starting dosages:
• Adults and adolescents ≥12 years: 110 mcg (2 sprays per nostril) once daily. (2.1)
• Children 2-11 years: 55 mcg (1 spray per nostril) once daily. (2.2)
• Priming Information: Prime VERAMYST Nasal Spray before using for the first time, when not used for more than 30 days, or if the cap has been left off the bottle for 5 days or longer. (2)

---DOSAGE FORMS AND STRENGTHS---
Nasal spray: 27.5 mcg of fluticasone furoate in each 50-microliter spray. (3)
Supplied in 10-g bottle containing 120 sprays. (16)

---CONTRAINDICATIONS---
Hypersensitivity to ingredients. (4)

---WARNINGS AND PRECAUTIONS---
• Epistaxis, nasal ulceration, *Candida albicans* infection, nasal septal perforation, impaired wound healing. Monitor patients periodically for signs of adverse effects on the nasal mucosa. Avoid use in patients with recent nasal ulcers, nasal surgery, or nasal trauma. (5.1)
• Development of glaucoma or posterior subcapsular cataracts. Monitor patients closely with a change in vision or with a history of increased intraocular pressure, glaucoma, and/or cataracts. (5.2)
• Hypersensitivity reactions, including anaphylaxis, angioedema, rash, and urticaria, may occur after administration of VERAMYST Nasal Spray. (5.3)
• Potential worsening of existing tuberculosis; fungal, bacterial, viral, or parasitic infections; or ocular herpes simplex. More serious or even fatal course of chickenpox or measles in susceptible patients. Use caution in patients with the above because of the potential for worsening of these infections. (5.4)
• Hypercorticism and adrenal suppression with very high dosages or at the regular dosage in susceptible individuals. If such changes occur, discontinue VERAMYST Nasal Spray slowly. (5.5)
• Potential reduction in growth velocity in children. Monitor growth routinely in pediatric patients receiving VERAMYST Nasal Spray. (5.7, 8.4)

---ADVERSE REACTIONS---
The most common adverse reactions (>1% incidence) included headache, epistaxis, pharyngolaryngeal pain, nasal ulceration, back pain, pyrexia, and cough. (6.1)
To report SUSPECTED ADVERSE REACTIONS, contact GlaxoSmithKline at 1-888-825-5249 or FDA at 1-800-FDA-1088 or www.fda.gov/medwatch.

---DRUG INTERACTIONS---
Potent inhibitors of cytochrome P450 (CYP) 3A4 may increase exposure to fluticasone furoate.
• Coadministration of ritonavir is not recommended. (5.5, 7)
• Use caution with coadministration of other potent CYP 3A4 inhibitors, such as ketoconazole. (5.6, 7)

---USE IN SPECIFIC POPULATIONS---
Hepatic impairment may increase exposure to fluticasone furoate. Use with caution in patients with severe hepatic impairment. (8.6)
See 17 for PATIENT COUNSELING INFORMATION and FDA-approved patient labeling

Revised: 04/2010

FULL PRESCRIBING INFORMATION: CONTENTS*
* Sections or subsections omitted from the full prescribing information are not listed

---

FULL PRESCRIBING INFORMATION

1   INDICATIONS AND USAGE
1.1   Treatment of Allergic Rhinitis
VERAMYST® (fluticasone furoate) Nasal Spray is indicated for the treatment of the symptoms of seasonal and perennial allergic rhinitis in patients aged 2 years and older.

2   DOSAGE AND ADMINISTRATION
Administer VERAMYST Nasal Spray by the intranasal route only. Prime VERAMYST Nasal Spray before using for the first time by shaking the contents well and releasing 6 sprays into the air away from the face. When VERAMYST Nasal Spray has not been used for more than 30 days or if the cap has been left off the bottle for 5 days or longer, prime the pump again until a fine mist appears. Shake VERAMYST Nasal Spray well before each use.
2.1   Adults and Adolescents Aged 12 Years and Older
The recommended starting dosage is 110 mcg once daily administered as 2 sprays (27.5 mcg/spray) in each nostril. Titrate an individual patient to the minimum effective dosage to reduce the possibility of side effects. When the maximum benefit has been achieved and symptoms have been controlled, reducing the dosage to 55 mcg (1 spray in each nostril) once daily may be effective in maintaining control of allergic rhinitis symptoms.
2.2   Children Aged 2 to 11 Years
The recommended starting dosage in children is 55 mcg once daily administered as 1 spray (27.5 mcg/spray) in each nostril. Children not adequately responding to 55 mcg may use 110 mcg (2 sprays in each nostril) once daily. Once symptoms have been controlled, the dosage may be decreased to 55 mcg once daily.

3   DOSAGE FORMS AND STRENGTHS
VERAMYST Nasal Spray is a nasal spray suspension. Each spray (50 microliters) delivers 27.5 mcg of fluticasone furoate.

4   CONTRAINDICATIONS
VERAMYST Nasal Spray is contraindicated in patients with hypersensitivity to any of its ingredients [see Warnings and Precautions (5.3)].

5   WARNINGS AND PRECAUTIONS
5.1   Local Nasal Effects
Epistaxis and Nasal Ulceration
In clinical studies of 2 to 52 weeks' duration, epistaxis and nasal ulcerations were observed more frequently and some epistaxis events were more severe in patients treated with VERAMYST Nasal Spray than those who received placebo [see Adverse Reactions (6)].
Candida Infection
Evidence of localized infections of the nose with *Candida albicans* was seen on nasal exams in 7 of 2,745 patients treated with VERAMYST Nasal Spray during clinical trials and was reported as an adverse event in 3 patients. When such an infection develops, it may require treatment with appropriate local therapy and discontinuation of VERAMYST Nasal Spray. Therefore, patients using VERAMYST Nasal Spray over several months or longer should be examined periodically for evidence of *Candida* infection or other signs of adverse effects on the nasal mucosa.
Nasal Septal Perforation
Instances of nasal septal perforation have been reported in patients following the intranasal application of corticosteroids. There were no instances of nasal septal perforation observed in clinical studies with VERAMYST Nasal Spray.

Impaired Wound Healing
Because of the inhibitory effect of corticosteroids on wound healing, patients who have experienced recent nasal ulcers, nasal surgery, or nasal trauma should not use VERAMYST Nasal Spray until healing has occurred.

5.2 Glaucoma and Cataracts
Nasal and inhaled corticosteroids may result in the development of glaucoma and/or cataracts. Therefore, close monitoring is warranted in patients with a change in vision or with a history of increased intraocular pressure, glaucoma, and/or cataracts.
Glaucoma and cataract formation was evaluated with intraocular pressure measurements and slit lamp examinations in 1 controlled 12-month study in 806 adolescent and adult patients aged 12 years and older and in 1 controlled 12-week study in 558 children aged 2 to 11 years. The patients had perennial allergic rhinitis and were treated with either VERAMYST Nasal Spray (110 mcg once daily in adult and adolescent patients and 55 or 110 mcg once daily in pediatric patients) or placebo. Intraocular pressure remained within the normal range (<21 mmHg) in ≥98% of the patients in any treatment group in both studies. However, in the 12-month study in adolescents and adults, 12 patients, all treated with VERAMYST Nasal Spray 110 mcg once daily, had intraocular pressure measurements that increased above normal levels (≥21 mmHg). In the same study, 7 patients (6 treated with VERAMYST Nasal Spray 110 mcg once daily and 1 patient treated with placebo) had cataracts identified during the study that were not present at baseline.

5.3 Hypersensitivity Reactions, Including Anaphylaxis
Hypersensitivity reactions, including anaphylaxis, angioedema, rash, and urticaria, may occur after administration of VERAMYST Nasal Spray. Discontinue VERAMYST Nasal Spray if such reactions occur *[see Contraindications (4)]*.

5.4 Immunosuppression
Persons who are using drugs that suppress the immune system are more susceptible to infections than healthy individuals. Chickenpox and measles, for example, can have a more serious or even fatal course in susceptible children or adults using corticosteroids. In children or adults who have not had these diseases or have not been properly immunized, particular care should be taken to avoid exposure. How the dose, route, and duration of corticosteroid administration affect the risk of developing a disseminated infection is not known. The contribution of the underlying disease and/or prior corticosteroid treatment to the risk is also not known. If a patient is exposed to chickenpox, prophylaxis with varicella zoster immune globulin (VZIG) may be indicated. If a patient is exposed to measles, prophylaxis with pooled intramuscular immunoglobulin (IG) may be indicated. (See the respective package inserts for complete VZIG and IG prescribing information.) If chickenpox or measles develops, treatment with antiviral agents may be considered.
Corticosteroids should be used with caution, if at all, in patients with active or quiescent tuberculous infections of the respiratory tract; untreated local or systemic fungal or bacterial infections; systemic viral or parasitic infections; or ocular herpes simplex because of the potential for worsening of these infections.

5.5 Hypothalamic-Pituitary-Adrenal Axis Effects
Hypercorticism and Adrenal Suppression
When intranasal steroids are used at higher than recommended dosages or in susceptible individuals at recommended dosages, systemic corticosteroid effects such as hypercorticism and adrenal suppression may appear. If such changes occur, the dosage of VERAMYST Nasal Spray should be discontinued slowly, consistent with accepted procedures for discontinuing oral corticosteroid therapy.
The replacement of a systemic corticosteroid with a topical corticosteroid can be accompanied by signs of adrenal insufficiency. In addition, some patients may experience symptoms of corticosteroid withdrawal, e.g., joint and/or muscular pain, lassitude, and depression. Patients previously treated for prolonged periods with systemic corticosteroids and transferred to topical corticosteroids should be carefully monitored for acute adrenal insufficiency in response to stress. In those patients who have asthma or other clinical conditions requiring long-term systemic corticosteroid treatment, rapid decreases in systemic corticosteroid dosages may cause a severe exacerbation of their symptoms.

5.6 Use of Cytochrome P450 3A4 Inhibitors
Co-administration with ritonavir is not recommended because of the risk of systemic effects secondary to increased exposure to fluticasone furoate. Use caution with the co-administration of VERAMYST Nasal Spray and other potent cytochrome P450 (CYP) 3A4 inhibitors, such as ketoconazole *[see Drug Interactions (7)]*.

5.7 Effect on Growth
Corticosteroids may cause a reduction in growth velocity when administered to pediatric patients. Monitor the growth routinely of pediatric patients receiving VERAMYST Nasal Spray. To minimize the systemic effects of intranasal corticosteroids, including VERAMYST Nasal Spray, titrate each patient's dose to the lowest dosage that effectively controls his/her symptoms *[see Use in Specific Populations (8.4)]*.

Table 2. Adverse Reactions With >3% Incidence in Controlled Clinical Trials of 2 to 12 Weeks' Duration With VERAMYST Nasal Spray in Pediatric Patients With Seasonal or Perennial Allergic Rhinitis

Adverse Event	Pediatric Patients Aged 2 to <12 Years		
	Vehicle Placebo (n = 429)	VERAMYST Nasal Spray 55 mcg Once Daily (n = 369)	VERAMYST Nasal Spray 110 mcg Once Daily (n = 426)
Headache	31 (7%)	28 (8%)	33 (8%)
Nasopharyngitis	21 (5%)	20 (5%)	21 (5%)
Epistaxis	19 (4%)	17 (5%)	17 (4%)
Pyrexia	7 (2%)	17 (5%)	19 (4%)
Pharyngolaryngeal pain	14 (3%)	16 (4%)	12 (3%)
Cough	12 (3%)	12 (3%)	16 (4%)

6 ADVERSE REACTIONS

Systemic and local corticosteroid use may result in the following:
- Epistaxis, ulcerations, *Candida albicans* infection, impaired wound healing *[see Warnings and Precautions (5.1)]*
- Cataracts and glaucoma *[see Warnings and Precautions (5.2)]*
- Immunosuppression *[see Warnings and Precautions (5.4)]*
- Hypothalamic-pituitary-adrenal (HPA) axis effects, including growth reduction *[see Warnings and Precautions (5.5), Use in Specific Populations (8.4)]*

6.1 Clinical Trials Experience
The safety data described below reflect exposure to VERAMYST Nasal Spray in 1,563 patients with seasonal or perennial allergic rhinitis in 9 controlled clinical trials of 2 to 12 weeks' duration. The data from adults and adolescents are based upon 6 clinical trials in which 768 patients with seasonal or perennial allergic rhinitis (473 females and 295 males aged 12 years and older) were treated with VERAMYST Nasal Spray 110 mcg once daily for 2 to 6 weeks. The racial distribution of adult and adolescent patients receiving VERAMYST Nasal Spray was 82% white, 5% black, and 13% other. The data from pediatric patients are based upon 3 clinical trials in which 795 children with seasonal or perennial rhinitis (352 females and 443 males aged 2 to 11 years) were treated with VERAMYST Nasal Spray 55 or 110 mcg once daily for 2 to 12 weeks. The racial distribution of pediatric patients receiving VERAMYST Nasal Spray was 75% white, 11% black, and 14% other.
Because clinical trials are conducted under widely varying conditions, adverse reaction rates observed in the clinical trials of a drug cannot be directly compared with rates in the clinical trials of another drug and may not reflect the rates observed in practice.
Adults and Adolescents Aged 12 Years and Older
Overall adverse reactions were reported with approximately the same frequency by patients treated with VERAMYST Nasal Spray and those receiving placebo. Less than 3% of patients in clinical trials discontinued treatment because of adverse reactions. The rate of withdrawal among patients receiving VERAMYST Nasal Spray was similar or lower than the rate among patients receiving placebo.
Table 1 displays the common adverse reactions (>1% in any patient group receiving VERAMYST Nasal Spray) that occurred more frequently in patients aged 12 years and older treated with VERAMYST Nasal Spray compared with placebo-treated patients.

Table 1. Adverse Reactions With >1% Incidence in Controlled Clinical Trials of 2 to 6 Weeks' Duration With VERAMYST Nasal Spray in Adult and Adolescent Patients With Seasonal or Perennial Allergic Rhinitis

Adverse Event	Adult and Adolescent Patients Aged 12 Years and Older	
	Vehicle Placebo (n = 774)	VERAMYST Nasal Spray 110 mcg Once Daily (n = 768)
Headache	54 (7%)	72 (9%)
Epistaxis	32 (4%)	45 (6%)
Pharyngolaryngeal pain	8 (1%)	15 (2%)
Nasal ulceration	3 (<1%)	11 (1%)
Back pain	7 (<1%)	9 (1%)

There were no differences in the incidence of adverse reactions based on gender or race. Clinical trials did not include sufficient numbers of patients aged 65 years and older to determine whether they respond differently from younger subjects.
Pediatric Patients Aged 2 to 11 Years
In the 3 clinical trials in pediatric patients aged 2 to <12 years, overall adverse reactions were reported with approximately the same frequency by patients treated with VERAMYST Nasal Spray and those receiving placebo. Table 2 displays the common adverse reactions (>3% in any patient group receiving VERAMYST Nasal Spray), that occurred more frequently in patients aged 2 to 11 years treated with VERAMYST Nasal Spray compared with placebo-treated patients.
[See table 2 above]
There were no differences in the incidence of adverse reactions based on gender or race. Pyrexia occurred more frequently in children aged 2 to <6 years compared with children aged 6 to <12 years.
Long-Term (52-Week) Safety Trial
In a 52-week, placebo-controlled, long-term safety trial, 605 patients (307 females and 298 males aged 12 years and older) with perennial allergic rhinitis were treated with VERAMYST Nasal Spray 110 mcg once daily for 12 months and 201 were treated with placebo nasal spray. While most adverse reactions were similar in type and rate between the treatment groups, epistaxis occurred more frequently in patients who received VERAMYST Nasal Spray (123/605, 20%) than in patients who received placebo (17/201, 8%). Epistaxis tended to be more severe in patients treated with VERAMYST Nasal Spray. All 17 reports of epistaxis that occurred in patients who received placebo were of mild intensity, while 83, 39, and 1 of the total 123 epistaxis events in patients treated with VERAMYST Nasal Spray were of mild, moderate, and severe intensity, respectively. No patient experienced a nasal septal perforation during this trial.

6.2 Postmarketing Experience
In addition to adverse reactions reported from clinical trials, the following adverse reactions have been identified during postmarketing use of VERAMYST Nasal Spray. Because these reactions are reported voluntarily from a population of uncertain size, it is not always possible to reliably estimate their frequency or establish a causal relationship to drug exposure. These events have been chosen for inclusion due to either their seriousness, frequency of reporting, or causal connection to fluticasone furoate or a combination of these factors.
Immune System Disorders: Hypersensitivity reactions, including anaphylaxis, angioedema, rash, and urticaria.

7 DRUG INTERACTIONS

Fluticasone furoate is cleared by extensive first-pass metabolism mediated by CYP3A4. In a drug interaction study of intranasal fluticasone furoate and the CYP3A4 inhibitor ketoconazole given as a 200-mg once-daily dose for 7 days, 6 of 20 subjects receiving fluticasone furoate and ketoconazole had measurable but low levels of fluticasone furoate compared with 1 of 20 receiving fluticasone furoate and placebo. Based on this study and the low systemic exposure, there was a 5% reduction in 24-hour serum cortisol levels with ketoconazole compared with placebo. The data from this study should be carefully interpreted because the study was conducted with ketoconazole 200 mg once daily rather than 400 mg, which is the maximum recommended dosage. Therefore, caution is required with the co-administration of VERAMYST Nasal Spray and ketoconazole or other potent CYP3A4 inhibitors.
Based on data with another glucocorticoid, fluticasone propionate, metabolized by CYP3A4, co-administration of VERAMYST Nasal Spray with the potent CYP3A4 inhibitor ritonavir is not recommended because of the risk of systemic effects secondary to increased exposure to fluticasone furoate. High exposure to corticosteroids increases the potential for systemic side effects, such as cortisol suppression.
Enzyme induction and inhibition data suggest that fluticasone furoate is unlikely to significantly alter the cytochrome P450-mediated metabolism of other compounds at clinically relevant intranasal dosages.

8 USE IN SPECIFIC POPULATIONS

8.1 Pregnancy

Teratogenic Effects

Pregnancy Category C. Corticosteroids have been shown to be teratogenic in laboratory animals when administered systemically at relatively low dosage levels.

There were no teratogenic effects in rats and rabbits at inhaled fluticasone furoate dosages of up to 91 and 8 mcg/kg/day, respectively (approximately 7 and 1 times, respectively, the maximum recommended daily intranasal dose in adults on a mcg/m^2 basis). There was also no effect on pre- or postnatal development in rats treated with up to 27 mcg/kg/day by inhalation during gestation and lactation (approximately 2 times the maximum recommended daily intranasal dose in adults on a mcg/m^2 basis).

There are no adequate and well-controlled studies in pregnant women. VERAMYST Nasal Spray should be used during pregnancy only if the potential benefit justifies the potential risk to the fetus.

Nonteratogenic Effects

Hypoadrenalism may occur in infants born of mothers receiving corticosteroids during pregnancy. Such infants should be carefully monitored.

8.3 Nursing Mothers

It is not known whether fluticasone furoate is excreted in human breast milk. However, other corticosteroids have been detected in human milk. Since there are no data from controlled trials on the use of intranasal fluticasone furoate by nursing mothers, caution should be exercised when VERAMYST Nasal Spray is administered to a nursing woman.

8.4 Pediatric Use

Controlled clinical trials with VERAMYST Nasal Spray included 1,224 patients aged 2 to 11 years and 344 adolescent patients aged 12 to 17 years *[see Clinical Studies (14)]*. The safety and effectiveness of VERAMYST Nasal Spray in children younger than 2 years have not been established.

Controlled clinical studies have shown that intranasal corticosteroids may cause a reduction in growth velocity in pediatric patients. This effect has been observed in the absence of laboratory evidence of HPA axis suppression, suggesting that growth velocity is a more sensitive indicator of systemic corticosteroid exposure in pediatric patients than some commonly used tests of HPA axis function. The long-term effects of reduction in growth velocity associated with intranasal corticosteroids, including the impact on final adult height, are unknown. The potential for "catch-up" growth following discontinuation of treatment with intranasal corticosteroids has not been adequately studied. The growth of pediatric patients receiving intranasal corticosteroids, including VERAMYST Nasal Spray, should be monitored routinely (e.g., via stadiometry). The potential growth effects of prolonged treatment should be weighed against the clinical benefits obtained and the risks/benefits of treatment alternatives. To minimize the systemic effects of intranasal corticosteroids, including VERAMYST Nasal Spray, each patient's dose should be titrated to the lowest dosage that effectively controls his/her symptoms.

The potential for VERAMYST Nasal Spray to cause growth suppression in susceptible patients or when given at higher than recommended dosages cannot be ruled out.

8.5 Geriatric Use

Clinical studies of VERAMYST Nasal Spray did not include sufficient numbers of subjects aged 65 years and older to determine whether they respond differently from younger subjects. Other reported clinical experience has not identified differences in responses between the elderly and younger patients. In general, dose selection for an elderly patient should be cautious, usually starting at the low end of the dosing range, reflecting the greater frequency of decreased hepatic, renal, or cardiac function, and of concomitant disease or other drug therapy.

8.6 Hepatic Impairment

Use VERAMYST Nasal Spray with caution in patients with severe hepatic impairment *[see Clinical Pharmacology (12.3)]*.

8.7 Renal Impairment

No dosage adjustment is required in patients with renal impairment *[see Clinical Pharmacology (12.3)]*.

10 OVERDOSAGE

Chronic overdosage may result in signs/symptoms of hypercorticism *[see Warnings and Precautions (5.4)]*. There are no data on the effects of acute or chronic overdosage with VERAMYST Nasal Spray. Because of low systemic bioavailability and an absence of acute drug-related systemic findings in clinical studies (with dosages of up to 440 mcg/day for 2 weeks [4 times the maximum recommended daily dose]), overdose is unlikely to require any therapy other than observation.

Intranasal administration of up to 2,640 mcg/day (24 times the recommended adult dose) of fluticasone furoate was administered to healthy human volunteers for 3 days. Single- and repeat-dose studies with orally inhaled fluticasone furoate doses of 50 to 4,000 mcg have shown decreased mean serum cortisol at doses of 500 mcg or higher. The oral median lethal dose in mice and rats was >2,000 mg/kg (approximately 74,000 and 147,000 times, respectively, the maximum recommended daily intranasal dose in adults and 52,000 and 105,000 times, respectively, the maximum recommended daily intranasal dose in children, on a mcg/m^2 basis).

Acute overdosage with the intranasal dosage form is unlikely since 1 bottle of VERAMYST Nasal Spray contains approximately 3 mg of fluticasone furoate, and the bioavailability of fluticasone furoate is <1% for 2.64 mg/day given intranasally and 1% for 2 mg/day given as an oral solution.

11 DESCRIPTION

Fluticasone furoate, the active component of VERAMYST Nasal Spray, is a synthetic fluorinated corticosteroid having the chemical name (6α,11β,16α,17α)-6,9-difluoro-17-{[(fluoro-methyl)thio]carbonyl}-11-hydroxy-16-methyl-3-oxoandrosta-1,4-dien-17-yl 2-furancarboxylate and the following chemical structure:

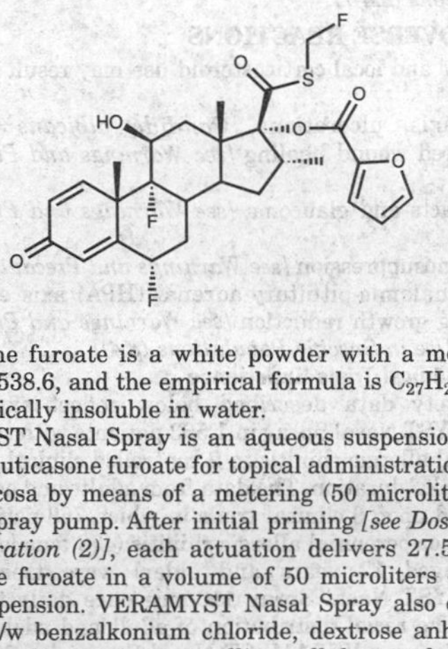

Fluticasone furoate is a white powder with a molecular weight of 538.6, and the empirical formula is $C_{27}H_{29}F_3O_6S$. It is practically insoluble in water.

VERAMYST Nasal Spray is an aqueous suspension of micronized fluticasone furoate for topical administration to the nasal mucosa by means of a metering (50 microliters), atomizing spray pump. After initial priming *[see Dosage and Administration (2)]*, each actuation delivers 27.5 mcg of fluticasone furoate in a volume of 50 microliters of nasal spray suspension. VERAMYST Nasal Spray also contains 0.015% w/w benzalkonium chloride, dextrose anhydrous, edetate disodium, microcrystalline cellulose and carboxymethylcellulose sodium, polysorbate 80, and purified water. It has a pH of approximately 6.

12 CLINICAL PHARMACOLOGY

12.1 Mechanism of Action

Fluticasone furoate is a synthetic trifluorinated corticosteroid with potent anti-inflammatory activity. The precise mechanism through which fluticasone furoate affects rhinitis symptoms is not known. Corticosteroids have been shown to have a wide range of actions on multiple cell types (e.g., mast cells, eosinophils, neutrophils, macrophages, lymphocytes) and mediators (e.g., histamine, eicosanoids, leukotrienes, cytokines) involved in inflammation. Specific effects of fluticasone furoate demonstrated in in vitro and in vivo models included activation of the glucocorticoid response element, inhibition of pro-inflammatory transcription factors such as NFkB, and inhibition of antigen-induced lung eosinophilia in sensitized rats.

Fluticasone furoate has been shown in vitro to exhibit a binding affinity for the human glucocorticoid receptor that is approximately 29.9 times that of dexamethasone and 1.7 times that of fluticasone propionate. The clinical relevance of these findings is unknown.

12.2 Pharmacodynamics

Adrenal Function

The effects of VERAMYST Nasal Spray on adrenal function have been evaluated in 4 controlled clinical trials in patients with perennial allergic rhinitis. Two 6-week clinical trials were designed specifically to assess the effect of VERAMYST Nasal Spray on the HPA axis with assessments of both 24-hour urinary cortisol excretion and serum cortisol levels in domiciled patients. In addition, one 52-week safety study and one 12-week safety and efficacy study included assessments of 24-hour urinary cortisol excretion. Details of the studies and results are described below. In all 4 studies, since serum fluticasone determinations were generally below the limit of quantification, compliance was assured by efficacy assessments.

Clinical Trials Specifically Designed to Assess Hypothalamic-Pituitary-Adrenal Axis Effect

In a 6-week randomized, double-blind, parallel-group study in adult and adolescent patients aged 12 years and older with perennial allergic rhinitis, VERAMYST Nasal Spray 110 mcg was compared with both placebo nasal spray and prednisone as a positive-control group that received prednisone 10 mg orally once daily for the final 7 days of the treatment period. Adrenal function was assessed by 24-hour urinary cortisol excretion before and after 6 weeks of treatment and by serial serum cortisol levels. Patients were domiciled for collection of 24-hour urinary cortisol. After 6 weeks of treatment, there was a change from baseline in the mean 24-hour urinary cortisol excretion in the group treated with VERAMYST Nasal Spray (n = 43) of -1.16 mcg/day compared with -3.48 mcg/day in the placebo group (n = 42). The difference from placebo in the group treated with VERAMYST Nasal Spray was 2.32 mcg/day (95% CI: -6.76, 11.39). Urinary cortisol data were not available for the positive-control (prednisone) treatment group. For serum cortisol levels, after 6 weeks of treatment there was a change from baseline in the mean (0-24 hours) of -0.38 and 0.08 mcg/dL for the group treated with VERAMYST Nasal Spray (n = 43) and the placebo group (n = 44), respectively, with a difference between the group treated with VERAMYST Nasal Spray and the placebo group of -0.47 mcg/dL (95% CI: -1.31, 0.37). For comparison, in the positive-control (prednisone, n = 12) treatment group, there was a change in mean serum cortisol (0-24 hours) from baseline of -4.49 mcg/dL with a difference between the prednisone and placebo group of -4.57 mcg/dL (95% CI: -5.83, -3.31).

The second 6-week study conducted in children aged 2 to 11 years was of similar design to the adult study, including adrenal function assessments, but did not include a prednisone positive-control arm. Patients were treated once daily with VERAMYST Nasal Spray 110 mcg or placebo nasal spray. After 6 weeks of treatment, there was a change in the mean 24-hour urinary cortisol excretion in the group treated with VERAMYST Nasal Spray (n = 43) of 0.49 mcg/day compared with 1.92 mcg/day in the placebo group (n = 41), with a difference between the group treated with VERAMYST Nasal Spray and the placebo group of -1.43 mcg/day (95% CI: -5.21, 2.35). For serum cortisol levels, after 6 weeks, there was a change from baseline in mean (0-24 hours) of -0.34 and -0.23 mcg/dL for the group treated with VERAMYST Nasal Spray (n = 48) and for the placebo group (n = 47), respectively, with a difference between the group treated with VERAMYST Nasal Spray and the placebo group of -0.11 mcg/dL (95% CI: -0.88, 0.66).

Additional Hypothalamic-Pituitary-Adrenal Axis Assessments

In the 52-week safety trial in adolescents and adults aged 12 years and older with perennial allergic rhinitis, VERAMYST Nasal Spray 110 mcg (n = 605) was compared with placebo nasal spray (n = 201). Adrenal function was assessed by 24-hour urinary cortisol excretion in a subset of patients who received VERAMYST Nasal Spray (n = 370) or placebo (n = 120) before and after 52 weeks of treatment. After 52 weeks of treatment, the mean change from baseline 24-hour urinary cortisol excretion was 5.84 mcg/day in the group treated with VERAMYST Nasal Spray and 3.34 mcg/day in the placebo group. The difference from placebo in mean change from baseline 24-hour urinary cortisol excretion was 2.50 mcg/day (95% CI: -5.49, 10.49).

In the 12-week safety and efficacy trial in children aged 2 to 11 years with perennial allergic rhinitis, VERAMYST Nasal Spray 55 mcg (n = 185) and VERAMYST Nasal Spray 110 mcg (n = 185) were compared with placebo nasal spray (n = 188). Adrenal function was assessed by measurement of 24-hour urinary free cortisol in a subset of patients who were aged 6 to 11 years (103 to 109 patients per group) before and after 12 weeks of treatment. After 12 weeks of treatment, there was a decrease in mean 24-hour urinary cortisol excretion from baseline in the group treated with VERAMYST Nasal Spray 55 mcg (n = 109) of -2.93 mcg/day and in the group treated with VERAMYST Nasal Spray 110 mcg (n = 103) of -2.07 mcg/day compared with an increase in the placebo group (n = 107) of 0.08 mcg/day. The difference from placebo in mean change from baseline in 24-hour urinary cortisol excretion for the group treated with VERAMYST Nasal Spray 55 mcg was -3.01 mcg/day (95% CI: -6.16, 0.13) and -2.14 mcg/day (95% CI: -5.33, 1.04) for the group treated with VERAMYST Nasal Spray 110 mcg. When the results of the HPA axis assessments described above are taken as a whole, an effect of intranasal fluticasone furoate on adrenal function cannot be ruled out, especially in pediatric patients.

Cardiac Effects

A QT/QTc study did not demonstrate an effect of fluticasone furoate administration on the QTc interval. The effect of a single dose of 4,000 mcg of orally inhaled fluticasone furoate on the QTc interval was evaluated over 24 hours in 40 healthy male and female subjects in a placebo and positive (a single dose of 400 mg oral moxifloxacin) controlled crossover study. The QTcF maximal mean change from baseline following fluticasone furoate was similar to that observed with placebo with a treatment difference of 0.788 msec, (90% CI: -1.802, 3.378). In contrast, moxifloxacin given as a 400-mg tablet resulted in prolongation of the QTcF maximal mean change from baseline compared with placebo with a treatment difference of 9.929 msec, (90% CI: 7.339, 12.520). While a single dose of fluticasone furoate had no effect on the QTc interval, the effects of fluticasone furoate may not be at steady state following single dose. The effect of fluticasone furoate on the QTc interval following multiple dose administration is unknown.

12.3 Pharmacokinetics

Absorption

Following intranasal administration of fluticasone furoate, most of the dose is eventually swallowed and undergoes incomplete absorption and extensive first-pass metabolism in the liver and gut, resulting in negligible systemic exposure. At the highest recommended intranasal dosage of 110 mcg once daily for up to 12 months in adults and up to 12 weeks in children, plasma concentrations of fluticasone furoate are typically not quantifiable despite the use of a sensitive HPLC-MS/MS assay with a lower limit of quantification (LOQ) of 10 pg/mL. However, in a few isolated cases (<0.3%) fluticasone furoate was detected in high concentrations above 500 pg/mL, and in a single case the concentration was as high as 1,430 pg/mL in the 52-week study. There was no relationship between these concentrations and cortisol levels in these subjects. The reasons for these high concentrations are unknown.

Absolute bioavailability was evaluated in 16 male and female subjects following supratherapeutic dosages of fluticasone furoate (880 mcg given intranasally at 8-hour intervals for 10 doses, or 2,640 mcg/day). The average absolute bioavailability was 0.50% (90% CI: 0.34%, 0.74%).

Due to the low bioavailability by the intranasal route, the majority of the pharmacokinetic data was obtained via other routes of administration. Studies using oral solution and intravenous dosing of radiolabeled drug have demonstrated that at least 30% of fluticasone furoate is absorbed and then rapidly cleared from plasma. Oral bioavailability is on average 1.26%, and the majority of the circulating radioactivity is due to inactive metabolites.

Distribution

Following intravenous administration, the mean volume of distribution at steady state is 608 L.

Binding of fluticasone furoate to human plasma proteins is greater than 99%.

Metabolism

In vivo studies have revealed no evidence of cleavage of the furoate moiety to form fluticasone. Fluticasone furoate is cleared (total plasma clearance of 58.7 L/h) from systemic circulation principally by hepatic metabolism via CYP3A4. The principal route of metabolism is hydrolysis of the S-fluoromethyl carbothioate function to form the inactive 17β-carboxylic acid metabolite.

Elimination

Fluticasone furoate and its metabolites are eliminated primarily in the feces, accounting for approximately 101% and 90% of the orally and intravenously administered dose, respectively. Urinary excretion accounted for approximately 1% and 2% of the orally and intravenously administered dose, respectively. The elimination phase half-life averaged 15.1 hours following intravenous administration.

Population Pharmacokinetics

Fluticasone furoate is typically not quantifiable in plasma following intranasal dosing of 110 mcg once daily with the exception of isolated cases of very high plasma levels (see Absorption). Overall, quantifiable levels (>10 pg/mL) were observed in <31% of patients aged 12 years and older and in <16% of children (aged 2 to 11 years) following intranasal dosing of 110 mcg once daily and in <7% of children following intranasal dosing of 55 mcg once daily. There was no evidence to suggest that the presence or absence of detectable levels of fluticasone furoate was related to gender, age, or race.

Hepatic Impairment

Reduced liver function may affect the elimination of corticosteroids. Since fluticasone furoate undergoes extensive first-pass metabolism by the hepatic CYP3A4, the pharmacokinetics of fluticasone furoate may be altered in patients with hepatic impairment. A study of a single 400-mcg dose of orally inhaled fluticasone furoate in patients with moderate hepatic impairment (Child-Pugh Class B) resulted in increased C_{max} (42%) and $AUC_{(0-\infty)}$ (172%), resulting in an approximately 20% reduction in serum cortisol level in patients with hepatic impairment compared with healthy subjects. The systemic exposure would be expected to be higher than that observed had the study been conducted after multiple doses and/or in patients with severe hepatic impairment. Therefore, use VERAMYST Nasal Spray with caution in patients with severe hepatic impairment.

Renal Impairment

Fluticasone furoate is not detectable in urine from healthy subjects following intranasal dosing. Less than 1% of dose-related material is excreted in urine. No dosage adjustment is required in patients with renal impairment.

13 NONCLINICAL TOXICOLOGY

13.1 Carcinogenesis, Mutagenesis, Impairment of Fertility

Fluticasone furoate produced no treatment-related increases in the incidence of tumors in 2-year inhalation studies in rats and mice at doses of up to 9 and 19 mcg/kg/day, respectively (less than the maximum recommended daily intranasal dose in adults and children on a mcg/m² basis).

Table 3. Mean Change From Baseline in Reflective Total Nasal Symptom Score Over 2 Weeks in Patients With Seasonal Allergic Rhinitis

Treatment	n	Baseline (AM + PM)	Change From Baseline	Difference From Placebo		
				LS Mean	95% CI	P Value
Fluticasone furoate 440 mcg	130	9.6	-4.02	-2.19	-2.75, -1.62	<0.001
Fluticasone furoate 220 mcg	129	9.5	-3.19	-1.36	-1.93, -0.79	<0.001
Fluticasone furoate 110 mcg	127	9.5	-3.84	-2.01	-2.58, -1.44	<0.001
Fluticasone furoate 55 mcg	125	9.6	-3.50	-1.68	-2.25, -1.10	<0.001
Placebo	128	9.6	-1.83			

Fluticasone furoate did not induce gene mutation in bacteria or chromosomal damage in a mammalian cell mutation test in mouse lymphoma L5178Y cells in vitro. There was also no evidence of genotoxicity in the in vivo micronucleus test in rats.

No evidence of impairment of fertility was observed in reproductive studies conducted in male and female rats at inhaled fluticasone furoate doses of up to 24 and 91 mcg/kg/day, respectively (approximately 2 and 7 times, respectively, the maximum recommended daily intranasal dose in adults on a mcg/m² basis).

14 CLINICAL STUDIES

14.1 Seasonal and Perennial Allergic Rhinitis

Adult and Adolescent Patients Aged 12 Years and Older

The efficacy and safety of VERAMYST Nasal Spray was evaluated in 5 randomized, double-blind, parallel-group, multicenter, placebo-controlled clinical trials of 2 to 4 weeks' duration in adult and adolescent patients aged 12 years and older with symptoms of seasonal or perennial allergic rhinitis. The 5 clinical trials included one 2-week dose-ranging trial in patients with seasonal allergic rhinitis, three 2-week confirmatory efficacy trials in patients with seasonal allergic rhinitis, and one 4-week efficacy trial in patients with perennial allergic rhinitis. These trials included 1,829 patients (697 males and 1,132 females). About 75% of patients were Caucasian, and the mean age was 36 years. Of these patients, 722 received VERAMYST Nasal Spray 110 mcg once daily administered as 2 sprays in each nostril.

Assessment of efficacy was based on total nasal symptom score (TNSS). TNSS is calculated as the sum of the patients' scoring of the 4 individual nasal symptoms (rhinorrhea, nasal congestion, sneezing, and nasal itching) on a 0 to 3 categorical severity scale (0 = absent, 1 = mild, 2 = moderate, 3 = severe) as reflective (rTNSS) or instantaneous (iTNSS). rTNSS required the patients to record symptom severity over the previous 12 hours; iTNSS required patients to record symptom severity at the time immediately prior to the next dose. Morning and evening rTNSS scores were averaged over the treatment period and the difference from placebo in the change from baseline rTNSS was the primary efficacy endpoint. The morning iTNSS (AM iTNSS) reflects the TNSS at the end of the 24-hour dosing interval and is an indication of whether the effect was maintained over the 24-hour dosing interval.

Additional secondary efficacy variables were assessed, including the total ocular symptom score (TOSS) and the Rhinoconjunctivitis Quality of Life Questionnaire (RQLQ). TOSS is calculated as the sum of the patients' scoring of the 3 individual ocular symptoms (itching/burning, tearing/watering, and redness) on a 0 to 3 categorical severity scale (0 = absent, 1 = mild, 2 = moderate, 3 = severe) as reflective (rTOSS) or instantaneous scores (iTOSS). To assess efficacy, rTOSS and AM iTOSS were evaluated as described above for the TNSS. Patients' perceptions of disease-specific quality of life were evaluated through use of the RQLQ, which assesses the impact of allergic rhinitis treatment through 28 items in 7 domains (activities, sleep, non-nose/eye symptoms, practical problems, nasal symptoms, eye symptoms, and emotional) on a 7-point scale where 0 = no impairment and 6 = maximum impairment. An overall RQLQ score is calculated from the mean of all items in the instrument. An absolute difference of ≥0.5 in mean change from baseline over placebo is considered the minimally important difference (MID) for the RQLQ.

Dose-Ranging Trial

The dose-ranging trial was a 2-week trial that evaluated the efficacy of 4 dosages of fluticasone furoate nasal spray (440, 220, 110, and 55 mcg) in patients with seasonal allergic rhinitis. In this trial, each of the 4 dosages of fluticasone furoate nasal spray demonstrated greater decreases in the rTNSS than placebo, and the difference was statistically significant (Table 3).

[See table 3 above]

Each of the 4 dosages of fluticasone furoate nasal spray also demonstrated greater decreases in the AM iTNSS than placebo, and the difference between each of the 4 fluticasone furoate treatment groups and placebo was statistically significant, indicating that the effect was maintained over the 24-hour dosing interval.

Seasonal Allergic Rhinitis Trials

Three clinical trials were designed to evaluate the efficacy of VERAMYST Nasal Spray 110 mcg once daily compared with placebo in patients with seasonal allergic rhinitis over a 2-week treatment period. In all 3 trials, VERAMYST Nasal Spray 110 mcg demonstrated a greater decrease from baseline in the rTNSS and AM iTNSS than placebo, and the difference from placebo was statistically significant. In terms of ocular symptoms, in all 3 seasonal allergic rhinitis trials, VERAMYST Nasal Spray 110 mcg demonstrated a greater decrease from baseline in the rTOSS than placebo and the difference from placebo was statistically significant. For the RQLQ in all 3 seasonal allergic rhinitis trials, VERAMYST Nasal Spray 110 mcg demonstrated greater decrease from baseline in the overall RQLQ than placebo, and the difference from placebo was statistically significant. The difference in the overall RQLQ score mean change from baseline between the groups treated with VERAMYST Nasal Spray and placebo ranged from -0.60 to -0.70 in the 3 trials, meeting the minimally important difference criterion. Table 4 displays the efficacy results from a representative trial in patients with seasonal allergic rhinitis.

Perennial Allergic Rhinitis Trials

One clinical trial was designed to evaluate the efficacy of VERAMYST Nasal Spray 110 mcg once daily compared with placebo in patients with perennial allergic rhinitis over a 4-week treatment period. VERAMYST Nasal Spray 110 mcg demonstrated a greater decrease from baseline in the rTNSS and AM iTNSS than placebo, and the difference from placebo was statistically significant. Similar to patients with seasonal allergic rhinitis, the improvement of nasal symptoms with VERAMYST Nasal Spray in patients with perennial allergic rhinitis persisted for a full 24 hours, as evaluated by AM iTNSS immediately prior to the next dose. However, unlike the trials in patients with seasonal allergic rhinitis, patients with perennial allergic rhinitis who were treated with VERAMYST Nasal Spray 110 mcg did not demonstrate statistically significant improvement from baseline in rTOSS or in disease-specific quality of life as measured by the RQLQ compared with placebo. In addition, the overall RQLQ score mean change from baseline difference between the group treated with VERAMYST Nasal Spray and the placebo group was -0.23, which did not meet the minimally important difference of ≥0.5. Table 4 displays the efficacy results from the clinical trial in patients with perennial allergic rhinitis.

[See table 4 at top of next page]

Onset of action was evaluated by frequent instantaneous TNSS assessments after the first dose in the clinical trials in patients with seasonal allergic rhinitis and perennial allergic rhinitis. Onset of action was generally observed within 24 hours in patients with seasonal allergic rhinitis. In patients with perennial rhinitis, onset of action was observed after 4 days of treatment. Continued improvement in symptoms was observed over approximately 1 and 3 weeks in patients with seasonal or perennial allergic rhinitis, respectively.

Pediatric Patients Aged 2 to 11 Years

The efficacy and safety of VERAMYST Nasal Spray were evaluated in 1,112 children (633 boys and 479 girls), mean age of 8 years with seasonal or perennial allergic rhinitis in 2 controlled clinical trials. The pediatric patients were treated with VERAMYST Nasal Spray 55 or 110 mcg once daily for 2 to 12 weeks (n = 369 for each dose). The trials were similar in design to the trials conducted in adolescents and adults; however, the efficacy determination was made from patient- or parent/guardian-reported TNSS for children aged 6 to <12 years. Children treated with VERAMYST Nasal Spray generally exhibited greater decreases in nasal symptoms than placebo-treated patients. In seasonal allergic rhinitis, the difference in rTNSS was statistically significant only for the 110-mcg dose. In perennial allergic rhinitis, the difference in rTNSS was statistically significant only for the 55-mcg dose. Changes in rTOSS in the seasonal allergic rhinitis trial were not statistically significant compared with placebo for either dose. rTOSS was not assessed in the perennial allergic rhinitis trial. Table 5 displays the efficacy results from the clinical trials in patients with perennial allergic rhinitis and seasonal allergic

Table 4. Mean Changes in Efficacy Variables in Adult and Adolescent Patients With Seasonal or Perennial Allergic Rhinitis

Treatment	n	Baseline	Change From Baseline – LS Mean	Difference From Placebo		
				LS Mean	95% CI	P Value
Reflective Total Nasal Symptom Scores						
Seasonal allergic rhinitis trial						
Fluticasone furoate 110 mcg	151	9.6	-3.55	-1.47	-2.01, -0.94	<0.001
Placebo	147	9.9	-2.07			
Perennnial allergic rhinitis trial						
Fluticasone furoate 110 mcg	149	8.6	-2.78	-0.71	-1.20, -0.21	0.005
Placebo	153	8.7	-2.08			
Instantaneous Total Nasal Symptom Scores						
Seasonal allergic rhinitis trial						
Fluticasone furoate 110 mcg	151	9.4	-2.90	-1.38	-1.90, -0.85	<0.001
Placebo	147	9.3	-1.53			
Perennnial allergic rhinitis trial						
Fluticasone furoate 110 mcg	149	8.2	-2.45	-0.71	-1.20, -0.21	0.006
Placebo	153	8.3	-1.75			
Reflective Total Ocular Symptom Scores						
Seasonal allergic rhinitis trial						
Fluticasone furoate 110 mcg	151	6.6	-2.23	-0.60	-1.01, -0.19	0.004
Placebo	147	6.5	-1.63			
Perennnial allergic rhinitis trial						
Fluticasone furoate 110 mcg	149	4.8	-1.39	-0.15	-0.52, 0.22	0.428
Placebo	153	5.0	-1.24			
Rhinoconjunctivitis Quality of Life Questionnaire						
Seasonal allergic rhinitis trial						
Fluticasone furoate 110 mcg	144	3.9	-1.77	-0.60	-0.93, -0.28	<0.001
Placebo	144	3.9	-1.16			
Perennnial allergic rhinitis trial						
Fluticasone furoate 110 mcg	143	3.5	-1.41	-0.23	-0.59, 0.13	0.214
Placebo	151	3.4	-1.18			

Table 5. Mean Changes in Efficacy Variables in Pediatric Patients Aged 6 to <12 Years With Seasonal or Perennial Allergic Rhinitis

Treatment	n	Baseline	Change From Baseline – LS Mean	Difference From Placebo		
				LS Mean	95% CI	P Value
Reflective Total Nasal Symptom Scores						
Seasonal allergic rhinitis trial						
Fluticasone furoate 55 mcg	151	8.6	-2.71	-0.16	-0.69, 0.37	0.553
Fluticasone furoate 110 mcg	146	8.5	-3.16	-0.62	-1.15, -0.08	0.025
Placebo	149	8.4	-2.54			
Perennnial allergic rhinitis trial						
Fluticasone furoate 55 mcg	144	8.5	-4.16	-0.75	-1.24, -0.27	0.003
Fluticasone furoate 110 mcg	140	8.6	-3.86	-0.45	-0.95, 0.04	0.073
Placebo	147	8.5	-3.41			
Instantaneous Total Nasal Symptom Scores						
Seasonal allergic rhinitis trial						
Fluticasone furoate 55 mcg	151	8.4	-2.37	-0.23	-0.77, 0.30	0.389
Fluticasone furoate 110 mcg	146	8.3	-2.80	-0.67	-1.21, -0.13	0.015
Placebo	149	8.4	-2.13			
Perennnial allergic rhinitis trial						
Fluticasone furoate 55 mcg	144	8.3	-3.62	-0.75	-1.24, -0.27	0.002
Fluticasone furoate 110 mcg	140	8.3	-3.52	-0.65	-1.14, -0.16	0.009
Placebo	147	8.3	-2.87			
Reflective Total Ocular Symptom Scores						
Seasonal allergic rhinitis trial						
Fluticasone furoate 55 mcg	151	4.4	-1.26	0.04	-0.33, 0.41	0.826
Fluticasone furoate 110 mcg	146	4.1	-1.45	-0.15	-0.52, 0.22	0.426
Placebo	149	3.8	-1.30			

rhinitis in children aged 6 to <12 years. Efficacy in children aged 2 to <6 years was supported by a numerical decrease in the rTNSS.
[See table 5 above]

16   HOW SUPPLIED/STORAGE AND HANDLING

VERAMYST Nasal Spray, 27.5 mcg per spray, is supplied in a brown glass bottle enclosed in a nasal device with a nozzle and a mist-release button to actuate the spray in a box of 1 (NDC 0173-0753-00) with FDA-Approved Patient Labeling (see Patient Instructions for Use for proper actuation of the device). Each bottle contains a net fill weight of 10 g of white, liquid suspension and will provide 120 metered sprays. After priming [see Dosage and Administration (2)], each spray delivers a fine mist containing 27.5 mcg of fluticasone furoate in 50 microliters of formulation through the nozzle. The contents of the bottle can be viewed through an indicator window. Shake the contents well before each use. The correct amount of medication in each spray cannot be assured before the initial priming and after 120 sprays have been used, even though the bottle is not completely empty. The nasal device should be discarded after 120 sprays have been used.

Store the device in the upright position with the cap in place between 15° and 30°C (59° and 86°F). Do not freeze or refrigerate.

17   PATIENT COUNSELING INFORMATION
See FDA-Approved Patient Labeling.
17.1   Local Nasal Effects
Patients should be informed that treatment with VERAMYST Nasal Spray may lead to adverse reactions, which include epistaxis and nasal ulceration. *Candida* infection may also occur with treatment with VERAMYST Nasal Spray. In addition, nasal corticosteroids are associated with nasal septal perforation and impaired wound healing. Patients who have experienced recent nasal ulcers, nasal surgery, or nasal trauma should not use VERAMYST Nasal Spray until healing has occurred [see Warnings and Precautions (5.1)].
17.2   Cataracts and Glaucoma
Patients should be informed that glaucoma and cataracts are associated with nasal and inhaled corticosteroid use. Patients should inform his/her health care provider if a change in vision is noted while using VERAMYST Nasal Spray [see Warnings and Precautions (5.2)].
17.3   Hypersensitivity Reactions, Including Anaphylaxis
Patients should be aware that hypersensitivity reactions, including anaphylaxis, angioedema, rash, and urticaria, may occur after administration of VERAMYST Nasal Spray. If such reactions occur, patients should discontinue use of VERAMYST Nasal Spray [see Warnings and Precautions (5.3)].
17.4   Immunosuppression
Patients who are on immunosuppressant doses of corticosteroids should be warned to avoid exposure to chickenpox or measles and, if exposed, to consult their physician without delay. Patients should be informed of potential worsening of existing tuberculosis, fungal, bacterial, viral or parasitic infections, or ocular herpes simplex [see Warnings and Precautions (5.4)].
17.5   Use Daily for Best Effect
Patients should use VERAMYST Nasal Spray on a regular once-daily basis for optimal effect. VERAMYST Nasal Spray, like other corticosteroids, does not have an immediate effect on rhinitis symptoms. Although significant improvement is usually achieved within 24 hours in patients with seasonal allergic rhinitis and 4 days in patients with perennial allergic rhinitis, maximum benefit may not be reached for several days. The patient should not increase the prescribed dosage but should contact the physician if symptoms do not improve or if the condition worsens.
17.6   Keep Spray Out of Eyes
Patients should be informed to avoid spraying VERAMYST Nasal Spray in their eyes.
17.7   Potential Drug Interactions
Patients should be advised that coadministration of VERAMYST Nasal Spray and ritonavir is not recommended and to be cautious if coadministrating with ketoconazole.

GlaxoSmithKline
Research Triangle Park, NC 27709
©2010, GlaxoSmithKline. All rights reserved.
March 2010
VRM:5PI

PATIENT INFORMATION
VERAMYST® [VAIR-uh-mist]
(fluticasone furoate)
Nasal Spray
FOR INTRANASAL USE ONLY
Read the Patient Information that comes with VERAMYST Nasal Spray carefully before you start using it and each time you get a refill. There may be new information. Keep the leaflet for reference because it gives you a summary of important information about VERAMYST Nasal Spray. This leaflet does not take the place of talking to your healthcare provider about your medical condition or your treatment.

What is VERAMYST Nasal Spray?
VERAMYST is a medicine that treats seasonal and year-round allergy symptoms in adults and children 2 years old and older.
VERAMYST contains fluticasone furoate, which is a man-made (synthetic) corticosteroid. Corticosteroids are natural substances found in the body that reduce inflammation. When you spray VERAMYST into your nose, it helps reduce the nasal symptoms of allergic rhinitis (inflammation of the lining of the nose), such as stuffy nose, runny nose, itching, and sneezing. VERAMYST may also help red, itchy, and watery eyes in adults and teenagers with seasonal allergic rhinitis.
Your healthcare provider has prescribed VERAMYST to treat your symptoms of allergic rhinitis.

What should I tell my healthcare provider before taking VERAMYST Nasal Spray?

Tell your healthcare provider about all of your medical conditions, including if you are:
• pregnant (or planning to become pregnant).
• breastfeeding a baby.

- allergic to any of the ingredients in VERAMYST or any other nasal corticosteroid. See "**What are the ingredients in VERAMYST Nasal Spray?**" below for a complete list of ingredients.
- exposed to chickenpox or measles.
- feeling unwell or have any symptoms that you do not understand.

Tell your healthcare provider about all the medicines you take, including prescription and non-prescription medicines, vitamins, and herbal products. VERAMYST and other medicines may affect each other, causing side effects. **Be certain to tell your healthcare provider if you are taking a medicine that contains ritonavir (commonly used to treat HIV infection or AIDS).**

How should I use VERAMYST Nasal Spray?
- This medicine is for use in the <u>nose only</u>. Do not spray it in your eyes or mouth.
- An adult should help a young child use this medicine.
- This medicine has been prescribed for you by your healthcare provider. DO NOT give this medicine to anyone else.
- Use VERAMYST exactly as your healthcare provider tells you to. DO NOT take more of your medicine or take it more often than your healthcare provider tells you. The prescription label will usually tell you how many sprays to take and how often. If it does not or if you are not sure, ask your healthcare provider or pharmacist.
- **For people aged 12 years and older,** the usual starting dosage is *2 sprays in each nostril, once a day.* After you begin to feel better, your healthcare provider may tell you that 1 spray in each nostril once a day may be enough for you.
- **For children aged 2 to 11 years,** the usual starting dosage is *1 spray in each nostril, once a day.* Your healthcare provider may tell you to take 2 sprays in each nostril once a day. After you begin to feel better, your healthcare provider may change the dosage to 1 spray in each nostril once a day. An adult should help a young child use this medicine.
- Do not use VERAMYST after 120 sprays (plus the initial priming sprays) have been used or after the expiration date, whichever comes first. (The sample bottle contains 30 sprays.) The bottle may not be completely empty. The expiration date is printed as "EXP" on the product label and box. Before you throw away VERAMYST, talk to your healthcare provider to see if you need a refill of your prescription. If your healthcare provider tells you to continue using VERAMYST, throw away the empty or expired bottle and use a new bottle of VERAMYST. Follow the **Patient Instructions for Use** below.
- Do not take extra doses or stop taking VERAMYST without telling your healthcare provider.
- VERAMYST may begin to work within 24 hours after you take your first dose. It may take several days before it has its greatest effect.
- You will get the best results if you keep using VERAMYST regularly each day without missing a dose. If you miss a dose by several hours, just take your next dose at the usual time. DO NOT take an extra dose.

What are the possible side effects of VERAMYST Nasal Spray?
Some patients taking VERAMYST had nosebleeds or nasal sores. These are not all of the possible side effects of VERAMYST. For more information, ask your healthcare provider or pharmacist.

What are other risks of using VERAMYST?
- Some patients may get a nasal fungal infection. This happened in about 1 out of 1,000 patients in clinical studies with VERAMYST.
- Corticosteroids can slow the healing of wounds. Do not use VERAMYST until your nose has healed if you have a sore in your nose, if you have surgery on your nose, or if your nose has been injured.
- Some patients may have eye problems, including glaucoma and cataracts. You should have regular eye exams.
- Immune system effects may increase the risk of infections.
- Corticosteroids may slow growth in children. A child taking VERAMYST should have his/her growth checked regularly.

What should I know about allergic rhinitis?
"Rhinitis" means inflammation of the lining of the nose. It is sometimes called "hay fever." Allergic rhinitis can be caused by allergies to pollen, animal dander, house dust mite, and mold spores. If you have allergic rhinitis, your nose becomes stuffy, runny, and itchy. You may also sneeze a lot. You may also have red, itchy, watery eyes; itchy throat; or blocked, itchy ears.

What are the ingredients in VERAMYST Nasal Spray?
Active ingredient: fluticasone furoate.
Inactive ingredients: 0.015% w/w benzalkonium chloride, dextrose anhydrous, edetate disodium, microcrystalline cellulose, carboxymethylcellulose sodium, polysorbate 80, and purified water.

Patient Instructions for Use
Read this leaflet carefully before you start to use VERAMYST Nasal Spray. If you have any questions, ask your healthcare provider or pharmacist.

The parts of the VERAMYST Nasal Spray
VERAMYST Nasal Spray comes in a brown glass bottle inside a nasal device. It contains 120 sprays (or 30 sprays if it is a sample) plus the first priming sprays. Be careful not to drop it. If you accidentally drop the device, check it for damage. If the device is damaged, return it to your pharmacist.

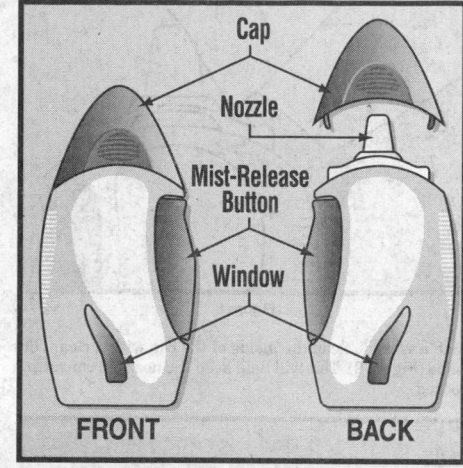

FRONT   BACK

The **Cap** has a tab that keeps the **Mist-Release Button** from being pressed accidentally. It also helps keep the nozzle clean. Do not throw the cap away. Always keep the cap on the device when you are not using it.
The **Nozzle** is small and short, so it will fit inside your nose. The medicine comes out of the nozzle.
Pressing the **Mist-Release Button** sprays a measured amount of medicine from the nozzle as a gentle, fine mist. Because the button is on the side of the device, you can keep the nozzle in the right place in your nose while you press the button.
The **Window** lets you see if there is medicine left in the bottle when you hold it in front of a bright light. (You may not be able to see the medicine in a full bottle because the liquid level is above the window.)

How to prime your VERAMYST Nasal Spray
Priming helps to make sure you always get the same full dose of medicine. You need to prime VERAMYST Nasal Spray:
- before you use a new bottle for the first time.
- if you have not used your VERAMYST Nasal Spray for 30 days or longer.
- if the cap has been left off the bottle for 5 days or longer.
- if the device does not seem to be working right.

To prime VERAMYST Nasal Spray:

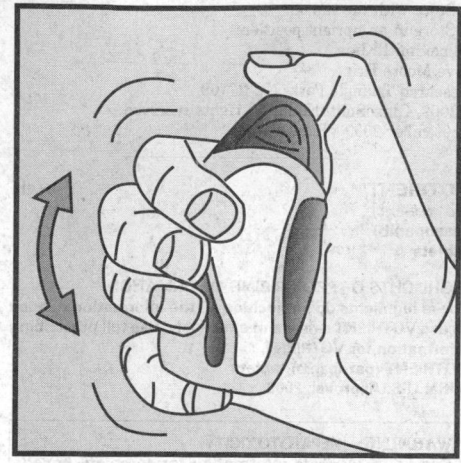

Figure 1

[See figure 2 at top of next column]
[See figure 3 in next column]
1. With the cap on, shake the device well (Figure 1). This is important to make the medicine a liquid that will spray.
2. Take the cap off by **squeezing** the finger grips and pulling it straight off (Figure 2).
3. Hold the device with the nozzle pointing up and away from you. Place your thumb or fingers on the button.

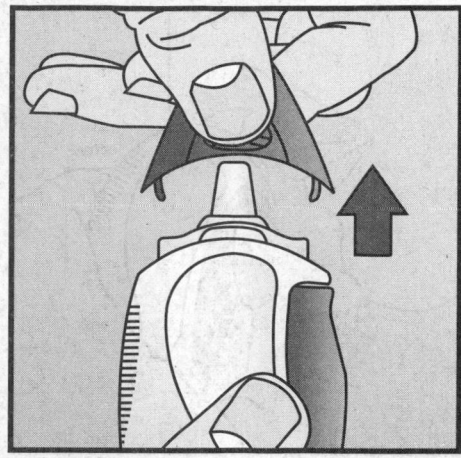

Figure 2

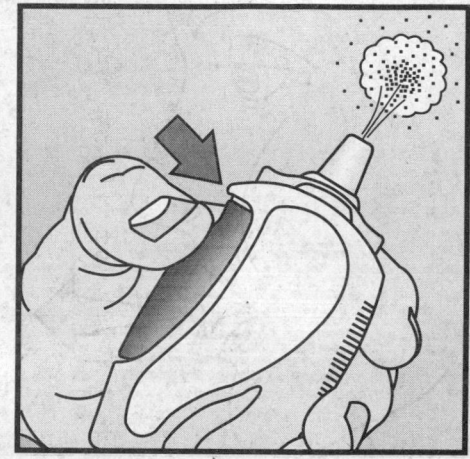

Figure 3

Press the button all the way in 6 times or until a fine mist sprays from the nozzle (Figure 3). Your VERAMYST Nasal Spray is now ready to use.

How to use your VERAMYST Nasal Spray
Follow the instructions below. If you have any questions, ask your healthcare provider or pharmacist.
Before taking a dose of VERAMYST Nasal Spray, gently blow your nose to clear your nostrils. Shake the bottle well. Then do these 3 simple steps: **Place, Press, Repeat.**

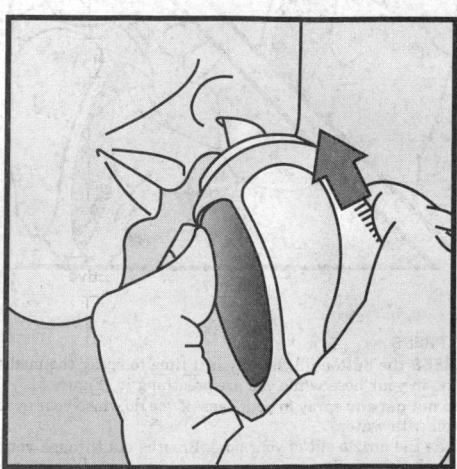

Figure 4

[See figure 5 at top of next column]
[See figure 6 in next column]
[See figure 7 in next column]
1. PLACE
Tilt your head forward a little bit. Hold the device upright. **PLACE** the nozzle in one of your nostrils (Figure 4).
Point the end of the nozzle toward the side of your nose, away from the center of your nose (septum). This helps get the medicine to the right part of your nose.

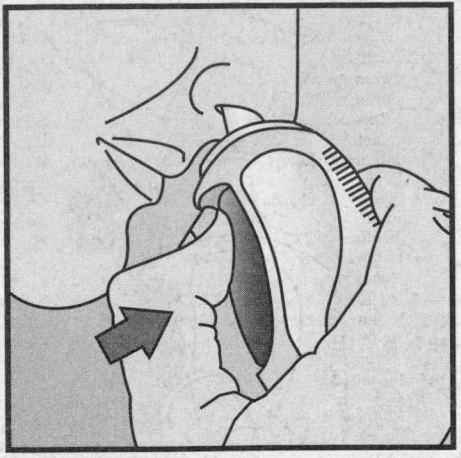

Figure 5

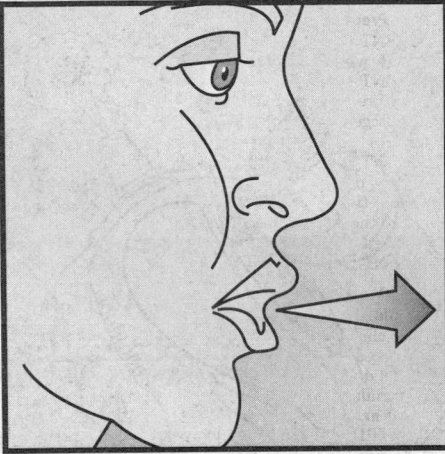

Figure 6

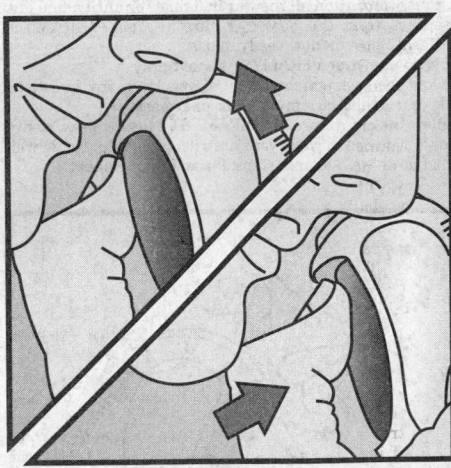

Figure 7

2. PRESS

PRESS the button all the way in 1 time to spray the medicine in your nose while you are breathing in (Figure 5).

Do not get any spray in your eyes. If you do, rinse your eyes well with water.

Take the nozzle out of your nose. Breathe out through your mouth (Figure 6).

3. REPEAT

To deliver the medicine to the other nostril, **REPEAT** Steps 1 and 2 in the other nostril (Figure 7).

If your healthcare provider has told you to take 2 sprays in each nostril, do Steps 1-3 again.

Put the cap back on the device after you have finished taking your dose.

How to clean your VERAMYST Nasal Spray

After each use: wipe the nozzle with a clean, dry tissue (Figure 8). **Never try to clean the nozzle with a pin or any-**

thing sharp because this will damage the nozzle. Do not use water to clean the nozzle.

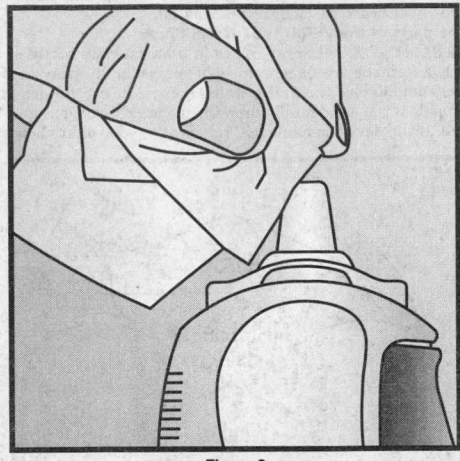

Figure 8

Once a week: clean the inside of the cap with a clean, dry tissue (Figure 9). This will help keep the nozzle from getting blocked.

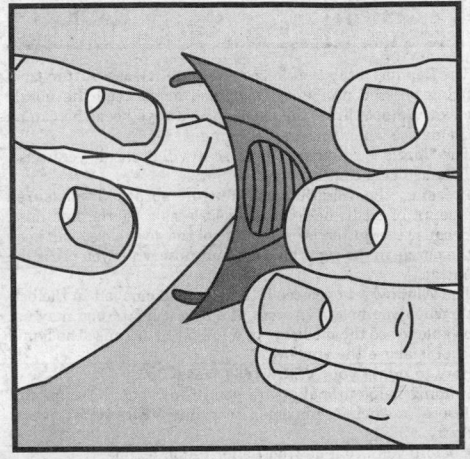

Figure 9

How to store your VERAMYST Nasal Spray

• Keep your VERAMYST Nasal Spray and all medicines out of the reach of children.
• Store between 59° and 86°F (15° and 30°C). Do not refrigerate or freeze.
• Store with the cap on.
• Store in an upright position.

GlaxoSmithKline
Five Moore Drive
Research Triangle Park, NC 27709
©2009, GlaxoSmithKline. All rights reserved.
September 2009 VRM:6PIL

VOTRIENT™ ℞

[vo' trē-ent]
(pazopanib)
tablets

HIGHLIGHTS OF PRESCRIBING INFORMATION
These highlights do not include all the information needed to use VOTRIENT safely and effectively. See full prescribing information for VOTRIENT.
VOTRIENT (pazopanib) tablets
Initial U.S. Approval: 2009

WARNING: HEPATOTOXICITY
See full prescribing information for complete boxed warning.
Severe and fatal hepatotoxicity has been observed in clinical studies. Monitor hepatic function and interrupt, reduce, or discontinue dosing as recommended. [See Warnings and Precautions (5.1).]

————INDICATIONS AND USAGE————
VOTRIENT is a kinase inhibitor indicated for the treatment of patients with advanced renal cell carcinoma. (1)

————DOSAGE AND ADMINISTRATION————
• 800 mg orally once daily without food (at least 1 hour before or 2 hours after a meal). (2.1)
• Baseline moderate hepatic impairment – 200 mg orally once daily. Not recommended in patients with severe hepatic impairment. (2.2)

————DOSAGE FORMS AND STRENGTHS————
200 mg tablets. (3)

————CONTRAINDICATIONS————
None. (4)

————WARNINGS AND PRECAUTIONS————
• Increases in serum transaminase levels and bilirubin were observed. Severe and fatal hepatotoxicity has occurred. Measure liver chemistries before the initiation of treatment and regularly during treatment. (5.1)
• Prolonged QT intervals and torsades de pointes have been observed. Use with caution in patients at higher risk of developing QT interval prolongation. Monitoring electrocardiograms and electrolytes should be considered. (5.2)
• Fatal hemorrhagic events have been reported. VOTRIENT has not been studied in patients who have a history of hemoptysis, cerebral, or clinically significant gastrointestinal hemorrhage in the past 6 months and should not be used in those patients. (5.3)
• Arterial thrombotic events have been observed and can be fatal. Use with caution in patients who are at increased risk for these events. (5.4)
• Gastrointestinal perforation or fistula has occurred. Fatal perforation events have occurred. Use with caution in patients at risk for gastrointestinal perforation or fistula. (5.5)
• Hypertension has been observed. Blood pressure should be well-controlled prior to initiating VOTRIENT. Monitor for hypertension and treat as needed. (5.6)
• Temporary interruption of therapy with VOTRIENT is recommended in patients undergoing surgical procedures. (5.7)
• Hypothyroidism may occur. Monitoring of thyroid function tests is recommended. (5.8)
• Proteinuria: Monitor urine protein. Discontinue for Grade 4 proteinuria. (5.9)
• VOTRIENT can cause fetal harm when administered to a pregnant woman. Women of childbearing potential should be advised of the potential hazard to the fetus and to avoid becoming pregnant while taking VOTRIENT. (5.10, 8.1)

————ADVERSE REACTIONS————
The most common adverse reactions (≥20%) are diarrhea, hypertension, hair color changes (depigmentation), nausea, anorexia, and vomiting. (6.1)

To report SUSPECTED ADVERSE REACTIONS, contact GlaxoSmithKline at 1-888-825-5249 or FDA at 1-800-FDA-1088 or www.fda.gov/medwatch

————DRUG INTERACTIONS————
• CYP3A4 Inhibitors: Avoid use of strong inhibitors. Consider dose reduction of VOTRIENT when administered with strong CYP3A4 inhibitors. (7.1)
• CYP3A4 Inducers: Consider an alternate concomitant medication with no or minimal enzyme induction potential or avoid VOTRIENT. (7.1)
• CYP Substrates: Concomitant use of VOTRIENT with agents with narrow therapeutic windows that are metabolized by CYP3A4, CYP2D6, or CYP2C8 is not recommended. (7.2)

See 17 for PATIENT COUNSELING INFORMATION and Medication Guide

Revised: 04/2010

*** Sections or subsections omitted from the full prescribing information are not listed**

FULL PRESCRIBING INFORMATION

WARNING: HEPATOTOXICITY
Severe and fatal hepatotoxicity has been observed in clinical studies. Monitor hepatic function and interrupt, reduce, or discontinue dosing as recommended. *[See Warnings and Precautions (5.1).]*

1 INDICATIONS AND USAGE

VOTRIENT™ is indicated for the treatment of patients with advanced renal cell carcinoma (RCC).

2 DOSAGE AND ADMINISTRATION

2.1 Recommended Dosing

The recommended dose of VOTRIENT is 800 mg orally once daily without food (at least 1 hour before or 2 hours after a meal) *[see Clinical Pharmacology (12.3)]*. The dose of VOTRIENT should not exceed 800 mg.

Do not crush tablets due to the potential for increased rate of absorption which may affect systemic exposure. *[See Clinical Pharmacology (12.3).]*

If a dose is missed, it should not be taken if it is less than 12 hours until the next dose.

2.2 Dose Modification Guidelines

Initial dose reduction should be 400 mg, and additional dose decrease or increase should be in 200 mg steps based on individual tolerability. The dose of VOTRIENT should not exceed 800 mg.

Hepatic Impairment: The dosage of VOTRIENT in patients with moderate hepatic impairment should be reduced to 200 mg per day. There are no data in patients with severe hepatic impairment; therefore, use of VOTRIENT is not recommended in these patients. *[See Use in Specific Populations (8.6).]*

Concomitant Strong CYP3A4 Inhibitors: The concomitant use of strong CYP3A4 inhibitors (e.g., ketoconazole, ritonavir, clarithromycin) may increase pazopanib concentrations and should be avoided. If coadministration of a strong CYP3A4 inhibitor is warranted, reduce the dose of VOTRIENT to 400 mg. Further dose reductions may be needed if adverse effects occur during therapy. This dose is predicted to adjust the pazopanib AUC to the range observed without inhibitors. However, there are no clinical data with this dose adjustment in patients receiving strong CYP3A4 inhibitors. *[See Drug Interactions (7.1).]*

Concomitant Strong CYP3A4 Inducer: The concomitant use of strong CYP3A4 inducers (e.g., rifampin) may decrease pazopanib concentrations and should be avoided. VOTRIENT should not be used in patients who can not avoid chronic use of strong CYP3A4 inducers. *[See Drug Interactions (7.1).]*

3 DOSAGE FORMS AND STRENGTHS

200 mg tablets of VOTRIENT—modified capsule-shaped, gray, film-coated with GS JT debossed on one side. Each tablet contains 216.7 mg of pazopanib hydrochloride equivalent to 200 mg of pazopanib.

4 CONTRAINDICATIONS

None.

5 WARNINGS AND PRECAUTIONS

5.1 Hepatic Effects

In clinical trials with VOTRIENT, hepatotoxicity, manifested as increases in serum transaminases (ALT, AST) and bilirubin, was observed *[see Adverse Reactions (6.1)]*. This hepatotoxicity can be severe and fatal. Transaminase elevations occur early in the course of treatment (92.5% of all transaminase elevations of any grade occurred in the first 18 weeks). Across all monotherapy studies with VOTRIENT, ALT >3 × upper limit of normal (ULN) was reported in 138/977 (14%) and ALT >8 × ULN was reported in 40/977 (4%) of patients who received VOTRIENT. Concurrent elevations in ALT >3 × ULN and bilirubin >2 × ULN regardless of alkaline phosphatase levels were detected in 13/977 (1%) of patients. Four of the 13 patients had no other explanation for these elevations.

Two of 977 (0.2%) patients died with disease progression and hepatic failure.

- Monitor serum liver tests before initiation of treatment with VOTRIENT and at least once every 4 weeks for at least the first 4 months of treatment or as clinically indicated. Periodic monitoring should then continue after this time period.
- Patients with isolated ALT elevations between 3 × ULN and 8 × ULN may be continued on VOTRIENT with weekly monitoring of liver function until ALT return to Grade 1 or baseline.
- Patients with isolated ALT elevations of >8 × ULN should have VOTRIENT interrupted until they return to Grade 1 or baseline. If the potential benefit for reinitiating treatment with VOTRIENT is considered to outweigh the risk for hepatotoxicity, then reintroduce VOTRIENT at a reduced dose of no more than 400 mg once daily and measure serum liver tests weekly for 8 weeks *[see Dosage and Administration (2.2)]*. Following reintroduction of VOTRIENT, if ALT elevations >3 × ULN recur, then VOTRIENT should be permanently discontinued.
- If ALT elevations >3 × ULN occur concurrently with bilirubin elevations >2 × ULN, VOTRIENT should be permanently discontinued. Patients should be monitored until resolution. VOTRIENT is a UGT1A1 inhibitor. Mild, indirect (unconjugated) hyperbilirubinemia may occur in patients with Gilbert's syndrome *[see Clinical Pharmacology (12.5)]*. Patients with only a mild indirect hyperbilirubinemia, known Gilbert's syndrome, and elevation in ALT >3 × ULN should be managed as per the recommendations outlined for isolated ALT elevations.

The safety of VOTRIENT in patients with pre-existing severe hepatic impairment, defined as total bilirubin >3 × ULN with any level of ALT, is unknown. Treatment with VOTRIENT is not recommended in patients with severe hepatic impairment. *[See Dosage and Administration (2.2) and Use in Specific Populations (8.6).]*

5.2 QT Prolongation and Torsades de Pointes

In clinical RCC studies of VOTRIENT, QT prolongation (≥500 msec) was identified on routine electrocardiogram monitoring in 11/558 (<2%) of patients. Torsades de pointes occurred in 2/977 (<1%) of patients who received VOTRIENT in the monotherapy studies.

In the randomized clinical trial, 3 of the 290 patients receiving VOTRIENT had post-baseline values between 500 to 549 msec. None of the 145 patients receiving placebo had post-baseline QTc values ≥500 msec.

VOTRIENT should be used with caution in patients with a history of QT interval prolongation, in patients taking antiarrhythmics or other medications that may prolong QT interval, and those with relevant pre-existing cardiac disease. When using VOTRIENT, baseline and periodic monitoring of electrocardiograms and maintenance of electrolytes (e.g., calcium, magnesium, potassium) within the normal range should be performed.

5.3 Hemorrhagic Events

In clinical RCC studies of VOTRIENT, hemorrhagic events have been reported [all Grades (16%) and Grades 3 to 5 (2%)]. Fatal hemorrhage has occurred in 5/586 (0.9%) *[see Adverse Reactions (6.1)]*. VOTRIENT has not been studied in patients who have a history of hemoptysis, cerebral, or clinically significant gastrointestinal hemorrhage in the past 6 months and should not be used in those patients.

5.4 Arterial Thrombotic Events

In clinical RCC studies of VOTRIENT, myocardial infarction, angina, ischemic stroke, and transient ischemic attack [all Grades (3%) and Grades 3 to 5 (2%)] were observed. Fatal events have been observed in 2/586 (0.3%). In the randomized study, these events were observed more frequently with VOTRIENT compared to placebo *[see Adverse Reactions (6.1)]*. VOTRIENT should be used with caution in patients who are at increased risk for these events or who have had a history of these events. VOTRIENT has not been studied in patients who have had an event within the previous 6 months and should not be used in those patients.

5.5 Gastrointestinal Perforation and Fistula

In clinical RCC studies of VOTRIENT, gastrointestinal perforation or fistula has been reported in 5 patients (0.9%). Fatal perforation events have occurred in 2/586 (0.3%). Monitor for symptoms of gastrointestinal perforation or fistula.

5.6 Hypertension

Blood pressure should be well-controlled prior to initiating VOTRIENT. Patients should be monitored for hypertension and treated as needed with anti-hypertensive therapy. Hypertension (systolic blood pressure ≥150 or diastolic blood pressure ≥100 mm Hg) was observed in 47% of patients with RCC treated with VOTRIENT. Hypertension occurs early in the course of treatment (88% occurred in the first 18 weeks). *[See Adverse Reactions (6.1).]* In the case of persistent hypertension despite anti-hypertensive therapy, the dose of VOTRIENT may be reduced *[see Dosage and Administration (2.2)]*. VOTRIENT should be discontinued if hypertension is severe and persistent despite anti-hypertensive therapy and dose reduction of VOTRIENT.

5.7 Wound Healing

No formal studies on the effect of VOTRIENT on wound healing have been conducted. Since vascular endothelial growth factor receptor (VEGFR) inhibitors such as pazopanib may impair wound healing, treatment with VOTRIENT should be stopped at least 7 days prior to scheduled surgery. The decision to resume VOTRIENT after surgery should be based on clinical judgment of adequate wound healing. VOTRIENT should be discontinued in patients with wound dehiscence.

5.8 Hypothyroidism

In clinical RCC studies of VOTRIENT, hypothyroidism reported as an adverse reaction in 26/586 (4%) *[see Adverse Reactions (6.1)]*. Proactive monitoring of thyroid function tests is recommended.

5.9 Proteinuria

In clinical RCC studies with VOTRIENT, proteinuria has been reported in 44/586 (8%) [Grade 3, 5/586 (<1%) and Grade 4, 1/586 (<1%)] *[see Adverse Reactions (6.1)]*. Baseline and periodic urinalysis during treatment is recommended. VOTRIENT should be discontinued if the patient develops Grade 4 proteinuria.

5.10 Pregnancy

VOTRIENT can cause fetal harm when administered to a pregnant woman. Based on its mechanism of action, VOTRIENT is expected to result in adverse reproductive effects. In pre-clinical studies in rats and rabbits, pazopanib was teratogenic, embryotoxic, fetotoxic, and abortifacient.

There are no adequate and well-controlled studies of VOTRIENT in pregnant women. If this drug is used during pregnancy, or if the patient becomes pregnant while taking this drug, the patient should be apprised of the potential hazard to the fetus. Women of childbearing potential should be advised to avoid becoming pregnant while taking VOTRIENT. *[See Use in Specific Populations (8.1).]*

6 ADVERSE REACTIONS

6.1 Clinical Trials Experience

Because clinical trials are conducted under widely varying conditions, adverse reaction rates observed in the clinical trials of a drug cannot be directly compared to rates in the clinical trials of another drug and may not reflect the rates observed in practice. Potentially serious adverse reactions with VOTRIENT included hepatotoxicity, QT prolongation and torsades de pointes, hemorrhagic events, arterial thrombotic events, and gastrointestinal perforation and fistula *[see Warnings and Precautions (5.1-5.5)]*.

The safety of VOTRIENT has been evaluated in 977 patients in the monotherapy studies which included 586 patients with RCC. With a median duration of treatment of 7.4 months (range 0.1 to 27.6), the most commonly observed adverse reactions (≥20%) in the 586 patients were diarrhea, hypertension, hair color change, nausea, fatigue, anorexia, and vomiting.

The data described below reflect the safety profile of VOTRIENT in 290 RCC patients who participated in a randomized, double-blind, placebo-controlled study *[see Clinical Studies (14)]*. The median duration of treatment was 7.4 months (range 0 to 23) for patients who received VOTRIENT and 3.8 months (range 0 to 22) for the placebo arm. Forty-two percent (42%) of patients on VOTRIENT required a dose interruption. Thirty-six percent (36%) of patients on VOTRIENT were dose reduced. Table 1 presents the most common adverse reactions occurring in ≥10% of patients who received VOTRIENT.

[See table 1 at top of next page]

Other adverse reactions observed more commonly in patients treated with VOTRIENT than placebo and that occurred in <10% (any grade) were alopecia (8% versus <1%), chest pain (5% versus 1%), dysgeusia (altered taste) (8% versus <1%), dyspepsia (5% versus <1%), facial edema (1% versus 0%), palmar-plantar erythrodysesthesia (hand-foot syndrome) (6% versus <1%), proteinuria (9% versus 0%), rash (8% versus 3%), skin depigmentation (3% versus 0%), and weight decreased (9% versus 3%).

Table 2 presents the most common laboratory abnormalities occurring in >10% of patients who received VOTRIENT and more commonly (≥5%) in patients who received VOTRIENT versus placebo.

[See table 2 on next page]

Hepatic Toxicity: In a controlled clinical study with VOTRIENT for the treatment of RCC, ALT >3 × ULN was reported in 18% and 3% of the VOTRIENT and placebo groups, respectively. ALT >10 × ULN was reported in 4% of patients who received VOTRIENT and in <1% of patients who received placebo. Concurrent elevation in ALT >3 × ULN and bilirubin >2 × ULN in the absence of significant alkaline phosphatase >3 × ULN occurred in 5/290 (2%) of patients on VOTRIENT and 2/145 (1%) on placebo. *[See*

Table 1. Adverse Reactions Occurring in ≥10% of Patients who Received VOTRIENT

Adverse Reactions	VOTRIENT (N = 290)			Placebo (N = 145)		
	All Grades[a]	Grade 3	Grade 4	All Grades[a]	Grade 3	Grade 4
	%	%	%	%	%	%
Diarrhea	52	3	<1	9	<1	0
Hypertension	40	4	0	10	<1	0
Hair color changes	38	<1	0	3	0	0
Nausea	26	<1	0	9	0	0
Anorexia	22	2	0	10	<1	0
Vomiting	21	2	<1	8	2	0
Fatigue	19	2	0	8	1	1
Asthenia	14	3	0	8	0	0
Abdominal pain	11	2	0	1	0	0
Headache	10	0	0	5	0	0

[a] National Cancer Institute Common Terminology Criteria for Adverse Events, version 3.

Table 2. Selected Laboratory Abnormalities Occurring in >10% of Patients who Received VOTRIENT and More Commonly (≥5%) in Patients who Received VOTRIENT Versus Placebo

Parameters	VOTRIENT (N = 290)			Placebo (N = 145)		
	All Grades[a]	Grade 3	Grade 4	All Grades[a]	Grade 3	Grade 4
	%	%	%	%	%	%
Hematologic						
Leukopenia	37	0	0	6	0	0
Neutropenia	34	1	<1	6	0	0
Thrombocytopenia	32	<1	<1	5	0	<1
Lymphocytopenia	31	4	<1	24	1	0
Chemistry						
ALT increased	53	10	2	22	1	0
AST increased	53	7	<1	19	<1	0
Glucose increased	41	<1	0	33	1	0
Total bilirubin increased	36	3	<1	10	1	<1
Phosphorus decreased	34	4	0	11	0	0
Sodium decreased	31	4	1	24	4	0
Magnesium decreased	26	<1	1	14	0	0
Glucose decreased	17	0	<1	3	0	0

[a] National Cancer Institute Common Terminology Criteria for Adverse Events, version 3.

Dosage and Administration (2.2) and Warnings and Precautions (5.1).]

Hypertension: In a controlled clinical study with VOTRIENT for the treatment of RCC, 115/290 patients (40%) receiving VOTRIENT compared with 15/145 patients (10%) on placebo experienced hypertension. Grade 3 hypertension was reported in 13/290 patients (4%) receiving VOTRIENT compared with 1/145 patients (<1%) on placebo. The majority of cases of hypertension were manageable with anti-hypertensive agents or dose reductions with 2/290 patients (<1%) permanently discontinuing treatment with VOTRIENT because of hypertension. In the overall safety population for RCC (N = 586), one patient had hypertensive crisis on VOTRIENT. *[See Warnings and Precautions (5.2).]*

QT Prolongation and Torsades de Pointes: In a controlled clinical study with VOTRIENT, QT prolongation (≥500 msec) was identified on routine electrocardiogram monitoring in 3/290 (1%) of patients treated with VOTRIENT compared with no patients on placebo. Torsades de pointes was reported in 2/586 (<1%) patients treated

with VOTRIENT in the RCC studies. *[See Warnings and Precautions (5.3).]*

Arterial Thrombotic Events: In a controlled clinical study with VOTRIENT, the incidences of arterial thrombotic events such as myocardial infarction/ischemia [5/290 (2%)], cerebral vascular accident [1/290 (<1%)], and transient ischemic attack [4/290 (1%)] were higher in patients treated with VOTRIENT compared to the placebo arm (0/145 for each event). *[See Warnings and Precautions (5.4).]*

Hemorrhagic Events: In a controlled clinical study with VOTRIENT, 37/290 patients (13%) treated with VOTRIENT and 7/145 patients (5%) on placebo experienced at least 1 hemorrhagic event. The most common hemorrhagic events in the patients treated with VOTRIENT were hematuria (4%), epistaxis (2%), hemoptysis (2%), and rectal hemorrhage (1%). Nine (9/37) patients treated with VOTRIENT who had hemorrhagic events experienced serious events including pulmonary, gastrointestinal, and genitourinary hemorrhage. Four (4/290) (1%) patients treated with VOTRIENT died from hemorrhage compared with no

(0/145) (0%) patients on placebo. *[See Warnings and Precautions (5.5).]* In the overall safety population in RCC (N = 586), cerebral/intracranial hemorrhage was observed in 2/586 (<1%) patients treated with VOTRIENT.

Hypothyroidism: In a controlled clinical study with VOTRIENT, more patients had a shift from thyroid stimulating hormone (TSH) within the normal range at baseline to above the normal range at any post-baseline visit in VOTRIENT compared with the placebo arm (27% compared with 5%, respectively). Hypothyroidism was reported as an adverse reaction in 19 patients (7%) treated with VOTRIENT and no patients (0%) in the placebo arm. *[See Warnings and Precautions (5.7).]*

Diarrhea: Diarrhea occurred frequently and was predominantly mild to moderate in severity. Patients should be advised how to manage mild diarrhea and to notify their healthcare provider if moderate to severe diarrhea occurs so appropriate management can be implemented to minimize its impact.

Proteinuria: In the controlled clinical study with VOTRIENT, proteinuria has been reported as an adverse reaction in 27 patients (9%) treated with VOTRIENT. In 2 patients, proteinuria led to discontinuation of treatment with VOTRIENT.

Lipase Elevations: In a single-arm clinical study, increases in lipase values were observed for 48/181 patients (27%). Elevations in lipase as an adverse reaction were reported for 10 patients (4%) and were Grade 3 for 6 patients and Grade 4 for 1 patient. In clinical RCC studies of VOTRIENT, clinical pancreatitis was observed in 4/586 patients (<1%).

Cardiac Dysfunction: Pazopanib has been associated with cardiac dysfunction (such as a decrease in ejection fraction and congestive heart failure) in patients with various cancer types, including RCC. In the overall safety population for RCC (N = 586), cardiac dysfunction was observed in 4/586 patients (<1%).

7 DRUG INTERACTIONS

7.1 Drugs That Inhibit or Induce Cytochrome P450 3A4 Enzymes

In vitro studies suggested that the oxidative metabolism of pazopanib in human liver microsomes is mediated primarily by CYP3A4, with minor contributions from CYP1A2 and CYP2C8. Therefore, inhibitors and inducers of CYP3A4 may alter the metabolism of pazopanib.

CYP3A4 Inhibitors: Coadministration of pazopanib with strong inhibitors of CYP3A4 (e.g., ketoconazole, ritonavir, clarithromycin) may increase pazopanib concentrations. A dose reduction for VOTRIENT should be considered when it must be coadministered with strong CYP3A4 inhibitors *[see Dosage and Administration (2.2)]*. Grapefruit juice should be avoided as it inhibits CYP3A4 activity and may also increase plasma concentrations of pazopanib.

CYP3A4 Inducers: CYP3A4 inducers such as rifampin may decrease plasma pazopanib concentrations. VOTRIENT should not be used if chronic use of strong CYP3A4 inducers can not be avoided *[see Dosage and Administration (2.2)]*.

7.2 Effects of Pazopanib on CYP Substrates

Results from drug-drug interaction studies conducted in cancer patients suggest that pazopanib is a weak inhibitor of CYP3A4, CYP2C8, and CYP2D6 in vivo, but had no effect on CYP1A2, CYP2C9, or CYP2C19 *[see Clinical Pharmacology (12.3)]*.

Concomitant use of VOTRIENT with agents with narrow therapeutic windows that are metabolized by CYP3A4, CYP2D6, or CYP2C8 is not recommended. Coadministration may result in inhibition of the metabolism of these products and create the potential for serious adverse events. *[See Clinical Pharmacology (12.3).]*

8 USE IN SPECIFIC POPULATIONS

8.1 Pregnancy

Pregnancy Category D *[see Warnings and Precautions (5.10)]*.

VOTRIENT can cause fetal harm when administered to a pregnant woman. There are no adequate and well-controlled studies of VOTRIENT in pregnant women.

In pre-clinical studies in rats and rabbits, pazopanib was teratogenic, embryotoxic, fetotoxic, and abortifacient. Administration of pazopanib to pregnant rats during organogenesis at a dose level of ≥3 mg/kg/day (approximately 0.1 times the human clinical exposure based on AUC) resulted in teratogenic effects including cardiovascular malformations (retroesophageal subclavian artery, missing innominate artery, changes in the aortic arch) and incomplete or absent ossification. In addition, there was reduced fetal body weight, and pre- and post-implantation embryolethality in rats administered pazopanib at doses ≥3 mg/kg/day. In rabbits, maternal toxicity (reduced food consumption, increased post-implantation loss, and abortion) was observed at doses ≥30 mg/kg/day (approximately 0.007 times the human clinical exposure). In addition, severe maternal body weight loss and 100% litter loss were observed at doses

≥100 mg/kg/day (0.02 times the human clinical exposure), while fetal weight was reduced at doses ≥3 mg/kg/day (AUC not calculated).

If this drug is used during pregnancy, or if the patient becomes pregnant while taking this drug, the patient should be apprised of the potential hazard to the fetus. Women of childbearing potential should be advised to avoid becoming pregnant while taking VOTRIENT.

8.3 Nursing Mothers

It is not known whether this drug is excreted in human milk. Because many drugs are excreted in human milk and because of the potential for serious adverse reactions in nursing infants from VOTRIENT, a decision should be made whether to discontinue nursing or to discontinue the drug, taking into account the importance of the drug to the mother.

8.4 Pediatric Use

The safety and effectiveness of VOTRIENT in pediatric patients have not been established.

In repeat-dose toxicology studies in rats including 4-week, 13-week, and 26-week administration, toxicities in bone, teeth, and nail beds were observed at doses ≥3 mg/kg/day (approximately 0.07 times the human clinical exposure based on AUC). Doses of 300 mg/kg/day (approximately 0.8 times the human clinical exposure based on AUC) were not tolerated in 13- and 26-week studies with rats. Body weight loss and morbidity were observed at these doses. Hypertrophy of epiphyseal growth plates, nail abnormalities (including broken, overgrown, or absent nails) and tooth abnormalities in growing incisor teeth (including excessively long, brittle, broken and missing teeth, and dentine and enamel degeneration and thinning) were observed in rats at ≥30 mg/kg/day (approximately 0.35 times the human clinical exposure based on AUC) at 26 weeks, with the onset of tooth and nail bed alterations noted clinically after 4 to 6 weeks.

8.5 Geriatric Use

In clinical trials with VOTRIENT for the treatment of RCC, 196 subjects (33%) were aged ≥65 years, and 34 subjects (6%) were aged >75 years. No overall differences in safety or effectiveness of VOTRIENT were observed between these subjects and younger subjects. However, patients >60 years of age may be at greater risk for an ALT >3 × ULN. Other reported clinical experience has not identified differences in responses between elderly and younger patients, but greater sensitivity of some older individuals cannot be ruled out.

8.6 Hepatic Impairment

The safety and pharmacokinetics of pazopanib in patients with hepatic impairment have not been fully established. In clinical studies for VOTRIENT, patients with total bilirubin ≤1.5 × ULN and AST and ALT ≤2 × ULN were included *[see Warnings and Precautions (5.1)]*.

An interim analysis of data from 12 patients with normal hepatic function and 9 with moderate hepatic impairment showed that the maximum tolerated dose in patients with moderate hepatic impairment was 200 mg per day *[see Clinical Pharmacology (12.3)]*. There are no data on patients with severe hepatic impairment *[see Dosage and Administration (2.2)]*.

8.7 Renal Impairment

Patients with renal cell cancer and mild/moderate renal impairment (creatinine clearance ≥30 mL/min) were included in clinical studies for VOTRIENT.

There are no clinical or pharmacokinetic data in patients with severe renal impairment or in patients undergoing peritoneal dialysis or hemodialysis. However, renal impairment is unlikely to significantly affect the pharmacokinetics of pazopanib since <4% of a radiolabeled oral dose was recovered in the urine. In a population pharmacokinetic analysis using 408 subjects with various cancers, creatinine clearance (30-150 mL/min) did not influence clearance of pazopanib. Therefore, renal impairment is not expected to influence pazopanib exposure, and dose adjustment is not necessary.

10 OVERDOSAGE

Pazopanib doses up to 2,000 mg have been evaluated in clinical trials. Dose-limiting toxicity (Grade 3 fatigue) and Grade 3 hypertension were each observed in 1 of 3 patients dosed at 2,000 mg daily and 1,000 mg daily, respectively.

Treatment of overdose with VOTRIENT should consist of general supportive measures. There is no specific antidote for overdosage of VOTRIENT.

Hemodialysis is not expected to enhance the elimination of VOTRIENT because pazopanib is not significantly renally excreted and is highly bound to plasma proteins.

11 DESCRIPTION

VOTRIENT (pazopanib) is a tyrosine kinase inhibitor (TKI). Pazopanib is presented as the hydrochloride salt, with the chemical name 5-[[4-[(2,3-dimethyl-2H-indazol-6-yl)methylamino]-2-pyrimidinyl]amino]-2-methylbenzenesulfonamide monohydrochloride. It has the molecular formula $C_{21}H_{23}N_7O_2S \cdot HCl$ and a molecular weight of 473.99. Pazopanib hydrochloride has the following chemical structure:

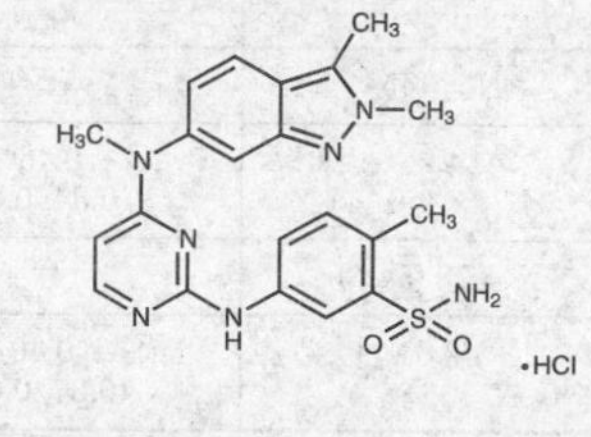

Pazopanib hydrochloride is a white to slightly yellow solid. It is very slightly soluble at pH 1 and practically insoluble above pH 4 in aqueous media.

Tablets of VOTRIENT are for oral administration. Each 200 mg tablet of VOTRIENT contains 216.7 mg of pazopanib hydrochloride, equivalent to 200 mg of pazopanib free base.

The inactive ingredients of VOTRIENT are: **Tablet Core:** Magnesium stearate, microcrystalline cellulose, povidone, sodium starch glycolate. **Coating**: Gray film-coat: Hypromellose, iron oxide black, macrogol/polyethylene glycol 400 (PEG 400), polysorbate 80, titanium dioxide.

12 CLINICAL PHARMACOLOGY

12.1 Mechanism of Action

Pazopanib is a multi-tyrosine kinase inhibitor of vascular endothelial growth factor receptor (VEGFR)-1, VEGFR-2, VEGFR-3, platelet-derived growth factor receptor (PDGFR)-α and -β, fibroblast growth factor receptor (FGFR) -1 and -3, cytokine receptor (Kit), interleukin-2 receptor inducible T-cell kinase (Itk), leukocyte-specific protein tyrosine kinase (Lck), and transmembrane glycoprotein receptor tyrosine kinase (c-Fms). In vitro, pazopanib inhibited ligand-induced autophosphorylation of VEGFR-2, Kit and PDGFR-β receptors. In vivo, pazopanib inhibited VEGF-induced VEGFR-2 phosphorylation in mouse lungs, angiogenesis in a mouse model, and the growth of some human tumor xenografts in mice.

12.2 Pharmacodynamics

Increases in blood pressure have been observed and are related to steady-state trough plasma pazopanib concentrations.

The QT prolongation potential of pazopanib was assessed as part of an uncontrolled. open-label, dose escalation study in advanced cancer patients. Sixty-three patients received doses of pazopanib ranging from 50 to 2,000 mg daily. Serial ECGs were collected on Day 1 and single pre-dose ECGs were collected on Days 8, 15, and 22 to evaluate the effect of pazopanib on QTc intervals. Two of the 63 patients had QTcF (corrected QT by the Fridericia method) >500 msec and three patients had an increase in QTcF >60 msec from baseline. *[See Warnings and Precautions (5.2).]*

12.3 Pharmacokinetics

Absorption: Pazopanib is absorbed orally with median time to achieve peak concentrations of 2 to 4 hours after the dose. Daily dosing at 800 mg results in geometric mean AUC and C_{max} of 1,037 hr•μg/mL and 58.1 μg/mL (equivalent to 132 μM), respectively. There was no consistent increase in AUC or C_{max} at pazopanib doses above 800 mg.

Administration of a single pazopanib 400 mg crushed tablet increased $AUC_{(0-72)}$ by 46% and C_{max} by approximately 2 fold and decreased t_{max} by approximately 2 hours compared to administration of the whole tablet. These results indicate that the bioavailability and the rate of pazopanib oral absorption are increased after administration of the crushed tablet relative to administration of the whole tablet. Therefore, due to this potential for increased exposure, tablets of VOTRIENT should not be crushed.

Systemic exposure to pazopanib is increased when administered with food. Administration of pazopanib with a high-fat or low-fat meal results in an approximately 2-fold increase in AUC and C_{max}. Therefore, pazopanib should be administered at least 1 hour before or 2 hours after a meal *[see Dosage and Administration (2.1)]*.

Distribution: Binding of pazopanib to human plasma protein in vivo was greater than 99% with no concentration dependence over the range of 10 to 100 μg/mL. In vitro studies suggest that pazopanib is a substrate for P-glycoprotein (Pgp) and breast cancer resistant protein (BCRP).

Metabolism: In vitro studies demonstrated that pazopanib is metabolized by CYP3A4 with a minor contribution from CYP1A2 and CYP2C8.

Elimination: Pazopanib has a mean half-life of 30.9 hours after administration of the recommended dose of 800 mg. Elimination is primarily via feces with renal elimination accounting for <4% of the administered dose.

Hepatic Impairment: Interim data from a dose escalation study assessed the influence of hepatic impairment on the safety and pharmacokinetics of pazopanib in cancer patients with normal hepatic function and in patients with mild, moderate, and severe hepatic impairment. The starting doses were 800, 400, 200, and 100 mg once daily for patients with normal hepatic function and patients with mild, moderate, and severe hepatic impairment, respectively.

Pharmacokinetic data from patients with normal hepatic function (n = 12) and moderate (n = 7) hepatic impairment indicate that pazopanib clearance was decreased by 50% in those with moderate hepatic impairment. The maximum tolerated pazopanib dose in patients with moderate hepatic impairment is 200 mg once daily. There are no data on patients with mild or severe hepatic impairment. *[See Use in Specific Populations (8.6).]*

Drug Interactions: Coadministration of oral pazopanib with CYP3A4 inhibitors has resulted in increased plasma pazopanib concentrations. Concurrent administration of a single dose of pazopanib eye drops with the strong CYP3A4 inhibitor and Pgp inhibitor, ketoconazole, in healthy volunteers resulted in 220% and 150% increase in mean $AUC_{(0-t)}$ and C_{max} values, respectively. *[See Dosage and Administration (2.2) and Drug Interactions (7.1).]*

Administration of 1,500 mg lapatinib, a substrate and weak inhibitor of CYP3A4, Pgp, and BCRP, with 800 mg pazopanib resulted in an approximately 50% to 60% increase in mean pazopanib $AUC_{(0-24)}$ and C_{max} compared to administration of 800 mg pazopanib alone.

In vitro studies with human liver microsomes showed that pazopanib inhibited the activities of CYP enzymes 1A2, 3A4, 2B6, 2C8, 2C9, 2C19, 2D6, and 2E1. Potential induction of human CYP3A4 was demonstrated in an in vitro human PXR assay. Clinical pharmacology studies, using pazopanib 800 mg once daily, have demonstrated that pazopanib does not have a clinically relevant effect on the pharmacokinetics of caffeine (CYP1A2 probe substrate), warfarin (CYP2C9 probe substrate), or omeprazole (CYP2C19 probe substrate) in cancer patients. Pazopanib resulted in an increase of approximately 30% in the mean AUC and C_{max} of midazolam (CYP3A4 probe substrate) and increases of 33% to 64% in the ratio of dextromethorphan to dextrorphan concentrations in the urine after oral administration of dextromethorphan (CYP2D6 probe substrate). Coadministration of pazopanib 800 mg once daily and paclitaxel 80 mg/m^2 (CYP3A4 and CYP2C8 substrate) once weekly resulted in a mean increase of 26% and 31% in paclitaxel AUC and C_{max}, respectively. *[See Drug Interactions (7.2).]*

In vitro studies also showed that pazopanib inhibits UGT1A1 and OATP1B1 with IC50s of 1.2 and 0.79 μM, respectively. Pazopanib may increase concentrations of drugs eliminated by UGT1A1 and OATP1B1.

12.5 Pharmacogenomics

Pazopanib can increase serum total bilirubin levels *[see Warnings and Precautions (5.1).]*. In vitro studies showed that pazopanib inhibits UGT1A1, which glucuronidates bilirubin for elimination. A pooled pharmacogenetic analysis of 236 Caucasian patients evaluated the TA repeat polymorphism of UGT1A1 and its potential association with hyperbilirubinemia during pazopanib treatment. In this analysis, the (TA)7/(TA)7 genotype (UGT1A1*28/*28) (underlying genetic susceptibility to Gilbert's syndrome) was associated with a statistically significant increase in the incidence of hyperbilirubinemia relative to the (TA)6/(TA)6 and (TA)6/(TA)7 genotypes.

13 NONCLINICAL TOXICOLOGY

13.1 Carcinogenesis, Mutagenesis, Impairment of Fertility

Carcinogenicity studies with pazopanib have not been conducted. However, in a 13-week study in mice, proliferative lesions in the liver including eosinophilic foci in 2 females and a single case of adenoma in another female was observed at doses of 1,000 mg/kg/ day (approximately 2.5 times the human clinical exposure based on AUC).

Pazopanib did not induce mutations in the microbial mutagenesis (Ames) assay and was not clastogenic in both the in vitro cytogenetic assay using primary human lymphocytes and in the in vivo rat micronucleus assay.

Pazopanib may impair fertility in humans. In female rats, reduced fertility including increased pre-implantation loss and early resorptions were noted at dosages ≥30 mg/kg/day (approximately 0.4 times the human clinical exposure based on AUC). Total litter resorption was seen at 300 mg/kg/day (approximately 0.8 times the human clinical exposure based on AUC). Post-implantation loss, embryolethality, and decreased fetal body weight were noted in females administered doses ≥10 mg/kg/day (approximately 0.3 times the human clinical exposure based on AUC). Decreased corpora lutea and increased cysts were noted in mice given ≥100 mg/kg/day for 13 weeks and ovarian atrophy was

Table 3. Efficacy Results by Independent Assessment

Endpoint/Study Population	VOTRIENT	Placebo	HR (95% CI)
PFS			
Overall ITT	N = 290	N = 145	
Median (months)	9.2	4.2	0.46[a] (0.34, 0.62)
Treatment-naïve subgroup	N = 155 (53%)	N = 78 (54%)	
Median (months)	11.1	2.8	0.40 (0.27, 0.60)
Cytokine pre-treated subgroup	N = 135 (47%)	N = 67 (46%)	
Median (months)	7.4	4.2	0.54 (0.35, 0.84)
Response Rate (CR + PR)	N = 290	N = 145	
% (95% CI)	30 (25.1, 35.6)	3 (0.5, 6.4)	–
Duration of response			
Median (weeks) (95% CI)	58.7 (52.1, 68.1)	_b	

HR = Hazard Ratio; ITT = Intent to Treat; PFS = Progression-free Survival; CR = Complete Response; PR = Partial Response
[a] P value <0.001
[b] There were only 5 objective responses.

noted in rats given ≥300 mg/kg/day for 26 weeks (approximately 1.3 and 0.85 times the human clinical exposure based on AUC, respectively). Decreased corpora lutea was also noted in monkeys given 500 mg/kg/day for up to 34 weeks (approximately 0.4 times the human clinical exposure based on AUC).

Pazopanib did not affect mating or fertility in male rats. However, there were reductions in sperm production rates and testicular sperm concentrations at doses ≥3 mg/kg/day, epididymal sperm concentrations at doses ≥30 mg/kg/day, and sperm motility at ≥100 mg/kg/day following 15 weeks of dosing. Following 15 and 26 weeks of dosing, there were decreased testicular and epididymal weights at doses of ≥30 mg/kg/day (approximately 0.35 times the human clinical exposure based on AUC); atrophy and degeneration of the testes with aspermia, hypospermia and cribiform change in the epididymis was also observed at this dose in the 6-month toxicity studies in male rats.

14 CLINICAL STUDIES

The safety and efficacy of VOTRIENT in renal cell carcinoma (RCC) were evaluated in a randomized, double-blind, placebo-controlled, multicenter, Phase 3 study. Patients (N = 435) with locally advanced and/or metastatic RCC who had received either no prior therapy or one prior cytokine-based systemic therapy were randomized (2:1) to receive VOTRIENT 800 mg once daily or placebo once daily. The primary objective of the study was to evaluate and compare the 2 treatment arms for progression-free survival (PFS); the secondary endpoints included overall survival (OS), overall response rate (RR), and duration of response.

Of the total of 435 patients enrolled in this study, 233 patients had no prior systemic therapy (treatment-naïve subgroup) and 202 patients received one prior IL-2 or INFα-based therapy (cytokine-pretreated subgroup). The baseline demographic and disease characteristics were balanced between the VOTRIENT and placebo arms. The majority of patients were male (71%) with a median age of 59 years. Eighty-six percent of patients were Caucasian, 14% were Asian and less than 1% were other. Forty-two percent were ECOG performance status 0 and 58% were ECOG performance status 1. All patients had clear cell histology (90%) or predominantly clear cell histology (10%). Approximately 50% of all patients had 3 or more organs involved with metastatic disease. The most common metastatic sites at baseline were lung (74%), lymph nodes (56%), bone (27%), and liver (25%).

A similar proportion of patients in each arm were treatment-naïve and cytokine-pretreated (see Table 3). In the cytokine-pretreated subgroup, the majority (75%) had received interferon-based treatment. Similar proportions of patients in each arm had prior nephrectomy (89% and 88% for VOTRIENT and placebo, respectively).

The analysis of the primary endpoint PFS was based on disease assessment by independent radiological review in the entire study population. OS data were not mature at the time of the interim survival analysis. Efficacy results are presented in Table 3 and Figure 1.

[See table 3 above]

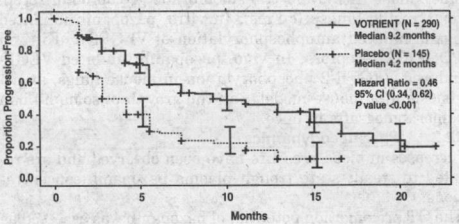

Figure 1. Kaplan-Meier Curve for Progression-Free Survival by Independent Assessment for the Overall Population (Treatment-Naïve and Cytokine Pre-Treated Populations)

16 HOW SUPPLIED/STORAGE AND HANDLING

The 200 mg tablets of VOTRIENT are modified capsule-shaped, gray, film-coated with GS JT debossed on one side and are available in:

Bottles of 120 tablets: NDC 0173-0804-09

Store at 25°C (77°F); excursions permitted to 15° to 30°C (59° to 86°F) [See USP Controlled Room Temperature].

17 PATIENT COUNSELING INFORMATION

See Medication Guide. The Medication Guide is contained in a separate leaflet that accompanies the product. However, inform patients of the following:

• Therapy with VOTRIENT may result in hepatobiliary laboratory abnormalities. Monitor serum liver tests (ALT, AST, and bilirubin) prior to initiation of VOTRIENT and at least once every 4 weeks for the first 4 months of treatment or as clinically indicated. Inform patients that they should report any of the following signs and symptoms of liver problems to their healthcare provider right away.

  • yellowing of the skin or the whites of the eyes (jaundice),
  • unusual darkening of the urine,
  • unusual tiredness,
  • right upper stomach area pain.

• Gastrointestinal adverse reactions such as diarrhea, nausea, and vomiting have been reported with VOTRIENT. Patients should be advised how to manage diarrhea and to notify their healthcare provider if moderate to severe diarrhea occurs.

• Women of childbearing potential should be advised of the potential hazard to the fetus and to avoid becoming pregnant.

• Patients should be advised to inform their healthcare providers of all concomitant medications, vitamins, or dietary and herbal supplements.

• Patients should be advised that depigmentation of the hair or skin may occur during treatment with VOTRIENT.

• Patients should be advised to take VOTRIENT without food (at least 1 hour before or 2 hours after a meal).

VOTRIENT is a trademark of GlaxoSmithKline.

GlaxoSmithKline
Research Triangle Park, NC 27709
©2010, GlaxoSmithKline. All rights reserved.
April 2010
VTR:3PI

MEDICATION GUIDE
VOTRIENT™ (VO-tree-ent)
(pazopanib)
tablets

Read the Medication Guide that comes with VOTRIENT before you start taking it and each time you get a refill. There may be new information. This Medication Guide does not take the place of talking with your healthcare provider about your medical condition or treatment.

What is the most important information I should know about VOTRIENT?

• **VOTRIENT can cause serious liver problems including death.** Your healthcare provider will do blood tests to check your liver before you start and while you take VOTRIENT.

Tell your healthcare provider right away if you have any of these signs of liver problems:

• yellowing of your skin or the whites of your eyes (jaundice)
• dark urine
• tiredness
• nausea or vomiting
• loss of appetite
• pain on the right side of your stomach
• bruise easily

What is VOTRIENT?

VOTRIENT is a prescription medicine used to treat advanced renal cell cancer in adults.

It is not known if VOTRIENT is safe or effective in children under 18 years of age.

What should I tell my healthcare provider before taking VOTRIENT?

Before you take VOTRIENT, tell your healthcare provider if you:

• have or had liver problems
• have high blood pressure
• have heart problems or an irregular heartbeat including QT prolongation
• have a history of a stroke
• have coughed up blood in the last 6 months
• had bleeding of your stomach or intestines in the last 6 months
• have a history of a tear (perforation) in your stomach or intestine, or an abnormal connection between two parts of your gastrointestinal tract (fistula)
• have thyroid problems
• had recent surgery (within the last 7 days) or are going to have surgery
• have any other medical conditions
• are pregnant or plan to become pregnant. VOTRIENT can harm your unborn baby. You should not become pregnant while you are taking VOTRIENT.
• are breast-feeding or plan to breast-feed. It is not known if VOTRIENT passes into your breast milk. You and your healthcare provider should decide if you will take VOTRIENT or breast-feed. You should not do both.

Tell your healthcare provider about all the medicines you take including prescription and non-prescription medicines, vitamins, and herbal supplements. VOTRIENT may affect the way other medicines work and other medicines may affect how VOTRIENT works.

Especially, tell your healthcare provider if you:

• take medicines that can affect enzyme metabolism such as:
  • some antibiotics (used to treat infections)
  • some drugs used to treat HIV
  • some drugs used to treat depression
  • drugs used to treat irregular heart beats
• drink grapefruit juice

Ask your healthcare provider if you are not sure if your medicine is one that is listed above.

Know the medicines you take. Keep a list of them and show it to your healthcare provider and pharmacist when you get a new medicine.

How should I take VOTRIENT?

• Take VOTRIENT exactly as your healthcare provider tells you. Your healthcare provider will tell you how much VOTRIENT to take.
• Your healthcare provider may change your dose.
• Take VOTRIENT on an empty stomach, at least 1 hour before or 2 hours after food.
• Do not crush tablets of VOTRIENT.
• Do not eat grapefruit or drink grapefruit juice at the same time as tablets of VOTRIENT. They may change the amount of VOTRIENT in your body.
• If you miss a dose, take it as soon as you remember. Do not take it if it is close (within 12 hours) to your next dose. Just take the next dose at your regular time. Do not take more than 1 dose of VOTRIENT at a time.
• Your healthcare provider will test your blood and heart before you start and while you take VOTRIENT.

What are the possible side effects of VOTRIENT?
VOTRIENT may cause serious side effects including:
- See "What is the most important information I should know about VOTRIENT?".
- **high blood pressure**
- **irregular or fast heartbeat or fainting**
- **heart attack or stroke:** chest pain or pressure, pain in your arms, back, neck or jaw, shortness of breath, numbness or weakness on one side of your body, trouble talking, headache, or dizziness.
- **bleeding problems:** unusual bleeding, bruising, wounds that do not heal.
- **tear in your stomach or intestinal wall (perforation) or bleeding:** pain, swelling in your stomach-area, vomiting blood, and black sticky stools.
- **thyroid problems**

Call your healthcare provider right away, if you have any of the symptoms listed above.
The most common side effects of VOTRIENT include:
- diarrhea
- change in hair color
- nausea or vomiting
- loss of appetite
- feeling tired

Tell your healthcare provider if you have any side effect that bothers you or that does not go away. These are not all the possible side effects of VOTRIENT. For more information, ask your healthcare provider or pharmacist.
Call your doctor for medical advice about side effects. You may report side effects to FDA at 1-800-FDA-1088.

How should I store VOTRIENT tablets?
Store VOTRIENT between 59°F to 86°F (15°C to 30°C).
Keep VOTRIENT and all medicines out of the reach of children.
General information about the safe and effective use of VOTRIENT:
Medicines are sometimes prescribed for purposes other than those listed in a Medication Guide. Do not use VOTRIENT for a condition for which it was not prescribed. Do not give VOTRIENT to other people even if they have the same symptoms that you have. It may harm them.
This Medication Guide summarizes the most important information about VOTRIENT. If you would like more information, talk with your healthcare provider. You can ask your pharmacist or healthcare provider for information about VOTRIENT that is written for healthcare professionals. For more information, go to www.VOTRIENT.com or call 1-888-825-5249.

What are the ingredients in VOTRIENT?
Active Ingredient: pazopanib.
Inactive Ingredients: hypromellose, iron oxide black, macrogol/polyethylene glycol 400 (PEG 400), magnesium stearate, microcrystalline cellulose, polysorbate 80, povidone, sodium starch glycolate, titanium dioxide.
VOTRIENT is a trademark of GlaxoSmithKline.
This Medication Guide has been approved by the U.S. Food and Drug Administration.
GlaxoSmithKline
Research Triangle Park, NC 27709
©2010, GlaxoSmithKline. All rights reserved.
Revised: April 2010
VTR:2MG

WELLBUTRIN®   ℞
[wel′byü-trin]
(bupropion hydrochloride)
Tablets

WARNING
Suicidality and Antidepressant Drugs
Use in Treating Psychiatric Disorders: Antidepressants increased the risk compared to placebo of suicidal thinking and behavior (suicidality) in children, adolescents, and young adults in short-term studies of major depressive disorder (MDD) and other psychiatric disorders. Anyone considering the use of WELLBUTRIN or any other antidepressant in a child, adolescent, or young adult must balance this risk with the clinical need. Short-term studies did not show an increase in the risk of suicidality with antidepressants compared to placebo in adults beyond age 24; there was a reduction in risk with antidepressants compared to placebo in adults aged 65 and older. Depression and certain other psychiatric disorders are themselves associated with increases in the risk of suicide. Patients of all ages who are started on antidepressant therapy should be monitored appropriately and observed closely for clinical worsening, suicidality, or unusual changes in behavior. Families and caregivers should be advised of the need for close observation and communication with the prescriber. WELLBUTRIN is not approved for use in pediatric patients. (See WARNINGS: Clinical Worsening and Suicide Risk in Treating Psychiatric Disorders, PRECAUTIONS: Information for Patients, and PRECAUTIONS: Pediatric Use.)

Use in Smoking Cessation Treatment: WELLBUTRIN®, WELLBUTRIN SR®, and WELLBUTRIN XL® are not approved for smoking cessation treatment, but bupropion under the name ZYBAN® is approved for this use. Serious neuropsychiatric events, including but not limited to depression, suicidal ideation, suicide attempt, and completed suicide have been reported in patients taking bupropion for smoking cessation. Some cases may have been complicated by the symptoms of nicotine withdrawal in patients who stopped smoking. Depressed mood may be a symptom of nicotine withdrawal. Depression, rarely including suicidal ideation, has been reported in smokers undergoing a smoking cessation attempt without medication. However, some of these symptoms have occurred in patients taking bupropion who continued to smoke. All patients being treated with bupropion for smoking cessation treatment should be observed for neuropsychiatric symptoms including changes in behavior, hostility, agitation, depressed mood, and suicide-related events, including ideation, behavior, and attempted suicide. These symptoms, as well as worsening of pre-existing psychiatric illness and completed suicide have been reported in some patients attempting to quit smoking while taking ZYBAN in the postmarketing experience. When symptoms were reported, most were during treatment with ZYBAN, but some were following discontinuation of treatment with ZYBAN. These events have occurred in patients with and without pre-existing psychiatric disease; some have experienced worsening of their psychiatric illnesses. Patients with serious psychiatric illness such as schizophrenia, bipolar disorder, and major depressive disorder did not participate in the premarketing studies of ZYBAN.
Advise patients and caregivers that the patient using bupropion for smoking cessation should stop taking bupropion and contact a healthcare provider immediately if agitation, hostility, depressed mood, or changes in thinking or behavior that are not typical for the patient are observed, or if the patient develops suicidal ideation or suicidal behavior. In many postmarketing cases, resolution of symptoms after discontinuation of ZYBAN was reported, although in some cases the symptoms persisted; therefore, ongoing monitoring and supportive care should be provided until symptoms resolve.
The risks of using bupropion for smoking cessation should be weighed against the benefits of its use. ZYBAN has been demonstrated to increase the likelihood of abstinence from smoking for as long as 6 months compared to treatment with placebo. The health benefits of quitting smoking are immediate and substantial. (See WARNINGS: Neuropsychiatric Symptoms and Suicide Risk in Smoking Cessation Treatment and PRECAUTIONS: Information for Patients.)

DESCRIPTION
WELLBUTRIN (bupropion hydrochloride), an antidepressant of the aminoketone class, is chemically unrelated to tricyclic, tetracyclic, selective serotonin re-uptake inhibitor, or other known antidepressant agents. Its structure closely resembles that of diethylpropion; it is related to phenylethylamines. It is designated as (±)-1-(3-chlorophenyl)-2-[(1,1-dimethylethyl)amino]-1-propanone hydrochloride. The molecular weight is 276.2. The empirical formula is $C_{13}H_{18}ClNO \cdot HCl$. Bupropion hydrochloride powder is white, crystalline, and highly soluble in water. It has a bitter taste and produces the sensation of local anesthesia on the oral mucosa. The structural formula is:

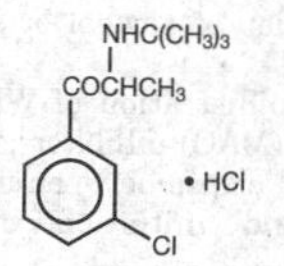

WELLBUTRIN is supplied for oral administration as 75-mg (yellow-gold) and 100-mg (red) film-coated tablets. Each tablet contains the labeled amount of bupropion hydrochloride and the inactive ingredients: 75-mg tablet – D&C Yellow No. 10 Lake, FD&C Yellow No. 6 Lake, hydroxypropyl cellulose, hypromellose, microcrystalline cellulose, polyethylene glycol, talc, and titanium dioxide; 100-mg tablet – FD&C Red No. 40 Lake, FD&C Yellow No. 6 Lake, hydroxypropyl cellulose, hypromellose, microcrystalline cellulose, polyethylene glycol, talc, and titanium dioxide.

CLINICAL PHARMACOLOGY
Pharmacodynamics
The neurochemical mechanism of the antidepressant effect of bupropion is not known. Bupropion is a relatively weak inhibitor of the neuronal uptake of norepinephrine and dopamine, and does not inhibit monoamine oxidase or the re-uptake of serotonin.
Bupropion produces dose-related central nervous system (CNS) stimulant effects in animals, as evidenced by increased locomotor activity, increased rates of responding in various schedule-controlled operant behavior tasks, and, at high doses, induction of mild stereotyped behavior.
Bupropion causes convulsions in rodents and dogs at doses approximately tenfold the dose recommended as the human antidepressant dose.
Pharmacokinetics
Bupropion is a racemic mixture. The pharmacological activity and pharmacokinetics of the individual enantiomers have not been studied. In humans, following oral administration of WELLBUTRIN, peak plasma bupropion concentrations are usually achieved within 2 hours, followed by a biphasic decline. The terminal phase has a mean half-life of 14 hours, with a range of 8 to 24 hours. The distribution phase has a mean half-life of 3 to 4 hours. The mean elimination half-life (±SD) of bupropion after chronic dosing is 21 (±9) hours, and steady-state plasma concentrations of bupropion are reached within 8 days. Plasma bupropion concentrations are dose-proportional following single doses of 100 to 250 mg; however, it is not known if the proportionality between dose and plasma level is maintained in chronic use.
Absorption
The absolute bioavailability of WELLBUTRIN in humans has not been determined because an intravenous formulation for human use is not available. However, it appears likely that only a small proportion of any orally administered dose reaches the systemic circulation intact.
Distribution
In vitro tests show that bupropion is 84% bound to human plasma protein at concentrations up to 200 mcg/mL. The extent of protein binding of the hydroxybupropion metabolite is similar to that for bupropion, whereas the extent of protein binding of the threohydrobupropion metabolite is about half that seen with bupropion.
Metabolism
Bupropion is extensively metabolized in humans. Three metabolites have been shown to be active: hydroxybupropion, which is formed via hydroxylation of the *tert*-butyl group of bupropion, and the amino-alcohol isomers threohydrobupropion and erythrohydrobupropion, which are formed via reduction of the carbonyl group. In vitro findings suggest that cytochrome P450IIB6 (CYP2B6) is the principal isoenzyme involved in the formation of hydroxybupropion, while cytochrome P450 isoenzymes are not involved in the formation of threohydrobupropion. Oxidation of the bupropion side chain results in the formation of a glycine conjugate of meta-chlorobenzoic acid, which is then excreted as the major urinary metabolite. The potency and toxicity of the metabolites relative to bupropion have not been fully characterized. However, it has been demonstrated in an antidepressant screening test in mice that hydroxybupropion is one-half as potent as bupropion, while threohydrobupropion and erythrohydrobupropion are 5-fold less potent than bupropion. This may be of clinical importance because their plasma concentrations are as high or higher than those of bupropion.
Because bupropion is extensively metabolized, there is the potential for drug-drug interactions, particularly with those agents that are metabolized by or which inhibit/induce the cytochrome P450IIB6 (CYP2B6) isoenzyme, such as ritonavir. In a healthy volunteer study, ritonavir at a dose of 100 mg twice daily reduced the AUC and C_{max} of bupropion by 22% and 21%, respectively. The exposure of the hydroxybupropion metabolite was decreased by 23%, the threohydrobupropion decreased by 38%, and the erythrohydrobupropion decreased by 48%.
In a second healthy volunteer study, ritonavir at a dose of 600 mg twice daily decreased the AUC and the C_{max} of bupropion by 66% and 62%, respectively. The exposure of the hydroxybupropion metabolite was decreased by 78%, the threohydrobupropion decreased by 50%, and the erythrohydrobupropion decreased by 68%.
In another healthy volunteer study, KALETRA® (lopinavir 400 mg/ritonavir 100 mg twice daily) decreased bupropion AUC and C_{max} by 57%. The AUC and C_{max} of hydroxybupropion were decreased by 50% and 31%, respectively (see PRECAUTIONS: Drug Interactions).
Although bupropion is not metabolized by cytochrome P450IID6 (CYP2D6), there is the potential for drug-drug interactions when bupropion is coadministered with drugs metabolized by this isoenzyme (see PRECAUTIONS: Drug Interactions).
Following a single dose in humans, peak plasma concentrations of hydroxybupropion occur approximately 3 hours after administration of WELLBUTRIN. Peak plasma concentrations of hydroxybupropion are approximately 10 times the peak level of the parent drug at steady state. The elimination half-life of hydroxybupropion is approximately 20

(±5) hours, and its AUC at steady state is about 17 times that of bupropion. The times to peak concentrations for the erythrohydrobupropion and threohydrobupropion metabolites are similar to that of the hydroxybupropion metabolite. However, their elimination half-lives are longer, 33 (±10) and 37 (±13) hours, respectively, and steady-state AUCs are 1.5 and 7 times that of bupropion, respectively.

Bupropion and its metabolites exhibit linear kinetics following chronic administration of 300 to 450 mg/day.

Elimination

Following oral administration of 200 mg of ^{14}C-bupropion in humans, 87% and 10% of the radioactive dose were recovered in the urine and feces, respectively. However, the fraction of the oral dose of WELLBUTRIN excreted unchanged was only 0.5%, a finding consistent with the extensive metabolism of bupropion.

Populations Subgroups

Factors or conditions altering metabolic capacity (e.g., liver disease, congestive heart failure [CHF], age, concomitant medications, etc.) or elimination may be expected to influence the degree and extent of accumulation of the active metabolites of bupropion. The elimination of the major metabolites of bupropion may be affected by reduced renal or hepatic function because they are moderately polar compounds and are likely to undergo further metabolism or conjugation in the liver prior to urinary excretion.

Hepatic

The effect of hepatic impairment on the pharmacokinetics of bupropion was characterized in 2 single-dose studies, one in patients with alcoholic liver disease and one in patients with mild-to-severe cirrhosis. The first study showed that the half-life of hydroxybupropion was significantly longer in 8 patients with alcoholic liver disease than in 8 healthy volunteers (32 ± 14 hours versus 21 ± 5 hours, respectively). Although not statistically significant, the AUCs for bupropion and hydroxybupropion were more variable and tended to be greater (by 53% to 57%) in volunteers with alcoholic liver disease. The differences in half-life for bupropion and the other metabolites in the 2 patient groups were minimal.

The second study showed that there were no statistically significant differences in the pharmacokinetics of bupropion and its active metabolites in 9 patients with mild-to-moderate hepatic cirrhosis compared to 8 healthy volunteers. However, more variability was observed in some of the pharmacokinetic parameters for bupropion (AUC, C_{max}, and T_{max}) and its active metabolites ($t_{1/2}$) in patients with mild-to-moderate hepatic cirrhosis. In addition, in patients with severe hepatic cirrhosis, the bupropion C_{max} and AUC were substantially increased (mean difference: by approximately 70% and 3-fold, respectively) and more variable when compared to values in healthy volunteers; the mean bupropion half-life was also longer (29 hours in patients with severe hepatic cirrhosis vs. 19 hours in healthy subjects). For the metabolite hydroxybupropion, the mean C_{max} was approximately 69% lower. For the combined amino-alcohol isomers threohydrobupropion and erythrohydrobupropion, the mean C_{max} was approximately 31% lower. The mean AUC increased by about 1½-fold for hydroxybupropion and about 2½-fold for threo/erythrohydrobupropion. The median T_{max} was observed 19 hours later for hydroxybupropion and 31 hours later for threo/erythrohydrobupropion. The mean half-lives for hydroxybupropion and threo/erythrohydrobupropion were increased 5- and 2-fold, respectively, in patients with severe hepatic cirrhosis compared to healthy volunteers (see WARNINGS, PRECAUTIONS, and DOSAGE AND ADMINISTRATION).

Renal

There is limited information on the pharmacokinetics of bupropion in patients with renal impairment. An inter-study comparison between normal subjects and patients with end-stage renal failure demonstrated that the parent drug C_{max} and AUC values were comparable in the 2 groups, whereas the hydroxybupropion and threohydrobupropion metabolites had a 2.3– and 2.8–fold increase, respectively, in AUC for patients with end-stage renal failure. A second study, comparing normal subjects and patients with moderate-to-severe renal impairment (GFR 30.9 ± 10.8 mL/min) showed that exposure to a single 150-mg dose of sustained-release bupropion was approximately 2-fold higher in patients with impaired renal function while levels of the hydroxybupropion and threo/erythrohydrobupropion (combined) metabolites were similar in the 2 groups. The elimination of bupropion and/or the major metabolites of bupropion may be reduced by impaired renal function (see PRECAUTIONS: Renal Impairment).

Left Ventricular Dysfunction

During a chronic dosing study in 14 depressed patients with left ventricular dysfunction (history of CHF or an enlarged heart on x-ray), no apparent effect on the pharmacokinetics of bupropion or its metabolites was revealed, compared to healthy volunteers.

Age

The effects of age on the pharmacokinetics of bupropion and its metabolites have not been fully characterized, but an ex-

ploration of steady-state bupropion concentrations from several depression efficacy studies involving patients dosed in a range of 300 to 750 mg/day, on a 3 times daily schedule, revealed no relationship between age (18 to 83 years) and plasma concentration of bupropion. A single-dose pharmacokinetic study demonstrated that the disposition of bupropion and its metabolites in elderly subjects was similar to that of younger subjects. These data suggest there is no prominent effect of age on bupropion concentration; however, another pharmacokinetic study, single and multiple dose, has suggested that the elderly are at increased risk for accumulation of bupropion and its metabolites (see PRECAUTIONS: Geriatric Use).

Gender

A single-dose study involving 12 healthy male and 12 healthy female volunteers revealed no sex-related differences in the pharmacokinetic parameters of bupropion.

Smokers

The effects of cigarette smoking on the pharmacokinetics of bupropion were studied in 34 healthy male and female volunteers; 17 were chronic cigarette smokers and 17 were nonsmokers. Following oral administration of a single 150-mg dose of bupropion, there were no statistically significant differences in C_{max}, half-life, T_{max}, AUC or clearance of bupropion or its active metabolites between smokers and nonsmokers.

INDICATIONS AND USAGE

WELLBUTRIN is indicated for the treatment of major depressive disorder. A physician considering WELLBUTRIN for the management of a patient's first episode of depression should be aware that the drug may cause generalized seizures in a dose-dependent manner with an approximate incidence of 0.4% (4/1,000). This incidence of seizures may exceed that of other marketed antidepressants by as much as 4-fold. This relative risk is only an approximate estimate because no direct comparative studies have been conducted (see WARNINGS).

The efficacy of WELLBUTRIN has been established in 3 placebo-controlled trials, including 2 of approximately 3 weeks' duration in depressed inpatients and one of approximately 6 weeks' duration in depressed outpatients. The depressive disorder of the patients studied corresponds most closely to the Major Depression category of the APA Diagnostic and Statistical Manual III.

Major Depression implies a prominent and relatively persistent depressed or dysphoric mood that usually interferes with daily functioning (nearly every day for at least 2 weeks); it should include at least 4 of the following 8 symptoms: change in appetite, change in sleep, psychomotor agitation or retardation, loss of interest in usual activities or decrease in sexual drive, increased fatigability, feelings of guilt or worthlessness, slowed thinking or impaired concentration, and suicidal ideation or attempts.

Effectiveness of WELLBUTRIN in long-term use, that is, for more than 6 weeks, has not been systematically evaluated in controlled trials. Therefore, the physician who elects to use WELLBUTRIN for extended periods should periodically reevaluate the long-term usefulness of the drug for the individual patient.

CONTRAINDICATIONS

WELLBUTRIN is contraindicated in patients with a seizure disorder.

WELLBUTRIN is contraindicated in patients treated with ZYBAN® (bupropion hydrochloride) Sustained-Release Tablets; WELLBUTRIN SR® (bupropion hydrochloride), the sustained-release formulation; WELLBUTRIN XL® (bupropion hydrochloride), the extended-release formulation; or any other medications that contain bupropion because the incidence of seizure is dose dependent.

WELLBUTRIN is contraindicated in patients with a current or prior diagnosis of bulimia or anorexia nervosa because of a higher incidence of seizures noted in such patients treated with WELLBUTRIN.

WELLBUTRIN is contraindicated in patients undergoing abrupt discontinuation of alcohol or sedatives (including benzodiazepines).

The concurrent administration of WELLBUTRIN and a monoamine oxidase (MAO) inhibitor is contraindicated. At least 14 days should elapse between discontinuation of an MAO inhibitor and initiation of treatment with WELLBUTRIN.

WELLBUTRIN is contraindicated in patients who have shown an allergic response to bupropion or the other ingredients that make up WELLBUTRIN.

WARNINGS

Clinical Worsening and Suicide Risk in Treating Psychiatric Disorders

Patients with major depressive disorder (MDD), both adult and pediatric, may experience worsening of their depression and/or the emergence of suicidal ideation and behavior (suicidality) or unusual changes in behavior, whether or not they are taking antidepressant medications, and this risk

may persist until significant remission occurs. Suicide is a known risk of depression and certain other psychiatric disorders, and these disorders themselves are the strongest predictors of suicide. There has been a long-standing concern, however, that antidepressants may have a role in inducing worsening of depression and the emergence of suicidality in certain patients during the early phases of treatment. Pooled analyses of short-term placebo-controlled trials of antidepressant drugs (SSRIs and others) showed that these drugs increase the risk of suicidal thinking and behavior (suicidality) in children, adolescents, and young adults (ages 18-24) with major depressive disorder (MDD) and other psychiatric disorders. Short-term studies did not show an increase in the risk of suicidality with antidepressants compared to placebo in adults beyond age 24; there was a reduction with antidepressants compared to placebo in adults aged 65 and older.

The pooled analyses of placebo-controlled trials in children and adolescents with MDD, obsessive compulsive disorder (OCD), or other psychiatric disorders included a total of 24 short-term trials of 9 antidepressant drugs in over 4,400 patients. The pooled analyses of placebo-controlled trials in adults with MDD or other psychiatric disorders included a total of 295 short-term trials (median duration of 2 months) of 11 antidepressant drugs in over 77,000 patients. There was considerable variation in risk of suicidality among drugs, but a tendency toward an increase in the younger patients for almost all drugs studied. There were differences in absolute risk of suicidality across the different indications, with the highest incidence in MDD. The risk differences (drug vs. placebo), however, were relatively stable within age strata and across indications. These risk differences (drug-placebo difference in the number of cases of suicidality per 1,000 patients treated) are provided in Table 1.

Table 1

Age Range	Drug-Placebo Difference in Number of Cases of Suicidality per 1,000 Patients Treated
Increases Compared to Placebo	
<18	14 additional cases
18-24	5 additional cases
Decreases Compared to Placebo	
25-64	1 fewer case
≥65	6 fewer cases

No suicides occurred in any of the pediatric trials. There were suicides in the adult trials, but the number was not sufficient to reach any conclusion about drug effect on suicide.

It is unknown whether the suicidality risk extends to longer-term use, i.e., beyond several months. However, there is substantial evidence from placebo-controlled maintenance trials in adults with depression that the use of antidepressants can delay the recurrence of depression.

All patients being treated with antidepressants for any indication should be monitored appropriately and observed closely for clinical worsening, suicidality, and unusual changes in behavior, especially during the initial few months of a course of drug therapy, or at times of dose changes, either increases or decreases.

The following symptoms, anxiety, agitation, panic attacks, insomnia, irritability, hostility, aggressiveness, impulsivity, akathisia (psychomotor restlessness), hypomania, and mania, have been reported in adult and pediatric patients being treated with antidepressants for major depressive disorder as well as for other indications, both psychiatric and nonpsychiatric. Although a causal link between the emergence of such symptoms and either the worsening of depression and/or the emergence of suicidal impulses has not been established, there is concern that such symptoms may represent precursors to emerging suicidality.

Consideration should be given to changing the therapeutic regimen, including possibly discontinuing the medication, in patients whose depression is persistently worse, or who are experiencing emergent suicidality or symptoms that might be precursors to worsening depression or suicidality, especially if these symptoms are severe, abrupt in onset, or were not part of the patient's presenting symptoms.

Families and caregivers of patients being treated with antidepressants for major depressive disorder or other indications, both psychiatric and nonpsychiatric, should be alerted about the need to monitor patients for the emergence of agitation, irritability, unusual changes in behavior, and the other symptoms described above, as well as the

emergence of suicidality, and to report such symptoms immediately to healthcare providers. Such monitoring should include daily observation by families and caregivers. Prescriptions for WELLBUTRIN should be written for the smallest quantity of tablets consistent with good patient management, in order to reduce the risk of overdose.

Neuropsychiatric Symptoms and Suicide Risk in Smoking Cessation Treatment: WELLBUTRIN, WELLBUTRIN SR, and WELLBUTRIN XL are not approved for smoking cessation treatment, but bupropion under the name ZYBAN is approved for this use. Serious neuropsychiatric symptoms have been reported in patients taking bupropion for smoking cessation (see BOXED WARNING, ADVERSE REACTIONS). These have included changes in mood (including depression and mania), psychosis, hallucinations, paranoia, delusions, homicidal ideation, hostility, agitation, aggression, anxiety, and panic, as well as suicidal ideation, suicide attempt, and completed suicide. Some reported cases may have been complicated by the symptoms of nicotine withdrawal in patients who stopped smoking. Depressed mood may be a symptom of nicotine withdrawal. Depression, rarely including suicidal ideation, has been reported in smokers undergoing a smoking cessation attempt without medication. However, some of these symptoms have occurred in patients taking bupropion who continued to smoke. When symptoms were reported, most were during bupropion treatment, but some were following discontinuation of bupropion therapy.

These events have occurred in patients with and without pre-existing psychiatric disease; some have experienced worsening of their psychiatric illnesses. All patients being treated with bupropion as part of smoking cessation treatment should be observed for neuropsychiatric symptoms or worsening of pre-existing psychiatric illness.

Patients with serious psychiatric illness such as schizophrenia, bipolar disorder, and major depressive disorder did not participate in the pre-marketing studies of ZYBAN.

Advise patients and caregivers that the patient using bupropion for smoking cessation should stop taking bupropion and contact a healthcare provider immediately if agitation, depressed mood, or changes in behavior or thinking that are not typical for the patient are observed, or if the patient develops suicidal ideation or suicidal behavior. In many postmarketing cases, resolution of symptoms after discontinuation of ZYBAN was reported, although in some cases the symptoms persisted; therefore, ongoing monitoring and supportive care should be provided until symptoms resolve.

The risks of using bupropion for smoking cessation should be weighed against the benefits of its use. ZYBAN has been demonstrated to increase the likelihood of abstinence from smoking for as long as six months compared to treatment with placebo. The health benefits of quitting smoking are immediate and substantial.

Screening Patients for Bipolar Disorder
A major depressive episode may be the initial presentation of bipolar disorder. It is generally believed (though not established in controlled trials) that treating such an episode with an antidepressant alone may increase the likelihood of precipitation of a mixed/manic episode in patients at risk for bipolar disorder. Whether any of the symptoms described above represent such a conversion is unknown. However, prior to initiating treatment with an antidepressant, patients with depressive symptoms should be adequately screened to determine if they are at risk for bipolar disorder; such screening should include a detailed psychiatric history, including a family history of suicide, bipolar disorder, and depression. It should be noted that WELLBUTRIN is not approved for use in treating bipolar depression.

Bupropion-Containing Products
Patients should be made aware that WELLBUTRIN contains the same active ingredient found in ZYBAN, used as an aid to smoking cessation treatment, and that WELLBUTRIN should not be used in combination with ZYBAN, or any other medications that contain bupropion, such as WELLBUTRIN SR (bupropion hydrochloride), the sustained-release formulation or WELLBUTRIN XL (bupropion hydrochloride), the extended-release formulation.

Seizures
Bupropion is associated with seizures in approximately 0.4% (4/1,000) of patients treated at doses up to 450 mg/day. This incidence of seizures may exceed that of other marketed antidepressants by as much as 4-fold. This relative risk is only an approximate estimate because no direct comparative studies have been conducted. The estimated seizure incidence for WELLBUTRIN increases almost tenfold between 450 and 600 mg/day, which is twice the usually required daily dose (300 mg) and one and one-third the maximum recommended daily dose (450 mg). Given the wide variability among individuals and their capacity to metabolize and eliminate drugs this disproportionate increase in seizure incidence with dose incrementation calls for caution in dosing.

During the initial development, 25 among approximately 2,400 patients treated with WELLBUTRIN experienced seizures. At the time of seizure, 7 patients were receiving daily doses of 450 mg or below for an incidence of 0.33% (3/1,000) within the recommended dose range. Twelve patients experienced seizures at 600 mg/day (2.3% incidence); 6 additional patients had seizures at daily doses between 600 and 900 mg (2.8% incidence).

A separate, prospective study was conducted to determine the incidence of seizure during an 8-week treatment exposure in approximately 3,200 additional patients who received daily doses of up to 450 mg. Patients were permitted to continue treatment beyond 8 weeks if clinically indicated. Eight seizures occurred during the initial 8-week treatment period and 5 seizures were reported in patients continuing treatment beyond 8 weeks, resulting in a total seizure incidence of 0.4%.

The risk of seizure appears to be strongly associated with dose. Sudden and large increments in dose may contribute to increased risk. While many seizures occurred early in the course of treatment, some seizures did occur after several weeks at fixed dose. WELLBUTRIN should be discontinued and not restarted in patients who experience a seizure while on treatment.

The risk of seizure is also related to patient factors, clinical situations, and concomitant medications, which must be considered in selection of patients for therapy with WELLBUTRIN.

* **Patient factors:** Predisposing factors that may increase the risk of seizure with bupropion use include history of head trauma or prior seizure, central nervous system (CNS) tumor, the presence of severe hepatic cirrhosis, and concomitant medications that lower seizure threshold.
* **Clinical situations:** Circumstances associated with an increased seizure risk include, among others, excessive use of alcohol or sedatives (including benzodiazepines); addiction to opiates, cocaine, or stimulants; use of over-the-counter stimulants and anorectics; and diabetes treated with oral hypoglycemics or insulin.
* **Concomitant medications:** Many medications (e.g., antipsychotics, antidepressants, theophylline, systemic steroids) are known to lower seizure threshold.

Recommendations for Reducing the Risk of Seizure: Retrospective analysis of clinical experience gained during the development of WELLBUTRIN suggests that the risk of seizure may be minimized if

* the total daily dose of WELLBUTRIN does *not* exceed 450 mg,
* the daily dose is administered 3 times daily, with each single dose *not* to exceed 150 mg to avoid high peak concentrations of bupropion and/or its metabolites, and
* the rate of incrementation of dose is very gradual.

WELLBUTRIN should be administered with extreme caution to patients with a history of seizure, cranial trauma, or other predisposition(s) toward seizure, or patients treated with other agents (e.g., antipsychotics, other antidepressants, theophylline, systemic steroids, etc.) that lower seizure threshold.

Hepatic Impairment
WELLBUTRIN should be used with extreme caution in patients with severe hepatic cirrhosis. In these patients a reduced dose and/or frequency is required, as peak bupropion, as well as AUC, levels are substantially increased and accumulation is likely to occur in such patients to a greater extent than usual. The dose should not exceed 75 mg once a day in these patients (see CLINICAL PHARMACOLOGY, PRECAUTIONS, and DOSAGE AND ADMINISTRATION).

Potential for Hepatotoxicity
In rats receiving large doses of bupropion chronically, there was an increase in incidence of hepatic hyperplastic nodules and hepatocellular hypertrophy. In dogs receiving large doses of bupropion chronically, various histologic changes were seen in the liver, and laboratory tests suggesting mild hepatocellular injury were noted.

PRECAUTIONS
General
Agitation and Insomnia

A substantial proportion of patients treated with WELLBUTRIN experience some degree of increased restlessness, agitation, anxiety, and insomnia, especially shortly after initiation of treatment. In clinical studies, these symptoms were sometimes of sufficient magnitude to require treatment with sedative/hypnotic drugs. In approximately 2% of patients, symptoms were sufficiently severe to require discontinuation of treatment with WELLBUTRIN. Psychosis, Confusion, and Other Neuropsychiatric Phenomena

Depressed patients treated with WELLBUTRIN have been reported to show a variety of neuropsychiatric signs and symptoms including delusions, hallucinations, psychosis, concentration disturbance, paranoia, and confusion. Be-

cause of the uncontrolled nature of many studies, it is impossible to provide a precise estimate of the extent of risk imposed by treatment with WELLBUTRIN. In several cases, neuropsychiatric phenomena abated upon dose reduction and/or withdrawal of treatment.
Activation of Psychosis and/or Mania

Antidepressants can precipitate manic episodes in bipolar disorder patients during the depressed phase of their illness and may activate latent psychosis in other susceptible patients. WELLBUTRIN is expected to pose similar risks.
Altered Appetite and Weight

A weight loss of greater than 5 lbs occurred in 28% of patients receiving WELLBUTRIN. This incidence is approximately double that seen in comparable patients treated with tricyclics or placebo. Furthermore, while 35% of patients receiving tricyclic antidepressants gained weight, only 9.4% of patients treated with WELLBUTRIN did. Consequently, if weight loss is a major presenting sign of a patient's depressive illness, the anorectic and/or weight reducing potential of WELLBUTRIN should be considered.
Allergic Reactions

Anaphylactoid/anaphylactic reactions characterized by symptoms such as pruritus, urticaria, angioedema, and dyspnea requiring medical treatment have been reported in clinical trials with bupropion. In addition, there have been rare spontaneous postmarketing reports of erythema multiforme, Stevens-Johnson syndrome, and anaphylactic shock associated with bupropion. A patient should stop taking WELLBUTRIN and consult a doctor if experiencing allergic or anaphylactoid/anaphylactic reactions (e.g., skin rash, pruritus, hives, chest pain, edema, and shortness of breath) during treatment.

Arthralgia, myalgia, and fever with rash and other symptoms suggestive of delayed hypersensitivity have been reported in association with bupropion. These symptoms may resemble serum sickness.
Cardiovascular Effects

In clinical practice, hypertension, in some cases severe, requiring acute treatment, has been reported in patients receiving bupropion alone and in combination with nicotine replacement therapy. These events have been observed in both patients with and without evidence of preexisting hypertension.

Data from a comparative study of the sustained-release formulation of bupropion (ZYBAN® Sustained-Release Tablets), nicotine transdermal system (NTS), the combination of sustained-release bupropion plus NTS, and placebo as an aid to smoking cessation suggest a higher incidence of treatment-emergent hypertension in patients treated with the combination of sustained-release bupropion and NTS. In this study, 6.1% of patients treated with the combination of sustained-release bupropion and NTS had treatment-emergent hypertension compared to 2.5%, 1.6%, and 3.1% of patients treated with sustained-release bupropion, NTS, and placebo, respectively. The majority of these patients had evidence of preexisting hypertension. Three patients (1.2%) treated with the combination of ZYBAN and NTS and 1 patient (0.4%) treated with NTS had study medication discontinued due to hypertension compared to none of the patients treated with ZYBAN or placebo. Monitoring of blood pressure is recommended in patients who receive the combination of bupropion and nicotine replacement.

There is no clinical experience establishing the safety of WELLBUTRIN in patients with a recent history of myocardial infarction or unstable heart disease. Therefore, care should be exercised if it is used in these groups. Bupropion was well tolerated in depressed patients who had previously developed orthostatic hypotension while receiving tricyclic antidepressants and was also generally well tolerated in a group of 36 depressed inpatients with stable congestive heart failure (CHF). However, bupropion was associated with a rise in supine blood pressure in the study of patients with CHF, resulting in discontinuation of treatment in 2 patients for exacerbation of baseline hypertension.
Hepatic Impairment

WELLBUTRIN should be used with extreme caution in patients with severe hepatic cirrhosis. In these patients, a reduced dose and frequency is required. WELLBUTRIN should be used with caution in patients with hepatic impairment (including mild-to-moderate hepatic cirrhosis) and a reduced frequency and/or dose should be considered in patients with mild-to-moderate hepatic cirrhosis.

All patients with hepatic impairment should be closely monitored for possible adverse effects that could indicate high drug and metabolite levels (see CLINICAL PHARMACOLOGY, WARNINGS, and DOSAGE AND ADMINISTRATION).
Renal Impairment

There is limited information on the pharmacokinetics of bupropion in patients with renal impairment. An interstudy comparison between normal subjects and patients with end-stage renal failure demonstrated that the parent drug C_{max} and AUC values were comparable in the 2 groups, whereas the hydroxybupropion and threohydrobupropion metabolites had a 2.3– and 2.8–fold increase, respectively, in AUC for patients with end-stage renal failure. A second study, comparing normal subjects and patients with moderate-to-severe renal impairment (GFR 30.9 ± 10.8 mL/min) showed that exposure to a single 150-mg dose of sustained-release bupropion was approximately 2-fold higher in patients with impaired renal function while levels of the hydroxybupropion and threo/erythrohydrobupropion (combined) metabolites were similar in the 2 groups. Bupropion is extensively metabolized in the liver to active metabolites, which are further metabolized and subsequently excreted by the kidneys. WELLBUTRIN should be used with caution in patients with renal impairment and a reduced frequency and/or dose should be considered as bupropion and the metabolites of bupropion may accumulate in such patients to a greater extent than usual. The patient should be closely monitored for possible adverse effects that could indicate high drug or metabolite levels.

Information for Patients

Prescribers or other health professionals should inform patients, their families, and their caregivers about the benefits and risks associated with treatment with WELLBUTRIN and should counsel them in its appropriate use. A patient Medication Guide about "Antidepressant Medicines, Depression and Other Serious Mental Illnesses, and Suicidal Thoughts or Actions," "Quitting Smoking, Quit-Smoking Medication, Changes in Thinking and Behavior, Depression, and Suicidal Thoughts or Actions," and "What Other Important Information Should I Know About WELLBUTRIN?" is available for WELLBUTRIN. The prescriber or health professional should instruct patients, their families, and their caregivers to read the Medication Guide and should assist them in understanding its contents. Patients should be given the opportunity to discuss the contents of the Medication Guide and to obtain answers to any questions they may have. The complete text of the Medication Guide is reprinted at the end of this document.

Patients should be advised of the following issues and asked to alert their prescriber if these occur while taking WELLBUTRIN.

Clinical Worsening and Suicide Risk in Treating Psychiatric Disorders

Patients, their families, and their caregivers should be encouraged to be alert to the emergence of anxiety, agitation, panic attacks, insomnia, irritability, hostility, aggressiveness, impulsivity, akathisia (psychomotor restlessness), hypomania, mania, other unusual changes in behavior, worsening of depression, and suicidal ideation, especially early during antidepressant treatment and when the dose is adjusted up or down. Families and caregivers of patients should be advised to look for the emergence of such symptoms on a day-to-day basis, since changes may be abrupt. Such symptoms should be reported to the patient's prescriber or health professional, especially if they are severe, abrupt in onset, or were not part of the patient's presenting symptoms. Symptoms such as these may be associated with an increased risk for suicidal thinking and behavior and indicate a need for very close monitoring and possibly changes in the medication.

Neuropsychiatric Symptoms and Suicide Risk in Smoking Cessation Treatment:

Although WELLBUTRIN is not indicated for smoking cessation treatment, it contains the same active ingredient as ZYBAN which is approved for this use. Patients should be informed that quitting smoking, with or without ZYBAN, may be associated with nicotine withdrawal symptoms (including depression or agitation), or exacerbation of pre-existing psychiatric illness. Furthermore, some patients have experienced changes in mood (including depression and mania), psychosis, hallucinations, paranoia, delusions, homicidal ideation aggression, anxiety, and panic, as well as suicidal ideation, suicide attempt, and completed suicide when attempting to quit smoking while taking ZYBAN. If patients develop agitation, hostility, depressed mood, or changes in thinking or behavior that are not typical for them, or if patients develop suicidal ideation or behavior, they should be urged to report these symptoms to their healthcare provider immediately.

Bupropion-Containing Products

Patients should be made aware that WELLBUTRIN contains the same active ingredient found in ZYBAN, used as an aid to smoking cessation, and that WELLBUTRIN should not be used in combination with ZYBAN or any other medications that contain bupropion hydrochloride (such as WELLBUTRIN SR, the sustained-release formulation and WELLBUTRIN XL, the extended-release formulation).

Patients should be instructed to take WELLBUTRIN in equally divided doses 3 or 4 times a day to minimize the risk of seizure.

Patients should be told that WELLBUTRIN should be discontinued and not restarted if they experience a seizure while on treatment.

Patients should be told that any CNS-active drug like WELLBUTRIN may impair their ability to perform tasks requiring judgment or motor and cognitive skills. Consequently, until they are reasonably certain that WELLBUTRIN does not adversely affect their performance, they should refrain from driving an automobile or operating complex, hazardous machinery.

Patients should be told that the excessive use or abrupt discontinuation of alcohol or sedatives (including benzodiazepines) may alter the seizure threshold. Some patients have reported lower alcohol tolerance during treatment with WELLBUTRIN. Patients should be advised that the consumption of alcohol should be minimized or avoided.

Patients should be advised to inform their physicians if they are taking or plan to take any prescription or over-the-counter drugs. Concern is warranted because WELLBUTRIN and other drugs may affect each other's metabolism.

Patients should be advised to notify their physicians if they become pregnant or intend to become pregnant during therapy.

Laboratory Tests

There are no specific laboratory tests recommended.

Drug Interactions

Few systemic data have been collected on the metabolism of bupropion following concomitant administration with other drugs or, alternatively, the effect of concomitant administration of bupropion on the metabolism of other drugs.

Because bupropion is extensively metabolized, the coadministration of other drugs may affect its clinical activity. In vitro studies indicate that bupropion is primarily metabolized to hydroxybupropion by the CYP2B6 isoenzyme. Therefore, the potential exists for a drug interaction between WELLBUTRIN and drugs that are substrates of or inhibitors/inducers of the CYP2B6 isoenzyme (e.g., orphenadrine, thiotepa, cyclophosphamide, ticlopidine, and clopidogrel). In addition, in vitro studies suggest that paroxetine, sertraline, norfluoxetine, and fluvoxamine as well as nelfinavir and efavirenz inhibit the hydroxylation of bupropion. No clinical studies have been performed to evaluate this finding. The threohydrobupropion metabolite of bupropion does not appear to be produced by the cytochrome P450 isoenzymes. The effects of concomitant administration of cimetidine on the pharmacokinetics of bupropion and its active metabolites were studied in 24 healthy young male volunteers. Following oral administration of two 150-mg sustained-release tablets with and without 800 mg of cimetidine, the pharmacokinetics of bupropion and hydroxybupropion were unaffected. However, there were 16% and 32% increases in the AUC and C_{max}, respectively, of the combined moieties of threohydrobupropion and erythrohydrobupropion.

In a series of studies in healthy volunteers, ritonavir (100 mg twice daily or 600 mg twice daily) or ritonavir 100 mg plus lopinavir 400 mg (KALETRA) twice daily reduced the exposure of bupropion and its major metabolites in a dose dependent manner by approximately 20% to 80%. This effect is thought to be due to the induction of bupropion metabolism. Patients receiving ritonavir may need increased doses of bupropion, but the maximum recommended dose of bupropion should not be exceeded (see CLINICAL PHARMACOLOGY: Metabolism).

While not systematically studied, certain drugs may induce the metabolism of bupropion (e.g., carbamazepine, phenobarbital, phenytoin).

Multiple oral doses of bupropion had no statistically significant effects on the single dose pharmacokinetics of lamotrigine in 12 healthy volunteers.

Animal data indicated that bupropion may be an inducer of drug-metabolizing enzymes in humans. In one study, following chronic administration of bupropion, 100 mg 3 times daily to 8 healthy male volunteers for 14 days, there was no evidence of induction of its own metabolism. Nevertheless, there may be the potential for clinically important alterations of blood levels of coadministered drugs.

Drugs Metabolized by Cytochrome P450IID6 (CYP2D6)

Many drugs, including most antidepressants (SSRIs, many tricyclics), beta-blockers, antiarrhythmics, and antipsychotics are metabolized by the CYP2D6 isoenzyme. Although bupropion is not metabolized by this isoenzyme, bupropion and hydroxybupropion are inhibitors of the CYP2D6 isoenzyme in vitro. In a study of 15 male subjects (ages 19 to 35 years) who were extensive metabolizers of the CYP2D6 isoenzyme, daily doses of bupropion given as 150 mg twice daily followed by a single dose of 50 mg desipramine increased the C_{max}, AUC, and $t_{1/2}$ of desipramine by an average of approximately 2-, 5- and 2-fold, respectively. The effect was present for at least 7 days after the last dose of bupropion. Concomitant use of bupropion with other drugs metabolized by CYP2D6 has not been formally studied.

Therefore, coadministration of bupropion with drugs that are metabolized by CYP2D6 isoenzyme including certain antidepressants (e.g., nortriptyline, imipramine, desipramine, paroxetine, fluoxetine, sertraline), antipsychotics (e.g., haloperidol, risperidone, thioridazine), beta-blockers (e.g., metoprolol), and Type 1C antiarrhythmics (e.g., propafenone, flecainide), should be approached with caution and should be initiated at the lower end of the dose range of the concomitant medication. If bupropion is added to the treatment regimen of a patient already receiving a drug metabolized by CYP2D6, the need to decrease the dose of the original medication should be considered, particularly for those concomitant medications with a narrow therapeutic index.

Although citalopram is not primarily metabolized by CYP2D6, in one study bupropion increased the C_{max} and AUC of citalopram by 30% and 40%, respectively. Citalopram did not affect the pharmacokinetics of bupropion and its 3 metabolites.

MAO Inhibitors

Studies in animals demonstrate that the acute toxicity of bupropion is enhanced by the MAO inhibitor phenelzine (see CONTRAINDICATIONS).

Levodopa and Amantadine

Limited clinical data suggest a higher incidence of adverse experiences in patients receiving bupropion concurrently with either levodopa or amantadine. Administration of WELLBUTRIN to patients receiving either levodopa or amantadine concurrently should be undertaken with caution, using small initial doses and small gradual dose increases.

Drugs that Lower Seizure Threshold

Concurrent administration of WELLBUTRIN and agents (e.g., antipsychotics, other antidepressants, theophylline, systemic steroids, etc.) that lower seizure threshold should be undertaken only with extreme caution (see WARNINGS). Low initial dosing and small gradual dose increases should be employed.

Nicotine Transdermal System

(see PRECAUTIONS: Cardiovascular Effects).

Alcohol

In postmarketing experience, there have been rare reports of adverse neuropsychiatric events or reduced alcohol tolerance in patients who were drinking alcohol during treatment with WELLBUTRIN. The consumption of alcohol during treatment with WELLBUTRIN should be minimized or avoided (also see CONTRAINDICATIONS).

Carcinogenesis, Mutagenesis, Impairment of Fertility

Lifetime carcinogenicity studies were performed in rats and mice at doses up to 300 and 150 mg/kg/day, respectively. In the rat study there was an increase in nodular proliferative lesions of the liver at doses of 100 to 300 mg/kg/day; lower doses were not tested. The question of whether or not such lesions may be precursors of neoplasms of the liver is currently unresolved. Similar liver lesions were not seen in the mouse study, and no increase in malignant tumors of the liver and other organs was seen in either study.

Bupropion produced a borderline positive response (2 to 3 times control mutation rate) in some strains in the Ames bacterial mutagenicity test, and a high oral dose (300 mg/kg, but not 100 or 200 mg/kg) produced a low incidence of chromosomal aberrations in rats. The relevance of these results in estimating the risk of human exposure to therapeutic doses is unknown.

A fertility study was performed in rats; no evidence of impairment of fertility was encountered at oral doses up to 300 mg/kg/day.

Pregnancy

Teratogenic Effects

Pregnancy Category C. In studies conducted in rats and rabbits, bupropion was administered orally at doses up to 450 and 150 mg/kg/day, respectively (approximately 11 and 7 times the MRHD, respectively, on a mg/m^2 basis), during the period of organogenesis. No clear evidence of teratogenic activity was found in either species; however, in rabbits, slightly increased incidences of fetal malformations and skeletal variations were observed at the lowest dose tested (25 mg/kg/day, approximately equal to the MRHD on a mg/m^2 basis) and greater. Decreased fetal weights were seen at 50 mg/kg and greater.

When rats were administered bupropion at oral doses of up to 300 mg/kg/day (approximately 7 times the MRHD on a mg/m^2 basis) prior to mating and throughout pregnancy and lactation, there were no apparent adverse effects on offspring development.

One study has been conducted in pregnant women. This retrospective, managed-care database study assessed the risk of congenital malformations overall and cardiovascular malformations specifically, following exposure to bupropion in the first trimester compared to the risk of these malformations following exposure to other antidepressants in the first trimester and bupropion outside of the first trimester. This study included 7,005 infants with antidepressant exposure during pregnancy, 1,213 of whom were exposed to bupropion in the first trimester. The study showed no greater risk for congenital malformations overall or cardiovascular malformations specifically, following first trimester bupropion exposure compared to exposure to all other antidepressants in the first trimester, or bupropion outside of the first trimester. The results of this study have not been corroborated. WELLBUTRIN should be used during pregnancy only if the potential benefit justifies the potential risk to the fetus.

Labor and Delivery
The effect of WELLBUTRIN on labor and delivery in humans is unknown.

Nursing Mothers
Like many other drugs, bupropion and its metabolites are secreted in human milk. Because of the potential for serious adverse reactions in nursing infants from WELLBUTRIN, a decision should be made whether to discontinue nursing or to discontinue the drug, taking into account the importance of the drug to the mother.

Pediatric Use
Safety and effectiveness in the pediatric population have not been established (see BOX WARNING and WARNINGS: Clinical Worsening and Suicide Risk in Treating Psychiatric Disorders). Anyone considering the use of WELLBUTRIN in a child or adolescent must balance the potential risks with the clinical need.

Geriatric Use
Of the approximately 6,000 patients who participated in clinical trials with bupropion sustained-release tablets (depression and smoking cessation studies), 275 were 65 and over and 47 were 75 and over. In addition, several hundred patients 65 and over participated in clinical trials using the immediate-release formulation of bupropion (depression studies). No overall differences in safety or effectiveness were observed between these subjects and younger subjects, and other reported clinical experience has not identified differences in responses between the elderly and younger patients, but greater sensitivity of some older individuals cannot be ruled out.

A single-dose pharmacokinetic study demonstrated that the disposition of bupropion and its metabolites in elderly subjects was similar to that of younger subjects; however, another pharmacokinetic study, single and multiple dose, has suggested that the elderly are at increased risk for accumulation of bupropion and its metabolites (see CLINICAL PHARMACOLOGY).

Bupropion is extensively metabolized in the liver to active metabolites, which are further metabolized and excreted by the kidneys. The risk of toxic reaction to this drug may be greater in patients with impaired renal function. Because elderly patients are more likely to have decreased renal function, care should be taken in dose selection, and it may be useful to monitor renal function (see PRECAUTIONS: Renal Impairment and DOSAGE AND ADMINISTRATION).

ADVERSE REACTIONS
(SEE ALSO WARNINGS AND PRECAUTIONS.)
Adverse events commonly encountered in patients treated with WELLBUTRIN are agitation, dry mouth, insomnia, headache/migraine, nausea/vomiting, constipation, and tremor.

Adverse events were sufficiently troublesome to cause discontinuation of treatment with WELLBUTRIN in approximately 10% of the 2,400 patients and volunteers who participated in clinical trials during the product's initial development. The more common events causing discontinuation include neuropsychiatric disturbances (3.0%), primarily agitation and abnormalities in mental status; gastrointestinal disturbances (2.1%), primarily nausea and vomiting; neurological disturbances (1.7%), primarily seizures, headaches, and sleep disturbances; and dermatologic problems (1.4%), primarily rashes. It is important to note, however, that many of these events occurred at doses that exceed the recommended daily dose.

Accurate estimates of the incidence of adverse events associated with the use of any drug are difficult to obtain. Estimates are influenced by drug dose, detection technique, setting, physician judgments, etc. Consequently, Table 2 is presented solely to indicate the relative frequency of adverse events reported in representative controlled clinical studies conducted to evaluate the safety and efficacy of WELLBUTRIN under relatively similar conditions of daily dosage (300 to 600 mg), setting, and duration (3 to 4 weeks). The figures cited cannot be used to predict precisely the incidence of untoward events in the course of usual medical practice where patient characteristics and other factors must differ from those which prevailed in the clinical trials. These incidence figures also cannot be compared with those obtained from other clinical studies involving related drug products as each group of drug trials is conducted under a different set of conditions.

Finally, it is important to emphasize that the tabulation does not reflect the relative severity and/or clinical importance of the events. A better perspective on the serious adverse events associated with the use of WELLBUTRIN is provided in WARNINGS and PRECAUTIONS.

Table 2. Treatment-Emergent Adverse Experience Incidence in Placebo-Controlled Clinical Trials[a] (Percent of Patients Reporting)

Adverse Experience	WELLBUTRIN Patients (n = 323)	Placebo Patients (n = 185)
Cardiovascular		
Cardiac arrhythmias	5.3	4.3
Dizziness	22.3	16.2
Hypertension	4.3	1.6
Hypotension	2.5	2.2
Palpitations	3.7	2.2
Syncope	1.2	0.5
Tachycardia	10.8	8.6
Dermatologic		
Pruritus	2.2	0.0
Rash	8.0	6.5
Gastrointestinal		
Anorexia	18.3	18.4
Appetite increase	3.7	2.2
Constipation	26.0	17.3
Diarrhea	6.8	8.6
Dyspepsia	3.1	2.2
Nausea/vomiting	22.9	18.9
Weight gain	13.6	22.7
Weight loss	23.2	23.2
Genitourinary		
Impotence	3.4	3.1
Menstrual complaints	4.7	1.1
Urinary frequency	2.5	2.2
Urinary retention	1.9	2.2
Musculoskeletal		
Arthritis	3.1	2.7
Neurological		
Akathisia	1.5	1.1
Akinesia/bradykinesia	8.0	8.6
Cutaneous temperature disturbance	1.9	1.6
Dry mouth	27.6	18.4
Excessive sweating	22.3	14.6
Headache/migraine	25.7	22.2
Impaired sleep quality	4.0	1.6
Increased salivary flow	3.4	3.8
Insomnia	18.6	15.7
Muscle spasms	1.9	3.2
Pseudoparkinsonism	1.5	1.6
Sedation	19.8	19.5
Sensory disturbance	4.0	3.2
Tremor	21.1	7.6
Neuropsychiatric		
Agitation	31.9	22.2
Anxiety	3.1	1.1
Confusion	8.4	4.9
Decreased libido	3.1	1.6
Delusions	1.2	1.1
Disturbed concentration	3.1	3.8
Euphoria	1.2	0.5
Hostility	5.6	3.8
Nonspecific		
Fatigue	5.0	8.6
Fever/chills	1.2	0.5
Respiratory		
Upper respiratory complaints	5.0	11.4
Special Senses		
Auditory disturbance	5.3	3.2
Blurred vision	14.6	10.3
Gustatory disturbance	3.1	1.1

[a] Events reported by at least 1% of patients receiving WELLBUTRIN are included.

Other Events Observed During the Development of WELLBUTRIN
The conditions and duration of exposure to WELLBUTRIN varied greatly, and a substantial proportion of the experience was gained in open and uncontrolled clinical settings. During this experience, numerous adverse events were reported; however, without appropriate controls, it is impossible to determine with certainty which events were or were not caused by WELLBUTRIN. The following enumeration is organized by organ system and describes events in terms of their relative frequency of reporting in the data base. Events of major clinical importance are also described in WARNINGS and PRECAUTIONS.

The following definitions of frequency are used: Frequent adverse events are defined as those occurring in at least 1/100 patients. Infrequent adverse events are those occurring in 1/100 to 1/1,000 patients, while rare events are those occurring in less than 1/1,000 patients.

Cardiovascular
Frequent was edema; infrequent were chest pain, electrocardiogram (ECG) abnormalities (premature beats and nonspecific ST-T changes), and shortness of breath/dyspnea; rare were flushing, pallor, phlebitis, and myocardial infarction.

Dermatologic
Frequent were nonspecific rashes; infrequent were alopecia and dry skin; rare were change in hair color, hirsutism, and acne.

Endocrine
Infrequent was gynecomastia; rare were glycosuria and hormone level change.

Gastrointestinal
Infrequent were dysphagia, thirst disturbance, and liver damage/jaundice; rare were rectal complaints, colitis, gastrointestinal bleeding, intestinal perforation, and stomach ulcer.

Genitourinary
Frequent was nocturia; infrequent were vaginal irritation, testicular swelling, urinary tract infection, painful erection, and retarded ejaculation; rare were dysuria, enuresis, urinary incontinence, menopause, ovarian disorder, pelvic infection, cystitis, dyspareunia, and painful ejaculation.

Hematologic/Oncologic
Rare were lymphadenopathy, anemia, and pancytopenia.

Musculoskeletal
Rare was musculoskeletal chest pain.

Neurological
(see WARNINGS) Frequent were ataxia/incoordination, seizure, myoclonus, dyskinesia, and dystonia; infrequent were mydriasis, vertigo, and dysarthria; rare were electroencephalogram (EEG) abnormality, abnormal neurological exam, impaired attention, sciatica, and aphasia.

Neuropsychiatric
(see PRECAUTIONS) Frequent were mania/hypomania, increased libido, hallucinations, decrease in sexual function, and depression; infrequent were memory impairment, depersonalization, psychosis, dysphoria, mood instability, paranoia, formal thought disorder, and frigidity; rare was suicidal ideation.

Oral Complaints
Frequent was stomatitis; infrequent were toothache, bruxism, gum irritation, and oral edema; rare was glossitis.

Respiratory
Infrequent were bronchitis and shortness of breath/dyspnea; rare were epistaxis, rate or rhythm disorder, pneumonia, and pulmonary embolism.

Special Senses
Infrequent was visual disturbance; rare was diplopia.

Nonspecific
Frequent were flu-like symptoms; infrequent was nonspecific pain; rare were body odor, surgically related pain, infection, medication reaction, and overdose.

Postintroduction Reports
Voluntary reports of adverse events temporally associated with bupropion that have been received since market introduction and which may have no causal relationship with the drug include the following:

Body (General)
arthralgia, myalgia, and fever with rash and other symptoms suggestive of delayed hypersensitivity. These symptoms may resemble serum sickness (see PRECAUTIONS).

Cardiovascular
hypertension (in some cases severe, see PRECAUTIONS), orthostatic hypotension, third degree heart block

Endocrine
syndrome of inappropriate antidiuretic hormone secretion, hyperglycemia, hypoglycemia

Gastrointestinal
esophagitis, hepatitis, liver damage

Hemic and Lymphatic
ecchymosis, leukocytosis, leukopenia, thrombocytopenia. Altered PT and/or INR, infrequently associated with hemorrhagic or thrombotic complications, were observed when bupropion was coadministered with warfarin.

Musculoskeletal
arthralgia, myalgia, muscle rigidity/fever/rhabdomyolysis, muscle weakness

Nervous
aggression, coma, completed suicide, delirium, dream abnormalities, paranoid ideation, paresthesia, restlessness, suicide attempt, unmasking of tardive dyskinesia

Skin and Appendages
Stevens-Johnson syndrome, angioedema, exfoliative dermatitis, urticaria

Table 3. Dosing Regimen

Treatment Day	Total Daily Dose	Tablet Strength	Number of Tablets		
			Morning	Midday	Evening
1	200 mg	100 mg	1	0	1
4	300 mg	100 mg	1	1	1

Special Senses
tinnitus, increased intraocular pressure

DRUG ABUSE AND DEPENDENCE

Humans

Controlled clinical studies conducted in normal volunteers, in subjects with a history of multiple drug abuse, and in depressed patients showed some increase in motor activity and agitation/excitement.

In a population of individuals experienced with drugs of abuse, a single dose of 400 mg of WELLBUTRIN produced mild amphetamine-like activity as compared to placebo on the Morphine-Benzedrine Subscale of the Addiction Research Center Inventories (ARCI) and a score intermediate between placebo and amphetamine on the Liking Scale of the ARCI. These scales measure general feelings of euphoria and drug desirability.

Findings in clinical trials, however, are not known to predict the abuse potential of drugs reliably. Nonetheless, evidence from single-dose studies does suggest that the recommended daily dosage of bupropion when administered in divided doses is not likely to be especially reinforcing to amphetamine or stimulant abusers. However, higher doses that could not be tested because of the risk of seizure might be modestly attractive to those who abuse stimulant drugs.

Animals

Studies in rodents have shown that bupropion exhibits some pharmacologic actions common to psychostimulants including increases in locomotor activity and the production of a mild stereotyped behavior and increases in rates of responding in several schedule-controlled behavior paradigms. Drug discrimination studies in rats showed stimulus generalization between bupropion and amphetamine and other psychostimulants. Rhesus monkeys have been shown to self-administer bupropion intravenously.

OVERDOSAGE

Human Overdose Experience

Overdoses of up to 30 g or more of bupropion have been reported. Seizure was reported in approximately one-third of all cases. Other serious reactions reported with overdoses of bupropion alone included hallucinations, loss of consciousness, sinus tachycardia, and ECG changes such as conduction disturbances (including QRS prolongation) or arrhythmias. Fever, muscle rigidity, rhabdomyolysis, hypotension, stupor, coma, and respiratory failure have been reported mainly when bupropion was part of multiple drug overdoses.

Although most patients recovered without sequelae, deaths associated with overdoses of bupropion alone have been reported in patients ingesting large doses of the drug. Multiple uncontrolled seizures, bradycardia, cardiac failure, and cardiac arrest prior to death were reported in these patients.

Overdosage Management

Ensure an adequate airway, oxygenation, and ventilation. Monitor cardiac rhythm and vital signs. EEG monitoring is also recommended for the first 48 hours post-ingestion. General supportive and symptomatic measures are also recommended. Induction of emesis is not recommended.

Activated charcoal should be administered. There is no experience with the use of forced diuresis, dialysis, hemoperfusion, or exchange transfusion in the management of bupropion overdoses. No specific antidotes for bupropion are known.

Due to the dose-related risk of seizures with WELLBUTRIN, hospitalization following suspected overdose should be considered. Based on studies in animals, it is recommended that seizures be treated with intravenous benzodiazepine administration and other supportive measures, as appropriate.

In managing overdosage, consider the possibility of multiple drug involvement. The physician should consider contacting a poison control center for additional information on the treatment of any overdose. Telephone numbers for certified poison control centers are listed in the *Physicians' Desk Reference* (PDR).

DOSAGE AND ADMINISTRATION

General Dosing Considerations

It is particularly important to administer WELLBUTRIN in a manner most likely to minimize the risk of seizure (see WARNINGS). Increases in dose should not exceed 100 mg/day in a 3-day period. Gradual escalation in dosage is also important if agitation, motor restlessness, and insomnia, often seen during the initial days of treatment, are to be minimized. If necessary, these effects may be managed by temporary reduction of dose or the short-term administration of an intermediate to long-acting sedative hypnotic. A sedative hypnotic usually is not required beyond the first week of treatment. Insomnia may also be minimized by avoiding bedtime doses. If distressing, untoward effects supervene, dose escalation should be stopped.

No single dose of WELLBUTRIN should exceed 150 mg. WELLBUTRIN should be administered 3 times daily, preferably with at least 6 hours between successive doses.

Usual Dosage for Adults

The usual adult dose is 300 mg/day, given 3 times daily. Dosing should begin at 200 mg/day, given as 100 mg twice daily. Based on clinical response, this dose may be increased to 300 mg/day, given as 100 mg 3 times daily, no sooner than 3 days after beginning therapy (see Table 3).

[See table 3 above]

Increasing the Dosage Above 300 mg/Day

As with other antidepressants, the full antidepressant effect of WELLBUTRIN may not be evident until 4 weeks of treatment or longer. An increase in dosage, up to a maximum of 450 mg/day, given in divided doses of not more than 150 mg each, may be considered for patients in whom no clinical improvement is noted after several weeks of treatment at 300 mg/day. Dosing above 300 mg/day may be accomplished using the 75- or 100-mg tablets. The 100-mg tablet must be administered 4 times daily with at least 4 hours between successive doses, in order not to exceed the limit of 150 mg in a single dose. WELLBUTRIN should be discontinued in patients who do not demonstrate an adequate response after an appropriate period of treatment at 450 mg/day.

Maintenance Treatment

The lowest dose that maintains remission is recommended. Although it is not known how long the patient should remain on WELLBUTRIN, it is generally recognized that acute episodes of depression require several months or longer of antidepressant drug treatment.

Dosage Adjustment for Patients with Impaired Hepatic Function

WELLBUTRIN should be used with extreme caution in patients with severe hepatic cirrhosis. The dose should not exceed 75 mg once a day in these patients. WELLBUTRIN should be used with caution in patients with hepatic impairment (including mild-to-moderate hepatic cirrhosis) and a reduced frequency and/or dose should be considered in patients with mild-to-moderate hepatic cirrhosis (see CLINICAL PHARMACOLOGY, WARNINGS, and PRECAUTIONS).

Dosage Adjustment for Patients with Impaired Renal Function

WELLBUTRIN should be used with caution in patients with renal impairment and a reduced frequency and/or dose should be considered (see CLINICAL PHARMACOLOGY and PRECAUTIONS).

HOW SUPPLIED

WELLBUTRIN Tablets, 75 mg of bupropion hydrochloride, are yellow-gold, round, biconvex tablets printed with "WELLBUTRIN 75" in bottles of 100 (NDC 0173-0177-55). WELLBUTRIN Tablets, 100 mg of bupropion hydrochloride, are red, round, biconvex tablets printed with "WELLBUTRIN 100" in bottles of 100 (NDC 0173-0178-55).

Store at 15° to 25°C (59° to 77°F). Protect from light and moisture.

WELLBUTRIN, WELLBUTRIN SR, and WELLBUTRIN XL are registered trademarks of GlaxoSmithKline.

KALETRA is a registered trademark of Abbott Laboratories.

Distributed by:
GlaxoSmithKline
Research Triangle Park, NC 27709
Manufactured by:
DSM Pharmaceuticals, Inc.
Greenville, NC 27834 for
GlaxoSmithKline
Research Triangle Park, NC 27709
©2010, GlaxoSmithKline. All rights reserved.
May 2010
WLT:5PI

MEDICATION GUIDE

**WELLBUTRIN® (WELL byu-trin)
(bupropion hydrochloride) Tablets**

Read this Medication Guide carefully before you start using WELLBUTRIN and each time you get a refill. There may be new information. This information does not take the place of talking with your doctor about your medical condition or your treatment. If you have any questions about WELLBUTRIN, ask your doctor or pharmacist.

IMPORTANT: Be sure to read the three sections of this Medication Guide. The first section is about the risk of suicidal thoughts and actions with antidepressant medicines; the second section is about the risk of changes in thinking and behavior, depression and suicidal thoughts or actions with medicines used to quit smoking; and the third section is entitled "What Other Important Information Should I Know About WELLBUTRIN?"

Antidepressant Medicines, Depression and Other Serious Mental Illnesses, and Suicidal Thoughts or Actions

This section of the Medication Guide is only about the risk of suicidal thoughts and actions with antidepressant medicines. Talk to your, or your family member's, healthcare provider about:

- all risks and benefits of treatment with antidepressant medicines
- all treatment choices for depression or other serious mental illness

What is the most important information I should know about antidepressant medicines, depression and other serious mental illnesses, and suicidal thoughts or actions?

1. Antidepressant medicines may increase suicidal thoughts or actions in some children, teenagers, and young adults within the first few months of treatment.
2. Depression and other serious mental illnesses are the most important causes of suicidal thoughts and actions. Some people may have a particularly high risk of having suicidal thoughts or actions. These include people who have (or have a family history of) bipolar illness (also called manic-depressive illness) or suicidal thoughts or actions.
3. How can I watch for and try to prevent suicidal thoughts and actions in myself or a family member?
   - Pay close attention to any changes, especially sudden changes, in mood, behaviors, thoughts, or feelings. This is very important when an antidepressant medicine is started or when the dose is changed.
   - Call the healthcare provider right away to report new or sudden changes in mood, behavior, thoughts, or feelings.
   - Keep all follow-up visits with the healthcare provider as scheduled. Call the healthcare provider between visits as needed, especially if you have concerns about symptoms.

Call a healthcare provider right away if you or your family member has any of the following symptoms, especially if they are new, worse, or worry you:

• thoughts about suicide or dying	• trouble sleeping (insomnia)
• attempts to commit suicide	• new or worse irritability
• new or worse depression	• acting aggressive, being angry, or violent
• new or worse anxiety	• acting on dangerous impulses
• feeling very agitated or restless	• an extreme increase in activity and talking (mania)
• panic attacks	• other unusual changes in behavior or mood

What else do I need to know about antidepressant medicines?

- **Never stop an antidepressant medicine without first talking to a healthcare provider.** Stopping an antidepressant medicine suddenly can cause other symptoms.
- **Antidepressants are medicines used to treat depression and other illnesses.** It is important to discuss all the risks of treating depression and also the risks of not treating it. Patients and their families or other caregivers should discuss all treatment choices with the healthcare provider, not just the use of antidepressants.
- **Antidepressant medicines have other side effects.** Talk to the healthcare provider about the side effects of the medicine prescribed for you or your family member.
- **Antidepressant medicines can interact with other medicines.** Know all of the medicines that you or your family member takes. Keep a list of all medicines to show the healthcare provider. Do not start new medicines without first checking with your healthcare provider.
- **Not all antidepressant medicines prescribed for children are FDA approved for use in children.** Talk to your child's healthcare provider for more information.

WELLBUTRIN has not been studied in children under the age of 18 and is not approved for use in children and teenagers.

Quitting Smoking, Quit-Smoking Medications, Changes in Thinking and Behavior, Depression, and Suicidal Thoughts or Actions

This section of the Medication Guide is only about the risk of changes in thinking and behavior, depression and suicidal thoughts or actions with drugs used to quit smoking. Although WELLBUTRIN is not a treatment for quitting smoking, it contains the same active ingredient (bupropion hydrochloride) as ZYBAN® which is used to help patients quit smoking.

Some people have had changes in behavior, hostility, agitation, depression, suicidal thoughts or actions while taking bupropion to help them quit smoking. These symptoms can develop during treatment with bupropion or after stopping treatment with bupropion.

If you, your family member, or your caregiver notice agitation, hostility, depression, or changes in thinking or behavior that are not typical for you, or you have any of the following symptoms, stop taking bupropion and call your healthcare provider right away:

- thoughts about suicide or dying
- attempts to commit suicide
- new or worse depression
- new or worse anxiety
- panic attacks
- feeling very agitated or restless
- acting aggressive, being angry, or violent
- acting on dangerous impulses

- an extreme increase in activity and talking (mania)
- abnormal thoughts or sensations
- seeing or hearing things that are not there (hallucinations)
- feeling people are against you (paranoia)
- feeling confused
- other unusual changes in behavior or mood

When you try to quit smoking, with or without bupropion, you may have symptoms that may be due to nicotine withdrawal, including urge to smoke, depressed mood, trouble sleeping, irritability, frustration, anger, feeling anxious, difficulty concentrating, restlessness, decreased heart rate, and increased appetite or weight gain. Some people have even experienced suicidal thoughts when trying to quit smoking without medication. Sometimes quitting smoking can lead to worsening of mental health problems that you already have, such as depression.

Before taking bupropion, tell your healthcare provider if you have ever had depression or other mental illnesses. You should also tell your doctor about any symptoms you had during other times you tried to quit smoking, with or without bupropion.

What Other Important Information Should I Know About WELLBUTRIN?

- **Seizures:** There is a chance of having a seizure (convulsion, fit) with WELLBUTRIN, especially in people:
  - with certain medical problems.
  - who take certain medicines.

The chance of having seizures increases with higher doses of WELLBUTRIN. For more information, see the sections "Who should not take WELLBUTRIN?" and "What should I tell my doctor before using WELLBUTRIN?" Tell your doctor about all of your medical conditions and all the medicines you take. **Do not take any other medicines while you are using WELLBUTRIN unless your doctor has said it is okay to take them.**

If you have a seizure while taking WELLBUTRIN, stop taking the tablets and call your doctor right away. Do not take WELLBUTRIN again if you have a seizure.

- **High blood pressure (hypertension).** Some people get high blood pressure, that can be severe, while taking WELLBUTRIN. The chance of high blood pressure may be higher if you also use nicotine replacement therapy (such as a nicotine patch) to help you stop smoking.
- **Severe allergic reactions.** Some people have severe allergic reaction to WELLBUTRIN. Stop taking WELLBUTRIN and call your doctor right away if you get a rash, itching, hives, fever, swollen lymph glands, painful sores in the mouth or around the eyes, swelling of the lips or tongue, chest pain, or have trouble breathing. These could be signs of a serious allergic reaction.
- **Unusual thoughts or behaviors.** Some patients have unusual thoughts or behaviors while taking WELLBUTRIN, including delusions (believe you are someone else), hallucinations (seeing or hearing things that are not there), paranoia (feeling that people are against you), or feeling confused. If this happens to you, call your doctor.

What is WELLBUTRIN?

WELLBUTRIN is a prescription medicine used to treat adults with a certain type of depression called major depressive disorder.

Who should not take WELLBUTRIN?

Do not take WELLBUTRIN if you
- have or had a seizure disorder or epilepsy.
- are taking ZYBAN (used to help people stop smoking) or any other medicines that contain bupropion hydrochloride, such as WELLBUTRIN SR Sustained-Release Tablets or WELLBUTRIN XL Extended-Release Tablets. Bupropion is the same ingredient that is in WELLBUTRIN.
- drink a lot of alcohol and abruptly stop drinking, or use medicines called sedatives (these make you sleepy) or benzodiazepines and you stop using them all of a sudden.
- have taken within the last 14 days medicine for depression called a monoamine oxidase inhibitor (MAOI), such as NARDIL® (phenelzine sulfate), PARNATE® (tranylcypromine sulfate), or MARPLAN® (isocarboxazid).
- have or had an eating disorder such as anorexia nervosa or bulimia.
- are allergic to the active ingredient in WELLBUTRIN, bupropion, or to any of the inactive ingredients. See the end of this leaflet for a complete list of ingredients in WELLBUTRIN.

What should I tell my doctor before using WELLBUTRIN?

Tell your doctor if you have ever had depression, suicidal thoughts or actions, or other mental health problems. See "Antidepressant Medicines, Depression and Other Serious Mental Illnesses, and Suicidal Thoughts or Actions."

- **Tell your doctor about your other medical conditions including if you:**
  - **are pregnant or plan to become pregnant.** It is not known if WELLBUTRIN can harm your unborn baby.
  - **are breastfeeding.** WELLBUTRIN passes through your milk. It is not known if WELLBUTRIN can harm your baby.
  - **have liver problems,** especially cirrhosis of the liver.
  - have kidney problems.
  - have an eating disorder, such as anorexia nervosa or bulimia.
  - have had a head injury.
  - have had a seizure (convulsion, fit).
  - have a tumor in your nervous system (brain or spine).
  - have had a heart attack, heart problems, or high blood pressure.
  - are a diabetic taking insulin or other medicines to control your blood sugar.
  - drink a lot of alcohol.
  - abuse prescription medicines or street drugs.
- **Tell your doctor about all the medicines you take,** including prescription and non-prescription medicines, vitamins, and herbal supplements. Many medicines increase your chances of having seizures or other serious side effects if you take them while you are using WELLBUTRIN.

How should I take WELLBUTRIN?

- Take WELLBUTRIN exactly as prescribed by your doctor.
- Take WELLBUTRIN at the same time each day.
- Take your doses of WELLBUTRIN at least 6 hours apart.
- You may take WELLBUTRIN with or without food.
- If you miss a dose, do not take an extra tablet to make up for the dose you forgot. Wait and take your next tablet at the regular time. **This is very important.** Too much WELLBUTRIN can increase your chance of having a seizure.
- If you take too much WELLBUTRIN, or overdose, call your local emergency room or poison control center right away.
- **Do not take any other medicines while using WELLBUTRIN unless your doctor has told you it is okay.**
- It may take several weeks for you to feel that WELLBUTRIN is working. Once you feel better, it is important to keep taking WELLBUTRIN exactly as directed by your doctor. Call your doctor if you do not feel WELLBUTRIN is working for you.
- Do not change your dose or stop taking WELLBUTRIN without talking with your doctor first.

What should I avoid while taking WELLBUTRIN?

- Do not drink a lot of alcohol while taking WELLBUTRIN. If you usually drink a lot of alcohol, talk with your doctor before suddenly stopping. If you suddenly stop drinking alcohol, you may increase your risk of having seizures.
- Do not drive a car or use heavy machinery until you know how WELLBUTRIN affects you. WELLBUTRIN can impair your ability to perform these tasks.

What are possible side effects of WELLBUTRIN?

WELLBUTRIN can cause serious side effects. Read this entire Medication Guide for more information about these serious side effects.

The most common side effects of WELLBUTRIN are nervousness, constipation, trouble sleeping, dry mouth, headache, nausea, vomiting, and shakiness (tremor).

If you have nausea, take your medicine with food. If you have trouble sleeping, do not take your medicine too close to bedtime.

These are not all the side effects of WELLBUTRIN. For a complete list, ask your doctor or pharmacist.

Call your doctor for medical advice about side effects. You may report side effects to FDA at 1-800-FDA-1088.

How should I store WELLBUTRIN?
- Store WELLBUTRIN at room temperature. Store out of direct sunlight. Keep WELLBUTRIN in its tightly closed bottle.

General Information about WELLBUTRIN.
- Medicines are sometimes prescribed for purposes other than those listed in a Medication Guide. Do not use WELLBUTRIN for a condition for which it was not prescribed. Do not give WELLBUTRIN to other people, even if they have the same symptoms you have. It may harm them. Keep WELLBUTRIN out of the reach of children. This Medication Guide summarizes important information about WELLBUTRIN. For more information, talk to your doctor. You can ask your doctor or pharmacist for information about WELLBUTRIN that is written for health professionals.

What are the ingredients in WELLBUTRIN?

Active ingredient: bupropion hydrochloride.

Inactive ingredients: 75-mg tablet – D&C Yellow No. 10 Lake, FD&C Yellow No. 6 Lake, hydroxypropyl cellulose, hypromellose, microcrystalline cellulose, polyethylene glycol, talc, and titanium dioxide; 100-mg tablet – FD&C Red No. 40 Lake, FD&C Yellow No. 6 Lake, hydroxypropyl cellulose, hypromellose, microcrystalline cellulose, polyethylene glycol, talc, and titanium dioxide.

Rx only

This Medication Guide has been approved by the U.S. Food and Drug Administration.

WELLBUTRIN, WELLBUTRIN SR, WELLBUTRIN XL, and PARNATE are registered trademarks of GlaxoSmithKline.

The following are registered trademarks of their respective manufacturers: NARDIL®/Warner Lambert Company; MARPLAN®/Oxford Pharmaceutical Services, Inc.

Distributed by:
GlaxoSmithKline
Research Triangle Park, NC 27709
Manufactured by:
DSM Pharmaceuticals, Inc.
Greenville, NC 27834 for
GlaxoSmithKline
Research Triangle Park, NC 27709
©2010, GlaxoSmithKline. All rights reserve.
May 2010
WLT:6MG

WELLBUTRIN SR®
[wel′byü-trin]
(bupropion hydrochloride)
Sustained-Release Tablets

℞

WARNING
Suicidality and Antidepressant Drugs
Use in Treating Psychiatric Disorders: Antidepressants increased the risk compared to placebo of suicidal thinking and behavior (suicidality) in children, adolescents, and young adults in short-term studies of major depressive disorder (MDD) and other psychiatric disorders. Anyone considering the use of WELLBUTRIN SR or any other antidepressant in a child, adolescent, or young adult must balance this risk with the clinical need. Short-term studies did not show an increase in the risk of suicidality with antidepressants compared to placebo in adults beyond age 24; there was a reduction in risk with antidepressants compared to placebo in adults aged 65 and older. Depression and certain other psychiatric disorders are themselves associated with increases in the risk of suicide. Patients of all ages who are started on antidepressant therapy should be monitored appropriately and observed closely for clinical worsening, suicidality, or unusual changes in behavior. Families and caregivers should be advised of the need for close observation and communication with the prescriber. WELLBUTRIN SR is not approved for use in pediatric patients. (See WARNINGS: Clinical Worsening and Suicide Risk in Treating Psychiatric Disorders, PRECAUTIONS: Information for Patients, and PRECAUTIONS: Pediatric Use.)
Use in Smoking Cessation Treatment: WELLBUTRIN®, WELLBUTRIN SR®, and WELLBUTRIN XL® are not approved for smoking cessation treatment, but bupropion under the name ZYBAN® is approved for this use. Serious neuropsychiatric events, including but not limited to depression, suicidal ideation, suicide attempt, and completed suicide have been reported in patients taking bupropion for smoking cessation. Some cases may have been complicated by the symptoms of nicotine withdrawal in patients who stopped smoking. Depressed mood may be a symptom of nicotine withdrawal. Depression, rarely including

suicidal ideation, has been reported in smokers undergoing a smoking cessation attempt without medication. However, some of these symptoms have occurred in patients taking bupropion who continued to smoke. All patients being treated with bupropion for smoking cessation treatment should be observed for neuropsychiatric symptoms including changes in behavior, hostility, agitation, depressed mood, and suicide-related events, including ideation, behavior, and attempted suicide. These symptoms, as well as worsening of pre-existing psychiatric illness and completed suicide have been reported in some patients attempting to quit smoking while taking ZYBAN in the postmarketing experience. When symptoms were reported, most were during treatment with ZYBAN, but some were following discontinuation of treatment with ZYBAN. These events have occurred in patients with and without pre-existing psychiatric disease; some have experienced worsening of their psychiatric illnesses. Patients with serious psychiatric illness such as schizophrenia, bipolar disorder, and major depressive disorder did not participate in the premarketing studies of ZYBAN.

Advise patients and caregivers that the patient using bupropion for smoking cessation should stop taking bupropion and contact a healthcare provider immediately if agitation, hostility, depressed mood, or changes in thinking or behavior that are not typical for the patient are observed, or if the patient develops suicidal ideation or suicidal behavior. In many postmarketing cases, resolution of symptoms after discontinuation of ZYBAN was reported, although in some cases the symptoms persisted; therefore, ongoing monitoring and supportive care should be provided until symptoms resolve.

The risks of using bupropion for smoking cessation should be weighed against the benefits of its use. ZYBAN has been demonstrated to increase the likelihood of abstinence from smoking for as long as 6 months compared to treatment with placebo. The health benefits of quitting smoking are immediate and substantial. (See WARNINGS: Neuropsychiatric Symptoms and Suicide Risk in Smoking Cessation Treatment and PRECAUTIONS: Information for Patients.)

DESCRIPTION

WELLBUTRIN SR (bupropion hydrochloride), an antidepressant of the aminoketone class, is chemically unrelated to tricyclic, tetracyclic, selective serotonin re-uptake inhibitor, or other known antidepressant agents. Its structure closely resembles that of diethylpropion; it is related to phenylethylamines. It is designated as (±)-1-(3-chlorophenyl)-2-[(1,1-dimethylethyl)amino]-1-propanone hydrochloride. The molecular weight is 276.2. The molecular formula is $C_{13}H_{18}ClNO \bullet HCl$. Bupropion hydrochloride powder is white, crystalline, and highly soluble in water. It has a bitter taste and produces the sensation of local anesthesia on the oral mucosa. The structural formula is:

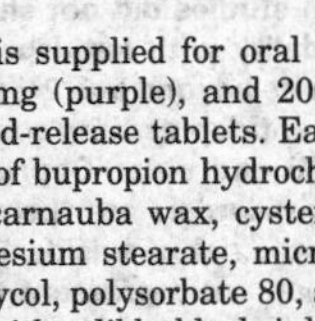

WELLBUTRIN SR is supplied for oral administration as 100-mg (blue), 150-mg (purple), and 200-mg (light pink), film-coated, sustained-release tablets. Each tablet contains the labeled amount of bupropion hydrochloride and the inactive ingredients: carnauba wax, cysteine hydrochloride, hypromellose, magnesium stearate, microcrystalline cellulose, polyethylene glycol, polysorbate 80, and titanium dioxide and is printed with edible black ink. In addition, the 100-mg tablet contains FD&C Blue No. 1 Lake, the 150-mg tablet contains FD&C Blue No. 2 Lake and FD&C Red No. 40 Lake, and the 200-mg tablet contains FD&C Red No. 40 Lake.

CLINICAL PHARMACOLOGY

Pharmacodynamics

Bupropion is a relatively weak inhibitor of the neuronal uptake of norepinephrine and dopamine, and does not inhibit monoamine oxidase or the re-uptake of serotonin. While the mechanism of action of bupropion, as with other antidepressants, is unknown, it is presumed that this action is mediated by noradrenergic and/or dopaminergic mechanisms.

Pharmacokinetics

Bupropion is a racemic mixture. The pharmacologic activity and pharmacokinetics of the individual enantiomers have not been studied. The mean elimination half-life (±SD) of bupropion after chronic dosing is 21 (±9) hours, and steady-state plasma concentrations of bupropion are reached within 8 days. In a study comparing chronic dosing with WELLBUTRIN SR 150 mg twice daily to the immediate-release formulation of bupropion at 100 mg 3 times daily, peak plasma concentrations of bupropion at steady state for WELLBUTRIN SR were approximately 85% of those achieved with the immediate-release formulation. There was equivalence for bupropion AUCs, as well as equivalence for both peak plasma concentration and AUCs for all 3 of the detectable bupropion metabolites. Thus, at steady state, WELLBUTRIN SR, given twice daily, and the immediate-release formulation of bupropion, given 3 times daily, are essentially bioequivalent for both bupropion and the 3 quantitatively important metabolites.

Absorption

Following oral administration of WELLBUTRIN SR to healthy volunteers, peak plasma concentrations of bupropion are achieved within 3 hours. Food increased C_{max} and AUC of bupropion by 11% and 17%, respectively, indicating that there is no clinically significant food effect.

Distribution

In vitro tests show that bupropion is 84% bound to human plasma proteins at concentrations up to 200 mcg/mL. The extent of protein binding of the hydroxybupropion metabolite is similar to that for bupropion, whereas the extent of protein binding of the threohydrobupropion metabolite is about half that seen with bupropion.

Metabolism

Bupropion is extensively metabolized in humans. Three metabolites have been shown to be active: hydroxybupropion, which is formed via hydroxylation of the *tert*-butyl group of bupropion, and the amino-alcohol isomers threohydrobupropion and erythrohydrobupropion, which are formed via reduction of the carbonyl group. In vitro findings suggest that cytochrome P450IIB6 (CYP2B6) is the principal isoenzyme involved in the formation of hydroxybupropion, while cytochrome P450 isoenzymes are not involved in the formation of threohydrobupropion. Oxidation of the bupropion side chain results in the formation of a glycine conjugate of meta-chlorobenzoic acid, which is then excreted as the major urinary metabolite. The potency and toxicity of the metabolites relative to bupropion have not been fully characterized. However, it has been demonstrated in an antidepressant screening test in mice that hydroxybupropion is one-half as potent as bupropion, while threohydrobupropion and erythrohydrobupropion are 5-fold less potent than bupropion. This may be of clinical importance because the plasma concentrations of the metabolites are as high or higher than those of bupropion.

Because bupropion is extensively metabolized, there is the potential for drug-drug interactions, particularly with those agents that are metabolized by or which inhibit/induce the cytochrome P450IIB6 (CYP2B6) isoenzyme, such as ritonavir. In a healthy volunteer study, ritonavir at a dose of 100 mg twice daily reduced the AUC and C_{max} of bupropion by 22% and 21%, respectively.

The exposure of the hydroxybupropion metabolite was decreased by 23%, the threohydrobupropion decreased by 38%, and the erythrohydrobupropion decreased by 48%.

In a second healthy volunteer study, ritonavir at a dose of 600 mg twice daily decreased the AUC and the C_{max} of bupropion by 66% and 62%, respectively. The exposure of the hydroxybupropion metabolite was decreased by 78%, the threohydrobupropion decreased by 50%, and the erythrohydrobupropion decreased by 68%.

In another healthy volunteer study, KALETRA® (lopinavir 400 mg/ritonavir 100 mg twice daily) decreased bupropion AUC and C_{max} by 57%. The AUC and C_{max} of hydroxybupropion were decreased by 50% and 31%, respectively (see PRECAUTIONS: Drug Interactions).

Although bupropion is not metabolized by cytochrome P450IID6 (CYP2D6), there is the potential for drug-drug interactions when bupropion is coadministered with drugs metabolized by this isoenzyme (see PRECAUTIONS: Drug Interactions).

Following a single dose in humans, peak plasma concentrations of hydroxybupropion occur approximately 6 hours after administration of WELLBUTRIN SR. Peak plasma concentrations of hydroxybupropion are approximately 10 times the peak level of the parent drug at steady state. The elimination half-life of hydroxybupropion is approximately 20 (±5) hours, and its AUC at steady state is about 17 times that of bupropion. The times to peak concentrations for the erythrohydrobupropion and threohydrobupropion metabolites are similar to that of the hydroxybupropion metabolite. However, their elimination half-lives are longer, 33 (±10) and 37 (±13) hours, respectively, and steady-state AUCs are 1.5 and 7 times that of bupropion, respectively.

Bupropion and its metabolites exhibit linear kinetics following chronic administration of 300 to 450 mg/day.

Elimination

Following oral administration of 200 mg of ^{14}C-bupropion in humans, 87% and 10% of the radioactive dose were recovered in the urine and feces, respectively. However, the fraction of the oral dose of bupropion excreted unchanged was only 0.5%, a finding consistent with the extensive metabolism of bupropion.

Population Subgroups

Factors or conditions altering metabolic capacity (e.g., liver disease, congestive heart failure [CHF], age, concomitant medications, etc.) or elimination may be expected to influence the degree and extent of accumulation of the active metabolites of bupropion. The elimination of the major metabolites of bupropion may be affected by reduced renal or hepatic function because they are moderately polar compounds and are likely to undergo further metabolism or conjugation in the liver prior to urinary excretion.

Hepatic

The effect of hepatic impairment on the pharmacokinetics of bupropion was characterized in 2 single-dose studies, one in patients with alcoholic liver disease and one in patients with mild-to-severe cirrhosis. The first study showed that the half-life of hydroxybupropion was significantly longer in 8 patients with alcoholic liver disease than in 8 healthy volunteers (32 ± 14 hours versus 21 ± 5 hours, respectively). Although not statistically significant, the AUCs for bupropion and hydroxybupropion were more variable and tended to be greater (by 53% to 57%) in patients with alcoholic liver disease. The differences in half-life for bupropion and the other metabolites in the 2 patient groups were minimal.

The second study showed no statistically significant differences in the pharmacokinetics of bupropion and its active metabolites in 9 patients with mild-to-moderate hepatic cirrhosis compared to 8 healthy volunteers. However, more variability was observed in some of the pharmacokinetic parameters for bupropion (AUC, C_{max}, and T_{max}) and its active metabolites ($t_{1/2}$) in patients with mild-to-moderate hepatic cirrhosis. In addition, in patients with severe hepatic cirrhosis, the bupropion C_{max} and AUC were substantially increased (mean difference: by approximately 70% and 3-fold, respectively) and more variable when compared to values in healthy volunteers; the mean bupropion half-life was also longer (29 hours in patients with severe hepatic cirrhosis vs. 19 hours in healthy subjects). For the metabolite hydroxybupropion, the mean C_{max} was approximately 69% lower. For the combined amino-alcohol isomers threohydrobupropion and erythrohydrobupropion, the mean C_{max} was approximately 31% lower. The mean AUC increased by about 1½-fold for hydroxybupropion and about 2½-fold for threo/erythrohydrobupropion. The median T_{max} was observed 19 hours later for hydroxybupropion and 31 hours later for threo/erythrohydrobupropion. The mean half-lives for hydroxybupropion and threo/erythrohydrobupropion were increased 5- and 2-fold, respectively, in patients with severe hepatic cirrhosis compared to healthy volunteers (see WARNINGS, PRECAUTIONS, and DOSAGE AND ADMINISTRATION).

Renal

There is limited information on the pharmacokinetics of bupropion in patients with renal impairment. An inter-study comparison between normal subjects and patients with end-stage renal failure demonstrated that the parent drug C_{max} and AUC values were comparable in the 2 groups, whereas the hydroxybupropion and threohydrobupropion metabolites had a 2.3– and 2.8–fold increase, respectively, in AUC for patients with end-stage renal failure. A second study, comparing normal subjects and patients with moderate-to-severe renal impairment (GFR 30.9 ± 10.8 mL/min) showed that exposure to a single 150-mg dose of sustained-release bupropion was approximately 2-fold higher in patients with impaired renal function while levels of the hydroxybupropion and threo/erythrohydrobupropion (combined) metabolites were similar in the 2 groups. The elimination of bupropion and/or the major metabolites of bupropion may be reduced by impaired renal function (see PRECAUTIONS: Renal Impairment).

Left Ventricular Dysfunction

During a chronic dosing study with bupropion in 14 depressed patients with left ventricular dysfunction (history of CHF or an enlarged heart on x-ray), no apparent effect on the pharmacokinetics of bupropion or its metabolites was revealed, compared to healthy volunteers.

Age

The effects of age on the pharmacokinetics of bupropion and its metabolites have not been fully characterized, but an exploration of steady-state bupropion concentrations from several depression efficacy studies involving patients dosed in a range of 300 to 750 mg/day, on a 3 times daily schedule, revealed no relationship between age (18 to 83 years) and plasma concentration of bupropion. A single-dose pharmacokinetic study demonstrated that the disposition of bupropion and its metabolites in elderly subjects was similar to that of younger subjects. These data suggest there is no prominent effect of age on bupropion concentration; however, another pharmacokinetic study, single and multiple dose, has suggested that the elderly are at increased risk for accumulation of bupropion and its metabolites (see PRECAUTIONS: Geriatric Use).

Gender

A single-dose study involving 12 healthy male and 12 healthy female volunteers revealed no sex-related differences in the pharmacokinetic parameters of bupropion.

Smokers

The effects of cigarette smoking on the pharmacokinetics of bupropion were studied in 34 healthy male and female volunteers; 17 were chronic cigarette smokers and 17 were nonsmokers. Following oral administration of a single 150-mg dose of bupropion, there was no statistically significant difference in C_{max}, half-life, T_{max}, AUC, or clearance of bupropion or its active metabolites between smokers and nonsmokers.

CLINICAL TRIALS

The efficacy of the immediate-release formulation of bupropion as a treatment for depression was established in two 4-week, placebo-controlled trials in adult inpatients with depression and in one 6-week, placebo-controlled trial in adult outpatients with depression. In the first study, patients were titrated in a bupropion dose range of 300 to 600 mg/day on a 3 times daily schedule; 78% of patients received maximum doses of 450 mg/day or less. This trial demonstrated the effectiveness of the immediate-release formulation of bupropion on the Hamilton Depression Rating Scale (HDRS) total score, the depressed mood item (item 1) from that scale, and the Clinical Global Impressions (CGI) severity score. A second study included 2 fixed doses of the immediate-release formulation of bupropion (300 and 450 mg/day) and placebo. This trial demonstrated the effectiveness of the immediate-release formulation of bupropion, but only at the 450-mg/day dose; the results were positive for the HDRS total score and the CGI severity score, but not for HDRS item 1. In the third study, outpatients received 300 mg/day of the immediate-release formulation of bupropion. This study demonstrated the effectiveness of the immediate-release formulation of bupropion on the HDRS total score, HDRS item 1, the Montgomery-Asberg Depression Rating Scale, the CGI severity score, and the CGI improvement score.

Although there are not as yet independent trials demonstrating the antidepressant effectiveness of the sustained-release formulation of bupropion, studies have demonstrated the bioequivalence of the immediate-release and sustained-release forms of bupropion under steady-state conditions, i.e., bupropion sustained-release 150 mg twice daily was shown to be bioequivalent to 100 mg 3 times daily of the immediate-release formulation of bupropion, with regard to both rate and extent of absorption, for parent drug and metabolites.

In a longer-term study, outpatients meeting DSM-IV criteria for major depressive disorder, recurrent type, who had responded during an 8-week open trial on WELLBUTRIN SR (150 mg twice daily) were randomized to continuation of their same dose of WELLBUTRIN SR or placebo, for up to 44 weeks of observation for relapse. Response during the open phase was defined as CGI Improvement score of 1 (very much improved) or 2 (much improved) for each of the final 3 weeks. Relapse during the double-blind phase was defined as the investigator's judgment that drug treatment was needed for worsening depressive symptoms. Patients receiving continued treatment with WELLBUTRIN SR experienced significantly lower relapse rates over the subsequent 44 weeks compared to those receiving placebo.

INDICATIONS AND USAGE

WELLBUTRIN SR is indicated for the treatment of major depressive disorder.

The efficacy of bupropion in the treatment of a major depressive episode was established in two 4-week controlled trials of depressed inpatients and in one 6-week controlled trial of depressed outpatients whose diagnoses corresponded most closely to the Major Depression category of the APA Diagnostic and Statistical Manual (DSM) (see CLINICAL PHARMACOLOGY).

A major depressive episode (DSM-IV) implies the presence of 1) depressed mood or 2) loss of interest or pleasure; in addition, at least 5 of the following symptoms have been present during the same 2-week period and represent a change from previous functioning: depressed mood, markedly diminished interest or pleasure in usual activities, significant change in weight and/or appetite, insomnia or hypersomnia, psychomotor agitation or retardation, increased fatigue, feelings of guilt or worthlessness, slowed thinking or impaired concentration, a suicide attempt or suicidal ideation.

The efficacy of WELLBUTRIN SR in maintaining an antidepressant response for up to 44 weeks following 8 weeks of acute treatment was demonstrated in a placebo-controlled trial (see CLINICAL PHARMACOLOGY). Nevertheless, the physician who elects to use WELLBUTRIN SR for extended periods should periodically reevaluate the long-term usefulness of the drug for the individual patient.

CONTRAINDICATIONS

WELLBUTRIN SR is contraindicated in patients with a seizure disorder.

WELLBUTRIN SR is contraindicated in patients treated with ZYBAN (bupropion hydrochloride) Sustained-Release Tablets; WELLBUTRIN (bupropion hydrochloride), the immediate-release formulation; WELLBUTRIN XL (bupropion hydrochloride), the extended-release formulation; or any other medications that contain bupropion because the incidence of seizure is dose dependent.

WELLBUTRIN SR is contraindicated in patients with a current or prior diagnosis of bulimia or anorexia nervosa because of a higher incidence of seizures noted in patients treated for bulimia with the immediate-release formulation of bupropion.

WELLBUTRIN SR is contraindicated in patients undergoing abrupt discontinuation of alcohol or sedatives (including benzodiazepines).

The concurrent administration of WELLBUTRIN SR and a monoamine oxidase (MAO) inhibitor is contraindicated. At least 14 days should elapse between discontinuation of an MAO inhibitor and initiation of treatment with WELLBUTRIN SR.

WELLBUTRIN SR is contraindicated in patients who have shown an allergic response to bupropion or the other ingredients that make up WELLBUTRIN SR.

WARNINGS

Clinical Worsening and Suicide Risk in Treating Psychiatric Disorders

Patients with major depressive disorder (MDD), both adult and pediatric, may experience worsening of their depression and/or the emergence of suicidal ideation and behavior (suicidality) or unusual changes in behavior, whether or not they are taking antidepressant medications, and this risk may persist until significant remission occurs. Suicide is a known risk of depression and certain other psychiatric disorders, and these disorders themselves are the strongest predictors of suicide. There has been a long-standing concern, however, that antidepressants may have a role in inducing worsening of depression and the emergence of suicidality in certain patients during the early phases of treatment. Pooled analyses of short-term placebo-controlled trials of antidepressant drugs (SSRIs and others) showed that these drugs increase the risk of suicidal thinking and behavior (suicidality) in children, adolescents, and young adults (ages 18-24) with major depressive disorder (MDD) and other psychiatric disorders. Short-term studies did not show an increase in the risk of suicidality with antidepressants compared to placebo in adults beyond age 24; there was a reduction with antidepressants compared to placebo in adults aged 65 and older.

The pooled analyses of placebo-controlled trials in children and adolescents with MDD, obsessive compulsive disorder (OCD), or other psychiatric disorders included a total of 24 short-term trials of 9 antidepressant drugs in over 4,400 patients. The pooled analyses of placebo-controlled trials in adults with MDD or other psychiatric disorders included a total of 295 short-term trials (median duration of 2 months) of 11 antidepressant drugs in over 77,000 patients. There was considerable variation in risk of suicidality among drugs, but a tendency toward an increase in the younger patients for almost all drugs studied. There were differences in absolute risk of suicidality across the different indications, with the highest incidence in MDD. The risk differences (drug vs. placebo), however, were relatively stable within age strata and across indications. These risk differences (drug-placebo difference in the number of cases of suicidality per 1,000 patients treated) are provided in Table 1.

Table 1

Age Range	Drug-Placebo Difference in Number of Cases of Suicidality per 1,000 Patients Treated
Increases Compared to Placebo	
<18	14 additional cases
18-24	5 additional cases
Decreases Compared to Placebo	
25-64	1 fewer case
≥65	6 fewer cases

No suicides occurred in any of the pediatric trials. There were suicides in the adult trials, but the number was not sufficient to reach any conclusion about drug effect on suicide.

It is unknown whether the suicidality risk extends to longer-term use, i.e., beyond several months. However,

there is substantial evidence from placebo-controlled maintenance trials in adults with depression that the use of antidepressants can delay the recurrence of depression.

All patients being treated with antidepressants for any indication should be monitored appropriately and observed closely for clinical worsening, suicidality, and unusual changes in behavior, especially during the initial few months of a course of drug therapy, or at times of dose changes, either increases or decreases.

The following symptoms, anxiety, agitation, panic attacks, insomnia, irritability, hostility, aggressiveness, impulsivity, akathisia (psychomotor restlessness), hypomania, and mania, have been reported in adult and pediatric patients being treated with antidepressants for major depressive disorder as well as for other indications, both psychiatric and nonpsychiatric. Although a causal link between the emergence of such symptoms and either the worsening of depression and/or the emergence of suicidal impulses has not been established, there is concern that such symptoms may represent precursors to emerging suicidality.

Consideration should be given to changing the therapeutic regimen, including possibly discontinuing the medication, in patients whose depression is persistently worse, or who are experiencing emergent suicidality or symptoms that might be precursors to worsening depression or suicidality, especially if these symptoms are severe, abrupt in onset, or were not part of the patient's presenting symptoms.

Families and caregivers of patients being treated with antidepressants for major depressive disorder or other indications, both psychiatric and nonpsychiatric, should be alerted about the need to monitor patients for the emergence of agitation, irritability, unusual changes in behavior, and the other symptoms described above, as well as the emergence of suicidality, and to report such symptoms immediately to healthcare providers. Such monitoring should include daily observation by families and caregivers. Prescriptions for WELLBUTRIN SR should be written for the smallest quantity of tablets consistent with good patient management, in order to reduce the risk of overdose.

Neuropsychiatric Symptoms and Suicide Risk in Smoking Cessation Treatment

WELLBUTRIN, WELLBUTRIN SR, and WELLBUTRIN XL are not approved for smoking cessation treatment, but bupropion under the name ZYBAN is approved for this use. Serious neuropsychiatric symptoms have been reported in patients taking bupropion for smoking cessation (see BOXED WARNING, ADVERSE REACTIONS). These have included changes in mood (including depression and mania), psychosis, hallucinations, paranoia, delusions, homicidal ideation, hostility, agitation, aggression, anxiety, and panic, as well as suicidal ideation, suicide attempt, and completed suicide. Some reported cases may have been complicated by the symptoms of nicotine withdrawal in patients who stopped smoking. Depressed mood may be a symptom of nicotine withdrawal. Depression, rarely including suicidal ideation, has been reported in smokers undergoing a smoking cessation attempt without medication. However, some of these symptoms have occurred in patients taking bupropion who continued to smoke. When symptoms were reported, most were during bupropion treatment, but some were following discontinuation of bupropion therapy. These events have occurred in patients with and without pre-existing psychiatric disease; some have experienced worsening of their psychiatric illnesses. All patients being treated with bupropion as part of smoking cessation treatment should be observed for neuropsychiatric symptoms or worsening of pre-existing psychiatric illness.

Patients with serious psychiatric illness such as schizophrenia, bipolar disorder, and major depressive disorder did not participate in the pre-marketing studies of ZYBAN.

Advise patients and caregivers that the patient using bupropion for smoking cessation should stop taking bupropion and contact a healthcare provider immediately if agitation, depressed mood, or changes in behavior or thinking that are not typical for the patient are observed, or if the patient develops suicidal ideation or suicidal behavior. In many postmarketing cases, resolution of symptoms after discontinuation of ZYBAN was reported, although in some cases the symptoms persisted, therefore, ongoing monitoring and supportive care should be provided until symptoms resolve.

The risks of using bupropion for smoking cessation should be weighed against the benefits of its use. ZYBAN has been demonstrated to increase the likelihood of abstinence from smoking for as long as six months compared to treatment with placebo. The health benefits of quitting smoking are immediate and substantial.

Screening Patients for Bipolar Disorder

A major depressive episode may be the initial presentation of bipolar disorder. It is generally believed (though not established in controlled trials) that treating such an episode with an antidepressant alone may increase the likelihood of precipitation of a mixed/manic episode in patients at risk for bipolar disorder. Whether any of the symptoms described above represent such a conversion is unknown. However, prior to initiating treatment with an antidepressant, patients with depressive symptoms should be adequately screened to determine if they are at risk for bipolar disorder; such screening should include a detailed psychiatric history, including a family history of suicide, bipolar disorder, and depression. It should be noted that WELLBUTRIN SR is not approved for use in treating bipolar depression.

Bupropion-Containing Products
Patients should be made aware that WELLBUTRIN SR contains the same active ingredient found in ZYBAN, used as an aid to smoking cessation treatment, and that WELLBUTRIN SR should not be used in combination with ZYBAN, or any other medications that contain bupropion, such as WELLBUTRIN (bupropion hydrochloride), the immediate-release formulation or WELLBUTRIN XL (bupropion hydrochloride), the extended-release formulation.

Seizures
Bupropion is associated with a dose-related risk of seizures. The risk of seizures is also related to patient factors, clinical situations, and concomitant medications, which must be considered in selection of patients for therapy with WELLBUTRIN SR. WELLBUTRIN SR should be discontinued and not restarted in patients who experience a seizure while on treatment.
* **Dose:** At doses of WELLBUTRIN SR up to a dose of 300 mg/day, the incidence of seizure is approximately 0.1% (1/1,000) and increases to approximately 0.4% (4/1,000) at the maximum recommended dose of 400 mg/day.

Data for the immediate-release formulation of bupropion revealed a seizure incidence of approximately 0.4% (i.e., 13 of 3,200 patients followed prospectively) in patients treated at doses in a range of 300 to 450 mg/day. The 450-mg/day upper limit of this dose range is close to the currently recommended maximum dose of 400 mg/day for WELLBUTRIN SR. This seizure incidence (0.4%) may exceed that of other marketed antidepressants and WELLBUTRIN SR up to 300 mg/day by as much as 4-fold. This relative risk is only an approximate estimate because no direct comparative studies have been conducted.

Additional data accumulated for the immediate-release formulation of bupropion suggested that the estimated seizure incidence increases almost tenfold between 450 and 600 mg/day, which is twice the usual adult dose and one and one-half the maximum recommended daily dose (400 mg) of WELLBUTRIN SR. This disproportionate increase in seizure incidence with dose incrementation calls for caution in dosing.

Data for WELLBUTRIN SR revealed a seizure incidence of approximately 0.1% (i.e., 3 of 3,100 patients followed prospectively) in patients treated at doses in a range of 100 to 300 mg/day. It is not possible to know if the lower seizure incidence observed in this study involving the sustained-release formulation of bupropion resulted from the different formulation or the lower dose used. However, as noted above, the immediate-release and sustained-release formulations are bioequivalent with regard to both rate and extent of absorption during steady state (the most pertinent condition to estimating seizure incidence), since most observed seizures occur under steady-state conditions.
* **Patient factors:** Predisposing factors that may increase the risk of seizure with bupropion use include history of head trauma or prior seizure, central nervous system (CNS) tumor, the presence of severe hepatic cirrhosis, and concomitant medications that lower seizure threshold.
* **Clinical situations:** Circumstances associated with an increased seizure risk include, among others, excessive use of alcohol or sedatives (including benzodiazepines); addiction to opiates, cocaine, or stimulants; use of over-the-counter stimulants and anorectics; and diabetes treated with oral hypoglycemics or insulin.
* **Concomitant medications:** Many medications (e.g., antipsychotics, antidepressants, theophylline, systemic steroids) are known to lower seizure threshold.

Recommendations for Reducing the Risk of Seizure
Retrospective analysis of clinical experience gained during the development of bupropion suggests that the risk of seizure may be minimized if
* the total daily dose of WELLBUTRIN SR does *not* exceed 400 mg,
* the daily dose is administered twice daily, and
* the rate of incrementation of dose is gradual.
* No single dose should exceed 200 mg to avoid high peak concentrations of bupropion and/or its metabolites.

WELLBUTRIN SR should be administered with extreme caution to patients with a history of seizure, cranial trauma, or other predisposition(s) toward seizure, or patients treated with other agents (e.g., antipsychotics, other antidepressants, theophylline, systemic steroids, etc.) that lower seizure threshold.

Hepatic Impairment
WELLBUTRIN SR should be used with extreme caution in patients with severe hepatic cirrhosis. In these patients a reduced frequency and/or dose is required, as peak bupropion, as well as AUC, levels are substantially increased and accumulation is likely to occur in such patients to a greater extent than usual. The dose should not exceed 100 mg every day or 150 mg every other day in these patients (see CLINICAL PHARMACOLOGY, PRECAUTIONS, and DOSAGE AND ADMINISTRATION).

Potential for Hepatotoxicity
In rats receiving large doses of bupropion chronically, there was an increase in incidence of hepatic hyperplastic nodules and hepatocellular hypertrophy. In dogs receiving large doses of bupropion chronically, various histologic changes were seen in the liver, and laboratory tests suggesting mild hepatocellular injury were noted.

PRECAUTIONS
General
Agitation and Insomnia
Patients in placebo-controlled trials with WELLBUTRIN SR experienced agitation, anxiety, and insomnia as shown in Table 2.

Table 2. Incidence of Agitation, Anxiety, and Insomnia in Placebo-Controlled Trials

Adverse Event Term	WELLBUTRIN SR 300 mg/day (n = 376)	WELLBUTRIN SR 400 mg/day (n = 114)	Placebo (n = 385)
Agitation	3%	9%	2%
Anxiety	5%	6%	3%
Insomnia	11%	16%	6%

In clinical studies, these symptoms were sometimes of sufficient magnitude to require treatment with sedative/hypnotic drugs.
Symptoms were sufficiently severe to require discontinuation of treatment in 1% and 2.6% of patients treated with 300 and 400 mg/day, respectively, of WELLBUTRIN SR and 0.8% of patients treated with placebo.
Psychosis, Confusion, and Other Neuropsychiatric Phenomena
Depressed patients treated with an immediate-release formulation of bupropion or with WELLBUTRIN SR have been reported to show a variety of neuropsychiatric signs and symptoms, including delusions, hallucinations, psychosis, concentration disturbance, paranoia, and confusion. In some cases, these symptoms abated upon dose reduction and/or withdrawal of treatment.
Activation of Psychosis and/or Mania
Antidepressants can precipitate manic episodes in bipolar disorder patients during the depressed phase of their illness and may activate latent psychosis in other susceptible patients. WELLBUTRIN SR is expected to pose similar risks.
Altered Appetite and Weight
In placebo-controlled studies, patients experienced weight gain or weight loss as shown in Table 3.

Table 3. Incidence of Weight Gain and Weight Loss in Placebo-Controlled Trials

Weight Change	WELLBUTRIN SR 300 mg/day (n = 339)	WELLBUTRIN SR 400 mg/day (n = 112)	Placebo (n = 347)
Gained >5 lbs	3%	2%	4%
Lost >5 lbs	14%	19%	6%

In studies conducted with the immediate-release formulation of bupropion, 35% of patients receiving tricyclic antidepressants gained weight, compared to 9% of patients treated with the immediate-release formulation of bupropion. If weight loss is a major presenting sign of a patient's depressive illness, the anorectic and/or weight-reducing potential of WELLBUTRIN SR should be considered.
Allergic Reactions
Anaphylactoid/anaphylactic reactions characterized by symptoms such as pruritus, urticaria, angioedema, and dyspnea requiring medical treatment have been reported in clinical trials with bupropion. In addition, there have been rare spontaneous postmarketing reports of erythema multiforme, Stevens-Johnson syndrome, and anaphylactic shock associated with bupropion. A patient should stop taking WELLBUTRIN SR and consult a doctor if experiencing allergic or anaphylactoid/anaphylactic reactions (e.g., skin rash, pruritus, hives, chest pain, edema, and shortness of breath) during treatment.
Arthralgia, myalgia, and fever with rash and other symptoms suggestive of delayed hypersensitivity have been reported in association with bupropion. These symptoms may resemble serum sickness.
Cardiovascular Effects
In clinical practice, hypertension, in some cases severe, requiring acute treatment, has been reported in patients receiving bupropion alone and in combination with nicotine replacement therapy. These events have been observed in both patients with and without evidence of preexisting hypertension.
Data from a comparative study of the sustained-release formulation of bupropion (ZYBAN® Sustained-Release Tablets), nicotine transdermal system (NTS), the combination of sustained-release bupropion plus NTS, and placebo as an aid to smoking cessation suggest a higher incidence of treatment-emergent hypertension in patients treated with the combination of sustained-release bupropion and NTS. In this study, 6.1% of patients treated with the combination of sustained-release bupropion and NTS had treatment-emergent hypertension compared to 2.5%, 1.6%, and 3.1% of patients treated with sustained-release bupropion, NTS, and placebo, respectively. The majority of these patients had evidence of preexisting hypertension. Three patients (1.2%) treated with the combination of ZYBAN and NTS and 1 patient (0.4%) treated with NTS had study medication discontinued due to hypertension compared to none of the patients treated with ZYBAN or placebo. Monitoring of blood pressure is recommended in patients who receive the combination of bupropion and nicotine replacement.
There is no clinical experience establishing the safety of WELLBUTRIN SR Tablets in patients with a recent history of myocardial infarction or unstable heart disease. Therefore, care should be exercised if it is used in these groups. Bupropion was well tolerated in depressed patients who had previously developed orthostatic hypotension while receiving tricyclic antidepressants, and was also generally well tolerated in a group of 36 depressed inpatients with stable congestive heart failure (CHF). However, bupropion was associated with a rise in supine blood pressure in the study of patients with CHF, resulting in discontinuation of treatment in 2 patients for exacerbation of baseline hypertension.
Hepatic Impairment
WELLBUTRIN SR should be used with extreme caution in patients with severe hepatic cirrhosis. In these patients, a reduced frequency and/or dose is required. WELLBUTRIN SR should be used with caution in patients with hepatic impairment (including mild-to-moderate hepatic cirrhosis) and reduced frequency and/or dose should be considered in patients with mild-to-moderate hepatic cirrhosis.
All patients with hepatic impairment should be closely monitored for possible adverse effects that could indicate high drug and metabolite levels (see CLINICAL PHARMACOLOGY, WARNINGS, and DOSAGE AND ADMINISTRATION).
Renal Impairment
There is limited information on the pharmacokinetics of bupropion in patients with renal impairment. An interstudy comparison between normal subjects and patients with end-stage renal failure demonstrated that the parent drug C_{max} and AUC values were comparable in the 2 groups, whereas the hydroxybupropion and threohydrobupropion metabolites had a 2.3– and 2.8–fold increase, respectively, in AUC for patients with end-stage renal failure. A second study, comparing normal subjects and patients with moderate-to-severe renal impairment (GFR 30.9 ± 10.8 mL/min) showed that exposure to a single 150-mg dose of sustained-release bupropion was approximately 2-fold higher in patients with impaired renal function while levels of the hydroxybupropion and threo/erythrohydrobupropion (combined) metabolites were similar in the 2 groups. Bupropion is extensively metabolized in the liver to active metabolites, which are further metabolized and subsequently excreted by the kidneys. WELLBUTRIN SR should be used with caution in patients with renal impairment and a reduced frequency and/or dose should be considered as bupropion and the metabolites of bupropion may accumulate in such patients to a greater extent than usual. The patient should be closely monitored for possible adverse effects that could indicate high drug or metabolite levels.
Information for Patients
Prescribers or other health professionals should inform patients, their families, and their caregivers about the benefits and risks associated with treatment with WELLBUTRIN SR and should counsel them in its appropriate use. A patient Medication Guide about "Antidepressant Medicines, Depression and Other Serious Mental Illnesses, and Suicidal Thoughts or Actions," "Quitting Smoking, Quit-Smoking Medication, Changes in Thinking and Behavior, Depression, and Suicidal Thoughts or Actions," and "What

Other Important Information Should I Know About WELLBUTRIN SR?" is available for WELLBUTRIN SR. The prescriber or health professional should instruct patients, their families, and their caregivers to read the Medication Guide and should assist them in understanding its contents. Patients should be given the opportunity to discuss the contents of the Medication Guide and to obtain answers to any questions they may have. The complete text of the Medication Guide is reprinted at the end of this document.

Patients should be advised of the following issues and asked to alert their prescriber if these occur while taking WELLBUTRIN SR.

Clinical Worsening and Suicide Risk in Treating Psychiatric Disorders

Patients, their families, and their caregivers should be encouraged to be alert to the emergence of anxiety, agitation, panic attacks, insomnia, irritability, hostility, aggressiveness, impulsivity, akathisia (psychomotor restlessness), hypomania, mania, other unusual changes in behavior, worsening of depression, and suicidal ideation, especially early during antidepressant treatment and when the dose is adjusted up or down. Families and caregivers of patients should be advised to look for the emergence of such symptoms on a day-to-day basis, since changes may be abrupt. Such symptoms should be reported to the patient's prescriber or health professional, especially if they are severe, abrupt in onset, or were not part of the patient's presenting symptoms. Symptoms such as these may be associated with an increased risk for suicidal thinking and behavior and indicate a need for very close monitoring and possibly changes in the medication.

Neuropsychiatric Symptoms and Suicide Risk in Smoking Cessation Treatment: Although WELLBUTRIN SR is not indicated for smoking cessation treatment, it contains the same active ingredient as ZYBAN which is approved for this use. Patients should be informed that quitting smoking, with or without ZYBAN, may be associated with nicotine withdrawal symptoms (including depression or agitation), or exacerbation of pre-existing psychiatric illness. Furthermore, some patients have experienced changes in mood (including depression and mania), psychosis, hallucinations, paranoia, delusions, homicidal ideation, aggression, anxiety, and panic, as well as suicidal ideation, suicide attempt, and completed suicide when attempting to quit smoking while taking ZYBAN. If patients develop agitation, hostility, depressed mood, or changes in thinking or behavior that are not typical for them, or if patients develop suicidal ideation or behavior, they should be urged to report these symptoms to their healthcare provider immediately.

Bupropion-Containing Products:

Patients should be made aware that WELLBUTRIN SR contains the same active ingredient found in ZYBAN, used as an aid to smoking cessation treatment, and that WELLBUTRIN SR should not be used in combination with ZYBAN or any other medications that contain bupropion hydrochloride (such as WELLBUTRIN, the immediate-release formulation and WELLBUTRIN XL, the extended-release formulation).

As dose is increased during initial titration to doses above 150 mg/day, patients should be instructed to take WELLBUTRIN SR in 2 divided doses, preferably with at least 8 hours between successive doses, to minimize the risk of seizures.

Patients should be told that WELLBUTRIN SR should be discontinued and not restarted if they experience a seizure while on treatment.

Patients should be told that any CNS-active drug like WELLBUTRIN SR may impair their ability to perform tasks requiring judgment or motor and cognitive skills. Consequently, until they are reasonably certain that WELLBUTRIN SR does not adversely affect their performance, they should refrain from driving an automobile or operating complex, hazardous machinery.

Patients should be told that the excessive use or abrupt discontinuation of alcohol or sedatives (including benzodiazepines) may alter the seizure threshold. Some patients have reported lower alcohol tolerance during treatment with WELLBUTRIN SR. Patients should be advised that the consumption of alcohol should be minimized or avoided.

Patients should be advised to inform their physicians if they are taking or plan to take any prescription or over-the-counter drugs. Concern is warranted because WELLBUTRIN SR and other drugs may affect each other's metabolism.

Patients should be advised to notify their physicians if they become pregnant or intend to become pregnant during therapy.

Patients should be advised to swallow WELLBUTRIN SR tablets whole so that the release rate is not altered. Do not chew, divide, or crush tablets, as this may lead to an increased risk of adverse effects, including seizures.

Laboratory Tests

There are no specific laboratory tests recommended.

Drug Interactions

Few systemic data have been collected on the metabolism of bupropion following concomitant administration with other drugs or, alternatively, the effect of concomitant administration of bupropion on the metabolism of other drugs.

Because bupropion is extensively metabolized, the coadministration of other drugs may affect its clinical activity. In vitro studies indicate that bupropion is primarily metabolized to hydroxybupropion by the CYP2B6 isoenzyme. Therefore, the potential exists for a drug interaction between WELLBUTRIN SR and drugs that are substrates of or inhibitors/inducers of the CYP2B6 isoenzyme (e.g., orphenadrine, thiotepa, cyclophosphamide, ticlopidine, and clopidogrel). In addition, in vitro studies suggest that paroxetine, sertraline, norfluoxetine, and fluvoxamine as well as nelfinavir and efavirenz inhibit the hydroxylation of bupropion. No clinical studies have been performed to evaluate this finding. The threohydrobupropion metabolite of bupropion does not appear to be produced by the cytochrome P450 isoenzymes. The effects of concomitant administration of cimetidine on the pharmacokinetics of bupropion and its active metabolites were studied in 24 healthy young male volunteers. Following oral administration of two 150-mg WELLBUTRIN SR Tablets with and without 800 mg of cimetidine, the pharmacokinetics of bupropion and hydroxybupropion were unaffected. However, there were 16% and 32% increases in the AUC and C_{max}, respectively, of the combined moieties of threohydrobupropion and erythrohydrobupropion.

In a series of studies in healthy volunteers, ritonavir (100 mg twice daily or 600 mg twice daily) or ritonavir 100 mg plus lopinavir 400 mg (KALETRA) twice daily reduced the exposure of bupropion and its major metabolites in a dose dependent manner by approximately 20% to 80%. This effect is thought to be due to the induction of bupropion metabolism. Patients receiving ritonavir may need increased doses of bupropion, but the maximum recommended dose of bupropion should not be exceeded (see CLINICAL PHARMACOLOGY: Metabolism).

While not systematically studied, certain drugs may induce the metabolism of bupropion (e.g., carbamazepine, phenobarbital, phenytoin).

Multiple oral doses of bupropion had no statistically significant effects on the single-dose pharmacokinetics of lamotrigine in 12 healthy volunteers.

Animal data indicated that bupropion may be an inducer of drug-metabolizing enzymes in humans. In one study, following chronic administration of bupropion, 100 mg 3 times daily to 8 healthy male volunteers for 14 days, there was no evidence of induction of its own metabolism. Nevertheless, there may be the potential for clinically important alterations of blood levels of coadministered drugs.

Drugs Metabolized By Cytochrome P450IID6 (CYP2D6)

Many drugs, including most antidepressants (SSRIs, many tricyclics), beta-blockers, antiarrhythmics, and antipsychotics are metabolized by the CYP2D6 isoenzyme. Although bupropion is not metabolized by this isoenzyme, bupropion and hydroxybupropion are inhibitors of CYP2D6 isoenzyme in vitro. In a study of 15 male subjects (aged 19 to 35 years) who were extensive metabolizers of the CYP2D6 isoenzyme, daily doses of bupropion given as 150 mg twice daily followed by a single dose of 50 mg desipramine increased the C_{max}, AUC, and $t_{1/2}$ of desipramine by an average of approximately 2-, 5-, and 2-fold, respectively. The effect was present for at least 7 days after the last dose of bupropion. Concomitant use of bupropion with other drugs metabolized by CYP2D6 has not been formally studied.

Therefore, coadministration of bupropion with drugs that are metabolized by CYP2D6 isoenzyme including certain antidepressants (e.g., nortriptyline, imipramine, desipramine, paroxetine, fluoxetine, sertraline), antipsychotics (e.g., haloperidol, risperidone, thioridazine), beta-blockers (e.g., metoprolol), and Type 1C antiarrhythmics (e.g., propafenone, flecainide), should be approached with caution and should be initiated at the lower end of the dose range of the concomitant medication. If bupropion is added to the treatment regimen of a patient already receiving a drug metabolized by CYP2D6, the need to decrease the dose of the original medication should be considered, particularly for those concomitant medications with a narrow therapeutic index.

Although citalopram is not primarily metabolized by CYP2D6, in one study bupropion increased the C_{max} and AUC of citalopram by 30% and 40%, respectively. Citalopram did not affect the pharmacokinetics of bupropion and its 3 metabolites.

MAO Inhibitors

Studies in animals demonstrate that the acute toxicity of bupropion is enhanced by the MAO inhibitor phenelzine (see CONTRAINDICATIONS).

Levodopa and Amantadine

Limited clinical data suggest a higher incidence of adverse experiences in patients receiving bupropion concurrently with either levodopa or amantadine. Administration of

WELLBUTRIN SR to patients receiving either levodopa or amantadine concurrently should be undertaken with caution, using small initial doses and gradual dose increases.

Drugs That Lower Seizure Threshold

Concurrent administration of WELLBUTRIN SR Tablets and agents (e.g., antipsychotics, other antidepressants, theophylline, systemic steroids, etc.) that lower seizure threshold should be undertaken only with extreme caution (see WARNINGS). Low initial dosing and gradual dose increases should be employed.

Nicotine Transdermal System

(see PRECAUTIONS: Cardiovascular Effects).

Alcohol

In postmarketing experience, there have been rare reports of adverse neuropsychiatric events or reduced alcohol tolerance in patients who were drinking alcohol during treatment with WELLBUTRIN SR. The consumption of alcohol during treatment with WELLBUTRIN SR should be minimized or avoided (also see CONTRAINDICATIONS).

Carcinogenesis, Mutagenesis, Impairment of Fertility

Lifetime carcinogenicity studies were performed in rats and mice at doses up to 300 and 150 mg/kg/day, respectively. These doses are approximately 7 and 2 times the maximum recommended human dose (MRHD), respectively, on a mg/m² basis. In the rat study there was an increase in nodular proliferative lesions of the liver at doses of 100 to 300 mg/kg/day (approximately 2 to 7 times the MRHD on a mg/m² basis); lower doses were not tested. The question of whether or not such lesions may be precursors of neoplasms of the liver is currently unresolved. Similar liver lesions were not seen in the mouse study, and no increase in malignant tumors of the liver and other organs was seen in either study.

Bupropion produced a positive response (2 to 3 times control mutation rate) in 2 of 5 strains in the Ames bacterial mutagenicity test and an increase in chromosomal aberrations in 1 of 3 in vivo rat bone marrow cytogenetic studies.

A fertility study in rats at doses up to 300 mg/kg/day revealed no evidence of impaired fertility.

Pregnancy

Teratogenic Effects

Pregnancy Category C. In studies conducted in rats and rabbits, bupropion was administered orally at doses up to 450 and 150 mg/kg/day, respectively (approximately 11 and 7 times the MRHD, respectively, on a mg/m² basis), during the period of organogenesis. No clear evidence of teratogenic activity was found in either species; however, in rabbits, slightly increased incidences of fetal malformations and skeletal variations were observed at the lowest dose tested (25 mg/kg/day, approximately equal to the MRHD on a mg/m² basis) and greater. Decreased fetal weights were seen at 50 mg/kg and greater.

When rats were administered bupropion at oral doses of up to 300 mg/kg/day (approximately 7 times the MRHD on a mg/m² basis) prior to mating and throughout pregnancy and lactation, there were no apparent adverse effects on offspring development.

One study has been conducted in pregnant women. This retrospective, managed-care database study assessed the risk of congenital malformations overall and cardiovascular malformations specifically, following exposure to bupropion in the first trimester compared to the risk of these malformations following exposure to other antidepressants in the first trimester and bupropion outside of the first trimester. This study included 7,005 infants with antidepressant exposure during pregnancy, 1,213 of whom were exposed to bupropion in the first trimester. The study showed no greater risk for congenital malformations overall or cardiovascular malformations specifically, following first trimester bupropion exposure compared to exposure to all other antidepressants in the first trimester, or bupropion outside of the first trimester. The results of this study have not been corroborated. WELLBUTRIN SR should be used during pregnancy only if the potential benefit justifies the potential risk to the fetus.

Labor and Delivery

The effect of WELLBUTRIN SR on labor and delivery in humans is unknown.

Nursing Mothers

Like many other drugs, bupropion and its metabolites are secreted in human milk. Because of the potential for serious adverse reactions in nursing infants from WELLBUTRIN SR, a decision should be made whether to discontinue nursing or to discontinue the drug, taking into account the importance of the drug to the mother.

Pediatric Use

Safety and effectiveness in the pediatric population have not been established (see BOX WARNING and WARNINGS: Clinical Worsening and Suicide Risk in Treating Psychiatric Disorders). Anyone considering the use of WELLBUTRIN

SR in a child or adolescent must balance the potential risks with the clinical need.

Geriatric Use

Of the approximately 6,000 patients who participated in clinical trials with bupropion sustained-release tablets (depression and smoking cessation studies), 275 were 65 and over and 47 were 75 and over. In addition, several hundred patients 65 and over participated in clinical trials using the immediate-release formulation of bupropion (depression studies). No overall differences in safety or effectiveness were observed between these subjects and younger subjects, and other reported clinical experience has not identified differences in responses between the elderly and younger patients, but greater sensitivity of some older individuals cannot be ruled out.

A single-dose pharmacokinetic study demonstrated that the disposition of bupropion and its metabolites in elderly subjects was similar to that of younger subjects; however, another pharmacokinetic study, single and multiple dose, has suggested that the elderly are at increased risk for accumulation of bupropion and its metabolites (see CLINICAL PHARMACOLOGY).

Bupropion is extensively metabolized in the liver to active metabolites, which are further metabolized and excreted by the kidneys. The risk of toxic reaction to this drug may be greater in patients with impaired renal function. Because elderly patients are more likely to have decreased renal function, care should be taken in dose selection, and it may be useful to monitor renal function (see PRECAUTIONS: Renal Impairment and DOSAGE AND ADMINISTRATION).

ADVERSE REACTIONS (SEE ALSO WARNINGS AND PRECAUTIONS.)

The information included under the Incidence in Controlled Trials subsection of ADVERSE REACTIONS is based primarily on data from controlled clinical trials with WELLBUTRIN SR. Information on additional adverse events associated with the sustained-release formulation of bupropion in smoking cessation trials, as well as the immediate-release formulation of bupropion, is included in a separate section (see Other Events Observed During the Clinical Development and Postmarketing Experience of Bupropion).

Incidence in Controlled Trials With WELLBUTRIN SR

Adverse Events Associated With Discontinuation of Treatment Among Patients Treated With WELLBUTRIN SR

In placebo-controlled clinical trials, 9% and 11% of patients treated with 300 and 400 mg/day, respectively, of WELLBUTRIN SR and 4% of patients treated with placebo discontinued treatment due to adverse events. The specific adverse events in these trials that led to discontinuation in at least 1% of patients treated with either 300 or 400 mg/day of WELLBUTRIN SR and at a rate at least twice the placebo rate are listed in Table 4.

Table 4. Treatment Discontinuations Due to Adverse Events in Placebo-Controlled Trials

Adverse Event Term	WELLBUTRIN SR 300 mg/day (n = 376)	WELLBUTRIN SR 400 mg/day (n = 114)	Placebo (n = 385)
Rash	2.4%	0.9%	0.0%
Nausea	0.8%	1.8%	0.3%
Agitation	0.3%	1.8%	0.3%
Migraine	0.0%	1.8%	0.3%

Adverse Events Occurring at an Incidence of 1% or More Among Patients Treated With WELLBUTRIN SR

Table 5 enumerates treatment-emergent adverse events that occurred among patients treated with 300 and 400 mg/day of WELLBUTRIN SR and with placebo in placebo-controlled trials. Events that occurred in either the 300- or 400-mg/day group at an incidence of 1% or more and were more frequent than in the placebo group are included. Reported adverse events were classified using a COSTART-based Dictionary.

Accurate estimates of the incidence of adverse events associated with the use of any drug are difficult to obtain. Estimates are influenced by drug dose, detection technique, setting, physician judgments, etc. The figures cited cannot be used to predict precisely the incidence of untoward events in the course of usual medical practice where patient characteristics and other factors differ from those that prevailed in the clinical trials. These incidence figures also cannot be compared with those obtained from other clinical studies involving related drug products as each group of drug trials is conducted under a different set of conditions. Finally, it is important to emphasize that the tabulation does not reflect the relative severity and/or clinical importance of the events. A better perspective on the serious adverse events associated with the use of WELLBUTRIN SR is provided in the WARNINGS and PRECAUTIONS sections.

[See table 5 at left]

Incidence of Commonly Observed Adverse Events in Controlled Clinical Trials

Adverse events from Table 5 occurring in at least 5% of patients treated with WELLBUTRIN SR and at a rate at least twice the placebo rate are listed below for the 300- and 400-mg/day dose groups.

WELLBUTRIN SR 300 mg/day

Anorexia, dry mouth, rash, sweating, tinnitus, and tremor.

WELLBUTRIN SR 400 mg/day

Abdominal pain, agitation, anxiety, dizziness, dry mouth, insomnia, myalgia, nausea, palpitation, pharyngitis, sweating, tinnitus, and urinary frequency.

Other Events Observed During the Clinical Development and Postmarketing Experience of Bupropion

In addition to the adverse events noted above, the following events have been reported in clinical trials and postmarketing experience with the sustained-release formulation of bupropion in depressed patients and in nondepressed smokers, as well as in clinical trials and postmarketing clinical experience with the immediate-release formulation of bupropion.

Adverse events for which frequencies are provided below occurred in clinical trials with the sustained-release formulation of bupropion. The frequencies represent the proportion of patients who experienced a treatment-emergent

Table 5. Treatment-Emergent Adverse Events in Placebo-Controlled Trials[a]

Body System/ Adverse Event	WELLBUTRIN SR 300 mg/day (n = 376)	WELLBUTRIN SR 400 mg/day (n = 114)	Placebo (n = 385)
Body (General)			
Headache	26%	25%	23%
Infection	8%	9%	6%
Abdominal pain	3%	9%	2%
Asthenia	2%	4%	1%
Chest pain	3%	4%	1%
Pain	2%	3%	2%
Fever	1%	2%	—
Cardiovascular			
Palpitation	2%	6%	2%
Flushing	1%	4%	—
Migraine	1%	4%	1%
Hot flashes	1%	3%	1%
Digestive			
Dry mouth	17%	24%	7%
Nausea	13%	18%	8%
Constipation	10%	5%	7%
Diarrhea	5%	7%	6%
Anorexia	5%	3%	2%
Vomiting	4%	2%	2%
Dysphagia	0%	2%	0%
Musculoskeletal			
Myalgia	2%	6%	3%
Arthralgia	1%	4%	1%
Arthritis	0%	2%	0%
Twitch	1%	2%	—
Nervous system			
Insomnia	11%	16%	6%
Dizziness	7%	11%	5%
Agitation	3%	9%	2%
Anxiety	5%	6%	3%
Tremor	6%	3%	1%
Nervousness	5%	3%	3%
Somnolence	2%	3%	2%
Irritability	3%	2%	2%
Memory decreased	—	3%	1%
Paresthesia	1%	2%	1%
Central nervous system stimulation	2%	1%	1%
Respiratory			
Pharyngitis	3%	11%	2%
Sinusitis	3%	1%	2%
Increased cough	1%	2%	1%
Skin			
Sweating	6%	5%	2%
Rash	5%	4%	1%
Pruritus	2%	4%	2%
Urticaria	2%	1%	0%
Special senses			
Tinnitus	6%	6%	2%
Taste perversion	2%	4%	—
Blurred vision or diplopia	3%	2%	2%
Urogenital			
Urinary frequency	2%	5%	2%
Urinary urgency	—	2%	0%
Vaginal hemorrhage[b]	0%	2%	—
Urinary tract infection	1%	0%	—

[a]Adverse events that occurred in at least 1% of patients treated with either 300 or 400 mg/day of WELLBUTRIN SR, but equally or more frequently in the placebo group, were: abnormal dreams, accidental injury, acne, appetite increased, back pain, bronchitis, dysmenorrhea, dyspepsia, flatulence, flu syndrome, hypertension, neck pain, respiratory disorder, rhinitis, and tooth disorder.

[b]Incidence based on the number of female patients.

— Hyphen denotes adverse events occurring in greater than 0 but less than 0.5% of patients.

adverse event on at least one occasion in placebo-controlled studies for depression (n = 987) or smoking cessation (n = 1,013), or patients who experienced an adverse event requiring discontinuation of treatment in an open-label surveillance study with WELLBUTRIN SR (n = 3,100). All treatment-emergent adverse events are included except those listed in Tables 2 through 5, those events listed in other safety-related sections, those adverse events subsumed under COSTART terms that are either overly general or excessively specific so as to be uninformative, those events not reasonably associated with the use of the drug, and those events that were not serious and occurred in fewer than 2 patients. Events of major clinical importance are described in the WARNINGS and PRECAUTIONS sections of the labeling.

Events are further categorized by body system and listed in order of decreasing frequency according to the following definitions of frequency: Frequent adverse events are defined as those occurring in at least 1/100 patients. Infrequent adverse events are those occurring in 1/100 to 1/1,000 patients, while rare events are those occurring in less than 1/1,000 patients.

Adverse events for which frequencies are not provided occurred in clinical trials or postmarketing experience with bupropion. Only those adverse events not previously listed for sustained-release bupropion are included. The extent to which these events may be associated with WELLBUTRIN SR is unknown.

Body (General)

Infrequent were chills, facial edema, musculoskeletal chest pain, and photosensitivity. Rare was malaise. Also observed were arthralgia, myalgia, and fever with rash and other symptoms suggestive of delayed hypersensitivity. These symptoms may resemble serum sickness (see PRECAUTIONS).

Cardiovascular

Infrequent were postural hypotension, stroke, tachycardia, and vasodilation. Rare was syncope. Also observed were complete atrioventricular block, extrasystoles, hypotension, hypertension (in some cases severe, see PRECAUTIONS), myocardial infarction, phlebitis, and pulmonary embolism.

Digestive

Infrequent were abnormal liver function, bruxism, gastric reflux, gingivitis, glossitis, increased salivation, jaundice, mouth ulcers, stomatitis, and thirst. Rare was edema of tongue. Also observed were colitis, esophagitis, gastrointestinal hemorrhage, gum hemorrhage, hepatitis, intestinal perforation, liver damage, pancreatitis, and stomach ulcer.

Endocrine

Also observed were hyperglycemia, hypoglycemia, and syndrome of inappropriate antidiuretic hormone.

Hemic and Lymphatic

Infrequent was ecchymosis. Also observed were anemia, leukocytosis, leukopenia, lymphadenopathy, pancytopenia, and thrombocytopenia. Altered PT and/or INR, infrequently associated with hemorrhagic or thrombotic complications, were observed when bupropion was coadministered with warfarin.

Metabolic and Nutritional

Infrequent were edema and peripheral edema. Also observed was glycosuria.

Musculoskeletal

Infrequent were leg cramps. Also observed were muscle rigidity/fever/rhabdomyolysis and muscle weakness.

Nervous System

Infrequent were abnormal coordination, decreased libido, depersonalization, dysphoria, emotional lability, hostility, hyperkinesia, hypertonia, hypesthesia, suicidal ideation, and vertigo. Rare were amnesia, ataxia, derealization, and hypomania. Also observed were abnormal electroencephalogram (EEG), akinesia, aggression, aphasia, coma, completed suicide, delirium, delusions, dysarthria, dyskinesia, dystonia, euphoria, extrapyramidal syndrome, hallucinations, hypokinesia, increased libido, manic reaction, neuralgia, neuropathy, paranoid ideation, restlessness, suicide attempt, and unmasking tardive dyskinesia.

Respiratory

Rare was bronchospasm. Also observed was pneumonia.

Skin

Rare was maculopapular rash. Also observed were alopecia, angioedema, exfoliative dermatitis, and hirsutism.

Special Senses

Infrequent were accommodation abnormality and dry eye. Also observed were deafness, diplopia, increased intraocular pressure, and mydriasis.

Urogenital

Infrequent were impotence, polyuria, and prostate disorder. Also observed were abnormal ejaculation, cystitis, dyspareunia, dysuria, gynecomastia, menopause, painful erection, salpingitis, urinary incontinence, urinary retention, and vaginitis.

DRUG ABUSE AND DEPENDENCE

Controlled Substance Class

Bupropion is not a controlled substance.

Humans

Controlled clinical studies of bupropion (immediate-release formulation) conducted in normal volunteers, in subjects with a history of multiple drug abuse, and in depressed patients showed some increase in motor activity and agitation/excitement.

In a population of individuals experienced with drugs of abuse, a single dose of 400 mg of bupropion produced mild amphetamine-like activity as compared to placebo on the Morphine-Benzedrine Subscale of the Addiction Research Center Inventories (ARCI), and a score intermediate between placebo and amphetamine on the Liking Scale of the ARCI. These scales measure general feelings of euphoria and drug desirability.

Findings in clinical trials, however, are not known to reliably predict the abuse potential of drugs. Nonetheless, evidence from single-dose studies does suggest that the recommended daily dosage of bupropion when administered in divided doses is not likely to be especially reinforcing to amphetamine or stimulant abusers. However, higher doses that could not be tested because of the risk of seizure might be modestly attractive to those who abuse stimulant drugs.

Animals

Studies in rodents and primates have shown that bupropion exhibits some pharmacologic actions common to psychostimulants. In rodents, it has been shown to increase locomotor activity, elicit a mild stereotyped behavioral response, and increase rates of responding in several schedule-controlled behavior paradigms. In primate models to assess the positive reinforcing effects of psychoactive drugs, bupropion was self-administered intravenously. In rats, bupropion produced amphetamine-like and cocaine-like discriminative stimulus effects in drug discrimination paradigms used to characterize the subjective effects of psychoactive drugs.

OVERDOSAGE

Human Overdose Experience

Overdoses of up to 30 g or more of bupropion have been reported. Seizure was reported in approximately one-third of all cases. Other serious reactions reported with overdoses of bupropion alone included hallucinations, loss of consciousness, sinus tachycardia, and ECG changes such as conduction disturbances (including QRS prolongation) or arrhythmias. Fever, muscle rigidity, rhabdomyolysis, hypotension, stupor, coma, and respiratory failure have been reported mainly when bupropion was part of multiple drug overdoses.

Although most patients recovered without sequelae, deaths associated with overdoses of bupropion alone have been reported in patients ingesting large doses of the drug. Multiple uncontrolled seizures, bradycardia, cardiac failure, and cardiac arrest prior to death were reported in these patients.

Overdosage Management

Ensure an adequate airway, oxygenation, and ventilation. Monitor cardiac rhythm and vital signs. EEG monitoring is also recommended for the first 48 hours post-ingestion. General supportive and symptomatic measures are also recommended. Induction of emesis is not recommended.

Activated charcoal should be administered. There is no experience with the use of forced diuresis, dialysis, hemoperfusion, or exchange transfusion in the management of bupropion overdoses. No specific antidotes for bupropion are known.

Due to the dose-related risk of seizures with WELLBUTRIN SR, hospitalization following suspected overdose should be considered. Based on studies in animals, it is recommended that seizures be treated with intravenous benzodiazepine administration and other supportive measures, as appropriate.

In managing overdosage, consider the possibility of multiple drug involvement. The physician should consider contacting a poison control center for additional information on the treatment of any overdose. Telephone numbers for certified poison control centers are listed in the *Physicians' Desk Reference* (PDR).

DOSAGE AND ADMINISTRATION

General Dosing Considerations

It is particularly important to administer WELLBUTRIN SR in a manner most likely to minimize the risk of seizure (see WARNINGS). Gradual escalation in dosage is also important if agitation, motor restlessness, and insomnia, often seen during the initial days of treatment, are to be minimized. If necessary, these effects may be managed by temporary reduction of dose or the short-term administration of an intermediate to long-acting sedative hypnotic. A sedative hypnotic usually is not required beyond the first week of treatment. Insomnia may also be minimized by avoiding bedtime doses. If distressing, untoward effects supervene, dose escalation should be stopped. WELLBUTRIN SR

should be swallowed whole and not crushed, divided, or chewed, as this may lead to an increase risk of adverse effects including seizures.

Initial Treatment

The usual adult target dose for WELLBUTRIN SR is 300 mg/day, given as 150 mg twice daily. Dosing with WELLBUTRIN SR should begin at 150 mg/day given as a single daily dose in the morning. If the 150-mg initial dose is adequately tolerated, an increase to the 300-mg/day target dose, given as 150 mg twice daily, may be made as early as day 4 of dosing. There should be an interval of at least 8 hours between successive doses.

Increasing the Dosage Above 300 mg/day

As with other antidepressants, the full antidepressant effect of WELLBUTRIN SR may not be evident until 4 weeks of treatment or longer. An increase in dosage to the maximum of 400 mg/day, given as 200 mg twice daily, may be considered for patients in whom no clinical improvement is noted after several weeks of treatment at 300 mg/day.

Maintenance Treatment

It is generally agreed that acute episodes of depression require several months or longer of sustained pharmacological therapy beyond response to the acute episode. In a study in which patients with major depressive disorder, recurrent type, who had responded during 8 weeks of acute treatment with WELLBUTRIN SR were assigned randomly to placebo or to the same dose of WELLBUTRIN SR (150 mg twice daily) during 44 weeks of maintenance treatment as they had received during the acute stabilization phase, longer-term efficacy was demonstrated (see CLINICAL TRIALS under CLINICAL PHARMACOLOGY). Based on these limited data, it is unknown whether or not the dose of WELLBUTRIN SR needed for maintenance treatment is identical to the dose needed to achieve an initial response. Patients should be periodically reassessed to determine the need for maintenance treatment and the appropriate dose for such treatment.

Dosage Adjustment for Patients with Impaired Hepatic Function

WELLBUTRIN SR should be used with extreme caution in patients with severe hepatic cirrhosis. The dose should not exceed 100 mg every day or 150 mg every other day in these patients. WELLBUTRIN SR should be used with caution in patients with hepatic impairment (including mild-to-moderate hepatic cirrhosis) and a reduced frequency and/or dose should be considered in patients with mild-to-moderate hepatic cirrhosis (see CLINICAL PHARMACOLOGY, WARNINGS, and PRECAUTIONS).

Dosage Adjustment for Patients with Impaired Renal Function

WELLBUTRIN SR should be used with caution in patients with renal impairment and a reduced frequency and/or dose should be considered (see CLINICAL PHARMACOLOGY and PRECAUTIONS).

HOW SUPPLIED

WELLBUTRIN SR Sustained-Release Tablets, 100 mg of bupropion hydrochloride, are blue, round, biconvex, film-coated tablets printed with "WELLBUTRIN SR 100" in bottles of 60 (NDC 0173-0947-55) tablets.

WELLBUTRIN SR Sustained-Release Tablets, 150 mg of bupropion hydrochloride, are purple, round, biconvex, film-coated tablets printed with "WELLBUTRIN SR 150" in bottles of 60 (NDC 0173-0135-55) tablets.

WELLBUTRIN SR Sustained-Release Tablets, 200 mg of bupropion hydrochloride, are light pink, round, biconvex, film-coated tablets printed with "WELLBUTRIN SR 200" in bottles of 60 (NDC 0173-0722-00) tablets.

Store at controlled room temperature, 20° to 25°C (68° to 77°F) [see USP]. Dispense in a tight, light-resistant container as defined in the USP.

WELLBUTRIN, WELLBUTRIN SR, WELLBUTRIN XL, and ZYBAN are registered trademarks of GlaxoSmithKline. KALETRA is a registered trademark of Abbott Laboratories.

Distributed by:
GlaxoSmithKline
Research Triangle Park, NC 27709
Manufactured by:
GlaxoSmithKline
Research Triangle Park, NC 27709
or DSM Pharmaceuticals, Inc.
Greenville, NC 27834
©2010, GlaxoSmithKline. All rights reserved
May 2010
WLS:5PI

MEDICATION GUIDE

WELLBUTRIN SR® (WELL byu-trin)
(bupropion hydrochloride) Sustained-Release Tablets

Read this Medication Guide carefully before you start using WELLBUTRIN SR and each time you get a refill. There may be new information. This information does not take the place of talking with your doctor about your medical condition or your treatment. If you have any questions about WELLBUTRIN SR, ask your doctor or pharmacist.

IMPORTANT: Be sure to read the three sections of this Medication Guide. The first section is about the risk of suicidal thoughts and actions with antidepressant medicines; the second section is about the risk of changes in thinking and behavior, depression and suicidal thoughts or actions with medicines used to quit smoking; and the third section is entitled "What Other Important Information Should I Know About WELLBUTRIN SR?"

Antidepressant Medicines, Depression and Other Serious Mental Illnesses, and Suicidal Thoughts or Actions

This section of the Medication Guide is only about the risk of suicidal thoughts and actions with antidepressant medicines. **Talk to your, or your family member's, healthcare provider about:**

- all risks and benefits of treatment with antidepressant medicines
- all treatment choices for depression or other serious mental illness

What is the most important information I should know about antidepressant medicines, depression and other serious mental illnesses, and suicidal thoughts or actions?

1. **Antidepressant medicines may increase suicidal thoughts or actions in some children, teenagers, and young adults within the first few months of treatment.**
2. **Depression and other serious mental illnesses are the most important causes of suicidal thoughts and actions. Some people may have a particularly high risk of having suicidal thoughts or actions.** These include people who have (or have a family history of) bipolar illness (also called manic-depressive illness) or suicidal thoughts or actions.
3. **How can I watch for and try to prevent suicidal thoughts and actions in myself or a family member?**
   - Pay close attention to any changes, especially sudden changes, in mood, behaviors, thoughts, or feelings. This is very important when an antidepressant medicine is started or when the dose is changed.
   - Call the healthcare provider right away to report new or sudden changes in mood, behavior, thoughts, or feelings.
   - Keep all follow-up visits with the healthcare provider as scheduled. Call the healthcare provider between visits as needed, especially if you have concerns about symptoms.

Call a healthcare provider right away if you or your family member has any of the following symptoms, especially if they are new, worse, or worry you:

• thoughts about suicide or dying	• new or worse irritability
• attempts to commit suicide	• acting aggressive, being angry, or violent
• new or worse depression	• acting on dangerous impulses
• new or worse anxiety	• an extreme increase in activity and talking (mania)
• feeling very agitated or restless	• other unusual changes in behavior or mood
• panic attacks	
• trouble sleeping (insomnia)	

What else do I need to know about antidepressant medicines?

- **Never stop an antidepressant medicine without first talking to a healthcare provider.** Stopping an antidepressant medicine suddenly can cause other symptoms.
- **Antidepressants are medicines used to treat depression and other illnesses.** It is important to discuss all the risks of treating depression and also the risks of not treating it. Patients and their families or other caregivers should discuss all treatment choices with the healthcare provider, not just the use of antidepressants.
- **Antidepressant medicines have other side effects.** Talk to the healthcare provider about the side effects of the medicine prescribed for you or your family member.
- **Antidepressant medicines can interact with other medicines.** Know all of the medicines that you or your family member takes. Keep a list of all medicines to show the healthcare provider. Do not start new medicines without first checking with your healthcare provider.
- **Not all antidepressant medicines prescribed for children are FDA approved for use in children.** Talk to your child's healthcare provider for more information.

WELLBUTRIN SR has not been studied in children under the age of 18 and is not approved for use in children and teenagers.

Quitting Smoking, Quit-Smoking Medications, Changes in Thinking and Behavior, Depression, and Suicidal Thoughts or Actions

This section of the Medication Guide is only about the risk of changes in thinking and behavior, depression and suicidal thoughts or actions with drugs used to quit smoking.

Although WELLBUTRIN SR is not a treatment for quitting smoking, it contains the same active ingredient (bupropion hydrochloride) as ZYBAN® which is used to help patients quit smoking.

Some people have had changes in behavior, hostility, agitation, depression, suicidal thoughts or actions while taking bupropion to help them quit smoking. These symptoms can develop during treatment with bupropion or after stopping treatment with bupropion.

If you, your family member, or your caregiver notice agitation, hostility, depression, or changes in thinking or behavior that are not typical for you, or you have any of the following symptoms, stop taking bupropion and call your healthcare provider right away:

• thoughts about suicide or dying	• an extreme increase in activity and talking (mania)
• attempts to commit suicide	• abnormal thoughts or sensations
• new or worse depression	• seeing or hearing things that are not there (hallucinations)
• new or worse anxiety	• feeling people are against you (paranoia)
• panic attacks	• feeling confused
• feeling very agitated or restless	• other unusual changes in behavior or mood
• acting aggressive, being angry, or violent	
• acting on dangerous	
• impulses	

When you try to quit smoking, with or without bupropion, you may have symptoms that may be due to nicotine withdrawal, including urge to smoke, depressed mood, trouble sleeping, irritability, frustration, anger, feeling anxious, difficulty concentrating, restlessness, decreased heart rate, and increased appetite or weight gain. Some people have even experienced suicidal thoughts when trying to quit smoking without medication. Sometimes quitting smoking can lead to worsening of mental health problems that you already have, such as depression.

Before taking bupropion, tell your healthcare provider if you have ever had depression or other mental illnesses. You should also tell your doctor about any symptoms you had during other times you tried to quit smoking, with or without bupropion.

What Other Important Information Should I Know About WELLBUTRIN SR?

- **Seizures: There is a chance of having a seizure (convulsion, fit) with WELLBUTRIN SR, especially in people:**
  - with certain medical problems.
  - who take certain medicines.

  The chance of having seizures increases with higher doses of WELLBUTRIN SR. For more information, see the sections "Who should not take WELLBUTRIN SR?" and "What should I tell my doctor before using WELLBUTRIN SR?" Tell your doctor about all of your medical conditions and all the medicines you take. **Do not take any other medicines while you are using WELLBUTRIN SR unless your doctor has said it is okay to take them.**

  If you have a seizure while taking WELLBUTRIN SR, stop taking the tablets and call your doctor right away. Do not take WELLBUTRIN SR again if you have a seizure.
- **High blood pressure (hypertension). Some people get high blood pressure, that can be severe, while taking WELLBUTRIN SR.** The chance of high blood pressure may be higher if you also use nicotine replacement therapy (such as a nicotine patch) to help you stop smoking.
- **Severe allergic reactions. Some people have severe allergic reaction to WELLBUTRIN SR. Stop taking WELLBUTRIN SR and call your doctor right away** if you get a rash, itching, hives, fever, swollen lymph glands, painful sores in the mouth or around the eyes, swelling of the lips or tongue, chest pain, or have trouble breathing. These could be signs of a serious allergic reaction.
- **Unusual thoughts or behaviors.** Some patients have unusual thoughts or behaviors while taking WELLBUTRIN SR, including delusions (believe you are someone else), hallucinations (seeing or hearing things that are not there), paranoia (feeling that people are against you), or feeling confused. If this happens to you, call your doctor.

What is WELLBUTRIN SR?

WELLBUTRIN SR is a prescription medicine used to treat adults with a certain type of depression called major depressive disorder.

Who should not take WELLBUTRIN SR?

Do not take WELLBUTRIN SR if you

- have or had a seizure disorder or epilepsy.
- **are taking ZYBAN® (used to help people stop smoking) or any other medicines that contain bupropion hydrochloride, such as WELLBUTRIN® Tablets or WELLBUTRIN XL® Extended-Release Tablets.** Bupropion is the same active ingredient that is in WELLBUTRIN SR.
- drink a lot of alcohol and abruptly stop drinking, or use medicines called sedatives (these make you sleepy) or benzodiazepines and you stop using them all of a sudden.
- have taken within the last 14 days medicine for depression called a monoamine oxidase inhibitor (MAOI), such as NARDIL® (phenelzine sulfate), PARNATE® (tranylcypromine sulfate), or MARPLAN® (isocarboxazid).
- have or had an eating disorder such as anorexia nervosa or bulimia.
- are allergic to the active ingredient in WELLBUTRIN SR, bupropion, or to any of the inactive ingredients. See the end of this leaflet for a complete list of ingredients in WELLBUTRIN SR.

What should I tell my doctor before using WELLBUTRIN SR?

Tell your doctor if you have ever had depression, suicidal thoughts or actions, or other mental health problems. See "Antidepressant Medicines, Depression and Other Serious Mental Illnesses, and Suicidal Thoughts or Actions."

- **Tell your doctor about your other medical conditions including if you:**
  - **are pregnant or plan to become pregnant.** It is not known if WELLBUTRIN SR can harm your unborn baby.
  - **are breastfeeding.** WELLBUTRIN SR passes through your milk. It is not known if WELLBUTRIN SR can harm your baby.
  - **have liver problems,** especially cirrhosis of the liver.
  - have kidney problems.
  - have an eating disorder such as anorexia nervosa or bulimia.
  - have had a head injury.
  - have had a seizure (convulsion, fit).
  - have a tumor in your nervous system (brain or spine).
  - have had a heart attack, heart problems, or high blood pressure.
  - are a diabetic taking insulin or other medicines to control your blood sugar.
  - drink a lot of alcohol.
  - abuse prescription medicines or street drugs.
- **Tell your doctor about all the medicines you take,** including prescription and non-prescription medicines, vitamins, and herbal supplements. Many medicines increase your chances of having seizures or other serious side effects if you take them while you are using WELLBUTRIN SR.

How should I take WELLBUTRIN SR?

- Take WELLBUTRIN SR exactly as prescribed by your doctor.
- **Do not chew, cut, or crush WELLBUTRIN SR tablets.** If you do, the medicine will be released into your body too quickly. If this happens you may be more likely to get side effects including seizures. You must swallow the tablets whole. **Tell your doctor if you cannot swallow medicine tablets.**
- Take WELLBUTRIN SR at the same time each day.
- Take your doses of WELLBUTRIN SR at least 8 hours apart.
- You may take WELLBUTRIN SR with or without food.
- If you miss a dose, do not take an extra tablet to make up for the dose you forgot. Wait and take your next tablet at the regular time. **This is very important.** Too much WELLBUTRIN SR can increase your chance of having a seizure.
- If you take too much WELLBUTRIN SR, or overdose, call your local emergency room or poison control center right away.
- **Do not take any other medicines while using WELLBUTRIN SR unless your doctor has told you it is okay.**
- It may take several weeks for you to feel that WELLBUTRIN SR is working. Once you feel better, it is important to keep taking WELLBUTRIN SR exactly as directed by your doctor. Call your doctor if you do not feel WELLBUTRIN SR is working for you.
- Do not change your dose or stop taking WELLBUTRIN SR without talking with your doctor first.

What should I avoid while taking WELLBUTRIN SR?

- Do not drink a lot of alcohol while taking WELLBUTRIN SR. If you usually drink a lot of alcohol, talk with your doctor before suddenly stopping. If you suddenly stop drinking alcohol, you may increase your chance of having seizures.
- Do not drive a car or use heavy machinery until you know how WELLBUTRIN SR affects you. WELLBUTRIN SR can impair your ability to perform these tasks.

What are possible side effects of WELLBUTRIN SR?

WELLBUTRIN SR can cause serious side effects. Read this entire Medication Guide for more information about these serious side effects.

The most common side effects of WELLBUTRIN SR are loss of appetite, dry mouth, skin rash, sweating, ringing in the ears, shakiness, stomach pain, agitation, anxiety, dizziness, trouble sleeping, muscle pain, nausea, fast heartbeat, sore throat, and urinating more often.

If you have nausea, take your medicine with food. If you have trouble sleeping, do not take your medicine too close to bedtime.

These are not all the side effects of WELLBUTRIN SR. For a complete list, ask your doctor or pharmacist.

Call your doctor for medical advice about side effects. You may report side effects to FDA at 1-800-FDA-1088.

How should I store WELLBUTRIN SR?

- Store WELLBUTRIN SR at room temperature. Store out of direct sunlight. Keep WELLBUTRIN SR in its tightly closed bottle.
- WELLBUTRIN SR tablets may have an odor.

General Information about WELLBUTRIN SR.

Medicines are sometimes prescribed for purposes other than those listed in a Medication Guide. Do not use WELLBUTRIN SR for a condition for which it was not prescribed. Do not give WELLBUTRIN SR to other people, even if they have the same symptoms you have. It may harm them. Keep WELLBUTRIN SR out of the reach of children.

This Medication Guide summarizes important information about WELLBUTRIN SR. For more information, talk with your doctor. You can ask your doctor or pharmacist for information about WELLBUTRIN SR that is written for health professionals.

What are the ingredients in WELLBUTRIN SR?

Active ingredient: bupropion hydrochloride.

Inactive ingredients: carnauba wax, cysteine hydrochloride, hypromellose, magnesium stearate, microcrystalline cellulose, polyethylene glycol, polysorbate 80, and titanium dioxide. In addition, the 100-mg tablet contains FD&C Blue No. 1 Lake, the 150-mg tablet contains FD&C Blue No. 2 Lake and FD&C Red No. 40 Lake, and the 200-mg tablet contains FD&C Red No. 40 Lake. The tablets are printed with edible black ink.

Rx only

This Medication Guide has been approved by the U.S. Food and Drug Administration.

WELLBUTRIN, WELLBUTRIN SR, WELLBUTRIN XL, ZYBAN, and PARNATE are registered trademarks of GlaxoSmithKline.

*The following are registered trademarks of their respective manufacturers: NARDIL®/Warner Lambert Company; MARPLAN®/Oxford Pharmaceutical Services, Inc.

Distributed by:
GlaxoSmithKline
Research Triangle Park, NC 27709
Manufactured by:
GlaxoSmithKline
Research Triangle Park, NC 27709
or DSM Pharmaceuticals, Inc.
Greenville, NC 27834
©2010, GlaxoSmithKline. All rights reserved.
May 2010
WLS:6MG

ZANTAC®   ℞
[zan' tak]
(ranitidine hydrochloride)
Injection
ZANTAC®   ℞
(ranitidine hydrochloride)
Injection Premixed

DESCRIPTION

The active ingredient in ZANTAC Injection and ZANTAC Injection Premixed is ranitidine hydrochloride (HCl), a histamine H$_2$-receptor antagonist. Chemically it is N[2-[[[5-[(dimethylamino)methyl]-2-furanyl]methyl]thio]ethyl]-N'-methyl-2-nitro-1,1-ethenediamine, hydrochloride. It has the following structure:

The empirical formula is $C_{13}H_{22}N_4O_3S \cdot HCl$, representing a molecular weight of 350.87.

Ranitidine HCl is a white to pale yellow, granular substance that is soluble in water.

ZANTAC Injection is a clear, colorless to yellow, nonpyrogenic liquid. The yellow color of the liquid tends to intensify without adversely affecting potency. The pH of the injection solution is 6.7 to 7.3.

Sterile Injection for Intramuscular or Intravenous Administration: Each 1 mL of aqueous solution contains ranitidine 25 mg (as the hydrochloride); phenol 5 mg as preservative;

and 0.96 mg of monobasic potassium phosphate and 2.4 mg of dibasic sodium phosphate as buffers.

Sterile, Premixed Solution for Intravenous Administration in Single-Dose, Flexible Plastic Containers: Each 50 mL contains ranitidine HCl equivalent to 50 mg of ranitidine, sodium chloride 225 mg, and citric acid 15 mg and dibasic sodium phosphate 90 mg as buffers in water for injection. It contains no preservatives. The osmolarity of this solution is 180 mOsm/L (approx.), and the pH is 6.7 to 7.3.

The flexible plastic container is fabricated from a specially formulated, nonplasticized, thermoplastic co-polyester (CR3). Water can permeate from inside the container into the overwrap but not in amounts sufficient to affect the solution significantly. Solutions inside the plastic container also can leach out certain of the chemical components in very small amounts before the expiration period is attained. However, the safety of the plastic has been confirmed by tests in animals according to USP biological standards for plastic containers.

CLINICAL PHARMACOLOGY

ZANTAC is a competitive, reversible inhibitor of the action of histamine at the histamine H$_2$-receptors, including receptors on the gastric cells. ZANTAC does not lower serum Ca++ in hypercalcemic states. ZANTAC is not an anticholinergic agent.

Pharmacokinetics: Absorption: ZANTAC is absorbed very rapidly after intramuscular (IM) injection. Mean peak levels of 576 ng/mL occur within 15 minutes or less following a 50-mg IM dose. Absorption from IM sites is virtually complete, with a bioavailability of 90% to 100% compared with intravenous (IV) administration. Following oral administration, the bioavailability of ZANTAC Tablets is 50%.

Distribution: The volume of distribution is about 1.4 L/kg. Serum protein binding averages 15%.

Metabolism: In humans, the N-oxide is the principal metabolite in the urine; however, this amounts to <4% of the dose. Other metabolites are the S-oxide (1%) and the desmethyl ranitidine (1%). The remainder of the administered dose is found in the stool. Studies in patients with hepatic dysfunction (compensated cirrhosis) indicate that there are minor, but clinically insignificant, alterations in ranitidine half-life, distribution, clearance, and bioavailability.

Excretion: Following IV injection, approximately 70% of the dose is recovered in the urine as unchanged drug. Renal clearance averages 530 mL/min, with a total clearance of 760 mL/min. The elimination half-life is 2.0 to 2.5 hours. Four patients with clinically significant renal function impairment (creatinine clearance 25 to 35 mL/min) administered 50 mg of ranitidine intravenously had an average plasma half-life of 4.8 hours, a ranitidine clearance of 29 mL/min, and a volume of distribution of 1.76 L/kg. In general, these parameters appear to be altered in proportion to creatinine clearance (see DOSAGE AND ADMINISTRATION).

Geriatrics: The plasma half-life is prolonged and total clearance is reduced in the elderly population due to a decrease in renal function. The elimination half-life is 3.1

hours (see PRECAUTIONS: Geriatric Use and DOSAGE AND ADMINISTRATION: Dosage Adjustment for Patients With Impaired Renal Function).

Pediatrics: There are no significant differences in the pharmacokinetic parameter values for ranitidine in pediatric patients (from 1 month up to 16 years of age) and healthy adults when correction is made for body weight. The pharmacokinetics of ZANTAC in pediatric patients are summarized in Table 1.

[See table 1 above]

Plasma clearance in neonatal patients (less than 1 month of age) receiving ECMO was considerably lower (3 to 4 mL/min/kg) than observed in children or adults. The elimination half-life in neonates averaged 6.6 hours as compared to approximately 2 hours in adults and pediatric patients.

Pharmacodynamics: Serum concentrations necessary to inhibit 50% of stimulated gastric acid secretion are estimated to be 36 to 94 ng/mL. Following single IV or IM 50-mg doses, serum concentrations of ranitidine are in this range for 6 to 8 hours.

Antisecretory Activity: 1. Effects on Acid Secretion: ZANTAC Injection inhibits basal gastric acid secretion as well as gastric acid secretion stimulated by betazole and pentagastrin, as shown in Table 2.

[See table 2 above]

In a group of 10 known hypersecretors, ranitidine plasma levels of 71, 180, and 376 ng/mL inhibited basal acid secretion by 76%, 90%, and 99.5%, respectively.

It appears that basal- and betazole-stimulated secretions are most sensitive to inhibition by ZANTAC, while pentagastrin-stimulated secretion is more difficult to suppress.

2. Effects on Other Gastrointestinal Secretions:

Pepsin: ZANTAC does not affect pepsin secretion. Total pepsin output is reduced in proportion to the decrease in volume of gastric juice.

Intrinsic Factor: ZANTAC has no significant effect on pentagastrin-stimulated intrinsic factor secretion.

Serum Gastrin: ZANTAC has little or no effect on fasting or postprandial serum gastrin.

Other Pharmacologic Actions:

1. Gastric bacterial flora—increase in nitrate-reducing organisms, significance not known.
2. Prolactin levels—no effect in recommended oral or IV dosage, but small, transient, dose-related increases in serum prolactin have been reported after IV bolus injections of 100 mg or more.
3. Other pituitary hormones—no effect on serum gonadotropins, TSH, or GH. Possible impairment of vasopressin release.
4. No change in cortisol, aldosterone, androgen, or estrogen levels.
5. No antiandrogenic action.
6. No effect on count, motility, or morphology of sperm.

Pediatrics: The ranitidine concentration necessary to suppress basal acid secretion by at least 90% has been reported to be 40 to 60 ng/mL in pediatric patients with duodenal or gastric ulcers.

Table 1. Ranitidine Pharmacokinetics in Pediatric Patients Following IV Dosing

Population (age)	n	Dose (mg/kg)	$t_{1/2}$ (hours)	Vd (L/kg)	CLp (mL/min/kg)
Peptic ulcer disease					
(<6 years)	6	1.25 or 2.5	2.2	1.29	11.41
(6–11.9 years)	11	1.25 or 2.5	2.1	1.14	8.96
(>12 years)	6	1.25 or 2.5	1.7	0.98	9.89
Adults	6	2.5	1.9	1.04	8.77
Peptic ulcer disease (3.5–16 years)	12	0.13–0.80	1.8	2.3	795 mL/min/1.73/m^2
Children in intensive care (1 day–12.6 years)	17	1.0	2.4	2	11.7
Neonates receiving ECMO	12	2	6.6	1.8	4.3

$T_{1/2}$ = Terminal half-life; CLp = Plasma clearance of ranitidine.
ECMO = extracorporeal membrane oxygenation.

Table 2. Effect of Intravenous ZANTAC on Gastric Acid Secretion

		% Inhibition of Gastric Acid Output by Intravenous Dose, mg		
	Time After Dose, hours	20 mg	60 mg	100 mg
Betazole	Up to 2	93	99	99
Pentagastrin	Up to 3	47	66	77

Table 3. Duodenal Ulcer Patient Healing Rates

	Oral ZANTAC*		Oral Placebo*	
	Number Entered	Healed/Evaluable	Number Entered	Healed/Evaluable
Outpatients Week 2	195	69/182 (38%)†	188	31/164 (19%)
Week 4		137/187 (73%)†		76/168 (45%)

*All patients were permitted antacids as needed for relief of pain.
†P<0.0001.

In a study of 20 critically ill pediatric patients receiving ranitidine IV at 1 mg/kg every 6 hours, 10 patients with a baseline pH ≥4 maintained this baseline throughout the study. Eight of the remaining 10 patients with a baseline of pH ≤2 achieved pH ≥4 throughout varying periods after dosing. It should be noted, however, that because these pharmacodynamic parameters were assessed in critically ill pediatric patients, the data should be interpreted with caution when dosing recommendations are made for a less seriously ill pediatric population.

In another small study of neonatal patients (n = 5) receiving ECMO, gastric pH <4 pretreatment increased to >4 after a 2-mg/kg dose and remained above 4 for at least 15 hours.

Clinical Trials: *Active Duodenal Ulcer:* In a multicenter, double-blind, controlled, US study of endoscopically diagnosed duodenal ulcers, earlier healing was seen in the patients treated with oral ZANTAC as shown in Table 3.
[See table 3 above]
In these studies, patients treated with oral ZANTAC reported a reduction in both daytime and nocturnal pain, and they also consumed less antacid than the placebo-treated patients.

Table 4. Mean Daily Doses of Antacid

	Ulcer Healed	Ulcer Not Healed
Oral ZANTAC	0.06	0.71
Oral placebo	0.71	1.43

Pathological Hypersecretory Conditions (such as Zollinger-Ellison syndrome): ZANTAC inhibits gastric acid secretion and reduces occurrence of diarrhea, anorexia, and pain in patients with pathological hypersecretion associated with Zollinger-Ellison syndrome, systemic mastocytosis, and other pathological hypersecretory conditions (e.g., postoperative, "short-gut" syndrome, idiopathic). Use of oral ZANTAC was followed by healing of ulcers in 8 of 19 (42%) patients who were intractable to previous therapy.
In a retrospective review of 52 Zollinger-Ellison patients given ZANTAC as a continuous IV infusion for up to 15 days, no patients developed complications of acid-peptic disease such as bleeding or perforation. Acid output was controlled to ≤10 mEq/h.

INDICATIONS AND USAGE

ZANTAC Injection and ZANTAC Injection Premixed are indicated in some hospitalized patients with pathological hypersecretory conditions or intractable duodenal ulcers, or as an alternative to the oral dosage form for short-term use in patients who are unable to take oral medication.

CONTRAINDICATIONS

ZANTAC Injection and ZANTAC Injection Premixed are contraindicated for patients known to have hypersensitivity to the drug.

PRECAUTIONS

General:
1. Symptomatic response to therapy with ZANTAC does not preclude the presence of gastric malignancy.
2. Since ZANTAC is excreted primarily by the kidney, dosage should be adjusted in patients with impaired renal function (see DOSAGE AND ADMINISTRATION). Caution should be observed in patients with hepatic dysfunction since ZANTAC is metabolized in the liver.
3. In controlled studies in normal volunteers, elevations in SGPT have been observed when H₂-antagonists have been administered intravenously at greater-than-recommended dosages for 5 days or longer. Therefore, it seems prudent in patients receiving IV ranitidine at dosages ≥100 mg 4 times daily for periods of 5 days or longer to monitor SGPT daily (from day 5) for the remainder of IV therapy.
4. Bradycardia in association with rapid administration of ZANTAC Injection has been reported rarely, usually in patients with factors predisposing to cardiac rhythm disturbances. Recommended rates of administration should not be exceeded (see DOSAGE AND ADMINISTRATION).
5. Rare reports suggest that ZANTAC may precipitate acute porphyric attacks in patients with acute porphyria. ZANTAC should therefore be avoided in patients with a history of acute porphyria.

Laboratory Tests: False-positive tests for urine protein with MULTISTIX® may occur during therapy with ZANTAC, and therefore testing with sulfosalicylic acid is recommended.

Drug Interactions: Ranitidine has been reported to affect the bioavailability of other drugs through several different mechanisms such as competition for renal tubular secretion, alteration of gastric pH, and inhibition of cytochrome P450 enzymes.

Procainamide: Ranitidine, a substrate of the renal organic cation transport system, may affect the clearance of other drugs eliminated by this route. High doses of ranitidine (e.g., such as those used in the treatment of Zollinger-Ellison syndrome) have been shown to reduce the renal excretion of procainamide and N-acetylprocainamide resulting in increased plasma levels of these drugs. Although this interaction is unlikely to be clinically relevant at usual ranitidine doses, it may be prudent to monitor for procainamide toxicity when administered with oral ranitidine at a dose exceeding 300 mg per day.

Warfarin: There have been reports of altered prothrombin time among patients on concomitant warfarin and ranitidine therapy. Due to the narrow therapeutic index, close monitoring of increased or decreased prothrombin time is recommended during concurrent treatment with ranitidine.

Ranitidine may alter the absorption of drugs in which gastric pH is an important determinant of bioavailability. This can result in either an increase in absorption (e.g., triazolam, midazolam, glipizide) or a decrease in absorption (e.g., ketoconazole, atazanavir, delavirdine, gefitinib). Appropriate clinical monitoring is recommended.

Atazanavir: Atazanavir absorption may be impaired based on known interactions with other agents that increase gastric pH. Use with caution. See atazanavir label for specific recommendations.

Delavirdine: Delavirdine absorption may be impaired based on known interactions with other agents that increase gastric pH. Chronic use of H₂-receptor antagonists with delavirdine is not recommended.

Gefitinib: Gefitinib exposure was reduced by 44% with the coadministration of ranitidine and sodium bicarbonate (dosed to maintain gastric pH above 5.0). Use with caution.

Glipizide: In diabetic patients, glipizide exposure was increased by 34% following a single 150-mg dose of oral ranitidine. Use appropriate clinical monitoring when initiating or discontinuing ranitidine.

Ketoconazole: Oral ketoconazole exposure was reduced by up to 95% when oral ranitidine was coadministered in a regimen to maintain a gastric pH of 6 or above. The degree of interaction with usual dose of ranitidine (150 mg twice daily) is unknown.

Midazolam: Oral midazolam exposure in 5 healthy volunteers was increased by up to 65% when administered with oral ranitidine at a dose of 150 mg twice daily. However, in another interaction study in 8 volunteers receiving IV midazolam, a 300 mg oral dose of ranitidine increased midazolam exposure by about 9%. Monitor patients for excessive or prolonged sedation when ranitidine is coadministered with oral midazolam.

Triazolam: Triazolam exposure in healthy volunteers was increased by approximately 30% when administered with oral ranitidine at a dose of 150 mg twice daily. Monitor patients for excessive or prolonged sedation.

Carcinogenesis, Mutagenesis, Impairment of Fertility: There was no indication of tumorigenic or carcinogenic effects in life-span studies in mice and rats at oral dosages up to 2,000 mg/kg/day.
Ranitidine was not mutagenic in standard bacterial tests (*Salmonella, Escherichia coli*) for mutagenicity at concentrations up to the maximum recommended for these assays. In a dominant lethal assay, a single oral dose of 1,000 mg/kg to male rats was without effect on the outcome of 2 matings per week for the next 9 weeks.

Pregnancy: *Teratogenic Effects:* Pregnancy Category B. Reproduction studies have been performed in rats and rabbits at oral doses up to 160 times the human oral dose and have revealed no evidence of impaired fertility or harm to the fetus due to ranitidine. There are, however, no adequate and well-controlled studies in pregnant women. Because animal reproduction studies are not always predictive of human response, this drug should be used during pregnancy only if clearly needed.

Nursing Mothers: Ranitidine is secreted in human milk. Caution should be exercised when ZANTAC is administered to a nursing mother.

Pediatric Use: The safety and effectiveness of ZANTAC Injection have been established in the age-group of 1 month to 16 years for the treatment of duodenal ulcer. Use of ZANTAC in this age-group is supported by adequate and well-controlled studies in adults, as well as additional pharmacokinetic data in pediatric patients, and an analysis of the published literature.
Safety and effectiveness in pediatric patients for the treatment of pathological hypersecretory conditions have not been established.
Limited data in neonatal patients (less than 1 month of age) receiving ECMO suggest that ZANTAC may be useful and safe for increasing gastric pH for patients at risk of gastrointestinal hemorrhage.

Geriatric Use: Clinical studies of ZANTAC Injection did not include sufficient numbers of subjects aged 65 and over to determine whether they responded differently from younger subjects. However, in clinical studies of oral formulations of ZANTAC, of the total number of subjects enrolled in US and foreign controlled clinical trials, for which there were subgroup analyses, 4,197 were 65 and over, while 899 were 75 and over. No overall differences in safety or effectiveness were observed between these subjects and younger subjects, and other reported clinical experience has not identified differences in responses between the elderly and younger patients, but greater sensitivity of some older individuals cannot be ruled out.
This drug is known to be substantially excreted by the kidney and the risk of toxic reactions to this drug may be greater in patients with impaired renal function. Because elderly patients are more likely to have decreased renal function, caution should be exercised in dose selection, and it may be useful to monitor renal function (see CLINICAL PHARMACOLOGY: Pharmacokinetics: Geriatric Use and DOSAGE AND ADMINISTRATION: Dosage Adjustment for Patients With Impaired Renal Function).

ADVERSE REACTIONS

Transient pain at the site of IM injection has been reported. Transient local burning or itching has been reported with IV administration of ZANTAC.
The following have been reported as events in clinical trials or in the routine management of patients treated with oral or parenteral ZANTAC. The relationship to therapy with ZANTAC has been unclear in many cases. Headache, sometimes severe, seems to be related to administration of ZANTAC.

Central Nervous System: Rarely, malaise, dizziness, somnolence, insomnia, and vertigo. Rare cases of reversible mental confusion, agitation, depression, and hallucinations have been reported, predominantly in severely ill elderly patients. Rare cases of reversible blurred vision suggestive of a change in accommodation have been reported. Rare reports of reversible involuntary motor disturbances have been received.

Cardiovascular: As with other H₂-blockers, rare reports of arrhythmias such as tachycardia, bradycardia, asystole, atrioventricular block, and premature ventricular beats.

Gastrointestinal: Constipation, diarrhea, nausea/vomiting, abdominal discomfort/pain, and rare reports of pancreatitis.

Hepatic: In normal volunteers, SGPT values were increased to at least twice the pretreatment levels in 6 of 12 subjects receiving 100 mg intravenously 4 times daily for 7 days, and in 4 of 24 subjects receiving 50 mg intravenously 4 times daily for 5 days. There have been occasional reports of hepatocellular, cholestatic, or mixed hepatitis, with or without jaundice. In such circumstances, ranitidine should be immediately discontinued. These events are usually reversible, but in rare circumstances death has occurred. Rare cases of hepatic failure have also been reported.

Musculoskeletal: Rare reports of arthralgias and myalgias.

Hematologic: Blood count changes (leukopenia, granulocytopenia, and thrombocytopenia) have occurred in a few patients. These were usually reversible. Rare cases of agranulocytosis, pancytopenia, sometimes with marrow hypoplasia, and aplastic anemia and exceedingly rare cases of acquired immune hemolytic anemia have been reported.

Endocrine: Controlled studies in animals and humans have shown no stimulation of any pituitary hormone by ZANTAC and no antiandrogenic activity, and cimetidine-induced gynecomastia and impotence in hypersecretory patients have resolved when ZANTAC has been substituted. However, occasional cases of impotence and loss of libido have been reported in male patients receiving ZANTAC, but the incidence did not differ from that in the general population. Rare cases of breast symptoms and conditions, including galactorrhea and gynecomastia, have been reported in both males and females.

Integumentary: Rash, including rare cases of erythema multiforme. Rare cases of alopecia and vasculitis.

Respiratory: A large epidemiological study suggested an increased risk of developing pneumonia in current users of histamine-2-receptor antagonists (H2RAs) compared to patients who had stopped H2RA treatment, with an observed adjusted relative risk of 1.63 (95% CI, 1.07-2.48). However, a causal relationship between use of H2RAs and pneumonia has not been established.

Other: Rare cases of hypersensitivity reactions (e.g., bronchospasm, fever, rash, eosinophilia), anaphylaxis, angioneurotic edema, acute interstitial nephritis, and small increases in serum creatinine.

OVERDOSAGE

There has been virtually no experience with overdosage with ZANTAC Injection and limited experience with oral doses of ranitidine. Reported acute ingestions of up to 18 g orally have been associated with transient adverse effects similar to those encountered in normal clinical experience (see ADVERSE REACTIONS). In addition, abnormalities of gait and hypotension have been reported.

When overdosage occurs, clinical monitoring and supportive therapy should be employed.

Studies in dogs receiving dosages of ZANTAC in excess of 225 mg/kg/day have shown muscular tremors, vomiting, and rapid respiration. Single oral doses of 1,000 mg/kg in mice and rats were not lethal. Intravenous LD_{50} values in mice and rats were 77 and 83 mg/kg, respectively.

DOSAGE AND ADMINISTRATION

Parenteral Administration: In some hospitalized patients with pathological hypersecretory conditions or intractable duodenal ulcers, or in patients who are unable to take oral medication, ZANTAC may be administered parenterally according to the following recommendations:

Intramuscular Injection: 50 mg (2 mL) every 6 to 8 hours. (No dilution necessary.)

Intermittent Intravenous Injection:

a. Intermittent Bolus: 50 mg (2 mL) every 6 to 8 hours. Dilute ZANTAC Injection, 50 mg, in 0.9% sodium chloride injection or other compatible IV solution (see Stability) to a concentration no greater than 2.5 mg/mL (20 mL). Inject at a rate no greater than 4 mL/min (5 minutes).

b. Intermittent Infusion: 50 mg (2 mL) every 6 to 8 hours. Dilute ZANTAC Injection, 50 mg, in 5% dextrose injection or other compatible IV solution (see Stability) to a concentration no greater than 0.5 mg/mL (100 mL). Infuse at a rate no greater than 5 to 7 mL/min (15 to 20 minutes).

ZANTAC Injection Premixed solution, 50 mg, in 0.45% sodium chloride, 50 mL, requires no dilution and should be infused over 15 to 20 minutes.

In some patients it may be necessary to increase dosage. When this is necessary, the increases should be made by more frequent administration of the dose, but generally should not exceed 400 mg/day.

Continuous Intravenous Infusion: Add ZANTAC Injection to 5% dextrose injection or other compatible IV solution (see Stability). Deliver at a rate of 6.25 mg/hour (e.g., 150 mg [6 mL] of ZANTAC Injection in 250 mL of 5% dextrose injection at 10.7 mL/hour).

For Zollinger-Ellison patients, dilute ZANTAC Injection in 5% dextrose injection or other compatible IV solution (see Stability) to a concentration no greater than 2.5 mg/mL. Start the infusion at a rate of 1.0 mg/kg/hour. If after 4 hours either a measured gastric acid output is >10 mEq/hour or the patient becomes symptomatic, the dose should be adjusted upward in 0.5-mg/kg/hour increments, and the acid output should be remeasured. Dosages up to 2.5 mg/kg/hour and infusion rates as high as 220 mg/hour have been used.

Pediatric Use: While limited data exist on the administration of IV ranitidine to children, the recommended dose in pediatric patients is for a total daily dose of 2 to 4 mg/kg, to be divided and administered every 6 to 8 hours, up to a maximum of 50 mg given every 6 to 8 hours. This recommendation is derived from adult clinical studies and pharmacokinetic data in pediatric patients. Limited data in neonatal patients (less than 1 month of age) receiving ECMO have shown that a dose of 2 mg/kg is usually sufficient to

increase gastric pH to >4 for at least 15 hours. Therefore, doses of 2 mg/kg given every 12 to 24 hours or as a continuous infusion should be considered.

ZANTAC Injection Premixed in Flexible Plastic Containers:

Instructions for Use: **To Open:** Tear outer wrap at notch and remove solution container. Check for minute leaks by squeezing container firmly. If leaks are found, discard unit as sterility may be impaired.

Preparation for Administration: Use aseptic technique.

1. Close flow control clamp of administration set.
2. Remove cover from outlet port at bottom of container.
3. Insert piercing pin of administration set into port with a twisting motion until the pin is firmly seated. NOTE: See full directions on administration set carton.
4. Suspend container from hanger.
5. Squeeze and release drip chamber to establish proper fluid level in chamber during infusion of ZANTAC Injection Premixed.
6. Open flow control clamp to expel air from set. Close clamp.
7. Attach set to venipuncture device. If device is not indwelling, prime and make venipuncture.
8. Perform venipuncture.
9. Regulate rate of administration with flow control clamp.

Caution: ZANTAC Injection Premixed in flexible plastic containers is to be administered by slow IV drip infusion only. **Additives should not be introduced into this solution.** If used with a primary IV fluid system, the primary solution should be discontinued during infusion of ZANTAC Injection Premixed.

Do not administer unless solution is clear and container is undamaged.

Warning: Do not use flexible plastic container in series connections.

Dosage Adjustment for Patients With Impaired Renal Function: The administration of ranitidine as a continuous infusion has not been evaluated in patients with impaired renal function. On the basis of experience with a group of subjects with severely impaired renal function treated with ZANTAC, the recommended dosage in patients with a creatinine clearance <50 mL/min is 50 mg every 18 to 24 hours. Should the patient's condition require, the frequency of dosing may be increased to every 12 hours or even further with caution. Hemodialysis reduces the level of circulating ranitidine. Ideally, the dosing schedule should be adjusted so that the timing of a scheduled dose coincides with the end of hemodialysis.

Elderly patients are more likely to have decreased renal function, therefore caution should be exercised in dose selection, and it may be useful to monitor renal function (see CLINICAL PHARMACOLOGY: Pharmacokinetics: Geriatric Use and PRECAUTIONS: Geriatric Use).

Stability: Undiluted, ZANTAC Injection tends to exhibit a yellow color that may intensify over time without adversely affecting potency. ZANTAC Injection is stable for 48 hours at room temperature when added to or diluted with most commonly used IV solutions, e.g., 0.9% sodium chloride injection, 5% dextrose injection, 10% dextrose injection, lactated ringer's injection, or 5% sodium bicarbonate injection. ZANTAC Injection Premixed in flexible plastic containers is sterile through the expiration date on the label when stored under recommended conditions.

Note: Parenteral drug products should be inspected visually for particulate matter and discoloration before administration whenever solution and container permit.

HOW SUPPLIED

ZANTAC Injection, 25 mg/mL, containing phenol 0.5% as preservative, is available as follows:
NDC 0173-0362-38, 2-mL single-dose vials (Tray of 10)
NDC 0173-0363-01, 6-mL multidose vials (Singles)
Store between 4° and 25°C (39° and 77°F); excursions permitted to 30°C (86°F). Protect from light.

ZANTAC Injection Premixed, 50 mg/50 mL, in 0.45% sodium chloride, is available as a sterile, premixed solution for IV administration in single-dose, flexible plastic containers (NDC 0173-0441-00) (case of 24). It contains no preservatives.

Store between 2° and 25°C (36° and 77°F). Protect from light.

Exposure of pharmaceutical products to heat should be minimized. Avoid excessive heat; however, brief exposure up to 40°C does not adversely affect the product. Protect from freezing.

ZANTAC® Injection:
GlaxoSmithKline
Research Triangle Park, NC 27709
ZANTAC® Injection Premixed:
Manufactured for GlaxoSmithKline
Research Triangle Park, NC 27709
by Hospira, Inc., Lake Forest, IL 60045
ZANTAC is a registered trademark of Warner-Lambert Company, used under license.

MULTISTIX is a registered trademark of Bayer Healthcare LLC.
©2009, GlaxoSmithKline. All rights reserved.
April 2009 ZNJ:5PI

ZANTAC® R_x
[zan' tak]
(ranitidine hydrochloride)
Injection

Pharmacy Bulk Package—Not for Direct Infusion

DESCRIPTION

The active ingredient in ZANTAC Injection is ranitidine hydrochloride (HCl), a histamine H2-receptor antagonist. Chemically it is N-[2-[[[5-[(dimethylamino)methyl]-2-furanyl]methyl]thio]ethyl]-N'-methyl-2-nitro-1,1-ethenediamine, hydrochloride. It has the following structure:

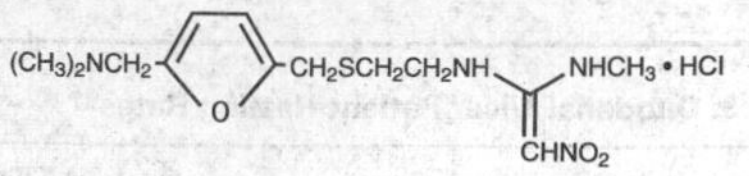

$$(CH_3)_2NCH_2 \quad CH_2SCH_2CH_2NH \quad NHCH_3 \cdot HCl$$
$$CHNO_2$$

The empirical formula is $C_{13}H_{22}N_4O_3S \bullet HCl$, representing a molecular weight of 350.87.

Ranitidine HCl is a white to pale yellow, granular substance that is soluble in water.

ZANTAC Injection is a clear, colorless to yellow, nonpyrogenic liquid. The yellow color of the liquid tends to intensify without adversely affecting potency. The pH of the injection solution is 6.7 to 7.3.

Each 1 mL of aqueous solution contains ranitidine 25 mg (as the hydrochloride); phenol 5 mg as preservative; and 0.96 mg of monobasic potassium phosphate and 2.4 mg of dibasic sodium phosphate as buffers.

A pharmacy bulk package is a container of a sterile preparation for parenteral use that contains many single doses. The contents are intended for use in a pharmacy admixture program and are restricted to the preparation of admixtures for intravenous (IV) infusion.

CLINICAL PHARMACOLOGY

ZANTAC is a competitive, reversible inhibitor of the action of histamine at the histamine H2-receptors, including receptors on the gastric cells. ZANTAC does not lower serum Ca++ in hypercalcemic states. ZANTAC is not an anticholinergic agent.

Pharmacokinetics: *Absorption:* ZANTAC is absorbed very rapidly after intramuscular (IM) injection. Mean peak levels of 576 ng/mL occur within 15 minutes or less following a 50-mg IM dose. Absorption from IM sites is virtually complete, with a bioavailability of 90% to 100% compared with intravenous (IV) administration. Following oral administration, the bioavailability of ZANTAC Tablets is 50%.

Distribution: The volume of distribution is about 1.4 L/kg. Serum protein binding averages 15%.

Metabolism: In humans, the N-oxide is the principal metabolite in the urine; however, this amounts to <4% of the dose. Other metabolites are the S-oxide (1%) and the desmethyl ranitidine (1%). The remainder of the administered dose is found in the stool. Studies in patients with hepatic dysfunction (compensated cirrhosis) indicate that there are minor, but clinically insignificant, alterations in ranitidine half-life, distribution, clearance, and bioavailability.

Excretion: Following IV injection, approximately 70% of the dose is recovered in the urine as unchanged drug. Renal clearance averages 530 mL/min, with a total clearance of 760 mL/min. The elimination half-life is 2.0 to 2.5 hours.

Four patients with clinically significant renal function impairment (creatinine clearance 25 to 35 mL/min) administered 50 mg of ranitidine intravenously had an average plasma half-life of 4.8 hours, a ranitidine clearance of 29 mL/min, and a volume of distribution of 1.76 L/kg. In general, these parameters appear to be altered in proportion to creatinine clearance (see DOSAGE AND ADMINISTRATION).

Geriatrics: The plasma half-life is prolonged and total clearance is reduced in the elderly population due to a decrease in renal function. The elimination half-life is 3.1 hours (see PRECAUTIONS: Geriatric Use and DOSAGE AND ADMINISTRATION: Dosage Adjustment for Patients With Impaired Renal Function).

Pediatrics: There are no significant differences in the pharmacokinetic parameter values for ranitidine in pediatric patients (from 1 month up to 16 years of age) and healthy adults when correction is made for body weight. The pharmacokinetics of ZANTAC in pediatric patients are summarized in Table 1.
[See table 1 at top of next page]

Table 1. Ranitidine Pharmacokinetics in Pediatric Patients Following IV Dosing

Population (age)	n	Dose (mg/kg)	$t_{1/2}$ (hours)	Vd (L/kg)	CLp (mL/min/kg)
Peptic ulcer disease					
(<6 years)	6	1.25 or 2.5	2.2	1.29	11.41
(6–11.9 years)	11	1.25 or 2.5	2.1	1.14	8.96
(>12 years)	6	1.25 or 2.5	1.7	0.98	9.89
Adults	6	2.5	1.9	1.04	8.77
Peptic ulcer disease (3.5–16 years)	12	0.13–0.80	1.8	2.3	795 mL/min/1.73m^2
Children in intensive care (1 day–12.6 years)	17	1.0	2.4	2	11.7
Neonates receiving ECMO	12	2	6.6	1.8	4.3

$T_{1/2}$ = Terminal half-life; CLp = Plasma clearance of ranitidine.
ECMO = extracorporeal membrane oxygenation.

Table 3. Duodenal Ulcer Patient Healing Rates

	Oral ZANTAC*		Oral Placebo*	
	Number Entered	Healed/Evaluable	Number Entered	Healed/Evaluable
Outpatients				
Week 2	195	69/182 (38%)†	188	31/164 (19%)
Week 4		137/187 (73%)†		76/168 (45%)

*All patients were permitted antacids as needed for relief of pain.
†P<0.0001.

Plasma clearance in neonatal patients (less than 1 month of age) receiving ECMO was considerably lower (3 to 4 mL/min/kg) than observed in children or adults. The elimination half-life in neonates averaged 6.6 hours as compared to approximately 2 hours in adults and pediatric patients.

Pharmacodynamics: Serum concentrations necessary to inhibit 50% of stimulated gastric acid secretion are estimated to be 36 to 94 ng/mL. Following single IV or IM 50-mg doses, serum concentrations of ranitidine are in this range for 6 to 8 hours.

Antisecretory Activity: 1. Effects on Acid Secretion: ZANTAC Injection inhibits basal gastric acid secretion as well as gastric acid secretion stimulated by betazole and pentagastrin, as shown in Table 2.

Table 2. Effect of Intravenous ZANTAC on Gastric Acid Secretion

	Time After Dose, hours	% Inhibition of Gastric Acid Output by Intravenous Dose, mg		
		20 mg	60 mg	100 mg
Betazole	Up to 2	93	99	99
Pentagastrin	Up to 3	47	66	77

In a group of 10 known hypersecretors, ranitidine plasma levels of 71, 180, and 376 ng/mL inhibited basal acid secretion by 76%, 90%, and 99.5%, respectively.

It appears that basal- and betazole-stimulated secretions are most sensitive to inhibition by ZANTAC, while pentagastrin-stimulated secretion is more difficult to suppress.

2. Effects on Other Gastrointestinal Secretions:
Pepsin: ZANTAC does not affect pepsin secretion. Total pepsin output is reduced in proportion to the decrease in volume of gastric juice.

Intrinsic Factor: ZANTAC has no significant effect on pentagastrin-stimulated intrinsic factor secretion.

Serum Gastrin: ZANTAC has little or no effect on fasting or postprandial serum gastrin.

Other Pharmacologic Actions:
1. Gastric bacterial flora—increase in nitrate-reducing organisms, significance not known.
2. Prolactin levels—no effect in recommended oral or IV dosage, but small, transient, dose-related increases in serum prolactin have been reported after IV bolus injections of 100 mg or more.
3. Other pituitary hormones—no effect on serum gonadotropins, TSH, or GH. Possible impairment of vasopressin release.

4. No change in cortisol, aldosterone, androgen, or estrogen levels.
5. No antiandrogenic action.
6. No effect on count, motility, or morphology of sperm.

Pediatrics: The ranitidine concentration necessary to suppress basal acid secretion by at least 90% has been reported to be 40 to 60 ng/mL in pediatric patients with duodenal or gastric ulcers.

In a study of 20 critically ill pediatric patients receiving ranitidine IV at 1 mg/kg every 6 hours, 10 patients with a baseline pH ≥4 maintained this baseline throughout the study. Eight of the remaining 10 patients with a baseline of pH ≤2 achieved pH ≥4 throughout varying periods after dosing. It should be noted, however, that because these pharmacodynamic parameters were assessed in critically ill pediatric patients, the data should be interpreted with caution when dosing recommendations are made for a less seriously ill pediatric population.

In another small study of neonatal patients (n = 5) receiving ECMO, gastric pH <4 pretreatment increased to >4 after a 2-mg/kg dose and remained above 4 for at least 15 hours.

Clinical Trials: *Active Duodenal Ulcer:* In a multicenter, double-blind, controlled, US study of endoscopically diagnosed duodenal ulcers, earlier healing was seen in the patients treated with oral ZANTAC as shown in Table 3. [See table 3 above]

In these studies, patients treated with oral ZANTAC reported a reduction in both daytime and nocturnal pain, and they also consumed less antacid than the placebo-treated patients.

Table 4. Mean Daily Doses of Antacid

	Ulcer Healed	Ulcer Not Healed
Oral ZANTAC	0.06	0.71
Oral placebo	0.71	1.43

Pathological Hypersecretory Conditions (such as Zollinger-Ellison syndrome): ZANTAC inhibits gastric acid secretion and reduces occurrence of diarrhea, anorexia, and pain in patients with pathological hypersecretion associated with Zollinger-Ellison syndrome, systemic mastocytosis, and other pathological hypersecretory conditions (e.g., postoperative, "short-gut" syndrome, idiopathic). Use of oral ZANTAC was followed by healing of ulcers in 8 of 19 (42%) patients who were intractable to previous therapy.

In a retrospective review of 52 Zollinger-Ellison patients given ZANTAC as a continuous IV infusion for up to 15 days, no patients developed complications of acid-peptic disease such as bleeding or perforation. Acid output was controlled to ≤10 mEq/h.

INDICATIONS AND USAGE

ZANTAC Injection is indicated in some hospitalized patients with pathological hypersecretory conditions or intractable duodenal ulcers, or as an alternative to the oral dosage form for short-term use in patients who are unable to take oral medication.

CONTRAINDICATIONS

ZANTAC Injection is contraindicated for patients known to have hypersensitivity to the drug.

PRECAUTIONS

General:
1. Symptomatic response to therapy with ZANTAC does not preclude the presence of gastric malignancy.
2. Since ZANTAC is excreted primarily by the kidney, dosage should be adjusted in patients with impaired renal function (see DOSAGE AND ADMINISTRATION). Caution should be observed in patients with hepatic dysfunction since ZANTAC is metabolized in the liver.
3. In controlled studies in normal volunteers, elevations in SGPT have been observed when H_2-antagonists have been administered intravenously at greater-than-recommended dosages for 5 days or longer. Therefore, it seems prudent in patients receiving IV ranitidine at dosages ≥100 mg 4 times daily for periods of 5 days or longer to monitor SGPT daily (from day 5) for the remainder of IV therapy.
4. Bradycardia in association with rapid administration of ZANTAC Injection has been reported rarely, usually in patients with factors predisposing to cardiac rhythm disturbances. Recommended rates of administration should not be exceeded (see DOSAGE AND ADMINISTRATION).
5. Rare reports suggest that ZANTAC may precipitate acute porphyric attacks in patients with acute porphyria. ZANTAC should therefore be avoided in patients with a history of acute porphyria.

Laboratory Tests: False-positive tests for urine protein with MULTISTIX® may occur during therapy with ZANTAC, and therefore testing with sulfosalicylic acid is recommended.

Drug Interactions: Ranitidine has been reported to affect the bioavailability of other drugs through several different mechanisms such as competition for renal tubular secretion, alteration of gastric pH, and inhibition of cytochrome P450 enzymes.

Procainamide: Ranitidine, a substrate of the renal organic cation transport system, may affect the clearance of other drugs eliminated by this route. High doses of ranitidine (e.g., such as those used in the treatment of Zollinger-Ellison syndrome) have been shown to reduce the renal excretion of procainamide and N-acetylprocainamide resulting in increased plasma levels of these drugs. Although this interaction is unlikely to be clinically relevant at usual ranitidine doses, it may be prudent to monitor for procainamide toxicity when administered with oral ranitidine at a dose exceeding 300 mg per day.

Warfarin: There have been reports of altered prothrombin time among patients on concomitant warfarin and ranitidine therapy. Due to the narrow therapeutic index, close monitoring of increased or decreased prothrombin time is recommended during concurrent treatment with ranitidine.

Ranitidine may alter the absorption of drugs in which gastric pH is an important determinant of bioavailability. This can result in either an increase in absorption (e.g., triazolam, midazolam, glipizide) or a decrease in absorption (e.g., ketoconazole, atazanavir, delavirdine, gefitinib). Appropriate clinical monitoring is recommended.

Atazanavir: Atazanavir absorption may be impaired based on known interactions with other agents that increase gastric pH. Use with caution. See atazanavir label for specific recommendations.

Delavirdine: Delavirdine absorption may be impaired based on known interactions with other agents that increase gastric pH. Chronic use of H_2-receptor antagonists with delavirdine is not recommended.

Gefitinib: Gefitinib exposure was reduced by 44% with the coadministration of ranitidine and sodium bicarbonate (dosed to maintain gastric pH above 5.0). Use with caution.

Glipizide: In diabetic patients, glipizide exposure was increased by 34% following a single 150-mg dose of oral ranitidine. Use appropriate clinical monitoring when initiating or discontinuing ranitidine.

Ketoconazole: Oral ketoconazole exposure was reduced by up to 95% when oral ranitidine was coadministered in a regimen to maintain a gastric pH of 6 or above. The degree of interaction with usual dose of ranitidine (150 mg twice daily) is unknown.

Midazolam: Oral midazolam exposure in 5 healthy volunteers was increased by up to 65% when administered with oral ranitidine at a dose of 150 mg twice daily. However, in another interaction study in 8 volunteers receiving IV midazolam, a 300 mg oral dose of ranitidine increased midazolam exposure by about 9%. Monitor patients for excessive or prolonged sedation when ranitidine is coadministered with oral midazolam.

Triazolam: Triazolam exposure in healthy volunteers was increased by approximately 30% when administered with oral ranitidine at a dose of 150 mg twice daily. Monitor patients for excessive or prolonged sedation.

Carcinogenesis, Mutagenesis, Impairment of Fertility: There was no indication of tumorigenic or carcinogenic effects in life-span studies in mice and rats at oral dosages up to 2,000 mg/kg/day.

Ranitidine was not mutagenic in standard bacterial tests (*Salmonella, Escherichia coli*) for mutagenicity at concentrations up to the maximum recommended for these assays. In a dominant lethal assay, a single oral dose of 1,000 mg/kg to male rats was without effect on the outcome of 2 matings per week for the next 9 weeks.

Pregnancy: *Teratogenic Effects:* Pregnancy Category B. Reproduction studies have been performed in rats and rabbits at oral doses up to 160 times the human oral dose and have revealed no evidence of impaired fertility or harm to the fetus due to ZANTAC. There are, however, no adequate and well-controlled studies in pregnant women. Because animal reproduction studies are not always predictive of human response, this drug should be used during pregnancy only if clearly needed.

Nursing Mothers: Ranitidine is secreted in human milk. Caution should be exercised when ZANTAC is administered to a nursing mother.

Pediatric Use: The safety and effectiveness of ZANTAC Injection have been established in the age-group of 1 month to 16 years for the treatment of duodenal ulcer. Use of ZANTAC in this age-group is supported by adequate and well-controlled studies in adults, as well as additional pharmacokinetic data in pediatric patients, and an analysis of the published literature.

Safety and effectiveness in pediatric patients for the treatment of pathological hypersecretory conditions have not been established.

Limited data in neonatal patients (less than 1 month of age) receiving ECMO suggest that ZANTAC may be useful and safe for increasing gastric pH for patients at risk of gastrointestinal hemorrhage.

Geriatric Use: Clinical studies of ZANTAC Injection did not include sufficient numbers of subjects aged 65 and over to determine whether they responded differently from younger subjects. However, in clinical studies of oral formulations of ZANTAC, of the total number of subjects enrolled in US and foreign controlled clinical trials, for which there were subgroup analyses, 4,197 were 65 and over, while 899 were 75 and over. No overall differences in safety or effectiveness were observed between these subjects and younger subjects, and other reported clinical experience has not identified differences in responses between the elderly and younger patients, but greater sensitivity of some older individuals cannot be ruled out.

This drug is known to be substantially excreted by the kidney, and the risk of toxic reactions to this drug may be greater in patients with impaired renal function. Because elderly patients are more likely to have decreased renal function, caution should be exercised in dose selection, and it may be useful to monitor renal function (see CLINICAL PHARMACOLOGY: Pharmacokinetics: Geriatric Use and DOSAGE AND ADMINISTRATION: Dosage Adjustment for Patients With Impaired Renal Function).

ADVERSE REACTIONS

Transient pain at the site of IM injection has been reported. Transient local burning or itching has been reported with IV administration of ZANTAC.

The following have been reported as events in clinical trials or in the routine management of patients treated with oral or parenteral ZANTAC. The relationship to therapy with ZANTAC has been unclear in many cases. Headache, sometimes severe, seems to be related to administration of ZANTAC.

Central Nervous System: Rarely, malaise, dizziness, somnolence, insomnia, and vertigo. Rare cases of reversible mental confusion, agitation, depression, and hallucinations have been reported, predominantly in severely ill elderly patients. Rare cases of reversible blurred vision suggestive of a change in accommodation have been reported. Rare reports of reversible involuntary motor disturbances have been received.

Cardiovascular: As with other H_2-blockers, rare reports of arrhythmias such as tachycardia, bradycardia, asystole, atrioventricular block, and premature ventricular beats.

Gastrointestinal: Constipation, diarrhea, nausea/vomiting, abdominal discomfort/pain, and rare reports of pancreatitis.

Hepatic: In normal volunteers, SGPT values were increased to at least twice the pretreatment levels in 6 of 12 subjects receiving 100 mg intravenously 4 times daily for 7 days, and in 4 of 24 subjects receiving 50 mg intravenously 4 times daily for 5 days. There have been occasional reports of hepatocellular, cholestatic, or mixed hepatitis, with or without jaundice. In such circumstances, ranitidine should be immediately discontinued. These events are usually reversible, but in rare circumstances death has occurred. Rare cases of hepatic failure have also been reported.

Musculoskeletal: Rare reports of arthralgias and myalgias.

Hematologic: Blood count changes (leukopenia, granulocytopenia, and thrombocytopenia) have occurred in a few patients. These were usually reversible. Rare cases of agranulocytosis, pancytopenia, sometimes with marrow hypoplasia, and aplastic anemia and exceedingly rare cases of acquired immune hemolytic anemia have been reported.

Endocrine: Controlled studies in animals and humans have shown no stimulation of any pituitary hormone by ZANTAC and no antiandrogenic activity, and cimetidine-induced gynecomastia and impotence in hypersecretory patients have resolved when ZANTAC has been substituted. However, occasional cases of impotence, and loss of libido have been reported in male patients receiving ZANTAC, but the incidence did not differ from that in the general population. Rare cases of breast symptoms and conditions, including galactorrhea and gynecomastia, have been reported in both males and females.

Integumentary: Rash, including rare cases of erythema multiforme. Rare cases of alopecia and vasculitis.

Respiratory: A large epidemiological study suggested an increased risk of developing pneumonia in current users of histamine-2-receptor antagonists (H_2RAs) compared to patients who had stopped H_2RA treatment, with an observed adjusted relative risk of 1.63 (95% CI, 1.07-2.48). However, a causal relationship between use of H_2RAs and pneumonia has not been established.

Other: Rare cases of hypersensitivity reactions (e.g., bronchospasm, fever, rash, eosinophilia), anaphylaxis, angioneurotic edema, acute interstitial nephritis, and small increases in serum creatinine.

OVERDOSAGE

There has been virtually no experience with overdosage with ZANTAC Injection and limited experience with oral doses of ranitidine. Reported acute ingestions of up to 18 g orally have been associated with transient adverse effects similar to those encountered in normal clinical experience (see ADVERSE REACTIONS). In addition, abnormalities of gait and hypotension have been reported.

When overdosage occurs, clinical monitoring and supportive therapy should be employed.

Studies in dogs receiving dosages of ZANTAC in excess of 225 mg/kg/day have shown muscular tremors, vomiting, and rapid respiration. Single oral doses of 1,000 mg/kg in mice and rats were not lethal. Intravenous LD_{50} values in mice and rats were 77 and 83 mg/kg, respectively.

DOSAGE AND ADMINISTRATION

Parenteral Administration: In some hospitalized patients with pathological hypersecretory conditions or intractable duodenal ulcers, or in patients who are unable to take oral medication, ZANTAC Injection may be administered parenterally according to the following recommendations:

Intramuscular Injection: 50 mg (2 mL) every 6 to 8 hours. (No dilution necessary.)

Intermittent Intravenous Injection:

a. Intermittent Bolus: 50 mg (2 mL) every 6 to 8 hours. Dilute ZANTAC Injection, 50 mg, in 0.9% sodium chloride injection or other compatible IV solution (see Stability) to a concentration no greater than 2.5 mg/mL (20 mL). Inject at a rate no greater than 4 mL/min (5 minutes).

b. Intermittent Infusion: 50 mg (2 mL) every 6 to 8 hours. Dilute ZANTAC Injection, 50 mg, in 5% dextrose injection or other compatible IV solution (see Stability) to a concentration no greater than 0.5 mg/mL (100 mL). Infuse at a rate no greater than 5 to 7 mL/min (15 to 20 minutes).

In some patients it may be necessary to increase dosage. When this is necessary, the increases should be made by more frequent administration of the dose, but generally should not exceed 400 mg/day.

Continuous Intravenous Infusion: Add ZANTAC Injection to 5% dextrose injection or other compatible IV solution (see Stability). Deliver at a rate of 6.25 mg/hour (e.g., 150 mg [6 mL] of ZANTAC Injection in 250 mL of 5% dextrose injection at 10.7 mL/hour).

For Zollinger-Ellison patients, dilute ZANTAC Injection in 5% dextrose injection or other compatible IV solution (see Stability) to a concentration no greater than 2.5 mg/mL. Start the infusion at a rate of 1.0 mg/kg/hour. If after 4 hours either a measured gastric acid output is >10 mEq/hour or the patient becomes symptomatic, the dose should be adjusted upward in 0.5-mg/kg/hour increments, and the acid output should be remeasured. Dosages up to 2.5 mg/kg/hour and infusion rates as high as 220 mg/hour have been used.

Pediatric Use: While limited data exist on the administration of IV ranitidine to children, the recommended dose in pediatric patients is for a total daily dose of 2 to 4 mg/kg, to be divided and administered every 6 to 8 hours, up to a maximum of 50 mg given every 6 to 8 hours. This recommendation is derived from adult clinical studies and pharmacokinetic data in pediatric patients. Limited data in neonatal patients (less than 1 month of age) receiving ECMO have shown that a dose of 2 mg/kg is usually sufficient to increase gastric pH to >4 for at least 15 hours. Therefore, doses of 2 mg/kg given every 12 to 24 hours or as a continuous infusion should be considered.

Dosage Adjustment for Patients With Impaired Renal Function: The administration of ranitidine as a continuous infusion has not been evaluated in patients with impaired renal function. On the basis of experience with a group of subjects with severely impaired renal function treated with ZANTAC, the recommended dosage in patients with a creatinine clearance <50 mL/min is 50 mg given every 18 to 24 hours. Should the patient's condition require, the frequency of dosing may be increased to every 12 hours or even further with caution. Hemodialysis reduces the level of circulating ranitidine. Ideally, the dosing schedule should be adjusted so that the timing of a scheduled dose coincides with the end of hemodialysis.

Elderly patients are more likely to have decreased renal function, therefore caution should be exercised in dose selection, and it may be useful to monitor renal function (see CLINICAL PHARMACOLOGY: Pharmacokinetics: Geriatric Use and PRECAUTIONS: Geriatric Use).

Stability: Undiluted, ZANTAC Injection tends to exhibit a yellow color that may intensify over time without adversely affecting potency. ZANTAC Injection is stable for 48 hours at room temperature when added to or diluted with most commonly used IV solutions, e.g., 0.9% sodium chloride injection, 5% dextrose injection, 10% dextrose injection, lactated ringer's injection, or 5% sodium bicarbonate injection.

Note: Parenteral drug products should be inspected visually for particulate matter and discoloration before administration whenever solution and container permit.

Directions for Dispensing: *Pharmacy Bulk Package—Not for Direct Infusion:* The pharmacy bulk package is for use in a pharmacy admixture service only under a laminar flow hood. The closure should be penetrated only once with a sterile transfer set or other sterile dispensing device, which allows measured distribution of the contents, and the contents dispensed in aliquots using aseptic technique. CONTENTS SHOULD BE USED AS SOON AS POSSIBLE FOLLOWING INITIAL CLOSURE PUNCTURE. DISCARD ANY UNUSED PORTION WITHIN 24 HOURS OF FIRST ENTRY. Following closure puncture, container should be maintained below 30°C (86°F) under a laminar flow hood until contents are dispensed.

HOW SUPPLIED

ZANTAC Injection, 25 mg/mL, containing phenol 0.5% as preservative, in a 40-mL pharmacy bulk package (NDC 0173-0363-00).

Store between 4° and 25°C (39° and 77°F); excursions permitted to 30°C (86°F). Protect from light. Store vial in carton until time of use.

GlaxoSmithKline
Research Triangle Park, NC 27709
ZANTAC is a registered trademark of Warner-Lambert Company, used under license.
MULTISTIX is a registered trademark of Bayer Healthcare LLC.
©2009, GlaxoSmithKline. All rights reserved.
April 2009 ZNP:4PI

ZANTAC® 150 ℞
[zan' tak]
(ranitidine hydrochloride)
Tablets, USP

ZANTAC® 300 ℞
(ranitidine hydrochloride)
Tablets, USP

ZANTAC® 25 ℞
(ranitidine hydrochloride effervescent)
EFFERdose® Tablets

ZANTAC® ℞
(ranitidine hydrochloride)
Syrup, USP

DESCRIPTION

The active ingredient in ZANTAC 150 Tablets, ZANTAC 300 Tablets, ZANTAC 25 EFFERdose Tablets, and ZANTAC Syrup is ranitidine hydrochloride (HCl), USP, a histamine H_2-receptor antagonist. Chemically it is N[2-[[[5-[(dimethylamino)methyl]-2-furanyl]methyl]thio]ethyl]-N'-

methyl-2-nitro-1,1-ethenediamine, HCl. It has the following structure:

(CH$_3$)$_2$NCH$_2$ — CH$_2$SCH$_2$CH$_2$NH — NHCH$_3$ • HCl
                                              CHNO$_2$

The empirical formula is C$_{13}$H$_{22}$N$_4$O$_3$S•HCl, representing a molecular weight of 350.87.

Ranitidine HCl is a white to pale yellow, granular substance that is soluble in water. It has a slightly bitter taste and sulfurlike odor.

Each ZANTAC 150 Tablet for oral administration contains 168 mg of ranitidine HCl equivalent to 150 mg of ranitidine. Each tablet also contains the inactive ingredients FD&C Yellow No. 6 Aluminum Lake, hypromellose, magnesium stearate, microcrystalline cellulose, titanium dioxide, triacetin, and yellow iron oxide.

Each ZANTAC 300 Tablet for oral administration contains 336 mg of ranitidine HCl equivalent to 300 mg of ranitidine. Each tablet also contains the inactive ingredients croscarmellose sodium, D&C Yellow No. 10 Aluminum Lake, hypromellose, magnesium stearate, microcrystalline cellulose, titanium dioxide, and triacetin.

ZANTAC 25 EFFERdose Tablets for oral administration is an effervescent formulation of ranitidine that must be dissolved in water before use. Each individual tablet contains 28 mg of ranitidine HCl equivalent to 25 mg of ranitidine and the following inactive ingredients: aspartame, monosodium citrate anhydrous, povidone, and sodium bicarbonate. Each tablet also contains sodium benzoate. The total sodium content of each tablet is 30.52 mg (1.33 mEq) per 25 mg of ranitidine.

Each 1 mL of ZANTAC Syrup contains 16.8 mg of ranitidine HCl equivalent to 15 mg of ranitidine. ZANTAC Syrup also contains the inactive ingredients alcohol (7.5%), butylparaben, dibasic sodium phosphate, hypromellose, peppermint flavor, monobasic potassium phosphate, propylparaben, purified water, saccharin sodium, sodium chloride, and sorbitol.

CLINICAL PHARMACOLOGY

ZANTAC is a competitive, reversible inhibitor of the action of histamine at the histamine H$_2$-receptors, including receptors on the gastric cells. ZANTAC does not lower serum Ca++ in hypercalcemic states. ZANTAC is not an anticholinergic agent.

Pharmacokinetics:

Absorption: ZANTAC is 50% absorbed after oral administration, compared to an intravenous (IV) injection with mean peak levels of 440 to 545 ng/mL occurring 2 to 3 hours after a 150-mg dose. The syrup and EFFERdose formulations are bioequivalent to the tablets. Absorption is not significantly impaired by the administration of food or antacids. Propantheline slightly delays and increases peak blood levels of ranitidine, probably by delaying gastric emptying and transit time. In one study, simultaneous administration of high-potency antacid (150 mmol) in fasting subjects has been reported to decrease the absorption of ZANTAC.

Distribution: The volume of distribution is about 1.4 L/kg. Serum protein binding averages 15%.

Metabolism: In humans, the N-oxide is the principal metabolite in the urine; however, this amounts to <4% of the dose. Other metabolites are the S-oxide (1%) and the desmethyl ranitidine (1%). The remainder of the administered dose is found in the stool. Studies in patients with hepatic dysfunction (compensated cirrhosis) indicate that there are minor, but clinically insignificant, alterations in ranitidine half-life, distribution, clearance, and bioavailability.

Excretion: The principal route of excretion is the urine, with approximately 30% of the orally administered dose collected in the urine as unchanged drug in 24 hours. Renal clearance is about 410 mL/min, indicating active tubular excretion. The elimination half-life is 2.5 to 3 hours. Four patients with clinically significant renal function impairment (creatinine clearance 25 to 35 mL/min) administered 50 mg of ranitidine intravenously had an average plasma half-life of 4.8 hours, a ranitidine clearance of 29 mL/min, and a volume of distribution of 1.76 L/kg. In general, these parameters appear to be altered in proportion to creatinine clearance (see DOSAGE AND ADMINISTRATION).

Geriatrics: The plasma half-life is prolonged and total clearance is reduced in the elderly population due to a decrease in renal function. The elimination half-life is 3 to 4 hours. Peak levels average 526 ng/mL following a 150-mg twice-daily dose and occur in about 3 hours (see PRECAUTIONS: Geriatric Use and DOSAGE AND ADMINISTRATION: Dosage Adjustment for Patients With Impaired Renal Function).

Pediatrics: There are no significant differences in the pharmacokinetic parameter values for ranitidine in pediatric patients (from 1 month up to 16 years of age) and healthy adults when correction is made for body weight. The average bioavailability of ranitidine given orally to pediatric

patients is 48% which is comparable to the bioavailability of ranitidine in the adult population. All other pharmacokinetic parameter values (t$_{1/2}$, Vd, and CL) are similar to those observed with intravenous ranitidine use in pediatric patients. Estimates of C$_{max}$ and T$_{max}$ are displayed in Table 1.

[See table 1 above]

Plasma clearance measured in 2 neonatal patients (less than 1 month of age) was considerably lower (3 mL/min/kg) than children or adults and is likely due to reduced renal function observed in this population (see PRECAUTIONS: Pediatric Use and DOSAGE AND ADMINISTRATION: Pediatric Use).

Pharmacodynamics: Serum concentrations necessary to inhibit 50% of stimulated gastric acid secretion are estimated to be 36 to 94 ng/mL. Following a single oral dose of 150 mg, serum concentrations of ranitidine are in this range up to 12 hours. However, blood levels bear no consistent relationship to dose or degree of acid inhibition.

In a pharmacodynamic comparison of the EFFERdose with the ZANTAC Tablets, during the first hour after administration, the EFFERdose tablet formulation gave a significantly higher intragastric pH, by approximately 1 pH unit, compared to the ZANTAC Tablets.

Antisecretory Activity: 1. Effects on Acid Secretion: ZANTAC inhibits both daytime and nocturnal basal gastric acid secretions as well as gastric acid secretion stimulated by food, betazole, and pentagastrin, as shown in Table 2.

[See table 2 above]

It appears that basal-, nocturnal-, and betazole-stimulated secretions are most sensitive to inhibition by ZANTAC, responding almost completely to doses of 100 mg or less, while pentagastrin- and food-stimulated secretions are more difficult to suppress.

2. Effects on Other Gastrointestinal Secretions:

Pepsin: Oral ZANTAC does not affect pepsin secretion. Total pepsin output is reduced in proportion to the decrease in volume of gastric juice.

Intrinsic Factor: Oral ZANTAC has no significant effect on pentagastrin-stimulated intrinsic factor secretion.

Serum Gastrin: ZANTAC has little or no effect on fasting or postprandial serum gastrin.

Other Pharmacologic Actions:

1. Gastric bacterial flora—increase in nitrate-reducing organisms, significance not known.

2. Prolactin levels—no effect in recommended oral or IV dosage, but small, transient, dose-related increases in serum prolactin have been reported after IV bolus injections of 100 mg or more.

3. Other pituitary hormones—no effect on serum gonadotropins, TSH, or GH. Possible impairment of vasopressin release.

4. No change in cortisol, aldosterone, androgen, or estrogen levels.

5. No antiandrogenic action.

6. No effect on count, motility, or morphology of sperm.

Pediatrics: Oral doses of 6 to 10 mg/kg/day in 2 or 3 divided doses maintain gastric pH >4 throughout most of the dosing interval.

Clinical Trials: Active Duodenal Ulcer: In a multicenter, double-blind, controlled, US study of endoscopically diagnosed duodenal ulcers, earlier healing was seen in the patients treated with ZANTAC as shown in Table 3.

[See table 3 above]

In these studies, patients treated with ZANTAC reported a reduction in both daytime and nocturnal pain, and they also consumed less antacid than the placebo-treated patients.

Foreign studies have shown that patients heal equally well with 150 mg twice daily and 300 mg at bedtime (85% versus 84%, respectively) during a usual 4-week course of therapy. If patients require extended therapy of 8 weeks, the healing rate may be higher for 150 mg twice daily as compared to 300 mg at bedtime (92% versus 87%, respectively).

Studies have been limited to short-term treatment of acute duodenal ulcer. Patients whose ulcers healed during therapy had recurrences of ulcers at the usual rates.

Maintenance Therapy in Duodenal Ulcer: Ranitidine has been found to be effective as maintenance therapy for patients following healing of acute duodenal ulcers. In 2 independent, double-blind, multicenter, controlled trials, the number of duodenal ulcers observed was significantly less

Table 1. Ranitidine Pharmacokinetics in Pediatric Patients Following Oral Dosing

Population (age)	n	Dosage Form (dose)	C$_{max}$ (ng/mL)	T$_{max}$ (hours)
Gastric or duodenal ulcer (3.5 to 16 years)	12	Tablets (1 to 2 mg/kg)	54 to 492	2.0
Otherwise healthy requiring ZANTAC (0.7 to 14 years, Single dose)	10	Syrup (2 mg/kg)	244	1.61
Otherwise healthy requiring ZANTAC (0.7 to 14 years, Multiple dose)	10	Syrup (2 mg/kg)	320	1.66

Table 2. Effect of Oral ZANTAC on Gastric Acid Secretion

| | Time After Dose, hours | % Inhibition of Gastric Acid Output by Dose, mg | | | |
		75-80	100	150	200
Basal	Up to 4		99	95	
Nocturnal	Up to 13	95	96	92	
Betazole	Up to 3		97	99	
Pentagastrin	Up to 5	58	72	72	80
Meal	Up to 3		73	79	95

Table 3. Duodenal Ulcer Patient Healing Rates

| | ZANTAC* | | Placebo* | |
	Number Entered	Healed/Evaluable	Number Entered	Healed/Evaluable
Outpatients				
Week 2	195	69/182 (38%)†	188	31/164 (19%)
Week 4		137/187 (73%)†		76/168 (45%)

* All patients were permitted antacids as needed for relief of pain.
† P<0.0001.

Table 4. Mean Daily Doses of Antacid

	Ulcer Healed	Ulcer Not Healed
ZANTAC	0.06	0.71
Placebo	0.71	1.43

in patients treated with ZANTAC (150 mg at bedtime) than in patients treated with placebo over a 12-month period. [See table 5 at right]

As with other H₂-antagonists, the factors responsible for the significant reduction in the prevalence of duodenal ulcers include prevention of recurrence of ulcers, more rapid healing of ulcers that may occur during maintenance therapy, or both.

Gastric Ulcer: In a multicenter, double-blind, controlled, US study of endoscopically diagnosed gastric ulcers, earlier healing was seen in the patients treated with ZANTAC as shown in Table 6.
[See table 6 at right]

In this multicenter trial, significantly more patients treated with ZANTAC became pain free during therapy.

Maintenance of Healing of Gastric Ulcers: In 2 multicenter, double-blind, randomized, placebo-controlled, 12-month trials conducted in patients whose gastric ulcers had been previously healed, ZANTAC 150 mg at bedtime was significantly more effective than placebo in maintaining healing of gastric ulcers.

Pathological Hypersecretory Conditions (such as Zollinger-Ellison syndrome): ZANTAC inhibits gastric acid secretion and reduces occurrence of diarrhea, anorexia, and pain in patients with pathological hypersecretion associated with Zollinger-Ellison syndrome, systemic mastocytosis, and other pathological hypersecretory conditions (e.g., postoperative, "short-gut" syndrome, idiopathic). Use of ZANTAC was followed by healing of ulcers in 8 of 19 (42%) patients who were intractable to previous therapy.

Gastroesophageal Reflux Disease (GERD): In 2 multicenter, double-blind, placebo-controlled, 6-week trials performed in the United States and Europe, ZANTAC 150 mg twice daily was more effective than placebo for the relief of heartburn and other symptoms associated with GERD. Ranitidine-treated patients consumed significantly less antacid than did placebo-treated patients.

The US trial indicated that ZANTAC 150 mg twice daily significantly reduced the frequency of heartburn attacks and severity of heartburn pain within 1 to 2 weeks after starting therapy. The improvement was maintained throughout the 6-week trial period. Moreover, patient response rates demonstrated that the effect on heartburn extends through both the day and night time periods.

In 2 additional US multicenter, double-blind, placebo-controlled, 2-week trials, ZANTAC 150 mg twice daily was shown to provide relief of heartburn pain within 24 hours of initiating therapy and a reduction in the frequency of severity of heartburn. In these trials, ZANTAC EFFERdose Tablets were shown to provide heartburn relief within 45 minutes of dosing.

Erosive Esophagitis: In 2 multicenter, double-blind, randomized, placebo-controlled, 12-week trials performed in the United States, ZANTAC 150 mg 4 times daily was significantly more effective than placebo in healing endoscopically diagnosed erosive esophagitis and in relieving associated heartburn. The erosive esophagitis healing rates were as follows:

Table 7. Erosive Esophagitis Patient Healing Rates

	Healed/Evaluable	
	Placebo* n = 229	ZANTAC 150 mg 4 times daily* n = 215
Week 4	43/198 (22%)	96/206 (47%)†
Week 8	63/176 (36%)	142/200 (71%)†
Week 12	92/159 (58%)	162/192 (84%)†

* All patients were permitted antacids as needed for relief of pain.
† P<0.001 versus placebo.

No additional benefit in healing of esophagitis or in relief of heartburn was seen with a ranitidine dose of 300 mg 4 times daily.

Maintenance of Healing of Erosive Esophagitis: In 2 multicenter, double-blind, randomized, placebo-controlled, 48-week trials conducted in patients whose erosive esophagitis had been previously healed, ZANTAC 150 mg twice daily was significantly more effective than placebo in maintaining healing of erosive esophagitis.

INDICATIONS AND USAGE

ZANTAC is indicated in:
1. Short-term treatment of active duodenal ulcer. Most patients heal within 4 weeks. Studies available to date have not assessed the safety of ranitidine in uncomplicated duodenal ulcer for periods of more than 8 weeks.
2. Maintenance therapy for duodenal ulcer patients at reduced dosage after healing of acute ulcers. No placebo-

Table 5. Duodenal Ulcer Prevalence

Multicenter Trial	Drug	Double-Blind, Multicenter, Placebo-Controlled Trials			
		Duodenal Ulcer Prevalence			No. of Patients
		0-4 Months	0-8 Months	0-12 Months	
USA	RAN	20%*	24%*	35%*	138
	PLC	44%	54%	59%	139
Foreign	RAN	12%*	21%*	28%*	174
	PLC	56%	64%	68%	165

% = Life table estimate.
* = P<0.05 (ZANTAC versus comparator).
RAN = ranitidine (ZANTAC).
PLC = placebo.

Table 6. Gastric Ulcer Patient Healing Rates

	ZANTAC*		Placebo*	
	Number Entered	Healed/Evaluable	Number Entered	Healed/Evaluable
Outpatients				
Week 2	92	16/83 (19%)	94	10/83 (12%)
Week 6		50/73 (68%)†		35/69 (51%)

* All patients were permitted antacids as needed for relief of pain.
† P = 0.009.

controlled comparative studies have been carried out for periods of longer than 1 year.
3. The treatment of pathological hypersecretory conditions (e.g., Zollinger-Ellison syndrome and systemic mastocytosis).
4. Short-term treatment of active, benign gastric ulcer. Most patients heal within 6 weeks and the usefulness of further treatment has not been demonstrated. Studies available to date have not assessed the safety of ranitidine in uncomplicated, benign gastric ulcer for periods of more than 6 weeks.
5. Maintenance therapy for gastric ulcer patients at reduced dosage after healing of acute ulcers. Placebo-controlled studies have been carried out for 1 year.
6. Treatment of GERD. Symptomatic relief commonly occurs within 24 hours after starting therapy with ZANTAC 150 mg twice daily.
7. Treatment of endoscopically diagnosed erosive esophagitis. Symptomatic relief of heartburn commonly occurs within 24 hours of therapy initiation with ZANTAC 150 mg 4 times daily.
8. Maintenance of healing of erosive esophagitis. Placebo-controlled trials have been carried out for 48 weeks.

Concomitant antacids should be given as needed for pain relief to patients with active duodenal ulcer; active, benign gastric ulcer; hypersecretory states; GERD; and erosive esophagitis.

CONTRAINDICATIONS

ZANTAC is contraindicated for patients known to have hypersensitivity to the drug or any of the ingredients (see PRECAUTIONS).

PRECAUTIONS

General:
1. Symptomatic response to therapy with ZANTAC does not preclude the presence of gastric malignancy.
2. Since ZANTAC is excreted primarily by the kidney, dosage should be adjusted in patients with impaired renal function (see DOSAGE AND ADMINISTRATION). Caution should be observed in patients with hepatic dysfunction since ZANTAC is metabolized in the liver.
3. Rare reports suggest that ZANTAC may precipitate acute porphyric attacks in patients with acute porphyria. ZANTAC should therefore be avoided in patients with a history of acute porphyria.

Information for Patients: *Phenylketonurics:* ZANTAC 25 EFFERdose Tablets contain phenylalanine 2.81 mg per 25 mg of ranitidine. ZANTAC EFFERdose Tablets should not be chewed, swallowed whole, or dissolved on the tongue.

Laboratory Tests: False-positive tests for urine protein with MULTISTIX® may occur during therapy with ZANTAC, and therefore testing with sulfosalicylic acid is recommended.

Drug Interactions: Ranitidine has been reported to affect the bioavailability of other drugs through several different mechanisms such as competition for renal tubular secretion, alteration of gastric pH, and inhibition of cytochrome P450 enzymes.

Procainamide: Ranitidine, a substrate of the renal organic cation transport system, may affect the clearance of other drugs eliminated by this route. High doses of ranitidine (e.g., such as those used in the treatment of Zollinger-Ellison syndrome) have been shown to reduce the renal excretion of procainamide and N-acetylprocainamide resulting in increased plasma levels of these drugs. Although this interaction is unlikely to be clinically relevant at usual ranitidine doses, it may be prudent to monitor for procainamide toxicity when administered with oral ranitidine at a dose exceeding 300 mg per day.

Warfarin: There have been reports of altered prothrombin time among patients on concomitant warfarin and ranitidine therapy. Due to the narrow therapeutic index, close monitoring of increased or decreased prothrombin time is recommended during concurrent treatment with ranitidine.

Ranitidine may alter the absorption of drugs in which gastric pH is an important determinant of bioavailability. This can result in either an increase in absorption (e.g., triazolam, midazolam, glipizide) or a decrease in absorption (e.g., ketoconazole, atazanavir, delavirdine, gefitinib). Appropriate clinical monitoring is recommended.

Atazanavir: Atazanavir absorption may be impaired based on known interactions with other agents that increase gastric pH. Use with caution. See atazanavir label for specific recommendations.

Delavirdine: Delavirdine absorption may be impaired based on known interactions with other agents that increase gastric pH. Chronic use of H₂-receptor antagonists with delavirdine is not recommended.

Gefitinib: Gefitinib exposure was reduced by 44% with the coadministration of ranitidine and sodium bicarbonate (dosed to maintain gastric pH above 5.0). Use with caution.

Glipizide: In diabetic patients, glipizide exposure was increased by 34% following a single 150-mg dose of oral ranitidine. Use appropriate clinical monitoring when initiating or discontinuing ranitidine.

Ketoconazole: Oral ketoconazole exposure was reduced by up to 95% when oral ranitidine was coadministered in a regimen to maintain a gastric pH of 6 or above. The degree of interaction with usual dose of ranitidine (150 mg twice daily) is unknown.

Midazolam: Oral midazolam exposure in 5 healthy volunteers was increased by up to 65% when administered with oral ranitidine at a dose of 150 mg twice daily. However, in another interaction study in 8 volunteers receiving IV midazolam, a 300 mg oral dose of ranitidine increased midazolam exposure by about 9%. Monitor patients for excessive or prolonged sedation when ranitidine is coadministered with oral midazolam.

Triazolam: Triazolam exposure in healthy volunteers was increased by approximately 30% when administered with oral ranitidine at a dose of 150 mg twice daily. Monitor patients for excessive or prolonged sedation.

Carcinogenesis, Mutagenesis, Impairment of Fertility: There was no indication of tumorigenic or carcinogenic effects in life-span studies in mice and rats at dosages up to 2,000 mg/kg/day.

Ranitidine was not mutagenic in standard bacterial tests (*Salmonella, Escherichia coli*) for mutagenicity at concentrations up to the maximum recommended for these assays.

In a dominant lethal assay, a single oral dose of 1,000 mg/kg to male rats was without effect on the outcome of 2 matings per week for the next 9 weeks.

Pregnancy: ***Teratogenic Effects:*** Pregnancy Category B. Reproduction studies have been performed in rats and rabbits at doses up to 160 times the human dose and have revealed no evidence of impaired fertility or harm to the fetus due to ZANTAC. There are, however, no adequate and well-controlled studies in pregnant women. Because animal reproduction studies are not always predictive of human response, this drug should be used during pregnancy only if clearly needed.

Nursing Mothers: Ranitidine is secreted in human milk. Caution should be exercised when ZANTAC is administered to a nursing mother.

Pediatric Use: The safety and effectiveness of ZANTAC have been established in the age-group of 1 month to 16 years for the treatment of duodenal and gastric ulcers, gastroesophageal reflux disease and erosive esophagitis, and the maintenance of healed duodenal and gastric ulcer. Use of ZANTAC in this age-group is supported by adequate and well-controlled studies in adults, as well as additional pharmacokinetic data in pediatric patients and an analysis of the published literature (see CLINICAL PHARMACOLOGY: Pediatrics and DOSAGE AND ADMINISTRATION: Pediatric Use).

Safety and effectiveness in pediatric patients for the treatment of pathological hypersecretory conditions or the maintenance of healing of erosive esophagitis have not been established.

Safety and effectiveness in neonates (less than 1 month of age) have not been established (see CLINICAL PHARMACOLOGY: Pediatrics).

Geriatric Use: Of the total number of subjects enrolled in US and foreign controlled clinical trials of oral formulations of ZANTAC, for which there were subgroup analyses, 4,197 were 65 and over, while 899 were 75 and over. No overall differences in safety or effectiveness were observed between these subjects and younger subjects, and other reported clinical experience has not identified differences in responses between the elderly and younger patients, but greater sensitivity of some older individuals cannot be ruled out.

This drug is known to be substantially excreted by the kidney and the risk of toxic reactions to this drug may be greater in patients with impaired renal function. Because elderly patients are more likely to have decreased renal function, caution should be exercised in dose selection, and it may be useful to monitor renal function (see CLINICAL PHARMACOLOGY: Pharmacokinetics: Geriatrics and DOSAGE AND ADMINISTRATION: Dosage Adjustment for Patients With Impaired Renal Function).

ADVERSE REACTIONS

The following have been reported as events in clinical trials or in the routine management of patients treated with ZANTAC. The relationship to therapy with ZANTAC has been unclear in many cases. Headache, sometimes severe, seems to be related to administration of ZANTAC.

Central Nervous System: Rarely, malaise, dizziness, somnolence, insomnia, and vertigo. Rare cases of reversible mental confusion, agitation, depression, and hallucinations have been reported, predominantly in severely ill elderly patients. Rare cases of reversible blurred vision suggestive of a change in accommodation have been reported. Rare reports of reversible involuntary motor disturbances have been received.

Cardiovascular: As with other H_2-blockers, rare reports of arrhythmias such as tachycardia, bradycardia, atrioventricular block, and premature ventricular beats.

Gastrointestinal: Constipation, diarrhea, nausea/vomiting, abdominal discomfort/pain, and rare reports of pancreatitis.

Hepatic: There have been occasional reports of hepatocellular, cholestatic, or mixed hepatitis, with or without jaundice. In such circumstances, ranitidine should be immediately discontinued. These events are usually reversible, but in rare circumstances death has occurred. Rare cases of hepatic failure have also been reported. In normal volunteers, SGPT values were increased to at least twice the pretreatment levels in 6 of 12 subjects receiving 100 mg intravenously 4 times daily for 7 days, and in 4 of 24 subjects receiving 50 mg intravenously 4 times daily for 5 days.

Musculoskeletal: Rare reports of arthralgias and myalgias.

Hematologic: Blood count changes (leukopenia, granulocytopenia, and thrombocytopenia) have occurred in a few patients. These were usually reversible. Rare cases of agranulocytosis, pancytopenia, sometimes with marrow hypoplasia, and aplastic anemia and exceedingly rare cases of acquired immune hemolytic anemia have been reported.

Endocrine: Controlled studies in animals and man have shown no stimulation of any pituitary hormone by ZANTAC and no antiandrogenic activity, and cimetidine-induced gynecomastia and impotence in hypersecretory patients have resolved when ZANTAC has been substituted. However, occasional cases of impotence and loss of libido have been reported in male patients receiving ZANTAC, but the incidence did not differ from that in the general population. Rare cases of breast symptoms and conditions, including galactorrhea and gynecomastia, have been reported in both males and females.

Integumentary: Rash, including rare cases of erythema multiforme. Rare cases of alopecia and vasculitis.

Respiratory: A large epidemiological study suggested an increased risk of developing pneumonia in current users of histamine-2-receptor antagonists (H_2RAs) compared to patients who had stopped H_2RA treatment, with an observed adjusted relative risk of 1.63 (95% CI, 1.07-2.48). However, a causal relationship between use of H_2RAs and pneumonia has not been established.

Other: Rare cases of hypersensitivity reactions (e.g., bronchospasm, fever, rash, eosinophilia), anaphylaxis, angioneurotic edema, acute interstitial nephritis, and small increases in serum creatinine.

OVERDOSAGE

There has been limited experience with overdosage. Reported acute ingestions of up to 18 g orally have been associated with transient adverse effects similar to those encountered in normal clinical experience (see ADVERSE REACTIONS). In addition, abnormalities of gait and hypotension have been reported.

When overdosage occurs, the usual measures to remove unabsorbed material from the gastrointestinal tract, clinical monitoring, and supportive therapy should be employed.

Studies in dogs receiving dosages of ZANTAC in excess of 225 mg/kg/day have shown muscular tremors, vomiting, and rapid respiration. Single oral doses of 1,000 mg/kg in mice and rats were not lethal. Intravenous LD_{50} values in mice and rats were 77 and 83 mg/kg, respectively.

DOSAGE AND ADMINISTRATION

Active Duodenal Ulcer: The current recommended adult oral dosage of ZANTAC for duodenal ulcer is 150 mg or 10 mL of syrup (2 teaspoonfuls of syrup equivalent to 150 mg of ranitidine) twice daily. An alternative dosage of 300 mg or 20 mL of syrup (4 teaspoonfuls of syrup equivalent to 300 mg of ranitidine) once daily after the evening meal or at bedtime can be used for patients in whom dosing convenience is important. The advantages of one treatment regimen compared to the other in a particular patient population have yet to be demonstrated (see Clinical Trials: *Active Duodenal Ulcer*). Smaller doses have been shown to be equally effective in inhibiting gastric acid secretion in US studies, and several foreign trials have shown that 100 mg twice daily is as effective as the 150-mg dose.

Antacid should be given as needed for relief of pain (see CLINICAL PHARMACOLOGY: Pharmacokinetics).

Maintenance of Healing of Duodenal Ulcers: The current recommended adult oral dosage is 150 mg or 10 mL of syrup (2 teaspoonfuls of syrup equivalent to 150 mg of ranitidine) at bedtime.

Pathological Hypersecretory Conditions (such as Zollinger-Ellison syndrome): The current recommended adult oral dosage is 150 mg or 10 mL of syrup (2 teaspoonfuls of syrup equivalent to 150 mg of ranitidine) twice daily. In some patients it may be necessary to administer ZANTAC 150-mg doses more frequently. Dosages should be adjusted to individual patient needs, and should continue as long as clinically indicated. Dosages up to 6 g/day have been employed in patients with severe disease.

Benign Gastric Ulcer: The current recommended adult oral dosage is 150 mg or 10 mL of syrup (2 teaspoonfuls of syrup equivalent to 150 mg of ranitidine) twice daily.

Maintenance of Healing of Gastric Ulcers: The current recommended adult oral dosage is 150 mg or 10 mL of syrup (2 teaspoonfuls of syrup equivalent to 150 mg of ranitidine) at bedtime.

GERD: The current recommended adult oral dosage is 150 mg or 10 mL of syrup (2 teaspoonfuls of syrup equivalent to 150 mg of ranitidine) twice daily.

Erosive Esophagitis: The current recommended adult oral dosage is 150 mg or 10 mL of syrup (2 teaspoonfuls of syrup equivalent to 150 mg of ranitidine) 4 times daily.

Maintenance of Healing of Erosive Esophagitis: The current recommended adult oral dosage is 150 mg or 10 mL of syrup (2 teaspoonfuls of syrup equivalent to 150 mg of ranitidine) twice daily.

Pediatric Use: The safety and effectiveness of ZANTAC have been established in the age-group of 1 month to 16 years. There is insufficient information about the pharmacokinetics of ZANTAC in neonatal patients (less than 1 month of age) to make dosing recommendations.

The following 3 subsections provide dosing information for each of the pediatric indications. Also, see the subsection on Preparation of ZANTAC 25 EFFERdose Tablets, below.

Treatment of Duodenal and Gastric Ulcers: The recommended oral dose for the treatment of active duodenal and gastric ulcers is 2 to 4 mg/kg twice daily to a maximum of 300 mg/day. This recommendation is derived from adult clinical studies and pharmacokinetic data in pediatric patients.

Maintenance of Healing of Duodenal and Gastric Ulcers: The recommended oral dose for the maintenance of healing of duodenal and gastric ulcers is 2 to 4 mg/kg once daily to a maximum of 150 mg/day. This recommendation is derived from adult clinical studies and pharmacokinetic data in pediatric patients.

Treatment of GERD and Erosive Esophagitis: Although limited data exist for these conditions in pediatric patients, published literature supports a dosage of 5 to 10 mg/kg/day, usually given as 2 divided doses.

Dosage Adjustment for Patients With Impaired Renal Function: On the basis of experience with a group of subjects with severely impaired renal function treated with ZANTAC, the recommended dosage in patients with a creatinine clearance <50 mL/min is 150 mg or 10 mL of syrup (2 teaspoonfuls of syrup equivalent to 150 mg of ranitidine) every 24 hours. Should the patient's condition require, the frequency of dosing may be increased to every 12 hours or even further with caution. Hemodialysis reduces the level of circulating ranitidine. Ideally, the dosing schedule should be adjusted so that the timing of a scheduled dose coincides with the end of hemodialysis.

Elderly patients are more likely to have decreased renal function, therefore caution should be exercised in dose selection, and it may be useful to monitor renal function (see CLINICAL PHARMACOLOGY: Pharmacokinetics: Geriatrics and PRECAUTIONS: Geriatric Use).

Preparation of ZANTAC 25 EFFERdose Tablets: Tablets should not be chewed, swallowed whole, or dissolved on the tongue. Dissolve 1 tablet in no less than 5 mL (1 teaspoonful) of water in an appropriate measuring cup. Wait until the tablet is completely dissolved before administering the solution to the infant/child. The solution may be administered to infants by medicine dropper or oral syringe.

HOW SUPPLIED

ZANTAC 150 Tablets (ranitidine HCl equivalent to 150 mg of ranitidine) are peach, film-coated, 5-sided tablets embossed with "ZANTAC 150" on one side and "Glaxo" on the other. They are available in bottles of 60 (NDC 0173-0344-42), 180 (NDC 0173-0344-17), and 500 (NDC 0173-0344-14) tablets.

ZANTAC 300 Tablets (ranitidine HCl equivalent to 300 mg of ranitidine) are yellow, film-coated, capsule-shaped tablets embossed with "ZANTAC 300" on one side and "Glaxo" on the other. They are available in bottles of 30 (NDC 0173-0393-40) tablets.

Store between 15° and 30°C (59° and 86°F) in a dry place. Protect from light. Replace cap securely after each opening.

ZANTAC 25 EFFERdose Tablets (ranitidine HCl equivalent to 25 mg of ranitidine) are white to pale yellow, round, flat-faced, bevel-edged tablets embossed with "GS" on one side and "25C" on the other side. They are packaged in foil strips and are available in a carton of 60 (NDC 0173-0734-00) tablets.

Store between 2° and 30°C (36° and 86°F).

ZANTAC Syrup, a clear, pale yellow, peppermint-flavored liquid, contains 16.8 mg of ranitidine HCl equivalent to 15 mg of ranitidine per 1 mL (75 mg/5 mL) in bottles of 16 fluid ounces (one pint) (NDC 0173-0383-54).

Store between 4° and 25°C (39° and 77°F). Dispense in tight, light-resistant containers as defined in the USP/NF.

GlaxoSmithKline
Research Triangle Park, NC 27709

ZANTAC and EFFERdose are registered trademarks of Warner-Lambert Company, used under license.

MULTISTIX is a registered trademark of Bayer Healthcare LLC.

©2009, GlaxoSmithKline. All rights reserved.

April 2009 ZNT:5PI

ZINACEF® ℞
[*zin'a-sef*]
(cefuroxime for injection)

ZINACEF® ℞
(cefuroxime injection)

To reduce the development of drug-resistant bacteria and maintain the effectiveness of ZINACEF and other antibacterial drugs, ZINACEF should be used only to treat or prevent infections that are proven or strongly suspected to be caused by bacteria.

DESCRIPTION

Cefuroxime is a semisynthetic, broad-spectrum, cephalosporin antibiotic for parenteral administration. It is the sodium salt of (6R,7R)-3-carbamoyloxymethyl-7-[Z-2-methoxyimino-2-(fur-2-yl)acetamido]ceph-3-em-4-carboxylate and it has the following chemical structure:

The empirical formula is $C_{16}H_{15}N_4NaO_8S$, representing a molecular weight of 446.4.

ZINACEF contains approximately 54.2 mg (2.4 mEq) of sodium per gram of cefuroxime activity.

ZINACEF in sterile crystalline form is supplied in vials equivalent to 750 mg, 1.5 g, or 7.5 g of cefuroxime as cefuroxime sodium and in ADD-Vantage® vials equivalent to 750 mg or 1.5 g of cefuroxime as cefuroxime sodium. Solutions of ZINACEF range in color from light yellow to amber, depending on the concentration and diluent used. The pH of freshly constituted solutions usually ranges from 6 to 8.5.

ZINACEF is available as a frozen, iso-osmotic, sterile, nonpyrogenic solution with 750 mg or 1.5 g of cefuroxime as cefuroxime sodium. Approximately 1.4 g of Dextrose Hydrous, USP has been added to the 750-mg dose to adjust the osmolality. Sodium Citrate Hydrous, USP has been added as a buffer (300 mg and 600 mg to the 750-mg and 1.5-g doses, respectively). ZINACEF contains approximately 111 mg (4.8 mEq) and 222 mg (9.7 mEq) of sodium in the 750-mg and 1.5-g doses, respectively. The pH has been adjusted with hydrochloric acid and may have been adjusted with sodium hydroxide. Solutions of premixed ZINACEF range in color from light yellow to amber. The solution is intended for intravenous (IV) use after thawing to room temperature. The osmolality of the solution is approximately 300 mOsmol/kg, and the pH of thawed solutions ranges from 5 to 7.5.

The plastic container for the frozen solution is fabricated from a specially designed multilayer plastic, PL 2040. Solutions are in contact with the polyethylene layer of this container and can leach out certain chemical components of the plastic in very small amounts within the expiration period. The suitability of the plastic has been confirmed in tests in animals according to USP biological tests for plastic containers as well as by tissue culture toxicity studies.

CLINICAL PHARMACOLOGY

After intramuscular (IM) injection of a 750-mg dose of cefuroxime to normal volunteers, the mean peak serum concentration was 27 mcg/mL. The peak occurred at approximately 45 minutes (range, 15 to 60 minutes). Following IV doses of 750 mg and 1.5 g, serum concentrations were approximately 50 and 100 mcg/mL, respectively, at 15 minutes. Therapeutic serum concentrations of approximately 2 mcg/mL or more were maintained for 5.3 hours and 8 hours or more, respectively. There was no evidence of accumulation of cefuroxime in the serum following IV administration of 1.5-g doses every 8 hours to normal volunteers. The serum half-life after either IM or IV injections is approximately 80 minutes.

Approximately 89% of a dose of cefuroxime is excreted by the kidneys over an 8-hour period, resulting in high urinary concentrations.

Following the IM administration of a 750-mg single dose, urinary concentrations averaged 1,300 mcg/mL during the first 8 hours. Intravenous doses of 750 mg and 1.5 g produced urinary levels averaging 1,150 and 2,500 mcg/mL, respectively, during the first 8-hour period.

The concomitant oral administration of probenecid with cefuroxime slows tubular secretion, decreases renal clearance by approximately 40%, increases the peak serum level by approximately 30%, and increases the serum half-life by approximately 30%. Cefuroxime is detectable in therapeutic concentrations in pleural fluid, joint fluid, bile, sputum, bone, and aqueous humor.

Cefuroxime is detectable in therapeutic concentrations in cerebrospinal fluid (CSF) of adults and pediatric patients with meningitis. The following table shows the concentrations of cefuroxime achieved in cerebrospinal fluid during multiple dosing of patients with meningitis.

[See table 1 above]

Cefuroxime is approximately 50% bound to serum protein.

Microbiology

Cefuroxime has in vitro activity against a wide range of gram-positive and gram-negative organisms, and it is

Table 1. Concentrations of Cefuroxime Achieved in Cerebrospinal Fluid During Multiple Dosing of Patients with Meningitis

Patients	Dose	Number of Patients	Mean (Range) CSF Cefuroxime Concentrations (mcg/mL) Achieved Within 8 Hours Post Dose
Pediatric patients (4 weeks to 6.5 years)	200 mg/kg/day, divided q 6 hours	5	6.6 (0.9-17.3)
Pediatric patients (7 months to 9 years)	200 to 230 mg/kg/day, divided q 8 hours	6	8.3 (<2-22.5)
Adults	1.5 grams q 8 hours	2	5.2 (2.7-8.9)
Adults	1.5 grams q 6 hours	10	6.0 (1.5-13.5)

highly stable in the presence of beta-lactamases of certain gram-negative bacteria. The bactericidal action of cefuroxime results from inhibition of cell-wall synthesis. Cefuroxime is usually active against the following organisms in vitro.

Aerobes, Gram-positive

Staphylococcus aureus, Staphylococcus epidermidis, Streptococcus pneumoniae, and *Streptococcus pyogenes* (and other streptococci).

NOTE: Most strains of enterococci, e.g., *Enterococcus faecalis* (formerly *Streptococcus faecalis*), are resistant to cefuroxime. Methicillin-resistant staphylococci and *Listeria monocytogenes* are resistant to cefuroxime.

Aerobes, Gram-negative

Citrobacter spp., *Enterobacter* spp., *Escherichia coli, Haemophilus influenzae* (including ampicillin-resistant strains), *Haemophilus parainfluenzae, Klebsiella* spp. (including *Klebsiella pneumoniae*), *Moraxella (Branhamella) catarrhalis* (including ampicillin- and cephalothin-resistant strains), *Morganella morganii* (formerly *Proteus morganii*), *Neisseria gonorrhoeae* (including penicillinase- and non–penicillinase-producing strains), *Neisseria meningitidis, Proteus mirabilis, Providencia rettgeri* (formerly *Proteus rettgeri*), *Salmonella* spp., and *Shigella* spp.

NOTE: Some strains of *Morganella morganii, Enterobacter cloacae,* and *Citrobacter* spp. have been shown by in vitro tests to be resistant to cefuroxime and other cephalosporins. *Pseudomonas* and *Campylobacter* spp., *Legionella* spp., *Acinetobacter calcoaceticus,* and most strains of *Serratia* spp. and *Proteus vulgaris* are resistant to most first- and second-generation cephalosporins.

Anaerobes

Gram-positive and gram-negative cocci (including *Peptococcus* and *Peptostreptococcus* spp.), gram-positive bacilli (including *Clostridium* spp.), and gram-negative bacilli (including *Bacteroides* and *Fusobacterium* spp.).

NOTE: *Clostridium difficile* and most strains of *Bacteroides fragilis* are resistant to cefuroxime.

Susceptibility Tests

Diffusion Techniques

Quantitative methods that require measurement of zone diameters give an estimate of antibiotic susceptibility. One such standard procedure[1] that has been recommended for use with disks to test susceptibility of organisms to cefuroxime uses the 30-mcg cefuroxime disk. Interpretation involves the correlation of the diameters obtained in the disk test with the minimum inhibitory concentration (MIC) for cefuroxime.

A report of "Susceptible" indicates that the pathogen is likely to be inhibited by generally achievable blood levels. A report of "Moderately Susceptible" suggests that the organism would be susceptible if high dosage is used or if the infection is confined to tissues and fluids in which high antibiotic levels are attained. A report of "Intermediate" suggests an equivocable or indeterminate result. A report of "Resistant" indicates that achievable concentrations of the antibiotic are unlikely to be inhibitory and other therapy should be selected.

Reports from the laboratory giving results of the standard single-disk susceptibility test for organisms other than *Haemophilus* spp. and *Neisseria gonorrhoeae* with a 30-mcg cefuroxime disk should be interpreted according to the following criteria:

Zone Diameter (mm)	Interpretation
≥18	(S) Susceptible
15-17	(MS) Moderately Susceptible
≤14	(R) Resistant

Results for *Haemophilus* spp. should be interpreted according to the following criteria:

Zone Diameter (mm)	Interpretation
≥24	(S) Susceptible

21-23	(I) Intermediate
≤20	(R) Resistant

Results for *Neisseria gonorrhoeae* should be interpreted according to the following criteria:

Zone Diameter (mm)	Interpretation
≥31	(S) Susceptible
26-30	(MS) Moderately Susceptible
≤25	(R) Resistant

Organisms should be tested with the cefuroxime disk since cefuroxime has been shown by in vitro tests to be active against certain strains found resistant when other beta-lactam disks are used. The cefuroxime disk should not be used for testing susceptibility to other cephalosporins. Standardized procedures require the use of laboratory control organisms. The 30-mcg cefuroxime disk should give the following zone diameters.

1. Testing for organisms other than *Haemophilus* spp. and *Neisseria gonorrhoeae*:

Organism	Zone Diameter (mm)
Staphylococcus aureus ATCC 25923	27-35
Escherichia coli ATCC 25922	20-26

2. Testing for *Haemophilus* spp.:

Organism	Zone Diameter (mm)
Haemophilus influenzae ATCC 49766	28-36

3. Testing for *Neisseria gonorrhoeae*:

Organism	Zone Diameter (mm)
Neisseria gonorrhoeae ATCC 49226	33-41
Staphylococcus aureus ATCC 25923	29-33

Dilution Techniques

Use a standardized dilution method[1] (broth, agar, microdilution) or equivalent with cefuroxime powder. The MIC values obtained for bacterial isolates other than *Haemophilus* spp. and *Neisseria gonorrhoeae* should be interpreted according to the following criteria:

MIC (mcg/mL)	Interpretation
≤8	(S) Susceptible
16	(MS) Moderately Susceptible
≥32	(R) Resistant

MIC values obtained for *Haemophilus* spp. should be interpreted according to the following criteria:

MIC (mcg/mL)	Interpretation
≤4	(S) Susceptible
8	(I) Intermediate
≥16	(R) Resistant

MIC values obtained for *Neisseria gonorrhoeae* should be interpreted according to the following criteria:

MIC (mcg/mL)	Interpretation
≤1	(S) Susceptible
2	(MS) Moderately Susceptible
≥4	(R) Resistant

As with standard diffusion techniques, dilution methods require the use of laboratory control organisms. Standard cefuroxime powder should provide the following MIC values.

1. For organisms other than *Haemophilus* spp. and *Neisseria gonorrhoeae*:

Organism	MIC (mcg/mL)
Staphylococcus aureus ATCC 29213	0.5-2.0
Escherichia coli ATCC 25922	2.0-8.0

2. For *Haemophilus* spp.:

Organism	MIC (mcg/mL)
Haemophilus influenzae ATCC 49766	0.25-1.0

3. For *Neisseria gonorrhoeae*:

Organism	MIC (mcg/mL)
Neisseria gonorrhoeae ATCC 49226	0.25-1.0
Staphylococcus aureus ATCC 29213	0.25-1.0

INDICATIONS AND USAGE

ZINACEF is indicated for the treatment of patients with infections caused by susceptible strains of the designated organisms in the following diseases:

1. Lower Respiratory Tract Infections, including pneumonia, caused by *Streptococcus pneumoniae, Haemophilus influenzae* (including ampicillin-resistant strains), *Klebsiella* spp., *Staphylococcus aureus* (penicillinase- and non–penicillinase-producing strains), *Streptococcus pyogenes,* and *Escherichia coli.*
2. Urinary Tract Infections caused by *Escherichia coli* and *Klebsiella* spp.
3. Skin and Skin-Structure Infections caused by *Staphylococcus aureus* (penicillinase- and non–penicillinase-producing strains), *Streptococcus pyogenes, Escherichia coli, Klebsiella* spp., and *Enterobacter* spp.
4. Septicemia caused by *Staphylococcus aureus* (penicillinase- and non–penicillinase-producing strains), *Streptococcus pneumoniae, Escherichia coli, Haemophilus influenzae* (including ampicillin-resistant strains), and *Klebsiella* spp.
5. Meningitis caused by *Streptococcus pneumoniae, Haemophilus influenzae* (including ampicillin-resistant strains), *Neisseria meningitidis,* and *Staphylococcus aureus* (penicillinase- and non–penicillinase-producing strains).
6. Gonorrhea: Uncomplicated and disseminated gonococcal infections due to *Neisseria gonorrhoeae* (penicillinase- and non–penicillinase-producing strains) in both males and females.
7. Bone and Joint Infections caused by *Staphylococcus aureus* (penicillinase- and non–penicillinase-producing strains).

Clinical microbiological studies in skin and skin-structure infections frequently reveal the growth of susceptible strains of both aerobic and anaerobic organisms. ZINACEF has been used successfully in these mixed infections in which several organisms have been isolated.

In certain cases of confirmed or suspected gram-positive or gram-negative sepsis or in patients with other serious infections in which the causative organism has not been identified, ZINACEF may be used concomitantly with an aminoglycoside (see PRECAUTIONS). The recommended doses of both antibiotics may be given depending on the severity of the infection and the patient's condition.

To reduce the development of drug-resistant bacteria and maintain the effectiveness of ZINACEF and other antibacterial drugs, ZINACEF should be used only to treat or prevent infections that are proven or strongly suspected to be caused by susceptible bacteria. When culture and susceptibility information are available, they should be considered in selecting or modifying antibacterial therapy. In the absence of such data, local epidemiology and susceptibility patterns may contribute to the empiric selection of therapy.

Prevention

The preoperative prophylactic administration of ZINACEF may prevent the growth of susceptible disease-causing bacteria and thereby may reduce the incidence of certain postoperative infections in patients undergoing surgical procedures (e.g., vaginal hysterectomy) that are classified as clean-contaminated or potentially contaminated procedures. Effective prophylactic use of antibiotics in surgery depends on the time of administration. ZINACEF should usually be given one-half to 1 hour before the operation to allow sufficient time to achieve effective antibiotic concentrations in the wound tissues during the procedure. The dose should be repeated intraoperatively if the surgical procedure is lengthy.

Prophylactic administration is usually not required after the surgical procedure ends and should be stopped within 24 hours. In the majority of surgical procedures, continuing prophylactic administration of any antibiotic does not reduce the incidence of subsequent infections but will increase the possibility of adverse reactions and the development of bacterial resistance.

The perioperative use of ZINACEF has also been effective during open heart surgery for surgical patients in whom infections at the operative site would present a serious risk. For these patients it is recommended that therapy with ZINACEF be continued for at least 48 hours after the surgical procedure ends. If an infection is present, specimens for culture should be obtained for the identification of the causative organism, and appropriate antimicrobial therapy should be instituted.

CONTRAINDICATIONS

ZINACEF is contraindicated in patients with known allergy to the cephalosporin group of antibiotics.

WARNINGS

BEFORE THERAPY WITH ZINACEF IS INSTITUTED, CAREFUL INQUIRY SHOULD BE MADE TO DETERMINE WHETHER THE PATIENT HAS HAD PREVIOUS HYPERSENSITIVITY REACTIONS TO CEPHALOSPORINS, PENICILLINS, OR OTHER DRUGS. THIS PRODUCT SHOULD BE GIVEN CAUTIOUSLY TO PENICILLIN-SENSITIVE PATIENTS. ANTIBIOTICS SHOULD BE ADMINISTERED WITH CAUTION TO ANY PATIENT WHO HAS DEMONSTRATED SOME FORM OF ALLERGY, PARTICULARLY TO DRUGS. IF AN ALLERGIC REACTION TO ZINACEF OCCURS, DISCONTINUE THE DRUG. SERIOUS ACUTE HYPERSENSITIVITY REACTIONS MAY REQUIRE EPINEPHRINE AND OTHER EMERGENCY MEASURES.

Clostridium difficile associated diarrhea (CDAD) has been reported with use of nearly all antibacterial agents, including ZINACEF, and may range in severity from mild diarrhea to fatal colitis. Treatment with antibacterial agents alters the normal flora of the colon leading to overgrowth of *C. difficile*

C. difficile produces toxins A and B which contribute to the development of CDAD. Hypertoxin producing strains of *C. difficile* cause increased morbidity and mortality, as these infections can be refractory to antimicrobial therapy and may require colectomy. CDAD must be considered in all patients who present with diarrhea following antibiotic use. Careful medical history is necessary since CDAD has been reported to occur over two months after the administration of antibacterial agents.

If CDAD is suspected or confirmed, ongoing antibiotic use not directed against *C. difficile* may need to be discontinued. Appropriate fluid and electrolyte management, protein supplementation, antibiotic treatment of *C. difficile,* and surgical evaluation should be instituted as clinically indicated.

When the colitis is not relieved by drug discontinuation or when it is severe, oral vancomycin is the treatment of choice for antibiotic-associated pseudomembranous colitis produced by *Clostridium difficile*. Other causes of colitis should also be considered.

PRECAUTIONS

General

Although ZINACEF rarely produces alterations in kidney function, evaluation of renal status during therapy is recommended, especially in seriously ill patients receiving the maximum doses. Cephalosporins should be given with caution to patients receiving concurrent treatment with potent diuretics as these regimens are suspected of adversely affecting renal function.

The total daily dose of ZINACEF should be reduced in patients with transient or persistent renal insufficiency (see DOSAGE AND ADMINISTRATION), because high and prolonged serum antibiotic concentrations can occur in such individuals from usual doses.

As with other antibiotics, prolonged use of ZINACEF may result in overgrowth of nonsusceptible organisms. Careful observation of the patient is essential. If superinfection occurs during therapy, appropriate measures should be taken.

Broad-spectrum antibiotics should be prescribed with caution in individuals with a history of gastrointestinal disease, particularly colitis.

Nephrotoxicity has been reported following concomitant administration of aminoglycoside antibiotics and cephalosporins.

As with other therapeutic regimens used in the treatment of meningitis, mild-to-moderate hearing loss has been reported in a few pediatric patients treated with cefuroxime. Persistence of positive CSF (cerebrospinal fluid) cultures at 18 to 36 hours has also been noted with cefuroxime injection, as well as with other antibiotic therapies; however, the clinical relevance of this is unknown.

Cephalosporins may be associated with a fall in prothrombin activity. Those at risk include patients with renal or hepatic impairment, or poor nutritional state, as well as patients receiving a protracted course of antimicrobial therapy, and patients previously stabilized on anticoagulant therapy. Prothrombin time should be monitored in patients at risk and exogenous Vitamin K administered as indicated.

Prescribing ZINACEF in the absence of a proven or strongly suspected bacterial infection or a prophylactic indication is unlikely to provide benefit to the patient and increases the risk of the development of drug-resistant bacteria.

Information for Patients

Patients should be counseled that antibacterial drugs, including ZINACEF, should only be used to treat bacterial infections. They do not treat viral infections (e.g., the common cold). When ZINACEF is prescribed to treat a bacterial infection, patients should be told that although it is common to feel better early in the course of therapy, the medication should be taken exactly as directed. Skipping doses or not completing the full course of therapy may: (1) decrease the effectiveness of the immediate treatment, and (2) increase the likelihood that bacteria will develop resistance and will not be treatable by ZINACEF or other antibacterial drugs in the future.

Diarrhea is a common problem caused by antibiotics which usually ends when the antibiotic is discontinued. Sometimes after starting treatment with antibiotics, patients can develop watery and bloody stools (with or without stomach cramps and fever) even as late as 2 or more months after having taken the last dose of the antibiotic. If this occurs, patients should contact their physician as soon as possible.

Drug Interactions

In common with other antibiotics, cefuroxime may affect the gut flora, leading to lower estrogen reabsorption and reduced efficacy of combined estrogen/progesterone oral contraceptives.

Drug/Laboratory Test Interactions

A false-positive reaction for glucose in the urine may occur with copper reduction tests (Benedict's or Fehling's solution or with CLINITEST® tablets) but not with enzyme-based tests for glycosuria. As a false-negative result may occur in the ferricyanide test, it is recommended that either the glucose oxidase or hexokinase method be used to determine blood plasma glucose levels in patients receiving ZINACEF. Cefuroxime does not interfere with the assay of serum and urine creatinine by the alkaline picrate method.

Carcinogenesis, Mutagenesis, Impairment of Fertility

Although lifetime studies in animals have not been performed to evaluate carcinogenic potential, no mutagenic activity was found for cefuroxime in the mouse lymphoma assay and a battery of bacterial mutation tests. Positive results were obtained in an in vitro chromosome aberration assay, however, negative results were found in an in vivo micronucleus test at doses up to 10 g/kg. Reproduction studies in mice at doses up to 3,200 mg/kg/day (3.1 times the recommended maximum human dose based on mg/m^2) have revealed no impairment of fertility.

Reproductive studies revealed no impairment of fertility in animals.

Pregnancy

Teratogenic Effects

Pregnancy Category B. Reproduction studies have been performed in mice at doses up to 6,400 mg/kg/day (6.3 times the recommended maximum human dose based on mg/m^2) and rabbits at doses up to 400 mg/kg/day (2.1 times the recommended maximum human dose based on mg/m^2) and have revealed no evidence of impaired fertility or harm to the fetus due to cefuroxime. There are, however, no adequate and well-controlled studies in pregnant women. Because animal reproduction studies are not always predictive of human response, this drug should be used during pregnancy only if clearly needed.

Nursing Mothers

Since cefuroxime is excreted in human milk, caution should be exercised when ZINACEF is administered to a nursing woman.

Pediatric Use

Safety and effectiveness in pediatric patients below 3 months of age have not been established. Accumulation of other members of the cephalosporin class in newborn infants (with resulting prolongation of drug half-life) has been reported.

Geriatric Use

Of the 1,914 subjects who received cefuroxime in 24 clinical studies of ZINACEF, 901 (47%) were 65 and over while 421 (22%) were 75 and over. No overall differences in safety or effectiveness were observed between these subjects and younger subjects, and other reported clinical experience has not identified differences in responses between the elderly and younger patients, but greater susceptibility of some older individuals to drug effects cannot be ruled out. This drug is known to be substantially excreted by the kidney, and the risk of toxic reactions to this drug may be greater in patients with impaired renal function. Because elderly patients are more likely to have decreased renal function, care should be taken in dose selection, and it may be useful to monitor renal function (see DOSAGE AND ADMINISTRATION).

ADVERSE REACTIONS

ZINACEF is generally well tolerated. The most common adverse effects have been local reactions following IV administration. Other adverse reactions have been encountered only rarely.

Local Reactions

Thrombophlebitis has occurred with IV administration in 1 in 60 patients.

Gastrointestinal

Gastrointestinal symptoms occurred in 1 in 150 patients and included diarrhea (1 in 220 patients) and nausea (1 in 440 patients). The onset of pseudomembranous colitis may occur during or after antibacterial treatment (see WARNINGS).

Hypersensitivity Reactions

Hypersensitivity reactions have been reported in fewer than 1% of the patients treated with ZINACEF and include rash (1 in 125). Pruritus, urticaria, and positive Coombs' test each occurred in fewer than 1 in 250 patients, and, as with other cephalosporins, rare cases of anaphylaxis, drug fever, erythema multiforme, interstitial nephritis, toxic epidermal necrolysis, and Stevens-Johnson syndrome have occurred.

Blood

A decrease in hemoglobin and hematocrit has been observed in 1 in 10 patients and transient eosinophilia in 1 in 14 patients. Less common reactions seen were transient neutropenia (fewer than 1 in 100 patients) and leukopenia (1 in 750 patients). A similar pattern and incidence were seen with other cephalosporins used in controlled studies. As with other cephalosporins, there have been rare reports of thrombocytopenia.

Hepatic

Transient rise in SGOT and SGPT (1 in 25 patients), alkaline phosphatase (1 in 50 patients), LDH (1 in 75 patients), and bilirubin (1 in 500 patients) levels has been noted.

Kidney

Elevations in serum creatinine and/or blood urea nitrogen and a decreased creatinine clearance have been observed, but their relationship to cefuroxime is unknown.

Postmarketing Experience with ZINACEF Products

In addition to the adverse events reported during clinical trials, the following events have been observed during clinical practice in patients treated with ZINACEF and were reported spontaneously. Data are generally insufficient to allow an estimate of incidence or to establish causation.

Immune System Disorders

Cutaneous vasculitis.

Neurologic

Seizure.

Non-site specific

Angioedema.

Cephalosporin-class Adverse Reactions

In addition to the adverse reactions listed above that have been observed in patients treated with cefuroxime, the following adverse reactions and altered laboratory tests have been reported for cephalosporin-class antibiotics:

Adverse Reactions

Vomiting, abdominal pain, colitis, vaginitis including vaginal candidiasis, toxic nephropathy, hepatic dysfunction including cholestasis, aplastic anemia, hemolytic anemia, hemorrhage.

Several cephalosporins, including ZINACEF, have been implicated in triggering seizures, particularly in patients with renal impairment when the dosage was not reduced (see DOSAGE AND ADMINISTRATION). If seizures associated with drug therapy should occur, the drug should be discontinued. Anticonvulsant therapy can be given if clinically indicated.

Altered Laboratory Tests

Prolonged prothrombin time, pancytopenia, agranulocytosis.

OVERDOSAGE

Overdosage of cephalosporins can cause cerebral irritation leading to convulsions. Serum levels of cefuroxime can be reduced by hemodialysis and peritoneal dialysis.

DOSAGE AND ADMINISTRATION

Dosage

Adults

The usual adult dosage range for ZINACEF is 750 mg to 1.5 grams every 8 hours, usually for 5 to 10 days. In uncomplicated urinary tract infections, skin and skin-structure infections, disseminated gonococcal infections, and uncomplicated pneumonia, a 750-mg dose every 8 hours is recommended. In severe or complicated infections, a 1.5-gram dose every 8 hours is recommended.

In bone and joint infections, a 1.5-gram dose every 8 hours is recommended. In clinical trials, surgical intervention was performed when indicated as an adjunct to therapy with

---

Males: Creatinine clearance (mL/min) = $\dfrac{\text{Weight (kg)} \times (140 - \text{age})}{72 \times \text{serum creatinine (mg/dL)}}$

Females: $0.85 \times$ male value

Table 3. Preparation of Solution and Suspension

Strength	Amount of Diluent to Be Added (mL)	Volume to Be Withdrawn	Approximate Cefuroxime Concentration (mg/mL)
750-mg Vial	3.0 (IM)	Total[a]	225
750-mg Vial	8.3 (IV)	Total	90
1.5-gram Vial	16.0 (IV)	Total	90
7.5-gram Pharmacy bulk package	77 (IV)	Amount Needed[b]	95

[a] **Note:** ZINACEF is a suspension at IM concentrations.
[b] 8 mL of solution contains 750 mg of cefuroxime; 16 mL of solution contains 1.5 grams of cefuroxime.

ZINACEF. A course of oral antibiotics was administered when appropriate following the completion of parenteral administration of ZINACEF.

In life-threatening infections or infections due to less susceptible organisms, 1.5 grams every 6 hours may be required. In bacterial meningitis, the dosage should not exceed 3 grams every 8 hours. The recommended dosage for uncomplicated gonococcal infection is 1.5 grams given intramuscularly as a single dose at 2 different sites together with 1 gram of oral probenecid. For preventive use for clean-contaminated or potentially contaminated surgical procedures, a 1.5-gram dose administered intravenously just before surgery (approximately one-half to 1 hour before the initial incision) is recommended. Thereafter, give 750 mg intravenously or intramuscularly every 8 hours when the procedure is prolonged.

For preventive use during open heart surgery, a 1.5-gram dose administered intravenously at the induction of anesthesia and every 12 hours thereafter for a total of 6 grams is recommended.

Impaired Renal Function

A reduced dosage must be employed when renal function is impaired. Dosage should be determined by the degree of renal impairment and the susceptibility of the causative organism (see Table 2).

Table 2. Dosage of ZINACEF in Adults With Reduced Renal Function

Creatinine Clearance (mL/min)	Dose	Frequency
>20	750 mg-1.5 grams	q8h
10-20	750 mg	q12h
<10	750 mg	q24h*

*Since ZINACEF is dialyzable, patients on hemodialysis should be given a further dose at the end of the dialysis.

When only serum creatinine is available, the following formula[2] (based on sex, weight, and age of the patient) may be used to convert this value into creatinine clearance. The serum creatinine should represent a steady state of renal function.

[See first table above]

Note: As with antibiotic therapy in general, administration of ZINACEF should be continued for a minimum of 48 to 72 hours after the patient becomes asymptomatic or after evidence of bacterial eradication has been obtained; a minimum of 10 days of treatment is recommended in infections caused by *Streptococcus pyogenes* in order to guard against the risk of rheumatic fever or glomerulonephritis; frequent bacteriologic and clinical appraisal is necessary during therapy of chronic urinary tract infection and may be required for several months after therapy has been completed; persistent infections may require treatment for several weeks; and doses smaller than those indicated above should not be used. In staphylococcal and other infections involving a collection of pus, surgical drainage should be carried out where indicated.

Pediatric Patients Above 3 Months of Age

Administration of 50 to 100 mg/kg/day in equally divided doses every 6 to 8 hours has been successful for most infections susceptible to cefuroxime. The higher dosage of 100 mg/kg/day (not to exceed the maximum adult dosage) should be used for the more severe or serious infections.

In bone and joint infections, 150 mg/kg/day (not to exceed the maximum adult dosage) is recommended in equally divided doses every 8 hours. In clinical trials, a course of oral antibiotics was administered to pediatric patients following the completion of parenteral administration of ZINACEF.

In cases of bacterial meningitis, a larger dosage of ZINACEF is recommended, 200 to 240 mg/kg/day intravenously in divided doses every 6 to 8 hours.

In pediatric patients with renal insufficiency, the frequency of dosing should be modified consistent with the recommendations for adults.

Preparation of Solution and Suspension

The directions for preparing ZINACEF for both IV and IM use are summarized in Table 3.

For Intramuscular Use

Each 750-mg vial of ZINACEF should be constituted with 3.0 mL of Sterile Water for Injection. Shake gently to disperse and withdraw completely the resulting suspension for injection.

For Intravenous Use

Each 750-mg vial should be constituted with 8.3 mL of Sterile Water for Injection. Withdraw completely the resulting solution for injection.

Each 1.5-gram vial should be constituted with 16.0 mL of Sterile Water for Injection, and the solution should be completely withdrawn for injection.

The 7.5-gram pharmacy bulk vial should be constituted with 77 mL of Sterile Water for Injection; each 8 mL of the resulting solution contains 750 mg of cefuroxime.

Each 750-mg and 1.5-gram infusion pack should be constituted with 100 mL of Sterile Water for Injection, 5% Dextrose Injection, 0.9% Sodium Chloride Injection, or any of the solutions listed under the Intravenous portion of the COMPATIBILITY AND STABILITY section.

[See table 3 above]

Administration

After constitution, ZINACEF may be given intravenously or by deep IM injection into a large muscle mass (such as the gluteus or lateral part of the thigh). Before injecting intramuscularly, aspiration is necessary to avoid inadvertent injection into a blood vessel.

Intravenous Administration

The IV route may be preferable for patients with bacterial septicemia or other severe or life-threatening infections or for patients who may be poor risks because of lowered resistance, particularly if shock is present or impending.

For direct intermittent IV administration, slowly inject the solution into a vein over a period of 3 to 5 minutes or give it through the tubing system by which the patient is also receiving other IV solutions.

For intermittent IV infusion with a Y-type administration set, dosing can be accomplished through the tubing system by which the patient may be receiving other IV solutions. However, during infusion of the solution containing ZINACEF, it is advisable to temporarily discontinue administration of any other solutions at the same site.

ADD-Vantage vials are to be constituted only with 50 or 100 mL of 5% Dextrose Injection, 0.9% Sodium Chloride Injection, or 0.45% Sodium Chloride Injection in Abbott ADD-Vantage flexible diluent containers (see Instructions for Constitution). ADD-Vantage vials that have been joined to Abbott ADD-Vantage diluent containers and activated to dissolve the drug are stable for 24 hours at room temperature or for 7 days under refrigeration. Joined vials that have not been activated may be used within a 14-day period; this period corresponds to that for use of Abbott ADD-Vantage containers following removal of the outer packaging (overwrap).

Freezing solutions of ZINACEF in the ADD-Vantage system is not recommended.

For continuous IV infusion, a solution of ZINACEF may be added to an IV infusion pack containing one of the following fluids: 0.9% Sodium Chloride Injection; 5% Dextrose Injection; 10% Dextrose Injection; 5% Dextrose and 0.9% Sodium Chloride Injection; 5% Dextrose and 0.45% Sodium Chloride Injection; or 1/6 M Sodium Lactate Injection.

Solutions of ZINACEF, like those of most beta-lactam antibiotics, should not be added to solutions of aminoglycoside antibiotics because of potential interaction.

However, if concurrent therapy with ZINACEF and an aminoglycoside is indicated, each of these antibiotics can be administered separately to the same patient.

Directions for Use of ZINACEF Frozen in Galaxy® Plastic Containers

ZINACEF supplied as a frozen, sterile, iso-osmotic, nonpyrogenic solution in plastic containers is to be administered after thawing either as a continuous or intermittent IV infusion. The thawed solution of the premixed product is stable for 28 days if stored under refrigeration (5°C) or for 24 hours if stored at room temperature (25°C). **Do not refreeze.** Thaw container at room temperature (25°C) or under refrigeration (5°C). Do not force thaw by immersion in water baths or by microwave irradiation. Components of the solution may precipitate in the frozen state and will dissolve upon reaching room temperature with little or no agitation. Potency is not affected. Mix after solution has reached room temperature. Check for minute leaks by squeezing bag firmly. Discard bag if leaks are found as sterility may be impaired. Do not add supplementary medication. Do not use unless solution is clear and seal is intact.

Use sterile equipment.

Caution

Do not use plastic containers in series connections. Such use could result in air embolism due to residual air being drawn from the primary container before administration of the fluid from the secondary container is complete.

Preparation for Administration

Suspend container from eyelet support.

Remove protector from outlet port at bottom of container.

Attach administration set. Refer to complete directions accompanying set.

COMPATIBILITY AND STABILITY

Intramuscular

When constituted as directed with Sterile Water for Injection, suspensions of ZINACEF for IM injection maintain satisfactory potency for 24 hours at room temperature and for 48 hours under refrigeration (5°C).

After the periods mentioned above any unused suspensions should be discarded.

Intravenous

When the 750-mg, 1.5-g, and 7.5-g pharmacy bulk vials are constituted as directed with Sterile Water for Injection, the solutions of ZINACEF for IV administration maintain satisfactory potency for 24 hours at room temperature and for 48 hours (750-mg and 1.5-g vials) or for 7 days (7.5-g pharmacy bulk vial) under refrigeration (5°C). More dilute solutions, such as 750 mg or 1.5 g plus 100 mL of Sterile Water for Injection, 5% Dextrose Injection, or 0.9% Sodium Chloride Injection, also maintain satisfactory potency for 24 hours at room temperature and for 7 days under refrigeration.

These solutions may be further diluted to concentrations of between 1 and 30 mg/mL in the following solutions and will lose not more than 10% activity for 24 hours at room temperature or for at least 7 days under refrigeration: 0.9% Sodium Chloride Injection; 1/6 M Sodium Lactate Injection; Ringer's Injection, USP; Lactated Ringer's Injection, USP; 5% Dextrose and 0.9% Sodium Chloride Injection; 5% Dextrose Injection; 5% Dextrose and 0.45% Sodium Chloride Injection; 5% Dextrose and 0.225% Sodium Chloride Injection; 10% Dextrose Injection; and 10% Invert Sugar in Water for Injection.

Unused solutions should be discarded after the time periods mentioned above.

ZINACEF has also been found compatible for 24 hours at room temperature when admixed in IV infusion with heparin (10 and 50 U/mL) in 0.9% Sodium Chloride Injection and Potassium Chloride (10 and 40 mEq/L) in 0.9% Sodium Chloride Injection. Sodium Bicarbonate Injection, USP is not recommended for the dilution of ZINACEF.

The 750-mg and 1.5-g ZINACEF ADD-Vantage vials, when diluted in 50 or 100 mL of 5% Dextrose Injection, 0.9% Sodium Chloride Injection, or 0.45% Sodium Chloride Injection, may be stored for up to 24 hours at room temperature or for 7 days under refrigeration.

Frozen Stability

Constitute the 750-mg, 1.5-g, or 7.5-g vial as directed for IV administration in Table 3. Immediately withdraw the total contents of the 750-mg or 1.5-g vial or 8 or 16 mL from the 7.5-g bulk vial and add to a Baxter VIAFLEX® MINI-BAG™ containing 50 or 100 mL of 0.9% Sodium Chloride Injection or 5% Dextrose Injection and freeze. Frozen solutions are stable for 6 months when stored at -20°C. Frozen solutions should be thawed at room temperature and not refrozen. Do not force thaw by immersion in water baths or by microwave irradiation. Thawed solutions may be stored for up to 24 hours at room temperature or for 7 days in a refrigerator.

Note: Parenteral drug products should be inspected visually for particulate matter and discoloration before administration whenever solution and container permit.

As with other cephalosporins, ZINACEF powder as well as solutions and suspensions tend to darken, depending on storage conditions, without adversely affecting product potency.

Directions for Dispensing

Pharmacy Bulk Package—Not for Direct Infusion

The pharmacy bulk package is for use in a pharmacy admixture service only under a laminar flow hood. Entry into the vial must be made with a sterile transfer set or other sterile dispensing device, and the contents dispensed in aliquots using aseptic technique. The use of syringe and needle is not recommended as it may cause leakage (see DOSAGE AND ADMINISTRATION). AFTER INITIAL WITHDRAWAL USE ENTIRE CONTENTS OF VIAL PROMPTLY. ANY UNUSED PORTION MUST BE DISCARDED WITHIN 24 HOURS.

HOW SUPPLIED

ZINACEF in the dry state should be stored between 15° and 30°C (59° and 86°F) and protected from light. ZINACEF is a dry, white to off-white powder supplied in vials as follows:
NDC 0173-0352-10 750-mg* Vial (Tray of 10)
NDC 0173-0354-10 1.5-g* Vial (Tray of 10)
NDC 0173-0400-00 7.5-g* Pharmacy Bulk Package (Tray of 6)
NDC 0173-0436-00 750-mg ADD-Vantage Vial (Tray of 25)
NDC 0173-0437-00 1.5-g ADD-Vantage Vial (Tray of 10)
(The above ADD-Vantage vials are to be used only with Abbott ADD-Vantage diluent containers.)
ZINACEF frozen as a premixed solution of cefuroxime injection should not be stored above -20°C. ZINACEF is supplied frozen in 50-mL, single-dose, plastic containers as follows:
NDC 0173-0424-00 750-mg* Plastic Container (Carton of 24)
NDC 0173-0425-00 1.5-g* Plastic Container (Carton of 24)
*Equivalent to cefuroxime.

REFERENCES

1. National Committee for Clinical Laboratory Standards. *Performance Standards for Antimicrobial Susceptibility Testing.* Third Informational Supplement. NCCLS Document M100-S3, Vol. 11, No. 17. Villanova, Pa: NCCLS; 1991.
2. Cockcroft DW, Gault MH. Prediction of creatinine clearance from serum creatinine. *Nephron.* 1976;16:31-41.

ZINACEF® (cefuroxime for injection):
GlaxoSmithKline
Research Triangle Park, NC 27709
ZINACEF® (cefuroxime injection):
Manufactured for GlaxoSmithKline
Research Triangle Park, NC 27709
by Baxter Healthcare Corporation, Deerfield, IL 60015
ZINACEF is a registered trademark of GlaxoSmithKline.
ADD-Vantage is a registered trademark of Abbott Laboratories.
CLINITEST is a registered trademark of Ames Division, Miles Laboratories, Inc.
GALAXY and VIAFLEX are registered trademarks of Baxter International Inc.
MINI-BAG is a trademark of Baxter International, Inc.
GlaxoSmithKline
Research Triangle Park, NC 27709
©2009, GlaxoSmithKline. All rights reserved.
November 2009   ZNF:1PI

Tear Away

ZINACEF®
(cefuroxime for injection)
Instructions for Constitution of ADD-Vantage® Vials
To Open Diluent Container:
Peel the corner of the ADD-Vantage diluent overwrap and remove flexible diluent container. Some opacity of the plastic flexible container due to moisture absorption during the sterilization process may be observed. This is normal and does not affect the solution quality or safety. The opacity will diminish gradually.

To Assemble Vial and Flexible Diluent Container (Use Aseptic Technique):
1. Remove the protective covers from the top of the vial and the vial port on the diluent container as follows:
a. To remove the breakaway vial cap, swing the pull ring over the top of the vial and pull down far enough to start the opening (see Figure 1), then pull straight up to remove the cap (see Figure 2). **Note:** Once the breakaway cap has been removed, do not access vial with syringe.
[See figure 1, 2 at top of next column]

b. To remove the vial port cover, grasp the tab on the pull ring, pull up to break the 3 tie strings, then pull back to remove the cover (see Figure 3).

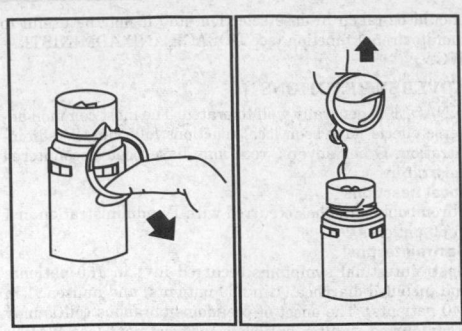

Figure 1   Figure 2

2. Screw the vial into the vial port until it will go no further. THE VIAL MUST BE SCREWED IN TIGHTLY TO ASSURE A SEAL. This occurs approximately one-half turn (180°) after the first audible click (see Figure 4). The clicking sound does not assure a seal; the vial must be turned as far as it will go. **Note:** Once vial is seated, do not attempt to remove (see Figure 4).

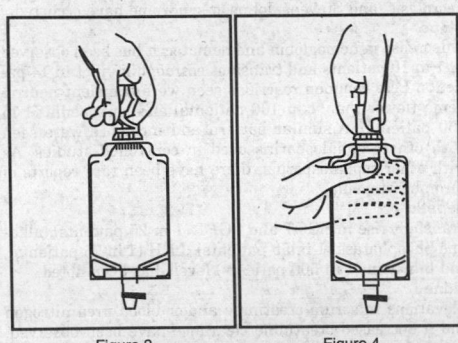

Figure 3   Figure 4

3. Recheck the vial to assure that it is tight by trying to turn it further in the direction of assembly.
4. Label appropriately.
To Prepare Admixture:
1. Squeeze the bottom of the diluent container gently to inflate the portion of the container surrounding the end of the drug vial.
2. With the other hand, push the drug vial down into the container, telescoping the walls of the container. Grasp the inner cap of the vial through the walls of the container (see Figure 5).
3. Pull the inner cap from the drug vial (see Figure 6). Verify that the rubber stopper has been pulled out, allowing the drug and diluent to mix.

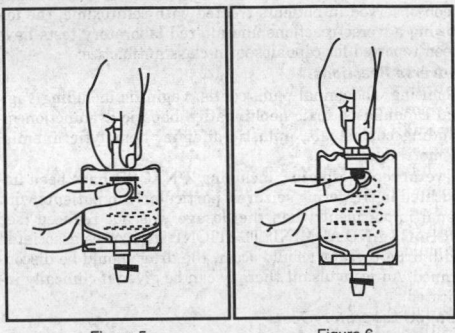

Figure 5   Figure 6

4. Mix container contents thoroughly and use within the specified time.
Preparation for Administration (Use Aseptic Technique):
1. Confirm the activation and admixture of vial contents.
2. Check for leaks by squeezing container firmly. If leaks are found, discard unit as sterility may be impaired.
3. Close flow control clamp of administration set.
4. Remove cover from outlet port at bottom of container.
5. Insert piercing pin of administration set into port with a twisting motion until the pin is firmly seated. **Note:** See full directions on administration set carton.
6. Lift the free end of the hanger loop on the bottom of the vial, breaking the 2 tie strings. Bend the loop outward to lock it in the upright position, then suspend container from hanger.
7. Squeeze and release drip chamber to establish proper fluid level in chamber.
8. Open flow control clamp and clear air from set. Close clamp.

---

9. Attach set to venipuncture device. If device is not indwelling, prime and make venipuncture.
10. Regulate rate of administration with flow control clamp.
WARNING: Do not use flexible container in series connections.
GlaxoSmithKline
Research Triangle Park, NC 27709
©2009, GlaxoSmithKline. All rights reserved.
November 2009 ZNF:1DIR

ZOFRAN®
[zō' fran]
(ondansetron hydrochloride)
Injection
℞

DESCRIPTION
The active ingredient in ZOFRAN Injection is ondansetron hydrochloride (HCl), the racemic form of ondansetron and a selective blocking agent of the serotonin 5-HT$_3$ receptor type. Chemically it is (±) 1, 2, 3, 9-tetrahydro-9-methyl-3-[(2-methyl-1H-imidazol-1-yl)methyl]-4H-carbazol-4-one, monohydrochloride, dihydrate. It has the following structural formula:

The empirical formula is C$_{18}$H$_{19}$N$_3$O•HCl•2H$_2$O, representing a molecular weight of 365.9.
Ondansetron HCl is a white to off-white powder that is soluble in water and normal saline.

Sterile Injection for Intravenous (I.V.) or Intramuscular (I.M.) Administration
Each 1 mL of aqueous solution in the 2-mL single-dose vial contains 2 mg of ondansetron as the hydrochloride dihydrate; 9.0 mg of sodium chloride, USP; and 0.5 mg of citric acid monohydrate, USP and 0.25 mg of sodium citrate dihydrate, USP as buffers in Water for Injection, USP.
Each 1 mL of aqueous solution in the 20-mL multidose vial contains 2 mg of ondansetron as the hydrochloride dihydrate; 8.3 mg of sodium chloride, USP; 0.5 mg of citric acid monohydrate, USP and 0.25 mg of sodium citrate dihydrate, USP as buffers; and 1.2 mg of methylparaben, NF and 0.15 mg of propylparaben, NF as preservatives in Water for Injection, USP.
ZOFRAN Injection is a clear, colorless, nonpyrogenic, sterile solution. The pH of the injection solution is 3.3 to 4.0.

CLINICAL PHARMACOLOGY
Pharmacodynamics
Ondansetron is a selective 5-HT$_3$ receptor antagonist. While ondansetron's mechanism of action has not been fully characterized, it is not a dopamine-receptor antagonist. Serotonin receptors of the 5-HT$_3$ type are present both peripherally on vagal nerve terminals and centrally in the chemoreceptor trigger zone of the area postrema. It is not certain whether ondansetron's antiemetic action in chemotherapy-induced nausea and vomiting is mediated centrally, peripherally, or in both sites. However, cytotoxic chemotherapy appears to be associated with release of serotonin from the enterochromaffin cells of the small intestine. In humans, urinary 5-HIAA (5-hydroxyindoleacetic acid) excretion increases after cisplatin administration in parallel with the onset of vomiting. The released serotonin may stimulate the vagal afferents through the 5-HT$_3$ receptors and initiate the vomiting reflex.
In animals, the emetic response to cisplatin can be prevented by pretreatment with an inhibitor of serotonin synthesis, bilateral abdominal vagotomy and greater splanchnic nerve section, or pretreatment with a serotonin 5-HT$_3$ receptor antagonist.
In normal volunteers, single I.V. doses of 0.15 mg/kg of ondansetron had no effect on esophageal motility, gastric motility, lower esophageal sphincter pressure, or small intestinal transit time. In another study in six normal male volunteers, a 16-mg dose infused over 5 minutes showed no effect of the drug on cardiac output, heart rate, stroke volume, blood pressure, or electrocardiogram (ECG). Multiday administration of ondansetron has been shown to slow colonic transit in normal volunteers. Ondansetron has no effect on plasma prolactin concentrations.
In a gender-balanced pharmacodynamic study (n = 56), ondansetron 4 mg administered intravenously or intramuscularly was dynamically similar in the prevention of nausea and vomiting using the ipecacuanha model of emesis.
Ondansetron does not alter the respiratory depressant effects produced by alfentanil or the degree of neuromuscular blockade produced by atracurium. Interactions with general or local anesthetics have not been studied.

Table 1. Pharmacokinetics in Normal Adult Volunteers

Age-group (years)	n	Peak Plasma Concentration (ng/mL)	Mean Elimination Half-life (h)	Plasma Clearance (L/h/kg)
19-40	11	102	3.5	0.381
61-74	12	106	4.7	0.319
≥ 75	11	170	5.5	0.262

Table 2. Pharmacokinetics in Pediatric Cancer Patients 1 Month to 18 Years of Age

Subjects and Age Group	N	CL (L/h/kg)	Vd$_{ss}$ (L/kg)	T½ (h)
		Geometric Mean		Mean
Pediatric Cancer Patients 4 to 18 years of age	N = 21	0.599	1.9	2.8
Population PK Patients[a] 1 month to 48 months of age	N = 115	0.582	3.65	4.9

[a] Population PK (Pharmacokinetic) Patients: 64% cancer patients and 36% surgery patients.

Table 3. Pharmacokinetics in Pediatric Surgery Patients 1 Month to 12 Years of Age

Subjects and Age Group	N	CL (L/h/kg)	Vd$_{ss}$ (L/kg)	T½ (h)
		Geometric Mean		Mean
Pediatric Surgery Patients 3 to 12 years of age	N = 21	0.439	1.65	2.9
Pediatric Surgery Patients 5 to 24 months of age	N = 22	0.581	2.3	2.9
Pediatric Surgery Patients 1 month to 4 months of age	N = 19	0.401	3.5	6.7

Pharmacokinetics
Ondansetron is extensively metabolized in humans, with approximately 5% of a radiolabeled dose recovered as the parent compound from the urine. The primary metabolic pathway is hydroxylation on the indole ring followed by glucuronide or sulfate conjugation.
Although some nonconjugated metabolites have pharmacologic activity, these are not found in plasma at concentrations likely to significantly contribute to the biological activity of ondansetron.
In vitro metabolism studies have shown that ondansetron is a substrate for human hepatic cytochrome P-450 enzymes, including CYP1A2, CYP2D6, and CYP3A4. In terms of overall ondansetron turnover, CYP3A4 played the predominant role. Because of the multiplicity of metabolic enzymes capable of metabolizing ondansetron, it is likely that inhibition or loss of one enzyme (e.g., CYP2D6 genetic deficiency) will be compensated by others and may result in little change in overall rates of ondansetron elimination. Ondansetron elimination may be affected by cytochrome P-450 inducers. In a pharmacokinetic study of 16 epileptic patients maintained chronically on CYP3A4 inducers, carbamazepine, or phenytoin, reduction in AUC, C$_{max}$, and T$_{1/2}$ of ondansetron was observed.[1] This resulted in a significant increase in clearance. However, on the basis of available data, no dosage adjustment for ondansetron is recommended (see PRECAUTIONS: Drug Interactions).
In humans, carmustine, etoposide, and cisplatin do not affect the pharmacokinetics of ondansetron.
In normal adult volunteers, the following mean pharmacokinetic data have been determined following a single 0.15-mg/kg I.V. dose.
[See table 1 above]
A reduction in clearance and increase in elimination half-life are seen in patients over 75 years of age. In clinical trials with cancer patients, safety and efficacy were similar in patients over 65 years of age and those under 65 years of age; there was an insufficient number of patients over 75 years of age to permit conclusions in that age-group. No dosage adjustment is recommended in the elderly.
In patients with mild-to-moderate hepatic impairment, clearance is reduced 2-fold and mean half-life is increased to 11.6 hours compared to 5.7 hours in normals. In patients with severe hepatic impairment (Child-Pugh[2] score of 10 or greater), clearance is reduced 2-fold to 3-fold and apparent volume of distribution is increased with a resultant increase in half-life to 20 hours. In patients with severe hepatic impairment, a total daily dose of 8 mg should not be exceeded.

Due to the very small contribution (5%) of renal clearance to the overall clearance, renal impairment was not expected to significantly influence the total clearance of ondansetron. However, ondansetron mean plasma clearance was reduced by about 41% in patients with severe renal impairment (creatinine clearance < 30 mL/min). This reduction in clearance is variable and was not consistent with an increase in half-life. No reduction in dose or dosing frequency in these patients is warranted.
In adult cancer patients, the mean elimination half-life was 4.0 hours, and there was no difference in the multidose pharmacokinetics over a 4-day period. In a study of 21 pediatric cancer patients (4 to 18 years of age) who received three I.V. doses of 0.15 mg/kg of ondansetron at 4-hour intervals, patients older than 15 years of age exhibited ondansetron pharmacokinetic parameters similar to those of adults. Patients 4 to 12 years of age generally showed higher clearance and somewhat larger volume of distribution than adults. Most pediatric patients younger than 15 years of age with cancer had a shorter (2.4 hours) ondansetron plasma half-life than patients older than 15 years of age. It is not known whether these differences in ondansetron plasma half-life may result in differences in efficacy between adults and some young pediatric patients (see CLINICAL TRIALS: Pediatric Studies).
Pharmacokinetic samples were collected from 74 cancer patients 6 to 48 months of age, who received a dose of 0.15 mg/kg of I.V. ondansetron every 4 hours for 3 doses during a safety and efficacy trial. These data were combined with sequential pharmacokinetics data from 41 surgery patients 1 month to 24 months of age, who received a single dose of 0.1 mg/kg of I.V. ondansetron prior to surgery with general anesthesia, and a population pharmacokinetic analysis was performed on the combined data set. The results of this analysis are included in Table 2 and are compared to the pharmacokinetic results in cancer patients 4 to 18 years of age.
[See table 2 above]
Based on the population pharmacokinetic analysis, cancer patients 6 to 48 months of age who receive a dose of 0.15 mg/kg of I.V. ondansetron every 4 hours for 3 doses would be expected to achieve a systemic exposure (AUC) consistent with the exposure achieved in previous pediatric studies in cancer patients (4 to 18 years of age) at similar doses.
In a study of 21 pediatric patients (3 to 12 years of age) who were undergoing surgery requiring anesthesia for a duration of 45 minutes to 2 hours, a single I.V. dose of

Table 4. Prevention of Chemotherapy-Induced Nausea and Vomiting in Single-Day Cisplatin Therapy[a] in Adults

	ZOFRAN Injection	Placebo	P Value[b]
Number of patients	14	14	
Treatment response			
0 Emetic episodes	2 (14%)	0 (0%)	
1-2 Emetic episodes	8 (57%)	0 (0%)	
3-5 Emetic episodes	2 (14%)	1 (7%)	
More than 5 emetic episodes/rescued	2 (14%)	13 (93%)	0.001
Median number of emetic episodes	1.5	Undefined[c]	
Median time to first emetic episode (h)	11.6	2.8	0.001
Median nausea scores (0-100)[d]	3	59	0.034
Global satisfaction with control of nausea and vomiting (0-100)[e]	96	10.5	0.009

[a] Chemotherapy was high dose (100 and 120 mg/m^2; ZOFRAN Injection n = 6, placebo n = 5) or moderate dose (50 and 80 mg/m^2; ZOFRAN Injection n = 8, placebo n = 9). Other chemotherapeutic agents included fluorouracil, doxorubicin, and cyclophosphamide. There was no difference between treatments in the types of chemotherapy that would account for differences in response.
[b] Efficacy based on "all patients treated" analysis.
[c] Median undefined since at least 50% of the patients were rescued or had more than five emetic episodes.
[d] Visual analog scale assessment of nausea: 0 = no nausea, 100 = nausea as bad as it can be.
[e] Visual analog scale assessment of satisfaction: 0 = not at all satisfied, 100 = totally satisfied.

Table 5. Prevention of Vomiting Induced by Cisplatin (≥ 100 mg/m^2) Single-Day Therapy[a] in Adults

	ZOFRAN Injection	Metoclopramide	P Value
Dose	0.15 mg/kg × 3	2 mg/kg × 6	
Number of patients in efficacy population	136	138	
Treatment response			
0 Emetic episodes	54 (40%)	41 (30%)	
1-2 Emetic episodes	34 (25%)	30 (22%)	
3-5 Emetic episodes	19 (14%)	18 (13%)	
More than 5 emetic episodes/rescued	29 (21%)	49 (36%)	
Comparison of treatments with respect to			
0 Emetic episodes	54/136	41/138	0.083
More than 5 emetic episodes/rescued	29/136	49/138	0.009
Median number of emetic episodes	1	2	0.005
Median time to first emetic episode (h)	20.5	4.3	< 0.001
Global satisfaction with control of nausea and vomiting (0-100)[b]	85	63	0.001
Acute dystonic reactions	0	8	0.005
Akathisia	0	10	0.002

[a] In addition to cisplatin, 68% of patients received other chemotherapeutic agents, including cyclophosphamide, etoposide, and fluorouracil. There was no difference between treatments in the types of chemotherapy that would account for differences in response.
[b] Visual analog scale assessment: 0 = not at all satisfied, 100 = totally satisfied.

ondansetron, 2 mg (3 to 7 years) or 4 mg (8 to 12 years), was administered immediately prior to anesthesia induction. Mean weight-normalized clearance and volume of distribution values in these pediatric surgical patients were similar to those previously reported for young adults. Mean terminal half-life was slightly reduced in pediatric patients (range, 2.5 to 3 hours) in comparison with adults (range, 3 to 3.5 hours).

In a study of 51 pediatric patients (1 month to 24 months of age) who were undergoing surgery requiring general anesthesia, a single I.V. dose of ondansetron, 0.1 or 0.2 mg/kg, was administered prior to surgery. As shown in Table 3, the 41 patients with pharmacokinetic data were divided into 2 groups, patients 1 month to 4 months of age and patients 5 to 24 months of age, and are compared to pediatric patients 3 to 12 years of age.

[See table 3 on previous page]

In general, surgical and cancer pediatric patients younger than 18 years tend to have a higher ondansetron clearance compared to adults leading to a shorter half-life in most pediatric patients. In patients 1 month to 4 months of age, a longer half-life was observed due to the higher volume of distribution in this age group.

In normal volunteers (19 to 39 years old, n = 23), the peak plasma concentration was 264 ng/mL following a single 32-mg dose administered as a 15-minute I.V. infusion. The mean elimination half-life was 4.1 hours. Systemic exposure to 32 mg of ondansetron was not proportional to dose as measured by comparing dose-normalized AUC values to an 8-mg dose. This is consistent with a small decrease in systemic clearance with increasing plasma concentrations.

A study was performed in normal volunteers (n = 56) to evaluate the pharmacokinetics of a single 4-mg dose administered as a 5-minute infusion compared to a single intramuscular injection. Systemic exposure as measured by mean AUC was equivalent, with values of 156 [95% CI 136, 180] and 161 [95% CI 137, 190] ng•h/mL for I.V. and I.M. groups, respectively. Mean peak plasma concentrations were 42.9 [95% CI 33.8, 54.4] ng/mL at 10 minutes after I.V. infusion and 31.9 [95% CI 26.3, 38.6] ng/mL at 41 minutes after I.M. injection. The mean elimination half-life was not affected by route of administration.

Plasma protein binding of ondansetron as measured in vitro was 70% to 76%, with binding constant over the pharmacologic concentration range (10 to 500 ng/mL). Circulating drug also distributes into erythrocytes.

A positive lymphoblast transformation test to ondansetron has been reported, which suggests immunologic sensitivity to ondansetron.

CLINICAL TRIALS
Chemotherapy-Induced Nausea and Vomiting
Adult Studies
In a double-blind study of three different dosing regimens of ZOFRAN Injection, 0.015 mg/kg, 0.15 mg/kg, and 0.30 mg/kg, each given three times during the course of cancer chemotherapy, the 0.15-mg/kg dosing regimen was more effective than the 0.015-mg/kg dosing regimen. The 0.30-mg/kg dosing regimen was not shown to be more effective than the 0.15-mg/kg dosing regimen.

Cisplatin-Based Chemotherapy
In a double-blind study in 28 patients, ZOFRAN Injection (three 0.15-mg/kg doses) was significantly more effective than placebo in preventing nausea and vomiting induced by cisplatin-based chemotherapy. Treatment response was as shown in Table 4.

[See table 4 at left]

Ondansetron was compared with metoclopramide in a single-blind trial in 307 patients receiving cisplatin ≥ 100 mg/m^2 with or without other chemotherapeutic agents. Patients received the first dose of ondansetron or metoclopramide 30 minutes before cisplatin. Two additional ondansetron doses were administered 4 and 8 hours later, or five additional metoclopramide doses were administered 2, 4, 7, 10, and 13 hours later. Cisplatin was administered over a period of 3 hours or less. Episodes of vomiting and retching were tabulated over the period of 24 hours after cisplatin. The results of this study are summarized in Table 5.

[See table 5 at left]

In a stratified, randomized, double-blind, parallel-group, multicenter study, a single 32-mg dose of ondansetron was compared with three 0.15-mg/kg doses in patients receiving cisplatin doses of either 50 to 70 mg/m^2 or ≥ 100 mg/m^2. Patients received the first ondansetron dose 30 minutes before cisplatin. Two additional ondansetron doses were administered 4 and 8 hours later to the group receiving three 0.15-mg/kg doses. In both strata, significantly fewer patients on the single 32-mg dose than those receiving the three-dose regimen failed.

[See table 6 at top of next page]

Cyclophosphamide-Based Chemotherapy
In a double-blind, placebo-controlled study of ZOFRAN Injection (three 0.15-mg/kg doses) in 20 patients receiving cyclophosphamide (500 to 600 mg/m^2) chemotherapy, ZOFRAN Injection was significantly more effective than placebo in preventing nausea and vomiting. The results are summarized in Table 7.

[See table 7 on next page]

Re-treatment
In uncontrolled trials, 127 patients receiving cisplatin (median dose, 100 mg/m^2) and ondansetron who had two or fewer emetic episodes were re-treated with ondansetron and chemotherapy, mainly cisplatin, for a total of 269 re-treatment courses (median, 2; range, 1 to 10). No emetic episodes occurred in 160 (59%), and two or fewer emetic episodes occurred in 217 (81%) re-treatment courses.

Pediatric Studies
Four open-label, noncomparative (one US, three foreign) trials have been performed with 209 pediatric cancer patients 4 to 18 years of age given a variety of cisplatin or noncisplatin regimens. In the three foreign trials, the initial ZOFRAN Injection dose ranged from 0.04 to 0.87 mg/kg for a total dose of 2.16 to 12 mg. This was followed by the oral administration of ondansetron ranging from 4 to 24 mg daily for 3 days. In the US trial, ZOFRAN was administered intravenously (only) in three doses of 0.15 mg/kg each for a total daily dose of 7.2 to 39 mg. In these studies, 58% of the 196 evaluable patients had a complete response (no emetic episodes) on day 1. Thus, prevention of vomiting in these pediatric patients was essentially the same as for patients older than 18 years of age.

An open-label, multicenter, noncomparative trial has been performed in 75 pediatric cancer patients 6 to 48 months of age receiving at least one moderately or highly emetogenic chemotherapeutic agent. Fifty-seven percent (57%) were females; 67% were white, 18% were American Hispanic, and 15% were black patients. ZOFRAN was administered intravenously over 15 minutes in three doses of 0.15 mg/kg. The first dose was administered 30 minutes before the start of chemotherapy, the second and third doses were administered 4 and 8 hours after the first dose, respectively. Eighteen patients (25%) received routine prophylactic dexamethasone (i.e., not given as rescue). Of the 75 evaluable patients, 56% had a complete response (no emetic episodes) on day 1. Thus, prevention of vomiting in these pediatric patients was comparable to the prevention of vomiting in patients 4 years of age and older.

Postoperative Nausea and Vomiting: Prevention of Postoperative Nausea and Vomiting
Adult Studies
Adult surgical patients who received ondansetron immediately before the induction of general balanced anesthesia (barbiturate: thiopental, methohexital, or thiamylal; opioid: alfentanil or fentanyl; nitrous oxide; neuromuscular blockade: succinylcholine/curare and/or vecuronium or atracurium; and supplemental isoflurane) were evaluated in two double-blind US studies involving 554 patients. ZOFRAN

Injection (4 mg) I.V. given over 2 to 5 minutes was significantly more effective than placebo. The results of these studies are summarized in Table 8.
[See table 8 at top of next page]
The study populations in Table 8 consisted mainly of females undergoing laparoscopic procedures.

In a placebo-controlled study conducted in 468 males undergoing outpatient procedures, a single 4-mg I.V. ondansetron dose prevented postoperative vomiting over a 24-hour study period in 79% of males receiving drug compared to 63% of males receiving placebo ($P < 0.001$).

Two other placebo-controlled studies were conducted in 2,792 patients undergoing major abdominal or gynecological surgeries to evaluate a single 4-mg or 8-mg I.V. ondansetron dose for prevention of postoperative nausea and vomiting over a 24-hour study period. At the 4-mg dosage, 59% of patients receiving ondansetron versus 45% receiving placebo in the first study ($P < 0.001$) and 41% of patients receiving ondansetron versus 30% receiving placebo in the second study ($P = 0.001$) experienced no emetic episodes. No additional benefit was observed in patients who received I.V. ondansetron 8 mg compared to patients who received I.V. ondansetron 4 mg.

Pediatric Studies
Three double-blind, placebo-controlled studies have been performed (one US, two foreign) in 1,049 male and female patients (2 to 12 years of age) undergoing general anesthesia with nitrous oxide. The surgical procedures included tonsillectomy with or without adenoidectomy, strabismus surgery, herniorrhaphy, and orchidopexy. Patients were randomized to either single I.V. doses of ondansetron (0.1 mg/kg for pediatric patients weighing 40 kg or less, 4 mg for pediatric patients weighing more than 40 kg) or placebo. Study drug was administered over at least 30 seconds, immediately prior to or following anesthesia induction. Ondansetron was significantly more effective than placebo in preventing nausea and vomiting. The results of these studies are summarized in Table 9.
[See table 9 on next page]
A double-blind, multicenter, placebo-controlled study was conducted in 670 pediatric patients 1 month to 24 months of age who were undergoing routine surgery under general anesthesia. Seventy-five percent (75%) were males; 64% were white, 15% were black, 13% were American Hispanic, 2% were Asian, and 6% were "other race" patients. A single 0.1-mg/kg I.V. dose of ondansetron administered within 5 minutes following induction of anesthesia was statistically significantly more effective than placebo in preventing vomiting. In the placebo group, 28% of patients experienced vomiting compared to 11% of subjects who received ondansetron ($P \leq 0.01$). Overall, 32 (10%) of placebo patients and 18 (5%) of patients who received ondansetron received antiemetic rescue medication(s) or prematurely withdrew from the study.

Prevention of Further Postoperative Nausea and Vomiting
Adult Studies
Adult surgical patients receiving general balanced anesthesia (barbiturate: thiopental, methohexital, or thiamylal; opioid: alfentanil or fentanyl; nitrous oxide; neuromuscular blockade: succinylcholine/curare and/or vecuronium or atracurium; and supplemental isoflurane) who received no prophylactic antiemetics and who experienced nausea and/or vomiting within 2 hours postoperatively were evaluated in two double-blind US studies involving 441 patients. Patients who experienced an episode of postoperative nausea and/or vomiting were given ZOFRAN Injection (4 mg) I.V. over 2 to 5 minutes, and this was significantly more effective than placebo. The results of these studies are summarized in Table 10.
[See table 10 at top of page 1645]
The study populations in Table 10 consisted mainly of women undergoing laparoscopic procedures.

Repeat Dosing in Adults
In patients who do not achieve adequate control of postoperative nausea and vomiting following a single, prophylactic, preinduction, I.V. dose of ondansetron 4 mg, administration of a second I.V. dose of ondansetron 4 mg postoperatively does not provide additional control of nausea and vomiting.

Pediatric Study
One double-blind, placebo-controlled, US study was performed in 351 male and female outpatients (2 to 12 years of age) who received general anesthesia with nitrous oxide and no prophylactic antiemetics. Surgical procedures were unrestricted. Patients who experienced two or more emetic episodes within 2 hours following discontinuation of nitrous oxide were randomized to either single I.V. doses of ondansetron (0.1 mg/kg for pediatric patients weighing 40 kg or less, 4 mg for pediatric patients weighing more than 40 kg) or placebo administered over at least 30 seconds. Ondansetron was significantly more effective than

Table 6. Prevention of Chemotherapy-Induced Nausea and Vomiting in Single-Dose Therapy in Adults

	Ondansetron Dose		
	0.15 mg/kg × 3	32 mg × 1	P Value
High-dose cisplatin ($\geq$ 100 mg/m^2)			
Number of patients	100	102	
Treatment response			
0 Emetic episodes	41 (41%)	49 (48%)	0.315
1-2 Emetic episodes	19 (19%)	25 (25%)	
3-5 Emetic episodes	4 (4%)	8 (8%)	
More than 5 emetic episodes/rescued	36 (36%)	20 (20%)	0.009
Median time to first emetic episode (h)	21.7	23	0.173
Median nausea scores (0-100)[a]	28	13	0.004
Medium-dose cisplatin (50-70 mg/m^2)			
Number of patients	101	93	
Treatment response			
0 Emetic episodes	62 (61%)	68 (73%)	0.083
1-2 Emetic episodes	11 (11%)	14 (15%)	
3-5 Emetic episodes	6 (6%)	3 (3%)	
More than 5 emetic episodes/rescued	22 (22%)	8 (9%)	0.011
Median time to first emetic episode (h)	Undefined[b]	Undefined	
Median nausea scores (0-100)[a]	9	3	0.131

[a] Visual analog scale assessment: 0 = no nausea, 100 = nausea as bad as it can be.
[b] Median undefined since at least 50% of patients did not have any emetic episodes.

Table 7. Prevention of Chemotherapy-Induced Nausea and Vomiting in Single-Day Cyclophosphamide Therapy[a] in Adults

	ZOFRAN Injection	Placebo	P Value[b]
Number of patients	10	10	
Treatment response			
0 Emetic episodes	7 (70%)	0 (0%)	0.001
1-2 Emetic episodes	0 (0%)	2 (20%)	
3-5 Emetic episodes	2 (20%)	4 (40%)	
More than 5 emetic episodes/rescued	1 (10%)	4 (40%)	0.131
Median number of emetic episodes	0	4	0.008
Median time to first emetic episode (h)	Undefined[c]	8.79	
Median nausea scores (0-100)[d]	0	60	0.001
Global satisfaction with control of nausea and vomiting (0-100)[e]	100	52	0.008

[a] Chemotherapy consisted of cyclophosphamide in all patients, plus other agents, including fluorouracil, doxorubicin, methotrexate, and vincristine. There was no difference between treatments in the type of chemotherapy that would account for differences in response.
[b] Efficacy based on "all patients treated" analysis.
[c] Median undefined since at least 50% of patients did not have any emetic episodes.
[d] Visual analog scale assessment of nausea: 0 = no nausea, 100 = nausea as bad as it can be.
[e] Visual analog scale assessment of satisfaction: 0 = not at all satisfied, 100 = totally satisfied.

placebo in preventing further episodes of nausea and vomiting. The results of the study are summarized in Table 11.
[See table 11 on page 1645]

INDICATIONS AND USAGE
1. Prevention of nausea and vomiting associated with initial and repeat courses of emetogenic cancer chemotherapy, including high-dose cisplatin. Efficacy of the 32-mg single dose beyond 24 hours in these patients has not been established.
2. Prevention of postoperative nausea and/or vomiting. As with other antiemetics, routine prophylaxis is not recommended for patients in whom there is little expectation that nausea and/or vomiting will occur postoperatively. In patients where nausea and/or vomiting must be avoided postoperatively, ZOFRAN Injection is recommended even where the incidence of postoperative nausea and/or vomiting is low. For patients who do not receive prophylactic ZOFRAN Injection and experience nausea and/or vomiting postoperatively, ZOFRAN Injection may be given to prevent further episodes (see CLINICAL TRIALS).

CONTRAINDICATIONS
The concomitant use of apomorphine with ondansetron is contraindicated based on reports of profound hypotension and loss of consciousness when apomorphine was administered with ondansetron.

ZOFRAN Injection is contraindicated for patients known to have hypersensitivity to the drug.

WARNINGS
Hypersensitivity reactions have been reported in patients who have exhibited hypersensitivity to other selective 5-HT$_3$ receptor antagonists.

PRECAUTIONS
General
Ondansetron is not a drug that stimulates gastric or intestinal peristalsis. It should not be used instead of nasogastric suction. The use of ondansetron in patients following abdominal surgery or in patients with chemotherapy-induced nausea and vomiting may mask a progressive ileus and/or gastric distention.

Rarely and predominantly with intravenous ondansetron, transient ECG changes including QT interval prolongation have been reported.

Drug Interactions
Ondansetron does not itself appear to induce or inhibit the cytochrome P-450 drug-metabolizing enzyme system of the liver (see CLINICAL PHARMACOLOGY: Pharmacokinetics). Because ondansetron is metabolized by hepatic cytochrome P-450 drug-metabolizing enzymes (CYP3A4, CYP2D6, CYP1A2), inducers or inhibitors of these enzymes may change the clearance and, hence, the half-life of

Table 8. Prevention of Postoperative Nausea and Vomiting in Adult Patients

	Ondansetron 4 mg I.V.	Placebo	P Value
Study 1			
Emetic episodes:			
Number of patients	136	139	
Treatment response over 24-h postoperative period			
0 Emetic episodes	103 (76%)	64 (46%)	< 0.001
1 Emetic episode	13 (10%)	17 (12%)	
More than 1 emetic episode/rescued	20 (15%)	58 (42%)	
Nausea assessments:			
Number of patients	134	136	
No nausea over 24-h postoperative period	56 (42%)	39 (29%)	
Study 2			
Emetic episodes:			
Number of patients	136	143	
Treatment response over 24-h postoperative period			
0 Emetic episodes	85 (63%)	63 (44%)	0.002
1 Emetic episode	16 (12%)	29 (20%)	
More than 1 emetic episode/rescued	35 (26%)	51 (36%)	
Nausea assessments:			
Number of patients	125	133	
No nausea over 24-h postoperative period	48 (38%)	42 (32%)	

Table 9. Prevention of Postoperative Nausea and Vomiting in Pediatric Patients 2 to 12 Years of Age

Treatment Response Over 24 Hours	Ondansetron n (%)	Placebo n (%)	P Value
Study 1			
Number of patients	205	210	
0 Emetic episodes	140 (68%)	82 (39%)	≤ 0.001
Failure[a]	65 (32%)	128 (61%)	
Study 2			
Number of patients	112	110	
0 Emetic episodes	68 (61%)	38 (35%)	≤ 0.001
Failure[a]	44 (39%)	72 (65%)	
Study 3			
Number of patients	206	206	
0 Emetic episodes	123 (60%)	96 (47%)	≤ 0.01
Failure[a]	83 (40%)	110 (53%)	
Nausea assessments[b]:			
Number of patients	185	191	
None	119 (64%)	99 (52%)	≤ 0.01

[a] Failure was one or more emetic episodes, rescued, or withdrawn.
[b] Nausea measured as none, mild, or severe.

ondansetron. On the basis of limited available data, no dosage adjustment is recommended for patients on these drugs.

Apomorphine
Based on reports of profound hypotension and loss of consciousness when apomorphine was administered with ondansetron, concomitant use of apomorphine with ondansetron is contraindicated (see CONTRAINDICATIONS).

Phenytoin, Carbamazepine, and Rifampicin
In patients treated with potent inducers of CYP3A4 (i.e., phenytoin, carbamazepine, and rifampicin), the clearance of ondansetron was significantly increased and ondansetron blood concentrations were decreased. However, on the basis of available data, no dosage adjustment for ondansetron is recommended for patients on these drugs.[1,3]

Tramadol
Although no pharmacokinetic drug interaction between ondansetron and tramadol has been observed, data from 2 small studies indicate that ondansetron may be associated with an increase in patient controlled administration of tramadol.[4,5]

Chemotherapy
Tumor response to chemotherapy in the P 388 mouse leukemia model is not affected by ondansetron. In humans, carmustine, etoposide, and cisplatin do not affect the pharmacokinetics of ondansetron.
In a crossover study in 76 pediatric patients, I.V. ondansetron did not increase blood levels of high-dose methotrexate.

Carcinogenesis, Mutagenesis, Impairment of Fertility
Carcinogenic effects were not seen in 2-year studies in rats and mice with oral ondansetron doses up to 10 and 30 mg/kg per day, respectively. Ondansetron was not mutagenic in standard tests for mutagenicity. Oral administration of ondansetron up to 15 mg/kg per day did not affect fertility or general reproductive performance of male and female rats.

Pregnancy
Teratogenic Effects
Pregnancy Category B. Reproduction studies have been performed in pregnant rats and rabbits at I.V. doses up to 4 mg/kg per day and have revealed no evidence of impaired fertility or harm to the fetus due to ondansetron. There are, however, no adequate and well-controlled studies in pregnant women. Because animal reproduction studies are not always predictive of human response, this drug should be used during pregnancy only if clearly needed.

Nursing Mothers
Ondansetron is excreted in the breast milk of rats. It is not known whether ondansetron is excreted in human milk. Because many drugs are excreted in human milk, caution should be exercised when ondansetron is administered to a nursing woman.

Pediatric Use
Little information is available about the use of ondansetron in pediatric surgical patients younger than 1 month of age. (See CLINICAL TRIALS section for studies of ondansetron in prevention of postoperative nausea and vomiting in pa-

tients 1 month of age and older.) Little information is available about the use of ondansetron in pediatric cancer patients younger than 6 months of age. (See CLINICAL TRIALS section for studies of ondansetron in chemotherapy-induced nausea and vomiting in pediatric patients 6 months of age and older.) (See DOSAGE AND ADMINISTRATION.)
The clearance of ondansetron in pediatric patients 1 month to 4 months of age is slower and the half-life is ~2.5 fold longer than patients who are > 4 to 24 months of age. As a precaution, it is recommended that patients less than 4 months of age receiving this drug be closely monitored. (See CLINICAL PHARMACOLOGY: Pharmacokinetics.)
The frequency and type of adverse events reported in pediatric patients receiving ondansetron were similar to those in patients receiving placebo. (See ADVERSE EVENTS.)

Geriatric Use
Of the total number of subjects enrolled in cancer chemotherapy-induced and postoperative nausea and vomiting in US- and foreign-controlled clinical trials, 862 were 65 years of age and over. No overall differences in safety or effectiveness were observed between these subjects and younger subjects, and other reported clinical experience has not identified differences in responses between the elderly and younger patients, but greater sensitivity of some older individuals cannot be ruled out. Dosage adjustment is not needed in patients over the age of 65 (see CLINICAL PHARMACOLOGY).

ADVERSE REACTIONS
Chemotherapy-Induced Nausea and Vomiting
The adverse events in Table 12 have been reported in adults receiving ondansetron at a dosage of three 0.15-mg/kg doses or as a single 32-mg dose in clinical trials. These patients were receiving concomitant chemotherapy, primarily cisplatin, and I.V. fluids. Most were receiving a diuretic.
[See table 12 on next page]
The following have been reported during controlled clinical trials:

Cardiovascular
Rare cases of angina (chest pain), electrocardiographic alterations, hypotension, and tachycardia have been reported. In many cases, the relationship to ZOFRAN Injection was unclear.

Gastrointestinal
Constipation has been reported in 11% of chemotherapy patients receiving multiday ondansetron.

Hepatic
In comparative trials in cisplatin chemotherapy patients with normal baseline values of aspartate transaminase (AST) and alanine transaminase (ALT), these enzymes have been reported to exceed twice the upper limit of normal in approximately 5% of patients. The increases were transient and did not appear to be related to dose or duration of therapy. On repeat exposure, similar transient elevations in transaminase values occurred in some courses, but symptomatic hepatic disease did not occur.

Integumentary
Rash has occurred in approximately 1% of patients receiving ondansetron.

Neurological
There have been rare reports consistent with, but not diagnostic of, extrapyramidal reactions in patients receiving ZOFRAN Injection, and rare cases of grand mal seizure. The relationship to ZOFRAN was unclear.

Other
Rare cases of hypokalemia have been reported. The relationship to ZOFRAN Injection was unclear.

Postoperative Nausea and Vomiting
The adverse events in Table 13 have been reported in ≥ 2% of adults receiving ondansetron at a dosage of 4 mg I.V. over 2 to 5 minutes in clinical trials. Rates of these events were not significantly different in the ondansetron and placebo groups. These patients were receiving multiple concomitant perioperative and postoperative medications.
[See table 13 at top of page 1646]

Pediatric Use
The adverse events in Table 14 were the most commonly reported adverse events in pediatric patients receiving ondansetron (a single 0.1-mg/kg dose for pediatric patients weighing 40 kg or less, or 4 mg for pediatric patients weighing more than 40 kg) administered intravenously over at least 30 seconds. Rates of these events were not significantly different in the ondansetron and placebo groups. These patients were receiving multiple concomitant perioperative and postoperative medications.
[See table 14 on page 1646]
The adverse events in Table 15 were the most commonly reported adverse events in pediatric patients, 1 month to 24 months of age, receiving a single 0.1-mg/kg I.V. dose of ondansetron. The incidence and type of adverse events were similar in both the ondansetron and placebo groups. These patients were receiving multiple concomitant perioperative and postoperative medications.

[See table 15 on next page]

Observed During Clinical Practice

In addition to adverse events reported from clinical trials, the following events have been identified during post-approval use of intravenous formulations of ZOFRAN. Because they are reported voluntarily from a population of unknown size, estimates of frequency cannot be made. The events have been chosen for inclusion due to a combination of their seriousness, frequency of reporting, or potential causal connection to ZOFRAN.

Cardiovascular

Arrhythmias (including ventricular and supraventricular tachycardia, premature ventricular contractions, and atrial fibrillation), bradycardia, electrocardiographic alterations (including second-degree heart block, QT interval prolongation, and ST segment depression), palpitations, and syncope.

General

Flushing. Rare cases of hypersensitivity reactions, sometimes severe (e.g., anaphylaxis/anaphylactoid reactions, angioedema, bronchospasm, cardiopulmonary arrest, hypotension, laryngeal edema, laryngospasm, shock, shortness of breath, stridor) have also been reported.

Hepatobiliary

Liver enzyme abnormalities have been reported. Liver failure and death have been reported in patients with cancer receiving concurrent medications including potentially hepatotoxic cytotoxic chemotherapy and antibiotics. The etiology of the liver failure is unclear.

Local Reactions

Pain, redness, and burning at site of injection.

Lower Respiratory

Hiccups

Neurological

Oculogyric crisis, appearing alone, as well as with other dystonic reactions.

Skin

Urticaria

Special Senses

Transient dizziness during or shortly after I.V. infusion.

Eye Disorders

Transient blurred vision, in some cases associated with abnormalities of accommodation. Cases of transient blindness, predominantly during intravenous administration, have been reported. These cases of transient blindness were reported to resolve within a few minutes up to 48 hours.

DRUG ABUSE AND DEPENDENCE

Animal studies have shown that ondansetron is not discriminated as a benzodiazepine nor does it substitute for benzodiazepines in direct addiction studies.

OVERDOSAGE

There is no specific antidote for ondansetron overdose. Patients should be managed with appropriate supportive therapy. Individual doses as large as 150 mg and total daily dosages (three doses) as large as 252 mg have been administered intravenously without significant adverse events. These doses are more than 10 times the recommended daily dose.

In addition to the adverse events listed above, the following events have been described in the setting of ondansetron overdose: "Sudden blindness" (amaurosis) of 2 to 3 minutes' duration plus severe constipation occurred in one patient that was administered 72 mg of ondansetron intravenously as a single dose. Hypotension (and faintness) occurred in another patient that took 48 mg of oral ondansetron. Following infusion of 32 mg over only a 4-minute period, a vasovagal episode with transient second-degree heart block was observed. In all instances, the events resolved completely.

DOSAGE AND ADMINISTRATION

Prevention of Chemotherapy-Induced Nausea and Vomiting

Adult Dosing

The recommended I.V. dosage of ZOFRAN for adults is a single 32-mg dose or three 0.15-mg/kg doses. A single 32-mg dose is infused over 15 minutes beginning 30 minutes before the start of emetogenic chemotherapy. The recommended infusion rate should not be exceeded (see OVERDOSAGE). With the three-dose (0.15-mg/kg) regimen, the first dose is infused over 15 minutes beginning 30 minutes before the start of emetogenic chemotherapy. Subsequent doses (0.15 mg/kg) are administered 4 and 8 hours after the first dose of ZOFRAN.

ZOFRAN Injection should not be mixed with solutions for which physical and chemical compatibility have not been established. In particular, this applies to alkaline solutions as a precipitate may form.

Vial

DILUTE BEFORE USE FOR PREVENTION OF CHEMOTHERAPY-INDUCED NAUSEA AND VOMITING.

ZOFRAN Injection should be diluted in 50 mL of 5% Dextrose Injection or 0.9% Sodium Chloride Injection before administration.

Pediatric Dosing

On the basis of the available information (see CLINICAL TRIALS: Pediatric Studies and CLINICAL PHARMACOLOGY: Pharmacokinetics), the dosage in pediatric cancer patients 6 months to 18 years of age should be three 0.15-mg/kg doses. The first dose is to be administered 30 minutes before the start of moderately to highly emetogenic chemotherapy, subsequent doses (0.15 mg/kg) are administered 4 and 8 hours after the first dose of ZOFRAN. The drug should be infused intravenously over 15 minutes. Little information is available about dosage in pediatric cancer patients younger than 6 months of age.

Vial

DILUTE BEFORE USE FOR PREVENTION OF CHEMOTHERAPY-INDUCED NAUSEA AND VOMITING.

ZOFRAN Injection should be diluted in 50 mL of 5% Dextrose Injection or 0.9% Sodium Chloride Injection before administration.

Geriatric Dosing

The dosage recommendation is the same as for the general population.

Prevention of Postoperative Nausea and Vomiting

Adult Dosing

The recommended I.V. dosage of ZOFRAN for adults is 4 mg **undiluted** administered intravenously in not less than 30 seconds, preferably over 2 to 5 minutes, immediately before induction of anesthesia, or postoperatively if the patient experiences nausea and/or vomiting occurring shortly after surgery. Alternatively, 4 mg **undiluted** may be administered intramuscularly as a single injection for adults. While recommended as a fixed dose for patients weighing more than 40 kg, few patients above 80 kg have been studied. In patients who do not achieve adequate control of postoperative nausea and vomiting following a single, prophylactic, preinduction, I.V. dose of ondansetron 4 mg, administration of a second I.V. dose of 4 mg ondansetron postoperatively does not provide additional control of nausea and vomiting.

Vial

REQUIRES NO DILUTION FOR ADMINISTRATION FOR POSTOPERATIVE NAUSEA AND VOMITING.

Table 10. Prevention of Further Postoperative Nausea and Vomiting in Adult Patients

	Ondansetron 4 mg I.V.	Placebo	P Value
Study 1			
Emetic episodes:			
Number of patients	104	117	
Treatment response 24 h after study drug			
0 Emetic episodes	49 (47%)	19 (16%)	<0.001
1 Emetic episode	12 (12%)	9 (8%)	
More than 1 emetic episode/rescued	43 (41%)	89 (76%)	
Median time to first emetic episode (min)[a]	55.0	43.0	
Nausea assessments:			
Number of patients	98	102	
Mean nausea score over 24-h postoperative period[b]	1.7	3.1	
Study 2			
Emetic episodes:			
Number of patients	112	108	
Treatment response 24 h after study drug			
0 Emetic episodes	49 (44%)	28 (26%)	0.006
1 Emetic episode	14 (13%)	3 (3%)	
More than 1 emetic episode/rescued	49 (44%)	77 (71%)	
Median time to first emetic episode (min)[a]	60.5	34.0	
Nausea assessments:			
Number of patients	105	85	
Mean nausea score over 24-h postoperative period[b]	1.9	2.9	

[a] After administration of study drug.

[b] Nausea measured on a scale of 0-10 with 0 = no nausea, 10 = nausea as bad as it can be.

Table 11. Prevention of Further Postoperative Nausea and Vomiting in Pediatric Patients 2 to 12 Years of Age

Treatment Response Over 24 Hours	Ondansetron n (%)	Placebo n (%)	P Value
Number of patients	180	171	
0 Emetic episodes	96 (53%)	29 (17%)	≤0.001
Failure[a]	84 (47%)	142 (83%)	

[a] Failure was one or more emetic episodes, rescued, or withdrawn.

Table 12. Principal Adverse Events in Comparative Trials in Adults

	Number of Adult Patients With Event			
	ZOFRAN Injection 0.15 mg/kg × 3 n = 419	ZOFRAN Injection 32 mg × 1 n = 220	Metoclopramide n = 156	Placebo n = 34
Diarrhea	16%	8%	44%	18%
Headache	17%	25%	7%	15%
Fever	8%	7%	5%	3%
Akathisia	0%	0%	6%	0%
Acute dystonic reactions[a]	0%	0%	5%	0%

[a] See Neurological.

Table 13. Adverse Events in ≥ 2% of Adults Receiving Ondansetron at a Dosage of 4 mg I.V. over 2 to 5 Minutes in Clinical Trials

	ZOFRAN Injection 4 mg I.V. n = 547 patients	Placebo n = 547 patients
Headache	92 (17%)	77 (14%)
Dizziness	67 (12%)	88 (16%)
Musculoskeletal pain	57 (10%)	59 (11%)
Drowsiness/sedation	44 (8%)	37 (7%)
Shivers	38 (7%)	39 (7%)
Malaise/fatigue	25 (5%)	30 (5%)
Injection site reaction	21 (4%)	18 (3%)
Urinary retention	17 (3%)	15 (3%)
Postoperative CO_2-related pain[a]	12 (2%)	16 (3%)
Chest pain (unspecified)	12 (2%)	15 (3%)
Anxiety/agitation	11 (2%)	16 (3%)
Dysuria	11 (2%)	9 (2%)
Hypotension	10 (2%)	12 (2%)
Fever	10 (2%)	6 (1%)
Cold sensation	9 (2%)	8 (1%)
Pruritus	9 (2%)	3 (< 1%)
Paresthesia	9 (2%)	2 (< 1%)

[a] Sites of pain included abdomen, stomach, joints, rib cage, shoulder.

Table 14. Frequency of Adverse Events From Controlled Studies in Pediatric Patients 2 to 12 Years of Age

Adverse Event	Ondansetron n = 755 Patients	Placebo n = 731 Patients
Wound problem	80 (11%)	86 (12%)
Anxiety/agitation	49 (6%)	47 (6%)
Headache	44 (6%)	43 (6%)
Drowsiness/sedation	41 (5%)	56 (8%)
Pyrexia	32 (4%)	41 (6%)

Table 15. Frequency of Adverse Events (Greater Than or Equal to 2% in Either Treatment Group) in Pediatric Patients 1 Month to 24 Months of Age

Adverse Event	Ondansetron n = 336 Patients	Placebo n = 334 Patients
Pyrexia	14 (4%)	14 (4%)
Bronchospasm	2 (< 1%)	6 (2%)
Post-procedural pain	4 (1%)	6 (2%)
Diarrhea	6 (2%)	3 (< 1%)

Pediatric Dosing
The recommended I.V. dosage of ZOFRAN for pediatric surgical patients (1 month to 12 years of age) is a single 0.1-mg/kg dose for patients weighing 40 kg or less, or a single 4-mg dose for patients weighing more than 40 kg. The rate of administration should not be less than 30 seconds, preferably over 2 to 5 minutes immediately prior to or following anesthesia induction, or postoperatively if the patient experiences nausea and/or vomiting occurring shortly after surgery. Prevention of further nausea and vomiting was only studied in patients who had not received prophylactic ZOFRAN.

Vial
REQUIRES NO DILUTION FOR ADMINISTRATION FOR POSTOPERATIVE NAUSEA AND VOMITING.

Geriatric Dosing
The dosage recommendation is the same as for the general population.

Dosage Adjustment for Patients With Impaired Renal Function
The dosage recommendation is the same as for the general population. There is no experience beyond first-day administration of ondansetron.

Dosage Adjustment for Patients With Impaired Hepatic Function
In patients with severe hepatic impairment (Child-Pugh[2] score of 10 or greater), a single maximal daily dose of 8 mg to be infused over 15 minutes beginning 30 minutes before the start of the emetogenic chemotherapy is recommended. There is no experience beyond first-day administration of ondansetron.

Stability
ZOFRAN Injection is stable at room temperature under normal lighting conditions for 48 hours after dilution with the following I.V. fluids: 0.9% Sodium Chloride Injection, 5% Dextrose Injection, 5% Dextrose and 0.9% Sodium Chloride Injection, 5% Dextrose and 0.45% Sodium Chloride Injection, and 3% Sodium Chloride Injection.

Although ZOFRAN Injection is chemically and physically stable when diluted as recommended, sterile precautions should be observed because diluents generally do not contain preservative. After dilution, do not use beyond 24 hours.

Note: Parenteral drug products should be inspected visually for particulate matter and discoloration before administration whenever solution and container permit.

Precaution: Occasionally, ondansetron precipitates at the stopper/vial interface in vials stored upright. Potency and safety are not affected. If a precipitate is observed, resolubilize by shaking the vial vigorously.

HOW SUPPLIED
ZOFRAN Injection, 2 mg/mL, is supplied as follows:
NDC 0173-0442-02   2-mL single-dose vials (Carton of 5)
NDC 0173-0442-00   20-mL multidose vials (Singles)
Store between 2° and 30°C (36° and 86°F). Protect from light.

REFERENCES
1. Britto MR, Hussey EK, Mydlow P, et al. Effect of enzyme inducers on ondansetron (OND) metabolism in humans. *Clin Pharmacol Ther.* 1997;61:228.
2. Pugh RNH, Murray-Lyon IM, Dawson JL, Pietroni MC, Williams R. Transection of the oesophagus for bleeding oesophageal varices. *Brit J Surg.* 1973;60:646-649.
3. Villikka K, Kivisto KT, Neuvonen PJ. The effect of rifampin on the pharmacokinetics of oral and intravenous ondansetron. *Clin Pharmacol Ther.* 1999;65: 377-381.
4. De Witte JL, Schoenmaekers B, Sessler DI, et al. *Anesth Analg.* 2001;92:1319-1321.
5. Arcioni R, della Rocca M, Romanò R, et al. *Anesth Analg.* 2002;94:1553-1557.

GlaxoSmithKline
Research Triangle Park, NC 27709
©2010, GlaxoSmithKline. All rights reserved.
May 2010
ZFJ:2PI

ZOFRAN® ℞
[zō'fran]
(ondansetron hydrochloride)
Tablets
ZOFRAN ODT® ℞
(ondansetron)
Orally Disintegrating Tablets
ZOFRAN® ℞
(ondansetron hydrochloride)
Oral Solution

DESCRIPTION
The active ingredient in ZOFRAN Tablets and ZOFRAN Oral Solution is ondansetron hydrochloride (HCl) as the dihydrate, the racemic form of ondansetron and a selective blocking agent of the serotonin 5-HT$_3$ receptor type. Chemically it is (±) 1, 2, 3, 9-tetrahydro-9-methyl-3-[(2-methyl-1H-imidazol-1-yl)methyl]-4H-carbazol-4-one, monohydrochloride, dihydrate. It has the following structural formula:

The empirical formula is $C_{18}H_{19}N_3O \cdot HCl \cdot 2H_2O$, representing a molecular weight of 365.9.

Ondansetron HCl dihydrate is a white to off-white powder that is soluble in water and normal saline.

The active ingredient in ZOFRAN ODT Orally Disintegrating Tablets is ondansetron base, the racemic form of ondansetron, and a selective blocking agent of the serotonin 5-HT$_3$ receptor type. Chemically it is (±) 1, 2, 3, 9-tetrahydro-9-methyl-3-[(2-methyl-1H-imidazol-1-yl)methyl]-4H-carbazol-4-one. It has the following structural formula:

The empirical formula is $C_{18}H_{19}N_3O$ representing a molecular weight of 293.4.

Each 4-mg ZOFRAN Tablet for oral administration contains ondansetron HCl dihydrate equivalent to 4 mg of ondansetron. Each 8-mg ZOFRAN Tablet for oral administration contains ondansetron HCl dihydrate equivalent to 8 mg of ondansetron. Each tablet also contains the inactive ingredients lactose, microcrystalline cellulose, pregelatinized starch, hypromellose, magnesium stearate, titanium dioxide, triacetin, and iron oxide yellow (8-mg tablet only).

Each 4-mg ZOFRAN ODT Orally Disintegrating Tablet for oral administration contains 4 mg ondansetron base. Each 8-mg ZOFRAN ODT Orally Disintegrating Tablet for oral administration contains 8 mg ondansetron base. Each ZOFRAN ODT Tablet also contains the inactive ingredients aspartame, gelatin, mannitol, methylparaben sodium, propylparaben sodium, and strawberry flavor. ZOFRAN ODT Tablets are a freeze-dried, orally disintegrating formulation of ondansetron which rapidly disintegrates on the tongue and does not require water to aid dissolution or swallowing. Each 5 mL of ZOFRAN Oral Solution contains 5 mg of ondansetron HCl dihydrate equivalent to 4 mg of ondansetron. ZOFRAN Oral Solution contains the inactive ingredients citric acid anhydrous, purified water, sodium benzoate, sodium citrate, sorbitol, and strawberry flavor.

CLINICAL PHARMACOLOGY
Pharmacodynamics
Ondansetron is a selective $5\text{-}HT_3$ receptor antagonist. While its mechanism of action has not been fully characterized, ondansetron is not a dopamine-receptor antagonist. Serotonin receptors of the $5\text{-}HT_3$ type are present both peripherally on vagal nerve terminals and centrally in the chemoreceptor trigger zone of the area postrema. It is not certain whether ondansetron's antiemetic action is mediated centrally, peripherally, or in both sites. However, cytotoxic chemotherapy appears to be associated with release of serotonin from the enterochromaffin cells of the small intestine. In humans, urinary 5-HIAA (5-hydroxyindoleacetic acid) excretion increases after cisplatin administration in parallel with the onset of emesis. The released serotonin may stimulate the vagal afferents through the $5\text{-}HT_3$ receptors and initiate the vomiting reflex.

In animals, the emetic response to cisplatin can be prevented by pretreatment with an inhibitor of serotonin synthesis, bilateral abdominal vagotomy and greater splanchnic nerve section, or pretreatment with a serotonin $5\text{-}HT_3$ receptor antagonist.

In normal volunteers, single intravenous doses of 0.15 mg/kg of ondansetron had no effect on esophageal motility, gastric emptying, lower esophageal sphincter pressure, or small intestinal transit time. Multiday administration of ondansetron has been shown to slow colonic transit in normal volunteers. Ondansetron has no effect on plasma prolactin concentrations.

Ondansetron does not alter the respiratory depressant effects produced by alfentanil or the degree of neuromuscular blockade produced by atracurium. Interactions with general or local anesthetics have not been studied.

Pharmacokinetics
Ondansetron is well absorbed from the gastrointestinal tract and undergoes some first-pass metabolism. Mean bioavailability in healthy subjects, following administration of a single 8-mg tablet, is approximately 56%.

Ondansetron systemic exposure does not increase proportionately to dose. AUC from a 16-mg tablet was 24% greater than predicted from an 8-mg tablet dose. This may reflect some reduction of first-pass metabolism at higher oral doses. Bioavailability is also slightly enhanced by the presence of food but unaffected by antacids.

Ondansetron is extensively metabolized in humans, with approximately 5% of a radiolabeled dose recovered as the parent compound from the urine. The primary metabolic pathway is hydroxylation on the indole ring followed by subsequent glucuronide or sulfate conjugation. Although some nonconjugated metabolites have pharmacologic activity, these are not found in plasma at concentrations likely to significantly contribute to the biological activity of ondansetron.

In vitro metabolism studies have shown that ondansetron is a substrate for human hepatic cytochrome P-450 enzymes, including CYP1A2, CYP2D6, and CYP3A4. In terms of overall ondansetron turnover, CYP3A4 played the predominant role. Because of the multiplicity of metabolic enzymes capable of metabolizing ondansetron, it is likely that inhibition or loss of one enzyme (e.g., CYP2D6 genetic deficiency) will be compensated by others and may result in little change in overall rates of ondansetron elimination. Ondansetron elimination may be affected by cytochrome P-450 inducers. In a pharmacokinetic study of 16 epileptic patients maintained chronically on CYP3A4 inducers, carbamazepine, or phenytoin, reduction in AUC, C_{max}, and $T_{1/2}$ of ondansetron was observed.[1] This resulted in a significant increase in clearance. However, on the basis of available data, no dosage adjustment for ondansetron is recommended (see PRECAUTIONS: Drug Interactions).

In humans, carmustine, etoposide, and cisplatin do not affect the pharmacokinetics of ondansetron.

Gender differences were shown in the disposition of ondansetron given as a single dose. The extent and rate of ondansetron's absorption is greater in women than men. Slower clearance in women, a smaller apparent volume of distribution (adjusted for weight), and higher absolute bioavailability resulted in higher plasma ondansetron levels. These higher plasma levels may in part be explained by differences in body weight between men and women. It is not known whether these gender-related differences were clinically important. More detailed pharmacokinetic information is contained in Tables 1 and 2 taken from 2 studies.
[See table 1 above]
[See table 2 above]

A reduction in clearance and increase in elimination half-life are seen in patients over 75 years of age. In clinical trials with cancer patients, safety and efficacy were similar in patients over 65 years of age and those under 65 years of age; there was an insufficient number of patients over 75 years of age to permit conclusions in that age-group. No dosage adjustment is recommended in the elderly.

In patients with mild-to-moderate hepatic impairment, clearance is reduced 2-fold and mean half-life is increased to 11.6 hours compared to 5.7 hours in normals. In patients with severe hepatic impairment (Child-Pugh[2] score of 10 or greater), clearance is reduced 2-fold to 3-fold and apparent volume of distribution is increased with a resultant increase in half-life to 20 hours. In patients with severe hepatic impairment, a total daily dose of 8 mg should not be exceeded.

Due to the very small contribution (5%) of renal clearance to the overall clearance, renal impairment was not expected to significantly influence the total clearance of ondansetron. However, ondansetron oral mean plasma clearance was reduced by about 50% in patients with severe renal impairment (creatinine clearance <30 mL/min). This reduction in clearance is variable and was not consistent with an increase in half-life. No reduction in dose or dosing frequency in these patients is warranted.

Plasma protein binding of ondansetron as measured in vitro was 70% to 76% over the concentration range of 10 to 500 ng/mL. Circulating drug also distributes into erythrocytes.

Four- and 8-mg doses of either ZOFRAN Oral Solution or ZOFRAN ODT Orally Disintegrating Tablets are bioequivalent to corresponding doses of ZOFRAN Tablets and may be used interchangeably. One 24-mg ZOFRAN Tablet is bioequivalent to and interchangeable with three 8-mg ZOFRAN Tablets.

CLINICAL TRIALS
Chemotherapy-Induced Nausea and Vomiting
Highly Emetogenic Chemotherapy
In 2 randomized, double-blind, monotherapy trials, a single 24-mg ZOFRAN Tablet was superior to a relevant historical placebo control in the prevention of nausea and vomiting associated with highly emetogenic cancer chemotherapy, including cisplatin ≥ 50 mg/m^2. Steroid administration was excluded from these clinical trials. More than 90% of patients receiving a cisplatin dose ≥ 50 mg/m^2 in the historical placebo comparator experienced vomiting in the absence of antiemetic therapy.

The first trial compared oral doses of ondansetron 24 mg once a day, 8 mg twice a day, and 32 mg once a day in 357 adult cancer patients receiving chemotherapy regimens containing cisplatin ≥ 50 mg/m^2. A total of 66% of patients in the ondansetron 24-mg once-a-day group, 55% in the ondansetron 8-mg twice-a-day group, and 55% in the ondansetron 32-mg once-a-day group completed the 24-hour study period with 0 emetic episodes and no rescue antiemetic medications, the primary endpoint of efficacy. Each of the 3 treatment groups was shown to be statistically significantly superior to a historical placebo control.

In the same trial, 56% of patients receiving oral ondansetron 24 mg once a day experienced no nausea during the 24-hour study period, compared with 36% of patients in the oral ondansetron 8-mg twice-a-day group ($P = 0.001$) and 50% in the oral ondansetron 32-mg once-a-day group.

In a second trial, efficacy of the oral ondansetron 24-mg once-a-day regimen in the prevention of nausea and vomiting associated with highly emetogenic cancer chemotherapy, including cisplatin ≥ 50 mg/m^2, was confirmed.

Moderately Emetogenic Chemotherapy
In 1 double-blind US study in 67 patients, ZOFRAN Tablets 8 mg administered twice a day were significantly more effective than placebo in preventing vomiting induced by cyclophosphamide-based chemotherapy containing doxorubicin. Treatment response was based on the total number of emetic episodes over the 3-day study period. The results of this study are summarized in Table 3:
[See table 3 above]

Table 1. Pharmacokinetics in Normal Volunteers: Single 8-mg ZOFRAN Tablet Dose

Age-group (years)		Mean Weight (kg)	n	Peak Plasma Concentration (ng/mL)	Time of Peak Plasma Concentration (h)	Mean Elimination Half-life (h)	Systemic Plasma Clearance L/h/kg	Absolute Bioavailability
18–40	M	69.0	6	26.2	2.0	3.1	0.403	0.483
	F	62.7	5	42.7	1.7	3.5	0.354	0.663
61–74	M	77.5	6	24.1	2.1	4.1	0.384	0.585
	F	60.2	6	52.4	1.9	4.9	0.255	0.643
≥75	M	78.0	5	37.0	2.2	4.5	0.277	0.619
	F	67.6	6	46.1	2.1	6.2	0.249	0.747

Table 2. Pharmacokinetics in Normal Volunteers: Single 24-mg ZOFRAN Tablet Dose

Age-group (years)		Mean Weight (kg)	n	Peak Plasma Concentration (ng/mL)	Time of Peak Plasma Concentration (h)	Mean Elimination Half-life (h)
18–43	M	84.1	8	125.8	1.9	4.7
	F	71.8	8	194.4	1.6	5.8

Table 3. Emetic Episodes: Treatment Response

	Ondansetron 8-mg b.i.d. ZOFRAN Tablets[a]	Placebo	P Value
Number of patients	33	34	
Treatment response			
0 Emetic episodes	20 (61%)	2 (6%)	<0.001
1-2 Emetic episodes	6 (18%)	8 (24%)	
More than 2 emetic episodes/withdrawn	7 (21%)	24 (71%)	<0.001
Median number of emetic episodes	0.0	Undefined[b]	
Median time to first emetic episode (h)	Undefined[c]	6.5	

[a] The first dose was administered 30 minutes before the start of emetogenic chemotherapy, with a subsequent dose 8 hours after the first dose. An 8-mg ZOFRAN Tablet was administered twice a day for 2 days after completion of chemotherapy.
[b] Median undefined since at least 50% of the patients were withdrawn or had more than 2 emetic episodes.
[c] Median undefined since at least 50% of patients did not have any emetic episodes.

Table 4. Emetic Episodes: Treatment Response

	Ondansetron	
	8-mg b.i.d. ZOFRAN Tablets[a]	8-mg t.i.d. ZOFRAN Tablets[b]
Number of patients	165	171
Treatment response		
0 Emetic episodes	101 (61%)	99 (58%)
1-2 Emetic episodes	16 (10%)	17 (10%)
More than 2 emetic episodes/withdrawn	48 (29%)	55 (32%)
Median number of emetic episodes	0.0	0.0
Median time to first emetic episode (h)	Undefined[c]	Undefined[c]
Median nausea scores (0-100)[d]	6	6

[a] The first dose was administered 30 minutes before the start of emetogenic chemotherapy, with a subsequent dose 8 hours after the first dose. An 8-mg ZOFRAN Tablet was administered twice a day for 2 days after completion of chemotherapy.
[b] The first dose was administered 30 minutes before the start of emetogenic chemotherapy, with subsequent doses 4 and 8 hours after the first dose. An 8-mg ZOFRAN Tablet was administered 3 times a day for 2 days after completion of chemotherapy.
[c] Median undefined since at least 50% of patients did not have any emetic episodes.
[d] Visual analog scale assessment: 0 = no nausea, 100 = nausea as bad as it can be.

In 1 double-blind US study in 336 patients, ZOFRAN Tablets 8 mg administered twice a day were as effective as ZOFRAN Tablets 8 mg administered 3 times a day in preventing nausea and vomiting induced by cyclophosphamide-based chemotherapy containing either methotrexate or doxorubicin. Treatment response is based on the total number of emetic episodes over the 3-day study period. The results of this study are summarized in Table 4:
[See table 4 above]

Re-treatment

In uncontrolled trials, 148 patients receiving cyclophosphamide-based chemotherapy were re-treated with ZOFRAN Tablets 8 mg 3 times daily during subsequent chemotherapy for a total of 396 re-treatment courses. No emetic episodes occurred in 314 (79%) of the re-treatment courses, and only 1 to 2 emetic episodes occurred in 43 (11%) of the re-treatment courses.

Pediatric Studies

Three open-label, uncontrolled, foreign trials have been performed with 182 pediatric patients 4 to 18 years old with cancer who were given a variety of cisplatin or noncisplatin regimens. In these foreign trials, the initial dose of ZOFRAN® (ondansetron HCl) Injection ranged from 0.04 to 0.87 mg/kg for a total dose of 2.16 to 12 mg. This was followed by the administration of ZOFRAN Tablets ranging from 4 to 24 mg daily for 3 days. In these studies, 58% of the 170 evaluable patients had a complete response (no emetic episodes) on day 1. Two studies showed the response rates for patients less than 12 years of age who received ZOFRAN Tablets 4 mg 3 times a day to be similar to those in patients 12 to 18 years of age who received ZOFRAN Tablets 8 mg 3 times daily. Thus, prevention of emesis in these pediatric patients was essentially the same as for patients older than 18 years of age. Overall, ZOFRAN Tablets were well tolerated in these pediatric patients.

Radiation-Induced Nausea and Vomiting

Total Body Irradiation

In a randomized, double-blind study in 20 patients, ZOFRAN Tablets (8 mg given 1.5 hours before each fraction of radiotherapy for 4 days) were significantly more effective than placebo in preventing vomiting induced by total body irradiation. Total body irradiation consisted of 11 fractions (120 cGy per fraction) over 4 days for a total of 1,320 cGy. Patients received 3 fractions for 3 days, then 2 fractions on day 4.

Single High-Dose Fraction Radiotherapy

Ondansetron was significantly more effective than metoclopramide with respect to complete control of emesis (0 emetic episodes) in a double-blind trial in 105 patients receiving single high-dose radiotherapy (800 to 1,000 cGy) over an anterior or posterior field size of ≥ 80 cm^2 to the abdomen. Patients received the first dose of ZOFRAN Tablets (8 mg) or metoclopramide (10 mg) 1 to 2 hours before radiotherapy. If radiotherapy was given in the morning, 2 additional doses of study treatment were given (1 tablet late afternoon and 1 tablet before bedtime). If radiotherapy was given in the afternoon, patients took only 1 further tablet that day before bedtime. Patients continued the oral medication on a 3 times a day basis for 3 days.

Daily Fractionated Radiotherapy

Ondansetron was significantly more effective than prochlorperazine with respect to complete control of emesis (0 emetic episodes) in a double-blind trial in 135 patients receiving a 1- to 4-week course of fractionated radiotherapy (180 cGy doses) over a field size of ≥ 100 cm^2 to the abdomen. Patients received the first dose of ZOFRAN Tablets (8 mg) or prochlorperazine (10 mg) 1 to 2 hours before the patient received the first daily radiotherapy fraction, with 2 subsequent doses on a 3 times a day basis. Patients continued the oral medication on a 3 times a day basis on each day of radiotherapy.

Postoperative Nausea and Vomiting

Surgical patients who received ondansetron 1 hour before the induction of general balanced anesthesia (barbiturate: thiopental, methohexital, or thiamylal; opioid: alfentanil, sufentanil, morphine, or fentanyl; nitrous oxide; neuromuscular blockade: succinylcholine/curare or gallamine and/or vecuronium, pancuronium, or atracurium; and supplemental isoflurane or enflurane) were evaluated in 2 double-blind studies (1 US study, 1 foreign) involving 865 patients. ZOFRAN Tablets (16 mg) were significantly more effective than placebo in preventing postoperative nausea and vomiting.

The study populations in all trials thus far consisted of women undergoing inpatient surgical procedures. No studies have been performed in males. No controlled clinical study comparing ZOFRAN Tablets to ZOFRAN Injection has been performed.

INDICATIONS AND USAGE

1. Prevention of nausea and vomiting associated with highly emetogenic cancer chemotherapy, including cisplatin ≥ 50 mg/m^2.
2. Prevention of nausea and vomiting associated with initial and repeat courses of moderately emetogenic cancer chemotherapy.
3. Prevention of nausea and vomiting associated with radiotherapy in patients receiving either total body irradiation, single high-dose fraction to the abdomen, or daily fractions to the abdomen.
4. Prevention of postoperative nausea and/or vomiting. As with other antiemetics, routine prophylaxis is not recommended for patients in whom there is little expectation that nausea and/or vomiting will occur postoperatively. In patients where nausea and/or vomiting must be avoided postoperatively, ZOFRAN Tablets, ZOFRAN ODT Orally Disintegrating Tablets, and ZOFRAN Oral Solution are recommended even where the incidence of postoperative nausea and/or vomiting is low.

CONTRAINDICATIONS

The concomitant use of apomorphine with ondansetron is contraindicated based on reports of profound hypotension and loss of consciousness when apomorphine was administered with ondansetron.

ZOFRAN Tablets, ZOFRAN ODT Orally Disintegrating Tablets, and ZOFRAN Oral Solution are contraindicated for patients known to have hypersensitivity to the drug.

WARNINGS

Hypersensitivity reactions have been reported in patients who have exhibited hypersensitivity to other selective 5-HT_3 receptor antagonists.

PRECAUTIONS

General

Ondansetron is not a drug that stimulates gastric or intestinal peristalsis. It should not be used instead of nasogastric suction. The use of ondansetron in patients following abdominal surgery or in patients with chemotherapy-induced nausea and vomiting may mask a progressive ileus and/or gastric distension.

Rarely and predominantly with intravenous ondansetron, transient ECG changes including QT interval prolongation have been reported.

Information for Patients

Phenylketonurics

Phenylketonuric patients should be informed that ZOFRAN ODT Orally Disintegrating Tablets contain phenylalanine (a component of aspartame). Each 4-mg and 8-mg orally disintegrating tablet contains < 0.03 mg phenylalanine.

Patients should be instructed not to remove ZOFRAN ODT Tablets from the blister until just prior to dosing. The tablet should not be pushed through the foil. With dry hands, the blister backing should be peeled completely off the blister. The tablet should be gently removed and immediately placed on the tongue to dissolve and be swallowed with the saliva. Peelable illustrated stickers are affixed to the product carton that can be provided with the prescription to ensure proper use and handling of the product.

Drug Interactions

Ondansetron does not itself appear to induce or inhibit the cytochrome P-450 drug-metabolizing enzyme system of the liver (see CLINICAL PHARMACOLOGY, Pharmacokinetics). Because ondansetron is metabolized by hepatic cytochrome P-450 drug-metabolizing enzymes (CYP3A4, CYP2D6, CYP1A2), inducers or inhibitors of these enzymes may change the clearance and, hence, the half-life of ondansetron. On the basis of available data, no dosage adjustment is recommended for patients on these drugs.

Apomorphine

Based on reports of profound hypotension and loss of consciousness when apomorphine was administered with ondansetron, concomitant use of apomorphine with ondansetron is contraindicated (see CONTRAINDICATIONS).

Phenytoin, Carbamazepine, and Rifampicin

In patients treated with potent inducers of CYP3A4 (i.e., phenytoin, carbamazepine, and rifampicin), the clearance of ondansetron was significantly increased and ondansetron blood concentrations were decreased. However, on the basis of available data, no dosage adjustment for ondansetron is recommended for patients on these drugs.[1,3]

Tramadol

Although no pharmacokinetic drug interaction between ondansetron and tramadol has been observed, data from 2 small studies indicate that ondansetron may be associated with an increase in patient controlled administration of tramadol.[4,5]

Chemotherapy

Tumor response to chemotherapy in the P-388 mouse leukemia model is not affected by ondansetron. In humans, carmustine, etoposide, and cisplatin do not affect the pharmacokinetics of ondansetron.

In a crossover study in 76 pediatric patients, I.V. ondansetron did not increase blood levels of high-dose methotrexate.

Use in Surgical Patients

The coadministration of ondansetron had no effect on the pharmacokinetics and pharmacodynamics of temazepam.

Carcinogenesis, Mutagenesis, Impairment of Fertility

Carcinogenic effects were not seen in 2-year studies in rats and mice with oral ondansetron doses up to 10 and 30 mg/kg/day, respectively. Ondansetron was not mutagenic in standard tests for mutagenicity. Oral administration of ondansetron up to 15 mg/kg/day did not affect fertility or general reproductive performance of male and female rats.

Pregnancy

Teratogenic Effects

Pregnancy Category B. Reproduction studies have been performed in pregnant rats and rabbits at daily oral doses up to 15 and 30 mg/kg/day, respectively, and have revealed no evidence of impaired fertility or harm to the fetus due to ondansetron. There are, however, no adequate and well-controlled studies in pregnant women. Because animal reproduction studies are not always predictive of human response, this drug should be used during pregnancy only if clearly needed.

Nursing Mothers

Ondansetron is excreted in the breast milk of rats. It is not known whether ondansetron is excreted in human milk. Because many drugs are excreted in human milk, caution should be exercised when ondansetron is administered to a nursing woman.

Pediatric Use

Little information is available about dosage in pediatric patients 4 years of age or younger (see CLINICAL PHARMACOLOGY and DOSAGE AND ADMINISTRATION sections for use in pediatric patients 4 to 18 years of age).

Geriatric Use

Of the total number of subjects enrolled in cancer chemotherapy-induced and postoperative nausea and vomiting in US- and foreign-controlled clinical trials, for which there were subgroup analyses, 938 were 65 years of age and over. No overall differences in safety or effectiveness were observed between these subjects and younger subjects, and other reported clinical experience has not identified differences in responses between the elderly and younger patients, but greater sensitivity of some older individuals cannot be ruled out. Dosage adjustment is not needed in patients over the age of 65 (see CLINICAL PHARMACOLOGY).

ADVERSE REACTIONS

The following have been reported as adverse events in clinical trials of patients treated with ondansetron, the active ingredient of ZOFRAN. A causal relationship to therapy with ZOFRAN has been unclear in many cases.

Chemotherapy-Induced Nausea and Vomiting

The adverse events in Table 5 have been reported in ≥ 5% of adult patients receiving a single 24-mg ZOFRAN Tablet in 2 trials. These patients were receiving concurrent highly emetogenic cisplatin-based chemotherapy regimens (cisplatin dose ≥ 50 mg/m²).

[See table 5 at right]

The adverse events in Table 6 have been reported in ≥ 5% of adults receiving either 8 mg of ZOFRAN Tablets 2 or 3 times a day for 3 days or placebo in 4 trials. These patients were receiving concurrent moderately emetogenic chemotherapy, primarily cyclophosphamide-based regimens.

[See table 6 at right]

Central Nervous System

There have been rare reports consistent with, but not diagnostic of, extrapyramidal reactions in patients receiving ondansetron.

Hepatic

In 723 patients receiving cyclophosphamide-based chemotherapy in US clinical trials, AST and/or ALT values have been reported to exceed twice the upper limit of normal in approximately 1% to 2% of patients receiving ZOFRAN Tablets. The increases were transient and did not appear to be related to dose or duration of therapy. On repeat exposure, similar transient elevations in transaminase values occurred in some courses, but symptomatic hepatic disease did not occur. The role of cancer chemotherapy in these biochemical changes cannot be clearly determined.

There have been reports of liver failure and death in patients with cancer receiving concurrent medications including potentially hepatotoxic cytotoxic chemotherapy and antibiotics. The etiology of the liver failure is unclear.

Integumentary

Rash has occurred in approximately 1% of patients receiving ondansetron.

Other

Rare cases of anaphylaxis, bronchospasm, tachycardia, angina (chest pain), hypokalemia, electrocardiographic alterations, vascular occlusive events, and grand mal seizures have been reported. Except for bronchospasm and anaphylaxis, the relationship to ZOFRAN was unclear.

Radiation-Induced Nausea and Vomiting

The adverse events reported in patients receiving ZOFRAN Tablets and concurrent radiotherapy were similar to those reported in patients receiving ZOFRAN Tablets and concurrent chemotherapy. The most frequently reported adverse events were headache, constipation, and diarrhea.

Postoperative Nausea and Vomiting

The adverse events in Table 7 have been reported in ≥ 5% of patients receiving ZOFRAN Tablets at a dosage of 16 mg orally in clinical trials. With the exception of headache, rates of these events were not significantly different in the ondansetron and placebo groups. These patients were receiving multiple concomitant perioperative and postoperative medications.

[See table 7 above]

Preliminary observations in a small number of subjects suggest a higher incidence of headache when ZOFRAN ODT Orally Disintegrating Tablets are taken with water, when compared to without water.

Observed During Clinical Practice

In addition to adverse events reported from clinical trials, the following events have been identified during postapproval use of oral formulations of ZOFRAN. Because they are reported voluntarily from a population of unknown size, estimates of frequency cannot be made. The events have been chosen for inclusion due to a combination of their seriousness, frequency of reporting, or potential causal connection to ZOFRAN.

Cardiovascular

Rarely and predominantly with intravenous ondansetron, transient ECG changes including QT interval prolongation have been reported.

General

Flushing. Rare cases of hypersensitivity reactions, sometimes severe (e.g., anaphylaxis/anaphylactoid reactions, angioedema, bronchospasm, shortness of breath, hypotension, laryngeal edema, stridor) have also been reported. Laryngospasm, shock, and cardiopulmonary arrest have occurred during allergic reactions in patients receiving injectable ondansetron.

Hepatobiliary

Liver enzyme abnormalities

Lower Respiratory

Hiccups

Neurology:

Oculogyric crisis, appearing alone, as well as with other dystonic reactions

Skin

Urticaria

Special Senses

Eye Disorders

Cases of transient blindness, predominantly during intravenous administration, have been reported. These cases of transient blindness were reported to resolve within a few minutes up to 48 hours.

DRUG ABUSE AND DEPENDENCE

Animal studies have shown that ondansetron is not discriminated as a benzodiazepine nor does it substitute for benzodiazepines in direct addiction studies.

OVERDOSAGE

There is no specific antidote for ondansetron overdose. Patients should be managed with appropriate supportive therapy. Individual intravenous doses as large as 150 mg and total daily intravenous doses as large as 252 mg have been inadvertently administered without significant adverse events. These doses are more than 10 times the recommended daily dose.

In addition to the adverse events listed above, the following events have been described in the setting of ondansetron overdose: "Sudden blindness" (amaurosis) of 2 to 3 minutes' duration plus severe constipation occurred in 1 patient that

Table 5. Principal Adverse Events in US Trials: Single Day Therapy With 24-mg ZOFRAN Tablets (Highly Emetogenic Chemotherapy)

Event	Ondansetron 24 mg q.d. n = 300	Ondansetron 8 mg b.i.d. n = 124	Ondansetron 32 mg q.d. n = 117
Headache	33 (11%)	16 (13%)	17 (15%)
Diarrhea	13 (4%)	9 (7%)	3 (3%)

Table 6. Principal Adverse Events in US Trials: 3 Days of Therapy With 8-mg ZOFRAN Tablets (Moderately Emetogenic Chemotherapy)

Event	Ondansetron 8 mg b.i.d. n = 242	Ondansetron 8 mg t.i.d. n = 415	Placebo n = 262
Headache	58 (24%)	113 (27%)	34 (13%)
Malaise/fatigue	32 (13%)	37 (9%)	6 (2%)
Constipation	22 (9%)	26 (6%)	1 (<1%)
Diarrhea	15 (6%)	16 (4%)	10 (4%)
Dizziness	13 (5%)	18 (4%)	12 (5%)

Table 7. Frequency of Adverse Events From Controlled Studies With ZOFRAN Tablets (Postoperative Nausea and Vomiting)

Adverse Event	Ondansetron 16 mg (n = 550)	Placebo (n = 531)
Wound problem	152 (28%)	162 (31%)
Drowsiness/sedation	112 (20%)	122 (23%)
Headache	49 (9%)	27 (5%)
Hypoxia	49 (9%)	35 (7%)
Pyrexia	45 (8%)	34 (6%)
Dizziness	36 (7%)	34 (6%)
Gynecological disorder	36 (7%)	33 (6%)
Anxiety/agitation	33 (6%)	29 (5%)
Bradycardia	32 (6%)	30 (6%)
Shiver(s)	28 (5%)	30 (6%)
Urinary retention	28 (5%)	18 (3%)
Hypotension	27 (5%)	32 (6%)
Pruritus	27 (5%)	20 (4%)

was administered 72 mg of ondansetron intravenously as a single dose. Hypotension (and faintness) occurred in a patient that took 48 mg of ZOFRAN Tablets. Following infusion of 32 mg over only a 4-minute period, a vasovagal episode with transient second-degree heart block was observed. In all instances, the events resolved completely.

DOSAGE AND ADMINISTRATION

Instructions for Use/Handling ZOFRAN ODT Orally Disintegrating Tablets

Do not attempt to push ZOFRAN ODT Tablets through the foil backing. With dry hands, PEEL BACK the foil backing of 1 blister and GENTLY remove the tablet. IMMEDIATELY place the ZOFRAN ODT Tablet on top of the tongue where it will dissolve in seconds, then swallow with saliva. Administration with liquid is not necessary.

Prevention of Nausea and Vomiting Associated With Highly Emetogenic Cancer Chemotherapy

The recommended adult oral dosage of ZOFRAN is 24 mg given as three 8-mg tablets administered 30 minutes before the start of single-day highly emetogenic chemotherapy, including cisplatin ≥ 50 mg/m². Multiday, single-dose administration of a 24 mg dosage has not been studied.

Pediatric Use

There is no experience with the use of a 24 mg dosage in pediatric patients.

Geriatric Use

The dosage recommendation is the same as for the general population.

Prevention of Nausea and Vomiting Associated With Moderately Emetogenic Cancer Chemotherapy

The recommended adult oral dosage is one 8-mg ZOFRAN Tablet or one 8-mg ZOFRAN ODT Tablet or 10 mL

(2 teaspoonfuls equivalent to 8 mg of ondansetron) of ZOFRAN Oral Solution given twice a day. The first dose should be administered 30 minutes before the start of emetogenic chemotherapy, with a subsequent dose 8 hours after the first dose. One 8-mg ZOFRAN Tablet or one 8-mg ZOFRAN ODT Tablet or 10 mL (2 teaspoonfuls equivalent to 8 mg of ondansetron) of ZOFRAN Oral Solution should be administered twice a day (every 12 hours) for 1 to 2 days after completion of chemotherapy.

Pediatric Use
For pediatric patients 12 years of age and older, the dosage is the same as for adults. For pediatric patients 4 through 11 years of age, the dosage is one 4-mg ZOFRAN Tablet or one 4-mg ZOFRAN ODT Tablet or 5 mL (1 teaspoonful equivalent to 4 mg of ondansetron) of ZOFRAN Oral Solution given 3 times a day. The first dose should be administered 30 minutes before the start of emetogenic chemotherapy, with subsequent doses 4 and 8 hours after the first dose. One 4-mg ZOFRAN Tablet or one 4-mg ZOFRAN ODT Tablet or 5 mL (1 teaspoonful equivalent to 4 mg of ondansetron) of ZOFRAN Oral Solution should be administered 3 times a day (every 8 hours) for 1 to 2 days after completion of chemotherapy.

Geriatric Use
The dosage is the same as for the general population.

Prevention of Nausea and Vomiting Associated With Radiotherapy, Either Total Body Irradiation, or Single High-Dose Fraction or Daily Fractions to the Abdomen
The recommended oral dosage is one 8-mg ZOFRAN Tablet or one 8-mg ZOFRAN ODT Tablet or 10 mL (2 teaspoonfuls equivalent to 8 mg of ondansetron) of ZOFRAN Oral Solution given 3 times a day.
For total body irradiation, one 8-mg ZOFRAN Tablet or one 8-mg ZOFRAN ODT Tablet or 10 mL (2 teaspoonfuls equivalent to 8 mg of ondansetron) of ZOFRAN Oral Solution should be administered 1 to 2 hours before each fraction of radiotherapy administered each day.
For single high-dose fraction radiotherapy to the abdomen, one 8-mg ZOFRAN Tablet or one 8-mg ZOFRAN ODT Tablet or 10 mL (2 teaspoonfuls equivalent to 8 mg of ondansetron) of ZOFRAN Oral Solution should be administered 1 to 2 hours before radiotherapy, with subsequent doses every 8 hours after the first dose for 1 to 2 days after completion of radiotherapy.
For daily fractionated radiotherapy to the abdomen, one 8-mg ZOFRAN Tablet or one 8-mg ZOFRAN ODT Tablet or 10 mL (2 teaspoonfuls equivalent to 8 mg of ondansetron) of ZOFRAN Oral Solution should be administered 1 to 2 hours before radiotherapy, with subsequent doses every 8 hours after the first dose for each day radiotherapy is given.

Pediatric Use
There is no experience with the use of ZOFRAN Tablets, ZOFRAN ODT Tablets, or ZOFRAN Oral Solution in the prevention of radiation-induced nausea and vomiting in pediatric patients.

Geriatric Use
The dosage recommendation is the same as for the general population.

Postoperative Nausea and Vomiting
The recommended dosage is 16 mg given as two 8-mg ZOFRAN Tablets or two 8-mg ZOFRAN ODT Tablets or 20 mL (4 teaspoonfuls equivalent to 16 mg of ondansetron) of ZOFRAN Oral Solution 1 hour before induction of anesthesia.

Pediatric Use
There is no experience with the use of ZOFRAN Tablets, ZOFRAN ODT Tablets, or ZOFRAN Oral Solution in the prevention of postoperative nausea and vomiting in pediatric patients.

Geriatric Use
The dosage is the same as for the general population.

Dosage Adjustment for Patients With Impaired Renal Function
The dosage recommendation is the same as for the general population. There is no experience beyond first-day administration of ondansetron.

Dosage Adjustment for Patients With Impaired Hepatic Function
In patients with severe hepatic impairment (Child-Pugh[2] score of 10 or greater), clearance is reduced and apparent volume of distribution is increased with a resultant increase in plasma half-life. In such patients, a total daily dose of 8 mg should not be exceeded.

HOW SUPPLIED
ZOFRAN Tablets, 4 mg (ondansetron HCl dihydrate equivalent to 4 mg of ondansetron), are white, oval, film-coated tablets engraved with "Zofran" on one side and "4" on the other in daily unit dose packs of 3 tablets (NDC 0173-0446-04), bottles of 30 tablets (NDC 0173-0446-00), and unit dose packs of 100 tablets (NDC 0173-0446-02).
Bottles: Store between 2° and 30°C (36° and 86°F). Protect from light. Dispense in tight, light-resistant container as defined in the USP.

Unit Dose Packs: Store between 2° and 30°C (36° and 86°F). Protect from light. Store blisters in cartons.
ZOFRAN Tablets, 8 mg (ondansetron HCl dihydrate equivalent to 8 mg of ondansetron), are yellow, oval, film-coated tablets engraved with "Zofran" on one side and "8" on the other in daily unit dose packs of 3 tablets (NDC 0173-0447-04), bottles of 30 tablets (NDC 0173-0447-00), and unit dose packs of 100 tablets (NDC 0173-0447-02).
Bottles: Store between 2° and 30°C (36° and 86°F). Dispense in tight container as defined in the USP.
Unit Dose Packs: Store between 2° and 30°C (36° and 86°F).
ZOFRAN ODT Orally Disintegrating Tablets, 4 mg (as 4 mg ondansetron base) are white, round and plano-convex tablets debossed with a "Z4" on one side in unit dose packs of 30 tablets (NDC 0173-0569-00).
ZOFRAN ODT Orally Disintegrating Tablets, 8 mg (as 8 mg ondansetron base) are white, round and plano-convex tablets debossed with a "Z8" on one side in unit dose packs of 10 tablets (NDC 0173-0570-04) and 30 tablets (NDC 0173-0570-00).
Store between 2° and 30°C (36° and 86°F).
ZOFRAN Oral Solution, a clear, colorless to light yellow liquid with a characteristic strawberry odor, contains 5 mg of ondansetron HCl dihydrate equivalent to 4 mg of ondansetron per 5 mL in amber glass bottles of 50 mL with child-resistant closures (NDC 0173-0489-00).
Store upright between 15° and 30°C (59° and 86°F). Protect from light. Store bottles upright in cartons.

REFERENCES
1. Britto MR, Hussey EK, Mydlow P, et al. Effect of enzyme inducers on ondansetron (OND) metabolism in humans. *Clin Pharmacol Ther.* 1997;61:228.
2. Pugh RNH, Murray-Lyon IM, Dawson JL, Pietroni MC, Williams R. Transection of the oesophagus for bleeding oesophageal varices. *Brit J Surg.* 1973;60:646-649.
3. Villikka K, Kivisto KT, Neuvonen PJ. The effect of rifampin on the pharmacokinetics of oral and intravenous ondansetron. *Clin Pharmacol Ther.* 1999;65:377-381.
4. De Witte JL, Schoenmaekers B, Sessler DI, et al. *Anesth Analg.* 2001;92:1319-1321.
5. Arcioni R, della Rocca M, Romanò R, et al. *Anesth Analg.* 2002;94:1553-1557.

GlaxoSmithKline
Research Triangle Park, NC 27709
ZOFRAN Tablets and Oral Solution:
GlaxoSmithKline
Research Triangle Park, NC 27709
ZOFRAN ODT Orally Disintegrating Tablets:
Manufactured for GlaxoSmithKline
Research Triangle Park, NC 27709
by Catalent UK Swindon Zydis Ltd.
Blagrove, Swindon, Wiltshire, UK SN5 8RU
©2010, GlaxoSmithKline. All rights reserved.
May 2010
ZFT:2PI

ZOVIRAX® ℞
[zō-vī' rax]
(acyclovir)
Capsules
ZOVIRAX® ℞
(acyclovir)
Tablets
ZOVIRAX® ℞
(acyclovir)
Suspension

DESCRIPTION
ZOVIRAX is the brand name for acyclovir, a synthetic nucleoside analogue active against herpesviruses. ZOVIRAX Capsules, Tablets, and Suspension are formulations for oral administration. Each capsule of ZOVIRAX contains 200 mg of acyclovir and the inactive ingredients corn starch, lactose, magnesium stearate, and sodium lauryl sulfate. The capsule shell consists of gelatin, FD&C Blue No. 2, and titanium dioxide. May contain one or more parabens. Printed with edible black ink.
Each 800-mg tablet of ZOVIRAX contains 800 mg of acyclovir and the inactive ingredients FD&C Blue No. 2, magnesium stearate, microcrystalline cellulose, povidone, and sodium starch glycolate.
Each 400-mg tablet of ZOVIRAX contains 400 mg of acyclovir and the inactive ingredients magnesium stearate, microcrystalline cellulose, povidone, and sodium starch glycolate.
Each teaspoonful (5 mL) of ZOVIRAX Suspension contains 200 mg of acyclovir and the inactive ingredients methylparaben 0.1% and propylparaben 0.02% (added as preservatives), carboxymethylcellulose sodium, flavor, glycerin, microcrystalline cellulose, and sorbitol.

Acyclovir is a white, crystalline powder with the molecular formula $C_8H_{11}N_5O_3$ and a molecular weight of 225. The maximum solubility in water at 37°C is 2.5 mg/mL. The pka's of acyclovir are 2.27 and 9.25.
The chemical name of acyclovir is 2-amino-1,9-dihydro-9-[(2-hydroxyethoxy)methyl]-6*H*-purin-6-one; it has the following structural formula:

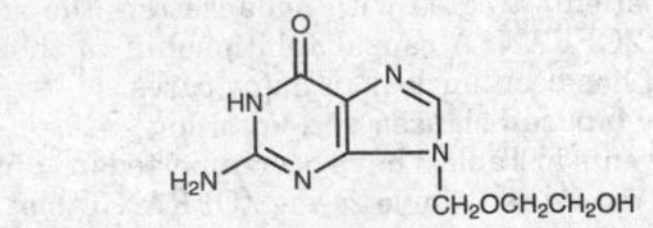

VIROLOGY
Mechanism of Antiviral Action: Acyclovir is a synthetic purine nucleoside analogue with in vitro and in vivo inhibitory activity against herpes simplex virus types 1 (HSV-1), 2 (HSV-2), and varicella-zoster virus (VZV).
The inhibitory activity of acyclovir is highly selective due to its affinity for the enzyme thymidine kinase (TK) encoded by HSV and VZV. This viral enzyme converts acyclovir into acyclovir monophosphate, a nucleotide analogue. The monophosphate is further converted into diphosphate by cellular guanylate kinase and into triphosphate by a number of cellular enzymes. In vitro, acyclovir triphosphate stops replication of herpes viral DNA. This is accomplished in 3 ways: 1) competitive inhibition of viral DNA polymerase, 2) incorporation into and termination of the growing viral DNA chain, and 3) inactivation of the viral DNA polymerase. The greater antiviral activity of acyclovir against HSV compared with VZV is due to its more efficient phosphorylation by the viral TK.
Antiviral Activities: The quantitative relationship between the in vitro susceptibility of herpes viruses to antivirals and the clinical response to therapy has not been established in humans, and virus sensitivity testing has not been standardized. Sensitivity testing results, expressed as the concentration of drug required to inhibit by 50% the growth of virus in cell culture (IC_{50}), vary greatly depending upon a number of factors. Using plaque-reduction assays, the IC_{50} against herpes simplex virus isolates ranges from 0.02 to 13.5 mcg/mL for HSV-1 and from 0.01 to 9.9 mcg/mL for HSV-2. The IC_{50} for acyclovir against most laboratory strains and clinical isolates of VZV ranges from 0.12 to 10.8 mcg/mL. Acyclovir also demonstrates activity against the Oka vaccine strain of VZV with a mean IC_{50} of 1.35 mcg/mL.
Drug Resistance: Resistance of HSV and VZV to acyclovir can result from qualitative and quantitative changes in the viral TK and/or DNA polymerase. Clinical isolates of HSV and VZV with reduced susceptibility to acyclovir have been recovered from immunocompromised patients, especially with advanced HIV infection. While most of the acyclovir-resistant mutants isolated thus far from immunocompromised patients have been found to be TK-deficient mutants, other mutants involving the viral TK gene (TK partial and TK altered) and DNA polymerase have been isolated. TK-negative mutants may cause severe disease in infants and immunocompromised adults. The possibility of viral resistance to acyclovir should be considered in patients who show poor clinical response during therapy.

CLINICAL PHARMACOLOGY
Pharmacokinetics: The pharmacokinetics of acyclovir after oral administration have been evaluated in healthy volunteers and in immunocompromised patients with herpes simplex or varicella-zoster virus infection. Acyclovir pharmacokinetic parameters are summarized in Table 1.

Table 1. Acyclovir Pharmacokinetic Characteristics (Range)

Parameter	Range
Plasma protein binding	9% to 33%
Plasma elimination half-life	2.5 to 3.3 hr
Average oral bioavailability	10% to 20%*

*Bioavailability decreases with increasing dose.

In one multiple-dose, crossover study in healthy subjects (n = 23), it was shown that increases in plasma acyclovir concentrations were less than dose proportional with increasing dose, as shown in Table 2. The decrease in bioavailability is a function of the dose and not the dosage form.

Table 2. Acyclovir Peak and Trough Concentrations at Steady State

Parameter	200 mg	400 mg	800 mg
C^{SS}_{max}	0.83 mcg/mL	1.21 mcg/mL	1.61 mcg/mL
C^{SS}_{trough}	0.46 mcg/mL	0.63 mcg/mL	0.83 mcg/mL

There was no effect of food on the absorption of acyclovir (n = 6); therefore, ZOVIRAX Capsules, Tablets, and Suspension may be administered with or without food.

The only known urinary metabolite is 9-[(carboxymethoxy)methyl]guanine.

Special Populations ***Adults With Impaired Renal Function:*** The half-life and total body clearance of acyclovir are dependent on renal function. A dosage adjustment is recommended for patients with reduced renal function (see DOSAGE AND ADMINISTRATION).

Geriatrics: Acyclovir plasma concentrations are higher in geriatric patients compared with younger adults, in part due to age-related changes in renal function. Dosage reduction may be required in geriatric patients with underlying renal impairment (see PRECAUTIONS: Geriatric Use).

Pediatrics: In general, the pharmacokinetics of acyclovir in pediatric patients is similar to that of adults. Mean half-life after oral doses of 300 mg/m^2 and 600 mg/m^2 in pediatric patients aged 7 months to 7 years was 2.6 hours (range 1.59 to 3.74 hours).

Drug Interactions: Coadministration of probenecid with intravenous acyclovir has been shown to increase the mean acyclovir half-life and the area under the concentration-time curve. Urinary excretion and renal clearance were correspondingly reduced.

Clinical Trials: ***Initial Genital Herpes:*** Double-blind, placebo-controlled studies have demonstrated that orally administered ZOVIRAX significantly reduced the duration of acute infection and duration of lesion healing. The duration of pain and new lesion formation was decreased in some patient groups.

Recurrent Genital Herpes: Double-blind, placebo-controlled studies in patients with frequent recurrences (6 or more episodes per year) have shown that orally administered ZOVIRAX given daily for 4 months to 10 years prevented or reduced the frequency and/or severity of recurrences in greater than 95% of patients.

In a study of patients who received ZOVIRAX 400 mg twice daily for 3 years, 45%, 52%, and 63% of patients remained free of recurrences in the first, second, and third years, respectively. Serial analyses of the 3-month recurrence rates for the patients showed that 71% to 87% were recurrence free in each quarter.

Herpes Zoster Infections: In a double-blind, placebo-controlled study of immunocompetent patients with localized cutaneous zoster infection, ZOVIRAX (800 mg 5 times daily for 10 days) shortened the times to lesion scabbing, healing, and complete cessation of pain, and reduced the duration of viral shedding and the duration of new lesion formation.

In a similar double-blind, placebo-controlled study, ZOVIRAX (800 mg 5 times daily for 7 days) shortened the times to complete lesion scabbing, healing, and cessation of pain; reduced the duration of new lesion formation; and reduced the prevalence of localized zoster-associated neurologic symptoms (paresthesia, dysesthesia, or hyperesthesia).

Treatment was begun within 72 hours of rash onset and was most effective if started within the first 48 hours.

Adults greater than 50 years of age showed greater benefit.

Chickenpox: Three randomized, double-blind, placebo-controlled trials were conducted in 993 pediatric patients aged 2 to 18 years with chickenpox. All patients were treated within 24 hours after the onset of rash. In 2 trials, ZOVIRAX was administered at 20 mg/kg 4 times daily (up to 3,200 mg per day) for 5 days. In the third trial, doses of 10, 15, or 20 mg/kg were administered 4 times daily for 5 to 7 days. Treatment with ZOVIRAX shortened the time to 50% healing; reduced the maximum number of lesions; reduced the median number of vesicles; decreased the median number of residual lesions on day 28; and decreased the proportion of patients with fever, anorexia, and lethargy by day 2. Treatment with ZOVIRAX did not affect varicella-zoster virus-specific humoral or cellular immune responses at 1 month or 1 year following treatment.

INDICATIONS AND USAGE

Herpes Zoster Infections: ZOVIRAX is indicated for the acute treatment of herpes zoster (shingles).

Genital Herpes: ZOVIRAX is indicated for the treatment of initial episodes and the management of recurrent episodes of genital herpes.

Chickenpox: ZOVIRAX is indicated for the treatment of chickenpox (varicella).

CONTRAINDICATIONS

ZOVIRAX is contraindicated for patients who develop hypersensitivity to acyclovir or valacyclovir.

WARNINGS

ZOVIRAX Capsules, Tablets, and Suspension are intended for oral ingestion only. Renal failure, in some cases resulting in death, has been observed with acyclovir therapy (see ADVERSE REACTIONS: Observed During Clinical Practice and OVERDOSAGE). Thrombotic thrombocytopenic purpura/hemolytic uremic syndrome (TTP/HUS), which has resulted in death, has occurred in immunocompromised patients receiving acyclovir therapy.

PRECAUTIONS

Dosage adjustment is recommended when administering ZOVIRAX to patients with renal impairment (see DOSAGE AND ADMINISTRATION). Caution should also be exercised when administering ZOVIRAX to patients receiving potentially nephrotoxic agents since this may increase the risk of renal dysfunction and/or the risk of reversible central nervous system symptoms such as those that have been reported in patients treated with intravenous acyclovir. Adequate hydration should be maintained.

Information for Patients: Patients are instructed to consult with their physician if they experience severe or troublesome adverse reactions, they become pregnant or intend to become pregnant, they intend to breastfeed while taking orally administered ZOVIRAX, or they have any other questions.

Patients should be advised to maintain adequate hydration.

Herpes Zoster: There are no data on treatment initiated more than 72 hours after onset of the zoster rash. Patients should be advised to initiate treatment as soon as possible after a diagnosis of herpes zoster.

Genital Herpes Infections: Patients should be informed that ZOVIRAX is not a cure for genital herpes. There are no data evaluating whether ZOVIRAX will prevent transmission of infection to others. Because genital herpes is a sexually transmitted disease, patients should avoid contact with lesions or intercourse when lesions and/or symptoms are present to avoid infecting partners. Genital herpes can also be transmitted in the absence of symptoms through asymptomatic viral shedding. If medical management of a genital herpes recurrence is indicated, patients should be advised to initiate therapy at the first sign or symptom of an episode.

Chickenpox: Chickenpox in otherwise healthy children is usually a self-limited disease of mild to moderate severity. Adolescents and adults tend to have more severe disease. Treatment was initiated within 24 hours of the typical chickenpox rash in the controlled studies, and there is no information regarding the effects of treatment begun later in the disease course.

Drug Interactions: See CLINICAL PHARMACOLOGY: Pharmacokinetics.

Carcinogenesis, Mutagenesis, Impairment of Fertility: The data presented below include references to peak steady-state plasma acyclovir concentrations observed in humans treated with 800 mg given orally 5 times a day (dosing appropriate for treatment of herpes zoster) or 200 mg given orally 5 times a day (dosing appropriate for treatment of genital herpes). Plasma drug concentrations in animal studies are expressed as multiples of human exposure to acyclovir at the higher and lower dosing schedules (see CLINICAL PHARMACOLOGY: Pharmacokinetics).

Acyclovir was tested in lifetime bioassays in rats and mice at single daily doses of up to 450 mg/kg administered by gavage. There was no statistically significant difference in the incidence of tumors between treated and control animals, nor did acyclovir shorten the latency of tumors. Maximum plasma concentrations were 3 to 6 times human levels in the mouse bioassay and 1 to 2 times human levels in the rat bioassay.

Acyclovir was tested in 16 in vitro and in vivo genetic toxicity assays. Acyclovir was positive in 5 of the assays.

Acyclovir did not impair fertility or reproduction in mice (450 mg/kg/day, p.o.) or in rats (25 mg/kg/day, s.c.). In the mouse study, plasma levels were 9 to 18 times human levels, while in the rat study, they were 8 to 15 times human levels. At higher doses (50 mg/kg/day, s.c.) in rats and rabbits (11 to 22 and 16 to 31 times human levels, respectively) implantation efficacy, but not litter size, was decreased. In a rat peri- and post-natal study at 50 mg/kg/day, s.c., there was a statistically significant decrease in group mean numbers of corpora lutea, total implantation sites, and live fetuses.

No testicular abnormalities were seen in dogs given 50 mg/kg/day, IV for 1 month (21 to 41 times human levels) or in dogs given 60 mg/kg/day orally for 1 year (6 to 12 times human levels). Testicular atrophy and aspermatogenesis were observed in rats and dogs at higher dose levels.

Pregnancy: ***Teratogenic Effects:*** Pregnancy Category B. Acyclovir administered during organogenesis was not teratogenic in the mouse (450 mg/kg/day, p.o.), rabbit (50 mg/kg/day, s.c. and IV), or rat (50 mg/kg/day, s.c.). These exposures resulted in plasma levels 9 and 18, 16 and 106, and 11 and 22 times, respectively, human levels.

There are no adequate and well-controlled studies in pregnant women. A prospective epidemiologic registry of acyclovir use during pregnancy was established in 1984 and completed in April 1999. There were 749 pregnancies followed in women exposed to systemic acyclovir during the first trimester of pregnancy resulting in 756 outcomes. The occurrence rate of birth defects approximates that found in the general population. However, the small size of the registry is insufficient to evaluate the risk for less common defects or to permit reliable or definitive conclusions regarding the safety of acyclovir in pregnant women and their developing fetuses. Acyclovir should be used during pregnancy only if the potential benefit justifies the potential risk to the fetus.

Nursing Mothers: Acyclovir concentrations have been documented in breast milk in 2 women following oral administration of ZOVIRAX and ranged from 0.6 to 4.1 times corresponding plasma levels. These concentrations would potentially expose the nursing infant to a dose of acyclovir up to 0.3 mg/kg/day. ZOVIRAX should be administered to a nursing mother with caution and only when indicated.

Pediatric Use: Safety and effectiveness of oral formulations of acyclovir in pediatric patients younger than 2 years of age have not been established.

Geriatric Use: Of 376 subjects who received ZOVIRAX in a clinical study of herpes zoster treatment in immunocompetent subjects ≥50 years of age, 244 were 65 and over while 111 were 75 and over. No overall differences in effectiveness for time to cessation of new lesion formation or time to healing were reported between geriatric subjects and younger adult subjects. The duration of pain after healing was longer in patients 65 and over. Nausea, vomiting, and dizziness were reported more frequently in elderly subjects. Elderly patients are more likely to have reduced renal function and require dose reduction. Elderly patients are also more likely to have renal or CNS adverse events. With respect to CNS adverse events observed during clinical practice, somnolence, hallucinations, confusion, and coma were reported more frequently in elderly patients (see CLINICAL PHARMACOLOGY, ADVERSE REACTIONS: Observed During Clinical Practice, and DOSAGE AND ADMINISTRATION).

ADVERSE REACTIONS

Herpes Simplex: ***Short-Term Administration:*** The most frequent adverse events reported during clinical trials of treatment of genital herpes with ZOVIRAX 200 mg administered orally 5 times daily every 4 hours for 10 days were nausea and/or vomiting in 8 of 298 patient treatments (2.7%). Nausea and/or vomiting occurred in 2 of 287 (0.7%) patients who received placebo.

Long-Term Administration: The most frequent adverse events reported in a clinical trial for the prevention of recurrences with continuous administration of 400 mg (two 200-mg capsules) 2 times daily for 1 year in 586 patients treated with ZOVIRAX were nausea (4.8%) and diarrhea (2.4%). The 589 control patients receiving intermittent treatment of recurrences with ZOVIRAX for 1 year reported diarrhea (2.7%), nausea (2.4%), and headache (2.2%).

Herpes Zoster: The most frequent adverse event reported during 3 clinical trials of treatment of herpes zoster (shingles) with 800 mg of oral ZOVIRAX 5 times daily for 7 to 10 days in 323 patients was malaise (11.5%). The 323 placebo recipients reported malaise (11.1%).

Chickenpox: The most frequent adverse event reported during 3 clinical trials of treatment of chickenpox with oral ZOVIRAX at doses of 10 to 20 mg/kg 4 times daily for 5 to 7 days or 800 mg 4 times daily for 5 days in 495 patients was diarrhea (3.2%). The 498 patients receiving placebo reported diarrhea (2.2%).

Observed During Clinical Practice: In addition to adverse events reported from clinical trials, the following events have been identified during post-approval use of ZOVIRAX. Because they are reported voluntarily from a population of unknown size, estimates of frequency cannot be made. These events have been chosen for inclusion due to either their seriousness, frequency of reporting, potential causal connection to ZOVIRAX, or a combination of these factors.

General: Anaphylaxis, angioedema, fever, headache, pain, peripheral edema.

Nervous: Aggressive behavior, agitation, ataxia, coma, confusion, decreased consciousness, delirium, dizziness, dysarthria, encephalopathy, hallucinations, paresthesia, psychosis, seizure, somnolence, tremors. These symptoms may be marked, particularly in older adults or in patients with renal impairment (see PRECAUTIONS).

Digestive: Diarrhea, gastrointestinal distress, nausea.

Table 3. Dosage Modification for Renal Impairment

Normal Dosage Regimen	Creatinine Clearance (mL/min/1.73 m^2)	Adjusted Dosage Regimen	
		Dose (mg)	Dosing Interval
200 mg every 4 hours	>10	200	every 4 hours, 5× daily
	0–10	200	every 12 hours
400 mg every 12 hours	>10	400	every 12 hours
	0–10	200	every 12 hours
800 mg every 4 hours	>25	800	every 4 hours, 5× daily
	10–25	800	every 8 hours
	0–10	800	every 12 hours

Hematologic and Lymphatic: Anemia, leukocytoclastic vasculitis, leukopenia, lymphadenopathy, thrombocytopenia.
Hepatobiliary Tract and Pancreas: Elevated liver function tests, hepatitis, hyperbilirubinemia, jaundice.
Musculoskeletal: Myalgia.
Skin: Alopecia, erythema multiforme, photosensitive rash, pruritus, rash, Stevens-Johnson syndrome, toxic epidermal necrolysis, urticaria.
Special Senses: Visual abnormalities.
Urogenital: Renal failure, renal pain (may be associated with renal failure), elevated blood urea nitrogen, elevated creatinine, hematuria (see WARNINGS).

OVERDOSAGE

Overdoses involving ingestion of up to 100 capsules (20 g) have been reported. Adverse events that have been reported in association with overdosage include agitation, coma, seizures, and lethargy. Precipitation of acyclovir in renal tubules may occur when the solubility (2.5 mg/mL) is exceeded in the intratubular fluid. Overdosage has been reported following bolus injections or inappropriately high doses and in patients whose fluid and electrolyte balance were not properly monitored. This has resulted in elevated BUN and serum creatinine and subsequent renal failure. In the event of acute renal failure and anuria, the patient may benefit from hemodialysis until renal function is restored (see DOSAGE AND ADMINISTRATION).

DOSAGE AND ADMINISTRATION

Acute Treatment of Herpes Zoster: 800 mg every 4 hours orally, 5 times daily for 7 to 10 days.
Genital Herpes: *Treatment of Initial Genital Herpes:* 200 mg every 4 hours, 5 times daily for 10 days.
Chronic Suppressive Therapy for Recurrent Disease: 400 mg 2 times daily for up to 12 months, followed by re-evaluation. Alternative regimens have included doses ranging from 200 mg 3 times daily to 200 mg 5 times daily. The frequency and severity of episodes of untreated genital herpes may change over time. After 1 year of therapy, the frequency and severity of the patient's genital herpes infection should be re-evaluated to assess the need for continuation of therapy with ZOVIRAX.
Intermittent Therapy: 200 mg every 4 hours, 5 times daily for 5 days. Therapy should be initiated at the earliest sign or symptom (prodrome) of recurrence.
Treatment of Chickenpox: *Children (2 years of age and older):* 20 mg/kg per dose orally 4 times daily (80 mg/kg/day) for 5 days. Children over 40 kg should receive the adult dose for chickenpox.
Adults and Children over 40 kg: 800 mg 4 times daily for 5 days.
Intravenous ZOVIRAX is indicated for the treatment of varicella-zoster infections in immunocompromised patients. When therapy is indicated, it should be initiated at the earliest sign or symptom of chickenpox. There is no information about the efficacy of therapy initiated more than 24 hours after onset of signs and symptoms.
Patients With Acute or Chronic Renal Impairment: In patients with renal impairment, the dose of ZOVIRAX Capsules, Tablets, or Suspension should be modified as shown in Table 3.
[See table above]
Hemodialysis: For patients who require hemodialysis, the mean plasma half-life of acyclovir during hemodialysis is approximately 5 hours. This results in a 60% decrease in plasma concentrations following a 6-hour dialysis period. Therefore, the patient's dosing schedule should be adjusted so that an additional dose is administered after each dialysis.
Peritoneal Dialysis: No supplemental dose appears to be necessary after adjustment of the dosing interval.
Bioequivalence of Dosage Forms: ZOVIRAX Suspension was shown to be bioequivalent to ZOVIRAX Capsules (n = 20) and 1 ZOVIRAX 800-mg tablet was shown to be bioequivalent to 4 ZOVIRAX 200-mg capsules (n = 24).

HOW SUPPLIED

ZOVIRAX Capsules (blue, opaque cap and body) containing 200 mg acyclovir and printed with "Wellcome ZOVIRAX 200."
Bottle of 100 (NDC 0173-0991-55).
Store at 15° to 25°C (59° to 77°F) and protect from moisture.
ZOVIRAX Tablets (light blue, oval) containing 800 mg acyclovir and engraved with "ZOVIRAX 800."
Bottle of 100 (NDC 0173-0945-55).
Store at 15° to 25°C (59° to 77°F) and protect from moisture.
ZOVIRAX Tablets (white, shield-shaped) containing 400 mg acyclovir and engraved with "ZOVIRAX" on one side and a triangle on the other side.
Bottle of 100 (NDC 0173-0949-55).
Store at 15° to 25°C (59° to 77°F) and protect from moisture.
ZOVIRAX Suspension (off-white, banana-flavored) containing 200 mg acyclovir in each teaspoonful (5 mL).
Bottle of 1 pint (473 mL) (NDC 0173-0953-96).
Store at 15° to 25°C (59° to 77°F).
ZOVIRAX is a registered trademark of GlaxoSmithKline.
GlaxoSmithKline
Research Triangle Park, NC 27709
©2007, GlaxoSmithKline. All rights reserved.
November 2007   ZVT:2PI

ZYBAN®   Rx
[zī'ban]
(bupropion hydrochloride)
Sustained-Release Tablets

WARNING

Serious neuropsychiatric events, including but not limited to depression, suicidal ideation, suicide attempt, and completed suicide have been reported in patients taking ZYBAN for smoking cessation. Some cases may have been complicated by the symptoms of nicotine withdrawal in patients who stopped smoking. Depressed mood may be a symptom of nicotine withdrawal. Depression, rarely including suicidal ideation, has been reported in smokers undergoing a smoking cessation attempt without medication. However, some of these symptoms have occurred in patients taking ZYBAN who continued to smoke.
All patients being treated with ZYBAN should be observed for neuropsychiatric symptoms including changes in behavior, hostility, agitation, depressed mood, and suicide-related events, including ideation, behavior, and attempted suicide. These symptoms, as well as worsening of pre-existing psychiatric illness and completed suicide have been reported in some patients attempting to quit smoking while taking ZYBAN in the postmarketing experience. When symptoms were reported, most were during treatment with ZYBAN, but some were following discontinuation of treatment with ZYBAN. These events have occurred in patients with and without pre-existing psychiatric disease; some have experienced worsening of their psychiatric illnesses. Patients with serious psychiatric illness such as schizophrenia, bipolar disorder, and major depressive disorder did not participate in the premarketing studies of ZYBAN.
Advise patients and caregivers that the patient should stop taking ZYBAN and contact a healthcare provider immediately if agitation, hostility, depressed mood, or changes in thinking or behavior that are not typical for the patient are observed, or if the patient develops suicidal ideation or suicidal behavior. In many postmarketing cases, resolution of symptoms after discontinuation of ZYBAN was reported, although in some cases the symptoms persisted; therefore, ongoing moni-

---

toring and supportive care should be provided until symptoms resolve.
The risks of ZYBAN should be weighed against the benefits of its use. ZYBAN has been demonstrated to increase the likelihood of abstinence from smoking for as long as 6 months compared to treatment with placebo. The health benefits of quitting smoking are immediate and substantial. (See WARNINGS: Neuropsychiatric Symptoms and Suicide Risk in Smoking Cessation Treatment and PRECAUTIONS: Information for Patients.)
Use in Treating Psychiatric Disorders: Although ZYBAN is not indicated for treatment of depression, it contains the same active ingredient as the antidepressant medications WELLBUTRIN®, WELLBUTRIN SR®, and WELLBUTRIN XL®. Antidepressants increased the risk compared to placebo of suicidal thinking and behavior (suicidality) in children, adolescents, and young adults in short-term studies of major depressive disorder (MDD) and other psychiatric disorders. Anyone considering the use of ZYBAN or any other antidepressant in a child, adolescent, or young adult must balance this risk with the clinical need. Short-term studies did not show an increase in the risk of suicidality with antidepressants compared to placebo in adults beyond age 24; there was a reduction in risk with antidepressants compared to placebo in adults aged 65 and older. Depression and certain other psychiatric disorders are themselves associated with increases in the risk of suicide. Patients of all ages who are started on antidepressant therapy should be monitored appropriately and observed closely for clinical worsening, suicidality, or unusual changes in behavior. Families and caregivers should be advised of the need for close observation and communication with the prescriber. ZYBAN is not approved for use in pediatric patients. (See WARNINGS: Clinical Worsening and Suicide Risk in Treating Psychiatric Disorders, PRECAUTIONS: Information for Patients, and PRECAUTIONS: Pediatric Use.)

DESCRIPTION

ZYBAN (bupropion hydrochloride) Sustained-Release Tablets are a non-nicotine aid to smoking cessation. ZYBAN is chemically unrelated to nicotine or other agents currently used in the treatment of nicotine addiction. Initially developed and marketed as an antidepressant (WELLBUTRIN [bupropion hydrochloride] Tablets and WELLBUTRIN SR [bupropion hydrochloride] Sustained-Release Tablets), ZYBAN is also chemically unrelated to tricyclic, tetracyclic, selective serotonin re-uptake inhibitor, or other known antidepressant agents. Its structure closely resembles that of diethylpropion; it is related to phenylethylamines. It is (±)-1-(3-chlorophenyl)-2-[(1,1-dimethylethyl)amino]-1-propanone hydrochloride. The molecular weight is 276.2. The molecular formula is $C_{13}H_{18}ClNO \bullet HCl$. Bupropion hydrochloride powder is white, crystalline, and highly soluble in water. It has a bitter taste and produces the sensation of local anesthesia on the oral mucosa. The structural formula is:

ZYBAN Tablets are supplied for oral administration as 150-mg (purple), film-coated, sustained-release tablets. Each tablet contains the labeled amount of bupropion hydrochloride and the inactive ingredients carnauba wax, cysteine hydrochloride, hypromellose, magnesium stearate, microcrystalline cellulose, polyethylene glycol, polysorbate 80 and titanium dioxide and is printed with edible black ink. In addition, the 150-mg tablet contains FD&C Blue No. 2 Lake and FD&C Red No. 40 Lake.

CLINICAL PHARMACOLOGY

Pharmacodynamics: Bupropion is a relatively weak inhibitor of the neuronal uptake of norepinephrine and dopamine, and does not inhibit monoamine oxidase or the re-uptake of serotonin. The mechanism by which ZYBAN enhances the ability of patients to abstain from smoking is unknown. However, it is presumed that this action is mediated by noradrenergic and/or dopaminergic mechanisms.
Pharmacokinetics: Bupropion is a racemic mixture. The pharmacologic activity and pharmacokinetics of the individual enantiomers have not been studied. Bupropion follows biphasic pharmacokinetics best described by a 2-compartment model. The terminal phase has a mean half-life (± % CV) of about 21 hours (±20%), while the distribution phase has a mean half-life of 3 to 4 hours.
Absorption: Bupropion has not been administered intravenously to humans; therefore, the absolute bioavailability

of ZYBAN Sustained-Release Tablets in humans has not been determined. In rat and dog studies, the bioavailability of bupropion ranged from 5% to 20%.

Following oral administration of ZYBAN to healthy volunteers, peak plasma concentrations of bupropion are achieved within 3 hours. The mean peak concentration (C_{max}) values were 91 and 143 ng/mL from 2 single-dose (150-mg) studies. At steady state, the mean C_{max} following a 150-mg dose every 12 hours is 136 ng/mL.

In a single-dose study, food increased the C_{max} of bupropion by 11% and the extent of absorption as defined by area under the plasma concentration-time curve (AUC) by 17%. The mean time to peak concentration (T_{max}) was prolonged by 1 hour. This effect was of no clinical significance.

Distribution: In vitro tests show that bupropion is 84% bound to human plasma proteins at concentrations up to 200 mcg/mL. The extent of protein binding of the hydroxybupropion metabolite is similar to that for bupropion, whereas the extent of protein binding of the threohydrobupropion metabolite is about half that seen with bupropion. The volume of distribution (V_{ss}/F) estimated from a single 150-mg dose given to 17 subjects is 1,950 L (20% CV).

Metabolism: Bupropion is extensively metabolized in humans. Three metabolites have been shown to be active: hydroxybupropion, which is formed via hydroxylation of the *tert*-butyl group of bupropion, and the amino-alcohol isomers threohydrobupropion and erythrohydrobupropion, which are formed via reduction of the carbonyl group. In vitro findings suggest that cytochrome P450IIB6 (CYP2B6) is the principal isoenzyme involved in the formation of hydroxybupropion, while cytochrome P450 isoenzymes are not involved in the formation of threohydrobupropion. Oxidation of the bupropion side chain results in the formation of a glycine conjugate of meta-chlorobenzoic acid, which is then excreted as the major urinary metabolite. The potency and toxicity of the metabolites relative to bupropion have not been fully characterized. However, it has been demonstrated in an antidepressant screening test in mice that hydroxybupropion is one half as potent as bupropion, while threohydrobupropion and erythrohydrobupropion are 5-fold less potent than bupropion. This may be of clinical importance because the plasma concentrations of the metabolites are as high or higher than those of bupropion.

Because bupropion is extensively metabolized, there is the potential for drug-drug interactions, particularly with those agents that are metabolized by the cytochrome P450IIB6 (CYP2B6) isoenzyme. Although bupropion is not metabolized by cytochrome P450IID6 (CYP2D6), there is the potential for drug-drug interactions when bupropion is coadministered with drugs metabolized by this isoenzyme (see PRECAUTIONS: Drug Interactions).

Following a single dose in humans, peak plasma concentrations of hydroxybupropion occur approximately 6 hours after administration of ZYBAN Tablets. Peak plasma concentrations of hydroxybupropion are approximately 10 times the peak level of the parent drug at steady state. The elimination half-life of hydroxybupropion is approximately 20 (±5) hours, and its AUC at steady state is about 17 times that of bupropion. The times to peak concentrations for the erythrohydrobupropion and threohydrobupropion metabolites are similar to that of the hydroxybupropion metabolite; however, their elimination half-lives are longer, 33 (±10) and 37 (±13) hours, respectively, and steady-state AUCs are 1.5 and 7 times that of bupropion, respectively.

Bupropion and its metabolites exhibit linear kinetics following chronic administration of 300 to 450 mg/day.

Elimination: The mean (±% CV) apparent clearance (Cl/F) estimated from 2 single-dose (150-mg) studies are 135 (±20%) and 209 L/hr (±21%). Following chronic dosing of 150 mg of ZYBAN every 12 hours for 14 days (n = 34), the mean Cl/F at steady state was 160 L/hr (±23%). The mean elimination half-life of bupropion estimated from a series of studies is approximately 21 hours. Estimates of the half-lives of the metabolites determined from a multiple-dose study were 20 hours (±25%) for hydroxybupropion, 37 hours (±35%) for threohydrobupropion, and 33 hours (±30%) for erythrohydrobupropion. Steady-state plasma concentrations of bupropion and metabolites are reached within 5 and 8 days, respectively.

Following oral administration of 200 mg of ^{14}C-bupropion in humans, 87% and 10% of the radioactive dose were recovered in the urine and feces, respectively. The fraction of the oral dose of bupropion excreted unchanged was only 0.5%.

The effects of cigarette smoking on the pharmacokinetics of bupropion were studied in 34 healthy male and female volunteers; 17 were chronic cigarette smokers and 17 were nonsmokers. Following oral administration of a single 150-mg dose of ZYBAN, there was no statistically significant difference in C_{max}, half-life, T_{max}, AUC, or clearance of bupropion or its major metabolites between smokers and nonsmokers.

In a study comparing the treatment combination of ZYBAN and nicotine transdermal system (NTS) versus ZYBAN alone, no statistically significant differences were observed between the 2 treatment groups of combination ZYBAN and NTS (n = 197) and ZYBAN alone (n = 193) in the plasma concentrations of bupropion or its active metabolites at weeks 3 and 6.

Population Subgroups: Factors or conditions altering metabolic capacity (e.g., liver disease, congestive heart failure [CHF], age, concomitant medications, etc.) or elimination may be expected to influence the degree and extent of accumulation of the active metabolites of bupropion. The elimination of the major metabolites of bupropion may be affected by reduced renal or hepatic function because they are moderately polar compounds and are likely to undergo further metabolism or conjugation in the liver prior to urinary excretion.

Hepatic: The effect of hepatic impairment on the pharmacokinetics of bupropion was characterized in 2 single-dose studies, one in patients with alcoholic liver disease and one in patients with mild-to-severe cirrhosis. The first study showed that the half-life of hydroxybupropion was significantly longer in 8 patients with alcoholic liver disease than in 8 healthy volunteers (32±14 hours versus 21±5 hours, respectively). Although not statistically significant, the AUCs for bupropion and hydroxybupropion were more variable and tended to be greater (by 53% to 57%) in patients with alcoholic liver disease. The differences in half-life for bupropion and the other metabolites in the 2 patient groups were minimal.

The second study showed that there were no statistically significant differences in the pharmacokinetics of bupropion and its active metabolites in 9 patients with mild to moderate hepatic cirrhosis compared to 8 healthy volunteers. However, more variability was observed in some of the pharmacokinetic parameters for bupropion (AUC, C_{max}, and T_{max}) and its active metabolites ($t_{½}$) in patients with mild to moderate hepatic cirrhosis. In addition, in patients with severe hepatic cirrhosis, the bupropion C_{max} and AUC were substantially increased (mean difference: by approximately 70% and 3-fold, respectively) and more variable when compared to values in healthy volunteers; the mean bupropion half-life was also longer (29 hours in patients with severe hepatic cirrhosis vs. 19 hours in healthy subjects). For the metabolite hydroxybupropion, the mean C_{max} was approximately 69% lower. For the combined amino-alcohol isomers threohydrobupropion and erythrohydrobupropion, the mean C_{max} was approximately 31% lower. The mean AUC increased by 28% for hydroxybupropion and 50% for threo/erythrohydrobupropion. The median T_{max} was observed 19 hours later for hydroxybupropion and 21 hours later for threo/erythrohydrobupropion. The mean half-lives for hydroxybupropion and threo/erythrohydrobupropion were increased 2- and 4-fold, respectively, in patients with severe hepatic cirrhosis compared to healthy volunteers (see WARNINGS, PRECAUTIONS, and DOSAGE AND ADMINISTRATION).

Renal: There is limited information on the pharmacokinetics of bupropion in patients with renal impairment. An inter-study comparison between normal subjects and patients with end-stage renal failure demonstrated that the parent drug C_{max} and AUC values were comparable in the 2 groups, whereas the hydroxybupropion and threohydrobupropion metabolites had a 2.3- and 2.8-fold increase, respectively, in AUC for patients with end-stage renal failure. A second study, comparing normal subjects and patients with moderate-to-severe renal impairment (GFR 30.9 ± 10.8 mL/min) showed that exposure to a single 150-mg dose of sustained-release bupropion was approximately 2-fold higher in patients with impaired renal function while levels of the hydroxybupropion and threo/erythrohydrobupropion (combined) metabolites were similar in the 2 groups. The elimination of bupropion and/or the major metabolites of bupropion may be reduced by impaired renal function (see PRECAUTIONS: Renal Impairment).

Left Ventricular Dysfunction: During a chronic dosing study with bupropion in 14 depressed patients with left ventricular dysfunction (history of CHF or an enlarged heart on x-ray), no apparent effect on the pharmacokinetics of bupropion or its metabolites, compared to healthy normal volunteers, was revealed.

Age: The effects of age on the pharmacokinetics of bupropion and its metabolites have not been fully characterized, but an exploration of steady-state bupropion concentrations from several depression efficacy studies involving patients dosed in a range of 300 to 750 mg/day, on a 3-times-a-day schedule, revealed no relationship between age (18 to 83 years) and plasma concentration of bupropion. A single-dose pharmacokinetic study demonstrated that the disposition of bupropion and its metabolites in elderly subjects was similar to that of younger subjects. These data suggest there is no prominent effect of age on bupropion concentration; however, another pharmacokinetic study, single and multiple dose, has suggested that the elderly are at increased risk for accumulation of bupropion and its metabolites (see PRECAUTIONS: Geriatric Use).

Gender: A single-dose study involving 12 healthy male and 12 healthy female volunteers revealed no sex-related differences in the pharmacokinetic parameters of bupropion.

CLINICAL TRIALS

The efficacy of ZYBAN as an aid to smoking cessation was demonstrated in 3 placebo-controlled, double-blind trials in nondepressed chronic cigarette smokers (n = 1,940, ≥15 cigarettes per day). In these studies, ZYBAN was used in conjunction with individual smoking cessation counseling.

The first study was a dose-response trial conducted at 3 clinical centers. Patients in this study were treated for 7 weeks with 1 of 3 doses of ZYBAN (100, 150, or 300 mg/day) or placebo; quitting was defined as total abstinence during the last 4 weeks of treatment (weeks 4 through 7). Abstinence was determined by patient daily diaries and verified by carbon monoxide levels in expired air.

Results of this dose-response trial with ZYBAN demonstrated a dose-dependent increase in the percentage of patients able to achieve 4-week abstinence (weeks 4 through 7). Treatment with ZYBAN at both 150 and 300 mg/day was significantly more effective than placebo in this study.

Table 1 presents quit rates over time in the multicenter trial by treatment group. The quit rates are the proportions of all persons initially enrolled (i.e., intent-to-treat analysis) who abstained from week 4 of the study through the specified week. Treatment with ZYBAN (150 or 300 mg/day) was more effective than placebo in helping patients achieve 4-week abstinence. In addition, treatment with ZYBAN (7 weeks at 300 mg/day) was more effective than placebo in helping patients maintain continuous abstinence through week 26 (6 months) of the study.

[See table 1 above]

Table 1. Dose-Response Trial: Quit Rates by Treatment Group

	Treatment Groups			
Abstinence From Week 4 Through Specified Week	Placebo (n = 151) % (95% CI)	ZYBAN 100 mg/day (n = 153) % (95% CI)	ZYBAN 150 mg/day (n = 153) % (95% CI)	ZYBAN 300 mg/day (n = 156) % (95% CI)
Week 7 (4-week quit)	17% (11-23)	22% (15-28)	27%[a] (20-35)	36%[a] (28-43)
Week 12	14% (8-19)	20% (13-26)	20% (14-27)	25%[a] (18-32)
Week 26	11% (6-16)	16% (11-22)	18% (12-24)	19%[a] (13-25)

[a] Significantly different from placebo ($P \leq 0.05$).

The second study was a comparative trial conducted at 4 clinical centers. Four treatments were evaluated: ZYBAN 300 mg/day, nicotine transdermal system (NTS) 21 mg/day, combination of ZYBAN 300 mg/day plus NTS 21 mg/day, and placebo. Patients were treated for 9 weeks. Treatment with ZYBAN was initiated at 150 mg/day while the patient was still smoking and was increased after 3 days to 300 mg/day given as 150 mg twice daily. NTS 21 mg/day was added to treatment with ZYBAN after approximately 1 week when the patient reached the target quit date. During weeks 8 and 9 of the study, NTS was tapered to 14 and 7 mg/day, respectively. Quitting, defined as total abstinence during weeks 4 through 7, was determined by patient daily diaries and verified by expired air carbon monoxide levels. In this study, patients treated with any of the 3 treatments achieved greater 4-week abstinence rates than patients treated with placebo.

Table 2 presents quit rates over time by treatment group for the comparative trial.
[See table 2 at right]
When patients in this study were followed out to one year, the superiority of ZYBAN and the combination of ZYBAN and NTS over placebo in helping patients to achieve abstinence from smoking was maintained. The continuous abstinence rate was 30% (95% CI 24-35) in the patients treated with ZYBAN, and 33% (95% CI 27-39) for patients treated with the combination at 26 weeks compared with 13% (95% CI 7-18) in the placebo group. At 52 weeks, the continuous abstinence rate was 23% (95% CI 18-28) in the patients treated with ZYBAN and 28% (95% CI 23-34) for patients treated with the combination, compared with 8% (95% CI 3-12) in the placebo group. Although the treatment combination of ZYBAN and NTS displayed the highest rates of continuous abstinence throughout the study, the quit rates for the combination were not significantly higher (*P*>0.05) than for ZYBAN alone.
The comparisons between ZYBAN, NTS, and combination treatment in this study have not been replicated, and, therefore should not be interpreted as demonstrating the superiority of any of the active treatment arms over any other.
The third study was a long-term maintenance trial conducted at 5 clinical centers. Patients in this study received open-label ZYBAN 300 mg/day for 7 weeks. Patients who quit smoking while receiving ZYBAN (n = 432) were then randomized to ZYBAN 300 mg/day or placebo for a total study duration of 1 year. Abstinence from smoking was determined by patient self-report and verified by expired air carbon monoxide levels. This trial demonstrated that at 6 months, continuous abstinence rates were significantly higher for patients continuing to receive ZYBAN than for those switched to placebo (*P*<0.05; 55% versus 44%).
Quit rates in clinical trials are influenced by the population selected. Quit rates in an unselected population may be lower than the above rates. Quit rates for ZYBAN were similar in patients with and without prior quit attempts using nicotine replacement therapy.
Treatment with ZYBAN reduced withdrawal symptoms compared to placebo. Reductions on the following withdrawal symptoms were most pronounced: irritability, frustration, or anger; anxiety; difficulty concentrating; restlessness; and depressed mood or negative affect. Depending on the study and the measure used, treatment with ZYBAN showed evidence of reduction in craving for cigarettes or urge to smoke compared to placebo.
Use In Patients With Chronic Obstructive Pulmonary Disease (COPD): ZYBAN was evaluated in a randomized, double-blind, comparative study of 404 patients with mild-to-moderate COPD, defined as $FEV_1 \geq 35\%$, $FEV_1/FVC \leq 70\%$ and a diagnosis of chronic bronchitis, emphysema and/or small airways disease. Patients aged 36 to 76 years were randomized to ZYBAN 300 mg/day (n = 204) or placebo (n = 200) and treated for 12 weeks. Treatment with ZYBAN was initiated at 150 mg/day for 3 days while the patient was still smoking and increased to 150 mg twice daily for the remaining treatment period. Abstinence from smoking was determined by patient daily diaries and verified by carbon monoxide levels in expired air. Quitters are defined as subjects who were abstinent during the last 4 weeks of treatment. Table 3 shows quit rates in the COPD Trial.

Table 3. COPD Trial: Quit Rates by Treatment Group

4-Week Abstinence Period	Treatment Groups	
	Placebo (n = 200) % (95% CI)	ZYBAN 300 mg/day (n = 204) % (95% CI)
Weeks 9 through 12	12% (8-16)	22%[a] (17-27)

[a] Significantly different from placebo (*P*<0.05).

INDICATIONS AND USAGE

ZYBAN is indicated as an aid to smoking cessation treatment.

CONTRAINDICATIONS

ZYBAN is contraindicated in patients with a seizure disorder.
ZYBAN is contraindicated in patients treated with WELLBUTRIN (bupropion hydrochloride), the immediate-release formulation; WELLBUTRIN SR (bupropion hydrochloride), the sustained-release formulation; WELLBUTRIN XL (bupropion hydrochloride), the extended-release formulation; or any other medications that contain bupropion because the incidence of seizure is dose dependent.

Table 2. Comparative Trial: Quit Rates by Treatment Group

Abstinence From Week 4 Through Specified Week	Treatment Groups			
	Placebo (n = 160) % (95% CI)	Nicotine Transdermal System (NTS) 21 mg/day (n = 244) % (95% CI)	ZYBAN 300 mg/day (n = 244) % (95% CI)	ZYBAN 300 mg/day and NTS 21 mg/day (n = 245) % (95% CI)
Week 7 (4-week quit)	23% (17-30)	36% (30-42)	49% (43-56)	58% (51-64)
Week 10	20% (14-26)	32% (26-37)	46% (39-52)	51% (45-58)

ZYBAN is contraindicated in patients with a current or prior diagnosis of bulimia or anorexia nervosa because of a higher incidence of seizures noted in patients treated for bulimia with the immediate-release formulation of bupropion.
ZYBAN is contraindicated in patients undergoing abrupt discontinuation of alcohol or sedatives (including benzodiazepines).
The concurrent administration of ZYBAN and a monoamine oxidase (MAO) inhibitor is contraindicated. At least 14 days should elapse between discontinuation of an MAO inhibitor and initiation of treatment with ZYBAN.
ZYBAN is contraindicated in patients who have shown an allergic response to bupropion or the other ingredients that make up ZYBAN.

WARNINGS

Neuropsychiatric Symptoms and Suicide Risk in Smoking Cessation Treatment: Serious neuropsychiatric symptoms have been reported in patients taking ZYBAN for smoking cessation **(see BOXED WARNING, ADVERSE REACTIONS). These have included changes in mood (including depression and mania), psychosis, hallucinations, paranoia, delusions, homicidal ideation, hostility, agitation, aggression, anxiety, and panic, as well as suicidal ideation, suicide attempt, and completed suicide.** Some reported cases may have been complicated by the symptoms of nicotine withdrawal in patients who stopped smoking. Depressed mood may be a symptom of nicotine withdrawal. Depression, rarely including suicidal ideation, has been reported in smokers undergoing a smoking cessation attempt without medication. However, some of these symptoms have occurred in patients taking ZYBAN who continued to smoke. When symptoms were reported, most were during treatment with ZYBAN, but some were following discontinuation of treatment with ZYBAN.
These events have occurred in patients with and without pre-existing psychiatric disease; some patients have experienced worsening of their psychiatric illnesses. All patients being treated with ZYBAN should be observed for neuropsychiatric symptoms or worsening of pre-existing psychiatric illness.
Patients with serious psychiatric illness such as schizophrenia, bipolar disorder, and major depressive disorder did not participate in the premarketing studies of ZYBAN.
Advise patients and caregivers that the patient should stop taking ZYBAN and contact a healthcare provider immediately if agitation, depressed mood, or changes in behavior or thinking that are not typical for the patient are observed, or if the patient develops suicidal ideation or suicidal behavior. In many post-marketing cases, resolution of symptoms after discontinuation of ZYBAN was reported, although in some cases the symptoms persisted, therefore, ongoing monitoring and supportive care should be provided until symptoms resolve.
The risks of ZYBAN should be weighed against the benefits of its use. ZYBAN has been demonstrated to increase the likelihood of abstinence from smoking for as long as six months compared to treatment with placebo. The health benefits of quitting smoking are immediate and substantial.
Clinical Worsening and Suicide Risk in Treating Psychiatric Disorders: Patients with major depressive disorder (MDD), both adult and pediatric, may experience worsening of their depression and/or the emergence of suicidal ideation and behavior (suicidality) or unusual changes in behavior, whether or not they are taking antidepressant medications, and this risk may persist until significant remission occurs. Suicide is a known risk of depression and certain other psychiatric disorders, and these disorders themselves are the strongest predictors of suicide. There has been a long-standing concern, however, that antidepressants may have a role in inducing worsening of depression and the emergence of suicidality in certain patients during the early phases of treatment. Pooled analyses of short-term placebo-controlled trials of antidepressant drugs (SSRIs and others) showed that these drugs increase the risk of suicidal thinking and behavior (suicidality) in children, adolescents, and young adults (ages 18-24) with major depressive disorder (MDD) and other psychiatric disorders. Short-term studies did not show an increase in the risk of suicidality with antidepressants compared to placebo in adults beyond age 24; there was a reduction with antidepressants compared to placebo in adults aged 65 and older.
The pooled analyses of placebo-controlled trials in children and adolescents with MDD, obsessive compulsive disorder (OCD), or other psychiatric disorders included a total of 24 short-term trials of 9 antidepressant drugs in over 4,400 patients. The pooled analyses of placebo-controlled trials in adults with MDD or other psychiatric disorders included a total of 295 short-term trials (median duration of 2 months) of 11 antidepressant drugs in over 77,000 patients. There was considerable variation in risk of suicidality among drugs, but a tendency toward an increase in the younger patients for almost all drugs studied. There were differences in absolute risk of suicidality across the different indications, with the highest incidence in MDD. The risk differences (drug vs placebo), however, were relatively stable within age strata and across indications. These risk differences (drug-placebo difference in the number of cases of suicidality per 1,000 patients treated) are provided in Table 4.

Table 4

Age Range	Drug-Placebo Difference in Number of Cases of Suicidality per 1,000 Patients Treated
Increases Compared to Placebo	
<18	14 additional cases
18-24	5 additional cases
Decreases Compared to Placebo	
25-64	1 fewer case
≥65	6 fewer cases

No suicides occurred in any of the pediatric trials. There were suicides in the adult trials, but the number was not sufficient to reach any conclusion about drug effect on suicide.
It is unknown whether the suicidality risk extends to longer-term use, i.e., beyond several months. However, there is substantial evidence from placebo-controlled maintenance trials in adults with depression that the use of antidepressants can delay the recurrence of depression.
All patients being treated with antidepressants for any indication should be monitored appropriately and observed closely for clinical worsening, suicidality, and unusual changes in behavior, especially during the initial few months of a course of drug therapy, or at times of dose changes, either increases or decreases.
The following symptoms, anxiety, agitation, panic attacks, insomnia, irritability, hostility, aggressiveness, impulsivity, akathisia (psychomotor restlessness), hypomania, and mania, have been reported in adult and pediatric patients being treated with antidepressants for major depressive disorder as well as for other indications, both psychiatric and nonpsychiatric. Although a causal link between the emergence of such symptoms and either the worsening of depression and/or the emergence of suicidal impulses has not been established, there is concern that such symptoms may represent precursors to emerging suicidality.
Consideration should be given to changing the therapeutic regimen, including possibly discontinuing the medication, in patients whose depression is persistently worse, or who

are experiencing emergent suicidality or symptoms that might be precursors to worsening depression or suicidality, especially if these symptoms are severe, abrupt in onset, or were not part of the patient's presenting symptoms.

Families and caregivers of patients being treated with antidepressants for major depressive disorder or other indications, both psychiatric and nonpsychiatric, should be alerted about the need to monitor patients for the emergence of agitation, irritability, unusual changes in behavior, and the other symptoms described above, as well as the emergence of suicidality, and to report such symptoms immediately to healthcare providers. Such monitoring should include daily observation by families and caregivers. Prescriptions for ZYBAN should be written for the smallest quantity of tablets consistent with good patient management, in order to reduce the risk of overdose.

Screening Patients for Bipolar Disorder: A major depressive episode may be the initial presentation of bipolar disorder. It is generally believed (though not established in controlled trials) that treating such an episode with an antidepressant alone may increase the likelihood of precipitation of a mixed/manic episode in patients at risk for bipolar disorder. Whether any of the symptoms described above represent such a conversion is unknown. However, prior to initiating treatment with an antidepressant, patients with depressive symptoms should be adequately screened to determine if they are at risk for bipolar disorder; such screening should include a detailed psychiatric history, including a family history of suicide, bipolar disorder, and depression. It should be noted that ZYBAN is not approved for use in treating bipolar depression.

Bupropion-Containing Products

Patients should be made aware that ZYBAN contains the same active ingredient found in WELLBUTRIN, WELLBUTRIN SR, and WELLBUTRIN XL used to treat depression, and that ZYBAN should not be used in combination with WELLBUTRIN (bupropion hydrochloride), the immediate release formulation; WELLBUTRIN SR (bupropion hydrochloride), the sustained-release formulation; WELLBUTRIN XL (bupropion hydrochloride), the extended-release formulation; or any other medications that contain bupropion.

Seizures: Because the use of bupropion is associated with a dose-dependent risk of seizures, *clinicians should not prescribe doses over 300 mg/day for smoking cessation.* The risk of seizures is also related to patient factors, clinical situation, and concomitant medications, which must be considered in selection of patients for therapy with ZYBAN. ZYBAN should be discontinued and not restarted in patients who experience a seizure while on treatment.

• **Dose:** *For smoking cessation, doses above 300 mg/day should not be used.* The seizure rate associated with doses of sustained-release bupropion up to 300 mg/day is approximately 0.1% (1/1,000). This incidence was prospectively determined during an 8-week treatment exposure in approximately 3,100 depressed patients.
Data for the immediate-release formulation of bupropion revealed a seizure incidence of approximately 0.4% (4/1,000) in depressed patients treated at doses in a range of 300 to 450 mg/day. In addition, the estimated seizure incidence increases almost tenfold between 450 and 600 mg/day.

• **Patient factors:** Predisposing factors that may increase the risk of seizure with bupropion use include history of head trauma or prior seizure, central nervous system (CNS) tumor, the presence of severe hepatic cirrhosis, and concomitant medications that lower seizure threshold.

• **Clinical situations:** Circumstances associated with an increased seizure risk include, among others, excessive use of alcohol or sedatives (including benzodiazepines); addiction to opiates, cocaine, or stimulants; use of over-the-counter stimulants and anorectics; and diabetes treated with oral hypoglycemics or insulin.

• **Concomitant medications:** Many medications (e.g., antipsychotics, antidepressants, theophylline, systemic steroids) are known to lower seizure threshold.

Recommendations for Reducing the Risk of Seizure: Retrospective analysis of clinical experience gained during the development of bupropion suggests that the risk of seizure may be minimized if

• the total daily dose of ZYBAN does *not* exceed 300 mg (the maximum recommended dose for smoking cessation), and

• the recommended daily dose for most patients (300 mg/day) is administered in divided doses (150 mg twice daily).

• No single dose should exceed 150 mg to avoid high peak concentrations of bupropion and/or its metabolites.

ZYBAN should be administered with extreme caution to patients with a history of seizure, cranial trauma, or other predisposition(s) toward seizure, or patients treated with other agents (e.g., antipsychotics, antidepressants, theophylline, systemic steroids, etc.) that lower seizure threshold.

Hepatic Impairment: ZYBAN should be used with extreme caution in patients with severe hepatic cirrhosis. In these patients a reduced frequency of dosing is required, as peak bupropion levels are substantially increased and accumulation is likely to occur in such patients to a greater extent than usual. The dose should not exceed 150 mg every other day in these patients (see **CLINICAL PHARMACOLOGY, PRECAUTIONS, and DOSAGE AND ADMINISTRATION**).

Potential for Hepatotoxicity: In rats receiving large doses of bupropion chronically, there was an increase in incidence of hepatic hyperplastic nodules and hepatocellular hypertrophy. In dogs receiving large doses of bupropion chronically, various histologic changes were seen in the liver, and laboratory tests suggesting mild hepatocellular injury were noted.

PRECAUTIONS

General: *Allergic Reactions:* Anaphylactoid/anaphylactic reactions characterized by symptoms such as pruritus, urticaria, angioedema, and dyspnea requiring medical treatment have been reported at a rate of about 1 to 3 per thousand in clinical trials of ZYBAN. In addition, there have been rare spontaneous postmarketing reports of erythema multiforme, Stevens-Johnson syndrome, and anaphylactic shock associated with bupropion. A patient should stop taking ZYBAN and consult a doctor if experiencing allergic or anaphylactoid/anaphylactic reactions (e.g., skin rash, pruritus, hives, chest pain, edema, and shortness of breath) during treatment.

Arthralgia, myalgia, and fever with rash and other symptoms suggestive of delayed hypersensitivity have been reported in association with bupropion. These symptoms may resemble serum sickness.

Insomnia: In the dose-response smoking cessation trial, 29% of patients treated with 150 mg/day of ZYBAN and 35% of patients treated with 300 mg/day of ZYBAN experienced insomnia, compared to 21% of placebo-treated patients. Symptoms were sufficiently severe to require discontinuation of treatment in 0.6% of patients treated with ZYBAN and none of the patients treated with placebo.

In the comparative trial, 40% of the patients treated with 300 mg/day of ZYBAN, 28% of the patients treated with 21 mg/day of NTS, and 45% of the patients treated with the combination of ZYBAN and NTS experienced insomnia compared to 18% of placebo-treated patients. Symptoms were sufficiently severe to require discontinuation of treatment in 0.8% of patients treated with ZYBAN and none of the patients in the other 3 treatment groups.

Insomnia may be minimized by avoiding bedtime doses and, if necessary, reduction in dose.

Psychosis, Confusion, and Other Neuropsychiatric Phenomena: Depressed patients treated with bupropion in depression trials have been reported to show a variety of neuropsychiatric signs and symptoms including delusions, hallucinations, psychosis, concentration disturbance, paranoia, and confusion. In some cases, these symptoms abated upon dose reduction and/or withdrawal of treatment. In clinical trials with ZYBAN conducted in nondepressed smokers, the incidence of neuropsychiatric side effects was generally comparable to placebo. However, in the postmarketing experience, patients taking ZYBAN to quit smoking have reported similar types of neuropsychiatric symptoms to those reported by patients in the clinical trials of bupropion for depression.

Activation of Psychosis and/or Mania: Antidepressants can precipitate manic episodes in bipolar disorder patients during the depressed phase of their illness and may activate latent psychosis in other susceptible individuals. The sustained-release formulation of bupropion is expected to pose similar risks. There were no reports of activation of psychosis or mania in clinical trials with ZYBAN conducted in nondepressed smokers.

Cardiovascular Effects: In clinical practice, hypertension, in some cases severe, requiring acute treatment, has been reported in patients receiving bupropion alone and in combination with nicotine replacement therapy. These events have been observed in both patients with and without evidence of preexisting hypertension.

Data from a comparative study of ZYBAN, nicotine transdermal system (NTS), the combination of sustained-release bupropion plus NTS, and placebo as an aid to smoking cessation suggest a higher incidence of treatment-emergent hypertension in patients treated with the combination of ZYBAN and NTS. In this study, 6.1% of patients treated with the combination of ZYBAN and NTS had treatment-emergent hypertension compared to 2.5%, 1.6%, and 3.1% of patients treated with ZYBAN, NTS, and placebo, respectively. The majority of these patients had evidence of preexisting hypertension. Three patients (1.2%) treated with the combination of ZYBAN and NTS and 1 patient (0.4%)

treated with NTS had study medication discontinued due to hypertension compared to none of the patients treated with ZYBAN or placebo. Monitoring of blood pressure is recommended in patients who receive the combination of bupropion and nicotine replacement.

There is no clinical experience establishing the safety of ZYBAN in patients with a recent history of myocardial infarction or unstable heart disease. Therefore, care should be exercised if it is used in these groups. Bupropion was well tolerated in depressed patients who had previously developed orthostatic hypotension while receiving tricyclic antidepressants, and was also generally well tolerated in a group of 36 depressed inpatients with stable congestive heart failure (CHF). However, bupropion was associated with a rise in supine blood pressure in the study of patients with CHF, resulting in discontinuation of treatment in 2 patients for exacerbation of baseline hypertension.

Hepatic Impairment: ZYBAN should be used with extreme caution in patients with severe hepatic cirrhosis. In these patients, a reduced frequency of dosing is required. ZYBAN should be used with caution in patients with hepatic impairment (including mild-to-moderate hepatic cirrhosis) and reduced frequency of dosing should be considered in patients with mild to moderate hepatic cirrhosis.

All patients with hepatic impairment should be closely monitored for possible adverse effects that could indicate high drug and metabolite levels (see CLINICAL PHARMACOLOGY, WARNINGS, and DOSAGE AND ADMINISTRATION).

Renal Impairment: There is limited information on the pharmacokinetics of bupropion in patients with renal impairment. An inter-study comparison between normal subjects and patients with end-stage renal failure demonstrated that the parent drug C_{max} and AUC values were comparable in the 2 groups, whereas the hydroxybupropion and threohydrobupropion metabolites had a 2.3- and 2.8-fold increase, respectively, in AUC for patients with end-stage renal failure. A second study, comparing normal subjects and patients with moderate-to-severe renal impairment (GFR 30.9 ± 10.8 mL/min) showed that exposure to a single 150-mg dose of sustained-release bupropion was approximately 2-fold higher in patients with impaired renal function while levels of the hydroxybupropion and threo/erythrohydrobupropion (combined) metabolites were similar in the 2 groups. Bupropion is extensively metabolized in the liver to active metabolites, which are further metabolized and subsequently excreted by the kidneys. ZYBAN should be used with caution in patients with renal impairment and a reduced frequency of dosing should be considered as bupropion and the metabolites of bupropion may accumulate in such patients to a greater extent than usual. The patient should be closely monitored for possible adverse effects that could indicate high drug or metabolite levels.

Information for Patients: Although ZYBAN is not indicated for treatment of depression, it contains the same active ingredient as the antidepressant medications WELLBUTRIN, WELLBUTRIN SR, and WELLBUTRIN XL. Prescribers or other health professionals should inform patients, their families, and their caregivers about the benefits and risks associated with treatment with ZYBAN and should counsel them in its appropriate use. A patient Medication Guide about "Quitting Smoking, Quit-Smoking Medication, Changes in Thinking and Behavior, Depression, and Suicidal Thoughts or Actions," "Antidepressant Medicines, Depression and Other Serious Mental Illnesses, and Suicidal Thoughts or Actions," and "What Other Important Information Should I Know About ZYBAN?" is available for ZYBAN. The prescriber or health professional should instruct patients, their families, and their caregivers to read the Medication Guide and should assist them in understanding its contents. Patients should be given the opportunity to discuss the contents of the Medication Guide and to obtain answers to any questions they may have. The complete text of the Medication Guide is reprinted at the end of this document.

Patients should be advised of the following issues and asked to alert their prescriber if these occur while taking ZYBAN.

Neuropsychiatric Symptoms and Suicide Risk in Smoking Cessation Treatment: Patients should be informed that quitting smoking, with or without ZYBAN, may be associated with nicotine withdrawal symptoms (including depression or agitation), or exacerbation of pre-existing psychiatric illness. Furthermore, some patients have experienced changes in mood (including depression and mania), psychosis, hallucinations, paranoia, delusions, homicidal ideation, aggression, anxiety, and panic, as well as suicidal ideation, suicide attempt, and completed suicide when attempting to quit smoking while taking ZYBAN. If patients develop agitation, hostility, depressed mood, or changes in thinking or

Table 5. Treatment-Emergent Adverse Event Incidence in the Dose-Response Trial[a]

Body System/ Adverse Experience	ZYBAN 100 to 300 mg/day (n = 461) %	Placebo (n = 150) %
Body (General)		
Neck pain	2	<1
Allergic reaction	1	0
Cardiovascular		
Hot flashes	1	0
Hypertension	1	<1
Digestive		
Dry mouth	11	5
Increased appetite	2	<1
Anorexia	1	<1
Musculoskeletal		
Arthralgia	4	3
Myalgia	2	1
Nervous system		
Insomnia	31	21
Dizziness	8	7
Tremor	2	1
Somnolence	2	1
Thinking abnormality	1	0
Respiratory		
Bronchitis	2	0
Skin		
Pruritus	3	<1
Rash	3	<1
Dry skin	2	0
Urticaria	1	0
Special senses		
Taste perversion	2	<1

[a] Selected adverse events with an incidence of at least 1% of patients treated with ZYBAN and more frequent than in the placebo group.

behavior that are not typical for them, or if patients develop suicidal ideation or behavior, they should be urged to report these symptoms to their healthcare provider immediately.

Clinical Worsening and Suicide Risk in Treating Psychiatric Disorders: Patients, their families, and their caregivers should be encouraged to be alert to the emergence of anxiety, agitation, panic attacks, insomnia, irritability, hostility, aggressiveness, impulsivity, akathisia (psychomotor restlessness), hypomania, mania, other unusual changes in behavior, worsening of depression, and suicidal ideation, especially early during antidepressant treatment and when the dose is adjusted up or down. Families and caregivers of patients should be advised to look for the emergence of such symptoms on a day-to-day basis, since changes may be abrupt. Such symptoms should be reported to the patient's prescriber or health professional, especially if they are severe, abrupt in onset, or were not part of the patient's presenting symptoms. Symptoms such as these may be associated with an increased risk for suicidal thinking and behavior and indicate a need for very close monitoring and possibly changes in the medication.

Bupropion-Containing Products: Patients should be made aware that ZYBAN contains the same active ingredient found in WELLBUTRIN, WELLBUTRIN SR, and WELLBUTRIN XL used to treat depression and that ZYBAN should not be used in conjunction with WELLBUTRIN, the immediate-release formulation; WELLBUTRIN SR, the sustained-release formulation; WELLBUTRIN XL, the extended-release formulation; or any other medications that contain bupropion hydrochloride.

Laboratory Tests: There are no specific laboratory tests recommended.

Drug Interactions: In vitro studies indicate that bupropion is primarily metabolized to hydroxybupropion by the CYP2B6 isoenzyme. Therefore, the potential exists for a drug interaction between ZYBAN and drugs that are substrates or inhibitors of the CYP2B6 isoenzyme (e.g., orphenadrine, thiotepa, and cyclophosphamide). In addition, in vitro studies suggest that paroxetine, sertraline, norfluoxetine, and fluvoxamine as well as nelfinavir, ritonavir, and efavirenz inhibit the hydroxylation of bupropion. No clinical studies have been performed to evaluate this finding. The threohydrobupropion metabolite of bupropion does not appear to be produced by the cytochrome P450 isoenzymes. Few systemic data have been collected on the metabolism of ZYBAN following concomitant administration with other drugs or, alternatively, the effect of con-

comitant administration of ZYBAN on the metabolism of other drugs.

Multiple oral doses of bupropion had no statistically significant effects on the single dose pharmacokinetics of lamotrigine in 12 healthy volunteers.

Animal data indicated that bupropion may be an inducer of drug-metabolizing enzymes in humans. However, following chronic administration of bupropion, 100 mg three times daily to 8 healthy male volunteers for 14 days, there was no evidence of induction of its own metabolism. Because bupropion is extensively metabolized, the coadministration of other drugs may affect its clinical activity. In particular, certain drugs may induce the metabolism of bupropion (e.g., carbamazepine, phenobarbital, phenytoin), while other drugs may inhibit the metabolism of bupropion (e.g., cimetidine). The effects of concomitant administration of cimetidine on the pharmacokinetics of bupropion and its active metabolites were studied in 24 healthy young male volunteers. Following oral administration of two 150-mg ZYBAN tablets with and without 800 mg of cimetidine, the pharmacokinetics of bupropion and its hydroxy metabolite were unaffected. However, there were 16% and 32% increases, respectively, in the AUC and C_{max} of the combined moieties of threohydro- and erythrohydro-bupropion.

Drugs Metabolized by Cytochrome P450IID6 (CYP2D6): Many drugs, including most antidepressants (SSRIs, many tricyclics), beta-blockers, antiarrhythmics, and antipsychotics are metabolized by the CYP2D6 isoenzyme. Although bupropion is not metabolized by this isoenzyme, bupropion and hydroxybupropion are inhibitors of the CYP2D6 isoenzyme in vitro. In a study of 15 male subjects (aged 19 to 35 years) who were extensive metabolizers of the CYP2D6 isoenzyme, daily doses of bupropion given as 150 mg twice daily followed by a single dose of 50 mg desipramine increased the C_{max}, AUC, and $t_{1/2}$ of desipramine by an average of approximately 2-, 5- and 2-fold, respectively. The effect was present for at least 7 days after the last dose of bupropion. Concomitant use of bupropion with other drugs metabolized by CYP2D6 has not been formally studied.

Therefore, coadministration of bupropion with drugs that are metabolized by CYP2D6 isoenzyme including certain antidepressants (e.g., nortriptyline, imipramine, desipramine, paroxetine, fluoxetine, sertraline), antipsychotics (e.g., haloperidol, risperidone, thioridazine), beta-blockers (e.g., metoprolol), and Type 1C antiarrhythmics (e.g., propafenone, flecainide), should be approached with caution and should be initiated at the lower end of the dose range of

the concomitant medication. If bupropion is added to the treatment regimen of a patient already receiving a drug metabolized by CYP2D6, the need to decrease the dose of the original medication should be considered, particularly for those concomitant medications with a narrow therapeutic index.

MAO Inhibitors: Studies in animals demonstrate that the acute toxicity of bupropion is enhanced by the MAO inhibitor phenelzine (see CONTRAINDICATIONS).

Levodopa and Amantadine: Limited clinical data suggest a higher incidence of adverse experiences in patients receiving bupropion concurrently with either levodopa or amantadine. Administration of ZYBAN to patients receiving either levodopa or amantadine concurrently should be undertaken with caution, using small initial doses and gradual dose increases.

Drugs that Lower Seizure Threshold: Concurrent administration of ZYBAN and agents (e.g., antipsychotics, antidepressants, theophylline, systemic steroids, etc.) that lower seizure threshold should be undertaken only with extreme caution (see WARNINGS).

Nicotine Transdermal System: (see PRECAUTIONS: Cardiovascular Effects).

Smoking Cessation: Physiological changes resulting from smoking cessation itself, with or without treatment with ZYBAN, may alter the pharmacokinetics of some concomitant medications, which may require dosage adjustment. Blood concentrations of concomitant medications that are extensively metabolized, such as theophylline and warfarin, may be expected to increase following smoking cessation due to de-induction of hepatic enzymes.

Alcohol: In post-marketing experience, there have been rare reports of adverse neuropsychiatric events or reduced alcohol tolerance in patients who were drinking alcohol during treatment with ZYBAN. The consumption of alcohol during treatment with ZYBAN should be minimized or avoided (also see CONTRAINDICATIONS).

Carcinogenesis, Mutagenesis, Impairment of Fertility: Lifetime carcinogenicity studies were performed in rats and mice at doses up to 300 and 150 mg/kg/day, respectively. These doses are approximately 10 and 2 times the maximum recommended human dose (MRHD), respectively, on a mg/m^2 basis. In the rat study, there was an increase in nodular proliferative lesions of the liver at doses of 100 to 300 mg/kg/day (approximately 3 to 10 times the MRHD on a mg/m^2 basis); lower doses were not tested. The question of whether or not such lesions may be precursors of neoplasms of the liver is currently unresolved. Similar liver lesions were not seen in the mouse study, and no increase in malignant tumors of the liver and other organs was seen in either study.

Bupropion produced a positive response (2 to 3 times control mutation rate) in 2 of 5 strains in the Ames bacterial mutagenicity test and an increase in chromosomal aberrations in 1 of 3 in vivo rat bone marrow cytogenetic studies.

A fertility study in rats at doses up to 300 mg/kg revealed no evidence of impaired fertility.

Pregnancy: Teratogenic Effects: Pregnancy Category C. In studies conducted in rats and rabbits, bupropion was administered orally at doses up to 450 and 150 mg/kg/day, respectively (approximately 14 and 10 times the MRHD, respectively, on a mg/m^2 basis), during the period of organogenesis. No clear evidence of teratogenic activity was found in either species; however, in rabbits, slightly increased incidences of fetal malformations and skeletal variations were observed at the lowest dose tested (25 mg/kg/day, approximately 2 times the MRHD on a mg/m^2 basis) and greater. Decreased fetal weights were seen at 50 mg/kg and greater.

When rats were administered bupropion at oral doses of up to 300 mg/kg/day (approximately 10 times the MRHD on a mg/m^2 basis) prior to mating and throughout pregnancy and lactation, there were no apparent adverse effects on offspring development.

One study has been conducted in pregnant women. This retrospective, managed-care database study assessed the risk of congenital malformations overall and cardiovascular malformations specifically, following exposure to bupropion in the first trimester compared to the risk of these malformations following exposure to other antidepressants in the first trimester and bupropion outside of the first trimester. This study included 7,005 infants with antidepressant exposure during pregnancy, 1,213 of whom were exposed to bupropion in the first trimester. The study showed no greater risk for congenital malformations overall or cardiovascular malformations specifically, following first trimester bupropion exposure compared to exposure to all other antidepressants in the first trimester, or bupropion outside of the first trimester. The results of this study have not been corroborated. ZYBAN should be used during pregnancy only if the potential benefit justifies the potential risk to the fetus. Pregnant smokers should be encouraged to attempt cessation using educational and behavioral interventions before pharmacological approaches are used.

Labor and Delivery: The effect of ZYBAN on labor and delivery in humans is unknown.

Nursing Mothers: Bupropion and its metabolites are secreted in human milk. Because of the potential for serious adverse reactions in nursing infants from ZYBAN, a decision should be made whether to discontinue nursing or to discontinue the drug, taking into account the importance of the drug to the mother.

Pediatric Use: Safety and effectiveness in the pediatric population have not been established (see BOX WARNING and WARNINGS: Clinical Worsening and Suicide Risk in Treating Psychiatric Disorders). Anyone considering the use of ZYBAN in a child or adolescent must balance the potential risks with the clinical need.

Geriatric Use: Of the approximately 6,000 patients who participated in clinical trials with bupropion sustained-release tablets (depression and smoking cessation studies), 275 were 65 and over and 47 were 75 and over. In addition, several hundred patients 65 and over participated in clinical trials using the immediate-release formulation of bupropion (depression studies). No overall differences in safety or effectiveness were observed between these subjects and younger subjects, and other reported clinical experience has not identified differences in responses between the elderly and younger patients, but greater sensitivity of some older individuals cannot be ruled out.

A single-dose pharmacokinetic study demonstrated that the disposition of bupropion and its metabolites in elderly subjects was similar to that of younger subjects; however, another pharmacokinetic study, single and multiple dose, has suggested that the elderly are at increased risk for accumulation of bupropion and its metabolites (see CLINICAL PHARMACOLOGY).

Bupropion is extensively metabolized in the liver to active metabolites, which are further metabolized and excreted by the kidneys. The risk of toxic reaction to this drug may be greater in patients with impaired renal function. Because elderly patients are more likely to have decreased renal function, care should be taken in dose selection, and it may be useful to monitor renal function (see PRECAUTIONS: Renal Impairment and DOSAGE AND ADMINISTRATION).

ADVERSE REACTIONS (See also WARNINGS and PRECAUTIONS)

The information included under ADVERSE REACTIONS is based primarily on data from the dose-response trial and the comparative trial that evaluated ZYBAN for smoking cessation (see CLINICAL TRIALS). Information on additional adverse events associated with the sustained-release formulation of bupropion in depression trials, as well as the immediate-release formulation of bupropion, is included in a separate section (see Other Events Observed During the Clinical Development and Postmarketing Experience of Bupropion).

Adverse Events Associated With the Discontinuation of Treatment: Adverse events were sufficiently troublesome to cause discontinuation of treatment in 8% of the 706 patients treated with ZYBAN and 5% of the 313 patients treated with placebo. The more common events leading to discontinuation of treatment with ZYBAN included nervous system disturbances (3.4%), primarily tremors, and skin disorders (2.4%), primarily rashes.

Incidence of Commonly Observed Adverse Events: The most commonly observed adverse events consistently associated with the use of ZYBAN were dry mouth and insomnia. The most commonly observed adverse events were defined as those that consistently occurred at a rate of 5 percentage points greater than that for placebo across clinical studies.

Dose Dependency of Adverse Events: The incidence of dry mouth and insomnia may be related to the dose of ZYBAN. The occurrence of these adverse events may be minimized by reducing the dose of ZYBAN. In addition, insomnia may be minimized by avoiding bedtime doses.

Adverse Events Occurring at an Incidence of 1% or More Among Patients Treated With ZYBAN: Table 5 enumerates selected treatment-emergent adverse events from the dose-response trial that occurred at an incidence of 1% or more and were more common in patients treated with ZYBAN compared to those treated with placebo. Table 6 enumerates selected treatment-emergent adverse events from the comparative trial that occurred at an incidence of 1% or more and were more common in patients treated with ZYBAN, NTS, or the combination of ZYBAN and NTS compared to those treated with placebo. Reported adverse events were classified using a COSTART-based dictionary.

[See table 5 at top of previous page]

[See table 6 above]

ZYBAN was well tolerated in the long-term maintenance trial that evaluated chronic administration of ZYBAN for up to 1 year and in the COPD trial that evaluated patients with mild-to-moderate COPD for a 12-week period. Adverse

Table 6. Treatment-Emergent Adverse Event Incidence in the Comparative Trial[a]

Adverse Experience (COSTART Term)	ZYBAN 300 mg/day (n = 243) %	Nicotine Transdermal System (NTS) 21 mg/day (n = 243) %	ZYBAN and NTS (n = 244) %	Placebo (n = 159) %
Body				
Abdominal pain	3	4	1	1
Accidental injury	2	2	1	1
Chest pain	<1	1	3	1
Neck pain	2	1	<1	0
Facial edema	<1	0	1	0
Cardiovascular				
Hypertension	1	<1	2	0
Palpitations	2	0	1	0
Digestive				
Nausea	9	7	11	4
Dry mouth	10	4	9	4
Constipation	8	4	9	3
Diarrhea	4	4	3	1
Anorexia	3	1	5	1
Mouth ulcer	2	1	1	1
Thirst	<1	<1	1	1
Musculoskeletal				
Myalgia	4	3	5	3
Arthralgia	5	3	3	2
Nervous system				
Insomnia	40	28	45	18
Dream abnormality	5	18	13	3
Anxiety	8	6	9	6
Disturbed concentration	9	3	9	4
Dizziness	10	2	8	6
Nervousness	4	<1	2	2
Tremor	1	<1	2	0
Dysphoria	<1	1	2	1
Respiratory				
Rhinitis	12	11	9	8
Increased cough	3	5	<1	1
Pharyngitis	3	2	3	0
Sinusitis	2	2	2	1
Dyspnea	1	0	2	0
Epistaxis	2	1	1	0
Skin				
Application site reaction[b]	11	17	15	7
Rash	4	3	3	2
Pruritus	3	1	5	1
Urticaria	2	0	2	0
Special Senses				
Taste perversion	3	1	3	2
Tinnitus	1	0	<1	0

[a]Selected adverse events with an incidence of at least 1% of patients treated with either ZYBAN, NTS, or the combination of ZYBAN and NTS and more frequent than in the placebo group.
[b]Patients randomized to ZYBAN or placebo received placebo patches.

events in both studies were quantitatively and qualitatively similar to those observed in the dose-response and comparative trials.

Other Events Observed During the Clinical Development and Postmarketing Experience of Bupropion: In addition to the adverse events noted above, the following events have been reported in clinical trials and postmarketing experience with the sustained-release formulation of bupropion in depressed patients and in nondepressed smokers, as well as in clinical trials and postmarketing clinical experience with the immediate-release formulation of bupropion.

Adverse events for which frequencies are provided below occurred in clinical trials with the sustained-release formulation of bupropion. The frequencies represent the proportion of patients who experienced a treatment-emergent adverse event on at least one occasion in placebo-controlled studies for depression (n = 987) or smoking cessation (n = 1,013), or patients who experienced an adverse event requiring discontinuation of treatment in an open-label surveillance study with bupropion sustained-release tablets (n = 3,100). All treatment-emergent adverse events are included except those listed in Tables 5 and 6, those events listed in other safety-related sections of the insert, those adverse events subsumed under COSTART terms that are either overly general or excessively specified so as to be uninformative, those events not reasonably associated with the use of the drug, and those events that were not serious and occurred in fewer than 2 patients.

Events are further categorized by body system and listed in order of decreasing frequency according to the following definitions of frequency: Frequent adverse events are defined as those occurring in at least 1/100 patients. Infrequent adverse events are those occurring in 1/100 to 1/1,000 patients, while rare events are those occurring in less than 1/1,000 patients.

Adverse events for which frequencies are not provided occurred in clinical trials or postmarketing experience with bupropion. Only those adverse events not previously listed for sustained-release bupropion are included. The extent to which these events may be associated with ZYBAN is unknown.

Body (General): Frequent were asthenia, fever, and headache. Infrequent were back pain, chills, inguinal hernia, musculoskeletal chest pain, pain, and photosensitivity. Rare was malaise. Also observed were arthralgia, myalgia, and fever with rash and other symptoms suggestive of delayed hypersensitivity. These symptoms may resemble serum sickness (see PRECAUTIONS).

Cardiovascular: Infrequent were flushing, migraine, postural hypotension, stroke, tachycardia, and vasodilation. Rare was syncope. Also observed were cardiovascular disorder, complete AV block, extrasystoles, hypotension, hypertension (in some cases severe, see PRECAUTIONS), myocardial infarction, phlebitis, and pulmonary embolism.

Digestive: Frequent were dyspepsia, flatulence, and vomiting. Infrequent were abnormal liver function, bruxism, dysphagia, gastric reflux, gingivitis, glossitis, jaundice, and stomatitis. Rare was edema of tongue. Also observed were colitis, esophagitis, gastrointestinal hemorrhage, gum hemorrhage, hepatitis, increased salivation, intestinal perforation, liver damage, pancreatitis, stomach ulcer, and stool abnormality.

Endocrine: Also observed were hyperglycemia, hypoglycemia, and syndrome of inappropriate antidiuretic hormone.

Hemic and Lymphatic: Infrequent was ecchymosis. Also observed were anemia, leukocytosis, leukopenia, lymphadenopathy, pancytopenia, and thrombocytopenia. Altered PT and/or INR, infrequently associated with hemorrhagic or thrombotic complications, were observed when bupropion was coadministered with warfarin.

Metabolic and Nutritional: Infrequent were edema, increased weight, and peripheral edema. Also observed was glycosuria.

Musculoskeletal: Infrequent were leg cramps and twitching. Also observed were arthritis and muscle rigidity/fever/rhabdomyolysis, and muscle weakness.

Nervous System: Frequent were agitation, depression, and irritability. Infrequent were abnormal coordination, CNS stimulation, confusion, decreased libido, decreased memory, depersonalization, emotional lability, hostility, hyperkinesia, hypertonia, hypesthesia, paresthesia, suicidal ideation, and vertigo. Rare were amnesia, ataxia, derealization, and hypomania. Also observed were abnormal electroencephalogram (EEG), aggression, akinesia, aphasia, coma, completed suicide, delirium, delusions, dysarthria, dyskinesia, dystonia, euphoria, extrapyramidal syndrome, hallucinations, hypokinesia, increased libido, manic reaction, neuralgia, neuropathy, paranoid ideation, restlessness, suicide attempt, and unmasking tardive dyskinesia.

Respiratory: Rare was bronchospasm. Also observed was pneumonia.

Skin: Frequent was sweating. Infrequent was acne and dry skin. Rare was maculopapular rash. Also observed were alopecia, angioedema, exfoliative dermatitis, and hirsutism.

Special Senses: Frequent was blurred vision or diplopia. Infrequent were accommodation abnormality and dry eye. Also observed were deafness, increased intraocular pressure, and mydriasis.

Urogenital: Frequent was urinary frequency. Infrequent were impotence, polyuria, and urinary urgency. Also observed were abnormal ejaculation, cystitis, dyspareunia, dysuria, gynecomastia, menopause, painful erection, prostate disorder, salpingitis, urinary incontinence, urinary retention, urinary tract disorder, and vaginitis.

DRUG ABUSE AND DEPENDENCE

ZYBAN is likely to have a low abuse potential.

Humans: There have been few reported cases of drug dependence and withdrawal symptoms associated with the immediate-release formulation of bupropion. In human studies of abuse liability, individuals experienced with drugs of abuse reported that bupropion produced a feeling of euphoria and desirability. In these subjects, a single dose of 400 mg (1.33 times the recommended daily dose) of bupropion produced mild amphetamine-like effects compared to placebo on the Morphine-Benzedrine Subscale of the Addiction Research Center Inventories (ARCI), which is indicative of euphorigenic properties and a score intermediate between placebo and amphetamine on the Liking Scale of the ARCI.

Animals: Studies in rodents and primates have shown that bupropion exhibits some pharmacologic actions common to psychostimulants. In rodents, it has been shown to increase locomotor activity, elicit a mild stereotyped behavioral response, and increase rates of responding in several schedule-controlled behavior paradigms. In primate models to assess the positive reinforcing effects of psychoactive drugs, bupropion was self-administered intravenously. In rats, bupropion produced amphetamine- and cocaine-like discriminative stimulus effects in drug discrimination paradigms used to characterize the subjective effects of psychoactive drugs.

The possibility that bupropion may induce dependence should be kept in mind when evaluating the desirability of including the drug in smoking cessation programs of individual patients.

OVERDOSAGE

Human Overdose Experience: Overdoses of up to 30 g or more of bupropion have been reported. Seizure was reported in approximately one third of all cases. Other serious reactions reported with overdoses of bupropion alone included hallucinations, loss of consciousness, sinus tachycardia, and ECG changes such as conduction disturbances (including QRS prolongation) or arrhythmias. Fever, muscle rigidity, rhabdomyolysis, hypotension, stupor, coma, and respiratory failure have been reported mainly when bupropion was part of multiple drug overdoses.

Although most patients recovered without sequelae, deaths associated with overdoses of bupropion alone have been reported in patients ingesting large doses of the drug. Multiple uncontrolled seizures, bradycardia, cardiac failure, and cardiac arrest prior to death were reported in these patients.

Overdosage Management: Ensure an adequate airway, oxygenation, and ventilation. Monitor cardiac rhythm and vital signs. EEG monitoring is also recommended for the first 48 hours post-ingestion. General supportive and symptomatic measures are also recommended. Induction of emesis is not recommended.

Activated charcoal should be administered. There is no experience with the use of forced diuresis, dialysis, hemoperfusion, or exchange transfusion in the management of bupropion overdoses. No specific antidotes for bupropion are known.

Due to the dose-related risk of seizures with ZYBAN, hospitalization following suspected overdose should be considered. Based on studies in animals, it is recommended that seizures be treated with intravenous benzodiazepine administration and other supportive measures, as appropriate.

In managing overdosage, consider the possibility of multiple drug involvement. The physician should consider contacting a poison control center for additional information on the treatment of any overdose. Telephone numbers for certified poison control centers are listed in the *Physicians' Desk Reference* (PDR).

DOSAGE AND ADMINISTRATION

Usual Dosage for Adults: The recommended and maximum dose of ZYBAN is 300 mg/day, given as 150 mg twice daily. Dosing should begin at 150 mg/day given every day for the first 3 days, followed by a dose increase for most patients to the recommended usual dose of 300 mg/day. There should be an interval of at least 8 hours between successive doses. Doses above 300 mg/day should not be used (see WARNINGS). ZYBAN should be swallowed whole and not crushed, divided, or chewed. Treatment with ZYBAN should be initiated **while the patient is still smoking,** since approximately 1 week of treatment is required to achieve steady-state blood levels of bupropion. Patients should set a "target quit date" within the first 2 weeks of treatment with ZYBAN, generally in the second week. Treatment with ZYBAN should be continued for 7 to 12 weeks; longer treatment should be guided by the relative benefits and risks for individual patients. If a patient has not made significant progress towards abstinence by the seventh week of therapy with ZYBAN, it is unlikely that he or she will quit during that attempt, and treatment should probably be discontinued. Conversely, a patient who successfully quits after 7 to 12 weeks of treatment should be considered for ongoing therapy with ZYBAN. Dose tapering of ZYBAN is not required when discontinuing treatment. It is important that patients continue to receive counseling and support throughout treatment with ZYBAN, and for a period of time thereafter.

Individualization of Therapy: Patients are more likely to quit smoking and remain abstinent if they are seen frequently and receive support from their physicians or other healthcare professionals. It is important to ensure that patients read the instructions provided to them and have their questions answered. Physicians should review the patient's overall smoking cessation program that includes treatment with ZYBAN. Patients should be advised of the importance of participating in the behavioral interventions, counseling, and/or support services to be used in conjunction with ZYBAN. See Medication Guide at the end of the prescribing information.

The goal of therapy with ZYBAN is complete abstinence. If a patient has not made significant progress towards abstinence by the seventh week of therapy with ZYBAN, it is unlikely that he or she will quit during that attempt, and treatment should probably be discontinued.

Patients who fail to quit smoking during an attempt may benefit from interventions to improve their chances for success on subsequent attempts. Patients who are unsuccessful should be evaluated to determine why they failed. A new quit attempt should be encouraged when factors that contributed to failure can be eliminated or reduced, and conditions are more favorable.

Maintenance: Nicotine dependence is a chronic condition. Some patients may need continuous treatment. Systematic evaluation of ZYBAN 300 mg/day for maintenance therapy demonstrated that treatment for up to 6 months was efficacious. Whether to continue treatment with ZYBAN for periods longer than 12 weeks for smoking cessation must be determined for individual patients.

Combination Treatment With ZYBAN and a Nicotine Transdermal System (NTS): Combination treatment with ZYBAN and NTS may be prescribed for smoking cessation. The prescriber should review the complete prescribing information for both ZYBAN and NTS before using combination treatment. See also CLINICAL TRIALS for methods and dosing used in the ZYBAN and NTS combination trial. Monitoring for treatment-emergent hypertension in patients treated with the combination of ZYBAN and NTS is recommended.

Dosage Adjustment for Patients with Impaired Hepatic Function: ZYBAN should be used with extreme caution in patients with severe hepatic cirrhosis. The dose should not exceed 150 mg every other day in these patients. ZYBAN should be used with caution in patients with hepatic impairment (including mild-to-moderate hepatic cirrhosis) and a reduced frequency of dosing should be considered in patients with mild-to-moderate hepatic cirrhosis (see CLINICAL PHARMACOLOGY, WARNINGS, and PRECAUTIONS).

Dosage Adjustment for Patients with Impaired Renal Function: ZYBAN should be used with caution in patients with renal impairment and a reduced frequency of dosing should be considered (see CLINICAL PHARMACOLOGY and PRECAUTIONS).

HOW SUPPLIED

ZYBAN Sustained-Release Tablets, 150 mg of bupropion hydrochloride, are purple, round, biconvex, film-coated tablets printed with "ZYBAN 150" in bottles of 60 (NDC 0173-0556-02) tablets and the ZYBAN Advantage Pack® containing 1 bottle of 60 (NDC 0173-0556-01) tablets.

Store at controlled room temperature, 20° to 25°C (68° to 77°F) (see USP). Dispense in tight, light-resistant containers as defined in the USP.

MEDICATION GUIDE

ZYBAN® (zi ban)

(bupropion hydrochloride) Sustained-Release Tablets

Read this Medication Guide carefully before you start using ZYBAN and each time you get a refill. There may be new information. This information does not take the place of talking with your doctor about your medical condition or your treatment. If you have any questions about ZYBAN, ask your doctor or pharmacist.

IMPORTANT: Be sure to read the three sections of this Medication Guide. The first section is about the risk of changes in thinking and behavior, depression and suicidal thoughts or actions with medicines used to quit smoking; the second section is about the risk of suicidal thoughts and actions with antidepressant medicines; and the third section is entitled "What Other Important Information Should I Know About ZYBAN?"

Quitting Smoking, Quit-Smoking Medications, Changes in Thinking and Behavior, Depression, and Suicidal Thoughts or Actions

This section of the Medication Guide is only about the risk of changes in thinking and behavior, depression and suicidal thoughts or actions with drugs used to quit smoking. Some people have had changes in behavior, hostility, agitation, depression, suicidal thoughts or actions while taking ZYBAN to help them quit smoking. These symptoms can develop during treatment with ZYBAN or after stopping treatment with ZYBAN.

If you, your family member, or your caregiver notice agitation, hostility, depression, or changes in thinking or behavior that are not typical for you, or you have any of the following symptoms, stop taking ZYBAN and call your healthcare provider right away: (this is a bulleted list in 2 columns, the 1st 8 items are column 1 & the next 6 are column 2)

- thoughts about suicide or dying
- attempts to commit suicide
- new or worse depression
- new or worse anxiety
- panic attacks
- feeling very agitated or restless
- acting aggressive, being angry, or violent
- acting on dangerous impulses
- an extreme increase in activity and talking (mania)
- abnormal thoughts or sensations
- seeing or hearing things that are not there (hallucinations)
- feeling people are against you (paranoia)
- feeling confused
- other unusual changes in behavior or mood

When you try to quit smoking, with or without ZYBAN, you may have symptoms that may be due to nicotine withdrawal, including urge to smoke, depressed mood, trouble sleeping, irritability, frustration, anger, feeling anxious, difficulty concentrating, restlessness, decreased heart rate, and increased appetite or weight gain. Some people have even experienced suicidal thoughts when trying to quit smoking without medication. Sometimes quitting smoking can lead to worsening of mental health problems that you already have, such as depression.

Before taking ZYBAN, tell your healthcare provider if you have ever had depression or other mental health problems. You should also tell your doctor about any symptoms you had during other times you tried to quit smoking, with or without ZYBAN.

Antidepressant Medicines, Depression and Other Serious Mental Illnesses, and Suicidal Thoughts or Actions

Although ZYBAN is not a treatment for depression, it contains bupropion, the same active ingredient as the antidepressant medications WELLBUTRIN®, WELLBUTRIN SR®, and WELLBUTRIN XL®. This section of the Medication Guide is only about the risk of suicidal thoughts and actions with antidepressant medicines. **Talk to your doctor, or your family member's healthcare provider about:**

- all risks and benefits of treatment with antidepressant medicines
- all treatment choices for depression or other serious mental illness

What is the most important information I should know about antidepressant medicines, depression and other serious mental illnesses, and suicidal thoughts or actions?

1. **Antidepressant medicines may increase suicidal thoughts or actions in some children, teenagers, and young adults within the first few months of treatment.**
2. **Depression and other serious mental illnesses are the most important causes of suicidal thoughts and actions.** Some people may have a particularly high risk of having suicidal thoughts or actions. These include people who have (or have a family history of) bipolar illness (also called manic-depressive illness) or suicidal thoughts or actions.
3. **How can I watch for and try to prevent suicidal thoughts and actions in myself or a family member?**
   - Pay close attention to any changes, especially sudden changes, in mood, behaviors, thoughts, or feelings. This is very important when an antidepressant medicine is started or when the dose is changed.
   - Call the healthcare provider right away to report new or sudden changes in mood, behavior, thoughts, or feelings.
   - Keep all follow-up visits with the healthcare provider as scheduled. Call the healthcare provider between visits as needed, especially if you have concerns about symptoms.

Call a healthcare provider right away if you or your family member has any of the following symptoms, especially if they are new, worse, or worry you:

- thoughts about suicide or dying
- attempts to commit suicide
- new or worse depression
- new or worse anxiety
- feeling very agitated or restless
- panic attacks
- trouble sleeping (insomnia)
- new or worse irritability
- acting aggressive, being angry, or violent
- acting on dangerous impulses
- an extreme increase in activity and talking (mania)
- other unusual changes in behavior or mood

What else do I need to know about antidepressant medicines?

- Never stop an antidepressant medicine without first talking to a healthcare provider. Stopping an antidepressant medicine suddenly can cause other symptoms.
- Antidepressants are medicines used to treat depression and other illnesses. It is important to discuss all the risks of treating depression and also the risks of not treating it. Patients and their families or other caregivers should discuss all treatment choices with the healthcare provider, not just the use of antidepressants.
- Antidepressant medicines have other side effects. Talk to the healthcare provider about the side effects of the medicine prescribed for you or your family member.
- Antidepressant medicines can interact with other medicines. Know all of the medicines that you or your family member takes. Keep a list of all medicines to show the healthcare provider. Do not start new medicines without first checking with your healthcare provider.
- Not all antidepressant medicines prescribed for children are FDA approved for use in children. Talk to your child's healthcare provider for more information.

ZYBAN has not been studied in children under the age of 18 and is not approved for use in children and teenagers.

What Other Important Information Should I Know About ZYBAN?

- **Seizures: There is a chance of having a seizure (convulsion, fit) with ZYBAN, especially in people:**
  - with certain medical problems
  - who take certain medicines

The chance of having seizures increases with higher doses of ZYBAN. For more information, see the sections "Who should not take ZYBAN?" and "What should I tell my doctor before using ZYBAN?" Tell your doctor about all of your

medical conditions and all the medicines you take. **Do not take any other medicines while you are using ZYBAN unless your doctor has said it is okay to take them.**

If you have a seizure while taking ZYBAN, stop taking the tablets and call your doctor right away. Do not take ZYBAN again if you have a seizure.

- **High blood pressure (hypertension): Some people get high blood pressure that can be severe, while taking ZYBAN.** The chance of high blood pressure may be higher if you also use nicotine replacement therapy (such as a nicotine patch) to help you stop smoking (see "Can ZYBAN be used at the same time as nicotine patches?").
- **Severe allergic reactions: Some people have severe allergic reactions to ZYBAN. Stop taking ZYBAN and call your doctor right away** if you get a rash, itching, hives, fever, swollen lymph glands, painful sores in your mouth or around your eyes, swelling of your lips or tongue, chest pain, or have trouble breathing. These could be signs of a serious allergic reaction.

What is ZYBAN?

ZYBAN is a prescription medicine to help people quit smoking. Studies have shown that more than one third of people quit smoking for at least 1 month while taking ZYBAN and participating in a patient support program. For many patients, ZYBAN reduces withdrawal symptoms and the urge to smoke. ZYBAN should be used with a patient support program. It is important to participate in the behavioral program, counseling, or other support program your healthcare professional recommends.

Who should not take ZYBAN?

Do not take ZYBAN if you:

- have or had a seizure disorder or epilepsy.
- **are taking WELLBUTRIN, WELLBUTRIN SR, WELLBUTRIN XL, or any other medicines that contain bupropion hydrochloride.** Bupropion is the same active ingredient that is in ZYBAN.
- drink a lot of alcohol and abruptly stop drinking, or use medicines called sedatives (these make you sleepy) or benzodiazepines and you stop using them all of a sudden.
- have taken within the last 14 days medicine for depression called a monoamine oxidase inhibitor (MAOI), such as NARDIL®* (phenelzine sulfate), PARNATE® (tranylcypromine sulfate), or MARPLAN®* (isocarboxazid).
- have or had an eating disorder such as anorexia nervosa or bulimia.
- are allergic to the active ingredient in ZYBAN, bupropion, or to any of the inactive ingredients. See the end of this leaflet for a complete list of ingredients in ZYBAN.

What should I tell my doctor before using ZYBAN?

Tell your doctor if you have ever had depression, suicidal thoughts or actions, or other mental health problems. You should also tell your doctor about any symptoms you had during other times you tried to quit smoking, with or without ZYBAN. See "Quitting Smoking, Quit-Smoking Medications, Changes in Thinking and Behavior, Depression, and Suicidal Thoughts or Actions."

- **Tell your doctor about your other medical conditions, including if you:**
  - **are pregnant or plan to become pregnant.** It is not known if ZYBAN can harm your unborn baby.
  - **are breastfeeding.** ZYBAN passes through your milk. It is not known if ZYBAN can harm your baby.
  - **have liver problems,** especially cirrhosis of the liver.
  - have kidney problems.
  - have an eating disorder such as anorexia nervosa or bulimia.
  - have had a head injury.
  - have had a seizure (convulsion, fit).
  - have a tumor in your nervous system (brain or spine).
  - have had a heart attack, heart problems, or high blood pressure.
  - are a diabetic taking insulin or other medicines to control your blood sugar.
  - drink a lot of alcohol.
  - abuse prescription medicines or street drugs.
- **Tell your doctor about all the medicines you take,** including prescription and non-prescription medicines, vitamins, and herbal supplements. Many medicines increase your chances of getting seizures or other serious side effects if you take them while you are using ZYBAN.

How should I take ZYBAN?

- Take ZYBAN exactly as prescribed by your doctor.
- **Do not chew, cut, or crush ZYBAN Tablets.** You must swallow the tablets whole. **Tell your doctor if you cannot swallow medicine tablets.**
- Take ZYBAN at the same time each day.
- Take your doses of ZYBAN at least 8 hours apart.
- If you miss a dose, do not take an extra tablet to make up for the dose you forgot. Wait and take your next tablet at the regular time. **This is very important.** Too much ZYBAN can increase your chance of having a seizure.
- If you take too much ZYBAN, or overdose, call your local emergency room or poison control center right away.

- **Do not take any other medicines while using ZYBAN unless your doctor has told you it is okay.**
- Do not change your dose or stop taking ZYBAN without talking with your doctor first.

How long should I take ZYBAN?

Most people should take ZYBAN for at least 7 to 12 weeks. Some people may need to take ZYBAN for a longer period of time to assist in their smoking cessation efforts. Follow your doctor's instructions.

When should I stop smoking?

It takes about 1 week for ZYBAN to start working. For your best chance of quitting, you should not stop smoking until you have been taking ZYBAN for 1 week. You should set a date to stop smoking during the second week you're taking ZYBAN.

Can I smoke while taking ZYBAN?

It is not physically dangerous to smoke and use ZYBAN at the same time. But you will seriously lower your chance of breaking your smoking habit if you smoke after the date you set to stop smoking.

Can ZYBAN be used at the same time as nicotine patches?

Yes, ZYBAN and nicotine patches can be used at the same time but should only be used together under the supervision of your doctor. Using ZYBAN and nicotine patches together may raise your blood pressure, sometimes severely. Tell your doctor if you are planning to use nicotine replacement therapy because your doctor should check your blood pressure regularly.

Do not smoke at any time if you are using a nicotine patch or any other nicotine product along with ZYBAN. It is possible to get too much nicotine and have serious side effects.

What should I avoid while taking ZYBAN?

- Do not drink a lot of alcohol while taking ZYBAN. If you usually drink a lot of alcohol, talk with your doctor before suddenly stopping. If you suddenly stop drinking alcohol, you may increase your chance of having seizures.
- Do not drive a car or use heavy machinery until you know how ZYBAN affects you. ZYBAN can affect your ability to do these things safely.

What are possible side effects of ZYBAN?

ZYBAN can cause serious side effects. Read this entire Medication Guide for more information about these serious side effects.

The most common side effects of ZYBAN are dry mouth and trouble sleeping. These side effects are generally mild and often disappear after a few weeks. If you have trouble sleeping, do not take ZYBAN too close to bedtime.

These are not all the side effects of ZYBAN. For a complete list, ask your doctor or pharmacist.

Call your doctor for medical advice about side effects. You may report side effects to FDA at 1-800-FDA-1088.

How should I store ZYBAN?

- Store ZYBAN at room temperature. Store out of direct sunlight. Keep ZYBAN in its tightly closed bottle.
- ZYBAN may have an odor.

General Information about ZYBAN.

- Medicines are sometimes prescribed for purposes other than those listed in a Medication Guide. Do not use ZYBAN for a condition for which it was not prescribed. Do not give ZYBAN to other people, even if they have the same symptoms you have. It may harm them. Keep ZYBAN out of the reach of children.

This Medication Guide summarizes important information about ZYBAN. For more information, talk with your doctor. You can ask your doctor or pharmacist for information about ZYBAN that is written for health professionals.

What are the ingredients in ZYBAN?

Active ingredient: bupropion hydrochloride.

Inactive ingredients: carnauba wax, cysteine hydrochloride, hypromellose, magnesium stearate, microcrystalline cellulose, polyethylene glycol, polysorbate 80 and titanium dioxide. The tablets are printed with edible black ink. In addition, the 150-mg tablet contains FD&C Blue No. 2 Lake and FD&C Red No. 40 Lake.

WELLBUTRIN, WELLBUTRIN SR, WELLBUTRIN XL, and PARNATE are registered trademarks of GlaxoSmithKline.

*The following are registered trademarks of their respective manufacturers: NARDIL®/Warner Lambert Company; MARPLAN®/Oxford Pharmaceutical Services, Inc.

℞ only

This Medication Guide has been approved by the U.S. Food and Drug Administration.

July 2009   ZYB:5MG

Distributed by:
GlaxoSmithKline, Research Triangle Park, NC 27709
Manufactured by:
GlaxoSmithKline, Research Triangle Park
or DSM Pharmaceuticals, Inc., Greenville, NC 27834
©2009, GlaxoSmithKline. All rights reserved.
July 2009   ZYB:4PI

Glenwood

111 CEDAR LANE
ENGLEWOOD, NJ 07631

Direct Inquiries to:
Professional Services Department
201 569-0050
800 542-0772
For Medical Information Contact:
In Emergencies:
Professional Services Department
201 569-0050
800 542-0772

POTABA® ℞
Aminobenzoate Potassium, USP
Systemic ANTIFIBROSIS THERAPY

PRODUCT OVERVIEW
KEY FACTS
Potaba® (Aminobenzoate Potassium, USP) is considered a member of the vitamin B complex. It has been suggested that the antifibrotic action of Potaba® is due to its mediation of increased oxygen uptake at the tissue level.
MAJOR USES
Potaba® offers a means of treatment of serious and often chronic entities, such as scleroderma and Peyronie's Disease.
SAFETY INFORMATION
Contraindicated in patients taking sulfonamides. Anorexia, nausea, fever and rash have occurred infrequently and subside with omission of the drug. Often, desensitization can be accomplished and treatment resumed.
FORMULA: POTABA is chemically pure potassium p-aminobenzoate.

DESCRIPTION
Aminobenzoate Potassium, Potaba is available in the following forms: Capsules and Tablets. Each Capsule contains the following inactive ingredients: Colloidal Silicon Dioxide, Stearic Acid. Capsule Shell contains: Gelatin and Titanium Dioxide. The imprinting ink contains Titanium Dioxide. Each Tablet contains the following inactive ingredients: Colloidal Silicon Dioxide, Magnesium Stearate, Microcrystalline Cellulose, and Sodium Starch Glycolate.

INDICATIONS
Based on a review of this drug by the National Academy of Sciences-National Research Council and/or other information, FDA has classified the indications as follows:
"Possibly" effective: Potassium aminobenzoate is possibly effective in the treatment of scleroderma, dermatomyositis, morphea, linear scleroderma, pemphigus, and Peyronie's disease.
Final classification of the less-than-effective indications requires further investigation.

ADVANTAGES: POTABA offers a means of treatment of serious and often chronic entities involving fibrosis and non-suppurative inflammation.

PHARMACOLOGY
p-Aminobenzoate is considered a member of the vitamin B complex. Small amounts are found in cereal, eggs, milk and meats. Detectable amounts are normally present in human blood, spinal fluid, urine, and sweat. PABA is a component of several biologically important systems, and it participates in a number of fundamental biological processes.
It has been suggested that the antifibrosis action of POTABA is due to its mediation of increased oxygen uptake at the tissue level. Fibrosis is believed to occur from either too much serotonin or too little monoamine oxidase (MAO) activity over a period of time. Monoamine oxidase requires an adequate supply of oxygen to function properly. By increasing oxygen supply at the tissue level POTABA may enhance MAO activity and prevent or bring about regression of fibrosis.[3]

CLINICAL USES
PEYRONIE'S DISEASE: 21 patients with Peyronie's disease were placed on POTABA therapy for periods ranging from 3 months to 2 years. Pain disappeared from 16 of 16 cases in which it had been present. There was objective improvement in penile deformity in 10 of 17 patients, and decrease in plaque size in 16 of 21. The authors suggest that this medication offers no hazard of further local injury as may result from other therapy. There were no significant

untoward effects encountered on long term POTABA therapy.[5,10]
SCLERODERMA: Of 135 patients with diffuse systemic sclerosis treated with POTABA every patient but one has shown softening of the involved skin if treatment has been continued for 3 months or longer. The responses have been reported in a number of publications.[9] The treatment program consists of systemic antifibrosis therapy with POTABA, physical therapy, including deep breathing exercises and dynamic traction splints where indicated, and bethanechol chloride for relief of dysphagia as well as small doses of reserpine for amelioration of Raynaud's phenomena.[1,3]
DERMATOMYOSITIS: Five patients with scleroderma and 2 with dermatomyositis were treated with POTABA. There was striking clinical improvement in each patient. Doses of 15-20 grams per day were well tolerated, and patients were easily able to take these doses.[6]
MORPHEA and LINEAR SCLERODERMA: All 14 patients with localized forms of scleroderma placed on long-term Potaba treatment showed softening of the sclerotic component of their disorder. Treatment is particularly indicated in patients where persistent compressive sclerosis may contribute even greater disfigurement or functional embarrassment from secondary pressure atrophy.[8,9]

DOSAGE & ADMINISTRATION
The average adult daily dose of POTABA is 12 grams, usually given in four to six divided doses. Tablets and capsules 0.5 grams are given at the rate of 4 tablets or capsules 6 times daily, or 6 given four times daily, usually with meals, and at bedtime with a snack. Tablets must be taken with an adequate amount of liquid to prevent gastrointestinal upset.
Children are given 1 gram of POTABA daily in divided doses for each 10 lbs. of body weight.
SIDE EFFECTS: Anorexia, nausea, fever and rash have occurred infrequently and subside with omission of the drug. Desensitization can be accomplished and treatment resumed.
USAGE IN PREGNANCY: Safety for use in pregnancy or during lactation has not been established.

PRECAUTIONS
Should anorexia or nausea occur, therapy is interrupted until the patient is eating normally again. This permits prompt subsidence of symptoms and also avoids the possible development of hypoglycemia. Give cautiously to patients with renal disease. If hypersensitivity reaction should occur, Potaba should be stopped.

CONTRAINDICATIONS
POTABA should not be administered to patients taking sulfonamides.

HOW SUPPLIED
POTABA Capsules 0.5 grams are supplied as number 0 white/white opaque hard gelatin capsules printed "Potaba 51" in black ink.
NDC-0516-0051-25 bottle of 250
NDC-0516-0051-10 bottle of 1000

POTABA Tablets 0.5 grams are supplied as white round tablets embossed "Potaba 54".
NDC-0516-0054-01 bottle of 100
NDC-0516-0054-10 bottle of 1000
Rx only.

REFERENCES
1. From: Inflammation and Diseases of Connective Tissue, Edited by Drs. Lewis C. Mills and John H. Moyer, Published by W. B. Saunders Company, Phila. 1961.
3. Zarafonetis, Chris J. D.: Treatment of Scleroderma, Annals of Int. Med. 50:343-365 (1959).
5. Zarafonetis, C. J. D., and Horrax, T.M.: Treatment of Peyronie's Disease with POTABA, Journ. of Urology 81:770-772 (June 1959).
6. Grace, William J., Kennedy, Richard J., Formato, Anthony: Therapy of Scleroderma and Dermatomyositis, N.Y. State J. of Med. 63:140-144, 1963.
8. Zarafonetis, C. J. D.: Treatment of Localized Forms of Scleroderma, Am. J. Med. Sci. 243:147-158. 1962.
9. Zarafonetis, Chris J. D.: Antifibrotic Therapy With POTABA, Amer. Jrnl. of Med. Sci. 248: No. 5/551-561 (Nov. 1964).
10. Horrax, Trudeau M.: Peyronie's Disease, Scientific Exhibit, Amer. Urological Assn. Annl. Meet., New Orleans, May 1965.

GLENWOOD, LLC
111 Cedar Lane
Englewood, NJ 07631

REV. 11/09
Shown in Product Identification Guide, page 310

Gordon Laboratories

6801 LUDLOW STREET
UPPER DARBY, PA 19082

Direct inquiries to:
Customer Service
(610) 734-2011
Fax (610) 734-2049
Website: http://www.gordonlabs.net
E-mail: gordonlabs@att.net
For medical emergencies contact:
David Dercher   (610) 734-2011
                                 Fax (610) 734-2049

FORMADON ℞

INDICATIONS
Used as a drying agent for pre and postsurgical removal of warts; and as an antiperspirant in the treatment of severe conditions of hyperhidrosis and bromidrosis.
ACTIVE INGREDIENT: Formaldehyde (10% of U.S.P. strength).

DESCRIPTION
Formadon provides a preferable vehicle for the topical application of formalin solution (10% U.S.P. strength formaldehyde). It is formulated with an aqueous perfumed base which helps minimize the characteristic pungent odor.

PHARMACOLOGY
Formalin, a solution of formaldehyde, has been extensively used as a drying agent as well as a disinfectant. Direct topical application of formalin solution has been an extremely useful way of dealing with odor-causing bacteria on the surface of the skin. The elimination of hyperhidrosis is of paramount importance in reducing bacteria associated with odor and wetness. Formalin, in drying the skin surface, reduces bacteria flora which can thrive in moisture.

CONTRAINDICATIONS/WARNINGS
Avoid excessive use. Avoid contact with eyes or mucous membranes. Discontinue use if any irritation occurs, avoid breathing vapor, and **keep out of reach of children. For external use only.** Harmful if swallowed. Contact a local Poison Control Center immediately. Do not induce vomiting. If conscious, give eight ounces (240 mL) of milk, water or water with activated charcoal. Keep well closed in a cool place. **Federal law prohibits dispensing without a prescription.**

DIRECTIONS
Apply to feet twice weekly or as prescribed by a Physician. Do not apply to open wounds.

HOW SUPPLIED
2 oz. sponge tip bottle NDC 10481-1050-05
4 oz. plastic bottle NDC 10481-1050-2
Shown in Product Identification Guide, page 310

GORDOCHOM™ Solution OTC
[gōrdō′kōm]

DESCRIPTION
Gordochom is an antifungal solution for topical use containing 25% Undecylenic Acid and 3% Chloroxylenol as its active ingredients in a penetrating oil base. Undecylenic Acid is chemically 10 hendecenoic acid having the empirical formula $C_{11}H_{20}O_2$ and the chemical bond structure $CH_2=CH$ $(CH_2)8$ CO_2H.
Undecylenic Acid is a colorless to pale yellow liquid. It is insoluble in water and soluble in alcohol, chloroform and ether.
Chloroxylenol is chemically 2-chloro-5-hydroxy-1,3-dimethylbenzene having the empirical formula C_8H_9ClO.

CLINICAL PHARMACOLOGY
Undecylenic Acid is a fungistatic agent employed in the treatment of tinea pedis, ringworm and dermatophytosis. Chloroxylenol is a topical antiseptic, germicide and antifungal agent effective against a wide variety of causative fungi and yeast organisms. Among those affected by chloroxylenol are candida albicans, aspergillus niger, aspergillus flavus, trichophyton rubrum, trichophyton mentagrophytes, penicillum luteum and epidermophyton floccosum.
The penetrating oil base vehicle serves as a delivery system, enhancing the impregnation of Undecylenic Acid and Chloroxylenol as antimicrobial agents.

INDICATIONS
Cures athlete's foot (tinea pedis), and ringworm (tinea corporis).

CONTRAINDICATIONS

Gordochom is contraindicated in patients who are sensitive to Undecylenic Acid or Chloroxylenol.

WARNINGS

FOR EXTERNAL USE ONLY. Not for opthalmic or optic use. Avoid inhaling and contact with eyes or other mucous membranes. Not to be applied over blistered, raw or oozing areas of skin or over deep puncture wounds.

PRECAUTIONS

If a reaction suggesting sensitivity or chemical irritation should occur with the use of Gordochom, treatment should be discontinued. Use of Gordochom in pregnancy has not been established.

ADVERSE REACTIONS

No significant adverse reactions have been reported. However, attention should be paid to localized hypersensitivity.

DOSAGE AND ADMINISTRATION

Cleanse and dry affected areas. Apply a thin application twice a day (morning and night) to the affected area, or as recommended by your physician. Supervise children in the use of this product. For athlete's foot, pay special attention to the spaces between the toes; wear well-fitting, ventilated shoes, and change shoes and socks at least once daily. For athlete's foot and ringworm, use daily for 4 weeks. If condition persists longer, consult a physician. This product has not been proven effective on the scalp or nails.

HOW SUPPLIED

Gordochom is available in 1 oz. bottles with special brush applicator. (NDC 10481-8010-2)
Store at controlled room temperatures (59°–86°F).
For external use only.
Keep out of reach of children.
Shown in Product Identification Guide, page 310

Graceway Pharmaceuticals, LLC

**340 MARTIN LUTHER KING JR. BLVD.,
SUITE 500
BRISTOL, TN 37620**

Direct Inquiries to:
800-328-0255
www.gracewaypharma.com

ZYCLARA™
[zi-cla-ra]
(imiquimod)
Cream 3.75%

℞

HIGHLIGHTS OF PRESCRIBING INFORMATION
**These highlights do not include all the information needed to use Zyclara™ safely and effectively. See full prescribing information for Zyclara Cream.
Zyclara (imiquimod), Cream, 3.75%
For topical use only
Initial U.S. Approval: 1997**

————INDICATIONS AND USAGE————
Zyclara Cream is indicated for:
The topical treatment of clinically typical, visible or palpable actinic keratoses (AK), of the full face or balding scalp in immunocompetent adults. (1.1)

————DOSAGE AND ADMINISTRATION————
Zyclara Cream is not for oral, ophthalmic, or intravaginal use. (2)
• Once daily to the skin of the affected area (either the entire face or balding scalp) for two 2-week treatment cycles separated by a 2-week no-treatment period. (2.1)

————DOSAGE FORMS AND STRENGTHS————
Cream, 3.75%, white to faintly yellow cream. (3)

————CONTRAINDICATIONS————
None (4)

————WARNINGS AND PRECAUTIONS————
• Intense local inflammatory reactions can occur (e.g., skin weeping, erosion). Dosing interruption may be required (2, 5.1, 6)
• Flu-like systemic signs and symptoms including fatigue, nausea, fever, myalgias, arthralgias, and chills. Dosing interruption may be required (2, 5.2, 6)
• Avoid exposure to sunlight and sunlamps (5.3). Wear sunscreen daily (17.4).
• Avoid concomitant use of Zyclara Cream and any other imiquimod cream.

————ADVERSE REACTIONS————
Most common Adverse Reactions (incidence >50%) are local skin reactions erythema, edema, weeping/exudate, flaking/scaling/dryness, scabbing/crusting and erosion/ulceration (6.2). Other reported reactions (occurring in ≥2% of ZYCLARA-Treated Subjects) include headache, fatigue, nausea and fever (see 6.1).

To report SUSPECTED ADVERSE REACTIONS, contact Graceway Pharmaceuticals, LLC at 1-800-328-0255 or FDA at 1-800-FDA-1088 or *www.fda.gov/medwatch*.

See 17 for PATIENT COUNSELING INFORMATION and FDA-approved patient labeling
Revised: 03/2010

FULL PRESCRIBING INFORMATION: CONTENTS*

FULL PRESCRIBING INFORMATION

1 INDICATIONS AND USAGE
1.1 Actinic Keratosis
ZYCLARA Cream is indicated for the topical treatment of clinically typical visible or palpable, actinic keratoses (AK), of the full face or balding scalp in immunocompetent adults.
1.2 Unevaluated Populations
Safety and efficacy have not been established for ZYCLARA Cream in the treatment of actinic keratosis, with more than one 2-cycle treatment course in the same area.
The safety and efficacy of ZYCLARA Cream in immunosuppressed patients have not been established.
The safety and efficacy have not been established for ZYCLARA Cream in the treatment of patients with xeroderma pigmentosum.
The safety and efficacy have not been established for ZYCLARA Cream in the treatment of superficial basal cell carcinoma.
The safety and efficacy have not been established for ZYCLARA Cream in the treatment of external genital warts.
ZYCLARA Cream should be used with caution in patients with pre-existing autoimmune conditions.

2 DOSAGE AND ADMINISTRATION
ZYCLARA Cream is not for oral, ophthalmic, or intravaginal use.
2.1 Actinic Keratosis
ZYCLARA Cream should be applied once daily before bedtime to the skin of the affected area (either entire face or balding scalp) for two 2-week treatment cycles separated by a 2-week no-treatment period. ZYCLARA Cream should be applied as a thin film to the entire treatment area and rubbed in until the cream is no longer visible. Up to 2 packets of ZYCLARA Cream may be applied to the treatment area at each application. **ZYCLARA Cream should be left on the skin for approximately 8 hours, after which time the cream should be removed by washing the area with mild soap and water.** The prescriber should demonstrate the proper application technique to maximize the benefit of ZYCLARA Cream therapy.
Patients should wash their hands before and after applying ZYCLARA cream.
Avoid use in or on the lips and nostrils. Do not use in or near the eyes.
Local skin reactions in the treatment area are common *[see Adverse Reactions (6.1, 6.2)]*. A rest period of several days may be taken if required by the patient's discomfort or severity of the local skin reaction. **However, neither 2-week**

---

treatment cycle should be extended due to missed doses or rest periods. A transient increase in AK lesion counts may be observed during treatment. Response to treatment cannot be adequately assessed until resolution of local skin reactions. The patient should continue dosing as prescribed. Treatment should continue for the full treatment course even if all actinic keratoses appear to be gone. Lesions that do not respond to treatment should be carefully re-evaluated and management reconsidered.
ZYCLARA Cream is packaged in single-use packets, with 28 packets supplied per box. Patients should be prescribed no more than 56 packets for the total 2-cycle treatment course. Unused packets should be discarded. Partially-used packets should be discarded and not reused.

3 DOSAGE FORMS AND STRENGTHS
Cream, 3.75%, white to faintly yellow cream.

4 CONTRAINDICATIONS
None.

5 WARNINGS AND PRECAUTIONS
5.1 Local Skin Reactions
Intense local skin reactions including skin weeping or erosion can occur after a few applications of ZYCLARA Cream and may require an interruption of dosing *[see Dosage and Administration (2) and Adverse Reactions (6)]*. ZYCLARA Cream has the potential to exacerbate inflammatory conditions of the skin, including chronic graft versus host disease.
Administration of ZYCLARA Cream is not recommended until the skin is healed from any previous drug or surgical treatment. Concomitant use of ZYCLARA and any other imiquimod creams, in the same treatment area, should be avoided since they contain the same active ingredient (imiquimod) and may increase the risk for and severity of local skin reactions.
5.2 Systemic Reactions
Flu-like signs and symptoms may accompany, or even precede, local skin reactions and may include fatigue, nausea, fever, myalgias, arthralgias, and chills. An interruption of dosing and an assessment of the patient should be considered *[see Adverse Reactions (6)]*. Lymphadenopathy occurred in 2% of subjects treated with ZYCLARA Cream *[see Adverse Reactions (6)]*. This reaction resolved in all subjects by 4 weeks after completion of treatment.
The safety of concomitant use of ZYCLARA Cream and any other imiquimod creams has not been established and should be avoided since they contain the same active ingredient (imiquimod) and may increase the risk for and severity of systemic reactions.
5.3 Ultraviolet Light Exposure
Exposure to sunlight (including sunlamps) should be avoided or minimized during use of ZYCLARA Cream because of concern for heightened sunburn susceptibility. Patients should be warned to use protective clothing (e.g., a hat) when using ZYCLARA Cream. Patients with sunburn should be advised not to use ZYCLARA Cream until fully recovered. Patients who may have considerable sun exposure, e.g. due to their occupation, and those patients with inherent sensitivity to sunlight should exercise caution when using ZYCLARA Cream.
In an animal photo-carcinogenicity study, imiquimod cream shortened the time to skin tumor formation *[see Nonclinical Toxicology (13.1)]*. The enhancement of ultraviolet carcinogenicity is not necessarily dependent on phototoxic mechanisms. Therefore, patients should minimize or avoid natural or artificial sunlight exposure.

6 ADVERSE REACTIONS
Because clinical trials are conducted under widely varying conditions, adverse reaction rates observed in the clinical trials of a drug cannot be directly compared to rates in the clinical trials of another drug and may not reflect the rates observed in practice.
6.1 Clinical Trials Experience
The data described below reflect exposure to ZYCLARA Cream or vehicle in 319 subjects enrolled in two double-blind, vehicle- controlled trials. Subjects applied up to two packets of ZYCLARA Cream or vehicle daily to the skin of the affected area (either entire face or balding scalp) for two 2-week treatment cycles separated by a 2-week no treatment period.
[See table 1 at top of next page]
[See table 2 on next page]
Local skin reactions may extend beyond treatment area. Overall, in the clinical trials, 11% (17/160) of subjects on ZYCLARA Cream and 0% on vehicle cream required rest periods due to adverse reactions.
Other adverse reactions observed in subjects treated with ZYCLARA Cream include: application site bleeding, application site swelling, arthralgia, cheilitis, chills, dermatitis, herpes zoster, influenza-like illness, insomnia, lethargy, myalgia, pancytopenia, pruritus, squamous cell carcinoma, and vomiting.
6.2 Postmarketing Experience
There are currently no postmarketing adverse reactions reported for ZYCLARA Cream.
The following adverse reactions have been identified during post-approval use of Aldara (imiquimod) Cream, 5%. Because these reactions are reported voluntarily from a

Table 1: Selected Adverse Reactions Occurring in ≥ 2% of ZYCLARA-Treated Subjects and at a Greater Frequency than with Vehicle in the Combined Studies

Preferred Term	Zyclara Cream 3.75% (N=160)	Placebo (N=159)
Headache	10 (6%)	5 (3%)
Application site pruritus	7 (4%)	1 (<1%)
Fatigue	7 (4%)	0 (0%)
Nausea	6 (4%)	2 (1%)
Application site irritation	5 (3%)	0 (0%)
Application site pain	5 (3%)	0 (0%)
Pyrexia	5 (3%)	0 (0%)
Anorexia	4 (3%)	0 (0%)
Dizziness	4 (3%)	0 (0%)
Herpes simplex	4 (3%)	1 (<1%)
Pain	4 (3%)	0 (0%)
Chest pain	3 (2%)	0 (0%)
Diarrhea	3 (2%)	0 (0%)
Lymphadenopathy	3 (2%)	0 (0%)

Table 2: Local Skin Reactions in the Treatment Area in ZYCLARA-Treated Subjects as Assessed by the Investigator

	ZYCLARA Cream 3.75% (N=160)		Vehicle (N=159)	
	All Grades*	Severe	All Grades*	Severe
Erythema	154 (96%)	40 (25%)	124 (78%)	0 (0%)
Scabbing/Crusting	149 (93%)	22 (14%)	72 (45%)	0 (0%)
Flaking/Scaling/Dryness	147 (92%)	13 (8%)	123 (77%)	2 (1%)
Edema	120 (75%)	9 (6%)	31 (19%)	0 (0%)
Erosion/Ulceration	99 (62%)	17 (11%)	14 (9%)	0 (0%)
Weeping/Exudate	81 (51%)	9 (6%)	6 (4%)	0 (0%)

* All Grades: mild, moderate or severe

population of uncertain size, it is not always possible to reliably estimate their frequency or establish a causal relationship to drug exposure.

Body as a Whole: angioedema.

Cardiovascular: capillary leak syndrome, cardiac failure, cardiomyopathy, pulmonary edema, arrhythmias (tachycardia, supraventricular tachycardia, atrial fibrillation, palpitations), chest pain, ischemia, myocardial infarction, syncope.

Endocrine: thyroiditis.

Gastro-Intestinal System Disorders: abdominal pain.

Hematological: decreases in red cell, white cell and platelet counts (including idiopathic thrombocytopenic purpura), lymphoma.

Hepatic: abnormal liver function.

Infections and Infestations: herpes simplex.

Neuropsychiatric: agitation, cerebrovascular accident, convulsions (including febrile convulsions), depression, insomnia, multiple sclerosis aggravation, paresis, suicide.

Respiratory: dyspnea.

Urinary System Disorders: proteinuria, urinary retention, dysuria.

Skin and Appendages: exfoliative dermatitis, erythema multiforme, hyperpigmentation, hypertrophic scar.

Vascular: Henoch-Schonlein purpura syndrome.

8 USE IN SPECIFIC POPULATIONS

8.1 Pregnancy

Pregnancy Category C:

There are no adequate and well-controlled studies in pregnant women. ZYCLARA Cream should be used during pregnancy only if the potential benefit justifies the potential risk to the fetus.

Note: The animal multiples of human exposure calculations were based on daily dose comparisons for the reproductive toxicology studies described in this label. The animal multiples of human exposure were based on weekly dose comparisons for the carcinogenicity studies described in this label. For the animal multiple of human exposure

ratios presented in this label, the Maximum Recommended Human Dose (MRHD) was set at 2 packets (500 mg cream) per treatment of ZYCLARA Cream (imiquimod 3.75%, 18.75 mg imiquimod).

Systemic embryofetal development studies were conducted in rats and rabbits. Oral doses of 1, 5 and 20 mg/kg/day imiquimod were administered during the period of organogenesis (gestational days 6–15) to pregnant female rats. In the presence of maternal toxicity, fetal effects noted at 20 mg/kg/day (190× MRHD based on AUC comparisons) included increased resorptions, decreased fetal body weights, delays in skeletal ossification, bent limb bones, and two fetuses in one litter (2 of 1567 fetuses) demonstrated exencephaly, protruding tongues and low-set ears. No treatment related effects on embryofetal toxicity or teratogenicity were noted at 5 mg/kg/day (32× MRHD based on AUC comparisons).

Intravenous doses of 0.5, 1 and 2 mg/kg/day imiquimod were administered during the period of organogenesis (gestational days 6–18) to pregnant female rabbits. No treatment related effects on embryofetal toxicity or teratogenicity were noted at 2 mg/kg/day (2.1× MRHD based on BSA comparisons), the highest dose evaluated in this study, or 1 mg/kg/day (134× MRHD based on AUC comparisons).

A combined fertility and peri- and post-natal development study was conducted in rats. Oral doses of 1, 1.5, 3 and 6 mg/kg/day imiquimod were administered to male rats from 70 days prior to mating through the mating period and to female rats from 14 days prior to mating through parturition and lactation. No effects on growth, fertility, reproduction or post-natal development were noted at doses up to 6 mg/kg/day (29× MRHD based on AUC comparisons), the highest dose evaluated in this study. In the absence of maternal toxicity, bent limb bones were noted in the F1 fetuses at a dose of 6 mg/kg/day (29× MRHD based on AUC comparisons). This fetal effect was also noted in the oral rat embryofetal development study conducted with imiquimod. No treatment related effects on teratogenicity were noted at 3 mg/kg/day (14× MRHD based on AUC comparisons).

8.3 Nursing Mothers

It is not known whether imiquimod is excreted in human milk following use of ZYCLARA Cream. Because many drugs are excreted in human milk, caution should be exercised when ZYCLARA Cream is administered to nursing women.

8.4 Pediatric Use

AK is a condition not generally seen within the pediatric population. The safety and efficacy of ZYCLARA Cream for AK in patients less than 18 years of age has not been established.

8.5 Geriatric Use

Of the 160 subjects treated with ZYCLARA Cream in the clinical studies, 78 subjects were 65 years or older. No overall differences in safety or effectiveness were observed between these subjects and younger subjects.

10 OVERDOSAGE

Topical overdosing of ZYCLARA Cream could result in an increased incidence of severe local skin reactions and may increase the risk for systemic reactions.

Hypotension was reported in a clinical trial following multiple oral imiquimod doses of >200 mg (equivalent to the ingestion of imiquimod content of > 21 packets of ZYCLARA). This resolved following oral or intravenous fluid administration.

11 DESCRIPTION

ZYCLARA Cream is intended for topical administration. Each gram contains 37.5 mg of imiquimod in a white to faintly yellow oil-in-water cream base consisting of isostearic acid, cetyl alcohol, stearyl alcohol, white petrolatum, polysorbate 60, sorbitan monostearate, glycerin, xanthan gum, purified water, benzyl alcohol, methylparaben, and propylparaben.

Chemically, imiquimod is 1-(2-methylpropyl)-1H-imidazo-[4,5-c]quinolin-4-amine. Imiquimod has a molecular formula of $C_{14}H_{16}N_4$ and a molecular weight of 240.3. Its structural formula is:

12 CLINICAL PHARMACOLOGY

12.1 Mechanism of Action

The mechanism of action of ZYCLARA Cream in treating AK lesions is unknown.

12.2 Pharmacodynamics

The pharmacodynamics of ZYCLARA are unknown.

Imiquimod is a Toll-like receptor 7 agonist that activates immune cells. Topical application to skin is associated with increases in markers for cytokines and immune cells.

In a study of 18 subjects with AK comparing Aldara (imiquimod) Cream, 5% to vehicle, increases from baseline in week 2 biomarker levels were reported for CD3, CD4, CD8, CD11c, and CD68 for Aldara (imiquimod) Cream, 5% treated subjects; however, the clinical relevance of these findings is unknown.

12.3 Pharmacokinetics

Following dosing with 2 packets once daily (18.75 mg imiquimod/day) for up to three weeks, systemic absorption of imiquimod was observed in all subjects when Zyclara Cream was applied to the face and/or scalp in 17 subjects with at least 10 AK lesions. The mean peak serum imiquimod concentration at the end of the trial was approximately 0.323 ng/mL. The median time to maximal concentrations (T_{max}) occurred at 9 hours after dosing. Based on the plasma half-life of imiquimod observed at the end of the study, 29.3±17.0 hours, steady-state concentrations can be anticipated to occur by day 7 with once daily dosing.

13 NONCLINICAL TOXICOLOGY

13.1 Carcinogenesis, Mutagenesis, Impairment of Fertility

In an oral (gavage) rat carcinogenicity study, imiquimod was administered to Wistar rats on a 2×/week (up to 6 mg/kg/day) or daily (3 mg/kg/day) dosing schedule for 24 months. No treatment related tumors were noted in the oral rat carcinogenicity study up to the highest doses tested in this study of 6 mg/kg administered 2×/week in female rats (8.2× MRHD based on weekly AUC comparisons), 4 mg/kg administered 2×/week in male rats (7.1× MRHD) based on weekly AUC comparisons) or 3 mg/kg administered 7×/week to male and female rats (14× MRHD based on weekly AUC comparisons).

In a dermal mouse carcinogenicity study, imiquimod cream (up to 5 mg/kg/application imiquimod or 0.3% imiquimod cream) was applied to the backs of mice 3×/week for 24 months. A statistically significant increase in the incidence of liver adenomas and carcinomas was noted in high dose male mice compared to control male mice (24× MRHD based on weekly AUC comparisons). An increased number of skin papillomas was observed in vehicle cream control group animals at the treated site only.

In a 52-week dermal photo-carcinogenicity study, the median time to onset of skin tumor formation was decreased in hairless mice following chronic topical dosing (3×/week; 40 weeks of treatment followed by 12 weeks of observation) with concurrent exposure to UV radiation (5 days per week) with vehicle alone. No additional effect on tumor development beyond the vehicle effect was noted with the addition of the active ingredient, imiquimod, to the vehicle cream.

Imiquimod revealed no evidence of mutagenic or clastogenic potential based on the results of five in vitro genotoxicity tests (Ames assay, mouse lymphoma L5178Y assay, Chinese hamster ovary cell chromosome aberration assay, human lymphocyte chromosome aberration assay and SHE cell transformation assay) and three in vivo genotoxicity tests (rat and hamster bone marrow cytogenetics assay and a mouse dominant lethal test).

Daily oral administration of imiquimod to rats, throughout mating, gestation, parturition and lactation, demonstrated no effects on growth, fertility or reproduction, at doses up to 29× MRHD based on AUC comparisons.

14 CLINICAL STUDIES

In two double-blind, randomized, vehicle-controlled clinical studies, 319 subjects with AK were treated with ZYCLARA Cream, or vehicle cream. Studies enrolled subjects >18 years of age with 5-20 typical visible or palpable AK lesions of the face or scalp. Study cream was applied to either the entire face (excluding ears) or balding scalp once daily for two 2-week treatment cycles separated by a 2-week no-treatment period. Subjects then continued in the study for an 8-week follow-up period during which they returned for clinical observations and safety monitoring. Study subjects ranged from 36 to 90 years of age and 54% had Fitzpatrick skin type I or II. All ZYCLARA Cream-treated subjects were Caucasians.

On a scheduled dosing day, up to two packets of the study cream were applied to the entire treatment area prior to normal sleeping hours and left on for approximately 8 hours. Efficacy was assessed by AK lesion counts at the 8-week post-treatment visit. All AKs in the treatment area were counted, including baseline lesions as well as lesions which appeared during therapy.

Complete clearance required absence of any lesions including those that appeared during therapy in the treatment area. Complete and partial clearance rates are shown in the tables below. Partial clearance rate was defined as the percentage of subjects in whom the number of baseline AKs was reduced by 75% or more. The partial clearance rate was measured relative to the numbers of AK lesions at Baseline.

Table 3: Rate of Subjects with Complete Clearance at 8 Weeks Post Treatment

	ZYCLARA Cream 3.75%	Vehicle Cream
Study 1	25.9% (21/81)	2.5% (2/80)
Study 2	45.6% (36/79)	10.1% (8/79)

Table 4: Rate of Subjects with Partial Clearance (≥75%) at 8 Weeks Post Treatment

	ZYCLARA Cream 3.75%	Vehicle Cream
Study 1	45.7 (37/81)	18.8 (15/80)
Study 2	73.4 (58/79)	26.6 (21/79)

During the course of treatment, 86% (138/160) of subjects experienced a transient increase in lesions evaluated as actinic keratoses relative to the number present at baseline within the treatment area.

16 HOW SUPPLIED/STORAGE AND HANDLING

ZYCLARA (imiquimod) Cream, 3.75%, is supplied in single-use packets which contain 250 mg of the cream. Available as: Box of 28 packets NDC 29336-710-28. Store at 25°C (77°F); excursions permitted to 15° to 30°C (59° to 86°F) [see USP Controlled Room Temperature].

Avoid freezing.

Keep out of reach of children.

17 PATIENT COUNSELING INFORMATION

See FDA-Approved Patient Labeling (17.7)

17.1 Instructions for Administration

Zyclara Cream should be used as directed by a physician [see Dosage and Administration (2)]. Zyclara Cream is for external use only. Contact with the eyes, lips and nostrils should be avoided [see Indications and Usage (1) and [Dosage and Administration (2)].

The treatment area should not be bandaged or otherwise occluded. Partially-used packets should be discarded and not reused. The prescriber should demonstrate the proper application technique to maximize the benefit of ZYCLARA Cream therapy.

It is recommended that patients wash their hands before and after applying Zyclara Cream.

17.2 Local Skin Reactions

Patients may experience local skin reactions during treatment with Zyclara Cream. Potential local skin reactions include erythema, edema, erosions/ulcerations, weeping/exudate, flaking/scaling/dryness, and scabbing/crusting. These reactions can range from mild to severe in intensity and may extend beyond the application site onto the surrounding skin. Patients may also experience application site reactions such as itching, irritation or pain [see Adverse Reactions (6)].

Local skin reactions may be of such an intensity that patients may require rest periods from treatment. Treatment with Zyclara Cream can be resumed after the skin reaction has subsided, as determined by the physician. However, each treatment cycle should not be extended beyond 2 weeks due to missed doses or rest periods. Patients should contact their physician promptly if they experience any sign or symptom at the application site that restricts or prohibits their daily activity or makes continued application of the cream difficult.

Because of local skin reactions, during treatment and until healed, the treatment area is likely to appear noticeably different from normal skin. Localized hypopigmentation and hyperpigmentation have been reported following use of imiquimod cream. These skin color changes may be permanent in some patients.

17.3 Systemic Reactions

Patients may experience flu-like systemic signs and symptoms during treatment with Zyclara Cream. Systemic signs and symptoms may include fatigue, nausea, fever, myalgia, arthralgia, and chills [see Adverse Reactions (6)]. An interruption of dosing or dose adjustment and an assessment of the patient should be considered.

17.4 Recommended Administration

Dosing is once daily before bedtime to the skin of the affected area (entire face or balding scalp) for two 2-week treatment cycles separated by a 2-week no-treatment period. However, the treatment period should not be extended beyond two 2-week treatment cycles due to missed doses or rest periods. Treatment should continue for the full treatment course even if all actinic keratoses appear to be gone [see Dosage and Administration (2.1)].

It is recommended that patients wash their hands before and after applying ZYCLARA Cream. Before applying the cream, the patient should wash the treatment area with mild soap and water and allow the area to dry thoroughly. It is recommended that the treatment area be washed with mild soap and water 8 hours following ZYCLARA Cream application.

Most patients using ZYCLARA Cream for the treatment of AK experience erythema, flaking/scaling/dryness and scabbing/crusting at the application site with normal dosing [see Adverse Reactions (6.1)].

Use of sunscreen is encouraged, and patients should minimize or avoid exposure to natural or artificial sunlight (tanning beds or UVA/ B treatment) while using ZYCLARA Cream [see Warnings and Precautions (5.3)].

Additional lesions may become apparent in the treatment area during treatment [see Clinical Studies (14.1)].

17.7 FDA-Approved Patient Labeling

Patient Information
Zyclara [imiquimod] **Cream, 3.75%**

IMPORTANT: For use on the skin only (topical). Do not use ZYCLARA cream in or on your eyes, nostrils, mouth or vagina.

Read the Patient Information that comes with ZYCLARA cream before you start using it and each time you get a refill. There may be new information. This leaflet does not take the place of talking with your healthcare provider about your medical condition or treatment. If you do not understand the information, or have any questions about ZYCLARA cream, talk with your healthcare provider or pharmacist.

What is ZYCLARA Cream?
ZYCLARA cream is a prescription medicine for use on the face or balding scalp only (a topical medicine) to treat actinic keratosis (AK).

Actinic keratosis is caused by too much sun exposure.

It is not known if ZYCLARA cream is safe and effective:

- in people who do not have a normal immune system.
- in the treatment of patients with xeroderma pigmentosum.
- in the treatment of superficial basal cell carcinoma.
- in the treatment of external genital warts.

It is not known if ZYCLARA cream is safe and effective in children younger than 18 years old.

What should I tell my healthcare provider before using ZYCLARA Cream?
Before you use ZYCLARA cream, tell your healthcare provider if you:

- have problems with your immune system
- are being treated or have been treated for actinic keratosis with other medicines or surgery. You should not use ZYCLARA cream until you have healed from other treatments
- have other skin problems
- have any other medical conditions
- are pregnant or planning to become pregnant. It is not known if ZYCLARA cream can harm your unborn baby. Talk to your healthcare provider if you are pregnant or plan to become pregnant.
- are breast-feeding or plan to breast-feed. It is not known if ZYCLARA cream passes into your breast milk and if it can harm your baby. Talk to your healthcare provider about the best way to feed your baby if you use ZYCLARA cream.

Tell your healthcare provider about all the medicines you take, including prescription and non-prescription medicines, vitamins and herbal supplements.

Especially tell your healthcare provider if you have had other treatments for actinic keratosis.

How should I use ZYCLARA Cream?
- **Do not** get ZYCLARA cream in or near your eyes.
- **Do not** get ZYCLARA cream in or on your nostrils, lips, or vagina.
- Use ZYCLARA cream exactly as your healthcare provider tells you to use it. Your healthcare provider will tell you where to apply ZYCLARA cream and how often and for how long to apply it for your condition. Do not apply ZYCLARA cream to other areas.
- Using too much ZYCLARA cream, or using it too often, or for too long can increase your chances for having a severe skin reaction or other side effects.
- Talk to your healthcare provider if you think ZYCLARA cream is not working for you.

Applying ZYCLARA Cream
Zyclara Cream should be applied just before your bedtime.

Do not use more ZYCLARA cream than you need to cover the treatment area.

Do not use more than two packets of ZYCLARA cream on the treatment area.

- Wash the area where the cream will be applied with mild soap and water.
- Allow the area to dry.
- Wash your hands.
- Open a packet of ZYLCARA cream and apply a thin layer to the affected area on the scalp or face to be treated. You may need to use more than one packet.
- Rub the cream into your skin until you can not see the ZYCLARA cream.
- After you apply ZYCLARA cream, wash your hands with mild soap and water.
- Leave the cream on the treated area for the amount of time your healthcare provider tells you (usually about 8 hours). Do not take a bath or get the treated area wet during this time.
- After the right amount of time has passed, wash the treated area with mild soap and water.
- If you forget to apply ZYCLARA cream, just apply the next dose of ZYCLARA cream at your regular time.
- If you get ZYCLARA cream in your mouth or in your eyes rinse well with water right away.

What should I avoid while using ZYCLARA Cream?
- **Do not** cover the treated area with bandages or other closed dressings.
- **Do not** use sunlamps or tanning beds, and avoid sunlight as much as possible during treatment with ZYCLARA cream. Use sunscreen and wear protective clothing if you go outside during daylight.

What are the possible side effects of ZYCLARA Cream?
ZYCLARA Cream may cause serious side effects, including:
- **Local Skin Reactions:** skin redness, scabbing or crusting, flaking, scaling or dryness, swelling, sores or blisters, draining (weeping)
- **Flu-like symptoms:** tiredness, nausea, vomiting, fever, chills, muscle pain, joint pain

The most common side effects of ZYCLARA cream include:
- headache
- itching at application site
- tiredness
- nausea
- skin irritation
- pain at the treatment area

- fever
- loss of appetite
- dizziness
- cold sores
- pain
- chest pain
- diarrhea
- swelling of lymph nodes

Tell your healthcare provider if you have any side effect that bothers you or that does not go away.

These are not all the possible side effects of ZYCLARA cream. For more information, ask your healthcare provider or pharmacist.

Call your doctor for medical advice about side effects. You may report side effects to FDA at 1-800-FDA-1088 or to Graceway Pharmaceuticals, LLC at 1-800-328-0255.

How do I store ZYCLARA Cream?
- Store ZYCLARA cream at 59°F to 86°F (15°C to 30°C).
- Do not freeze.

Keep ZYCLARA cream and all medicines out of the reach of children.

General information about ZYCLARA Cream
Medicines are sometimes prescribed for purposes other than those listed in the patient information. Do not use ZYCLARA cream for a condition for which it was not prescribed. Do not give ZYCLARA cream to other people, even if they have the same symptoms you have. It may harm them.

This patient information leaflet summarizes the most important information about ZYCLARA cream. If you would like more information, talk with your healthcare provider. You can ask your pharmacist or healthcare provider for information about ZYCLARA cream that is written for the health professionals.

What are the ingredients in ZYCLARA Cream?
Active Ingredient: imiquimod
Inactive ingredients: isostearic acid, cetyl alcohol, stearyl alcohol, white petrolatum, polysorbate 60, sorbitan monostearate, glycerin, xanthan gum, purified water, benzyl alcohol, methylparaben, and propylparaben.

Rx Only
Manufactured by
3M Health Care Limited
Loughborough LE11 1EP England
Distributed by
Graceway Pharmaceuticals, LLC
Bristol, TN 37620

Grifols Biologicals Inc.
5555 VALLEY BOULEVARD
LOS ANGELES, CA 90032

Direct Inquiries to:
CONTACTS:
All services, incl.
24 hr. ordering	888 GRIFOLS or 888 474 3657
Direct Inquiries:	323 225 2221
Fax:	323-441-7968
Website	www.grifolsusa.com

ALBUTEIN® 5% SOLUTION   ℞
Albumin (Human) U.S.P.

HIGHLIGHTS OF PRESCRIBING INFORMATION
These highlights do not include all the information needed to use Albutein® 5% safely and effectively. See full prescribing information for Albutein® 5%.
Albutein® 5% [Albumin (Human) U.S.P.] sterile, aqueous solution for single dose intravenous administration
Initial U.S. Approval: 1978

─────INDICATIONS AND USAGE─────
Albumin (Human) U.S.P., Albutein® 5% Solution is indicated (1):
- For treatment of hypovolemic shock.
- In conditions in which there is severe hypoalbuminemia. However, unless the pathologic condition responsible for the hypoalbuminemia can be corrected, administration of albumin can afford only symptomatic or supportive relief.
- As an adjunct in hemodialysis and in cardiopulmonary bypass procedures.
In those conditions in which the colloid requirement is high and there is less need for fluid, albumin should be administered as a 25% solution.

─────DOSAGE AND ADMINISTRATION─────
Albutein® 5% is administered intravenously. The total dosage will vary with the individual. In adults, an initial infusion of 500 mL is suggested. Additional amounts may be administered as clinically indicated.
- When an administration set is used (2.1)
- When an administration set is not used (2.2)

─────DOSAGE FORMS AND STRENGTHS─────
Albutein® 5% is a sterile, aqueous solution for single dose intravenous administration containing 5% human albumin (weight/volume), provided in the following presentations: (3)

- 12.5 g albumin/250 mL single dose
- 25 g albumin/500 mL single dose

─────CONTRAINDICATIONS─────
- Patients with severe anemia or cardiac failure in the presence of normal or increased intravascular volume (4)
- Patients with a history of allergic reactions to albumin (4)

─────WARNINGS AND PRECAUTIONS─────
- Risk of infectious agents (5.1)
- Patients with low cardiac reserve (5.2)

─────ADVERSE REACTIONS─────
The most common adverse reactions include fever and chills, rash, nausea, vomiting, tachycardia and hypotension (6)

To report SUSPECTED ADVERSE REACTIONS, contact Grifols Biologicals Inc. at 1-888-GRIFOLS (1-888-474-3657) or FDA at 1-800-FDA-1088 or www.fda.gov/medwatch.

─────USE IN SPECIFIC POPULATIONS─────
- Unknown whether can cause fetal harm or affect reproduction capacity (8.1)
- The pediatric use has not been clinically evaluated (8.4)

See 17 for PATIENT COUNSELING INFORMATION
Revised: 07/2008

FULL PRESCRIBING INFORMATION: CONTENTS*
1 INDICATIONS AND USAGE
2 DOSAGE AND ADMINISTRATION
  2.1   When an Administration Set is Used
  2.2   When an Administration Set is Not Used
3 DOSAGE FORMS AND STRENGTHS
4 CONTRAINDICATIONS
5 WARNINGS AND PRECAUTIONS
  5.1   Warnings
  5.2   Precautions
6 ADVERSE REACTIONS
8 USE IN SPECIFIC POPULATIONS
  8.1   Pregnancy
  8.4   Pediatric Use
11 DESCRIPTION
12 CLINICAL PHARMACOLOGY
  12.1   Mechanism of Action
15 REFERENCES
16 HOW SUPPLIED/STORAGE AND HANDLING
17 PATIENT COUNSELING INFORMATION
* Sections or subsections omitted from the full prescribing information are not listed.

FULL PRESCRIBING INFORMATION

1. INDICATIONS AND USAGE
Albumin (Human) U.S.P., Albutein® 5% Solution is indicated:
1. For treatment of hypovolemic shock.[1,2]
2. In conditions in which there is severe hypoalbuminemia. However, unless the pathologic condition responsible for the hypoalbuminemia can be corrected, administration of albumin can afford only symptomatic or supportive relief.
3. As an adjunct in hemodialysis and in cardiopulmonary bypass procedures.
In those conditions in which the colloid requirement is high and there is less need for fluid, albumin should be administered as a 25% solution.

2. DOSAGE AND ADMINISTRATION
Albutein® 5% is administered intravenously. The total dosage will vary with the individual. In adults, an initial infusion of 500 mL is suggested. Additional amounts may be administered as clinically indicated.
In the treatment of the patient in shock with greatly reduced blood volume, Albutein® 5% may be administered as rapidly as necessary in order to improve the clinical condition and restore normal blood volume. This may be repeated in 15-30 minutes if the initial dose fails to prove adequate. In the patient with a slightly low or normal blood volume, the rate of administration should be 1-2 mL per minute.
DIRECTIONS FOR USE: (250 mL and 500 mL)
2.1 When an Administration Set is Used
Flip off plastic cap on top of the vial and expose rubber stopper. Cleanse exposed rubber stopper with suitable germicidal solution, being sure to remove any excess. Observe aseptic technique and prepare sterile intravenous equipment as follows:
1. Close clamp on administration set.
2. With bottle upright, squeeze drip chamber, thrust piercing pin straight through stopper center. Do not twist or angle.
3. Immediately invert bottle, release drip chamber to automatically establish proper fluid level in drip chamber (half full).
4. Attach infusion set to administration set, open clamp and allow solution to expel air from tubing and needle, then close clamp.
5. Make venipuncture and adjust flow.
6. Discard all administration equipment after use. Discard any unused contents.
2.2 When an Administration Set is Not Used
Flip off plastic cap on top of the vial and expose rubber stopper. Cleanse exposed rubber stopper with suitable germi-

cidal solution, being sure to remove any excess. Observe aseptic technique and prepare sterile intravenous equipment as follows:
1. Using aseptic technique, attach filter needle to a sterile disposable plastic syringe.
2. Insert filter needle into Albutein® 5%.
3. Aspirate Albutein® 5% from the vial into the syringe.
4. Remove and discard the filter needle from the syringe.
5. Attach desired size needle to syringe.
6. Discard all administration equipment after use. Discard any unused contents.

3. DOSAGE FORMS AND STRENGTHS
Albutein® 5% is a sterile, aqueous solution for single dose intravenous administration containing 5% human albumin (weight/volume). It is available in the following presentations:
- 12.5 g albumin/250 mL single dose vial.
- 25 g albumin/500 mL single dose vial.

4. CONTRAINDICATIONS
Albutein® 5% is contraindicated in patients with severe anemia or cardiac failure in the presence of normal or increased intravascular volume.
The use of Albutein® 5% is contraindicated in patients with a history of allergic reactions to albumin.

5. WARNINGS AND PRECAUTIONS
5.1 Warnings
Albutein® 5% is made from pooled human plasma. Based on effective donor screening and product manufacturing processes, it carries an extremely remote risk for transmission of viral diseases, including a theoretical risk for transmission of Creutzfeldt-Jakob disease (CJD). Although no cases of transmission of viral diseases or CJD have ever been identified for albumin, the risk of infectious agents cannot be totally eliminated. The physician should weigh the risks and benefits of the use of this product and should discuss these with the patient.
Solutions of Albutein® 5% should not be used if they appear turbid or if there is sediment in the bottle. Do not begin administration more than 4 hours after the container has been entered. Discard unused portion.

5.2 Precautions
Albutein® 5% should be administered with caution to patients with low cardiac reserve.
Rapid infusion may cause vascular overload with resultant pulmonary edema. Patients should be closely monitored for signs of increased venous pressure.
A rapid rise in blood pressure following infusion necessitates careful observation of injured or postoperative patients to detect and treat severed blood vessels that may not have bled at a lower pressure.
Patients with marked dehydration require administration of additional fluids. Albutein® 5% may be administered with the usual dextrose and saline intravenous solutions. However, solutions containing protein hydrolysates or alcohol must not be infused through the same administration set in conjunction with Albutein® 5% since these combinations may cause the proteins to precipitate. See also **PATIENT COUNSELING INFORMATION (17)**.

6. ADVERSE REACTIONS
The most common adverse reactions include fever and chills, rash, nausea, vomiting, tachycardia and hypotension. Should an adverse reaction occur, slow or stop the infusion for a period of time which may result in the disappearance of the symptoms. If administration has been stopped and the patient requires additional Albutein® 5%, material from a different lot should be used.
Albutein® 5%, particularly if administered rapidly, may result in vascular overload with resultant pulmonary edema.
To report SUSPECTED ADVERSE REACTIONS, contact Grifols Biologicals Inc. at 1-888-GRIFOLS (1-888-474-3657) or FDA at 1-800-FDA-1088 or www.fda.gov/medwatch.

8. USE IN SPECIFIC POPULATIONS
8.1 Pregnancy
Pregnancy Category C. Animal reproduction studies have not been conducted with Albutein® 5%. It is also not known whether Albutein® 5% can cause fetal harm when administered to a pregnant woman or can affect reproductive capacity. Albutein® 5% should be given to a pregnant woman only if clearly needed.
8.4 Pediatric Use
The pediatric use of Albutein® 5% has not been clinically evaluated. The dosage will vary with the clinical state and body weight of the individual. Typically, a dose one-quarter to one-half the adult dose may be administered, or dosage may be calculated on the basis of 0.6 to 1.0 gram per kilogram of body weight (12 to 20 mL of Albutein® 5%). The usual rate of administration in children should be one-quarter the adult rate. Therefore, physicians should weigh the risks and benefits of the use of Albutein® 5% in the pediatric population.

Parenteral drug products should be inspected visually for particulate matter and discoloration prior to administration, whenever solution and container permit.

11. DESCRIPTION

Albutein® 5% is a sterile, aqueous solution for single dose intravenous administration containing 5% human albumin (weight/volume). Albutein® 5% is prepared by a cold alcohol fractionation method from pooled human plasma obtained from venous blood. The product is stabilized with 0.08 millimole sodium caprylate and 0.08 millimole sodium acetyltryptophanate per gram of albumin. Albutein® 5% is osmotically and isotonically equivalent to an equal volume of normal human plasma. Albutein® 5% contains 130-160 milliequivalents of sodium ion per liter and has a pH of 7.0 ± 0.3. The aluminum content of the solution is not more than 200 micrograms per liter during the shelf life of the product. The product contains no preservatives.

Albutein® 5% is heated at 60 °C for ten hours. No positive assertion can be made, however, that this heat treatment completely destroys the causative agents of viral hepatitis.

12. CLINICAL PHARMACOLOGY

12.1 Mechanism of Action

There are no known cases of viral hepatitis which have resulted from the administration of Albutein® 5%. Albumin is a highly soluble, globular protein (MW 66,500), accounting for 70-80% of the colloid osmotic pressure of plasma. Therefore, it is important in regulating the osmotic pressure of plasma.[1,3] Albutein® 5% supplies the oncotic equivalent of approximately its volume of human plasma. It will increase the circulating plasma volume by an amount approximately equal to the volume infused. This extra fluid reduces hemoconcentration and decreases blood viscosity.[4] The degree and duration of volume expansion depend upon the initial blood volume. When treating patients with diminished blood volume, the effect of infused albumin may persist for many hours. The hemodilution lasts for a shorter time when albumin is administered to individuals with normal blood volume.

Albumin is also a transport protein and binds naturally occurring, therapeutic, and toxic materials in the circulation.[1] The binding properties of albumin may, in special circumstances, provide an indication for its clinical use. For such purposes, however, the 25% solution should be used.

Albumin is distributed throughout the extracellular water and more than 60% of the body albumin pool is located in the extravascular fluid compartment. The total body albumin in a 70 kg man is approximately 320 g. Albumin has a circulating life span of 15-20 days, with a turnover of approximately 15 g per day.[3]

15. REFERENCES

1. Finlayson, J.S., Albumin Products, *Semin Thromb Hemo*, 6:85-120, 1980.
2. Hauser, C.J., et. al., Oxygen Transport Responses to Colloids and Crystalloids in Critically Ill Surgical Patients, *Surg Gyn Obs*, 150:811-816, June 1980.
3. Tullis, J.L., Albumin: 1. Background and Use, 2. Guidelines for Clinical Use, *JAMA*, 237:355-360, 460-463, 1977.
4. Janeway, C.A., Human Serum Albumin: Historical Review in *Proceedings of the Workshop on Albumin*, Sgouris, J.T. and Rene A. (eds), DHEW Publication No. (NIH) 76-925, Washington, D.C., U.S. Government Printing Office, 1976, pp. 3-21.

16. HOW SUPPLIED/STORAGE AND HANDLING

Albutein® 5% is supplied as a sterile, aqueous solution for single dose intravenous administration containing 5% human albumin (weight/volume). It is available in the following vial sizes:
• 250 mL vial Albutein® 5% (NDC 68516-5214-1).
• 500 mL vial Albutein® 5% (NDC 68516-5214-2).

Storage

Albutein® 5% is stable for three years provided that storage temperature does not exceed 30 °C. Protect from freezing.

17. PATIENT COUNSELING INFORMATION

The most common adverse reactions include fever and chills, rash, nausea, vomiting, tachycardia and hypotension. Depending on the severity of the reaction, patients should be advised to discontinue use of the product and contact their physician and/or seek immediate emergency care.

Albutein® 5% should be administered with caution to patients with low cardiac reserve.

Rapid infusion may cause vascular overload with resultant pulmonary edema. Patients should be closely monitored for signs of increased venous pressure.

A rapid rise in blood pressure following infusion necessitates careful observation of injured or postoperative patients to detect and treat severed blood vessels that may not have bled at a lower pressure.

Patients with marked dehydration require administration of additional fluids. Albutein® 5% may be administered

with the usual dextrose and saline intravenous solutions. However, solutions containing protein hydrolysates or alcohol must not be infused through the same administration set in conjunction with Albutein® 5% since these combinations may cause the proteins to precipitate. See also **WARNINGS AND PRECAUTIONS (5.2)**.

Manufactured and Distributed by:
Grifols Biologicals Inc.
Los Angeles, CA 90032, U.S.A.
U.S. License No. 1694
DATE OF REVISION: 07/2008

ALBUTEIN® 25% SOLUTION ℞
[ăl-bū-tān]
Albumin (Human) U.S.P.

HIGHLIGHTS OF PRESCRIBING INFORMATION

These highlights do not include all the information needed to use Albutein® 25% safely and effectively. See full prescribing information for Albutein® 25%.

Albutein® 25% [Albumin (Human) U.S.P.] sterile, aqueous solution for single dose intravenous administration

Initial U.S. Approval: 1978

———————INDICATIONS AND USAGE———————

Albumin (Human) U.S.P., Albutein® 25% Solution is indicated (1):
• For treatment of hypovolemic shock.
• As an adjunct in hemodialysis for patients undergoing long-term dialysis or for those patients who are fluid-overloaded and cannot tolerate substantial volumes of salt solution for therapy of shock or hypotension.
• In cardiopulmonary bypass procedures; however, the optimum regimen of fluids has not been established.

Conditions in which Albutein® 25% **MAY BE** indicated:
• Adult respiratory distress syndrome (ARDS).
• Major injury or surgery resulting in increased albumin loss or inadequate synthesis.
• Acute nephrosis not responding to cyclophosphamide or steroid therapy. Steroid therapy may increase edema which may respond to combined therapy of albumin with a diuretic.
• Acute liver failure or ascites where the therapeutic use is regulated by the individual circumstances.

Unless the pathologic condition responsible for hypoalbuminemia can be corrected, administration of albumin can afford only symptomatic relief. There is **NO** valid reason for the use of albumin as an intravenous nutrient.

———————DOSAGE AND ADMINISTRATION———————

Albutein® 25% is administered intravenously. The total dosage will vary with the individual. In adults, an initial infusion of 100 mL is suggested. Additional amounts may be administered as clinically indicated.
• When an administration set is used (2.1)
• When an administration set is not used (2.2)

———————DOSAGE FORMS AND STRENGTHS———————

Albutein® 25% is a sterile, aqueous solution for single dose intravenous administration containing 25% human albumin (weight/volume), provided in the following presentations: (3)
• 12.5 g albumin/50 mL single dose vial
• 25 g albumin/100 mL single dose vial

———————CONTRAINDICATIONS———————

• Patients with severe anemia or cardiac failure in the presence of normal or increased intravascular volume (4)
• Patients with a history of allergic reactions to albumin (4)

———————WARNINGS AND PRECAUTIONS———————

• Risk of infectious agents (5.1)
• Patients with low cardiac reserve (5.2)

———————ADVERSE REACTIONS———————

The most common adverse reactions include fever and chills, rash, nausea, vomiting, tachycardia and hypotension (6)

To report SUSPECTED ADVERSE REACTIONS, contact Grifols Biologicals Inc. at 1-888-GRIFOLS (1-888-474-3657) or FDA at 1-800-FDA-1088 or www.fda.gov/medwatch.

———————USE IN SPECIFIC POPULATIONS———————

• Unknown whether can cause fetal harm or affect reproduction capacity (8.1)
• The pediatric use has not been clinically evaluated (8.4)

See 17 for PATIENT COUNSELING INFORMATION

Revised: 07/2008

FULL PRESCRIBING INFORMATION:
CONTENTS*
1   INDICATIONS AND USAGE
2   DOSAGE AND ADMINISTRATION
      2.1   When an Administration Set is Used
      2.2   When an Administration Set is Not Used
3   DOSAGE FORMS AND STRENGTH
4   CONTRAINDICATIONS
5   WARNINGS AND PRECAUTIONS
      5.1   Warnings
      5.2   Precautions

6   ADVERSE REACTIONS
8   USE IN SPECIFIC POPULATIONS
      8.1   Pregnancy
      8.4   Pediatric Use
11   DESCRIPTION
12   CLINICAL PHARMACOLOGY
      12.1   Mechanism of Action
15   REFERENCES
16   HOW SUPPLIED/STORAGE AND HANDLING
17   PATIENT COUNSELING INFORMATION
*Sections or subsections omitted from the full prescribing information are not listed.

FULL PRESCRIBING INFORMATION

1. INDICATIONS AND USAGE

Albumin (Human) U.S.P., Albutein® 25% Solution is indicated:
1. For treatment of hypovolemic shock.[1,2]
2. As an adjunct in hemodialysis for patients undergoing long-term dialysis or for those patients who are fluid-overloaded and cannot tolerate substantial volumes of salt solution for therapy of shock or hypotension.[3]
3. In cardiopulmonary bypass procedures; however, the optimum regimen of fluids has not been established.

Conditions in which Albutein® 25% **MAY BE** indicated:
• Adult respiratory distress syndrome (ARDS).[3,4]
• Major injury or surgery resulting in increased albumin loss or inadequate synthesis.[3,5]
• Acute nephrosis not responding to cyclophosphamide or steroid therapy. Steroid therapy may increase edema which may respond to combined therapy of albumin with a diuretic.[3]
• Acute liver failure or ascites where the therapeutic use is regulated by the individual circumstances.[3]

Unless the pathologic condition responsible for hypoalbuminemia can be corrected, administration of albumin can afford only symptomatic relief. There is **NO** valid reason for the use of albumin as an intravenous nutrient.

2. DOSAGE AND ADMINISTRATION

Albutein® 25% is administered intravenously. The total dosage will vary with the individual. In adults, an initial infusion of 100 mL is suggested. Additional amounts may be administered as clinically indicated.

In the treatment of the patient in shock with greatly reduced blood volume, Albutein® 25% may be administered as rapidly as necessary in order to improve the clinical condition and restore normal blood volume. This may be repeated in 15-30 minutes if the initial dose fails to prove adequate. In the patient with a slightly low or normal blood volume, the rate of administration should be 1 mL per minute.

If dilution of Albutein® 25% is clinically desirable, compatible diluents include sterile 0.9% Sodium Chloride solution or sterile 5% Dextrose in Water.[6]

DIRECTIONS FOR USE: (50 mL and 100 mL)

2.1 When an Administration Set is Used

Flip off plastic cap on top of the vial and expose rubber stopper. Cleanse exposed rubber stopper with suitable germicidal solution, being sure to remove any excess. Observe aseptic technique and prepare sterile intravenous equipment as follows:
1. Close clamp on administration set.
2. With bottle upright, squeeze drip chamber, thrust piercing pin straight through stopper center. Do not twist or angle.
3. Immediately invert bottle, release drip chamber to automatically establish proper fluid level in drip chamber (half full).
4. Attach infusion set to administration set, open clamp and allow solution to expel air from tubing and needle, then close clamp.
5. Make venipuncture and adjust flow.
6. Discard all administration equipment after use. Discard any unused contents.

2.2 When an Administration Set is Not Used

Flip off plastic cap on top of the vial and expose rubber stopper. Cleanse exposed rubber stopper with suitable germicidal solution, being sure to remove any excess. Observe aseptic technique and prepare sterile intravenous equipment as follows:
1. Using aseptic technique, attach filter needle to a sterile disposable plastic syringe.
2. Insert filter needle into Albutein® 25%.
3. Aspirate Albutein® 25% from the vial into the syringe.
4. Remove and discard the filter needle from the syringe.
5. Attach desired size needle to syringe.
6. Discard all administration equipment after use. Discard any unused contents.

3. DOSAGE FORMS AND STRENGTHS

Albutein® 25% is a sterile, aqueous solution for single dose intravenous administration containing 25% human albumin (weight/volume). It is available in the following presentations:

- 12.5 g albumin/50 mL single dose vial.
- 25 g albumin/100 mL single dose vial.

4. CONTRAINDICATIONS

Albutein® 25% is contraindicated in patients with severe anemia or cardiac failure in the presence of normal or increased intravascular volume.

The use of Albutein® 25% is contraindicated in patients with a history of allergic reactions to albumin.

5. WARNINGS AND PRECAUTIONS

5.1 Warnings

Following reports that there exists a risk of potentially fatal hemolysis and acute renal failure from the inappropriate use of Sterile Water for Injection as a diluent for Albumin (Human)[7], if dilution is required, acceptable diluents include 0.9% Sodium Chloride or 5% Dextrose in Water.[6]

Albutein® 25% is made from pooled human plasma. Based on effective donor screening and product manufacturing processes, it carries an extremely remote risk for transmission of viral diseases, including a theoretical risk for transmission of Creutzfeldt-Jakob disease (CJD). Although no cases of transmission of viral diseases or CJD have ever been identified for albumin, the risk of infectious agents cannot be totally eliminated. The physician should weigh the risks and benefits of the use of this product and should discuss these with the patient.

Solutions of Albutein® 25% should not be used if they appear turbid or if there is sediment in the bottle. Do not begin administration more than 4 hours after the container has been entered. Discard unused portion.

5.2 Precautions

Albutein® 25% should be administered with caution to patients with low cardiac reserve.

Rapid infusion may cause vascular overload with resultant pulmonary edema. Patients should be closely monitored for signs of increased venous pressure.

A rapid rise in blood pressure following infusion necessitates careful observation of injured or postoperative patients to detect and treat severed blood vessels that may not have bled at a lower pressure.

Patients with marked dehydration require administration of additional fluids. Albutein® 25% may be administered with the usual dextrose and saline intravenous solutions. However, certain solutions containing protein hydrolysates or alcohol must not be infused through the same administration set in conjunction with Albutein® 25% since these combinations may cause the proteins to precipitate. See also PATIENT COUNSELING INFORMATION (17).

6. ADVERSE REACTIONS

The most common adverse reactions include fever and chills, rash, nausea, vomiting, tachycardia and hypotension. Should an adverse reaction occur, slow or stop the infusion for a short period of time which may result in the disappearance of the symptoms. If administration has been stopped and the patient requires additional Albutein® 25%, material from a different lot should be used. Albutein® 25%, particularly if administered rapidly, may result in vascular overload with resultant pulmonary edema.

To report SUSPECTED ADVERSE REACTIONS, contact Grifols Biologicals Inc. at 1-888-GRIFOLS (1-888-474-3657) or FDA at 1-800-FDA-1088 or www.fda.gov/medwatch.

8. USE IN SPECIFIC POPULATIONS

8.1 Pregnancy

Pregnancy Category C. Animal reproduction studies have not been conducted with Albutein® 25%. It is also not known whether Albutein® 25% can cause fetal harm when administered to a pregnant woman or can affect reproductive capacity. Albutein® 25% should be given to a pregnant woman only if clearly needed.

8.4 Pediatric Use

Albutein® 25% is indicated in conjunction with exchange transfusion in the treatment of neonatal hyperbilirubinemia. The pediatric use of Albutein® 25% has not been clinically evaluated. The dosage will vary with the clinical state and body weight of the individual. Typically, a dose one-quarter to one-half the adult dose may be administered, or dosage may be calculated on the basis of 0.6 to 1.0 gram per kilogram of body weight (2.4 to 4 mL of Albutein® 25%). For jaundiced infants suffering from hemolytic disease of the newborn, the appropriate dose for binding of free serum bilirubin is 1 gram per kilogram of body weight which may be administered during the procedure.[8] The usual rate of administration in children should be one-quarter the adult rate. Therefore, physicians should weigh the risks and benefits of the use of Albutein® 25% in the pediatric population. Parenteral drug products should be inspected visually for particulate matter and discoloration prior to administration, whenever solution and container permit.

11. DESCRIPTION

Albutein® 25% is a sterile, aqueous solution for single dose intravenous administration containing 25% human albumin (weight/volume). Albutein® 25% is prepared by a cold alcohol fractionation method from pooled human plasma obtained from venous blood. The product is stabilized with 0.08 millimole sodium caprylate and 0.08 millimole sodium acetyltryptophanate per gram of albumin. Albutein® 25% is osmotically equivalent to five times its volume of normal human plasma. Albutein® 25% contains 130-160 milliequivalents of sodium ion per liter and has a pH of 7.0 ± 0.3. The aluminum content of the solution is not more than 200 micrograms per liter during the shelf life of the product. The product contains no preservatives.

Albutein® 25% is heated at 60 °C for ten hours. No positive assertion can be made, however, that this heat treatment completely destroys the causative agents of viral hepatitis.

12. CLINICAL PHARMACOLOGY

12.1 Mechanism of Action

There are no known cases of viral hepatitis which have resulted from the administration of Albutein® 25%. Albumin is a highly soluble, globular protein (MW 66,500), accounting for 70-80% of the colloid osmotic pressure of plasma. Therefore, it is important in regulating the osmotic pressure of plasma.[1,3] Albutein® 25% supplies the oncotic equivalent of approximately 5 times its volume of human plasma. It will increase the circulating plasma volume by an amount approximately 3.5 times the volume infused within 15 minutes, if the recipient is adequately hydrated.[9] This extra fluid reduces hemoconcentration and decreases blood viscosity. The degree and duration of volume expansion depend upon the initial blood volume. When treating patients with diminished blood volume, the effect of infused albumin may persist for many hours. The hemodilution lasts for a shorter time when albumin is administered to individuals with normal blood volume.

Albumin is also a transport protein and binds naturally occurring, therapeutic, and toxic materials in the circulation.[1] Albumin is distributed throughout the extracellular water and more than 60% of the body albumin pool is located in the extravascular fluid compartment. The total body albumin in a 70 kg man is approximately 320 g. Albumin has a circulating life span of 15-20 days, with a turnover of approximately 15 g per day.[3]

15. REFERENCES

1. Finlayson, J.S., Albumin Products, *Semin Thromb Hemo*, 6:85-120, 1980.
2. Hauser, C.J., et. al., Oxygen Transport Responses to Colloids and Crystalloids in Critically Ill Surgical Patients, *Surg Gyn Obs*, 150:811-816, June 1980.
3. Tullis, J.L., Albumin: 1. Background and Use, 2. Guidelines for Clinical Use, *JAMA*, 237:355-360, 460-463, 1977.
4. Shoemaker, W.C., et. al., Comparison of the Relative Effectiveness of Colloids and Crystalloids in Emergency Resuscitation, *Am J Surg*, 142:73-84, July 1981.
5. Peters, T., Jr., Serum Albumin in: *The Plasma Proteins*, 2nd Ed., Putnam F.W. (ed), New York, Academic Press, 1:133-181, 1975.
6. Albumin Human. In AHFS Drug Information, 1144-1146, 1998.
7. Data on File, FDA.
8. Tsao, Y.C., Yu, V.Y.H., Albumin in the Management of Neonatal Hyperbilirubinemia, *Arch Dis Childhood*, 47: 250-256, 1972.
9. Janeway, C.A., Human Serum Albumin: Historical Review in *Proceedings of the Workshop on Albumin*, Sgouris, J.T. and Rene A. (eds), DHEW Publication No. (NIH) 76-925, Washington, D.C., U.S. Government Printing Office, 1976, pp. 3-21.

16. HOW SUPPLIED/STORAGE AND HANDLING

Albutein® 25% is supplied as a sterile, aqueous solution for single dose intravenous administration containing 25% human albumin (weight/volume). It is available in the following vial sizes:

- 50 mL vial Albutein® 25%
  (NDC 68516-5216-1).
- 100 mL vial Albutein® 25%
  (NDC 68516-5216-2).

Storage

Albutein® 25% is stable for three years provided that storage temperature does not exceed 30 °C. Protect from freezing.

17. PATIENT COUNSELING INFORMATION

The most common adverse reactions include fever and chills, rash, nausea, vomiting, tachycardia and hypotension. Depending on the severity of the reaction, patients should be advised to discontinue use of the product and contact their physician and/or seek immediate emergency care.

Albutein® 25% should be administered with caution to patients with low cardiac reserve.

Rapid infusion may cause vascular overload with resultant pulmonary edema. Patients should be closely monitored for signs of increased venous pressure.

A rapid rise in blood pressure following infusion necessitates careful observation of injured or postoperative patients to detect and treat severed blood vessels that may not have bled at a lower pressure.

Patients with marked dehydration require administration of additional fluids. Albutein® 25% may be administered with the usual dextrose and saline intravenous solutions. However, solutions containing protein hydrolysates or alcohol must not be infused through the same administration set in conjunction with Albutein® 25% since these combinations may cause the proteins to precipitate. See also WARNINGS AND PRECAUTIONS (5.2).

Manufactured and Distributed by:
Grifols Biologicals Inc.
Los Angeles, CA 90032, U.S.A.
U.S. License No. 1694
DATE OF REVISION: 07/2008

ALPHANATE®   ℞
[al-fan-ate]
(Antihemophilic Factor/von WillebrandFactor Complex [Human])
sterile, lyophilized powder for injection

HIGHLIGHTS OF PRESCRIBING INFORMATION

These highlights do not include all the information needed to use Alphanate® safely and effectively. See full prescribing information for Alphanate®.

ALPHANATE® (ANTIHEMOPHILIC FACTOR/VON WILLEBRAND FACTOR COMPLEX [HUMAN]) sterile, lyophilized powder for injection

Initial U.S. Approval: 1978

—————RECENT MAJOR CHANGES—————
von Willebrand Disease (for surgical and/or invasive procedures) (1.2) 03/2010

—————INDICATIONS AND USAGE—————
Alphanate® is an Antihemophilic Factor/von Willebrand Factor Complex (Human) indicated for:
- the prevention and control of bleeding in patients with Factor VIII deficiency due to Hemophilia A or acquired Factor VIII deficiency (1.1)
- for surgical and/or invasive procedures in patients with von Willebrand Disease in whom desmopressin (DDAVP) is either ineffective or contraindicated. It is not indicated for patients with severe VWD (Type 3) undergoing major surgery (1.2)

—————DOSAGE AND ADMINISTRATION—————
Antihemophilic factor potency (Factor VIII:C activity) is expressed in International Units (IU) on the product label. Additionally, each vial of Alphanate® also contains VWF:RCo activity in IU for the treatment of VWD (2).
Hemophilia A (2.1)
- As a general rule, dosing requirements and frequency of dosing is calculated on the basis of an expected initial response of 2% of normal FVIII:C increase per FVIII:C IU/kg body weight administered.

von Willebrand Disease (2.2)
- Adults: 40-60 VWF:RCo IU/kg body weight
- Pediatric: 50-75 VWF:RCo IU/kg body weight

—————DOSAGE FORMS AND STRENGTHS—————
- Alphanate® is a sterile, lyophilized powder for injection, provided in the following potencies: (3)
- 250 IU FVIII/5 mL single dose vial
- 500 IU FVIII/5 mL single dose vial
- 1000 IU FVIII/10 mL single dose vial
- 1500 IU FVIII/10 mL single dose vial

—————CONTRAINDICATIONS—————
- None known (4)

—————WARNINGS AND PRECAUTIONS—————
- Thromboembolic events associated with AHF/VWF products (5.1)
- Theoretical risk of infectious agents transmission as the product is made from human plasma (5.2)
- Factor VIII antibodies (inhibitors) and alloantibodies to VWF (5.3)
- Symptoms and signs of hypersensitivity reaction (5.4)

—————ADVERSE REACTIONS—————
The most common adverse reactions include: urticaria, fever, chills, nausea, vomiting, headache, somnolence, or lethargy (6.1).

To report SUSPECTED ADVERSE REACTIONS, contact Grifols Biologicals at 1-888-GRIFOLS (1-888-474-3657) or FDA at 1-800-FDA-1088 or www.fda.gov/medwatch.

—————DRUG INTERACTIONS—————
- None known (7)

—————USE IN SPECIFIC POPULATIONS—————
- Unknown whether can cause fetal harm or affect reproduction capacity (8.1)
- Clinical trials for safety and effectiveness in pediatric Hemophilia A patients have not been conducted (8.4)

See 17 for PATIENT COUNSELING INFORMATION
Revised: 03/2010

FULL PRESCRIBING INFORMATION: CONTENTS*

FULL PRESCRIBING INFORMATION

1.   INDICATIONS AND USAGE
1.1   Hemophilia A or Acquired Factor VIII Deficiency
Antihemophilic Factor/von Willebrand Factor Complex (Human), Alphanate®, is indicated for the prevention and control of bleeding in patients with Factor VIII deficiency due to hemophilia A or acquired Factor VIII deficiency.[1]
1.2   von Willebrand Disease
Antihemophilic Factor/von Willebrand Factor Complex (Human), Alphanate®, is also indicated for surgical and/or invasive procedures in patients with von Willebrand Disease (VWD) in whom desmopressin (DDAVP®) is either ineffective or contraindicated. It is not indicated for patients with severe VWD (Type 3) undergoing major surgery.

2.   DOSAGE AND ADMINISTRATION
Following reconstitution with the supplied diluent, Alphanate® should be administered intravenously within three hours after reconstitution to avoid the potential ill effect of any inadvertent bacterial contamination occurring during reconstitution. Alphanate® is administered by injection (plastic disposable syringes are recommended). Administer at room temperature, do not refrigerate after reconstitution, and discard any unused contents into the appropriate safety container.
Antihemophilic Factor (AHF) potency (Factor VIII:C activity) is expressed in International Units (IU) on the product label. Each vial of Alphanate® also contains von Willebrand Factor:Ristocetin Cofactor (VWF:RCo) activity in IU for the treatment of VWD.
2.1   Hemophilia A
Dosing requirements and frequency of dosing is calculated on the basis of an expected initial response of 2% of normal FVIII:C increase per FVIII:C IU/kg body weight administered.[2,3] The *in vivo* increase in plasma Factor VIII can therefore be estimated by multiplying the dose of AHF per kilogram of body weight (FVIII:C IU/kg) by 2%. Thus, an administered AHF dose of 50 IU/kg will be expected to increase the circulating Factor VIII level by 100% of normal (100 IU/dL). The following formulas and examples illustrate these principles:
[See first table above]
The following dosages are presented as general guidance. It should be emphasized that the dosage of Alphanate® required for hemostasis must be individualized according to the needs of the patient, the severity of the deficiency, the severity of the hemorrhage, the presence of inhibitors, and the FVIII level desired. Adequacy of treatment must be judged by the clinical effects and situation and thus, the dosage may vary with individual cases.
[See table 1 above]
Dosing requirements and frequency of dosing is calculated on the basis of an expected initial response of 2% FVIII:C increase per FVIII:C IU/kg body weight (i.e., 2% per IU/kg)

a) Expected plasma Factor VIII:C increase (% normal) = $\dfrac{\text{Number of FVIII:C IU administered} \times 2\%/\text{IU/kg}}{\text{body weight (kg)}}$

  Example: A 70 kg adult administered AHF 2100 IU:
  Plasma FVIII:C increase (% normal) = $\dfrac{2100\ \text{IU} \times 2\%/\text{IU/kg}}{70\ \text{kg}}$ = 60% normal plasma FVIII:C level

b) Dosage required (IU) = $\dfrac{\text{desired plasma Factor VIII increase (\% normal)} \times \text{body weight (kg)}}{2\%/\text{IU/kg}}$

  Example: A 15 kg child with a baseline plasma FVIII level of 0%. To increase the plasma Factor VIII concentration to 100% of normal, the dosage required is as follows:
  Dosage required (IU) = $\dfrac{100\%}{2\%/\text{IU/kg}} \times 15\ \text{kg}$ = 50 IU/kg × 15 kg = 750 IU

Table 1: Dosage Guidelines for the Treatment of Hemophilia A

Hemorrhagic event	Dosage (AHF FVIII:C IU/kg Body Weight)
Minor hemorrhage: • Bruises • Cuts or scrapes • Uncomplicated joint hemorrhage	FVIII:C levels should be brought to 30% of normal (15 FVIII IU/kg twice daily) until hemorrhage stops and healing has been achieved (1-2 days).
Moderate hemorrhage: • Nose, mouth and gum bleeds • Dental extractions • Hematuria	FVIII:C levels should be brought to 50% (25 FVIII IU/kg twice daily). Treatment should continue until healing has been achieved (2-7 days, on average).
Major hemorrhage: • Joint hemorrhage • Muscle hemorrhage • Major trauma • Hematuria • Intracranial and intraperitoneal bleeding	FVIII:C levels should be brought to 80-100% for at least 3-5 days (40-50 FVIII IU/kg twice daily). Following this treatment period, FVIII levels should be maintained at 50% (25 FVIII IU/kg twice daily) until healing has been achieved. Major hemorrhages may require treatment for up to 10 days.
Surgery	Prior to surgery, the levels of FVIII:C should be brought to 80-100% of normal (40-50 FVIII IU/kg). For the next 7-10 days, or until healing has been achieved, the patient should be maintained at 60-100% FVIII levels (25-50 FVIII IU/kg twice daily).

Table 2: Dosage Guidelines for the Prophylaxis During Surgery and Invasive Procedure of von Willebrand Disease (Except Type 3 Subjects Undergoing Major Surgery)

Bleeding Prophylaxis for Surgical or Invasive Procedures	Dosage (AHF VWF:RCo IU/kg Body Weight)
Adult	Pre-operative dosage: 60 VWF:RCo IU/kg body weight. Subsequent infusions: 40 to 60 VWF:RCo IU/kg body weight at 8 to 12 hour intervals as clinically needed. Dosing may be reduced after the third postoperative day. Continue treatment until healing is complete.
	Minor procedure: VWF activity of 40%-50% during 1 to 3 days postoperative.
	Major procedure: VWF activity of 40%-50% during at least 3 to 7 days postoperative.
Pediatric	Initial dosage: 75 VWF:RCo IU/kg body weight. Subsequent infusions: 50 to 75 VWF:RCo IU/kg body weight at 8 to 12 hour intervals as clinically needed. Dosing may be reduced after the third postoperative day. Continue treatment until healing is complete.

and an average half-life for FVIII:C of 12 hours.[4,5] If dosing studies have determined that a particular patient exhibits a lower than expected response, the dose should be adjusted accordingly. Failure to achieve the expected plasma FVIII:C level or to control bleeding after an appropriately calculated dosage may be indicative of the development of an inhibitor (an antibody to FVIII:C). Its presence should be documented and the inhibitor level quantitated by appropriate laboratory procedures. Treatment with AHF in such cases must be individualized.[6-8]
Plasma factor VIII levels should be monitored periodically to evaluate individual patient response to the dosage regime.
2.2   von Willebrand Disease
The following table provides dosing guidelines for pediatric and adult patients with von Willebrand Disease.[9-12]
The amount of VWF:RCo and Factor VIII contained in each vial of Alphanate® is indicated on the vial's label. The ratio of VWF:RCo to Factor VIII in Alphanate® varies by lot, so dosage should be re-evaluated whenever lot selection is changed.
[See table 2 above]
2.3   Reconstitution
Always Use Aseptic Technique
1. Warm diluent (Sterile Water for Injection, USP) and concentrate (Alphanate®) to at least room temperature (but not above 37 °C).

2. Remove the plastic flip off cap from the diluent vial.
3. Gently swab the exposed stopper surface with a cleansing agent such as alcohol trying to avoid leaving any excess cleansing agent on the stopper.
4. Open the Mix2Vial™ package by peeling away the lid (Figure 1). Leave the Mix2Vial™ in the clear outer packaging.
5. Place the diluent vial upright on an even surface and hold the vial tight and pick up the Mix2Vial™ in its clear outer packaging. Holding the diluent vial securely, push the **blue** end of the Mix2Vial™ vertically down through the diluent vial stopper (Figure 2).
6. While holding onto the diluent vial, carefully remove the clear outer packaging from the Mix2Vial™ set, ensuring the Mix2Vial™ remains attached to the diluent vial (Figure 3).
7. Place the product vial upright on an even surface, invert the diluent vial with the Mix2Vial™ attached.
8. While holding the product vial securely on a flat surface, push the **clear** end of the Mix2Vial™ set **vertically** down through the product vial stopper (Figure 4). The diluent will automatically transfer out of its vial into the product vial. (NOTE: If the Mix2Vial™ is connected at an angle, the vacuum may be released from the product vial and the diluent will not transfer into the product vial.)
9. With the diluent and product vials still attached to the Mix2Vial™, gently swirl the product vial to ensure the

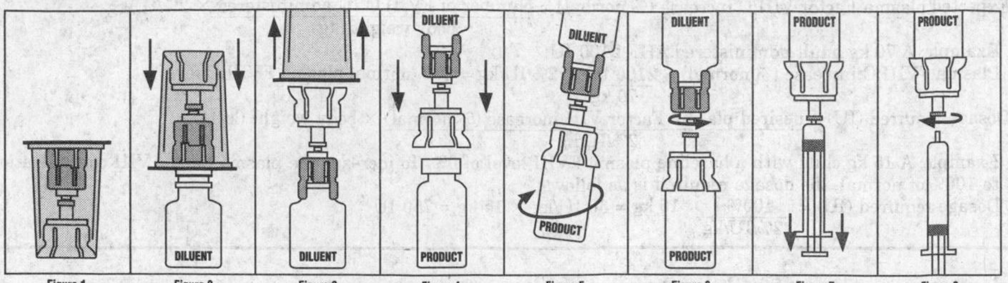

Figure 1 Figure 2 Figure 3 Figure 4 Figure 5 Figure 6 Figure 7 Figure 8

product is fully dissolved (Figure 5). Reconstitution requires less than 5 minutes. Do not shake the vial.

10. Disconnect the Mix2Vial™ into two separate pieces (Figure 6) by holding each vial adapter and twisting counterclockwise. After separating, discard the diluent vial with the **blue** end of the Mix2Vial™.
11. Draw air into an empty, sterile syringe. Keeping the product vial upright with the **clear** end of the Mix2Vial™ attached, screw the disposable syringe onto the luer lock portion of the Mix2Vial™ device by pressing and twisting clockwise. Inject air into the product vial.
12. While keeping the syringe plunger depressed, invert the system upside down and draw the reconstituted product into the syringe by pulling the plunger back slowly (Figure 7).
13. When the reconstituted product has been transferred into the syringe, firmly hold the barrel of the syringe and the clear vial adapter (keeping the syringe plunger facing down) and unscrew the syringe from the Mix2Vial™ (Figure 8). Hold the syringe upright and push the plunger until no air is left in the syringe. Attach the syringe to a venipuncture set.
14. NOTE: If the same patient is to receive more than one vial of concentrate, the contents of two vials may be drawn into the same syringe through a separate unused Mix2Vial™ set before attaching to the venipuncture set.
15. Use prepared drug as soon as possible after reconstitution.
16. After reconstitution, parenteral drug products should be inspected visually for particulate matter and discoloration prior to administration, whenever solution and container permit. When reconstitution procedure is strictly followed, a few small particles may occasionally remain. The Mix2Vial™ set will remove particles and the labeled potency will not be reduced.
17. Discard all administration equipment after use into the appropriate safety container. Do not reuse.

[See figure above]

3. DOSAGE FORMS AND STRENGTHS

Alphanate® is a sterile, lyophilized powder for injection. It is available in the following potencies:

- 250 IU FVIII/5 mL single dose vial
- 500 IU FVIII/5 mL single dose vial
- 1000 IU FVIII/10 mL single dose vial
- 1500 IU FVIII/10 mL single dose vial

4. CONTRAINDICATIONS

None.

5. WARNINGS AND PRECAUTIONS

5.1 Thromboembolic Events

Thromboembolic events have been reported in von Willebrand Disease patients receiving Antihemophilic Factor/von Willebrand Factor Complex replacement therapy, especially in the setting of known risk factors for thrombosis.[13,14] Early reports might indicate a higher incidence in females. In addition, endogenous high levels of FVIII have also been associated with thrombosis but no causal relationship has been established. In all VWD patients in situations of high thrombotic risk receiving coagulation factor replacement therapy, caution should be exercised and antithrombotic measures should be considered. See also **ADVERSE REACTIONS (6.1) and PATIENT COUNSELING INFORMATION (17.1).**

5.2 Infections

Because Antihemophilic Factor/von Willebrand Factor Complex (Human), Alphanate® is made from pooled human plasma, it may carry a risk of transmitting infectious agents, e.g., viruses, and theoretically, the Creutzfeldt-Jakob disease (CJD) agent. Stringent procedures designed to reduce the risk of adventitious agent transmission have been employed in the manufacture of this product, from the screening of plasma donors and the collection and testing of plasma, through the application of viral elimination/reduction steps such as solvent detergent and heat treatment in the manufacturing process. Despite these measures, such products can still potentially transmit disease; therefore, the risk of infectious agents cannot be totally eliminated. The physician should weigh the risks and benefits of the use of this product and should discuss these with the patient. See also **PATIENT COUNSELING INFORMATION (17.2).**

Individuals who receive infusions of blood or plasma products may develop signs and/or symptoms of some viral infections, particularly hepatitis C.[15,16] Incubation in a solvent detergent mixture during the manufacturing process is designed to reduce the risk of transmitting viral infection.[15,16] However, medical opinion encourages hepatitis A and hepatitis B vaccinations for patients with hemophilia at birth or at the time of diagnosis.

Nursing personnel, and others who administer this material, should exercise appropriate caution when handling due to the risk of exposure to viral infection.

5.3 Inhibitor Formation

Rapid administration of a Factor VIII concentrate may result in vasomotor reactions. Alphanate® should not be administered at a rate exceeding 10 mL/minute.

Some patients develop inhibitors to Factor VIII. These inhibitors are circulating antibodies (i.e., globulins) that neutralize the procoagulant activity of Factor VIII. No studies have been conducted with Alphanate® to evaluate inhibitor formation. Therefore, it is not known whether there are greater, lesser or the same risks of developing inhibitors due to the use of this product than there are with other antihemophilic factor preparations. Patients with these inhibitors may not respond to treatment with Antihemophilic Factor/von Willebrand Factor Complex (Human), or the response may be much less than would otherwise be expected; therefore, larger doses of Antihemophilic Factor/von Willebrand Factor Complex (Human) are often required. The management of bleeding in patients with inhibitors requires careful monitoring, especially if surgical procedures are indicated.[6-8] See also **PATIENT COUNSELING INFORMATION (17.3).**

Reports in the literature suggest that patients with Type 3, severe von Willebrand Disease, may occasionally develop alloantibodies to von Willebrand factor after replacement therapy.[17] The risk of developing alloantibodies in patients with von Willebrand disease due to the use of this product is not known.

Unused contents should be discarded into the appropriate safety container. Administration equipment should be discarded after single use into the appropriate safety container. Components should not be re-sterilized.

5.4 Information for Patients

Patients should be informed of the early symptoms and signs of hypersensitivity reaction, including hives, generalized urticaria, chest tightness, dyspnea, wheezing, faintness, hypotension, and anaphylaxis. Patients should be advised to discontinue use of the product and contact their physician and/or seek immediate emergency care, depending on the severity of the reaction, if these symptoms occur.

Patients should be informed of a potential for viral infection such as parvovirus B19 or hepatitis A. Parvovirus B19 may most seriously affect seronegative pregnant women, or immunocompromised individuals. Patients should report any signs and symptoms of fever, sore throat, or joint soreness to the physician immediately.

6. ADVERSE REACTIONS

6.1 General

The most common adverse reactions may include urticaria, fever, chills, nausea, vomiting, headache, somnolence, or lethargy.

Occasionally, mild reactions occur following the administration of Antihemophilic Factor/von Willebrand Factor Complex (Human), such as allergic reactions, chills, nausea, or stinging at the infusion site.[4] If a reaction is experienced, and the patient requires additional Antihemophilic Factor/von Willebrand Factor Complex (Human), product from a different lot should be administered.

Massive doses of Antihemophilic Factor/von Willebrand Factor Complex (Human) have rarely resulted in acute hemolytic anemia, increased bleeding tendency or hyperfibrinogenemia.[5] Alphanate® contains blood group specific isoagglutinins and, when large and/or frequent doses are required in patients of blood groups A, B, or AB, the patient should be monitored for signs of intravascular hemolysis and falling hematocrit. Should this condition occur, thus leading to progressive hemolytic anemia, the administration of serologically compatible Type O red blood cells should be considered, the administration of Alphanate® should be discontinued, and alternative therapy should be considered.

Reports of thromboembolic events in VWD patients with other thrombotic risk factors receiving coagulation factor replacement therapy have been obtained from published literature. Early reports might indicate a higher incidence in females. Caution should be exercised and antithrombotic measures should be considered in all VWD patients in situations of high thrombotic risk. See **WARNINGS AND PRECAUTIONS (5.1).**

6.2 Adverse Reactions in VWD Patients from Clinical Studies

In clinical studies of Alphanate® (A-SD/HT) in patients with VWD, adverse reactions occurred in 6 of 38 (15.8%) subjects and 17 of 299 (5.7%) infusions. The most common adverse events were pruritus, pharyngitis (throat tightness), paresthesia and headache, edema of the face, rash and chills. Except for one instance of pruritus, which was considered moderate in severity, all the adverse events were assessed as mild in severity.

A single incident of pulmonary embolus was reported that was considered to have a possible relationship to the product. This subject received the dose of 60 VWF:RCo IU/kg body weight and the FVIII:C level achieved was 290%.

In the retrospective study, 3 out of 39 subjects (7.7%) experienced 6 adverse drug reactions. Four were considered mild and 2 were considered moderate; and no subject discontinued their treatment due to an adverse reaction. The adverse drug reactions were pruritus, paresthesia (2 events) and hemorrhage (all considered mild), and one event each of moderate hematocrit decrease and orthostatic hypotension.

Only one adverse event (pain) related to the treatment with heat-treated Alphanate® (A-SD/HT) was reported on the four pediatric patients with von Willebrand Disease during the course of the prospective study and none of the five subjects in the retrospective clinical study.[18]

6.3 Adverse Reaction Information from Spontaneous Reports

The following adverse reactions have been identified during post-approval use of Alphanate® (A-SD/HT). Because these reactions are reported voluntarily from a population of uncertain size, it is not always possible to reliably estimate their frequency or establish a causal relationship to drug exposure.

These adverse reactions have been reported as swelling of the parotid gland, urticaria, nausea, shortness of breath, chest tightness, chills, fever, rigors, headache, flushing, vomiting, joint pain, seizure, pulmonary embolus, femoral venous thrombosis, itching and cardiorespiratory arrest.

To report SUSPECTED ADVERSE REACTIONS, contact Grifols Biologicals Inc. at 1-888-GRIFOLS (1-888-474-3657) or FDA at 1-800-FDA-1088 or www.fda.gov/medwatch.

7. DRUG INTERACTIONS

None known.

8. USE IN SPECIFIC POPULATIONS

8.1 Pregnancy

Pregnancy Category C. Animal reproduction studies have not been conducted with Alphanate®. It is also not known whether Alphanate® can cause fetal harm when administered to a pregnant woman or affect reproductive capacity. Alphanate® should be given to a pregnant woman only if clearly needed.

8.4 Pediatric Use

8.4.1 Hemophilia A Indication

Clinical trials for safety and effectiveness in pediatric Hemophilia A patients 16 years of age and younger have not been conducted. During a well controlled half-life and recovery clinical trial in patients previously treated with Factor VIII concentrates for Hemophilia A, the single pediatric patient receiving Alphanate® (solvent detergent non-heat treated) responded similarly when compared with 12 adult patients.[4] No adverse events were reported in either pediatric or adult patients with Alphanate®.

8.4.2 VWD Indication

Fifteen pediatric patients with von Willebrand Disease younger than 18 years of age were treated with non-heat (A-SD) and heat-treated (A-SD/HT) Alphanate® during the course of clinical studies.[18] In the retrospective study, five patients younger than 18 years of age were treated with heat-treated (A-SD/HT) Alphanate®.

11. DESCRIPTION

Antihemophilic Factor/von Willebrand Factor Complex (Human), Alphanate® sterile, lyophilized concentrate of Factor VIII (AHF) and von Willebrand Factor (VWF), is intended for intravenous administration in the treatment of hemophilia A, acquired Factor VIII deficiency, and von Willebrand Disease (VWD).

Alphanate® is prepared from pooled human plasma by cryoprecipitation of Factor VIII, fractional solubilization, and further purification employing heparin-coupled, cross-linked agarose which has an affinity to the heparin binding domain of VWF/FVIII:C complex.[19] The product is treated with a mixture of tri-n-butyl phosphate (TNBP) and polysorbate 80 to reduce the risks of transmission of viral infection. In order to provide an additional safeguard against potential non-lipid enveloped viral contaminants, the product is also subjected to an 80 °C heat treatment step for 72 hours. However, no procedure has been shown to be totally effective in removing viral infectivity from coagulation factor products.

Alphanate® is labeled with the antihemophilic factor potency (Factor VIII:C activity) in International Units (IU) per vial. Each vial of Alphanate® also contains the labeled amount of von Willebrand Factor:Ristocetin Cofactor (VWF:RCo) activity expressed in IU. An IU is defined by the current international standard established by the World Health Organization. One IU of Factor VIII or one IU of VWF:RCo is approximately equal to the amount of Factor VIII or VWF:RCo in 1 mL of freshly-pooled human plasma. Alphanate® contains Albumin (Human) as a stabilizer, resulting in a final container concentrate with a specific activity of at least 5 FVIII:C IU/mg total protein. Prior to the addition of the Albumin (Human) stabilizer, the specific activity is significantly higher.

When reconstituted as directed, the composition of Alphanate® is as follows:

Component	Concentration
Factor VIII:C activity	40-180 IU/mL
VWF:RCo activity	NLT 0.4 VWF:RCo IU per 1 IU of FVIII:C
Albumin (Human)	0.3-0.9 g/100 mL
Calcium	NMT 5 mmol/L
Glycine	NMT 750 µg per FVIII:C IU
Heparin	NMT 1.0 U/mL
Histidine	10-40 mmol/L
Imidazole	NMT 0.1 mg/mL
Arginine	50-200 mmol/L
Polyethylene Glycol and Polysorbate 80	NMT 1.0 µg per FVIII:C IU
Sodium	NLT 10 mEq/vial
Tri-n-butyl Phosphate (TNBP)	NMT 0.1 µg per FVIII:C IU

NMT = not more than
NLT = not less than

Viral Reduction Capacity

The solvent detergent treatment process has been shown by Horowitz, et al., to provide a high level of viral inactivation without compromising protein structure and function.[20] The susceptibility of human pathogenic viruses such as Human Immunodeficiency viruses (HIV), hepatitis viruses, as well as marker viruses such as Sindbis virus (SIN, a model for Hepatitis C virus) and Vesicular Stomatitis virus (VSV, a model for large, enveloped RNA virus), to inactivation by organic solvent detergent treatment has been discussed in the literature.[21]

In vitro inactivation studies to evaluate the solvent detergent treatment (0.3% Tri-n-butyl Phosphate and 1.0% Polysorbate 80) step in the manufacture of Alphanate® demonstrated a log inactivation of ≥ 11.1 for HIV-1, ≥ 6.1 for HIV-2, ≥ 4.1 for VSV and ≥ 4.7 for SIN. Since the number of virus particles inactivated by the process represents the maximum amount of virus added initially to the sample, these results indicate that all the virus added was killed to the assay limit of detection.[18]

Additional steps in the manufacturing process of Alphanate® were evaluated for virus elimination capability. The dry heat cycle of 80 °C for 72 hours was shown to inactivate greater than 5.8 logs of Hepatitis A virus (HAV).[18] Precipitation with 3.5% polyethylene glycol (PEG) and heparin-actigel-ALD chromatography are additional steps studied using Bovine Herpes virus (BHV, a model for Hepatitis B virus), Bovine Viral Diarrhea virus (BVD, a second model for Hepatitis C virus), human Poliovirus Sabin type 2 (POL, a model for Hepatitis A virus), Canine Parvovirus (CPV, a model for Parvovirus B19) and HIV-1.

Table 3 summarizes the reduction factors for each virus validation study performed for the manufacturing process of Alphanate®.[18] It must be stated that no treatment method has yet been shown capable of totally eliminating all potential infectious virus in preparations of coagulation factor concentrates.

[See table 3 above]

12. CLINICAL PHARMACOLOGY
12.1 Mechanism of Action
Antihemophilic Factor/von Willebrand Factor Complex (Human) (Factor VIII) and von Willebrand Factor (VWF) are constituents of normal plasma and are required for clot-

Table 3: Virus Log Reduction

Virus (Model Virus for)	3.5% PEG Precipitation	Solvent–Detergent	Column Chromatography	Lyophilization	Dry Heat Cycle (80 °C, 72 h)	Total Log Removal
BHV (HBV)	< 1.0	≥ 8.0	7.6	1.3	2.1	≥ 19.0
BVD (HCV)	< 1.0	≥ 4.5	< 1.0	< 1.0	≥ 4.9	≥ 9.4
POL (HAV)	3.3	—	< 1.0	3.4	≥ 2.5	≥ 9.2
CPV (B19)	1.2	—	< 1.0	< 1.0	4.1	5.3
VSV	—	≥ 4.1	—	—	—	≥ 4.1
SIN (HCV)	—	≥ 4.7	—	—	—	≥ 4.7
HIV-1	< 1.0	≥ 11.1	≥ 2.0	—	—	≥ 13.1
HIV-2	—	≥ 6.1	—	—	—	≥ 6.1
HAV	—	—	—	2.1	≥ 5.8	≥ 7.9

ting. The administration of Alphanate® temporarily increases the plasma level of Factor VIII, thus minimizing the hazard of hemorrhage.[22,23] Factor VIII is an essential cofactor in activation of Factor X leading to formation of thrombin and fibrin. VWF promotes platelet aggregation and platelet adhesion on damaged vascular endothelium; it also serves as a stabilizing carrier protein for the procoagulant protein Factor VIII.[24,25]

12.3 Pharmacokinetics
12.3.1 Pharmacokinetics in Hemophilia A
Following the administration of Alphanate® during clinical trials, the mean *in vivo* half-life of Factor VIII observed in 12 adult subjects with severe hemophilia A was 17.9 ± 9.6 hours. In this same study, the *in vivo* recovery was 96.7 ± 14.5% at 10 minutes postinfusion.[18] Recovery at 10 minutes post-infusion was also determined as 2.4 ± 0.4 IU FVIII rise/dL plasma per IU FVIII infused/kg body weight.[18]

12.3.2 Pharmacokinetics in von Willebrand Disease (VWD)
A pharmacokinetic crossover study was conducted in 14 non-bleeding subjects with VWD (1 type 1, 2 type 2A, and 11 type 3) comparing the pharmacokinetics of Alphanate® SD/HT (A-SD/HT) and an earlier formulation, Alphanate® SD (A-SD), which was treated with solvent-detergent but was not heat-treated.[18] Subjects received, in random order at least seven days apart, a single intravenous dose each of A-SD and A-SD/HT, 60 VWF:RCo IU/kg (75 VWF:RCo IU/kg in subjects younger than 18 years of age). Pharmacokinetic parameters were similar for the two preparations and indicated that they were biochemically equivalent. Pharmacokinetic analysis of A-SD/HT in the 14 subjects revealed the following results[18]: the median plasma levels of VWF:RCo rose from 0.17 IU/dL [mean, 0.2 ± 0.08 IU/dL; range: 0.1 to 0.5 IU/dL] at baseline to 3.43 IU/dL [mean, 3.5 ± 1.47 IU/dL; range: 1.5 to 5.9 IU/dL] 15 minutes post-infusion; median plasma levels of FVIII:C rose from 0.08 IU/dL [mean, 0.2 ± 0.34 IU/dL; range: 0.0 to 1.2 IU/dL] to 2.14 IU/dL [mean, 2.4 ± 0.72 IU/dL; range: 1.4 to 3.9 IU/dL]. The median bleeding time (BT) prior to infusion was 30 minutes (mean, 28.8 ± 4.41 minutes; range: 13.5 to 30 minutes), which shortened to 10.38 minutes (mean, 10.4 ± 3.20 minutes; range: 6 to 16 minutes) 1 hour post-infusion.

Following infusion of A-SD/HT, the median half-lives for VWF:RCo, FVIII:C and VWF:Ag were 6.91 hours (mean, 7.46 ± 3.20 hours, range, 3.68 to 16.22 hours), 20.87 hours (mean, 21.52 ± 7.21 hours; range: 7.19 to 32.20 hours), and 12.66 hours (mean, 13.03 ± 2.12 hours: range: 10.34 to 17.45 hours), respectively. The median incremental *in vivo* recoveries of VWF:RCo and FVIII:C were 3.12 (IU/dL)/(IU/kg) [mean, 3.29 ± 1.46 (IU/dL)/(IU/kg); range: 1.3 to 5.7 (IU/dL)/(IU/kg)] for VWF:RCo and 1.94 (IU/dL)/(IU/kg) [mean, 2.14 ± 0.58 (IU/dL)/(IU/kg); range: 1.3 to 3.3 (IU/dL)/(IU/kg)] for FVIII:C.

Following infusion of both A-SD and A-SD/HT, an increase in the size of VWF multimers was seen and persisted for at least 24 hours. The shortening of the BT was transient, lasting less than 6 hours following treatment and did not correlate with the presence of large and intermediate size VWF multimers.[26]

14. CLINICAL STUDIES
Prophylaxis for Elective Surgery
Thirty seven subjects with VWD (6 Type 1, 16 Type 2A, 3 Type 2B, 12 Type 3) underwent 59 surgical procedures that included 20 dental, 7 orthopedic, 8 gastrointestinal, 6 gastrointestinal (diagnostic), 9 vascular, 3 gynecologic, 2 genitourinary, 2 dermatologic and 2 head and neck procedures administering A-SD or A-SD/HT (21 subjects were administered A-SD and 18 were administered A-SD/HT, 2 received

both products) for bleeding prophylaxis (see **Table 4**). Prior to each surgical procedure, the investigators provided an estimation of the expected blood loss during surgery for a normal person of the same sex and of similar stature and age as the subject undergoing the same type of surgical procedure. An initial preoperative infusion of 60 VWF:RCo IU/kg (75 VWF:RCo IU/kg for patients less than 18 years of age), was administered one hour preoperatively. A sample was obtained 15 minutes after the initial infusion for the determination of the plasma FVIII:C level. The level had to equal or exceed 100% of normal for an operation to proceed. No cryoprecipitate or alternative FVIII product was administered during these surgical procedures. Platelets were required in only two subjects. Intra-operative infusions of A-SD and A-SD/HT at 60 VWF:RCo IU/kg (75 VWF:RCo IU/kg for patients less than 18 years of age) was administered according to the judgment of the investigator.

Table 4. Number of and Types of Surgical Procedures

Type of Surgical Procedure	Treatment		
	A-SD	A-SD/HT	Total
Number of Subjects	21	18	37^
Dental	14	6	20
Dermatologic	1	1	2
Gastrointestinal	4	4	8
Gastrointestinal (diagnostic)	6	0	6
Genitourinary	0	2	2
Gynecologic	2	1	3
Head and neck	1	1	2
Orthopedic	4	3	7
Vascular	3	6	9
Total number of procedures	35	24	59

^ Two patients received both preparations; the total number of subjects is therefore less than the sum of the columns.

Postoperative infusions at doses of 40 to 60 VWF:RCo IU/kg (50 to 75 VWF:RCo IU/kg for pediatric patients) was administered at 8- to 12-hour intervals until healing had occurred. After achieving primary hemostasis, for maintenance of secondary hemostasis the dose was reduced after the third postoperative day. See **DOSAGE AND ADMINISTRATION (2.2)**.

Overall, in 55 surgical procedures undertaken with a prolonged BT pre-infusion, the BT at 30 minutes post-infusion was fully corrected in 18 (32.7%) cases, partially corrected in 24 (43.6%) cases, demonstrated no correction in 12 (21.8%) cases, and was not done in one case (1.8%).

The mean blood loss was lower than predicted prospectively. Bleeding exceeding the predicted value did not correlate with correction of the BT. Three patients had bleeding which exceeded by more than 50 mL the amount predicted prospectively. Among the latter subjects, the BT 30 minutes post-infusion was normal in one and only slightly lengthened in two cases.

Surgical infusion summary data are included in **Table 5**.

Table 5: Prophylaxis with A-SD and/or A-SD/HT in Surgery

	A-SD	A-SD/HT	Total
Number of patients	21	18	37*
Number of surgical procedures	35	24	59
Median number of infusions per surgical procedure (range)	3 (1-13)	4 (1–18)	4 (1-18)
Median dosage VWF:RCo IU/kg			
Infusion #1 (range)	59.8 (19.8-75.1)	59.9 (40.6-75.0)	59.9 (19.8-75.1)
Infusion ≥ #2 combined (range)	40.0 (4.5-75.1)	40.0 (10.0-63.1)	40.0 (4.5-75.1)

* Two subjects received both products

Table 6. Effect of Treatment on Surgical Prophylaxis (Investigator Evaluation): Analysis per Treated Event (A-SD/HT)

Investigator's Outcome Evaluation	Type of von Willebrand Disease											
	Type 1 (4 Subjects, 4 Procedures)			Type 2 (9 Subjects, 13 Procedures)			Type 3 (5 Subjects, 7 Procedures)			Total (18 Subjects, 24 Procedures)		
	Procedure			Procedure			Procedure			Procedure		
	1	2	3	1	2	3	1	2	3	1	2	3
Excellent	1	0	2	5	1	5	5	0	1	11	1	8
Good	0	0	1	0	0	1	0	0	0	0	0	2
Poor	0	0	0	0	0	0	0	0	0	0	0	0
None	0	0	0	0	1	0	0	1	0	0	2	0

Procedure 1=Minor, 2=Major, 3=Invasive
Absolute frequency & proportion of successful outcomes = 22/24 (91.66%)
95% Confidence Interval (CI) for the proportion of subjects with successful prophylaxis = 0.7300 to 0.9897

Table 9. Proportion of Procedures (N = 61) With a Daily Investigator Rating of Effective versus Non-effective

Study Day[a]	Outcome of Alphanate® Treatment	Proportion of Procedures (%)	95% Confidence Interval	P Value[b]
0	Effective[c]	95.1	87.8-8.6	< 0.0001
	Non-effective[d]	4.9	1.4-12.2	
1	Effective	91.8	83.5-96.7	< 0.0001
	Non-effective	8.2	3.3-16.5	

[a] Study Day 0 = day of surgery.
[b] Binomial test (H_0: < 70% of procedures have an overall rating of effective).
[c] Effective = Investigator rating of "excellent" or "good."
[d] Non-effective = Investigator rating of "poor" or "none."

[See table 5 above]
Additionally, the surgeries were categorized as major, minor or invasive procedures according to definitions used in the study. The outcome of each surgery was evaluated according to a clinical rating scale (excellent, good, poor or none) and was considered successful if the outcome was excellent or good. These outcomes are presented in **Table 6**.
[See table 6 above]
The study results were also evaluated independently by two referees with clinical experience in this field in the same way (surgery categorization and outcome of each surgery according to a clinical rating scale).
The results for the effect of treatment on surgical prophylaxis (Referee Evaluation) per treated subject are summarized in **Table 7**. There is a high level of agreement between the referee evaluations and the analyzed outcome data, with a decrease of only a single success (21/24 vs. 22/24).

Table 7. Effect of Treatment on Surgical Prophylaxis (Referee Evaluation): Analysis per Treated Event (A-SD/HT)

	Referee 1	Referee 2
Number of Treated Subjects	18	18
Number of Treated Events	24	24
Success Absolute Frequency & Proportion (%)	22 (0.9166)	21 (0.8750)

* 95% CI for the Proportion	0.7300 to 0.9897	0.6763 to 0.9734

* 95% confidence interval for the proportion of subjects with successful prophylaxis, exact estimation.

A retrospective study was performed to assess the efficacy of Alphanate® (A-SD/HT) as replacement therapy in preventing excessive bleeding in subjects with congenital VWD undergoing surgical or invasive procedures, for whom DDAVP® was ineffective or inadequate. The study was performed between September 2004 and December 2005, and 61 surgeries/procedures (in 39 subjects) were evaluated.
Of the 39 subjects, 18 had Type 1 VWD (46.2%); 12 subjects (30.8%) had Type 2 VWD, and 9 subjects (23.1%) had Type 3 VWD. The median age for subjects overall was 40 years; approximately one-half of the subjects overall were male.
The primary efficacy variable was the overall treatment outcome for each surgical or invasive procedure, as rated by the investigator using a 4-point verbal rating scale (VRS): "excellent," "good," "poor," or "none." The categorization of the replacement treatment outcome according to the proposed scale was based upon the investigator's clinical experience. The secondary efficacy variables were:
• Daily (Day 0 and Day 1) treatment outcome for each surgical or invasive procedure, rated by the investigator using the same 4-point VRS used for the primary efficacy variable. Day 0 was the day of surgery, and Day 1 was the day following surgery.
• Overall treatment outcome for each surgical or invasive procedure, rated by an independent referee committee using the same 4-point VRS used for the primary efficacy variable.

In addition, an independent referee committee was convened to evaluate the efficacy outcomes. The committee was composed of 2 physicians with demonstrated clinical expertise treating subjects with similar medical characteristics to those of the study population. The committee was blinded to the investigator ratings; and each referee evaluated the outcomes independent of one another.
More than 90% received an investigator and referee's overall and daily rating of "effective" ("excellent" or "good"). The results of the primary efficacy analysis are in **Table 8**.

Table 8. Proportion of Procedures (N = 61) With an Overall Investigator Rating of Effective versus Non-effective

Outcome of Alphanate® Treatment	Proportion of Procedures (%)	95% Confidence Interval	P Value[a]
Effective[b]	95.1	87.8-98.6	< 0.0001
Non-effective[c]	4.9	1.4-12.2	

[a] Binomial test (H_0: < 70% of procedures have an overall rating of effective).
[b] Effective = Investigator rating of "excellent" or "good."
[c] Non-effective = Investigator rating of "poor" or "none."

The results of the analysis of daily investigator ratings are in **Table 9**.
[See table 9 at left]
The results of the analysis of overall referee ratings are in **Table 10**.

Table 10. Proportion of Procedures (N = 61) With an Overall Referee Rating of Effective versus Non-effective

Outcome of Alphanate® Treatment	Proportion of Procedures (%)	95% Confidence Interval	P Value[a]
Effective[b]	91.8	83.5-96.7	< 0.0001
Non-effective[c]	8.2	3.3-16.5	

[a] Binomial test (H_0: < 70% of procedures have an overall rating of effective).
[b] Effective = Referee rating of "excellent" or "good."
[c] Non-effective = Referee rating of "poor" or "none."

The overall investigator ratings are summarized by type of VWD in **Table 11**.
[See table 11 at top of next page]
The majority of ratings were "excellent" (≥ 81.3% in each VWD type). Only 2 procedures in 1 subject with Type 3 VWD received an overall efficacy rating of "none," and 1 procedure in 1 subject with Type 2 VWD received an overall efficacy rating of "poor."
The total dose of Alphanate® received over the entire perioperative period of the retrospective study is summarized in **Table 12**.

Table 12: Alphanate® Received (VWF:RCo) by Category of Procedure

	A-SD/HT
Number of patients	39
Number of surgical procedures	61
Mean number of infusions	5.9
Median number of infusions per surgical procedure (range)	3 (1-27)

15. REFERENCES

1. Eyster, M.E. Hemophilia: A Guide for the Primary Care Physician. Postgrad Med 1978; 64:75-81.
2. Shanbrom, E., Thelin, M. Experimental Prophylaxis of Severe Hemophilia with a Factor VIII Concentrate. JAMA 1969; 208(9):1853-1856.
3. Levine, P.H. Hemophilia and Allied Conditions. In: Brain, M.C. ed. Current Therapy in Hematology-Oncology: 1983-1984, New York: BC Decker, 1983, pp. 147-152.
4. Rizza, C.R., Biggs, R. Blood Products in the Management of Haemophilia and Christmas Disease. In: Poller, L., ed. Recent Advances in Blood Coagulation, Boston: Little Brown, 1969, pp. 179-195.
5. Hathaway, W.E., Mahasandana, C., Clarke, S. Alteration of Platelet Function After Transfusion in Hemophilia. Proc 14th Ann Mtg, Am Soc Hematol 1971, Abstracts, 58, No. 88.

Table 11. Number (%) of Investigator's Overall Efficacy Ratings by Type of VWD

Investigator's Overall Rating	Type 1 (18 Subjects, 22 Procedures)		Type 2 (12 Subjects, 23 Procedures)		Type 3 (9 Subjects, 16 Procedures)		Total (39 Subjects, 61 Procedures)	
	Major	Minor[a]	Major	Minor	Major	Minor	Major	Minor
Excellent	6 (85.7%)	12 (80.0%)	2 (50.0%)	18 (94.7%)	0 (0.0%)	13 (86.7%)	8 (66.7%)	43 (87.8%)
Good	1 (14.3%)	3 (20.0%)	2 (50.0%)	0 (0.0%)	0 (0.0%)	1 (6.7%)	3 (25.0%)	4 (8.2%)
Poor	0 (0.0%)	0 (0.0%)	0 (0.0%)	1 (5.3%)	0 (0.0%)	0 (0.0%)	0 (0.0%)	1 (2.0%)
None	0 (0.0%)	0 (0.0%)	0 (0.0%)	0 (0.0%)	1 (100%)	1 (6.7%)	1 (8.3%)	1 (2.0%)

[a] Minor surgery also includes invasive procedures.

6. Kasper, C.K. Incidence and Course of Inhibitors Among Patients with classic Hemophilia. Thromb Diath Haemorrh 1973; 30:263-271.
7. Rizza, C.R., Biggs, R. The Treatment of Patients Who Have Factor VIII Antibodies Br J Haematol 1973; 24:65-82.
8. Roberts, H.R., Knowles, M.R., Jones, T.L., McMillan, C. The Use of Factor VIII in the Management of Patients with Factor VIII Inhibitors. In: Brinkhous, K.M., ed. Hemophilia and New Hemorrhagic States, International Symposium, New York, University of North Carolina Press, 1970, pp. 152-163.
9. Federici, A.B., Baudo, F., Caracciolo, C., Mancuso, G., Mazzucconi, M.G., Musso, R., Schinco, P.C., Targhetta. R., Mannucci, P.M. Clinical efficacy of highly purified, doubly virus-inactivated factor VIII/von Willebrand factor concentrate (Fanhdi®) in the treatment of von Willebrand disease: a retrospective clinical study. Haemophilia 2002; 8:761-767.
10. Federici, A.B. Managment of von Willebrand disease with FVIII/von Willebrand factor concentrates: results from current studies and surveys. Blood Coagul Fibrinolysis 2005;16(Suppl 1):S17-S21.
11. Mannucci, P.M. How I treat patients with von Willebrand disease. Blood 2001; 97:1915-1919.
12. Mannucci, P.M. Treatment of von Willebrand's Disease. N Engl J Med 2004;351:683-694.
13. Mannucci, P.M. Venous Thromboembolism in von Willebrand Disease. Thromb Haemost 2002; 88:378-379.
14. Markis, M., Colvin, B., Gupta, V., Shields, M.L., Smith, M.P. Venous Thrombosis Following the Use of Intermediate Purity FVIII Concentrate to Treat Patients with von Willebrand Disease. Thromb Haemost 2002; 88: 387-388.
15. Biggs, R. Jaundice and Antibodies Directed Against Factors VIII and IX in Patients Treated for Haemophilia or Christmas Disease in the United Kingdom. Br J Haematol 1974; 26:313-329.
16. Kasper, C.K., Kipnis, S.A. Hepatitis and Clotting Factor Concentrates. JAMA 1972; 221:510.
17. Mannucci, P.M., Federici, A.B. Antibodies to von Willebrand Factor in von Willebrand Disease. In: Aledort L.M., Hoyer L.W., Reisener J.M., White II, G.C. eds. Inhibitors to coagulation factor in the 1990s, 1995, Plenum Press, pp. 87-92.
18. Data on file at Grifols Biologicals Inc.
19. Fujimura, Y., Titani, K., Holland, L.Z., Roberts, J.R., Kostel, P., Ruggeri, Z.M., Zimmerman, T.S. A heparin-binding domain of human von Willebrand factor: Characterization and localization to a tryptic fragment extending from amino acid residue Val-449 to Lys-728. J Biol Chem 1987; 262(4):1734-1739.
20. Horowitz, B. Investigations into the Application of Tri (n-Butyl) Phosphate/Detergent Mixture to Blood Derivatives. In: Morgenthaler, J-J ed. Viral Inactivation in Plasma Products, Karger, 1989, 56:83-96.
21. Edwards, C.A., Piet, M.P.J., Chin, S., Horowitz, B. Tri (n-Butyl) Phosphate/Detergent Treatment of Licensed Therapeutic and Experimental Blood Derivatives. Vox Sang 1987; 52:53-59.
22. Hershgold, E.J. Properties of Factor VIII (Antihaemophilic Factor). In: Spaet, T.H., ed. Progress in Hemostasis and Thrombosis, Grune and Stratton Publisher, 1974, 2:99-139.
23. Ashenhurst, J.B., Langehenning, P.L., Seeler, R.A. Early Treatment of Bleeding Episodes with 10 U/Kg of Factor VIII. Blood 1977:50:181.
24. Hoyer, L.W. The Factor VIII complex: Structure and function. Blood 1981; 58:1-13.
25. Meyer, D., and Girma, J-P. von Willebrand factor: Structure and function. Thromb Haemost 1983; 70:99-104.
26. Mannucci, P.M., Chediak, J., Hanna, W. Byrnes, J.J., Kessler, C.M, Ledford, M., Retzios, A.D., Kapelan, B.A., Gallagher, P., Schwartz, R.S., and the Alphanate®Study Group. Treatment of von Willebrand's Disease (VWD) with a high purity factor VIII concentrate: Dissociation between correction of the bleeding time (BT), VWF multimer pattern, and treatment efficacy. Blood 1999; 94 (Suppl 1, Part 2 of 2):98b.

16. HOW SUPPLIED/STORAGE AND HANDLING

Alphanate® is supplied in sterile, lyophilized form in a single dose vial with a vial of diluent (Sterile Water for Injection, USP), a Mix2Vial™ filter transfer set for use in administration. International unit activity of Factor VIII and VWF:RCo are stated on the carton and label of each vial. It is available in the following potencies, and the product is also color coded based upon assay on the carton and label as follows:

Potency	NDC	Assay Color Code
250 IU FVIII/5 mL single dose vial	68516-4601-1	LOW in grey box
500 IU FVIII/5 mL single dose vial	68516-4602-1	MID in blue box
1000 IU FVIII/ 10 mL single dose vial	68516-4603-2	HIGH in red box
1500 IU FVIII/ 10 mL single dose vial	68516-4604-2	SUPER HIGH in black box

Storage

Alphanate® should be stored at temperatures between 2 and 8 °C. Do not freeze to prevent damage to diluent vial. Alphanate® may be stored at room temperature not to exceed 30 °C for up to 2 months. When removed from refrigeration, record the date removed on the space provided on the carton.

17. PATIENT COUNSELING INFORMATION

Patients should be informed of the early symptoms and signs of hypersensitivity reaction, including hives, generalized urticaria, chest tightness, dyspnea, wheezing, faintness, hypotension, and anaphylaxis. Patients should be advised to discontinue use of the product and contact their physician and/or seek immediate emergency care, depending on the severity of the reaction, if these symptoms occur. It is recommended that the lot number of the vials used be recorded when Alphanate® is administered.

17.1 Thromboembolic Events

Thromboembolic events have been reported in von Willebrand Disease patients receiving Antihemophilic Factor/von Willebrand Factor Complex replacement therapy, especially in the setting of known risk factors for thrombosis.[13,14] Early reports might indicate a higher incidence in females. In addition, endogenous high levels of FVIII have also been associated with thrombosis but no causal relationship has been established. In all VWD patients in situations of high thrombotic risk receiving coagulation factor replacement therapy, caution should be exercised and antithrombotic measures should be considered. See also **WARNINGS AND PRECAUTIONS (5.1)**.

17.2 Infections

Because Antihemophilic Factor/von Willebrand Factor Complex (Human), Alphanate® is made from pooled human plasma, it may carry a risk of transmitting infectious agents, e.g., viruses, and theoretically, the Creutzfeldt-Jakob disease (CJD) agent. Stringent procedures designed to reduce the risk of adventitious agent transmission have been employed in the manufacture of this product, from the screening of plasma donors and the collection and testing of plasma, through the application of viral elimination/reduction steps such as solvent detergent and heat treatment in the manufacturing process. Despite these measures, such products can still potentially transmit disease; therefore, the risk of infectious agents cannot be totally eliminated. The physician should weigh the risks and benefits of the use of this product and should discuss these with the patient. See also **WARNINGS AND PRECAUTIONS (5.2)**.

17.3 Inhibitor Formation

Some patients develop inhibitors to Factor VIII. These inhibitors are circulating antibodies (i.e., globulins) that neutralize the procoagulant activity of Factor VIII. No studies have been conducted with Alphanate® to evaluate inhibitor formation. Therefore, it is not known whether there are greater, lesser or the same risks of developing inhibitors due to the use of this product than there are with other antihemophilic factor preparations. Patients with these inhibitors may not respond to treatment with Antihemophilic Factor/von Willebrand Factor Complex (Human), or the response may be much less than would otherwise be expected; therefore, larger doses of Antihemophilic Factor/von Willebrand Factor Complex (Human) are often required. The management of bleeding in patients with inhibitors requires careful monitoring, especially if surgical procedures are indicated.[6-8] See also **WARNINGS AND PRECAUTIONS (5.3)**.

Manufactured and Distributed by:
Grifols Biologicals Inc.
Los Angeles, CA 90032, U.S.A.
U. S. License No. 1694
DATE OF REVISION: March 2010

ALPHANINE® SD ℞

[al-fa-nine]
Coagulation Factor IX (Human)
Solvent Detergent Treated/Virus Filtered

DESCRIPTION

Coagulation Factor IX (Human), AlphaNine® SD, is a purified, solvent detergent treated, virus filtered preparation of Factor IX derived from human plasma.[1] It contains a minimum of 150 IU Factor IX/mg protein; levels of Factor VII (proconvertin), Factor II (prothrombin) and Factor X (Stuart-Prower Factor) which are below the limit of detection (less than 0.04 Factor VII unit, less than 0.05 Factor II unit, and less than 0.05 Factor X unit per IU Factor IX). AlphaNine® SD is a sterile, lyophilized preparation intended for intravenous administration only. Each vial is a single dose container.

AlphaNine® SD is labeled with the Factor IX potency expressed in International Units (IU). AlphaNine® SD contains not more than (NMT) 0.04 unit of heparin, NMT 0.2 mg of dextrose, NMT 1.0 µg polysorbate 80 and NMT 0.10 µg tri(n-butyl) phosphate/IU of Factor IX.

CLINICAL PHARMACOLOGY

AlphaNine® SD is a purified formulation of Factor IX containing not less than 150 IU Factor IX activity/mg of total protein.[2] AlphaNine® SD contains non-therapeutic levels of Factor II, Factor VII and Factor X.

Thrombogenicity of AlphaNine® SD in animals is markedly lower than that of Factor IX Complex, Profilnine® Heat-Treated. Five lots of AlphaNine® SD (three lots of non-virus filtered product and two lots of virus filtered product) failed to show any evidence of thrombogenicity when tested directly in the Wessler rabbit stasis model for thrombogenicity[3-6] at a dose of 200 IU Factor IX/kg body weight. When various lots of AlphaNine® SD were further tested at doses between 300 and 650 IU Factor IX/kg, only 5 out of 40 animals (12.5%) showed evidence of thrombus formation (Wessler scores of +1, +2, +1, +1, +1 out of +4 maximum). In comparison, Factor IX Complex concentrate, Profilnine®, was thrombogenic in 100% of the animals tested at a dose of 100 IU Factor IX/kg.

At a dose of 200 IU Factor IX/kg body weight in a porcine model, the heptane heat-treated formulation of this product (AlphaNine®) showed little evidence of disseminated intravascular coagulation (DIC) following infusion.[7] This model exhibited no depletion of coagulation factors, a minimal increase in fibrin monomer (+1 in protamine test), a slight temporary decrease in platelet counts, and no evidence of intravascular coagulation upon gross autopsy.[8] In contrast, Harrison, et al., report that all Factor IX Complex concentrates studied in the same porcine model were thrombogenic at doses between 50 and 100 IU of Factor IX/kg animal weight.[9]

A clinical evaluation of AlphaNine® SD half-life and recovery characteristics was performed. A total of 18 patients with severe to moderate hemophilia B each received a single infusion of 40 to 50 IU Factor IX/kg body weight of AlphaNine® SD. Following the administration of AlphaNine® SD, the mean half-life of Factor IX observed was approximately 21 hours.[2] This half-life value was computed using the biphasic linear regression model recommended by the International Society of Thrombosis and Haemostasis.[10] The half-life obtained for the solvent detergent treated product is comparable to that of AlphaNine®

(approximately 19 hours) as well as the range of 18 to 36 hours reported for Factor IX Complex preparations.[11] The mean recovery observed in clinical trials was approximately 48% and was comparable to that of AlphaNine® (approximately 51%).[2]

A clinical trial was conducted using the heptane heat-treated product, AlphaNine®, to evaluate the efficacy of the product in providing hemostatic protection during and after surgery in 13 patients with hemophilia B. The types of surgical procedures performed included bilateral knee replacement (1), total knee replacement with synovectomy (2), hip replacement (1), below the knee amputation (1), herniorrhaphy (2), hemorrhoidectomy (1), rhinoplasty (2), oral surgery (2) and Hickman catheter insertion with temporalis muscle transfer (1). Presurgery doses ranged from 30.1 to 65.0 IU Factor IX/kg; postsurgery replacement therapy doses ranged from approximately 9.4 to 52.0 IU Factor IX/kg. The number of postsurgery days of treatment ranged from 1 to 23; the number of postsurgery infusions ranged from 2 to 26. No bleeding episodes were reported and hemostasis was maintained during the course of postsurgery therapy. None of the hematologic parameters examined (hematocrit, partial thromboplastin time, prothrombin time, fibrinogen/fibrin degradation products, fibrin monomers, D-dimers and platelet counts) provided any evidence that AlphaNine® possessed thrombogenic potential.[12]

A randomized crossover study with 11 hemophilia B patients was conducted with the heptane heat-treated version of the product, AlphaNine®, to determine whether an infusion of AlphaNine® caused less activation of the hemostatic system than the Factor IX Complex concentrate preparation, Profilnine® Heat-Treated. Each subject received a single infusion of either AlphaNine® or Profilnine® Heat-Treated for the treatment of a bleeding episode, at a dose of 50 IU Factor IX/kg body weight. Each subject received the other Factor IX concentrate for the treatment of a subsequent bleeding episode, separated by an interval of not less than 10 days. The level of prothrombin fragment 1+2 (F_{1+2}) is a sensitive index of the cleavage of prothrombin by activated Factor X. The level of fibrinopeptide A (FPA) released into the plasma measures the activity of thrombin on fibrinogen in the formation of fibrin. Following infusion of Factor IX Complex, statistically significant increases in F_{1+2} and in FPA were detected at all monitored time points (15, 60, 90, 120 and 240 minutes postinfusion). The statistically significant elevation in these two hemostatic parameters indicates increased activation of the coagulation cascade. Administration of AlphaNine® resulted in no increase in F_{1+2} at any monitored time points, and a statistically nonsignificant increase in FPA at 15, 60, and 90 minutes following infusion. Only at 120 and 240 minutes after infusion of AlphaNine® were statistically significant increases in FPA levels detected. These results suggest that the infusion of a high purity factor IX, such as AlphaNine®, may result in a lower level of activation of the coagulation cascade than does Factor IX Complex.[13]

The ability of the manufacturing process to inactivate and eliminate virus from the Coagulation Factor IX (Human) products was evaluated at key stages in the process (see Table 1). Known amounts of different viruses were added to samples obtained prior to those steps most likely to reduce virus load (DEAE Chromatography, Solvent Detergent, Dual Affinity Chromatography and nanofiltration) in the AlphaNine® and AlphaNine® SD processes to determine the level of viral inactivation/elimination of these specific steps in the process.

[See table 1 below]

The retrovirus known as human immunodeficiency virus (HIV) has been identified as a causative agent of Acquired Immunodeficiency Syndrome (AIDS) and has been shown to be transmissible via blood or blood products. The solvent detergent process used in the manufacture of AlphaNine® SD, was shown to inactivate greater than 12.2 logs of HIV-1 when the retrovirus was intentionally added to product samples under laboratory evaluation (as measured by virus antigen capture and reverse transcriptase assays). In addition, this process was shown to inactivate 6 logs of HIV-2 (as measured by reverse transcriptase assays) when the retrovirus was intentionally added to product samples.[2] In an on going efficacy and safety study of 26 patients, no subjects tested positive for HIV or viral hepatitis in relation to the investigation drug.[2]

In order to assess the ability of the solvent detergent treatment process to inactivate other viruses such as hepatitis B and C virus, the inactivation of the model viruses, Sindbis virus, a model virus for hepatitis C virus, and vesicular stomatitis virus (VSV), a model RNA virus for lipid enveloped viruses, by solvent detergent treatment was studied. Prior to solvent detergent treatment, samples were inoculated with a titer of either Sindbis or VSV. The results demonstrated that a minimum of 5.3 logs of Sindbis and a minimum of 4.9 logs of VSV were inactivated after 180 minutes of incubation with solvent detergent (when compared to an untreated control). It should be noted that the incubation time in the actual AlphaNine® SD process is twice (360 minutes total) that used in the model virus studies.

The ability of the AlphaNine® SD process to eliminate virus, by physically partitioning virus from product, was evaluated at key stages of the manufacturing process. Studies were performed using a lipid-enveloped model virus (Sindbis) and non-lipid model viruses (porcine parvovirus, encephalomyocarditis virus, and reovirus). Known amounts of these viruses were added to samples obtained from the AlphaNine® SD process. The amount of virus removed at each subsequent purification step was then determined by plaque assay.

Addition of Sindbis or porcine parvovirus prior to Factor IX Complex adsorption by DEAE chromatography showed this step to eliminate 1.4 logs of Sindbis and 1.5 logs (95% confidence. interval: 1.51-2.33) of added porcine parvovirus. When Sindbis or parvovirus was introduced into the process after the barium citrate precipitation step of the AlphaNine® SD process, the subsequent dual affinity chromatography step was found to eliminate 4.7 logs of Sindbis and 2.2 logs (95% confidence interval: 2.25-2.75) of added parvovirus. When parvovirus, encephalomyocarditis virus (EMC), or Reovirus was introduced into the process after the dual affinity chromatography step, the subsequent nanofiltration step of the AlphaNine® SD process was found to eliminate 3.6 logs of parvovirus, 3.4 logs of EMC and 4.1 logs of added Reovirus. The studies mentioned above indicate that the manufacturing process of AlphaNine® SD is capable of reducing viruses by approximately 6 logs, in addition to virus reduction achieved by the solvent detergent process.[14] In another study, the nanofiltration step removed ≥ 4.4 logs of hepatitis A virus (HAV), a non-lipid enveloped virus. Table 1 summarizes the reduction factors obtained for each virus when individual steps in the manufacturing process for AlphaNine® SD were validated for virus removal/inactivation.

INDICATIONS AND USAGE

AlphaNine® SD is indicated for the prevention and control of bleeding in patients with Factor IX deficiency due to hemophilia B. AlphaNine® SD contains low, non-therapeutic levels of Factors II, VII, and X, and, therefore, is *not* indicated for the treatment of Factor II, VII or X deficiencies. This product is also *not* indicated for the reversal of coumarin anticoagulant-induced hemorrhage, nor in the treatment of hemophilia A patients with inhibitors to Factor VIII.

CONTRAINDICATIONS

None known.

WARNINGS

Because Coagulation Factor IX (Human), AlphaNine® SD is made from pooled human plasma, it may carry a risk of transmitting infectious agents, e.g., viruses, and theoretically, the Creutzfeldt-Jakob disease (CJD) agent. Stringent procedures designed to reduce the risk of adventitious agent transmission have been employed in the manufacture of this product, from the screening of plasma donors and the collection and testing of plasma to the application of viral elimination/reduction steps such as column chromatography, solvent detergent treatment and nanofiltration in the manufacturing process. Despite these measures, such product can potentially transmit disease, therefore the risk of infectious agents cannot be totally eliminated. The physician should weigh the risks and benefits of the use of this product and should discuss these with the patient.

Individuals who receive infusions of blood or plasma products may develop signs and/or symptoms of some viral infections. Scientific opinion encourages hepatitis B and hepatitis A vaccinations at birth or diagnosis for patients with hemophilia.

Incidences of thrombosis or disseminated intravascular coagulation (DIC), have been reported following administration of Factor IX Complex concentrates which contain high amounts of Factor II, VII and X.

Following administration of Coagulation Factor IX (Human), AlphaNine® SD in surgery patients and individuals with known liver disease, the physician should closely observe the patient for signs or symptoms of potential disseminated intravascular coagulation (DIC). Continued administration of the product should be left to the discretion of the physician.

Allergic type hypersensitivity reactions, including anaphylaxis, have been reported for all factor IX products. Frequently these events have occurred in close temporal association with the development of factor IX inhibitors. Patients should be informed of the early symptoms and signs of hypersensitivity reactions, including hives, generalized urticaria, angioedema, chest tightness, dyspnea, wheezing, faintness, hypotension, tachycardia and anaphylaxis. Patients should be advised to discontinue use of the product and contact physician and/or seek immediate emergency care, depending on the severity of the reactions, if any of these symptoms occur.

Nephrotic syndrome has been reported following attempted immune tolerance induction with factor IX products in Hemophilia B patients with factor IX inhibitors and a history of severe allergic reactions to Factor IX. The safety and efficacy of using AlphaNine® SD in attempted immune tolerance induction has not been established.

In Previously Untreated Patients (PUPs), it is possible that anaphylaxis may occur after a median exposure of eleven (11) days.[15] It is recommended that these patients are monitored closely between the tenth and twentieth exposure day.

PRECAUTIONS

General

In order to minimize the possibility of thrombogenic complications, dosing guidelines should be *strictly* followed. Refer to "Dosage and Administration" section for recommended amount of product to be administered.

AlphaNine® SD should *not* be administered at a rate exceeding 10 mL/minute. Rapid administration may result in vasomotor reactions.

Nursing personnel and others who administer this material should exercise appropriate caution in handling due to the risk of exposure to viral infection.

Discard any unused contents into the appropriate safety container. Discard administration equipment after single use into the appropriate safety container. Do not resterilize components.

Information for Patients

Patients should be informed of the early symptoms and signs of hypersensitivity reaction, including hives, generalized urticaria, chest tightness, dyspnea, wheezing, faintness, hypotension, and anaphylaxis. Patients should be advised to discontinue use of the product and contact their physician and/or seek immediate emergency care, depending on the severity of the reaction, if these symptoms occur.

Some viruses, such as parvovirus B19 or hepatitis A, are particularly difficult to remove or inactivate at this time. Parvovirus B19 may most seriously affect sero-negative pregnant women, or immunocompromised individuals. The majority of parvovirus B19 and hepatitis A infections are acquired by environmental (natural) sources.

Preliminary information suggests a relationship may exist between the presence of major deletion mutations in the Factor IX gene and an increased risk of inhibitor formation and of acute hypersensitivity reactions. Patients known to have major deletion mutations of the Factor IX gene should be observed closely for signs and symptoms of acute hypersensitivity reactions, particularly during the early phases of initial exposure to product.

Pregnancy Category C

Animal reproduction studies have not been conducted with AlphaNine® SD. It is also not known whether AlphaNine® SD can cause fetal harm when administered to a pregnant woman or can affect reproduction capacity. AlphaNine® SD should be given to a pregnant woman only if clearly indicated.

Pediatric Use

Clinical trials for safety and effectiveness in pediatric patients 16 years of age and younger have not been conducted. Across a well controlled half-life and recovery clinical trial in patients previously treated with Factor IX concentrates

Table 1

Process Step	Virus Reduction (log_{10})							
	Sindbis	VSV	HIV-1	HIV-2	Parvo**	EMC	Reo	HAV
DEAE Chromatography	1.4	NT	NT	NT	1.5*	NT	NT	NT
Solvent-Detergent	NLT 5.3	NLT 4.9	NLT 12.2	6.0	NT	NT	NT	NT
Dual Affinity Chromatography	4.7	NT	NT	NT	2.2*	NT	NT	NT
Nanofiltration	NT	NT	NT	NT	3.6	3.4	4.1	≥ 4.4

** Porcine NT=Not tested NLT=Not less than *Lower 95% confidence interval

of Hemophilia B, the three pediatric patients receiving AlphaNine® SD (solvent detergent treated) responded similarly when compared with 15 adult patients.[2] In an ongoing safety and efficacy clinical trial in patients not previously treated with Factor IX concentrates for Hemophilia B, 21 pediatric patients received AlphaNine® SD (solvent detergent treated) responded similarly when compared with the five adult patients above the age of 16 years. Adverse events were similar in this group compared to the patients above the age of 16 years. Anecdotal evaluation of the results indicates no safety and efficacy differences between pediatric and adult populations.

ADVERSE REACTIONS

The administration of plasma preparations may cause allergic reactions, mild chills, nausea or stinging at the infusion site. For most reactive individuals, slowing the infusion rate relieves the symptoms. For those highly reactive individuals, a different lot may be satisfactory.

Adverse reactions, characterized by either thrombosis or disseminated intravascular coagulation (DIC), have been reported following administration of Factor IX Complex concentrates. Patients who receive Coagulation Factor IX (Human), AlphaNine® SD, following operation, or those with known liver disease, should be kept under close observation for potential signs or symptoms of intravascular coagulation. Continued administration should be left to the discretion of the physician.

In the clinical study that compared the *in vivo* half-life and recovery of AlphaNine® SD and HT products, no adverse events were associated with 18 infusions of AlphaNine® SD administered to 18 individuals with severe to moderate hemophilia B.[2] Short term safety of the earlier version of this product, AlphaNine®, was demonstrated by an absence of adverse events after 225 infusions of this product were received by 31 patients participating in three clinical trials. In the clinical trial to evaluate efficacy of AlphaNine® in providing hemostatic protection during and after surgery, 13 patients received a total of 370,655 IU of AlphaNine®. In 208 total infusions, each patient received approximately 15,000 IU (range 3,295 to 52,200 IU Factor IX) in an average of 16 infusions (range 2 to 26 infusions). Results from this study showed no bleeding episodes during the course of postsurgery therapy. There was no hematological evidence (measured by hematocrit, partial thromboplastin time, prothrombin time, fibrinogen/fibrin degradation products, fibrin monomers, D-dimers and platelet counts) of thrombogenicity.[12]

To report SUSPECTED ADVERSE REACTIONS, contact Grifols at 1-888-GRIFOLS (1-888-474-3657) or FDA at 1-800-FDA-1088 or www.fda.gov/medwatch.

DOSAGE AND ADMINISTRATION

For adult usage:

AlphaNine® SD should be administered intravenously promptly following reconstitution. Administration of AlphaNine® SD within three hours after reconstitution is recommended to avoid the potential ill effect of any inadvertent bacterial contamination occurring during reconstitution. Discard any unused contents into the appropriate safety container.

Each vial of AlphaNine® SD is labeled with the total units expressed as International Units (IU) of Factor IX, which is referenced to the WHO International Standard. One unit approximates the activity in one mL of pooled normal human plasma.

The amount of AlphaNine® SD required to establish hemostasis will vary with each patient and depend upon the circumstances. The following formula may be used as a guide in determining the number of units to be administered.[16]

[See first table above]

In clinical practice there is variability between patients and their clinical response. Therefore, the Factor IX level of each patient should be monitored frequently during replacement therapy.

For pediatric usage: See PRECAUTIONS

[See second table above]

Dosing requirements and frequency of dosing is calculated on the basis of an initial response of 1% FIX increase achieved per IU of FIX infused per kg body weight and an average half-life for FIX of 18 hours. If dosing studies have revealed that a particular patient exhibits a lower response, the dose should be adjusted accordingly.

For pediatric usage: See PRECAUTIONS

RECONSTITUTION

Use Aseptic Technique

1. Warm diluent (Sterile Water for Injection, USP) and concentrate (AlphaNine® SD) to at least room temperature (but not above 37 °C).
2. Remove the plastic flip off cap from the diluent vial.
3. Gently swab the exposed stopper surface with a cleansing agent such as alcohol trying to avoid leaving any excess cleansing agent on the stopper.

Body weight (in kg)	×	Desired increase in Plasma Factor IX (Percent)	×	1.0 IU/kg	=	Number of Factor IX IU Required
Example:						
70 kg	×	40 (% increase)	×	1.0 IU/kg	=	2,800 IU AlphaNine® SD

Treatment Guidelines for Hemorrhagic Events and Surgery in Patients Diagnosed with Hemophilia B

Type of Hemorrhage or Surgical Procedure	Examples	Treatment Guidelines
Minor Hemorrhages	Bruises, cuts or scrapes, uncomplicated joint hemorrhage	FIX levels should be brought to at least 20-30% (20-30 IU FIX/kg/twice daily) until hemorrhage stops and healing has been achieved (1-2 days).[17,18,19]
Moderate Hemorrhages	Nose bleeds, mouth and gum bleeds, dental extractions, hematuria	FIX levels should be brought to 25-50% (25-50 IU FIX/kg/twice daily) until healing has been achieved (2-7 days, on average).[17,18,19,20,21]
Major Hemorrhages	Joint and muscle hemorrhages (especially in the large muscles), major trauma, hematuria, intracranial and intraperitoneal bleeding	FIX levels should be brought 50% for at least 3-5 days (30-50 IU FIX/kg/twice daily). Following this treatment period, FIX levels should be maintained at 20% (20 IU FIX/kg/twice daily) until healing has been achieved. Major hemorrhages may require treatment for up to 10 days.[17,18,19,20,21]
Surgery		Prior to surgery, FIX should be brought to 50-100% of normal (50-100 IU FIX/kg/twice daily). For the next 7 to 10 days, or until healing has been achieved, the patient should be maintained at 50-100% FIX levels (50-100 IU FIX/kg/twice daily).[17,18,19,20,21]

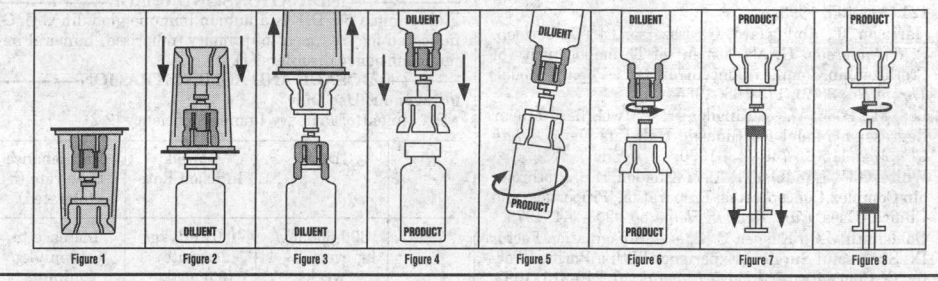

Figure 1 Figure 2 Figure 3 Figure 4 Figure 5 Figure 6 Figure 7 Figure 8

4. Open the Mix2Vial™ package by peeling away the lid (Figure 1). Leave the Mix2Vial™ in the clear outer packaging.
5. Place the diluent vial upright on an even surface and hold the vial tight and pick up the Mix2Vial™ in its clear outer packaging. Holding the diluent securely, push the **blue** end of the Mix2Vial™ vertically down through the diluent vial stopper (Figure 2).
6. While holding onto the diluent vial, carefully remove the clear outer packaging from the Mix2Vial™ set, ensuring the Mix2Vial™ remains attached to the diluent vial (Figure 3).
7. Place the product vial upright on an even surface, invert the diluent vial with the Mix2Vial™ attached.
8. While holding the product vial securely on a flat surface, push the **clear** end of the Mix2Vial™ set **vertically** down through the product vial stopper (Figure 4). The diluent will automatically transfer out of its vial into the product vial. (NOTE: If the Mix2Vial™ is connected at an angle, the vacuum may be released from the product vial and the diluent will not transfer into the product vial.)
9. With the diluent and product vials still attached to the Mix2Vial™, gently swirl the product vial to ensure the product is fully dissolved (Figure 5). Reconstitution requires less than 5 minutes. Do not shake the vial.
10. Disconnect the Mix2Vial™ into two separate pieces (Figure 6) by holding each vial adapter and twisting counterclockwise. After separating, discard the diluent vial with the **blue** end of the Mix2Vial™.
11. Draw air into an empty, sterile syringe. Keeping the product vial upright with the **clear** end of the Mix2Vial™ attached, screw the disposable syringe onto the luer lock portion of the Mix2Vial™ device by pressing and twisting clockwise. Inject air into the product vial.
12. While keeping the syringe plunger depressed, invert the system upside down and draw the reconstituted product into the syringe by pulling the plunger back slowly (Figure 7).
13. When the reconstituted product has been transferred into the syringe, firmly hold the barrel of the syringe

and the clear vial adapter (keeping the syringe plunger facing down) and unscrew the syringe from the Mix2Vial™ (Figure 8). Hold the syringe upright and push the plunger until no air is left in the syringe. Attach the syringe to a venipuncture set.
14. NOTE: If the same patient is to receive more than one vial of concentrate, the contents of two vials may be drawn into the same syringe through a separate unused Mix2Vial™ set before attaching to the venipuncture set.
15. Use prepared drug as soon as possible after reconstitution.
16. After reconstitution, parenteral drug products should be inspected visually for particulate matter and discoloration prior to administration, whenever solution and container permit. When reconstitution procedure is strictly followed, a few small particles may occasionally remain. The Mix2Vial™ set will remove particles and the labeled potency will not be reduced.
17. Discard all administration equipment after use into the appropriate safety container. Do not reuse.

[See figure above]

HOW SUPPLIED

AlphaNine® SD is supplied in sterile, lyophilized form in single dose vials accompanied by 10 mL diluent (Sterile Water for Injection, USP). Factor IX activity, expressed in International Units (IU) which is referenced to WHO International Standard, is stated on the label of each concentrate vial. AlphaNine® SD is packaged with a Mix2Vial™ filter transfer set for use in administration.

It is available in the following potencies, and the product is also color coded based upon assay on the carton and vial label as follows:

[See table at top of next page]

STORAGE

AlphaNine® SD should be stored at temperatures between 2 and 8 °C. Do not freeze to prevent damage to diluent vial. May be stored at room temperature not to exceed 30 °C for 1 month. When removed from refrigeration, record the date removed on the space provided on the carton.

Rx only

Potency	NDC	Assay Color Code
500 IU FIX/10 mL single dose vial	68516-3601-2	MID in blue box
1000 IU FIX/10 mL single dose vial	68516-3602-2	HIGH in red box
1500 IU FIX/10 mL single dose vial	68516-3603-2	SUPER HIGH in black box

REFERENCES

1. Plasma Fraction Purification Serial No. 902.155 Patent issued.
2. Data on file at Grifols Biologicals Inc.
3. Giles, A.R., Johnston, M., Hoogendoorn, H., Blajchman, M. & Hirsch, J. The Thrombogenicity of Prothrombin Complex Concentrates: I. The Relationship Between *In Vitro* Characteristics and *In Vivo* Thrombogenicity in Rabbits. *Thromb Res* 17:353-366, 1980.
4. Kingdon, H.S., Lundblad, R.L., Veltkamp, J.J. & Aronson, D.L. Potentially Thrombogenic Materials in Factor IX Concentrates. *Thromb Diath Haemorrh* (Stuttg) 33:617-631, 1975.
5. Prowse, C.V. & Williams, A.E. A Comparison of the *In Vitro* and *In Vivo* Thrombogenic Activity of Factor IX Concentrate Using Stasis (Wessler) and Non-Stasis Rabbit Models. *Thromb Hemostas* 44:81-86, 1980.
6. Wessler, S., Reimer, S.M. & Sheps, M.C. Biologic Assay of a Thrombosis-Inducing Activity in Human Serum. *J Appl Physiol* 14:943-946, 1959.
7. Herring, S.W. & Heldebrant, C.M. Heat-Treated Pure Factor IX. *Proc 5th Int Symp HT*, 1986, pp. 151-158.
8. Herring, S.W., Abildgaard, C., Shitanishi, K.T., Harrison, J., Gendler, S. & Heldebrant, C.M. Human Coagulation Factor IX Assessment of Thrombogenicity in Animal Models and Viral Safety. *J. Lab. Clin Med.* 121: 394-405, 1993.
9. Harrison, J., Abildgaard, C., Lazerson, J., Culbertson, R. & Anderson, G. Assessment of Thrombogenicity of Prothrombin Complex Concentrates in a Porcine Model. *Throm Res* 38(2): 173-188, 1985.
10. Lee, M., Poon, W., & Kingdon, H. A Two-Phase Linear Regression Model for Biologic Half-Life Data. *J Lab Clin Med* 115(6): 745-748, 1990.
11. White, G.C., Lundblad, R.L., & Kingdon, H.S. Prothrombin Complex Concentrates: Preparation, Properties, and Clinical Uses. *Curr Topic in Hematol* 2:203-244, 1979.
12. Goldsmith, J.C., Kasper, C.K., et al. Coagulation Factor IX: Successful Surgical Experience With a Purified Factor IX Concentrate. *Amer J Hematol* 40: 210-215, 1992.
13. Mannucci, P.M., Bauer, K.A., Gringeri, A., Barzegar, S., Bottasso, B., Simoni L. & Rosenberg, R.D. Thrombin Generation Is Not Increased in the Blood of Hemophilia B Patients After the Infusion of a Purified Factor IX Concentrate. *Blood* 76(12): 2540-2545, December 15, 1990.
14. Herring, S., Peddada, L., Shitanishi, K., Chavez, D., Chio, A., & Heldebrant, C. Elimination of Virus During Manufacture of a Coagulation Factor IX Concentrate. Abstract presented at XIX *International Congress World Federation of Hemophilia,* Washington, DC, USA, August 14-19, 1990.
15. Warrier, I., Ewenstein, B.M., Koerper, M.A., Shapiro, A., Key, N., DiMichele, D., Miller, R.T., Pasi, J., Rivard, G.E., Sommer, S.S., Katz, J., Bergmann, F., Ljung, R., Petrini, P., Lusher, J.M. *Journal of Pediatric Hematology/Oncology* 19(1):23-27, 1997.
16. Zauber, N.P. & Levine, J. Factor IX Levels in Patients with Hemophilia B (Christmas Disease) Following Transfusion with Concentrates of Factor IX or Fresh Frozen Plasma (FFP). *Medicine* 56:213-224, 1977.
17. Nillson, I.M.: Hemorrhagic and Thrombotic Diseases: London, John Wiley and Sons, 1974.
18. Roberts, H.R. and Eberst, M.E.: Current Management of Hemophilia B. Hematology/Oncology Clinics of North America 7(6): 1269-1280, 1993.
19. Roberts, H.R. and Gray, T.F.: Clinical Aspects of Hemophilia B. In Hematology: Basic Principles and Practice, 2nd Edition, pp 1678-1685, Churchill Livingston.
20. Hedner, U. and Davie, E.W.: In "Hemostasis and Thrombosis: Basic Principles and Clinical Practice", eds. Colman, R.W., Hirsh, J., Marder, V.J., Salzman, E.W., 2nd Edition, Philadelphia, J.B. Lippincot Co, 1987.
21. Levin, P.H.: In "Hemostasis and Thrombosis: Basic Principles and Clinical Practice", eds. Colman, R.W., Hirsh, J., Marder, V.J., Salzman, E.W., 2nd Edition, Philadelphia, J.B, Lippincot Co, 1987.

Manufactured and Distributed by:
Grifols Biologicals Inc.
Los Angeles, CA 90032, U.S.A.
U.S. License No. 1694
DATE OF REVISION: March 2010
3030397

FLEBOGAMMA® 5% DIF
Immune Globulin Intravenous (Human) ℞
5% Liquid Preparation

HIGHLIGHTS OF PRESCRIBING INFORMATION
These highlights do not include all the information needed to use Flebogamma 5% DIF safely and effectively. See full prescribing information for Flebogamma 5% DIF.
Immune Globulin Intravenous (Human)
Flebogamma 5% DIF
5% Liquid Preparation
Initial U.S. Approval: 2006

> **WARNING: ACUTE RENAL DYSFUNCTION AND FAILURE**
> *See full prescribing information for complete boxed warning.*
> • Immune globulin intravenous (IGIV) products, particularly those with sucrose, have been reported to be associated with renal dysfunction, acute renal failure, osmotic nephrosis, and death.
> • For patients pre-disposed to renal dysfunction or failure, administer Flebogamma 5% DIF at the minimum concentration available and the minimum infusion rate practicable.
> • Flebogamma 5% DIF does not contain sucrose.

INDICATIONS AND USAGE
Flebogamma 5% DIF is a human immune globulin G (IgG) indicated for treatment of primary (inherited) humoral immunodeficiency disorders (1).

DOSAGE AND ADMINISTRATION
Intravenous Use Only
• Treatment of Primary Immunodeficiency (2.2)

	Dose	Initial Infusion Rate	Maintenance Dose rate (if tolerated)
PI	300-600 mg/kg every 3 - 4 weeks	0.01 mL/kg/minute (0.5 mg/kg/min)	Increase to 0.10 mL/kg/minute (5 mg/kg/min)

• For patients at risk of renal dysfunction or thrombotic events, administer Flebogamma 5% DIF at the minimum infusion rate practicable. [5.2, 5.4]
• Ensure that patients with pre-existing renal insufficiency are not volume-depleted and discontinue Flebogamma 5% DIF if renal function deteriorates. [5.2]

DOSAGE FORMS AND STRENGTHS
Flebogamma 5% DIF is supplied in 0.5, 2.5, 5, 10 and 20 g single use bottles. [3]

0.5 g	10 mL
2.5 g	50 mL
5 g	100 mL
10 g	200 mL
20 g	400 mL

CONTRAINDICATIONS
• Anaphylactic or severe systemic reactions to human immunoglobulin.
• IgA deficient patients with antibodies against IgA and a history of hypersensitivity.

WARNINGS AND PRECAUTIONS
• IgA deficient patients with antibodies against IgA are at greater risk of developing severe hypersensitivity and anaphylactic reactions. Have Epinephrine immediately available to treat any acute severe hypersensitivity reactions. [5.1]
• Monitor renal function, including blood urea nitrogen, serum creatinine and urine output in patients at risk of developing acute renal failure. [5.2]
• Hyperproteinemia, with resultant changes in serum osmolarity and electrolyte imbalances may occur in patients receiving IGIV therapy. [5.3]
• Thrombotic events have occurred in patients receiving IGIV therapy. Monitor patients with known risk factors for thrombotic events and consider baseline assessment of blood viscosity for those at risk of hyperviscosity. [5.4]

• Aseptic Meningitis Syndrome (AMS) has been reported with IGIV treatments, especially with high doses or rapid infusion. [5.5]
• Hemolytic anemia can develop subsequent to IGIV therapy due to enhanced RBC sequestration. Monitor patients for hemolysis and hemolytic anemia. [5.6]
• Monitor patients for pulmonary adverse reactions (TRALI). [5.7]
• Flebogamma 5% DIF is made from human plasma may contain infectious agents, e.g., viruses and, theoretically, the Creutzfeldt-Jakob disease agent. [5.8]
• Transitory rise of various passively transferred antibodies in patient blood may yield positive serological testing results. [5.9]
• Patients receiving Flebogamma 5% DIF for first time or being restarted on product after treatment hiatus of more than 8 weeks may be at higher risk for development fever, chills, nausea, and vomiting. [5.10]

ADVERSE REACTIONS
The most common temporally related adverse reactions with an incidence ≥ 5% include: headache, chills, fever, shaking, fatigue, malaise, anxiety, back pain, muscle cramps, abdominal cramps, blood pressure changes, chest tightness, palpitations, tachycardia, nausea, vomiting, cutaneous reactions, wheezing, rash, arthralgia, and edema. [6]
To report SUSPECTED ADVERSE REACTIONS, contact Grifols Biologicals at 1-888-GRIFOLS (1-888-474-3657) or FDA at 1-800-FDA-1 088 or www.fda.gov/medwatch.

DRUG INTERACTIONS
Passive transfer of antibodies may transiently interfere with the immune response to live virus vaccines and confound results of serological testing [7].

USE IN SPECIFIC POPULATIONS
• Pregnancy: No human or animal data. Use only if clearly needed. [8.1]
• Geriatric: In patients over age 65 or in any patients at risk of developing renal insufficiency, do not exceed the recommended dose, and infuse Flebogamma 5% DIF at the minimum infusion rate practicable. [8.5]

See 17 for PATIENT COUNSELING INFORMATION
Revised: 01/2010

FULL PRESCRIBING INFORMATION: CONTENTS*
WARNING: ACUTE RENAL DYSFUNCTION AND ACUTE RENAL FAILURE

* Sections or subsections omitted from the full prescribing information are not listed.

FULL PRESCRIBING INFORMATION
Immune Globulin Intravenous (Human)
Flebogamma® 5% DIF
5% Liquid Preparation

WARNING: ACUTE RENAL DYSFUNCTION AND ACUTE RENAL FAILURE
Immune Globulin Intravenous (Human) (IGIV) products have been reported to be associated with renal dysfunction, acute renal failure, osmotic nephrosis, and death (*1*). Patients predisposed to acute renal failure include patients with any degree of pre-existing renal insufficiency, diabetes mellitus, age greater than 65, volume depletion, sepsis, paraproteinemia, or patients receiving known nephrotoxic drugs. Especially in such patients, IGIV products should be administered at the minimum concentration available and the minimum rate of infusion practicable. While these reports of renal dysfunction and acute renal failure have been associated with the use of many of the licensed IGIV products, those containing sucrose as a stabilizer accounted for a disproportionate share of the total number. Flebogamma® 5% DIF does not contain sucrose.
(See *Dosage and Administration [2.3]* and *Warnings and Precautions [5.2]* for important information intended to reduce the risk of acute renal failure.)

1 INDICATIONS AND USAGE
Flebogamma® 5% DIF is an immune globulin intravenous (Human) 5% preparation that is indicated for the treatment of primary immune deficiency, such as common variable immunodeficiency, x-linked agammaglobulinemia, severe combined immunodeficiency, and Wiskott-Aldrich syndrome.

2 DOSAGE AND ADMINISTRATION
Intravenous Use Only

2.1 Preparation and Handling
- Flebogamma® 5% DIF should be inspected visually for particulate matter and color prior to administration. If particles are detected the vial shall not be used. Do not use if turbid.
- If large doses are to be administered, several vials of Flebogamma® 5% DIF may be pooled into an empty sterile IV solution container by using aseptic technique.
- Dilution with IV fluids is not recommended. Injection of other medications into intravenous tubing being used for Flebogamma® 5% DIF is not recommended.
- Specific drug interactions and incompatibilities have not been studied.
- Flebogamma® 5% DIF should be infused through a separate intravenous line. Do not add any medications or IV fluids to the Flebogamma® 5% DIF infusion container. Do not mix IGIV products of different formulations or from different manufacturers.
- According to international recommendations for infusion equipment for medical use, an in-line filter with a pore size of 15 to 20 microns is recommended for the infusion. Antibacterial filters (0.2 micron) may also be used, although they may slow infusions.
- Discard unused contents and administration devices after use.

2.2 Treatment of Primary Humoral Immunodeficiency (PI)
As there are significant differences in the half-life of IgG among patients with primary immunodeficiency, the frequency and amount of immunoglobulin therapy may vary from patient to patient. The proper amount can be determined by monitoring clinical response.

The usual dose of Flebogamma® 5% DIF for patients with PI is 300 to 600 mg/kg body weight (6.0 to 12.0 mL/kg) administered every 3 to 4 weeks. The dosage may be adjusted over time to achieve the desired trough IgG levels and clinical responses. No randomized controlled trial data are available to determine an optimum target trough serum IgG level.

2.3 Administration
The recommended initial infusion rate of Flebogamma® 5% DIF is 0.01 mL/kg body weight/minute (0.5 mg/kg/minute). If the infusion is well-tolerated, during the first 30 minutes, the rate may be gradually increased to a maximum of 0.10 mL/kg/minute (5 mg/kg/minute).

For patients judged to be at risk for developing renal dysfunction or thromboembolic events, Flebogamma® 5% DIF should be administered at the minimum infusion rate practicable. [See *Warnings and Precautions (5.2, 5.4)*]

Monitor patient vital signs throughout the infusion. Slow or stop infusion if adverse reactions occur. If symptoms subside promptly, the infusion may be resumed at a lower rate that is comfortable for the patient.

Any vial that has been entered should be used promptly. Partially used vials should be discarded and not saved for future use because the solution contains no preservative. Do not use if turbid. Solution that has been frozen should not be used.

3 DOSAGE FORMS AND STRENGTHS
- 0.5 g protein in 10 mL solution
- 2.5 g protein in 50 mL solution
- 5 g protein in 100 mL solution
- 10 g protein in 200 mL solution
- 20 g protein in 400 mL solution

4 CONTRAINDICATIONS
- Anaphylactic or severe reactions to human immune globulin.
- IgA deficient patients with antibodies against IgA and a history of hypersensitivity. (See *Warnings and Precautions [5.1]*)

5 WARNINGS AND PRECAUTIONS

5.1 Hypersensitivity
Severe hypersensitivity reactions may occur. In case of hypersensitivity, discontinue Flebogamma® 5% DIF infusion immediately and institute appropriate treatment. Have Epinephrine immediately available for treatment of acute severe hypersensitivity reactions.

Flebogamma® 5% DIF contains trace amounts of IgA (less than 50 µg/mL). Patients with known antibodies to IgA may have a greater risk of developing potentially severe hypersensitivity and anaphylactic reactions. Flebogamma® 5% DIF is contraindicated in patients with antibodies against IgA and a history of hypersensitivity reaction.

Rarely, Immune Globulin Intravenous (Human) can induce a severe fall in blood pressure with anaphylactic reaction, even in patients who had tolerated previous treatment with IGIV. In the case of shock, the current standard medical treatment for shock should be implemented.

5.2 Renal Failure
Assure that patients are not volume depleted prior to the initiation of the infusion of Flebogamma® 5% DIF.

Periodic monitoring of renal function and urine output is particularly important in patients judged to have a potential increased risk for developing acute renal failure *(1)*. Assess renal function, including measurement of BUN/serum creatinine, before the initial infusion of Flebogamma® 5% DIF and at appropriate intervals thereafter. If renal function deteriorates, consider discontinue use of the product.

For patients judged to be at risk for developing renal dysfunction, including patients with any degree of pre-existing renal insufficiency, diabetes mellitus, age greater than 65, volume depletion, sepsis, paraproteinemia, or patients receiving known nephrotoxic drugs, administer Flebogamma® 5% DIF at the minimum rate of infusion practicable (2). (See Boxed Warning) (See *Dosing and Administration [2.3]*)

5.3 Hyperproteinemia
Hyperproteinemia, increased serum viscosity and hyponatremia may occur in patients receiving Flebogamma® 5% DIF. It is clinically critical to distinguishing true hyponatremia from a pseudohyponatremia that is caused by a decreased calculated serum osmolarity or elevated osmolar gap because treatment aimed at decreasing serum free water in patients with pseudohyponatremia may lead to volume depletion, a further increase in serum viscosity and a higher risk of thrombotic events.

5.4 Thromboembolic Events
Thrombotic events may occur during or following IGIV treatment *(11 – 13)*. Patients at risk may include those with a history of atherosclerosis, multiple cardiovascular risk factors, advanced age, impaired cardiac output, coagulation disorders, prolonged periods of immobilization, or known/suspected hyperviscosity. Consider baseline assessment of blood viscosity in patients at risk for hyperviscosity, including those with cryoglobulins, fasting chylomicronemia/markedly high triacylglycerols (triglycerides), or monoclonal gammopathies. For patients judged to be at risk of developing thrombotic events, administer Flebogamma® 5% DIF at the minimum rate of infusion practicable.

5.5 Aseptic Meningitis Syndrome (AMS)
AMS may occur infrequently with IGIV treatment. Discontinuation of IGIV treatment has resulted in remission of AMS within several days without sequelae *(3 – 6)*. AMS usually begins within several hours to 2 days following IGIV treatment.

AMS is characterized by the following symptoms and signs: severe headache, nuchal rigidity, drowsiness, fever, photophobia, painful eye movements, nausea and vomiting. Cerebrospinal fluid (CSF) studies are frequently positive with pleocytosis up to several thousand cells per cubic milliliter, predominantly from the granulocytic series, and with elevated protein levels up to several hundred mg/dL. Provide a thorough neurological examination to patients exhibiting such symptoms and signs, including CSF studies, to rule out other causes of meningitis.

AMS may occur more frequently following high-dose (e.g., > 1.0 g/kg body weight) and/or rapid-infusion IGIV treatment. Patients with a history of migraine may be more susceptible. (See *Patient Counseling Information [17]*)

5.6 Hemolysis
Flebogamma® 5% DIF may contain blood group antibodies which may act as hemolysins and induce *in vivo* coating of red blood cells (RBC) with immunoglobulin, causing a positive direct antiglobulin reaction and, rarely, hemolysis (7 – 9). Hemolytic anemia may develop subsequent to Flebogamma® 5% DIF therapy due to enhanced RBC sequestration *(10)*.

Monitor patients for clinical signs and symptoms of hemolysis. If these are present after Flebogamma® 5% DIF infusion, perform appropriate confirmatory laboratory testing. (See *Patient Counseling Information [17]*)

5.7 Transfusion-Related Acute Lung Injury (TRALI)
Non-cardiogenic pulmonary edema may occur in patients following IGIV treatment *(14)*. This Transfusion-Related Acute Lung Injury (TRALI) is characterized by severe respiratory distress, pulmonary edema, hypoxemia, normal left ventricular function, and fever. Symptoms typically appear within 1 to 6 hours after transfusion.

Monitor patients for pulmonary adverse reactions. (See *Patient Counseling Information [17]*) If TRALI is suspected, perform appropriate tests for the presence of antineutrophil antibodies in both the product and patient serum.

Patients with TRALI may be managed by using oxygen therapy with adequate ventilatory support.

5.8 Infectious Disease Transmission
Flebogamma® 5% DIF is made from human plasma. Based on effective donor screening and product manufacturing processes, it carries an extremely remote risk of transmission of viral diseases. A theoretical risk for transmission of Creutzfeldt-Jakob disease (CJD) also is considered extremely remote. No cases of transmission of viral diseases or CJD have ever been identified for Flebogamma® 5% DIF. (See *Patient Counseling Information [17]*)

5.9 Laboratory Tests
After infusion of IgG, the transitory rise of the various passively transferred antibodies in the patient's blood may yield positive serological testing results, with the potential for misleading interpretation. Passive transmission of antibodies to erythrocyte antigens (e.g., A, B, and D) may cause a positive direct or indirect antiglobulin (Coombs') test.

Assess renal function, including measurement of BUN and serum creatinine, before the initial infusion of Flebogamma® 5% DIF and at appropriate intervals thereafter.

Consider baseline assessment of blood viscosity should be considered in patients at risk for hyperviscosity, including those with cryoglobulins, fasting chylomicronemia/markedly high triacylglycerols (triglycerides), or monoclonal gammopathies.

5.10 Special Care Precautions
All patients, but especially individuals receiving Flebogamma® 5% DIF for the first time or being restarted on the product after a treatment hiatus of more than 8 weeks, may be at a higher risk for the development of inflammatory reactions characterized by fever, chills, nausea, and vomiting. Careful monitoring of recipients and adherence to recommendations regarding information in the *Dosage and Administration [2.3]* section may reduce the risk of these types of events.

6 ADVERSE REACTIONS
The most common temporally related adverse reactions (≥ 5%) occurring during or within 72 hours of the end of an infusion observed for PI were: headache, chills, fever, shaking, fatigue, malaise, anxiety, back pain, muscle cramps, abdominal cramps, blood pressure changes, chest tightness, palpitations, tachycardia, nausea, vomiting, cutaneous reactions, wheezing, rash, arthralgia, and edema (see Table 1). The adverse reactions often begin within 60 minutes of the start of the infusion.

To report SUSPECTED ADVERSE REACTIONS, contact Grifols Biologicals at 1-888-GRIFOLS (1-888–474–3657) or FDA at 1-800-FDA-1 088 or www.fda.gov/medwatch.

6.1 Clinical Studies Experience
Because clinical trials are conducted under widely varying conditions, adverse reaction rates observed in the clinical trials of a drug cannot be directly compared to rates in the clinical trials of another drug and may not reflect the rates observed in clinical practice.

Adverse events were reported in a study of 46 individuals with primary humoral immunodeficiency diseases receiving infusions every 3 to 4 weeks of 300 to 600 mg/kg body weight. Forty-three (94%) subjects experienced at least 1 adverse event irrespective of the relationship with the product, and these subjects reported a total of 595 adverse events. None of the 46 subjects who participated in this study discontinued the study prematurely due to an adverse event considered related to the study drug. One subject had treatment-emergent bronchiestasis, mild, ongoing, after infusion #10; and one subject had recurrent moderate leucopenia after the 7th and 12th infusions.

Adverse events that occurred with an incidence of ≥ 5% on a per subject basis are summarized in Table 1.

Table 1. Adverse Events Occurring with an Incidence of ≥ 5% Irrespective of Causality

Adverse Event	Subjects (%) [N = 46]	Infusions* (%) [N = 709]
Sinusitis	20 (44)	5 (0.7)
Pyrexia	17 (37)	15 (2)
Headache	16 (35)	26 (4)
Upper respiratory tract infection	15 (33)	6 (0.8)
Combined bronchitis [1]	14 (30)	9 (1)
Cough or Productive cough	10 (22)	3 (0.4)
Diarrhoea	9 (20)	7 (1)
Pharyngitis	8 (17)	3 (0.4)
Asthma	8 (17)	0 (0)
Infusion site reaction [2]	7 (15)	13 (2)
Nasal congestion	7 (15)	0 (0)
Arthralgia	7 (15)	1 (0.1)
Nausea	6 (13)	3 (0.4)
Postnasal drip	6 (13)	2 (0.3)
Dizziness	6 (13)	1 (0.1)
Joint problems [3]	5 (11)	0 (0)
Rigors	5 (11)	6 (0.8)
Conjunctivitis	5 (11)	2 (0.3)
Nasopharyngitis	5 (11)	2 (0.3)
Rhinorrhea	5 (11)	3 (0.4)
Back pain	4 (9)	5 (0.7)
Dyspnoea	4 (9)	1 (0.1)
Abdominal pain	4 (9)	1 (0.1)
Gastroenteritis	4 (9)	0 (0)
Dermatitis contact	4 (9)	2 (0.3)
Urticaria	4 (9)	3 (0.4)
Anemia	4 (9)	1 (0.1)
Erythema	4 (9)	4 (0.6)
Myalgia	3 (7)	2 (0.3)
Pain	3 (7)	5 (0.7)
Fatigue	3 (7)	1 (0.1)
Wheezing	3 (7)	1 (0.1)
Dyspepsia	3 (7)	0 (0)
Toothache	3 (7)	1 (0.1)
Sinus congestion	3 (7)	1 (0.1)
Muscle strain	3 (7)	1 (0.1)
Thermal burn	3 (7)	1 (0.1)
Abrasion	3 (7)	0 (0)
Eczema	3 (7)	1 (0.1)
Rash papular	3 (7)	1 (0.1)

* Number of infusions for which AE onset occurred during an infusion or within 72 hours post-infusion.

[1] Includes reported preferred terms of Bronchiectasis NOS, Bronchitis NOS, and Bronchitis acute NOS.
[2] Corresponds to preferred term of Injection site reaction NOS. If combined to include Infusion site inflammation, Injection site oedema, Injection site pain, Injection site pruritis, Injection site reaction NOS, and Injection site swelling, there are 9 (20) subjects and 17 (2) infusions.
[3] Includes reported preferred terms of Bursitis, Chondromalacia patellae, Epicondylitis, Joint sprain, Joint swelling, Tenosynovitis, and Trigger finger.

The total number of AEs (regardless of attribution) reported whose onset were within 72 hours after the end of an infusion of Flebogamma® 5% DIF was 216. There were a total of 709 infusions, resulting in a rate of 0.305 (upper bound 95% CI=41.2%) temporally associated AEs per infusion. There were 144 infusions (20.1%, 1-sided 95% upper bound CI = 24.4%) associated with 1 or more AEs that began within 72 hours after the completion of an infusion.

A summary of infusions with mild, moderate, and severe treatment-related adverse events is in Table 2.

Table 2. Summary of Infusions with Mild, Moderate, and Severe Treatment-Related Adverse Events

Severity of AE	No. Infusions with AE	Adjusted %*	Confidence Interval†
Mild	58	7.9	10.4
Moderate	25	3.6	4.9
Severe	1	0.1	0.3

* Adjusted % = average of the % of infusions with a treatment-related adverse event for each individual subject.
† The 95% upper bound for the adjusted % of infusions for which at least 1 treatment-related adverse event was reported was derived by using the t-statistic.

The number and percent of subjects with treatment-emergent rises in AST or ALT are in Table 3.

Table 3. Number (%) of Subjects with Treatment-Emergent Rises in AST or ALT (N = 46)

Laboratory Test	Assessment Criteria	n	%
AST	Above 3× the ULN*	3	6.5
ALT	Above 3× the ULN	1	2.2

* ULN = upper limit of normal.

None of these subjects had a concomitant treatment-emergent rise in total bilirubin.

6.2 Post-marketing Experience

The following adverse reactions have been identified during the post-approval use of IGIV products, including Flebogamma® 5% DIF [see References [15]]. Because these reactions are reported voluntarily from a population of uncertain size, it is not always possible to reliably estimate the frequency or establish a casual relationship to exposure to the product.

Respiratory	Apnea, Acute Respiratory Distress Syndrome (ARDS), Transfusion-Related Acute Lung Injury (TRALI), cyanosis, hypoxemia, pulmonary edema, dyspnea, bronchospasm
Cardiovascular	Cardiac arrest, thromboembolism, vascular collapse, hypotension
Neurological	Coma, loss of consciousness, seizures, tremor
Integumentary	Stevens-Johnson Syndrome, epidermolysis, erythema multiformae, bullous dermatitis
Hematologic	Pancytopenia, leukopenia, hemolysis, positive direct antiglobulin (Coombs) test
Musculoskeletal	Back pain
Gastrointestinal	Hepatic dysfunction, abdominal pain
General/Body as a Whole	Pyrexia, rigors

7 DRUG INTERACTIONS

Immunoglobulin administration may transiently impair the efficacy of live viral vaccines, such as measles, mumps, and rubella. The immunizing physician should be informed of recent therapy with Flebogamma® 5% DIF so that appropriate measures may be taken. (See Patient Counseling Information [17])

8 USE IN SPECIFIC POPULATIONS

8.1 Pregnancy

Pregnancy Category C. Animal reproduction studies have not been performed with Flebogamma® 5% DIF. It is also not known whether Flebogamma® 5% DIF can cause fetal harm when administered to a pregnant woman or can affect reproduction capacity. Flebogamma® 5% DIF should be given to a pregnant woman only if clearly needed. Immunoglobulins cross the placenta from maternal circulation increasingly after 30 weeks of gestation.

8.4 Pediatric Use

Efficacy and safety in pediatric patients have not been established.

8.5 Geriatric Use

Subjects over 65 are at increased risk of renal failure with IGIV treatment. (See Boxed Warnings and Precautions [5.2]). For these subjects, and for any other subjects at risk of renal failure, the infusion rate of Flebogamma® 5% DIF should be limited to < 0.06 mL/kg/min (3 mg/kg/minute). Clinical studies of Flebogamma® 5% DIF did not include sufficient numbers of subjects over the age of 65, and therefore, the information available on these subjects is limited.

In patients over age 65 or in any patient at risk of developing renal insufficiency, do not exceed the recommended dose, and infuse Flebogamma® 5% DIF at the minimum infusion rate practicable.

11 DESCRIPTION

Immune Globulin Intravenous (Human), Flebogamma® 5% DIF (dual inactivation plus nanofiltration) (IGIV) is a ready to use, sterile, clear or slightly opalescent and colorless to pale yellow, liquid, preparation of highly purified immunoglobulin (IgG) obtained from human plasma pools. The purification process includes cold ethanol fractionation, polyethylene glycol precipitation, ion exchange chromatography, low pH treatment, pasteurization, solvent detergent treatment and Planova nanofiltration down to 20 nm filters.

Flebogamma® 5% DIF is a highly purified (≥ 97% IgG), unmodified, human IgG that contains the antibody specificities found in the donor population. IgG subclasses are fully represented with the following approximate percents of total IgG: IgG_1 is 66.6%, IgG_2, 28.5%, IgG_3, 2.7%, and IgG_4, 2.2%. Flebogamma® 5% DIF contains trace amounts of IgA (typically < 50 μg/mL) and IgM.

In the final formulation, Flebogamma® 5% DIF contains 5 g human normal immunoglobulin and 5 g D-sorbitol (as stabilizer) in 100 mL of water for injection, and ≤ 3 mg/mL polyethylene glycol. There is no preservative in the formulation. The pH of the solution ranges from 5 to 6 and the osmolarity from 240 to 370 mOsm/L, which is within the normal physiological range. The Fc and Fab functionality is maintained in Flebogamma® 5% DIF.

All Source Plasma used in the manufacture of Flebogamma® 5% DIF was collected only at FDA approved plasmapheresis centers in the United States and tested by FDA-licensed serological tests and found to be non-reactive (negative) for Hepatitis B Surface Antigen (HBsAg), antibodies to Hepatitis C Virus (HCV) and Human Immunodeficiency Virus (HIV) and negative on Nucleic Acid Test (NAT) for HCV and HIV. Additionally, NAT testing for the presence of HCV and HIV in the manufacturing plasma pool is also performed and found to be negative.

In addition, several manufacturing steps can contribute towards the safety of the final product. The effectiveness of these steps to remove or inactivate viruses from the product is evaluated through virus spiking experiments using a scaled down version of the manufacturing process. Virus elimination experiments have been performed on 7 steps of the production process.

Flebogamma® 5% DIF production process includes the following specific virus inactivation/removal steps:
• Pasteurization at 60 °C, 10 hours
• Solvent-Detergent treatment for 6 hours
• Nanofiltration down to 20 nm Planova filters

Grifols has developed a pasteurization method (heat treatment at 60 °C, 10 hours) using sorbitol as a stabilizer, which avoids denaturation of proteins and preserves antibody activity. Pasteurization achieves significant inactivation of both enveloped and non-enveloped viruses.

Solvent detergent treatment inactivates lipid coated potential viral contaminants such as HIV, HBV and HCV by destroying the lipid coat and the associated virus binding sites. By using this method, infection of the target cells and in-vivo virus replication is prevented.

Planova nanofiltration down to 20 nm pore size filter is included in the production process. This procedure eliminates potential viruses by a specific size exclusion mechanism. This has been shown to be effective in removing by more than $4 \log_{10}$ the virus of the smallest size assayed (porcine Parvovirus) by the smallest pore size nanofilter (20 nm).

Table 4. Flebogamma® 5% DIF: viral reduction capacity of combined steps (log₁₀)

Target virus	HIV-1, HIV-2 (env. RNA)	HBV, Herpesvirus (env. DNA)		HCV (env. RNA)		WNV (env. RNA)	HAV (non-env. RNA)	Virus B19 (non-env. DNA)
Model virus	HIV-1	PRV	IBR	BVDV	SINDBIS	WNV	EMC	PPV
Fraction I precipitation	< 1.00*	nd	nd	nd	nd	2.78	nd	< 1.00*
Ethanol incubation (Fraction II+III)	1.48	nd	nd	nd	nd	< 1.00*	nd	nd
PEG precipitation	≥ 6.10	≥ 5.92	nd	≥ 5.78	nd	nd	≥ 6.41	6.35
Acid pH treatment	2.47	≥ 5.32	nd	< 1.00*	nd	nd	1.36	na
Pasteurization	≥ 5.64	≥ 4.96	≥ 6.33	≥ 4.69	≥ 6.49	≥ 5.42	≥ 5.56	4.08
Solvent Detergent	≥ 4.61	≥ 6.95	nd	≥ 6.14	nd	≥ 5.59	na	na
Nanofiltration 20 nm	a	a	a	a	a	a	a	4.61
Overall Reduction Capacity	≥ 20.30	≥ 23.15	≥ 6.33	≥ 16.61	≥ 6.49	≥ 13.79	≥ 13.33	15.04

* When the RF is < 1 log₁₀, it is not taken into account for the calculation of the overall reduction capacity.
≥: No residual infectivity detected / nd: not done / na: non-applicable, since the virus is theoretically resistant to this treatment.
a) During the nanofiltration validation, 9 different viruses (HIV, PRV, BVDV, WNV, EMC, SV40, BEV, Echo 11 and PPV) were evaluated. Eight of these viruses were inactivated by the process conditions and/or removed by prefiltration. Only PPV, the virus of smallest size, was affected neither by the filtration conditions nor by the prefiltration and it was able to be assayed with the nanofilters.
Abbreviations: HIV; Human Immunodeficiency Virus, PRV; Pseudorabies Virus, IBR; Infectious Bovine Rhinotracheitis Virus, BVDV; Bovine Viral Diarrhoea Virus, SINDBIS; Sindbis Virus, WNV; West Nile Virus, EMC; Encephalomyocarditis Virus, PPV; Porcine Parvovirus.

Table 5. Pharmacokinetic Variables of Total IgG in Patients with PID

Variable	3-Week Dosing Interval (n=8)		4-Week Dosing Interval (n=12)	
	Mean	SD	Mean	SD
Cmax (mg/dL)	1,929	441	2,069	338
	[1,300-2,420]ᵃ		[1,590-2,800]	
AUC₀-last (day·mg/dL)	31,159	6,572	32,894	3,886
	[20,458-40,104]		[27,650-41,814]	
Clearance (mL/day)	139	57	109	33
	[81-243]		[59-161]	
Half-life (days)ᵇ	30	9	32	5
	[19-41]		[25-39]	
Trough IgG level (mg/dL)ᶜ	951.38	132.42	899.89	92.03
	[773.17-1,143.15]		[776.70-1,137.14]	

a. The numbers in brackets are the minimum and maximum values.
b. This half-life is an apparent value derived from a period of measurement of 28 days.
c. For subjects on the 3-week schedule, the average of the trough levels from Infusion 7 to the end of the study was calculated; for those on a 4-week schedule, the average of the trough levels from Infusion 5 to the end of the study was calculated. The means of the subject means are presented in this table.

The following purification processes can eliminate or inactivate a theoretical viral load as well:
• Fraction I precipitation
• Fraction II+III precipitation
• 4% PEG precipitation
• pH 4 treatment for 4 hours at 37 °C
The viral reduction data (in log₁₀) from these experiments are summarized in Table 4.
[See table 4 above]
Additionally, the manufacturing process was investigated for its capacity to decrease infectivity of an experimental agent of transmissible spongiform encephalopathy (TSE), considered as a model for the vCJD and CJD agents. Several of the individual production steps in Flebogamma® 5% DIF manufacturing process have been shown to decrease TSE infectivity of an experimental model agent. TSE reduction steps include: 4% Polyethylene glycol precipitation [≥ 6.19 log₁₀] and Planova nanofiltration down to 20 nm [≥ 5.45 log₁₀]. These studies provide reasonable assurance that low levels of CJD/vCJD agent infectivity, if present in the starting material, would be removed.

12 CLINICAL PHARMACOLOGY

12.1 Mechanism of Action
Flebogamma® 5% DIF supplies a broad spectrum of opsonic and neutralizing IgG antibodies against bacteria, viral, parasitic, and mycoplasma agents and their toxins. The mechanism of action in PI has not been fully elucidated.

12.2 Pharmacodynamics
Immunoglobulins are fractionated blood products made from pooled human plasma. Immunoglobulins are endogenous proteins produced by B lymphocyte cells. The main component of Flebogamma® 5% DIF is IgG (≥ 97%) and a sub-class distribution of IgG₁, IgG₂, IgG₃ and IgG₄ of approximately 66.6%, 28.5%, 2.7% and 2.2%, respectively.

12.3 Pharmacokinetics
In the clinical study assessing safety and efficacy in primary immunodeficiency disease (PI), Flebogamma® 5% DIF was administered as an IV infusion (300 to 600 mg/kg) to subjects with PI every 3 (n = 8) or 4 (n = 12) weeks for 12 months. The pharmacokinetics of total IgG was determined after the 7th infusion for the 3-week dosing interval and after the 5th infusion for the 4-week dosing interval (Table 5).

[See table 5 below]
There were 3 adolescent (≤ 16 years of age) subjects who underwent pharmacokinetic testing, all of whom were on the 3-week infusion schedule. There were no clinically relevant differences among the adults and adolescents that were tested.

13 NONCLINICAL TOXICOLOGY

13.1 Carcinogenity, Mutagenesis, Impairment of Fertility
No animal studies were conducted to evaluate the carcinogenic or mutagenic effect of Flebogamma® 5% DIF or its effects on fertility.

13.2 Toxicology and/or Pharmacology
Acute toxicity studies were performed in mice and rats at doses up to 2.5 g/kg body weight with infusion rates 6 to 30 times higher than the maximum rates recommended for humans. Although the NOAEL was not determined, no relevant adverse effects could be confirmed affecting respiratory, circulatory, renal, autonomic and central nervous systems, somatomotor activity, and behavior of the treated mice and rats.
Five out of the 25 rats treated with the highest dose at approximately 8 times the maximum infusion rate recommended for humans, showed a transient "reddish urine" sign which was not confirmed as a relevant toxicity causing phenomenon after renal macro and microscopical analysis. This phenomenon was associated to hemolysis when serum was analyzed, suggesting a possible relation to cross reactivity of rodent red cells with human antibodies. No "reddish urine" was detected in any mouse, a much smaller animal where the rate of infusion is comparatively much higher than in rats. The macroscopic inspection of all treated mice did not show any renal alteration either.

14 CLINICAL STUDIES
A multicenter, open-label, historically controlled study was conducted in the United States to assess the efficacy, safety and pharmacokinetics of Flebogamma® 5% DIF in adult and pediatric subjects with PI. A total of 46 patients aged 15-75 years (63% male, 37% female) were enrolled, and were treated with Flebogamma® 5% DIF at a dose of 300-600 mg/kg per infusion every 3 or 4 weeks for 12-months.
During the study period, the annual rate of acute serious bacterial infection, the key efficacy variable, defined as bacterial pneumonia, bacteremia or sepsis, osteomyelitis/septic arthritis, visceral abscesses and bacterial meningitis per subject per year, was 0.021 (with an upper 1-sided 98% confidence interval of 0.001 to 0.112). One subject had one episode of bacterial pneumonia and there were no other episodes of serious bacterial infections reported (Table 6).
[See table 6 at top of next page]
The number of days of work/school missed, the number of hospitalizations and the number of days of each hospitalization, the number of visits to physicians or emergency rooms, the number of other infections documented by positive radiographic findings and fever, and the number of days of therapeutic and prophylactic oral/parenteral antibiotic use was also monitored. These additional efficacy variables were annualized by using the subject-years exposure data only of those subjects experiencing the endpoints, not the entire study cohort. With regard to the number of other validated infections, the mean rate was less than 2 days/subject/year. (The calculation uses all subjects, including those who had no infections, see Table 7)

Table 7. Summary of Secondary Efficacy Variables

Variable	Subjects		Mean number of events, days or visits/ subject/year [1]
	N	%	
Work/school days missed	23	50.0	12.95
Days of normal activities missed	18	39.1	7.28
Days in hospital	4	8.7	0.77
Visits to physician/ER	29	63.0	4.31
Number of other documented infectious episodes	33	71.7	1.96
Days of therapeutic oral antibiotic use	35	76.1	55.52
Days of therapeutic parenteral antibiotic use	2	4.3	0.14

Table 6. Summary of Bacterial Infections (Intention-to-Treat Population, N = 46)

Infections	Patients (N=46) N (%)	Episodes	Estimates [1]	98% CI [2]
Bacterial pneumonia	1 (2.2)	1		
Bacteremia or sepsis	0 (0.0)	0		
Osteomyelitis/septic arthritis	0 (0.0)	0		
Bacterial meningitis	0 (0.0)	0		
Total Patients	1 (2.2)	1	0.021	(0.001-0.112)

[1] Estimate = Total episodes/Total patient years.
[2] The confidence interval is obtained by using a generalized linear model procedure for Poisson distribution.

Days of other therapeutic antibiotic use	16	34.8	44.30
Days of prophylactic oral antibiotic use	19	41.3	81.08
Days of prophylactic parenteral antibiotic use	1	2.3	0.02
Days of other prophylactic antibiotic use	0	0.0	0.00

[1] Days of work/school missed per patient year are derived as total days of work/school missed divided by total days in study multiplied by 365. If data are missing for a period (e.g., between Infusion 2 and Infusion 3), then number of days in this period is not counted in the denominator. All other endpoints are derived similarly.

The dosing statistics for this study are in Table 8.

Table 8. Statistical Summary of the Mean Total Dose (mg/kg) of Flebogamma® 5% DIF Administered Per Infusion

Statistic	3-Week Dosing Interval	4-Week Dosing Interval	Total
N	13	33	46
Mean (SD)	451 (98.72)	448 (81.93)	449 (85.96)
Median	440	453	449
Q1, Q3[a]	384.2, 540.5	379.5, 511.1	380.9, 518.8
Min, Max	288.4, 588.2	298.2, 591.1	288.4, 591.1

a. Q1 is the 25th percentile, and Q3 is the 75th percentile.

15　REFERENCES

1. Cayco AV, Perazella MA, Hayslett JP. Renal insufficiency after intravenous immune globulin therapy: a report of two cases and an analysis of the literature. *J Am Soc Nephrol* 1997; 8:1788-94.
2. Tan E, Hajinazarian M, Bay W, et al. Acute renal failure resulting from intravenous immunoglobulin therapy. *Arch Neurol* 1993; 50:137-9.
3. Sekul EA, Cupler EJ, Dalakas MC. Aseptic meningitis associated with high-dose intravenous immunoglobulin therapy: frequency and risk factors. *Ann Intern Med* 1994; 121:259-62.
4. Kato E, Shindo S, Eto Y, et al. Administration of immune globulin associated with aseptic meningitis. *JAMA* 1988; 259:3269-71.
5. Casteels-Van Daele M, Wijndaele L, Hanninck K, et al. Intravenous immune globulin and acute aseptic meningitis. *N Engl J Med* 1990; 323:614-5.
6. Scribner CL, Kapit RM, Phillips ET, et al. Aseptic meningitis and intravenous immunoglobulin therapy. *Ann Intern Med* 1994; 121:305-6.
7. Copelan EA, Strohm PL, Kennedy MS, et al. Hemolysis following intravenous immune globulin therapy. *Transfusion* 1986; 26:410-2.
8. Thomas MJ, Misbah SA, Chapel HM, et al. Hemolysis after high-dose intravenous Ig. *Blood* 1993; 15:3789.
9. Reinhart WH, Berchtold PE. Effect of high-dose intravenous immunoglobulin therapy on blood rheology. *Lancet* 1992; 339:662-4.
10. Kessary-Shoham H, Levy Y, Shoenfeld Y, et al. In vivo administration of intravenous immunoglobulin (IVIG) can lead to enhanced erythrocyte sequestration. *J Autoimmune* 1999; 13:129-35.
11. Dalakas MC. High-dose intravenous immunoglobulin and serum viscosity: risk of precipitating thromboembolic events. *Neurology* 1994; 44:223-6.
12. Woodruff RK, Grigg AP, Firkin FC, et al. Fatal thrombotic events during treatment of autoimmune thrombocytopenia with intravenous immunoglobulin in elderly patients. *Lancet* 1986; ii:217-8.
13. Wolberg AS, Kon RH, Monroe DM, et al. Coagulation factor XI is a contaminant in intravenous immunoglobulin preparations. *Am J Hematol* 2000; 65:30-4.
14. Rizk A, Gorson KC, Kenney L, et al. Transfusion-related acute lung injury after the infusion of IVIG. *Transfusion* 2001; 41:264-8.
15. Winward DB, Brophy MT. Acute renal failure after administration of intravenous immunoglobulin: review of the literature and case report. *Pharmacotherapy* 1995; 15:765-72.
16. Phillips AO. Renal failure and intravenous immunoglobulin. *Clin Nephrol* 1992; 37:217.
17. Pierce LR, Jain N. Risks associated with the use of intravenous immunoglobulin. *Transfus Med Rev* 2003; 17:241-51.
18. Waldmann TA, Strober W. Metabolism of immunoglobulins. *Prog Allergy* 1969; 13:1-110.
19. Morrell A, Riesen W. Structure, function and catabolism of immunoglobulins. In: Nydegger UE, editor. Immunohemotherapy. London: Academic Press; 1981, p. 17-26.
20. Stiehm ER. Standard and special human immune serum globulins as therapeutic agents. *Pediatrics* 1979; 63:301–19.
21. Buckley RH. Immunoglobulin replacement therapy: indications and contraindications for use and variable IgG levels achieved. In: Alving BM, Finlayson JS, editors. Immunoglobulins: characteristics and use of intravenous preparations. Washington DC: US Department of Health and Human Services; 1979, p. 3-8.

16　HOW SUPPLIED/STORAGE AND HANDLING

Flebogamma® 5% DIF is supplied in single-use, individually laser etched vials containing the labeled amount of functionally active IgG.
The following dosage forms are available:

NDC Number	Size	Grams Protein
61953-0004-1	10 mL	0.5 g
61953-0004-2	50 mL	2.5 g
61953-0004-3	100 mL	5.0 g
61953-0004-4	200 mL	10.0 g
61953-0004-5	400 mL	20.0 g

Each vial has an integral suspension band and a label with two peel-off strips showing the product name and lot number.
When stored at room temperature (up to 25 °C [77 °F]), Flebogamma® 5% DIF is stable for 24 months, as indicated by the expiration date printed on the outer carton and container label. Store at +2 to +25 °C (36 to 77 °F). Do not freeze. Discard after expiration date.

17　PATIENT COUNSELING INFORMATION

Inform patients to immediately report the following to their physician:
- Decreased urine output, sudden weight gain, fluid retention/edema, and/or shortness of breath. (See *Renal Failure [5.2]*)
- Severe headache, neck stiffness, drowsiness, fever, sensitivity to light, painful eye movements, nausea, and vomiting. (See *Aseptic Meningitis Syndrom [5.5]*)
- Fatigue, increased heart rate, yellowing of the skin or eyes, and dark-colored urine. (See Hemolysis *[5.6]*)
- Trouble breathing, chest pain, blue lips or extremities, fever. (See TRALI *[5.7]*)

Inform patients that Flebogamma® 5% DIF is made from human plasma and may contain infectious agents that can cause disease. Explain that the risk Flebogamma® 5% DIF may transmit an infectious agent has been reduced by screening plasma donors for prior exposure to certain viruses, by testing the donated plasma for certain virus infections and by inactivating and/or removing certain viruses during manufacturing (see *Warnings and Precautions [5.8]*). Patients should report any symptoms that concern them.
Inform patients that Flebogamma® 5% DIF may interfere with their immune response to live viral vaccines (i.e., MMR) and instruct patients to notify their health care provider of this potential interaction when they are receiving vaccinations. It is recommended that the lot number of the vials used be recorded when Flebogamma® 5% DIF is administered.

Manufactured by INSTITUTO GRIFOLS, S.A.
BARCELONA - SPAIN
U.S. License No. 1181
Distributed by GRIFOLS BIOLOGICALS Inc.
LOS ANGELES - CA 90032
Phone: 1-888-GRIFOLS (1-888-474-3657)

Flebogamma® 10% DIF　　　　Ŗ

[fle-bo-gam-ma]
Immune Globulin Intravenous (Human), 10% Liquid preparation

HIGHLIGHTS OF PRESCRIBING INFORMATION
These highlights do not include all the information needed to use Flebogamma® 10% DIF safely and effectively. See full prescribing information for Flebogamma® 10% DIF, Immune Globulin Intravenous (Human), 10% Liquid preparation
Initial U.S. Approval: 2010

> **WARNING: ACUTE RENAL DYSFUNCTION AND FAILURE**
> *See full prescribing information for complete boxed warning.*
> - Renal dysfunction, acute renal failure, osmotic nephrosis, and death may occur with the administration of human immune globulin intravenous (IGIV) products.
> - Renal dysfunction and acute renal failure occur more commonly in patients receiving IGIV products that contain sucrose. Flebogamma® 10% DIF does not contain sucrose.
> - For patients at risk of renal dysfunction or failure, administer Flebogamma® 10% DIF at the minimum infusion rate practicable.

INDICATIONS AND USAGE
Flebogamma® 10% DIF is a human immune globulin intravenous (IGIV) indicated for the treatment of primary humoral immunodeficiency (PI).

DOSAGE AND ADMINISTRATION

For Intravenous Use Only

Indication	Dose	Initial Infusion Rate	Maintenance Infusion Rate (if tolerated)
PI	300-600 mg/kg every 3 - 4 weeks	0.01 mL/kg/minute (1 mg/kg/min)	0.08 mL/kg/minute (8 mg/kg/min)

Ensure that patients with pre-existing renal insufficiency are not volume depleted; discontinue Flebogamma® 10% DIF if renal function deteriorates. [5.2]
For patients at risk of renal dysfunction or thrombotic events, administer Flebogamma® 10% DIF at the minimum infusion rate practicable. [5.2, 5.4]

DOSAGE FORMS AND STRENGTHS
Flebogamma® 10% DIF is a liquid solution containing 10% IgG (100 mg/mL).

CONTRAINDICATIONS
- History of anaphylactic or severe systemic reactions to human immunoglobulin. [4]
- IgA deficient patients with antibodies against IgA and a history of hypersensitivity. [4]

WARNINGS AND PRECAUTIONS
- IgA deficient patients with antibodies to IgA are at greater risk of developing severe hypersensitivity and anaphylactic reactions. [5.1]

- Monitor renal function, including blood urea nitrogen, serum creatinine, and urine output in patients at risk of developing acute renal failure. [5.2]
- Hyperproteinemia, increased serum viscosity and hyponatremia may occur in patients receiving Flebogamma® 10% DIF therapy. [5.3]
- Thrombotic events may occur. Monitor patients with known risk factors for thrombotic events; consider baseline assessment of blood viscosity for those at risk for hyperviscosity. [5.4]
- Aseptic Meningitis Syndrome (AMS) may occur in patients receiving Flebogamma® 10% DIF therapy, especially with high doses or rapid infusion. [5.5]
- Hemolytic anemia can develop subsequent to Flebogamma® 10% DIF treatment. Monitor patients for hemolysis and hemolytic anemia. [5.6]
- Monitor patients for pulmonary adverse reactions (transfusion-related acute lung injury, TRALI). [5.7]
- Patients receiving Flebogamma® 10% DIF for the first time or being restarted on the product after a treatment hiatus of more than 8 weeks may be at a higher risk for development of fever, chills, nausea, and vomiting. [5.8]
- Flebogamma® 10% DIF is made from human plasma and may contain infectious agents, e.g., viruses and, theoretically, the Creutzfeldt-Jakob disease (CJD) agent. [5.9]
- Passive transfer of antibodies may confound serologic testing. [5.11]

ADVERSE REACTIONS

The most common adverse reactions reported in greater than 5% of subjects were headache, chills, fever, shaking, fatigue, malaise, anxiety, back pain, muscle cramps, abdominal cramps, blood pressure changes, chest tightness, palpitations, tachycardia, nausea, vomiting, cutaneous reactions, wheezing, rash, arthralgia and edema. [6]

Serious adverse reactions included back pain, chest discomfort, headache, chest pain, maculopathy, rigors, tachycardia, and vasovagal syncope.

To report SUSPECTED ADVERSE REACTIONS, contact Grifols Biologicals at 1-888-GRIFOLS (1-888-474-3657) or FDA at 1-800-FDA-1088 or www.fda.gov/medwatch.

DRUG INTERACTIONS

Passive transfer of antibodies may transiently interfere with the immune response to live virus vaccines, such as measles, mumps, and rubella. [7]

USE IN SPECIFIC POPULATIONS

- Pregnancy: No human or animal data. Use only if clearly needed. [8.1]
- Geriatric: In patients over age 65 or in any patient at risk of developing renal insufficiency, do not exceed the recommended dose, and infuse Flebogamma® 10% DIF at the minimum infusion rate practicable. [8.5]

See 17 for PATIENT COUNSELING INFORMATION

Revised: 07/2010

FULL PRESCRIBING INFORMATION: CONTENTS*

WARNING: ACUTE RENAL DYSFUNCTION AND ACUTE RENAL FAILURE

* Sections or subsections omitted from the full prescribing information are not listed.

FULL PRESCRIBING INFORMATION

Flebogamma® 10% DIF
Immune Globulin Intravenous (Human)
10% Liquid Preparation

> **WARNING: ACUTE RENAL DYSFUNCTION AND ACUTE RENAL FAILURE**
>
> - Use of immune globulin intravenous (IGIV) products, particularly those containing sucrose, has been reported to be associated with renal dysfunction, acute renal failure, osmotic nephropathy, and death (1). Patients at risk of acute renal failure include those with any degree of pre-existing renal insufficiency, diabetes mellitus, advanced age (above 65 years of age), volume depletion, sepsis, paraproteinemia, or those receiving known nephrotoxic drugs (see Warnings and Precautions [5.2]). Flebogamma® 10% DIF does not contain sucrose.
> - For patients at risk of renal dysfunction or failure, administer Flebogamma® 10% DIF at the minimum infusion rate practicable (see Dosage and Administration [2.3], Warnings and Precautions [5.2]).

1   INDICATIONS AND USAGE

Flebogamma® 10% DIF is a human immune globulin intravenous (IGIV) that is indicated for the treatment of primary immune deficiency (PI) including the humoral immune defect in common variable immunodeficiency, x-linked agammaglobulinemia, severe combined immunodeficiency, and Wiskott-Aldrich syndrome.

2.   DOSAGE AND ADMINISTRATION

For Intravenous Use Only

2.1   Preparation and Handling

- Flebogamma® 10% DIF is a clear or slightly opalescent, colorless solution. Inspect the drug product visually for particulate matter and discoloration prior to administration, whenever solution and container permit. Do not use if the solution is cloudy, turbid, or if it contains particulates.
- Do not shake.
- Do not freeze.
- Flebogamma® 10% DIF should be administered at room temperature.
- The vial is for single use only.
- Flebogamma® 10% DIF contains no preservative. Once the vial has been entered under aseptic conditions, its contents should be used promptly. Because the solution contains no preservative, Flebogamma® 10% DIF should be infused as soon as possible.
- Do not mix Flebogamma® 10% DIF with other IGIV products or other intravenous medications.
- Infuse Flebogamma® 10% DIF using a separate infusion line.
- If larger doses of Flebogamma® 10% DIF are to be administered, several vials may be pooled into sterile infusion bags using aseptic technique.

2.2   Dose

As there are significant differences in the half-life of IgG among patients with PI, the frequency and amount of immunoglobulin therapy may vary from patient to patient. Dosing should be adjusted according to the clinical response.

The recommended dose of Flebogamma® 10% DIF for patients with PI is 300 to 600 mg/kg body weight (3.0 to 6.0 mL/kg), administered every 3 to 4 weeks. Adjust the dosage over time to achieve the desired serum trough levels and clinical responses. No randomized controlled trial data are available to determine an optimum target trough serum IgG level.

2.3   Administration

It has been reported that the frequency of adverse drug reactions to IGIV increases with the infusion rate. Initial infusion rates should be slow. If there are no adverse drug reactions, the infusion rate for subsequent infusions can be slowly increased to the maximum rate. For patients experiencing adverse drug reactions, it is advisable to reduce the infusion rate in subsequent infusions, or administer IGIV at a 5% concentration.

Table 1. Recommended Infusion Rates for Flebogamma® 10% DIF

Indication	Dose	Initial Infusion Rate	Maintenance Infusion Rate (if tolerated)
PI	300-600 mg/kg every 3 - 4 weeks	0.01 mL/kg/minute (1 mg/kg/min)	0.08 mL/kg/minute (8 mg/kg/min)

Monitor patient vital signs throughout the infusion. Slow or stop infusion if adverse reactions occur. If symptoms subside promptly, the infusion may be resumed at a lower rate that is comfortable for the patient.

Ensure that patients with pre-existing renal insufficiency are not volume depleted. For patients judged to be at risk for renal dysfunction or thrombotic events, administer Flebogamma® 10% DIF at the minimum infusion rate practicable, and consider discontinuation of administration if renal function deteriorates (see Warnings and Precautions [5.2, 5.4]).

3.   DOSAGE FORMS AND STRENGTHS

Flebogamma® 10% DIF is a liquid solution containing 10% IgG (100 mg/mL).

4   CONTRAINDICATIONS

- Flebogamma® 10% DIF is contraindicated in patients who have had a history of anaphylactic or severe systemic reactions to the administration of human immune globulin.
- Flebogamma® 10% DIF is contraindicated in IgA deficient patients with antibodies to IgA and a history of hypersensitivity.

5   WARNINGS AND PRECAUTIONS

- Weigh the potential risks and benefits of Flebogamma® 10% DIF against those of alternative therapies in all patients for whom Flebogamma® 10% DIF is being considered.
- Before prescribing Flebogamma® 10% DIF, the physician should discuss risks and benefits of its use with patients.

5.1   Hypersensitivity

Severe hypersensitivity reactions may occur (see Contraindications [4]). In case of hypersensitivity, discontinue Flebogamma® 10% DIF infusion immediately and institute appropriate treatment. Medications such as epinephrine should be available for immediate treatment of acute hypersensitivity reactions.

Flebogamma® 10% DIF contains trace amounts of IgA (less than 100 µg/mL) (see Description [11]). Patients with antibodies to IgA have a greater risk of developing potentially severe hypersensitivity and anaphylactic reactions. Flebogamma® 10% DIF is contraindicated in patients with antibodies against IgA and a history of hypersensitivity reaction (see Contraindications [4]).

5.2   Renal Dysfunction/Failure

Acute renal dysfunction/failure, osmotic nephropathy, and death may occur upon use of Flebogamma® 10% DIF. Ensure that patients are not volume-depleted before administering Flebogamma® 10% DIF. In patients who are at risk of developing renal dysfunction because of pre-existing renal insufficiency or predisposition to acute renal failure (such as diabetes mellitus, age greater than 65 years, volume depletion, sepsis, paraproteinemia, use of concomitant nephrotoxic drugs, etc.), administer Flebogamma® 10% DIF at the minimum rate of infusion practicable (2) (see Dosage and Administration [2.3]).

Periodic monitoring of renal function and urine output is particularly important in patients judged to be at increased risk of developing acute renal failure (1). Assess renal function, including measurement of blood urea nitrogen (BUN) and serum creatinine, before the initial infusion of Flebogamma® 10% DIF and at appropriate intervals thereafter. If renal function deteriorates, consider discontinue use of Flebogamma® 10% DIF.

5.3   Hyperproteinemia, Increased Serum Viscosity, and Hyponatremia

Hyperproteinemia, increased serum viscosity and hyponatremia may occur in patients receiving Flebogamma® 10% DIF therapy. It is clinically critical to distinguish true hyponatremia from a pseudohyponatremia that is temporally or causally related to hyperproteinemia with concomitant decreased calculated serum osmolarity or elevated osmolar gap, because treatment aimed at decreasing serum free water in patients with pseudohyponatremia may lead to volume depletion, a further increase in serum viscosity and a higher risk of thrombotic events.

5.4   Thrombotic Events

Thrombotic events may occur during or following treatment with Flebogamma® 10% DIF (8-10). Patients at risk include those with a history of atherosclerosis, multiple cardiovascular risk factors, advanced age, impaired cardiac output, coagulation disorders, prolonged periods of immobilization, and known or suspected hyperviscosity.

Consider baseline assessment of blood viscosity in patients at risk for hyperviscosity, including those with cryoglobulins, fasting chylomicronemia/markedly high triacylglycerols (triglycerides), or monoclonal gammopathies. For patients judged to be at risk of developing thrombotic events, administer Flebogamma® 10% DIF at the minimum rate of infusion practicable (see Dosage and Administration [2.3]).

5.5   Aseptic Meningitis Syndrome (AMS)
AMS may occur infrequently with Flebogamma® 10% DIF treatment. Discontinuation of IGIV treatment has resulted in remission of AMS within several days without sequelae (3-4).

AMS is characterized by the following signs and symptoms: severe headache, nuchal rigidity, drowsiness, fever, photophobia, painful eye movements, nausea, and vomiting (see Patient Counseling Information [17]). Cerebrospinal fluid (CSF) studies frequently reveal pleocytosis up to several thousand cells per cubic millimeter, predominantly from the granulocytic series and elevated protein levels up to several hundred mg/dL, but negative culture results. Conduct a thorough neurological examination to patients exhibiting such signs and symptoms, including CSF studies, to rule out other causes of meningitis.

AMS may occur more frequently following high doses (2 g/kg) and/or rapid infusion of IGIV.

5.6   Hemolysis
Flebogamma® 10% DIF may contain blood group antibodies that can act as hemolysins and induce in vivo coating of red blood cells (RBCs) with immunoglobulin, causing a positive direct antiglobulin reaction and hemolysis (5-6). Delayed hemolytic anemia may develop subsequent to Flebogamma® 10% DIF therapy due to enhanced RBC sequestration (7), and acute hemolysis, consistent with intravascular hemolysis, has been reported.

Monitor patients for clinical signs and symptoms of hemolysis. If signs and/or symptoms of hemolysis are present after Flebogamma® 10% DIF infusion, perform appropriate confirmatory laboratory testing (see Patient Counseling Information [17]).

5.7   Transfusion-Related Acute Lung Injury (TRALI)
Non-cardiogenic pulmonary edema may occur in patients following Flebogamma® 10% DIF treatment (11). TRALI is characterized by severe respiratory distress, pulmonary edema, hypoxemia, normal left ventricular function, and fever. Symptoms typically appear within 1 to 6 hours following treatment.

Monitor patients for pulmonary adverse reactions (see Patient Counseling Information [17]). If TRALI is suspected, perform appropriate tests for the presence of anti-neutrophil antibodies and anti-HLA antibodies in both the product and patient serum. TRALI may be managed using oxygen therapy with adequate ventilatory support.

5.8   Infusion Reactions
All patients, but especially individuals receiving Flebogamma® 10% DIF for the first time or being restarted on the product after a treatment hiatus of more than 8 weeks, may be at a higher risk for the development of fever, chills, nausea, and vomiting. Careful monitoring of recipients and adherence to recommendations regarding dosage and administration may reduce the risk of these types of events (see Dosage and Administration [2.3]).

5.9   Transmissible Infectious Agents
Because Flebogamma® 10% DIF is made from human plasma, it may carry a risk of transmitting infectious agents, e.g., viruses, and theoretically, the Creutzfeldt-Jakob (CJD) agent. No cases of transmission of viral diseases or CJD have ever been identified for Flebogamma® 10% DIF. All infections suspected by a physician possibly to have been transmitted by this product should be reported by the physician or other healthcare provider to Grifols Biologicals at 1-888-474-3657. Before prescribing or administering Flebogamma® 10% DIF, the physician should discuss the risks and benefits of its use with the patient (see Patient Counseling Information [17]).

5.10   Monitoring: Laboratory Tests
• Periodic monitoring of renal function and urine output is particularly important in patients judged to be at increased risk of developing acute renal failure. Assess renal function, including measurement of BUN and serum creatinine, before the initial infusion of Flebogamma® 10% DIF and at appropriate intervals thereafter.
• Consider baseline assessment of blood viscosity in patients at risk for hyperviscosity, including those with cryoglobulins, fasting chylomicronemia/markedly high triacylglycerols (triglycerides), or monoclonal gammopathies, because of the potentially increased risk of thrombosis.
• If signs and/or symptoms of hemolysis are present after an infusion of Flebogamma® 10% DIF, perform appropriate laboratory testing for confirmation.

• If TRALI is suspected, perform appropriate tests for the presence of anti-neutrophil antibodies and anti-HLA antibodies in both the product and patient's serum.

5.11   Interference with Laboratory Tests
After infusion of IgG, the transitory rise of the various passively transferred antibodies in the patient's blood may yield positive serological testing results, with the potential for misleading interpretation. Passive transmission of antibodies to erythrocyte antigens (e.g., A, B, and D) may cause a positive direct or indirect antiglobulin (Coombs') test.

6   ADVERSE REACTIONS
Serious adverse reactions observed with Flebogamma® 10% DIF were back pain, chest discomfort, headache, chest pain, maculopathy, rigors, tachycardia, bacterial pneumonia, and vasovagal syncope.

The most common adverse reactions (reported in ≥ 5% of clinical trial subjects) occurring during or within 72 hours of the end of an infusion were headache, chills, fever, shaking, fatigue, malaise, anxiety, back pain, muscle cramps, abdominal cramps, blood pressure changes, chest tightness, palpitations, tachycardia, nausea, vomiting, cutaneous reactions, wheezing, rash, arthralgia, and edema (see Tables 2 and 3).

6.1   Clinical Trials Experience
Because clinical trials are conducted under widely varying conditions, adverse reaction rates observed in the clinical trials of a drug cannot be directly compared to rates in the clinical trials of another drug and may not reflect the rates observed in clinical practice.

In a multicenter, open-label, non-randomized, historically controlled clinical study, 46 individuals with primary humoral immunodeficiency received infusion doses of Flebogamma® 10% DIF at 300 to 600 mg/kg body weight every 3 weeks (mean dose 469 mg/kg) or 4 weeks (mean dose 457 mg/kg) for up to 12 months (see Clinical Studies [14.1]). Routine pre-medication was not allowed. Of the 601 infusions administered, 130 infusions (22%) in 21 (47%) subjects were given pre-medications (antipyretic, antihistamine, or antiemetic agent) because of experience with consecutive infusion-related adverse reactions.

One subject experienced four serious adverse events (AEs, bacterial pneumonia, subcutaneous abscess and two episodes of cellulitis) and withdrew from the study. Two other subjects who participated in the study discontinued prematurely due to AEs (back pain/chest pain/headache; and chills/tachycardia). Three subjects experienced four serious non-related AEs (drug abuse/depression; hernia; and sinusitis).

Forty-five (98%) subjects experienced at least 1 AE irrespective of the relationship with the product, and these subjects reported a total of 723 AEs. Thirty-eight subjects (83%) had an adverse reaction at some time during the study that was considered product-related. Of the 21 subjects receiving premedications, 12 (57%) subjects reported adverse reactions during or within 72 hours after the infusion in 48 of the 130 pre-medicated infusions (37%).

Table 2. Treatment-related Adverse Events Occurring in ≥ 5% of Subjects with PI during a Flebogamma® 10% DIF Infusion or within 72 Hours after the End of an infusion

Adverse Event	Subjects (%) [N=46]	Infusions (%) [N=601]
Headache	24 (52%)	67 (11%)
Rigors	17 (37%)	37 (6%)
Pyrexia	15 (33%)	27 (5%)
Tachycardia	10 (22%)	18 (3%)
Hypotension	9 (20%)	11 (2%)
Back pain	8 (17%)	27 (5%)
Myalgia	8 (17%)	17 (3%)
Body temperature increased	4 (9%)	6 (1%)
Nausea	4 (9%)	6 (1%)
Pain	4 (9%)	8 (1%)
Chest discomfort	3 (7%)	4 (1%)
Chest pain	3 (7%)	5 (1%)
Infusion site reaction	3 (7%)	4 (1%)
Pain in extremity	3 (7%)	3 (0.5%)

The total number of adverse events occurring during or within 72 hours after the end of an infusion, irrespective of causality, was 359, excluding non-serious infections.

Table 3 lists the AEs that occurred in greater than 5% of subjects during a Flebogamma® 10% DIF infusion or within 72 hours after the end of an infusion, irrespective of causality.

Table 3. Adverse Events Occurring in ≥ 5% of Subjects with PI during a Flebogamma® 10% DIF Infusion or within 72 Hours after the End of an infusion, Irrespective of Causality

Adverse Event	Subjects (%) [N=46]	Infusions (%) [N=601]
Headache	28 (61%)	71 (12%)
Pyrexia	17 (37%)	27 (5%)
Rigors	17 (37%)	37 (6%)
Back pain	13 (28%)	29 (5%)
Cough or Productive cough	12 (26%)	5 (1%)
Nausea	12 (26%)	8 (1%)
Hypotension	10 (22%)	13 (2%)
Tachycardia	10 (22%)	19 (3%)
Myalgia	9 (20%)	17 (3%)
Diarrhea	8 (17%)	2 (0.3%)
Infusion site reaction	8 (17%)	8 (1%)
Pharyngolaryngeal pain	7 (15%)	3 (1%)
Nasal congestion	7 (15%)	2 (0.3%)
Postnasal drip	7 (15%)	4 (1%)
Arthralgia	6 (13%)	2 (0.3%)
Conjunctivitis	6 (13%)	2 (0.3%)
Pain	6 (13%)	10 (2%)
Vomiting	6 (13%)	0 (0%)
Dizziness	5 (11%)	3 (1%)
Fatigue	5 (11%)	1 (0.2%)
Urinary tract infection	5 (11%)	4 (1%)
Chest pain	5 (11%)	4 (1%)
Ear pain	5 (11%)	1 (0.2%)
Pain in extremity	5 (11%)	2 (0.3%)
Dyspnea	5 (11%)	0 (0%)
Rhinorrhea	4 (9%)	1 (0.2%)
Wheezing	4 (9%)	4 (1%)
Body temperature increased	4 (9%)	6 (1%)
Neck pain	4 (9%)	2 (0.3%)
Sinus pain	4 (9%)	1 (0.2%)
Chest discomfort	4 (9%)	4 (1%)
Crackles lung	4 (9%)	2 (0.3%)
Abdominal pain	3 (7%)	2 (0.3%)
Dyspepsia	3 (7%)	1 (0.2%)
Toothache	3 (7%)	0 (0%)
Gastroesophageal reflux disease	3 (7%)	0 (0%)
Lymphadenopathy	3 (7%)	3 (1%)
Respiratory tract congestion	3 (7%)	0 (0%)
Fall	3 (7%)	1 (0.2%)
Hypertension	3 (7%)	4 (1%)

In this study, the upper bound of the 1-sided 95% confidence interval for the proportion of Flebogamma® 10% DIF infusions associated with one or more AEs was 37.8% (total infusions: 208; actual proportions: 34.6%). The average percent of infusions with AEs during or within 72 hours after the end of an infusion for each individual subject was 36.7% and the upper bound of the 1-sided 95% confidence interval was 43.9%.

AE reporting was based upon a clinical protocol precluding pre-medication against AEs. Pre-medication could be utilized only after the first 2 infusions only in those patients that exhibited adverse events.

Forty-three of the 46 subjects enrolled in this study had a negative Coombs test at baseline. Of these 43 subjects, 10 (23.3%) developed a positive Coombs test at some time during the study. However, no subjects showed evidence of hemolytic anemia.

6.2 Postmarketing Experience

Because adverse reactions are reported voluntarily post-approval from a population of uncertain size, it is not always possible to reliably estimate their frequency or establish a causal relationship to product exposure. The following adverse reactions have been identified during post-approval use of intravenous immune globulins, including Flebogamma® 5% (see References [15]).

Infusion reactions	Hypersensitivity (e.g., anaphylaxis), headache, diarrhea, tachycardia, fever, fatigue, dizziness, malaise, chills, flushing, urticaria or other skin reactions, wheezing or other chest discomfort, nausea, vomiting, rigors, back pain, myalgia, arthralgia, and changes in blood pressure
Renal	Acute renal dysfunction/failure, osmotic nephropathy
Respiratory	Apnea, Acute Respiratory Distress Syndrome (ARDS), Transfusion-Related Acute Lung Injury (TRALI), cyanosis, hypoxemia, pulmonary edema, dyspnea, bronchospasm
Cardiovascular	Cardiac arrest, thromboembolism, vascular collapse, hypotension
Neurological	Coma, loss of consciousness, seizures, tremor, aseptic meningitis syndrome
Integumentary	Stevens-Johnson Syndrome, epidermolysis, erythema multiformae, dermatitis (e.g., bullous dermatitis)
Hematologic	Pancytopenia, leukopenia, hemolysis, positive direct antiglobulin (Coombs) test
Musculoskeletal	Back pain
Gastrointestinal	Hepatic dysfunction, abdominal pain
General/Body as a Whole	Pyrexia, rigors

7 DRUG INTERACTIONS

Passive transfer of antibodies may transiently impair the immune response to live attenuated virus vaccines such as measles, mumps, and rubella. Inform the immunizing physician of recent therapy with Flebogamma® 10% DIF so that appropriate measures may be taken (*see Patient Counseling Information [17]*).

8 USE IN SPECIFIC POPULATIONS

8.1 Pregnancy

Pregnancy Category C. Animal reproduction studies have not been performed with Flebogamma® 10% DIF. It is also not known whether Flebogamma® 10% DIF can cause fetal harm when administered to a pregnant woman or can affect reproduction capacity. Flebogamma® 10% DIF should be given to a pregnant woman only if clearly needed. Immunoglobulins cross the placenta from maternal circulation increasingly after 30 weeks of gestation.

8.3 Nursing Mothers

Use of Flebogamma® 10% DIF has not been evaluated in nursing mothers.

8.4 Pediatric Use

Three (3) pediatric patients with primary humoral immunodeficiency (two between the ages of 6 and 10, and one 16 year old) were included in the clinical evaluation of Flebogamma® 10% DIF. This number of subjects is too small to establish safety and efficacy in the pediatric population (*see Clinical Studies [14]*).

Table 4. Flebogamma® 10% DIF: viral reduction capacity of combined steps (log$_{10}$)

Target virus	HIV-1, HIV-2 (env. RNA)	HBV, Herpesvirus (env. DNA)		HCV (env. RNA)		WNV (env. RNA)	HAV (non-env. RNA)	Virus B19 (non-env. DNA)
Model virus	HIV-1	PRV	IBR	BVDV	SINDBIS	WNV	EMC	PPV
Fraction I precipitation	< 1.00*	nd	nd	nd	nd	2.78	nd	< 1.00*
Ethanol incubation (Fraction II+III)	1.48	nd	nd	nd	nd	< 1.00*	nd	nd
PEG precipitation	≥ 6.10	≥ 5.92	nd	≥ 5.78	nd	nd	≥ 6.41	6.35
Acid pH treatment	2.47	≥ 5.32	nd	< 1.00*	nd	nd	1.36	na
Pasteurization	≥ 5.64	≥ 4.96	≥ 6.33	≥ 4.69	≥ 6.49	≥ 5.42	≥ 5.56	4.08
Solvent Detergent	≥ 4.61	≥ 6.95	nd	≥ 6.14	nd	≥ 5.59	na	na
Nanofiltration 20 nanometer	a	a	a	a	a	a	a	4.61
Overall Reduction Capacity	≥ 20.30	≥ 23.15	≥ 6.33	≥ 16.61	≥ 6.49	≥ 13.79	≥ 13.33	15.04

* When the RF is <1 log$_{10}$, it is not taken into account for the calculation of the overall reduction capacity.
≥: No residual infectivity detected / nd: not done / na: non-applicable, since the virus is theoretically resistant to this treatment.
a) During the nanofiltration validation, 9 different viruses (HIV, PRV, BVDV, WNV, EMC, SV40, BEV, Echo 11 and PPV) were evaluated. Eight of these viruses were inactivated by the process conditions and/or removed by prefiltration. Only PPV was affected neither by the filtration conditions nor by the prefiltration and could be assayed and efficiently removed in these experiments.
Abbreviations: HIV; Human Immunodeficiency Virus, PRV; Pseudorabies Virus, IBR; Infectious Bovine Rhinotracheitis Virus, BVDV; Bovine Viral Diarrhoea Virus, SINDBIS; Sindbis Virus, WNV; West Nile Virus, EMC; Encephalomyocarditis Virus, PPV; Porcine Parvovirus.

8.5 Geriatric Use

Use caution when administering Flebogamma® 10% DIF to patients over 65 years of age who are judged to be at increased risk for developing certain adverse reactions such as thromboembolic events and acute renal failure (*see Boxed Warning, Warnings and Precautions [5.2]*). Do not exceed the recommended dose, and infuse Flebogamma® 10% DIF at the minimum infusion rate practicable.

One (1) patient with primary humoral immunodeficiency at or over the age of 65 was included within the clinical evaluation of Flebogamma® 10% DIF. This number of geriatric patients was too small for separate evaluation from the younger patients for safety or efficacy (*see Clinical Studies [14]*).

11 DESCRIPTION

Flebogamma® 10% DIF is a ready to use, sterile, clear or slightly opalescent and colorless to pale yellow, liquid preparation of highly purified immunoglobulin (IgG) obtained from human plasma pools. The purification process includes cold ethanol fractionation, polyethylene glycol precipitation, ion exchange chromatography, low pH treatment, pasteurization, solvent detergent treatment and Planova nanofiltration using 20 nanometer (nm) filters.

Flebogamma® 10% DIF is a purified (≥ 97% IgG), unmodified, human IgG. The distribution of the four IgG subclasses is approximately 66.6% IgG$_1$, 27.9% IgG$_2$, 3.0% IgG$_3$ and 2.5% IgG$_4$. Flebogamma® 10% DIF contains trace amounts of IgA (typically < 100 µg/mL) and trace amounts of sodium and IgM.

Flebogamma® 10% DIF contains 10 g human normal immunoglobulin and 5 g D-sorbitol (as stabilizer) in 100 mL of water for injection, and ≤ 6 mg/mL polyethylene glycol. There is no preservative in the formulation. The pH of the solution ranges from 5 to 6 and the osmolality from 240 to 370 mOsm/kg, which is within the normal physiological range. The Fc and Fab functionality is maintained in Flebogamma® 10% DIF.

All Source Plasma used in the manufacture of Flebogamma® 10% DIF was collected only at FDA approved plasmapheresis centers in the United States and tested by FDA-licensed serological tests and found to be non-reactive (negative) for Hepatitis B Surface Antigen (HBsAg), antibodies to Hepatitis C Virus (HCV) and Human Immunodeficiency Virus (HIV) and negative on Nucleic Acid Test (NAT) for HCV and HIV. An investigational NAT for HBV is also performed on all Source Plasma and found to be negative; however, the significance of a negative result has not been established. Additionally, plasma is tested by in-process NAT testing for hepatitis A virus (HAV) and parvovirus B19 (B19) on minipools and the viral load limit for B19 in the manufacturing pool is set not to exceed 10^4 IU/ml. NAT testing for the presence of HCV and HIV in the manufacturing plasma pool is also performed and found to be negative.

In addition, several manufacturing steps can contribute towards viral safety of the final product. The effectiveness of these steps to remove or inactivate viruses from the product was evaluated through virus spiking experiments using a scaled down version of the manufacturing process. Virus elimination experiments have been performed on 7 steps of the production process.

Flebogamma® 10% DIF production process includes the following specific virus inactivation/removal steps:
• Pasteurization at 60 °C, 10 hours
• Solvent-Detergent treatment for 6 hours
• Nanofiltration down to 20 nm Planova filters

The following purification processes can also reduce the risk of viral transmission:
• Fraction I precipitation
• Fraction II+III precipitation
• 4% PEG precipitation
• pH 4 treatment for 4 hours at 37 °C

The viral reduction data (in log$_{10}$) from these experiments are summarized in Table 4.
[See table 4 above]

Additionally, the manufacturing process was investigated for its capacity to decrease infectivity of an experimental agent of transmissible spongiform encephalopathy (TSE), considered as a model for the vCJD and CJD agents.

Several individual production steps in the Flebogamma® 10% DIF manufacturing process have been shown to decrease TSE infectivity of an experimental model agent. TSE reduction steps include: 4% Polyethylene glycol precipitation [≥ 6.19 log$_{10}$] and Planova nanofiltration using a 20 nanometer filter [≥ 5.45 log$_{10}$]. These studies provide reasonable assurance that low levels of CJD/vCJD agent infectivity, if present in the starting material, would be removed.

12 CLINICAL PHARMACOLOGY

12.1 Mechanism of Action

Flebogamma® 10% DIF is a replacement therapy for PI. It supplies a broad spectrum of opsonizing and neutralizing antibodies against a wide variety of bacterial and viral agents. However, the mechanism of action in PI has not been fully elucidated.

12.3 Pharmacokinetics

In the clinical study assessing safety and efficacy in primary immunodeficiency disease (PI), the pharmacokinetics of Flebogamma® 10% DIF was assessed for 21 or 28 days after administration in 19 subjects. PK analysis was performed for 10 subjects receiving Flebogamma® 10% DIF on a 21-day schedule and for 9 subjects receiving treatment on a 28-day schedule. The mean dose (range) for those on the 21-day schedule was 476 mg/kg (range: 339-597), and for those on the 28-day schedule was 496 mg/kg (range: 434-588). Blood samples for PK analysis were obtained after Infusion 7 for subjects on a 28-day schedule and after Infusion

Table 5. Pharmacokinetic Variables of Total IgG in Patients with PI

Variable	3-Week Dosing Interval (n=10)		4-Week Dosing Interval (n=9)	
	Mean ± SD	Range	Mean ± SD	Range
Cmax (mg/dL)	1,950 ± 283	1,510 – 2,440	2,092 ± 366	1,680 – 2,920
AUC_{0-last} (day·mg/dL)	33,951 ± 4,527	24,112 – 38,021	34,237 ± 3,972	27,683 – 40,825
Clearance (mL/day)	115 ± 31	81 – 186	144 ± 47	77 – 237
Half-life (days)[a]	34 ± 10	21 – 58	37 ± 13	24 – 59
Trough IgG level (mg/dL)[b]	976 ± 165	645 – 1,140	877 ± 126	759 – 1,170

a. This half-life is an apparent value derived from a period of measurement of 28 days.
b. For subjects on the 3-week schedule, the average of the trough levels from Infusion 9 to the end of the study was calculated; for those on a 4-week schedule, the average of the trough levels from Infusion 7 to the end of the study was calculated. The means of the subject means are presented in this table.

Table 6. Summary of Bacterial Infections (Intention-to-Treat Population, N = 46)

Infections	Patients (N=46) N (%)	Episodes	Estimates [1]	98% CI [2]
Bacterial pneumonia	1 (2.2)	1		
Bacteremia or sepsis	0 (0.0)	0		
Osteomyelitis/septic arthritis	0 (0.0)	0		
Visceral abscess	0 (0.0)	0		
Bacterial meningitis	0 (0.0)	0		
Patients with at least 1 serious bacterial infection	1 (2.2)	1	0.025	(0.001, 0.133)

[1] Estimate = Total episodes/Total patient years.
[2] The confidence interval is obtained by using a generalized linear model procedure for Poisson distribution.

9 for subjects on a 21-day schedule. Table 5 summarizes the pharmacokinetic parameters of Flebogamma® 10% DIF, measured as serum concentrations of total IgG.
[See table 5 above]
The half-life of IgG can vary considerably among patients.

13 NONCLINICAL TOXICOLOGY

13.1 Carcinogenity, Mutagenesis, Impairment of Fertility

No animal studies were conducted to evaluate the carcinogenic or mutagenic effect of Flebogamma® 10% DIF or its effects on fertility

13.2 Animal Toxicology and/or Pharmacology

Acute toxicity studies were performed in mice and rats at doses up to 2.5 g/kg body weight with infusion rates 6 to 37 times higher than the maximum rates recommended for humans. The most common clinical observations in mice studies were piloerection, ptosis, ataxia and increase in respiration all lasting 90 minutes or less. No relevant adverse effects could be confirmed affecting respiratory, circulatory, renal, autonomic and central nervous systems, somatomotor activity, and behavior of the treated mice and rats.

Five out of the 25 rats treated with the highest dose at approximately 8 times the maximum infusion rate recommended for humans, showed a transient "reddish urine" sign which was not confirmed as a relevant toxicity causing phenomenon after renal macro and microscopic analysis. This phenomenon was ascribed to hemolysis when serum was analyzed, suggesting a possible relation to cross-reactivity of rodent red cells with human antibodies. No "reddish urine" was detected in any mouse, a much smaller animal where the rate of infusion was comparatively much higher than in rats. The macroscopic inspection of all treated mice did not show any renal alteration.

14 CLINICAL STUDIES

A phase 3, multicenter, open-label, historically controlled study to assess the efficacy, safety and pharmacokinetics of Flebogamma® 10% DIF in subjects with PI was conducted in the United States. Forty-six subjects were treated with Flebogamma® 10% DIF for 12 months at a 3-week or 4-week dosing interval. Subjects ranged in age from 6 to 65 years; 65% were male and 35% were female; 96% were Caucasian and 4% were Hispanic.
The study included 46 subjects, 16 on a 3-week dosing interval and 30 on a 4-week dosing interval. Doses ranged from 307 mg/kg to 597 mg/kg. The median dose for the 3-week interval was 462.8 mg/kg; the median dose for the 4-week interval was 444 mg/kg. Subjects received a total of 601 infusions of Flebogamma® 10% DIF. The maximum infusion rate allowed during the study was 0.08 mL/kg/min. During the study period, the annual rate of acute serious bacterial infection, defined as bacterial pneumonia, bacteremia or sepsis, osteomyelitis/septic arthritis, visceral ab-

scesses and bacterial meningitis per subject per year, was 0.025 (with an upper 1-sided 98% confidence interval of 0.001 to 0.133). One subject had one episode of bacterial pneumonia. There were no other episodes of serious bacterial infections (Table 6).
[See table 6 above]
The other efficacy variables were the number of days of work/school missed, the number of hospitalizations and the number of days of each hospitalization, the number of visits to physicians or emergency rooms, the number of other infections documented by positive radiographic findings, fever, and the number of days of therapeutic and prophylactic oral and parenteral antibiotic use. These additional efficacy variables were annualized by using the subject-years exposure data only of those subjects experiencing the endpoints, not the entire study cohort. With regard to the number of other validated infections, the mean rate was less than 2 days/subject/year (The calculation uses all subjects, including those who had no infections, see Table 7).

Table 7. Summary of Annualized Efficacy Variables

Variable	Subjects		Mean number of events, days or visits/ subject/year [1]
	N	%	
Work/school days missed	20	43.5	3.0
Days in hospital	5	11.0	0.6
Visits to physician/ER	24	52.2	2.1
Number of other documented infectious episodes	7	15.2	0.2
Days of therapeutic oral antibiotic use	36	78.3	56.4
Days of therapeutic parenteral antibiotic use	2	4.3	1.3
Days of other therapeutic antibiotic use	14	30.4	60.5
Days of prophylactic oral antibiotic use	19	41.3	45.8
Days of prophylactic parenteral antibiotic use	1	2.2	0.02
Days of other prophylactic antibiotic use	1	2.2	3.3

[1] Days of work/school missed per patient year are derived as total days of work/school missed divided by total days in study multiplied by 365. If data are missing for a period (e.g., between Infusion 2 and Infusion 3), then number of days in this period is not counted in the denominator. All other endpoints are derived similarly.

15 REFERENCES

1. Cayco AV, Perazella MA, Hayslett JP. Renal insufficiency after intravenous immune globulin therapy: a report of two cases and an analysis of the literature. *J Am Soc Nephrol* 1997; 8:1788-94.
2. Tan E, Hajinazarian M, Bay W, et al. Acute renal failure resulting from intravenous immunoglobulin therapy. *Arch Neurol* 1993; 50:137-9.
3. Sekul EA, Cupler EJ, Dalakas MC. Aseptic meningitis associated with high-dose intravenous immunoglobulin therapy: frequency and risk factors. *Ann Intern Med* 1994; 121:259-62.
4. Scribner CL, Kapit RM, Phillips ET, et al. Aseptic meningitis and intravenous immunoglobulin therapy. *Ann Intern Med* 1994; 121:305-6.
5. Thomas MJ, Misbah SA, Chapel HM, et al. Hemolysis after high-dose intravenous Ig. *Blood* 1993; 15:3789.
6. Reinhart WH, Berchtold PE. Effect of high-dose intravenous immunoglobulin therapy on blood rheology. *Lancet* 1992; 339:662-4.
7. Kessary-Shoham H, Levy Y, Shoenfeld Y, et al. In vivo administration of intravenous immunoglobulin (IVIG) can lead to enhanced erythrocyte sequestration. *J Autoimmun* 1999; 13:129-35.
8. Dalakas MC. High-dose intravenous immunoglobulin and serum viscosity: risk of precipitating thromboembolic events. *Neurology* 1994; 44:223-6.
9. Woodruff RK, Grigg AP, Firkin FC, et al. Fatal thrombotic events during treatment of autoimmune thrombocytopenia with intravenous immunoglobulin in elderly patients. *Lancet* 1986; ii:217-8.
10. Wolberg AS, Kon RH, Monroe DM, et al. Coagulation factor XI is a contaminant in intravenous immunoglobulin preparations. *Am J Hematol* 2000; 65:30-4.
11. Rizk A, Gorson KC, Kenney L, et al. Transfusion-related acute lung injury after the infusion of IVIG. *Transfusion* 2001; 41:264-8.

16 HOW SUPPLIED/STORAGE AND HANDLING

Flebogamma® 10% DIF is supplied in single-use, individually laser etched vials containing the labeled amount of functionally active IgG.
The following presentations of Flebogamma® 10% DIF are available:

NDC Number	Fill Size	Grams Protein
61953-0005-1	50 mL	5 g
61953-0005-2	100 mL	10 g
61953-0005-3	200 mL	20 g

Each vial has an integral suspension band and a label with two peel-off strips showing the product name and lot number.
DO NOT FREEZE.
When stored at room temperature (up to 25 °C [77 °F]), Flebogamma® 10% DIF is stable for up to 24 months, as indicated by the expiration date printed on the outer carton and container label.
Keep Flebogamma® 10% DIF in its original carton to protect it from light.

17 PATIENT COUNSELING INFORMATION

Inform patients to immediately report the following signs and symptoms to their physician:
• Decreased urine output, sudden weight gain, fluid retention/edema, and/or shortness of breath (*see Warnings and Precautions [5.2]*)
• Acute chest pain, shortness of breath, leg pain, and swelling of the legs/feet (*see Warnings and Precautions [5.4]*)
• Severe headache, neck stiffness, drowsiness, fever, sensitivity to light, painful eye movements, nausea and vomiting (*see Warnings and Precautions [5.5]*)
• Increased heart rate, fatigue, yellowing of skin or eyes, dark-colored urine (*see Warnings and Precautions [5.6]*)
• Trouble breathing, chest pain, blue lips or extremities, fever (*see Warnings and Precautions [5.7]*)

Inform patients that Flebogamma® 10% DIF is made from human plasma and may contain infectious agents that can cause disease (e.g., viruses, and, theoretically, the CJD agent). While the risk that Flebogamma® 10% DIF may transmit an infection has been reduced by screening plasma donors for prior exposure, testing donated plasma, and inactivating and/or removing certain viruses during manufacturing, patients should report any symptoms that concern them (see *Warnings and Precautions [5.8]*).

Inform patients that Flebogamma® 10% DIF can interfere with the response to live viral vaccines such as measles, mumps and rubella, and instruct patients to notify their healthcare professional of this potential interaction when they are receiving vaccinations (see *Drug Interactions [7]*).

Manufactured by:
INSTITUTO GRIFOLS, S.A.
BARCELONA – SPAIN
U.S. License No. 1181
U.S. Distributor
GRIFOLS BIOLOGICALS Inc.
LOS ANGELES - CA 90032, U.S.A.
U.S. License No. 1694

PROFILNINE® SD ℞
[*PRO-fil-nine*]
Factor IX Complex
Solvent Detergent Treated

DESCRIPTION

Factor IX Complex, Profilnine® SD, Solvent Detergent Treated, is a sterile, lyophilized concentrate of Factor IX (antihemophilic factor B), Factor II (prothrombin), Factor X (Stuart-Prower Factor), and low levels of Factor VII (proconvertin) derived from human plasma. Factor II content has been assayed at no more than (NMT) 150 Units per 100 Factor IX Units, Factor X at NMT 100 Units per 100 Factor IX Units, and Factor VII at NMT 35 Units per 100 Factor IX Units. Profilnine® SD is intended for intravenous administration only. Each vial is a single dose container.

Profilnine® SD is a non-activated Factor IX Complex prepared from pooled human plasma and purified by DEAE cellulose adsorption. Profilnine® SD is treated with a mixture of the organic solvent tri(n-butyl)phosphate (TNBP) and the nonionic detergent polysorbate 80 (Solvent Detergent Mixture) to reduce risks of transmission of viral infection. However, no procedure has been shown to be totally effective in removing viral infectivity from coagulation factor products. Each vial of Profilnine® SD is labeled with the Factor IX potency expressed in International Units (IU). Profilnine® SD does not contain heparin. Profilnine® SD contains low levels of activated coagulation factors, as indicated by the non-activated Partial Thromboplastin Time Test.[1,2] Profilnine® SD contains no preservatives.

When reconstituted with the appropriate volume of Sterile Water for Injection, USP, Profilnine® SD contains not more than 2.5 µg polysorbate 80 and 0.40 µg TNBP per IU of Factor IX.

CLINICAL PHARMACOLOGY

Profilnine® SD is a mixture of vitamin K-dependent clotting factors. The administration of Factor IX Complex, Profilnine® SD, temporarily increases the plasma levels of Factor IX, thus minimizing the hazards of hemorrhage. A clinical study, which evaluated twelve subjects with hemophilia B, indicated that, following administration of Profilnine® SD, Factor IX *in vivo* half-life is 24.68 ± 8.29 hours and recovery is 1.15 ± 0.16 IU/dL per IU infused per kg body weight.[3]

Administration of Factor IX Complex can result in higher than normal levels of Factor II due to its significantly longer half-life.[4]

The retrovirus known as Human Immunodeficiency Virus (HIV-1) has been identified as the causative agent of Acquired Immunodeficiency Syndrome (AIDS) and has been shown to be transmissible via blood or blood products. The solvent detergent process used in the manufacture of Profilnine® SD has been shown to provide a very high level of virus kill without compromising protein structure and function.[5] The susceptibility of human pathogenic viruses such as HIV-1, hepatitis B virus, hepatitis C virus and marker viruses such as Sindbis and Vesicular Stomatitis Virus (VSV) to inactivation by organic solvent detergent treatment has been discussed in the literature.[6-8]

The solvent detergent process used in the manufacture of Profilnine® SD was shown to inactivate greater than 12.2 logs of HIV-1 when the retrovirus was intentionally added to product samples under laboratory evaluation (as measured by virus antigen capture and reverse transcriptase assays). In addition, this process was shown to inactivate 6.0 logs of HIV-2 (as measured by reverse transcriptase assays) when the retrovirus was intentionally added to product samples.

In order to assess the ability of the solvent detergent process to inactivate other viruses such as hepatitis B and C virus, the inactivation of the model viruses, Sindbis virus and vesicular stomatitis virus (VSV), by solvent detergent treatment was studied. Prior to solvent detergent treatment, samples were inoculated with a titer of either Sindbis or VSV. The results demonstrated that a minimum of 5.3 logs of Sindbis and a minimum of 4.9 logs of VSV were removed after 180 minutes of incubation with solvent detergent (when compared to an untreated control). It should be noted that the incubation time in the actual Profilnine® SD process is twice (360 minutes total) that used in the model virus studies.

The ability of the Profilnine® SD process to eliminate virus, by physically partitioning virus from product, was evaluated at the DEAE chromatography step. Addition of Sindbis virus prior to Factor IX Complex adsorption by DEAE chromatography showed this step to eliminate 1.4 logs of added virus.

However, no treatment method has yet been shown capable of totally eliminating all potential infective virus in preparations of coagulation factor concentrates.

INDICATIONS AND USAGE

Factor IX Complex, Profilnine® SD is indicated for the prevention and control of bleeding in patients with Factor IX deficiency due to hemophilia B.

This product contains non-therapeutic levels of Factor VII, and is *not* indicated for use in the treatment of Factor VII deficiency.

CONTRAINDICATIONS

None known.

WARNINGS

Because Factor IX Complex, Profilnine® SD is made from pooled human plasma, it may carry a risk of transmitting infectious agents, e.g., viruses, and theoretically, the Creutzfeldt-Jakob disease (CJD) agent. Stringent procedures designed to reduce the risk of adventitious agent transmission have been employed in the manufacture of this product, from the screening of plasma donors and the collection and testing of plasma to the application of viral elimination/reduction steps such as DEAE chromatography and solvent detergent treatment in the manufacturing process.[9-10] Despite these measures, such product can potentially transmit disease, therefore the risk of infectious agents cannot be totally eliminated. The physician should weigh the risks and benefits of the use of this product and should discuss these with the patient.

Individuals who receive infusions of blood or plasma products may develop signs and/or symptoms of some viral infections. Scientific opinion encourages hepatitis B and hepatitis A vaccinations for patients with hemophilia at birth or diagnosis.

In patients undergoing surgery and in patients with known liver disease, thrombosis or disseminated intravascular coagulation (DIC) are serious and potentially fatal adverse reactions associated with the administration of Factor IX Complex concentrates.[11-13] Infrequent but consistent reports have been described which indicate that patients are at greater risk of developing thrombosis and DIC in the period following surgery. Cases have also been cited which indicate that patients with liver disease may be predisposed to thrombosis or DIC when treated with Factor IX Complex. Although the available data is limited, Profilnine® SD should only be administered to patients when the beneficial effects of use outweigh the serious risk of potential hypercoagulation.

PRECAUTIONS

General

Factor IX Complex, Profilnine® SD should *not* be administered at a rate exceeding 10 mL/minute. Rapid administration may result in vasomotor reactions.

Nursing personnel, and others who administer this material, should exercise appropriate caution in handling due to the risk of exposure to viral infection.

Discard any unused contents. Discard administration equipment after single use. Do *not* resterilize components. Do *not* reuse components.

Information for Patients

Patients should be informed of the early symptoms and signs of hypersensitivity reaction, including hives, generalized urticaria, chest tightness, dyspnea, wheezing, faintness, hypotension, and anaphylaxis. Patients should be advised to discontinue use of the product and contact their physician and/or seek immediate emergency care, depending on the severity of the reaction, if these symptoms occur.

Some viruses, such as parvovirus B19 or hepatitis A, are particularly difficult to remove or inactivate at this time. Parvovirus B19 may most seriously affect sero-negative pregnant women, or immunocompromised individuals. The majority of parvovirus B19 and hepatitis A infections are acquired by environmental (natural) sources.

Pregnancy Category C

Animal reproduction studies have not been conducted with Profilnine® SD. It is also not known whether Profilnine® SD can cause fetal harm when administered to a pregnant woman or can affect reproduction capacity. Profilnine® SD should be given to a pregnant woman only if clearly indicated.

Pediatric Use

Clinical Trials for safety and effectiveness in pediatric patients 16 years of age and younger have not been conducted. Across a well controlled half-life and recovery clinical trial in patients previously treated with factor IX concentrates for Hemophilia B, the two pediatric patients receiving Profilnine® SD (solvent detergent treated) responded similarly when compared with the adult patients. There were no adverse events in the pediatric patients and one mild adverse event in the adult population (headache). Anecdotal evaluation of the results indicate no safety and efficacy differences between pediatric and adult populations.[3]

ADVERSE REACTIONS

Adverse reactions characterized by either thrombosis or disseminated intravascular coagulation (DIC) are associated with administration of Factor IX Complex concentrates.[11-14] In particular, patients who receive prolonged treatment with Factor IX Complex concentrates postoperatively or with known liver disease should be kept under close observation for signs or symptoms of intravascular coagulation. Continued administration should be left to the discretion of the physician.

Adverse reactions may include urticaria, fever, chills, nausea, vomiting, headache, somnolence, lethargy, flushing or tingling. For most reactive individuals, slowing the rate of infusion relieves the symptoms. For those highly reactive individuals, a different lot may be satisfactory.

To report SUSPECTED ADVERSE REACTIONS, contact Grifols at 1-888-GRIFOLS (1-888-474-3657) or FDA at 1-800-FDA-1088 or www.fda.gov/medwatch.

DOSAGE AND ADMINISTRATION

For adult usage:

Factor IX Complex, Profilnine® SD should be administered intravenously, promptly following reconstitution with the supplied diluent. Although Profilnine® SD is stable for at least three (3) hours at room temperature after reconstitution, prompt administration is recommended to avoid the ill effect of any inadvertent bacterial contamination occurring during reconstitution. Profilnine® SD may be administered by injection (plastic disposable syringe only) or infusion. Administer at room temperature, do not refrigerate after reconstitution and discard any unused contents.

Each vial of Profilnine® SD is labeled with the total units expressed as International Units (IU) which is referenced to the WHO International Standard. One unit approximates the activity in one mL of normal plasma.

A 1.0% increase in Factor IX (0.01 IU/IU administered/kg) can be expected.[15] The amount of Profilnine® SD required to establish hemostasis will vary with each patient and depend on the circumstances. The following formula may be used as a guide in determining the number of units to be administered:

Body Weight (in kg)	×	Desired increase in Plasma Factor IX (Percent)	×	1.0 IU/kg	=	Number of Factor IX IU Required

Example:

50 kg	×	25 (% increase)	×	1.0 IU/kg	=	1,250 IU Factor IX

In normal clinical practice there is variability among patients and their clinical condition. Therefore, the Factor IX level of each patient should be monitored frequently during replacement therapy.

Mild to moderate hemorrhages may usually be treated with a single administration sufficient to raise the plasma Factor IX level to 20 to 30 percent. In the event of more serious hemorrhage, the patient's plasma Factor IX level should be raised to 30 to 50 percent. Infusions are generally required daily.

Surgery in patients with Factor IX deficiency requires that the Factor IX level should be raised to 30 to 50 percent for at least one week following operation. For dental extractions, the Factor IX level should be raised to 50 percent immediately prior to the procedure; additional Factor IX Complex may be given if bleeding recurs.

For pediatric usage: See PRECAUTIONS

RECONSTITUTION

Use Aseptic Technique

1. Warm diluent (Sterile Water for Injection, USP) and concentrate (Profilnine® SD) to at least room temperature (but not above 37 °C).

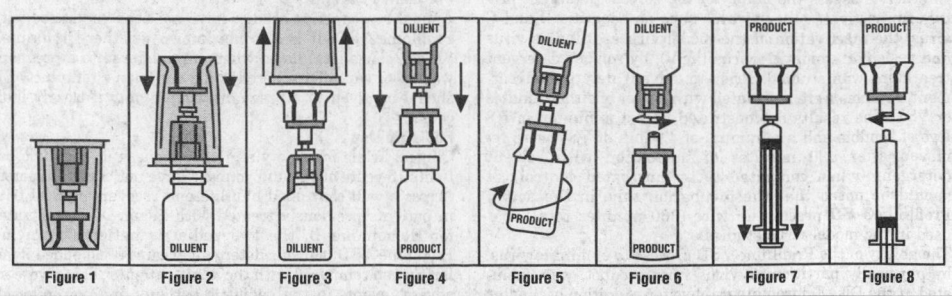

| Figure 1 | Figure 2 | Figure 3 | Figure 4 | Figure 5 | Figure 6 | Figure 7 | Figure 8 |

Potency	NDC	Assay Color Code
500 IU FIX/5 mL single dose vial	68516-3201-1	MID in blue box
1000 IU FIX/10 mL single dose vial	68516-3202-2	HIGH in red box
1500 IU FIX/10 mL single dose vial	68516-3203-2	SUPER HIGH in black box

2. Remove the plastic flip off cap from the diluent vial.
3. Gently swab the exposed stopper surface with a cleansing agent such as alcohol trying to avoid leaving any excess cleansing agent on the stopper.
4. Open the Mix2Vial™ package by peeling away the lid (Figure 1). Leave the Mix2Vial™ in the clear outer packaging.
5. Place the diluent vial upright on an even surface and hold the vial tight and pick up the Mix2Vial™ in its clear outer packaging. Holding the diluent vial securely, push the **blue** end of the Mix2Vial™ vertically down through the diluent vial stopper (Figure 2).
6. While holding onto the diluent vial, carefully remove the clear outer packaging from the Mix2Vial™ set, ensuring the Mix2Vial™ remains attached to the diluent vial (Figure 3).
7. Place the product vial upright on an even surface, invert the diluent vial with the Mix2Vial™ attached.
8. While holding the product vial securely on a flat surface, push the **clear** end of the Mix2Vial™ set **vertically** down through the product vial stopper (Figure 4). The diluent will automatically transfer out of its vial into the product vial. (NOTE: If the Mix2Vial™ is connected at an angle, the vacuum may be released from the product vial and the diluent will not transfer into the product vial.)
9. With the diluent and product vials still attached to the Mix2Vial™, gently swirl the product vial to ensure the product is fully dissolved (Figure 5). Reconstitution requires less than 10 minutes. Do not shake the vial.
10. Disconnect the Mix2Vial™ into two separate pieces (Figure 6) by holding each vial adapter and twisting counterclockwise. After separating, discard the diluent vial with the **blue** end of the Mix2Vial™.
11. Draw air into an empty, sterile syringe. Keeping the product vial upright with the **clear** end of the Mix2Vial™ attached, screw the disposable syringe onto the luer lock portion of the Mix2Vial™ device by pressing and twisting clockwise. Inject air into the product vial.
12. While keeping the syringe plunger depressed, invert the system upside down and draw the reconstituted product into the syringe by pulling the plunger back slowly (Figure 7).
13. When the reconstituted product has been transferred into the syringe, firmly hold the barrel of the syringe and the clear vial adapter (keeping the syringe plunger facing down) and unscrew the syringe from the Mix2Vial™ (Figure 8). Hold the syringe upright and push the plunger until no air is left in the syringe. Attach the syringe to a venipuncture set.
14. NOTE: If the same patient is to receive more than one vial of concentrate, the contents of two vials may be drawn into the same syringe through a separate unused Mix2Vial™ set before attaching to the venipuncture set.
15. Use prepared drug as soon as possible after reconstitution.
16. After reconstitution, parenteral drug products should be inspected visually for particulate matter and discoloration prior to administration, whenever solution and container permit. When reconstitution procedure is strictly followed, a few small particles may occasionally remain. The Mix2Vial™ set will remove particles and the labeled potency will not be reduced.
17. Discard all administration equipment after use into the appropriate safety container. Do not reuse.

[See figure above]

HOW SUPPLIED
Profilnine® SD is supplied in sterile lyophilized form in single dose vials accompanied by a suitable volume of diluent (Sterile Water for Injection, USP), according to Factor IX potency.
Each vial is labeled with the Factor IX potency expressed in International Units which is referenced to the WHO International Standard. Profilnine® SD is packaged with a Mix2Vial™ filter transfer set for use in administration.
It is available in the following potencies, and the product is also color coded based upon assay on the carton and vial label as follows:
[See table above]

STORAGE
Profilnine® SD should be stored at temperatures between 2 and 8 °C. Do not freeze diluent. May be stored at room temperature not to exceed 30 °C for up to 3 months. When removed from refrigeration, record the date on the vial or carton.

Rx only

REFERENCES
1. Kingdon, H.S., Lundblad, R.L., Veltkamp, J.J., Aronson, D.L. Potentially thrombogenic materials in Factor IX Concentrates. *Thromb Diath Haemorrh* 33:617-631, 1975.
2. Middleton, S.M., Forbes, C.D., Prentice, C.R.M. Thrombogenic Potential in Factor IX Concentrates Comparison of Tests. *Thromb Haemost* (Stuttg) 40:574-576, 1979.
3. Data on file at Grifols Biologicals Inc.
4. Aronson, D.L. Factor IX Complex. *Semin Thromb Hemostas* 6(1):28-43, 1979.
5. Horowitz, B. Investigations into the Application of Tri(n-butyl) phosphate/Detergent Mixtures to Blood Derivatives. In *Viral Inactivation of Plasma Products*, Morgenthaler J.J. (ed), Karger.
6. Horowitz, B., Wiebe, M.E. et al. Inactivation of viruses in labile blood derivatives. *Transfusion* 25:516-522, 1985.
7. Edward, C.A., Piet, M.P.J. et al. Tri(n-butyl)phosphate/detergent treatment of licensed therapeutic and experimental blood derivatives. *Vox Sang* 52:53-59, 1987.
8. Prince, A.M., Horowitz, B., Horowitz, M. et al. The development of virus-free labile blood derivatives-a review. *Eur J Epidemiology*, 3:103-118, 1987.
9. Menache, D., Roberts, H.R. Summary Report and Recommendations of the Task Force Members and Consultants. *Thromb Diath Haemorrh* 33:645-647, 1975.
10. Carnelli, V., Gomperts, E.D., Friedman, A., et al. Assessment for Evidence of Non A-Non B Hepatitis in Patients Given n-Heptane-Suspended Heat-Treated Clotting Factor Concentrate. *Thromb Res*, 46:827-834, 1987.
11. Lusher, J.M. Management of Hemophiliacs with Inhibitors. *Hemophilia in the Child and Adult*. Raven Press, Ltd., New York, 1989, pp. 121-136.
12. Aledort, L.M. Factor IX and Thrombosis. *Scand J Haematol*, Suppl 30:40-42, 1977.
13. Kasper, C.K. Thromboembolic Complications. *Thromb Diath Haemorrh* (Stuttg) 33:640-644, 1975.
14. Chistolini, A., Mazzucconi, M.G., Tirindelli, M.L., LaVerde, G., Ferrari, A., Mandelli, F. Disseminated intravascular coagulation and myocardial infarction in a haemophilia B patient during therapy with prothrombin complex concentrate. *Acta Haematol* 83:163-165, 1990.
15. Zauber, N.P., Levin, J. Factor IX Levels in Patients with Hemophilia B (Christmas Disease) Following Transfusion with Concentrates of Factor IX or Fresh Frozen Plasma (FFP). *Medicine* 56(3):213-224, 1977.

Manufactured and Distributed by:
Grifols Biologicals Inc.
Los Angeles, CA 90032, U.S.A.
U.S. License No. 1694
DATE OF REVISION: March 2010

EDUCATIONAL MATERIAL

Scientific publications, monographs, product literature, brochures and formulary kits available upon request.

Heel Inc.
10421 RESEARCH RD. SE
ALBUQUERQUE, NM 87123

Direct Inquiries to:
Medical Department
800-621-7644
Fax: (800) 217-6934
www.heelusa.com
info@heelusa.com

TRAUMEEL® Gel	OTC
Anti-inflammatory	
TRAUMEEL® Tablets	OTC
Anti-inflammatory	
TRAUMEEL® Ointment	OTC
Anti-inflammatory	
TRAUMEEL® Oral Drops	OTC
Anti-inflammatory	
TRAUMEEL® Oral Liquid in Vials	OTC
Anti-inflammatory	
TRAUMEEL® Ear Drops	OTC
Anti-inflammatory	
TRAUMEEL® Injection Solution	℞
Anti-inflammatory	

TRAUMEEL® ℞
Injection Solution

HIGHLIGHTS OF PRESCRIBING INFORMATION
DESCRIPTION
• Injection Solution Ingredient Information: Each 2,2 ml ampule contains: Arnica montana, radix 2X, Belladonna 2X, Calendula officinalis 2X, Chamomilla 3X, Millefolium 3X, Hepar sulphuris calcareum 6X, Symphytum officinale 6X 2.2 mcl each; Aconitum napellus 2X 1.32 mcl; Bellis perennis 2X, Mercurius solubilis 6X, 1.1 mcl each; Hypericum perforatum 2X 0.66 mcl; Echinacea 2X, Echinacea purpurea 2X 0.55 mcl each; Hamamelis virginiana 1X 0.22 mcl. Inactive ingredient: Sterile isotonic sodium chloride solution
INDICATIONS AND USAGE
• Traumeel® Injection Solution is indicated for the temporary relief of muscular pain, inflammation, sports injuries and bruising. (1.1)
DOSAGE AND ADMINISTRATION
• *Adults* in acute disorders, 1 ampule per day, otherwise 1 ampule, 1 to 3 times per week IM/SC/IV/ID or periarticular. *Children ages 2 to 6* receive ½ the adult dosage. (2.1)
DOSAGE FORM AND STRENGTH
• Injections: 2.2 ml ampule
CONTRAINDICATIONS
• Traumeel® Injection Solution is contraindicated in patients with known hypersensitivity to Traumeel® Injection Solution or any of its ingredients (see Adverse Reactions).
WARNINGS AND PRECAUTIONS
If pain persists or worsens, if new symptoms occur, or if redness or swelling is present, the patient should be carefully re-evaluated because these could be signs of a serious condition.
• Pregnancy Category C. Animal reproduction studies have not been conducted with this drug. It is also not known whether this drug can cause fetal harm when administered to a pregnant woman or can affect reproduction capacity. This drug should be given to a pregnant woman only if clearly needed.
ADVERSE REACTIONS
• In rare cases, patients with hypersensitivity to botanicals of the Compositae family may experience an allergic reaction after the administration of Traumeel® Injection

Solution. Traumeel® Injection Solution ingredients of the Compositae familiar are: Arnica montana, radix (mountain arnica), Calendula officinalis (marigold), Millefolium (milfoil), Chamomilla (chamomile), Bellis perennis (daisy), Echinacea angustifolia (narrow-lead cone flower), Echinacea purpurea (purple cone flower). (3.1)
To report SUSPECTED ADVERSE REACTIONS, contact Heel Inc. at 505-293-3843, info@heelusa.com or FDA at 1-800-FDA-1088 or www.fda.gov/medwatch
FULL PRESCRIBING INFORMATION

1. INDICATIONS AND USAGE

1.1 Traumeel® Injection Solution is an anti-inflammatory, analgesic, anti-edematous, anti-exudative combination formulation of 12 botanical substances, 1 mineral substance and 1 animal derived substance. Traumeel® Injection Solution is officially classified as a homeopathic combination drug.[1]
1.2 Botanical ingredients:
Arnica montana, radix (mountain arnica)
Calendula officinalis (marigold)
Hamamelis virginiana (witch hazel)
Millefolium (milfoil)
Belladonna (deadly nightshade)
Aconitum napellus (monkshood)
Chamomilla (chamomile)
Symphytum officinale (comfrey)
Bellis perennis (daisy)
Echinacea angustifolia (narrow-leafed cone flower)
Echinacea purpurea (purple cone flower)
Hypericum perforatum (St. John's wort)
1.3 Mineral ingredient:
Mercurius solubilis (Hahnemann's soluble mercury)
1.4 Animal derived ingredient:
Hepar sulphuris calcareum (calcium sulfide-made with oyster shells)
1.5 Traumeel® Injection Solution is indicated for the temporary relief of muscular pain, joint pain, sports injuries and bruising.

2. DOSAGE AND ADMINISTRATION

2.1 The dosage schedules listed below can be used as a general guide for the administration of Traumeel® Injection Solution. Traumeel® Injection Solution shows individual differences in clinical response. Therefore, the dosage for each patient should be individualized according to the patient's response therapy. For best results, treatment with Traumeel® Injection Solution should be initiated immediately following injury or at the first sign of symptoms. Traumeel® Injection Solution may be administered until symptoms disappear.
Adults and children 7 years and older: in acute disorders, 1 ampule per day, otherwise 1 ampule, 1 to 3 times weekly. *Children ages 2 to 6* receive ½ the adult dosage. Discard unused solution.
Traumeel® Injection Solution may be administered intravenously, intramuscularly, subcutaneously, or intradermally. Traumeel® Injection Solution is indicated for intra-articular use under sterile conditions. If coadminstration with local anesthetic is desired, Traumeel® Injection Solution may be mixed in a 1:1 ratio with 1% or 2% lidocaine hydrochloride. Similar local anesthetics may also be used. The required dose of Traumeel® Injection Solution is first withdrawn from the ampule into the syringe, and the syringe is then shaken briefly. Normally, about 0.5 to 1.0 milliliters of each drug is withdrawn into the syringe. Traumeel® Injection Solution should be administered using a narrow gauge needle (e.g. 22 to 30 gauge). Note: Parental drug products like Traumeel® Injection Solution should be inspected visually for particulate matter and discoloration prior to administration when ever solution and container permit. Traumeel® Injection Solution is a clear, colorless solution. Discolored solutions should be discarded.

3. WARNINGS AND PRECAUTIONS

3.1 Adverse effects with Traumeel® Injection Solution are extremely rare. Traumeel® Injection Solution exhibits no known adverse renal, hepatic, cardiovascular, gastrointestinal or central nervous system effects.
3.2 No harmful or potentially harmful side effects such as central nervous system depression are known. Traumeel® Injection Solution is generally well-tolerated, however, if symptoms persist or worsen, a physician should be consulted.
3.3 Teratogenic effects: In general, homeopathic drugs are not known to cause direct or indirect harm to the fetus.
3.4 Drug Interactions: None known
3.5 Drug / Laboratory Test Interaction: None known
3.6 Carcinogenesis, mutagenesis, impairment of fertility: Not applicable

4. USE IN SPECIFIC POPULATIONS

4.1 Pediatric Use: Traumeel® Injection Solution can safely be administered to children as young as 2 years (see Dosage and Administration).
4.2 Nursing Mothers: It is not known whether any of the ingredients in Traumeel® Injection Solution are excreted in human milk. However, because many drugs are excreted in human milk, Traumeel® Injection Solution should be administered with caution to nursing mothers.
4.3 Geriatric use: Traumeel® Injection Solution is safe to use in adults 12 years and older (see Dosage and Administration)

5. CLINICAL PHARMACOLOGY

5.1 The exact mechanism of action of Traumeel® Injection Solution is not fully understood. Various cellular and biochemical pathways appear to be modulated by the product ingredients. The mechanism or action of Traumeel® Injection Solution does not appear to be the result of cyclooxygenase or lipoxygenase enzyme inhibition, as is the case with nonsteroidal anti-inflammatory drugs (NSAIDS). Traumeel® Injection Solution does not inhibit the arachidonic acid pathway of prostaglandin synthesis. Instead, the mechanism of action of Traumeel® Injection Solution appears to be the result of modulation of the release of oxygen radicals from activated neutrophils, and inhibition of the release of inflammatory mediators (possibly interleukin-1 from activated macrophages) and neuropepetides.[2]
5.2 *In-vitro* studies show that the ingredients of Traumeel® Injection Solution are noncytotoxic to granulocytes, lymphocytes, platelets, and endothelia, which indicates that the defensive functions of these cells are preserved during treatment with Traumeel® Injection Solution.[3]
5.3 The anti-inflammatory, analgesic, anti-edematous, and anti-exudative effects of Traumeel® Injection Solution have been demonstrated in clinical trials as well as in *in vivo* experimental models including the carrageenin-induced edema test and the adjuvant arthritis test.[3]

6. DRUG ABUSE AND DEPENDENCE

6.1 Not applicable for homeopathic drugs

7. OVERDOSAGE

7.1 Due to the low concentration of active ingredients in homeopathic preparations such as Traumeel® Injection Solution, adverse reactions following over dosage are extremely unlikely. However, care must be taken not to exceed the recommended dosage.

8. HOW SUPPLIED

8.1 Traumeel® Injection Solution 2.2 ml ampules: Packs of 10 ampules: NDC 50114-7004-1

9. STORAGE CONDITIONS

9.1 Avoid freezing and excessive heat. Store at room temperature. Protect from light.

REFERENCES

1. The Homeopathic Pharmacopoeia of the United States (HPUS), 8th edition, Falls Church, Virginia, 1979; and the Homeopathic Pharmacopoeia of the United States Revision Service (HPRS), 1988.
2. Data on file, Heel GmbH, Baden-Baden, Germany.
3. Conforti A, *et al.* Experimental Studies on the Anti-inflammatory Activity of a Homeopathic Preparation. *Biomedical Therapy* XV No.1:28–31, 1997.

This full prescribing information has been compiled in accordance with the Code of Federal Regulations (CFR), 21 sections 201.56 and 201.57.

ZEEL® ℞
Injection Solution
Rx only

Package Insert Information for Zeel® Injection Solution
Homeopathic Medicine
HIGHLIGHTS OF PRESCRIBING INFORMATION

DESCRIPTION

• Injection Solution Ingredient Information: Each 2.0 ml ampule contains: Arnica montana, radix 4× 200 mcl, Rhus toxicodendron 2× 10 mcl, Dulcamara 3× 10 mcl, Symphytum officinale 6× 10 mcl, Sulphur 6× 3.6 mcl, Sanguinaria canadensis 4× 3 mcl, Cartilago suis 6× 2 mcl, Embryo suis 6× 2 mcl, Funiculus umbilicalis suis 6× 2 mcl, Placenta suis 6× 2 mcl, α-Lipoicum acidum 8× 2 mcl, Coenzyme A 8× 2 mcl, Nadidum 8× 2 mcl, Natrum oxalaceticum 8× 2 mcl. Inactive ingredient: Sterile isotonic sodium chloride solution.

INDICATIONS AND USAGE

• Zeel® Injection Solution is indicated for the temporary relief of mild to moderate arthritic pain, osteoarthritis and joint stiffness.

DOSAGE AND ADMINISTRATION

• *Adults and children 7 years and older:* in acute disorders, 1 ampule per day, otherwise 1 ampule, 1 to 3 times per week IM/SC/IV/ID. *Children* ages 2 to 6 receive ½ the adult dosage. (2.1)

DOSAGE FORM AND STRENGTH

• *Injections: 2.0 ml ampule*

WARNINGS AND PRECAUTIONS

Zeel® Injection Solution should not be administered for pain for more than 10 days for adults or five days for children. If new symptoms occur, or if redness, pain or swelling at the puncture site persists, the patient should be carefully re-evaluated because these could be signs of a more serious condition. Zeel® Injection Solution should not be administered to children for the pain of arthritis unless directed by a physician.
• Pregnancy Category C. Animal reproduction studies have not been conducted with this drug. It is also not known whether this drug can cause fetal harm when administered to a pregnant woman or can affect reproduction capacity. This drug should be given to a pregnant woman only if clearly needed.
• To report SUSPECTED ADVERSE REACTIONS, contact Heel Inc. at 1.800.920.9203 or info@heelusa.com or FDA at 1-800-FDA-1088 or www.fda.gov/medwatch
Revised 09/2009
FULL PRESCRIBING INFORMATION

1 INDICATIONS AND USAGE

1.1 Zeel® Injection Solution is classified as a homeopathic combination drug.[1]
1.2 Botanical ingredients:
Arnica montana, radix (Mountain arnica)
Dulcamara (Bittersweet)
Rhus toxicodendron (Poison oak)
Sanguinaria canadensis (Blood root)
Symphytum officinale (Comfrey)
1.3 Mineral ingredients:
Sulphur (Sulfur)
α-Lipoicum acid (Thioctic acid)
Coenzyme A (Coenzyme A)
Nadidum (Nicotinamide adenine dinucleotide)
Natrum oxalaceticum (Disodium oxaloacetate)
1.4 Animal-derived ingredients
Cartilago suis (Porcine cartilage)
Embryo totalis suis (Porcine embryo)
Funiculus umbilicalis suis (Porcine umbilical cord)
Placenta suis (porcine placenta)
1.5 Zeel® Injection Solution is indicated for the temporary relief of mild to moderate arthritic pain, osteoarthritis and joint stiffness.

2 DOSAGE AND ADMINISTRATION

2.1 The dosage schedules listed below can be used as a general guide for the administration of Zeel® Injection Solution. Zeel® Injection Solution shows individual differences in clinical response. Therefore, the dosage for each patient should be individualized according to the patient's response to therapy.
Adults and children 7 years and older: 1 ampule daily for acute disorders, or 1 ampule 1 to 3 times per week. *Children ages 2 to 6 years receive:* ½ the adult dosage.
Discard unused solution.
Zeel® Injection Solution may be administered intravenously, intramuscularly, subcutaneously, or intradermally. The required dose of Zeel® Injection Solution is first withdrawn from the ampule into the syringe, and the syringe is then shaken briefly. Zeel® Injection Solution should be administered using a narrow gauge needle (e.g. 22 to 30 gauge). Note: Parental drug products like Zeel® Injection Solution should be inspected visually for particulate matter and discoloration prior to administration whenever solution and container permit. Zeel® Injection Solution is a clear, colorless solution. Discolored solutions should be discarded.

3 WARNINGS AND PRECAUTIONS

3.1 Zeel® Injection Solution exhibits no known adverse renal, hepatic, cardiovascular, gastrointestinal or central nervous system effects.
3.2 No harmful or potentially harmful side effects such as central nervous system depression are known. Zeel® Injection Solution is generally well-tolerated, however, if symptoms persist or worsen discontinue use.
3.3 Teratogenic effects: In general, homeopathic drugs are not known to cause direct or indirect harm to the fetus. Pregnancy Category C. Animal reproduction studies have not been conducted with this drug. It is also not known whether this drug can cause fetal harm when administered to a pregnant woman or can affect reproduction capacity. This drug should be given to a pregnant woman only if clearly needed.
3.4 Drug Interactions: None known
3.5 Drug / Laboratory Test Interaction: None known
3.6 Carcinogenesis, mutagenesis, impairment of fertility: Not applicable

4 USE IN SPECIFIC POPULATIONS

4.1 Pediatric Use: Zeel® Injection Solution can be safely administered to children as young as 2 years (see Dosage and Administration).
4.2 Nursing Mothers: It is not known whether any of the ingredients in Zeel® Injection Solution are excreted in

human milk. However, because many drugs are excreted in human milk, Zeel® Injection Solution should be administered with caution to nursing mothers.

4.3   Geriatric use: Zeel® Injection Solution is safe to use in adults 12 years and older (see Dosage and Administration).

5   CLINICAL PHARMACOLOGY

5.1   The exact mechanism of action of Zeel® Injection Solution is not fully understood. In-vitro data indicates that the ingredients in Zeel® Injection Solution may reduce pain, stiffness and inflammation in arthritic joints via immunomodulation. Hence, it has been shown that Zeel® Injection Solution inhibits activity of the leukocyte elastase. This enzyme is released during inflammatory reactions and attacks the articular cartilage which is rich in proteoglycans.[2] A study of human whole blood cultures demonstrated that certain plant extracts contained in Zeel® Injection Solution (e.g. Rhus toxicodendron, Arnica montana) stimulates lymphocytes to release the transforming growth factor β.[3] The protective effect of Zeel® Injection Solution upon cartilage has also been demonstrated by in-vitro and in-vivo studies.[4,5] The clinical effectiveness and tolerance of Zeel® Injection Solution has also been demonstrated in a drug monitoring study.[6]

6   DRUG ABUSE AND DEPENDENCE

6.1   Not applicable for homeopathic drugs

7   OVERDOSAGE

7.1   Due to the low concentration of active ingredients in homeopathic preparations such as Zeel® Injection Solution, adverse reactions following over dosage are extremely unlikely. However, care must be taken not to exceed the recommended dosage.

8   HOW SUPPLIED

8.1   Zeel® Injection Solution 2.0 ml ampules: Packs of 10 ampules: NDC 50114-7030-1

9   STORAGE CONDITIONS

9.1   Avoid freezing and excessive heat. Store at room temperature. Protect from light.

Rx only

REFERENCES

1. The Homeopathic Pharmacopoeia of the United States (HPUS), 8th edition, Falls Church, Virginia, 1979; and the Homeopathic Pharmacopoeia of the United States Revision Service (HPRS), 1988.
2. Stancikova M. Inhibition of leucyte elastasis in vitro with Zeel and its various potentized components—a preliminary report. Biological Medicine. Vol 28(2) 1999, 83-4.
3. Heine H. The working mechanisms of Antihomotoxic Potentized Preparations. Biomedical Therapy. XVII (4) 1999, 117-20.
4. Weh L, Froeschle G. Incubation in Preparations as a Means of Influencing cartilage mechanics: A mechanical study. Biological Therapy. VIII (4) 1990, 91-3.
5. Orlandini A, Rossi M, Setti M. The Effectiveness of Zeel and new Research Methods in Rheumatology. Biological Medicine. Vol 26(4) 1997, 164-65.
6. Rainer Gottwald and Michael Weiser. Treatment of Osteoarthritis of the Knee with Zeel. Medicina Biológica Vol. 13, No. 4, 2000, pp. 109-13.

Hemispherx Biopharma, Inc.

ONE PENN CENTER
1617 JFK BOULEVARD
PHILADELPHIA, PA 19103-1806

Direct Inquiries to:
Alferon Access Program™
Phone 1 888 ALFERON
Fax 1 888 FAXX AFN
website: www.hemispherx.net

ALFERON N INJECTION®   ℞
Interferon alfa-n3
(human leukocyte derived)

DESCRIPTION

Alferon N Injection® [Interferon alfa-n3 (human leukocyte derived)] is a sterile aqueous formulation of purified, natural, human interferon alpha proteins for use by injection. Alferon N Injection® consists of interferon alpha proteins comprising approximately 166 amino acids ranging in molecular weights from 16,000 to 27,000 daltons. The specific activity of Interferon alfa-n3 is approximately equal to, or greater than, 2×10^8 IU/mg of protein.
Alferon N Injection® is manufactured from pooled units of human leukocytes which have been induced by incomplete infection with a murine virus (Sendai virus) to produce Interferon alfa-n3. The manufacturing process includes immunoaffinity chromatography with a murine monoclonal antibody, acidification (pH 2) for 5 days at 4°C, and gel filtration chromatography.
Since Alferon N Injection® is manufactured using source leukocytes, human donor screening is performed to minimize the risk that the leukocytes could contain infectious agents. In addition, the manufacturing process contains steps which have been shown to inactivate known viruses. There has been no evidence of infection transmission to recipients in clinical trials (See **WARNINGS**).
The Alferon N Injection® manufacturing process was evaluated for quantitative removal or inactivation of model pathogenic viruses. The viruses were deliberately added to the leukocytes in amounts far exceeding those present in contaminated blood, i.e., $\geq 10^9$ infectious units per milliliter. The manufacturing process yielded a cumulative reduction of $\geq 10^{14}$ of infectious HIV-1, i.e., $\geq 10^{6.5}$ removal by acid inactivation and $\geq 10^{7.9}$ removal by the purification process. In the validation studies, there was 10^8 reduction in the titer of hepatitis B virus as determined by HBsAg assay, and a 10^9 reduction in the infectious titer of herpes simplex virus-1 (HSV-1). Cultivation of Alferon N Injection® [Interferon alfa-n3 (human leukocyte derived)] Purified Drug Concentrate with human indicator cells, i.e., MRC-5 cells, peripheral blood leukocytes in the presence of Cyclosporin A, and fetal cord blood cells, did not detect the presence of infectious viruses.
As part of a validation study, Alferon N Injection® was examined for the presence of the following viruses; Sendai virus (SV), HIV-1, HTLV-1, HBV, HSV-1, CMV, and EBV. Alferon N Injection® contained no detectable quantities of these viruses. In addition, other studies, i.e., Polymerase Chain Reaction (PCR) and Dot Blot Hybridization (DBH), have shown no detectable genetic material from these viruses in Alferon N Injection®. The sensitivity of the PCR was 10 copies for HIV-1 (env gene probe) and 10 copies for HBV (S/P gene probe). The sensitivity of the DBH was 1 pg for EBV, < 10 pg for CMV, < 10 pg for HSV-1, and < 2 pg for SV. Furthermore, sera from 105 patients treated with Alferon N Injection® (95 with condylomata acuminata and 10 with cancer) were tested for antibody to HIV-1 and HIV p24 antigen. There was no evidence to suggest transmission of HIV-1 by Alferon N Injection®. Sera from 135 patients with condylomata acuminata treated with Alferon N Injection® were tested to determine abnormal SGOT laboratory values. There was no evidence to suggest transmission of hepatitis by Alferon N Injection® based on both SGOT results and patient data collected during clinical trials.
Alferon N Injection® has been extensively purified using immunoaffinity chromatography with a murine monoclonal antibody, acidification (pH 2) for 5 days at 4°C, and gel filtration chromatography. Alferon N Injection® has been subjected to the acid treatment for five days during its manufacture in order to reduce the risk of viral transmission. Subsequent analyses of the Alferon N Injection® Purified Drug Concentrate confirm the absence of detectable infectious or non-infectious viral particles.
The leukocyte nutrient medium contains the antibiotic neomycin sulfate at a concentration of 35 mg/L; however, neomycin sulfate is not detectable in the final product, i.e., < 0.64 µg/ml.
Murine immunoglobulin (IgG) is detected in the Alferon N Injection® [Interferon alfa-n3 (human leukocyte derived)] Purified Drug Concentrate at levels below 0.15% of the Interferon alfa-n3 protein. This equates to levels less than 8 ng of murine IgG per million of IU Interferon alfa-n3 (range of 0.9 to 5.6 ng typically found).
Alferon N Injection® is available in an injectable solution containing 5 million IU Interferon alfa-n3 per vial for intralesional injection. The solution is clear and colorless. Each milliliter (ml) contains five million IU of Interferon alfa-n3 in phosphate-buffered saline (8.0 mg sodium chloride, 1.74 mg sodium phosphate dibasic, 0.20 mg potassium phosphate monobasic, and 0.20 mg potassium chloride) containing 3.3 mg phenol as a preservative and 1 mg Albumin (Human) as a stabilizer.

CLINICAL PHARMACOLOGY

General—Interferons are naturally occurring proteins with antiviral, antiproliferative, and immunoregulatory properties. They are produced and secreted in response to viral infections and to a variety of other synthetic and biological inducers. Four major families of interferons have been identified: alpha, beta, gamma, and omega. The interferon alpha family contains 13 different non-allelic molecular species. Their molecular weights range from 16,000 to 27,000 daltons.
Interferons bind to specific membrane receptors on cell surfaces. Interferon alfa-n3 has been shown to bind to the same receptors as Interferon alfa-2b. The receptors have a high degree of selectivity for the binding of human but not mouse interferon. This correlates with the high species specificity found in laboratory studies.
Binding of interferon to membrane receptors initiates a series of events including induction of protein synthesis. These actions are followed by a variety of cellular responses, including inhibition of virus replication and suppression of cell proliferation. Immunomodulation, including enhancement of phagocytosis by macrophages, augmentation of the cytotoxicity of lymphocytes and enhancement of human leukocyte antigen expression occurs in response to exposure to interferons. One or more of these activities may contribute to the therapeutic effect of interferon.
Pharmacokinetics—In a study of intralesional use of Alferon N Injection® [Interferon alfa-n3 (human leukocyte derived)] for the treatment of condylomata acuminata, plasma concentrations of interferon were below the detection limit of the assay, i.e., ≤ 3 IU/ml. Minor systemic effects (e.g., myalgias, fever, and headaches) were noted, indicating that some of the injected interferon entered the systemic circulation (See **ADVERSE REACTIONS**).
Condylomata Acuminata—Condylomata acuminata (venereal or genital warts) are associated with infections of human papilloma virus (HPV), especially HPV type-6 and possibly type-11. Given the antiviral and antiproliferative activities of interferons and the viral etiology of condylomata, a placebo-controlled clinical trial was conducted to evaluate the safety and efficacy of intralesional injection of Alferon N Injection® in the treatment of condylomata acuminata.
In a multicenter, randomized, double-blind, placebo-controlled, clinical trial, intralesional administration of Alferon N Injection® was an effective treatment for condylomata acuminata.[1-4] One hundred fifty-six (156) patients were evaluable for efficacy (81 Alferon N Injection® patients and 75 placebo patients). Patients had a mean of five warts (range was 2-14) and all warts were treated. Patients were injected intralesionally with a mean of 225,000 IU of Alferon N Injection® [Interferon alfa-n3 (human leukocyte derived)] per wart 2 times a week for up to 8 weeks.
Overall, 80% ($^{65}/_{81}$) of patients treated with Alferon N Injection® had a complete or partial resolution of warts compared with 44% ($^{33}/_{75}$) of placebo-treated patients (p < 0.001). Alferon N Injection® was significantly more effective than placebo in producing a complete resolution of warts (p < 0.001), as shown by Table 1.
[See table 1 above]
Of the patients who had a complete resolution of warts, approximately half ($^{21}/_{44}$) the patients had complete resolution of warts by the end of treatment, and half ($^{23}/_{44}$) had complete resolution of warts during the three months after the cessation of treatment. Patients with complete resolution of warts were followed for a median of 48 weeks. Overall, 76% ($^{31}/_{41}$) of Alferon N Injection® [Interferon alfa-n3 (human leukocyte derived)]-treated patients who achieved complete resolution of warts remained clear of all treated lesions during follow-up, while 79% ($^{11}/_{14}$) of the placebo patients remained clear of all treated lesions during follow-up. A total of 762 evaluable warts were injected in this trial. Of the 407 Alferon N Injection®-treated warts, 73% ($^{297}/_{407}$) completely resolved, as compared to 35% ($^{125}/_{355}$) of the placebo-treated warts (p < 0.0001). Alferon N Injection® was effective in treating lesions of all sizes, and there was no difference in resolution for perianal, penile, or vulvar lesions.

Table 1
Degree of Resolution as Measured By Total Wart Volume per Patient

	Complete Resolution	Partial Resolution (≥50% resolution)	Minor Resolution (<50% resolution)	Progression/ No change
		Percent of Patients with:		
Alferon (n = 81)	54%	26%	15%	5%
Placebo (n = 75)	20%	24%	13%	43%

There was no difference in resolution for patients who had received prior treatment of their warts and for those who had not. Among patients with recalcitrant warts (i.e., warts that were refractory to previous treatment or recurring), 82% ($^{58}/_{71}$) of the evaluable patients had complete or partial resolution of warts due to intralesional administration of Alferon N Injection® as compared to 43% ($^{29}/_{67}$) of placebo patients (p <0.001). Fifty-four percent ($^{38}/_{71}$) of the evaluable Alferon N Injection® patients had complete resolution of warts as compared to 18% ($^{12}/_{67}$) of placebo patients (p < 0.001). Patients with primary occurrence of genital warts (i.e., no prior treatment of warts) had a similar resolution rate compared to the patients with recalcitrant warts: 70% ($^{7}/_{10}$) had complete or partial resolution of warts due to Alferon N Injection® treatment and 60% ($^{6}/_{10}$) had complete resolution of warts, as compared to 50% ($^{4}/_{8}$) of placebo recipients who had complete or partial resolution of warts and 38% ($^{3}/_{8}$) who had complete resolution. Overall, 83% ($^{5}/_{6}$) of Alferon N Injection® [Interferon alfa-n3 (human leukocyte derived)]-treated patients with primary occurrence, who achieved complete resolution of warts, remained clear of all treated lesions during a median follow-up of 52 weeks. Because the number of patients with primary occurrence of warts was small (10 Alferon N Injection® recipients and 8 placebo recipients), the difference between Alferon N Injection® and placebo treatment was not statistically significant. However, when the resolution of primary warts was examined, 75% ($^{33}/_{44}$) of the Alferon N Injection®-treated primary warts resolved completely as compared to 39% ($^{11}/_{28}$) of the placebo-treated primary warts (p = 0.003).

In an open clinical trial using a once-a-week treatment schedule for up to 16 weeks, 28 patients were evaluable for efficacy. Eighty-nine percent ($^{25}/_{28}$) of patients had a complete or partial resolution of warts following treatment with Alferon N Injection®. The condylomata acuminata resolved completely in 46% ($^{13}/_{28}$) of the patients. Of the 154 warts treated, 77% ($^{118}/_{154}$) resolved completely.

After injections of Alferon N Injection®, side effects were minor and transient. After 4 weeks of treatment, the frequency of adverse reactions was similar in Alferon N Injection® and placebo treatment groups. The most frequent side effects were myalgias, fever, and headache (See **ADVERSE REACTIONS**).

Antigenicity

1. Alferon N Injection®
   One hundred five (105) patients treated with Alferon N Injection® [Interferon alfa-n3 (human leukocyte derived)] during clinical trials were tested for the presence of anti-interferon antibodies using three different antibody assays: Immunoradiometric Assay (IRMA), Enzyme Linked Immunosorbent Assay (ELISA), and neutralization by the Cytopathic Effect Assay (CPE). To date, no antibodies to Interferon alfa-n3 have been detected in any of the patients.
2. Mouse Proteins
   No hypersensitivity reactions to the components in Alferon N Injection® [Interferon alfa-n3 (human leukocyte derived)] have been observed. Alferon N Injection® uses a murine monoclonal antibody in one of the purification procedures. A possibility exists that patients treated with Alferon N Injection® may develop hypersensitivity to the mouse proteins. However, none of the patients receiving Alferon N Injection® during clinical trials developed antibodies or hypersensitivity to mouse proteins (See **CONTRAINDICATIONS**).
3. Egg Protein
   The initial stage in the manufacture of Alferon N Injection® uses Sendai virus which was grown in chicken-embryonated eggs as the specific Interferon alfa-n3 inducer. Although no egg protein (ovalbumin) has been detected in the initial stage of interferon manufacture using an ELISA (sensitivity of 16 ng/ml), a possibility exists that patients treated with Alferon N Injection® may develop hypersensitivity to egg protein (See **CONTRAINDICATIONS**).

INDICATIONS AND USAGE

Alferon N Injection® [Interferon alfa-n3 (human leukocyte derived)] is indicated for the intralesional treatment of refractory or recurring external condylomata acuminata.

CONTRAINDICATIONS

Alferon N Injection® [Interferon alfa-n3 (human leukocyte derived)] is contraindicated in patients with known hypersensitivity to human interferon alpha proteins or any component of the product. The product is also contraindicated in patients who have anaphylactic sensitivity to mouse immunoglobulin (IgG), egg protein or neomycin.

WARNINGS

Because of the fever and other "flu-like" symptoms associated with Alferon N Injection® [Interferon alfa-n3 (human leukocyte derived)] (See **ADVERSE REACTIONS**), it should be used cautiously in patients with debilitating medical conditions such as cardiovascular disease (e.g., unstable angina and uncontrolled congestive heart failure), severe pulmonary disease (e.g., chronic obstructive pulmonary disease), or diabetes mellitus with ketoacidosis. Alferon N Injection® should be used cautiously in patients with coagulation disorders (e.g., thrombophlebitis, pulmonary embolism and hemophilia), severe myelosuppression, or seizure disorders. Acute, serious hypersensitivity reactions (e.g., urticaria, angioedema, bronchoconstriction, and anaphylaxis) have not been observed in patients receiving Alferon N Injection® [Interferon alfa-n3 (human leukocyte derived)]. However, if such reactions develop, drug administration should be discontinued immediately and appropriate medical therapy should be instituted.

Because this product is made from human blood, it may carry a risk of transmitting infectious agents, e.g., viruses, and theoretically, the Creutzfeldt Jakob disease (CJD) agent.

PRECAUTIONS

General—Patients being treated with Alferon N Injection® should be informed of the benefits and risks associated with the treatment. Because the manufacturing process, strength, and type of interferon (e.g., natural, human leukocyte interferon versus single-species recombinant interferon) may vary for different interferon formulations, changing brands may require a change in dosage. Therefore, physicians are cautioned not to change from one interferon product to another without considering these factors. The physician should select patients for treatment with Alferon N Injection® after consideration of the locations and sizes of the lesions, response to previous treatment, and the patient's ability to comply with the treatment regimen. Data on Alferon N Injection® as initial treatment are limited. There are no data on a second course of Alferon N Injection® treatment. The mean number of warts treated in one treatment cycle was five.

Information for Patients—Patients should be informed of the early signs of hypersensitivity reactions including hives, generalized urticaria, tightness of the chest, wheezing, hypotension, and anaphylaxis, and should be advised to contact their physician if these symptoms occur.

Patients being treated with Alferon N Injection® [Interferon alfa-n3 (human leukocyte derived)] should be informed of benefits and risks associated with treatment.

Patients should be cautioned not to change brands of interferon without medical consultation, as a change in dosage may occur.

Carcinogenesis, Mutagenesis, Impairment of Fertility—Studies with Alferon N Injection® [Interferon alfa-n3 (human leukocyte derived)] have not been performed to determine carcinogenicity, mutagenicity, or the effect on fertility. In studies with adult females, interferon alpha has been shown to affect the menstrual cycle and decrease serum estradiol and progesterone levels[5].

Alferon N Injection® should be used with caution in fertile men. Fertile women should be cautioned to use effective contraception while being treated with Alferon N Injection®.

Changes in the menstrual cycle and abortions have been reported to occur in non-human primates given extremely high doses of recombinant interferon alpha[6]. In these studies, Macaca mulatta (rhesus monkeys) were given interferon daily by intramuscular injection. When given at daily intramuscular doses 326 times the average intralesional dose of Alferon N Injection® (120 times the maximum recommended dose), this recombinant interferon formulation produced menstrual cycle changes in the monkeys.

In human clinical trials with Alferon N Injection®, menstrual cycle data were reported by 51 patients (36 Alferon N Injection® and 15 placebo). There was no significant difference between Alferon N Injection® and placebo treatment groups with regard to menstrual cycle changes.

PREGNANCY Pregnancy Category C—Animal reproduction studies have not been conducted with Alferon N Injection® [Interferon alfa-n3 (human leukocyte derived)]. It is also not known whether Alferon N Injection® [Interferon alfa-n3 (human leukocyte derived)] can cause fetal harm when administered to a pregnant woman or can affect reproductive capacity. Alferon N Injection® should be given to a pregnant woman only if clearly needed.

Changes in the menstrual cycle and abortions have been reported to occur in non-human primates given extremely high doses of recombinant interferon alpha. In these studies, Macaca mulatta (rhesus monkeys) were given interferon daily by intramuscular injection. Abortifacient effects were noted when the recombinant interferon alpha was given daily during early to mid-gestation at intramuscular doses of 978 times the average intralesional dose of Alferon N Injection® (360 times the maximum recommended dose).

Nursing Mothers—It is not known whether Alferon N Injection® [Interferon alfa-n3 (human leukocyte derived)] is excreted in human milk. Studies in mice have shown that mouse interferons are excreted in milk[7]. Because many drugs are excreted in human milk and because of the potential for serious adverse reactions in nursing infants, a decision should be made whether to discontinue nursing or to not initiate drug treatment, taking into account the importance of the drug to the mother and the potential risks to the infant.

Pediatric Use—There have been no studies with this product in adolescents.

ADVERSE REACTIONS

Adverse reactions were evaluated in 202 patients with condylomata acuminata receiving Alferon N Injection® by intralesional administration and in 31 patients with cancer receiving Alferon N Injection® by systemic administration. In the double-blind efficacy trial for the treatment of condylomata acuminata, 104 patients were treated with doses of Alferon N Injection® of 0.05 million to 2.5 million IU per treatment session (average dose = 0.92 million IU per treatment session) by intralesional injection. In open trials, an additional 98 patients received a dose range of 0.05 to 4.6 million IU of Alferon N Injection® per treatment session (average dose = 1.12 million IU per treatment session). Patients with cancer were given doses of Alferon N Injection® [Interferon alfa-n3 (human leukocyte derived)] of 3 million, 9 million, or 15 million IU per day for ten days by intramuscular injection.

Adverse Reactions in Patients with Condylomata Acuminata—A total of 104 patients with condylomata acuminata was treated with Alferon N Injection® [Interferon alfa-n3 (human leukocyte derived)] during the double-blind clinical trial. Adverse reactions were reported to be likely, unlikely, or not known to be related to Alferon N Injection®. Adverse reactions consisted primarily of "flu-like" symptoms (myalgias, fever, and/or headache) which were in most cases mild or moderate, and transient, and did not interfere with treatment.

The "flu-like" adverse reactions, consisting of fever, myalgias, and/or headache, occurred primarily after the first treatment session and were reported by 30% of the patients. The frequency of "flu-like" adverse reactions abated with repeated dosing of Alferon N Injection® so that the incidences due to Alferon N Injection® [Interferon alfa-n3 (human leukocyte derived)] and placebo were similar after three to four weeks of treatment (after six to eight treatment sessions). "Flu-like" symptoms were relieved by administration of acetaminophen.

Adverse reactions were reported at least once during the course of treatment in the following percentages of patients in each treatment group:

Table 2

Percent of Patients with Adverse Reactions

Adverse Reactions:	Alferon (n = 104)	Placebo (n = 85)
Autonomic Nervous System		
Sweating	2%	1%
Vasovagal Reaction	2%	0%
Body as a Whole		
Fever	40%	19%
Chills	14%	2%
Fatigue	14%	6%
Malaise	9%	9%
Skin		
Generalized Pruritus	2%	0%
Central & Peripheral Nervous System		
Dizziness	9%	4%
Insomnia	2%	1%
Gastrointestinal System		
Nausea	4%	7%
Vomiting	3%	0%
Dyspepsia/Heartburn	3%	1%
Diarrhea	2%	2%
Musculoskeletal System		
Arthralgia	5%	1%
Back Pain	4%	1%
Myalgias	45%	15%
Headache	31%	15%

Psychiatric Disorders

Depression	2%	1%

Nasopharyngeal

Nose/sinus drainage	2%	2%

Most of the systemic adverse reactions were mild or moderate. Severe systemic adverse reactions were reported by 18% of Alferon N Injection® [Interferon alfa-n3 (human leukocyte derived)]-treated patients and 13% of placebo-treated patients (not a statistically significant difference). Most of the severe systemic adverse reactions reported were "flu-like". Other severe systemic adverse reactions included back pain, insomnia, and sensitivity to allergens. Those adverse reactions which were reported by 1% of patients treated with Alferon N Injection® in the double-blind trial include: left groin lymph node swelling, tongue hyperaesthesia, thirst, tingling of legs/feet, hot sensation on bottom of feet, strange taste in mouth, increased salivation, heat intolerance, visual disturbances, pharyngitis, sensitivity to allergens, muscle cramps, nosebleed, throat tightness, and papular rash on neck. Additional adverse reactions which were reported by 1% of patients treated with placebo include: pharyngitis, oral pain, penile discharge, cold, knuckle stiffness, herpes outbreak, cough, disorientation, and weight/appetite loss.

Additional adverse reactions which occurred only in open clinical trials of intralesional use of Alferon N Injection® [Interferon alfa-n3 (human leukocyte derived)] for treatment of condylomata acuminata were herpes labialis, hot flashes, nervousness, decrease in concentration, dysuria, photosensitivity, and swollen lymph nodes. These reactions occurred in 1% of the patients. One patient with a history of epilepsy, who was not taking anticonvulsant medication, had a grand mal seizure while being treated with Alferon N Injection®; this seizure was judged to be unrelated to Alferon N Injection® administration.

Application Site Disorders—The frequency of application site disorders (such as itching and pain) for patients treated with Alferon N Injection® was significantly less than that reported with placebo (12% versus 26%). No severe application site disorders were reported by patients treated with Alferon N Injection® [Interferon alfa-n3 (human leukocyte derived)], while 7% of placebo-treated patients reported severe disorders.

Laboratory Test Values—Abnormalities were seen with statistically equivalent frequencies in both the Alferon N Injection® and placebo groups. None of the laboratory abnormalities were considered clinically significant. The abnormalities in the Alferon N Injection®-treated patients consisted primarily of decreased WBC (11%). Decreases also occurred in 4% of the placebo patients (not a statistically significant difference). The abnormalities in Alferon N Injection®-treated patients involved increases of only one WHO grade.

Adverse Reactions in Patients with Cancer—Thirty-one (31) patients with cancer were treated with a maximum of ten intramuscular injections of Alferon N Injection® in doses of 3 million IU, 9 million IU, or 15 million IU per treatment session. The occurrence of adverse reactions was judged to be unrelated to the dose of Alferon N Injection®. The following adverse reactions were reported at least once (the percentage of patients experiencing the reaction is indicated in parentheses): chills (87%), fever (81%), anorexia (68%), malaise (65%), nausea (48%), vomiting (29%), myalgias (16%), arthralgia (10%), chest pains (10%), soreness at injection site (10%), sleepiness (10%), headache (10%), diarrhea (6%), fatigue (6%), low blood pressure (6%), sore mouth/stomatitis (6%), and blurred vision (6%). Those adverse reactions which were each reported by only one patient treated with Alferon N Injection® [Interferon alfa-n3 (human leukocyte derived)] include: stiff shoulders, flushed face, edema, dry mouth, mucositis, coughing, numbness, numbness in hands, numbness in fingers, pain on ocular rotation, shakes/shivers, ringing in ears, cramps, constipation, muscle soreness, confusion, light-headedness, depression, upset stomach, and sweating. The following adverse reactions were reported as severe by at least one patient (the percentage of patients experiencing the reaction is indicated in parentheses): fever (55%), malaise (54%), anorexia (45%), chills (45%), nausea (16%), myalgias (13%), vomiting (10%), fatigue (6%), low blood pressure (6%), chest pains (6%), sore mouth/stomatitis (6%), headache (3%), diarrhea (3%), sleepiness (3%), arthralgia (3%), blurred vision (3%), stiff shoulders (3%), numbness (3%), pain on ocular rotation (3%), muscle soreness (3%), confusion (3%), light-headedness (3%), depression (3%), and sweating (3%).

The number and percentage of patients with cancer who experienced a significant abnormal laboratory test value (values that changed from WHO Grades 0, 1, or 2 at baseline to WHO Grades 3 or 4 during or after treatment) at least once during the trials are shown in the following table:

Table 3
Abnormal Laboratory Test Values

	Cancer (n = 31)
Hemoglobin Level	2 (7%)
White Blood Cell Count	1 (3%)
Platelet Count	1 (3%)
GGT	1 (6%)
SGOT	1 (3%)
Alkaline Phosphatase	2 (8%)
Total Bilirubin	1 (4%)

DOSAGE AND ADMINISTRATION

The recommended dose of Alferon N Injection® for the treatment of condylomata acuminata is 0.05 ml (250,000 IU) per wart. Alferon N Injection® should be administered twice weekly for up to 8 weeks. The maximum recommended dose per treatment session is 0.5 ml (2.5 million IU). Alferon N Injection® should be injected into the base of each wart, preferably using a 30 gauge needle. For large warts, Alferon N Injection® [Interferon alfa-n3 (human leukocyte derived)] may be injected at several points around the periphery of the wart, using a total dose of 0.05 ml per wart.

The minimum effective dose of Alferon N Injection® [Interferon alfa-n3 (human leukocyte derived)] for the treatment of condylomata acuminata has not been established. Moderate to severe adverse experiences may require modification of the dosage regimen or, in some cases, termination of therapy with Alferon N Injection®.

Genital warts usually begin to disappear after several weeks of treatment with Alferon N Injection®. Treatment should continue for a maximum of 8 weeks. In clinical trials with Alferon N Injection®, many patients who had partial resolution of warts during treatment experienced further resolution of their warts after cessation of treatment. Of the patients who had complete resolution of warts due to treatment, half the patients had complete resolution of warts by the end of the treatment and half had complete resolution of warts during the 3 months after cessation of treatment. Thus, it is recommended that no further therapy (Alferon N Injection® or conventional therapy) be administered for 3 months after the initial 8-week course of treatment unless the warts enlarge or new warts appear. Studies to determine the safety and efficacy of a second course of treatment with Alferon N Injection® have not been conducted.

Parenteral drug products should be inspected visually for particulate matter and discoloration prior to administration, whenever solution and container permit.

HOW SUPPLIED

Injectable Solution: Each vial contains 1 ml of Alferon N Injection®. Each ml of Alferon N Injection® contains 5 million IU of Interferon alfa-n3, 3.3 mg of phenol, and 1 mg of Albumin (Human) in a pH 7.4 phosphate-buffered saline solution (8.0 mg/ml sodium chloride, 1.74 mg/ml sodium phosphate dibasic, 0.20 mg/ml potassium phosphate monobasic, and 0.20 mg/ml potassium chloride). One vial per box. (NDC 54746-001-01).

STORAGE

Alferon N Injection® [Interferon alfa-n3 (human leukocyte derived)] should be stored at 2° to 8°C (36° to 46°F). Do not freeze. Do not shake.

℞ Only

REFERENCES

1. Friedman-Kien, AE; Eron, LJ; Conant, M; et al., *JAMA* 1988; *259*: 533–538.
2. Kirby, P; (editorial comment), *JAMA* 1988; *259*: 570–572.
3. Friedman-Kien, AE; Plasse, TF; et al., *Papilloma Viruses: Molecular and Clinical Aspects*[Howley, PM, Broker, TR (eds)], New York, Alan R. Liss, Inc.; 1986; 217–233.
4. Geffen, JR; Klein, RJ; Friedman-Kien, AE; *J. Infect. Dis.* 1984; *150*: 612–615.
5. Kauppila, A; et al., *Int. J. Cancer* 1982; *29*: 291–294.
6. Trown, PW; et al., *Cancer* 1986; *57* (Suppl): 1648–1656.
7. Schafer, TW; et al., *Science* 1972; *176*: 1326–1327.

Manufactured and Distributed by:
Hemispherx Biopharma, Inc.
One Penn Center
1617 JFK Boulevard
Philadelphia, PA 19103-1806
U.S. Lic. 1703
Copyright © 1989, 1990, 1997, 2000, 2003, 2004

Hemispherx Biopharma, Inc.
Philadelphia, PA
All rights reserved.
09/04
Shown in Product Identification Guide, page 310

High Chemical Company
3901-A NEBRASKA STREET
LEVITTOWN, PA 19056
www.sarapin.com

Phone: 800-447-8792, 215-788-3113
Email: sarapin@gmail.com

SARAPIN ℞

DESCRIPTION

A sterile aqueous solution of soluble salts of the volatile bases from Sarraceniaceae (Pitcher Plant). Benzyl Alcohol 0.75%.

ACTIONS

The painful syndromes most commonly encountered in general practice which are relieved by SARAPIN® treatment are as follows:
Sciatic Pain
Intercostal Neuralgia
Alcoholic Neuritis
Occipital Neuritis
Brachial Plexus Neuralgia
Meralgia Paresthetica
Lumbar Neuralgia
Trigeminal Neuralgia

ADMINISTRATION

These and allied conditions may be treated with success in a majority of cases by nerve block or local infiltration:
Paravertebral—Careful localization of the zone of tenderness permits a determination of the corresponding trunk levels to be injected.
Perineural—In some instances, as in sciatica, the affected nerve can be injected at a site distant from its origin.
Local Infiltration—Multiple injections throughout an area of tenderness provide for diffusion into all the affected parts.

DOSAGE AND ADMINISTRATION

Paravertebral Injections

Cervical	2–3 ml
Dorsal	5–10 ml
Lumbar	5–10 ml
Sacral	3–5 ml
Caudal Canal	10 ml
Sciatic Nerve	10 ml
Local Infiltration	5–10 ml

WARNINGS

Withdraw plunger of syringe to make sure the needle point is not in a blood vessel.

PRECAUTIONS

Procedure should be gentle and unhurried.
SARAPIN® is intended only for professional use. Its successful employment depends upon a thorough knowledge of the anatomy involved.

ADVERSE REACTIONS

Patients should be maintained in a recumbent position for 10 to 15 minutes following injection. A local sensation is to be expected, limited to the distribution of the nerve injected, and usually appearing as a temporary feeling of heaviness, although some cases will feel heat or a transitory aggravation of symptoms.

CONTRAINDICATIONS

SARAPIN® is non-toxic, has no side effects other than above and is contraindicated only in areas of infection.

HOW SUPPLIED

50 ml Multiple Dose Vial.
NDC-10541-492-50
CAUTION: Federal law prohibits dispensing without prescription.
HIGH CHEMICAL COMPANY
3901-A Nebraska Street
Levittown, PA 19056-3333
800-447-8792, 215-788-3113
www.sarapin.com
Shown in Product Identification Guide, page 310

Inspire Pharmaceuticals
4222 EMPEROR BOULEVARD, #200
DURHAM, NC 27703

Direct Inquiries to:
Telephone: 919-941-9777
Fax: 919-941-9797
E-mail: info@inspirepharm.com
For AzaSite:
Patient/Physician Questions: 1-888-881-4696

AZASITE®
[āz-ə-sīt]
(azithromycin ophthalmic solution) 1%
Sterile topical ophthalmic drops

HIGHLIGHTS OF PRESCRIBING INFORMATION
These highlights do not include all the information needed to use AzaSite safely and effectively. See full prescribing information for AzaSite.
AZASITE (azithromycin) solution for ophthalmic use
Initial U.S. Approval: 2007

——————INDICATIONS AND USAGE——————
AzaSite® is a macrolide antibiotic indicated for the treatment of bacterial conjunctivitis caused by susceptible isolates of the following microorganisms: CDC coryneform group G, *Haemophilus influenzae*, *Staphylococcus aureus*, *Streptococcus mitis* group, and *Streptococcus pneumoniae*. (1)

——————DOSAGE AND ADMINISTRATION——————
Instill 1 drop in the affected eye(s) twice daily, eight to twelve hours apart for the first two days and then instill 1 drop in the affected eye(s) once daily for the next five days. (2)

——————DOSAGE FORMS AND STRENGTHS——————
5 mL size bottle filled with 2.5 mL of 1% sterile topical ophthalmic solution. (3)

——————CONTRAINDICATIONS——————
None (4)

——————WARNING AND PRECAUTIONS——————
• For topical ophthalmic use only. (5.1)
• Anaphylaxis and hypersensitivity have been reported with systemic use of azithromycin. (5.2)
• Growth of resistant organisms may occur with prolonged use. (5.3)
• Patients should not wear contact lenses if they have signs or symptoms of bacterial conjunctivitis. (5.4)

——————ADVERSE REACTIONS——————
Most common adverse reaction reported in patients was eye irritation (1-2% of patients). (6)

To report SUSPECTED ADVERSE REACTIONS, contact Inspire Pharmaceuticals, Inc. at 1-888-881-4696 or FDA at 1-800-FDA-1088 or www.fda.gov/medwatch

See 17 for PATIENT COUNSELING INFORMATION.
Revised: 11/2008

FULL PRESCRIBING INFORMATION: CONTENTS*

FULL PRESCRIBING INFORMATION

1   INDICATIONS AND USAGE
AzaSite is indicated for the treatment of bacterial conjunctivitis caused by susceptible isolates of the following microorganisms:

CDC coryneform group G*
Haemophilus influenzae
Staphylococcus aureus
Streptococcus mitis group
Streptococcus pneumoniae

*Efficacy for this organism was studied in fewer than 10 infections.

2   DOSAGE AND ADMINISTRATION
The recommended dosage regimen for the treatment of bacterial conjunctivitis is: Instill 1 drop in the affected eye(s) twice daily, eight to twelve hours apart for the first two days and then instill 1 drop in the affected eye(s) once daily for the next five days.

3   DOSAGE FORMS AND STRENGTHS
5 mL bottle containing 2.5 mL of a 1% sterile topical ophthalmic solution.

4   CONTRAINDICATIONS
None

5   WARNINGS AND PRECAUTIONS
5.1   Topical Ophthalmic Use Only
NOT FOR INJECTION. AzaSite is indicated for topical ophthalmic use only, and should not be administered systemically, injected subconjunctivally, or introduced directly into the anterior chamber of the eye.

5.2   Anaphylaxis and Hypersensitivity with Systemic Use of Azithromycin
In patients receiving systemically administered azithromycin, serious allergic reactions, including angioedema, anaphylaxis, and dermatologic reactions including Stevens Johnson Syndrome and toxic epidermal necrolysis have been reported rarely in patients on azithromycin therapy. Although rare, fatalities have been reported. The potential for anaphylaxis or other hypersensitivity reactions should be considered since patients with a known hypersensitivity to azithromycin or erythromycin were excluded from study.

5.3   Growth of Resistant Organisms with Prolonged Use
As with other anti-infectives, prolonged use may result in overgrowth of non-susceptible organisms, including fungi. If super-infection occurs, discontinue use and institute alternative therapy. Whenever clinical judgment dictates, the patient should be examined with the aid of magnification, such as slit-lamp biomicroscopy, and where appropriate, fluorescein staining.

5.4   Avoidance of Contact Lenses
Patients should be advised not to wear contact lenses if they have signs or symptoms of bacterial conjunctivitis.

6   ADVERSE REACTIONS
6.1   Clinical Trials Experience
Because clinical trials are conducted under widely varying conditions, adverse reaction rates observed in one clinical trial of a drug cannot be directly compared with the rates in the clinical trials of the same or another drug and may not reflect the rates observed in practice.

The data described below reflect exposure to AzaSite in 698 patients. The population was between 1 and 87 years old with clinical signs and symptoms of bacterial conjunctivitis. The most frequently reported ocular adverse reaction reported in patients receiving AzaSite was eye irritation. This reaction occurred in approximately 1-2% of patients. Other adverse reactions associated with the use of AzaSite were reported in less than 1% of patients and included: burning, stinging and irritation upon instillation, contact dermatitis, corneal erosion, dry eye, dysgeusia, nasal congestion, ocular discharge, punctate keratitis, and sinusitis.

6.2   Postmarketing Experience
In addition to adverse events reported from clinical trials, the following events have been identified during post approval use of AzaSite. These events were reported voluntarily from a population of unknown size, and the frequency of occurrence cannot be determined precisely. These events have been chosen for inclusion due to either their seriousness, frequency of reporting, or causal connection to AzaSite or a combination of these factors.

Eye: blurring, eyelid swelling, itching, pain, visual acuity reduction.

General: allergic reactions including facial swelling, hives, periocular swelling, rash, urticaria.

7   DRUG INTERACTIONS
Drug interaction studies have not been conducted with AzaSite ophthalmic solution.

8   USE IN SPECIFIC POPULATIONS
8.1   Pregnancy
Pregnancy Category B. Reproduction studies have been performed in rats and mice at doses up to 200 mg/kg/d. The highest dose was associated with moderate maternal toxicity. These doses are estimated to be approximately 5000 times, the maximum human ocular daily dose of 2 mg. In the animal studies, no evidence of harm to the fetus due to azithromycin was found. There are, however, no adequate and well-controlled studies in pregnant women. Because animal reproduction studies are not always predictive of human response, azithromycin should be used during pregnancy only if clearly needed.

8.3   Nursing Mothers
It is not known whether azithromycin is excreted in human milk. Because many drugs are excreted in human milk, caution should be exercised when azithromycin is administered to a nursing woman.

8.4   Pediatric Use
The safety and effectiveness of AzaSite solution in pediatric patients below 1 year of age have not been established. The efficacy of AzaSite in treating bacterial conjunctivitis in pediatric patients one year or older has been demonstrated in controlled clinical trials. [see Clinical Studies (14)].

8.5   Geriatric Use
No overall differences in safety or effectiveness have been observed between elderly and younger patients.

11   DESCRIPTION
AzaSite (azithromycin ophthalmic solution) is a 1% sterile aqueous topical ophthalmic solution of azithromycin formulated in DuraSite® (polycarbophil, edetate disodium, sodium chloride). AzaSite is an off-white, viscous liquid with an osmolality of approximately 290 mOsm/kg.

Preservative: 0.003% benzalkonium chloride.

Inactives: mannitol, citric acid, sodium citrate, poloxamer 407, polycarbophil, edetate disodium (EDTA), sodium chloride, water for injection, and sodium hydroxide to adjust pH to 6.3.

Azithromycin is a macrolide antibiotic with a 15-membered ring. Its chemical name is (2R,3S,4R,5R,8R,10R,11R,12S,13S,14R)-13-[(2,6-dideoxy-3-C-methyl-3-O-methyl-α-L-ribo-hexopyranosyl)oxy]-2-ethyl-3,4,10-trihydroxy-3,5,6,8,10,12,14-heptamethyl-11-[[3,4,6-trideoxy-3-(dimethylamino)-ß-D-xylo-hexopyranosyl]oxy]-1-oxa-6-aza-cyclopentadecan-15-one, and the structural formula is:

Azithromycin has a molecular weight of 749, and its empirical formula is $C_{38}H_{72}N_2O_{12}$.

12   CLINICAL PHARMACOLOGY
12.1   Mechanism of Action
Azithromycin is a macrolide antibiotic [see Clinical Pharmacology, Microbiology (12.4)].

12.3   Pharmacokinetics
The plasma concentration of azithromycin following ocular administration of AzaSite (azithromycin ophthalmic solution) in humans is unknown. Based on the proposed dose of one drop to each eye (total dose of 100 mcL or 1 mg) and exposure information from systemic administration, the systemic concentration of azithromycin following ocular administration is estimated to be below quantifiable limits (≤10 ng/mL) at steady-state in humans, assuming 100% systemic availability.

12.4   Microbiology
Azithromycin acts by binding to the 50S ribosomal subunit of susceptible microorganisms and interfering with microbial protein synthesis.

Azithromycin has been shown to be active against most isolates of the following microorganisms, both *in vitro* and clinically in conjunctival infections as described in the INDICATIONS AND USAGE section:

CDC coryneform group G*
Haemophilus influenzae
Staphylococcus aureus
Streptococcus mitis group
Streptococcus pneumoniae

The following *in vitro* data are also available, **but their clinical significance in ophthalmic infections is unknown.** The safety and effectiveness of AzaSite in treating ophthalmological infections due to these microorganisms have not been established.

The following microorganisms are considered susceptible when evaluated using systemic breakpoints. However, a correlation between the *in vitro* systemic breakpoint and ophthalmological efficacy has not been established. This list of microorganisms is provided as an aid only in assessing the potential treatment of conjunctival infections. Azithromycin exhibits *in vitro* minimal inhibitory concentrations (MICs) of equal or less (systemic susceptible breakpoint) against most (≥90%) of isolates of the following ocular pathogens:

Chlamydia pneumoniae
Chlamydia trachomatis
Legionella pneumophila
Moraxella catarrhalis
Mycoplasma hominis
Mycoplasma pneumoniae
Neisseria gonorrhoeae
Peptostreptococcus species
Streptococci (Groups C, F, G)
Streptococcus pyogenes
Streptococcus agalactiae
Ureaplasma urealyticum
Viridans group streptococci

Efficacy for this organism was studied in fewer than 10 infections.

13 NONCLINICAL TOXICOLOGY

13.1 Carcinogenesis, Mutagenesis, Impairment of Fertility

Long term studies in animals have not been performed to evaluate carcinogenic potential. Azithromycin has shown no mutagenic potential in standard laboratory tests: mouse lymphoma assay, human lymphocyte clastogenic assay, and mouse bone marrow clastogenic assay. No evidence of impaired fertility due to azithromycin was found in mice or rats that received oral doses of up to 200 mg/kg/day.

13.2 Animal Toxicology and/or Pharmacology

Phospholipidosis (intracellular phospholipid accumulation) has been observed in some tissues of mice, rats, and dogs given multiple systemic doses of azithromycin. Cytoplasmic microvacuolation, which is likely a manifestation of phospholipidosis, has been observed in the corneas of rabbits given multiple ocular doses of AzaSite. This effect was reversible upon cessation of AzaSite treatment. The significance of this toxicological finding for animals and for humans is unknown.

14 CLINICAL STUDIES

In a randomized, vehicle-controlled, double-blind, multicenter clinical study in which patients were dosed twice daily for the first two days, then once daily on days 3, 4, and 5, AzaSite solution was superior to vehicle on days 6-7 in patients who had a confirmed clinical diagnosis of bacterial conjunctivitis. Clinical resolution was achieved in 63% (82/130) of patients treated with AzaSite versus 50% (74/149) of patients treated with vehicle. The p value for the comparison was 0.03 and the 95% confidence interval around the 13% (63%-50%) difference was 2% to 25%. The microbiological success rate for the eradication of the baseline pathogens was approximately 88% compared to 66% of patients treated with vehicle (p<.001, confidence interval around the 22% difference was 13% to 31%). Microbiologic eradication does not always correlate with clinical outcome in anti-infective trials.

16 HOW SUPPLIED/STORAGE AND HANDLING

AzaSite is a sterile aqueous topical ophthalmic formulation of 1% azithromycin in a white, round, low-density polyethylene (LDPE) bottle, with a natural LDPE dropper tip, and a tan colored high density polyethylene (HDPE) eyedropper cap. A white tamper evident overcap is provided.
2.5 mL in 5 mL bottle containing a total of 25 mg of azithromycin
(NDC 31357-040-25)

Storage and Handling:

Store unopened bottle under refrigeration at 2°C to 8°C (36°F to 46°F). Once the bottle is opened, store at 2°C to 25°C (36°F to 77°F) for up to 14 days. Discard after the 14 days.

17 PATIENT COUNSELING INFORMATION

Patients should be advised to avoid contaminating the applicator tip by allowing it to touch the eye, fingers or other sources.

Patients should be directed to discontinue use and contact a physician if any signs of an allergic reaction occur.

Patients should be told that although it is common to feel better early in the course of the therapy, the medication should be taken exactly as directed. Skipping doses or not completing the full course of therapy may (1) decrease the effectiveness of the immediate treatment and (2) increase

---

the likelihood that bacteria will develop resistance and will not be treatable by AzaSite (azithromycin ophthalmic solution) or other antibacterial drugs in the future.

Patients should be advised not to wear contact lenses if they have signs or symptoms of bacterial conjunctivitis.

Patients are advised to thoroughly wash hands prior to using AzaSite.

Invert closed bottle (upside down) and shake once before each use. Remove cap with bottle still in the inverted position. Tilt head back, and with bottle inverted, gently squeeze bottle to instill one drop into the affected eye(s).

Inspire Pharmaceuticals Inc.

Licensee of InSite Vision Incorporated

Manufactured by Catalent Pharma Solutions, LLC

U.S. PAT NO. 5,192,535; 6,239,113; 6,569,443; 6,861,411; 7,056,893; and Patents Pending

AZA-0289

ISV06-42-0004

Intendis, Inc.

36 COLUMBIA ROAD
P.O. BOX 1941
MORRISTOWN, NJ 07962-1941

Direct Inquiries to:
1-(866) 463-3634
For Medical Information and to report adverse drug events contact:
1-(866) 463-3634

DESONATE®   ℞
[de-son-ate]
(desonide)
Gel for topical use only

HIGHLIGHTS OF PRESCRIBING INFORMATION

These highlights do not include all the information needed to use DESONATE® Gel safely and effectively. See full prescribing information for DESONATE® Gel.

DESONATE® (desonide) Gel for topical use only

Initial U.S. Approval: 1972

————————INDICATIONS AND USAGE————————

Desonate is a corticosteroid indicated for the topical treatment of mild to moderate atopic dermatitis in patients 3 months of age and older. (1)

————DOSAGE AND ADMINISTRATION————

- Apply as a thin layer to the affected areas two times daily and rub in gently. (2)
- Therapy should be discontinued when control is achieved. (2)
- If no improvement is seen within 4 weeks, reassessment of diagnosis may be necessary. (2)
- Should not be used with occlusive dressings. (2)
- Treatment beyond 4 consecutive weeks is not recommended. (2)
- For topical use only. Not for oral, ophthalmic, or intravaginal use. (2)

————DOSAGE FORMS AND STRENGTHS————

Gel, 0.05%; (0.5mg/g) desonide in a translucent to opaque gel

————————CONTRAINDICATIONS————————

History of hypersensitivity to any of the components of the preparation.

————WARNINGS AND PRECAUTIONS————

- Topical corticosteroids can produce reversible hypothalamic pituitary adrenal (HPA) axis suppression, Cushing's syndrome and unmask latent diabetes. (5.1)
- Systemic absorption may require evaluation for HPA axis suppression (5.1).
- Modify use should HPA axis suppression develop (5.1)
- Potent corticosteroids, use on large areas, prolonged use or occlusive use may increase systemic absorption (5.1)
- Local adverse reactions may include atrophy, striae, irritation, acneiform eruptions, hypopigmentation, and allergic contact dermatitis and may be more likely with occlusive use or more potent corticosteroids. (5.2, 5.4, 6)
- Children may be more susceptible to systemic toxicity when treated with topical corticosteroids. (5.1, 8.4)

————————ADVERSE REACTIONS————————

The most common adverse reactions (incidence ≥ 1%) are headache and application site burning. (6)

To report SUSPECTED ADVERSE REACTIONS, contact Intendis, Inc. at 1-866-463-3634 or FDA at 1-800-FDA-1088 or www.fda.gov/medwatch.

————USE IN SPECIFIC POPULATIONS————

Safety and effectiveness of Desonate in pediatric patients less than 3 months of age have not been evaluated, and therefore its use in this age group is not recommended. (8.4)

See 17 for PATIENT COUNSELING INFORMATION

Revised: 6/2010

FULL PRESCRIBING INFORMATION: CONTENTS*

1 INDICATIONS AND USAGE
2 DOSAGE AND ADMINISTRATION
3 DOSAGE FORMS AND STRENGTHS
4 CONTRAINDICATIONS
5 WARNINGS AND PRECAUTIONS
   5.1   Effects on Endocrine System
   5.2   Local Adverse Reactions with Topical Corticosteroids
   5.3   Concomitant Skin Infections
   5.4   Skin Irritation
6 ADVERSE REACTIONS
8 USE IN SPECIFIC POPULATIONS
   8.1   Pregnancy
   8.3   Nursing Mothers
   8.4   Pediatric Use
   8.5   Geriatric Use
10 OVERDOSAGE
11 DESCRIPTION
12 CLINICAL PHARMACOLOGY
   12.1   Mechanism of Action
   12.2   Pharmacodynamics
   12.3   Pharmacokinetics
13 NONCLINICAL TOXICOLOGY
   13.1   Carcinogenesis, Mutagenesis, Impairment of Fertility
14 CLINICAL STUDIES
16 HOW SUPPLIED/STORAGE AND HANDLING
17 PATIENT COUNSELING INFORMATION
*Sections or subsections omitted from the full prescribing information are not listed

---

FULL PRESCRIBING INFORMATION

1 INDICATIONS AND USAGE

Desonate is indicated for the treatment of mild to moderate atopic dermatitis in patients 3 months of age and older.

Patients should be instructed to use Desonate for the minimum amount of time as necessary to achieve the desired results because of the potential for Desonate to suppress the hypothalamic-pituitary-adrenal (HPA) axis *[see Warnings and Precautions (5.1)]*. Treatment should not exceed 4 consecutive weeks *[see Dosage and Administration (2)]*.

2 DOSAGE AND ADMINISTRATION

Apply a thin layer to the affected areas two times daily and rub in gently. Discontinue use when control is achieved. If no improvement is seen within 4 weeks, reassessment of diagnosis may be necessary. Treatment beyond 4 consecutive weeks is not recommended. Do not use with occlusive dressings. Avoid contact with eyes or other mucous membranes. For topical use only. Not for oral, ophthalmic, or intravaginal use.

3 DOSAGE FORMS AND STRENGTHS

Gel, 0.05%; (0.5mg/g) desonide in a translucent to opaque gel

4 CONTRAINDICATIONS

Desonate is contraindicated in those patients with a history of hypersensitivity to any of the components of the preparation.

5 WARNINGS AND PRECAUTIONS

5.1 Effects on Endocrine System

Systemic absorption of topical corticosteroids can produce reversible hypothalamic-pituitary-adrenal (HPA) axis suppression with the potential for clinical glucocorticosteroid insufficiency. This may occur during treatment or upon withdrawal of the topical corticosteroid.

The effect of Desonate on HPA axis function was investigated in pediatric subjects, 6 months to 6 years old, with atopic dermatitis covering at least 35% of their body, who were treated with Desonate twice daily for 4 weeks. One of 37 subjects (3%) displayed adrenal suppression after 4 weeks of use, based on the cosyntropin stimulation test. As follow-up evaluation of the subject's adrenal axis was not performed, it is unknown whether the suppression was reversible *[see Use In Specific Populations (8.4) and Clinical Pharmacology (12.2)]*.

Pediatric patients may be more susceptible than adults to systemic toxicity from equivalent doses of Desonate due to their larger skin surface-to-body mass ratios *[see Use In Specific Populations (8.4)]*.

Because of the potential for systemic absorption, use of topical corticosteroids may require that patients be periodically evaluated for HPA axis suppression. Factors that predispose a patient using a topical corticosteroid to HPA axis suppression include the use of more potent steroids, use over large surface areas, use over prolonged periods, use under occlusion, use on an altered skin barrier, and use in patients with liver failure.

An ACTH stimulation test may be helpful in evaluating patients for HPA axis suppression. If HPA axis suppression is documented, an attempt should be made to gradually withdraw the drug, to reduce the frequency of application, or to substitute a less potent steroid. Manifestations of adrenal insufficiency may require supplemental systemic corticosteroids. Recovery of HPA axis function is generally prompt and complete upon discontinuation of topical corticosteroids.

Cushing's syndrome, hyperglycemia, and unmasking of latent diabetes mellitus can also result from systemic absorption of topical corticosteroids.

Use of more than one corticosteroid-containing product at the same time may increase the total systemic corticosteroid exposure.

5.2 Local Adverse Reactions with Topical Corticosteroids

Local adverse reactions may be more likely to occur with occlusive use, prolonged use or use of higher potency corticosteroids. Reactions may include skin atrophy, striae, telangiectasias, burning, itching, irritation, dryness, folliculitis, acneiform eruptions, hypopigmentation, perioral dermatitis, allergic contact dermatitis, secondary infection, and miliaria. Some local adverse reactions may be irreversible.

5.3 Concomitant Skin Infections

If concomitant skin infections are present or develop during treatment, an appropriate antifungal or antibacterial agent should be used. If a favorable response does not occur promptly, use of Desonate should be discontinued until the infection is adequately controlled.

5.4 Skin Irritation

If irritation develops, Desonate should be discontinued and appropriate therapy instituted. Allergic contact dermatitis with corticosteroids is usually diagnosed by observing failure to heal rather than noting a clinical exacerbation as with most topical products not containing corticosteroids. Such an observation should be corroborated with appropriate diagnostic patch testing.

6 ADVERSE REACTIONS

Because clinical trials are conducted under widely varying conditions, adverse reaction rates observed in the clinical trials of a drug cannot be directly compared to rates in the clinical trials of another drug and may not reflect the rates observed in practice.

In controlled clinical studies of 425 Desonate-treated subjects and 157 Vehicle-treated subjects, adverse events occurred at the application site in 3% of subjects treated with Desonate and the incidence rate was not higher compared with vehicle-treated subjects. The most common local adverse events in Desonate treated subjects were application site burning in 1% (4/425) and rash in 1% (3/425) followed by application site pruritus in <1% (2/425).

Adverse events that resulted in premature discontinuation of study drug in Desonate treated subjects were telangiectasia and worsening of atopic dermatitis in one subject each.

Additional adverse events observed during clinical trials for patients treated with Desonate included headache in 2% (8/425) compared with 1% (2/157) in those treated with vehicle.

The following additional local adverse reactions have been reported infrequently with topical corticosteroids. They may occur more frequently with the use of occlusive dressings, especially with higher potency corticosteroids. These reactions are listed in an approximate decreasing order of occurrence: folliculitis, acneiform eruptions, hypopigmentation, perioral dermatitis, secondary infection, skin atrophy, striae, and miliaria.

8 USE IN SPECIFIC POPULATIONS

8.1 Pregnancy

Teratogenic effects: Pregnancy Category C:

There are no adequate and well-controlled studies in pregnant women. Therefore, Desonate should be used during pregnancy only if the potential benefit justifies the potential risk to the fetus.

Corticosteroids have been shown to be teratogenic in laboratory animals when administered systemically at relatively low dosage levels. Some corticosteroids have been shown to be teratogenic after dermal application in laboratory animals.

No reproductive studies in animals have been performed with Desonate. Dermal embryofetal development studies were conducted in rats and rabbits with a desonide cream, 0.05% formulation. Topical doses of 0.2, 0.6, and 2.0 g cream/kg/day of a desonide cream, 0.05% formulation or 2.0 g/kg of the cream base were administered topically to pregnant rats (gestational days 6-15) and pregnant rabbits (gestational days 6-18). Maternal body weight loss was noted at all dose levels of the desonide cream, 0.05% formulation in rats and rabbits. Teratogenic effects characteristic of corticosteroids were noted in both species. The desonide cream, 0.05% formulation was teratogenic in rats at topical doses of 0.6 and 2.0 g cream/kg/day and in rabbits at a topical dose of 2.0 g cream/kg/day. No teratogenic effects were noted for the desonide cream, 0.05% formulation at a topical dose of 0.2 g cream/kg/day in rats and 0.6 g cream/kg/day in rabbits. These doses (0.2 g cream/kg/day and 0.6 g cream/kg/day) are similar to the maximum recommended human dose based on body surface area comparisons.

8.3 Nursing Mothers

Systemically administered corticosteroids appear in human milk and could suppress growth, interfere with endogenous corticosteroid production, or cause other untoward effects. It is not known whether topical administration of corticosteroids could result in sufficient systemic absorption to produce detectable quantities in human milk. Because many drugs are excreted in human milk, caution should be exercised when Desonate is administered to a nursing woman.

8.4 Pediatric Use

Safety and effectiveness of Desonate in pediatric patients less than 3 months of age have not been evaluated, and therefore its use in this age group is not recommended.

The effect of Desonate on HPA axis function was investigated in pediatric subjects, with atopic dermatitis covering at least 35% of their body, who were treated with Desonate twice daily for 4 weeks. One of 37 subjects (3%) displayed adrenal suppression after 4 weeks of use, based on the cosyntropin stimulation test *[see Warnings and Precautions (5.1)]*.

In controlled clinical studies in subjects 3 months to 18 years of age, 425 subjects were treated with Desonate and 157 subjects were treated with vehicle *[see Adverse Reactions (6) and Clinical Studies (14)]*.

Because of a higher ratio of skin surface area to body mass, pediatric patients are at a greater risk than adults of HPA axis suppression when they are treated with topical corticosteroids. They are therefore also at greater risk of glucocorticosteroid insufficiency after withdrawal of treatment and of Cushing's syndrome while on treatment.

Adverse effects, including striae, have been reported with inappropriate use of topical corticosteroids in infants and children. HPA axis suppression, Cushing's syndrome, linear growth retardation, delayed weight gain and intracranial hypertension have been reported in children receiving topical corticosteroids. Manifestations of adrenal suppression in children include low plasma cortisol levels and absence of response to ACTH stimulation. Manifestations of intracranial hypertension include bulging fontanelles, headaches, and bilateral papilledema.

8.5 Geriatric Use

Clinical studies of Desonate did not include patients aged 65 and older to determine if they respond differently than younger patients. Treatment of this patient population should reflect the greater frequency of decreased hepatic, renal, or cardiac function, and of concomitant disease or other drug therapy.

10 OVERDOSAGE

Topically applied Desonate can be absorbed in sufficient amounts to produce systemic effects *[see Warnings and Precautions (5.1)]*.

11 DESCRIPTION

Desonate contains desonide [(pregna-1, 4-diene-3, 20-dione, 11, 21-dihydroxy-16, 17-[(1-methylethylidene) bis(oxy)]-, (11β,16α)]- a synthetic nonfluorinated corticosteroid for topical dermatologic use. Chemically, desonide is $C_{24}H_{32}O_6$. It has the following structural formula:

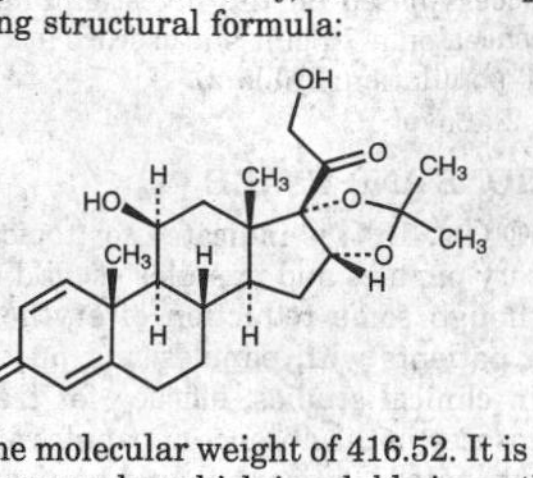

Desonide has the molecular weight of 416.52. It is a white to off-white odorless powder which is soluble in methanol and practically insoluble in water. Each gram of Desonate contains 0.5 mg of desonide in an aqueous gel base of purified water, glycerin, propylene glycol, edetate disodium dihydrate, methylparaben, propylparaben, sodium hydroxide, and Carbopol® 981.

12 CLINICAL PHARMACOLOGY

12.1 Mechanism of Action

The mechanism of action of desonide is unknown.

12.2 Pharmacodynamics

In an HPA axis suppression study, one of 37 (3%) pediatric subjects, 6 months to 6 years old, with moderate to severe atopic dermatitis covering at least 35% body surface area who applied Desonate experienced suppression of the adrenal glands following 4 weeks of therapy *[see Warnings And Precautions (5.1) and Use In Specific Populations (8.4)]*. A follow-up evaluation of the subject's adrenal axis was not performed; it is unknown whether the suppression was reversible.

12.3 Pharmacokinetics

The extent of percutaneous absorption of topical corticosteroids is determined by many factors, including product formulation and the integrity of the epidermal barrier. Occlusion, inflammation and/or other disease processes in the skin may also increase percutaneous absorption. Once absorbed through the skin, topical corticosteroids are handled through pharmacokinetic pathways similar to systemically administered corticosteroids. They are metabolized primarily in the liver and then are excreted by the kidneys. Some corticosteroids and their metabolites are also excreted in the bile.

13 NONCLINICAL TOXICOLOGY

13.1 Carcinogenesis, Mutagenesis, Impairment of Fertility

Long-term animal studies have not been performed to evaluate the carcinogenic or photoco-carcinogenic potential of Desonate or the effect of desonide on fertility. Desonide revealed no evidence of mutagenic potential based on the results of an *in vitro* genotoxicity test (Ames assay) and an *in vivo* genotoxicity test (mouse micronucleus assay). Desonide was positive without S9 activation and was equivocal with S9 activation in an in vitro mammalian cell mutagenesis assay (L5178YITK+ mouse lymphoma assay). A dose response trend was not noted in this assay.

14 CLINICAL STUDIES

In two randomized vehicle-controlled clinical studies, subjects 3 months to 18 years of age with mild to moderate atopic dermatitis were treated twice daily for 4 weeks with either Desonate or vehicle. Treatment success was defined as achieving clear or almost clear on the Investigator's Global Severity Score (IGSS) with at least a 2-point change (decrease) from the subject's baseline IGSS when compared to the Week 4 IGSS. The results of the 2 clinical trials are summarized in Table 1:

Table 1: Subjects Achieving Treatment Success

Clinical Trial 1	
Desonate N = 289	Vehicle N = 92
128 (44%)	13 (14%)
Clinical Trial 2	
Desonate N = 136	Vehicle N = 65
38 (28%)	4 (6%)

16 HOW SUPPLIED/STORAGE AND HANDLING

Desonate is a translucent to opaque gel supplied in 60g tubes in cartons containing 1× 60g tube (NDC 10922-828-06), or a 2 × 60g tube Twin Pack (NDC 10922-828-12).

Storage:

Store at 25°C (77°F); excursions permitted to 15-30°C (59-86°F). [See USP Controlled Room Temperature].

Keep out of reach of children.

17 PATIENT COUNSELING INFORMATION

Patients using topical corticosteroids should receive the following information and instructions:

- This medication is to be used as directed by the physician. It is for external use only. Avoid contact with the eyes.
- This medication should not be used for any disorder other than that for which it was prescribed.
- Unless directed by the physician, the treated skin area should not be bandaged or otherwise covered or wrapped so as to be occlusive.
- Unless directed by a physician, this medication should not be used on the underarm or groin areas of pediatric patients.
- Parents of pediatric patients should be advised not to use Desonate in the treatment of diaper dermatitis. Desonate should not be applied in the diaper area, as diapers or plastic pants may constitute occlusive dressing [see Dosage and Administration (2)].
- Patients should report to their physician any signs of local adverse reactions.
- Other corticosteroid-containing products should not be used with Desonate without first consulting with the physician.
- As with other corticosteroids, therapy should be discontinued when control is achieved. If no improvement is seen within 4 weeks, contact the physician.

© 2010, Intendis, Inc. All rights reserved. June 2010

Manufactured by Contract Pharmaceuticals Limited, Buffalo, NY 14213

Distributed by:

INTENDIS Morristown, NJ 07962

Intendis is part of the Bayer Group

6706903 09-0081

The Desonate logo is a registered trademark of Intendis, Inc.
Covered by US Patent No. 6,387,383
Shown in Product Identification Guide, page 310

FINACEA® ℞

[fi'nā-shē-ə]
(azelaic acid) Gel, 15%
For Dermatologic Use Only–Not for Ophthalmic, Oral, or Intravaginal Use
Rx only

DESCRIPTION

FINACEA® (azelaic acid) Gel, 15%, contains azelaic acid, a naturally occurring saturated dicarboxylic acid. Chemically, azelaic acid is 1,7-heptanedicarboxylic acid, with the molecular formula $C_9H_{16}O_4$, a molecular weight of 188.22, and the structural formula:

$[HOOC-(CH_2)_7-COOH]$

Azelaic acid is a white, odorless crystalline solid that is poorly soluble in water at 20°C (0.24%), but freely soluble in boiling water and in ethanol.
Each gram of FINACEA® Gel, 15%, contains 0.15 gm azelaic acid (15% w/w) as the active ingredient in an aqueous gel base containing benzoic acid (as a preservative), disodium-EDTA, lecithin, medium-chain triglycerides, polyacrylic acid, polysorbate 80, propylene glycol, purified water, and sodium hydroxide to adjust pH.

CLINICAL PHARMACOLOGY

The mechanism(s) by which azelaic acid interferes with the pathogenic events in rosacea are unknown.
Pharmacokinetics: The percutaneous absorption of azelaic acid after topical application of FINACEA® Gel, 15%, could not be reliably determined. Mean plasma azelaic acid concentrations in rosacea patients treated with FINACEA® Gel, 15%, twice daily for at least 8 weeks are in the range of 42 to 63.1 ng/mL. These values are within the maximum concentration range of 24.0 to 90.5 ng/mL observed in rosacea patients treated with vehicle only. This indicates that FINACEA® Gel, 15%, does not increase plasma azelaic acid concentration beyond the range derived from nutrition and endogenous metabolism.
In vitro and human data suggest negligible cutaneous metabolism of ³H-azelaic acid 20% cream after topical application. Azelaic acid is mainly excreted unchanged in the urine, but undergoes some β-oxidation to shorter chain dicarboxylic acids.

CLINICAL STUDIES

FINACEA® Gel, 15%, was evaluated for the treatment of mild to moderate papulopustular rosacea in 2 clinical trials comprising a total of 664 (333 active to 331 vehicle) patients. Both trials were multicenter, randomized, double-blind, vehicle-controlled 12-week studies with identical protocols. Overall, 92.5% of patients were Caucasian and 73% of patients were women, and the mean age was 49 (range 21 to 86) years. Enrolled patients had mild to moderate rosacea with a mean lesion count of 18 (range 8 to 60) inflammatory papules and pustules. Subjects without papules and pustules, with nodules, rhinophyma, or ocular involvement, and a history of hypersensitivity to propylene glycol or to any other ingredients of the study drug were excluded. FINACEA® Gel, 15%, or its vehicle were to be applied twice daily for 12 weeks; no other topical or systemic medication affecting the course of rosacea and/or evaluability was to be used during the studies. Patients were instructed to avoid spicy foods, thermally hot foods and drinks, and alcoholic beverages during the study, and to use only very mild soaps or soapless cleansing lotion for facial cleansing.
The primary efficacy endpoints were both 1) change from baseline in inflammatory lesion counts and 2) success defined as a score of clear or minimal with at least a 2 step reduction from baseline on the Investigator's Global Assessment (IGA):
CLEAR:
No papules and/or pustules; no or residual erythema; no or mild to moderate telangiectasia
MINIMAL:
Rare papules and/or pustules; residual to mild erythema; mild to moderate telangiectasia
MILD:
Few papules and/or pustules; mild erythema; mild to moderate telangiectasia
MILD TO MODERATE:
Distinct number of papules and/or pustules; mild to moderate erythema; mild to moderate telangiectasia

MODERATE:
Pronounced number of papules and/or pustules; moderate erythema; mild to moderate telangiectasia
MODERATE TO SEVERE:
Many papules and/or pustules, occasionally with large inflamed lesions; moderate erythema; moderate degree of telangiectasia
SEVERE:
Numerous papules and/or pustules, occasionally with confluent areas of inflamed lesions; moderate or severe erythema; moderate or severe telangiectasia
Primary efficacy assessment was based on the intent-to-treat (ITT) population with last observation carried forward (LOCF).
Both studies demonstrated a statistically significant difference in favor of FINACEA® Gel, 15%, over its vehicle in reducing the number of inflammatory papules and pustules associated with rosacea (Table 1) and with success on the IGA in the ITT-LOCF population at the end of treatment.
[See table 1 above]
Although some reduction of erythema which was present in patients with papules and pustules of rosacea occurred in clinical studies, efficacy for treatment of erythema in rosacea in the absence of papules and pustules has not been evaluated.
FINACEA® Gel, 15%, was superior to the vehicle with regard to success based on the investigator's global assessment of rosacea on a 7-point static score at the end of treatment, (ITT population; Table 2).
[See table 2 above]

INDICATIONS AND USAGE

FINACEA® Gel, 15%, is indicated for topical treatment of inflammatory papules and pustules of mild to moderate rosacea. Although some reduction of erythema which was present in patients with papules and pustules of rosacea occurred in clinical studies, efficacy for treatment of erythema in rosacea in the absence of papules and pustules has not been evaluated. Patients should be instructed to avoid spicy foods, thermally hot foods and drinks, alcoholic beverages and to use only very mild soaps or soapless cleansing lotion for facial cleansing.

CONTRAINDICATIONS

FINACEA® Gel, 15%, is contraindicated in individuals with a history of hypersensitivity to propylene glycol or any other component of the formulation.

WARNINGS

FINACEA® Gel, 15%, is for dermatologic use only, and not for ophthalmic, oral or intravaginal use.
There have been isolated reports of hypopigmentation after use of azelaic acid. Since azelaic acid has not been well studied in patients with dark complexion, these patients should be monitored for early signs of hypopigmentation.

PRECAUTIONS

General: Contact with the eyes should be avoided. If sensitivity or severe irritation develops with the use of FINACEA® Gel, 15%, treatment should be discontinued and appropriate therapy instituted.

Information for Patients: Patients using FINACEA® Gel, 15%, should receive the following information and instructions:
• FINACEA® Gel, 15%, is to be used only as directed by the physician.
• FINACEA® Gel, 15%, is for external use only. It is not to be used orally, intravaginally, or for the eyes.
• Cleanse affected area(s) with a very mild soap or a soapless cleansing lotion and pat dry with a soft towel before applying FINACEA® Gel, 15%. Avoid alcoholic cleansers, tinctures and astringents, abrasives and peeling agents.
• Avoid contact of FINACEA® Gel, 15%, with the mouth, eyes and other mucous membranes. If it does come in contact with the eyes, wash the eyes with large amounts of water and consult a physician if eye irritation persists.
• The hands should be washed following application of FINACEA® Gel, 15%.
• Cosmetics may be applied after FINACEA® Gel, 15%, has dried.
• Skin irritation (e.g., pruritus, burning, or stinging) may occur during use of FINACEA® Gel, 15%, usually during the first few weeks of treatment. If irritation is excessive or persists, use of FINACEA® Gel, 15%, should be discontinued, and patients should consult their physician (See **ADVERSE REACTIONS**).
• Avoid any foods and beverages that might provoke erythema, flushing, and blushing (including spicy food, alcoholic beverages, and thermally hot drinks, including hot coffee and tea).
• Patients should report abnormal changes in skin color to their physician.
• Avoid the use of occlusive dressings or wrappings.
Drug Interactions: There have been no formal studies of the interaction of FINACEA® Gel, 15%, with other drugs.
Carcinogenesis, Mutagenesis, Impairment of Fertility: Long-term animal studies have not been performed to evaluate the carcinogenic potential of FINACEA® Gel, 15%. Azelaic acid was not mutagenic or clastogenic in a battery of in vitro (Ames assay, HGPRT in V79 cells {Chinese hamster lung cells}, and chromosomal aberration assay in human lymphocytes) and in vivo (dominant lethal assay in mice and mouse micronucleus assay) genotoxicity tests.
Oral administration of azelaic acid at dose levels up to 2500 mg/kg/day (162 times the maximum recommended human dose based on body surface area) did not affect fertility or reproductive performance in male or female rats.
Pregnancy: Teratogenic Effects: Pregnancy Category B
There are no adequate and well-controlled studies of topically administered azelaic acid in pregnant women. The experience with FINACEA® Gel, 15%, when used by pregnant women is too limited to permit assessment of the safety of its use during pregnancy.
Dermal embryofetal developmental toxicology studies have not been performed with azelaic acid, 15%, gel. Oral embryofetal developmental studies were conducted with azelaic acid in rats, rabbits, and cynomolgus monkeys. Azelaic acid was administered during the period of organogenesis in all three animal species. Embryotoxicity was ob-

---

Table 1. Inflammatory Papules and Pustules (ITT population)[1]

	Study One FINACEA® Gel, 15% N = 164	Study One VEHICLE N = 165	Study Two FINACEA® Gel, 15% N = 167	Study Two VEHICLE N = 166
Mean Lesion Count Baseline	17.5	17.6	17.9	18.5
End of Treatment[1]	6.8	10.5	9.0	12.1
Mean Percent Reduction End of Treatment[1]	57.9%	39.9%	50.0%	38.2%

[1] ITT population with last observation carried forward (LOCF);

Table 2. Investigator's Global Assessment at the End of Treatment[1]

	Study One FINACEA® Gel, 15% N = 164	Study One VEHICLE N = 165	Study Two FINACEA® Gel, 15% N = 167	Study Two VEHICLE N = 166
CLEAR, MINIMAL or MILD at End of Treatment (% of Patients)	61%	40%	61%	48%

[1] ITT population with last observation carried forward (LOCF);

---

served in rats, rabbits, and monkeys at oral doses of azelaic acid that generated some maternal toxicity. Embryotoxicity was observed in rats given 2500 mg/kg/day (162 times the maximum recommended human dose based on body surface area), rabbits given 150 or 500 mg/kg/day (19 or 65 times the maximum recommended human dose based on body surface area) and cynomolgus monkeys given 500 mg/kg/day (65 times the maximum recommended human dose based on body surface area) azelaic acid. No teratogenic effects were observed in the oral embryofetal developmental studies conducted in rats, rabbits and cynomolgus monkeys. An oral peri- and post-natal developmental study was conducted in rats. Azelaic acid was administered from gestational day 15 through day 21 postpartum up to a dose level of 2500 mg/kg/day. Embryotoxicity was observed in rats at an oral dose that generated some maternal toxicity (2500 mg/kg/day; 162 times the maximum recommended human dose based on body surface area). In addition, slight disturbances in the postnatal development of fetuses was noted in rats at oral doses that generated some maternal toxicity (500 and 2500 mg/kg/day; 32 and 162 times the maximum recommended human dose based on body surface area). No effects on sexual maturation of the fetuses were noted in this study.

Because animal reproduction studies are not always predictive of human response, this drug should be used only if clearly needed during pregnancy.

Nursing Mothers: Equilibrium dialysis was used to assess human milk partitioning *in vitro.* At an azelaic acid concentration of 25 µg/mL, the milk/plasma distribution coefficient was 0.7 and the milk/buffer distribution was 1.0, indicating that passage of drug into maternal milk may occur. Since less than 4% of a topically applied dose of azelaic acid cream, 20%, is systemically absorbed, the uptake of azelaic acid into maternal milk is not expected to cause a significant change from baseline azelaic acid levels in the milk. However, caution should be exercised when FINACEA® Gel, 15%, is administered to a nursing mother.

Pediatric Use: Safety and effectiveness of FINACEA® Gel, 15%, in pediatric patients have not been established.

Geriatric: Clinical studies of FINACEA® Gel, 15%, did not include sufficient numbers of subjects aged 65 and over to determine whether they respond differently from younger subjects.

ADVERSE REACTIONS

Overall, treatment related adverse events, including burning, stinging/tingling, dryness/tightness/scaling, itching, and erythema/irritation/redness, were 19.4% (24/124) for FINACEA® Gel, 15%, and 7.1% (9/127) for the active comparator gel at 15 weeks.

In two vehicle controlled, and one active controlled U.S. clinical studies, treatment safety was monitored in 788 patients who used twice daily FINACEA® Gel, 15%, for 12 weeks (N=333) or for 15 weeks (N=124), or the gel vehicle (N=331) for 12 weeks.

[See table 3 at top right]

FINACEA® Gel, 15%, and its vehicle caused irritant reactions at the application site in human dermal safety studies. FINACEA® Gel, 15%, caused significantly more irritation than its vehicle in a cumulative irritation study. Some improvement in irritation was demonstrated over the course of the clinical studies, but this improvement might be attributed to subject dropouts. No phototoxicity or photoallergenicity were reported in human dermal safety studies.

In patients using azelaic acid formulations, the following additional adverse experiences have been reported rarely: worsening of asthma, vitiligo depigmentation, small depigmented spots, hypertrichosis, reddening (signs of keratosis pilaris), and exacerbation of recurrent herpes labialis.

Post-marketing safety—Skin: facial burning and irritation; Eyes: iridocyclitis on accidental exposure with FINACEA® Gel, 15%, to the eye (see **PRECAUTIONS**).

OVERDOSAGE

FINACEA® Gel, 15%, is intended for cutaneous use only. If pronounced local irritation occurs, patients should be directed to discontinue use and appropriate therapy should be instituted (See **PRECAUTIONS**).

DOSAGE AND ADMINISTRATION

A thin layer of FINACEA® Gel, 15%, should be gently massaged into the affected areas on the face twice daily, in the morning and evening. Patients should be reassessed if no improvement is observed upon completing 12 weeks of therapy.

HOW SUPPLIED

FINACEA® Gel, 15%, is supplied in tubes in the following size:

50 g – NDC 10922-825-02

Storage

Store at 25°C (77°F); excursions permitted between 15-30°C (59-86°F) [See USP Controlled Room Temperature].

Distributed under license; *U.S. Patent No 4,713,394*

Table 3. Cutaneous Adverse Events Occurring in ≥1% of Subjects in the Rosacea Trials by Treatment Group and Maximum Intensity*

	FINACEA® Gel, 15% N = 457 (100%)			VEHICLE N = 331 (100%)		
	Mild n = 99 (22%)	Moderate n = 61 (13%)	Severe n = 27 (6%)	Mild n = 46 (14%)	Moderate n = 30 (9%)	Severe n = 5 (2%)
Burning/ stinging/ tingling	71 (16%)	42 (9%)	17 (4%)	8 (2%)	6 (2%)	2 (1%)
Pruritus	29 (6%)	18 (4%)	5 (1%)	9 (3%)	6 (2%)	0 (0%)
Scaling/dry Skin/xerosis	21 (5%)	10 (2%)	5 (1%)	31 (9%)	14 (4%)	1 (<1%)
Erythema/ irritation	6 (1%)	7 (2%)	2 (<1%)	8 (2%)	4 (1%)	2 (1%)
Contact dermatitis	2 (<1%)	3 (1%)	0 (0%)	1 (<1%)	0 (0%)	0 (0%)
Edema	3 (1%)	2 (<1%)	0 (0%)	3 (1%)	0 (0%)	0 (0%)
Acne	3 (1%)	1 (<1%)	0 (0%)	1 (<1%)	0 (0%)	0 (0%)

*Subjects may have >1 cutaneous adverse event; thus, the sum of the frequencies of preferred terms may exceed the number of subjects with at least 1 cutaneous adverse event.

Manufactured by Intendis Manufacturing S.p.A., Segrate, Milan, Italy
Distributed by:
INTENDIS Pine Brook, NJ 07058
Intendis is part of the Bayer Group
6706800   80660910
Shown in Product Identification Guide, page 310

NEOBENZ® MICRO SD   ℞
[ne-O-benz]
(benzoyl peroxide cream 5.5%)
Pre-filled Sponge Applicator
NEOBENZ® MICRO WASH
(benzoyl peroxide 7%)
Rx ONLY.
FOR EXTERNAL USE ONLY.

I. DESCRIPTION

NeoBenz® *Micro* SD 5.5% single dose cream pre-filled sponge applicator and NeoBenz® *Micro* Wash 7% are topical preparations containing benzoyl peroxide as the active ingredient incorporated into patented porous microspheres (MICROSPONGE®* delivery system) composed of methyl methacrylate/glycol dimethacrylate crosspolymer. This polymeric system has been shown to provide gradual release of active ingredient into the skin[1] and absorb natural skin oils[2]. Ingredients for the SD include C13-14 isoparaffin, cetyl alcohol, citric acid, ethylhexyl palmitate, glycerin, glyceryl dilaurate, laureth-7, magnesium aluminum silicate, methyl methacrylate/glycol dimethacrylate crosspolymer, methylparaben, polyacrylamide, propylparaben, silica, sodium citrate, sodium lauryl sulfate, sorbitol, stearyl alcohol, water, and xanthan gum. Ingredients for the Wash include citric acid, cocamidopropyl betaine, cocamine oxide, disodium laureth sulfosuccinate, edetate disodium, fragrance, glycerin, hydrogenated castor oil, hypromellose, magnesium aluminum silicate, methyl methacrylate/glycol dimethacrylate crosspolymer, methylparaben, PEG-150 pentaerythrityl tetrastearate (and) PEG-6 caprylic/capric glycerides, PEG-40 hydrogenated castor oil, poloxamer 182, purified water, and xanthan gum.

Benzoyl peroxide is an oxidizing agent that possesses antibacterial properties and is classified as a keratolytic. Benzoyl peroxide ($C_{14}H_{10}O_4$) is represented by the following structure:

II. CLINICAL PHARMACOLOGY

The exact method of action of benzoyl peroxide in acne vulgaris is not known. Benzoyl peroxide is an antibacterial agent with demonstrated activity against *Propionibacterium acnes.* This action, combined with the mild keratolytic effect of benzoyl peroxide, is believed to be responsible for its usefulness in acne. Benzoyl peroxide is absorbed by the skin where it is metabolized to benzoic acid and excreted as benzoate in the urine.

III. INDICATIONS AND USAGE

NeoBenz® *Micro* SD and NeoBenz® *Micro* Wash are indicated for use in the topical treatment of mild to moderate acne vulgaris.

IV. CONTRAINDICATIONS

NeoBenz® *Micro* SD and NeoBenz® *Micro* Wash should not be used in patients who have shown hypersensitivity to benzoyl peroxide or to any of the other ingredients in the products.

V. WARNINGS

When using this product, avoid unnecessary sun exposure and use a sunscreen. Keep out of reach of children.

VI. PRECAUTIONS (SEE WARNINGS):

General—For external use only. Avoid contact with eyes and mucous membranes. If severe irritation develops, discontinue use and institute appropriate therapy.

Information for Patients: Avoid contact with eyes, eyelids, lips and mucous membranes. If accidental contact occurs, rinse with water. Avoid contact with hair, fabrics or carpeting as benzoyl peroxide will cause bleaching or discoloration. If excessive irritation develops, discontinue use and consult your physician.

Carcinogenesis, Mutagenesis, Impairment of Fertility: Based upon all available evidence, benzoyl peroxide is not considered to be a carcinogen. However, data from a study using mice known to be highly susceptible to cancer suggest that benzoyl peroxide acts as a tumor promoter. The clinical significance of this finding is not known.

Pregnancy: Category C - Animal reproduction studies have not been conducted with benzoyl peroxide. It is also not known whether benzoyl peroxide can cause fetal harm when administered to a pregnant woman or can affect reproduction capacity. Benzoyl peroxide should be used by a pregnant woman only if clearly needed.

Nursing Mothers: It is not known whether this drug is excreted in human milk. Because many drugs are excreted in human milk, caution should be exercised when benzoyl peroxide is administered to a nursing woman.

Pediatric Use: Safety and effectiveness in children below the age of 12 have not been established.

VII. ADVERSE REACTIONS

Allergic contact dermatitis and dryness have been reported with topical benzoyl peroxide therapy.

VIII. OVERDOSAGE

If excessive scaling, erythema or edema occurs, the use of these preparations should be discontinued. To hasten resolution of the adverse effects, cool compresses may be used. After symptoms and signs subside, a reduced dosage schedule may be cautiously tried if the reaction is judged to be due to excessive use and not allergenicity.

IX. DOSAGE AND ADMINISTRATION

NeoBenz® *Micro* SD and NeoBenz® *Micro* Wash should be used once or twice daily on the affected areas. Frequency of use should be adjusted to obtain the desired clinical response. If you see medication or white residue on skin after application of NeoBenz® *Micro* SD, you are applying too much. Gentle cleansing of the affected areas with a mild cleanser prior to application of NeoBenz® *Micro* SD may be beneficial. Clinically visible improvement will normally occur by the third week of therapy. Maximum lesion reduction may be expected after approximately eight to twelve weeks of drug use. Continuing use of the drug is normally required to maintain a satisfactory clinical response.

NeoBenz® Micro SD: Firmly squeeze applicator until seal between applicator and sponge has broken. Apply medication by rubbing sponge in small circular motions on affected areas. Dispose of each applicator after single use only.

NeoBenz® Micro Wash: Shake well before using. Wet skin areas to be treated; apply NeoBenz® Micro Wash by massaging gently into skin for 10-20 seconds, working into a full lather. Rinse thoroughly and pat dry.

X. HOW SUPPLIED

NeoBenz® Micro SD is supplied as follows:
SIZE: 1 box of thirty 0.5 gram applicators
NDC NUMBER: 10922-821-30
(benzoyl peroxide cream 5.5%) Pre-filled Sponge Applicator
NeoBenz® Micro Wash Plus Pack
NDC NUMBER: 10922-822-23
Contains:
1 tottle (180 gram), NeoBenz® Micro Wash (benzoyl peroxide 7%)
1 convenient travel case containing seven 0.5 gram applicators, NeoBenz® Micro SD (benzoyl peroxide cream 5.5%) Pre-filled Sponge Applicator
Store between 15°- 25°C (59°-77°F)

REFERENCES

1. Wester RC, Patel R, Nacht S, Leyden J, Melendres J, Maibach H. Controlled release of benzoyl peroxide from a porous microsphere polymeric system can reduce topical irritancy. *J. Am. Acad. Dermatol.* 1991; 24: 720-726.
2. Meyer R. Rosen (ed.), *Delivery System Handbook for Personal Care and Cosmetic Products,* 332-352 (2005).
Covered by US Patents: 5,879,716; 6,007,264.
*MICROSPONGE® is a registered trademark of AMCOL Health and Beauty Solutions, Inc, a subsidiary of AMCOL International Corporation.
www.neobenz.com
© 2010, Intendis, Inc. All rights reserved. August 2010
Made in USA
Distributed by:
INTENDIS, Morristown, NJ 07962
Intendis is part of the Bayer Group
6707302   129445

Shown in Product Identification Guide, page 310

InterMune, Inc.
3280 BAYSHORE BOULEVARD
BRISBANE, CA 94005

For Direct Inquiries Contact:
Medical Information:
(888) 486-6411
Corporate Offices:
(415) 466-2200
Corporate Fax:
(415) 466-2300

ACTIMMUNE®   ℞
[ăk-tĭ-mewn]
(Interferon gamma-1b)

DESCRIPTION

ACTIMMUNE® (Interferon gamma-1b), a biologic response modifier, is a single-chain polypeptide containing 140 amino acids. Production of *ACTIMMUNE* is achieved by fermentation of a genetically engineered *Escherichia coli* bacterium containing the DNA which encodes for the human protein. Purification of the product is achieved by conventional column chromatography. *ACTIMMUNE* is a highly purified sterile solution consisting of non-covalent dimers of two identical 16,465 dalton monomers; with a specific activity of 20 million International Units (IU)/mg (2×10^6 IU per 0.5 mL) which is equivalent to 30 million units/mg.

ACTIMMUNE is a sterile, clear, colorless solution filled in a single-use vial for subcutaneous injection. Each 0.5 mL of *ACTIMMUNE* contains: **100 mcg (2 million IU)** of Interferon gamma-1b formulated in 20 mg mannitol, 0.36 mg sodium succinate, 0.05 mg polysorbate 20 and Sterile Water for Injection. *Note that the above activity is expressed in International Units (1 million IU/50mcg). This is equivalent to what was previously expressed as units (1.5 million U/50mcg).*

CLINICAL PHARMACOLOGY
General
Interferons bind to specific cell surface receptors and initiate a sequence of intracellular events that lead to the transcription of interferon-stimulated genes. The three major groups of interferons (alpha, beta, gamma) have partially overlapping biological activities that include immunoregulation such as increased resistance to microbial pathogens and inhibition of cell proliferation. Type 1 interferons (alpha and beta) bind to the alpha/beta receptor. Interferon-gamma binds to a different cell surface receptor and is classified as Type 2 interferon. Specific effects of interferon-gamma include the enhancement of the oxidative metabolism of macrophages, antibody dependent cellular cytotoxicity (ADCC), activation of natural killer (NK) cells, and the expression of Fc receptors and major histocompatibility antigens.

Chronic Granulomatous Disease (CGD) is an inherited disorder of leukocyte function caused by defects in the enzyme complex responsible for phagocyte superoxide generation. *ACTIMMUNE* does not increase phagocyte superoxide production even in treatment responders.[1]

In severe, malignant osteopetrosis (an inherited disorder characterized by an osteoclast defect, leading to bone overgrowth, and by deficient phagocyte oxidative metabolism), a treatment-related enhancement of superoxide production by phagocytes was observed. *ACTIMMUNE* was found to enhance osteoclast function *in vivo.*[2-4]

In both disorders, the exact mechanism(s) by which *ACTIMMUNE* has a treatment effect has not been established. Changes in superoxide levels during *ACTIMMUNE* therapy do not predict efficacy and should not be used to assess patient response to therapy.

Pharmacokinetics
The intravenous, intramuscular, and subcutaneous pharmacokinetics of *ACTIMMUNE* have been investigated in 24 healthy male subjects following single-dose administration of 100 mcg/m². *ACTIMMUNE* is rapidly cleared after intravenous administration (1.4 liters/minute) and slowly absorbed after intramuscular or subcutaneous injection. After intramuscular or subcutaneous injection, the apparent fraction of dose absorbed was greater than 89%. The mean elimination half-life after intravenous administration of 100 mcg/m² in healthy male subjects was 38 minutes. The mean elimination half-lives for intramuscular and subcutaneous dosing with 100 mcg/m² were 2.9 and 5.9 hours, respectively. Peak plasma concentrations, determined by ELISA, occurred approximately 4 hours (1.5 ng/mL) after intramuscular dosing and 7 hours (0.6 ng/mL) after subcutaneous dosing. Multiple dose subcutaneous pharmacokinetic studies were conducted in 38 healthy male subjects. There was no accumulation of *ACTIMMUNE* after 12 consecutive daily injections of 100 mcg/m². Pharmacokinetic studies in patients with Chronic Granulomatous Disease have not been performed.

Trace amounts of interferon-gamma were detected in the urine of squirrel monkeys following intravenous administration of 500 mcg/kg. Interferon-gamma was not detected in the urine of healthy human volunteers following administration of 100 mcg/m² of *ACTIMMUNE* by the intravenous, intramuscular and subcutaneous routes. *In vitro* perfusion studies utilizing rabbit livers and kidneys demonstrate that these organs are capable of clearing interferon-gamma from perfusate. Studies of the administration of interferon-gamma to nephrectomized mice and squirrel monkeys demonstrate a reduction in clearance of interferon-gamma from blood; however, prior nephrectomy did not prevent elimination.

Effects in Chronic Granulomatous Disease
A randomized, double-blind, placebo-controlled study of *ACTIMMUNE* (Interferon gamma-1b) in patients with Chronic Granulomatous Disease (CGD) was performed to determine whether *ACTIMMUNE* administered subcutaneously on a three times weekly schedule could decrease the incidence of serious infectious episodes and improve existing infectious and inflammatory conditions in patients with Chronic Granulomatous Disease. One hundred twenty-eight eligible patients were enrolled on this study including patients with different patterns of inheritance. Most patients received prophylactic antibiotics. Patients ranged in age from 1 to 44 years with the mean age being 14.6 years. The study was terminated early following demonstration of a highly statistically significant benefit of *ACTIMMUNE* therapy compared to placebo with respect to time to serious infection (p=0.0036), the primary endpoint of the investigation. Serious infection was defined as a clinical event requiring hospitalization and the use of parenteral antibiotics. The final analysis provided further support for the primary endpoint (p=0.0006). There was a 67 percent reduction in relative risk of serious infection in patients receiving *ACTIMMUNE* (n=63) compared to placebo (n=65). Additional supportive evidence in the number of primary serious infections in the *ACTIMMUNE* group (30 on placebo versus 14 on *ACTIMMUNE*, p=0.002) and the total number and rate of serious infections including recurrent events (56 on placebo versus 20 on *ACTIMMUNE*, p=<0.0001). Moreover, the length of hospitalization for the treatment of all clinical events provided evidence highly supportive of an *ACTIMMUNE* treatment benefit. Placebo patients required three times as many inpatient hospitalization days for treatment of clinical events compared to patients receiving *ACTIMMUNE* (1493 versus 497 total days, p=0.02). An *ACTIMMUNE* treatment benefit with respect to time to serious infection was consistently demonstrated in all subgroup analyses according to stratification factors, including pattern of inheritance, use of prophylactic antibiotics, as well as age. There was a 67 percent reduction in relative risk of serious infection in patients receiving *ACTIMMUNE* compared to placebo across all groups. The beneficial effect of *ACTIMMUNE* therapy was observed throughout the entire study, in which the mean duration of *ACTIMMUNE* administration was 8.9 months/patient.

Effects in Osteopetrosis
A controlled, randomized study in patients with severe, malignant osteopetrosis was conducted with *ACTIMMUNE* administered subcutaneously three times weekly. Sixteen patients were randomized to receive either *ACTIMMUNE* plus calcitriol (n=11), or calcitriol alone (n=5). Patients ranged in age from 1 month to 8 years, mean 1.5 years. Treatment failure was considered to be disease progression as defined by 1) death, 2) significant reduction in hemoglobin or platelet counts, 3) a serious bacterial infection requiring antibiotics, or 4) a 50 dB decrease in hearing or progressive optic atrophy. The median time to disease progression was significantly delayed in the *ACTIMMUNE* plus calcitriol arm versus calcitriol alone. In the treatment arm, the median was not reached. Based on the observed data, however, the median time to progression in this arm was at least 165 days versus a median of 65 days in the calcitriol alone arm. In an analysis which combined data from a second study, 19 of 24 patients treated with *ACTIMMUNE* plus or minus calcitriol for at least 6 months had reduced trabecular bone volume compared to baseline.

INDICATIONS AND USAGE

ACTIMMUNE is indicated for reducing the frequency and severity of serious infections associated with Chronic Granulomatous Disease.

ACTIMMUNE is indicated for delaying time to disease progression in patients with severe, malignant osteopetrosis.

CONTRAINDICATIONS

ACTIMMUNE is contraindicated in patients who develop or have known hypersensitivity to interferon-gamma, *E. coli* derived products, or any component of the product.

WARNINGS
Cardiovascular Disorders
Acute and transient "flu-like" symptoms such as fever and chills induced by *ACTIMMUNE* at doses of 250 mcg/m²/day (greater than 10 times the weekly recommended dose) or higher may exacerbate pre-existing cardiac conditions. *ACTIMMUNE* should be used with caution in patients with pre-existing cardiac conditions, including ischemia, congestive heart failure or arrhythmia.

Neurologic Disorders
Decreased mental status, gait disturbance and dizziness have been observed, particularly in patients receiving *ACTIMMUNE* doses greater than 250 mcg/m²/day (greater than 10 times the weekly recommended dose). Most of these abnormalities were mild and reversible within a few days upon dose reduction or discontinuation of therapy. Caution should be exercised when administering *ACTIMMUNE* to patients with seizure disorders or compromised central nervous system function.

Bone Marrow Toxicity
Reversible neutropenia and thrombocytopenia that can be severe and may be dose related have been observed during *ACTIMMUNE* therapy. Caution should be exercised when administering *ACTIMMUNE* to patients with myelosuppression.

Hepatic Toxicity
Elevations of AST and/or ALT (up to 25-fold) have been observed during *ACTIMMUNE* therapy. The incidence appeared to be higher in patients less than 1 year of age compared to older children. The transaminase elevations were reversible with reduction in dosage or interruption of *ACTIMMUNE* treatment. Patients begun on *ACTIMMUNE* before age one year should receive monthly assessments of liver function. If severe hepatic enzyme elevations develop, *ACTIMMUNE* dosage should be modified (see **DOSAGE AND ADMINISTRATION: Dose Modification**).

PRECAUTIONS
General
Isolated cases of acute serious hypersensitivity reactions have been observed in patients receiving *ACTIMMUNE*. If such an acute reaction develops the drug should be discontinued immediately and appropriate medical therapy instituted. Transient cutaneous rashes have occurred in some patients following injection but have rarely necessitated treatment interruption.

Information for Patients
Patients being treated with *ACTIMMUNE* and/or their parents should be informed regarding the potential benefits and risks associated with treatment. If home use is deter-

mined to be desirable by the physician, instructions on appropriate use should be given, including review of the contents of the Patient Information Insert. This information is intended to aid in the safe and effective use of the medication. It is not a disclosure of all possible adverse or intended effects.

If home use is prescribed, a puncture resistant container for the disposal of used syringes and needles should be supplied to the patient. Patients should be thoroughly instructed in the importance of proper disposal and cautioned against any reuse of needles and syringes. The full container should be disposed of according to the directions provided by the physician (see **Patient Information Insert**).

The most common adverse experiences occurring with *ACTIMMUNE* therapy are "flu-like" or constitutional symptoms such as fever, headache, chills, myalgia or fatigue (see **ADVERSE REACTIONS**) which may decrease in severity as treatment continues. Some of the "flu-like" symptoms may be minimized by bedtime administration. Acetaminophen may be used to prevent or partially alleviate the fever and headache.

Laboratory Tests

In addition to those tests normally required for monitoring patients with Chronic Granulomatous Disease and osteopetrosis, the following laboratory tests are recommended for all patients on *ACTIMMUNE* (Interferon gamma-1b) therapy prior to the beginning of and at three month intervals during treatment (see **WARNINGS: Bone Marrow** and **Hepatic Toxicity**).

* Hematologic tests - including complete blood counts, differential and platelet counts
* Blood chemistries - including renal and liver function tests. In patients less than 1 year of age, liver function tests should be measured monthly (see **ADVERSE REACTIONS: Post-Marketing Experience**).
* Urinalysis

Drug Interactions

Interactions between *ACTIMMUNE* and other drugs have not been fully evaluated. Caution should be exercised when administering *ACTIMMUNE* in combination with other potentially myelosuppressive agents (see **WARNINGS**).

Preclinical studies in rodents using species-specific interferon-gamma have demonstrated a decrease in hepatic microsomal cytochrome P-450 concentrations. This could potentially lead to a depression of the hepatic metabolism of certain drugs that utilize this degradative pathway.

Carcinogenesis, Mutagenesis and Impairment of Fertility

Carcinogenesis: *ACTIMMUNE* has not been tested for its carcinogenic potential.

Mutagenesis: Ames tests using five different tester strains of bacteria with and without metabolic activation revealed no evidence of mutagenic potential. *ACTIMMUNE* was tested in a micronucleus assay for its ability to induce chromosomal damage in bone marrow cells of mice following two intravenous doses of 20 mg/kg. No evidence of chromosomal damage was noted.

Impairment of Fertility: Female cynomolgus monkeys treated with daily subcutaneous doses of 30 or 150 mcg/kg *ACTIMMUNE* (approximately 20 and 100 times the human dose) exhibited irregular menstrual cycles or absence of cyclicity during treatment. Similar findings were not observed in animals treated with 3 mcg/kg *ACTIMMUNE*.

Female mice receiving recombinant murine IFN-gamma (rmuIFN-gamma) at 32 times the maximum recommended clinical dose of *ACTIMMUNE* for 4 weeks via intramuscular injection exhibited an increased incidence of atretic ovarian follicles.

Male cynomolgus monkeys treated intravenously for 4 weeks with 8 times the maximum recommended clinical dose of *ACTIMMUNE* exhibited decreased spermatogenesis. The impact of this finding on fertility is not known. Male mice receiving rmuIFN-gamma at 32 times the maximum recommended clinical dose of *ACTIMMUNE* for 4 weeks via intramuscular injection exhibited decreased spermatogenesis. Male mice treated subcutaneously with rmuIFN-gamma from shortly after birth through puberty with 280 times the maximum recommended clinical dose of ACTIMMUNE exhibited profound yet reversible decreases in sperm counts and fertility, and an increase in the number of abnormal sperm.

The clinical significance of these findings observed following treatment of mice with rmuIFN-gamma is uncertain.

Pregnancy

Teratogenic Effects: Pregnancy Category C. *ACTIMMUNE* has shown an increased incidence of abortions in primates when given in doses approximately 100 times the human dose. A study in pregnant primates treated with subcutaneous doses 2-100 times the human dose failed to demonstrate teratogenic activity for *ACTIMMUNE*.

Female mice treated subcutaneously with rmuIFN-gamma at 280 times the maximum recommended clinical dose of *ACTIMMUNE* from shortly after birth through puberty but not during pregnancy had offspring which exhibited decreased body weight during the lactation period. The clinical significance of this finding observed following treatment of mice with rmuIFN-gamma is uncertain.

There are no adequate and well-controlled studies in pregnant women. *ACTIMMUNE* should be used during pregnancy only if the potential benefit justifies the potential risk to the fetus.

Nursing Mothers

It is not known whether *ACTIMMUNE* is excreted in human milk. Because many drugs are excreted in human milk and because of the potential for serious adverse reactions in nursing infants from *ACTIMMUNE*, a decision should be made whether to discontinue nursing or to discontinue the drug, dependent upon the importance of the drug to the mother.

ADVERSE REACTIONS

The following data on adverse reactions are based on the subcutaneous administration of *ACTIMMUNE* at a dose of 50 mcg/m², three times weekly, in patients with Chronic Granulomatous Disease (CGD) during an investigational trial in the United States and Europe.

The most common adverse events observed in patients with CGD are shown in the following table:

Clinical Toxicity	Percent of Patients	
	ACTIMMUNE CGD (n=63)	Placebo CGD (n=65)
Fever	52	28
Headache	33	9
Rash	17	6
Chills	14	0
Injection site erythema or tenderness	14	2
Fatigue	14	11
Diarrhea	14	12
Vomiting	13	5
Nausea	10	2
Myalgia	6	0
Arthralgia	2	0
Injection site pain	0	2

Miscellaneous adverse events which occurred infrequently in patients with CGD and may have been related to underlying disease included back pain (2 percent versus 0 percent), abdominal pain (8 percent versus 3 percent) and depression (3 percent versus 0 percent) for *ACTIMMUNE* and placebo treated patients, respectively.

Similar safety data were observed in 34 patients with severe malignant osteopetrosis.

ACTIMMUNE has also been evaluated in additional disease states in studies in which patients have generally received higher doses (>100 mcg/m²/three times weekly) administered by intramuscular or subcutaneous injection, or intravenous infusion. All of the previously described adverse reactions which occurred in patients with Chronic Granulomatous Disease have also been observed in patients receiving higher doses. Adverse reactions not observed in patients with Chronic Granulomatous Disease but reported in patients receiving *ACTIMMUNE* (Interferon gamma-1b) in other studies include: *Cardiovascular*—hypotension, syncope, tachyarrhythmia, heart block, heart failure, and myocardial infarction. *Central Nervous System*—confusion, disorientation, gait disturbance, Parkinsonian symptoms, seizure, hallucinations, and transient ischemic attacks. *Gastrointestinal*—dyspepsia, hepatic insufficiency, gastrointestinal bleeding, and pancreatitis, including pancreatitis with fatal outcome. *General Disorders and Administration Site Conditions*—malaise, injection site hemorrhage. *Hematologic*—deep venous thrombosis and pulmonary embolism. *Immunological*—increased autoantibodies, lupus-like syndrome. *Metabolic*— hyponatremia, hyperglycemia, and hypertriglyceridemia. *Musculoskeletal*—clubbing, muscle spasms. *Pulmonary*—tachypnea, bronchospasm, and interstitial pneumonitis. *Renal*—reversible renal insufficiency. *Other*—chest discomfort, exacerbation of dermatomyositis.

Abnormal Laboratory Test Values: Elevations of ALT and AST, neutropenia, thrombocytopenia, and proteinuria have been observed (see **WARNINGS** and **PRECAUTIONS: Laboratory Tests**).

No neutralizing antibodies to *ACTIMMUNE* have been detected in any Chronic Granulomatous Disease patients receiving *ACTIMMUNE*.

Post-Marketing Experience

Children with CGD less than 3 years of age: Data on the safety and activity of *ACTIMMUNE* in 37 patients under the age of 3 years was pooled from four uncontrolled post-marketing studies. The rate of serious infections per patient-year in this uncontrolled group was similar to the rate observed in the *ACTIMMUNE* treatment groups in controlled trials. Developmental parameters (height, weight and endocrine maturation) for this uncontrolled group conformed to national normative scales before and during *ACTIMMUNE* therapy.

In 6 of the 10 patients receiving *ACTIMMUNE* therapy before age one year 2-fold to 25-fold elevations from baseline of AST and/or ALT were observed. These elevations occurred as early as 7 days after starting treatment. Treatment with *ACTIMMUNE* was interrupted in all 6 of these patients and was restarted at a reduced dosage in 4. Liver transaminase values returned to baseline in all patients and transaminase elevation recurred in one patient upon *ACTIMMUNE* rechallenge. An 11-fold alkaline phosphatase elevation and hypokalemia in one patient and neutropenia (ANC=525 cells/mm³) in another patient resolved with interruption of *ACTIMMUNE* treatment and did not recur with rechallenge.

In the post-marketing safety database clinically significant adverse events observed during *ACTIMMUNE* therapy in children under the age of three years (n=14) included: two cases of hepatomegaly, and one case each of Stevens-Johnson syndrome, granulomatous colitis, urticaria, and atopic dermatitis.

OVERDOSAGE

Central nervous system adverse reactions including decreased mental status, gait disturbance and dizziness have been observed, particularly in cancer patients receiving doses greater than 100 mcg/m²/day by intravenous or intramuscular administration. These abnormalities were reversible within a few days upon dose reduction or discontinuation of therapy. Reversible neutropenia, elevation of hepatic enzymes and of triglycerides, and thrombocytopenia have also been observed.

DOSAGE AND ADMINISTRATION

The recommended dosage of *ACTIMMUNE* for the treatment of patients with Chronic Granulomatous Disease and severe, malignant osteopetrosis is 50 mcg/m² (1 million IU/m²) for patients whose body surface area is greater than 0.5 m² and 1.5 mcg/kg/dose for patients whose body surface area is equal to or less than 0.5 m². *Note that the above activity is expressed in International Units (1 million IU/50 mcg). This is equivalent to what was previously expressed as units (1.5 million U/50 mcg).* Injections should be administered subcutaneously three times weekly (for example, Monday, Wednesday, Friday). The optimum sites of injection are the right and left deltoid and anterior thigh. *ACTIMMUNE* can be administered by a physician, nurse, family member or patient when trained in the administration of subcutaneous injections. Parenteral drug products should be inspected visually for particulate matter and discoloration prior to administration, whenever solution and container permit.

The formulation does not contain a preservative. A vial of *ACTIMMUNE* is suitable for a single use only. The unused portion of any vial should be discarded. Higher doses are not recommended. Safety and efficacy has not been established for *ACTIMMUNE* given in doses greater or less than the recommended dose of 50 mcg/m². The minimum effective dose of *ACTIMMUNE* has not been established.

ACTIMMUNE should not be mixed with other drugs in the same syringe.

Dose Modification

If severe reactions occur, the dosage should be reduced by 50 percent or therapy should be interrupted until the adverse reaction abates.

ACTIMMUNE may be administered using either sterilized glass or plastic disposable syringes.

HOW SUPPLIED

ACTIMMUNE (Interferon gamma-1b) is a sterile, clear, colorless solution filled in a single-use vial for subcutaneous injection. Each 0.5 mL of *ACTIMMUNE* contains: **100 mcg (2 million IU)** of Interferon gamma-1b, formulated in 20 mg mannitol, 0.36 mg sodium succinate, 0.05 mg polysorbate 20 and Sterile Water for Injection.

Single vial (NDC 64116-011-01)

Cartons of 12 (NDC 64116-011-12)

Stability and Storage

Vials of *ACTIMMUNE* must be placed in a 2–8°C (36–46°F) refrigerator immediately upon receipt to ensure optimal retention of physical and biochemical integrity. DO NOT FREEZE. Avoid excessive or vigorous agitation. DO NOT SHAKE. An unentered vial of *ACTIMMUNE* should not be left at room temperature for a total time exceeding 12 hours prior to use. Vials exceeding this time period should not be returned to the refrigerator; such vials should be discarded. Do not use beyond the expiration date stamped on the vial.

REFERENCES

1. The International Chronic Granulomatous Disease Cooperative Study Group. A controlled trial of interferon gamma to prevent infection in chronic granulomatous disease. N Engl J Med 324: 509–516,1991.

2. Beard CJ, Key L, Newburger PE, Ezekowitz RAB, *et al.* Neutrophil defect associated with malignant infantile osteopetrosis. J Lab Clin Med *108*: 498–505, 1986.
3. Shankar L, Gerritsen EJA, and Key LL. Osteopetrosis: pathogenesis and rationale for the use of interferon-γ-1b. Biodrugs *7*: 23–29, 1997.
4. Key LL, Rodriguiz RM, Willi SM. Long-term treatment of osteopetrosis with recombinant human interferon gamma. N Engl J Med *24*: 1594–1599, 1995.

Manufactured by:
InterMune, Inc.
Brisbane, CA 94005
U.S. License No. 1626
Revised January 2009
 PH01037.04

Jacobus Pharmaceutical Co., Inc.

37 CLEVELAND LANE
P.O. BOX 5290
PRINCETON, NJ 08540

Direct All Inquiries to:
(609) 921-7447
FAX: (609) 799-1176

DAPSONE ℞

[*dap 'sōne*]
Tablets, USP
25 mg & 100 mg

DESCRIPTION

Dapsone-USP, 4,4′-diaminodiphenylsulfone (DDS), is a primary treatment for Dermatitis herpetiformis. It is an antibacterial drug for susceptible cases of leprosy. It is a white, odorless crystalline powder, practically insoluble in water and insoluble in fixed and vegetable oils.

Dapsone is issued on prescription in tablets of 25 and 100 mg for oral use.

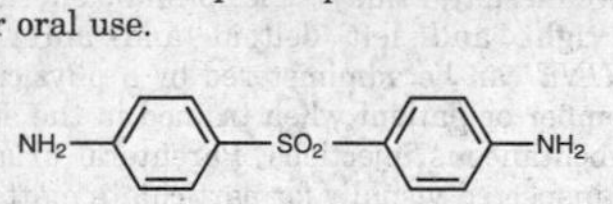

Inactive Ingredients: Colloidal silicone dioxide, magnesium stearate, microcrystalline cellulose and corn starch.

CLINICAL PHARMACOLOGY

Actions: The mechanism of action in Dermatitis herpetiformis has not been established. By the kinetic method in mice, Dapsone is bactericidal as well as bacteriostatic against *Mycobacterium leprae.*

Absorption and Excretion: Dapsone, when given orally, is rapidly and almost completely absorbed. About 85 percent of the daily intake is recoverable from the urine mainly in the form of water-soluble metabolites. Excretion of the drug is slow and a constant blood level can be maintained with the usual dosage.

Blood Levels: Detected a few minutes after ingestion, the drug reaches peak concentration in 4-8 hours. Daily administration for at least eight days is necessary to achieve a plateau level. With doses of 200 mg daily, this level averaged 2.3 µg/ml with a range of 0.1-7.0 µg/ml. The half-life in the plasma in different individuals varies from ten hours to fifty hours and averages twenty-eight hours. Repeat tests in the same individual are constant. Daily administration (50-100 mg) in leprosy patients will provide blood levels in excess of the usual minimum inhibitory concentration even for patients with a short Dapsone half-life.

INDICATIONS AND USAGE

Dermatitis herpetiformis: (D.H.)
Leprosy: All forms of leprosy except for cases of proven Dapsone resistance.

CONTRAINDICATION

Hypersensitivity to Dapsone and/or its derivatives.

WARNINGS

The patient should be warned to respond to the presence of clinical signs such as sore throat, fever, pallor, purpura or jaundice. Deaths associated with the administration of Dapsone have been reported from agranulocytosis, aplastic anemia and other blood dyscrasias. Complete blood counts should be done frequently in patients receiving Dapsone. The FDA Dermatology Advisory Committee recommended that, when feasible, counts should be done weekly for the first month, monthly for six months and semi-annually thereafter. If a significant reduction in leucocytes, platelets or hemopoiesis is noted, Dapsone should be discontinued and the patient followed intensively. Folic acid antagonists have similar effects and may increase the incidence of hematologic reactions; if co-administered with Dapsone the patient should be monitored more frequently. Patients on weekly pyrimethamine and Dapsone have developed agranulocytosis during the second and third month of therapy.

Severe anemia should be treated prior to initiation of therapy and hemoglobin monitored. Hemolysis and methemoglobin may be poorly tolerated by patients with severe cardiopulmonary disease.

Cutaneous reactions, especially bullous, include exfoliative dermatitis and are probably one of the most serious, though rare, complications of sulfone therapy. They are directly due to drug sensitization. Such reactions include toxic erythema, erythema multiforme, toxic epidermal necrolysis, morbilliform and scarlatiniform reactions, urticaria and erythema nodosum. If new or toxic dermatologic reactions occur, sulfone therapy must be promptly discontinued and appropriate therapy instituted. Leprosy reactional states, including cutaneous, are not hypersensitivity reactions to Dapsone and do not require discontinuation. See special section.

PRECAUTIONS

General: Hemolysis and Heinz body formation may be exaggerated in individuals with a glucose-6-phosphate dehydrogenase (G6PD) deficiency, or methemoglobin reductase deficiency, or hemoglobin M. This reaction is frequently dose-related. Dapsone should be given with caution to these patients or if the patient is exposed to other agents or conditions such as infection or diabetic ketosis capable of producing hemolysis. Drugs or chemicals which have produced significant hemolysis in G6PD or methemoglobin reductase deficient patients include Dapsone, sulfanilamide, nitrite, aniline, phenylhydrazine, napthalene, niridazole, nitrofurantoin and 8-amino-antimalarials such as primaquine.

Toxic hepatitis and cholestatic jaundice have been reported early in therapy. Hyperbilirubinemia may occur more often in G6PD deficient patients. When feasible, baseline and subsequent monitoring of liver function is recommended; if abnormal, Dapsone should be discontinued until the source of the abnormality is established.

Drug Interactions: Rifampin lowers Dapsone levels 7 to 10-fold by accelerating plasma clearance; in leprosy this reduction has not required a change in dosage. Folic acid antagonists such as pyrimethamine may increase the likelihood of hematologic reactions.

A modest interaction has been reported for patients receiving 100 mg Dapsone daily in combination with trimethoprim 5 mg/kg q6h. On Day 7, the serum Dapsone levels averaged 2.1 ± 1.0 µg/mL in comparison to 1.5 ± 0.5 µg/mL for Dapsone alone. On Day 7, trimethoprim levels averaged 18.4 ± 5.2 µg/mL in comparison to 12.4 ± 4.5 µg/mL for patients not receiving Dapsone. Thus, there is a mutual interaction between Dapsone and trimethoprim in which each raises the level of the other about 1.5 times.

A crossover study[1] designed to assess the potential of a drug interaction between Dapsone, 100 mg/day and trimethoprim, 200 mg every 12 hours, in eight asymptomatic HIV positive volunteers (average CD4 count 524 cells/mm^3) demonstrated that there was not a significant drug intreraction between Dapsone and trimethoprim. However, an earlier report[2] also by Lee et al, in 78 HIV infected patients with acute *Pneumocystis carinii* pneumonia, receiving Dapsone, 100 mg/day and higher trimethoprim dose, 20 mg/kg/day, demonstrated that the serum levels of Dapsone were increased by 40% and trimethoprim levels were increased by 48% when the drugs were administered concurrently.

Carcinogenesis, mutagenesis: Dapsone has been found carcinogenic (sarcomagenic) for male rats and female mice causing mesenchymal tumors in the spleen and peritoneum, and thyroid carcinoma in female rats. Dapsone is not mutagenic with or without microsomal activation in *S. typhimurium* tester strains 1535, 1537, 1538, 98, or 100.

Pregnancy: Teratogenic Effects. Pregnancy Category C: Animal reproduction studies have not been conducted with Dapsone. Extensive, but uncontrolled experience and two published surveys on the use of Dapsone in pregnant women have not shown that Dapsone increases the risk of fetal abnormalities if administered during all trimesters of pregnancy or can affect reproduction capacity. Because of the lack of animal studies or controlled human experience, Dapsone should be given to a pregnant woman only if clearly needed. In general, for leprosy, USPHS at Carville recommends maintenance of Dapsone. Dapsone has been important for the management of some pregnant D.H. patients.

Nursing Mothers: Dapsone is excreted in breast milk in substantial amounts. Hemolytic reactions can occur in neonates. See section on hemolysis. Because of the potential for tumorgenicity shown for Dapsone in animal studies a decision should be made whether to discontinue nursing or discontinue the drug taking into account the importance of drug to the mother.

Pediatric Use: Pediatric patients are treated on the same schedule as adults but with correspondingly smaller doses. Dapsone is generally not considered to have an effect on the later growth, development and functional development of the pediatric patient.

ADVERSE REACTIONS

In addition to the warnings listed above, the following syndromes and serious reactions have been reported in patients on Dapsone.

Hematologic Effects: Dose-related hemolysis is the most common adverse effect and is seen in patients with or without G6PD deficiency. Almost all patients demonstrate the inter-related changes of a loss of 1-2g of hemoglobin, an increase in the reticulocytes (2-12%), a shortened red cell life span and a rise in methemoglobin. G6PD deficient patients have greater responses.

Nervous System Effects: Peripheral neuropathy is a definite but unusual complication of Dapsone therapy in nonleprosy patients. Motor loss is predominant. If muscle weakness appears, Dapsone should be withdrawn. Recovery on withdrawal is usually substantially complete. The mechanism of recovery is reported by axonal regeneration. Some recovered patients have tolerated retreatment at reduced dosage. In leprosy this complication may be difficult to distinguish from a leprosy reactional state.

Body As A Whole: In addition to the warnings and adverse effects reported above, additional adverse reactions include: nausea, vomiting, abdominal pains, pancreatitis, vertigo, blurred vision, tinnitus, insomnia, fever, headache, psychosis, phototoxicity, pulmonary eosinophilia, tachycardia, albuminuria, the nephrotic syndrome, hypoalbuminemia without proteinuria, renal papillary necrosis, male infertility, drug-induced Lupus erythematosus and an infectious mononucleosis-like syndrome. In general, with the exception of the complications of severe anoxia from overdosage (retinal and optic nerve damage, etc.) these adverse reactions have regressed off drug.

OVERDOSAGE

Nausea, vomiting, hyperexcitability can appear a few minutes up to 24 hours after ingestion of an overdosage. Methemoglobin induced depression, convulsions or severe cyanosis requires prompt treatment. In normal and methemoglobin reductase deficient patients, methylene blue, 1-2 mg/kg of body weight, given slowly intravenously, is the treatment of choice. The effect is complete in 30 minutes, but may have to be repeated if methemoglobin reaccumulates. For non-emergencies, if treatment is needed, methylene blue may be given orally in doses of 3-5 mg/kg every 4-6 hours. Methylene blue reduction depends on G6PD and should not be given to fully expressed G6PD deficient patients.

DOSAGE AND ADMINISTRATION

Dermatitis herpetiformis: The dosage should be individually titrated starting in adults with 50 mg daily and correspondingly smaller doses in children. If full control is not achieved within the range of 50-300 mg daily, higher doses may be tried. Dosage should be reduced to a minimum maintenance level as soon as possible. In responsive patients there is a prompt reduction in pruritus followed by clearance of skin lesions. There is no effect on the gastrointestinal component of the disease. Dapsone levels are influenced by acetylation rates. Patients with high acetylation rates, or who are receiving treatment affecting acetylation may require an adjustment in dosage.

A strict gluten free diet is an option for the patient to elect, permitting many to reduce or eliminate the need for Dapsone; the average time for dosage reduction is 8 months with a range of 4 months to 2 1/2 years and for dosage elimination 29 months with a range of 6 months to 9 years.

Leprosy: In order to reduce secondary Dapsone resistance, the WHO Expert Committee on Leprosy and the USPHS at Carville, LA, recommended that Dapsone should be commenced in combination with one or more anti-leprosy drugs. In the multidrug program Dapsone should be maintained at the full dosage of 100 mg daily without interruption (with corresponding smaller doses for children) and provided to all patients who have sensitive organisms with new or recrudescent disease or who have not yet completed a two year course of Dapsone monotherapy. For advice and other drugs, the USPHS at Carville, LA (1-800-642-2477) should be contacted. Before using other drugs consult appropriate product labeling.

In bacteriologically negative tuberculoid and indeterminate disease, the recommendation is the coadministration of Dapsone 100 mg daily with six months of Rifampin 600 mg daily. Under WHO, daily Rifampin may be replaced by 600 mg Rifampin monthly, if supervised. The Dapsone is continued until all signs of clinical activity are controlled - usually after an additional six months. Then Dapsone

should be continued for an additional three years for tuberculoid and indeterminate patients and for five years for borderline tuberculoid patients.
In lepromatous and borderline lepromatous patients, the recommendation is the co-administration of Dapsone 100 mg daily with two years of Rifampin 600 mg daily. Under WHO daily Rifampin may be replaced by 600 mg Rifampin monthly, if supervised. One may elect the concurrent administration of a third anti-leprosy drug, usually either Clofazamine 50-100 mg daily or Ethionamide 250-500 mg daily. Dapsone 100 mg daily is continued 3-10 years until all signs of clinical activity are controlled with skin scrapings and biopsies negative for one year. Dapsone should then be continued for an additional 10 years for borderline patients and for life for lepromatous patients.
Secondary Dapsone resistance should be suspected whenever a lepromatous or borderline lepromatous patient receiving Dapsone treatment relapses clinically and bacteriologically, solid staining bacilli being found in the smears taken from the new active lesions. If such cases show no response to regular and supervised Dapsone therapy within three to six months or good compliance for the past 3-6 months can be assured, Dapsone resistance should be considered confirmed clinically. Determination of drug sensitivity using the mouse footpad method is recommended and, after prior arrangement, is available without charge from the USPHS, Carville, LA. Patients with proven Dapsone resistance should be treated with other drugs.

LEPROSY REACTIONAL STATES

Abrupt changes in clinical activity occur in leprosy with any effective treatment and are known as reactional states. The majority can be classified into two groups. The "Reversal" reaction (Type 1) may occur in borderline or tuberculoid leprosy patients often soon after chemotherapy is started. The mechanism is presumed to result from a reduction in the antigenic load: the patient is able to mount an enhanced delayed hypersensitivity response to residual infection leading to swelling ("Reversal") of existing skin and nerve lesions. If severe, or if neuritis is present, large doses of steroids should always be used. If severe, the patient should be hospitalized. In general anti leprosy treatment is continued and therapy to suppress the reaction is indicated such as analgesics, steroids, or surgical decompression of swollen nerve trunks. USPHS at Carville, LA should be contacted for advice in management.
Erythema nodosum leprosum (ENL) (lepromatous reaction) (Type 2 reaction) occurs mainly in lepromatous patients and small numbers of borderline patients. Approximately 50% of treated patients show this reaction in the first year. The principal clinical features are fever and tender erythematous skin nodules sometimes associated with malaise, neuritis, orchitis, albuminuria, joint swelling, iritis, epistaxis or depression. Skin lesions can become pustular and/or ulcerate. Histologically there is a vasculitis with an intense polymorphonuclear infiltrate. Elevated circulating immune complexes are considered to be the mechanism of reaction. If severe, patients should be hospitalized. In general, anti-leprosy treatment is continued. Analgesics, steroids, and other agents available from USPHS, Carville, LA, are used to suppress the reaction.

HOW SUPPLIED

Dapsone Tablets USP, 25 mg are available as round white scored tablets, debossed "25" above and "102" below the score and on the obverse "JACOBUS" in a Unit of Use carton of 30 tablets (2 × 15). The blisters are light and child-resistant. NDC 49938-102-30.
Dapsone Tablets USP, 100 mg are available as round white scored tablets, debossed "100" above and "101" below the score and on the obverse "JACOBUS" in a Unit of Use carton of 30 tablets (2 × 15). The blisters are light and child-resistant. NDC 49938-101-30.
Dapsone Tablets USP, 25 mg are available as round white scored tablets, debossed "25" above and "102" below the score and on the obverse "JACOBUS" in a Unit of Use carton of 28 tablets (2 × 14). The blisters are light and child-resistant. NDC 49938-102-28.
Dapsone Tablets USP, 100 mg are available as round white scored tablets, debossed "100" above and "101" below the score and on the obverse "JACOBUS" in a Unit of Use carton of 28 tablets (2 × 14). The blisters are light and child-resistant. NDC 49938-101-28.

REFERENCES

1. Lee, B., et al., Zidovudine, Trimethoprim, and Dapsone Pharmacokinetic Interactions in Patients with HIV Infection. *Antimicrobial Agents and Chemotherapy*, May 1996; 1231-1236.
2. Lee, B., et al., Dapsone, Trimethoprim, and Sulfamethoxazole Plasma Levels During Treatment of Pneumocystis Carinii Pneumonia in Patients with AIDS, *Annals of Internal Medicine*, 1989; 110:606-611.

Store at 20°-25° C (68°-77°F). [see USP Controlled Room Temperature]. Protect from light.
Rx only. Keep this and all medication out of the reach of children.
JACOBUS PHARMACEUTICAL CO., INC.
P.O. Box 5290
Princeton, NJ 08540
Revised August 2009
0826A09

PASER® GRANULES ℞

[*Pa - ser*]
(4 grams aminosalicylic acid delayed-release granules)

DESCRIPTION

PASER granules are a delayed release granule preparation of aminosalicylic acid (p-aminosalicylic acid; 4-aminosalicylic acid) for use with other anti-tuberculosis drugs for the treatment of all forms of active tuberculosis due to susceptible strains of tubercle bacilli. The granules are designed for gradual release to avoid high peak levels not useful (and perhaps toxic) with bacteriostatic drugs. Aminosalicylic acid is rapidly degraded in acid media; the protective acid-resistant outer coating is rapidly dissolved in neutral media so a mildly acidic food such as orange, apple or tomato juice, yogurt or apple sauce should be used.
Aminosalicylic acid (p-aminosalicylic acid) is 4-Amino-2-hydroxybenzoic acid. PASER granules are the free base of aminosalicylic acid and do NOT contain sodium or a sugar. The molecular formula is $C_7H_7NO_3$ with a molecular weight of 153.14. With heat p-aminosalicylic acid is decarboxylated to produce CO_2 and m-aminophenol. If the airtight packets are swollen, storage has been improper. DO NOT USE if packets are swollen or the granules have lost their tan color and are dark brown or purple.
The structural formula is:

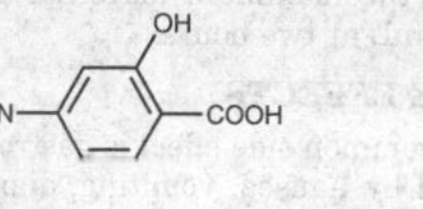

PASER granules are supplied as off-white tan colored granules with an average diameter of 1.5 mm and an average content of 60% aminosalicylic acid by weight. The acid resistant outer coating will be completely removed by a few minutes at a neutral pH. The inert ingredients are:

- colloidal silicon dioxide
- dibutyl sebacate
- hydroxypropyl methyl cellulose
- methacrylic acid copolymer
- microcrystalline cellulose
- talc

The packets contain 4 grams of aminosalicylic acid for oral administration three times a day by sprinkling on apple sauce or yogurt to be eaten without chewing. Suspension in an acidic fruit drink such as orange juice or tomato juice will protect the coating for at least 2 hours. Swirling the juice in the glass will help resuspend the granules if they sink.

CLINICAL PHARMACOLOGY

Mechanism of Action: Aminosalicylic acid is bacteriostatic against Mycobacterium tuberculosis. It inhibits the onset of bacterial resistance to streptomycin and isoniazid. The mechanism of action has been postulated to be inhibition of folic acid synthesis (but without potentiation with antifolic compounds) and/or inhibition of synthesis of the cell wall component, mycobactin, thus reducing iron uptake by M. tuberculosis.
Characteristics: The two major considerations in the clinical pharmacology of aminosalicylic acid are the prompt production of a toxic inactive metabolite under acid conditions and the short serum half life of one hour for the free drug. Both are discussed below.
After two hours in simulated gastric fluid, 10% of unprotected aminosalicylic acid is decarboxylated to form meta-aminophenol, a known hepatotoxin. The acid-resistant coating of the PASER granules protects against degradation in the stomach. The small granules are designed to escape the usual restriction on gastric emptying of large particles. Under neutral conditions such as are found in the small intestine or in neutral foods, the acid-resistant coating is dissolved within one minute. Care must be taken in the administration of these granules to protect the acid-resistant coating by maintaining the granules in an acidic food during dosage administration. Patients who have neutralized gastric acid with antacids will not need to protect the acid resistant coating with an acidic food since no acid is present to spoil the drug. Antacids may influence the absorption of other medications and are not necessary for PASER consumed with an acidic food.
Because PASER granules are protected by an enteric coating absorption does not commence until they leave the stomach; the soft skeletons of the granules remain and may be seen in the stool.
Absorption and excretion: In a single 4 gram pharmacokinetic study with food in normal volunteers the initial time to a 2µg/mL serum level of aminosalicylic acid was 2 hours with a range of 45 minutes to 24 hours; the median time to peak was 6 hours with a range of 1.5 to 24 hours; the mean peak level was 20 µg/mL with a range of 9 to 35 µg/mL; a level of 2 µg/mL was maintained for an average of 7.9 hours with a range of 5 to 9; a level of 1 µg/mL was maintained for an average of 8.8 hours with a range of 6 to 11.5 hours. The recommended schedule is 4 grams every 8 hours.
80% of aminosalicylic acid is excreted in the urine, with 50% or more of the dosage excreted in acetylated form. The acetylation process is not genetically determined as is the case for isoniazid. Aminosalicylic acid is excreted by glomerular filtration; although previously reported otherwise, probenecid, a tubular blocking agent, does not enhance plasma concentration. In a 1954 study thyroxine synthesis but not iodide uptake was reported reduced about 40% when the sodium salt (not PASER granules) of aminosalicylic acid was administered one hour before radio-iodine; the sodium salt typically produces a serum level over 120 µg/mL at one hour lasting one hour. Occasional goiter development can be prevented by the administration of thyroxine but not iodide. Penetration into the cerebrospinal fluid occurs only if the meminges are inflamed.
Approximately 50-60% of aminosalicylic acid is protein bound; binding is reported to be reduced 50% in kwashiorkor.
Microbiology: The aminosalicylic acid MIC for M. tuberculosis in 7H11 agar was less than 1.0 µg/mL for nine strains including three multidrug resistant strains, but 4 and 8 µg/mL for two other multidrug resistant strains. The 90% inhibition in 7H12 broth (Bactec) showed little dose response but was interpreted as being less than or equal to 0.12-0.25 µg/mL for eight strains of which three were multi-resistant, 0.50 µg/mL for one resistant strain, questionable for four non-resistant strains and greater than 1µg/mL for one non-resistant and three resistant strains. Aminosalicylic acid is not active in vitro against M. avium.

INDICATIONS AND USAGE

PASER is indicated for the treatment of tuberculosis in combination with other active agents. It is most commonly used in patients with Multi-drug Resistant TB (MDR-TB) or in situations when therapy with isoniazid and rifampin is not possible due to a combination of resistance and/or intolerance. When PASER is added to the treatment regimen in patients proven or suspected drug resistance, it should be accompanied by at least one and preferably two other new agents to which the patient's organism is known or expected to be susceptible.

CONTRAINDICATIONS

Hypersensitivity to any component of this medication.
Severe renal disease.
Patients with severe renal disease will accumulate aminosalicylic acid and its acetyl metabolite but will continue to acetylate, thus leading exclusively to the inactive acetylated form; deacetylation, if any, is not significant.
The half life of free aminosalicylic acid in renal disease is 30.8 minutes in comparison to 26.4 minutes in normal volunteers. but the half life of the inactive metabolite is 309 minutes in uremic patients in comparison to 51 minutes in normal volunteers. Although aminosalicylic acid passes dialysis membranes, the frequency of dialysis usually is not comparable to the half-life of 50 minutes for the free acid. Patients with end stage renal disease should not receive aminosalicylic acid.

WARNINGS

Liver Function
In one retrospective study of 7492 patients on rapidly absorbed aminosalicylic acid preparations, drug-induced hepatitis occurred in 38 patients (0.5%); in these 38 the first symptom usually appeared within three months of the start of therapy with a rash as the most common event followed by fever and much less frequently by GI disturbances of anorexia, nausea or diarrhea. Only one patient was diagnosed on routine biochemistry.
Premonitory symptoms in 90% of these 38 patients preceded jaundice by a few days to several weeks with the mean time of onset 33 days with a range of 7-90 days. Half of the adverse reactions occurred during the third, fourth or fifth weeks. When aminosalicylic acid-induced hepatitis was diagnosed, hepatomegaly was invariably present with lymphadenopathy in 46%, leucocytosis in 79%, and eosinophilia in 55%. Prompt recognition with discontinuation led to the recovery of all 38 patients. If recognized in the premonitory stage, the reaction is reported to "settle" in 24 hours and no jaundice ensues. From other reported studies failure to recognize the reaction can result in a mortality of

up to 21%. The patient must be monitored carefully during the first three months of therapy and treatment must be discontinued immediately at the first sign of a rash, fever or other premonitory signs of intolerance.

PRECAUTIONS

(1) General:

All drugs should be stopped at the first sign suggesting a hypersensitivity reaction. They may be restarted one at a time in very small but gradually increasing doses to determine whether the manifestations are drug-induced and, if so, which drug is responsible.

Desensitization has been accomplished successfully in 15 of 17 patients starting with 10 mg aminosalicylic acid given as a single dose. The dosage is doubled every 2 days until reaching a total of 1 gram after which the dosage is divided to follow the regular schedule of administration. If a mild temperature rise or skin reaction develops, the increment is to be dropped back one level or the progression held for one cycle. Reactions are rare after a total dosage of 1.5 grams.

Patients with hepatic disease may not tolerate aminosalicylic acid as well as normal patients, even though the metabolism in patients with hepatic disease has been reported to be comparable to that in normal volunteers.

(2) Information for Patients:

The patient should be advised that the first signs of hypersensitivity include a rash, often followed by fever, and much less frequently, GI disturbances of anorexia, nausea or diarrhea. If such symptoms develop, the patient should immediately cease taking the medication and arrange for a prompt clinical visit.

Patients should be advised that poor compliance in taking anti-TB medication often leads to treatment failure, and, not infrequently, to the development of resistance of the organisms in the individual patient.

Patients should be advised that the skeleton of the granules may be seen in the stool.

The coating to protect the PASER granules dissolves promptly under neutral conditions; the granules therefore should be administered by sprinkling on acidic foods such as apple sauce or yogurt or by suspension in a fruit drink which will protect the coating, but the granules sink and will have to be swirled. The coating will last at least 2 hours in either system. All juices tested to date have been satisfactory; tested are: tomato, orange, grapefruit, grape, cranberry, apple, "fruit punch".

Patients should be advised to store PASER in a refrigerator or freezer. PASER packets may be stored at room temperature for short periods of time.

Patients should be advised NOT to use if the packets are swollen or the granules have lost their tan color and are dark brown or purple. The patient should inform the pharmacist or physician immediately and return the medication.

(3) Laboratory Tests:

Aminosalicylic acid has been reported to interfere technically with the serum determinations of albumin by dye-binding, SGOT by the azoene dye method and with qualitative urine tests for ketones, bilirubin, urobilinogen or porphobilinogen.

(4) Drug Interactions:

Aminosalicylic acid at a dosage of 12 grams in a rapidly available form has been reported to produce a 20 percent reduction in the acetylation of isoniazid, especially in patients who are rapid acetylators; INH serum levels, half lives and excretions in fast acetylators still remain half of the levels seen in slow acetylators with or without p-aminosalicylic acid. The effect is dose related and, while it has not been studied with the current delayed release preparation, the lower serum levels with this preparation will result in a reduced effect on the acetylation of INH.

Aminosalicylic acid has previously been reported to block the absorption of rifampin. A subsequent report has shown that this blockade was due to an excipient not included in PASER granules. Oral administration of a solution containing both aminosalicylic acid and rifampin showed full absorption of each product.

As a result of competition, Vitamin B_{12} absorption has been reduced 55% by 5 grams of aminosalicylic acid with clinically significant erythrocyte abnormalities developing after depletion; patients on therapy of more than one month should be considered for maintenance B_{12}.

A malabsorption syndrome can develop in patients on aminosalicylic acid but is usually not complete. The complete syndrome includes steatorrhea, an abnormal small bowel pattern on x-ray, villus atrophy, depressed cholesterol, reduced D-xylose and iron absorption. Triglyceride absorption always is normal.

In one literature report 8 hours after the last dosage of aminosalicylic acid at 2 gm qid serum digoxin levels were reduced 40% in two of ten patients but not changed in the remaining eight.

(5) Carcinogenesis, mutagenesis, impairment of fertility:

Sodium aminosalicylate produced an occipital bone defect, probably with a dose response, when administered to ten pregnant Wistar rats at five doses from 3.85 to 385 mg/kg from days 6 to 14. There were no significant changes from controls in any group in corpora lutea, early resorptions, total resorptions, fetal death, litter size, or hematomas. For all except the 77 mg/kg group, fetal weights were significantly greater than controls. Chinchilla rabbits on 5 mg/kg from days 7 to 14 did not show any significant differences as compared to controls for the same parameters studied.

Sodium aminosalicylic acid was not mutagenic in Ames tester strain TA 100. In human lymphocyte cultures in-vitro clastogenic effects of achromatic, chromatid, isochromatic breaks or chromatid translocations were not seen at 153 or 600 µg/mL. At 1500 and 3000 µg/mL there was a dose related increase in chromatid aberrations.

Patients on isoniazid and aminosalicylic acid have been reported to have an increased number of chromosomal aberrations as compared to controls.

(6) Pregnancy: Pregnancy Category C:

Aminosalicylic acid has been reported to produce occipital malformations in rats when given at doses within the human dose range. Although there probably is a dose response, the frequency of abnormalities was comparable to controls at the highest level tested (two times the human dosage). When administered to rabbits at 5 mg/kg, throughout all three trimesters, no teratologic or embryocidal effects were seen. Literature reports on aminosalicylic acid in pregnant women always report coadministration of other medications. Because there are no adequate and well controlled studies of aminosalicylic acid in humans, PASER granules should be given to a pregnant woman only if clearly needed.

(8) Nursing mothers:

After administration of a different preparation of aminosalicylic acid to one patient, the maximum concentration in the milk was 1 µg/mL at 3 hours with a half-life of 2.5 hours; the maximum maternal plasma concentration was 70 µg/mL at two hours.

ADVERSE EFFECTS

The most common side effect is gastrointestinal intolerance manifested by nausea, vomiting, diarrhea, and abdominal pain.

Hypersensitivity reactions: Fever, skin eruptions of various types, including exfoliative dermatitis, infectious mononucleosis-like, or lymphoma-like syndrome, leucopenia, agranulocytosis, thrombocytopenia, Coombs' positive hemolytic anemia, jaundice, hepatitis, pericarditis, hypoglycemia, optic neuritis, encephalopathy, Leoffler's syndrome, vasculitis and a reduction in prothrombin.

Crystalluria may be prevented by the maintenance of urine at a neutral or an alkaline pH.

OVERDOSAGE

Overdosage has not been reported.

DOSAGE AND ADMINISTRATION

PASER granules should be administered with other drugs to which the organism is known or expected to be susceptible. It is most commonly administered to patients with Multi-drug Resistant TB (MDR-TB) or in other situations in which therapy with isoniazid or rifampin is not possible due to a combination of resistance and/or intolerance. The adult dosage of four grams (one packet) three times per day or correspondingly smaller doses in children should be given by sprinkling on apple sauce or yogurt or by swirling in the glass to suspend the granules in an acidic drink such as tomato or orange juice.

DO NOT USE if packet is swollen or the granules have lost their tan color, turning dark brown or purple.

HOW SUPPLIED

Carton of 30 PASER packets (NDC 49938-107-04).

Each packet contains four grams aminosalicylic acid.

PASER granules are supplied in packets containing 4 grams of aminosalicylic acid for administration three times a day by suspension in an acidic drink or food with a pH less than 5. Examples include apple sauce, yogurt, tomato or orange juice.

Distributors and Pharmacists: Store below 59°F (15°C) (in a refrigerator or freezer).

Patients are urged to store PASER in a refrigerator or freezer. PASER packets may be stored at room temperature for short periods of time.

AVOID EXCESSIVE HEAT. DO NOT USE if packet is swollen or the granules have lost their tan color, turning dark brown or purple.

JACOBUS PHARMACEUTICAL CO. INC.
P.O. Box 5290
Princeton, NJ 08540
2A JULY, 1996

Jazz Pharmaceuticals, Inc.

3180 PORTER DRIVE
PALO ALTO, CA 94304

Direct Inquiries to:
Phone: (650) 496-3777
Fax: (650) 496-3781
E-mail: customercare@jazzpharma.com
For medical information:
E-mail: jazzpharma@medcomsol.com
For media information:
E-mail: mediainfo@jazzpharma.com

XYREM®

(sodium oxybate) oral solution
Rx only

!WARNING: Central nervous system depressant with abuse potential. Should not be used with alcohol or other CNS depressants.

Sodium oxybate is GHB, a known drug of abuse. Abuse has been associated with some important central nervous system (CNS) adverse events (including death). Even at recommended doses, use has been associated with confusion, depression and other neuropsychiatric events. Reports of respiratory depression occurred in clinical trials. Almost all of the patients who received sodium oxybate during clinical trials were receiving CNS stimulants.

Important CNS adverse events associated with abuse of GHB include seizure, respiratory depression and profound decreases in level of consciousness, with instances of coma and death. For events that occurred outside of clinical trials, in people taking GHB for recreational purposes, the circumstances surrounding the events are often unclear (e.g., dose of GHB taken, the nature and amount of alcohol or any concomitant drugs).

Xyrem is available through the Xyrem Success Program, using a centralized pharmacy 1-866-XYREM88® (1-866-997-3688). The Success Program provides educational materials to the prescriber and the patient explaining the risks and proper use of sodium oxybate, and the required prescription form. Once it is documented that the patient has read and/or understood the materials, the drug will be shipped to the patient. The Xyrem Success Program also recommends patient follow-up every 3 months. Physicians are expected to report all serious adverse events to the manufacturer. (See WARNINGS).

DESCRIPTION

Xyrem (sodium oxybate) is a central nervous system depressant that reduces excessive daytime sleepiness and cataplexy in patients with narcolepsy. Sodium oxybate is intended for oral administration. The chemical name for sodium oxybate is sodium 4-hydroxybutyrate. The molecular formula is $C_4H_7NaO_3$ and the molecular weight is 126.09 grams/mole. The chemical structure is:

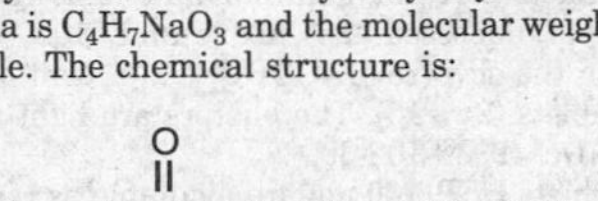

Sodium oxybate is a white to off-white, crystalline powder that is very soluble in aqueous solutions. Xyrem oral solution contains 500 mg of sodium oxybate per milliliter of USP Purified Water, neutralized to pH 7.5 with malic acid.

CLINICAL PHARMACOLOGY

Mechanism of Action

The precise mechanism by which sodium oxybate produces an effect on cataplexy is unknown.

Pharmacokinetics

Sodium oxybate is rapidly but incompletely absorbed after oral administration; absorption is delayed and decreased by a high fat meal. It is eliminated mainly by metabolism with a half-life of 0.5 to 1 hour. Pharmacokinetics are nonlinear with blood levels increasing 3.7-fold as dose is doubled from 4.5 to 9 grams (g). The pharmacokinetics are not altered with repeat dosing.

Absorption

Sodium oxybate is absorbed rapidly following oral administration with an absolute bioavailability of about 25%. The average peak plasma concentrations (1st and 2nd peak) following administration of a 9 g daily dose divided into two equivalent doses given four hours apart were 78 and 142 micrograms/milliliter (mcg/mL), respectively. The average time to peak plasma concentration (T_{max}) ranged from 0.5 to 1.25 hours in eight pharmacokinetic studies. Following oral administration, the plasma levels of sodium oxybate increase more than proportionally with increasing dose. Single doses greater than 4.5 g have not been studied. Administration of sodium oxybate immediately after a high fat meal resulted in delayed absorption (average T_{max} increased from 0.75 hr to 2.0 hr) and a reduction in peak plasma level (C_{max}) by a mean of 58% and of systemic exposure (AUC) by 37%.

Distribution

Sodium oxybate is a hydrophilic compound with an apparent volume of distribution averaging 190–384 mL/kg. At sodium oxybate concentrations ranging from 3 to 300 mcg/mL, less than 1% is bound to plasma proteins.

Metabolism

Animal studies indicate that metabolism is the major elimination pathway for sodium oxybate, producing carbon dioxide and water via the tricarboxylic acid (Krebs) cycle and secondarily by beta-oxidation. The primary pathway involves a cytosolic $NADP^+$-linked enzyme, GHB dehydrogenase, that catalyses the conversion of sodium oxybate to succinic semialdehyde, which is then biotransformed to succinic acid by the enzyme succinic semialdehyde dehydrogenase. Succinic acid enters the Krebs cycle where it is metabolized to carbon dioxide and water. A second mitochondrial oxidoreductase enzyme, a transhydrogenase, also catalyses the conversion to succinic semialdehyde in the presence of α-ketoglutarate. An alternate pathway of biotransformation involves β-oxidation via 3,4-dihydroxybutyrate to carbon dioxide and water. No active metabolites have been identified.

Studies in vitro with pooled human liver microsomes indicate that sodium oxybate does not significantly inhibit the activities of the human isoenzymes: CYP1A2, CYP2C9, CYP2C19, CYP2D6, CYP2E1, or CYP3A up to the concentration of 3 mM (378 mcg/mL). These levels are considerably higher than levels achieved with therapeutic doses.

Elimination

The clearance of sodium oxybate is almost entirely by biotransformation to carbon dioxide, which is then eliminated by expiration. On average, less than 5% of unchanged drug appears in human urine within 6 to 8 hours after dosing. Fecal excretion is negligible.

Special Populations

Geriatric

The pharmacokinetics of sodium oxybate in patients greater than the age of 65 years have not been studied.

Pediatric

The pharmacokinetics of sodium oxybate in patients under the age of 18 years have not been studied.

Gender

In a study of 18 female and 18 male healthy adult volunteers, no gender differences were detected in the pharmacokinetics of sodium oxybate following a single oral dose of 4.5 g.

Race

There are insufficient data to evaluate any pharmacokinetic differences among races.

Renal Disease

Because the kidney does not have a significant role in the excretion of sodium oxybate, no pharmacokinetic study in patients with renal dysfunction has been conducted; no effect of renal function on sodium oxybate pharmacokinetics would be expected.

Hepatic Disease

Sodium oxybate undergoes significant presystemic (hepatic first-pass) metabolism. The kinetics of sodium oxybate in 16 cirrhotic patients, half without ascites, (Child's Class A) and half with ascites (Child's Class C) were compared to the kinetics in 8 healthy adults after a single oral dose of 25 mg/kg. AUC values were double in the cirrhotic patients, with apparent oral clearance reduced from 9.1 in healthy adults to 4.5 and 4.1 mL/min/kg in Class A and Class C patients, respectively. Elimination half-life was significantly longer in Class C and Class A patients than in control subjects (mean $t_{1/2}$ of 59 and 32 versus 22 minutes). It is prudent to reduce the starting dose of sodium oxybate by one-half in patients with liver dysfunction (see Dosage and Administration).

Drug-Drug Interaction

Drug interaction studies in healthy adults demonstrated no pharmacokinetic interactions between sodium oxybate and protriptyline hydrochloride, zolpidem tartrate, and modafinil. However, pharmacodynamic interactions with these drugs cannot be ruled out. Alteration of gastric pH with omeprazole produced no significant change in the oxybate kinetics.

CLINICAL TRIALS

Cataplexy

The effectiveness of sodium oxybate in the treatment of cataplexy was established in two randomized, double-blind,

placebo-controlled trials (Trials 1 and 2) in patients with narcolepsy, 85% and 80%, respectively, of whom were also being treated with CNS stimulants. The high percentages of concomitant stimulant use make it impossible to assess the efficacy and safety of Xyrem independent of stimulant use. In each trial, the treatment period was 4 weeks and the total daily doses ranged from 3 to 9 g, with the daily dose divided into two equal doses. The first dose each night was taken at bedtime and the second dose was taken 2.5 to 4 hours later. There were no restrictions on the time between food consumption and dosing.

Trial 1 was a multi-center, double-blind, placebo-controlled, parallel-group trial that enrolled 136 narcoleptic patients with moderate to severe cataplexy (median of 21 cataplexy attacks per week) at baseline. Prior to randomization, medications with possible effects on cataplexy were withdrawn, but stimulants were continued at stable doses. Patients were randomized to receive placebo, sodium oxybate 3 g/night, sodium oxybate 6 g/night, or sodium oxybate 9 g/night.

Trial 2 was a multi-center, double-blind, placebo-controlled, parallel-group, randomized withdrawal trial that enrolled 55 narcoleptic patients who had been taking open-label sodium oxybate for 7 to 44 months. To be included, patients were required to have a history of at least 5 cataplexy attacks per week prior to any treatment for cataplexy. Patients were randomized to continued treatment with sodium oxybate at their stable dose or to placebo. Trial 2 was designed specifically to evaluate the continued efficacy of sodium oxybate after long-term use.

The primary efficacy measure in Trials 1 and 2 was the frequency of cataplexy attacks.

[See table 1 above]

In Trial 1, both the 6 g/night and 9 g/night doses gave statistically significant reductions in the frequency of cataplexy attacks. The 3 g/night dose had little effect. In Trial 2, following the discontinuation of long-term open-label sodium oxybate therapy, patients randomized to placebo experienced a significant increase in cataplexy (p <0.001), providing evidence of long-term efficacy of sodium oxybate. In Trial 2, the response was numerically similar for patients treated with doses of 6 to 9 g/night, but there was no effect seen in patients treated with doses less than 6 g/night, suggesting little effect at these doses.

Excessive Daytime Sleepiness

The effectiveness of sodium oxybate in the treatment of excessive daytime sleepiness in narcolepsy was established in two randomized, double-blind, placebo-controlled trials (Trials 3 and 4) in patients with narcolepsy. Seventy-eight percent of patients in Trial 3 were also being treated with CNS stimulants.

Trial 3 was a multi-center, randomized, double-blind, placebo-controlled, parallel-arm trial that evaluated 228 pa-

tients with moderate to severe symptoms at entry into the study including a median Epworth Sleepiness Scale (see below) score of 18, and Maintenance of Wakefulness Test (see below) score of 8.25 minutes. These patients were randomized to one of 4 treatment groups: placebo; sodium oxybate 4.5 g/night; sodium oxybate 6 g/night; and sodium oxybate 9 g/night. The period of double-blind treatment in this trial was 8 weeks. Antidepressants were withdrawn prior to randomization; stimulants were continued at stable doses.

The primary efficacy measures in Trial 3 were the Epworth Sleepiness Scale and the Clinical Global Impression of Change. The Epworth Sleepiness Scale is intended to evaluate the extent of sleepiness in everyday situations by asking the patient a series of questions. In these questions, patients are asked to rate their chances of dozing during each of 8 activities on a scale from 0–3 (0=never; 1=slight; 2=moderate; 3=high). Higher total scores indicate a greater tendency to sleepiness. The Clinical Global Impression of Change is a 7-point scale, centered at No Change, and ranging from Very Much Worse to Very Much Improved. In Trial 3, patients were rated by evaluators who based their assessments on the severity of narcolepsy at baseline.

Trial 4 was a multi-center randomized, double-blind, double-dummy placebo-controlled, parallel-arm trial that evaluated 222 patients with moderate to severe symptoms at entry into the study including a median Epworth Sleepiness Scale score of 15, and Maintenance of Wakefulness Test (see below) score of 10.25 minutes. At entry, patients had to be taking modafinil for ≥1 month and at stable doses of 200, 400, or 600 mg daily for at least 1 month prior to randomization. The patients enrolled in the study were randomized to one of 4 treatment groups: placebo; sodium oxybate; modafinil; and sodium oxybate plus modafinil. Sodium oxybate was administered in a dose of 6 g/night for 4 weeks, followed by 9 g/night for 4 weeks. Modafinil was continued at the prior dose. Patients taking antidepressants could continue these medications at stable doses.

The only primary efficacy measure in Trial 4 was the Maintenance of Wakefulness Test. The Maintenance of Wakefulness Test measures latency (in minutes) to sleep onset averaged over 4 sessions at 2 hour intervals following nocturnal polysomnography. For each test session, the subject is asked to remain awake without using extraordinary measures. Each test session is terminated after 20 minutes if no sleep occurs, or after 10 minutes, if sleep occurs. The overall score is the mean sleep latency for the 4 sessions.

In Trial 3, statistically significant improvements were seen on the Epworth Sleepiness Scale and on the Clinical Global Impression of Change at the 6 g/night and 9 g/night doses of sodium oxybate.

[See table 2 above]

Table 1
Summary of Outcomes in Clinical Trials Supporting the Efficacy of Sodium Oxybate

Trial/Dosage Group (n)	Baseline	Median Change From Baseline	Comparison to Placebo p-value
CATAPLEXY ATTACKS			
Trial 1		(median attacks/week)	
Placebo (33)	20.5	−4	------
6.0 g/night (31)	23.0	−10	0.0451
9.0 g/night (33)	23.5	−16	0.0016
Trial 2		(median attacks/two weeks)	
Placebo (29)	4.0	21.0	–
Sodium oxybate (26)	1.9	0	<0.001

Table 2
Daytime Sleepiness in Trial 3

Dose Group [g/night (n)]	Epworth Sleepiness Scale (Range 0–24)			
	Baseline	Endpoint	Median Change from Baseline	Change from Baseline Compared to Placebo (p-value)
Placebo (59)	17.5	17.0	−0.5	--
6 (58)	19.0	16.0	−2.0	< 0.001
9 (47)	19.0	12.0	−5.0	< 0.001

Table 3
Clinical Global Impression of Change in Day and Nighttime Symptoms (Responder Analysis) in Trial 3

Dose Group [g/night (n)]	Percent Responders (Very Much Improved or Much Improved)	Significance Compared to Placebo (p-value) Change from Baseline
Placebo (59)	22%	–
6 (58)	52%	<0.001
9 (47)	64%	<0.001

In Trial 4, a statistically significant improvement on the Maintenance of Wakefulness Test score was seen in the sodium oxybate and sodium oxybate plus modafinil groups.

Table 4
Daytime Sleepiness as Evaluated in Trial 4

	Maintenance of Wakefulness Test (minutes)			
Dose Group (n)	Baseline	Endpoint	Mean Change from Baseline	Endpoint Compared to Placebo
Placebo (55)	9.7	6.9	−2.7	--
Sodium Oxybate (50)	11.3	12.0	0.6	<0.001
Sodium Oxybate plus Modafinil (54)	10.4	13.2	2.7	<0.001

This trial was not capable by design of comparing the effects of sodium oxybate to modafinil, because patients receiving modafinil were not titrated to a maximally effective dose.

INDICATIONS AND USAGE

Xyrem (sodium oxybate) oral solution is indicated for the treatment of excessive daytime sleepiness and cataplexy in patients with narcolepsy.

In Xyrem clinical trials, approximately 80% of patients maintained concomitant stimulant use (see BLACK BOX WARNINGS).

CONTRAINDICATIONS

Sodium oxybate is contraindicated in patients being treated with sedative hypnotic agents.

Sodium oxybate is contraindicated in patients with succinic semialdehyde dehydrogenase deficiency. This rare disorder is an inborn error of metabolism variably characterized by mental retardation, hypotonia, and ataxia.

WARNINGS

SEE BOXED WARNING

Due to the rapid onset of its CNS depressant effects, sodium oxybate should only be ingested at bedtime, and while in bed. For at least 6 hours after ingesting sodium oxybate, patients must not engage in hazardous occupations or activities requiring complete mental alertness or motor coordination, such as operating machinery, driving a motor vehicle, or flying an airplane. When patients first start taking Xyrem or any other sleep medicine, until they know whether the medicine will still have some carryover effect on them the next day, they should use extreme care while performing any task that could be dangerous or requires full mental alertness.

The combined use of alcohol (ethanol) with sodium oxybate may result in potentiation of the central nervous system-depressant effects of sodium oxybate and alcohol. Therefore, patients should be warned strongly against the use of any alcoholic beverages in conjunction with sodium oxybate. Sodium oxybate should not be used in combination with sedative hypnotics or other CNS depressants.

Central Nervous System Depression/Respiratory Depression

Sodium oxybate is a CNS depressant with the potential to impair respiratory drive, especially in patients with already-compromised respiratory function. In overdoses, life-threatening respiratory depression has been reported (see OVERDOSAGE). In clinical trials two subjects had profound CNS depression. A 39 year-old woman, a healthy volunteer received a single 4.5 g dose of sodium oxybate after fasting for 10 hours. An hour later, while asleep, she developed decreased respiration and was treated with an oxygen mask. An hour later, this event recurred. She also vomited

and had fecal incontinence. In another case, a 64 year-old narcoleptic man was found unresponsive on the floor on Day 170 of treatment with sodium oxybate at a total daily dose of 4.5 g/night. He was taken to an emergency room where he was intubated. He improved and was able to return home later the same day. Two other patients discontinued sodium oxybate because of severe difficulty breathing and an increase in obstructive sleep apnea.

The respiratory depressant effects of Xyrem, at recommended doses, were assessed in 21 patients with narcolepsy, and no dose-related changes in oxygen saturation were demonstrated in the group as a whole. One of these patients had significant concomitant pulmonary illness, and 4 of the 21 had moderate-to-severe sleep apnea. One of the 4 patients with sleep apnea had significant worsening of the apnea/hypopnea index during treatment, but worsening did not increase at higher doses. Another patient discontinued treatment because of a perceived increase in clinical apnea events. In the randomized controlled Trials 3 and 4, a total of 40 narcolepsy patients were included with a baseline apnea/hypopnea index of 16 to 67 events per hour indicative of mild to severe sleep disordered breathing. None of the 40 patients had a clinically significant worsening of their respiratory function as measured by apnea/hypopnea index and pulse oximetry while receiving sodium oxybate at dosages of 4.5 to 9 g/night in divided dosages. Nevertheless, caution should be observed if Xyrem is prescribed to patients with compromised respiratory function. Prescribers should be aware that sleep apnea has been reported with a high incidence (even 50%) in some cohorts of narcoleptic patients.

Confusion/Neuropsychiatric Adverse Events

During clinical trials, 2.6% of patients treated with sodium oxybate experienced confusion. Fewer than 1% of patients discontinued the drug because of confusion. Confusion was reported at all recommended doses from 6 to 9 g/night. In a controlled trial where patients were randomized to fixed total daily doses of 3, 6, and 9 g/night or placebo, a dose-response relationship for confusion was demonstrated with 17% of patients at 9 g/night experiencing confusion. In all cases in that controlled trial, the confusion resolved soon after termination of treatment. In Trial 3 where sodium oxybate was titrated from an initial 4.5 g/night dose, there was a single event of confusion in one patient at the 9 g/night dose. In the majority of cases in all clinical trials, confusion resolved either soon after termination of dosing or with continued treatment. However, patients treated with Xyrem who become confused should be evaluated fully, and appropriate intervention considered on an individual basis. Other neuropsychiatric events included psychosis, paranoia, hallucinations, and agitation. The emergence of thought disorders and/or behavior abnormalities when patients are treated with sodium oxybate requires careful and immediate evaluation.

Depression

In clinical trials, 3.2% of patients treated with sodium oxybate reported depressive symptoms. In the majority of cases, no change in sodium oxybate treatment was required. Four patients (<1%) discontinued because of depressive symptoms. In the controlled clinical trial where patients were randomized to fixed doses of 3, 6, 9 g/night or placebo, there was a single event of depression at the 3 g/night dose. In Trial 3, where patients were titrated from an initial 4.5 g/night starting dose, the incidence of depression was 1 (1.7%), 1 (1.5%), 2 (3.2%), and 2 (3.6%) for the placebo, 4.5 g, 6 g, and 9 g/night doses respectively.

In the 717 patient dataset, there were two suicides and one attempted suicide recorded in patients with a previous history of depressive psychiatric disorder. Of the two suicides, one patient used sodium oxybate in conjunction with other drugs. Sodium oxybate was not involved in the second suicide. Sodium oxybate was the only drug involved in the attempted suicide. A fourth patient without a previous history of depression attempted suicide by taking an overdose of a drug other than sodium oxybate.

The emergence of depression when patients are treated with Xyrem requires careful and immediate evaluation. Patients with a previous history of a depressive illness and/or suicide attempt should be monitored especially carefully for the emergence of depressive symptoms while taking Xyrem.

Usage in the Elderly

There is very limited experience with sodium oxybate in the elderly. Therefore, elderly patients should be monitored closely for impaired motor and/or cognitive function when taking sodium oxybate.

PRECAUTIONS

Incontinence

During clinical trials, 7% of narcoleptic patients treated with sodium oxybate experienced either a single episode or sporadic nocturnal urinary incontinence and <1% experienced a single episode of nocturnal fecal incontinence. Less than 1% of patients discontinued as a result of incontinence. Incontinence has been reported at all doses tested.

In a controlled trial where patients were randomized to fixed total daily doses of 3, 6, and 9 g/night or placebo, a dose-response relationship for urinary incontinence was demonstrated with 14% of patients initiated at 9 g/night experiencing urinary incontinence. In the same trial, one patient experienced fecal incontinence when initiated at a dose of 9 g/night and discontinued treatment as a result.

If a patient experiences urinary or fecal incontinence during Xyrem therapy, the prescriber should consider pursuing investigations to rule out underlying etiologies, including worsening sleep apnea or nocturnal seizures, although there is no evidence to suggest that incontinence has been associated with seizures in patients being treated with Xyrem.

Sleepwalking

The term "sleepwalking" in this section refers to confused behavior occurring at night and, at times, associated with wandering. It is unclear if some or all of these episodes correspond to true somnambulism, which is a parasomnia occurring during non-REM sleep, or to any other specific medical disorder. Sleepwalking was reported in 4% of 717 patients treated in clinical trials with sodium oxybate. In sodium oxybate-treated patients <1% discontinued due to sleepwalking. In controlled trials of up to 4 weeks duration, the incidence of sleepwalking was 1% in both placebo and sodium oxybate-treated patients. Sleepwalking was reported by 32% of patients treated with sodium oxybate for periods up to 16 years in one independent uncontrolled trial. Fewer than 1% of the patients in that trial discontinued due to sleepwalking. Five instances of significant injury or potential injury were associated with sleepwalking during a clinical trial of sodium oxybate including a fall, clothing set on fire while attempting to smoke, attempted ingestion of nail polish remover, and overdose of oxybate. Therefore, episodes of sleepwalking should be fully evaluated and appropriate interventions considered.

Sodium Intake

Daily sodium intake in patients taking sodium oxybate is provided below and should be considered in patients with heart failure, hypertension or compromised renal function.

Table 5
Sodium Content per Total Nightly Dose

Xyrem Dose (g)	Xyrem (mL)	Sodium Content/Dose
3	6	546 mg
4.5	9	819 mg
6	12	1092 mg
7.5	15	1365 mg
9	18	1638 mg

Hepatic Insufficiency

Patients with compromised liver function will have an increased elimination half-life and systemic exposure to sodium oxybate (see Pharmacokinetics). The starting dose should therefore be decreased by one-half in such patients, and response to dose increments monitored closely (see Dosage and Administration).

Renal Insufficiency

No studies have been conducted in patients with renal failure. Because less than 5% of sodium oxybate is excreted via the kidney, no dose adjustment should be necessary in patients with renal impairment. The sodium load associated with administration of sodium oxybate should be considered in patients with renal insufficiency.

Information for Patients

The Xyrem Patient Success Program® includes detailed information about the safe and proper use of sodium oxybate, as well as information to help the patient prevent accidental use or abuse of sodium oxybate by others. Patients must read and/or understand the materials before initiating therapy. Prescribers will discuss dosing (including the procedure for preparing the dose to be administered) prior to the initiation of treatment. Patients should also be informed that they should be seen by the prescriber frequently during the course of their treatment to review dose titration, symptom response and adverse reactions. Food significantly decreases the bioavailability of sodium oxybate (see Pharmacokinetics). Whether sodium oxybate is taken in the fed or fasted state may affect both the efficacy and safety of sodium oxybate for a given patient. Patients should be made aware of this and try to take the first dose several hours after a meal. Patients should be informed that sodium oxybate is associated with urinary and, less frequently, fecal incontinence. As a safety precaution, patients should be instructed to lie down and sleep after each dose of sodium oxybate, and not to take sodium oxybate at any time other than at night, immediately before bedtime and again 2.5 to 4 hours later. Patients should be instructed that they should not take alcohol or other sedative hypnotics with sodium oxybate.

For additional information, patients should see the Medication Guide for Xyrem.

Laboratory Tests

Laboratory tests are not required to monitor patient response or adverse events resulting from sodium oxybate administration.

In an open-label trial of long term exposure to sodium oxybate, which extended as long as 16 years for some patients, 30% (26/87) of patients tested had at least one positive anti-nuclear antibody (ANA) test. Of the 26, 17 patients had multiple positive ANA tests over time. The clinical course of these patients was not always clearly recorded, but one patient was clearly diagnosed with rheumatoid arthritis at the time of the first recorded positive ANA test. No instances of systemic lupus erythematosus have been reported in patients taking sodium oxybate.

Drug Interactions

Interactions between sodium oxybate and three drugs commonly used in patients with narcolepsy (zolpidem tartrate, protriptyline HCl, and modafinil) have been evaluated in formal studies. Sodium oxybate, in combination with these drugs, produced no significant pharmacokinetic changes for either drug (see Pharmacokinetics). However, pharmacodynamic interactions cannot be ruled out. Nonetheless, sodium oxybate should not be used in combination with sedative hypnotics or other CNS depressants. Alteration of gastric pH with omeprazole produced no significant change in the oxybate kinetics.

Carcinogenicity, Mutagenicity, Impairment of Fertility

Sodium oxybate was not carcinogenic in rats administered oral doses of up to 1000 mg/kg/day (2 times the exposure in humans receiving the maximum recommended dose (MRHD) of 9 g/day, on an AUC basis) for 83 weeks in the male rats and for 104 weeks in female rats. The results of 2-year carcinogenicity studies in mouse and rat with gamma-butyrolactone, a compound that is metabolized to sodium oxybate in vivo, showed no clear evidence of carcinogenic activity. The plasma AUCs of sodium oxybate achieved at the high doses in these studies were 1/2 (mice and female rats) and 1/10 (male rats) the plasma AUCs at the MRHD.

Sodium oxybate was negative in the Ames microbial mutagen test, an in vitro chromosomal aberration assay in CHO cells, and an in vivo rat micronucleus assay.

Sodium oxybate did not impair fertility in rats at doses up to 1000 mg/kg (approximately equal to the maximum recommended human daily dose on a mg/m² basis).

Pregnancy

Pregnancy Category B: Reproduction studies conducted in pregnant rats at doses up to 1000 mg/kg (approximately equal to the maximum recommended human daily dose on a mg/m² basis) and in pregnant rabbits at doses up to 1200 mg/kg (approximately 3 times the maximum recommended human daily dose on a mg/m² basis) revealed no evidence of teratogenicity. In a study in which rats were given sodium oxybate from Day 6 of gestation through Day 21 post-partum, slight decreases in pup and maternal weight gains were seen at 1000 mg/kg; there were no drug effects on other developmental parameters. There are, however, no adequate and well-controlled studies in pregnant women. Because animal reproduction studies are not always predictive of human response, this drug should be used during pregnancy only if clearly needed.

Labor and Delivery

Sodium oxybate has not been studied in labor or delivery. In obstetric anesthesia using an injectable formulation of sodium oxybate newborns had stable cardiovascular and respiratory measures but were very sleepy, causing a slight decrease in Apgar scores. There was a fall in the rate of uterine contractions 20 minutes after injection. Placental transfer is rapid, but umbilical vein levels of sodium oxybate were no more than 25% of the maternal concentration. No sodium oxybate was detected in the infant's blood 30 minutes after delivery. Elimination curves of sodium oxybate between a 2-day old infant and a 15-year old patient were similar. Subsequent effects of sodium oxybate on later growth, development and maturation in humans are unknown.

Nursing Mothers

It is not known whether sodium oxybate is excreted in human milk. Because many drugs are excreted in human milk, caution should be exercised when sodium oxybate is administered to a nursing woman.

Pediatric Use

Safety and effectiveness in patients under 16 years of age have not been established.

Race and Gender Effects

There were too few non-Caucasian patients to permit evaluation of racial effects on safety or efficacy. More than 90% of the subjects in clinical trials were Caucasian.

Table 6
Incidence (%) of Treatment-Emergent Adverse Events in Trial 1

System Organ Class	Placebo	Sodium Oxybate Dosage (g/night) at Onset		
MedDRA Preferred Term	N = 34	3 N = 34	6 N = 33	9 N = 35
Ear and labyrinth disorders				
Tinnitus	0	2 (5.9%)	0	0
Eye disorders				
Vision blurred	1 (2.9%)	2 (5.9%)	0	0
Gastrointestinal disorders				
Abdominal Pain Upper	0	0	1 (3.0%)	4 (11.4%)
Diarrhea	0	0	2 (6.1%)	3 (8.6%)
Dyspepsia	2 (5.9%)	1 (2.9%)	3 (9.1%)	3 (8.6%)
Nausea	2 (5.9%)	3 (8.8%)	8 (24.2%)	14 (40.0%)
Vomiting	0	0	3 (9.1%)	8 (22.9%)
General disorders and administration site conditions				
Feeling Drunk	0	0	0	3 (8.6%)
Lethargy	0	2 (5.9%)	0	0
Pain	1 (2.9%)	1 (2.9%)	1 (3.0%)	2 (5.7%)
Infections and infestations				
Gastroenteritis viral	0	0	2 (6.1%)	0
Nasopharyngitis	1 (2.9%)	1 (2.9%)	2 (6.1%)	2 (5.7%)
Upper respiratory tract infection	1 (2.9%)	1 (2.9%)	2 (6.1%)	0
Injury, poisoning and procedural complications				
Post procedural pain	0	0	0	2 (5.7%)
Investigations				
Blood pressure increased	1 (2.9%)	0	2 (6.1%)	0
Musculoskeletal and connective tissue disorders				
Back Pain	2 (5.9%)	0	2 (6.1%)	2 (5.7%)
Cataplexy	0	0	0	3 (8.6%)
Muscular weakness	0	2 (5.9%)	1 (3.0%)	0
Nervous system disorders				
Disturbance in attention	0	1 (2.9%)	0	3 (8.6%)
Dizziness	2 (5.9%)	8 (23.5%)	10 (30.3%)	13 (37.1%)
Headache	8 (23.5%)	3 (8.8%)	7 (21.2%)	13 (37.1%)
Hypoaesthesia	0	2 (5.9%)	0	0
Sleep Paralysis	1 (2.9%)	1 (2.9%)	2 (6.1%)	5 (14.3%)
Somnolence	3 (8.8%)	4 (11.8%)	4 (12.1%)	5 (14.3%)

(Table continued on next page)

The database was 58% female. No important differences in safety or efficacy of Xyrem were noted between men and women. The overall percentage of patients with at least one adverse event was slightly higher in women (80%) than in men (69%). The incidence of serious adverse events and discontinuations due to adverse events were similar in both men and women.

ADVERSE REACTIONS

A total of 717 narcoleptic patients were exposed to sodium oxybate in clinical trials. The most commonly observed adverse events associated with the use of sodium oxybate were:

Headache (22%), nausea (21%), dizziness (17%), nasopharyngitis (8%), somnolence (8%), vomiting (8%), and urinary incontinence (7%).

Two deaths occurred in these clinical trials, both from drug overdoses. Both of these deaths resulted from ingestion of multiple drugs, including sodium oxybate in one patient.

In these clinical trials, **10%** of patients discontinued because of adverse events. **The most frequent reasons for discontinuation (>1%) were nausea (2%), dizziness (2%) and vomiting (1%).**

Approximately 9% of patients receiving sodium oxybate in 5 placebo-controlled clinical trials (n=443) withdrew due to an adverse event, compared to 1% receiving placebo (n=79). The reasons for discontinuation that occurred more frequently in sodium oxybate-treated patients than placebo-treated patients were: nausea (2%), dizziness (2%), vomiting (1%); as well as urinary incontinence, confusional state, dyspnea, hypesthesia, paresthesia, somnolence, tremor, vertigo, and blurred vision, all occurring in <1% of patients.

Table 6 (cont.)
Incidence (%) of Treatment-Emergent Adverse Events in Trial 1

System Organ Class	Placebo	Sodium Oxybate Dosage (g/night) at Onset		
MedDRA Preferred Term	N = 34	3 N = 34	6 N = 33	9 N = 35
Psychiatric disorders				
Confusional state	0	2 (5.9%)	1 (3.0%)	2 (5.7%)
Depression	0	2 (5.9%)	0	0
Disorientation	1 (2.9%)	1 (2.9%)	0	3 (8.6%)
Nightmare	0	1 (2.9%)	2 (6.1%)	0
Sleep disorder	0	0	2 (6.1%)	1 (2.9%)
Sleep walking	0	0	0	2 (5.7%)
Renal and urinary disorders				
Enuresis	0	0	1 (3.0%)	6 (17.1%)
Respiratory, thoracic and mediastinal disorders				
Pharyngolaryngeal pain	2 (5.9%)	0	3 (9.1%)	1 (2.9%)
Skin and subcutaneous tissue disorders				
Hyperhidrosis	0	1 (2.9%)	1 (3.0%)	2 (5.7%)

Table 7
Incidence (%) of Treatment-Emergent Adverse Events in Trial 3
where dose titration from 4.5 to 9 grams occurred in weekly intervals

System Organ Class	Placebo	Sodium Oxybate Dosage (g/night) at Onset		
MedDRA Preferred Term	N = 60	4.5 N = 185	6 N = 114	9 N = 46
Gastrointestinal disorders				
Nausea	2 (3.3%)	14 (7.6%)	12 (10.5%)	9 (19.6%)
Vomiting	1 (1.7%)	3 (1.6%)	4 (3.5%)	4 (8.7%)
Nervous system disorders				
Disturbance in Attention	0	2 (1.1%)	0	3 (6.5%)
Dizziness	1 (1.7%)	17 (9.2%)	9 (7.9%)	4 (8.7%)
Somnolence	0	2 (1.1%)	0	5 (10.9%)
Renal and urinary disorders				
Enuresis	1 (1.7%)	6 (3.2%)	4 (3.5%)	6 (13.0%)

Incidence in Controlled Clinical Trials

Most Commonly Reported Adverse Events in Controlled Clinical Trials

The most commonly reported adverse events (≥5%) in placebo controlled clinical trials associated with the use of sodium oxybate and occurring more frequently than seen in placebo-treated patients were: nausea (19%), dizziness (18%), headache (18%), vomiting (8%), somnolence (6%), urinary incontinence (6%), and nasopharyngitis (6%). These incidences are based on combined data from Trial 1, Trial 2, Trial 3, and two smaller randomized, double-blind, placebo-controlled, cross-over trials (n=655).

Because clinical trials are conducted under widely varying conditions, adverse reaction rates observed in the clinical trials of a drug cannot be directly compared to rates in the clinical trials of another drug and may not reflect the rates observed in practice. The adverse reaction information from clinical trials does, however, provide a basis for identifying the adverse events that appear to be related to drug use and for approximating incidence rates.

The data presented below come from two placebo-controlled clinical trials, Trial 1 and Trial 3.

Tables 6 and 7 list the incidence of treatment-emergent adverse events in Trials 1 and 3, respectively, for which there was an incidence of ≥5% and the incidence in at least one dosage group on sodium oxybate was greater than placebo. The number of patients in each dosage group represents the total number of patients treated at each dose. Treatment was initiated at assigned doses of 3, 6, and 9 g in Trial 1.
[See table 6 on previous page and above]

[See table 7 above]

Dose Response Information

Discontinuations of treatment due to adverse events were most common at the highest dose of sodium oxybate. A dose-response relationship was observed for nausea, vomiting, paresthesia, disorientation, irritability, disturbance in attention, feeling drunk, sleepwalking and enuresis. The incidence of all these events was notably higher at 9 g/d. Dizziness was most common at 3 and 9 g/night.

Less Common Adverse Events

During clinical trials sodium oxybate was administered to 717 patients with narcolepsy, and 182 healthy volunteers. A total of 283 patients and 25 healthy volunteers received 9 g/night, the maximum recommended dose. A total of 334 patients received sodium oxybate for at least one year. To establish the rate of adverse events, data from all subjects receiving any dose of sodium oxybate were pooled. All adverse events reported by at least two people are included except for those already listed elsewhere in the labeling, terms too general to be informative, or events unlikely to be drug induced. Events are classified by body system and listed under the following definitions: frequent adverse events (those occurring in at least 1/100 people); infrequent events (those occurring in 1/100 to 1/1000 people). These events are not necessarily related to sodium oxybate treatment.

Blood and lymphatic system disorders
Frequent: none; **Infrequent:** leukopenia, lymphadenopathy.
Cardiac disorders
Frequent: none; **Infrequent:** tachycardia.

Ear and labyrinth disorders
Frequent: ear pain, vertigo; **Infrequent:** ear discomfort, tinnitus.
Eye disorders
Frequent: vision blurred; **Infrequent:** conjunctivitis, eye irritation, eye pain, eye redness, eye swelling, keratoconjunctivitis sicca, miosis.
Gastrointestinal disorders
Frequent: constipation, dyspepsia, toothache; **Infrequent:** abdominal distension, dysphagia, eructation, fecal incontinence, flatulence, gastroesophageal reflux disease, oral pain, retching, salivary hypersecretion, stomach discomfort.
General disorders and administration site conditions
Frequent: asthenia, chest pain, fatigue, influenza like illness, malaise, pyrexia; **Infrequent:** chest discomfort, discomfort, edema, feeling abnormal, feeling cold, feeling hot, feeling hot and cold, feeling jittery, gait abnormal, hangover, lethargy, sensation of foreign body, sluggishness.
Immune system disorders
Frequent: none; **Infrequent:** hypersensitivity, multiple allergies.
Infections and infestations
Frequent: bronchitis, gastroenteritis viral, influenza, nasopharyngitis, sinusitis, upper respiratory tract infection, urinary tract infection; **Infrequent:** bladder infection, bronchial infection, cellulitis, dental caries, ear infection, fungal infection, gastroenteritis, herpes simplex, herpes zoster, laryngitis, localized infection, otitis externa, pharyngitis, pneumonia, tinea pedis, tooth abscess, tooth infection, vaginal infection, vaginal mycosis.
Injury, poisoning and procedural complications
Frequent: contusion, fall, pain trauma activated; **Infrequent:** ankle fracture, back injury, concussion, head injury, joint sprain, limb injury, muscle strain, post procedural pain, road traffic accident, skin laceration, tooth injury.
Investigations
Frequent: weight decreased; **Infrequent:** alanine aminotransferase increased, blood alkaline phosphatase increased, blood calcium decreased, blood cholesterol increased, blood glucose increased, blood uric acid increased, blood urine, electrocardiogram abnormal, heart rate increased, liver function test abnormal, protein urine, respiratory rate increased, urine analysis abnormal.
Metabolism and nutrition disorders
Frequent: anorexia; **Infrequent:** decreased appetite, hypernatremia, hypocalcemia, increased appetite.
Musculoskeletal and connective tissue disorders
Frequent: arthralgia, back pain, myalgia, neck pain; **Infrequent:** arthritis, chest wall pain, joint stiffness, joint swelling, muscle tightness, muscle twitching, muscular weakness, musculoskeletal discomfort, musculoskeletal stiffness, polyarthritis, sensation of heaviness, tendonitis.
Neoplasms benign, malignant and unspecified
Frequent: none; **Infrequent:** cyst.
Nervous system disorders
Frequent: balance disorder, headache, hypoesthesia, memory impairment; **Infrequent:** coordination abnormal, depressed level of consciousness, dizziness postural, dysarthria, dysgeusia, dyskinesia, dysstasia, head discomfort, hyperaesthesia, mental impairment, migraine, myoclonus, paralysis, psychomotor hyperactivity, restless leg syndrome, sedation, sinus headache, sleep talking, sudden onset of sleep, syncope, tension headache.
Psychiatric disorders
Frequent: abnormal dreams, confusional state, depression, insomnia, nervousness, nightmare, sleep disorder; **Infrequent:** affect lability, crying, emotional disorder, euphoric mood, fear, hallucination-auditory, hypnagogic hallucination, initial insomnia, libido increased, middle insomnia, mood altered, panic disorder, paranoia, restlessness, sleep attacks, stress symptoms.
Renal and urinary disorders
Frequent: none; **Infrequent:** chromaturia, hematuria, incontinence, micturition urgency, nocturia, pollakiuria, proteinuria, urinary incontinence.
Reproductive system and breast disorders
Frequent: none; **Infrequent:** ovarian cyst, vaginal hemorrhage.
Respiratory, thoracic and mediastinal disorders
Frequent: cough, dyspnea, nasal congestion, pharyngolaryngeal pain, sinus congestion; **Infrequent:** allergic sinusitis, apnea, asthma, dry throat, hiccups, hyperventilation, nocturnal dyspnea, oropharyngeal swelling, respiratory disorder, rhinitis, rhinitis allergic, sinus disorder, snoring, throat secretion increased, upper respiratory tract congestion.
Skin and subcutaneous tissue disorders
Frequent: pruritus; **Infrequent:** acne, alopecia, cold sweat, dermatitis contact, night sweats, rosacea, skin irritation, urticaria.
Surgical and medical procedures
Frequent: none; **Infrequent:** endodontic procedure.
Vascular disorders
Frequent: hypertension; **Infrequent:** hypotension, peripheral coldness.

DRUG ABUSE AND DEPENDENCE

Controlled Substance Class

Xyrem is classified as a Schedule III controlled substance by Federal law. The active ingredient, sodium oxybate or gamma-hydroxybutyrate (GHB), is listed in the most restrictive schedule of the Controlled Substances Act (Schedule I). Thus, non-medical uses of sodium oxybate (Xyrem or GHB) are classified under Schedule I.

Abuse, Dependence, and Tolerance

Abuse

See applicable directions for use under **HANDLING AND DISPOSAL** below. Although sodium oxybate (also known as GHB) has not been systematically studied in clinical trials for its potential for abuse, illicit use and abuse have been reported. Sodium oxybate is a psychoactive drug that produces a wide range of pharmacological effects. It is a sedative-hypnotic that produces dose and concentration dependent central nervous system effects in humans. The onset of effect is rapid, enhancing its desirability as a drug of abuse or misuse.

The rapid onset of sedation, coupled with the amnestic features of sodium oxybate, particularly when combined with alcohol, has proven to be dangerous for the voluntary and involuntary (assault victim) user.

GHB is abused in social settings primarily by young adults. GHB has some commonalties with ethanol over a limited dose range and some cross tolerance with ethanol has been reported as well. Cases of severe dependence and craving for GHB have been reported. Dependence is indicated by the use of increasingly large doses, increased frequency of use, and continued use despite adverse consequences. Some of the doses reported abused in the "rave" setting have been similar to the dose range studied for therapeutic treatment of cataplexy.

Hospital emergency department reports increased 100-fold from 1992 to 1999 (source: Substance Abuse Mental Health Services Administration, Drug Abuse Warning Network [DAWN]). Sixty percent of the ED reports involved individuals 25 years and younger. Numerous deaths had been reported over that period of time, typically involving GHB in combination with alcohol and other drugs, including five in the DAWN system in which GHB was the only drug that could be identified. However, the incidence of hospital emergency department reports of events involving GHB and GHB-related analogs has decreased by about 33% since 2000, and reports to the American Association of Poison Control Centers of GHB exposures has decreased from 1916 (involving 6 deaths) in 2001 to 800 (without any deaths) in 2003.

Dependence

There have been case reports of dependence after illicit use of GHB at frequent repeated doses (18 to 250 g/day), in excess of the therapeutic dose range. In these cases, the signs and symptoms of abrupt discontinuation included an abstinence syndrome consisting of insomnia, restlessness, anxiety, psychosis, lethargy, nausea, tremor, sweating, muscle cramps, and tachycardia. These symptoms generally abated in 3 to 14 days. The discontinuation effects of sodium oxybate have not been systematically evaluated in controlled clinical trials. An abstinence syndrome has not been reported in clinical investigations. Although the clinical trial experience with sodium oxybate in narcolepsy/cataplexy patients at therapeutic doses does not show clear evidence of a withdrawal syndrome, two patients reported anxiety and one reported insomnia following abrupt discontinuation at the termination of the clinical trial; in the two patients with anxiety, the frequency of cataplexy had increased markedly at the same time.

Tolerance

Tolerance to sodium oxybate has not been systematically studied in controlled clinical trials. Open-label, long-term (≥6 months) clinical trials did not demonstrate development of tolerance. There have been some case reports of symptoms of tolerance developing after illicit use at dosages far in excess of the recommended Xyrem dosage regimen. Clinical studies of sodium oxybate in the treatment of alcohol withdrawal suggest a potential cross-tolerance with alcohol. Because illicit use and abuse of GHB have been reported, physicians should carefully evaluate patients for a history of drug abuse and follow such patients closely, observing them for signs of misuse or abuse of GHB (e.g. increase in size or frequency of dosing, drug-seeking behavior). Physicians should document the diagnosis and indication for Xyrem, being alert to drug-seeking behavior and/or feigned cataplexy.

OVERDOSAGE

Human Experience

Information regarding overdose with sodium oxybate is derived largely from reports in the medical literature that describe symptoms and signs in individuals who have ingested GHB illicitly. In these circumstances the co-ingestion of other drugs and alcohol is common, and may influence the presentation and severity of clinical manifestations of overdose. In addition, overdose with GHB may be indistinguishable from overdose with other drugs, or from several other medical conditions that result in similar symptoms.

In clinical trials two cases of overdose with Xyrem were reported. In the first case, an estimated dose of 150 g, more than 15 times the maximum recommended dose, caused a patient to be unresponsive with brief periods of apnea and to be incontinent of urine and feces. This individual recovered without sequelae. In the second case, death was reported following a multiple drug overdose consisting of Xyrem and numerous other drugs.

Signs and Symptoms

Information about signs and symptoms associated with overdosage with sodium oxybate derives from reports of its illicit use. Patient presentation following overdose is influenced by the dose ingested, the time since ingestion, the co-ingestion of other drugs and alcohol, and the fed or fasted state. Patients have exhibited varying degrees of depressed consciousness that may fluctuate rapidly between a confusional, agitated combative state with ataxia and coma. Emesis (even when obtunded), diaphoresis, headache, and impaired psychomotor skills may be observed. No typical pupillary changes have been described to assist in diagnosis; pupillary reactivity to light is maintained. Blurred vision has been reported. An increasing depth of coma has been observed at higher doses. Myoclonus and tonic-clonic seizures have been reported. Respiration may be unaffected or compromised in rate and depth. Cheyne-Stokes respiration and apnea have been observed. Bradycardia and hypothermia may accompany unconsciousness, as well as muscular hypotonia, but tendon reflexes remain intact.

Recommended Treatment of Overdose

General symptomatic and supportive care should be instituted immediately, and gastric decontamination may be considered if co-ingestants are suspected. Because emesis may occur in the presence of obtundation, appropriate posture (left lateral recumbent position) and protection of the airway by intubation may be warranted. Although the gag reflex may be absent in deeply comatose patients, even unconscious patients may become combative to intubation, and rapid-sequence induction (without the use of a sedative) should be considered. Vital signs and consciousness should be closely monitored. The bradycardia reported with GHB overdose has been responsive to atropine intravenous administration. No reversal of the central depressant effects of sodium oxybate can be expected from naloxone or flumazenil administration. The use of hemodialysis and other forms of extracorporeal drug removal have not been studied in GHB overdose. However, due to the rapid metabolism of sodium oxybate, these measures are not warranted.

Poison Control Center

As with the management of all cases of drug overdosage, the possibility of multiple drug ingestion should be considered. The physician is encouraged to collect urine and blood samples for routine toxicologic screening, and to consult with a regional poison control center (1-800-222-1222) for current treatment recommendations.

DOSAGE AND ADMINISTRATION

Xyrem is required to be taken at bedtime while in bed and again 2.5 to 4 hours later. The dose of Xyrem should be titrated to effect. The recommended starting dose is 4.5 g/night divided into two equal doses of 2.25 g. The starting dosage can then be increased to a maximum of 9 g/night in increments of 1.5 g/night (0.75 g per dose). One to two weeks are recommended between dosage increases to evaluate clinical response and minimize adverse effects. The effective dose range of Xyrem is 6 to 9 g/night. The efficacy and safety of Xyrem at doses higher than 9 g/night have not been investigated, and doses greater than 9 g/night ordinarily should not be administered.

Prepare both doses of Xyrem prior to bedtime. Each dose of Xyrem must be diluted with two ounces (60 mL, 1/4 cup, or 4 tablespoons) of water in the child-resistant dosing cups provided prior to ingestion. The first dose is to be taken at bedtime and the second taken 2.5 to 4 hours later; both doses should be taken while seated in bed. Patients will probably need to set an alarm to awaken for the second dose. The second dose must be prepared prior to ingesting the first dose, and should be placed in close proximity to the patient's bed. After ingesting each dose patients should then lie down and remain in bed.

Because food significantly reduces the bioavailability of sodium oxybate, the patient should allow at least 2 hours after eating before taking the first dose of sodium oxybate. Patients should try to minimize variability in the timing of dosing in relation to meals.

Hepatic Insufficiency

Patients with compromised liver function will have increased elimination half-life and systemic exposure along with reduced clearance (see Pharmacokinetics). As a result, the starting dose should be decreased by one-half and dose increments should be titrated to effect while closely monitoring potential adverse events.

Preparation and Administration Precautions

Each bottle of Xyrem is provided with a child resistant cap. The pharmacy provides two dosing cups with child-resistant caps with each Xyrem shipment.

Care should be taken to prevent access to this medication by children and pets.

See the Medication Guide for a complete description.

HOW SUPPLIED

Xyrem (sodium oxybate) is a clear to slightly opalescent oral solution. It is supplied in kits containing one bottle of Xyrem, a press-in-bottle-adaptor, a 10 mL oral measuring device (plastic syringe), a Medication Guide and a professional insert. The pharmacy provides two 90 mL dosing cups with child-resistant caps with each Xyrem shipment. Each amber oval PET bottle contains 180 mL of Xyrem oral solution at a concentration of 500 mg/mL and is sealed with a child resistant cap.

NDC 68727-100-01: Each tamper evident single unit carton contains one 180 mL bottle (500 mg/mL) of Xyrem, one press-in-bottle-adaptor and one oral dispensing syringe.

STORAGE

Store at 25°C (77°F); excursions permitted up to 15°–30°C (59°–86°F). See USP Controlled Room Temperature.

Solutions prepared following dilution should be consumed within 24 hours to minimize bacterial growth and contamination.

HANDLING AND DISPOSAL

Xyrem is a Schedule III drug under the Controlled Substances Act. Xyrem should be handled according to state and federal regulations. It is safe to dispose of Xyrem oral solution down the sanitary sewer.

Rx only

CAUTION

Federal law prohibits the transfer of this drug to any person other than the patient for whom it was prescribed.

Distributed By:

Jazz Pharmaceuticals, Inc.
Palo Alto, CA 94304

For questions of a medical nature or to order Xyrem call the Xyrem Success Program® at 1-866-XYREM88 (1-866-997-3688).

Protected by US Patent Numbers 6780889, 6472431; Additional US Patents Pending

PI-8511 REV1105

Johnson & Johnson · MERCK

Consumer Pharmaceuticals Co.
CAMP HILL ROAD
FORT WASHINGTON, PA 19034

Direct Inquiries to:
Consumer Relationship Center
Fort Washington, PA 19034
1-800-755-4008

PEPCID® AC® — OTC

Original Strength PEPCID® AC® Tablets
Maximum Strength PEPCID® AC® Tablets
Acid reducer

DESCRIPTION

Each Original Strength PEPCID® AC® Tablet contains famotidine 10 mg as an active ingredient.

Each Maximum Strength PEPCID® AC® Tablet contains famotidine 20 mg as an active ingredient.

INACTIVE INGREDIENTS (Orig. Strength PEPCID® AC®)

TABLETS: hydroxypropyl cellulose, hypromellose, magnesium stearate, microcrystalline cellulose, red iron oxide, starch, talc, titanium dioxide

INACTIVE INGREDIENTS (Max. Strength PEPCID® AC®.)

carnauba wax, hydroxypropyl cellulose, hypromellose, magnesium stearate, microcrystalline cellulose, pregelatinized starch, talc, titanium dioxide

Product Benefits:

- **1 Tablet** relieves heartburn associated with acid indigestion and sour stomach.
- Original Strength and Maximum Strength PEPCID® AC® prevent heartburn associated with acid indigestion and sour stomach brought on by eating or drinking certain food and beverages.
- They contain famotidine, a prescription-proven medicine.

The ingredient in Original Strength PEPCID® AC® and Maximum Strength PEPCID® AC®, famotidine, has been prescribed by doctors for years to treat millions of patients safely and effectively. The active ingredient in Original Strength PEPCID® AC® and Maximum Strength PEPCID® AC® has been taken safely with many frequently prescribed medications.

ACTION

It is normal for the stomach to produce acid, especially after consuming food and beverages. However, acid in the wrong place (the esophagus), or too much acid, can cause burning pain and discomfort that interfere with everyday activities.

•Heartburn—Caused by acid in the esophagus

A valve-like muscle called the lower esophageal sphincter (LES) is relaxed in an open position

Burning pain/discomfort

Excess acid moves up into esophagus

USE
• **Relieves heartburn associated with acid indigestion and sour stomach;**
• **Prevents heartburn associated with acid indigestion and sour stomach brought on by eating or drinking certain food and beverages.**

Tips for Managing Heartburn:
• Do not lie flat or bend over soon after eating.
• Do not eat late at night, or just before bedtime.
• Certain foods or drinks are more likely to cause heartburn, such as rich, spicy, fatty, and fried foods, chocolate, caffeine, alcohol, and even some fruits and vegetables.
• Eat slowly and do not eat big meals.
• If you are overweight, lose weight.
• If you smoke, quit smoking.
• Raise the head of your bed.
• Wear loose fitting clothing around your stomach.

WARNINGS
Allergy alert: Do not use if you are allergic to famotidine or other acid reducers

Do not use:
• if you have trouble or pain swallowing food, vomiting with blood, or bloody or black stools. These may be signs of a serious condition. See your doctor.
• if you have kidney disease, except under the advice and supervision of a doctor (Maximum Strength PEPCID® AC®)
• with other acid reducers

Ask a doctor before use if you have
• had heartburn over 3 months. This may be a sign of a more serious condition.
• heartburn with **lightheadedness, sweating, or dizziness**
• chest pain or shoulder pain with shortness of breath; sweating; pain spreading to arms, neck or shoulder; or lightheadedness
• frequent **chest pain**
• frequent wheezing, particularly with heartburn
• unexplained weight loss
• nausea or vomiting
• stomach pain

Stop use and ask a doctor if
• your heartburn continues or worsens
• you need to take this product for more than 14 days

If pregnant or breast-feeding, ask a health professional before use.

Keep out of reach of children. In case of overdose, get medical help or contact a Poison Control Center right away. (1-800-222-1222)

DIRECTIONS
Original Strength PEPCID® AC®:
• adults and children 12 years and over:
• Tablet: To **relieve** symptoms, swallow 1 tablet with a glass of water. Do not chew.
• Tablet: To **prevent** symptoms, swallow 1 tablet with a glass of water at any time from **15 to 60 minutes before** eating food or drinking beverages that cause heartburn
• do not use more than 2 tablets in 24 hours
• children under 12 years: ask a doctor

Maximum Strength PEPCID® AC®:
• adults and children 12 years and over:
• to **relieve** symptoms, swallow 1 tablet with a glass of water. Do not chew.
• to **prevent** symptoms, swallow 1 tablet with a glass of water at any time from **10 to 60 minutes before** eating food or drinking beverages that cause heartburn
• do not use more than 2 tablets in 24 hours
• children under 12 years: ask a doctor

OTHER INFORMATION
• read the directions and warnings before use
• keep the carton. It contains important information.
• store at 20°–30°C (68°–86°F)
• protect from moisture

HOW SUPPLIED
Original Strength PEPCID® AC® Tablet is available as a rose-colored tablet identified as 'PEPCID® AC®'.
Maximum Strength PEPCID® AC® Tablet is a white, "D" shaped, film coated tablet identified as "PAC 20."

PEPCID® COMPLETE®   OTC
Acid Reducer + Antacid Chewable Tablets
DUAL ACTION:
Reduces and Neutralizes Acid

DESCRIPTION
Active Ingredients   **Purpose:**
(in each chewable tablet):
Famotidine 10 mg   Acid Reducer
Calcium carbonate 800 mg   Antacid
Magnesium hydroxide 165 mg   Antacid
Inactive Ingredients:
Mint flavor: Cellulose acetate, corn starch, crospovidone, D&C yellow #10 aluminum lake, dextrose, FD&C blue #1 aluminum lake, flavors, gum arabic, hydroxypropyl cellulose, hypromellose, lactose, magnesium stearate, maltodextrin, mineral oil, sucralose.
Berry flavor: Cellulose acetate, corn starch, crospovidone, D&C red #7 calcium lake, dextrose, FD&C blue #1 aluminum lake, FD&C red #40 aluminum lake, flavors, gum arabic, hydroxypropyl cellulose, hypromellose, lactose, magnesium stearate, maltodextrin, mineral oil, sucralose
Tropical Fruit flavor: Cellulose acetate, corn starch, corn syrup solids, crospovidone, dextrose, FD&C yellow #5 aluminum lake (tartrazine), FD&C yellow #6 aluminum lake, flavors, gum arabic, hydroxypropyl cellulose, hypromellose, lactose, magnesium stearate, maltodextrin, mineral oil, sucralose, triacetin
Product Benefits: PEPCID® COMPLETE® combines an acid reducer (famotidine) with antacids (calcium carbonate and magnesium hydroxide) to relieve heartburn in two different ways: Acid reducers decrease the production of new stomach acid; antacids neutralize acid that is already in the stomach. The active ingredients in PEPCID® COMPLETE® have been used for years to treat acid-related problems in millions of people safely and effectively.

USE: **Relieves heartburn associated with acid indigestion and sour stomach.**

ACTION
It is normal for the stomach to produce acid, especially after consuming food and beverages. However, acid in the stomach may move up into the wrong place (the esophagus), causing burning pain and discomfort that interfere with everyday activities.

Heartburn—Caused by acid in the esophagus

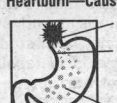

Burning pain/discomfort in esophagus
A valve-like muscle called the lower esophageal sphincter (LES) is relaxed in an open position
Acid moves up from stomach

Tips For Managing Heartburn
• Do not lie flat or bend over soon after eating.
• Do not eat late at night, or just before bedtime.
• Certain foods or drinks are more likely to cause heartburn, such as rich, spicy, fatty, and fried foods, chocolate, caffeine, alcohol, and even some fruits and vegetables.
• Eat slowly and do not eat big meals.
• If you are overweight, lose weight.
• If you smoke, quit smoking.
• Raise the head of your bed.
• Wear loose fitting clothing around your stomach.

WARNINGS
Allergy alert: Do not use if you are allergic to famotidine or other acid reducers

Do not use
• if you have trouble or pain swallowing food, vomiting with blood, or bloody or black stools. These may be signs of a serious condition. See your doctor.
• with other acid reducers

Ask a doctor before use if you have
• had heartburn over 3 months. This may be a sign of a more serious condition.
• heartburn with **lightheadedness, sweating, or dizziness**
• chest pain or shoulder pain with shortness of breath; sweating; pain spreading to arms, neck or shoulders; or lightheadedness
• frequent **chest pain**
• frequent wheezing, particularly with heartburn
• unexplained weight loss
• nausea or vomiting
• stomach pain

Ask a doctor or pharmacist before use if you are presently taking a prescription drug. Antacids may interact with certain prescription drugs.

Stop use and ask a doctor if
• your heartburn continues or worsens
• you need to take this product for more than 14 days
• **If pregnant or breast-feeding,** ask a health professional before use.
• **Keep out of reach of children.** In case of overdose, get medical help or contact a Poison Control Center right away. (1-800-222-1222)

DIRECTIONS
• adults and children 12 years and over:
• **do not swallow tablet whole; chew completely**
• to relieve symptoms, **chew** 1 tablet before swallowing
• do not use more than 2 chewable tablets in 24 hours
• children under 12 years: ask a doctor

OTHER INFORMATION:
• each tablet contains: **calcium 320 mg; magnesium 70 mg.**
• keep the carton. It contains important information.
• read the directions and warnings before use
• read the bottle label. It contains important information.
• store at 20°–30°C (68°–86°F).
• protect from moisture

HOW SUPPLIED
PEPCID® COMPLETE® Mint flavor is available as a green-colored chewable tablet. PEPCID® COMPLETE® Berry flavor is available as a pink-colored chewable tablet. PEPCID® COMPLETE® Tropical Fruit flavor is available as a yellow-colored chewable tablet.

King Pharmaceuticals®, Inc.
501 FIFTH STREET
BRISTOL, TN 37620

Direct Inquiries to:
Customer Service:
Tel: 1 (888) 358-6436
Fax: 1 (866) 990-0545
To report an Adverse Drug Experience:
Tel: 1 (800) 546-4905
Fax: 1 (423) 990-8351
www.kingpharm.com

ALTACE®   ℞
[al-ta-ce]
(ramipril)
Capsules

USE IN PREGNANCY

> When used in pregnancy during the second and third trimesters, ACE inhibitors can cause injury and even death to the developing fetus. When pregnancy is detected, ALTACE® should be discontinued as soon as possible. See WARNINGS: Fetal/neonatal morbidity and mortality.

DESCRIPTION
Ramipril is a 2-aza-bicyclo [3.3.0]-octane-3-carboxylic acid derivative. It is a white, crystalline substance soluble in polar organic solvents and buffered aqueous solutions. Ramipril melts between 105°C and 112°C.
The CAS Registry Number is 87333-19-5. Ramipril's chemical name is $(2S,3aS,6aS)$-1[(S)-N-[(S)-1-Carboxy-3-phenylpropyl] alanyl] octahydrocyclopenta [b]pyrrole-2-carboxylic acid, 1-ethyl ester; its structural formula is:

Its empiric formula is $C_{23}H_{32}N_2O_5$, and its molecular weight is 416.5.
Ramiprilat, the diacid metabolite of ramipril, is a nonsulfhydryl angiotensin converting enzyme inhibitor. Ramipril is converted to ramiprilat by hepatic cleavage of the ester group.
ALTACE (ramipril) is supplied as hard shell capsules for oral administration containing 1.25 mg, 2.5 mg, 5 mg, and 10 mg of ramipril. The inactive ingredients present are pregelatinized starch NF, gelatin, and titanium dioxide. The 1.25 mg capsule shell contains yellow iron oxide, the 2.5 mg capsule shell contains D&C yellow #10 and FD&C red #40, the 5 mg capsule shell contains FD&C blue #1 and FD&C red #40, and the 10 mg capsule shell contains FD&C blue #1.

CLINICAL PHARMACOLOGY
Mechanism of Action
Ramipril and ramiprilat inhibit angiotensin-converting enzyme (ACE) in human subjects and animals. ACE is a peptidyl dipeptidase that catalyzes the conversion of angiotensin I to the vasoconstrictor substance, angiotensin II. Angiotensin II also stimulates aldosterone secretion by the

adrenal cortex. Inhibition of ACE results in decreased plasma angiotensin II, which leads to decreased vasopressor activity and to decreased aldosterone secretion. The latter decrease may result in a small increase of serum potassium. In hypertensive patients with normal renal function treated with ALTACE alone for up to 56 weeks, approximately 4% of patients during the trial had an abnormally high serum potassium and an increase from baseline greater than 0.75 mEq/L, and none of the patients had an abnormally low potassium and a decrease from baseline greater than 0.75 mEq/L. In the same study, approximately 2% of patients treated with ALTACE and hydrochlorothiazide for up to 56 weeks had abnormally high potassium values and an increase from baseline of 0.75 mEq/L or greater, and approximately 2% had abnormally low values and decreases from baseline of 0.75 mEq/L or greater. (See **PRECAUTIONS**.) Removal of angiotensin II negative feedback on renin secretion leads to increased plasma renin activity.

The effect of ramipril on hypertension appears to result at least in part from inhibition of both tissue and circulating ACE activity, thereby reducing angiotensin II formation in tissue and plasma.

ACE is identical to kininase, an enzyme that degrades bradykinin. Whether increased levels of bradykinin, a potent vasodepressor peptide, play a role in the therapeutic effects of ALTACE remains to be elucidated.

While the mechanism through which ALTACE lowers blood pressure is believed to be primarily suppression of the renin-angiotensin- aldosterone system, ALTACE has an antihypertensive effect even in patients with low-renin hypertension. Although ALTACE was antihypertensive in all races studied, black hypertensive patients (usually a low-renin hypertensive population) had a smaller average response to monotherapy than non-black patients.

Pharmacokinetics and Metabolism

Following oral administration of ALTACE, peak plasma concentrations of ramipril are reached within one hour. The extent of absorption is at least 50–60% and is not significantly influenced by the presence of food in the GI tract, although the rate of absorption is reduced.

In a trial in which subjects received ALTACE capsules or the contents of identical capsules dissolved in water, dissolved in apple juice, or suspended in apple sauce, serum ramiprilat levels were essentially unrelated to the use or nonuse of the concomitant liquid or food.

Cleavage of the ester group (primarily in the liver) converts ramipril to its active diacid metabolite, ramiprilat. Peak plasma concentrations of ramiprilat are reached 2–4 hours after drug intake. The serum protein binding of ramipril is about 73% and that of ramiprilat about 56%; in vitro, these percentages are independent of concentration over the range of 0.01 to 10μg/ml.

Ramipril is almost completely metabolized to ramiprilat, which has about 6 times the ACE inhibitory activity of ramipril, and to the diketopiperazine ester, the diketopiperazine acid, and the glucuronides of ramipril and ramiprilat, all of which are inactive. After oral administration of ramipril, about 60% of the parent drug and its metabolites is eliminated in the urine, and about 40% is found in the feces. Drug recovered in the feces may represent both biliary excretion of metabolites and/or unabsorbed drug, however the proportion of a dose eliminated by the bile has not been determined. Less than 2% of the administered dose is recovered in urine as unchanged ramipril.

Blood concentrations of ramipril and ramiprilat increase with increased dose, but are not strictly dose-proportional. The 24-hour AUC for ramiprilat, however, is dose-proportional over the 2.5–20 mg dose range. The absolute bioavailabilities of ramipril and ramiprilat were 28% and 44%, respectively, when 5 mg of oral ramipril was compared with the same dose of ramipril given intravenously. Plasma concentrations of ramiprilat decline in a triphasic manner (initial rapid decline, apparent elimination phase, terminal elimination phase). The initial rapid decline, which represents distribution of the drug into a large peripheral compartment and subsequent binding to both plasma and tissue ACE, has a half-life of 2–4 hours. Because of its potent binding to ACE and slow dissociation from the enzyme, ramiprilat shows two elimination phases. The apparent elimination phase corresponds to the clearance of free ramiprilat and has a half-life of 9–18 hours. The terminal elimination phase has a prolonged half-life (>50 hours) and probably represents the binding/dissociation kinetics of the ramiprilat/ACE complex. It does not contribute to the accumulation of the drug. After multiple daily doses of ramipril 5–10 mg, the half-life of ramiprilat concentrations within the therapeutic range was 13–17 hours.

After once-daily dosing, steady-state plasma concentrations of ramiprilat are reached by the fourth dose. Steady-state concentrations of ramiprilat are somewhat higher than those seen after the first dose of ALTACE, especially at low doses (2.5 mg), but the difference is clinically insignificant. In patients with creatinine clearance less than 40 ml/min/1.73m², peak levels of ramiprilat are approxi-

mately doubled, and trough levels may be as much as quintupled. In multiple-dose regimens, the total exposure to ramiprilat (AUC) in these patients is 3–4 times as large as it is in patients with normal renal function who receive similar doses.

The urinary excretion of ramipril, ramiprilat, and their metabolites is reduced in patients with impaired renal function. Compared to normal subjects, patients with creatinine clearance less than 40 ml/min/1.73m² had higher peak and trough ramiprilat levels and slightly longer times to peak concentrations. (See **DOSAGE AND ADMINISTRATION**.)

In patients with impaired liver function, the metabolism of ramipril to ramiprilat appears to be slowed, possibly because of diminished activity of hepatic esterases, and plasma ramipril levels in these patients are increased about 3-fold. Peak concentrations of ramiprilat in these patients, however, are not different from those seen in subjects with normal hepatic function, and the effect of a given dose on plasma ACE activity does not vary with hepatic function.

Pharmacodynamics

Single doses of ramipril of 2.5–20 mg produce approximately 60–80% inhibition of ACE activity 4 hours after dosing with approximately 40–60% inhibition at 24 hours. Multiple oral doses of ramipril of 2.0 mg or more cause plasma ACE activity to fall by more than 90% 4 hours after dosing, with over 80% inhibition of ACE activity remaining 24 hours after dosing. The more prolonged effect of even small multiple doses presumably reflects saturation of ACE binding sites by ramiprilat and relatively slow release from those sites.

Pharmacodynamics and Clinical Effects
Reduction in Risk of Myocardial Infarction, Stroke, and Death from Cardiovascular Causes

The Heart Outcomes Prevention Evaluation study (HOPE study) was a large, multi-center, randomized, placebo controlled, 2×2 factorial design, double-blind study conducted in 9,541 patients (4,645 on ALTACE) who were 55 years or older and considered at high risk of developing a major cardiovascular event because of a history of coronary artery disease, stroke, peripheral vascular disease, or diabetes that was accompanied by at least one other cardiovascular risk factor (hypertension, elevated total cholesterol levels, low HDL levels, cigarette smoking, or documented microalbuminuria). Patients were either normotensive or under treatment with other antihypertensive agents. Patients were excluded if they had clinical heart failure or were known to have a low ejection fraction (<0.40). This study was designed to examine the long-term (mean of five years) effects of ALTACE (10 mg orally once a day) on the combined endpoint of myocardial infarction, stroke or death from cardiovascular causes.

The HOPE study results showed that ALTACE (10 mg/day) significantly reduced the rate of myocardial infarction, stroke or death from cardiovascular causes (651/4645 vs. 826/4652, relative risk 0.78) as well as the rates of the 3 components of the combined endpoint.

[See first table above]

This effect was evident after about one year of treatment.

[See figure 1 in next column]

Ramipril was effective in different demographic subgroups, (i.e., gender, age), subgroups defined by underlying disease (e.g., cardiovascular disease, hypertension), and subgroups defined by concomitant medication. There were insufficient data to determine whether or not ramipril was equally effective in ethnic subgroups.

This study was designed with a prespecified substudy in diabetics with at least one other cardiovascular risk factor.

Outcome	ALTACE (N=4645) no. (%)	Placebo (N=4652) no. (%)	Relative Risk (95% CI) P value
Combined End-Point			
(MI, stroke, or death from CV cause)	651 (14.0%)	826 (17.8%)	0.78 (0.70-0.86), P=0.0001
Component End-Point			
Death from Cardiovascular Causes	282 (6.1%)	377 (8.1%)	0.74 (0.64-0.87), P=0.0002
Myocardial infarction	459 (9.9%)	570 (12.3%)	0.80(0.70-0.90), P=0.0003
Stroke	156 (3.4%)	226 (4.9%)	0.68 (0.56-0.84), P=0.0002
Overall Mortality			
(Death from any Cause)	482 (10.4%)	569 (12.2%)	0.84 (0.75-0.95), P=0.005

Outcome	ALTACE (N=1808) no. (%)	Placebo (N=1769) no. (%)	Relative Risk Reduction (95% CI)
Combined End-Point			
(MI, stroke, or death from CV cause)	277 (15.3%)	351 (19.8%)	0.25 (0.12-0.36), P=0.0004
Component End-Point			
Death from Cardiovascular Causes	112 (6.2%)	172 (9.7%)	0.37 (0.21-0.51), P=0.0001
Myocardial infarction	185 (10.2%)	229 (12.9%)	0.22(0.06-0.36), P=0.01
Stroke	76 (4.2%)	108 (6.1%)	0.33 (0.10-0.50), P=0.007

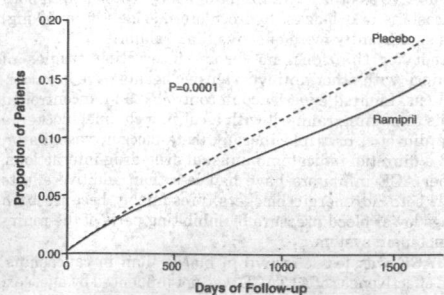

Figure 1: Kaplan-Meier Estimates of the composite outcome of MI, Stroke, or Death from CV causes in the Ramipril Group and the Placebo Group. The relative risk of the composite outcomes in the Ramipril Group as compared with the Placebo Group was 0.78% (95% confidence interval, 0.70–0.86).

Effects of ramipril on the combined endpoint and its components were similar in diabetics (n=3,577) to those in the overall study population.

[See second table above]

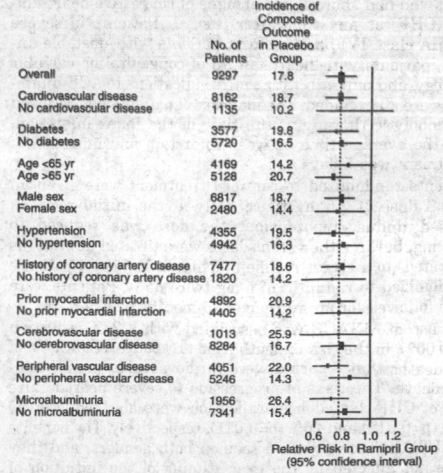

Figure 2: The Beneficial Effect of Treatment with Ramipril on the Composite Outcome of Myocardial Infarction, Stroke, or Death from Cardiovascular Causes Overall and in Various Subgroups. Cerebrovascular disease was defined as stroke or transient ischemic attacks. The size of each symbol is proportional to the number of patients in each group. The dashed line indicates overall relative risk.

The benefits of Altace were observed among patients who were taking aspirin or other anti-platelet agents, beta-blockers, and lipid-lowering agents as well as diuretics and calcium channel blockers.

Hypertension

Administration of ALTACE to patients with mild to moderate hypertension results in a reduction of both supine and standing blood pressure to about the same extent with no compensatory tachycardia. Symptomatic postural hypotension is infrequent, although it can occur in patients who are salt- and/or volume-depleted. (See **WARNINGS**.) Use of

ALTACE in combination with thiazide diuretics gives a blood pressure lowering effect greater than that seen with either agent alone.

In single-dose studies, doses of 5–20 mg of ALTACE lowered blood pressure within 1–2 hours, with peak reductions achieved 3–6 hours after dosing. The antihypertensive effect of a single dose persisted for 24 hours. In longer term (4–12 weeks) controlled studies, once-daily doses of 2.5–10 mg were similar in their effect, lowering supine or standing systolic and diastolic blood pressures 24 hours after dosing by about 6/4 mm Hg more than placebo. In comparisons of peak vs. trough effect, the trough effect represented about 50–60% of the peak response. In a titration study comparing divided (bid) vs. qd treatment, the divided regimen was superior, indicating that for some patients the antihypertensive effect with once-daily dosing is not adequately maintained. (See **DOSAGE AND ADMINISTRATION.**)

In most trials, the antihypertensive effect of ALTACE increased during the first several weeks of repeated measurements. The antihypertensive effect of ALTACE has been shown to continue during long-term therapy for at least 2 years. Abrupt withdrawal of ALTACE has not resulted in a rapid increase in blood pressure.

ALTACE has been compared with other ACE inhibitors, beta-blockers, and thiazide diuretics. It was approximately as effective as other ACE inhibitors and as atenolol. In both caucasians and blacks, hydrochlorothiazide (25 or 50 mg) was significantly more effective than ramipril.

Except for thiazides, no formal interaction studies of ramipril with other antihypertensive agents have been carried out. Limited experience in controlled and uncontrolled trials combining ramipril with a calcium channel blocker, a loop diuretic, or triple therapy (beta-blocker, vasodilator, and a diuretic) indicate no unusual drug-drug interactions. Other ACE inhibitors have had less than additive effects with beta adrenergic blockers, presumably because both drugs lower blood pressure by inhibiting parts of the renin-angiotensin system.

ALTACE was less effective in blacks than in caucasians. The effectiveness of ALTACE was not influenced by age, sex, or weight. In a baseline controlled study of 10 patients with mild essential hypertension, blood pressure reduction was accompanied by a 15% increase in renal blood flow. In healthy volunteers, glomerular filtration rate was unchanged.

Heart Failure Post Myocardial Infarction

ALTACE was studied in the Acute Infarction Ramipril Efficacy (AIRE) trial. This was a multinational (mainly European) 161-center, 2006-patient, double-blind, randomized, parallel-group study comparing ALTACE to placebo in stable patients, 2–9 days after an acute myocardial infarction (MI), who had shown clinical signs of congestive heart failure (CHF) at any time after the MI. Patients in severe (NYHA class IV) heart failure, patients with unstable angina, patients with heart failure of congenital or valvular etiology, and patients with contraindications to ACE inhibitors were all excluded. The majority of patients had received thrombolytic therapy at the time of the index infarction, and the average time between infarction and initiation of treatment was 5 days.

Patients randomized to ramipril treatment were given an initial dose of 2.5 mg twice daily. If the initial regimen caused undue hypotension, the dose was reduced to 1.25 mg, but in either event doses were titrated upward (as tolerated) to a target regimen (achieved in 77% of patients randomized to ramipril) of 5 mg twice daily. Patients were then followed for an average of 15 months (range 6–46).

The use of ALTACE was associated with a 27% reduction (p=0.002) in the risk of death from any cause; about 90% of the deaths that occurred were cardiovascular, mainly sudden death. The risks of progression to severe heart failure and of CHF-related hospitalization were also reduced, by 23% (p=0.017) and 26% (p=0.011), respectively. The benefits of ALTACE therapy were seen in both genders, and they were not affected by the exact timing of the initiation of therapy, but older patients may have had a greater benefit than those under 65. The benefits were seen in patients on, and not on, various concomitant medications; at the time of randomization these included aspirin (about 80% of patients), diuretics (about 60%), organic nitrates (about 55%), beta-blockers (about 20%), calcium channel blockers (about 15%), and digoxin (about 12%).

INDICATIONS AND USAGE

Reduction in Risk of Myocardial Infarction, Stroke, and Death from Cardiovascular Causes

Altace is indicated in patients 55 years or older at high risk of developing a major cardiovascular event because of a history of coronary artery disease, stroke, peripheral vascular disease, or diabetes that is accompanied by at least one other cardiovascular risk factor (hypertension, elevated total cholesterol levels, low HDL levels, cigarette smoking, or documented microalbuminuria), to reduce the risk of myocardial infarction, stroke, or death from cardiovascular

causes. Altace can be used in addition to other needed treatment (such as antihypertensive, antiplatelet or lipid-lowering therapy).

Hypertension

ALTACE is indicated for the treatment of hypertension. It may be used alone or in combination with thiazide diuretics. In using ALTACE, consideration should be given to the fact that another angiotensin converting enzyme inhibitor, captopril, has caused agranulocytosis, particularly in patients with renal impairment or collagen-vascular disease. Available data are insufficient to show that ALTACE does not have a similar risk. (See **WARNINGS.**)

In considering use of ALTACE, it should be noted that in controlled trials ACE inhibitors have an effect on blood pressure that is less in black patients than in non-blacks. In addition, ACE inhibitors (for which adequate data are available) cause a higher rate of angioedema in black than in non-black patients. (See **WARNINGS, Angioedema.**)

Heart Failure Post Myocardial Infarction

Ramipril is indicated in stable patients who have demonstrated clinical signs of congestive heart failure within the first few days after sustaining acute myocardial infarction. Administration of ramipril to such patients has been shown to decrease the risk of death (principally cardiovascular death) and to decrease the risks of failure-related hospitalization and progression to severe/resistant heart failure. (See **CLINICAL PHARMACOLOGY, Heart Failure Post Myocardial Infarction** for details and limitations of the survival trial.)

CONTRAINDICATIONS

ALTACE is contraindicated in patients who are hypersensitive to this product or any other angiotensin converting enzyme inhibitor (e.g., a patient who has experienced angioedema during therapy with any other ACE inhibitor).

WARNINGS

Anaphylactoid and Possibly Related Reactions

Presumably because angiotensin-converting enzyme inhibitors affect the metabolism of eicosanoids and polypeptides, including endogenous bradykinin, patients receiving ACE inhibitors (including ALTACE) may be subject to a variety of adverse reactions, some of them serious.

Head and Neck Angioedema

Patients with a history of angioedema unrelated to ACE inhibitor therapy may be at increased risk of angioedema while receiving an ACE inhibitor. (See also **CONTRAINDICATIONS.**)

Angioedema of the face, extremities, lips, tongue, glottis, and larynx has been reported in patients treated with angiotensin converting enzyme inhibitors. Angioedema associated with laryngeal edema can be fatal. If laryngeal stridor or angioedema of the face, tongue, or glottis occurs, treatment with ALTACE should be discontinued and appropriate therapy instituted immediately. **Where there is involvement of the tongue, glottis, or larynx, likely to cause airway obstruction, appropriate therapy, e.g., subcutaneous epinephrine solution 1:1,000 (0.3 ml to 0.5 ml) should be promptly administered.** (See **ADVERSE REACTIONS.**)

Intestinal Angioedema

Intestinal angioedema has been reported in patients treated with ACE inhibitors. These patients presented with abdominal pain (with or without nausea or vomiting); in some cases there was no prior history of facial angioedema and C-1 esterase levels were normal. The angioedema was diagnosed by procedures including abdominal CT scan or ultrasound, or at surgery, and symptoms resolved after stopping the ACE inhibitor. Intestinal angioedema should be included in the differential diagnosis of patients on ACE inhibitors presenting with abdominal pain.

In a large U.S. postmarketing study, angioedema (defined as reports of angio, face, larynx, tongue, or throat edema) was reported in 3/1523 (0.20%) of black patients and in 8/8680 (0.09%) of white patients. These rates were not different statistically.

Anaphylactoid reactions during desensitization: Two patients undergoing desensitizing treatment with hymenoptera venom while receiving ACE inhibitors sustained life-threatening anaphylactoid reactions. In the same patients, these reactions were avoided when ACE inhibitors were temporarily withheld, but they reappeared upon inadvertent rechallenge.

Anaphylactoid reactions during membrane exposure: Anaphylactoid reactions have been reported in patients dialyzed with high-flux membranes and treated concomitantly with an ACE inhibitor. Anaphylactoid reactions have also been reported in patients undergoing low-density lipoprotein apheresis with dextran sulfate absorption.

Hypotension

ALTACE can cause symptomatic hypotension, after either the initial dose or a later dose when the dosage has been increased. Like other ACE inhibitors, ramipril has been only rarely associated with hypotension in uncomplicated hypertensive patients. Symptomatic hypotension is most likely to occur in patients who have been volume- and/or

salt-depleted as a result of prolonged diuretic therapy, dietary salt restriction, dialysis, diarrhea, or vomiting. Volume and/or salt depletion should be corrected before initiating therapy with ALTACE.

In patients with congestive heart failure, with or without associated renal insufficiency, ACE inhibitor therapy may cause excessive hypotension, which may be associated with oliguria or azotemia and, rarely, with acute renal failure and death. In such patients, ALTACE therapy should be started under close medical supervision; they should be followed closely for the first 2 weeks of treatment and whenever the dose of ramipril or diuretic is increased.

If hypotension occurs, the patient should be placed in a supine position and, if necessary, treated with intravenous infusion of physiological saline. ALTACE treatment usually can be continued following restoration of blood pressure and volume.

Hepatic Failure

Rarely, ACE inhibitors, including Altace, have been associated with a syndrome that starts with cholestatic jaundice and progresses to fulminant hepatic necrosis and (sometimes) death. The mechanism of this syndrome is not understood. Patients receiving ACE inhibitors who develop jaundice or marked elevations of hepatic enzymes should discontinue the ACE inhibitor and receive appropriate medical follow-up.

Neutropenia/Agranulocytosis

As with other ACE inhibitors, rarely, a mild – in isolated cases severe – reduction in the red blood cell count and hemoglobin content, white blood cell or platelet count may develop. In isolated cases, agranulocytosis, pancytopenia, and bone marrow depression may occur. Hematological reactions to ACE inhibitors are more likely to occur in patients with collagen vascular disease (e.g. systemic lupus erythematosus, scleroderma) and renal impairment. Monitoring of white blood cell counts should be considered in patients with collagen-vascular disease, especially if the disease is associated with impaired renal function.

Fetal/Neonatal Morbidity and Mortality

ACE inhibitors can cause fetal and neonatal morbidity and death when administered to pregnant women. Several dozen cases have been reported in the world literature. When pregnancy is detected, ACE inhibitors should be discontinued as soon as possible. The use of ACE inhibitors during the second and third trimesters of pregnancy has been associated with fetal and neonatal injury, including hypotension, neonatal skull hypoplasia, anuria, reversible or irreversible renal failure, and death. Oligohydramnios has also been reported, presumably resulting from decreased fetal renal function; oligohydramnios in this setting has been associated with fetal limb contractures, craniofacial deformation, and hypoplastic lung development. Prematurity, intrauterine growth retardation, and patent ductus arteriosus have also been reported, although it is not clear whether these occurrences were due to the ACE inhibitor exposure.

In a published retrospective epidemiological study, infants whose mothers had taken an ACE inhibitor during their first trimester of pregnancy appeared to have an increased risk of major congenital malformations compared with infants whose mothers had not undergone first trimester exposure to ACE inhibitor drugs. The number of cases of birth defects is small and the findings of this study have not yet been confirmed.

Rarely (probably less often than once in every thousand pregnancies), no alternative to ACE inhibitors will be found. In these rare cases, the mothers should be apprised of the potential hazards to their fetuses, and serial ultrasound examinations should be performed to assess the intraamniotic environment.

If oligohydramnios is observed, ALTACE should be discontinued unless it is considered life-saving for the mother. Contraction stress testing (CST), a non-stress test (NST), or biophysical profiling (BPP) may be appropriate, depending upon the week of pregnancy. Patients and physicians should be aware, however, that oligohydramnios may not appear until after the fetus has sustained irreversible injury.

Infants with histories of *in utero* exposure to ACE inhibitors should be closely observed for hypotension, oliguria, and hyperkalemia. If oliguria occurs, attention should be directed toward support of blood pressure and renal perfusion. Exchange transfusion or dialysis may be required as means of reversing hypotension and/or substituting for disordered renal function. ALTACE which crosses the placenta can be removed from the neonatal circulation by these means, but limited experience has not shown that such removal is central to the treatment of these infants.

No teratogenic effects of ALTACE were seen in studies of pregnant rats, rabbits, and cynomolgus monkeys. On a body surface area basis, the doses used were up to approximately 400 times (in rats and monkeys) and 2 times (in rabbits) the recommended human dose.

PRECAUTIONS

Impaired Renal Function: As a consequence of inhibiting the renin-angiotensin-aldosterone system, changes in renal function may be anticipated in susceptible individuals. In patients with severe congestive heart failure whose renal function may depend on the activity of the renin-angiotensin-aldosterone system, treatment with angiotensin converting enzyme inhibitors, including ALTACE, may be associated with oliguria and/or progressive azotemia and (rarely) with acute renal failure and/or death.

In hypertensive patients with unilateral or bilateral renal artery stenosis, increases in blood urea nitrogen and serum creatinine may occur. Experience with another angiotensin converting enzyme inhibitor suggests that these increases are usually reversible upon discontinuation of ALTACE and/or diuretic therapy. In such patients renal function should be monitored during the first few weeks of therapy. Some hypertensive patients with no apparent pre-existing renal vascular disease have developed increases in blood urea nitrogen and serum creatinine, usually minor and transient, especially when ALTACE has been given concomitantly with a diuretic. This is more likely to occur in patients with pre-existing renal impairment. Dosage reduction of ALTACE and/or discontinuation of the diuretic may be required.

Evaluation of the hypertensive patient should always include assessment of renal function. (See **DOSAGE AND ADMINISTRATION.**)

Hyperkalemia: In clinical trials, hyperkalemia (serum potassium greater than 5.7 mEq/L) occurred in approximately 1% of hypertensive patients receiving ALTACE (ramipril). In most cases, these were isolated values, which resolved despite continued therapy. None of these patients was discontinued from the trials because of hyperkalemia. Risk factors for the development of hyperkalemia include renal insufficiency, diabetes mellitus, and the concomitant use of potassium-sparing diuretics, potassium supplements, and/or potassium-containing salt substitutes, which should be used cautiously, if at all, with ALTACE. (See **Drug Interactions.**)

Cough: Presumably due to the inhibition of the degradation of endogenous bradykinin, persistent nonproductive cough has been reported with all ACE inhibitors, always resolving after discontinuation of therapy. ACE inhibitor-induced cough should be considered in the differential diagnosis of cough.

Impaired Liver Function: Since ramipril is primarily metabolized by hepatic esterases to its active moiety, ramiprilat, patients with impaired liver function could develop markedly elevated plasma levels of ramipril. No formal pharmacokinetic studies have been carried out in hypertensive patients with impaired liver function. However, since the renin-angiotensin system may be activated in patients with severe liver cirrhosis and/or ascites, particular caution should be exercised in treating these patients.

Surgery/Anesthesia: In patients undergoing surgery or during anesthesia with agents that produce hypotension, ramipril may block angiotensin II formation that would otherwise occur secondary to compensatory renin release. Hypotension that occurs as a result of this mechanism can be corrected by volume expansion.

Information for Patients

Pregnancy: Female patients of childbearing age should be told about the consequences of exposure to ACE inhibitors during pregnancy. These patients should be asked to report pregnancies to their physicians as soon as possible.

Angioedema: Angioedema, including laryngeal edema, can occur with treatment with ACE inhibitors, especially following the first dose. Patients should be so advised and told to report immediately any signs or symptoms suggesting angioedema (swelling of face, eyes, lips, or tongue, or difficulty in breathing) and to take no more drug until they have consulted with the prescribing physician.

Symptomatic Hypotension: Patients should be cautioned that lightheadedness can occur, especially during the first days of therapy, and it should be reported. Patients should be told that if syncope occurs, ALTACE should be discontinued until the physician has been consulted.

All patients should be cautioned that inadequate fluid intake or excessive perspiration, diarrhea, or vomiting can lead to an excessive fall in blood pressure, with the same consequences of lightheadedness and possible syncope.

Hyperkalemia: Patients should be told not to use salt substitutes containing potassium without consulting their physician.

Neutropenia: Patients should be told to promptly report any indication of infection (e.g., sore throat, fever), which could be a sign of neutropenia.

Drug Interactions

Gold: Nitritoid reactions (symptoms include facial flushing, nausea, vomiting and hypotension) have been reported rarely in patients on therapy with injectable gold (sodium aurothiomalate) and concomitant ACE inhibitor therapy including ALTACE.

With nonsteroidal anti-inflammatory agents: Rarely, concomitant treatment with ACE inhibitors and nonsteroidal anti-inflammatory agents have been associated with worsening of renal failure and an increase in serum potassium.

With diuretics: Patients on diuretics, especially those in whom diuretic therapy was recently instituted, may occasionally experience an excessive reduction of blood pressure after initiation of therapy with ALTACE. The possibility of hypotensive effects with ALTACE can be minimized by either discontinuing the diuretic or increasing the salt intake prior to initiation of treatment with ALTACE. If this is not possible, the starting dose should be reduced. (See **DOSAGE AND ADMINISTRATION.**)

With potassium supplements and potassium-sparing diuretics: ALTACE can attenuate potassium loss caused by thiazide diuretics. Potassium-sparing diuretics (spironolactone, amiloride, triamterene, and others) or potassium supplements can increase the risk of hyperkalemia. Therefore, if concomitant use of such agents is indicated, they should be given with caution, and the patient's serum potassium should be monitored frequently.

With lithium: Increased serum lithium levels and symptoms of lithium toxicity have been reported in patients receiving ACE inhibitors during therapy with lithium. These drugs should be coadministered with caution, and frequent monitoring of serum lithium levels is recommended. If a diuretic is also used, the risk of lithium toxicity may be increased.

Other: Neither ALTACE nor its metabolites have been found to interact with food, digoxin, antacid, furosemide, cimetidine, indomethacin, and simvastatin. The combination of ALTACE and propranolol showed no adverse effects on dynamic parameters (blood pressure and heart rate). The co-administration of ALTACE and warfarin did not adversely affect the anticoagulant effects of the latter drug. Additionally, co-administration of ALTACE with phenprocoumon did not affect minimum phenprocoumon levels or interfere with the subjects' state of anti-coagulation.

Carcinogenesis, Mutagenesis, Impairment of Fertility

No evidence of a tumorigenic effect was found when ramipril was given by gavage to rats for up to 24 months at doses of up to 500 mg/kg/day or to mice for up to 18 months at doses of up to 1000 mg/kg/day. (For either species, these doses are about 200 times the maximum recommended human dose when compared on the basis of body surface area.) No mutagenic activity was detected in the Ames test in bacteria, the micronucleus test in mice, unscheduled DNA synthesis in a human cell line, or a forward gene-mutation assay in a Chinese hamster ovary cell line. Several metabolites and degradation products of ramipril were also negative in the Ames test. A study in rats with dosages as great as 500 mg/kg/day did not produce adverse effects on fertility.

Pregnancy

Pregnancy Categories C (first trimester) and D (second and third trimesters). See **WARNINGS: Fetal/Neonatal Morbidity and Mortality.**

Nursing Mothers

Ingestion of single 10 mg oral dose of ALTACE resulted in undetectable amounts of ramipril and its metabolites in breast milk. However, because multiple doses may produce low milk concentrations that are not predictable from single doses, women receiving ALTACE should not breast feed.

Geriatric Use

Of the total number of patients who received ramipril in US clinical studies of ALTACE 11.0% were 65 and over while 0.2% were 75 and over. No overall differences in effectiveness or safety were observed between these patients and younger patients, and other reported clinical experience has not identified differences in responses between the elderly and younger patients, but greater sensitivity of some older individuals cannot be ruled out.

One pharmacokinetic study conducted in hospitalized elderly patients indicated that peak ramiprilat levels and area under the plasma concentration time curve (AUC) for ramiprilat are higher in older patients.

Pediatric Use

Safety and effectiveness in pediatric patients have not been established. Irreversible kidney damage has been observed in very young rats given a single dose of ramipril.

ADVERSE REACTIONS

Hypertension

ALTACE has been evaluated for safety in over 4,000 patients with hypertension; of these, 1,230 patients were studied in US controlled trials, and 1,107 were studied in foreign controlled trials. Almost 700 of these patients were treated for at least one year. The overall incidence of reported adverse events was similar in ALTACE and placebo patients. The most frequent clinical side effects (possibly or probably related to study drug) reported by patients receiving ALTACE in US placebo-controlled trials were: headache (5.4%), "dizziness" (2.2%) and fatigue or asthenia (2.0%), but only the last was more common in ALTACE patients than in patients given placebo. Generally, the side effects were mild and transient, and there was no relation to total dosage within the range of 1.25 to 20 mg. Discontinuation of therapy because of a side effect was required in approximately 3% of US patients treated with ALTACE. The most common reasons for discontinuation were: cough (1.0%), "dizziness" (0.5%), and impotence (0.4%).

Of observed side effects considered possibly or probably related to study drug that occurred in US placebo-controlled trials in more than 1% of patients treated with ALTACE, only asthenia (fatigue) was more common on Altace than placebo (2% vs. 1%).

PATIENTS IN US PLACEBO CONTROLLED STUDIES

	ALTACE (n=651)		Placebo (n=286)	
	n	%	n	%
Asthenia (Fatigue)	13	2	2	1

In placebo-controlled trials, there was also an excess of upper respiratory infection and flu syndrome in the ramipril group, not attributed at that time to ramipril. As these studies were carried out before the relationship of cough to ACE inhibitors was recognized, some of these events may represent ramipril-induced cough. In a later 1-year study, increased cough was seen in almost 12% of ramipril patients, with about 4% of patients requiring discontinuation of treatment.

Heart Failure Post Myocardial Infarction

Adverse reactions (except laboratory abnormalities) considered possibly/probably related to study drug that occurred in more than one percent of patients and more frequently on ramipril are shown below. The incidences represent the experiences from the AIRE study. The follow-up time was between 6 and 46 months for this study.

Percentage of Patients with Adverse Events Possibly/Probably Related to Study Drug
Placebo-Controlled (AIRE) Mortality Study

Adverse Event	Ramipril (n=1004)	Placebo (n=982)
Hypotension	11	5
Cough Increased	8	4
Dizziness	4	3
Angina Pectoris	3	2
Nausea	2	1
Postural Hypotension	2	1
Syncope	2	1
Vomiting	2	0.5
Vertigo	2	0.7
Abnormal Kidney Function	1	0.5
Diarrhea	1	0.4

HOPE Study:
Safety data in the HOPE trial were collected as reasons for discontinuation or temporary interruption of treatment. The incidence of cough was similar to that seen in the AIRE trial. The rate of angioedema was the same as in previous clinical trials (see WARNINGS).

	RAMIPRIL (N=4645) %	PLACEBO (N=4652) %
Discontinuation at any time	34	32
Permanent discontinuation	29	28
Reasons for stopping Cough	7	2
Hypotension or Dizziness	1.9	1.5
Angioedema	0.3	0.1

Other adverse experiences reported in controlled clinical trials (in less than 1% of ramipril patients), or rarer events seen in postmarketing experience, include the following (in some, a causal relationship to drug use is uncertain):

Body As a Whole: Anaphylactoid reactions. (See **WARNINGS.**)

Cardiovascular: Symptomatic hypotension (reported in 0.5% of patients in US trials) (See **WARNINGS** and **PRECAUTIONS**), syncope and palpitations.

Hematologic: Pancytopenia, hemolytic anemia and thrombocytopenia.

Renal: Some hypertensive patients with no apparent pre-existing renal disease have developed minor, usually transient, increases in blood urea nitrogen and serum creatinine when taking ALTACE, particularly when ALTACE was given concomitantly with a diuretic. (See **WARNINGS.**) Acute renal failure.

Angioneurotic Edema: Angioneurotic edema has been reported in 0.3% of patients in US clinical trials. (See **WARNINGS.**)

Gastrointestinal: Hepatic failure, hepatitis, jaundice, pancreatitis, abdominal pain (sometimes with enzyme changes suggesting pancreatitis), anorexia, constipation, diarrhea, dry mouth, dyspepsia, dysphagia, gastroenteritis, increased salivation and taste disturbance.

Dermatologic: Apparent hypersensitivity reactions (manifested by urticaria, pruritus, or rash, with or without fever), photosensitivity, purpura, onycholysis, pemphigus, pemphigoid, erythema multiforme, toxic epidermal necrolysis, and Stevens-Johnson syndrome.

Neurologic and Psychiatric: Anxiety, amnesia, convulsions, depression, hearing loss, insomnia, nervousness, neuralgia, neuropathy, paresthesia, somnolence, tinnitus, tremor, vertigo, and vision disturbances.

Miscellaneous: As with other ACE inhibitors, a symptom complex has been reported which may include a positive ANA, an elevated erythrocyte sedimentation rate, arthralgia/arthritis, myalgia, fever, vasculitis, eosinophilia, photosensitivity, rash and other dermatologic manifestations. Additionally, as with other ACE inhibitors, eosinophilic pneumonitis has been reported.

Fetal/Neonatal Morbidity and Mortality. See **WARNINGS: Fetal/Neonatal Morbidity and Mortality.**

Other: arthralgia, arthritis, dyspnea, edema, epistaxis, impotence, increased sweating, malaise, myalgia, and weight gain.

Post-Marketing Experience: In addition to adverse events reported from clinical trials, there have been rare reports of hypoglycemia reported during ALTACE therapy when given to patients concomitantly taking oral hypoglycemic agents or insulin. The causal relationship is unknown.

Clinical Laboratory Test Findings:

Creatinine and Blood Urea Nitrogen: Increases in creatinine levels occurred in 1.2% of patients receiving ALTACE alone, and in 1.5% of patients receiving ALTACE and a diuretic. Increases in blood urea nitrogen levels occurred in 0.5% of patients receiving ALTACE alone and in 3% of patients receiving ALTACE with a diuretic. None of these increases required discontinuation of treatment. Increases in these laboratory values are more likely to occur in patients with renal insufficiency or those pretreated with a diuretic and, based on experience with other ACE inhibitors, would be expected to be especially likely in patients with renal artery stenosis. (See **WARNINGS** and **PRECAUTIONS**.)

Since ramipril decreases aldosterone secretion, elevation of serum potassium can occur. Potassium supplements and potassium-sparing diuretics should be given with caution, and the patient's serum potassium should be monitored frequently. (See **WARNINGS** and **PRECAUTIONS**.)

Hemoglobin and Hematocrit: Decreases in hemoglobin or hematocrit (a low value and a decrease of 5 g/dl or 5% respectively) were rare, occurring in 0.4% of patients receiving ALTACE alone and in 1.5% of patients receiving ALTACE plus a diuretic. No US patients discontinued treatment because of decreases in hemoglobin or hematocrit.

Other (causal relationships unknown): Clinically important changes in standard laboratory tests were rarely associated with ALTACE administration. Elevations of liver enzymes, serum bilirubin, uric acid, and blood glucose have been reported, as have cases of hyponatremia and scattered incidents of leukopenia, eosinophilia, and proteinuria. In US trials, less than 0.2% of patients discontinued treatment for laboratory abnormalities; all of these were cases of proteinuria or abnormal liver-function tests.

OVERDOSAGE

Single oral doses in rats and mice of 10–11 g/kg resulted in significant lethality. In dogs, oral doses as high as 1 g/kg induced only mild gastrointestinal distress. Limited data on human overdosage are available. The most likely clinical manifestations would be symptoms attributable to hypotension.

Laboratory determinations of serum levels of ramipril and its metabolites are not widely available, and such determinations have, in any event, no established role in the management of ramipril overdose.

No data are available to suggest physiological maneuvers (e.g., maneuvers to change the pH of the urine) that might accelerate elimination of ramipril and its metabolites. Similarly, it is not known which, if any, of these substances can be usefully removed from the body by hemodialysis.

Angiotensin II could presumably serve as a specific antagonist-antidote in the setting of ramipril overdose, but angiotensin II is essentially unavailable outside of scattered research facilities. Because the hypotensive effect of ramipril is achieved through vasodilation and effective hypovolemia, it is reasonable to treat ramipril overdose by infusion of normal saline solution.

DOSAGE AND ADMINISTRATION

Blood pressure decreases associated with any dose of ALTACE depend, in part, on the presence or absence of volume depletion (e.g., past and current diuretic use) or the presence or absence of renal artery stenosis. If such circumstances are suspected to be present, the initial starting dose should be 1.25 mg once daily.

Reduction in Risk of Myocardial Infarction, Stroke, and Death from Cardiovascular Causes

ALTACE should be given at an initial dose of 2.5 mg, once a day for 1 week, 5 mg, once a day for the next 3 weeks, and then increased as tolerated, to a maintenance dose of 10 mg, once a day. If the patient is hypertensive or recently post myocardial infarction, it can also be given as a divided dose.

Hypertension

The recommended initial dose for patients not receiving a diuretic is 2.5 mg once a day. Dosage should be adjusted according to the blood pressure response. The usual maintenance dosage range is 2.5 to 20 mg per day administered as a single dose or in two equally divided doses. In some patients treated once daily, the antihypertensive effect may diminish toward the end of the dosing interval. In such patients, an increase in dosage or twice daily administration should be considered. If blood pressure is not controlled with ALTACE alone, a diuretic can be added.

Heart Failure Post Myocardial Infarction

For the treatment of post-infarction patients who have shown signs of congestive failure, the recommended starting dose of ALTACE is 2.5 mg twice daily (5 mg per day). A patient who becomes hypotensive at this dose may be switched to 1.25 mg twice daily, and after one week at the starting dose, patients should then be titrated (if tolerated) toward a target dose of 5 mg twice daily, with dosage increases being about 3 weeks apart.

After the initial dose of ALTACE, the patient should be observed under medical supervision for at least two hours and until blood pressure has stabilized for at least an additional hour. (See **WARNINGS** and **PRECAUTIONS, Drug Interactions.**) If possible, the dose of any concomitant diuretic should be reduced which may diminish the likelihood of hypotension. The appearance of hypotension after the initial dose of ALTACE does not preclude subsequent careful dose titration with the drug, following effective management of the hypotension.

The ALTACE Capsule is usually swallowed whole. The ALTACE Capsule can also be opened and the contents sprinkled on a small amount (about 4 oz.) of apple sauce or mixed in 4 oz. (120 ml) of water or apple juice. To be sure that ramipril is not lost when such a mixture is used, the mixture should be consumed in its entirety. The described mixtures can be pre-prepared and stored for up to 24 hours at room temperature or up to 48 hours under refrigeration.

Concomitant administration of ALTACE with potassium supplements, potassium salt substitutes, or potassium-sparing diuretics can lead to increases of serum potassium. (See **PRECAUTIONS**.)

In patients who are currently being treated with a diuretic, symptomatic hypotension occasionally can occur following the initial dose of ALTACE. To reduce the likelihood of hypotension, the diuretic should, if possible, be discontinued two to three days prior to beginning therapy with ALTACE. (See WARNINGS.) Then, if blood pressure is not controlled with ALTACE alone, diuretic therapy should be resumed.

If the diuretic cannot be discontinued, an initial dose of 1.25 mg ALTACE should be used to avoid excess hypotension.

Dosage Adjustment in Renal Impairment

In patients with creatinine clearance <40 ml/min/1.73m^2 (serum creatinine approximately >2.5 mg/dl) doses only 25% of those normally used should be expected to induce full therapeutic levels of ramiprilat. (See **CLINICAL PHARMACOLOGY**.)

Hypertension: For patients with hypertension and renal impairment, the recommended initial dose is 1.25 mg ALTACE once daily. Dosage may be titrated upward until blood pressure is controlled or to a maximum total daily dose of 5 mg.

Heart Failure Post Myocardial Infarction: For patients with heart failure and renal impairment, the recommended initial dose is 1.25 mg ALTACE once daily. The dose may be increased to 1.25 mg b.i.d. and up to a maximum dose of 2.5 mg b.i.d. depending upon clinical response and tolerability.

HOW SUPPLIED

ALTACE is available in potencies of 1.25 mg, 2.5 mg, 5 mg, and 10 mg in hard gelatin capsules.

ALTACE 1.25 mg capsules are supplied as yellow, hard gelatin capsules in bottles of 100 (NDC 61570-110-01).

ALTACE 2.5 mg capsules are supplied as orange, hard gelatin capsules in bottles of 100 (NDC 61570-111-01).

ALTACE 5 mg capsules are supplied as red, hard gelatin capsules in bottles of 100 (NDC 61570-112-01).

ALTACE 10 mg capsules are supplied as Process Blue, hard gelatin capsules in bottles of 100 (NDC 61570-120-01).

Dispense in well-closed container with safety closure.

Store at controlled room temperature (59° to 86°F).

Rx only.

Distributed by: Monarch Pharmaceuticals, Inc., Bristol, TN 37620

(A wholly owned subsidiary of King Pharmaceuticals, Inc.)

Manufactured by: King Pharmaceuticals, Inc., Bristol, TN 37620

Prescribing Information as of July 2010.

AVINZA® Ⓒ℞

[*ă-vĭn-ză*]

(morphine sulfate extended-release capsules)

30 mg, 45 mg, 60 mg, 75 mg, 90 mg, 120 mg

℞ Only

> **WARNING:**
> **AVINZA capsules are a modified-release formulation of morphine sulfate indicated for once daily administration for the relief of moderate to severe pain requiring continuous, around-the-clock opioid therapy for an extended period of time. AVINZA CAPSULES ARE TO BE SWALLOWED WHOLE OR THE CONTENTS OF THE CAPSULES SPRINKLED ON APPLESAUCE. THE CAPSULE BEADS ARE NOT TO BE CHEWED, CRUSHED, OR DISSOLVED DUE TO THE RISK OF RAPID RELEASE AND ABSORPTION OF A POTENTIALLY FATAL DOSE OF MORPHINE. PATIENTS MUST NOT CONSUME ALCOHOLIC BEVERAGES WHILE ON AVINZA THERAPY. ADDITIONALLY, PATIENTS MUST NOT USE PRESCRIPTION OR NON-PRESCRIPTION MEDICATIONS CONTAINING ALCOHOL WHILE ON AVINZA THERAPY. CONSUMPTION OF ALCOHOL WHILE TAKING AVINZA MAY RESULT IN THE RAPID RELEASE AND ABSORPTION OF A POTENTIALLY FATAL DOSE OF MORPHINE.**

DESCRIPTION

AVINZA (morphine sulfate extended-release capsules) 30, 45, 60, 75, 90, and 120 mg contain both immediate release and extended release beads of morphine sulfate for once daily oral administration.

Chemically, morphine sulfate is 7,8-didehydro-4,5 alpha-epoxy-17-methylmorphinan-3,6 alpha-diol sulfate (2:1) (salt) pentahydrate with a molecular weight of 758. Morphine sulfate occurs as white, feathery, silky crystals; cubical masses of crystal; or white crystalline powder. It is soluble in water and slightly soluble in alcohol, but is practically insoluble in chloroform or ether. The octanol:water partition coefficient of morphine is 1.42 at physiologic pH and the pK$_a$ is 7.9 for the tertiary nitrogen (the majority is ionized at pH 7.4).

Each AVINZA Capsule contains either 30, 45, 60, 75, 90, or 120 mg of morphine sulfate, USP and the following inactive ingredients: ammoniomethacrylate copolymers, NF, fumaric acid, NF, povidone, USP, sodium lauryl sulfate, NF, sugar starch spheres, NF, and talc, USP. The capsule shell contains black ink, gelatin, titanium dioxide, D&C yellow No. 10 (30 mg), FD&C blue No. 2 (45 mg), FD&C green No. 3 (60 mg), FDA iron oxide and FDA yellow iron oxide (75 mg), FD&C red No. 40 (90 mg), FD&C red No. 3 (120 mg), and FD&C blue No. 1 (120 mg).

Structure:

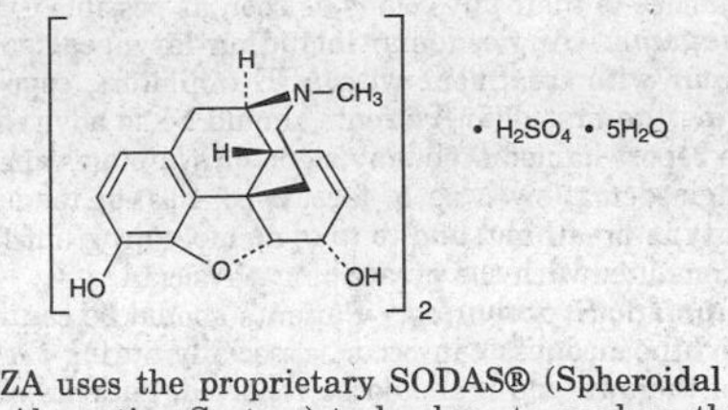

AVINZA uses the proprietary SODAS® (Spheroidal Oral Drug Absorption System) technology to produce the extended release component of AVINZA, which combined with an immediate release component achieves the desired release profile characteristics of AVINZA capsules. Within the gastrointestinal tract, due to the permeability of the ammoniomethacrylate copolymers of the beads, fluid enters the beads and solubilizes the drug. This is mediated by fumaric acid, which acts as an osmotic agent and a local pH modifier. The resultant solution then diffuses out in a predetermined manner which prolongs the *in vivo* dissolution and absorption phases. (see **Pharmacokinetics**)

CLINICAL PHARMACOLOGY

Morphine, a pure opioid agonist, is relatively selective for the mu receptor, although it can interact with other opioid receptors at higher doses. In addition to analgesia, the widely diverse effects of morphine include drowsiness, changes in mood, respiratory depression, decreased gastrointestinal motility, nausea, vomiting, and alterations of the endocrine and autonomic nervous system.

Effects on the Central Nervous System (CNS): The principal therapeutic action of morphine is analgesia. Other therapeutic effects of morphine include anxiolysis, euphoria and feelings of relaxation. Although the precise mechanism of the analgesic action is unknown, specific CNS opiate receptors and endogenous compounds with morphine-like activity have been identified throughout the brain and spinal cord and are likely to play a role in the expression and perception of analgesic effects. In common with other opioids, morphine causes respiratory depression, in part by a direct effect on the brainstem respiratory centers. Morphine and related opioids depress the cough reflex by direct effect on the cough center in the medulla. Antitussive effects may occur with doses lower than those usually required for analgesia. Morphine causes miosis, even in total darkness. Pinpoint pupils are a sign of opioid overdose; however, when asphyxia is present during opioid overdose, marked mydriasis occurs.

Effects on the Gastrointestinal Tract and on Other Smooth Muscle: Gastric, biliary and pancreatic secretions are decreased by morphine. Morphine causes a reduction in motility and is associated with an increase in tone in the antrum of the stomach and duodenum. Digestion of food in the small intestine is delayed and propulsive contractions are decreased. Propulsive peristaltic waves in the colon are decreased, while tone is increased to the point of spasm. The end result may be constipation. Morphine can cause a marked increase in biliary tract pressure as a result of spasm of the sphincter of Oddi. Morphine may also cause spasm of the sphincter of the urinary bladder.

Effects on the Cardiovascular System: In therapeutic doses, morphine does not usually exert major effects on the cardiovascular system. Morphine produces peripheral vasodilation which may result in orthostatic hypotension and fainting. Release of histamine can occur, which may play a role in opioid-induced hypotension. Manifestations of histamine release and/or peripheral vasodilation may include pruritus, flushing, red eyes and sweating.

Pharmacodynamics

Morphine concentrations are not predictive of analgesic response, especially in patients previously treated with opioids. The minimum effective concentration varies widely and is influenced by a variety of factors, including the extent of previous opioid use, age, and general medical condition. Effective doses in tolerant patients may be significantly higher than in opioid-naïve patients.

In all patients, the dose of morphine should be titrated on the basis of clinical evaluation of the patient and to achieve a balance between therapeutic and adverse effects.

Pharmacokinetics

AVINZA consists of two components, an immediate release component that rapidly achieves plateau morphine plasma concentrations and an extended release component that maintains plasma concentrations throughout the 24-hour dosing interval. The amount of morphine absorbed from AVINZA following oral administration is similar to that absorbed from other oral morphine formulations.

The oral bioavailability of morphine is less than 40% and shows large inter-individual variability due to extensive pre-systemic metabolism.

Absorption

Following single-dose oral administration of a 60 mg dose of AVINZA under fasting conditions, morphine concentrations of approximately 3 to 6 ng/ml were achieved within 30 minutes after dosing and maintained for the 24-hour dosing interval. The pharmacokinetics of AVINZA were shown to be dose-proportional over a single oral dose range of 30 to 120 mg in healthy volunteers and a multiple oral dose range of at least 30 to 180 mg in patients with chronic moderate to severe pain.

Food Effects: When a 60 mg dose of AVINZA was administered immediately following a high fat meal, peak morphine concentrations and AUC values were similar to those observed when the dose of AVINZA was administered in a fasting state, although achievement of initial concentrations was delayed by approximately 1 hour under fed conditions. Therefore, AVINZA can be administered without regard to food. When the contents of AVINZA were administered by sprinkling on applesauce, the rate and extent of morphine absorption were found to be bioequivalent to the same dose when administered as an intact capsule.

Steady State: When dosed once-daily, AVINZA steady-state pharmacokinetics are characterized by a plateau-like plasma concentration profile. Steady-state plasma concentrations of morphine are achieved 2 to 3 days after initiation of once-daily administration of AVINZA.

AVINZA 60 mg Capsules (once-daily) and 10 mg morphine oral solution (6 times daily) were equally bioavailable.

[See Graph 1 at top of next column]

A once-daily dose of AVINZA provided similar C_{max}, C_{min}, and AUC values and peak-trough fluctuations (% FL, C_{max}-C_{min}/C_{av}) compared to 6-times daily administration of the same total daily dose of morphine oral solution (Table 1).

Graph 1
Mean Steady-State Plasma Morphine Concentrations Following Once-Daily Administration of AVINZA Capsules or 6-Times Daily Administration of Morphine Solution

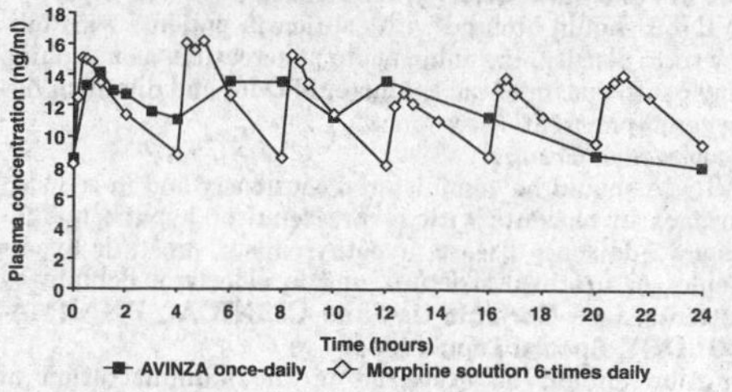

Table 1 Pharmacokinetic Data Mean ± SD

Parameter	AVINZA Capsules Once-Daily	Morphine Oral Solution 6-Times Daily
AUC (ng/ml.h)	273.25 ± 81.24	279.11 ± 63.00
C_{max} (ng/ml)	18.65 ± 7.13	19.96 ± 4.82
C_{min} (ng/ml)	6.98 ± 2.44	6.61 ± 2.15
% FL	106.38 ± 78.14	116.22 ± 26.67

Distribution

Once absorbed, morphine is distributed to skeletal muscle, kidneys, liver, intestinal tract, lungs, spleen and brain. Although the primary site of action is the CNS, only small quantities cross the blood-brain barrier. Morphine also crosses the placental membranes and has been found in breast milk. The volume of distribution of morphine is approximately 1 to 6 L/kg, and morphine is 20 to 35% reversibly bound to plasma proteins.

Metabolism

The major pathway of morphine detoxification is conjugation, either with D-glucuronic acid to produce glucuronides or with sulfuric acid to produce morphine-3-etheral sulfate. While a small fraction (less than 5%) of morphine is demethylated, virtually all morphine is converted by hepatic metabolism to the 3- and 6-glucuronide metabolites (M3G and M6G; about 50% and 15%, respectively). M6G has been shown to have analgesic activity but crosses the blood-brain barrier poorly, while M3G has no significant analgesic activity.

Excretion

Most of a dose of morphine is excreted in urine as M3G and M6G, with elimination of morphine occurring primarily as renal excretion of M3G. Approximately 10% of the dose is excreted unchanged in urine. A small amount of the glucuronide conjugates are excreted in bile, with minor enterohepatic recycling. Seven to 10% of administered morphine is excreted in the feces.

The mean adult plasma clearance is approximately 20 to 30 ml/min/kg. The effective terminal half-life of morphine after IV administration is reported to be approximately 2 hours. In some studies involving longer periods of plasma sampling, a longer terminal half-life of morphine of about 15 hours was reported.

In Vitro AVINZA-Alcohol Interaction

In vitro studies performed by the FDA demonstrated that when AVINZA 30 mg was mixed with 900 mL of buffer solutions containing ethanol (20% and 40%), the dose of morphine that was released was alcohol concentration-dependent, leading to a more rapid release of morphine. While the relevance of *in vitro* lab tests regarding AVINZA to the clinical setting remains to be determined, this acceleration of release may correlate with *in vivo* rapid release of the total morphine dose, which could result in the absorption of a potentially fatal dose of morphine.

Special Populations

Geriatric: Elderly patients (aged 65 years or older) may have increased sensitivity to morphine. AVINZA pharmacokinetics have not been studied specifically in elderly patients.

Nursing Mothers: Low levels of morphine sulfate have been detected in maternal milk. The milk:plasma morphine AUC ratio is about 2.5:1. The amount of morphine delivered to the infant depends on the plasma concentration of the mother, the amount of milk ingested by the infant, and the extent of first-pass metabolism.

Pediatric: The pharmacokinetics of AVINZA have not been studied in pediatric patients below the age of 18. The range of dose strengths available may not be appropriate for treatment of very young pediatric patients. Sprinkling on applesauce is NOT a suitable alternative for these patients.

Gender: A gender analysis of pharmacokinetic data from healthy subjects taking AVINZA indicated that morphine concentrations were similar in males and females.

Race: There may be some pharmacokinetic differences associated with race. In one published study, Chinese subjects given intravenous morphine had a higher clearance when compared to Caucasian subjects (1852 +/- 116 ml/min compared to 1495 +/- 80 ml/min).

Hepatic Failure: Morphine pharmacokinetics have been reported to be significantly altered in patients with cirrhosis. Clearance was found to decrease with a corresponding increase in half-life. The M3G and M6G to morphine plasma AUC ratios also decreased in these subjects, indicating diminished metabolic activity.

Renal Insufficiency: Morphine pharmacokinetics are altered in patients with renal failure. Clearance is decreased and the metabolites, M3G and M6G, may accumulate to much higher plasma levels in patients with renal failure as compared to patients with normal renal function.

Drug-Drug Interactions: Known drug-drug interactions involving morphine are pharmacodynamic, not pharmacokinetic. (see **PRECAUTIONS, Drug Interactions**)

Clinical Studies

AVINZA was studied in over 140 healthy volunteers and 560 patients with chronic, moderate to severe pain who participated in 6 pharmacokinetic studies, 4 clinical studies and 3 studies which provided both pharmacokinetic and clinical data. The patient population included those who were either receiving chronic opioid therapy or had a prior sub-optimal response to acetaminophen and/or NSAID therapy, as well as patients who previously received intermittent opioid analgesic therapy. In the controlled clinical studies, patients were followed from 7 days to up to 4 weeks, and in the open label studies, patients were followed for up to 6 to 12 months.

AVINZA was studied in a double-blind, placebo-controlled, fixed-dose, parallel group trial in 295 patients with moderate to severe pain due to osteoarthritis. These patients had either a prior sub-optimal response to acetaminophen, NSAID therapy, or previously received intermittent opioid analgesic therapy. Thirty-milligrams AVINZA capsules administered once-daily, either in the morning or the evening, were more effective than placebo in reducing pain.

Table 2 Change from Baseline in WOMAC OA Index Pain VAS Subscale Score

Overall	Placebo	AVINZA QAM	AVINZA QPM
LS Mean	-36.23	-75.26*	-75.39*
Std. Error	11.482	11.305	11.747

*P<0.05; REPEATED MEASURES ANALYSIS

This study was not designed to assess the effects of AVINZA on the course of the osteoarthritis.

INDICATIONS AND USAGE

AVINZA capsules are a modified-release formulation of morphine sulfate intended for once daily administration indicated for the relief of moderate to severe pain requiring continuous, around-the-clock opioid therapy for an extended period of time.

AVINZA is **NOT** intended for use as a prn analgesic.

The safety and efficacy of using AVINZA in the postoperative setting has not been evaluated. AVINZA is not indicated for postoperative use. If the patient has been receiving the drug prior to surgery, resumption of the pre-surgical dose may be appropriate once the patient is able to take the drug by mouth. Physicians should individualize treatment, moving from parenteral to oral analgesics as appropriate. (see American Pain Society guidelines)

CONTRAINDICATIONS

AVINZA is contraindicated in patients with known hypersensitivity to morphine, morphine salts, or any components of the product. AVINZA, like all opioids, is contraindicated in patients with respiratory depression in the absence of resuscitative equipment and in patients with acute or severe bronchial asthma.

AVINZA, like all opioids, is contraindicated in any patient who has or is suspected of having paralytic ileus.

WARNINGS

AVINZA must be swallowed whole (not chewed, crushed, or dissolved) or AVINZA may be opened and the entire bead contents sprinkled on a small amount of applesauce immediately prior to ingestion. **THE CAPSULES MUST NOT BE CHEWED, CRUSHED, OR DISSOLVED DUE TO THE RISK OF RAPID RELEASE AND ABSORPTION OF A POTENTIALLY FATAL DOSE OF MORPHINE.** (see **BOX WARNING, CLINICAL PHARMACOLOGY**)

Patients must not consume alcoholic beverages while on AVINZA therapy. Additionally, patients must not use prescription or non-prescription medications containing alcohol while on AVINZA therapy. Consumption of alcohol while taking AVINZA may result in the rapid release and absorption of a potentially fatal dose of morphine.

THE DAILY DOSE OF AVINZA MUST BE LIMITED TO A MAXIMUM OF 1600 MG/DAY. AVINZA DOSES OF OVER

1600 MG/DAY CONTAIN A QUANTITY OF FUMARIC ACID THAT HAS NOT BEEN DEMONSTRATED TO BE SAFE, AND WHICH MAY RESULT IN SERIOUS RENAL TOXICITY.

Misuse, Abuse and Diversion of Opioids

Morphine is an opioid agonist and a Schedule II controlled substance. Such drugs are sought by drug abusers and people with addiction disorders. Diversion of Schedule II products is an act subject to criminal penalty.

Morphine can be abused in a manner similar to other opioid agonists, legal or illicit. This should be considered when prescribing or dispensing AVINZA in situations where the physician or pharmacist is concerned about an increased risk of misuse, abuse, or diversion.

Abuse of AVINZA by crushing, chewing, snorting, or injecting the dissolved product will result in the immediate release of the entire daily dose of the opioid and pose a significant risk to the abuser that could result in overdose and death. Intravenous abuse of a water extract of AVINZA may lead to serious pulmonary complications due to the extraction of talc along with morphine sulfate. (see DRUG ABUSE AND ADDICTION)

Concerns about abuse, addiction, and diversion should not prevent the proper management of pain. Healthcare professionals should contact their State Professional Licensing Board, or State Controlled Substances Authority for information on how to prevent and detect abuse or diversion of this product.

Interactions with Alcohol and Drugs of Abuse

Morphine may be expected to have additive effects when used in conjunction with alcohol, other opioids, or illicit drugs that cause central nervous system depression. *In vitro* studies performed by the FDA demonstrated that when AVINZA 30 mg was mixed with 900 mL of buffer solutions containing ethanol (20% and 40%), the dose of morphine that was released was alcohol concentration-dependent, leading to a more rapid release of morphine. While the relevance of *in vitro* lab tests regarding AVINZA to the clinical setting remains to be determined, this acceleration of release may correlate with *in vivo* rapid release of the total morphine dose, which could result in the absorption of a potentially fatal dose of morphine.

Impaired Respiration

Respiratory depression is the chief hazard of all morphine preparations. Respiratory depression occurs more frequently in elderly or debilitated patients and in those suffering from conditions accompanied by hypoxia, hypercapnia, or upper airway obstruction, in whom even moderate therapeutic doses may significantly decrease pulmonary ventilation.

Morphine should be used with extreme caution in patients with chronic obstructive pulmonary disease or cor pulmonale and in patients having a substantially decreased respiratory reserve (e.g., severe kyphoscoliosis), hypoxia, hypercapnia, or pre-existing respiratory depression. In such patients, even usual therapeutic doses of morphine may increase airway resistance and decrease respiratory drive to the point of apnea.

Head Injury and Increased Intracranial Pressure

The respiratory depressant effects of morphine with carbon dioxide retention and secondary elevation of cerebrospinal fluid pressure may be markedly exaggerated in the presence of head injury, other intracranial lesions, or a pre-existing increase in intracranial pressure. Morphine produces effects which may obscure neurologic signs of further increases in intracranial pressure in patients with head injuries. Morphine should only be administered under such circumstances when considered essential and then with extreme care.

Hypotensive Effect

AVINZA, like all morphine products, may cause severe hypotension in an individual whose ability to maintain blood pressure has already been compromised by a depleted blood volume or concurrent administration of drugs such as phenothiazines or general anesthetics. (see also PRECAUTIONS, Drug Interactions) AVINZA may produce orthostatic hypotension and syncope in ambulatory patients.

AVINZA is an opioid analgesic which should be administered with caution to patients in circulatory shock, as vasodilation produced by the drug may further reduce cardiac output and blood pressure.

Gastrointestinal Obstruction

AVINZA should not be administered to patients with gastrointestinal obstruction, especially paralytic ileus because AVINZA, like all morphine preparations, diminishes propulsive peristaltic waves in the gastrointestinal tract and may prolong the obstruction.

PRECAUTIONS

General

AVINZA is intended for use in patients requiring continuous around-the-clock treatment with an opioid analgesic. It is not appropriate as a prn treatment for pain. As with any opioid, it is critical to adjust the dose of AVINZA for each individual patient, taking into account the patient's prior experience with analgesics. (see DOSAGE AND ADMINISTRATION)

Use in Pancreatic/Biliary Tract Disease

AVINZA should be used with caution in patients with biliary tract disease, including acute pancreatitis, as morphine may cause spasm of the sphincter of Oddi and diminish biliary and pancreatic secretions.

Special Risk Groups

AVINZA should be administered cautiously and in reduced dosages in patients with severe renal or hepatic insufficiency, Addison's disease, hypothyroidism, prostatic hypertrophy, or urethral stricture, and in elderly or debilitated patients. (see Geriatric Use and CLINICAL PHARMACOLOGY, Special Populations)

Caution should be exercised in the administration of morphine to patients with CNS depression, toxic psychosis, acute alcoholism and delirium tremens, and seizure disorders.

Driving and Operating Machinery

Patients should be cautioned that AVINZA could impair the mental and/or physical abilities needed to perform potentially hazardous activities such as driving a car or operating machinery.

Patients should also be cautioned about the potential combined effects of AVINZA with other CNS depressants, including other opioids, phenothiazines, sedative/hypnotics and alcohol. (see PRECAUTIONS, Drug Interactions)

Tolerance and Physical Dependence

Tolerance is the need for increasing doses of opioids to maintain a defined effect such as analgesia (in the absence of disease progression or other external factors). Physical dependence is manifested by withdrawal symptoms after abrupt discontinuation of a drug or upon administration of an antagonist. Physical dependence and tolerance are not unusual during chronic opioid therapy.

The opioid abstinence or withdrawal syndrome is characterized by some or all of the following: restlessness, lacrimation, rhinorrhea, yawning, perspiration, chills, myalgia, and mydriasis. Other symptoms also may develop, including irritability, anxiety, backache, joint pain, weakness, abdominal cramps, insomnia, nausea, anorexia, vomiting, diarrhea, or increased blood pressure, respiratory rate, or heart rate.

In general, opioids should not be abruptly discontinued. (see DOSAGE AND ADMINISTRATION, Cessation of Therapy)

Information for Patients

Patients receiving AVINZA (morphine sulfate extended-release capsules) should be given the following instructions by the physician:

1. Patients should be advised that AVINZA capsules contain morphine and should be taken once daily.
2. AVINZA must be swallowed whole (not chewed, crushed, or dissolved) or AVINZA may be opened and the entire bead contents sprinkled on a small amount of applesauce immediately prior to ingestion. **The beads must NOT be chewed, crushed, or dissolved due to the risk of exposure to a potentially toxic dose of morphine.**
3. **Patients should be informed that they must not consume alcoholic beverages while on AVINZA therapy. Additionally, patients should be informed that they must not use prescription or non-prescription medication containing alcohol while on AVINZA therapy. Consumption of alcohol while taking AVINZA may result in the rapid release and absorption of a potentially fatal dose of morphine.**
4. The dose of AVINZA should not be adjusted without consulting with a physician or other healthcare professional.
5. Patients should be advised that AVINZA may impair mental and/or physical ability required for the performance of potentially hazardous tasks (e.g., driving, operating machinery). Patients started on AVINZA or patients whose dose has been adjusted should refrain from any potentially dangerous activity until it is established that they are not adversely affected.
6. Patients should be advised that AVINZA should not be combined with alcohol or other CNS depressants (e.g., sleep medications, tranquilizers). A physician should be consulted if other medications are currently being used or are added in the future.
7. Women of childbearing potential who become or are planning to become pregnant should consult a physician prior to initiating or continuing therapy with AVINZA.
8. If patients have been receiving treatment with AVINZA for more than a few weeks and cessation of therapy is indicated, they should be counseled on the importance of safely tapering the dose and that abruptly discontinuing the medication could precipitate withdrawal symptoms. The physician should provide a dose schedule to accomplish a gradual discontinuation of the medication.
9. Patients should be advised that AVINZA is a potential drug of abuse. They should protect it from theft. It should never be given to anyone other than the individual for whom it was prescribed.
10. Patients should be instructed to keep AVINZA in a secure place out of the reach of children. When AVINZA is no longer needed, the unused capsules should be destroyed by flushing down the toilet.

As with other opioids, patients taking AVINZA should be advised of the potential for severe constipation; appropriate laxatives, and/or stool softeners as well as other appropriate treatments should be initiated from the onset of opioid therapy.

Drug Interactions

CNS Depressants: The concurrent use of other central nervous system (CNS) depressants including sedatives, hypnotics, general anesthetics, antiemetics, phenothiazines, or other tranquilizers or alcohol increases the risk of respiratory depression, hypotension, profound sedation, or coma. Use with caution and in reduced dosages in patients taking these agents.

Muscle Relaxants: Morphine may enhance the neuromuscular blocking action of skeletal muscle relaxants and produce an increased degree of respiratory depression.

Mixed Agonist/Antagonist Opioid Analgesics: Mixed agonist/antagonist analgesics (i.e., pentazocine, nalbuphine and butorphanol) should NOT be administered to patients who have received or are receiving a course of therapy with a pure opioid agonist analgesic. In these patients, mixed agonist/antagonist analgesics may reduce the analgesic effect and/or may precipitate withdrawal symptoms.

Monoamine Oxidase Inhibitors (MAOIs): MAOIs markedly potentiate the action of morphine. AVINZA should not be used in patients taking MAOIs or within 14 days of stopping such treatment.

Cimetidine: Concomitant administration of morphine and cimetidine has been reported to precipitate apnea, confusion and muscle twitching in an isolated report. Patients should be monitored for increased respiratory and CNS depression when receiving cimetidine concomitantly with AVINZA.

Food: AVINZA can be administered without regard to food. (see CLINICAL PHARMACOLOGY, Food Effects).

Carcinogenicity/Mutagenicity/Impairment of Fertility

Studies in animals to evaluate the carcinogenic potential of morphine sulfate have not been conducted. No formal studies to assess the mutagenic potential of morphine have been conducted. In the published literature, the results of *in vitro* studies showed that morphine is non-mutagenic in the *Drosophila melanogaster* lethal mutation assay and produced no evidence of chromosomal aberrations when incubated with murine splenocytes. Contrary to these results, morphine was found to increase DNA fragmentation when incubated *in vitro* with a human lymphoma cell line. *In vivo*, morphine has been reported to produce an increase in the frequency of micronuclei in bone marrow cells and immature red blood cells in the mouse micronucleus test and to induce chromosomal aberrations in murine lymphocytes and spermatids. Some of the *in vivo* clastogenic effects reported with morphine in mice may be directly related to increases in glucocorticoid levels produced by morphine in this species.

Pregnancy

Teratogenic Effects (Pregnancy Category C)

No formal studies to assess the teratogenic effects of morphine in animals have been performed. Several literature reports indicate that morphine administered subcutaneously during the early gestational period in mice and hamsters produced neurological, soft tissue and skeletal abnormalities. With one exception, the effects that have been reported were following doses that were maternally toxic and the abnormalities noted were characteristic of those observed when maternal toxicity is present. In one study, following subcutaneous infusion of doses greater than or equal to 0.15 mg/kg to mice, exencephaly, hydronephrosis, intestinal hemorrhage, split supraoccipital, malformed sternebrae, and malformed xiphoid were noted in the absence of maternal toxicity. In the hamster, morphine sulfate given subcutaneously on gestation day 8 produced exencephaly and cranioschisis. Morphine was not a significant teratogen in the rat at exposure levels significantly beyond that normally encountered in clinical practice. In one study however, decreased litter size and viability were observed in the offspring of male rats administered morphine at doses approximately 3-fold the maximum recommended human daily dose (MRHDD) for 10 days prior to mating. In two studies performed in the rabbit, no evidence of teratogenicity was reported at subcutaneous doses up to 100 mg/kg.

In humans, the frequency of congenital anomalies has been reported to be no greater than expected among the children of 70 women who were treated with morphine during the first four months of pregnancy or in 448 women treated with this drug anytime during pregnancy. Furthermore, no malformations were observed in the infant of a woman who attempted suicide by taking an overdose of morphine and other medication during the first trimester of pregnancy.

Nonteratogenic Effects

Published literature has reported that exposure to morphine during pregnancy is associated with reduction in growth and a host of behavioral abnormalities in the off-spring of animals. Morphine treatment during gestational periods of organogenesis in rats, hamsters, guinea pigs and rabbits resulted in the following treatment-related embryo-toxicity and neonatal toxicity in one or more studies: decreased litter size, embryo-fetal viability, fetal and neonatal body weights, absolute brain and cerebellar weights, lengths or widths at birth and during the neonatal period, delayed motor and sexual maturation, and increased neonatal mortality, cyanosis and hypothermia. Decreased fertility in female offspring, and decreased plasma and testicular levels of luteinizing hormone and testosterone, decreased testes weights, seminiferous tubule shrinkage, germinal cell aplasia, and decreased spermatogenesis in male offspring were also observed. Behavioral abnormalities resulting from chronic morphine exposure of fetal animals included altered reflex and motor skill development, mild withdrawal, and altered responsiveness to morphine persisting into adulthood.

Controlled studies of chronic *in utero* morphine exposure in pregnant women have not been conducted. Infants born to mothers who have taken opioids chronically may exhibit withdrawal symptoms, reversible reduction in brain volume, small size, decreased ventilatory response to CO_2 and increased risk of sudden infant death syndrome. Morphine sulfate should be used by a pregnant woman only if the need for opioid analgesia clearly outweighs the potential risks to the fetus.

Labor and Delivery

Opioids cross the placenta and may produce respiratory depression and psycho-physiologic effects in neonates. AVINZA is not recommended for use in women during and immediately prior to labor, when use of shorter acting analgesics or other analgesic techniques are more appropriate. Occasionally, opioid analgesics may prolong labor through actions which temporarily reduce the strength, duration and frequency of uterine contractions. However this effect is not consistent and may be offset by an increased rate of cervical dilatation, which tends to shorten labor. Neonates whose mothers received opioid analgesics during labor should be observed closely for signs of respiratory depression. A specific opioid antagonist, such as naloxone or nalmefene, should be available for reversal of opioid-induced respiratory depression in the neonate.

Neonatal Withdrawal Syndrome

Chronic maternal use of opioids during pregnancy may cause newborns to suffer from neonatal withdrawal syndrome (NWS) following birth. Manifestations of this syndrome include irritability, hyperactivity, abnormal sleep pattern, high-pitched cry, tremor, vomiting, diarrhea, weight loss, and failure to gain weight. The time and amount of the mother's last dose, and the rate of elimination of the drug from the newborn may affect the onset, duration, and severity of the disorder. When severe symptoms occur, pharmacologic intervention may be required.

Nursing Mothers

Low levels of morphine sulfate have been detected in human milk. Breast-feeding infants might experience withdrawal symptoms upon cessation of AVINZA administration to the mother. Because of the potential for nursing infants to experience adverse reactions, a decision should be made whether to discontinue nursing or discontinue AVINZA, taking into account the benefit of the drug to the mother.

Pediatric Use

Safety and effectiveness of AVINZA in pediatric patients below the age of 18 have not been established. The range of dose strengths available may not be appropriate for treatment of very young pediatric patients. Sprinkling on applesauce is NOT a suitable alternative for these patients.

Geriatric Use

Of the total number of subjects in clinical studies of AVINZA, there were 168 patients age 65 and over, including 64 patients over the age of 74, 100 of whom were treated with AVINZA. Subgroup analyses comparing efficacy were not possible given the small number of subjects in each treatment group. No overall differences in safety were observed between these subjects and younger subjects. In general, caution should be exercised in the selection of the starting dose of AVINZA for an elderly patient, usually starting at the low end of the dosing range. As with all opioids, the starting dose should be reduced in debilitated and non-tolerant patients. (see **CLINICAL PHARMACOLOGY, Special Populations, Geriatric**, and **PRECAUTIONS, Special Risk Groups**)

ADVERSE REACTIONS

In controlled and open label clinical studies, 560 patients with chronic malignant or non-malignant pain were treated with AVINZA. The most common serious adverse events reported with administration of AVINZA were vomiting, nausea, death, dehydration, dyspnea, and sepsis. (Deaths

occurred in patients treated for pain due to underlying malignancy.) Serious adverse events caused by morphine include respiratory depression, apnea, and to a lesser degree, circulatory depression, respiratory arrest, shock and cardiac arrest.

Adverse Events

The common adverse events seen on initiation of therapy with morphine are dose-dependent and are typical opioid-related side effects. The most frequent of these include constipation, nausea and somnolence. The frequency of these events depends upon several factors including the clinical setting, the patient's level of opioid tolerance, and host factors specific to the individual. These events should be anticipated and managed as part of opioid analgesia therapy. The most common adverse events (seen in greater than 10%) reported by patients treated with AVINZA during the clinical trials at least once during therapy were constipation, nausea, somnolence, vomiting, and headache. Adverse events occurring in 5-10% of study patients were peripheral edema, diarrhea, abdominal pain, infection, urinary tract infection, accidental injury, flu syndrome, back pain, rash, sweating, fever, insomnia, depression, paresthesia, anorexia, dry mouth, asthenia and dyspnea. Other less common side effects expected from opioid analgesics, including morphine, or seen in fewer than 5% of patients taking AVINZA in the clinical trials were:

Body as a Whole: malaise, withdrawal syndrome.
Cardiovascular System: bradycardia, hypertension, hypotension, palpitations, syncope, tachycardia.
Digestive System: biliary pain, dyspepsia, dysphagia, gastroenteritis, abnormal liver function tests, rectal disorder, thirst.
Hemic and Lymphatic System: anemia, thrombocytopenia.
Metabolic and Nutritional Disorders: edema, weight loss.
Musculoskeletal: skeletal muscle rigidity.
Nervous System: abnormal dreams, abnormal gait, agitation, amnesia, anxiety, ataxia, confusion, convulsions, coma, delirium, euphoria, hallucinations, lethargy, nervousness, abnormal thinking, tremor, vasodilation, vertigo.
Respiratory System: hiccup, hypoventilation, voice alteration.
Skin and Appendages: dry skin, urticaria.
Special Senses: amblyopia, eye pain, taste perversion.
Urogenital System: abnormal ejaculation, dysuria, impotence, decreased libido, oliguria, urinary retention.

DRUG ABUSE AND ADDICTION

AVINZA is a mu-agonist opioid and is a Schedule II controlled substance. Morphine, like other opioids used in analgesia, can be abused and is subject to criminal diversion.

Drug addiction is characterized by compulsive use, use for non-medical purposes, and continued use despite harm or risk of harm. Drug addiction is a treatable disease, utilizing a multi-disciplinary approach, but relapse is common. "Drug-seeking" behavior is very common in addicts and drug abusers. Drug-seeking tactics include emergency calls or visits near the end of office hours, refusal to undergo appropriate examination, testing or referral, repeated "loss" of prescriptions, tampering with prescriptions and reluctance to provide prior medical records or contact information for other treating physician(s). "Doctor shopping" to obtain additional prescriptions is common among drug abusers and people suffering from untreated addiction.

Abuse and addiction are separate and distinct from physical dependence and tolerance. Physicians should be aware that addiction may not be accompanied by concurrent tolerance and symptoms of physical dependence. The converse is also true. In addition, abuse of opioids can occur in the absence of true addiction and is characterized by misuse for non-medical purposes, often in combination with other psychoactive substances. Careful record-keeping of prescribing information, including quantity, frequency, and renewal requests is strongly advised.

Proper assessment of the patient, proper prescribing practices, periodic re-evaluation of therapy, and proper dispensing and storage are appropriate measures that help to limit abuse of opioid drugs.

AVINZA is intended for oral use only. Abuse of the crushed capsule poses a hazard of overdose and death. This risk is increased with concurrent abuse of alcohol and other substances. With parenteral abuse, the capsule excipients, especially talc, can be expected to result in local tissue necrosis, infection, pulmonary granulomas, and increased risk of endocarditis and valvular heart injury. Parenteral drug abuse is commonly associated with transmission of infectious diseases such as hepatitis and HIV.

AVINZA OVERDOSAGE

Symptoms

Acute overdosage with morphine is manifested by respiratory depression, somnolence progressing to stupor or coma, skeletal muscle flaccidity, cold and clammy skin, constricted pupils, and, in some cases, pulmonary edema, bradycardia, hypotension, and death.

Treatment

Primary attention should be given to re-establishment of a patent airway and institution of assisted or controlled ventilation when overdose of an extended-release formulation such as AVINZA has been ingested. Elimination or evacuation of gastric contents may be necessary in order to eliminate unabsorbed drug. Before attempting treatment by gastric emptying or activated charcoal, care should be taken to secure the airway. Pure opioid antagonists, naloxone or nalmefene, are specific antidotes to respiratory depression resulting from opioid overdose. Since the duration of reversal is expected to be less than the duration of action of AVINZA, the patient must be carefully monitored until spontaneous respiration is reliably re-established. AVINZA, as with other controlled delivery preparations in overdose situations, may continue to release morphine for 36 to 48 hours or longer following ingestion, and management of an overdose should be monitored accordingly. If the response to opioid antagonists is suboptimal or only brief in nature, additional antagonist should be administered as directed by the manufacturer of the product.

Opioid antagonists should not be administered in the absence of clinically significant respiratory or circulatory depression secondary to morphine overdose. Such agents should be administered cautiously to persons who are known, or suspected to be physically dependent on AVINZA. In such cases, an abrupt or complete reversal of opioid effects may precipitate an acute abstinence syndrome.

Opioid-Tolerant Individuals: In an individual physically dependent on opioids, administration of the usual dose of the antagonist will precipitate an acute withdrawal syndrome. The severity of the withdrawal symptoms experienced will depend on the degree of physical dependence and the dose of the antagonist administered. Use of an opioid antagonist should be reserved for cases where such treatment is clearly needed. If it is necessary to treat serious respiratory depression in the physically dependent patient, administration of the antagonist should be initiated with care and titrated with smaller than usual doses.

Supportive measures (including oxygen, vasopressors) should be employed in the management of circulatory shock and pulmonary edema as indicated. Cardiac arrest or arrhythmias may require cardiac massage or defibrillation.

DOSAGE AND ADMINISTRATION

AVINZA MUST BE SWALLOWED WHOLE (NOT CHEWED, CRUSHED, OR DISSOLVED) OR AVINZA MAY BE OPENED AND THE ENTIRE BEAD CONTENTS SPRINKLED ON A SMALL AMOUNT OF APPLESAUCE IMMEDIATELY PRIOR TO INGESTION. THE BEADS MUST NOT BE CHEWED, CRUSHED, OR DISSOLVED DUE TO RISK OF ACUTE OVERDOSE. INGESTING CHEWED OR CRUSHED AVINZA BEADS WILL LEAD TO THE RAPID RELEASE AND ABSORPTION OF A POTENTIALLY TOXIC DOSE OF MORPHINE.

Patients must not consume alcoholic beverages while on AVINZA therapy. Additionally, patients must not use prescription or non-prescription medicine containing alcohol while on AVINZA therapy. Consumption of alcohol while taking AVINZA may result in the rapid release and absorption of a potentially fatal dose of morphine.

The daily dose of AVINZA must be limited to a maximum of 1600 mg/day. AVINZA doses of over 1600 mg/day contain a quantity of fumaric acid that has not been demonstrated to be safe, and which may result in serious renal toxicity. (see **WARNINGS**)

The 45, 60, 75, 90, and 120 mg capsules are for use only in opioid-tolerant patients.

All doses are intended to be administered once daily. As with any opioid drug product, it is necessary to adjust the dosing regimen for each patient individually, taking into account the patient's prior analgesic treatment experience. In the selection of the initial dose of AVINZA, attention should be given to the following:

1. the total daily dose, potency and specific characteristics of the opioid the patient has been taking previously;
2. the reliability of the relative potency estimate used to calculate the equivalent morphine dose needed;
3. the patient's degree of opioid tolerance;
4. the general condition and medical status of the patient;
5. concurrent medications;
6. the type and severity of the patient's pain.

The following dosing recommendations, therefore, can only be considered suggested approaches to what is actually a series of clinical decisions over time in the management of the pain of each individual patient.

Conversion from Other Oral Morphine Formulations to AVINZA

Patients receiving other oral morphine formulations may be converted to AVINZA by administering the patient's total daily oral morphine dose as AVINZA once-daily. AVINZA should not be given more frequently than every 24 hours. As with conversion from any oral morphine formulation to another, supplemental pain medication may be required until the response to the patient's daily AVINZA dosage has stabilized (up to 4 days).

Conversion from Parenteral Morphine or Other Non-Morphine Opioids (Parenteral or Oral) to AVINZA

There is inter-patient variability in the potency of opioid drugs and opioid formulations. Therefore, a conservative approach is advised when determining the total daily dose of AVINZA. It is better to underestimate a patient's 24-hour oral morphine dose and make available rescue medication than to overestimate the 24-hour oral morphine dose and manage an adverse experience or overdose. The following general points should be considered regarding opioid conversions.

Parenteral to oral morphine ratio: Anywhere from 3 to 6 mg of oral morphine may be required to provide pain relief equivalent to 1 mg of parenteral morphine. Based on this rationale, a reasonable starting dose of AVINZA would be approximately three times the previous daily parenteral morphine requirement.

Other parenteral or oral non-morphine opioids to oral morphine sulfate: Physicians and other healthcare professionals are advised to refer to published relative potency information, keeping in mind that conversion ratios are only approximate. In general, it is safest to administer half of the estimated daily morphine requirement as the initial AVINZA dose once per day and then manage insufficient pain relief by supplementation with immediate-release morphine or other short-acting analgesics. (see **Individualization of Dosage**)

Individualization of Dosage

Physicians should individualize treatment using a progressive plan of pain management such as outlined by the World Health Organization, the American Pain Society and the Federation of State Medical Boards Model Guidelines. Healthcare professionals should follow appropriate pain management principles of careful assessment and ongoing monitoring. AVINZA (morphine sulfate) is on the third step of the WHO three step analgesic ladder and is of most benefit when a constant level of opioid analgesia is used as a platform from which break-through pain is managed. Once acceptable pain relief is no longer achieved from combinations of non-opioid medications (NSAIDs and acetaminophen) and intermittent usage of moderate or strong opioids, conversion to a 24-hour oral morphine equivalent is warranted.

The dose may be titrated as frequently as every other day to control analgesia. In the event that break-through pain occurs, AVINZA may be supplemented with a small dose (5-15% of the total daily dose of morphine) of a short-acting analgesic.

When AVINZA is chosen as the initial opioid for patients who do not have a proven tolerance to opioids, patients should be treated initially at a dose of 30 mg once-daily (at 24-hour intervals). For opioid-naïve patients, the dose should be increased conservatively. For such patients, it is recommended that the dose of AVINZA be adjusted in increments not greater than 30 mg every 4 days. Some degree of tolerance may occur, requiring dosage adjustment until the achievement of a balance between analgesia and opioid side effects. When necessary, the total dose of AVINZA should be increased until pain relief is reached or clinically significant opioid-related adverse reactions occur.

Alternative Methods of Administration

AVINZA beads sprinkled over applesauce were found to be bioequivalent to AVINZA capsules swallowed whole under fasting conditions in a study of healthy volunteers. Absorption of the beads sprinkled on other foods has not been tested. This method of administration may be beneficial for patients who have difficulty swallowing whole capsules or tablets.

1. Sprinkle the entire contents of the capsule(s) onto a small amount of applesauce. The applesauce should be at room temperature or cooler. Use immediately. (see also **CLINICAL PHARMACOLOGY, Food Effects**)
2. Swallow mixture without chewing or crushing beads.
3. Rinse mouth and swallow to ensure all beads have been ingested.
4. Patients should consume the entire portion and should not divide applesauce into separate doses.

Conversion from AVINZA to Other Pain Control Therapies

It is important to remember that the persistence of AVINZA-derived plasma morphine concentrations may be in excess of 36 hours when making a conversion to other pain control therapies.

Conversion from AVINZA to Other Controlled-Release Oral Morphine Formulations

For a given dose, the same total amount of morphine is available from AVINZA as from oral morphine solution or controlled-release morphine tablets. The extended duration of release of morphine from AVINZA results in reduced maximum and increased minimum plasma morphine concentrations than with shorter acting morphine products. Conversion from AVINZA to the same total daily dose of another controlled-release morphine formulation could lead to either excessive sedation at peak serum levels or inadequate analgesia at trough serum levels. Dosage adjustment with close observation is recommended.

Conversion from AVINZA to Parenteral Opioids

When converting from AVINZA to parenteral opioids, it is best to calculate an equivalent parenteral dose and then initiate treatment at half of this calculated value. As an example, an estimated total 24-hour parenteral morphine requirement of a patient receiving AVINZA is one-third of the dose of AVINZA. This is because the oral bioavailability of morphine is one-third that of parenteral morphine. This estimated dose should then be divided in half, and this last calculated dose is the total daily dose. This value should be further divided by six if the desire is to dose with parenteral morphine every four hours.

Consider a patient taking 360 mg of AVINZA daily. First, divide by 3, to account for differences in bioavailability between oral and parenteral morphine. This new figure, 120 mg, is the estimated total 24-hour requirement of parenteral morphine. Dividing by 2, the result gives the total daily dose of 60 mg. If it is decided to administer the drug at four-hour intervals, then administer 10 mg (60 divided by 6) every four hours.

Although this approach may require a dosage increase in the first 24 hours for many patients, this method is recommended, as it is less likely to result in overdose. Overdose is more likely to occur when administering an equivalent dose of parenteral morphine without titration. Provision for break-through pain should be made.

Cessation of Therapy

When the patient no longer requires therapy with AVINZA capsules, doses should be tapered gradually to prevent signs and symptoms of withdrawal in the physically dependent patient.

SAFETY AND HANDLING

AVINZA consists of hard gelatin capsules containing polymer-coated morphine sulfate beads that pose no known risk of handling to healthcare workers. All opioids are liable to diversion and misuse both by the general public and healthcare workers and should be handled accordingly.

HOW SUPPLIED

30 mg Capsule: size 3 capsule, yellow cap imprinted ***AVINZA*** and white, opaque body imprinted 30 mg and 505. NDC 60793-605-01: Bottles of 100 capsules.

45 mg Capsule: size 3 capsule, light blue cap imprinted ***AVINZA*** and white, opaque body imprinted 45 mg and 509. NDC 60793-603-01: Bottles of 100 capsules.

60 mg Capsule: size 3 capsule, bluish-green cap imprinted ***AVINZA*** and white, opaque body imprinted 60 mg and 506. NDC 60793-606-01: Bottles of 100 capsules.

75 mg Capsule: size 1 capsule, orange cap imprinted ***AVINZA*** and white, opaque body imprinted 75 mg and 510. NDC 60793-604-01: Bottles of 100 capsules.

90 mg Capsule: size 1 capsule, red cap imprinted ***AVINZA*** and white, opaque body imprinted 90 mg and 507. NDC 60793-607-01: Bottles of 100 capsules.

120 mg Capsule: size 1 capsule, blue-violet cap imprinted ***AVINZA*** and white, opaque body imprinted 120 mg and 508. NDC 60793-608-01: Bottles of 100 capsules.

Store at 25°C (77°F); excursions permitted to 15-30°C (59-86°F). [see USP Controlled Room Temperature]

Protect from light and moisture.

Dispense in a tight, light-resistant container as defined in USP.

CAUTION: DEA Order Form Required.

℞ Only.

Prescribing Information as of April 2008.

Manufactured for:
King Pharmaceuticals, Inc.
Bristol, TN 37620

AVINZA® Information Service: 1-800-776-3637

Utilizing technology developed by:
Elan Pharma International, Ltd.,
Monksland, Athlone
Co Westmeath, Ireland

AVINZA® is a registered trademark of King Pharmaceuticals Research and Development, Inc.

SODAS® is a registered trademark of Elan Pharma International, Ltd.,

U.S. Patent No.: 6,066,339

Revised: 05/2010 King Pharmaceuticals, Inc.

Shown in Product Identification Guide, page 310

BICILLIN® L-A ℞

[bī-sil 'in]

(penicillin G benzathine injectable suspension)
Disposable Syringe

for deep **IM** injection only

WARNING: NOT FOR INTRAVENOUS USE. DO NOT INJECT INTRAVENOUSLY OR ADMIX WITH OTHER INTRAVENOUS SOLUTIONS. THERE HAVE BEEN REPORTS OF INADVERTENT INTRAVENOUS ADMINISTRATION OF PENICILLIN G BENZATHINE WHICH HAS BEEN ASSOCIATED WITH CARDIORESPIRATORY ARREST AND DEATH. Prior to administration of this drug, carefully read the WARNINGS, ADVERSE REACTIONS, and DOSAGE AND ADMINISTRATION sections of the labeling.

To reduce the development of drug-resistant bacteria and maintain the effectiveness of Bicillin L-A and other antibacterial drugs, Bicillin L-A should be used only to treat or prevent infections that are proven or strongly suspected to be caused by bacteria.

DESCRIPTION

Bicillin L-A (penicillin G benzathine injectable suspension) is available for deep intramuscular injection. Penicillin G benzathine is prepared by the reaction of dibenzylethylene diamine with two molecules of penicillin G. It is chemically designated as (2*S*, 5*R*, 6*R*)-3,3-Dimethyl-7-oxo-6-(2-phenylacetamido)-4-thia-1-azabicyclo[3.2.0]heptane-2-carboxylic acid compound with *N,N'*-dibenzylethylenediamine (2:1), tetrahydrate. It occurs as a white, crystalline powder and is very slightly soluble in water and sparingly soluble in alcohol. Its chemical structure is as follows:

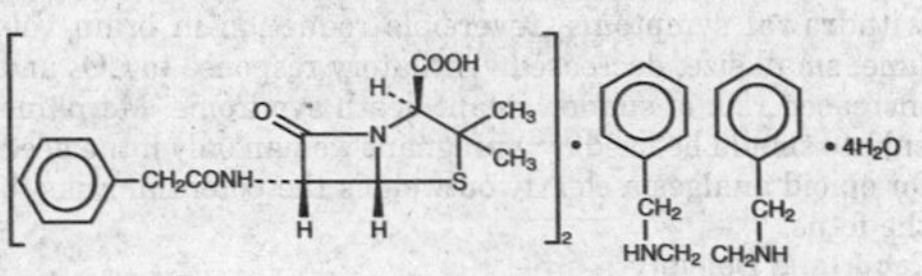

Bicillin L-A contains penicillin G benzathine in aqueous suspension with sodium citrate buffer and, as w/v, approximately 0.5% lecithin, 0.6% carboxymethylcellulose, 0.6% povidone, 0.1% methylparaben, and 0.01% propylparaben.

Bicillin L-A suspension in the disposable-syringe formulation is viscous and opaque. It is available in a 1 mL, 2 mL, and 4 mL sizes containing the equivalent of 600,000, 1,200,000 and 2,400,000 units respectively of penicillin G as the benzathine salt. Read **CONTRAINDICATIONS, WARNINGS, PRECAUTIONS,** and **DOSAGE AND ADMINISTRATION** sections prior to use.

CLINICAL PHARMACOLOGY

General

Penicillin G benzathine has an extremely low solubility and, thus, the drug is slowly released from intramuscular injection sites. The drug is hydrolyzed to penicillin G. This combination of hydrolysis and slow absorption results in blood serum levels much lower but much more prolonged than other parenteral penicillins.

Intramuscular administration of 300,000 units of penicillin G benzathine in adults results in blood levels of 0.03 to 0.05 units per mL, which are maintained for 4 to 5 days. Similar blood levels may persist for 10 days following administration of 600,000 units and for 14 days following administration of 1,200,000 units. Blood concentrations of 0.003 units per mL may still be detectable 4 weeks following administration of 1,200,000 units.

Approximately 60% of penicillin G is bound to serum protein. The drug is distributed throughout the body tissues in widely varying amounts. Highest levels are found in the kidneys with lesser amounts in the liver, skin, and intestines. Penicillin G penetrates into all other tissues and the spinal fluid to a lesser degree. With normal kidney function, the drug is excreted rapidly by tubular excretion. In neonates and young infants and in individuals with impaired kidney function, excretion is considerably delayed.

Microbiology

Penicillin G exerts a bactericidal action against penicillin-susceptible microorganisms during the stage of active multiplication. It acts through the inhibition of biosynthesis of cell-wall mucopeptide. It is not active against the penicillinase-producing bacteria, which include many strains of staphylococci.

The following *in vitro* data are available, but their clinical significance is unknown. Penicillin G exerts high in vitro activity against staphylococci (except penicillinase-producing strains), streptococci (Groups A, C, G, H, L, and M), and pneumococci. Other organisms susceptible to penicillin G are *Neisseria gonorrhoeae, Corynebacterium diphtheriae, Bacillus anthracis,* Clostridia species, *Actinomyces bovis, Streptobacillus moniliformis, Listeria monocytogenes,* and Leptospira species. *Treponema pallidum* is extremely susceptible to the bactericidal action of penicillin G.

Susceptibility Test: If the Kirby-Bauer method of disc susceptibility is used, a 20-unit penicillin disc should give a zone greater than 28 mm when tested against a penicillin-susceptible bacterial strain.

INDICATIONS AND USAGE

To reduce the development of drug-resistant bacteria and maintain the effectiveness of Bicillin L-A and other antibacterial drugs, Bicillin L-A should be used only to treat or prevent infections that are proven or strongly suspected to be caused by bacteria. When culture and susceptibility information are available, they should be considered in selecting or modifying antibacterial therapy. In the absence of such data, local epidemiology and susceptibility patterns may contribute to the empiric selection of therapy.

Intramuscular penicillin G benzathine is indicated in the treatment of infections due to penicillin-G-sensitive microorganisms that are susceptible to the low and very prolonged serum levels common to this particular dosage form. Therapy should be guided by bacteriological studies (including sensitivity tests) and by clinical response.

The following infections will usually respond to adequate dosage of intramuscular penicillin G benzathine:

Mild-to-moderate infections of the upper-respiratory tract due to susceptible streptococci.

Venereal infections—Syphilis, yaws, bejel, and pinta.

Medical Conditions in which Penicillin G Benzathine Therapy is Indicated as Prophylaxis:

Rheumatic fever and/or chorea—Prophylaxis with penicillin G benzathine has proven effective in preventing recurrence of these conditions. It has also been used as follow-up prophylactic therapy for rheumatic heart disease and acute glomerulonephritis.

CONTRAINDICATIONS

A history of a previous hypersensitivity reaction to any of the penicillins is a contraindication.

WARNINGS

> **WARNING: NOT FOR INTRAVENOUS USE. DO NOT INJECT INTRAVENOUSLY OR ADMIX WITH OTHER INTRAVENOUS SOLUTIONS. THERE HAVE BEEN REPORTS OF INADVERTENT INTRAVENOUS ADMINISTRATION OF PENICILLIN G BENZATHINE WHICH HAS BEEN ASSOCIATED WITH CARDIORESPIRATORY ARREST AND DEATH. Prior to administration of this drug, carefully read the WARNINGS, ADVERSE REACTIONS, and DOSAGE AND ADMINISTRATION sections of the labeling.**

Penicillin G benzathine should only be prescribed for the indications listed in this insert.

Anaphylaxis

SERIOUS AND OCCASIONALLY FATAL HYPERSENSITIVITY (ANAPHYLACTIC) REACTIONS HAVE BEEN REPORTED IN PATIENTS ON PENICILLIN THERAPY. THESE REACTIONS ARE MORE LIKELY TO OCCUR IN INDIVIDUALS WITH A HISTORY OF PENICILLIN HYPERSENSITIVITY AND/OR A HISTORY OF SENSITIVITY TO MULTIPLE ALLERGENS. THERE HAVE BEEN REPORTS OF INDIVIDUALS WITH A HISTORY OF PENICILLIN HYPERSENSITIVITY WHO HAVE EXPERIENCED SEVERE REACTIONS WHEN TREATED WITH CEPHALOSPORINS. BEFORE INITIATING THERAPY WITH BICILLIN L-A, CAREFUL INQUIRY SHOULD BE MADE CONCERNING PREVIOUS HYPERSENSITIVITY REACTIONS TO PENICILLINS, CEPHALOSPORINS, OR OTHER ALLERGENS. IF AN ALLERGIC REACTION OCCURS, BICILLIN L-A SHOULD BE DISCONTINUED AND APPROPRIATE THERAPY INSTITUTED. SERIOUS ANAPHYLACTIC REACTIONS REQUIRE IMMEDIATE EMERGENCY TREATMENT WITH EPINEPHRINE. OXYGEN, INTRAVENOUS STEROIDS AND AIRWAY MANAGEMENT, INCLUDING INTUBATION, SHOULD ALSO BE ADMINISTERED AS INDICATED.

Clostridium difficile associated diarrhea (CDAD) has been reported with use of nearly all antibacterial agents, including Bicillin L-A, and may range in severity from mild diarrhea to fatal colitis. Treatment with antibacterial agents alters the normal flora of the colon leading to overgrowth of *C. difficile.*

C. difficile produces toxins A and B which contribute to the development of CDAD. Hypertoxin producing strains of *C. difficile* cause increased morbidity and mortality, as these infections can be refractory to antimicrobial therapy and may require colectomy. CDAD must be considered in all patients who present with diarrhea following antibacterial use. Careful medical history is necessary since CDAD has been reported to occur over two months after the administration of antibacterial agents.

If CDAD is suspected or confirmed, ongoing antibiotic use not directed against *C. difficile* may need to be discontinued. Appropriate fluid and electrolyte management, protein supplementation, antibiotic treatment of *C. difficile*, and surgical evaluation should be instituted as clinically indicated.

Method of Administration

Do not inject into or near an artery or nerve.

Injection into or near a nerve may result in permanent neurological damage.

Inadvertent intravascular administration, including inadvertent direct intra-arterial injection or injection immediately adjacent to arteries, of Bicillin L-A and other penicillin preparations has resulted in severe neurovascular damage, including transverse myelitis with permanent paralysis, gangrene requiring amputation of digits and more proximal portions of extremities, and necrosis and sloughing at and surrounding the injection site. Such severe effects have been reported following injections into the buttock, thigh, and deltoid areas. Other serious complications of suspected intravascular administration which have been reported include immediate pallor, mottling, or cyanosis of the extremity both distal and proximal to the injection site, followed by bleb formation; severe edema requiring anterior and/or posterior compartment fasciotomy in the lower extremity. The above-described severe effects and complications have most often occurred in infants and small children. Prompt consultation with an appropriate specialist is indicated if any evidence of compromise of the blood supply occurs at, proximal to, or distal to the site of injection.[1-9] (See **PRECAUTIONS**, and **DOSAGE AND ADMINISTRATION** sections.)

Do not inject intravenously or admix with other intravenous solutions. There have been reports of inadvertent intravenous administration of penicillin G benzathine which has been associated with cardiorespiratory arrest and death. (See **DOSAGE AND ADMINISTRATION** section.) Quadriceps femoris fibrosis and atrophy have been reported following repeated intramuscular injections of penicillin preparations into the anterolateral thigh.

PRECAUTIONS

General

Prescribing Bicillin L-A in the absence of a proven or strongly suspected bacterial infection or a prophylactic indication is unlikely to provide benefit to the patient and increases the risk of a development of drug-resistant bacteria. Penicillin should be used with caution in individuals with histories of significant allergies and/or asthma.

Care should be taken to avoid intravenous or intra-arterial administration, or injection into or near major peripheral nerves or blood vessels, since such injection may produce neurovascular damage. (See **WARNINGS**, and **DOSAGE AND ADMINISTRATION** sections.)

Prolonged use of antibiotics may promote the overgrowth of nonsusceptible organisms, including fungi. Should superinfection occur, appropriate measures should be taken.

Information for Patients

Diarrhea is a common problem caused by antibiotics which usually ends when the antibiotic is discontinued. Sometimes after starting treatment with antibiotics, patients can develop watery and bloody stools (with or without stomach cramps and fever) even as late as two or more months after having taken the last dose of the antibiotic. If this occurs, patients should contact their physician as soon as possible. Patients should be counseled that antibacterial drugs including Bicillin L-A should only be used to treat bacterial infections. They do not treat viral infections (e.g., the common cold). When Bicillin L-A is prescribed to treat a bacterial infection, patients should be told that although it is common to feel better early in the course of therapy, the medication should be taken exactly as directed. Skipping doses or not completing the full course of therapy may (1) decrease the effectiveness of the immediate treatment and (2) increase the likelihood that bacteria will develop resistance and will not be treatable by Bicillin L-A or other antibacterial drugs in the future.

Laboratory Tests

In streptococcal infections, therapy must be sufficient to eliminate the organism; otherwise, the sequelae of streptococcal disease may occur. Cultures should be taken following completion of treatment to determine whether streptococci have been eradicated.

Drug Interactions

Tetracycline, a bacteriostatic antibiotic, may antagonize the bactericidal effect of penicillin, and concurrent use of these drugs should be avoided.

Concurrent administration of penicillin and probenecid increases and prolongs serum penicillin levels by decreasing the apparent volume of distribution and slowing the rate of excretion by competitively inhibiting renal tubular secretion of penicillin.

Pregnancy Category B

Reproduction studies performed in the mouse, rat, and rabbit have revealed no evidence of impaired fertility or harm to the fetus due to penicillin G. Human experience with the penicillins during pregnancy has not shown any positive evidence of adverse effects on the fetus. There are, however, no adequate and well-controlled studies in pregnant women showing conclusively that harmful effects of these drugs on the fetus can be excluded. Because animal reproduction studies are not always predictive of human response, this drug should be used during pregnancy only if clearly needed.

Nursing Mothers

Soluble penicillin G is excreted in breast milk. Caution should be exercised when penicillin G benzathine is administered to a nursing woman.

Carcinogenesis, Mutagenesis, Impairment of Fertility

No long-term animal studies have been conducted with this drug.

Pediatric Use

(See **INDICATIONS AND USAGE** and **DOSAGE AND ADMINISTRATION** sections.)

Geriatric Use

Clinical studies of penicillin G benzathine did not include sufficient numbers of subjects aged 65 and over to determine whether they respond differently from younger subjects. Other reported clinical experience has not identified differences in responses between the elderly and younger patients. In general, dose selection for an elderly patient should be cautious, usually starting at the low end of the dosing range, reflecting the greater frequency of decreased hepatic, renal, or cardiac function, and of concomitant disease or other drug therapy. This drug is known to be substantially excreted by the kidney, and the risk of toxic reactions to this drug may be greater in patients with impaired renal function (see **CLINICAL PHARMACOLOGY**). Because elderly patients are more likely to have decreased renal function, care should be taken in dose selection, and it may be useful to monitor renal function.

ADVERSE REACTIONS

As with other penicillins, untoward reactions of the sensitivity phenomena are likely to occur, particularly in individuals who have previously demonstrated hypersensitivity to penicillins or in those with a history of allergy, asthma, hay fever, or urticaria.

As with other treatments for syphilis, the Jarisch-Herxheimer reaction has been reported.

The following have been reported with parenteral penicillin G:

General: Hypersensitivity reactions including the following: skin eruptions (maculopapular to exfoliative dermatitis), urticaria, laryngeal edema, fever, eosinophilia; other serum sickness-like reactions (including chills, fever, edema, arthralgia, and prostration); and anaphylaxis including shock and death. Note: Urticaria, other skin rashes, and serum sickness-like reactions may be controlled with antihistamines and, if necessary, systemic corticosteroids. Whenever such reactions occur, penicillin G should be discontinued unless, in the opinion of the physician, the condition being treated is life-threatening and amenable only to therapy with penicillin G. Serious anaphylactic reactions require immediate emergency treatment with epinephrine. Oxygen, intravenous steroids, and airway management, including intubation, should also be administered as indicated.

Gastrointestinal: Pseudomembranous colitis. Onset of pseudomembranous colitis symptoms may occur during or after antibacterial treatment. (See **WARNINGS** section.)

Hematologic: Hemolytic anemia, leukopenia, thrombocytopenia.

Neurologic: Neuropathy.

Urogenital: Nephropathy.

The following adverse events have been temporally associated with parenteral administration of penicillin G benzathine:

Body as a Whole: Hypersensitivity reactions including allergic vasculitis, pruritus, fatigue, asthenia, and pain; aggravation of existing disorder; headache.

Cardiovascular: Cardiac arrest; hypotension; tachycardia; palpitations; pulmonary hypertension; pulmonary embolism; vasodilatation; vasovagal reaction; cerebrovascular accident; syncope.

Gastrointestinal: Nausea, vomiting; blood in stool; intestinal necrosis.

Hemic and Lymphatic: Lymphadenopathy.

Injection Site: Injection site reactions including pain, inflammation, lump, abscess, necrosis, edema, hemorrhage, cellulitis, hypersensitivity, atrophy, ecchymosis, and skin ulcer. Neurovascular reactions including warmth, vasospasm, pallor, mottling, gangrene, numbness of the extremities, cyanosis of the extremities, and neurovascular damage.

Metabolic: Elevated BUN, creatinine, and SGOT.

Musculoskeletal: Joint disorder; periostitis; exacerbation of arthritis; myoglobinuria; rhabdomyolysis.

Nervous System: Nervousness; tremors; dizziness; somnolence; confusion; anxiety; euphoria; transverse myelitis; seizures; coma. A syndrome manifested by a variety of CNS symptoms such as severe agitation with confusion, visual and auditory hallucinations, and a fear of impending death (Hoigne's syndrome), has been reported after administration of penicillin G procaine and, less commonly, after injection of the combination of penicillin G benzathine and penicillin G procaine. Other symptoms associated with this syndrome, such as psychosis, seizures, dizziness, tinnitus, cyanosis, palpitations, tachycardia, and/or abnormal perception in taste, also may occur.

Respiratory: Hypoxia; apnea; dyspnea.

Skin: Diaphoresis.

Special Senses: Blurred vision; blindness.

Urogenital: Neurogenic bladder; hematuria; proteinuria; renal failure; impotence; priapism.

OVERDOSAGE

Penicillin in overdosage has the potential to cause neuromuscular hyperirritability or convulsive seizures.

DOSAGE AND ADMINISTRATION

Streptococcal (Group A) Upper Respiratory Infections (for example, pharyngitis)
Adults—a single injection of 1,200,000 units; older pediatric patients—a single injection of 900,000 units; infants and pediatric patients under 60 lbs.—300,000 to 600,000 units.

Syphilis
Primary, secondary, and latent—2,400,000 units (1 dose).
Late (tertiary and neurosyphilis)—2,400,000 units at 7-day intervals for three doses.
Congenital—under 2 years of age: 50,000 units/kg/body weight; ages 2 to 12 years: adjust dosage based on adult dosage schedule.

Yaws, Bejel, and Pinta—1,200,000 units (1 injection).
Prophylaxis—for rheumatic fever and glomerulonephritis.
Following an acute attack, penicillin G benzathine (parenteral) may be given in doses of 1,200,000 units once a month or 600,000 units every 2 weeks.

METHOD OF ADMINISTRATION
BICILLIN L-A IS INTENDED FOR INTRAMUSCULAR INJECTION ONLY. DO NOT INJECT INTO OR NEAR AN ARTERY OR NERVE, OR INTRAVENOUSLY OR ADMIX WITH OTHER INTRAVENOUS SOLUTIONS. (SEE **WARNINGS** SECTION.)
Administer by DEEP INTRAMUSCULAR INJECTION in the upper, outer quadrant of the buttock. In neonates, infants and small children, the midlateral aspect of the thigh may be preferable. When doses are repeated, vary the injection site.
Because of the high concentration of suspended material in this product, the needle may be blocked if the injection is not made at a slow, steady rate.
Parenteral drug products should be inspected visually for particulate matter and discoloration prior to administration whenever solution and container permit.

HOW SUPPLIED

Bicillin L-A (penicillin G benzathine injectable suspension) is supplied in packages of 10 disposable syringes as follows:
1 mL size, containing 600,000 units per syringe, (21 gauge, thin-wall 1 inch needle for pediatric use), NDC 60793-700-10.
2 mL size, containing 1,200,000 units per syringe, (21 gauge, thin-wall 1-1/2 inch needle), NDC 60793-701-10.
4 mL size, containing 2,400,000 units per syringe (18 gauge × 1–1/2 inch needle), NDC 60793-702-10.
Store in a refrigerator, 2° to 8°C (36° to 46°F).
Keep from freezing.

REFERENCES

1. SHAW, E.: Transverse myelitis from injection of penicillin. *Am. J. Dis. Child., 111*:548, 1966.
2. KNOWLES, J.: Accidental intra-arterial injection of penicillin. *Am. J. Dis. Child., 111*:552, 1966.
3. DARBY, C. et al: Ischemia following an intragluteal injection of benzathine-procaine penicillin G mixture in a one-year-old boy. *Clin. Pediatrics, 12*:485, 1973.
4. BROWN, L. & NELSON, A.: Postinfectious intravascular thrombosis with gangrene. *Arch. Surg., 94*:652, 1967.
5. BORENSTINE, J.: Transverse myelitis and penicillin (Correspondence). *Am. J. Dis. Child., 112*:166, 1966.
6. ATKINSON, J.: Transverse myelopathy secondary to penicillin injection. *J. Pediatrics, 75*:867, 1969.
7. TALBERT, J. et al: Gangrene of the foot following intramuscular injection in the lateral thigh: A case report with recommendations for prevention. *J. Pediatrics, 70*:110, 1967.
8. FISHER, T.: Medicolegal affairs. *Canad. Med. Assoc. J., 112*:395, 1975.
9. SCHANZER, H. et al: Accidental intra-arterial injection of penicillin G. *JAMA, 242*:1289, 1979.

Rx only
Prescribing Information as of September 2009.
Manufactured and Distributed by: King Pharmaceuticals, Inc., Bristol, TN 37620

CYTOMEL® ℞

[*sī'tō-mĕl*]
brand of liothyronine sodium tablets

DESCRIPTION

Thyroid hormone drugs are natural or synthetic preparations containing tetraiodothyronine (T_4, levothyroxine) sodium or triiodothyronine (T_3, liothyronine) sodium or both. T_4 and T_3 are produced in the human thyroid gland by the iodination and coupling of the amino acid tyrosine. T_4 contains four iodine atoms and is formed by the coupling of two molecules of diiodotyrosine (DIT). T_3 contains three atoms of iodine and is formed by the coupling of one molecule of DIT with one molecule of monoiodotyrosine (MIT). Both hormones are stored in the thyroid colloid as thyroglobulin. Thyroid hormone preparations belong to two categories: (1) natural hormonal preparations derived from animal thyroid, and (2) synthetic preparations. Natural preparations include desiccated thyroid and thyroglobulin. Desiccated thyroid is derived from domesticated animals that are used for food by man (either beef or hog thyroid), and thyroglobulin is derived from thyroid glands of the hog. The United States Pharmacopeia (USP) has standardized the total iodine content of natural preparations. Thyroid USP contains not less than (NLT) 0.17 percent and not more than (NMT) 0.23 percent iodine, and thyroglobulin contains not less than (NLT) 0.7 percent of organically bound iodine. Iodine content is only an indirect indicator of true hormonal biologic activity.
Cytomel (liothyronine sodium) Tablets contain liothyronine (L-triiodothyronine or LT_3), a synthetic form of a natural thyroid hormone, and is available as the sodium salt.
The structural and empirical formulas and molecular weight of liothyronine sodium are given below.

Liothyronine Sodium

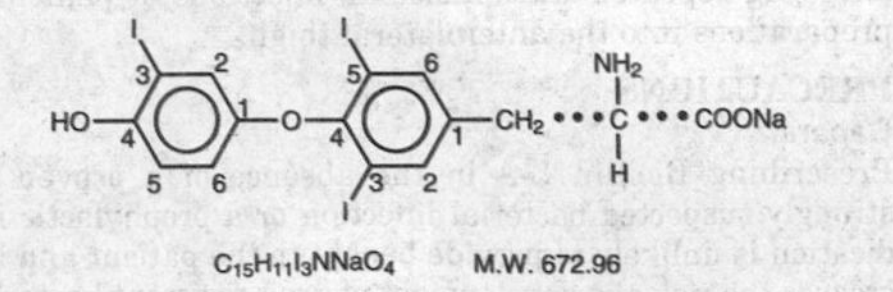

$C_{15}H_{11}I_3NNaO_4$ M.W. 672.96

L-Tyrosine, *O*-(4-hydroxy-3-iodophenyl)-3,5-diiodo-, monosodium salt

Twenty-five mcg of liothyronine is equivalent to approximately 1 grain of desiccated thyroid or thyroglobulin and 0.1 mg of L-thyroxine.
Each round, white to off-white Cytomel (liothyronine sodium) tablet contains liothyronine sodium equivalent to liothyronine as follows: 5 mcg debossed KPI and 115; 25 mcg scored and debossed KPI and 116; 50 mcg scored and debossed KPI and 117. Inactive ingredients consist of calcium sulfate, gelatin, starch, stearic acid, sucrose and talc.

CLINICAL PHARMACOLOGY

The mechanisms by which thyroid hormones exert their physiologic action are not well understood. These hormones enhance oxygen consumption by most tissues of the body, increase the basal metabolic rate and the metabolism of carbohydrates, lipids and proteins. Thus, they exert a profound influence on every organ system in the body and are of particular importance in the development of the central nervous system.

Pharmacokinetics
Since liothyronine sodium (T_3) is not firmly bound to serum protein, it is readily available to body tissues. The onset of activity of liothyronine sodium is rapid, occurring within a few hours. Maximum pharmacologic response occurs within 2 or 3 days, providing early clinical response. The biological half-life is about 2-1/2 days.
T_3 is almost totally absorbed, 95 percent in 4 hours. The hormones contained in the natural preparations are absorbed in a manner similar to the synthetic hormones.
Liothyronine sodium has a rapid cutoff of activity which permits quick dosage adjustment and facilitates control of the effects of overdosage, should they occur.
The higher affinity of levothyroxine (T_4) for both thyroid-binding globulin and thyroid-binding prealbumin as compared to triiodothyronine (T_3) partially explains the higher serum levels and longer half-life of the former hormone. Both protein-bound hormones exist in reverse equilibrium with minute amounts of free hormone, the latter accounting for the metabolic activity.

INDICATIONS AND USAGE

Thyroid hormone drugs are indicated:

1. As replacement or supplemental therapy in patients with hypothyroidism of any etiology, except transient hypothyroidism during the recovery phase of subacute thyroiditis. This category includes cretinism, myxedema and ordinary hypothyroidism in patients of any age (pediatric patients, adults, the elderly), or state (including pregnancy); primary hypothyroidism resulting from functional deficiency, primary atrophy, partial or total absence of thyroid gland, or the effects of surgery, radiation, or drugs, with or without the presence of goiter; and secondary (pituitary) or tertiary (hypothalamic) hypothyroidism (see **WARNINGS**).
2. As pituitary thyroid-stimulating hormone (TSH) suppressants, in the treatment or prevention of various types of euthyroid goiters, including thyroid nodules, subacute or chronic lymphocytic thyroiditis (Hashimoto's) and multinodular goiter.
3. As diagnostic agents in suppression tests to differentiate suspected mild hyperthyroidism or thyroid gland autonomy.

Cytomel (liothyronine sodium) Tablets can be used in patients allergic to desiccated thyroid or thyroid extract derived from pork or beef.

CONTRAINDICATIONS

Thyroid hormone preparations are generally contraindicated in patients with diagnosed but as yet uncorrected adrenal cortical insufficiency, untreated thyrotoxicosis and apparent hypersensitivity to any of their active or extraneous constituents. There is no well-documented evidence from the literature, however, of true allergic or idiosyncratic reactions to thyroid hormone.

WARNINGS

Drugs with thyroid hormone activity, alone or together with other therapeutic agents, have been used for the treatment of obesity. In euthyroid patients, doses within the range of daily hormonal requirements are ineffective for weight reduction. Larger doses may produce serious or even life-threatening manifestations of toxicity, particularly when given in association with sympathomimetic amines such as those used for their anorectic effects.

The use of thyroid hormones in the therapy of obesity, alone or combined with other drugs, is unjustified and has been shown to be ineffective. Neither is their use justified for the treatment of male or female infertility unless this condition is accompanied by hypothyroidism.
Thyroid hormones should be used with great caution in a number of circumstances where the integrity of the cardiovascular system, particularly the coronary arteries, is suspected. These include patients with angina pectoris or the elderly, in whom there is a greater likelihood of occult cardiac disease. In these patients, liothyronine sodium therapy should be initiated with low doses, with due consideration for its relatively rapid onset of action. Starting dosage of Cytomel (liothyronine sodium) Tablets is 5 mcg daily, and should be increased by no more than 5 mcg increments at 2-week intervals. When, in such patients, a euthyroid state can only be reached at the expense of an aggravation of the cardiovascular disease, thyroid hormone dosage should be reduced.
Morphologic hypogonadism and nephrosis should be ruled out before the drug is administered. If hypopituitarism is present, the adrenal deficiency must be corrected prior to starting the drug. Myxedematous patients are very sensitive to thyroid; dosage should be started at a very low level and increased gradually.
Severe and prolonged hypothyroidism can lead to a decreased level of adrenocortical activity commensurate with the lowered metabolic state. When thyroid-replacement therapy is administered, the metabolism increases at a greater rate than adrenocortical activity. This can precipitate adrenocortical insufficiency. Therefore, in severe and prolonged hypothyroidism, supplemental adrenocortical steroids may be necessary. In rare instances the administration of thyroid hormone may precipitate a hyperthyroid state or may aggravate existing hyperthyroidism.

PRECAUTIONS

General
Thyroid hormone therapy in patients with concomitant diabetes mellitus or insipidus or adrenal cortical insufficiency aggravates the intensity of their symptoms. Appropriate adjustments of the various therapeutic measures directed at these concomitant endocrine diseases are required.
The therapy of myxedema coma requires simultaneous administration of glucocorticoids.
Hypothyroidism decreases and hyperthyroidism increases the sensitivity to oral anticoagulants. Prothrombin time should be closely monitored in thyroid-treated patients on oral anticoagulants and dosage of the latter agents adjusted on the basis of frequent prothrombin time determinations.
In infants, excessive doses of thyroid hormone preparations may produce craniosynostosis.

Information for Patients
Patients on thyroid hormone preparations and parents of pediatric patients on thyroid therapy should be informed that:

1. Replacement therapy is to be taken essentially for life, with the exception of cases of transient hypothyroidism, usually associated with thyroiditis, and in those patients receiving a therapeutic trial of the drug.
2. They should immediately report during the course of therapy any signs or symptoms of thyroid hormone toxicity, e.g., chest pain, increased pulse rate, palpitations, excessive sweating, heat intolerance, nervousness, or any other unusual event.
3. In case of concomitant diabetes mellitus, the daily dosage of antidiabetic medication may need readjustment as thy-

roid hormone replacement is achieved. If thyroid medication is stopped, a downward readjustment of the dosage of insulin or oral hypoglycemic agent may be necessary to avoid hypoglycemia. At all times, close monitoring of urinary glucose levels is mandatory in such patients.

4. In case of concomitant oral anticoagulant therapy, the prothrombin time should be measured frequently to determine if the dosage of oral anticoagulants is to be readjusted.
5. Partial loss of hair may be experienced by pediatric patients in the first few months of thyroid therapy, but this is usually a transient phenomenon and later recovery is usually the rule.

Laboratory Tests

Treatment of patients with thyroid hormones requires the periodic assessment of thyroid status by means of appropriate laboratory tests besides the full clinical evaluation. The TSH suppression test can be used to test the effectiveness of any thyroid preparation, bearing in mind the relative insensitivity of the infant pituitary to the negative feedback effect of thyroid hormones. Serum T_4 levels can be used to test the effectiveness of all thyroid medications except products containing liothyronine sodium. When the total serum T_4 is low but TSH is normal, a test specific to assess unbound (free) T_4 levels is warranted. Specific measurements of T_4 and T_3 by competitive protein binding or radioimmunoassay are not influenced by blood levels of organic or inorganic iodine and have essentially replaced older tests of thyroid hormone measurements, i.e., PBI, BEI and T_4 by column.

Drug Interactions

Oral Anticoagulants

Thyroid hormones appear to increase catabolism of vitamin K-dependent clotting factors. If oral anticoagulants are also being given, compensatory increases in clotting factor synthesis are impaired. Patients stabilized on oral anticoagulants who are found to require thyroid replacement therapy should be watched very closely when thyroid is started. If a patient is truly hypothyroid, it is likely that a reduction in anticoagulant dosage will be required. No special precautions appear to be necessary when oral anticoagulant therapy is begun in a patient already stabilized on maintenance thyroid replacement therapy.

Insulin or Oral Hypoglycemics

Initiating thyroid replacement therapy may cause increases in insulin or oral hypoglycemic requirements. The effects seen are poorly understood and depend upon a variety of factors such as dose and type of thyroid preparations and endocrine status of the patient. Patients receiving insulin or oral hypoglycemics should be closely watched during initiation of thyroid replacement therapy.

Cholestyramine

Cholestyramine binds both T_4 and T_3 in the intestine, thus impairing absorption of these thyroid hormones. *In vitro* studies indicate that the binding is not easily removed. Therefore, 4 to 5 hours should elapse between administration of cholestyramine and thyroid hormones.

Estrogen, Oral Contraceptives

Estrogens tend to increase serum thyroxine-binding globulin (TBg). In a patient with a nonfunctioning thyroid gland who is receiving thyroid replacement therapy, free levothyroxine may be decreased when estrogens are started thus increasing thyroid requirements. However, if the patient's thyroid gland has sufficient function, the decreased free thyroxine will result in a compensatory increase in thyroxine output by the thyroid. Therefore, patients without a functioning thyroid gland who are on thyroid replacement therapy may need to increase their thyroid dose if estrogens or estrogen-containing oral contraceptives are given.

Tricyclic Antidepressants

Use of thyroid products with imipramine and other tricyclic antidepressants may increase receptor sensitivity and enhance antidepressant activity; transient cardiac arrhythmias have been observed. Thyroid hormone activity may also be enhanced.

Digitalis

Thyroid preparations may potentiate the toxic effects of digitalis. Thyroid hormonal replacement increases metabolic rate, which requires an increase in digitalis dosage.

Ketamine

When administered to patients on a thyroid preparation, this parenteral anesthetic may cause hypertension and tachycardia. Use with caution and be prepared to treat hypertension, if necessary.

Vasopressors

Thyroxine increases the adrenergic effect of catecholamines such as epinephrine and norepinephrine. Therefore, injection of these agents into patients receiving thyroid preparations increases the risk of precipitating coronary insufficiency, especially in patients with coronary artery disease. Careful observation is required.

Drug and Laboratory Test Interactions

The following drugs or moieties are known to interfere with laboratory tests performed in patients on thyroid hormone therapy: androgens, corticosteroids, estrogens, oral contraceptives containing estrogens, iodine-containing preparations and the numerous preparations containing salicylates.

1. Changes in TBg concentration should be taken into consideration in the interpretation of T_4 and T_3 values. In such cases, the unbound (free) hormone should be measured. Pregnancy, estrogens and estrogen-containing oral contraceptives increase TBg concentrations. TBg may also be increased during infectious hepatitis. Decreases in TBg concentrations are observed in nephrosis, acromegaly and after androgen or corticosteroid therapy. Familial hyper- or hypo-thyroxine-binding-globulinemias have been described. The incidence of TBg deficiency approximates 1 in 9000. The binding of thyroxine by thyroxine-binding prealbumin (TBPA) is inhibited by salicylates.
2. Medicinal or dietary iodine interferes with all *in vivo* tests of radioiodine uptake, producing low uptakes which may not be reflective of a true decrease in hormone synthesis.
3. The persistence of clinical and laboratory evidence of hypothyroidism in spite of adequate dosage replacement indicates either poor patient compliance, poor absorption, excessive fecal loss, or inactivity of the preparation. Intracellular resistance to thyroid hormone is quite rare.

Carcinogenesis, Mutagenesis, Impairment of Fertility

A reportedly apparent association between prolonged thyroid therapy and breast cancer has not been confirmed and patients on thyroid for established indications should not discontinue therapy. No confirmatory long-term studies in animals have been performed to evaluate carcinogenic potential, mutagenicity, or impairment of fertility in either males or females.

Pregnancy

Category A

Thyroid hormones do not readily cross the placental barrier. The clinical experience to date does not indicate any adverse effect on fetuses when thyroid hormones are administered to pregnant women. On the basis of current knowledge, thyroid replacement therapy to hypothyroid women should not be discontinued during pregnancy.

Nursing Mothers

Minimal amounts of thyroid hormones are excreted in human milk. Thyroid is not associated with serious adverse reactions and does not have a known tumorigenic potential. However, caution should be exercised when thyroid is administered to a nursing woman.

Geriatric Use

Clinical studies of liothyronine sodium did not include sufficient numbers of subjects aged 65 and over to determine whether they respond differently from younger subjects. Other reported clinical experience has not identified differences in responses between the elderly and younger patients. In general, dose selection for an elderly patient should be cautious, usually starting at the low end of the dosing range, reflecting the greater frequency of decreased hepatic, renal, or cardiac function, and of concomitant disease or other drug therapy. This drug is known to be substantially excreted by the kidney, and the risk of toxic reactions to this drug may be greater in patients with impaired renal function. Because elderly patients are more likely to have decreased renal function, care should be taken in dose selection, and it may be useful to monitor renal function.

Pediatric Use

Pregnant mothers provide little or no thyroid hormone to the fetus. The incidence of congenital hypothyroidism is relatively high (1:4000) and the hypothyroid fetus would not derive any benefit from the small amounts of hormone crossing the placental barrier. Routine determinations of serum T_4 and/or TSH is strongly advised in neonates in view of the deleterious effects of thyroid deficiency on growth and development.

Treatment should be initiated immediately upon diagnosis and maintained for life, unless transient hypothyroidism is suspected, in which case, therapy may be interrupted for 2 to 8 weeks after the age of 3 years to reassess the condition. Cessation of therapy is justified in patients who have maintained a normal TSH during those 2 to 8 weeks.

ADVERSE REACTIONS

Adverse reactions, other than those indicative of hyperthyroidism because of therapeutic overdosage, either initially or during the maintenance period are rare (see **OVERDOSAGE**).

In rare instances, allergic skin reactions have been reported with Cytomel (liothyronine sodium) Tablets.

OVERDOSAGE

Signs and Symptoms

Headache, irritability, nervousness, sweating, arrhythmia (including tachycardia), increased bowel motility and menstrual irregularities. Angina pectoris or congestive heart failure may be induced or aggravated. Shock may also develop. Massive overdosage may result in symptoms resembling thyroid storm. Chronic excessive dosage will produce the signs and symptoms of hyperthyroidism.

Treatment Of Overdosage

Dosage should be reduced or therapy temporarily discontinued if signs and symptoms of overdosage appear. Treatment may be reinstituted at a lower dosage. In normal individuals, normal hypothalamic-pituitary-thyroidaxis function is restored in 6 to 8 weeks after thyroid suppression.

Treatment of acute massive thyroid hormone overdosage is aimed at reducing gastrointestinal absorption of the drugs and counteracting central and peripheral effects, mainly those of increased sympathetic activity. Vomiting may be induced initially if further gastrointestinal absorption can reasonably be prevented and barring contraindications such as coma, convulsions, or loss of the gagging reflex. Treatment is symptomatic and supportive. Oxygen may be administered and ventilation maintained. Cardiac glycosides may be indicated if congestive heart failure develops. Measures to control fever, hypoglycemia, or fluid loss should be instituted if needed. Antiadrenergic agents, particularly propranolol, have been used advantageously in the treatment of increased sympathetic activity. Propranolol may be administered intravenously at a dosage of 1 to 3 mg over a 10-minute period or orally, 80 to 160 mg/day, especially when no contraindications exist for its use.

DOSAGE AND ADMINISTRATION

The dosage of thyroid hormones is determined by the indication and must in every case be individualized according to patient response and laboratory findings.

Cytomel (liothyronine sodium) Tablets are intended for oral administration; once-a-day dosage is recommended. Although liothyronine sodium has a rapid cutoff, its metabolic effects persist for a few days following discontinuance.

Mild Hypothyroidism

Recommended starting dosage is 25 mcg daily. Daily dosage then may be increased by up to 25 mcg every 1 or 2 weeks. Usual maintenance dose is 25 to 75 mcg daily.

The rapid onset and dissipation of action of liothyronine sodium (T_3), as compared with levothyroxine sodium (T_4), has led some clinicians to prefer its use in patients who might be more susceptible to the untoward effects of thyroid medication. However, the wide swings in serum T_3 levels that follow its administration and the possibility of more pronounced cardiovascular side effects tend to counterbalance the stated advantages.

Cytomel (liothyronine sodium) Tablets may be used in preference to levothyroxine (T_4) during radioisotope scanning procedures, since induction of hypothyroidism in those cases is more abrupt and can be of shorter duration. It may also be preferred when impairment of peripheral conversion of T_4 to T_3 is suspected.

Myxedema

Recommended starting dosage is 5 mcg daily. This may be increased by 5 to 10 mcg daily every 1 or 2 weeks. When 25 mcg daily is reached, dosage may be increased by 5 to 25 mcg every 1 or 2 weeks until a satisfactory therapeutic response is attained. Usual maintenance dose is 50 to 100 mcg daily.

Myxedema Coma

Myxedema coma is usually precipitated in the hypothyroid patient of long standing by intercurrent illness or drugs such as sedatives and anesthetics and should be considered a medical emergency.

An intravenous preparation of liothyronine sodium is marketed by JONES PHARMA INCORPORATED, under the trade name Triostat® for use in myxedema coma/precoma.

Congenital Hypothyroidism

Recommended starting dosage is 5 mcg daily, with a 5 mcg increment every 3 to 4 days until the desired response is achieved. Infants a few months old may require only 20 mcg daily for maintenance. At 1 year, 50 mcg daily may be required. Above 3 years, full adult dosage may be necessary (see **PRECAUTIONS; Pediatric Use**).

Simple (non-toxic) Goiter

Recommended starting dosage is 5 mcg daily. This dosage may be increased by 5 to 10 mcg daily every 1 or 2 weeks. When 25 mcg daily is reached, dosage may be increased every week or two by 12.5 or 25 mcg. Usual maintenance dosage is 75 mcg daily.

In the elderly or in pediatric patients, therapy should be started with 5 mcg daily and increased only by 5 mcg increments at the recommended intervals.

When switching a patient to Cytomel (liothyronine sodium) Tablets from thyroid, L-thyroxine or thyroglobulin, discontinue the other medication, initiate Cytomel at a low dosage, and increase gradually according to the patient's response. When selecting a starting dosage, bear in mind that this drug has a rapid onset of action, and that residual effects of the other thyroid preparation may persist for the first several weeks of therapy.

Thyroid Suppression Therapy

Administration of thyroid hormone in doses higher than those produced physiologically by the gland results in suppression of the production of endogenous hormone. This is the basis for the thyroid suppression test and is used as an aid in the diagnosis of patients with signs of mild hyperthyroidism in whom baseline laboratory tests appear normal or to demonstrate thyroid gland autonomy in patients with Graves' ophthalmopathy. ^{131}I uptake is determined before and after the administration of the exogenous hormone. A 50% or greater suppression of uptake indicates a normal thyroid-pituitary axis and thus rules out thyroid gland autonomy.

Cytomel (liothyronine sodium) Tablets are given in doses of 75 to 100 mcg/day for 7 days, and radioactive iodine uptake is determined before and after administration of the hormone. If thyroid function is under normal control, the radio-iodine uptake will drop significantly after treatment. Cytomel (liothyronine sodium) Tablets should be administered cautiously to patients in whom there is a strong suspicion of thyroid gland autonomy, in view of the fact that the exogenous hormone effects will be additive to the endogenous source.

HOW SUPPLIED

Cytomel (liothyronine sodium) Tablets: 5 mcg in bottles of 100; 25 mcg in bottles of 100; and 50 mcg in bottles of 100.

5 mcg 100's: NDC 60793-115-01
25 mcg 100's: NDC 60793-116-01
50 mcg 100's: NDC 60793-117-01

Store between 15° and 30°C (59° and 86°F).
Prescribing Information as of March 2004.
Manufactured by: King Pharmaceuticals, Inc., Bristol, TN 37620

EMBEDA™   CⅡ ℞

[im-bed-a]
(morphine sulfate and naltrexone hydrochloride)
extended release capsules for oral use

HIGHLIGHTS OF PRESCRIBING INFORMATION

These highlights do not include all the information needed to use EMBEDA safely and effectively. See full prescribing information for EMBEDA.

EMBEDA ((morphine sulfate and naltrexone hydrochloride) extended release capsules) capsules for oral use - CII
Initial U.S. Approval: 2009

> **WARNING**
>
> *See full prescribing information for complete boxed warning.*
>
> - EMBEDA capsules contain pellets of morphine sulfate, an opioid receptor agonist with a sequestered core of naltrexone hydrochloride, an opioid receptor antagonist, and is indicated for the management of moderate to severe pain when a continuous, around-the-clock opioid analgesic is needed for an extended period of time. (5)
> - EMBEDA is to be swallowed whole or the contents of the capsules sprinkled on apple sauce. The pellets in the capsules are not to be crushed, dissolved, or chewed. Misuse or abuse of EMBEDA by tampering with the formulation, crushing or chewing the pellets, causes the rapid release and absorption of both morphine and naltrexone. The resulting morphine dose may be fatal, particularly in opioid-naïve individuals. In opioid-tolerant individuals, the absorption of naltrexone may increase the risk of precipitating withdrawal. (5)
> - EMBEDA is NOT intended for use as a prn analgesic. (5)
> - EMBEDA 100 mg/4mg capsules ARE FOR USE IN OPIOID-TOLERANT PATIENTS ONLY (2).
> - Patients should not consume alcoholic beverages or use prescription or non-prescription medications containing alcohol while on EMBEDA therapy. (5.2)

INDICATIONS AND USAGE

EMBEDA is indicated for:
- the management of moderate to severe pain when a continuous, around-the-clock opioid analgesic is needed for an extended period of time (1)
- EMBEDA is NOT intended for use as a prn analgesic

DOSAGE AND ADMINISTRATION

- EMBEDA may be administered once or twice daily. (2)
- Alternatively, EMBEDA may be sprinkled on apple sauce. (2.3)

DOSAGE FORMS AND STRENGTHS

- Capsules: 20 mg/0.8 mg, 30 mg/1.2 mg, 50 mg/2 mg, 60 mg/2.4 mg, 80 mg/3.2 mg, 100 mg/4 mg (morphine sulfate/naltrexone hydrochloride) (3)

CONTRAINDICATIONS

- Known hypersensitivity to morphine, morphine salts, naltrexone, or in any situation where opioids are contraindicated. (4)
- Respiratory depression (4.1)
- Patients with acute or severe bronchial asthma or hypercarbia. (4.1)

- Paralytic ileus (4.2)

WARNINGS AND PRECAUTIONS

- EMBEDA may be associated with clinically significant respiratory depression. Monitor patients accordingly. (5.3)
- EMBEDA may have additive effects when used in conjunction with alcohol and other CNS depressants. (5.6)
- EMBEDA should be used with extreme caution in patients susceptible to intracranial effects of CO_2 retention. (5.4)

ADVERSE REACTIONS

Most common (≥10%) adverse reactions are constipation, nausea, and somnolence. (6.1)

To report SUSPECTED ADVERSE REACTIONS, contact King Pharmaceuticals, Inc. at 1-800-546-4905 or DSP@Kingpharm.com or FDA at 1-800-FDA-1088 or www.fda.gov/medwatch

DRUG INTERACTIONS

- CNS Depressants should be used with caution and in reduced dosage in patients who are receiving EMBEDA Capsules. (7.1)
- Muscle Relaxants may enhance the action of EMBEDA Capsules and produce an increased degree of respiratory depression. (7.2)
- Mixed Agonist/Antagonist Opioid Analgesics may reduce the analgesic effect of EMBEDA Capsules and/or may precipitate withdrawal symptoms. (7.3)
- Monoamine Oxidase Inhibitors should not be used in patients taking EMBEDA Capsules or within 14 days of stopping such treatment. (7.4)

USE IN SPECIFIC POPULATIONS

Administered with caution, and in reduced dosages in elderly or debilitated patients, and patients with severe renal or hepatic insufficiency. (5.11)

See 17 for PATIENT COUNSELING INFORMATION and Medication Guide

                          Revised: 07/2010

FULL PRESCRIBING INFORMATION

> **WARNING**
>
> EMBEDA™ capsules contain morphine, an opioid agonist and a Schedule II controlled substance with an abuse liability similar to other opioid agonists. EMBEDA can be abused in a manner similar to other opioid agonists, legal or illicit. This should be considered when prescribing or dispensing EMBEDA in situations where the physician or pharmacist is concerned about an increased risk of misuse, abuse, or diversion. EMBEDA contains pellets of an extended-release oral formulation of morphine sulfate, an opioid receptor agonist, surrounding an inner core of naltrexone hydrochloride, an opioid receptor antagonist indicated for the management of moderate to severe pain when a continuous, around-the-clock opioid analgesic is needed for an extended period of time.
>
> EMBEDA is NOT intended for use as a prn analgesic. EMBEDA 100 mg/4 mg IS FOR USE IN OPIOID-TOLERANT PATIENTS ONLY. Ingestion of these capsules or the pellets within the capsules may cause fatal respiratory depression when administered to patients not already tolerant to high doses of opioids.
>
> Patients should not consume alcoholic beverages while on EMBEDA therapy. Additionally, patients must not use prescription or non-prescription medications containing alcohol while on EMBEDA therapy. The co-ingestion of alcohol with EMBEDA may result in an increase of plasma levels and potentially fatal overdose of morphine. EMBEDA is to be swallowed whole or the contents of the capsules sprinkled on apple sauce. The pellets in the capsules are not to be crushed, dissolved, or chewed due to the risk of rapid release and absorption of a potentially fatal dose of morphine.
>
> Crushing, chewing, or dissolving EMBEDA will also result in the release of naltrexone which may precipitate withdrawal in opioid-tolerant individuals.

1 INDICATIONS AND USAGE

EMBEDA is an extended-release oral formulation of morphine sulfate and naltrexone hydrochloride indicated for the management of moderate to severe pain when a continuous, around-the-clock opioid analgesic is needed for an extended period of time.

EMBEDA is NOT intended for use as a prn analgesic.

EMBEDA is not indicated for acute/postoperative pain or if the pain is mild or not expected to persist for an extended period of time.

EMBEDA is only indicated for postoperative use if the patient is already receiving chronic opioid therapy prior to surgery or if the postoperative pain is expected to be moderate to severe and persist for an extended period of time. Physicians should individualize treatment, moving from parenteral to oral analgesics as appropriate.

2 DOSAGE AND ADMINISTRATION

Selection of patients for treatment with morphine sulfate should be governed by the same principles that apply to the use of similar opioid analgesics. Physicians should individualize treatment in every case, using non-opioid analgesics, opioids on an as needed basis and/or combination products, and chronic opioid therapy in a progressive plan of pain management such as outlined by the World Health Organization and Federation of State Medical Boards Model Guidelines.

Care should be taken to use low initial doses of EMBEDA in patients who are not already opioid-tolerant, especially those who are receiving concurrent treatment with muscle relaxants, sedatives, or other CNS active medications.

The 100 mg/4 mg capsules are for use only in opioid-tolerant patients.

EMBEDA is to be swallowed whole or the contents of the capsules sprinkled on apple sauce and taken by mouth. The pellets in the capsules are not to be crushed, dissolved, or chewed before swallowing.

2.1 Initiating Therapy with EMBEDA

It is critical to adjust the dosing regimen for each patient individually, taking into account the patient's prior analgesic treatment experience. In the selection of the initial dose of EMBEDA, attention should be given to:

1) the total daily dose, potency, and kind of opioid the patient has been taking previously;
2) the reliability of the relative potency estimate used to calculate the equivalent dose of morphine needed (Note: potency estimates may vary with the route of administration);
3) the patient's degree of opioid experience and opioid tolerance;
4) the general condition and medical status of the patient;
5) concurrent medication;
6) the type and severity of the patient's pain.

The following dosing recommendations can be considered approaches to what is actually a series of clinical decisions over time in the management of the pain of an individual patient:

Use of EMBEDA as the First Opioid Analgesic
The lowest dose of EMBEDA should be used as the initial opioid analgesic in patients with chronic pain. Patients may subsequently be titrated to a once or twice a day dosage which adequately manages their pain.

Conversion from Other Oral Morphine Formulations to EMBEDA
Patients on other oral morphine formulations may be converted to EMBEDA by administering one-half of the patient's total daily oral morphine dose as EMBEDA every 12 hours (twice-a-day) or by administering the total daily oral morphine dose as EMBEDA every 24 hours (once-a-day). EMBEDA should not be given more frequently than every 12 hours.

Conversion from Oral Opioids, Parenteral Morphine, or Other Parenteral Opioids to EMBEDA
EMBEDA can be administered to patients previously receiving treatment with parenteral morphine or other opioids. While there are useful tables of oral and parenteral equivalents in cancer analgesia, there is substantial inter-patient variation in the relative potency of different opioid drugs and formulations. For these reasons, it is better to underestimate the patient's 24-hour oral morphine requirement and provide rescue medication than to overestimate and manage an adverse event. The following general points should be considered:

1. Parenteral to Oral Morphine Ratio: It may take anywhere from 2-6 mg of oral morphine to provide analgesia equivalent to 1 mg of parenteral morphine. A dose of oral morphine three times the daily parenteral morphine requirement may be sufficient in chronic use settings.
2. Other Oral or Parenteral Opioids to Oral Morphine Sulfate: There is lack of systematic evidence bearing on these types of analgesic substitutions. Therefore, specific recommendations are not possible. Physicians are advised to refer to published relative potency data, keeping in mind that such ratios are only approximate. In general, it is safest to give half of the estimated daily morphine demand as the initial dose and to manage inadequate analgesia by supplementation with immediate-release morphine.

The first dose of EMBEDA may be taken with the last dose of any immediate-release (short-acting) opioid medication due to the extended-release characteristics of EMBEDA.

2.2 Individualization of Dosage

Patients may develop some degree of tolerance, requiring dosage adjustment until they have achieved their individual balance between effective analgesia and opioid side effects such as confusion, sedation, and constipation.

• EMBEDA should be titrated no more frequently than every-other-day to allow patients to stabilize before escalating the dose.
• If breakthrough pain occurs, the dose may be supplemented with a small dose (less than 20% of the total daily dose) of a short-acting analgesic.
• Patients who exhibit signs of excessive opioid side effects such as sedation should have their dose reduced.
• Patients who experience inadequate analgesia on once-daily dosing should be switched to twice-a-day.
• EMBEDA should not be dosed more frequently than every 12 hours.

During periods of changing analgesic requirements including initial titration, frequent communication is recommended between physician, other members of the healthcare team, the patient, and the caregiver/family.

2.3 Alternative Methods of Administration

Patients who have difficulty swallowing whole capsules or tablets may benefit from an alternative method of administration. EMBEDA pellets may be sprinkled over apple sauce. Other foods have not been tested and should not be substituted for apple sauce.

1. Sprinkle the pellets onto a small amount of apple sauce and use immediately.
2. The patient must be cautioned not to chew the pellets [see WARNINGS AND PRECAUTIONS (5)].
3. Rinse mouth to ensure all pellets have been swallowed.
4. Patients should consume entire portion and should not divide apple sauce into separate doses.

Do not administer EMBEDA pellets through a nasogastric or gastric tubes.

2.4 Maintenance of Therapy

Continual re-evaluation of the patient receiving morphine sulfate is important, with special attention to the maintenance of pain control and the relative incidence of side effects associated with therapy. If the level of pain increases, effort should be made to identify the source of increased pain, while adjusting the dose as described above to decrease the level of pain. During chronic therapy, especially for non-cancer-related pain (or pain associated with other terminal illnesses), the continued need for the use of opioid analgesics should be re-assessed as appropriate.

2.5 Cessation of Therapy

In general, EMBEDA should not be abruptly discontinued. However, EMBEDA, like other opioids, can be safely discontinued without the development of withdrawal symptoms by slowly tapering the daily dose.

3 DOSAGE FORMS AND STRENGTHS

EMBEDA contains creamy white to light tan spheroidal pellets, have an outer opaque capsule with colors as identified below and are available in six dosage strengths:

Each 20 mg/0.8 mg capsule contains 20 mg of morphine sulfate and 0.8 mg of naltrexone hydrochloride in a two-toned yellow opaque capsule with "EMBEDA" printed in grey ink on the darker-toned cap and a single grey band around ¾ of the circumference and the lighter-toned body has "20" reverse-printed in a grey circle.

Each 30 mg/1.2 mg capsule contains 30 mg of morphine sulfate and 1.2 mg of naltrexone hydrochloride in a two-toned blue violet opaque capsule with "EMBEDA" printed in grey ink on the darker-toned cap and a single grey band around ¾ of the circumference and the lighter-toned body has "30" reverse-printed in a grey circle.

Each 50 mg/2 mg capsule contains 50 mg of morphine sulfate and 2 mg of naltrexone hydrochloride in a two-toned blue opaque capsule with "EMBEDA" printed in grey ink on the darker-toned cap and a single grey band around ¾ of the circumference and the lighter-toned body has "50" reverse-printed in a grey circle.

Each 60 mg/2.4 mg capsule contains 60 mg of morphine sulfate and 2.4 mg of naltrexone hydrochloride in a two-toned pink opaque capsule with "EMBEDA" printed in grey ink on the darker-toned cap and a single grey band around ¾ of the circumference and the lighter-toned body has "60" reverse-printed in a grey circle.

Each 80 mg/3.2 mg capsule contains 80 mg of morphine sulfate and 3.2 mg of naltrexone hydrochloride in a two-toned light peach opaque elongated capsule with "EMBEDA" printed in grey ink on the darker-toned cap and a single grey band around ¾ of the circumference and the lighter-toned body has "80" reverse-printed in a grey circle.

Each 100 mg/4 mg capsule contains 100 mg of morphine sulfate and 4 mg of naltrexone hydrochloride in a two-toned green opaque capsule with "EMBEDA" printed in grey ink on the darker-toned cap and a single grey band around ¾ of the circumference and the lighter-toned body has "100" reverse-printed in a grey circle.

4 CONTRAINDICATIONS

EMBEDA is contraindicated in patients with a known hypersensitivity to morphine, morphine salts, naltrexone, or in any situation where opioids are contraindicated.

4.1 Impaired Pulmonary Function

EMBEDA is contraindicated in patients with significant respiratory depression in unmonitored settings or the absence of resuscitative equipment.

EMBEDA is contraindicated in patients with acute or severe bronchial asthma or hypercapnia in unmonitored settings or the absence of resuscitative equipment [see WARNINGS AND PRECAUTIONS (5.1)].

4.2 Paralytic Ileus

• EMBEDA is contraindicated in any patient who has or is suspected of having paralytic ileus.

5 WARNINGS AND PRECAUTIONS

EMBEDA is to be swallowed whole or the contents of the capsules sprinkled on apple sauce. The pellets in the capsules are not to be crushed, dissolved, or chewed. The resulting morphine dose may be fatal, particularly in opioid-naïve individuals. In opioid-tolerant individuals, the absorption of naltrexone may increase the risk of precipitating withdrawal.

EMBEDA 100 mg/4 mg is for use in opioid-tolerant patients only. Ingestion of these capsules or of the pellets within the capsules may cause fatal respiratory depression when administered to patients not already tolerant to high doses of opioids.

5.1 Misuse, Abuse, and Diversion of Opioids

EMBEDA contains morphine, an opioid agonist, and is a Schedule II controlled substance. Opioid agonists have the potential for being abused and are sought by drug abusers and people with addiction disorders and are subject to criminal diversion.

Morphine can be abused in a manner similar to other opioid agonists, legal or illicit. This should be considered when prescribing or dispensing EMBEDA in situations where the physician or pharmacist is concerned about an increased risk of misuse, abuse, or diversion.

Abuse of EMBEDA by crushing, chewing, snorting, or injecting the dissolved product will result in the uncontrolled delivery of the opioid and pose a significant risk to the abuser that could result in overdose and death [see DRUG ABUSE AND DEPENDENCE (9)].

Concerns about abuse and addiction should not prevent the proper management of pain. Healthcare professionals should contact their State Professional Licensing Board or State Controlled Substances Authority for information on how to prevent and detect abuse of this product.

5.2 Interactions with Alcohol and Drugs of Abuse

EMBEDA may be expected to have additive effects when used in conjunction with alcohol, other opioids, or illicit drugs that cause central nervous system depression because respiratory depression, hypotension, and profound sedation or coma may result.

Patients should not consume alcoholic beverages, prescription or non-prescription medications containing alcohol while on EMBEDA therapy. The co-ingestion of alcohol with EMBEDA can result in an increase of morphine plasma levels and potentially fatal overdose of morphine [see CLINICAL PHARMACOLOGY (12.3)].

5.3 Impaired Respiration

Respiratory depression is the chief hazard of all morphine preparations such as EMBEDA. Respiratory depression occurs more frequently and is more dangerous in elderly and debilitated patients, and those suffering from conditions accompanied by hypoxia, hypercapnia, or upper airway obstruction (when even moderate therapeutic doses may significantly decrease pulmonary ventilation).

EMBEDA should be used with extreme caution in patients with chronic obstructive pulmonary disease or cor pulmonale, and in patients having a substantially decreased respiratory reserve (e.g., severe kyphoscoliosis), hypoxia, hypercapnia, or pre-existing respiratory depression. In such patients, even usual therapeutic doses of morphine may increase airway resistance and decrease respiratory drive to the point of apnea. In these patients, alternative non-opioid analgesics should be considered, and opioids should be employed only under careful medical supervision at the lowest effective dose.

5.4 Head Injury and Increased Intracranial Pressure

The respiratory depressant effects of morphine with carbon dioxide retention and secondary elevation of cerebrospinal fluid pressure may be markedly exaggerated in the presence of head injury, other intracranial lesions, or a pre-existing increase in intracranial pressure. EMBEDA can produce effects on pupillary response and consciousness, which may obscure neurologic signs of further increases in pressure in patients with head injuries. EMBEDA should only be administered under such circumstances when considered essential and then with extreme care.

5.5 Hypotensive Effect

EMBEDA may cause severe hypotension. There is an added risk to individuals whose ability to maintain blood pressure has already been compromised by a reduced blood volume or a concurrent administration of drugs such as phenothiazines or general anesthetics [see DRUG INTERACTIONS (7.1)]. EMBEDA may produce orthostatic hypotension and syncope in ambulatory patients.

EMBEDA should be administered with caution to patients in circulatory shock, as vasodilation produced by the drug may further reduce cardiac output and blood pressure.

5.6 Interactions with other CNS Depressants

EMBEDA should be used with caution and in reduced dosage in patients who are concurrently receiving other central nervous system depressants including sedatives or hypnotics, general anesthetics, phenothiazines, other tranquiliz-

Table 1: Adverse Reactions Reported by ≥2.0% of Subjects in 12-Week Efficacy Study – Safety Population

System Organ Class Preferred Term	Titration EMBEDA (N=547) n (%)*	Maintenance EMBEDA (N=171) n (%)	Maintenance Placebo (N=173) n (%)
Subjects With At Least One TEAE	313 (57.2%)	56 (32.7%)	45 (26.0%)
Gastrointestinal disorders	260 (47.5%)	41 (24.0%)	28 (16.2%)
Abdominal pain upper	6 (1.1%)	4 (2.3%)	3 (1.7%)
Constipation	165 (30.2%)	12 (7.0%)	7 (4.0%)
Diarrhoea	6 (1.1%)	12 (7.0%)	12 (6.9%)
Dry mouth	31 (5.7%)	3 (1.8%)	2 (1.2%)
Nausea	106 (19.4%)	19 (11.1%)	11 (6.4%)
Vomiting	46 (8.4%)	7 (4.1%)	2 (1.2%)
General disorders and administration site conditions	39 (7.1%)	9 (5.3%)	10 (5.8%)
Fatigue	16 (2.9%)	1 (0.6%)	2 (1.2%)
Nervous system disorders	135 (24.7%)	12 (7.0%)	11 (6.4%)
Dizziness	42 (7.7%)	2 (1.2%)	2 (1.2%)
Headache	22 (4.0%)	4 (2.3%)	2 (1.2%)
Somnolence	76 (13.9%)	2 (1.2%)	5 (2.9%)
Psychiatric disorders	34 (6.2%)	10 (5.8%)	9 (5.2%)
Insomnia	7 (1.3%)	5 (2.9%)	4 (2.3%)
Skin and subcutaneous tissue disorders	46 (8.4%)	7 (4.1%)	7 (4.0%)
Pruritus	34 (6.2%)	0	1 (0.6%)
Vascular disorders	4 (0.7%)	5 (2.9%)	2 (1.2%)
Flushing	0	4 (2.3%)	1 (0.6%)

*Adverse reactions are classified by System Organ Class and Preferred Term as defined by the Medical Dictionary of Regulatory Affairs (MedDRA) v9.1. If a subject had more than one AE that codes to the same Preferred Term, the subject was counted only once for that Preferred Term.

ers, and alcohol because respiratory depression, hypotension, and profound sedation or coma may result [see DRUG INTERACTIONS (7.1)].

5.7 Gastrointestinal Effects
EMBEDA should not be given to patients with gastrointestinal obstruction, particularly paralytic ileus, as there is a risk of the product remaining in the stomach for an extended period and the subsequent release of a bolus of morphine when normal gut motility is restored. As with other solid morphine formulations diarrhea may reduce morphine absorption.
The administration of morphine may obscure the diagnosis or clinical course in patients with acute abdominal condition.

5.8 Cordotomy
Patients taking EMBEDA who are scheduled for cordotomy or other interruption of pain transmission pathways should have EMBEDA ceased 24 hours prior to the procedure and the pain controlled by parenteral short-acting opioids. In addition, the post-procedure titration of analgesics for such patients should be individualized to avoid either oversedation or withdrawal syndromes.

5.9 Use in Pancreatic/Biliary Tract Disease
EMBEDA may cause spasm of the sphincter of Oddi and should be used with caution in patients with biliary tract disease, including acute pancreatitis. Opioids may cause increases in the serum amylase level.

5.10 Tolerance and Physical Dependence
Tolerance is the need for increasing doses of opioids to maintain a defined effect such as analgesia (in the absence of disease progression or other external factors). Physical dependence is manifested by withdrawal symptoms after abrupt discontinuation of a drug or upon administration of an antagonist. Physical dependence and tolerance are common during chronic opioid therapy.
The opioid abstinence or withdrawal syndrome is characterized by some or all of the following: restlessness, lacrimation, rhinorrhea, yawning, perspiration, chills, myalgia, and mydriasis. Other symptoms also may develop, including: irritability, anxiety, backache, joint pain, weakness, abdomi-

nal cramps, insomnia, nausea, anorexia, vomiting, diarrhea, or increased blood pressure, respiratory rate, or heart rate.
EMBEDA should not be abruptly discontinued [see DOSAGE AND ADMINISTRATION (2.5)].

5.11 Special Risk Groups
EMBEDA should be administered with caution, and in reduced dosages in elderly or debilitated patients; patients with severe renal or hepatic insufficiency; patients with Addison's disease; myxedema; hypothyroidism; prostatic hypertrophy or urethral stricture.
Caution should also be exercised in the administration of EMBEDA to patients with CNS depression, toxic psychosis, acute alcoholism, and delirium tremens.
All opioids may aggravate convulsions in patients with convulsive disorders, and all opioids may induce or aggravate seizures in some clinical settings.

5.12 Driving and Operating Machinery
EMBEDA may impair the mental and/or physical abilities needed to perform potentially hazardous activities such as driving a car or operating machinery. Patients must be cautioned accordingly. Patients should also be warned about the potential combined effects of EMBEDA with other CNS depressants, including other opioids, phenothiazines, sedative/hypnotics, and alcohol [see DRUG INTERACTIONS (7.1)].

5.13 Anaphylaxis
Although extremely rare, cases of anaphylaxis have been reported with the use of a similar extended release morphine formulation.

5.14 Accidentally Precipitated Withdrawal
Agonist/antagonist analgesics (i.e., pentazocine, nalbuphine, butorphanol) should be administered with caution to a patient who has received or is receiving a course of therapy with EMBEDA. In this situation, mixed agonist/antagonist analgesics may reduce the analgesic effect of EMBEDA and/or may precipitate withdrawal symptoms in these patients.
Consuming EMBEDA that have been tampered by crushing, chewing, or dissolving the extended-release formulation

can release sufficient naltrexone to precipitate withdrawal in opioid-dependent individuals. Symptoms of withdrawal usually appear within five minutes of ingestion of naltrexone and can last for up to 48 hours. Mental status changes can include confusion, somnolence, and visual hallucinations. Significant fluid losses from vomiting and diarrhea can require intravenous fluid administration. Patients should be closely monitored and therapy with non-opioid medications tailored to meet individual requirements.

5.15 Laboratory Tests
Naltrexone does not interfere with thin-layer, gas-liquid, and high pressure liquid chromatographic methods which may be used for the separation and detection of morphine, methadone, or quinine in the urine. Naltrexone may or may not interfere with enzymatic methods for the detection of opioids depending on the specificity of the test. Please consult the test manufacturer for specific details.

6 ADVERSE REACTIONS
Serious adverse reactions that may be associated with EMBEDA therapy in clinical use include: respiratory depression, respiratory arrest, apnea, circulatory depression, cardiac arrest, hypotension, and/or shock [see OVERDOSAGE (10), WARNINGS AND PRECAUTIONS (5)].
The common adverse events seen on initiation of therapy with EMBEDA are dose dependent, and their frequency depends on the clinical setting, the patient's level of opioid tolerance, and host factors specific to the individual. They should be expected and managed as a part of opioid analgesia. The most frequent of these include drowsiness, dizziness, constipation, and nausea.

6.1 Clinical Studies Experience
Because clinical trials are conducted under widely varying conditions, adverse reaction rates observed in the clinical trials of a drug cannot be directly compared with rates in the clinical trials of another drug and may not reflect the rates observed in practice.
There were 1251 subjects exposed to at least one dose of EMBEDA in the clinical program. During late phase clinical development, 618 subjects received EMBEDA in two randomized, controlled, double-blind studies in subjects with osteoarthritis of the hip or knee. An additional 465 subjects received EMBEDA in an open-label, year-long safety study of subjects with chronic, non-cancer pain, 208 subjects for at least six months and 124 for 12 months. The remaining 168 subjects were exposed to a single dose of EMBEDA in early PK/PD studies.
Short-Term (12-Week) Randomized Study
Adverse reactions observed in at least 2% of subjects treated with EMBEDA
This study utilized an enriched enrollment with a randomized withdrawal design in which subjects were titrated to effect on open-label EMBEDA for up to 45 days. Once their pain was controlled, subjects were randomized to either active treatment with EMBEDA or were tapered off EMBEDA using a double-dummy design and placed on placebo. The Maintenance Period was 12 weeks. The most common adverse reactions leading to study discontinuation were nausea, constipation, vomiting, fatigue, dizziness, pruritus, and somnolence. Adverse reactions, defined as treatment-related adverse events assessed by the investigators, reported by ≥2.0% of subjects in either the titration or maintenance phase of the 12-week study are presented in Table 1.
[See table 1 at top left]
Long-Term Open-Label Safety Study
In the long-term open-label safety study, 465 patients with chronic non-malignant pain were enrolled and 124 patients were treated for up to 1 year. The distributions of adverse events were similar to that of the randomized, controlled studies, and were consistent with the most common opioid related adverse events. Adverse reactions, defined as treatment-related adverse events assessed by the investigators, reported by ≥ 2.0% of subjects are presented in Table 2.

Table 2: Adverse Reactions Reported by ≥2.0% of Subjects in Long-Term Safety Study – Safety Population

System Organ Class Preferred Term	EMBEDA (N=465) n (%)*
Any Related AE	288 (61.9%)
Gastrointestinal disorders	219 (47.1%)
Constipation	145 (31.2%)
Diarrhoea	10 (2.2%)
Dry mouth	17 (3.7%)
Nausea	103 (22.2%)

Vomiting	37 (8.0%)
General disorders and administration site conditions	51 (11.0%)
Fatigue	19 (4.1%)
Nervous system disorders	99 (21.3%)
Dizziness	19 (4.1%)
Headache	32 (6.9%)
Somnolence	34 (7.3%)
Psychiatric disorders	42 (9.0%)
Anxiety	10 (2.2%)
Insomnia	13 (2.8%)
Skin and subcutaneous tissue disorders	52 (11.2%)
Hyperhidrosis	16 (3.4%)
Pruritus	26 (5.6%)

*Adverse reactions are classified by System Organ Class and Preferred Term as defined by the Medical Dictionary of Regulatory Affairs (MedDRA) v9.1. If a subject had more than one AE that codes to the same Preferred Term, the subject was counted only once for that Preferred Term.

Adverse Reactions Observed in the Phase 2/3 Studies
Most common (≥10%): constipation, nausea, somnolence
Common (≥1% to <10%): vomiting, headache, dizziness, pruritus, dry mouth, diarrhea, fatigue, insomnia, hyperhidrosis, anxiety, chills, abdominal pain, lethargy, edema peripheral, dyspepsia, anorexia, muscle spasms, depression, flatulence, restlessness, decreased appetite, irritability, stomach discomfort, tremor, arthralgia, hot flush, sedation

Adverse Reactions Observed in the Phase 2/3 Studies
Most common (≥10%):
Gastrointestinal disorders: constipation, nausea;
Nervous system disorders: somnolence.
Common (≥1% to <10%):
Gastrointestinal disorders: abdominal pain, diarrhea, dry mouth, dyspepsia, flatulence, stomach discomfort, vomiting;
General disorders and administration site conditions: chills, edema peripheral, fatigue, irritability;
Metabolism and nutrition disorders: anorexia, decreased appetite;
Musculoskeletal and connective tissue disorders: arthralgia, muscle spasms;
Nervous system disorders: dizziness, headache, lethargy, sedation, tremor;
Psychiatric disorders: anxiety, depression, insomnia, restlessness;
Skin and subcutaneous tissue disorders: hyperhidrosis, pruritus;
Vascular disorders: hot flush.
Less Common (<1%):
Eye disorders: vision blurred, orthostatic hypotension;
Gastrointestinal disorders: abdominal distension, pancreatitis, abdominal discomfort, fecaloma, abdominal pain lower, abdominal tenderness;
General disorders and administration site conditions: malaise, asthenia, feeling jittery, drug withdrawal syndrome;
Hepatobiliary disorders: cholecystitis;
Investigations: alanine aminotransferase increased, aspartate aminotransferase increased;
Musculoskeletal and connective tissue disorders: myalgia, muscular weakness;
Nervous system disorders: depressed level of consciousness, mental impairment, memory impairment, disturbance in attention, stupor, paraesthesia, coordination abnormal;
Psychiatric disorders: disorientation, thinking abnormal, mental status changes, confusional state, euphoric mood, hallucination, abnormal dreams, mood swings, nervousness;
Renal and urinary disorders: urinary retention, dysuria;
Reproductive system and breast disorders: erectile dysfunction;
Respiratory, thoracic and mediastinal disorders: dyspnea, rhinorrhoea;
Skin and subcutaneous tissue disorders: rash, piloerection, cold sweat, night sweats;
Vascular disorders: hypotension, flushing.

7 DRUG INTERACTIONS

7.1 CNS Depressants

EMBEDA should be used with great caution and in reduced dosage in patients who are concurrently receiving other central nervous system (CNS) depressants including sedatives, hypnotics, general anesthetics, antiemetics, phenothiazines, other tranquilizers, and alcohol because of the risk of respiratory depression, hypotension, and profound sedation or coma. When such combined therapy is contemplated, the initial dose of one or both agents should be reduced by at least 50%.

7.2 Muscle Relaxants

EMBEDA may enhance the neuromuscular blocking action of skeletal relaxants and produce an increased degree of respiratory depression.

7.3 Mixed Agonist/Antagonist Opioid Analgesics

Agonist/antagonist analgesics (i.e., pentazocine, nalbuphine, butorphanol) should be administered with caution to a patient who has received or is receiving a course of therapy with EMBEDA. In this situation, mixed agonist/antagonist analgesics may reduce the analgesic effect of EMBEDA and/or may precipitate withdrawal symptoms in these patients.

7.4 Monoamine Oxidase Inhibitors (MAOIs)

MAOIs have been reported to potentiate the effects of morphine anxiety, confusion, and significant depression of respiration or coma. EMBEDA should not be used in patients taking MAOIs or within 14 days of stopping such treatment.

7.5 Cimetidine

There is an isolated report of confusion and severe respiratory depression when a hemodialysis patient was concurrently administered morphine and cimetidine.

7.6 Diuretics

Morphine can reduce the efficacy of diuretics by inducing the release of antidiuretic hormone. Morphine may also lead to acute retention of urine by causing spasm of the sphincter of the bladder, particularly in men with prostatism.

7.7 Anticholinergics

Anticholinergics or other medications with anticholinergic activity when used concurrently with opioid analgesics may result in increased risk of urinary retention and/or severe constipation, which may lead to paralytic ileus.

7.8 P-Glycoprotein (PGP) Inhibitors

Based on published reports, PGP inhibitors (e.g. quinidine) may increase the absorption/exposure of morphine sulfate by about two fold. Therefore, caution should be exercised when morphine sulfate is co-administered with PGP inhibitors.

8 USE IN SPECIFIC POPULATIONS

8.1 Pregnancy

Teratogenic Effects

Pregnancy Category C: Teratogenic effects of morphine have been reported in the animal literature. High parental doses during the second trimester were teratogenic in neurological, soft and skeletal tissue. The abnormalities included encephalopathy and axial skeletal fusions. These doses were often maternally toxic and were 0.3 to 3-fold the maximum recommended human dose (MRHD) on a mg/m^2 basis. The relative contribution of morphine-induced maternal hypoxia and malnutrition, each of which can be teratogenic, has not been clearly defined. Treatment of male rats with approximately 3-fold the MRHD for 10 days prior to mating decreased litter size and viability.

Nonteratogenic Effects

Morphine given subcutaneously, at non-maternally toxic doses, to rats during the third trimester with approximately 0.15-fold the MRHD caused reversible reductions in brain and spinal cord volume, and testes size and body weight in the offspring, and decreased fertility in female offspring. The offspring of rats and hamsters treated orally or intraperitoneally throughout pregnancy with 0.04- to 0.3-fold the MRHD of morphine have demonstrated delayed growth, motor and sexual maturation, and decreased male fertility. Chronic morphine exposure of fetal animals resulted in mild withdrawal, altered reflex and motor skill development, and altered responsiveness to morphine that persisted into adulthood.

There are no well-controlled studies of chronic *in utero* exposure to morphine sulfate in human subjects. However, uncontrolled retrospective studies of human neonates chronically exposed to other opioids *in utero*, demonstrated reduced brain volume which normalized over the first month of life. Infants born to opioid-abusing mothers are more often small for gestational age, have a decreased ventilatory response to CO_2, and increased risk of sudden infant death syndrome.

There are no adequate and well-controlled studies of naltrexone in pregnant women.

EMBEDA should only be used during pregnancy if the need for strong opioid analgesia justifies the potential risk to the fetus.

8.2 Labor and Delivery

EMBEDA is not recommended for use in women during and immediately prior to labor, where shorter acting analgesics or other analgesic techniques are more appropriate. Occasionally, opioid analgesics may prolong labor through actions which temporarily reduce the strength, duration, and frequency of uterine contractions. However, this effect is not consistent and may be offset by an increased rate of cervical dilatation which tends to shorten labor. Neonates whose mothers received opioid analgesics during labor should be observed closely for signs of respiratory depression. A specific opioid antagonist, such as naloxone or nalmefene, should be available for reversal of opioid-induced respiratory depression in the neonate.

8.3 Nursing Mothers

Morphine is excreted in the maternal milk, and the milk to plasma morphine AUC ratio is about 2.5:1. The amount of morphine received by the infant depends on the maternal plasma concentration, amount of milk ingested by the infant, and the extent of first pass metabolism.

Withdrawal symptoms can occur in breast-feeding infants when maternal administration of morphine sulfate is stopped. Because of the potential for adverse reactions in nursing infants from EMBEDA, a decision should be made whether to discontinue nursing or discontinue the drug, taking into account the importance of the drug to the mother.

8.4 Pediatric Use

The safety and efficacy of EMBEDA in individuals less than 18 years of age have not been established.

8.5 Geriatric Use

Clinical studies of EMBEDA did not include sufficient numbers of subjects aged 65 and over to determine whether they respond differently from younger subjects. The pharmacokinetics of EMBEDA have not been investigated in elderly patients (>65 years) although such patients were included in clinical studies. In a long-term open label safety study, the pre-dose plasma morphine concentrations after dose normalization were similar for subjects <65 years and those ≥65 years of age. Other reported clinical experience has not identified differences in responses between the elderly and younger patients. In general, dose selection for an elderly patient should be cautious, usually starting at the low end of the dosing range, reflecting the greater frequency of decreased hepatic, renal, or cardiac function, and of concomitant disease or other drug therapy.

8.6 Neonatal Withdrawal Syndrome

Chronic maternal use of opiates or opioids during pregnancy coexposes the fetus. The newborn may experience subsequent neonatal withdrawal syndrome (NWS). Manifestations of NWS include irritability, hyperactivity, abnormal sleep pattern, high-pitched cry, tremor, vomiting, diarrhea, weight loss, and failure to gain weight. The onset, duration, and severity of the disorder differ based on such factors as the addictive drug used, time and amount of mother's last dose, and rate of elimination of the drug from the newborn. Approaches to the treatment of this syndrome have included supportive care and, when indicated, drugs such as paregoric or phenobarbital.

8.7 Race

Pharmacokinetic differences due to race may exist. Chinese subjects given intravenous morphine in one study had a higher clearance when compared to Caucasian subjects (1852 ± 116 mL/min versus 1495 ± 80 mL/min).

8.8 Hepatic Failure

The pharmacokinetics of morphine was found to be significantly altered in individuals with alcoholic cirrhosis. The clearance was found to decrease with a corresponding increase in half-life. The morphine-3-glucuronide (M3G) and morphine-6-glucuronide (M6G) to morphine plasma AUC ratios also decreased in these patients indicating a decrease in metabolic activity.

8.9 Renal Insufficiency

The pharmacokinetics of morphine is altered in renal failure patients. AUC is increased and clearance is decreased. The metabolites, M3G and M6G, accumulate several fold in renal failure patients compared with healthy subjects.

Adequate studies of naltrexone in patients with severe hepatic or renal impairment have not been conducted.

9 DRUG ABUSE AND DEPENDENCE

9.1 Controlled Substance

EMBEDA contains morphine, a mu-opioid agonist, and is a Schedule II controlled substance. EMBEDA can be abused and is subject to criminal diversion.

9.2 Abuse

Drug addiction is characterized by compulsive use, use for non-medical purposes, and continued use despite harm or risk of harm. Drug addiction is a treatable disease, utilizing a multi-disciplinary approach, but relapse is common.

"Drug-seeking" behavior and attempts at wrongful procurement of prescription medicines are very common in addicts and drug abusers. Drug-seeking tactics include emergency calls or visits near the end of office hours, refusal to undergo appropriate examination, testing or referral, repeated "loss" of prescriptions, tampering with prescriptions and reluctance to provide prior medical records or contact information for other treating physician(s). "Doctor shopping" to obtain additional prescriptions is common among drug abusers. However, it is important to note that "drug-seeking behavior" may also be exhibited by patients who are experiencing under-treatment for their moderate to severe chronic pain.

Abuse and addiction are separate and distinct from physical dependence and tolerance. Physicians should be aware that addiction may not be accompanied by concurrent tolerance and symptoms of physical dependence in all addicts. In addition, abuse of opioids can occur in the absence of true addiction and is characterized by misuse for non-medical purposes, often in combination with other psychoactive substances. EMBEDA, like other opioids, can be diverted for non-medical use into illicit channels of distribution. Careful record-keeping of prescribing information, including quantity, frequency, and renewal requests is strongly advised.

Proper assessment of the patient, proper prescribing practices, periodic re-evaluation of therapy, and proper dispensing and storage are appropriate measures that help to reduce abuse of opioid drugs.

EMBEDA is intended for oral use only. Misuse or abuse of EMBEDA by crushing or chewing the pellets will result in the uncontrolled release of both morphine and naltrexone, posing the risk of overdose and death. In opioid-tolerant individuals, the absorption of naltrexone may increase the risk of precipitating withdrawal. The risk of overdose and death is increased with concurrent abuse of alcohol and other central nervous system depressants. The sequestered naltrexone is intended to have no clinical effect when EMBEDA is taken as directed; however, if crushed or chewed, up to 100% of the sequestered naltrexone dose could be released, bioequivalent to an immediate release naltrexone oral solution of the same dose.

Due to the presence of talc as one of the excipients in EMBEDA, parenteral abuse can be expected to result in local tissue necrosis, infection, pulmonary granulomas, and increased risk of endocarditis and valvular heart injury. Parenteral drug abuse is commonly associated with transmission of infectious diseases such as hepatitis and HIV.

9.3 Dependence

Tolerance is the need for increasing doses of opioids to maintain a defined effect such as analgesia (in the absence of disease progression or other external factors). Physical dependence is manifested by withdrawal symptoms after abrupt discontinuation of a drug or upon administration of an antagonist. Physical dependence and tolerance are not unusual during chronic opioid therapy.

The opioid abstinence or withdrawal syndrome is characterized by some or all of the following: restlessness, lacrimation, rhinorrhea, yawning, perspiration, chills, myalgia, and mydriasis. Other symptoms also may develop, including irritability, anxiety, backache, joint pain, weakness, abdominal cramps, insomnia, nausea, anorexia, vomiting, diarrhea, or increased blood pressure, respiratory rate, or heart rate.

In general, opioids should not be abruptly discontinued *[see DOSAGE AND ADMINISTRATION (2.5)]*.

10 OVERDOSAGE

10.1 Symptoms

Acute overdosage with morphine is manifested by respiratory depression, somnolence progressing to stupor or coma, skeletal muscle flaccidity, cold and clammy skin, constricted pupils, and, sometimes, pulmonary edema, bradycardia, hypotension, and death. Marked mydriasis rather than miosis may be seen due to severe hypoxia in overdose situations.

10.2 Treatment

Primary attention should be given to the re-establishment of a patent and protected airway and institution of assisted or controlled ventilation if needed. Other supportive measures (including oxygen, vasopressors) should be employed in the management of circulatory shock and pulmonary edema accompanying overdose as indicated. Cardiac arrest or arrhythmias will require advanced life support techniques.

The pure opioid antagonists, naloxone or nalmefene, are specific antidotes to respiratory depression which results from opioid overdose. Since the duration of reversal would be expected to be less than the duration of action of morphine in EMBEDA, the patient must be carefully monitored until spontaneous respiration is reliably re-established. EMBEDA will continue to release and add to the morphine load for up to 24 hours after administration and the management of an overdose should be monitored accordingly. If the response to opioid antagonists is suboptimal or not sustained, additional antagonist should be given as directed by the manufacturer of the product.

Opioid antagonists should not be administered in the absence of clinically significant respiratory or circulatory depression secondary to morphine overdose. Such agents should be administered cautiously to persons who are known, or suspected to be physically dependent on EMBEDA. In such cases, an abrupt or complete reversal of opioid effects may precipitate an acute withdrawal syndrome.

The sequestered naltrexone in EMBEDA has no role in the treatment of opioid overdose.

In an individual physically dependent on opioids, administration of an opioid receptor antagonist may precipitate an acute withdrawal. The severity of the withdrawal produced will depend on the degree of physical dependence and the dose of the antagonist administered. Use of an opioid antagonist should be reserved for cases where such treatment is clearly needed. If it is necessary to treat serious respiratory depression in the physically dependent patient, administration of the antagonist should be begun with care and by titration with smaller than usual doses of the antagonist.

11 DESCRIPTION

EMBEDA Capsules contain pellets of morphine sulfate and naltrexone hydrochloride at a ratio of 100:4. Morphine sulfate is an agonist and naltrexone hydrochloride is an antagonist at the mu-opioid receptor.

The chemical name of morphine sulfate is 7,8-didehydro-4,5 α-epoxy-17-methyl-morphinan-3,6 α-diol sulfate (2:1) (salt) pentahydrate. The empirical formula is $(C_{17}H_{19}NO_3)_2 \bullet H_2SO_4 \bullet 5H_2O$ and its molecular weight is 758.85.

Morphine sulfate is an odorless, white, crystalline powder with a bitter taste. It has a solubility of 1 in 21 parts of water and 1 in 1000 parts of alcohol, but is practically insoluble in chloroform or ether. The octanol: water partition coefficient of morphine is 1.42 at physiologic pH and the pK_b is 7.9 for the tertiary nitrogen (mostly ionized at pH 7.4). Its structural formula is:

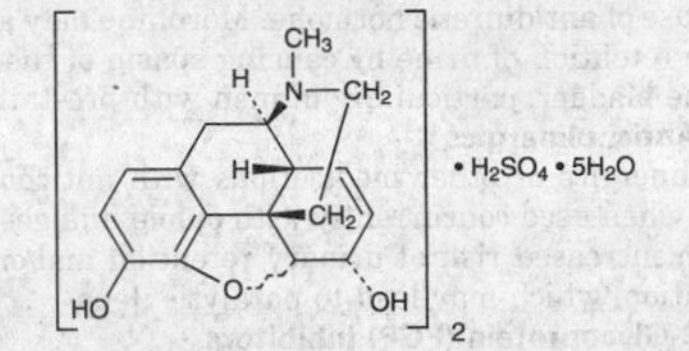

The chemical name of naltrexone hydrochloride is (5α)-17-(Cyclopropylmethyl)-4,5-epoxy-3,14-dihydroxymorphinan-6-one hydrochloride. The empirical formula is $C_{20}H_{23}NO_4 \bullet HCl$ and its molecular weight is 377.46.

Naltrexone hydrochloride is a white to slightly off-white powder that is soluble in water. Its structural formula is:

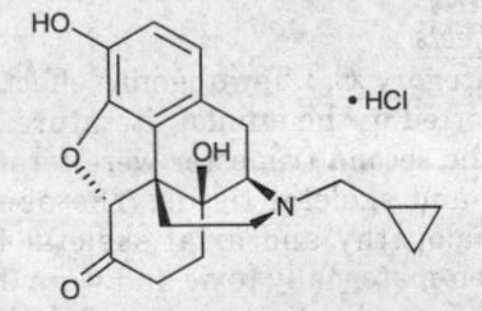

Each capsule contains the following inactive ingredients common to all strengths: talc, ammonio methacrylate copolymer, sugar spheres, ethylcellulose, sodium chloride, polyethylene glycol, hydroxypropyl cellulose, dibutyl sebacate, methacrylic acid copolymer, diethyl phthalate, magnesium stearate, sodium lauryl sulfate, and ascorbic acid. The capsule shells contain gelatin, titanium dioxide, and grey ink, D&C yellow #10 (EMBEDA 20 mg/0.8 mg), FD&C red #3, FD&C blue #1 (EMBEDA 30 mg/1.2 mg), D&C red #28, FD&C red #40, FD&C blue #1 (EMBEDA 50 mg/2 mg), D&C red #28, FD&C red #40, FD&C blue #1 (EMBEDA 60 mg/2.4 mg), FD&C blue #1, FD&C red #40, FD&C yellow #6 (EMBEDA 80 mg/3.2 mg), D&C yellow #10, FD&C blue #1 (EMBEDA 100 mg/4 mg).

EMBEDA contains no gluten.

12 CLINICAL PHARMACOLOGY

12.1 Mechanism of Action

Morphine sulfate, a pure opioid agonist, is relatively selective for the mu receptor, although it can interact with other opioid receptors at higher doses. In addition to analgesia, the widely diverse effects of morphine sulfate include analgesia, dysphoria, euphoria, somnolence, respiratory depression, diminished gastrointestinal motility, altered circulatory dynamics, histamine release, physical dependence, and alterations of the endocrine and autonomic nervous systems.

Morphine produces both its therapeutic and its adverse effects by interaction with one or more classes of specific opioid receptors located throughout the body. Morphine acts as a pure agonist, binding with and activating opioid receptors at sites in the peri-aqueductal and peri-ventricular grey matter, the ventro-medial medulla and the spinal cord to produce analgesia.

Effects on the Central Nervous System

The principal actions of therapeutic value of morphine are analgesia and sedation (i.e., sleepiness and anxiolysis). Specific CNS opiate receptors and endogenous compounds with morphine-like activity have been identified throughout the brain and spinal cord and are likely to play a role in the expression of analgesic effects. In addition, when morphine binds to mu-opioid receptors, it results in positive subjective effects, such as drug liking, euphoria, and high. Morphine produces respiratory depression by direct action on brainstem respiratory centers. The mechanism of respiratory depression involves a reduction in the responsiveness of the brainstem respiratory centers to increases in carbon dioxide tension, and to electrical stimulation. Morphine depresses the cough reflex by direct effect on the cough center in the medulla. Antitussive effects may occur with doses lower than those usually required for analgesia. Morphine causes miosis, even in total darkness, and little tolerance develops to this effect. Pinpoint pupils are a sign of opioid overdose but are not pathognomonic (e.g., pontine lesions of hemorrhagic or ischemic origins may produce similar findings). Marked mydriasis rather than miosis may be seen with worsening hypoxia in the setting of EMBEDA overdose *[see OVERDOSAGE (10)]*.

Effects on the Gastrointestinal Tract and Other Smooth Muscle

Gastric, biliary, and pancreatic secretions are decreased by morphine. Morphine causes a reduction in motility associated with an increase in tone in the antrum of the stomach and duodenum. Digestion of food in the small intestine is delayed and propulsive contractions are decreased. Propulsive peristaltic waves in the colon are decreased, while tone is increased to the point of spasm. The end result is constipation. Morphine can cause a marked increase in biliary tract pressure as a result of spasm of the sphincter of Oddi.

Effects on the Cardiovascular System

Morphine produces peripheral vasodilation which may result in orthostatic hypotension or syncope. Release of histamine may be induced by morphine and can contribute to opioid-induced hypotension. Manifestations of histamine release and/or peripheral vasodilation may include pruritus, flushing, red eyes and sweating.

Mechanism of Action of Naltrexone

Naltrexone is a pure, centrally acting mu-opioid antagonist that reverses the subjective and analgesic effects of mu-opioid receptor agonists by competitively binding at mu-opioid receptors.

12.2 Pharmacodynamics

Plasma Level-Analgesia Relationships

In any particular patient, both analgesic effects and plasma morphine concentrations are related to the morphine dose. While plasma morphine-efficacy relationships can be demonstrated in non-tolerant individuals, they are influenced by a wide variety of factors and are not generally useful as a guide to the clinical use of morphine. The effective dose in opioid-tolerant patients may be 10-50 times as great (or greater) than the appropriate dose for opioid-naïve individuals. Dosages of morphine should be chosen and must be titrated on the basis of clinical evaluation of the patient and the balance between therapeutic and adverse effects.

For any fixed dose and dosing interval, EMBEDA will have, at steady-state, a lower C_{max} and a higher C_{min} than conventional immediate-release morphine.

The pharmacodynamic effect of naltrexone in the setting of crushed EMBEDA was examined in two clinical trials. In a randomized double-blind, triple-dummy, four-way crossover study, 32 non-dependent recreational opioid users received 120 mg of EMBEDA whole and crushed, 120 mg of immediate-release morphine sulfate and placebo. Overall, 87.5% of subjects had some degree of reduced drug liking after receiving crushed EMBEDA, while 12.5% had no reduction in drug liking. There was considerable individual variability in the degree of reduction in drug liking, ranging between 10 and 50%. Similarly, 69% of subjects showed some degree of a decrease in euphoria with crushed EMBEDA compared to IR morphine and 31% of subjects did not report a reduction in euphoria. There was similar individual variability in the degree of reduction in euphoria.

A randomized double-blind, placebo-controlled, three-way cross-over trial in 28 non-dependent recreational opioid-users was performed using 30 mg of IV morphine alone and 30 mg of IV morphine in combination with 1.2 mg of IV naltrexone to simulate parenteral use of crushed EMBEDA. The combination of morphine with naltrexone resulted in 71% of subjects reporting a reduction in euphoria compared to morphine alone. Note that the intravenous injection of crushed EMBEDA may result in serious injury and death due to a morphine overdose or an embolic event. Intravenous injection of crushed EMBEDA may preciptitate a severe withdrawal syndrome in opioid-dependent patients.

The clinical significance of the degree of reduction in drug liking and euphoria reported in these studies has not yet been established. There is no evidence that the naltrexone in EMBEDA reduces the abuse liability of EMBEDA.

12.3 Pharmacokinetics

Absorption

EMBEDA Capsules contain extended-release pellets of morphine sulfate that release morphine slowly compared to an oral morphine solution. Following the administration of oral morphine solution, approximately 50% of the morphine absorbed reaches the systemic circulation within 30 minutes. However, following the administration of an equal amount of EMBEDA to healthy volunteers, this occurs, on average, after 8 hours. As with most forms of oral morphine, because of pre-systemic elimination, only about 20 to 40% of the administered dose reaches the systemic circulation.

EMBEDA is bioequivalent to a similar morphine sulfate extended release capsules product with regard to rate and extent of plasma morphine absorption. The median time to peak plasma morphine levels (T_{max}) was shorter for EMBEDA (7.5 hrs) compared to KADIAN® (10 hrs). Dose-related increase in steady-state pre-dose plasma concentrations of morphine were noted following multiple dose administration of EMBEDA in patients.

Food effect: While concurrent administration of high fat food decreases the rate and extent of morphine absorption from EMBEDA, the total bioavailability is not affected. Co-administration of a high-fat meal with EMBEDA did not compromise sequestration of naltrexone.

When taken as directed, the sequestered naltrexone in EMBEDA is not consistently absorbed into systemic circulation following single dose administration. In some subjects, a limited number (~2%) of blood samples had low and highly variable plasma naltrexone levels (median = 7.74 pg/mL, range 4.05-132 pg/mL) following single dose administration of 60–120 mg EMBEDA compared to oral naltrexone solution. In patients titrated up to 60–80 mg BID EMBEDA, naltrexone levels (4-25.5 pg/mL) were detected in 13 out of 67 patients at steady-state. In a long-term safety study where an average dose of EMBEDA was up to 860 mg administered twice a day for 12 months, 11.0% of blood samples at pre-dose timepoints at steady-state had detectable plasma naltrexone concentrations ranging from 4.03 to 145 pg/mL.

Compared to 2.4 mg naltrexone oral solution, which produced mean (SD) naltrexone plasma levels of 689 (± 429 pg/mL) and mean (SD) 6β-naltrexol plasma levels of 3920 (± 1350 pg/mL), administration of intact 60 mg EMBEDA produced no naltrexone plasma levels and mean (SD) 6β-naltrexol plasma levels of 16.7 (± 13.5 pg/mL). Trough levels of plasma naltrexone and 6-β-naltrexol did not accumulate upon repeated administration of EMBEDA.

Tampering with the EMBEDA formulation by crushing or chewing the pellets, results in the rapid release and absorption of both morphine and naltrexone comparable to an oral solution. This has not been shown to reduce the abuse liability of EMBEDA.

Distribution

Once absorbed, morphine is distributed to skeletal muscle, kidneys, liver, intestinal tract, lungs, spleen, and brain. The volume of distribution of morphine is approximately 3 to 4 L/kg. Morphine is 30 to 35% reversibly bound to plasma proteins. Although the primary site of action of morphine is in the CNS, only small quantities pass the blood brain barrier. Morphine also crosses the placental membranes *[see USE IN SPECIFIC POPULATIONS (8.1)]* and has been found in breast milk *[see USE IN SPECIFIC POPULATIONS (8.3)]*.

Metabolism

Major pathways of morphine metabolism include glucuronidation and sulfation in the liver to produce including morphine-3-glucuronide, M3G (about 50%) and morphine-6-glucuronide, M6G (about 5 to 15%) or morphine-3-etheral sulfate. A small fraction (less than 5%) of morphine is demethylated. M3G has no significant contribution to the analgesic activity. Although M6G does not readily cross the blood-brain barrier, it has been shown to have opioid agonist and analgesic activity in humans.

Naltrexone is extensively metabolized into 6-β-naltrexol.

Excretion

Approximately 10% of morphine dose is excreted unchanged in the urine. Elimination of morphine is primarily via hepatic metabolism to glucuronide metabolites M3G and M6G (55 to 65%) which are then renally excreted. A small amount of the glucuronide metabolites is excreted in the bile and there is some minor enterohepatic cycling.

The mean adult plasma clearance is about 20-30 mL/minute/kg. The effective half-life of morphine after IV administration is reported to be approximately 2.0 hours. The terminal elimination half-life of morphine following single dose EMBEDA administration is approximately 29 hours.

Special Populations

Geriatric: Pharmacokinetics of EMBEDA have not been investigated in elderly patients (>65 years) although such patients were included in clinical studies. However, in a long-term open label safety study, the pre-dose plasma morphine concentrations after dose normalization were similar for subjects <65 years and those ≥65 years of age *[see USE IN SPECIFIC POPULATIONS (8.5)]*.

Pediatric: Pharmacokinetics of EMBEDA were not evaluated in pediatric population.

	EMBEDA 20 mg/0.8 mg	EMBEDA 30 mg/1.2 mg	EMBEDA 50 mg/2 mg	EMBEDA 60 mg/2.4 mg	EMBEDA 80 mg/3.2 mg	EMBEDA 100 mg/4 mg
Morphine sulfate	20 mg	30 mg	50 mg	60 mg	80 mg	100 mg
Sequestered naltrexone hydrochloride	0.8 mg	1.2 mg	2 mg	2.4 mg	3.2 mg	4 mg
Capsule Description	size 4, two-toned, yellow opaque hard gelatin capsule. The darker-toned cap has "EMBEDA" printed in grey ink and a single grey band around ¾ of the circumference. The lighter-toned body has "20" reverse-printed in a grey circle.	size 3, two-toned, blue violet opaque hard gelatin capsule. The darker-toned cap has "EMBEDA" printed in grey ink and a single grey band around ¾ of the circumference. The lighter-toned body has "30" reverse-printed in a grey circle.	size 1, two-toned, blue opaque hard gelatin capsule. The darker-toned cap has "EMBEDA" printed in grey ink and a single grey band around ¾ of the circumference. The lighter-toned body has "50" reverse-printed in a grey circle.	size 0, two-toned, pink opaque hard gelatin capsule. The darker-toned cap has "EMBEDA" printed in grey ink and a single grey band around ¾ of the circumference. The lighter-toned body has "60" reverse-printed in a grey circle.	size 0, two-toned, light peach opaque elongated hard gelatin capsule. The darker-toned cap has "EMBEDA" printed in grey ink and a single grey band around ¾ of the circumference. The lighter-toned body has "80" reverse-printed in a grey circle.	size 00, two-toned, green opaque hard gelatin capsule. The darker-toned cap has "EMBEDA" printed in grey ink and a single grey band around ¾ of the circumference. The lighter-toned body has "100" reverse-printed in a grey circle.
Bottle Size	100	100	100	100	100	100
NDC #	60793-430-01	60793-431-01	60793-433-01	60793-434-01	60793-435-01	60793-437-01

Gender: No meaningful differences were noted between male and female patients in the analysis of pharmacokinetic data of morphine from clinical studies.

Race: Pharmacokinetic differences due to race may exist. Additionally, Chinese subjects given intravenous morphine in one study had a higher clearance when compared to Caucasian subjects (1852 ± 116 mL/min versus 1495 ± 80 mL/min).

Hepatic Failure: The pharmacokinetics of morphine was found to be significantly altered in individuals with alcoholic cirrhosis. The clearance was found to decrease with a corresponding increase in half-life. The morphine-3-glucuronide (M3G) and morphine-6-glucuronide (M6G) to morphine plasma AUC ratios also decreased in these patients indicating a decrease in metabolic activity.

Renal Insufficiency: The pharmacokinetics of morphine is altered in renal failure patients. AUC is increased and clearance is decreased. The metabolites, M3G and M6G, accumulate several fold in renal failure patients compared with healthy subjects.

Drug Interaction/Alcohol Interaction: As such additive pharmacodynamic effects may be expected when EMBEDA is used in conjunction with alcohol, other opioids, or illicit drugs that cause central nervous system depression. Additionally, a pharmacokinetic drug interaction is noted with concomitant administration of 40% alcohol and EMBEDA, where an average 2-fold (range 1.4- to 5-fold increase) higher C_{max} of morphine was noted compared to EMBEDA consumed with water.

13 NONCLINICAL TOXICOLOGY

13.1 Carcinogenesis, Mutagenesis, Impairment of Fertility

Carcinogenesis: Studies in animals to evaluate the carcinogenic potential of morphine have not been conducted.

Mutagenesis: No formal studies to assess the mutagenic potential of morphine have been conducted. In the published literature, *in vitro* studies have reported that morphine is non-mutagenic in *Drosophila* (no lethal mutation induction), in the Ames test with *Salmonella*, and induces chromosomal aberrations in human leukocytes. Morphine was found to be mutagenic *in vitro* in human T-cells, increasing the DNA fragmentation. *In vivo*, morphine was mutagenic in the mouse micronucleus test and induced chromosomal aberrations in spermatids and murine lymphocytes. Chronic opioid abusers (e.g., heroin abusers) and their offspring display higher rates of chromosomal damage. However, the rates of chromosomal abnormalities were similar in nonexposed individuals and in heroin users enrolled in long term opioid maintenance programs.

Impairment of Fertility: No formal nonclinical studies to assess the potential of morphine to impair fertility have been conducted. Several nonclinical studies from the literature have demonstrated adverse effects on male fertility in the rat from exposure to morphine. Studies from the literature have also reported changes in hormonal levels (i.e. testosterone, luteinizing hormone, serum corticosterone) following treatment with morphine. These changes may be associated with the reported effects on fertility in the rat.

14 CLINICAL STUDIES

The analgesic efficacy of EMBEDA has been evaluated in one randomized, double-blind, placebo-controlled clinical trial in osteoarthritis patients with moderate to severe pain (Study ALO-KNT-301). This study, with a randomized withdrawal design, was conducted in subjects with moderate to severe pain from osteoarthritis of the hip or knee over a 12-week treatment period. Subjects started open-label treatment with EMBEDA and titrated to effect. Once their pain was controlled (Brief Pain Inventory Average 24-hour Pain Intensity ≤ 4 AND at least a 2-point drop from screening baseline), they were randomized to either active treatment with EMBEDA or were tapered off EMBEDA using a double-dummy design and placed on placebo. Of these, 75.1% of the randomized subjects were opioid naïve and distributed evenly between the 2 groups.

The mean change in the weekly diary BPI average pain score from randomization baseline (Visit Y) to the end of study (Visit Y + 12 Weeks/Early Termination) was statistically significantly superior for those treated with EMBEDA compared to the placebo group.

16 HOW SUPPLIED/STORAGE AND HANDLING

[See table above]

Store at 25°C (77°F); excursions permitted between 15° and 30°C (59° and 86°F). Dispense in a sealed, tamper-evident, childproof, light-resistant container.

17 PATIENT COUNSELING INFORMATION

Patients receiving EMBEDA should be given the following instructions by the physician:

- Patients should be advised that EMBEDA contains morphine and naltrexone and should be taken only as directed.
- The dose of morphine sulfate should not be adjusted without consulting with a physician or other healthcare professional. EMBEDA should be swallowed whole (not crushed, dissolved, or chewed) due to a risk of fatal morphine overdose or naltrexone precipitated withdrawal symptoms. Alternately, EMBEDA Capsules may be opened and the entire contents sprinkled on a small amount of apple sauce immediately prior to ingestion *[see DOSAGE AND ADMINISTRATION (2.3)]*.
- Patients should not consume alcoholic beverages while on EMBEDA therapy. Additionally, patients must not use prescription or non-prescription medications containing alcohol while on EMBEDA therapy. The co-ingestion of alcohol with EMBEDA may result in an increase of plasma levels and potentially fatal overdose of morphine.
- Patients should be advised of the most common adverse reactions that may occur while taking EMBEDA: constipation, nausea, somnolence, vomiting, dizziness, pruritus, and headache.
- Patients should be advised that EMBEDA may cause drowsiness, dizziness, or lightheadedness and may impair

mental and/or physical ability required for the performance of potentially hazardous tasks (e.g., driving, operating machinery). Patients started on EMBEDA or patients whose dose has been adjusted should refrain from any potentially dangerous activity until it is established that they are not adversely affected.

- Patients should not combine EMBEDA with central nervous system depressants (sleep aids, tranquilizers) except by the orders of the prescribing physician because dangerous additive effects may occur resulting in serious injury or death.
- Patients should be advised that EMBEDA is a potential drug of abuse. They should protect it from theft.
- Special care must be taken to avoid accidental ingestion or use by individuals (including children) other than the patient for whom it was originally prescribed, as such unsupervised use may have severe, even fatal, consequences [see WARNINGS AND PRECAUTIONS (5)].
- Patients should be advised that EMBEDA 100 mg/4 mg is for use only in opioid-tolerant patients.
- Women of childbearing potential who become or are planning to become pregnant should consult a physician prior to initiating or continuing therapy with EMBEDA.
- Safe use in pregnancy has not been established. Prolonged use of opioid analgesics during pregnancy may cause fetal neonatal physical dependence, and neonatal withdrawal may occur.
- As with other opioids, patients taking EMBEDA should be advised of the potential for severe constipation; appropriate laxatives and/or stool softeners as well as other appropriate treatments should be initiated from the onset of opioid therapy.
- Patients should be advised to seek medical attention immediately if signs of a serious allergic reaction occur, such as swelling of the face, throat, or tongue, trouble breathing, feeling dizzy or faint, pounding heart beat, chest pain or feeling of doom [see WARNINGS AND PRECAUTIONS (5.13)].

17.1 Breakthrough Pain/Adverse Experiences
Patients should be advised to report episodes of breakthrough pain and adverse experiences occurring during therapy. Individualization of dosage is essential to make optimal use of this medication.

17.2 Mental and/or Physical Ability
Patients should be advised that EMBEDA may impair mental and/or physical ability required for the performance of potentially hazardous tasks (e.g., driving, operating machinery). Patients started on EMBEDA or whose dose has been changed should refrain from dangerous activity until it is established that they are not adversely affected [see WARNINGS AND PRECAUTIONS (5.12)].

17.3 Avoidance of Alcohol or Other CNS Depressants
Patients should be advised that EMBEDA should not be taken with alcohol, prescription or non-prescription medications containing alcohol, or other CNS depressants (sleeping medication, tranquilizers) except by the orders of the prescribing healthcare provider because dangerous additive effects may occur resulting in serious injury or death [see WARNINGS AND PRECAUTIONS (5.2), (5.6)].

17.4 Pregnancy
Women of childbearing potential who become or are planning to become pregnant, should consult their prescribing healthcare provider prior to initiating or continuing therapy with EMBEDA [see USE IN SPECIFIC POPULATIONS (8.1)].

17.5 Cessation of Therapy
Patients should be advised that if they have been receiving treatment with EMBEDA for more than a few weeks and cessation of therapy is indicated, it may be appropriate to taper the EMBEDA dose, rather than abruptly discontinue it, due to the risk of precipitating withdrawal symptoms. Their prescribing healthcare provider should provide a dose schedule to accomplish a gradual discontinuation of the medication.

17.6 Drug of Abuse
Patients should be advised that EMBEDA is a potential drug of abuse. They should protect it from theft, and it should never be given to anyone other than the individual for whom it was prescribed [see WARNINGS AND PRECAUTIONS (5.1)].

17.7 Constipation
Patients should be advised that severe constipation could occur as a result of taking EMBEDA and appropriate laxatives, stool softeners and other appropriate treatments should be initiated from the beginning of opioid therapy.

17.8 Storage/Destruction of Unused EMBEDA
Patients should be instructed to keep EMBEDA in a secure place out of the reach of children. When EMBEDA is no longer needed, the unused capsules should be destroyed by flushing down the toilet.

17.9 FDA-APPROVED PATIENT LABELING
[See separate leaflet.]
Manufactured for: **King Pharmaceuticals, Inc.,** 501 Fifth Street, Bristol, TN 37620

(Telephone: 1-800-776-3637)
by: Actavis Elizabeth LLC, 200 Elmora Avenue, Elizabeth, NJ 07207 USA
EMBEDA is a trademark of Alpharma Pharmaceuticals LLC, a wholly owned subsidiary of King Pharmaceuticals, Inc.
KADIAN is a registered trademark of Actavis Elizabeth LLC
To report SUSPECTED ADVERSE REACTIONS, contact King Pharmaceuticals, Inc. at 1-800-546-4905 or DSP@Kingpharm.com or FDA at 1-800-FDA-1088 or www.fda. gov/medwatch
U.S. Patent Numbers:
5,202,128
5,378,474
5,330,766
40-9096
Revised – June 2009
v.10

MEDICATION GUIDE
EMBEDA™ (im-bed-a)
(morphine sulfate and naltrexone hydrochloride)
Extended Release Capsules CII

> **IMPORTANT: Keep EMBEDA in a safe place away from children. Accidental use by a child is a medical emergency and can result in death. If a child accidentally takes EMBEDA, get emergency help right away.**

Read the Medication Guide that comes with EMBEDA before you start taking it and each time you get a new prescription. There may be new information. This information does not take the place of talking with your healthcare provider about your medical condition or your treatment. Share this important information with members of your household.

What Is the Most Important Information I Should Know About EMBEDA?
- **Do not crush, dissolve, or chew EMBEDA capsules or the capsule contents before swallowing. If EMBEDA is taken in this way, both the morphine and naltrexone in EMBEDA will be released too fast. This is dangerous. It may cause you to have trouble breathing, and lead to death.**
  - If your body is not used to taking opioids and your body absorbs too much morphine, you could overdose and die.
  - If you have been taking opioids (narcotics) for a period of time, and your body absorbs the naltrexone in EMBEDA, this could cause you to have uncomfortable withdrawal symptoms.
- Take EMBEDA exactly as prescribed by your healthcare provider.
- EMBEDA is not for use to treat pain that you only have once in a while ("as needed").
- If you cannot swallow capsules, tell your healthcare provider. There may be another way to take EMBEDA that may be right for you. See "How should I take EMBEDA?"
- **Do not take the highest dose of EMBEDA (morphine sulfate 100 mg and naltrexone hydrochloride 4 mg) unless you are "opioid tolerant."** Opioid tolerant means that you regularly use another opioid medicine for your constant (around the clock) pain and your body is used to it.
- **Do not drink alcohol, or use prescription or non-prescription medicines that contain alcohol while you are being treated with EMBEDA.** Alcohol can cause very high levels of morphine in your blood and you can die due to an overdose of morphine.
- **Prevent theft, misuse or abuse.** Keep EMBEDA in a safe place to protect it from being stolen. EMBEDA can be a target for people who misuse or abuse prescription medicines or street drugs.
- **Never give EMBEDA to anyone else,** even if they have the same symptoms you have. It may harm them or even cause death.

See the section "What are the possible side effects of EMBEDA?" for more information about side effects.

What is EMBEDA?
- EMBEDA is a prescription medicine that contains morphine sulfate, an opioid receptor agonist (narcotic pain medicine) and naltrexone hydrochloride, an opioid receptor antagonist. Naltrexone hydrochloride is in the middle of each pellet and has a special coating to protect it from being released. If you crush or chew EMBEDA, the naltrexone will be released all at one time. **See "What is the most important information I should know about EMBEDA?"**
- **EMBEDA is a federally controlled substance** (CII) because it is a strong opioid pain medicine that can be abused by people who abuse prescription medicines or street drugs.

- EMBEDA is used to manage moderate to severe pain that continues around-the-clock and is expected to last for a long period of time.
- It is not known if EMBEDA is safe and works in children under the age of 18.

Who Should Not Take EMBEDA?
Do not take EMBEDA if you:
- are having an asthma attack or have severe asthma, trouble breathing, or lung problems.
- have a bowel blockage called paralytic ileus.
- are allergic to morphine, morphine salts, naltrexone, or any of the ingredients in EMBEDA. See the end of this Medication Guide for a complete list of ingredients in EMBEDA.

What Should I Tell My Healthcare Provider Before Starting EMBEDA?
- **EMBEDA may not be right for you. Tell your healthcare provider about all of your medical conditions, especially if you:**
  - have trouble breathing or lung problems
  - have a head injury or brain problem
  - have liver or kidney problems
  - have adrenal gland problems, such as Addison's disease
  - have convulsions or seizures
  - have thyroid problems
  - have problems urinating or prostate problems
  - have constipation or other bowel problems
  - have problems with your pancreas or gallbladder
  - have severe scoliosis
  - have a drinking problem or alcoholism
  - have severe mental problems or hallucinations (see or hear things that are not really there)
  - have or have had drug abuse or drug addiction problems
  - are planning to have surgery (cordotomy) or another procedure that will interrupt the pain signals to your body.
  - **are pregnant or plan to become pregnant.** EMBEDA may harm your unborn baby.
  - **are breastfeeding.** EMBEDA may pass through your milk and may harm your baby. You should not breastfeed while taking EMBEDA.
- **Tell your healthcare provider about all the medicines you take,** including prescription and nonprescription medicines, vitamins, and herbal supplements. Some medicines may cause serious problems when taken with EMBEDA. Sometimes, the doses of certain medicines and EMBEDA may need to be changed if used together.
- Be especially careful about taking other medicines that make you sleepy such as:
  - other pain medicines
  - anti-depressant medicines
  - sleeping pills
  - anti-anxiety medicines
  - muscle relaxants
  - antihistamines
  - anti-nausea medicines
  - tranquilizers
  Also tell your healthcare provider if you take:
  - cimetidine (Tagamet)
  - a water pill (diuretic)
  - an anticholinergic medicine
- Do not take EMBEDA if you already take a monoamine oxidase inhibitor medicine (MAOI) or within 14 days after you stop taking an MAOI medicine.
- **Do not take any new medicine while using EMBEDA until you have talked to your healthcare provider or pharmacist. They will tell you if it is safe to take other medicines with EMBEDA.**

Ask your healthcare provider if you are not sure if your medicine is one listed above.
Know the medicines you take. Keep a list of them to show your healthcare provider and pharmacist when you get a new medicine.

How Should I Take EMBEDA?
- **Take EMBEDA exactly as prescribed by your healthcare provider.** Do not change your dose unless your healthcare provider tells you to.
- You can take EMBEDA with or without food.
- **Swallow EMBEDA capsule whole.** Do not crush, dissolve, or chew EMBEDA or the pellets in the capsules before swallowing. See "What is the most important information I should know about EMBEDA?"
- If you cannot swallow capsules, tell your healthcare provider. There may be another way to take EMBEDA that may be right for you. If your doctor tells you that you can take EMBEDA using this other way, follow these steps:
EMBEDA can be opened and the pellets inside the capsule can be sprinkled over apple sauce, as follows:
- Open the EMBEDA capsule and sprinkle the pellets over approximately one tablespoon of apple sauce (Figure 1).

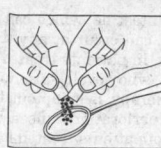

Figure 1

- Swallow all of the apple sauce and pellets right away. Do not save any of the apple sauce and pellets for another dose (*Figure 2*).

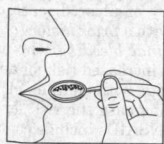

Figure 2

- Rinse your mouth to make sure you have swallowed all of the pellets. Do not chew the pellets (*Figure 3*).

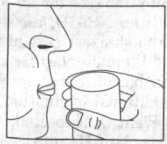

Figure 3

- Flush the empty capsule down the toilet right away (*Figure 4*).

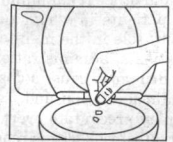

Figure 4

- You should not receive EMBEDA through a nasogastric tube or gastric tube (stomach tube).
- **If you miss a dose**, take it as soon as possible. If it is almost time for your next dose, skip the missed dose. Just take the next dose at your regular time. **Do not take 2 doses at the same time unless your healthcare provider tells you to.** If you are not sure about your dosing, call your healthcare provider.
- **If you take too much EMBEDA or overdose,** call 911 or poison control center right away.
- Call your healthcare provider if the dose of EMBEDA that you are taking does not relieve your pain.

What Should I Avoid While Taking EMBEDA?
- **Do not drive, operate heavy machinery, or do other dangerous activities, especially when you start taking EMBEDA and when your dose is changed,** until you know how you react to this medicine. EMBEDA can make you sleepy, and also cause you to feel dizzy and lightheaded. Ask your healthcare provider to tell you when it is okay to do these activities.

What are the Possible Side Effects of EMBEDA?
EMBEDA can cause serious side effects, including:
- See "What is the most important information I should know about EMBEDA?"
- **EMBEDA can cause serious breathing problems that can become life-threatening, especially if used the wrong way.**

Call your healthcare provider or get medical help right away if:
- your breathing slows down
- you have shallow breathing (little chest movement with breathing)
- you feel faint, dizzy, confused, or
- have any other unusual symptoms

These can be symptoms that you have taken too much EMBEDA (overdose) or the dose is too high for you. **These symptoms may lead to serious problems or death if not treated right away.**
- **EMBEDA can cause your blood pressure to drop.** This can make you feel dizzy and faint if you get up too fast from sitting or lying down. Low blood pressure is also more likely to happen if you take other medicines that can also lower your blood pressure. Severe low blood pressure can happen if you lose blood or take certain other medicines.
- **EMBEDA can cause physical dependence.** Do not stop taking EMBEDA or any other opioid without talking to your healthcare provider. You could become sick with un-

comfortable withdrawal symptoms because your body has become used to these medicines. Physical dependence is not the same as drug addiction.
- **There is a chance of abuse or addiction with EMBEDA.** The chance is higher if you are or have been addicted to or abused other medicines, street drugs, or alcohol, or if you have a history of mental problems.
- **Serious allergic reactions.** Rarely, severe allergic reactions happen in people who take a long-acting morphine medicine that is like EMBEDA. Get medical help right away if you have any of these symptoms of a severe allergic reaction:
  - feel dizzy or faint
  - trouble breathing
  - pounding heart beat
  - chest pain
  - swelling of the face, throat, or tongue
  - feeling of doom

The most common side effects of EMBEDA are
- constipation
- nausea
- sleepiness
- vomiting
- dizziness
- itching
- headache

These side effects may decrease with continued use. Talk to your healthcare provider if you continue to have these side effects. These are not all the possible side effects of EMBEDA. For a complete list, ask your healthcare provider or pharmacist.

Constipation (not often enough or hard bowel movements) is a common side effect of pain medicines (opioids) including EMBEDA and is unlikely to go away without treatment. Talk to your healthcare provider about dietary changes, and the use of laxatives (medicines to treat constipation) and stool softeners to prevent or treat constipation while taking EMBEDA.

Talk to your healthcare provider if you have any side effects that bother you or do not go away.

These are not all the possible side effects of EMBEDA. For more information, ask your healthcare provider or pharmacist.

Call your doctor for medical advice about side effects. You may report side effects to FDA at 1-800-FDA-1088.
- Selling or giving away this medicine is against the law

How should I store EMBEDA?
- See "What is the most important information I should know about EMBEDA?"
- **Keep EMBEDA out of the reach of children.**
- Keep EMBEDA in the container it comes in.
- Keep EMBEDA at room temperature between 59° to 86°F (15° to 30°C).
- **After you stop taking EMBEDA, flush the unused capsules down the toilet.**

General Information about EMBEDA
Medicines are sometimes prescribed for purposes other than those listed in a Medication Guide. Do not use EMBEDA for conditions for which it was not prescribed. Do not give EMBEDA to other people, even if they have the same symptoms you have. It may harm them and even cause death.

Sharing EMBEDA is against the law.
This medication guide summarizes the most important information about EMBEDA. If you would like more information, talk with your healthcare provider. Also, you can ask your pharmacist or healthcare provider for information about EMBEDA that is written for healthcare professionals. For more information call 1-800-776-3637 or go to www.kingpharm.com.

What are the ingredients in EMBEDA?
Active Ingredients: pellets of morphine sulfate and naltrexone hydrochloride

Inactive Ingredients common to all strengths: talc, ammonio methacrylate copolymer, sugar spheres, ethylcellulose, sodium chloride, polyethylene glycol, hydroxypropyl cellulose, dibutyl sebacate, methacrylic acid copolymer, diethyl phthalate, magnesium stearate, sodium lauryl sulfate, and ascorbic acid. The capsule shells contain gelatin, titanium dioxide, and grey ink, D&C yellow #10 (EMBEDA 20 mg/0.8 mg), FD&C red #3, FD&C blue #1 (EMBEDA 30 mg/1.2 mg), D&C red #28, FD&C red #40, FD&C blue #1 (EMBEDA 50 mg/2 mg), D&C red #28, FD&C red #40, FD&C blue #1 (EMBEDA 60 mg/2.4 mg), FD&C blue #1, FD&C red #40, FD&C yellow #6 (EMBEDA 80 mg/3.2 mg), D&C yellow #10, FD&C blue #1 (EMBEDA 100 mg/4 mg).

Manufactured for: King Pharmaceuticals, Inc., 501 Fifth Street, Bristol, TN 37620
(Telephone: 1-800-776-3637)
by: Actavis Elizabeth LLC, 200 Elmora Avenue, Elizabeth, NJ 07207 USA
EMBEDA is a trademark of Alpharma Pharmaceuticals LLC, a wholly owned subsidiary of King Pharmaceuticals, Inc.
41-1126

Revision: June 2009
This Medication Guide has been approved by the U.S. Food and Drug Administration
v.10
Shown in Product Identification Guide, page 310

FLECTOR® PATCH ℞
(diclofenac epolamine topical patch) 1.3%
Rx Only

BOXED WARNING
Cardiovascular Risk
- **NSAIDs may cause an increased risk of serious cardiovascular thrombotic events, myocardial infarction, and stroke, which can be fatal. This risk may increase with duration of use. Patients with cardiovascular disease or risk factors for cardiovascular disease may be at greater risk. (See WARNINGS and CLINICAL TRIALS).**
- **Flector® Patch is contraindicated for the treatment of peri-operative pain in the setting of coronary artery bypass graft (CABG) surgery (see WARNINGS).**

Gastrointestinal Risk
- **NSAIDs cause an increased risk of serious gastrointestinal adverse events including bleeding, ulceration, and perforation of the stomach or intestines, which can be fatal. These events can occur at any time during use and without warning symptoms. Elderly patients are at greater risk for serious gastrointestinal events. (See WARNINGS).**

DESCRIPTION
Flector® Patch (10 cm x 14 cm) is comprised of an adhesive material containing 1.3% diclofenac epolamine which is applied to a non-woven polyester felt backing and covered with a polypropylene film release liner. The release liner is removed prior to topical application to the skin.
Diclofenac epolamine is a non-opioid analgesic chemically designated as 2-[(2,6-dichlorophenyl) amino]benzeneacetic acid, (2-(pyrrolidin-1-yl) ethanol salt, with a molecular formula of $C_{20}H_{24}Cl_2N_2O_3$ (molecular weight 411.3), an n-octanol/water partition coefficient of 8 at pH 8.5, and the following structure:

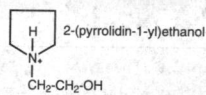

Each adhesive patch contains 180 mg of diclofenac epolamine (13 mg per gram adhesive) in an aqueous base. It also contains the following inactive ingredients: 1,3-butylene glycol, dihydroxyaluminum aminoacetate, disodium edetate, D-sorbitol, fragrance (Dalin PH), gelatin, kaolin, methylparaben, polysorbate 80, povidone, propylene glycol, propylparaben, sodium carboxymethylcellulose, sodium polyacrylate, tartaric acid, titanium dioxide, and purified water.

CLINICAL PHARMACOLOGY

Pharmacodynamics
Flector® Patch applied to intact skin provides local analgesia by releasing diclofenac epolamine from the patch into the skin. Diclofenac is a nonsteroidal anti-inflammatory drug (NSAID). In pharmacologic studies, diclofenac has shown anti-inflammatory, analgesic, and antipyretic activity. As with other NSAIDs, its mode of action is not known; its ability to inhibit prostaglandin synthesis, however, may be involved in its anti-inflammatory activity, as well as contribute to its efficacy in relieving pain associated with inflammation.

Pharmacokinetics
Absorption
Following a single application of the Flector® Patch on the upper inner arm, peak plasma concentrations of diclofenac (range 0.7–6 ng/mL) were noted between 10–20 hours of application. Plasma concentrations of diclofenac in the range of 1.3–8.8 ng/mL were noted after five days with twice-a-day Flector® Patch application.

Systemic exposure (AUC) and maximum plasma concentrations of diclofenac, after repeated dosing for four days with Flector® Patch, were lower (<1%) than after a single oral 50-mg diclofenac sodium tablet.

The pharmacokinetics of Flector® Patch has been tested in healthy volunteers at rest or undergoing moderate exercise (cycling 20 min/h for 12 h at a mean HR of 100.3 bpm). No clinically relevant differences in systemic absorption were observed, with peak plasma concentrations in the range of 2.2–8.1 ng/mL while resting, and 2.7–7.2 ng/mL during exercise.

Distribution
Diclofenac has a very high affinity (>99%) for human serum albumin.

Metabolism and Excretion
The plasma elimination half-life of diclofenac after application of Flector® Patch is approximately 12 hours. Diclofenac is eliminated through metabolism and subsequent urinary and biliary excretion of the glucuronide and the sulfate conjugates of the metabolites.

CLINICAL STUDIES
Efficacy of Flector® Patch was demonstrated in two of four studies of patients with minor sprains, strains, and contusions. Patients were randomly assigned to treatment with the Flector® Patch, or a placebo patch identical to the Flector® Patch minus the active ingredient. In the first of these two studies, patients with ankle sprains were treated once daily for a week. In the second study, patients with sprains, strains and contusions were treated twice daily for up to two weeks. Pain was assessed over the period of treatment. Patients treated with the Flector® Patch experienced a greater reduction in pain as compared to patients randomized to placebo patch as evidenced by the responder curves presented below.

Figure 1: Patients Achieving Various Levels of Pain Relief at Day 3; 14-Day Study

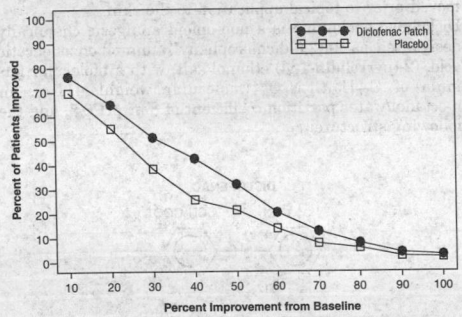

Figure 2: Patients Achieving Various Levels of Pain Relief at End of Study; 14-Day Study

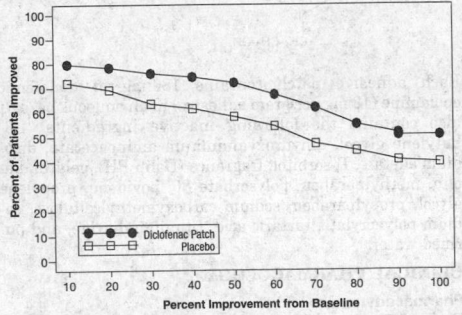

[See figure 3 at top of next column]
[See figure 4 at next column]

INDICATION AND USAGE
Carefully consider the potential benefits and risks of Flector® Patch and other treatment options before deciding to use Flector® Patch. Use the lowest effective dose for the shortest duration consistent with individual patient treatment goals (see **WARNINGS**).

Flector® Patch is indicated for the topical treatment of acute pain due to minor strains, sprains, and contusions.

CONTRAINDICATIONS
Flector® Patch is contraindicated in patients with known hypersensitivity to diclofenac.

Flector® Patch should not be given to patients who have experienced asthma, urticaria, or allergic-type reactions after taking aspirin or other NSAIDs. Severe, rarely fatal,

Figure 3: Patients Achieving Various Levels of Pain Relief at Day 3; 7-Day Study

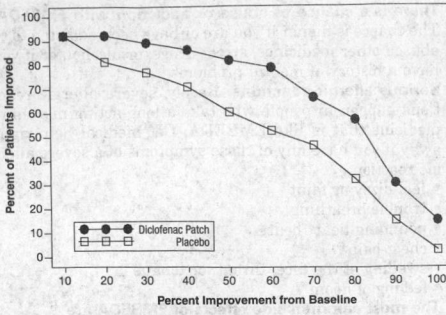

Figure 4: Patients Achieving Various Levels of Pain Relief at End of Study; 7-Day Study

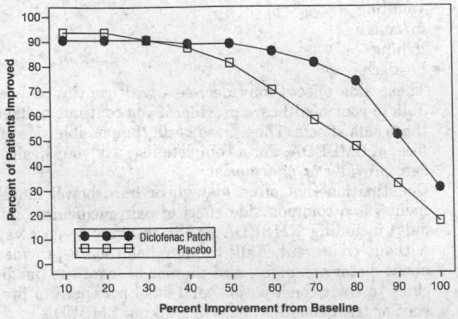

anaphylactic-like reactions to NSAIDs have been reported in such patients (see **WARNINGS - Anaphylactoid Reactions**, and **PRECAUTIONS - Preexisting Asthma**).

Flector® Patch is contraindicated for the treatment of perioperative pain in the setting of coronary artery bypass graft (CABG) surgery (see **WARNINGS**).

Flector® Patch should not be applied to non-intact or damaged skin resulting from any etiology e.g. exudative dermatitis, eczema, infected lesion, burns or wounds.

WARNINGS
CARDIOVASCULAR EFFECTS
Cardiovascular Thrombotic Events
Clinical trials of several COX-2 selective and nonselective NSAIDs of up to three years duration have shown an increased risk of serious cardiovascular (CV) thrombotic events, myocardial infarction, and stroke, which can be fatal. All NSAIDs, both COX-2 selective and nonselective, may have a similar risk. Patients with known CV disease or risk factors for CV disease may be at greater risk. To minimize the potential risk for an adverse CV event in patients treated with an NSAID, the lowest effective dose should be used for the shortest duration possible. Physicians and patients should remain alert for the development of such events, even in the absence of previous CV symptoms. Patients should be informed about the signs and/or symptoms of serious CV events and the steps to take if they occur.

There is no consistent evidence that concurrent use of aspirin mitigates the increased risk of serious CV thrombotic events associated with NSAID use. The concurrent use of aspirin and an NSAID does increase the risk of serious GI events (see **GI WARNINGS**).

Two large, controlled, clinical trials of a COX-2 selective NSAID for the treatment of pain in the first 10-14 days following CABG surgery found an increased incidence of myocardial infarction and stroke (see **CONTRAINDICATIONS**).

Hypertension
NSAIDs, including Flector® Patch, can lead to onset of new hypertension or worsening of pre-existing hypertension, either of which may contribute to the increased incidence of CV events. Patients taking thiazides or loop diuretics may have impaired response to these therapies when taking NSAIDs. NSAIDs, including Flector® Patch, should be used with caution in patients with hypertension. Blood pressure (BP) should be monitored closely during the initiation of NSAID treatment and throughout the course of therapy.

Congestive Heart Failure and Edema
Fluid retention and edema have been observed in some patients taking NSAIDs. Flector® Patch should be used with caution in patients with fluid retention or heart failure.

Gastrointestinal Effects- Risk of Ulceration, Bleeding, and Perforation
NSAIDs, including Flector® Patch, can cause serious gastrointestinal (GI) adverse events including inflammation, bleeding, ulceration, and perforation of the stomach, small

intestine, or large intestine, which can be fatal. These serious adverse events can occur at any time, with or without warning symptoms, in patients treated with NSAIDs. Only one in five patients, who develop a serious upper GI adverse event on NSAID therapy, is symptomatic. Upper GI ulcers, gross bleeding, or perforation caused by NSAIDs occur in approximately 1% of patients treated for 3-6 months, and in about 2-4% of patients treated for one year. These trends continue with longer duration of use, increasing the likelihood of developing a serious GI event at some time during the course of therapy. However, even short-term therapy is not without risk.

NSAIDs should be prescribed with extreme caution in those with a prior history of ulcer disease or gastrointestinal bleeding. Patients with a *prior history of peptic ulcer disease and/or gastrointestinal bleeding* who use NSAIDs have a greater than 10-fold increased risk for developing a GI bleed compared to patients with neither of these risk factors. Other factors that increase the risk for GI bleeding in patients treated with NSAIDs include concomitant use of oral corticosteroids or anticoagulants, longer duration of NSAID therapy, smoking, use of alcohol, older age, and poor general health status. Most spontaneous reports of fatal GI events are in elderly or debilitated patients and therefore, special care should be taken in treating this population.

To minimize the potential risk for an adverse GI event in patients treated with an NSAID, the lowest effective dose should be used for the shortest possible duration. Patients and physicians should remain alert for signs and symptoms of GI ulceration and bleeding during NSAID therapy and promptly initiate additional evaluation and treatment if a serious GI adverse event is suspected. This should include discontinuation of the NSAID until a serious GI adverse event is ruled out. For high risk patients, alternate therapies that do not involve NSAIDs should be considered.

Renal Effects
Long-term administration of NSAIDs has resulted in renal papillary necrosis and other renal injury. Renal toxicity has also been seen in patients in whom renal prostaglandins have a compensatory role in the maintenance of renal perfusion. In these patients, administration of a nonsteroidal anti-inflammatory drug may cause a dose-dependent reduction in prostaglandin formation and, secondarily, in renal blood flow, which may precipitate overt renal decompensation. Patients at greatest risk of this reaction are those with impaired renal function, heart failure, liver dysfunction, those taking diuretics and ACE inhibitors, and the elderly. Discontinuation of NSAID therapy is usually followed by recovery to the pretreatment state.

Hepatic Effects
Elevations of one or more liver tests may occur during therapy with Flector® Patch. These laboratory abnormalities may progress, may remain unchanged, or may be transient with continued therapy. Borderline elevations (i.e., less than 3 times the ULN [ULN = the upper limit of the normal range]) or greater elevations of transaminases occurred in about 15% of diclofenac-treated patients. Of the markers of hepatic function, ALT (SGPT) is recommended for the monitoring of liver injury.

In clinical trials, meaningful elevations (i.e., more than 3 times the ULN) of AST (GOT) (ALT was not measured in all studies) occurred in about 2% of approximately 5,700 patients at some time during diclofenac treatment. In a large, open-label, controlled trial of 3,700 patients treated for 2-6 months, patients were monitored first at 8 weeks and 1,200 patients were monitored again at 24 weeks. Meaningful elevations of ALT and/or AST occurred in about 4% of patients and included marked elevations (i.e., more than 8 times the ULN) in about 1% of the 3,700 patients. In that open-label study, a higher incidence of borderline (less than 3 times the ULN), moderate (3-8 times the ULN), and marked (>8 times the ULN) elevations of ATL or AST was observed in patients receiving diclofenac when compared to other NSAIDs. Elevations in transaminases were seen more frequently in patients with osteoarthritis than in those with rheumatoid arthritis.

Almost all meaningful elevations in transaminases were detected before patients became symptomatic. Abnormal tests occurred during the first 2 months of therapy with diclofenac in 42 of the 51 patients in all trials who developed marked transaminase elevations.

In postmarketing reports, cases of drug-induced hepatotoxicity have been reported in the first month, and in some cases, the first 2 months of therapy, but can occur at any time during treatment with diclofenac. Postmarketing surveillance has reported cases of severe hepatic reactions, including liver necrosis, jaundice, fulminant hepatitis with and without jaundice, and liver failure. Some of these reported cases resulted in fatalities or liver transplantation. Physicians should measure transaminases periodically in patients receiving long-term therapy with diclofenac, because severe hepatotoxicity may develop without a prodrome of distinguishing symptoms. The optimum times for making the first and subsequent transaminase measurements are not known. Based on clinical trial data and post-marketing experiences, transaminases should be monitored within 4 to 8 weeks after initiating treatment with diclofenac. However, severe hepatic reactions can occur at any time during treatment with diclofenac.

If abnormal liver tests persist or worsen, if clinical signs and/or symptoms consistent with liver disease develop, or if systemic manifestations occur (e.g. eosinophilia, rash, abdominal pain, diarrhea, dark urine, etc.), Flector® Patch should be discontinued immediately. To minimize the possibility that hepatic injury will become severe between transaminase measurements, physicians should inform patients of the warning signs and symptoms of hepatotoxicity (e.g., nausea, fatigue, lethargy, diarrhea, pruritus, jaundice, right upper quadrant tenderness, and "flu-like" symptoms), and the appropriate action patients should take if these signs and symptoms appear.

To minimize the potential risk for an adverse liver related event in patients treated with Flector® Patch, the lowest effective dose should be used for the shortest duration possible. Caution should be exercised in prescribing Flector® Patch with concomitant drugs that are known to be potentially hepatotoxic (e.g., antibiotics, anti-epileptics).

Advanced Renal Disease
No information is available from controlled clinical studies regarding the use of Flector® Patch in patients with advanced renal disease. Therefore, treatment with Flector® Patch is not recommended in these patients with advanced renal disease. If Flector® Patch therapy is initiated, close monitoring of the patient's renal function is advisable.

Anaphylactoid Reactions
As with other NSAIDs, anaphylactoid reactions may occur in patients without known prior exposure to Flector® Patch. Flector® Patch should not be given to patients with the aspirin triad. This symptom complex typically occurs in asthmatic patients who experience rhinitis with or without nasal polyps, or who exhibit severe, potentially fatal bronchospasm after taking aspirin or other NSAIDs (see **CONTRAINDICATIONS** and **PRECAUTIONS - Pre-existing Asthma**). Emergency help should be sought in cases where an anaphylactoid reaction occurs.

Skin Reactions
NSAIDs, including Flector® Patch, can cause serious skin adverse events such as exfoliative dermatitis, Stevens-Johnson Syndrome (SJS), and toxic epidermal necrolysis (TEN), which can be fatal. These serious events may occur without warning. Patients should be informed about the signs and symptoms of serious skin manifestations and use of the drug should be discontinued at the first appearance of skin rash or any other sign of hypersensitivity.

Pregnancy
In late pregnancy, as with other NSAIDs, Flector® Patch should be avoided because it may cause premature closure of the ductus arteriosus.

PRECAUTIONS
General
Flector® Patch cannot be expected to substitute for corticosteroids or to treat corticosteroid insufficiency. Abrupt discontinuation of corticosteroids may lead to disease exacerbation. Patients on prolonged corticosteroid therapy should have their therapy tapered slowly if a decision is made to discontinue corticosteroids.

The pharmacological activity of Flector® Patch in reducing inflammation may diminish the utility of these diagnostic signs in detecting complications of presumed noninfectious, painful conditions.

Hematological Effects
Anemia is sometimes seen in patients receiving NSAIDs. This may be due to fluid retention, occult or gross GI blood loss, or an incompletely described effect upon erythropoiesis. Patients on long-term treatment with NSAIDs, including Flector® Patch, should have their hemoglobin or hematocrit checked if they exhibit any signs or symptoms of anemia.

NSAIDs inhibit platelet aggregation and have been shown to prolong bleeding time in some patients. Unlike aspirin, their effect on platelet function is quantitatively less, of shorter duration, and reversible. Patients receiving Flector® Patch who may be adversely affected by alterations in platelet function, such as those with coagulation disorders or patients receiving anticoagulants, should be carefully monitored.

Preexisting Asthma
Patients with asthma may have aspirin-sensitive asthma. The use of aspirin in patients with aspirin-sensitive asthma has been associated with severe bronchospasm which can be fatal. Since cross reactivity, including bronchospasm, between aspirin and other nonsteroidal anti-inflammatory drugs has been reported in such aspirin-sensitive patients, Flector® Patch should not be administered to patients with this form of aspirin sensitivity and should be used with caution in patients with preexisting asthma.

Eye Exposure
Contact of Flector® Patch with eyes and mucosa, although not studied, should be avoided. If eye contact occurs, immediately wash out the eye with water or saline. Consult a physician if irritation persists for more than an hour.

Accidental Exposure in Children
Even a used Flector® Patch contains a large amount of diclofenac epolamine (as much as 170 mg). The potential therefore exists for a small child or pet to suffer serious adverse effects from chewing or ingesting a new or used Flector® Patch. It is important for patients to store and dispose of Flector® Patch out of the reach of children and pets.

Information for Patients
Patients should be informed of the following information before initiating therapy with an NSAID and periodically during the course of ongoing therapy. Patients should also be encouraged to read the NSAID Medication Guide that accompanies each prescription dispensed.

1. Flector® Patch, like other NSAIDs, may cause serious CV side effects, such as MI or stroke, which may result in hospitalization and even death. Although serious CV events can occur without warning symptoms, patients should be alert for the signs and symptoms of chest pain, shortness of breath, weakness, slurring of speech, and should ask for medical advice when observing any indicative sign or symptoms. Patients should be apprised of the importance of this follow-up (see **WARNINGS, Cardiovascular Effects**).

2. Flector® Patch, like other NSAIDs, may cause GI discomfort and, rarely, serious GI side effects, such as ulcers and bleeding, which may result in hospitalization and even death. Although serious GI tract ulcerations and bleeding can occur without warning symptoms, patients should be alert for the signs and symptoms of ulcerations and bleeding, and should ask for medical advice when observing any indicative sign or symptoms including epigastric pain, dyspepsia, melena, and hematemesis. Patients should be apprised of the importance of this follow-up (see **WARNINGS, Gastrointestinal Effects: Risk of Ulceration, Bleeding, and Perforation**).

3. Flector® Patch, like other NSAIDs, may cause serious skin side effects such as exfoliative dermatitis, SJS, and TEN, which may result in hospitalizations and even death. Although serious skin reactions may occur without warning, patients should be alert for the signs and symptoms of skin rash and blisters, fever, or other signs of hypersensitivity such as itching, and should ask for medical advice when observing any indicative signs or symptoms. Patients should be advised to stop the drug immediately if they develop any type of rash and contact their physicians as soon as possible.

4. Patients should be instructed to promptly report signs or symptoms of unexplained weight gain or edema to their physicians (see **WARNINGS, Cardiovascular Effects**).

5. Patients should be informed of the warning signs and symptoms of hepatotoxicity (e.g., nausea, fatigue, lethargy, pruritus, jaundice, right upper quadrant tenderness, and "flu-like" symptoms). If these occur, patients should be instructed to stop therapy and seek immediate medical therapy

6. Patients should be informed of the signs of an anaphylactoid reaction (e.g. difficulty breathing, swelling of the face or throat). If these occur, patients should be instructed to seek immediate emergency help (see **WARNINGS**).

7. In late pregnancy, as with other NSAIDs, Flector® Patch should be avoided because it may cause premature closure of the ductus arteriosus.

8. Patients should be advised not to use Flector® Patch if they have an aspirin-sensitive asthma. Flector® Patch, like other NSAIDs, could cause severe and even fatal bronchospasm in these patients (see **PRECAUTIONS, Preexisting asthma**). Patients should discontinue use of Flector® Patch and should immediately seek emergency help if they experience wheezing or shortness of breath

9. Patients should be informed that Flector® Patch should be used only on intact skin.

10. Patients should be advised to avoid contact of Flector® Patch with eyes and mucosa. Patients should be instructed that if eye contact occurs, they should immediately wash out the eye with water or saline, and consult a physician if irritation persists for more than an hour

11. Patients and caregivers should be instructed to wash their hands after applying, handling or removing the patch.

12. Patients should be informed that, if Flector® Patch begins to peel off, the edges of the patch may be taped down.

13. Patients should be instructed not to wear Flector® Patch during bathing or showering. Bathing should take place in between scheduled patch removal and application (see **DOSAGE AND ADMINISTRATION**).

14. Patients should be advised to store Flector® Patch and to discard used patches out of the reach of children and pets. If a child or pet accidentally ingests Flector® Patch, medical help should be sought immediately (see **PRECAUTIONS, Accidental Exposure in Children**).

Laboratory Tests
Because serious GI tract ulcerations and bleeding can occur without warning symptoms, physicians should monitor for signs or symptoms of GI bleeding. Patients on long-term treatment with NSAIDs, should have their CBC and a chemistry profile checked periodically. If clinical signs and symptoms consistent with liver or renal disease develop, systemic manifestations occur (e.g., eosinophilia, rash, etc.) or if abnormal liver tests persist or worsen, Flector® Patch should be discontinued.

Drug Interactions
ACE-inhibitors
Reports suggest that NSAIDs may diminish the antihypertensive effect of ACE-inhibitors. This interaction should be given consideration in patients taking NSAIDs concomitantly with ACE-inhibitors.

Aspirin
When Flector® Patch is administered with aspirin, the binding of diclofenac to protein is reduced, although the clearance of free diclofenac is not altered. The clinical significance of this interaction is not known; however, as with other NSAIDs, concomitant administration of diclofenac and aspirin is not generally recommended because of the potential of increased adverse effects.

Diuretics
Clinical studies, as well as post marketing observations, have shown that Flector® Patch may reduce the natriuretic effect of furosemide and thiazides in some patients. This response has been attributed to inhibition of renal prostaglandin synthesis. During concomitant therapy with NSAIDs, the patient should be observed closely for signs of renal failure (see **WARNINGS, Renal Effects**), as well as to assure diuretic efficacy.

Lithium
NSAIDs have produced an elevation of plasma lithium levels and a reduction in renal lithium clearance. The mean minimum lithium concentration increased 15% and the renal clearance was decreased by approximately 20%. These effects have been attributed to inhibition of renal prostaglandin synthesis by the NSAID. Thus, when NSAIDs and lithium are administered concurrently, subjects should be observed carefully for signs of lithium toxicity.

Methotrexate
NSAIDs have been reported to competitively inhibit methotrexate accumulation in rabbit kidney slices. This may indicate that they could enhance the toxicity of methotrexate. Caution should be used when NSAIDs are administered concomitantly with methotrexate.

Warfarin
The effects of warfarin and NSAIDs on GI bleeding are synergistic, such that users of both drugs together have a risk of serious GI bleeding higher than users of either drug alone.

Carcinogenesis, Mutagenesis, Impairment of Fertility
Carcinogenesis
Long-term studies in animals have not been performed to evaluate the carcinogenic potential of either diclofenac epolamine or Flector® Patch.

Mutagenesis
Diclofenac epolamine is not mutagenic in *Salmonella Typhimurium* strains, nor does it induce an increase in metabolic aberrations in cultured human lymphocytes, or the frequency of micronucleated cells in the bone marrow micronucleus test performed in rats.

Impairment of Fertility
Male and female Sprague Dawley rats were administered 1, 3, or 6 mg/kg/day diclofenac epolamine via oral gavage (males treated for 60 days prior to conception and during mating period, females treated for 14 days prior to mating through day 19 of gestation). Diclofenac epolamine treatment with 6 mg/kg/day resulted in increased early resorptions and postimplantation losses; however, no effects on the mating and fertility indices were found. The 6 mg/kg/day dose corresponds to 3-times the maximum recommended daily exposure in humans based on a body surface area comparison.

Pregnancy
Teratogenic Effects. Pregnancy Category C.
Pregnant Sprague Dawley rats were administered 1, 3, or 6 mg/kg diclofenac epolamine via oral gavage daily from gestation days 6-15. Maternal toxicity, embryotoxicity, and increased incidence of skeletal anomalies were noted with 6 mg/kg/day diclofenac epolamine, which corresponds to 3-times the maximum recommended daily exposure in humans based on a body surface area comparison. Pregnant New Zealand White rabbits were administered 1, 3, or 6 mg/kg diclofenac epolamine via oral gavage daily from gestation days 6-18. No maternal toxicity was noted; however, embryotoxicity was evident at 6 mg/kg/day group

which corresponds to 6.5-times the maximum recommended daily exposure in humans based on a body surface area comparison.

There are no adequate and well-controlled studies in pregnant women. Flector® Patch should be used during pregnancy only if the potential benefit justifies the potential risk to the fetus.

Nonteratogenic Effects

Because of the known effects of nonsteroidal anti-inflammatory drugs on the fetal cardiovascular system (closure of ductus arteriosus), use during pregnancy (particularly late pregnancy) should be avoided.

Male rats were orally administered diclofenac epolamine (1, 3, 6 mg/kg) for 60 days prior to mating and throughout the mating period, and females were given the same doses 14 days prior to mating and through mating, gestation, and lactation. Embryotoxicity was observed at 6 mg/kg diclofenac epolamine (3-times the maximum recommended daily exposure in humans based on a body surface area comparison), and was manifested as an increase in early resorptions, post-implantation losses, and a decrease in live fetuses. The number of live born and total born were also reduced as was F1 postnatal survival, but the physical and behavioral development of surviving F1 pups in all groups was the same as the deionized water control, nor was reproductive performance adversely affected despite a slight treatment-related reduction in body weight.

Labor and Delivery

In rat studies with NSAIDs, as with other drugs known to inhibit prostaglandin synthesis, an increased incidence of dystocia, delayed parturition, and decreased pup survival occurred. The effects of Flector® Patch on labor and delivery in pregnant women are unknown.

Nursing Mothers

It is not known whether this drug is excreted in human milk. Because many drugs are excreted in human-milk and because of the potential for serious adverse reactions in nursing infants from Flector® Patch, a decision should be made whether to discontinue nursing or to discontinue the drug, taking into account the importance of the drug to the mother.

Pediatric Use

Safety and effectiveness in pediatric patients have not been established.

Geriatric Use

Clinical studies of Flector® Patch did not include sufficient numbers of subjects aged 65 and over to determine whether they respond differently from younger subjects. Other reported clinical experience has not identified differences in responses between the elderly and younger patients.

Diclofenac, as with any NSAID, is known to be substantially excreted by the kidney, and the risk of toxic reactions to Flector® Patch may be greater in patients with impaired renal function. Because elderly patients are more likely to have decreased renal function, care should be taken when using Flector® Patch in the elderly, and it may be useful to monitor renal function.

ADVERSE REACTIONS

In controlled trials during the premarketing development of Flector® Patch, approximately 600 patients with minor sprains, strains, and contusions have been treated with Flector® Patch for up to two weeks.

Adverse Events Leading to Discontinuation of Treatment

In the controlled trials, 3% of patients in both the Flector® Patch and placebo patch groups discontinued treatment due to an adverse event. The most common adverse events leading to discontinuation were application site reactions, occurring in 2% of both the Flector® Patch and placebo patch groups. Application site reactions leading to dropout included pruritus, dermatitis, and burning.

Common Adverse Events

Localized Reactions

Overall, the most common adverse events associated with Flector® Patch treatment were skin reactions at the site of treatment.

Table 1 lists all adverse events, regardless of causality, occurring in ≥ 1% of patients in controlled trials of Flector® Patch. A majority of patients treated with Flector® Patch had adverse events with a maximum intensity of "mild" or "moderate."

[See table 1 below]

Foreign labeling describes that dermal allergic reactions may occur with Flector® Patch treatment. Additionally, the treated area may become irritated or develop itching, erythema, edema, vesicles, or abnormal sensation.

DRUG ABUSE AND DEPENDENCE

Controlled Substance Class

Flector® Patch is not a controlled substance.

Physical and Psychological Dependence

Diclofenac, the active ingredient in Flector® Patch, is an NSAID that does not lead to physical or psychological dependence.

OVERDOSAGE

There is limited experience with overdose of Flector® Patch. In clinical studies, the maximum single dose administered was one Flector® Patch containing 180 mg of diclofenac epolamine. There were no serious adverse events.

Should systemic side effects occur due to incorrect use or accidental overdose of this product, the general measures recommended for intoxication with non-steroidal anti-inflammatory drugs should be taken.

DOSAGE AND ADMINISTRATION

Carefully consider the potential benefits and risks of Flector® Patch and other treatment options before deciding to use Flector® Patch. Use the lowest effective dose for the shortest duration consistent with individual patient treatment goals (see **WARNINGS**).

The recommended dose of Flector® Patch is one (1) patch to the most painful area twice a day.

Flector® patch should not be applied to damaged or non-intact skin.

Flector® patch should not be worn when bathing or showering.

HANDLING AND DISPOSAL

Patients and caregivers should wash their hands after applying, handling or removing the patch. Eye contact should be avoided.

HOW SUPPLIED

The Flector® Patch is supplied in resealable envelopes, each containing 5 patches (10 cm × 14 cm), with 6 envelopes per box (NDC 60793-411-30). Each individual patch is embossed with "FLECTOR PATCH <DICLOFENAC EPOLAMINE TOPICAL PATCH> 1.3%".

- Each patch contains 180 mg of diclofenac epolamine in an aqueous base (13 mg of active per gram of adhesive or 1.3%).
- The product is intended for topical use only.
- Keep out of reach of children and pets.
- THE ENVELOPES SHOULD BE SEALED AT ALL TIMES WHEN NOT IN USE.
- Store at 25°C (77°F); excursions permitted to 15°-30°C (59°-86°F). [See USP Controlled Room Temperature].

Distributed by: King Pharmaceuticals, Inc.
501 Fifth Street
Bristol, TN 37620, USA
Telephone:1-888-840-8884
www.FlectorPatch.com

Manufactured for: IBSA Institut Biochimique SA, CH-6903 Lugano, Switzerland
Manufactured by: Teikoku Seiyaku Co., Ltd., Sanbonmatsu, Kagawa 769-2695 Japan
Version October 2009
FI/161 1086
Ed V/10.09

Medication Guide for Non-Steroidal Anti-Inflammatory Drugs (NSAIDs)

(See the end of this Medication Guide for a list of prescription NSAID medicines.)

What is the most important information I should know about medicines called Non-Steroidal Anti-Inflammatory Drugs (NSAIDs)?

NSAID medicines may increase the chance of a heart attack or stroke that can lead to death. This chance increases:
- with longer use of NSAID medicines
- in people who have heart disease

NSAID medicines should never be used right before or after a heart surgery called a "coronary artery bypass graft" (CABG).

NSAID medicines can cause ulcers and bleeding in the stomach and intestines at any time during treatment. Ulcers and bleeding:
- can happen without warning symptom
- may cause death

The chance of a person getting an ulcer or bleeding increases with:
- taking medicines called "corticosteroids" and "anticoagulants"
- longer use
- smoking
- drinking alcohol
- older age
- having poor health

NSAID medicines should only be used:
- exactly as prescribed
- at the lowest dose possible for your treatment
- for the shortest time needed

What are Non-Steroidal Anti-Inflammatory Drugs (NSAIDs)?

NSAID medicines are used to treat pain and redness, swelling, and heat (inflammation) from medical conditions such as:
- different types of arthritis
- menstrual cramps and other types of short-term pain

Who should not take a Non-Steroidal Anti-Inflammatory Drug (NSAID)?

Do not take an NSAID medicine:
- if you had an asthma attack, hives, or other allergic reaction with aspirin or any other NSAID medicine

Table 1. Common Adverse Events (by body system and preferred term) in ≥1% of Patients treated with Flector® Patch or Placebo Patch[1]

	Diclofenac N=572		Placebo N=564	
	N	Percent	N	Percent
Application Site Conditions	64	11	70	12
Pruritus	31	5	44	8
Dermatitis	9	2	3	<1
Burning	2	<1	8	1
Other[2]	22	4	15	3
Gastrointestinal Disorders	49	9	33	6
Nausea	17	3	11	2
Dysgeusia	10	2	3	<1
Dyspepsia	7	1	8	1
Other[3]	15	3	11	2
Nervous System Disorders	13	2	18	3
Headache	7	1	10	2
Paresthesia	6	1	8	1
Somnolence	4	1	6	1
Other[4]	4	1	3	<1

[1] The table lists adverse events occurring in placebo-treated patients because the placebo-patch was comprised of the same ingredients as Flector® Patch except for diclofenac. Adverse events in the placebo group may therefore reflect effects of the non-active ingredients.
[2] Includes: application site dryness, irritation, erythema, atrophy, discoloration, hyperhidriosis, and vesicles.
[3] Includes: gastritis, vomiting, diarrhea, constipation, upper abdominal pain, and dry mouth.
[4] Includes: hypoaesthesia, dizziness, and hyperkinesias.

• for pain right before or after heart bypass surgery

Tell your healthcare provider:
• about all of your medical conditions.
• about all of the medicines you take. NSAIDs and some other medicines can interact with each other and cause serious side effects.
Keep a list of your medicines to show to your healthcare provider and pharmacist.
• if you are pregnant.
NSAID medicines should not be used by pregnant women late in their pregnancy.
• if you are breastfeeding.
Talk to your doctor.

What are the possible side effects of Non-Steroidal Anti-Inflammatory Drugs (NSAIDs)?

Serious side effects include:	Other side effects include:
• heart attack	• stomach pain
• stroke	• constipation
• high blood pressure	• diarrhea
• heart failure from body swelling (fluid retention)	• gas
• kidney problems including kidney failure	• heartburn
• bleeding and ulcers in the stomach and intestine	• nausea
• low red blood cells (anemia)	• vomiting
• life-threatening skin reactions	• dizziness
• life-threatening allergic reactions	
• liver problems including liver failure	
• asthma attacks in people who have asthma	

Get emergency help right away if you have any of the following symptoms:
• shortness of breath or trouble breathing
• chest pain
• weakness in one part or side of your body
• slurred speech
• swelling of the face or throat

Stop your NSAID medicine and call your healthcare provider right away if you have any of the following symptoms:
• nausea
• more tired or weaker than usual
• itching
• your skin or eyes look yellow
• stomach pain
• flu-like symptoms
• vomit blood
• there is blood in your bowel movement or it is black and sticky like tar
• unusual weight gain
• skin rash or blisters with fever
• swelling of the arms and legs, hands and feet

These are not all the side effects with NSAID medicines. Talk to your healthcare provided or pharmacist for more information about NSAID medicines.
Call your doctor for medical advice about side effects. You may report side effects to FDA at 1-800-FDA-1088.

Other information about Non-Steroidal Anti-Inflammatory Drugs (NSAIDs)
• Aspirin is an NSAID medicine but it does not increase the chance of a heart attack. Aspirin can cause bleeding in the brain, stomach, and intestines. Aspirin can also cause ulcers in the stomach and intestines.
• Some of these NSAID medicines are sold in lower doses without a prescription (over–the–counter). Talk to your healthcare provider before using over–the–counter NSAIDs for more than 10 days.

NSAID medicines that need a prescription

Generic Name	Tradename
Celecoxib	Celebrex
Diclofenac	Flector, Cataflam, Voltaren, Arthrotec (combined with misoprostol)
Diflunisal	Dolobid
Etodolac	Lodine, Lodine XL
Fenoprofen	Nalfon, Nalfon 200
Flurbirofen	Ansaid
Ibuprofen	Motrin, Tab-Profen, Vicoprofen (combined with hydrocodone), Combunox (combined with oxycodone)
Indomethacin	Indocin, Indocin SR, Indo-Lemmon, Indomethagan
Ketoprofen	Oruvail
Ketorolac	Toradol
Mefenamic Acid	Ponstel
Meloxicam	Mobic
Nabumetone	Relafen
Naproxen	Naprosyn, Anaprox, Anaprox DS, EC-Naproxyn, Naprelan, Naprapac (copackaged with lansoprazole)
Oxaprozin	Daypro
Piroxicam	Feldene
Sulindac	Clinoril
Tolmetin	Tolectin, Tolectin DS, Tolectin 600

This Medication Guide has been approved by the U.S. Food and Drug Administration.
Distributed by: King Pharmaceuticals, Inc.
501 Fifth Street
Bristol, TN 37620, USA
Telephone:1-888-840-8884
www.FlectorPatch.com
Manufactured for: IBSA Institut Biochimique SA, CH-6903 Lugano, Switzerland
Manufactured by: Teikoku Seiyaku Co., Ltd., Sanbonmatsu, Kagawa 769-2695 Japan
Version October 2009
FI/161 1086
Ed. V/10.09
Shown in Product Identification Guide, page 310

LEVOXYL® ℞
[lĕ-vŏks-əl]
(levothyroxine sodium tablets, USP)

DESCRIPTION

–LEVOXYL® (levothyroxine sodium tablets, USP) contain synthetic crystalline L-3,3′,5,5′-tetraiodothyronine sodium salt [levothyroxine (T_4) sodium]. Synthetic T_4 is identical to that produced in the human thyroid gland. Levothyroxine (T_4) sodium has an empirical formula of $C_{15}H_{10}I_4N$ NaO_4 • H_2O, molecular weight of 798.86 g/mol (anhydrous), and structural formula as shown:

Inactive Ingredients
Microcrystalline cellulose, croscarmellose sodium and magnesium stearate. The following are the coloring additives per tablet strength:

Strength (mcg)	Color additive(s)
25	FD&C Yellow No. 6 Aluminum Lake
50	None
75	FD&C Blue No. 1 Aluminum Lake, D&C Red No. 30 Aluminum Lake
88	FD&C Yellow No. 6 Aluminum Lake, FD&C Blue No. 1 Aluminum Lake, D&C Yellow No. 10 Aluminum Lake
100	FD&C Yellow No. 6 Aluminum Lake, D&C Yellow No. 10 Aluminum Lake
112	FD&C Yellow No. 6 Aluminum Lake, FD&C Red No. 40 Aluminum Lake, D&C Red No. 30 Aluminum Lake
125	FD&C Red No. 40 Aluminum Lake, D&C Yellow No. 10 Aluminum Lake
137	FD&C Blue No. 1 Aluminum Lake
150	FD&C Blue No. 1 Aluminum Lake, D&C Red No. 30 Aluminum Lake
175	FD&C Blue No. 1 Aluminum Lake, D&C Yellow No. 10 Aluminum Lake
200	D&C Red No. 30 Aluminum Lake, D&C Yellow No. 10 Aluminum Lake

CLINICAL PHARMACOLOGY

Thyroid hormone synthesis and secretion is regulated by the hypothalamic-pituitary-thyroid axis. Thyrotropin-releasing hormone (TRH) released from the hypothalamus stimulates secretion of thyroid-stimulating hormone, TSH, from the anterior pituitary. TSH, in turn, is the physiologic stimulus for the synthesis and secretion of thyroid hormones, L-thyroxine (T_4) and L-triiodothyronine (T_3), by the thyroid gland. Circulating serum T_3 and T_4 levels exert a feedback effect on both TRH and TSH secretion. When serum T_3 and T_4 levels increase, TRH and TSH secretion decrease. When thyroid hormone levels decrease, TRH and TSH secretion increase.

The mechanisms by which thyroid hormones exert their physiologic actions are not completely understood, but it is thought that their principal effects are exerted through control of DNA transcription and protein synthesis. T_3 and T_4 diffuse into the cell nucleus and bind to thyroid receptor proteins attached to DNA. This hormone nuclear receptor complex activates gene transcription and synthesis of messenger RNA and cytoplasmic proteins.

Thyroid hormones regulate multiple metabolic processes and play an essential role in normal growth and development, and normal maturation of the central nervous system and bone. The metabolic actions of thyroid hormones include augmentation of cellular respiration and thermogenesis, as well as metabolism of proteins, carbohydrates and lipids. The protein anabolic effects of thyroid hormones are essential to normal growth and development.

The physiologic actions of thyroid hormones are produced predominantly by T_3, the majority of which (approximately 80%) is derived from T_4 by deiodination in peripheral tissues.

Levothyroxine, at doses individualized according to patient response, is effective as replacement or supplemental therapy in hypothyroidism of any etiology, except transient hypothyroidism during the recovery phase of subacute thyroiditis.

Levothyroxine is also effective in the suppression of pituitary TSH secretion in the treatment or prevention of various types of euthyroid goiters, including thyroid nodules, Hashimoto's thyroiditis, multinodular goiter and, as adjunctive therapy in the management of thyrotropin-dependent well-differentiated thyroid cancer (see **INDICATIONS AND USAGE, PRECAUTIONS, DOSAGE AND ADMINISTRATION**).

Pharmacokinetics

Absorption—Absorption of orally administered T_4 from the gastrointestinal (GI) tract ranges from 40% to 80%. The majority of the levothyroxine dose is absorbed from the jejunum and upper ileum. The relative bioavailability of LEVOXYL® tablets, compared to an equal nominal dose of oral levothyroxine sodium solution, is approximately 98%. T_4 absorption is increased by fasting, and decreased in malabsorption syndromes and by certain foods such as soybean infant formula. Dietary fiber decreases bioavailability of T_4. Absorption may also decrease with age. In addition, many drugs and foods affect T_4 absorption (see **PRECAUTIONS, Drug Interactions** and **Drug-Food Interactions**).

Distribution—Circulating thyroid hormones are greater than 99% bound to plasma proteins, including thyroxine-binding globulin (TBG), thyroxine-binding prealbumin (TBPA), and albumin (TBA), whose capacities and affinities vary for each hormone. The higher affinity of both TBG and TBPA for T_4 partially explains the higher serum levels, slower metabolic clearance, and longer half-life of T_4 compared to T_3. Protein-bound thyroid hormones exist in reverse equilibrium with small amounts of free hormone. Only unbound hormone is metabolically active. Many drugs and physiologic conditions affect the binding of thyroid hormones to serum proteins (see **PRECAUTIONS, Drug Interactions** and **Drug-Laboratory Test Interactions**). Thyroid hormones do not readily cross the placental barrier (see **PRECAUTIONS, Pregnancy**).

Metabolism—T_4 is slowly eliminated (see **TABLE 1**). The major pathway of thyroid hormone metabolism is through sequential deiodination. Approximately eighty-percent of circulating T_3 is derived from peripheral T_4 by monodeiodi-

Table 1: Pharmacokinetic Parameters of Thyroid Hormones in Euthyroid Patients

Hormone	Ratio in Thyroglobulin	Biologic Potency	$t_{1/2}$(days)	Protein Binding (%)[2]
Levothyroxine (T_4)	10—20	1	6—7[1]	99.96
Liothyronine (T_3)	1	4	≤ 2	99.5

[1] 3 to 4 days in hyperthyroidism, 9 to 10 days in hypothyroidism; [2] Includes TBG, TBPA, and TBA.

nation. The liver is the major site of degradation for both T_4 and T_3, with T_4 deiodination also occurring at a number of additional sites, including the kidney and other tissues. Approximately 80% of the daily dose of T_4 is deiodinated to yield equal amounts of T_3 and reverse T_3 (rT_3). T_3 and rT_3 are further deiodinated to diiodothyronine. Thyroid hormones are also metabolized via conjugation with glucuronides and sulfates and excreted directly into the bile and gut where they undergo enterohepatic recirculation.

Elimination—Thyroid hormones are primarily eliminated by the kidneys. A portion of the conjugated hormone reaches the colon unchanged and is eliminated in the feces. Approximately 20% of T_4 is eliminated in the stool. Urinary excretion of T_4 decreases with age.
[See table 1 above]

INDICATIONS AND USAGE

Levothyroxine sodium is used for the following indications:
Hypothyroidism—As replacement or supplemental therapy in congenital or acquired hypothyroidism of any etiology, except transient hypothyroidism during the recovery phase of subacute thyroiditis. Specific indications include: primary (thyroidal), secondary (pituitary), and tertiary (hypothalamic) hypothyroidism and subclinical hypothyroidism. Primary hypothyroidism may result from functional deficiency, primary atrophy, partial or total congenital absence of the thyroid gland, or from the effects of surgery, radiation, or drugs, with or without the presence of goiter.
Pituitary TSH Suppression—In the treatment or prevention of various types of euthyroid goiters (see **WARNINGS** and **PRECAUTIONS**), including thyroid nodules (see **WARNINGS** and **PRECAUTIONS**), subacute or chronic lymphocytic thyroiditis (Hashimoto's thyroiditis), multinodular goiter (see **WARNINGS and PRECAUTIONS**) and, as an adjunct to surgery and radioiodine therapy in the management of thyrotropin-dependent well-differentiated thyroid cancer.

CONTRAINDICATIONS

Levothyroxine is contraindicated in patients with untreated subclinical (suppressed serum TSH level with normal T_3 and T_4 levels) or overt thyrotoxicosis of any etiology and in patients with acute myocardial infarction. Levothyroxine is contraindicated in patients with uncorrected adrenal insufficiency since thyroid hormones may precipitate an acute adrenal crisis by increasing the metabolic clearance of glucocorticoids (see **PRECAUTIONS**). LEVOXYL® is contraindicated in patients with hypersensitivity to any of the inactive ingredients in LEVOXYL® tablets (see **DESCRIPTION, Inactive Ingredients**).

WARNINGS

WARNING: Thyroid hormones, including LEVOXYL®, either alone or with other therapeutic agents, should not be used for the treatment of obesity or for weight loss. In euthyroid patients, doses within the range of daily hormonal requirements are ineffective for weight reduction. Larger doses may produce serious or even life threatening manifestations of toxicity, particularly when given in association with sympathomimetic amines such as those used for their anorectic effects.

Levothyroxine sodium should not be used in the treatment of male or female infertility unless this condition is associated with hypothyroidism.
In patients with nontoxic diffuse goiter or nodular thyroid disease, particularly the elderly or those with underlying cardiovascular disease, levothyroxine sodium therapy is contraindicated if the serum TSH level is already suppressed due to the risk of precipitating overt thyrotoxicosis (see **CONTRAINDICATIONS**). If the serum TSH level is not suppressed, LEVOXYL® should be used with caution in conjunction with careful monitoring of thyroid function for evidence of hyperthyroidism and clinical monitoring for potential associated adverse cardiovascular signs and symptoms of hyperthyroidism.

PRECAUTIONS

General
Levothyroxine has a narrow therapeutic index. Regardless of the indication for use, careful dosage titration is necessary to avoid the consequences of over- or under-treatment. These consequences include, among others, effects on growth and development, cardiovascular function, bone metabolism, reproductive function, cognitive function, emotional state, gastrointestinal function, and on glucose and lipid metabolism. Many drugs interact with levothyroxine sodium necessitating adjustments in dosing to maintain therapeutic response (see **Drug Interactions**).
Effects on bone mineral density—In women, long-term levothyroxine sodium therapy has been associated with decreased bone mineral density, especially in postmenopausal women on greater than replacement doses or in women who are receiving suppressive doses of levothyroxine sodium. Therefore, it is recommended that patients receiving levothyroxine sodium be given the minimum dose necessary to achieve the desired clinical and biochemical response.

Patients with underlying cardiovascular disease—Exercise caution when administering levothyroxine to patients with cardiovascular disorders and to the elderly in whom there is an increased risk of occult cardiac disease. In these patients, levothyroxine therapy should be initiated at lower doses than those recommended in younger individuals or in patients without cardiac disease (see **WARNINGS; PRECAUTIONS, Geriatric Use**; and **DOSAGE AND ADMINISTRATION**). If cardiac symptoms develop or worsen, the levothyroxine dose should be reduced or withheld for one week and then cautiously restarted at a lower dose. Overtreatment with levothyroxine sodium may have adverse cardiovascular effects such as an increase in heart rate, cardiac wall thickness, and cardiac contractility and may precipitate angina or arrhythmias. Patients with coronary artery disease who are receiving levothyroxine therapy should be monitored closely during surgical procedures, since the possibility of precipitating cardiac arrhythmias may be greater in those treated with levothyroxine. Concomitant administration of levothyroxine and sympathomimetic agents to patients with coronary artery disease may precipitate coronary insufficiency.

Patients with nontoxic diffuse goiter or nodular thyroid disease—Exercise caution when administering levothyroxine to patients with nontoxic diffuse goiter or nodular thyroid disease in order to prevent precipitation of thyrotoxicosis (see **WARNINGS**). If the serum TSH is already suppressed, levothyroxine sodium should not be administered (see **CONTRAINDICATIONS**)

Associated endocrine disorders

Hypothalamic/pituitary hormone deficiencies—In patients with secondary or tertiary hypothyroidism, additional hypothalamic/pituitary hormone deficiencies should be considered, and, if diagnosed, treated (see **PRECAUTIONS, Autoimmune polyglandular syndrome**) for adrenal insufficiency.
Autoimmune polyglandular syndrome—Occasionally, chronic autoimmune thyroiditis may occur in association with other autoimmune disorders such as adrenal insufficiency, pernicious anemia, and insulin-dependent diabetes mellitus. Patients with concomitant adrenal insufficiency should be treated with replacement glucocorticoids prior to initiation of treatment with levothyroxine sodium. Failure to do so may precipitate an acute adrenal crisis when thyroid hormone therapy is initiated, due to increased metabolic clearance of glucocorticoids by thyroid hormone. Patients with diabetes mellitus may require upward adjustments of their antidiabetic therapeutic regimens when treated with levothyroxine (see **PRECAUTIONS, Drug Interactions**).

Other associated medical conditions

Infants with congenital hypothyroidism appear to be at increased risk for other congenital anomalies, with cardiovascular anomalies (pulmonary stenosis, atrial septal defect, and ventricular septal defect), being the most common association.

Information for Patients

Patients should be informed of the following information to aid in the safe and effective use of LEVOXYL®:
1. Notify your physician if you are allergic to any foods or medicines, are pregnant or intend to become pregnant, are breast-feeding or are taking any other medications, including prescription and over-the-counter preparations.
2. Notify your physician of any other medical conditions you may have, particularly heart disease, diabetes, clotting disorders, and adrenal or pituitary gland problems. Your dose of medications used to control these other conditions may need to be adjusted while you are taking LEVOXYL®. If you have diabetes, monitor your blood and/or urinary glucose levels as directed by your physician and immediately report any changes to your physician. If you are taking anticoagulants (blood thinners), your clotting status should be checked frequently.
3. Use LEVOXYL® only as prescribed by your physician. Do not discontinue or change the amount you take or how often you take it, unless directed to do so by your physician.
4. The levothyroxine in LEVOXYL® is intended to replace a hormone that is normally produced by your thyroid gland. Generally, replacement therapy is to be taken for life, except in cases of transient hypothyroidism, which is usually associated with an inflammation of the thyroid gland (thyroiditis).
5. Take LEVOXYL® in the morning on an empty stomach, at least one-half hour before eating any food.
6. LEVOXYL® may rapidly swell and disintegrate resulting in choking, gagging, the tablet getting stuck in your throat or difficulty swallowing. It is very important that you take the tablet with a full glass of water. Most of these problems disappeared when Levoxyl® tablets were taken with water.
7. It may take several weeks before you notice an improvement in your symptoms.
8. Notify your physician if you experience any of the following symptoms: rapid or irregular heartbeat, chest pain, shortness of breath, leg cramps, headache, nervousness, irritability, sleeplessness, tremors, change in appetite, weight gain or loss, vomiting, diarrhea, excessive sweating, heat intolerance, fever, changes in menstrual periods, hives or skin rash, or any other unusual medical event.
9. Notify your physician if you become pregnant while taking LEVOXYL®. It is likely that your dose of LEVOXYL® will need to be increased while you are pregnant.
10. Notify your physician or dentist that you are taking LEVOXYL® prior to any surgery.
11. Partial hair loss may occur rarely during the first few months of LEVOXYL® therapy, but this is usually temporary.
12. LEVOXYL® should not be used as a primary or adjunctive therapy in a weight control program.
13. Keep LEVOXYL® out of the reach of children. Store LEVOXYL® away from heat, moisture, and light.

Laboratory Tests
General
The diagnosis of hypothyroidism is confirmed by measuring TSH levels using a sensitive assay (second generation assay sensitivity ≤0.1 mIU/L or third generation assay sensitivity ≤0.01 mIU/L) and measurement of free-T_4.
The adequacy of therapy is determined by periodic assessment of appropriate laboratory tests and clinical evaluation. The choice of laboratory tests depends on various factors including the etiology of the underlying thyroid disease, the presence of concomitant medical conditions, including pregnancy, and the use of concomitant medications (see **PRECAUTIONS, Drug Interactions** and **Drug-Laboratory Test Interactions**). Persistent clinical and laboratory evidence of hypothyroidism despite an apparent adequate replacement dose of LEVOXYL® may be evidence of inadequate absorption, poor compliance, drug interactions, or decreased T_4 potency of the drug product.
Adults
In adult patients with primary (thyroidal) hypothyroidism, serum TSH levels (using a sensitive assay) alone may be used to monitor therapy. The frequency of TSH monitoring during levothyroxine dose titration depends on the clinical situation but it is generally recommended at 6—8 week intervals until normalization. For patients who have recently initiated levothyroxine therapy and whose serum TSH has normalized or in patients who have had their dosage or brand of levothyroxine changed, the serum TSH concentration should be measured after 8—12 weeks. When the optimum replacement dose has been attained, clinical (physical examination) and biochemical monitoring may be performed every 6—12 months, depending on the clinical situation, and whenever there is a change in the patient's status. It is recommended that a physical examination and a serum TSH measurement be performed at least annually in patients receiving LEVOXYL® (see **WARNINGS, PRECAUTIONS,** and **DOSAGE AND ADMINISTRATION**).
Pediatrics
In patients with congenital hypothyroidism, the adequacy of replacement therapy should be assessed by measuring both serum TSH (using a sensitive assay) and total- or free-T_4. During the first three years of life, the serum total- or free-T_4 should be maintained at all times in the upper half of the normal range. While the aim of therapy is to also normalize the serum TSH level, this is not always possible in a small percentage of patients, particularly in the first few months of therapy. TSH may not normalize due to a resetting of the pituitary-thyroid feedback threshold as a result of *in utero* hypothyroidism. Failure of the serum T_4 to increase into the upper half of the normal range within 2 weeks of initiation

of LEVOXYL® therapy and/or of the serum TSH to decrease below 20 mU/L within 4 weeks should alert the physician to the possibility that the child is not receiving adequate therapy. Careful inquiry should then be made regarding compliance, dose of medication administered, and method of administration prior to raising the dose of LEVOXYL®.

The recommended frequency of monitoring of TSH and total or free T_4 in children is as follows: at 2 and 4 weeks after the initiation of treatment; every 1—2 months during the first year of life; every 2—3 months between 1 and 3 years of age; and every 3 to 12 months thereafter until growth is completed. More frequent intervals of monitoring may be necessary if poor compliance is suspected or abnormal values are obtained. It is recommended that TSH and T_4 levels, and a physical examination, if indicated, be performed 2 weeks after any change in LEVOXYL® dosage. Routine clinical examination, including assessment of mental and physical growth and development, and bone maturation, should be performed at regular intervals (see **PRECAUTIONS, Pediatric Use** and **DOSAGE AND ADMINISTRATION**).

Secondary (pituitary) and tertiary (hypothalamic) hypothyroidism
Adequacy of therapy should be assessed by measuring serum free-T_4 levels, which should be maintained in the upper half of the normal range in these patients.

Drug Interactions
Many drugs affect thyroid hormone pharmacokinetics and metabolism (e.g., absorption, synthesis, secretion, catabolism, protein binding, and target tissue response) and may alter the therapeutic response to LEVOXYL®. In addition, thyroid hormones and thyroid status have varied effects on the pharmacokinetics and action of other drugs. A listing of drug-thyroidal axis interactions is contained in Table 2.

The list of drug-thyroidal axis interactions in Table 2 may not be comprehensive due to the introduction of new drugs that interact with the thyroidal axis or the discovery of previously unknown interactions. The prescriber should be aware of this fact and should consult appropriate reference sources. (e.g., package inserts of newly approved drugs, medical literature) for additional information if a drug-drug interaction with levothyroxine is suspected.
[See table 2 at right and on next page]

Oral anticoagulants—Levothyroxine increases the response to oral anticoagulant therapy. Therefore, a decrease in the dose of anticoagulant may be warranted with correction of the hypothyroid state or when the LEVOXYL® dose is increased. Prothrombin time should be closely monitored to permit appropriate and timely dosage adjustments (see **Table 2**).

Digitalis glycosides—The therapeutic effects of digitalis glycosides may be reduced by levothyroxine. Serum digitalis glycoside levels may be decreased when a hypothyroid patient becomes euthyroid, necessitating an increase in the dose of digitalis glycosides (see **Table 2**).

Drug-Food Interactions
Consumption of certain foods may affect levothyroxine absorption thereby necessitating adjustments in dosing. Soybean flour (infant formula), cotton seed meal, walnuts, and dietary fiber may bind and decrease the absorption of levothyroxine sodium from the GI tract.

Drug-Laboratory Test Interactions
Changes in TBG concentration must be considered when interpreting T_4 and T_3 values, which necessitates measurement and evaluation of unbound (free) hormone and/or determination of the free T_4 index (FT_4I). Pregnancy, infectious hepatitis, estrogens, estrogen-containing oral contraceptives, and acute intermittent porphyria increase TBG concentrations. Decreases in TBG concentrations are observed in nephrosis, severe hypoproteinemia, severe liver disease, acromegaly, and after androgen or corticosteroid therapy (see also **Table 2**). Familial hyper- or hypothyroxine binding globulinemias have been described, with the incidence of TBG deficiency approximating 1 in 9000.

Carcinogenesis, Mutagenesis, and Impairment of Fertility
Animal studies have not been performed to evaluate the carcinogenic potential, mutagenic potential or effects on fertility of levothyroxine. The synthetic T_4 in LEVOXYL® is identical to that produced naturally by the human thyroid gland. Although there has been a reported association between prolonged thyroid hormone therapy and breast cancer, this has not been confirmed. Patients receiving LEVOXYL® for appropriate clinical indications should be titrated to the lowest effective replacement dose.

Pregnancy—Category A
Studies in women taking levothyroxine sodium during pregnancy have not shown an increased risk of congenital abnormalities. Therefore, the possibility of fetal harm appears remote. LEVOXYL® should not be discontinued during pregnancy and hypothyroidism diagnosed during pregnancy should be promptly treated.

Table 2: Drug — Thyroidal Axis Interactions

Drug or Drug Class	Effect
Drugs that may reduce TSH secretion -the reduction is not sustained; therefore, hypothyroidism does not occur	
Dopamine/Dopamine Agonists Glucocorticoids Octreotide	Use of these agents may result in a transient reduction in TSH secretion when administered at the following doses: Dopamine ($\geq$1 mcg/kg/min); Glucocorticoids (hydrocortisone $\geq$100 mg/day or equivalent); Octreotide (>100 mcg/day).
Drugs that alter thyroid hormone secretion	
Drugs that may decrease thyroid hormone secretion, which may result in hypothyroidism	
Aminoglutethimide Amiodarone Iodine (including iodine-Containing Radiographic contrast agents) Lithium Methimazole Propylthiouracil (PTU) Sulfonamides Tolbutamide	Long-term lithium therapy can result in goiter in up to 50% of patients, and either subclinical or overt hypothyroidism, each in up to 20% of patients. The fetus, neonate, elderly and euthyroid patients with underlying thyroid disease (e.g., Hashimoto's thyroiditis or with Grave's disease previously treated with radioiodine or surgery) are among those individuals who are particularly susceptible to iodine-induced hypothyroidism. Oral cholecystographic agents and amiodarone are slowly excreted, producing more prolonged hypothyroidism than parenterally administered iodinated contrast agents. Long-term aminoglutethimide therapy may minimally decrease T_4 and T_3 levels and increase TSH, although all values remain within normal limits in most patients.
Drugs that may increase thyroid hormone secretion, which may result in hyperthyroidism	
Amiodarone Iodine (including iodine-containing Radiographic contrast agents)	Iodide and drugs that contain pharmacologic amounts of iodide may cause hyperthyroidism in euthyroid patients with Grave's disease previously treated with antithyroid drugs or in euthyroid patients with thyroid autonomy (e.g., multinodular goiter or hyperfunctioning thyroid adenoma). Hyperthyroidism may develop over several weeks and may persist for several months after therapy discontinuation. Amiodarone may induce hyperthyroidism by causing thyroiditis.
Drugs that may decrease T_4 absorption, which may result in hypothyroidism	
Antacids - Aluminum & Magnesium Hydroxides - Simethicone Bile Acid Sequestrants - Cholestyramine - Colestipol Calcium Carbonate Cation Exchange Resins - Kayexalate Ferrous Sulfate Orlistat Sucralfate	Concurrent use may reduce the efficacy of levothyroxine by binding and delaying or preventing absorption, potentially resulting in hypothyroidism. Calcium carbonate may form an insoluble chelate with levothyroxine, and ferrous sulfate likely forms a ferric-thyroxine complex. Administer levothyroxine at least 4 hours apart from these agents. Patients treated concomitantly with orlistat and levothyroxine should be monitored for changes in thyroid function.

Drugs that may alter T_4 and T_3 serum transport — but FT_4 concentration remains normal; and, therefore, the patient remains euthyroid

Drugs that may increase serum TBG concentration	Drugs that may decrease serum TBG concentration
Clofibrate Estrogen-containing oral contraceptives Estrogens (oral) Heroin/Methadone 5-Fluorouracil Mitotane Tamoxifen	Androgens/Anabolic Steroids Asparaginase Glucocorticoids Slow-Release Nicotinic Acid

Drugs that may cause protein-binding site displacement	
Furosemide (>80 mg IV) Heparin Hydantoins Non-Steroidal Anti-Inflammatory Drugs - Fenamates - Phenylbutazone Salicylates (> 2 g/day)	Administration of these agents with levothyroxine results in an initial transient increase in FT_4. Continued administration results in a decrease in serum T_4 and normal FT_4 and TSH concentrations and, therefore, patients are clinically euthyroid. Salicylates inhibit binding of T_4 and T_3 to TBG and transthyretin. An initial increase in serum FT_4 is followed by return of FT_4 to normal levels with sustained therapeutic serum salicylate concentrations, although total-T_4 levels may decrease by as much as 30%.
Drugs that may alter T_4 and T_3 metabolism	
Drugs that may increase hepatic metabolism, which may result in hypothyroidism	
Carbamazepine Hydantoins Phenobarbital Rifampin	Stimulation of hepatic microsomal drug-metabolizing enzyme activity may cause increased hepatic degradation of levothyroxine, resulting in increased levothyroxine requirements. Phenytoin and carbamazepine reduce serum protein binding of levothyroxine, and total- and free-T_4 may be reduced by 20% to 40%, but most patients have normal serum TSH levels and are clinically euthyroid.

(Table continued on next page)

Hypothyroidism during pregnancy is associated with a higher rate of complications, including spontaneous abortion, pre-eclampsia, stillbirth and premature delivery. Maternal hypothyroidism may have an adverse effect on fetal and childhood growth and development. During pregnancy, serum T_4 levels may decrease and serum TSH levels increase to values outside the normal range. Since elevations in serum TSH may occur as early as 4 weeks gestation, pregnant women taking LEVOXYL® should have their TSH measured during each trimester. An elevated serum TSH level should be corrected by an increase in the dose of LEVOXYL®. Since postpartum TSH levels are similar to preconception values, the LEVOXYL® dosage should return to the pre-pregnancy dose immediately after delivery. A serum TSH level should be obtained 6—8 weeks postpartum.

Thyroid hormones do not readily cross the placental barrier; however, some transfer does occur as evidenced by levels in cord blood of athyreotic fetuses being approximately one-third maternal levels. Transfer of thyroid hormone from the mother to the fetus, however, may not be adequate to prevent in utero hypothyroidism.

Nursing Mothers

Although thyroid hormones are excreted only minimally in human milk, caution should be exercised when LEVOXYL® is administered to a nursing woman. However, adequate replacement doses of levothyroxine are generally needed to maintain normal lactation.

Pediatric Use

General

The goal of treatment in pediatric patients with hypothyroidism is to achieve and maintain normal intellectual and physical growth and development.

The initial dose of levothyroxine varies with age and body weight (see **DOSAGE AND ADMINISTRATION, Table 3**). Dosing adjustments are based on an assessment of the individual patient's clinical and laboratory parameters (see **PRECAUTIONS, Laboratory Tests**).

In children in whom a diagnosis of permanent hypothyroidism has not been established, it is recommended that levothyroxine administration be discontinued for a 30-day trial period, but only after the child is at least 3 years of age. Serum T_4 and TSH levels should then be obtained. If the T_4 is low and the TSH high, the diagnosis of permanent hypothyroidism is established, and levothyroxine therapy should be reinstituted. If the T_4 and TSH levels are normal, euthyroidism may be assumed and, therefore, the hypothyroidism can be considered to have been transient. In this instance, however, the physician should carefully monitor the child and repeat the thyroid function tests if any signs or symptoms of hypothyroidism develop. In this setting, the clinician should have a high index of suspicion of relapse. If the results of the levothyroxine withdrawal test are inconclusive, careful follow-up and subsequent testing will be necessary.

Since some more severely affected children may become clinically hypothyroid when treatment is discontinued for 30 days, an alternate approach is to reduce the replacement dose of levothyroxine by half during the 30-day trial period. If, after 30 days, the serum TSH is elevated above 20 mU/L, the diagnosis of permanent hypothyroidism is confirmed, and full replacement therapy should be resumed. However, if the serum TSH has not risen to greater than 20mU/L, levothyroxine treatment should be discontinued for another 30-day trial period followed by repeat serum T_4 and TSH. The presence of concomitant medical conditions should be considered in certain clinical circumstances and, if present, appropriately treated (see **PRECAUTIONS**).

*Congenital Hypothyroidism (see **PRECAUTIONS, Laboratory Tests** and **DOSAGE AND ADMINISTRATION**)*

Rapid restoration of normal serum T_4 concentrations is essential for preventing the adverse effects of congenital hypothyroidism on intellectual development as well as on overall physical growth and maturation. Therefore, LEVOXYL® therapy should be initiated immediately upon diagnosis and is generally continued for life.

During the first 2 weeks of LEVOXYL® therapy, infants should be closely monitored for cardiac overload, arrhythmias, and aspiration from avid suckling.

The patient should be monitored closely to avoid undertreatment or overtreatment. Undertreatment may have deleterious effects on intellectual development and linear growth. Overtreatment has been associated with craniosynostosis in infants, and may adversely affect the tempo of brain maturation and accelerate the bone age with resultant premature closure of the epiphyses and compromised adult stature.

Acquired Hypothyroidism in Pediatric Patients

The patient should be monitored closely to avoid undertreatment and overtreatment. Undertreatment may result in poor school performance due to impaired concentration and slowed mentation and in reduced adult height. Overtreatment may accelerate the bone age and result in premature epiphyseal closure and compromised adult stature. Treated children may manifest a period of catch-up growth, which may be adequate in some cases to normalize adult height. In children with severe or prolonged hypothyroidism, catch-up growth may not be adequate to normalize adult height.

Geriatric Use

Because of the increased prevalence of cardiovascular disease among the elderly, levothyroxine therapy should not

Table 2 *(cont.)*: Drug — Thyroidal Axis Interactions

Drug or Drug Class	Effect
Drugs that may decrease T_4 5′-deiodinase activity	
Amiodarone Beta-adrenergic antagonists - (e.g., Propranolol >160 mg/day) Glucocorticoids - (e.g., Dexamethasone > 4 mg/day) Propylthiouracil (PTU)	Administration of these enzyme inhibitors decreases the peripheral conversion of T_4 to T_3, leading to decreased T_3 levels. However, serum T_4 levels are usually normal but may occasionally be slightly increased. In patients treated with large doses of propranolol (>160 mg/day), T_3 and T_4 levels change slightly, TSH levels remain normal, and patients are clinically euthyroid. It should be noted that actions of particular beta-adrenergic antagonists may be impaired when the hypothyroid patient is converted to the euthyroid state. Short-term administration of large doses of glucocorticoids may decrease serum T_3 concentrations by 30% with minimal change in serum T_4 levels. However, long-term glucocorticoid therapy may result in slightly decreased T_3 and T_4 levels due to decreased TBG production (see above).
Miscellaneous	
Anticoagulants (oral) - Coumarin Derivatives - Indandione Derivatives	Thyroid hormones appear to increase the catabolism of vitamin K-dependent clotting factors, thereby increasing the anticoagulant activity of oral anticoagulants. Concomitant use of these agents impairs the compensatory increases in clotting factor synthesis. Prothrombin time should be carefully monitored in patients taking levothyroxine and oral anticoagulants and the dose of anticoagulant therapy adjusted accordingly.
Antidepressants - Tricyclics (e.g., Amitriptyline) - Tetracyclics (e.g., Maprotiline) - Selective Serotonin Reuptake Inhibitors (SSRIs; e.g., Sertraline)	Concurrent use of tri/tetracyclic antidepressants and levothyroxine may increase the therapeutic and toxic effects of both drugs, possibly due to increased receptor sensitivity to catecholamines. Toxic effects may include increased risk of cardiac arrhythmias and CNS stimulation; onset of action of tricyclics may be accelerated. Administration of sertraline in patients stabilized on levothyroxine may result in increased levothyroxine requirements.
Antidiabetic Agents - Biguanides - Meglitinides - Sulfonylureas - Thiazolidinediones - Insulin	Addition of levothyroxine to antidiabetic or insulin therapy may result in increased antidiabetic agent or insulin requirements. Careful monitoring of diabetic control is recommended, especially when thyroid therapy is started, changed, or discontinued.
Cardiac Glycosides	Serum digitalis glycoside levels may be reduced in hyperthyroidism or when the hypothyroid patient is converted to the euthyroid state. Therapeutic effect of digitalis glycosides may be reduced.
Cytokines - Interferon-α - Interleukin-2	Therapy with interferon-α has been associated with the development of antithyroid microsomal antibodies in 20% of patients and some have transient hypothyroidism, hyperthyroidism, or both. Patients who have antithyroid antibodies before treatment are at higher risk for thyroid dysfunction during treatment. Interleukin-2 has been associated with transient painless thyroiditis in 20% of patients. Interferon-β and -γ have not been reported to cause thyroid dysfunction.
Growth Hormones - Somatrem - Somatropin	Excessive use of thyroid hormones with growth hormones may accelerate epiphyseal closure. However, untreated hypothyroidism may interfere with growth response to growth hormone.
Ketamine	Concurrent use may produce marked hypertension and tachycardia; cautious administration to patients receiving thyroid hormone therapy is recommended.
Methylxanthine Bronchodilators - (e.g., Theophylline)	Decreased theophylline clearance may occur in hypothyroid patients; clearance returns to normal when the euthyroid state is achieved.
Radiographic Agents	Thyroid hormones may reduce the uptake of ^{123}I, ^{131}I, and ^{99m}Tc.
Sympathomimetics	Concurrent use may increase the effects of sympathomimetics or thyroid hormone. Thyroid hormones may increase the risk of coronary insufficiency when sympathomimetic agents are administered to patients with coronary artery disease.
Chloral Hydrate Diazepam Ethionamide Lovastatin Metoclopramide 6-Mercaptopurine Nitroprusside Para-aminosalicylate sodium Perphenazine Resorcinol (excessive topical use) Thiazide Diuretics	These agents have been associated with thyroid hormone and/or TSH level alterations by various mechanisms.

be initiated at the full replacement dose (see **WARNINGS, PRECAUTIONS, and DOSAGE AND ADMINISTRATION**).

ADVERSE REACTIONS

Adverse reactions associated with levothyroxine therapy are primarily those of hyperthyroidism due to therapeutic overdosage. They include the following:

General: fatigue, increased appetite, weight loss, heat intolerance, fever, excessive sweating;
Central nervous system: headache, hyperactivity, nervousness, anxiety, irritability, emotional lability, insomnia;
Musculoskeletal: tremors, muscle weakness;
Cardiac: palpitations, tachycardia, arrhythmias, increased pulse and blood pressure, heart failure, angina, myocardial infarction, cardiac arrest;

Pulmonary: dyspnea;
GI: diarrhea, vomiting, abdominal cramps;
Dermatologic: hair loss, flushing;
Reproductive: menstrual irregularities, impaired fertility.

Pseudotumor cerebri and slipped capital femoral epiphysis have been reported in children receiving levothyroxine therapy. Overtreatment may result in craniosynostosis in infants and premature closure of the epiphyses in children with resultant compromised adult height.

Seizures have been reported rarely with the institution of levothyroxine therapy.

Inadequate levothyroxine dosage will produce or fail to ameliorate the signs and symptoms of hypothyroidism.

Hypersensitivity reactions to inactive ingredients have occurred in patients treated with thyroid hormone products. These include urticaria, pruritus, skin rash, flushing, angioedema, various GI symptoms (abdominal pain, nausea, vomiting and diarrhea), fever, arthralgia, serum sickness and wheezing. Hypersensitivity to levothyroxine itself is not known to occur.

In addition to the above events, the following have been reported, predominately when Levoxyl® tablets were not taken with water: choking, gagging, tablet stuck in throat and dysphagia (see **Information for Patients**).

Strength (mcg)	Color	NDC # for bottles of 100	NDC # for bottles of 1000
25	Orange	NDC 60793-850-01	NDC 60793-850-10
50	White	NDC 60793-851-01	NDC 60793-851-10
75	Purple	NDC 60793-852-01	NDC 60793-852-10
88	Olive	NDC 60793-853-01	NDC 60793-853-10
100	Yellow	NDC 60793-854-01	NDC 60793-854-10
112	Rose	NDC 60793-855-01	NDC 60793-855-10
125	Brown	NDC 60793-856-01	NDC 60793-856-10
137	Dark Blue	NDC 60793-857-01	NDC 60793-857-10
150	Blue	NDC 60793-858-01	NDC 60793-858-10
175	Turquoise	NDC 60793-859-01	NDC 60793-859-10
200	Pink	NDC 60793-860-01	NDC 60793-860-10

OVERDOSAGE

The signs and symptoms of overdosage are those of hyperthyroidism (see **PRECAUTIONS** and **ADVERSE REACTIONS**). In addition, confusion and disorientation may occur. Cerebral embolism, shock, coma, and death have been reported. Seizures have occurred in a child ingesting approximately 20 mg of levothyroxine. Symptoms may not necessarily be evident or may not appear until several days after ingestion of levothyroxine sodium.

Treatment of Overdosage

Levothyroxine sodium should be reduced in dose or temporarily discontinued if signs or symptoms of overdosage occur.

• **Acute Massive Overdosage**—This may be a life-threatening emergency, therefore, symptomatic and supportive therapy should be instituted immediately. If not contraindicated (e.g., by seizures, coma, or loss of the gag reflex), the stomach should be emptied by emesis or gastric lavage to decrease gastrointestinal absorption. Activated charcoal or cholestyramine may also be used to decrease absorption. Central and peripheral increased sympathetic activity may be treated by administering B-receptor antagonists, e.g., propranolol (1 to 3 mg intravenously over a 10-minute period, or orally, 80 to 160 mg/day). Provide respiratory support as needed; control congestive heart failure; control fever, hypoglycemia, and fluid loss as necessary. Glucocorticoids may be given to inhibit the conversion of T_4 to T_3. Because T_4 is highly protein bound, very little drug will be removed by dialysis.

DOSAGE AND ADMINISTRATION

General Principles:

The goal of replacement therapy is to achieve and maintain a clinical and biochemical euthyroid state. The goal of suppressive therapy is to inhibit growth and/or function of abnormal thyroid tissue. The dose of LEVOXYL® that is adequate to achieve these goals depends on a variety of factors including the patient's age, body weight, cardiovascular status, concomitant medical conditions, including pregnancy, concomitant medications, and the specific nature of the condition being treated (see **WARNINGS** and **PRECAUTIONS**). Hence, the following recommendations serve only as dosing guidelines. Dosing must be individualized and adjustments made based on periodic assessment of the patient's clinical response and laboratory parameters (see **PRECAUTIONS, Laboratory Tests**).

The LEVOXYL® should be taken in the morning on an empty stomach, at least one-half hour before any food is eaten. LEVOXYL® should be taken at least 4 hours apart from drugs that are known to interfere with its absorption (see **PRECAUTIONS, Drug Interactions**).

LEVOXYL® should be taken with water (see **Information for Patients** and **ADVERSE REACTIONS**).

Due to the long half-life of levothyroxine, the peak therapeutic effect at a given dose of levothyroxine sodium may not be attained for 4—6 weeks.

Caution should be exercised when administering LEVOXYL® to patients with underlying cardiovascular disease, to the elderly, and to those with concomitant adrenal insufficiency (see **PRECAUTIONS**).

Specific Patient Populations:

Hypothyroidism in Adults and in Children in Whom Growth and Puberty are Complete (see **WARNINGS** and **PRECAUTIONS, Laboratory Tests**). Therapy may begin at full replacement doses in otherwise healthy individuals less than 50 years old and in those older than 50 years who have been recently treated for hyperthyroidism or who have been hypothyroid for only a short time (such as a few months).

The average full replacement dose of levothyroxine sodium is approximately 1.7 mcg/kg/day (e.g., **100—125 mcg/day** for a 70 kg adult). Older patients may require less than 1 mcg/kg/day. Levothyroxine sodium doses greater than 200 mcg/day are seldom required. An inadequate response to daily doses ≥300 mcg/day is rare and may indicate poor compliance, malabsorption, and/or drug interactions.

For most patients older than 50 years or for patients under 50 years of age with underlying cardiac disease, an initial starting dose of **25—50 mcg/day** of levothyroxine sodium is recommended, with gradual increments in dose at 6—8 week intervals, as needed. The recommended starting dose of levothyroxine sodium in elderly patients with cardiac disease is **12.5—25 mcg/day**, with gradual dose increments at 4—6 week intervals. The levothyroxine sodium dose is generally adjusted in 12.5—25 mcg increments until the patient with primary hypothyroidism is clinically euthyroid and the serum TSH has normalized.

In patients with severe hypothyroidism, the recommended initial levothyroxine sodium dose is **12.5—25 mcg/day** with increases of 25 mcg/day every 2—4 weeks, accompanied by clinical and laboratory assessment, until the TSH level is normalized.

In patients with secondary (pituitary) or tertiary (hypothalamic) hypothyroidism, the levothyroxine sodium dose should be titrated until the patient is clinically euthyroid and the serum free-T_4 level is restored to the upper half of the normal range.

Pediatric Dosage—Congenital or Acquired Hypothyroidism (see **PRECAUTIONS, Laboratory Tests**)

General Principles

In general, levothyroxine therapy should be instituted at full replacement doses as soon as possible. Delays in diagnosis and institution of therapy may have deleterious effects on the child's intellectual and physical growth and development.

Undertreatment and overtreatment should be avoided (see **PRECAUTIONS, Pediatric Use**).

LEVOXYL® may be administered to infants and children who cannot swallow intact tablets by crushing the tablet and suspending the freshly crushed tablet in a small amount (5—10 mL or 1—2 teaspoons) of water. This suspension can be administered by spoon or dropper. **DO NOT STORE THE SUSPENSION.** Foods that decrease absorption of levothyroxine, such as soybean infant formula, should not be used for administering levothyroxine sodium tablets. (see **PRECAUTIONS, Drug-Food Interactions**).

Newborns

The recommended starting dose of levothyroxine sodium in newborn infants is **10—15 mcg/kg/day**. A lower starting dose (e.g., 25 mcg/day) should be considered in infants at risk for cardiac failure, and the dose should be increased in 4—6 weeks as needed based on clinical and laboratory response to treatment. In infants with very low (< 5 mcg/dL) or undetectable serum T_4 concentrations, the recommended initial starting dose is **50 mcg/day** of levothyroxine sodium.

Infants and Children

Levothyroxine therapy is usually initiated at full replacement doses, with the recommended dose per body weight decreasing with age (see **TABLE 3**). However, in children with chronic or severe hypothyroidism, an initial dose of **25 mcg/day** of levothyroxine sodium is recommended with increments of 25 mcg every 2—4 weeks until the desired effect is achieved.

Hyperactivity in an older child can be minimized if the starting dose is one-fourth of the recommended full replacement dose, and the dose is then increased on a weekly basis by an amount equal to one-fourth the full recommended replacement dose until the full recommended replacement dose is reached.

Table 3: Levothyroxine Sodium Dosing Guidelines for Pediatric Hypothyroidism

AGE	Daily Dose Per Kg Body Weight[a]
0—3 months	10—15 mcg/kg/day
3—6 months	8—10 mcg/kg/day
6—12 months	6—8 mcg/kg/day
1—5 years	5—6 mcg/kg/day
6—12 years	4—5 mcg/kg/day
>12 years	2—3 mcg/kg/day
Growth and puberty complete	1.7 mcg/kg/day

a - The dose should be adjusted based on clinical response and laboratory parameters (see **PRECAUTIONS, Laboratory Tests** and **Pediatric Use**).

Pregnancy—Pregnancy may increase levothyroxine requirements (see **PREGNANCY**).

Subclinical Hypothyroidism—If this condition is treated, a lower levothyroxine sodium dose (e.g., **1 mcg/kg/day**) than that used for full replacement may be adequate to normalize the serum TSH level. Patients who are not treated should be monitored yearly for changes in clinical status and thyroid laboratory parameters.

TSH Suppression in Well-differentiated Thyroid Cancer and Thyroid Nodules—The target level for TSH suppression in these conditions has not been established with controlled studies. In addition, the efficacy of TSH suppression for benign nodular disease is controversial. Therefore, the dose of LEVOXYL® used for TSH suppression should be individualized based on the specific disease and the patient being treated.

In the treatment of well differentiated (papillary and follicular) thyroid cancer, levothyroxine is used as an adjunct to surgery and radioiodine therapy. Generally, TSH is suppressed to <0.1 mU/L, and this usually requires a levothyroxine sodium dose of **greater than 2 mcg/kg/day**. However, in patients with high-risk tumors, the target level for TSH suppression may be <0.01 mU/L.

In the treatment of benign nodules and nontoxic multinodular goiter, TSH is generally suppressed to a higher target (e.g., 0.1—0.5 mU/L for nodules and 0.5—1.0 mU/L for multinodular goiter) than that used for the treatment of thyroid cancer. Levothyroxine sodium is contraindicated if the serum TSH is already suppressed due to the risk of precipitating overt thyrotoxicosis (see **CONTRAINDICATIONS, WARNINGS** and **PRECAUTIONS**).

Myxedema Coma—Myxedema coma is a life-threatening emergency characterized by poor circulation and hypometabolism, and may result in unpredictable absorption of levothyroxine sodium from the gastrointestinal tract. Therefore, oral thyroid hormone drug products are not recommended to treat this condition. Thyroid hormone products formulated for intravenous administration should be administered.

HOW SUPPLIED

–LEVOXYL® (levothyroxine sodium tablets, USP) are supplied as oval, color-coded, potency marked tablets in 11 strengths:
[See table at top of previous page]

STORAGE CONDITIONS

20°—25°C (68°—77°F) with excursions permitted between 15°—30°C (59°—86°F).
Meets USP Dissolution Tests 1 and 2.

Rx ONLY
Manufactured and Distributed by:
King Pharmaceuticals, Inc.
Bristol, TN 37620
Prescribing Information as of October 2007
3000000-D
Shown in Product Identification Guide, page 310

SKELAXIN® TABLETS ℞

[skĕ-lăks-ĭn]
(metaxalone)
Tablets

DESCRIPTION

SKELAXIN® (metaxalone) is available as an 800 mg oval, scored pink tablet.

Chemically, metaxalone is 5-[(3,5- dimethylphenoxy) methyl]-2-oxazolidinone. The empirical formula is $C_{12}H_{15}NO_3$, which corresponds to a molecular weight of 221.25. The structural formula is:

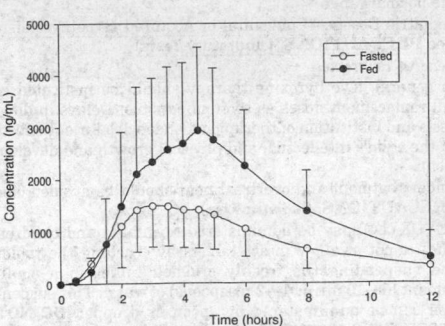

Metaxalone is a white to almost white, odorless crystalline powder freely soluble in chloroform, soluble in methanol and in 96% ethanol, but practically insoluble in ether or water.

Each tablet contains 800 mg metaxalone and the following inactive ingredients: alginic acid, ammonium calcium alginate, B-Rose Liquid, corn starch, and magnesium stearate.

CLINICAL PHARMACOLOGY

Mechanism of Action
The mechanism of action of metaxalone in humans has not been established, but may be due to general central nervous system depression. Metaxalone has no direct action on the contractile mechanism of striated muscle, the motor end plate, or the nerve fiber.

Pharmacokinetics
The pharmacokinetics of metaxalone have been evaluated in healthy adult volunteers after single dose administration of SKELAXIN under fasted and fed conditions at doses ranging from 400 mg to 800 mg.

Absorption
Peak plasma concentrations of metaxalone occur approximately 3 hours after a 400 mg oral dose under fasted conditions. Thereafter, metaxalone concentrations decline loglinearly with a terminal half-life of 9.0 ± 4.8 hours. Doubling the dose of SKELAXIN from 400 mg to 800 mg results in a roughly proportional increase in metaxalone exposure as indicated by peak plasma concentrations (C_{max}) and area under the curve (AUC). Dose proportionality at doses above 800 mg has not been studied. The absolute bioavailability of metaxalone is not known.

The single-dose pharmacokinetic parameters of metaxalone in two groups of healthy volunteers are shown in Table 1.

Table 1: Mean (%CV) Metaxalone Pharmacokinetic Parameters

Dose (mg)	C_{max} (ng/mL)	T_{max} (h)	AUC_∞ (ng•h/mL)	$t_{1/2}$ (h)	CL/F (L/h)
400[1]	983 (53)	3.3 (35)	7479 (51)	9.0 (53)	68 (50)
800[2]	1816 (43)	3.0 (39)	15044 (46)	8.0 (58)	66 (51)

[1] Subjects received 1×400 mg tablet under fasted conditions (N=42)
[2] Subjects received 2×400 mg tablets under fasted conditions (N=59)

Food Effects
A randomized, two-way, crossover study was conducted in 42 healthy volunteers (31 males, 11 females) administered one 400 mg SKELAXIN tablet under fasted conditions and following a standard high-fat breakfast. Subjects ranged in age from 18 to 48 years (mean age = 23.5 ± 5.7 years). Compared to fasted conditions, the presence of a high fat meal at the time of drug administration increased C_{max} by 177.5% and increased AUC (AUC_{0-t}, AUC_∞) by 123.5% and 115.4%, respectively. Time-to-peak concentration (T_{max}) was also delayed (4.3 h *versus* 3.3 h) and terminal half-life was decreased (2.4 h *versus* 9.0 h) under fed conditions compared to fasted.

In a second food effect study of similar design, two 400 mg SKELAXIN tablets (800 mg) were administered to healthy volunteers (N=59, 37 males, 22 females), ranging in age from 18-50 years (mean age = 25.6± 8.7 years). Compared to fasted conditions, the presence of a high fat meal at the time of drug administration increased C_{max} by 193.6% and increased AUC (AUC_{0-t}, AUC_∞) by 146.4% and 142.2%, respectively. Time-to-peak concentration (T_{max}) was also delayed (4.9 h *versus* 3.0 h) and terminal half-life was decreased (4.2 h *versus* 8.0 h) under fed conditions compared to fasted conditions. Similar food effect results were observed in the above study when one SKELAXIN 800 mg tablet was administered in place of two SKELAXIN 400 mg tablets. The increase in metaxalone exposure coinciding with a reduction in half-life may be attributed to more complete absorption of metaxalone in the presence of a high fat meal (Figure 1).

Figure 1. Mean (SD) Concentrations of Metaxalone following an 800 mg Dose under Fasted and Fed Conditions

Distribution, Metabolism, and Excretion
Although plasma protein binding and absolute bioavailability of metaxalone are not known, the apparent volume of distribution (V/F ~ 800 L) and lipophilicity (log P = 2.42) of metaxalone suggest that the drug is extensively distributed in the tissues. Metaxalone is metabolized by the liver and excreted in the urine as unidentified metabolites. Hepatic Cytochrome P450 enzymes play a role in the metabolism of metaxalone. Specifically, CYP1A2, CYP2D6, CYP2E1, and CYP3A4 and, to a lesser extent, CYP2C8, CYP2C9, and CYP2C19 appear to metabolize metaxalone.

Metaxalone does not significantly inhibit major CYP enzymes such as CYP1A2, CYP2A6, CYP2B6, CYP2C8, CYP2C9, CYP2C19, CYP2D6, CYP2E1, and CYP3A4. Metaxalone does not significantly induce major CYP enzymes such as CYP1A2, CYP2B6, and CYP3A4 *in vitro*.

Pharmacokinetics in Special Populations
Age:
The effects of age on the pharmacokinetics of metaxalone were determined following single administration of two 400 mg tablets (800 mg) under fasted and fed conditions. The results were analyzed separately, as well as in combination with the results from three other studies. Using the combined data, the results indicate that the pharmacokinetics of metaxalone are significantly more affected by age under fasted conditions than under fed conditions, with bioavailability under fasted conditions increasing with age. The bioavailability of metaxalone under fasted and fed conditions in three groups of healthy volunteers of varying age is shown in Table 2.
[See table 2 above]

Gender:
The effect of gender on the pharmacokinetics of metaxalone was assessed in an open label study, in which 48 healthy adult volunteers (24 males, 24 females) were administered two SKELAXIN 400 mg tablets (800 mg) under fasted conditions. The bioavailability of metaxalone was significantly higher in females compared to males as evidenced by C_{max} (2115 ng/mL *versus* 1335 ng/mL) and AUC_∞ (17884 ng•h/mL *versus* 10328 ng•h/mL). The mean half-life was 11.1 hours in females and 7.6 hours in males. The apparent volume of distribution of metaxalone was approximately 22% higher in males than in females, but not significantly different when adjusted for body weight. Similar findings were also seen when the previously described combined dataset was used in the analysis.

Hepatic/Renal Insufficiency:
The impact of hepatic and renal disease on the pharmacokinetics of metaxalone has not been determined. In the absence of such information, SKELAXIN should be used with caution in patients with hepatic and/or renal impairment.

INDICATIONS AND USAGE

SKELAXIN (metaxalone) is indicated as an adjunct to rest, physical therapy, and other measures for the relief of discomforts associated with acute, painful musculoskeletal conditions. The mode of action of this drug has not been clearly identified, but may be related to its sedative properties. Metaxalone does not directly relax tense skeletal muscles in man.

CONTRAINDICATIONS

Known hypersensitivity to any components of this product.
Known tendency to drug induced, hemolytic, or other anemias.
Significantly impaired renal or hepatic function.

WARNINGS

SKELAXIN may enhance the effects of alcohol and other CNS depressants.

PRECAUTIONS

Metaxalone should be administered with great care to patients with pre-existing liver damage. Serial liver function studies should be performed in these patients.

False-positive Benedict's tests, due to an unknown reducing substance, have been noted. A glucose-specific test will differentiate findings.

Taking SKELAXIN with food may enhance general CNS depression; elderly patients may be especially susceptible to this CNS effect. (See **CLINICAL PHARMACOLOGY: Pharmacokinetics** and **PRECAUTIONS: Information for Patients**).

Information for Patients
SKELAXIN may impair mental and/or physical abilities required for performance of hazardous tasks, such as operating machinery or driving a motor vehicle, especially when used with alcohol or other CNS depressants.

Drug Interactions
The sedative effects of SKELAXIN and other CNS depressants (e.g., alcohol, benzodiazepines, opioids, tricyclic antidepressants) may be additive. Therefore, caution should be exercised with patients who take more than one of these CNS depressants simultaneously.

Table 2: Mean (%CV) Pharmacokinetic Parameters Following Single Administration of Two 400 mg SKELAXIN Tablets (800 mg) under Fasted and Fed Conditions

	Younger Volunteers		Older Volunteers			
Age (years)	25.6 ± 8.7		39.3 ± 10.8		71.5 ± 5.0	
N	59		21		23	
Food	Fasted	Fed	Fasted	Fed	Fasted	Fed
C_{max} (ng/mL)	1816 (43)	3510 (41)	2719 (46)	2915 (55)	3168 (43)	3680 (59)
T_{max} (h)	3.0 (39)	4.9 (48)	3.0 (40)	8.7 (91)	2.6 (30)	6.5 (67)
AUC_{0-t} (ng•h/mL)	14531 (47)	20683 (41)	19836 (40)	20482 (37)	23797 (45)	24340 (48)
AUC_∞ (ng•h/mL)	15045 (46)	20833 (41)	20490 (39)	20815 (37)	24194 (44)	24704 (47)

Carcinogenesis, Mutagenesis, Impairment of Fertility

The carcinogenic potential of metaxalone has not been determined.

Pregnancy

Reproduction studies in rats have not revealed evidence of impaired fertility or harm to the fetus due to metaxalone. Post marketing experience has not revealed evidence of fetal injury, but such experience cannot exclude the possibility of infrequent or subtle damage to the human fetus. Safe use of metaxalone has not been established with regard to possible adverse effects upon fetal development. Therefore, metaxalone tablets should not be used in women who are or may become pregnant and particularly during early pregnancy unless, in the judgement of the physician, the potential benefits outweigh the possible hazards.

Nursing Mothers

It is not known whether this drug is secreted in human milk. As a general rule, nursing should not be undertaken while a patient is on a drug since many drugs are excreted in human milk.

Pediatric Use

Safety and effectiveness in children 12 years of age and below have not been established.

ADVERSE REACTIONS

The most frequent reactions to metaxalone include:

CNS: drowsiness, dizziness, headache, and nervousness or "irritability";

Digestive: nausea, vomiting, gastrointestinal upset.

Other adverse reactions are:

Immune System: hypersensitivity reaction, rash with or without pruritus;

Hematologic: leukopenia; hemolytic anemia;

Hepatobiliary: jaundice.

Though rare, anaphylactoid reactions have been reported with metaxalone.

OVERDOSAGE

Deaths by deliberate or accidental overdose have occurred with metaxalone, particularly in combination with antidepressants, and have been reported with this class of drug in combination with alcohol.

When determining the LD_{50} in rats and mice, progressive sedation, hypnosis, and finally respiratory failure were noted as the dosage increased. In dogs, no LD_{50} could be determined as the higher doses produced an emetic action in 15 to 30 minutes.

Treatment - Gastric lavage and supportive therapy. Consultation with a regional poison control center is recommended.

DOSAGE AND ADMINISTRATION

The recommended dose for adults and children over 12 years of age is one 800 mg tablet three to four times a day.

HOW SUPPLIED

SKELAXIN (metaxalone) is available as an 800 mg oval, scored pink tablet inscribed with 8667 on the scored side and "S" on the other. Available in bottles of 100 (NDC 60793-136-01) and in bottles of 500 (NDC 60793-136-05).

Store at Controlled Room Temperature, between 15°C and 30°C (59°F and 86°F).

Rx Only

Prescribing Information as of April 2008.

Distributed by: King Pharmaceuticals, Inc., Bristol, TN 37620

Manufactured by: Corepharma LLC, Middlesex, NJ 08846

Shown in Product Identification Guide, page 310

Kowa Pharmaceuticals America, Inc.

**530 INDUSTRIAL PARK BOULEVARD
MONTGOMERY, AL 36117**

Direct Inquiries:
Tel: 334-288-1288
Fax: 334-288-2788
info@kowapharma.com

LIVALO®   Rx

[li-va-lo]

(pitavastatin)

Tablet, Film Coated for Oral use

HIGHLIGHTS OF PRESCRIBING INFORMATION

These highlights do not include all the information needed to use LIVALO® safely and effectively. See full prescribing information for LIVALO.

LIVALO (pitavastatin) Tablet, Film Coated for Oral use

Initial U.S. Approval: 2009

---RECENT MAJOR CHANGES---

None

---INDICATIONS AND USAGE---

LIVALO is a HMG-CoA reductase inhibitor indicated for:

• Patients with primary hyperlipidemia and mixed dyslipidemia as an adjunctive therapy to diet to reduce elevated total cholesterol (TC), low-density lipoprotein cholesterol (LDL-C), apolipoprotein B (Apo B), triglycerides (TG), and to increase high-density lipoprotein cholesterol (HDL-C) (1.1)

Limitations of Use (1.2):

• Doses of LIVALO greater than 4 mg once daily were associated with an increased risk for severe myopathy in premarketing clinical studies. Do not exceed 4 mg once daily dosing of LIVALO.

• The effect of LIVALO on cardiovascular morbidity and mortality has not been determined.

• LIVALO has not been studied in patients with severe renal impairment (glomerular filtration rate < 30 mL/min/1.73 m²), not yet on hemodialysis. LIVALO should not be used in this patient population.

• LIVALO has not been studied with the protease inhibitor combination lopinavir/ritonavir. LIVALO should not be used with this combination of protease inhibitors

• LIVALO has not been studied in Fredrickson Type I, III, and V dyslipidemias

---DOSAGE AND ADMINISTRATION---

• LIVALO can be taken with or without food, at any time of day (2.1) Dose Range: 1 mg to 4 mg once daily (2.1)

• **Primary hyperlipidemia and mixed dyslipidemia:** Starting dose 2 mg. When lowering of LDL-C is insufficient, the dosage may be increased to a maximum of 4 mg per day. (2.1)

• **Moderate renal impairment (glomerular filtration rate 30 < 60 mL/min/1.73 m²) and end-stage renal disease on hemodialysis:** Starting dose of 1 mg once daily and maximum dose of 2 mg once daily (2.2)

---DOSAGE FORMS AND STRENGTHS---

• Tablets: 1 mg, 2 mg, and 4 mg (3)

---CONTRAINDICATIONS---

• Known hypersensitivity to product components (4)

• Active liver disease, which may include unexplained persistent elevations in hepatic transaminase levels (4)

• Women who are pregnant or may become pregnant (4, 8.1)

• Nursing mothers (4, 8.3)

• Co-administration with cyclosporine (4, 7.1, 12.3)

---WARNINGS AND PRECAUTIONS---

• **Skeletal muscle effects (e.g., myopathy and rhabdomyolysis):** Risks increase in a dose-dependent manner, with advanced age (>65), renal impairment, inadequately treated hypothyroidism, and combination use with fibrates. Advise patients to promptly report unexplained muscle pain, tenderness, or weakness, and discontinue LIVALO if signs or symptoms appear (5.1)

• **Liver enzymes abnormalities and monitoring:** Persistent elevations in hepatic transaminases can occur. Monitor liver enzymes before and during treatment (5.2)

---ADVERSE REACTIONS---

The most frequent adverse reactions (rate ≥2.0% in at least one marketed dose) were myalgia, back pain, diarrhea, constipation and pain in extremity. (6)

To report SUSPECTED ADVERSE REACTIONS, contact Kowa Pharmaceuticals America, Inc. at 1-877-334-3464 or FDA at 1-800-FDA-1088 or www.fda.gov/medwatch.

---DRUG INTERACTIONS---

• **Lopinavir/Ritonavir:** This combination should not be used with LIVALO (1.2, 7.2)

• **Erythromycin:** Combination increases pitavastatin exposure. Limit LIVALO to 1 mg once daily (2.3, 7.3)

• **Rifampin:** Combination increases pitavastatin exposure. Limit LIVALO to 2 mg once daily (2.4, 7.4)

• **Fibrates:** Use with fibrate products may increase the risk of adverse skeletal muscle effects (5.1, 7.5)

---USE IN SPECIFIC POPULATIONS---

• **Pediatric use:** Safety and effectiveness have not been established. (8.4)

• **Renal impairment:** Limitation of a starting dose of LIVALO 1 mg once daily and a maximum dose of LIVALO 2 mg once daily for patients with moderate renal impairment and patients receiving hemodialysis (2.2, 8.6) Patients with severe renal impairment not receiving hemodialysis have not been studied. LIVALO should not be used in this patient population (5.1, 8.6)

See 17 for PATIENT COUNSELING INFORMATION

Revised: 08/2009

FULL PRESCRIBING INFORMATION: CONTENTS*

* Sections or subsections omitted from the full prescribing information are not listed

---

FULL PRESCRIBING INFORMATION

1   INDICATIONS AND USAGE

Drug therapy should be one component of multiple-risk-factor intervention in individuals who require modifications of their lipid profile. Lipid-altering agents should be used in addition to a diet restricted in saturated fat and cholesterol only when the response to diet and other nonpharmacological measures has been inadequate.

1.1   Primary Hyperlipidemia and Mixed Dyslipidemia

LIVALO® is indicated as an adjunctive therapy to diet to reduce elevated total cholesterol (TC), low-density lipoprotein cholesterol (LDL-C), apolipoprotein B (Apo B), triglycerides (TG), and to increase HDL-C in adult patients with primary hyperlipidemia or mixed dyslipidemia.

1.2   Limitations of Use

Doses of LIVALO greater than 4 mg once daily were associated with an increased risk for severe myopathy in premarketing clinical studies. Do not exceed 4 mg once daily dosing of LIVALO.

The effect of LIVALO on cardiovascular morbidity and mortality has not been determined.

LIVALO has not been studied in patients with severe renal impairment (glomerular filtration rate < 30 mL/min/1.73 m²) not on hemodialysis. LIVALO should not be used in this patient population.

LIVALO has not been studied with the protease inhibitor combination lopinavir/ritonavir. LIVALO should not be used with this combination of protease inhibitors.

LIVALO has not been studied in Fredrickson Type I, III, and V dyslipidemias.

2   DOSAGE AND ADMINISTRATION

2.1   General Dosing Information

The dose range for LIVALO is 1 to 4 mg orally once daily at any time of the day with or without food. The recommended starting dose is 2 mg and the maximum dose is 4 mg. The starting dose and maintenance doses of LIVALO should be individualized according to patient characteristics, such as goal of therapy and response.

After initiation or upon titration of LIVALO, lipid levels should be analyzed after 4 weeks and the dosage adjusted accordingly.

2.2   Dosage in Patients with Renal Impairment

Patients with moderate renal impairment (glomerular filtration rate 30 to < 60 mL/min/1.73 m²) and end-stage renal disease receiving hemodialysis should receive a starting dose of LIVALO 1 mg once daily and a maximum dose of LIVALO 2 mg once daily. LIVALO should not be used in patients with severe renal impairment (glomerular filtration rate < 30 mL/min/1.73 m²) not yet on hemodialysis.

2.3   Use with Erythromycin

In patients taking erythromycin, a dose of LIVALO 1 mg once daily should not be exceeded [*see Drug Interactions (7.3)*].

2.4 Use with Rifampin

In patients taking rifampin, a dose of LIVALO 2 mg once daily should not be exceeded [see Drug Interactions (7.4)].

3 DOSAGE FORMS AND STRENGTHS

1 mg: Round white film-coated tablet. Debossed "KC" on one side and "1" on the other side of the tablet.

2 mg: Round white film-coated tablet. Debossed "KC" on one side and "2" on the other side of the tablet.

4 mg: Round white film-coated tablet. Debossed "KC" on one side and "4" on the other side of the tablet.

4 CONTRAINDICATIONS

The use of LIVALO is contraindicated in the following conditions:

- Patients with a known hypersensitivity to any component of this product. Hypersensitivity reactions including rash, pruritus, and urticaria have been reported with LIVALO [see Adverse Reactions (6.1)].
- Patients with active liver disease which may include unexplained persistent elevations of hepatic transaminase levels [see Warnings and Precautions (5.2), Use in Specific Populations (8.7)].
- Women who are pregnant or may become pregnant. Because HMG-CoA reductase inhibitors decrease cholesterol synthesis and possibly the synthesis of other biologically active substances derived from cholesterol, LIVALO may cause fetal harm when administered to pregnant women. Additionally, there is no apparent benefit to therapy during pregnancy, and safety in pregnant women has not been established. If the patient becomes pregnant while taking this drug, the patient should be apprised of the potential hazard to the fetus and the lack of known clinical benefit with continued use during pregnancy [see Use in Specific Populations (8.1) and Nonclinical Toxicology (13.2)].
- Nursing mothers. Animal studies have shown that LIVALO passes into breast milk. Since HMG-CoA reductase inhibitors have the potential to cause serious adverse reactions in nursing infants, LIVALO, like other HMG-CoA reductase inhibitors, is contraindicated in pregnant or nursing mothers [see Use in Specific Populations (8.3) and Nonclinical Toxicology (13.2)].
- Co-administration with cyclosporine [see Drug Interactions (7.1) and Clinical Pharmacology (12.3)].

5 WARNINGS AND PRECAUTIONS

5.1 Skeletal Muscle Effects

Cases of myopathy and rhabdomyolysis with acute renal failure secondary to myoglobinuria have been reported with HMG-CoA reductase inhibitors, including LIVALO. These risks can occur at any dose level, but increase in a dose-dependent manner. LIVALO should be prescribed with caution in patients with predisposing factors for myopathy. These factors include advanced age (>65 years), renal impairment, and inadequately treated hypothyroidism. The risk of myopathy may also be increased with concurrent administration of fibrates or lipid-modifying doses of niacin. LIVALO should be administered with caution in patients with impaired renal function, in elderly patients, or when used concomitantly with fibrates or lipid-modifying doses of niacin [see Drug Interactions (7.6), Use in Specific Populations (8.5, 8.6) and Clinical Pharmacology (12.3)].

LIVALO therapy should be discontinued if markedly elevated creatine kinase (CK) levels occur or myopathy is diagnosed or suspected. LIVALO therapy should also be temporarily withheld in any patient with an acute, serious condition suggestive of myopathy or predisposing to the development of renal failure secondary to rhabdomyolysis (e.g., sepsis, hypotension, dehydration, major surgery, trauma, severe metabolic, endocrine, and electrolyte disorders, or uncontrolled seizures). All patients should be advised to promptly report unexplained muscle pain, tenderness, or weakness, particularly if accompanied by malaise or fever.

5.2 Liver Enzyme Abnormalities and Monitoring

Increases in serum transaminases (aspartate aminotransferase [AST]/serum glutamic-oxaloacetic transaminase, or alanine aminotransferase [ALT]/serum glutamic-pyruvic transaminase) have been reported with HMG-CoA reductase inhibitors, including LIVALO. In most cases, the elevations were transient and resolved or improved on continued therapy or after a brief interruption in therapy.

In placebo-controlled Phase 2 studies, ALT >3 times the upper limit of normal was not observed in the placebo, LIVALO 1 mg, or LIVALO 2 mg groups. One out of 202 patients (0.5%) administered LIVALO 4 mg had ALT >3 times the upper limit of normal. It is recommended that liver enzyme tests be performed before and at 12 weeks following both the initiation of therapy and any elevation of dose and periodically (e.g., semiannually) thereafter.

Patients who develop increased transaminase levels should be monitored until the abnormalities have resolved. Should

an increase in ALT or AST of >3 times upper limit of normal persist, reduction of dose or withdrawal of LIVALO is recommended.

As with other HMG-CoA reductase inhibitors, LIVALO should be used with caution in patients who consume substantial quantities of alcohol. Active liver disease, which may include unexplained persistent transaminase elevations, is a contraindication to the use of LIVALO [see Contraindications (4)].

6 ADVERSE REACTIONS

The following serious adverse reactions are discussed in greater detail in other sections of the label:

- Rhabdomyolysis with myoglobinuria and acute renal failure and myopathy (including myositis) [see Warnings and Precautions (5.1)].
- Liver Enzyme Abnormalities [see Warning and Precautions (5.2)].

Of 4,798 patients enrolled in 10 controlled clinical studies and 4 subsequent open-label extension studies, 3,291 patients were administered pitavastatin 1 mg to 4 mg daily. The mean continuous exposure of pitavastatin (1 mg to 4 mg) was 36.7 weeks (median 51.1 weeks). The mean age of the patients was 60.9 years (range; 18 years–89 years) and the gender distribution was 48% males and 52% females. Approximately 93% of the patients were Caucasian, 7% were Asian/Indian, 0.2% were African American and 0.3% were Hispanic and other.

6.1 Clinical Studies Experience

Because clinical studies on LIVALO are conducted in varying study populations and study designs, the frequency of adverse reactions observed in the clinical studies of LIVALO cannot be directly compared with that in the clinical studies of other HMG-CoA reductase inhibitors and may not reflect the frequency of adverse reactions observed in clinical practice.

Adverse reactions reported in ≥ 2% of patients in controlled clinical studies and at a rate greater than or equal to placebo are shown in Table 1. These studies had treatment duration of up to 12 weeks.

Table 1. Adverse Reactions* Reported by ≥2.0% of Patients Treated with LIVALO and > Placebo in Short-Term Controlled Studies

Adverse Reactions*	Placebo N= 208	LIVALO 1 mg N=309	LIVALO 2 mg N=951	LIVALO 4 mg N=1540
Back Pain	2.9%	3.9%	1.8%	1.4%
Constipation	1.9%	3.6%	1.5%	2.2%
Diarrhea	1.9%	2.6%	1.5%	1.9%
Myalgia	1.4%	1.9%	2.8%	3.1%
Pain in extremity	1.9%	2.3%	0.6%	0.9%

*Adverse reactions by MedDRA preferred term.

Other adverse reactions reported from clinical studies were arthralgia, headache, influenza, and nasopharyngitis.

The following laboratory abnormalities have also been reported: elevated creatine phosphokinase, transaminases, alkaline phosphatase, bilirubin, and glucose.

In controlled clinical studies and their open-label extensions, 3.9% (1 mg), 3.3% (2 mg), and 3.7% (4 mg) of pitavastatin-treated patients were discontinued due to adverse reactions. The most common adverse reactions that led to treatment discontinuation were: elevated creatine phosphokinase (0.6% on 4 mg) and myalgia (0.5% on 4 mg).

Hypersensitivity reactions including rash, pruritus, and urticaria have been reported with LIVALO.

7 DRUG INTERACTIONS

7.1 Cyclosporine

Cyclosporine significantly increased pitavastatin exposure. Co-administration of cyclosporine with LIVALO is contraindicated [see Contraindications (4), and Clinical Pharmacology (12.3)].

7.2 Lopinavir/Ritonavir

Based on data with another HMG-CoA reductase inhibitor that has a similar pharmacokinetic profile to that of pitavastatin, co-administration of the protease inhibitor combination, lopinavir/ritonavir, with LIVALO may significantly increase pitavastatin exposure. Therefore, LIVALO should not be used with this combination of protease inhibitors. [see Limitations of Use (1.2)].

7.3 Erythromycin

Erythromycin significantly increased pitavastatin exposure. In patients taking erythromycin, a dose of LIVALO 1 mg once daily should not be exceeded [see Dosage and Administration (2.3) and Clinical Pharmacology (12.3)].

7.4 Rifampin

Rifampin significantly increased pitavastatin exposure. In patients taking rifampin, a dose of LIVALO 2 mg once daily should not be exceeded [see Dosage and Administration (2.4) and Clinical Pharmacology (12.3)].

7.5 Fibrates

Because it is known that the risk of myopathy during treatment with HMG-CoA reductase inhibitors may be increased with concurrent administration of fibrates, LIVALO should be administered with caution when used concomitantly with gemfibrozil or other fibrates [see Warnings and Precautions (5.1), and Clinical Pharmacology (12.3)].

7.6 Niacin

The risk of skeletal muscle effects may be enhanced when LIVALO is used in combination with niacin; a reduction in LIVALO dosage should be considered in this setting [see Warnings and Precautions (5.1)].

7.7 Warfarin

LIVALO had no significant pharmacokinetic interaction with R- and S- warfarin. LIVALO had no significant effect on prothrombin time (PT) and international normalized ratio (INR) when administered to patients receiving chronic warfarin treatment [see Clinical Pharmacology (12.3)]. However, patients receiving warfarin should have their PT and INR monitored when pitavastatin is added to their therapy.

8 USE IN SPECIFIC POPULATIONS

8.1 Pregnancy

Teratogenic effects: Pregnancy Category X

LIVALO is contraindicated in women who are or may become pregnant. Serum cholesterol and TG increase during normal pregnancy, and cholesterol products are essential for fetal development. Atherosclerosis is a chronic process and discontinuation of lipid-lowering drugs during pregnancy should have little impact on long-term outcomes of primary hyperlipidemia therapy [see Contraindications (4)].

There are no adequate and well-controlled studies of LIVALO in pregnant women, although, there have been rare reports of congenital anomalies following intrauterine exposure to HMG-CoA reductase inhibitors. In a review of about 100 prospectively followed pregnancies in women exposed to other HMG-CoA reductase inhibitors, the incidences of congenital anomalies, spontaneous abortions, and fetal deaths/stillbirths did not exceed the rate expected in the general population. However, this study was only able to exclude a three-to-four-fold increased risk of congenital anomalies over background incidence. In 89% of these cases, drug treatment started before pregnancy and stopped during the first trimester when pregnancy was identified.

Reproductive toxicity studies have shown that pitavastatin crosses the placenta in rats and is found in fetal tissues at ≤36% of maternal plasma concentrations following a single dose of 1 mg/kg/day during gestation.

Embryo-fetal developmental studies were conducted in pregnant rats treated with 3, 10, 30 mg/kg/day pitavastatin by oral gavage during organogenesis. No adverse effects were observed at 3 mg/kg/day, systemic exposures 22 times human systemic exposure at 4 mg/day based on AUC.

Embryo-fetal developmental studies were conducted in pregnant rabbits treated with 0.1, 0.3, 1 mg/kg/day pitavastatin by oral gavage during the period of fetal organogenesis. Maternal toxicity consisting of reduced body weight and abortion was observed at all doses tested (4 times human systemic exposure at 4 mg/day based on AUC).

In perinatal/postnatal studies in pregnant rats given oral gavage doses of pitavastatin at 0.1, 0.3, 1, 3, 10, 30 mg/kg/day from organogenesis through weaning, maternal toxicity consisting of mortality at ≥0.3 mg/kg/day and impaired lactation at all doses contributed to the decreased survival of neonates in all dose groups (0.1 mg/kg/day represents approximately 1 time human systemic exposure at 4 mg/day dose based on AUC).

LIVALO may cause fetal harm when administered to a pregnant woman. If the patient becomes pregnant while taking LIVALO, the patient should be apprised of the potential risks to the fetus and the lack of known clinical benefit with continued use during pregnancy.

8.3 Nursing Mothers

It is not known whether pitavastatin is excreted in human milk, however, it has been shown that a small amount of another drug in this class passes into human milk. Rat studies have shown that pitavastatin is excreted into breast milk. Because another drug in this class passes into human milk and HMG-CoA reductase inhibitors have a potential to cause serious adverse reactions in nursing infants, women who require LIVALO treatment should be advised not to nurse their infants or to discontinue LIVALO [see Contraindications (4)].

8.4 Pediatric Use

Safety and effectiveness of LIVALO in pediatric patients have not been established.

8.5 Geriatric Use
Of the 2,800 patients randomized to LIVALO 1 mg to 4 mg in controlled clinical studies, 1,209 (43%) were 65 years and older. No significant differences in efficacy or safety were observed between elderly patients and younger patients. However, greater sensitivity of some older individuals cannot be ruled out.

8.6 Renal Impairment
Patients with moderate renal impairment (glomerular filtration rate 30 to < 60 mL/min/1.73 m^2) and end-stage renal disease receiving hemodialysis should receive a starting dose of LIVALO 1 mg once daily and a maximum dose of LIVALO 2 mg once daily *[see Dosage and Administration (2.2) and Clinical Pharmacology (12.3)]*.

8.7 Hepatic Impairment
LIVALO is contraindicated in patients with active liver disease which may include unexplained persistent elevations of hepatic transaminase levels.

10 OVERDOSAGE
There is no known specific treatment in the event of overdose of pitavastatin. In the event of overdose, the patient should be treated symptomatically and supportive measures instituted as required. Hemodialysis is unlikely to be of benefit due to high protein binding ratio of pitavastatin.

11 DESCRIPTION
LIVALO (pitavastatin) is an inhibitor of HMG-CoA reductase. It is a synthetic lipid-lowering agent for oral administration. The chemical name for pitavastatin is (+)monocalcium *bis*{(3R, 5S, 6E)-7-[2-cyclopropyl-4-(4-fluorophenyl)-3-quinolyl]-3,5-dihydroxy-6-heptenoate}. The structural formula is:

The empirical formula for pitavastatin is $C_{50}H_{46}CaF_2N_2O_8$ and the molecular weight is 880.98. Pitavastatin is odorless and occurs as white to pale-yellow powder. It is freely soluble in pyridine, chloroform, dilute hydrochloric acid, and tetrahydrofuran, soluble in ethylene glycol, sparingly soluble in octanol, slightly soluble in methanol, very slightly soluble in water or ethanol, and practically insoluble in acetonitrile or diethyl ether. Pitavastatin is hygroscopic and slightly unstable in light.

Each film-coated tablet of LIVALO contains 1.045 mg, 2.09 mg, or 4.18 mg of pitavastatin calcium, which is equivalent to 1 mg, 2 mg, or 4 mg, respectively of free base and the following inactive ingredients: lactose monohydrate, low substituted hydroxypropylcellulose, hypromellose, magnesium aluminometasilicate, magnesium stearate, and film coating containing the following inactive ingredients: hypromellose, titanium dioxide, triethyl citrate, and colloidal anhydrous silica.

12 CLINICAL PHARMACOLOGY
12.1 Mechanism of Action
Pitavastatin competitively inhibits HMG-CoA reductase, which is a rate-determining enzyme involved with biosynthesis of cholesterol, in a manner of competition with the substrate so that it inhibits cholesterol synthesis in the liver. As a result, the expression of LDL-receptors followed by the uptake of LDL from blood to liver is accelerated and then the plasma TC decreases. Further, the sustained inhibition of cholesterol synthesis in the liver decreases levels of very low density lipoproteins.

12.2 Pharmacodynamics
In a randomized, double-blind, placebo-controlled, 4-way parallel, active-comparator study in 174 healthy participants, LIVALO was not associated with clinically meaningful prolongation of the QTc interval or heart rate at daily doses up to 16 mg (4 times the recommended maximum daily dose).

12.3 Pharmacokinetics
Absorption: Pitavastatin peak plasma concentrations are achieved about 1 hour after oral administration. Both C_{max} and AUC_{0-inf} increased in an approximately dose-proportional manner for single LIVALO doses from 1 to 24 mg once daily. The absolute bioavailability of pitavastatin oral solution is 51%. Administration of LIVALO with a high fat meal (50% fat content) decreases pitavastatin C_{max} by 43% but does not significantly reduce pitavastatin AUC. The C_{max} and AUC of pitavastatin did not differ following evening or morning drug administration. In healthy volunteers receiving 4 mg pitavastatin, the percent change from baseline for LDL-C following evening dosing was slightly greater than that following morning dosing. Pitavastatin was absorbed in the small intestine but very little in the colon.

Distribution: Pitavastatin is more than 99% protein bound in human plasma, mainly to albumin and alpha 1-acid glycoprotein, and the mean volume of distribution is approximately 148 L. Association of pitavastatin and/or its metabolites with the blood cells is minimal.

Metabolism:. Pitavastatin is marginally metabolized by CYP2C9 and to a lesser extent by CYP2C8. The major metabolite in human plasma is the lactone which is formed via an ester-type pitavastatin glucuronide conjugate by uridine 5'-diphosphate (UDP) glucuronosyltransferase (UGT1A3 and UGT2B7).

Excretion: A mean of 15% of radioactivity of orally administered single 32 mg ^{14}C-labeled pitavastatin dose was excreted in urine, whereas a mean of 79% of the dose was excreted in feces within 7 days. The mean plasma elimination half-life is approximately 12 hours.

Race: In pharmacokinetic studies pitavastatin C_{max} and AUC were 21 and 5% lower, respectively in Black or African American healthy volunteers compared with those of Caucasian healthy volunteers. In pharmacokinetic comparison between Caucasian volunteers and Japanese volunteers, there were no significant differences in C_{max} and AUC.

Gender: In a pharmacokinetic study which compared healthy male and female volunteers, pitavastatin C_{max} and AUC were 60 and 54% higher, respectively in females. This had no effect on the efficacy or safety of LIVALO in women in clinical studies.

Geriatric: In a pharmacokinetic study which compared healthy young and elderly (≥65 years) volunteers, pitavastatin C_{max} and AUC were 10 and 30% higher, respectively, in the elderly. This had no effect on the efficacy or safety of LIVALO in elderly subjects in clinical studies.

Renal Impairment: In patients with moderate renal impairment (glomerular filtration rate of 30 to <60 mL/min/1.73 m^2) and end stage renal disease receiving hemodialysis, pitavastatin AUC_{0-inf} is 79 and 86% higher than those of healthy volunteers, respectively, while pitavastatin C_{max} is 60 and 40% higher than those of healthy volunteers, respectively. Patients received hemodialysis immediately before pitavastatin dosing and did not undergo hemodialysis during the pharmacokinetic study. Hemodialysis patients have 33 and 36% increases in the mean unbound fraction of pitavastatin as compared to healthy volunteers and patients with moderate renal impairment, respectively. The effect of mild and severe renal impairment on pitavastatin exposure is unknown.

Hepatic Impairment: The disposition of pitavastatin was compared in healthy volunteers and patients with various degrees of hepatic impairment. The ratio of pitavastatin C_{max} between patients with moderate hepatic impairment (Child-Pugh B disease) and healthy volunteers was 2.7. The ratio of pitavastatin AUC_{inf} between patients with moderate hepatic impairment and healthy volunteers was 3.8. The ratio of pitavastatin C_{max} between patients with mild hepatic impairment (Child-Pugh A disease) and healthy volunteers was 1.3. The ratio of pitavastatin AUC_{inf} between patients with mild hepatic impairment and healthy volunteers was 1.6. Mean pitavastatin $t_{1/2}$ for moderate hepatic impairment, mild hepatic impairment, and healthy were 15, 10, and 8 hours, respectively.

Drug-Drug Interactions: The principal route of pitavastatin metabolism is glucuronidation via liver UGTs with subsequent formation of pitavastatin lactone. There is only minimal metabolism by the cytochrome P450 system.

Table 2. Effect of Co-Administered Drugs on Pitavastatin Systemic Exposure

Co-administered drug	Dose regimen	Change in AUC*	Change in C_{max}*
Cyclosporine	Pitavastatin 2 mg QD for 6 days + cyclosporine 2 mg/kg on Day 6	↑ 4.6 fold†	↑ 6.6 fold†
Erythromycin	Pitavastatin 4 mg single dose on Day 4 + erythromycin 500 mg 4 times daily for 6 days	↑ 2.8 fold†	↑ 3.6 fold†
Rifampin	Pitavastatin 4 mg QD + rifampin 600 mg QD for 5 days	↑ 29%	↑ 2.0 fold
Atazanavir	Pitavastatin 4 mg QD + atazanavir 300 mg daily for 5 days	↑ 31%	↑ 60%
Gemfibrozil	Pitavastatin 4 mg QD + gemfibrozil 600 mg BID for 7 days	↑ 45%	↑ 31%
Fenofibrate	Pitavastatin 4 mg QD + fenofibrate 160 mg QD for 7 days	↑18%	↑ 11%
Ezetimibe	Pitavastatin 2 mg QD + ezetimibe 10 mg for 7 days	↓ 2%	↓0.2%
Enalapril	Pitavastatin 4 mg QD + enalapril 20 mg daily for 5 days	↑ 6%	↓ 7%
Digoxin	Pitavastatin 4 mg QD + digoxin 0.25 mg for 7 days	↑ 4%	↓ 9%
Grapefruit Juice	Pitavastatin 2 mg single dose on Day 3 + grapefruit juice for 4 days	↑ 15%	↓ 12%
Itraconazole	Pitavastatin 4 mg single dose on Day 4 + itraconazole 200 mg daily for 5 days	↓ 23%	↓ 22%

* Data presented as x-fold change represent the ratio between co-administration and pitavastatin alone (i.e., 1-fold = no change). Data presented as % change represent % difference relative to pitavastatin alone (i.e., 0% = no change).
† Considered clinically significant *[see Dosage and Administration (2) and Drug Interactions (7)]*

Table 3. Effect of Pitavastatin Co-Administration on Systemic Exposure to Other Drugs

Co-administered drug	Dose regimen		Change in AUC*	Change in C_{max}*
Atazanavir	Pitavastatin 4 mg QD + atazanavir 300 mg daily for 5 days		↑ 6%	↑ 13%
Enalapril	Pitavastatin 4 mg QD + enalapril 20 mg daily for 5 days	Enalapril	↑ 12%	↑ 12%
		Enalaprilat	↓ 1%	↓ 1%
Warfarin	Individualized maintenance dose of warfarin (2-7 mg) for 8 days + pitavastatin 4 mg QD for 9 days	R-warfarin	↑ 7%	↑ 3%
		S-warfarin	↑ 6%	↑ 3%
Ezetimibe	Pitavastatin 2 mg QD + ezetimibe 10 mg for 7 days		↑ 9%	↑ 2%
Digoxin	Pitavastatin 4 mg QD + digoxin 0.25 mg for 7 days		↓ 3%	↓ 4%
Rifampin	Pitavastatin 4 mg QD + rifampin 600 mg QD for 5 days		↓ 15%	↓ 18%

* Data presented as % change represent % difference relative to the investigated drug alone (i.e., 0% = no change).

Table 5. Response by Dose of LIVALO and Atorvastatin in Patients with Primary Hyperlipidemia or Mixed Dyslipidemia (Mean % Change from Baseline at Week 12)

Treatment	N	LDL-C	Apo-B	TC	TG	HDL-C	non-HDL-C
LIVALO 2 mg daily	315	-38	-30	-28	-14	4	-35
LIVALO 4 mg daily	298	-45	-35	-32	-19	5	-41
Atorvastatin 10 mg daily	102	-38	-29	-28	-18	3	-35
Atorvastatin 20 mg daily	102	-44	-36	-33	-22	2	-41
Atorvastatin 40 mg daily	----------------------------Not Studied----------------------------						
Atorvastatin 80 mg daily	----------------------------Not Studied----------------------------						

Table 6. Response by Dose of LIVALO and Simvastatin in Patients with Primary Hyperlipidemia or Mixed Dyslipidemia (Mean % Change from Baseline at Week 12)

Treatment	N	LDL-C	Apo-B	TC	TG	HDL-C	non-HDL-C
LIVALO 2 mg daily	307	-39	-30	-28	-16	6	-36
LIVALO 4 mg daily	319	-44	-35	-32	-17	6	-41
Simvastatin 20 mg daily	107	-35	-27	-25	-16	6	-32
Simvastatin 40 mg daily	110	-43	-34	-31	-16	7	-39
Simvastatin 80 mg	----------------------------Not Studied----------------------------						

Table 7. Response by Dose of LIVALO and Pravastatin in Patients with Primary Hyperlipidemia or Mixed Dyslipidemia (Mean % Change from Baseline at Week 12)

Treatment	N	LDL-C	Apo-B	TC	TG	HDL-C	non-HDL-C
LIVALO 1 mg daily	207	-31	-25	-22	-13	1	-29
LIVALO 2 mg daily	224	-39	-31	-27	-15	2	-36
LIVALO 4 mg daily	210	-44	-37	-31	-22	4	-41
Pravastatin 10 mg daily	103	-22	-17	-15	-5	-0	-20
Pravastatin 20 mg daily	96	-29	-22	-21	-11	-1	-27
Pravastatin 40 mg daily	102	-34	-28	-24	-15	1	-32
Pravastatin 80 mg daily	----------------------------Not Studied----------------------------						

Warfarin: The steady-state pharmacodynamics (international normalized ratio [INR] and prothrombin time [PT]) and pharmacokinetics of warfarin in healthy volunteers were unaffected by the co-administration of LIVALO 4 mg daily. However, patients receiving warfarin should have their PT time or INR monitored when pitavastatin is added to their therapy.
[See table 2 at top of previous page]
[See table 3 on previous page]

13   NONCLINICAL TOXICOLOGY
13.1   Carcinogenesis, Mutagenesis, Impairment of Fertility
In a 92-week carcinogenicity study in mice given pitavastatin, at the maximum tolerated dose of 75 mg/kg/day with systemic maximum exposures (AUC) 26 times the clinical maximum exposure at 4 mg/day, there was an absence of drug-related tumors. In a 92-week carcinogenicity study in rats given pitavastatin at 1, 5, 25 mg/kg/day by oral gavage there was a significant increase in the incidence of thyroid follicular cell tumors at 25 mg/kg/day, which represents 295 times human systemic exposures based on AUC at the 4 mg/day maximum human dose.
In a 26-week transgenic mouse (Tg rasH2) carcinogenicity study where animals were given pitavastatin at 30, 75, and 150 mg/kg/day by oral gavage, no clinically significant tumors were observed.
Pitavastatin was not mutagenic in the Ames test with *Salmonella typhimurium* and *Escherichia coli* with and without metabolic activation, the micronucleus test following a single administration in mice and multiple administrations

in rats, the unscheduled DNA synthesis test in rats, and a Comet assay in mice. In the chromosomal aberration test, clastogenicity was observed at the highest doses tested which also elicited high levels of cytotoxicity.
Pitavastatin had no adverse effects on male and female rat fertility at oral doses of 10 and 30 mg/kg/day, respectively, at systemic exposures 56- and 354-times clinical exposure at 4 mg/day based on AUC.
Pitavastatin treatment in rabbits resulted in mortality in males and females given 1 mg/kg/day (30-times clinical systemic exposure at 4 mg/day based on AUC) and higher during a fertility study. Although the cause of death was not determined, rabbits had gross signs of renal toxicity (kidneys whitened) indicative of possible ischemia. Lower doses (15-times human systemic exposure) did not show significant toxicity in adult males and females. However, decreased implantations, increased resorptions, and decreased viability of fetuses were observed.

13.2   Animal Toxicology and/or Pharmacology
Central Nervous System Toxicity
CNS vascular lesions, characterized by perivascular hemorrhages, edema, and mononuclear cell infiltration of perivascular spaces, have been observed in dogs treated with several other members of this drug class. A chemically similar drug in this class produced dose-dependent optic nerve degeneration (Wallerian degeneration of retinogeniculate fibers) in dogs, at a dose that produced plasma drug levels about 30 times higher than the mean drug level in humans taking the highest recommended dose. Wallerian degeneration has not been observed with pitavastatin. Cataracts and lens opacities were seen in dogs treated for 52 weeks at a

dose level of 1 mg/kg/day (9 times clinical exposure at the maximum human dose of 4 mg/day based on AUC comparisons.

14   CLINICAL STUDIES
14.1   Primary Hyperlipidemia or Mixed Dyslipidemia
Dose-ranging study: A multicenter, randomized, double-blind, placebo-controlled, dose-ranging study was performed to evaluate the efficacy of LIVALO compared with placebo in 251 patients with primary hyperlipidemia (Table 4). LIVALO given as a single daily dose for 12 weeks significantly reduced plasma LDL-C, TC, TG, and Apo-B compared to placebo and was associated with variable increases in HDL-C across the dose range.

Table 4. Dose-Response in Patients with Primary Hypercholesterolemia (Adjusted Mean % Change from Baseline at Week 12)

Treatment	N	LDL-C	Apo-B	TC	TG	HDL-C
Placebo	53	-3	-2	-2	1	0
LIVALO 1mg	52	-32	-25	-23	-15	8
LIVALO 2mg	49	-36	-30	-26	-19	7
LIVALO 4mg	51#	-43	-35	-31	-18	5

The number of subjects for Apo-B was 49

Active-controlled study with atorvastatin (NK-104-301): LIVALO was compared with the HMG-CoA reductase inhibitor atorvastatin in a randomized, multicenter, double-blind, double-dummy, active-controlled, non-inferiority Phase 3 study of 817 patients with primary hyperlipidemia or mixed dyslipidemia. Patients entered a 6- to 8-week wash-out/dietary lead-in period and then were randomized to a 12-week treatment with either LIVALO or atorvastatin (Table 5). Non-inferiority of pitavastatin to a given dose of atorvastatin was considered to be demonstrated if the lower bound of the 95% CI for the mean treatment difference was greater than -6% for the mean percent change in LDL-C. Lipid results are shown in Table 5. For the percent change from baseline to endpoint in LDL-C, LIVALO was non-inferior to atorvastatin for the two pairwise comparisons: LIVALO 2 mg vs. atorvastatin 10 mg and LIVALO 4 mg vs. atorvastatin 20 mg. Mean treatment differences (95% CI) were 0% (-3%, 3%) and 1% (-2%, 4%), respectively.
[See table 5 at top left]
Active-controlled study with simvastatin (NK-104-302): LIVALO was compared with the HMG-CoA reductase inhibitor simvastatin in a randomized, multicenter, double-blind, double-dummy, active-controlled, non-inferiority Phase 3 study of 843 patients with primary hyperlipidemia or mixed dyslipidemia. Patients entered a 6- to 8-week wash-out/dietary lead-in period and then were randomized to a 12 week treatment with either LIVALO or simvastatin (Table 6). Non-inferiority of pitavastatin to a given dose of simvastatin was considered to be demonstrated if the lower bound of the 95% CI for the mean treatment difference was greater than -6% for the mean percent change in LDL-C.
Lipid results are shown in Table 6. For the percent change from baseline to endpoint in LDL-C, LIVALO was non-inferior to simvastatin for the two pairwise comparisons: LIVALO 2 mg vs. simvastatin 20 mg and LIVALO 4 mg vs. simvastatin 40 mg. Mean treatment differences (95% CI) were 4% (1%, 7%) and 1% (-2%, 4%), respectively.
[See table 6 above]
Active-controlled study with pravastatin in elderly (NK-104-306): LIVALO was compared with the HMG-CoA reductase inhibitor pravastatin in a randomized, multicenter, double-blind, double-dummy, parallel group, active-controlled non-inferiority Phase 3 study of 942 elderly patients (≥65 years) with primary hyperlipidemia or mixed dyslipidemia. Patients entered a 6- to 8-week wash-out/dietary lead-in period, and then were randomized to a once daily dose of LIVALO or pravastatin for 12 weeks (Table 7). Non-inferiority of LIVALO to a given dose of pravastatin was assumed if the lower bound of the 95% CI for the treatment difference was greater than -6% for the mean percent change in LDL-C.
Lipid results are shown in Table 7. LIVALO significantly reduced LDL-C compared to pravastatin as demonstrated by the following pairwise dose comparisons: LIVALO 1 mg vs. pravastatin 10 mg, LIVALO 2 mg vs. pravastatin 20 mg and LIVALO 4 mg vs. pravastatin 40 mg. Mean treatment differences (95% CI) were 9% (6%, 12%), 10% (7%, 13%) and 10% (7%, 13%), respectively.
[See table 7 above]
Active-controlled study with simvastatin in patients with ≥ 2 risk factors for coronary heart disease (NK-104-304): LIVALO was compared with the HMG-CoA reductase inhibitor simvastatin in a randomized, multicenter, double-blind, double-dummy, active-controlled, non-inferiority Phase 3 study of 351 patients with primary hyperlipidemia or mixed dyslipidemia with ≥2 risk factors for coronary heart disease. After a 6- to 8-week wash-out/dietary lead-in period, patients were randomized to a 12-week treatment with either LIVALO or simvastatin (Table 8). Non-inferiority of

Table 8. Response by Dose of LIVALO and Simvastatin in Patients with Primary Hyperlipidemia or Mixed Dyslipidemia with ≥2 Risk Factors for Coronary Heart Disease (Mean % Change from Baseline at Week 12)

Treatment	N	LDL-C	Apo-B	TC	TG	HDL-C	non-HDL-C
LIVALO 4 mg daily	233	-44	-34	-31	-20	7	-40
Simvastatin 40 mg daily	118	-44	-34	-31	-15	5	-39
Simvastatin 80 mg daily		--------------------------------------Not Studied--------------------------------						

Table 9. Response by Dose of LIVALO and Atorvastatin in Patients with Type II Diabetes Mellitus and Combined Dyslipidemia (Mean % Change from Baseline at Week 12)

Treatment	N	LDL-C	Apo-B	TC	TG	HDL-C	non-HDL-C
LIVALO 4 mg daily	274	-41	-32	-28	-20	7	-36
Atorvastatin 20 mg daily	136	-43	-34	-32	-27	8	-40
Atorvastatin 40 mg daily		--------------------------------------Not Studied--------------------------------						
Atorvastatin 80 mg daily		--------------------------------------Not Studied--------------------------------						

LIVALO to simvastatin was considered to be demonstrated if the lower bound of the 95% CI for the mean treatment difference was greater than -6% for the mean percent change in LDL-C.

Lipid results are shown in Table 8. LIVALO 4 mg was non-inferior to simvastatin 40 mg for percent change from baseline to endpoint in LDL-C. The mean treatment difference (95% CI) was 0% (-2%, 3%).

[See table 8 above]

Active-controlled study with atorvastatin in patients with type II diabetes mellitus (NK-104-305): LIVALO was compared with the HMG-CoA reductase inhibitor atorvastatin in a randomized, multicenter, double-blind, double-dummy, parallel group, active-controlled, non-inferiority Phase 3 study of 410 subjects with type II diabetes mellitus and combined dyslipidemia. Patients entered a 6- to 8-week washout/dietary lead-in period and were randomized to a once daily dose of LIVALO or atorvastatin for 12 weeks. Non-inferiority of LIVALO was considered to be demonstrated if the lower bound of the 95% CI for the mean treatment difference was greater than -6% for the mean percent change in LDL-C.

Lipid results are shown in Table 9. The treatment difference (95% CI) for LDL-C percent change from baseline was -2% (-6.2%, 1.5%). The two treatment groups were not statistically different on LDL-C. However, the lower limit of the CI was -6.2%, slightly exceeding the -6% non-inferiority limit so that the non-inferiority objective was not achieved.

[See table 9 above]

The treatment differences in efficacy in LDL-C change from baseline between LIVALO and active controls in the Phase 3 studies are summarized in Figure 1.

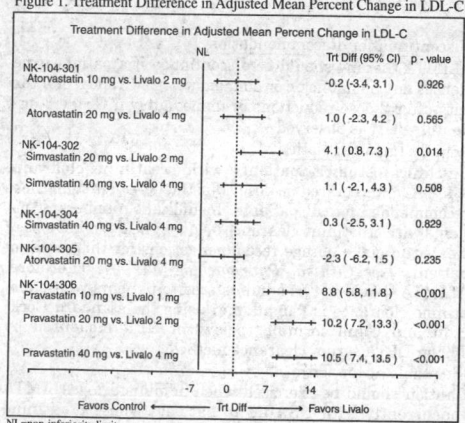

Figure 1. Treatment Difference in Adjusted Mean Percent Change in LDL-C

NL=non-inferiority limit.

16 HOW SUPPLIED/STORAGE AND HANDLING

LIVALO tablets for oral administration are provided as white, film-coated tablets that contain 1 mg, 2 mg, or 4 mg of pitavastatin. Each tablet has "KC" debossed on one side and a code number specific to the tablet strength on the other.

Packaging

LIVALO (pitavastatin) Tablets are supplied as;

- NDC 0002-4770-90 : 1 mg. Round white film-coated tablet debossed "KC" on one face and "1" on the reverse; HDPE bottles of 90 tablets
- NDC 0002-4771-90 : 2 mg. Round white film-coated tablet debossed "KC" on one face and "2" on the reverse; HDPE bottles of 90 tablets
- NDC 0002-4772-90 : 4 mg. Round white film-coated tablet debossed "KC" on one face and "4" on the reverse; HDPE bottles of 90 tablets

Storage

Store at room temperature between 15°C and 30°C (59° to 86° F) [see USP]. Protect from light.

17 PATIENT COUNSELING INFORMATION

The patient should be informed of the following:

17.1 Dosing Time

LIVALO can be taken at any time of the day with or without food.

17.2 Muscle Pain

Patients should be advised to promptly notify their physician of any unexplained muscle pain, tenderness, or weakness. They should discuss all medication, both prescription and over the counter, with their physician.

17.3 Pregnancy

Women of childbearing age should use an effective method of birth control to prevent pregnancy while using LIVALO. Discuss future pregnancy plans with your healthcare professional, and discuss when to stop LIVALO if you are trying to conceive. If you are pregnant, stop taking LIVALO and call your healthcare professional.

17.4 Breastfeeding

Women who are breastfeeding should not use LIVALO. If you have a lipid disorder and are breastfeeding, stop taking LIVALO and consult with your healthcare professional.

17.5 Liver Enzymes

It is recommended that liver enzymes be checked before and at 12 weeks following both the initiation of therapy and any elevation of dose, and periodically (e.g., semiannually) thereafter.

LIVALO is a trademark of the Kowa group of companies.

© Kowa Pharmaceuticals America, Inc. (2009)

Manufactured under license from: Kowa Company, Limited Tokyo 103-8433 Japan

Manufactured by: Patheon, Inc. Cincinnati, OH 45237 USA

Marketed by: Kowa Pharmaceuticals America, Inc. Montgomery, AL 36117 USA

and Lilly USA, LLC. Indianapolis, IN 46285 USA

To request additional information or if you have questions concerning LIVALO please phone Kowa Pharmaceuticals America, Inc. at 877-8-LIVALO (877-854-8256) or fax your inquiry to 800-689-0244

Rev: 1/10

Shown in Product Identification Guide, page 310

Eli Lilly and Company
LILLY CORPORATE CENTER
INDIANAPOLIS, IN 46285

Direct Inquiries to:
Lilly Corporate Center
Indianapolis, IN 46285
(317) 276-2000
www.lilly.com
For Medical Information Contact:
Lilly Research Laboratories
Lilly Corporate Center
Indianapolis, IN 46285
(800) 545-5979
lillymedical.com (US HCP registration required)

ALIMTA®   R
[*uh-LIM-tuh*]
(pemetrexed disodium)
Injection, Powder, Lyophilized, For Solution for Intravenous Use

HIGHLIGHTS OF PRESCRIBING INFORMATION

These highlights do not include all the information needed to use ALIMTA safely and effectively. See full prescribing information for ALIMTA.

ALIMTA (pemetrexed disodium) Injection, Powder, Lyophilized, For Solution for Intravenous Use
Initial U.S. Approval: 2004

———————INDICATIONS AND USAGE———————

ALIMTA® is a folate analog metabolic inhibitor indicated for:

- Locally Advanced or Metastatic Nonsquamous Non-Small Cell Lung Cancer:
  - Initial treatment in combination with cisplatin. (1.1)
  - Maintenance treatment of patients whose disease has not progressed after four cycles of platinum-based first-line chemotherapy. (1.2)
  - After prior chemotherapy as a single-agent. (1.3)
- Mesothelioma: in combination with cisplatin. (1.4)

Limitations of Use:

- ALIMTA is not indicated for the treatment of patients with squamous cell non-small cell lung cancer. (1.5)

————DOSAGE AND ADMINISTRATION————

- Combination use in Non-Small Cell Lung Cancer and Mesothelioma: Recommended dose of ALIMTA is 500 mg/m² i.v. on Day 1 of each 21-day cycle in combination with cisplatin 75 mg/m² i.v. beginning 30 minutes after ALIMTA administration. (2.1)
- Single-Agent use in Non-Small Cell Lung Cancer: Recommended dose of ALIMTA is 500 mg/m² i.v. on Day 1 of each 21-day cycle. (2.2)
- Dose Reductions: Dose reductions or discontinuation may be needed based on toxicities from the preceding cycle of therapy. (2.4)

————DOSAGE FORMS AND STRENGTHS————

- 100 mg vial for injection (3)
- 500 mg vial for injection (3)

—————————CONTRAINDICATIONS—————————

History of severe hypersensitivity reaction to pemetrexed. (4)

————WARNINGS AND PRECAUTIONS————

- Premedication regimen: Instruct patients to take folic acid and vitamin B_{12}. Pretreatment with dexamethasone or equivalent reduces cutaneous reaction. (5.1)
- Bone marrow suppression: Reduce doses for subsequent cycles based on hematologic and nonhematologic toxicities. (5.2)
- Renal function: Do not administer when CrCl <45 mL/min. (2.4, 5.3)
- NSAIDs with renal insufficiency: Use caution in patients with mild to moderate renal insufficiency (CrCl 45-79 mL/min). (5.4)
- Lab monitoring: Do not begin next cycle unless ANC ≥1500 cells/mm³, platelets ≥100,000 cells/mm³, and CrCl ≥45 mL/min. (5.5)
- Pregnancy: Fetal harm can occur when administered to a pregnant woman. Women should be advised to use effective contraception measures to prevent pregnancy during treatment with ALIMTA. (5.6)

————————ADVERSE REACTIONS————————

The most common adverse reactions (incidence ≥20%) with single-agent use are fatigue, nausea, and anorexia. Additional common adverse reactions when used in combination with cisplatin include vomiting, neutropenia, leukopenia, anemia, stomatitis/pharyngitis, thrombocytopenia, and constipation. (6.1)

To report SUSPECTED ADVERSE REACTIONS, contact Eli Lilly and Company at 1-800-LillyRx (1-800-545-5979) or FDA at 1-800-FDA-1088 or www.fda.gov/medwatch

—————————DRUG INTERACTIONS—————————

- NSAIDs: Use caution with ibuprofen or other NSAIDs. (7.1)

Males:	$\dfrac{[140 - \text{Age in years}] \times \text{Actual Body Weight (kg)}}{72 \times \text{Serum Creatinine (mg/dL)}}$	= mL/min
Females:	Estimated creatinine clearance for males × 0.85	

• Nephrotoxic drugs: Concomitant use of these drugs and/or substances which are tubularly secreted may result in delayed clearance. (7.2)

See 17 for PATIENT COUNSELING INFORMATION and FDA-approved patient labeling

Revised: 8/2010

FULL PRESCRIBING INFORMATION: CONTENTS*

FULL PRESCRIBING INFORMATION

1 INDICATIONS AND USAGE

1.1 Nonsquamous Non-Small Cell Lung Cancer – Combination with Cisplatin
ALIMTA is indicated in combination with cisplatin therapy for the initial treatment of patients with locally advanced or metastatic nonsquamous non-small cell lung cancer.

1.2 Nonsquamous Non-Small Cell Lung Cancer – Maintenance
ALIMTA is indicated for the maintenance treatment of patients with locally advanced or metastatic nonsquamous non-small cell lung cancer whose disease has not progressed after four cycles of platinum-based first-line chemotherapy.

1.3 Nonsquamous Non-Small Cell Lung Cancer – After Prior Chemotherapy
ALIMTA is indicated as a single-agent for the treatment of patients with locally advanced or metastatic nonsquamous non-small cell lung cancer after prior chemotherapy.

1.4 Mesothelioma
ALIMTA in combination with cisplatin is indicated for the treatment of patients with malignant pleural mesothelioma whose disease is unresectable or who are otherwise not candidates for curative surgery.

1.5 Limitations of Use
ALIMTA is not indicated for the treatment of patients with squamous cell non-small cell lung cancer. *[see Clinical Studies (14.1, 14.2, 14.3)]*

2 DOSAGE AND ADMINISTRATION

2.1 Combination Use with Cisplatin
Nonsquamous Non-Small Cell Lung Cancer and Malignant Pleural Mesothelioma
The recommended dose of ALIMTA is 500 mg/m² administered as an intravenous infusion over 10 minutes on Day 1 of each 21-day cycle. The recommended dose of cisplatin is 75 mg/m² infused over 2 hours beginning approximately 30 minutes after the end of ALIMTA administration. Patients should receive appropriate hydration prior to and/or after receiving cisplatin. See cisplatin package insert for more information.

2.2 Single-Agent Use
Nonsquamous Non-Small Cell Lung Cancer
The recommended dose of ALIMTA is 500 mg/m² administered as an intravenous infusion over 10 minutes on Day 1 of each 21-day cycle.

2.3 Premedication Regimen
Vitamin Supplementation
To reduce toxicity, patients treated with ALIMTA must be instructed to take a low-dose oral folic acid preparation or multivitamin with folic acid on a daily basis. At least 5 daily doses of folic acid must be taken during the 7-day period preceding the first dose of ALIMTA; and dosing should continue during the full course of therapy and for 21 days after the last dose of ALIMTA. Patients must also receive one (1) intramuscular injection of vitamin B$_{12}$ during the week preceding the first dose of ALIMTA and every 3 cycles thereafter. Subsequent vitamin B$_{12}$ injections may be given the same day as ALIMTA. In clinical trials, the dose of folic acid studied ranged from 350 to 1000 mcg, and the dose of vitamin B$_{12}$ was 1000 mcg. The most commonly used dose of oral folic acid in clinical trials was 400 mcg *[see Warnings and Precautions (5.1)]*.
Corticosteroid
Skin rash has been reported more frequently in patients not pretreated with a corticosteroid. Pretreatment with dexamethasone (or equivalent) reduces the incidence and severity of cutaneous reaction. In clinical trials, dexamethasone 4 mg was given by mouth twice daily the day before, the day of, and the day after ALIMTA administration *[see Warnings and Precautions (5.1)]*.

2.4 Laboratory Monitoring and Dose Reduction/Discontinuation Recommendations
Monitoring
Complete blood cell counts, including platelet counts, should be performed on all patients receiving ALIMTA. Patients should be monitored for nadir and recovery, which were tested in the clinical study before each dose and on days 8 and 15 of each cycle. Patients should not begin a new cycle of treatment unless the ANC is ≥1500 cells/mm³, the platelet count is ≥100,000 cells/mm³, and creatinine clearance is ≥45 mL/min. Periodic chemistry tests should be performed to evaluate renal and hepatic function *[see Warnings and Precautions (5.5)]*.
Dose Reduction Recommendations
Dose adjustments at the start of a subsequent cycle should be based on nadir hematologic counts or maximum nonhe-

matologic toxicity from the preceding cycle of therapy. Treatment may be delayed to allow sufficient time for recovery. Upon recovery, patients should be retreated using the guidelines in Tables 1-3, which are suitable for using ALIMTA as a single-agent or in combination with cisplatin.

Table 1: Dose Reduction for ALIMTA (single-agent or in combination) and Cisplatin - Hematologic Toxicities

Nadir ANC <500/mm³ and nadir platelets ≥50,000/mm³.	75% of previous dose (pemetrexed and cisplatin).
Nadir platelets <50,000/mm³ without bleeding regardless of nadir ANC.	75% of previous dose (pemetrexed and cisplatin).
Nadir platelets <50,000/mm³ with bleeding[a], regardless of nadir ANC.	50% of previous dose (pemetrexed and cisplatin).

[a] These criteria meet the CTC version 2.0 (NCI 1998) definition of ≥CTC Grade 2 bleeding.

If patients develop nonhematologic toxicities (excluding neurotoxicity) ≥Grade 3, treatment should be withheld until resolution to less than or equal to the patient's pretherapy value. Treatment should be resumed according to guidelines in Table 2.

Table 2: Dose Reduction for ALIMTA (single-agent or in combination) and Cisplatin - Nonhematologic Toxicities[a],[b]

	Dose of ALIMTA (mg/m²)	Dose of Cisplatin (mg/m²)
Any Grade 3 or 4 toxicities except mucositis	75% of previous dose	75% of previous dose
Any diarrhea requiring hospitalization (irrespective of Grade) or Grade 3 or 4 diarrhea	75% of previous dose	75% of previous dose
Grade 3 or 4 mucositis	50% of previous dose	100% of previous dose

[a] NCI Common Toxicity Criteria (CTC).
[b] Excluding neurotoxicity (see Table 3).

In the event of neurotoxicity, the recommended dose adjustments for ALIMTA and cisplatin are described in Table 3. Patients should discontinue therapy if Grade 3 or 4 neurotoxicity is experienced.

Table 3: Dose Reduction for ALIMTA (single-agent or in combination) and Cisplatin - Neurotoxicity

CTC Grade	Dose of ALIMTA (mg/m²)	Dose of Cisplatin (mg/m²)
0-1	100% of previous dose	100% of previous dose
2	100% of previous dose	50% of previous dose

Discontinuation Recommendation
ALIMTA therapy should be discontinued if a patient experiences any hematologic or nonhematologic Grade 3 or 4 toxicity after 2 dose reductions or immediately if Grade 3 or 4 neurotoxicity is observed.
Renally Impaired Patients
In clinical studies, patients with creatinine clearance ≥45 mL/min required no dose adjustments other than those recommended for all patients. Insufficient numbers of patients with creatinine clearance below 45 mL/min have been treated to make dosage recommendations for this group of patients *[see Clinical Pharmacology (12.3)]*. Therefore, ALIMTA should not be administered to patients whose creatinine clearance is <45 mL/min using the standard Cockcroft and Gault formula (below) or GFR measured by Tc99m-DPTA serum clearance method:
[See table at top left]
Caution should be exercised when administering ALIMTA concurrently with NSAIDs to patients whose creatinine clearance is <80 mL/min *[see Drug Interactions (7.1)]*.

2.5 Preparation and Administration Precautions
As with other potentially toxic anticancer agents, care should be exercised in the handling and preparation of infusion solutions of ALIMTA. The use of gloves is recommended. If a solution of ALIMTA contacts the skin, wash the

skin immediately and thoroughly with soap and water. If ALIMTA contacts the mucous membranes, flush thoroughly with water. Several published guidelines for handling and disposal of anticancer agents are available *[see References (15)]*.

ALIMTA is not a vesicant. There is no specific antidote for extravasation of ALIMTA. To date, there have been few reported cases of ALIMTA extravasation, which were not assessed as serious by the investigator. ALIMTA extravasation should be managed with local standard practice for extravasation as with other non-vesicants.

2.6   Preparation for Intravenous Infusion Administration
1. Use aseptic technique during the reconstitution and further dilution of ALIMTA for intravenous infusion administration.
2. Calculate the dose of ALIMTA and determine the number of vials needed. Vials contain either 100 mg or 500 mg of ALIMTA. The vials contain an excess of ALIMTA to facilitate delivery of label amount.
3. Reconstitute each 100-mg vial with 4.2 ml of 0.9% Sodium Chloride Injection (preservative free). Reconstitute each 500-mg vial with 20 mL of 0.9% Sodium Chloride Injection (preservative free). Reconstitution of either size vial gives a solution containing 25 mg/mL ALIMTA. Gently swirl each vial until the powder is completely dissolved. The resulting solution is clear and ranges in color from colorless to yellow or green-yellow without adversely affecting product quality. The pH of the reconstituted ALIMTA solution is between 6.6 and 7.8. FURTHER DILUTION IS REQUIRED.
4. Parenteral drug products should be inspected visually for particulate matter and discoloration prior to administration, whenever solution and container permit. If particulate matter is observed, do not administer.
5. An appropriate quantity of the reconstituted ALIMTA solution must be further diluted into a solution of 0.9% Sodium Chloride Injection (preservative free), so that the total volume of solution is 100 ml. ALIMTA is administered as an intravenous infusion over 10 minutes.
6. Chemical and physical stability of reconstituted and infusion solutions of ALIMTA were demonstrated for up to 24 hours following initial reconstitution, when stored at refrigerated or ambient room temperature *[see USP Controlled Room Temperature]* and lighting. When prepared as directed, reconstitution and infusion solutions of ALIMTA contain no antimicrobial preservatives. Discard any unused portion.

Reconstitution and further dilution prior to intravenous infusion is only recommended with 0.9% Sodium Chloride Injection (preservative free). ALIMTA is physically incompatible with diluents containing calcium, including Lactated Ringer's Injection, USP and Ringer's Injection, USP and therefore these should not be used. Coadministration of ALIMTA with other drugs and diluents has not been studied, and therefore is not recommended. ALIMTA is compatible with standard polyvinyl chloride (PVC) administration sets and intravenous solution bags.

3   DOSAGE FORMS AND STRENGTHS

ALIMTA, pemetrexed for injection, is a white to either light-yellow or green-yellow lyophilized powder available in sterile single-use vials containing 100 mg or 500 mg pemetrexed.

4   CONTRAINDICATIONS

ALIMTA is contraindicated in patients who have a history of severe hypersensitivity reaction to pemetrexed or to any other ingredient used in the formulation.

5   WARNINGS AND PRECAUTIONS
5.1   Premedication Regimen
Need for Folate and Vitamin B$_{12}$ Supplementation
Patients treated with ALIMTA must be instructed to take folic acid and vitamin B$_{12}$ as a prophylactic measure to reduce treatment-related hematologic and GI toxicity *[see Dosage and Administration (2.3)]*. In clinical studies, less overall toxicity and reductions in Grade 3/4 hematologic and nonhematologic toxicities such as neutropenia, febrile neutropenia, and infection with Grade 3/4 neutropenia were reported when pretreatment with folic acid and vitamin B$_{12}$ was administered.
Corticosteroid Supplementation
Skin rash has been reported more frequently in patients not pretreated with a corticosteroid in clinical trials. Pretreatment with dexamethasone (or equivalent) reduces the incidence and severity of cutaneous reaction *[see Dosage and Administration (2.3)]*.
5.2   Bone Marrow Suppression
ALIMTA can suppress bone marrow function, as manifested by neutropenia, thrombocytopenia, and anemia (or pancytopenia) *[see Adverse Reactions (6.1)]*, myelosuppression is usually the dose-limiting toxicity. Dose reductions for subsequent cycles are based on nadir ANC, platelet count, and maximum nonhematologic toxicity seen in the previous cycle *[see Dosage and Administration (2.4)]*.
5.3   Decreased Renal Function
ALIMTA is primarily eliminated unchanged by renal excretion. No dosage adjustment is needed in patients with creatinine clearance ≥45 mL/min. Insufficient numbers of patients have been studied with creatinine clearance <45 mL/min to give a dose recommendation. Therefore, ALIMTA should not be administered to patients whose creatinine clearance is <45 mL/min *[see Dosage and Administration (2.4)]*.

One patient with severe renal impairment (creatinine clearance 19 mL/min) who did not receive folic acid and vitamin B$_{12}$ died of drug-related toxicity following administration of ALIMTA alone.
5.4   Use with Non-Steroidal Anti-Inflammatory Drugs with Mild to Moderate Renal Insufficiency
Caution should be used when administering ibuprofen concurrently with ALIMTA to patients with mild to moderate renal insufficiency (creatinine clearance from 45 to 79 mL/min). Other NSAIDs should also be used with caution *[see Drug Interactions (7.1)]*.
5.5   Required Laboratory Monitoring
Patients should not begin a new cycle of treatment unless the ANC is ≥1500 cells/mm³, the platelet count is ≥100,000 cells/mm³, and creatinine clearance is ≥45 mL/min *[see Dosage and Administration (2.4)]*.
5.6   Pregnancy Category D
Based on its mechanism of action, ALIMTA can cause fetal harm when administered to a pregnant woman. Pemetrexed administered intraperitoneally to mice during organogenesis was embryotoxic, fetotoxic and teratogenic in mice at greater than 1/833rd the recommended human dose. If ALIMTA is used during pregnancy, or if the patient becomes pregnant while taking this drug, the patient should be apprised of the potential hazard to the fetus. Women of childbearing potential should be advised to avoid becoming pregnant. Women should be advised to use effective contraceptive measures to prevent pregnancy during treatment with ALIMTA *[see Use in Specific Populations (8.1)]*.
5.7   Third Space Fluid
The effect of third space fluid, such as pleural effusion and ascites, on ALIMTA is unknown. In patients with clinically significant third space fluid, consideration should be given to draining the effusion prior to ALIMTA administration.

6   ADVERSE REACTIONS
6.1   Clinical Trials Experience
Because clinical trials are conducted under widely varying conditions, adverse reactions rates cannot be directly compared to rates in other clinical trials and may not reflect the rates observed in clinical practice.

Table 4: Adverse Reactions in Fully Supplemented Patients Receiving ALIMTA plus Cisplatin in NSCLC[a]

Reaction[b]	ALIMTA/cisplatin (N=839)		Gemcitabine/cisplatin (N=830)	
	All Grades Toxicity (%)	Grade 3-4 Toxicity (%)	All Grades Toxicity (%)	Grade 3-4 Toxicity (%)
All Adverse Reactions	90	37	91	53
Laboratory				
Hematologic				
Anemia	33	6	46	10
Neutropenia	29	15	38	27
Leukopenia	18	5	21	8
Thrombocytopenia	10	4	27	13
Renal				
Creatinine elevation	10	1	7	1
Clinical				
Constitutional Symptoms				
Fatigue	43	7	45	5
Gastrointestinal				
Nausea	56	7	53	4
Vomiting	40	6	36	6
Anorexia	27	2	24	1
Constipation	21	1	20	0
Stomatitis/Pharyngitis	14	1	12	0
Diarrhea	12	1	13	2
Dyspepsia/Heartburn	5	0	6	0
Neurology				
Neuropathy-sensory	9	0	12	1
Taste disturbance	8	0[c]	9	0[c]
Dermatology/Skin				
Alopecia	12	0[c]	21	1[c]
Rash/Desquamation	7	0	8	1

[a] For the purpose of this table a cut off of 5% was used for inclusion of all events where the reporter considered a possible relationship to ALIMTA.
[b] Refer to NCI CTC Criteria version 2.0 for each Grade of toxicity.
[c] According to NCI CTC Criteria version 2.0, this adverse event term should only be reported as Grade 1 or 2.

Table 5: Adverse Reactions in Patients Receiving ALIMTA versus Placebo in NSCLC[a]

Reaction[b]	ALIMTA (N=438)		Placebo (N=218)	
	All Grades Toxicity (%)	Grade 3-4 Toxicity (%)	All Grades Toxicity (%)	Grade 3-4 Toxicity (%)
All Adverse Reactions	66	16	37	4
Laboratory				
Hematologic				
Anemia	15	3	6	1
Neutropenia	6	3	0	0
Leukopenia	6	2	1	1
Hepatic				
Increased ALT	10	0	4	0
Increased AST	8	0	4	0
Clinical				
Constitutional Symptoms				
Fatigue	25	5	11	1
Gastrointestinal				
Nausea	19	1	6	1
Anorexia	19	2	5	0
Vomiting	9	0	1	0
Mucositis/stomatitis	7	1	2	0
Diarrhea	5	1	3	0
Infection	5	2	2	0
Neurology				
Neuropathy-sensory	9	1	4	0
Dermatology/Skin				
Rash/Desquamation	10	0	3	0

[a] For the purpose of this table a cut off of 5% was used for inclusion of all events where the reporter considered a possible relationship to ALIMTA.
[b] Refer to NCI CTCAE Criteria version 3.0 for each Grade of toxicity.

Table 6: Adverse Reactions in Fully Supplemented Patients Receiving ALIMTA versus Docetaxel in NSCLC[a]

Reaction[b]	ALIMTA (N=265)		Docetaxel (N=276)	
	All Grades Toxicity (%)	Grades 3-4 Toxicity (%)	All Grades Toxicity (%)	Grades 3-4 Toxicity (%)
Laboratory				
Hematologic				
Anemia	19	4	22	4
Leukopenia	12	4	34	27
Neutropenia	11	5	45	40
Thrombocytopenia	8	2	1	0
Hepatic				
Increased ALT	8	2	1	0
Increased AST	7	1	1	0

(Table continued on next page)

In clinical trials, the most common adverse reactions (incidence ≥20%) during therapy with ALIMTA as a single-agent were fatigue, nausea, and anorexia. Additional common adverse reactions (incidence ≥20%) during therapy with ALIMTA when used in combination with cisplatin included vomiting, neutropenia, leukopenia, anemia, stomatitis/pharyngitis, thrombocytopenia, and constipation.

Non-Small Cell Lung Cancer (NSCLC) — Combination with Cisplatin
Table 4 provides the frequency and severity of adverse reactions that have been reported in >5% of 839 patients with NSCLC who were randomized to study and received ALIMTA plus cisplatin and 830 patients with NSCLC who were randomized to study and received gemcitabine plus cisplatin. All patients received study therapy as initial treatment for locally advanced or metastatic NSCLC and patients in both treatment groups were fully supplemented with folic acid and vitamin B_{12}.
[See table 4 at top of previous page]
No clinically relevant differences in adverse reactions were seen in patients based on histology.
In addition to the lower incidence of hematologic toxicity on the ALIMTA and cisplatin arm, use of transfusions (RBC and platelet) and hematopoietic growth factors was lower in the ALIMTA and cisplatin arm compared to the gemcitabine and cisplatin arm.
The following additional adverse reactions were observed in patients with non-small cell lung cancer randomly assigned to receive ALIMTA plus cisplatin.
Incidence 1% to 5%
Body as a Whole—febrile neutropenia, infection, pyrexia
General Disorders—dehydration
Metabolism and Nutrition—increased AST, increased ALT
Renal—creatinine clearance decrease, renal failure
Special Senses—conjunctivitis
Incidence Less than 1%
Cardiovascular—arrhythmia
General Disorders—chest pain
Metabolism and Nutrition—increased GGT
Neurology—motor neuropathy
Non-Small Cell Lung Cancer (NSCLC) — Maintenance
Table 5 provides the frequency and severity of adverse reactions that have been reported in >5% of 438 patients with NSCLC who received ALIMTA and 218 patients with NSCLC who received placebo. All patients received study therapy immediately following 4 cycles of platinum-based treatment for locally advanced or metastatic NSCLC. Patients in both study arms were fully supplemented with folic acid and vitamin B_{12}.
[See table 5 at top left]
No clinically relevant differences in Grade 3/4 adverse reactions were seen in patients based on age, gender, ethnic origin, or histology except a higher incidence of Grade 3/4 fatigue for Caucasian patients compared to non-Caucasian patients (6.5% versus 0.6%).
Safety was assessed by exposure for patients who received at least one dose of ALIMTA (N=438). The incidence of adverse reactions was evaluated for patients who received ≤6 cycles of ALIMTA, and compared to patients who received >6 cycles of ALIMTA. Increases in adverse reactions (all grades) were observed with longer exposure; however no clinically relevant differences in Grade 3/4 adverse reactions were seen.
Consistent with the higher incidence of anemia (all grades) on the ALIMTA arm, use of transfusions (mainly RBC) and erythropoiesis stimulating agents (ESAs; erythropoietin and darbepoetin) were higher in the ALIMTA arm compared to the placebo arm (transfusions 9.5% versus 3.2%, ESAs 5.9% versus 1.8%).
The following additional adverse reactions were observed in patients with non-small cell lung cancer who received ALIMTA.
Incidence 1% to 5%
Dermatology/Skin—alopecia, pruritus/itching
Gastrointestinal—constipation
General Disorders—edema, fever (in the absence of neutropenia)
Hematologic—thrombocytopenia
Renal—decreased creatinine clearance, increased creatinine, decreased glomerular filtration rate
Special Senses—ocular surface disease (including conjunctivitis), increased lacrimation
Incidence Less than 1%
Cardiovascular—supraventricular arrhythmia
Dermatology/Skin—erythema multiforme
General Disorders—febrile neutropenia, allergic reaction/hypersensitivity
Neurology—motor neuropathy
Renal—renal failure
Non-Small Cell Lung Cancer (NSCLC) – After Prior Chemotherapy
Table 6 provides the frequency and severity of adverse reactions that have been reported in >5% of 265 patients randomly assigned to receive single-agent ALIMTA with folic acid and vitamin B_{12} supplementation and 276 patients randomly assigned to receive single-agent docetaxel. All patients were diagnosed with locally advanced or metastatic NSCLC and received prior chemotherapy.
[See table 6 at left and on next page]
No clinically relevant differences in adverse reactions were seen in patients based on histology.
Clinically relevant adverse reactions occurring in <5% of patients that received ALIMTA treatment but >5% of patients that received docetaxel include CTC Grade 3/4 febrile neutropenia (1.9% ALIMTA, 12.7% docetaxel).
The following additional adverse reactions were observed in patients with non-small cell lung cancer randomly assigned to receive ALIMTA.

Incidence 1% to 5%
Body as a Whole—abdominal pain, allergic reaction/hypersensitivity, febrile neutropenia, infection
Dermatology/Skin—erythema multiforme
Neurology—motor neuropathy, sensory neuropathy
Renal—increased creatinine

Incidence Less than 1%
Cardiovascular—supraventricular arrhythmias

Malignant Pleural Mesothelioma (MPM)
Table 7 provides the frequency and severity of adverse reactions that have been reported in >5% of 168 patients with mesothelioma who were randomly assigned to receive cisplatin and ALIMTA and 163 patients with mesothelioma randomly assigned to receive single-agent cisplatin. In both treatment arms, these chemonaive patients were fully supplemented with folic acid and vitamin B_{12}.
[See table 7 at right and on next page]
The following additional adverse reactions were observed in patients with malignant pleural mesothelioma randomly assigned to receive ALIMTA plus cisplatin.

Incidence 1% to 5%
Body as a Whole—febrile neutropenia, infection, pyrexia
Dermatology/Skin—urticaria
General Disorders—chest pain
Metabolism and Nutrition—increased AST, increased ALT, increased GGT
Renal—renal failure

Incidence Less than 1%
Cardiovascular—arrhythmia
Neurology—motor neuropathy

Effects of Vitamin Supplementations
Table 8 compares the incidence (percentage of patients) of CTC Grade 3/4 toxicities in patients who received vitamin supplementation with daily folic acid and vitamin B_{12} from the time of enrollment in the study (fully supplemented) with the incidence in patients who never received vitamin supplementation (never supplemented) during the study in the ALIMTA plus cisplatin arm.

Table 8: Selected Grade 3/4 Adverse Events Comparing Fully Supplemented versus Never Supplemented Patients in the ALIMTA plus Cisplatin arm (% incidence)

Adverse Event[a] (%)	Fully Supplemented Patients (N=168)	Never Supplemented Patients (N=32)
Neutropenia/granulocytopenia	23	38
Thrombocytopenia	5	9
Vomiting	11	31
Febrile neutropenia	1	9
Infection with Grade 3/4 neutropenia	0	6
Diarrhea	4	9

[a] Refer to NCI CTC criteria for lab and non-laboratory values for each grade of toxicity (Version 2.0).

The following adverse events were greater in the fully supplemented group compared to the never supplemented group: hypertension (11%, 3%), chest pain (8%, 6%), and thrombosis/embolism (6%, 3%).

Subpopulations
No relevant effect for ALIMTA safety due to gender or race was identified, except an increased incidence of rash in men (24%) compared to women (16%).

6.2   Additional Clinical Trials Experience
Across clinical trials, sepsis, which in some cases was fatal, occurred in approximately 1% of patients.

6.3   Post-Marketing Experience
The following adverse reactions have been identified during post-approval use of ALIMTA. Because these reactions are reported voluntarily from a population of uncertain size, it is not always possible to reliably estimate their frequency or establish a causal relationship to drug exposure.
These reactions have occurred with ALIMTA when used as a single-agent and in combination therapies.

Gastrointestinal—colitis

General Disorders and Administration Site Conditions—edema

Injury, poisoning, and procedural complications—Radiation recall has been reported in patients who have previously received radiotherapy.

Respiratory—interstitial pneumonitis

Table 6 (cont.): Adverse Reactions in Fully Supplemented Patients Receiving ALIMTA versus Docetaxel in NSCLC[a]

Reaction[b]	ALIMTA (N=265)		Docetaxel (N=276)	
	All Grades Toxicity (%)	Grades 3-4 Toxicity (%)	All Grades Toxicity (%)	Grades 3-4 Toxicity (%)
Clinical				
Gastrointestinal				
Nausea	31	3	17	2
Anorexia	22	2	24	3
Vomiting	16	2	12	1
Stomatitis/Pharyngitis	15	1	17	1
Diarrhea	13	0	24	3
Constipation	6	0	4	0
Constitutional Symptoms				
Fatigue	34	5	36	5
Fever	8	0	8	0
Dermatology/Skin				
Rash/Desquamation	14	0	6	0
Pruritis	7	0	2	0
Alopecia	6	1[c]	38	2[c]

[a] For the purpose of this table a cut off of 5% was used for inclusion of all events where the reporter considered a possible relationship to ALIMTA.
[b] Refer to NCI CTC Criteria for lab values for each Grade of toxicity (version 2.0).
[c] According to NCI CTC Criteria version 2.0, this adverse event term should only be reported as Grade 1 or 2.

Table 7: Adverse Reactions in Fully Supplemented Patients Receiving ALIMTA plus Cisplatin in MPM[a]

Reaction[b]	ALIMTA/cisplatin (N=168)		Cisplatin (N=163)	
	All Grades Toxicity (%)	Grade 3-4 Toxicity (%)	All Grades Toxicity (%)	Grade 3-4 Toxicity (%)
Laboratory				
Hematologic				
Neutropenia	56	23	13	3
Leukopenia	53	15	17	1
Anemia	26	4	10	0
Thrombocytopenia	23	5	9	0
Renal				
Creatinine elevation	11	1	10	1
Creatinine clearance decreased	16	1	18	2

(Table continued on next page)

Skin—Bullous conditions have been reported including Stevens-Johnson Syndrome and Toxic epidermal necrolysis, which in some cases were fatal.

7   DRUG INTERACTIONS
7.1   Non-Steroidal Anti-Inflammatory Drugs (NSAIDs)
Ibuprofen
Although ibuprofen (400 mg four times a day) can decrease the clearance of pemetrexed, it can be administered with ALIMTA in patients with normal renal function (creatinine clearance ≥80 mL/min). Caution should be used when administering ibuprofen concurrently with ALIMTA to patients with mild to moderate renal insufficiency (creatinine clearance from 45 to 79 mL/min) *[see Clinical Pharmacology (12.3)]*.
Other NSAIDs
Patients with mild to moderate renal insufficiency should avoid taking NSAIDs with short elimination half-lives for a period of 2 days before, the day of, and 2 days following administration of ALIMTA.
In the absence of data regarding potential interaction between ALIMTA and NSAIDs with longer half-lives, all patients taking these NSAIDs should interrupt dosing for at least 5 days before, the day of, and 2 days following ALIMTA administration. If concomitant administration of an NSAID is necessary, patients should be monitored closely for toxicity, especially myelosuppression, renal, and gastrointestinal toxicity.

7.2   Nephrotoxic Drugs
ALIMTA is primarily eliminated unchanged renally as a result of glomerular filtration and tubular secretion. Concomitant administration of nephrotoxic drugs could result in delayed clearance of ALIMTA. Concomitant administration of substances that are also tubularly secreted (e.g., probenecid) could potentially result in delayed clearance of ALIMTA.

8   USE IN SPECIFIC POPULATIONS
8.1   Pregnancy
Teratogenic Effects—Pregnancy Category D *[see Warnings and Precautions (5.6)]*
Based on its mechanism of action, ALIMTA can cause fetal harm when administered to a pregnant woman. There are no adequate and well controlled studies of ALIMTA in preg-

Table 7 (cont.): Adverse Reactions in Fully Supplemented Patients Receiving ALIMTA plus Cisplatin in MPM[a]

Reaction[b]	ALIMTA/cisplatin (N=168)		Cisplatin (N=163)	
	All Grades Toxicity (%)	Grade 3-4 Toxicity (%)	All Grades Toxicity (%)	Grade 3-4 Toxicity (%)
Clinical				
Eye Disorder				
Conjunctivitis	5	0	1	0
Gastrointestinal				
Nausea	82	12	77	6
Vomiting	57	11	50	4
Stomatitis/Pharyngitis	23	3	6	0
Anorexia	20	1	14	1
Diarrhea	17	4	8	0
Constipation	12	1	7	1
Dyspepsia	5	1	1	0
Constitutional Symptoms				
Fatigue	48	10	42	9
Metabolism and Nutrition				
Dehydration	7	4	1	1
Neurology				
Neuropathy-sensory	10	0	10	1
Taste Disturbance	8	0[c]	6	0[c]
Dermatology/Skin				
Rash	16	1	5	0
Alopecia	11	0[c]	6	0[c]

[a] For the purpose of this table a cut off of 5% was used for inclusion of all events where the reporter considered a possible relationship to ALIMTA.
[b] Refer to NCI CTC Criteria version 2.0 for each Grade of toxicity except the term "creatinine clearance decreased" which is derived from the CTC term "renal/genitourinary-other".
[c] According to NCI CTC Criteria version 2.0, this adverse event term should only be reported as Grade 1 or 2.

nant women. Pemetrexed was embryotoxic, fetotoxic, and teratogenic in mice. In mice, repeated intraperitoneal doses of pemetrexed when given during organogenesis caused fetal malformations (incomplete ossification of talus and skull bone; about 1/833rd the recommended intravenous human dose on a mg/m² basis), and cleft palate (1/33rd the recommended intravenous human dose on a mg/m² basis). Embryotoxicity was characterized by increased embryo-fetal deaths and reduced litter sizes. If ALIMTA is used during pregnancy, or if the patient becomes pregnant while taking this drug, the patient should be apprised of the potential hazard to the fetus. Women of childbearing potential should be advised to use effective contraceptive measures to prevent pregnancy during the treatment with ALIMTA.

8.3 Nursing Mothers
It is not known whether ALIMTA or its metabolites are excreted in human milk. Because many drugs are excreted in human milk, and because of the potential for serious adverse reactions in nursing infants from ALIMTA, a decision should be made to discontinue nursing or discontinue the drug, taking into account the importance of the drug for the mother.

8.4 Pediatric Use
The safety and effectiveness of ALIMTA in pediatric patients have not been established.

8.5 Geriatric Use
ALIMTA is known to be substantially excreted by the kidney, and the risk of adverse reactions to this drug may be greater in patients with impaired renal function. Because elderly patients are more likely to have decreased renal function, care should be taken in dose selection. Renal function monitoring is recommended with administration of ALIMTA. No dose reductions other than those recommended for all patients are necessary for patients 65 years of age or older [see Dosage and Administration (2.4)].
In the initial treatment non-small cell lung cancer clinical trial, 37.7% of patients treated with ALIMTA plus cisplatin were ≥65 years and Grade 3/4 neutropenia was greater as compared to patients <65 years (19.9% versus 12.2%). For patients <65 years, the HR for overall survival was 0.96 (95% CI: 0.83, 1.10) and for patients ≥65 years the HR was 0.88 (95% CI: 0.74, 1.06) in the intent to treat population.
In the maintenance non-small cell lung cancer trial 33.3% of patients treated with ALIMTA were ≥65 years and no differences were seen in Grade 3/4 adverse reactions as compared to patients <65 years. For patients <65 years, the HR for overall survival was 0.74 (95% CI: 0.58, 0.93) and for patients ≥65 years the HR was 0.88 (95% CI: 0.65, 1.21) in the intent to treat population.
In the non-small cell lung cancer trial after prior chemotherapy, 29.7% patients treated with ALIMTA were ≥65 years and Grade 3/4 hypertension was greater as compared to patients <65 years. For patients <65 years, the HR for overall survival was 0.95 (95% CI: 0.76, 1.19), and for patients ≥65 years the HR was 1.15 (95% CI: 0.79, 1.68) in the intent to treat population.
The mesothelioma trial included 36.7% patients treated with ALIMTA plus cisplatin that were ≥65 years, and Grade 3/4 fatigue, leukopenia, neutropenia, and thrombocytopenia were greater as compared to patients <65 years. For patients <65 years, the HR for overall survival was 0.71 (95% CI: 0.53, 0.96) and for patients ≥65 years, the HR was 0.85 (95% CI: 0.59, 1.22) in the intent to treat population.

8.6 Patients with Hepatic Impairment
There was no effect of elevated AST, ALT, or total bilirubin on the pharmacokinetics of pemetrexed [see Clinical Pharmacology (12.3)].
Dose adjustments based on hepatic impairment experienced during treatment with ALIMTA are provided in Table 2 [see Dosage and Administration (2.4)].

8.7 Patients with Renal Impairment
ALIMTA is known to be primarily excreted by the kidneys. Decreased renal function will result in reduced clearance and greater exposure (AUC) to ALIMTA compared with patients with normal renal function [see Dosage and Adminis-

tration (2.4) and Clinical Pharmacology (12.3)]. Cisplatin coadministration with ALIMTA has not been studied in patients with moderate renal impairment.

8.8 Gender
In the initial treatment non-small cell lung cancer trial, 70% of patients were males and 30% females. For males the HR for overall survival was 0.97 (95% CI: 0.85, 1.10) and for females the HR was 0.86 (95% CI: 0.70, 1.06) in the intent to treat population.
In the maintenance non-small cell lung cancer trial, 73% of patients were males and 27% females. For males the HR for overall survival was 0.78 (95% CI: 0.63, 0.96) and for females the HR was 0.83 (95% CI: 0.56, 1.21) in the intent to treat population.
In the non-small cell lung cancer trial after prior chemotherapy, 72% of patients were males and 28% females. For males the HR for overall survival was 0.95 (95% CI: 0.76, 1.19) and for females the HR was 1.28 (95% CI: 0.86, 1.91) in the intent to treat population.
In the mesothelioma trial, 82% of patients were males and 18% females. For males the HR for overall survival was 0.85 (95% CI: 0.66, 1.09) and for females the HR was 0.48 (95% CI: 0.27, 0.85) in the intent to treat population.

8.9 Race
In the initial treatment non-small cell lung cancer trial, 78% of patients were Caucasians, 13% East/Southeast Asians, and 9% others. For Caucasians, the HR for overall survival was 0.92 (95% CI: 0.82, 1.04), for East/Southeast Asians the HR was 0.86 (95% CI: 0.61, 1.21), and for others the HR was 1.24 (95% CI: 0.84, 1.84) in the intent to treat population.
In the maintenance non-small cell lung cancer trial, 65% of patients were Caucasians, 23% East Asian, and 12% others. For Caucasians the HR for overall survival was 0.77 (95% CI: 0.62, 0.97), for East Asians was 1.05 (95% CI: 0.70, 1.59) and for others the HR was 0.46 (95% CI: 0.26, 0.79) in the intent to treat population.
In the non-small cell lung cancer trial after prior chemotherapy, 71% of patients were Caucasians and 29% others. For Caucasians the HR for overall survival was 0.91 (95% CI: 0.73, 1.15) and for others the HR was 1.27 (95% CI: 0.87, 1.87) in the intent to treat population.
In the mesothelioma trial, 92% of patients were Caucasians and 8% others. For Caucasians, the HR for overall survival was 0.77 (95% CI: 0.61, 0.97) and for others the HR was 0.86 (95% CI: 0.39, 1.90) in the intent to treat population.

10 OVERDOSAGE
There have been few cases of ALIMTA overdose. Reported toxicities included neutropenia, anemia, thrombocytopenia, mucositis, and rash. Anticipated complications of overdose include bone marrow suppression as manifested by neutropenia, thrombocytopenia, and anemia. In addition, infection with or without fever, diarrhea, and mucositis may be seen. If an overdose occurs, general supportive measures should be instituted as deemed necessary by the treating physician.
In clinical trials, leucovorin was permitted for CTC Grade 4 leukopenia lasting ≥3 days, CTC Grade 4 neutropenia lasting ≥3 days, and immediately for CTC Grade 4 thrombocytopenia, bleeding associated with Grade 3 thrombocytopenia, or Grade 3 or 4 mucositis. The following intravenous doses and schedules of leucovorin were recommended for intravenous use: 100 mg/m², intravenously once, followed by leucovorin, 50 mg/m², intravenously every 6 hours for 8 days.
The ability of ALIMTA to be dialyzed is unknown.

11 DESCRIPTION
Pemetrexed disodium heptahydrate has the chemical name L-Glutamic acid, N-[4-[2-(2-amino-4,7-dihydro-4-oxo-1H-pyrrolo[2,3-d]pyrimidin-5-yl)ethyl]benzoyl]-, disodium salt, heptahydrate. It is a white to almost-white solid with a molecular formula of $C_{20}H_{19}N_5Na_2O_6 \cdot 7H_2O$ and a molecular weight of 597.49. The structural formula is as follows:

ALIMTA is supplied as a sterile lyophilized powder for intravenous infusion available in single-dose vials. The product is a white to either light yellow or green-yellow lyophilized solid. Each 100-mg or 500-mg vial of ALIMTA contains pemetrexed disodium equivalent to 100 mg pemetrexed and 106 mg mannitol or 500 mg pemetrexed and 500 mg mannitol, respectively. Hydrochloric acid and/or sodium hydroxide may have been added to adjust pH.

12 CLINICAL PHARMACOLOGY

12.1 Mechanism of Action

ALIMTA, pemetrexed for injection, is a folate analog metabolic inhibitor that exerts its action by disrupting folate-dependent metabolic processes essential for cell replication. In vitro studies have shown that pemetrexed inhibits thymidylate synthase (TS), dihydrofolate reductase (DHFR), and glycinamide ribonucleotide formyltransferase (GARFT), which are folate-dependent enzymes involved in the de novo biosynthesis of thymidine and purine nucleotides. Pemetrexed is taken into cells by membrane carriers such as the reduced folate carrier and membrane folate binding protein transport systems. Once in the cell, pemetrexed is converted to polyglutamate forms by the enzyme folylpolyglutamate synthetase. The polyglutamate forms are retained in cells and are inhibitors of TS and GARFT. Polyglutamation is a time- and concentration-dependent process that occurs in tumor cells and, is thought to occur to a lesser extent, in normal tissues. Polyglutamated metabolites are thought to have an increased intracellular half-life resulting in prolonged drug action in malignant cells.

12.2 Pharmacodynamics

Preclinical studies have shown that pemetrexed inhibits the in vitro growth of mesothelioma cell lines (MSTO-211H, NCI-H2052). Studies with the MSTO-211H mesothelioma cell line showed synergistic effects when pemetrexed was combined concurrently with cisplatin.

Absolute neutrophil counts (ANC) following single-agent administration of ALIMTA to patients not receiving folic acid and vitamin B_{12} supplementation were characterized using population pharmacodynamic analyses. Severity of hematologic toxicity, as measured by the depth of the ANC nadir, correlates with the systemic exposure, or area under the curve (AUC) of pemetrexed. It was also observed that lower ANC nadirs occurred in patients with elevated baseline cystathionine or homocysteine concentrations. The levels of these substances can be reduced by folic acid and vitamin B_{12} supplementation. There is no cumulative effect of pemetrexed exposure on ANC nadir over multiple treatment cycles.

Time to ANC nadir with pemetrexed systemic exposure (AUC), varied between 8 to 9.6 days over a range of exposures from 38.3 to 316.8 mcg•hr/mL. Return to baseline ANC occurred 4.2 to 7.5 days after the nadir over the same range of exposures.

12.3 Pharmacokinetics

Absorption

The pharmacokinetics of ALIMTA administered as a single-agent in doses ranging from 0.2 to 838 mg/m^2 infused over a 10-minute period have been evaluated in 426 cancer patients with a variety of solid tumors. Pemetrexed total systemic exposure (AUC) and maximum plasma concentration (C_{max}) increase proportionally with dose. The pharmacokinetics of pemetrexed do not change over multiple treatment cycles.

Distribution

Pemetrexed has a steady-state volume of distribution of 16.1 liters. In vitro studies indicate that pemetrexed is approximately 81% bound to plasma proteins. Binding is not affected by degree of renal impairment.

Metabolism and Excretion

Pemetrexed is not metabolized to an appreciable extent and is primarily eliminated in the urine, with 70% to 90% of the dose recovered unchanged within the first 24 hours following administration. The clearance decreases, and exposure (AUC) increases, as renal function decreases. The total systemic clearance of pemetrexed is 91.8 mL/min and the elimination half-life of pemetrexed is 3.5 hours in patients with normal renal function (creatinine clearance of 90 mL/min). The pharmacokinetics of pemetrexed in special populations were examined in about 400 patients in controlled and single arm studies.

Effect of Age

No effect of age on the pharmacokinetics of pemetrexed was observed over a range of 26 to 80 years.

Effect of Gender

The pharmacokinetics of pemetrexed were not different in male and female patients.

Effect of Race

The pharmacokinetics of pemetrexed were similar in Caucasians and patients of African descent. Insufficient data are available to compare pharmacokinetics for other ethnic groups.

Effect of Hepatic Insufficiency

There was no effect of elevated AST, ALT, or total bilirubin on the pharmacokinetics of pemetrexed. However, studies of hepatically impaired patients have not been conducted [see Dosage and Administration (2.4) and Use in Specific Populations (8.6)].

Effect of Renal Insufficiency

Pharmacokinetic analyses of pemetrexed included 127 patients with reduced renal function. Plasma clearance of pemetrexed decreases as renal function decreases, with a resultant increase in systemic exposure. Patients with creatinine clearances of 45, 50, and 80 mL/min had 65%, 54%, and 13% increases, respectively in pemetrexed total systemic exposure (AUC) compared to patients with creatinine clearance of 100 mL/min [see Warnings and Precautions (5.4) and Dosage and Administration (2.4)].

Pediatric

Pediatric patients were not included in clinical trials.

Effect of Ibuprofen

Ibuprofen doses of 400 mg four times a day reduce pemetrexed's clearance by about 20% (and increase AUC by 20%) in patients with normal renal function. The effect of greater doses of ibuprofen on pemetrexed pharmacokinetics is unknown [see Drug Interactions (7.1)].

Effect of Aspirin

Aspirin, administered in low to moderate doses (325 mg every 6 hours), does not affect the pharmacokinetics of pemetrexed. The effect of greater doses of aspirin on pemetrexed pharmacokinetics is unknown.

Effect of Cisplatin

Cisplatin does not affect the pharmacokinetics of pemetrexed and the pharmacokinetics of total platinum are unaltered by pemetrexed.

Effect of Vitamins

Coadministration of oral folic acid or intramuscular vitamin B_{12} does not affect the pharmacokinetics of pemetrexed.

Drugs Metabolized by Cytochrome P450 Enzymes

Results from in vitro studies with human liver microsomes predict that pemetrexed would not cause clinically significant inhibition of metabolic clearance of drugs metabolized by CYP3A, CYP2D6, CYP2C9, and CYP1A2.

13 NONCLINICAL TOXICOLOGY

13.1 Carcinogenesis, Mutagenesis, Impairment of Fertility

No carcinogenicity studies have been conducted with pemetrexed. Pemetrexed was clastogenic in the in vivo micronucleus assay in mouse bone marrow but was not mutagenic in multiple in vitro tests (Ames assay, CHO cell assay). Pemetrexed administered at i.v. doses of 0.1 mg/kg/day or greater to male mice (about 1/1666 the recommended human dose on a mg/m^2 basis) resulted in reduced fertility, hypospermia, and testicular atrophy.

14 CLINICAL STUDIES

14.1 Non-Small Cell Lung Cancer (NSCLC) – Combination with Cisplatin

A multi-center, randomized, open-label study in 1725 chemonaive patients with Stage IIIb/IV NSCLC was conducted to compare the overall survival following treatment with ALIMTA in combination with cisplatin (AC) versus gemcitabine in combination with cisplatin (GC). ALIMTA was administered intravenously over 10 minutes at a dose of 500 mg/m^2 with cisplatin administered intravenously at a dose of 75 mg/m^2 after ALIMTA administration, on Day 1 of each 21-day cycle. Gemcitabine was administered at a dose of 1250 mg/m^2 on Day 1 and Day 8, and cisplatin was administered intravenously at a dose of 75 mg/m^2 after administration of gemcitabine, on Day 1 of each 21-day cycle. Treatment was administered up to a total of 6 cycles, and patients in both treatment arms received folic acid, vitamin B_{12}, and dexamethasone [see Dosage and Administration (2.3)].

Patient demographics of the intent to treat (ITT) population are shown in Table 9. The demographics and disease characteristics were well balanced.

Table 9: First-Line Therapy: Summary of Patient Characteristics in Study of NSCLC

Patient characteristic	ALIMTA plus Cisplatin (AC) (N=862)	Gemcitabine plus Cisplatin (GC) (N=863)
Age (yrs)		
Median (range)	61.1 (28.8-83.2)	61.0 (26.4-79.4)
Gender		
Male/Female	70.2%/29.8%	70.1%/29.9%
Origin		
Caucasian	669 (77.6%)	680 (78.8%)
Hispanic	27 (3.1%)	23 (2.7%)
Asian	146 (16.9%)	141 (16.3%)
African descent	18 (2.1%)	18 (2.1%)
Stage at Entry		
IIIb/IV	23.8%/76.2%	24.3%/75.7%
Histology		
Nonsquamous NSCLC[a]	618 (71.7%)	634 (73.5%)
Adenocarcinoma	436 (50.6%)	411 (47.6%)
Large cell	76 (8.8%)	77 (8.9%)
Other[b]	106 (12.3%)	146 (16.9%)
Squamous	244 (28.3%)	229 (26.5%)
ECOG PS[c,d]		
0/1	35.4%/64.6%	35.6%/64.3%
Smoking History[e]		
Ever/never smoker	83.1%/16.9%	83.9%/16.1%

[a] Includes adenocarcinoma, large cell, and other histologies except those with squamous cell type.

[b] The subgroup of "other" represents patients with a primary diagnosis of NSCLC whose disease did not clearly qualify as adenocarcinoma, squamous cell carcinoma, or large cell carcinoma.

[c] Eastern Cooperative Oncology Group Performance Status.

[d] ECOG PS was not reported for all randomized patients. Percentages are representative of N=861 for the ALIMTA plus cisplatin arm, and N=861 for the gemcitabine plus cisplatin arm.

[e] Smoking history was collected for 88% of randomized patients (N=757 for the ALIMTA plus cisplatin arm and N=759 for the gemcitabine plus cisplatin arm).

Patients received a median of 5 cycles of treatment in both study arms. Patients treated with ALIMTA plus cisplatin received a relative dose intensity of 94.8% of the protocol-specified ALIMTA dose intensity and 95.0% of the protocol-specified cisplatin dose intensity. Patients treated with gemcitabine plus cisplatin received a relative dose intensity of 85.8% of the protocol-specified gemcitabine dose intensity and 93.5% of the protocol-specified cisplatin dose intensity. The primary endpoint in this study was overall survival. The median survival time was 10.3 months in the ALIMTA plus cisplatin treatment arm and 10.3 months in the gemcitabine plus cisplatin arm, with an adjusted hazard ratio of 0.94.

Table 10: First-Line Therapy: Efficacy in NSCLC—ITT Population

	ALIMTA plus Cisplatin (N=862)	Gemcitabine plus Cisplatin (N=863)
Median overall survival (95% CI)	10.3 mos (9.8-11.2)	10.3 mos (9.6-10.9)
Adjusted hazard ratio (HR)[a,b] (95% CI)	0.94 (0.84-1.05)	
Median progression-free survival (95% CI)	4.8 mos (4.6-5.3)	5.1 mos (4.6-5.5)
Adjusted hazard ratio (HR)[a,b] (95% CI)	1.04 (0.94-1.15)	
Overall response rate (95% CI)	27.1% (24.2-30.1)	24.7% (21.8-27.6)

[a] Adjusted for gender, stage, basis of diagnosis, and performance status.

[b] A HR that is less than 1.0 indicates that survival is better in the AC arm than in the GC arm. Alternatively, a HR that is greater than 1.0 indicates survival is better in the GC arm than in the AC arm.

[See figure 1 on next page]

A pre-specified analysis of the impact of NSCLC histology on overall survival was examined. Clinically relevant differences in survival according to histology were observed and are shown in Table 11. This difference in treatment effect for ALIMTA based on histology demonstrating a lack of efficacy in squamous cell histology was also observed in the single-

Table 11: First-Line Therapy: Overall Survival in NSCLC Histologic Subgroups

Histology Subgroup	Median Overall Survival in Months (95% CI)				Unadjusted Hazard Ratio (HR)[a,b] (95% CI)	Adjusted Hazard Ratio (HR)[a,b,c] (95% CI)
	ALIMTA plus Cisplatin		Gemcitabine plus Cisplatin			
Nonsquamous NSCLC[d] (N=1252)	11.0 (10.1-12.5)	N=618	10.1 (9.3-10.9)	N=634	0.84 (0.74-0.96)	0.84 (0.74-0.96)
Adenocarcinoma (N=847)	12.6 (10.7-13.6)	N=436	10.9 (10.2-11.9)	N=411	0.84 (0.71-0.98)	0.84 (0.71-0.99)
Large Cell (N=153)	10.4 (8.6-14.1)	N=76	6.7 (5.5-9.0)	N=77	0.68 (0.48-0.97)	0.67 (0.48-0.96)
Other[e] (N=252)	8.6 (6.8-10.2)	N=106	9.2 (8.1-10.6)	N=146	1.12 (0.84-1.49)	1.08 (0.81-1.45)
Squamous Cell (N=473)	9.4 (8.4-10.2)	N=244	10.8 (9.5-12.1)	N=229	1.22 (0.99-1.50)	1.23 (1.00-1.51)

[a] A HR that is less than 1.0 indicates that survival is better in the AC arm than in the GC arm. Alternatively, a HR that is greater than 1.0 indicates survival is better in the GC arm than in the AC arm.
[b] Unadjusted for multiple comparisons.
[c] HRs adjusted for ECOG PS, gender, disease stage, and basis for pathological diagnosis (histopathological/cytopathological).
[d] Includes adenocarcinoma, large cell, and other histologies except those with squamous cell type.
[e] The subgroup of "other" represents patients with a primary diagnosis of NSCLC whose disease did not clearly qualify as adenocarcinoma, squamous cell carcinoma, or large cell carcinoma.

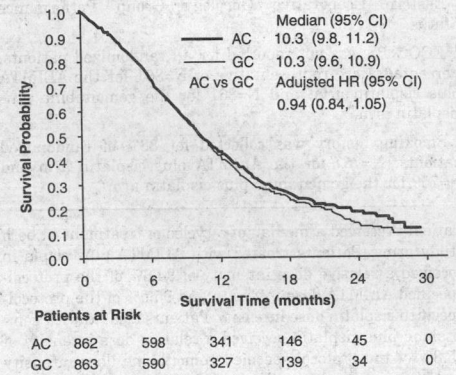

Figure 1: Kaplan-Meier Curves for Overall Survival ALIMTA plus Cisplatin (AC) versus Gemcitabine plus Cisplatin (GC) in NSCLC — ITT Population.

agent, second-line study and the maintenance study [see Clinical Studies (14.2, 14.3)].
[See table 11 above]

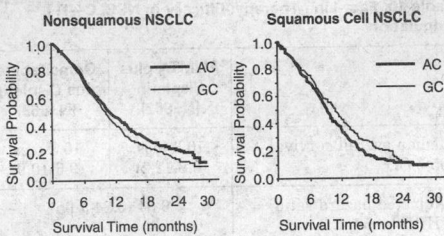

Figure 2: Kaplan-Meier Curves for Overall Survival ALIMTA plus Cisplatin (AC) versus Gemcitabine plus Cisplatin (GC) in NSCLC — Nonsquamous NSCLC and Squamous Cell NSCLC.

14.2 Non-Small Cell Lung Cancer – Maintenance

A multi-center, randomized, double-blind, placebo-controlled study was conducted in 663 patients with Stage IIIb/IV NSCLC who did not progress after four cycles of platinum-based chemotherapy. Patients who did not progress were randomized 2:1 to receive ALIMTA or placebo immediately following platinum-based chemotherapy. ALIMTA was administered intravenously over 10 minutes at a dose of 500 mg/m² on Day 1 of each 21-day cycle, until disease progression. Patients in both study arms received folic acid, vitamin B12, and dexamethasone [see Dosage and Administration (2.3)].
The study was designed to demonstrate superior progression-free survival and overall survival of ALIMTA over placebo. Progression-free survival (PFS) was assessed by independent review. Patient characteristics of the intent to treat (ITT) population are shown in Table 12. The demographics and baseline disease characteristics were well-balanced between study arms.

Table 12: Maintenance Therapy: Summary of Patient Characteristics in Study of NSCLC

Patient characteristic	ALIMTA (N=441)	Placebo (N=222)
Age (yrs)		
Median (range)	60.6 (25.6-82.6)	60.4 (35.4-78.5)
Gender		
Male/Female	73.0%/27.0%	72.5%/27.5%
Ethnic Origin		
Caucasian	279 (63.3%)	149 (67.1%)
East Asian	104 (23.6%)	50 (22.5%)
Other	58 (13.2%)	23 (10.4%)
Stage at Entry[a]		
IIIb/IV	18.0%/82.0%	21.2%/78.8%
Histology (%)		
Nonsquamous NSCLC[b]	325 (73.7%)	156 (70.3%)
Adenocarcinoma	222 (50.3%)	106 (47.7%)
Large cell	10 (2.3%)	10 (4.5%)
Other[c]	93 (21.1%)	40 (18.0%)
Squamous	116 (26.3%)	66 (29.7%)
ECOG PS[d]		
0/1	40.1%/59.9%	38.3%/61.7%
Smoking History[e]		
Ever/never smoker	74.1%/25.9%	71.5%/28.5%
Time from start of induction therapy to study randomization (months)		
Median (range)	3.25 (1.6-4.8)	3.29 (2.7-5.1)

[a] Stage at Entry was not reported for all randomized patients. Percentages are representative of N=440 for the ALIMTA arm and N=222 for the placebo arm.
[b] Includes patients with adenocarcinoma, large cell, and other histologic diagnoses.
[c] The subgroup of "Other" represents patients with a primary diagnosis of NSCLC whose disease did not clearly qualify as adenocarcinoma, large cell carcinoma, or squamous cell carcinoma.

[d] Eastern Cooperative Oncology Group Performance Status (ECOG PS) was not reported for all randomized patients. Percentages are representative of N=439 for the ALIMTA arm, and N=222 for the placebo arm.
[e] Smoking history was not reported for all randomized patients. Percentages are representative of N=437 for the ALIMTA arm and N=221 for the placebo arm.

Patients received a median of 5 cycles of ALIMTA and 3.5 cycles of placebo. Patients randomized to ALIMTA received a relative dose intensity of 95.7%. A total of 213 patients (48.3%) completed ≥6 cycles and a total of 98 patients (22.6%) completed ≥10 cycles of treatment with ALIMTA. In the overall study population, ALIMTA was statistically superior to placebo in terms of overall survival (OS) (median 13.4 months versus 10.6 months, HR=0.79 (95% CI: 0.65-0.95), p-value=0.012) and PFS (median 4.0 months versus 2.0 months, HR=0.60 (95% CI: 0.49-0.73), p-value<0.00001). A difference in treatment outcomes was observed according to histologic classification. For the population of patients with nonsquamous NSCLC, ALIMTA was superior to placebo for OS (median 15.5 months versus 10.3 months, HR=0.70 (95% CI: 0.56-0.88)) and PFS (median 4.4 months versus 1.8 months, HR=0.47 (95% CI: 0.37-0.60)). For the population of patients with squamous NSCLC, ALIMTA did not improve OS compared to placebo (median 9.9 months versus 10.8 months, HR=1.07 (95% CI: 0.77-1.50)) or PFS (median 2.4 months versus 2.5 months, HR=1.03 (95% CI: 0.71-1.49)). This difference in treatment effect for ALIMTA based on histology demonstrating lack of benefit in squamous cell histology was also observed in the first-line and second line studies. [see Clinical Studies (14.1, 14.3)]
Efficacy results for the overall patient population are presented in Table 13 and Figure 3, and efficacy results by pre-specified histologic subgroups are presented in Table 14 and Figure 4, below.

Table 13: Maintenance Therapy: Efficacy of ALIMTA versus Placebo in NSCLC - ITT Population

Efficacy Parameter[a,b]	ALIMTA (N=441)	Placebo (N=222)
Median overall survival[c] (95% CI)	13.4 mos (11.9-15.9)	10.6 mos (8.7-12.0)
Hazard ratio (HR)[c] (95% CI)	0.79 (0.65-0.95)	
p-value	p=0.012	
Median progression-free survival (95% CI)	4.0 mos (3.1-4.4)	2.0 mos (1.5-2.8)
Hazard ratio (HR)[c] (95% CI)	0.60 (0.49-0.73)	
p-value	p<0.00001	

[a] PFS and OS were calculated from time of randomization, after completion of 4 cycles of induction platinum-based chemotherapy.
[b] Values for PFS given based on independent review (ALIMTA N=387, Placebo N=194).
[c] Unadjusted hazard ratios are provided. A HR <1.0 indicates that the result is better in the ALIMTA arm than in the placebo arm.

[See table 14 at top of next page]

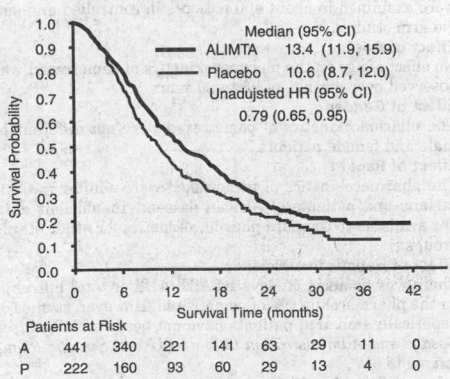

Figure 3: Kaplan-Meier Curve for Overall Survival ALIMTA (A) versus Placebo (P) in NSCLC - ITT Population.

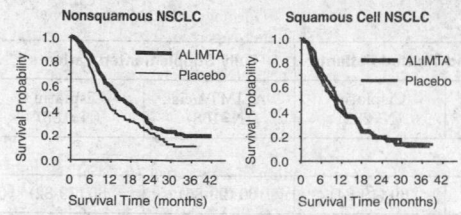

Figure 4: Kaplan-Meier Curves for Overall Survival ALIMTA versus Placebo in NSCLC - Nonsquamous NSCLC and Squamous Cell NSCLC.

14.3 Non-Small Cell Lung Cancer – After Prior Chemotherapy

A multi-center, randomized, open label study was conducted in patients with Stage III or IV NSCLC after prior chemotherapy to compare the overall survival following treatment with ALIMTA versus docetaxel. ALIMTA was administered intravenously over 10 minutes at a dose of 500 mg/m² and docetaxel was administered at 75 mg/m² as a 1-hour intravenous infusion. Both drugs were given on Day 1 of each 21-day cycle. All patients treated with ALIMTA received vitamin supplementation with folic acid and vitamin B₁₂. The study was intended to show either an overall survival superiority or non-inferiority of ALIMTA to docetaxel. Patient demographics of the intent to treat (ITT) population are shown in Table 15.

Table 15: Second-Line Therapy: Summary of Patient Characteristics in NSCLC Study

Patient characteristic	ALIMTA (N=283)	Docetaxel (N=288)
Age (yrs)		
Median (range)	59 (22-81)	57 (28-87)
Gender (%)		
Male/Female	68.6/31.4	75.3/24.7
Stage at Entry (%)		
III/IV	25.1/74.9	25.3/74.7
Diagnosis/Histology (%)		
Adenocarcinoma	154 (54.4)	142 (49.3)
Squamous	78 (27.6)	94 (32.6)
Bronchoalveolar	4 (1.4)	1 (0.3)
Other	47 (16.6)	51 (17.7)
Performance Status (%)ᵃ		
0-1	234 (88.6)	240 (87.6)
2	30 (11.4)	34 (12.4)

ᵃ Performance status was not reported for all randomized patients. Percentages are representative of N=264 for the ALIMTA arm and N=274 for the docetaxel arm.

The primary endpoint in this study was overall survival. The median survival time was 8.3 months in the ALIMTA treatment arm and 7.9 months in the docetaxel arm, with a hazard ratio of 0.99 (see Table 16). The study did not show an overall survival superiority of ALIMTA.

Table 16: Efficacy of ALIMTA versus Docetaxel in Non-Small Cell Lung Cancer - ITT Population

	ALIMTA (N=283)	Docetaxel (N=288)
Median overall survival (95% CI)	8.3 mos (7.0-9.4)	7.9 mos (6.3-9.2)
Hazard ratio (HR) (95% CI)	0.99 (0.82-1.20)	
Median progression-free survival (95% CI)	2.9 mos (2.4-3.1)	2.9 mos (2.7-3.4)
Hazard ratio (HR) (95% CI)	0.97 (0.82-1.16)	
Overall response rate (95% CI)	8.5% (5.2-11.7)	8.3% (5.1-11.5)

Table 14: Maintenance Therapy: Efficacy in NSCLC by Histologic Subgroupsᵃ

	Overall Survival		Progression-Free Survivalᵇ	
	ALIMTA	Placebo	ALIMTA	Placebo
	Median (months) HRᶜ (95% CI)	Median (months)	Median (months) HRᶜ (95% CI)	Median (months)
Nonsquamous NSCLCᵈ N=481	15.5 0.70 (0.56-0.88)	10.3	4.4 0.47 (0.37-0.60)	1.8
Adenocarcinoma N=328	16.8 0.73 (0.56-0.96)	11.5	4.6 0.51 (0.38-0.68)	2.7
Large cell carcinoma N=20	8.4 0.98 (0.36-2.65)	7.9	4.5 0.40 (0.12-1.29)	1.5
Otherᵉ N=133	11.3 0.61 (0.40-0.94)	7.7	4.1 0.44 (0.28-0.68)	1.6
Squamous cell N=182	9.9 1.07 (0.77-1.50)	10.8	2.4 1.03 (0.71-1.49)	2.5

ᵃ PFS and OS were calculated from time of randomization, after completion of 4 cycles of induction platinum-based chemotherapy. All results unadjusted for multiple comparisons.
ᵇ Values for PFS are given based on independent review (ALIMTA N=387, Placebo N=194).
ᶜ Unadjusted hazard ratios are provided. A HR <1.0 indicates that the result is better in the ALIMTA arm than in the placebo arm. A HR >1.0 indicates that the result is better in the placebo arm than in the ALIMTA arm.
ᵈ Includes patients with adenocarcinoma, large cell carcinoma, and other histology.
ᵉ The subgroup of "Other" represents patients with a primary diagnosis of NSCLC whose disease did not clearly qualify as adenocarcinoma, large cell carcinoma, or squamous cell carcinoma.

Table 17: Second Line Therapy: Overall Survival of ALIMTA versus Docetaxel in NSCLC by Histologic Subgroups

Histology Subgroup	Median Overall Survival in Months (95% CI)				Unadjusted Hazard Ratio (HR)ᵃ·ᵇ (95% CI)	Adjusted Hazard Ratio (HR)ᵃ·ᵇ·ᶜ (95% CI)
	ALIMTA		Docetaxel			
Nonsquamous NSCLCᵈ (N=399)	9.3 (7.8-9.7)	N=205	8.0 (6.3-9.3)	N=194	0.89 (0.71-1.13)	0.78 (0.61-1.00)
Adenocarcinoma (N=301)	9.0 (7.6-9.6)	N=158	9.2 (7.5-11.3)	N=143	1.09 (0.83-1.44)	0.92 (0.69-1.22)
Large Cell (N=47)	12.8 (5.8-14.0)	N=18	4.5 (2.3-9.1)	N=29	0.38 (0.18-0.78)	0.27 (0.11-0.63)
Otherᵉ (N=51)	9.4 (6.0-10.1)	N=29	7.9 (4.0-8.9)	N=22	0.62 (0.32-1.23)	0.57 (0.27-1.20)
Squamous Cell (N=172)	6.2 (4.9-8.0)	N=78	7.4 (5.6-9.5)	N=94	1.32 (0.93-1.86)	1.56 (1.08-2.26)

ᵃ A HR that is less than 1.0 indicates that survival is better in the ALIMTA arm than in the docetaxel arm. Alternatively, a HR that is greater than 1.0 indicates survival is better in the docetaxel arm than in the ALIMTA arm.
ᵇ Unadjusted for multiple comparisons.
ᶜ HRs adjusted for ECOG PS, time since prior chemotherapy, disease stage, and gender.
ᵈ Includes adenocarcinoma, large cell, and other histologies except those with squamous cell type.
ᵉ The subgroup of "other" represents patients with a primary diagnosis of NSCLC whose disease did not clearly qualify as adenocarcinoma, squamous cell carcinoma, or large cell carcinoma.

A retrospective analysis of the impact of NSCLC histology on overall survival was examined. Clinically relevant differences in survival according to histology were observed and are shown in Table 17. This difference in treatment effect for ALIMTA based on histology demonstrating a lack of efficacy in squamous cell histology was also observed in the first-line combination study and in the maintenance study *[see Clinical Studies (14.1, 14.2)]*.
[See table 17 above]

14.4 Malignant Pleural Mesothelioma

A multi-center, randomized, single-blind study in 448 chemonaive patients with malignant pleural mesothelioma (MPM) compared survival in patients treated with ALIMTA in combination with cisplatin to survival in patients receiving cisplatin alone. ALIMTA was administered intravenously over 10 minutes at a dose of 500 mg/m² and cisplatin was administered intravenously over 2 hours at a dose of 75 mg/m² beginning approximately 30 minutes after the end of administration of ALIMTA. Both drugs were given on Day 1 of each 21-day cycle. After 117 patients were treated, white cell and GI toxicity led to a change in protocol whereby all patients were given folic acid and vitamin B₁₂ supplementation.
The primary analysis of this study was performed on the population of all patients randomly assigned to treatment who received study drug (randomized and treated). An analysis was also performed on patients who received folic acid and vitamin B₁₂ supplementation during the entire course of study therapy (fully supplemented), as supplementation is recommended *[see Dosage and Administration (2.3)]*. Results in all patients and those fully supplemented were similar. Patient demographics are shown in Table 18.
[See table 18 at top of next page]
Table 19 and Figure 5 summarize the survival results for all randomized and treated patients regardless of vitamin supplementation status and those patients receiving vitamin supplementation from the time of enrollment in the trial.
[See table 19 on next page]
Similar results were seen in the analysis of patients (N=303) with confirmed histologic diagnosis of malignant pleural mesothelioma. There were too few non-white patients to assess possible ethnic differences. The effect in women (median survival 15.7 months with the combination versus 7.5 months on cisplatin alone), however, was larger than the effect in males (median survival 11 versus 9.4 respectively). As with any exploratory analysis, it is not clear whether this difference is real or is a chance finding.
[See figure 5 at top of next page]
Objective tumor response for malignant pleural mesothelioma is difficult to measure and response criteria are not universally agreed upon. However, based upon prospectively defined criteria, the objective tumor response rate for ALIMTA plus cisplatin was greater than the objective tumor response rate for cisplatin alone. There was also improvement in lung function (forced vital capacity) in the ALIMTA plus cisplatin arm compared to the control arm.

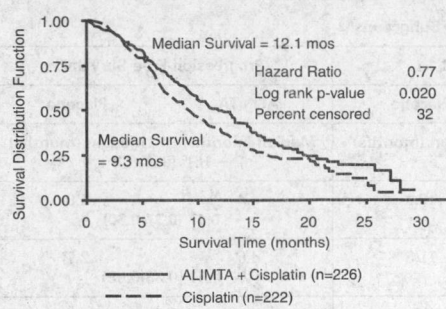

Figure 5: Kaplan-Meier Estimates of Survival Time for ALIMTA plus Cisplatin and Cisplatin Alone in all Randomized and Treated Patients.

Patients who received full supplementation with folic acid and vitamin B_{12} during study therapy received a median of 6 and 4 cycles in the ALIMTA/cisplatin (N=168) and cisplatin (N=163) arms, respectively. Patients who never received folic acid and vitamin B_{12} during study therapy received a median of 2 cycles in both treatment arms (N=32 and N=38 for the ALIMTA/cisplatin and cisplatin arm, respectively). Patients receiving ALIMTA in the fully supplemented group received a relative dose intensity of 93% of the protocol specified ALIMTA dose intensity; patients treated with cisplatin in the same group received 94% of the projected dose intensity. Patients treated with cisplatin alone had a dose intensity of 96%.

15   REFERENCES

1. Preventing Occupational Exposures to Antineoplastic and Other Hazardous Drugs in Health Care Settings. NIOSH Alert 2004-165.
2. OSHA Technical Manual, TED 1-0.15A, Section VI: Chapter 2. Controlling Occupational Exposure to Hazardous Drugs. OSHA, 1999. http://www.osha.gov/dts/osta/otm/otm_vi/otm_vi_2.html
3. American Society of Health-System Pharmacists. ASHP guidelines on handling hazardous drugs. *Am J Health-Syst Pharm.* 2006; 63:1172-1193.
4. Polovich, M., White, J. M., & Kelleher, L. O. (eds.) 2005. Chemotherapy and biotherapy guidelines and recommendations for practice (2nd. ed.) Pittsburgh, PA: Oncology Nursing Society.

16   HOW SUPPLIED/STORAGE AND HANDLING

16.1   How Supplied

ALIMTA, pemetrexed for injection, is available in sterile single-use vials containing 100 mg pemetrexed.
NDC 0002-7640-01 (VL7640): single-use vial with ivory flip-off cap individually packaged in a carton.
ALIMTA, pemetrexed for injection, is available in sterile single-use vials containing 500 mg pemetrexed.
NDC 0002-7623-01 (VL7623): single-use vial with ivory flip-off cap individually packaged in a carton.

16.2   Storage and Handling

ALIMTA, pemetrexed for injection, should be stored at 25°C (77°F); excursions permitted to 15-30°C (59-86°F) [see USP Controlled Room Temperature].
Chemical and physical stability of reconstituted and infusion solutions of ALIMTA were demonstrated for up to 24 hours following initial reconstitution, when stored refrigerated, 2-8°C (36-46°F), or at 25°C (77°F), excursions permitted to 15-30°C (59-86°F) [see USP Controlled Room Temperature]. When prepared as directed, reconstituted and infusion solutions of ALIMTA contain no antimicrobial preservatives. Discard unused portion [see Dosage and Administration (2.5)].
ALIMTA is not light sensitive.

17   PATIENT COUNSELING INFORMATION

See FDA-Approved Patient Labeling
Patients should be instructed to read the patient package insert carefully.

17.1   Need for Folic Acid and Vitamin B_{12}

Patients treated with ALIMTA must be instructed to take folic acid and vitamin B_{12} as a prophylactic measure to reduce treatment-related hematologic and gastrointestinal toxicity [see Dosage and Administration (2.3)].

17.2   Low Blood Cell Counts

Patients should be adequately informed of the risk of low blood cell counts and instructed to immediately contact their physician should any sign of infection develop including fever. Patients should also contact their physician if bleeding or symptoms of anemia occur.

17.3   Gastrointestinal Effects

Patients should be instructed to contact their physician if persistent vomiting, diarrhea, or signs of dehydration appear.

17.4   Concomitant Medications

Patients should be instructed to inform the physician if they are taking any concomitant prescription or over-the-counter

medications including those for pain or inflammation such as non-steroidal anti-inflammatory drugs [see Drug Interactions (7.1)].
Literature revised August 9, 2010
Eli Lilly and Company
Indianapolis, IN 46285, USA

INFORMATION FOR PATIENTS AND CAREGIVERS
ALIMTA® (uh-LIM-tuh)
(pemetrexed for injection)
Read the Patient Information that comes with ALIMTA before you start treatment and each time you get treated with ALIMTA. There may be new information. This leaflet does not take the place of talking to your doctor about your medical condition or treatment. Talk to your doctor if you have any questions about ALIMTA.

What is ALIMTA?
ALIMTA is a treatment for:
- **Malignant pleural mesothelioma.** This cancer affects the inside lining of the chest cavity. ALIMTA is given with cisplatin, another anti-cancer medicine (chemotherapy).
- **Nonsquamous non-small cell lung cancer.** This cancer is a disease in which malignant (cancer) cells form in the tissues of the lung. If you are having initial treatment for your lung cancer, ALIMTA may be given alone or in combination with another chemotherapy drug. If this is the first time you have been treated for your lung cancer, ALIMTA may be given with another anti-cancer drug called cisplatin. If you have completed initial treatment for your lung cancer, ALIMTA may be given alone immediately following your initial treatment. If you are being treated because your cancer has come back or you had trouble tolerating a prior treatment, ALIMTA may be given alone. Your doctor will speak to you about whether ALIMTA is appropriate for your specific type of non-small cell lung cancer.

Table 18: Summary of Patient Characteristics in MPM Study

Patient characteristic	Randomized and Treated Patients		Fully Supplemented Patients	
	ALIMTA/cis (N=226)	Cisplatin (N=222)	ALIMTA/cis (N=168)	Cisplatin (N=163)
Age (yrs)				
Median (range)	61 (29-85)	60 (19-84)	60 (29-85)	60 (19-82)
Gender (%)				
Male	184 (81.4)	181 (81.5)	136 (81.0)	134 (82.2)
Female	42 (18.6)	41 (18.5)	32 (19.0)	29 (17.8)
Origin (%)				
Caucasian	204 (90.3)	206 (92.8)	150 (89.3)	153 (93.9)
Hispanic	11 (4.9)	12 (5.4)	10 (6.0)	7 (4.3)
Asian	10 (4.4)	4 (1.9)	7 (4.2)	3 (1.8)
African descent	1 (0.4)	0	1 (0.6)	0
Stage at Entry (%)				
I	16 (7.1)	14 (6.3)	15 (8.9)	12 (7.4)
II	35 (15.6)	33 (15.0)	27 (16.2)	27 (16.8)
III	73 (32.4)	68 (30.6)	51 (30.5)	49 (30.4)
IV	101 (44.9)	105 (47.2)	74 (44.3)	73 (45.3)
Unspecified	1 (0.4)	2 (0.9)	1 (0.6)	2 (1.2)
Diagnosis/Histology[a] (%)				
Epithelial	154 (68.1)	152 (68.5)	117 (69.6)	113 (69.3)
Mixed	37 (16.4)	36 (16.2)	25 (14.9)	25 (15.3)
Sarcomatoid	18 (8.0)	25 (11.3)	14 (8.3)	17 (10.4)
Other	17 (7.5)	9 (4.1)	12 (7.1)	8 (4.9)
Baseline KPS[b] (%)				
70-80	109 (48.2)	97 (43.7)	83 (49.4)	69 (42.3)
90-100	117 (51.8)	125 (56.3)	85 (50.6)	94 (57.7)

[a] Only 67% of the patients had the histologic diagnosis of malignant mesothelioma confirmed by independent review.
[b] Karnofsky Performance Scale.

Table 19: Efficacy of ALIMTA plus Cisplatin versus Cisplatin in Malignant Pleural Mesothelioma

Efficacy Parameter	Randomized and Treated Patients		Fully Supplemented Patients	
	ALIMTA/cis (N=226)	Cisplatin (N=222)	ALIMTA/cis (N=168)	Cisplatin (N=163)
Median overall survival (95% CI)	12.1 mos (10.0-14.4)	9.3 mos (7.8-10.7)	13.3 mos (11.4-14.9)	10.0 mos (8.4-11.9)
Hazard ratio	0.77		0.75	
Log rank p-value[a]	0.020		0.051	

[a] p-value refers to comparison between arms.

To lower your chances of side effects of ALIMTA, you must also take folic acid and vitamin B_{12} prior to and during your treatment with ALIMTA. Your doctor will prescribe a medicine called a "corticosteroid" to take for 3 days during your treatment with ALIMTA. Corticosteroid medicines lower your chances of getting skin reactions with ALIMTA.
ALIMTA has not been studied in children.

What should I tell my doctor before taking ALIMTA?
Tell your doctor about all of your medical conditions, including if you:

- **are pregnant or planning to become pregnant.** ALIMTA may harm your unborn baby.
- **are breastfeeding.** It is not known if ALIMTA passes into breast milk. You should stop breastfeeding once you start treatment with ALIMTA.
- **are taking other medicines,** including prescription and nonprescription medicines, vitamins, and herbal supplements. ALIMTA and other medicines may affect each other causing serious side effects. Especially, tell your doctor if you are taking medicines called "nonsteroidal anti-inflammatory drugs" (NSAIDs) for pain or swelling. There are many NSAID medicines. If you are not sure, ask your doctor or pharmacist if any of your medicines are NSAIDs.

How is ALIMTA given?

- ALIMTA is slowly infused (injected) into a vein. The injection or infusion will last about 10 minutes. You will usually receive ALIMTA once every 21 days (3 weeks).
- If you are being treated with ALIMTA and cisplatin for the initial treatment of either mesothelioma or non-small cell lung cancer, ALIMTA will be given first as a 10 minute infusion into your vein and cisplatin (another anti-cancer drug) will also be given through your vein starting about 30 minutes after ALIMTA and ending about 2 hours later.
- If you have completed initial treatment for your non-small cell lung cancer, you may receive ALIMTA alone, given as a 10 minute infusion into your vein.
- If you are being treated because your non-small cell lung cancer has returned, you may receive ALIMTA alone, given as a 10 minute infusion into your vein.
- Your doctor will prescribe a medicine called a "corticosteroid" to take for 3 days during your treatment with ALIMTA. Corticosteroid medicines lower your chances for getting skin reactions with ALIMTA.
- **It is very important to take folic acid and vitamin B_{12} during your treatment with ALIMTA to lower your chances of harmful side effects.** You must start taking 350-1000 micrograms of folic acid every day for at least 5 days out of the 7 days before your first dose of ALIMTA. You must keep taking folic acid every day during the time you are getting treatment with ALIMTA, and for 21 days after your last treatment. You can get folic acid vitamins over-the-counter. Folic acid is also found in many multivitamin pills. Ask your doctor or pharmacist for help if you are not sure how to choose a folic acid product. Your doctor will give you vitamin B_{12} injections while you are getting treatment with ALIMTA. You will get your first vitamin B_{12} injection during the week before your first dose of ALIMTA, and then about every 9 weeks during treatment.
- You will have regular blood tests before and during your treatment with ALIMTA. Your doctor may adjust your dose of ALIMTA or delay treatment based on the results of your blood tests and on your general condition.

What should I avoid while taking ALIMTA?

- **Women who can become pregnant should not become pregnant during treatment with ALIMTA.** ALIMTA may harm the unborn baby.
- **Ask your doctor before taking medicines called NSAIDs.** There are many NSAID medicines. If you are not sure, ask your doctor or pharmacist if any of your medicines are NSAIDs.

What are the possible side effects of ALIMTA?
Most patients taking ALIMTA will have side effects. Sometimes it is not always possible to tell whether ALIMTA, another medicine, or the cancer itself is causing these side effects. **Call your doctor right away if you have a fever, chills, diarrhea, or mouth sores.** These symptoms could mean you have an infection which may be severe and could lead to death.
The most common side effects of ALIMTA when given alone or in combination with cisplatin are:

- **Stomach upset, including nausea, vomiting, and diarrhea.** You can obtain medicines to help control some of these symptoms. Call your doctor if you get any of these symptoms.
- **Low blood cell counts:**
  - **Low red blood cells.** Low red blood cells may make you feel tired, get tired easily, appear pale, and become short of breath.
  - **Low white blood cells.** Low white blood cells may give you a greater chance for infection. If you have a fever (temperature above 100.4°F) or other signs of infection, call your doctor right away.
  - **Low platelets.** Low platelets give you a greater chance for bleeding. Your doctor will do blood tests to check your blood counts before and during treatment with ALIMTA.
- **Tiredness.** You may feel tired or weak for a few days after your ALIMTA treatments. If you have severe weakness or tiredness, call your doctor.
- **Mouth, throat, or lip sores** (stomatitis, pharyngitis). You may get redness or sores in your mouth, throat, or on your lips. These symptoms may happen a few days after ALIMTA treatment. Talk with your doctor about proper mouth and throat care.
- **Loss of appetite.** You may lose your appetite and lose weight during your treatment. Talk to your doctor if this is a problem for you.
- **Rash.** You may get a rash or itching during treatment. These usually appear between treatments with ALIMTA and usually go away before the next treatment. Rarely, these reactions may be severe (can lead to Stevens-Johnson Syndrome or Toxic epidermal necrolysis) and could lead to death. Call your doctor if you get a severe rash, itching, or blistering.

Talk with your doctor, nurse or pharmacist about any side effect that bothers you or that doesn't go away.
These are not all the side effects of ALIMTA. For more information, ask your doctor, nurse or pharmacist.

General information about ALIMTA
Medicines are sometimes prescribed for conditions other than those listed in patient information leaflets. ALIMTA was prescribed for your medical condition.
This leaflet summarizes the most important information about ALIMTA. If you would like more information, talk with your doctor. You can ask your doctor or pharmacist for information about ALIMTA that is written for health professionals. You can also call 1-800-LILLY-RX (1-800-545-5979) or visit www.ALIMTA.com.
Patient information revised August 9, 2010

Eli Lilly and Company
Indianapolis, IN 46285, USA
www.ALIMTA.com

PV 6753 AMP

BYETTA® ℞
[*bye-A-tuh*]
exenatide injection

For full prescribing information see listing under Amylin Pharmaceuticals, Inc.

CAPASTAT® SULFATE ℞
[*cap-uh-stat*]
Capreomycin For Injection, USP
For Intramuscular & Intravenous Injection Only
Not For Pediatric Use

WARNINGS
The use of Capastat® Sulfate (Capreomycin for Injection, USP) in patients with renal insufficiency or preexisting auditory impairment must be undertaken with great caution, and the risk of additional cranial nerve VIII impairment or renal injury should be weighed against the benefits to be derived from therapy. *Refer to* **ANIMAL PHARMACOLOGY** *for additional information.*
Since other parenteral antituberculosis agents (streptomycin, viomycin) also have similar and sometimes irreversible toxic effects, particularly on cranial nerve VIII and renal function, simultaneous administration of these agents with Capastat Sulfate is not recommended. Use with nonantituberculosis drugs (polymyxin A sulfate, colistin sulfate, amikacin, gentamicin, tobramycin, vancomycin, kanamycin, and neomycin) having ototoxic or nephrotoxic potential should be undertaken only with great caution.

Usage in Pregnancy: The safety of the use of Capastat Sulfate in pregnancy has not been determined.

Pediatric Usage: Safety and effectiveness in pediatric patients have not been established.

DESCRIPTION
Capastat Sulfate is a polypeptide antibiotic isolated from *Streptomyces capreolus*. It is a complex of 4 microbiologically active components which have been characterized in part; however, complete structural determination of all the components has not been established.
Capreomycin is supplied as the disulfate salt and is soluble in water. In complete solution, it is almost colorless.
Each vial contains the equivalent of 1 g capreomycin activity.
The structural formula is as follows:

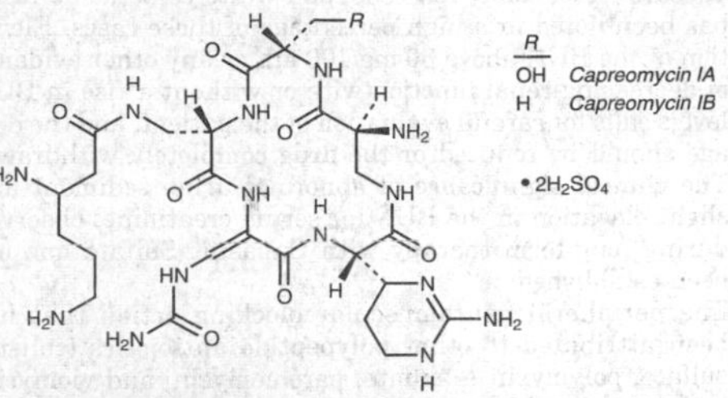

CLINICAL PHARMACOLOGY
Human Pharmacology
Capreomycin is not absorbed in significant quantities from the gastrointestinal tract and must be administered parenterally. In 2 studies of 10 patients each, peak serum concentrations following 1 g of capreomycin given intramuscularly were achieved 1 to 2 hours after administration, and average peak levels reached were 28 and 32 µg/mL respectively (range, 20 to 47 µg/mL). Low serum concentrations were present at 24 hours. However, 1 g of capreomycin daily for 30 days or more produced no significant accumulation in subjects with normal renal function. Two patients with marked reduction of renal function had high serum concentrations 24 hours after administration of the drug. When a 1–g dose of capreomycin was given intramuscularly to normal volunteers, 52% was excreted in the urine within 12 hours.
Lehmann, et al, examined the pharmacokinetics of single dose capreomycin (1.0 g) administered intramuscularly and by intravenous infusion (1 hour) in 6 healthy volunteers. The area under the serum concentration versus time curve was similar for the two routes of administration. Capreomycin peak concentrations after intravenous infusion were 30 ± 47% higher than after intramuscular administration.[1,2]
Paper chromatographic studies indicated that capreomycin is excreted essentially unaltered. Urine concentrations averaged 1.68 mg/mL (average urine volume, 228 mL) during the 6 hours following a 1–g dose.

Microbiology
Capreomycin is active against strains of *Mycobacterium tuberculosis* found in humans.

Susceptibility Tests
The *in vitro* susceptibility of strains of *M. tuberculosis* to capreomycin varies with the media and techniques employed. In general, the minimum inhibitory concentrations for *M. tuberculosis* are lowest in liquid media that are free of egg protein (7H10 or Dubos) and range from 1 to 5 µg/mL when the indirect method is used. Comparable inhibitory concentrations are obtained when 7H10 agar is used for direct susceptibility testing. When indirect susceptibility tests are performed on standard tube slants with 7H10 media, susceptible strains are inhibited by 10 to 25 µg/mL capreomycin. Egg-containing media, such as Löwenstein-Jensen or ATS, require concentrations of 25 to 50 µg/mL to inhibit susceptible strains.

Cross–Resistance
Frequent cross-resistance occurs between capreomycin and viomycin. Varying degrees of cross-resistance between capreomycin and kanamycin and neomycin have been reported. No cross-resistance has been observed between capreomycin and isoniazid, aminosalicylic acid, cycloserine, streptomycin, ethionamide, or ethambutol.

INDICATIONS AND USAGE
Capastat Sulfate, which is to be used concomitantly with other appropriate antituberculosis agents, is indicated in pulmonary infections caused by capreomycin–susceptible strains of *M. tuberculosis* when the primary agents (isoniazid, rifampin, ethambutol, aminosalicylic acid, and streptomycin) have been ineffective or cannot be used because of toxicity or the presence of resistant tubercle bacilli.
Susceptibility studies should be performed to determine the presence of a capreomycin–susceptible strain of *M. tuberculosis*.

CONTRAINDICATION
Capastat Sulfate is contraindicated in patients who are hypersensitive to capreomycin.

PRECAUTIONS
General
Audiometric measurements and assessment of vestibular function should be performed prior to initiation of therapy with Capastat Sulfate and at regular intervals during treatment.
Renal injury, with tubular necrosis, elevation of the blood urea nitrogen (BUN) or serum creatinine, and abnormal

urinary sediment, has been noted. Slight elevation of the BUN and serum creatinine has been observed in a significant number of patients receiving prolonged therapy. The appearance of casts, red cells, and white cells in the urine has been noted in a high percentage of these cases. Elevation of the BUN above 30 mg/100 mL or any other evidence of decreasing renal function with or without a rise in BUN levels calls for careful evaluation of the patient, and the dosage should be reduced or the drug completely withdrawn. The clinical significance of abnormal urine sediment and slight elevation in the BUN (or serum creatinine) observed during long-term therapy with Capastat Sulfate has not been established.

The peripheral neuromuscular blocking action that has been attributed to other polypeptide antibiotics (colistin sulfate, polymyxin A sulfate, paromomycin, and viomycin) and to aminoglycoside antibiotics (streptomycin, dihydrostreptomycin, neomycin, and kanamycin) has been studied with Capastat Sulfate. A partial neuromuscular blockade was demonstrated after large intravenous doses of Capastat Sulfate. This action was enhanced by ether anesthesia (as has been reported for neomycin) and was antagonized by neostigmine.

Caution should be exercised in the administration of antibiotics, including Capastat Sulfate, to any patient who has demonstrated some form of allergy, particularly to drugs.

Laboratory Tests

Regular tests of renal function should be made throughout the period of treatment, and reduced dosage should be employed in patients with known or suspected renal impairment.

Renal function studies should be made both before therapy with Capastat Sulfate is started and on a weekly basis during treatment.

Since hypokalemia, hypomagnesemia and hypocalcemia may occur during therapy, these serum electrolyte levels should be determined frequently.

Drug Interactions

For neuromuscular blocking action of this drug, *see* **PRECAUTIONS, General.**

Carcinogenesis, Mutagenesis, Impairment of Fertility

Studies have not been performed to determine potential for carcinogenicity, mutagenicity, or impairment of fertility.

Usage in Pregnancy — Pregnancy Category C

Capastat Sulfate has been shown to be teratogenic in rats when given in doses 3 1/2 times the human dose. There are no adequate and well-controlled studies in pregnant women. Capastat Sulfate should be used during pregnancy only if the potential benefit justifies the potential risk to the fetus (*see boxed* **WARNINGS** *and* ANIMAL PHARMACOLOGY).

Nursing Mothers

It is not known whether this drug is excreted in human milk. Because many drugs are excreted in human milk, caution should be exercised when Capastat Sulfate is administered to a nursing woman.

Pediatric Use

Safety and effectiveness in pediatric patients have not been established (*see boxed* **WARNINGS**).

Geriatric Use

Clinical studies of Capastat Sulfate did not analyze the safety and efficacy of patients aged 65 and over to determine whether they respond differently from younger patients. Other reported clinical experience has not identified differences in responses between the elderly and younger patients. In general, dose selection for an elderly patient should be cautious, usually starting at the low end of the dosing range, reflecting the greater frequency of decreased hepatic, renal, or cardiac function, and of concomitant disease or other drug therapy.

Capastat Sulfate is known to be substantially excreted by the kidney (*see* **CLINICAL PHARMACOLOGY**), and the risk of toxic reactions to this drug may be greater in patients with impaired renal function. Because elderly patients are more likely to have decreased renal function, care should be taken in dose selection, and it may be useful to monitor renal function (*see* **PRECAUTIONS**, Laboratory Tests). Patients with reduced renal function should have dosage reduction based on creatinine clearance using the guidelines included in Table 1 (*see* **DOSAGE AND ADMINISTRATION**).

The geriatric population is also more likely to have impaired hearing at baseline. Audiometric measurements and assessment of vestibular function should be performed prior to initiation of therapy with Capastat Sulfate and at regular intervals during treatment (*see* **PRECAUTIONS**, General).

ADVERSE REACTIONS

Nephrotoxicity: In 36% of 722 patients treated with Capastat Sulfate, elevation of the BUN above 20 mg/100 mL has been observed. In many instances, there was also depression of PSP excretion and abnormal urine sediment. In 10% of this series, the BUN elevation exceeded 30 mg/100 mL.

Toxic nephritis was reported in 1 patient with tuberculosis and portal cirrhosis who was treated with Capastat Sulfate (1 g) and aminosalicylic acid daily for 1 month. This patient developed renal insufficiency and oliguria and died. Autopsy showed subsiding acute tubular necrosis.

Electrolyte disturbances including hypokalemia, hypomagnesemia and hypocalcemia, sometimes serious in nature, have been reported.

Ototoxicity: Subclinical auditory loss was noted in approximately 11% of 722 patients undergoing treatment with Capastat Sulfate. This was a 5– to 10–decibel loss in the 4000– to 8000–CPS range. Clinically apparent hearing loss occurred in 3% of the 722 subjects. Some audiometric changes were reversible. Other cases with permanent loss were not progressive following withdrawal of Capastat Sulfate.

Tinnitus and vertigo have occurred.

Liver: Serial tests of liver function have demonstrated a decrease in BSP excretion without change in AST (SGOT) or ALT (SGPT) in the presence of preexisting liver disease. Abnormal results in liver function tests have occurred in many persons receiving Capastat Sulfate in combination with other antituberculosis agents that also are known to cause changes in hepatic function. The role of Capastat Sulfate in producing these abnormalities is not clear; however, periodic determinations of liver function are recommended.

Blood: Leukocytosis and leukopenia have been observed. The majority of patients treated have had eosinophilia exceeding 5% while receiving daily injections of Capastat Sulfate. This has subsided with reduction of the Capastat Sulfate dosage to 2 or 3 g weekly.

Pain and induration at the injection site have been observed. Excessive bleeding at the injection site has been reported. Sterile abscesses have been noted. Rare cases of thrombocytopenia have been reported.

Hypersensitivity: Urticaria and maculopapular skin rashes associated in some cases with febrile reactions have been reported when Capastat Sulfate and other antituberculosis drugs were given concomitantly.

OVERDOSAGE

Signs and Symptoms

Nephrotoxicity following the parenteral administration of Capastat Sulfate is most closely related to the area under the curve of the serum concentration versus time graph. The elderly patient, patients with abnormal renal function or dehydration, and patients receiving other nephrotoxic drugs are at much greater risk for developing acute tubular necrosis.

Damage to the auditory and vestibular divisions of cranial nerve VIII has been associated with Capastat Sulfate given to patients with abnormal renal function or dehydration and in those receiving medications with additive auditory toxicities. These patients often experience dizziness, tinnitus, vertigo, and a loss of high–tone acuity.

Neuromuscular blockage or respiratory paralysis may occur following rapid intravenous infusion.

If capreomycin is ingested, toxicity would be unlikely because it is poorly absorbed (less than 1%) from an intact gastrointestinal system.

Hypokalemia, hypocalcemia, hypomagnesemia, and an electrolyte disturbance resembling Bartter's syndrome have been reported to occur in patients with capreomycin toxicity.

The subcutaneous median lethal dose in mice was 514 mg/kg.

Treatment

To obtain up-to-date information about the treatment of overdose, a good resource is your certified Regional Poison Control Center. Telephone numbers of certified poison control centers are listed in the *Physicians' Desk Reference (PDR)*. In managing overdosage, consider the possibility of multiple drug overdoses, interaction among drugs, and unusual drug kinetics in your patient.

Protect the patient's airway and support ventilation and perfusion. Meticulously monitor and maintain, within acceptable limits, the patient's vital signs, blood gases, serum electrolytes, etc. Absorption of drugs from the gastrointestinal tract may be decreased by giving activated charcoal, which, in many cases, is more effective than emesis or lavage; consider charcoal instead of or in addition to gastric emptying. Repeated doses of charcoal over time may hasten elimination of some drugs that have been absorbed. Safeguard the patient's airway when employing gastric emptying or charcoal.

Patients who have received an overdose of capreomycin and have normal renal function should be carefully hydrated to maintain a urine output of 3 to 5 mL/kg/h. Fluid balance, electrolytes, and creatinine clearance should be carefully monitored.

Hemodialysis may be effectively used to remove capreomycin in patients with significant renal disease.

DOSAGE AND ADMINISTRATION

Capastat Sulfate may be administered intramuscularly or intravenously following reconstitution. Reconstitution is achieved by dissolving the vial contents (1 g) in 2 mL of 0.9% Sodium Chloride Injection or Sterile Water for Injection. Two to 3 minutes should be allowed for complete dissolution.

Intravenously—For intravenous infusion, reconstituted Capastat Sulfate should be diluted in 100 mL of 0.9% Sodium Chloride Injection and administered over 60 minutes.

Intramuscularly—Reconstituted Capastat Sulfate should be given by deep intramuscular injection into a large muscle mass, since superficial injection may be associated with increased pain and the development of sterile abscesses.

For administration of a 1–g dose, the entire contents of the vial should be given. For doses lower than 1 g, the following dilution table may be used.

DILUTION TABLE

Diluent Added to 1-g, 10-mL Vial	Volume of Capastat Sulfate Solution	Concentration (Approx)
2.15 mL	2.85 mL	370 mg*/mL
2.63 mL	3.33 mL	315 mg*/mL
3.3 mL	4 mL	260 mg*/mL
4.3 mL	5 mL	210 mg*/mL

*Equivalent to capreomycin activity. Approximated concentration takes into account the retention volume.

The solution may acquire a pale straw color and darken with time, but this is not associated with loss of potency or the development of toxicity. After reconstitution, all solutions of Capastat Sulfate may be stored for up to 24 hours under refrigeration.

Capreomycin is always administered in combination with at least 1 other antituberculosis agent to which the patient's strain of tubercle bacilli is susceptible. The usual dose is 1 g daily (not to exceed 20 mg/kg/day) given intramuscularly or intravenously for 60 to 120 days, followed by 1 g by either route 2 or 3 times weekly. (Note — Therapy for tuberculosis should be maintained for 12 to 24 months. If facilities for administering injectable medication are not available, a change to appropriate oral therapy is indicated on the patient's release from the hospital.)

Patients with reduced renal function should have dosage reduction based on creatinine clearance using the guidelines included in Table 1. These dosages are designed to achieve a mean steady–state capreomycin level of 10 µg/mL.

Table 1. Estimated Dosages to Attain Mean Steady-State Serum Capreomycin Concentration of 10 µg/mL (Based on Creatinine Clearance)

CrCl (mL/min)	Capreomycin Clearance (L/kg/h × 10^{-2})	Half-life (hours)	Dose* (mg/kg) for the Following Dosing Intervals 24 h	48 h	72 h
0	0.54	55.5	1.29	2.58	3.87
10	1.01	29.4	2.43	4.87	7.30
20	1.49	20.0	3.58	7.16	10.7
30	1.97	15.1	4.72	9.45	14.2
40	2.45	12.2	5.87	11.7	
50	2.92	10.2	7.01	14.0	
60	3.40	8.8	8.16		
80	4.35	6.8	10.4†		
100	5.31	5.6	12.7†		
110	5.78	5.2	13.9†		

*For patients with renal impairment, initial maintenance dose estimates are given for optional dosing intervals; longer dosing intervals are expected to provide greater peak and lower trough serum capreomycin levels than shorter dosing intervals.

† The usual dosage for patients with normal renal function is 1000 mg daily, not to exceed 20 mg/kg/day, for 60 to 120 days, then 1000 mg 2 to 3 times weekly.

Parenteral drug products should be inspected visually for particulate matter and discoloration prior to administration, whenever solution and container permit.

HOW SUPPLIED

Capastat® Sulfate, Capreomycin for Injection, USP, is available in:

Vials: 1 g[1], 10 mL size (No. 718) (1s) NDC 0002-1485-01

[1] Equivalent to capreomycin activity.

Store at controlled room temperature 15° to 30°C (59° to 86°F) prior to reconstitution.

ANIMAL PHARMACOLOGY

In addition to renal and cranial nerve VIII toxicity demonstrated in animal toxicology studies, cataracts developed in 2 dogs on doses of 62 mg/kg and 100 mg/kg for prolonged periods.

In teratology studies, a low incidence of "wavy ribs" was noted in litters of female rats treated with daily doses of 50 mg/kg or more of capreomycin.

REFERENCES

1. Lehmann CR, Garrett LE, Winn RE, Springberg PD, Vicks S, Porter DK, Pierson WP, Wolny JD, Brier GL, Black HR. Capreomycin kinetics in renal impairment and clearance by hemodialysis. Am Rev Respir Dis 1988;138/5:1312–3.
2. Unpublished data on file at Lilly.

Literature revised January 14, 2008
Eli Lilly and Company
Indianapolis, IN 46285, USA
PV 4801 AMP

CIALIS®   ℞

[See-AL-iss]
(tadalafil)
tablet, film coated for oral use

HIGHLIGHTS OF PRESCRIBING INFORMATION

These highlights do not include all the information needed to use CIALIS safely and effectively. See full prescribing information for CIALIS.

CIALIS (tadalafil) tablet, film coated for oral use
Initial U.S. Approval: 2003

————————RECENT MAJOR CHANGES————————

Contraindications, Hypersensitivity Reactions (4.2) 07/2009
Warnings and Precautions, Combination With Other PDE5 Inhibitors or Erectile Dysfunction Therapies (5.11) 02/2010

————————INDICATIONS AND USAGE————————

CIALIS® is a phosphodiesterase 5 (PDE5) inhibitor indicated for erectile dysfunction (ED) (1.1).

——————DOSAGE AND ADMINISTRATION——————

• CIALIS for use as needed: Starting dose: 10 mg up to once daily. Increase to 20 mg or decrease to 5 mg based upon efficacy/tolerability. Improves erectile function compared to placebo up to 36 hours post dose (2.1).
• CIALIS for once daily use: 2.5 mg taken once daily, without regard to timing of sexual activity. May increase to 5 mg based upon efficacy and tolerability (2.1).
• CIALIS may be taken without regard to food (2.2).

——————DOSAGE FORMS AND STRENGTHS——————

Tablets (not scored): 2.5 mg, 5 mg, 10 mg, 20 mg (3).

————————CONTRAINDICATIONS————————

• Administration of CIALIS to patients using any form of organic nitrate is contraindicated. CIALIS was shown to potentiate the hypotensive effect of nitrates (4.1).
• History of known serious hypersensitivity reaction to CIALIS or ADCIRCA™ (4.2).

——————WARNINGS AND PRECAUTIONS——————

• Patients should not use CIALIS if sex is inadvisable due to cardiovascular status (5.1).
• Use of CIALIS with alpha blockers, antihypertensives or substantial amounts of alcohol (≥5 units) may lead to hypotension (5.6, 5.9).
• If taking potent inhibitors of CYP3A4, dose should be adjusted: CIALIS for use as needed: ≤10 mg every 72 hours. For once daily use: dose not to exceed 2.5 mg (5.10).
• Patients should seek emergency treatment if an erection lasts >4 hours. Use CIALIS with caution in patients predisposed to priapism (5.3).
• Patients should stop CIALIS and seek medical care if a sudden loss of vision occurs in one or both eyes, which could be a sign of Non Arteritic Ischemic Optic Neuropathy (NAION). Discuss increased risk of NAION in patients with history of NAION (5.4).
• Patients should stop CIALIS and seek prompt medical attention in the event of sudden decrease or loss of hearing (5.5).

————————ADVERSE REACTIONS————————

Most common adverse reactions (≥2%) include headache, dyspepsia, back pain, myalgia, nasal congestion, flushing, and pain in limb (6.1, 6.2).

To report SUSPECTED ADVERSE REACTIONS, contact Eli Lilly and Company at 1-800-LillyRx (1-800-545-5979) or FDA at 1-800-FDA-1088 or www.fda.gov/medwatch

————————DRUG INTERACTIONS————————

• CIALIS can potentiate the hypotensive effects of nitrates, alpha blockers, antihypertensives or alcohol (7.1).
• CYP3A4 inhibitors (e.g. ketoconazole, ritonavir) increase CIALIS exposure (7.2).
• CYP3A4 inducers (e.g. rifampin) decrease CIALIS exposure (7.2).

——————USE IN SPECIFIC POPULATIONS——————

Hepatic Impairment (2.3, 5.8, 8.6):
• Mild or Moderate: Dosage adjustment may be needed (2.3).
• Severe: Use is not recommended (2.3).

Renal Insufficiency (2.3, 5.7, 8.7):
• Moderate: For use as needed: Dosage adjustment may be needed. For once daily use: No dose adjustment is needed (2.3).
• Severe: For use as needed: Dose should not exceed 5 mg every 72 hours. Once daily use is not recommended (2.3).

See 17 for PATIENT COUNSELING INFORMATION and FDA-approved patient labeling

Revised: 02/2010

FULL PRESCRIBING INFORMATION: CONTENTS*

* Sections or subsections omitted from the full prescribing information are not listed

---

FULL PRESCRIBING INFORMATION

1   INDICATIONS AND USAGE

1.1   Erectile Dysfunction

CIALIS is indicated for the treatment of erectile dysfunction.

2   DOSAGE AND ADMINISTRATION

2.1   Erectile Dysfunction

CIALIS for Use as Needed
• The recommended starting dose of CIALIS for use as needed in most patients is 10 mg, taken prior to anticipated sexual activity.
• The dose may be increased to 20 mg or decreased to 5 mg, based on individual efficacy and tolerability. The maximum recommended dosing frequency is once per day in most patients.
• CIALIS for use as needed was shown to improve erectile function compared to placebo up to 36 hours following dosing. Therefore, when advising patients on optimal use of CIALIS, this should be taken into consideration.

CIALIS for Once Daily Use
• The recommended starting dose of CIALIS for once daily use is 2.5 mg, taken at approximately the same time every day, without regard to timing of sexual activity.
• The CIALIS dose for once daily use may be increased to 5 mg, based on individual efficacy and tolerability.

2.2   Use with Food

CIALIS may be taken without regard to food.

2.3   Use in Special Populations

Renal Insufficiency
CIALIS for Use as Needed
• Mild (creatinine clearance 51 to 80 mL/min): No dose adjustment is required.
• Moderate (creatinine clearance 31 to 50 mL/min): A starting dose of 5 mg not more than once per day is recommended, and the maximum dose should be limited to 10 mg not more than once in every 48 hours.
• Severe (creatinine clearance <30 mL/min and on hemodialysis): The maximum recommended dose is 5 mg not more than once in every 72 hours [see Warnings and Precautions (5.7) and Use In Specific Populations (8.7)].

CIALIS for Once Daily Use
• Mild (creatinine clearance 51 to 80 mL/min): No dose adjustment is required.
• Moderate (creatinine clearance 31 to 50 mL/min): No dose adjustment is required.
• Severe (creatinine clearance <30 mL/min and on hemodialysis): CIALIS for once daily use is not recommended [see Warnings and Precautions (5.7) and Use In Specific Populations (8.7)].

Hepatic Impairment
CIALIS for Use as Needed
• Mild or moderate (Child Pugh Class A or B): The dose of CIALIS should not exceed 10 mg once per day. The use of CIALIS once per day has not been extensively evaluated in patients with hepatic insufficiency and therefore, caution is advised.
• Severe (Child Pugh Class C): The use of CIALIS is not recommended [see Warnings and Precautions (5.8) and Use in Specific Populations (8.6)].

CIALIS for Once Daily Use
• Mild or moderate (Child Pugh Class A or B): CIALIS for once daily use has not been extensively evaluated in patients with hepatic insufficiency. Therefore, caution is advised if CIALIS for once daily use is prescribed to these patients.
• Severe (Child Pugh Class C): The use of CIALIS is not recommended [see Warnings and Precautions (5.8) and Use in Specific Populations (8.6)].

Geriatrics
• No dose adjustment is required in patients >65 years of age.

2.4   Concomitant Medications

Nitrates
• Concomitant use of nitrates in any form is contraindicated [see Contraindications (4.1)].

Alpha Blockers
• When CIALIS is coadministered with an alpha blocker, patients should be stable on alpha-blocker therapy prior to initiating treatment with CIALIS, and CIALIS should be initiated at the lowest recommended dose [see Warnings and Precautions (5.6), Drug Interactions (7.1) and Clinical Pharmacology (12.2)].

CYP3A4 Inhibitors
CIALIS for Use as Needed—For patients taking concomitant potent inhibitors of CYP3A4, such as ketoconazole or ritonavir, the maximum recommended dose of CIALIS is 10 mg, not to exceed once every 72 hours [see Warnings and Precautions (5.10) and Drug Interactions (7.2)].
CIALIS for Once Daily Use—For patients taking concomitant potent inhibitors of CYP3A4, such as ketoconazole or ritonavir, the dose should not exceed 2.5 mg [see Warnings and Precautions (5.10) and Drug Interactions (7.2)].

3   DOSAGE FORMS AND STRENGTHS

Four strengths of film-coated, almond-shaped tablets (not scored) are available in different sizes and different shades of yellow:
• 2.5-mg tablets debossed with "C 2 1/2"
• 5-mg tablets debossed with "C 5"

- 10-mg tablets debossed with "C 10"
- 20-mg tablets debossed with "C 20"

4 CONTRAINDICATIONS

4.1 Nitrates

Administration of CIALIS to patients who are using any form of organic nitrate, either regularly and/or intermittently, is contraindicated. In clinical pharmacology studies, CIALIS was shown to potentiate the hypotensive effect of nitrates. This is thought to result from the combined effects of nitrates and CIALIS on the nitric oxide/cGMP pathway [see Clinical Pharmacology (12.2)].

4.2 Hypersensitivity Reactions

CIALIS is contraindicated in patients with a known serious hypersensitivity to tadalafil (CIALIS or ADCIRCA™). Hypersensitivity reactions have been reported, including Stevens-Johnson syndrome and exfoliative dermatitis [see Adverse Reactions (6.2)].

5 WARNINGS AND PRECAUTIONS

Evaluation of erectile dysfunction should include an appropriate medical assessment to identify potential underlying causes, as well as treatment options.

Before prescribing CIALIS, it is important to note the following:

5.1 Cardiovascular

Physicians should consider the cardiovascular status of their patients, since there is a degree of cardiac risk associated with sexual activity. Therefore, treatments for erectile dysfunction, including CIALIS, should not be used in men for whom sexual activity is inadvisable as a result of their underlying cardiovascular status. Patients who experience symptoms upon initiation of sexual activity should be advised to refrain from further sexual activity and seek immediate medical attention.

Physicians should discuss with patients the appropriate action in the event that they experience anginal chest pain requiring nitroglycerin following intake of CIALIS. In such a patient, who has taken CIALIS, where nitrate administration is deemed medically necessary for a life-threatening situation, at least 48 hours should have elapsed after the last dose of CIALIS before nitrate administration is considered. In such circumstances, nitrates should still only be administered under close medical supervision with appropriate hemodynamic monitoring. Therefore, patients who experience anginal chest pain after taking CIALIS should seek immediate medical attention. [See Contraindications (4.1) and Patient Counseling Information (17.1)].

Patients with left ventricular outflow obstruction, (e.g., aortic stenosis and idiopathic hypertrophic subaortic stenosis) can be sensitive to the action of vasodilators, including PDE5 inhibitors.

The following groups of patients with cardiovascular disease were not included in clinical safety and efficacy trials for CIALIS, and therefore until further information is available, CIALIS is not recommended for the following groups of patients:

- myocardial infarction within the last 90 days
- unstable angina or angina occurring during sexual intercourse
- New York Heart Association Class 2 or greater heart failure in the last 6 months
- uncontrolled arrhythmias, hypotension (<90/50 mm Hg), or uncontrolled hypertension (>170/100 mm Hg)
- stroke within the last 6 months.

As with other PDE5 inhibitors, tadalafil has mild systemic vasodilatory properties that may result in transient decreases in blood pressure. In a clinical pharmacology study, tadalafil 20 mg resulted in a mean maximal decrease in supine blood pressure, relative to placebo, of 1.6/0.8 mm Hg in healthy subjects [see Clinical Pharmacology (12.2)]. While this effect should not be of consequence in most patients, prior to prescribing CIALIS, physicians should carefully consider whether their patients with underlying cardiovascular disease could be affected adversely by such vasodilatory effects. Patients with severely impaired autonomic control of blood pressure may be particularly sensitive to the actions of vasodilators, including PDE5 inhibitors.

5.2 Potential for Drug Interactions When Taking CIALIS for Once Daily Use

Physicians should be aware that CIALIS for once daily use provides continuous plasma tadalafil levels and should consider this when evaluating the potential for interactions with medications (e.g., nitrates, alpha-blockers, antihypertensives and potent inhibitors of CYP3A4) and with substantial consumption of alcohol [see Drug Interactions (7.1), (7.2), (7.3)].

5.3 Prolonged Erection

There have been rare reports of prolonged erections greater than 4 hours and priapism (painful erections greater than 6 hours in duration) for this class of compounds. Priapism, if not treated promptly, can result in irreversible damage to the erectile tissue. Patients who have an erection lasting greater than 4 hours, whether painful or not, should seek emergency medical attention.

CIALIS should be used with caution in patients who have conditions that might predispose them to priapism (such as sickle cell anemia, multiple myeloma, or leukemia), or in patients with anatomical deformation of the penis (such as angulation, cavernosal fibrosis, or Peyronie's disease).

5.4 Eye

Physicians should advise patients to stop use of all PDE5 inhibitors, including CIALIS, and seek medical attention in the event of a sudden loss of vision in one or both eyes. Such an event may be a sign of non-arteritic anterior ischemic optic neuropathy (NAION), a cause of decreased vision, including permanent loss of vision that has been reported rarely postmarketing in temporal association with the use of all PDE5 inhibitors. It is not possible to determine whether these events are related directly to the use of PDE5 inhibitors or other factors. Physicians should also discuss with patients the increased risk of NAION in individuals who have already experienced NAION in one eye, including whether such individuals could be adversely affected by use of vasodilators such as PDE5 inhibitors [see Adverse Reactions (6.2)].

Patients with known hereditary degenerative retinal disorders, including retinitis pigmentosa, were not included in the clinical trials, and use in these patients is not recommended.

5.5 Sudden Hearing Loss

Physicians should advise patients to stop taking PDE5 inhibitors, including CIALIS, and seek prompt medical attention in the event of sudden decrease or loss of hearing. These events, which may be accompanied by tinnitus and dizziness, have been reported in temporal association to the intake of PDE5 inhibitors, including CIALIS. It is not possible to determine whether these events are related directly to the use of PDE5 inhibitors or to other factors [see Adverse Reactions (6.1) and (6.2)].

5.6 Alpha blockers and Antihypertensives

Physicians should discuss with patients the potential for CIALIS to augment the blood-pressure-lowering effect of alpha blockers and antihypertensive medications [see Drug Interactions (7.1) and Clinical Pharmacology (12.2)].

Caution is advised when PDE5 inhibitors are coadministered with alpha blockers. PDE5 inhibitors, including CIALIS, and alpha-adrenergic blocking agents are both vasodilators with blood-pressure-lowering effects. When vasodilators are used in combination, an additive effect on blood pressure may be anticipated. In some patients, concomitant use of these two drug classes can lower blood pressure significantly [see Clinical Pharmacology (12.2) and Drug Interactions (7.1)], which may lead to symptomatic hypotension (e.g., fainting). Consideration should be given to the following:

- Patients should be stable on alpha-blocker therapy prior to initiating a PDE5 inhibitor. Patients who demonstrate hemodynamic instability on alpha-blocker therapy alone are at increased risk of symptomatic hypotension with concomitant use of PDE5 inhibitors.
- In those patients who are stable on alpha-blocker therapy, PDE5 inhibitors should be initiated at the lowest recommended dose.
- In those patients already taking an optimized dose of PDE5 inhibitor, alpha-blocker therapy should be initiated at the lowest dose. Stepwise increase in alpha-blocker dose may be associated with further lowering of blood pressure when taking a PDE5 inhibitor.
- Safety of combined use of PDE5 inhibitors and alpha blockers may be affected by other variables, including intravascular volume depletion and other antihypertensive drugs.

[See Dosage and Administration (2.4) and Drug Interactions (7.1)].

5.7 Renal Insufficiency

CIALIS for Use as Needed

CIALIS should be limited to 5 mg not more than once in every 72 hours in patients with severe renal insufficiency or end-stage renal disease on hemodialysis. The starting dose of CIALIS in patients with a moderate degree of renal insufficiency should be 5 mg not more than once per day, and the maximum dose should be limited to 10 mg not more than once in every 48 hours. No dose adjustment is required in patients with mild renal insufficiency [see Use in Specific Populations (8.7)].

CIALIS for Once Daily Use

Due to increased tadalafil exposure (AUC), limited clinical experience, and the lack of ability to influence clearance by dialysis, CIALIS for once daily use is not recommended in patients with severe renal insufficiency. No dose adjustment is required in patients with mild or moderate renal insufficiency [see Use in Specific Populations (8.7)].

5.8 Hepatic Impairment

CIALIS for Use as Needed

In patients with mild or moderate hepatic impairment, the dose of CIALIS should not exceed 10 mg. Because of insufficient information in patients with severe hepatic impairment, use of CIALIS in this group is not recommended [see Use In Specific Populations (8.6)].

CIALIS for Once Daily Use

CIALIS for once daily use has not been extensively evaluated in patients with mild or moderate hepatic insufficiency. Therefore, caution is advised if CIALIS for once daily use is prescribed to these patients. Because of insufficient information in patients with severe hepatic impairment, use of CIALIS in this group is not recommended [see Use In Specific Populations (8.6)].

5.9 Alcohol

Patients should be made aware that both alcohol and CIALIS, a PDE5 inhibitor, act as mild vasodilators. When mild vasodilators are taken in combination, blood-pressure-lowering effects of each individual compound may be increased. Therefore, physicians should inform patients that substantial consumption of alcohol (e.g., 5 units or greater) in combination with CIALIS can increase the potential for orthostatic signs and symptoms, including increase in heart rate, decrease in standing blood pressure, dizziness, and headache [see Dosage and Administration (2.4) and Clinical Pharmacology (12.2)].

5.10 Concomitant Use of Potent Inhibitors of Cytochrome P450 3A4 (CYP3A4)

CIALIS is metabolized predominantly by CYP3A4 in the liver. The dose of CIALIS should be limited to 10 mg no more than once every 72 hours in patients taking potent inhibitors of CYP3A4 such as ritonavir, ketoconazole, and itraconazole [see Drug Interactions (7.2)]. In patients taking potent inhibitors of CYP3A4 and CIALIS for once daily use, the dose of CIALIS should not exceed 2.5 mg [see Dosage and Administration (2.4)].

5.11 Combination With Other PDE5 Inhibitors or Erectile Dysfunction Therapies

The safety and efficacy of combinations of CIALIS and other PDE5 inhibitors or treatments for erectile dysfunction have not been studied. Inform patients not to take CIALIS with other PDE5 inhibitors, including ADCIRCA.

5.12 Effects on Bleeding

Studies in vitro have demonstrated that tadalafil is a selective inhibitor of PDE5. PDE5 is found in platelets. When administered in combination with aspirin, tadalafil 20 mg did not prolong bleeding time, relative to aspirin alone. CIALIS has not been administered to patients with bleeding disorders or significant active peptic ulceration. Although CIALIS has not been shown to increase bleeding times in healthy subjects, use in patients with bleeding disorders or significant active peptic ulceration should be based upon a careful risk-benefit assessment and caution.

5.13 Counseling Patients About Sexually Transmitted Diseases

The use of CIALIS offers no protection against sexually transmitted diseases. Counseling patients about the protective measures necessary to guard against sexually transmitted diseases, including Human Immunodeficiency Virus (HIV) should be considered.

6 ADVERSE REACTIONS

6.1 Clinical Studies Experience

Because clinical trials are conducted under widely varying conditions, adverse reaction rates observed in the clinical trials of a drug cannot be directly compared to rates in the clinical trials of another drug and may not reflect the rates observed in practice.

Tadalafil was administered to over 6550 men during clinical trials worldwide. In trials of CIALIS for once daily use, a total of 716, 389, and 115 were treated for at least 6 months, 1 year, and 2 years, respectively. For CIALIS for use as needed, over 1300 and 1000 subjects were treated for at least 6 months and 1 year, respectively.

CIALIS for Use as Needed

In eight primary placebo-controlled Phase 3 studies of 12 weeks duration, mean age was 59 years (range 22 to 88) and the discontinuation rate due to adverse events in patients treated with tadalafil 10 or 20 mg was 3.1%, compared to 1.4% in placebo treated patients.

When taken as recommended in the placebo-controlled clinical trials, the following adverse events were reported (see Table 1) for CIALIS for use as needed:

[See table 1 at top of next page]

CIALIS for Once Daily Use

In three placebo-controlled Phase 3 clinical trials of 12 or 24 weeks duration, mean age was 58 years (range 21 to 82) and the discontinuation rate due to adverse events in patients treated with tadalafil was 4.1%, compared to 2.8% in placebo-treated patients.

The following adverse events were reported (see Table 2) in clinical trials of 12 weeks duration:

Table 1: Treatment-Emergent Adverse Events Reported by ≥2% of Patients Treated with CIALIS (10 or 20 mg) and More Frequent on Drug than Placebo in the Eight Primary Placebo-Controlled Phase 3 Studies (Including a Study in Patients with Diabetes) for CIALIS for Use as Needed

Adverse Event	Placebo (N=476)	Tadalafil 5 mg (N=151)	Tadalafil 10 mg (N=394)	Tadalafil 20 mg (N=635)
Headache	5%	11%	11%	15%
Dyspepsia	1%	4%	8%	10%
Back pain	3%	3%	5%	6%
Myalgia	1%	1%	4%	3%
Nasal congestion	1%	2%	3%	3%
Flushing[a]	1%	2%	3%	3%
Pain in limb	1%	1%	3%	3%

[a] The term flushing includes: facial flushing and flushing

Table 2: Treatment-Emergent Adverse Events Reported by ≥2% of Patients Treated with CIALIS for Once Daily Use (2.5 or 5 mg) and More Frequent on Drug than Placebo in the Three Primary Placebo-Controlled Phase 3 Studies at 12 weeks (Including a Study in Patients with Diabetes) for CIALIS for Once Daily Use

Adverse Event	Placebo (N=248)	Tadalafil 2.5 mg (N=196)	Tadalafil 5 mg (N=304)
Headache	5%	3%	6%
Dyspepsia	2%	3%	5%
Nasopharyngitis	4%	4%	3%
Back pain	1%	3%	3%
Upper respiratory tract infection	1%	3%	3%
Flushing	1%	1%	3%
Influenza	2%	3%	2%
Myalgia	1%	2%	2%
Cough	0%	4%	2%
Diarrhea	0%	1%	2%
Nasal congestion	0%	2%	2%
Pain in extremity	0%	1%	2%
Bronchitis	1%	2%	0%
Urinary tract infection	0%	2%	0%
Gastroesophageal reflux	0%	2%	1%
Abdominal pain	0%	2%	1%
Upper Respiratory Tract Infection	0%	3%	4%
Dyspepsia	1%	4%	1%
Gastroesophageal Reflux Disease	0%	3%	2%
Myalgia	2%	4%	1%
Hypertension	0%	1%	3%
Nasal Congestion	0%	0%	4%

The following adverse events were reported (see Table 3) over 24 weeks treatment duration in one placebo-controlled Phase 3 clinical study:

Table 3: Treatment-Emergent Adverse Events Reported by ≥2% of Patients Treated with CIALIS for Once Daily Use (2.5 or 5 mg) and More Frequent on Drug than Placebo in One Placebo-Controlled Phase 3 Study of 24 Weeks Treatment Duration for CIALIS for Once Daily Use

Adverse Event	Placebo (N=94)	Tadalafil 2.5 mg (N=96)	Tadalafil 5 mg (N=97)
Nasopharyngitis	5%	6%	6%
Gastroenteritis viral	2%	3%	5%
Influenza	3%	5%	3%
Back Pain	3%	5%	2%

Back pain or myalgia was reported at incidence rates described in Tables 1 and 2. In tadalafil clinical pharmacology trials, back pain or myalgia generally occurred 12 to 24 hours after dosing and typically resolved within 48 hours. The back pain/myalgia associated with tadalafil treatment was characterized by diffuse bilateral lower lumbar, gluteal, thigh, or thoracolumbar muscular discomfort and was exacerbated by recumbancy. In general, pain was reported as mild or moderate in severity and resolved without medical treatment, but severe back pain was reported with a low frequency (<5% of all reports). When medical treatment was necessary, acetaminophen or non-steroidal anti-inflammatory drugs were generally effective; however, in a small percentage of subjects who required treatment, a mild narcotic (e.g., codeine) was used. Overall, approximately 0.5% of all subjects treated with CIALIS for on demand use discontinued treatment as a consequence of back pain/myalgia. In the 1-year open label extension study, back pain and myalgia were reported in 5.5% and 1.3% of patients, respectively. Diagnostic testing, including measures for inflammation, muscle injury, or renal damage revealed no evidence of medically significant underlying pathology. Incidence rates for CIALIS for once daily use are described in Table 2. In studies of CIALIS for once daily use, events of back pain and myalgia were generally mild or moderate with a discontinuation rate of 0.3%.

Across all studies with any CIALIS dose, reports of changes in color vision were rare (<0.1% of patients).

The following section identifies additional, less frequent events (<2%) reported in controlled clinical trials of CIALIS for once daily use or use as needed. Excluded from this list are those events that were minor, those with no plausible relation to drug use, and reports too imprecise to be meaningful:

Body as a whole—asthenia, face edema, fatigue, pain
Cardiovascular—angina pectoris, chest pain, hypotension, myocardial infarction, postural hypotension, palpitations, syncope, tachycardia
Digestive—abnormal liver function tests, dry mouth, dysphagia, esophagitis, gastritis, GGTP increased, loose stools, nausea, upper abdominal pain, vomiting
Musculoskeletal—arthralgia, neck pain
Nervous—dizziness, hypesthesia, insomnia, paresthesia, somnolence, vertigo
Respiratory—dyspnea, epistaxis, pharyngitis
Skin and Appendages—pruritus, rash, sweating
Ophthalmologic—blurred vision, changes in color vision, conjunctivitis (including conjunctival hyperemia), eye pain, lacrimation increase, swelling of eyelids
Otologic—sudden decrease or loss of hearing, tinnitus
Urogenital—erection increased, spontaneous penile erection

6.2 Postmarketing Experience

The following adverse reactions have been identified during post approval use of CIALIS. These events have been chosen for inclusion either due to their seriousness, reporting frequency, lack of clear alternative causation, or a combination of these factors. Because these reactions are reported voluntarily from a population of uncertain size, it is not always possible to reliably estimate their frequency or establish a causal relationship to drug exposure. The list does not include adverse events that are reported from clinical trials and that are listed elsewhere in this section.

Cardiovascular and cerebrovascular—Serious cardiovascular events, including myocardial infarction, sudden cardiac death, stroke, chest pain, palpitations, and tachycardia, have been reported postmarketing in temporal association with the use of tadalafil. Most, but not all, of these patients had preexisting cardiovascular risk factors. Many of these events were reported to occur during or shortly after sexual activity, and a few were reported to occur shortly after the use of CIALIS without sexual activity. Others were reported to have occurred hours to days after the use of CIALIS and sexual activity. It is not possible to determine whether these events are related directly to CIALIS, to sexual activity, to the patient's underlying cardiovascular disease, to a combination of these factors, or to other factors [see Warnings and Precautions (5.1)].

Body as a whole—hypersensitivity reactions including urticaria, Stevens-Johnson syndrome, and exfoliative dermatitis

Nervous—migraine, seizure and seizure recurrence, transient global amnesia

Ophthalmologic—visual field defect, retinal vein occlusion, retinal artery occlusion

Non-arteritic anterior ischemic optic neuropathy (NAION), a cause of decreased vision including permanent loss of vision, has been reported rarely postmarketing in temporal association with the use of phosphodiesterase type 5 (PDE5) inhibitors, including CIALIS. Most, but not all, of these patients had underlying anatomic or vascular risk factors for development of NAION, including but not necessarily limited to: low cup to disc ratio ("crowded disc"), age over 50, diabetes, hypertension, coronary artery disease, hyperlipidemia, and smoking. It is not possible to determine whether these events are related directly to the use of PDE5 inhibitors, to the patient's underlying vascular risk factors or anatomical defects, to a combination of these factors, or to other factors [see Warnings and Precautions (5.4) and Patient Counseling Information (17.6)].

Otologic—Cases of sudden decrease or loss of hearing have been reported postmarketing in temporal association with the use of PDE5 inhibitors, including CIALIS. In some of the cases, medical conditions and other factors were reported that may have also played a role in the otologic adverse events. In many cases, medical follow-up information was limited. It is not possible to determine whether these reported events are related directly to the use of CIALIS, to the patient's underlying risk factors for hearing loss, a combination of these factors, or to other factors [see Warnings and Precautions (5.5) and Patient Counseling Information (17.7)].

Urogenital—priapism [see Warnings and Precautions (5.3)].

7 DRUG INTERACTIONS

7.1 Potential for Pharmacodynamic Interactions with CIALIS

Nitrates—Administration of CIALIS to patients who are using any form of organic nitrate, is contraindicated. In clinical pharmacology studies, CIALIS was shown to potentiate the hypotensive effect of nitrates. In a patient who has taken CIALIS, where nitrate administration is deemed medically necessary in a life-threatening situation, at least 48 hours should elapse after the last dose of CIALIS before nitrate administration is considered. In such circumstances, nitrates should still only be administered under close medical supervision with appropriate hemodynamic monitoring [see Contraindications (4.1), Dosage and Administration (2.4) and Clinical Pharmacology (12.2)].

Alpha Blockers—Caution is advised when PDE5 inhibitors are coadministered with alpha blockers. PDE5 inhibitors, including CIALIS, and alpha-adrenergic blocking agents are both vasodilators with blood-pressure-lowering effects. When vasodilators are used in combination, an additive effect on blood pressure may be anticipated. Clinical pharmacology studies have been conducted with coadministration of tadalafil with doxazosin or tamsulosin [see Warnings and Precautions (5.6), Dosage and Administration (2.4) and Clinical Pharmacology (12.2)].

Antihypertensives—PDE5 inhibitors, including tadalafil, are mild systemic vasodilators. Clinical pharmacology studies were conducted to assess the effect of tadalafil on the potentiation of the blood-pressure-lowering effects of selected antihypertensive medications (amlodipine, angiotensin II receptor blockers, bendrofluazide, enalapril, and metoprolol). Small reductions in blood pressure occurred following coadministration of tadalafil with these agents compared with placebo. [See Warnings and Precautions (5.6) and Clinical Pharmacology (12.2)].

Alcohol—Both alcohol and tadalafil, a PDE5 inhibitor, act as mild vasodilators. When mild vasodilators are taken in combination, blood-pressure-lowering effects of each individual compound may be increased. Substantial consumption of alcohol (e.g., 5 units or greater) in combination with CIALIS can increase the potential for orthostatic signs and symptoms, including increase in heart rate, decrease in standing blood pressure, dizziness, and headache. Tadalafil did not affect alcohol plasma concentrations and alcohol did not affect tadalafil plasma concentrations. *[See Warnings and Precautions (5.9) and Clinical Pharmacology (12.2)].*

7.2 Potential for Other Drugs to Affect CIALIS

[See Dosage and Administration (2.4) and Warnings and Precautions (5.10)].

Antacids—Simultaneous administration of an antacid (magnesium hydroxide/aluminum hydroxide) and tadalafil reduced the apparent rate of absorption of tadalafil without altering exposure (AUC) to tadalafil.

H_2 Antagonists (e.g. Nizatidine)—An increase in gastric pH resulting from administration of nizatidine had no significant effect on pharmacokinetics.

Cytochrome P450 Inhibitors—CIALIS is a substrate of and predominantly metabolized by CYP3A4. Studies have shown that drugs that inhibit CYP3A4 can increase tadalafil exposure.

CYP3A4 (e.g., Ketoconazole)—Ketoconazole (400 mg daily), a selective and potent inhibitor of CYP3A4, increased tadalafil 20 mg single-dose exposure (AUC) by 312% and C_{max} by 22%, relative to the values for tadalafil 20 mg alone. Ketoconazole (200 mg daily) increased tadalafil 10-mg single-dose exposure (AUC) by 107% and C_{max} by 15%, relative to the values for tadalafil 10 mg alone *[see Dosage and Administration (2.4)].*

Although specific interactions have not been studied, other CYP3A4 inhibitors, such as erythromycin, itraconazole, and grapefruit juice, would likely increase tadalafil exposure.

HIV Protease inhibitor—Ritonavir (500 mg or 600 mg twice daily at steady state), an inhibitor of CYP3A4, CYP2C9, CYP2C19, and CYP2D6, increased tadalafil 20-mg single-dose exposure (AUC) by 32% with a 30% reduction in C_{max}, relative to the values for tadalafil 20 mg alone. Ritonavir (200 mg twice daily), increased tadalafil 20-mg single-dose exposure (AUC) by 124% with no change in C_{max}, relative to the values for tadalafil 20 mg alone. Although specific interactions have not been studied, other HIV protease inhibitors would likely increase tadalafil exposure *[see Dosage and Administration (2.4)].*

Cytochrome P450 Inducers—Studies have shown that drugs that induce CYP3A4 can decrease tadalafil exposure.

CYP3A4 (e.g., Rifampin)—Rifampin (600 mg daily), a CYP3A4 inducer, reduced tadalafil 10-mg single-dose exposure (AUC) by 88% and C_{max} by 46%, relative to the values for tadalafil 10 mg alone. Although specific interactions have not been studied, other CYP3A4 inducers, such as carbamazepine, phenytoin, and phenobarbital, would likely decrease tadalafil exposure. No dose adjustment is warranted. The reduced exposure of tadalafil with the coadministration of rifampin or other CYP3A4 inducers can be anticipated to decrease the efficacy of CIALIS for once daily use; the magnitude of decreased efficacy is unknown.

7.3 Potential for CIALIS to Affect Other Drugs

Aspirin—Tadalafil did not potentiate the increase in bleeding time caused by aspirin.

Cytochrome P450 Substrates—CIALIS is not expected to cause clinically significant inhibition or induction of the clearance of drugs metabolized by cytochrome P450 (CYP) isoforms. Studies have shown that tadalafil does not inhibit or induce P450 isoforms CYP1A2, CYP3A4, CYP2C9, CYP2C19, CYP2D6, and CYP2E1.

CYP1A2 (e.g. Theophylline)—Tadalafil had no significant effect on the pharmacokinetics of theophylline. When tadalafil was administered to subjects taking theophylline, a small augmentation (3 beats per minute) of the increase in heart rate associated with theophylline was observed.

CYP2C9 (e.g. Warfarin)—Tadalafil had no significant effect on exposure (AUC) to S-warfarin or R-warfarin, nor did tadalafil affect changes in prothrombin time induced by warfarin.

CYP3A4 (e.g. Midazolam or Lovastatin)—Tadalafil had no significant effect on exposure (AUC) to midazolam or lovastatin.

P-glycoprotein *(e.g. Digoxin)*—Coadministration of tadalafil (40 mg once per day) for 10 days did not have a significant effect on the steady-state pharmacokinetics of digoxin (0.25 mg/day) in healthy subjects.

8 USE IN SPECIFIC POPULATIONS

8.1 Pregnancy

Pregnancy Category B—CIALIS (tadalafil) is not indicated for use in women. There are no adequate and well controlled studies of CIALIS use in pregnant women. Animal reproduction studies in rats and mice revealed no evidence of fetal harm.

Non-teratogenic effects—Animal reproduction studies showed no evidence of teratogenicity, embryotoxicity, or fetotoxicity when tadalafil was given to pregnant rats or mice at exposures up to 11 times the maximum recommended human dose (MRHD) of 20 mg/day during organogenesis. In one of two perinatal/postnatal developmental studies in rats, postnatal pup survival decreased following maternal exposure to tadalafil doses greater than 10 times the MRHD based on AUC. Signs of maternal toxicity occurred at doses greater than 16 times the MRHD based on AUC. Surviving offspring had normal development and reproductive performance. *(See Animal Toxicology and/or Pharmacology Section 13.2)*

8.3 Nursing Mothers

CIALIS is not indicated for use in women. It is not known whether tadalafil is excreted into human milk. While tadalafil or some metabolite of tadalafil was excreted into rat milk, drug levels in animal breast milk may not accurately predict levels of drug in human breast milk.

8.4 Pediatric Use

CIALIS is not indicated for use in pediatric patients. Safety and efficacy in patients below the age of 18 years has not been established.

8.5 Geriatric Use

Of the total number of subjects in clinical studies of tadalafil, approximately 25 percent were 65 and over, while approximately 3 percent were 75 and over. No overall differences in efficacy or safety were observed between subjects over 65 years of age compared to younger subjects, therefore no dose adjustment is warranted based on age alone. However, a greater sensitivity to medications in some older individuals should be considered. *[See Clinical Pharmacology (12.3)].*

8.6 Hepatic Impairment

In clinical pharmacology studies, tadalafil exposure (AUC) in subjects with mild or moderate hepatic impairment (Child-Pugh Class A or B) was comparable to exposure in healthy subjects when a dose of 10 mg was administered. There are no available data for doses higher than 10 mg of tadalafil in patients with hepatic impairment. Insufficient data are available for subjects with severe hepatic impairment (Child-Pugh Class C). *[See Dosage and Administration (2.3) and Warnings and Precautions (5.8)].*

8.7 Renal Insufficiency

In clinical pharmacology studies using single-dose tadalafil (5 to 10 mg), tadalafil exposure (AUC) doubled in subjects with mild (creatinine clearance 51 to 80 mL/min) or moderate (creatinine clearance 31 to 50 mL/min) renal insufficiency. In subjects with end-stage renal disease on hemodialysis, there was a two-fold increase in C_{max} and 2.7- to 4.1-fold increase in AUC following single-dose administration of 10 or 20 mg tadalafil. Exposure to total methylcatechol (unconjugated plus glucuronide) was 2- to 4-fold higher in subjects with renal impairment, compared to those with normal renal function. Hemodialysis (performed between 24 and 30 hours post-dose) contributed negligibly to tadalafil or metabolite elimination. In a clinical pharmacology study (N=28) at a dose of 10 mg, back pain was reported as a limiting adverse event in male patients with moderate renal impairment. At a dose of 5 mg, the incidence and severity of back pain was not significantly different than in the general population. In patients on hemodialysis taking 10- or 20-mg tadalafil, there were no reported cases of back pain. *[See Dosage and Administration (2.3) and Warnings and Precautions (5.7)].*

10 OVERDOSAGE

Single doses up to 500 mg have been given to healthy subjects, and multiple daily doses up to 100 mg have been given to patients. Adverse events were similar to those seen at lower doses. In cases of overdose, standard supportive measures should be adopted as required. Hemodialysis contributes negligibly to tadalafil elimination.

11 DESCRIPTION

CIALIS (tadalafil), an oral treatment for erectile dysfunction, is a selective inhibitor of cyclic guanosine monophosphate (cGMP)-specific phosphodiesterase type 5 (PDE5). Tadalafil has the empirical formula $C_{22}H_{19}N_3O_4$ representing a molecular weight of 389.41. The structural formula is:

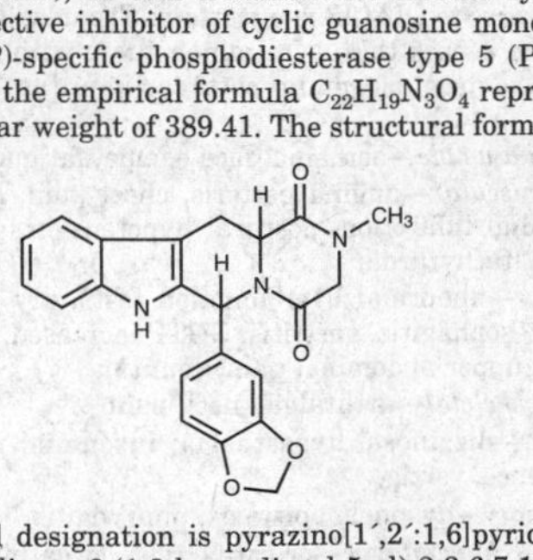

The chemical designation is pyrazino[1´,2´:1,6]pyrido[3,4-b]indole-1,4-dione, 6-(1,3-benzodioxol-5-yl)-2,3,6,7,12,12a-hexahydro-2-methyl-, (6R,12aR)-. It is a crystalline solid that is practically insoluble in water and very slightly soluble in ethanol.

CIALIS is available as film-coated, almond-shaped tablets for oral administration. Each tablet contains 2.5, 5, 10, or 20 mg of tadalafil and the following inactive ingredients: croscarmellose sodium, hydroxypropyl cellulose, hypromellose, iron oxide, lactose monohydrate, magnesium stearate, microcrystalline cellulose, sodium lauryl sulfate, talc, titanium dioxide, and triacetin.

12 CLINICAL PHARMACOLOGY

12.1 Mechanism of Action

Penile erection during sexual stimulation is caused by increased penile blood flow resulting from the relaxation of penile arteries and corpus cavernosal smooth muscle. This response is mediated by the release of nitric oxide (NO) from nerve terminals and endothelial cells, which stimulates the synthesis of cGMP in smooth muscle cells. Cyclic GMP causes smooth muscle relaxation and increased blood flow into the corpus cavernosum. The inhibition of phosphodiesterase type 5 (PDE5) enhances erectile function by increasing the amount of cGMP. Tadalafil inhibits PDE5. Because sexual stimulation is required to initiate the local release of nitric oxide, the inhibition of PDE5 by tadalafil has no effect in the absence of sexual stimulation.

Studies *in vitro* have demonstrated that tadalafil is a selective inhibitor of PDE5. PDE5 is found in corpus cavernosum smooth muscle, vascular and visceral smooth muscle, skeletal muscle, platelets, kidney, lung, cerebellum, and pancreas.

In vitro studies have shown that the effect of tadalafil is more potent on PDE5 than on other phosphodiesterases. These studies have shown that tadalafil is >10,000-fold more potent for PDE5 than for PDE1, PDE2, PDE4, and PDE7 enzymes, which are found in the heart, brain, blood vessels, liver, leukocytes, skeletal muscle, and other organs. Tadalafil is >10,000-fold more potent for PDE5 than for PDE3, an enzyme found in the heart and blood vessels. Additionally, tadalafil is 700-fold more potent for PDE5 than for PDE6, which is found in the retina and is responsible for phototransduction. Tadalafil is >9,000-fold more potent for PDE5 than for PDE8, PDE9, and PDE10. Tadalafil is 14-fold more potent for PDE5 than for PDE11A1 and 40-fold more potent for PDE5 than for PDE11A4, two of the four known forms of PDE11. PDE11 is an enzyme found in human prostate, testes, skeletal muscle and in other tissues. *In vitro,* tadalafil inhibits human recombinant PDE11A1 and, to a lesser degree, PDE11A4 activities at concentrations within the therapeutic range. The physiological role and clinical consequence of PDE11 inhibition in humans have not been defined.

12.2 Pharmacodynamics

Effects on Blood Pressure

Tadalafil 20 mg administered to healthy male subjects produced no significant difference compared to placebo in supine systolic and diastolic blood pressure (difference in the mean maximal decrease of 1.6/0.8 mm Hg, respectively) and in standing systolic and diastolic blood pressure (difference in the mean maximal decrease of 0.2/4.6 mm Hg, respectively). In addition, there was no significant effect on heart rate.

Effects on Blood Pressure When Administered with Nitrates

In clinical pharmacology studies, tadalafil (5 to 20 mg) was shown to potentiate the hypotensive effect of nitrates. Therefore, the use of CIALIS in patients taking any form of nitrates is contraindicated *[see Contraindications (4.1)].*

A study was conducted to assess the degree of interaction between nitroglycerin and tadalafil, should nitroglycerin be required in an emergency situation after tadalafil was taken. This was a double-blind, placebo-controlled, crossover study in 150 male subjects at least 40 years of age (including subjects with diabetes mellitus and/or controlled hypertension) and receiving daily doses of tadalafil 20 mg or matching placebo for 7 days. Subjects were administered a single dose of 0.4 mg sublingual nitroglycerin (NTG) at prespecified timepoints, following their last dose of tadalafil (2, 4, 8, 24, 48, 72, and 96 hours after tadalafil). The objective of the study was to determine when, after tadalafil dosing, no apparent blood pressure interaction was observed. In this study, a significant interaction between tadalafil and NTG was observed at each timepoint up to and including 24 hours. At 48 hours, by most hemodynamic measures, the interaction between tadalafil and NTG was not observed, although a few more tadalafil subjects compared to placebo experienced greater blood-pressure lowering at this timepoint. After 48 hours, the interaction was not detectable *(see Figure 1).*

[See figure 1 at top of next page]

Therefore, CIALIS administration with nitrates is contraindicated. In a patient who has taken CIALIS, where nitrate administration is deemed medically necessary in a life-threatening situation, at least 48 hours should elapse after the last dose of CIALIS before nitrate administration is considered. In such circumstances, nitrates should still only be administered under close medical supervision with appropriate hemodynamic monitoring *[see Contraindications (4.1)].*

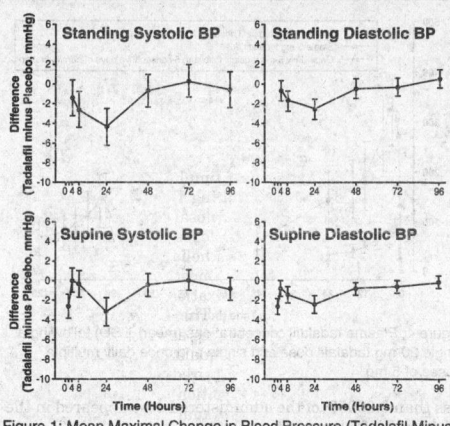

Figure 1: Mean Maximal Change in Blood Pressure (Tadalafil Minus Placebo, Point Estimate with 90% CI) in Response to Sublingual Nitroglycerin at 2 (Supine Only), 4, 8, 24, 48, 72, and 96 Hours after the Last Dose of Tadalafil 20 mg or Placebo

Effect on Blood Pressure When Administered With Alpha Blockers

Six randomized, double-blinded, crossover clinical pharmacology studies were conducted to investigate the potential interaction of tadalafil with alpha-blocker agents in healthy male subjects [see Dosage and Administration (2.4) and Warnings and Precautions (5.6)]. In four studies, a single oral dose of tadalafil was administered to healthy male subjects taking daily (at least 7 days duration) oral alpha blocker. In two studies, daily oral alpha blocker (at least 7 days duration) was administered to healthy male subjects taking repeated daily doses of tadalafil.

Doxazosin—Three clinical pharmacology studies were conducted with tadalafil and doxazosin, an alpha[1]-adrenergic blocker.

In the first doxazosin study, a single oral dose of tadalafil 20 mg or placebo was administered in a 2-period, crossover design to healthy subjects taking oral doxazosin 8 mg daily (N=18 subjects). Doxazosin was administered at the same time as tadalafil or placebo after a minimum of seven days of doxazosin dosing (see Table 4 and Figure 2).

Table 4: Doxazosin Study 1: Mean Maximal Decrease (95% CI) in Systolic Blood Pressure

Placebo-subtracted mean maximal decrease in systolic blood pressure (mm Hg)	Tadalafil 20 mg
Supine	3.6 (-1.5, 8.8)
Standing	9.8 (4.1, 15.5)

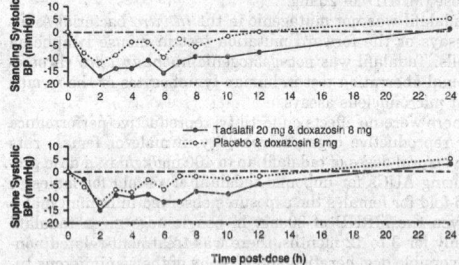

Figure 2: Doxazosin Study 1: Mean Change from Baseline in Systolic Blood Pressure

Blood pressure was measured manually at 1, 2, 3, 4, 5, 6, 7, 8, 10, 12, and 24 hours after tadalafil or placebo administration. Outliers were defined as subjects with a standing systolic blood pressure of <85 mm Hg or a decrease from baseline in standing systolic blood pressure of >30 mm Hg at one or more time points. There were nine and three outliers following administration of tadalafil 20 mg and placebo, respectively. Five and two subjects were outliers due to a decrease from baseline in standing systolic BP of >30 mm Hg, while five and one subject were outliers due to standing systolic BP <85 mm Hg following tadalafil and placebo, respectively. Severe adverse events potentially related to blood-pressure effects were assessed. No such events were reported following placebo. Two such events were reported following administration of tadalafil. Vertigo was reported in one subject that began 7 hours after dosing and

lasted about 5 days. This subject previously experienced a mild episode of vertigo on doxazosin and placebo. Dizziness was reported in another subject that began 25 minutes after dosing and lasted 1 day. No syncope was reported.

In the second doxazosin study, a single oral dose of tadalafil 20 mg was administered to healthy subjects taking oral doxazosin, either 4 or 8 mg daily. The study (N=72 subjects) was conducted in three parts, each a 3-period crossover.

In part A (N=24), subjects were titrated to doxazosin 4 mg administered daily at 8 a.m. Tadalafil was administered at either 8 a.m., 4 p.m., or 8 p.m. There was no placebo control.

In part B (N=24), subjects were titrated to doxazosin 4 mg administered daily at 8 p.m. Tadalafil was administered at either 8 a.m., 4 p.m., or 8 p.m. There was no placebo control.

In part C (N=24), subjects were titrated to doxazosin 8 mg administered daily at 8 a.m. In this part, tadalafil or placebo were administered at either 8 a.m. or 8 p.m.

The placebo-subtracted mean maximal decreases in systolic blood pressure over a 12-hour period after dosing in the placebo-controlled portion of the study (part C) are shown in Table 5 and Figure 3.

Table 5: Doxazosin Study 2 (Part C): Mean Maximal Decrease in Systolic Blood Pressure

Placebo-subtracted mean maximal decrease in systolic blood pressure (mm Hg)	Tadalafil 20 mg at 8 a.m.	Tadalafil 20 mg at 8 p.m.
Ambulatory Blood-Pressure Monitoring (ABPM)	7	8

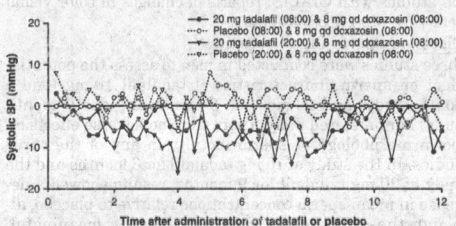

Figure 3: Doxazosin Study 2 (Part C): Mean Change from Time-Matched Baseline in Systolic Blood Pressure

Blood pressure was measured by ABPM every 15 to 30 minutes for up to 36 hours after tadalafil or placebo. Subjects were categorized as outliers if one or more systolic blood pressure readings of <85 mm Hg were recorded or one or more decreases in systolic blood pressure of >30 mm Hg from a time-matched baseline occurred during the analysis interval.

Of the 24 subjects in part C, 16 subjects were categorized as outliers following administration of tadalafil and 6 subjects were categorized as outliers following placebo during the 24-hour period after 8 a.m. dosing of tadalafil or placebo. Of these, 5 and 2 were outliers due to systolic BP <85 mm Hg, while 15 and 4 were outliers due to a decrease from baseline in systolic BP of >30 mm Hg following tadalafil and placebo, respectively.

During the 24-hour period after 8 p.m. dosing, 17 subjects were categorized as outliers following administration of tadalafil and 7 subjects following placebo. Of these, 10 and 2 subjects were outliers due to systolic BP <85 mm Hg, while 15 and 5 subjects were outliers due to a decrease from baseline in systolic BP of >30 mm Hg, following tadalafil and placebo, respectively.

Some additional subjects in both the tadalafil and placebo groups were categorized as outliers in the period beyond 24 hours.

Severe adverse events potentially related to blood-pressure effects were assessed. In the study (N=72 subjects), 2 such events were reported following administration of tadalafil (symptomatic hypotension in one subject that began 10 hours after dosing and lasted approximately 1 hour, and dizziness in another subject that began 11 hours after dosing and lasted 2 minutes). No such events were reported following placebo. In the period prior to tadalafil dosing, one severe event (dizziness) was reported in a subject during the doxazosin run-in phase.

In the third doxazosin study, healthy subjects (N=45 treated; 37 completed) received 28 days of once per day dosing of tadalafil 5 mg or placebo in a two-period crossover design. After 7 days, doxazosin was initiated at 1 mg and titrated up to 4 mg daily over the last 21 days of each period (7 days on 1 mg; 7 days of 2 mg; 7 days of 4 mg doxazosin). The results are shown in Table 6.

Table 6: Doxazosin Study 3: Mean Maximal Decrease (95% CI) in Systolic Blood Pressure

Placebo-subtracted mean maximal decrease in systolic blood pressure		Tadalafil 5 mg
Day 1 of 4 mg Doxazosin	Supine	2.4 (-0.4, 5.2)
	Standing	-0.5 (-4.0, 3.1)
Day 7 of 4 mg Doxazosin	Supine	2.8 (-0.1, 5.7)
	Standing	1.1 (-2.9, 5.0)

Blood pressure was measured manually pre-dose at two time points (-30 and -15 minutes) and then at 1, 2, 3, 4, 5, 6, 7, 8, 10, 12 and 24 hours post dose on the first day of each doxazosin dose, (1 mg, 2 mg, 4 mg), as well as on the seventh day of 4 mg doxazosin administration.

Following the first dose of doxazosin 1 mg, there were no outliers on tadalafil 5 mg and one outlier on placebo due to a decrease from baseline in standing systolic BP of >30 mm Hg.

There were 2 outliers on tadalafil 5 mg and none on placebo following the first dose of doxazosin 2 mg due to a decrease from baseline in standing systolic BP of >30 mm Hg.

There were no outliers on tadalafil 5 mg and two on placebo following the first dose of doxazosin 4 mg due to a decrease from baseline in standing systolic BP of >30 mm Hg. There was one outlier on tadalafil 5 mg and three on placebo following standing systolic BP <85 mm Hg. Following the seventh day of doxazosin 4 mg, there were no outliers on tadalafil 5 mg, one subject on placebo had a decrease >30 mm Hg in standing systolic blood pressure, and one subject on placebo had standing systolic blood pressure <85 mm Hg. All adverse events potentially related to blood pressure effects were rated as mild or moderate. There were two episodes of syncope in this study, one subject following a dose of tadalafil 5 mg alone, and another subject following coadministration of tadalafil 5 mg and doxazosin 4 mg.

Tamsulosin—In the first tamsulosin study, a single oral dose of tadalafil 10, 20 mg, or placebo was administered in a 3 period, crossover design to healthy subjects taking 0.4 mg once per day tamsulosin, a selective alpha[1A]-adrenergic blocker (N=18 subjects). Tadalafil or placebo was administered 2 hours after tamsulosin following a minimum of seven days of tamsulosin dosing.

Table 7: Tamsulosin Study 1: Mean Maximal Decrease (95% CI) in Systolic Blood Pressure

Placebo-subtracted mean maximal decrease in systolic blood pressure (mm Hg)	Tadalafil 10 mg	Tadalafil 20 mg
Supine	3.2 (-2.3, 8.6)	3.2 (-2.3, 8.7)
Standing	1.7 (-4.7, 8.1)	2.3 (-4.1, 8.7)

Blood pressure was measured manually at 1, 2, 3, 4, 5, 6, 7, 8, 10, 12, and 24 hours after tadalafil or placebo dosing. There were 2, 2, and 1 outliers (subjects with a decrease from baseline in standing systolic blood pressure of >30 mm Hg at one or more time points) following administration of tadalafil 10 mg, 20 mg, and placebo, respectively. There were no subjects with a standing systolic blood pressure <85 mm Hg. No severe adverse events potentially related to blood-pressure effects were reported. No syncope was reported.

In the second tamsulosin study, healthy subjects (N=39 treated; and 35 completed) received 14 days of once per day dosing of tadalafil 5 mg or placebo in a two-period crossover design. Daily dosing of tamsulosin 0.4 mg was added for the last seven days of each period.

Table 8: Tamsulosin Study 2: Mean Maximal Decrease (95% CI) in Systolic Blood Pressure

Placebo-subtracted mean maximal decrease in systolic blood pressure		Tadalafil 5 mg
Day 1 of Tamsulosin	Supine	-0.1 (-2.2, 1.9)
	Standing	0.9 (-1.4, 3.2)
Day 7 of Tamsulosin	Supine	1.2 (-1.2, 3.6)
	Standing	1.2 (-1.0, 3.5)

Blood pressure was measured manually pre-dose at two time points (-30 and -15 minutes) and then at 1, 2, 3, 4, 5, 6, 7, 8, 10, 12, and 24 hours post dose on the first, sixth and seventh days of tamsulosin administration. There were no outliers (subjects with a decrease from baseline in standing systolic blood pressure of >30 mm Hg at one or more time points). One subject on placebo plus tamsulosin (Day 7) and one subject on tadalafil plus tamsulosin (Day 6) had standing systolic blood pressure <85 mm Hg. No severe adverse events potentially related to blood pressure were reported. No syncope was reported.

Alfuzosin—A single oral dose of tadalafil 20 mg or placebo was administered in a 2-period, crossover design to healthy subjects taking once-daily alfuzosin HCl 10 mg extended-release tablets, an alpha[1]-adrenergic blocker (N=17 completed subjects). Tadalafil or placebo was administered 4 hours after alfuzosin following a minimum of seven days of alfuzosin dosing.

Table 9: Alfuzosin Study: Mean Maximal Decrease (95% CI) in Systolic Blood Pressure

Placebo-subtracted mean maximal decrease in systolic blood pressure (mm Hg)	Tadalafil 20 mg
Supine	2.2 (-0.9, -5.2)
Standing	4.4 (-0.2, 8.9)

Blood pressure was measured manually at 1, 2, 3, 4, 6, 8, 10, 20, and 24 hours after tadalafil or placebo dosing. There was 1 outlier (subject with a standing systolic blood pressure <85 mm Hg) following administration of tadalafil 20 mg. There were no subjects with a decrease from baseline in standing systolic blood pressure of >30 mm Hg at one or more time points. No severe adverse events potentially related to blood pressure effects were reported. No syncope was reported.

Effects on Blood Pressure When Administered with Antihypertensives

Amlodipine—A study was conducted to assess the interaction of amlodipine (5 mg daily) and tadalafil 10 mg. There was no effect of tadalafil on amlodipine blood levels and no effect of amlodipine on tadalafil blood levels. The mean reduction in supine systolic/diastolic blood pressure due to tadalafil 10 mg in subjects taking amlodipine was 3/2 mm Hg, compared to placebo. In a similar study using tadalafil 20 mg, there were no clinically significant differences between tadalafil and placebo in subjects taking amlodipine.

Angiotensin II receptor blockers (with and without other antihypertensives)—A study was conducted to assess the interaction of angiotensin II receptor blockers and tadalafil 20 mg. Subjects in the study were taking any marketed angiotensin II receptor blocker, either alone, as a component of a combination product, or as part of a multiple antihypertensive regimen. Following dosing, ambulatory measurements of blood pressure revealed differences between tadalafil and placebo of 8/4 mm Hg in systolic/diastolic blood pressure.

Bendrofluazide—A study was conducted to assess the interaction of bendrofluazide (2.5 mg daily) and tadalafil 10 mg. Following dosing, the mean reduction in supine systolic/diastolic blood pressure due to tadalafil 10 mg in subjects taking bendrofluazide was 6/4 mm Hg, compared to placebo.

Enalapril—A study was conducted to assess the interaction of enalapril (10 to 20 mg daily) and tadalafil 10 mg. Following dosing, the mean reduction in supine systolic/diastolic blood pressure due to tadalafil 10 mg in subjects taking enalapril was 4/1 mm Hg, compared to placebo.

Metoprolol—A study was conducted to assess the interaction of sustained-release metoprolol (25 to 200 mg daily) and tadalafil 10 mg. Following dosing, the mean reduction in supine systolic/diastolic blood pressure due to tadalafil 10 mg in subjects taking metoprolol was 5/3 mm Hg, compared to placebo.

Effects on Blood Pressure When Administered with Alcohol

Alcohol and PDE5 inhibitors, including tadalafil, are mild systemic vasodilators. The interaction of tadalafil with alcohol was evaluated in 3 clinical pharmacology studies. In 2 of these, alcohol was administered at a dose of 0.7 g/kg, which is equivalent to approximately 6 ounces of 80-proof vodka in an 80-kg male, and tadalafil was administered at a dose of 10 mg in one study and 20 mg in another. In both these studies, all patients imbibed the entire alcohol dose within 10 minutes of starting. In one of these two studies, blood alcohol levels of 0.08% were confirmed. In these two studies, more patients had clinically significant decreases in blood pressure on the combination of tadalafil and alcohol as compared to alcohol alone. Some subjects reported postural dizziness, and orthostatic hypotension was observed in some subjects. When tadalafil 20 mg was administered with a lower dose of alcohol (0.6 g/kg, which is equivalent to approximately 4 ounces of 80-proof vodka, administered in less than 10 minutes), orthostatic hypotension was not observed, dizziness occurred with similar frequency to alcohol alone, and the hypotensive effects of alcohol were not potentiated.

Tadalafil did not affect alcohol plasma concentrations and alcohol did not affect tadalafil plasma concentrations.

Effects on Exercise Stress Testing

The effects of tadalafil on cardiac function, hemodynamics, and exercise tolerance were investigated in a single clinical pharmacology study. In this blinded crossover trial, 23 subjects with stable coronary artery disease and evidence of exercise-induced cardiac ischemia were enrolled. The primary endpoint was time to cardiac ischemia. The mean difference in total exercise time was 3 seconds (tadalafil 10 mg minus placebo), which represented no clinically meaningful difference. Further statistical analysis demonstrated that tadalafil was non-inferior to placebo with respect to time to ischemia. Of note, in this study, in some subjects who received tadalafil followed by sublingual nitroglycerin in the post-exercise period, clinically significant reductions in blood pressure were observed, consistent with the augmentation by tadalafil of the blood-pressure-lowering effects of nitrates.

Effects on Vision

Single oral doses of phosphodiesterase inhibitors have demonstrated transient dose-related impairment of color discrimination (blue/green), using the Farnsworth-Munsell 100-hue test, with peak effects near the time of peak plasma levels. This finding is consistent with the inhibition of PDE6, which is involved in phototransduction in the retina. In a study to assess the effects of a single dose of tadalafil 40 mg on vision (N=59), no effects were observed on visual acuity, intraocular pressure, or pupilometry. Across all clinical studies with CIALIS, reports of changes in color vision were rare (<0.1% of patients).

Effects on Sperm Characteristics

Three studies were conducted in men to assess the potential effect on sperm characteristics of tadalafil 10 mg (one 6 month study) and 20 mg (one 6 month and one 9 month study) administered daily. There were no adverse effects on sperm morphology or sperm motility in any of the three studies. In the study of 10 mg tadalafil for 6 months and the study of 20 mg tadalafil for 9 months, results showed a decrease in mean sperm concentrations relative to placebo, although these differences were not clinically meaningful. This effect was not seen in the study of 20 mg tadalafil taken for 6 months. In addition there was no adverse effect on mean concentrations of reproductive hormones, testosterone, luteinizing hormone or follicle stimulating hormone with either 10 or 20 mg of tadalafil compared to placebo.

Effects on Cardiac Electrophysiology

The effect of a single 100-mg dose of tadalafil on the QT interval was evaluated at the time of peak tadalafil concentration in a randomized, double-blinded, placebo, and active (intravenous ibutilide) -controlled crossover study in 90 healthy males aged 18 to 53 years. The mean change in QT_c (Fridericia QT correction) for tadalafil, relative to placebo, was 3.5 milliseconds (two-sided 90% CI=1.9, 5.1). The mean change in QT_c (Individual QT correction) for tadalafil, relative to placebo, was 2.8 milliseconds (two-sided 90% CI=1.2, 4.4). A 100-mg dose of tadalafil (5 times the highest recommended dose) was chosen because this dose yields exposures covering those observed upon coadministration of tadalafil with potent CYP3A4 inhibitors or those observed in renal impairment. In this study, the mean increase in heart rate associated with a 100-mg dose of tadalafil compared to placebo was 3.1 beats per minute.

12.3 Pharmacokinetics

Over a dose range of 2.5 to 20 mg, tadalafil exposure (AUC) increases proportionally with dose in healthy subjects. Steady-state plasma concentrations are attained within 5 days of once per day dosing and exposure is approximately 1.6-fold greater than after a single dose. Mean tadalafil concentrations measured after the administration of a single oral dose of 20 mg and single and once daily multiple doses of 5 mg, from a separate study, *(see Figure 4)* to healthy male subjects are depicted in Figure 4.

[See figure 4 at top of next column]

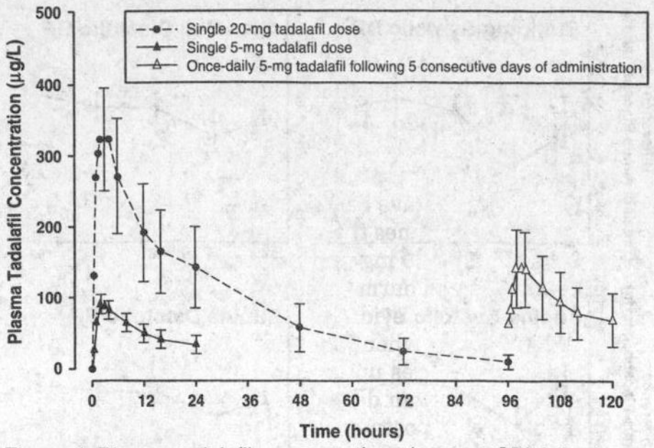

Figure 4: Plasma tadalafil concentrations (mean ± SD) following a single 20-mg tadalafil dose and single and once daily multiple doses of 5 mg

Absorption—After single oral-dose administration, the maximum observed plasma concentration (C_{max}) of tadalafil is achieved between 30 minutes and 6 hours (median time of 2 hours). Absolute bioavailability of tadalafil following oral dosing has not been determined.

The rate and extent of absorption of tadalafil are not influenced by food; thus CIALIS may be taken with or without food.

Distribution—The mean apparent volume of distribution following oral administration is approximately 63 L, indicating that tadalafil is distributed into tissues. At therapeutic concentrations, 94% of tadalafil in plasma is bound to proteins.

Less than 0.0005% of the administered dose appeared in the semen of healthy subjects.

Metabolism—Tadalafil is predominantly metabolized by CYP3A4 to a catechol metabolite. The catechol metabolite undergoes extensive methylation and glucuronidation to form the methylcatechol and methylcatechol glucuronide conjugate, respectively. The major circulating metabolite is the methylcatechol glucuronide. Methylcatechol concentrations are less than 10% of glucuronide concentrations. *In vitro* data suggests that metabolites are not expected to be pharmacologically active at observed metabolite concentrations.

Elimination—The mean oral clearance for tadalafil is 2.5 L/hr and the mean terminal half-life is 17.5 hours in healthy subjects. Tadalafil is excreted predominantly as metabolites, mainly in the feces (approximately 61% of the dose) and to a lesser extent in the urine (approximately 36% of the dose).

Geriatric—Healthy male elderly subjects (65 years or over) had a lower oral clearance of tadalafil, resulting in 25% higher exposure (AUC) with no effect on C_{max} relative to that observed in healthy subjects 19 to 45 years of age. No dose adjustment is warranted based on age alone. However, greater sensitivity to medications in some older individuals should be considered *[see Use in Specific Populations (8.5)]*.

Pediatric—Tadalafil has not been evaluated in individuals less than 18 years old *[see Use in Specific Populations (8.4)]*.

Patients with Diabetes Mellitus—In male patients with diabetes mellitus after a 10 mg tadalafil dose, exposure (AUC) was reduced approximately 19% and C_{max} was 5% lower than that observed in healthy subjects. No dose adjustment is warranted.

13 NONCLINICAL TOXICOLOGY

13.1 Carcinogenesis, Mutagenesis, Impairment of Fertility

Tadalafil was not carcinogenic to rats or mice when administered daily for 2 years at doses up to 400 mg/kg/day. Systemic drug exposures, as measured by AUC of unbound tadalafil, were approximately 10-fold for mice, and 14- and 26-fold for male and female rats, respectively, the exposures in human males given Maximum Recommended Human Dose (MRHD) of 20 mg.

Tadalafil was not mutagenic in the *in vitro* bacterial Ames assays or the forward mutation test in mouse lymphoma cells. Tadalafil was not clastogenic in the *in vitro* chromosomal aberration test in human lymphocytes or the *in vivo* rat micronucleus assays.

There were no effects on fertility, reproductive performance or reproductive organ morphology in male or female rats given oral doses of tadalafil up to 400 mg/kg/day, a dose producing AUCs for unbound tadalafil of 14-fold for males or 26-fold for females the exposures observed in human males given the MRHD of 20 mg. In beagle dogs given tadalafil daily for 3 to 12 months, there was treatment-related non-reversible degeneration and atrophy of the seminiferous tubular epithelium in the testes in 20-100% of the dogs that resulted in a decrease in spermatogenesis in 40-75% of the dogs at doses of ≥10 mg/kg/day. Systemic exposure (based on AUC) at no-observed-adverse-effect-level (NOAEL) (10 mg/kg/day) for unbound tadalafil was similar to that expected in humans at the MRHD of 20 mg.

There were no treatment-related testicular findings in rats or mice treated with doses up to 400 mg/kg/day for 2 years.

13.2 Animal Toxicology and/or Pharmacology

Animal studies showed vascular inflammation in tadalafil-treated mice, rats, and dogs. In mice and rats, lymphoid necrosis and hemorrhage were seen in the spleen, thymus, and mesenteric lymph nodes at unbound tadalafil exposure of 2- to 33-fold above the human exposure (AUCs) at the MRHD of 20 mg. In dogs, an increased incidence of disseminated arteritis was observed in 1- and 6-month studies at unbound tadalafil exposure of 1- to 54-fold above the human exposure (AUC) at the MRHD of 20 mg. In a 12-month dog study, no disseminated arteritis was observed, but 2 dogs exhibited marked decreases in white blood cells (neutrophils) and moderate decreases in platelets with inflammatory signs at unbound tadalafil exposures of approximately 14- to 18-fold the human exposure at the MRHD of 20 mg. The abnormal blood-cell findings were reversible within 2 weeks upon removal of the drug.

Reproductive Toxicology Studies

Reproduction studies have been performed in rats and mice at exposures up to 11 times the maximum recommended human dose (MRHD) of 20 mg and have revealed no evidence of impaired fertility or harm to the fetus due to tadalafil. In addition, there was no evidence of teratogenicity, embryotoxicity, or fetotoxicity when tadalafil was given to pregnant rats or mice at exposures up to 11 times the MRHD during the period of major organ development.

In a rat prenatal and postnatal development study at doses of 60, 200, and 1000 mg/kg, a reduction in postnatal survival of pups was observed. The no observed effect level (NOEL) for maternal toxicity was 200 mg/kg/day and for developmental toxicity was 30 mg/kg/day. This gives approximately 16 and 10 fold exposure multiples, respectively, of the human AUC for the MRHD of 20 mg. Tadalafil and/or its metabolites cross the placenta, resulting in fetal exposure in rats.

Tadalafil and/or its metabolites were secreted into the milk in lactating rats at concentrations approximately 2.4-fold greater than found in the plasma.

14   CLINICAL STUDIES

14.1   CIALIS for Use as Needed

The efficacy and safety of tadalafil in the treatment of erectile dysfunction has been evaluated in 22 clinical trials of up to 24-weeks duration, involving over 4000 patients. CIALIS, when taken as needed up to once per day, was shown to be effective in improving erectile function in men with erectile dysfunction (ED).

CIALIS was studied in the general ED population in 7 randomized, multicenter, double-blinded, placebo-controlled, parallel-arm design, primary efficacy and safety studies of 12-weeks duration. Two of these studies were conducted in the United States and 5 were conducted in centers outside the US. Additional efficacy and safety studies were performed in ED patients with diabetes mellitus and in patients who developed ED status post bilateral nerve-sparing radical prostatectomy.

In these 7 trials, CIALIS was taken as needed, at doses ranging from 2.5 to 20 mg, up to once per day. Patients were free to choose the time interval between dose administration and the time of sexual attempts. Food and alcohol intake were not restricted.

Several assessment tools were used to evaluate the effect of CIALIS on erectile function. The 3 primary outcome measures were the Erectile Function (EF) domain of the International Index of Erectile Function (IIEF) and Questions 2 and 3 from Sexual Encounter Profile (SEP). The IIEF is a 4-week recall questionnaire that was administered at the end of a treatment-free baseline period and subsequently at follow-up visits after randomization. The IIEF EF domain has a 30-point total score, where higher scores reflect better erectile function. SEP is a diary in which patients recorded each sexual attempt made throughout the study. SEP Question 2 asks, "Were you able to insert your penis into the partner's vagina?" SEP Question 3 asks, "Did your erection last long enough for you to have successful intercourse?" The overall percentage of successful attempts to insert the penis into the vagina (SEP2) and to maintain the erection for successful intercourse (SEP3) is derived for each patient.

Results in ED Population in US Trials—The 2 primary US efficacy and safety trials included a total of 402 men with erectile dysfunction, with a mean age of 59 years (range 27 to 87 years). The population was 78% White, 14% Black, 7% Hispanic, and 1% of other ethnicities, and included patients with ED of various severities, etiologies (organic, psychogenic, mixed), and with multiple co-morbid conditions, including diabetes mellitus, hypertension, and other cardiovascular disease. Most (>90%) patients reported ED of at least 1-year duration. Study A was conducted primarily in academic centers. Study B was conducted primarily in community-based urology practices. In each of these 2 trials, CIALIS 20 mg showed clinically meaningful and statistically significant improvements in all 3 primary efficacy variables (see Table 10). The treatment effect of CIALIS did not diminish over time.

[See table 10 at top right]

Results in General ED Population in Trials Outside the US—The 5 primary efficacy and safety studies conducted in the general ED population outside the US included 1112 patients, with a mean age of 59 years (range 21 to 82 years). The population was 76% White, 1% Black, 3% Hispanic, and 20% of other ethnicities, and included patients with ED of various severities, etiologies (organic, psychogenic, mixed), and with multiple co-morbid conditions, including diabetes mellitus, hypertension, and other cardiovascular disease. Most (90%) patients reported ED of at least 1-year duration.

Table 10: Mean Endpoint and Change from Baseline for the Primary Efficacy Variables in the Two Primary US Trials

	Study A			Study B		
	Placebo	CIALIS 20 mg		Placebo	CIALIS 20 mg	
	(N=49)	(N=146)	p-value	(N=48)	(N=159)	p-value
EF Domain Score						
Endpoint	13.5	19.5		13.6	22.5	
Change from baseline	-0.2	6.9	<.001	0.3	9.3	<.001
Insertion of Penis (SEP2)						
Endpoint	39%	62%		43%	77%	
Change from baseline	2%	26%	<.001	2%	32%	<.001
Maintenance of Erection (SEP3)						
Endpoint	25%	50%		23%	64%	
Change from baseline	5%	34%	<.001	4%	44%	<.001

Table 11: Mean Endpoint and Change from Baseline for the EF Domain of the IIEF in the General ED Population in Five Primary Trials Outside the US

	Placebo	CIALIS 5 mg	CIALIS 10 mg	CIALIS 20 mg
Study C				
Endpoint [Change from baseline]	15.0 [0.7]	17.9 [4.0]	20.0 [5.6]	
		p=.006	p<.001	
Study D				
Endpoint [Change from baseline]	14.4 [1.1]	17.5 [5.1]	20.6 [6.0]	
		p=.002	p<.001	
Study E				
Endpoint [Change from baseline]	18.1 [2.6]		22.6 [8.1]	25.0 [8.0]
			p<.001	p<.001
Study F[a]				
Endpoint [Change from baseline]	12.7 [-1.6]			22.8 [6.8]
				p<.001
Study G				
Endpoint [Change from baseline]	14.5 [-0.9]		21.2 [6.6]	23.3 [8.0]
			p<.001	p<.001

[a] Treatment duration in Study F was 6 months

In these 5 trials, CIALIS 5, 10, and 20 mg showed clinically meaningful and statistically significant improvements in all 3 primary efficacy variables (see Tables 11, 12 and 13). The treatment effect of CIALIS did not diminish over time.

[See table 11 above]
[See table 12 at top of next page]
[See table 13 on next page]

In addition, there were improvements in EF domain scores, success rates based upon SEP Questions 2 and 3, and patient-reported improvement in erections across patients with ED of all degrees of disease severity while taking CIALIS, compared to patients on placebo.

Therefore, in all 7 primary efficacy and safety studies, CIALIS showed statistically significant improvement in patients' ability to achieve an erection sufficient for vaginal penetration and to maintain the erection long enough for successful intercourse, as measured by the IIEF questionnaire and by SEP diaries.

Efficacy Results in ED Patients with Diabetes Mellitus—CIALIS was shown to be effective in treating ED in patients with diabetes mellitus. Patients with diabetes were included in all 7 primary efficacy studies in the general ED population (N=235) and in one study that specifically assessed CIALIS in ED patients with type 1 or type 2 diabetes (N=216). In this randomized, placebo-controlled, double-blinded, parallel-arm design prospective trial, CIALIS demonstrated clinically meaningful and statistically significant improvement in erectile function, as measured by the EF

domain of the IIEF questionnaire and Questions 2 and 3 of the SEP diary (see Table 14).

[See table 14 at top of page 1757]

Efficacy Results in ED Patients following Radical Prostatectomy—CIALIS was shown to be effective in treating patients who developed ED following bilateral nerve-sparing radical prostatectomy. In 1 randomized, placebo-controlled, double-blinded, parallel-arm design prospective trial in this population (N=303), CIALIS demonstrated clinically meaningful and statistically significant improvement in erectile function, as measured by the EF domain of the IIEF questionnaire and Questions 2 and 3 of the SEP diary (see Table 15).

[See table 15 on page 1757]

Results in Studies to Determine the Optimal Use of CIALIS—Several studies were conducted with the objective of determining the optimal use of CIALIS in the treatment of ED. In one of these studies, the percentage of patients reporting successful erections within 30 minutes of dosing was determined. In this randomized, placebo-controlled, double-blinded trial, 223 patients were randomized to placebo, CIALIS 10, or 20 mg. Using a stopwatch, patients recorded the time following dosing at which a successful erection was obtained. A successful erection was defined as at least 1 erection in 4 attempts that led to successful intercourse. At or prior to 30 minutes, 35% (26/74), 38% (28/74), and 52% (39/75) of patients in the placebo, 10-, and 20-mg groups, respectively, reported successful erections as defined above.

Two studies were conducted to assess the efficacy of CIALIS at a given timepoint after dosing, specifically at 24 hours and at 36 hours after dosing.

In the first of these studies, 348 patients with ED were randomized to placebo or CIALIS 20 mg. Patients were encouraged to make 4 total attempts at intercourse; 2 attempts were to occur at 24 hours after dosing and 2 completely separate attempts were to occur at 36 hours after dosing. The results demonstrated a difference between the placebo group and the CIALIS group at each of the pre-specified timepoints. At the 24-hour timepoint, (more specifically, 22 to 26 hours), 53/144 (37%) patients reported at least 1 successful intercourse in the placebo group versus 84/138 (61%) in the CIALIS 20-mg group. At the 36-hour timepoint (more specifically, 33 to 39 hours), 49/133 (37%) of patients reported at least 1 successful intercourse in the placebo group versus 88/137 (64%) in the CIALIS 20-mg group.

In the second of these studies, a total of 483 patients were evenly randomized to 1 of 6 groups: 3 different dosing groups (placebo, CIALIS 10, or 20 mg) that were instructed to attempt intercourse at 2 different times (24 and 36 hours post-dosing). Patients were encouraged to make 4 separate attempts at their assigned dose and assigned timepoint. In this study, the results demonstrated a statistically significant difference between the placebo group and the CIALIS groups at each of the pre-specified timepoints. At the 24-hour timepoint, the mean, per patient percentage of attempts resulting in successful intercourse were 42, 56, and 67% for the placebo, CIALIS 10-, and 20-mg groups, respectively. At the 36-hour timepoint, the mean, per-patient percentage of attempts resulting in successful intercourse were 33, 56, and 62% for placebo, CIALIS 10-, and 20-mg groups, respectively.

14.2 CIALIS for Once Daily Use

The efficacy and safety of CIALIS for once daily use in the treatment of erectile dysfunction has been evaluated in 2 clinical trials of 12-weeks duration and 1 clinical trial of 24-weeks duration, involving a total of 853 patients. CIALIS, when taken once daily, was shown to be effective in improving erectile function in men with erectile dysfunction (ED). CIALIS was studied in the general ED population in 2 randomized, multicenter, double-blinded, placebo-controlled, parallel-arm design, primary efficacy and safety studies of 12- and 24-weeks duration, respectively. One of these studies was conducted in the United States and one was conducted in centers outside the US. An additional efficacy and safety study was performed in ED patients with diabetes mellitus. CIALIS was taken once daily at doses ranging from 2.5 to 10 mg. Food and alcohol intake were not restricted. Timing of sexual activity was not restricted relative to when patients took Cialis.

Results in General ED Population—The primary US efficacy and safety trial included a total of 287 patients, with a mean age of 59 years (range 25 to 82 years). The population was 86% White, 6% Black, 6% Hispanic, and 2% of other ethnicities, and included patients with ED of various severities, etiologies (organic, psychogenic, mixed), and with multiple co-morbid conditions, including diabetes mellitus, hypertension, and other cardiovascular disease. Most (>96%) patients reported ED of at least 1-year duration.

The primary efficacy and safety study conducted outside the US included 268 patients, with a mean age of 56 years (range 21 to 78 years). The population was 86% White, 3% Black, 0.4% Hispanic, and 10% of other ethnicities, and included patients with ED of various severities, etiologies (organic, psychogenic, mixed), and with multiple co-morbid conditions, including diabetes mellitus, hypertension, and other cardiovascular disease. Ninety-three percent of patients reported ED of at least 1-year duration.

In each of these trials, conducted without regard to the timing of dose and sexual intercourse, CIALIS demonstrated clinically meaningful and statistically significant improvement in erectile function, as measured by the EF domain of the IIEF questionnaire and Questions 2 and 3 of the SEP diary (see Table 16). When taken as directed, CIALIS was effective at improving erectile function.

In the 6 month double blind study, the treatment effect of CIALIS did not diminish over time.

[See table 16 on next page]

Efficacy Results in ED Patients with Diabetes Mellitus—CIALIS for once daily use was shown to be effective in treating ED in patients with diabetes mellitus. Patients with diabetes were included in both studies in the general ED population (N=79). A third randomized, multicenter, double-blinded, placebo-controlled, parallel-arm design trial included only ED patients with type 1 or type 2 diabetes (N=298). In this third trial, CIALIS demonstrated clinically meaningful and statistically significant improvement in erectile function, as measured by the EF domain of the IIEF questionnaire and Questions 2 and 3 of the SEP diary (see Table 17).

[See table 17 at top of page 1758]

16 HOW SUPPLIED/STORAGE AND HANDLING

16.1 How Supplied

CIALIS (tadalafil) is supplied as follows:

Table 12: Mean Post-Baseline Success Rate and Change from Baseline for SEP Question 2 ("Were you able to insert your penis into the partner's vagina?") in the General ED Population in Five Pivotal Trials Outside the US

	Placebo	CIALIS 5 mg	CIALIS 10 mg	CIALIS 20 mg
Study C				
Endpoint [Change from baseline]	49% [6%]	57% [15%]	73% [29%]	
		p=.063	p<.001	
Study D				
Endpoint [Change from baseline]	46% [2%]	56% [18%]	68% [15%]	
		p=.008	p<.001	
Study E				
Endpoint [Change from baseline]	55% [10%]		77% [35%]	85% [35%]
			p<.001	p<.001
Study F[a]				
Endpoint [Change from baseline]	42% [-8%]			81% [27%]
				p<.001
Study G				
Endpoint [Change from baseline]	45% [-6%]		73% [21%]	76% [21%]
			p<.001	p<.001

[a] Treatment duration in Study F was 6 months

Table 13: Mean Post-Baseline Success Rate and Change from Baseline for SEP Question 3 ("Did your erection last long enough for you to have successful intercourse?") in the General ED Population in Five Pivotal Trials Outside the US

	Placebo	CIALIS 5 mg	CIALIS 10 mg	CIALIS 20 mg
Study C				
Endpoint [Change from baseline]	26% [4%]	38% [19%]	58% [32%]	
		p=.040	p<.001	
Study D				
Endpoint [Change from baseline]	28% [4%]	42% [24%]	51% [26%]	
		p<.001	p<.001	
Study E				
Endpoint [Change from baseline]	43% [15%]		70% [48%]	78% [50%]
			p<.001	p<.001
Study F[a]				
Endpoint [Change from baseline]	27% [1%]			74% [40%]
				p<.001
Study G				
Endpoint [Change from baseline]	32% [5%]		57% [33%]	62% [29%]
			p<.001	p<.001

[a] Treatment duration in Study F was 6 months

Four strengths of film-coated, almond-shaped tablets (not scored) are available in different sizes and different shades of yellow, and supplied in the following package sizes:

2.5 mg tablets debossed with "C 2 1/2"
Blisters of 2 × 15   NDC 0002-4465-34
5-mg tablets debossed with "C 5"
Bottles of 10   NDC 0002-4462-10
Bottles of 30   NDC 0002-4462-30
Blisters of 2 × 15   NDC 0002-4462-34
10-mg tablets debossed with "C 10"
Bottles of 30   NDC 0002-4463-30
20-mg tablets debossed with "C 20"
Bottles of 30   NDC 0002-4464-30

16.2 Storage

Store at 25°C (77°F); excursions permitted to 15-30°C (59-86°F) [see USP Controlled Room Temperature]. Keep out of reach of children.

17 PATIENT COUNSELING INFORMATION

See FDA approved Patient Labeling

17.1 Nitrates

Physicians should discuss with patients the contraindication of CIALIS with regular and/or intermittent use of organic nitrates. Patients should be counseled that concomitant use of CIALIS with nitrates could cause blood pressure to suddenly drop to an unsafe level, resulting in dizziness, syncope, or even heart attack or stroke.

Physicians should discuss with patients the appropriate action in the event that they experience anginal chest pain requiring nitroglycerin following intake of CIALIS. In such a patient, who has taken CIALIS, where nitrate administration is deemed medically necessary for a life-threatening situation, at least 48 hours should have elapsed after the last dose of CIALIS before nitrate administration is considered. In such circumstances, nitrates should still only be administered under close medical supervision with appropriate hemodynamic monitoring. Therefore, patients who experience anginal chest pain after taking CIALIS should seek immediate medical attention [see Contraindications (4.1) and Warnings and Precautions (5.1)].

17.2   Cardiovascular Considerations
Physicians should consider the potential cardiac risk of sexual activity in patients with preexisting cardiovascular disease. Physicians should advise patients who experience symptoms upon initiation of sexual activity to refrain from further sexual activity and seek immediate medical attention [see Warnings and Precautions (5.1)].

17.3   Concomitant Use with Drugs Which Lower Blood Pressure
Physicians should discuss with patients the potential for CIALIS to augment the blood-pressure-lowering effect of alpha blockers and antihypertensive medications [see Warnings and Precautions (5.6), Drug Interactions (7.1), and Clinical Pharmacology (12.2)].

17.4   Potential for Drug Interactions When Taking CIALIS for Once Daily Use
Physicians should discuss with patients the clinical implications of continuous exposure to tadalafil when prescribing CIALIS for once daily use, especially the potential for interactions with medications (e.g., nitrates, alpha blockers, antihypertensives and potent inhibitors of cytochrome P450 3A4) and with substantial consumption of alcohol.

17.5   Priapism
There have been rare reports of prolonged erections greater than 4 hours and priapism (painful erections greater than 6 hours in duration) for this class of compounds. Priapism, if not treated promptly, can result in irreversible damage to the erectile tissue. Physicians should advise patients who have an erection lasting greater than 4 hours, whether painful or not, to seek emergency medical attention.

17.6   Vision
Physicians should advise patients to stop use of all PDE5 inhibitors, including CIALIS, and seek medical attention in the event of a sudden loss of vision in one or both eyes. Such an event may be a sign of non-arteritic anterior ischemic optic neuropathy (NAION), a cause of decreased vision, including permanent loss of vision that has been reported rarely postmarketing in temporal association with the use of all PDE5 inhibitors. It is not possible to determine whether these events are related directly to the use of PDE5 inhibitors or other factors. Physicians should also discuss with patients the increased risk of NAION in individuals who have already experienced NAION in one eye, including whether such individuals could be adversely affected by use of vasodilators such as PDE5 inhibitors [see Clinical Studies (6.2)].

17.7   Sudden Hearing Loss
Physicians should advise patients to stop taking PDE5 inhibitors, including CIALIS, and seek prompt medical attention in the event of sudden decrease or loss of hearing. These events, which may be accompanied by tinnitus and dizziness, have been reported in temporal association to the intake of PDE5 inhibitors, including CIALIS. It is not possible to determine whether these events are related directly to the use of PDE5 inhibitors or to other factors [see Adverse Reactions (6.1) and (6.2)].

17.8   Alcohol
Patients should be made aware that both alcohol and CIALIS, a PDE5 inhibitor, act as mild vasodilators. When mild vasodilators are taken in combination, blood-pressure-lowering effects of each individual compound may be increased. Therefore, physicians should inform patients that substantial consumption of alcohol (e.g., 5 units or greater) in combination with CIALIS can increase the potential for orthostatic signs and symptoms, including increase in heart rate, decrease in standing blood pressure, dizziness, and headache [see Warnings and Precautions (5.9), Drug Interactions (7.1), and Clinical Pharmacology (12.2)].

17.9   Sexually Transmitted Disease
The use of CIALIS offers no protection against sexually transmitted diseases. Counseling of patients about the protective measures necessary to guard against sexually transmitted diseases, including Human Immunodeficiency Virus (HIV) should be considered.

17.10   Recommended Administration
CIALIS is available in two dosing regimens; therefore, physicians should instruct patients on the appropriate administration to allow optimal use.
For CIALIS for use as needed, patients should be instructed to take one tablet at least 30 minutes before anticipated sexual activity. In most patients, the ability to have sexual intercourse is improved for up to 36 hours.

Table 14: Mean Endpoint and Change from Baseline for the Primary Efficacy Variables in a Study in ED Patients with Diabetes

	Placebo	CIALIS 10 mg	CIALIS 20 mg	
	(N=71)	(N=73)	(N=72)	p-value
EF Domain Score				
Endpoint [Change from baseline]	12.2 [0.1]	19.3 [6.4]	18.7 [7.3]	<.001
Insertion of Penis (SEP2)				
Endpoint [Change from baseline]	30% [-4%]	57% [22%]	54% [23%]	<.001
Maintenance of Erection (SEP3)				
Endpoint [Change from baseline]	20% [2%]	48% [28%]	42% [29%]	<.001

Table 15: Mean Endpoint and Change from Baseline for the Primary Efficacy Variables in a Study in Patients who Developed ED Following Bilateral Nerve-Sparing Radical Prostatectomy

	Placebo	CIALIS 20 mg	
	(N=102)	(N=201)	p-value
EF Domain Score			
Endpoint [Change from baseline]	13.3 [1.1]	17.7 [5.3]	<.001
Insertion of Penis (SEP2)			
Endpoint [Change from baseline]	32% [2%]	54% [22%]	<.001
Maintenance of Erection (SEP3)			
Endpoint [Change from baseline]	19% [4%]	41% [23%]	<.001

Table 16: Mean Endpoint and Change from Baseline for the Primary Efficacy Variables in the Two CIALIS for Once Daily Use Studies

	Study H[a]				Study I[b]		
	Placebo	CIALIS 2.5 mg	CIALIS 5 mg		Placebo	CIALIS 5 mg	
	(N=94)	(N=96)	(N=97)	p-value	(N=54)	(N=109)	p-value
EF Domain Score							
Endpoint	14.6	19.1	20.8		15.0	22.8	
Change from baseline	1.2	6.1[c]	7.0[c]	<.001	0.9	9.7[c]	<.001
Insertion of Penis (SEP2)							
Endpoint	51%	65%	71%		52%	79%	
Change from baseline	5%	24%[c]	26%[c]	<.001	11%	37%[c]	<.001
Maintenance of Erection (SEP3)							
Endpoint	31%	50%	57%		37%	67%	
Change from baseline	10%	31%[c]	35%[c]	<.001	13%	46%[c]	<.001

[a] Twenty-four-week study conducted in the US.
[b] Twelve-week study conducted outside the US.
[c] Statistically significantly different from placebo

For CIALIS for once daily use, patients should be instructed to take one tablet at approximately the same time every day without regard for the timing of sexual activity. Cialis is effective at improving erectile function over the course of therapy.
Literature revised February 1, 2010

Eli Lilly and Company
Indianapolis, IN 46285, USA
www.cialis.com
Copyright © 2003, 2010, Eli Lilly and Company. All rights reserved.
PV 6603 AMP

Patient Information
CIALIS® (See-AL-iss)
(tadalafil) tablets
Read this important information before you start taking CIALIS and each time you get a refill. There may be new information. You may also find it helpful to share this information with your partner. This information does not take the place of talking with your healthcare provider. You and your healthcare provider should talk about CIALIS when you start taking it and at regular checkups. If you do not understand the information, or have questions, talk with your healthcare provider or pharmacist.
What Is The Most Important Information I Should Know About CIALIS?
CIALIS can cause your blood pressure to drop suddenly to an unsafe level if it is taken with certain other medicines. You could get dizzy, faint, or have a heart attack or stroke. Do not take CIALIS if you take any medicines called "nitrates." Nitrates are commonly used to treat angina. Angina is a symptom of heart disease and can cause pain in your chest, jaw, or down your arm.
● Medicines called nitrates include nitroglycerin that is found in tablets, sprays, ointments, pastes, or patches. Ni-

Table 17: Mean Endpoint and Change from Baseline for the Primary Efficacy Variables in a CIALIS for Once Daily Use Study in ED Patients with Diabetes

	Placebo	CIALIS 2.5 mg	CIALIS 5 mg	
	(N=100)	(N=100)	(N=98)	p-value
EF Domain Score				
Endpoint	14.7	18.3	17.2	
Change from baseline	1.3	4.8[a]	4.5[a]	<.001
Insertion of Penis (SEP2)				
Endpoint	43%	62%	61%	
Change from baseline	5%	21%[a]	29%[a]	<.001
Maintenance of Erection (SEP3)				
Endpoint	28%	46%	41%	
Change from baseline	8%	26%[a]	25%[a]	<.001

[a] Statistically significantly different from placebo

trates can also be found in other medicines such as isosorbide dinitrate or isosorbide mononitrate. Some recreational drugs called "poppers" also contain nitrates, such as amyl nitrite and butyl nitrite.

* Ask your healthcare provider or pharmacist if you are not sure if any of your medicines are nitrates. (See "**Who should not take CIALIS?**")

Tell all of your healthcare providers that you take CIALIS. If you need emergency medical care for a heart problem, it will be important for your healthcare provider to know when you last took CIALIS.

After taking a single tablet, some of the active ingredient of CIALIS remains in your body for more than 2 days. The active ingredient can remain longer if you have problems with your kidneys or liver, or you are taking certain other medications (see "**Can Other Medicines Affect CIALIS?**").

Stop sexual activity and get medical help right away if you get symptoms such as chest pain, dizziness, or nausea during sex. Sexual activity can put an extra strain on your heart, especially if your heart is already weak from a heart attack or heart disease.

See also "**What Are The Possible Side Effects Of CIALIS?**"

What Is CIALIS?

CIALIS is a prescription medicine taken by mouth for the treatment of erectile dysfunction (ED) in men.

ED is a condition where the penis does not fill with enough blood to harden and expand when a man is sexually excited, or when he cannot keep an erection. A man who has trouble getting or keeping an erection should see his healthcare provider for help if the condition bothers him. CIALIS helps increase blood flow to the penis and may help men with ED get and keep an erection satisfactory for sexual activity. Once a man has completed sexual activity, blood flow to his penis decreases, and his erection goes away.

Some form of sexual stimulation is needed for an erection to happen with CIALIS.

CIALIS does not:

* cure ED
* increase a man's sexual desire
* protect a man or his partner from sexually transmitted diseases, including HIV. Speak to your healthcare provider about ways to guard against sexually transmitted diseases.
* serve as a male form of birth control

CIALIS is only for men over the age of 18 who have ED, including men with diabetes or who have undergone prostatectomy

CIALIS is not for women or children.

CIALIS must be used only under a healthcare provider's care.

Who Should Not Take CIALIS?

Do not take CIALIS if you:

* **take any medicines called "nitrates".**
* use recreational drugs called "poppers" like amyl nitrite and butyl nitrite. (See "**What Is The Most Important Information I Should Know About CIALIS?**")

What Should I Tell My Healthcare Provider Before Taking CIALIS?

CIALIS is not right for everyone. **Only your healthcare provider and you can decide if CIALIS is right for you.** Before taking CIALIS, tell your healthcare provider about all your medical problems, including if you:

* **are allergic to CIALIS or ADCIRCA™ or any of its ingredients.** See the end of this leaflet for a complete list of ingredients in CIALIS.
* **have heart problems** such as angina, heart failure, irregular heartbeats, or have had a heart attack. Ask your

healthcare provider if it is safe for you to have sexual activity. You should not take CIALIS if your healthcare provider has told you not to have sexual activity because of your health problems.

* **have low blood pressure** or have high blood pressure that is not controlled
* **have had a stroke**
* **have liver problems**
* **have kidney problems or require dialysis**
* have retinitis pigmentosa, a rare genetic (runs in families) eye disease
* **have ever had severe vision loss, including a condition called NAION**
* **have stomach ulcers**
* **have a bleeding problem**
* **have a deformed penis shape** or Peyronie's disease
* **have had an erection that lasted more than 4 hours**
* **have blood cell problems** such as sickle cell anemia, multiple myeloma, or leukemia

Can Other Medicines Affect CIALIS?

Tell your healthcare provider about all the medicines you take including prescription and non-prescription medicines, vitamins, and herbal supplements. CIALIS and other medicines may affect each other. Always check with your healthcare provider before starting or stopping any medicines. Especially tell your healthcare provider if you take any of the following:*

* medicines called nitrates (see "**What Is The Most Important Information I Should Know About CIALIS?**")
* medicines called alpha blockers. These include Hytrin® (terazosin HCl), Flomax® (tamsulosin HCl), Cardura® (doxazosin mesylate), Minipress® (prazosin HCl) or Uroxatral® (alfuzosin HCl). Alpha blockers are sometimes prescribed for prostate problems or high blood pressure. If CIALIS is taken with certain alpha blockers, your blood pressure could suddenly drop. You could get dizzy or faint.
* other medicines to treat high blood pressure (hypertension)
* medicines called HIV protease inhibitors, such as ritonavir (Norvir®, Kaletra®)
* ketoconazole (Nizoral®)
* itraconazole (Sporanox®)
* erythromycin
* other medicines or treatments for ED.
* CIALIS is also marketed as ADCIRCA for the treatment of pulmonary arterial hypertension. Do not take both CIALIS and ADCIRCA. Do not take sildenafil citrate (Revatio™) with CIALIS.

How Should I Take CIALIS?

* Take CIALIS exactly as your healthcare provider prescribes it. Your healthcare provider will prescribe the dose that is right for you.
* Some men can only take a low dose of CIALIS or may have to take it less often, because of medical conditions or medicines they take.
* Do not change your dose or the way you take CIALIS without talking to your healthcare provider. Your healthcare provider may lower or raise your dose, depending on how your body reacts to CIALIS and your health condition.
* CIALIS may be taken with or without meals.
* If you take too much CIALIS, call your healthcare provider or emergency room right away.

There are two ways to take CIALIS:

CIALIS for use as needed:

* **Do not take CIALIS more than one time each day.**
* Take one CIALIS tablet before you expect to have sexual activity. You may be able to have sexual activity at 30 minutes after taking CIALIS and up to 36 hours after taking it. You and your healthcare provider should consider this in deciding when you should take CIALIS before sexual activity. Some form of sexual stimulation is needed for an erection to happen with CIALIS.
* Your healthcare provider may change your dose of CIALIS depending on how you respond to the medicine, and on your health condition.

OR

CIALIS for once daily use:

* **Do not take CIALIS more than one time each day.**
* Take one CIALIS tablet every day at about the same time of day. You may attempt sexual activity at any time between doses.
* If you miss a dose, you may take it when you remember but do not take more than one dose per day.
* Some form of sexual stimulation is needed for an erection to happen with CIALIS.
* Your healthcare provider may change your dose of CIALIS depending on how you respond to the medicine, and on your health condition.

What Should I Avoid While Taking CIALIS?

* Do not use other ED medicines or ED treatments while taking CIALIS.
* Do not drink too much alcohol when taking CIALIS (for example, 5 glasses of wine or 5 shots of whiskey). Drinking too much alcohol can increase your chances of getting a headache or getting dizzy, increasing your heart rate, or lowering your blood pressure.

What Are The Possible Side Effects Of CIALIS?

See "**What Is The Most Important Information I Should Know About CIALIS?**"

The most common side effects with CIALIS are: headache, indigestion, back pain, muscle aches, flushing, and stuffy or runny nose. These side effects usually go away after a few hours. Men who get back pain and muscle aches usually get it 12 to 24 hours after taking CIALIS. Back pain and muscle aches usually go away within 2 days.

Call your healthcare provider if you get any side effect that bothers you or one that does not go away.

Uncommon side effects include:

An erection that won't go away (priapism). If you get an erection that lasts more than 4 hours, get medical help right away. Priapism must be treated as soon as possible or lasting damage can happen to your penis, including the inability to have erections.

Color vision changes, such as seeing a blue tinge (shade) to objects or having difficulty telling the difference between the colors blue and green.

In rare instances, men taking PDE5 inhibitors (oral erectile dysfunction medicines, including CIALIS) reported a sudden decrease or loss of vision in one or both eyes. It is not possible to determine whether these events are related directly to these medicines, to other factors such as high blood pressure or diabetes, or to a combination of these. If you experience sudden decrease or loss of vision, stop taking PDE5 inhibitors, including CIALIS, and call a healthcare provider right away.

Sudden loss or decrease in hearing, sometimes with ringing in the ears and dizziness, has been rarely reported in people taking PDE5 inhibitors, including CIALIS. It is not possible to determine whether these events are related directly to the PDE5 inhibitors, to other diseases or medications, to other factors, or to a combination of factors. If you experience these symptoms, stop taking CIALIS and contact a healthcare provider right away.

These are not all the possible side effects of CIALIS. For more information, ask your healthcare provider or pharmacist.

How Should I Store CIALIS?

Store CIALIS at room temperature between 59° and 86°F (15° and 30°C).

Keep CIALIS and all medicines out of the reach of children.

General Information About CIALIS:

Medicines are sometimes prescribed for conditions other than those described in patient information leaflets. Do not use CIALIS for a condition for which it was not prescribed. Do not give CIALIS to other people, even if they have the same symptoms that you have. It may harm them.

This is a summary of the most important information about CIALIS. If you would like more information, talk with your healthcare provider. You can ask your healthcare provider or pharmacist for information about CIALIS that is written for health providers. You can also visit www.cialis.com, or call 1-877-CIALIS1 (1-877-242-5471).

What Are The Ingredients In CIALIS?

Active Ingredient: tadalafil

Inactive Ingredients: croscarmellose sodium, hydroxypropyl cellulose, hypromellose, iron oxide, lactose monohydrate, magnesium stearate, microcrystalline cellulose, sodium lauryl sulfate, talc, titanium dioxide, and triacetin.

Rx only

CIALIS® (tadalafil) is a registered trademark of Eli Lilly and Company.

Eli Lilly and Company
Indianapolis, IN 46285, USA
www.cialis.com
PV 5226 AMP

Shown in Product Identification Guide, page 310

CYMBALTA® ℞
[sǐm-bǎl-tǎ]
(duloxetine hydrochloride)
Capsule, Delayed Release for Oral Use

HIGHLIGHTS OF PRESCRIBING INFORMATION
These highlights do not include all the information needed to use CYMBALTA safely and effectively. See full prescribing information for CYMBALTA.
CYMBALTA (duloxetine hydrochloride) capsule, delayed release for oral use
Initial U.S. Approval: 2004

> **WARNING: Suicidality and Antidepressant Drugs**
> *See full prescribing information for complete boxed warning.*
> • **Increased risk of suicidal thinking and behavior in children, adolescents, and young adults taking antidepressants for major depressive disorder (MDD) and other psychiatric disorders. Cymbalta is not approved for use in pediatric patients (5.1).**

-------RECENT MAJOR CHANGES-------
Indications and Usage, Generalized Anxiety Disorder (1.2) 11/2009
Dosage and Administration, Maintenance/Continuation/Extended Treatment (2.2) 11/2009
Warnings and Precautions, Serotonin Syndrome or Neuroleptic Malignant Syndrome (NMS)-like Reactions (5.4) 01/2009

-------INDICATIONS AND USAGE-------
Cymbalta® is a serotonin and norepinephrine reuptake inhibitor (SNRI) indicated for:
• Major Depressive Disorder (MDD) (1.1)
  Efficacy was established in 4 short-term and one maintenance trial in adults (14.1).
• Generalized Anxiety Disorder (GAD) (1.2)
  Efficacy was established in 3 short-term and one maintenance trial in adults (14.2).
• Diabetic Peripheral Neuropathic Pain (DPNP) (1.3).
• Fibromyalgia (FM) (1.4)

-------DOSAGE AND ADMINISTRATION-------
• Cymbalta should generally be administered once daily without regard to meals. Cymbalta should be swallowed whole and should not be chewed or crushed, nor should the capsule be opened and its contents be sprinkled on food or mixed with liquids (2.1).

Indication	Starting Dose	Target Dose	Maximum Dose
MDD (2.1, 2.2)	40 mg/day to 60 mg/day	Acute Treatment: 40 mg/day (20 mg twice daily) to 60 mg/day (once daily or as 30 mg twice daily); Maintenance Treatment: 60 mg/day	120 mg/day
GAD (2.1)	60 mg/day	60 mg/day (once daily)	120 mg/day
DPNP (2.1)	60 mg/day	60 mg/day (once daily)	60 mg/day
FM (2.1)	30 mg/day	60 mg/day (once daily)	60 mg/day

• Some patients may benefit from starting at 30 mg once daily.

• There is no evidence that doses greater than 60 mg/day confers additional benefit, while some adverse reactions were observed to be dose-dependent.
• Discontinuing Cymbalta: A gradual dose reduction is recommended to avoid discontinuation symptoms (5.6).

-------DOSAGE FORMS AND STRENGTHS-------
• 20 mg, 30 mg, and 60 mg capsules (3)

-------CONTRAINDICATIONS-------
• Use of a monoamine oxidase inhibitor concomitantly or in close temporal proximity (4.1)
• Use in patients with uncontrolled narrow-angle glaucoma (4.2)

-------WARNINGS AND PRECAUTIONS-------
• Suicidality: Monitor for clinical worsening and suicide risk (5.1).
• Hepatotoxicity: Hepatic failure, sometimes fatal, has been reported in patients treated with Cymbalta. Cymbalta should be discontinued in patients who develop jaundice or other evidence of clinically significant liver dysfunction and should not be resumed unless another cause can be established. Cymbalta should ordinarily not be prescribed to patients with substantial alcohol use or evidence of chronic liver disease (5.2).
• Orthostatic Hypotension and Syncope: Cases have been reported with duloxetine therapy (5.3).
• Serotonin Syndrome, or Neuroleptic Malignant Syndrome (NMS)-like reactions: Serotonin syndrome or NMS-like reactions have been reported with SSRIs and SNRIs. Discontinue Cymbalta and initiate supportive treatment (5.4, 7.14).
• Abnormal Bleeding: Cymbalta may increase the risk of bleeding events. Patients should be cautioned about the risk of bleeding associated with the concomitant use of duloxetine and NSAIDs, aspirin, or other drugs that affect coagulation (5.5, 7.4).
• Discontinuation: May result in symptoms, including dizziness, nausea, headache, fatigue, paresthesia, vomiting, irritability, nightmares, insomnia, diarrhea, anxiety, hyperhidrosis, and vertigo (5.6).
• Activation of mania or hypomania has occurred (5.7).
• Seizures: Prescribe with care in patients with a history of seizure disorder (5.8).
• Blood Pressure: Monitor blood pressure prior to initiating treatment and periodically throughout treatment (5.9).
• Inhibitors of CYP1A2 or Thioridazine: Should not administer with Cymbalta (5.10).
• Hyponatremia: Cases of hyponatremia have been reported (5.11).
• Hepatic Insufficiency and Severe Renal Impairment: Should ordinarily not be administered to these patients (5.12).
• Controlled Narrow-Angle Glaucoma: Use cautiously in these patients (5.12).
• Glucose Control in Diabetes: In diabetic peripheral neuropathic pain patients, small increases in fasting blood glucose, HbA_{1c}, and total cholesterol have been observed (5.12).
• Conditions that Slow Gastric Emptying: Use cautiously in these patients (5.12).
• Urinary Hesitation and Retention (5.13).

-------ADVERSE REACTIONS-------
• Most common adverse reactions (≥5% and at least twice the incidence of placebo patients): nausea, dry mouth, constipation, somnolence, hyperhidrosis, and decreased appetite (6.3).

To report SUSPECTED ADVERSE REACTIONS, contact Eli Lilly and Company at 1-800-LillyRx or FDA at 1-800-FDA-1088 or www.fda.gov/medwatch

-------DRUG INTERACTIONS-------
• Potent inhibitors of CYP1A2 should be avoided (7.1).
• Potent inhibitors of CYP2D6 may increase duloxetine concentrations (7.2).
• Duloxetine is a moderate inhibitor of CYP2D6 (7.9).

-------USE IN SPECIFIC POPULATIONS-------
• Pregnancy and Nursing Mothers: Use only if the potential benefit justifies the potential risk to the fetus or child (2.3, 8.1, 8.3).

See 17 for PATIENT COUNSELING INFORMATION and Medication Guide

Revised: 03/2010

FULL PRESCRIBING INFORMATION: CONTENTS*
1 INDICATIONS AND USAGE
   1.1 Major Depressive Disorder
   1.2 Generalized Anxiety Disorder
   1.3 Diabetic Peripheral Neuropathic Pain
   1.4 Fibromyalgia
2 DOSAGE AND ADMINISTRATION
   2.1 Initial Treatment
   2.2 Maintenance/Continuation/Extended Treatment
   2.3 Dosing in Special Populations
   2.4 Discontinuing Cymbalta

   2.5 Switching Patients to or from a Monoamine Oxidase Inhibitor
3 DOSAGE FORMS AND STRENGTHS
4 CONTRAINDICATIONS
   4.1 Monoamine Oxidase Inhibitors
   4.2 Uncontrolled Narrow-Angle Glaucoma
5 WARNINGS AND PRECAUTIONS
   5.1 Clinical Worsening and Suicide Risk
   5.2 Hepatotoxicity
   5.3 Orthostatic Hypotension and Syncope
   5.4 Serotonin Syndrome or Neuroleptic Malignant Syndrome (NMS)-like Reactions
   5.5 Abnormal Bleeding
   5.6 Discontinuation of Treatment with Cymbalta
   5.7 Activation of Mania/Hypomania
   5.8 Seizures
   5.9 Effect on Blood Pressure
   5.10 Clinically Important Drug Interactions
   5.11 Hyponatremia
   5.12 Use in Patients with Concomitant Illness
   5.13 Urinary Hesitation and Retention
   5.14 Laboratory Tests
6 ADVERSE REACTIONS
   6.1 Clinical Trial Data Sources
   6.2 Adverse Reactions Reported as Reasons for Discontinuation of Treatment in Placebo-Controlled Trials
   6.3 Adverse Reactions Occurring at an Incidence of 5% or More and at least Twice Placebo Among Duloxetine-Treated Patients in Placebo-Controlled Trials
   6.4 Adverse Reactions Occurring at an Incidence of 5% or More Among Duloxetine-Treated Patients in Placebo-Controlled Trials
   6.5 Adverse Reactions Occurring at an Incidence of 2% or More Among Duloxetine-Treated Patients in Placebo-Controlled Trials
   6.6 Effects on Male and Female Sexual Function
   6.7 Vital Sign Changes
   6.8 Weight Changes
   6.9 Laboratory Changes
   6.10 Electrocardiogram Changes
   6.11 Other Adverse Reactions Observed During the Premarketing and Postmarketing Clinical Trial Evaluation of Duloxetine
   6.12 Postmarketing Spontaneous Reports
7 DRUG INTERACTIONS
   7.1 Inhibitors of CYP1A2
   7.2 Inhibitors of CYP2D6
   7.3 Dual Inhibition of CYP1A2 and CYP2D6
   7.4 Drugs that Interfere with Hemostasis (e.g., NSAIDs, Aspirin, and Warfarin)
   7.5 Lorazepam
   7.6 Temazepam
   7.7 Drugs that Affect Gastric Acidity
   7.8 Drugs Metabolized by CYP1A2
   7.9 Drugs Metabolized by CYP2D6
   7.10 Drugs Metabolized by CYP2C9
   7.11 Drugs Metabolized by CYP3A
   7.12 Drugs Metabolized by CYP2C19
   7.13 Monoamine Oxidase Inhibitors
   7.14 Serotonergic Drugs
   7.15 Triptans
   7.16 Alcohol
   7.17 CNS Drugs
   7.18 Drugs Highly Bound to Plasma Protein
8 USE IN SPECIFIC POPULATIONS
   8.1 Pregnancy
   8.2 Labor and Delivery
   8.3 Nursing Mothers
   8.4 Pediatric Use
   8.5 Geriatric Use
   8.6 Gender
   8.7 Smoking Status
   8.8 Race
   8.9 Hepatic Insufficiency
   8.10 Severe Renal Impairment
9 DRUG ABUSE AND DEPENDENCE
   9.2 Abuse
   9.3 Dependence
10 OVERDOSAGE
   10.1 Signs and Symptoms
   10.2 Management of Overdose
11 DESCRIPTION
12 CLINICAL PHARMACOLOGY
   12.1 Mechanism of Action
   12.2 Pharmacodynamics
   12.3 Pharmacokinetics
13 NONCLINICAL TOXICOLOGY
   13.1 Carcinogenesis, Mutagenesis, and Impairment of Fertility
14 CLINICAL STUDIES
   14.1 Major Depressive Disorder
   14.2 Generalized Anxiety Disorder

*** Sections or subsections omitted from the full prescribing information are not listed**

FULL PRESCRIBING INFORMATION

WARNING: SUICIDALITY AND ANTIDEPRESSANT DRUGS

Antidepressants increased the risk compared to placebo of suicidal thinking and behavior (suicidality) in children, adolescents, and young adults in short-term studies of major depressive disorder (MDD) and other psychiatric disorders. Anyone considering the use of Cymbalta or any other antidepressant in a child, adolescent, or young adult must balance this risk with the clinical need. Short-term studies did not show an increase in the risk of suicidality with antidepressants compared to placebo in adults beyond age 24; there was a reduction in risk with antidepressants compared to placebo in adults aged 65 and older. Depression and certain other psychiatric disorders are themselves associated with increases in the risk of suicide. Patients of all ages who are started on antidepressant therapy should be monitored appropriately and observed closely for clinical worsening, suicidality, or unusual changes in behavior. Families and caregivers should be advised of the need for close observation and communication with the prescriber. Cymbalta is not approved for use in pediatric patients. *[see Warnings and Precautions (5.1), Use in Specific Populations (8.4), and Information for Patients (17.2).]*

1 INDICATIONS AND USAGE

1.1 Major Depressive Disorder

Cymbalta is indicated for the treatment of major depressive disorder (MDD). The efficacy of Cymbalta was established in four short term and one maintenance trial in adults *[see Clinical Studies (14.1)]*.

A major depressive episode (DSM-IV) implies a prominent and relatively persistent (nearly every day for at least 2 weeks) depressed or dysphoric mood that usually interferes with daily functioning, and includes at least 5 of the following 9 symptoms: depressed mood, loss of interest in usual activities, significant change in weight and/or appetite, insomnia or hypersomnia, psychomotor agitation or retardation, increased fatigue, feelings of guilt or worthlessness, slowed thinking or impaired concentration, or a suicide attempt or suicidal ideation.

1.2 Generalized Anxiety Disorder

Cymbalta is indicated for the treatment of generalized anxiety disorder (GAD). The efficacy of Cymbalta was established in three short-term trials and one maintenance trial in adults *[see Clinical Studies (14.2)]*.

Generalized anxiety disorder is defined by the DSM-IV as excessive anxiety and worry, present more days than not, for at least 6 months. The excessive anxiety and worry must be difficult to control and must cause significant distress or impairment in normal functioning. It must be associated with at least 3 of the following 6 symptoms: restlessness or feeling keyed up or on edge, being easily fatigued, difficulty concentrating or mind going blank, irritability, muscle tension, and/or sleep disturbance.

1.3 Diabetic Peripheral Neuropathic Pain

Cymbalta is indicated for the management of neuropathic pain (DPNP) associated with diabetic peripheral neuropathy *[see Clinical Studies (14.3)]*.

1.4 Fibromyalgia

Cymbalta is indicated for the management of fibromyalgia (FM) *[see Clinical Studies (14.4)]*.

2 DOSAGE AND ADMINISTRATION

Cymbalta should be swallowed whole and should not be chewed or crushed, nor should the capsule be opened and its contents sprinkled on food or mixed with liquids. All of these might affect the enteric coating. Cymbalta should be given without regard to meals.

2.1 Initial Treatment

Major Depressive Disorder—Cymbalta should be administered at a total dose of 40 mg/day (given as 20 mg twice daily) to 60 mg/day (given either once daily or as 30 mg twice daily). For some patients, it may be desirable to start at 30 mg once daily for 1 week, to allow patients to adjust to the medication before increasing to 60 mg once daily. While a 120 mg/day dose was shown to be effective, there is no evidence that doses greater than 60 mg/day confer any additional benefits. The safety of doses above 120 mg/day has not been adequately evaluated *[see Clinical Studies (14.1)]*.

Generalized Anxiety Disorder—For most patients, the recommended starting dose for Cymbalta is 60 mg administered once daily. For some patients, it may be desirable to start at 30 mg once daily for 1 week, to allow patients to adjust to the medication before increasing to 60 mg once daily. While a 120 mg once daily dose was shown to be effective, there is no evidence that doses greater than 60 mg/day confer additional benefit. Nevertheless, if a decision is made to increase the dose beyond 60 mg once daily, dose increases should be in increments of 30 mg once daily. The safety of doses above 120 mg once daily has not been adequately evaluated *[see Clinical Studies (14.2)]*.

Diabetic Peripheral Neuropathic Pain—The recommended dose for Cymbalta is 60 mg administered once daily. There is no evidence that doses higher than 60 mg confer additional significant benefit and the higher dose is clearly less well tolerated *[see Clinical Studies (14.3)]*. For patients for whom tolerability is a concern, a lower starting dose may be considered.

Since diabetes is frequently complicated by renal disease, a lower starting dose and gradual increase in dose should be considered for patients with renal impairment *[see Clinical Pharmacology (12.3) and Dosage and Administration (2.3)]*.

Fibromyalgia—The recommended dose for Cymbalta is 60 mg administered once daily. Treatment should begin at 30 mg once daily for 1 week, to allow patients to adjust to the medication before increasing to 60 mg once daily. Some patients may respond to the starting dose. There is no evidence that doses greater than 60 mg/day confer additional benefit, even in patients who do not respond to a 60 mg dose, and higher doses are associated with a higher rate of adverse reactions *[see Clinical Studies (14.4)]*.

2.2 Maintenance/Continuation/Extended Treatment

Major Depressive Disorder—It is generally agreed that acute episodes of major depression require several months or longer of sustained pharmacologic therapy. Maintenance of efficacy in MDD was demonstrated with Cymbalta as monotherapy. Cymbalta should be administered at a total dose of 60 mg once daily. Patients should be periodically reassessed to determine the need for maintenance treatment and the appropriate dose for such treatment *[see Clinical Studies (14.1)]*.

Generalized Anxiety Disorder—It is generally agreed that episodes of generalized anxiety disorder require several months or longer of sustained pharmacological therapy. Maintenance of efficacy in GAD was demonstrated with Cymbalta as monotherapy. Cymbalta should be administered in a dose range of 60-120 mg once daily. Patients should be periodically reassessed to determine the continued need for maintenance treatment and the appropriate dose for such treatment *[see Clinical Studies (14.2)]*.

Diabetic Peripheral Neuropathic Pain—As the progression of diabetic peripheral neuropathy is highly variable and management of pain is empirical, the effectiveness of Cymbalta must be assessed individually. Efficacy beyond 12 weeks has not been systematically studied in placebo-controlled trials.

Fibromyalgia—Fibromyalgia is recognized as a chronic condition. The efficacy of Cymbalta in the management of fibromyalgia has been demonstrated in placebo-controlled studies up to 3 months. The efficacy of Cymbalta was not demonstrated in longer studies; however, continued treatment should be based on individual patient response.

2.3 Dosing in Special Populations

Hepatic Insufficiency—It is recommended that Cymbalta should ordinarily not be administered to patients with any hepatic insufficiency *[see Warnings and Precautions (5.12) and Use in Specific Populations (8.9)]*.

Severe Renal Impairment—Cymbalta is not recommended for patients with end-stage renal disease or severe renal impairment (estimated creatinine clearance <30 mL/min) *[see Warnings and Precautions (5.12) and Use in Specific Populations (8.10)]*.

Elderly Patients—No dose adjustment is recommended for elderly patients on the basis of age. As with any drug, caution should be exercised in treating the elderly. When individualizing the dosage in elderly patients, extra care should be taken when increasing the dose *[see Use in Specific Populations (8.5)]*.

Pregnant Women—There are no adequate and well-controlled studies in pregnant women; therefore, Cymbalta should be used during pregnancy only if the potential benefit justifies the potential risk to the fetus *[see Use in Specific Populations (8.1)]*.

Nursing Mothers—Because the safety of duloxetine in infants is not known, nursing while on Cymbalta is not recommended *[see Use in Specific Populations (8.3)]*.

2.4 Discontinuing Cymbalta

Symptoms associated with discontinuation of Cymbalta and other SSRIs and SNRIs have been reported. A gradual reduction in the dose rather than abrupt cessation is recommended whenever possible *[see Warnings and Precautions (5.6)]*.

2.5 Switching Patients to or from a Monoamine Oxidase Inhibitor

At least 14 days should elapse between discontinuation of an MAOI and initiation of therapy with Cymbalta. In addition, at least 5 days should be allowed after stopping Cymbalta before starting an MAOI *[see Contraindications (4.1) and Warnings and Precautions (5.4)]*.

3 DOSAGE FORMS AND STRENGTHS

Cymbalta is available as delayed release capsules:

- 20mg opaque green capsules imprinted with "Lilly 3235 20mg"
- 30mg opaque white and blue capsules imprinted with "Lilly 3240 30mg"
- 60mg opaque green and blue capsules imprinted with "Lilly 3237 60mg"
- 60mg opaque green and blue capsules imprinted with "Lilly 3270 60mg"

4 CONTRAINDICATIONS

4.1 Monoamine Oxidase Inhibitors

Concomitant use in patients taking monoamine oxidase inhibitors (MAOIs) is contraindicated due to the risk of serious, sometimes fatal, drug interactions with serotonergic drugs. These interactions may include hyperthermia, rigidity, myoclonus, autonomic instability with possible rapid fluctuations of vital signs, and mental status changes that include extreme agitation progressing to delirium and coma. These reactions have also been reported in patients who have recently discontinued serotonin reuptake inhibitors and are then started on an MAOI. Some cases presented with features resembling neuroleptic malignant syndrome *[see Dosage and Administration (2.5) and Warnings and Precautions (5.4)]*.

4.2 Uncontrolled Narrow-Angle Glaucoma

In clinical trials, Cymbalta use was associated with an increased risk of mydriasis; therefore, its use should be avoided in patients with uncontrolled narrow-angle glaucoma *[see Warnings and Precautions (5.12)]*.

5 WARNINGS AND PRECAUTIONS

5.1 Clinical Worsening and Suicide Risk

Patients with major depressive disorder (MDD), both adult and pediatric, may experience worsening of their depression and/or the emergence of suicidal ideation and behavior (suicidality) or unusual changes in behavior, whether or not they are taking antidepressant medications, and this risk may persist until significant remission occurs. Suicide is a known risk of depression and certain other psychiatric disorders, and these disorders themselves are the strongest predictors of suicide. There has been a long-standing concern, however, that antidepressants may have a role in inducing worsening of depression and the emergence of suicidality in certain patients during the early phases of treatment.

Pooled analyses of short-term placebo-controlled trials of antidepressant drugs (SSRIs and others) showed that these drugs increase the risk of suicidal thinking and behavior (suicidality) in children, adolescents, and young adults (ages 18-24) with major depressive disorder (MDD) and other psychiatric disorders. Short-term studies did not show an increase in the risk of suicidality with antidepressants compared to placebo in adults beyond age 24; there was a reduction with antidepressants compared to placebo in adults aged 65 and older.

The pooled analyses of placebo-controlled trials in children and adolescents with MDD, obsessive compulsive disorder (OCD), or other psychiatric disorders included a total of 24 short-term trials of 9 antidepressant drugs in over 4400 patients. The pooled analyses of placebo-controlled trials in adults with MDD or other psychiatric disorders included a total of 295 short-term trials (median duration of 2 months) of 11 antidepressant drugs in over 77,000 patients. There was considerable variation in risk of suicidality among drugs, but a tendency toward an increase in the younger patients for almost all drugs studied. There were differences in absolute risk of suicidality across the different indications, with the highest incidence in MDD. The risk of differences (drug vs placebo), however, were relatively stable within age strata and across indications. These risk differences (drug-placebo difference in the number of cases of suicidality per 1000 patients treated) are provided in Table 1.

Table 1

Age Range	Drug-Placebo Difference in Number of Cases of Suicidality per 1000 Patients Treated
	Increases Compared to Placebo
<18	14 additional cases
18-24	5 additional cases
	Decreases Compared to Placebo
25-64	1 fewer case
≥65	6 fewer cases

No suicides occurred in any of the pediatric trials. There were suicides in the adult trials, but the number was not sufficient to reach any conclusion about drug effect on suicide.

It is unknown whether the suicidality risk extends to longer-term use, i.e., beyond several months. However, there is substantial evidence from placebo-controlled maintenance trials in adults with depression that the use of antidepressants can delay the recurrence of depression.

All patients being treated with antidepressants for any indication should be monitored appropriately and observed closely for clinical worsening, suicidality, and unusual changes in behavior, especially during the initial few months of a course of drug therapy, or at times of dose changes, either increases or decreases.

The following symptoms, anxiety, agitation, panic attacks, insomnia, irritability, hostility, aggressiveness, impulsivity, akathisia (psychomotor restlessness), hypomania, and mania, have been reported in adult and pediatric patients being treated with antidepressants for major depressive disorder as well as for other indications, both psychiatric and nonpsychiatric. Although a causal link between the emergence of such symptoms and either the worsening of depression and/or the emergence of suicidal impulses has not been established, there is concern that such symptoms may represent precursors to emerging suicidality.

Consideration should be given to changing the therapeutic regimen, including possibly discontinuing the medication, in patients whose depression is persistently worse, or who are experiencing emergent suicidality or symptoms that might be precursors to worsening depression or suicidality, especially if these symptoms are severe, abrupt in onset, or were not part of the patient's presenting symptoms.

If the decision has been made to discontinue treatment, medication should be tapered, as rapidly as is feasible, but with recognition that discontinuation can be associated with certain symptoms [see Dosage and Administration (2.4) and Warnings and Precautions (5.6) for descriptions of the risks of discontinuation of Cymbalta].

Families and caregivers of patients being treated with antidepressants for major depressive disorder or other indications, both psychiatric and nonpsychiatric, should be alerted about the need to monitor patients for the emergence of agitation, irritability, unusual changes in behavior, and the other symptoms described above, as well as the emergence of suicidality, and to report such symptoms immediately to health care providers. Such monitoring should include daily observation by families and caregivers. Prescriptions for Cymbalta should be written for the smallest quantity of capsules consistent with good patient management, in order to reduce the risk of overdose.

Screening Patients for Bipolar Disorder—A major depressive episode may be the initial presentation of bipolar disorder. It is generally believed (though not established in controlled trials) that treating such an episode with an antidepressant alone may increase the likelihood of precipitation of a mixed/manic episode in patients at risk for bipolar disorder. Whether any of the symptoms described above represent such a conversion is unknown. However, prior to initiating treatment with an antidepressant, patients with depressive symptoms should be adequately screened to determine if they are at risk for bipolar disorder; such screening should include a detailed psychiatric history, including a family history of suicide, bipolar disorder, and depression. It should be noted that Cymbalta (duloxetine) is not approved for use in treating bipolar depression.

5.2 Hepatotoxicity

There have been reports of hepatic failure, sometimes fatal, in patients treated with Cymbalta. These cases have presented as hepatitis with abdominal pain, hepatomegaly, and elevation of transaminase levels to more than twenty times the upper limit of normal with or without jaundice, reflecting a mixed or hepatocellular pattern of liver injury. Cymbalta should be discontinued in patients who develop jaundice or other evidence of clinically significant liver dysfunction and should not be resumed unless another cause can be established.

Cases of cholestatic jaundice with minimal elevation of transaminase levels have also been reported. Other post-marketing reports indicate that elevated transaminases, bilirubin, and alkaline phosphatase have occurred in patients with chronic liver disease or cirrhosis.

Cymbalta increased the risk of elevation of serum transaminase levels in development program clinical trials. Liver transaminase elevations resulted in the discontinuation of 0.3% (82/27,229) of Cymbalta-treated patients. In these patients, the median time to detection of the transaminase elevation was about two months. In placebo-controlled trials in any indication, elevation of ALT >3 times the upper limit of normal occurred in 1.1% (85/7,632) of Cymbalta-treated patients compared to 0.2% (13/5,578) of placebo-treated patients. In placebo-controlled studies using a fixed dose design, there was evidence of a dose response relationship for ALT and AST elevation of >3 times the upper limit of normal and >5 times the upper limit of normal, respectively.

Because it is possible that duloxetine and alcohol may interact to cause liver injury or that duloxetine may aggravate pre-existing liver disease, Cymbalta should ordinarily not be prescribed to patients with substantial alcohol use or evidence of chronic liver disease.

5.3 Orthostatic Hypotension and Syncope

Orthostatic hypotension and syncope have been reported with therapeutic doses of duloxetine. Syncope and orthostatic hypotension tend to occur within the first week of therapy but can occur at any time during duloxetine treatment, particularly after dose increases. The risk of blood pressure decreases may be greater in patients taking concomitant medications that induce orthostatic hypotension (such as antihypertensives) or are potent CYP1A2 inhibitors [see Warnings and Precautions (5.10) and Drug Interactions (7.1)] and in patients taking duloxetine at doses above 60 mg daily. Consideration should be given to discontinuing duloxetine in patients who experience symptomatic orthostatic hypotension and/or syncope during duloxetine therapy.

5.4 Serotonin Syndrome or Neuroleptic Malignant Syndrome (NMS)-like Reactions

The development of a potentially life-threatening serotonin syndrome or Neuroleptic Malignant Syndrome (NMS)-like reactions have been reported with SNRIs and SSRIs alone, including Cymbalta treatment, but particularly with concomitant use of serotonergic drugs (including triptans) with drugs which impair metabolism of serotonin (including MAOIs), or with antipsychotics or other dopamine antagonists. Serotonin syndrome symptoms may include mental status changes (e.g., agitation, hallucinations, coma), autonomic instability (e.g., tachycardia, labile blood pressure, hyperthermia), neuromuscular aberrations (e.g., hyperreflexia, incoordination) and/or gastrointestinal symptoms (e.g., nausea, vomiting, diarrhea). Serotonin syndrome, in its most severe form can resemble neuroleptic malignant syndrome, which includes hyperthermia, muscle rigidity, autonomic instability with possible rapid fluctuation of vital signs, and mental status changes. Patients should be monitored for the emergence of serotonin syndrome or NMS-like signs and symptoms.

The concomitant use of Cymbalta with MAOIs intended to treat depression is contraindicated [see Contraindications (4.1)].

If concomitant treatment of Cymbalta with a 5-hydroxytryptamine receptor agonist (triptan) is clinically warranted, careful observation of the patient is advised, particularly during treatment initiation and dose increases [see Drug Interactions (7.15)].

The concomitant use of Cymbalta with serotonin precursors (such as tryptophan) is not recommended [see Drug Interactions (7.14)].

Treatment with duloxetine and any concomitant serotonergic or antidopaminergic agents, including antipsychotics, should be discontinued immediately if the above events occur and supportive symptomatic treatment should be initiated.

5.5 Abnormal Bleeding

SSRIs and SNRIs, including duloxetine, may increase the risk of bleeding events. Concomitant use of aspirin, nonsteroidal anti-inflammatory drugs, warfarin, and other anticoagulants may add to this risk. Case reports and epidemiological studies (case-control and cohort design) have demonstrated an association between use of drugs that interfere with serotonin reuptake and the occurrence of gastrointestinal bleeding. Bleeding events related to SSRIs and SNRIs use have ranged from ecchymoses, hematomas, epistaxis, and petechiae to life-threatening hemorrhages.

Patients should be cautioned about the risk of bleeding associated with the concomitant use of duloxetine and NSAIDs, aspirin, or other drugs that affect coagulation.

5.6 Discontinuation of Treatment with Cymbalta

Discontinuation symptoms have been systematically evaluated in patients taking duloxetine. Following abrupt or tapered discontinuation in placebo-controlled clinical trials, the following symptoms occurred at a rate greater than or equal to 1% and at a significantly higher rate in duloxetine-treated patients compared to those discontinuing from placebo: dizziness, nausea, headache, fatigue, paresthesia, vomiting, irritability, nightmares, insomnia, diarrhea, anxiety, hyperhidrosis and vertigo.

During marketing of other SSRIs and SNRIs (serotonin and norepinephrine reuptake inhibitors), there have been spontaneous reports of adverse events occurring upon discontinuation of these drugs, particularly when abrupt, including the following: dysphoric mood, irritability, agitation, dizziness, sensory disturbances (e.g., paresthesias such as electric shock sensations), anxiety, confusion, headache, lethargy, emotional lability, insomnia, hypomania, tinnitus, and seizures. Although these events are generally self-limiting, some have been reported to be severe.

Patients should be monitored for these symptoms when discontinuing treatment with Cymbalta. A gradual reduction in the dose rather than abrupt cessation is recommended whenever possible. If intolerable symptoms occur following a decrease in the dose or upon discontinuation of treatment, then resuming the previously prescribed dose may be considered. Subsequently, the physician may continue decreasing the dose but at a more gradual rate [see Dosage and Administration (2.4)].

5.7 Activation of Mania/Hypomania

In placebo-controlled trials in patients with major depressive disorder, activation of mania or hypomania was reported in 0.1% (2/2,489) of duloxetine-treated patients and 0.1% (1/1,625) of placebo-treated patients. No activation of mania or hypomania was reported in DPNP, GAD, or fibromyalgia placebo-controlled trials. Activation of mania or hypomania has been reported in a small proportion of patients with mood disorders who were treated with other marketed drugs effective in the treatment of major depressive disorder. As with these other agents, Cymbalta should be used cautiously in patients with a history of mania.

5.8 Seizures

Duloxetine has not been systematically evaluated in patients with a seizure disorder, and such patients were excluded from clinical studies. In placebo-controlled clinical trials, seizures/convulsions occurred in 0.03% (3/9,445) of patients treated with duloxetine and 0.01% (1/6,770) of patients treated with placebo. Cymbalta should be prescribed with care in patients with a history of a seizure disorder.

5.9 Effect on Blood Pressure

In clinical trials across indications, relative to placebo, duloxetine treatment was associated with mean increases of up to 2.1 mm Hg in systolic blood pressure and up to 2.3 mm Hg in diastolic blood pressure. There was no significant difference in the frequency of sustained (3 consecutive visits) elevated blood pressure. In a clinical pharmacology study designed to evaluate the effects of duloxetine on various parameters, including blood pressure at supratherapeutic doses with an accelerated dose titration, there was evidence of increases in supine blood pressure at doses up to 200 mg twice daily. At the highest 200 mg twice daily dose, the increase in mean pulse rate was 5.0 to 6.8 beats and increases in mean blood pressure were 4.7 to 6.8 mm Hg (systolic) and 4.5 to 7 mm Hg (diastolic) up to 12 hours after dosing.

Blood pressure should be measured prior to initiating treatment and periodically measured throughout treatment [see Adverse Reactions (6.7)].

5.10 Clinically Important Drug Interactions

Both CYP1A2 and CYP2D6 are responsible for duloxetine metabolism.

Potential for Other Drugs to Affect Cymbalta

CYP1A2 Inhibitors—Co-administration of Cymbalta with potent CYP1A2 inhibitors should be avoided [see Drug Interactions (7.1)].

CYP2D6 Inhibitors—Because CYP2D6 is involved in duloxetine metabolism, concomitant use of duloxetine with potent inhibitors of CYP2D6 would be expected to, and does, result in higher concentrations (on average of 60%) of duloxetine [see Drug Interactions (7.2)].

Potential for Cymbalta to Affect Other Drugs

Drugs Metabolized by CYP2D6—Co-administration of Cymbalta with drugs that are extensively metabolized by CYP2D6 and that have a narrow therapeutic index, including certain antidepressants (tricyclic antidepressants [TCAs], such as nortriptyline, amitriptyline, and imipramine), phenothiazines and Type 1C antiarrhythmics (e.g., propafenone, flecainide), should be approached with caution. Plasma TCA concentrations may need to be monitored and the dose of the TCA may need to be reduced if a TCA is co-administered with Cymbalta. Because of the risk of serious ventricular arrhythmias and sudden death potentially associated with elevated plasma levels of thioridazine,

Cymbalta and thioridazine should not be co-administered [see Drug Interactions (7.9)].

Other Clinically Important Drug Interactions

Alcohol—Use of Cymbalta concomitantly with heavy alcohol intake may be associated with severe liver injury. For this reason, Cymbalta should ordinarily not be prescribed for patients with substantial alcohol use [see Warnings and Precautions (5.2) and Drug Interactions (7.16)].

CNS Acting Drugs—Given the primary CNS effects of Cymbalta, it should be used with caution when it is taken in combination with or substituted for other centrally acting drugs, including those with a similar mechanism of action [see Warnings and Precautions (5.10) and Drug Interactions (7.17)].

5.11   Hyponatremia

Hyponatremia may occur as a result of treatment with SSRIs and SNRIs, including Cymbalta. In many cases, this hyponatremia appears to be the result of the syndrome of inappropriate antidiuretic hormone secretion (SIADH). Cases with serum sodium lower than 110 mmol/L have been reported and appeared to be reversible when Cymbalta was discontinued. Elderly patients may be at greater risk of developing hyponatremia with SSRIs and SNRIs. Also, patients taking diuretics or who are otherwise volume depleted may be at greater risk [see Use in Specific Populations (8.5)]. Discontinuation of Cymbalta should be considered in patients with symptomatic hyponatremia and appropriate medical intervention should be instituted.

Signs and symptoms of hyponatremia include headache, difficulty concentrating, memory impairment, confusion, weakness, and unsteadiness, which may lead to falls. More severe and/or acute cases have been associated with hallucination, syncope, seizure, coma, respiratory arrest, and death.

5.12   Use in Patients with Concomitant Illness

Clinical experience with Cymbalta in patients with concomitant systemic illnesses is limited. There is no information on the effect that alterations in gastric motility may have on the stability of Cymbalta's enteric coating. In extremely acidic conditions, Cymbalta, unprotected by the enteric coating, may undergo hydrolysis to form naphthol. Caution is advised in using Cymbalta in patients with conditions that may slow gastric emptying (e.g., some diabetics).

Cymbalta has not been systematically evaluated in patients with a recent history of myocardial infarction or unstable coronary artery disease. Patients with these diagnoses were generally excluded from clinical studies during the product's premarketing testing.

Hepatic Insufficiency—Cymbalta should ordinarily not be used in patients with hepatic insufficiency [see Dosage and Administration (2.3), Warnings and Precautions (5.2), and Use in Specific Populations (8.9)].

Severe Renal Impairment—Cymbalta should ordinarily not be used in patients with end-stage renal disease or severe renal impairment (creatinine clearance <30 mL/min). Increased plasma concentration of duloxetine, and especially of its metabolites, occur in patients with end-stage renal disease (requiring dialysis) [see Dosage and Administration (2.3) and Use in Specific Populations (8.10)].

Controlled Narrow-Angle Glaucoma—In clinical trials, Cymbalta was associated with an increased risk of mydriasis; therefore, it should be used cautiously in patients with controlled narrow-angle glaucoma [see Contraindications (4.2)].

Glycemic Control in Patients with Diabetes—As observed in DPNP trials, Cymbalta treatment worsens glycemic control in some patients with diabetes. In three clinical trials of Cymbalta for the management of neuropathic pain associated with diabetic peripheral neuropathy, the mean duration of diabetes was approximately 12 years, the mean baseline fasting blood glucose was 176 mg/dL, and the mean baseline hemoglobin A_{1c} (HbA_{1c}) was 7.8%. In the 12-week acute treatment phase of these studies, Cymbalta was associated with a small increase in mean fasting blood glucose as compared to placebo. In the extension phase of these studies, which lasted up to 52 weeks, mean fasting blood glucose increased by 12 mg/dL in the Cymbalta group and decreased by 11.5 mg/dL in the routine care group. HbA_{1c} increased by 0.5% in the Cymbalta and by 0.2% in the routine care groups.

5.13   Urinary Hesitation and Retention

Cymbalta is in a class of drugs known to affect urethral resistance. If symptoms of urinary hesitation develop during treatment with Cymbalta, consideration should be given to the possibility that they might be drug-related.

In post marketing experience, cases of urinary retention have been observed. In some instances of urinary retention associated with duloxetine use, hospitalization and/or catheterization has been needed.

5.14   Laboratory Tests

No specific laboratory tests are recommended.

6   ADVERSE REACTIONS

6.1   Clinical Trial Data Sources

The data described below reflect exposure to duloxetine in placebo-controlled trials for MDD (N=2,327), GAD (N=668), DPNP (N=568), and FM (N=876). The population studied was 17 to 89 years of age; 64.8%, 64.7%, 38.7%, and 94.6% female; and 85.5%, 84.6%, 77.6%, and 88% Caucasian for MDD, GAD, DPNP, and FM, respectively. Most patients received doses of a total of 60 to 120 mg per day [see Clinical Studies (14)].

The stated frequencies of adverse reactions represent the proportion of individuals who experienced, at least once, a treatment-emergent adverse reaction of the type listed. A reaction was considered treatment-emergent if it occurred for the first time or worsened while receiving therapy following baseline evaluation. Reactions reported during the studies were not necessarily caused by the therapy, and the frequencies do not reflect investigator impression (assessment) of causality.

Because clinical trials are conducted under widely varying conditions, adverse reaction rates observed in the clinical trials of a drug cannot be directly compared to rates in the clinical trials of another drug and may not reflect the rates observed in practice.

6.2   Adverse Reactions Reported as Reasons for Discontinuation of Treatment in Placebo-Controlled Trials

Major Depressive Disorder—Approximately 9% (209/2,327) of the patients who received duloxetine in placebo-controlled trials for MDD discontinued treatment due to an adverse reaction, compared with 4.7% (68/1,460) of the patients receiving placebo. Nausea (duloxetine 1.3%, placebo 0.5%) was the only common adverse reaction reported as a reason for discontinuation and considered to be drug-related (i.e., discontinuation occurring in at least 1% of the duloxetine-treated patients and at a rate of at least twice that of placebo).

Generalized Anxiety Disorder—Approximately 15.3% (102/668) of the patients who received duloxetine in placebo-controlled trials for GAD discontinued treatment due to an adverse reaction, compared with 4.0% (20/495) for placebo. Common adverse reactions reported as a reason for discontinuation and considered to be drug-related (as defined above) included nausea (duloxetine 3.7%, placebo 0.2%), vomiting (duloxetine 1.3%, placebo 0.0%), and dizziness (duloxetine 1.0%, placebo 0.2%).

Diabetic Peripheral Neuropathic Pain—Approximately 14.3% (81/568) of the patients who received duloxetine in placebo-controlled trials for DPNP discontinued treatment due to an adverse reaction, compared with 7.2% (16/223) for placebo. Common adverse reactions reported as a reason for discontinuation and considered to be drug-related (as defined above) were nausea (duloxetine 3.5%, placebo 0.4%), dizziness (duloxetine 1.6%, placebo 0.4%), somnolence (duloxetine 1.6%, placebo 0.0%), and fatigue (duloxetine 1.1%, placebo 0.0%).

Fibromyalgia—Approximately 19.5% (171/876) of the patients who received duloxetine in 3 to 6 month placebo-controlled trials for FM discontinued treatment due to an adverse reaction, compared with 11.8% (63/535) for placebo. Common adverse reactions reported as a reason for discontinuation and considered to be drug-related (as defined above) included nausea (duloxetine 1.9%, placebo 0.7%), somnolence (duloxetine 1.5%, placebo 0.0%), and fatigue (duloxetine 1.3%, placebo 0.2%).

6.3   Adverse Reactions Occurring at an Incidence of 5% or More and at least Twice Placebo Among Duloxetine-Treated Patients in Placebo-Controlled Trials

Pooled Trials for all Approved Indications—The most commonly observed adverse reactions in Cymbalta-treated patients (incidence of at least 5% and at least twice the incidence in placebo patients) were nausea, dry mouth, constipation, somnolence, hyperhidrosis, and decreased appetite.

In addition to the adverse reactions listed above, DPNP trials also included dizziness and asthenia.

6.4   Adverse Reactions Occurring at an Incidence of 5% or More Among Duloxetine-Treated Patients in Placebo-Controlled Trials

Table 2 gives the incidence of treatment-emergent adverse reactions in placebo-controlled trials for approved indications that occurred in 5% or more of patients treated with duloxetine and with an incidence greater than placebo.

Table 2: Treatment-Emergent Adverse Reactions: Incidence of 5% or More in Placebo-Controlled Trials of Approved Indications

Adverse Reaction	Percentage of Patients Reporting Reaction	
	Cymbalta (N=4843)	Placebo (N=3048)
Nausea	25	9
Headache	16	15
Dry mouth	14	6
Fatigue[b]	11	6
Insomnia[a,c]	11	7
Dizziness	11	6
Somnolence[a,d]	11	3
Constipation[a]	11	4
Diarrhea	10	7
Decreased appetite[a,e]	8	2
Hyperhidrosis	7	2

[a] Events for which there was a significant dose-dependent relationship in fixed-dose studies, excluding three MDD studies which did not have a placebo lead-in period or dose titration.
[b] Also includes asthenia
[c] Also includes middle insomnia, early morning awakening, and initial insomnia
[d] Also includes hypersomnia and sedation
[e] Also includes anorexia

6.5   Adverse Reactions Occurring at an Incidence of 2% or More Among Duloxetine-Treated Patients in Placebo-Controlled Trials

Pooled MDD and GAD Trials—Table 3 gives the incidence of treatment-emergent adverse reactions in MDD and GAD placebo-controlled trials for approved indications that occurred in 2% or more of patients treated with duloxetine and with an incidence greater than placebo.

Table 3: Treatment-Emergent Adverse Reactions: Incidence of 2% or More in MDD and GAD Placebo-Controlled Trials

System Organ Class/ Adverse Reaction	Percentage of Patients Reporting Reaction	
	Cymbalta (N=2995)	Placebo (N=1955)
Cardiac Disorders		
Palpitations	2	2
Eye Disorders		
Vision blurred	3	2
Gastrointestinal Disorders		
Nausea	25	9
Dry mouth	15	6
Diarrhea	10	7
Constipation[a]	10	4
Abdominal pain[b]	4	4
Vomiting	5	2
General Disorders and Administration Site Conditions		
Fatigue[c]	10	6
Investigations		
Weight decreased[a]	2	<1
Metabolism and Nutrition Disorders		
Decreased appetite[d]	7	2
Nervous System Disorders		
Dizziness	10	6
Somnolence[e]	10	4
Tremor	3	<1
Psychiatric Disorders		
Insomnia[f]	10	6
Agitation[g]	5	3
Anxiety	3	2
Libido decreased[h]	4	1
Orgasm abnormal[j]	3	<1
Abnormal dreams[j]	2	1
Reproductive System and Breast Disorders		
Erectile dysfunction[k]	5	1
Ejaculation delayed[a,k]	3	<1
Ejaculation disorder[k,l]	2	<1
Respiratory, Thoracic, and Mediastinal Disorders		
Yawning	2	<1

Skin and Subcutaneous Tissue Disorders		
Hyperhidrosis	6	2

Vascular Disorders		
Hot flush	2	<1

[a] Events for which there was a significant dose-dependent relationship in fixed-dose studies, excluding three MDD studies which did not have a placebo lead-in period or dose titration.
[b] Also includes abdominal pain upper, abdominal pain lower, abdominal tenderness, abdominal discomfort, and gastrointestinal pain
[c] Also includes asthenia
[d] Also includes anorexia
[e] Also includes hypersomnia and sedation
[f] Also includes middle insomnia, early morning awakening, and initial insomnia
[g] Also includes feeling jittery, nervousness, restlessness, tension, and psychomotor agitation
[h] Also includes loss of libido
[i] Also includes anorgasmia
[j] Also includes nightmare
[k] Male patients only
[l] Also includes ejaculation failure and ejaculation dysfunction

Diabetic Peripheral Neuropathic Pain—Table 4 gives the incidence of treatment-emergent adverse events that occurred in 2% or more of patients treated with Cymbalta in the premarketing acute phase of DPNP placebo-controlled trials (doses of 20 to 120 mg/day) and with an incidence greater than placebo.
[See table 4 at top right]
Fibromyalgia—Table 5 gives the incidence of treatment-emergent adverse events that occurred in 2% or more of patients treated with Cymbalta in the premarketing acute phase of FM placebo-controlled trials and with an incidence greater than placebo.

Table 5: Treatment-Emergent Adverse Reactions: Incidence of 2% or More in Fibromyalgia Placebo-Controlled Trials

System Organ Class/Adverse Reaction	Percentage of Patients Reporting Reaction	
	Cymbalta (N=876)	Placebo (N=535)
Cardiac Disorders		
Palpitations	2	2
Eye Disorders		
Vision blurred	2	1
Gastrointestinal Disorders		
Nausea	29	11
Dry mouth	18	5
Constipation	15	4
Diarrhea	12	8
Dyspepsia	5	3
General Disorders and Administration Site Conditions		
Fatigue[b]	15	8
Immune System Disorders		
Seasonal allergy	3	2
Infections and Infestations		
Upper respiratory tract infection	7	6
Urinary tract infection	3	3
Influenza	2	2
Gastroenteritis viral	2	2
Investigations		
Weight increased	2	1
Metabolism and Nutrition Disorders		
Decreased appetite[c]	11	2
Musculoskeletal and Connective Tissue Disorders		
Musculoskeletal pain	5	4
Muscle spasms	4	3
Nervous System Disorders		
Headache	20	12
Dizziness	11	7
Somnolence[d]	11	3
Tremor	4	1
Paraesthesia	4	4
Migraine	3	3
Dysgeusia	3	1
Psychiatric Disorders		
Insomnia[e]	16	10
Agitation[f]	6	2
Sleep disorder	3	2
Abnormal dreams[g]	3	1
Orgasm abnormal[h]	3	<1
Libido decreased[i]	2	<1
Reproductive System and Breast Disorders		
Ejaculation disorder[a,j]	4	0
Penis disorder[a]	2	0
Respiratory, Thoracic, and Mediastinal Disorders		
Cough	4	3
Pharyngolaryngeal pain	3	3
Skin and Subcutaneous Tissue Disorders		
Hyperhidrosis	7	1
Rash	4	2
Pruritis	3	2
Vascular Disorders		
Hot flush	3	2

Table 4: Treatment-Emergent Adverse Reactions Incidence of 2% or More in DPNP Placebo-Controlled Trials

System Organ Class/Adverse Reaction	Percentage of Patients Reporting Reaction			
	Cymbalta 20 mg once daily (N=115)	Cymbalta 60 mg once daily (N=228)	Cymbalta 60 mg twice daily (N=225)	Placebo (N=223)
Gastrointestinal Disorders				
Nausea	14	22	30	9
Constipation	5	11	15	3
Diarrhea	13	11	7	6
Dry mouth	5	7	12	4
Vomiting	6	5	5	4
Dyspepsia	4	4	4	3
Loose stools	2	3	2	1
General Disorders and Administration Site Conditions				
Fatigue	2	10	12	5
Asthenia	2	4	8	1
Pyrexia	2	1	3	1
Infections and Infestations				
Nasopharyngitis	9	7	9	5
Metabolism and Nutrition Disorders				
Decreased appetite	3	4	11	<1
Anorexia	3	3	5	<1
Musculoskeletal and Connective Tissue Disorders				
Muscle cramp	5	4	4	3
Myalgia	3	1	4	<1
Nervous System Disorders				
Somnolence	7	15	21	5
Headache	13	13	15	10
Dizziness	6	14	17	6
Tremor	0	1	5	0
Psychiatric Disorders				
Insomnia	9	8	13	7
Renal and Urinary Disorders				
Pollakiuria	3	1	5	2
Reproductive System and Breast Disorders				
Erectile dysfunction[a]	0	1	4	0
Respiratory, Thoracic and Mediastinal Disorders				
Cough	6	3	5	4
Pharyngolaryngeal pain	3	1	6	1
Skin and Subcutaneous Tissue Disorders				
Hyperhidrosis	6	6	8	2

[a] Male patients only.

[a] Male patients only (N = 46 duloxetine-treated patients versus 26 placebo patients)
[b] Also includes asthenia
[c] Also includes anorexia
[d] Also includes hypersomnia and sedation
[e] Also includes middle insomnia, early morning awakening, and initial insomnia
[f] Also includes feeling jittery, nervousness, restlessness, tension, and psychomotor agitation
[g] Also includes nightmare
[h] Also includes anorgasmia
[i] Also includes loss of libido
[j] Also includes ejaculation failure and ejaculation dysfunction

6.6   Effects on Male and Female Sexual Function
Changes in sexual desire, sexual performance and sexual satisfaction often occur as manifestations of psychiatric disorders or diabetes, but they may also be a consequence of pharmacologic treatment. Because adverse sexual reactions are presumed to be voluntarily underreported, the Arizona Sexual Experience Scale (ASEX), a validated measure designed to identify sexual side effects, was used prospectively in 4 MDD placebo-controlled trials. In these trials, as shown in Table 6 below, patients treated with Cymbalta experienced significantly more sexual dysfunction, as measured by the total score on the ASEX, than did patients treated with placebo. Gender analysis showed that this difference occurred only in males. Males treated with Cymbalta experienced more difficulty with ability to reach orgasm (ASEX Item 4) than males treated with placebo. Females did not experience more sexual dysfunction on Cymbalta than on

Table 6: Mean Change in ASEX Scores by Gender in MDD Placebo-Controlled Trials

	Male Patients[a]		Female Patients[a]	
	Cymbalta (n=175)	Placebo (n=83)	Cymbalta (n=241)	Placebo (n=126)
ASEX Total (Items 1-5)	0.56[b]	-1.07	-1.15	-1.07
Item 1—Sex drive	-0.07	-0.12	-0.32	-0.24
Item 2—Arousal	0.01	-0.26	-0.21	-0.18
Item 3—Ability to achieve erection (men); Lubrication (women)	0.03	-0.25	-0.17	-0.18
Item 4—Ease of reaching orgasm	0.40[c]	-0.24	-0.09	-0.13
Item 5—Orgasm satisfaction	0.09	-0.13	-0.11	-0.17

[a] n=Number of patients with non-missing change score for ASEX total
[b] p=0.013 versus placebo
[c] p<0.001 versus placebo

placebo as measured by ASEX total score. Negative numbers signify an improvement from a baseline level of dysfunction, which is commonly seen in depressed patients. Physicians should routinely inquire about possible sexual side effects.
[See table 6 above]

6.7 Vital Sign Changes
In clinical trials across indications, relative to placebo, duloxetine treatment was associated with mean increases of up to 2.1 mm Hg in systolic blood pressure and up to 2.3 mm Hg in diastolic blood pressure. There was no significant difference in the frequency of sustained (3 consecutive visits) elevated blood pressure [see Warnings and Precautions (5.3 and 5.9)].
Duloxetine treatment, for up to 26 weeks in placebo-controlled trials typically caused a small increase in heart rate compared to placebo of up to 3-4 beats per minute.

6.8 Weight Changes
In placebo-controlled clinical trials, MDD and GAD patients treated with Cymbalta for up to 10 weeks experienced a mean weight loss of approximately 0.5 kg, compared with a mean weight gain of approximately 0.2 kg in placebo-treated patients. In DPN placebo-controlled clinical trials, patients treated with Cymbalta for up to 13-weeks experienced a mean weight loss of approximately 1.1 kg, compared with a mean weight gain of approximately 0.2 kg in placebo-treated patients. In fibromyalgia studies, patients treated with Cymbalta for up to 26 weeks experienced a mean weight loss of approximately 0.4 kg compared with a mean weight gain of approximately 0.3 kg in placebo-treated patients. In one long-term fibromyalgia 60-week uncontrolled study, duloxetine patients had a mean weight increase of 0.7 kg.

6.9 Laboratory Changes
Cymbalta treatment in placebo-controlled clinical trials, was associated with small mean increases from baseline to endpoint in ALT, AST, CPK, and alkaline phosphatase; infrequent, modest, transient, abnormal values were observed for these analytes in Cymbalta-treated patients when compared with placebo-treated patients [see Warnings and Precautions (5.2)].

6.10 Electrocardiogram Changes
Electrocardiograms were obtained from duloxetine-treated patients and placebo-treated patients in clinical trials lasting up to 13 weeks. No clinically significant differences were observed for QTc, QT, PR, and QRS intervals between duloxetine-treated and placebo-treated patients. There were no differences in clinically meaningful QTcF elevations between duloxetine and placebo. In a positive-controlled study in healthy volunteers using duloxetine up to 200 mg twice daily, no prolongation of the corrected QT interval was observed.

6.11 Other Adverse Reactions Observed During the Pre-marketing and Postmarketing Clinical Trial Evaluation of Duloxetine
Following is a list of treatment-emergent adverse reactions reported by patients treated with duloxetine in clinical trials. In clinical trials of all indications, 27,229 patients were treated with duloxetine. Of these, 29% (7,886) took duloxetine for at least 6 months, and 13.3% (3,614) for at least one year. The following listing is not intended to include reactions (1) already listed in previous tables or elsewhere in labeling, (2) for which a drug cause was remote, (3) which were so general as to be uninformative, (4) which were not considered to have significant clinical implications, or (5) which occurred at a rate equal to or less than placebo. Reactions are categorized by body system according to the following definitions: frequent adverse reactions are those occurring in at least 1/100 patients; infrequent adverse reactions are those occurring in 1/100 to 1/1000 patients; rare reactions are those occurring in fewer than 1/1000 patients.

Cardiac Disorders—*Frequent:* palpitations; *Infrequent:* myocardial infarction and tachycardia.

Ear and Labyrinth Disorders—*Frequent:* vertigo; *Infrequent:* ear pain and tinnitus.
Endocrine Disorders—*Infrequent:* hypothyroidism.
Eye Disorders—*Frequent:* vision blurred; *Infrequent:* diplopia and visual disturbance.
Gastrointestinal Disorders—*Frequent:* flatulence; *Infrequent:* eructation, gastritis, halitosis, and stomatitis; *Rare:* gastric ulcer, hematochezia, and melena.
General Disorders and Administration Site Conditions—*Frequent:* chills/rigors; *Infrequent:* feeling abnormal, feeling hot and/or cold, malaise, and thirst; *Rare:* gait disturbance.
Infections and Infestations—*Infrequent:* gastroenteritis and laryngitis.
Investigations—*Frequent:* weight increased; *Infrequent:* blood cholesterol increased.
Metabolism and Nutrition Disorders—*Infrequent:* dehydration and hyperlipidemia; *Rare:* dyslipidemia.
Musculoskeletal and Connective Tissue Disorders—*Frequent:* musculoskeletal pain; *Infrequent:* muscle tightness and muscle twitching.
Nervous System Disorders—*Frequent:* dysgeusia, lethargy, and parasthesia/hypoesthesia; *Infrequent:* disturbance in attention, dyskinesia, myoclonus, and poor quality sleep; *Rare:* dysarthria.
Psychiatric Disorders—*Frequent:* abnormal dreams and sleep disorder; *Infrequent:* apathy, bruxism, disorientation/confusional state, irritability, mood swings, and suicide attempt; *Rare:* completed suicide.
Renal and Urinary Disorders—*Infrequent:* dysuria, micturition urgency, nocturia, polyuria, and urine odor abnormal.
Reproductive System and Breast Disorders—*Frequent:* anorgasmia/orgasm abnormal; *Infrequent:* menopausal symptoms, and sexual dysfunction.
Respiratory, Thoracic and Mediastinal Disorders—*Frequent:* yawning; *Infrequent:* throat tightness.
Skin and Subcutaneous Tissue Disorders—*Infrequent:* cold sweat, dermatitis contact, erythema, increased tendency to bruise, night sweats, and photosensitivity reaction; *Rare:* ecchymosis.
Vascular Disorders—*Frequent:* hot flush; *Infrequent:* flushing, orthostatic hypotension, and peripheral coldness.

6.12 Postmarketing Spontaneous Reports
The following adverse reactions have been identified during postapproval use of Cymbalta. Because these reactions are reported voluntarily from a population of uncertain size, it is not always possible to reliably estimate their frequency or establish a causal relationship to drug exposure.

Adverse reactions reported since market introduction that were temporally related to duloxetine therapy and not mentioned elsewhere in labeling include: anaphylactic reaction, aggression and anger (particularly early in treatment or after treatment discontinuation), angioneurotic edema, erythema multiforme, extrapyramidal disorder, glaucoma, gynecological bleeding, hallucinations, hyperglycemia, hypersensitivity, hypertensive crisis, muscle spasm, rash, restless legs syndrome, seizures upon treatment discontinuation, supraventricular arrhythmia, tinnitus (upon treatment discontinuation), trismus, and urticaria.

Serious skin reactions including Stevens-Johnson Syndrome that have required drug discontinuation and/or hospitalization have been reported with duloxetine.

7 DRUG INTERACTIONS
Both CYP1A2 and CYP2D6 are responsible for duloxetine metabolism.

7.1 Inhibitors of CYP1A2
When duloxetine 60 mg was co-administered with fluvoxamine 100 mg, a potent CYP1A2 inhibitor, to male subjects (n=14) duloxetine AUC was increased approximately 6-fold, the C_{max} was increased about 2.5-fold, and duloxetine $t_{1/2}$ was increased approximately 3-fold. Other drugs that in-

hibit CYP1A2 metabolism include cimetidine and quinolone antimicrobials such as ciprofloxacin and enoxacin [see Warnings and Precautions (5.10)].

7.2 Inhibitors of CYP2D6
Concomitant use of duloxetine (40 mg once daily) with paroxetine (20 mg once daily) increased the concentration of duloxetine AUC by about 60%, and greater degrees of inhibition are expected with higher doses of paroxetine. Similar effects would be expected with other potent CYP2D6 inhibitors (e.g., fluoxetine, quinidine) [see Warnings and Precautions (5.10)].

7.3 Dual Inhibition of CYP1A2 and CYP2D6
Concomitant administration of duloxetine 40 mg twice daily with fluvoxamine 100 mg, a potent CYP1A2 inhibitor, to CYP2D6 poor metabolizer subjects (n=14) resulted in a 6-fold increase in duloxetine AUC and C_{max}.

7.4 Drugs that Interfere with Hemostasis (e.g., NSAIDs, Aspirin, and Warfarin)
Serotonin release by platelets plays an important role in hemostasis. Epidemiological studies of the case-control and cohort design that have demonstrated an association between use of psychotropic drugs that interfere with serotonin reuptake and the occurrence of upper gastrointestinal bleeding have also shown that concurrent use of an NSAID or aspirin may potentiate this risk of bleeding. Altered anticoagulant effects, including increased bleeding, have been reported when SSRIs or SNRIs are coadministered with warfarin. Patients receiving warfarin therapy should be carefully monitored when duloxetine is initiated or discontinued [see Warnings and Precautions (5.5)].

7.5 Lorazepam
Under steady-state conditions for duloxetine (60 mg Q 12 hours) and lorazepam (2 mg Q 12 hours), the pharmacokinetics of duloxetine were not affected by co-administration.

7.6 Temazepam
Under steady-state conditions for duloxetine (20 mg qhs) and temazepam (30 mg qhs), the pharmacokinetics of duloxetine were not affected by co-administration.

7.7 Drugs that Affect Gastric Acidity
Cymbalta has an enteric coating that resists dissolution until reaching a segment of the gastrointestinal tract where the pH exceeds 5.5. In extremely acidic conditions, Cymbalta, unprotected by the enteric coating, may undergo hydrolysis to form naphthol. Caution is advised in using Cymbalta in patients with conditions that may slow gastric emptying (e.g., some diabetics). Drugs that raise the gastrointestinal pH may lead to an earlier release of duloxetine. However, co-administration of Cymbalta with aluminum- and magnesium-containing antacids (51 mEq) or Cymbalta with famotidine, had no significant effect on the rate or extent of duloxetine absorption after administration of a 40 mg oral dose. It is unknown whether the concomitant administration of proton pump inhibitors affects duloxetine absorption [see Warnings and Precautions (5.12)].

7.8 Drugs Metabolized by CYP1A2
In vitro drug interaction studies demonstrate that duloxetine does not induce CYP1A2 activity. Therefore, an increase in the metabolism of CYP1A2 substrates (e.g., theophylline, caffeine) resulting from induction is not anticipated, although clinical studies of induction have not been performed. Duloxetine is an inhibitor of the CYP1A2 isoform in *in vitro* studies, and in two clinical studies the average (90% confidence interval) increase in theophylline AUC was 7% (1%-15%) and 20% (13%-27%) when co-administered with duloxetine (60 mg twice daily).

7.9 Drugs Metabolized by CYP2D6
Duloxetine is a moderate inhibitor of CYP2D6. When duloxetine was administered (at a dose of 60 mg twice daily) in conjunction with a single 50 mg dose of desipramine, a CYP2D6 substrate, the AUC of desipramine increased 3-fold [see Warnings and Precautions (5.10)].

7.10 Drugs Metabolized by CYP2C9
Duloxetine does not inhibit the *in vitro* enzyme activity of CYP2C9. Inhibition of the metabolism of CYP2C9 substrates is therefore not anticipated, although clinical studies have not been performed.

7.11 Drugs Metabolized by CYP3A
Results of *in vitro* studies demonstrate that duloxetine does not inhibit or induce CYP3A activity. Therefore, an increase or decrease in the metabolism of CYP3A substrates (e.g., oral contraceptives and other steroidal agents) resulting from induction or inhibition is not anticipated, although clinical studies have not been performed.

7.12 Drugs Metabolized by CYP2C19
Results of *in vitro* studies demonstrate that duloxetine does not inhibit CYP2C19 activity at therapeutic concentrations. Inhibition of the metabolism of CYP2C19 substrates is therefore not anticipated, although clinical studies have not been performed.

7.13 Monoamine Oxidase Inhibitors
[see Dosage and Administration (2.5), Contraindications (4.1), and Warnings and Precautions (5.4)].

7.14 Serotonergic Drugs

Based on the mechanism of action of SNRIs and SSRIs, including Cymbalta, and the potential for serotonin syndrome, caution is advised when Cymbalta is co-administered with other drugs that may affect the serotonergic neurotransmitter systems, such as triptans, linezolid (an antibiotic which is a reversible non-selective MAOI), lithium, tramadol, or St. John's Wort. The concomitant use of Cymbalta with other SSRIs, SNRIs or tryptophan is not recommended *[see Warnings and Precautions (5.4)]*.

7.15 Triptans

There have been rare postmarketing reports of serotonin syndrome with use of an SSRI and a triptan. If concomitant treatment of Cymbalta with a triptan is clinically warranted, careful observation of the patient is advised, particularly during treatment initiation and dose increases *[see Warnings and Precautions (5.4)]*.

7.16 Alcohol

When Cymbalta and ethanol were administered several hours apart so that peak concentrations of each would coincide, Cymbalta did not increase the impairment of mental and motor skills caused by alcohol.

In the Cymbalta clinical trials database, three Cymbalta-treated patients had liver injury as manifested by ALT and total bilirubin elevations, with evidence of obstruction. Substantial intercurrent ethanol use was present in each of these cases, and this may have contributed to the abnormalities seen *[see Warnings and Precautions (5.2 and 5.10)]*.

7.17 CNS Drugs

[see Warnings and Precautions (5.10)].

7.18 Drugs Highly Bound to Plasma Protein

Because duloxetine is highly bound to plasma protein, administration of Cymbalta to a patient taking another drug that is highly protein bound may cause increased free concentrations of the other drug, potentially resulting in adverse reactions.

8 USE IN SPECIFIC POPULATIONS

8.1 Pregnancy

Teratogenic Effects, Pregnancy Category C—In animal reproduction studies, duloxetine has been shown to have adverse effects on embryo/fetal and postnatal development.

When duloxetine was administered orally to pregnant rats and rabbits during the period of organogenesis, there was no evidence of teratogenicity at doses up to 45 mg/kg/day (7 times the maximum recommended human dose [MRHD, 60 mg/day] and 4 times the human dose of 120 mg/day on a mg/m^2 basis, in rat; 15 times the MRHD and 7 times the human dose of 120 mg/day on a mg/m^2 basis in rabbit). However, fetal weights were decreased at this dose, with a no-effect dose of 10 mg/kg/day (2 times the MRHD and $\approx$1 times the human dose of 120 mg/day on a mg/m^2 basis in rat; 3 times the MRHD and 2 times the human dose of 120 mg/day on a mg/m^2 basis in rabbits).

When duloxetine was administered orally to pregnant rats throughout gestation and lactation, the survival of pups to 1 day postpartum and pup body weights at birth and during the lactation period were decreased at a dose of 30 mg/kg/day (5 times the MRHD and 2 times the human dose of 120 mg/day on a mg/m^2 basis); the no-effect dose was 10 mg/kg/day. Furthermore, behaviors consistent with increased reactivity, such as increased startle response to noise and decreased habituation of locomotor activity, were observed in pups following maternal exposure to 30 mg/kg/day. Post-weaning growth and reproductive performance of the progeny were not affected adversely by maternal duloxetine treatment.

There are no adequate and well-controlled studies in pregnant women; therefore, duloxetine should be used during pregnancy only if the potential benefit justifies the potential risk to the fetus.

Nonteratogenic Effects—Neonates exposed to SSRIs or serotonin and norepinephrine reuptake inhibitors (SNRIs), late in the third trimester have developed complications requiring prolonged hospitalization, respiratory support, and tube feeding. Such complications can arise immediately upon delivery. Reported clinical findings have included respiratory distress, cyanosis, apnea, seizures, temperature instability, feeding difficulty, vomiting, hypoglycemia, hypotonia, hypertonia, hyperreflexia, tremor, jitteriness, irritability, and constant crying. These features are consistent with either a direct toxic effect of SSRIs and SNRIs or, possibly, a drug discontinuation syndrome. It should be noted that, in some cases, the clinical picture is consistent with serotonin syndrome *[see Warnings and Precautions (5.4)]*.

When treating pregnant women with Cymbalta during the third trimester, the physician should carefully consider the potential risks and benefits of treatment. The physician may consider tapering Cymbalta in the third trimester *[see Dosage and Administration (2.3)]*.

8.2 Labor and Delivery

The effect of duloxetine on labor and delivery in humans is unknown. Duloxetine should be used during labor and delivery only if the potential benefit justifies the potential risk to the fetus.

8.3 Nursing Mothers

Duloxetine is excreted into the milk of lactating women. The estimated daily infant dose on a mg/kg basis is approximately 0.14% of the maternal dose. Because the safety of duloxetine in infants is not known, nursing while on Cymbalta is not recommended. However, if the physician determines that the benefit of duloxetine therapy for the mother outweighs any potential risk to the infant, no dosage adjustment is required as lactation did not influence duloxetine pharmacokinetics.

The disposition of duloxetine was studied in 6 lactating women who were at least 12 weeks postpartum. Duloxetine 40 mg twice daily was given for 3.5 days. Like many other drugs, duloxetine is detected in breast milk, and steady state concentrations in breast milk are about one-fourth those in plasma. The amount of duloxetine in breast milk is approximately 7 µg/day while on 40 mg BID dosing. The excretion of duloxetine metabolites into breast milk was not examined. Because the safety of duloxetine in infants is not known, nursing while on Cymbalta is not recommended *[see Dosage and Administration (2.3)]*.

8.4 Pediatric Use

Safety and effectiveness in the pediatric population have not been established *[see Boxed Warning and Warnings and Precautions (5.1)]*. Anyone considering the use of Cymbalta in a child or adolescent must balance the potential risks with the clinical need.

8.5 Geriatric Use

Of the 2,418 patients in premarketing clinical studies of Cymbalta for MDD, 5.9% (143) were 65 years of age or over. Of the 1,074 patients in the DPNP premarketing studies, 33% (357) were 65 years of age or over. Of the 1,761 patients in FM premarketing studies, 7.9% (140) were 65 years of age or over. Premarketing clinical studies of GAD did not include sufficient numbers of subjects age 65 or over to determine whether they respond differently from younger subjects. In the MDD, DPNP, and FM studies, no overall differences in safety or effectiveness were observed between these subjects and younger subjects, and other reported clinical experience has not identified differences in responses between the elderly and younger patients, but greater sensitivity of some older individuals cannot be ruled out. SSRIs and SNRIs, including Cymbalta have been associated with cases of clinically significant hyponatremia in elderly patients, who may be at greater risk for this adverse event *[see Warnings and Precautions (5.11)]*.

The pharmacokinetics of duloxetine after a single dose of 40 mg were compared in healthy elderly females (65 to 77 years) and healthy middle-age females (32 to 50 years). There was no difference in the C_{max}, but the AUC of duloxetine was somewhat (about 25%) higher and the half-life about 4 hours longer in the elderly females. Population pharmacokinetic analyses suggest that the typical values for clearance decrease by approximately 1% for each year of age between 25 to 75 years of age; but age as a predictive factor only accounts for a small percentage of between-patient variability. Dosage adjustment based on the age of the patient is not necessary *[see Dosage and Administration (2.3)]*.

8.6 Gender

Duloxetine's half-life is similar in men and women. Dosage adjustment based on gender is not necessary.

8.7 Smoking Status

Duloxetine bioavailability (AUC) appears to be reduced by about one-third in smokers. Dosage modifications are not recommended for smokers.

8.8 Race

No specific pharmacokinetic study was conducted to investigate the effects of race.

8.9 Hepatic Insufficiency

Patients with clinically evident hepatic insufficiency have decreased duloxetine metabolism and elimination. After a single 20 mg dose of Cymbalta, 6 cirrhotic patients with moderate liver impairment (Child-Pugh Class B) had a mean plasma duloxetine clearance about 15% that of age- and gender-matched healthy subjects, with a 5-fold increase in mean exposure (AUC). Although C_{max} was similar to normals in the cirrhotic patients, the half-life was about 3 times longer *[see Dosage and Administration (2.3) and Warnings and Precautions (5.12)]*.

8.10 Severe Renal Impairment

Limited data are available on the effects of duloxetine in patients with end-stage renal disease (ESRD). After a single 60 mg dose of duloxetine, C_{max} and AUC values were approximately 100% greater in patients with end-stage renal disease receiving chronic intermittent hemodialysis than in subjects with normal renal function. The elimination half-life, however, was similar in both groups. The AUCs of the major circulating metabolites, 4-hydroxy duloxetine glucuronide and 5-hydroxy, 6-methoxy duloxetine sulfate, largely excreted in urine, were approximately 7- to 9-fold higher and would be expected to increase further with multiple dosing. Population PK analyses suggest that mild to moderate degrees of renal dysfunction (estimated CrCl 30-80 mL/min) have no significant effect on duloxetine apparent clearance *[see Dosage and Administration (2.3) and Warnings and Precautions (5.12)]*.

9 DRUG ABUSE AND DEPENDENCE

9.2 Abuse

In animal studies, duloxetine did not demonstrate barbiturate-like (depressant) abuse potential.

While Cymbalta has not been systematically studied in humans for its potential for abuse, there was no indication of drug-seeking behavior in the clinical trials. However, it is not possible to predict on the basis of premarketing experience the extent to which a CNS active drug will be misused, diverted, and/or abused once marketed. Consequently, physicians should carefully evaluate patients for a history of drug abuse and follow such patients closely, observing them for signs of misuse or abuse of Cymbalta (e.g., development of tolerance, incrementation of dose, drug-seeking behavior).

9.3 Dependence

In drug dependence studies, duloxetine did not demonstrate dependence-producing potential in rats.

10 OVERDOSAGE

10.1 Signs and Symptoms

In postmarketing experience, fatal outcomes have been reported for acute overdoses, primarily with mixed overdoses, but also with duloxetine only, at doses as low as 1000 mg. Signs and symptoms of overdose (duloxetine alone or with mixed drugs) included somnolence, coma, serotonin syndrome, seizures, syncope, tachycardia, hypotension, hypertension, and vomiting.

10.2 Management of Overdose

There is no specific antidote to Cymbalta, but if serotonin syndrome ensues, specific treatment (such as with cyproheptadine and/or temperature control) may be considered. In case of acute overdose, treatment should consist of those general measures employed in the management of overdose with any drug.

An adequate airway, oxygenation, and ventilation should be assured, and cardiac rhythm and vital signs should be monitored. Induction of emesis is not recommended. Gastric lavage with a large-bore orogastric tube with appropriate airway protection, if needed, may be indicated if performed soon after ingestion or in symptomatic patients.

Activated charcoal may be useful in limiting absorption of duloxetine from the gastrointestinal tract. Administration of activated charcoal has been shown to decrease AUC and C_{max} by an average of one-third, although some subjects had a limited effect of activated charcoal. Due to the large volume of distribution of this drug, forced diuresis, dialysis, hemoperfusion, and exchange transfusion are unlikely to be beneficial.

In managing overdose, the possibility of multiple drug involvement should be considered. A specific caution involves patients who are taking or have recently taken Cymbalta and might ingest excessive quantities of a TCA. In such a case, decreased clearance of the parent tricyclic and/or its active metabolite may increase the possibility of clinically significant sequelae and extend the time needed for close medical observation *[see Warnings and Precautions (5.4) and Drug Interactions (7)]*. The physician should consider contacting a poison control center for additional information on the treatment of any overdose. Telephone numbers for certified poison control centers are listed in the *Physicians' Desk Reference* (PDR).

11 DESCRIPTION

Cymbalta® (duloxetine hydrochloride) is a selective serotonin and norepinephrine reuptake inhibitor (SSNRI) for oral administration. Its chemical designation is (+)-(*S*)-*N*-methyl-γ-(1-naphthyloxy)-2-thiophenepropylamine hydrochloride. The empirical formula is $C_{18}H_{19}NOS \bullet HCl$, which corresponds to a molecular weight of 333.88. The structural formula is:

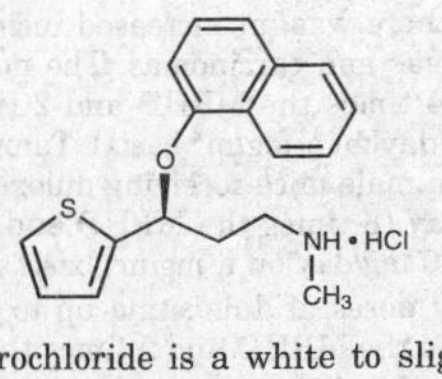

Duloxetine hydrochloride is a white to slightly brownish white solid, which is slightly soluble in water.

Each capsule contains enteric-coated pellets of 22.4, 33.7, or 67.3 mg of duloxetine hydrochloride equivalent to 20, 30, or 60 mg of duloxetine, respectively. These enteric-coated pellets are designed to prevent degradation of the drug in the acidic environment of the stomach. Inactive ingredients include FD&C Blue No. 2, gelatin, hypromellose, hydroxypropyl methylcellulose acetate succinate, sodium lauryl sulfate, sucrose, sugar spheres, talc, titanium dioxide, and triethyl citrate. The 20 and 60 mg capsules also contain iron oxide yellow.

12 CLINICAL PHARMACOLOGY

12.1 Mechanism of Action

Although the exact mechanisms of the antidepressant, central pain inhibitory and anxiolytic actions of duloxetine in humans are unknown, these actions are believed to be related to its potentiation of serotonergic and noradrenergic activity in the CNS.

12.2 Pharmacodynamics

Preclinical studies have shown that duloxetine is a potent inhibitor of neuronal serotonin and norepinephrine reuptake and a less potent inhibitor of dopamine reuptake. Duloxetine has no significant affinity for dopaminergic, adrenergic, cholinergic, histaminergic, opioid, glutamate, and GABA receptors *in vitro*. Duloxetine does not inhibit monoamine oxidase (MAO).

Cymbalta is in a class of drugs known to affect urethral resistance. If symptoms of urinary hesitation develop during treatment with Cymbalta, consideration should be given to the possibility that they might be drug-related.

12.3 Pharmacokinetics

Duloxetine has an elimination half-life of about 12 hours (range 8 to 17 hours) and its pharmacokinetics are dose proportional over the therapeutic range. Steady-state plasma concentrations are typically achieved after 3 days of dosing. Elimination of duloxetine is mainly through hepatic metabolism involving two P450 isozymes, CYP1A2 and CYP2D6.

Absorption and Distribution—Orally administered duloxetine hydrochloride is well absorbed. There is a median 2 hour lag until absorption begins (T_{lag}), with maximal plasma concentrations (C_{max}) of duloxetine occurring 6 hours post dose. Food does not affect the C_{max} of duloxetine, but delays the time to reach peak concentration from 6 to 10 hours and it marginally decreases the extent of absorption (AUC) by about 10%. There is a 3 hour delay in absorption and a one-third increase in apparent clearance of duloxetine after an evening dose as compared to a morning dose.

The apparent volume of distribution averages about 1640 L. Duloxetine is highly bound (>90%) to proteins in human plasma, binding primarily to albumin and α_1-acid glycoprotein. The interaction between duloxetine and other highly protein bound drugs has not been fully evaluated. Plasma protein binding of duloxetine is not affected by renal or hepatic impairment.

Metabolism and Elimination—Biotransformation and disposition of duloxetine in humans have been determined following oral administration of ^{14}C-labeled duloxetine. Duloxetine comprises about 3% of the total radiolabeled material in the plasma, indicating that it undergoes extensive metabolism to numerous metabolites. The major biotransformation pathways for duloxetine involve oxidation of the naphthyl ring followed by conjugation and further oxidation. Both CYP1A2 and CYP2D6 catalyze the oxidation of the naphthyl ring *in vitro*. Metabolites found in plasma include 4-hydroxy duloxetine glucuronide and 5-hydroxy, 6-methoxy duloxetine sulfate. Many additional metabolites have been identified in urine, some representing only minor pathways of elimination. Only trace (<1% of the dose) amounts of unchanged duloxetine are present in the urine. Most (about 70%) of the duloxetine dose appears in the urine as metabolites of duloxetine; about 20% is excreted in the feces. Duloxetine undergoes extensive metabolism, but the major circulating metabolites have not been shown to contribute significantly to the pharmacologic activity of duloxetine.

13 NONCLINICAL TOXICOLOGY

13.1 Carcinogenesis, Mutagenesis, and Impairment of Fertility

Carcinogenesis—Duloxetine was administered in the diet to mice and rats for 2 years.

In female mice receiving duloxetine at 140 mg/kg/day (11 times the maximum recommended human dose [MRHD, 60 mg/day] and 6 times the human dose of 120 mg/day on a mg/m^2 basis), there was an increased incidence of hepatocellular adenomas and carcinomas. The no-effect dose was 50 mg/kg/day (4 times the MRHD and 2 times the human dose of 120 mg/day on a mg/m^2 basis). Tumor incidence was not increased in male mice receiving duloxetine at doses up to 100 mg/kg/day (8 times the MRHD and 4 times the human dose of 120 mg/day on a mg/m^2 basis).

In rats, dietary doses of duloxetine up to 27 mg/kg/day in females (4 times the MRHD and 2 times the human dose of 120 mg/day on a mg/m^2 basis) and up to 36 mg/kg/day in males (6 times the MRHD and 3 times the human dose of 120 mg/day on a mg/m^2 basis) did not increase the incidence of tumors.

Mutagenesis—Duloxetine was not mutagenic in the *in vitro* bacterial reverse mutation assay (Ames test) and was not clastogenic in an *in vivo* chromosomal aberration test in mouse bone marrow cells. Additionally, duloxetine was not genotoxic in an *in vitro* mammalian forward gene mutation assay in mouse lymphoma cells or in an *in vitro* unscheduled DNA synthesis (UDS) assay in primary rat hepatocytes, and did not induce sister chromatid exchange in Chinese hamster bone marrow *in vivo*.

Impairment of Fertility—Duloxetine administered orally to either male or female rats prior to and throughout mating at doses up to 45 mg/kg/day (7 times the maximum recommended human dose of 60 mg/day and 4 times the human dose of 120 mg/day on a mg/m^2 basis) did not alter mating or fertility.

14 CLINICAL STUDIES

14.1 Major Depressive Disorder

The efficacy of Cymbalta as a treatment for depression was established in 4 randomized, double-blind, placebo-controlled, fixed-dose studies in adult outpatients (18 to 83 years) meeting DSM-IV criteria for major depression. In 2 studies, patients were randomized to Cymbalta 60 mg once daily (N=123 and N=128, respectively) or placebo (N=122 and N=139, respectively) for 9 weeks; in the third study, patients were randomized to Cymbalta 20 or 40 mg twice daily (N=86 and N=91, respectively) or placebo (N=89) for 8 weeks; in the fourth study, patients were randomized to Cymbalta 40 or 60 mg twice daily (N=95 and N=93, respectively) or placebo (N=93) for 8 weeks. There is no evidence that doses greater than 60 mg/day confer additional benefits.

In all 4 studies, Cymbalta demonstrated superiority over placebo as measured by improvement in the 17-item Hamilton Depression Rating Scale (HAMD-17) total score.

In all of these clinical studies, analyses of the relationship between treatment outcome and age, gender, and race did not suggest any differential responsiveness on the basis of these patient characteristics.

In another study, 533 patients meeting DSM-IV criteria for MDD received Cymbalta 60 mg once daily during an initial 12-week open-label treatment phase. Two hundred and seventy-eight patients who responded to open label treatment (defined as meeting the following criteria at weeks 10 and 12: a HAMD-17 total score ≤9, Clinical Global Impressions of Severity (CGI-S) ≤2, and not meeting the DSM-IV criteria for MDD) were randomly assigned to continuation of Cymbalta at the same dose (N=136) or to placebo (N=142) for 6 months. Patients on Cymbalta experienced a statistically significantly longer time to relapse of depression than did patients on placebo. Relapse was defined as an increase in the CGI-S score of ≥2 points compared with that obtained at week 12, as well as meeting the DSM-IV criteria for MDD at 2 consecutive visits at least 2 weeks apart, where the 2-week temporal criterion had to be satisfied at only the second visit. The effectiveness of Cymbalta in hospitalized patients with major depressive disorder has not been studied.

14.2 Generalized Anxiety Disorder

The efficacy of Cymbalta in the treatment of generalized anxiety disorder (GAD) was established in 1 fixed-dose randomized, double-blind, placebo-controlled trial and 2 flexible-dose randomized, double-blind, placebo-controlled trials in adult outpatients between 18 and 83 years of age meeting the DSM-IV criteria for GAD.

In 1 flexible-dose study and in the fixed-dose study, the starting dose was 60 mg once daily where down titration to 30 mg once daily was allowed for tolerability reasons before increasing it to 60 mg once daily. Fifteen percent of patients were down titrated. One flexible-dose study had a starting dose of 30 mg once daily for 1 week before increasing it to 60 mg once daily.

The 2 flexible-dose studies involved dose titration with Cymbalta doses ranging from 60 mg once daily to 120 mg once daily (N=168 and N=162) compared to placebo (N=159 and N=161) over a 10-week treatment period. The mean dose for completers at endpoint in the flexible-dose studies was 104.75 mg/day. The fixed-dose study evaluated Cymbalta doses of 60 mg once daily (N=168) and 120 mg once daily (N=170) compared to placebo (N=175) over a 9-week treatment period. While a 120 mg/day dose was shown to be effective, there is no evidence that doses greater than 60 mg/day confer additional benefit.

In all 3 studies, Cymbalta demonstrated superiority over placebo as measured by greater improvement in the Hamilton Anxiety Scale (HAM-A) total score and by the Sheehan Disability Scale (SDS) global functional impairment score. The SDS is a widely used and well-validated scale that measures the extent emotional symptoms disrupt patient functioning in 3 life domains: work/school, social life/leisure activities, and family life/home responsibilities.

In another study, 887 patients meeting DSM-IV-TR criteria for GAD received Cymbalta 60 mg to 120 mg once daily during an initial 26-week open-label treatment phase. Four hundred and twenty-nine patients who responded to open-label treatment (defined as meeting the following criteria at weeks 24 and 26: a decrease from baseline HAM-A total score by at least 50% to a score no higher than 11, and a Clinical Global Impressions of Improvement [CGI-Improvement] score of 1 or 2) were randomly assigned to continuation of Cymbalta at the same dose (N = 216) or to placebo (N = 213) and were observed for relapse. Of the patients randomized, 73% had been in a responder status for at least 10 weeks. Relapse was defined as an increase in CGI-Severity score at least 2 points to a score ≥4 and a MINI (Mini-International Neuropsychiatric Interview) diagnosis of GAD (excluding duration), or discontinuation due to lack of efficacy. Patients taking Cymbalta experienced a statistically significantly longer time to relapse of GAD than did patients taking placebo.

Subgroup analyses did not indicate that there were any differences in treatment outcomes as a function of age or gender.

14.3 Diabetic Peripheral Neuropathic Pain

The efficacy of Cymbalta for the management of neuropathic pain associated with diabetic peripheral neuropathy was established in 2 randomized, 12-week, double-blind, placebo-controlled, fixed-dose studies in adult patients having diabetic peripheral neuropathic pain for at least 6 months. Study 1 and 2 enrolled a total of 791 patients of whom 592 (75%) completed the studies. Patients enrolled had Type I or II diabetes mellitus with a diagnosis of painful distal symmetrical sensorimotor polyneuropathy for at least 6 months. The patients had a baseline pain score of ≥4 on an 11-point scale ranging from 0 (no pain) to 10 (worst possible pain). Patients were permitted up to 4 g of acetaminophen per day as needed for pain, in addition to Cymbalta. Patients recorded their pain daily in a diary.

Both studies compared Cymbalta 60 mg once daily or 60 mg twice daily with placebo. Study 1 additionally compared Cymbalta 20 mg with placebo. A total of 457 patients (342 Cymbalta, 115 placebo) were enrolled in Study 1 and a total of 334 patients (226 Cymbalta, 108 placebo) were enrolled in Study 2. Treatment with Cymbalta 60 mg one or two times a day statistically significantly improved the endpoint mean pain scores from baseline and increased the proportion of patients with at least a 50% reduction in pain score from baseline. For various degrees of improvement in pain from baseline to study endpoint, Figures 1 and 2 show the fraction of patients achieving that degree of improvement. The figures are cumulative, so that patients whose change from baseline is, for example, 50%, are also included at every level of improvement below 50%. Patients who did not complete the study were assigned 0% improvement. Some patients experienced a decrease in pain as early as week 1, which persisted throughout the study.

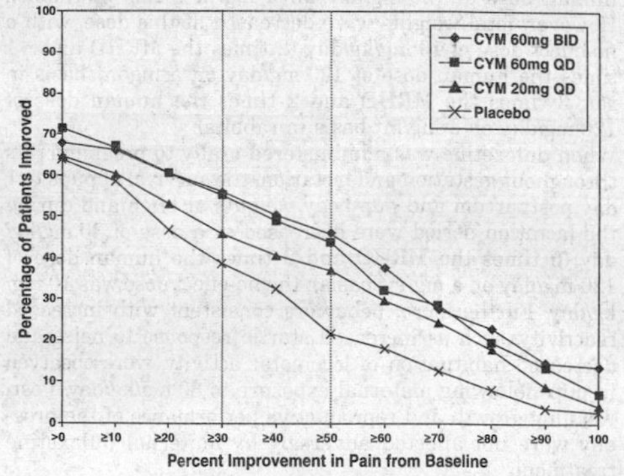

Figure 1: Percentage of Patients Achieving Various Levels of Pain Relief as Measured by 24-Hour Average Pain Severity - Study 1

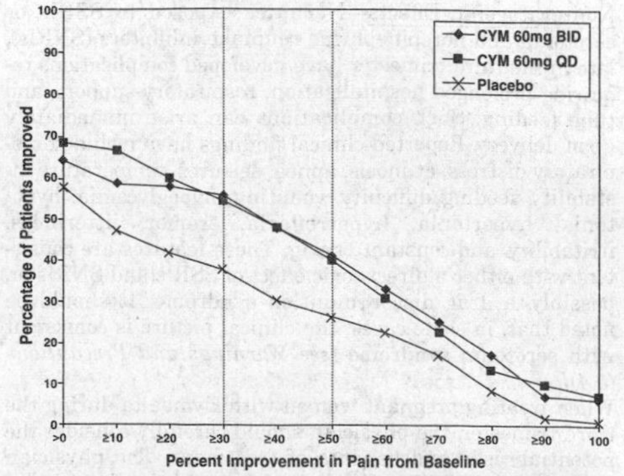

Figure 2: Percentage of Patients Achieving Various Levels of Pain Relief as Measured by 24-Hour Average Pain Severity - Study 2

14.4 Fibromyalgia

The efficacy of Cymbalta for the management of fibromyalgia was established in two randomized, double-blind, placebo-controlled, fixed-dose studies in adult patients meeting the American College of Rheumatology criteria for fibromyalgia (a history of widespread pain for 3 months, and pain present at 11 or more of the 18 specific tender point sites). Study 1 was three months in duration and enrolled female patients only. Study 2 was six months in duration and enrolled male and female patients. Approximately 25% of participants had a comorbid diagnosis of major depressive disorder (MDD). Study 1 and 2 enrolled a total of 874 patients of whom 541 (62%) completed the studies. The patients had a baseline pain score of 6.5 on an 11-point scale ranging from 0 (no pain) to 10 (worse possible pain).

Both studies compared Cymbalta 60 mg once daily or 120 mg daily (given in divided doses in Study 1 and as a single daily dose in Study 2) with placebo. Study 2 additionally compared Cymbalta 20 mg with placebo during the initial three months of a six-month study. A total of 354 patients (234 Cymbalta, 120 placebo) were enrolled in Study 1 and a total of 520 patients (376 Cymbalta, 144 placebo) were enrolled in Study 2 (5% male, 95% female). Treatment with Cymbalta 60 mg or 120 mg daily statistically significantly improved the endpoint mean pain scores from baseline and increase the proportion of patients with at least a 50% reduction in pain score from baseline. Pain reduction was observed in patients both with and without comorbid MDD. However, the degree of pain reduction may be greater in patients with comorbid MDD. For various degrees of improvement in pain from baseline to study endpoint, Figures 3 and 4 show the fraction of patients achieving that degree of improvement. The figures are cumulative so that patients whose change from baseline is, for example, 50%, are also included at every level of improvement below 50%. Patients who did not complete the study were assigned 0% improvement. Some patients experienced a decrease in pain as early as week 1, which persisted throughout the study. Improvement was also demonstrated on measures of function (Fibromyalgia Impact Questionnaires) and patient global impression of change (PGI). Neither study demonstrated a benefit of 120 mg compared to 60 mg, and a higher dose was associated with more adverse reactions and premature discontinuations of treatment.

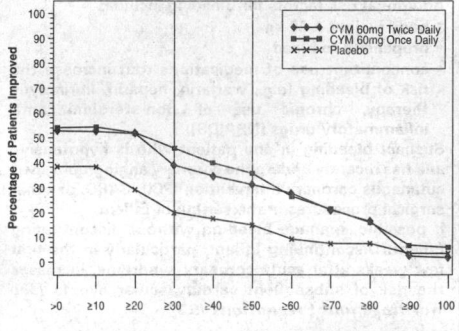

Figure 3: Percentage of Patients Achieving Various Levels of Pain Relief as Measured by 24-Hour Average Pain Severity - Study 1

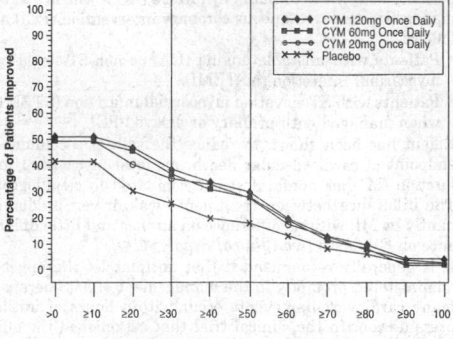

Figure 4: Percentage of Patients Achieving Various Levels of Pain Relief as Measured by 24-Hour Average Pain Severity - Study 2

Additionally, the benefit of up-titration in non-responders to Cymbalta at 60 mg/day was evaluated in a separate study. Patients were initially treated with Cymbalta 60 mg once daily for eight weeks in open-label fashion. Subsequently, completers of this phase were randomized to double-blind treatment with Cymbalta at either 60 mg once daily or 120 mg once daily. Those patients who were considered non-responders, where response was defined as at least a 30%

Features	Strengths			
	20 mg[a]	30 mg[a]	60 mg[a]	
Body color	Opaque green	Opaque white	Opaque green	
Cap color	Opaque green	Opaque blue	Opaque blue	
Cap imprint	Lilly 3235	Lilly 3240	Lilly 3237	Lilly 3270
Body imprint	20mg	30mg	60mg	60mg
Capsule number	PU3235	PU3240	PU3237	PU3270
Presentations and NDC Codes				
Bottles of 30	NA	0002-3240-30	0002-3237-30	0002-3270-30
Bottles of 60	0002-3235-60	NA	NA	NA
Bottles of 90	NA	0002-3240-90	NA	NA
Bottles of 1000	NA	0002-3240-04	0002-3237-04	0002-3270-04
Blisters ID† 100	NA	0002-3240-33	0002-3237-33	0002-3270-33

[a] equivalent to duloxetine base
† Identi-Dose® (unit dose medication, Lilly)

reduction in pain score from baseline at the end of the 8-week treatment, were no more likely to meet response criteria at the end of 60 weeks of treatment if blindly titrated to Cymbalta 120 mg as compared to those who were blindly continued on Cymbalta 60 mg.

16 HOW SUPPLIED/STORAGE AND HANDLING
16.1 How Supplied
Cymbalta is available as delayed release capsules in the following strengths, colors, imprints, and presentations:
[See table above]
16.2 Storage
Store at 25°C (77°F); excursions permitted to 15-30°C (59-86°F) [see USP Controlled Room Temperature].

17 PATIENT COUNSELING INFORMATION
See FDA-approved Medication Guide
17.1 Information on Medication Guide
Prescribers or other health professionals should inform patients, their families, and their caregivers about the benefits and risks associated with treatment with Cymbalta and should counsel them in its appropriate use. A patient Medication Guide About Using Antidepressants in Children and Teenagers is available for Cymbalta. The prescriber or health professional should instruct patients, their families, and their caregivers to read the Medication Guide and should assist them in understanding its contents. Patients should be given the opportunity to discuss the contents of the Medication Guide and to obtain answers to any questions they may have. The complete text of the Medication Guide is reprinted at the end of this document.
Patients should be advised of the following issues and asked to alert their prescriber if these occur while taking Cymbalta.
17.2 Clinical Worsening and Suicide Risk
Patients, their families, and their caregivers should be encouraged to be alert to the emergence of anxiety, agitation, panic attacks, insomnia, irritability, hostility, aggressiveness, impulsivity, akathisia (psychomotor restlessness), hypomania, mania, other unusual changes in behavior, worsening of depression, and suicidal ideation, especially early during antidepressant treatment and when the dose is adjusted up or down. Families and caregivers of patients should be advised to observe for the emergence of such symptoms on a day-to-day basis, since changes may be abrupt. Such symptoms should be reported to the patient's prescriber or health professional, especially if they are severe, abrupt in onset, or were not part of the patient's presenting symptoms. Symptoms such as these may be associated with an increased risk for suicidal thinking and behavior and indicate a need for very close monitoring and possibly changes in the medication [see Boxed Warning, and Warnings and Precautions (5.1)].
17.3 Medication Administration
Cymbalta should be swallowed whole and should not be chewed or crushed, nor should the capsule be opened and its contents be sprinkled on food or mixed with liquids. All of these might affect the enteric coating.
17.4 Continuing the Therapy Prescribed
While patients may notice improvement with Cymbalta therapy in 1 to 4 weeks, they should be advised to continue therapy as directed.
17.5 Abnormal Bleeding
Patients should be cautioned about the concomitant use of duloxetine and NSAIDs, aspirin, warfarin, or other drugs

that affect coagulation since combined use of psychotropic drugs that interfere with serotonin reuptake and these agents has been associated with an increased risk of bleeding [see Warnings and Precautions (5.5)].
17.6 Concomitant Medications
Patients should be advised to inform their physicians if they are taking, or plan to take, any prescription or over-the-counter medications, since there is a potential for interactions [see Dosage and Administration (2.5), Contraindications (4.1), Warnings and Precautions (5.4 and 5.10), and Drug Interactions (7)].
17.7 Serotonin Syndrome
Patients should be cautioned about the risk of serotonin syndrome with the concomitant use of Cymbalta and triptans, tramadol or other serotonergic agents [see Warnings and Precautions (5.4) and Drug Interactions (7.14)].
17.8 Pregnancy and Breast Feeding
Patients should be advised to notify their physician if they
• become pregnant during therapy
• intend to become pregnant during therapy
• are breast feeding [see Dosage and Administration (2.3) and Use in Specific Populations (8.1, 8.2, and 8.3)].
17.9 Alcohol
Although Cymbalta does not increase the impairment of mental and motor skills caused by alcohol, use of Cymbalta concomitantly with heavy alcohol intake may be associated with severe liver injury. For this reason, Cymbalta should ordinarily not be prescribed for patients with substantial alcohol use [see Warnings and Precautions (5.2) and Drug Interactions (7.16)].
17.10 Orthostatic Hypotension and Syncope
Patients should be advised of the risk of orthostatic hypotension and syncope, especially during the period of initial use and subsequent dose escalation, and in association with the use of concomitant drugs that might potentiate the orthostatic effect of duloxetine [see Warnings and Precautions (5.3)].
17.11 Interference with Psychomotor Performance
Any psychoactive drug may impair judgment, thinking, or motor skills. Although in controlled studies Cymbalta has not been shown to impair psychomotor performance, cognitive function, or memory, it may be associated with sedation and dizziness. Therefore, patients should be cautioned about operating hazardous machinery including automobiles, until they are reasonably certain that Cymbalta therapy does not affect their ability to engage in such activities.
Literature revised: January 13, 2010

Eli Lilly and Company
Indianapolis, IN 46285, USA

PV 7211 AMP
MEDICATION GUIDE
Antidepressant Medicines, Depression and other Serious Mental Illnesses, and Suicidal Thoughts or Actions
Read the Medication Guide that comes with your or your family member's antidepressant medicine. This Medication Guide is only about the risk of suicidal thoughts and actions with antidepressant medicines. **Talk to your, or your family member's, healthcare provider about:**
• all risks and benefits of treatment with antidepressant medicines
• all treatment choices for depression or other serious mental illness

What is the most important information I should know about antidepressant medicines, depression and other serious mental illnesses, and suicidal thoughts or actions?

1. Antidepressant medicines may increase suicidal thoughts or actions in some children, teenagers, and young adults within the first few months of treatment.
2. Depression and other serious mental illnesses are the most important causes of suicidal thoughts and actions. Some people may have a particularly high risk of having suicidal thoughts or actions. These include people who have (or have a family history of) bipolar illness (also called manic-depressive illness) or suicidal thoughts or actions.
3. How can I watch for and try to prevent suicidal thoughts and actions in myself or a family member?
   - Pay close attention to any changes, especially sudden changes, in mood, behaviors, thoughts, or feelings. This is very important when an antidepressant medicine is started or when the dose is changed.
   - Call the healthcare provider right away to report new or sudden changes in mood, behavior, thoughts, or feelings.
   - Keep all follow-up visits with the healthcare provider as scheduled. Call the healthcare provider between visits as needed, especially if you have concerns about symptoms.

Call a healthcare provider right away if you or your family member has any of the following symptoms, especially if they are new, worse, or worry you:

- thoughts about suicide or dying
- attempts to commit suicide
- new or worse depression
- new or worse anxiety
- feeling very agitated or restless
- panic attacks
- trouble sleeping (insomnia)
- new or worse irritability
- acting aggressive, being angry, or violent
- acting on dangerous impulses
- an extreme increase in activity and talking (mania)
- other unusual changes in behavior or mood

What else do I need to know about antidepressant medicines?

- **Never stop an antidepressant medicine without first talking to a healthcare provider.** Stopping an antidepressant medicine suddenly can cause other symptoms.
- **Antidepressants are medicines used to treat depression and other illnesses.** It is important to discuss all the risks of treating depression and also the risks of not treating it. Patients and their families or other caregivers should discuss all treatment choices with the healthcare provider, not just the use of antidepressants.
- **Antidepressant medicines have other side effects.** Talk to the healthcare provider about the side effects of the medicine prescribed for you or your family member.
- **Antidepressant medicines can interact with other medicines.** Know all of the medicines that you or your family member takes. Keep a list of all medicines to show the healthcare provider. Do not start new medicines without first checking with your healthcare provider.
- **Not all antidepressant medicines prescribed for children are FDA approved for use in children.** Talk to your child's healthcare provider for more information.

These are not all the possible side effects. Call your doctor for medical advice about side effects. You may report side effects to FDA at 1-800-FDA-1088.

This Medication Guide has been approved by the US Food and Drug Administration for all antidepressants.

Patient Information revised December 4, 2008
PV 7090 AMP

Shown in Product Identification Guide, page 310

EFFIENT™   ℞
[*Ef´-fee-ent*]
(prasugrel)
Tablets

HIGHLIGHTS OF PRESCRIBING INFORMATION
These highlights do not include all the information needed to use Effient safely and effectively. See full prescribing information for Effient.
EFFIENT (prasugrel) tablets
Initial U.S. Approval: 2009

WARNING: BLEEDING RISK
See full prescribing information for complete boxed warning
Effient can cause significant, sometimes fatal, bleeding (5.1, 5.2, and 6.1).
Do not use Effient in patients with active pathological bleeding or a history of transient ischemic attack or stroke (4.1 and 4.2).

In patients ≥ 75 years of age, Effient is generally not recommended because of the increased risk of fatal and intracranial bleeding and uncertain benefit, except in high-risk patients (diabetes or prior MI), where its effect appears to be greater and its use may be considered (8.5).
Do not start Effient in patients likely to undergo urgent coronary artery bypass graft surgery (CABG). When possible, discontinue Effient at least 7 days prior to any surgery.
Additional risk factors for bleeding include:
- body weight < 60 kg
- propensity to bleed
- concomitant use of medications that increase the risk of bleeding
Suspect bleeding in any patient who is hypotensive and has recently undergone coronary angiography, percutaneous coronary intervention (PCI), CABG, or other surgical procedures in the setting of Effient.
If possible, manage bleeding without discontinuing Effient. Stopping Effient, particularly in the first few weeks after acute coronary syndrome, increases the risk of subsequent cardiovascular events (5.3).

---INDICATIONS AND USAGE---

Effient is a $P2Y_{12}$ platelet inhibitor indicated for the reduction of thrombotic cardiovascular events (including stent thrombosis) in patients with acute coronary syndrome who are to be managed with PCI as follows:
- Patients with unstable angina or, non-ST-elevation myocardial infarction (NSTEMI) (1.1).
- Patients with ST-elevation myocardial infarction (STEMI) when managed with either primary or delayed PCI (1.1).

---DOSAGE AND ADMINISTRATION---

- Initiate treatment with a single 60 mg oral loading dose (2).
- Continue at 10 mg once daily with or without food. Consider 5 mg once daily for patients <60 kg (2).
- Patients should also take aspirin (75 mg to 325 mg) daily (2).

---DOSAGE FORMS AND STRENGTHS---

5 mg and 10 mg tablets (3)

---CONTRAINDICATIONS---

- Active pathological bleeding (4.1)
- Prior transient ischemic attack or stroke (4.2)

---WARNINGS AND PRECAUTIONS---

- CABG-related bleeding: Risk increases in patients receiving Effient who undergo CABG (5.2).
- Discontinuation of Effient: Premature discontinuation increases risk of stent thrombosis, MI, and death (5.3).

---ADVERSE REACTIONS---

Bleeding, including life-threatening and fatal bleeding, is the most commonly reported adverse reaction (6.1).
To report SUSPECTED ADVERSE REACTIONS, contact Eli Lilly and Company at 1-800-545-5979 or FDA at 1-800-FDA-1088 or www.fda.gov/medwatch
See 17 for PATIENT COUNSELING INFORMATION and Medication Guide

Revised: 07/2009

FULL PRESCRIBING INFORMATION: CONTENTS*
* Sections or subsections omitted from the full prescribing information are not listed

---

FULL PRESCRIBING INFORMATION

WARNING: BLEEDING RISK
Effient can cause significant, sometimes fatal, bleeding *[see Warnings and Precautions (5.1 and 5.2) and Adverse Reactions (6.1)]*.
Do not use Effient in patients with active pathological bleeding or a history of transient ischemic attack or stroke *[see Contraindications (4.1 and 4.2)]*.
In patients ≥ 75 years of age, Effient is generally not recommended, because of the increased risk of fatal and intracranial bleeding and uncertain benefit, except in high-risk situations (patients with diabetes or a history of prior MI) where its effect appears to be greater and its use may be considered *[see Use in Specific Populations (8.5)]*.
Do not start Effient in patients likely to undergo urgent coronary artery bypass graft surgery (CABG). When possible, discontinue Effient at least 7 days prior to any surgery.
Additional risk factors for bleeding include:
- body weight < 60 kg
- propensity to bleed
- concomitant use of medications that increase the risk of bleeding (e.g., warfarin, heparin, fibrinolytic therapy, chronic use of non-steroidal anti-inflammatory drugs [NSAIDS])
Suspect bleeding in any patient who is hypotensive and has recently undergone coronary angiography, percutaneous coronary intervention (PCI), CABG, or other surgical procedures in the setting of Effient.
If possible, manage bleeding without discontinuing Effient. Discontinuing Effient, particularly in the first few weeks after acute coronary syndrome, increases the risk of subsequent cardiovascular events *[see Warnings and Precautions (5.3)]*.

---

1   INDICATIONS AND USAGE

1.1   Acute Coronary Syndrome

Effient™ is indicated to reduce the rate of thrombotic cardiovascular (CV) events (including stent thrombosis) in patients with acute coronary syndrome (ACS) who are to be managed with percutaneous coronary intervention (PCI) as follows:
- Patients with unstable angina (UA) or non-ST-elevation myocardial infarction (NSTEMI).
- Patients with ST-elevation myocardial infarction (STEMI) when managed with primary or delayed PCI.

Effient has been shown to reduce the rate of a combined endpoint of cardiovascular death, nonfatal myocardial infarction (MI), or nonfatal stroke compared to clopidogrel. The difference between treatments was driven predominantly by MI, with no difference on strokes and little difference on CV death *[see Clinical Studies (14)]*.
It is generally recommended that antiplatelet therapy be administered promptly in the management of ACS because many cardiovascular events occur within hours of initial presentation. In the clinical trial that established the efficacy of Effient, Effient and the control drug were not administered to UA/NSTEMI patients until coronary anatomy was established. For the small fraction of patients that required urgent CABG after treatment with Effient, the risk of significant bleeding was substantial *[see Warnings and Precautions (5.2)]*. Because the large majority of patients are managed without CABG, however, treatment can be considered before determining coronary anatomy if need for CABG is considered unlikely. The advantages of earlier treatment with Effient must then be balanced against the increased rate of bleeding in patients who do need to undergo urgent CABG.

2 DOSAGE AND ADMINISTRATION

Initiate Effient treatment as a single 60 mg oral loading dose and then continue at 10 mg orally once daily. Patients taking Effient should also take aspirin (75 mg to 325 mg) daily [see Drug Interactions (7) and Clinical Pharmacology (12.3)]. Effient may be administered with or without food [see Clinical Pharmacology (12.3) and Clinical Studies (14)].
Dosing in Low Weight Patients
Compared to patients weighing ≥ 60 kg, patients weighing < 60 kg have an increased exposure to the active metabolite of prasugrel and an increased risk of bleeding on a 10 mg once daily maintenance dose. Consider lowering the maintenance dose to 5 mg in patients < 60 kg. The effectiveness and safety of the 5 mg dose have not been prospectively studied.

3 DOSAGE FORMS AND STRENGTHS

Effient 5 mg is a yellow, elongated hexagonal, film-coated, non-scored tablet debossed with "5 MG" on one side and "4760" on the other side.
Effient 10 mg is a beige, elongated hexagonal, film-coated, non-scored tablet debossed with "10 MG" on one side and with "4759" on the other side.

4 CONTRAINDICATIONS

4.1 Active Bleeding

Effient is contraindicated in patients with active pathological bleeding such as peptic ulcer or intracranial hemorrhage [see Warnings and Precautions (5.1) and Adverse Reactions (6.1)].

4.2 Prior Transient Ischemic Attack or Stroke

Effient is contraindicated in patients with a history of prior transient ischemic attack (TIA) or stroke. In TRITON-TIMI 38 (TRial to Assess Improvement in Therapeutic Outcomes by Optimizing Platelet InhibitioN with Prasugrel), patients with a history of TIA or ischemic stroke (> 3 months prior to enrollment) had a higher rate of stroke on Effient (6.5%; of which 4.2% were thrombotic stroke and 2.3% were intracranial hemorrhage [ICH]) than on clopidogrel (1.2%; all thrombotic). In patients without such a history, the incidence of stroke was 0.9% (0.2% ICH) and 1.0% (0.3% ICH) with Effient and clopidogrel, respectively. Patients with a history of ischemic stroke within 3 months of screening and patients with a history of hemorrhagic stroke at any time were excluded from TRITON-TIMI 38. Patients who experience a stroke or TIA while on Effient generally should have therapy discontinued [see Adverse Reactions (6.1) and Clinical Studies (14)].

5 WARNINGS AND PRECAUTIONS

5.1 General Risk of Bleeding

Thienopyridines, including Effient, increase the risk of bleeding. With the dosing regimens used in TRITON-TIMI 38, TIMI (Thrombolysis in Myocardial Infarction) Major (clinically overt bleeding associated with a fall in hemoglobin ≥ 5 g/dL, or intracranial hemorrhage) and TIMI Minor (overt bleeding associated with a fall in hemoglobin of ≥ 3 g/dL but < 5 g/dL) bleeding events were more common on Effient than on clopidogrel [see Adverse Reactions (6.1)]. The bleeding risk is highest initially, as shown in Figure 1 (events through 450 days; inset shows events through 7 days).

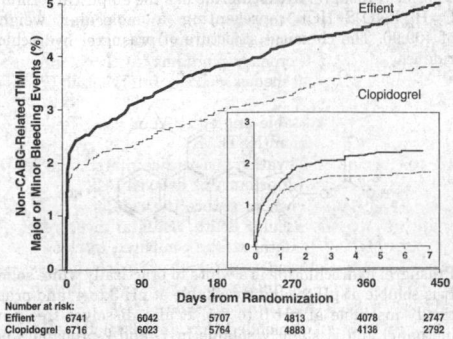

Number at risk:
Effient	6741	6042	5707	4813	4078	2747
Clopidogrel	6716	6023	5764	4883	4136	2792

Figure 1: Non-CABG-Related TIMI Major or Minor Bleeding Events

Suspect bleeding in any patient who is hypotensive and has recently undergone coronary angiography, PCI, CABG, or other surgical procedures even if the patient does not have overt signs of bleeding.
Do not use Effient in patients with active bleeding, prior TIA or stroke [see Contraindications (4.1 and 4.2)].
Other risk factors for bleeding are:
• Age ≥ 75 years. Because of the risk of bleeding (including fatal bleeding) and uncertain effectiveness in patients ≥ 75 years of age, use of Effient is generally not recommended in these patients, except in high-risk situations (patients with diabetes or history of myocardial infarction) where its effect appears to be greater and its use

may be considered [see Adverse Reactions (6.1), Use in Specific Populations (8.5), Clinical Pharmacology (12.3), and Clinical Trials (14)].
• CABG or other surgical procedure [see Warnings and Precautions (5.2)].
• Body weight < 60 kg. Consider a lower (5 mg) maintenance dose [see Dosage and Administration (2), Adverse Reactions (6.1), Use in Specific Populations (8.6)].
• Propensity to bleed (e.g., recent trauma, recent surgery, recent or recurrent gastrointestinal (GI) bleeding, active peptic ulcer disease, or severe hepatic impairment) [see Adverse Reactions (6.1) and Use in Specific Populations (8.8)].
• Medications that increase the risk of bleeding (e.g., oral anticoagulants, chronic use of non-steroidal anti-inflammatory drugs [NSAIDs], and fibrinolytic agents). Aspirin and heparin were commonly used in TRITON-TIMI 38 [see Drug Interactions (7), Clinical Studies (14)].
Thienopyridines inhibit platelet aggregation for the lifetime of the platelet (7-10 days), so withholding a dose will not be useful in managing a bleeding event or the risk of bleeding associated with an invasive procedure. Because the half-life of prasugrel's active metabolite is short relative to the lifetime of the platelet, it may be possible to restore hemostasis by administering exogenous platelets; however, platelet transfusions within 6 hours of the loading dose or 4 hours of the maintenance dose may be less effective.

5.2 Coronary Artery Bypass Graft Surgery-Related Bleeding

The risk of bleeding is increased in patients receiving Effient who undergo CABG. If possible, Effient should be discontinued at least 7 days prior to CABG.
Of the 437 patients who underwent CABG during TRITON-TIMI 38, the rates of CABG-related TIMI Major or Minor bleeding were 14.1% in the Effient group and 4.5% in the clopidogrel group [see Adverse Reactions (6.1)]. The higher risk for bleeding events in patients treated with Effient persisted up to 7 days from the most recent dose of study drug. For patients receiving a thienopyridine within 3 days prior to CABG, the frequencies of TIMI Major or Minor bleeding were 26.7% (12 of 45 patients) in the Effient group, compared with 5.0% (3 of 60 patients) in the clopidogrel group. For patients who received their last dose of thienopyridine within 4 to 7 days prior to CABG, the frequencies decreased to 11.3% (9 of 80 patients) in the prasugrel group and 3.4% (3 of 89 patients) in the clopidogrel group.
Do not start Effient in patients likely to undergo urgent CABG. CABG-related bleeding may be treated with transfusion of blood products, including packed red blood cells and platelets; however, platelet transfusions within 6 hours of the loading dose or 4 hours of the maintenance dose may be less effective.

5.3 Discontinuation of Effient

Discontinue thienopyridines, including Effient, for active bleeding, elective surgery, stroke, or TIA. The optimal duration of thienopyridine therapy is unknown. In patients who are managed with PCI and stent placement, premature discontinuation of any antiplatelet medication, including thienopyridines, conveys an increased risk of stent thrombosis, myocardial infarction, and death. Patients who require premature discontinuation of a thienopyridine will be at increased risk for cardiac events. Lapses in therapy should be avoided, and if thienopyridines must be temporarily discontinued because of an adverse event(s), they should

be restarted as soon as possible. [see Contraindications (4.1 and 4.2) and Warnings and Precautions (5.1)].

5.4 Thrombotic Thrombocytopenic Purpura

Thrombotic thrombocytopenic purpura (TTP) has been reported with the use of other thienopyridines, sometimes after a brief exposure (< 2 weeks). TTP is a serious condition that can be fatal and requires urgent treatment, including plasmapheresis (plasma exchange). TTP is characterized by thrombocytopenia, microangiopathic hemolytic anemia (schistocytes [fragment red blood cells] seen on peripheral smear), neurological findings, renal dysfunction, and fever.

6 ADVERSE REACTIONS

6.1 Clinical Trials Experience

The following serious adverse reactions are also discussed elsewhere in the labeling:
• Bleeding [see Boxed Warning and Warnings and Precautions (5.1, 5.2)]
• Thrombotic thrombocytopenic purpura [see Warnings and Precautions (5.4)]
Safety in patients with ACS undergoing PCI was evaluated in a clopidogrel-controlled study, TRITON-TIMI 38, in which 6741 patients were treated with Effient (60 mg loading dose and 10 mg once daily) for a median of 14.5 months (5802 patients were treated for over 6 months; 4136 patients were treated for more than 1 year). The population treated with Effient was 27 to 96 years of age, 25% female, and 92% Caucasian. All patients in the TRITON-TIMI 38 study were to receive aspirin. The dose of clopidogrel in this study was a 300 mg loading dose and 75 mg once daily.
Because clinical trials are conducted under widely varying conditions, adverse reaction rates observed in the clinical trials cannot be directly compared with the rates observed in other clinical trials of another drug and may not reflect the rates observed in practice.

Drug Discontinuation
The rate of study drug discontinuation because of adverse reactions was 7.2% for Effient and 6.3% for clopidogrel. Bleeding was the most common adverse reaction leading to study drug discontinuation for both drugs (2.5% for Effient and 1.4% for clopidogrel).

Bleeding
Bleeding Unrelated to CABG Surgery—In TRITON-TIMI 38, overall rates of TIMI Major or Minor bleeding adverse reactions unrelated to coronary artery bypass graft surgery (CABG) were significantly higher on Effient than on clopidogrel, as shown in Table 1.
[See table 1 above]

Figure 1 demonstrates non-CABG related TIMI Major or Minor bleeding. The bleeding rate is highest initially, as shown in Figure 1 (inset: Days 0 to 7) [see Warnings and Precautions (5.1)].

Bleeding rates in patients with the risk factors of age ≥ 75 years and weight < 60 kg are shown in Table 2.
[See table 2 at top of next page]

Bleeding Related to CABG—In TRITON-TIMI 38, 437 patients who received a thienopyridine underwent CABG during the course of the study. The rate of CABG-related TIMI Major or Minor bleeding was 14.1% in the Effient group and 4.5% in the clopidogrel group (Table 3). The higher risk for bleeding adverse reactions in patients treated with Effient persisted up to 7 days from the most recent dose of study drug.

Table 1: Non-CABG-Related Bleeding[a] (TRITON-TIMI 38)

	Effient (%) (N=6741)	Clopidogrel (%) (N=6716)	p-value
TIMI Major or Minor bleeding	4.5	3.4	p=0.002
TIMI Major bleeding[b]	2.2	1.7	p=0.029
Life-threatening	1.3	0.8	p=0.015
Fatal	0.3	0.1	
Symptomatic intracranial hemorrhage (ICH)	0.3	0.3	
Requiring inotropes	0.3	0.1	
Requiring surgical intervention	0.3	0.3	
Requiring transfusion (≥4 units)	0.7	0.5	
TIMI Minor bleeding[b]	2.4	1.9	p=0.022

[a] Patients may be counted in more than one row.
[b] See 5.1 for definition.

Table 2: Bleeding Rates for Non-CABG-Related Bleeding by Weight and Age (TRITON-TIMI 38)

	Major/Minor		Fatal	
	Effient (%)	Clopidogrel (%)	Effient (%)	Clopidogrel (%)
Weight < 60 kg (N=308 Effient, N=356 clopidogrel)	10.1	6.5	0.0	0.3
Weight ≥ 60 kg (N=6373 Effient, N=6299 clopidogrel)	4.2	3.3	0.3	0.1
Age < 75 years (N=5850 Effient, N=5822 clopidogrel)	3.8	2.9	0.2	0.1
Age ≥ 75 years (N=891 Effient, N=894 clopidogrel)	9.0	6.9	1.0	0.1

Table 3: CABG-Related Bleeding[a] (TRITON-TIMI 38)

	Effient (%) (N=213)	Clopidogrel (%) (N=224)
TIMI Major or Minor bleeding	14.1	4.5
TIMI Major bleeding	11.3	3.6
Fatal	0.9	0
Reoperation	3.8	0.5
Transfusion of ≥5 units	6.6	2.2
Intracranial hemorrhage	0	0
TIMI Minor bleeding	2.8	0.9

[a] Patients may be counted in more than one row.

Bleeding Reported as Adverse Reactions—Hemorrhagic events reported as adverse reactions in TRITON-TIMI 38 were, for Effient and clopidogrel, respectively: epistaxis (6.2%, 3.3%), gastrointestinal hemorrhage (1.5%, 1.0%), hemoptysis (0.6%, 0.5%), subcutaneous hematoma (0.5%, 0.2%), post-procedural hemorrhage (0.5%, 0.2%), retroperitoneal hemorrhage (0.3%, 0.2%), and retinal hemorrhage (0.0%, 0.1%).
Malignancies
During TRITON-TIMI 38, newly diagnosed malignancies were reported in 1.6% and 1.2% of patients treated with prasugrel and clopidogrel, respectively. The sites contributing to the differences were primarily colon and lung. It is unclear if these observations are causally-related or are random occurrences.
Other Adverse Events
In TRITON-TIMI 38, common and other important nonhemorrhagic adverse events were, for Effient and clopidogrel, respectively: severe thrombocytopenia (0.06%, 0.04%), anemia (2.2%, 2.0%), abnormal hepatic function (0.22%, 0.27%), allergic reactions (0.36%, 0.36%), and angioedema (0.06%, 0.04%). Table 4 summarizes the adverse events reported by at least 2.5% of patients.

Table 4: Non-Hemorrhagic Treatment Emergent Adverse Events Reported by at Least 2.5% of Patients in Either Group

	Effient (%) (N=6741)	Clopidogrel (%) (N=6716)
Hypertension	7.5	7.1
Hypercholesterolemia/Hyperlipidemia	7.0	7.4
Headache	5.5	5.3
Back pain	5.0	4.5
Dyspnea	4.9	4.5
Nausea	4.6	4.3
Dizziness	4.1	4.6
Cough	3.9	4.1
Hypotension	3.9	3.8
Fatigue	3.7	4.8
Non-cardiac chest pain	3.1	3.5
Atrial fibrillation	2.9	3.1
Bradycardia	2.9	2.4
Leukopenia (< 4 × 10⁹ WBC/L)	2.8	3.5
Rash	2.8	2.4
Pyrexia	2.7	2.2
Peripheral edema	2.7	3.0
Pain in extremity	2.6	2.6
Diarrhea	2.3	2.6

7 DRUG INTERACTIONS
7.1 Warfarin
Coadministration of Effient and warfarin increases the risk of bleeding [see Warnings and Precautions (5.1) and Clinical Pharmacology (12.3)].
7.2 Non-Steroidal Anti-Inflammatory Drugs
Coadministration of Effient and NSAIDs (used chronically) may increase the risk of bleeding [see Warnings and Precautions (5.1)].
7.3 Other Concomitant Medications
Effient can be administered with drugs that are inducers or inhibitors of cytochrome P450 enzymes [see Clinical Pharmacology (12.3)].
Effient can be administered with aspirin (75 mg to 325 mg per day), heparin, GPIIb/IIIa inhibitors, statins, digoxin, and drugs that elevate gastric pH, including proton pump inhibitors and H₂ blockers [see Clinical Pharmacology (12.3)].

8 USE IN SPECIFIC POPULATIONS
8.1 Pregnancy
Pregnancy Category B—There are no adequate and well-controlled studies of Effient use in pregnant women. Reproductive and developmental toxicology studies in rats and rabbits at doses of up to 30 times the recommended therapeutic exposures in humans (based on plasma exposures to the major circulating human metabolite) revealed no evidence of fetal harm; however, animal studies are not always predictive of a human response. Effient should be used during pregnancy only if the potential benefit to the mother justifies the potential risk to the fetus.
In embryo fetal developmental toxicology studies, pregnant rats and rabbits received prasugrel at maternally toxic oral doses equivalent to more than 40 times the human exposure. A slight decrease in pup body weight was observed; but, there were no structural malformations in either species. In prenatal and postnatal rat studies, maternal treatment with prasugrel had no effect on the behavioral or reproductive development of the offspring at doses greater than 150 times the human exposure [see Nonclinical Toxicology (13.1)].
8.3 Nursing Mothers
It is not known whether Effient is excreted in human milk; however, metabolites of Effient were found in rat milk. Because many drugs are excreted in human milk, prasugrel should be used during nursing only if the potential benefit to the mother justifies the potential risk to the nursing infant.
8.4 Pediatric Use
Safety and effectiveness in pediatric patients have not been established [see Clinical Pharmacology (12.3)].
8.5 Geriatric Use
In TRITON-TIMI 38, 38.5% of patients were ≥65 years of age and 13.2% were ≥75 years of age. The risk of bleeding increased with advancing age in both treatment groups, although the relative risk of bleeding (Effient compared with clopidogrel) was similar across age groups.
Patients ≥ 75 years of age who received Effient had an increased risk of fatal bleeding events (1.0%) compared to patients who received clopidogrel (0.1%). In patients ≥ 75 years of age, symptomatic intracranial hemorrhage occurred in 7 patients (0.8%) who received Effient and in 3

patients (0.3%) who received clopidogrel. Because of the risk of bleeding, and because effectiveness is uncertain in patients ≥ 75 years of age [see Clinical Studies (14)], use of Effient is generally not recommended in these patients, except in high-risk situations (diabetes and past history of myocardial infarction) where its effect appears to be greater and its use may be considered [see Warnings and Precautions (5.1), Clinical Pharmacology (12.3), and Clinical Studies (14)].
8.6 Low Body Weight
In TRITON-TIMI 38, 4.6% of patients treated with Effient had body weight <60 kg. Individuals with body weight < 60 kg had an increased risk of bleeding and an increased exposure to the active metabolite of prasugrel [see Dosage and Administration (2), Warnings and Precautions (5.1), and Clinical Pharmacology (12.3)]. Consider lowering the maintenance dose to 5 mg in patients <60 kg. The effectiveness and safety of the 5 mg dose have not been prospectively studied.
8.7 Renal Impairment
No dosage adjustment is necessary for patients with renal impairment. There is limited experience in patients with end-stage renal disease [see Clinical Pharmacology (12.3)].
8.8 Hepatic Impairment
No dosage adjustment is necessary in patients with mild to moderate hepatic impairment (Child-Pugh Class A and B). The pharmacokinetics and pharmacodynamics of prasugrel in patients with severe hepatic disease have not been studied, but such patients are generally at higher risk of bleeding [see Warnings and Precautions (5.1) and Clinical Pharmacology (12.3)].
8.9 Metabolic Status
In healthy subjects, patients with stable atherosclerosis, and patients with ACS receiving prasugrel, there was no relevant effect of genetic variation in CYP2B6, CYP2C9, CYP2C19, or CYP3A5 on the pharmacokinetics of prasugrel's active metabolite or its inhibition of platelet aggregation.

10 OVERDOSAGE
10.1 Signs and Symptoms
Platelet inhibition by prasugrel is rapid and irreversible, lasting for the life of the platelet, and is unlikely to be increased in the event of an overdose. In rats, lethality was observed after administration of 2000 mg/kg. Symptoms of acute toxicity in dogs included emesis, increased serum alkaline phosphatase, and hepatocellular atrophy. Symptoms of acute toxicity in rats included mydriasis, irregular respiration, decreased locomotor activity, ptosis, staggering gait, and lacrimation.
10.2 Recommendations about Specific Treatment
Platelet transfusion may restore clotting ability. The prasugrel active metabolite is not likely to be removed by dialysis.

11 DESCRIPTION
Effient contains prasugrel, a thienopyridine class inhibitor of platelet activation and aggregation mediated by the P2Y₁₂ ADP receptor. Effient is formulated as the hydrochloride salt, a racemate, which is chemically designated as 5-[(1RS)-2-cyclopropyl-1-(2-fluorophenyl)-2-oxoethyl]-4,5,6,7-tetrahydrothieno[3,2-c]pyridin-2-yl acetate hydrochloride. Prasugrel hydrochloride has the empirical formula $C_{20}H_{20}FNO_3S \bullet HCl$ representing a molecular weight of 409.90. The chemical structure of prasugrel hydrochloride is:

Prasugrel hydrochloride is a white to practically white solid. It is soluble at pH 2, slightly soluble at pH 3 to 4, and practically insoluble at pH 6 to 7.5. It also dissolves freely in methanol and is slightly soluble in 1- and 2-propanol and acetone. It is practically insoluble in diethyl ether and ethyl acetate.
Effient is available for oral administration as 5 mg or 10 mg elongated hexagonal, film-coated, non-scored tablets, debossed on each side. Each yellow 5 mg tablet is manufactured with 5.49 mg prasugrel hydrochloride, equivalent to 5 mg prasugrel and each beige 10 mg tablet with 10.98 mg prasugrel hydrochloride, equivalent to 10 mg of prasugrel. During manufacture and storage, partial conversion from prasugrel hydrochloride to prasugrel free base may occur. Other ingredients include mannitol, hypromellose, croscarmellose sodium, microcrystalline cellulose, and vegetable magnesium stearate. The color coatings contain lactose, hypromellose, titanium dioxide, triacetin, iron oxide yellow, and iron oxide red (only in Effient 10 mg tablet).

12 CLINICAL PHARMACOLOGY

12.1 Mechanism of Action

Prasugrel is an inhibitor of platelet activation and aggregation through the irreversible binding of its active metabolite to the $P2Y_{12}$ class of ADP receptors on platelets.

12.2 Pharmacodynamics

Prasugrel produces inhibition of platelet aggregation to 20 µM or 5 µM ADP, as measured by light transmission aggregometry. Following a 60-mg loading dose of Effient, approximately 90% of patients had at least 50% inhibition of platelet aggregation by 1 hour. Maximum platelet inhibition was about 80% (Figure 2). Mean steady-state inhibition of platelet aggregation was about 70% following 3 to 5 days of dosing at 10 mg daily after a 60-mg loading dose of Effient.

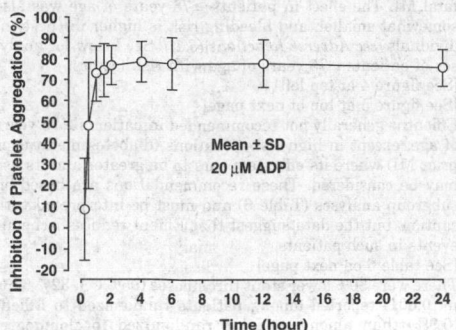

Figure 2: Inhibition (Mean±SD) of 20 µM ADP-induced Platelet Aggregation (IPA) Measured by Light Transmission Aggregometry after Prasugrel 60 mg

Platelet aggregation gradually returns to baseline values over 5-9 days after discontinuation of prasugrel, this time course being a reflection of new platelet production rather than pharmacokinetics of prasugrel. Discontinuing clopidogrel 75 mg and initiating prasugrel 10 mg with the next dose resulted in increased inhibition of platelet aggregation, but not greater than that typically produced by a 10 mg maintenance dose of prasugrel alone. The relationship between inhibition of platelet aggregation and clinical activity has not been established.

12.3 Pharmacokinetics

Prasugrel is a prodrug and is rapidly metabolized to a pharmacologically active metabolite and inactive metabolites. The active metabolite has an elimination half-life of about 7 hours (range 2-15 hours). Healthy subjects, patients with stable atherosclerosis, and patients undergoing PCI show similar pharmacokinetics.

Absorption and Binding—Following oral administration, ≥ 79% of the dose is absorbed. The absorption and metabolism are rapid, with peak plasma concentrations (C_{max}) of the active metabolite occurring approximately 30 minutes after dosing. The active metabolite's exposure (AUC) increases slightly more than proportionally over the dose range of 5 to 60 mg. Repeated daily doses of 10 mg do not lead to accumulation of the active metabolite. In a study of healthy subjects given a single 15 mg dose, the AUC of the active metabolite was unaffected by a high fat, high calorie meal, but C_{max} was decreased by 49% and T_{max} was increased from 0.5 to 1.5 hours. Effient can be administered without regard to food. The active metabolite is bound about 98% to human serum albumin.

Metabolism and Elimination—Prasugrel is not detected in plasma following oral administration. It is rapidly hydrolyzed in the intestine to a thiolactone, which is then converted to the active metabolite by a single step, primarily by CYP3A4 and CYP2B6 and to a lesser extent by CYP2C9 and CYP2C19. The estimates of apparent volume of distribution of prasugrel's active metabolite ranged from 44 to 68 L and the estimates of apparent clearance ranged from 112 to 166 L/hr in healthy subjects and patients with stable atherosclerosis. The active metabolite is metabolized to two inactive compounds by S-methylation or conjugation with cysteine. The major inactive metabolites are highly bound to human plasma proteins. Approximately 68% of the prasugrel dose is excreted in the urine and 27% in the feces as inactive metabolites.

Specific Populations

Pediatric—Pharmacokinetics and pharmacodynamics of prasugrel have not been evaluated in a pediatric population [*see Use in Specific Populations (8.4)*].

Geriatric—In a study of 32 healthy subjects between the ages of 20 and 80 years, age had no significant effect on pharmacokinetics of prasugrel's active metabolite or its inhibition of platelet aggregation. In TRITON-TIMI 38, the mean exposure (AUC) of the active metabolite was 19% higher in patients ≥75 years of age than in patients <75 years of age [*see Warnings and Precautions (5.1), Adverse Reactions (6.1), and Use in Specific Populations (8.5)*].

Body Weight—The mean exposure (AUC) to the active metabolite is approximately 30 to 40% higher in subjects with a body weight of <60 kg than in those weighing ≥60 kg [*see Dosage and Administration (2), Warnings and Precautions (5.1), Adverse Reactions (6.1), and Use in Specific Populations (8.6)*].

Gender—Pharmacokinetics of prasugrel's active metabolite are similar in men and women.

Ethnicity—Exposure in subjects of African and Hispanic descent is similar to that in Caucasians. In clinical pharmacology studies, after adjusting for body weight, the AUC of the active metabolite was approximately 19% higher in Chinese, Japanese, and Korean subjects than in Caucasian subjects.

Smoking—Pharmacokinetics of prasugrel's active metabolite are similar in smokers and nonsmokers.

Renal Impairment—Pharmacokinetics of prasugrel's active metabolite and its inhibition of platelet aggregation are similar in patients with moderate renal impairment (CrCL=30 to 50 mL/min) and healthy subjects. In patients with end stage renal disease, exposure to the active metabolite (both C_{max} and AUC (0-t_{last})) was about half that in healthy controls and patients with moderate renal impairment [*see Use in Specific Populations (8.7)*].

Hepatic Impairment—Pharmacokinetics of prasugrel's active metabolite and inhibition of platelet aggregation were similar in patients with mild to moderate hepatic impairment compared to healthy subjects. The pharmacokinetics and pharmacodynamics of prasugrel's active metabolite in patients with severe hepatic disease have not been studied [*see Warnings and Precautions (5.1) and Use in Specific Populations (8.8)*].

Drug Interactions

Potential for Other Drugs to Affect Prasugrel

Inhibitors of CYP3A—Ketoconazole (400 mg daily), a selective and potent inhibitor of CYP3A4 and CYP3A5, did not affect prasugrel-mediated inhibition of platelet aggregation or the active metabolite's AUC and T_{max}, but decreased the C_{max} by 34% to 46%. Therefore, CYP3A inhibitors such as verapamil, diltiazem, indinavir, ciprofloxacin, clarithromycin, and grapefruit juice are not expected to have a significant effect on the pharmacokinetics of the active metabolite of prasugrel [*see Drug Interactions (7.3)*].

Inducers of Cytochromes P450—Rifampicin (600 mg daily), a potent inducer of CYP3A and CYP2B6 and an inducer of CYP2C9, CYP2C19, and CYP2C8, did not significantly change the pharmacokinetics of prasugrel's active metabolite or its inhibition of platelet aggregation. Therefore, known CYP3A inducers such as rifampicin, carbamazepine, and other inducers of cytochromes P450 are not expected to have significant effect on the pharmacokinetics of the active metabolite of prasugrel [*see Drug Interactions (7.3)*].

Drugs that Elevate Gastric pH—Daily coadministration of ranitidine (an H_2 blocker) or lansoprazole (a proton pump inhibitor) decreased the C_{max} of the prasugrel active metabolite by 14% and 29%, respectively, but did not change the active metabolite's AUC and T_{max}. In TRITON-TIMI 38, Effient was administered without regard to coadministration of a proton pump inhibitor or H_2 blocker [*see Drug Interactions (7.3)*].

Statins—Atorvastatin (80 mg daily), a drug metabolized by CYP450 3A4, did not alter the pharmacokinetics of prasugrel's active metabolite or its inhibition of platelet aggregation [*see Drug Interactions (7.3)*].

Heparin—A single intravenous dose of unfractionated heparin (100 U/kg) did not significantly alter coagulation or the prasugrel-mediated inhibition of platelet aggregation; however, bleeding time was increased compared with either drug alone [*see Drug Interactions (7.3)*].

Aspirin—Aspirin 150 mg daily did not alter prasugrel-mediated inhibition of platelet aggregation; however, bleeding time was increased compared with either drug alone [*see Drug Interactions (7.3)*].

Warfarin—A significant prolongation of the bleeding time was observed when prasugrel was coadministered with 15 mg of warfarin [*see Drug Interactions (7.1)*].

Potential for Prasugrel to Affect Other Drugs

In vitro metabolism studies demonstrate that prasugrel's main circulating metabolites are not likely to cause clinically significant inhibition of CYP1A2, CYP2C9, CYP2C19, CYP2D6, or CYP3A, or induction of CYP1A2 or CYP3A.

Drugs Metabolized by CYP2B6—Prasugrel is a weak inhibitor of CYP2B6. In healthy subjects, prasugrel decreased exposure to hydroxybupropion, a CYP2B6-mediated metabolite of bupropion, by 23%, an amount not considered clinically significant. Prasugrel is not anticipated to have significant effect on the pharmacokinetics of drugs that are primarily metabolized by CYP2B6, such as halothane, cyclophosphamide, propofol, and nevirapine.

Effect on Digoxin—The potential role of prasugrel as a Pgp substrate was not evaluated. Prasugrel is not an inhibitor of Pgp, as digoxin clearance was not affected by prasugrel coadministration [*see Drug Interactions (7.3)*].

12.5 Pharmacogenomics

There is no relevant effect of genetic variation in CYP2B6, CYP2C9, CYP2C19, or CYP3A5 on the pharmacokinetics of prasugrel's active metabolite or its inhibition of platelet aggregation.

13 NONCLINICAL TOXICOLOGY

13.1 Carcinogenesis, Mutagenesis, Impairment of Fertility

Carcinogenesis—No compound-related tumors were observed in a 2-year rat study with prasugrel at oral doses up to 100 mg/kg/day (>100 times the recommended therapeutic exposures in humans) (based on plasma exposures to the major circulating human metabolite). There was an increased incidence of tumors (hepatocellular adenomas) in mice exposed for 2 years to high doses (>250 times the human metabolite exposure).

Mutagenesis—Prasugrel was not genotoxic in two *in vitro* tests (Ames bacterial gene mutation test, clastogenicity assay in Chinese hamster fibroblasts) and in one *in vivo* test (micronucleus test by intraperitoneal route in mice).

Impairment of Fertility—Prasugrel had no effect on fertility of male and female rats at oral doses up to 300 mg/kg/day (80 times the human major metabolite exposure at daily dose of 10 mg prasugrel).

14 CLINICAL STUDIES

The clinical evidence for the effectiveness of Effient is derived from the TRITON-TIMI 38 (TRial to Assess Improvement in Therapeutic Outcomes by Optimizing Platelet InhibitioN with Prasugrel) study, a 13,608-patient, multicenter, international, randomized, double-blind, parallel-group study comparing Effient to a regimen of clopidogrel, each added to aspirin and other standard therapy, in patients

Table 5: Patients with Outcome Events (CV Death, MI, Stroke) in TRITON-TIMI 38

	Patients with events		From Kaplan-Meier analysis	
	Effient (%)	Clopidogrel (%)	Relative Risk Reduction (%)[a] (95% CI)	p-value
UA/NSTEMI	**N=5044**	**N=5030**		
CV death, nonfatal MI, or nonfatal stroke	9.3	11.2	18.0 (7.3, 27.4)	0.002
CV death	1.8	1.8	2.1 (-30.9, 26.8)	0.885
Nonfatal MI	7.1	9.2	23.9 (12.7, 33.7)	<0.001
Nonfatal Stroke	0.8	0.8	2.1 (-51.3, 36.7)	0.922
STEMI	**N=1769**	**N=1765**		
CV death, nonfatal MI, or nonfatal stroke	9.8	12.2	20.7 (3.2, 35.1)	0.019
CV death	2.4	3.3	26.2 (-9.4, 50.3)	0.129
Nonfatal MI	6.7	8.8	25.4 (5.2, 41.2)	0.016
Nonfatal Stroke	1.2	1.1	-9.7 (-104.0, 41.0)	0.77

[a] RRR = (1-Hazard Ratio) × 100%. Values with a negative relative risk reduction indicate a relative risk increase.

Baseline Characteristics		N	Percent Events	
			Effient	Clopidogrel
OVERALL-UA/NSTEMI		10074	9.9	12.1
Age	<65 y	5987	7.5	10.0
	≥65 y	4087	11.9	13.1
	<75 y	8672	8.2	10.5
	≥75 y	1402	15.8	16.2
Gender	Female	2724	10.3	11.4
	Male	7350	8.9	11.2
Body Weight	<60 kg	503	9.2	9.8
	≥60 kg	9458	9.2	11.1
Region	North America	3538	9.6	11.9
	United States	3382	9.7	12.2
	South America	534	13.3	15.2
	Western Europe	2527	8.8	9.8
	Eastern Europe	2300	8.5	10.0
	Rest of World	1175	9.1	13.1
Diabetes Mellitus	Yes	2472	10.8	15.0
	No	7602	8.8	10.0
Metabolic Syndrome	Yes	4511	9.1	11.5
	No	5563	9.5	11.1
Previous MI	Yes	2075	12.9	15.8
	No	7999	8.3	10.1
Previous PCI	Yes	1597	12.0	14.8
	No	8477	8.8	10.6
Previous CABG	Yes	957	16.0	18.2
	No	9117	8.6	10.5
Previous TIA/Stroke	Yes	405	18.3	12.5
	No	9669	8.9	11.2
Time From Symptom Onset	≤24 h	3902	8.3	10.8
	>24 h	5976	10.1	11.5
Stent Type	Drug-eluting ≥1	5225	9.2	10.9
	Bare Metal Only	4362	9.2	11.6
	None	401	11.7	14.9
GP IIb/IIIa Inhibitor Use	Yes	5183	9.9	11.9
	No	4891	8.7	10.5

Hazard Ratio

0.2   0.5   1   2

← Effient better   Clopidogrel better →

Figure 4: Subgroup analyses for time to first event of CV death, MI, or stroke (HR and 95% CI; TRITON-TIMI 38) – UA/NSTEMI Patients.

with ACS (UA, NSTEMI, or STEMI) who were to be managed with PCI. Randomization was stratified for UA/NSTEMI and STEMI.

Patients with UA/NSTEMI presenting within 72 hours of symptom onset were to be randomized after undergoing coronary angiography. Patients with STEMI presenting within 12 hours of symptom onset could be randomized prior to coronary angiography. Patients with STEMI presenting between 12 hours and 14 days of symptom onset were to be randomized after undergoing coronary angiography. Patients underwent PCI, and for both UA/NSTEMI and STEMI patients, the loading dose was to be administered anytime between randomization and 1 hour after the patient left the catheterization lab. If patients with STEMI were treated with thrombolytic therapy, randomization could not occur until at least 24 hours (for tenecteplase, reteplase or alteplase) or 48 hours (for streptokinase) after the thrombolytic was given.

Patients were randomized to receive Effient (60 mg loading dose followed by 10 mg once daily) or clopidogrel (300 mg loading dose followed by 75 mg once daily), with administration and follow-up for a minimum of 6 months (actual median 14.5 months). Patients also received aspirin (75 mg to 325 mg once daily). Other therapies, such as heparin and intravenous glycoprotein IIb/IIIa (GPIIb/IIIa) inhibitors, were administered at the discretion of the treating physician. Oral anticoagulants, other platelet inhibitors, and chronic NSAIDs were not allowed.

The primary outcome measure was the composite of cardiovascular death, nonfatal MI, or nonfatal stroke in the UA/NSTEMI population. Success in this group allowed analysis of the same endpoint in the overall ACS and STEMI populations. Nonfatal MIs included both MIs detected solely through analysis of creatine kinase muscle-brain (CK-MB) changes and clinically apparent (investigator-reported) MIs.

The patient population was 92% Caucasian, 26% female, and 39% ≥65 years of age. The median time from symptom onset to study drug administration was 7 hours for patients with STEMI and 30 hours for patients with UA/NSTEMI. Approximately 99% of patients underwent PCI. The study drug was administered after the first coronary guidewire was placed in approximately 75% of patients.

Effient significantly reduced total endpoint events compared to clopidogrel (*see* Table 5 and Figure 3). The reduction of total endpoint events was driven primarily by a decrease in nonfatal MIs, both those occurring early (through 3 days) and later (after 3 days). Approximately 40% of MIs occurred peri-procedurally and were detected solely by changes in CK-MB. Administration of the clopidogrel loading dose in TRITON-TIMI 38 was delayed relative to the placebo-controlled trials that supported its approval for

ACS. Effient produced higher rates of clinically significant bleeding than clopidogrel in TRITON-TIMI 38 *[see Adverse Reactions (6.1)]*. Choice of therapy requires balancing these differences in outcome.

The treatment effect of Effient was apparent within the first few days, and persisted to the end of the study (Figure 3). The inset shows results over the first 7 days.

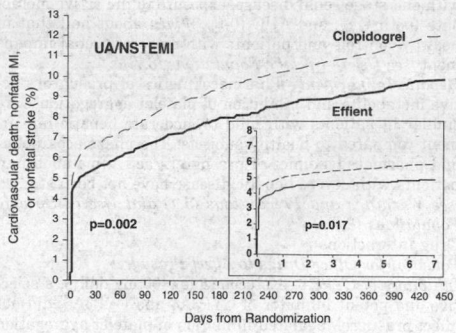

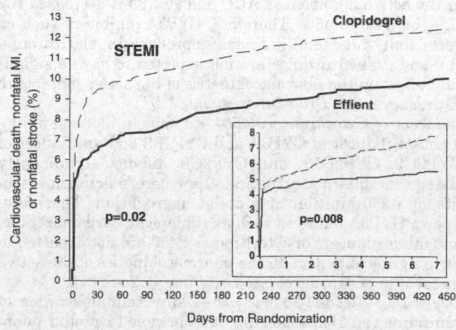

Figure 3: Time to first event of CV death, MI, or stroke (TRITON-TIMI 38)

The Kaplan-Meier curves (Figure 3) show the primary composite endpoint of CV death, nonfatal MI, or nonfatal stroke over time in the UA/NSTEMI and STEMI populations. In both populations, the curves separate within the first few hours. In the UA/NSTEMI population, the curves continue to diverge throughout the 15 month follow-up period. In the

STEMI population, the early separation was maintained throughout the 15 month follow-up period, but there was no progressive divergence after the first few weeks.

Effient reduced the occurrence of the primary composite endpoint compared to clopidogrel in both the UA/NSTEMI and STEMI populations (*see* Table 5). In patients who survived an on-study myocardial infarction, the incidence of subsequent events was also lower in the Effient group.

[See table 5 at top of previous page]

The effect of Effient in various subgroups is shown in Figures 4 and 5. Results are generally consistent across prespecified subgroups, with the exception of patients with a history of TIA or stroke *[see Contraindications (4.2)]*. The treatment effect was driven primarily by a reduction in nonfatal MI. The effect in patients ≥75 years of age was also somewhat smaller, and bleeding risk is higher in these individuals *[see Adverse Reactions (6.1)]*. See below for analyses of patients ≥75 years of age with risk factors.

[See figure 4 at top left]

[See figure 5 at top of next page]

Effient is generally not recommended in patients ≥75 years of age, except in high-risk situations (diabetes mellitus or prior MI) where its effect appears to be greater and its use may be considered. These recommendations are based on subgroup analyses (Table 6) and must be interpreted with caution, but the data suggest that Effient reduces ischemic events in such patients.

[See table 6 on next page]

There were 50% fewer stent thromboses (95% C.I. 32%-64%; p< 0.001) reported among patients randomized to Effient (0.9%) than among patients randomized to clopidogrel (1.8%). The difference manifested early and was maintained through one year of follow-up. Findings were similar with bare metal and drug-eluting stents.

In TRITON-TIMI 38, prasugrel reduced ischemic events (mainly nonfatal MIs) and increased bleeding events *[see Adverse Reactions (6.1)]* relative to clopidogrel. The findings are consistent with the intended greater inhibition of platelet aggregation by prasugrel at the doses used in the study *[see Clinical Pharmacology (12.2)]*. There is, however, an alternative explanation: both prasugrel and clopidogrel are pro-drugs that must be metabolized to their active moieties. Whereas the pharmacokinetics of prasugrel's active metabolite are not known to be affected by genetic variations in CYP2B6, CYP2C9, CYP2C19, or CYP3A5, the pharmacokinetics of clopidogrel's active metabolite are affected by CYP2C19 genotype, and approximately 30% of Caucasians are reduced-metabolizers. Moreover, certain proton pump inhibitors, widely used in the ACS patient population and used in TRITON-TIMI 38, inhibit CYP2C19, thereby decreasing formation of clopidogrel's active metabolite. Thus, reduced metabolizer status and use of proton pump inhibitors may diminish clopidogrel's activity in a fraction of the population, and may have contributed to prasugrel's greater treatment effect and greater bleeding rate in TRITON-TIMI 38. The extent to which these factors were operational, however, is unknown.

16 HOW SUPPLIED/STORAGE AND HANDLING

Effient (prasugrel) 5 mg is supplied as a yellow, elongated hexagonal, film-coated, non-scored tablet debossed with "5 MG" on one side and with "4760" on the other side.

    5 mg tablets are supplied as follows:
    Bottles of 7 - NDC 0002-4760-76
    Bottles of 30 - NDC 0002-4760-30

Effient (prasugrel) 10 mg is supplied as a beige, elongated hexagonal, film-coated, non-scored tablet debossed with "10 MG" on one side and "4759" on the other side.

    10 mg tablets are supplied as follows:
    Bottles of 30 – NDC 0002-4759-30
    Blisters ID 90* NDC 0002-4759-77

(*Identi Dose®, unit dose medication, Lilly)

Store at 25°C (77°F); excursions permitted to 15° to 30°C (59° to 86°F).

Dispense and keep product in original container. Keep container closed and do not remove desiccant from bottle. Do not break the tablet.

17 PATIENT COUNSELING INFORMATION

See Medication Guide

17.1 Benefits and Risks

• Summarize the effectiveness features and potential side effects of Effient.
• Tell patients to take Effient exactly as prescribed.
• Remind patients not to discontinue Effient without first discussing it with the physician who prescribed Effient.
• Recommend that patients read the Medication Guide.

17.2 Bleeding

Inform patients that they:
• will bruise and bleed more easily.
• will take longer than usual to stop bleeding.
• should report any unanticipated, prolonged, or excessive bleeding, or blood in their stool or urine.

17.3 Other Signs and Symptoms Requiring Medical Attention

- Inform patients that TTP is a rare but serious condition that has been reported with medications in this class of drugs.
- Instruct patients to get prompt medical attention if they experience any of the following symptoms that cannot otherwise be explained: fever, weakness, extreme skin paleness, purple skin patches, yellowing of the skin or eyes, or neurological changes.

17.4 Invasive Procedures

Instruct patients to:

- inform physicians and dentists that they are taking Effient before any invasive procedure is scheduled.
- tell the doctor performing the invasive procedure to talk to the prescribing health care professional before stopping Effient.

17.5 Concomitant Medications

Ask patients to list all prescription medications, over-the-counter medications, or dietary supplements they are taking or plan to take so the physician knows about other treatments that may affect bleeding risk (*e.g.*, warfarin and NSAIDs).

Literature Issued: July 10, 2009

Manufactured by Eli Lilly and Company, Indianapolis, IN, 46285

Marketed by Daiichi Sankyo, Inc. and Eli Lilly and Company
Copyright ©2009, Daiichi Sankyo, Inc. and Eli Lilly and Company. All rights reserved.
PV 7310 AMP

MEDICATION GUIDE

Effient™ (Ef´-fee-ent)
(prasugrel)
Tablets

Read this Medication Guide before you start taking Effient and each time you get a refill. There may be new information. This Medication Guide does not take the place of talking with your doctor about your medical condition or your treatment.

What is the most important information I should know about Effient?

- Effient is used to lower your chance of having a heart attack or other serious problems with your heart or blood vessels. But, Effient can cause bleeding, which can be serious, and sometimes lead to death. You should not start to take Effient if it is likely that you will have heart bypass surgery (coronary artery bypass graft surgery or CABG) right away. You have a higher risk of bleeding if you take Effient and then have heart bypass surgery.
- **Do not take Effient if you:**
  - currently have abnormal bleeding, such as stomach or intestinal bleeding, or bleeding in your head
  - have a history of stroke, or "mini-stroke" (transient ischemic attack or TIA)
  - You should stop taking Effient if you have a stroke.
- **Whenever possible, you should stop taking Effient at least 7 days before any surgery, as instructed by the doctor who prescribed Effient for you.**

You may also have a higher risk of bleeding if you take Effient and:

- have had trauma, such as an accident or surgery
- have stomach or intestine bleeding that is recent or keeps coming back, or you have a stomach ulcer
- have severe liver problems
- weigh less than 132 pounds
- take other medicines that increase your risk of bleeding, including:
  - warfarin sodium (Coumadin*, Jantoven*)
  - a medicine that contains heparin
  - other medicines to prevent or treat blood clots
  - non-steroidal anti-inflammatory drugs (NSAIDs) for a long time

Tell your doctor if you take any of these medicines. Ask your doctor if you are not sure if your medicine is one listed above.

- Effient increases your risk of bleeding because it lessens the ability of your blood to clot. While you take Effient:
  - you will bruise and bleed more easily
  - you are more likely to have nose bleeds
  - it will take longer for any bleeding to stop
- Call your doctor right away if you have any of these signs or symptoms of bleeding:
  - unexpected bleeding or bleeding that lasts a long time
  - bleeding that is severe or you can not control
  - pink or brown urine
  - red or black stools (looks like tar)
  - bruises that happen without a known cause or get larger
  - cough up blood or blood clots
  - vomit blood or your vomit looks like "coffee grounds"
- **Do not stop taking Effient without talking to the doctor who prescribes it for you. People who are treated with angioplasty and have a stent, and stop taking Effient too**

soon, have a higher risk of a blood clot in the stent, having a heart attack, or dying. If you must stop Effient because of bleeding, your risk of a heart attack may be higher. See "What are the possible side effects of Effient?" for more information about side effects.

What is Effient?

Effient is a prescription medicine used to treat people who:

- have had a heart attack or severe chest pain that happens when your heart does not get enough oxygen, and
- have been treated with a procedure called "angioplasty" (also called balloon angioplasty).

Effient is used to lower your chance of having another serious problem with your heart or blood vessels, such as another heart attack, a stroke, blood clots in your stent, or death.

Platelets are blood cells that help with normal blood clotting. Effient helps prevent platelets from sticking together and forming a clot that can block an artery or a stent.

It is not known if Effient is safe and works in children.

What should I tell my doctor before taking Effient?

Effient may not be right for you. Tell your doctor about all of your medical conditions, including if you:

- have any bleeding problems
- have a history of stomach ulcers, colon polyps, diverticulosis
- have liver problems
- have had any recent severe injury or surgery
- plan to have surgery or a dental procedure. See "What is the most important information I should know about Effient?"
- pregnant, or are planning to get pregnant. It is not known if Effient will harm your baby.
- if you are breast-feeding. It is not known if Effient passes into your breast-milk. You and your doctor should decide if you will take Effient or breast-feed. You should not do both without talking with your doctor.

Tell all of your doctors and dentists that you are taking Effient. They should talk to the doctor who prescribed

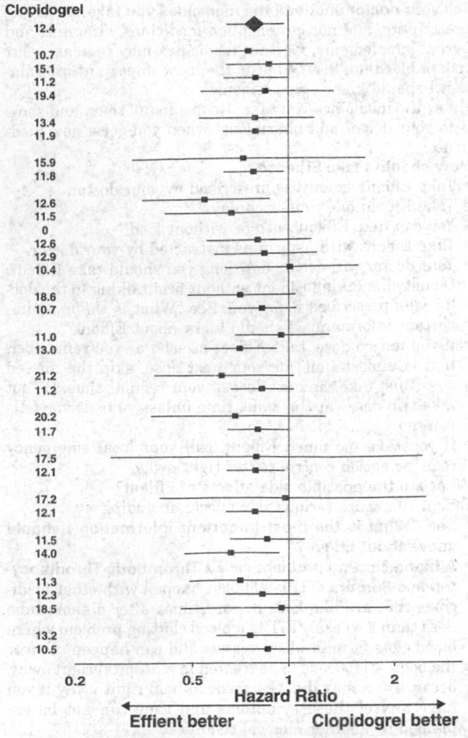

Figure 5: Subgroup analyses for time to first event of CV death, MI, or stroke (HR and 95% CI; TRITON-TIMI 38) – STEMI Patients.

Baseline Characteristics		N	Percent Events	
			Effient	Clopidogrel
OVERALL-STEMI		3534	10.0	12.4
Age	<65 y	2335	8.2	10.7
	≥65 y	1199	13.4	15.1
	<75 y	3127	9.0	11.2
	≥75 y	407	16.8	19.4
Gender	Female	799	10.8	13.4
	Male	2735	9.6	11.9
Body Weight	<60 kg	165	12.1	15.9
	≥60 kg	3311	9.4	11.8
Region	North America	772	7.2	12.6
	United States	677	7.8	11.5
	South America	0	0	0
	Western Europe	1026	10.3	12.6
	Eastern Europe	1022	10.9	12.9
	Rest of World	714	10.6	10.4
Diabetes Mellitus	Yes	674	13.6	18.6
	No	2860	9.0	10.7
Metabolic Syndrome	Yes	1393	10.4	11.0
	No	2141	9.4	13.0
Previous MI	Yes	359	14.3	21.2
	No	3175	9.4	11.2
Previous PCI	Yes	233	14.9	20.2
	No	3301	9.5	11.7
Previous CABG	Yes	81	14.6	17.5
	No	3453	9.7	12.1
Previous TIA/Stroke	Yes	113	16.3	17.2
	No	3421	9.7	12.1
Time From Symptom Onset	≤12 h	2438	10.1	11.5
	>12 h	1094	9.4	14.0
Stent Type	Drug-eluting ≥1	1158	8.2	11.3
	Bare Metal Only	2099	10.3	12.3
	None	168	17.2	18.5
GP IIb/IIIa Inhibitor Use	Yes	2220	10.3	13.2
	No	1314	9.1	10.5

Table 6: Subgroup Analyses for Time to First Event of CV Death, MI, or Stroke: Patients < or ≥75 Years of Age, ± Diabetes, ± Prior History of MI, All ACS Patient Population

	Effient		Clopidogrel		Hazard Ratio (95% CI)	p-value
	N	% with events	N	% with events		
Age ≥75						
Diabetes - yes	249	14.9	234	21.8	0.64 (0.42, 0.97)	0.034
Diabetes - no	652	16.4	674	15.3	1.1 (0.83, 1.43)	NS
Age <75						
Diabetes - yes	1327	10.8	1336	14.8	0.72 (0.58, 0.89)	0.002
Diabetes - no	4585	7.8	4551	9.5	0.82 (0.71, 0.94)	0.004
Age ≥75						
Prior MI - yes	220	17.3	212	22.6	0.72 (0.47, 1.09)	0.12
Prior MI - no	681	15.6	696	15.2	1.05 (0.80, 1.37)	NS
Age <75						
Prior MI - yes	1006	12.2	996	15.4	0.78 (0.62, 0.99)	0.04
Prior MI - no	4906	7.7	4891	9.7	0.78 (0.68, 0.90)	<0.001

Effient for you, before you have any surgery or invasive procedure.

Tell your doctor about all the medicines you take, including prescription and non-prescription medicines, vitamins, and herbal supplements. Certain medicines may increase your risk of bleeding. See "What is the most important information I should know about Effient?"

Know the medicines you take. Keep a list of them and show it to your doctor and pharmacist when you get a new medicine.

How should I take Effient?
• Take Effient exactly as prescribed by your doctor.
• Take Effient one time each day.
• You can take Effient with or without food.
• Take Effient with aspirin as instructed by your doctor.
• Your doctor will decide how long you should take Effient. Do not stop taking Effient without first talking to the doctor who prescribed it for you. See "What is the most important information I should know about Effient?"
• If you miss a dose, take Effient as soon as you remember. If it is almost time for your next dose, skip the missed dose. Just take the next dose at your regular time. Do not take two doses at the same time unless your doctor tells you to.
• If you take too much Effient, call your local emergency room or poison control center right away.

What are the possible side effects of Effient?
Effient can cause serious side effects, including:
• **See "What is the most important information I should know about Effient?"**
• **A blood clotting problem called Thrombotic Thrombocytopenic Purpura (TTP).** TTP can happen with other medicines that are like Effient, sometimes after a short time (less than 2 weeks). TTP is a blood clotting problem where blood clots form in blood vessels and can happen all over the body. TTP needs to be treated in a hospital right away, because you may die. Get medical help right away if you have any of these symptoms and they can not be explained by another medical condition:
• purplish spots called purpura on the skin or mucous membranes (such as on the mouth) due to bleeding under the skin
• paleness or jaundice (a yellowish color of the skin or eyes)
• feeling tired or weak
• fever
• fast heart rate or feeling short of breath
• headache, speech changes, confusion, coma, stroke, or seizure
• low amount of urine, or urine that is pink-tinged or has blood in it
• stomach area (abdominal) pain, nausea, vomiting, or diarrhea
• visual changes
Tell your doctor if you have any side effect that bothers you or that does not go away.

These are not all of the possible side effects of Effient. For more information, ask your doctor or pharmacist.

Call your doctor for medical advice about side effects. You may report side effects to FDA at 1-800-FDA-1088.

How should I store Effient?
• Keep Effient at room temperature between 59°F to 86°F (15°C to 30°C).
• Keep Effient in the container it comes in.
• Keep the container closed tightly with the gray cylinder inside.
• Protect Effient from moisture.
Keep Effient and all medicines out of the reach of children.

General Information about Effient
Medicines are sometimes prescribed for purposes other than those listed in a Medication Guide. Do not use Effient for a condition for which it was not prescribed. Do not give your Effient to other people, even if they have similar symptoms. It may harm them.

This Medication Guide summarizes the most important information about Effient. If you would like more information about Effient, talk with your doctor or pharmacist. For more information, call 1-800-545-5979 or go to the following website: www.Effient.com

What are the ingredients in Effient?
Active Ingredient: prasugrel
Inactive Ingredients: mannitol, hypromellose, croscarmellose sodium, microcrystalline cellulose, and vegetable magnesium stearate. The color coatings contain lactose, hypromellose, titanium dioxide, triacetin, iron oxide yellow, and iron oxide red (only in Effient 10 mg tablet).

*The brands listed are trademarks of their respective owners and are not trademarks of Daiichi Sankyo, Inc. or Eli Lilly and Company.

Issued July 10, 2009
Manufactured by Eli Lilly and Company, Indianapolis, IN, 46285
Marketed by Daiichi Sankyo, Inc and Eli Lilly and Company
This Medication Guide has been approved by the U.S. Food and Drug Administration.

EVISTA®
[É-VISS-tah]
(raloxifene hydrochloride)
Tablet for Oral use   ℞

HIGHLIGHTS OF PRESCRIBING INFORMATION
These highlights do not include all the information needed to use EVISTA safely and effectively. See full prescribing information for EVISTA.

EVISTA (raloxifene hydrochloride) Tablet for Oral use
Initial U.S. Approval: 1997

WARNING: INCREASED RISK OF VENOUS THROMBOEMBOLISM AND DEATH FROM STROKE
See full prescribing information for complete boxed warning.
• **Increased risk of deep vein thrombosis and pulmonary embolism have been reported with EVISTA (5.1). Women with active or past history of venous thromboembolism should not take EVISTA (4.1).**
• **Increased risk of death due to stroke occurred in a trial in postmenopausal women with documented coronary heart disease or at increased risk for major coronary events. Consider risk-benefit balance in women at risk for stroke (5.2, 14.5).**

————RECENT MAJOR CHANGES————
————INDICATIONS AND USAGE————
EVISTA® is an estrogen agonist/antagonist indicated for:
• Treatment and prevention of osteoporosis in postmenopausal women. (1.1)
• Reduction in risk of invasive breast cancer in postmenopausal women with osteoporosis. (1.2)
• Reduction in risk of invasive breast cancer in postmenopausal women at high risk for invasive breast cancer. (1.3)
Important Limitations: EVISTA is not indicated for the treatment of invasive breast cancer, reduction of the risk of recurrence of breast cancer, or reduction of risk of noninvasive breast cancer. (1.3)

————DOSAGE AND ADMINISTRATION————
60 mg tablet orally once daily. (2.1)

————DOSAGE FORMS AND STRENGTHS————
Tablets (not scored): 60 mg (3)

————CONTRAINDICATIONS————
• Active or past history of venous thromboembolism, including deep vein thrombosis, pulmonary embolism, and retinal vein thrombosis. (4.1)
• Pregnancy, women who may become pregnant, and nursing mothers. (4.2, 8.1, 8.3)

————WARNINGS AND PRECAUTIONS————
• *Venous Thromboembolism:* Increased risk of deep vein thrombosis, pulmonary embolism, and retinal vein thrombosis. Discontinue use 72 hours prior to and during prolonged immobilization. (5.1, 6.1)
• *Death Due to Stroke:* Increased risk of death due to stroke occurred in a trial in postmenopausal women with documented coronary heart disease or at increased risk for major coronary events. No increased risk of stroke was seen in this trial. Consider risk-benefit balance in women at risk for stroke. (5.2, 14.5)
• *Cardiovascular Disease:* EVISTA should not be used for the primary or secondary prevention of cardiovascular disease. (5.3, 14.5)
• *Premenopausal Women:* Use is not recommended. (5.4)
• *Hepatic Impairment:* Use with caution. (5.5)
• *Concomitant Use with Systemic Estrogens:* Not recommended. (5.6)
• *Hypertriglyceridemia:* If previous treatment with estrogen resulted in hypertriglyceridemia, monitor serum triglycerides. (5.7)

————ADVERSE REACTIONS————
Adverse reactions (>2% and more common than with placebo) include: hot flashes, leg cramps, peripheral edema, flu syndrome, arthralgia, sweating. (6.1)
To report SUSPECTED ADVERSE REACTIONS, contact Eli Lilly and Company at 1-800-545-5979 or FDA at 1-800-FDA-1088 or www.fda.gov/medwatch

————DRUG INTERACTIONS————
• *Cholestyramine:* Use with EVISTA is not recommended. Reduces the absorption and enterohepatic cycling of raloxifene. (7.1, 12.3)
• *Warfarin:* Monitor prothrombin time when starting or stopping EVISTA. (7.2, 12.3)
• *Highly Protein-Bound Drugs:* Use with EVISTA with caution. Highly protein-bound drugs include diazepam, diazoxide, and lidocaine. EVISTA is more than 95% bound to plasma proteins. (7.3, 12.3)

————USE IN SPECIFIC POPULATIONS————
• *Pediatric Use:* Safety and effectiveness not established. (8.4)

See 17 for PATIENT COUNSELING INFORMATION and Medication Guide

Revised: 11/2009

FULL PRESCRIBING INFORMATION

WARNING: INCREASED RISK OF VENOUS THROMBOEMBOLISM AND DEATH FROM STROKE

- **Increased risk of deep vein thrombosis and pulmonary embolism have been reported with EVISTA *[see Warnings and Precautions (5.1)]*. Women with active or past history of venous thromboembolism should not take EVISTA *[see Contraindications (4.1)]*.**
- **Increased risk of death due to stroke occurred in a trial in postmenopausal women with documented coronary heart disease or at increased risk for major coronary events. Consider risk-benefit balance in women at risk for stroke *[see Warnings and Precautions (5.2) and Clinical Studies (14.5)]*.**

1 INDICATIONS AND USAGE

1.1 Treatment and Prevention of Osteoporosis in Postmenopausal Women

EVISTA is indicated for the treatment and prevention of osteoporosis in postmenopausal women *[see Clinical Studies (14.1, 14.2)]*.

1.2 Reduction in the Risk of Invasive Breast Cancer in Postmenopausal Women with Osteoporosis

EVISTA is indicated for the reduction in risk of invasive breast cancer in postmenopausal women with osteoporosis *[see Clinical Studies (14.3)]*.

1.3 Reduction in the Risk of Invasive Breast Cancer in Postmenopausal Women at High Risk of Invasive Breast Cancer

EVISTA is indicated for the reduction in risk of invasive breast cancer in postmenopausal women at high risk of invasive breast cancer *[see Clinical Studies (14.4)]*.

The effect in the reduction in the incidence of breast cancer was shown in a study of postmenopausal women at high risk for breast cancer with a 5-year planned duration with a median follow-up of 4.3 years *[see Clinical Studies (14.4)]*. Twenty-seven percent of the participants received drug for 5 years. The long-term effects and the recommended length of treatment are not known.

High risk of breast cancer is defined as at least one breast biopsy showing lobular carcinoma in situ (LCIS) or atypical hyperplasia, one or more first-degree relatives with breast cancer, or a 5-year predicted risk of breast cancer ≥1.66% (based on the modified Gail model). Among the factors included in the modified Gail model are the following: current age, number of first-degree relatives with breast cancer, number of breast biopsies, age at menarche, nulliparity or age of first live birth. Healthcare professionals can obtain a Gail Model Risk Assessment Tool by dialing 1-800-545-5979. Currently, no single clinical finding or test result can quantify risk of breast cancer with certainty.

After an assessment of the risk of developing breast cancer, the decision regarding therapy with EVISTA should be based upon an individual assessment of the benefits and risks.

EVISTA does not eliminate the risk of breast cancer. Patients should have breast exams and mammograms before starting EVISTA and should continue regular breast exams and mammograms in keeping with good medical practice after beginning treatment with EVISTA.

Important Limitations of Use for Breast Cancer Risk Reduction

- There are no data available regarding the effect of EVISTA on invasive breast cancer incidence in women with inherited mutations (BRCA1, BRCA2) to be able to make specific recommendations on the effectiveness of EVISTA.
- EVISTA is not indicated for the treatment of invasive breast cancer or reduction of the risk of recurrence.
- EVISTA is not indicated for the reduction in the risk of noninvasive breast cancer.

2 DOSAGE AND ADMINISTRATION

2.1 Recommended Dosing

The recommended dosage is one 60 mg EVISTA (raloxifene hydrochloride tablets) tablet daily, which may be administered any time of day without regard to meals *[see Clinical Pharmacology (12.3)]*.

For the indications in risk of invasive breast cancer the optimum duration of treatment is not known *[see Clinical Studies (14.3, 14.4)]*.

2.2 Recommendations for Calcium and Vitamin D Supplementation

For either osteoporosis treatment or prevention, supplemental calcium and/or vitamin D should be added to the diet if daily intake is inadequate. Postmenopausal women require an average of 1500 mg/day of elemental calcium. Total daily intake of calcium above 1500 mg has not demonstrated additional bone benefits while daily intake above 2000 mg has been associated with increased risk of adverse effects, including hypercalcemia and kidney stones. The recommended intake of vitamin D is 400-800 IU daily. Patients at increased risk for vitamin D insufficiency (e.g., over the age of 70 years, nursing home bound, or chronically ill) may need additional vitamin D supplements. Patients with gastrointestinal malabsorption syndromes may require higher doses of vitamin D supplementation and measurement of 25-hydroxyvitamin D should be considered.

3 DOSAGE FORMS AND STRENGTHS

60 mg, white, elliptical, film-coated tablets (not scored). They are imprinted on one side with LILLY and the tablet code 4165 in edible blue ink.

4 CONTRAINDICATIONS

4.1 Venous Thromboembolism

EVISTA is contraindicated in women with active or past history of venous thromboembolism (VTE), including deep vein thrombosis, pulmonary embolism, and retinal vein thrombosis *[see Warnings and Precautions (5.1)]*.

4.2 Pregnancy, Women Who May Become Pregnant, and Nursing Mothers

EVISTA is contraindicated in pregnancy, in women who may become pregnant, and in nursing mothers *[see Use in Specific Populations (8.1, 8.3)]*. EVISTA may cause fetal harm when administered to a pregnant woman. If this drug is used during pregnancy, or if the patient becomes pregnant while taking this drug, the patient should be apprised of the potential hazard to the fetus.

In rabbit studies, abortion and a low rate of fetal heart anomalies (ventricular septal defects) occurred in rabbits at doses ≥0.1 mg/kg (≥0.04 times the human dose based on surface area, mg/m^2), and hydrocephaly was observed in fetuses at doses ≥10 mg/kg (≥4 times the human dose based on surface area, mg/m^2). In rat studies, retardation of fetal development and developmental abnormalities (wavy ribs, kidney cavitation) occurred at doses ≥1 mg/kg (≥0.2 times the human dose based on surface area, mg/m^2). Treatment of rats at doses of 0.1 to 10 mg/kg (0.02 to 1.6 times the human dose based on surface area, mg/m^2) during gestation and lactation produced effects that included delayed and disrupted parturition; decreased neonatal survival and altered physical development; sex- and age-specific reductions in growth and changes in pituitary hormone content; and decreased lymphoid compartment size in offspring. At 10 mg/kg, raloxifene disrupted parturition, which resulted in maternal and progeny death and morbidity. Effects in adult offspring (4 months of age) included uterine hypoplasia and reduced fertility; however, no ovarian or vaginal pathology was observed.

5 WARNINGS AND PRECAUTIONS

5.1 Venous Thromboembolism

In clinical trials, EVISTA-treated women had an increased risk of venous thromboembolism (deep vein thrombosis and pulmonary embolism). Other venous thromboembolic events also could occur. A less serious event, superficial thrombophlebitis, also has been reported more frequently with EVISTA than with placebo. The greatest risk for deep vein thrombosis and pulmonary embolism occurs during the first 4 months of treatment, and the magnitude of risk appears to be similar to the reported risk associated with use of hormone therapy. Because immobilization increases the risk for venous thromboembolic events independent of therapy, EVISTA should be discontinued at least 72 hours prior to and during prolonged immobilization (e.g., post-surgical recovery, prolonged bed rest), and EVISTA therapy should be resumed only after the patient is fully ambulatory. In addition, women taking EVISTA should be advised to move about periodically during prolonged travel. The risk-benefit balance should be considered in women at risk of thromboembolic disease for other reasons, such as congestive heart failure, superficial thrombophlebitis, and active malignancy *[see Contraindications (4.1) and Adverse Reactions (6.1)]*.

5.2 Death Due to Stroke

In a clinical trial of postmenopausal women with documented coronary heart disease or at increased risk for coronary events, an increased risk of death due to stroke was observed after treatment with EVISTA. During an average follow-up of 5.6 years, 59 (1.2%) EVISTA-treated women died due to a stroke compared to 39 (0.8%) placebo-treated women (22 versus 15 per 10,000 women-years; hazard ratio 1.49; 95% confidence interval, 1.00-2.24; p=0.0499). There was no statistically significant difference between treatment groups in the incidence of stroke (249 in EVISTA [4.9%] versus 224 placebo [4.4%]). EVISTA had no significant effect on all-cause mortality. The risk-benefit balance should be considered in women at risk for stroke, such as prior stroke or transient ischemic attack (TIA), atrial fibrillation, hypertension, or cigarette smoking *[see Clinical Studies (14.5)]*.

5.3 Cardiovascular Disease

EVISTA should not be used for the primary or secondary prevention of cardiovascular disease. In a clinical trial of postmenopausal women with documented coronary heart disease or at increased risk for coronary events, no cardiovascular benefit was demonstrated after treatment with raloxifene for 5 years *[see Clinical Studies (14.5)]*.

5.4 Premenopausal Use

There is no indication for premenopausal use of EVISTA. Safety of EVISTA in premenopausal women has not been established and its use is not recommended.

5.5 Hepatic Impairment

EVISTA should be used with caution in patients with hepatic impairment. Safety and efficacy have not been established in patients with hepatic impairment *[see Clinical Pharmacology (12.3)]*.

5.6 Concomitant Estrogen Therapy

The safety of concomitant use of EVISTA with systemic estrogens has not been established and its use is not recommended.

5.7 History of Hypertriglyceridemia when Treated with Estrogens

Limited clinical data suggest that some women with a history of marked hypertriglyceridemia (>5.6 mmol/L or >500 mg/dL) in response to treatment with oral estrogen or estrogen plus progestin may develop increased levels of triglycerides when treated with EVISTA. Women with this medical history should have serum triglycerides monitored when taking EVISTA.

5.8 Renal Impairment

EVISTA should be used with caution in patients with moderate or severe renal impairment. Safety and efficacy have not been established in patients with moderate or severe renal impairment *[see Clinical Pharmacology (12.3)]*.

5.9 History of Breast Cancer

EVISTA has not been adequately studied in women with a prior history of breast cancer.

5.10 Use in Men

There is no indication for the use of EVISTA in men. EVISTA has not been adequately studied in men and its use is not recommended.

5.11 Unexplained Uterine Bleeding

Any unexplained uterine bleeding should be investigated as clinically indicated. EVISTA-treated and placebo-treated groups had similar incidences of endometrial proliferation *[see Clinical Studies (14.1, 14.2)]*.

5.12 Breast Abnormalities

Any unexplained breast abnormality occurring during EVISTA therapy should be investigated. EVISTA does not eliminate the risk of breast cancer *[see Clinical Studies (14.4)]*.

6 ADVERSE REACTIONS

6.1 Clinical Trials Experience

Because clinical studies are conducted under widely varying conditions, adverse reaction rates observed in the clinical trials of a drug cannot be directly compared to rates in the clinical trials of another drug and may not reflect the rates observed in practice.

The data described below reflect exposure to EVISTA in 8429 patients who were enrolled in placebo-controlled trials, including 6666 exposed for 1 year and 5685 for at least 3 years.

Osteoporosis Treatment Clinical Trial (MORE)—The safety of raloxifene in the treatment of osteoporosis was assessed in a large (7705 patients) multinational, placebo-controlled trial. Duration of treatment was 36 months, and 5129 postmenopausal women were exposed to raloxifene hydrochloride (2557 received 60 mg/day, and 2572 received 120 mg/day). The incidence of all-cause mortality was similar among groups: 23 (0.9%) placebo, 13 (0.5%) EVISTA-treated (raloxifene HCl 60 mg), and 28 (1.1%) raloxifene HCl 120 mg women died. Therapy was discontinued due to an adverse reaction in 10.9% of EVISTA-treated women and 8.8% of placebo-treated women.

Venous Thromboembolism: The most serious adverse reaction related to EVISTA was VTE (deep venous thrombosis, pulmonary embolism, and retinal vein thrombosis). During an average of study-drug exposure of 2.6 years, VTE occurred in about 1 out of 100 patients treated with EVISTA. Twenty-six EVISTA-treated women had a VTE compared to 11 placebo-treated women, the hazard ratio was 2.4 (95% confidence interval, 1.2, 4.5), and the highest VTE risk was during the initial months of treatment.

Common adverse reactions considered to be related to EVISTA therapy were hot flashes and leg cramps. Hot flashes occurred in about one in 10 patients on EVISTA and were most commonly reported during the first 6 months of treatment and were not different from placebo thereafter. Leg cramps occurred in about one in 14 patients on EVISTA.

Placebo-Controlled Osteoporosis Prevention Clinical Trials—The safety of raloxifene has been assessed primarily in 12 Phase 2 and Phase 3 studies with placebo, estrogen, and estrogen-progestin therapy control groups. The duration of treatment ranged from 2 to 30 months, and 2036 women were exposed to raloxifene HCl (371 patients received 10 to 50 mg/day, 828 received 60 mg/day, and 837 received from 120 to 600 mg/day).

Therapy was discontinued due to an adverse reaction in 11.4% of 581 EVISTA-treated women and 12.2% of 584 placebo-treated women. Discontinuation rates due to hot flashes did not differ significantly between EVISTA and placebo groups (1.7% and 2.2%, respectively).

Table 1: Adverse Reactions Occurring in Placebo–Controlled Osteoporosis Clinical Trials at a Frequency ≥2.0% and in More EVISTA-Treated (60 mg Once Daily) Women than Placebo–Treated Women*

	Treatment		Prevention	
	EVISTA N=2557 %	Placebo N=2576 %	EVISTA N=581 %	Placebo N=584 %
Body as a Whole				
Infection	A	A	15.1	14.6
Flu Syndrome	13.5	11.4	14.6	13.5
Headache	9.2	8.5	A	A
Leg Cramps	7.0	3.7	5.9	1.9
Chest Pain	A	A	4.0	3.6
Fever	3.9	3.8	3.1	2.6
Cardiovascular System				
Hot Flashes	9.7	6.4	24.6	18.3
Migraine	A	A	2.4	2.1
Syncope	2.3	2.1	B	B
Varicose Vein	2.2	1.5	A	A
Digestive System				
Nausea	8.3	7.8	8.8	8.6
Diarrhea	7.2	6.9	A	A
Dyspepsia	A	A	5.9	5.8
Vomiting	4.8	4.3	3.4	3.3
Flatulence	A	A	3.1	2.4
Gastrointestinal Disorder	A	A	3.3	2.1
Gastroenteritis	B	B	2.6	2.1
Metabolic and Nutritional				
Weight Gain	A	A	8.8	6.8
Peripheral Edema	5.2	4.4	3.3	1.9
Musculoskeletal System				
Arthralgia	15.5	14.0	10.7	10.1
Myalgia	A	A	7.7	6.2
Arthritis	A	A	4.0	3.6
Tendon Disorder	3.6	3.1	A	A
Nervous System				
Depression	A	A	6.4	6.0
Insomnia	A	A	5.5	4.3
Vertigo	4.1	3.7	A	A
Neuralgia	2.4	1.9	B	B
Hypesthesia	2.1	2.0	B	B
Respiratory System				
Sinusitis	7.9	7.5	10.3	6.5
Rhinitis	10.2	10.1	A	A
Bronchitis	9.5	8.6	A	A
Pharyngitis	5.3	5.1	7.6	7.2
Cough Increased	9.3	9.2	6.0	5.7
Pneumonia	A	A	2.6	1.5
Laryngitis	B	B	2.2	1.4
Skin and Appendages				
Rash	A	A	5.5	3.8
Sweating	2.5	2.0	3.1	1.7
Special Senses				
Conjunctivitis	2.2	1.7	A	A
Urogenital System				
Vaginitis	A	A	4.3	3.6
Urinary Tract Infection	A	A	4.0	3.9
Cystitis	4.6	4.5	3.3	3.1
Leukorrhea	A	A	3.3	1.7
Uterine Disorder†‡	3.3	2.3	A	A
Endometrial Disorder†	B	B	3.1	1.9
Vaginal Hemorrhage	2.5	2.4	A	A
Urinary Tract Disorder	2.5	2.1	A	A

*A: Placebo incidence greater than or equal to EVISTA incidence; B: Less than 2% incidence and more frequent with EVISTA.

†Includes only patients with an intact uterus: Prevention Trials: EVISTA, n=354, Placebo, n=364; Treatment Trial: EVISTA, n=1948, Placebo, n=1999.

‡Actual terms most frequently referred to endometrial fluid.

Common adverse reactions considered to be drug-related were hot flashes and leg cramps. Hot flashes occurred in about one in four patients on EVISTA versus about one in six on placebo. The first occurrence of hot flashes was most commonly reported during the first 6 months of treatment. Table 1 lists adverse reactions occurring in either the osteoporosis treatment or in five prevention placebo-controlled clinical trials at a frequency ≥2.0% in either group and in more EVISTA-treated women than in placebo-treated women. Adverse reactions are shown without attribution of causality. The majority of adverse reactions occurring during the studies were mild and generally did not require discontinuation of therapy.
[See table 1 above]

Comparison of EVISTA and Hormone Therapy—EVISTA was compared with estrogen-progestin therapy in three clinical trials for prevention of osteoporosis. Table 2 shows adverse reactions occurring more frequently in one treatment group and at an incidence ≥2.0% in any group. Adverse reactions are shown without attribution of causality.
[See table 2 at top of next page]

Breast Pain—Across all placebo-controlled trials, EVISTA was indistinguishable from placebo with regard to fre-quency and severity of breast pain and tenderness. EVISTA was associated with less breast pain and tenderness than reported by women receiving estrogens with or without added progestin.

Gynecologic Cancers—EVISTA-treated and placebo-treated groups had similar incidences of endometrial cancer and ovarian cancer.

Placebo-Controlled Trial of Postmenopausal Women at Increased Risk for Major Coronary Events (RUTH)—The safety of EVISTA (60 mg once daily) was assessed in a placebo-controlled multinational trial of 10,101 postmeno-pausal women (age range 55-92) with documented coronary heart disease (CHD) or multiple CHD risk factors. Median study drug exposure was 5.1 years for both treatment groups [see Clinical Studies (14.3)]. Therapy was discontinued due to an adverse reaction in 25% of 5044 EVISTA-treated women and 24% of 5057 placebo-treated women. The incidence per year of all-cause mortality was similar between the raloxifene (2.07%) and placebo (2.25%) groups. Adverse reactions reported more frequently in EVISTA-treated women than in placebo-treated women included peripheral edema (14.1% raloxifene versus 11.7% placebo), muscle spasms/leg cramps (12.1% raloxifene versus 8.3%

placebo), hot flashes (7.8% raloxifene versus 4.7% placebo), venous thromboembolic events (2.0% raloxifene versus 1.4% placebo), and cholelithiasis (3.3% raloxifene versus 2.6% placebo) [see Clinical Studies (14.3, 14.5)].

Tamoxifen-Controlled Trial of Postmenopausal Women at Increased Risk for Invasive Breast Cancer (STAR)—The safety of EVISTA 60 mg/day versus tamoxifen 20 mg/day over 5 years was assessed in 19,747 postmenopausal women (age range 35-83 years) in a randomized, double-blind trial. As of 31 December 2005, the median follow-up was 4.3 years. The safety profile of raloxifene was similar to that in the placebo-controlled raloxifene trials [see Clinical Studies (14.4)].

6.2   Postmarketing Experience

Because these reactions are reported voluntarily from a population of uncertain size, it is not always possible to reliably estimate their frequency or establish a causal rela-tionship to drug exposure.

Adverse reactions reported very rarely since market intro-duction include retinal vein occlusion, stroke, and death associated with venous thromboembolism (VTE).

7   DRUG INTERACTIONS

7.1   Cholestyramine

Concomitant administration of cholestyramine with EVISTA is not recommended. Although not specifically studied, it is anticipated that other anion exchange resins would have a similar effect. EVISTA should not be co-administered with other anion exchange resins [see Clinical Pharmacology (12.3)].

7.2   Warfarin

If EVISTA is given concomitantly with warfarin or other warfarin derivatives, prothrombin time should be moni-tored more closely when starting or stopping therapy with EVISTA [see Clinical Pharmacology (12.3)].

7.3   Other Highly Protein-Bound Drugs

EVISTA should be used with caution with certain other highly protein-bound drugs such as diazepam, diazoxide, and lidocaine. Although not examined, EVISTA might affect the protein binding of other drugs. Raloxifene is more than 95% bound to plasma proteins [see Clinical Pharmacology (12.3)].

7.4   Systemic Estrogens

The safety of concomitant use of EVISTA with systemic es-trogens has not been established and its use is not recom-mended.

7.5   Other Concomitant Medications

EVISTA can be concomitantly administered with ampicillin, amoxicillin, antacids, corticosteroids, and digoxin [see Clin-ical Pharmacology (12.3)].

The concomitant use of EVISTA and lipid-lowering agents has not been studied.

8   USE IN SPECIFIC POPULATIONS

8.1   Pregnancy

Pregnancy Category X. EVISTA should not be used in women who are or may become pregnant [see Contraindica-tions (4.2)].

8.3   Nursing Mothers

EVISTA should not be used by lactating women [see Contra-indications (4.2)]. It is not known whether this drug is ex-creted in human milk. Because many drugs are excreted in human milk, caution should be exercised when raloxifene is administered to a nursing woman.

8.4   Pediatric Use

Safety and effectiveness in pediatric patients have not been established.

8.5   Geriatric Use

Of the total number of patients in placebo-controlled clinical studies of EVISTA, 61% were 65 and over, while 15.5% were 75 and over. No overall differences in safety or effectiveness were observed between these subjects and younger subjects, and other reported clinical experience has not identified dif-ferences in responses between the elderly and younger pa-tients, but greater sensitivity of some older individuals can-not be ruled out. Based on clinical trials, there is no need for dose adjustment for geriatric patients [see Clinical Pharma-cology (12.3)].

8.6   Renal Impairment

EVISTA should be used with caution in patients with moderate or severe renal impairment [see Warnings and Precautions (5.8) and Clinical Pharmacology (12.3)].

8.7   Hepatic Impairment

EVISTA should be used with caution in patients with hepatic impairment [see Warnings and Precautions (5.5) and Clinical Pharmacology (12.3)].

10   OVERDOSAGE

In an 8-week study of 63 postmenopausal women, a dose of raloxifene hydrochloride (HCl) 600 mg/day was safely toler-ated. In clinical trials, no raloxifene overdose has been reported.

In postmarketing spontaneous reports, raloxifene overdose has been reported very rarely (less than 1 out of 10,000 [<0.01%] patients treated). The highest overdose has been approximately 1.5 grams. No fatalities associated with raloxifene overdose have been reported. Adverse reactions were reported in approximately half of the adults who took ≥180 mg raloxifene HCl and included leg cramps and dizziness.

Two 18-month-old children each ingested raloxifene HCl 180 mg. In these two children, symptoms reported included ataxia, dizziness, vomiting, rash, diarrhea, tremor, and flushing, as well as elevation in alkaline phosphatase. There is no specific antidote for raloxifene.

No mortality was seen after a single oral dose in rats or mice at 5000 mg/kg (810 times the human dose for rats and 405 times the human dose for mice based on surface area, mg/m^2) or in monkeys at 1000 mg/kg (80 times the AUC in humans).

11   DESCRIPTION

EVISTA (raloxifene hydrochloride) is an estrogen agonist/ antagonist, commonly referred to as a selective estrogen receptor modulator (SERM) that belongs to the benzothiophene class of compounds. The chemical structure is:

The chemical designation is methanone, [6-hydroxy-2-(4-hydroxyphenyl)benzo[b]thien-3-yl]-[4-[2-(1-piperidinyl)ethoxy]phenyl]-, hydrochloride. Raloxifene hydrochloride (HCl) has the empirical formula $C_{28}H_{27}NO_4S \cdot HCl$, which corresponds to a molecular weight of 510.05. Raloxifene HCl is an off-white to pale-yellow solid that is very slightly soluble in water.

EVISTA is supplied in a tablet dosage form for oral administration. Each EVISTA tablet contains 60 mg of raloxifene HCl, which is the molar equivalent of 55.71 mg of free base. Inactive ingredients include anhydrous lactose, carnauba wax, crospovidone, FD&C Blue No. 2 aluminum lake, hypromellose, lactose monohydrate, magnesium stearate, modified pharmaceutical glaze, polyethylene glycol, polysorbate 80, povidone, propylene glycol, and titanium dioxide.

12   CLINICAL PHARMACOLOGY

12.1   Mechanism of Action

Raloxifene is an estrogen agonist/antagonist, commonly referred to as a selective estrogen receptor modulator (SERM). The biological actions of raloxifene are largely mediated through binding to estrogen receptors. This binding results in activation of estrogenic pathways in some tissues (agonism) and blockade of estrogenic pathways in others (antagonism). The agonistic or antagonistic action of raloxifene depends on the extent of recruitment of coactivators and corepressors to estrogen receptor (ER) target gene promotors.

Raloxifene appears to act as an estrogen agonist in bone. It decreases bone resorption and bone turnover, increases bone mineral density (BMD) and decreases fracture incidence. Preclinical data demonstrate that raloxifene is an estrogen antagonist in uterine and breast tissues. These results are consistent with findings in clinical trials, which suggest that EVISTA lacks estrogen-like effects on the uterus and breast tissue.

12.2   Pharmacodynamics

Decreases in estrogen levels after oophorectomy or menopause lead to increases in bone resorption and accelerated bone loss. Bone is initially lost rapidly because the compensatory increase in bone formation is inadequate to offset resorptive losses. In addition to loss of estrogen, this imbalance between resorption and formation may be due to age-related impairment of osteoblasts or their precursors. In some women, these changes will eventually lead to decreased bone mass, osteoporosis, and increased risk for fractures, particularly of the spine, hip, and wrist. Vertebral fractures are the most common type of osteoporotic fracture in postmenopausal women.

In both the osteoporosis treatment and prevention trials, EVISTA therapy resulted in consistent, statistically significant suppression of bone resorption and bone formation, as reflected by changes in serum and urine markers of bone turnover (e.g., bone-specific alkaline phosphatase, osteocalcin, and collagen breakdown products). The suppression of bone turnover markers was evident by 3 months and persisted throughout the 36-month and 24-month observation periods.

In a 31-week, open-label, radiocalcium kinetics study, 33 early postmenopausal women were randomized to treatment with once-daily EVISTA 60 mg, cyclic estrogen/progestin (0.625 mg conjugated estrogens daily with 5 mg medroxyprogesterone acetate daily for the first 2 weeks of each month [hormone therapy]), or no treatment. Treatment with either EVISTA or hormone therapy was associated with reduced bone resorption and a positive shift in calcium balance (-82 mg Ca/day and +60 mg Ca/day, respectively, for EVISTA and −162 mg Ca/day and +91 mg Ca/day, respectively, for hormone therapy).

There were small decreases in serum total calcium, inorganic phosphate, total protein, and albumin, which were generally of lesser magnitude than decreases observed during estrogen or hormone therapy. Platelet count was also decreased slightly and was not different from estrogen therapy.

12.3   Pharmacokinetics

The disposition of raloxifene has been evaluated in more than 3000 postmenopausal women in selected raloxifene osteoporosis treatment and prevention clinical trials, using a population approach. Pharmacokinetic data also were obtained in conventional pharmacology studies in 292 postmenopausal women. Raloxifene exhibits high within-subject variability (approximately 30% coefficient of variation) of most pharmacokinetic parameters. Table 3 summarizes the pharmacokinetic parameters of raloxifene.

Absorption—Raloxifene is absorbed rapidly after oral administration. Approximately 60% of an oral dose is absorbed, but presystemic glucuronide conjugation is extensive. Absolute bioavailability of raloxifene is 2%. The time to reach average maximum plasma concentration and bioavailability are functions of systemic interconversion and enterohepatic cycling of raloxifene and its glucuronide metabolites.

Administration of raloxifene HCl with a standardized, high-fat meal increases the absorption of raloxifene (C_{max} 28% and AUC 16%), but does not lead to clinically meaningful changes in systemic exposure. EVISTA can be administered without regard to meals.

Distribution—Following oral administration of single doses ranging from 30 to 150 mg of raloxifene HCl, the apparent volume of distribution is 2348 L/kg and is not dose dependent.

Raloxifene and the monoglucuronide conjugates are highly (95%) bound to plasma proteins. Raloxifene binds to both albumin and α_1-acid glycoprotein, but not to sex-steroid binding globulin.

Metabolism—Biotransformation and disposition of raloxifene in humans have been determined following oral administration of ^{14}C-labeled raloxifene. Raloxifene undergoes extensive first-pass metabolism to the glucuronide conjugates: raloxifene-4'-glucuronide, raloxifene-6-glucuronide, and raloxifene-6, 4'-diglucuronide. No other metabolites have been detected, providing strong evidence that raloxifene is not metabolized by cytochrome P450 pathways. Unconjugated raloxifene comprises less than 1% of the total radiolabeled material in plasma. The terminal log-linear portions of the plasma concentration curves for raloxifene and the glucuronides are generally parallel. This is consistent with interconversion of raloxifene and the glucuronide metabolites.

Following intravenous administration, raloxifene is cleared at a rate approximating hepatic blood flow. Apparent oral clearance is 44.1 L/kg•hr. Raloxifene and its glucuronide conjugates are interconverted by reversible systemic metabolism and enterohepatic cycling, thereby prolonging its plasma elimination half-life to 27.7 hours after oral dosing. Results from single oral doses of raloxifene predict multiple-dose pharmacokinetics. Following chronic dosing, clearance ranges from 40 to 60 L/kg•hr. Increasing doses of raloxifene HCl (ranging from 30 to 150 mg) result in slightly less than a proportional increase in the area under the plasma time concentration curve (AUC).

Excretion—Raloxifene is primarily excreted in feces, and less than 0.2% is excreted unchanged in urine. Less than 6% of the raloxifene dose is eliminated in urine as glucuronide conjugates.

[See table 3 above]

Special Populations

Pediatric—The pharmacokinetics of raloxifene has not been evaluated in a pediatric population [see Use in Specific Populations (8.4)].

Geriatric—No differences in raloxifene pharmacokinetics were detected with regard to age (range 42 to 84 years) [see Use in Specific Populations (8.5)].

Gender—Total extent of exposure and oral clearance, normalized for lean body weight, are not significantly different between age-matched female and male subjects.

Race—Pharmacokinetic differences due to race have been studied in 1712 women, including 97.5% White, 1.0% Asian, 0.7% Hispanic, and 0.5% Black in the osteoporosis treatment trial and in 1053 women, including 93.5% White, 4.3% Hispanic, 1.2% Asian, and 0.5% Black in the osteoporosis prevention trials. There were no discernible differences in raloxifene plasma concentrations among these groups; however, the influence of race cannot be conclusively determined.

Table 2: Adverse Reactions Reported in the Clinical Trials for Osteoporosis Prevention with EVISTA (60 mg Once Daily) and Continuous Combined or Cyclic Estrogen Plus Progestin (Hormone Therapy) at an Incidence ≥2.0% in any Treatment Group*

	EVISTA (N=317) %	Hormone Therapy– Continuous Combined[†] (N=96) %	Hormone Therapy–Cyclic[‡] (N=219) %
Urogenital			
Breast Pain	4.4	37.5	29.7
Vaginal Bleeding[§]	6.2	64.2	88.5
Digestive			
Flatulence	1.6	12.5	6.4
Cardiovascular			
Hot Flashes	28.7	3.1	5.9
Body as a Whole			
Infection	11.0	0	6.8
Abdominal Pain	6.6	10.4	18.7
Chest Pain	2.8	0	0.5

*These data are from both blinded and open–label studies.
†Continuous Combined Hormone Therapy = 0.625 mg conjugated estrogens plus 2.5 mg medroxyprogesterone acetate.
‡Cyclic Hormone Therapy = 0.625 mg conjugated estrogens for 28 days with concomitant 5 mg medroxyprogesterone acetate or 0.15 mg norgestrel on Days 1 through 14 or 17 through 28.
§Includes only patients with an intact uterus: EVISTA, n=290; Hormone Therapy–Continuous Combined, n=67; Hormone Therapy-Cyclic, n=217.

Table 3: Summary of Raloxifene Pharmacokinetic Parameters in the Healthy Postmenopausal Woman

	C_{max}[*,†] (ng/mL)/ (mg/kg)	$t_{1/2}$ (hr)*	AUC_∞[*,†] (ng•hr/mL)/ (mg/kg)	CL/F* (L/kg•hr)	V/F* (L/kg)
Single Dose					
Mean	0.50	27.7	27.2	44.1	2348
CV* (%)	52	10.7 to 273[‡]	44	46	52
Multiple Dose					
Mean	1.36	32.5	24.2	47.4	2853
CV* (%)	37	15.8 to 86.6[‡]	36	41	56

*Abbreviations: C_{max}= maximum plasma concentration, $t_{1/2}$ = half-life, AUC = area under the curve, CL = clearance, V = volume of distribution, F = bioavailability, CV= coefficient of variation.
†Data normalized for dose in mg and body weight in kg.
‡Range of observed half–life.

Renal Impairment—In the osteoporosis treatment and prevention trials, raloxifene concentrations in women with mild renal impairment are similar to women with normal creatinine clearance. When a single dose of 120 mg raloxifene HCl was administered to 10 renally impaired males [7 moderate impairment (CrCl = 31–50 mL/min); 3 severe impairment (CrCl ≤30 mL/min)] and to 10 healthy males (CrCl >80 mL/min), plasma raloxifene concentrations were 122% ($AUC_{0-\infty}$) higher in renally impaired patients than those of healthy volunteers. Raloxifene should be used with caution in patients with moderate or severe renal impairment *[see Warnings and Precautions (5.8) and Use in Specific Populations (8.6)]*.

Hepatic Impairment—The disposition of raloxifene was compared in 9 patients with mild (Child-Pugh Class A) hepatic impairment (total bilirubin ranging from 0.6 to 2 mg/dL) to 8 subjects with normal hepatic function following a single dose of 60 mg raloxifene HCl. Apparent clearance of raloxifene was reduced 56% and the half-life of raloxifene was not altered in patients with mild hepatic impairment. Plasma raloxifene concentrations were approximately 150% higher than those in healthy volunteers and correlated with total bilirubin concentrations. The pharmacokinetics of raloxifene has not been studied in patients with moderate or severe hepatic impairment. Raloxifene should be used with caution in patients with hepatic impairment *[see Warnings and Precautions (5.5) and Use in Specific Populations (8.7)]*.

Drug Interactions

Cholestyramine—Cholestyramine, an anion exchange resin, causes a 60% reduction in the absorption and enterohepatic cycling of raloxifene after a single dose. Although not specifically studied, it is anticipated that other anion exchange resins would have a similar effect *[see Drug Interactions (7.1)]*.

Warfarin—In vitro, raloxifene did not interact with the binding of warfarin. The concomitant administration of EVISTA and warfarin, a coumarin derivative, has been assessed in a single-dose study. In this study, raloxifene had no effect on the pharmacokinetics of warfarin. However, a 10% decrease in prothrombin time was observed in the single-dose study. In the osteoporosis treatment trial, there were no clinically relevant effects of warfarin co-administration on plasma concentrations of raloxifene *[see Drug Interactions (7.2)]*.

Other Highly Protein-Bound Drugs—In the osteoporosis treatment trial, there were no clinically relevant effects of co-administration of other highly protein-bound drugs (e.g., gemfibrozil) on plasma concentrations of raloxifene. In vitro, raloxifene did not interact with the binding of phenytoin, tamoxifen, or warfarin (*see* above) *[see Drug Interactions (7.3)]*.

Ampicillin and Amoxicillin—Peak concentrations of raloxifene and the overall extent of absorption are reduced 28% and 14%, respectively, with co-administration of ampicillin. These reductions are consistent with decreased enterohepatic cycling associated with antibiotic reduction of enteric bacteria. However, the systemic exposure and the elimination rate of raloxifene were not affected. In the osteoporosis treatment trial, co-administration of amoxicillin had no discernible differences in plasma raloxifene concentrations *[see Drug Interactions (7.5)]*.

Antacids—Concomitant administration of calcium carbonate or aluminum and magnesium hydroxide-containing antacids does not affect the systemic exposure of raloxifene *[see Drug Interactions (7.5)]*.

Corticosteroids—The chronic administration of raloxifene in postmenopausal women has no effect on the pharmacokinetics of methylprednisolone given as a single oral dose *[see Drug Interactions (7.5)]*.

Digoxin—Raloxifene has no effect on the pharmacokinetics of digoxin *[see Drug Interactions (7.5)]*.

Cyclosporine—Concomitant administration of EVISTA with cyclosporine has not been studied.

Lipid-Lowering Agents—Concomitant administration of EVISTA with lipid-lowering agents has not been studied.

13 NONCLINICAL TOXICOLOGY

13.1 Carcinogenesis, Mutagenesis, Impairment of Fertility

Carcinogenesis—In a 21-month carcinogenicity study in mice, there was an increased incidence of ovarian tumors in female animals given 9 to 242 mg/kg, which included benign and malignant tumors of granulosa/theca cell origin and benign tumors of epithelial cell origin. Systemic exposure (AUC) of raloxifene in this group was 0.3 to 34 times that in postmenopausal women administered a 60 mg dose. There was also an increased incidence of testicular interstitial cell tumors and prostatic adenomas and adenocarcinomas in male mice given 41 or 210 mg/kg (4.7 or 24 times the AUC in humans) and prostatic leiomyoblastoma in male mice given 210 mg/kg.

In a 2-year carcinogenicity study in rats, an increased incidence in ovarian tumors of granulosa/theca cell origin was observed in female rats given 279 mg/kg (approximately 400 times the AUC in humans). The female rodents in these studies were treated during their reproductive lives when their ovaries were functional and responsive to hormonal stimulation.

Mutagenesis—Raloxifene HCl was not genotoxic in any of the following test systems: the Ames test for bacterial mutagenesis with and without metabolic activation, the unscheduled DNA synthesis assay in rat hepatocytes, the mouse lymphoma assay for mammalian cell mutation, the chromosomal aberration assay in Chinese hamster ovary cells, the in vivo sister chromatid exchange assay in Chinese hamsters, and the in vivo micronucleus test in mice.

Impairment of Fertility—When male and female rats were given daily doses ≥5 mg/kg (≥0.8 times the human dose based on surface area, mg/m^2) prior to and during mating, no pregnancies occurred. In male rats, daily doses up to 100 mg/kg (16 times the human dose based on surface area, mg/m^2) for at least 2 weeks did not affect sperm production or quality or reproductive performance. In female rats, at doses of 0.1 to 10 mg/kg/day (0.02 to 1.6 times the human dose based on surface area, mg/m^2), raloxifene disrupted estrous cycles and inhibited ovulation. These effects of raloxifene were reversible. In another study in rats in which raloxifene was given during the preimplantation period at doses ≥0.1 mg/kg (≥0.02 times the human dose based on surface area, mg/m^2), raloxifene delayed and disrupted embryo implantation, resulting in prolonged gestation and reduced litter size. The reproductive and developmental effects observed in animals are consistent with the estrogen receptor activity of raloxifene.

13.2 Animal Toxicology and/or Pharmacology

The skeletal effects of raloxifene treatment were assessed in ovariectomized rats and monkeys. In rats, raloxifene prevented increased bone resorption and bone loss after ovariectomy. There were positive effects of raloxifene on bone strength, but the effects varied with time. Cynomolgus monkeys were treated with raloxifene or conjugated estrogens for 2 years. In terms of bone cycles, this is equivalent to approximately 6 years in humans. Raloxifene and estrogen suppressed bone turnover and increased BMD in the lumbar spine and in the central cancellous bone of the proximal tibia. In this animal model, there was a positive correlation between vertebral compressive breaking force and BMD of the lumbar spine.

Histologic examination of bone from rats and monkeys treated with raloxifene showed no evidence of woven bone, marrow fibrosis, or mineralization defects.

These results are consistent with data from human studies of radiocalcium kinetics and markers of bone metabolism, and are consistent with the action of EVISTA as a skeletal antiresorptive agent.

Table 4: Effect of EVISTA on Risk of Vertebral Fractures

	Number of Patients		Absolute Risk Reduction (ARR)	Relative Risk Reduction (95% CI)
	EVISTA	Placebo		
Fractures diagnosed radiographically				
Patients with no baseline fracture*	n=1401	n=1457		
Number (%) of patients with ≥1 new vertebral fracture	27 (1.9%)	62 (4.3%)	2.4%	55% (29%, 71%)
Patients with ≥1 baseline fracture*	n=858	n=835		
Number (%) of patients with ≥1 new vertebral fracture	121 (14.1%)	169 (20.2%)	6.1%	30% (14%, 44%)
Symptomatic vertebral fractures				
All randomized patients	n=2557	n=2576		
Number (%) of patients with ≥1 new	47 (1.8%)	81 (3.1%)	1.3%	.41%
clinical (painful) vertebral fracture				(17%, 59%)

*Includes all patients with baseline and at least one follow-up radiograph.

14 CLINICAL STUDIES

14.1 Treatment of Postmenopausal Osteoporosis

Effect on Fracture Incidence

The effects of EVISTA on fracture incidence and BMD in postmenopausal women with osteoporosis were examined at 3 years in a large randomized, placebo-controlled, double-blind, multinational osteoporosis treatment trial (MORE). All vertebral fractures were diagnosed radiographically; some of these fractures also were associated with symptoms (i.e., clinical fractures). The study population consisted of 7705 postmenopausal women with osteoporosis as defined by: a) low BMD (vertebral or hip BMD at least 2.5 standard deviations below the mean value for healthy young women) without baseline vertebral fractures or b) one or more baseline vertebral fractures. Women enrolled in this study had a median age of 67 years (range 31 to 80) and a median time since menopause of 19 years.

Effect on Bone Mineral Density

EVISTA, 60 mg administered once daily, increased spine and hip BMD by 2 to 3%. EVISTA decreased the incidence of the first vertebral fracture from 4.3% for placebo to 1.9% for EVISTA (relative risk reduction = 55%) and subsequent vertebral fractures from 20.2% for placebo to 14.1% for EVISTA (relative risk reduction = 30%) (*see* Table 4). All women in the study received calcium (500 mg/day) and vitamin D (400 to 600 IU/day). EVISTA reduced the incidence of vertebral fractures whether or not patients had a vertebral fracture upon study entry. The decrease in incidence of vertebral fracture was greater than could be accounted for by increase in BMD alone.

[See table 4 at bottom left]

The mean percentage change in BMD from baseline for EVISTA was statistically significantly greater than for placebo at each skeletal site (*see* Table 5).

Table 5: EVISTA- (60 mg Once Daily) Related Increases in BMD* for the Osteoporosis Treatment Study Expressed as Mean Percentage Increase vs. Placebo†,‡

	Time		
Site	**12 Months %**	**24 Months %**	**36 Months %**
Lumbar Spine	2.0	2.6	2.6
Femoral Neck	1.3	1.9	2.1
Ultradistal Radius	ND§	2.2	ND§
Distal Radius	ND§	0.9	ND§
Total Body	ND§	1.1	ND§

*Note: all BMD increases were significant (p<0.001).

†Intent-to-treat analysis; last observation carried forward.

‡All patients received calcium and vitamin D.

§ND = not done (total body and radius BMD were measured only at 24 months).

Discontinuation from the study was required when excessive bone loss or multiple incident vertebral fractures occurred. Such discontinuation was statistically significantly more frequent in the placebo group (3.7%) than in the EVISTA group (1.1%).

Bone Histology

Bone biopsies for qualitative and quantitative histomorphometry were obtained at baseline and after 2 years of treatment. There were 56 paired biopsies evaluable for all indices. In EVISTA-treated patients, there were statistically significant decreases in bone formation rate per tissue volume, consistent with a reduction in bone turnover. Normal bone quality was maintained; specifically, there was no evidence of osteomalacia, marrow fibrosis, cellular toxicity, or woven bone after 2 years of treatment.

Effect on Endometrium

Endometrial thickness was evaluated annually in a subset of the study population (1781 patients) for 3 years. Placebo-treated women had a 0.27 mm mean decrease from baseline in endometrial thickness over 3 years, whereas the EVISTA-treated women had a 0.06 mm mean increase. Patients in the osteoporosis treatment study were not screened at baseline or excluded for pre-existing endometrial or uterine disease. This study was not specifically designed to detect endometrial polyps. Over the 36 months of the study, clinically or histologically benign endometrial polyps were reported in 17 of 1999 placebo-treated women, 37 of 1948 EVISTA-treated women, and in 31 of 2010 women treated with raloxifene HCl 120 mg/day. There was no difference between EVISTA- and placebo-treated women in the incidences of endometrial carcinoma, vaginal bleeding, or vaginal discharge.

14.2 Prevention of Postmenopausal Osteoporosis

The effects of EVISTA on BMD in postmenopausal women were examined in three randomized, placebo-controlled, double-blind osteoporosis prevention trials: (1) a North American trial enrolled 544 women; (2) a European trial, 601 women; and (3) an international trial, 619 women who had undergone hysterectomy. In these trials, all women received calcium supplementation (400 to 600 mg/day). Women enrolled in these trials had a median age of 54 years and a median time since menopause of 5 years (less than 1 year up to 15 years postmenopause). The majority of the women were White (93.5%). Women were included if they had spine BMD between 2.5 standard deviations below and 2 standard deviations above the mean value for healthy young women. The mean T scores (number of standard deviations above or below the mean in healthy young women) for the three trials ranged from -1.01 to -0.74 for spine BMD and included women both with normal and low BMD. EVISTA, 60 mg administered once daily, produced increases in bone mass versus calcium supplementation alone, as reflected by dual-energy x-ray absorptiometric (DXA) measurements of hip, spine, and total body BMD.

Effect on Bone Mineral Density

Compared with placebo, the increases in BMD for each of the three studies were statistically significant at 12 months and were maintained at 24 months (*see* Table 6). The placebo groups lost approximately 1% of BMD over 24 months.

Table 6: EVISTA- (60 mg Once Daily) Related Increases in BMD* for the Three Osteoporosis Prevention Studies Expressed as Mean Percentage Increase vs. Placebo† at 24 Months‡

		Study	
Site	**NA§ %**	**EU§ %**	**INT§,¶ %**
Total Hip	2.0	2.4	1.3
Femoral Neck	2.1	2.5	1.6
Trochanter	2.2	2.7	1.3
Intertrochanter	2.3	2.4	1.3
Lumbar Spine	2.0	2.4	1.8

*Note: all BMD increases were significant ($p \leq 0.001$).
†All patients received calcium.
‡Intent-to-treat analysis; last observation carried forward.
§Abbreviations: NA = North American, EU = European, INT = International.
¶All women in the study had previously undergone hysterectomy.

EVISTA also increased BMD compared with placebo in the total body by 1.3% to 2.0% and in Ward's Triangle (hip) by 3.1% to 4.0%. The effects of EVISTA on forearm BMD were inconsistent between studies. In Study EU, EVISTA prevented bone loss at the ultradistal radius, whereas in Study NA, it did not (*see* Figure 1).

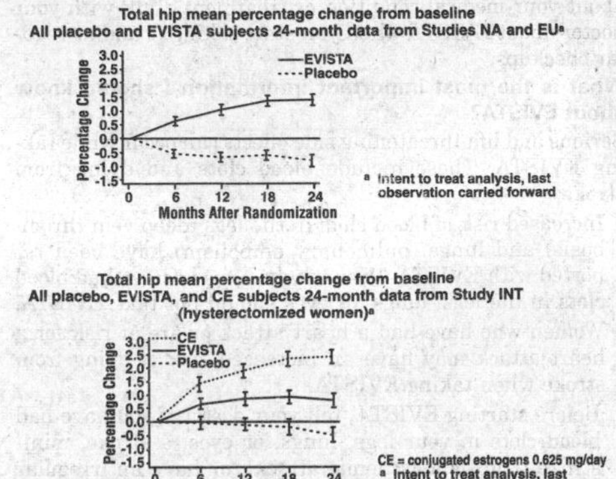
Total hip mean percentage change from baseline
All placebo and EVISTA subjects 24-month data from Studies NA and EUa
EVISTA
Placebo
Percentage Change
3.0
2.5
2.0
1.5
1.0
0.5
0.0
-0.5
-1.0
-1.5
0
6
12
18
24
Months After Randomization
a Intent to treat analysis, last observation carried forward
Total hip mean percentage change from baseline
All placebo, EVISTA, and CE subjects 24-month data from Study INT (hysterectomized women)a
CE
EVISTA
Placebo
Percentage Change
Months After Randomization
CE = conjugated estrogens 0.625 mg/day
a Intent to treat analysis, last observation carried forward

Figure 1: Total hip bone mineral density mean percentage change from baseline

Effect on Endometrium

In placebo-controlled osteoporosis prevention trials, endometrial thickness was evaluated every 6 months (for 24 months) by transvaginal ultrasonography (TVU). A total of 2978 TVU measurements were collected from 831 women in all dose groups. Placebo-treated women had a 0.04 mm mean increase from baseline in endometrial thickness over 2 years, whereas the EVISTA-treated women had a 0.09 mm mean increase. Endometrial thickness measurements in raloxifene-treated women were indistinguishable from placebo. There were no differences between the raloxifene and placebo groups with respect to the incidence of reported vaginal bleeding.

14.3 Reduction in Risk of Invasive Breast Cancer in Postmenopausal Women with Osteoporosis

MORE Trial

The effect of EVISTA on the incidence of breast cancer was assessed as a secondary safety endpoint in a randomized, placebo-controlled, double-blind, multinational osteoporosis treatment trial in postmenopausal women *[see Clinical Studies (14.1)]*. After 4 years, EVISTA, 60 mg administered once daily, reduced the incidence of all breast cancers by 62%, compared with placebo (HR 0.38, 95% CI 0.22-0.67). EVISTA reduced the incidence of invasive breast cancer by 71%, compared with placebo (ARR 3.1 per 1000 women-years); this was primarily due to an 80% reduction in the incidence of ER-positive invasive breast cancer in the EVISTA group compared with placebo. Table 7 presents efficacy and selected safety outcomes.

Table 7: EVISTA (60 mg Once Daily) vs. Placebo on Outcomes in Postmenopausal Women with Osteoporosis

	MORE 4 years					CORE* 4 years				
	Placebo (N=2576)		EVISTA (N=2557)		HR (95% CI)†	Placebo (N=1286)		EVISTA (N=2725)		HR (95% CI)†
Outcomes	n	IR†	n	IR†		n	IR†	n	IR†	
Invasive‡ breast cancer	38	4.36	11	1.26	0.29 (0.15, 0.56)§	20	5.41	19	2.43	0.44 (0.24, 0.83)§
ER†,‡ positive	29	3.33	6	0.69	0.20 (0.08, 0.49)	15	4.05	12	1.54	0.37 (0.17, 0.79)
ER†,‡ negative	4	0.46	5	0.57	1.23 (0.33, 4.60)	3	0.81	6	0.77	0.95 (0.24, 3.79)
ER†,‡ unknown	5	0.57	0	0.00	N/A†	2	0.54	1	0.13	N/A†
Noninvasive‡,¶ breast cancer	5	0.57	3	0.34	0.59 (0.14, 2.47)	2	0.54	5	0.64	1.18 (0.23, 6.07)
Clinical vertebral fractures	107	12.27	62	7.08	0.57 (0.42, 0.78)	N/A†	N/A†	N/A†	N/A†	N/A†
Death	36	4.13	23	2.63	0.63 (0.38, 1.07)	29	7.76	47	5.99	0.77 (0.49, 1.23)
Death due to stroke	6	0.69	3	0.34	0.49 (0.12, 1.98)	1	0.27	6	0.76	2.87 (0.35, 23.80)
Stroke	56	6.42	43	4.91	0.76 (0.51, 1.14)	14	3.75	49	6.24	1.67 (0.92, 3.03)
Deep vein thrombosis	8	0.92	20	2.28	2.50 (1.10, 5.68)	4	1.07	17	2.17	2.03 (0.68, 6.03)
Pulmonary embolism	4	0.46	11	1.26	2.76 (0.88, 8.67)	0	0.00	9	1.15	N/A†
Endometrial and uterine cancer#	5	0.74	5	0.74	1.01 (0.29, 3.49)	3	1.02	4	0.65	0.64 (0.14, 2.85)
Ovarian cancer	6	0.69	3	0.34	0.49 (0.12, 1.95)	2	0.54	2	0.25	0.47 (0.07, 3.36)
Hot flashes	151	17.31	237	27.06	1.61 (1.31, 1.97)	11	2.94	26	3.31	1.12 (0.55, 2.27)
Peripheral edema	134	15.36	164	18.73	1.23 (0.98, 1.54)	30	8.03	61	7.77	0.96 (0.62, 1.49)
Cholelithiasis	45	5.16	53	6.05	1.18 (0.79, 1.75)	12	3.21	35	4.46	1.39 (0.72, 2.67)

*CORE was a follow-up study conducted in a subset of 4011 postmenopausal women who originally enrolled in MORE. Women were not re-randomized; the treatment assignment from MORE was carried forward to this study. At CORE enrollment, the EVISTA group included 2725 total patients with 1355 patients who were originally assigned to raloxifene HCl 60 mg once daily and 1370 patients who were originally assigned to raloxifene HCl 120 mg at MORE randomization.
†Abbreviations: CI = confidence interval; ER = estrogen receptor; HR = hazard ratio; IR = annual incidence rate per 1000 women; N/A = not applicable.
‡Included 1274 patients in placebo and 2716 patients in EVISTA who were not diagnosed with breast cancer prior to CORE enrollment.
§$p<0.05$, obtained from the log-rank test, and not adjusted for multiple comparisons in MORE.
¶ All cases were ductal carcinoma in situ.
#Only patients with an intact uterus were included (MORE: placebo = 1999, EVISTA = 1950; CORE: placebo = 1008, EVISTA = 2138).

CORE Trial

The effect of EVISTA on the incidence of invasive breast cancer was evaluated for 4 additional years in a follow-up study conducted in a subset of postmenopausal women originally enrolled in the MORE osteoporosis treatment trial. Women were not re-randomized; the treatment assignment from the osteoporosis treatment trial was carried forward to this study. EVISTA, 60 mg administered once daily, reduced the incidence of invasive breast cancer by 56%, compared with placebo (ARR 3.0 per 1000 women-years); this was primarily due to a 63% reduction in the incidence of ER-positive invasive breast cancer in the EVISTA group compared with placebo. There was no reduction in the incidence of ER-negative breast cancer. In the osteoporosis treatment trial and the follow-up study, there was no difference in incidence of noninvasive breast cancer between the EVISTA and placebo groups. Table 7 presents efficacy and selected safety outcomes.

In a subset of postmenopausal women followed for up to 8 years from randomization in MORE to the end of CORE, EVISTA, 60 mg administered once daily, reduced the incidence of invasive breast cancer by 60% in women assigned EVISTA (N=1355) compared with placebo (N=1286) (HR 0.40, 95% CI 0.21, 0.77; ARR 1.95 per 1000 women-years); this was primarily due to a 65% reduction in the incidence of ER-positive invasive breast cancer in the EVISTA group compared with placebo.

[See table 7 above]

RUTH Trial

The effect of EVISTA on the incidence of invasive breast cancer was assessed in a randomized, placebo-controlled, double-blind, multinational study in 10,101 postmenopausal women at increased risk of coronary events. Women in this study had a median age of 67.6 years (range 55-92) and were followed for a median of 5.6 years (range 0.01–7.1). Eighty-four percent were White, 9.8% of women reported a first-degree relative with a history of breast cancer, and 41.4% of the women had a 5-year predicted risk of invasive breast cancer ≥1.66%, based on the modified Gail model.

EVISTA, 60 mg administered once daily, reduced the incidence of invasive breast cancer by 44% compared with placebo [absolute risk reduction (ARR) 1.2 per 1000 women-years]; this was primarily due to a 55% reduction in estrogen receptor (ER)-positive invasive breast cancer in the EVISTA group compared with placebo (ARR 1.2 per 1000 women-years). There was no reduction in ER-negative invasive breast cancer. Table 8 presents efficacy and selected safety outcomes.

[See table 8 at top of next page]

The effect of EVISTA in reducing the incidence of invasive breast cancer was consistent among women above or below age 65 or with a 5-year predicted invasive breast cancer risk, based on the modified Gail model, <1.66%, or ≥1.66%.

14.4 Reduction in Risk of Invasive Breast Cancer in Postmenopausal Women at High Risk of Invasive Breast Cancer

STAR Trial

The effects of EVISTA 60 mg/day versus tamoxifen 20 mg/day over 5 years on reducing the incidence of invasive breast cancer were assessed in 19,747 postmenopausal women in a randomized, double-blind trial conducted in North America by the National Surgical Adjuvant Breast and Bowel Project and sponsored by the National Cancer Institute. Women in this study had a mean age of 58.5 years (range 35-83), a mean 5-year predicted invasive breast cancer risk of 4.03% (range 1.66-23.61%), and 9.1% had a history of lobular carcinoma in situ (LCIS). More than 93% of participants were White. As of 31 December 2005, the median time of follow-up was 4.3 years (range 0.07-6.50 years).

EVISTA was not superior to tamoxifen in reducing the incidence of invasive breast cancer. The observed incidence rates of invasive breast cancer were EVISTA 4.4 and tamoxifen 4.3 per 1000 women per year. The results from a non-inferiority analysis are consistent with EVISTA potentially losing up to 35% of the tamoxifen effect on reduction of invasive breast cancer. The effect of each treatment on invasive breast cancer was consistent when women were compared by baseline age, history of LCIS, history of atypical hyperplasia, 5-year predicted risk of breast cancer by the modified Gail model, or the number of relatives with a history of breast cancer. Fewer noninvasive breast cancers occurred in the tamoxifen group compared to the EVISTA group. Table 9 presents efficacy and selected safety outcomes.

[See table 9 on next page]

14.5 Effects on Cardiovascular Disease

In a randomized, placebo-controlled, double-blind, multinational clinical trial (RUTH) of 10,101 postmenopausal women with documented coronary heart disease or at increased risk for coronary events, no cardiovascular benefit was demonstrated after treatment with EVISTA 60 mg once daily for a median follow-up of 5.6 years. No significant increase or decrease was observed for coronary events (death from coronary causes, nonfatal myocardial infarction, or hospitalization for an acute coronary syndrome). An increased risk of death due to stroke after treatment with EVISTA was observed: 59 (1.2%) EVISTA-treated women died due to a stroke compared to 39 (0.8%) placebo-treated

Table 8: EVISTA (60 mg Once Daily) vs. Placebo on Outcomes in Postmenopausal Women at Increased Risk for Major Coronary Events

Outcomes	Placebo* (N=5057) n	IR[†]	EVISTA* (N=5044) n	IR[†]	HR (95% CI)[†]
Invasive breast cancer	70	2.66	40	1.50	0.56 (0.38, 0.83)[‡]
ER[†] positive	55	2.09	25	0.94	0.45 (0.28, 0.72)
ER[†] negative	9	0.34	13	0.49	1.44 (0.61, 3.36)
ER[†] unknown	6	0.23	2	0.07	0.33 (0.07, 1.63)
Noninvasive[§] breast cancer	5	0.19	11	0.41	2.17 (0.75, 6.24)
Clinical vertebral fractures	97	3.70	64	2.40	0.65 (0.47, 0.89)
Death	595	22.45	554	20.68	0.92 (0.82, 1.03)
Death due to stroke	39	1.47	59	2.20	1.49 (1.00, 2.24)
Stroke	224	8.60	249	9.46	1.10 (0.92, 1.32)
Deep vein thrombosis	47	1.78	65	2.44	1.37 (0.94, 1.99)
Pulmonary embolism	24	0.91	36	1.35	1.49 (0.89, 2.49)
Endometrial and uterine cancer[¶]	17	0.83	21	1.01	1.21 (0.64-2.30)
Ovarian cancer[#]	10	0.41	17	0.70	1.69 (0.78, 3.70)
Hot flashes	241	9.09	397	14.82	1.68 (1.43, 1.97)
Peripheral edema	583	22.00	706	26.36	1.22 (1.09, 1.36)
Cholelithiasis[Þ]	131	6.20	168	7.83	1.26 (1.01, 1.59)

*Note: There were a total of 76 breast cancer cases in the placebo group and 52 in the EVISTA group. For two cases, one in each treatment group, invasive status was unknown.
†Abbreviations: CI = confidence interval; ER = estrogen receptor; HR = hazard ratio; IR = annual incidence rate per 1000 women.
‡p<0.05, obtained from the log-rank test, after adjusting for the co-primary endpoint of major coronary events.
§All cases were ductal carcinoma in situ.
¶Only patients with an intact uterus were included (placebo = 3882, EVISTA = 3900).
#Only patients with at least one ovary were included (placebo = 4606, EVISTA = 4559).
ÞOnly patients with an intact gallbladder at baseline were included (placebo = 4111, EVISTA = 4144).

Table 9: EVISTA (60 mg Once Daily) vs. Tamoxifen (20 mg Once Daily) on Outcomes in Postmenopausal Women at Increased Risk for Invasive Breast Cancer

Outcomes	EVISTA (N=9751) n	IR*	Tamoxifen (N=9736) n	IR*	RR (95% CI)*
Invasive breast cancer	173	4.40	168	4.30	1.02 (0.82, 1.27)
ER* positive	115	2.93	120	3.07	0.95 (0.73, 1.24)
ER* negative	52	1.32	46	1.18	1.12 (0.74, 1.71)
ER* unknown	6	0.15	2	0.05	2.98 (0.53, 30.21)
Noninvasive breast cancer[†]	83	2.12	60	1.54	1.38 (0.98, 1.95)
DCIS*	47	1.20	32	0.82	1.46 (0.91, 2.37)
LCIS*	29	0.74	23	0.59	1.26 (0.70, 2.27)
Uterine cancer[‡]	23	1.21	37	1.99	0.61 (0.34, 1.05)
Endometrial hyperplasia[‡]	17	0.90	100	5.42	0.17 (0.09, 0.28)
Hysterectomy[‡]	92	4.84	246	13.25	0.37 (0.28, 0.47)
Ovarian cancer[§]	18	0.66	14	0.52	1.27 (0.60, 2.76)
Ischemic heart disease[¶]	138	3.50	125	3.19	1.10 (0.86, 1.41)
Stroke	54	1.36	56	1.42	0.96 (0.65, 1.42)
Deep vein thrombosis	67	1.69	92	2.35	0.72 (0.52, 1.00)
Pulmonary embolism	38	0.96	58	1.47	0.65 (0.42, 1.00)
Clinical vertebral fractures	58	1.46	58	1.47	0.99 (0.68, 1.46)
Cataracts[#]	343	10.34	435	13.19	0.78 (0.68, 0.91)
Cataract surgery[#]	240	7.17	295	8.85	0.81 (0.68, 0.96)
Death	104	2.62	109	2.76	0.95 (0.72, 1.25)
Edema[Þ]	741	18.66	664	16.83	1.11 (1.00, 1.23)
Hot flashes	6748	169.91	7170	181.71	0.94 (0.90, 0.97)

*Abbreviations: CI = confidence interval; DCIS = ductal carcinoma in situ; ER = estrogen receptor; IR = annual incidence rate per 1000 women; LCIS = lobular carcinoma in situ; RR = risk ratio for women in the EVISTA group compared with those in the tamoxifen group.
†Of the 60 noninvasive breast cases in the tamoxifen group, 5 were mixed types. Of the 83 noninvasive breast cancers in the raloxifene group, 7 were mixed types.
‡Only patients with an intact uterus at baseline were included (tamoxifen = 4739, EVISTA = 4715).
§Only patients with at least one intact ovary at baseline were included (tamoxifen = 6813, EVISTA = 6787).
¶Defined as myocardial infarction, severe angina, or acute ischemic syndromes.
#Only patients who were free of cataracts at baseline were included (tamoxifen = 8342, EVISTA = 8333).
ÞPeripheral edema events are included in the term edema.

women (2.2 versus 1.5 per 1000 women-years; hazard ratio 1.49; 95% confidence interval, 1.00-2.24; p=0.0499). The incidence of stroke did not differ significantly between treatment groups (249 with EVISTA [4.9%] versus 224 with placebo [4.4%]; hazard ratio 1.10; 95% confidence interval 0.92-1.32; p=0.30; 9.5 versus 8.6 per 1000 women-years) [see Warnings and Precautions (5.2, 5.3)].

16 HOW SUPPLIED/STORAGE AND HANDLING
16.1 How Supplied
EVISTA 60 mg tablets are white, elliptical, and film coated. They are imprinted on one side with LILLY and the tablet code 4165 in edible blue ink. They are available as follows:

Bottles of 30 (unit of use)	NDC 0002–4165–30
Blisters of 2 × 15	NDC 0002–4165–34
Bottles of 100 (unit of use)	NDC 0002–4165–02
Bottles of 2000	NDC 0002–4165–07

16.2 Storage and Handling
Store at controlled room temperature, 20° to 25°C (68° to 77°F) [see USP]. The USP defines controlled room temperature as a temperature maintained thermostatically that encompasses the usual and customary working environment of 20° to 25°C (68° to 77°F); that results in a mean kinetic temperature calculated to be not more than 25°C; and that allows for excursions between 15° and 30°C (59° and 86°F) that are experienced in pharmacies, hospitals, and warehouses.

17 PATIENT COUNSELING INFORMATION
See FDA-approved Medication Guide.
Physicians should instruct their patients to read the Medication Guide before starting therapy with EVISTA and to reread it each time the prescription is renewed.
17.1 Osteoporosis Recommendations, Including Calcium and Vitamin D Supplementation
For osteoporosis treatment or prevention, patients should be instructed to take supplemental calcium and/or vitamin D if intake is inadequate. Patients at increased risk for vitamin D insufficiency (e.g., over the age of 70 years, nursing home bound, chronically ill, or with gastrointestinal malabsorption syndromes) should be instructed to take additional vitamin D if needed. Weight-bearing exercises should be considered along with the modification of certain behavioral factors, such as cigarette smoking and/or excessive alcohol consumption, if these factors exist.
17.2 Patient Immobilization
EVISTA should be discontinued at least 72 hours prior to and during prolonged immobilization (e.g., post-surgical recovery, prolonged bed rest), and patients should be advised to avoid prolonged restrictions of movement during travel because of the increased risk of venous thromboembolic events [see Warnings and Precautions (5.1)].
17.3 Hot Flashes or Flushes
EVISTA may increase the incidence of hot flashes and is not effective in reducing hot flashes or flushes associated with estrogen deficiency. In some asymptomatic patients, hot flashes may occur upon beginning EVISTA therapy.
17.4 Reduction in Risk of Invasive Breast Cancer in Postmenopausal Women with Osteoporosis or at High Risk of Invasive Breast Cancer
Use of EVISTA is associated with the reduction of the risk of invasive breast cancer in postmenopausal women. EVISTA has not been shown to reduce the risk of noninvasive breast cancer. When considering treatment, physicians need to discuss the potential benefits and risks of EVISTA treatment with the patient.
EVISTA is not indicated for the treatment of invasive breast cancer or reduction of the risk of recurrence.
Patients should have breast exams and mammograms before starting EVISTA and should continue regular breast exams and mammograms in keeping with good medical practice after beginning treatment with EVISTA.
Literature revised October 30, 2008
Eli Lilly and Company, Indianapolis, IN 46285, USA
Copyright © 1997, 2008, Eli Lilly and Company. All rights reserved.
PV 6770 AMP
Medication Guide
EVISTA® (Ē-VISS-tah)
(raloxifene hydrochloride tablets)
Tablets for Oral Use
Read the Medication Guide that comes with EVISTA before you start taking it and each time you refill your prescription. The information may have changed. This Medication Guide does not take the place of talking with your doctor about your medical condition or treatment. Talk with your doctor about EVISTA when you start taking it and at regular checkups.
What is the most important information I should know about EVISTA?
Serious and life-threatening side effects can occur while taking EVISTA. These include blood clots and dying from stroke:
- Increased risk of blood clots in the legs (deep vein thrombosis) and lungs (pulmonary embolism) have been reported with EVISTA. Women who have or have had blood clots in the legs, lungs, or eyes should not take EVISTA.
- Women who have had a heart attack or are at risk for a heart attack may have an increased risk of dying from stroke when taking EVISTA.
1. Before starting EVISTA, tell your doctor if you have had blood clots in your legs, lungs, or eyes, a stroke, mini-stroke (transient ischemic attack), or have an irregular heartbeat.
2. Stop taking EVISTA and call your doctor if you have:
   - leg pain or a feeling of warmth in the lower leg (calf).
   - swelling of the legs, hands, or feet.
   - sudden chest pain, shortness of breath, or coughing up blood.
   - sudden change in your vision, such as loss of vision or blurred vision.
3. Being still for a long time (such as sitting still during a long car or airplane trip or being in bed after surgery) can increase your risk of blood clots. (See "What should I avoid if I am taking EVISTA?")
What is EVISTA?
EVISTA is a type of prescription medicine called a Selective Estrogen Receptor Modulator (SERM). EVISTA is for women after menopause, and has more than one use:
- **Osteoporosis:** EVISTA treats and prevents osteoporosis by helping make your bones stronger and less likely to break.
- **Invasive Breast Cancer:** If you have osteoporosis or are at high risk for breast cancer, EVISTA can be used to lower your chance of getting invasive breast cancer. EVISTA will not totally get rid of your chance of getting breast cancer. Your doctor can estimate your risk of breast cancer by asking you about risk factors, including:

- your age (getting older).
- family history of breast cancer in your mother, sister, or daughter.
- a history of any breast biopsy, especially an abnormal biopsy.

You and your doctor should talk about whether the possible benefit of EVISTA in lowering your chance of getting invasive breast cancer is greater than its possible risks. EVISTA is not for use in premenopausal women (women who have not passed menopause).

Who should not take EVISTA?
Do not take EVISTA if you:
- have or have had blood clots in your legs, lungs, or eyes. Taking EVISTA may increase the risk of getting blood clots.
- are pregnant or could become pregnant. EVISTA could harm your unborn child.
- are nursing a baby. It is not known if EVISTA passes into breast milk or what effect it might have on the baby.

What should I tell my doctor before taking EVISTA?
EVISTA may not be right for you. Before taking EVISTA, tell your doctor about all your medical conditions, including if you:
- have had blood clots in your legs, lungs, or eyes, a stroke, mini-stroke (TIA/transient ischemic attack), or a type of irregular heartbeat (atrial fibrillation).
- have had breast cancer. EVISTA has not been fully studied in women who have a history of breast cancer.
- have liver or kidney problems.
- have taken estrogen in the past and had a high increase of triglycerides (a kind of fat in the blood).
- are pregnant, planning to become pregnant, or breastfeeding (see "**Who should not take EVISTA?**").

Tell your doctor about all medicines you take, including prescription and non-prescription medicines, vitamins, and herbal supplements. Know the medicines you take. Keep a list of them and show it to your doctor and pharmacist each time you get a new medicine. Especially tell your doctor if you take*:
- warfarin (Coumadin®, Jantoven®)
  If you are taking warfarin or other coumarin blood thinners, your doctor may need to do a blood test when you first start or if you need to stop taking EVISTA. Names for this test include "prothrombin time," "pro-time," or "INR." Your doctor may need to adjust the dose of your warfarin or other coumarin blood thinner.
- cholestyramine
- estrogens

EVISTA should not be taken with cholestyramine or estrogens.

How should I take EVISTA?
- Take EVISTA exactly how your doctor tells you to.
- Keep taking EVISTA for as long as your doctor prescribes it for you. It is not known how long you should keep taking EVISTA to lower your chance of getting invasive breast cancers.
- It is important to get your refills on time so you do not run out of the medicine.
- Take one EVISTA tablet each day.
- Take EVISTA at any time of the day, with or without food.
- To help you remember to take EVISTA, it may be best to take it at about the same time each day.
- Calcium and vitamin D may be taken at the same time as EVISTA. It is important to take calcium and vitamin D, as directed by your physician, to prevent or treat osteoporosis.
- If you miss a dose, take it as soon as you remember. However, if it is almost time for your next dose, skip the missed dose and take only your next regularly scheduled dose. Do not take two doses at the same time.

What should I avoid while taking EVISTA?
- Being still for a long time (such as during long trips or being in bed after surgery) can increase the risk of blood clots. EVISTA may add to this risk. If you will need to be still for a long time, talk with your doctor about ways to reduce the risk of blood clots. On long trips, move around periodically. Stop taking EVISTA at least 3 days before a planned surgery or before you plan on being still for a long time. You should start taking EVISTA again when you return to your normal activities.
- Some medicines should not be taken with EVISTA (see "What should I tell my doctor before taking EVISTA?").

What are the possible side effects of EVISTA?
Serious and life-threatening side effects can occur while taking EVISTA. These include blood clots and dying from stroke:
- Increased risk of blood clots in the legs (deep vein thrombosis) and lungs (pulmonary embolism) have been reported with EVISTA. Women who have or have had blood clots in the legs, lungs, or eyes should not take EVISTA.
- Women who have had a heart attack or are at risk for a heart attack may have an increased risk of dying from stroke when taking EVISTA.

See "What is the most important information I should know about EVISTA?"
The most common side effects of EVISTA are hot flashes, leg cramps, swelling of the feet, ankles, and legs, flu syndrome, joint pain, and sweating. Hot flashes are more common during the first 6 months after starting treatment.
These are not all the side effects of EVISTA. Tell your doctor about any side effect that bothers you or that does not go away. Call your doctor for medical advice about side effects. You may report side effects to FDA at 1-800-FDA-1088.

What else should I know about EVISTA?
- Do not use EVISTA to prevent heart disease, heart attack, or strokes.
- To get the calcium and vitamin D you need, your doctor may advise you to change your diet and/or take supplemental calcium and vitamin D. Your doctor may suggest other ways to help treat or prevent osteoporosis, in addition to taking EVISTA and getting the calcium and vitamin D you need. These may include regular exercise, stopping smoking, and drinking less alcohol.
- Women who have hot flashes can take EVISTA. EVISTA does not treat hot flashes, and it may cause hot flashes in some women. (See "What are the possible side effects of EVISTA?")
- EVISTA has not been found to cause breast tenderness or enlargement. If you notice any changes in your breasts, call your doctor to find out the cause. Before starting and while taking EVISTA you should have breast exams and mammograms, as directed by your doctor. Because EVISTA does not eliminate the chance of developing breast cancers, you need these examinations to find any breast cancers as early as possible.
- EVISTA should not cause spotting or menstrual-type bleeding. If you have any vaginal bleeding, call your doctor to find out the cause. EVISTA has not been found to increase the risk for cancer of the lining of the uterus.
- Women in clinical trials have taken EVISTA for up to eight years.

How should I store EVISTA?
- Store EVISTA at 68°F to 77°F (20°C-25°C).
- **Keep EVISTA and all medicines out of the reach of children.**

General Information about the safe and effective use of EVISTA
Medicines are sometimes prescribed for purposes other than those listed in a Medication Guide. Do not use EVISTA for a condition for which it was not prescribed. Do not give your EVISTA to other people, even if they have the same symptoms you have. It may harm them.
This Medication Guide is a summary of the most important information about EVISTA. If you would like more information about EVISTA, talk with your doctor. You can ask your doctor or pharmacist for information about EVISTA that is written for health professionals. For more information, call 1-800-545-5979 (toll-free) or go to the following website: www.evista.com.

What are the ingredients in EVISTA?
Active Ingredient: raloxifene hydrochloride
Inactive Ingredients: anhydrous lactose, carnauba wax, crospovidone, FD&C Blue No. 2 aluminum lake, hypromellose, lactose monohydrate, magnesium stearate, modified pharmaceutical glaze, polyethylene glycol, polysorbate 80, povidone, propylene glycol, and titanium dioxide.
This Medication Guide has been approved by the U.S. Food and Drug Administration.

*The brands listed are trademarks of their respective owners and are not trademarks of Eli Lilly and Company. The makers of these brands are not affiliated with and do not endorse Eli Lilly and Company or its products.
Medication Guide revised October 30, 2008
Eli Lilly and Company, Indianapolis, IN 46285, USA
Copyright © 1997, 2008, Eli Lilly and Company. All rights reserved.
PV 3125 AMP
Revised: 11/2009   Distributed by: Eli Lilly and Company
Shown in Product Identification Guide, page 310

FORTEO®   ℞
[for-tay-o]
(teriparatide [rDNA origin] injection)
for subcutaneous use

HIGHLIGHTS OF PRESCRIBING INFORMATION
These highlights do not include all the information needed to use FORTEO safely and effectively. See full prescribing information for FORTEO.
FORTEO (teriparatide [rDNA origin] injection) for subcutaneous use
Initial U.S. Approval: 2002

WARNING: POTENTIAL RISK OF OSTEOSARCOMA
See full prescribing information for complete boxed warning.

- In rats, teriparatide caused an increase in the incidence of osteosarcoma, a malignant bone tumor. (5.1, 13.1)
- Because of the uncertain relevance of the rat osteosarcoma finding to humans, prescribe FORTEO only for patients for whom potential benefits outweigh potential risk. (5.1)
- FORTEO should not be prescribed for patients at increased baseline risk for osteosarcoma (e.g., those with Paget's disease of bone or unexplained elevations of alkaline phosphatase, pediatric and young adult patients with open epiphyses, or prior external beam or implant radiation therapy involving the skeleton). (5.1)

---RECENT MAJOR CHANGES---
Indications and Usage, Treatment of Men and Women with Glucocorticoid-Induced Osteoporosis (1.3)	07/2009
Dosage and Administration, Treatment of Men and Women with Glucocorticoid-Induced Osteoporosis (2.3)	07/2009

---INDICATIONS AND USAGE---
FORTEO is recombinant human parathyroid hormone analog (1-34), [rhPTH(1-34)] indicated for:
- Treatment of postmenopausal women with osteoporosis at high risk for fracture (1.1)
- Increase of bone mass in men with primary or hypogonadal osteoporosis at high risk for fracture (1.2)
- Treatment of men and women with osteoporosis associated with sustained systemic glucocorticoid therapy at high risk for fracture (1.3)

---DOSAGE AND ADMINISTRATION---
- Recommended dose is 20 mcg subcutaneously once a day (2.1, 2.2, 2.3)
- Administer as a subcutaneous injection into the thigh or abdominal wall (2.4)
- Administer initially under circumstances in which the patient can sit or lie down if symptoms of orthostatic hypotension occur (2.4)
- Use of the drug for more than 2 years during a patient's lifetime is not recommended (2.5)

---DOSAGE FORMS AND STRENGTHS---
Multi-dose prefilled delivery device (pen) containing 28 daily doses of 20 mcg (3)

---CONTRAINDICATIONS---
- Patients with hypersensitivity to teriparatide or to any of its excipients (4)

---WARNINGS AND PRECAUTIONS---
- Patients with Paget's disease of bone, pediatric and young adult patients with open epiphyses, and patients with prior external beam or implant radiation involving the skeleton: Should not be treated with FORTEO (5.1, 8.4)
- Treatment duration: Use of FORTEO for more than 2 years during a patient's lifetime is not recommended. (5.2)
- Patients with bone metastases, history of skeletal malignancies, metabolic bone diseases other than osteoporosis, or hypercalcemic disorders: Should not be treated with FORTEO (5.3, 5.4, 5.5)
- Laboratory alterations: FORTEO may increase serum calcium, urinary calcium, and serum uric acid (5.5, 5.6)
- Urolithiasis: Use with caution in patients with active or recent urolithiasis because of risk of exacerbation (5.6)
- Orthostatic hypotension: Transient orthostatic hypotension may occur with initial doses of FORTEO (5.7)

---ADVERSE REACTIONS---
Most common adverse reactions (>10%) include: arthralgia, pain, and nausea (6.1)
To report SUSPECTED ADVERSE REACTIONS, contact Eli Lilly and Company at 1-800-545-5979 or FDA at 1-800-FDA-1088 or www.fda.gov/medwatch

---DRUG INTERACTIONS---
Digoxin: Use FORTEO with caution in patients receiving digoxin. Transient hypercalcemia may predispose patients to digitalis toxicity (5.8, 7.1, 12.3)

---USE IN SPECIFIC POPULATIONS---
- Pregnancy: Based on animal studies, may cause fetal harm (8.1)
- Nursing Mothers: Discontinue nursing or FORTEO, taking into account the importance of treatment to the mother (8.3)
- Pediatric Use: FORTEO should not be used in pediatric and young adult patients with open epiphyses due to increased baseline risk of osteosarcoma (5.1, 8.4)

See 17 for PATIENT COUNSELING INFORMATION and Medication Guide

Revised: 11/2009

FULL PRESCRIBING INFORMATION: CONTENTS*
WARNING: POTENTIAL RISK OF OSTEOSARCOMA
1   **INDICATIONS AND USAGE**
    1.1   Treatment of Postmenopausal Women with Osteoporosis at High Risk for Fracture

1.2 Increase of Bone Mass in Men with Primary or Hypogonadal Osteoporosis at High Risk for Fracture

1.3 Treatment of Men and Women with Glucocorticoid-Induced Osteoporosis at High Risk for Fracture

2 DOSAGE AND ADMINISTRATION

2.1 Treatment of Postmenopausal Women with Osteoporosis at High Risk for Fracture

2.2 Increase of Bone Mass in Men with Primary or Hypogonadal Osteoporosis at High Risk for Fracture

2.3 Treatment of Men and Women with Glucocorticoid-Induced Osteoporosis at High Risk for Fracture

2.4 Administration

2.5 Treatment Duration

3 DOSAGE FORMS AND STRENGTHS

4 CONTRAINDICATIONS

5 WARNINGS AND PRECAUTIONS

5.1 Osteosarcoma

5.2 Treatment Duration

5.3 Bone Metastases and Skeletal Malignances

5.4 Metabolic Bone Diseases

5.5 Hypercalcemia and Hypercalcemic Disorders

5.6 Urolithiasis or Pre-existing Hypercalciuria

5.7 Orthostatic Hypotension

5.8 Drug Interactions

6 ADVERSE REACTIONS

6.1 Clinical Trials Experience

6.2 Postmarketing Experience

7 DRUG INTERACTIONS

7.1 Digoxin

7.2 Hydrochlorothiazide

7.3 Furosemide

8 USE IN SPECIFIC POPULATIONS

8.1 Pregnancy

8.3 Nursing Mothers

8.4 Pediatric Use

8.5 Geriatric Use

8.6 Hepatic Impairment

8.7 Renal Impairment

10 OVERDOSAGE

11 DESCRIPTION

12 CLINICAL PHARMACOLOGY

12.1 Mechanism of Action

12.2 Pharmacodynamics

12.3 Pharmacokinetics

13 NONCLINICAL TOXICOLOGY

13.1 Carcinogenesis, Mutagenesis, Impairment of Fertility

13.2 Animal Toxicology

14 CLINICAL STUDIES

14.1 Treatment of Osteoporosis in Postmenopausal Women

14.2 Treatment to Increase Bone Mass in Men with Primary or Hypogonadal Osteoporosis

14.3 Treatment of Men and Women with Glucocorticoid-Induced Osteoporosis

16 HOW SUPPLIED/STORAGE AND HANDLING

16.1 How Supplied

16.2 Storage and Handling

17 PATIENT COUNSELING INFORMATION

17.1 Potential Risk of Osteosarcoma and Voluntary FORTEO Patient Registry

17.2 Orthostatic Hypotension

17.3 Hypercalcemia

17.4 Other Osteoporosis Treatment Modalities

17.5 Use of Delivery Device

17.6 Availability of Medication Guide and User Manual

* Sections or subsections omitted from the full prescribing information are not listed

FULL PRESCRIBING INFORMATION

WARNING: POTENTIAL RISK OF OSTEOSARCOMA

In male and female rats, teriparatide caused an increase in the incidence of osteosarcoma (a malignant bone tumor) that was dependent on dose and treatment duration. The effect was observed at systemic exposures to teriparatide ranging from 3 to 60 times the exposure in humans given a 20-mcg dose. Because of the uncertain relevance of the rat osteosarcoma finding to humans, prescribe FORTEO® only for patients for whom the potential benefits are considered to outweigh the potential risk. FORTEO should not be prescribed for patients who are at increased baseline risk for osteosarcoma (including those with Paget's disease of bone or unexplained elevations of alkaline phosphatase, pediatric and young adult patients with open epiphyses, or prior external beam or implant radiation therapy involving

---

the skeleton) *[see Warnings and Precautions (5.1), Adverse Reactions (6.2), and Nonclinical Toxicology (13.1)].*

1 INDICATIONS AND USAGE

1.1 Treatment of Postmenopausal Women with Osteoporosis at High Risk for Fracture

FORTEO is indicated for the treatment of postmenopausal women with osteoporosis at high risk for fracture, defined as a history of osteoporotic fracture, multiple risk factors for fracture, or patients who have failed or are intolerant to other available osteoporosis therapy. In postmenopausal women with osteoporosis, FORTEO reduces the risk of vertebral and nonvertebral fractures *[see Clinical Studies (14.1)].*

1.2 Increase of Bone Mass in Men with Primary or Hypogonadal Osteoporosis at High Risk for Fracture

FORTEO is indicated to increase bone mass in men with primary or hypogonadal osteoporosis at high risk for fracture, defined as a history of osteoporotic fracture, multiple risk factors for fracture, or patients who have failed or are intolerant to other available osteoporosis therapy *[see Clinical Studies (14.2)].*

1.3 Treatment of Men and Women with Glucocorticoid-Induced Osteoporosis at High Risk for Fracture

FORTEO is indicated for the treatment of men and women with osteoporosis associated with sustained systemic glucocorticoid therapy (daily dosage equivalent to 5 mg or greater of prednisone) at high risk for fracture, defined as a history of osteoporotic fracture, multiple risk factors for fracture, or patients who have failed or are intolerant to other available osteoporosis therapy *[see Clinical Studies (14.3)].*

2 DOSAGE AND ADMINISTRATION

2.1 Treatment of Postmenopausal Women with Osteoporosis at High Risk for Fracture

The recommended dose is 20 mcg subcutaneously once a day.

2.2 Increase of Bone Mass in Men with Primary or Hypogonadal Osteoporosis at High Risk for Fracture

The recommended dose is 20 mcg subcutaneously once a day.

2.3 Treatment of Men and Women with Glucocorticoid-Induced Osteoporosis at High Risk for Fracture

The recommended dose is 20 mcg subcutaneously once a day.

2.4 Administration

• FORTEO should be administered as a subcutaneous injection into the thigh or abdominal wall. There are no data available on the safety or efficacy of intravenous or intramuscular injection of FORTEO.

• FORTEO should be administered initially under circumstances in which the patient can sit or lie down if symptoms of orthostatic hypotension occur *[see Warnings and Precautions (5.7)].*

• Parenteral drug products should be inspected visually for particulate matter and discoloration prior to administration, whenever solution and container permit. FORTEO is a clear and colorless liquid. Do not use if solid particles appear or if the solution is cloudy or colored.

• Patients and caregivers who administer FORTEO should receive appropriate training and instruction on the proper use of the FORTEO delivery device from a qualified health professional *[see Patient Counseling Information (17.5)].*

2.5 Treatment Duration

The safety and efficacy of FORTEO have not been evaluated beyond 2 years of treatment. Consequently, use of the drug for more than 2 years during a patient's lifetime is not recommended.

3 DOSAGE FORMS AND STRENGTHS

Multi-dose prefilled delivery device (pen) for subcutaneous injection containing 28 daily doses of 20 mcg.

4 CONTRAINDICATIONS

Do not use FORTEO in patients with:

• Hypersensitivity to teriparatide or to any of its excipients. Reactions have included angioedema and anaphylaxis *[see Adverse Reactions (6.2)].*

5 WARNINGS AND PRECAUTIONS

5.1 Osteosarcoma

In male and female rats, teriparatide caused an increase in the incidence of osteosarcoma (a malignant bone tumor) that was dependent on dose and treatment duration *[see Boxed Warning and Nonclinical Toxicology (13.1)].* FORTEO should not be prescribed for patients at increased baseline risk of osteosarcoma. These include:

• Paget's disease of bone. Unexplained elevations of alkaline phosphatase may indicate Paget's disease of bone.

• Pediatric and young adult patients with open epiphyses.

• Prior external beam or implant radiation therapy involving the skeleton.

Patients should be encouraged to enroll in the voluntary FORTEO Patient Registry, which is designed to collect information about any potential risk of osteosarcoma in patients who have taken FORTEO. Enrollment information can be obtained by calling 1-866-382-6813, or by visiting www.forteoregistry.rti.org

5.2 Treatment Duration

The safety and efficacy of FORTEO have not been evaluated beyond 2 years of treatment. Consequently, use of the drug for more than 2 years during a patients' lifetime is not recommended.

5.3 Bone Metastases and Skeletal Malignancies

Patients with bone metastases or a history of skeletal malignancies should not be treated with FORTEO.

5.4 Metabolic Bone Diseases

Patients with metabolic bone diseases other than osteoporosis should not be treated with FORTEO.

5.5 Hypercalcemia and Hypercalcemic Disorders

FORTEO has not been studied in patients with pre-existing hypercalcemia. These patients should not be treated with FORTEO because of the possibility of exacerbating hypercalcemia. Patients known to have an underlying hypercalcemic disorder, such as primary hyperparathyroidism, should not be treated with FORTEO.

5.6 Urolithiasis or Pre-existing Hypercalciuria

In clinical trials, the frequency of urolithiasis was similar in patients treated with FORTEO and placebo. However, FORTEO has not been studied in patients with active urolithiasis. If active urolithiasis or pre-existing hypercalciuria are suspected, measurement of urinary calcium excretion should be considered. FORTEO should be used with caution in patients with active or recent urolithiasis because of the potential to exacerbate this condition.

5.7 Orthostatic Hypotension

FORTEO should be administered initially under circumstances in which the patient can sit or lie down if symptoms of orthostatic hypotension occur. In short-term clinical pharmacology studies with teriparatide, transient episodes of symptomatic orthostatic hypotension were observed in 5% of patients. Typically, an event began within 4 hours of dosing and spontaneously resolved within a few minutes to a few hours. When transient orthostatic hypotension occurred, it happened within the first several doses, it was relieved by placing the person in a reclining position, and it did not preclude continued treatment.

5.8 Drug Interactions

Hypercalcemia may predispose patients to digitalis toxicity. Because FORTEO transiently increases serum calcium, patients receiving digoxin should use FORTEO with caution *[see Drug Interactions (7.1) and Clinical Pharmacology (12.3)].*

6 ADVERSE REACTIONS

6.1 Clinical Trials Experience

Because clinical studies are conducted under widely varying conditions, adverse reaction rates observed in the clinical studies of a drug cannot be directly compared to rates in the clinical studies of another drug and may not reflect the rates observed in practice.

Treatment of Osteoporosis in Men and Postmenopausal Women

The safety of FORTEO in the treatment of osteoporosis in men and postmenopausal women was assessed in two randomized, double-blind, placebo-controlled trials of 1382 patients (21% men, 79% women) aged 28 to 86 years (mean 67 years). The median durations of the trials were 11 months for men and 19 months for women, with 691 patients exposed to FORTEO and 691 patients to placebo. All patients received 1000 mg of calcium plus at least 400 IU of vitamin D supplementation per day.

The incidence of all cause mortality was 1% in the FORTEO group and 1% in the placebo group. The incidence of serious adverse events was 16% in FORTEO patients and 19% in placebo patients. Early discontinuation due to adverse events occurred in 7% of FORTEO patients and 6% of placebo patients.

Table 1 lists adverse events from the two principal osteoporosis trials in men and postmenopausal women that occurred in ≥2% of FORTEO-treated and more frequently than placebo-treated patients.

Table 1. Percentage of Patients with Adverse Events Reported by at Least 2% of FORTEO-Treated Patients and in More FORTEO-Treated Patients than Placebo-Treated Patients from the Two Principal Osteoporosis Trials in Women and Men Adverse Events are Shown Without Attribution of Causality

	FORTEO N=691	Placebo N=691
Event Classification	(%)	(%)
Body as a Whole		
Pain	21.3	20.5

Headache	7.5	7.4
Asthenia	8.7	6.8
Neck pain	3.0	2.7
Cardiovascular		
Hypertension	7.1	6.8
Angina pectoris	2.5	1.6
Syncope	2.6	1.4
Digestive System		
Nausea	8.5	6.7
Constipation	5.4	4.5
Diarrhea	5.1	4.6
Dyspepsia	5.2	4.1
Vomiting	3.0	2.3
Gastrointestinal disorder	2.3	2.0
Tooth disorder	2.0	1.3
Musculoskeletal		
Arthralgia	10.1	8.4
Leg cramps	2.6	1.3
Nervous System		
Dizziness	8.0	5.4
Depression	4.1	2.7
Insomnia	4.3	3.6
Vertigo	3.8	2.7
Respiratory System		
Rhinitis	9.6	8.8
Cough increased	6.4	5.5
Pharyngitis	5.5	4.8
Dyspnea	3.6	2.6
Pneumonia	3.9	3.3
Skin and Appendages		
Rash	4.9	4.5
Sweating	2.2	1.7

Immunogenicity—In the clinical trial, antibodies that cross-reacted with teriparatide were detected in 3% of women (15/541) receiving FORTEO. Generally, antibodies were first detected following 12 months of treatment and diminished after withdrawal of therapy. There was no evidence of hypersensitivity reactions or allergic reactions among these patients. Antibody formation did not appear to have effects on serum calcium, or on bone mineral density (BMD) response.

Laboratory Findings

Serum Calcium—FORTEO transiently increased serum calcium, with the maximal effect observed at approximately 4 to 6 hours post-dose. Serum calcium measured at least 16 hours post-dose was not different from pretreatment levels. In clinical trials, the frequency of at least 1 episode of transient hypercalcemia in the 4 to 6 hours after FORTEO administration was increased from 2% of women and none of the men treated with placebo to 11% of women and 6% of men treated with FORTEO. The number of patients treated with FORTEO whose transient hypercalcemia was verified on consecutive measurements was 3% of women and 1% of men.

Urinary Calcium—FORTEO increased urinary calcium excretion, but the frequency of hypercalciuria in clinical trials was similar for patients treated with FORTEO and placebo *[see Clinical Pharmacology (12.2)].*

Serum Uric Acid—FORTEO increased serum uric acid concentrations. In clinical trials, 3% of FORTEO patients had serum uric acid concentrations above the upper limit of nor-

mal compared with 1% of placebo patients. However, the hyperuricemia did not result in an increase in gout, arthralgia, or urolithiasis.

Renal Function—No clinically important adverse renal effects were observed in clinical studies. Assessments included creatinine clearance; measurements of blood urea nitrogen (BUN), creatinine, and electrolytes in serum; urine specific gravity and pH; and examination of urine sediment.

Studies in Men and Women with Glucocorticoid-Induced Osteoporosis

The safety of FORTEO in the treatment of men and women with glucocorticoid-induced osteoporosis was assessed in a randomized, double-blind, active-controlled trial of 428 patients (19% men, 81% women) aged 22 to 89 years (mean 57 years) treated with ≥ 5mg per day prednisone or equivalent for a minimum of 3 months. The duration of the trial was 18 months with 214 patients exposed to FORTEO and 214 patients exposed to oral daily bisphosphonate (active control). All patients received 1000 mg of calcium plus 800 IU of vitamin D supplementation per day.

The incidence of all cause mortality was 4% in the FORTEO group and 6% in the active control group. The incidence of serious adverse events was 21% in FORTEO patients and 18% in active control patients, and included pneumonia (3% FORTEO, 1% active control). Early discontinuation because of adverse events occurred in 15% of FORTEO patients and 12% of active control patients, and included dizziness (2% FORTEO, 0% active control).

Adverse events reported at a higher incidence in the FORTEO group and with at least a 2% difference in FORTEO-treated patients compared with active control-treated patients were: nausea (14%, 7%), gastritis (7%, 3%), pneumonia (6%, 3%), dyspnea (6%, 3%), insomnia (5%, 1%), anxiety (4%, 1%), and herpes zoster (3%, 1%), respectively.

6.2   Postmarketing Experience

The following adverse reactions have been identified during postapproval use of FORTEO. Because these reactions are reported voluntarily from a population of uncertain size, it is not always possible to reliably estimate their frequency or establish a causal relationship to drug exposure.

- Osteosarcoma: Cases of bone tumor and osteosarcoma have been reported rarely in the postmarketing period. The causality to FORTEO use is unclear. Long term osteosarcoma surveillance studies are ongoing *[see Warnings and Precautions (5.1)]*
- Hypercalcemia: Hypercalcemia greater than 13.0 mg/dL has been reported with FORTEO use.

Adverse events reported since market introduction that were temporally (but not necessarily causally) related to FORTEO therapy include the following:

- Allergic Reactions: Anaphylactic reactions, drug hypersensitivity, angioedema, urticaria
- Investigations: Hyperuricemia
- Respiratory System: Acute dyspnea, chest pain
- Musculoskeletal: Muscle spasms of the leg or back
- Other: Injection site reactions including injection site pain, swelling and bruising; oro-facial edema

7   DRUG INTERACTIONS

7.1   Digoxin

A single FORTEO dose did not alter the effect of digoxin on the systolic time interval (from electrocardiographic Q-wave onset to aortic valve closure, a measure of digoxin's calcium-mediated cardiac effect). However, because FORTEO may transiently increase serum calcium, FORTEO should be used with caution in patients taking digoxin *[see Warnings and Precaution (5.8) and Clinical Pharmacology (12.3)].*

7.2   Hydrochlorothiazide

The coadministration of hydrochlorothiazide 25 mg with teriparatide did not affect the serum calcium response to teriparatide 40 mcg. The effect of coadministration of a higher dose of hydrochlorothiazide with teriparatide on serum calcium levels has not been studied *[see Clinical Pharmacology (12.3)].*

7.3   Furosemide

Coadministration of intravenous furosemide (20 to 100 mg) with teriparatide 40 mcg in healthy people and patients with mild, moderate, or severe renal impairment (CrCl 13 to 72 mL/min) resulted in small increases in the serum calcium (2%) and 24-hour urine calcium (37%) responses to teriparatide that did not appear to be clinically important *[see Clinical Pharmacology (12.3)].*

8   USE IN SPECIFIC POPULATIONS

8.1   Pregnancy

Pregnancy Category C—There are no adequate and well-controlled studies of FORTEO in pregnant women. In animal studies, teriparatide increased skeletal deviations and variations in mouse offspring at doses more than 60 times the equivalent human dose and produced mild growth retardation and reduced motor activity in rat offspring at doses more than 120 times the equivalent human dose. FORTEO should be used during pregnancy only if the potential benefit justifies the potential risk to the fetus.

In animal studies, pregnant mice received teriparatide during organogenesis at subcutaneous doses 8 to 267 times the human dose. At doses ≥ 60 times the human dose, the fetuses showed an increased incidence of skeletal deviations or variations (interrupted rib, extra vertebra or rib). When pregnant rats received subcutaneous teriparatide during organogenesis at doses 16 to 540 times the human dose, the fetuses showed no abnormal findings.

In a perinatal/postnatal study, pregnant rats received subcutaneous teriparatide from organogenesis through lactation. Mild growth retardation in female offspring at doses ≥120 times the human dose (based on surface area, mcg/m²). Mild growth retardation in male offspring and reduced motor activity in both male and female offspring occurred at maternal doses 540 times the human dose. There were no developmental or reproductive effects in mice or rats at doses 8 or 16 times the human dose, respectively.

Exposure multiples were normalized based on body surface area (mcg/m²). Actual animal doses: mice (30 to 1000 mcg/kg/day); rats (30 to 1000 mcg/kg/day).

8.3   Nursing Mothers

It is not known whether teriparatide is excreted in human milk. Because of the potential for tumorigenicity shown for teriparatide in animal studies, a decision should be made whether to discontinue nursing or to discontinue the drug, taking into account the importance of the drug to the mother.

8.4   Pediatric Use

The safety and efficacy of FORTEO have not been established in any pediatric population. FORTEO should not be prescribed in patients at an increased baseline risk of osteosarcoma which include pediatric and young adult patients with open epiphyses. Therefore, FORTEO is not indicated for use in pediatric or young adult patients with open epiphyses *[see Warnings and Precautions (5.1)].*

8.5   Geriatric Use

Of the patients receiving FORTEO in the osteoporosis trial of 1637 postmenopausal women, 75% were 65 years of age and over and 23% were 75 years of age and over. Of the patients receiving FORTEO in the osteoporosis trial of 437 men, 39% were 65 years of age and over and 13% were 75 years of age and over. No overall differences in safety or effectiveness were observed between these subjects and younger subjects, and other reported clinical experience has not identified differences in responses between the elderly and younger patients, but greater sensitivity of some older individuals cannot be ruled out.

8.6   Hepatic Impairment

No studies have been performed in patients with hepatic impairment. *[see Clinical Pharmacology (12.3)].*

8.7   Renal Impairment

In 5 patients with severe renal impairment (CrCl<30 mL/min), the AUC and $T_{1/2}$ of teriparatide were increased by 73% and 77%, respectively. Maximum serum concentration of teriparatide was not increased *[see Clinical Pharmacology (12.3)].*

10   OVERDOSAGE

Incidents of overdose in humans have not been reported in clinical trials. Teriparatide has been administered in single doses of up to 100 mcg and in repeated doses of up to 60 mcg/day for 6 weeks. The effects of overdose that might be expected include a delayed hypercalcemic effect and risk of orthostatic hypotension. Nausea, vomiting, dizziness, and headache might also occur.

In postmarketing spontaneous reports, there have been cases of medication errors in which the entire contents (up to 800 mcg) of the FORTEO delivery device (pen) have been administered as a single dose. Transient events reported have included nausea, weakness/lethargy and hypotension. In some cases, no adverse events occurred as a result of the overdose. No fatalities associated with overdose have been reported.

Overdose Management—There is no specific antidote for teriparatide. Treatment of suspected overdose should include discontinuation of FORTEO, monitoring of serum calcium and phosphorus, and implementation of appropriate supportive measures, such as hydration.

11   DESCRIPTION

FORTEO (teriparatide [rDNA origin] injection) contains recombinant human parathyroid hormone (1-34), and is also called rhPTH (1-34). It has an identical sequence to the 34 N-terminal amino acids (the biologically active region) of the 84-amino acid human parathyroid hormone.

Teriparatide has a molecular weight of 4117.8 daltons and its amino acid sequence is shown below:

[See chemical structure at top of next column]

Teriparatide (rDNA origin) is manufactured using a strain of *Escherichia coli* modified by recombinant DNA technology. FORTEO is supplied as a sterile, colorless, clear, isotonic solution in a glass cartridge which is pre-assembled into a disposable delivery device (pen) for subcutaneous injection. Each prefilled delivery device is filled with 2.7 mL to

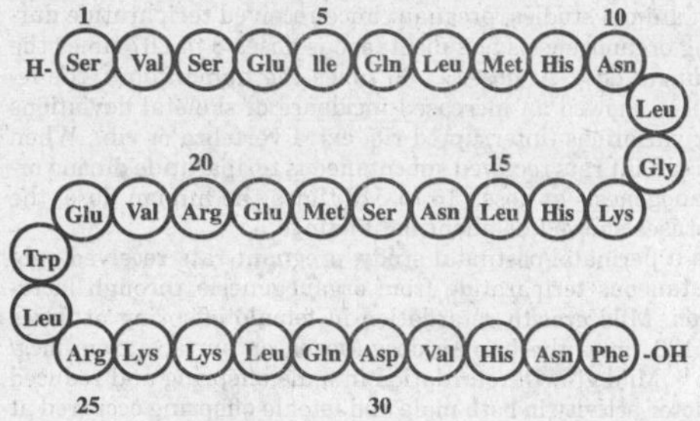

deliver 2.4 mL. Each mL contains 250 mcg teriparatide (corrected for acetate, chloride, and water content), 0.41 mg glacial acetic acid, 0.1 mg sodium acetate (anhydrous), 45.4 mg mannitol, 3 mg Metacresol, and Water for Injection. In addition, hydrochloric acid solution 10% and/or sodium hydroxide solution 10% may have been added to adjust the product to pH 4.

Each cartridge, pre-assembled into a delivery device, delivers 20 mcg of teriparatide per dose each day for up to 28 days.

12 CLINICAL PHARMACOLOGY

12.1 Mechanism of Action

Endogenous 84-amino acid parathyroid hormone (PTH) is the primary regulator of calcium and phosphate metabolism in bone and kidney. Physiological actions of PTH include regulation of bone metabolism, renal tubular reabsorption of calcium and phosphate, and intestinal calcium absorption. The biological actions of PTH and teriparatide are mediated through binding to specific high-affinity cell-surface receptors. Teriparatide and the 34 N-terminal amino acids of PTH bind to these receptors with the same affinity and have the same physiological actions on bone and kidney. Teriparatide is not expected to accumulate in bone or other tissues.

The skeletal effects of teriparatide depend upon the pattern of systemic exposure. Once-daily administration of teriparatide stimulates new bone formation on trabecular and cortical (periosteal and/or endosteal) bone surfaces by preferential stimulation of osteoblastic activity over osteoclastic activity. In monkey studies, teriparatide improved trabecular microarchitecture and increased bone mass and strength by stimulating new bone formation in both cancellous and cortical bone. In humans, the anabolic effects of teriparatide manifest as an increase in skeletal mass, an increase in markers of bone formation and resorption, and an increase in bone strength. By contrast, continuous excess of endogenous PTH, as occurs in hyperparathyroidism, may be detrimental to the skeleton because bone resorption may be stimulated more than bone formation.

12.2 Pharmacodynamics

Pharmacodynamics in Men and Postmenopausal Women with Osteoporosis

Effects on Mineral Metabolism—Teriparatide affects calcium and phosphorus metabolism in a pattern consistent with the known actions of endogenous PTH (e.g., increases serum calcium and decreases serum phosphorus).

Serum Calcium Concentrations—When teriparatide 20 mcg is administered once daily, the serum calcium concentration increases transiently, beginning approximately 2 hours after dosing and reaching a maximum concentration between 4 and 6 hours (median increase, 0.4 mg/dL). The serum calcium concentration begins to decline approximately 6 hours after dosing and returns to baseline by 16 to 24 hours after each dose.

In a clinical study of postmenopausal women with osteoporosis, the median peak serum calcium concentration measured 4 to 6 hours after dosing with FORTEO (teriparatide 20 mcg) was 2.42 mmol/L (9.68 mg/dL) at 12 months. The peak serum calcium remained below 2.76 mmol/L (11.0 mg/dL) in >99% of women at each visit. Sustained hypercalcemia was not observed.

In this study, 11.1% of women treated with FORTEO had at least 1 serum calcium value above the upper limit of normal [2.64 mmol/L (10.6 mg/dL)] compared with 1.5% of women treated with placebo. The percentage of women treated with FORTEO whose serum calcium was above the upper limit of normal on consecutive 4- to 6-hour post-dose measurements was 3.0% compared with 0.2% of women treated with placebo. In these women, calcium supplements and/or FORTEO doses were reduced. The timing of these dose reductions was at the discretion of the investigator. FORTEO dose adjustments were made at varying intervals after the first observation of increased serum calcium (median 21 weeks). During these intervals, there was no evidence of progressive increases in serum calcium.

In a clinical study of men with either primary or hypogonadal osteoporosis, the effects on serum calcium were similar to those observed in postmenopausal women. The median peak serum calcium concentration measured 4 to 6 hours after dosing with FORTEO was 2.35 mmol/L (9.44 mg/dL) at 12 months. The peak serum calcium remained below 2.76 mmol/L (11.0 mg/dL) in 98% of men at each visit. Sustained hypercalcemia was not observed.

In this study, 6.0% of men treated with FORTEO daily had at least 1 serum calcium value above the upper limit of normal [2.64 mmol/L (10.6 mg/dL)] compared with none of the men treated with placebo. The percentage of men treated with FORTEO whose serum calcium was above the upper limit of normal on consecutive measurements was 1.3% (2 men) compared with none of the men treated with placebo. Although calcium supplements and/or FORTEO doses could have been reduced in these men, only calcium supplementation was reduced *[see Warnings and Precautions (5.5) and Adverse Reactions (6.1)]*.

In a clinical study of women previously treated for 18 to 39 months with raloxifene (n=26) or alendronate (n=33), mean serum calcium >12 hours after FORTEO injection was increased by 0.09 to 0.14 mmol/L (0.36 to 0.56 mg/dL), after 1 to 6 months of FORTEO treatment compared with baseline. Of the women pretreated with raloxifene, 3 (11.5%) had a serum calcium >2.76 mmol/L (11.0 mg/dL), and of those pretreated with alendronate, 3 (9.1%) had a serum calcium >2.76 mmol/L (11.0 mg/dL). The highest serum calcium reported was 3.12 mmol/L (12.5 mg/dL). None of the women had symptoms of hypercalcemia. There were no placebo controls in this study.

In the study of patients with glucocorticoid-induced osteoporosis, the effects of FORTEO on serum calcium were similar to those observed in postmenopausal women with osteoporosis not taking glucocorticoids.

Urinary Calcium Excretion—In a clinical study of postmenopausal women with osteoporosis who received 1000 mg of supplemental calcium and at least 400 IU of vitamin D, daily FORTEO increased urinary calcium excretion. The median urinary excretion of calcium was 4.8 mmol/day (190 mg/day) at 6 months and 4.2 mmol/day (170 mg/day) at 12 months. These levels were 0.76 mmol/day (30 mg/day) and 0.3 mmol/day (12 mg/day) higher, respectively, than in women treated with placebo. The incidence of hypercalciuria (>7.5 mmol Ca/day or 300 mg/day) was similar in the women treated with FORTEO or placebo.

In a clinical study of men with either primary or hypogonadal osteoporosis who received 1000 mg of supplemental calcium and at least 400 IU of vitamin D, daily FORTEO had inconsistent effects on urinary calcium excretion. The median urinary excretion of calcium was 5.6 mmol/day (220 mg/day) at 1 month and 5.3 mmol/day (210 mg/day) at 6 months. These levels were 0.5 mmol/day (20 mg/day) higher and 0.2 mmol/day (8.0 mg/day) lower, respectively, than in men treated with placebo. The incidence of hypercalciuria (>7.5 mmol Ca/day or 300 mg/day) was similar in the men treated with FORTEO or placebo.

Phosphorus and Vitamin D—In single-dose studies, teriparatide produced transient phosphaturia and mild transient reductions in serum phosphorus concentration. However, hypophosphatemia (<0.74 mmol/L or 2.4 mg/dL) was not observed in clinical trials with FORTEO.

In clinical trials of daily FORTEO, the median serum concentration of 1,25-dihydroxyvitamin D was increased at 12 months by 19% in women and 14% in men, compared with baseline. In the placebo group, this concentration decreased by 2% in women and increased by 5% in men. The median serum 25-hydroxyvitamin D concentration at 12 months was decreased by 19% in women and 10% in men compared with baseline. In the placebo group, this concentration was unchanged in women and increased by 1% in men.

In the study of patients with glucocorticoid-induced osteoporosis, the effects of FORTEO on serum phosphorus were similar to those observed in postmenopausal women with osteoporosis not taking glucocorticoids.

Effects on Markers of Bone Turnover—Daily administration of FORTEO to men and postmenopausal women with osteoporosis in clinical studies stimulated bone formation, as shown by increases in the formation markers serum bone-specific alkaline phosphatase (BSAP) and procollagen I carboxy-terminal propeptide (PICP). Data on biochemical markers of bone turnover were available for the first 12 months of treatment. Peak concentrations of PICP at 1 month of treatment were approximately 41% above baseline, followed by a decline to near-baseline values by 12 months. BSAP concentrations increased by 1 month of treatment and continued to rise more slowly from 6 through 12 months. The maximum increases of BSAP were 45% above baseline in women and 23% in men. After discontinuation of therapy, BSAP concentrations returned toward baseline. The increases in formation markers were accompanied by secondary increases in the markers of bone resorption: urinary N-telopeptide (NTX) and urinary deoxypyridinoline (DPD), consistent with the physiological coupling of bone formation and resorption in skeletal remodeling. Changes in BSAP, NTX, and DPD were lower in men than in women, possibly because of lower systemic exposure to teriparatide in men.

In the study of patients with glucocorticoid-induced osteoporosis, the effects of FORTEO on serum markers of bone turnover were similar to those observed in postmenopausal women with osteoporosis not taking glucocorticoids.

12.3 Pharmacokinetics

Absorption—Teriparatide is absorbed after subcutaneous injection; the absolute bioavailability is approximately 95% based on pooled data from 20-, 40-, and 80- mcg doses. The rates of absorption and elimination are rapid. The peptide reaches peak serum concentrations about 30 minutes after subcutaneous injection of a 20-mcg dose and declines to non-quantifiable concentrations within 3 hours.

Distribution—Systemic clearance of teriparatide (approximately 62 L/hr in women and 94 L/hr in men) exceeds the rate of normal liver plasma flow, consistent with both hepatic and extra-hepatic clearance. Volume of distribution, following intravenous injection, is approximately 0.12 L/kg. Intersubject variability in systemic clearance and volume of distribution is 25% to 50%. The half-life of teriparatide in serum is 5 minutes when administered by intravenous injection and approximately 1 hour when administered by subcutaneous injection. The longer half-life following subcutaneous administration reflects the time required for absorption from the injection site.

Metabolism and Excretion—No metabolism or excretion studies have been performed with teriparatide. However, the mechanisms of metabolism and elimination of PTH(1-34) and intact PTH have been extensively described in published literature. Peripheral metabolism of PTH is believed to occur by non-specific enzymatic mechanisms in the liver followed by excretion via the kidneys.

Pediatric Patients—Pharmacokinetic data in pediatric patients are not available *[see Warnings and Precautions (5.1)]*.

Geriatric Patients—No age-related differences in teriparatide pharmacokinetics were detected (range 31 to 85 years).

Gender—Although systemic exposure to teriparatide was approximately 20% to 30% lower in men than women, the recommended dose for both genders is 20 mcg/day.

Race—The populations included in the pharmacokinetic analyses were 98.5% Caucasian. The influence of race has not been determined.

Renal Impairment—No pharmacokinetic differences were identified in 11 patients with mild or moderate renal impairment [creatinine clearance (CrCl) 30 to 72 mL/min] administered a single dose of teriparatide. In 5 patients with severe renal impairment (CrCl<30 mL/min), the AUC and $T_{1/2}$ of teriparatide were increased by 73% and 77%, respectively. Maximum serum concentration of teriparatide was not increased. No studies have been performed in patients undergoing dialysis for chronic renal failure *[see Use in Specific Populations (8.7)]*.

Hepatic Impairment—No studies have been performed in patients with hepatic impairment. Non-specific proteolytic enzymes in the liver (possibly Kupffer cells) cleave PTH(1-34) and PTH(1-84) into fragments that are cleared from the circulation mainly by the kidney *[see Use in Specific Populations (8.6)]*.

Drug Interactions

Digoxin—In a study of 15 healthy people administered digoxin daily to steady state, a single FORTEO dose did not alter the effect of digoxin on the systolic time interval (from electrocardiographic Q-wave onset to aortic valve closure, a measure of digoxin's calcium-mediated cardiac effect). However, sporadic case reports have suggested that hypercalcemia may predispose patients to digitalis toxicity. Because FORTEO may transiently increase serum calcium, FORTEO should be used with caution in patients taking digoxin *[see Drug Interactions (7.1)]*.

Hydrochlorothiazide—In a study of 20 healthy people, the coadministration of hydrochlorothiazide 25 mg with teriparatide did not affect the serum calcium response to teriparatide 40 mcg. The 24-hour urine excretion of calcium was reduced by a clinically unimportant amount (15%). The effect of coadministration of a higher dose of hydrochlorothiazide with teriparatide on serum calcium levels has not been studied *[see Drug Interactions (7.2)]*.

Furosemide—In a study of 9 healthy people and 17 patients with mild, moderate, or severe renal impairment (CrCl 13 to 72 mL/min), coadministration of intravenous furosemide (20 to 100 mg) with teriparatide 40 mcg resulted in small increases in the serum calcium (2%) and 24-hour urine calcium (37%) responses to teriparatide that did not appear to be clinically important *[see Drug Interactions (7.3)]*.

13 NONCLINICAL TOXICOLOGY

13.1 Carcinogenesis, Mutagenesis, Impairment of Fertility

Carcinogenesis—Two carcinogenicity bioassays were conducted in Fischer 344 rats. In the first study, male and female rats were given daily subcutaneous teriparatide injections of 5, 30, or 75 mcg/kg/day for 24 months from 2 months of age. These doses resulted in systemic exposures that were, respectively, 3, 20, and 60 times higher than the systemic exposure observed in humans following a subcutaneous dose of 20 mcg (based on AUC comparison). Teriparatide treatment resulted in a marked dose-related increase in the incidence of osteosarcoma, a rare malignant bone tumor, in both male and female rats. Osteosarcomas were observed at all doses and the incidence reached 40% to 50% in the high-dose groups. Teriparatide also caused a dose-related increase in osteoblastoma and osteoma in both sexes. No osteosarcomas, osteoblastomas or osteomas were observed in untreated control rats. The bone tumors in rats occurred in association with a large increase in bone mass and focal osteoblast hyperplasia.

The second 2-year study was carried out in order to determine the effect of treatment duration and animal age on the development of bone tumors. Female rats were treated for different periods between 2 and 26 months of age with subcutaneous doses of 5 and 30 mcg/kg (equivalent to 3 and 20 times the human exposure at the 20-mcg dose, based on AUC comparison). The study showed that the occurrence of osteosarcoma, osteoblastoma and osteoma was dependent upon dose and duration of exposure. Bone tumors were observed when immature 2-month old rats were treated with 30 mcg/kg/day for 24 months or with 5 or 30 mcg/kg/day for 6 months. Bone tumors were also observed when mature 6-month old rats were treated with 30 mcg/kg/day for 6 or 20 months. Tumors were not detected when mature 6-month old rats were treated with 5 mcg/kg/day for 6 or 20 months. The results did not demonstrate a difference in susceptibility to bone tumor formation, associated with teriparatide treatment, between mature and immature rats.

The relevance of these animal findings to humans is uncertain.

Mutagenesis—Teriparatide was not genotoxic in any of the following test systems: the Ames test for bacterial mutagenesis; the mouse lymphoma assay for mammalian cell mutation; the chromosomal aberration assay in Chinese hamster ovary cells, with and without metabolic activation; and the in vivo micronucleus test in mice.

Impairment of Fertility—No effects on fertility were observed in male and female rats given subcutaneous teriparatide doses of 30, 100, or 300 mcg/kg/day prior to mating and in females continuing through gestation Day 6 (16 to 160 times the human dose of 20 mcg based on surface area, mcg/m²).

13.2 Animal Toxicology

In single-dose rodent studies using subcutaneous injection of teriparatide, no mortality was seen in rats given doses of 1000 mcg/kg (540 times the human dose based on surface area, mcg/m²) or in mice given 10,000 mcg/kg (2700 times the human dose based on surface area, mcg/m²).

In a long-term study, skeletally mature ovariectomized female monkeys (N=30 per treatment group) were given either daily subcutaneous teriparatide injections of 5 mcg/kg or vehicle. Following the 18-month treatment period, the monkeys were removed from teriparatide treatment and were observed for an additional 3 years. The 5 mcg/kg dose resulted in systemic exposures that were approximately 6 times higher than the systemic exposure observed in humans following a subcutaneous dose of 20 mcg (based on AUC comparison). Bone tumors were not detected by radiographic or histologic evaluation in any monkey in the study.

14   CLINICAL STUDIES

14.1   Treatment of Osteoporosis in Postmenopausal Women

The safety and efficacy of once-daily FORTEO, median exposure of 19 months, were examined in a double-blind, multicenter, placebo-controlled clinical study of 1637 postmenopausal women with osteoporosis (FORTEO 20 mcg, n=541).

All women received 1000 mg of calcium and at least 400 IU of vitamin D per day. Baseline and endpoint spinal radiographs were evaluated using the semiquantitative scoring. Ninety percent of the women in the study had 1 or more radiographically diagnosed vertebral fractures at baseline. The primary efficacy endpoint was the occurrence of new radiographically diagnosed vertebral fractures defined as changes in the height of previously undeformed vertebrae. Such fractures are not necessarily symptomatic.

Effect on Fracture Incidence

New Vertebral Fractures—FORTEO, when taken with calcium and vitamin D and compared with calcium and vitamin D alone, reduced the risk of 1 or more new vertebral fractures from 14.3% of women in the placebo group to 5.0% in the FORTEO group. This difference was statistically significant (p<0.001); the absolute reduction in risk was 9.3% and the relative reduction was 65%. FORTEO was effective in reducing the risk for vertebral fractures regardless of age, baseline rate of bone turnover, or baseline BMD (see Table 2).

[See table 2 at top right]

Table 2. Effect of FORTEO on Risk of Vertebral Fractures in Postmenopausal Women with Osteoporosis

	Percent of Women With Fracture			
	FORTEO (N=444)	Placebo (N=448)	Absolute Risk Reduction (%, 95% CI)	Relative Risk Reduction (%, 95% CI)
New fracture (≥1)	5.0[a]	14.3	9.3 (5.5-13.1)	65 (45-78)
1 fracture	3.8	9.4		
2 fractures	0.9	2.9		
≥3 fractures	0.2	2.0		

[a] p≤0.001 compared with placebo.

New Nonvertebral Osteoporotic Fractures—FORTEO significantly reduced the risk of any nonvertebral fracture from 5.5% in the placebo group to 2.6% in the FORTEO group (p<0.05). The absolute reduction in risk was 2.9% and the relative reduction was 53%. The incidence of new nonvertebral fractures in the FORTEO group compared with the placebo group was ankle/foot (0.2%, 0.7%), hip (0.2%, 0.7%), humerus (0.4%, 0.4%), pelvis (0%, 0.6%), ribs (0.6%, 0.9%), wrist (0.4%, 1.3%), and other sites (1.1%, 1.5%), respectively.

The cumulative percentage of postmenopausal women with osteoporosis who sustained new nonvertebral fractures was lower in women treated with FORTEO than in women treated with placebo (see Figure 1).

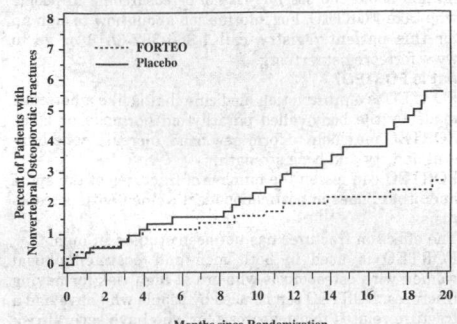

Figure 1. Cumulative Percentage of Postmenopausal Women with Osteoporosis Sustaining New Nonvertebral Osteoporotic Fractures

Effect on Bone Mineral Density (BMD)

FORTEO increased lumbar spine BMD in postmenopausal women with osteoporosis. Statistically significant increases were seen at 3 months and continued throughout the treatment period. Postmenopausal women with osteoporosis who were treated with FORTEO had statistically significant increases in BMD from baseline to endpoint at the lumbar spine, femoral neck, total hip, and total body (see Table 3).

Table 3. Mean Percent Change in BMD from Baseline to Endpoint[a] in Postmenopausal Women with Osteoporosis, Treated with FORTEO or Placebo for a Median of 19 Months

	FORTEO N=541	Placebo N=544
Lumbar spine BMD	9.7[b]	1.1
Femoral neck BMD	2.8[c]	-0.7
Total hip BMD	2.6[c]	-1.0
Trochanter BMD	3.5[c]	-0.2
Intertrochanter BMD	2.6[c]	-1.3
Ward's triangle BMD	4.2[c]	-0.8
Total body BMD	0.6[c]	-0.5
Distal 1/3 radius BMD	-2.1	-1.3
Ultradistal radius BMD	-0.1	-1.6

[a] Intent-to-treat analysis, last observation carried forward.
[b] p<0.001 compared with placebo.
[c] p<0.05 compared with placebo.

FORTEO treatment increased lumbar spine BMD from baseline in 96% of postmenopausal women treated. Seventy-two percent of patients treated with FORTEO achieved at least a 5% increase in spine BMD, and 44% gained 10% or more.

Both treatment groups lost height during the trial. The mean decreases were 3.61 and 2.81 mm in the placebo and FORTEO groups, respectively.

Bone Histology

The effects of teriparatide on bone histology were evaluated in iliac crest biopsies of 35 postmenopausal women treated for 12 to 24 months with calcium and vitamin D and teriparatide 20 or 40 mcg/day. Normal mineralization was observed with no evidence of cellular toxicity. The new bone formed with teriparatide was of normal quality (as evidenced by the absence of woven bone and marrow fibrosis).

14.2   Treatment to Increase Bone Mass in Men with Primary or Hypogonadal Osteoporosis

The safety and efficacy of once-daily FORTEO, median exposure of 10 months, were examined in a double-blind, multicenter, placebo-controlled clinical study of 437 men with either primary (idiopathic) or hypogonadal osteoporosis (FORTEO 20 mcg, n=151). All men received 1000 mg of calcium and at least 400 IU of vitamin D per day. The primary efficacy endpoint was change in lumbar spine BMD.

FORTEO increased lumbar spine BMD in men with primary or hypogonadal osteoporosis. Statistically significant increases were seen at 3 months and continued throughout the treatment period. FORTEO was effective in increasing lumbar spine BMD regardless of age, baseline rate of bone turnover, and baseline BMD. The effects of FORTEO at additional skeletal sites are shown in Table 4.

FORTEO treatment for a median of 10 months increased lumbar spine BMD from baseline in 94% of men treated. Fifty-three percent of patients treated with FORTEO achieved at least a 5% increase in spine BMD, and 14% gained 10% or more.

Table 4. Mean Percent Change in BMD from Baseline to Endpoint[a] in Men with Primary or Hypogonadal Osteoporosis, Treated with FORTEO or Placebo for a Median of 10 Months

	FORTEO N=151	Placebo N=147
Lumbar spine BMD	5.9[b]	0.5
Femoral neck BMD	1.5[c]	0.3
Total hip BMD	1.2	0.5
Trochanter BMD	1.3	1.1
Intertrochanter BMD	1.2	0.6
Ward's triangle BMD	2.8	1.1
Total body BMD	0.4	-0.4
Distal 1/3 radius BMD	-0.5	-0.2
Ultradistal radius BMD	-0.5	-0.3

[a] Intent-to-treat analysis, last observation carried forward.
[b] p<0.001 compared with placebo.
[c] p<0.05 compared with placebo.

14.3   Treatment of Men and Women with Glucocorticoid-Induced Osteoporosis

The efficacy of FORTEO for treating glucocorticoid-induced osteoporosis was assessed in a randomized, double-blind, active-controlled trial of 428 patients (19% men, 81% women) aged 22 to 89 years (mean 57 years) treated with ≥5 mg/day prednisone or equivalent for a minimum of 3 months. The duration of the trial was 18 months with 214 patients exposed to FORTEO. In the FORTEO group, the baseline median glucocorticoid dose was 7.5 mg/day and the median duration of glucocorticoid use was 1.5 years. The mean (SD) baseline lumbar spine BMD was 0.85 ± 0.13 g/cm² and lumbar spine BMD T-score was −2.5 ± 1 (number of standard deviations below the mean BMD value for healthy adults). A total of 30% of patients had prevalent vertebral fracture(s) and 43% had prior non-vertebral fracture(s). The patients had chronic rheumatologic, respiratory or other diseases that required sustained glucocorticoid therapy. All patients received 1000 mg of calcium plus 800 IU of vitamin D supplementation per day.

Because of differences in mechanism of action (anabolic vs. anti-resorptive) and lack of clarity regarding differences in BMD as an adequate predictor of fracture efficacy, data on the active comparator are not presented.

Effect on Bone Mineral Density (BMD)

In patients with glucocorticoid-induced osteoporosis, FORTEO increased lumbar spine BMD compared with baseline at 3 months through 18 months of treatment. In patients treated with FORTEO, the mean percent change in BMD from baseline to endpoint was 7.2% at the lumbar spine, 3.6% at the total hip, and 3.7% at the femoral neck (p<0.001 all sites). The relative treatment effects of FORTEO were consistent in subgroups defined by gender, age, geographic region, body mass index, underlying disease, prevalent vertebral fracture, baseline glucocorticoid dose, prior bisphosphonate use, and glucocorticoid discontinuation during trial.

16   HOW SUPPLIED/STORAGE AND HANDLING

16.1   How Supplied

The FORTEO delivery device (pen) is available in the following package size:
- 2.4 mL prefilled delivery device NDC 0002-8400-01 (MS8400).

16.2   Storage and Handling

- The FORTEO delivery device should be stored under refrigeration at 2° to 8°C (36° to 46°F) at all times.
- Recap the delivery device when not in use to protect the cartridge from physical damage and light.
- During the use period, time out of the refrigerator should be minimized; the dose may be delivered immediately following removal from the refrigerator.
- Do not freeze. Do not use FORTEO if it has been frozen.

17   PATIENT COUNSELING INFORMATION

See Medication Guide.

17.1   Potential Risk of Osteosarcoma and Voluntary FORTEO Patient Registry

Patients should be made aware that in rats, teriparatide caused an increase in the incidence of osteosarcoma (a malignant bone tumor) that was dependent on dose and treatment duration. Patients should be encouraged to enroll in the voluntary FORTEO Patient Registry, which is designed to collect information about any potential risk of osteosarcoma in patients who have taken FORTEO. Enrollment information can be obtained by calling 1-866-382-6813, or by visiting www.forteoregistry.rti.org.

17.2   Orthostatic Hypotension

FORTEO should be administered initially under circumstances where the patient can immediately sit or lie down if symptoms occur. Patients should be instructed that if they feel lightheaded or have palpitations after the injection, they should sit or lie down until the symptoms resolve. If symptoms persist or worsen, patients should be instructed to consult a physician before continuing treatment *[see Warnings and Precautions (5.7)].*

17.3   Hypercalcemia

Although symptomatic hypercalcemia was not observed in clinical trials, physicians should instruct patients taking FORTEO to contact a health care provider if they develop persistent symptoms of hypercalcemia (e.g., nausea, vomiting, constipation, lethargy, muscle weakness).

17.4   Other Osteoporosis Treatment Modalities

Patients should be informed regarding the roles of supplemental calcium and/or vitamin D, weight-bearing exercise, and modification of certain behavioral factors such as cigarette smoking and/or alcohol consumption.

17.5   Use of Delivery Device

Patients and caregivers who administer FORTEO should be instructed on how to properly use the delivery device (refer to *User Manual*), properly dispose of needles, and be advised not to share their delivery device with other patients. The contents of the delivery device should NOT be transferred to a syringe.

Each FORTEO delivery device can be used for up to 28 days including the first injection from the delivery device. After the 28-day use period, discard the FORTEO delivery device, even if it still contains some unused solution.

17.6   Availability of Medication Guide and User Manual

Patients should read the *Medication Guide* and delivery device (pen) *User Manual* before starting therapy with FORTEO and re-read them each time the prescription is renewed. Patients need to understand and follow the instructions in the FORTEO delivery device *User Manual*. Failure to do so may result in inaccurate dosing.

Literature revised January 25, 2010

Manufactured by Lilly France - F-67640 Fegersheim, France for Eli Lilly and Company - Indianapolis, IN 46285, USA
www.forteo.com

PV 9401 PA097FSAM00

MEDICATION GUIDE
FORTEO® (for-TAY-o)
teriparatide (rDNA origin)
injection

Read this Medication Guide before you start taking FORTEO and each time you get a refill. There may be new information. Also, read the User Manual that comes with the FORTEO delivery device (pen) for information on how to use the device to inject your medicine the right way. This Medication Guide does not take the place of talking with your healthcare provider about your medical condition or your treatment.

What is the most important information I should know about FORTEO?

- During the drug testing process, the medicine in FORTEO caused some rats to develop a bone cancer called osteosarcoma. In people, osteosarcoma is a serious but rare cancer. Osteosarcoma has been reported rarely in people who took FORTEO. It is not known if people who take FORTEO have a higher chance of getting osteosarcoma.
- You should not take FORTEO for more than 2 years over your lifetime.
- There is a voluntary Patient Registry for people who take FORTEO. The purpose of the registry is to collect information about the possible risk of osteosarcoma in people who take FORTEO. For information about how to sign up for this patient registry, call 1-866-382-6813 or go to www.forteoregistry.rti.org.

What is FORTEO?

- FORTEO is a prescription medicine that is like a hormone made by the body called parathyroid hormone or PTH. FORTEO may help to form new bone, increase bone mineral density and bone strength.
- FORTEO can lessen the number of fractures of the spine and other bones in postmenopausal women with osteoporosis.
- The effect on fractures has not been studied in men.
- FORTEO is used in both men and postmenopausal women with osteoporosis who are at high risk for having fractures. FORTEO can be used by people who have had a fracture related to osteoporosis, or who have several risk factors for fracture, or who can not use other osteoporosis treatments.
- FORTEO is used in both men and women with osteoporosis due to use of glucocorticoid medicines, such as prednisone, for several months, who are at high risk for having broken bones (fractures). These include men and women with either a history of broken bones, who have several risk factors for fracture, or who can not use other osteoporosis treatments.

It is not known if FORTEO is safe and effective in children. FORTEO should not be used in children and young adults whose bones are still growing.

Who should not use FORTEO?
Do not use FORTEO if you:
- are allergic to any of the ingredients in FORTEO. See the end of this Medication Guide for a complete list of the ingredients in FORTEO.

What should I tell my healthcare provider before taking FORTEO?
Before you take FORTEO, tell your healthcare provider if you:
- have the condition listed in the section "Who should not use FORTEO?"
- have Paget's disease or other bone disease
- have cancer in your bones
- have trouble injecting yourself and do not have someone who can help you
- are a child or young adult whose bones are still growing
- have or have had kidney stones
- have had radiation therapy
- have or had too much calcium in your blood
- have any other medical conditions
- are pregnant or thinking about becoming pregnant. It is not known if FORTEO will harm your unborn baby.
- are breast-feeding or plan to breast-feed. It is not known if FORTEO passes into your breast milk. You and your doctor should decide if you will take FORTEO or breast feed. You should not do both.

Tell your healthcare provider about all the medicines you take including prescription and non-prescription medicines, vitamins, and herbal supplements. Your healthcare provider needs this information to help keep you from taking FORTEO with other medicines that may harm you.
- Especially tell your doctor if you take medicines that contain digoxin (Digoxin, Lanoxicaps, Lanoxin).

How should I use FORTEO?
- Inject FORTEO one time each day in your thigh or abdomen (lower stomach area). Talk to a healthcare provider about how to rotate injection sites.
- Before you try to inject FORTEO yourself, a healthcare provider should teach you how to use the FORTEO delivery device to give your injection the right way.
- Read the detailed User Manual at the end of this Medication Guide.
- You can take FORTEO with or without food or drink.
- The FORTEO delivery device has enough medicine for 28 days. It is set to give a 20 microgram dose of medicine each day. Do not inject all the medicine in the FORTEO delivery device at any one time.
- Do not transfer the medicine from the FORTEO delivery device to a syringe. This can result in taking the wrong dose of FORTEO. If you do not have pen needles to use with your FORTEO delivery device, talk with your healthcare provider.
- FORTEO should look clear and colorless. Do not use FORTEO if it has particles in it, or if it is cloudy or colored.
- Inject FORTEO right away after you take the delivery device out of the refrigerator.
- After each use, safely remove the needle, recap the delivery device, and put it back in the refrigerator right away.
- You can take FORTEO at any time of the day. To help you remember to take FORTEO, take it at about the same time each day.
- If you forget or can not take FORTEO at your usual time, take it as soon as you can on that day. Do not take more than one injection in the same day.
- If you take more FORTEO than prescribed, call your healthcare provider. If you take too much FORTEO, you may have nausea, vomiting, weakness or dizziness.

Follow your healthcare provider's instructions about other ways you can help your osteoporosis, such as exercise, diet, and reducing or stopping your use of tobacco and alcohol. If your healthcare provider recommends calcium and vitamin D supplements, you can take them at the same time you take FORTEO.

What are the possible side effects of FORTEO?
FORTEO can cause serious side effects including:
- See "What is the most important information I should know about FORTEO?"
- **Decrease in blood pressure when you change positions.** Some people feel dizzy, get a fast heartbeat, or feel faint right after the first few doses. This usually happens within 4 hours of taking FORTEO and goes away within a few hours. For the first few doses, take your injections of FORTEO in a place where you can sit or lie down right away if you get these symptoms. If your symptoms get worse or do not go away, stop taking FORTEO and call your healthcare provider.
- **Increased calcium in your blood.** Tell your healthcare provider if you have nausea, vomiting, constipation, low energy, or muscle weakness. These may be signs there is too much calcium in your blood.

Common side effects of FORTEO include:
- nausea
- joint aches
- pain

Your healthcare provider may take samples of blood and urine during treatment to check your response to FORTEO. Also, your healthcare provider may ask you to have follow-up tests of bone mineral density.

Tell your healthcare provider if you have any side effect that bothers you or that does not go away.

These are not all the possible side effects of FORTEO. For more information, ask your doctor or pharmacist.

Call your doctor for medical advice about side effects. You may report side effects to FDA at 1-800-FDA-1088.

How should I store FORTEO?
- Keep your FORTEO delivery device in the refrigerator between 36° to 46°F (2° to 8°C).
- Do not freeze the FORTEO delivery device. Do not use FORTEO if it has been frozen.
- Do not use FORTEO after the expiration date printed on the delivery device and packaging.
- Throw away the FORTEO delivery device after 28 days even if it has medicine in it (see the User Manual).

Keep FORTEO and all medicines out of the reach of children.

General information about FORTEO
Medicines are sometimes prescribed for purposes other than those listed in a Medication Guide. Do not use FORTEO for a condition for which it was not prescribed. Do not give FORTEO to other people, even if they have the same condition you have.

This Medication Guide summarizes the most important information about FORTEO. If you would like more information, talk with your healthcare provider. You can ask your pharmacist or healthcare provider for information about

FORTEO that is written for healthcare professionals. For more information, go to www.FORTEO.com or call Lilly at 1-866-436-7836.

What are the ingredients in FORTEO?
Active ingredient:　teriparatide
Inactive ingredients:　glacial acetic acid, sodium acetate (anhydrous), mannitol, metacresol, and water for injection. In addition, hydrochloric acid solution 10% and/or sodium hydroxide solution 10% may have been added to adjust the product to pH 4.

What is Osteoporosis?
Osteoporosis is a disease in which the bones become thin and weak, increasing the chance of having a broken bone. Osteoporosis usually causes no symptoms until a fracture happens. The most common fractures are in the spine (backbone). They can shorten height, even without causing pain. Over time, the spine can become curved or deformed and the body bent over. Fractures from osteoporosis can also happen in almost any bone in the body, for example, the wrist, rib, or hip. Once you have had a fracture, the chance for more fractures greatly increases.

The following risk factors increase your chance of getting fractures from osteoporosis:
- past broken bones from osteoporosis.
- very low bone mineral density (BMD).
- frequent falls.
- limited movement, such as using a wheelchair.
- medical conditions likely to cause bone loss, such as some kinds of arthritis.
- taking steroid medicines called glucocorticoids, such as prednisone.
- other medicines that may cause bone loss, for example: seizure medicines (such as phenytoin), blood thinners (such as heparin), high doses of vitamin A.

This Medication Guide has been approved by the U.S. Food and Drug Administration.
Medication Guide revised July 22, 2009
Manufactured by Lilly France - F-67640 Fegersheim, France
for Eli Lilly and Company - Indianapolis, IN 46285, USA
Copyright © 2002, 2009, Eli Lilly and Company. All rights reserved.
PV 9411 FSAMP
Shown in Product Identification Guide, page 310

GEMZAR®　　　　　　　　　　　　　　　　℞
[jĕm-zar]
(gemcitabine hydrochloride)
Injection, Powder, Lyophilized, For Solution For Intravenous Use

HIGHLIGHTS OF PRESCRIBING INFORMATION
These highlights do not include all the information needed to use GEMZAR safely and effectively. See full prescribing information for GEMZAR.
GEMZAR (gemcitabine hydrochloride) Injection, Powder, Lyophilized, For Solution For Intravenous Use
Initial U.S. Approval: 1996

─────────INDICATIONS AND USAGE─────────
Gemzar® is a nucleoside metabolic inhibitor indicated for:
- Ovarian Cancer in combination with carboplatin (1.1)
- Breast Cancer in combination with paclitaxel (1.2)
- Non-Small Cell Lung Cancer in combination with cisplatin (1.3)
- Pancreatic Cancer as a single-agent (1.4)
─────────DOSAGE AND ADMINISTRATION─────────
Gemzar is for intravenous use only.
- Ovarian:　1000 mg/m² over 30 minutes on Days 1 and 8 of each 21-day cycle (2.1)
- Breast Cancer:　1250 mg/m² over 30 minutes on Days 1 and 8 of each 21-day cycle (2.2)
- Non-Small Cell Lung Cancer: 4-week schedule, 1000 mg/m² over 30 minutes on Days 1, 8, and 15 of each 28-day cycle: 3-week schedule; 1250 mg/m² over 30 minutes on Days 1 and 8 of each 21-day cycle (2.3)
- Pancreatic:　1000 mg/m² over 30 minutes once weekly for up to 7 weeks (or until toxicity necessitates reducing or holding a dose), followed by a week of rest from treatment. Subsequent cycles should consist of infusions once weekly for 3 consecutive weeks out of every 4 weeks (2.4)
- Dose Reductions or discontinuation may be needed based on toxicities (2.1-2.4)
─────────DOSAGE FORMS AND STRENGTHS─────────
- 200 mg vial for injection (3)
- 1 g vial for injection (3)
─────────CONTRAINDICATIONS─────────
Patients with a known hypersensitivity to Gemcitabine (4)
─────────WARNINGS AND PRECAUTIONS─────────
- Infusion time and dose frequency:　Increased toxicity with infusion time >60 minutes or dosing more frequently than once weekly. (5.1)
- Hematology:　Monitor for myelosuppression, which can be dose-limiting. (5.2, 5.7)

- Pulmonary toxicity:　Discontinue Gemzar immediately for severe pulmonary toxicity. (5.3)
- Renal:　Monitor renal function prior to initiation of therapy and periodically thereafter. Use with caution in patients with renal impairment. Cases of hemolytic uremic syndrome (HUS) and/or renal failure, some fatal, have occurred. Discontinue Gemzar for HUS or severe renal toxicity. (5.4)
- Hepatic:　Monitor hepatic function prior to initiation of therapy and periodically thereafter. Use with caution in patients with hepatic impairment. Serious hepatotoxicity, including liver failure and death, have occurred. Discontinue Gemzar for severe hepatic toxicity. (5.5)
- Pregnancy:　Can cause fetal harm. Advise women of potential risk to the fetus. (5.6, 8.1)
- Radiation toxicity. May cause severe and life-threatening toxicity. (5.8)
─────────ADVERSE REACTIONS─────────
The most common adverse reactions for the single-agent (≥20%) are nausea and vomiting, anemia, ALT, AST, neutropenia, leukopenia, alkaline phosphatase, proteinuria, fever, hematuria, rash, thrombocytopenia, dyspnea (6.1)
To report SUSPECTED ADVERSE REACTIONS, contact Eli Lilly and Company at 1-800-LillyRx (1-800-545 5979) or FDA at 1-800-FDA-1088 or www.fda.gov/medwatch.

See 17 for PATIENT COUNSELING INFORMATION
Revised: 05/2010

FULL PRESCRIBING INFORMATION: CONTENTS*

FULL PRESCRIBING INFORMATION

1　INDICATIONS AND USAGE
1.1　Ovarian Cancer
Gemzar in combination with carboplatin is indicated for the treatment of patients with advanced ovarian cancer that has relapsed at least 6 months after completion of platinum-based therapy.
1.2　Breast Cancer
Gemzar in combination with paclitaxel is indicated for the first-line treatment of patients with metastatic breast cancer after failure of prior anthracycline-containing adjuvant chemotherapy, unless anthracyclines were clinically contraindicated.
1.3　Non-Small Cell Lung Cancer
Gemzar is indicated in combination with cisplatin for the first-line treatment of patients with inoperable, locally advanced (Stage IIIA or IIIB), or metastatic (Stage IV) non-small cell lung cancer.
1.4　Pancreatic Cancer
Gemzar is indicated as first-line treatment for patients with locally advanced (nonresectable Stage II or Stage III) or metastatic (Stage IV) adenocarcinoma of the pancreas. Gemzar is indicated for patients previously treated with 5-FU.

2　DOSAGE AND ADMINISTRATION
Gemzar is for intravenous use only. Gemzar may be administered on an outpatient basis.
2.1　Ovarian Cancer
Gemzar should be administered intravenously at a dose of 1000 mg/m² over 30 minutes on Days 1 and 8 of each 21-day cycle. Carboplatin AUC 4 should be administered intravenously on Day 1 after Gemzar administration. Patients should be monitored prior to each dose with a complete blood count, including differential counts. Patients should have an absolute granulocyte count ≥1500 × 10⁶/L and a platelet count ≥100,000 × 10⁶/L prior to each cycle.
Dose Modifications
Gemzar dosage adjustments for hematological toxicity within a cycle of treatment is based on the granulocyte and platelet counts taken on Day 8 of therapy. If marrow suppression is detected, Gemzar dosage should be modified according to guidelines in Table 1.

Table 1: Day 8 Dosage Reduction Guidelines for Gemzar in Combination with Carboplatin

Absolute granulocyte count (× 10⁶/L)		Platelet count (× 10⁶/L)	% of full dose
≥1500	and	≥100,000	100
1000-1499	and/or	75,000-99,999	50
<1000	and/or	<75,000	Hold

In general, for severe (Grade 3 or 4) non-hematological toxicity, except nausea/vomiting, therapy with Gemzar should be held or decreased by 50% depending on the judgment of the treating physician. For carboplatin dosage adjustment, see manufacturer's prescribing information.

Dose adjustment for Gemzar in combination with carboplatin for subsequent cycles is based upon observed toxicity. The dose of Gemzar in subsequent cycles should be reduced to 800 mg/m² on Days 1 and 8 in case of any of the following hematologic toxicities:
- Absolute granulocyte count <500 × 10⁶/L for more than 5 days
- Absolute granulocyte count <100 × 10⁶/L for more than 3 days
- Febrile neutropenia
- Platelets <25,000 × 10⁶/L
- Cycle delay of more than one week due to toxicity
If any of the above toxicities recur after the initial dose reduction, for the subsequent cycle, Gemzar should be given on Day 1 only at 800 mg/m².
2.2　Breast Cancer
Gemzar should be administered intravenously at a dose of 1250 mg/m² over 30 minutes on Days 1 and 8 of each 21-day cycle. Paclitaxel should be administered at 175 mg/m² on Day 1 as a 3-hour intravenous infusion before Gemzar administration. Patients should be monitored prior to each dose with a complete blood count, including differential counts. Patients should have an absolute granulocyte count ≥1500 × 10⁶/L and a platelet count ≥100,000 × 10⁶/L prior to each cycle.
Dose Modifications
Gemzar dosage adjustments for hematological toxicity is based on the granulocyte and platelet counts taken on Day 8 of therapy. If marrow suppression is detected, Gemzar dosage should be modified according to the guidelines in Table 2.

Table 2: Day 8 Dosage Reduction Guidelines for Gemzar in Combination with Paclitaxel

Absolute granulocyte count ($\times 10^6$/L)		Platelet count ($\times 10^6$/L)	% of full dose
≥1200	and	>75,000	100
1000-1199	or	50,000-75,000	75
700-999	and	≥50,000	50
<700	or	<50,000	Hold

In general, for severe (Grade 3 or 4) non-hematological toxicity, except alopecia and nausea/vomiting, therapy with Gemzar should be held or decreased by 50% depending on the judgment of the treating physician. For paclitaxel dosage adjustment, see manufacturer's prescribing information.

2.3 Non-Small Cell Lung Cancer

Two schedules have been investigated and the optimum schedule has not been determined [see Clinical Studies (14.3)]. With the 4-week schedule, Gemzar should be administered intravenously at 1000 mg/m^2 over 30 minutes on Days 1, 8, and 15 of each 28-day cycle. Cisplatin should be administered intravenously at 100 mg/m^2 on Day 1 after the infusion of Gemzar. With the 3-week schedule, Gemzar should be administered intravenously at 1250 mg/m^2 over 30 minutes on Days 1 and 8 of each 21-day cycle. Cisplatin at a dose of 100 mg/m^2 should be administered intravenously after the infusion of Gemzar on Day 1. See prescribing information for cisplatin administration and hydration guidelines.

Dose Modifications

Dosage adjustments for hematologic toxicity may be required for Gemzar and for cisplatin. Gemzar dosage adjustment for hematological toxicity is based on the granulocyte and platelet counts taken on the day of therapy. Patients receiving Gemzar should be monitored prior to each dose with a complete blood count (CBC), including differential and platelet counts. If marrow suppression is detected, therapy should be modified or suspended according to the guidelines in Table 3. For cisplatin dosage adjustment, see manufacturer's prescribing information.

In general, for severe (Grade 3 or 4) non-hematological toxicity, except alopecia and nausea/vomiting, therapy with Gemzar plus cisplatin should be held or decreased by 50% depending on the judgment of the treating physician. During combination therapy with cisplatin, serum creatinine, serum potassium, serum calcium, and serum magnesium should be carefully monitored (Grade 3/4 serum creatinine toxicity for Gemzar plus cisplatin was 5% versus 2% for cisplatin alone).

2.4 Pancreatic Cancer

Gemzar should be administered by intravenous infusion at a dose of 1000 mg/m^2 over 30 minutes once weekly for up to 7 weeks (or until toxicity necessitates reducing or holding a dose), followed by a week of rest from treatment. Subsequent cycles should consist of infusions once weekly for 3 consecutive weeks out of every 4 weeks.

Dose Modifications

Dosage adjustment is based upon the degree of hematologic toxicity experienced by the patient [see Warnings and Precautions (5.2)]. Clearance in women and the elderly is reduced and women were somewhat less able to progress to subsequent cycles [see Warnings and Precautions (5.2) and Clinical Pharmacology (12.3)].

Patients receiving Gemzar should be monitored prior to each dose with a complete blood count (CBC), including differential and platelet count. If marrow suppression is detected, therapy should be modified or suspended according to the guidelines in Table 3.

Table 3: Dosage Reduction Guidelines

Absolute granulocyte count ($\times 10^6$/L)		Platelet count ($\times 10^6$/L)	% of full dose
≥1000	and	≥100,000	100
500-999	or	50,000-99,999	75
<500	or	<50,000	Hold

Laboratory evaluation of renal and hepatic function, including transaminases and serum creatinine, should be performed prior to initiation of therapy and periodically thereafter. Gemzar should be administered with caution in patients with evidence of significant renal or hepatic impairment as there is insufficient information from clinical studies to allow clear dose recommendation for these patient populations.

Patients treated with Gemzar who complete an entire cycle of therapy may have the dose for subsequent cycles in-

creased by 25%, provided that the absolute granulocyte count (AGC) and platelet nadirs exceed 1500 × 10^6/L and 100,000 × 10^6/L, respectively, and if non-hematologic toxicity has not been greater than WHO Grade 1. If patients tolerate the subsequent course of Gemzar at the increased dose, the dose for the next cycle can be further increased by 20%, provided again that the AGC and platelet nadirs exceed 1500 × 10^6/L and 100,000 × 10^6/L, respectively, and that non-hematologic toxicity has not been greater than WHO Grade 1.

2.5 Preparation and Administration Precautions

Caution should be exercised in handling and preparing Gemzar solutions. The use of gloves is recommended. If Gemzar solution contacts the skin or mucosa, immediately wash the skin thoroughly with soap and water or rinse the mucosa with copious amounts of water. Although acute dermal irritation has not been observed in animal studies, 2 of 3 rabbits exhibited drug-related systemic toxicities (death, hypoactivity, nasal discharge, shallow breathing) due to dermal absorption.

Procedures for proper handling and disposal of anti-cancer drugs should be considered. Several guidelines on this subject have been published [see References (15)].

2.6 Preparation for Intravenous Infusion Administration

The recommended diluent for reconstitution of Gemzar is 0.9% Sodium Chloride Injection without preservatives. Due to solubility considerations, the maximum concentration for Gemzar upon reconstitution is 40 mg/mL. Reconstitution at concentrations greater than 40 mg/mL may result in incomplete dissolution, and should be avoided.

To reconstitute, add 5 mL of 0.9% Sodium Chloride Injection to the 200-mg vial or 25 mL of 0.9% Sodium Chloride Injection to the 1-g vial. Shake to dissolve. These dilutions each yield a gemcitabine concentration of 38 mg/mL which includes accounting for the displacement volume of the lyophilized powder (0.26 mL for the 200-mg vial or 1.3 mL for the 1-g vial). The total volume upon reconstitution will be 5.26 mL or 26.3 mL, respectively. Complete withdrawal of the vial contents will provide 200 mg or 1 g of gemcitabine, respectively. The appropriate amount of drug may be administered as prepared or further diluted with 0.9% Sodium Chloride Injection to concentrations as low as 0.1 mg/mL. Reconstituted Gemzar is a clear, colorless to light straw-colored solution. After reconstitution with 0.9% Sodium Chloride Injection, the pH of the resulting solution lies in

the range of 2.7 to 3.3. The solution should be inspected visually for particulate matter and discoloration prior to administration, whenever solution or container permit. If particulate matter or discoloration is found, do not administer.

When prepared as directed, Gemzar solutions are stable for 24 hours at controlled room temperature 20° to 25°C (68° to 77°F) [see USP Controlled Room Temperature]. Discard unused portion. Solutions of reconstituted Gemzar should not be refrigerated, as crystallization may occur.

The compatibility of Gemzar with other drugs has not been studied. No incompatibilities have been observed with infusion bottles or polyvinyl chloride bags and administration sets.

3 DOSAGE FORMS AND STRENGTHS

GEMZAR (gemcitabine for injection, USP) is a white to off-white lyophilized powder available in sterile single-use vials containing 200 mg or 1 g gemcitabine.

4 CONTRAINDICATIONS

Gemzar is contraindicated in those patients with a known hypersensitivity to the drug.

5 WARNINGS AND PRECAUTIONS

Patients receiving therapy with Gemzar should be monitored closely by a physician experienced in the use of cancer chemotherapeutic agents.

5.1 Infusion Time

Caution—Prolongation of the infusion time beyond 60 minutes and more frequent than weekly dosing have been shown to increase toxicity [see Clinical Studies (14.5)].

5.2 Hematology

Gemzar can suppress bone marrow function as manifested by leukopenia, thrombocytopenia, and anemia [see Adverse Reactions (6.1)], and myelosuppression is usually the dose-limiting toxicity. Patients should be monitored for myelosuppression during therapy. [see Dosage and Administration (2.1, 2.2, 2.3, and 2.4)]

5.3 Pulmonary

Pulmonary toxicity has been reported with the use of Gemzar. In cases of severe lung toxicity, Gemzar therapy should be discontinued immediately and appropriate supportive care measures instituted [see Adverse Reactions (6.1 and 6.2)].

Table 4: Selected WHO-Graded Adverse Reactions in Patients Receiving Single-Agent Gemzar WHO Grades (% incidence)[a]

	All Patients[b]			Pancreatic Cancer Patients[c]			Discontinuations (%)[d]
	All Grades	Grade 3	Grade 4	All Grades	Grade 3	Grade 4	All Patients
Laboratory[e]							
Hematologic							
Anemia	68	7	1	73	8	2	<1
Leukopenia	62	9	<1	64	8	1	<1
Neutropenia	63	19	6	61	17	7	-
Thrombocytopenia	24	4	1	36	7	<1	<1
Hepatic							<1
ALT	68	8	2	72	10	1	
AST	67	6	2	78	12	5	
Alkaline Phosphatase	55	7	2	77	16	4	
Bilirubin	13	2	<1	26	6	2	
Renal							<1
Proteinuria	45	<1	0	32	<1	0	
Hematuria	35	<1	0	23	0	0	
BUN	16	0	0	15	0	0	
Creatinine	8	<1	0	6	0	0	
Non-laboratory[f]							
Nausea and Vomiting	69	13	1	71	10	2	<1
Fever	41	2	0	38	2	0	<1
Rash	30	<1	0	28	<1	0	<1
Dyspnea	23	3	<1	10	0	<1	<1
Diarrhea	19	1	0	30	3	0	0
Hemorrhage	17	<1	<1	4	2	<1	<1
Infection	16	1	<1	10	2	<1	<1
Alopecia	15	<1	0	16	0	0	0
Stomatitis	11	<1	0	10	<1	0	<1
Somnolence	11	<1	<1	11	2	<1	<1
Paresthesias	10	<1	0	10	<1	0	0

[a] Grade based on criteria from the World Health Organization (WHO).
[b] N=699-974; all patients with laboratory or non-laboratory data.
[c] N=161-241; all pancreatic cancer patients with laboratory or non-laboratory data.
[d] N=979.
[e] Regardless of causality.
[f] Table includes non-laboratory data with incidence for all patients ≥10%. For approximately 60% of the patients, non-laboratory adverse reactions were graded only if assessed to be possibly drug-related.

5.4 Renal

Hemolytic Uremic Syndrome (HUS) and/or renal failure have been reported following one or more doses of Gemzar. Renal failure leading to death or requiring dialysis, despite discontinuation of therapy, has been reported. The majority of the cases of renal failure leading to death were due to HUS [see Adverse Reactions (6.1 and 6.2)]. Gemzar should be used with caution in patients with preexisting renal impairment as there is insufficient information from clinical studies to allow clear dose recommendation for these patient populations. [see Use In Specific Populations (8.6)]

5.5 Hepatic

Serious hepatotoxicity, including liver failure and death, has been reported in patients receiving Gemzar alone or in combination with other potentially hepatotoxic drugs [see Adverse Reactions (6.1 and 6.2)]. Gemzar should be used with caution in patients with preexisting hepatic insufficiency as there is insufficient information from clinical studies to allow clear dose recommendation for these patient populations. Administration of Gemzar in patients with concurrent liver metastases or a preexisting medical history of hepatitis, alcoholism, or liver cirrhosis may lead to exacerbation of the underlying hepatic insufficiency. [see Use In Specific Populations (8.7)]

5.6 Pregnancy

Gemzar can cause fetal harm when administered to a pregnant woman. In pre-clinical studies in mice and rabbits, gemcitabine was teratogenic, embryotoxic, and fetotoxic. There are no adequate and well-controlled studies of Gemzar in pregnant women. If this drug is used during pregnancy, or if the patient becomes pregnant while taking this drug, the patient should be apprised of the potential hazard to the fetus. [see Use In Specific Populations (8.1)]

5.7 Laboratory Tests

Patients receiving Gemzar should be monitored prior to each dose with a complete blood count (CBC), including differential and platelet count. Suspension or modification of therapy should be considered when marrow suppression is detected. [see Dosage and Administration (2.1, 2.2, 2.3, and 2.4)]

Laboratory evaluation of renal and hepatic function should be performed prior to initiation of therapy and periodically thereafter [see Dosage and Administration (2.4)].

5.8 Radiation Therapy

A pattern of tissue injury typically associated with radiation toxicity has been reported in association with concurrent and non-concurrent use of Gemzar.

Non-concurrent (given >7 days apart)—Analysis of the data does not indicate enhanced toxicity when Gemzar is administered more than 7 days before or after radiation, other than radiation recall. Data suggest that Gemzar can be started after the acute effects of radiation have resolved or at least one week after radiation.

Concurrent (given together or ≤7 days apart)—Preclinical and clinical studies have shown that Gemzar has radiosensitizing activity. Toxicity associated with this multimodality therapy is dependent on many different factors, including dose of Gemzar, frequency of Gemzar administration, dose of radiation, radiotherapy planning technique, the target tissue, and target volume. In a single trial, where Gemzar at a dose of 1000 mg/m^2 was administered concurrently for up to 6 consecutive weeks with therapeutic thoracic radiation to patients with non-small cell lung cancer, significant toxicity in the form of severe, and potentially life-threatening mucositis, especially esophagitis and pneumonitis was observed, particularly in patients receiving large volumes of radiotherapy [median treatment volumes 4795 cm^3]. Subsequent studies have been reported and suggest that Gemzar administered at lower doses with concurrent radiotherapy has predictable and less severe toxicity. However, the optimum regimen for safe administration of Gemzar with therapeutic doses of radiation has not yet been determined in all tumor types.

6 ADVERSE REACTIONS

6.1 Clinical Trials Experience

Because clinical trials are conducted under widely varying conditions, adverse reaction rates observed in the clinical trials of a drug cannot be directly compared to rates in the clinical trials of another drug and may not reflect the rates observed in practice. Most adverse reactions are reversible and do not need to result in discontinuation, although doses may need to be withheld or reduced. Gemzar has been used in a wide variety of malignancies, both as a single-agent and in combination with other cytotoxic drugs.

Single-Agent Use:

Myelosuppression is the principal dose-limiting toxicity with Gemzar therapy. Dosage adjustments for hematologic toxicity are frequently needed [see Dosage and Administration (2.1, 2.2, 2.3, and 2.4)].

The data in Table 4 are based on 979 patients receiving Gemzar as a single-agent administered weekly as a 30-minute infusion for treatment of a wide variety of malignancies. The Gemzar starting doses ranged from 800 to 1250 mg/m^2. Data are also shown for the subset of patients with pancreatic cancer treated in 5 clinical studies. The frequency of all grades and severe (WHO Grade 3 or 4) adverse reactions were generally similar in the single-agent safety database of 979 patients and the subset of patients with pancreatic cancer. Adverse reactions reported in the single-agent safety database resulted in discontinuation of Gemzar therapy in about 10% of patients. In the comparative trial in pancreatic cancer, the discontinuation rate for adverse reactions was 14.3% for the Gemzar arm and 4.8% for the 5-FU arm. All WHO-graded laboratory adverse reactions are listed in Table 4, regardless of causality. Non-laboratory adverse reactions listed in Table 4 or discussed below were those reported, regardless of causality, for at least 10% of all patients, except the categories of Extravasation, Allergic, and Cardiovascular and certain specific adverse reactions under the Renal, Pulmonary, and Infection categories.

[See table 4 at top of previous page]

Hematologic—In studies in pancreatic cancer myelosuppression is the dose-limiting toxicity with Gemzar, but <1% of patients discontinued therapy for either anemia, leukopenia, or thrombocytopenia. Red blood cell transfusions were required by 19% of patients. The incidence of sepsis was less than 1%. Petechiae or mild blood loss (hemorrhage), from any cause, was reported in 16% of patients; less than 1% of patients required platelet transfusions. Patients should be monitored for myelosuppression during Gemzar therapy and dosage modified or suspended according to the degree of hematologic toxicity. [see Dosage and Administration (2.1, 2.2, 2.3, and 2.4)]

Gastrointestinal—Nausea and vomiting were commonly reported (69%) but were usually of mild to moderate severity. Severe nausea and vomiting (WHO Grade 3/4) occurred in <15% of patients. Diarrhea was reported by 19% of patients, and stomatitis by 11% of patients.

Hepatic—In clinical trials, Gemzar was associated with transient elevations of one or both serum transaminases in approximately 70% of patients, but there was no evidence of increasing hepatic toxicity with either longer duration of exposure to Gemzar or with greater total cumulative dose. Serious hepatotoxicity, including liver failure and death, has been reported very rarely in patients receiving Gemzar alone or in combination with other potentially hepatotoxic drugs. [see Adverse Reactions (6.2)]

Renal—In clinical trials, mild proteinuria and hematuria were commonly reported. Clinical findings consistent with the Hemolytic Uremic Syndrome (HUS) were reported in 6 of 2429 patients (0.25%) receiving Gemzar in clinical trials. Four patients developed HUS on Gemzar therapy, 2 immediately posttherapy. The diagnosis of HUS should be considered if the patient develops anemia with evidence of microangiopathic hemolysis, elevation of bilirubin or LDH, reticulocytosis, severe thrombocytopenia, and/or evidence of renal failure (elevation of serum creatinine or BUN). Gemzar therapy should be discontinued immediately. Renal failure may not be reversible even with discontinuation of therapy and dialysis may be required. [see Adverse Reactions (6.2)]

Fever—The overall incidence of fever was 41%. This is in contrast to the incidence of infection (16%) and indicates that Gemzar may cause fever in the absence of clinical in-

Table 5: Selected CTC-Graded Adverse Reactions From Comparative Trial of Gemzar Plus Cisplatin Versus Single-Agent Cisplatin in NSCLC CTC Grades (% incidence)[a]

	Gemzar plus Cisplatin[b]			Cisplatin[c]		
	All Grades	Grade 3	Grade 4	All Grades	Grade 3	Grade 4
Laboratory[d]						
Hematologic						
Anemia	89	22	3	67	6	1
RBC Transfusion[e]	39			13		
Leukopenia	82	35	11	25	2	1
Neutropenia	79	22	35	20	3	1
Thrombocytopenia	85	25	25	13	3	1
Platelet Transfusions[e]	21			<1		
Lymphocytes	75	25	18	51	12	5
Hepatic						
Transaminase	22	2	1	10	1	0
Alkaline Phosphatase	19	1	0	13	0	0
Renal						
Proteinuria	23	0	0	18	0	0
Hematuria	15	0	0	13	0	0
Creatinine	38	4	<1	31	2	<1
Other Laboratory						
Hyperglycemia	30	4	0	23	3	0
Hypomagnesemia	30	4	3	17	2	0
Hypocalcemia	18	2	0	7	0	<1
Non-laboratory[f]						
Nausea	93	25	2	87	20	<1
Vomiting	78	11	12	71	10	9
Alopecia	53	1	0	33	0	0
Neuro Motor	35	12	0	15	3	0
Neuro Hearing	25	6	0	21	6	0
Diarrhea	24	2	2	13	0	0
Neuro Sensory	23	1	0	18	1	0
Infection	18	3	2	12	1	0
Fever	16	0	0	5	0	0
Neuro Cortical	16	3	1	9	1	0
Neuro Mood	16	1	0	10	1	0
Local	15	0	0	6	0	0
Neuro Headache	14	0	0	7	0	0
Stomatitis	14	1	0	5	0	0
Hemorrhage	14	1	0	4	0	0
Dyspnea	12	4	3	11	3	2
Hypotension	12	1	0	7	1	0
Rash	11	0	0	3	0	0

[a] Grade based on Common Toxicity Criteria (CTC). Table includes data for adverse reactions with incidence ≥10% in either arm.

[b] N=217-253; all Gemzar plus cisplatin patients with laboratory or non-laboratory data. Gemzar at 1000 mg/m^2 on Days 1, 8, and 15 and cisplatin at 100 mg/m^2 on Day 1 every 28 days.

[c] N=213-248; all cisplatin patients with laboratory or non-laboratory data. Cisplatin at 100 mg/m^2 on Day 1 every 28 days.

[d] Regardless of causality.

[e] Percent of patients receiving transfusions. Percent transfusions are not CTC-graded events.

[f] Non-laboratory events were graded only if assessed to be possibly drug-related.

Table 6: Selected WHO-Graded Adverse Reactions From Comparative Trial of Gemzar Plus Cisplatin Versus Etoposide Plus Cisplatin in NSCLC WHO Grades (% incidence)[a]

	Gemzar plus Cisplatin[b]			Etoposide plus Cisplatin[c]		
	All Grades	Grade 3	Grade 4	All Grades	Grade 3	Grade 4
Laboratory[d]						
Hematologic						
Anemia	88	22	0	77	13	2
RBC Transfusions[e]	29			21		
Leukopenia	86	26	3	87	36	7
Neutropenia	88	36	28	87	20	56
Thrombocytopenia	81	39	16	45	8	5
Platelet Transfusions[e]	3			8		
Hepatic						
ALT	6	0	0	12	0	0
AST	3	0	0	11	0	0
Alkaline Phosphatase	16	0	0	11	0	0
Bilirubin	0	0	0	0	0	0
Renal						
Proteinuria	12	0	0	5	0	0
Hematuria	22	0	0	10	0	0
BUN	6	0	0	4	0	0
Creatinine	2	0	0	2	0	0
Non-laboratory[f,g]						
Nausea and Vomiting	96	35	4	86	19	7
Fever	6	0	0	3	0	0
Rash	10	0	0	3	0	0
Dyspnea	1	0	1	3	0	0
Diarrhea	14	1	1	13	0	2
Hemorrhage	9	0	3	3	0	3
Infection	28	3	1	21	8	0
Alopecia	77	13	0	92	51	0
Stomatitis	20	4	0	18	2	0
Somnolence	3	0	0	3	2	0
Paresthesias	38	0	0	16	2	0

[a] Grade based on criteria from the World Health Organization (WHO).

[b] N=67-69; all Gemzar plus cisplatin patients with laboratory or non-laboratory data. Gemzar at 1250 mg/m² on Days 1 and 8 and cisplatin at 100 mg/m² on Day 1 every 21 days.

[c] N=57-63; all cisplatin plus etoposide patients with laboratory or non-laboratory data. Cisplatin at 100 mg/m² on Day 1 and IV etoposide at 100 mg/m² on Days 1, 2, and 3 every 21 days.

[d] Regardless of causality.

[e] Percent of patients receiving transfusions. Percent transfusions are not WHO-graded events.

[f] Non-laboratory events were graded only if assessed to be possibly drug-related.

[g] Pain data were not collected.

fection. Fever was frequently associated with other flu-like symptoms and was usually mild and clinically manageable.

Rash—Rash was reported in 30% of patients. The rash was typically a macular or finely granular maculopapular pruritic eruption of mild to moderate severity involving the trunk and extremities. Pruritus was reported for 13% of patients.

Pulmonary—In clinical trials, dyspnea, unrelated to underlying disease, has been reported in association with Gemzar therapy. Dyspnea was occasionally accompanied by bronchospasm. Pulmonary toxicity has been reported with the use of Gemzar. [see Adverse Reactions (6.2)] The etiology of these effects is unknown. If such effects develop, Gemzar should be discontinued. Early use of supportive care measures may help ameliorate these conditions.

Edema—Edema (13%), peripheral edema (20%), and generalized edema (<1%) were reported. Less than 1% of patients discontinued due to edema.

Flu-like Symptoms—"Flu syndrome" was reported for 19% of patients. Individual symptoms of fever, asthenia, anorexia, headache, cough, chills, and myalgia were commonly reported. Fever and asthenia were also reported frequently as isolated symptoms. Insomnia, rhinitis, sweating, and malaise were reported infrequently. Less than 1% of patients discontinued due to flu-like symptoms.

Infection—Infections were reported for 16% of patients. Sepsis was rarely reported (<1%).

Alopecia—Hair loss, usually minimal, was reported by 15% of patients.

Neurotoxicity—There was a 10% incidence of mild paresthesias and a <1% rate of severe paresthesias.

Extravasation—Injection-site related events were reported for 4% of patients. There were no reports of injection site necrosis. Gemzar is not a vesicant.

Allergic—Bronchospasm was reported for less than 2% of patients. Anaphylactoid reaction has been reported rarely. Gemzar should not be administered to patients with a known hypersensitivity to this drug [see Contraindications (4)].

Cardiovascular—During clinical trials, 2% of patients discontinued therapy with Gemzar due to cardiovascular events such as myocardial infarction, cerebrovascular accident, arrhythmia, and hypertension. Many of these patients had a prior history of cardiovascular disease [see Adverse Reactions (6.2)].

Combination Use in Non-Small Cell Lung Cancer:

In the Gemzar plus cisplatin versus cisplatin study, dose adjustments occurred with 35% of Gemzar injections and 17% of cisplatin injections on the combination arm, versus 6% on the cisplatin-only arm. Dose adjustments were required in greater than 90% of patients on the combination, versus 16% on cisplatin. Study discontinuations for possibly drug-related adverse reactions occurred in 15% of patients on the combination arm and 8% of patients on the cisplatin arm. With a median of 4 cycles of Gemzar plus cisplatin treatment, 94 of 262 patients (36%) experienced a total of 149 hospitalizations due to possibly treatment-related adverse reactions. With a median of 2 cycles of cisplatin treatment, 61 of 260 patients (23%) experienced 78 hospitalizations due to possibly treatment-related adverse reactions.

In the Gemzar plus cisplatin versus etoposide plus cisplatin study, dose adjustments occurred with 20% of Gemzar injections and 16% of cisplatin injections in the Gemzar plus cisplatin arm compared with 20% of etoposide injections and 15% of cisplatin injections in the etoposide plus cisplatin arm. With a median of 5 cycles of Gemzar plus cisplatin treatment, 15 of 69 patients (22%) experienced 15 hospitalizations due to possibly treatment-related adverse reactions. With a median of 4 cycles of etoposide plus cisplatin treatment, 18 of 66 patients (27%) experienced 22 hospitalizations due to possibly treatment-related adverse reactions. In patients who completed more than one cycle, dose adjustments were reported in 81% of the Gemzar plus cisplatin patients, compared with 68% on the etoposide plus cisplatin arm. Study discontinuations for possibly drug-related adverse reactions occurred in 14% of patients on the Gemzar plus cisplatin arm and in 8% of patients on the etoposide plus cisplatin arm. The incidence of myelosuppression was increased in frequency with Gemzar plus cisplatin treatment (~90%) compared to that with the Gemzar monotherapy (~60%). With combination therapy Gemzar dosage adjustments for hematologic toxicity were required more often while cisplatin dose adjustments were less frequently required.

Table 5 presents the safety data from the Gemzar plus cisplatin versus cisplatin study in non-small cell lung cancer. The NCI Common Toxicity Criteria (CTC) were used. The two-drug combination was more myelosuppressive with 4 (1.5%) possibly treatment-related deaths, including 3 resulting from myelosuppression with infection and one case of renal failure associated with pancytopenia and infection. No deaths due to treatment were reported on the cisplatin arm. Nine cases of febrile neutropenia were reported on the combination therapy arm compared to 2 on the cisplatin arm. More patients required RBC and platelet transfusions on the Gemzar plus cisplatin arm.

Myelosuppression occurred more frequently on the combination arm, and in 4 possibly treatment-related deaths myelosuppression was observed. Sepsis was reported in 4% of patients on the Gemzar plus cisplatin arm compared to 1% on the cisplatin arm. Platelet transfusions were required in 21% of patients on the combination arm and <1% of patients on the cisplatin arm. Hemorrhagic events occurred in 14% of patients on the combination arm and 4% on the cisplatin arm. However, severe hemorrhagic events were rare. Red blood cell transfusions were required in 39% of the patients on the Gemzar plus cisplatin arm, versus 13% on the cisplatin arm. The data suggest cumulative anemia with continued Gemzar plus cisplatin use.

Nausea and vomiting despite the use of antiemetics occurred more often with Gemzar plus cisplatin therapy (78%) than with cisplatin alone (71%). In studies with single-agent Gemzar, a lower incidence of nausea and vomiting (58% to 69%) was reported. Renal function abnormalities, hypomagnesemia, neuromotor, neurocortical, and neurocerebellar toxicity occurred more often with Gemzar plus cisplatin than with cisplatin monotherapy. Neurohearing toxicity was similar on both arms.

Cardiac dysrrhythmias of Grade 3 or greater were reported in 7 (3%) patients treated with Gemzar plus cisplatin compared to one (<1%) Grade 3 dysrrhythmia reported with cisplatin therapy. Hypomagnesemia and hypokalemia were associated with one Grade 4 arrhythmia on the Gemzar plus cisplatin combination arm.

Table 6 presents data from the randomized study of Gemzar plus cisplatin versus etoposide plus cisplatin in 135 patients with NSCLC. One death (1.5%) was reported on the Gemzar plus cisplatin arm due to febrile neutropenia associated with renal failure which was possibly treatment-related. No deaths related to treatment occurred on the etoposide plus cisplatin arm. The overall incidence of Grade 4 neutropenia on the Gemzar plus cisplatin arm was less than on the etoposide plus cisplatin arm (28% versus 56%). Sepsis was experienced by 2% of patients on both treatment arms. Grade 3 anemia and Grade 3/4 thrombocytopenia were more common on the Gemzar plus cisplatin arm. RBC transfusions were given to 29% of the patients who received Gemzar plus cisplatin versus 21% of patients who received etoposide plus cisplatin. Platelet transfusions were given to 3% of the patients who received Gemzar plus cisplatin versus 8% of patients who received etoposide plus cisplatin. Grade 3/4 nausea and vomiting were also more common on the Gemzar plus cisplatin arm. On the Gemzar plus cisplatin arm, 7% of participants were hospitalized due to febrile neutropenia compared to 12% on the etoposide plus cisplatin arm. More than twice as many patients had dose reductions or omissions of a scheduled dose of Gemzar as compared to etoposide, which may explain the differences in the incidence of neutropenia and febrile neutropenia between treatment arms. Flu syndrome was reported by 3% of patients on the Gemzar plus cisplatin arm with none reported on the comparator arm. Eight patients (12%) on the Gemzar plus cisplatin arm reported edema compared to one patient (2%) on the etoposide plus cisplatin arm.

[See table 5 at top of previous page]

[See table 6 at top left]

Combination Use in Breast Cancer:

In the Gemzar plus paclitaxel versus paclitaxel study, dose reductions occurred with 8% of Gemzar injections and 5% of paclitaxel injections on the combination arm, versus 2% on the paclitaxel arm. On the combination arm, 7% of Gemzar doses were omitted and <1% of paclitaxel doses were omitted, compared to <1% of paclitaxel doses on the paclitaxel arm. A total of 18 patients (7%) on the Gemzar plus paclitaxel arm and 12 (5%) on the paclitaxel arm discontinued the study because of adverse reactions. There were two deaths on study or within 30 days after study drug discontinuation that were possibly drug-related, one on each arm. Table 7 presents the safety data occurrences of ≥10% (all grades) from the Gemzar plus paclitaxel versus paclitaxel study in breast cancer.

[See table 7 at top of next page]

The following are the clinically relevant adverse reactions that occurred in >1% and <10% (all grades) of patients on either arm. In parentheses are the incidences of Grade 3 and 4 adverse reactions (Gemzar plus paclitaxel versus paclitaxel): febrile neutropenia (5.0% versus 1.2%), infection (0.8% versus 0.8%), dyspnea (1.9% versus 0) and allergic reaction/hypersensitivity (0 versus 0.8%).

No differences in the incidence of laboratory and non-laboratory events were observed in patients 65 years or older, as compared to patients younger than 65.

Combination Use in Ovarian Cancer:
In the Gemzar plus carboplatin versus carboplatin study, dose reductions occurred with 10.4% of Gemzar injections and 1.8% of carboplatin injections on the combination arm, versus 3.8% on the carboplatin alone arm. On the combination arm, 13.7% of Gemzar doses were omitted and 0.2% of carboplatin doses were omitted, compared to 0% of carboplatin doses on the carboplatin alone arm. There were no differences in discontinuations due to adverse reactions between arms (10.9% versus 9.8%, respectively).

Table 8 presents the adverse reactions (all grades) occurring in ≥10% of patients in the ovarian cancer study.

[See table 8 at right]

In addition to blood product transfusions as listed in Table 8, myelosuppression was also managed with hematopoietic agents. These agents were administered more frequently with combination therapy than with monotherapy (granulocyte growth factors: 23.6% and 10.1%, respectively; erythropoietic agents: 7.3% and 3.9%, respectively).

The following are the clinically relevant adverse reactions, regardless of causality, that occurred in >1% and <10% (all grades) of patients on either arm. In parentheses are the incidences of Grade 3 and 4 adverse reactions (Gemzar plus carboplatin versus carboplatin): AST or ALT elevation (0 versus 1.2%), dyspnea (3.4% versus 2.9%), febrile neutropenia (1.1% versus 0), hemorrhagic event (2.3% versus 1.1%), hypersensitivity reaction (2.3% versus 2.9%), motor neuropathy (1.1% versus 0.6%), and rash/desquamation (0.6% versus 0).

No differences in the incidence of laboratory and non-laboratory events were observed in patients 65 years or older, as compared to patients younger than 65.

6.2 Post-Marketing Experience

The following adverse reactions have been identified during post-approval use of Gemzar. Because these reactions are reported voluntarily from a population of uncertain size, it is not always possible to reliably estimate their frequency or establish a causal relationship to drug exposure.

These adverse reactions have occurred after Gemzar single-agent use and Gemzar in combination with other cytotoxic agents. Decisions to include these events are based on the seriousness of the event, frequency of reporting, or potential causal connection to Gemzar.

Cardiovascular—Congestive heart failure and myocardial infarction have been reported very rarely with the use of Gemzar. Arrhythmias, predominantly supraventricular in nature, have been reported very rarely.

Vascular Disorders—Clinical signs of peripheral vasculitis and gangrene have been reported very rarely.

Skin—Cellulitis and non-serious injection site reactions in the absence of extravasation have been rarely reported. Severe skin reactions, including desquamation and bullous skin eruptions, have been reported very rarely.

Hepatic—Increased liver function tests including elevations in aspartate aminotransferase (AST), alanine aminotransferase (ALT), gamma-glutamyl transferase (GGT), alkaline phosphatase, and bilirubin levels have been reported rarely. Serious hepatotoxicity including liver failure and death has been reported very rarely in patients receiving Gemzar alone or in combination with other potentially hepatotoxic drugs.

Pulmonary—Parenchymal toxicity, including interstitial pneumonitis, pulmonary fibrosis, pulmonary edema, and adult respiratory distress syndrome (ARDS), has been reported rarely following one or more doses of Gemzar administered to patients with various malignancies. Some patients experienced the onset of pulmonary symptoms up to 2 weeks after the last Gemzar dose. Respiratory failure and death occurred very rarely in some patients despite discontinuation of therapy.

Renal—Hemolytic Uremic Syndrome (HUS) and/or renal failure have been reported following one or more doses of Gemzar. Renal failure leading to death or requiring dialysis, despite discontinuation of therapy, has been rarely reported. The majority of the cases of renal failure leading to death were due to HUS.

Injury, Poisoning, and Procedural Complications—Radiation recall reactions have been reported. [see Warnings and Precautions (5.8)]

7 DRUG INTERACTIONS

No specific drug interaction studies have been conducted. Information is available on the pharmacodynamics and pharmacokinetics of Gemzar in combination with cisplatin, paclitaxel, or carboplatin. [see Clinical Pharmacology (12.2 and 12.3)]

8 USE IN SPECIFIC POPULATIONS

8.1 Pregnancy

Pregnancy Category D [see Warnings and Precautions (5.6)]
Gemzar can cause fetal harm when administered to a pregnant woman. Based on its mechanism of action, Gemzar is expected to result in adverse reproductive effects. There are no adequate and well-controlled studies of Gemzar in pregnant women. Gemcitabine is embryotoxic causing fetal malformations (cleft palate, incomplete ossification) at doses of 1.5 mg/kg/day in mice (about 1/200 the recommended human dose on a mg/m² basis). Gemcitabine is fetotoxic causing fetal malformations (fused pulmonary artery, absence of gall bladder) at doses of 0.1 mg/kg/day in rabbits (about 1/600 the recommended human dose on a mg/m² basis). Embryotoxicity was characterized by decreased fetal viability, reduced live litter sizes, and developmental delays. If this drug is used during pregnancy, or if the patient becomes pregnant while taking this drug, the patient should be apprised of the potential hazard to the fetus. [see Warnings and Precautions (5.6)]

8.3 Nursing Mothers

It is not known whether this drug is excreted in human milk. Because many drugs are excreted in human milk and because of the potential for serious adverse reactions in nursing infants from Gemzar, a decision should be made whether to discontinue nursing or to discontinue the drug, taking into account the importance of the drug to the mother.

8.4 Pediatric Use

The safety and effectiveness of Gemzar in pediatric patients has not been established. Gemzar was evaluated in a Phase 1 trial in pediatric patients with refractory leukemia and determined that the maximum tolerated dose was 10 mg/m²/min for 360 minutes three times weekly followed by a one-week rest period. Gemzar was also evaluated in a Phase 2 trial in patients with relapsed acute lymphoblastic leukemia (22 patients) and acute myelogenous leukemia (10 patients) using 10 mg/m²/min for 360 minutes three times weekly followed by a one-week rest period. Toxicities observed included bone marrow suppression, febrile neutropenia, elevation of serum transaminases, nausea, and rash/desquamation, which were similar to those reported in adults. No meaningful clinical activity was observed in this Phase 2 trial.

Table 7: Adverse Reactions From Comparative Trial of Gemzar Plus Paclitaxel Versus Single-Agent Paclitaxel in Breast Cancer[a] CTC Grades (% incidence)

	Gemzar plus Paclitaxel (N=262)			Paclitaxel (N=259)		
	All Grades	Grade 3	Grade 4	All Grades	Grade 3	Grade 4
Laboratory[b]						
Hematologic						
Anemia	69	6	1	51	3	<1
Neutropenia	69	31	17	31	4	7
Thrombocytopenia	26	5	<1	7	<1	<1
Leukopenia	21	10	1	12	2	0
Hepatobiliary						
ALT	18	5	<1	6	<1	0
AST	16	2	0	5	<1	0
Non-laboratory[c]						
Alopecia	90	14	4	92	19	3
Neuropathy-sensory	64	5	<1	58	3	0
Nausea	50	1	0	31	2	0
Fatigue	40	6	<1	28	1	<1
Myalgia	33	4	0	33	3	<1
Vomiting	29	2	0	15	2	0
Arthralgia	24	3	0	22	2	<1
Diarrhea	20	3	0	13	2	0
Anorexia	17	0	0	12	<1	0
Neuropathy-motor	15	2	<1	10	<1	0
Stomatitis/pharyngitis	13	1	<1	8	<1	0
Fever	13	<1	0	3	0	0
Rash/desquamation	11	<1	<1	5	0	0

[a] Grade based on Common Toxicity Criteria (CTC) Version 2.0 (all grades ≥10%).
[b] Regardless of causality.
[c] Non-laboratory events were graded only if assessed to be possibly drug-related.

Table 8: Adverse Reactions From Comparative Trial of Gemzar Plus Carboplatin Versus Single-Agent Carboplatin in Ovarian Cancer[a] CTC Grades (% incidence)

	Gemzar plus Carboplatin (N=175)			Carboplatin (N=174)		
	All Grades	Grade 3	Grade 4	All Grades	Grade 3	Grade 4
Laboratory[b]						
Hematologic						
Neutropenia	90	42	29	58	11	1
Anemia	86	22	6	75	9	2
Leukopenia	86	48	5	70	6	<1
Thrombocytopenia	78	30	5	57	10	1
RBC Transfusions[c]	38			15		
Platelet Transfusions[c]	9			3		
Non-laboratory[b]						
Nausea	69	6	0	61	3	0
Alopecia	49	0	0	17	0	0
Vomiting	46	6	0	36	2	<1
Constipation	42	6	1	37	3	0
Fatigue	40	3	<1	32	5	0
Neuropathy-sensory	29	1	0	27	2	0
Diarrhea	25	3	0	14	<1	0
Stomatitis/pharyngitis	22	<1	0	13	0	0
Anorexia	16	1	0	13	0	0

[a] Grade based on Common Toxicity Criteria (CTC) Version 2.0 (all grades ≥10%).
[b] Regardless of causality.
[c] Percent of patients receiving transfusions. Transfusions are not CTC-graded events. Blood transfusions included both packed red blood cells and whole blood.

8.5 Geriatric Use

Gemzar clearance is affected by age *[see Clinical Pharmacology (12.3)]*. There is no evidence, however, that unusual dose adjustments *[see Dosage and Administration (2.1, 2.2, 2.3, and 2.4)]* are necessary in patients over 65, and in general, adverse reaction rates in the single-agent safety database of 979 patients were similar in patients above and below 65. Grade 3/4 thrombocytopenia was more common in the elderly. In the randomized clinical trial of Gemzar in combination with carboplatin for recurrent ovarian cancer *[see Clinical Studies (14.1)]*, 125 women treated with Gemzar plus carboplatin were <65 years and 50 were ≥65 years. Similar effectiveness was observed between older and younger women. There was significantly higher Grade 3/4 neutropenia in women 65 years of age or older. Overall, there were no other substantial differences in toxicity profile of Gemzar plus carboplatin based on age.

8.6 Renal

Hemolytic Uremic Syndrome (HUS) and/or renal failure have been reported following one or more doses of Gemzar. Renal failure leading to death or requiring dialysis, despite discontinuation of therapy, has been reported. The majority of the cases of renal failure leading to death were due to HUS *[see Adverse Reactions (6.1 and 6.2)]*. Gemzar should be used with caution in patients with preexisting renal impairment as there is insufficient information from clinical studies to allow clear dose recommendation for these patient populations. *[see Warnings and Precautions (5.4)]*

8.7 Hepatic

Serious hepatotoxicity, including liver failure and death, has been reported in patients receiving Gemzar alone or in combination with other potentially hepatotoxic drugs *[see Adverse Reactions (6.1 and 6.2)]*. Gemzar should be used with caution in patients with preexisting hepatic insufficiency as there is insufficient information from clinical studies to allow clear dose recommendation for these patient populations. Administration of Gemzar in patients with concurrent liver metastases or a preexisting medical history of hepatitis, alcoholism, or liver cirrhosis may lead to exacerbation of the underlying hepatic insufficiency. *[see Warnings and Precautions (5.5)]*

8.8 Gender

Gemzar clearance is affected by gender. *[see Clinical Pharmacology (12.3)]* In the single-agent safety database (N=979 patients), however, there is no evidence that unusual dose adjustments *[see Dosage and Administration (2)]* are necessary in women. In general, in single-agent studies of Gemzar, adverse reaction rates were similar in men and women, but women, especially older women, were more likely not to proceed to a subsequent cycle and to experience Grade 3/4 neutropenia and thrombocytopenia. There was a greater tendency in women, especially older women, not to proceed to the next cycle.

10 OVERDOSAGE

There is no known antidote for overdoses of Gemzar. Myelosuppression, paresthesias, and severe rash were the principal toxicities seen when a single dose as high as 5700 mg/m^2 was administered by IV infusion over 30 minutes every 2 weeks to several patients in a Phase 1 study. In the event of suspected overdose, the patient should be monitored with appropriate blood counts and should receive supportive therapy, as necessary.

11 DESCRIPTION

Gemzar (gemcitabine for injection, USP) is a nucleoside metabolic inhibitor that exhibits antitumor activity. Gemcitabine HCl is 2′-deoxy-2′,2′-difluorocytidine monohydrochloride (β-isomer).

The structural formula is as follows:

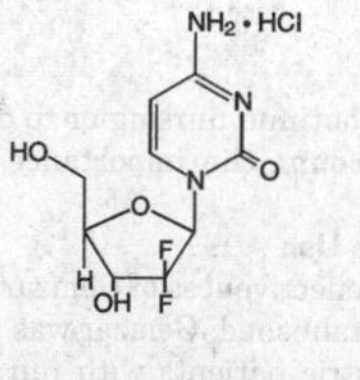

The empirical formula for gemcitabine HCl is $C_9H_{11}F_2N_3O_4$ • HCl. It has a molecular weight of 299.66.

Gemcitabine HCl is a white to off-white solid. It is soluble in water, slightly soluble in methanol, and practically insoluble in ethanol and polar organic solvents.

The clinical formulation is supplied in a sterile form for intravenous use only. Vials of Gemzar contain either 200 mg or 1 g of gemcitabine HCl (expressed as free base) formulated with mannitol (200 mg or 1 g, respectively) and sodium acetate (12.5 mg or 62.5 mg, respectively) as a sterile lyophilized powder. Hydrochloric acid and/or sodium hydroxide may have been added for pH adjustment.

Table 9: Gemcitabine Clearance and Half-Life for the "Typical" Patient

Age	Clearance Men (L/hr/m^2)	Clearance Women (L/hr/m^2)	Half-Life[a] Men (min)	Half-Life[a] Women (min)
29	92.2	69.4	42	49
45	75.7	57.0	48	57
65	55.1	41.5	61	73
79	40.7	30.7	79	94

[a] Half-life for patients receiving a short infusion (<70 min).

12 CLINICAL PHARMACOLOGY

12.1 Mechanism of Action

Gemcitabine exhibits cell phase specificity, primarily killing cells undergoing DNA synthesis (S-phase) and also blocking the progression of cells through the G1/S-phase boundary. Gemcitabine is metabolized intracellularly by nucleoside kinases to the active diphosphate (dFdCDP) and triphosphate (dFdCTP) nucleosides. The cytotoxic effect of gemcitabine is attributed to a combination of two actions of the diphosphate and the triphosphate nucleosides, which leads to inhibition of DNA synthesis. First, gemcitabine diphosphate inhibits ribonucleotide reductase, which is responsible for catalyzing the reactions that generate the deoxynucleoside triphosphates for DNA synthesis. Inhibition of this enzyme by the diphosphate nucleoside causes a reduction in the concentrations of deoxynucleotides, including dCTP. Second, gemcitabine triphosphate competes with dCTP for incorporation into DNA. The reduction in the intracellular concentration of dCTP (by the action of the diphosphate) enhances the incorporation of gemcitabine triphosphate into DNA (self-potentiation). After the gemcitabine nucleotide is incorporated into DNA, only one additional nucleotide is added to the growing DNA strands. After this addition, there is inhibition of further DNA synthesis. DNA polymerase epsilon is unable to remove the gemcitabine nucleotide and repair the growing DNA strands (masked chain termination). In CEM T lymphoblastoid cells, gemcitabine induces internucleosomal DNA fragmentation, one of the characteristics of programmed cell death.

12.2 Pharmacodynamics

Gemcitabine demonstrated dose-dependent synergistic activity with cisplatin *in vitro*. No effect of cisplatin on gemcitabine triphosphate accumulation or DNA double-strand breaks was observed. *In vivo*, gemcitabine showed activity in combination with cisplatin against the LX-1 and CALU-6 human lung xenografts, but minimal activity was seen with the NCI-H460 or NCI-H520 xenografts. Gemcitabine was synergistic with cisplatin in the Lewis lung murine xenograft. Sequential exposure to gemcitabine 4 hours before cisplatin produced the greatest interaction.

12.3 Pharmacokinetics

Absorption and Distribution

The pharmacokinetics of gemcitabine were examined in 353 patients, with various solid tumors. Pharmacokinetic parameters were derived using data from patients treated for varying durations of therapy given weekly with periodic rest weeks and using both short infusions (<70 minutes) and long infusions (70 to 285 minutes). The total Gemzar dose varied from 500 to 3600 mg/m^2.

The volume of distribution was increased with infusion length. Volume of distribution of gemcitabine was 50 L/m^2 following infusions lasting <70 minutes. For long infusions, the volume of distribution rose to 370 L/m^2.

Gemcitabine pharmacokinetics are linear and are described by a 2-compartment model. Population pharmacokinetic analyses of combined single and multiple dose studies showed that the volume of distribution of gemcitabine was significantly influenced by duration of infusion and gender. Gemcitabine plasma protein binding is negligible.

Metabolism

Gemcitabine disposition was studied in 5 patients who received a single 1000 mg/m^2/30 minute infusion of radiolabeled drug. Within one (1) week, 92% to 98% of the dose was recovered, almost entirely in the urine. Gemcitabine (<10%) and the inactive uracil metabolite, 2′-deoxy-2′,2′-difluorouridine (dFdU), accounted for 99% of the excreted dose. The metabolite dFdU is also found in plasma.

The active metabolite, gemcitabine triphosphate, can be extracted from peripheral blood mononuclear cells. The half-life of the terminal phase for gemcitabine triphosphate from mononuclear cells ranges from 1.7 to 19.4 hours.

Excretion

Clearance of gemcitabine was affected by age and gender. The lower clearance in women and the elderly results in higher concentrations of gemcitabine for any given dose. Differences in either clearance or volume of distribution based on patient characteristics or the duration of infusion result in changes in half-life and plasma concentrations. Table 9 shows plasma clearance and half-life of gemcitabine following short infusions for typical patients by age and gender.

[See table 9 above]

Gemcitabine half-life for short infusions ranged from 42 to 94 minutes, and the value for long infusions varied from 245 to 638 minutes, depending on age and gender, reflecting a greatly increased volume of distribution with longer infusions.

Drug Interactions

When Gemzar (1250 mg/m^2 on Days 1 and 8) and cisplatin (75 mg/m^2 on Day 1) were administered in NSCLC patients, the clearance of gemcitabine on Day 1 was 128 L/hr/m^2 and on Day 8 was 107 L/hr/m^2. The clearance of cisplatin in the same study was reported to be 3.94 mL/min/m^2 with a corresponding half-life of 134 hours *[see Drug Interactions (7)]*. Analysis of data from metastatic breast cancer patients shows that, on average, Gemzar has little or no effect on the pharmacokinetics (clearance and half-life) of paclitaxel and paclitaxel has little or no effect on the pharmacokinetics of Gemzar. Data from NSCLC patients demonstrate that Gemzar and carboplatin given in combination does not alter the pharmacokinetics of Gemzar or carboplatin compared to administration of either single-agent. However, due to wide confidence intervals and small sample size, interpatient variability may be observed.

13 NONCLINICAL TOXICOLOGY

13.1 Carcinogenesis, Mutagenesis, Impairment of Fertility

Long-term animal studies to evaluate the carcinogenic potential of Gemzar have not been conducted. Gemcitabine induced forward mutations *in vitro* in a mouse lymphoma (L5178Y) assay and was clastogenic in an *in vivo* mouse micronucleus assay. Gemcitabine was negative when tested using the Ames, *in vivo* sister chromatid exchange, and *in vitro* chromosomal aberration assays, and did not cause unscheduled DNA synthesis *in vitro*. Gemcitabine IP doses of 0.5 mg/kg/day (about 1/700 the human dose on a mg/m^2 basis) in male mice had an effect on fertility with moderate to severe hypospermatogenesis, decreased fertility, and decreased implantations. In female mice, fertility was not affected but maternal toxicities were observed at 1.5 mg/kg/day IV (about 1/200 the human dose on a mg/m^2 basis) and fetotoxicity or embryolethality was observed at 0.25 mg/kg/day IV (about 1/1300 the human dose on a mg/m^2 basis).

14 CLINICAL STUDIES

14.1 Ovarian Cancer

Gemzar was studied in a randomized Phase 3 study of 356 patients with advanced ovarian cancer that had relapsed at least 6 months after first-line platinum-based therapy. Patients were randomized to receive either Gemzar 1000 mg/m^2 on Days 1 and 8 of a 21-day cycle and carboplatin AUC 4 administered after Gemzar on Day 1 of each cycle or single-agent carboplatin AUC 5 administered on Day 1 of each 21-day cycle as the control arm. The primary endpoint of this study was progression free survival (PFS). Patient characteristics are shown in Table 10. The addition of Gemzar to carboplatin resulted in statistically significant improvement in PFS and overall response rate as shown in Table 11 and Figure 1. Approximately 75% of patients in each arm received poststudy chemotherapy. Only 13 of 120 patients with documented poststudy chemotherapy regimen in the carboplatin arm received Gemzar after progression. There was not a significant difference in overall survival between arms.

[See table 10 at top of next page]
[See table 11 on next page]
[See figure 1 at top of next page]

14.2 Breast Cancer

Data from a multi-national, randomized Phase 3 study (529 patients) support the use of Gemzar in combination with paclitaxel for treatment of breast cancer patients who have received prior adjuvant/neoadjuvant anthracycline chemotherapy unless clinically contraindicated. Gemzar 1250 mg/m^2 was administered on Days 1 and 8 of a 21-day

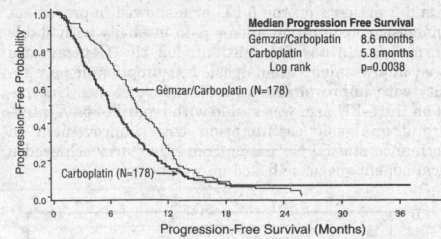

Figure 1: Kaplan-Meier Curve of Progression Free Survival in Gemzar Plus Carboplatin Versus Carboplatin in Ovarian Cancer (N=356)

cycle with paclitaxel 175 mg/m² administered prior to Gemzar on Day 1 of each cycle. Single-agent paclitaxel 175 mg/m² was administered on Day 1 of each 21-day cycle as the control arm.

The addition of Gemzar to paclitaxel resulted in statistically significant improvement in time to documented disease progression and overall response rate compared to monotherapy with paclitaxel as shown in Table 12 and Figure 2. Final survival analysis results at 440 events were Hazard Ratio of 0.86 (95%, CI: 0.71–1.04) for the ITT population, as shown in Table 12.

[See table 12 at top of next page]

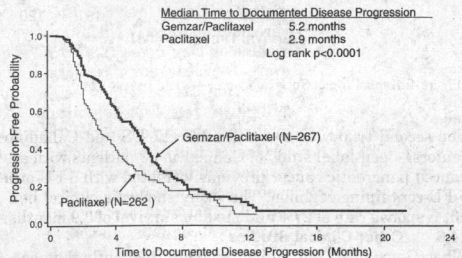

Figure 2: Kaplan-Meier Curve of Time to Documented Disease Progression in Gemzar Plus Paclitaxel Versus Paclitaxel Breast Cancer Study (N=529)

14.3 Non-Small Cell Lung Cancer (NSCLC)

Data from 2 randomized clinical studies (657 patients) support the use of Gemzar in combination with cisplatin for the first-line treatment of patients with locally advanced or metastatic NSCLC.

Gemzar plus cisplatin versus cisplatin: This study was conducted in Europe, the US, and Canada in 522 patients with inoperable Stage IIIA, IIIB, or IV NSCLC who had not received prior chemotherapy. Gemzar 1000 mg/m² was administered on Days 1, 8, and 15 of a 28-day cycle with cisplatin 100 mg/m² administered on Day 1 of each cycle. Single-agent cisplatin 100 mg/m² was administered on Day 1 of each 28-day cycle. The primary endpoint was survival. Patient demographics are shown in Table 13. An imbalance with regard to histology was observed with 48% of patients on the cisplatin arm and 37% of patients on the Gemzar plus cisplatin arm having adenocarcinoma.

The Kaplan-Meier survival curve is shown in Figure 3. Median survival time on the Gemzar plus cisplatin arm was 9.0 months compared to 7.6 months on the single-agent cisplatin arm (Log rank p=0.008, two-sided). Median time to disease progression was 5.2 months on the Gemzar plus cisplatin arm compared to 3.7 months on the cisplatin arm (Log rank p=0.009, two-sided). The objective response rate on the Gemzar plus cisplatin arm was 26% compared to 10% with cisplatin (Fisher's Exact p<0.0001, two-sided). No difference between treatment arms with regard to duration of response was observed.

Gemzar plus cisplatin versus etoposide plus cisplatin: A second, multicenter, study in Stage IIIB or IV NSCLC randomized 135 patients to Gemzar 1250 mg/m² on Days 1 and 8, and cisplatin 100 mg/m² on Day 1 of a 21-day cycle or to etoposide 100 mg/m² IV on Days 1, 2, and 3 and cisplatin 100 mg/m² on Day 1 of a 21-day cycle (Table 13).

There was no significant difference in survival between the two treatment arms (Log rank p=0.18, two-sided). The median survival was 8.7 months for the Gemzar plus cisplatin arm versus 7.0 months for the etoposide plus cisplatin arm. Median time to disease progression for the Gemzar plus cisplatin arm was 5.0 months compared to 4.1 months on the etoposide plus cisplatin arm (Log rank p=0.015, two-sided). The objective response rate for the Gemzar plus cisplatin arm was 33% compared to 14% on the etoposide plus cisplatin arm (Fisher's Exact p=0.01, two-sided).

Quality of Life (QOL): QOL was a secondary endpoint in both randomized studies. In the Gemzar plus cisplatin study, QOL was measured using the FACT-L, which assessed physical, social, emotional and functional well-being, and lung cancer symptoms. In the study of Gemzar plus cisplatin versus etoposide plus cisplatin, QOL

Table 10: Gemzar Plus Carboplatin Versus Carboplatin in Ovarian Cancer - Baseline Demographics and Clinical Characteristics

	Gemzar/Carboplatin	Carboplatin
Number of randomized patients	178	178
Median age, years	59	58
Range	36 to 78	21 to 81
Baseline ECOG performance status 0-1[a]	94%	95%
Disease Status		
Evaluable	7.9%	2.8%
Bidimensionally measurable	91.6%	95.5%
Platinum-free interval[b]		
6-12 months	39.9%	39.9%
>12 months	59.0%	59.6%
First-line therapy		
Platinum-taxane combination	70.2%	71.3%
Platinum-non-taxane combination	28.7%	27.5%
Platinum monotherapy	1.1%	1.1%

[a] Nine patients (5 on the Gemzar plus carboplatin arm and 4 on the carboplatin arm) did not have baseline Eastern Cooperative Oncology Group (ECOG) performance status recorded.
[b] Three patients (2 on the Gemzar plus carboplatin arm and 1 on the carboplatin arm) had a platinum-free interval of less than 6 months.

Table 11: Gemzar Plus Carboplatin Versus Carboplatin in Ovarian Cancer - Results of Efficacy Analysis

	Gemzar/Carboplatin (N=178)	Carboplatin (N=178)	
PFS			
Median (95%, C.I.) months	8.6 (8.0, 9.7)	5.8 (5.2, 7.1)	p=0.0038[d]
Hazard Ratio (95%, C.I.)	0.72 (0.57, 0.90)		
Overall Survival			
Median (95%, C.I.) months	18.0 (16.2, 20.3)	17.3 (15.2, 19.3)	p=0.8977[d]
Hazard Ratio (95%, C.I.)	0.98 (0.78, 1.24)		
Adjusted[a] Hazard Ratio (95%, C.I.)	0.86 (0.67, 1.10)		
Investigator Reviewed Overall Response Rate	47.2%	30.9%	p=0.0016[e]
CR	14.6%	6.2%	
PR+PRNM[b]	32.6%	24.7%	
Independently Reviewed Overall Response Rate[c,f]	46.3%	35.6%	p=0.11[e]
CR	9.1%	4.0%	
PR+PRNM	37.2%	31.7%	

[a] Treatment adjusted for performance status, tumor area, and platinum-free interval.
[b] Partial response non-measurable disease
[c] Independent reviewers could not evaluate disease demonstrated by sonography or physical exam.
[d] Log Rank, unadjusted
[e] Chi Square
[f] Independently reviewed cohort - Gemzar/Carboplatin N=121, Carboplatin N=101

was measured using the EORTC QLQ-C30 and LC13, which assessed physical and psychological functioning and symptoms related to both lung cancer and its treatment. In both studies no significant differences were observed in QOL between the Gemzar plus cisplatin arm and the comparator arm.

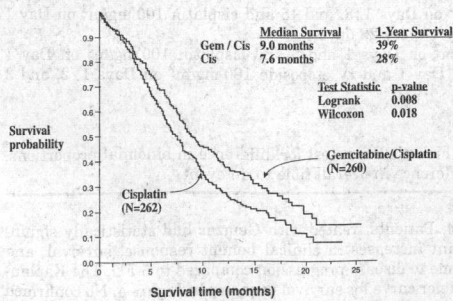

Figure 3: Kaplan-Meier Survival Curve in Gemzar Plus Cisplatin Versus Cisplatin NSCLC Study (N=522)

[See table 13 on next page]

14.4 Pancreatic Cancer

Data from 2 clinical trials evaluated the use of Gemzar in patients with locally advanced or metastatic pancreatic cancer. The first trial compared Gemzar to 5-Fluorouracil (5-FU) in patients who had received no prior chemotherapy. A second trial studied the use of Gemzar in pancreatic cancer patients previously treated with 5-FU or a 5-FU-containing regimen. In both studies, the first cycle of Gemzar was administered intravenously at a dose of 1000 mg/m² over 30 minutes once weekly for up to 7 weeks (or until toxicity necessitated holding a dose) followed by a week of rest from treatment with Gemzar. Subsequent cycles consisted of injections once weekly for 3 consecutive weeks out of every 4 weeks.

The primary efficacy parameter in these studies was "clinical benefit response," which is a measure of clinical improvement based on analgesic consumption, pain intensity, performance status, and weight change. Definitions for improvement in these variables were formulated prospectively during the design of the 2 trials. A patient was considered a clinical benefit responder if either:

i) the patient showed a ≥50% reduction in pain intensity (Memorial Pain Assessment Card) or analgesic consumption, or a 20-point or greater improvement in performance status (Karnofsky Performance Status) for a period of at least 4 consecutive weeks, without showing any sustained worsening in any of the other parameters. Sustained worsening was defined as 4 consecutive weeks with either any increase in pain intensity or analgesic consumption or a 20-point decrease in performance status occurring during the first 12 weeks of therapy.

Table 12: Gemzar Plus Paclitaxel Versus Paclitaxel in Breast Cancer

	Gemzar/Paclitaxel	Paclitaxel	
Number of patients	267	262	
Median age, years	53	52	
Range	26 to 83	26 to 75	
Metastatic disease	97.0%	96.9%	
Baseline KPS[a] ≥90	70.4%	74.4%	
Number of tumor sites			
1-2	56.6%	58.8%	
≥3	43.4%	41.2%	
Visceral disease	73.4%	72.9%	
Prior anthracycline	96.6%	95.8%	
Overall Survival[b]			
Median (95%, CI)	18.6 (16.5, 20.7)	15.8 (14.1, 17.3)	
Hazard Ratio (95%, CI)	0.86 (0.71, 1.04)		
Time to Documented Disease Progression[c]			p<0.0001
Median (95%, C.I.), months	5.2 (4.2, 5.6)	2.9 (2.6, 3.7)	
Hazard Ratio (95%, C.I.)	0.650 (0.524, 0.805)		p<0.0001
Overall Response Rate[c] (95%, C.I.)	40.8% (34.9, 46.7)	22.1% (17.1, 27.2)	p<0.0001

[a] Karnofsky Performance Status.
[b] Based on the ITT population
[c] These represent reconciliation of investigator and Independent Review Committee assessments according to a predefined algorithm.

Table 13: Randomized Trials of Combination Therapy With Gemzar Plus Cisplatin in NSCLC

Trial	28-day Schedule[a]			21-day Schedule[b]		
Treatment Arm	Gemzar/ Cisplatin	Cisplatin		Gemzar/ Cisplatin	Cisplatin/ Etoposide	
Number of patients	260	262		69	66	
Male	182	186		64	61	
Female	78	76		5	5	
Median age, years	62	63		58	60	
Range	36 to 88	35 to 79		33 to 76	35 to 75	
Stage IIIA	7%	7%		N/A[c]	N/A[c]	
Stage IIIB	26%	23%		48%	52%	
Stage IV	67%	70%		52%	49%	
Baseline KPS[d] 70 to 80	41%	44%		45%	52%	
Baseline KPS[d] 90 to 100	57%	55%		55%	49%	
Survival			p=0.008			p=0.18
Median, months	9.0	7.6		8.7	7.0	
(95%, C.I.) months	8.2, 11.0	6.6, 8.8		7.8, 10.1	6.0, 9.7	
Time to Disease Progression			p=0.009			p=0.015
Median, months	5.2	3.7		5.0	4.1	
(95%, C.I.) months	4.2, 5.7	3.0, 4.3		4.2, 6.4	2.4, 4.5	
Tumor Response	26%	10%	p<0.0001[e]	33%	14%	p=0.01[e]

[a] 28-day schedule — Gemzar plus cisplatin: Gemzar 1000 mg/m² on Days 1, 8, and 15 and cisplatin 100 mg/m² on Day 1 every 28 days; Single-agent cisplatin: cisplatin 100 mg/m² on Day 1 every 28 days.
[b] 21-day schedule — Gemzar plus cisplatin: Gemzar 1250 mg/m² on Days 1 and 8 and cisplatin 100 mg/m² on Day 1 every 21 days; Etoposide plus Cisplatin: cisplatin 100 mg/m² on Day 1 and IV etoposide 100 mg/m² on Days 1, 2, and 3 every 21 days.
[c] N/A Not applicable.
[d] Karnofsky Performance Status.
[e] p-value for tumor response was calculated using the two-sided Fisher's Exact test for difference in binomial proportions. All other p-values were calculated using the Log rank test for difference in overall time to an event.

OR:
ii) the patient was stable on all of the aforementioned parameters, and showed a marked, sustained weight gain (≥7% increase maintained for ≥4 weeks) not due to fluid accumulation.

The first study was a multicenter (17 sites in US and Canada), prospective, single-blinded, two-arm, randomized, comparison of Gemzar and 5-FU in patients with locally advanced or metastatic pancreatic cancer who had received no prior treatment with chemotherapy. 5-FU was administered intravenously at a weekly dose of 600 mg/m² for 30 minutes. The results from this randomized trial are shown in Table

14. Patients treated with Gemzar had statistically significant increases in clinical benefit response, survival, and time to disease progression compared to 5-FU. The Kaplan-Meier curve for survival is shown in Figure 4. No confirmed objective tumor responses were observed with either treatment.

[See table 14 at top of next page]

Clinical benefit response was achieved by 14 patients treated with Gemzar and 3 patients treated with 5-FU. One patient on the Gemzar arm showed improvement in all 3 primary parameters (pain intensity, analgesic consumption, and performance status). Eleven patients on the Gemzar

arm and 2 patients on the 5-FU arm showed improvement in analgesic consumption and/or pain intensity with stable performance status. Two patients on the Gemzar arm showed improvement in analgesic consumption or pain intensity with improvement in performance status. One patient on the 5-FU arm was stable with regard to pain intensity and analgesic consumption with improvement in performance status. No patient on either arm achieved a clinical benefit response based on weight gain.

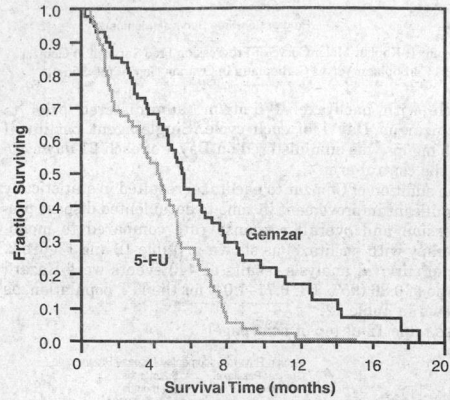

Figure 4: Kaplan-Meier Survival Curve

The second trial was a multicenter (17 US and Canadian centers), open-label study of Gemzar in 63 patients with advanced pancreatic cancer previously treated with 5-FU or a 5-FU-containing regimen. The study showed a clinical benefit response rate of 27% and median survival of 3.9 months.

14.5 Other Clinical Studies

When Gemzar was administered more frequently than once weekly or with infusions longer than 60 minutes, increased toxicity was observed. Results of a Phase 1 study of Gemzar to assess the maximum tolerated dose (MTD) on a daily × 5 schedule showed that patients developed significant hypotension and severe flu-like symptoms that were intolerable at doses above 10 mg/m². The incidence and severity of these events were dose-related. Other Phase 1 studies using a twice-weekly schedule reached MTDs of only 65 mg/m² (30-minute infusion) and 150 mg/m² (5-minute bolus). The dose-limiting toxicities were thrombocytopenia and flu-like symptoms, particularly asthenia. In a Phase 1 study to assess the maximum tolerated infusion time, clinically significant toxicity, defined as myelosuppression, was seen with weekly doses of 300 mg/m² at or above a 270-minute infusion time. The half-life of gemcitabine is influenced by the length of the infusion [see Clinical Pharmacology (12.3)] and the toxicity appears to be increased if Gemzar is administered more frequently than once weekly or with infusions longer than 60 minutes [see Warnings and Precautions (5.1)].

15 REFERENCES

1. NIOSH Alert: Preventing occupational exposures to antineoplastic and other hazardous drugs in healthcare settings. 2004. U.S. Department of Health and Human Services, Public Health Service, Centers for Disease Control and Prevention, National Institute for Occupational Safety and Health, DHHS (NIOSH) Publication No. 2004-165.
2. OSHA Technical Manual, TED 1-0.15A, Section VI: Chapter 2. Controlling Occupational Exposure to Hazardous Drugs. OSHA, 1999. http://www.osha.gov/dts/osta/otm/otm_vi/otm_vi_2.html
3. American Society of Health-System Pharmacists. ASHP Guidelines on Handling Hazardous Drugs: Am J Health-Syst Pharm. 2006;63:1172-1193.
4. Polovich, M., White, J. M., & Kelleher, L. O. (eds.) 2005. Chemotherapy and biotherapy guidelines and recommendations for practice (2nd. ed.) Pittsburgh, PA: Oncology Nursing Society.

16 HOW SUPPLIED/STORAGE AND HANDLING

16.1 How Supplied

GEMZAR (gemcitabine for injection, USP), is available in sterile single-use vials individually packaged in a carton containing:
200 mg white to off-white, lyophilized powder in a 10-mL size sterile single-use vial - NDC 0002-7501-01 (No. 7501)
1 g white to off-white, lyophilized powder in a 50-mL size sterile single-use vial - NDC 0002-7502-01 (No. 7502)

16.2 Storage and Handling

Unopened vials of Gemzar are stable until the expiration date indicated on the package when stored at controlled room temperature 20° to 25°C (68° to 77°F) and that allows

Table 14: Gemzar Versus 5-FU in Pancreatic Cancer

	Gemzar	5-FU	
Number of patients	63	63	
Male	34	34	
Female	29	29	
Median age	62 years	61 years	
Range	37 to 79	36 to 77	
Stage IV disease	71.4%	76.2%	
Baseline KPS[a] ≤70	69.8%	68.3%	
Clinical benefit response	22.2%	4.8%	p=0.004[e]
	(N[c]=14)	(N[c]=3)	
Survival			p=0.0009
Median	5.7 months	4.2 months	
6-month probability[b]	(N=30) 46%	(N=19) 29%	
9-month probability[b]	(N=14) 24%	(N=4) 5%	
1-year probability[b]	(N=9) 18%	(N=2) 2%	
Range	0.2 to 18.6 months	0.4 to 15.1+[d] months	
95% C.I. of the median	4.7 to 6.9 months	3.1 to 5.1 months	
Time to Disease Progression			p=0.0013
Median	2.1 months	0.9 months	
Range	0.1+[d] to 9.4 months	0.1 to 12.0+[d] months	
95% C.I. of the median	1.9 to 3.4 months	0.9 to 1.1 months	

[a] Karnofsky Performance Status.
[b] Kaplan-Meier estimates.
[c] N=number of patients.
[d] No progression at last visit; remains alive.
[e] The p-value for clinical benefit response was calculated using the two-sided test for difference in binomial proportions. All other p-values were calculated using the Log rank test for difference in overall time to an event.

for excursions between 15° and 30°C (59° and 86°F) [See USP Controlled Room Temperature]. *[see Dosage and Administration (2.5 and 2.6)]*

17 PATIENT COUNSELING INFORMATION

17.1 Low Blood Cell Counts
Patients should be adequately informed of the risk of low blood cell counts and instructed to immediately contact their physician should any sign of infection develop including fever. Patients should also contact their physician if bleeding or symptoms of anemia occur. *[see Warnings and Precautions (5.2)]*

17.2 Pregnancy
There are no adequate and well-controlled studies of Gemzar in pregnant women. Based on animal studies Gemzar can cause fetal harm when administered to a pregnant woman. If this drug is used during pregnancy, or if the patient becomes pregnant while taking this drug, the risks to the fetus need to be discussed with their physician. *[see Warnings and Precautions (5.6) and Use in Specific Populations (8.1)]*

17.3 Nursing Mothers
It is not known whether this drug is excreted in human milk. Because many drugs are excreted in human milk and because of the potential for serious adverse reactions in nursing infants from Gemzar, a decision should be made whether to discontinue nursing or to discontinue the drug, taking into account the importance of the drug to the mother. *[see Use in Specific Populations (8.3)]*
Literature revised March 19, 2010
Eli Lilly and Company, Indianapolis, IN 46285, USA
Copyright © 1996, 2010, Eli Lilly and Company. All rights reserved.
PV 4068 AMP

GLUCAGON
[glōō ′ka-gŏn]
FOR INJECTION
(rDNAORIGIN)

℞

DESCRIPTION
Glucagon for Injection (rDNA origin) is a polypeptide hormone identical to human glucagon that increases blood glucose and relaxes smooth muscle of the gastrointestinal tract. Glucagon is synthesized in a special non-pathogenic laboratory strain of *Escherichia coli* bacteria that has been genetically altered by the addition of the gene for glucagon. Glucagon is a single-chain polypeptide that contains 29 amino acid residues and has a molecular weight of 3483. The empirical formula is $C_{153}H_{225}N_{43}O_{49}S$. The primary sequence of glucagon is shown below.

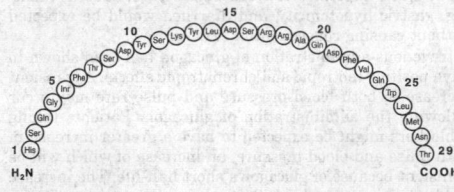

Crystalline glucagon is a white to off-white powder. It is relatively insoluble in water but is soluble at a pH of less than 3 or more than 9.5.
Glucagon is available for use intravenously, intramuscularly, or subcutaneously in a kit that contains a vial of sterile glucagon and a syringe of sterile diluent. The vial contains 1 mg (1 unit) of glucagon and 49 mg of lactose. Hydrochloric acid may have been added during manufacture to adjust the pH of the glucagon. One International Unit of glucagon is equivalent to 1 mg of glucagon.[1] The diluent syringe contains 12 mg/mL of glycerin, Water For Injection, and hydrochloric acid.

CLINICAL PHARMACOLOGY
Glucagon increases blood glucose concentration and is used in the treatment of hypoglycemia. Glucagon acts only on liver glycogen, converting it to glucose.
Glucagon administered through a parenteral route relaxes smooth muscle of the stomach, duodenum, small bowel, and colon.

Pharmacokinetics
Glucagon has been studied following intramuscular, subcutaneous, and intravenous administration in adult volunteers. Administration of the intravenous glucagon showed dose proportionality of the pharmacokinetics between 0.25 and 2.0 mg. Calculations from a 1 mg dose showed a small volume of distribution (mean, 0.25 L/kg) and a moderate clearance (mean, 13.5 mL/min/kg). The half-life was short, ranging from 8 to 18 minutes.
Maximum plasma concentrations of 7.9 ng/mL were achieved approximately 20 minutes after subcutaneous administration (see Figure 1A). With intramuscular dosing, maximum plasma concentrations of 6.9 ng/mL were attained approximately 13 minutes after dosing.
Glucagon is extensively degraded in liver, kidney, and plasma. Urinary excretion of intact glucagon has not been measured.

Pharmacodynamics
In a study of 25 volunteers, a subcutaneous dose of 1 mg glucagon resulted in a mean peak dose glucose concentration of 136 mg/dL 30 minutes after injection (see Figure 1B). Similarly, following intramuscular injection, the mean peak glucose level was 138 mg/dL, which occurred at 26 minutes after injection. No difference in maximum blood glucose

concentration between animal-sourced and rDNA glucagon was observed after subcutaneous and intramuscular injection.

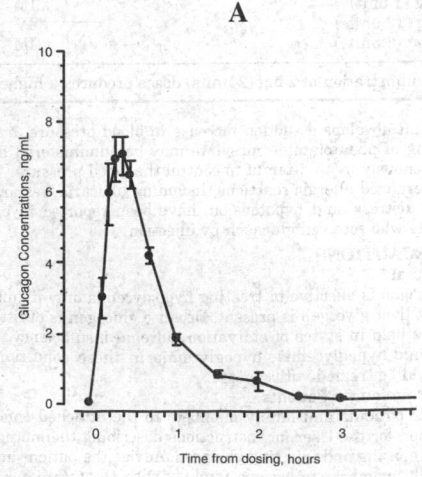

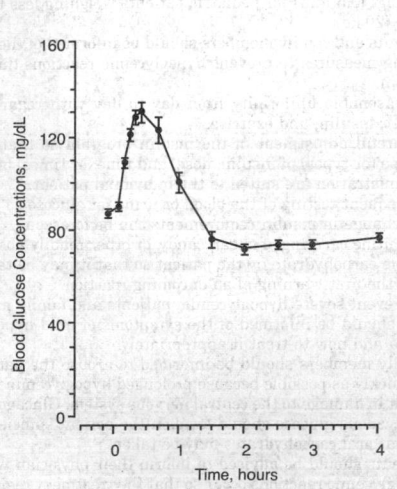

Figure 1 Mean (±SE) serum glucagon and blood glucose levels after subcutaneous injection of glucagon (1 mg) in 25 normal volunteers

INDICATIONS AND USAGE

For the treatment of hypoglycemia:
Glucagon is indicated as a treatment for severe hypoglycemia.
Because patients with type 1 diabetes may have less of an increase in blood glucose levels compared with a stable type 2 patient, supplementary carbohydrate should be given as soon as possible, especially to a pediatric patient.

For use as a diagnostic aid:
Glucagon is indicated as a diagnostic aid in the radiologic examination of the stomach, duodenum, small bowel, and colon when diminished intestinal motility would be advantageous.
Glucagon is as effective for this examination as are the anticholinergic drugs. However, the addition of the anticholinergic agent may result in increased side effects.

CONTRAINDICATIONS
Glucagon is contraindicated in patients with known hypersensitivity to it or in patients with known pheochromocytoma.

WARNINGS
Glucagon should be administered cautiously to patients with a history suggestive of insulinoma, pheochromocytoma, or both. In patients with insulinoma, intravenous administration of glucagon may produce an initial increase in blood glucose; however, because of glucagon's hyperglycemic effect the insulinoma may release insulin and cause subsequent hypoglycemia. A patient developing symptoms of hypoglycemia after a dose of glucagon should be given glucose orally, intravenously, or by gavage, whichever is most appropriate.
Exogenous glucagon also stimulates the release of catecholamines. In the presence of pheochromocytoma, glucagon can cause the tumor to release catecholamines, which may result in a sudden and marked increase in blood pressure. If a

Dose	Route of Administration	Time of Onset of Action	Approximate Duration of Effect
0.25-0.5 mg (0.25-0.5 units)	IV	1 minute	9-17 minutes
1-mg (1 unit)	IM	8-10 minutes	12-27 minutes
2 mg* (2 units)	IV	1 minute	22-25 minutes
2 mg* (2 units)	IM	4-7 minutes	21-32 minutes

*Administration of 2 mg (2 units) doses produces a higher incidence of nausea and vomiting than do lower doses.

patient develops a sudden increase in blood pressure, 5 to 10 mg of phentolamine mesylate may be administered intravenously in an attempt to control the blood pressure.
Generalized allergic reactions, including urticaria, respiratory distress, and hypotension, have been reported in patients who received glucagon by injection.

PRECAUTIONS

General

Glucagon is effective in treating hypoglycemia only if sufficient liver glycogen is present. Because glucagon is of little or no help in states of starvation, adrenal insufficiency, or chronic hypoglycemia, hypoglycemia in these conditions should be treated with glucose.

Information for Patients

Refer patients and family members to the attached Information for the User for instructions describing the method of preparing and injecting glucagon. Advise the patient and family members to become familiar with the technique of preparing glucagon before an emergency arises. Instruct patients to use 1 mg (1 unit) for adults and 1/2 the adult dose (0.5 mg) [0.5 unit] for pediatric patients weighing less than 44 lb (20 kg).

Patients and family members should be informed of the following measures to prevent hypoglycemic reactions due to insulin:

1. Reasonable uniformity from day to day with regard to diet, insulin, and exercise.
2. Careful adjustment of the insulin program so that the type (or types) of insulin, dose, and time (or times) of administration are suited to the individual patient.
3. Frequent testing of the blood or urine for glucose so that a change in insulin requirements can be foreseen.
4. Routine carrying of sugar, candy, or other readily absorbable carbohydrate by the patient so that it may be taken at the first warning of an oncoming reaction.

To prevent severe hypoglycemia, patients and family members should be informed of the symptoms of mild hypoglycemia and how to treat it appropriately.

Family members should be informed to arouse the patient as quickly as possible because prolonged hypoglycemia may result in damage to the central nervous system. Glucagon or intravenous glucose should awaken the patient sufficiently so that oral carbohydrates may be taken.

Patients should be advised to inform their physician when hypoglycemic reactions occur so that the treatment regimen may be adjusted if necessary.

Laboratory Tests

Blood glucose determinations should be obtained to follow the patient with hypoglycemia until patient is asymptomatic.

Carcinogenesis, Mutagenesis, Impairment of Fertility

Because glucagon is usually given in a single dose and has a very short half-life, no studies have been done regarding carcinogenesis. In a series of studies examining effects on the bacterial mutagenesis (Ames) assay, it was determined that *an increase* in colony counts was related to technical difficulties in running this assay with peptides and was not due to mutagenic activities of the glucagon.

Reproduction studies have been performed in rats at doses up to 2 mg/kg glucagon administered two times a day (up to 40 times the human dose based on body surface area, mg/m^2) and have revealed no evidence of impaired fertility.

Pregnancy

Pregnancy Category B—Reproduction studies have not been performed with recombinant glucagon. However, studies with animal-sourced glucagon were performed in rats at doses up to 2 mg/kg glucagon administered two times a day (up to 40 times the human dose based on body surface area, mg/m^2), and have revealed no evidence of impaired fertility or harm to the fetus due to glucagon. There are, however, no adequate and well-controlled studies in pregnant women. Because animal reproduction studies are not always predictive of human response, this drug should be used during pregnancy only if clearly needed.

Nursing Mothers

It is not known whether this drug is excreted in human milk. Because many drugs are excreted in human milk, caution should be exercised when glucagon is administered to a nursing woman. If the drug is excreted in human milk during its short half-life, it will be hydrolyzed and absorbed like any other polypeptide. Glucagon is not active when taken orally because it is destroyed in the gastrointestinal tract before it can be absorbed.

Pediatric Use

For the treatment of hypoglycemia: The use of glucagon in pediatric patients has been reported to be safe and effective.[2-6]

For use as a diagnostic aid: Effectiveness has not been established in pediatric patients.

Geriatric Use

Clinical studies of glucagon did not include sufficient numbers of subjects aged 65 and over to determine whether they respond differently from younger subjects. Other reported clinical experience has not identified differences in responses between the elderly and younger patients. In general, dose selection for an elderly patient should be cautious, usually starting at the low end of the dosing range, reflecting the greater frequency of decreased hepatic, renal, or cardiac function, and of concomitant disease or other drug therapy.

ADVERSE REACTIONS

Severe adverse reactions are very rare, although nausea and vomiting may occur occasionally. These reactions may also occur with hypoglycemia. Generalized allergic reactions have been reported (*see* WARNINGS). In a three month controlled study of 75 volunteers comparing animal-sourced glucagon with glucagon manufactured through rDNA technology, no glucagon-specific antibodies were detected in either treatment group.

OVERDOSAGE

Signs and Symptoms—If overdosage occurs, nausea, vomiting, gastric hypotonicity, and diarrhea would be expected without causing consequential toxicity.

Intravenous administration of glucagon has been shown to have positive inotropic and chronotropic effects. A transient increase in both blood pressure and pulse rate may occur following the administration of glucagon. Patients taking β-blockers might be expected to have a greater increase in both pulse and blood pressure, an increase of which will be transient because of glucagon's short half-life. The increase in blood pressure and pulse rate may require therapy in patients with pheochromocytoma or coronary artery disease.

When glucagon was given in large doses to patients with cardiac disease, investigators reported a positive inotropic effect. These investigators administered glucagon in doses of 0.5 to 16 mg/hour by continuous infusion for periods of 5 to 166 hours. Total doses ranged from 25 to 996 mg, and a 21-month-old infant received approximately 8.25 mg in 165 hours. Side effects included nausea, vomiting, and decreasing serum potassium concentration. Serum potassium concentration could be maintained within normal limits with supplemental potassium.

The intravenous median lethal dose for glucagon in mice and rats is approximately 300 mg/kg and 38.6 mg/kg, respectively.

Because glucagon is a polypeptide, it would be rapidly destroyed in the gastrointestinal tract if it were to be accidentally ingested.

Treatment—To obtain up-to-date information about the treatment of overdose, a good resource is your certified Regional Poison Control Center. Telephone numbers of certified poison control centers are listed in the *Physicians' Desk Reference (PDR)*. In managing overdosage, consider the possibility of multiple drug overdoses, interaction among drugs, and unusual drug kinetics in your patient.

In view of the extremely short half-life of glucagon and its prompt destruction and excretion, the treatment of overdosage is symptomatic, primarily for nausea, vomiting, and possible hypokalemia.

If the patient develops a dramatic increase in blood pressure, 5 to 10 mg of phentolamine mesylate has been shown to be effective in lowering blood pressure for the short time that control would be needed.

Forced diuresis, peritoneal dialysis, hemodialysis, or charcoal hemoperfusion have not been established as beneficial for an overdose of glucagon; it is extremely unlikely that one of these procedures would ever be indicated.

DOSAGE AND ADMINISTRATION

General Instructions for Use:

- The diluent is provided for use only in the preparation of glucagon for parenteral injection and for no other use.
- Glucagon should not be used at concentrations greater than 1 mg/mL (1 unit/mL).
- Reconstituted glucagon should be used immediately. **Discard any unused portion.**
- Reconstituted glucagon solutions should be used only if they are clear and of a water-like consistency.
- Parenteral drug products should be inspected visually for particulate matter and discoloration prior to administration.

Directions for Treatment of Severe Hypoglycemia:

Severe hypoglycemia should be treated initially with intravenous glucose, if possible.

1. If parenteral glucose can not be used, dissolve the lyophilized glucagon using the accompanying diluting solution and use immediately.
2. For adults and for pediatric patients weighing more than 44 lb (20 kg), give 1 mg (1 unit) by subcutaneous, intramuscular, or intravenous injection.
3. For pediatric patients weighing less than 44 lb (20 kg), give 0.5 mg (0.5 unit) or a dose equivalent to 20 to 30 μg/kg.[2-6]
4. **Discard any unused portion.**
5. An unconscious patient will usually awaken within 15 minutes following the glucagon injection. If the response is delayed, there is no contraindication to the administration of an additional dose of glucagon; however, in view of the deleterious effects of cerebral hypoglycemia emergency aid should be sought so that parenteral glucose can be given.
6. After the patient responds, supplemental carbohydrate should be given to restore liver glycogen and to prevent secondary hypoglycemia.

Directions for Use as a Diagnostic Aid:

Dissolve the lyophilized glucagon using the accompanying diluting solution and use immediately. **Discard any unused portion.**

The doses in the following table may be administered for relaxation of the stomach, duodenum, and small bowel, depending on the onset and duration of effect required for the examination. Since the stomach is less sensitive to the effect of glucagon, 0.5 mg (0.5 units) IV or 2 mg (2 units) IM are recommended.

[See table at top left]

For examination of the colon, it is recommended that a 2 mg (2 units) dose be administered intramuscularly approximately 10 minutes prior to the procedure. Colon relaxation and reduction of patient discomfort may allow the radiologist to perform a more satisfactory examination.

HOW SUPPLIED

Glucagon Emergency Kit for Low Blood Sugar (Glucagon for Injection [rDNA origin]) (MS8031):

- 1 mg (1 unit)—(VL7529), with 1 mL of diluting solution (Hyporet®[1] HY7530) (1s) NDC 0002-8031-01

[1]Hyporet® (disposable syringe, Lilly).

Stability and Storage:

Before Reconstitution—Vials of Glucagon, as well as the Diluting Solution for Glucagon, may be stored at controlled room temperature 20° to 25°C (68° to 77°F)[see USP].

The USP defines controlled room temperature by the following: A temperature maintained thermostatically that encompasses the usual and customary working environment of 20° to 25°C (68° to 77°F); that results in a mean kinetic temperature calculated to be not more than 25°C; and that allows for excursions between 15° and 30°C (59° and 86°F) that are experienced in pharmacies, hospitals, and warehouses.

After Reconstitution—Glucagon for Injection (rDNA origin) should be used immediately. **Discard any unused portion.**

REFERENCES

1. *Drug Information for the Health Care Professional.* 18th ed. Rockville, Maryland: The United States Pharmacopeial Convention, Inc; 1998; I:1512.
2. Gibbs et al: Use of glucagon to terminate insulin reactions in diabetic children. *Nebr Med J* 1958;43:56-57.
3. Cornblath M, et al: Studies of carbohydrate metabolism in the newborn: Effect of glucagon on concentration of sugar in capillary blood of newborn infant. *Pediatrics* 1958;21:885-892.
4. Carson MJ, Koch R: Clinical studies with glucagon in children. *J Pediatr* 1955;47:161-170.
5. Shipp JC, et al: Treatment of insulin hypoglycemia in diabetic campers. *Diabetes* 1964;13:645-648.
6. Aman J, Wranne L: Hypoglycemia in childhood diabetes II: Effect of subcutaneous or intramuscular injection of different doses of glucagon. *Acta Pediatr Scand* 1988;77: 548-553.

Literature revised February 18, 2005

Eli Lilly and Company
Indianapolis, IN 46285, USA

INFORMATION FOR THE USER
GLUCAGON
FOR INJECTION
(rDNA ORIGIN)

BECOME FAMILIAR WITH THE FOLLOWING INSTRUCTIONS BEFORE AN EMERGENCY ARISES. DO NOT USE THIS KIT AFTER DATE STAMPED ON THE BOTTLE LABEL. IF YOU HAVE QUESTIONS CONCERNING THE USE OF THIS PRODUCT, CONSULT A DOCTOR, NURSE OR PHARMACIST.

Make sure that your relatives or close friends know that if you become unconscious, medical assistance must always be sought. Glucagon may have been prescribed so that members of your household can give the injection if you become hypoglycemic and are unable to take sugar by mouth. If you are unconscious, glucagon can be given while awaiting medical assistance.

Show your family members and others where you keep this kit and how to use it. They need to know how to use it before you need it. They can practice giving a shot by giving you your normal insulin shots. It is important that they practice. A person who has never given a shot probably will not be able to do it in an emergency.

IMPORTANT
- Act quickly. Prolonged unconsciousness may be harmful.
- These simple instructions will help you give glucagon successfully.
- Turn patient on his/her side to prevent patient from choking.
- The contents of the syringe are inactive. You must mix the contents of the syringe with the glucagon in the accompanying bottle before giving injection. (*See* DIRECTIONS FOR USE below.)
- Do not prepare Glucagon for Injection until you are ready to use it.

WARNING: THE PATIENT MAY BE IN A COMA FROM SEVERE HYPERGLYCEMIA (HIGH BLOOD GLUCOSE) RATHER THAN HYPOGLYCEMIA. IN SUCH A CASE, THE PATIENT WILL **NOT** RESPOND TO GLUCAGON AND REQUIRES IMMEDIATE MEDICAL ATTENTION.

INDICATIONS FOR USE
Use glucagon to treat insulin coma or insulin reaction resulting from severe hypoglycemia (low blood sugar). Symptoms of severe hypoglycemia include disorientation, unconsciousness, and seizures or convulsions. Give glucagon if (1) the patient is unconscious (2) the patient is unable to eat sugar or a sugar-sweetened product (3) the patient is having a seizure, or (4) repeated administration of sugar or a sugar-sweetened product such as a regular soft drink or fruit juice does not improve the patient's condition. Milder cases of hypoglycemia should be treated promptly by eating sugar or a sugar-sweetened product. (*See* INFORMATION ON HYPOGLYCEMIA below for more information on the symptoms of hypoglycemia.) Glucagon is not active when taken orally.

DIRECTIONS FOR USE
TO PREPARE GLUCAGON FOR INJECTION
1. Remove the flip-off seal from the bottle of glucagon. Wipe rubber stopper on bottle with alcohol swab.

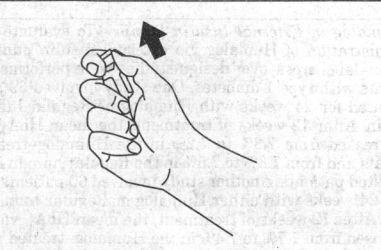

2. Remove the needle protector from the syringe, and inject the entire contents of the syringe into the bottle of glucagon. DO NOT REMOVE THE PLASTIC CLIP FROM THE SYRINGE. Remove syringe from the bottle.

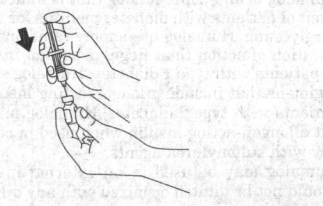

3. Swirl bottle gently until glucagon dissolves completely. GLUCAGON SHOULD NOT BE USED UNLESS THE SOLUTION IS CLEAR AND OF A WATER-LIKE CONSISTENCY.

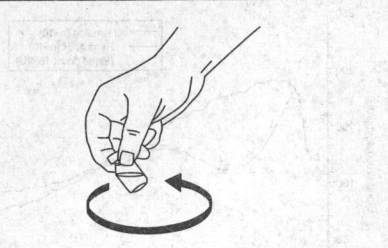

TO INJECT GLUCAGON
Use Same Technique as for Injecting Insulin
4. Using the same syringe, hold bottle upside down and, making sure the needle tip remains in solution, gently withdraw all of the solution (1 mg mark on syringe) from bottle. The plastic clip on the syringe will prevent the rubber stopper from being pulled out of the syringe; however, if the plastic plunger rod separates from the rubber stopper, simply reinsert the rod by turning it clockwise. The usual adult dose is 1 mg (1 unit). For children weighing less than 44 lb (20 kg), give 1/2 adult dose (0.5 mg). For children, withdraw 1/2 of the solution from the bottle (0.5 mg mark on syringe). DISCARD UNUSED PORTION.

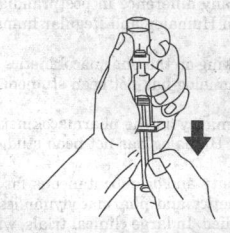

USING THE FOLLOWING DIRECTIONS, INJECT GLUCAGON IMMEDIATELY AFTER MIXING.
5. Cleanse injection site on buttock, arm, or thigh with alcohol swab.
6. Insert the needle into the loose tissue under the cleansed injection site, and inject all (or 1/2 for children weighing less than 44 lb) of the glucagon solution. THERE IS NO DANGER OF OVERDOSE. Apply light pressure at the injection site, and withdraw the needle. Press an alcohol swab against the injection site.
7. Turn the patient on his/her side. When an unconscious person awakens, he/she may vomit. Turning the patient on his/her side will prevent him/her from choking.
8. FEED THE PATIENT AS SOON AS HE/SHE AWAKENS AND IS ABLE TO SWALLOW. Give the patient a fast-acting source of sugar (such as a regular soft drink or fruit juice) and a long-acting source of sugar (such as crackers and cheese or a meat sandwich). If the patient does not awaken within 15 minutes, give another dose of glucagon and INFORM A DOCTOR OR EMERGENCY SERVICES IMMEDIATELY.
9. Even if the glucagon revives the patient, his/her doctor should be promptly notified. A doctor should be notified whenever severe hypoglycemic reactions occur.

INFORMATION ON HYPOGLYCEMIA
Early symptoms of hypoglycemia (low blood glucose) include:

- sweating
- dizziness
- palpitation
- tremor
- hunger
- restlessness
- tingling in the hands, feet, lips, or tongue
- lightheadedness
- inability to concentrate
- headache
- drowsiness
- sleep disturbances
- anxiety
- blurred vision
- slurred speech
- depressed mood
- irritability
- abnormal behavior
- unsteady movement
- personality changes

If not treated, the patient may progress to severe hypoglycemia that can include:

- disorientation
- unconsciousness
- seizures
- death

The occurrence of early symptoms calls for prompt and, if necessary, repeated administration of some form of carbohydrate. Patients should always carry a quick source of sugar, such as candy mints or glucose tablets. The prompt treatment of mild hypoglycemic symptoms can prevent severe hypoglycemic reactions. If the patient does not improve or if administration of carbohydrate is impossible, glucagon should be given or the patient should be treated with intravenous glucose at a medical facility. Glucagon, a naturally occurring substance produced by the pancreas, is helpful because it enables the patient to produce his/her own blood glucose to correct the hypoglycemia.

POSSIBLE PROBLEMS WITH GLUCAGON TREATMENT
Severe side effects are very rare, although nausea and vomiting may occur occasionally.

A few people may be allergic to glucagon or to one of the inactive ingredients in glucagon, or may experience rapid heart beat for a short while.

If you experience any other reactions which are likely to have been caused by glucagon, please contact your doctor.

STORAGE
Before dissolving glucagon with diluting solution—Store the kit at controlled room temperature between 20° to 25°C (68° to 77°F).

After dissolving glucagon with diluting solution—Should be used immediately. **Discard any unused portion.** Solutions should be clear and of a water-like consistency at time of use.

Literature revised February 18, 2005
Eli Lilly and Company
Indianapolis, IN 46285, USA
Copyright © 1999, 2005, Eli Lilly and Company. All rights reserved.

HUMALOG®
[hū′mă-lŏg]
INSULIN LISPRO INJECTION, USP
(rDNA ORIGIN)
100 UNITS PER ML (U-100)

℞

DESCRIPTION
Humalog® [insulin lispro injection, USP (rDNA origin)] is a human insulin analog that is a rapid–acting, parenteral blood glucose–lowering agent. Chemically, it is Lys(B28), Pro(B29) human insulin analog, created when the amino acids at positions 28 and 29 on the insulin B-chain are reversed. Humalog is synthesized in a special non–pathogenic laboratory strain of *Escherichia coli* bacteria that has been genetically altered to produce insulin lispro.
Humalog has the following primary structure:

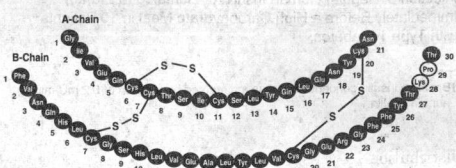

Insulin lispro has the empirical formula $C_{257}H_{383}N_{65}O_{77}S_6$ and a molecular weight of 5808, both identical to that of human insulin.

The vials, cartridges, Humalog® KwikPen™ and Pens contain a sterile solution of Humalog for use as an injection. Humalog injection consists of zinc–insulin lispro crystals dissolved in a clear aqueous fluid.

Each milliliter of Humalog injection contains insulin lispro 100 units, 16 mg glycerin, 1.88 mg dibasic sodium phosphate, 3.15 mg Metacresol, zinc oxide content adjusted to provide 0.0197 mg zinc ion, trace amounts of phenol, and Water for Injection. Insulin lispro has a pH of 7.0 to 7.8. Hydrochloric acid 10% and/or sodium hydroxide 10% may be added to adjust pH.

CLINICAL PHARMACOLOGY
Antidiabetic Activity
The primary activity of insulin, including Humalog, is the regulation of glucose metabolism. In addition, all insulins have several anabolic and anti–catabolic actions on many tissues in the body. In muscle and other tissues (except the brain), insulin causes rapid transport of glucose and amino acids intracellularly, promotes anabolism, and inhibits protein catabolism. In the liver, insulin promotes the uptake and storage of glucose in the form of glycogen, inhibits gluconeogenesis, and promotes the conversion of excess glucose into fat.

Humalog has been shown to be equipotent to human insulin on a molar basis. One unit of Humalog has the same glucose–lowering effect as one unit of Regular human insulin, but its effect is more rapid and of shorter duration. The glucose–lowering activity of Humalog and Regular human insulin is comparable when administered to nondiabetic subjects by the intravenous route.

Pharmacokinetics

Absorption and Bioavailability
Humalog is as bioavailable as Regular human insulin, with absolute bioavailability ranging between 55% to 77% with doses between 0.1 to 0.2 U/kg, inclusive. Studies in nondiabetic subjects and patients with type 1 (insulin–dependent) diabetes demonstrated that Humalog is absorbed faster than Regular human insulin (U–100) (see Figure 1). In nondiabetic subjects given subcutaneous doses of Humalog ranging from 0.1 to 0.4 U/kg, peak serum concentrations were observed 30 to 90 minutes after dosing. When nondiabetic subjects received equivalent doses of Regular human insulin, peak insulin concentrations occurred between 50 to 120 minutes after dosing. Similar results were seen in patients with type 1 diabetes. The pharmacokinetic profiles of Humalog and Regular human insulin are comparable to one another when administered to nondiabetic subjects by the intravenous route. Humalog was absorbed at a consistently faster rate than Regular human insulin in healthy male volunteers given 0.2 U/kg Regular human insulin or Humalog at abdominal, deltoid, or femoral subcutaneous sites, the three sites often used by patients with diabetes. After abdominal administration of Humalog, serum drug levels are higher and the duration of action is slightly shorter than after deltoid or thigh administration (see DOSAGE AND ADMINISTRATION). Humalog has less intra– and inter-patient variability compared with Regular human insulin.

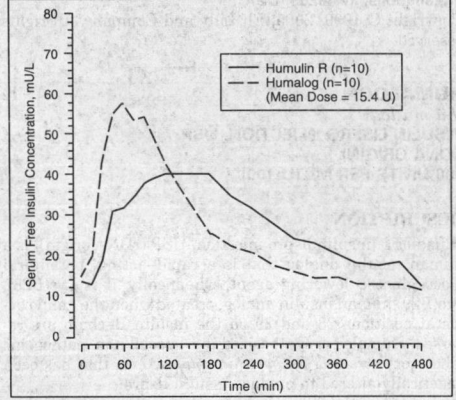

Figure 1: Serum Humalog and Insulin Levels After Subcutaneous Injection of Regular Human Insulin or Humalog (0.2 U/kg) Immediately Before a High Carbohydrate Meal in 10 Patients with Type 1 Diabetes.[1]

[1]Baseline insulin concentration was maintained by infusion of 0.2 mU/min/kg human insulin.

Distribution
The volume of distribution following injection of Humalog is identical to that of Regular human insulin, with a range of 0.26 to 0.36 L/kg.

Metabolism
Human metabolism studies have not been conducted. However, animal studies indicate that the metabolism of Humalog is identical to that of Regular human insulin.

Elimination
When Humalog is given subcutaneously, its $t_{1/2}$ is shorter than that of Regular human insulin (1 versus 1.5 hours, respectively). When given intravenously, Humalog and Regular human insulin show identical dose–dependent elimination, with a $t_{1/2}$ of 26 and 52 minutes at 0.1 U/kg and 0.2 U/kg, respectively.

Pharmacodynamics
Studies in nondiabetic subjects and patients with diabetes demonstrated that Humalog has a more rapid onset of glucose–lowering activity, an earlier peak for glucose–lowering, and a shorter duration of glucose–lowering activity than Regular human insulin (see Figure 2). The earlier onset of activity of Humalog is directly related to its more rapid rate of absorption. The time course of action of insulin and insulin analogs, such as Humalog, may vary considerably in different individuals or within the same individual. The parameters of Humalog activity (time of onset, peak time, and duration) as presented in Figure 2 should be considered only as general guidelines. The rate of insulin absorption and consequently the onset of activity is known to be affected by the site of injection, exercise, and other variables (see General under PRECAUTIONS).

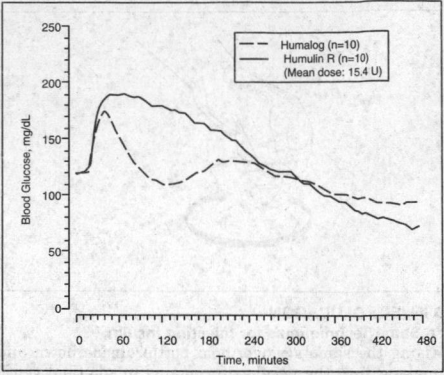

Figure 2: Blood Glucose Levels After Subcutaneous Injection of Regular Human Insulin or Humalog (0.2 U/kg) Immediately Before a High Carbohydrate Meal in 10 Patients with Type 1 Diabetes.[2]

[2]Baseline insulin concentration was maintained by infusion of 0.2 mU/min/kg human insulin.

Special Populations
Age and Gender
Information on the effect of age and gender on the pharmacokinetics of Humalog is unavailable. However, in large clinical trials, sub–group analysis based on age and gender did not indicate any difference in postprandial glucose parameters between Humalog and Regular human insulin.

Smoking
The effect of smoking on the pharmacokinetics and pharmacodynamics of Humalog has not been studied.

Pregnancy
The effect of pregnancy on the pharmacokinetics and pharmacodynamics of Humalog has not been studied.

Obesity
The effect of obesity and/or subcutaneous fat thickness on the pharmacokinetics and pharmacodynamics of Humalog has not been studied. In large clinical trials, which included patients with Body Mass Index up to and including 35 kg/m^2, no consistent differences were observed between Humalog and Humulin® R with respect to postprandial glucose parameters.

Renal Impairment
Some studies with human insulin have shown increased circulating levels of insulin in patients with renal failure. In a study of 25 patients with type 2 diabetes and a wide range of renal function, the pharmacokinetic differences between Humalog and Regular human insulin were generally maintained. However, the sensitivity of the patients to insulin did change, with an increased response to insulin as the renal function declined. Careful glucose monitoring and dose reductions of insulin, including Humalog, may be necessary in patients with renal dysfunction.

Hepatic Impairment
Some studies with human insulin have shown increased circulating levels of insulin in patients with hepatic failure. In a study of 22 patients with type 2 diabetes, impaired hepatic function did not affect the subcutaneous absorption or general disposition of Humalog when compared with patients with no history of hepatic dysfunction. In that study, Humalog maintained its more rapid absorption and elimination when compared with Regular human insulin. Careful glucose monitoring and dose adjustments of insulin, including Humalog, may be necessary in patients with hepatic dysfunction.

CLINICAL STUDIES
In open–label, cross–over studies of 1008 patients with type 1 diabetes and 722 patients with type 2 (non–insulin–dependent) diabetes, Humalog reduced postprandial glucose compared with Regular human insulin (see Table 1). The clinical significance of improvement in postprandial hyperglycemia has not been established.

Table 1: Comparison of Means of Glycemic Parameters at the End of Combined Treatment Periods. All Randomized Patients in Cross–Over Studies (3 Months for Each Treatment)

Type 1, N=1008 Glycemic Parameter, (mg/dL)	Humalog*	Humulin R*[†]
Fasting Blood Glucose	209.5 ± 91.6	204.1 ± 89.3
1–Hour Postprandial	232.4 ± 97.7	250.0 ± 96.7
2–Hour Postprandial	200.9 ± 95.4	231.7 ± 103.9
HbA$_{1c}$ (%)	8.2 ± 1.5	8.2 ± 1.5
Type 2, N=722 Glycemic Parameter, (mg/dL)	Humalog*	Humulin R*
Fasting Blood Glucose	192.1 ± 67.9	183.1 ± 66.1
1–Hour Postprandial	238.1 ± 79.7	250.0 ± 75.2
2–Hour Postprandial	217.4 ± 83.2	236.5 ± 80.6
HbA$_{1c}$ (%)	8.2 ± 1.3	8.2 ± 1.4

*Mean ± Standard Deviation.
†REGULAR insulin human injection, USP (rDNA origin).

In 12–month parallel studies in patients with type 1 and type 2 diabetes, HbA$_{1c}$ did not differ between patients treated with Regular human insulin and those treated with Humalog.

Hypoglycemia—While the overall rate of hypoglycemia did not differ between patients with type 1 and type 2 diabetes treated with Humalog compared with Regular human insulin, patients with type 1 diabetes treated with Humalog had fewer hypoglycemic episodes between midnight and 6 a.m. The lower rate of hypoglycemia in the Humalog–treated group may have been related to higher nocturnal blood glucose levels, as reflected by a small increase in mean fasting blood glucose levels.

Humalog in Combination with Sulfonylurea Agents—In a two–month study in patients with fasting hyperglycemia despite maximal dosing with sulfonylureas (SU), patients were randomized to one of three treatment regimens; Humulin® NPH at bedtime plus SU, Humalog three times a day before meals plus SU, or Humalog three times a day before meals and Humulin NPH at bedtime. The combination of Humalog and SU resulted in an improvement in HbA$_{1c}$ accompanied by a weight gain (see Table 2).

Table 2: Results of a Two–Month Study in Which Humalog Was Added to Sulfonylurea Therapy in Patients Not Adequately Controlled on Sulfonylurea Alone

	Humulin N h.s.+ SU*	Humalog a.c. + SU	Humalog a.c. + Humulin N h.s.
Randomized (n)	135	139	149
HbA$_{1c}$ (%) at baseline	9.9	10.0	10.0
HbA$_{1c}$ (%) at 2–months	8.7	8.4	8.5
HbA$_{1c}$ (%) change from baseline	−1.2	−1.6	−1.4
Weight gain at 2–months (kg)	0.6	1.2	1.5
Hypoglycemia[†] (events/mo)	0.11	0.03	0.09
Number of injections	1	3	4
Total insulin dose (U/kg) at 2–months	0.23	0.33	0.52

*a.c.–three times a day before meals. h.s.–at bedtime. SU–oral sulfonylurea agent.
†blood glucose ≤36 mg/dL or needing assistance from third party.

Humalog in External Insulin Pumps—To evaluate the administration of Humalog via external insulin pumps, two open–label cross–over design studies were performed in patients with type 1 diabetes. One study involved 39 patients treated for 24 weeks with Humalog or Regular human insulin. After 12 weeks of treatment, the mean HbA$_{1c}$ values decreased from 7.8% to 7.2% in the Humalog–treated patients and from 7.8% to 7.5% in the Regular human insulin–treated patients. Another study involved 60 patients treated for 24 weeks with either Humalog or Regular human insulin. After 12 weeks of treatment, the mean HbA$_{1c}$ values decreased from 7.7% to 7.4% in the Humalog–treated patients and remained unchanged from 7.7% in the Regular human insulin–treated patients. Rates of hypoglycemia were comparable between treatment groups in both studies. Humalog administration in insulin pumps has not been studied in patients with type 2 diabetes.

INDICATIONS AND USAGE
Humalog is an insulin analog that is indicated in the treatment of patients with diabetes mellitus for the control of hyperglycemia. Humalog has a more rapid onset and a shorter duration of action than Regular human insulin. Therefore, in patients with type 1 diabetes, Humalog should be used in regimens that include a longer–acting insulin. However, in patients with type 2 diabetes, Humalog may be used without a longer–acting insulin when used in combination therapy with sulfonylurea agents.

Humalog may be used in an external insulin pump, but should not be diluted or mixed with any other insulin when used in the pump.

CONTRAINDICATIONS
Humalog is contraindicated during episodes of hypoglycemia and in patients sensitive to Humalog or any of its excipients.

WARNINGS

This human insulin analog differs from Regular human insulin by its rapid onset of action as well as a shorter duration of activity. When used as a meal-time insulin, the dose of Humalog should be given within 15 minutes before or immediately after the meal. Because of the short duration of action of Humalog, patients with type 1 diabetes also require a longer–acting insulin to maintain glucose control (except when using an external insulin pump). Glucose monitoring is recommended for all patients with diabetes and is particularly important for patients using an external insulin pump.

Hypoglycemia is the most common adverse effect associated with insulins, including Humalog. As with all insulins, the timing of hypoglycemia may differ among various insulin formulations. Glucose monitoring is recommended for all patients with diabetes.

Any change of insulin should be made cautiously and only under medical supervision. Changes in insulin strength, manufacturer, type (e.g., Regular, NPH, analog), species, or method of manufacture may result in the need for a change in dosage.

External Insulin Pumps: When used in an external insulin pump, Humalog should not be diluted or mixed with any other insulin. Patients should carefully read and follow the external insulin pump manufacturer's instructions and the Patient Information leaflet before using Humalog.

Physicians should carefully evaluate information on external insulin pump use in this Humalog physician package insert and in the external insulin pump manufacturer's instructions. If unexplained hyperglycemia or ketosis occurs during external insulin pump use, prompt identification and correction of the cause is necessary. The patient may require interim therapy with subcutaneous insulin injections (*see* PRECAUTIONS, *For Patients Using External Insulin Pumps, and* DOSAGE AND ADMINISTRATION).

PRECAUTIONS

General

Hypoglycemia and hypokalemia are among the potential clinical adverse effects associated with the use of all insulins. Because of differences in the action of Humalog and other insulins, care should be taken in patients in whom such potential side effects might be clinically relevant (e.g., patients who are fasting, have autonomic neuropathy, or are using potassium–lowering drugs or patients taking drugs sensitive to serum potassium level). Lipodystrophy and hypersensitivity are among other potential clinical adverse effects associated with the use of all insulins.

As with all insulin preparations, the time course of Humalog action may vary in different individuals or at different times in the same individual and is dependent on site of injection, blood supply, temperature, and physical activity.

Adjustment of dosage of any insulin may be necessary if patients change their physical activity or their usual meal plan. Insulin requirements may be altered during illness, emotional disturbances, or other stress.

Hypoglycemia—As with all insulin preparations, hypoglycemic reactions may be associated with the administration of Humalog. Rapid changes in serum glucose concentrations may induce symptoms of hypoglycemia in persons with diabetes, regardless of the glucose value. Early warning symptoms of hypoglycemia may be different or less pronounced under certain conditions, such as long duration of diabetes, diabetic nerve disease, use of medications such as beta–blockers, or intensified diabetes control.

Renal Impairment—The requirements for insulin may be reduced in patients with renal impairment.

Hepatic Impairment—Although impaired hepatic function does not affect the absorption or disposition of Humalog, careful glucose monitoring and dose adjustments of insulin, including Humalog, may be necessary.

Allergy—Local Allergy—As with any insulin therapy, patients may experience redness, swelling, or itching at the site of injection. These minor reactions usually resolve in a few days to a few weeks. In some instances, these reactions may be related to factors other than insulin, such as irritants in the skin cleansing agent or poor injection technique.

Systemic Allergy—Less common, but potentially more serious, is generalized allergy to insulin, which may cause rash (including pruritus) over the whole body, shortness of breath, wheezing, reduction in blood pressure, rapid pulse, or sweating. Severe cases of generalized allergy, including anaphylactic reaction, may be life threatening. In controlled clinical trials, pruritus (with or without rash) was seen in 17 patients receiving Humulin R (N=2969) and 30 patients receiving Humalog (N=2944) (p=0.053). Localized reactions and generalized myalgias have been reported with the use of cresol as an injectable excipient.

Antibody Production—In large clinical trials, antibodies that cross–react with human insulin and insulin lispro were observed in both Humulin R– and Humalog–treatment groups. As expected, the largest increase in the antibody levels during the 12–month clinical trials was observed with patients new to insulin therapy.

Usage in External Insulin Pumps—The infusion set (reservoir syringe, tubing, and catheter), Disetronic® D–TRON®[2,3] or D–TRON®[2,3] plus cartridge adapter, and Humalog in the external insulin pump reservoir should be replaced and a new infusion site selected every 48 hours or less. Humalog in the external insulin pump should not be exposed to temperatures above 37°C (98.6°F).

In the D–TRON®[2,3] or D–TRON®[2,3] plus pump, Humalog 3 mL cartridges may be used for up to 7 days. However, as with other external insulin pumps, the infusion set should be replaced and a new infusion site should be selected every 48 hours or less.

When used in an external insulin pump, Humalog should not be diluted or mixed with any other insulin (*see* INDICATIONS AND USAGE, WARNINGS, PRECAUTIONS, *For Patients Using External Insulin Pumps, Mixing of Insulins*, DOSAGE AND ADMINISTRATION, *and Storage)*.

Information for Patients

Patients should be informed of the potential risks and advantages of Humalog and alternative therapies. Patients should also be informed about the importance of proper insulin storage, injection technique, timing of dosage, adherence to meal planning, regular physical activity, regular blood glucose monitoring, periodic hemoglobin A_{1c} testing, recognition and management of hypo– and hyperglycemia, and periodic assessment for diabetes complications.

Patients should be advised to inform their physician if they are pregnant or intend to become pregnant.

Refer patients to the Patient Information leaflet for timing of Humalog dosing (≤15 minutes before or immediately after a meal), storing insulin, and common adverse effects.

For Patients Using Insulin Pen Delivery Devices: Before starting therapy, patients should read the Patient Information leaflet that accompanies the drug product and the User Manual that accompanies the delivery device and re-read them each time the prescription is renewed. Patients should be instructed on how to properly use the delivery device, prime the Pen to a stream of insulin, and properly dispose of needles. Patients should be advised not to share their Pens with others.

For Patients Using External Insulin Pumps: Patients using an external infusion pump should be trained in intensive insulin therapy and in the function of their external insulin pump and pump accessories. Humalog was tested in the MiniMed®[1] Models 506, 507, and 508 insulin pumps using MiniMed®[1] Polyfin®[1] infusion sets. Humalog was also tested in Disetronic®[2] H–TRONplus® V100 insulin pump (with plastic 3.15 mL insulin reservoir), and the Disetronic D–TRON®[2,3] and D–TRON®[2,3] plus insulin pumps (with Humalog 3 mL cartridges) using Disetronic Rapid®[2] infusion sets.

The infusion set (reservoir syringe, tubing, catheter), D–TRON®[2,3] or D–TRON®[2,3] plus cartridge adapter, and Humalog in the external insulin pump reservoir should be replaced, and a new infusion site selected every 48 hours or less. Humalog in the external pump should not be exposed to temperatures above 37°C (98.6°F). A Humalog 3 mL cartridge used in the D–TRON®[2,3] or D–TRON®[2,3] plus pump should be discarded after 7 days, even if it still contains Humalog. Infusion sites that are erythematous, pruritic, or thickened should be reported to medical personnel, and a new site selected.

Humalog should not be diluted or mixed with any other insulin when used in an external insulin pump.

Laboratory Tests

As with all insulins, the therapeutic response to Humalog should be monitored by periodic blood glucose tests. Periodic measurement of hemoglobin A_{1c} is recommended for the monitoring of long–term glycemic control.

Drug Interactions

Insulin requirements may be increased by medications with hyperglycemic activity such as corticosteroids, isoniazid, certain lipid–lowering drugs (e.g., niacin), estrogens, oral contraceptives, phenothiazines, and thyroid replacement therapy (*see* CLINICAL PHARMACOLOGY).

Insulin requirements may be decreased in the presence of drugs that increase insulin sensitivity or have hypoglycemic activity, such as oral antidiabetic agents, salicylates, sulfa antibiotics, certain antidepressants (monoamine oxidase inhibitors), angiotensin–converting–enzyme inhibitors, angiotensin II receptor blocking agents, beta–adrenergic blockers, inhibitors of pancreatic function (e.g., octreotide), and alcohol. Beta–adrenergic blockers may mask the symptoms of hypoglycemia in some patients.

Mixing of Insulins—Care should be taken when mixing all insulins as a change in peak action may occur. The American Diabetes Association warns in its Position Statement on Insulin Administration, "On mixing, physiochemical changes in the mixture may occur (either immediately or over time). As a result, the physiological response to the insulin mixture may differ from that of the injection of the insulins separately." Mixing Humalog with Humulin N or Humulin® U does not decrease the absorption rate or the total bioavailability of Humalog. Given alone or mixed with Humulin N, Humalog results in a more rapid absorption and glucose–lowering effect compared with Regular human insulin.

The effects of mixing Humalog with insulins of animal source or insulin preparations produced by other manufacturers have not been studied (*see* WARNINGS).

If Humalog is mixed with a longer–acting insulin, such as Humulin N or Humulin U, Humalog should be drawn into the syringe first to prevent clouding of the Humalog by the longer–acting insulin. Injection should be made immediately after mixing. Mixtures should not be administered intravenously.

The cartridge containing Humalog is not designed to allow any other insulin to be mixed in the cartridge, for the Humalog in the cartridge to be diluted or for the cartridge to be refilled with insulin. Humalog should not be diluted or mixed with any other insulin when used in an external insulin pump.

Carcinogenesis, Mutagenesis, Impairment of Fertility

Long–term studies in animals have not been performed to evaluate the carcinogenic potential of Humalog, Humalog Mix75/25, or Humalog Mix50/50. Insulin lispro was not mutagenic in a battery of *in vitro* and *in vivo* genetic toxicity assays (bacterial mutation tests, unscheduled DNA synthesis, mouse lymphoma assay, chromosomal aberration tests, and a micronucleus test). There is no evidence from animal studies of impairment of fertility induced by insulin lispro.

Pregnancy

Teratogenic Effects—Pregnancy Category B

Reproduction studies have been performed in pregnant rats and rabbits at parenteral doses up to 4 and 0.3 times, respectively, the average human dose (40 units/day) based on body surface area. The results have revealed no evidence of impaired fertility or harm to the fetus due to Humalog. There are, however, no adequate and well–controlled studies with Humalog, Humalog Mix75/25, or Humalog Mix50/50 in pregnant women. Because animal reproduction studies are not always predictive of human response, this drug should be used during pregnancy only if clearly needed.

Although there are limited clinical studies of the use of Humalog in pregnancy, published studies with human insulins suggest that optimizing overall glycemic control, including postprandial control, before conception and during pregnancy improves fetal outcome. Although the fetal complications of maternal hyperglycemia have been well documented, fetal toxicity also has been reported with maternal hypoglycemia. Insulin requirements usually fall during the first trimester and increase during the second and third trimesters. Careful monitoring of the patient is required throughout pregnancy. During the perinatal period, careful monitoring of infants born to mothers with diabetes is warranted.

Nursing Mothers

It is unknown whether Humalog is excreted in significant amounts in human milk. Many drugs, including human insulin, are excreted in human milk. For this reason, caution should be exercised when Humalog is administered to a nursing woman. Patients with diabetes who are lactating may require adjustments in Humalog dose, meal plan, or both.

Pediatric Use

In a 9–month, cross–over study of pre–pubescent children (n=60), aged 3 to 11 years, comparable glycemic control as measured by HbA_{1c} was achieved regardless of treatment group: Regular human insulin 30 minutes before meals 8.4%, Humalog immediately before meals 8.4%, and Humalog immediately after meals 8.5%. In an 8–month, cross–over study of adolescents (n=463), aged 9 to 19 years, comparable glycemic control as measured by HbA_{1c} was achieved regardless of treatment group: Regular human insulin 30 to 45 minutes before meals 8.7% and Humalog immediately before meals 8.7%. The incidence of hypoglycemia was similar for all three treatment regimens. Adjustment of basal insulin may be required. To improve accuracy in dosing in pediatric patients, a diluent may be used. If the diluent is added directly to the Humalog vial, the shelf–life may be reduced (*see* DOSAGE AND ADMINISTRATION).

Geriatric Use

Of the total number of subjects (n=2834) in eight clinical studies of Humalog, twelve percent (n=338) were 65 years of age or over. The majority of these were patients with type 2 diabetes. HbA_{1c} values and hypoglycemia rates did not differ by age. Pharmacokinetic/pharmacodynamic studies to assess the effect of age on the onset of Humalog action have not been performed.

ADVERSE REACTIONS

Clinical studies comparing Humalog with Regular human insulin did not demonstrate a difference in frequency of adverse events between the two treatments.

Adverse events commonly associated with human insulin therapy include the following:

Body as a Whole—allergic reactions (*see* PRECAUTIONS).

Skin and Appendages—injection site reaction, lipodystrophy, pruritus, rash.
Other—hypoglycemia (see WARNINGS and PRECAUTIONS).

OVERDOSAGE

Hypoglycemia may occur as a result of an excess of insulin relative to food intake, energy expenditure, or both. Mild episodes of hypoglycemia usually can be treated with oral glucose. Adjustments in drug dosage, meal patterns, or exercise, may be needed. More severe episodes with coma, seizure, or neurologic impairment may be treated with intramuscular/subcutaneous glucagon or concentrated intravenous glucose. Sustained carbohydrate intake and observation may be necessary because hypoglycemia may recur after apparent clinical recovery.

DOSAGE AND ADMINISTRATION

Humalog is intended for subcutaneous administration, including use in select external insulin pumps (see DOSAGE AND ADMINISTRATION, *External Insulin Pumps*). Dosage regimens of Humalog will vary among patients and should be determined by the healthcare provider familiar with the patient's metabolic needs, eating habits, and other lifestyle variables. Pharmacokinetic and pharmacodynamic studies showed Humalog to be equipotent to Regular human insulin (i.e., one unit of Humalog has the same glucose–lowering effect as one unit of Regular human insulin), but with more rapid activity. The quicker glucose–lowering effect of Humalog is related to the more rapid absorption rate from subcutaneous tissue. An adjustment of dose or schedule of basal insulin may be needed when a patient changes from other insulins to Humalog, particularly to prevent pre–meal hyperglycemia.

When used as a meal–time insulin, Humalog should be given within 15 minutes before or immediately after a meal. Regular human insulin is best given 30 to 60 minutes before a meal. To achieve optimal glucose control, the amount of longer–acting insulin being given may need to be adjusted when using Humalog.

The rate of insulin absorption and consequently the onset of activity are known to be affected by the site of injection, exercise, and other variables. Humalog was absorbed at a consistently faster rate than Regular human insulin in healthy male volunteers given 0.2 U/kg Regular human insulin or Humalog at abdominal, deltoid, or femoral sites, the three sites often used by patients with diabetes. When not mixed in the same syringe with other insulins, Humalog maintains its rapid onset of action and has less variability in its onset of action among injection sites compared with Regular human insulin (see PRECAUTIONS). After abdominal administration, Humalog concentrations are higher than those following deltoid or thigh injections. Also, the duration of action of Humalog is slightly shorter following abdominal injection, compared with deltoid and femoral injections. As with all insulin preparations, the time course of action of Humalog may vary considerably in different individuals or within the same individual. Patients must be educated to use proper injection techniques.

Humalog in a vial may be diluted with STERILE DILUENT for Humalog®, Humulin® N, Humulin® R, Humulin® 70/30, and Humulin® R U-500 to a concentration of 1:10 (equivalent to U–10) or 1:2 (equivalent to U–50). Diluted Humalog may remain in patient use for 28 days when stored at 5°C (41°F) and for 14 days when stored at 30°C (86°F). Do not dilute Humalog contained in a cartridge or Humalog used in an external insulin pump.

Parenteral drug products should be inspected visually before use whenever the solution and the container permit. If the solution is cloudy, contains particulate matter, is thickened, or is discolored, the contents must not be injected. Humalog should not be used after its expiration date.

The cartridge containing Humalog is not designed to allow any other insulin to be mixed in the cartridge or for the cartridge to be refilled with insulin.

External Insulin Pumps—Humalog was tested in MiniMed®[1] Models 506, 507, and 508 insulin pumps using MiniMed®[1] Polyfin®[1] infusion sets. Humalog was also tested in the Disetronic®[2] H–TRONplus® V100 insulin pump (with plastic 3.15 mL insulin reservoir) and the Disetronic D–TRON®[2,3] and D–TRON®[2,3] plus pumps (with Humalog 3 mL cartridges) using Disetronic Rapid®[2] infusion sets.

Humalog should not be diluted or mixed with any other insulin when used in an external insulin pump.

HOW SUPPLIED

Humalog [insulin lispro injection, USP (rDNA origin)] is available in the following package sizes: each presentation containing 100 units insulin lispro per mL (U-100).

10 mL vials	NDC 0002–7510–01 (VL-7510)
3 mL vials	NDC 0002–7510–17 (VL-7533)
5 × 3 mL cartridges[3]	NDC 0002–7516–59 (VL-7516)
5 × 3 mL prefilled insulin delivery devices (Pen)	NDC 0002–8725–59 (HP-8725)
5 × 3 mL prefilled insulin delivery devices (Humalog KwikPen)	NDC 0002–8799–59 (HP-8799)

[1] MiniMed® and Polyfin® are registered trademarks of MiniMed, Inc.
[2] Disetronic®, H–TRONplus®, D–TRON®, and Rapid® are registered trademarks of Roche Diagnostics GMBH.
[3] 3 mL cartridge is for use in Eli Lilly and Company's HumaPen® MEMOIR™ and HumaPen® LUXURA™ HD insulin delivery devices, Owen Mumford, Ltd.'s Autopen® 3 mL insulin delivery device and Disetronic D–TRON® and D–TRON®plus pumps. Autopen® is a registered trademark of Owen Mumford, Ltd. HumaPen®, Humalog®, Humalog® KwikPen™, HumaPen® MEMOIR™ and HumaPen® LUXURA™ HD are trademarks of Eli Lilly and Company.

Other product and company names may be the trademarks of their respective owners.

Storage—Unopened Humalog should be stored in a refrigerator [2° to 8°C (36° to 46°F)], but not in the freezer. Do not use Humalog if it has been frozen. Unrefrigerated [below 30°C (86°F)] vials, cartridges, Pens, and Humalog KwikPen must be used within 28 days or be discarded, even if they still contain Humalog. Protect from direct heat and light. See table below:
[See table below]
Use in an External Insulin Pump—A Humalog 3 mL cartridge used in the D–TRON®[2,3] or D–TRON®[2,3] plus should be discarded after 7 days, even if it still contains Humalog. Infusion sets, D–TRON®[2,3] and D–TRON®[2,3] plus cartridge adapters, and Humalog in the external insulin pump reservoir should be discarded every 48 hours or less.

Literature revised September 2, 2009
Humalog KwikPen manufactured by
Eli Lilly and Company, Indianapolis, IN 46285, USA
Pens manufactured by
Eli Lilly and Company, Indianapolis, IN 46285, USA or Lilly France, F-67640 Fegersheim, France
10 mL Vials manufactured by
Eli Lilly and Company, Indianapolis, IN 46285, USA or Hospira, Inc., Lake Forest, IL 60045, USA or Lilly France, F-67640 Fegersheim, France
3 mL Vials manufactured by
Eli Lilly and Company, Indianapolis, IN 46285, USA
Cartridges manufactured by
Lilly France, F-67640 Fegersheim, France
for Eli Lilly and Company, Indianapolis, IN 46285, USA
www.humalog.com

Copyright © 2007, 2009, Eli Lilly and Company. All rights reserved.
PV 5532 AMP

Patient Information

HUMALOG® (HU-ma-log)
insulin lispro injection, USP (rDNA origin)

Important:
Know your insulin. Do not change the type of insulin you use unless told to do so by your healthcare provider. Your insulin dose and the time you take your dose can change with different types of insulin.
Make sure you have the right type and strength of insulin prescribed for you.

Read the Patient Information that comes with Humalog before you start using it and each time you get a refill. There may be new information. This leaflet does not take the place of talking with your healthcare provider about your diabe-

tes or treatment. Make sure that you know how to manage your diabetes. Ask your healthcare provider if you have questions about managing your diabetes.
What is Humalog?
Humalog is an injectable fast-acting man-made insulin. Humalog is used to control high blood sugar (glucose) in people with diabetes.
Humalog comes in:
- 10 mL vials (bottles) for use with a syringe or external insulin pump
- 3 mL vials (bottles) for use with a syringe or external insulin pump
- 3 mL prefilled pens
- 3 mL cartridges for use with a reusable pen or external insulin pump
Who should not take Humalog?
Do not take Humalog if:
- your blood sugar is too low (hypoglycemia). After treating your low blood sugar, follow your healthcare provider's instructions on the use of Humalog.
- you are allergic to anything in Humalog. See the end of this leaflet for a complete list of ingredients in Humalog.
Tell your healthcare provider:
- **about all your medical conditions.** Medical conditions can affect your insulin needs and your dose of Humalog.
- **if you are pregnant or breastfeeding.** You and your healthcare provider should talk about the best way to manage your diabetes while you are pregnant or breastfeeding. Humalog has not been studied in pregnant or nursing women.
- **about all the medicines you take, including prescription and non-prescription medicines, vitamins and herbal supplements.** Many medicines can affect your blood sugar levels and insulin needs. Your Humalog dose may need to change if you take other medicines.
Know the medicines you take. Keep a list of your medicines with you to show to all of your healthcare providers.
How should I use Humalog?
Humalog can be used with a syringe, prefilled pen, reusable pen or external insulin pump. Talk to your healthcare provider if you have any questions. Your healthcare provider will tell you the right syringes to use with Humalog vials. Your healthcare provider should show you how to inject Humalog before you start using it.
- **Read the User Manual that comes with your Humalog prefilled pen and the manufacturer's instructions that comes with your external insulin pump. Use Humalog exactly as prescribed by your healthcare provider.**
- **If you have type 1 diabetes, you need to take a longer-acting insulin in addition to Humalog (except when using an external insulin pump).**
- **If you have type 2 diabetes, you may be taking diabetes pills and/or a longer-acting insulin in addition to Humalog.**
- **Humalog starts working faster than other insulins that contain regular human insulin. Inject Humalog within fifteen minutes before eating or right after eating a meal.**
- **Check your blood sugar levels as told by your healthcare provider.**
- Look at your Humalog before using. Humalog should be clear, have no color and look like water. If your Humalog is cloudy, thickened, even slightly colored, or has solid particles or clumps in it, do not use. Return it to your pharmacy for new Humalog.
- Humalog can be mixed with a longer-acting human insulin, but only if you are told to do so by your healthcare provider. If you are mixing two types of insulin, always draw Humalog into the syringe first. Talk with your healthcare provider about how to properly mix Humalog with a different insulin.
- Humalog can be used in an external insulin pump either by withdrawing Humalog from a vial or using a 3 mL Humalog cartridge that is inserted into the pump.
- Humalog was tested with MiniMed®[1] Models 506, 507, and 508 insulin pumps using MiniMed Polyfin®[1] infusion sets. Humalog was also tested with the Disetronic®[2] H-TRONplus®[2] V100 insulin pump (with plastic 3.15 mL insulin reservoir), using the Disetronic Rapid®[2] infusion set.
- A Humalog cartridge used in the D-TRON[2] or D-TRONplus[2] pump, may be used for up to 7 days. Humalog in the external insulin pump reservoir and the complete infusion set should be replaced and a new infusion site selected every 48 hours or less.
- Humalog in an external insulin pump should not be exposed to temperature above 98.6°F (37°C), such as in a sauna or hot tub, hot showers, direct sunlight, or radiant heaters.
- **Inject your dose of Humalog under the skin of your stomach area, upper arm, upper leg, or buttocks. Never inject Humalog into a muscle or vein.**
- Change (rotate) your injection site with each dose.
- Your insulin needs may change because of:
  - illness

	Not In-Use (Unopened) Room Temperature [Below 30°C (86°F)]	Not In-Use (Unopened) Refrigerated	In-Use (Opened) Room Temperature, [Below 30°C (86°F)]
10 mL Vial and 3 mL Vial	28 days	Until expiration date	28 days, refrigerated/room temperature
3 mL Cartridge	28 days	Until expiration date	28 days, **Do not refrigerate.**
3 mL Pen and Humalog KwikPen (prefilled)	28 days	Until expiration date	28 days, **Do not refrigerate.**

- stress
- other medicines you take
- changes in eating
- physical activity changes

Follow your healthcare provider's instructions to make changes in your insulin dose.

- **Never dilute or mix Humalog with another insulin in the same prefilled pen, cartridge or external insulin pump.**
- **Always carry a quick source of sugar to treat low blood sugar, such as glucose tablets, hard candy, or juice.**

What are the possible side effects of Humalog?
Low Blood Sugar (Hypoglycemia). Symptoms of low blood sugar include:

- hunger
- dizziness
- feeling shaky or shakiness
- lightheadedness
- sweating
- irritability
- headache
- fast heartbeat
- confusion

Low blood sugar symptoms can happen suddenly. Symptoms of low blood sugar may be different for each person and may change from time to time. Severe low blood sugar can cause seizures and death. Low blood sugar may affect your ability to drive a car or use mechanical equipment, risking injury to yourself or others. Know your symptoms of low blood sugar. Low blood sugar can be treated by drinking juice or regular soda or eating glucose tablets, sugar, or hard candy. Follow your healthcare provider's instructions for treating low blood sugar. Talk to your healthcare provider if low blood sugar is a problem for you.

- **Serious allergic reactions** (whole body allergic reaction). Severe, life-threatening allergic reactions can happen with insulin. Get medical help right away if you develop a rash over your whole body, have trouble breathing, wheezing, a fast heartbeat, or sweating.
- **Reactions at the injection site** (local allergic reaction). You may get redness, swelling, and itching at the injection site. If you keep having injection site reactions or they are serious, you need to call your healthcare provider. Do not inject insulin into a skin area that is red, swollen, or itchy.
- **Skin thickens or pits at the injection site (lipodystrophy).** This can happen if you don't change (rotate) your injection sites enough.

These are not all the side effects from Humalog. Ask your healthcare provider or pharmacist for more information.

How should I store Humalog?

- **Store all unopened (unused) Humalog in the original carton in a refrigerator at 36°F to 46°F (2°C to 8°C).** Do not freeze.
- Do not use Humalog that has been frozen.
- Do not use after the expiration date printed on the carton and label.
- Protect Humalog from extreme heat, cold or light.

After starting use (open):

- **Vials:** Keep in the refrigerator or at room temperature below 86°F (30°C) for up to 28 days. Keep open vials away from direct heat or light. Throw away an opened vial 28 days after first use, even if there is insulin left in the vial.
- **Cartridge and Prefilled Pens:** Do not store a cartridge or prefilled pen that you are using in the refrigerator. Keep at room temperature below 86°F (30°C) for up to 28 days. Throw away a cartridge or prefilled pen 28 days after first use, even if there is insulin left in the cartridge or the pen.

General information about Humalog
Use Humalog only to treat your diabetes. Do not share it with anyone else, even if they also have diabetes. It may harm them.

This leaflet summarized the most important information about Humalog. If you would like more information about Humalog or diabetes, talk with your healthcare provider. You can ask your healthcare provider or pharmacist for information about Humalog that is written for health professionals.

For questions you may call 1–800–LillyRx (1–800–545–5979) or visit www.humalog.com.

What are the ingredients in Humalog?
Active ingredient: insulin lispro.
Inactive ingredients: glycerin, dibasic sodium phosphate, metacresol, zinc oxide (zinc ion), trace amounts of phenol and water for injection.

[1] MiniMed® and Polyfin® are registered trademarks of MiniMed, Inc.
[2] Disetronic®, H-TRONplus®, D-TRON®, D-TRONplus and Rapid® are registered trademarks of Roche Diagnostics GMBH.

Humalog® and Humalog® KwikPen™ are registered trademarks of Eli Lilly and Company.
Patient Information revised September 2, 2009
Humalog KwikPen manufactured by
Eli Lilly and Company, Indianapolis, IN 46285, USA

Pens manufactured by
Eli Lilly and Company, Indianapolis, IN 46285, USA or
Lilly France, F-67640 Fegersheim, France
10 mL Vials manufactured by
Eli Lilly and Company, Indianapolis, IN 46285, USA or
Hospira, Inc., Lake Forest, IL 60045, USA or
Lilly France, F-67640 Fegersheim, France
3 mL Vials manufactured by
Eli Lilly and Company, Indianapolis, IN 46285, USA
Cartridges manufactured by
Lilly France, F-67640 Fegersheim, France
for Eli Lilly and Company, Indianapolis, IN 46285, USA
www.humalog.com
Copyright © 2007, 2009, Eli Lilly and Company. All rights reserved.
PV 5561 AMP
Revised: 02-2010   Distributed by: Eli Lilly and Company
Shown in Product Identification Guide, page 311

HUMALOG® Mix50/50™ ℞
[hū'mă-lŏg]
50% INSULIN LISPRO PROTAMINE SUSPENSIONAND 50% INSULIN LISPRO INJECTION
(rDNA ORIGIN)
100 UNITS PER ML (U-100)

DESCRIPTION
Humalog® Mix50/50™ [50% insulin lispro protamine suspension and 50% insulin lispro injection, (rDNA origin)] is a mixture of insulin lispro solution, a rapid-acting blood glucose-lowering agent and insulin lispro protamine suspension, an intermediate-acting blood glucose-lowering agent. Chemically, insulin lispro is Lys(B28), Pro(B29) human insulin analog, created when the amino acids at positions 28 and 29 on the insulin B-chain are reversed. Insulin lispro is synthesized in a special non-pathogenic laboratory strain of *Escherichia coli* bacteria that has been genetically altered to produce insulin lispro. Insulin lispro protamine suspension (NPL component) is a suspension of crystals produced from combining insulin lispro and protamine sulfate under appropriate conditions for crystal formation.
Insulin lispro has the following primary structure:

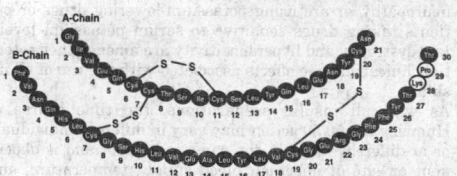

Insulin lispro has the empirical formula $C_{257}H_{383}N_{65}O_{77}S_6$ and a molecular weight of 5808, both identical to that of human insulin.
Humalog Mix50/50 vials and Pens contain a sterile suspension of insulin lispro protamine suspension mixed with soluble insulin lispro for use as an injection.
Each milliliter of Humalog Mix50/50 injection contains insulin lispro 100 units, 0.19 mg protamine sulfate, 16 mg glycerin, 3.78 mg dibasic sodium phosphate, 2.20 mg Metacresol, zinc oxide content adjusted to provide 0.0305 mg zinc ion, 0.89 mg phenol, and Water for Injection. Humalog Mix50/50 has a pH of 7.0 to 7.8. Hydrochloric acid 10% and/or sodium hydroxide 10% may have been added to adjust pH.

CLINICAL PHARMACOLOGY
Antidiabetic Activity
The primary activity of insulin, including Humalog Mix50/50, is the regulation of glucose metabolism. In addition, all insulins have several anabolic and anti-catabolic actions on many tissues in the body. In muscle and other tissues (except the brain), insulin causes rapid transport of glucose and amino acids intracellularly, promotes anabolism, and inhibits protein catabolism. In the liver, insulin promotes the uptake and storage of glucose in the form of glycogen, inhibits gluconeogenesis, and promotes the conversion of excess glucose into fat.
Insulin lispro, the rapid-acting component of Humalog Mix50/50, has been shown to be equipotent to Regular human insulin on a molar basis. One unit of Humalog® has the same glucose-lowering effect as one unit of Regular human insulin, but its effect is more rapid and of shorter duration.

Pharmacokinetics
Absorption
Studies in nondiabetic subjects and patients with type 1 (insulin-dependent) diabetes demonstrated that Humalog, the rapid-acting component of Humalog Mix50/50, is absorbed faster than Regular human insulin (U-100). In nondiabetic subjects given subcutaneous doses of Humalog

ranging from 0.1 to 0.4 U/kg, peak serum concentrations were observed 30 to 90 minutes after dosing. When nondiabetic subjects received equivalent doses of Regular human insulin, peak insulin concentrations occurred between 50 to 120 minutes after dosing. Similar results were seen in patients with type 1 diabetes.

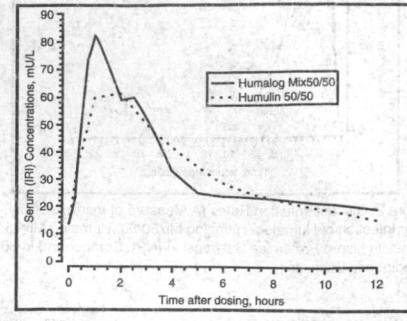

Figure 1: Serum Immunoreactive Insulin (IRI) Concentrations, After Subcutaneous Injection of Humalog Mix50/50 or Humulin 50/50 in Healthy Nondiabetic Subjects.

Humalog Mix50/50 has two phases of absorption. The early phase represents insulin lispro and its distinct characteristics of rapid onset. The late phase represents the prolonged action of insulin lispro protamine suspension. In 30 healthy nondiabetic subjects given subcutaneous doses (0.3 U/kg) of Humalog Mix50/50, peak serum concentrations were observed 45 minutes to 13.5 hours (median, 60 minutes) after dosing (*see* Figure 1). In patients with type 1 diabetes, peak serum concentrations were observed 45 minutes to 120 minutes (median, 60 minutes) after dosing. The rapid absorption characteristics of Humalog are maintained with Humalog Mix50/50 (*see* Figure 1).
Direct comparison of Humalog Mix50/50 and Humulin 50/50 was not performed. However, a cross-study comparison shown in Figure 1 suggests that Humalog Mix50/50 has a more rapid absorption than Humulin 50/50.
Distribution
Radiolabeled distribution studies of Humalog Mix50/50 have not been conducted. However, the volume of distribution following injection of Humalog is identical to that of Regular human insulin, with a range of 0.26 to 0.36 L/kg.
Metabolism
Human metabolism studies of Humalog Mix50/50 have not been conducted. Studies in animals indicate that the metabolism of Humalog, the rapid-acting component of Humalog Mix50/50, is identical to that of Regular human insulin.
Elimination
Humalog Mix50/50 has two absorption phases, a rapid and a prolonged phase, representative of the insulin lispro and insulin lispro protamine suspension components of the mixture. As with other intermediate-acting insulins, a meaningful terminal phase half-life cannot be calculated after administration of Humalog Mix50/50 because of the prolonged insulin lispro protamine suspension absorption.

Pharmacodynamics
Studies in nondiabetic subjects and patients with diabetes demonstrated that Humalog has a more rapid onset of glucose-lowering activity, an earlier peak for glucose-lowering, and a shorter duration of glucose-lowering activity than Regular human insulin. The early onset of activity of Humalog Mix50/50 is directly related to the rapid absorption of Humalog. The time course of action of insulin and insulin analogs, such as Humalog (and hence Humalog Mix50/50), may vary considerably in different individuals or within the same individual. The parameters of Humalog Mix50/50 activity (time of onset, peak time, and duration) as presented in Figures 2 and 3 should be considered only as general guidelines. The rate of insulin absorption and consequently the onset of activity is known to be affected by the site of injection, exercise, and other variables (*see* General *under* PRECAUTIONS).
In a glucose clamp study performed in 30 nondiabetic subjects, the onset of action and glucose-lowering activity of Humalog, Humalog Mix50/50, Humalog® Mix75/25™, and insulin lispro protamine suspension (NPL component) were compared (*see* Figure 2). Graphs of mean glucose infusion rate versus time showed a distinct insulin activity profile for each formulation. The rapid onset of glucose-lowering activity characteristic of Humalog was maintained in Humalog Mix50/50.
Direct comparison between Humalog Mix50/50 and Humulin 50/50 was not performed. However, a cross-study comparison shown on Figure 3 suggests that Humalog Mix50/50 has a duration of activity that is similar to Humulin 50/50.

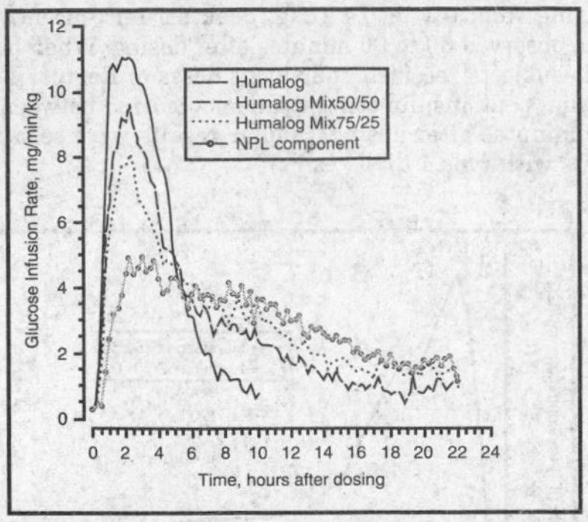

Figure 2: Glucose Infusion Rates (A Measure of Insulin Activity) After Injection of Humalog, Humalog Mix50/50, Humalog Mix75/25, or Insulin Lispro Protamine Suspension (NPL Component) in 30 Nondiabetic Subjects.

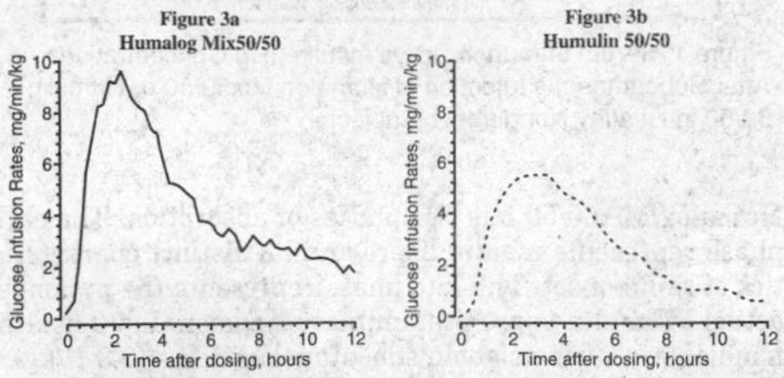

Figure 3: Insulin Activity After Subcutaneous Injection of Humalog Mix50/50 and Humulin 50/50 in Nondiabetic Subjects.

Figures 2 and 3 represent insulin activity profiles as measured by glucose clamp studies in healthy nondiabetic subjects.

Figure 2 shows the time activity profiles of Humalog, Humalog Mix75/25, Humalog Mix50/50, and insulin lispro protamine suspension (NPL component).

Figure 3 is a comparison of the time activity profiles of Humalog Mix50/50 (*see* Figure 3a) and of Humulin 50/50 (*see* Figure 3b) from two different studies.

Special Populations

Age and Gender

Information on the effect of age on the pharmacokinetics of Humalog Mix50/50 is unavailable. Pharmacokinetic and pharmacodynamic comparisons between men and women administered Humalog Mix50/50 showed no gender differences. In large Humalog clinical trials, sub-group analysis based on age and gender demonstrated that differences between Humalog and Regular human insulin in postprandial glucose parameters are maintained across sub-groups.

Smoking

The effect of smoking on the pharmacokinetics and pharmacodynamics of Humalog Mix50/50 has not been studied.

Pregnancy

The effect of pregnancy on the pharmacokinetics and pharmacodynamics of Humalog Mix50/50 has not been studied.

Obesity

The effect of obesity and/or subcutaneous fat thickness on the pharmacokinetics and pharmacodynamics of Humalog Mix50/50 has not been studied. In large clinical trials, which included patients with Body Mass Index up to and including 35 kg/m^2, no consistent differences were observed between Humalog and Humulin® R with respect to postprandial glucose parameters.

Renal Impairment

The effect of renal impairment on the pharmacokinetics and pharmacodynamics of Humalog Mix50/50 has not been studied. In a study of 25 patients with type 2 diabetes and a wide range of renal function, the pharmacokinetic differences between Humalog and Regular human insulin were generally maintained. However, the sensitivity of the patients to insulin did change, with an increased response to insulin as the renal function declined. Careful glucose monitoring and dose reductions of insulin, including Humalog Mix50/50, may be necessary in patients with renal dysfunction.

Hepatic Impairment

Some studies with human insulin have shown increased circulating levels of insulin in patients with hepatic failure. The effect of hepatic impairment on the pharmacokinetics and pharmacodynamics of Humalog Mix50/50 has not been studied. However, in a study of 22 patients with type 2 diabetes, impaired hepatic function did not affect the subcutaneous absorption or general disposition of Humalog when compared with patients with no history of hepatic dysfunction. In that study, Humalog maintained its more rapid absorption and elimination when compared with Regular human insulin. Careful glucose monitoring and dose adjustments of insulin, including Humalog Mix50/50, may be necessary in patients with hepatic dysfunction.

INDICATIONS AND USAGE

Humalog Mix50/50, a mixture of 50% insulin lispro protamine suspension and 50% insulin lispro injection, (rDNA origin), is indicated in the treatment of patients with diabetes mellitus for the control of hyperglycemia. Based on cross-study comparisons of the pharmacodynamics of Humalog Mix50/50 and Humulin 50/50, it is likely that Humalog Mix50/50 has a more rapid onset of glucose-lowering activity compared with Humulin 50/50 while having a similar duration of action. This profile is achieved by combining the rapid onset of Humalog with the intermediate action of insulin lispro protamine suspension.

CONTRAINDICATIONS

Humalog Mix50/50 is contraindicated during episodes of hypoglycemia and in patients sensitive to insulin lispro or any of the excipients contained in the formulation.

WARNINGS

Humalog differs from Regular human insulin by its rapid onset of action as well as a shorter duration of activity. Therefore, the dose of Humalog Mix50/50 should be given within 15 minutes before a meal.

Hypoglycemia is the most common adverse effect associated with the use of insulins, including Humalog Mix50/50. As with all insulins, the timing of hypoglycemia may differ among various insulin formulations. Glucose monitoring is recommended for all patients with diabetes.

Any change of insulin should be made cautiously and only under medical supervision. Changes in insulin strength, manufacturer, type (e.g., Regular, NPH, analog), species, or method of manufacture may result in the need for a change in dosage.

PRECAUTIONS

General

Hypoglycemia and hypokalemia are among the potential clinical adverse effects associated with the use of all insulins. Because of differences in the action of Humalog Mix50/50 and other insulins, care should be taken in patients in whom such potential side effects might be clinically relevant (e.g., patients who are fasting, have autonomic neuropathy, or are using potassium-lowering drugs or patients taking drugs sensitive to serum potassium level). Lipodystrophy and hypersensitivity are among other potential clinical adverse effects associated with the use of all insulins.

As with all insulin preparations, the time course of Humalog Mix50/50 action may vary in different individuals or at different times in the same individual and is dependent on site of injection, blood supply, temperature, and physical activity.

Adjustment of dosage of any insulin may be necessary if patients change their physical activity or their usual meal plan. Insulin requirements may be altered during illness, emotional disturbances, or other stress.

Hypoglycemia—As with all insulin preparations, hypoglycemic reactions may be associated with the administration of Humalog Mix50/50. Rapid changes in serum glucose concentrations may induce symptoms of hypoglycemia in persons with diabetes, regardless of the glucose value. Early warning symptoms of hypoglycemia may be different or less pronounced under certain conditions, such as long duration of diabetes, diabetic nerve disease, use of medications such as beta-blockers, or intensified diabetes control.

Renal Impairment—As with other insulins, the requirements for Humalog Mix50/50 may be reduced in patients with renal impairment.

Hepatic Impairment—Although impaired hepatic function does not affect the absorption or disposition of Humalog, careful glucose monitoring and dose adjustments of insulin, including Humalog Mix50/50, may be necessary.

Allergy—Local Allergy—As with any insulin therapy, patients may experience redness, swelling, or itching at the site of injection. These minor reactions usually resolve in a few days to a few weeks. In some instances, these reactions may be related to factors other than insulin, such as irritants in the skin cleansing agent or poor injection technique.

Systemic Allergy—Less common, but potentially more serious, is generalized allergy to insulin, which may cause rash (including pruritus) over the whole body, shortness of breath, wheezing, reduction in blood pressure, rapid pulse, or sweating. Severe cases of generalized allergy, including anaphylactic reaction, may be life threatening. Localized reactions and generalized myalgias have been reported with the use of cresol as an injectable excipient.

Antibody Production—In clinical trials, antibodies that cross-react with human insulin and insulin lispro were observed in both human insulin mixtures and insulin lispro mixtures treatment groups.

Information for Patients

Patients should be informed of the potential risks and advantages of Humalog Mix50/50 and alternative therapies. Patients should not mix Humalog Mix50/50 with any other insulin. They should also be informed about the importance of proper insulin storage, injection technique, timing of dosage, adherence to meal planning, regular physical activity, regular blood glucose monitoring, periodic hemoglobin A_{1c} testing, recognition and management of hypo- and hyperglycemia, and periodic assessment for diabetes complications.

Patients should be advised to inform their physician if they are pregnant or intend to become pregnant.

Refer patients to the Patient Information leaflet for information on normal appearance, timing of dosing (within 15 minutes before a meal), storage, and common adverse effects.

For Patients Using Insulin Pen Delivery Devices: Before starting therapy, patients should read the Patient Information leaflet that accompanies the drug product and the User Manual that accompanies the delivery device and re-read them each time the prescription is renewed. Patients should be instructed on how to properly use the delivery device, prime the Pen to a stream of insulin, and properly dispose of needles. Patients should be advised not to share their Pens with others.

Laboratory Tests

As with all insulins, the therapeutic response to Humalog Mix50/50 should be monitored by periodic blood glucose tests. Periodic measurement of hemoglobin A_{1c} is recommended for the monitoring of long-term glycemic control.

Drug Interactions

Insulin requirements may be increased by medications with hyperglycemic activity such as corticosteroids, isoniazid, certain lipid-lowering drugs (e.g., niacin), estrogens, oral contraceptives, phenothiazines, and thyroid replacement therapy.

Insulin requirements may be decreased in the presence of drugs that increase insulin sensitivity or have hypoglycemic activity, such as oral antidiabetic agents, salicylates, sulfa antibiotics, certain antidepressants (monoamine oxidase inhibitors), angiotensin-converting-enzyme inhibitors, angiotensin II receptor blocking agents, beta-adrenergic blockers, inhibitors of pancreatic function (e.g., octreotide), and alcohol. Beta-adrenergic blockers may mask the symptoms of hypoglycemia in some patients.

Carcinogenesis, Mutagenesis, Impairment of Fertility

Long-term studies in animals have not been performed to evaluate the carcinogenic potential of Humalog, Humalog Mix75/25, or Humalog Mix50/50. Insulin lispro was not mutagenic in a battery of *in vitro* and *in vivo* genetic toxicity assays (bacterial mutation tests, unscheduled DNA synthesis, mouse lymphoma assay, chromosomal aberration tests, and a micronucleus test). There is no evidence from animal studies of impairment of fertility induced by insulin lispro.

Pregnancy

Teratogenic Effects—Pregnancy Category B

Reproduction studies with insulin lispro have been performed in pregnant rats and rabbits at parenteral doses up to 4 and 0.3 times, respectively, the average human dose (40 units/day) based on body surface area. The results have revealed no evidence of impaired fertility or harm to the fetus due to insulin lispro. There are, however, no adequate and well-controlled studies with Humalog, Humalog Mix75/25, or Humalog Mix50/50 in pregnant women. Because animal reproduction studies are not always predictive of human response, this drug should be used during pregnancy only if clearly needed.

Nursing Mothers

It is unknown whether insulin lispro is excreted in significant amounts in human milk. Many drugs, including human insulin, are excreted in human milk. For this reason, caution should be exercised when Humalog Mix50/50 is administered to a nursing woman. Patients with diabetes who are lactating may require adjustments in Humalog Mix50/50 dose, meal plan, or both.

Pediatric Use

Safety and effectiveness of Humalog Mix50/50 in patients less than 18 years of age have not been established.

Geriatric Use

Clinical studies of Humalog Mix50/50 did not include sufficient numbers of patients aged 65 and over to determine whether they respond differently than younger patients. In general, dose selection for an elderly patient should take into consideration the greater frequency of decreased hepatic, renal, or cardiac function, and of concomitant disease or other drug therapy in this population.

ADVERSE REACTIONS

Clinical studies comparing Humalog Mix50/50 with human insulin mixtures did not demonstrate a difference in frequency of adverse events between the two treatments.

Adverse events commonly associated with human insulin therapy include the following:

Body as a Whole—allergic reactions (see PRECAUTIONS).
Skin and Appendages—injection site reaction, lipodystrophy, pruritus, rash.
Other—hypoglycemia (see WARNINGS and PRECAUTIONS).

OVERDOSAGE

Hypoglycemia may occur as a result of an excess of insulin relative to food intake, energy expenditure, or both. Mild episodes of hypoglycemia usually can be treated with oral glucose. Adjustments in drug dosage, meal patterns, or exercise, may be needed. More severe episodes with coma, seizure, or neurologic impairment may be treated with intramuscular/subcutaneous glucagon or concentrated intravenous glucose. Sustained carbohydrate intake and observation may be necessary because hypoglycemia may recur after apparent clinical recovery.

DOSAGE AND ADMINISTRATION

[See table 1 at right]
Humalog Mix50/50 is intended only for subcutaneous administration. Humalog Mix50/50 should not be administered intravenously. Dosage regimens of Humalog Mix50/50 will vary among patients and should be determined by the healthcare provider familiar with the patient's metabolic needs, eating habits, and other lifestyle variables. Humalog has been shown to be equipotent to Regular human insulin on a molar basis. One unit of Humalog has the same glucose-lowering effect as one unit of Regular human insulin, but its effect is more rapid and of shorter duration. The quicker glucose-lowering effect of Humalog is related to the more rapid absorption rate of insulin lispro from subcutaneous tissue.

Direct comparison between Humalog Mix50/50 and Humulin 50/50 was not performed. However, a cross-study comparison shown in Figure 3 suggests that Humalog Mix50/50 has a duration of activity that is similar to Humulin 50/50.

The rate of insulin absorption and consequently the onset of activity are known to be affected by the site of injection, exercise, and other variables. As with all insulin preparations, the time course of action of Humalog Mix50/50 may vary considerably in different individuals or within the same individual. Patients must be educated to use proper injection techniques.

Humalog Mix50/50 should be inspected visually before use. Humalog Mix50/50 should be used only if it appears uniformly cloudy after mixing. Humalog Mix50/50 should not be used after its expiration date.

HOW SUPPLIED

Humalog Mix50/50 [50% insulin lispro protamine suspension and 50% insulin lispro injection, (rDNA origin)] is available in the following package sizes: each presentation containing 100 units insulin lispro per mL (U-100).
[See second table above]
Storage—Humalog Mix50/50 should be stored in a refrigerator [2° to 8°C (36° to 46°F)], but not in the freezer. Do not use Humalog Mix50/50 if it has been frozen. Unrefrigerated [below 30°C (86°F)] vials must be used within 28 days or be discarded, even if they still contain Humalog Mix50/50. Unrefrigerated [below 30°C (86°F)] Pens, and KwikPens must be used within 10 days or be discarded, even if they still contain Humalog Mix50/50. Protect from direct heat and light. See table below:
[See third table above]
Literature revised March 16, 2009
KwikPens manufactured by
Eli Lilly and Company, Indianapolis, IN 46285, USA
Pens manufactured by
Eli Lilly and Company, Indianapolis, IN 46285, USA or
Lilly France, F-67640 Fegersheim, France
Vials manufactured by
Eli Lilly and Company, Indianapolis, IN 46285, USA or
Lilly France, F-67640 Fegersheim, France
for Eli Lilly and Company, Indianapolis, IN 46285, USA
www.humalog.com
PV 5542 AMP

Patient Information

HUMALOG® (HU-ma-log) Mix50/50™
50% insulin lispro protamine suspension and
50% insulin lispro injection (rDNA origin)

Important:
Know your insulin. Do not change the type of insulin you use unless told to do so by your healthcare provider. Your insulin dose and the time you take your dose can change with different types of insulin.
Make sure you have the right type and strength of insulin prescribed for you.

Table 1*: Summary of Pharmacodynamic Properties of Insulin Products (Pooled Cross-Study Comparison)

Insulin Products	Dose, U/kg	Time of Peak Activity, Hours After Dosing	Percent of Total Activity Occurring in the First 4 Hours
Humalog	0.3	2.4 (0.8-4.3)	70% (49-89%)
Humulin R	0.32 (0.26-0.37)	4.4 (4.0-5.5)	54% (38-65%)
Humalog Mix75/25	0.3	2.6 (1.0-6.5)	35% (21-56%)
Humulin 70/30	0.3	4.4 (1.5-16)	32% (14-60%)
Humalog Mix50/50	0.3	2.3 (0.8-4.8)	45% (27-69%)
Humulin 50/50	0.3	3.3 (2.0-5.5)	44% (21-60%)
NPH	0.32 (0.27-0.40)	5.5 (3.5-9.5)	14% (3.0-48%)
NPL component	0.3	5.8 (1.3-18.3)	22% (6.3-40%)

*The information supplied in Table 1 indicates when peak insulin activity can be expected and the percent of the total insulin activity occurring during the first 4 hours. The information was derived from 3 separate glucose clamp studies in nondiabetic subjects. Values represent means, with ranges provided in parentheses.

10 mL vials	NDC 0002-7512-01	(VL-7512)
5 × 3 mL prefilled insulin delivery devices (Pen)	NDC 0002-8793-59	(HP-8793)
5 × 3 mL prefilled insulin delivery devices (KwikPen™)	NDC 0002-8798-59	(HP-8798)

	Not In-Use (Unopened) Room Temperature [Below 30°C (86°F)]	Not In-Use (Unopened) Refrigerated	In-Use (Opened) Room Temperature [Below 30°C (86°F)]
10 mL Vial	28 days	Until expiration date	28 days, refrigerated/room temperature
3 mL Pen and KwikPen (prefilled)	10 days	Until expiration date	10 days. **Do not refrigerate.**

Read the Patient Information that comes with Humalog Mix50/50 before you start using it and each time you get a refill. There may be new information. This leaflet does not take the place of talking with your healthcare provider about your diabetes or treatment. Make sure that you know how to manage your diabetes. Ask your healthcare provider if you have questions about managing your diabetes.
What is Humalog Mix50/50?
Humalog Mix50/50 is a mixture of fast-acting and longer-acting man-made insulins. Humalog Mix50/50 is used to control high blood sugar (glucose) in people with diabetes.
Humalog Mix50/50 comes in:
• 10 mL vials (bottles) for use with a syringe
• Prefilled pens
Who should not take Humalog Mix50/50?
Do not take Humalog Mix50/50 if:
• your blood sugar is too low (hypoglycemia). After treating your low blood sugar, follow your healthcare provider's instructions on the use of Humalog Mix50/50.
• you are allergic to anything in Humalog Mix50/50. See the end of this leaflet for a complete list of ingredients in Humalog Mix50/50.
Tell your healthcare provider:
• **about all your medical conditions.** Medical conditions can affect your insulin needs and your dose of Humalog Mix50/50.
• **if you are pregnant or breastfeeding.** You and your healthcare provider should talk about the best way to manage your diabetes while you are pregnant or breastfeeding. Humalog Mix50/50 has not been studied in pregnant or nursing women.
• **about all the medicines you take, including prescription and non-prescription medicines, vitamins and herbal supplements.** Many medicines can affect your blood sugar levels and insulin needs. Your Humalog Mix50/50 dose may need to change if you take other medicines.
Know the medicines you take. Keep a list of your medicines with you to show to all of your healthcare providers.
How should I use Humalog Mix50/50?
Talk to your healthcare provider if you have any questions. Your healthcare provider will tell you the right syringes to use with Humalog Mix50/50 vials. Your healthcare provider should show you how to inject Humalog Mix50/50 before you start using it. **Read the User Manual that comes with your Humalog Mix50/50 prefilled pen.**
• **Use Humalog Mix50/50 exactly as prescribed by your healthcare provider.**
• **Humalog Mix50/50 starts working faster than other insulins that contain regular human insulin.** Inject Humalog Mix50/50 fifteen minutes or less before a meal. If you do not plan to eat within 15 minutes, delay the injection until the correct time (15 minutes before eating).

• **Check your blood sugar levels as told by your healthcare provider.**
• **Mix Humalog Mix50/50 well before each use.** For Humalog Mix50/50 in a vial, carefully shake or rotate the vial until completely mixed. For prefilled pens, carefully follow the User Manual for instructions on mixing the pen. Humalog Mix50/50 should be cloudy or milky after mixing well.
• Look at your Humalog Mix50/50 before each injection. If it is not evenly mixed or has solid particles or clumps in it, do not use. Return it to your pharmacy for new Humalog Mix50/50.
• **Inject your dose of Humalog Mix50/50 under the skin of your stomach area, upper arm, upper leg, or buttocks.** Never inject Humalog Mix50/50 into a muscle or vein.
• **Change (rotate) your injection site with each dose.**
• **Your insulin needs may change because of:**
 • illness
 • stress
 • other medicines you take
 • changes in eating
 • physical activity changes
Follow your healthcare provider's instructions to make changes in your insulin dose.
• **Never mix Humalog Mix50/50 in the same syringe with other insulin products.**
• **Never use Humalog Mix50/50 in an insulin pump.**
• **Always carry a quick source of sugar to treat low blood sugar, such as glucose tablets, hard candy, or juice.**
What are the possible side effects of Humalog Mix50/50?
Low Blood Sugar (Hypoglycemia). Symptoms of low blood sugar include:
• hunger
• dizziness
• feeling shaky or shakiness
• lightheadedness
• sweating
• irritability
• headache
• fast heartbeat
• confusion
Low blood sugar symptoms can happen suddenly. Symptoms of low blood sugar may be different for each person and may change from time to time. Severe low blood sugar can cause seizures and death. Low blood sugar may affect your ability to drive a car or use mechanical equipment, risking injury to yourself or others. Know your symptoms of low blood sugar. Low blood sugar can be treated by drinking juice or regular soda or eating glucose tablets, sugar, or hard candy. Follow your healthcare provider's instructions for treating low blood sugar. Talk to your healthcare provider if low blood sugar is a problem for you.

- **Serious allergic reactions** (whole body allergic reaction). Severe, life-threatening allergic reactions can happen with insulin. Get medical help right away if you develop a rash over your whole body, have trouble breathing, wheezing, a fast heartbeat, or sweating.
- **Reactions at the injection site** (local allergic reaction). You may get redness, swelling, and itching at the injection site. If you keep having injection site reactions or they are serious, you need to call your healthcare provider. Do not inject insulin into a skin area that is red, swollen, or itchy.
- **Skin thickens or pits at the injection site (lipodystrophy).** This can happen if you don't change (rotate) your injection sites enough.

These are not all the side effects from Humalog Mix50/50. Ask your healthcare provider or pharmacist for more information.

How should I store Humalog Mix50/50?
- **Store all unopened (unused) Humalog Mix50/50 in the original carton in a refrigerator at 36°F to 46°F (2°C to 8°C).** Do not freeze.
- Do not use Humalog Mix50/50 that has been frozen.
- Do not use after the expiration date printed on the carton and label.
- Protect Humalog Mix50/50 from extreme heat, cold or light.

After starting use (open):
- **Vials:** Keep in the refrigerator or at room temperature below 86°F (30°C) for up to 28 days. Keep open vials away from direct heat or light. Throw away an opened vial 28 days after first use, even if there is insulin left in the vial.
- **Prefilled Pens:** Do not store a prefilled pen that you are using in the refrigerator. Keep at room temperature below 86°F (30°C) for up to 10 days. Throw away a prefilled pen 10 days after first use, even if there is insulin left in the pen.

General information about Humalog Mix50/50
Use Humalog Mix50/50 only to treat your diabetes. Do not share it with anyone else, even if they also have diabetes. It may harm them.

This leaflet summarized the most important information about Humalog Mix50/50. If you would like more information about Humalog Mix50/50 or diabetes, talk with your healthcare provider. You can ask your healthcare provider or pharmacist for information about Humalog Mix50/50 that is written for health professionals.

For questions you may call 1-800-LillyRx (1-800-545-5979) or visit www.humalog.com.

What are the ingredients in Humalog Mix50/50?
Active ingredients: insulin lispro protamine suspension and insulin lispro.
Inactive ingredients: protamine sulfate, glycerin, dibasic sodium phosphate, metacresol, zinc oxide (zinc ion), phenol and water for injection.

Patient Information revised March 16, 2009
KwikPens manufactured by
Eli Lilly and Company, Indianapolis, IN 46285, USA
Pens manufactured by
Eli Lilly and Company, Indianapolis, IN 46285, USA or
Lilly France, F-67640 Fegersheim, France
Vials manufactured by
Eli Lilly and Company, Indianapolis, IN 46285, USA or
Lilly France, F-67640 Fegersheim, France
for Eli Lilly and Company, Indianapolis, IN 46285, USA
www.humalog.com
Copyright © 2007, 2009, Eli Lilly and Company. All rights reserved.
PV 5571 AMP
Shown in Product Identification Guide, page 311

HUMALOG® Mix75/25™　　℞

[*hū'mă-lŏg*]
75% INSULIN LISPRO PROTAMINE SUSPENSION AND 25% INSULIN LISPRO INJECTION
(rDNA ORIGIN)
100 UNITS PER ML (U-100)

DESCRIPTION

Humalog® Mix75/25™ [75% insulin lispro protamine suspension and 25% insulin lispro injection, (rDNA origin)] is a mixture of insulin lispro solution, a rapid-acting blood glucose-lowering agent and insulin lispro protamine suspension, an intermediate-acting blood glucose-lowering agent. Chemically, insulin lispro is Lys(B28), Pro(B29) human insulin analog, created when the amino acids at positions 28 and 29 on the insulin B-chain are reversed. Insulin lispro is synthesized in a special non-pathogenic laboratory strain of *Escherichia coli* bacteria that has been genetically altered to produce insulin lispro. Insulin lispro protamine suspension (NPL component) is a suspension of crystals produced from combining insulin lispro and protamine sulfate under appropriate conditions for crystal formation.

Insulin lispro has the following primary structure:

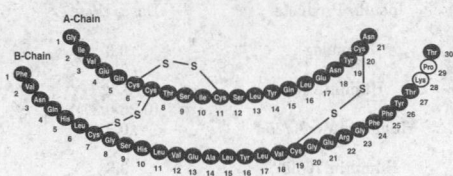

Insulin lispro has the empirical formula $C_{257}H_{383}N_{65}O_{77}S_6$ and a molecular weight of 5808, both identical to that of human insulin.

Humalog Mix75/25 vials and Pens contain a sterile suspension of insulin lispro protamine suspension mixed with soluble insulin lispro for use as an injection.

Each milliliter of Humalog Mix75/25 injection contains insulin lispro 100 units, 0.28 mg protamine sulfate, 16 mg glycerin, 3.78 mg dibasic sodium phosphate, 1.76 mg Metacresol, zinc oxide content adjusted to provide 0.025 mg zinc ion, 0.715 mg phenol, and Water for Injection. Humalog Mix75/25 has a pH of 7.0 to 7.8. Hydrochloric acid 10% and/or sodium hydroxide 10% may have been added to adjust pH.

CLINICAL PHARMACOLOGY

Antidiabetic Activity

The primary activity of insulin, including Humalog Mix75/25, is the regulation of glucose metabolism. In addition, all insulins have several anabolic and anti-catabolic actions on many tissues in the body. In muscle and other tissues (except the brain), insulin causes rapid transport of glucose and amino acids intracellularly, promotes anabolism, and inhibits protein catabolism. In the liver, insulin promotes the uptake and storage of glucose in the form of glycogen, inhibits gluconeogenesis, and promotes the conversion of excess glucose into fat.

Insulin lispro, the rapid-acting component of Humalog Mix75/25, has been shown to be equipotent to Regular human insulin on a molar basis. One unit of Humalog® has the same glucose-lowering effect as one unit of Regular human insulin, but its effect is more rapid and of shorter duration. Humalog Mix75/25 has a similar glucose-lowering effect as compared with Humulin® 70/30 on a unit for unit basis.

Pharmacokinetics

Absorption

Studies in nondiabetic subjects and patients with type 1 (insulin-dependent) diabetes demonstrated that Humalog, the rapid-acting component of Humalog Mix75/25, is absorbed faster than Regular human insulin (U-100). In nondiabetic subjects given subcutaneous doses of Humalog ranging from 0.1 to 0.4 U/kg, peak serum concentrations were observed 30 to 90 minutes after dosing. When nondiabetic subjects received equivalent doses of Regular human insulin, peak insulin concentrations occurred between 50 to 120 minutes after dosing. Similar results were seen in patients with type 1 diabetes.

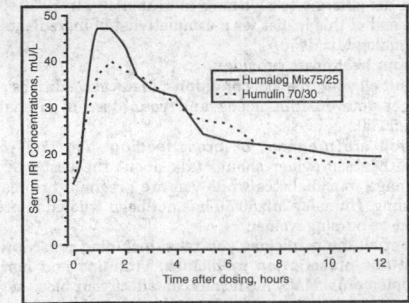

Figure 1: Serum Immunoreactive Insulin (IRI) Concentrations, After Subcutaneous Injection of Humalog Mix75/25 or Humulin 70/30 in Healthy Nondiabetic Subjects.

Humalog Mix75/25 has two phases of absorption. The early phase represents insulin lispro and its distinct characteristics of rapid onset. The late phase represents the prolonged action of insulin lispro protamine suspension. In 30 healthy nondiabetic subjects given subcutaneous doses (0.3 U/kg) of Humalog Mix75/25, peak serum concentrations were observed 30 to 240 minutes (median, 60 minutes) after dosing (*see* Figure 1). Identical results were found in patients with type 1 diabetes. The rapid absorption characteristics of Humalog are maintained with Humalog Mix75/25 (*see* Figure 1).

Figure 1 represents serum insulin concentration versus time curves of Humalog Mix75/25 and Humulin 70/30.

Humalog Mix75/25 has a more rapid absorption than Humulin 70/30, which has been confirmed in patients with type 1 diabetes.
Distribution
Radiolabeled distribution studies of Humalog Mix75/25 have not been conducted. However, the volume of distribution following injection of Humalog is identical to that of Regular human insulin, with a range of 0.26 to 0.36 L/kg.
Metabolism
Human metabolism studies of Humalog Mix75/25 have not been conducted. Studies in animals indicate that the metabolism of Humalog, the rapid-acting component of Humalog Mix75/25, is identical to that of Regular human insulin.
Elimination
Humalog Mix75/25 has two absorption phases, a rapid and a prolonged phase, representative of the insulin lispro and insulin lispro protamine suspension components of the mixture. As with other intermediate-acting insulins, a meaningful terminal phase half-life cannot be calculated after administration of Humalog Mix75/25 because of the prolonged insulin lispro protamine suspension absorption.

Pharmacodynamics

Studies in nondiabetic subjects and patients with diabetes demonstrated that Humalog has a more rapid onset of glucose-lowering activity, an earlier peak for glucose-lowering, and a shorter duration of glucose-lowering activity than Regular human insulin. The early onset of activity of Humalog Mix75/25 is directly related to the rapid absorption of Humalog. The time course of action of insulin and insulin analogs, such as Humalog (and hence Humalog Mix75/25), may vary considerably in different individuals or within the same individual. The parameters of Humalog Mix75/25 activity (time of onset, peak time, and duration) as presented in Figures 2 and 3 should be considered only as general guidelines. The rate of insulin absorption and consequently the onset of activity is known to be affected by the site of injection, exercise, and other variables (*see* General *under* PRECAUTIONS).

In a glucose clamp study performed in 30 nondiabetic subjects, the onset of action and glucose-lowering activity of Humalog, Humalog® Mix50/50™, Humalog Mix75/25, and insulin lispro protamine suspension (NPL component) were compared (*see* Figure 2). Graphs of mean glucose infusion rate versus time showed a distinct insulin activity profile for each formulation. The rapid onset of glucose-lowering activity characteristic of Humalog was maintained in Humalog Mix75/25.

In separate glucose clamp studies performed in nondiabetic subjects, pharmacodynamics of Humalog Mix75/25 and Humulin 70/30 were assessed and are presented in Figure 3. Humalog Mix75/25 has a duration of activity similar to that of Humulin 70/30.

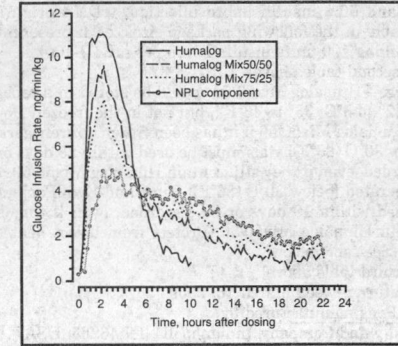

Figure 2: Insulin Activity After Injection of Humalog, Humalog Mix50/50, Humalog Mix75/25, or Insulin Lispro Protamine Suspension (NPL Component) in 30 Nondiabetic Subjects.

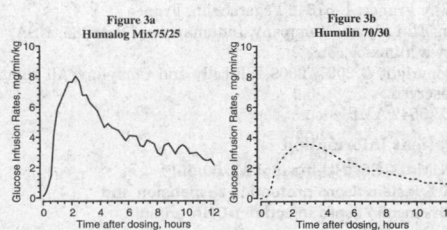

Figure 3: Insulin Activity After Injection of Humalog Mix75/25 and Humulin 70/30 in Nondiabetic Subjects.

Figures 2 and 3 represent insulin activity profiles as measured by glucose clamp studies in healthy nondiabetic subjects.

Figure 2 shows the time activity profiles of Humalog, Humalog Mix50/50, Humalog Mix75/25, and insulin lispro protamine suspension (NPL component).

Figure 3 is a comparison of the time activity profiles of Humalog Mix75/25 (*see* Figure 3a) and of Humulin 70/30 (*see* Figure 3b) from two different studies.

Special Populations

Age and Gender

Information on the effect of age on the pharmacokinetics of Humalog Mix75/25 is unavailable. Pharmacokinetic and pharmacodynamic comparisons between men and women administered Humalog Mix75/25 showed no gender differences. In large Humalog clinical trials, sub-group analysis based on age and gender demonstrated that differences between Humalog and Regular human insulin in postprandial glucose parameters are maintained across sub-groups.

Smoking

The effect of smoking on the pharmacokinetics and pharmacodynamics of Humalog Mix75/25 has not been studied.

Pregnancy

The effect of pregnancy on the pharmacokinetics and pharmacodynamics of Humalog Mix75/25 has not been studied.

Obesity

The effect of obesity and/or subcutaneous fat thickness on the pharmacokinetics and pharmacodynamics of Humalog Mix75/25 has not been studied. In large clinical trials, which included patients with Body Mass Index up to and including 35 kg/m^2, no consistent differences were observed between Humalog and Humulin® R with respect to postprandial glucose parameters.

Renal Impairment

The effect of renal impairment on the pharmacokinetics and pharmacodynamics of Humalog Mix75/25 has not been studied. In a study of 25 patients with type 2 diabetes and a wide range of renal function, the pharmacokinetic differences between Humalog and Regular human insulin were generally maintained. However, the sensitivity of the patients to insulin did change, with an increased response to insulin as the renal function declined. Careful glucose monitoring and dose reductions of insulin, including Humalog Mix75/25, may be necessary in patients with renal dysfunction.

Hepatic Impairment

Some studies with human insulin have shown increased circulating levels of insulin in patients with hepatic failure. The effect of hepatic impairment on the pharmacokinetics and pharmacodynamics of Humalog Mix75/25 has not been studied. However, in a study of 22 patients with type 2 diabetes, impaired hepatic function did not affect the subcutaneous absorption or general disposition of Humalog when compared with patients with no history of hepatic dysfunction. In that study, Humalog maintained its more rapid absorption and elimination when compared with Regular human insulin. Careful glucose monitoring and dose adjustments of insulin, including Humalog Mix75/25, may be necessary in patients with hepatic dysfunction.

INDICATIONS AND USAGE

Humalog Mix75/25, a mixture of 75% insulin lispro protamine suspension and 25% insulin lispro injection, (rDNA origin), is indicated in the treatment of patients with diabetes mellitus for the control of hyperglycemia. Humalog Mix75/25 has a more rapid onset of glucose–lowering activity compared with Humulin 70/30 while having a similar duration of action. This profile is achieved by combining the rapid onset of Humalog with the intermediate action of insulin lispro protamine suspension.

CONTRAINDICATIONS

Humalog Mix75/25 is contraindicated during episodes of hypoglycemia and in patients sensitive to insulin lispro or any of the excipients contained in the formulation.

WARNINGS

Humalog differs from Regular human insulin by its rapid onset of action as well as a shorter duration of activity. Therefore, the dose of Humalog Mix75/25 should be given within 15 minutes before a meal.

Hypoglycemia is the most common adverse effect associated with the use of insulins, including Humalog Mix75/25. As with all insulins, the timing of hypoglycemia may differ among various insulin formulations. Glucose monitoring is recommended for all patients with diabetes.

Any change of insulin should be made cautiously and only under medical supervision. Changes in insulin strength, manufacturer, type (e.g., Regular, NPH, analog), species, or method of manufacture may result in the need for a change in dosage.

PRECAUTIONS

General

Hypoglycemia and hypokalemia are among the potential clinical adverse effects associated with the use of all insulins. Because of differences in the action of Humalog Mix75/25 and other insulins, care should be taken in patients in whom such potential side effects might be clinically relevant (e.g., patients who are fasting, have autonomic neuropathy, or are using potassium–lowering drugs or patients taking drugs sensitive to serum potassium level).

Lipodystrophy and hypersensitivity are among other potential clinical adverse effects associated with the use of all insulins.

As with all insulin preparations, the time course of Humalog Mix75/25 action may vary in different individuals or at different times in the same individual and is dependent on site of injection, blood supply, temperature, and physical activity.

Adjustment of dosage of any insulin may be necessary if patients change their physical activity or their usual meal plan. Insulin requirements may be altered during illness, emotional disturbances, or other stress.

Hypoglycemia—As with all insulin preparations, hypoglycemic reactions may be associated with the administration of Humalog Mix75/25. Rapid changes in serum glucose concentrations may induce symptoms of hypoglycemia in persons with diabetes, regardless of the glucose value. Early warning symptoms of hypoglycemia may be different or less pronounced under certain conditions, such as long duration of diabetes, diabetic nerve disease, use of medications such as beta–blockers, or intensified diabetes control.

Renal Impairment—As with other insulins, the requirements for Humalog Mix75/25 may be reduced in patients with renal impairment.

Hepatic Impairment—Although impaired hepatic function does not affect the absorption or disposition of Humalog, careful glucose monitoring and dose adjustments of insulin, including Humalog Mix75/25, may be necessary.

Allergy—Local Allergy—As with any insulin therapy, patients may experience redness, swelling, or itching at the site of injection. These minor reactions usually resolve in a few days to a few weeks. In some instances, these reactions may be related to factors other than insulin, such as irritants in the skin cleansing agent or poor injection technique.

Systemic Allergy—Less common, but potentially more serious, is generalized allergy to insulin, which may cause rash (including pruritus) over the whole body, shortness of breath, wheezing, reduction in blood pressure, rapid pulse, or sweating. Severe cases of generalized allergy, including anaphylactic reaction, may be life threatening. Localized reactions and generalized myalgias have been reported with the use of cresol as an injectable excipient.

Antibody Production—In clinical trials, antibodies that cross-react with human insulin and insulin lispro were observed in both human insulin mixtures and insulin lispro mixtures treatment groups.

Information for Patients

Patients should be informed of the potential risks and advantages of Humalog Mix75/25 and alternative therapies. Patients should not mix Humalog Mix75/25 with any other insulin. They should also be informed about the importance of proper insulin storage, injection technique, timing of dosage, adherence to meal planning, regular physical activity, regular blood glucose monitoring, periodic hemoglobin A$_{1c}$ testing, recognition and management of hypo- and hyperglycemia, and periodic assessment for diabetes complications.

Patients should be advised to inform their physician if they are pregnant or intend to become pregnant.

Refer patients to the Patient Information leaflet for information on normal appearance, timing of dosing (within 15 minutes before a meal), storing, and common adverse effects.

For Patients Using Insulin Pen Delivery Devices: Before starting therapy, patients should read the Patient Information leaflet that accompanies the drug product and the User Manual that accompanies the delivery device and re-read them each time the prescription is renewed. Patients should be instructed on how to properly use the delivery device, prime the Pen to a stream of insulin, and properly dispose of needles. Patients should be advised not to share their Pens with others.

Laboratory Tests

As with all insulins, the therapeutic response to Humalog Mix75/25 should be monitored by periodic blood glucose tests. Periodic measurement of hemoglobin A$_{1c}$ is recommended for the monitoring of long–term glycemic control.

Drug Interactions

Insulin requirements may be increased by medications with hyperglycemic activity such as corticosteroids, isoniazid, certain lipid-lowering drugs (e.g., niacin), estrogens, oral contraceptives, phenothiazines, and thyroid replacement therapy.

Insulin requirements may be decreased in the presence of drugs that increase insulin sensitivity or have hypoglycemic activity, such as oral antidiabetic agents, salicylates, sulfa antibiotics, certain antidepressants (monoamine oxidase inhibitors), angiotensin-converting-enzyme inhibitors, angiotensin II receptor blocking agents, beta-adrenergic blockers, inhibitors of pancreatic function (e.g., octreotide), and alcohol. Beta–adrenergic blockers may mask the symptoms of hypoglycemia in some patients.

Carcinogenesis, Mutagenesis, Impairment of Fertility

Long-term studies in animals have not been performed to evaluate the carcinogenic potential of Humalog, Humalog Mix75/25, or Humalog Mix50/50. Insulin lispro was not mutagenic in a battery of *in vitro* and *in vivo* genetic toxicity assays (bacterial mutation tests, unscheduled DNA synthesis, mouse lymphoma assay, chromosomal aberration tests, and a micronucleus test). There is no evidence from animal studies of impairment of fertility induced by insulin lispro.

Pregnancy

Teratogenic Effects—Pregnancy Category B

Reproduction studies with insulin lispro have been performed in pregnant rats and rabbits at parenteral doses up to 4 and 0.3 times, respectively, the average human dose (40 units/day) based on body surface area. The results have revealed no evidence of impaired fertility or harm to the fetus due to insulin lispro. There are, however, no adequate and well–controlled studies with Humalog, Humalog Mix75/25, or Humalog Mix50/50 in pregnant women. Because animal reproduction studies are not always predictive of human response, this drug should be used during pregnancy only if clearly needed.

Nursing Mothers

It is unknown whether insulin lispro is excreted in significant amounts in human milk. Many drugs, including human insulin, are excreted in human milk. For this reason, caution should be exercised when Humalog Mix75/25 is administered to a nursing woman. Patients with diabetes who are lactating may require adjustments in Humalog Mix75/25 dose, meal plan, or both.

Pediatric Use

Safety and effectiveness of Humalog Mix75/25 in patients less than 18 years of age have not been established.

Geriatric Use

Clinical studies of Humalog Mix75/25 did not include sufficient numbers of patients aged 65 and over to determine whether they respond differently than younger patients. In general, dose selection for an elderly patient should take into consideration the greater frequency of decreased hepatic, renal, or cardiac function, and of concomitant disease or other drug therapy in this population.

ADVERSE REACTIONS

Clinical studies comparing Humalog Mix75/25 with human insulin mixtures did not demonstrate a difference in frequency of adverse events between the two treatments.

Adverse events commonly associated with human insulin therapy include the following:

Body as a Whole—allergic reactions (*see* PRECAUTIONS).

Skin and Appendages—injection site reaction, lipodystrophy, pruritus, rash.

Other—hypoglycemia (*see* WARNINGS *and* PRECAUTIONS).

OVERDOSAGE

Hypoglycemia may occur as a result of an excess of insulin relative to food intake, energy expenditure, or both. Mild episodes of hypoglycemia usually can be treated with oral glucose. Adjustments in drug dosage, meal patterns, or exercise, may be needed. More severe episodes with coma, seizure, or neurologic impairment may be treated with intramuscular/subcutaneous glucagon or concentrated intravenous glucose. Sustained carbohydrate intake and observation may be necessary because hypoglycemia may recur after apparent clinical recovery.

DOSAGE AND ADMINISTRATION

[See table 1 at top of next page]

Humalog Mix75/25 is intended only for subcutaneous administration. Humalog Mix75/25 should not be administered intravenously. Dosage regimens of Humalog Mix75/25 will vary among patients and should be determined by the healthcare provider familiar with the patient's metabolic needs, eating habits, and other lifestyle variables. Humalog has been shown to be equipotent to Regular human insulin on a molar basis. One unit of Humalog has the same glucose–lowering effect as one unit of Regular human insulin, but its effect is more rapid and of shorter duration. Humalog Mix75/25 has a similar glucose–lowering effect as compared with Humulin 70/30 on a unit for unit basis. The quicker glucose–lowering effect of Humalog is related to the more rapid absorption rate of insulin lispro from subcutaneous tissue.

Humalog Mix75/25 starts lowering blood glucose more quickly than Regular human insulin, allowing for convenient dosing immediately before a meal (within 15 minutes). In contrast, mixtures containing Regular human insulin should be given 30 to 60 minutes before a meal.

The rate of insulin absorption and consequently the onset of activity are known to be affected by the site of injection, exercise, and other variables. As with all insulin preparations, the time course of action of Humalog Mix75/25 may vary considerably in different individuals or within the same individual. Patients must be educated to use proper injection techniques.

Humalog Mix75/25 should be inspected visually before use. Humalog Mix75/25 should be used only if it appears uniformly cloudy after mixing. Humalog Mix75/25 should not be used after its expiration date.

HOW SUPPLIED

Humalog Mix75/25 [75% insulin lispro protamine suspension and 25% insulin lispro injection, (rDNA origin)] is available in the following package sizes: each presentation containing 100 units insulin lispro per mL (U-100).

10 mL vials	NDC 0002–7511–01 (VL-7511)
5 × 3 mL prefilled insulin delivery devices (Pen)	NDC 0002–8794–59 (HP-8794)
5 × 3 mL prefilled insulin delivery devices (KwikPen™)	NDC 0002–8797–59 (HP-8797)

Storage—Humalog Mix75/25 should be stored in a refrigerator [2° to 8°C (36° to 46°F)], but not in the freezer. Do not use Humalog Mix75/25 if it has been frozen. Unrefrigerated [below 30°C (86°F)] vials must be used within 28 days or be discarded, even if they still contain Humalog Mix75/25. Unrefrigerated [below 30°C (86°F)] Pens, and KwikPens must be used within 10 days or be discarded, even if they still contain Humalog Mix75/25. Protect from direct heat and light. See table below:
[See second table at right]
Literature revised March 16, 2009
KwikPens manufactured by
Eli Lilly and Company, Indianapolis, IN 46285, USA
Pens manufactured by
Eli Lilly and Company, Indianapolis, IN 46285, USA or Lilly France, F-67640 Fegersheim, France
Vials manufactured by
Eli Lilly and Company, Indianapolis, IN 46285, USA or Lilly France, F-67640 Fegersheim, France
for Eli Lilly and Company, Indianapolis, IN 46285, USA
www.humalog.com
Copyright © 2007, 2009, Eli Lilly and Company. All rights reserved.
PV 5551 AMP

Patient Information
HUMALOG® (HU-ma-log) Mix75/25™
75% insulin lispro protamine suspension and
25% insulin lispro injection (rDNA origin)

Important:
Know your insulin. Do not change the type of insulin you use unless told to do so by your healthcare provider. Your insulin dose and the time you take your dose can change with different types of insulin.
Make sure you have the right type and strength of insulin prescribed for you.

Read the Patient Information that comes with Humalog Mix75/25 before you start using it and each time you get a refill. There may be new information. This leaflet does not take the place of talking with your healthcare provider about your diabetes or treatment. Make sure that you know how to manage your diabetes. Ask your healthcare provider if you have questions about managing your diabetes.
What is Humalog Mix75/25?
Humalog Mix75/25 is a mixture of fast-acting and longer-acting man-made insulins. Humalog Mix75/25 is used to control high blood sugar (glucose) in people with diabetes.
Humalog Mix75/25 comes in:
• 10 mL vials (bottles) for use with a syringe
• Prefilled pens
Who should not take Humalog Mix75/25?
Do not take Humalog Mix75/25 if:
• your blood sugar is too low (hypoglycemia). After treating your low blood sugar, follow your healthcare provider's instructions on the use of Humalog Mix75/25.
• you are allergic to anything in Humalog Mix75/25. See the end of this leaflet for a complete list of ingredients in Humalog Mix75/25.
Tell your healthcare provider:
• **about all your medical conditions.** Medical conditions can affect your insulin needs and your dose of Humalog Mix75/25.
• **if you are pregnant or breastfeeding.** You and your healthcare provider should talk about the best way to manage your diabetes while you are pregnant or breastfeeding. Humalog Mix75/25 has not been studied in pregnant or nursing women.
• **about all the medicines you take, including prescription and non-prescription medicines, vitamins and herbal supplements.** Many medicines can affect your blood sugar levels and insulin needs. Your Humalog Mix75/25 dose may need to change if you take other medicines.
Know the medicines you take. Keep a list of your medicines with you to show to all of your healthcare providers.

Table 1*: Summary of Pharmacodynamic Properties of Insulin Products (Pooled Cross-Study Comparison)

Insulin Products	Dose, U/kg	Time of Peak Activity, Hours After Dosing	Percent of Total Activity Occurring in the First 4 Hours
Humalog	0.3	2.4 (0.8–4.3)	70% (49–89%)
Humulin R	0.32 (0.26–0.37)	4.4 (4.0–5.5)	54% (38–65%)
Humalog Mix75/25	0.3	2.6 (1.0–6.5)	35% (21–56%)
Humulin 70/30	0.3	4.4 (1.5–16)	32% (14–60%)
Humalog Mix50/50	0.3	2.3 (0.8–4.8)	45% (27–69%)
Humulin 50/50	0.3	3.3 (2.0–5.5)	44% (21–60%)
NPH	0.32 (0.27–0.40)	5.5 (3.5–9.5)	14% (3.0–48%)
NPL component	0.3	5.8 (1.3–18.3)	22% (6.3–40%)

*The information supplied in Table 1 indicates when peak insulin activity can be expected and the percent of the total insulin activity occurring during the first 4 hours. The information was derived from 3 separate glucose clamp studies in nondiabetic subjects. Values represent means, with ranges provided in parentheses.

	Not In-Use (Unopened) Room Temperature [Below 30°C (86°F)]	Not In-Use (Unopened) Refrigerated	In-Use (Opened) Room Temperature [Below 30°C (86°F)]
10 mL Vial	28 days	Until expiration date	28 days, refrigerated/room temperature
3 mL Pen and KwikPen (prefilled)	10 days	Until expiration date	10 days. Do not refrigerate.

How should I use Humalog Mix75/25?
Talk to your healthcare provider if you have any questions. Your healthcare provider will tell you the right syringes to use with Humalog Mix75/25 vials. Your healthcare provider should show you how to inject Humalog Mix75/25 before you start using it. **Read the User Manual that comes with your Humalog Mix75/25 prefilled pen.**
• **Use Humalog Mix75/25 exactly as prescribed by your healthcare provider.**
• **Humalog Mix75/25 starts working faster than other insulins that contain regular human insulin.** Inject Humalog Mix75/25 fifteen minutes or less before a meal. If you do not plan to eat within 15 minutes, delay the injection until the correct time (15 minutes before eating).
• **Check your blood sugar levels as told by your healthcare provider.**
• **Mix Humalog Mix75/25 well before each use.** For Humalog Mix75/25 in a vial, carefully shake or rotate the vial until completely mixed. For prefilled pens, carefully follow the User Manual for instructions on mixing the pen. Humalog Mix75/25 should be cloudy or milky after mixing well.
• Look at your Humalog Mix75/25 before each injection. If it is not evenly mixed or has solid particles or clumps in it, do not use. Return it to your pharmacy for new Humalog Mix75/25.
• **Inject your dose of Humalog Mix75/25 under the skin of your stomach area, upper arm, upper leg, or buttocks. Never inject Humalog Mix75/25 into a muscle or vein.**
• **Change (rotate) your injection site with each dose.**
• **Your insulin needs may change because of:**
  • illness
  • stress
  • other medicines you take
  • changes in eating
  • physical activity changes
  Follow your healthcare provider's instructions to make changes in your insulin dose.
• **Never mix Humalog Mix75/25 in the same syringe with other insulin products.**
• **Never use Humalog Mix75/25 in an insulin pump.**
• **Always carry a quick source of sugar to treat low blood sugar, such as glucose tablets, hard candy, or juice.**
What are the possible side effects of Humalog Mix75/25?
Low Blood Sugar (Hypoglycemia). Symptoms of low blood sugar include:
• hunger
• dizziness
• feeling shaky or shakiness
• lightheadedness
• sweating
• irritability
• headache
• fast heartbeat
• confusion
Low blood sugar symptoms can happen suddenly. Symptoms of low blood sugar may be different for each person and

may change from time to time. Severe low blood sugar can cause seizures and death. Low blood sugar may affect your ability to drive a car or use mechanical equipment, risking injury to yourself or others. Know your symptoms of low blood sugar. Low blood sugar can be treated by drinking juice or regular soda or eating glucose tablets, sugar, or hard candy. Follow your healthcare provider's instructions for treating low blood sugar. Talk to your healthcare provider if low blood sugar is a problem for you.
• **Serious allergic reactions** (whole body allergic reaction). Severe, life-threatening allergic reactions can happen with insulin. Get medical help right away if you develop a rash over your whole body, have trouble breathing, wheezing, a fast heartbeat, or sweating.
• **Reactions at the injection site** (local allergic reaction). You may get redness, swelling, and itching at the injection site. If you keep having injection site reactions or they are serious, you need to call your healthcare provider. Do not inject insulin into a skin area that is red, swollen, or itchy.
• **Skin thickens or pits at the injection site (lipodystrophy).** This can happen if you don't change (rotate) your injection sites enough.
These are not all the side effects from Humalog Mix75/25. Ask your healthcare provider or pharmacist for more information.
How should I store Humalog Mix75/25?
• **Store all unopened (unused) Humalog Mix75/25 in the original carton in a refrigerator at 36°F to 46°F (2°C to 8°C).** Do not freeze.
• Do not use Humalog Mix75/25 that has been frozen.
• Do not use after the expiration date printed on the carton and label.
• Protect Humalog Mix75/25 from extreme heat, cold or light.
After starting use (open):
• **Vials:** Keep in the refrigerator or at room temperature below 86°F (30°C) for up to 28 days. Keep open vials away from direct heat or light. Throw away an opened vial 28 days after first use, even if there is insulin left in the vial.
• **Prefilled Pens:** Do not store a prefilled pen that you are using in the refrigerator. Keep at room temperature below 86°F (30°C) for up to 10 days. Throw away a prefilled pen 10 days after first use, even if there is insulin left in the pen.
General information about Humalog Mix75/25
Use Humalog Mix75/25 only to treat your diabetes. Do not share it with anyone else, even if they also have diabetes. It may harm them.
This leaflet summarized the most important information about Humalog Mix75/25. If you would like more information about Humalog Mix75/25 or diabetes, talk with your healthcare provider. You can ask your healthcare provider or pharmacist for information about Humalog Mix75/25 that is written for health professionals.
For questions you may call 1–800–LillyRx (1–800–545–5979) or visit www.humalog.com.

What are the ingredients in Humalog Mix75/25?
Active ingredients: insulin lispro protamine suspension and insulin lispro.
Inactive ingredients: protamine sulfate, glycerin, dibasic sodium phosphate, metacresol, zinc oxide (zinc ion), phenol and water for injection.
Patient Information issued September 6, 2007
KwikPens manufactured by
Eli Lilly and Company, Indianapolis, IN 46285, USA
Pens manufactured by
Eli Lilly and Company, Indianapolis, IN 46285, USA or
Lilly France, F-67640 Fegersheim, France
Vials manufactured by
Eli Lilly and Company, Indianapolis, IN 46285, USA or
Lilly France, F-67640 Fegersheim, France
for Eli Lilly and Company, Indianapolis, IN 46285, USA
www.humalog.com
Copyright © 2007, Eli Lilly and Company. All rights reserved.
PV 5580 AMP
Shown in Product Identification Guide, page 311

HUMULIN® 70/30 OTC

[*hū'mū-lĭn*]
70% HUMAN INSULIN ISOPHANESUSPENSION AND
30% HUMAN INSULIN INJECTION (rDNA ORIGIN)
100 UNITS PER ML (U-100)

INFORMATION FOR THE PATIENT
10 mL Vial (1000 Units per vial)

WARNINGS

THIS LILLY HUMAN INSULIN PRODUCT DIFFERS FROM ANIMAL–SOURCE INSULINS BECAUSE IT IS STRUCTURALLY IDENTICAL TO THE INSULIN PRODUCED BY YOUR BODY'S PANCREAS AND BECAUSE OF ITS UNIQUE MANUFACTURING PROCESS.
ANY CHANGE OF INSULIN SHOULD BE MADE CAUTIOUSLY AND ONLY UNDER MEDICAL SUPERVISION. CHANGES IN STRENGTH, MANUFACTURER, TYPE (E.G., REGULAR, NPH, ANALOG), SPECIES, OR METHOD OF MANUFACTURE MAY RESULT IN THE NEED FOR A CHANGE IN DOSAGE.
SOME PATIENTS TAKING HUMULIN® (HUMAN INSULIN, rDNA ORIGIN) MAY REQUIRE A CHANGE IN DOSAGE FROM THAT USED WITH OTHER INSULINS. IF AN ADJUSTMENT IS NEEDED, IT MAY OCCUR WITH THE FIRST DOSE OR DURING THE FIRST SEVERAL WEEKS OR MONTHS.

DIABETES

Insulin is a hormone produced by the pancreas, a large gland that lies near the stomach. This hormone is necessary for the body's correct use of food, especially sugar. Diabetes occurs when the pancreas does not make enough insulin to meet your body's needs.
To control your diabetes, your doctor has prescribed injections of insulin products to keep your blood glucose at a near–normal level. You have been instructed to test your blood and/or your urine regularly for glucose. Studies have shown that some chronic complications of diabetes such as eye disease, kidney disease, and nerve disease can be significantly reduced if the blood sugar is maintained as close to normal as possible. The American Diabetes Association recommends that if your pre–meal glucose levels are consistently above 130 mg/dL or your hemoglobin A_{1c} (HbA_{1c}) is more than 7%, you should talk to your doctor. A change in your diabetes therapy may be needed. If your blood tests consistently show below–normal glucose levels, you should also let your doctor know. Proper control of your diabetes requires close and constant cooperation with your doctor. Despite diabetes, you can lead an active and healthy life if you eat a balanced diet, exercise regularly, and take your insulin injections as prescribed by your doctor.
Always keep an extra supply of insulin as well as a spare syringe and needle on hand. Always wear diabetic identification so that appropriate treatment can be given if complications occur away from home.

70/30 HUMAN INSULIN

Description
Humulin is synthesized in a special non–disease–producing laboratory strain of *Escherichia coli* bacteria that has been genetically altered to produce human insulin. Humulin 70/30 is a mixture of 70% Human Insulin Isophane Suspension and 30% Human Insulin Injection (rDNA origin). It is an intermediate-acting insulin combined with the more rapid onset of action of Regular human insulin. The duration of activity may last up to 24 hours following injection. The time course of action of any insulin may vary considerably in different individuals or at different times in the same individual. As with all insulin preparations, the duration of action of Humulin 70/30 is dependent on dose, site of injection, blood supply, temperature, and physical activity. Humulin 70/30 is a sterile suspension and is for subcutaneous injection only. It should not be used intravenously or intramuscularly. The concentration of Humulin 70/30 is 100 units/mL (U–100).
Identification
Human insulin from Eli Lilly and Company has the trademark Humulin. Your doctor has prescribed the type of insulin that he/she believes is best for you.
DO NOT USE ANY OTHER INSULIN EXCEPT ON YOUR DOCTOR'S ADVICE AND DIRECTION.
Always check the carton and the bottle label for the name and letter designation of the insulin you receive from your pharmacy to make sure it is the same as prescribed by your doctor.
Always check the appearance of your bottle of Humulin 70/30 before withdrawing each dose. Before each injection the Humulin 70/30 bottle must be carefully shaken or rotated several times to completely mix the insulin. Humulin 70/30 suspension should look uniformly cloudy or milky after mixing. If not, repeat the above steps until contents are mixed.
Do not use Humulin 70/30:
- if the insulin substance (the white material) remains at the bottom of the bottle after mixing or
- if there are clumps in the insulin after mixing, or
- if solid white particles stick to the bottom or wall of the bottle, giving a frosted appearance.

If you see anything unusual in the appearance of Humulin 70/30 suspension in your bottle or notice your insulin requirements changing, talk to your doctor.
Storage
Not in-use (unopened): Humulin 70/30 bottles not in-use should be stored in a refrigerator, but not in the freezer.
In-use (opened): The Humulin 70/30 bottle you are currently using can be kept unrefrigerated as long as it is kept as cool as possible [below 86°F (30°C)] away from heat and light.
Do not use Humulin 70/30 after the expiration date stamped on the label or if it has been frozen.

INSTRUCTIONS FOR INSULIN VIAL USE

NEVER SHARE NEEDLES AND SYRINGES
Correct Syringe Type
Doses of insulin are measured in **units**. U–100 insulin contains 100 units/mL (1 mL=1 cc). With Humulin 70/30, it is important to use a syringe that is marked for U–100 insulin preparations. Failure to use the proper syringe can lead to a mistake in dosage, causing serious problems for you, such as a blood glucose level that is too low or too high.
Syringe Use
To help avoid contamination and possible infection, follow these instructions exactly.
Disposable syringes and needles should be used only once and then discarded by placing the used needle in a puncture-resistant disposable container. Properly dispose of the puncture-resistant container as directed by your Health Care Professional.
Preparing the Dose
1. Wash your hands.
2. Carefully shake or rotate the bottle of insulin several times to completely mix the insulin.
3. Inspect the insulin. Humulin 70/30 suspension should look uniformly cloudy or milky. Do not use Humulin 70/30 if you notice anything unusual in its appearance.
4. If using a new Humulin 70/30 bottle, flip off the plastic protective cap, but **do not** remove the stopper. Wipe the top of the bottle with an alcohol swab.
5. Draw an amount of air into the syringe that is equal to the Humulin 70/30 dose. Put the needle through rubber top of the Humulin 70/30 bottle and inject the air into the bottle.
6. Turn the Humulin 70/30 bottle and syringe upside down. Hold the bottle and syringe firmly in one hand and shake gently.
7. Making sure the tip of the needle is in the Humulin 70/30 suspension, withdraw the correct dose of Humulin 70/30 into the syringe.
8. Before removing the needle from the Humulin 70/30 bottle, check the syringe for air bubbles. If bubbles are present, hold the syringe straight up and tap its side until the bubbles float to the top. Push the bubbles out with the plunger and then withdraw the correct dose.
9. Remove the needle from the bottle and lay the syringe down so that the needle does not touch anything.

Injection Instructions
1. To avoid tissue damage, choose a site for each injection that is at least 1/2 inch from the previous injection site. The usual sites of injection are abdomen, thighs, and arms.
2. Cleanse the skin with alcohol where the injection is to be made.
3. With one hand, stabilize the skin by spreading it or pinching up a large area.
4. Insert the needle as instructed by your doctor.
5. Push the plunger in as far as it will go.
6. Pull the needle out and apply gentle pressure over the injection site for several seconds. **Do not rub the area.**
7. Place the used needle in a puncture-resistant disposable container and properly dispose of the puncture-resistant container as directed by your Health Care Professional.

DOSAGE

Your doctor has told you which insulin to use, how much, and when and how often to inject it. Because each patient's diabetes is different, this schedule has been individualized for you.
Your usual dose of Humulin 70/30 may be affected by changes in your diet, activity, or work schedule. Carefully follow your doctor's instructions to allow for these changes. Other things that may affect your Humulin 70/30 dose are:
Illness
Illness, especially with nausea and vomiting, may cause your insulin requirements to change. Even if you are not eating, you will still require insulin. You and your doctor should establish a sick day plan for you to use in case of illness. When you are sick, test your blood glucose frequently. If instructed by your doctor, test your ketones and report the results to your doctor.
Pregnancy
Good control of diabetes is especially important for you and your unborn baby. Pregnancy may make managing your diabetes more difficult. If you are planning to have a baby, are pregnant, or are nursing a baby, talk to your doctor.
Medication
Insulin requirements may be increased if you are taking other drugs with blood–glucose–raising activity, such as oral contraceptives, corticosteroids, or thyroid replacement therapy. Insulin requirements may be reduced in the presence of drugs that lower blood glucose or affect how your body responds to insulin, such as oral antidiabetic agents, salicylates (for example, aspirin), sulfa antibiotics, alcohol, certain antidepressants and some kidney and blood pressure medicines. Your Health Care Professional may be aware of other medications that may affect your diabetes control. Therefore, always discuss any medications you are taking with your doctor.
Exercise
Exercise may lower your body's need for insulin during and for some time after the physical activity. Exercise may also speed up the effect of an insulin dose, especially if the exercise involves the area of injection site (for example, the leg should not be used for injection just prior to running). Discuss with your doctor how you should adjust your insulin regimen to accommodate exercise.
Travel
When traveling across more than 2 time zones, you should talk to your doctor concerning adjustments in your insulin schedule.

COMMON PROBLEMS OF DIABETES

Hypoglycemia (Low Blood Sugar)
Hypoglycemia (too little glucose in the blood) is one of the most frequent adverse events experienced by insulin users. It can be brought about by:
1. **Missing or delaying meals.**
2. Taking too much insulin.
3. Exercising or working more than usual.
4. An infection or illness associated with diarrhea or vomiting.
5. A change in the body's need for insulin.
6. Diseases of the adrenal, pituitary, or thyroid gland, or progression of kidney or liver disease.
7. Interactions with certain drugs, such as oral antidiabetic agents, salicylates (for example, aspirin), sulfa antibiotics, certain antidepressants and some kidney and blood pressure medicines.
8. Consumption of alcoholic beverages.

Symptoms of mild to moderate hypoglycemia may occur suddenly and can include:

• sweating	• drowsiness
• dizziness	• sleep disturbances
• palpitation	• anxiety
• tremor	• blurred vision
• hunger	• slurred speech
• restlessness	• depressed mood
• tingling in the hands, feet, lips, or tongue	• irritability
• lightheadedness	• abnormal behavior
• inability to concentrate	• unsteady movement
• headache	• personality changes

Signs of severe hypoglycemia can include:

• disorientation	• seizures
• unconsciousness	• death

Therefore, it is important that assistance be obtained immediately.
Early warning symptoms of hypoglycemia may be different or less pronounced under certain conditions, such as long duration of diabetes, diabetic nerve disease, use of medications such as beta–blockers, changing insulin preparations, or intensified control (3 or more insulin injections per day) of diabetes.
A few patients who have experienced hypoglycemic reactions after transfer from animal–source insulin to human insulin have reported that the early warning symptoms of hypoglycemia were less pronounced or different from those experienced with their previous insulin.
Without recognition of early warning symptoms, you may not be able to take steps to avoid more serious hypoglycemia. Be alert for all of the various types of symptoms that may indicate hypoglycemia. Patients who experience hypoglycemia without early warning symptoms should monitor their blood glucose frequently, especially prior to activities such as driving. If the blood glucose is below your normal fasting glucose, you should consider eating or drinking sugar–containing foods to treat your hypoglycemia.
Mild to moderate hypoglycemia may be treated by eating foods or drinks that contain sugar. Patients should always carry a quick source of sugar, such as hard candy or glucose tablets. More severe hypoglycemia may require the assistance of another person. Patients who are unable to take sugar orally or who are unconscious require an injection of glucagon or should be treated with intravenous administration of glucose at a medical facility.
You should learn to recognize your own symptoms of hypoglycemia. If you are uncertain about these symptoms, you should monitor your blood glucose frequently to help you learn to recognize the symptoms that you experience with hypoglycemia.
If you have frequent episodes of hypoglycemia or experience difficulty in recognizing the symptoms, you should talk to your doctor to discuss possible changes in therapy, meal plans, and/or exercise programs to help you avoid hypoglycemia.

Hyperglycemia (High Blood Sugar) and Diabetic Ketoacidosis (DKA)
Hyperglycemia (too much glucose in the blood) may develop if your body has too little insulin. Hyperglycemia can be brought about by any of the following:
1. Omitting your insulin or taking less than your doctor has prescribed.
2. Eating significantly more than your meal plan suggests.
3. Developing a fever, infection, or other significant stressful situation.

In patients with type 1 or insulin–dependent diabetes, prolonged hyperglycemia can result in DKA (a life-threatening emergency). The first symptoms of DKA usually come on gradually, over a period of hours or days, and include a drowsy feeling, flushed face, thirst, loss of appetite, and fruity odor on the breath. With DKA, blood and urine tests show large amounts of glucose and ketones. Heavy breathing and a rapid pulse are more severe symptoms. If uncorrected, prolonged hyperglycemia or DKA can lead to nausea, vomiting, stomach pain, dehydration, loss of consciousness, or death. Therefore, it is important that you obtain medical assistance immediately.

Lipodystrophy
Rarely, administration of insulin subcutaneously can result in lipoatrophy (seen as an apparent depression of the skin) or lipohypertrophy (seen as a raised area of the skin). If you notice either of these conditions, talk to your doctor. A change in your injection technique may help alleviate the problem.

Allergy
Local Allergy—Patients occasionally experience redness, swelling, and itching at the site of injection. This condition, called local allergy, usually clears up in a few days to a few weeks. In some instances, this condition may be related to factors other than insulin, such as irritants in the skin cleansing agent or poor injection technique. If you have local reactions, talk to your doctor.
Systemic Allergy—Less common, but potentially more serious, is generalized allergy to insulin, which may cause rash over the whole body, shortness of breath, wheezing, reduction in blood pressure, fast pulse, or sweating. Severe cases of generalized allergy may be life threatening. If you think you are having a generalized allergic reaction to insulin, call your doctor immediately.

ADDITIONAL INFORMATION
Information about diabetes may be obtained from your diabetes educator.
Additional information about diabetes and Humulin can be obtained by calling The Lilly Answers Center at 1-800-LillyRx (1-800-545-5979) or by visiting www.LillyDiabetes.com.
Patient Information revised August 22, 2007

Vials manufactured by
Eli Lilly and Company, Indianapolis, IN 46285, USA or
Lilly France, F-67640 Fegersheim, France
for Eli Lilly and Company, Indianapolis, IN 46285, USA
Copyright © 1992, 2007, Eli Lilly and Company. All rights reserved.
PV 5722 AMP

INFORMATION FOR THE PATIENT
3 ML PREFILLED INSULIN DELIVERY DEVICE
HUMULIN® 70/30 Pen
70% HUMAN INSULIN
ISOPHANE SUSPENSION
AND
30% HUMAN INSULIN INJECTION
(rDNA ORIGIN)
100 UNITS PER ML (U-100)

WARNINGS
THIS LILLY HUMAN INSULIN PRODUCT DIFFERS FROM ANIMAL–SOURCE INSULINS BECAUSE IT IS STRUCTURALLY IDENTICAL TO THE INSULIN PRODUCED BY YOUR BODY'S PANCREAS AND BECAUSE OF ITS UNIQUE MANUFACTURING PROCESS.
ANY CHANGE OF INSULIN SHOULD BE MADE CAUTIOUSLY AND ONLY UNDER MEDICAL SUPERVISION. CHANGES IN STRENGTH, MANUFACTURER, TYPE (E.G., REGULAR, NPH, ANALOG), SPECIES, OR METHOD OF MANUFACTURE MAY RESULT IN THE NEED FOR A CHANGE IN DOSAGE.
SOME PATIENTS TAKING HUMULIN® (HUMAN INSULIN, rDNA ORIGIN) MAY REQUIRE A CHANGE IN DOSAGE FROM THAT USED WITH OTHER INSULINS. IF AN ADJUSTMENT IS NEEDED, IT MAY OCCUR WITH THE FIRST DOSE OR DURING THE FIRST SEVERAL WEEKS OR MONTHS.
TO OBTAIN AN ACCURATE DOSE, CAREFULLY READ AND FOLLOW THE INSULIN DELIVERY DEVICE USER MANUAL AND THIS "INFORMATION FOR THE PATIENT" INSERT BEFORE USING THIS PRODUCT.
THE PEN MUST BE PRIMED TO A STREAM OF INSULIN (NOT JUST A FEW DROPS) BEFORE EACH INJECTION TO MAKE SURE THE PEN IS READY TO DOSE. YOU MAY NEED TO PRIME A NEW PEN UP TO SIX TIMES BEFORE A STREAM OF INSULIN APPEARS.
PRIMING THE PEN IS IMPORTANT TO CONFIRM THAT INSULIN COMES OUT WHEN YOU PUSH THE INJECTION BUTTON AND TO REMOVE AIR THAT MAY COLLECT IN THE INSULIN CARTRIDGE DURING NORMAL USE. IF YOU DO NOT PRIME, YOU MAY RECEIVE TOO MUCH OR TOO LITTLE INSULIN (*see also* INSTRUCTIONS FOR INSULIN PEN USE section).

DIABETES
Insulin is a hormone produced by the pancreas, a large gland that lies near the stomach. This hormone is necessary for the body's correct use of food, especially sugar. Diabetes occurs when the pancreas does not make enough insulin to meet your body's needs.
To control your diabetes, your doctor has prescribed injections of insulin products to keep your blood glucose at a near–normal level. You have been instructed to test your blood and/or your urine regularly for glucose. Studies have shown that some chronic complications of diabetes such as eye disease, kidney disease, and nerve disease can be significantly reduced if the blood sugar is maintained as close to normal as possible. The American Diabetes Association recommends that if your pre-meal glucose levels are consistently above 130 mg/dL or your hemoglobin A_{1c} (HbA_{1c}) is more than 7%, you should talk to your doctor. A change in your diabetes therapy may be needed. If your blood tests consistently show below–normal glucose levels, you should also let your doctor know. Proper control of your diabetes requires close and constant cooperation with your doctor. Despite diabetes, you can lead an active and healthy life if you eat a balanced diet, exercise regularly, and take your insulin injections as prescribed by your doctor.
Always keep an extra supply of insulin as well as a spare syringe and needle on hand. Always wear diabetic identification so that appropriate treatment can be given if complications occur away from home.

70/30 HUMAN INSULIN
Description
Humulin is synthesized in a special non–disease–producing laboratory strain of *Escherichia coli* bacteria that has been genetically altered to produce human insulin. Humulin 70/30 is a mixture of 70% Human Insulin Isophane Suspension and 30% Human Insulin Injection, (rDNA origin). It is an intermediate-acting insulin combined with the more rapid onset of action of Regular human insulin. The duration of activity may last up to 24 hours following injection. The time course of action of any insulin may vary considerably in different individuals or at different times in the same individual. As with all insulin preparations, the duration of action of Humulin 70/30 is dependent on dose, site of injection, blood supply, temperature, and physical activity. Humulin 70/30 is a sterile suspension and is for subcutaneous injection only. It should not be used intravenously or intramuscularly. The concentration of Humulin 70/30 is 100 units/mL (U–100).

Identification
Human insulin from Eli Lilly and Company has the trademark Humulin.
Your doctor has prescribed the type of insulin that he/she believes is best for you.
DO NOT USE ANY OTHER INSULIN EXCEPT ON YOUR DOCTOR'S ADVICE AND DIRECTION.
The Humulin 70/30 Pen is available in boxes of 5 prefilled insulin delivery devices ("insulin Pens"). The Humulin 70/30 Pen is not designed to allow any other insulin to be mixed in its cartridge, or for the cartridge to be removed.
Always check the carton and the Pen label for the name and letter designation of the insulin you receive from your pharmacy to make sure it is the same as prescribed by your doctor.
Always check the appearance of Humulin 70/30 suspension in your insulin Pen before using. A cartridge of Humulin 70/30 contains a small glass bead to assist in mixing. Roll the Pen back and forth between the palms 10 times (*see* Figure 1). Gently turn the Pen up and down 10 times until the insulin is evenly mixed (see Figure 2).

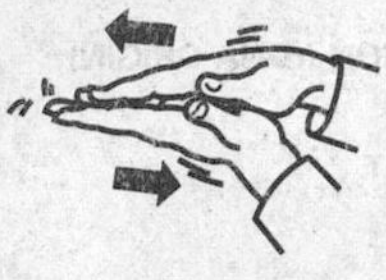

Figure 1.

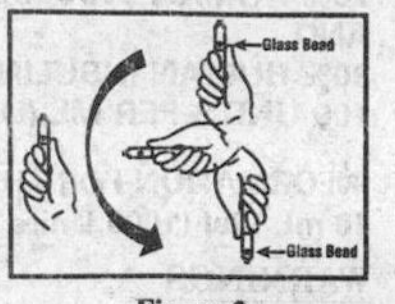

Figure 2.

If not evenly mixed, repeat the above steps until contents are mixed. Pens containing Humulin 70/30 suspension should be examined frequently.
Do not use Humulin 70/30:
- if the insulin substance (the white material) remains visibly separated from the liquid after mixing or
- if there are clumps in the insulin after mixing, or
- if solid white particles stick to the walls of the cartridge, giving a frosted appearance.

If you see anything unusual in the appearance of the Humulin 70/30 suspension in your Pen or notice your insulin requirements changing, talk to your doctor.
Never attempt to remove the cartridge from the Humulin 70/30 Pen. Inspect the cartridge through the clear cartridge holder.

Storage
Not in-use (unopened): Humulin 70/30 Pens not in-use should be stored in a refrigerator, but not in the freezer.
In-use (opened): Humulin 70/30 Pens in-use should **NOT** be refrigerated but should be kept at room temperature [below 86°F (30°C)] away from direct heat and light. The Humulin 70/30 Pen you are currently using must be discarded **10 days** after the first use, even if it still contains Humulin 70/30.
Do not use Humulin 70/30 after the expiration date stamped on the label or if it has been frozen.

INSTRUCTIONS FOR INSULIN PEN USE
It is important to read, understand, and follow the instructions in the Insulin Delivery Device User Manual before using. Failure to follow instructions may result in getting too much or too little insulin. The needle must be changed and the Pen must be primed to a stream of insulin (not just a few drops) before each injection to make sure the Pen is ready to dose. You may need to prime a new Pen up to six times before a stream of insulin appears. Performing these steps before each injection is important to confirm that insulin comes out when you push the injection button, and to remove air that may collect in the insulin cartridge during normal use.
Every time you inject:
- **Use a new needle.**
- **Prime to a stream of insulin (not just a few drops) to make sure the Pen is ready to dose.**
- **Make sure you got your full dose.**

NEVER SHARE INSULIN PENS, CARTRIDGES, OR NEEDLES.

PREPARING FOR INJECTION
1. Wash your hands.
2. To avoid tissue damage, choose a site for each injection that is at least 1/2 inch from the previous injection site. The usual sites of injection are abdomen, thighs, and arms.
3. Follow the instructions in your Insulin Delivery Device User Manual to prepare for injection.
4. After injecting the dose, pull the needle out and apply gentle pressure over the injection site for several seconds. **Do not rub the area.**
5. After the injection, remove the needle from the Humulin 70/30 Pen. **Do not reuse needles.**

6. Place the used needle in a puncture-resistant disposable container and properly dispose of the puncture-resistant container as directed by your Health Care Professional.

DOSAGE

Your doctor has told you which insulin to use, how much, and when and how often to inject it. Because each patient's diabetes is different, this schedule has been individualized for you.

Your usual dose of Humulin 70/30 may be affected by changes in your diet, activity, or work schedule. Carefully follow your doctor's instructions to allow for these changes. Other things that may affect your Humulin 70/30 dose are:

Illness

Illness, especially with nausea and vomiting, may cause your insulin requirements to change. Even if you are not eating, you will still require insulin. You and your doctor should establish a sick day plan for you to use in case of illness. When you are sick, test your blood glucose frequently. If instructed by your doctor, test your ketones and report the results to your doctor.

Pregnancy

Good control of diabetes is especially important for you and your unborn baby. Pregnancy may make managing your diabetes more difficult. If you are planning to have a baby, are pregnant, or are nursing a baby, talk to your doctor.

Medication

Insulin requirements may be increased if you are taking other drugs with blood–glucose–raising activity, such as oral contraceptives, corticosteroids, or thyroid replacement therapy. Insulin requirements may be reduced in the presence of drugs that lower blood glucose or affect how your body responds to insulin, such as oral antidiabetic agents, salicylates (for example, aspirin); sulfa antibiotics, alcohol, certain antidepressants and some kidney and blood pressure medicines. Your Health Care Professional may be aware of other medications that may affect your diabetes control. Therefore, always discuss any medications you are taking with your doctor.

Exercise

Exercise may lower your body's need for insulin during and for some time after the physical activity. Exercise may also speed up the effect of an insulin dose, especially if the exercise involves the area of injection site (for example, the leg should not be used for injection just prior to running). Discuss with your doctor how you should adjust your insulin regimen to accommodate exercise.

Travel

When traveling across more than 2 time zones, you should talk to your doctor concerning adjustments in your insulin schedule.

COMMON PROBLEMS OF DIABETES

Hypoglycemia (Low Blood Sugar)

Hypoglycemia (too little glucose in the blood) is one of the most frequent adverse events experienced by insulin users. It can be brought about by:

1. **Missing or delaying meals.**
2. Taking too much insulin.
3. Exercising or working more than usual.
4. An infection or illness associated with diarrhea or vomiting.
5. A change in the body's need for insulin.
6. Diseases of the adrenal, pituitary, or thyroid gland, or progression of kidney or liver disease.
7. Interactions with certain drugs, such as oral antidiabetic agents, salicylates (for example, aspirin), sulfa antibiotics, certain antidepressants and some kidney and blood pressure medicines.
8. Consumption of alcoholic beverages.

Symptoms of mild to moderate hypoglycemia may occur suddenly and can include:

• sweating	• drowsiness
• dizziness	• sleep disturbances
• palpitation	• anxiety
• tremor	• blurred vision
• hunger	• slurred speech
• restlessness	• depressed mood
• tingling in the hands, feet, lips, or tongue	• irritability
	• abnormal behavior
• lightheadedness	• unsteady movement
• inability to concentrate	• personality changes
• headache	

Signs of severe hypoglycemia can include:

• disorientation	• seizures
• unconsciousness	• death

Therefore, it is important that assistance be obtained immediately.

Early warning symptoms of hypoglycemia may be different or less pronounced under certain conditions, such as long duration of diabetes, diabetic nerve disease, use of medications such as beta–blockers, changing insulin preparations, or intensified control (3 or more insulin injections per day) of diabetes.

A few patients who have experienced hypoglycemic reactions after transfer from animal–source insulin to human insulin have reported that the early warning symptoms of hypoglycemia were less pronounced or different from those experienced with their previous insulin.

Without recognition of early warning symptoms, you may not be able to take steps to avoid more serious hypoglycemia. Be alert for all of the various types of symptoms that may indicate hypoglycemia. Patients who experience hypoglycemia without early warning symptoms should monitor their blood glucose frequently, especially prior to activities such as driving. If the blood glucose is below your normal fasting glucose, you should consider eating or drinking sugar–containing foods to treat your hypoglycemia.

Mild to moderate hypoglycemia may be treated by eating foods or drinks that contain sugar. Patients should always carry a quick source of sugar, such as hard candy or glucose tablets. More severe hypoglycemia may require the assistance of another person. Patients who are unable to take sugar orally or who are unconscious require an injection of glucagon or should be treated with intravenous administration of glucose at a medical facility.

You should learn to recognize your own symptoms of hypoglycemia. If you are uncertain about these symptoms, you should monitor your blood glucose frequently to help you learn to recognize the symptoms that you experience with hypoglycemia.

If you have frequent episodes of hypoglycemia or experience difficulty in recognizing the symptoms, you should talk to your doctor to discuss possible changes in therapy, meal plans, and/or exercise programs to help you avoid hypoglycemia.

Hyperglycemia (High Blood Sugar) and Diabetic Ketoacidosis (DKA)

Hyperglycemia (too much glucose in the blood) may develop if your body has too little insulin. Hyperglycemia can be brought about by any of the following:

1. Omitting your insulin or taking less than your doctor has prescribed.
2. Eating significantly more than your meal plan suggests.
3. Developing a fever, infection, or other significant stressful situation.

In patients with type 1 or insulin–dependent diabetes, prolonged hyperglycemia can result in DKA (a life-threatening emergency). The first symptoms of DKA usually come on gradually, over a period of hours or days, and include a drowsy feeling, flushed face, thirst, loss of appetite, and fruity odor on the breath. With DKA, blood and urine tests show large amounts of glucose and ketones. Heavy breathing and a rapid pulse are more severe symptoms. If uncorrected, prolonged hyperglycemia or DKA can lead to nausea, vomiting, stomach pain, dehydration, loss of consciousness, or death. Therefore, it is important that you obtain medical assistance immediately.

Lipodystrophy

Rarely, administration of insulin subcutaneously can result in lipoatrophy (seen as an apparent depression of the skin) or lipohypertrophy (seen as a raised area of the skin). If you notice either of these conditions, talk to your doctor. A change in your injection technique may help alleviate the problem.

Allergy

Local Allergy—Patients occasionally experience redness, swelling, and itching at the site of injection. This condition, called local allergy, usually clears up in a few days to a few weeks. In some instances, this condition may be related to factors other than insulin, such as irritants in the skin cleansing agent or poor injection technique. If you have local reactions, talk to your doctor.

Systemic Allergy—Less common, but potentially more serious, is generalized allergy to insulin, which may cause rash over the whole body, shortness of breath, wheezing, reduction in blood pressure, fast pulse, or sweating. Severe cases of generalized allergy may be life threatening. If you think you are having a generalized allergic reaction to insulin, call your doctor immediately.

ADDITIONAL INFORMATION

Information about diabetes may be obtained from your diabetes educator.

Additional information about diabetes and Humulin can be obtained by calling The Lilly Answers Center at 1–800–LillyRx (1–800–545–5979) or by visiting www.LillyDiabetes.com.

Patient Information revised March 16, 2009

Pens manufactured by
Eli Lilly and Company, Indianapolis, IN 46285, USA or
Lilly France, F-67640 Fegersheim, France
for Eli Lilly and Company, Indianapolis, IN 46285, USA

HUMULIN® N   OTC
[*hū ′mŭ-lĭn ĕn*]
NPH
HUMAN INSULIN (rDNA ORIGIN)
ISOPHANE SUSPENSION
100 UNITS PER ML (U-100)

INFORMATION FOR THE PATIENT
10 mL Vial (1000 Units per vial)

WARNINGS

**THIS LILLY HUMAN INSULIN PRODUCT DIFFERS FROM ANIMAL–SOURCE INSULINS BECAUSE IT IS STRUCTURALLY IDENTICAL TO THE INSULIN PRODUCED BY YOUR BODY'S PANCREAS AND BECAUSE OF ITS UNIQUE MANUFACTURING PROCESS.
ANY CHANGE OF INSULIN SHOULD BE MADE CAUTIOUSLY AND ONLY UNDER MEDICAL SUPERVISION. CHANGES IN STRENGTH, MANUFACTURER, TYPE (E.G., REGULAR, NPH, ANALOG), SPECIES, OR METHOD OF MANUFACTURE MAY RESULT IN THE NEED FOR A CHANGE IN DOSAGE.
SOME PATIENTS TAKING HUMULIN® (HUMAN INSULIN, rDNA ORIGIN) MAY REQUIRE A CHANGE IN DOSAGE FROM THAT USED WITH OTHER INSULINS. IF AN ADJUSTMENT IS NEEDED, IT MAY OCCUR WITH THE FIRST DOSE OR DURING THE FIRST SEVERAL WEEKS OR MONTHS.**

DIABETES

Insulin is a hormone produced by the pancreas, a large gland that lies near the stomach. This hormone is necessary for the body's correct use of food, especially sugar. Diabetes occurs when the pancreas does not make enough insulin to meet your body's needs.

To control your diabetes, your doctor has prescribed injections of insulin products to keep your blood glucose at a near–normal level. You have been instructed to test your blood and/or your urine regularly for glucose. Studies have shown that some chronic complications of diabetes such as eye disease, kidney disease, and nerve disease can be significantly reduced if the blood sugar is maintained as close to normal as possible. The American Diabetes Association recommends that if your pre–meal glucose levels are consistently above 130 mg/dL or your hemoglobin A_{1c} (HbA_{1c}) is more than 7%, you should talk to your doctor. A change in your diabetes therapy may be needed. If your blood tests consistently show below–normal glucose levels, you should also let your doctor know. Proper control of your diabetes requires close and constant cooperation with your doctor. Despite diabetes, you can lead an active and healthy life if you eat a balanced diet, exercise regularly, and take your insulin injections as prescribed by your doctor.

Always keep an extra supply of insulin as well as a spare syringe and needle on hand. Always wear diabetic identification so that appropriate treatment can be given if complications occur away from home.

NPH HUMAN INSULIN
Description

Humulin is synthesized in a special non–disease–producing laboratory strain of *Escherichia coli* bacteria that has been genetically altered to produce human insulin. Humulin N [Human insulin (rDNA origin) isophane suspension] is a crystalline suspension of human insulin with protamine and zinc providing an intermediate-acting insulin with a slower onset of action and a longer duration of activity (up to 24 hours) than that of Regular human insulin. The time course of action of any insulin may vary considerably in different individuals or at different times in the same individual. As with all insulin preparations, the duration of action of Humulin N is dependent on dose, site of injection, blood supply, temperature, and physical activity. Humulin N is a sterile suspension and is for subcutaneous injection only. It should not be used intravenously or intramuscularly. The concentration of Humulin N is 100 units/mL (U-100).

Identification

Human insulin from Eli Lilly and Company has the trademark Humulin. Your doctor has prescribed the type of insulin that he/she believes is best for you.
DO NOT USE ANY OTHER INSULIN EXCEPT ON YOUR DOCTOR'S ADVICE AND DIRECTION.

Always check the carton and the bottle label for the name and letter designation of the insulin you receive from your pharmacy to make sure it is the same as prescribed by your doctor.

Always check the appearance of your bottle of Humulin N before withdrawing each dose. Before each injection the Humulin N bottle must be carefully shaken or rotated several times to completely mix the insulin. Humulin N suspension should look uniformly cloudy or milky after mixing. If not, repeat the above steps until contents are mixed.

Do not use Humulin N:

- if the insulin substance (the white material) remains at the bottom of the bottle after mixing or
- if there are clumps in the insulin after mixing, or
- if solid white particles stick to the bottom or wall of the bottle, giving a frosted appearance.

If you see anything unusual in the appearance of Humulin N suspension in your bottle or notice your insulin requirements changing, talk to your doctor.

Storage

Not in-use (unopened): Humulin N bottles not in-use should be stored in a refrigerator, but not in the freezer.

In-use (opened): The Humulin N bottle you are currently using can be kept unrefrigerated as long as it is kept as cool as possible [below 86°F (30°C)] away from heat and light.

Do not use Humulin N after the expiration date stamped on the label or if it has been frozen.

INSTRUCTIONS FOR INSULIN VIAL USE

NEVER SHARE NEEDLES AND SYRINGES.

Correct Syringe Type

Doses of insulin are measured in **units**. U–100 insulin contains 100 units/mL (1 mL=1 cc). With Humulin N, it is important to use a syringe that is marked for U–100 insulin preparations. Failure to use the proper syringe can lead to a mistake in dosage, causing serious problems for you, such as a blood glucose level that is too low or too high.

Syringe Use

To help avoid contamination and possible infection, follow these instructions exactly.

Disposable syringes and needles should be used only once and then discarded by placing the used needle in a puncture-resistant disposable container. Properly dispose of the puncture-resistant container as directed by your Health Care Professional.

Preparing the Dose

1. Wash your hands.
2. Carefully shake or rotate the bottle of insulin several times to completely mix the insulin.
3. Inspect the insulin. Humulin N suspension should look uniformly cloudy or milky. Do not use Humulin N if you notice anything unusual in its appearance.
4. If using a new Humulin N bottle, flip off the plastic protective cap, but **do not** remove the stopper. Wipe the top of the bottle with an alcohol swab.
5. If you are mixing insulins, refer to the "Mixing Humulin N and Regular Human Insulin" section below.
6. Draw an amount of air into the syringe that is equal to the Humulin N dose. Put the needle through rubber top of the Humulin N bottle and inject the air into the bottle.
7. Turn the Humulin N bottle and syringe upside down. Hold the bottle and syringe firmly in one hand and shake gently.
8. Making sure the tip of the needle is in the Humulin N suspension, withdraw the correct dose of Humulin N into the syringe.
9. Before removing the needle from the Humulin N bottle, check the syringe for air bubbles. If bubbles are present, hold the syringe straight up and tap its side until the bubbles float to the top. Push the bubbles out with the plunger and then withdraw the correct dose.
10. Remove the needle from the bottle and lay the syringe down so that the needle does not touch anything.
11. If you do not need to mix your Humulin N with Regular human insulin, go to the "Injection Instructions" section below and follow the directions.

Mixing Humulin N and Regular Human Insulin (Humulin R)

1. Humulin N should be mixed with Humulin R only on the advice of your doctor.
2. Draw an amount of air into the syringe that is equal to the amount of Humulin N you are taking. Insert the needle into the Humulin N bottle and inject the air. Withdraw the needle.
3. Draw an amount of air into the syringe that is equal to the amount of Humulin R you are taking. Insert the needle into the Humulin R bottle and inject the air, but **not** withdraw the needle.
4. Turn the Humulin R bottle and syringe upside down.
5. Making sure the tip of the needle is in the Humulin R solution, withdraw the correct dose of Humulin R into the syringe.
6. Before removing the needle from the Humulin R bottle, check the syringe for air bubbles. If bubbles are present, hold the syringe straight up and tap its side until the bubbles float to the top. Push the bubbles out with the plunger and then withdraw the correct dose.
7. Remove the syringe with the needle from the Humulin R bottle and insert it into the Humulin N bottle. Turn the Humulin N bottle and syringe upside down. Hold the bottle and syringe firmly in one hand and shake gently. Making sure the tip of the needle is in the Humulin N, withdraw the correct dose of Humulin N.
8. Remove the needle from the bottle and lay the syringe down so that the needle does not touch anything.

9. Follow the directions under "Injection Instructions" section below.

Follow your doctor's instructions on whether to mix your insulins ahead of time or just before giving your injection. It is important to be consistent in your method.

Syringes from different manufacturers may vary in the amount of space between the bottom line and the needle. Because of this, do not change:

- the sequence of mixing, or
- the model and brand of syringe or needle that your doctor has prescribed.

Injection Instructions

1. To avoid tissue damage, choose a site for each injection that is at least 1/2 inch from the previous injection site. The usual sites of injection are abdomen, thighs, and arms.
2. Cleanse the skin with alcohol where the injection is to be made.
3. With one hand, stabilize the skin by spreading it or pinching up a large area.
4. Insert the needle as instructed by your doctor.
5. Push the plunger in as far as it will go.
6. Pull the needle out and apply gentle pressure over the injection site for several seconds. **Do not rub the area.**
7. Place the used needle in a puncture-resistant disposable container and properly dispose of the puncture-resistant container as directed by your Health Care Professional.

DOSAGE

Your doctor has told you which insulin to use, how much, and when and how often to inject it. Because each patient's diabetes is different, this schedule has been individualized for you.

Your usual dose of Humulin N may be affected by changes in your diet, activity, or work schedule. Carefully follow your doctor's instructions to allow for these changes. Other things that may affect your Humulin N dose are:

Illness

Illness, especially with nausea and vomiting, may cause your insulin requirements to change. Even if you are not eating, you will still require insulin. You and your doctor should establish a sick day plan for you to use in case of illness. When you are sick, test your blood glucose frequently. If instructed by your doctor, test your ketones and report the results to your doctor.

Pregnancy

Good control of diabetes is especially important for you and your unborn baby. Pregnancy may make managing your diabetes more difficult. If you are planning to have a baby, are pregnant, or are nursing a baby, talk to your doctor.

Medication

Insulin requirements may be increased if you are taking other drugs with blood–glucose–raising activity, such as oral contraceptives, corticosteroids, or thyroid replacement therapy. Insulin requirements may be reduced in the presence of drugs that lower blood glucose or affect how your body responds to insulin, such as oral antidiabetic agents, salicylates (for example, aspirin), sulfa antibiotics, alcohol, certain antidepressants and some kidney and blood pressure medicines. Your Health Care Professional may be aware of other medications that may affect your diabetes control. Therefore, always discuss any medications you are taking with your doctor.

Exercise

Exercise may lower your body's need for insulin during and for some time after the physical activity. Exercise may also speed up the effect of an insulin dose, especially if the exercise involves the area of injection site (for example, the leg should not be used for injection just prior to running). Discuss with your doctor how you should adjust your insulin regimen to accommodate exercise.

Travel

When traveling across more than 2 time zones, you should talk to your doctor concerning adjustments in your insulin schedule.

COMMON PROBLEMS OF DIABETES

Hypoglycemia (Low Blood Sugar)

Hypoglycemia (too little glucose in the blood) is one of the most frequent adverse events experienced by insulin users. It can be brought about by:

1. **Missing or delaying meals.**
2. Taking too much insulin.
3. Exercising or working more than usual.
4. An infection or illness associated with diarrhea or vomiting.
5. A change in the body's need for insulin.
6. Diseases of the adrenal, pituitary, or thyroid gland, or progression of kidney or liver disease.
7. Interactions with certain drugs, such as oral antidiabetic agents, salicylates (for example, aspirin), sulfa antibiotics, certain antidepressants and some kidney and blood pressure medicines.
8. Consumption of alcoholic beverages.

Symptoms of mild to moderate hypoglycemia may occur suddenly and can include:

• sweating	• drowsiness
• dizziness	• sleep disturbances
• palpitation	• anxiety
• tremor	• blurred vision
• hunger	• slurred speech
• restlessness	• depressed mood
• tingling in the hands, feet, lips, or tongue	• irritability
	• abnormal behavior
• lightheadedness	• unsteady movement
• inability to concentrate	• personality changes
• headache	

Signs of severe hypoglycemia can include:

• disorientation	• seizures
• unconsciousness	• death

Therefore, it is important that assistance be obtained immediately.

Early warning symptoms of hypoglycemia may be different or less pronounced under certain conditions, such as long duration of diabetes, diabetic nerve disease, use of medications such as beta–blockers, changing insulin preparations, or intensified control (3 or more insulin injections per day) of diabetes.

A few patients who have experienced hypoglycemic reactions after transfer from animal–source insulin to human insulin have reported that the early warning symptoms of hypoglycemia were less pronounced or different from those experienced with their previous insulin.

Without recognition of early warning symptoms, you may not be able to take steps to avoid more serious hypoglycemia. Be alert for all of the various types of symptoms that may indicate hypoglycemia. Patients who experience hypoglycemia without early warning symptoms should monitor their blood glucose frequently, especially prior to activities such as driving. If the blood glucose is below your normal fasting glucose, you should consider eating or drinking sugar–containing foods to treat your hypoglycemia.

Mild to moderate hypoglycemia may be treated by eating foods or drinks that contain sugar. Patients should always carry a quick source of sugar, such as hard candy or glucose tablets. More severe hypoglycemia may require the assistance of another person. Patients who are unable to take sugar orally or who are unconscious require an injection of glucagon or should be treated with intravenous administration of glucose at a medical facility.

You should learn to recognize your own symptoms of hypoglycemia. If you are uncertain about these symptoms, you should monitor your blood glucose frequently to help you learn to recognize the symptoms that you experience with hypoglycemia.

If you have frequent episodes of hypoglycemia or experience difficulty in recognizing the symptoms, you should talk to your doctor to discuss possible changes in therapy, meal plans, and/or exercise programs to help you avoid hypoglycemia.

Hyperglycemia (High Blood Sugar) and Diabetic Ketoacidosis (DKA)

Hyperglycemia (too much glucose in the blood) may develop if your body has too little insulin. Hyperglycemia can be brought about by any of the following:

1. Omitting your insulin or taking less than your doctor has prescribed.
2. Eating significantly more than your meal plan suggests.
3. Developing a fever, infection, or other significant stressful situation.

In patients with type 1 or insulin–dependent diabetes, prolonged hyperglycemia can result in DKA (a life-threatening emergency). The first symptoms of DKA usually come on gradually, over a period of hours or days, and include a drowsy feeling, flushed face, thirst, loss of appetite, and fruity odor on the breath. With DKA, blood and urine tests show large amounts of glucose and ketones. Heavy breathing and a rapid pulse are more severe symptoms. If uncorrected, prolonged hyperglycemia or DKA can lead to nausea, vomiting, stomach pain, dehydration, loss of consciousness, or death. Therefore, it is important that you obtain medical assistance immediately.

Lipodystrophy

Rarely, administration of insulin subcutaneously can result in lipoatrophy (seen as an apparent depression of the skin) or lipohypertrophy (seen as a raised area of the skin). If you notice either of these conditions, talk to your doctor. A change in your injection technique may help alleviate the problem.

Allergy

Local Allergy—Patients occasionally experience redness, swelling, and itching at the site of injection. This condition, called local allergy, usually clears up in a few days to a few weeks. In some instances, this condition may be related to factors other than insulin, such as irritants in the skin cleansing agent or poor injection technique. If you have local reactions, talk to your doctor.

Systemic Allergy—Less common, but potentially more serious, is generalized allergy to insulin, which may cause rash over the whole body, shortness of breath, wheezing, reduction in blood pressure, fast pulse, or sweating. Severe cases of generalized allergy may be life threatening. If you think you are having a generalized allergic reaction to insulin, call your doctor immediately.

ADDITIONAL INFORMATION

Information about diabetes may be obtained from your diabetes educator.

Additional information about diabetes and Humulin can be obtained by calling The Lilly Answers Center at 1-800-LillyRx (1-800-545-5979) or by visiting www.LillyDiabetes.com.

Patient Information revised August 22, 2007

Vials manufactured by

Eli Lilly and Company, Indianapolis, IN 46285, USA or

Lilly France, F-67640 Fegersheim, France

for Eli Lilly and Company, Indianapolis, IN 46285, USA

Copyright © 1997, 2007, Eli Lilly and Company. All rights reserved.

PV 5712 AMP

INFORMATION FOR THE PATIENT

3 ML PREFILLED INSULIN DELIVERY DEVICE
HUMULIN® N Pen
NPH
HUMAN INSULIN
(rDNA ORIGIN) ISOPHANE SUSPENSION
100 UNITS PER ML (U-100)

WARNINGS

THIS LILLY HUMAN INSULIN PRODUCT DIFFERS FROM ANIMAL-SOURCE INSULINS BECAUSE IT IS STRUCTURALLY IDENTICAL TO THE INSULIN PRODUCED BY YOUR BODY'S PANCREAS AND BECAUSE OF ITS UNIQUE MANUFACTURING PROCESS.

ANY CHANGE OF INSULIN SHOULD BE MADE CAUTIOUSLY AND ONLY UNDER MEDICAL SUPERVISION. CHANGES IN STRENGTH, MANUFACTURER, TYPE (E.G., REGULAR, NPH, ANALOG), SPECIES, OR METHOD OF MANUFACTURE MAY RESULT IN THE NEED FOR A CHANGE IN DOSAGE.

SOME PATIENTS TAKING HUMULIN® (HUMAN INSULIN, rDNA ORIGIN) MAY REQUIRE A CHANGE IN DOSAGE FROM THAT USED WITH OTHER INSULINS. IF AN ADJUSTMENT IS NEEDED, IT MAY OCCUR WITH THE FIRST DOSE OR DURING THE FIRST SEVERAL WEEKS OR MONTHS.

TO OBTAIN AN ACCURATE DOSE, CAREFULLY READ AND FOLLOW THE INSULIN DELIVERY DEVICE USER MANUAL AND THIS "INFORMATION FOR THE PATIENT" INSERT BEFORE USING THIS PRODUCT. THE PEN MUST BE PRIMED TO A STREAM OF INSULIN (NOT JUST A FEW DROPS) BEFORE EACH INJECTION TO MAKE SURE THE PEN IS READY TO DOSE. YOU MAY NEED TO PRIME A NEW PEN UP TO SIX TIMES BEFORE A STREAM OF INSULIN APPEARS.

PRIMING THE PEN IS IMPORTANT TO CONFIRM THAT INSULIN COMES OUT WHEN YOU PUSH THE INJECTION BUTTON AND TO REMOVE AIR THAT MAY COLLECT IN THE INSULIN CARTRIDGE DURING NORMAL USE. IF YOU DO NOT PRIME, YOU MAY RECEIVE TOO MUCH OR TOO LITTLE INSULIN *(see also* INSTRUCTIONS FOR INSULIN PEN USE section).

DIABETES

Insulin is a hormone produced by the pancreas, a large gland that lies near the stomach. This hormone is necessary for the body's correct use of food, especially sugar. Diabetes occurs when the pancreas does not make enough insulin to meet your body's needs.

To control your diabetes, your doctor has prescribed injections of insulin products to keep your blood glucose at a near–normal level. You have been instructed to test your blood and/or your urine regularly for glucose. Studies have shown that some chronic complications of diabetes such as eye disease, kidney disease, and nerve disease can be significantly reduced if the blood sugar is maintained as close to normal as possible. The American Diabetes Association recommends that if your pre-meal glucose levels are consistently above 130 mg/dL or your hemoglobin A_{1c} (HbA_{1c}) is more than 7%, you should talk to your doctor. A change in your diabetes therapy may be needed. If your blood tests consistently show below–normal glucose levels, you should also let your doctor know. Proper control of your diabetes requires close and constant cooperation with your doctor. Despite diabetes, you can lead an active and healthy life if you eat a balanced diet, exercise regularly, and take your insulin injections as prescribed by your doctor.

Always keep an extra supply of insulin as well as a spare syringe and needle on hand. Always wear diabetic identification so that appropriate treatment can be given if complications occur away from home.

NPH HUMAN INSULIN

Description

Humulin is synthesized in a special non–disease–producing laboratory strain of *Escherichia coli* bacteria that has been genetically altered to produce human insulin. Humulin N [Human insulin (rDNA origin) isophane suspension] is a crystalline suspension of human insulin with protamine and zinc providing an intermediate-acting insulin with a slower onset of action and a longer duration of activity (up to 24 hours) than that of Regular human insulin. The time course of action of any insulin may vary considerably in different individuals or at different times in the same individual. As with all insulin preparations, the duration of action of Humulin N is dependent on dose, site of injection, blood supply, temperature, and physical activity. Humulin N is a sterile suspension and is for subcutaneous injection only. It should not be used intravenously or intramuscularly. The concentration of Humulin N is 100 units/mL (U–100).

Identification

Human insulin from Eli Lilly and Company has the trademark Humulin. Your doctor has prescribed the type of insulin that he/she believes is best for you.

DO NOT USE ANY OTHER INSULIN EXCEPT ON YOUR DOCTOR'S ADVICE AND DIRECTION.

The Humulin N Pen is available in boxes of 5 prefilled insulin delivery devices ("insulin Pens"). The Humulin N Pen is not designed to allow any other insulin to be mixed in its cartridge, or for the cartridge to be removed.

Always check the carton and the Pen label for the name and letter designation of the insulin you receive from your pharmacy to make sure it is the same as prescribed by your doctor.

Always check the appearance of Humulin N suspension in your insulin Pen before using. A cartridge of Humulin N contains a small glass bead to assist in mixing. Roll the Pen back and forth between the palms 10 times (see Figure 1). Gently turn the Pen up and down 10 times until the insulin is evenly mixed (see Figure 2).

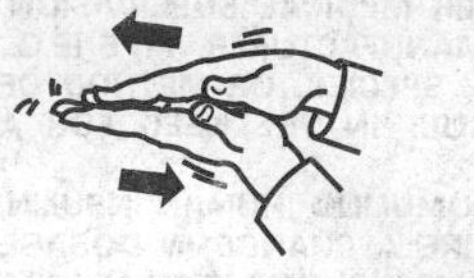

Figure 1.

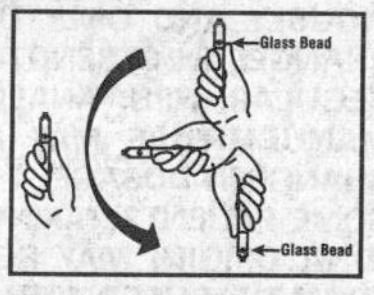

Figure 2.

If not evenly mixed, repeat the above steps until contents are mixed. Pens containing Humulin N suspension should be examined frequently.

Do not use Humulin N:

- if the insulin substance (the white material) remains visibly separated from the liquid after mixing or
- if there are clumps in the insulin after mixing, or
- if solid white particles stick to the walls of the cartridge, giving a frosted appearance.

If you see anything unusual in the appearance of the Humulin N suspension in your Pen or notice your insulin requirements changing, talk to your doctor.

Never attempt to remove the cartridge from the Humulin N Pen. Inspect the cartridge through the clear cartridge holder.

Storage

Not in-use (unopened): Humulin N Pens not in-use should be stored in a refrigerator, but not in the freezer.

In-use (opened): Humulin N Pens in-use should **NOT** be refrigerated but should be kept at room temperature [below 86°F (30°C)] away from direct heat and light. The Humulin N Pen you are currently using must be discarded **2 weeks** after the first use, even if it still contains Humulin N.

Do not use Humulin N after the expiration date stamped on the label or if it has been frozen.

INSTRUCTIONS FOR INSULIN PEN USE

It is important to read, understand, and follow the instructions in the Insulin Delivery Device User Manual before using. Failure to follow instructions may result in getting too much or too little insulin. The needle must be changed and the Pen must be primed to a stream of insulin (not just a few drops) before each injection to make sure the Pen is ready to dose. You may need to prime a new Pen up to six times before a stream of insulin appears. Performing these steps before each injection is important to confirm that insulin comes out when you push the injection button, and to remove air that may collect in the insulin cartridge during normal use.

Every time you inject:

- **Use a new needle.**
- **Prime to a stream of insulin (not just a few drops) to make sure the Pen is ready to dose.**
- **Make sure you got your full dose.**

NEVER SHARE INSULIN PENS, CARTRIDGES, OR NEEDLES.

PREPARING FOR INJECTION

1. Wash your hands.
2. To avoid tissue damage, choose a site for each injection that is at least 1/2 inch from the previous injection site. The usual sites of injection are abdomen, thighs, and arms.
3. Follow the instructions in your Insulin Delivery Device User Manual to prepare for injection.
4. After injecting the dose, pull the needle out and apply gentle pressure over the injection site for several seconds. **Do not rub the area.**
5. After the injection, remove the needle from the Humulin N Pen. **Do not reuse needles.**
6. Place the used needle in a puncture-resistant disposable container and properly dispose of the puncture-resistant container as directed by your Health Care Professional.

DOSAGE

Your doctor has told you which insulin to use, how much, and when and how often to inject it. Because each patient's diabetes is different, this schedule has been individualized for you.

Your usual dose of Humulin N may be affected by changes in your diet, activity, or work schedule. Carefully follow your doctor's instructions to allow for these changes. Other things that may affect your Humulin N dose are:

Illness

Illness, especially with nausea and vomiting, may cause your insulin requirements to change. Even if you are not eating, you will still require insulin. You and your doctor should establish a sick day plan for you to use in case of illness. When you are sick, test your blood glucose frequently. If instructed by your doctor, test your ketones and report the results to your doctor.

Pregnancy

Good control of diabetes is especially important for you and your unborn baby. Pregnancy may make managing your diabetes more difficult. If you are planning to have a baby, are pregnant, or are nursing a baby, talk to your doctor.

Medication

Insulin requirements may be increased if you are taking other drugs with blood–glucose–raising activity, such as oral contraceptives, corticosteroids, or thyroid replacement therapy. Insulin requirements may be reduced in the presence of drugs that lower blood glucose or affect how your body responds to insulin, such as oral antidiabetic agents, salicylates (for example, aspirin), sulfa antibiotics, alcohol, certain antidepressants and some kidney and blood pressure medicines. Your Health Care Professional may be aware of other medications that may affect your diabetes control. Therefore, always discuss any medications you are taking with your doctor.

Exercise

Exercise may lower your body's need for insulin during and for some time after the physical activity. Exercise may also speed up the effect of an insulin dose, especially if the exercise involves the area of injection site (for example, the leg should not be used for injection just prior to running). Discuss with your doctor how you should adjust your insulin regimen to accommodate exercise.

Travel

When traveling across more than 2 time zones, you should talk to your doctor concerning adjustments in your insulin schedule.

COMMON PROBLEMS OF DIABETES

Hypoglycemia (Low Blood Sugar)

Hypoglycemia (too little glucose in the blood) is one of the most frequent adverse events experienced by insulin users. It can be brought about by:

1. **Missing or delaying meals.**
2. Taking too much insulin.
3. Exercising or working more than usual.
4. An infection or illness associated with diarrhea or vomiting.
5. A change in the body's need for insulin.
6. Diseases of the adrenal, pituitary, or thyroid gland, or progression of kidney or liver disease.
7. Interactions with certain drugs, such as oral antidiabetic agents, salicylates (for example, aspirin), sulfa antibiotics, certain antidepressants and some kidney and blood pressure medicines.
8. Consumption of alcoholic beverages.

Symptoms of mild to moderate hypoglycemia may occur suddenly and can include:

- sweating
- dizziness
- palpitation
- tremor
- hunger
- restlessness
- tingling in the hands, feet, lips, or tongue
- lightheadedness
- inability to concentrate
- headache
- drowsiness
- sleep disturbances
- anxiety
- blurred vision
- slurred speech
- depressed mood
- irritability
- abnormal behavior
- unsteady movement
- personality changes

Signs of severe hypoglycemia can include:

- disorientation
- unconsciousness
- seizures
- death

Therefore, it is important that assistance be obtained immediately.

Early warning symptoms of hypoglycemia may be different or less pronounced under certain conditions, such as long duration of diabetes, diabetic nerve disease, use of medications such as beta-blockers, changing insulin preparations, or intensified control (3 or more insulin injections per day) of diabetes.

A few patients who have experienced hypoglycemic reactions after transfer from animal-source insulin to human insulin have reported that the early warning symptoms of hypoglycemia were less pronounced or different from those experienced with their previous insulin.

Without recognition of early warning symptoms, you may not be able to take steps to avoid more serious hypoglycemia. Be alert for all of the various types of symptoms that may indicate hypoglycemia. Patients who experience hypoglycemia without early warning symptoms should monitor their blood glucose frequently, especially prior to activities such as driving. If the blood glucose is below your normal fasting glucose, you should consider eating or drinking sugar-containing foods to treat your hypoglycemia.

Mild to moderate hypoglycemia may be treated by eating foods or drinks that contain sugar. Patients should always carry a quick source of sugar, such as hard candy or glucose tablets. More severe hypoglycemia may require the assistance of another person. Patients who are unable to take sugar orally or who are unconscious require an injection of glucagon or should be treated with intravenous administration of glucose at a medical facility.

You should learn to recognize your own symptoms of hypoglycemia. If you are uncertain about these symptoms, you should monitor your blood glucose frequently to help you learn to recognize the symptoms that you experience with hypoglycemia.

If you have frequent episodes of hypoglycemia or experience difficulty in recognizing the symptoms, you should talk to your doctor to discuss possible changes in therapy, meal plans, and/or exercise programs to help you avoid hypoglycemia.

Hyperglycemia (High Blood Sugar) and Diabetic Ketoacidosis (DKA)

Hyperglycemia (too much glucose in the blood) may develop if your body has too little insulin. Hyperglycemia can be brought about by any of the following:

1. Omitting your insulin or taking less than your doctor has prescribed.
2. Eating significantly more than your meal plan suggests.
3. Developing a fever, infection, or other significant stressful situation.

In patients with type 1 or insulin-dependent diabetes, prolonged hyperglycemia can result in DKA (a life-threatening emergency). The first symptoms of DKA usually come on gradually, over a period of hours or days, and include a drowsy feeling, flushed face, thirst, loss of appetite, and fruity odor on the breath. With DKA, blood and urine tests show large amounts of glucose and ketones. Heavy breathing and a rapid pulse are more severe symptoms. If uncorrected, prolonged hyperglycemia or DKA can lead to nausea, vomiting, stomach pain, dehydration, loss of consciousness, or death. Therefore, it is important that you obtain medical assistance immediately.

Lipodystrophy

Rarely, administration of insulin subcutaneously can result in lipoatrophy (seen as an apparent depression of the skin) or lipohypertrophy (seen as a raised area of the skin). If you notice either of these conditions, talk to your doctor. A change in your injection technique may help alleviate the problem.

Allergy

Local Allergy—Patients occasionally experience redness, swelling, and itching at the site of injection. This condition,

called local allergy, usually clears up in a few days to a few weeks. In some instances, this condition may be related to factors other than insulin, such as irritants in the skin cleansing agent or poor injection technique. If you have local reactions, talk to your doctor.

Systemic Allergy—Less common, but potentially more serious, is generalized allergy to insulin, which may cause rash over the whole body, shortness of breath, wheezing, reduction in blood pressure, fast pulse, or sweating. Severe cases of generalized allergy may be life threatening. If you think you are having a generalized allergic reaction to insulin, call your doctor immediately.

ADDITIONAL INFORMATION

Information about diabetes may be obtained from your diabetes educator.

Additional information about diabetes and Humulin can be obtained by calling The Lilly Answers Center at 1-800-LillyRx (1-800-545-5979) or by visiting www.LillyDiabetes.com.

Patient Information revised March 16, 2009

Pens manufactured by

Eli Lilly and Company, Indianapolis, IN 46285, USA or Lilly France, F-67640 Fegersheim, France

for Eli Lilly and Company, Indianapolis, IN 46285, USA

Copyright © 1998, 2009, Eli Lilly and Company. All rights reserved.

PA 9135 FSAMP

Revised: 02/2010   Distributed by: Eli Lilly and Company

HUMULIN® R REGULAR   OTC

[hū' mŭ-lĭn-ar]

INSULIN HUMAN INJECTION, USP

(rDNA ORIGIN)

100 UNITS PER ML (U-100)

INFORMATION FOR THE PATIENT

10 mL Vial (1000 Units per vial)

3 mL Vial (300 Units per vial)

WARNINGS

THIS LILLY HUMAN INSULIN PRODUCT DIFFERS FROM ANIMAL-SOURCE INSULINS BECAUSE IT IS STRUCTURALLY IDENTICAL TO THE INSULIN PRODUCED BY YOUR BODY'S PANCREAS AND BECAUSE OF ITS UNIQUE MANUFACTURING PROCESS.

ANY CHANGE OF INSULIN SHOULD BE MADE CAUTIOUSLY AND ONLY UNDER MEDICAL SUPERVISION. CHANGES IN STRENGTH, MANUFACTURER, TYPE (E.G., REGULAR, NPH, ANALOG), SPECIES, OR METHOD OF MANUFACTURE MAY RESULT IN THE NEED FOR A CHANGE IN DOSAGE.

SOME PATIENTS TAKING HUMULIN® (HUMAN INSULIN, rDNA ORIGIN) MAY REQUIRE A CHANGE IN DOSAGE FROM THAT USED WITH OTHER INSULINS. IF AN ADJUSTMENT IS NEEDED, IT MAY OCCUR WITH THE FIRST DOSE OR DURING THE FIRST SEVERAL WEEKS OR MONTHS.

DIABETES

Insulin is a hormone produced by the pancreas, a large gland that lies near the stomach. This hormone is necessary for the body's correct use of food, especially sugar. Diabetes occurs when the pancreas does not make enough insulin to meet your body's needs.

To control your diabetes, your doctor has prescribed injections of insulin products to keep your blood glucose at a near-normal level. You have been instructed to test your blood and/or your urine regularly for glucose. Studies have shown that some chronic complications of diabetes such as eye disease, kidney disease, and nerve disease can be significantly reduced if the blood sugar is maintained as close to normal as possible. The American Diabetes Association recommends that if your pre-meal glucose levels are consistently above 130 mg/dL or your hemoglobin A_{1c} (HbA_{1c}) is more than 7%, you should talk to your doctor. A change in your diabetes therapy may be needed. If your blood tests consistently show below-normal glucose levels, you should also let your doctor know. Proper control of your diabetes requires close and constant cooperation with your doctor. Despite diabetes, you can lead an active and healthy life if you eat a balanced diet, exercise regularly, and take your insulin injections as prescribed by your doctor.

Always keep an extra supply of insulin as well as a spare syringe and needle on hand. Always wear diabetic identification so that appropriate treatment can be given if complications occur away from home.

REGULAR HUMAN INSULIN

Description

Humulin is synthesized in a special non-disease-producing laboratory strain of *Escherichia coli* bacteria that has been genetically altered to produce human insulin. Humulin R [Regular insulin human injection, USP (rDNA origin)] consists of zinc-insulin crystals dissolved in a clear fluid. Humulin R has had nothing added to change the speed or length of its action. It takes effect rapidly and has a rela-

tively short duration of activity (4 to 12 hours) as compared with other insulins. The time course of action of any insulin may vary considerably in different individuals or at different times in the same individual. As with all insulin preparations, the duration of action of Humulin R is dependent on dose, site of injection, blood supply, temperature, and physical activity. Humulin R is a sterile solution and is for subcutaneous injection. It should not be used intramuscularly. The concentration of Humulin R is 100 units/mL (U-100).

Identification

Human insulin from Eli Lilly and Company has the trademark Humulin. Your doctor has prescribed the type of insulin that he/she believes is best for you.

DO NOT USE ANY OTHER INSULIN EXCEPT ON YOUR DOCTOR'S ADVICE AND DIRECTION.

Always check the carton and the bottle label for the name and letter designation of the insulin you receive from your pharmacy to make sure it is the same as prescribed by your doctor.

Always check the appearance of your bottle of Humulin R before withdrawing each dose. Humulin R is a clear and colorless liquid with a water-like appearance and consistency. Do not use Humulin R:

- if it appears cloudy, thickened, or slightly colored, or
- if solid particles are visible.

If you see anything unusual in the appearance of Humulin R solution in your bottle or notice your insulin requirements changing, talk to your doctor.

Storage

Not in-use (unopened): Humulin R bottles not in-use should be stored in a refrigerator, but not in the freezer.

In-use (opened): The Humulin R bottle you are currently using can be kept unrefrigerated as long as it is kept as cool as possible [below 86°F (30°C)] away from heat and light.

Do not use Humulin R after the expiration date stamped on the label or if it has been frozen.

INSTRUCTIONS FOR INSULIN VIAL USE

NEVER SHARE NEEDLES AND SYRINGES.

Correct Syringe Type

Doses of insulin are measured in **units**. U-100 insulin contains 100 units/mL (1 mL=1 cc). With Humulin R, it is important to use a syringe that is marked for U-100 insulin preparations. Failure to use the proper syringe can lead to a mistake in dosage, causing serious problems for you, such as a blood glucose level that is too low or too high.

Syringe Use

To help avoid contamination and possible infection, follow these instructions exactly.

Disposable syringes and needles should be used only once and then discarded by placing the used needle in a puncture-resistant disposable container. Properly dispose of the puncture-resistant container as directed by your Health Care Professional.

Preparing the Dose

1. Wash your hands.
2. Inspect the insulin. Humulin R solution should look clear and colorless. Do not use Humulin R if it appears cloudy, thickened, or slightly colored, or if you see particles in the solution. Do not use Humulin R if you notice anything unusual in its appearance.
3. If using a new Humulin R bottle, flip off the plastic protective cap, but **do not** remove the stopper. Wipe the top of the bottle with an alcohol swab.
4. If you are mixing insulins, refer to the "Mixing Humulin R with Longer-Acting Human Insulins" section below.
5. Draw an amount of air into the syringe that is equal to the Humulin R dose. Put the needle through rubber top of the Humulin R bottle and inject the air into the bottle.
6. Turn the Humulin R bottle and syringe upside down. Hold the bottle and syringe firmly in one hand.
7. Making sure the tip of the needle is in the Humulin R solution, withdraw the correct dose of Humulin R into the syringe.
8. Before removing the needle from the Humulin R bottle, check the syringe for air bubbles. If bubbles are present, hold the syringe straight up and tap its side until the bubbles float to the top. Push the bubbles out with the plunger and then withdraw the correct dose.
9. Remove the needle from the bottle and lay the syringe down so that the needle does not touch anything.
10. If you do not need to mix your Humulin R with a longer-acting insulin, go to the "Injection Instructions" section below and follow the directions.

Mixing Humulin R with Longer-Acting Human Insulins

1. Humulin R should be mixed with longer-acting human insulins only on the advice of your doctor.
2. Draw an amount of air into the syringe that is equal to the amount of longer-acting insulin you are taking. Insert the needle into the longer-acting insulin bottle and inject the air. Withdraw the needle.
3. Draw an amount of air into the syringe that is equal to the amount of Humulin R you are taking. Insert the needle into the Humulin R bottle and inject the air, but **do not** withdraw the needle.
4. Turn the Humulin R bottle and syringe upside down.

5. Making sure the tip of the needle is in the Humulin R solution, withdraw the correct dose of Humulin R into the syringe.

6. Before removing the needle from the Humulin R bottle, check the syringe for air bubbles. If bubbles are present, hold the syringe straight up and tap its side until the bubbles float to the top. Push the bubbles out with the plunger and then withdraw the correct dose.

7. Remove the syringe with the needle from the Humulin R bottle and insert it into the longer–acting insulin bottle. Turn the longer-acting insulin bottle and syringe upside down. Hold the bottle and syringe firmly in one hand and shake gently. Making sure the tip of the needle is in the longer–acting insulin, withdraw the correct dose of longer-acting insulin.

8. Remove the needle from the bottle and lay the syringe down so that the needle does not touch anything.

9. Follow the directions under "Injection Instructions" section below.

Follow your doctor's instructions on whether to mix your insulins ahead of time or just before giving your injection. It is important to be consistent in your method.

Syringes from different manufacturers may vary in the amount of space between the bottom line and the needle. Because of this, do not change:
• the sequence of mixing, or
• the model and brand of syringe or needle that your doctor has prescribed.

Injection Instructions

1. To avoid tissue damage, choose a site for each injection that is at least 1/2 inch from the previous injection site. The usual sites of injection are abdomen, thighs, and arms.

2. Cleanse the skin with alcohol where the injection is to be made.

3. With one hand, stabilize the skin by spreading it or pinching up a large area.

4. Insert the needle as instructed by your doctor.

5. Push the plunger in as far as it will go.

6. Pull the needle out and apply gentle pressure over the injection site for several seconds. **Do not rub the area.**

7. Place the used needle in a puncture-resistant disposable container and properly dispose of the puncture-resistant container as directed by your Health Care Professional.

DOSAGE

Your doctor has told you which insulin to use, how much, and when and how often to inject it. Because each patient's diabetes is different, this schedule has been individualized for you.

Your usual dose of Humulin R may be affected by changes in your diet, activity, or work schedule. Carefully follow your doctor's instructions to allow for these changes. Other things that may affect your Humulin R dose are:

Illness

Illness, especially with nausea and vomiting, may cause your insulin requirements to change. Even if you are not eating, you will still require insulin. You and your doctor should establish a sick day plan for you to use in case of illness. When you are sick, test your blood glucose frequently. If instructed by your doctor, test your ketones and report the results to your doctor.

Pregnancy

Good control of diabetes is especially important for you and your unborn baby. Pregnancy may make managing your diabetes more difficult. If you are planning to have a baby, are pregnant, or are nursing a baby, talk to your doctor.

Medication

Insulin requirements may be increased if you are taking other drugs with blood–glucose–raising activity, such as oral contraceptives, corticosteroids, or thyroid replacement therapy. Insulin requirements may be reduced in the presence of drugs that lower blood glucose or affect how your body responds to insulin, such as oral antidiabetic agents, salicylates (for example, aspirin), sulfa antibiotics, alcohol, certain antidepressants and some kidney and blood pressure medicines. Your Health Care Professional may be aware of other medications that may affect your diabetes control. Therefore, always discuss any medications you are taking with your doctor.

Exercise

Exercise may lower your body's need for insulin during and for some time after the physical activity. Exercise may also speed up the effect of an insulin dose, especially if the exercise involves the area of injection site (for example, the leg should not be used for injection just prior to running). Discuss with your doctor how you should adjust your insulin regimen to accommodate exercise.

Travel

When traveling across more than 2 time zones, you should talk to your doctor concerning adjustments in your insulin schedule.

COMMON PROBLEMS OF DIABETES

Hypoglycemia (Low Blood Sugar)

Hypoglycemia (too little glucose in the blood) is one of the most frequent adverse events experienced by insulin users. It can be brought about by:

1. **Missing or delaying meals.**
2. Taking too much insulin.
3. Exercising or working more than usual.
4. An infection or illness associated with diarrhea or vomiting.
5. A change in the body's need for insulin.
6. Diseases of the adrenal, pituitary, or thyroid gland, or progression of kidney or liver disease.
7. Interactions with certain drugs, such as oral antidiabetic agents, salicylates (for example, aspirin), sulfa antibiotics, certain antidepressants and some kidney and blood pressure medicines.
8. Consumption of alcoholic beverages.

Symptoms of mild to moderate hypoglycemia may occur suddenly and can include:

• sweating
• dizziness
• palpitation
• tremor
• hunger
• restlessness
• tingling in the hands, feet, lips, or tongue
• lightheadedness
• inability to concentrate
• headache

• drowsiness
• sleep disturbances
• anxiety
• blurred vision
• slurred speech
• depressed mood
• irritability
• abnormal behavior
• unsteady movement
• personality changes

Symptoms of severe hypoglycemia can include:

• disorientation
• unconsciousness

• seizures
• death

Therefore, it is important that assistance be obtained immediately.

Early warning symptoms of hypoglycemia may be different or less pronounced under certain conditions, such as long duration of diabetes, diabetic nerve disease, use of medications such as beta–blockers, changing insulin preparations, or intensified control (3 or more insulin injections per day) of diabetes.

A few patients who have experienced hypoglycemic reactions after transfer from animal–source insulin to human insulin have reported that the early warning symptoms of hypoglycemia were less pronounced or different from those experienced with their previous insulin.

Without recognition of early warning symptoms, you may not be able to take steps to avoid more serious hypoglycemia. Be alert for all of the various types of symptoms that may indicate hypoglycemia. Patients who experience hypoglycemia without early warning symptoms should monitor their blood glucose frequently, especially prior to activities such as driving. If the blood glucose is below your normal fasting glucose, you should consider eating or drinking sugar–containing foods to treat your hypoglycemia.

Mild to moderate hypoglycemia may be treated by eating foods or drinks that contain sugar. Patients should always carry a quick source of sugar, such as hard candy or glucose tablets. More severe hypoglycemia may require the assistance of another person. Patients who are unable to take sugar orally or who are unconscious require an injection of glucagon or should be treated with intravenous administration of glucose at a medical facility.

You should learn to recognize your own symptoms of hypoglycemia. If you are uncertain about these symptoms, you should monitor your blood glucose frequently to help you learn to recognize the symptoms that you experience with hypoglycemia.

If you have frequent episodes of hypoglycemia or experience difficulty in recognizing the symptoms, you should talk to your doctor to discuss possible changes in therapy, meal plans, and/or exercise programs to help you avoid hypoglycemia.

Hyperglycemia (High Blood Sugar) and Diabetic Ketoacidosis (DKA)

Hyperglycemia (too much glucose in the blood) may develop if your body has too little insulin. Hyperglycemia can be brought about by any of the following:

1. Omitting your insulin or taking less than your doctor has prescribed.
2. Eating significantly more than your meal plan suggests.
3. Developing a fever, infection, or other significant stressful situation.

In patients with type 1 or insulin–dependent diabetes, prolonged hyperglycemia can result in DKA (a life-threatening emergency). The first symptoms of DKA usually come on gradually, over a period of hours or days, and include a drowsy feeling, flushed face, thirst, loss of appetite, and fruity odor on the breath. With DKA, blood and urine tests show large amounts of glucose and ketones. Heavy breathing and a rapid pulse are more severe symptoms. If uncorrected, prolonged hyperglycemia or DKA can lead to nausea, vomiting, stomach pain, dehydration, loss of consciousness, or death. Therefore, it is important that you obtain medical assistance immediately.

Lipodystrophy

Rarely, administration of insulin subcutaneously can result in lipoatrophy (seen as an apparent depression of the skin) or lipohypertrophy (seen as a raised area of the skin). If you notice either of these conditions, talk to your doctor. A change in your injection technique may help alleviate the problem.

Allergy

Local Allergy—Patients occasionally experience redness, swelling, and itching at the site of injection. This condition, called local allergy, usually clears up in a few days to a few weeks. In some instances, this condition may be related to factors other than insulin, such as irritants in the skin cleansing agent or poor injection technique. If you have local reactions, talk to your doctor.

Systemic Allergy—Less common, but potentially more serious, is generalized allergy to insulin, which may cause rash over the whole body, shortness of breath, wheezing, reduction in blood pressure, fast pulse, or sweating. Severe cases of generalized allergy may be life threatening. If you think you are having a generalized allergic reaction to insulin, call your doctor immediately.

ADDITIONAL INFORMATION

Information about diabetes may be obtained from your diabetes educator.

Additional information about diabetes and Humulin can be obtained by calling The Lilly Answers Center at 1-800-LillyRx (1-800-545-5979) or by visiting www.LillyDiabetes.com.

Patient Information revised September 2, 2009

10 mL Vials manufactured by
Eli Lilly and Company, Indianapolis, IN 46285, USA or
Hospira, Inc., Lake Forest, IL 60045, USA or
Lilly France, F-67640 Fegersheim, France
3 mL Vials manufactured by
Eli Lilly and Company, Indianapolis, IN 46285, USA
for Eli Lilly and Company, Indianapolis, IN 46285, USA
Copyright © 1997, 2009, Eli Lilly and Company. All rights reserved.
PV 5693 AMP

HUMULIN® R

[hū'mū-lĭn är]
REGULAR
U-500 (CONCENTRATED)
INSULIN HUMAN INJECTION, USP
(rDNA ORIGIN)
INFORMATION FOR THE PHYSICIAN

DESCRIPTION

Humulin is synthesized in a special non–disease–producing laboratory strain of *Escherichia coli* bacteria that has been genetically altered by the addition of the gene for human insulin production. Humulin R (U–500) consists of zinc–insulin crystals dissolved in a clear fluid. Humulin R (U–500) is a sterile solution and is for subcutaneous injection. It should not be used intravenously or intramuscularly. The concentration of Humulin R (U–500) is 500 units/mL. Each milliliter contains 500 units of biosynthetic human insulin, 16 mg glycerin, 2.5 mg Metacresol as a preservative, and zinc–oxide calculated to supplement endogenous zinc to obtain a total zinc content of 0.017 mg/100 units. Sodium hydroxide and/or hydrochloric acid may be added during manufacture to adjust the pH.

CLINICAL PHARMACOLOGY

Adequate insulin dosage permits the diabetic patient to utilize carbohydrates and fats in a comparatively satisfactory manner. Regardless of concentration, the action of insulin is basically the same: to enable carbohydrate metabolism to occur and thus to prevent the production of ketone bodies by the liver. Although, under usual circumstances, diabetes can be controlled with doses in the vicinity of 40 to 60 units or less, an occasional patient develops such resistance or becomes so unresponsive to the effect of insulin that daily doses of several hundred, or even several thousand, units are required. Patients who require doses in excess of 300 to 500 units daily usually have impaired insulin receptor function.

Occasionally, a cause of the insulin resistance can be found (such as hemochromatosis, cirrhosis of the liver, some complicating disease of the endocrine glands other than the pancreas, allergy, or infection), but in other cases, no cause of the high insulin requirement can be determined.

Humulin R (U–500) is unmodified by any agent that might prolong its action; however, clinical experience has shown that it frequently has a time action similar to a repository insulin preparation. It takes effect rapidly but has a relatively long duration of activity following a single dose (up to 24 hours) as compared with other Regular insulins. This effect has been credited to the high concentration of the preparation. The time course of action of any insulin may vary considerably in different individuals or at different times in the same individual. As with all insulin preparations, the duration of action of Humulin R (U–500) is dependent on dose, site of injection, blood supply, temperature, and physical activity.

INDICATIONS AND USAGE

Humulin R (U–500) is especially useful for the treatment of diabetic patients with marked insulin resistance (daily requirements more than 200 units), since a large dose may be administered subcutaneously in a reasonable volume.

CONTRAINDICATIONS

Humulin R (U–500) is contraindicated in hypoglycemia.

WARNINGS

THIS LILLY HUMAN INSULIN PRODUCT DIFFERS FROM ANIMAL–SOURCE INSULINS BECAUSE IT IS STRUCTURALLY IDENTICAL TO THE INSULIN PRODUCED BY YOUR BODY'S PANCREAS AND BECAUSE OF ITS UNIQUE MANUFACTURING PROCESS.

ANY CHANGE OF INSULIN SHOULD BE MADE CAUTIOUSLY AND ONLY UNDER MEDICAL SUPERVISION. CHANGES IN PURITY, STRENGTH, BRAND (MANUFACTURER), TYPE (REGULAR, NPH, LENTE®, ETC), SPECIES (BEEF, PORK, BEEF–PORK, HUMAN), AND/OR METHOD OF MANUFACTURE (rDNA VERSUS ANIMAL–SOURCE INSULIN) MAY RESULT IN THE NEED FOR A CHANGE IN DOSAGE.

SOME PATIENTS TAKING HUMULIN® (HUMAN INSULIN, rDNA ORIGIN, LILLY) MAY REQUIRE A CHANGE IN DOSAGE FROM THAT USED WITH ANIMAL–SOURCE INSULINS. IF AN ADJUSTMENT IS NEEDED, IT MAY OCCUR WITH THE FIRST DOSE OR DURING THE FIRST SEVERAL WEEKS OR MONTHS.

This insulin preparation contains 500 units of insulin in each milliliter. Extreme caution must be observed in the measurement of dosage because inadvertent overdose may result in irreversible insulin shock. Serious consequences may result if it is used other than under constant medical supervision.

PRECAUTIONS

General
Every patient exhibiting insulin resistance who requires Humulin R (U–500) for control of diabetes should be under close observation until appropriate dosage is established. The response will vary among patients. Some patients can be controlled with a single dose daily; others may require 2 or 3 injections per day. Most patients will show a "tolerance" to insulin, so that minor variations in dosage can occur without the development of untoward symptoms of insulin shock.

Insulin resistance is frequently self–limited; after several weeks or months during which high dosage is required, responsiveness to the pharmacologic effect of insulin may be regained and dosage can be reduced.

Information for Patients
Patients should be instructed regarding their dosage and should be reminded that this formulation requires the administration of a smaller volume of solution than is the case with less concentrated formulations.

Laboratory Tests
Blood and urine glucose, glycohemoglobin, and urine ketones should be monitored frequently.

Drug Interactions
The concurrent use of oral hypoglycemic agents with Humulin R (U–500) is not recommended since there are no data to support such use.

Insulin requirements may be increased by medications with hyperglycemic activity such as corticosteroids, isoniazid, certain lipid-lowering drugs (e.g., niacin), estrogens, oral contraceptives, phenothiazines, and thyroid replacement therapy (see CLINICAL PHARMACOLOGY).

Insulin requirements may be decreased in the presence of drugs that increase insulin sensitivity or have hypoglycemic activity, such as oral antidiabetic agents, salicylates, sulfa antibiotics, certain antidepressants (monoamine oxidase inhibitors), angiotensin-converting-enzyme inhibitors, angiotensin II receptor blocking agents, beta-adrenergic blockers, inhibitors of pancreatic function (e.g., octreotide), and alcohol. Beta-adrenergic blockers may mask the symptoms of hypoglycemia in some patients.

Pregnancy
Teratogenic Effects—No reproduction studies have been conducted in animals, and there are no adequate and well–controlled studies in pregnant women. It would be anticipated that the benefits of this insulin preparation would outweigh any risk to the developing fetus.
Nonteratogenic Effects—Insulin does not cross the placenta as does glucose.

Labor and Delivery
Careful monitoring of the patient is required, since the insulin requirement may decrease following delivery.

Nursing Mothers
It is not known whether insulin is excreted in significant amounts in human milk. Because many drugs are excreted in human milk, caution should be exercised when Humulin R (U–500) insulin injection is administered to a nursing woman.

Pediatric Use
There are no special precautions relating to the use of this insulin formulation in the pediatric age group.

ADVERSE REACTIONS
As with other human insulin preparations, hypoglycemic reactions may be associated with the administration of Humulin R (U–500). However, deep secondary hypoglycemic reactions may develop 18 to 24 hours after the original injection of Humulin R (U–500). Consequently, patients should be carefully observed, and prompt treatment of such reactions should be initiated with glucagon injections and/or with glucose by intravenous injection or gavage.

Hypoglycemia
Hypoglycemia is one of the most frequent adverse events experienced by insulin users.

Symptoms of mild to moderate hypoglycemia may occur suddenly and can include:

- sweating
- dizziness
- palpitation
- tremor
- hunger
- restlessness
- tingling in the hands, feet, lips, or tongue
- lightheadedness
- inability to concentrate
- headache
- drowsiness
- sleep disturbances
- anxiety
- blurred vision
- slurred speech
- depressive mood
- irritability
- abnormal behavior
- unsteady movement
- personality changes

Signs of severe hypoglycemia can include:

- disorientation
- unconsciousness
- seizures
- death

Early warning symptoms of hypoglycemia may be different or less pronounced under certain conditions, such as long duration of diabetes, diabetic nerve disease, medications such as beta–blockers, change in insulin preparations, or intensified control (3 or more insulin injections per day) of diabetes.

A few patients who have experienced hypoglycemic reactions after transfer from animal–source insulin to human insulin have reported that the early warning symptoms of hypoglycemia were less pronounced or different from those experienced with their previous insulin.

Without recognition of early warning symptoms, the patient may not be able to take steps to avoid more serious hypoglycemia. Patients who experience hypoglycemia without early warning symptoms should monitor their blood glucose frequently, especially prior to activities such as driving. Mild to moderate hypoglycemia may be treated by eating foods or taking drinks that contain sugar. Patients should always carry a quick source of sugar, such as candy mints or glucose tablets.

Hypoglycemia when using Humulin R (U–500) can be prolonged and severe.

Lipodystrophy
Rarely, administration of insulin subcutaneously can result in lipoatrophy (depression in the skin) or lipohypertrophy (enlargement or thickening of tissue).

Allergy to Insulin
Local Allergy—Patients occasionally experience erythema, local edema, and pruritus at the site of injection of insulin. This condition usually is self–limiting. In some instances, this condition may be related to factors other than insulin, such as irritants in the skin cleansing agent or poor injection technique.
Systemic Allergy—Less common, but potentially more serious, is generalized allergy to insulin, which may cause rash over the whole body, shortness of breath, wheezing, reduction in blood pressure, fast pulse, or sweating. Severe cases of generalized allergy (anaphylaxis) may be life threatening.

DOSAGE AND ADMINISTRATION
Humulin R (U–500) should only be administered subcutaneously. It is inadvisable to inject Humulin R (U–500) intravenously because of possible inadvertent overdosage.

It is recommended that an insulin syringe or tuberculin–type syringe be used for the measurement of dosage. Variations in dosage are frequently possible in the insulin-resistant patient, since the individual is unresponsive to the pharmacologic effect of the insulin. Nevertheless, accuracy of measurement is to be encouraged because of the potential danger of the preparation.

STORAGE
Insulin should be kept in a cold place, preferably in a refrigerator, but must not be frozen.

Do not inject insulin that is not water–clear. Discoloration, turbidity, or unusual viscosity indicates deterioration or contamination.

Use of a package of insulin should not be started after the expiration date stamped on it.

HOW SUPPLIED
Vials, 500 units/mL, 20 mL (HI–500) (1s), NDC 0002–8501–01

Literature revised September 10, 2007
Eli Lilly and Company, Indianapolis, IN 46285, USA
Copyright © 1996, 2007, Eli Lilly and Company. All rights reserved.
PA 3053 AMP

INFORMATION FOR THE PATIENT
HUMULIN® R
REGULAR
U–500 (CONCENTRATED)
INSULIN HUMAN INJECTION, USP
(rDNA ORIGIN)
WARNINGS
THIS LILLY HUMAN INSULIN PRODUCT DIFFERS FROM ANIMAL–SOURCE INSULINS BECAUSE IT IS STRUCTURALLY IDENTICAL TO THE INSULIN PRODUCED BY YOUR BODY'S PANCREAS AND BECAUSE OF ITS UNIQUE MANUFACTURING PROCESS.

ANY CHANGE OF INSULIN SHOULD BE MADE CAUTIOUSLY AND ONLY UNDER MEDICAL SUPERVISION. CHANGES IN PURITY, STRENGTH, BRAND (MANUFACTURER), TYPE (REGULAR, NPH, E.G., LENTE), SPECIES (BEEF, PORK, BEEF–PORK, HUMAN), AND/OR METHOD OF MANUFACTURE (rDNA VERSUS ANIMAL–SOURCE INSULIN) MAY RESULT IN THE NEED FOR A CHANGE IN DOSAGE.

SOME PATIENTS TAKING HUMULIN® (HUMAN INSULIN, rDNA ORIGIN, LILLY) MAY REQUIRE A CHANGE IN DOSAGE FROM THAT USED WITH ANIMAL–SOURCE INSULINS. IF AN ADJUSTMENT IS NEEDED, IT MAY OCCUR WITH THE FIRST DOSE OR DURING THE FIRST SEVERAL WEEKS OR MONTHS.

This insulin preparation contains 500 units of insulin in each milliliter. Extreme caution must be observed in the measurement of dosage because inadvertent overdose may result in irreversible insulin shock. Serious consequences may result if it is used other than under constant medical supervision.

DIABETES
Insulin is a hormone produced by the pancreas, a large gland that lies near the stomach. This hormone is necessary for the body's correct use of food, especially sugar. Diabetes occurs when the pancreas does not make enough insulin to meet your body's needs.

To control your diabetes, your doctor has prescribed injections of insulin products to keep your blood glucose at a near–normal level. You have been instructed to test your blood and/or your urine regularly for glucose. Studies have shown that some chronic complications of diabetes such as eye disease, kidney disease, and nerve disease can be significantly reduced if the blood sugar is maintained as close to normal as possible. The American Diabetes Association recommends that if your pre-meal glucose levels are consistently above 130 mg/dL or your hemoglobin A_{1c} (HbA_{1c}) is more than 7%, consult your doctor. A change in your diabetes therapy may be needed. If your blood tests consistently show below–normal glucose levels you should also let your doctor know. Proper control of your diabetes requires close and constant cooperation with your doctor. Despite diabetes, you can lead an active and healthy life if you eat a balanced diet, exercise regularly, and take your insulin injections as prescribed.

Always keep an extra supply of insulin as well as a spare syringe and needle on hand. Always wear diabetic identification so that appropriate treatment can be given if complications occur away from home.

REGULAR HUMAN INSULIN
Description
Humulin is synthesized in a special non–disease–producing laboratory strain of *Escherichia coli* bacteria that has been genetically altered by the addition of the gene for human

insulin production. Humulin R (U–500) consists of zinc–insulin crystals dissolved in a clear fluid. Humulin R (U–500) has had nothing added to change the speed or length of its action. It takes effect rapidly but has a relatively long duration of activity (up to 24 hours) as compared with other Regular insulins. The time course of action of any insulin may vary considerably in different individuals or at different times in the same individual. As with all insulin preparations, the duration of action of Humulin R (U–500) is dependent on dose, site of injection, blood supply, temperature, and physical activity. Humulin R (U–500), is a sterile solution and is for subcutaneous injection only. It should not be used intravenously or intramuscularly. The concentration of Humulin R (U–500) is 500 units/mL.

Identification

Human insulin by Eli Lilly and Company has the trademark Humulin and is available in 6 formulations—Regular (**R**), NPH (**N**), Lente (**L**), Ultralente® (**U**), 50% Human Insulin Isophane Suspension [NPH]/50% Human Insulin Injection [regular] (**50/50**), and 70% Human Insulin Isophane Suspension [NPH]/30% Human Insulin Injection [regular] (**70/30**). Humulin R (U–500) is the only human insulin by Eli Lilly and Company that has a concentration of 500 units/mL. Your doctor has prescribed the type of insulin that he/she believes is best for you. **DO NOT USE ANY OTHER INSULIN EXCEPT ON HIS/HER ADVICE AND DIRECTION.**

Always check the carton and the bottle label for the name and letter designation of the insulin you receive from your pharmacy to make sure it is the same as that your doctor has prescribed.

Always examine the appearance of your bottle of insulin before withdrawing each dose. Humulin R (U–500) is a clear and colorless liquid with a water–like appearance and consistency. Do not use if it appears cloudy, thickened, or slightly colored or if solid particles are visible. Always check the appearance of your bottle of insulin before using, and if you note anything unusual in the appearance of your insulin or notice your insulin requirements changing markedly, consult your doctor.

Storage

Insulin should be stored in a refrigerator but not in the freezer. If refrigeration is not possible, the bottle of insulin that you are currently using can be kept unrefrigerated as long as it is kept as cool as possible (below 30°C [86°F]) and away from heat and light. Do not use insulin if it has been frozen. Do not use a bottle of Humulin R (U-500) after the expiration date stamped on the label.

INJECTION PROCEDURES

Correct Syringe Type

Doses of insulin are measured in **units**. U–500 insulin contains 500 units/mL (1 mL=1 cc). With Humulin R (U–500), it is important to use a tuberculin (or similar) syringe as instructed by your doctor. Failure to use the proper syringe type can lead to a mistake in dosage, causing serious problems for you, such as a blood glucose level that is too low or too high.

Syringe Use

To help avoid contamination and possible infection, follow these instructions exactly.

Disposable plastic syringes and needles should be used only once and then discarded in a responsible manner. **NEEDLES AND SYRINGES MUST NOT BE SHARED.**

Reusable glass syringes and needles must be sterilized before each injection. **Follow the package directions supplied with your syringe.** Described below are 2 methods of sterilizing.

Boiling

1. Put syringe, plunger, and needle in strainer, place in saucepan, and cover with water. Boil for 5 minutes.
2. Remove articles from water. When they have cooled, insert plunger into barrel, and fasten needle to syringe with a slight twist.
3. Push plunger in and out several times until water is completely removed.

Isopropyl Alcohol

If the syringe, plunger, and needle cannot be boiled, as when you are traveling, they may be sterilized by immersion for at least 5 minutes in Isopropyl Alcohol, 91%. Do not use bathing, rubbing, or medicated alcohol for this sterilization. If the syringe is sterilized with alcohol, it must be absolutely dry before use.

Preparing the Dose

1. Wash your hands.
2. Inspect the insulin. Humulin R (U–500) should look clear and colorless. Do not use Humulin R (U–500) if it appears cloudy, thickened, or slightly colored or if solid particles are visible.
3. If using a new bottle, flip off the plastic protective cap, but **do not** remove the stopper. When using a new bottle, wipe the top of the bottle with an alcohol swab.
4. Draw air into the syringe equal to your insulin dose. Put the needle through the rubber top of the insulin bottle and inject the air into the bottle.
5. Turn the bottle and syringe upside down. Hold the bottle and syringe firmly in one hand.
6. Making sure the tip of the needle is in the insulin, withdraw the correct dose of insulin into the syringe.
7. Before removing the needle from the bottle, check your syringe for air bubbles which reduce the amount of insulin in it. If bubbles are present, hold the syringe straight up and tap its side until the bubbles float to the top. Push them out with the plunger and withdraw the correct dose.
8. Remove the needle from the bottle and lay the syringe down so that the needle does not touch anything.

Injection

Once you have chosen an injection site, cleanse the skin with alcohol where the injection is to be made. Stabilize the skin by spreading it or pinching up a large area. Insert the needle as instructed by your doctor. Push the plunger in as far as it will go. Pull the needle out and apply gentle pressure over the injection site for several seconds. **Do not rub the area.** To avoid tissue damage, give the next injection at a site at least 1/2 inch from the previous site.

DOSAGE

Your doctor has told you which insulin to use, how much, and when and how often to inject it. Because each patient's case of diabetes is different, this schedule has been individualized for you.

Your usual insulin dose may be affected by changes in your food, activity, or work schedule. Carefully follow your doctor's instructions to allow for these changes. Other things that may affect your insulin dose are:

Illness

Illness, especially with nausea and vomiting, may cause your insulin requirements to change. Even if you are not eating, you will still require insulin. You and your doctor should establish a sick day plan for you to use in case of illness. When you are sick, test your blood glucose/urine glucose and ketones frequently and call your doctor as instructed.

Pregnancy

Good control of diabetes is especially important for you and your unborn baby. Pregnancy may make managing your diabetes more difficult. If you are planning to have a baby, are pregnant, or are nursing a baby, consult your doctor.

Medication

Insulin requirements may be increased if you are taking other drugs with blood–glucose–raising activity, such as oral contraceptives, corticosteroids, or thyroid replacement therapy. Insulin requirements may be reduced in the presence of drugs that lower blood glucose or affect how your body responds to insulin, such as oral antidiabetic agents, salicylates (for example, aspirin), sulfa antibiotics, alcohol, certain antidepressants and some kidney and blood pressure medicines. Your Health Care Professional may be aware of other medications that may affect your diabetes control. Therefore, always discuss any medications you are taking with your doctor.

Exercise

Exercise may lower your body's need for insulin during and for some time after the activity. Exercise may also speed up the effect of an insulin dose, especially if the exercise involves the area of injection site (for example, the leg should not be used for injection just prior to running). Discuss with your doctor how you should adjust your regimen to accommodate exercise.

Travel

Persons traveling across more than 2 time zones should consult their doctor concerning adjustments in their insulin schedule.

COMMON PROBLEMS OF DIABETES

Hypoglycemia (Low Blood Sugar)

Hypoglycemia (too little glucose in the blood) is one of the most frequent adverse events experienced by insulin users. It can be brought about by:

1. **Missing or delaying meals.**
2. Taking too much insulin.
3. Exercising or working more than usual.
4. An infection or illness (especially with diarrhea or vomiting).
5. A change in the body's need for insulin.
6. Diseases of the adrenal, pituitary, or thyroid gland, or progression of kidney or liver disease.
7. Interactions with certain drugs, such as oral antidiabetic agents, salicylates (for example, aspirin), sulfa antibiotics, certain antidepressants and some kidney and blood pressure medicines.
8. Consumption of alcoholic beverages.

Symptoms of mild to moderate hypoglycemia may occur suddenly and can include:

• sweating	• drowsiness
• dizziness	• sleep disturbances
• palpitation	• anxiety
• tremor	• blurred vision
• hunger	• slurred speech
• restlessness	• depressive mood
• tingling in the hands, feet, lips, or tongue	• irritability
• lightheadedness	• abnormal behavior
• inability to concentrate	• unsteady movement
• headache	• personality changes

Signs of severe hypoglycemia can include:

• disorientation	• seizures
• unconsciousness	• death

Therefore, it is important that assistance be obtained immediately.

Early warning symptoms of hypoglycemia may be different or less pronounced under certain conditions, such as long duration of diabetes, diabetic nerve disease, medications such as beta–blockers, change in insulin preparations, or intensified control (3 or more insulin injections per day) of diabetes.

A few patients who have experienced hypoglycemic reactions after transfer from animal–source insulin to human insulin have reported that the early warning symptoms of hypoglycemia were less pronounced or different from those experienced with their previous insulin.

Without recognition of early warning symptoms, you may not be able to take steps to avoid more serious hypoglycemia. Be alert for all of the various types of symptoms that may indicate hypoglycemia. Patients who experience hypoglycemia without early warning symptoms should monitor their blood glucose frequently, especially prior to activities such as driving. If the blood glucose is below your normal fasting glucose, you should consider eating or drinking sugar–containing foods to treat your hypoglycemia.

Mild to moderate hypoglycemia may be treated by eating foods or taking drinks that contain sugar. Patients should always carry a quick source of sugar, such as candy mints or glucose tablets. More severe hypoglycemia may require the assistance of another person. Patients who are unable to take sugar orally or who are unconscious require an injection of glucagon or should be treated with intravenous administration of glucose at a medical facility.

Hypoglycemia when using Humulin R (U–500) can be prolonged and severe. All hypoglycemic episodes should be reported to your doctor.

You should learn to recognize your own symptoms of hypoglycemia. If you are uncertain about these symptoms, you should monitor your blood glucose frequently to help you learn to recognize the symptoms that you experience with hypoglycemia.

If you have frequent episodes of hypoglycemia or experience difficulty in recognizing the symptoms, you should consult your doctor to discuss possible changes in therapy, meal plans, and/or exercise programs to help you avoid hypoglycemia.

Hyperglycemia and Diabetic Ketoacidosis (DKA)

Hyperglycemia (too much glucose in the blood) may develop if your body has too little insulin. Hyperglycemia can be brought about by:

1. Omitting your insulin or taking less than the doctor has prescribed.
2. Eating significantly more than your meal plan suggests.
3. Developing a fever, infection, or other significant stressful situation.

In patients with type 1 or insulin–dependent diabetes, prolonged hyperglycemia can result in DKA. The first symptoms of DKA usually come on gradually, over a period of hours or days, and include a drowsy feeling, flushed face, thirst, loss of appetite, and fruity odor on the breath. With DKA, urine tests show large amounts of glucose and ketones. Heavy breathing and a rapid pulse are more severe symptoms. If uncorrected, prolonged hyperglycemia or DKA can lead to nausea, vomiting, dehydration, loss of consciousness or death. Therefore, it is important that you obtain medical assistance immediately.

Lipodystrophy

Rarely, administration of insulin subcutaneously can result in lipoatrophy (depression in the skin) or lipohypertrophy (enlargement or thickening of tissue). If you notice either of these conditions, consult your doctor. A change in your injection technique may help alleviate the problem.

Allergy to Insulin

Local Allergy—Patients occasionally experience redness, swelling, and itching at the site of injection of insulin. This condition, called local allergy, usually clears up in a few days to a few weeks. In some instances, this condition may be related to factors other than insulin, such as irritants in the skin cleansing agent or poor injection technique. If you have local reactions, contact your doctor.

Systemic Allergy—Less common, but potentially more serious, is generalized allergy to insulin, which may cause rash over the whole body, shortness of breath, wheezing, reduction in blood pressure, fast pulse, or sweating. Severe cases of generalized allergy may be life threatening. If you think you are having a generalized allergic reaction to insulin, notify a doctor immediately.

ADDITIONAL INFORMATION

Additional information about diabetes may be obtained from your diabetes educator.

DIABETES FORECAST is a magazine designed especially for people with diabetes and their families. It is available by subscription from the American Diabetes Association (ADA), P.O. Box 363, Mt. Morris, IL 61054-0363, 1-800-DIABETES (1-800-342-2383).

Another publication, **COUNTDOWN**, is available from the Juvenile Diabetes Research Foundation International (JDRFI), 120 Wall Street 19th Floor, New York, NY 10005, 1-800-533-CURE (1-800-533-2873).

Additional information about Humulin can be obtained by calling The Lilly Answers Center at 1-800-LillyRx (1-800-545-5979).

Patient Information revised September 10, 2007
Eli Lilly and Company, Indianapolis, IN 46285, USA
PA 3053 AMP

PROZAC® ℞

[prō-zăk]
(fluoxetine hydrochloride)
Pulvules for oral use

PROZAC®
(fluoxetine hydrochloride)
delayed-release capsules for oral use

HIGHLIGHTS OF PRESCRIBING INFORMATION
These highlights do not include all the information needed to use PROZAC safely and effectively. See full prescribing information for PROZAC.
PROZAC (fluoxetine hydrochloride) Pulvules for oral use
PROZAC (fluoxetine hydrochloride) delayed-release capsules for oral use
Initial U.S. Approval: 1987

WARNING: SUICIDALITY AND ANTIDEPRESSANT DRUGS
See full prescribing information for complete boxed warning.
Increased risk of suicidal thinking and behavior in children, adolescents, and young adults taking antidepressants for Major Depressive Disorder (MDD) and other psychiatric disorders (5.1).
When using PROZAC and olanzapine in combination, also refer to Boxed Warning section of the package insert for Symbyax.

——RECENT MAJOR CHANGES——
Indications and Usage, PROZAC and olanzapine in combination:
Depressive Episodes Associated with Bipolar I Disorder (1.5) 03/2009
Treatment Resistant Depression (1.6) 03/2009
Dosage and Administration, PROZAC and olanzapine in combination:
Depressive Episodes Associated with Bipolar I Disorder (2.5) 03/2009
Treatment Resistant Depression (2.6) 03/2009
Warnings and Precautions:
Serotonin Syndrome or Neuroleptic Malignant Syndrome (NMS)-like Reactions (5.2) 01/2009

——INDICATIONS AND USAGE——
PROZAC is a selective serotonin reuptake inhibitor indicated for:
- Acute and maintenance treatment of Major Depressive Disorder (MDD) in adult and pediatric patients aged 8 to 18 years (1.1)
- Acute and maintenance treatment of Obsessive Compulsive Disorder (OCD) in adult and pediatric patients aged 7-17 years (1.2)
- Acute and maintenance treatment of Bulimia Nervosa in adult patients (1.3)
- Acute treatment of Panic Disorder, with or without agoraphobia, in adult patients (1.4)
PROZAC and olanzapine in combination for:
- Acute treatment of Depressive Episodes Associated with Bipolar I Disorder in adults (1.5)
- Acute treatment of Treatment Resistant Depression in adults (Major Depressive Disorder in adult patients who do not respond to 2 separate trials of different antidepressants of adequate dose and duration in the current episode) (1.6)

——DOSAGE AND ADMINISTRATION——

Indication	Adult	Pediatric
MDD (2.1)	20 mg/day in am (initial dose)	10 to 20 mg/day (initial dose)
OCD (2.2)	20 mg/day in am (initial dose)	10 mg/day (initial dose)
Bulimia Nervosa (2.3)	60 mg/day in am	-
Panic Disorder (2.4)	10 mg/day (initial dose)	-
Depressive Episodes Associated with Bipolar I Disorder (2.5)	Oral in combination with olanzapine: 5 mg of oral olanzapine and 20 mg of fluoxetine once daily (initial dose)	-
Treatment Resistant Depression (2.6)	Oral in combination with olanzapine: 5 mg of oral olanzapine and 20 mg of fluoxetine once daily (initial dose)	-

- Consider tapering the dose of fluoxetine for pregnant women during the third trimester (2.7)
- A lower or less frequent dosage should be used in patients with hepatic impairment, the elderly, and for patients with concurrent disease or on multiple concomitant medications (2.7)
- Dosing with PROZAC Weekly capsules - initiate 7 days after the last daily dose of PROZAC 20 mg (2.1)
PROZAC and olanzapine in combination:
- Dosage adjustments, if indicated, should be made with the individual components according to efficacy and tolerability (2.5, 2.6)
- Fluoxetine monotherapy is not indicated for the treatment of Depressive Episodes associated with Bipolar I Disorder or treatment resistant depression (2.5, 2.6)
- Safety of the coadministration of doses above 18 mg olanzapine with 75 mg fluoxetine has not been evaluated (2.5, 2.6)

——DOSAGE FORMS AND STRENGTHS——
- Pulvules: 10 mg, 20 mg, 40 mg (3)
- Weekly capsules: 90 mg (3)

——CONTRAINDICATIONS——
- Do not use with an MAOI or within 14 days of discontinuing an MAOI due to risk of drug interaction. At least 5 weeks should be allowed after stopping PROZAC before treatment with an MAOI (4, 7.1)
- Do not use with pimozide due to risk of drug interaction or QT$_c$ prolongation (4, 7.9)
- Do not use with thioridazine due to QT$_c$ interval prolongation or potential for elevated thioridazine plasma levels. Do not use thioridazine within 5 weeks of discontinuing PROZAC (4, 7.9)
- When using PROZAC and olanzapine in combination, also refer to the Contraindications section of the package insert for Symbyax (4)

——WARNINGS AND PRECAUTIONS——
- *Clinical Worsening and Suicide Risk:* Monitor for clinical worsening and suicidal thinking and behavior (5.1)
- *Serotonin Syndrome or Neuroleptic Malignant Syndrome (NMS)-like Reactions:* Have been reported with PROZAC. Discontinue PROZAC and initiate supportive treatment (5.2)
- *Allergic Reactions and Rash:* Discontinue upon appearance of rash or allergic phenomena (5.3)
- *Activation of Mania/Hypomania:* Screen for Bipolar Disorder and monitor for mania/hypomania (5.4)
- *Seizures:* Use cautiously in patients with a history of seizures or with conditions that potentially lower the seizure threshold (5.5)
- *Altered Appetite and Weight:* Significant weight loss has occurred (5.6)
- *Abnormal Bleeding:* May increase the risk of bleeding. Use with NSAIDs, aspirin, warfarin, or drugs that affect coagulation may potentiate the risk of gastrointestinal or other bleeding (5.7)
- *Hyponatremia:* Has been reported with PROZAC in association with syndrome of inappropriate antidiuretic hormone (SIADH) (5.8)
- *Anxiety and Insomnia:* May occur (5.9)
- *Potential for Cognitive and Motor Impairment:* Has potential to impair judgment, thinking, and motor skills. Use caution when operating machinery (5.11)

- *Long Half-Life:* Changes in dose will not be fully reflected in plasma for several weeks (5.12)
- *PROZAC and Olanzapine in Combination:* When using PROZAC and olanzapine in combination, also refer to the Warnings and Precautions section of the package insert for Symbyax (5.14)

——ADVERSE REACTIONS——
Most common adverse reactions (≥5% and at least twice that for placebo) associated with:
Major Depressive Disorder, Obsessive Compulsive Disorder, Bulimia, and Panic Disorder: abnormal dreams, abnormal ejaculation, anorexia, anxiety, asthenia, diarrhea, dry mouth, dyspepsia, flu syndrome, impotence, insomnia, libido decreased, nausea, nervousness, pharyngitis, rash, sinusitis, somnolence, sweating, tremor, vasodilatation, and yawn (6.1)
PROZAC and olanzapine in combination—Also refer to the Adverse Reactions section of the package insert for Symbyax (6)
To report SUSPECTED ADVERSE REACTIONS, contact Eli Lilly and Company at 1-800-LillyRx or FDA at 1-800-FDA-1088 or *www.fda.gov/medwatch.*

——DRUG INTERACTIONS——
- *Monoamine Oxidase Inhibitors (MAOI):* PROZAC is contraindicated for use with MAOI's, or within 14 days of discontinuing an MAOI due to risk of drug interaction. At least 5 weeks should be allowed after stopping PROZAC before starting treatment with an MAOI (4, 7.1)
- *Pimozide:* PROZAC is contraindicated for use with pimozide due to risk of drug interaction or QT$_c$ prolongation (4, 7.9)
- *Thioridazine:* PROZAC is contraindicated for use with thioridazine due to QT$_c$ interval prolongation or potential for elevated thioridazine plasma levels. Do not use thioridazine within 5 weeks of discontinuing PROZAC (4, 7.9)
- *Drugs Metabolized by CYP2D6:* Fluoxetine is a potent inhibitor of CYP2D6 enzyme pathway (7.9)
- *Tricyclic Antidepressants (TCAs):* Monitor TCA levels during coadministration with PROZAC or when PROZAC has been recently discontinued (7.9)
- *CNS Acting Drugs:* Caution should be used when taken in combination with other centrally acting drugs (7.2)
- *Benzodiazepines:* Diazepam – increased t½, alprazolam-further psychomotor performance decrement due to increased levels (7.9)
- *Antipsycotics:* Potential for elevation of haloperidol and clozapine levels (7.9)
- *Anticonvulsants:* Potential for elevated phenytoin and carbamazepine levels and clinical anticonvulsant toxicity (7.9)
- *Serotonergic Drugs:* Potential for Serotonin Syndrome (5.2, 7.3)
- *Triptans:* There have been rare postmarketing reports of Serotonin Syndrome with use of an SSRI and a triptan (5.2, 7.4)
- *Tryptophan:* Concomitant use with tryptophan is not recommended (5.2, 7.5)
- *Drugs that Interfere with Hemostasis (e.g. NSAIDs, Aspirin, Warfarin):* May potentiate the risk of bleeding (7.6)
- *Drugs Tightly Bound to Plasma Proteins:* May cause a shift in plasma concentrations (7.8, 7.9)
- *Olanzapine:* When used in combination with PROZAC, also refer to the Drug Interactions section of the package insert for Symbyax (7.9)

——USE IN SPECIFIC POPULATIONS——
- *Pregnancy:* PROZAC should be used during pregnancy only if the potential benefit justifies the potential risks to the fetus (8.1)
- *Nursing Mothers:* Breast feeding is not recommended (8.3)
- *Pediatric Use:* Safety and effectiveness of PROZAC and olanzapine in combination have not been established in patients less than 18 years of age (8.4)
- *Hepatic Impairment:* Lower or less frequent dosing may be appropriate in patients with cirrhosis (8.6)
See 17 for PATIENT COUNSELING INFORMATION and Medication Guide

Revised: 10/2009

FULL PRESCRIBING INFORMATION: CONTENTS*
WARNING: SUICIDALITY AND ANTIDEPRESSANT DRUGS
1 INDICATIONS AND USAGE
  1.1 Major Depressive Disorder
  1.2 Obsessive Compulsive Disorder
  1.3 Bulimia Nervosa
  1.4 Panic Disorder
  1.5 PROZAC and Olanzapine in Combination: Depressive Episodes Associated with Bipolar I Disorder
  1.6 PROZAC and Olanzapine in Combination: Treatment Resistant Depression
2 DOSAGE AND ADMINISTRATION
  2.1 Major Depressive Disorder

FULL PRESCRIBING INFORMATION

WARNING: SUICIDALITY AND ANTIDEPRESSANT DRUGS

Antidepressants increased the risk compared to placebo of suicidal thinking and behavior (suicidality) in children, adolescents, and young adults in short-term studies of Major Depressive Disorder (MDD) and other psychiatric disorders. Anyone considering the use of PROZAC or any other antidepressant in a child, adolescent, or young adult must balance this risk with the clinical need. Short-term studies did not show an increase in the risk of suicidality with antidepressants compared to placebo in adults beyond age 24; there was a reduction in risk with antidepressants compared to placebo in adults aged 65 and older. Depression and certain other psychiatric disorders are themselves associated with increases in the risk of suicide. Patients of all ages who are started on antidepressant therapy should be monitored appropriately and observed closely for clinical worsening, suicidality, or unusual changes in behavior. Families and caregivers should be advised of the need for close observation and communication with the prescriber. PROZAC is approved for use in pediatric patients with MDD and Obsessive Compulsive Disorder (OCD) [see Warnings and Precautions (5.1) and Use in Specific Populations (8.4)].

When using PROZAC and olanzapine in combination, also refer to Boxed Warning section of the package insert for Symbyax.

1   INDICATIONS AND USAGE

1.1   Major Depressive Disorder

PROZAC® is indicated for the acute and maintenance treatment of Major Depressive Disorder in adult patients and in pediatric patients aged 8 to 18 years [see Clinical Studies (14.1)].

The usefulness of the drug in adult and pediatric patients receiving fluoxetine for extended periods, should periodically be re-evaluated [see Dosage and Administration (2.1)].

1.2   Obsessive Compulsive Disorder

PROZAC is indicated for the acute and maintenance treatment of obsessions and compulsions in adult patients and in pediatric patients aged 7 to 17 years with Obsessive Compulsive Disorder (OCD) [see Clinical Studies (14.2)].

The effectiveness of PROZAC in long-term use, i.e., for more than 13 weeks, has not been systematically evaluated in placebo-controlled trials. Therefore, the physician who elects to use PROZAC for extended periods, should periodically re-evaluate the long-term usefulness of the drug for the individual patient [see Dosage and Administration (2.2)].

1.3   Bulimia Nervosa

PROZAC is indicated for the acute and maintenance treatment of binge-eating and vomiting behaviors in adult patients with moderate to severe Bulimia Nervosa [see Clinical Studies (14.3)].

The physician who elects to use PROZAC for extended periods should periodically re-evaluate the long-term usefulness of the drug for the individual patient [see Dosage and Administration (2.3)].

1.4   Panic Disorder

PROZAC is indicated for the acute treatment of Panic Disorder, with or without agoraphobia, in adult patients [see Clinical Studies (14.4)].

The effectiveness of PROZAC in long-term use, i.e., for more than 12 weeks, has not been established in placebo-controlled trials. Therefore, the physician who elects to use PROZAC for extended periods, should periodically re-evaluate the long-term usefulness of the drug for the individual patient [see Dosage and Administration (2.4)].

1.5   PROZAC and Olanzapine in Combination: Depressive Episodes Associated with Bipolar I Disorder

When using PROZAC and olanzapine in combination, also refer to the Clinical Studies section of the package insert for Symbyax®.

PROZAC and olanzapine in combination is indicated for the acute treatment of depressive episodes associated with Bipolar I Disorder in adult patients.

PROZAC monotherapy is not indicated for the treatment of depressive episodes associated with Bipolar I Disorder.

1.6   PROZAC and Olanzapine in Combination: Treatment Resistant Depression

When using PROZAC and olanzapine in combination, also refer to the Clinical Studies section of the package insert for Symbyax.

PROZAC and olanzapine in combination is indicated for the acute treatment of treatment resistant depression (Major Depressive Disorder in adult patients, who do not respond to 2 separate trials of different antidepressants of adequate dose and duration in the current episode).

PROZAC monotherapy is not indicated for the treatment of treatment resistant depression.

2   DOSAGE AND ADMINISTRATION

2.1   Major Depressive Disorder

Initial Treatment

Adult—In controlled trials used to support the efficacy of fluoxetine, patients were administered morning doses ranging from 20 to 80 mg/day. Studies comparing fluoxetine 20, 40, and 60 mg/day to placebo indicate that 20 mg/day is sufficient to obtain a satisfactory response in Major Depressive Disorder in most cases. Consequently, a dose of 20 mg/day, administered in the morning, is recommended as the initial dose.

A dose increase may be considered after several weeks if insufficient clinical improvement is observed. Doses above 20 mg/day may be administered on a once-a-day (morning) or BID schedule (i.e., morning and noon) and should not exceed a maximum dose of 80 mg/day.

Pediatric (children and adolescents)—In the short-term (8 to 9 week) controlled clinical trials of fluoxetine supporting its effectiveness in the treatment of Major Depressive Disorder, patients were administered fluoxetine doses of 10 to 20 mg/day [see Clinical Studies (14.1)]. Treatment should be initiated with a dose of 10 or 20 mg/day. After 1 week at 10 mg/day, the dose should be increased to 20 mg/day.

However, due to higher plasma levels in lower weight children, the starting and target dose in this group may be 10 mg/day. A dose increase to 20 mg/day may be considered after several weeks if insufficient clinical improvement is observed.

All patients—As with other drugs effective in the treatment of Major Depressive Disorder, the full effect may be delayed until 4 weeks of treatment or longer.

Maintenance/Continuation/Extended Treatment—It is generally agreed that acute episodes of Major Depressive Disorder require several months or longer of sustained pharmacologic therapy. Whether the dose needed to induce remission is identical to the dose needed to maintain and/or sustain euthymia is unknown.

Daily Dosing—Systematic evaluation of PROZAC in adult patients has shown that its efficacy in Major Depressive Disorder is maintained for periods of up to 38 weeks following 12 weeks of open-label acute treatment (50 weeks total) at a dose of 20 mg/day [see Clinical Studies (14.1)].

Weekly Dosing—Systematic evaluation of PROZAC® Weekly™ in adult patients has shown that its efficacy in Major Depressive Disorder is maintained for periods of up to 25 weeks with once-weekly dosing following 13 weeks of open-label treatment with PROZAC 20 mg once daily. However, therapeutic equivalence of PROZAC Weekly given on a once-weekly basis with PROZAC 20 mg given daily for delaying time to relapse has not been established [see Clinical Studies (14.1)].

Weekly dosing with PROZAC Weekly capsules is recommended to be initiated 7 days after the last daily dose of PROZAC 20 mg [see Clinical Pharmacology (12.3)].

If satisfactory response is not maintained with PROZAC Weekly, consider reestablishing a daily dosing regimen [see Clinical Studies (14.1)].

Switching Patients to a Tricyclic Antidepressant (TCA)—Dosage of a TCA may need to be reduced, and plasma TCA concentrations may need to be monitored temporarily when fluoxetine is coadministered or has been recently discontinued [see Drug Interactions (7.9)].

Switching Patients to or from a Monoamine Oxidase Inhibitor (MAOI)—At least 14 days should elapse between discontinuation of an MAOI and initiation of therapy with PROZAC. In addition, at least 5 weeks, perhaps longer, should be allowed after stopping PROZAC before starting an MAOI [see Contraindications (4) and Drug Interactions (7.1)].

2.2   Obsessive Compulsive Disorder

Initial Treatment

Adult—In the controlled clinical trials of fluoxetine supporting its effectiveness in the treatment of OCD, patients were administered fixed daily doses of 20, 40, or 60 mg of fluoxetine or placebo [see Clinical Studies (14.2)]. In one of these studies, no dose-response relationship for effectiveness was demonstrated. Consequently, a dose of 20 mg/day, administered in the morning, is recommended as the initial dose. Since there was a suggestion of a possible dose-response relationship for effectiveness in the second study, a dose increase may be considered after several weeks if insufficient clinical improvement is observed. The full therapeutic effect may be delayed until 5 weeks of treatment or longer.

Doses above 20 mg/day may be administered on a once daily (i.e., morning) or BID schedule (i.e., morning and noon). A dose range of 20 to 60 mg/day is recommended; however, doses of up to 80 mg/day have been well tolerated in open studies of OCD. The maximum fluoxetine dose should not exceed 80 mg/day.

Pediatric (children and adolescents)—In the controlled clinical trial of fluoxetine supporting its effectiveness in the treatment of OCD, patients were administered fluoxetine doses in the range of 10 to 60 mg/day *[see Clinical Studies (14.2)]*.

In adolescents and higher weight children, treatment should be initiated with a dose of 10 mg/day. After 2 weeks, the dose should be increased to 20 mg/day. Additional dose increases may be considered after several more weeks if insufficient clinical improvement is observed. A dose range of 20 to 60 mg/day is recommended.

In lower weight children, treatment should be initiated with a dose of 10 mg/day. Additional dose increases may be considered after several more weeks if insufficient clinical improvement is observed. A dose range of 20 to 30 mg/day is recommended. Experience with daily doses greater than 20 mg is very minimal, and there is no experience with doses greater than 60 mg.

Maintenance/Continuation Treatment—While there are no systematic studies that answer the question of how long to continue PROZAC, OCD is a chronic condition and it is reasonable to consider continuation for a responding patient. Although the efficacy of PROZAC after 13 weeks has not been documented in controlled trials, adult patients have been continued in therapy under double-blind conditions for up to an additional 6 months without loss of benefit. However, dosage adjustments should be made to maintain the patient on the lowest effective dosage, and patients should be periodically reassessed to determine the need for treatment.

2.3 Bulimia Nervosa

Initial Treatment—In the controlled clinical trials of fluoxetine supporting its effectiveness in the treatment of Bulimia Nervosa, patients were administered fixed daily fluoxetine doses of 20 or 60 mg, or placebo *[see Clinical Studies (14.3)]*. Only the 60 mg dose was statistically significantly superior to placebo in reducing the frequency of binge-eating and vomiting. Consequently, the recommended dose is 60 mg/day, administered in the morning. For some patients it may be advisable to titrate up to this target dose over several days. Fluoxetine doses above 60 mg/day have not been systematically studied in patients with bulimia.

Maintenance/Continuation Treatment—Systematic evaluation of continuing PROZAC 60 mg/day for periods of up to 52 weeks in patients with bulimia who have responded while taking PROZAC 60 mg/day during an 8-week acute treatment phase has demonstrated a benefit of such maintenance treatment *[see Clinical Studies (14.3)]*. Nevertheless, patients should be periodically reassessed to determine the need for maintenance treatment.

2.4 Panic Disorder

Initial Treatment—In the controlled clinical trials of fluoxetine supporting its effectiveness in the treatment of Panic Disorder, patients were administered fluoxetine doses in the range of 10 to 60 mg/day *[see Clinical Studies (14.4)]*. Treatment should be initiated with a dose of 10 mg/day. After one week, the dose should be increased to 20 mg/day. The most frequently administered dose in the 2 flexible-dose clinical trials was 20 mg/day.

A dose increase may be considered after several weeks if no clinical improvement is observed. Fluoxetine doses above 60 mg/day have not been systematically evaluated in patients with Panic Disorder.

Maintenance/Continuation Treatment—While there are no systematic studies that answer the question of how long to continue PROZAC, panic disorder is a chronic condition and it is reasonable to consider continuation for a responding patient. Nevertheless, patients should be periodically reassessed to determine the need for continued treatment.

2.5 PROZAC and Olanzapine in Combination: Depressive Episodes Associated with Bipolar I Disorder

When using PROZAC and olanzapine in combination, also refer to the Clinical Studies section of the package insert for Symbyax.

Fluoxetine should be administered in combination with oral olanzapine once daily in the evening, without regard to meals, generally beginning with 5 mg of oral olanzapine and 20 mg of fluoxetine. Dosage adjustments, if indicated, can be made according to efficacy and tolerability within dose ranges of fluoxetine 20 to 50 mg and oral olanzapine 5 to 12.5 mg. Antidepressant efficacy was demonstrated with olanzapine and fluoxetine in combination with a dose range of olanzapine 6 to 12 mg and fluoxetine 25 to 50 mg.

Safety and efficacy of fluoxetine in combination with olanzapine was determined in clinical trials supporting approval of Symbyax (fixed-dose combination of olanzapine and fluoxetine). Symbyax is dosed between 3 mg/25 mg (olanzapine/fluoxetine) per day and 12 mg/50 mg (olanzapine/fluoxetine) per day. The following table demonstrates the appropriate individual component doses of PROZAC and olanzapine versus Symbyax. Dosage adjustments, if indicated, should be made with the individual components according to efficacy and tolerability.

Table 1: Approximate Dose Correspondence Between Symbyax[1] and the Combination of PROZAC and Olanzapine

	Use in Combination	
For Symbyax (mg/day)	Olanzapine (mg/day)	PROZAC (mg/day)
3 mg olanzapine/ 25 mg fluoxetine	2.5	20
6 mg olanzapine/ 25 mg fluoxetine	5	20
12 mg olanzapine/ 25 mg fluoxetine	10+2.5	20
6 mg olanzapine/ 50 mg fluoxetine	5	40+10
12 mg olanzapine/ 50 mg fluoxetine	10+2.5	40+10

[1] Symbyax (olanzapine/fluoxetine HCl) is a fixed-dose combination of PROZAC and olanzapine.

While there is no body of evidence to answer the question of how long a patient treated with PROZAC and olanzapine in combination should remain on it, it is generally accepted that Bipolar I Disorder, including the depressive episodes associated with Bipolar I Disorder, is a chronic illness requiring chronic treatment. The physician should periodically re-examine the need for continued pharmacotherapy.

Safety of coadministration of doses above 18 mg olanzapine with 75 mg fluoxetine has not been evaluated in clinical studies.

PROZAC monotherapy is not indicated for the treatment of depressive episodes associated with Bipolar I Disorder.

2.6 PROZAC and Olanzapine in Combination: Treatment Resistant Depression

When using PROZAC and olanzapine in combination, also refer to the Clinical Studies section of the package insert for Symbyax.

Fluoxetine should be administered in combination with oral olanzapine once daily in the evening, without regard to meals, generally beginning with 5 mg of oral olanzapine and 20 mg of fluoxetine. Dosage adjustments, if indicated, can be made according to efficacy and tolerability within dose ranges of fluoxetine 20 to 50 mg and oral olanzapine 5 to 20 mg. Antidepressant efficacy was demonstrated with olanzapine and fluoxetine in combination with a dose range of olanzapine 6 to 18 mg and fluoxetine 25 to 50 mg.

Safety and efficacy of fluoxetine in combination with olanzapine was determined in clinical trials supporting approval of Symbyax (fixed dose combination of olanzapine and fluoxetine). Symbyax is dosed between 3 mg/25 mg (olanzapine/fluoxetine) per day and 12 mg/50 mg (olanzapine/fluoxetine) per day. Table 1 demonstrates the appropriate individual component doses of PROZAC and olanzapine versus Symbyax. Dosage adjustments, if indicated, should be made with the individual components according to efficacy and tolerability.

While there is no body of evidence to answer the question of how long a patient treated with PROZAC and olanzapine in combination should remain on it, it is generally accepted that treatment resistant depression (Major Depressive Disorder in adult patients who do not respond to 2 separate trials of different antidepressants of adequate dose and duration in the current episode) is a chronic illness requiring chronic treatment. The physician should periodically reexamine the need for continued pharmacotherapy.

Safety of coadministration of doses above 18 mg olanzapine with 75 mg fluoxetine has not been evaluated in clinical studies.

PROZAC monotherapy is not indicated for the treatment of treatment resistant depression (Major Depressive Disorder in patients who do not respond to 2 antidepressants of adequate dose and duration in the current episode) have not been established.

2.7 Dosing in Specific Populations

Treatment of pregnant Women During the Third Trimester—When treating pregnant women with PROZAC during the third trimester, the physician should carefully consider the potential risks and potential benefits of treatment. Neonates exposed to SNRIs or SSRIs late in the third trimester have developed complications requiring prolonged hospitalization, respiratory support, and tube feeding. The physician may consider tapering PROZAC in the third trimester *[see Use in Specific Populations (8.1)]*.

Geriatric—A lower or less frequent dosage should be considered for the elderly *[see Use in Specific Populations (8.5)]*

Hepatic Impairment—As with many other medications, a lower or less frequent dosage should be used in patients with hepatic impairment *[see Clinical Pharmacology (12.4) and Use in Specific Populations (8.6)]*.

Concomitant Illness—Patients with concurrent disease or on multiple concomitant medications may require dosage adjustments *[see Clinical Pharmacology (12.4) and Warnings and Precautions (5.10)]*.

PROZAC and Olanzapine in Combination—The starting dose of oral olanzapine 2.5 to 5 mg with fluoxetine 20 mg should be used for patients with a predisposition to hypotensive reactions, patients with hepatic impairment, or patients who exhibit a combination of factors that may slow the metabolism of olanzapine or fluoxetine in combination (female gender, geriatric age, non-smoking status), or those patients who may be pharmacodynamically sensitive to olanzapine. Dosing modifications may be necessary in patients who exhibit a combination of factors that may slow metabolism. When indicated, dose escalation should be performed with caution in these patients. PROZAC and olanzapine in combination have not been systematically studied in patients over 65 years of age or in patients less than 18 years of age *[see Warnings and Precautions (5.14) and Drug Interactions (7.9)]*.

2.8 Discontinuation of Treatment

Symptoms associated with discontinuation of fluoxetine, SNRIs, and SSRIs, have been reported *[see Warnings and Precautions (5.13)]*.

3 DOSAGE FORMS AND STRENGTHS

- 10 mg Pulvule is an opaque green cap and opaque green body, imprinted with DISTA 3104 on the cap and Prozac 10 mg on the body
- 20 mg Pulvule is an opaque green cap and opaque yellow body, imprinted with DISTA 3105 on the cap and Prozac 20 mg on the body
- 40 mg Pulvule is an opaque green cap and opaque orange body, imprinted with DISTA 3107 on the cap and Prozac 40 mg on the body
- 90 mg Prozac Weekly™ Capsule is an opaque green cap and clear body containing discretely visible white pellets through the clear body of the capsule, imprinted with Lilly on the cap and 3004 and 90 mg on the body

4 CONTRAINDICATIONS

When using PROZAC and olanzapine in combination, also refer to the Contraindications section of the package insert for Symbyax.

The use of PROZAC is contraindicated with the following:

- Monoamine Oxidase Inhibitors *[see Drug Interactions (7.1)]*
- Pimozide *[see Drug Interactions (7.9)]*
- Thioridazine *[see Drug Interactions (7.9)]*

5 WARNINGS AND PRECAUTIONS

When using PROZAC and olanzapine in combination, also refer to the Warnings and Precautions section of the package insert for Symbyax.

5.1 Clinical Worsening and Suicide Risk

Patients with Major Depressive Disorder (MDD), both adult and pediatric, may experience worsening of their depression and/or the emergence of suicidal ideation and behavior (suicidality) or unusual changes in behavior, whether or not they are taking antidepressant medications, and this risk may persist until significant remission occurs. Suicide is a known risk of depression and certain other psychiatric disorders, and these disorders themselves are the strongest predictors of suicide. There has been a long-standing concern, however, that antidepressants may have a role in inducing worsening of depression and the emergence of suicidality in certain patients during the early phases of treatment. Pooled analyses of short-term placebo-controlled trials of antidepressant drugs (SSRIs and others) showed that these drugs increase the risk of suicidal thinking and behavior (suicidality) in children, adolescents, and young adults (ages 18-24) with Major Depressive Disorder (MDD) and other psychiatric disorders. Short-term studies did not show an increase in the risk of suicidality with antidepressants compared to placebo in adults beyond age 24; there was a reduction with antidepressants compared to placebo in adults aged 65 and older.

The pooled analyses of placebo-controlled trials in children and adolescents with MDD, Obsessive Compulsive Disorder (OCD), or other psychiatric disorders included a total of 24 short-term trials of 9 antidepressant drugs in over 4400 patients. The pooled analyses of placebo-controlled trials in adults with MDD or other psychiatric disorders included a total of 295 short-term trials (median duration of 2 months) of 11 antidepressant drugs in over 77,000 patients. There was considerable variation in risk of suicidality among drugs, but a tendency toward an increase in the younger patients for almost all drugs studied. There were differences in absolute risk of suicidality across the different indications, with the highest incidence in MDD. The risk differences (drug versus placebo), however, were relatively stable within age strata and across indications. These risk differences (drug-placebo difference in the number of cases of suicidality per 1000 patients treated) are provided in Table 2.

Table 2: Suicidality per 1000 Patients Treated

Age Range	Drug-Placebo Difference in Number of Cases of Suicidality per 1000 Patients Treated
	Increases Compared to Placebo
<18	14 additional cases
18-24	5 additional cases
	Decreases Compared to Placebo
25-64	1 fewer case
≥65	6 fewer cases

No suicides occurred in any of the pediatric trials. There were suicides in the adult trials, but the number was not sufficient to reach any conclusion about drug effect on suicide.

It is unknown whether the suicidality risk extends to longer-term use, i.e., beyond several months. However, there is substantial evidence from placebo-controlled maintenance trials in adults with depression that the use of antidepressants can delay the recurrence of depression.

All patients being treated with antidepressants for any indication should be monitored appropriately and observed closely for clinical worsening, suicidality, and unusual changes in behavior, especially during the initial few months of a course of drug therapy, or at times of dose changes, either increases or decreases.

The following symptoms, anxiety, agitation, panic attacks, insomnia, irritability, hostility, aggressiveness, impulsivity, akathisia (psychomotor restlessness), hypomania, and mania, have been reported in adult and pediatric patients being treated with antidepressants for Major Depressive Disorder as well as for other indications, both psychiatric and nonpsychiatric. Although a causal link between the emergence of such symptoms and either the worsening of depression and/or the emergence of suicidal impulses has not been established, there is concern that such symptoms may represent precursors to emerging suicidality.

Consideration should be given to changing the therapeutic regimen, including possibly discontinuing the medication, in patients whose depression is persistently worse, or who are experiencing emergent suicidality or symptoms that might be precursors to worsening depression or suicidality, especially if these symptoms are severe, abrupt in onset, or were not part of the patient's presenting symptoms.

If the decision has been made to discontinue treatment, medication should be tapered, as rapidly as is feasible, but with recognition that abrupt discontinuation can be associated with certain symptoms *[see Warnings and Precautions (5.13)]*.

Families and caregivers of patients being treated with antidepressants for Major Depressive Disorder or other indications, both psychiatric and nonpsychiatric, should be alerted about the need to monitor patients for the emergence of agitation, irritability, unusual changes in behavior, and the other symptoms described above, as well as the emergence of suicidality, and to report such symptoms immediately to health care providers. Such monitoring should include daily observation by families and caregivers. Prescriptions for PROZAC should be written for the smallest quantity of capsules consistent with good patient management, in order to reduce the risk of overdose.

It should be noted that PROZAC is approved in the pediatric population only for Major Depressive Disorder and Obsessive Compulsive Disorder. Safety and effectiveness of PROZAC and olanzapine in combination in patients less than 18 years of age have not been established.

5.2 Serotonin Syndrome or Neuroleptic Malignant Syndrome (NMS)-like Reactions

The development of a potentially life-threatening serotonin syndrome or neuroleptic malignant syndrome (NMS)-like reactions have been reported with SNRIs and SSRIs alone, including PROZAC treatment, but particularly with concomitant use of serotonergic drugs (including triptans) with drugs which impair metabolism of serotonin (including MAOIs), or with antipsychotics or other dopamine antagonists. Serotonin syndrome symptoms may include mental status changes (e.g., agitation, hallucinations, coma), autonomic instability (e.g., tachycardia, labile blood pressure, hyperthermia), neuromuscular aberrations (e.g., hyperreflexia, incoordination) and/or gastrointestinal symptoms (e.g., nausea, vomiting, diarrhea). Serotonin syndrome, in its most severe form can resemble neuroleptic malignant syndrome, which includes hyperthermia, muscle rigidity, autonomic instability with possible rapid fluctuation of vital signs, and mental status changes. Patients should be monitored for the emergence of serotonin syndrome or NMS-like signs and symptoms.

The concomitant use of PROZAC with MAOIs intended to treat depression is contraindicated *[see Contraindications (4) and Drug Interactions (7.1)]*.

If concomitant treatment of PROZAC with a 5-hydroxytryptamine receptor agonist (triptan) is clinically warranted, careful observation of the patient is advised, particularly during treatment initiation and dose increases *[see Drug Interactions (7.4)]*.

The concomitant use of PROZAC with serotonin precursors (such as tryptophan) is not recommended *[see Drug Interactions (7.3)]*.

Treatment with fluoxetine and any concomitant serotonergic or antidopaminergic agents, including antipsychotics, should be discontinued immediately if the above reactions occur and supportive symptomatic treatment should be initiated.

5.3 Allergic Reactions and Rash

In US fluoxetine clinical trials as of May 8, 1995, 7% of 10,782 patients developed various types of rashes and/or urticaria. Among the cases of rash and/or urticaria reported in premarketing clinical trials, almost a third were withdrawn from treatment because of the rash and/or systemic signs or symptoms associated with the rash. Clinical findings reported in association with rash include fever, leukocytosis, arthralgias, edema, carpal tunnel syndrome, respiratory distress, lymphadenopathy, proteinuria, and mild transaminase elevation. Most patients improved promptly with discontinuation of fluoxetine and/or adjunctive treatment with antihistamines or steroids, and all patients experiencing these reactions were reported to recover completely.

In premarketing clinical trials, 2 patients are known to have developed a serious cutaneous systemic illness. In neither patient was there an unequivocal diagnosis, but one was considered to have a leukocytoclastic vasculitis, and the other, a severe desquamating syndrome that was considered variously to be a vasculitis or erythema multiforme. Other patients have had systemic syndromes suggestive of serum sickness.

Since the introduction of PROZAC, systemic reactions, possibly related to vasculitis and including lupus-like syndrome, have developed in patients with rash. Although these reactions are rare, they may be serious, involving the lung, kidney, or liver. Death has been reported to occur in association with these systemic reactions.

Anaphylactoid reactions, including bronchospasm, angioedema, laryngospasm, and urticaria alone and in combination, have been reported.

Pulmonary reactions, including inflammatory processes of varying histopathology and/or fibrosis, have been reported rarely. These reactions have occurred with dyspnea as the only preceding symptom.

Whether these systemic reactions and rash have a common underlying cause or are due to different etiologies or pathogenic processes is not known. Furthermore, a specific underlying immunologic basis for these reactions has not been identified. Upon the appearance of rash or of other possibly allergic phenomena for which an alternative etiology cannot be identified, PROZAC should be discontinued.

5.4 Screening Patients for Bipolar Disorder and Monitoring for Mania/Hypomania

A major depressive episode may be the initial presentation of Bipolar Disorder. It is generally believed (though not established in controlled trials) that treating such an episode with an antidepressant alone may increase the likelihood of precipitation of a mixed/manic episode in patients at risk for Bipolar Disorder. Whether any of the symptoms described for clinical worsening and suicide risk represent such a conversion is unknown. However, prior to initiating treatment with an antidepressant, patients with depressive symptoms should be adequately screened to determine if they are at risk for Bipolar Disorder; such screening should include a detailed psychiatric history, including a family history of suicide, Bipolar Disorder, and depression. It should be noted that PROZAC and olanzapine in combination is approved for the acute treatment of depressive episodes associated with Bipolar I Disorder [*see Warnings and Precautions section of the package insert for Symbyax*]. PROZAC monotherapy is not indicated for the treatment of depressive episodes associated with Bipolar I Disorder.

In US placebo-controlled clinical trials for Major Depressive Disorder, mania/hypomania was reported in 0.1% of patients treated with PROZAC and 0.1% of patients treated with placebo. Activation of mania/hypomania has also been reported in a small proportion of patients with Major Affective Disorder treated with other marketed drugs effective in the treatment of Major Depressive Disorder *[see Use in Specific Populations (8.4)]*.

In US placebo-controlled clinical trials for OCD, mania/hypomania was reported in 0.8% of patients treated with PROZAC and no patients treated with placebo. No patients reported mania/hypomania in US placebo-controlled clinical trials for bulimia. In all US PROZAC clinical trials as of May 8, 1995, 0.7% of 10,782 patients reported mania/hypomania *[see Use in Specific Populations (8.4)]*.

5.5 Seizures

In US placebo-controlled clinical trials for Major Depressive Disorder, convulsions (or reactions described as possibly having been seizures) were reported in 0.1% of patients treated with PROZAC and 0.2% of patients treated with placebo. No patients reported convulsions in US placebo-controlled clinical trials for either OCD or bulimia. In all US PROZAC clinical trials as of May 8, 1995, 0.2% of 10,782 patients reported convulsions. The percentage appears to be similar to that associated with other marketed drugs effective in the treatment of Major Depressive Disorder. PROZAC should be introduced with care in patients with a history of seizures.

5.6 Altered Appetite and Weight

Significant weight loss, especially in underweight depressed or bulimic patients, may be an undesirable result of treatment with PROZAC.

In US placebo-controlled clinical trials for Major Depressive Disorder, 11% of patients treated with PROZAC and 2% of patients treated with placebo reported anorexia (decreased appetite). Weight loss was reported in 1.4% of patients treated with PROZAC and in 0.5% of patients treated with placebo. However, only rarely have patients discontinued treatment with PROZAC because of anorexia or weight loss *[see Use in Specific Populations (8.4)]*.

In US placebo-controlled clinical trials for OCD, 17% of patients treated with PROZAC and 10% of patients treated with placebo reported anorexia (decreased appetite). One patient discontinued treatment with PROZAC because of anorexia *[see Use in Specific Populations (8.4)]*.

In US placebo-controlled clinical trials for Bulimia Nervosa, 8% of patients treated with PROZAC 60 mg and 4% of patients treated with placebo reported anorexia (decreased appetite). Patients treated with PROZAC 60 mg on average lost 0.45 kg compared with a gain of 0.16 kg by patients treated with placebo in the 16-week double-blind trial. Weight change should be monitored during therapy.

5.7 Abnormal Bleeding

SNRIs and SSRIs, including fluoxetine, may increase the risk of bleeding reactions. Concomitant use of aspirin, nonsteroidal anti-inflammatory drugs, warfarin, and other anticoagulants may add to this risk. Case reports and epidemiological studies (case-control and cohort design) have demonstrated an association between use of drugs that interfere with serotonin reuptake and the occurrence of gastrointestinal bleeding. Bleeding reactions related to SNRIs and SSRIs use have ranged from ecchymoses, hematomas, epistaxis, and petechiae to life-threatening hemorrhages. Patients should be cautioned about the risk of bleeding associated with the concomitant use of fluoxetine and NSAIDs, aspirin, warfarin, or other drugs that affect coagulation *[see Drug Interactions (7.6)]*.

5.8 Hyponatremia

Hyponatremia has been reported during treatment with SNRIs and SSRIs, including PROZAC. In many cases, this hyponatremia appears to be the result of the syndrome of inappropriate antidiuretic hormone secretion (SIADH). Cases with serum sodium lower than 110 mmol/L have been reported and appeared to be reversible when PROZAC was discontinued. Elderly patients may be at greater risk of developing hyponatremia with SNRIs and SSRIs. Also, patients taking diuretics or who are otherwise volume depleted may be at greater risk *[see Use in Specific Populations (8.5)]*. Discontinuation of PROZAC should be considered in patients with symptomatic hyponatremia and appropriate medical intervention should be instituted.

Signs and symptoms of hyponatremia include headache, difficulty concentrating, memory impairment, confusion, weakness, and unsteadiness, which may lead to falls. More severe and/or acute cases have been associated with hallucination, syncope, seizure, coma, respiratory arrest, and death.

5.9 Anxiety and Insomnia

In US placebo-controlled clinical trials for Major Depressive Disorder, 12% to 16% of patients treated with PROZAC and 7% to 9% of patients treated with placebo reported anxiety, nervousness, or insomnia.

In US placebo-controlled clinical trials for OCD, insomnia was reported in 28% of patients treated with PROZAC and in 22% of patients treated with placebo. Anxiety was reported in 14% of patients treated with PROZAC and in 7% of patients treated with placebo.

In US placebo-controlled clinical trials for Bulimia Nervosa, insomnia was reported in 33% of patients treated with PROZAC 60 mg, and 13% of patients treated with placebo. Anxiety and nervousness were reported, respectively, in 15% and 11% of patients treated with PROZAC 60 mg and in 9% and 5% of patients treated with placebo.

Among the most common adverse reactions associated with discontinuation (incidence at least twice that for placebo

Table 3: Most Common Treatment-Emergent Adverse Reactions: Incidence in Major Depressive Disorder, OCD, Bulimia, and Panic Disorder Placebo-Controlled Clinical Trials[1,2]

Body System/ Adverse Reaction	Major Depressive Disorder		OCD		Bulimia		Panic Disorder	
	PROZAC (N=1728)	Placebo (N=975)	PROZAC (N=266)	Placebo (N=89)	PROZAC (N=450)	Placebo (N=267)	PROZAC (N=425)	Placebo (N=342)
Body as a Whole								
Asthenia	9	5	15	11	21	9	7	7
Flu syndrome	3	4	10	7	8	3	5	5
Cardiovascular System								
Vasodilatation	3	2	5	—	2	1	1	—
Digestive System								
Nausea	21	9	26	13	29	11	12	7
Diarrhea	12	8	18	13	8	6	9	4
Anorexia	11	2	17	10	8	4	4	1
Dry mouth	10	7	12	3	9	6	4	4
Dyspepsia	7	5	10	4	10	6	6	2
Nervous System								
Insomnia	16	9	28	22	33	13	10	7
Anxiety	12	7	14	7	15	9	6	2
Nervousness	14	9	14	15	11	5	8	6
Somnolence	13	6	17	7	13	5	5	2
Tremor	10	3	9	1	13	1	3	1
Libido decreased	3	—	11	2	5	1	1	2
Abnormal dreams	1	1	5	2	5	3	1	1
Respiratory System								
Pharyngitis	3	3	11	9	10	5	3	3
Sinusitis	1	4	5	2	6	4	2	3
Yawn	—	—	7	—	11	—	1	—
Skin and Appendages								
Sweating	8	3	7	—	8	3	2	2
Rash	4	3	6	3	4	4	2	2
Urogenital System								
Impotence[3]	2	—			7	—	1	—
Abnormal ejaculation[3]	—	—	7	—	7	—	2	1

[1] Incidence less than 1%.
[2] Includes US data for Major Depressive Disorder, OCD, Bulimia, and Panic Disorder clinical trials, plus non-US data for Panic Disorder clinical trials.
[3] Denominator used was for males only (N=690 PROZAC Major Depressive Disorder; N=410 placebo Major Depressive Disorder; N=116 PROZAC OCD; N=43 placebo OCD; N=14 PROZAC bulimia; N=1 placebo bulimia; N=162 PROZAC panic; N=121 placebo panic).

and at least 1% for PROZAC in clinical trials collecting only a primary reaction associated with discontinuation) in US placebo-controlled fluoxetine clinical trials were anxiety (2% in OCD), insomnia (1% in combined indications and 2% in bulimia), and nervousness (1% in Major Depressive Disorder) [see Table 5].

5.10   Use in Patients with Concomitant Illness
Clinical experience with PROZAC in patients with concomitant systemic illness is limited. Caution is advisable in using PROZAC in patients with diseases or conditions that could affect metabolism or hemodynamic responses.
Cardiovascular—Fluoxetine has not been evaluated or used to any appreciable extent in patients with a recent history of myocardial infarction or unstable heart disease. Patients with these diagnoses were systematically excluded from clinical studies during the product's premarket testing. However, the electrocardiograms of 312 patients who received PROZAC in double-blind trials were retrospectively

evaluated; no conduction abnormalities that resulted in heart block were observed. The mean heart rate was reduced by approximately 3 beats/min.
Glycemic Control—In patients with diabetes, PROZAC may alter glycemic control. Hypoglycemia has occurred during therapy with PROZAC, and hyperglycemia has developed following discontinuation of the drug. As is true with many other types of medication when taken concurrently by patients with diabetes, insulin and/or oral hypoglycemic, dosage may need to be adjusted when therapy with PROZAC is instituted or discontinued.

5.11   Potential for Cognitive and Motor Impairment
As with any CNS-active drug, PROZAC has the potential to impair judgment, thinking, or motor skills. Patients should be cautioned about operating hazardous machinery, including automobiles, until they are reasonably certain that the drug treatment does not affect them adversely.

5.12   Long Elimination Half-Life
Because of the long elimination half-lives of the parent drug and its major active metabolite, changes in dose will not be fully reflected in plasma for several weeks, affecting both strategies for titration to final dose and withdrawal from treatment. This is of potential consequence when drug discontinuation is required or when drugs are prescribed that might interact with fluoxetine and norfluoxetine following the discontinuation of fluoxetine [see Clinical Pharmacology (12.3)].

5.13   Discontinuation of Treatment
During marketing of PROZAC, SNRIs, and SSRIs, there have been spontaneous reports of adverse reactions occurring upon discontinuation of these drugs, particularly when abrupt, including the following: dysphoric mood, irritability, agitation, dizziness, sensory disturbances (e.g., paresthesias such as electric shock sensations), anxiety, confusion, headache, lethargy, emotional lability, insomnia, and hypomania. While these reactions are generally self-limiting, there have been reports of serious discontinuation symptoms. Patients should be monitored for these symptoms when discontinuing treatment with PROZAC. A gradual reduction in the dose rather than abrupt cessation is recommended whenever possible. If intolerable symptoms occur following a decrease in the dose or upon discontinuation of treatment, then resuming the previously prescribed dose may be considered. Subsequently, the physician may continue decreasing the dose but at a more gradual rate. Plasma fluoxetine and norfluoxetine concentration decrease gradually at the conclusion of therapy which may minimize the risk of discontinuation symptoms with this drug.

5.14   PROZAC and Olanzapine in Combination
When using PROZAC and olanzapine in combination, also refer to the Warnings and Precautions section of the package insert for Symbyax.

6   ADVERSE REACTIONS
When using PROZAC and olanzapine in combination, also refer to the Adverse Reactions section of the package insert for Symbyax.

6.1   Clinical Trials Experience
Because clinical trials are conducted under widely varying conditions, adverse reaction rates observed in the clinical trials of a drug cannot be directly compared to rates in the clinical trials of another drug and may not reflect or predict the rates observed in practice.
Multiple doses of PROZAC had been administered to 10,782 patients with various diagnoses in US clinical trials as of May 8, 1995. In addition, there have been 425 patients administered PROZAC in panic clinical trials. Adverse reactions were recorded by clinical investigators using descriptive terminology of their own choosing. Consequently, it is not possible to provide a meaningful estimate of the proportion of individuals experiencing adverse reactions without first grouping similar types of reactions into a limited (i.e., reduced) number of standardized reaction categories.
In the tables and tabulations that follow, COSTART Dictionary terminology has been used to classify reported adverse reactions. The stated frequencies represent the proportion of individuals who experienced, at least once, a treatment-emergent adverse reaction of the type listed. A reaction was considered treatment-emergent if it occurred for the first time or worsened while receiving therapy following baseline evaluation. It is important to emphasize that reactions reported during therapy were not necessarily caused by it.
The prescriber should be aware that the figures in the tables and tabulations cannot be used to predict the incidence of side effects in the course of usual medical practice where patient characteristics and other factors differ from those that prevailed in the clinical trials. Similarly, the cited frequencies cannot be compared with figures obtained from other clinical investigations involving different treatments, uses, and investigators. The cited figures, however, do provide the prescribing physician with some basis for estimating the relative contribution of drug and nondrug factors to the side effect incidence rate in the population studied.
Incidence in Major Depressive Disorder, OCD, bulimia, and Panic Disorder placebo-controlled clinical trials (excluding data from extensions of trials)—Table 3 enumerates the most common treatment-emergent adverse reactions associated with the use of PROZAC (incidence of at least 5% for PROZAC and at least twice that for placebo within at least 1 of the indications) for the treatment of Major Depressive Disorder, OCD, and bulimia in US controlled clinical trials and Panic Disorder in US plus non-US controlled trials. Table 5 enumerates treatment-emergent adverse reactions that occurred in 2% or more patients treated with PROZAC and with incidence greater than placebo who participated in US Major Depressive Disorder, OCD, and bulimia controlled clinical trials and US plus non-US Panic Disorder controlled clinical trials. Table 4 provides combined data for the pool of studies that are provided separately by indication in Table 3.
[See table 3 at top left]

Table 4: Treatment-Emergent Adverse Reactions: Incidence in Major Depressive Disorder, OCD, Bulimia, and Panic Disorder Placebo-Controlled Clinical Trials[1,2]

Body System/ Adverse Reaction	PROZAC (N=2869)	Placebo (N=1673)
Body as a Whole		
Headache	21	19
Asthenia	11	6
Flu syndrome	5	4
Fever	2	1
Cardiovascular System		
Vasodilatation	2	1
Digestive System		
Nausea	22	9
Diarrhea	11	7
Anorexia	10	3
Dry mouth	9	6
Dyspepsia	8	4
Constipation	5	4
Flatulence	3	2
Vomiting	3	2
Metabolic and Nutritional Disorders		
Weight loss	2	1
Nervous System		
Insomnia	19	10
Nervousness	13	8
Anxiety	12	6
Somnolence	12	5
Dizziness	9	6
Tremor	9	2
Libido decreased	4	1
Thinking abnormal	2	1
Respiratory System		
Yawn	3	—
Skin and Appendages		
Sweating	7	3
Rash	4	3
Pruritus	3	2
Special Senses		
Abnormal vision	2	1

The table above shows "Percentage of Patients Reporting Event" for "Major Depressive Disorder, OCD, Bulimia, and Panic Disorder Combined".

[1] Incidence less than 1%.
[2] Includes US data for Major Depressive Disorder, OCD, bulimia, and Panic Disorder clinical trials, plus non-US data for Panic Disorder clinical trials.

Associated with discontinuation in Major Depressive Disorder, OCD, bulimia, and Panic Disorder placebo-controlled clinical trials (excluding data from extensions of trials)— Table 5 lists the adverse reactions associated with discontinuation of PROZAC treatment (incidence at least twice that for placebo and at least 1% for PROZAC in clinical trials collecting only a primary reaction associated with discontinuation) in Major Depressive Disorder, OCD, bulimia, and Panic Disorder clinical trials, plus non-US Panic Disorder clinical trials.
[See table 5 above]

Table 5: Most Common Adverse Reactions Associated with Discontinuation in Major Depressive Disorder, OCD, Bulimia, and Panic Disorder Placebo-Controlled Clinical Trials[1]

Major Depressive Disorder, OCD, Bulimia, and Panic Disorder Combined (N=1533)	Major Depressive Disorder (N=392)	OCD (N=266)	Bulimia (N=450)	Panic Disorder (N=425)
Anxiety (1%)	—	Anxiety (2%)	—	Anxiety (2%)
—	—	—	Insomnia (2%)	—
—	Nervousness (1%)	—	—	Nervousness (1%)
—	—	Rash (1%)	—	—

[1] Includes US Major Depressive Disorder, OCD, bulimia, and Panic Disorder clinical trials, plus non-US Panic Disorder clinical trials.

*Other adverse reactions in pediatric patients (children and adolescents)—*Treatment-emergent adverse reactions were collected in 322 pediatric patients (180 fluoxetine-treated, 142 placebo-treated). The overall profile of adverse reactions was generally similar to that seen in adult studies, as shown in Tables 4 and 5. However, the following adverse reactions (excluding those which appear in the body or footnotes of Tables 4 and 5 and those for which the COSTART terms were uninformative or misleading) were reported at an incidence of at least 2% for fluoxetine and greater than placebo: thirst, hyperkinesia, agitation, personality disorder, epistaxis, urinary frequency, and menorrhagia.

The most common adverse reaction (incidence at least 1% for fluoxetine and greater than placebo) associated with discontinuation in 3 pediatric placebo-controlled trials (N=418 randomized; 228 fluoxetine-treated; 190 placebo-treated) was mania/hypomania (1.8% for fluoxetine-treated, 0% for placebo-treated). In these clinical trials, only a primary reaction associated with discontinuation was collected.

*Reactions observed in PROZAC Weekly clinical trials—*Treatment-emergent adverse reactions in clinical trials with PROZAC Weekly were similar to the adverse reactions reported by patients in clinical trials with PROZAC daily. In a placebo-controlled clinical trial, more patients taking PROZAC Weekly reported diarrhea than patients taking placebo (10% versus 3%, respectively) or taking PROZAC 20 mg daily (10% versus 5%, respectively).

*Male and female sexual dysfunction with SSRIs—*Although changes in sexual desire, sexual performance, and sexual satisfaction often occur as manifestations of a psychiatric disorder, they may also be a consequence of pharmacologic treatment. In particular, some evidence suggests that SSRIs can cause such untoward sexual experiences. Reliable estimates of the incidence and severity of untoward experiences involving sexual desire, performance, and satisfaction are difficult to obtain, however, in part because patients and physicians may be reluctant to discuss them. Accordingly, estimates of the incidence of untoward sexual experience and performance, cited in product labeling, are likely to underestimate their actual incidence. In patients enrolled in US Major Depressive Disorder, OCD, and bulimia placebo-controlled clinical trials, decreased libido was the only sexual side effect reported by at least 2% of patients taking fluoxetine (4% fluoxetine, <1% placebo). There have been spontaneous reports in women taking fluoxetine of orgasmic dysfunction, including anorgasmia.

There are no adequate and well-controlled studies examining sexual dysfunction with fluoxetine treatment.

Priapism has been reported with all SSRIs.

While it is difficult to know the precise risk of sexual dysfunction associated with the use of SSRIs, physicians should routinely inquire about such possible side effects.

6.2 Other Reactions

Following is a list of treatment-emergent adverse reactions reported by patients treated with fluoxetine in clinical trials. This listing is not intended to include reactions (1) already listed in previous tables or elsewhere in labeling, (2) for which a drug cause was remote, (3) which were so general as to be uninformative, (4) which were not considered to have significant clinical implications, or (5) which occurred at a rate equal to or less than placebo.

Reactions are classified by body system using the following definitions: frequent adverse reactions are those occurring in at least 1/100 patients; infrequent adverse reactions are those occurring in 1/100 to 1/1000 patients; rare reactions are those occurring in fewer than 1/1000 patients.

Body as a Whole—*Frequent:* chills; *Infrequent:* suicide attempt; *Rare:* acute abdominal syndrome, photosensitivity reaction.
Cardiovascular System—*Frequent:* palpitation; *Infrequent:* arrhythmia.
Digestive System—*Infrequent:* dysphagia, gastritis, gastroenteritis, melena, stomach ulcer; *Rare:* bloody diarrhea, duodenal ulcer, esophageal ulcer, gastrointestinal hemorrhage, hematemesis, hepatitis, peptic ulcer, stomach ulcer hemorrhage.
Hemic and Lymphatic System—*Infrequent:* ecchymosis; *Rare:* petechia, purpura.
Nervous System—*Frequent:* emotional lability; *Infrequent:* akathisia, ataxia, buccoglossal syndrome, euphoria, hypertonia, libido increased, myoclonus, paranoid reaction; *Rare:* delusions.
Respiratory System—*Rare:* larynx edema.
Skin and Appendages—*Rare:* purpuric rash.
Special Senses—*Frequent:* taste perversion; *Infrequent:* mydriasis.

6.3 Postmarketing Experience

The following adverse reactions have been identified during post approval use of PROZAC. Because these reactions are reported voluntarily from a population of uncertain size, it is difficult to reliably estimate their frequency or evaluate a causal relationship to drug exposure.

Voluntary reports of adverse reactions temporally associated with PROZAC that have been received since market introduction and that may have no causal relationship with the drug include the following: aplastic anemia, atrial fibrillation[1], cataract, cerebrovascular accident[1], cholestatic jaundice, dyskinesia (including, for example, a case of buccal-lingual-masticatory syndrome with involuntary tongue protrusion reported to develop in a 77-year-old female after 5 weeks of fluoxetine therapy and which completely resolved over the next few months following drug discontinuation), eosinophilic pneumonia[1], epidermal necrolysis, erythema multiforme, erythema nodosum, exfoliative dermatitis, gynecomastia, heart arrest[1], hepatic failure/necrosis, hyperprolactinemia, hypoglycemia, immune-related hemolytic anemia, kidney failure, movement disorders developing in patients with risk factors including drugs associated with such reactions and worsening of pre-existing movement disorders optic neuritis, pancreatitis[1], pancytopenia, pulmonary embolism, pulmonary hypertension, QT prolongation, Stevens-Johnson syndrome, thrombocytopenia[1], thrombocytopenic purpura, ventricular tachycardia (including torsades de pointes–type arrhythmias), vaginal bleeding, and violent behaviors[1].

[1] These terms represent serious adverse events, but do not meet the definition for adverse drug reactions. They are included here because of their seriousness.

7 DRUG INTERACTIONS

As with all drugs, the potential for interaction by a variety of mechanisms (e.g., pharmacodynamic, pharmacokinetic drug inhibition or enhancement, etc.) is a possibility.

7.1 Monoamine Oxidase Inhibitors (MAOI)

There have been reports of serious, sometimes fatal, reactions (including hyperthermia, rigidity, myoclonus, autonomic instability with possible rapid fluctuations of vital signs, and mental status changes that include extreme agitation progressing to delirium and coma) in patients receiving fluoxetine in combination with a monoamine oxidase inhibitor (MAOI), and in patients who have recently discontinued fluoxetine and are then started on an MAOI. Some cases presented with features resembling neuroleptic malignant syndrome. Therefore, PROZAC should not be used in combination with an MAOI, or within a minimum of 14 days of discontinuing therapy with an MAOI *[see Contraindications (4)]*. Since fluoxetine and its major metabolite have very long elimination half-lives, at least 5 weeks perhaps longer, especially if fluoxetine has been prescribed chronically and/or at higher doses should be allowed after stopping PROZAC before starting an MAOI *[see Clinical Pharmacology (12.3)]*.

7.2 CNS Acting Drugs

Caution is advised if the concomitant administration of PROZAC and such drugs is required. In evaluating individual cases, consideration should be given to using lower initial doses of the concomitantly administered drugs, using conservative titration schedules, and monitoring of clinical status *[see Clinical Pharmacology (12.3)]*.

7.3 Serotonergic Drugs

Based on the mechanism of action of SNRIs and SSRIs, including PROZAC, and the potential for serotonin syndrome, caution is advised when PROZAC is coadministered with other drugs that may affect the serotonergic neurotransmitter systems, such as triptans, linezolid (an antibiotic which is a reversible non-selective MAOI), lithium, tramadol, or St. John's Wort *[see Warnings and Precautions (5.2)]*. The concomitant use of PROZAC with SNRIs, SSRIs, or tryptophan is not recommended *[see Drug Interactions (7.4), (7.5)]*.

7.4 Triptans

There have been rare postmarketing reports of serotonin syndrome with use of an SSRI and a triptan. If concomitant treatment of PROZAC with a triptan is clinically warranted, careful observation of the patient is advised, particularly during treatment initiation and dose increases *[see Warnings and Precautions (5.2) and Drug Interactions (7.3)]*.

7.5 Tryptophan

Five patients receiving PROZAC in combination with tryptophan experienced adverse reactions, including agitation, restlessness, and gastrointestinal distress. The concomitant use with tryptophan is not recommended *[see Warnings and Precautions (5.2) and Drug Interactions (7.3)]*.

7.6 Drugs that Interfere with Hemostasis (e.g., NSAIDS, Aspirin, Warfarin)

Serotonin release by platelets plays an important role in hemostasis. Epidemiological studies of the case-control and cohort design that have demonstrated an association between use of psychotropic drugs that interfere with serotonin reuptake and the occurrence of upper gastrointestinal bleeding have also shown that concurrent use of an NSAID or aspirin may potentiate this risk of bleeding. Altered anticoagulant effects, including increased bleeding, have been reported when SNRIs or SSRIs are coadministered with warfarin. Patients receiving warfarin therapy should be carefully monitored when fluoxetine is initiated or discontinued *[see Warnings and Precautions (5.7)]*.

7.7 Electroconvulsive Therapy (ECT)

There are no clinical studies establishing the benefit of the combined use of ECT and fluoxetine. There have been rare reports of prolonged seizures in patients on fluoxetine receiving ECT treatment.

7.8 Potential for Other Drugs to affect PROZAC

Drugs Tightly Bound to Plasma Proteins—Because fluoxetine is tightly bound to plasma protein, adverse effects may result from displacement of protein-bound fluoxetine by other tightly-bound drugs *[see Clinical Pharmacology (12.3)]*.

7.9 Potential for PROZAC to affect Other Drugs

Pimozide—Concomitant use in patients taking pimozide is contraindicated. Clinical studies of pimozide with other antidepressants demonstrate an increase in drug interaction or QT_c prolongation. While a specific study with pimozide and fluoxetine has not been conducted, the potential for drug interactions or QT_c prolongation warrants restricting the concurrent use of pimozide and PROZAC *[see Contraindications (4)]*.

Thioridazine—Thioridazine should not be administered with PROZAC or within a minimum of 5 weeks after PROZAC has been discontinued *[see Contraindications (4)]*.

In a study of 19 healthy male subjects, which included 6 slow and 13 rapid hydroxylators of debrisoquin, a single 25 mg oral dose of thioridazine produced a 2.4-fold higher C_{max} and a 4.5-fold higher AUC for thioridazine in the slow hydroxylators compared with the rapid hydroxylators. The rate of debrisoquin hydroxylation is felt to depend on the level of CYP2D6 isozyme activity. Thus, this study suggests that drugs which inhibit CYP2D6, such as certain SSRIs, including fluoxetine, will produce elevated plasma levels of thioridazine.

Thioridazine administration produces a dose-related prolongation of the QT_c interval, which is associated with serious ventricular arrhythmias, such as torsades de pointes-type arrhythmias, and sudden death. This risk is expected to increase with fluoxetine-induced inhibition of thioridazine metabolism.

Drugs Metabolized by CYP2D6—Fluoxetine inhibits the activity of CYP2D6, and may make individuals with normal CYP2D6 metabolic activity resemble a poor metabolizer. Coadministration of fluoxetine with other drugs that are metabolized by CYP2D6, including certain antidepressants (e.g., TCAs), antipsychotics (e.g., phenothiazines and most atypicals), and antiarrhythmics (e.g., propafenone, flecainide, and others) should be approached with caution. Therapy with medications that are predominantly metabolized by the CYP2D6 system and that have a relatively narrow therapeutic index (see list below) should be initiated at the low end of the dose range if a patient is receiving fluoxetine concurrently or has taken it in the previous 5 weeks. Thus, his/her dosing requirements resemble those of poor metabolizers. If fluoxetine is added to the treatment regimen of a patient already receiving a drug metabolized by CYP2D6, the need for decreased dose of the original medication should be considered. Drugs with a narrow therapeutic index represent the greatest concern (e.g., flecainide, propafenone, vinblastine, and TCAs). Due to the risk of serious ventricular arrhythmias and sudden death potentially associated with elevated plasma levels of thioridazine, thioridazine should not be administered with fluoxetine or within a minimum of 5 weeks after fluoxetine has been discontinued *[see Contraindications (4)]*.

Tricyclic Antidepressants (TCAs)—In 2 studies, previously stable plasma levels of imipramine and desipramine have increased greater than 2- to 10-fold when fluoxetine has been administered in combination. This influence may persist for 3 weeks or longer after fluoxetine is discontinued. Thus, the dose of TCAs may need to be reduced and plasma TCA concentrations may need to be monitored temporarily when fluoxetine is coadministered or has been recently discontinued *[see Clinical Pharmacology (12.3)]*.

Benzodiazapines—The half-life of concurrently administered diazepam may be prolonged in some patients *[see Clinical Pharmacology (12.3)]*. Coadministration of alprazolam and fluoxetine has resulted in increased alprazolam plasma concentrations and in further psychomotor performance decrement due to increased alprazolam levels.

Antipsychotics—Some clinical data suggests a possible pharmacodynamic and/or pharmacokinetic interaction between SSRIs and antipsychotics. Elevation of blood levels of haloperidol and clozapine has been observed in patients receiving concomitant fluoxetine *[see Contraindications (4)]*.

Anticonvulsants—Patients on stable doses of phenytoin and carbamazepine have developed elevated plasma anticonvulsant concentrations and clinical anticonvulsant toxicity following initiation of concomitant fluoxetine treatment.

Lithium—There have been reports of both increased and decreased lithium levels when lithium was used concomitantly with fluoxetine. Cases of lithium toxicity and increased serotonergic effects have been reported. Lithium levels should be monitored when these drugs are administered concomitantly.

Drugs Tightly Bound to Plasma Proteins—Because fluoxetine is tightly bound to plasma protein, the administration of fluoxetine to a patient taking another drug that is tightly bound to protein (e.g., Coumadin, digitoxin) may cause a shift in plasma concentrations potentially resulting in an adverse effect *[see Clinical Pharmacology (12.3)]*.

Drugs Metabolized by CYP3A4—In an in vivo interaction study involving coadministration of fluoxetine with single doses of terfenadine (a CYP3A4 substrate), no increase in plasma terfenadine concentrations occurred with concomitant fluoxetine.

Additionally, in vitro studies have shown ketoconazole, a potent inhibitor of CYP3A4 activity, to be at least 100 times more potent than fluoxetine or norfluoxetine as an inhibitor of the metabolism of several substrates for this enzyme, including astemizole, cisapride, and midazolam. These data indicate that fluoxetine's extent of inhibition of CYP3A4 activity is not likely to be of clinical significance.

Olanzapine—Fluoxetine (60 mg single dose or 60 mg daily dose for 8 days) causes a small (mean 16%) increase in the maximum concentration of olanzapine and a small (mean 16%) decrease in olanzapine clearance. The magnitude of the impact of this factor is small in comparison to the overall variability between individuals, and therefore dose modification is not routinely recommended.

When using PROZAC and olanzapine and in combination, also refer to the Drug Interactions section of the package insert for Symbyax.

8 USE IN SPECIFIC POPULATIONS

When using PROZAC and olanzapine in combination, also refer to the Use in Specific Populations section of the package insert for Symbyax.

8.1 Pregnancy

Pregnancy Category C—PROZAC should be used during pregnancy only if the potential benefit justifies the potential risk to the fetus. All pregnancies have a background risk of birth defects, loss, or other adverse outcome regardless of drug exposure.

Treatment of Pregnant Women During the First Trimester—There are no adequate and well-controlled clinical studies on the use of fluoxetine in pregnant women. Results of a number of epidemiological studies assessing the risk of fluoxetine exposure in early pregnancy have been inconsistent and have not provided conclusive evidence of an increased risk of congenital malformations. However, one meta-analysis suggests a potential risk of cardiovascular defects in infants of women exposed to fluoxetine during the first trimester of pregnancy compared to infants of women who were not exposed to fluoxetine.

Treatment of Pregnant Women During the Third Trimester—Neonates exposed to PROZAC, SNRIs, or SSRIs late in the third trimester have developed complications requiring prolonged hospitalization, respiratory support, and tube feeding. Such complications can arise immediately upon delivery. Reported clinical findings have included respiratory distress, cyanosis, apnea, seizures, temperature instability, feeding difficulty, vomiting, hypoglycemia, hypotonia, hypertonia, hyperreflexia, tremor, jitteriness, irritability, and constant crying. These features are consistent with either a direct toxic effect of SNRIs and SSRIs or, possibly, a drug discontinuation syndrome. It should be noted that, in some cases, the clinical picture is consistent with serotonin syndrome.

Infants exposed to SSRIs in late pregnancy may have an increased risk for persistent pulmonary hypertension of the newborn (PPHN). PPHN occurs in 1 to 2 per 1000 live births in the general population and is associated with substantial neonatal morbidity and mortality. In a retrospective case-control study of 377 women whose infants were born with PPHN and 836 women whose infants were born healthy, the risk for developing PPHN was approximately six-fold higher for infants exposed to SSRIs after the 20th week of gestation compared to infants who had not been exposed to antidepressants during pregnancy. There is currently no corroborative evidence regarding the risk for PPHN following exposure to SSRIs in pregnancy; this is the first study that has investigated the potential risk. The study did not include enough cases with exposure to individual SSRIs to determine if all SSRIs posed similar levels of PPHN risk.

Clinical Considerations—When treating pregnant women with PROZAC, the physician should carefully consider both the potential risks and potential benefits of treatment, taking into account the risk of untreated depression during pregnancy. Physicians should note that in a prospective longitudinal study of 201 women with a history of major depression who were euthymic at the beginning of pregnancy, women who discontinued antidepressant medication during pregnancy were more likely to experience a relapse of major depression than women who continued antidepressant medication.

The physician may consider tapering PROZAC in the third trimester *[see Dosage and Administration (2.7)]*.

Animal Data—In embryo-fetal development studies in rats and rabbits, there was no evidence of teratogenicity following administration of fluoxetine at doses up to 12.5 and 15 mg/kg/day, respectively (1.5 and 3.6 times, respectively, the maximum recommended human dose (MRHD) of 80 mg on a mg/m^2 basis) throughout organogenesis. However, in rat reproduction studies, an increase in stillborn pups, a decrease in pup weight, and an increase in pup deaths during the first 7 days postpartum occurred following maternal exposure to 12 mg/kg/day (1.5 times MRHD on a mg/m^2 basis) during gestation or 7.5 mg/kg/day (0.9 times the MRHD on a mg/m^2 basis) during gestation and lactation. There was no evidence of developmental neurotoxicity in the surviving offspring of rats treated with 12 mg/kg/day during gestation. The no-effect dose for rat pup mortality was 5 mg/kg/day (0.6 times the MRHD on a mg/m^2 basis).

8.2 Labor and Delivery

The effect of PROZAC on labor and delivery in humans is unknown. However, because fluoxetine crosses the placenta and because of the possibility that fluoxetine may have adverse effects on the newborn, fluoxetine should be used during labor and delivery only if the potential benefit justifies the potential risk to the fetus.

8.3 Nursing Mothers

Because PROZAC is excreted in human milk, nursing while on PROZAC is not recommended. In one breast-milk sample, the concentration of fluoxetine plus norfluoxetine was 70.4 ng/mL. The concentration in the mother's plasma was 295.0 ng/mL. No adverse effects on the infant were reported. In another case, an infant nursed by a mother on PROZAC developed crying, sleep disturbance, vomiting, and watery stools. The infant's plasma drug levels were 340 ng/mL of fluoxetine and 208 ng/mL of norfluoxetine on the second day of feeding.

8.4 Pediatric Use

The efficacy of PROZAC for the treatment of Major Depressive Disorder was demonstrated in two 8- to 9-week placebo-controlled clinical trials with 315 pediatric outpatients ages 8 to ≤18 *[see Clinical Studies (14.1)]*.

The efficacy of PROZAC for the treatment of OCD was demonstrated in one 13-week placebo-controlled clinical trial with 103 pediatric outpatients ages 7 to <18 *[see Clinical Studies (14.2)]*.

The safety and effectiveness in pediatric patients <8 years of age in Major Depressive Disorder and <7 years of age in OCD have not been established.

Fluoxetine pharmacokinetics were evaluated in 21 pediatric patients (ages 6 to ≤18) with Major Depressive Disorder or OCD *[see Clinical Pharmacology (12.3)]*.

The acute adverse reaction profiles observed in the 3 studies (N=418 randomized; 228 fluoxetine-treated, 190 placebo-treated) were generally similar to that observed in adult studies with fluoxetine. The longer-term adverse reaction profile observed in the 19-week Major Depressive Disorder study (N=219 randomized; 109 fluoxetine-treated, 110 placebo-treated) was also similar to that observed in adult trials with fluoxetine *[see Adverse Reactions (6.1)]*.

Manic reaction, including mania and hypomania, was reported in 6 (1 mania, 5 hypomania) out of 228 (2.6%) fluoxetine-treated patients and in 0 out of 190 (0%) placebo-treated patients. Mania/hypomania led to the discontinuation of 4 (1.8%) fluoxetine-treated patients from the acute phases of the 3 studies combined. Consequently, regular monitoring for the occurrence of mania/hypomania is recommended.

As with other SSRIs, decreased weight gain has been observed in association with the use of fluoxetine in children and adolescent patients. After 19 weeks of treatment in a clinical trial, pediatric subjects treated with fluoxetine gained an average of 1.1 cm less in height and 1.1 kg less in weight than subjects treated with placebo. In addition, fluoxetine treatment was associated with a decrease in alkaline phosphatase levels. The safety of fluoxetine treatment for pediatric patients has not been systematically assessed for chronic treatment longer than several months in duration. In particular, there are no studies that directly evaluate the longer-term effects of fluoxetine on the growth, development and maturation of children and adolescent patients. Therefore, height and weight should be monitored periodically in pediatric patients receiving fluoxetine *[see Warnings and Precautions (5.6)]*.

PROZAC is approved for use in pediatric patients with MDD and OCD *[see Box Warning and Warnings and Precautions (5.1)]*. Anyone considering the use of PROZAC in a child or adolescent must balance the potential risks with the clinical need.

Significant toxicity, including myotoxicity, long-term neurobehavioral and reproductive toxicity, and impaired bone development, has been observed following exposure of juvenile animals to fluoxetine. Some of these effects occurred at clinically relevant exposures.

In a study in which fluoxetine (3, 10, or 30 mg/kg) was orally administered to young rats from weaning (Postnatal Day 21) through adulthood (Day 90), male and female sexual development was delayed at all doses, and growth (body weight gain, femur length) was decreased during the dosing period in animals receiving the highest dose. At the end of the treatment period, serum levels of creatine kinase (marker of muscle damage) were increased at the intermediate and high doses, and abnormal muscle and reproductive organ histopathology (skeletal muscle degeneration and necrosis, testicular degeneration and necrosis, epididymal vacuolation and hypospermia) was observed at the high dose. When animals were evaluated after a recovery period (up to 11 weeks after cessation of dosing), neurobehavioral abnormalities (decreased reactivity at all doses and learning deficit at the high dose) and reproductive functional impairment (decreased mating at all doses and impaired fertility at the high dose) were seen; in addition, testicular and epididymal microscopic lesions and decreased sperm concentrations were found in the high dose group, indicating that the reproductive organ effects seen at the end of treatment were irreversible. The reversibility of fluoxetine-induced muscle damage was not assessed. Adverse effects similar to those observed in rats treated with fluoxetine during the juvenile period have not been reported after administration of fluoxetine to adult animals. Plasma exposures (AUC) to fluoxetine in juvenile rats receiving the low, intermediate, and high dose in this study were approximately 0.1-0.2, 1-2, and 5-10 times, respectively, the average exposure in pediatric patients receiving the maximum recommended dose (MRD) of 20 mg/day. Rat exposures to the major metabolite, norfluoxetine, were approximately 0.3-0.8, 1-8, and 3-20 times, respectively, pediatric exposure at the MRD.

A specific effect of fluoxetine on bone development has been reported in mice treated with fluoxetine during the juvenile period. When mice were treated with fluoxetine (5 or 20 mg/kg, intraperitoneal) for 4 weeks starting at 4 weeks of age, bone formation was reduced resulting in decreased bone mineral content and density. These doses did not affect overall growth (body weight gain or femoral length). The doses administered to juvenile mice in this study are approximately 0.5 and 2 times the MRD for pediatric patients on a body surface area (mg/m^2) basis.

In another mouse study, administration of fluoxetine (10 mg/kg intraperitoneal) during early postnatal development (Postnatal Days 4 to 21) produced abnormal emotional behaviors (decreased exploratory behavior in elevated plus-maze, increase shock avoidance latency) in adulthood (12 weeks of age). The dose used in this study is approximately equal to the pediatric MRD on a mg/m^2 basis. Because of the early dosing period in this study, the significance of these findings to the approved pediatric use in humans is uncertain.

Safety and effectiveness of PROZAC and olanzapine in combination in patients less than 18 years of age have not been established.

8.5 Geriatric Use

US fluoxetine clinical trials included 687 patients ≥65 years of age and 93 patients ≥75 years of age. The efficacy in geriatric patients has been established *[see Clinical Studies (14.1)]*. For pharmacokinetic information in geriatric patients, *[see Clinical Pharmacology (12.4)]*. No overall differences in safety or effectiveness were observed between these subjects and younger subjects, and other reported clinical experience has not identified differences in responses between the elderly and younger patients, but greater sensitivity of some older individuals cannot be ruled out. SNRIs and SSRIs, including fluoxetine, have been associated with cases of clinically significant hyponatremia in elderly patients, who may be at greater risk for this adverse reaction *[see Warnings and Precautions (5.8)]*.

Clinical studies of olanzapine and fluoxetine in combination did not include sufficient numbers of patients ≥65 years of age to determine whether they respond differently from younger patients.

8.6 Hepatic Impairment

In subjects with cirrhosis of the liver, the clearances of fluoxetine and its active metabolite, norfluoxetine, were decreased, thus increasing the elimination half-lives of these substances. A lower or less frequent dose of fluoxetine should be used in patients with cirrhosis. Caution is advised when using PROZAC in patients with diseases or conditions that could affect its metabolism *[see Dosage and Administration (2.7) and Clinical Pharmacology (12.4)]*.

9 DRUG ABUSE AND DEPENDENCE

9.3 Dependence

PROZAC has not been systematically studied, in animals or humans, for its potential for abuse, tolerance, or physical dependence. While the premarketing clinical experience with PROZAC did not reveal any tendency for a withdrawal syndrome or any drug seeking behavior, these observations were not systematic and it is not possible to predict on the basis of this limited experience the extent to which a CNS active drug will be misused, diverted, and/or abused once marketed. Consequently, physicians should carefully evaluate patients for history of drug abuse and follow such patients closely, observing them for signs of misuse or abuse of PROZAC (e.g., development of tolerance, incrementation of dose, drug-seeking behavior).

10 OVERDOSAGE

10.1 Human Experience

Worldwide exposure to fluoxetine hydrochloride is estimated to be over 38 million patients (circa 1999). Of the 1578 cases of overdose involving fluoxetine hydrochloride, alone or with other drugs, reported from this population, there were 195 deaths.

Among 633 adult patients who overdosed on fluoxetine hydrochloride alone, 34 resulted in a fatal outcome, 378 completely recovered, and 15 patients experienced sequelae after overdosage, including abnormal accommodation, abnormal gait, confusion, unresponsiveness, nervousness, pulmonary dysfunction, vertigo, tremor, elevated blood pressure, impotence, movement disorder, and hypomania. The remaining 206 patients had an unknown outcome. The most common signs and symptoms associated with non-fatal overdosage were seizures, somnolence, nausea, tachycardia, and vomiting. The largest known ingestion of fluoxetine hydrochloride in adult patients was 8 grams in a patient who took fluoxetine alone and who subsequently recovered. However, in an adult patient who took fluoxetine alone, an ingestion as low as 520 mg has been associated with lethal outcome, but causality has not been established.

Among pediatric patients (ages 3 months to 17 years), there were 156 cases of overdose involving fluoxetine alone or in combination with other drugs. Six patients died, 127 patients completely recovered, 1 patient experienced renal failure, and 22 patients had an unknown outcome. One of the six fatalities was a 9-year-old boy who had a history of OCD, Tourette's syndrome with tics, attention deficit disorder, and fetal alcohol syndrome. He had been receiving 100 mg of fluoxetine daily for 6 months in addition to clonidine, methylphenidate, and promethazine. Mixed-drug ingestion or other methods of suicide complicated all 6 overdoses in children that resulted in fatalities. The largest ingestion in pediatric patients was 3 grams which was nonlethal.

Other important adverse reactions reported with fluoxetine overdose (single or multiple drugs) include coma, delirium, ECG abnormalities (such as QT interval prolongation and ventricular tachycardia, including torsades de pointes-type arrhythmias), hypotension, mania, neuroleptic malignant syndrome-like reactions, pyrexia, stupor, and syncope.

10.2 Animal Experience

Studies in animals do not provide precise or necessarily valid information about the treatment of human overdose. However, animal experiments can provide useful insights into possible treatment strategies.

The oral median lethal dose in rats and mice was found to be 452 and 248 mg/kg, respectively. Acute high oral doses produced hyperirritability and convulsions in several animal species.

Among 6 dogs purposely overdosed with oral fluoxetine, 5 experienced grand mal seizures. Seizures stopped immediately upon the bolus intravenous administration of a standard veterinary dose of diazepam. In this short-term study, the lowest plasma concentration at which a seizure occurred was only twice the maximum plasma concentration seen in humans taking 80 mg/day, chronically.

In a separate single-dose study, the ECG of dogs given high doses did not reveal prolongation of the PR, QRS, or QT intervals. Tachycardia and an increase in blood pressure were observed. Consequently, the value of the ECG in predicting cardiac toxicity is unknown. Nonetheless, the ECG should ordinarily be monitored in cases of human overdose *[see Overdosage (10.3)]*.

10.3 Management of Overdose

Treatment should consist of those general measures employed in the management of overdosage with any drug effective in the treatment of Major Depressive Disorder.

Ensure an adequate airway, oxygenation, and ventilation. Monitor cardiac rhythm and vital signs. General supportive and symptomatic measures are also recommended. Induction of emesis is not recommended. Gastric lavage with a large-bore orogastric tube with appropriate airway protection, if needed, may be indicated if performed soon after ingestion, or in symptomatic patients.

Activated charcoal should be administered. Due to the large volume of distribution of this drug, forced diuresis, dialysis, hemoperfusion, and exchange transfusion are unlikely to be of benefit. No specific antidotes for fluoxetine are known.

A specific caution involves patients who are taking or have recently taken fluoxetine and might ingest excessive quantities of a TCA. In such a case, accumulation of the parent tricyclic and/or an active metabolite may increase the possibility of clinically significant sequelae and extend the time needed for close medical observation *[see Drug Interactions (7.9)]*.

Based on experience in animals, which may not be relevant to humans, fluoxetine-induced seizures that fail to remit spontaneously may respond to diazepam.

In managing overdosage, consider the possibility of multiple drug involvement. The physician should consider contacting a poison control center for additional information on the treatment of any overdose. Telephone numbers for certified poison control centers are listed in the *Physicians' Desk Reference (PDR)*.

For specific information about overdosage with olanzapine and fluoxetine in combination, refer to the Overdosage section of the Symbyax package insert.

11 DESCRIPTION

PROZAC® (fluoxetine capsules, USP) is a selective serotonin reuptake inhibitor for oral administration. It is also marketed for the treatment of premenstrual dysphoric disorder (Sarafem®, fluoxetine hydrochloride). It is designated (±)-N-methyl-3-phenyl-3-[(α,α,α-trifluoro-*p*-tolyl)oxy]propylamine hydrochloride and has the empirical formula of $C_{17}H_{18}F_3NO \bullet HCl$. Its molecular weight is 345.79. The structural formula is:

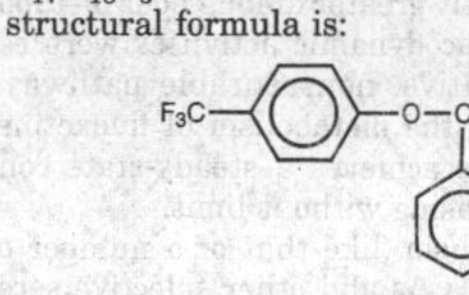

F3C
O—CHCH2CH2NHCH3
• HCl

Fluoxetine hydrochloride is a white to off-white crystalline solid with a solubility of 14 mg/mL in water.

Each Pulvule® contains fluoxetine hydrochloride equivalent to 10 mg (32.3 μmol), 20 mg (64.7 μmol), or 40 mg (129.3 μmol) of fluoxetine. The Pulvules also contain starch, gelatin, silicone, titanium dioxide, iron oxide, and other inactive ingredients. The 10 and 20 mg Pulvules also contain FD&C Blue No. 1, and the 40 mg Pulvule also contains FD&C Blue No. 1 and FD&C Yellow No. 6.

PROZAC Weekly™ capsules, a delayed-release formulation, contain enteric-coated pellets of fluoxetine hydrochloride equivalent to 90 mg (291 μmol) of fluoxetine. The capsules also contain D&C Yellow No. 10, FD&C Blue No. 2, gelatin, hypromellose, hypromellose acetate succinate, sodium lauryl sulfate, sucrose, sugar spheres, talc, titanium dioxide, triethyl citrate, and other inactive ingredients.

12 CLINICAL PHARMACOLOGY

12.1 Mechanism of Action

Although the exact mechanism of PROZAC is unknown, it is presumed to be linked to its inhibition of CNS neuronal uptake of serotonin.

12.2 Pharmacodynamics

Studies at clinically relevant doses in man have demonstrated that fluoxetine blocks the uptake of serotonin into human platelets. Studies in animals also suggest that fluoxetine is a much more potent uptake inhibitor of serotonin than of norepinephrine.

Antagonism of muscarinic, histaminergic, and α_1-adrenergic receptors has been hypothesized to be associated with various anticholinergic, sedative, and cardiovascular effects of classical tricyclic antidepressant (TCA) drugs. Fluoxetine binds to these and other membrane receptors from brain tissue much less potently in vitro than do the tricyclic drugs.

12.3 Pharmacokinetics

Systemic Bioavailability—In man, following a single oral 40 mg dose, peak plasma concentrations of fluoxetine from 15 to 55 ng/mL are observed after 6 to 8 hours.

The Pulvule and PROZAC Weekly capsule dosage forms of fluoxetine are bioequivalent. Food does not appear to affect the systemic bioavailability of fluoxetine, although it may delay its absorption by 1 to 2 hours, which is probably not clinically significant. Thus, fluoxetine may be administered with or without food. PROZAC Weekly capsules, a delayed-release formulation, contain enteric-coated pellets that resist dissolution until reaching a segment of the gastrointestinal tract where the pH exceeds 5.5. The enteric coating delays the onset of absorption of fluoxetine 1 to 2 hours relative to the immediate-release formulations.

Protein Binding—Over the concentration range from 200 to 1000 ng/mL, approximately 94.5% of fluoxetine is bound in vitro to human serum proteins, including albumin and α_1-glycoprotein. The interaction between fluoxetine and other highly protein-bound drugs has not been fully evaluated, but may be important.

Enantiomers—Fluoxetine is a racemic mixture (50/50) of *R*-fluoxetine and *S*-fluoxetine enantiomers. In animal models, both enantiomers are specific and potent serotonin uptake inhibitors with essentially equivalent pharmacologic activity. The *S*-fluoxetine enantiomer is eliminated more slowly and is the predominant enantiomer present in plasma at steady state.

Metabolism—Fluoxetine is extensively metabolized in the liver to norfluoxetine and a number of other unidentified metabolites. The only identified active metabolite, norfluoxetine, is formed by demethylation of fluoxetine. In animal models, *S*-norfluoxetine is a potent and selective inhibitor of serotonin uptake and has activity essentially equivalent to *R*- or *S*-fluoxetine. *R*-norfluoxetine is significantly less potent than the parent drug in the inhibition of serotonin uptake. The primary route of elimination appears to be hepatic metabolism to inactive metabolites excreted by the kidney.

Variability in Metabolism—A subset (about 7%) of the population has reduced activity of the drug metabolizing enzyme cytochrome P450 2D6 (CYP2D6). Such individuals are referred to as "poor metabolizers" of drugs such as debrisoquin, dextromethorphan, and the TCAs. In a study involving labeled and unlabeled enantiomers administered as a racemate, these individuals metabolized *S*-fluoxetine at a slower rate and thus achieved higher concentrations of *S*-fluoxetine. Consequently, concentrations of *S*-norfluoxetine at steady state were lower. The metabolism of *R*-fluoxetine in these poor metabolizers appears normal. When compared with normal metabolizers, the total sum at steady state of the plasma concentrations of the 4 active enantiomers was not significantly greater among poor metabolizers. Thus, the net pharmacodynamic activities were essentially the same. Alternative, nonsaturable pathways (non-2D6) also contribute to the metabolism of fluoxetine. This explains how fluoxetine achieves a steady-state concentration rather than increasing without limit.

Because fluoxetine's metabolism, like that of a number of other compounds including TCAs and other selective serotonin reuptake inhibitors (SSRIs), involves the CYP2D6 system, concomitant therapy with drugs also metabolized by this enzyme system (such as the TCAs) may lead to drug interactions *[see Drug Interactions (7.9)]*.

Accumulation and Slow Elimination—The relatively slow elimination of fluoxetine (elimination half-life of 1 to 3 days after acute administration and 4 to 6 days after chronic administration) and its active metabolite, norfluoxetine (elimination half-life of 4 to 16 days after acute and chronic administration), leads to significant accumulation of these active species in chronic use and delayed attainment of steady state, even when a fixed dose is used *[see Warnings and Precautions (5.12)]*. After 30 days of dosing at 40 mg/day, plasma concentrations of fluoxetine in the range of 91 to 302 ng/mL and norfluoxetine in the range of 72 to 258 ng/mL have been observed. Plasma concentrations of fluoxetine were higher than those predicted by single-dose studies, because fluoxetine's metabolism is not proportional to dose. Norfluoxetine, however, appears to have linear pharmacokinetics. Its mean terminal half-life after a single dose was 8.6 days and after multiple dosing was 9.3 days. Steady-state levels after prolonged dosing are similar to levels seen at 4 to 5 weeks.

The long elimination half-lives of fluoxetine and norfluoxetine assure that, even when dosing is stopped, active drug substance will persist in the body for weeks (primarily depending on individual patient characteristics, previous dosing regimen, and length of previous therapy at discontinuation). This is of potential consequence when drug discontinuation is required or when drugs are prescribed that might interact with fluoxetine and norfluoxetine following the discontinuation of PROZAC.

Weekly Dosing—Administration of PROZAC Weekly once weekly results in increased fluctuation between peak and trough concentrations of fluoxetine and norfluoxetine compared with once-daily dosing [for fluoxetine: 24% (daily) to 164% (weekly) and for norfluoxetine: 17% (daily) to 43% (weekly)]. Plasma concentrations may not necessarily be predictive of clinical response. Peak concentrations from once-weekly doses of PROZAC Weekly capsules of fluoxetine are in the range of the average concentration for 20 mg once-daily dosing. Average trough concentrations are 76% lower for fluoxetine and 47% lower for norfluoxetine than the concentrations maintained by 20 mg once-daily dosing. Average steady-state concentrations of either once-daily or once-weekly dosing are in relative proportion to the total dose administered. Average steady-state fluoxetine concentrations are approximately 50% lower following the once-weekly regimen compared with the once-daily regimen.

C_{max} for fluoxetine following the 90 mg dose was approximately 1.7-fold higher than the C_{max} value for the established 20 mg once-daily regimen following transition the next day to the once-weekly regimen. In contrast, when the first 90 mg once-weekly dose and the last 20 mg once-daily dose were separated by 1 week, C_{max} values were similar. Also, there was a transient increase in the average steady-state concentrations of fluoxetine observed following transition the next day to the once-weekly regimen. From a pharmacokinetic perspective, it may be better to separate the first 90 mg weekly dose and the last 20 mg once-daily dose by 1 week *[see Dosage and Administration (2.1)]*.

12.4 Specific Populations

Liver Disease—As might be predicted from its primary site of metabolism, liver impairment can affect the elimination of fluoxetine. The elimination half-life of fluoxetine was prolonged in a study of cirrhotic patients, with a mean of 7.6 days compared with the range of 2 to 3 days seen in subjects without liver disease; norfluoxetine elimination was also delayed, with a mean duration of 12 days for cirrhotic patients compared with the range of 7 to 9 days in normal subjects. This suggests that the use of fluoxetine in patients with liver disease must be approached with caution. If fluoxetine is administered to patients with liver disease, a lower or less frequent dose should be used *[see Dosage and Administration (2.7), Use in Specific Populations (8.6)]*.

Renal Disease—In depressed patients on dialysis (N=12), fluoxetine administered as 20 mg once daily for 2 months produced steady-state fluoxetine and norfluoxetine plasma concentrations comparable with those seen in patients with normal renal function. While the possibility exists that renally excreted metabolites of fluoxetine may accumulate to higher levels in patients with severe renal dysfunction, use of a lower or less frequent dose is not routinely necessary in renally impaired patients.

Geriatric Pharmacokinetics—The disposition of single doses of fluoxetine in healthy elderly subjects (>65 years of age) did not differ significantly from that in younger normal subjects. However, given the long half-life and nonlinear disposition of the drug, a single-dose study is not adequate to rule out the possibility of altered pharmacokinetics in the elderly, particularly if they have systemic illness or are receiving multiple drugs for concomitant diseases. The effects of age upon the metabolism of fluoxetine have been investigated in 260 elderly but otherwise healthy depressed patients (≥60 years of age) who received 20 mg fluoxetine for 6 weeks. Combined fluoxetine plus norfluoxetine plasma concentrations were 209.3 ± 85.7 ng/mL at the end of 6 weeks. No unusual age-associated pattern of adverse reactions was observed in those elderly patients.

Pediatric Pharmacokinetics (children and adolescents)—Fluoxetine pharmacokinetics were evaluated in 21 pediatric patients (10 children ages 6 to <13, 11 adolescents ages 13 to <18) diagnosed with Major Depressive Disorder or Obsessive Compulsive Disorder (OCD). Fluoxetine 20 mg/day was administered for up to 62 days. The average steady-state concentrations of fluoxetine in these children were 2-fold higher than in adolescents (171 and 86 ng/mL, respectively). The average norfluoxetine steady-state concentrations in these children were 1.5-fold higher than in adolescents (195 and 113 ng/mL, respectively). These differences can be almost entirely explained by differences in weight. No gender-associated difference in fluoxetine pharmacokinetics was observed. Similar ranges of fluoxetine and norfluoxetine plasma concentrations were observed in another study in 94 pediatric patients (ages 8 to <18) diagnosed with Major Depressive Disorder.

Higher average steady-state fluoxetine and norfluoxetine concentrations were observed in children relative to adults; however, these concentrations were within the range of concentrations observed in the adult population. As in adults, fluoxetine and norfluoxetine accumulated extensively following multiple oral dosing; steady-state concentrations were achieved within 3 to 4 weeks of daily dosing.

13 NONCLINICAL TOXICOLOGY

13.1 Carcinogenesis, Mutagenesis, Impairment of Fertility

Carcinogenicity—The dietary administration of fluoxetine to rats and mice for 2 years at doses of up to 10 and 12 mg/kg/day, respectively [approximately 1.2 and 0.7 times, respectively, the maximum recommended human dose (MRHD) of 80 mg on a mg/m^2 basis], produced no evidence of carcinogenicity.

Mutagenicity—Fluoxetine and norfluoxetine have been shown to have no genotoxic effects based on the following assays: bacterial mutation assay, DNA repair assay in cultured rat hepatocytes, mouse lymphoma assay, and in vivo sister chromatid exchange assay in Chinese hamster bone marrow cells.

Impairment of Fertility—Two fertility studies conducted in adult rats at doses of up to 7.5 and 12.5 mg/kg/day (approximately 0.9 and 1.5 times the MRHD on a mg/m^2 basis) indicated that fluoxetine had no adverse effects on fertility. However, adverse effects on fertility were seen when juvenile rats were treated with fluoxetine *[see Use in Specific Populations (8.4)]*.

13.2 Animal Toxicology and/or Pharmacology

Phospholipids are increased in some tissues of mice, rats, and dogs given fluoxetine chronically. This effect is reversible after cessation of fluoxetine treatment. Phospholipid accumulation in animals has been observed with many cationic amphiphilic drugs, including fenfluramine, imipramine, and ranitidine. The significance of this effect in humans is unknown.

14 CLINICAL STUDIES

When using PROZAC and olanzapine in combination, also refer to the Clinical Studies section of the package insert for Symbyax.

14.1 Major Depressive Disorder

Daily Dosing

Adult—The efficacy of PROZAC was studied in 5- and 6-week placebo-controlled trials with depressed adult and geriatric outpatients (≥18 years of age) whose diagnoses corresponded most closely to the DSM-III (currently DSM-IV) category of Major Depressive Disorder. PROZAC was shown to be significantly more effective than placebo as measured by the Hamilton Depression Rating Scale (HAM-D). PROZAC was also significantly more effective than placebo on the HAM-D subscores for depressed mood, sleep disturbance, and the anxiety subfactor.

Two 6-week controlled studies (N=671, randomized) comparing PROZAC 20 mg and placebo have shown PROZAC 20 mg daily to be effective in the treatment of elderly patients (≥60 years of age) with Major Depressive Disorder. In these studies, PROZAC produced a significantly higher rate of response and remission as defined, respectively, by a 50% decrease in the HAM-D score and a total endpoint HAM-D score of ≤8. PROZAC was well tolerated and the rate of treatment discontinuations due to adverse reactions did not differ between PROZAC (12%) and placebo (9%).

A study was conducted involving depressed outpatients who had responded (modified HAMD-17 score of ≤7 during each of the last 3 weeks of open-label treatment and absence of Major Depressive Disorder by DSM-III-R criteria) by the end of an initial 12-week open-treatment phase on PROZAC 20 mg/day. These patients (N=298) were randomized to continuation on double-blind PROZAC 20 mg/day or placebo. At 38 weeks (50 weeks total), a statistically significantly lower relapse rate (defined as symptoms sufficient to meet a diagnosis of Major Depressive Disorder for 2 weeks or a modified HAMD-17 score of ≥14 for 3 weeks) was observed for patients taking PROZAC compared with those on placebo.

Pediatric (children and adolescents)—The efficacy of PROZAC 20 mg/day in children and adolescents (N=315 randomized; 170 children ages 8 to <13, 145 adolescents ages 13 to ≤18) was studied in two 8- to 9-week placebo-controlled clinical trials in depressed outpatients whose diagnoses corresponded most closely to the DSM-III-R or DSM-IV category of Major Depressive Disorder.

In both studies independently, PROZAC produced a statistically significantly greater mean change on the Childhood Depression Rating Scale-Revised (CDRS-R) total score from baseline to endpoint than did placebo.

Subgroup analyses on the CDRS-R total score did not suggest any differential responsiveness on the basis of age or gender.

Weekly dosing for Maintenance / Continuation Treatment
A longer-term study was conducted involving adult outpatients meeting DSM-IV criteria for Major Depressive Disorder who had responded (defined as having a modified HAMD-17 score of ≤9, a CGI-Severity rating of ≤2, and no longer meeting criteria for Major Depressive Disorder) for 3 consecutive weeks at the end of 13 weeks of open-label treatment with PROZAC 20 mg once daily. These patients were randomized to double-blind, once-weekly continuation treatment with PROZAC Weekly, PROZAC 20 mg once daily, or placebo. PROZAC Weekly once weekly and PROZAC 20 mg once daily demonstrated superior efficacy (having a significantly longer time to relapse of depressive symptoms) compared with placebo for a period of 25 weeks. However, the equivalence of these 2 treatments during continuation therapy has not been established.

14.2 Obsessive Compulsive Disorder
Adult—The effectiveness of PROZAC for the treatment of Obsessive Compulsive Disorder (OCD) was demonstrated in two 13-week, multicenter, parallel group studies (Studies 1 and 2) of adult outpatients who received fixed PROZAC doses of 20, 40, or 60 mg/day (on a once-a-day schedule, in the morning) or placebo. Patients in both studies had moderate to severe OCD (DSM-III-R), with mean baseline ratings on the Yale-Brown Obsessive Compulsive Scale (YBOCS, total score) ranging from 22 to 26. In Study 1, patients receiving PROZAC experienced mean reductions of approximately 4 to 6 units on the YBOCS total score, compared with a 1-unit reduction for placebo patients. In Study 2, patients receiving PROZAC experienced mean reductions of approximately 4 to 9 units on the YBOCS total score, compared with a 1-unit reduction for placebo patients. While there was no indication of a dose-response relationship for effectiveness in Study 1, a dose-response relationship was observed in Study 2, with numerically better responses in the 2 higher dose groups. The following table provides the outcome classification by treatment group on the Clinical Global Impression (CGI) improvement scale for Studies 1 and 2 combined:

Table 6

Outcome Classification (%) on CGI Improvement Scale for Completers in Pool of Two OCD Studies

		PROZAC		
Outcome Classification	Placebo	20 mg	40 mg	60 mg
Worse	8%	0%	0%	0%
No change	64%	41%	33%	29%
Minimally improved	17%	23%	28%	24%
Much improved	8%	28%	27%	28%
Very much improved	3%	8%	12%	19%

Exploratory analyses for age and gender effects on outcome did not suggest any differential responsiveness on the basis of age or sex.
Pediatric (children and adolescents)—In one 13-week clinical trial in pediatric patients (N=103 randomized; 75 children ages 7 to <13, 28 adolescents ages 13 to <18) with OCD (DSM-IV), patients received PROZAC 10 mg/day for 2 weeks, followed by 20 mg/day for 2 weeks. The dose was then adjusted in the range of 20 to 60 mg/day on the basis of clinical response and tolerability. PROZAC produced a statistically significantly greater mean change from baseline to endpoint than did placebo as measured by the Children's Yale-Brown Obsessive Compulsive Scale (CY-BOCS).
Subgroup analyses on outcome did not suggest any differential responsiveness on the basis of age or gender.

14.3 Bulimia Nervosa
The effectiveness of PROZAC for the treatment of bulimia was demonstrated in two 8-week and one 16-week, multicenter, parallel group studies of adult outpatients meeting DSM-III-R criteria for bulimia. Patients in the 8-week studies received either 20 or 60 mg/day of PROZAC or placebo in the morning. Patients in the 16-week study received a fixed PROZAC dose of 60 mg/day (once a day) or placebo. Patients in these 3 studies had moderate to severe bulimia with median binge-eating and vomiting frequencies ranging from 7 to 10 per week and 5 to 9 per week, respectively. In these 3 studies, PROZAC 60 mg, but not 20 mg, was statistically significantly superior to placebo in reducing the number of binge-eating and vomiting episodes per week. The statistically significantly superior effect of 60 mg versus placebo was present as early as Week 1 and persisted throughout each study. The PROZAC-related reduction in bulimic episodes appeared to be independent of baseline depression as assessed by the Hamilton Depression Rating Scale. In each of these 3 studies, the treatment effect, as measured by differences between PROZAC 60 mg and placebo on median reduction from baseline in frequency of bulimic behaviors at endpoint, ranged from 1 to 2 episodes per week for binge-eating and 2 to 4 episodes per week for vomiting. The size of the effect was related to baseline frequency, with greater reductions seen in patients with higher baseline frequencies. Although some patients achieved freedom from binge-eating and purging as a result of treatment, for the majority, the benefit was a partial reduction in the frequency of binge-eating and purging.
In a longer-term trial, 150 patients meeting DSM-IV criteria for Bulimia Nervosa, purging subtype, who had responded during a single-blind, 8-week acute treatment phase with PROZAC 60 mg/day, were randomized to continuation of PROZAC 60 mg/day or placebo, for up to 52 weeks of observation for relapse. Response during the single-blind phase was defined by having achieved at least a 50% decrease in vomiting frequency compared with baseline. Relapse during the double-blind phase was defined as a persistent return to baseline vomiting frequency or physician judgment that the patient had relapsed. Patients receiving continued PROZAC 60 mg/day experienced a significantly longer time to relapse over the subsequent 52 weeks compared with those receiving placebo.

14.4 Panic Disorder
The effectiveness of PROZAC in the treatment of Panic Disorder was demonstrated in 2 double-blind, randomized, placebo-controlled, multicenter studies of adult outpatients who had a primary diagnosis of Panic Disorder (DSM-IV), with or without agoraphobia.
Study 1 (N=180 randomized) was a 12-week flexible-dose study. PROZAC was initiated at 10 mg/day for the first week, after which patients were dosed in the range of 20 to 60 mg/day on the basis of clinical response and tolerability. A statistically significantly greater percentage of PROZAC-treated patients were free from panic attacks at endpoint than placebo-treated patients, 42% versus 28%, respectively.
Study 2 (N=214 randomized) was a 12-week flexible-dose study. PROZAC was initiated at 10 mg/day for the first week, after which patients were dosed in a range of 20 to 60 mg/day on the basis of clinical response and tolerability. A statistically significantly greater percentage of PROZAC-treated patients were free from panic attacks at endpoint than placebo-treated patients, 62% versus 44%, respectively.

16 HOW SUPPLIED/STORAGE AND HANDLING

16.1 How Supplied
The following products are manufactured by Eli Lilly and Company for Dista Products Company:
Pulvule are available in 10mg, 20mg and 40mg capsule strengths and packages as follows:

	Pulvule Strength		
	10 mg[1]	20 mg[1]	40 mg[1]
Pulvule No.[2]	PU3104	PU3105	PU3107
Cap Color	Opaque green	Opaque green	Opaque green
Body Color	Opaque green	Opaque yellow	Opaque orange
Identification	DISTA 3104 Prozac 10 mg	DISTA 3105 Prozac 20 mg	DISTA 3107 Prozac 40 mg
NDC Codes:			
Bottles of 30		0777-3105-30	0777-3107-30
Bottles 100	0777-3104-02	0777-3105-02	
Bottles of 2000		0777-3105-07	

The following product is manufactured and distributed by Eli Lilly and Company:
PROZAC® Weekly™ Capsules are available in:
The 90 mg[1] capsule is an opaque green cap and clear body containing discretely visible white pellets through the clear body of the capsule, imprinted with Lilly on the cap and 3004 and 90 mg on the body.
• NDC 0002-3004-75 (PU3004) – Blister package of 4

[1] Fluoxetine base equivalent.
[2] Protect from light.

16.2 Storage and Handling
Store at Controlled Room Temperature, 15° to 30°C (59° to 86°F).

17 PATIENT COUNSELING INFORMATION

See the FDA-approved Medication Guide.
Patients should be advised of the following issues and asked to alert their prescriber if these occur while taking PROZAC as monotherapy or in combination with olanzapine. When using PROZAC and olanzapine in combination, also refer to the Patient Counseling Information section of the package insert for Symbyax.

17.1 General Information
Healthcare providers should instruct their patients to read the Medication Guide before starting therapy with PROZAC and to reread it each time the prescription is renewed.
Healthcare providers should inform patients, their families, and their caregivers about the benefits and risks associated with treatment with PROZAC and should counsel them in its appropriate use. Healthcare providers should instruct patients, their families, and their caregivers to read the Medication Guide and should assist them in understanding its contents. Patients should be given the opportunity to discuss the contents of the Medication Guide and to obtain answers to any questions they may have.
Patients should be advised of the following issues and asked to alert their healthcare provider if these occur while taking PROZAC.
When using PROZAC and olanzapine in combination, also refer to the Medication Guide for Symbyax.

17.2 Clinical Worsening and Suicide Risk
Patients, their families, and their caregivers should be encouraged to be alert to the emergence of anxiety, agitation, panic attacks, insomnia, irritability, hostility, aggressiveness, impulsivity, akathisia (psychomotor restlessness), hypomania, mania, other unusual changes in behavior, worsening of depression, and suicidal ideation, especially early during antidepressant treatment and when the dose is adjusted up or down. Families and caregivers of patients should be advised to look for the emergence of such symptoms on a day-to-day basis, since changes may be abrupt. Such symptoms should be reported to the patient's prescriber or health professional, especially if they are severe, abrupt in onset, or were not part of the patient's presenting symptoms. Symptoms such as these may be associated with an increased risk for suicidal thinking and behavior and indicate a need for very close monitoring and possibly changes in the medication *[see Box Warning and Warnings and Precautions (5.1)]*.

17.3 Serotonin Syndrome or Neuroleptic Malignant Syndrome (NMS)-like Reactions
Patients should be cautioned about the risk of serotonin syndrome or NMS-like reactions with the concomitant use of PROZAC and triptans, tramadol, or other serotonergic agents *[see Warnings and Precautions (5.2) and Drug Interactions (7.3)]*.
Patients should be advised of the signs and symptoms associated with serotonin syndrome or NMS-like reactions that may include mental status changes (e.g., agitation, hallucinations, coma), autonomic instability (e.g., tachycardia, labile blood pressure, hyperthermia), neuromuscular aberrations (e.g., hyperreflexia, incoordination) and/or gastrointestinal symptoms (e.g., nausea, vomiting, diarrhea). Serotonin syndrome, in its most severe form can resemble neuroleptic malignant syndrome, in which the symptoms may include hyperthermia, muscle rigidity, autonomic instability with possible rapid fluctuation of vital signs, and mental status changes. Patients should be cautioned to seek medical care immediately if they experience these symptoms.

17.4 Allergic Reactions and Rash
Patients should be advised to notify their physician if they develop a rash or hives *[see Warnings and Precautions (5.3)]*. Patients should also be advised of the signs and symptoms associated with a severe allergic reaction, including swelling of the face, eyes, or mouth, or have trouble breathing. Patients should be cautioned to seek medical care immediately if they experience these symptoms.

17.5 Abnormal Bleeding
Patients should be cautioned about the concomitant use of fluoxetine and NSAIDs, aspirin, warfarin, or other drugs that affect coagulation since combined use of psychotropic drugs that interfere with serotonin reuptake and these agents have been associated with an increased risk of bleeding *[see Warnings and Precautions (5.7) and Drug Interactions (7.6)]*. Patients should be advised to call their doctor if they experience any increased or unusual bruising or bleeding while taking PROZAC.

17.6 Hyponatremia
Patients should be advised that hyponatremia has been reported as a result of treatment with SNRIs and SSRIs, including PROZAC. Signs and symptoms of hyponatremia include headache, difficulty concentrating, memory impair-

ment, confusion, weakness, and unsteadiness, which may lead to falls. More severe and/or acute cases have been associated with hallucination, syncope, seizure, coma, respiratory arrest, and death [see Warnings and Precautions (5.8)].

17.7 Potential for Cognitive and Motor Impairment

PROZAC may impair judgment, thinking, or motor skills. Patients should be advised to avoid driving a car or operating hazardous machinery until they are reasonably certain that their performance is not affected [see Warnings and Precautions (5.11)].

17.8 Use of Concomitant Medications

Patients should be advised to inform their physician if they are taking, or plan to take, any prescription medication, including Symbyax, Sarafem, or over-the-counter drugs, including herbal supplements or alcohol. Patients should also be advised to inform their physicians if they plan to discontinue any medications they are taking while on PROZAC.

17.9 Discontinuation of Treatment

Patients should be advised to take PROZAC exactly as prescribed, and to continue taking PROZAC as prescribed even after their symptoms improve. Patients should be advised that they should not alter their dosing regimen, or stop taking PROZAC without consulting their physician [see Warnings and Precautions (5.13)]. Patients should be advised to consult with their healthcare provider if their symptoms do not improve with PROZAC.

17.10 Use in Specific Populations

Pregnancy—Patients should be advised to notify their physician if they become pregnant or intend to become pregnant during therapy. Prozac should be used during pregnancy only if the potential benefit justifies the potential risk to the fetus [see Use in Specific Populations (8.1)].

Nursing Mothers—Patients should be advised to notify their physician if they intend to breast-feed an infant during therapy. Because PROZAC is excreted in human milk, nursing while taking PROZAC is not recommended [see Use in Specific Populations (8.3)].

Pediatric Use—PROZAC is approved for use in pediatric patients with MDD and OCD [see Box Warning and Warnings and Precautions (5.1)]. Limited evidence is available concerning the longer-term effects of fluoxetine on the development and maturation of children and adolescent patients. Height and weight should be monitored periodically in pediatric patients receiving fluoxetine. Safety and effectiveness of PROZAC and olanzapine in combination in patients less than 18 years of age have not been established [see Warnings and Precautions (5.6) and Use in Specific Populations (8.4)].

Literature revised October 29, 2009

Eli Lilly and Company, Indianapolis, IN 46285, USA

Copyright © 1987, 2009, Eli Lilly and Company. All rights reserved.

PV 7430 DPP

Medication Guide

PROZAC® (PRO-zac)
(fluoxetine hydrochloride)
Pulvule® and Weekly™ Capsule

Read the Medication Guide that comes with PROZAC before you start taking it and each time you get a refill. There may be new information. This Medication Guide does not take the place of talking to your doctor about your medical condition or treatment. Talk with your doctor or pharmacist if there is something you do not understand or you want to learn more about PROZAC.

What is the most important information I should know about PROZAC?

Antidepressant medicines, depression and other serious mental illnesses, and suicidal thoughts or actions:

Talk to your, or your family member's, healthcare provider about:

• all risks and benefits of treatment with antidepressant medicines
• all treatment choices for depression or other serious mental illness

1. **Antidepressant medicines may increase suicidal thoughts or actions in some children, teenagers, and young adults within the first few months of treatment.**
2. **Depression and other serious mental illnesses are the most important causes of suicidal thoughts and actions. Some people may have a particularly high risk of having suicidal thoughts or actions.** These include people who have (or have a family history of) bipolar illness (also called manic-depressive illness) or suicidal thoughts or actions.
3. **How can I watch for and try to prevent suicidal thoughts and actions in myself or a family member?**
   • Pay close attention to any changes, especially sudden changes, in mood, behaviors, thoughts, or feelings. This is very important when an antidepressant medicine is started or when the dose is changed.
   • Call the healthcare provider right away to report new or sudden changes in mood, behavior, thoughts, or feelings.
   • Keep all follow-up visits with the healthcare provider as scheduled. Call the healthcare provider between vis-

its as needed, especially if you have concerns about symptoms.

Call a healthcare provider right away if you or your family member has any of the following symptoms, especially if they are new, worse, or worry you:

• thoughts about suicide or dying
• attempts to commit suicide
• new or worse depression
• new or worse anxiety
• feeling very agitated or restless
• panic attacks
• trouble sleeping (insomnia)
• new or worse irritability
• acting aggressive, being angry, or violent
• acting on dangerous impulses
• an extreme increase in activity and talking (mania)
• or other unusual changes in behavior or mood

What else do I need to know about antidepressant medicines?

• **Never stop an antidepressant medicine without first talking to a healthcare provider.** Stopping an antidepressant medicine suddenly can cause other symptoms.
• **Antidepressants are medicines used to treat depression and other illnesses.** It is important to discuss all the risks of treating depression and also the risks of not treating it. Patients and their families or other caregivers should discuss all treatment choices with the healthcare provider, not just the use of antidepressants.
• **Antidepressant medicines have other side effects.** Talk to the healthcare provider about the side effects of the medicine prescribed for you or your family member.
• **Antidepressant medicines can interact with other medicines.** Know all of the medicines that you or your family member takes. Keep a list of all medicines to show the healthcare provider. Do not start new medicines without first checking with your healthcare provider.
• **Not all antidepressant medicines prescribed for children are FDA approved for use in children.** Talk to your child's healthcare provider for more information.

What is PROZAC?

PROZAC is a prescription medicine used:
• for short and long-term treatment of depression in adults and children over the age of 8.
• for short and long-term treatment of Obsessive Compulsive Disorder (OCD) in adults and children over the age of 7.
• for short and long-term treatment of Bulimia Nervosa in adults.
• for short-term treatment of Panic Disorder, with or without agoraphobia, in adults.
• with the medicine olanzapine (Zyprexa), for the short-term treatment of episodes of depression that happen with Bipolar I Disorder.
• with the medicine olanzapine (Zyprexa), for the short-term treatment of episodes of depression that do not respond to 2 other medicines, also called treatment resistant depression.

It is not known if PROZAC and olanzapine (Zyprexa) taken together is safe and works in children under 18 years of age. The symptoms of depression (Major Depressive Disorder, Bipolar I Disorder and Treatment Resistant Depression) include decreased mood, decreased interest, increased guilty feelings, decreased energy, decreased concentration, changes in appetite, and suicidal thoughts or behavior. With treatment, some of your symptoms of depression may improve.

OCD is an anxiety disorder and is characterized by recurrent, unwanted thoughts (obsessions) and/or repetitive behaviors (compulsions). With treatment, some of your symptoms of OCD may improve.

Panic Disorder is an anxiety disorder that includes panic attacks, which are sudden feelings of terror for no reason. You may also have physical symptoms, such as; fast heartbeat, chest pain, breathing difficulty, dizziness. With treatment, some of your symptoms of Panic Disorder may improve.

Bulimia Nervosa, involves periods of overeating followed by purging (e.g. vomiting, excessive laxative use). With treatment, some of your symptoms of Bulimia Nervosa may improve.

If you do not think you are getting better, call your doctor.

Who should not take PROZAC?

• Do not take PROZAC if you take a Monoamine Oxidase Inhibitor (MAOI) or if you stopped taking an MAOI in the last 2 weeks.
• Do not take an MAOI **within 5 weeks of stopping PROZAC.** People who take PROZAC close in time to an MAOI can have serious and life-threatening side effects, with symptoms including:
   • high fever
   • continued muscle spasms that you can not control
   • rigid muscles

   • changes in heart rate and blood pressure that happen fast
   • confusion
   • unconsciousness

Ask your doctor or pharmacist if you are not sure if your medicine is an MAOI.
• Do not take PROZAC if you take Mellaril® (thioridazine). Do not take Mellaril **within 5 weeks of stopping PROZAC. Mellaril can cause serious heart rhythm problems and you could die suddenly.**
• Do not take PROZAC if you take the antipsychotic medicine pimozide (Orap®).

What should I tell my doctor before taking PROZAC?

PROZAC may not be right for you. Before starting PROZAC, tell your doctor about all your medical conditions, including if you have or had any of the following:
• seizures (convulsions)
• bipolar disorder (mania)
• are pregnant or plan to become pregnant. It is not known if PROZAC will harm your unborn baby.
• are breast-feeding or plan to breast-feed. PROZAC can pass into your breast milk and may harm your baby. You should not breast-feed while taking PROZAC. Talk to your doctor about the best way to feed your baby if you take PROZAC.

Tell your doctor about all the medicines that you take, including prescription and non-prescription medicines, vitamins, and herbal supplements. PROZAC and some medicines may interact with each other and may not work as well, or cause possible serious side effects. Your doctor can tell you if it is safe to take PROZAC with your other medicines. Do not start or stop any medicine while taking PROZAC without talking to your doctor first.

If you take PROZAC, you should not take any other medicines that contain fluoxetine hydrochloride:
• Symbyax
• Sarafem
• Prozac Weekly

You could take too much medicine (overdose).

How should I take PROZAC?

• Take PROZAC exactly as prescribed. Your doctor may need to change (adjust) the dose of PROZAC until it is right for you.
• If you miss a dose of PROZAC, take the missed dose as soon as you remember. If it is almost time for the next dose, skip the missed dose and take your next dose at the regular time. Do not take two doses of PROZAC at the same time.
• **To prevent serious side effects, do not stop taking PROZAC suddenly. If you need to stop taking PROZAC, your doctor can tell you how to safely stop taking it.**
• **If you take too much PROZAC, call your doctor or poison control center right away, or get emergency treatment.**
• PROZAC can be taken with or without food.
• PROZAC is usually taken once a day or once weekly, depending on how your doctor prescribes your medicine.
• If you do not think you are getting better or have any concerns about your condition while taking PROZAC, call your doctor.

What should I avoid while taking PROZAC?

• PROZAC can cause sleepiness and may affect your ability to make decisions, think clearly, or react quickly. You should not drive, operate heavy machinery, or do other dangerous activities until you know how PROZAC affects you.

What are the possible side effects of PROZAC?

PROZAC may be associated with the following serious risks:
• **Serotonin Syndrome:** This is a condition that can be life threatening. Call your doctor right away if you become severely ill and have some or all of these symptoms:
   • agitation
   • hallucinations
   • problems with coordination
   • racing heart beat
   • over-active reflexes
   • fever
   • nausea, vomiting, and diarrhea
• **Severe allergic reactions:** Tell your doctor right away if you get red itchy welts (hives) or, a rash alone or with fever and joint pain, while taking PROZAC. Call your doctor right away if you become severely ill and have some or all of these symptoms:
   • swelling of your face, eyes, or mouth
   • trouble breathing
• **Abnormal bleeding:** Tell your doctor if you notice any increased or unusual bruising or bleeding while taking PROZAC, especially if you take one of these medicines:
   • the blood thinner warfarin (Coumadin, Jantoven)
   • a non-steroidal anti-inflammatory drug (NSAID)
   • aspirin
• **Mania:** You may have a high mood, become extremely irritable, have too much energy, feel pressure to keep talking, or have a decreased need for sleep.
• Seizures

- Loss of appetite
- **Low salt (sodium) levels in the blood (hyponatremia):** Call your doctor right away if you become severely ill and have some or all of these symptoms:
  - headache
  - feel weak
  - confusion
  - problems concentrating
  - memory problems
  - feel unsteady

Common possible side effects of PROZAC include: abnormal dreams, orgasm problems, decreased appetite, anxiety, weakness, diarrhea, dry mouth, indigestion, flu, difficulty maintaining an erection for sexual activity, trouble sleeping, decreased sex drive, feeling sick to your stomach, nervousness, sore throat, rash, watery nasal discharge, sleepiness, sweating, tremor (shakes), hot flashes, and yawn.

Tell your doctor about any side effect that bothers you or that does not go away.

These are not all the possible side effects with PROZAC. For more information, ask your doctor or pharmacist.

Call your doctor for medical advice about side effects. You may report side effects to FDA at 1-800-FDA-1088.

How should I store PROZAC?
- Store PROZAC at room temperature, between 59°F to 86°F (15°C to 30°C).
- Keep PROZAC away from light.

Keep PROZAC and all medicines out of the reach of children.

General information about PROZAC
Medicines are sometimes prescribed for purposes other than those listed in a Medication Guide. Do not use PROZAC for a condition for which it was not prescribed. Do not give PROZAC to other people, even if they have the same condition. It may harm them.

This Medication Guide summarizes the most important information about PROZAC. If you would like more information, talk with your doctor. You can ask your doctor or pharmacist for information about PROZAC that was written for healthcare professionals. For more information about PROZAC call 1-800-Lilly-Rx (1-800-545-5979) or visit www.prozac.com.

What are the Ingredients in PROZAC?
Active ingredients: fluoxetine hydrochloride
Inactive ingredients in pulvules: starch, gelatin, silicone, titanium dioxide, iron oxide, and other inactive ingredients. The 10 and 20 mg pulvules also contain FD&C Blue No. 1, and the 40 mg pulvules also contains FD&C Blue No. 1 and FD&C Yellow No. 6.
Inactive ingredients in PROZAC Weekly™ capsules: D&C Yellow No. 10, FD&C Blue No. 2, gelatin, hypromellose, hypromellose acetate succinate, sodium lauryl sulfate, sucrose, sugar spheres, talc, titanium oxide, triethyl citrate, and other inactive ingredients.

This Medication Guide has been approved by the U.S. Food and Drug Administration.
Medication Guide revised June 23, 2009
Eli Lilly and Company
Indianapolis, IN 46285, USA
www.prozac.com
Copyright © 2009, Eli Lilly and Company. All rights reserved.
PV 7101 AMP
Shown in Product Identification Guide, page 311

SEROMYCIN®
[cero-mi-cin]
(Cycloserine) Capsules, USP
℞

DESCRIPTION
Seromycin® (Cycloserine Capsules, USP), 3-isoxazolidinone, 4-amino-, (R)- is a broad-spectrum antibiotic that is produced by a strain of *Streptomyces orchidaceus* and has also been synthesized. Cycloserine is a white to off-white powder that is soluble in water and stable in alkaline solution. It is rapidly destroyed at a neutral or acid pH.

Cycloserine has a pH between 5.5 and 6.5 in a solution containing 100 mg/mL. The molecular weight of cycloserine is 102.09, and it has an empirical formula of $C_3H_6N_2O_2$. The structural formula of cycloserine is as follows:

Each capsule contains cycloserine, 250 mg (2.45 mmol); D&C Yellow No. 10, FD&C Blue No. 1, FD&C Red No. 3, FD&C Yellow No. 6, gelatin, iron oxide, talc, titanium dioxide, and other inactive ingredients.

CLINICAL PHARMACOLOGY
After oral administration, cycloserine is readily absorbed from the gastrointestinal tract, with peak blood levels occurring in 4 to 8 hours. Blood levels of 25 to 30 µg/mL can generally be maintained with the usual dosage of 250 mg twice a day, although the relationship of plasma levels to dosage is not always consistent. Concentrations in the cerebrospinal fluid, pleural fluid, fetal blood, and mother's milk approach those found in the serum. Detectable amounts are found in ascitic fluid, bile, sputum, amniotic fluid, and lung and lymph tissues. Approximately 65% of a single dose of cycloserine can be recovered in the urine within 72 hours after oral administration. The remaining 35% is apparently metabolized to unknown substances. The maximum excretion rate occurs 2 to 6 hours after administration, with 50% of the drug eliminated in 12 hours.

Microbiology
Cycloserine inhibits cell–wall synthesis in susceptible strains of gram–positive and gram–negative bacteria and in *Mycobacterium tuberculosis.*

Susceptibility Tests
Cycloserine clinical laboratory standard powder is available for both direct and indirect methods[1] of determining the susceptibility of strains of mycobacteria. Cycloserine MICs for susceptible strains are 25 µg/mL or lower.

INDICATIONS AND USAGE
Seromycin is indicated in the treatment of active pulmonary and extrapulmonary tuberculosis (including renal disease) when the causative organisms are susceptible to this drug and when treatment with the primary medications (streptomycin, isoniazid, rifampin, and ethambutol) has proved inadequate. Like all antituberculosis drugs, Seromycin should be administered in conjunction with other effective chemotherapy and not as the sole therapeutic agent.

Seromycin may be effective in the treatment of acute urinary tract infections caused by susceptible strains of gram–positive and gram–negative bacteria, especially *Enterobacter* spp. and *Escherichia coli.* It is generally no more and is usually less effective than other antimicrobial agents in the treatment of urinary tract infections caused by bacteria other than mycobacteria. Use of Seromycin in these infections should be considered only when more conventional therapy has failed and when the organism has been demonstrated to be susceptible to the drug.

CONTRAINDICATIONS
Administration is contraindicated in patients with any of the following:
  Hypersensitivity to cycloserine
  Epilepsy
  Depression, severe anxiety, or psychosis
  Severe renal insufficiency
  Excessive concurrent use of alcohol

WARNINGS
Administration of Seromycin should be discontinued or the dosage reduced if the patient develops allergic dermatitis or symptoms of CNS toxicity, such as convulsions, psychosis, somnolence, depression, confusion, hyperreflexia, headache, tremor, vertigo, paresis, or dysarthria.

The toxicity of Seromycin is closely related to excessive blood levels (above 30 µg/mL), as determined by high dosage or inadequate renal clearance. The ratio of toxic dose to effective dose in tuberculosis is small.

The risk of convulsions is increased in chronic alcoholics. Patients should be monitored by hematologic, renal excretion, blood level, and liver function studies.

PRECAUTIONS
General
Before treatment with Seromycin is initiated, cultures should be taken and the organism's susceptibility to the drug should be established. In tuberculous infections, the organism's susceptibility to the other antituberculosis agents in the regimen should also be demonstrated.

Anticonvulsant drugs or sedatives may be effective in controlling symptoms of CNS toxicity, such as convulsions, anxiety, and tremor. Patients receiving more than 500 mg of Seromycin daily should be closely observed for such symptoms. The value of pyridoxine in preventing CNS toxicity from Seromycin has not been proved.

Administration of Seromycin and other antituberculosis drugs has been associated in a few instances with vitamin B_{12} and/or folic–acid deficiency, megaloblastic anemia, and sideroblastic anemia. If evidence of anemia develops during treatment, appropriate studies and therapy should be instituted.

Laboratory Tests
Blood levels should be determined at least weekly for patients with reduced renal function, for individuals receiving a daily dosage of more than 500 mg, and for those showing signs and symptoms suggestive of toxicity. The dosage should be adjusted to keep the blood level below 30 µg/mL.

Drug Interactions
Concurrent administration of ethionamide has been reported to potentiate neurotoxic side effects.

Alcohol and Seromycin are incompatible, especially during a regimen calling for large doses of the latter. Alcohol increases the possibility and risk of epileptic episodes.

Concurrent administration of isoniazid may result in increased incidence of CNS effects, such as dizziness or drowsiness. Dosage adjustments may be necessary and patients should be monitored closely for signs of CNS toxicity.

Carcinogenesis, Mutagenicity, and Impairment of Fertility
Studies have not been performed to determine potential for carcinogenicity. The Ames test and unscheduled DNA repair test were negative. A study in 2 generations of rats showed no impairment of fertility relative to controls for the first mating but somewhat lower fertility in the second mating.

Pregnancy Category C
A study in 2 generations of rats given doses up to 100 mg/kg/day demonstrated no teratogenic effect in offspring. It is not known whether Seromycin can cause fetal harm when administered to a pregnant woman or can affect reproduction capacity. Seromycin should be given to a pregnant woman only if clearly needed.

Nursing Mothers
Because of the potential for serious adverse reactions in nursing infants from Seromycin, a decision should be made whether to discontinue nursing or to discontinue the drug, taking into account the importance of the drug to the mother.

Usage in Pediatric Patients
Safety and effectiveness in pediatric patients have not been established.

ADVERSE REACTIONS
Most adverse reactions occurring during therapy with Seromycin involve the nervous system or are manifestations of drug hypersensitivity. The following side effects have been observed in patients receiving Seromycin:

Nervous system symptoms (which appear to be related to higher dosages of the drug, i.e., more than 500 mg daily)
  Convulsions
  Drowsiness and somnolence
  Headache
  Tremor
  Dysarthria
  Vertigo
  Confusion and disorientation with loss of memory
  Psychoses, possibly with suicidal tendencies
  Character changes
  Hyperirritability
  Aggression
  Paresis
  Hyperreflexia
  Paresthesia
  Major and minor (localized) clonic seizures
  Coma

Cardiovascular
  Sudden development of congestive heart failure in patients receiving 1 to 1.5 g of Seromycin daily has been reported

Allergy (apparently not related to dosage)

Skin rash

Miscellaneous
  Elevated serum transaminase, especially in patients with preexisting liver disease

OVERDOSAGE
Signs and Symptoms
Acute toxicity from cycloserine can occur if more than 1 g is ingested by an adult. Chronic toxicity from cycloserine is dose related and can occur if more than 500 mg is administered daily. Patients with renal impairment will accumulate cycloserine and may develop toxicity if the dosing regimen is not modified. Patients with severe renal impairment should not receive the drug. The central nervous system is the most common organ system involved with toxicity. Toxic effects may include headache, vertigo, confusion, drowsiness, hyperirritability, paresthesias, dysarthria, and psychosis. Following larger ingestions, paresis, convulsions, and coma often occur. Ethyl alcohol may increase the risk of seizures in patients receiving cycloserine.

The oral median lethal dose in mice is 5290 mg/kg.

Treatment
To obtain up–to–date information about the treatment of overdose, a good resource is your certified Regional Poison Control Center. Telephone numbers of certified poison control centers are listed in the *Physicians' Desk Reference (PDR).* In managing overdosage, consider the possibility of multiple drug overdoses, interaction among drugs, and unusual drug kinetics in your patient.

Overdoses of cycloserine have been reported rarely. The following is provided to serve as a guide should such an overdose be encountered.

Protect the patient's airway and support ventilation and perfusion. Meticulously monitor and maintain, within acceptable limits, the patient's vital signs, blood gases, serum electrolytes, etc. Absorption of drugs from the gastrointestinal tract may be decreased by giving activated charcoal, which, in many cases, is more effective than emesis or lavage; consider charcoal instead of or in addition to gastric emptying. Repeated doses of charcoal over time may hasten elimination of some drugs that have been absorbed. Safeguard the patient's airway when employing gastric emptying or charcoal.

In adults, many of the neurotoxic effects of cycloserine can be both treated and prevented with the administration of 200 to 300 mg of pyridoxine daily.

The use of hemodialysis has been shown to remove cycloserine from the bloodstream. This procedure should be reserved for patients with life-threatening toxicity that is unresponsive to less invasive therapy.

DOSAGE AND ADMINISTRATION

Seromycin is effective orally and is currently administered only by this route. The usual dosage is 500 mg to 1 g daily in divided doses monitored by blood levels.[2] The initial adult dosage most frequently given is 250 mg twice daily at 12–hour intervals for the first 2 weeks. A daily dosage of 1 g should not be exceeded.

HOW SUPPLIED

Seromycin® is available as a 250 mg capsule with an opaque red cap and opaque gray body imprinted with "Lilly" and "F04" in edible black ink on both the cap and the body.
  Bottles of 40 (No.12) NDC 0002-0604-40
Store at controlled room temperature, 20° to 25°C (68° to 77°F) [see USP].

REFERENCES

1. Kubica GP, Dye WE: Laboratory methods for clinical and public health — mycobacteriology. US Department of Health, Education and Welfare, Public Health Service, 1967, pp 47–55, 66–70.
2. Jones LR: Colorimetric determination of cycloserine, a new antibiotic. *Anal Chem* 1956;28:39.
Literature revised April 28, 2005
Eli Lilly and Company
Indianapolis, IN 46285, USA

STRATTERA®   ℞

[strä-tĕr-ă]
(atomoxetine hydrochloride)
Capsules for Oral Use

HIGHLIGHTS OF PRESCRIBING INFORMATION
These highlights do not include all the information needed to use STRATTERA safely and effectively. See full prescribing information for STRATTERA.
STRATTERA® (atomoxetine hydrochloride) Capsules for Oral Use
Initial U.S. Approval: 2002

WARNING: SUICIDAL IDEATION IN CHILDREN AND ADOLESCENTS
See full prescribing information for complete boxed warning.
- **Increased risk of suicidal ideation in children or adolescents (5.1)**
- **No suicides occurred in clinical trials (5.1)**
- **Patients started on therapy should be monitored closely (5.1)**

————RECENT MAJOR CHANGES————
Warning and Precautions, Severe Liver Injury (5.2) 06/2009
  Warnings and Precautions, Effects on Blood
Pressure and Heart Rate (5.4)   09/2008
Boxed Warning   07/2008
Warnings and Precautions, Suicidal Ideation (5.1),
  Effects on Blood Pressure and Heart Rate (5.4),
  Effects on Urine Outflow from the Bladder (5.9) 07/2008
————INDICATIONS AND USAGE————
STRATTERA® is a selective norepinephrine reuptake inhibitor indicated for the treatment of Attention–Deficit/Hyperactivity Disorder (ADHD). (1.1)
————DOSAGE AND ADMINISTRATION————
Initial, Target and Maximum Daily Dose (2.1)
[See table below]
Dosing adjustment—Hepatic Impairment, Strong CYP2D6 Inhibitor, and in patients known to be CYP2D6 poor metabolizers (PMs). (2.4, 12.3)
————DOSAGE FORMS AND STRENGTHS————
Each capsule contains atomoxetine HCl equivalent to 10, 18, 25, 40, 60, 80, or 100 mg of atomoxetine. (3, 11, 16)
————CONTRAINDICATIONS————
- Hypersensitivity to atomoxetine or other constituents of product. (4.1)

- STRATTERA use within 2 weeks after discontinuing MAOI or other drugs that affect brain monoamine concentrations. (4.2, 7.1)
- Narrow Angle Glaucoma. (4.3)
————WARNINGS AND PRECAUTIONS————
- Suicidal Ideation—Monitor for suicidality, clinical worsening, and unusual changes in behavior. (5.1)
- Severe Liver Injury—Should be discontinued and not restarted in patients with jaundice or laboratory evidence of liver injury. (5.2)
- Serious Cardiovascular Events—Sudden death, stroke and myocardial infarction have been reported in association with atomoxetine treatment. Patients should have a careful history and physical exam to assess for presence of cardiovascular disease. STRATTERA generally should not be used in children or adolescents with known serious structural cardiac abnormalities, cardiomyopathy, serious heart rhythm abnormalities, or other serious cardiac problems that may place them at increased vulnerability to its noradrenergic effects. Consideration should be given to not using STRATTERA in adults with clinically significant cardiac abnormalities. (5.3)
- Emergent Cardiovascular Symptoms—Patients should undergo prompt cardiac evaluation. (5.3)
- Effects on Blood Pressure and Heart Rate—Can increase blood pressure and heart rate; orthostasis, syncope and Raynaud's phenomenon may occur. Use with caution in patients with hypertension, tachycardia, or cardiovascular or cerebrovascular disease. (5.4)
- Emergent Psychotic or Manic Symptoms—Consider discontinuing treatment if such new symptoms occur. (5.5)
- Bipolar Disorder—Screen patients to avoid possible induction of a mixed/manic episode. (5.6)
- Aggressive behavior or hostility should be monitored. (5.7)
- Possible allergic reactions, including angioneurotic edema, urticaria, and rash. (5.8)
- Effects on Urine Outflow—Urinary hesitancy and retention may occur. (5.9)
- Priapism—Prompt medical attention is required in the event of suspected priapism. (5.10, 17.5)
- Growth—Height and weight should be monitored in pediatric patients. (5.11)
- Concomitant Use of Potent CYP2D6 Inhibitors or Use in patients known to be CYP2D6 PMs—Dose adjustment of STRATTERA may be necessary. (5.13)
————ADVERSE REACTIONS————
Most common adverse reactions (≥5% and at least twice the incidence of placebo patients)
- Child and Adolescent Clinical Trials—Nausea, vomiting, fatigue, decreased appetite, abdominal pain, and somnolence. (6.1)
- Adult Clinical Trials—Constipation, dry mouth, nausea, fatigue, decreased appetite, insomnia, erectile dysfunction, urinary hesitation and/or urinary retention and/or dysuria, dysmenorrhea, and hot flush. (6.1)
To report SUSPECTED ADVERSE REACTIONS, contact Eli Lilly and Company at 1-800-LillyRx (1-800-545-5979) or FDA at 1-800-FDA-1088 or www.fda.gov/medwatch
————DRUG INTERACTIONS————
- Monoamine Oxidase Inhibitors. (4.2, 7.1)
- CYP2D6 Inhibitors—Concomitant use may increase atomoxetine steady–state plasma concentrations in EMs. (7.2)
- Pressor Agents—Possible effects on blood pressure. (7.3)
- Albuterol (or other beta₂ agonists)—Action of albuterol on cardiovascular system can be potentiated. (7.4)
————USE IN SPECIFIC POPULATIONS————
- Pregnancy/Lactation—Pregnant or nursing women should not use unless potential benefit justifies potential risk to fetus or infant. (8.1, 8.3)
- Hepatic Insufficiency—Increased exposure (AUC) to atomoxetine than with normal subjects in EM subjects with moderate (Child–Pugh Class B) (2-fold increase) and severe (Child–Pugh Class C) (4-fold increase). (8.6)
- Renal Insufficiency—Higher systemic exposure to atomoxetine than healthy subjects for EM subjects with end stage renal disease - no difference when exposure corrected for mg/kg dose. (8.7)
- Patients with Concomitant Illness—Does not worsen tics in patients with ADHD and comorbid Tourette's Disorder. (8.10)
- Patients with Concomitant Illness—Does not worsen anxiety in patients with ADHD and comorbid Anxiety Disorders. (8.10)
See 17 for PATIENT COUNSELING INFORMATION and Medication Guide

Revised: 11/2009

FULL PRESCRIBING INFORMATION: CONTENTS*
WARNING: SUICIDAL IDEATION IN CHILDREN AND ADOLESCENTS
* Sections or subsections omitted from the full prescribing information are not listed

Body Weight	Initial Daily Dose	Target Total Daily Dose	Maximum Total Daily Dose
Children and adolescents up to 70 kg	0.5 mg/kg	1.2 mg/kg	1.4 mg/kg
Children and adolescents over 70 kg and adults	40 mg	80 mg	100 mg

FULL PRESCRIBING INFORMATION

WARNING: SUICIDAL IDEATION IN CHILDREN AND ADOLESCENTS

STRATTERA (atomoxetine) increased the risk of suicidal ideation in short-term studies in children or adolescents with Attention-Deficit/Hyperactivity Disorder (ADHD). Anyone considering the use of STRATTERA in a child or adolescent must balance this risk with the clinical need. Co-morbidities occurring with ADHD may be associated with an increase in the risk of suicidal ideation and/or behavior. Patients who are started on therapy should be monitored closely for suicidality (suicidal thinking and behavior), clinical worsening, or unusual changes in behavior. Families and caregivers should be advised of the need for close observation and communication with the prescriber. STRATTERA is approved for ADHD in pediatric and adult patients. STRATTERA is not approved for major depressive disorder.

Pooled analyses of short-term (6 to 18 weeks) placebo-controlled trials of STRATTERA in children and adolescents (a total of 12 trials involving over 2200 patients, including 11 trials in ADHD and 1 trial in enuresis) have revealed a greater risk of suicidal ideation early during treatment in those receiving STRATTERA compared to placebo. The average risk of suicidal ideation in patients receiving STRATTERA was 0.4% (5/1357 patients), compared to none in placebo-treated patients (851 patients). No suicides occurred in these trials *[see Warnings and Precautions (5.1)]*.

1 INDICATIONS AND USAGE

1.1 Attention-Deficit/Hyperactivity Disorder (ADHD)

STRATTERA is indicated for the treatment of Attention-Deficit/Hyperactivity Disorder (ADHD).

The efficacy of STRATTERA Capsules was established in seven clinical trials in outpatients with ADHD: four 6 to 9-week trials in pediatric patients (ages 6 to 18), two 10-week trial in adults, and one maintenance trial in pediatrics (ages 6 to 15) *[see Clinical Studies (14)]*.

1.2 Diagnostic Considerations

A diagnosis of ADHD (DSM-IV) implies the presence of hyperactive-impulsive or inattentive symptoms that cause impairment and that were present before age 7 years. The symptoms must be persistent, must be more severe than is typically observed in individuals at a comparable level of development, must cause clinically significant impairment, e.g., in social, academic, or occupational functioning, and must be present in 2 or more settings, e.g., school (or work) and at home. The symptoms must not be better accounted for by another mental disorder.

The specific etiology of ADHD is unknown, and there is no single diagnostic test. Adequate diagnosis requires the use not only of medical but also of special psychological, educational, and social resources. Learning may or may not be impaired. The diagnosis must be based upon a complete history and evaluation of the patient and not solely on the presence of the required number of DSM-IV characteristics.

For the Inattentive Type, at least 6 of the following symptoms must have persisted for at least 6 months: lack of attention to details/careless mistakes, lack of sustained attention, poor listener, failure to follow through on tasks, poor organization, avoids tasks requiring sustained mental effort, loses things, easily distracted, forgetful. For the Hyperactive-Impulsive Type, at least 6 of the following symptoms must have persisted for at least 6 months: fidgeting/squirming, leaving seat, inappropriate running/climbing, difficulty with quiet activities, "on the go," excessive talking, blurting answers, can't wait turn, intrusive. For a Combined Type diagnosis, both inattentive and hyperactive-impulsive criteria must be met.

1.3 Need for Comprehensive Treatment Program

STRATTERA is indicated as an integral part of a total treatment program for ADHD that may include other measures (psychological, educational, social) for patients with this syndrome. Drug treatment may not be indicated for all patients with this syndrome. Drug treatment is not intended for use in the patient who exhibits symptoms secondary to environmental factors and/or other primary psychiatric disorders, including psychosis. Appropriate educational placement is essential in children and adolescents with this diagnosis and psychosocial intervention is often helpful. When remedial measures alone are insufficient, the decision to prescribe drug treatment medication will depend upon the physician's assessment of the chronicity and severity of the patient's symptoms.

2 DOSAGE AND ADMINISTRATION

2.1 Acute Treatment

Dosing of children and adolescents up to 70 kg body weight—STRATTERA should be initiated at a total daily dose of approximately 0.5 mg/kg and increased after a minimum of 3 days to a target total daily dose of approximately 1.2 mg/kg administered either as a single daily dose in the morning or as evenly divided doses in the morning and late afternoon/early evening. No additional benefit has been demonstrated for doses higher than 1.2 mg/kg/day *[see Clinical Studies (14)]*.

The total daily dose in children and adolescents should not exceed 1.4 mg/kg or 100 mg, whichever is less.

Dosing of children and adolescents over 70 kg body weight and adults—STRATTERA should be initiated at a total daily dose of 40 mg and increased after a minimum of 3 days to a target total daily dose of approximately 80 mg administered either as a single daily dose in the morning or as evenly divided doses in the morning and late afternoon/early evening. After 2 to 4 additional weeks, the dose may be increased to a maximum of 100 mg in patients who have not achieved an optimal response. There are no data that support increased effectiveness at higher doses *[see Clinical Studies (14)]*.

The maximum recommended total daily dose in children and adolescents over 70 kg and adults is 100 mg.

2.2 Maintenance/Extended Treatment

It is generally agreed that pharmacological treatment of ADHD may be needed for extended periods. The benefit of maintaining pediatric patients (ages 6-15 years) with ADHD on STRATTERA after achieving a response in a dose range of 1.2 to 1.8 mg/kg/day was demonstrated in a controlled trial. Patients assigned to STRATTERA in the maintenance phase were generally continued on the same dose used to achieve a response in the open label phase. The physician who elects to use STRATTERA for extended periods should periodically reevaluate the long-term usefulness of the drug for the individual patient *[see Clinical Studies (14.1)]*.

2.3 General Dosing Information

STRATTERA may be taken with or without food.

STRATTERA can be discontinued without being tapered.

STRATTERA capsules are not intended to be opened, they should be taken whole *[see Patient Counseling Information (17.6)]*.

The safety of single doses over 120 mg and total daily doses above 150 mg have not been systematically evaluated.

2.4 Dosing in Specific Populations

Dosing adjustment for hepatically impaired patients—For those ADHD patients who have hepatic insufficiency (HI), dosage adjustment is recommended as follows: For patients with moderate HI (Child-Pugh Class B), initial and target doses should be reduced to 50% of the normal dose (for patients without HI). For patients with severe HI (Child-Pugh Class C), initial dose and target doses should be reduced to 25% of normal *[see Use In Specific Populations (8.6)]*.

Dosing adjustment for use with a strong CYP2D6 inhibitor or in patients who are known to be CYP2D6 PMs—In children and adolescents up to 70 kg body weight administered strong CYP2D6 inhibitors, e.g., paroxetine, fluoxetine, and quinidine, or in patients who are known to be CYP2D6 PMs, STRATTERA should be initiated at 0.5 mg/kg/day and only increased to the usual target dose of 1.2 mg/kg/day if symptoms fail to improve after 4 weeks and the initial dose is well tolerated.

In children and adolescents over 70 kg body weight and adults administered strong CYP2D6 inhibitors, e.g., paroxetine, fluoxetine, and quinidine, STRATTERA should be initiated at 40 mg/day and only increased to the usual target dose of 80 mg/day if symptoms fail to improve after 4 weeks and the initial dose is well tolerated.

3 DOSAGE FORMS AND STRENGTHS

Each capsule contains atomoxetine HCl equivalent to 10 mg (Opaque White, Opaque White), 18 mg (Gold, Opaque White), 25 mg (Opaque Blue, Opaque White), 40 mg (Opaque Blue, Opaque Blue), 60 mg (Opaque Blue, Gold), 80 mg (Opaque Brown, Opaque White), or 100 mg (Opaque Brown, Opaque Brown) of atomoxetine.

4 CONTRAINDICATIONS

4.1 Hypersensitivity

STRATTERA is contraindicated in patients known to be hypersensitive to atomoxetine or other constituents of the product *[see Warnings and Precautions (5.7)]*.

4.2 Monoamine Oxidase Inhibitors (MAOI)

STRATTERA should not be taken with an MAOI, or within 2 weeks after discontinuing an MAOI. Treatment with an MAOI should not be initiated within 2 weeks after discontinuing STRATTERA. With other drugs that affect brain monoamine concentrations, there have been reports of serious, sometimes fatal reactions (including hyperthermia, rigidity, myoclonus, autonomic instability with possible rapid fluctuations of vital signs, and mental status changes that include extreme agitation progressing to delirium and coma) when taken in combination with an MAOI. Some cases presented with features resembling neuroleptic malignant syndrome. Such reactions may occur when these drugs are given concurrently or in close proximity *[see Drug Interactions (7.1)]*.

4.3 Narrow Angle Glaucoma

In clinical trials, STRATTERA use was associated with an increased risk of mydriasis and therefore its use is not recommended in patients with narrow angle glaucoma.

5 WARNINGS AND PRECAUTIONS

5.1 Suicidal Ideation

STRATTERA increased the risk of suicidal ideation in short-term studies in children and adolescents with Attention-Deficit/Hyperactivity Disorder (ADHD). Pooled analyses of short-term (6 to 18 weeks) placebo-controlled trials of STRATTERA in children and adolescents have revealed a greater risk of suicidal ideation early during treatment in those receiving STRATTERA. There were a total of 12 trials (11 in ADHD and 1 in enuresis) involving over 2200 patients (including 1357 patients receiving STRATTERA and 851 receiving placebo). The average risk of suicidal ideation in patients receiving STRATTERA was 0.4% (5/1357 patients), compared to none in placebo-treated patients. There was 1 suicide attempt among these approximately 2200 patients, occurring in a patient treated with STRATTERA. **No suicides occurred in these trials.** All reactions occurred in children 12 years of age or younger. All reactions occurred during the first month of treatment. It is unknown whether the risk of suicidal ideation in pediatric patients extends to longer-term use. A similar analysis in adult patients treated with STRATTERA for either ADHD or major depressive disorder (MDD) did not reveal an increased risk of suicidal ideation or behavior in association with the use of STRATTERA.

All pediatric patients being treated with STRATTERA should be monitored appropriately and observed closely for clinical worsening, suicidality, and unusual changes in behavior, especially during the initial few months of a course of drug therapy, or at times of dose changes, either increases or decreases.

The following symptoms have been reported with STRATTERA: anxiety, agitation, panic attacks, insomnia, irritability, hostility, aggressiveness, impulsivity, akathisia (psychomotor restlessness), hypomania and mania. Although a causal link between the emergence of such symptoms and the emergence of suicidal impulses has not been established, there is a concern that such symptoms may represent precursors to emerging suicidality. Thus, patients being treated with STRATTERA should be observed for the emergence of such symptoms.

Consideration should be given to changing the therapeutic regimen, including possibly discontinuing the medication, in patients who are experiencing emergent suicidality or symptoms that might be precursors to emerging suicidality, especially if these symptoms are severe or abrupt in onset, or were not part of the patient's presenting symptoms.

Families and caregivers of pediatric patients being treated with STRATTERA should be alerted about the need to monitor patients for the emergence of agitation, irritability, unusual changes in behavior, and the other symptoms described above, as well as the emergence of suicidality, and to report such symptoms immediately to healthcare providers. Such monitoring should include daily observation by families and caregivers.

5.2 Severe Liver Injury

Postmarketing reports indicate that STRATTERA can cause severe liver injury. Although no evidence of liver injury was detected in clinical trials of about 6000 patients, there have been rare cases of clinically significant liver injury that were considered probably or possibly related to STRATTERA use in postmarketing experience. Because of probable underreporting, it is impossible to provide an accurate estimate of the true incidence of these reactions. Reported cases of liver injury occurred within 120 days of initiation of atomoxetine in the majority of cases and some patients presented with markedly elevated liver enzymes [>20 × upper limit of normal (ULN)], and jaundice with significantly elevated bilirubin levels (>2 × ULN), followed by recovery upon atomoxetine discontinuation. In one patient, liver injury, manifested by elevated hepatic enzymes up to 40 × upper limit of normal ULN and jaundice with bilirubin up to 12 × ULN, recurred upon rechallenge, and was followed by recovery upon drug discontinuation, providing evidence that STRATTERA likely caused the liver injury. Such reactions may occur several months after therapy is started, but laboratory abnormalities may continue to worsen for several weeks after drug is stopped. The patient described above recovered from his liver injury, and did not require a liver transplant. However, severe liver injury due to any drug may potentially progress to acute liver failure resulting in death or the need for a liver transplant.

STRATTERA should be discontinued in patients with jaundice or laboratory evidence of liver injury, and should not be restarted. Laboratory testing to determine liver enzyme levels should be done upon the first symptom or sign of liver dysfunction (e.g., pruritus, dark urine, jaundice, right upper quadrant tenderness, or unexplained "flu like" symptoms) *[see Warnings and Precautions (5.12); Patient Counseling Information (17.3)].*

5.3 Serious Cardiovascular Events

Sudden Death and Pre-existing Structural Cardiac Abnormalities or Other Serious Heart Problems

Children and Adolescents—Sudden death has been reported in association with atomoxetine treatment at usual doses in children and adolescents with structural cardiac abnormalities or other serious heart problems. Although some serious heart problems alone carry an increased risk of sudden death, atomoxetine generally should not be used in children or adolescents with known serious structural cardiac abnormalities, cardiomyopathy, serious heart rhythm abnormalities, or other serious cardiac problems that may place them at increased vulnerability to the noradrenergic effects of atomoxetine.

Adults—Sudden deaths, stroke, and myocardial infarction have been reported in adults taking atomoxetine at usual doses for ADHD. Although the role of atomoxetine in these adult cases is also unknown, adults have a greater likelihood than children of having serious structural cardiac abnormalities, cardiomyopathy, serious heart rhythm abnormalities, coronary artery disease, or other serious cardiac problems. Consideration should be given to not treating adults with clinically significant cardiac abnormalities.

Assessing Cardiovascular Status in Patients being Treated with Atomoxetine

Children, adolescents, or adults who are being considered for treatment with atomoxetine should have a careful history (including assessment for a family history of sudden death or ventricular arrhythmia) and physical exam to assess for the presence of cardiac disease, and should receive further cardiac evaluation if findings suggest such disease (e.g., electrocardiogram and echocardiogram). Patients who develop symptoms such as exertional chest pain, unexplained syncope, or other symptoms suggestive of cardiac disease during atomoxetine treatment should undergo a prompt cardiac evaluation.

5.4 Effects on Blood Pressure and Heart Rate

STRATTERA should be used with caution in patients with hypertension, tachycardia, or cardiovascular or cerebrovascular disease because it can increase blood pressure and heart rate. Pulse and blood pressure should be measured at baseline, following STRATTERA dose increases, and periodically while on therapy.

In pediatric placebo–controlled trials, STRATTERA–treated subjects experienced a mean increase in heart rate of about 6 beats/minute compared with placebo subjects. At the final study visit before drug discontinuation, 2.5% (36/1434) of STRATTERA–treated subjects had heart rate increases of at least 25 beats/minute and a heart rate of at least 110 beats/minute, compared with 0.2% (2/850) of placebo subjects. There were 1.1% (15/1417) pediatric STRATTERA-treated subjects with a heart rate increase of at least 25 beats/minute and a heart rate of at least 110 beats/minute on more than one occasion. Tachycardia was identified as an adverse event for 0.3% (5/1597) of these pediatric subjects compared with 0% (0/934) of placebo subjects. The mean heart rate increase in extensive metabolizer (EM) patients was 5.0 beats/minute, and in poor metabolizer (PM) patients 9.4 beats/minute.

STRATTERA–treated pediatric subjects experienced mean increases of about 1.6 and 2.4 mm Hg in systolic and diastolic blood pressures, respectively compared with placebo. At the final study visit before drug discontinuation, 4.8% (59/1226) of STRATTERA–treated pediatric subjects had high systolic blood pressure measurements compared with 3.5% (26/748) of placebo subjects. High systolic blood pressures were measured on 2 or more occasions in 4.4% (54/1226) of STRATTERA–treated subjects and 1.9% (14/748) of placebo subjects. At the final study visit before drug discontinuation, 4.0% (50/1262) of STRATTERA–treated pediatric subjects had high diastolic blood pressure measurements compared with 1.1% (8/759) of placebo subjects. High diastolic blood pressures were measured on 2 or more occasions in 3.5% (44/1262) of STRATTERA–treated subjects and 0.5% (4/759) of placebo subjects. (High systolic and diastolic blood pressure measurements were defined as those exceeding the 95th percentile, stratified by age, gender, and height percentile – National High Blood Pressure Education Working Group on Hypertension Control in Children and Adolescents.)

In adult placebo–controlled trials, STRATTERA–treated subjects experienced a mean increase in heart rate of 5 beats/minute compared with placebo subjects. Tachycardia was identified as an adverse event for 1.5% (8/540) of these adult atomoxetine subjects compared with 0.5% (2/402) of placebo subjects.

STRATTERA–treated adult subjects experienced mean increases in systolic (about 2.0 mm Hg) and diastolic (about 1.0 mm Hg) blood pressures compared with placebo. At the final study visit before drug discontinuation, 2.2% (11/510) of STRATTERA–treated adult subjects had systolic blood pressure measurements ≥150 mm Hg compared with 1.0% (4/393) of placebo subjects. At the final study visit before drug discontinuation, 0.4% (2/510) of STRATTERA–treated adult subjects had diastolic blood pressure measurements ≥100 mm Hg compared with 0.5% (2/393) of placebo subjects. No adult subject had a high systolic or diastolic blood pressure detected on more than one occasion.

Orthostatic hypotension and syncope have been reported in patients taking STRATTERA. In child and adolescent trials, 0.2% (12/5596) of STRATTERA-treated patients experienced orthostatic hypotension and 0.8% (46/5596) experienced syncope. In short-term child and adolescent controlled trials, 1.8% (6/340) of STRATTERA–treated patients experienced orthostatic hypotension compared with 0.5% (1/207) of placebo-treated patients. Syncope was not reported during short-term child and adolescent placebo-controlled ADHD trials. STRATTERA should be used with caution in any condition that may predispose patients to hypotension, or conditions associated with abrupt heart rate or blood pressure changes.

Peripheral vascular effects—There have been spontaneous postmarketing reports of Raynaud's phenomenon (new onset and exacerbation of preexisting condition).

5.5 Emergence of New Psychotic or Manic Symptoms

Treatment emergent psychotic or manic symptoms, e.g., hallucinations, delusional thinking, or mania in children and adolescents without a prior history of psychotic illness or mania can be caused by atomoxetine at usual doses. If such symptoms occur, consideration should be given to a possible causal role of atomoxetine, and discontinuation of treatment should be considered. In a pooled analysis of multiple short–term, placebo–controlled studies, such symptoms occurred in about 0.2% (4 patients with reactions out of 1939 exposed to atomoxetine for several weeks at usual doses) of atomoxetine–treated patients compared to 0 out of 1056 placebo–treated patients.

5.6 Screening Patients for Bipolar Disorder

In general, particular care should be taken in treating ADHD in patients with comorbid bipolar disorder because of concern for possible induction of a mixed/manic episode in patients at risk for bipolar disorder. Whether any of the symptoms described above represent such a conversion is unknown. However, prior to initiating treatment with STRATTERA, patients with comorbid depressive symptoms should be adequately screened to determine if they are at risk for bipolar disorder; such screening should include a detailed psychiatric history, including a family history of suicide, bipolar disorder, and depression.

5.7 Aggressive Behavior or Hostility

Patients beginning treatment for ADHD should be monitored for the appearance or worsening of aggressive behavior or hostility. Aggressive behavior or hostility is often observed in children and adolescents with ADHD. In short–term controlled clinical trials, 21/1308 (1.6%) of atomoxetine patients versus 9/806 (1.1%) of placebo–treated patients spontaneously reported treatment emergent hostility-related adverse events. Although this is not conclusive evidence that STRATTERA causes aggressive behavior or hostility, these behaviors were more frequently observed in clinical trials among children and adolescents treated with STRATTERA compared to placebo (overall risk ratio of 1.33 [95% C.I. 0.67–2.64–not statistically significant]).

5.8 Allergic Events

Although uncommon, allergic reactions, including angioneurotic edema, urticaria, and rash, have been reported in patients taking STRATTERA.

5.9 Effects on Urine Outflow from the Bladder

In adult ADHD controlled trials, the rates of urinary retention (1.7%, 9/540) and urinary hesitation (5.6%, 30/540) were increased among atomoxetine subjects compared with placebo subjects (0%, 0/402 ; 0.5%, 2/402, respectively). Two adult atomoxetine subjects and no placebo subjects discontinued from controlled clinical trials because of urinary retention. A complaint of urinary retention or urinary hesitancy should be considered potentially related to atomoxetine.

5.10 Priapism

Rare postmarketing cases of priapism, defined as painful and nonpainful penile erection lasting more than 4 hours, have been reported for pediatric and adult patients treated with STRATTERA. The erections resolved in cases in which follow-up information was available, some following discontinuation of STRATTERA. Prompt medical attention is required in the event of suspected priapism.

5.11 Effects on Growth

Data on the long–term effects of STRATTERA on growth come from open–label studies, and weight and height changes are compared to normative population data. In general, the weight and height gain of pediatric patients treated with STRATTERA lags behind that predicted by normative population data for about the first 9–12 months of treatment. Subsequently, weight gain rebounds and at about 3 years of treatment, patients treated with STRATTERA have gained 17.9 kg on average, 0.5 kg more than predicted by their baseline data. After about 12 months, gain in height stabilizes, and at 3 years, patients treated with STRATTERA have gained 19.4 cm on average, 0.4 cm less than predicted by their baseline data (*see* Figure 1 below).

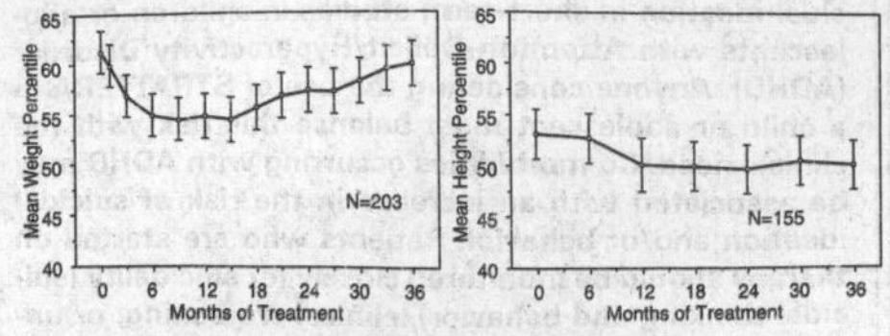

Figure 1: Mean Weight and Height Percentiles Over Time for Patients With Three Years of STRATTERA Treatment

This growth pattern was generally similar regardless of pubertal status at the time of treatment initiation. Patients who were pre–pubertal at the start of treatment (girls ≤8 years old, boys ≤9 years old) gained an average of 2.1 kg and 1.2 cm less than predicted after three years. Patients who were pubertal (girls >8 to ≤13 years old, boys >9 to ≤14 years old) or late pubertal (girls >13 years old, boys >14 years old) had average weight and height gains that were close to or exceeded those predicted after three years of treatment.

Growth followed a similar pattern in both extensive and poor metabolizers (EMs, PMs). PMs treated for at least two years gained an average of 2.4 kg and 1.1 cm less than predicted, while EMs gained an average of 0.2 kg and 0.4 cm less than predicted.

In short–term controlled studies (up to 9 weeks), STRATTERA–treated patients lost an average of 0.4 kg and gained an average of 0.9 cm, compared to a gain of 1.5 kg and 1.1 cm in the placebo–treated patients. In a fixed–dose controlled trial, 1.3%, 7.1%, 19.3%, and 29.1% of patients lost at least 3.5% of their body weight in the placebo, 0.5, 1.2, and 1.8 mg/kg/day dose groups.

Growth should be monitored during treatment with STRATTERA.

5.12 Laboratory Tests

Routine laboratory tests are not required.

CYP2D6 metabolism—Poor metabolizers (PMs) of CYP2D6 have a 10–fold higher AUC and a 5–fold higher peak concentration to a given dose of STRATTERA compared with extensive metabolizers (EMs). Approximately 7% of a Caucasian population are PMs. Laboratory tests are available to identify CYP2D6 PMs. The blood levels in PMs are similar to those attained by taking strong inhibitors of CYP2D6. The higher blood levels in PMs lead to a higher rate of some adverse effects of STRATTERA *[see Adverse Reactions (6.1)].*

5.13 Concomitant Use of Potent CYP2D6 Inhibitors or Use in patients who are known to be CYP2D6 PMs

Atomoxetine is primarily metabolized by the CYP2D6 pathway to 4–hydroxyatomoxetine. Dosage adjustment of STRATTERA may be necessary when coadministered with potent CYP2D6 inhibitors (e.g., paroxetine, fluoxetine, and quinidine) or when administered to CYP2D6 PMs. *[see Dosage and Administration (2.3) and Drug Interactions (7.2)].*

6 ADVERSE REACTIONS

6.1 Clinical Trials Experience

STRATTERA was administered to 5382 children or adolescent patients with ADHD and 1007 adults with ADHD in clinical studies. During the ADHD clinical trials, 1625 children and adolescent patients were treated for longer than 1 year and 2529 children and adolescent patients were treated for over 6 months.

Because clinical trials are conducted under widely varying conditions, adverse reaction rates observed in the clinical trials of a drug cannot be directly compared to rates in the clinical trials of another drug and may not reflect the rates observed in practice.

Child and Adolescent Clinical Trials

Reasons for discontinuation of treatment due to adverse reactions in child and adolescent clinical trials—In acute child and adolescent placebo–controlled trials, 3.0% (48/1613) of atomoxetine subjects and 1.4% (13/945) placebo subjects discontinued for adverse reactions. For all studies, (including open–label and long–term studies), 6.3% of extensive metabolizer (EM) patients and 11.2% of poor metabolizer (PM) patients discontinued because of an adverse reaction. Among STRATTERA–treated patients, irritability (0.3%, N=5); somnolence (0.3%, N=5); aggression (0.2%, N=4); nausea (0.2%, N=4); vomiting (0.2%, N=4); abdominal pain (0.2%, N=4); constipation (0.1%, N=2); fatigue (0.1%, N=2); feeling abnormal (0.1%, N=2); and headache (0.1%, N=2) were the reasons for discontinuation reported by more than 1 patient.

Seizures—STRATTERA has not been systematically evaluated in pediatric patients with seizure disorder as these patients were excluded from clinical studies during the product's premarket testing. In the clinical development program, seizures were reported in 0.2% (12/5073) of children whose average age was 10 years (range 6 to 16 years). In these clinical trials, the seizure risk among poor metabolizers was 0.3% (1/293) compared to 0.2% (11/4741) for extensive metabolizers.

Commonly observed adverse reactions in acute child and adolescent, placebo–controlled trials—Commonly observed adverse reactions associated with the use of STRATTERA (incidence of 2% or greater) and not observed at an equivalent incidence among placebo–treated patients (STRATTERA incidence greater than placebo) are listed in Table 1. Results were similar in the BID and the QD trial except as shown in Table 2, which shows both BID and QD results for selected adverse reactions based on statistically significant Breslow-Day tests. The most commonly observed adverse reactions in patients treated with STRATTERA (incidence of 5% or greater and at least twice the incidence in placebo patients, for either BID or QD dosing) were: nausea, vomiting, fatigue, decreased appetite, abdominal pain, and somnolence (see Tables 1 and 2).

Table 1: Common Treatment–Emergent Adverse Reactions Associated with the Use of STRATTERA in Acute (up to 18 weeks) Child and Adolescent Trials

Adverse Reaction*	Percentage of Patients Reporting Reaction	
	STRATTERA (N=1597)	Placebo (N=934)
Gastrointestinal Disorders		
Abdominal pain†	18	10
Vomiting	11	6
Nausea	10	5
General Disorders and Administration Site Conditions		
Fatigue	8	3
Irritability	6	3
Therapeutic response unexpected	2	1
Investigations		
Weight decreased	3	0
Metabolism and Nutritional Disorders		
Decreased appetite	16	4
Anorexia	3	1
Nervous System Disorders		
Headache	19	15
Somnolence‡	11	4
Dizziness	5	2
Skin and Subcutaneous Tissue Disorders		
Rash	2	1

*Reactions reported by at least 2% of patients treated with atomoxetine, and greater than placebo. The following reactions did not meet this criterion but were reported by more atomoxetine–treated patients than placebo–treated patients and are possibly related to atomoxetine treatment: blood pressure increased, early morning awakening, flushing, mydriasis, sinus tachycardia, asthenia, palpitations, mood swings, constipation. The following reactions were reported by at least 2% of patients treated with atomoxetine, and equal to or less than placebo: pharyngolaryngeal pain, insomnia (insomnia includes the terms, insomnia, initial insomnia, middle insomnia). The following reaction did not meet this criterion but shows a statistically significant dose relationship: pruritus.
†Abdominal pain includes the terms: abdominal pain upper, abdominal pain, stomach discomfort, abdominal discomfort, epigastric discomfort.
‡Somnolence includes the terms: sedation, somnolence.

[See table 2 at top right]
The following adverse reactions occurred in at least 2% of PM patients and were either twice as frequent or statistically significantly more frequent in PM patients compared with EM patients: insomnia (15% of PMs, 10% of EMs); weight decreased (7% of PMs, 4% of EMs); constipation (7% of PMs, 4% of EMs); depression[1] (7% of PMs, 4% of EMs); tremor (5% of PMs, 1% of EMs); excoriation (4% of PMs, 2% of EMs); conjunctivitis 3% of PMs, 1% of EMs); syncope (3% of PMs, 1% of EMs); early morning awakening (2% of PMs, 1% of EMs); mydriasis (2% of PMs, 1% of EMs).

[1] Depression includes the following terms: depression, major depression, depressive symptoms, depressed mood, dysphoria.
Adult Clinical Trials
Reasons for discontinuation of treatment due to adverse reactions in acute adult placebo–controlled trials—In the

Table 2: Common Treatment-Emergent Adverse Reactions Associated with the Use of STRATTERA in Acute (up to 18 weeks) Child and Adolescent Trials

Adverse Reaction	Percentage of Patients Reporting Reaction from BID Trials		Percentage of Patients Reporting Reaction from QD Trials	
	STRATTERA (N=715)	Placebo (N=434)	STRATTERA (N=882)	Placebo (N=500)
Gastrointestinal Disorders				
Abdominal pain*	17	13	18	7
Vomiting	11	8	11	4
Nausea	7	6	13	4
Constipation†	2	1	1	0
General Disorders				
Fatigue	6	4	9	2
Psychiatric Disorders				
Mood swings‡	2	0	1	1

*Abdominal pain includes the terms: abdominal pain upper, abdominal pain, stomach discomfort, abdominal discomfort, epigastric discomfort.
†Constipation didn't meet the statistical significance on Breslow-Day test but is included in the table because of pharmacologic plausibility.
‡Mood swings didn't meet the statistical significance on Breslow-Day test at 0.05 level but p-value was <0.1 (trend).

acute adult placebo–controlled trials, 11.3% (61/541) atomoxetine subjects and 3.0% (12/405) placebo subjects discontinued for adverse reactions. Among STRATTERA-treated patients, insomnia (0.9%, N=5); nausea (0.9%, N=5); chest pain (0.6%, N=3); fatigue (0.6%, N=3); anxiety (0.4%, N=2); erectile dysfunction (0.4%, N=2); mood swings (0.4%, N=2); nervousness (0.4%, N=2); palpitations (0.4%, N=2); and urinary retention (0.4%, N=2) were the reasons for discontinuation reported by more than 1 patient.
Seizures—STRATTERA has not been systematically evaluated in adult patients with a seizure disorder as these patients were excluded from clinical studies during the product's premarket testing. In the clinical development program, seizures were reported on 0.1% (1/748) of adult patients. In these clinical trials, no poor metabolizers (0/43) reported seizures compared to 0.1% (1/705) for extensive metabolizers.
Commonly observed adverse reactions in acute adult placebo–controlled trials—Commonly observed adverse reactions associated with the use of STRATTERA (incidence of 2% or greater) and not observed at an equivalent incidence among placebo–treated patients (STRATTERA incidence greater than placebo) are listed in Table 3. The most commonly observed adverse reactions in patients treated with STRATTERA (incidence of 5% or greater and at least twice the incidence in placebo patients) were: constipation, dry mouth, nausea, fatigue, decreased appetite, insomnia, erectile dysfunction, urinary hesitation and/or urinary retention and/or dysuria, dysmenorrhea, and hot flush (see Table 3).

Table 3: Common Treatment-Emergent Adverse Reactions Associated with the Use of STRATTERA in Acute (up to 25 weeks) Adult Trials

Adverse Reaction* System Organ Class/ Adverse Reaction	Percentage of Patients Reporting Reaction	
	STRATTERA (N=540)	Placebo (N=402)
Cardiac Disorders		
Palpitations	3	1
Gastrointestinal Disorders		
Dry mouth	21	7
Nausea	21	5
Constipation	9	3
Abdominal pain†	7	5
Dyspepsia	4	2
Vomiting	3	2
General Disorders and Administration Site Conditions		
Fatigue	9	4
Chills	3	1
Therapeutic response unexpected	3	1
Feeling jittery	2	0
Investigations		
Weight decreased	2	1
Metabolism and Nutritional Disorders		
Decreased appetite	11	4
Nervous System Disorders		
Dizziness	6	4
Somnolence‡	4	3
Sinus headache	3	1
Tremor	2	0
Psychiatric Disorders		
Insomnia§	15	7
Libido decreased	4	2
Sleep disorder	3	1
Renal and Urinary Disorders		
Urinary hesitation and/or urinary retention	7	1
Dysuria	3	0
Reproductive System and Breast Disorders		
Erectile dysfunction¶	9	1
Dysmenorrhea#	6	2
Ejaculation delayed¶ and/or ejaculation disorder¶	3	1
Menstruation irregular#	2	0
Skin and Subcutaneous Tissue Disorders		
Hyperhidrosis	4	1
Rash	2	1
Vascular Disorders		
Hot flush	8	1

*Reactions reported by at least 2% of patients treated with atomoxetine, and greater than placebo. The following reactions did not meet this criterion but were reported by more atomoxetine–treated patients than placebo–treated patients and are possibly related to atomoxetine treatment: early morning awakening, peripheral coldness, tachycardia, prostatitis, testicular pain, and orgasm abnormal. The following reactions were reported by at least 2% of patients treated with atomoxetine, and equal to or less than placebo: headache, pharyngolaryngeal pain, irritability.
†Abdominal pain includes the terms: abdominal pain upper, abdominal pain, stomach discomfort, abdominal discomfort, epigastric discomfort.
‡Somnolence includes the terms: sedation, somnolence.
§Insomnia includes the terms: insomnia, initial insomnia, middle insomnia.
¶Based on total number of males (STRATTERA, N=326; placebo, N=260).
#Based on total number of females (STRATTERA, N=214; placebo, N=142).

Male and female sexual dysfunction—Atomoxetine appears to impair sexual function in some patients. Changes in sexual desire, sexual performance, and sexual satisfaction are not well assessed in most clinical trials because they need special attention and because patients and physicians may be reluctant to discuss them. Accordingly, estimates of the incidence of untoward sexual experience and performance cited in product labeling are likely to underestimate the actual incidence. Table 3 above displays the incidence of sexual side effects reported by at least 2% of adult patients taking STRATTERA in placebo-controlled trials.
There are no adequate and well–controlled studies examining sexual dysfunction with STRATTERA treatment. While it is difficult to know the precise risk of sexual dysfunction associated with the use of STRATTERA, physicians should routinely inquire about such possible side effects.
6.2   Postmarketing Spontaneous Reports
The following adverse reactions have been identified during post approval use of STRATTERA. Unless otherwise specified, these adverse reactions have occurred in adults and children and adolescents. Because these reactions are reported voluntarily from a population of uncertain size, it is not always possible to reliably estimate their frequency or establish a causal relationship to drug exposure.
Cardiovascular system—QT prolongation, syncope.
General disorders and administration site conditions—Lethargy.

Nervous system disorders—Hypoaesthesia; paraesthesia in children and adolescents; sensory disturbances.

Seizures—Seizures have been reported in the postmarketing period. The postmarketing seizure cases include patients with pre-existing seizure disorders and those with identified risk factors for seizures, as well as patients with neither a history of nor identified risk factors for seizures. The exact relationship between STRATTERA and seizures is difficult to evaluate due to uncertainty about the background risk of seizures in ADHD patients.

Urogenital system—Male pelvic pain; urinary hesitation in children and adolescents; urinary retention in children and adolescents.

7 DRUG INTERACTIONS

7.1 Monoamine Oxidase Inhibitors

With other drugs that affect brain monoamine concentrations, there have been reports of serious, sometimes fatal reactions (including hyperthermia, rigidity, myoclonus, autonomic instability with possible rapid fluctuations of vital signs, and mental status changes that include extreme agitation progressing to delirium and coma) when taken in combination with an MAOI. Some cases presented with features resembling neuroleptic malignant syndrome. Such reactions may occur when these drugs are given concurrently or in close proximity [see Contraindications (4.2)].

7.2 Effect of CYP2D6 Inhibitors on Atomoxetine

In extensive metabolizers (EMs), inhibitors of CYP2D6 (e.g., paroxetine, fluoxetine, and quinidine) increase atomoxetine steady-state plasma concentrations to exposures similar to those observed in poor metabolizers (PMs). In EM individuals treated with paroxetine or fluoxetine, the AUC of atomoxetine is approximately 6– to 8-fold and $C_{ss,max}$ is about 3– to 4-fold greater than atomoxetine alone.

In vitro studies suggest that coadministration of cytochrome P450 inhibitors to PMs will not increase the plasma concentrations of atomoxetine.

7.3 Pressor Agents

Because of possible effects on blood pressure, STRATTERA should be used cautiously with pressor agents (e.g., dopamine, dobutamine).

7.4 Albuterol

STRATTERA should be administered with caution to patients being treated with systemically-administered (oral or intravenous) albuterol (or other beta$_2$ agonists) because the action of albuterol on the cardiovascular system can be potentiated resulting in increases in heart rate and blood pressure. Albuterol (600 mcg iv over 2 hours) induced increases in heart rate and blood pressure. These effects were potentiated by atomoxetine (60 mg BID for 5 days) and were most marked after the initial coadministration of albuterol and atomoxetine. However, these effects on heart rate and blood pressure were not seen in another study after the coadministration with inhaled dose of albuterol (200-800 mcg) and atomoxetine (80 mg QD for 5 days) in 21 healthy Asian subjects who were excluded for poor metabolizer status.

7.5 Effect of Atomoxetine on P450 Enzymes

Atomoxetine did not cause clinically important inhibition or induction of cytochrome P450 enzymes, including CYP1A2, CYP3A, CYP2D6, and CYP2C9.

CYP3A Substrate (e.g., Midazolam)—Coadministration of STRATTERA (60 mg BID for 12 days) with midazolam, a model compound for CYP3A4 metabolized drugs (single dose of 5 mg), resulted in 15% increase in AUC of midazolam. No dose adjustment is recommended for drugs metabolized by CYP3A.

CYP2D6 Substrate (e.g., Desipramine)—Coadministration of STRATTERA (40 or 60 mg BID for 13 days) with desipramine, a model compound for CYP2D6 metabolized drugs (single dose of 50 mg), did not alter the pharmacokinetics of desipramine. No dose adjustment is recommended for drugs metabolized by CYP2D6.

7.6 Alcohol

Consumption of ethanol with STRATTERA did not change the intoxicating effects of ethanol.

7.7 Methylphenidate

Coadministration of methylphenidate with STRATTERA did not increase cardiovascular effects beyond those seen with methylphenidate alone.

7.8 Drugs Highly Bound to Plasma Protein

In vitro drug-displacement studies were conducted with atomoxetine and other highly-bound drugs at therapeutic concentrations. Atomoxetine did not affect the binding of warfarin, acetylsalicylic acid, phenytoin, or diazepam to human albumin. Similarly, these compounds did not affect the binding of atomoxetine to human albumin.

7.9 Drugs that Affect Gastric pH

Drugs that elevate gastric pH (magnesium hydroxide/aluminum hydroxide, omeprazole) had no effect on STRATTERA bioavailability.

8 USE IN SPECIFIC POPULATIONS

8.1 Pregnancy

Pregnancy Category C—Pregnant rabbits were treated with up to 100 mg/kg/day of atomoxetine by gavage throughout the period of organogenesis. At this dose, in 1 of 3 studies, a decrease in live fetuses and an increase in early resorptions was observed. Slight increases in the incidences of atypical origin of carotid artery and absent subclavian artery were observed. These findings were observed at doses that caused slight maternal toxicity. The no-effect dose for these findings was 30 mg/kg/day. The 100 mg/kg dose is approximately 23 times the maximum human dose on a mg/m^2 basis; plasma levels (AUC) of atomoxetine at this dose in rabbits are estimated to be 3.3 times (extensive metabolizers) or 0.4 times (poor metabolizers) those in humans receiving the maximum human dose.

Rats were treated with up to approximately 50 mg/kg/day of atomoxetine (approximately 6 times the maximum human dose on a mg/m^2 basis) in the diet from 2 weeks (females) or 10 weeks (males) prior to mating through the periods of organogenesis and lactation. In 1 of 2 studies, decreases in pup weight and pup survival were observed. The decreased pup survival was also seen at 25 mg/kg (but not at 13 mg/kg). In a study in which rats were treated with atomoxetine in the diet from 2 weeks (females) or 10 weeks (males) prior to mating throughout the period of organogenesis, a decrease in fetal weight (female only) and an increase in the incidence of incomplete ossification of the vertebral arch in fetuses were observed at 40 mg/kg/day (approximately 5 times the maximum human dose on a mg/m^2 basis) but not at 20 mg/kg/day.

No adverse fetal effects were seen when pregnant rats were treated with up to 150 mg/kg/day (approximately 17 times the maximum human dose on a mg/m^2 basis) by gavage throughout the period of organogenesis.

No adequate and well-controlled studies have been conducted in pregnant women. STRATTERA should not be used during pregnancy unless the potential benefit justifies the potential risk to the fetus.

8.2 Labor and Delivery

Parturition in rats was not affected by atomoxetine. The effect of STRATTERA on labor and delivery in humans is unknown.

8.3 Nursing Mothers

Atomoxetine and/or its metabolites were excreted in the milk of rats. It is not known if atomoxetine is excreted in human milk. Caution should be exercised if STRATTERA is administered to a nursing woman.

8.4 Pediatric Use

Anyone considering the use of STRATTERA in a child or adolescent must balance the potential risks with the clinical need [see Boxed Warning and Warnings and Precautions (5.1)].

The pharmacokinetics of atomoxetine in children and adolescents are similar to those in adults. The safety, efficacy, and pharmacokinetics of STRATTERA in pediatric patients less than 6 years of age have not been evaluated.

A study was conducted in young rats to evaluate the effects of atomoxetine on growth and neurobehavioral and sexual development. Rats were treated with 1, 10, or 50 mg/kg/day (approximately 0.2, 2, and 8 times, respectively, the maximum human dose on a mg/m^2 basis) of atomoxetine given by gavage from the early postnatal period (Day 10 of age) through adulthood. Slight delays in onset of vaginal patency (all doses) and preputial separation (10 and 50 mg/kg), slight decreases in epididymal weight and sperm number (10 and 50 mg/kg), and a slight decrease in corpora lutea (50 mg/kg) were seen, but there were no effects on fertility or reproductive performance. A slight delay in onset of incisor eruption was seen at 50 mg/kg. A slight increase in motor activity was seen on Day 15 (males at 10 and 50 mg/kg and females at 50 mg/kg) and on Day 30 (females at 50 mg/kg) but not on Day 60 of age. There were no effects on learning and memory tests. The significance of these findings to humans is unknown.

8.5 Geriatric Use

The safety, efficacy and pharmacokinetics of STRATTERA in geriatric patients have not been evaluated.

8.6 Hepatic Insufficiency

Atomoxetine exposure (AUC) is increased, compared with normal subjects, in EM subjects with moderate (Child-Pugh Class B) (2-fold increase) and severe (Child-Pugh Class C) (4-fold increase) hepatic insufficiency. Dosage adjustment is recommended for patients with moderate or severe hepatic insufficiency [see Dosage and Administration (2.3)].

8.7 Renal Insufficiency

EM subjects with end stage renal disease had higher systemic exposure to atomoxetine than healthy subjects (about a 65% increase), but there was no difference when exposure was corrected for mg/kg dose. STRATTERA can therefore be administered to ADHD patients with end stage renal disease or lesser degrees of renal insufficiency using the normal dosing regimen.

8.8 Gender

Gender did not influence atomoxetine disposition.

8.9 Ethnic Origin

Ethnic origin did not influence atomoxetine disposition (except that PMs are more common in Caucasians).

8.10 Patients with Concomitant Illness

Tics in patients with ADHD and comorbid Tourette's Disorder—Atomoxetine administered in a flexible dose range of 0.5 to 1.5 mg/kg/day (mean dose of 1.3 mg/kg/day) and placebo were compared in 148 randomized pediatric (age 7-17 years) subjects with a DSM-IV diagnosis of ADHD and comorbid tic disorder in an 18 week, double-blind, placebo-controlled study in which the majority (80%) enrolled in this trial with Tourette's Disorder (Tourette's Disorder: 116 subjects; chronic motor tic disorder: 29 subjects). A non-inferiority analysis revealed that STRATTERA did not worsen tics in these patients as determined by the Yale Global Tic Severity Scale Total Score (YGTSS). Out of 148 patients who entered the acute treatment phase, 103 (69.6%) patients discontinued the study. The primary reason for discontinuation in both the atomoxetine (38 of 76 patients, 50.0%) and placebo (45 of 72 patients, 62.5%) treatment groups was identified as lack of efficacy with most of the patients discontinuing at Week 12. This was the first visit where patients with a CGI-S ≥4 could also meet the criteria for "clinical non-responder" (CGI-S remained the same or increased from study baseline) and be eligible to enter an open-label extension study with atomoxetine.

Anxiety in patients with ADHD and comorbid Anxiety Disorders—In two post-marketing, double-blind, placebo-controlled trials, it has been demonstrated that treating patients with ADHD and comorbid anxiety disorders with STRATTERA does not worsen their anxiety.

In a 12-week double-blind, placebo-controlled trial, 176 patients, aged 8-17, who met DSM-IV criteria for ADHD and at least one of the anxiety disorders of separation anxiety disorder, generalized anxiety disorder or social phobia were randomized. Following a 2-week double-blind placebo lead-in, STRATTERA was initiated at 0.8 mg/kg/day with increase to a target dose of 1.2 mg/kg/day (median dose 1.30 mg/kg/day +/- 0.29 mg/kg/day). STRATTERA did not worsen anxiety in these patients as determined by the Pediatric Anxiety Rating Scale (PARS). Of the 158 patients who completed the double-blind placebo lead-in, 26 (16%) patients discontinued the study.

In a separate 16-week, double-blind, placebo-controlled trial, 442 patients aged 18-65, who met DSM-IV criteria for adult ADHD and social anxiety disorder (23% of whom also had Generalized Anxiety Disorder) were randomized. Following a 2-week double-blind placebo lead-in, STRATTERA was initiated at 40 mg/day to a maximum dose of 100 mg/day (mean daily dose 83 mg/day +/- 19.5 mg/day). STRATTERA did not worsen anxiety in these patients as determined by the Liebowitz Social Anxiety Scale (LSAS). Of the 436 patients who completed the double-blind placebo lead-in, 172 (39.4%) patients discontinued the study.

9 DRUG ABUSE AND DEPENDENCE

9.1 Controlled Substance

STRATTERA is not a controlled substance.

9.2 Abuse

In a randomized, double-blind, placebo-controlled, abuse-potential study in adults comparing effects of STRATTERA and placebo, STRATTERA was not associated with a pattern of response that suggested stimulant or euphoriant properties.

9.3 Dependence

Clinical study data in over 2000 children, adolescents, and adults with ADHD and over 1200 adults with depression showed only isolated incidents of drug diversion or inappropriate self-administration associated with STRATTERA. There was no evidence of symptom rebound or adverse reactions suggesting a drug-discontinuation or withdrawal syndrome.

Animal Experience—Drug discrimination studies in rats and monkeys showed inconsistent stimulus generalization between atomoxetine and cocaine.

10 OVERDOSAGE

10.1 Human Experience

No fatal overdoses occurred in clinical trials. There is limited clinical trial experience with STRATTERA overdose. During postmarketing, there have been fatalities reported involving a mixed ingestion overdose of STRATTERA and at least one other drug. There have been no reports of death involving overdose of STRATTERA alone, including intentional overdoses at amounts up to 1400 mg. In some cases of overdose involving STRATTERA, seizures have been reported. The most commonly reported symptoms accompanying acute and chronic overdoses of STRATTERA were somnolence, agitation, hyperactivity, abnormal behavior, and gastrointestinal symptoms. Signs and symptoms consistent with mild to moderate sympathetic nervous system activation (e.g., mydriasis, tachycardia, dry mouth) have also been observed. Less commonly, there have been reports of QT prolongation and mental changes, including disorientation and hallucinations.

10.2 Management of Overdose

An airway should be established. Monitoring of cardiac and vital signs is recommended, along with appropriate symptomatic and supportive measures. Gastric lavage may be indicated if performed soon after ingestion. Activated charcoal may be useful in limiting absorption. Because atomoxetine is highly protein–bound, dialysis is not likely to be useful in the treatment of overdose.

11 DESCRIPTION

STRATTERA® (atomoxetine HCl) is a selective norepinephrine reuptake inhibitor. Atomoxetine HCl is the *R*(-) isomer as determined by x–ray diffraction. The chemical designation is (-)-*N*-Methyl-3-phenyl-3-(*o*-tolyloxy)-propylamine hydrochloride. The molecular formula is $C_{17}H_{21}NO \bullet HCl$, which corresponds to a molecular weight of 291.82. The chemical structure is:

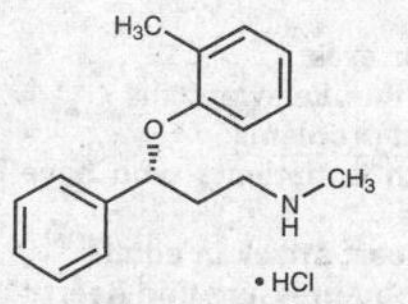

Atomoxetine HCl is a white to practically white solid, which has a solubility of 27.8 mg/mL in water.

STRATTERA capsules are intended for oral administration only.

Each capsule contains atomoxetine HCl equivalent to 10, 18, 25, 40, 60, 80, or 100 mg of atomoxetine. The capsules also contain pregelatinized starch and dimethicone. The capsule shells contain gelatin, sodium lauryl sulfate, and other inactive ingredients. The capsule shells also contain one or more of the following:

FD&C Blue No. 2, synthetic yellow iron oxide, titanium dioxide, red iron oxide. The capsules are imprinted with edible black ink.

12 CLINICAL PHARMACOLOGY

12.1 Mechanism of Action

The precise mechanism by which atomoxetine produces its therapeutic effects in Attention–Deficit/Hyperactivity Disorder (ADHD) is unknown, but is thought to be related to selective inhibition of the pre–synaptic norepinephrine transporter, as determined in ex vivo uptake and neurotransmitter depletion studies.

12.2 Pharmacodynamics

An exposure–response analysis encompassing doses of atomoxetine (0.5, 1.2 or 1.8 mg/kg/day) or placebo demonstrated atomoxetine exposure correlates with efficacy as measured by the Attention–Deficit/Hyperactivity Disorder Rating Scale–IV–Parent Version: Investigator administered and scored. The exposure-efficacy relationship was similar to that observed between dose and efficacy with median exposures at the two highest doses resulting in near maximal changes from baseline *[see Clinical Studies (14.2)]*.

12.3 Pharmacokinetics

Atomoxetine is well–absorbed after oral administration and is minimally affected by food. It is eliminated primarily by oxidative metabolism through the cytochrome P450 2D6 (CYP2D6) enzymatic pathway and subsequent glucuronidation. Atomoxetine has a half–life of about 5 hours. A fraction of the population (about 7% of Caucasians and 2% of African Americans) are poor metabolizers (PMs) of CYP2D6 metabolized drugs. These individuals have reduced activity in this pathway resulting in 10–fold higher AUCs, 5–fold higher peak plasma concentrations, and slower elimination (plasma half–life of about 24 hours) of atomoxetine compared with people with normal activity [extensive metabolizers (EMs)]. Drugs that inhibit CYP2D6, such as fluoxetine, paroxetine, and quinidine, cause similar increases in exposure.

The pharmacokinetics of atomoxetine have been evaluated in more than 400 children and adolescents in selected clinical trials, primarily using population pharmacokinetic studies. Single–dose and steady–state individual pharmacokinetic data were also obtained in children, adolescents, and adults. When doses were normalized to a mg/kg basis, similar half–life, C_{max}, and AUC values were observed in children, adolescents, and adults. Clearance and volume of distribution after adjustment for body weight were also similar.

Absorption and distribution—Atomoxetine is rapidly absorbed after oral administration, with absolute bioavailability of about 63% in EMs and 94% in PMs. Maximal plasma concentrations (C_{max}) are reached approximately 1 to 2 hours after dosing.

STRATTERA can be administered with or without food. Administration of STRATTERA with a standard high–fat meal in adults did not affect the extent of oral absorption of atomoxetine (AUC), but did decrease the rate of absorption, resulting in a 37% lower C_{max}, and delayed T_{max} by 3 hours. In clinical trials with children and adolescents, administration of STRATTERA with food resulted in a 9% lower C_{max}. The steady–state volume of distribution after intravenous administration is 0.85 L/kg indicating that atomoxetine distributes primarily into total body water. Volume of distribution is similar across the patient weight range after normalizing for body weight.

At therapeutic concentrations, 98% of atomoxetine in plasma is bound to protein, primarily albumin.

Metabolism and elimination—Atomoxetine is metabolized primarily through the CYP2D6 enzymatic pathway. People with reduced activity in this pathway (PMs) have higher plasma concentrations of atomoxetine compared with people with normal activity (EMs). For PMs, AUC of atomoxetine is approximately 10–fold and $C_{ss,max}$ is about 5–fold greater than EMs. Laboratory tests are available to identify CYP2D6 PMs. Coadministration of STRATTERA with potent inhibitors of CYP2D6, such as fluoxetine, paroxetine, or quinidine, results in a substantial increase in atomoxetine plasma exposure, and dosing adjustment may be necessary *[see Warnings and Precautions (5.13)]*. Atomoxetine did not inhibit or induce the CYP2D6 pathway.

The major oxidative metabolite formed, regardless of CYP2D6 status, is 4–hydroxyatomoxetine, which is glucuronidated. 4–Hydroxyatomoxetine is equipotent to atomoxetine as an inhibitor of the norepinephrine transporter but circulates in plasma at much lower concentrations (1% of atomoxetine concentration in EMs and 0.1% of atomoxetine concentration in PMs). 4–Hydroxyatomoxetine is primarily formed by CYP2D6, but in PMs, 4–hydroxyatomoxetine is formed at a slower rate by several other cytochrome P450 enzymes. N–Desmethylatomoxetine is formed by CYP2C19 and other cytochrome P450 enzymes, but has substantially less pharmacological activity compared with atomoxetine and circulates in plasma at lower concentrations (5% of atomoxetine concentration in EMs and 45% of atomoxetine concentration in PMs).

Mean apparent plasma clearance of atomoxetine after oral administration in adult EMs is 0.35 L/hr/kg and the mean half–life is 5.2 hours. Following oral administration of atomoxetine to PMs, mean apparent plasma clearance is 0.03 L/hr/kg and mean half–life is 21.6 hours. For PMs, AUC of atomoxetine is approximately 10–fold and $C_{ss,max}$ is about 5–fold greater than EMs. The elimination half–life of 4–hydroxyatomoxetine is similar to that of N–desmethylatomoxetine (6 to 8 hours) in EM subjects, while the half–life of N–desmethylatomoxetine is much longer in PM subjects (34 to 40 hours).

Atomoxetine is excreted primarily as 4–hydroxyatomoxetine-*O*-glucuronide, mainly in the urine (greater than 80% of the dose) and to a lesser extent in the feces (less than 17% of the dose). Only a small fraction of the STRATTERA dose is excreted as unchanged atomoxetine (less than 3% of the dose), indicating extensive biotransformation.

[See Use In Specific Populations (8.4, 8.5, 8.6, 8.7, 8.8, 8.9)].

13 NONCLINICAL TOXICOLOGY

13.1 Carcinogenesis, Mutagenesis, Impairment of Fertility

Carcinogenesis—Atomoxetine HCl was not carcinogenic in rats and mice when given in the dict for 2 years at time–weighted average doses up to 47 and 458 mg/kg/day, respectively. The highest dose used in rats is approximately 8 and 5 times the maximum human dose in children and adults, respectively, on a mg/m^2 basis. Plasma levels (AUC) of atomoxetine at this dose in rats are estimated to be 1.8 times (extensive metabolizers) or 0.2 times (poor metabolizers) those in humans receiving the maximum human dose. The highest dose used in mice is approximately 39 and 26 times the maximum human dose in children and adults, respectively, on a mg/m^2 basis.

Mutagenesis—Atomoxetine HCl was negative in a battery of genotoxicity studies that included a reverse point mutation assay (Ames Test), an in vitro mouse lymphoma assay, a chromosomal aberration test in Chinese hamster ovary cells, an unscheduled DNA synthesis test in rat hepatocytes, and an in vivo micronucleus test in mice. However, there was a slight increase in the percentage of Chinese hamster ovary cells with diplochromosomes, suggesting endoreduplication (numerical aberration).

The metabolite N–desmethylatomoxetine HCl was negative in the Ames Test, mouse lymphoma assay, and unscheduled DNA synthesis test.

Impairment of fertility—Atomoxetine HCl did not impair fertility in rats when given in the diet at doses of up to 57 mg/kg/day, which is approximately 6 times the maximum human dose on a mg/m^2 basis.

14 CLINICAL STUDIES

14.1 ADHD studies in Children and Adolescents

Acute Studies—The effectiveness of STRATTERA in the treatment of ADHD was established in 4 randomized, double–blind, placebo–controlled studies of pediatric patients (ages 6 to 18). Approximately one–third of the patients met DSM–IV criteria for inattentive subtype and two–thirds met criteria for both inattentive and hyperactive/impulsive subtypes.

Signs and symptoms of ADHD were evaluated by a comparison of mean change from baseline to endpoint for STRATTERA- and placebo–treated patients using an intent–to–treat analysis of the primary outcome measure, the investigator administered and scored ADHD Rating Scale–IV–Parent Version (ADHDRS) total score including hyperactive/impulsive and inattentive subscales. Each item on the ADHDRS maps directly to one symptom criterion for ADHD in the DSM–IV.

In Study 1, an 8–week randomized, double–blind, placebo–controlled, dose–response, acute treatment study of children and adolescents aged 8 to 18 (N=297), patients received either a fixed dose of STRATTERA (0.5, 1.2, or 1.8 mg/kg/day) or placebo. STRATTERA was administered as a divided dose in the early morning and late afternoon/early evening. At the 2 higher doses, improvements in ADHD symptoms were statistically significantly superior in STRATTERA–treated patients compared with placebo–treated patients as measured on the ADHDRS scale. The 1.8 mg/kg/day STRATTERA dose did not provide any additional benefit over that observed with the 1.2 mg/kg/day dose. The 0.5 mg/kg/day STRATTERA dose was not superior to placebo.

In Study 2, a 6–week randomized, double–blind, placebo–controlled, acute treatment study of children and adolescents aged 6 to 16 (N=171), patients received either STRATTERA or placebo. STRATTERA was administered as a single dose in the early morning and titrated on a weight–adjusted basis according to clinical response, up to a maximum dose of 1.5 mg/kg/day. The mean final dose of STRATTERA was approximately 1.3 mg/kg/day. ADHD symptoms were statistically significantly improved on STRATTERA compared with placebo, as measured on the ADHDRS scale. This study shows that STRATTERA is effective when administered once daily in the morning.

In 2 identical, 9–week, acute, randomized, double–blind, placebo–controlled studies of children aged 7 to 13 (Study 3, N=147; Study 4, N=144), STRATTERA and methylphenidate were compared with placebo. STRATTERA was administered as a divided dose in the early morning and late afternoon (after school) and titrated on a weight–adjusted basis according to clinical response. The maximum recommended STRATTERA dose was 2.0 mg/kg/day. The mean final dose of STRATTERA for both studies was approximately 1.6 mg/kg/day. In both studies, ADHD symptoms statistically significantly improved more on STRATTERA than on placebo, as measured on the ADHDRS scale.

Examination of population subsets based on gender and age (<12 and 12 to 17) did not reveal any differential responsiveness on the basis of these subgroupings. There was not sufficient exposure of ethnic groups other than Caucasian to allow exploration of differences in these subgroups.

Maintenance Study—The effectiveness of STRATTERA in the maintenance treatment of ADHD was established in an outpatient study of children and adolescents (ages 6-15 years). Patients meeting DSM-IV criteria for ADHD who showed continuous response for about 4 weeks during an initial 10 week open-label treatment phase with STRATTERA (1.2 to 1.8 mg/kg/day) were randomized to continuation of their current dose of STRATTERA (N=292) or to placebo (N=124) under double-blind treatment for observation of relapse. Response during the open-label phase was defined as CGI-ADHD-S score ≤2 and a reduction of at least 25% from baseline in ADHDRS-IV-Parent:Inv total score. Patients who were assigned to STRATTERA and showed continuous response for approximately 8 months during the first double-blind treatment phase were again randomized to continuation of their current dose of STRATTERA (N=81) or to placebo (N=82) under double-blind treatment for observation of relapse. Relapse during the double-blind phase was defined as CGI-ADHD-S score increases of at least 2 from the end of open-label phase and ADHDRS-IV-Parent:Inv total score returns to ≥90% of study entry score for 2 consecutive visits. In both double-blind phases, patients receiving continued STRATTERA treatment experienced significantly longer times to relapse than those receiving placebo.

14.2 ADHD studies in Adults

The effectiveness of STRATTERA in the treatment of ADHD was established in 2 randomized, double–blind, placebo–controlled clinical studies of adult patients, age 18 and older, who met DSM–IV criteria for ADHD.

Signs and symptoms of ADHD were evaluated using the investigator–administered Conners Adult ADHD Rating Scale Screening Version (CAARS), a 30–item scale. The primary effectiveness measure was the 18–item Total ADHD Symptom score (the sum of the inattentive and hyperactivity/impulsivity subscales from the CAARS) evaluated by a comparison of mean change from baseline to endpoint using an intent–to–treat analysis.

In 2 identical, 10–week, randomized, double–blind, placebo–controlled acute treatment studies (Study 5, N=280; Study 6, N=256), patients received either STRATTERA or placebo. STRATTERA was administered as

STRATTERA® Capsules	10 mg*	18 mg*	25 mg*	40 mg*	60 mg*	80 mg*	100 mg*
Color	Opaque White, Opaque White	Gold, Opaque White	Opaque Blue, Opaque White	Opaque Blue, Opaque Blue	Opaque Blue, Gold	Opaque Brown, Opaque White	Opaque Brown, Opaque Brown
Identification	LILLY 3227 10 mg	LILLY 3238 18 mg	LILLY 3228 25 mg	LILLY 3229 40 mg	LILLY 3239 60 mg	LILLY 3250 80 mg	LILLY 3251 100 mg
NDC Codes: Bottles of 30	0002-3227-30	0002-3238-30	0002-3228-30	0002-3229-30	0002-3239-30	0002-3250-30	0002-3251-30

*Atomoxetine base equivalent.

a divided dose in the early morning and late afternoon/early evening and titrated according to clinical response in a range of 60 to 120 mg/day. The mean final dose of STRATTERA for both studies was approximately 95 mg/day. In both studies, ADHD symptoms were statistically significantly improved on STRATTERA, as measured on the ADHD Symptom score from the CAARS scale.

Examination of population subsets based on gender and age (<42 and ≥42) did not reveal any differential responsiveness on the basis of these subgroupings. There was not sufficient exposure of ethnic groups other than Caucasian to allow exploration of differences in these subgroups.

16 HOW SUPPLIED/STORAGE AND HANDLING

16.1 How Supplied
[See table above]

16.2 Storage and Handling
Store at 25°C (77°F); excursions permitted to 15° to 30°C (59° to 86°F) [see USP Controlled Room Temperature].

17 PATIENT COUNSELING INFORMATION
See FDA-approved Medication Guide.

17.1 General Information
Physicians should instruct their patients to read the Medication Guide before starting therapy with STRATTERA and to reread it each time the prescription is renewed.

Prescribers or other health professionals should inform patients, their families, and their caregivers about the benefits and risks associated with treatment with STRATTERA and should counsel them in its appropriate use. The prescriber or health professional should instruct patients, their families, and their caregivers to read the Medication Guide and should assist them in understanding its contents. Patients should be given the opportunity to discuss the contents of the Medication Guide and to obtain answers to any questions they may have.

Patients should be advised of the following issues and asked to alert their prescriber if these occur while taking STRATTERA.

17.2 Suicide Risk
Patients, their families, and their caregivers should be encouraged to be alert to the emergence of anxiety, agitation, panic attacks, insomnia, irritability, hostility, aggressiveness, impulsivity, akathisia (psychomotor restlessness), hypomania, mania, other unusual changes in behavior, depression, and suicidal ideation, especially early during STRATTERA treatment and when the dose is adjusted. Families and caregivers of patients should be advised to observe for the emergence of such symptoms on a day-to-day basis, since changes may be abrupt. Such symptoms should be reported to the patient's prescriber or health professional, especially if they are severe, abrupt in onset, or were not part of the patient's presenting symptoms. Symptoms such as these may be associated with an increased risk for suicidal thinking and behavior and indicate a need for very close monitoring and possibly changes in the medication.

17.3 Severe Liver Injury
Patients initiating STRATTERA should be cautioned that severe liver injury may develop. Patients should be instructed to contact their physician immediately should they develop pruritus, dark urine, jaundice, right upper quadrant tenderness, or unexplained "flu-like" symptoms [see Warnings and Precautions (5.2)].

17.4 Aggression or Hostility
Patients should be instructed to call their doctor as soon as possible should they notice an increase in aggression or hostility.

17.5 Priapism
Rare postmarketing cases of priapism, defined as painful and nonpainful penile erection lasting more than 4 hours, have been reported for pediatric and adult patients treated with STRATTERA. The parents or guardians of pediatric patients taking STRATTERA and adult patients taking STRATTERA should be instructed that priapism requires prompt medical attention.

17.6 Ocular Irritant
STRATTERA is an ocular irritant. STRATTERA capsules are not intended to be opened. In the event of capsule content coming in contact with the eye, the affected eye should be flushed immediately with water, and medical advice obtained. Hands and any potentially contaminated surfaces should be washed as soon as possible.

17.7 Drug-Drug Interaction
Patients should be instructed to consult a physician if they are taking or plan to take any prescription or over-the-counter medicines, dietary supplements, or herbal remedies.

17.8 Pregnancy
Patients should be instructed to consult a physician if they are nursing, pregnant, or thinking of becoming pregnant while taking STRATTERA.

17.9 Food
Patients may take STRATTERA with or without food.

17.10 Missed Dose
If patients miss a dose, they should be instructed to take it as soon as possible, but should not take more than the prescribed total daily amount of STRATTERA in any 24-hour period.

17.11 Interference with Psychomotor Performance
Patients should be instructed to use caution when driving a car or operating hazardous machinery until they are reasonably certain that their performance is not affected by atomoxetine.

Literature revised June 3, 2009
Eli Lilly and Company
Indianapolis, IN 46285, USA
Copyright © 2002, 2009, Eli Lilly and Company. All rights reserved.
PV 6264 AMP
www.strattera.com

MEDICATION GUIDE
STRATTERA® (Stra-TAIR-a)
(atomoxetine hydrochloride)

Read the Medication Guide that comes with STRATTERA® before you or your child starts taking it and each time you get a refill. There may be new information. This Medication Guide does not take the place of talking to your doctor about your treatment or your child's treatment with STRATTERA.

What is the most important information I should know about STRATTERA?
The following have been reported with use of STRATTERA:
1. Suicidal thoughts and actions in children and teenagers: Children and teenagers sometimes think about suicide, and many report trying to kill themselves. Results from STRATTERA clinical studies with over 2200 child or teenage ADHD patients suggest that some children and teenagers may have a higher chance of having suicidal thoughts or actions. Although no suicides occurred in these studies, 4 out of every 1000 patients developed suicidal thoughts. Tell your child or teenager's doctor if your child or teenager (or there is a family history of):
- has bipolar illness (manic-depressive illness)
- had suicide thoughts or actions before starting STRATTERA

The chance for suicidal thoughts and actions may be higher:
- early during STRATTERA treatment
- during dose adjustments

Prevent suicidal thoughts and action in your child or teenager by:
- paying close attention to your child or teenager's moods, behaviors, thoughts, and feelings during STRATTERA treatment
- keeping all follow-up visits with your child or teenager's doctor as scheduled

Watch for the following signs in your child or teenager during STRATTERA treatment:
- anxiety
- agitation
- panic attacks
- trouble sleeping
- irritability
- hostility
- aggressiveness
- impulsivity
- restlessness
- mania
- depression
- suicide thoughts

Call your child or teenager's doctor right away if they have any of the above signs, especially if they are new, sudden, or severe. Your child or teenager may need to be closely watched for suicidal thoughts and actions or need a change in medicine.

2. Severe liver damage:
STRATTERA can cause liver injury in some patients. Call your doctor right away if you or your child has the following signs of liver problems:
- itching
- right upper belly pain
- dark urine
- yellow skin or eyes
- unexplained flu-like symptoms

3. Heart-related problems:
- **sudden death in patients who have heart problems or heart defects**
- **stroke and heart attack in adults**
- **increased blood pressure and heart rate**

Tell your doctor if you or your child has any heart problems, heart defects, high blood pressure, or a family history of these problems. Your doctor should check you or your child carefully for heart problems before starting STRATTERA. Your doctor should check your blood pressure or your child's blood pressure and heart rate regularly during treatment with STRATTERA.

Call your doctor right away if you or your child has any signs of heart problems such as chest pain, shortness of breath, or fainting while taking STRATTERA.

4. New mental (psychiatric) problems in children and teenagers:
- new psychotic symptoms (such as hearing voices, believing things that are not true, being suspicious) or new manic symptoms

Call your child or teenager's doctor right away about any new mental symptoms because adjusting or stopping STRATTERA treatment may need to be considered.

What is STRATTERA?
STRATTERA is a selective norepinephrine reuptake inhibitor medicine. It is used for the treatment of attention deficit and hyperactivity disorder (ADHD). STRATTERA may help increase attention and decrease impulsiveness and hyperactivity in patients with ADHD.

STRATTERA should be used as a part of a total treatment program for ADHD that may include counseling or other therapies.

STRATTERA has not been studied in children less than 6 years old.

Who should not take STRATTERA?
STRATTERA should not be taken if you or your child:
- are taking or have taken within the past 14 days an antidepression medicine called a monoamine oxidase inhibitor or MAOI. Some names of MAOI medicines are Nardil® (phenelzine sulfate), Parnate® (tranylcypromine sulfate) and Emsam® (selegiline transdermal system).
- have an eye problem called narrow angle glaucoma
- are allergic to anything in STRATTERA. See the end of this Medication Guide for a complete list of ingredients.

STRATTERA may not be right for you or your child. Before starting STRATTERA tell your doctor or your child's doctor about all health conditions (or a family history of) including:
- have or had suicide thoughts or actions
- heart problems, heart defects, irregular heart beat, high blood pressure, or low blood pressure
- mental problems, psychosis, mania, bipolar illness, or depression
- liver problems

Tell your doctor if you or your child is pregnant, planning to become pregnant, or breastfeeding.

Can STRATTERA be taken with other medicines?
Tell your doctor about all the medicines that you or your child takes including prescription and nonprescription medicines, vitamins, and herbal supplements. STRATTERA and some medicines may interact with each other and cause serious side effects. Your doctor will decide whether STRATTERA can be taken with other medicines.

Especially tell your doctor if you or your child takes:
- asthma medicines
- anti-depression medicines including MAOIs
- blood pressure medicines
- cold or allergy medicines that contain decongestants

Know the medicines that you or your child takes. Keep a list of your medicines with you to show your doctor and pharmacist.

Do not start any new medicine while taking STRATTERA without talking to your doctor first.

How should STRATTERA be taken?
- **Take STRATTERA exactly as prescribed. STRATTERA comes in different dose strength capsules. Your doctor may adjust the dose until it is right for you or your child.**

- Do not chew, crush, or open the capsules. Swallow STRATTERA capsules whole with water or other liquids. Tell your doctor if you or your child cannot swallow STRATTERA whole. A different medicine may need to be prescribed.
- Avoid touching a broken STRATTERA capsule. Wash hands and surfaces that touched an open STRATTERA capsule. If any of the powder gets in your eyes or your child's eyes, rinse them with water right away and call your doctor.
- STRATTERA can be taken with or without food.
- STRATTERA is usually taken once or twice a day. Take STRATTERA at the same time each day to help you remember. If you miss a dose of STRATTERA, take it as soon as you remember that day. If you miss a day of STRATTERA, do not double your dose the next day. Just skip the day you missed.
- From time to time, your doctor may stop STRATTERA treatment for a while to check ADHD symptoms.
- Your doctor may do regular checks of the blood, heart, and blood pressure while taking STRATTERA. Children should have their height and weight checked often while taking STRATTERA. STRATTERA treatment may be stopped if a problem is found during these check-ups.
- If you or your child takes too much STRATTERA or overdoses, call your doctor or poison control center right away, or get emergency treatment.

What are possible side effects of STRATTERA?

See "What is the most important information I should know about STRATTERA?" for information on reported suicidal thoughts and actions, other mental problems, severe liver damage, and heart problems.

Other serious side effects include:

- serious allergic reactions (call your doctor if you see swelling, hives, or experience other allergic reactions)
- slowing of growth (height and weight) in children
- problems passing urine including
  - trouble starting or keeping a urine stream
  - cannot fully empty the bladder

Common side effects in children and teenagers include:

- upset stomach
- decreased appetite
- nausea or vomiting
- dizziness
- tiredness
- mood swings

Common side effects in adults include:

- constipation
- dry mouth
- nausea
- decreased appetite
- dizziness
- trouble sleeping
- sexual side effects
- menstrual cramps
- problems passing urine

Other information for children, teenagers, and adults:

- Erections that won't go away (priapism) have occurred rarely during treatment with STRATTERA. If you have an erection that lasts more than 4 hours, seek medical help right away. Because of the potential for lasting damage, including the potential inability to have erections, priapism should be evaluated by a doctor immediately.
- STRATTERA may affect your ability or your child's ability to drive or operate heavy machinery. Be careful until you know how STRATTERA affects you or your child.
- Talk to your doctor if you or your child has side effects that are bothersome or do not go away.

This is not a complete list of possible side effects. Call your doctor for medical advice about side effects. You may report side effects to FDA at 1-800-FDA-1088.

How should I store STRATTERA?

- Store STRATTERA in a safe place at room temperature, 59 to 86°F (15 to 30°C).
- Keep STRATTERA and all medicines out of the reach of children.

General information about STRATTERA

Medicines are sometimes prescribed for purposes other than those listed in a Medication Guide. Do not use STRATTERA for a condition for which it was not prescribed. Do not give STRATTERA to other people, even if they have the same condition. It may harm them.

This Medication Guide summarizes the most important information about STRATTERA. If you would like more information, talk with your doctor. You can ask your doctor or pharmacist for information about STRATTERA that was written for healthcare professionals. For more information about STRATTERA call 1–800–Lilly–Rx (1–800–545–5979) or visit www.strattera.com.

What are the ingredients in STRATTERA?

Active ingredient: atomoxetine hydrochloride.

Inactive ingredients: pregelatinized starch, dimethicone, gelatin, sodium lauryl sulfate, FD&C Blue No. 2, synthetic

yellow iron oxide, titanium dioxide, red iron oxide, and edible black ink.

Nardil® is a registered trademark of Pfizer Inc.

Parnate® is a registered trademark of GlaxoSmithKline.

Emsam® is a registered trademark of Somerset Pharmaceuticals Inc.

This Medication Guide has been approved by the US Food and Drug Administration.

Patient Information revised July 23, 2008

Eli Lilly and Company

Indianapolis, IN 46285, USA

www.strattera.com

Copyright © 2003, 2008, Eli Lilly and Company. All rights reserved.

PV 5854 AMP

Shown in Product Identification Guide, page 311

SYMBYAX® ℞

[*sim-bee-ax*]

(olanzapine and fluoxetine hydrochloride) capsule for oral use

HIGHLIGHTS OF PRESCRIBING INFORMATION

These highlights do not include all the information needed to use SYMBYAX safely and effectively. See full prescribing information for SYMBYAX.

SYMBYAX (olanzapine and fluoxetine hydrochloride) capsule for oral use

Initial U.S. Approval: 2003

WARNING: SUICIDALITY AND ANTIDEPRESSANT DRUGS AND INCREASED MORTALITY IN ELDERLY PATIENTS WITH DEMENTIA-RELATED PSYCHOSIS

See full prescribing information for complete boxed warning.

- **Increased risk of suicidal thinking and behavior in children, adolescents, and young adults taking antidepressants for Major Depressive Disorder (MDD) and other psychiatric disorders. SYMBYAX is not approved for use in children and adolescents (5.1, 8.4, 17.2).**
- **Elderly patients with dementia-related psychosis treated with antipsychotic drugs are at an increased risk of death. SYMBYAX is not approved for the treatment of patients with dementia-related psychosis (5.2, 5.19, 17.3).**

———RECENT MAJOR CHANGES———

Indications and Usage:	
Depressive Episodes Associated with Bipolar I Disorder (1.1)	03/2009
Treatment Resistant Depression (1.2)	03/2009
Dosage and Administration:	
Depressive Episodes Associated with Bipolar I Disorder (2.1)	03/2009
Treatment Resistant Depression (2.2)	03/2009
Specific Populations (2.3)	03/2009
Warnings and Precautions:	
Hyperglycemia (5.4)	03/2009
Hyperlipidemia (5.5)	03/2009
Weight Gain (5.6)	03/2009
Serotonin Syndrome or Neuroleptic Malignant Syndrome (NMS)-like Reactions (5.7)	03/2009
Activation of Mania/Hypomania (5.9)	03/2009
Orthostatic Hypotension (5.11)	03/2009
Leukopenia, Neutropenia, and Agranulocytosis (5.12)	08/2009
Seizures (5.14)	03/2009
Hyponatremia (5.16)	03/2009
Potential for Cognitive and Motor Impairment (5.17)	03/2009
Use in Patients with Concomitant Illness (5.19)	03/2009
Hyperprolactinemia (5.20)	01/2010
Laboratory Tests (5.24)	03/2009

———INDICATIONS AND USAGE———

SYMBYAX® combines olanzapine, an atypical antipsychotic and fluoxetine, a selective serotonin reuptake inhibitor, indicated for acute treatment of:

- Depressive Episodes Associated with Bipolar I Disorder in adults (1.1)
- Treatment Resistant Depression (Major Depressive Disorder in adults who do not respond to 2 separate trials of different antidepressants of adequate dose and duration in the current episode) (1.2)

———DOSAGE AND ADMINISTRATION———

- Once daily in the evening, generally beginning with 6 mg/25 mg (2.1, 2.2)
- The starting dose of SYMBYAX 3 mg/25 mg–6 mg/25 mg should be used in patients predisposed to hypotensive reactions, hepatic impairment, or with potential for slowed metabolism. Escalate dose cautiously (2.3)
- Consider using a lower dose for pregnant women during the third trimester (2.3)
- Discontinue gradually (2.4)
- The safety of doses above 18 mg olanzapine with 75 mg fluoxetine has not been evaluated in clinical trials (2.1, 2.2)

———DOSAGE FORMS AND STRENGTHS———

- Capsules: 3 mg/25 mg, 6 mg/25 mg, 6 mg/50 mg, 12 mg/25 mg, and 12 mg/50 mg (mg equivalent olanzapine/mg equivalent fluoxetine) (3)

———CONTRAINDICATIONS———

- Do not use with an MAOI or within 14 days of discontinuing an MAOI due to risk of drug interaction. At least 5 weeks should be allowed after stopping SYMBYAX before starting treatment with an MAOI (4, 7.1)
- Do not use with pimozide due to risk of drug interaction or QT$_c$ prolongation (4, 7.9)
- Do not use with thioridazine due to QT$_c$ interval prolongation or potential for elevated thioridazine plasma levels. Do not use thioridazine within 5 weeks of discontinuing SYMBYAX (4, 7.9)

———WARNINGS AND PRECAUTIONS———

- *Clinical Worsening and Suicide Risk:* Monitor for clinical worsening and suicidal thinking and behavior (5.1)
- *Elderly Patients with Dementia-Related Psychosis:* Increased risk of death and increased incidence of cerebrovascular adverse events (e.g., stroke, transient ischemic attack) (5.2)
- *Neuroleptic Malignant Syndrome:* Manage with immediate discontinuation and close monitoring (5.3)
- *Hyperglycemia:* In some cases extreme and associated with ketoacidosis or hyperosmolar coma or death, has been reported in patients taking olanzapine. Patients taking SYMBYAX should be monitored for symptoms of hyperglycemia and undergo fasting blood glucose testing at the beginning of, and periodically during, treatment. (5.4)
- *Hyperlipidemia:* Undesirable alterations in lipids have been observed. Appropriate clinical monitoring is recommended, including fasting blood lipid testing at the beginning of, and periodically during, treatment (5.5)
- *Weight gain:* Potential consequences of weight gain should be considered. Patients should receive regular monitoring of weight (5.6)
- *Serotonin Syndrome and Neuroleptic Malignant Syndrome (NMS)-like Reactions:* Have been reported with SYMBYAX. Discontinue and initiate supportive treatment (5.7)
- *Allergic Reactions and Rash:* Discontinue upon appearance of rash or allergic phenomena (5.8)
- *Activation of Mania/Hypomania:* Screen for Bipolar Disorder and monitor for activation of mania/hypomania (5.9)
- *Tardive Dyskinesia:* Discontinue if clinically appropriate (5.10)
- *Orthostatic Hypotension:* Orthostatic hypotension associated with dizziness, tachycardia, bradycardia and, in some patients, syncope, may occur especially during initial dose titration. Use caution in patients with cardiovascular disease or cerebrovascular disease, and those conditions that could affect hemodynamic responses (5.11)
- *Leukopenia, Neutropenia, and Agranulocytosis:* Has been reported with antipsychotics, including SYMBYAX. Patients with a history of a clinically significant low white blood cell count (WBC) or drug induced leukopenia/neutropenia should have their complete blood count (CBC) monitored frequently during the first few months of therapy and discontinuation of SYMBYAX should be considered at the first sign of a clinically significant decline in WBC in the absence of other causative factors (5.12)
- *Seizures:* Use cautiously in patients with a history of seizures or with conditions that potentially lower the seizure threshold (5.14)
- *Abnormal Bleeding:* May increase the risk of bleeding. Use with NSAIDs, aspirin, warfarin, or drugs that affect coagulation may potentiate the risk of gastrointestinal or other bleeding (5.15)
- *Hyponatremia:* Has been reported with SYMBYAX in association with syndrome of inappropriate antidiuretic hormone (SIADH) (5.16)
- *Potential for Cognitive and Motor Impairment:* Has potential to impair judgment, thinking, and motor skills. Use caution when operating machinery (5.17)
- *Hyperprolactinemia:* May elevate prolactin levels (5.20)

- *Long Elimination Half-Life of Fluoxetine:* Changes in dose will not be fully reflected in plasma for several weeks (5.22)
- *Laboratory Tests:* Monitor fasting blood glucose and lipid profiles at the beginning of, and periodically during, treatment (5.24)

ADVERSE REACTIONS

Most common adverse reactions (≥5% and at least twice that for placebo) are disturbance in attention, dry mouth, fatigue, hypersomnia, increased appetite, peripheral edema, sedation, somnolence, tremor, vision blurred, and weight increased (6.1)

To report SUSPECTED ADVERSE REACTIONS, contact Eli Lilly and Company at 1-800-LillyRx (1-800-545-5979) or FDA at 1-800-FDA-1088 or www.fda.gov/medwatch

DRUG INTERACTIONS

- *Monoamine Oxidase Inhibitor (MAOI):* SYMBYAX is contraindicated for use with MAOI's, or within 14 days of discontinuing an MAOI due to risk of drug interaction. At least 5 weeks should be allowed after stopping SYMBYAX before starting treatment with an MAOI (4, 7.1)
- *Pimozide:* SYMBYAX is contraindicated for use with pimozide due to risk of drug interaction or QT_c prolongation (4, 7.9)
- *Thioridazine:* SYMBYAX is contraindicated for use with thioridazine due to QT_c interval prolongation or potential for elevated thioridazine plasma levels. Do not use thioridazine within 5 weeks of discontinuing SYMBYAX (4, 7.9)
- *Drugs Metabolized by CYP2D6:* Fluoxetine is a potent inhibitor of CYP2D6 enzyme pathway (7.9)
- *Tricyclic Antidepressants (TCAs):* Monitor TCA levels during coadministration with SYMBYAX or when SYMBYAX has been recently discontinued (7.9)
- *CNS Acting Drugs:* Caution is advised if the concomitant administration of SYMBYAX and other CNS-active drugs is required (7.2)
- *Antihypertensive Agent:* Enhanced antihypertensive effect (7.9)
- *Levodopa and Dopamine Agonists:* May antagonize levodopa/dopamine agonists (7.9)
- *Benzodiazepines:* May potentiate orthostatic hypotension and sedation (7.8, 7.9)
- *Clozapine:* May elevate clozapine levels (7.9)
- *Haloperidol:* Elevated haloperidol levels have been observed (7.9)
- *Carbamazepine:* Potential for elevated carbamazepine levels and clinical anticonvulsant toxicity (7.9)
- *Phenytoin:* Potential for elevated phenytoin levels and clinical anticonvulsant toxicity (7.9)
- *Alcohol:* May potentiate sedation and orthostatic hypotension (7.9)
- *Serotonergic Drugs:* Potential for Serotonin Syndrome (5.7, 7.3)
- *Triptans:* There have been rare postmarketing reports of Serotonin Syndrome with use of an SSRI and a triptan (5.7, 7.4)
- *Tryptophan:* Concomitant use with tryptophan is not recommended (5.7, 7.5)
- *Fluvoxamine:* May increase olanzapine levels; a lower dose of the olanzapine component of SYMBYAX should be considered (7.8)
- *Drugs that Interfere with Hemostasis (e.g., NSAIDs, Aspirin, Warfarin, etc.):* May potentiate the risk of bleeding (7.6)
- *Drugs Tightly Bound to Plasma Proteins:* Fluoxetine may cause shift in plasma concentrations (7.9)

USE IN SPECIFIC POPULATIONS

- *Pregnancy:* SYMBYAX should be used during pregnancy only if the potential benefit justifies the potential risk to the fetus (8.1)
- *Nursing Mothers:* Breast feeding is not recommended (8.3)
- *Pediatric Use:* Safety and effectiveness of SYMBYAX in children and adolescent patients have not been established (8.4)
- *Hepatic Impairment:* Use a lower or less frequent dose in patients with cirrhosis (8.6)

See 17 for PATIENT COUNSELING INFORMATION and Medication Guide

Revised: 01/2010

FULL PRESCRIBING INFORMATION: CONTENTS*

FULL PRESCRIBING INFORMATION

> **WARNING: SUICIDALITY AND ANTIDEPRESSANT DRUGS AND INCREASED MORTALITY IN ELDERLY PATIENTS WITH DEMENTIA-RELATED PSYCHOSIS**
> **Suicidality and Antidepressant Drugs**—Antidepressants increased the risk compared to placebo of suicidal thinking and behavior (suicidality) in children, adolescents, and young adults in short-term studies of Major Depressive Disorder (MDD) and other psychiatric disorders. Anyone considering the use of SYMBYAX or any other antidepressant in a child, adolescent, or young adult must balance this risk with the clinical need. Short-term studies did not show an increase in the risk of suicidality with antidepressants compared to placebo in adults beyond age 24; there was a reduction in risk with antidepressants compared to placebo in adults aged 65 and older. Depression and certain other psychiatric disorders are themselves associated with increases in the risk of suicide. Patients of all ages who are started on antidepressant therapy should be monitored appropriately and observed closely for clinical worsening, suicidality, or unusual changes in behavior. Families and caregivers should be advised of the need for close observation and communication with the prescriber. SYMBYAX is not approved for use in pediatric patients. *[See Warnings and Precautions (5.1), Use in Specific Populations (8.4), and Patient Counseling Information (17.2)].*
> **Increased Mortality in Elderly Patients with Dementia-Related Psychosis**—Elderly patients with dementia-related psychosis treated with antipsychotic drugs are at an increased risk of death. Analyses of seventeen placebo-controlled trials (modal duration of 10 weeks), largely in patients taking atypical antipsychotic drugs, revealed a risk of death in drug-treated patients of between 1.6 to 1.7 times the risk of death in placebo-treated patients. Over the course of a typical 10-week controlled trial, the rate of death in drug-treated patients was about 4.5%, compared to a rate of about 2.6% in the placebo group. Although the causes of death were varied, most of the deaths appeared to be either cardiovascular (e.g., heart failure, sudden death) or infectious (e.g., pneumonia) in nature. Observational studies suggest that, similar to atypical antipsychotic drugs, treatment with conventional antipsychotic drugs may increase mortality. The extent to which the findings of increased mortality in observational studies may be attributed to the antipsychotic drug as opposed to some characteristic(s) of the patients is not clear. SYMBYAX (olanzapine and fluoxetine HCl) is not approved for the treatment of patients with dementia-related psychosis *[see Warnings and Precautions (5.2, 5.19) and Patient Counseling Information (17.3)].*

1 INDICATIONS AND USAGE

1.1 Depressive Episodes Associated with Bipolar I Disorder

SYMBYAX is indicated for the acute treatment of depressive episodes associated with Bipolar I Disorder in adults *[see Clinical Studies (14.1)].*

1.2 Treatment Resistant Depression

SYMBYAX is indicated for the acute treatment of treatment resistant depression (Major Depressive Disorder in adults who do not respond to 2 separate trials of different antidepressants of adequate dose and duration in the current episode) *[see Clinical Studies (14.2)].*

2 DOSAGE AND ADMINISTRATION

2.1 Depressive Episodes Associated with Bipolar I Disorder

SYMBYAX should be administered once daily in the evening, generally beginning with the 6-mg/25-mg capsule. While food has no appreciable effect on the absorption of olanzapine and fluoxetine given individually, the effect of food on the absorption of SYMBYAX has not been studied. Dosage adjustments, if indicated, can be made according to efficacy and tolerability. Antidepressant efficacy was demonstrated with SYMBYAX in a dose range of olanzapine 6 to 12 mg and fluoxetine 25 to 50 mg *[see Clinical Studies (14.1)].* The safety of doses above 18 mg per 75 mg has not been evaluated in clinical studies.

While there is no body of evidence to answer the question of how long a patient treated with SYMBYAX should remain on it, it is generally accepted that Bipolar I Disorder, including the depressive episodes associated with Bipolar I Disorder, is a chronic illness requiring chronic treatment. The physician should periodically reexamine the need for continued pharmacotherapy.

2.2 Treatment Resistant Depression

SYMBYAX should be administered once daily in the evening, generally beginning with the 6-mg/25-mg capsule. While food has no appreciable effect on the absorption of olanzapine and fluoxetine given individually, the effect of food on the absorption of SYMBYAX has not been studied. Dosage adjustments, if indicated, can be made according to efficacy and tolerability. Antidepressant efficacy was demonstrated with SYMBYAX in a dose range of olanzapine 6 to 18 mg and fluoxetine 25 to 50 mg *[see Clinical Studies (14.2)]*. The safety of doses above 18 mg per 75 mg has not been evaluated in clinical studies.

While there is no body of evidence to answer the question of how long a patient treated with SYMBYAX should remain on it, it is generally accepted that treatment resistant depression (Major Depressive Disorder in adult patients who do not respond to 2 separate trials of different antidepressants of adequate dose and duration in the current episode) is a chronic illness requiring chronic treatment. The physician should periodically reexamine the need for continued pharmacotherapy.

2.3 Specific Populations

The starting dose of SYMBYAX 3 mg/25 mg to 6 mg/25 mg should be used for patients with a predisposition to hypotensive reactions, patients with hepatic impairment, or patients who exhibit a combination of factors that may slow the metabolism of SYMBYAX (female gender, geriatric age, nonsmoking status) or those patients who may be pharmacodynamically sensitive to olanzapine. Dosing modification may be necessary in patients who exhibit a combination of factors that may slow metabolism. When indicated, dose escalation should be performed with caution in these patients. SYMBYAX has not been systematically studied in patients >65 years of age or in patients <18 years of age *[see Warnings and Precautions (5.19), Use in Specific Populations (8.5), and Clinical Pharmacology (12.3, 12.4)]*.

Treatment of Pregnant Women During the Third Trimester—When treating pregnant women with fluoxetine, a component of SYMBYAX, during the third trimester, the physician should carefully consider the potential risks and potential benefits of treatment. Neonates exposed to SNRIs or SSRIs late in the third trimester have developed complications requiring prolonged hospitalizations, respiratory support, and tube feeding. The physician may consider using a lower dose in the third trimester *[see Use in Specific Populations (8.1)]*.

2.4 Discontinuation of Treatment with SYMBYAX

Symptoms associated with discontinuation of fluoxetine, a component of SYMBYAX, SNRIs, and SSRIs, have been reported *[see Warnings and Precautions (5.23)]*.

3 DOSAGE FORMS AND STRENGTHS

Capsules (mg equivalent olanzapine/mg equivalent fluoxetine):
- 3 mg/25 mg
- 6 mg/25 mg
- 6 mg/50 mg
- 12 mg/25 mg
- 12 mg/50 mg

4 CONTRAINDICATIONS

The use of SYMBYAX is contraindicated with the following:
- Monoamine Oxidase Inhibitors (MAOI)—*[see Drug Interactions (7.1)]*
- Pimozide—*[see Drug Interactions (7.9)]*
- Thioridazine—*[see Drug Interactions (7.9)]*

5 WARNINGS AND PRECAUTIONS

5.1 Clinical Worsening and Suicide Risk

Patients with Major Depressive Disorder (MDD), both adult and pediatric, may experience worsening of their depression and/or the emergence of suicidal ideation and behavior (suicidality) or unusual changes in behavior, whether or not they are taking antidepressant medications, and this risk may persist until significant remission occurs. Suicide is a known risk of depression and certain other psychiatric disorders, and these disorders themselves are the strongest predictors of suicide. There has been a long-standing concern, however, that antidepressants may have a role in inducing worsening of depression and the emergence of suicidality in certain patients during the early phases of treatment. Pooled analyses of short-term placebo-controlled trials of antidepressant drugs (SSRIs and others) showed that these drugs increase the risk of suicidal thinking and behavior (suicidality) in children, adolescents, and young adults (ages 18 to 24) with Major Depressive Disorder (MDD) and other psychiatric disorders. Short-term studies did not show an increase in the risk of suicidality with antidepressants compared to placebo in adults beyond age 24; there was a reduction with antidepressants compared to placebo in adults aged 65 and older.

Table 2: Changes in Random Glucose Levels from Adult SYMBYAX Studies

Laboratory Analyte	Category Change (at least once) from Baseline	Treatment Arm	Up to 12 weeks exposure: N	Up to 12 weeks exposure: Patients	At least 48 weeks exposure: N	At least 48 weeks exposure: Patients
Random Glucose	Normal to High (<140 mg/dL to ≥200 mg/dL)	Symbyax	609	2.3%	382	3.1%
		Placebo	346	0.3%	NA[a]	NA[a]
	Borderline to High (≥140 mg/dL and <200 mg/dL to ≥200 mg/dL)	Symbyax	44	34.1%	27	37.0%
		Placebo	28	3.6%	NA[a]	NA[a]

[a]Not Applicable.

The pooled analyses of placebo-controlled trials in children and adolescents with MDD, Obsessive Compulsive Disorder (OCD), or other psychiatric disorders included a total of 24 short-term trials of 9 antidepressant drugs in over 4400 patients. The pooled analyses of placebo-controlled trials in adults with MDD or other psychiatric disorders included a total of 295 short-term trials (median duration of 2 months) of 11 antidepressant drugs in over 77,000 patients. There was considerable variation in risk of suicidality among drugs, but a tendency toward an increase in the younger patients for almost all drugs studied. There were differences in absolute risk of suicidality across the different indications, with the highest incidence in MDD. The risk differences (drug versus placebo), however, were relatively stable within age strata and across indications. These risk differences (drug-placebo difference in the number of cases of suicidality per 1000 patients treated) are provided in Table 1.

Table 1: Suicidality per 1000 Patients Treated

Age Range	Drug-Placebo Difference in Number of Cases of Suicidality per 1000 Patients Treated
	Increases Compared to Placebo
<18	14 additional cases
18-24	5 additional cases
	Decreases Compared to Placebo
25-64	1 fewer case
≥65	6 fewer cases

No suicides occurred in any of the pediatric trials. There were suicides in the adult trials, but the number was not sufficient to reach any conclusion about drug effect on suicide.

It is unknown whether the suicidality risk extends to longer-term use, i.e., beyond several months. However, there is substantial evidence from placebo-controlled maintenance trials in adults with depression that the use of antidepressants can delay the recurrence of depression.

All patients being treated with antidepressants for any indication should be monitored appropriately and observed closely for clinical worsening, suicidality, and unusual changes in behavior, especially during the initial few months of a course of drug therapy, or at times of dose changes, either increases or decreases.

The following symptoms, anxiety, agitation, panic attacks, insomnia, irritability, hostility, aggressiveness, impulsivity, akathisia (psychomotor restlessness), hypomania, and mania, have been reported in adult and pediatric patients being treated with antidepressants for Major Depressive Disorder as well as for other indications, both psychiatric and nonpsychiatric. Although a causal link between the emergence of such symptoms and either the worsening of depression and/or the emergence of suicidal impulses has not been established, there is concern that such symptoms may represent precursors to emerging suicidality.

Consideration should be given to changing the therapeutic regimen, including possibly discontinuing the medication, in patients whose depression is persistently worse, or who are experiencing emergent suicidality or symptoms that might be precursors to worsening depression or suicidality, especially if these symptoms are severe, abrupt in onset, or were not part of the patient's presenting symptoms.

If the decision has been made to discontinue treatment, medication should be tapered, as rapidly as is feasible, but with recognition that abrupt discontinuation can be associated with certain symptoms *[see Warnings and Precautions (5.23)]*.

Families and caregivers of patients being treated with antidepressants for Major Depressive Disorder or other indications, both psychiatric and nonpsychiatric, should be alerted about the need to monitor patients for the emergence of agitation, irritability, unusual changes in behavior, and the other symptoms described above, as well as the emergence of suicidality, and to report such symptoms immediately to health care providers. Such monitoring should include daily observation by families and caregivers. Prescriptions for SYMBYAX should be written for the smallest quantity of capsules consistent with good patient management, in order to reduce the risk of overdose.

It should be noted that SYMBYAX is not approved for use in treating any indications in the pediatric population *[see Use in Specific Populations (8.4)]*.

5.2 Elderly Patients with Dementia-Related Psychosis

Increased Mortality—Elderly patients with dementia-related psychosis treated with antipsychotic drugs are at an increased risk of death. SYMBYAX is not approved for the treatment of patients with dementia-related psychosis *[see Boxed Warning, Warnings and Precautions (5.19), and Patient Counseling Information (17.3)]*.

In olanzapine placebo-controlled clinical trials of elderly patients with dementia-related psychosis, the incidence of death in olanzapine-treated patients was significantly greater than placebo-treated patients (3.5% vs 1.5%, respectively).

Cerebrovascular Adverse Events (CVAE), Including Stroke—Cerebrovascular adverse events (e.g., stroke, transient ischemic attack), including fatalities, were reported in patients in trials of olanzapine in elderly patients with dementia-related psychosis. In placebo-controlled trials, there was a significantly higher incidence of cerebrovascular adverse events in patients treated with olanzapine compared to patients treated with placebo. Olanzapine and SYMBYAX are not approved for the treatment of patients with dementia-related psychosis *[see Boxed Warning and Patient Counseling Information (17.3)]*.

5.3 Neuroleptic Malignant Syndrome (NMS)

A potentially fatal symptom complex sometimes referred to as NMS has been reported in association with administration of antipsychotic drugs, including olanzapine. Clinical manifestations of NMS are hyperpyrexia, muscle rigidity, altered mental status, and evidence of autonomic instability (irregular pulse or blood pressure, tachycardia, diaphoresis, and cardiac dysrhythmia). Additional signs may include elevated creatinine phosphokinase, myoglobinuria (rhabdomyolysis), and acute renal failure.

The diagnostic evaluation of patients with this syndrome is complicated. In arriving at a diagnosis, it is important to exclude cases where the clinical presentation includes both serious medical illness (e.g., pneumonia, systemic infection, etc.) and untreated or inadequately treated extrapyramidal signs and symptoms (EPS). Other important considerations in the differential diagnosis include central anticholinergic toxicity, heat stroke, drug fever, and primary central nervous system pathology.

The management of NMS should include: 1) immediate discontinuation of antipsychotic drugs and other drugs not essential to concurrent therapy, 2) intensive symptomatic treatment and medical monitoring, and 3) treatment of any concomitant serious medical problems for which specific treatments are available. There is no general agreement about specific pharmacological treatment regimens for NMS.

If after recovering from NMS, a patient requires treatment with an antipsychotic, the patient should be carefully mon-

Table 3: Changes in Fasting Glucose Levels from Adolescent Olanzapine Monotherapy Studies

Laboratory Analyte	Category Change (at least once) from Baseline	Treatment Arm	Up to 12 weeks exposure		At least 24 weeks exposure	
			N	Patients	N	Patients
Fasting Glucose	Normal to High (<100 mg/dL to ≥126 mg/dL)	Olanzapine	124	0%	108	0.9%
		Placebo	53	1.9%	NA[a]	NA[a]
	Borderline to High (≥100 mg/dL and <126 mg/dL to ≥126 mg/dL)	Olanzapine	14	14.3%	13	23.1%
		Placebo	13	0%	NA[a]	NA[a]

[a]Not Applicable.

Table 4: Changes in Nonfasting Lipids Values from Controlled Clinical Studies with Treatment Duration up to 12 Weeks

Laboratory Analyte	Category Change (at least once) from Baseline	Treatment Arm	N	Patients
Nonfasting Triglycerides	Increase by ≥50 mg/dL	OFC	174	67.8%
		Olanzapine	172	72.7%
	Normal to High (<150 mg/dL to ≥500 mg/dL)	OFC	57	0%
		Olanzapine	58	0%
	Borderline to High (≥150 mg/dL and <500 mg/dL to ≥500 mg/dL)	OFC	106	15.1%
		Olanzapine	103	8.7%
Nonfasting Total Cholesterol	Increase by ≥40 mg/dL	OFC	685	35%
		Olanzapine	749	22.7%
		Placebo	390	9%
	Normal to High (<200 mg/dL to ≥240 mg/dL)	OFC	256	8.2%
		Olanzapine	279	2.9%
		Placebo	175	1.7%
	Borderline to High (≥200 mg/dL and <240 mg/dL to ≥240 mg/dL)	OFC	213	36.2%
		Olanzapine	261	27.6%
		Placebo	111	9.9%

Table 5: Changes in Fasting Lipids Values from Adult Olanzapine Monotherapy Studies

Laboratory Analyte	Category Change (at least once) from Baseline	Treatment Arm	Up to 12 weeks exposure		At least 48 weeks exposure	
			N	Patients	N	Patients
Fasting Triglycerides	Increase by ≥50 mg/dL	Olanzapine	745	39.6%	487	61.4%
		Placebo	402	26.1%	NA[a]	NA[a]
	Normal to High (<150 mg/dL to ≥200 mg/dL)	Olanzapine	457	9.2%	293	32.4%
		Placebo	251	4.4%	NA[a]	NA[a]
	Borderline to High (≥150 mg/dL and <200 mg/dL to ≥200 mg/dL)	Olanzapine	135	39.3%	75	70.7%
		Placebo	65	20.0%	NA[a]	NA[a]
	Increase by ≥40 mg/dL	Olanzapine	745	21.6%	489	32.9%
		Placebo	402	9.5%	NA[a]	NA[a]

(Table continued on next page)

itored, since recurrences of NMS have been reported [see *Warnings and Precautions (5.7)* and *Patient Counseling Information (17.4, 17.8)*].

5.4   Hyperglycemia
Physicians should consider the risks and benefits when prescribing SYMBYAX to patients with an established diagnosis of diabetes mellitus, or having borderline increased blood glucose level (fasting 100-126 mg/dL, nonfasting 140-200 mg/dL). Patients taking SYMBYAX should be mon-

itored regularly for worsening of glucose control. Patients starting treatment with SYMBYAX should undergo fasting blood glucose testing at the beginning of treatment and periodically during treatment. Any patient treated with atypical antipsychotics should be monitored for symptoms of hyperglycemia including polydipsia, polyuria, polyphagia, and weakness. Patients who develop symptoms of hyperglycemia during treatment with atypical antipsychotics should undergo fasting blood glucose testing. In some cases, hyper-

glycemia has resolved when the atypical antipsychotic was discontinued; however, some patients required continuation of anti-diabetic treatment despite discontinuation of the suspect drug [see *Patient Counseling Information (17.5)*]. Hyperglycemia, in some cases extreme and associated with ketoacidosis or hyperosmolar coma or death, has been reported in patients treated with atypical antipsychotics, including olanzapine alone, as well as olanzapine taken concomitantly with fluoxetine. Assessment of the relationship between atypical antipsychotic use and glucose abnormalities is complicated by the possibility of an increased background risk of diabetes mellitus in patients with schizophrenia and the increasing incidence of diabetes mellitus in the general population. Epidemiological studies suggest an increased risk of treatment-emergent hyperglycemia-related adverse reactions in patients treated with the atypical antipsychotics. While relative risk estimates are inconsistent, the association between atypical antipsychotics and increases in glucose levels appears to fall on a continuum and olanzapine appears to have a greater association than some other atypical antipsychotics.

Mean increases in blood glucose have been observed in patients treated (median exposure of 9.2 months) with olanzapine in phase 1 of the Clinical Antipsychotic Trials of Intervention Effectiveness (CATIE). The mean increase of serum glucose (fasting and nonfasting samples) from baseline to the average of the 2 highest serum concentrations was 15.0 mg/dL.

In a study of healthy volunteers, subjects who received olanzapine (N=22) for 3 weeks had a mean increase compared to baseline in fasting blood glucose of 2.3 mg/dL. Placebo-treated subjects (N=19) had a mean increase in fasting blood glucose compared to baseline of 0.34 mg/dL.

In an analysis of 7 controlled clinical studies, 2 of which were placebo-controlled, with treatment duration up to 12 weeks, SYMBYAX was associated with a greater mean change in random glucose compared to placebo (8.65 mg/dL vs -3.86 mg/dL). The difference in mean changes between SYMBYAX and placebo was greater in patients with evidence of glucose dysregulation at baseline (including those patients diagnosed with diabetes mellitus or related adverse reactions, patients treated with anti-diabetic agents, patients with a baseline random glucose level ≥200 mg/dL, or a baseline fasting glucose level ≥126 mg/dL). SYMBYAX-treated patients had a greater mean HbA$_{1c}$ increase from baseline of 0.15% (median exposure 63 days), compared to a mean HbA$_{1c}$ decrease of 0.04% in fluoxetine-treated subjects (median exposure 57 days) and a mean HbA$_{1c}$ increase of 0.12% in olanzapine-treated patients (median exposure 56 days).

In an analysis of 6 controlled clinical studies, a larger proportion of SYMBYAX-treated subjects had glycosuria (4.4%) compared to placebo-treated subjects (1.4%).

The mean change in nonfasting glucose in patients exposed at least 48 weeks was 5.9 mg/dL (N=425).

Table 2 shows short-term and long-term changes in random glucose levels from adult SYMBYAX studies.

[See table 2 at top of previous page]

Controlled fasting glucose data is limited for SYMBYAX; however, in an analysis of 5 placebo-controlled olanzapine monotherapy studies with treatment duration up to 12 weeks, olanzapine was associated with a greater mean change in fasting glucose levels compared to placebo (2.76 mg/dL vs 0.17 mg/dL).

The mean change in fasting glucose for olanzapine-treated patients exposed at least 48 weeks was 4.2 mg/dL (N=487). In analyses of patients who completed 9-12 months of olanzapine therapy, mean change in fasting and nonfasting glucose levels continued to increase over time.

Olanzapine Monotherapy in Adolescents—The safety and efficacy of olanzapine and fluoxetine in combination have not been established in patients under the age of 18 years. The safety and efficacy of olanzapine have not been established in patients under the age of 18 years. In an analysis of 3 placebo-controlled olanzapine monotherapy studies of adolescent patients, including those with Schizophrenia (6 weeks) or Bipolar I Disorder (manic or mixed episodes) (3 weeks), olanzapine was associated with a greater mean change from baseline in fasting glucose levels compared to placebo (2.68 mg/dL vs -2.59 mg/dL). The mean change in fasting glucose for adolescents exposed at least 24 weeks was 3.1 mg/dL (N=121). Table 3 shows short-term and long-term changes in fasting blood glucose from adolescent olanzapine monotherapy studies.

[See table 3 at top left]

5.5   Hyperlipidemia
Undesirable alterations in lipids have been observed with SYMBYAX use. Clinical monitoring, including baseline and periodic follow-up lipid evaluations in patients using SYMBYAX, is recommended [see *Patient Counseling Information (17.6)*].

Clinically meaningful, and sometimes very high (>500 mg/dL), elevations in triglyceride levels have been observed with SYMBYAX use. Clinically meaningful increases in total cholesterol have also been seen with SYMBYAX use.

In an analysis of 7 controlled clinical studies, 2 of which were placebo-controlled, with treatment duration up to 12 weeks, SYMBYAX-treated patients had an increase from baseline in mean random total cholesterol of 12.1 mg/dL compared to an increase from baseline in mean random total cholesterol of 4.8 mg/dL for olanzapine-treated patients and a decrease in mean random total cholesterol of 5.5 mg/dL for placebo-treated patients. Table 4 shows categorical changes in nonfasting lipid values.

In long-term olanzapine and fluoxetine in combination studies (at least 48 weeks), changes (at least once) in nonfasting total cholesterol from normal at baseline to high occurred in 12% (N=150) and changes from borderline to high occurred in 56.6% (N=143) of patients. The mean change in nonfasting total cholesterol was 11.3 mg/dL (N= 426).
[See table 4 on previous page]

Fasting lipid data is limited for SYMBYAX; however, in an analysis of 5 placebo-controlled olanzapine monotherapy studies with treatment duration up to 12 weeks, olanzapine-treated patients had increases from baseline in mean fasting total cholesterol, LDL cholesterol, and triglycerides of 5.3 mg/dL, 3.0 mg/dL, and 20.8 mg/dL respectively compared to decreases from baseline in mean fasting total cholesterol, LDL cholesterol, and triglycerides of 6.1 mg/dL, 4.3 mg/dL, and 10.7 mg/dL for placebo-treated patients. For fasting HDL cholesterol, no clinically meaningful differences were observed between olanzapine-treated patients and placebo-treated patients. Mean increases in fasting lipid values (total cholesterol, LDL cholesterol, and triglycerides) were greater in patients without evidence of lipid dysregulation at baseline, where lipid dysregulation was defined as patients diagnosed with dyslipidemia or related adverse reactions, patients treated with lipid lowering agents, patients with high baseline lipid levels.

In long-term olanzapine studies (at least 48 weeks), patients had increases from baseline in mean fasting total cholesterol, LDL cholesterol, and triglycerides of 5.6 mg/dL, 2.5 mg/dL, and 18.7 mg/dL, respectively, and a mean decrease in fasting HDL cholesterol of 0.16 mg/dL. In an analysis of patients who completed 12 months of therapy, the mean nonfasting total cholesterol did not increase further after approximately 4-6 months.

The proportion of olanzapine-treated patients who had changes (at least once) in total cholesterol, LDL cholesterol or triglycerides from normal or borderline to high, or changes in HDL cholesterol from normal or borderline to low, was greater in long-term studies (at least 48 weeks) as compared with short-term studies. Table 5 shows categorical changes in fasting lipids values.
[See table 5 on previous page and at top right]

In phase 1 of the Clinical Antipsychotic Trials of Intervention Effectiveness (CATIE), over a median exposure of 9.2 months, the mean increase in triglycerides in patients taking olanzapine was 40.5 mg/dL. In phase 1 of CATIE, the median increase in total cholesterol was 9.4 mg/dL.

Olanzapine Monotherapy in Adolescents—The safety and efficacy of olanzapine and fluoxetine in combination have not been established in patients under the age of 18 years. The safety and efficacy of olanzapine have not been established in patients under the age of 18 years.

In an analysis of 3 placebo-controlled olanzapine monotherapy studies of adolescents, including those with Schizophrenia (6 weeks) or Bipolar I Disorder (manic or mixed episodes) (3 weeks), olanzapine-treated adolescents had increases from baseline in mean fasting total cholesterol, LDL cholesterol, and triglycerides of 12.9 mg/dL, 6.5 mg/dL, and 28.4 mg/dL, respectively, compared to increases from baseline in mean fasting total cholesterol and LDL cholesterol of 1.3 mg/dL and 1.0 mg/dL, and a decrease in triglycerides of 1.1 mg/dL for placebo-treated adolescents. For fasting HDL cholesterol, no clinically meaningful differences were observed between olanzapine-treated adolescents and placebo-treated adolescents.

In long-term olanzapine studies (at least 24 weeks), adolescents had increases from baseline in mean fasting total cholesterol, LDL cholesterol, and triglycerides of 5.5 mg/dL, 5.4 mg/dL, and 20.5 mg/dL, respectively, and a mean decrease in fasting HDL cholesterol of 4.5 mg/dL. Table 6 shows categorical changes in fasting lipids values in adolescents.
[See table 6 at right]

5.6 Weight Gain

Potential consequences of weight gain should be considered prior to starting SYMBYAX. Patients receiving SYMBYAX should receive regular monitoring of weight [see Patient Counseling Information (17.7)].

In an analysis of 7 controlled clinical studies, 2 of which were placebo-controlled, the mean weight increase for SYMBYAX-treated patients was greater than placebo-treated patients [4 kg (8.8 lb) vs -0.3 kg (-0.7 lb)]. Twenty-two percent of SYMBYAX-treated patients gained at least 7% of their baseline weight, with a median exposure of 6 weeks. This was greater than placebo-treated patients (1.8%). Approximately 3% of SYMBYAX-treated patients gained at least 15% of their baseline weight, with a median exposure of 8 weeks. This was greater than in placebo-treated patients (0%). Clinically significant weight gain was observed across all baseline Body Mass Index (BMI) categories. Discontinuation due to weight gain occurred in 2.5% of SYMBYAX-treated patients and 0% of placebo-treated patients.

In long-term olanzapine and fluoxetine in combination studies (at least 48 weeks), the mean weight gain was 6.7 kg (14.7 lb) (median exposure of 448 days, N=431). The percentages of patients who gained at least 7%, 15% or 25% of their baseline body weight with long-term exposure were 66%, 33%, and 10%, respectively. Discontinuation due to weight gain occurred in 1.2% of patients treated with olanzapine and fluoxetine in combination following at least 48 weeks of exposure.

In long-term olanzapine studies (at least 48 weeks), the mean weight gain was 5.6 kg (12.3 lb) (median exposure of 573 days, N=2021). The percentages of patients who gained at least 7%, 15%, or 25% of their baseline body weight with

Table 5 (cont.): Changes in Fasting Lipids Values from Adult Olanzapine Monotherapy Studies

Laboratory Analyte	Category Change (at least once) from Baseline	Treatment Arm	Up to 12 weeks exposure		At least 48 weeks exposure	
			N	Patients	N	Patients
Fasting Total Cholesterol	Normal to High	Olanzapine	392	2.8%	283	14.8%
	(<200 mg/dL to ≥240 mg/dL)	Placebo	207	2.4%	NAa	NAa
	Borderline to High	Olanzapine	222	23.0%	125	55.2%
	(≥200 mg/dL and <240 mg/dL to ≥240 mg/dL)	Placebo	112	12.5%	NAa	NAa
	Increase by ≥30 mg/dL	Olanzapine	536	23.7%	483	39.8%
		Placebo	304	14.1%	NAa	NAa
Fasting LDL Cholesterol	Normal to High	Olanzapine	154	0%	123	7.3%
	(<100 mg/dL to ≥160 mg/dL)	Placebo	82	1.2%	NAa	NAa
	Borderline to High	Olanzapine	302	10.6%	284	31.0%
	(≥100 mg/dL and <160 mg/dL to ≥160 mg/dL)	Placebo	173	8.1%	NAa	NAa

aNot Applicable.

Table 6: Changes in Fasting Lipids Values from Adolescent Olanzapine Monotherapy Studies

Laboratory Analyte	Category Change (at least once) from Baseline	Treatment Arm	Up to 6 weeks exposure		At least 24 weeks exposure	
			N	Patients	N	Patients
	Increase by ≥50 mg/dL	Olanzapine	138	37.0%	122	45.9%
		Placebo	66	15.2%	NAa	NAa
Fasting Triglycerides	Normal to High	Olanzapine	67	26.9%	66	36.4%
	(<90 mg/dL to >130 mg/dL)	Placebo	28	10.7%	NAa	NAa
	Borderline to High	Olanzapine	37	59.5%	31	64.5%
	(≥90 mg/dL and ≤130 mg/dL to >130 mg/dL)	Placebo	17	35.3%	NAa	NAa
	Increase by ≥40 mg/dL	Olanzapine	138	14.5%	122	14.8%
		Placebo	66	4.5%	NAa	NAa
Fasting Total Cholesterol	Normal to High	Olanzapine	87	6.9%	78	7.7%
	(<170 mg/dL to ≥200 mg/dL)	Placebo	43	2.3%	NAa	NAa
	Borderline to High	Olanzapine	36	38.9%	33	57.6%
	(≥170 mg/dL and <200 mg/dL to ≥200 mg/dL)	Placebo	13	7.7%	NAa	NAa
	Increase by ≥30 mg/dL	Olanzapine	137	17.5%	121	22.3%
		Placebo	63	11.1%	NAa	NAa
Fasting LDL Cholesterol	Normal to High	Olanzapine	98	5.1%	92	10.9%
	(<110 mg/dL to ≥130 mg/dL)	Placebo	44	4.5%	NAa	NAa
	Borderline to High	Olanzapine	29	48.3%	21	47.6%
	(≥110 mg/dL and <130 mg/dL to ≥130 mg/dL)	Placebo	9	0%	NAa	NAa

aNot Applicable.

Table 7: Weight Gain with Olanzapine Use in Adults

Amount Gained kg (lb)	6 Weeks (N=7465) (%)	6 Months (N=4162) (%)	12 Months (N=1345) (%)	24 Months (N=474) (%)	36 Months (N=147) (%)
≤0	26.2	24.3	20.8	23.2	17.0
0 to ≤5 (0-11 lb)	57.0	36.0	26.0	23.4	25.2
>5 to ≤10 (11-22 lb)	14.9	24.6	24.2	24.1	18.4
>10 to ≤15 (22-33 lb)	1.8	10.9	14.9	11.4	17.0
>15 to ≤20 (33-44 lb)	0.1	3.1	8.6	9.3	11.6
>20 to ≤25 (44-55 lb)	0	0.9	3.3	5.1	4.1
>25 to ≤30 (55-66 lb)	0	0.2	1.4	2.3	4.8
>30 (>66 lb)	0	0.1	0.8	1.2	2

Table 8: Weight Gain with Olanzapine Use in Adolescents from 4 Placebo-Controlled Trials

	Olanzapine-treated patients	Placebo-treated patients
Mean change in body weight from baseline (median exposure = 3 weeks)	4.6 kg (10.1 lb)	0.3 kg (0.7 lb)
Percentage of patients who gained at least 7% of baseline body weight	40.6% (median exposure to 7% = 4 weeks)	9.8% (median exposure to 7% = 8 weeks)
Percentage of patients who gained at least 15% of baseline body weight	7.1% (median exposure to 15% = 19 weeks)	2.7% (median exposure to 15% = 8 weeks)

long-term exposure were 64%, 32%, and 12%, respectively. Discontinuation due to weight gain occurred in 0.4% of olanzapine-treated patients following at least 48 weeks of exposure.

Table 7 includes data on adult weight gain with olanzapine pooled from 86 clinical trials. The data in each column represent data for those patients who completed treatment periods of the durations specified.
[See table 7 above]

Olanzapine Monotherapy in Adolescents—The safety and efficacy of olanzapine and fluoxetine in combination have not been established in patients under the age of 18 years. The safety and efficacy of olanzapine have not been established in patients under the age of 18 years. Mean increase in weight in adolescents was greater than in adults. In 4 placebo-controlled trials, discontinuation due to weight gain occurred in 1% of olanzapine-treated patients, compared to 0% of placebo-treated patients.
[See table 8 above]

In long-term olanzapine studies (at least 24 weeks), the mean weight gain was 11.2 kg (24.6 lb) (median exposure of 201 days, N=179). The percentages of adolescents who gained at least 7%, 15%, or 25% of their baseline body weight with long-term exposure were 89%, 55%, and 29%, respectively. Among adolescent patients, mean weight gain by baseline BMI category was 11.5 kg (25.3 lb), 12.1 kg (26.6 lb), and 12.7 kg (27.9 lb), respectively, for normal (N=106), overweight (N=26) and obese (N=17). Discontinuation due to weight gain occurred in 2.2% of olanzapine-treated patients following at least 24 weeks of exposure.

Table 9 shows data on adolescent weight gain with olanzapine pooled from 6 clinical trials. The data in each column represent data for those patients who completed treatment periods of the durations specified. Little clinical trial data is available on weight gain in adolescents with olanzapine beyond 6 months of treatment.

Table 9: Weight Gain with Olanzapine Use in Adolescents

Amount Gained kg (lb)	6 Weeks (N=243) (%)	6 Months (N=191) (%)
≤0	2.9	2.1
0 to ≤5 (0-11 lb)	47.3	24.6
>5 to ≤10 (11-22 lb)	42.4	26.7
>10 to ≤15 (22-33 lb)	5.8	22.0
>15 to ≤20 (33-44 lb)	0.8	12.6
>20 to ≤25 (44-55 lb)	0.8	9.4
>25 to ≤30 (55-66 lb)	0	2.1
>30 to ≤35 (66-77 lb)	0	0
>35 to ≤40 (77-88 lb)	0	0
>40 (>88 lb)	0	0.5

5.7   Serotonin Syndrome or Neuroleptic Malignant Syndrome (NMS)-like Reactions
The development of a potentially life-threatening serotonin syndrome or neuroleptic malignant syndrome (NMS)-like reactions have been reported with SNRIs and SSRIs alone but particularly with concomitant use of serotonergic drugs (including triptans) with drugs which impair metabolism of serotonin (including MAOIs), or with antipsychotics or other dopamine antagonists. Serotonin syndrome symptoms may include mental status changes (e.g., agitation, hallucinations, coma), autonomic instability (e.g., tachycardia, labile blood pressure, hyperthermia), neuromuscular aberrations (e.g., hyperreflexia, incoordination) and/or gastrointestinal symptoms (e.g., nausea, vomiting, diarrhea). Serotonin syndrome, in its most severe form can resemble neuroleptic malignant syndrome, which includes hyperthermia, muscle rigidity, autonomic instability with possible rapid fluctuation of vital signs, and mental status changes. Patients should be monitored for the emergence of serotonin syndrome or NMS-like signs and symptoms.

The concomitant use of SYMBYAX with MAOIs intended to treat depression is contraindicated [see Contraindications (4) and Drug Interactions (7.1)].

If concomitant treatment of SYMBYAX with a 5-hydroxytryptamine receptor agonist (triptan) is clinically warranted, careful observation of the patient is advised, particularly during treatment initiation and dose increases [see Drug Interactions (7.4)].

The concomitant use of SYMBYAX with serotonin precursors (such as tryptophan) is not recommended [see Drug Interactions (7.5)].

Treatment with SYMBYAX and any concomitant serotonergic or antidopaminergic agents, including antipsychotics, should be discontinued immediately, if the above reactions occur, and supportive symptomatic treatment should be initiated [see Warnings and Precautions (5.3) and Patient Counseling Information (17.4, 17.8)].

5.8   Allergic Reactions and Rash
In SYMBYAX premarketing controlled clinical studies, the overall incidence of rash or allergic reactions in SYMBYAX-treated patients [4.6% (26/571)] was similar to that of placebo [5.2% (25/477)]. The majority of the cases of rash and/or urticaria were mild; however, 3 patients discontinued (1 due to rash, which was moderate in severity and 2 due to allergic reactions, 1 of which included face edema).

In fluoxetine US clinical studies, 7% of 10,782 fluoxetine-treated patients developed various types of rashes and/or urticaria. Among the cases of rash and/or urticaria reported in premarketing clinical studies, almost a third were withdrawn from treatment because of the rash and/or systemic signs or symptoms associated with the rash. Clinical findings reported in association with rash include fever, leukocytosis, arthralgias, edema, carpal tunnel syndrome, respiratory distress, lymphadenopathy, proteinuria, and mild transaminase elevation. Most patients improved promptly with discontinuation of fluoxetine and/or adjunctive treatment with antihistamines or steroids, and all patients experiencing these reactions were reported to recover completely.

In fluoxetine premarketing clinical studies, 2 patients are known to have developed a serious cutaneous systemic illness. In neither patient was there an unequivocal diagnosis, but 1 was considered to have a leukocytoclastic vasculitis, and the other, a severe desquamating syndrome that was considered variously to be a vasculitis or erythema multiforme. Other patients have had systemic syndromes suggestive of serum sickness.

Since the introduction of fluoxetine, systemic reactions, possibly related to vasculitis, have developed in patients with rash. Although these reactions are rare, they may be serious, involving the lung, kidney, or liver. Death has been reported to occur in association with these systemic reactions. Anaphylactoid reactions, including bronchospasm, angioedema, and urticaria alone and in combination, have been reported.

Pulmonary reactions, including inflammatory processes of varying histopathology and/or fibrosis, have been reported rarely. These reactions have occurred with dyspnea as the only preceding symptom.

Whether these systemic reactions and rash have a common underlying cause or are due to different etiologies or pathogenic processes is not known. Furthermore, a specific underlying immunologic basis for these reactions has not been identified. Upon the appearance of rash or of other possible allergic phenomena for which an alternative etiology cannot be identified, SYMBYAX should be discontinued.

5.9   Activation of Mania/Hypomania
A major depressive episode may be the initial presentation of Bipolar Disorder. It is generally believed (though not established in controlled trials) that treating such an episode with an antidepressant alone may increase the likelihood of precipitation of a manic episode in patients at risk for Bipolar Disorder. Whether any of the symptoms described for clinical worsening and suicide risk represent such a conversion is unknown. However, prior to initiating treatment with an antidepressant, patients with depressive symptoms should be adequately screened to determine if they are at risk for Bipolar Disorder; such screening should include a detailed psychiatric history, including a family history of suicide, Bipolar Disorder, and depression. It should be noted that SYMBYAX is approved for the acute treatment of depressive episodes associated with Bipolar I Disorder.

In the 2 controlled bipolar depression studies there was no statistically significant difference in the incidence of manic reactions (manic reaction or manic depressive reaction) between SYMBYAX- and placebo-treated patients. In 1 of the studies, the incidence of manic reactions was (7% [3/43]) in SYMBYAX-treated patients compared to (3% [5/184]) in placebo-treated patients. In the other study, the incidence of manic reactions was (2% [1/43]) in SYMBYAX-treated patients compared to (8% [15/193]) in placebo-treated patients. This limited controlled trial experience of SYMBYAX in the acute treatment of depressive episodes associated with Bipolar I Disorder makes it difficult to interpret these findings until additional data is obtained. Because of this and the cyclical nature of Bipolar I Disorder, patients should be monitored closely for the development of symptoms of mania/hypomania during treatment with SYMBYAX.

5.10   Tardive Dyskinesia
A syndrome of potentially irreversible, involuntary, dyskinetic movements may develop in patients treated with antipsychotic drugs. Although the prevalence of the syndrome appears to be highest among the elderly, especially elderly women, it is impossible to rely upon prevalence estimates to predict, at the inception of antipsychotic treatment, which patients are likely to develop the syndrome. Whether antipsychotic drug products differ in their potential to cause tardive dyskinesia is unknown.

The risk of developing tardive dyskinesia and the likelihood that it will become irreversible are believed to increase as the duration of treatment and the total cumulative dose of antipsychotic drugs administered to the patient increase. However, the syndrome can develop, although much less commonly, after relatively brief treatment periods at low doses or may even arise after discontinuation of treatment. There is no known treatment for established cases of tardive dyskinesia, although the syndrome may remit, partially or completely, if antipsychotic treatment is withdrawn. Antipsychotic treatment itself, however, may suppress (or partially suppress) the signs and symptoms of the syndrome and thereby may possibly mask the underlying process. The effect that symptomatic suppression has upon the long-term course of the syndrome is unknown.

The incidence of dyskinetic movement in SYMBYAX-treated patients was infrequent. The mean score on the Abnormal Involuntary Movement Scale (AIMS) in the SYMBYAX-controlled database across clinical studies involving SYMBYAX-treated patients decreased from baseline. Nonetheless, SYMBYAX should be prescribed in a manner that is most likely to minimize the risk of tardive dyskinesia. If signs and symptoms of tardive dyskinesia appear in a patient on SYMBYAX, drug discontinuation should be considered. However, some patients may require treatment with SYMBYAX despite the presence of the syndrome. The need for continued treatment should be reassessed periodically.

5.11 Orthostatic Hypotension

SYMBYAX may induce orthostatic hypotension associated with dizziness, tachycardia, bradycardia and, in some patients, syncope, especially during the initial dose-titration period *[see Patient Counseling Information (17.10)]*.

In the SYMBYAX-controlled clinical trials across all indications, there were no significant differences between SYMBYAX-treated patients and olanzapine, fluoxetine- or placebo-treated patients in exposure-adjusted rates of orthostatic systolic blood pressure decreases of at least 30 mm Hg. Orthostatic systolic blood pressure decreases of at least 30 mm Hg occurred in 4.0% (28/705), 2.3% (19/831), 4.5% (18/399), and 1.8% (8/442) of the SYMBYAX, olanzapine, fluoxetine, and placebo groups, respectively. In this group of studies, the incidence of syncope-related adverse reactions (i.e., syncope and/or loss of consciousness) in SYMBYAX-treated patients was 0.4% (3/771) compared to placebo 0.2% (1/477).

In a clinical pharmacology study of SYMBYAX, 3 healthy subjects were discontinued from the trial after experiencing severe, but self-limited, hypotension and bradycardia that occurred 2 to 9 hours following a single 12-mg/50-mg dose of SYMBYAX. Reactions consisting of this combination of hypotension and bradycardia (and also accompanied by sinus pause) have been observed in at least 3 other healthy subjects treated with various formulations of olanzapine (1 oral, 2 intramuscular). In controlled clinical studies, the incidence of patients with a ≥20 bpm decrease in orthostatic pulse concomitantly with a ≥20 mm Hg decrease in orthostatic systolic blood pressure was 0.3% (2/706) in the SYMBYAX group, 0.2% (1/445) in the placebo group, 0.7% (6/837) in the olanzapine group, and 0% (0/404) in the fluoxetine group.

SYMBYAX should be used with particular caution in patients with known cardiovascular disease (history of myocardial infarction or ischemia, heart failure, or conduction abnormalities), cerebrovascular disease, or conditions that would predispose patients to hypotension (dehydration, hypovolemia, and treatment with antihypertensive medications).

5.12 Leukopenia, Neutropenia, and Agranulocytosis

Class Effect—In clinical trial and/or postmarketing experience, events of leukopenia/neutropenia have been reported temporally related to antipsychotic agents, including SYMBYAX. Agranulocytosis has also been reported.

Possible risk factors for leukopenia/neutropenia include preexisting low white blood cell count (WBC) and history of drug induced leukopenia/neutropenia. Patients with a history of a clinically significant low WBC or drug induced leukopenia/neutropenia should have their complete blood count (CBC) monitored frequently during the first few months of therapy and discontinuation of SYMBYAX should be considered at the first sign of a clinically significant decline in WBC in the absence of other causative factors. Patients with clinically significant neutropenia should be carefully monitored for fever or other symptoms or signs of infection and treated promptly if such symptoms or signs occur. Patients with severe neutropenia (absolute neutrophil count <1000/mm^3) should discontinue SYMBYAX and have their WBC followed until recovery.

5.13 Dysphagia

Esophageal dysmotility and aspiration have been associated with antipsychotic drug use. Aspiration pneumonia is a common cause of morbidity and mortality in patients with advanced Alzheimer's disease. SYMBYAX is not approved for the treatment of patients with Alzheimer's disease.

5.14 Seizures

Seizures occurred in 0.2% (4/2547) of SYMBYAX-treated patients during open-label clinical studies. No seizures occurred in the controlled SYMBYAX studies. Seizures have also been reported with both olanzapine and fluoxetine monotherapy. SYMBYAX should be used cautiously in patients with a history of seizures or with conditions that potentially lower the seizure threshold, e.g., Alzheimer's dementia. SYMBYAX is not approved for the treatment of patients with Alzheimer's disease. Conditions that lower the seizure threshold may be more prevalent in a population of ≥65 years of age.

5.15 Abnormal Bleeding

SNRIs and SSRIs, including fluoxetine, may increase the risk of bleeding reactions. Concomitant use of aspirin, nonsteroidal anti-inflammatory drugs, warfarin, and other anticoagulants may add to this risk. Case reports and epidemiological studies (case-control and cohort design) have demonstrated an association between use of drugs that interfere with serotonin reuptake and the occurrence of gastrointestinal bleeding. Bleeding reactions related to SNRIs and SSRIs use have ranged from ecchymoses, hematomas, epistaxis, and petechiae to life-threatening hemorrhages.

Patients should be cautioned about the risk of bleeding associated with the concomitant use of SYMBYAX and NSAIDs, aspirin, or other drugs that affect coagulation *[see Drug Interactions (7.6) and Patient Counseling Information (17.11)]*.

5.16 Hyponatremia

Hyponatremia has been reported during treatment with SNRIs and SSRIs, including fluoxetine and SYMBYAX. In many cases, this hyponatremia appears to be the result of the syndrome of inappropriate antidiuretic hormone secretion (SIADH). Cases with serum sodium lower than 110 mmol/L have been reported and appeared to be reversible when SYMBYAX was discontinued. Elderly patients may be at greater risk of developing hyponatremia with SNRIs and SSRIs. Also, patients taking diuretics or who are otherwise volume depleted may be at greater risk *[see Use in Specific Populations (8.5)]*. Discontinuation of SYMBYAX should be considered in patients with symptomatic hyponatremia and appropriate medical intervention should be instituted.

Signs and symptoms of hyponatremia include headache, difficulty concentrating, memory impairment, confusion, weakness, and unsteadiness, which may lead to falls. More severe and/or acute cases have been associated with hallucination, syncope, seizure, coma, respiratory arrest, and death. *[See Patient Counseling Information (17.12)]*.

5.17 Potential for Cognitive and Motor Impairment

Sedation-related adverse reactions were commonly reported with SYMBYAX treatment occurring at an incidence of 26.6% in SYMBYAX-treated patients compared with 10.9% in placebo-treated patients. Sedation-related adverse reactions (sedation, somnolence, hypersomnia, and lethargy) led to discontinuation in 2% (15/771) of patients in the controlled clinical studies. As with any CNS-active drug, SYMBYAX has the potential to impair judgment, thinking, or motor skills. Patients should be cautioned about operating hazardous machinery, including automobiles, until they are reasonably certain that SYMBYAX therapy does not affect them adversely *[see Patient Counseling Information (17.13)]*.

5.18 Body Temperature Regulation

Disruption of the body's ability to reduce core body temperature has been attributed to antipsychotic drugs. Appropriate care is advised when prescribing SYMBYAX for patients who will be experiencing conditions which may contribute to an elevation in core body temperature (e.g., exercising strenuously, exposure to extreme heat, receiving concomitant medication with anticholinergic activity, or being subject to dehydration). *[See Patient Counseling Information (17.13)]*.

5.19 Use in Patients with Concomitant Illness

Clinical experience with SYMBYAX in patients with concomitant systemic illnesses is limited *[see Clinical Pharmacology (12.4)]*. The following precautions for the individual components may be applicable to SYMBYAX.

Olanzapine exhibits in vitro muscarinic receptor affinity. In premarketing clinical studies, SYMBYAX was associated with constipation, dry mouth, and tachycardia, all adverse reactions possibly related to cholinergic antagonism. Such adverse reactions were not often the basis for study discontinuations; SYMBYAX should be used with caution in patients with clinically significant prostatic hypertrophy, narrow angle glaucoma, a history of paralytic ileus, or related conditions.

In 5 placebo-controlled studies of olanzapine in elderly patients with dementia-related psychosis (n=1184), the following treatment-emergent adverse reactions were reported in olanzapine-treated patients at an incidence of at least 2% and significantly greater than placebo-treated patients: falls, somnolence, peripheral edema, abnormal gait, urinary incontinence, lethargy, increased weight, asthenia, pyrexia, pneumonia, dry mouth, and visual hallucinations. The rate of discontinuation due to adverse reactions was significantly greater with olanzapine than placebo (13% vs 7%). Elderly patients with dementia-related psychosis treated with olanzapine are at an increased risk of death compared to placebo. Olanzapine is not approved for the treatment of patients with dementia-related psychosis *[see Boxed Warning, Warnings and Precautions (5.2), and Patient Counseling Information (17.3)]*.

As with other CNS-active drugs, SYMBYAX should be used with caution in elderly patients with dementia. Olanzapine is not approved for the treatment of patients with dementia-related psychosis. If the prescriber elects to treat elderly patients with dementia-related psychosis, vigilance should be exercised *[see Boxed Warning and Warnings and Precautions (5.2), and Patient Counseling Information (17.3)]*.

SYMBYAX has not been evaluated or used to any appreciable extent in patients with a recent history of myocardial infarction or unstable heart disease. Patients with these diagnoses were excluded from clinical studies during the premarket testing.

Caution is advised when using SYMBYAX in cardiac patients and in patients with diseases or conditions that could affect hemodynamic responses *[see Warnings and Precautions (5.11)]*.

5.20 Hyperprolactinemia

As with other drugs that antagonize dopamine D_2 receptors, SYMBYAX elevates prolactin levels, and the elevation persists during administration. Hyperprolactinemia may suppress hypothalamic GnRH, resulting in reduced pituitary gonadotropin secretion. This, in turn, may inhibit reproductive function by impairing gonadal steroidogenesis in both female and male patients. Galactorrhea, amenorrhea, gynecomastia, and impotence have been reported in patients receiving prolactin-elevating compounds. Long-standing hyperprolactinemia when associated with hypogonadism may lead to decreased bone density in both female and male subjects.

Tissue culture experiments indicate that approximately one-third of human breast cancers are prolactin dependent in vitro, a factor of potential importance if the prescription of these drugs is contemplated in a patient with previously detected breast cancer. As is common with compounds that increase prolactin release, an increase in mammary gland neoplasia was observed in the olanzapine carcinogenicity studies conducted in mice and rats *[see Nonclinical Toxicology (13.1)]*. Neither clinical studies nor epidemiologic studies conducted to date have shown an association between chronic administration of this class of drugs and tumorigenesis in humans; the available evidence is considered too limited to be conclusive at this time.

In controlled clinical studies of SYMBYAX (up to 12 weeks), changes from normal to high in prolactin concentrations were observed in 28% of adults treated with SYMBYAX as compared to 5% of placebo-treated patients. The elevations persisted throughout administration of SYMBYAX. In a pooled analysis from clinical studies including 2929 adults treated with SYMBYAX, potentially associated clinical manifestations included menstrual-related events[1] (1% [20/1946] of females), sexual function-related events[2] (7% [192/2929] of females and males), and breast-related events[3] (0.8% [16/1946] of females, 0.2% [2/983] of males).

In placebo-controlled olanzapine clinical studies (up to 12 weeks), changes from normal to high in prolactin concentrations were observed in 30% of adults treated with olanzapine as compared to 10.5% of adults treated with placebo. In a pooled analysis from clinical studies including 8136 adults treated with olanzapine, potentially associated clinical manifestations included menstrual-related events[1] (2% [49/3240] of females), sexual function-related events[2] (2% [150/8136] of females and males), and breast-related events[3] (0.7% [23/3240] of females, 0.2% [9/4896] of males).

In placebo-controlled olanzapine monotherapy studies in adolescent patients (up to 6 weeks) with schizophrenia or bipolar I disorder (manic or mixed episodes), changes from normal to high in prolactin concentrations were observed in 47% of olanzapine-treated patients compared to 7% of placebo-treated patients. In a pooled analysis from clinical trials including 454 adolescents treated with olanzapine, potentially associated clinical manifestations included menstrual-related events[1] (1% [2/168] of females), sexual function-related events[2] (0.7% [3/454] of females and males), and breast-related events[3] (2% [3/168] of females, 2% [7/286] of males); *[see Use in Specific Populations (8.4)]*.

[1] Based on a search of the following terms: amenorrhea, hypomenorrhea, menstruation delayed, and oligomenorrhea.

[2] Based on a search of the following terms: anorgasmia, delayed ejaculation, erectile dysfunction, decreased libido, loss of libido, abnormal orgasm, and sexual dysfunction.

[3] Based on a search of the following terms: breast discharge, enlargement or swelling, galactorrhea, gynecomastia, and lactation disorder.

5.21 Concomitant Use of Olanzapine and Fluoxetine Products

SYMBYAX contains the same active ingredients that are in Zyprexa®, Zyprexa® Zydis® (olanzapine), and in Prozac®, Prozac® Weekly™, and Sarafem® (fluoxetine HCl). Caution should be exercised when prescribing these medications concomitantly with SYMBYAX *[see Overdosage (10)]*.

5.22 Long Elimination Half-Life of Fluoxetine

Because of the long elimination half-lives of fluoxetine and its major active metabolite, changes in dose will not be fully reflected in plasma for several weeks, affecting both strategies for titration to final dose and withdrawal from treatment. This is of potential consequence when drug discontinuation is required or when drugs are prescribed that might interact with fluoxetine and norfluoxetine following the discontinuation of fluoxetine [see Clinical Pharmacology (12.3)].

5.23 Discontinuation of Treatment with SYMBYAX

During marketing of fluoxetine, a component of SYMBYAX, SNRIs, and SSRIs, there have been spontaneous reports of adverse reactions occurring upon discontinuation of these drugs, particularly when abrupt, including the following: dysphoric mood, irritability, agitation, dizziness, sensory disturbances (e.g., paresthesias such as electric shock sensations), anxiety, confusion, headache, lethargy, emotional lability, insomnia, and hypomania. While these reactions are generally self-limiting, there have been reports of serious discontinuation symptoms. Patients should be monitored for these symptoms when discontinuing treatment with fluoxetine. A gradual reduction in the dose rather than abrupt cessation is recommended whenever possible. If intolerable symptoms occur following a decrease in the dose or upon discontinuation of treatment, then resuming the previously prescribed dose may be considered. Subsequently, the physician may continue decreasing the dose but at a more gradual rate. Plasma fluoxetine and norfluoxetine concentration decrease gradually at the conclusion of therapy, which may minimize the risk of discontinuation symptoms with this drug [see Dosage and Administration (2.4) and Patient Counseling Information (17.16)].

5.24 Laboratory Tests

Fasting blood glucose testing and lipid profile at the beginning of, and periodically during, treatment is recommended [see Warnings and Precautions (5.4, 5.5) and Patient Counseling Information (17.5, 17.6)].

6 ADVERSE REACTIONS

Because clinical trials are conducted under widely varying conditions, adverse reaction rates observed in the clinical trials of a drug cannot be directly compared to rates in the clinical trials of another drug and may not reflect or predict the rates observed in practice.

6.1 Clinical Trials Experience

The information below is derived from a clinical study database for SYMBYAX consisting of 2547 patients with treatment resistant depression, depressive episodes associated with Bipolar I Disorder, Major Depressive Disorder with psychosis, or sexual dysfunction with approximately 1085 patient-years of exposure. The conditions and duration of treatment with SYMBYAX varied greatly and included (in overlapping categories) open-label and double-blind phases of studies, inpatients and outpatients, fixed-dose and dose-titration studies, and short-term or long-term exposure.

Adverse reactions were recorded by clinical investigators using descriptive terminology of their own choosing. Consequently, it is not possible to provide a meaningful estimate of the proportion of individuals experiencing adverse reactions without first grouping similar types of reactions into a limited (i.e., reduced) number of standardized reaction categories.

In the tables and tabulations that follow, MedDRA or COSTART Dictionary terminology has been used to classify reported adverse reactions. The data in the tables represent the proportion of individuals who experienced, at least once, a treatment-emergent adverse reaction of the type listed. A reaction was considered treatment-emergent if it occurred for the first time or worsened while receiving therapy following baseline evaluation. It is possible that reactions reported during therapy were not necessarily related to drug exposure.

The prescriber should be aware that the figures in the tables and tabulations cannot be used to predict the incidence of side effects in the course of usual medical practice where patient characteristics and other factors differ from those that prevailed in the clinical studies. Similarly, the cited frequencies cannot be compared with figures obtained from other clinical investigations involving different treatments, uses, and investigators. The cited figures, however, do provide the prescribing clinician with some basis for estimating the relative contribution of drug and nondrug factors to the side effect incidence rate in the population studied.

Adverse Reactions Associated with Discontinuation of Treatment in Short-Term, Controlled Studies Including Depressive Episodes Associated with Bipolar I Disorder and Treatment Resistant Depression—Overall, 11.3% of the 771 patients in the SYMBYAX group discontinued due to adverse reactions compared with 4.4% of the 477 patients for placebo. Adverse reactions leading to discontinuation associated with the use of SYMBYAX (incidence of at least 1% for SYMBYAX and greater than that for placebo) using MedDRA Dictionary coding were weight increased (2%) and sedation (1%) versus placebo patients which had 0% incidence of weight increased and sedation.

Commonly Observed Adverse Reactions in Short-Term, Controlled Studies Including Depressive Episodes Associated with Bipolar I Disorder and Treatment Resistant Depression—The most commonly observed adverse reactions associated with the use of SYMBYAX (incidence ≥5% and at least twice that for placebo in the SYMBYAX-controlled database) using MedDRA Dictionary coding were: disturbance in attention, dry mouth, fatigue, hypersomnia, increased appetite, peripheral edema, sedation, somnolence, tremor, vision blurred, and weight increased. Adverse reactions reported in clinical trials of olanzapine and fluoxetine in combination are generally consistent with treatment-emergent adverse reactions during olanzapine or fluoxetine monotherapy.

Adverse Reactions Occurring at an Incidence of 2% or More in Short-Term Controlled Studies Including Depressive Episodes Associated with Bipolar I Disorder and Treatment Resistant Depression—Table 10 enumerates the treatment-emergent adverse reactions associated with the use of SYMBYAX (incidence of at least 2% for SYMBYAX and twice or more than for placebo). The SYMBYAX-controlled column includes patients with various diagnoses while the placebo column includes only patients with bipolar depression and major depression with psychotic features. [See table 10 at left]

Extrapyramidal Symptoms

Dystonia, Class Effect for Antipsychotics—Symptoms of dystonia, prolonged abnormal contractions of muscle groups, may occur in susceptible individuals during the first few days of treatment. Dystonic symptoms include: spasm of the neck muscles, sometimes progressing to tightness of the throat, swallowing difficulty, difficulty breathing, and/or protrusion of the tongue. While these symptoms can occur at low doses, the frequency and severity are greater with high potency and at higher doses of first generation antipsychotic drugs. In general, an elevated risk of acute dystonia may be observed in males and younger age groups receiving antipsychotics; however, events of dystonia have been reported infrequently (<1%) with the olanzapine and fluoxetine combination.

Additional Findings Observed in Clinical Studies

Sexual Dysfunction—In the pool of controlled SYMBYAX studies in patients with bipolar depression, there were higher rates of the treatment-emergent adverse reactions decreased libido, anorgasmia, impotence and abnormal ejaculation in the SYMBYAX group than in the placebo group. One case of decreased libido led to discontinuation in the SYMBYAX group. In the controlled studies that contained a fluoxetine arm, the rates of decreased libido and abnormal ejaculation in the SYMBYAX group were less than the rates in the fluoxetine group. None of the differences were statistically significant.

Sexual dysfunction, including priapism, has been reported with all SSRIs. While it is difficult to know the precise risk of sexual dysfunction associated with the use of SSRIs, physicians should routinely inquire about such possible side effects.

Difference Among Dose Levels Observed in Other Olanzapine Clinical Trials

In a single 8-week randomized, double-blind, fixed-dose study comparing 10 (N=199), 20 (N=200), and 40 (N=200) mg/day of olanzapine in patients with Schizophrenia or Schizoaffective Disorder, statistically significant differences among 3 dose groups were observed for the following safety outcomes: weight gain, prolactin elevation, fatigue, and dizziness. Mean baseline to endpoint increase in weight (10 mg/day: 1.9 kg; 20 mg/day: 2.3 kg; 40 mg/day: 3 kg) was observed with significant differences between 10 vs 40 mg/day. Incidence of treatment-emergent prolactin elevation >24.2 ng/mL (female) or >18.77 ng/mL (male) at any time during the trial (10 mg/day: 31.2%; 20 mg/day: 42.7%;

Table 10: Treatment-Emergent Adverse Reactions: Incidence in Controlled Clinical Studies

System Organ Class	Adverse Reaction	Percentage of Patients Reporting Event	
		SYMBYAX-Controlled (N=771)	Placebo (N=477)
Eye disorders	Vision blurred	5	2
Gastrointestinal disorders	Dry mouth	15	6
	Flatulence	3	1
	Abdominal distension	2	0
General disorders and administration site conditions	Fatigue	12	2
	Edema peripheral	9	0
	Edema	3	0
	Asthenia	3	1
	Pain	2	1
	Pyrexia	2	1
Infections and infestations	Sinusitis	2	1
Investigations	Weight increased	25	3
Metabolism and nutrition disorders	Increased appetite	20	4
Musculoskeletal and connective tissue disorders	Arthralgia	4	1
	Pain in extremity	3	1
	Musculoskeletal stiffness	2	1
Nervous system disorders	Somnolence	14	6
	Tremor	9	3
	Sedation	8	4
	Hypersomnia	5	1
	Disturbance in attention	5	1
	Lethargy	3	1
Psychiatric disorders	Restlessness	4	1
	Thinking abnormal	2	1
	Nervousness	2	1
Reproductive system and breast disorders	Erectile dysfunction	2	1

40 mg/day: 61.1%) with significant differences between 10 vs 40 mg/day and 20 vs 40 mg/day; fatigue (10 mg/day: 1.5%; 20 mg/day: 2.1%; 40 mg/day: 6.6%) with significant differences between 10 vs 40 and 20 vs 40 mg/day; and dizziness (10 mg/day: 2.6%; 20 mg/day: 1.6%; 40 mg/day: 6.6%) with significant differences between 20 vs 40 mg, was observed.

Other Adverse Reactions Observed in Clinical Studies

Following is a list of treatment-emergent adverse reactions reported by patients treated with SYMBYAX in clinical trials. This listing is not intended to include reactions (1) already listed in previous tables or elsewhere in labeling, (2) for which a drug cause was remote, (3) which were so general as to be uninformative, (4) which were not considered to have significant clinical implications, or (5) which occurred at a rate equal to or less than placebo.

Reactions are classified by body system using the following definitions: frequent adverse reactions are those occurring in at least 1/100 patients; infrequent adverse reactions are those occurring in 1/100 to 1/1000 patients; and rare reactions are those occurring in fewer than 1/1000 patients.

- **Body as a Whole**—*Frequent:* chills, neck rigidity, photosensitivity reaction; *Rare:* death[1].
- **Cardiovascular System**—*Frequent:* vasodilatation; *Infrequent:* QT-interval prolonged.
- **Digestive System**—*Frequent:* diarrhea; *Infrequent:* gastritis, gastroenteritis, nausea and vomiting, peptic ulcer; *Rare:* gastrointestinal hemorrhage, intestinal obstruction, liver fatty deposit, pancreatitis.
- **Hemic and Lymphatic System**—*Frequent:* ecchymosis; *Infrequent:* anemia, thrombocytopenia; *Rare:* leukopenia, purpura.
- **Metabolic and Nutritional**—*Frequent:* generalized edema, weight loss; *Rare:* bilirubinemia, creatinine increased, gout.
- **Musculoskeletal System**—*Rare:* osteoporosis.
- **Nervous System**—*Frequent:* amnesia; *Infrequent:* ataxia, buccoglossal syndrome, coma, dysarthria, emotional lability, euphoria, hypokinesia, movement disorder, myoclonus; *Rare:* hyperkinesia, libido increased, withdrawal syndrome.
- **Respiratory System**—*Infrequent:* epistaxis, yawn; *Rare:* laryngismus.
- **Skin and Appendages**—*Infrequent:* alopecia, dry skin, pruritis; *Rare:* exfoliative dermatitis.
- **Special Senses**—*Frequent:* taste perversion; *Infrequent:* abnormality of accommodation, dry eyes.
- **Urogenital System**—*Frequent:* breast pain, menorrhagia[2], urinary frequency, urinary incontinence; *Infrequent:* amenorrhea[2], female lactation[2], hypomenorrhea[2], metrorrhagia[2], urinary retention, urinary urgency, urination impaired; *Rare:* breast engorgement[2].

[1]This term represents a serious adverse event but does not meet the definition for adverse drug reactions. It is included here because of its seriousness.

[2]Adjusted for gender.

Other Adverse Reactions Observed with Olanzapine or Fluoxetine Monotherapy

The following adverse reactions were not observed in SYMBYAX-treated patients during premarketing clinical studies but have been reported with olanzapine or fluoxetine monotherapy: aplastic anemia, cholestatic jaundice, diabetic coma, dyskinesia, eosinophilic pneumonia[3], erythema multiforme, jaundice, neutropenia, sudden unexpected death[3], and violent behaviors[3]. Random triglyceride levels of ≥1000 mg/dL have been reported.

[3] These terms represent serious adverse events but do not meet the definition for adverse drug reactions. They are included here because of their seriousness.

6.2 Vital Signs and Laboratory Studies

Vital Signs—Tachycardia, bradycardia, and orthostatic hypotension have occurred in SYMBYAX-treated patients [see *Warnings and Precautions (5.11)*]. The mean standing pulse rate of SYMBYAX-treated patients was reduced by 0.7 beats/min.

Laboratory Changes—In SYMBYAX clinical studies, (including treatment resistant depression, depressive episodes associated with Bipolar I Disorder, Major Depressive Disorder with psychosis, or sexual dysfunction) SYMBYAX was associated with statistically significantly greater frequencies for the following treatment-emergent findings in laboratory analytes (normal at baseline to abnormal at any time during the trial) compared to placebo: elevated prolactin (27.6% vs 4.8%); elevated urea nitrogen (2.8% vs 0.8%); elevated uric acid (2.9% vs 0.5%); low albumin (2.7% vs 0.3%); low bicarbonate (14.1% vs 8.8%); low hemoglobin (2.6% vs 0%); low inorganic phosphorus (1.9% vs 0.3%); low lymphocytes (1.9% vs 0%); and low total bilirubin (15.3% vs 3.9%). As with olanzapine, asymptomatic elevations of hepatic transaminases [ALT, AST, and GGT] and alkaline phosphatase have been observed with SYMBYAX. In the SYMBYAX-controlled database, ALT elevations (normal baseline and ≥3 times the upper limit of the normal range post-baseline) were observed in 3.4% (20/586) of patients exposed to

SYMBYAX compared with none of the 342 placebo patients and 3.5% (23/665) of olanzapine-treated patients. The difference between SYMBYAX and placebo was statistically significant. Of the SYMBYAX patients who started normal at baseline and had increases in ALT ≥5 times the upper limit of normal range, none experienced jaundice and 4 had transient elevations >200 IU/L [see *Adverse Reactions (6.1)*].

In olanzapine placebo-controlled studies, clinically significant ALT elevations (≥3 times the upper limit of the normal range) were observed in 2% (6/243) of patients exposed to olanzapine compared with 0% (0/115) of the placebo patients. None of these patients experienced jaundice. In 2 of these patients, liver enzymes decreased toward normal despite continued treatment and, in 2 others, enzymes decreased upon discontinuation of olanzapine. In the remaining 2 patients, 1, seropositive for hepatitis C, had persistent enzyme elevations for 4 months after discontinuation, and the other had insufficient follow-up to determine if enzymes normalized.

Within the larger olanzapine premarketing database of about 2400 patients with baseline ALT ≤90 IU/L, the incidence of ALT elevation to >200 IU/L was 2% (50/2381). Again, none of these patients experienced jaundice or other symptoms attributable to liver impairment and most had transient changes that tended to normalize while olanzapine treatment was continued.

Among all 2500 patients in olanzapine clinical studies, approximately 1% (23/2500) discontinued treatment due to transaminase increases.

Rare postmarketing reports of hepatitis have been received. Very rare cases of cholestatic or mixed liver injury have also been reported in the postmarketing period.

Caution should be exercised in patients with signs and symptoms of hepatic impairment, in patients with pre-existing conditions associated with limited hepatic functional reserve, and in patients who are being treated with potentially hepatotoxic drugs.

An increase in creatine phosphokinase has been reported very rarely in SYMBYAX-treated patients and infrequently in clinical trials of olanzapine-treated patients.

Effect on Cardiac Repolarization—The mean increase in QT_c interval for SYMBYAX-treated patients (4.4 msec) in clinical studies was significantly greater than that for placebo-treated (-0.8 msec), olanzapine-treated (-0.3 msec) patients, and fluoxetine-treated (1.7 msec) patients. There were no significant differences between patients treated with SYMBYAX, placebo, olanzapine, or fluoxetine in the incidence of QT_c outliers (>500 msec).

6.3 Postmarketing Experience

The following adverse reactions have been identified during post-approval use of SYMBYAX. Because these reactions are reported voluntarily from a population of uncertain size, it is difficult to reliably estimate their frequency or evaluate a causal relationship to drug exposure.

Adverse reactions reported since market introduction that were temporally (but not necessarily causally) related to SYMBYAX therapy include the following: rhabdomyolysis and venous thromboembolic events (including pulmonary embolism and deep venous thrombosis).

7 DRUG INTERACTIONS

The risks of using SYMBYAX in combination with other drugs have not been extensively evaluated in systematic studies. The drug-drug interactions sections of fluoxetine and olanzapine are applicable to SYMBYAX. As with all drugs, the potential for interaction by a variety of mechanisms (e.g., pharmacodynamic, pharmacokinetic drug inhibition or enhancement, etc.) is a possibility. In evaluating individual cases, consideration should be given to using lower initial doses of the concomitantly administered drugs, using conservative titration schedules, and monitoring of clinical status [see *Clinical Pharmacology (12.3)*].

7.1 Monoamine Oxidase Inhibitors (MAOI)

SYMBYAX should not be used in combination with an MAOI, or within a minimum of 14 days of discontinuing therapy with an MAOI. There have been reports of serious, sometimes fatal reactions (including hyperthermia, rigidity, myoclonus, autonomic instability with possible rapid fluctuations of vital signs, and mental status changes that include extreme agitation progressing to delirium and coma) in patients receiving fluoxetine in combination with an MAOI, and in patients who have recently discontinued fluoxetine and are then started on an MAOI. Some cases presented with features resembling neuroleptic malignant syndrome [see *Warnings and Precautions (5.3)*]. Since fluoxetine and its major metabolite have very long elimination half-lives, at least 5 weeks (perhaps longer, especially if fluoxetine has been prescribed chronically and/or at higher doses) should be allowed after stopping SYMBYAX before starting an MAOI. [See *Contraindications (4), Warnings and Precautions (5.22), and Clinical Pharmacology (12.3)*].

7.2 CNS Acting Drugs

Caution is advised if the concomitant administration of SYMBYAX and other CNS-active drugs is required. In eval-

uating individual cases, consideration should be given to using lower initial doses of the concomitantly administered drugs, using conservative titration schedules, and monitoring of clinical status [see *Clinical Pharmacology (12.3)*].

7.3 Serotonergic Drugs

Based on the mechanism of action of SNRIs and SSRIs, including SYMBYAX, and the potential for serotonin syndrome, caution is advised when SYMBYAX is coadministered with other drugs that may affect the serotonergic neurotransmitter systems, such as triptans, linezolid (an antibiotic which is a reversible non-selective MAOI), lithium, tramadol, or St. John's Wort [see *Warnings and Precautions (5.7)*]. The concomitant use of SYMBYAX with SNRIs, SSRIs, or tryptophan is not recommended [see *Drug Interactions (7.5)*].

7.4 Triptans

There have been rare postmarketing reports of serotonin syndrome with use of an SSRI and a triptan. If concomitant treatment of SYMBYAX with a triptan is clinically warranted, careful observation of the patient is advised, particularly during treatment initiation and dose increases [see *Warnings and Precautions (5.7)*].

7.5 Tryptophan

Five patients receiving fluoxetine in combination with tryptophan experienced adverse reactions, including agitation, restlessness, and gastrointestinal distress. Concomitant use with tryptophan is not recommended [see *Warnings and Precautions (5.7)*].

7.6 Drugs that Interfere with Hemostasis (e.g., NSAIDs, Aspirin, Warfarin)

Serotonin release by platelets plays an important role in hemostasis. Epidemiological studies of the case-control and cohort design that have demonstrated an association between use of psychotropic drugs that interfere with serotonin reuptake and the occurrence of upper gastrointestinal bleeding have also shown that concurrent use of an NSAID or aspirin may potentiate this risk of bleeding. Altered anticoagulant effects, including increased bleeding, have been reported when SNRIs or SSRIs are coadministered with warfarin [see *Warnings and Precautions (5.15)*]. Warfarin (20-mg single dose) did not affect olanzapine pharmacokinetics. Single doses of olanzapine did not affect the pharmacokinetics of warfarin. Patients receiving warfarin therapy should be carefully monitored when SYMBYAX is initiated or discontinued.

7.7 Electroconvulsive Therapy (ECT)

There are no clinical studies establishing the benefit of the combined use of ECT and fluoxetine. There have been rare reports of prolonged seizures in patients on fluoxetine receiving ECT treatment [see *Warnings and Precautions (5.14)*].

7.8 Potential for Other Drugs to Affect SYMBYAX

Benzodiazepines—Co-administration of diazepam with olanzapine potentiated the orthostatic hypotension observed with olanzapine [see *Drug Interactions (7.9)*].

Inducers of 1A2—Carbamazepine therapy (200 mg BID) causes an approximate 50% increase in the clearance of olanzapine. This increase is likely due to the fact that carbamazepine is a potent inducer of CYP1A2 activity. Higher daily doses of carbamazepine may cause an even greater increase in olanzapine clearance [see *Drug Interactions (7.9)*].

Alcohol—Ethanol (45 mg/70 kg single dose) did not have an effect on olanzapine pharmacokinetics [see *Drug Interactions (7.9)*].

Inhibitors of CYP1A2—Fluvoxamine decreases the clearance of olanzapine. This results in a mean increase in olanzapine C_{max} following fluvoxamine administration of 54% in female nonsmokers and 77% in male smokers. The mean increase in olanzapine AUC is 52% and 108%, respectively. Lower doses of the olanzapine component of SYMBYAX should be considered in patients receiving concomitant treatment with fluvoxamine.

The Effect of Other Drugs on Olanzapine—Fluoxetine, an inhibitor of CYP2D6, decreases olanzapine clearance a small amount [see *Clinical Pharmacology (12.3)*]. Agents that induce CYP1A2 or glucuronyl transferase enzymes, such as omeprazole and rifampin, may cause an increase in olanzapine clearance. The effect of CYP1A2 inhibitors, such as fluvoxamine and some fluoroquinolone antibiotics, on SYMBYAX has not been evaluated. Although olanzapine is metabolized by multiple enzyme systems, induction or inhibition of a single enzyme may appreciably alter olanzapine clearance. Therefore, a dosage increase (for induction) or a dosage decrease (for inhibition) may need to be considered with specific drugs.

7.9 Potential for SYMBYAX to Affect Other Drugs

Pimozide—Concomitant use of fluoxetine and pimozide is contraindicated. Clinical studies of pimozide with other antidepressants demonstrate an increase in drug interaction or QT_c prolongation. While a specific study with pimozide and fluoxetine has not been conducted, the potential for drug interactions or QT_c prolongation warrants restricting the concurrent use of pimozide and fluoxetine. [See *Contraindications (4)*].

Carbamazepine—Patients on stable doses of carbamazepine have developed elevated plasma anticonvulsant concentrations and clinical anticonvulsant toxicity following initiation of concomitant fluoxetine treatment.

Alcohol—The coadministration of ethanol with SYMBYAX may potentiate sedation and orthostatic hypotension [see Drug Interactions (7.8)].

Thioridazine—Thioridazine should not be administered with SYMBYAX or administered within a minimum of 5 weeks after discontinuation of SYMBYAX.

In a study of 19 healthy male subjects, which included 6 slow and 13 rapid hydroxylators of debrisoquin, a single 25-mg oral dose of thioridazine produced a 2.4-fold higher C_{max} and a 4.5-fold higher AUC for thioridazine in the slow hydroxylators compared with the rapid hydroxylators. The rate of debrisoquin hydroxylation is felt to depend on the level of CYP2D6 isozyme activity. Thus, this study suggests that drugs that inhibit CYP2D6, such as certain SSRIs, including fluoxetine, will produce elevated plasma levels of thioridazine [see Contraindications (4)].

Thioridazine administration produces a dose-related prolongation of the QT_c interval, which is associated with serious ventricular arrhythmias, such as torsades de pointes-type arrhythmias and sudden death. This risk is expected to increase with fluoxetine-induced inhibition of thioridazine metabolism [see Contraindications (4)].

Due to the risk of serious ventricular arrhythmias and sudden death potentially associated with elevated thioridazine plasma levels, thioridazine should not be administered with fluoxetine or within a minimum of 5 weeks after fluoxetine has been discontinued [see Contraindications (4)].

Tricyclic Antidepressants (TCAs)—Single doses of olanzapine did not affect the pharmacokinetics of imipramine or its active metabolite desipramine.

In 2 fluoxetine studies, previously stable plasma levels of imipramine and desipramine have increased >2- to 10-fold when fluoxetine has been administered in combination. This influence may persist for 3 weeks or longer after fluoxetine is discontinued. Thus, the dose of TCA may need to be reduced and plasma TCA concentrations may need to be monitored temporarily when SYMBYAX is coadministered or has been recently discontinued [see Clinical Pharmacology (12.3)].

Antihypertensive Agents—Because of the potential for olanzapine to induce hypotension, SYMBYAX may enhance the effects of certain antihypertensive agents [see Warnings and Precautions (5.11)].

Levodopa and Dopamine Agonists—The olanzapine component of SYMBYAX may antagonize the effects of levodopa and dopamine agonists.

Benzodiazepines—Multiple doses of olanzapine did not influence the pharmacokinetics of diazepam and its active metabolite N-desmethyldiazepam.

When concurrently administered with fluoxetine, the half-life of diazepam may be prolonged in some patients [see Clinical Pharmacology (12.3)]. Coadministration of alprazolam and fluoxetine has resulted in increased alprazolam plasma concentrations and in further psychomotor performance decrement due to increased alprazolam levels.

Clozapine—Elevation of blood levels of clozapine has been observed in patients receiving concomitant fluoxetine.

Haloperidol—Elevation of blood levels of haloperidol has been observed in patients receiving concomitant fluoxetine.

Phenytoin—Patients on stable doses of phenytoin have developed elevated plasma levels of phenytoin with clinical phenytoin toxicity following initiation of concomitant fluoxetine.

Drugs Metabolized by CYP2D6—In vitro studies utilizing human liver microsomes suggest that olanzapine has little potential to inhibit CYP2D6. Thus, olanzapine is unlikely to cause clinically important drug interactions mediated by this enzyme.

Fluoxetine inhibits the activity of CYP2D6 and may make individuals with normal CYP2D6 metabolic activity resemble a poor metabolizer. Coadministration of fluoxetine with other drugs that are metabolized by CYP2D6, including certain antidepressants (e.g., TCAs), antipsychotics (e.g., phenothiazines and most atypicals), and antiarrhythmics (e.g., propafenone, flecainide, and others) should be approached with caution. Therapy with medications that are predominantly metabolized by the CYP2D6 system and that have a relatively narrow therapeutic index should be initiated at the low end of the dose range if a patient is receiving fluoxetine concurrently or has taken it in the previous 5 weeks. If fluoxetine is added to the treatment regimen of a patient already receiving a drug metabolized by CYP2D6, the need for a decreased dose of the original medication should be considered. Drugs with a narrow therapeutic index represent the greatest concern (including but not limited to, flecainide, propafenone, vinblastine, and TCAs).

Drugs Metabolized by CYP3A—In vitro studies utilizing human liver microsomes suggest that olanzapine has little potential to inhibit CYP3A. Thus, olanzapine is unlikely to cause clinically important drug interactions mediated by these enzymes.

In an in vivo interaction study involving the coadministration of fluoxetine with single doses of terfenadine (a CYP3A substrate), no increase in plasma terfenadine concentrations occurred with concomitant fluoxetine. In addition, in vitro studies have shown ketoconazole, a potent inhibitor of CYP3A activity, to be at least 100 times more potent than fluoxetine or norfluoxetine as an inhibitor of the metabolism of several substrates for this enzyme, including astemizole, cisapride, and midazolam. These data indicate that fluoxetine's extent of inhibition of CYP3A activity is not likely to be of clinical significance.

Effect of Olanzapine on Drugs Metabolized by Other CYP Enzymes—In vitro studies utilizing human liver microsomes suggest that olanzapine has little potential to inhibit CYP1A2, CYP2C9, and CYP2C19. Thus, olanzapine is unlikely to cause clinically important drug interactions mediated by these enzymes.

Lithium—Multiple doses of olanzapine did not influence the pharmacokinetics of lithium.

There have been reports of both increased and decreased lithium levels when lithium was used concomitantly with fluoxetine. Cases of lithium toxicity and increased serotonergic effects have been reported. Lithium levels should be monitored in patients taking SYMBYAX concomitantly with lithium.

Drugs Tightly Bound to Plasma Proteins—The in vitro binding of SYMBYAX to human plasma proteins is similar to the individual components. The interaction between SYMBYAX and other highly protein-bound drugs has not been fully evaluated. Because fluoxetine is tightly bound to plasma protein, the administration of fluoxetine to a patient taking another drug that is tightly bound to protein (e.g., Coumadin, digitoxin) may cause a shift in plasma concentrations potentially resulting in an adverse effect. Conversely, adverse effects may result from displacement of protein-bound fluoxetine by other tightly bound drugs [see Clinical Pharmacology (12.3)].

Valproate—In vitro studies using human liver microsomes determined that olanzapine has little potential to inhibit the major metabolic pathway, glucuronidation, of valproate. Further, valproate has little effect on the metabolism of olanzapine in vitro. Thus, a clinically significant pharmacokinetic interaction between olanzapine and valproate is unlikely.

Biperiden—Multiple doses of olanzapine did not influence the pharmacokinetics of biperiden.

Theophylline—Multiple doses of olanzapine did not affect the pharmacokinetics of theophylline or its metabolites.

8 USE IN SPECIFIC POPULATIONS

8.1 Pregnancy

Teratogenic Effects—Pregnancy Category C

SYMBYAX—Embryo fetal development studies were conducted in rats and rabbits with olanzapine and fluoxetine in low-dose and high-dose combinations. In rats, the doses were: 2 and 4 mg/kg/day (low-dose) [1 and 0.5 times the maximum recommended human dose (MRHD) on a mg/m² basis, respectively], and 4 and 8 mg/kg/day (high-dose) [2 and 1 times the MRHD on a mg/m² basis, respectively]. In rabbits, the doses were 4 and 4 mg/kg/day (low-dose) [4 and 1 times the MRHD on a mg/m² basis, respectively], and 8 and 8 mg/kg/day (high-dose) [9 and 2 times the MRHD on a mg/m² basis, respectively]. In these studies, olanzapine and fluoxetine were also administered alone at the high-doses (4 and 8 mg/kg/day, respectively, in the rat; 8 and 8 mg/kg/day, respectively, in the rabbit). In the rabbit, there was no evidence of teratogenicity; however, the high-dose combination produced decreases in fetal weight and retarded skeletal ossification in conjunction with maternal toxicity. Similarly, in the rat there was no evidence of teratogenicity; however, a decrease in fetal weight was observed with the high-dose combination.

In a pre- and postnatal study conducted in rats, olanzapine and fluoxetine were administered during pregnancy and throughout lactation in combination (low-dose: 2 and 4 mg/kg/day [1 and 0.5 times the MRHD on a mg/m² basis], respectively, high-dose: 4 and 8 mg/kg/day [2 and 1 times the MRHD on a mg/m² basis], respectively, and alone: 4 and 8 mg/kg/day [2 and 1 times the MRHD on a mg/m² basis], respectively). Administration of the high-dose combination resulted in a marked elevation in offspring mortality and growth retardation in comparison to the same doses of olanzapine and fluoxetine administered alone. These effects were not observed with the low-dose combination; however, there were a few cases of testicular degeneration and atrophy, depletion of epididymal sperm and infertility in the male progeny. The effects of the high-dose combination on postnatal endpoints could not be assessed due to high progeny mortality.

There are no adequate and well-controlled studies with SYMBYAX in pregnant women.

SYMBYAX should be used during pregnancy only if the potential benefit justifies the potential risk to the fetus.

Olanzapine—In oral reproduction studies in rats at doses up to 18 mg/kg/day and in rabbits at doses up to 30 mg/kg/day (9 and 30 times the MRHD on a mg/m² basis, respectively), no evidence of teratogenicity was observed. In a rat teratology study, early resorptions and increased numbers of nonviable fetuses were observed at a dose of 18 mg/kg/day (9 times the MRHD on a mg/m² basis). Gestation was prolonged at 10 mg/kg/day (5 times the MRHD on a mg/m² basis). In a rabbit teratology study, fetal toxicity (manifested as increased resorptions and decreased fetal weight) occurred at a maternally toxic dose of 30 mg/kg/day (30 times the MRHD on a mg/m² basis). Because animal reproduction studies are not always predictive of human response, this drug should be used during pregnancy only if the potential benefit justifies the potential risk to the fetus. Placental transfer of olanzapine occurs in rat pups.

There are no adequate and well-controlled clinical studies with olanzapine in pregnant women. Seven pregnancies were observed during premarketing clinical studies with olanzapine, including 2 resulting in normal births, 1 resulting in neonatal death due to a cardiovascular defect, 3 therapeutic abortions, and 1 spontaneous abortion.

Fluoxetine—In oral embryo fetal development studies in rats and rabbits, there was no evidence of teratogenicity following administration of up to 12.5 and 15 mg/kg/day, respectively (1.5 and 3.6 times the MRHD on a mg/m² basis, respectively) throughout organogenesis. However, in rat reproduction studies, an increase in stillborn pups, a decrease in pup weight, and an increase in pup deaths during the first 7 days postpartum occurred following maternal exposure to 12 mg/kg/day (1.5 times the MRHD on a mg/m² basis) during gestation or 7.5 mg/kg/day (0.9 times the MRHD on a mg/m² basis) during gestation and lactation. There was no evidence of developmental neurotoxicity in the surviving offspring of rats treated with 12 mg/kg/day during gestation. The no-effect dose for rat pup mortality was 5 mg/kg/day (0.6 times the MRHD on a mg/m² basis).

Treatment of Pregnant Women During the Third Trimester—Neonates exposed to fluoxetine, a component of SYMBYAX, SNRIs, or SSRIs, late in the third trimester have developed complications requiring prolonged hospitalization, respiratory support, and tube feeding. Such complications can arise immediately upon delivery. Reported clinical findings have included respiratory distress, cyanosis, apnea, seizures, temperature instability, feeding difficulty, vomiting, hypoglycemia, hypotonia, hypertonia, hyperreflexia, tremor, jitteriness, irritability, and constant crying. These features are consistent with either a direct toxic effect of SNRIs and SSRIs or, possibly, a drug discontinuation syndrome. It should be noted that, in some cases, the clinical picture is consistent with serotonin syndrome [see Dosage and Administration (2.3), Contraindications (4), Warnings and Precautions (5.7), and Drug Interactions (7.3)].

Infants exposed to SSRIs in late pregnancy may have an increased risk for persistent pulmonary hypertension of the newborn (PPHN). PPHN occurs in 1–2 per 1000 live births in the general population and is associated with substantial neonatal morbidity and mortality. In a retrospective case-control study of 377 women whose infants were born with PPHN and 836 women whose infants were born healthy, the risk for developing PPHN was approximately 6-fold higher for infants exposed to SSRIs after the 20th week of gestation compared to infants who had not been exposed to antidepressants during pregnancy. There is currently no corroborative evidence regarding the risk for PPHN following exposure to SSRIs in pregnancy; this is the first study that has investigated the potential risk. The study did not include enough cases with exposure to individual SSRIs to determine if all SSRIs posed similar levels of PPHN risk.

When treating pregnant women with fluoxetine during the third trimester, the physician should carefully consider both the potential risks and benefits of treatment. Physicians should note that in a prospective longitudinal study of 201 women with a history of major depression who were euthymic at the beginning of pregnancy, women who discontinued antidepressant medication during pregnancy were more likely to experience a relapse of major depression than women who continued antidepressant medication. The physician may consider tapering fluoxetine in the third trimester.

8.2 Labor and Delivery

SYMBYAX—The effect of SYMBYAX on labor and delivery in humans is unknown. Parturition in rats was not affected by SYMBYAX. SYMBYAX should be used during labor and delivery only if the potential benefit justifies the potential risk.

Olanzapine—The effect of olanzapine on labor and delivery in humans is unknown. Parturition in rats was not affected by olanzapine.

Fluoxetine—The effect of fluoxetine on labor and delivery in humans is unknown. Fluoxetine crosses the placenta; therefore, there is a possibility that fluoxetine may be associated with adverse effects on the newborn.

8.3 Nursing Mothers

SYMBYAX— Studies evaluating the individual components of SYMBYAX (olanzapine and fluoxetine) in nursing mothers are described below. Because of the potential for serious adverse reactions in nursing infants from SYMBYAX, a decision should be made whether to discontinue nursing or to discontinue the drug, taking into account the importance of the drug to the mother. It is recommended that women not breast-feed when receiving SYMBYAX.

Olanzapine— In a study in lactating, healthy women, olanzapine was excreted in breast milk. Mean infant dose at steady state was estimated to be 1.8% of the maternal olanzapine dose. It is recommended that women receiving olanzapine should not breast-feed.

Fluoxetine— Fluoxetine is excreted in human breast milk. In 1 breast milk sample, the concentration of fluoxetine plus norfluoxetine was 70.4 ng/mL. The concentration in the mother's plasma was 295.0 ng/mL. No adverse effects on the infant were reported. In another case, an infant nursed by a mother on fluoxetine developed crying, sleep disturbance, vomiting, and watery stools. The infant's plasma drug levels were 340 ng/mL of fluoxetine and 208/mL of norfluoxetine on the 2nd day of feeding.

8.4 Pediatric Use

SYMBYAX— Safety and effectiveness in children and adolescent patients have not been established [see Boxed Warning and Warnings and Precautions (5.1)]. Anyone considering the use of SYMBYAX in a child or adolescent must balance the potential risks with the clinical need.

Safety and effectiveness of olanzapine and fluoxetine in combination in children and adolescent patients have not been established.

Fluoxetine— Significant toxicity, including myotoxicity, long-term neurobehavioral and reproductive toxicity, and impaired bone development, has been observed following exposure of juvenile animals to fluoxetine. Some of these effects occurred at clinically relevant exposures.

In a study in which fluoxetine (3, 10, or 30 mg/kg) was orally administered to young rats from weaning (Postnatal Day 21) through adulthood (Day 90), male and female sexual development was delayed at all doses, and growth (body weight gain, femur length) was decreased during the dosing period in animals receiving the highest dose. At the end of the treatment period, serum levels of creatine kinase (marker of muscle damage) were increased at the intermediate and high doses, and abnormal muscle and reproductive organ histopathology (skeletal muscle degeneration and necrosis, testicular degeneration and necrosis, epididymal vacuolation and hypospermia) was observed at the high dose. When animals were evaluated after a recovery period (up to 11 weeks after cessation of dosing), neurobehavioral abnormalities (decreased reactivity at all doses and learning deficit at the high dose) and reproductive functional impairment (decreased mating at all doses and impaired fertility at the high dose) were seen; in addition, testicular and epididymal microscopic lesions and decreased sperm concentrations were found in the high dose group, indicating that the reproductive organ effects seen at the end of treatment were irreversible. The reversibility of fluoxetine-induced muscle damage was not assessed. Adverse effects similar to those observed in rats treated with fluoxetine during the juvenile period have not been reported after administration of fluoxetine to adult animals. Plasma exposures (AUC) to fluoxetine in juvenile rats receiving the low, intermediate, and high dose in this study were approximately 0.1-0.2, 1-2, and 5-10 times, respectively, the average exposure in pediatric patients receiving the maximum recommended dose (MRD) of 20 mg/day. Rat exposures to the major metabolite, norfluoxetine, were approximately 0.3-0.8, 1-8, and 3-20 times, respectively, pediatric exposure at the MRD.

A specific effect of fluoxetine on bone development has been reported in mice treated with fluoxetine during the juvenile period. When mice were treated with fluoxetine (5 or 20 mg/kg, intraperitoneal) for 4 weeks starting at 4 weeks of age, bone formation was reduced resulting in decreased bone mineral content and density. These doses did not affect overall growth (body weight gain or femoral length). The doses administered to juvenile mice in this study are approximately 0.5 and 2 times the MRD for pediatric patients on a body surface area (mg/m²) basis.

In another mouse study, administration of fluoxetine (10 mg/kg intraperitoneal) during early postnatal development (Postnatal Days 4 to 21) produced abnormal emotional behaviors (decreased exploratory behavior in elevated plus-maze, increased shock avoidance latency) in adulthood (12 weeks of age). The dose used in this study is approximately equal to the pediatric MRD on a mg/m² basis. Because of the early dosing period in this study, the significance of these findings to the approved pediatric use in humans is uncertain.

8.5 Geriatric Use

SYMBYAX— Clinical studies of SYMBYAX did not include sufficient numbers of patients ≥65 years of age to determine whether they respond differently from younger patients. Other reported clinical experience has not identified differences in responses between the elderly and younger patients. In general, dose selection for an elderly patient should be cautious, usually starting at the low end of the dosing range, reflecting the greater frequency of decreased hepatic, renal, or cardiac function, and of concomitant disease or other drug therapy [see Dosage and Administration (2.3)].

Olanzapine— Of the 2500 patients in premarketing clinical studies with olanzapine, 11% (263 patients) were ≥65 years of age. In patients with Schizophrenia, there was no indication of any different tolerability of olanzapine in the elderly compared with younger patients. Studies in patients with dementia-related psychosis have suggested that there may be a different tolerability profile in this population compared with younger patients with Schizophrenia. Elderly patients with dementia-related psychosis treated with olanzapine are at an increased risk of death compared to placebo. In placebo-controlled studies of olanzapine in elderly patients with dementia-related psychosis, there was a higher incidence of cerebrovascular adverse reactions (e.g., stroke, transient ischemic attack) in patients treated with olanzapine compared to patients treated with placebo. Olanzapine is not approved for the treatment of patients with dementia-related psychosis [see Boxed Warning, Dosage and Administration (2.3), and Warnings and Precautions (5.2)].

Also, the presence of factors that might decrease pharmacokinetic clearance or increase the pharmacodynamic response to olanzapine should lead to consideration of a lower starting dose for any geriatric patient.

Fluoxetine— US fluoxetine clinical studies included 687 patients ≥65 years of age and 93 patients ≥75 years of age. No overall differences in safety or effectiveness were observed between these subjects and younger subjects, and other reported clinical experience has not identified differences in responses between the elderly and younger patients, but greater sensitivity of some older individuals cannot be ruled out. SNRIs and SSRIs, including SYMBYAX, have been associated with cases of clinically significant hyponatremia in elderly patients, who may be at greater risk for this adverse reaction [see Warnings and Precautions (5.16)].

8.6 Hepatic Impairment

In subjects with cirrhosis of the liver, the clearances of fluoxetine and its active metabolite, norfluoxetine, were decreased, thus increasing the elimination half-lives of these substances. A lower or less frequent dose of the fluoxetine-component of SYMBYAX should be used in patients with cirrhosis. Caution is advised when using SYMBYAX in patients with diseases or conditions that could affect its metabolism [see Dosage and Administration (2.3) and Clinical Pharmacology (12.4)].

9 DRUG ABUSE AND DEPENDENCE

9.3 Dependence

SYMBYAX, as with fluoxetine and olanzapine, has not been systematically studied in humans for its potential for abuse, tolerance, or physical dependence. While the clinical studies did not reveal any tendency for any drug-seeking behavior, these observations were not systematic, and it is not possible to predict on the basis of this limited experience the extent to which a CNS-active drug will be misused, diverted, and/or abused once marketed. Consequently, physicians should carefully evaluate patients for history of drug abuse and follow such patients closely, observing them for signs of misuse or abuse of SYMBYAX (e.g., development of tolerance, incrementation of dose, drug-seeking behavior).

In studies in rats and rhesus monkeys designed to assess abuse and dependence potential, olanzapine alone was shown to have acute depressive CNS effects but little or no potential of abuse or physical dependence at oral doses up to 15 (rat) and 8 (monkey) times the MRHD (20 mg) on a mg/m² basis.

10 OVERDOSAGE

SYMBYAX— During premarketing clinical studies of olanzapine and fluoxetine in combination, overdose of both fluoxetine and olanzapine were reported in 5 study subjects. Four of the 5 subjects experienced loss of consciousness (3) or coma (1). No fatalities occurred.

Adverse reactions involving overdose of fluoxetine and olanzapine in combination, and SYMBYAX, have been reported spontaneously to Eli Lilly and Company. An overdose of combination therapy is defined as confirmed or suspected ingestion of a dose of >20 mg olanzapine in combination with a dose of >80 mg fluoxetine. Adverse reactions associated with these reports included somnolence (sedation), impaired consciousness (coma), impaired neurologic function (ataxia, confusion, convulsions, dysarthria), arrhythmias, lethargy, essential tremor, agitation, acute psychosis, hypo-

tension, hypertension, and aggression. Fatalities have been confounded by exposure to additional substances including alcohol, thioridazine, oxycodone, and propoxyphene.

Olanzapine— In postmarketing reports of overdose with olanzapine alone, symptoms have been reported in the majority of cases. In symptomatic patients, symptoms with ≥10% incidence included agitation/aggressiveness, dysarthria, tachycardia, various extrapyramidal symptoms, and reduced level of consciousness ranging from sedation to coma. Among less commonly reported symptoms were the following potentially medically serious reactions: aspiration, cardiopulmonary arrest, cardiac arrhythmias (such as supraventricular tachycardia as well as a patient that experienced sinus pause with spontaneous resumption of normal rhythm), delirium, possible neuroleptic malignant syndrome, respiratory depression/arrest, convulsion, hypertension, and hypotension. Eli Lilly and Company has received reports of fatality in association with overdose of olanzapine alone. In 1 case of death, the amount of acutely ingested olanzapine was reported to be possibly as low as 450 mg of oral olanzapine; however, in another case, a patient was reported to survive an acute olanzapine ingestion of approximately 2 g of oral olanzapine.

Fluoxetine— Worldwide exposure to fluoxetine is estimated to be over 38 million patients (circa 1999). Of the 1578 cases of overdose involving fluoxetine, alone or with other drugs, reported from this population, there were 195 deaths.

Among 633 adult patients who overdosed on fluoxetine alone, 34 resulted in a fatal outcome, 378 completely recovered, and 15 patients experienced sequelae after overdose, including abnormal accommodation, abnormal gait, confusion, unresponsiveness, nervousness, pulmonary dysfunction, vertigo, tremor, elevated blood pressure, impotence, movement disorder, and hypomania. The remaining 206 patients had an unknown outcome. The most common signs and symptoms associated with non-fatal overdose were seizures, somnolence, nausea, tachycardia, and vomiting. The largest known ingestion of fluoxetine in adult patients was 8 grams in a patient who took fluoxetine alone and who subsequently recovered. However, in an adult patient who took fluoxetine alone, an ingestion as low as 520 mg has been associated with lethal outcome, but causality has not been established.

Among pediatric patients (ages 3 months to 17 years), there were 156 cases of overdose involving fluoxetine alone or in combination with other drugs. Six patients died, 127 patients completely recovered, 1 patient experienced renal failure, and 22 patients had an unknown outcome. One of the 6 fatalities was a 9-year-old boy who had a history of OCD, Tourette's Syndrome with tics, attention deficit disorder, and fetal alcohol syndrome. He had been receiving 100 mg of fluoxetine daily for 6 months in addition to clonidine, methylphenidate, and promethazine. Mixed-drug ingestion or other methods of suicide complicated all 6 overdoses in children that resulted in fatalities. The largest ingestion in pediatric patients was 3 grams, which was non-lethal.

Other important adverse reactions reported with fluoxetine overdose (single or multiple drugs) included coma, delirium, ECG abnormalities (such as QT-interval prolongation and ventricular tachycardia, including torsades de pointes-type arrhythmias), hypotension, mania, neuroleptic malignant syndrome-like reactions, pyrexia, stupor, and syncope.

10.1 Management of Overdose

In managing overdose, the possibility of multiple drug involvement should be considered. In case of acute overdose, establish and maintain an airway and ensure adequate ventilation, which may include intubation. Induction of emesis is not recommended as the possibility of obtundation, seizures, or dystonic reactions of the head and neck following overdose may create a risk for aspiration. Gastric lavage (after intubation, if patient is unconscious) and administration of activated charcoal together with a laxative should be considered. Cardiovascular monitoring should commence immediately and should include continuous electrocardiographic monitoring to detect possible arrhythmias.

A specific precaution involves patients who are taking or have recently taken SYMBYAX and may have ingested excessive quantities of a TCA (tricyclic antidepressant). In such cases, accumulation of the parent TCA and/or an active metabolite may increase the possibility of serious sequelae and extend the time needed for close medical observation. Due to the large volume of distribution of olanzapine and fluoxetine, forced diuresis, dialysis, hemoperfusion, and exchange transfusion are unlikely to be of benefit. No specific antidote for either fluoxetine or olanzapine overdose is known. Hypotension and circulatory collapse should be treated with appropriate measures such as intravenous fluids and/or sympathomimetic agents. Do not use epinephrine, dopamine, or other sympathomimetics with β-agonist activity, since beta stimulation may worsen hypotension in the setting of olanzapine-induced alpha blockade.

The physician should consider contacting a poison control center for additional information on the treatment of any overdose. Telephone numbers for certified poison control centers are listed in the *Physicians' Desk Reference (PDR)*.

11 DESCRIPTION

SYMBYAX (olanzapine and fluoxetine HCl capsules) combines an atypical antipsychotic and a selective serotonin reuptake inhibitor, olanzapine (the active ingredient in Zyprexa, and Zyprexa Zydis) and fluoxetine hydrochloride (the active ingredient in Prozac, Prozac Weekly, and Sarafem).

Olanzapine belongs to the thienobenzodiazepine class. The chemical designation is 2-methyl-4-(4-methyl-1-piperazinyl)-10*H*-thieno[2,3-*b*] [1,5]benzodiazepine. The molecular formula is $C_{17}H_{20}N_4S$, which corresponds to a molecular weight of 312.44.

Fluoxetine hydrochloride is a selective serotonin reuptake inhibitor (SSRI). The chemical designation is (±)-N-methyl-3-phenyl-3-[(α,α,α-trifluoro-*p*-tolyl)oxy]propylamine hydrochloride. The molecular formula is $C_{17}H_{18}F_3NO \cdot HCl$, which corresponds to a molecular weight of 345.79.

The chemical structures are:

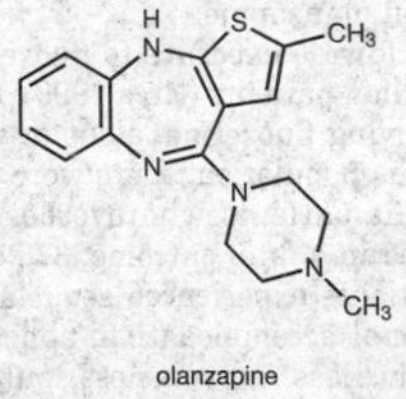

olanzapine

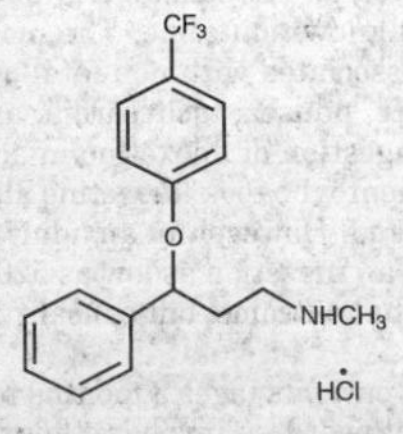

fluoxetine hydrochloride

Olanzapine is a yellow crystalline solid, which is practically insoluble in water.

Fluoxetine hydrochloride is a white to off-white crystalline solid with a solubility of 14 mg/mL in water.

SYMBYAX capsules are available for oral administration in the following strength combinations:

[See table below]

Each capsule also contains pregelatinized starch, gelatin, dimethicone, titanium dioxide, sodium lauryl sulfate, edible black ink, red iron oxide, yellow iron oxide, and/or black iron oxide.

	3 mg/25 mg	6 mg/25 mg	6 mg/50 mg	12 mg/25 mg	12 mg/50 mg
olanzapine equivalent	3	6	6	12	12
fluoxetine base equivalent	25	25	50	25	50

12 CLINICAL PHARMACOLOGY

12.1 Mechanism of Action

Although the exact mechanism of SYMBYAX is unknown, it has been proposed that the activation of 3 monoaminergic neural systems (serotonin, norepinephrine, and dopamine) is responsible for its enhanced antidepressant effect. In animal studies, ZYPREXA and fluoxetine in combination has been shown to produce synergistic increases in norepinephrine and dopamine release in the prefrontal cortex compared with either component alone, as well as increases in serotonin.

12.2 Pharmacodynamics

Olanzapine binds with high affinity to the following receptors: serotonin $5HT_{2A2C}$, $5HT_6$ (K_i=4, 11, and 5 nM, respectively), dopamine $D_{1\text{-}4}$ (K_i=11 to 31 nM), histamine H_1 (K_i=7 nM), and adrenergic α_1 receptors (K_i=19 nM). Olanzapine is an antagonist with moderate affinity binding for serotonin $5HT_3$ (K_i=57 nM) and muscarinic $M_{1\text{-}5}$ (K_i=73, 96, 132, 32, and 48 nM, respectively). Olanzapine binds weakly to $GABA_A$, BZD, and β-adrenergic receptors (K_i>10 μM). Fluoxetine is an inhibitor of the serotonin transporter and is a weak inhibitor of the norepinephrine and dopamine transporters.

Antagonism at receptors other than dopamine and $5HT_2$ may explain some of the other therapeutic and side effects of olanzapine. Olanzapine's antagonism of muscarinic $M_{1\text{-}5}$ receptors may explain its anticholinergic-like effects. The antagonism of histamine H_1 receptors by olanzapine may explain the somnolence observed with this drug. The antagonism of α_1-adrenergic receptors by olanzapine may explain the orthostatic hypotension observed with this drug. Fluoxetine has relatively low affinity for muscarinic, α_1-adrenergic, and histamine H_1 receptors.

12.3 Pharmacokinetics

SYMBYAX—Fluoxetine (administered as a 60-mg single dose or 60 mg daily for 8 days) caused a small increase in the mean maximum concentration of olanzapine (16%) following a 5-mg dose, an increase in the mean area under the curve (17%) and a small decrease in mean apparent clearance of olanzapine (16%). In another study, a similar decrease in apparent clearance of olanzapine of 14% was observed following olanzapine doses of 6 or 12 mg with concomitant fluoxetine doses of 25 mg or more. The decrease in clearance reflects an increase in bioavailability. The terminal half-life is not affected, and therefore the time to reach steady state should not be altered. The overall steady-state plasma concentrations of olanzapine and fluoxetine when given as the combination in the therapeutic dose ranges were comparable with those typically attained with each of the monotherapies. The small change in olanzapine clearance, observed in both studies, likely reflects the inhibition of a minor metabolic pathway for olanzapine via CYP2D6 by fluoxetine, a potent CYP2D6 inhibitor, and was not deemed clinically significant. Therefore, the pharmacokinetics of the individual components is expected to reasonably characterize the overall pharmacokinetics of the combination.

Absorption and Bioavailability

SYMBYAX—Following a single oral 12-mg/50-mg dose of SYMBYAX, peak plasma concentrations of olanzapine and fluoxetine occur at approximately 4 and 6 hours, respectively. The effect of food on the absorption and bioavailability of SYMBYAX has not been evaluated. The bioavailability of olanzapine given as Zyprexa, and the bioavailability of fluoxetine given as Prozac were not affected by food. It is unlikely that there would be a significant food effect on the bioavailability of SYMBYAX.

Olanzapine—Olanzapine is well absorbed and reaches peak concentration approximately 6 hours following an oral dose. Food does not affect the rate or extent of olanzapine absorption when olanzapine is given as Zyprexa. It is eliminated extensively by first pass metabolism, with approximately 40% of the dose metabolized before reaching the systemic circulation.

Fluoxetine—Following a single oral 40-mg dose, peak plasma concentrations of fluoxetine from 15 to 55 ng/mL are observed after 6 to 8 hours. Food does not appear to affect the systemic bioavailability of fluoxetine given as Prozac, although it may delay its absorption by 1 to 2 hours, which is probably not clinically significant.

Distribution

SYMBYAX—The in vitro binding to human plasma proteins of olanzapine and fluoxetine in combination is similar to the binding of the individual components.

Olanzapine—Olanzapine is extensively distributed throughout the body, with a volume of distribution of approximately 1000 L. It is 93% bound to plasma proteins over the concentration range of 7 to 1100 ng/mL, binding primarily to albumin and α_1-acid glycoprotein.

Fluoxetine—Over the concentration range from 200 to 1000 ng/mL, approximately 94.5% of fluoxetine is bound in vitro to human serum proteins, including albumin and α_1-glycoprotein. The interaction between fluoxetine and other highly protein-bound drugs has not been fully evaluated *[see Drug Interactions (7.9)]*.

Metabolism and Elimination

SYMBYAX—SYMBYAX therapy yielded steady-state concentrations of norfluoxetine similar to those seen with fluoxetine in the therapeutic dose range.

Olanzapine—Olanzapine displays linear pharmacokinetics over the clinical dosing range. Its half-life ranges from 21 to 54 hours (5th to 95th percentile; mean of 30 hr), and apparent plasma clearance ranges from 12 to 47 L/hr (5th to 95th percentile; mean of 25 L/hr). Administration of olanzapine once daily leads to steady-state concentrations in about 1 week that are approximately twice the concentrations after single doses. Plasma concentrations, half-life, and clearance of olanzapine may vary between individuals on the basis of smoking status, gender, and age *[see Dosage and Administration (2.3) and Clinical Pharmacology (12.4)]*.

Following a single oral dose of ^{14}C-labeled olanzapine, 7% of the dose of olanzapine was recovered in the urine as unchanged drug, indicating that olanzapine is highly metabolized. Approximately 57% and 30% of the dose was recovered in the urine and feces, respectively. In the plasma, olanzapine accounted for only 12% of the AUC for total radioactivity, indicating significant exposure to metabolites. After multiple dosing, the major circulating metabolites were the 10-N-glucuronide, present at steady state at 44% of the concentration of olanzapine, and 4′-N-desmethyl olanzapine, present at steady state at 31% of the concentration of olanzapine. Both metabolites lack pharmacological activity at the concentrations observed.

Direct glucuronidation and CYP450-mediated oxidation are the primary metabolic pathways for olanzapine. In vitro studies suggest that CYP1A2, CYP2D6, and the flavin-containing monooxygenase system are involved in olanzapine oxidation. CYP2D6-mediated oxidation appears to be a minor metabolic pathway in vivo, because the clearance of olanzapine is not reduced in subjects who are deficient in this enzyme.

Fluoxetine—Fluoxetine is a racemic mixture (50/50) of *R*-fluoxetine and *S*-fluoxetine enantiomers. In animal models, both enantiomers are specific and potent serotonin uptake inhibitors with essentially equivalent pharmacologic activity. The *S*-fluoxetine enantiomer is eliminated more slowly and is the predominant enantiomer present in plasma at steady state.

Fluoxetine is extensively metabolized in the liver to its only identified active metabolite, norfluoxetine, via the CYP2D6 pathway. A number of unidentified metabolites exist.

In animal models, *S*-norfluoxetine is a potent and selective inhibitor of serotonin uptake and has activity essentially equivalent to *R*- or *S*-fluoxetine. *R*-norfluoxetine is significantly less potent than the parent drug in the inhibition of serotonin uptake. The primary route of elimination appears to be hepatic metabolism to inactive metabolites excreted by the kidney.

Clinical Issues Related to Metabolism and Elimination

The complexity of the metabolism of fluoxetine has several consequences that may potentially affect the clinical use of SYMBYAX.

Variability in Metabolism—A subset (about 7%) of the population has reduced activity of the drug metabolizing enzyme CYP2D6. Such individuals are referred to as "poor metabolizers" of drugs such as debrisoquin, dextromethorphan, and the tricyclic antidepressants (TCAs). In a study involving labeled and unlabeled enantiomers administered as a racemate, these individuals metabolized *S*-fluoxetine at a slower rate and thus achieved higher concentrations of *S*-fluoxetine. Consequently, concentrations of *S*-norfluoxetine at steady state were lower. The metabolism of *R*-fluoxetine in these poor metabolizers appears normal. When compared with normal metabolizers, the total sum at steady state of the plasma concentrations of the 4 enantiomers was not significantly greater among poor metabolizers. Thus, the net pharmacodynamic activities were essentially the same. Alternative nonsaturable pathways (non-CYP2D6) also contribute to the metabolism of fluoxetine. This explains how fluoxetine achieves a steady-state concentration rather than increasing without limit.

Because the metabolism of fluoxetine, like that of a number of other compounds including TCAs and other selective serotonin antidepressants, involves the CYP2D6 system, concomitant therapy with drugs also metabolized by this enzyme system (such as the TCAs) may lead to drug interactions *[see Drug Interactions (7.9)]*.

Accumulation and Slow Elimination—The relatively slow elimination of fluoxetine (elimination half-life of 1 to 3 days after acute administration and 4 to 6 days after chronic administration) and its active metabolite, norfluoxetine (elimination half-life of 4 to 16 days after acute and chronic administration), leads to significant accumulation of these active species in chronic use and delayed attainment of steady state, even when a fixed dose is used. After 30 days of dosing at 40 mg/day, plasma concentrations of fluoxetine in the range of 91 to 302 ng/mL and norfluoxetine in the range of 72 to 258 ng/mL have been observed. Plasma concentrations of fluoxetine were higher than those predicted by single-dose studies, because the metabolism of fluoxetine is not proportional to dose. However, norfluoxetine appears to have linear pharmacokinetics. Its mean terminal half-life after a single dose was 8.6 days and after multiple dosing was 9.3 days. Steady-state levels after prolonged dosing are similar to levels seen at 4 to 5 weeks.

The long elimination half-lives of fluoxetine and norfluoxetine assure that, even when dosing is stopped, active drug substance will persist in the body for weeks (primarily depending on individual patient characteristics, previous dosing regimen, and length of previous therapy at discontinuation). This is of potential consequence when drug discontinuation is required or when drugs are prescribed that might interact with fluoxetine and norfluoxetine following the discontinuation of fluoxetine.

12.4 Specific Populations

Geriatric—Based on the individual pharmacokinetic profiles of olanzapine and fluoxetine, the pharmacokinetics of

SYMBYAX may be altered in geriatric patients. Caution should be used in dosing the elderly, especially if there are other factors that might additively influence drug metabolism and/or pharmacodynamic sensitivity.

In a study involving 24 healthy subjects, the mean elimination half-life of olanzapine was about 1.5 times greater in elderly subjects (≥65 years of age) than in non-elderly subjects (<65 years of age).

The disposition of single doses of fluoxetine in healthy elderly subjects (≥65 years of age) did not differ significantly from that in younger normal subjects. However, given the long half-life and nonlinear disposition of the drug, a single-dose study is not adequate to rule out the possibility of altered pharmacokinetics in the elderly, particularly if they have systemic illness or are receiving multiple drugs for concomitant diseases. The effects of age upon the metabolism of fluoxetine have been investigated in 260 elderly but otherwise healthy depressed patients (≥60 years of age) who received 20 mg fluoxetine for 6 weeks. Combined fluoxetine plus norfluoxetine plasma concentrations were 209.3 ± 85.7 ng/mL at the end of 6 weeks. No unusual age-associated pattern of adverse reactions was observed in those elderly patients.

Renal Impairment—The pharmacokinetics of SYMBYAX has not been studied in patients with renal impairment. However, olanzapine and fluoxetine individual pharmacokinetics do not differ significantly in patients with renal impairment. SYMBYAX dosing adjustment based upon renal impairment is not routinely required.

Because olanzapine is highly metabolized before excretion and only 7% of the drug is excreted unchanged, renal dysfunction alone is unlikely to have a major impact on the pharmacokinetics of olanzapine. The pharmacokinetic characteristics of olanzapine were similar in patients with severe renal impairment and normal subjects, indicating that dosage adjustment based upon the degree of renal impairment is not required. In addition, olanzapine is not removed by dialysis. The effect of renal impairment on olanzapine metabolite elimination has not been studied.

In depressed patients on dialysis (N=12), fluoxetine administered as 20 mg once daily for 2 months produced steady-state fluoxetine and norfluoxetine plasma concentrations comparable with those seen in patients with normal renal function. While the possibility exists that renally excreted metabolites of fluoxetine may accumulate to higher levels in patients with severe renal dysfunction, use of a lower or less frequent dose is not routinely necessary in renally impaired patients.

Hepatic Impairment—Based on the individual pharmacokinetic profiles of olanzapine and fluoxetine, the pharmacokinetics of SYMBYAX may be altered in patients with hepatic impairment. The lowest starting dose should be considered for patients with hepatic impairment *[see Dosage and Administration (2.3) and Warnings and Precautions (5.19)]*.

Although the presence of hepatic impairment may be expected to reduce the clearance of olanzapine, a study of the effect of impaired liver function in subjects (N=6) with clinically significant cirrhosis (Childs-Pugh Classification A and B) revealed little effect on the pharmacokinetics of olanzapine.

As might be predicted from its primary site of metabolism, liver impairment can affect the elimination of fluoxetine. The elimination half-life of fluoxetine was prolonged in a study of cirrhotic patients, with a mean of 7.6 days compared with the range of 2 to 3 days seen in subjects without liver disease; norfluoxetine elimination was also delayed, with a mean duration of 12 days for cirrhotic patients compared with the range of 7 to 9 days in normal subjects.

Gender—Clearance of olanzapine is approximately 30% lower in women than in men. There were, however, no apparent differences between men and women in effectiveness or adverse effects. Dosage modifications based on gender should not be needed.

Smoking Status—Olanzapine clearance is about 40% higher in smokers than in nonsmokers, although dosage modifications are not routinely required.

Race—No SYMBYAX pharmacokinetic study was conducted to investigate the effects of race. In vivo studies have shown that exposures to olanzapine are similar among Japanese, Chinese and Caucasians, especially after normalization for body weight differences. Dosage modifications for race, therefore, are not routinely required.

Combined Effects—The combined effects of age, smoking, and gender could lead to substantial pharmacokinetic differences in populations. The clearance of olanzapine in young smoking males, for example, may be 3 times higher than that in elderly nonsmoking females. SYMBYAX dosing modification may be necessary in patients who exhibit a combination of factors that may result in slower metabolism of the olanzapine component *[see Dosage and Administration (2.3)]*.

13 NONCLINICAL TOXICOLOGY

13.1 Carcinogenesis, Mutagenesis, Impairment of Fertility

No carcinogenicity, mutagenicity, or fertility studies were conducted with SYMBYAX. The following data are based on findings in studies performed with the individual components.

Carcinogenesis

Olanzapine—Oral carcinogenicity studies were conducted in mice and rats. Olanzapine was administered to mice in two 78-week studies at doses of 3, 10, and 30/20 mg/kg/day [equivalent to 0.8 to 5 times the maximum recommended human daily dose (MRHD) on a mg/m_2 basis] and 0.25, 2, and 8 mg/kg/day (equivalent to 0.06 to 2 times the MRHD on a mg/m^2 basis). Rats were dosed for 2 years at doses of 0.25, 1, 2.5, and 4 mg/kg/day (males) and 0.25, 1, 4, and 8 mg/kg/day (females) (equivalent to 0.1 to 2 and 0.1 to 4 times the MRHD on a mg/m^2 basis, respectively). The incidence of liver hemangiomas and hemangiosarcomas was significantly increased in 1 mouse study in females dosed at 8 mg/kg/day (2 times the MRHD on a mg/m^2 basis). These tumors were not increased in another mouse study in females dosed at 10 or 30/20 mg/kg/day (2 to 5 times the MRHD on a mg/m^2 basis); in this study, there was a high incidence of early mortalities in males of the 30/20 mg/kg/day group. The incidence of mammary gland adenomas and adenocarcinomas was significantly increased in female mice dosed at ≥2 mg/kg/day and in female rats dosed at ≥4 mg/kg/day (0.5 and 2 times the MRHD on a mg/m^2 basis, respectively). Antipsychotic drugs have been shown to chronically elevate prolactin levels in rodents. Serum prolactin levels were not measured during the olanzapine carcinogenicity studies; however, measurements during subchronic toxicity studies showed that olanzapine elevated serum prolactin levels up to 4-fold in rats at the same doses used in the carcinogenicity study. An increase in mammary gland neoplasms has been found in rodents after chronic administration of other antipsychotic drugs and is considered to be prolactin-mediated. The relevance for human risk of the finding of prolactin-mediated endocrine tumors in rodents is unknown *[see Warnings and Precautions (5.20)]*.

Fluoxetine—The dietary administration of fluoxetine to rats and mice for 2 years at doses of up to 10 and 12 mg/kg/day, respectively (approximately 1.2 and 0.7 times, respectively, the MRHD on a mg/m^2 basis), produced no evidence of carcinogenicity.

Mutagenesis

Olanzapine—No evidence of genotoxic potential for olanzapine was found in the Ames reverse mutation test, in vivo micronucleus test in mice, the chromosomal aberration test in Chinese hamster ovary cells, unscheduled DNA synthesis test in rat hepatocytes, induction of forward mutation test in mouse lymphoma cells, or in vivo sister chromatid exchange test in bone marrow of Chinese hamsters.

Fluoxetine—Fluoxetine and norfluoxetine have been shown to have no genotoxic effects based on the following assays: bacterial mutation assay, DNA repair assay in cultured rat hepatocytes, mouse lymphoma assay, and in vivo sister chromatid exchange assay in Chinese hamster bone marrow cells.

Impairment of Fertility

SYMBYAX—Fertility studies were not conducted with SYMBYAX. However, in a repeat-dose rat toxicology study of 3 months duration, ovary weight was decreased in females treated with the low-dose [2 and 4 mg/kg/day (1 and 0.5 times the MRHD on a mg/m^2 basis), respectively] and high-dose [4 and 8 mg/kg/day (2 and 1 times the MRHD on a mg/m^2 basis), respectively] combinations of olanzapine and fluoxetine. Decreased ovary weight, and corpora luteal depletion and uterine atrophy were observed to a greater extent in the females receiving the high-dose combination than in females receiving either olanzapine or fluoxetine alone. In a 3-month repeat-dose dog toxicology study, reduced epididymal sperm and reduced testicular and prostate weights were observed with the high-dose combination of olanzapine and fluoxetine [5 and 5 mg/kg/day (9 and 2 times the MRHD on a mg/m^2 basis), respectively] and with olanzapine alone (5 mg/kg/day or 9 times the MRHD on a mg/m^2 basis).

Olanzapine—In an oral fertility and reproductive performance study in rats, male mating performance, but not fertility, was impaired at a dose of 22.4 mg/kg/day and female fertility was decreased at a dose of 3 mg/kg/day (11 and 1.5 times the MRHD on a mg/m^2 basis, respectively). Discontinuance of olanzapine treatment reversed the effects on male-mating performance. In female rats, the precoital period was increased and the mating index reduced at 5 mg/kg/day (2.5 times the MRHD on a mg/m^2 basis). Diestrous was prolonged and estrous was delayed at 1.1 mg/kg/day (0.6 times the MRHD on a mg/m^2 basis); therefore, olanzapine may produce a delay in ovulation.

Fluoxetine—Two fertility studies conducted in adult rats at doses of up to 7.5 and 12.5 mg/kg/day (approximately 0.9 and 1.5 times the MRHD on a mg/m^2 basis) indicated that fluoxetine had no adverse effects on fertility. However, adverse effects on fertility were seen when juvenile rats were treated with fluoxetine at a high dose (30 mg/kg) associated with significant toxicity *[see Use in Specific Populations (8.4)]*.

14 CLINICAL STUDIES

14.1 Depressive Episodes Associated with Bipolar I Disorder

The efficacy of SYMBYAX for the acute treatment of depressive episodes associated with Bipolar I Disorder was established in 2 identically designed, 8-week, randomized, double-blind, controlled studies of patients who met Diagnostic and Statistical Manual 4th edition (DSM-IV) criteria for Bipolar I Disorder, Depressed utilizing flexible dosing of SYMBYAX (6/25, 6/50, or 12/50 mg/day), olanzapine (5 to 20 mg/day), and placebo. These studies included patients (≥18 years of age [n=788]) with or without psychotic symptoms and with or without a rapid cycling course.

The primary rating instrument used to assess depressive symptoms in these studies was the Montgomery-Asberg Depression Rating Scale (MADRS), a 10-item clinician-rated scale with total scores ranging from 0 to 60. The primary outcome measure of these studies was the change from baseline to endpoint in the MADRS total score. In both studies, SYMBYAX was statistically significantly superior to both olanzapine monotherapy and placebo in reduction of the MADRS total score.

14.2 Treatment Resistant Depression

The efficacy of SYMBYAX in acute treatment resistant depression was demonstrated with data from 3 clinical studies (n=579). Doses evaluated in these studies ranged from 6 to 18 mg for olanzapine and 25 to 50 mg for fluoxetine.

An 8-week randomized, double-blind controlled study was conducted to evaluate the efficacy of SYMBYAX in patients (n=300) who met DSM-IV criteria for Major Depressive Disorder and did not respond to 2 antidepressants of adequate dose and duration in their current episode. Patients who were not responding to an antidepressant in their current episode entered an 8-week open-label fluoxetine lead-in; non-responders were randomized (1:1:1) to receive SYMBYAX, olanzapine, or fluoxetine, and were treated for 8 weeks. SYMBYAX was flexibly dosed between 6/50 mg, 12/50 mg, and 18/50 mg. Results from this study yielded statistically significant greater reduction in mean total MADRS scores from baseline to endpoint for SYMBYAX versus fluoxetine and olanzapine. A second study with the same treatment-resistant patient population (n=28), when analyzed with change in MADRS as the outcome measure, demonstrated statistically significantly greater reduction in MADRS scores for SYMBYAX versus fluoxetine and olanzapine. A third study demonstrated statistically significantly greater reduction in total MADRS scores for SYMBYAX versus fluoxetine or olanzapine alone, when analyzed in a subpopulation of depressed patients (n=251) who met the definition of treatment resistance (patients who had not responded to 2 antidepressants of adequate dose and duration in the current episode).

16 HOW SUPPLIED/STORAGE AND HANDLING

16.1 How Supplied

[See table at top of next page]

16.2 Storage and Handling

Store at 25°C (77°F); excursions permitted to 15-30°C (59-86°F) [see USP Controlled Room Temperature].

Keep tightly closed and protect from moisture.

17 PATIENT COUNSELING INFORMATION

See FDA-approved Medication Guide.

Patients should be advised of the following issues and asked to alert their prescriber if these occur while taking SYMBYAX.

17.1 Information on Medication Guide

Prescribers or other health professionals should inform patients, their families, and their caregivers about the potential benefits and potential risks associated with treatment with SYMBYAX and should counsel them in its appropriate use. A patient Medication Guide is available for SYMBYAX. The prescribers or other health professionals should instruct patients, their families, and their caregivers to read the Medication Guide and should assist them in understanding its contents. Patients should be given the opportunity to discuss the contents of the Medication Guide and to obtain answers to any questions they may have.

17.2 Clinical Worsening and Suicide Risk

Patients, their families, and their caregivers should be encouraged to be alert to the emergence of anxiety, agitation, panic attacks, insomnia, irritability, hostility, aggressiveness, impulsivity, akathisia (psychomotor restlessness), hypomania, mania, other unusual changes in behavior, worsening of depression, and suicidal ideation, especially early during antidepressant treatment and when the dose is adjusted up or down. Families and caregivers of patients should be advised to look for the emergence of such symptoms on a day-to-day basis, since changes may be abrupt. Such symptoms should be reported to the patient's prescriber or health professional, especially if they are severe, abrupt in onset, or were not part of the patient's presenting symptoms. Symptoms such as these may be associated with an increased risk for suicidal thinking and behavior and indicate a need for very close monitoring and possibly changes in the medication *[see Boxed Warning and Warnings and Precautions (5.1)]*.

17.3 Elderly Patients with Dementia-Related Psychosis: Increased Mortality and Cerebrovascular Adverse Events (CVAE), Including Stroke

Patients and caregivers should be advised that elderly patients with dementia-related psychosis treated with antipsychotic drugs are at increased risk of death. Patients and caregivers should be advised that elderly patients with dementia-related psychosis treated with olanzapine had a significantly higher incidence of cerebrovascular adverse events (e.g., stroke, transient ischemic attack) compared with placebo. SYMBYAX is not approved for elderly patients with dementia-related psychosis *[see Boxed Warning and Warnings and Precautions (5.2)].*

17.4 Neuroleptic Malignant Syndrome (NMS)

Patients and caregivers should be counseled that a potentially fatal symptom complex sometimes referred to as NMS has been reported in association with administration of antipsychotic drugs, including olanzapine, a component of SYMBYAX. Signs and symptoms of NMS include hyperpyrexia, muscle rigidity, altered mental status, and evidence of autonomic instability (irregular pulse or blood pressure, tachycardia, diaphoresis, and cardiac dysrhythmia) *[see Warnings and Precautions (5.3)].*

17.5 Hyperglycemia

Patients should be advised of the potential risk of hyperglycemia-related adverse reactions. Patients should be monitored regularly for worsening of glucose control. Patients and caregivers should be counseled that metabolic changes have occurred during treatment with SYMBYAX. Patients who have diabetes should follow their doctor's instructions about how often to check their blood sugar while taking SYMBYAX *[see Warnings and Precautions (5.4)].*

17.6 Hyperlipidemia

Patients should be counseled that hyperlipidemia has occurred during treatment with SYMBYAX. Patients should have their lipid profile monitored regularly *[see Warnings and Precautions (5.5)].*

17.7 Weight Gain

Patients should be counseled that weight gain has occurred during treatment with SYMBYAX. Patients should have their weight monitored regularly *[see Warnings and Precautions (5.6)].*

17.8 Serotonin Syndrome or Neuroleptic Malignant Syndrome (NMS)-like Reactions

Patients should be cautioned about the risk of serotonin syndrome or NMS-like reactions with the concomitant use of SYMBYAX and triptans, tryptophan, tramadol, or other serotonergic agents *[see Warnings and Precautions (5.7) and Drug Interactions (7.3)].* Patients should be advised of the signs and symptoms associated with serotonin syndrome or NMS-like reactions that may include mental status changes (e.g., agitation, hallucinations, coma), autonomic instability (e.g., tachycardia, labile blood pressure, hyperthermia), neuromuscular aberrations (e.g., hyperreflexia, incoordination) and/or gastrointestinal symptoms (e.g., nausea, vomiting, diarrhea). Serotonin syndrome, in its most severe form can resemble neuroleptic malignant syndrome, in which the symptoms may include hyperthermia, muscle rigidity, autonomic instability with possible rapid fluctuation of vital signs, and mental status changes. Patients should be cautioned to seek medical care immediately if they experience these symptoms.

17.9 Allergic Reactions and Rash

Patients should be advised to notify their physician if they develop a rash or hives *[see Warnings and Precautions (5.8)].* Patients should also be advised of the signs and symptoms associated with a severe allergic reaction, including swelling of the face, eyes, or mouth, or have trouble breathing. Patients should be cautioned to seek medical care immediately if they experience these symptoms.

17.10 Orthostatic Hypotension

Patients should be advised of the risk of orthostatic hypotension, especially during the period of initial dose titration and in association with the use of concomitant drugs that may potentiate the orthostatic effect of olanzapine, e.g., diazepam or alcohol *[see Warnings and Precautions (5.11) and Drug Interactions (7.8, 7.9)].* Patients should be advised to change positions carefully to help prevent orthostatic hypotension, and to lie down if they feel dizzy or faint, until they feel better. Patients should be advised to call their doctor if they experience any of the following signs and symptoms associated with orthostatic hypotension: dizziness, fast or slow heart beat, or fainting.

17.11 Abnormal Bleeding

Patients should be cautioned about the concomitant use of SYMBYAX and NSAIDs, aspirin, warfarin, or other drugs that affect coagulation since the combined use of psychotropic drugs that interfere with serotonin reuptake and these agents have been associated with an increased risk of bleeding *[see Warnings and Precautions (5.15)].* Patients should be advised to call their doctor if they experience any increased or unusual bruising or bleeding while taking Symbyax.

17.12 Hyponatremia

Patients should be advised that hyponatremia has been reported during treatment with SNRIs and SSRIs, including SYMBYAX. Signs and symptoms of hyponatremia include headache, difficulty concentrating, memory impairment, confusion, weakness, and unsteadiness, which may lead to

SYMBYAX capsules are supplied in 3/25-, 6/25-, 6/50-, 12/25-, and 12/50-mg (mg equivalent olanzapine/mg equivalent fluoxetine[a]) strengths.

SYMBYAX	CAPSULE STRENGTH				
	3 mg/25 mg	6 mg/25 mg	6 mg/50 mg	12 mg/25 mg	12 mg/50 mg
Color	Peach & Light Yellow	Mustard Yellow & Light Yellow	Mustard Yellow & Light Grey	Red & Light Yellow	Red & Light Grey
Capsule No.	PU3230	PU3231	PU3233	PU3232	PU3234
Identification	Lilly 3230 3/25	Lilly 3231 6/25	Lilly 3233 6/50	Lilly 3232 12/25	Lilly 3234 12/50
NDC Codes					
Bottles 30	0002-3230-30	0002-3231-30	0002-3233-30	0002-3232-30	0002-3234-30
Bottles 100		0002-3231-02	0002-3233-02	0002-3232-02	0002-3234-02
Bottles 1000		0002-3231-04	0002-3233-04	0002-3232-04	0002-3234-04
Blisters ID[b] 100		0002-3231-33	0002-3233-33	0002-3232-33	0002-3234-33

[a] Fluoxetine base equivalent.
[b] IDENTI–DOSE®, Unit Dose Medication, Lilly.

falls. More severe and/or acute cases have been associated with hallucination, syncope, seizure, coma, respiratory arrest, and death *[see Warnings and Precautions (5.16)].*

17.13 Potential for Cognitive and Motor Impairment

As with any CNS-active drug, SYMBYAX has the potential to impair judgment, thinking, or motor skills. Patients should be cautioned about operating hazardous machinery, including automobiles, until they are reasonably certain that SYMBYAX therapy does not affect them adversely *[see Warnings and Precautions (5.17)].*

17.14 Body Temperature Regulation

Patients should be advised regarding appropriate care in avoiding overheating and dehydration. Patients should be advised to call their doctor right away if they become severely ill and have some or all of these symptoms of dehydration: sweating too much or not at all, dry mouth, feeling very hot, feeling thirsty, not able to produce urine *[see Warnings and Precautions (5.18)].*

17.15 Concomitant Medication

Patients should be advised to inform their physician if they are taking Prozac, Prozac Weekly, Sarafem, fluoxetine, Zyprexa, or Zyprexa Zydis. Patients should be advised to inform their physicians if they are taking, plan to take, or have stopped taking any prescription or over-the-counter drugs, including herbal supplements, since there is a potential for interactions. Patients should also be advised to inform their physicians if they plan to discontinue any medications they are taking while taking SYMBYAX, as stopping a medication may also impact the overall blood level of SYMBYAX *[see Warnings and Precautions (5.21)].*

17.16 Discontinuation of Treatment with SYMBYAX

Patients should be advised to take SYMBYAX exactly as prescribed, and to continue taking SYMBYAX as prescribed even after their mood symptoms improve. Patients should be advised that they should not alter their dosing regimen, or stop taking SYMBYAX, without consulting their physician *[see Warnings and Precautions (5.23)].*

17.17 Alcohol

Patients should be advised to avoid alcohol while taking SYMBYAX *[see Drug Interactions (7.8, 7.9)].*

17.18 Use in Specific Populations

• Pregnancy—Patients should be advised to notify their physician if they become pregnant or intend to become pregnant during SYMBYAX therapy *[see Use in Specific Populations (8.1)].*

• Nursing Mothers—Patients, if taking SYMBYAX, should be advised not to breast-feed *[see Use in Specific Populations (8.3)].*

Literature revised January 27, 2010

Eli Lilly and Company
Indianapolis, IN 46285, USA

PV 6235 AMP

MEDICATION GUIDE

SYMBYAX® (SIM-be-ax)
(olanzapine and fluoxetine hydrochloride)
Capsule

Read the Medication Guide that comes with SYMBYAX before you start taking it and each time you get a refill. There may be new information. This Medication Guide does not take the place of talking to your doctor about your medical condition or treatment. Talk with your doctor or pharmacist if there is something you do not understand or you want to learn more about SYMBYAX.

What is the most important information I should know about SYMBYAX?

Antidepressant medicines, depression and other serious mental illnesses, and suicidal thoughts or actions:
Talk to your, or your family member's, healthcare provider about:

• all risks and benefits of treatment with antidepressant medicines.

• all treatment choices for depression or other serious mental illness.

1. **Antidepressant medicines may increase suicidal thoughts or actions in some children, teenagers, and young adults within the first few months of treatment.**

2. **Depression and other serious mental illnesses are the most important causes of suicidal thoughts and actions. Some people may have a particularly high risk of having suicidal thoughts or actions.** These include people who have (or have a family history of) bipolar illness (also called manic-depressive illness) or suicidal thoughts or actions.

3. **How can I watch for and try to prevent suicidal thoughts and actions in myself or a family member?**

• Pay close attention to any changes, especially sudden changes, in mood, behaviors, thoughts, or feelings. This is very important when an antidepressant medicine is started or when the dose is changed.

• Call the healthcare provider right away to report new or sudden changes in mood, behavior, thoughts, or feelings.

• Keep all follow-up visits with the healthcare provider as scheduled. Call the healthcare provider between visits as needed, especially if you have concerns about symptoms.

Call a healthcare provider right away if you or your family member has any of the following symptoms, especially if they are new, worse, or worry you:

• thoughts about suicide or dying
• attempts to commit suicide
• new or worse depression
• new or worse anxiety
• feeling very agitated or restless
• panic attacks
• trouble sleeping (insomnia)
• new or worse irritability
• acting aggressive, being angry, or violent
• acting on dangerous impulses
• an extreme increase in activity and talking (mania)
• or other unusual changes in behavior or mood

What else do I need to know about antidepressant medicines?

• **Never stop an antidepressant medicine without first talking to a healthcare provider.** Stopping an antidepressant medicine suddenly can cause other symptoms.

• **Antidepressants are medicines used to treat depression and other illnesses.** It is important to discuss all the risks of treating depression and also the risks of not treating it. Patients and their families or other caregivers should discuss all treatment choices with the healthcare provider, not just the use of antidepressants.

- **Antidepressant medicines have other side effects.** Talk to the healthcare provider about the side effects of the medicine prescribed for you or your family member.
- **Antidepressant medicines can interact with other medicines.** Know all of the medicines that you or your family member takes. Keep a list of all medicines to show the healthcare provider. Do not start new medicines without first checking with your healthcare provider.
- **Not all antidepressant medicines prescribed for children are FDA approved for use in children.** Talk to your child's healthcare provider for more information.

SYMBYAX may be associated with the following serious risks:

High blood sugar (hyperglycemia): High blood sugar can occur if you have diabetes already or even if you have never had diabetes. In rare cases, this could lead to ketoacidosis (build up of acid in the blood due to ketones), coma, or death. Your doctor should do lab tests to check your blood sugar before you start taking SYMBYAX and during treatment. In people who do not have diabetes, sometimes high blood sugar goes away when SYMBYAX is stopped. People with diabetes and some people who did not have diabetes before taking SYMBYAX need to take medicine for high blood sugar even after they stop taking SYMBYAX.

If you have diabetes, follow your doctor's instructions about how often to check your blood sugar while taking SYMBYAX.

Call your doctor if you have any of these symptoms of high blood sugar (hyperglycemia) while taking SYMBYAX:
- feel very thirsty
- need to urinate more than usual
- feel very hungry
- feel weak or tired
- feel sick to your stomach
- feel confused, or your breath smells fruity.

High cholesterol and triglyceride levels in the blood (fat in the blood): These have been observed in patients treated with SYMBYAX, especially in teenagers (13-17 years old) who received olanzapine, one of the components of SYMBYAX. SYMBYAX is not approved for use in patients less than 18 years old. You may not have any symptoms, so your doctor should do blood tests to check your cholesterol and triglyceride levels before you start taking SYMBYAX and during treatment.

Increase in weight (weight gain): Weight gain is very commonly seen in patients who take SYMBYAX. Teenagers (13-17 years old) who received olanzapine, one of the components of SYMBYAX, are more likely to gain weight and to gain more weight than adults. SYMBYAX is not approved for use in patients less than 18 years old. Some patients may gain a lot of weight while taking SYMBYAX, so you and your doctor should check your weight regularly. Talk to your doctor about ways to control weight gain, such as eating a healthy, balanced diet, and exercising.

What is SYMBYAX?

SYMBYAX is a prescription medicine approved for use in adults:
- for short-term treatment of episodes of depression that happen with Bipolar I Disorder.
- for short-term treatment of episodes of depression that do not respond to 2 other medicines, also called treatment resistant depression.

SYMBYAX contains two medicines, olanzapine and fluoxetine hydrochloride.

It is not known if olanzapine is safe and works in children under 18 years of age.

It is not known if olanzapine and fluoxetine hydrochloride taken together, or as SYMBYAX, is safe and works in children under 18 years of age.

The symptoms of Bipolar I Disorder include alternating periods of depression and high or irritable mood, increased activity and restlessness, racing thoughts, talking fast, impulsive behavior, and a decreased need for sleep. With treatment, some of your symptoms of Bipolar I Disorder may improve.

The symptoms of treatment resistant depression include decreased mood, decreased interest, increased guilty feelings, decreased energy, decreased concentration, changes in appetite, and suicidal thoughts or behavior. With treatment, some of your symptoms of treatment resistant depression may improve.

If you do not think you are getting better, call your doctor.

Who should not take SYMBYAX?
- Do not take SYMBYAX if you take a Monoamine Oxidase Inhibitor (MAOI) or if you stopped taking an MAOI in the last 2 weeks.
- Do not take an MAOI within 5 weeks of stopping SYMBYAX. People who take SYMBYAX close in time to an MAOI can have serious and life-threatening side effects, with symptoms including:
  - high fever
  - continued muscle spasms that you cannot control
  - rigid muscles

- changes in heart rate and blood pressure that happen fast
- confusion
- unconsciousness.

Ask your doctor or pharmacist if you are not sure if your medicine is an MAOI.
- Do not take SYMBYAX if you take Mellaril® (thioridazine). Do not take Mellaril within 5 weeks of stopping SYMBYAX. Mellaril can cause serious heart rhythm problems and you could die suddenly.
- Do not take SYMBYAX if you take the antipsychotic medicine pimozide (Orap®).

What should I tell my doctor before taking SYMBYAX?

SYMBYAX may not be right for you. Before starting SYMBYAX, tell your doctor about all your medical conditions, including if you have or had any of the following:
- heart problems
- seizures (convulsions)
- diabetes or high blood sugar levels (hyperglycemia)
- high cholesterol or triglyceride levels in your blood
- liver problems
- low or high blood pressure
- strokes or "mini-strokes" also called transient ischemic attacks (TIAs)
- bleeding problems
- Alzheimer's disease
- narrow-angle glaucoma
- enlarged prostate in men
- bowel obstruction
- breast cancer
- are pregnant or plan to become pregnant. It is not known if SYMBYAX will harm your unborn baby.
- are breast-feeding or plan to breast-feed. Olanzapine and fluoxetine can pass into your breast milk and may harm your baby. You should not breast-feed while taking SYMBYAX. Talk to your doctor about the best way to feed your baby if you take SYMBYAX.

Tell your doctor about all the medicines that you take, including prescription and non-prescription medicines, vitamins, and herbal supplements. SYMBYAX and some medicines may interact with each other and may not work as well, or cause possible serious side effects. Your doctor can tell you if it is safe to take SYMBYAX with your other medicines. Do not start or stop any medicine while taking SYMBYAX without talking to your doctor first.

If you take SYMBYAX, you should not take any other medicines that contain:
- olanzapine (the active ingredient in Zyprexa® and Zyprexa® Zydis) or
- fluoxetine hydrochloride (the active ingredient in Prozac®, Prozac® Weekly™, and Sarafem®).

You could take too much medicine (overdose).

How should I take SYMBYAX?
- Take SYMBYAX exactly as prescribed. Your doctor may need to change (adjust) the dose of SYMBYAX until it is right for you.
- If you miss a dose of SYMBYAX, take the missed dose as soon as you remember. If it is almost time for the next dose, skip the missed dose and take your next dose at the regular time. Do not take two doses of SYMBYAX at the same time.
- **To prevent serious side effects, do not stop taking SYMBYAX suddenly. If you need to stop taking SYMBYAX, your doctor can tell you how to safely stop taking it.**
- **If you take too much SYMBYAX, call your doctor or poison control center right away, or get emergency treatment.**
- SYMBYAX can be taken with or without food.
- SYMBYAX is usually taken one time each day, in the evening.
- If you do not think you are getting better or have any concerns about your condition while taking SYMBAX, call your doctor.

What should I avoid while taking SYMBYAX?
- SYMBYAX can cause sleepiness and may affect your ability to make decisions, think clearly, or react quickly. You should not drive, operate heavy machinery, or do other dangerous activities until you know how SYMBYAX affects you.
- Avoid drinking alcohol while taking SYMBYAX. Drinking alcohol while you take SYMBYAX may make you sleepier than if you take SYMBYAX alone.

What are the possible side effects of SYMBYAX?

Other possible serious risks:
- **Increased risk of death and increased incidence of stroke or "mini-strokes" called transient ischemic attacks (TIAs) in elderly people with psychosis related to dementia** (a brain disorder that lessens the ability to remember, think, and reason). SYMBYAX is not approved for these patients.
- **Severe allergic reactions:** Tell your doctor right away if you get red itchy welts (hives) or, a rash alone or with fe-

ver and joint pain, while taking SYMBYAX. Call your doctor right away if you become severely ill and have some or all of these symptoms:
- swelling of your face, eyes, or mouth
- trouble breathing
- **Neuroleptic malignant syndrome (NMS):** NMS is a rare but very serious condition that can happen in people who take antipsychotic medicines, including SYMBYAX. NMS can cause death and must be treated in a hospital. Call your doctor right away if you become severely ill and have some or all of these symptoms:
  - high fever
  - excessive sweating
  - rigid muscles
  - confusion
  - changes in your breathing, heartbeat, and blood pressure
- **Tardive Dyskinesia:** This condition causes body movements that keep happening and that you cannot control. These movements usually affect the face and tongue. Tardive dyskinesia may not go away, even if you stop taking SYMBYAX. It may also start after you stop taking SYMBYAX. Tell your doctor if you get any body movements that you cannot control.
- **Serotonin Syndrome:** This is a condition that can be life threatening. Call your doctor right away if you become severely ill and have some or all of these symptoms:
  - agitation
  - hallucinations
  - problems with coordination
  - racing heart beat
  - over-active reflexes
  - fever
  - nausea, vomiting, and diarrhea
- **Abnormal bleeding:** Tell your doctor if you notice any increased or unusual bruising or bleeding while taking SYMBYAX, especially if you take one of these medicines:
  - the blood thinner warfarin (Coumadin, Jantoven)
  - a non-steroidal anti-inflammatory drug (NSAID)
  - aspirin
- **Low salt (sodium) levels in the blood (hyponatremia):** Call your doctor right away if you become severely ill and have some or all of these symptoms:
  - headache
  - feel weak
  - confusion
  - problems concentrating
  - memory problems
  - feel unsteady
- **Decreased blood pressure when you change positions, with symptoms of dizziness, fast or slow heart beat, or fainting**
- Difficulty swallowing
- Seizures
- Problems with control of body temperature: You could become very hot, for instance when you exercise a lot or stay in an area that is very hot. It is important for you to drink water to avoid dehydration. Call your doctor right away if you become severely ill and have some or all of these symptoms of dehydration:
  - sweating too much or not at all
  - dry mouth
  - feeling very hot
  - feeling thirsty
  - not able to produce urine

Common possible side effects of SYMBYAX include: dry mouth, tiredness, sleeping for long period of time, increased appetite, swelling of your hands and feet, drowsiness, tremors (shakes), or blurred vision.

Tell your doctor about any side effect that bothers you or that does not go away.

These are not all the possible side effects with SYMBYAX. For more information, ask your doctor or pharmacist.

Call your doctor for medical advice about side effects. You may report side effects to FDA at 1-800-FDA-1088.

How should I store SYMBYAX?
- Store SYMBYAX at room temperature, between 59°F to 86°F (15°C to 30°C).
- Keep SYMBYAX away from light.
- Keep SYMBYAX dry and away from moisture. Keep the bottle closed tightly.

Keep SYMBYAX and all medicines out of the reach of children.

General information about SYMBYAX

Medicines are sometimes prescribed for purposes other than those listed in a Medication Guide. Do not use SYMBYAX for a condition for which it was not prescribed. Do not give SYMBYAX to other people, even if they have the same condition. It may harm them.

This Medication Guide summarizes the most important information about SYMBYAX. If you would like more information, talk with your doctor. You can ask your doctor or pharmacist for information about SYMBYAX that was written for healthcare professionals. For more information about SYMBYAX call 1-800-Lilly-Rx (1-800-545-5979) or visit www.symbyax.com.

What are the ingredients in SYMBYAX?
Active ingredients: olanzapine and fluoxetine hydrochloride
Inactive ingredients: pregelatinized starch, gelatin, dimethicone, titanium dioxide, sodium lauryl sulfate, edible black ink, red iron oxide, yellow iron oxide, and/or black iron oxide.
This Medication Guide has been approved by the U.S. Food and Drug Administration.
Medication Guide revised March 19, 2009
Eli Lilly and Company
Indianapolis, IN 46285, USA
www.symbyax.com
Copyright © 2009, Eli Lilly and Company. All rights reserved.
PV 7110 AMP
Shown in Product Identification Guide, page 311

ZYPREXA® ℞
[*zī-prex-ah*]
(olanzapine)
Tablet for Oral Use
ZYPREXA® ZYDIS®
(olanzapine)
Tablet, Orally Disintegrating for Oral Use
ZYPREXA® IntraMuscular
(olanzapine)
Injection, Powder, For Solution for Intramuscular Use

HIGHLIGHTS OF PRESCRIBING INFORMATION
These highlights do not include all the information needed to use ZYPREXA safely and effectively. See full prescribing information for ZYPREXA.
ZYPREXA (olanzapine) Tablet for Oral use
ZYPREXA ZYDIS (olanzapine) Tablet, Orally Disintegrating for Oral use
ZYPREXA IntraMuscular (olanzapine) Injection, Powder, For Solution for Intramuscular use
Initial U.S. Approval: 1996

WARNING: INCREASED MORTALITY IN ELDERLY PATIENTS WITH DEMENTIA-RELATED PSYCHOSIS
See full prescribing information for complete boxed warning.
• Elderly patients with dementia-related psychosis treated with antipsychotic drugs are at an increased risk of death. ZYPREXA is not approved for the treatment of patients with dementia-related psychosis. (5.1, 5.14, 17.2)
When using ZYPREXA and fluoxetine in combination, also refer to the Boxed Warning section of the package insert for Symbyax.

RECENT MAJOR CHANGES

Indications and Usage:	
Schizophrenia (1.1)	12/2009
Bipolar I Disorder (Manic or Mixed Episodes) (1.2)	12/2009
Special Considerations in Treating Pediatric Schizophrenia and Bipolar I Disorder (1.3)	12/2009
ZYPREXA IntraMuscular: Agitation Associated with Schizophrenia and Bipolar I Mania (1.4)	12/2009
Dosage and Administration:	
Schizophrenia (2.1)	12/2009
Bipolar I Disorder (Manic or Mixed Episodes) (2.2)	12/2009
Warnings and Precautions:	
Orthostatic Hypotension (5.8)	05/2010
Leukopenia, Neutropenia, and Agranulocytosis (5.9)	08/2009
Hyperprolactinemia (5.15)	01/2010

INDICATIONS AND USAGE

ZYPREXA® (olanzapine) is an atypical antipsychotic indicated:
As oral formulation for the:
• Treatment of schizophrenia. (1.1)
  • Adults: Efficacy was established in three clinical trials in patients with schizophrenia: two 6-week trials and one maintenance trial. (14.1)
  • Adolescents (ages 13-17): Efficacy was established in one 6-week trial in patients with schizophrenia (14.1). The increased potential (in adolescents compared with adults) for weight gain and hyperlipidemia may lead clinicians to consider prescribing other drugs first in adolescents. (1.1)

• Acute treatment of manic or mixed episodes associated with bipolar I disorder and maintenance treatment of bipolar I disorder. (1.2)
  • Adults: Efficacy was established in three clinical trials in patients with manic or mixed episodes of bipolar I disorder: two 3- to 4-week trials and one maintenance trial. (14.2)
  • Adolescents (ages 13-17): Efficacy was established in one 3-week trial in patients with manic or mixed episodes associated with bipolar I disorder (14.2). The increased potential (in adolescents compared with adults) for weight gain and hyperlipidemia may lead clinicians to consider prescribing other drugs first in adolescents. (1.2)
• Medication therapy for pediatric patients with schizophrenia or bipolar I disorder should be undertaken only after a thorough diagnostic evaluation and with careful consideration of the potential risks. (1.3)
• Adjunct to valproate or lithium in the treatment of manic or mixed episodes associated with bipolar I disorder. (1.2)
  • Efficacy was established in two 6-week clinical trials in adults (14.2). Maintenance efficacy has not been systematically evaluated.
As ZYPREXA IntraMuscular for the:
• Treatment of acute agitation associated with schizophrenia and bipolar I mania. (1.4)
  • Efficacy was established in three 1-day trials in adults. (14.3)
As ZYPREXA and Fluoxetine in Combination for the:
• Treatment of depressive episodes associated with bipolar I disorder. (1.5)
  • Efficacy was established with Symbyax (olanzapine and fluoxetine in combination) in adults; refer to the product label for Symbyax.
• Treatment of treatment resistant depression (major depressive disorder in patients who do not respond to 2 separate trials of different antidepressants of adequate dose and duration in the current episode). (1.6)
  • Efficacy was established with Symbyax (olanzapine and fluoxetine in combination) in adults; refer to the product label for Symbyax.

DOSAGE AND ADMINISTRATION

Schizophrenia in adults (2.1)	Oral: Start at 5-10 mg once daily; Target: 10 mg/day within several days
Schizophrenia in adolescents (2.1)	Oral: Start at 2.5-5 mg once daily; Target: 10 mg/day
Bipolar I Disorder (manic or mixed episodes) in adults (2.2)	Oral: Start at 10 or 15 mg once daily
Bipolar I Disorder (manic or mixed episodes) in adolescents (2.2)	Oral: Start at 2.5-5 mg once daily; Target: 10 mg/day
Bipolar I Disorder (manic or mixed episodes) with lithium or valproate in adults (2.2)	Oral: Start at 10 mg once daily
Agitation associated with Schizophrenia and Bipolar I Mania in adults (2.4)	IM: 10 mg (5 mg or 7.5 mg when clinically warranted) Assess for orthostatic hypotension prior to subsequent dosing (max. 3 doses 2-4 hrs apart)
Depressive Episodes associated with Bipolar I Disorder in adults (2.5)	Oral in combination with fluoxetine: Start at 5 mg of oral olanzapine and 20 mg of fluoxetine once daily
Treatment Resistant Depression in adults (2.6)	Oral in combination with fluoxetine: Start at 5 mg of oral olanzapine and 20 mg of fluoxetine once daily

• Lower starting dose recommended in debilitated or pharmacodynamically sensitive patients or patients with predisposition to hypotensive reactions, or with potential for slowed metabolism. (2.1)
• Olanzapine may be given without regard to meals. (2.1)
ZYPREXA and Fluoxetine in Combination:
• Dosage adjustments, if indicated, should be made with the individual components according to efficacy and tolerability. (2.5, 2.6)
• Olanzapine monotherapy is not indicated for the treatment of depressive episodes associated with bipolar I disorder or treatment resistant depression. (2.5, 2.6)

• Safety of co-administration of doses above 18 mg olanzapine with 75 mg fluoxetine has not been evaluated. (2.5, 2.6)

DOSAGE FORMS AND STRENGTHS

• Tablets (not scored): 2.5, 5, 7.5, 10, 15, 20 mg (3)
• Orally Disintegrating Tablets (not scored): 5, 10, 15, 20 mg (3)
• Intramuscular Injection: 10 mg vial (3)

CONTRAINDICATIONS

• None with ZYPREXA monotherapy.
• When using ZYPREXA and fluoxetine in combination, also refer to the Contraindications section of the package insert for Symbyax®. (4)
• When using ZYPREXA in combination with lithium or valproate, refer to the Contraindications section of the package inserts for those products. (4)

WARNINGS AND PRECAUTIONS

• *Elderly Patients with Dementia-Related Psychosis:* Increased risk of death and increased incidence of cerebrovascular adverse events (e.g., stroke, transient ischemic attack). (5.1)
• *Suicide:* The possibility of a suicide attempt is inherent in schizophrenia and in bipolar I disorder, and close supervision of high-risk patients should accompany drug therapy; when using in combination with fluoxetine, also refer to the Boxed Warning and Warnings and Precautions sections of the package insert for Symbyax. (5.2)
• *Neuroleptic Malignant Syndrome:* Manage with immediate discontinuation and close monitoring. (5.3)
• *Hyperglycemia:* In some cases extreme and associated with ketoacidosis or hyperosmolar coma or death, has been reported in patients taking olanzapine. Patients taking olanzapine should be monitored for symptoms of hyperglycemia and undergo fasting blood glucose testing at the beginning of, and periodically during, treatment. (5.4)
• *Hyperlipidemia:* Undesirable alterations in lipids have been observed. Appropriate clinical monitoring is recommended, including fasting blood lipid testing at the beginning of, and periodically during, treatment. (5.5)
• *Weight Gain:* Potential consequences of weight gain should be considered. Patients should receive regular monitoring of weight. (5.6)
• *Tardive Dyskinesia:* Discontinue if clinically appropriate. (5.7)
• *Orthostatic Hypotension:* Orthostatic hypotension associated with dizziness, tachycardia, bradycardia and, in some patients, syncope, may occur especially during initial dose titration. Use caution in patients with cardiovascular disease, cerebrovascular disease, and those conditions that could affect hemodynamic responses. (5.8)
• *Leukopenia, Neutropenia, and Agranulocytosis:* Has been reported with antipsychotics, including ZYPREXA. Patients with a history of a clinically significant low white blood cell count (WBC) or drug induced leukopenia/neutropenia should have their complete blood count (CBC) monitored frequently during the first few months of therapy and discontinuation of ZYPREXA should be considered at the first sign of a clinically significant decline in WBC in the absence of other causative factors. (5.9)
• *Seizures:* Use cautiously in patients with a history of seizures or with conditions that potentially lower the seizure threshold. (5.11)
• *Potential for Cognitive and Motor Impairment:* Has potential to impair judgment, thinking, and motor skills. Use caution when operating machinery. (5.12)
• *Hyperprolactinemia:* May elevate prolactin levels. (5.15)
• *Use in Combination with Fluoxetine, Lithium or Valproate:* Also refer to the package inserts for Symbyax, lithium, or valproate. (5.16)
• *Laboratory Tests:* Monitor fasting blood glucose and lipid profiles at the beginning of, and periodically during, treatment. (5.17)

ADVERSE REACTIONS

Most common adverse reactions (≥5% and at least twice that for placebo) associated with:
Oral Olanzapine Monotherapy:
• Schizophrenia (Adults)—postural hypotension, constipation, weight gain, dizziness, personality disorder, akathisia (6.1)
• Schizophrenia (Adolescents)—sedation, weight increased, headache, increased appetite, dizziness, abdominal pain, pain in extremity, fatigue, dry mouth (6.1)
• Manic or Mixed Episodes, Bipolar I Disorder (Adults)—asthenia, dry mouth, constipation, increased appetite, somnolence, dizziness, tremor (6.1)
• Manic or Mixed Episodes, Bipolar I Disorder (Adolescents)—sedation, weight increased, increased appetite, headache, fatigue, dizziness, dry mouth, abdominal pain, pain in extremity (6.1)
Combination of ZYPREXA and Lithium or Valproate:
• Manic or Mixed Episodes, Bipolar I Disorder (Adults)—dry mouth, weight gain, increased appetite, dizziness,

back pain, constipation, speech disorder, increased salivation, amnesia, paresthesia (6.1)

ZYPREXA and Fluoxetine in Combination: Also refer to the Adverse Reactions section of the package insert for Symbyax. (6)

ZYPREXA IntraMuscular for Injection:
• Agitation with Schizophrenia and Bipolar I Mania (Adults)—somnolence (6.1)

To report SUSPECTED ADVERSE REACTIONS, contact Eli Lilly and Company at 1-800-LillyRx (1-800-545-5979) or FDA at 1-800-FDA-1088 or www.fda.gov/medwatch

————————DRUG INTERACTIONS————————

• *Diazepam:* May potentiate orthostatic hypotension. (7.1, 7.2)
• *Alcohol:* May potentiate orthostatic hypotension. (7.1)
• *Carbamazepine:* Increased clearance of olanzapine. (7.1)
• *Fluvoxamine:* May increase olanzapine levels. (7.1)
• *ZYPREXA and Fluoxetine in Combination:* Also refer to the Drug Interactions section of the package insert for Symbyax. (7.1)
• *CNS Acting Drugs:* Caution should be used when taken in combination with other centrally acting drugs and alcohol. (7.2)
• *Antihypertensive Agents:* Enhanced antihypertensive effect. (7.2)
• *Levodopa and Dopamine Agonists:* May antagonize levodopa/dopamine agonists. (7.2)
• *Lorazepam (IM):* Increased somnolence with IM olanzapine. (7.2)
• *Other Concomitant Drug Therapy:* When using olanzapine in combination with lithium or valproate, refer to the Drug Interactions sections of the package insert for those products. (7.2)

————————USE IN SPECIFIC POPULATIONS————————

• *Pregnancy:* ZYPREXA should be used during pregnancy only if the potential benefit justifies the potential risk to the fetus. (8.1)
• *Nursing Mothers:* Breast-feeding is not recommended. (8.3)
• *Pediatric Use:* Safety and effectiveness of ZYPREXA in children <13 years of age have not been established. (8.4)

See 17 for PATIENT COUNSELING INFORMATION and Medication Guide

Revised: 05/2010

FULL PRESCRIBING INFORMATION: CONTENTS*
WARNING: INCREASED MORTALITY IN ELDERLY PATIENTS WITH DEMENTIA-RELATED PSYCHOSIS

* Sections or subsections omitted from the full prescribing information are not listed

FULL PRESCRIBING INFORMATION

WARNING: INCREASED MORTALITY IN ELDERLY PATIENTS WITH DEMENTIA-RELATED PSYCHOSIS
Elderly patients with dementia-related psychosis treated with antipsychotic drugs are at an increased risk of death. Analyses of seventeen placebo-controlled trials (modal duration of 10 weeks), largely in patients taking atypical antipsychotic drugs, revealed a risk of death in drug-treated patients of between 1.6 to 1.7 times the risk of death in placebo-treated patients. Over the course of a typical 10-week controlled trial, the rate of death in drug-treated patients was about 4.5%, compared to a rate of about 2.6% in the placebo group. Although the causes of death were varied, most of the deaths appeared to be either cardiovascular (e.g., heart failure, sudden death) or infectious (e.g., pneumonia) in nature. Observational studies suggest that, similar to atypical antipsychotic drugs, treatment with conventional antipsychotic drugs may increase mortality. The extent to which the findings of increased mortality in observational studies may be attributed to the antipsychotic drug as opposed to some characteristic(s) of the patients is not clear. ZYPREXA (olanzapine) is not approved for the treatment of patients with dementia-related psychosis [see Warnings and Precautions (5.1, 5.14) and Patient Counseling Information (17.2)].
When using ZYPREXA and fluoxetine in combination, also refer to the Boxed Warning section of the package insert for Symbyax.

1 INDICATIONS AND USAGE

1.1 Schizophrenia
Oral ZYPREXA is indicated for the treatment of schizophrenia. Efficacy was established in three clinical trials in adult patients with schizophrenia: two 6-week trials and one maintenance trial. In adolescent patients with schizophrenia (ages 13-17), efficacy was established in one 6-week trial [see Clinical Studies (14.1)].
When deciding among the alternative treatments available for adolescents, clinicians should consider the increased potential (in adolescents as compared with adults) for weight gain and hyperlipidemia. Clinicians should consider the potential long-term risks when prescribing to adolescents, and in many cases this may lead them to consider prescribing other drugs first in adolescents [see Warnings and Precautions (5.5, 5.6)].

1.2 Bipolar I Disorder (Manic or Mixed Episodes)
Monotherapy—Oral ZYPREXA is indicated for the acute treatment of manic or mixed episodes associated with bipolar I disorder and maintenance treatment of bipolar I disorder. Efficacy was established in three clinical trials in adult patients with manic or mixed episodes of bipolar I disorder: two 3- to 4-week trials and one monotherapy maintenance trial. In adolescent patients with manic or mixed episodes associated with bipolar I disorder (ages 13-17), efficacy was established in one 3-week trial [see Clinical Studies (14.2)].
When deciding among the alternative treatments available for adolescents, clinicians should consider the increased potential (in adolescents as compared with adults) for weight gain and hyperlipidemia. Clinicians should consider the potential long-term risks when prescribing to adolescents, and in many cases this may lead them to consider prescribing other drugs first in adolescents [see Warnings and Precautions (5.5, 5.6)].
Adjunctive Therapy to Lithium or Valproate—Oral ZYPREXA is indicated for the treatment of manic or mixed episodes associated with bipolar I disorder as an adjunct to lithium or valproate. Efficacy was established in two 6-week clinical trials in adults. The effectiveness of adjunctive therapy for longer-term use has not been systematically evaluated in controlled trials [see Clinical Studies (14.2)].

1.3 Special Considerations in Treating Pediatric Schizophrenia and Bipolar I Disorder
Pediatric schizophrenia and bipolar I disorder are serious mental disorders; however, diagnosis can be challenging. For pediatric schizophrenia, symptom profiles can be variable, and for bipolar I disorder, pediatric patients may have variable patterns of periodicity of manic or mixed symptoms. It is recommended that medication therapy for pediatric schizophrenia and bipolar I disorder be initiated only after a thorough diagnostic evaluation has been performed and careful consideration given to the risks associated with medication treatment. Medication treatment for both pediatric schizophrenia and bipolar I disorder should be part of a total treatment program that often includes psychological, educational and social interventions.

1.4 ZYPREXA IntraMuscular: Agitation Associated with Schizophrenia and Bipolar I Mania
ZYPREXA IntraMuscular is indicated for the treatment of acute agitation associated with schizophrenia and bipolar I mania.
Efficacy was demonstrated in 3 short-term (24 hours of IM treatment) placebo-controlled trials in agitated adult inpatients with: schizophrenia or bipolar I disorder (manic or mixed episodes) [see Clinical Studies (14.3)].
"Psychomotor agitation" is defined in DSM-IV as "excessive motor activity associated with a feeling of inner tension." Patients experiencing agitation often manifest behaviors that interfere with their diagnosis and care, e.g., threatening behaviors, escalating or urgently distressing behavior, or self-exhausting behavior, leading clinicians to the use of intramuscular antipsychotic medications to achieve immediate control of the agitation.

1.5 ZYPREXA and Fluoxetine in Combination: Depressive Episodes Associated with Bipolar I Disorder
Oral ZYPREXA and fluoxetine in combination is indicated for the treatment of depressive episodes associated with bipolar I disorder, based on clinical studies in adult patients. When using ZYPREXA and fluoxetine in combination, refer to the Clinical Studies section of the package insert for Symbyax.
ZYPREXA monotherapy is not indicated for the treatment of depressive episodes associated with bipolar I disorder.

1.6 ZYPREXA and Fluoxetine in Combination: Treatment Resistant Depression
Oral ZYPREXA and fluoxetine in combination is indicated for the treatment of treatment resistant depression (major depressive disorder in patients who do not respond to 2 separate trials of different antidepressants of adequate dose and duration in the current episode), based on clinical studies in adult patients. When using ZYPREXA and fluoxetine in combination, refer to the Clinical Studies section of the package insert for Symbyax.

ZYPREXA monotherapy is not indicated for the treatment of treatment resistant depression.

2 DOSAGE AND ADMINISTRATION

2.1 Schizophrenia

Adults

Dose Selection—Oral olanzapine should be administered on a once-a-day schedule without regard to meals, generally beginning with 5 to 10 mg initially, with a target dose of 10 mg/day within several days. Further dosage adjustments, if indicated, should generally occur at intervals of not less than 1 week, since steady state for olanzapine would not be achieved for approximately 1 week in the typical patient. When dosage adjustments are necessary, dose increments/decrements of 5 mg QD are recommended.

Efficacy in schizophrenia was demonstrated in a dose range of 10 to 15 mg/day in clinical trials. However, doses above 10 mg/day were not demonstrated to be more efficacious than the 10 mg/day dose. An increase to a dose greater than the target dose of 10 mg/day (i.e., to a dose of 15 mg/day or greater) is recommended only after clinical assessment. Olanzapine is not indicated for use in doses above 20 mg/day.

Dosing in Special Populations—The recommended starting dose is 5 mg in patients who are debilitated, who have a predisposition to hypotensive reactions, who otherwise exhibit a combination of factors that may result in slower metabolism of olanzapine (e.g., nonsmoking female patients ≥65 years of age), or who may be more pharmacodynamically sensitive to olanzapine *[see Warnings and Precautions (5.14), Drug Interactions (7), and Clinical Pharmacology (12.3)]*. When indicated, dose escalation should be performed with caution in these patients.

Maintenance Treatment—The effectiveness of oral olanzapine, 10 mg/day to 20 mg/day, in maintaining treatment response in schizophrenic patients who had been stable on ZYPREXA for approximately 8 weeks and were then followed for relapse has been demonstrated in a placebo-controlled trial *[see Clinical Studies (14.1)]*. The physician who elects to use ZYPREXA for extended periods should periodically reevaluate the long-term usefulness of the drug for the individual patient.

Adolescents

Dose Selection—Oral olanzapine should be administered on a once-a-day schedule without regard to meals with a recommended starting dose of 2.5 or 5 mg, with a target dose of 10 mg/day. Efficacy in adolescents with schizophrenia was demonstrated based on a flexible dose range of 2.5 to 20 mg/day in clinical trials, with a mean modal dose of 12.5 mg/day (mean dose of 11.1 mg/day). When dosage adjustments are necessary, dose increments/decrements of 2.5 or 5 mg are recommended.

The safety and effectiveness of doses above 20 mg/day have not been evaluated in clinical trials *[see Clinical Studies (14.1)]*.

Maintenance Treatment—The efficacy of ZYPREXA for the maintenance treatment of schizophrenia in the adolescent population has not been systematically evaluated; however, maintenance efficacy can be extrapolated from adult data along with comparisons of olanzapine pharmacokinetic parameters in adult and adolescent patients. Thus, it is generally recommended that responding patients be continued beyond the acute response, but at the lowest dose needed to maintain remission. Patients should be periodically reassessed to determine the need for maintenance treatment.

2.2 Bipolar I Disorder (Manic or Mixed Episodes)

Adults

Dose Selection for Monotherapy—Oral olanzapine should be administered on a once-a-day schedule without regard to meals, generally beginning with 10 or 15 mg. Dosage adjustments, if indicated, should generally occur at intervals of not less than 24 hours, reflecting the procedures in the placebo-controlled trials. When dosage adjustments are necessary, dose increments/decrements of 5 mg QD are recommended.

Short-term (3-4 weeks) antimanic efficacy was demonstrated in a dose range of 5 mg to 20 mg/day in clinical trials. The safety of doses above 20 mg/day has not been evaluated in clinical trials *[see Clinical Studies (14.2)]*.

Maintenance Monotherapy—The benefit of maintaining bipolar I patients on monotherapy with oral ZYPREXA at a dose of 5 to 20 mg/day, after achieving a responder status for an average duration of 2 weeks, was demonstrated in a controlled trial *[see Clinical Studies (14.2)]*. The physician who elects to use ZYPREXA for extended periods should periodically reevaluate the long-term usefulness of the drug for the individual patient.

Dose Selection for Adjunctive Treatment—When administered as adjunctive treatment to lithium or valproate, oral olanzapine dosing should generally begin with 10 mg once-a-day without regard to meals.

Antimanic efficacy was demonstrated in a dose range of 5 mg to 20 mg/day in clinical trials *[see Clinical Studies (14.2)]*. The safety of doses above 20 mg/day has not been evaluated in clinical trials.

Adolescents

Dose Selection—Oral olanzapine should be administered on a once-a-day schedule without regard to meals with a recommended starting dose of 2.5 or 5 mg, with a target dose of 10 mg/day. Efficacy in adolescents with bipolar I disorder (manic or mixed episodes) was demonstrated based on a flexible dose range of 2.5 to 20 mg/day in clinical trials, with a mean modal dose of 10.7 mg/day (mean dose of 8.9 mg/day). When dosage adjustments are necessary, dose increments/decrements of 2.5 or 5 mg are recommended.

The safety and effectiveness of doses above 20 mg/day have not been evaluated in clinical trials *[see Clinical Studies (14.2)]*.

Maintenance Treatment—The efficacy of ZYPREXA for the maintenance treatment of bipolar I disorder in the adolescent population has not been evaluated; however, maintenance efficacy can be extrapolated from adult data along with comparisons of olanzapine pharmacokinetic parameters in adult and adolescent patients. Thus, it is generally recommended that responding patients be continued beyond the acute response, but at the lowest dose needed to maintain remission. Patients should be periodically reassessed to determine the need for maintenance treatment.

2.3 Administration of ZYPREXA ZYDIS (olanzapine orally disintegrating tablets)

After opening sachet, peel back foil on blister. Do not push tablet through foil. Immediately upon opening the blister, using dry hands, remove tablet and place entire ZYPREXA ZYDIS in the mouth. Tablet disintegration occurs rapidly in saliva so it can be easily swallowed with or without liquid.

2.4 ZYPREXA IntraMuscular: Agitation Associated with Schizophrenia and Bipolar I Mania

Dose Selection for Agitated Adult Patients with Schizophrenia and Bipolar I Mania—The efficacy of intramuscular olanzapine for injection in controlling agitation in these disorders was demonstrated in a dose range of 2.5 mg to 10 mg. The recommended dose in these patients is 10 mg. A lower dose of 5 or 7.5 mg may be considered when clinical factors warrant *[see Clinical Studies (14.3)]*. If agitation warranting additional intramuscular doses persists following the initial dose, subsequent doses up to 10 mg may be given. However, the efficacy of repeated doses of intramuscular olanzapine for injection in agitated patients has not been systematically evaluated in controlled clinical trials. Also, the safety of total daily doses greater than 30 mg, or 10 mg injections given more frequently than 2 hours after the initial dose, and 4 hours after the second dose have not been evaluated in clinical trials. Maximal dosing of intramuscular olanzapine (e.g., 3 doses of 10 mg administered 2-4 hours apart) may be associated with a substantial occurrence of significant orthostatic hypotension *[see Warnings and Precautions (5.8)]*. Thus, it is recommended that patients requiring subsequent intramuscular injections be assessed for orthostatic hypotension prior to the administration of any subsequent doses of intramuscular olanzapine for injection. The administration of an additional dose to a patient with a clinically significant postural change in systolic blood pressure is not recommended.

If ongoing olanzapine therapy is clinically indicated, oral olanzapine may be initiated in a range of 5-20 mg/day as soon as clinically appropriate *[see Dosage and Administration (2.1, 2.2)]*.

Intramuscular Dosing in Special Populations—A dose of 5 mg/injection should be considered for geriatric patients or when other clinical factors warrant. A lower dose of 2.5 mg/injection should be considered for patients who otherwise might be debilitated, be predisposed to hypotensive reactions, or be more pharmacodynamically sensitive to olanzapine *[see Warnings and Precautions (5.14), Drug Interactions (7), and Clinical Pharmacology (12.3)]*.

Administration of ZYPREXA IntraMuscular—ZYPREXA IntraMuscular is intended for intramuscular use only. Do not administer intravenously or subcutaneously. Inject slowly, deep into the muscle mass.

Parenteral drug products should be inspected visually for particulate matter and discoloration prior to administration, whenever solution and container permit.

Directions for Preparation of ZYPREXA IntraMuscular with Sterile Water for Injection—Dissolve the contents of the vial using 2.1 mL of Sterile Water for Injection to provide a solution containing approximately 5 mg/mL of olanzapine. The resulting solution should appear clear and yellow. ZYPREXA IntraMuscular reconstituted with Sterile Water for Injection should be used immediately (within 1 hour) after reconstitution. *Discard any unused portion.*

The following table provides injection volumes for delivering various doses of intramuscular olanzapine for injection reconstituted with Sterile Water for Injection.

Dose, mg Olanzapine	Volume of Injection, mL
10	Withdraw total contents of vial
7.5	1.5
5	1
2.5	0.5

Physical Incompatibility Information—ZYPREXA IntraMuscular should be reconstituted only with Sterile Water for Injection. ZYPREXA IntraMuscular should not be combined in a syringe with diazepam injection because precipitation occurs when these products are mixed. Lorazepam injection should not be used to reconstitute ZYPREXA IntraMuscular as this combination results in a delayed reconstitution time. ZYPREXA IntraMuscular should not be combined in a syringe with haloperidol injection because the resulting low pH has been shown to degrade olanzapine over time.

2.5 ZYPREXA and Fluoxetine in Combination: Depressive Episodes Associated with Bipolar I Disorder

When using ZYPREXA and fluoxetine in combination, also refer to the Clinical Studies section of the package insert for Symbyax.

Oral olanzapine should be administered in combination with fluoxetine once daily in the evening, without regard to meals, generally beginning with 5 mg of oral olanzapine and 20 mg of fluoxetine. Dosage adjustments, if indicated, can be made according to efficacy and tolerability within dose ranges of oral olanzapine 5 to 12.5 mg and fluoxetine 20 to 50 mg. Antidepressant efficacy was demonstrated with ZYPREXA and fluoxetine in combination in adult patients with a dose range of olanzapine 6 to 12 mg and fluoxetine 25 to 50 mg.

Safety and efficacy of ZYPREXA and fluoxetine in combination was determined in clinical trials supporting approval of Symbyax (fixed dose combination of ZYPREXA and fluoxetine). Symbyax is dosed between 3 mg/25 mg (olanzapine/fluoxetine) per day and 12 mg/50 mg (olanzapine/fluoxetine) per day. The following table demonstrates the appropriate individual component doses of ZYPREXA and fluoxetine versus Symbyax. Dosage adjustments, if indicated, should be made with the individual components according to efficacy and tolerability.

[See table 1 at bottom left]

Table 1: Approximate Dose Correspondence Between Symbyax[a] and the Combination of ZYPREXA and Fluoxetine

For Symbyax (mg/day)	Use in Combination	
	ZYPREXA (mg/day)	Fluoxetine (mg/day)
3 mg olanzapine/25 mg fluoxetine	2.5	20
6 mg olanzapine/25 mg fluoxetine	5	20
12 mg olanzapine/25 mg fluoxetine	10+2.5	20
6 mg olanzapine/50 mg fluoxetine	5	40+10
12 mg olanzapine/50 mg fluoxetine	10+2.5	40+10

[a] Symbyax (olanzapine/fluoxetine HCl) is a fixed-dose combination of ZYPREXA and fluoxetine.

While there is no body of evidence to answer the question of how long a patient treated with ZYPREXA and fluoxetine in combination should remain on it, it is generally accepted that bipolar I disorder, including the depressive episodes associated with bipolar I disorder, is a chronic illness requiring chronic treatment. The physician should periodically reexamine the need for continued pharmacotherapy.

Safety of co-administration of doses above 18 mg olanzapine with 75 mg fluoxetine has not been evaluated in clinical studies.

ZYPREXA monotherapy is not indicated for the treatment of depressive episodes associated with bipolar I disorder.

2.6 ZYPREXA and Fluoxetine in Combination: Treatment Resistant Depression

When using ZYPREXA and fluoxetine in combination, also refer to the Clinical Studies section of the package insert for Symbyax.

Oral olanzapine should be administered in combination with fluoxetine once daily in the evening, without regard to meals, generally beginning with 5 mg of oral olanzapine and 20 mg of fluoxetine. Dosage adjustments, if indicated, can be made according to efficacy and tolerability within dose ranges of oral olanzapine 5 to 20 mg and fluoxetine 20 to 50 mg. Antidepressant efficacy was demonstrated with olanzapine and fluoxetine in combination in adult patients with a dose range of olanzapine 6 to 18 mg and fluoxetine 25 to 50 mg.

Safety and efficacy of olanzapine in combination with fluoxetine was determined in clinical trials supporting approval of Symbyax (fixed dose combination of olanzapine and fluoxetine). Symbyax is dosed between 3 mg/25 mg (olanzapine/fluoxetine) per day and 12 mg/50 mg (olanzapine/fluoxetine) per day. Table 1 above demonstrates the appropriate individual component doses of ZYPREXA and fluoxetine versus Symbyax. Dosage adjustments, if indicated, should be made with the individual components according to efficacy and tolerability.

While there is no body of evidence to answer the question of how long a patient treated with ZYPREXA and fluoxetine in combination should remain on it, it is generally accepted that treatment resistant depression (major depressive disorder in adult patients who do not respond to 2 separate trials of different antidepressants of adequate dose and duration in the current episode) is a chronic illness requiring chronic treatment. The physician should periodically reexamine the need for continued pharmacotherapy.

Safety of co-administration of doses above 18 mg olanzapine with 75 mg fluoxetine has not been evaluated in clinical studies.

ZYPREXA monotherapy is not indicated for treatment of treatment resistant depression (major depressive disorder in patients who do not respond to 2 antidepressants of adequate dose and duration in the current episode).

2.7 ZYPREXA and Fluoxetine in Combination: Dosing in Special Populations

The starting dose of oral olanzapine 2.5-5 mg with fluoxetine 20 mg should be used for patients with a predisposition to hypotensive reactions, patients with hepatic impairment, or patients who exhibit a combination of factors that may slow the metabolism of olanzapine or fluoxetine in combination (female gender, geriatric age, nonsmoking status), or those patients who may be pharmacodynamically sensitive to olanzapine. Dosing modification may be necessary in patients who exhibit a combination of factors that may slow metabolism. When indicated, dose escalation should be performed with caution in these patients. ZYPREXA and fluoxetine in combination have not been systematically studied in patients over 65 years of age or in patients <18 years of age *[see Warnings and Precautions (5.14), Drug Interactions (7), and Clinical Pharmacology (12.3)]*.

3 DOSAGE FORMS AND STRENGTHS

The ZYPREXA 2.5 mg, 5 mg, 7.5 mg, and 10 mg tablets are white, round, and imprinted in blue ink with LILLY and tablet number. The 15 mg tablets are elliptical, blue, and debossed with LILLY and tablet number. The 20 mg tablets are elliptical, pink, and debossed with LILLY and tablet number. Tablets are not scored. The tablets are available as follows:

[See first table at top right]

	TABLET STRENGTH 2.5 mg	5 mg	7.5 mg	10 mg	15 mg	20 mg
Tablet No.	4112	4115	4116	4117	4415	4420
Identification	LILLY 4112	LILLY 4115	LILLY 4116	LILLY 4117	LILLY 4415	LILLY 4420

ZYPREXA ZYDIS (olanzapine orally disintegrating tablets) are yellow, round, and debossed with the tablet strength. Tablets are not scored. The tablets are available as follows:

[See second table above]

ZYPREXA ZYDIS Tablets	TABLET STRENGTH 5 mg	10 mg	15 mg	20 mg
Tablet No.	4453	4454	4455	4456
Debossed	5	10	15	20

ZYPREXA IntraMuscular is available in 10 mg vial (1s).

4 CONTRAINDICATIONS

- None with ZYPREXA monotherapy.
- When using ZYPREXA and fluoxetine in combination, also refer to the Contraindications section of the package insert for Symbyax.
- For specific information about the contraindications of lithium or valproate, refer to the Contraindications section of the package inserts for these other products.

5 WARNINGS AND PRECAUTIONS

When using ZYPREXA and fluoxetine in combination, also refer to the Warnings and Precautions section of the package insert for Symbyax.

5.1 Elderly Patients with Dementia-Related Psychosis

Increased Mortality—Elderly patients with dementia-related psychosis treated with antipsychotic drugs are at an increased risk of death. ZYPREXA is not approved for the treatment of patients with dementia-related psychosis *[see Boxed Warning, Warnings and Precautions (5.14), and Patient Counseling Information (17.2)]*.

In placebo-controlled clinical trials of elderly patients with dementia-related psychosis, the incidence of death in olanzapine-treated patients was significantly greater than placebo-treated patients (3.5% vs 1.5%, respectively).

Cerebrovascular Adverse Events (CVAE), Including Stroke—Cerebrovascular adverse events (e.g., stroke, transient ischemic attack), including fatalities, were reported in patients in trials of olanzapine in elderly patients with dementia-related psychosis. In placebo-controlled trials, there was a significantly higher incidence of cerebrovascular adverse events in patients treated with olanzapine compared to patients treated with placebo. Olanzapine is not approved for the treatment of patients with dementia-related psychosis *[see Boxed Warning and Patient Counseling Information (17.2)]*.

5.2 Suicide

The possibility of a suicide attempt is inherent in schizophrenia and in bipolar I disorder, and close supervision of high-risk patients should accompany drug therapy. Prescriptions for olanzapine should be written for the smallest quantity of tablets consistent with good patient management, in order to reduce the risk of overdose.

5.3 Neuroleptic Malignant Syndrome (NMS)

A potentially fatal symptom complex sometimes referred to as Neuroleptic Malignant Syndrome (NMS) has been reported in association with administration of antipsychotic drugs, including olanzapine. Clinical manifestations of NMS are hyperpyrexia, muscle rigidity, altered mental status and evidence of autonomic instability (irregular pulse or blood pressure, tachycardia, diaphoresis and cardiac dysrhythmia). Additional signs may include elevated creatinine phosphokinase, myoglobinuria (rhabdomyolysis), and acute renal failure.

The diagnostic evaluation of patients with this syndrome is complicated. In arriving at a diagnosis, it is important to exclude cases where the clinical presentation includes both serious medical illness (e.g., pneumonia, systemic infection, etc.) and untreated or inadequately treated extrapyramidal signs and symptoms (EPS). Other important considerations in the differential diagnosis include central anticholinergic toxicity, heat stroke, drug fever, and primary central nervous system pathology.

The management of NMS should include: 1) immediate discontinuation of antipsychotic drugs and other drugs not essential to concurrent therapy; 2) intensive symptomatic treatment and medical monitoring; and 3) treatment of any concomitant serious medical problems for which specific treatments are available. There is no general agreement about specific pharmacological treatment regimens for NMS.

If a patient requires antipsychotic drug treatment after recovery from NMS, the potential reintroduction of drug therapy should be carefully considered. The patient should be carefully monitored, since recurrences of NMS have been reported *[see Patient Counseling Information (17.3)]*.

5.4 Hyperglycemia

Physicians should consider the risks and benefits when prescribing olanzapine to patients with an established diagnosis of diabetes mellitus, or having borderline increased blood glucose level (fasting 100-126 mg/dL, nonfasting 140-200 mg/dL). Patients taking olanzapine should be monitored regularly for worsening of glucose control. Patients starting treatment with olanzapine should undergo fasting blood glucose testing at the beginning of treatment and periodically during treatment. Any patient treated with atypical antipsychotics should be monitored for symptoms of hyperglycemia including polydipsia, polyuria, polyphagia, and weakness. Patients who develop symptoms of hyperglycemia during treatment with atypical antipsychotics should undergo fasting blood glucose testing. In some cases, hyperglycemia has resolved when the atypical antipsychotic was discontinued; however, some patients required continuation of anti-diabetic treatment despite discontinuation of the suspect drug *[see Patient Counseling Information (17.4)]*.

Hyperglycemia, in some cases extreme and associated with ketoacidosis or hyperosmolar coma or death, has been reported in patients treated with atypical antipsychotics including olanzapine. Assessment of the relationship between atypical antipsychotic use and glucose abnormalities is complicated by the possibility of an increased background risk of diabetes mellitus in patients with schizophrenia and the increasing incidence of diabetes mellitus in the general population. Epidemiological studies suggest an increased risk of treatment-emergent hyperglycemia-related adverse reactions in patients treated with the atypical antipsychotics. While relative risk estimates are inconsistent, the association between atypical antipsychotics and increases in glucose levels appears to fall on a continuum and olanzapine appears to have a greater association than some other atypical antipsychotics.

Mean increases in blood glucose have been observed in patients treated (median exposure of 9.2 months) with olanzapine in phase 1 of the Clinical Antipsychotic Trials of Intervention Effectiveness (CATIE). The mean increase of serum glucose (fasting and nonfasting samples) from baseline to the average of the 2 highest serum concentrations was 15.0 mg/dL.

In a study of healthy volunteers, subjects who received olanzapine (N=22) for 3 weeks had a mean increase compared to baseline in fasting blood glucose of 2.3 mg/dL. Placebo-treated subjects (N=19) had a mean increase in fasting blood glucose compared to baseline of 0.34 mg/dL.

Olanzapine Monotherapy in Adults—In an analysis of 5 placebo-controlled adult olanzapine monotherapy studies with a median treatment duration of approximately 3 weeks, olanzapine was associated with a greater mean change in fasting glucose levels compared to placebo (2.76 mg/dL versus 0.17 mg/dL). The difference in mean changes between olanzapine and placebo was greater in patients with evidence of glucose dysregulation at baseline (patients diagnosed with diabetes mellitus or related adverse reactions, patients treated with anti-diabetic agents, patients with a baseline random glucose level ≥200 mg/dL, and/or a baseline fasting glucose level ≥126 mg/dL). Olanzapine-treated patients had a greater mean HbA1c increase from baseline of 0.04% (median exposure 21 days), compared to a mean HbA1c decrease of 0.06% in placebo-treated subjects (median exposure 17 days).

In an analysis of 8 placebo-controlled studies (median treatment exposure 4-5 weeks), 6.1% of olanzapine-treated subjects (N=855) had treatment-emergent glycosuria compared to 2.8% of placebo-treated subjects (N=599). Table 2 shows short-term and long-term changes in fasting glucose levels from adult olanzapine monotherapy studies.

[See table 2 above]

Table 2: Changes in Fasting Glucose Levels from Adult Olanzapine Monotherapy Studies

Laboratory Analyte	Category Change (at least once) from Baseline	Treatment Arm	Up to 12 weeks exposure N	Patients	At least 48 weeks exposure N	Patients
Fasting Glucose	Normal to High (<100 mg/dL to ≥126 mg/dL)	Olanzapine	543	2.2%	345	12.8%
		Placebo	293	3.4%	NA[a]	NA[a]
	Borderline to High (≥100 mg/dL and <126 mg/dL to ≥126 mg/dL)	Olanzapine	178	17.4%	127	26.0%
		Placebo	96	11.5%	NA[a]	NA[a]

[a] Not Applicable.

The mean change in fasting glucose for patients exposed at least 48 weeks was 4.2 mg/dL (N=487). In analyses of patients who completed 9-12 months of olanzapine therapy, mean change in fasting and nonfasting glucose levels continued to increase over time.

Table 3: Changes in Fasting Glucose Levels from Adolescent Olanzapine Monotherapy Studies

Laboratory Analyte	Category Change (at least once) from Baseline	Treatment Arm	Up to 12 weeks exposure		At least 24 weeks exposure	
			N	Patients	N	Patients
Fasting Glucose	Normal to High (<100 mg/dL to ≥126 mg/dL)	Olanzapine	124	0%	108	0.9%
		Placebo	53	1.9%	NA[a]	NA[a]
	Borderline to High (≥100 mg/dL and <126 mg/dL to ≥126 mg/dL)	Olanzapine	14	14.3%	13	23.1%
		Placebo	13	0%	NA[a]	NA[a]

[a] Not Applicable.

Table 4: Changes in Fasting Lipids Values from Adult Olanzapine Monotherapy Studies

Laboratory Analyte	Category Change (at least once) from Baseline	Treatment Arm	Up to 12 weeks exposure		At least 48 weeks exposure	
			N	Patients	N	Patients
Fasting Triglycerides	Increase by ≥50 mg/dL	Olanzapine	745	39.6%	487	61.4%
		Placebo	402	26.1%	NA[a]	NA[a]
	Normal to High (<150 mg/dL to ≥200 mg/dL)	Olanzapine	457	9.2%	293	32.4%
		Placebo	251	4.4%	NA[a]	NA[a]
	Borderline to High (≥150 mg/dL and <200 mg/dL to ≥200 mg/dL)	Olanzapine	135	39.3%	75	70.7%
		Placebo	65	20.0%	NA[a]	NA[a]
Fasting Total Cholesterol	Increase by ≥40 mg/dL	Olanzapine	745	21.6%	489	32.9%
		Placebo	402	9.5%	NA[a]	NA[a]
	Normal to High (<200 mg/dL to ≥240 mg/dL)	Olanzapine	392	2.8%	283	14.8%
		Placebo	207	2.4%	NA[a]	NA[a]
	Borderline to High (≥200 mg/dL and <240 mg/dL to ≥240 mg/dL)	Olanzapine	222	23.0%	125	55.2%
		Placebo	112	12.5%	NA[a]	NA[a]
Fasting LDL Cholesterol	Increase by ≥30 mg/dL	Olanzapine	536	23.7%	483	39.8%
		Placebo	304	14.1%	NA[a]	NA[a]
	Normal to High (<100 mg/dL to ≥160 mg/dL)	Olanzapine	154	0%	123	7.3%
		Placebo	82	1.2%	NA[a]	NA[a]
	Borderline to High (≥100 mg/dL and <160 mg/dL to ≥160 mg/dL)	Olanzapine	302	10.6%	284	31.0%
		Placebo	173	8.1%	NA[a]	NA[a]

[a] Not Applicable.

Olanzapine Monotherapy in Adolescents—The safety and efficacy of olanzapine have not been established in patients under the age of 13 years. In an analysis of 3 placebo-controlled olanzapine monotherapy studies of adolescent patients, including those with schizophrenia (6 weeks) or bipolar I disorder (manic or mixed episodes) (3 weeks), olanzapine was associated with a greater mean change from baseline in fasting glucose levels compared to placebo (2.68 mg/dL versus -2.59 mg/dL). The mean change in fasting glucose for adolescents exposed at least 24 weeks was 3.1 mg/dL (N=121). Table 3 shows short-term and long-term changes in fasting blood glucose from adolescent olanzapine monotherapy studies.
[See table 3 above]

5.5 Hyperlipidemia
Undesirable alterations in lipids have been observed with olanzapine use. Clinical monitoring, including baseline and periodic follow-up lipid evaluations in patients using olanzapine, is recommended [see Patient Counseling Information (17.5)].
Clinically significant, and sometimes very high (>500 mg/dL), elevations in triglyceride levels have been observed with olanzapine use. Modest mean increases in total cholesterol have also been seen with olanzapine use.
Olanzapine Monotherapy in Adults—In an analysis of 5 placebo-controlled olanzapine monotherapy studies with treatment duration up to 12 weeks, olanzapine-treated patients had increases from baseline in mean fasting total cho-

lesterol, LDL cholesterol, and triglycerides of 5.3 mg/dL, 3.0 mg/dL, and 20.8 mg/dL respectively compared to decreases from baseline in mean fasting total cholesterol, LDL cholesterol, and triglycerides of 6.1 mg/dL, 4.3 mg/dL, and 10.7 mg/dL for placebo-treated patients. For fasting HDL cholesterol, no clinically meaningful differences were observed between olanzapine-treated patients and placebo-treated patients. Mean increases in fasting lipid values (total cholesterol, LDL cholesterol, and triglycerides) were greater in patients without evidence of lipid dysregulation at baseline, where lipid dysregulation was defined as patients diagnosed with dyslipidemia or related adverse reactions, patients treated with lipid lowering agents, or patients with high baseline lipid levels.
In long-term studies (at least 48 weeks), patients had increases from baseline in mean fasting total cholesterol, LDL cholesterol, and triglycerides of 5.6 mg/dL, 2.5 mg/dL, and 18.7 mg/dL, respectively, and a mean decrease in fasting HDL cholesterol of 0.16 mg/dL. In an analysis of patients who completed 12 months of therapy, the mean nonfasting total cholesterol did not increase further after approximately 4-6 months.
The proportion of patients who had changes (at least once) in total cholesterol, LDL cholesterol or triglycerides from normal or borderline to high, or changes in HDL cholesterol from normal or borderline to low, was greater in long-term studies (at least 48 weeks) as compared with short-term studies. Table 4 shows categorical changes in fasting lipids values.

[See table 4 at left]
In phase 1 of the Clinical Antipsychotic Trials of Intervention Effectiveness (CATIE), over a median exposure of 9.2 months, the mean increase in triglycerides in patients taking olanzapine was 40.5 mg/dL. In phase 1 of CATIE, the mean increase in total cholesterol was 9.4 mg/dL.
Olanzapine Monotherapy in Adolescents—The safety and efficacy of olanzapine have not been established in patients under the age of 13 years. In an analysis of 3 placebo-controlled olanzapine monotherapy studies of adolescents, including those with schizophrenia (6 weeks) or bipolar I disorder (manic or mixed episodes) (3 weeks), olanzapine-treated adolescents had increases from baseline in mean fasting total cholesterol, LDL cholesterol, and triglycerides of 12.9 mg/dL, 6.5 mg/dL, and 28.4 mg/dL, respectively, compared to increases from baseline in mean fasting total cholesterol and LDL cholesterol of 1.3 mg/dL and 1.0 mg/dL, and a decrease in triglycerides of 1.1 mg/dL for placebo-treated adolescents. For fasting HDL cholesterol, no clinically meaningful differences were observed between olanzapine-treated adolescents and placebo-treated adolescents.
In long-term studies (at least 24 weeks), adolescents had increases from baseline in mean fasting total cholesterol, LDL cholesterol, and triglycerides of 5.5 mg/dL, 5.4 mg/dL, and 20.5 mg/dL, respectively, and a mean decrease in fasting HDL cholesterol of 4.5 mg/dL. Table 5 shows categorical changes in fasting lipids values in adolescents.
[See table 5 at top of next page]

5.6 Weight Gain
Potential consequences of weight gain should be considered prior to starting olanzapine. Patients receiving olanzapine should receive regular monitoring of weight [see Patient Counseling Information (17.6)].
Olanzapine Monotherapy in Adults—In an analysis of 13 placebo-controlled olanzapine monotherapy studies, olanzapine-treated patients gained an average of 2.6 kg (5.7 lb) compared to an average 0.3 kg (0.6 lb) weight loss in placebo-treated patients with a median exposure of 6 weeks; 22.2% of olanzapine-treated patients gained at least 7% of their baseline weight, compared to 3% of placebo-treated patients, with a median exposure to event of 8 weeks; 4.2% of olanzapine-treated patients gained at least 15% of their baseline weight, compared to 0.3% of placebo-treated patients, with a median exposure to event of 12 weeks. Clinically significant weight gain was observed across all baseline Body Mass Index (BMI) categories. Discontinuation due to weight gain occurred in 0.2% of olanzapine-treated patients and in 0% of placebo-treated patients.
In long-term studies (at least 48 weeks), the mean weight gain was 5.6 kg (12.3 lb) (median exposure of 573 days, N=2021). The percentages of patients who gained at least 7%, 15%, or 25% of their baseline body weight with long-term exposure were 64%, 32%, and 12%, respectively. Discontinuation due to weight gain occurred in 0.4% of olanzapine-treated patients following at least 48 weeks of exposure.
Table 6 includes data on adult weight gain with olanzapine pooled from 86 clinical trials. The data in each column represent data for those patients who completed treatment periods of the durations specified.
[See table 6 on next page]
Olanzapine Monotherapy in Adolescents—The safety and efficacy of olanzapine have not been established in patients under the age of 13 years. Mean increase in weight in adolescents was greater than in adults. In 4 placebo-controlled trials, discontinuation due to weight gain occurred in 1% of olanzapine-treated patients, compared to 0% of placebo-treated patients.
[See table 7 on next page]
In long-term studies (at least 24 weeks), the mean weight gain was 11.2 kg (24.6 lb); (median exposure of 201 days, N=179). The percentages of adolescents who gained at least 7%, 15%, or 25% of their baseline body weight with long-term exposure were 89%, 55%, and 29%, respectively. Among adolescent patients, mean weight gain by baseline BMI category was 11.5 kg (25.3 lb), 12.1 kg (26.6 lb), and 12.7 kg (27.9 lb), respectively, for normal (N=106), overweight (N=26) and obese (N=17). Discontinuation due to weight gain occurred in 2.2% of olanzapine-treated patients following at least 24 weeks of exposure.
Table 8 shows data on adolescent weight gain with olanzapine pooled from 6 clinical trials. The data in each column represent data for those patients who completed treatment periods of the durations specified. Little clinical trial data is available on weight gain in adolescents with olanzapine beyond 6 months of treatment.

Table 8: Weight Gain with Olanzapine Use in Adolescents

Amount Gained kg (lb)	6 Weeks (N=243) (%)	6 Months (N=191) (%)
≤0	2.9	2.1
0 to ≤5 (0-11 lb)	47.3	24.6
>5 to ≤10 (11-22 lb)	42.4	26.7
>10 to ≤15 (22-33 lb)	5.8	22.0
>15 to ≤20 (33-44 lb)	0.8	12.6
>20 to ≤25 (44-55 lb)	0.8	9.4
>25 to ≤30 (55-66 lb)	0	2.1
>30 to ≤35 (66-77 lb)	0	0
>35 to ≤40 (77-88 lb)	0	0
>40 (>88 lb)	0	0.5

5.7 Tardive Dyskinesia

A syndrome of potentially irreversible, involuntary, dyskinetic movements may develop in patients treated with antipsychotic drugs. Although the prevalence of the syndrome appears to be highest among the elderly, especially elderly women, it is impossible to rely upon prevalence estimates to predict, at the inception of antipsychotic treatment, which patients are likely to develop the syndrome. Whether antipsychotic drug products differ in their potential to cause tardive dyskinesia is unknown.

The risk of developing tardive dyskinesia and the likelihood that it will become irreversible are believed to increase as the duration of treatment and the total cumulative dose of antipsychotic drugs administered to the patient increase. However, the syndrome can develop, although much less commonly, after relatively brief treatment periods at low doses or may even arise after discontinuation of treatment. There is no known treatment for established cases of tardive dyskinesia, although the syndrome may remit, partially or completely, if antipsychotic treatment is withdrawn. Antipsychotic treatment, itself, however, may suppress (or partially suppress) the signs and symptoms of the syndrome and thereby may possibly mask the underlying process. The effect that symptomatic suppression has upon the long-term course of the syndrome is unknown.

Given these considerations, olanzapine should be prescribed in a manner that is most likely to minimize the occurrence of tardive dyskinesia. Chronic antipsychotic treatment should generally be reserved for patients (1) who suffer from a chronic illness that is known to respond to antipsychotic drugs, and (2) for whom alternative, equally effective, but potentially less harmful treatments are not available or appropriate. In patients who do require chronic treatment, the smallest dose and the shortest duration of treatment producing a satisfactory clinical response should be sought. The need for continued treatment should be reassessed periodically.

If signs and symptoms of tardive dyskinesia appear in a patient on olanzapine, drug discontinuation should be considered. However, some patients may require treatment with olanzapine despite the presence of the syndrome.

For specific information about the warnings of lithium or valproate, refer to the Warnings section of the package inserts for these other products.

5.8 Orthostatic Hypotension

Olanzapine may induce orthostatic hypotension associated with dizziness, tachycardia, bradycardia and, in some patients, syncope, especially during the initial dose-titration period, probably reflecting its α_1-adrenergic antagonistic properties [see Patient Counseling Information (17.7)].

For oral olanzapine therapy, the risk of orthostatic hypotension and syncope may be minimized by initiating therapy with 5 mg QD [see Dosage and Administration (2)]. A more gradual titration to the target dose should be considered if hypotension occurs.

Hypotension, bradycardia with or without hypotension, tachycardia, and syncope were also reported during the clinical trials with intramuscular olanzapine for injection. In an open-label clinical pharmacology study in nonagitated patients with schizophrenia in which the safety and tolerability of intramuscular olanzapine were evaluated under a maximal dosing regimen (three 10 mg doses administered 4 hours apart), approximately one-third of these patients experienced a significant orthostatic decrease in systolic blood pressure (i.e., decrease ≥30 mmHg) [see Dosage and Administration (2.4)]. Syncope was reported in 0.6% (15/2500) of olanzapine-treated patients in phase 2-3 oral olanzapine

Table 5: Changes in Fasting Lipids Values from Adolescent Olanzapine Monotherapy Studies

Laboratory Analyte	Category Change (at least once) from Baseline	Treatment Arm	Up to 6 weeks exposure N	Up to 6 weeks exposure Patients	At least 24 weeks exposure N	At least 24 weeks exposure Patients
Fasting Triglycerides	Increase by ≥50 mg/dL	Olanzapine	138	37.0%	122	45.9%
		Placebo	66	15.2%	NA[a]	NA[a]
	Normal to High (<90 mg/dL to >130 mg/dL)	Olanzapine	67	26.9%	66	36.4%
		Placebo	28	10.7%	NA[a]	NA[a]
	Borderline to High (≥90 mg/dL and ≤130 mg/dL to >130 mg/dL)	Olanzapine	37	59.5%	31	64.5%
		Placebo	17	35.3%	NA[a]	NA[a]
Fasting Total Cholesterol	Increase by ≥40 mg/dL	Olanzapine	138	14.5%	122	14.8%
		Placebo	66	4.5%	NA[a]	NA[a]
	Normal to High (<170 mg/dL to ≥200 mg/dL)	Olanzapine	87	6.9%	78	7.7%
		Placebo	43	2.3%	NA[a]	NA[a]
	Borderline to High (≥170 mg/dL and <200 mg/dL to ≥200 mg/dL)	Olanzapine	36	38.9%	33	57.6%
		Placebo	13	7.7%	NA[a]	NA[a]
Fasting LDL Cholesterol	Increase by ≥30 mg/dL	Olanzapine	137	17.5%	121	22.3%
		Placebo	63	11.1%	NA[a]	NA[a]
	Normal to High (<110 mg/dL to ≥130 mg/dL)	Olanzapine	98	5.1%	92	10.9%
		Placebo	44	4.5%	NA[a]	NA[a]
	Borderline to High (≥110 mg/dL and <130 mg/dL to ≥130 mg/dL)	Olanzapine	29	48.3%	21	47.6%
		Placebo	9	0%	NA[a]	NA[a]

[a] Not Applicable.

Table 6: Weight Gain with Olanzapine Use in Adults

Amount Gained kg (lb)	6 Weeks (N=7465) (%)	6 Months (N=4162) (%)	12 Months (N=1345) (%)	24 Months (N=474) (%)	36 Months (N=147) (%)
≤0	26.2	24.3	20.8	23.2	17.0
0 to ≤5 (0-11 lb)	57.0	36.0	26.0	23.4	25.2
>5 to ≤10 (11-22 lb)	14.9	24.6	24.2	24.1	18.4
>10 to ≤15 (22-33 lb)	1.8	10.9	14.9	11.4	17.0
>15 to ≤20 (33-44 lb)	0.1	3.1	8.6	9.3	11.6
>20 to ≤25 (44-55 lb)	0	0.9	3.3	5.1	4.1
>25 to ≤30 (55-66 lb)	0	0.2	1.4	2.3	4.8
>30 (>66 lb)	0	0.1	0.8	1.2	2

Table 7: Weight Gain with Olanzapine Use in Adolescents from 4 Placebo-Controlled Trials

	Olanzapine-treated patients	Placebo-treated patients
Mean change in body weight from baseline (median exposure = 3 weeks)	4.6 kg (10.1 lb)	0.3 kg (0.7 lb)
Percentage of patients who gained at least 7% of baseline body weight	40.6% (median exposure to 7% = 4 weeks)	9.8% (median exposure to 7% = 8 weeks)
Percentage of patients who gained at least 15% of baseline body weight	7.1% (median exposure to 15% = 19 weeks)	2.7% (median exposure to 15% = 8 weeks)

studies and in 0.3% (2/722) of olanzapine-treated patients with agitation in the intramuscular olanzapine for injection studies. Three normal volunteers in phase 1 studies with intramuscular olanzapine experienced hypotension, bradycardia, and sinus pauses of up to 6 seconds that spontaneously resolved (in 2 cases the reactions occurred on intramuscular olanzapine, and in 1 case, on oral olanzapine). The risk for this sequence of hypotension, bradycardia, and sinus pause may be greater in nonpsychiatric patients compared to psychiatric patients who are possibly more adapted

to certain effects of psychotropic drugs. For intramuscular olanzapine for injection therapy, patients should remain recumbent if drowsy or dizzy after injection until examination has indicated that they are not experiencing postural hypotension, bradycardia, and/or hypoventilation.

Olanzapine should be used with particular caution in patients with known cardiovascular disease (history of myocardial infarction or ischemia, heart failure, or conduction abnormalities), cerebrovascular disease, and conditions which would predispose patients to hypotension (dehydration, hypovolemia, and treatment with antihypertensive medications) where the occurrence of syncope, or hypotension and/or bradycardia might put the patient at increased medical risk.

Caution is necessary in patients who receive treatment with other drugs having effects that can induce hypotension, bradycardia, respiratory or central nervous system depression [see Drug Interactions (7)]. Concomitant administration of intramuscular olanzapine and parenteral benzodiazepine is not recommended due to the potential for excessive sedation and cardiorespiratory depression.

5.9 Leukopenia, Neutropenia, and Agranulocytosis

Class Effect—In clinical trial and/or postmarketing experience, events of leukopenia/neutropenia have been reported temporally related to antipsychotic agents, including ZYPREXA. Agranulocytosis has also been reported.

Possible risk factors for leukopenia/neutropenia include pre-existing low white blood cell count (WBC) and history of drug induced leukopenia/neutropenia. Patients with a history of a clinically significant low WBC or drug induced leukopenia/neutropenia should have their complete blood count (CBC) monitored frequently during the first few months of therapy and discontinuation of ZYPREXA should be considered at the first sign of a clinically significant decline in WBC in the absence of other causative factors. Patients with clinically significant neutropenia should be carefully monitored for fever or other symptoms or signs of infection and treated promptly if such symptoms or signs occur. Patients with severe neutropenia (absolute neutrophil count <1000/mm^3) should discontinue ZYPREXA and have their WBC followed until recovery.

5.10 Dysphagia

Esophageal dysmotility and aspiration have been associated with antipsychotic drug use. Aspiration pneumonia is a common cause of morbidity and mortality in patients with advanced Alzheimer's disease. Olanzapine is not approved for the treatment of patients with Alzheimer's disease.

5.11 Seizures

During premarketing testing, seizures occurred in 0.9% (22/2500) of olanzapine-treated patients. There were confounding factors that may have contributed to the occurrence of seizures in many of these cases. Olanzapine should be used cautiously in patients with a history of seizures or with conditions that potentially lower the seizure threshold, e.g., Alzheimer's dementia. Olanzapine is not approved for the treatment of patients with Alzheimer's disease. Conditions that lower the seizure threshold may be more prevalent in a population of 65 years or older.

5.12 Potential for Cognitive and Motor Impairment

Somnolence was a commonly reported adverse reaction associated with olanzapine treatment, occurring at an incidence of 26% in olanzapine patients compared to 15% in placebo patients. This adverse reaction was also dose related. Somnolence led to discontinuation in 0.4% (9/2500) of patients in the premarketing database.

Since olanzapine has the potential to impair judgment, thinking, or motor skills, patients should be cautioned about operating hazardous machinery, including automobiles, until they are reasonably certain that olanzapine therapy does not affect them adversely [see Patient Counseling Information (17.8)].

5.13 Body Temperature Regulation

Disruption of the body's ability to reduce core body temperature has been attributed to antipsychotic agents. Appropriate care is advised when prescribing olanzapine for patients who will be experiencing conditions which may contribute to an elevation in core body temperature, e.g., exercising strenuously, exposure to extreme heat, receiving concomitant medication with anticholinergic activity, or being subject to dehydration [see Patient Counseling Information (17.9)].

5.14 Use in Patients with Concomitant Illness

Clinical experience with olanzapine in patients with certain concomitant systemic illnesses is limited [see Clinical Pharmacology (12.3)].

Olanzapine exhibits in vitro muscarinic receptor affinity. In premarketing clinical trials with olanzapine, olanzapine was associated with constipation, dry mouth, and tachycardia, all adverse reactions possibly related to cholinergic antagonism. Such adverse reactions were not often the basis for discontinuations from olanzapine, but olanzapine should be used with caution in patients with clinically significant prostatic hypertrophy, narrow angle glaucoma, or a history of paralytic ileus or related conditions.

In 5 placebo-controlled studies of olanzapine in elderly patients with dementia-related psychosis (n=1184), the following treatment-emergent adverse reactions were reported in olanzapine-treated patients at an incidence of at least 2% and significantly greater than placebo-treated patients:

falls, somnolence, peripheral edema, abnormal gait, urinary incontinence, lethargy, increased weight, asthenia, pyrexia, pneumonia, dry mouth and visual hallucinations. The rate of discontinuation due to adverse reactions was greater with olanzapine than placebo (13% vs 7%). Elderly patients with dementia-related psychosis treated with olanzapine are at an increased risk of death compared to placebo. Olanzapine is not approved for the treatment of patients with dementia-related psychosis [see Boxed Warning, Warnings and Precautions (5.1), and Patient Counseling Information (17.2)]. Olanzapine has not been evaluated or used to any appreciable extent in patients with a recent history of myocardial infarction or unstable heart disease. Patients with these diagnoses were excluded from premarketing clinical studies. Because of the risk of orthostatic hypotension with olanzapine, caution should be observed in cardiac patients [see Warnings and Precautions (5.8)].

5.15 Hyperprolactinemia

As with other drugs that antagonize dopamine D$_2$ receptors, olanzapine elevates prolactin levels, and the elevation persists during chronic administration. Hyperprolactinemia may suppress hypothalamic GnRH, resulting in reduced pituitary gonadotropin secretion. This, in turn, may inhibit reproductive function by impairing gonadal steroidogenesis in both female and male patients. Galactorrhea, amenorrhea, gynecomastia, and impotence have been reported in patients receiving prolactin-elevating compounds. Longstanding hyperprolactinemia when associated with hypogonadism may lead to decreased bone density in both female and male subjects.

Tissue culture experiments indicate that approximately one-third of human breast cancers are prolactin dependent in vitro, a factor of potential importance if the prescription of these drugs is contemplated in a patient with previously detected breast cancer. As is common with compounds which increase prolactin release, an increase in mammary gland neoplasia was observed in the olanzapine carcinogenicity studies conducted in mice and rats [see Nonclinical Toxicology (13.1)]. Neither clinical studies nor epidemiologic studies conducted to date have shown an association between chronic administration of this class of drugs and tumorigenesis in humans; the available evidence is considered too limited to be conclusive at this time.

In placebo-controlled olanzapine clinical studies (up to 12 weeks), changes from normal to high in prolactin concentrations were observed in 30% of adults treated with olanzapine as compared to 10.5% of adults treated with placebo. In a pooled analysis from clinical studies including 8136 adults treated with olanzapine, potentially associated clinical manifestations included menstrual-related events[1] (2% [49/3240] of females), sexual function-related events[2] (2% [150/8136] of females and males), and breast-related events[3] (0.7% [23/3240] of females, 0.2% [9/4896] of males). In placebo-controlled olanzapine monotherapy studies in adolescent patients (up to 6 weeks) with schizophrenia or bipolar I disorder (manic or mixed episodes), changes from normal to high in prolactin concentrations were observed in 47% of olanzapine-treated patients compared to 7% of placebo-treated patients. In a pooled analysis from clinical trials including 454 adolescents treated with olanzapine, potentially associated clinical manifestations included menstrual-related events[1] (1% [2/168] of females), sexual function-related events[2] (0.7% [3/454] of females and males), and breast-related events[3] (2% [3/168] of females, 2% [7/286] of males) [see Use in Specific Populations (8.4)].

[1] Based on a search of the following terms: amenorrhea, hypomenorrhea, menstruation delayed, and oligomenorrhea.

[2] Based on a search of the following terms: anorgasmia, delayed ejaculation, erectile dysfunction, decreased libido, loss of libido, abnormal orgasm, and sexual dysfunction.

[3] Based on a search of the following terms: breast discharge, enlargement or swelling, galactorrhea, gynecomastia, and lactation disorder.

5.16 Use in Combination with Fluoxetine, Lithium, or Valproate

When using ZYPREXA and fluoxetine in combination, the prescriber should also refer to the Warnings and Precautions section of the package insert for Symbyax. When using ZYPREXA in combination with lithium or valproate, the prescriber should refer to the Warnings and Precautions sections of the package inserts for lithium or valproate [see Drug Interactions (7)].

5.17 Laboratory Tests

Fasting blood glucose testing and lipid profile at the beginning of, and periodically during, treatment is recommended [see Warnings and Precautions (5.4, 5.5) and Patient Counseling Information (17.4, 17.5)].

6 ADVERSE REACTIONS

When using ZYPREXA and fluoxetine in combination, also refer to the Adverse Reactions section of the package insert for Symbyax.

6.1 Clinical Trials Experience

Because clinical trials are conducted under widely varying conditions, adverse reaction rates observed in the clinical trials of a drug cannot be directly compared to rates in the clinical trials of another drug and may not reflect or predict the rates observed in practice.

Clinical Trials in Adults

The information below for olanzapine is derived from a clinical trial database for olanzapine consisting of 8661 adult patients with approximately 4165 patient-years of exposure to oral olanzapine and 722 patients with exposure to intramuscular olanzapine for injection. This database includes: (1) 2500 patients who participated in multiple-dose oral olanzapine premarketing trials in schizophrenia and Alzheimer's disease representing approximately 1122 patient-years of exposure as of February 14, 1995; (2) 182 patients who participated in oral olanzapine premarketing bipolar I disorder (manic or mixed episodes) trials representing approximately 66 patient-years of exposure; (3) 191 patients who participated in an oral olanzapine trial of patients having various psychiatric symptoms in association with Alzheimer's disease representing approximately 29 patient-years of exposure; (4) 5788 patients from 88 additional oral olanzapine clinical trials as of December 31, 2001; and (5) 722 patients who participated in intramuscular olanzapine for injection premarketing trials in agitated patients with schizophrenia, bipolar I disorder (manic or mixed episodes), or dementia. In addition, information from the premarketing 6-week clinical study database for olanzapine in combination with lithium or valproate, consisting of 224 patients who participated in bipolar I disorder (manic or mixed episodes) trials with approximately 22 patient-years of exposure, is included below.

The conditions and duration of treatment with olanzapine varied greatly and included (in overlapping categories) open-label and double-blind phases of studies, inpatients and outpatients, fixed-dose and dose-titration studies, and short-term or longer-term exposure. Adverse reactions were assessed by collecting adverse reactions, results of physical examinations, vital signs, weights, laboratory analytes, ECGs, chest x-rays, and results of ophthalmologic examinations.

Certain portions of the discussion below relating to objective or numeric safety parameters, namely, dose-dependent adverse reactions, vital sign changes, weight gain, laboratory changes, and ECG changes are derived from studies in patients with schizophrenia and have not been duplicated for bipolar I disorder (manic or mixed episodes) or agitation. However, this information is also generally applicable to bipolar I disorder (manic or mixed episodes) and agitation.

Adverse reactions during exposure were obtained by spontaneous report and recorded by clinical investigators using terminology of their own choosing. Consequently, it is not possible to provide a meaningful estimate of the proportion of individuals experiencing adverse reactions without first grouping similar types of reactions into a smaller number of standardized reaction categories. In the tables and tabulations that follow, MedDRA and COSTART Dictionary terminology has been used to classify reported adverse reactions. The stated frequencies of adverse reactions represent the proportion of individuals who experienced, at least once, a treatment-emergent adverse reaction of the type listed. A reaction was considered treatment emergent if it occurred for the first time or worsened while receiving therapy following baseline evaluation. The reported reactions do not include those reaction terms that were so general as to be uninformative. Reactions listed elsewhere in labeling may not be repeated below. It is important to emphasize that, although the reactions occurred during treatment with olanzapine, they were not necessarily caused by it. The entire label should be read to gain a complete understanding of the safety profile of olanzapine.

The prescriber should be aware that the figures in the tables and tabulations cannot be used to predict the incidence of side effects in the course of usual medical practice where patient characteristics and other factors differ from those that prevailed in the clinical trials. Similarly, the cited frequencies cannot be compared with figures obtained from other clinical investigations involving different treatments, uses, and investigators. The cited figures, however, do provide the prescribing physician with some basis for estimating the relative contribution of drug and nondrug factors to the adverse reactions incidence in the population studied.

Incidence of Adverse Reactions in Short-Term, Placebo-Controlled and Combination Trials

The following findings are based on premarketing trials of (1) oral olanzapine for schizophrenia, bipolar I disorder (manic or mixed episodes), a subsequent trial of patients having various psychiatric symptoms in association with Alzheimer's disease, and premarketing combination trials, and (2) intramuscular olanzapine for injection in agitated patients with schizophrenia or bipolar I mania.

Adverse Reactions Associated with Discontinuation of Treatment in Short-Term, Placebo-Controlled Trials

Schizophrenia—Overall, there was no difference in the incidence of discontinuation due to adverse reactions (5% for oral olanzapine vs 6% for placebo). However, discontinuations due to increases in ALT were considered to be drug related (2% for oral olanzapine vs 0% for placebo).

Bipolar I Disorder (Manic or Mixed Episodes) Monotherapy—Overall, there was no difference in the incidence of discontinuation due to adverse reactions (2% for oral olanzapine vs 2% for placebo).

Agitation—Overall, there was no difference in the incidence of discontinuation due to adverse reactions (0.4% for intramuscular olanzapine for injection vs 0% for placebo).

Adverse Reactions Associated with Discontinuation of Treatment in Short-Term Combination Trials

Bipolar I Disorder (Manic or Mixed Episodes), Olanzapine as Adjunct to Lithium or Valproate—In a study of patients who were already tolerating either lithium or valproate as monotherapy, discontinuation rates due to adverse reactions were 11% for the combination of oral olanzapine with lithium or valproate compared to 2% for patients who remained on lithium or valproate monotherapy. Discontinuations with the combination of oral olanzapine and lithium or valproate that occurred in more than 1 patient were: somnolence (3%), weight gain (1%), and peripheral edema (1%).

Commonly Observed Adverse Reactions in Short-Term, Placebo-Controlled Trials

The most commonly observed adverse reactions associated with the use of oral olanzapine (incidence of 5% or greater) and not observed at an equivalent incidence among placebo-treated patients (olanzapine incidence at least twice that for placebo) were:

Table 9: Common Treatment-Emergent Adverse Reactions Associated with the Use of Oral Olanzapine in 6-Week Trials — SCHIZOPHRENIA

Adverse Reaction	Percentage of Patients Reporting Event	
	Olanzapine (N=248)	Placebo (N=118)
Postural hypotension	5	2
Constipation	9	3
Weight gain	6	1
Dizziness	11	4
Personality disorder[a]	8	4
Akathisia	5	1

[a] Personality disorder is the COSTART term for designating nonaggressive objectionable behavior.

Table 10: Common Treatment-Emergent Adverse Reactions Associated with the Use of Oral Olanzapine in 3-Week and 4-Week Trials — Bipolar I Disorder (Manic or Mixed Episodes)

Adverse Reaction	Percentage of Patients Reporting Event	
	Olanzapine (N=125)	Placebo (N=129)
Asthenia	15	6
Dry mouth	22	7
Constipation	11	5
Dyspepsia	11	5
Increased appetite	6	3
Somnolence	35	13
Dizziness	18	6
Tremor	6	3

Olanzapine Intramuscular—There was 1 adverse reaction (somnolence) observed at an incidence of 5% or greater among intramuscular olanzapine for injection-treated patients and not observed at an equivalent incidence among placebo-treated patients (olanzapine incidence at least twice that for placebo) during the placebo-controlled premarketing studies. The incidence of somnolence during the 24 hour IM treatment period in clinical trials in agitated patients with schizophrenia or bipolar I mania was 6% for intramuscular olanzapine for injection and 3% for placebo.

Adverse Reactions Occurring at an Incidence of 2% or More among Oral Olanzapine-Treated Patients in Short-Term, Placebo-Controlled Trials

Table 11 enumerates the incidence, rounded to the nearest percent, of treatment-emergent adverse reactions that occurred in 2% or more of patients treated with oral olanzapine (doses ≥2.5 mg/day) and with incidence greater than placebo who participated in the acute phase of placebo-controlled trials.

Table 11: Treatment-Emergent Adverse Reactions: Incidence in Short-Term, Placebo-Controlled Clinical Trials with Oral Olanzapine

Body System/Adverse Reaction	Percentage of Patients Reporting Event	
	Olanzapine (N=532)	Placebo (N=294)
Body as a Whole		
Accidental injury	12	8
Asthenia	10	9
Fever	6	2
Back pain	5	2
Chest pain	3	1
Cardiovascular System		
Postural hypotension	3	1
Tachycardia	3	1
Hypertension	2	1
Digestive System		
Dry mouth	9	5
Constipation	9	4
Dyspepsia	7	5
Vomiting	4	3
Increased appetite	3	2
Hemic and Lymphatic System		
Ecchymosis	5	3
Metabolic and Nutritional Disorders		
Weight gain	5	3
Peripheral edema	3	1
Musculoskeletal System		
Extremity pain (other than joint)	5	3
Joint pain	5	3
Nervous System		
Somnolence	29	13
Insomnia	12	11
Dizziness	11	4
Abnormal gait	6	1
Tremor	4	3
Akathisia	3	2
Hypertonia	3	2
Articulation impairment	2	1
Respiratory System		
Rhinitis	7	6
Cough increased	6	3
Pharyngitis	4	3
Special Senses		
Amblyopia	3	2
Urogenital System		
Urinary incontinence	2	1
Urinary tract infection	2	1

Commonly Observed Adverse Reactions in Short-Term Trials of Oral Olanzapine as Adjunct to Lithium or Valproate

In the bipolar I disorder (manic or mixed episodes) adjunct placebo-controlled trials, the most commonly observed adverse reactions associated with the combination of olanzapine and lithium or valproate (incidence of ≥5% and at least twice placebo) were:

Table 12: Common Treatment-Emergent Adverse Reactions Associated with the Use of Oral Olanzapine in 6-Week Adjunct to Lithium or Valproate Trials — Bipolar I Disorder (Manic or Mixed Episodes)

Adverse Reaction	Percentage of Patients Reporting Event	
	Olanzapine with lithium or valproate (N=229)	Placebo with lithium or valproate (N=115)
Dry mouth	32	9
Weight gain	26	7
Increased appetite	24	8
Dizziness	14	7
Back pain	8	4
Constipation	8	4

Speech disorder	7	1
Increased salivation	6	2
Amnesia	5	2
Paresthesia	5	2

Adverse Reactions Occurring at an Incidence of 2% or More among Oral Olanzapine-Treated Patients in Short-Term Trials of Olanzapine as Adjunct to Lithium or Valproate

Table 13 enumerates the incidence, rounded to the nearest percent, of treatment-emergent adverse reactions that occurred in 2% or more of patients treated with the combination of olanzapine (doses ≥5 mg/day) and lithium or valproate and with incidence greater than lithium or valproate alone who participated in the acute phase of placebo-controlled combination trials.

Table 13: Treatment-Emergent Adverse Reactions: Incidence in Short-Term, Placebo-Controlled Clinical Trials of Oral Olanzapine as Adjunct to Lithium or Valproate

Body System/Adverse Reaction	Percentage of Patients Reporting Event	
	Olanzapine with lithium or valproate (N=229)	Placebo with lithium or valproate (N=115)
Body as a Whole		
Asthenia	18	13
Back pain	8	4
Accidental injury	4	2
Chest pain	3	2
Cardiovascular System		
Hypertension	2	1
Digestive System		
Dry mouth	32	9
Increased appetite	24	8
Thirst	10	6
Constipation	8	4
Increased salivation	6	2
Metabolic and Nutritional Disorders		
Weight gain	26	7
Peripheral edema	6	4
Edema	2	1
Nervous System		
Somnolence	52	27
Tremor	23	13
Depression	18	17
Dizziness	14	7
Speech disorder	7	1
Amnesia	5	2
Paresthesia	5	2
Apathy	4	3
Confusion	4	1
Euphoria	3	2
Incoordination	2	0
Respiratory System		
Pharyngitis	4	1
Dyspnea	3	1
Skin and Appendages		
Sweating	3	1
Acne	2	0
Dry skin	2	0
Special Senses		
Amblyopia	9	5
Abnormal vision	2	0
Urogenital System		
Dysmenorrhea[a]	2	0
Vaginitis[a]	2	0

[a] Denominator used was for females only (olanzapine, N=128; placebo, N=51).

For specific information about the adverse reactions observed with lithium or valproate, refer to the Adverse Reactions section for these other products.

Adverse Reactions Occurring at an Incidence of 1% or More among Intramuscular Olanzapine for Injection-Treated Patients in Short-Term, Placebo-Controlled Trials

Table 14 enumerates the incidence, rounded to the nearest percent, of treatment-emergent adverse reactions that occurred in 1% or more of patients treated with intramuscular olanzapine for injection (dose range of

2.5-10 mg/injection) and with incidence greater than placebo who participated in the short-term, placebo-controlled trials in agitated patients with schizophrenia or bipolar I mania.

Table 14: Treatment-Emergent Adverse Reactions: Incidence in Short-Term (24 Hour), Placebo-Controlled Clinical Trials with Intramuscular Olanzapine for Injection in Agitated Patients with Schizophrenia or Bipolar I Mania

	Percentage of Patients Reporting Event	
Body System/Adverse Reaction	Olanzapine (N=415)	Placebo (N=150)
Body as a Whole		
Asthenia	2	1
Cardiovascular System		
Hypotension	2	0
Postural hypotension	1	0
Nervous System		
Somnolence	6	3
Dizziness	4	2
Tremor	1	0

Additional Findings Observed in Clinical Trials

Dose Dependency of Adverse Reactions in Short-Term, Placebo-Controlled Trials

Extrapyramidal Symptoms: The following table enumerates the percentage of patients with treatment-emergent extrapyramidal symptoms as assessed by categorical analyses of formal rating scales during acute therapy in a controlled clinical trial comparing oral olanzapine at 3 fixed doses with placebo in the treatment of schizophrenia in a 6-week trial.

[See table 15 at top right]

The following table enumerates the percentage of patients with treatment-emergent extrapyramidal symptoms as assessed by spontaneously reported adverse reactions during acute therapy in the same controlled clinical trial comparing olanzapine at 3 fixed doses with placebo in the treatment of schizophrenia in a 6-week trial.

[See table 16 above]

The following table enumerates the percentage of adolescent patients with treatment-emergent extrapyramidal symptoms as assessed by spontaneously reported adverse reactions during acute therapy (dose range: 2.5 to 20 mg/day).

Table 17: Treatment-Emergent Extrapyramidal Symptoms Assessed by Adverse Reactions Incidence in Placebo-Controlled Clinical Trials of Oral Olanzapine in Schizophrenia and Bipolar I Disorder — Adolescents

	Percentage of Patients Reporting Event	
Categories[a]	Placebo (N=89)	Olanzapine (N=179)
Dystonic events	0	1
Parkinsonism events	2	1
Akathisia events	4	6
Dyskinetic events	0	1
Nonspecific events	0	4
Any extrapyramidal event	6	10

[a] Categories are based on Standard MedDRA Queries (SMQ) for extrapyramidal symptoms as defined in MedDRA version 12.0.

The following table enumerates the percentage of patients with treatment-emergent extrapyramidal symptoms as assessed by categorical analyses of formal rating scales during controlled clinical trials comparing fixed doses of intramuscular olanzapine for injection with placebo in agitation. Patients in each dose group could receive up to 3 injections during the trials *[see Clinical Studies (14.3)]*. Patient assessments were conducted during the 24 hours following the initial dose of intramuscular olanzapine for injection.

[See table 18 above]

The following table enumerates the percentage of patients with treatment-emergent extrapyramidal symptoms as assessed by spontaneously reported adverse reactions in the same controlled clinical trial comparing fixed doses of intramuscular olanzapine for injection with placebo in agitated patients with schizophrenia.

[See table 19 at top of next page]

Dystonia, Class Effect: Symptoms of dystonia, prolonged abnormal contractions of muscle groups, may occur in susceptible individuals during the first few days of treatment. Dystonic symptoms include: spasm of the neck muscles, sometimes progressing to tightness of the throat, swallowing difficulty, difficulty breathing, and/or protrusion of the tongue. While these symptoms can occur at low doses, the frequency and severity are greater with high potency and at higher doses of first generation antipsychotic drugs. In general, an elevated risk of acute dystonia may be observed in males and younger age groups receiving antipsychotics; however, events of dystonia have been reported infrequently (<1%) with olanzapine use.

Other Adverse Reactions: The following table addresses dose relatedness for other adverse reactions using data from a schizophrenia trial involving fixed dosage ranges of oral olanzapine. It enumerates the percentage of patients with treatment-emergent adverse reactions for the 3 fixed-dose range groups and placebo. The data were analyzed using the Cochran-Armitage test, excluding the placebo group, and the table includes only those adverse reactions for which there was a trend.

[See table 20 on next page]

Table 15: Treatment-Emergent Extrapyramidal Symptoms Assessed by Rating Scales Incidence in a Fixed Dosage Range, Placebo-Controlled Clinical Trial of Oral Olanzapine in Schizophrenia — Acute Phase

	Percentage of Patients Reporting Event			
	Placebo	Olanzapine 5 ± 2.5 mg/day	Olanzapine 10 ± 2.5 mg/day	Olanzapine 15 ± 2.5 mg/day
Parkinsonism[a]	15	14	12	14
Akathisia[b]	23	16	19	27

[a] Percentage of patients with a Simpson-Angus Scale total score >3.
[b] Percentage of patients with a Barnes Akathisia Scale global score ≥2.

Table 16: Treatment-Emergent Extrapyramidal Symptoms Assessed by Adverse Reactions Incidence in a Fixed Dosage Range, Placebo-Controlled Clinical Trial of Oral Olanzapine in Schizophrenia — Acute Phase

	Percentage of Patients Reporting Event			
	Placebo (N=68)	Olanzapine 5 ± 2.5 mg/day (N=65)	Olanzapine 10 ± 2.5 mg/day (N=64)	Olanzapine 15 ± 2.5 mg/day (N=69)
Dystonic events[a]	1	3	2	3
Parkinsonism events[b]	10	8	14	20
Akathisia events[c]	1	5	11	10
Dyskinetic events[d]	4	0	2	1
Residual events[e]	1	2	5	1
Any extrapyramidal event	16	15	25	32

[a] Patients with the following COSTART terms were counted in this category: dystonia, generalized spasm, neck rigidity, oculogyric crisis, opisthotonos, torticollis.
[b] Patients with the following COSTART terms were counted in this category: akinesia, cogwheel rigidity, extrapyramidal syndrome, hypertonia, hypokinesia, masked facies, tremor.
[c] Patients with the following COSTART terms were counted in this category: akathisia, hyperkinesia.
[d] Patients with the following COSTART terms were counted in this category: buccoglossal syndrome, choreoathetosis, dyskinesia, tardive dyskinesia.
[e] Patients with the following COSTART terms were counted in this category: movement disorder, myoclonus, twitching.

Table 18: Treatment-Emergent Extrapyramidal Symptoms Assessed by Rating Scales Incidence in a Fixed Dose, Placebo-Controlled Clinical Trial of Intramuscular Olanzapine for Injection in Agitated Patients with Schizophrenia

	Percentage of Patients Reporting Event				
	Placebo	Olanzapine IM 2.5 mg	Olanzapine IM 5 mg	Olanzapine IM 7.5 mg	Olanzapine IM 10 mg
Parkinsonism[a]	0	0	0	0	3
Akathisia[b]	0	0	5	0	0

[a] Percentage of patients with a Simpson-Angus Scale total score >3.
[b] Percentage of patients with a Barnes Akathisia Scale global score ≥2.

Differences among Fixed-Dose Groups Observed in Other Olanzapine Clinical Trials

In a single 8-week randomized, double-blind, fixed-dose study comparing 10 (N=199), 20 (N=200) and 40 (N=200) mg/day of oral olanzapine in patients with schizophrenia or schizoaffective disorder, differences among 3 dose groups were observed for the following safety outcomes: weight gain, prolactin elevation, fatigue and dizziness. Mean baseline to endpoint increase in weight (10 mg/day: 1.9 kg; 20 mg/day: 2.3 kg; 40 mg/day: 3 kg) was observed with significant differences between 10 vs 40 mg/day. Incidence of treatment-emergent prolactin elevation >24.2 ng/mL (female) or >18.77 ng/mL (male) at any time during the trial (10 mg/day: 31.2%; 20 mg/day: 42.7%; 40 mg/day: 61.1%) with significant differences between 10 vs 40 mg/day and 20 vs 40 mg/day; fatigue (10 mg/day: 1.5%; 20 mg/day: 2.1%; 40 mg/day: 6.6%) with significant differences between 10 vs 40 and 20 vs 40 mg/day; and dizziness (10 mg/day: 2.6%; 20 mg/day: 1.6%; 40 mg/day: 6.6%) with significant differences between 20 vs 40 mg/day, was observed.

Other Adverse Reactions Observed During the Clinical Trial Evaluation of Oral Olanzapine

Following is a list of treatment-emergent adverse reactions reported by patients treated with oral olanzapine (at multiple doses ≥1 mg/day) in clinical trials. This listing is not in-

Table 19: Treatment-Emergent Extrapyramidal Symptoms Assessed by Adverse Reactions Incidence in a Fixed Dose, Placebo-Controlled Clinical Trial of Intramuscular Olanzapine for Injection in Agitated Patients with Schizophrenia

	Percentage of Patients Reporting Event				
	Placebo (N=45)	Olanzapine IM 2.5 mg (N=48)	Olanzapine IM 5 mg (N=45)	Olanzapine IM 7.5 mg (N=46)	Olanzapine IM 10 mg (N=46)
Dystonic events[a]	0	0	0	0	0
Parkinsonism events[b]	0	4	2	0	0
Akathisia events[c]	0	2	0	0	0
Dyskinetic events[d]	0	0	0	0	0
Residual events[e]	0	0	0	0	0
Any extrapyramidal events	0	4	2	0	0

[a] Patients with the following COSTART terms were counted in this category: dystonia, generalized spasm, neck rigidity, oculogyric crisis, opisthotonos, torticollis.
[b] Patients with the following COSTART terms were counted in this category: akinesia, cogwheel rigidity, extrapyramidal syndrome, hypertonia, hypokinesia, masked facies, tremor.
[c] Patients with the following COSTART terms were counted in this category: akathisia, hyperkinesia.
[d] Patients with the following COSTART terms were counted in this category: buccoglossal syndrome, choreoathetosis, dyskinesia, tardive dyskinesia.
[e] Patients with the following COSTART terms were counted in this category: movement disorder, myoclonus, twitching.

Table 20: Percentage of Patients from a Schizophrenia Trial with Treatment-Emergent Adverse Reactions for the 3 Dose Range Groups and Placebo

Adverse Reaction	Percentage of Patients Reporting Event			
	Placebo (N=68)	Olanzapine 5 ± 2.5 mg/day (N=65)	Olanzapine 10 ± 2.5 mg/day (N=64)	Olanzapine 15 ± 2.5 mg/day (N=69)
Asthenia	15	8	9	20
Dry mouth	4	3	5	13
Nausea	9	0	2	9
Somnolence	16	20	30	39
Tremor	3	0	5	7

Table 21: Treatment-Emergent Adverse Reactions of ≥5% Incidence among Adolescents (13-17 Years Old) with Schizophrenia or Bipolar I Disorder (Manic or Mixed Episodes)

	Percentage of Patients Reporting Event			
	6 Week Trial % Schizophrenia Patients		3 Week Trial % Bipolar Patients	
Adverse Reactions	Olanzapine (N=72)	Placebo (N=35)	Olanzapine (N=107)	Placebo (N=54)
Sedation[a]	39	9	48	9
Weight increased	31	9	29	4
Headache	17	6	17	17
Increased appetite	17	9	29	4
Dizziness	8	3	7	2
Abdominal pain[b]	6	3	6	7
Pain in extremity	6	3	5	0
Fatigue	3	3	14	6
Dry mouth	4	0	7	0

[a] Patients with the following MedDRA terms were counted in this category: hypersomnia, lethargy, sedation, somnolence.
[b] Patients with the following MedDRA terms were counted in this category: abdominal pain, abdominal pain lower, abdominal pain upper.

tended to include reactions (1) already listed in previous tables or elsewhere in labeling, (2) for which a drug cause was remote, (3) which were so general as to be uninformative, (4) which were not considered to have significant clinical implications, or (5) which occurred at a rate equal to or less than placebo. Reactions are classified by body system using the following definitions: frequent adverse reactions are those occurring in at least 1/100 patients; infrequent adverse reactions are those occurring in 1/100 to 1/1000 patients; rare reactions are those occurring in fewer than 1/1000 patients.
  Body as a Whole—*Infrequent:* chills, face edema, photosensitivity reaction, suicide attempt[1]; *Rare:* chills and fever, hangover effect, sudden death[1].
  Cardiovascular System—*Infrequent:* cerebrovascular accident, vasodilatation.

Digestive System—*Infrequent:* nausea and vomiting, tongue edema; *Rare:* ileus, intestinal obstruction, liver fatty deposit.
  Hemic and Lymphatic System—*Infrequent:* leukopenia, thrombocytopenia.
  Metabolic and Nutritional Disorders—*Infrequent:* alkaline phosphatase increased, bilirubinemia, hypoproteinemia.
  Musculoskeletal System—*Rare:* osteoporosis.
  Nervous System—*Infrequent:* ataxia, dysarthria, libido decreased, stupor; *Rare:* coma.
  Respiratory System—*Infrequent:* epistaxis; *Rare:* lung edema.
  Skin and Appendages—*Infrequent:* alopecia.
  Special Senses—*Infrequent:* abnormality of accommodation, dry eyes; *Rare:* mydriasis.
  Urogenital System—*Infrequent:* amenorrhea[2], breast pain, decreased menstruation, impotence[2], increased menstruation[2], menorrhagia[2], metrorrhagia[2], polyuria[2], urinary frequency, urinary retention, urinary urgency, urination impaired.
[1] These terms represent serious adverse events but do not meet the definition for adverse drug reactions. They are included here because of their seriousness.
[2] Adjusted for gender.

<u>Other Adverse Reactions Observed During the Clinical Trial Evaluation of Intramuscular Olanzapine for Injection</u>
Following is a list of treatment-emergent adverse reactions reported by patients treated with intramuscular olanzapine for injection (at 1 or more doses ≥2.5 mg/injection) in clinical trials. This listing is not intended to include reactions (1) already listed in previous tables or elsewhere in labeling, (2) for which a drug cause was remote, (3) which were so general as to be uninformative, (4) which were not considered to have significant clinical implications, or (5) for which occurred at a rate equal to or less than placebo. Reactions are classified by body system using the following definitions: frequent adverse reactions are those occurring in at least 1/100 patients; infrequent adverse reactions are those occurring in 1/100 to 1/1000 patients.
  Body as a Whole—*Frequent:* injection site pain.
  Cardiovascular System—*Infrequent:* syncope.
  Digestive System—*Infrequent:* nausea.
  Metabolic and Nutritional Disorders—*Infrequent:* creatine phosphokinase increased.

Clinical Trials in Adolescent Patients (age 13 to 17 years)
Commonly Observed Adverse Reactions in Oral Olanzapine Short-Term, Placebo-Controlled Trials
Adverse reactions in adolescent patients treated with oral olanzapine (doses ≥2.5 mg) reported with an incidence of 5% or more and reported at least twice as frequently as placebo-treated patients are listed in Table 21.
[See table 21 at left]

Adverse Reactions Occurring at an Incidence of 2% or More among Oral Olanzapine-Treated Patients in Short-Term (3-6 weeks), Placebo-Controlled Trials
Adverse reactions in adolescent patients treated with oral olanzapine (doses ≥2.5 mg) reported with an incidence of 2% or more and greater than placebo are listed in Table 22.

Table 22: Treatment-Emergent Adverse Reactions of ≥2% Incidence among Adolescents (13-17 Years Old) (Combined Incidence from Short-Term, Placebo-Controlled Clinical Trials of Schizophrenia or Bipolar I Disorder [Manic or Mixed Episodes])

	Percentage of Patients Reporting Event	
Adverse Reaction	Olanzapine (N=179)	Placebo (N=89)
Sedation[a]	44	9
Weight increased	30	6
Increased appetite	24	6
Headache	17	12
Fatigue	9	4
Dizziness	7	2
Dry mouth	6	0
Pain in extremity	5	1
Constipation	4	0
Nasopharyngitis	4	2
Diarrhea	3	0
Restlessness	3	2
Liver enzymes increased[b]	8	1
Dyspepsia	3	1
Epistaxis	3	0
Respiratory tract infection[c]	3	2
Sinusitis	3	0
Arthralgia	2	0
Musculoskeletal stiffness	2	0

[a] Patients with the following MedDRA terms were counted in this category: hypersomnia, lethargy, sedation, somnolence.

[b] The terms alanine aminotransferase (ALT), aspartate aminotransferase (AST), and hepatic enzyme were combined under liver enzymes.
[c] Patients with the following MedDRA terms were counted in this category: lower respiratory tract infection, respiratory tract infection, respiratory tract infection viral, upper respiratory tract infection, viral upper respiratory tract infection.

6.2 Vital Signs and Laboratory Studies

Vital Sign Changes—Oral olanzapine was associated with orthostatic hypotension and tachycardia in clinical trials. Intramuscular olanzapine for injection was associated with bradycardia, hypotension, and tachycardia in clinical trials *[see Warnings and Precautions (5)]*.

Laboratory Changes

Olanzapine Monotherapy in Adults: An assessment of the premarketing experience for olanzapine revealed an association with asymptomatic increases in ALT, AST, and GGT. Within the original premarketing database of about 2400 adult patients with baseline ALT ≤90 IU/L, the incidence of ALT elevations to >200 IU/L was 2% (50/2381). None of these patients experienced jaundice or other symptoms attributable to liver impairment and most had transient changes that tended to normalize while olanzapine treatment was continued.

In placebo-controlled olanzapine monotherapy studies in adults, clinically significant ALT elevations (change from <3 times the upper limit of normal [ULN] at baseline to ≥3 times ULN) were observed in 5% (77/1426) of patients exposed to olanzapine compared to 1% (10/1187) of patients exposed to placebo. ALT elevations ≥5 times ULN were observed in 2% (29/1438) of olanzapine-treated patients, compared to 0.3% (4/1196) of placebo-treated patients. ALT values returned to normal, or were decreasing, at last follow-up in the majority of patients who either continued treatment with olanzapine or discontinued olanzapine. No patient with elevated ALT values experienced jaundice, liver failure, or met the criteria for Hy's Rule.

Rare postmarketing reports of hepatitis have been received. Very rare cases of cholestatic or mixed liver injury have also been reported in the postmarketing period.

Caution should be exercised in patients with signs and symptoms of hepatic impairment, in patients with pre-existing conditions associated with limited hepatic functional reserve, and in patients who are being treated with potentially hepatotoxic drugs.

Olanzapine administration was also associated with increases in serum prolactin *[see Warnings and Precautions (5.15)]*, with an asymptomatic elevation of the eosinophil count in 0.3% of patients, and with an increase in CPK.

Olanzapine Monotherapy in Adolescents: In placebo-controlled clinical trials of adolescent patients with schizophrenia or bipolar I disorder (manic or mixed episodes), greater frequencies for the following treatment-emergent findings, at anytime, were observed in laboratory analytes compared to placebo: elevated ALT (≥3× ULN in patients with ALT at baseline <3× ULN), (12% vs 2%); elevated AST (28% vs 4%); low total bilirubin (22% vs 7%); elevated GGT (10% vs 1%); and elevated prolactin (47% vs 7%).

In placebo-controlled olanzapine monotherapy studies in adolescents, clinically significant ALT elevations (change from <3 times ULN at baseline to ≥3 times ULN) were observed in 12% (22/192) of patients exposed to olanzapine compared to 2% (2/109) of patients exposed to placebo. ALT elevations ≥5 times ULN were observed in 4% (8/192) of olanzapine-treated patients, compared to 1% (1/109) of placebo-treated patients. ALT values returned to normal, or were decreasing, at last follow-up in the majority of patients who either continued treatment with olanzapine or discontinued olanzapine. No adolescent patient with elevated ALT values experienced jaundice, liver failure, or met the criteria for Hy's Rule.

ECG Changes—In pooled studies of adults as well as pooled studies of adolescents, there were no significant differences between olanzapine and placebo in the proportions of patients experiencing potentially important changes in ECG parameters, including QT, QTc (Fridericia corrected), and PR intervals. Olanzapine use was associated with a mean increase in heart rate compared to placebo (adults: +2.4 beats per minute vs no change with placebo; adolescents: +6.3 beats per minute vs -5.1 beats per minute with placebo). This increase in heart rate may be related to olanzapine's potential for inducing orthostatic changes *[see Warnings and Precautions (5.8)]*.

6.3 Postmarketing Experience

The following adverse reactions have been identified during post-approval use of ZYPREXA. Because these reactions are reported voluntarily from a population of uncertain size, it is difficult to reliably estimate their frequency or evaluate a causal relationship to drug exposure.

Adverse reactions reported since market introduction that were temporally (but not necessarily causally) related to ZYPREXA therapy include the following: allergic reaction (e.g., anaphylactoid reaction, angioedema, pruritus or urticaria), diabetic coma, diabetic ketoacidosis, discontinuation reaction (diaphoresis, nausea or vomiting), jaundice, neutropenia, pancreatitis, priapism, rash, rhabdomyolysis, and venous thromboembolic events (including pulmonary embolism and deep venous thrombosis). Random cholesterol levels of ≥240 mg/dL and random triglyceride levels of ≥1000 mg/dL have been reported.

7 DRUG INTERACTIONS

The risks of using olanzapine in combination with other drugs have not been extensively evaluated in systematic studies.

7.1 Potential for Other Drugs to Affect Olanzapine

Diazepam—The co-administration of diazepam with olanzapine potentiated the orthostatic hypotension observed with olanzapine *[see Drug Interactions (7.2)]*.

Cimetidine and Antacids—Single doses of cimetidine (800 mg) or aluminum- and magnesium-containing antacids did not affect the oral bioavailability of olanzapine.

Inducers of CYP1A2—Carbamazepine therapy (200 mg bid) causes an approximately 50% increase in the clearance of olanzapine. This increase is likely due to the fact that carbamazepine is a potent inducer of CYP1A2 activity. Higher daily doses of carbamazepine may cause an even greater increase in olanzapine clearance.

Alcohol—Ethanol (45 mg/70 kg single dose) did not have an effect on olanzapine pharmacokinetics. The co-administration of alcohol (i.e., ethanol) with olanzapine potentiated the orthostatic hypotension observed with olanzapine *[see Drug Interactions (7.2)]*.

Inhibitors of CYP1A2

Fluvoxamine: Fluvoxamine, a CYP1A2 inhibitor, decreases the clearance of olanzapine. This results in a mean increase in olanzapine Cmax following fluvoxamine of 54% in female nonsmokers and 77% in male smokers. The mean increase in olanzapine AUC is 52% and 108%, respectively. Lower doses of olanzapine should be considered in patients receiving concomitant treatment with fluvoxamine.

Inhibitors of CYP2D6

Fluoxetine: Fluoxetine (60 mg single dose or 60 mg daily dose for 8 days) causes a small (mean 16%) increase in the maximum concentration of olanzapine and a small (mean 16%) decrease in olanzapine clearance. The magnitude of the impact of this factor is small in comparison to the overall variability between individuals, and therefore dose modification is not routinely recommended. When using ZYPREXA and fluoxetine in combination, also refer to the Drug Interactions section of the package insert for Symbyax.

Warfarin—Warfarin (20 mg single dose) did not affect olanzapine pharmacokinetics *[see Drug Interactions (7.2)]*.

Inducers of CYP1A2 or Glucuronyl Transferase—Omeprazole and rifampin may cause an increase in olanzapine clearance.

Charcoal—The administration of activated charcoal (1 g) reduced the Cmax and AUC of oral olanzapine by about 60%. As peak olanzapine levels are not typically obtained until about 6 hours after dosing, charcoal may be a useful treatment for olanzapine overdose.

7.2 Potential for Olanzapine to Affect Other Drugs

CNS Acting Drugs—Given the primary CNS effects of olanzapine, caution should be used when olanzapine is taken in combination with other centrally acting drugs and alcohol.

Antihypertensive Agents—Olanzapine, because of its potential for inducing hypotension, may enhance the effects of certain antihypertensive agents.

Levodopa and Dopamine Agonists—Olanzapine may antagonize the effects of levodopa and dopamine agonists.

Lorazepam (IM)—Administration of intramuscular lorazepam (2 mg) 1 hour after intramuscular olanzapine for injection (5 mg) did not significantly affect the pharmacokinetics of olanzapine, unconjugated lorazepam, or total lorazepam. However, this co-administration of intramuscular lorazepam and intramuscular olanzapine for injection added to the somnolence observed with either drug alone *[see Warnings and Precautions (5.8)]*.

Lithium—Multiple doses of olanzapine (10 mg for 8 days) did not influence the kinetics of lithium. Therefore, concomitant olanzapine administration does not require dosage adjustment of lithium *[see Warnings and Precautions (5.16)]*.

Valproate—Olanzapine (10 mg daily for 2 weeks) did not affect the steady state plasma concentrations of valproate. Therefore, concomitant olanzapine administration does not require dosage adjustment of valproate *[see Warnings and Precautions (5.16)]*.

Effect of Olanzapine on Drug Metabolizing Enzymes—In vitro studies utilizing human liver microsomes suggest that olanzapine has little potential to inhibit CYP1A2, CYP2C9, CYP2C19, CYP2D6, and CYP3A. Thus, olanzapine is unlikely to cause clinically important drug interactions mediated by these enzymes.

Imipramine—Single doses of olanzapine did not affect the pharmacokinetics of imipramine or its active metabolite desipramine.

Warfarin—Single doses of olanzapine did not affect the pharmacokinetics of warfarin *[see Drug Interactions (7.1)]*.

Diazepam—Olanzapine did not influence the pharmacokinetics of diazepam or its active metabolite N-desmethyldiazepam. However, diazepam co-administered with olanzapine increased the orthostatic hypotension observed with either drug given alone *[see Drug Interactions (7.1)]*.

Alcohol—Multiple doses of olanzapine did not influence the kinetics of ethanol *[see Drug Interactions (7.1)]*.

Biperiden—Multiple doses of olanzapine did not influence the kinetics of biperiden.

Theophylline—Multiple doses of olanzapine did not affect the pharmacokinetics of theophylline or its metabolites.

8 USE IN SPECIFIC POPULATIONS

When using ZYPREXA and fluoxetine in combination, also refer to the Use in Specific Populations section of the package insert for Symbyax.

8.1 Pregnancy

Teratogenic Effects, Pregnancy Category C—In oral reproduction studies in rats at doses up to 18 mg/kg/day and in rabbits at doses up to 30 mg/kg/day (9 and 30 times the maximum recommended human daily oral dose on a mg/m^2 basis, respectively) no evidence of teratogenicity was observed. In an oral rat teratology study, early resorptions and increased numbers of nonviable fetuses were observed at a dose of 18 mg/kg/day (9 times the maximum recommended human daily oral dose on a mg/m^2 basis). Gestation was prolonged at 10 mg/kg/day (5 times the maximum recommended human daily oral dose on a mg/m^2 basis). In an oral rabbit teratology study, fetal toxicity (manifested as increased resorptions and decreased fetal weight) occurred at a maternally toxic dose of 30 mg/kg/day (30 times the maximum recommended human daily oral dose on a mg/m^2 basis). Because animal reproduction studies are not always predictive of human response, this drug should be used during pregnancy only if the potential benefit justifies the potential risk to the fetus.

Placental transfer of olanzapine occurs in rat pups.

There are no adequate and well-controlled trials with olanzapine in pregnant females. Seven pregnancies were observed during clinical trials with olanzapine, including 2 resulting in normal births, 1 resulting in neonatal death due to a cardiovascular defect, 3 therapeutic abortions, and 1 spontaneous abortion.

8.2 Labor and Delivery

The effect of olanzapine on labor and delivery in humans is unknown. Parturition in rats was not affected by olanzapine.

8.3 Nursing Mothers

In a study in lactating, healthy women, olanzapine was excreted in breast milk. Mean infant dose at steady state was estimated to be 1.8% of the maternal olanzapine dose. It is recommended that women receiving olanzapine should not breast-feed.

8.4 Pediatric Use

The safety and effectiveness of oral ZYPREXA in the treatment of schizophrenia and manic or mixed episodes associated with bipolar I disorder were established in short-term studies in adolescents (ages 13 to 17 years). Use of ZYPREXA in adolescents is supported by evidence from adequate and well-controlled studies of ZYPREXA in which 268 adolescents received ZYPREXA in a range of 2.5 to 20 mg/day *[see Clinical Studies (14.1, 14.2)]*. Recommended starting dose for adolescents is lower than that for adults *[see Dosage and Administration (2.1, 2.2)]*. Compared to patients from adult clinical trials, adolescents were likely to gain more weight, experience increased sedation, and have greater increases in total cholesterol, triglycerides, LDL cholesterol, prolactin and hepatic transaminase levels *[see Warnings and Precautions (5.5, 5.6, 5.15, 5.17) and Adverse Reactions (6.2)]*. When deciding among the alternative treatments available for adolescents, clinicians should consider the increased potential (in adolescents as compared with adults) for weight gain and hyperlipidemia. Clinicians should consider the potential long-term risks when prescribing to adolescents, and in many cases this may lead them to consider prescribing other drugs first in adolescents *[see Indications and Usage (1.1, 1.2)]*. Safety and effectiveness of olanzapine in children <13 years of age have not been established *[see Patient Counseling Information (17.13)]*.

Safety and effectiveness of ZYPREXA and fluoxetine in combination in children and adolescents <18 years of age have not been established.

8.5 Geriatric Use

Of the 2500 patients in premarketing clinical studies with oral olanzapine, 11% (263) were 65 years of age or over. In patients with schizophrenia, there was no indication of any different tolerability of olanzapine in the elderly compared to younger patients. Studies in elderly patients with dementia-related psychosis have suggested that there may be a different tolerability profile in this population compared to younger patients with schizophrenia. Elderly patients with dementia-related psychosis treated with olanzapine are at an increased risk of death compared to placebo. In placebo-controlled studies of olanzapine in elderly patients with dementia-related psychosis, there was a higher incidence of cerebrovascular adverse events (e.g., stroke, transient ischemic attack) in patients treated with olanzapine compared to patients treated with placebo. Olanzapine is not approved for the treatment of patients with dementia-related psychosis. Also, the presence of factors that might decrease pharmacokinetic clearance or increase the pharmacodynamic response to olanzapine should lead to consideration of a lower starting dose for any geriatric patient *[see Boxed Warning, Dosage and Administration (2.1), and Warnings and Precautions (5.1)]*.

Clinical studies of ZYPREXA and fluoxetine in combination did not include sufficient numbers of patients ≥65 years of age to determine whether they respond differently from younger patients.

9 DRUG ABUSE AND DEPENDENCE

9.3 Dependence

In studies prospectively designed to assess abuse and dependence potential, olanzapine was shown to have acute depressive CNS effects but little or no potential of abuse or physical dependence in rats administered oral doses up to 15 times the maximum recommended human daily oral dose (20 mg) and rhesus monkeys administered oral doses up to 8 times the maximum recommended human daily oral dose on a mg/m^2 basis.

Olanzapine has not been systematically studied in humans for its potential for abuse, tolerance, or physical dependence. While the clinical trials did not reveal any tendency for any drug-seeking behavior, these observations were not systematic, and it is not possible to predict on the basis of this limited experience the extent to which a CNS-active drug will be misused, diverted, and/or abused once marketed. Consequently, patients should be evaluated carefully for a history of drug abuse, and such patients should be observed closely for signs of misuse or abuse of olanzapine (e.g., development of tolerance, increases in dose, drug-seeking behavior).

10 OVERDOSAGE

10.1 Human Experience

In premarketing trials involving more than 3100 patients and/or normal subjects, accidental or intentional acute overdosage of olanzapine was identified in 67 patients. In the patient taking the largest identified amount, 300 mg, the only symptoms reported were drowsiness and slurred speech. In the limited number of patients who were evaluated in hospitals, including the patient taking 300 mg, there were no observations indicating an adverse change in laboratory analytes or ECG. Vital signs were usually within normal limits following overdoses.

In postmarketing reports of overdose with olanzapine alone, symptoms have been reported in the majority of cases. In symptomatic patients, symptoms with ≥10% incidence included agitation/aggressiveness, dysarthria, tachycardia, various extrapyramidal symptoms, and reduced level of consciousness ranging from sedation to coma. Among less commonly reported symptoms were the following potentially medically serious reactions: aspiration, cardiopulmonary arrest, cardiac arrhythmias (such as supraventricular tachycardia and 1 patient experiencing sinus pause with spontaneous resumption of normal rhythm), delirium, possible neuroleptic malignant syndrome, respiratory depression/arrest, convulsion, hypertension, and hypotension. Eli Lilly and Company has received reports of fatality in association with overdose of olanzapine alone. In 1 case of death, the amount of acutely ingested olanzapine was reported to be possibly as low as 450 mg of oral olanzapine; however, in another case, a patient was reported to survive an acute olanzapine ingestion of approximately 2 g of oral olanzapine.

10.2 Management of Overdose

The possibility of multiple drug involvement should be considered. In case of acute overdosage, establish and maintain an airway and ensure adequate oxygenation and ventilation, which may include intubation. Gastric lavage (after intubation, if patient is unconscious) and administration of activated charcoal together with a laxative should be considered. The administration of activated charcoal (1 g) reduced the Cmax and AUC of oral olanzapine by about 60%. As peak olanzapine levels are not typically obtained until about 6 hours after dosing, charcoal may be a useful treatment for olanzapine overdose.

The possibility of obtundation, seizures, or dystonic reaction of the head and neck following overdose may create a risk of aspiration with induced emesis. Cardiovascular monitoring should commence immediately and should include continuous electrocardiographic monitoring to detect possible arrhythmias.

There is no specific antidote to olanzapine. Therefore, appropriate supportive measures should be initiated. Hypotension and circulatory collapse should be treated with appropriate measures such as intravenous fluids and/or sympathomimetic agents. (Do not use epinephrine, dopamine, or other sympathomimetics with beta-agonist activity, since beta stimulation may worsen hypotension in the setting of olanzapine-induced alpha blockade.) Close medical supervision and monitoring should continue until the patient recovers.

For specific information about overdosage with lithium or valproate, refer to the Overdosage section of the package inserts for these products. For specific information about overdosage with olanzapine and fluoxetine in combination, refer to the Overdosage section of the Symbyax package insert.

11 DESCRIPTION

ZYPREXA (olanzapine) is an atypical antipsychotic that belongs to the thienobenzodiazepine class. The chemical designation is 2-methyl-4-(4-methyl-1-piperazinyl)-10*H*-thieno[2,3-*b*] [1,5]benzodiazepine. The molecular formula is $C_{17}H_{20}N_4S$, which corresponds to a molecular weight of 312.44. The chemical structure is:

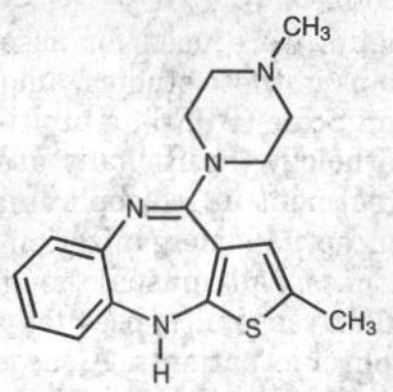

Olanzapine is a yellow crystalline solid, which is practically insoluble in water.

ZYPREXA tablets are intended for oral administration only.

Each tablet contains olanzapine equivalent to 2.5 mg (8 µmol), 5 mg (16 µmol), 7.5 mg (24 µmol), 10 mg (32 µmol), 15 mg (48 µmol), or 20 mg (64 µmol). Inactive ingredients are carnauba wax, crospovidone, hydroxypropyl cellulose, hypromellose, lactose, magnesium stearate, microcrystalline cellulose, and other inactive ingredients. The color coating contains Titanium Dioxide (all strengths), FD&C Blue No. 2 Aluminum Lake (15 mg), or Synthetic Red Iron Oxide (20 mg). The 2.5, 5, 7.5, and 10 mg tablets are imprinted with edible ink which contains FD&C Blue No. 2 Aluminum Lake.

ZYPREXA ZYDIS (olanzapine orally disintegrating tablets) is intended for oral administration only.

Each orally disintegrating tablet contains olanzapine equivalent to 5 mg (16 µmol), 10 mg (32 µmol), 15 mg (48 µmol) or 20 mg (64 µmol). It begins disintegrating in the mouth within seconds, allowing its contents to be subsequently swallowed with or without liquid. ZYPREXA ZYDIS (olanzapine orally disintegrating tablets) also contains the following inactive ingredients: gelatin, mannitol, aspartame, sodium methyl paraben, and sodium propyl paraben.

ZYPREXA IntraMuscular (olanzapine for injection) is intended for intramuscular use only.

Each vial provides for the administration of 10 mg (32 µmol) olanzapine with inactive ingredients 50 mg lactose monohydrate and 3.5 mg tartaric acid. Hydrochloric acid and/or sodium hydroxide may have been added during manufacturing to adjust pH.

12 CLINICAL PHARMACOLOGY

12.1 Mechanism of Action

The mechanism of action of olanzapine, as with other drugs having efficacy in schizophrenia, is unknown. However, it has been proposed that this drug's efficacy in schizophrenia is mediated through a combination of dopamine and serotonin type 2 (5HT2) antagonism. The mechanism of action of olanzapine in the treatment of acute manic or mixed episodes associated with bipolar I disorder is unknown.

12.2 Pharmacodynamics

Olanzapine binds with high affinity to the following receptors: serotonin $5HT_{2A/2C}$, $5HT_6$ (K_i=4, 11, and 5 nM, respectively), dopamine $D_{1\text{-}4}$ (K_i=11-31 nM), histamine H_1 (K_i=7 nM), and adrenergic α_1 receptors (K_i=19 nM). Olanzapine is an antagonist with moderate affinity binding for serotonin $5HT_3$ (K_i=57 nM) and muscarinic $M_{1\text{-}5}$ (K_i=73, 96, 132, 32, and 48 nM, respectively). Olanzapine binds weakly to $GABA_A$, BZD, and β-adrenergic receptors (K_i>10 µM).

Antagonism at receptors other than dopamine and $5HT_2$ may explain some of the other therapeutic and side effects of olanzapine. Olanzapine's antagonism of muscarinic $M_{1\text{-}5}$ receptors may explain its anticholinergic-like effects. Olanzapine's antagonism of histamine H_1 receptors may explain the somnolence observed with this drug. Olanzapine's antagonism of adrenergic α_1 receptors may explain the orthostatic hypotension observed with this drug.

12.3 Pharmacokinetics

Oral Administration, Monotherapy—Olanzapine is well absorbed and reaches peak concentrations in approximately 6 hours following an oral dose. It is eliminated extensively by first pass metabolism, with approximately 40% of the dose metabolized before reaching the systemic circulation. Food does not affect the rate or extent of olanzapine absorption. Pharmacokinetic studies showed that ZYPREXA tablets and ZYPREXA ZYDIS (olanzapine orally disintegrating tablets) dosage forms of olanzapine are bioequivalent.

Olanzapine displays linear kinetics over the clinical dosing range. Its half-life ranges from 21 to 54 hours (5th to 95th percentile; mean of 30 hr), and apparent plasma clearance ranges from 12 to 47 L/hr (5th to 95th percentile; mean of 25 L/hr).

Administration of olanzapine once daily leads to steady-state concentrations in about 1 week that are approximately twice the concentrations after single doses. Plasma concentrations, half-life, and clearance of olanzapine may vary between individuals on the basis of smoking status, gender, and age.

Olanzapine is extensively distributed throughout the body, with a volume of distribution of approximately 1000 L. It is 93% bound to plasma proteins over the concentration range of 7 to 1100 ng/mL, binding primarily to albumin and α_1-acid glycoprotein.

Metabolism and Elimination—Following a single oral dose of ^{14}C labeled olanzapine, 7% of the dose of olanzapine was recovered in the urine as unchanged drug, indicating that olanzapine is highly metabolized. Approximately 57% and 30% of the dose was recovered in the urine and feces, respectively. In the plasma, olanzapine accounted for only 12% of the AUC for total radioactivity, indicating significant exposure to metabolites. After multiple dosing, the major circulating metabolites were the 10-N-glucuronide, present at steady state at 44% of the concentration of olanzapine, and 4′-N-desmethyl olanzapine, present at steady state at 31% of the concentration of olanzapine. Both metabolites lack pharmacological activity at the concentrations observed.

Direct glucuronidation and cytochrome P450 (CYP) mediated oxidation are the primary metabolic pathways for olanzapine. In vitro studies suggest that CYPs 1A2 and 2D6, and the flavin-containing monooxygenase system are involved in olanzapine oxidation. CYP2D6 mediated oxidation appears to be a minor metabolic pathway in vivo, because the clearance of olanzapine is not reduced in subjects who are deficient in this enzyme.

Intramuscular Administration—ZYPREXA IntraMuscular results in rapid absorption with peak plasma concentrations occurring within 15 to 45 minutes. Based upon a pharmacokinetic study in healthy volunteers, a 5 mg dose of intramuscular olanzapine for injection produces, on average, a maximum plasma concentration approximately 5 times higher than the maximum plasma concentration produced by a 5 mg dose of oral olanzapine. Area under the curve achieved after an intramuscular dose is similar to that achieved after oral administration of the same dose. The half-life observed after intramuscular administration is similar to that observed after oral dosing. The pharmacokinetics are linear over the clinical dosing range. Metabolic profiles after intramuscular administration are qualitatively similar to metabolic profiles after oral administration.

Specific Populations

Renal Impairment—Because olanzapine is highly metabolized before excretion and only 7% of the drug is excreted unchanged, renal dysfunction alone is unlikely to have a major impact on the pharmacokinetics of olanzapine. The pharmacokinetic characteristics of olanzapine were similar in patients with severe renal impairment and normal subjects, indicating that dosage adjustment based upon the degree of renal impairment is not required. In addition, olanzapine is not removed by dialysis. The effect of renal impairment on metabolite elimination has not been studied.

Hepatic Impairment—Although the presence of hepatic impairment may be expected to reduce the clearance of olanzapine, a study of the effect of impaired liver function in subjects (n=6) with clinically significant (Childs Pugh Classification A and B) cirrhosis revealed little effect on the pharmacokinetics of olanzapine.

Geriatric—In a study involving 24 healthy subjects, the mean elimination half-life of olanzapine was about 1.5 times greater in elderly (≥65 years) than in nonelderly subjects (<65 years). Caution should be used in dosing the elderly, especially if there are other factors that might additively influence drug metabolism and/or pharmacodynamic sensitivity *[see Dosage and Administration (2)]*.

Gender—Clearance of olanzapine is approximately 30% lower in women than in men. There were, however, no apparent differences between men and women in effectiveness or adverse effects. Dosage modifications based on gender should not be needed.

Smoking Status—Olanzapine clearance is about 40% higher in smokers than in nonsmokers, although dosage modifications are not routinely recommended.

Race—In vivo studies have shown that exposures are similar among Japanese, Chinese and Caucasians, especially after normalization for body weight differences. Dosage modifications for race are, therefore, not recommended.

Combined Effects—The combined effects of age, smoking, and gender could lead to substantial pharmacokinetic differences in populations. The clearance in young smoking males, for example, may be 3 times higher than that in elderly nonsmoking females. Dosing modification may be necessary in patients who exhibit a combination of factors that may result in slower metabolism of olanzapine *[see Dosage and Administration (2)]*.

Adolescents (ages 13 to 17 years)—In clinical studies, most adolescents were nonsmokers and this population had a lower average body weight, which resulted in higher average olanzapine exposure compared to adults.

13 NONCLINICAL TOXICOLOGY

13.1 Carcinogenesis, Mutagenesis, Impairment of Fertility

Carcinogenesis—Oral carcinogenicity studies were conducted in mice and rats. Olanzapine was administered to mice in two 78-week studies at doses of 3, 10, 30/20 mg/kg/day (equivalent to 0.8-5 times the maximum recommended human daily oral dose on a mg/m^2 basis) and 0.25, 2, 8 mg/kg/day (equivalent to 0.06-2 times the maximum recommended human daily oral dose on a mg/m^2 basis). Rats were dosed for 2 years at doses of 0.25, 1, 2.5, 4 mg/kg/day (males) and 0.25, 1, 4, 8 mg/kg/day (females) (equivalent to 0.13-2 and 0.13-4 times the maximum recommended human daily oral dose on a mg/m^2 basis, respectively). The incidence of liver hemangiomas and hemangiosarcomas was significantly increased in 1 mouse study in female mice dosed at 8 mg/kg/day (2 times the maximum recommended human daily oral dose on a mg/m^2 basis). These tumors were not increased in another mouse study in females dosed at 10 or 30/20 mg/kg/day (2-5 times the maximum recommended human daily oral dose on a mg/m^2 basis); in this study, there was a high incidence of early mortalities in males of the 30/20 mg/kg/day group. The incidence of mammary gland adenomas and adenocarcinomas was significantly increased in female mice dosed at ≥2 mg/kg/day and in female rats dosed at ≥4 mg/kg/day (0.5 and 2 times the maximum recommended human daily oral dose on a mg/m^2 basis, respectively). Antipsychotic drugs have been shown to chronically elevate prolactin levels in rodents. Serum prolactin levels were not measured during the olanzapine carcinogenicity studies; however, measurements during subchronic toxicity studies showed that olanzapine elevated serum prolactin levels up to 4-fold in rats at the same doses used in the carcinogenicity study. An increase in mammary gland neoplasms has been found in rodents after chronic administration of other antipsychotic drugs and is considered to be prolactin mediated. The relevance for human risk of the finding of prolactin mediated endocrine tumors in rodents is unknown *[see Warnings and Precautions (5.15)]*.

Mutagenesis—No evidence of genotoxic potential for olanzapine was found in the Ames reverse mutation test, in vivo micronucleus test in mice, the chromosomal aberration test in Chinese hamster ovary cells, unscheduled DNA synthesis test in rat hepatocytes, induction of forward mutation test in mouse lymphoma cells, or in vivo sister chromatid exchange test in bone marrow of Chinese hamsters.

Impairment of Fertility—In an oral fertility and reproductive performance study in rats, male mating performance, but not fertility, was impaired at a dose of 22.4 mg/kg/day and female fertility was decreased at a dose of 3 mg/kg/day (11 and 1.5 times the maximum recommended human daily oral dose on a mg/m^2 basis, respectively). Discontinuance of olanzapine treatment reversed the effects on male mating performance. In female rats, the precoital period was increased and the mating index reduced at 5 mg/kg/day (2.5 times the maximum recommended human daily oral dose on a mg/m^2 basis). Diestrous was prolonged and estrous delayed at 1.1 mg/kg/day (0.6 times the maximum recommended human daily oral dose on a mg/m^2 basis); therefore olanzapine may produce a delay in ovulation.

13.2 Animal Toxicology and/or Pharmacology

In animal studies with olanzapine, the principal hematologic findings were reversible peripheral cytopenias in individual dogs dosed at 10 mg/kg (17 times the maximum recommended human daily oral dose on a mg/m^2 basis), dose-related decreases in lymphocytes and neutrophils in mice, and lymphopenia in rats. A few dogs treated with 10 mg/kg developed reversible neutropenia and/or reversible hemolytic anemia between 1 and 10 months of treatment. Dose-related decreases in lymphocytes and neutrophils were seen in mice given doses of 10 mg/kg (equal to 2 times the maximum recommended human daily oral dose on a mg/m^2 basis) in studies of 3 months' duration. Nonspecific lymphopenia, consistent with decreased body weight gain, occurred in rats receiving 22.5 mg/kg (11 times the maximum recommended human daily oral dose on a mg/m^2 basis) for 3 months or 16 mg/kg (8 times the maximum recommended human daily oral dose on a mg/m^2 basis) for 6 or 12 months. No evidence of bone marrow cytotoxicity was found in any of the species examined. Bone marrows were normocellular or hypercellular, indicating that the reductions in circulating blood cells were probably due to peripheral (non-marrow) factors.

14 CLINICAL STUDIES

When using ZYPREXA and fluoxetine in combination, also refer to the Clinical Studies section of the package insert for Symbyax.

14.1 Schizophrenia

Adults

The efficacy of oral olanzapine in the treatment of schizophrenia was established in 2 short-term (6-week) controlled trials of adult inpatients who met DSM III-R criteria for schizophrenia. A single haloperidol arm was included as a comparative treatment in 1 of the 2 trials, but this trial did not compare these 2 drugs on the full range of clinically relevant doses for both.

Several instruments were used for assessing psychiatric signs and symptoms in these studies, among them the Brief Psychiatric Rating Scale (BPRS), a multi-item inventory of general psychopathology traditionally used to evaluate the effects of drug treatment in schizophrenia. The BPRS psychosis cluster (conceptual disorganization, hallucinatory behavior, suspiciousness, and unusual thought content) is considered a particularly useful subset for assessing actively psychotic schizophrenic patients. A second traditional assessment, the Clinical Global Impression (CGI), reflects the impression of a skilled observer, fully familiar with the manifestations of schizophrenia, about the overall clinical state of the patient. In addition, 2 more recently developed scales were employed; these included the 30-item Positive and Negative Symptoms Scale (PANSS), in which are embedded the 18 items of the BPRS, and the Scale for Assessing Negative Symptoms (SANS). The trial summaries below focus on the following outcomes: PANSS total and/or BPRS total; BPRS psychosis cluster; PANSS negative subscale or SANS; and CGI Severity. The results of the trials follow:

(1) In a 6-week, placebo-controlled trial (n=149) involving 2 fixed olanzapine doses of 1 and 10 mg/day (once daily schedule), olanzapine, at 10 mg/day (but not at 1 mg/day), was superior to placebo on the PANSS total score (also on the extracted BPRS total), on the BPRS psychosis cluster, on the PANSS Negative subscale, and on CGI Severity.

(2) In a 6-week, placebo-controlled trial (n=253) involving 3 fixed dose ranges of olanzapine (5 ± 2.5 mg/day, 10 ± 2.5 mg/day, and 15 ± 2.5 mg/day) on a once daily schedule, the 2 highest olanzapine dose groups (actual mean doses of 12 and 16 mg/day, respectively) were superior to placebo on BPRS total score, BPRS psychosis cluster, and CGI severity score; the highest olanzapine dose group was superior to placebo on the SANS. There was no clear advantage for the high-dose group over the medium-dose group.

(3) In a longer-term trial, adult outpatients (n=326) who predominantly met DSM-IV criteria for schizophrenia and who remained stable on olanzapine during open-label treatment for at least 8 weeks were randomized to continuation on their current olanzapine doses (ranging from 10 to 20 mg/day) or to placebo. The follow-up period to observe patients for relapse, defined in terms of increases in BPRS positive symptoms or hospitalization, was planned for 12 months, however, criteria were met for stopping the trial early due to an excess of placebo relapses compared to olanzapine relapses, and olanzapine was superior to placebo on time to relapse, the primary outcome for this study. Thus, olanzapine was more effective than placebo at maintaining efficacy in patients stabilized for approximately 8 weeks and followed for an observation period of up to 8 months.

Examination of population subsets (race and gender) did not reveal any differential responsiveness on the basis of these subgroupings.

Adolescents

The efficacy of oral olanzapine in the acute treatment of schizophrenia in adolescents (ages 13 to 17 years) was established in a 6-week double-blind, placebo-controlled, randomized trial of inpatients and outpatients with schizophrenia (n=107) who met diagnostic criteria according to DSM-IV-TR and confirmed by the Kiddie Schedule for Affective Disorders and Schizophrenia for School Aged Children-Present and Lifetime Version (K-SADS-PL).

The primary rating instrument used for assessing psychiatric signs and symptoms in this trial was the Anchored Version of the Brief Psychiatric Rating Scale for Children (BPRS-C) total score.

In this flexible-dose trial, olanzapine 2.5 to 20 mg/day (mean modal dose 12.5 mg/day, mean dose of 11.1 mg/day) was more effective than placebo in the treatment of adolescents diagnosed with schizophrenia, as supported by the statistically significantly greater mean reduction in BPRS-C total score for patients in the olanzapine treatment group than in the placebo group.

While there is no body of evidence available to answer the question of how long the adolescent patient treated with ZYPREXA should be maintained, maintenance efficacy can be extrapolated from adult data along with comparisons of olanzapine pharmacokinetic parameters in adult and adolescent patients. It is generally recommended that responding patients be continued beyond the acute response, but at the lowest dose needed to maintain remission. Patients should be periodically reassessed to determine the need for maintenance treatment.

14.2 Bipolar I Disorder (Manic or Mixed Episodes)

Adults

Monotherapy—The efficacy of oral olanzapine in the treatment of manic or mixed episodes was established in 2 short-term (one 3-week and one 4-week) placebo-controlled trials in adult patients who met the DSM-IV criteria for bipolar I disorder with manic or mixed episodes. These trials included patients with or without psychotic features and with or without a rapid-cycling course.

The primary rating instrument used for assessing manic symptoms in these trials was the Young Mania Rating Scale (Y-MRS), an 11-item clinician-rated scale traditionally used to assess the degree of manic symptomatology (irritability, disruptive/aggressive behavior, sleep, elevated mood, speech, increased activity, sexual interest, language/thought disorder, thought content, appearance, and insight) in a range from 0 (no manic features) to 60 (maximum score). The primary outcome in these trials was change from baseline in the Y-MRS total score. The results of the trials follow:

(1) In one 3-week placebo-controlled trial (n=67) which involved a dose range of olanzapine (5-20 mg/day, once daily, starting at 10 mg/day), olanzapine was superior to placebo in the reduction of Y-MRS total score. In an identically designed trial conducted simultaneously with the first trial, olanzapine demonstrated a similar treatment difference, but possibly due to sample size and site variability, was not shown to be superior to placebo on this outcome.

(2) In a 4-week placebo-controlled trial (n=115) which involved a dose range of olanzapine (5-20 mg/day, once daily, starting at 15 mg/day), olanzapine was superior to placebo in the reduction of Y-MRS total score.

(3) In another trial, 361 patients meeting DSM-IV criteria for a manic or mixed episode of bipolar I disorder who had responded during an initial open-label treatment phase for about 2 weeks, on average, to olanzapine 5 to 20 mg/day were randomized to either continuation of olanzapine at their same dose (n=225) or to placebo (n=136), for observation of relapse. Approximately 50% of the patients had discontinued from the olanzapine group by day 59 and 50% of the placebo group had discontinued by day 23 of double-blind treatment. Response during the open-label phase was defined by having a decrease of the Y-MRS total score to ≤12 and HAM-D 21 to ≤8. Relapse during the double-blind phase was defined as an increase of the Y-MRS or HAM-D 21 total score to ≥15, or being hospitalized for either mania or depression. In the randomized phase, patients receiving continued olanzapine experienced a significantly longer time to relapse.

Adjunct to Lithium or Valproate—The efficacy of oral olanzapine with concomitant lithium or valproate in the treatment of manic or mixed episodes was established in 2 controlled trials in patients who met the DSM-IV criteria for bipolar I disorder with manic or mixed episodes. These trials included patients with or without psychotic features and with or without a rapid-cycling course. The results of the trials follow:

(1) In one 6-week placebo-controlled combination trial, 175 outpatients on lithium or valproate therapy with inadequately controlled manic or mixed symptoms (Y-MRS ≥16) were randomized to receive either olanzapine or placebo, in combination with their original therapy. Olanzapine (in a dose range of 5-20 mg/day, once daily, starting at 10 mg/day) combined with lithium or valproate (in a therapeutic range of 0.6 mEq/L to 1.2 mEq/L or 50 µg/mL to 125 µg/mL, respectively) was superior to lithium or valproate alone in the reduction of Y-MRS total score.

(2) In a second 6-week placebo-controlled combination trial, 169 outpatients on lithium or valproate therapy with inadequately controlled manic or mixed symptoms (Y-MRS ≥16) were randomized to receive either olanzapine or placebo, in combination with their original therapy. Olanzapine (in a dose range of 5-20 mg/day, once daily, starting at 10 mg/day) combined with lithium or valproate (in a therapeutic range of 0.6 mEq/L to 1.2 mEq/L or 50 µg/mL to 125 µg/mL, respectively) was superior to lithium or valproate alone in the reduction of Y-MRS total score.

Adolescents

Acute Monotherapy—The efficacy of oral olanzapine in the treatment of acute manic or mixed episodes in adolescents (ages 13 to 17 years) was established in a 3-week, double-blind, placebo-controlled, randomized trial of adolescent inpatients and outpatients who met the diagnostic criteria for manic or mixed episodes associated with bipolar I disorder (with or without psychotic features) according to the DSM-IV-TR (n=161). Diagnosis was confirmed by the K-SADS-PL. The primary rating instrument used for assessing manic symptoms in this trial was the Adolescent Structured Young-Mania Rating Scale (Y-MRS) total score.

In this flexible-dose trial, olanzapine 2.5 to 20 mg/day (mean modal dose 10.7 mg/day, mean dose of 8.9 mg/day) was more effective than placebo in the treatment of adolescents with manic or mixed episodes associated with bipolar I disorder, as supported by the statistically significantly greater mean reduction in Y-MRS total score for patients in the olanzapine treatment group than in the placebo group.

While there is no body of evidence available to answer the question of how long the adolescent patient treated with ZYPREXA should be maintained, maintenance efficacy can be extrapolated from adult data along with comparisons of olanzapine pharmacokinetic parameters in adult and adolescent patients. It is generally recommended that responding patients be continued beyond the acute response, but at the lowest dose needed to maintain remission. Patients should be periodically reassessed to determine the need for maintenance treatment.

14.3 Agitation Associated with Schizophrenia and Bipolar I Mania

The efficacy of intramuscular olanzapine for injection for the treatment of agitation was established in 3 short-term (24 hours of IM treatment) placebo-controlled trials in agitated adult inpatients from 2 diagnostic groups: schizophrenia and bipolar I disorder (manic or mixed episodes). Each of the trials included a single active comparator treatment arm of either haloperidol injection (schizophrenia studies) or lorazepam injection (bipolar I mania study). Patients enrolled in the trials needed to be: (1) judged by the clinical investigators as clinically agitated and clinically appropriate candidates for treatment with intramuscular medication, and (2) exhibiting a level of agitation that met or exceeded a threshold score of ≥14 on the 5 items comprising the Positive and Negative Syndrome Scale (PANSS) Excited Component (i.e., poor impulse control, tension, hostility, uncooperativeness and excitement items) with at least 1 individual item score ≥4 using a 1-7 scoring system (1=absent, 4=moderate, 7=extreme). In the studies, the mean baseline PANSS Excited Component score was 18.4, with scores ranging from 13 to 32 (out of a maximum score of 35), thus suggesting predominantly moderate levels of agitation with some patients experiencing mild or severe levels of agitation. The primary efficacy measure used for assessing agitation signs and symptoms in these trials was the change from baseline in the PANSS Excited Component at 2 hours post-injection. Patients could receive up to 3 injections during the 24 hour IM treatment periods; however, patients could not receive the second injection until after the initial 2 hour period when the primary efficacy measure was assessed. The results of the trials follow:

(1) In a placebo-controlled trial in agitated inpatients meeting DSM-IV criteria for schizophrenia (n=270), 4 fixed intramuscular olanzapine for injection doses of 2.5 mg, 5 mg, 7.5 mg and 10 mg were evaluated. All doses were statistically superior to placebo on the PANSS Excited Component at 2 hours post-injection. However, the effect was larger and more consistent for the 3 highest doses. There were no significant pairwise differences for the 7.5 and 10 mg doses over the 5 mg dose.

(2) In a second placebo-controlled trial in agitated inpatients meeting DSM-IV criteria for schizophrenia (n=311), 1 fixed intramuscular olanzapine for injection dose of 10 mg was evaluated. Olanzapine for injection was statistically superior to placebo on the PANSS Excited Component at 2 hours post-injection.

(3) In a placebo-controlled trial in agitated inpatients meeting DSM-IV criteria for bipolar I disorder (and currently displaying an acute manic or mixed episode with or without psychotic features) (n=201), 1 fixed intramuscular olanzapine for injection dose of 10 mg was evaluated. Olanzapine for injection was statistically superior to placebo on the PANSS Excited Component at 2 hours post-injection.

Examination of population subsets (age, race, and gender) did not reveal any differential responsiveness on the basis of these subgroupings.

16 HOW SUPPLIED/STORAGE AND HANDLING

16.1 How Supplied

The ZYPREXA 2.5 mg, 5 mg, 7.5 mg, and 10 mg tablets are white, round, and imprinted in blue ink with LILLY and tablet number. The 15 mg tablets are elliptical, blue, and debossed with LILLY and tablet number. The 20 mg tablets are elliptical, pink, and debossed with LILLY and tablet number. The tablets are available as follows:

	TABLET STRENGTH 2.5 mg	5 mg	7.5 mg	10 mg	15 mg	20 mg
Tablet No.	4112	4115	4116	4117	4415	4420
Identification	LILLY 4112	LILLY 4115	LILLY 4116	LILLY 4117	LILLY 4415	LILLY 4420
NDC Codes:						
Bottles 30	NDC 0002-4112-30	NDC 0002-4115-30	NDC 0002-4116-30	NDC 0002-4117-30	NDC 0002-4415-30	NDC 0002-4420-30
Blisters – ID[a] 100	NDC 0002-4112-33	NDC 0002-4115-33	NDC 0002-4116-33	NDC 0002-4117-33	NDC 0002-4415-33	NDC 0002-4420-33
Bottles 1000	NDC 0002-4112-04	NDC 0002-4115-04	NDC 0002-4116-04	NDC 0002-4117-04	NDC 0002-4415-04	NDC 0002-4420-04

[a] Identi-Dose® (unit dose medication, Lilly).

ZYPREXA ZYDIS Tablets[a]	TABLET STRENGTH 5 mg	10 mg	15 mg	20 mg
Tablet No.	4453	4454	4455	4456
Debossed	5	10	15	20
NDC Codes:				
Dose Pack 30 (Child Resistant)	NDC 0002-4453-85	NDC 0002-4454-85	NDC 0002-4455-85	NDC 0002-4456-85

ZYPREXA is a registered trademark of Eli Lilly and Company.
ZYDIS is a registered trademark of Catalent Pharma Solutions.
[a] ZYPREXA ZYDIS (olanzapine orally disintegrating tablets) is manufactured for Eli Lilly and Company by Catalent Pharma Solutions, United Kingdom, SN5 8RU.

[See first table above]

ZYPREXA ZYDIS (olanzapine orally disintegrating tablets) are yellow, round, and debossed with the tablet strength. The tablets are available as follows:

[See second table above]

ZYPREXA IntraMuscular is available in:

NDC 0002-7597-01 (No. VL7597) – 10 mg vial (1s)

16.2 Storage and Handling

Store ZYPREXA tablets, ZYPREXA ZYDIS, and ZYPREXA IntraMuscular vials (before reconstitution) at controlled room temperature, 20° to 25°C (68° to 77°F) [*see* USP]. Reconstituted ZYPREXA IntraMuscular may be stored at controlled room temperature, 20° to 25°C (68° to 77°F) [*see* USP] for up to 1 hour if necessary. *Discard any unused portion of reconstituted ZYPREXA IntraMuscular*. The USP defines controlled room temperature as a temperature maintained thermostatically that encompasses the usual and customary working environment of 20° to 25°C (68° to 77°F); that results in a mean kinetic temperature calculated to be not more than 25°C; and that allows for excursions between 15° and 30°C (59° and 86°F) that are experienced in pharmacies, hospitals, and warehouses.

Protect ZYPREXA tablets and ZYPREXA ZYDIS from light and moisture. Protect ZYPREXA IntraMuscular from light, do not freeze.

17 PATIENT COUNSELING INFORMATION

See FDA-approved Medication Guide for the oral formulations.

Patients should be advised of the following issues and asked to alert their prescriber if these occur while taking ZYPREXA as monotherapy or in combination with fluoxetine. If you do not think you are getting better or have any concerns about your condition while taking ZYPREXA, call your doctor. When using ZYPREXA and fluoxetine in combination, also refer to the Patient Counseling Information section of the package insert for Symbyax.

17.1 Information on Medication Guide

Prescribers or other health professionals should inform patients, their families, and their caregivers about the potential benefits and potential risks associated with treatment with ZYPREXA, and should counsel them in its appropriate use. A patient Medication Guide is available for ZYPREXA. Prescribers or other health professionals should instruct patients, their families, and their caregivers to read the Medication Guide and should assist them in understanding its contents. Patients should be given the opportunity to discuss the contents of the Medication Guide and to obtain answers to any questions they may have. When using ZYPREXA and fluoxetine in combination, also refer to the Medication Guide for Symbyax.

17.2 Elderly Patients with Dementia-Related Psychosis: Increased Mortality and Cerebrovascular Adverse Events (CVAE), Including Stroke

Patients and caregivers should be advised that elderly patients with dementia-related psychosis treated with antipsychotic drugs are at an increased risk of death. Patients and caregivers should be advised that elderly patients with dementia-related psychosis treated with ZYPREXA had a significantly higher incidence of cerebrovascular adverse events (e.g., stroke, transient ischemic attack) compared with placebo.

ZYPREXA is not approved for elderly patients with dementia-related psychosis *[see Boxed Warning and Warnings and Precautions (5.1)]*.

17.3 Neuroleptic Malignant Syndrome (NMS)

Patients and caregivers should be counseled that a potentially fatal symptom complex sometimes referred to as NMS has been reported in association with administration of antipsychotic drugs, including ZYPREXA. Signs and symptoms of NMS include hyperpyrexia, muscle rigidity, altered mental status, and evidence of autonomic instability (irregular pulse or blood pressure, tachycardia, diaphoresis, and cardiac dysrhythmia) *[see Warnings and Precautions (5.3)]*.

17.4 Hyperglycemia

Patients should be advised of the potential risk of hyperglycemia-related adverse reactions. Patients should be monitored regularly for worsening of glucose control. Patients who have diabetes should follow their doctor's instructions about how often to check their blood sugar while taking ZYPREXA *[see Warnings and Precautions (5.4)]*.

17.5 Hyperlipidemia

Patients should be counseled that hyperlipidemia has occurred during treatment with ZYPREXA. Patients should have their lipid profile monitored regularly *[see Warnings and Precautions (5.5)]*.

17.6 Weight Gain

Patients should be counseled that weight gain has occurred during treatment with ZYPREXA. Patients should have their weight monitored regularly *[see Warnings and Precautions (5.6)]*.

17.7 Orthostatic Hypotension

Patients should be advised of the risk of orthostatic hypotension, especially during the period of initial dose titration and in association with the use of concomitant drugs that may potentiate the orthostatic effect of ZYPREXA, e.g., diazepam or alcohol *[see Warnings and Precautions (5.8) and Drug Interactions (7)]*. Patients should be advised to change positions carefully to help prevent orthostatic hypotension, and to lie down if they feel dizzy or faint, until they feel better. Patients should be advised to call their doctor if they experience any of the following signs and symptoms associated with orthostatic hypotension: dizziness, fast or slow heart beat, or fainting.

17.8 Potential for Cognitive and Motor Impairment

Because ZYPREXA has the potential to impair judgment, thinking, or motor skills, patients should be cautioned about operating hazardous machinery, including automobiles, until they are reasonably certain that ZYPREXA therapy does not affect them adversely *[see Warnings and Precautions (5.12)]*.

17.9 Body Temperature Regulation

Patients should be advised regarding appropriate care in avoiding overheating and dehydration. Patients should be advised to call their doctor right away if they become severely ill and have some or all of these symptoms of dehydration: sweating too much or not at all, dry mouth, feeling very hot, feeling thirsty, not able to produce urine *[see Warnings and Precautions (5.13)]*.

17.10 Concomitant Medication

Patients should be advised to inform their physicians if they are taking, or plan to take, Symbyax. Patients should also be advised to inform their physicians if they are taking, plan to take, or have stopped taking any prescription or over-the-counter drugs, including herbal supplements, since there is a potential for interactions [see Drug Interactions (7)].

17.11 Alcohol

Patients should be advised to avoid alcohol while taking ZYPREXA [see Drug Interactions (7)].

17.12 Phenylketonurics

ZYPREXA ZYDIS (olanzapine orally disintegrating tablets) contains phenylalanine (0.34, 0.45, 0.67, or 0.90 mg per 5, 10, 15, or 20 mg tablet, respectively) [see Description (11)].

17.13 Use in Specific Populations

Pregnancy—Patients should be advised to notify their physician if they become pregnant or intend to become pregnant during therapy with ZYPREXA [see Use in Specific Populations (8.1)].

Nursing Mothers—Patients should be advised not to breast-feed an infant if they are taking ZYPREXA [see Use in Specific Populations (8.3)].

Pediatric Use—ZYPREXA is indicated for treatment of schizophrenia and manic or mixed episodes associated with bipolar I disorder in adolescents 13 to 17 years of age. Compared to patients from adult clinical trials, adolescents were likely to gain more weight, experience increased sedation, and have greater increases in total cholesterol, triglycerides, LDL cholesterol, prolactin, and hepatic transaminase levels. Patients should be counseled about the potential long-term risks associated with ZYPREXA and advised that these risks may lead them to consider other drugs first [see Indications and Usage (1.1, 1.2)]. Safety and effectiveness of ZYPREXA in patients under 13 years of age have not been established. Safety and effectiveness of ZYPREXA and fluoxetine in combination in patients <18 years of age have not been established [see Warnings and Precautions (5.5, 5.6) and Use in Specific Populations (8.4)].

17.14 Need for Comprehensive Treatment Program in Pediatric Patients

ZYPREXA is indicated as an integral part of a total treatment program for pediatric patients with schizophrenia and bipolar disorder that may include other measures (psychological, educational, social) for patients with the disorder. Effectiveness and safety of ZYPREXA have not been established in pediatric patients less than 13 years of age. Atypical antipsychotics are not intended for use in the pediatric patient who exhibits symptoms secondary to environmental factors and/or other primary psychiatric disorders. Appropriate educational placement is essential and psychosocial intervention is often helpful. The decision to prescribe atypical antipsychotic medication will depend upon the physician's assessment of the chronicity and severity of the patient's symptoms [see Indications and Usage (1.3)].

Literature revised May 27, 2010

Eli Lilly and Company, Indianapolis, IN 46285, USA

Copyright © 1997, 2010, Eli Lilly and Company. All rights reserved.

PV 6246 AMP

Medication Guide

ZYPREXA® (zy-PREX-a)

(olanzapine)

Tablet

ZYPREXA® ZYDIS® (zy-PREX-a ZY-dis)

(olanzapine)

Tablet, Orally Disintegrating

Read the Medication Guide that comes with ZYPREXA before you start taking it and each time you get a refill. There may be new information. This Medication Guide does not take the place of talking to your doctor about your medical condition or treatment. Talk with your doctor or pharmacist if there is something you do not understand or you want to learn more about ZYPREXA.

What is the most important information I should know about ZYPREXA?

Serious side effects may happen when you take ZYPREXA, including:

Increased risk of death in elderly patients with dementia-related psychosis: Medicines like ZYPREXA can raise the risk of death in elderly people who have lost touch with reality (psychosis) due to confusion and memory loss (dementia). ZYPREXA is not approved for treating psychosis in the elderly with dementia.

High blood sugar (hyperglycemia): High blood sugar can happen if you have diabetes already or even if you have never had diabetes. In rare cases, this could lead to ketoacidosis (build up of acid in the blood due to ketones), coma, or death. Your doctor should do lab tests to check your blood sugar before you start taking ZYPREXA and during treatment. In people who do not have diabetes, sometimes high blood sugar goes away when ZYPREXA is stopped. People with diabetes and some people who did not have diabetes before taking ZYPREXA need to take medicine for high blood sugar even after they stop taking ZYPREXA.

If you have diabetes, follow your doctor's instructions about how often to check your blood sugar while taking ZYPREXA.

Call your doctor if you have any of these symptoms of high blood sugar (hyperglycemia) while taking ZYPREXA:

- feel very thirsty
- need to urinate more than usual
- feel very hungry
- feel weak or tired
- feel sick to your stomach
- feel confused, or your breath smells fruity.

High cholesterol and triglyceride levels in the blood (fat in the blood) may happen in people treated with ZYPREXA, especially in teenagers (13-17 years old). You may not have any symptoms, so your doctor should do blood tests to check your cholesterol and triglyceride levels before you start taking ZYPREXA and during treatment.

Increase in weight (weight gain): Weight gain is very common in people who take ZYPREXA. Teenagers (13-17 years old) are more likely to gain weight and to gain more weight than adults. Some people may gain a lot of weight while taking ZYPREXA, so you and your doctor should check your weight regularly. Talk to your doctor about ways to control weight gain, such as eating a healthy, balanced diet, and exercising.

Increased risk in teenagers (13-17 years old): Possible serious risks of weight gain and increases in cholesterol and triglycerides are more common in teenagers than in adults. You and your doctor should decide if other available treatments should be used first. Before your teenager takes ZYPREXA, talk with your doctor about the possible long-term risks of teenagers taking ZYPREXA.

What is ZYPREXA?

ZYPREXA is a prescription medicine used to treat:

- schizophrenia in people age 13 or older.
- bipolar disorder, including:
  - manic or mixed episodes that happen with bipolar I disorder in people age 13 or older.
  - manic or mixed episodes that happen with bipolar I disorder, when used with the medicine lithium or valproate, in adults.
  - long-term treatment of bipolar I disorder in adults.
- episodes of depression that happen with bipolar I disorder, when used with the medicine fluoxetine (Prozac®), in adults.
- episodes of depression that do not get better after 2 other medicines, also called treatment resistant depression, when used with the medicine fluoxetine (Prozac), in adults.

ZYPREXA has not been approved for use in children under 13 years of age.

The symptoms of schizophrenia include hearing voices, seeing things that are not there, having beliefs that are not true, and being suspicious or withdrawn.

The symptoms of bipolar I disorder include alternating periods of depression and high or irritable mood, increased activity and restlessness, racing thoughts, talking fast, impulsive behavior, and a decreased need for sleep.

The symptoms of treatment resistant depression include decreased mood, decreased interest, increased guilty feelings, decreased energy, decreased concentration, changes in appetite, and suicidal thoughts or behavior.

Some of your symptoms may improve with treatment. If you do not think you are getting better, call your doctor.

What should I tell my doctor before taking ZYPREXA?

ZYPREXA may not be right for you. Before starting ZYPREXA, tell your doctor if you have or had:

- heart problems
- seizures
- diabetes or high blood sugar levels (hyperglycemia)
- high cholesterol or triglyceride levels in your blood
- liver problems
- low or high blood pressure
- strokes or "mini-strokes" also called transient ischemic attacks (TIAs)
- Alzheimer's disease
- narrow-angle glaucoma
- enlarged prostate in men
- bowel obstruction
- phenylketonuria, because ZYPREXA ZYDIS contains phenylalanine
- breast cancer
- thoughts of suicide or hurting yourself
- any other medical condition
- are pregnant or plan to become pregnant. It is not known if ZYPREXA will harm your unborn baby.
- are breast-feeding or plan to breast-feed. ZYPREXA can pass into your breast milk and may harm your baby. You should not breast-feed while taking ZYPREXA. Talk to your doctor about the best way to feed your baby if you take ZYPREXA.

Tell your doctor if you exercise a lot or are in hot places often.

The symptoms of bipolar I disorder, treatment resistant depression, or schizophrenia may include **thoughts of suicide** or of hurting yourself or others. If you have these thoughts at any time, tell your doctor or go to an emergency room right away.

Tell your doctor about all the medicines that you take, including prescription and nonprescription medicines, vitamins, and herbal supplements. ZYPREXA and some medicines may interact with each other and may not work as well, or cause possible serious side effects. Your doctor can tell you if it is safe to take ZYPREXA with your other medicines. Do not start or stop any medicine while taking ZYPREXA without talking to your doctor first.

How should I take ZYPREXA?

- Take ZYPREXA exactly as prescribed. Your doctor may need to change (adjust) the dose of ZYPREXA until it is right for you.
- If you miss a dose of ZYPREXA, take the missed dose as soon as you remember. If it is almost time for the next dose, just skip the missed dose and take your next dose at the regular time. Do not take two doses of ZYPREXA at the same time.
- **To prevent serious side effects, do not stop taking ZYPREXA suddenly. If you need to stop taking ZYPREXA, your doctor can tell you how to safely stop taking it.**
- **If you take too much ZYPREXA, call your doctor or poison control center at 1-800-222-1222 right away, or get emergency treatment.**
- ZYPREXA can be taken with or without food.
- ZYPREXA is usually taken one time each day.
- Take ZYPREXA ZYDIS as follows:
  - Be sure that your hands are dry.
  - Open the sachet and peel back the foil on the blister. Do not push the tablet through the foil.
  - As soon as you open the blister, remove the tablet and put it into your mouth.
  - The tablet will disintegrate quickly in your saliva so that you can easily swallow it with or without drinking liquid.
- Call your doctor if you do not think you are getting better or have any concerns about your condition while taking ZYPREXA.

What should I avoid while taking ZYPREXA?

- ZYPREXA can cause sleepiness and may affect your ability to make decisions, think clearly, or react quickly. You should not drive, operate heavy machinery, or do other dangerous activities until you know how ZYPREXA affects you.
- Avoid drinking alcohol while taking ZYPREXA. Drinking alcohol while you take ZYPREXA may make you sleepier than if you take ZYPREXA alone.

What are the possible side effects of ZYPREXA?

Serious side effects may happen when you take ZYPREXA, including:

- See "What is the most important information I should know about ZYPREXA?", which describes the increased risk of death in elderly people with dementia-related psychosis and the risks of high blood sugar, high cholesterol and triglyceride levels, and weight gain.
- **Increased incidence of stroke or "mini-strokes" called transient ischemic attacks (TIAs) in elderly people with dementia-related psychosis** (elderly people who have lost touch with reality due to confusion and memory loss). ZYPREXA is not approved for these patients.
- **Neuroleptic Malignant Syndrome (NMS):** NMS is a rare but very serious condition that can happen in people who take antipsychotic medicines, including ZYPREXA. NMS can cause death and must be treated in a hospital. Call your doctor right away if you become severely ill and have any of these symptoms:
  - high fever
  - excessive sweating
  - rigid muscles
  - confusion
  - changes in your breathing, heartbeat, and blood pressure.
- **Tardive Dyskinesia:** This condition causes body movements that keep happening and that you can not control. These movements usually affect the face and tongue. Tardive dyskinesia may not go away, even if you stop taking ZYPREXA. It may also start after you stop taking ZYPREXA. Tell your doctor if you get any body movements that you can not control.
- **Decreased blood pressure when you change positions, with symptoms of dizziness, fast or slow heartbeat, or fainting.**
- **Difficulty swallowing, that can cause food or liquid to get into your lungs.**
- **Seizures:** Tell your doctor if you have a seizure during treatment with ZYPREXA.
- **Problems with control of body temperature:** You could become very hot, for instance when you exercise a lot or

stay in an area that is very hot. It is important for you to drink water to avoid dehydration. Call your doctor right away if you become severely ill and have any of these symptoms of dehydration:

- sweating too much or not at all
- dry mouth
- feeling very hot
- feeling thirsty
- not able to produce urine.

Common side effects of ZYPREXA include: lack of energy, dry mouth, increased appetite, sleepiness, tremor (shakes), having hard or infrequent stools, dizziness, changes in behavior, or restlessness.

Other common side effects in teenagers (13-17 years old) include: headache, stomach-area (abdominal) pain, pain in your arms or legs, or tiredness. Teenagers experienced greater increases in prolactin, liver enzymes, and sleepiness, as compared with adults.

Tell your doctor about any side effect that bothers you or that does not go away.

These are not all the possible side effects with ZYPREXA. For more information, ask your doctor or pharmacist.

Call your doctor for medical advice about side effects. You may report side effects to FDA at 1-800-FDA-1088.

How should I store ZYPREXA?

- Store ZYPREXA at room temperature, between 68°F to 77°F (20°C to 25°C).
- Keep ZYPREXA away from light.
- Keep ZYPREXA dry and away from moisture.

Keep ZYPREXA and all medicines out of the reach of children.

General information about ZYPREXA

Medicines are sometimes prescribed for purposes other than those listed in a Medication Guide. Do not use ZYPREXA for a condition for which it was not prescribed. Do not give ZYPREXA to other people, even if they have the same condition. It may harm them.

This Medication Guide summarizes the most important information about ZYPREXA. If you would like more information, talk with your doctor. You can ask your doctor or pharmacist for information about ZYPREXA that was written for healthcare professionals. For more information about ZYPREXA call 1-800-Lilly-Rx (1-800-545-5979) or visit www.zyprexa.com.

What are the ingredients in ZYPREXA?

Active ingredient: olanzapine

Inactive ingredients:

Tablets—carnauba wax, crospovidone, hydroxypropyl cellulose, hypromellose, lactose, magnesium stearate, microcrystalline cellulose, and other inactive ingredients. The color coating contains: Titanium Dioxide, FD&C Blue No. 2 Aluminum Lake, or Synthetic Red Iron Oxide.

ZYDIS—gelatin, mannitol, aspartame, sodium methyl paraben, and sodium propyl paraben.

This Medication Guide has been approved by the U.S. Food and Drug Administration.

Medication Guide revised January 5, 2010

Eli Lilly and Company
Indianapolis, IN 46285, USA
www.zyprexa.com

PV 6922 AMP

Shown in Product Identification Guide, page 311

ZYPREXA® RELPREVV™   ℞
[zī-prex-ah]
(olanzapine)
For Extended Release Injectable Suspension

HIGHLIGHTS OF PRESCRIBING INFORMATION
These highlights do not include all the information needed to use ZYPREXA RELPREVV safely and effectively. See full prescribing information for ZYPREXA RELPREVV.
ZYPREXA RELPREVV (olanzapine) For Extended Release Injectable Suspension
Initial U.S. Approval: 1996

WARNING: POST-INJECTION DELIRIUM/SEDATION SYNDROME AND INCREASED MORTALITY IN ELDERLY PATIENTS WITH DEMENTIA-RELATED PSYCHOSIS
See full prescribing information for complete boxed warning.

- **Patients are at risk for severe sedation (including coma) and/or delirium after each injection and must be observed for at least 3 hours in a registered facility with ready access to emergency response services. Because of this risk, ZYPREXA RELPREVV is available only through a restricted distribution program called ZYPREXA RELPREVV Patient Care Program and requires prescriber, healthcare facility, patient, and pharmacy enrollment. (2.1, 5.1, 5.2, 10.2, 17.2)**

- **Elderly patients with dementia-related psychosis treated with antipsychotic drugs are at an increased risk of death. ZYPREXA RELPREVV is not approved for the treatment of patients with dementia-related psychosis. (5.3, 5.16, 17.3)**

——————RECENT MAJOR CHANGES——————

Warnings and Precautions:	
Hyperprolactinemia (5.17)	03/2010

——————INDICATIONS AND USAGE——————
ZYPREXA® RELPREVV™ is a long-acting atypical antipsychotic for intramuscular injection indicated for the treatment of schizophrenia. (1.1)
Efficacy was established in two clinical trials in patients with schizophrenia: one 8-week trial in adults and one maintenance trial in adults. (14.1)

——————DOSAGE AND ADMINISTRATION——————
150 mg/2 wks, 300 mg/4 wks, 210 mg/2 wks, 405 mg/4 wks, or 300 mg/2 wks. See Table 1 for dosing recommendations. (2.1)
ZYPREXA RELPREVV is intended for deep intramuscular gluteal injection only.

- Do not administer intravenously or subcutaneously. (2.1)
- Be aware that there are two ZYPREXA intramuscular formulations with different dosing schedules. ZYPREXA IntraMuscular (10 mg/vial) is a short-acting formulation and should not be confused with ZYPREXA RELPREVV. (2.1)
- Establish tolerability with oral olanzapine prior to initiating treatment. (2.1)
- ZYPREXA RELPREVV doses above 405 mg every 4 weeks or 300 mg every 2 weeks have not been evaluated in clinical trials. (2.1)
- Use in specific populations (including renal and hepatic impaired, and pediatric population) has not been studied. (2.1)
- Must be suspended using only the diluent for ZYPREXA RELPREVV provided in the convenience kit. (2.2)

——————DOSAGE FORMS AND STRENGTHS——————
Powder for suspension for intramuscular use only:
210 mg/vial, 300 mg/vial, and 405 mg/vial (3, 11, 16)

——————CONTRAINDICATIONS——————
None.

——————WARNINGS AND PRECAUTIONS——————

- *Elderly Patients with Dementia-Related Psychosis:* Increased risk of death and increased incidence of cerebrovascular adverse events (e.g. stroke, transient ischemic attack). (5.3)
- *Suicide:* The possibility of a suicide attempt is inherent in schizophrenia, and close supervision of high-risk patients should accompany drug therapy. (5.4)
- *Neuroleptic Malignant Syndrome:* Manage with immediate discontinuation and close monitoring. (5.5)
- *Hyperglycemia:* In some cases extreme and associated with ketoacidosis or hyperosmolar coma or death, has been reported in patients taking olanzapine. Patients taking olanzapine should be monitored for symptoms of hyperglycemia and undergo fasting blood glucose testing at the beginning of, and periodically during, treatment. (5.6)
- *Hyperlipidemia:* Undesirable alterations in lipids have been observed. Appropriate clinical monitoring is recommended, including fasting blood lipid testing at the beginning of, and periodically during, treatment. (5.7)
- *Weight Gain:* Potential consequences of weight gain should be considered. Patients should receive regular monitoring of weight. (5.8)
- *Tardive Dyskinesia:* Discontinue if clinically appropriate. (5.9)
- *Orthostatic Hypotension:* Orthostatic hypotension associated with dizziness, tachycardia, bradycardia and, in some patients, syncope, may occur especially during initial dose titration. Use caution in patients with cardiovascular disease, cerebrovascular disease, and those conditions that could affect hemodynamic responses. (5.10)
- *Leukopenia, Neutropenia, and Agranulocytosis:* Has been reported with antipsychotics, including ZYPREXA. Patients with a history of a clinically significant low white blood cell count (WBC) or drug induced leukopenia/neutropenia should have their complete blood count (CBC) monitored frequently during the first few months of therapy and discontinuation of ZYPREXA RELPREVV should be considered at the first sign of a clinically significant decline in WBC in the absence of other causative factors. (5.11)
- *Seizures:* Use cautiously in patients with a history of seizures or with conditions that potentially lower the seizure threshold. (5.13)
- *Potential for Cognitive and Motor Impairment:* Has potential to impair judgment, thinking, and motor skills. Use caution when operating machinery. (5.14)

- *Hyperprolactinemia:* May elevate prolactin levels. (5.17)
- *Laboratory Tests:* Monitor fasting blood glucose and lipid profiles at the beginning of, and periodically during, treatment. (5.18)

——————ADVERSE REACTIONS——————
Most common adverse reactions (≥5% in at least one of the treatment groups and greater than placebo) associated with ZYPREXA RELPREVV treatment: headache, sedation, weight gain, cough, diarrhea, back pain, nausea, somnolence, dry mouth, nasopharyngitis, increased appetite, and vomiting. (6.1)

To report SUSPECTED ADVERSE REACTIONS, contact Eli Lilly and Company at 1-800-LillyRx (1-800-545-5979) or FDA at 1-800-FDA-1088 or www.fda.gov/medwatch

——————DRUG INTERACTIONS——————

- *CNS Acting Drugs:* Caution should be used when used in combination with other centrally acting drugs and alcohol. (7.2)
- *Antihypertensive Agents:* Enhanced antihypertensive effect. (7.2)
- *Levodopa and Dopamine Agonists:* May antagonize levodopa/dopamine agonists. (7.2)
- *Diazepam:* May potentiate orthostatic hypotension. (7.1, 7.2)
- *Alcohol:* May potentiate orthostatic hypotension. (7.1)
- *Carbamazepine:* Increased clearance of olanzapine. (7.1)
- *Fluvoxamine:* May increase olanzapine levels. (7.1)

——————USE IN SPECIFIC POPULATIONS——————

- *Pregnancy:* ZYPREXA RELPREVV should be used during pregnancy only if the potential benefit justifies the potential risk to the fetus. (8.1)
- *Nursing Mothers:* Breast-feeding is not recommended. (8.3)
- *Pediatric Use:* Safety and effectiveness of ZYPREXA RELPREVV in children <18 years of age have not been established. (8.4)

See 17 for PATIENT COUNSELING INFORMATION and Medication Guide

Revised: 05/2010

FULL PRESCRIBING INFORMATION: CONTENTS*
WARNING: POST-INJECTION DELIRIUM/SEDATION SYNDROME AND INCREASED MORTALITY IN ELDERLY PATIENTS WITH DEMENTIA-RELATED PSYCHOSIS

FULL PRESCRIBING INFORMATION

WARNING: POST-INJECTION DELIRIUM/SEDATION SYNDROME AND INCREASED MORTALITY IN ELDERLY PATIENTS WITH DEMENTIA-RELATED PSYCHOSIS

Post-Injection Delirium/Sedation Syndrome—Adverse events with signs and symptoms consistent with olanzapine overdose, in particular, sedation (including coma) and/or delirium, have been reported following injections of ZYPREXA RELPREVV. ZYPREXA RELPREVV must be administered in a registered healthcare facility with ready access to emergency response services. After each injection, patients must be observed at the healthcare facility by a healthcare professional for at least 3 hours. Because of this risk, ZYPREXA RELPREVV is available only through a restricted distribution program called ZYPREXA RELPREVV Patient Care Program and requires prescriber, healthcare facility, patient, and pharmacy enrollment [see Dosage and Administration (2.1), Warnings and Precautions (5.1, 5.2), Overdosage (10.2), and Patient Counseling Information (17.2)].

Increased Mortality in Elderly Patients with Dementia-Related Psychosis—Elderly patients with dementia-related psychosis treated with antipsychotic drugs are at an increased risk of death. Analyses of seventeen placebo-controlled trials (modal duration of 10 weeks), largely in patients taking atypical antipsychotic drugs, revealed a risk of death in drug-treated patients of between 1.6 to 1.7 times the risk of death in placebo-treated patients. Over the course of a typical 10-week controlled trial, the rate of death in drug-treated patients was about 4.5%, compared to a rate of about 2.6% in the placebo group. Although the causes of death were varied, most of the deaths appeared to be either cardiovascular (e.g., heart failure, sudden death) or infectious (e.g., pneumonia) in nature. Observational studies suggest that, similar to atypical antipsychotic drugs, treatment with conventional antipsychotic drugs may increase mortality. The extent to which the findings of increased mortality in observational studies may be attributed to the antipsychotic drug as opposed to some characteristic(s) of the patients is not clear. ZYPREXA RELPREVV is not approved for the treatment of patients with dementia-related psychosis [see Warnings and Precautions (5.3, 5.16) and Patient Counseling Information (17.3)].

---

1 INDICATIONS AND USAGE

ZYPREXA RELPREVV is available only through a restricted distribution program [see Warnings and Precautions (5.2)]. ZYPREXA RELPREVV must not be dispensed directly to a patient. For a patient to receive treatment, the prescriber, healthcare facility, patient, and pharmacy must all be enrolled in the ZYPREXA RELPREVV Patient Care Program. To enroll, call 1-877-772-9390.

1.1 Schizophrenia

ZYPREXA RELPREVV is indicated for the treatment of schizophrenia. Efficacy was established in two clinical trials in patients with schizophrenia: one 8-week trial in adults and one maintenance trial in adults [see Clinical Studies (14.1)].

2 DOSAGE AND ADMINISTRATION

2.1 Dosage

ZYPREXA RELPREVV is intended for deep intramuscular gluteal injection only and should not be administered intravenously or subcutaneously.

Be aware that there are two ZYPREXA intramuscular formulations with different dosing schedules. ZYPREXA IntraMuscular (10 mg/vial) is a short-acting formulation and should not be confused with ZYPREXA RELPREVV. Refer to the package insert for ZYPREXA IntraMuscular for more information about that product.

Establish tolerability with oral olanzapine prior to initiating treatment.

ZYPREXA RELPREVV should be administered by a healthcare professional every 2 to 4 weeks by deep intramuscular gluteal injection using a 19-gauge, 1.5-inch needle. Following insertion of the needle into the muscle, aspiration should be maintained for several seconds to ensure that no blood is drawn into the syringe. If any blood is aspirated into the syringe, it should be discarded and fresh drug should be prepared using a new convenience kit. The injection should be performed at a steady, continuous pressure. Do not massage the injection site.

Dose Selection—The efficacy of ZYPREXA RELPREVV has been demonstrated within the range of 150 mg to 300 mg administered every 2 weeks and with 405 mg administered every 4 weeks. Dose recommendations considering oral ZYPREXA and ZYPREXA RELPREVV are shown in Table 1.

[See table 1 below]

ZYPREXA RELPREVV doses greater than 405 mg every 4 weeks or 300 mg every 2 weeks have not been evaluated in clinical trials.

Post-Injection Delirium/Sedation Syndrome—During premarketing clinical studies, adverse events that presented with signs and symptoms consistent with olanzapine overdose, in particular, sedation (including coma) and/or delirium, were reported in patients following an injection of ZYPREXA RELPREVV [see Boxed Warning, Warnings and Precautions (5.1), and Overdosage (10.1)]. Patients should be informed of this risk and how to recognize related symptoms [see Patient Counseling Information (17.1, 17.2)]. ZYPREXA RELPREVV must be administered in a registered healthcare facility with ready access to emergency response services. After each ZYPREXA RELPREVV injection, a healthcare professional must continuously observe the patient at the healthcare facility for at least 3 hours for symptoms consistent with olanzapine overdose, including sedation (ranging from mild in severity to coma) and/or delirium (including confusion, disorientation, agitation, anxiety, and other cognitive impairment). Other symptoms noted include extrapyramidal symptoms, dysarthria, ataxia, aggression, dizziness, weakness, hypertension, and convulsion. The potential for onset of an event is greatest within the first hour. The majority of cases have occurred within the first 3 hours after injection; however, the event has occurred after 3 hours. Following the 3-hour observation period, healthcare professionals must confirm that the patient is alert, oriented, and absent of any signs and symptoms of post-injection delirium/sedation syndrome prior to being released. All patients must be accompanied to their destination upon leaving the facility. For the remainder of the day of each injection, patients should not drive or operate heavy machinery, and should be advised to be vigilant for symptoms of post-injection delirium/sedation syndrome

and be able to obtain medical assistance if needed. If post-injection delirium/sedation syndrome is suspected, close medical supervision and monitoring should be instituted in a facility capable of resuscitation [see Overdosage (10)].

Dosing in Specific Populations—Tolerance of oral ZYPREXA should be established prior to initiating treatment with ZYPREXA RELPREVV. The recommended starting dose is ZYPREXA RELPREVV 150 mg/4 wks in patients who are debilitated, who have a predisposition to hypotensive reactions, who otherwise exhibit a combination of factors that may result in slower metabolism of olanzapine (e.g., nonsmoking female patients ≥65 years of age), or who may be more pharmacodynamically sensitive to olanzapine. When indicated, dose escalation should be undertaken with caution in these patients [see Warnings and Precautions (5.4), Drug Interactions (7), and Clinical Pharmacology (12.3)]. ZYPREXA RELPREVV has not been studied in subjects under 18 years of age [see Warnings and Precautions (5.6, 5.7, and 5.8)].

Maintenance Treatment—Although no controlled studies have been conducted to determine how long patients should be treated with ZYPREXA RELPREVV, efficacy has been demonstrated over a period of 24 weeks in patients with stabilized schizophrenia. Additionally, oral ZYPREXA has been shown to be effective in maintenance of treatment response in schizophrenia in longer-term use. Patients should be periodically reassessed to determine the need for continued treatment.

Switching from Other Antipsychotics—There are no systematically collected data to specifically address how to switch patients with schizophrenia from other antipsychotics to ZYPREXA RELPREVV.

2.2 Instructions to Reconstitute and Administer ZYPREXA RELPREVV

For deep intramuscular gluteal injection only. Not to be injected intravenously or subcutaneously.

Step 1: Preparing Materials

Convenience kit includes:
- Vial of ZYPREXA RELPREVV powder
- 3-mL vial of diluent
- One 3-mL syringe with pre-attached 19-gauge, 1.5-inch (38 mm) Hypodermic Needle-Pro® needle with needle protection device
- Two 19-gauge, 1.5-inch (38 mm) Hypodermic Needle-Pro needles with needle protection device
  - For obese patients, a 2-inch (50 mm), 19-gauge or larger needle (not included in convenience kit) may be used for administration.

ZYPREXA RELPREVV must be suspended using only the diluent supplied in the convenience kit.

It is recommended that gloves are used when reconstituting, as ZYPREXA RELPREVV may be irritating to the skin. Flush with water if contact is made with skin.

See additional insert entitled "Instructions to Reconstitute and Administer ZYPREXA RELPREVV" (included) for more information regarding the safe and effective use of the Hypodermic Needle-Pro syringe and needle.

Step 2: Determining Reconstitution Volume

Refer to the table below to determine the amount of diluent to be added to powder for reconstitution of each vial strength.

It is important to note that there is more diluent in the vial than is needed to reconstitute.

Dose	Vial Strength	Diluent to Add
150 mg	210 mg	1.3 mL
210 mg	210 mg	1.3 mL
300 mg	300 mg	1.8 mL
405 mg	405 mg	2.3 mL

Step 3: Reconstituting ZYPREXA RELPREVV

Please read the Hypodermic Needle-Pro Instructions for Use before proceeding with Step 3. Failure to follow these instructions may result in a needlestick injury.

Loosen the powder by lightly tapping the vial.

Open the prepackaged Hypodermic Needle-Pro syringe and needle with needle protection device.

Withdraw the pre-determined diluent volume (Step 2) into the syringe.

Inject the diluent into the powder vial.

Withdraw air to equalize the pressure in the vial by pulling back slightly on the plunger in the syringe.

Remove the needle from the vial, holding the vial upright to prevent any loss of material.

Engage the needle safety device (refer to complete Hypodermic Needle-Pro Instructions for Use).

Table 1: Recommended Dosing for ZYPREXA RELPREVV Based on Correspondence to Oral ZYPREXA Doses

Target Oral ZYPREXA Dose	Dosing of ZYPREXA RELPREVV During the First 8 Weeks	Maintenance Dose After 8 Weeks of ZYPREXA RELPREVV Treatment
10 mg/day	210 mg/2 weeks or 405 mg/4 weeks	150 mg/2 weeks or 300 mg/4 weeks
15 mg/day	300 mg/2 weeks	210 mg/2 weeks or 405 mg/4 weeks
20 mg/day	300 mg/2 weeks	300 mg/2 weeks

Pad a hard surface to cushion impact (*see* Figure 1). Tap the vial firmly and repeatedly on the surface until no powder is visible.

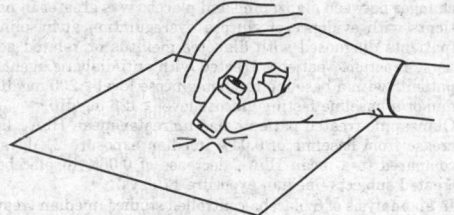

Figure 1: Tap firmly to mix.

Visually check the vial for clumps. Unsuspended powder appears as yellow, dry clumps clinging to the vial. Additional tapping may be required if large clumps remain (*see* Figure 2).

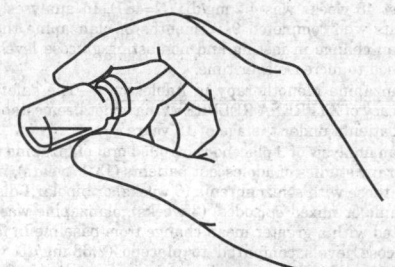

Figure 2: Check for unsuspended powder and repeat tapping if needed.

Shake the vial vigorously until the suspension appears smooth and is consistent in color and texture. The suspended product will be yellow and opaque (*see* Figure 3).

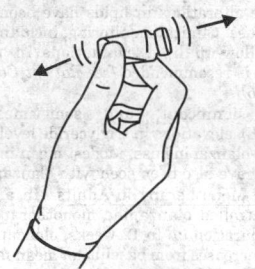

Figure 3: Vigorously shake vial.

If foam forms, let vial stand to allow foam to dissipate.
If the product is not used right away, it should be shaken vigorously to re-suspend. Reconstituted ZYPREXA RELPREVV remains stable for up to 24 hours in the vial.
Step 4: Injecting ZYPREXA RELPREVV
Before administering the injection, confirm there will be someone to accompany the patient after the 3-hour observation period. If this cannot be confirmed, do not give the injection.
Refer to the table below to determine the final volume to inject. **Suspension concentration is 150 mg/mL ZYPREXA RELPREVV.**

Dose	Final Volume to Inject
150 mg	1 mL
210 mg	1.4 mL
300 mg	2 mL
405 mg	2.7 mL

Attach a new safety needle to the syringe.
Slowly withdraw the desired amount into the syringe.
Some excess product will remain in the vial.
Engage the needle safety device and remove needle from syringe.
For administration, select the 19-gauge, 1.5-inch (38 mm) Hypodermic Needle-Pro needle with needle protection device. For obese patients, a 2-inch (50 mm), 19-gauge or larger needle (not included in convenience kit) may be used.
To help prevent clogging, a 19-gauge or larger needle must be used.

Attach the new safety needle to the syringe prior to injection. Once the suspension has been removed from the vial, it should be injected immediately.
For deep intramuscular gluteal injection only. Do not inject intravenously or subcutaneously.
Select and prepare a site for injection in the **gluteal** area. After insertion of the needle into the muscle, **aspirate for several seconds to ensure that no blood appears**. If any blood is drawn into the syringe, discard the syringe and the dose and begin with a new convenience kit. The injection should be performed with steady, continuous pressure.
Do not massage the injection site.
Engage the needle safety device.
Dispose of the vials, needles, and syringe appropriately after injection. The vial is for single-use only.

3 DOSAGE FORMS AND STRENGTHS
ZYPREXA RELPREVV is a powder for suspension for intramuscular use only. ZYPREXA RELPREVV is present as a yellow solid in a glass vial equivalent to 210, 300, or 405 mg olanzapine per vial. The diluent is a clear, colorless to slightly yellow solution in a glass vial [*see Description (11) and How Supplied/Storage and Handling (16)*]. The reconstituted suspension is yellow and opaque [*see Dosage and Administration (2.2)*].

4 CONTRAINDICATIONS
None.

5 WARNINGS AND PRECAUTIONS
5.1 Post-Injection Delirium/Sedation Syndrome
During premarketing clinical studies of ZYPREXA RELPREVV, adverse events that presented with signs and symptoms consistent with olanzapine overdose, in particular, sedation (including coma) and/or delirium, were reported in patients following an injection of ZYPREXA RELPREVV [*see Boxed Warning and Dosage and Administration (2.1)*]. These events occurred in <0.1% of injections and in approximately 2% of patients who received injections for up to 46 months. These events were correlated with an unintentional rapid increase in serum olanzapine concentrations to supra-therapeutic ranges in some cases. While a rapid and greater than expected increase in serum olanzapine concentration has been observed in some patients with these events, the exact mechanism by which the drug was unintentionally introduced into the blood stream is not known. Clinical signs and symptoms included dizziness, confusion, disorientation, slurred speech, altered gait, difficulty ambulating, weakness, agitation, extrapyramidal symptoms, hypertension, convulsion, and reduced level of consciousness ranging from mild sedation to coma. Time after injection to event ranged from soon after injection to greater than 3 hours after injection. The majority of patients were hospitalized and some required supportive care, including intubation, in several cases. All patients had largely recovered by 72 hours. The risk of an event is the same at each injection, so the risk per patient is cumulative (i.e., increases with the number of injections) [*see Overdosage (10.1)*].
Healthcare professionals are advised to discuss this potential risk with patients each time they prescribe and administer ZYPREXA RELPREVV [*see Patient Counseling Information (17.1, 17.2)*].
5.2 Prescribing and Distribution Program for ZYPREXA RELPREVV
ZYPREXA RELPREVV is available only through a restricted distribution program [*see Boxed Warning, Indications and Usage (1), and Patient Counseling Information (17.2)*]. ZYPREXA RELPREVV must not be dispensed directly to a patient. For a patient to receive treatment, the prescriber, healthcare facility, patient, and pharmacy must all be enrolled in the ZYPREXA RELPREVV Patient Care Program. To enroll, call 1-877-772-9390.
ZYPREXA RELPREVV must be administered in a registered healthcare facility (such as a hospital, clinic, residential treatment center, or community healthcare center) with

ready access to emergency response services. After each ZYPREXA RELPREVV injection, a healthcare professional must continuously observe the patient at the healthcare facility for at least 3 hours and must confirm that the patient is alert, oriented, and absent of any signs and symptoms of post-injection delirium/sedation syndrome prior to being released. All patients must be accompanied to their destination upon leaving the facility. For the remainder of the day of each injection, patients should not drive or operate heavy machinery, and should be advised to be vigilant for symptoms of post-injection delirium/sedation syndrome and be able to obtain medical assistance if needed. If post-injection delirium/sedation syndrome is suspected, close medical supervision and monitoring should be instituted in a facility capable of resuscitation [*see Overdosage (10)*]. If parenteral benzodiazepines are required for patient management during an event of post-injection delirium/sedation syndrome, careful evaluation of clinical status for excessive sedation and cardiorespiratory depression is recommended.
5.3 Elderly Patients with Dementia-Related Psychosis
Increased Mortality
Elderly patients with dementia-related psychosis treated with antipsychotic drugs are at an increased risk of death. ZYPREXA RELPREVV is not approved for the treatment of patients with dementia-related psychosis [*see Boxed Warning, Warnings and Precautions (5.16), and Patient Counseling Information (17.3)*].
In placebo-controlled oral olanzapine clinical trials of elderly patients with dementia-related psychosis, the incidence of death in olanzapine-treated patients was significantly greater than placebo-treated patients (3.5% vs 1.5%, respectively).
Cerebrovascular Adverse Events (CVAE), Including Stroke
Cerebrovascular adverse events (e.g., stroke, transient ischemic attack), including fatalities, were reported in patients in trials of oral olanzapine in elderly patients with dementia-related psychosis. In placebo-controlled trials, there was a significantly higher incidence of cerebrovascular adverse events in patients treated with oral olanzapine compared to patients treated with placebo. ZYPREXA RELPREVV is not approved for the treatment of patients with dementia-related psychosis [*see Boxed Warning and Patient Counseling Information (17.3)*].
5.4 Suicide
The possibility of a suicide attempt is inherent in schizophrenia, and close supervision of high-risk patients should accompany drug therapy.
5.5 Neuroleptic Malignant Syndrome (NMS)
A potentially fatal symptom complex sometimes referred to as Neuroleptic Malignant Syndrome (NMS) has been reported in association with administration of antipsychotic drugs, including olanzapine. Clinical manifestations of NMS are hyperpyrexia, muscle rigidity, altered mental status and evidence of autonomic instability (irregular pulse or blood pressure, tachycardia, diaphoresis and cardiac dysrhythmia). Additional signs may include elevated creatinine phosphokinase, myoglobinuria (rhabdomyolysis), and acute renal failure.
The diagnostic evaluation of patients with this syndrome is complicated. In arriving at a diagnosis, it is important to exclude cases where the clinical presentation includes both serious medical illness (e.g., pneumonia, systemic infection, etc.) and untreated or inadequately treated extrapyramidal signs and symptoms (EPS). Other important considerations in the differential diagnosis include central anticholinergic toxicity, heat stroke, drug fever, and primary central nervous system pathology.
The management of NMS should include: 1) immediate discontinuation of antipsychotic drugs and other drugs not essential to concurrent therapy; 2) intensive symptomatic treatment and medical monitoring; and 3) treatment of any concomitant serious medical problems for which specific treatments are available. There is no general agreement about specific pharmacological treatment regimens for NMS.

Table 2: Changes in Fasting Glucose Levels from Adult Olanzapine Monotherapy Studies

Laboratory Analyte	Category Change (at least once) from Baseline	Treatment Arm	Up to 12 weeks exposure		At least 48 weeks exposure	
			N	Patients	N	Patients
Fasting Glucose	Normal to High (<100 mg/dL to ≥126 mg/dL)	Olanzapine	543	2.2%	345	12.8%
		Placebo	293	3.4%	NA[a]	NA[a]
	Borderline to High (≥100 mg/dL and <126 mg/dL to ≥126 mg/dL)	Olanzapine	178	17.4%	127	26.0%
		Placebo	96	11.5%	NA[a]	NA[a]

[a] Not Applicable.

Table 3: Changes in Fasting Glucose Levels from Adolescent Oral Olanzapine Monotherapy Studies

Laboratory Analyte	Category Change (at least once) from Baseline	Treatment Arm	Up to 12 weeks exposure		At least 24 weeks exposure	
			N	Patients	N	Patients
Fasting Glucose	Normal to High (<100 mg/dL to ≥126 mg/dL)	Olanzapine	124	0%	108	0.9%
		Placebo	53	1.9%	NA[a]	NA[a]
	Borderline to High (≥100 mg/dL and <126 mg/dL to ≥126 mg/dL)	Olanzapine	14	14.3%	13	23.1%
		Placebo	13	0%	NA[a]	NA[a]

[a] Not Applicable.

Table 4: Changes in Fasting Lipids Values from Adult Olanzapine Monotherapy Studies

Laboratory Analyte	Category Change (at least once) from Baseline	Treatment Arm	Up to 12 weeks exposure		At least 48 weeks exposure	
			N	Patients	N	Patients
Fasting Triglycerides	Increase by ≥50 mg/dL	Olanzapine	745	39.6%	487	61.4%
		Placebo	402	26.1%	NA[a]	NA[a]
	Normal to High (<150 mg/dL to ≥200 mg/dL)	Olanzapine	457	9.2%	293	32.4%
		Placebo	251	4.4%	NA[a]	NA[a]
	Borderline to High (≥150 mg/dL and <200 mg/dL to ≥200 mg/dL)	Olanzapine	135	39.3%	75	70.7%
		Placebo	65	20.0%	NA[a]	NA[a]
Fasting Total Cholesterol	Increase by ≥40 mg/dL	Olanzapine	745	21.6%	489	32.9%
		Placebo	402	9.5%	NA[a]	NA[a]
	Normal to High (<200 mg/dL to ≥240 mg/dL)	Olanzapine	392	2.8%	283	14.8%
		Placebo	207	2.4%	NA[a]	NA[a]
	Borderline to High (≥200 mg/dL and <240 mg/dL to ≥240 mg/dL)	Olanzapine	222	23.0%	125	55.2%
		Placebo	112	12.5%	NA[a]	NA[a]
Fasting LDL Cholesterol	Increase by ≥30 mg/dL	Olanzapine	536	23.7%	483	39.8%
		Placebo	304	14.1%	NA[a]	NA[a]
	Normal to High (<100 mg/dL to ≥160 mg/dL)	Olanzapine	154	0%	123	7.3%
		Placebo	82	1.2%	NA[a]	NA[a]
	Borderline to High (≥100 mg/dL and <160 mg/dL to ≥160 mg/dL)	Olanzapine	302	10.6%	284	31.0%
		Placebo	173	8.1%	NA[a]	NA[a]

[a] Not Applicable.

If a patient requires antipsychotic drug treatment after recovery from NMS, the potential reintroduction of drug therapy should be carefully considered and tolerability with oral olanzapine should be established prior to initiating treatment with ZYPREXA RELPREVV [see Dosage and Administration (2.1)]. The patient should be carefully monitored, since recurrences of NMS have been reported [see Patient Counseling Information (17.4)].

5.6 Hyperglycemia

Physicians should consider the risks and benefits when prescribing olanzapine to patients with an established diagnosis of diabetes mellitus, or having borderline increased blood glucose level (fasting 100-126 mg/dL, nonfasting 140-200 mg/dL). Patients taking olanzapine should be monitored regularly for worsening of glucose control. Patients starting treatment with olanzapine should undergo fasting blood glucose testing at the beginning of treatment and periodically during treatment. Any patient treated with atypical antipsychotics should be monitored for symptoms of hyperglycemia including polydipsia, polyuria, polyphagia, and weakness. Patients who develop symptoms of hyperglycemia during treatment with atypical antipsychotics should undergo fasting blood glucose testing. In some cases, hyperglycemia has resolved when the atypical antipsychotic was discontinued; however, some patients required continuation of anti-diabetic treatment despite discontinuation of the suspect drug [see Patient Counseling Information (17.5)]. Hyperglycemia, in some cases extreme and associated with ketoacidosis or hyperosmolar coma or death, has been reported in patients treated with atypical antipsychotics including olanzapine. Assessment of the relationship between atypical antipsychotic use and glucose abnormalities is complicated by the possibility of an increased background risk of diabetes mellitus in patients with schizophrenia and the increasing incidence of diabetes mellitus in the general population. Epidemiological studies suggest an increased risk of treatment-emergent hyperglycemia-related adverse reactions in patients treated with the atypical antipsychotics. While relative risk estimates are inconsistent, the association between atypical antipsychotics and increases in glucose levels appears to fall on a continuum and olanzapine appears to have a greater association than some other atypical antipsychotics.

Mean increases in blood glucose have been observed in patients treated (median exposure of 9.2 months) with olanzapine in phase 1 of the Clinical Antipsychotic Trials of Intervention Effectiveness (CATIE). The mean increase of serum glucose (fasting and nonfasting samples) from baseline to the average of the 2 highest serum concentrations was 15.0 mg/dL.

In a study of healthy volunteers, subjects who received olanzapine (N=22) for 3 weeks had a mean increase compared to baseline in fasting blood glucose of 2.3 mg/dL. Placebo-treated subjects (N=19) had a mean increase in fasting blood glucose compared to baseline of 0.34 mg/dL.

Olanzapine Monotherapy in Adults—In an analysis of 5 placebo-controlled adult olanzapine monotherapy studies with a median treatment duration of approximately 3 weeks, olanzapine was associated with a greater mean change in fasting glucose levels compared to placebo (2.76 mg/dL versus 0.17 mg/dL). The difference in mean changes between olanzapine and placebo was greater in patients with evidence of glucose dysregulation at baseline (patients diagnosed with diabetes mellitus or related adverse reactions, patients treated with anti-diabetic agents, patients with a baseline random glucose level ≥200 mg/dL, and/or a baseline fasting glucose level ≥126 mg/dL).

Olanzapine-treated patients had a greater mean HbA$_{1c}$ increase from baseline of 0.04% (median exposure 21 days), compared to a mean HbA$_{1c}$ decrease of 0.06% in placebo-treated subjects (median exposure 17 days).

In an analysis of 8 placebo-controlled studies (median treatment exposure 4-5 weeks), 6.1% of olanzapine-treated subjects (N=855) had treatment-emergent glycosuria compared to 2.8% of placebo-treated subjects (N=599). Table 2 shows short-term and long-term changes in fasting glucose levels from adult olanzapine monotherapy studies.

[See table 2 at top of previous page]

The mean change in fasting glucose for patients exposed at least 48 weeks was 4.2 mg/dL (N=487). In analyses of patients who completed 9-12 months of olanzapine therapy, mean change in fasting and nonfasting glucose levels continued to increase over time.

Olanzapine Monotherapy in Adolescents—The safety and efficacy of ZYPREXA RELPREVV have not been established in patients under the age of 18 years.

In an analysis of 3 placebo-controlled oral olanzapine monotherapy studies of adolescent patients (13-17 years), including those with schizophrenia (6 weeks) or bipolar I disorder (manic or mixed episodes) (3 weeks), olanzapine was associated with a greater mean change from baseline in fasting glucose levels compared to placebo (2.68 mg/dL versus -2.59 mg/dL). The mean change in fasting glucose for adolescents exposed at least 24 weeks was 3.1 mg/dL (N=121). Table 3 shows short-term and long-term changes in fasting blood glucose from adolescent oral olanzapine monotherapy studies.

[See table 3 at top left]

5.7 Hyperlipidemia

Undesirable alterations in lipids have been observed with olanzapine use. Clinical monitoring, including baseline and periodic follow-up lipid evaluations in patients using olanzapine, is recommended [see Patient Counseling Information (17.6)].

Clinically significant, and sometimes very high (>500 mg/dL), elevations in triglyceride levels have been observed with olanzapine use. Modest mean increases in total cholesterol have also been seen with olanzapine use.

Olanzapine Monotherapy in Adults—In an analysis of 5 placebo-controlled olanzapine monotherapy studies with treatment duration up to 12 weeks, olanzapine-treated patients had increases from baseline in mean fasting total cholesterol, LDL cholesterol, and triglycerides of 5.3 mg/dL, 3.0 mg/dL, and 20.8 mg/dL respectively compared to decreases from baseline in mean fasting total cholesterol, LDL cholesterol, and triglycerides of 6.1 mg/dL, 4.3 mg/dL, and 10.7 mg/dL for placebo-treated patients. For fasting HDL cholesterol, no clinically meaningful differences were observed between olanzapine-treated patients and placebo-treated patients. Mean increases in fasting lipid values (total cholesterol, LDL cholesterol, and triglycerides) were greater in patients without evidence of lipid dysregulation at baseline, where lipid dysregulation was defined as patients diagnosed with dyslipidemia or related adverse reactions, patients treated with lipid lowering agents, or patients with high baseline lipid levels.

In long-term studies (at least 48 weeks), patients had increases from baseline in mean fasting total cholesterol, LDL cholesterol, and triglycerides of 5.6 mg/dL, 2.5 mg/dL, and 18.7 mg/dL, respectively, and a mean decrease in fasting HDL cholesterol of 0.16 mg/dL. In an analysis of patients who completed 12 months of therapy, the mean nonfasting total cholesterol did not increase further after approximately 4-6 months.

The proportion of patients who had changes (at least once) in total cholesterol, LDL cholesterol or triglycerides from normal or borderline to high, or changes in HDL cholesterol from normal or borderline to low, was greater in long-term studies (at least 48 weeks) as compared with short-term studies. Table 4 shows categorical changes in fasting lipids values.

[See table 4 above]

In phase 1 of the Clinical Antipsychotic Trials of Intervention Effectiveness (CATIE), over a median exposure of 9.2 months, the mean increase in triglycerides in patients taking olanzapine was 40.5 mg/dL. In phase 1 of CATIE, the mean increase in total cholesterol was 9.4 mg/dL.

Olanzapine Monotherapy in Adolescents—The safety and efficacy of ZYPREXA RELPREVV have not been established in patients under the age of 18 years.

Table 5: Changes in Fasting Lipids Values from Adolescent Oral Olanzapine Monotherapy Studies

Laboratory Analyte	Category Change (at least once) from Baseline	Treatment Arm	Up to 6 weeks exposure N	Up to 6 weeks exposure Patients	At least 24 weeks exposure N	At least 24 weeks exposure Patients
Fasting Triglycerides	Increase by ≥50 mg/dL	Olanzapine	138	37.0%	122	45.9%
		Placebo	66	15.2%	NA[a]	NA[a]
	Normal to High (<90 mg/dL to >130 mg/dL)	Olanzapine	67	26.9%	66	36.4%
		Placebo	28	10.7%	NA[a]	NA[a]
	Borderline to High (≥90 mg/dL and ≤130 mg/dL to >130 mg/dL)	Olanzapine	37	59.5%	31	64.5%
		Placebo	17	35.3%	NA[a]	NA[a]
Fasting Total Cholesterol	Increase by ≥40 mg/dL	Olanzapine	138	14.5%	122	14.8%
		Placebo	66	4.5%	NA[a]	NA[a]
	Normal to High (<170 mg/dL to ≥200 mg/dL)	Olanzapine	87	6.9%	78	7.7%
		Placebo	43	2.3%	NA[a]	NA[a]
	Borderline to High (≥170 mg/dL and <200 mg/dL to ≥200 mg/dL)	Olanzapine	36	38.9%	33	57.6%
		Placebo	13	7.7%	NA[a]	NA[a]
Fasting LDL Cholesterol	Increase by ≥30 mg/dL	Olanzapine	137	17.5%	121	22.3%
		Placebo	63	11.1%	NA[a]	NA[a]
	Normal to High (<110 mg/dL to ≥130 mg/dL)	Olanzapine	98	5.1%	92	10.9%
		Placebo	44	4.5%	NA[a]	NA[a]
	Borderline to High (≥110 mg/dL and <130 mg/dL to ≥130 mg/dL)	Olanzapine	29	48.3%	21	47.6%
		Placebo	9	0%	NA[a]	NA[a]

[a] Not Applicable.

Table 6: Weight Gain with Olanzapine Use in Adults

Amount Gained kg (lb)	6 Weeks (N=7465) (%)	6 Months (N=4162) (%)	12 Months (N=1345) (%)	24 Months (N=474) (%)	36 Months (N=147) (%)
≤0	26.2	24.3	20.8	23.2	17.0
0 to ≤5 (0-11 lb)	57.0	36.0	26.0	23.4	25.2
>5 to ≤10 (11-22 lb)	14.9	24.6	24.2	24.1	18.4
>10 to ≤15 (22-33 lb)	1.8	10.9	14.9	11.4	17.0
>15 to ≤20 (33-44 lb)	0.1	3.1	8.6	9.3	11.6
>20 to ≤25 (44-55 lb)	0	0.9	3.3	5.1	4.1
>25 to ≤30 (55-66 lb)	0	0.2	1.4	2.3	4.8
>30 (>66 lb)	0	0.1	0.8	1.2	2

Table 7: Weight Gain with Oral Olanzapine Use in Adolescents from 4 Placebo-Controlled Trials

	Olanzapine-treated patients	Placebo-treated patients
Mean change in body weight from baseline (median exposure = 3 weeks)	4.6 kg (10.1 lb)	0.3 kg (0.7 lb)
Percentage of patients who gained at least 7% of baseline body weight	40.6% (median exposure to 7% = 4 weeks)	9.8% (median exposure to 7% = 8 weeks)
Percentage of patients who gained at least 15% of baseline body weight	7.1% (median exposure to 15% = 19 weeks)	2.7% (median exposure to 15% = 8 weeks)

In an analysis of 3 placebo-controlled oral olanzapine monotherapy studies of adolescents (13-17 years), including those with schizophrenia (6 weeks) or bipolar I disorder (manic or mixed episodes) (3 weeks), olanzapine-treated adolescents had increases from baseline in mean fasting total cholesterol, LDL cholesterol, and triglycerides of 12.9 mg/dL, 6.5 mg/dL, and 28.4 mg/dL, respectively, compared to increases from baseline in mean fasting total cholesterol and LDL cholesterol of 1.3 mg/dL and 1.0 mg/dL, and a decrease in triglycerides of 1.1 mg/dL for placebo-treated adolescents.

For fasting HDL cholesterol, no clinically meaningful differences were observed between olanzapine-treated adolescents and placebo-treated adolescents.

In long-term studies (at least 24 weeks), adolescents had increases from baseline in mean fasting total cholesterol, LDL cholesterol, and triglycerides of 5.5 mg/dL, 5.4 mg/dL, and 20.5 mg/dL, respectively, and a mean decrease in fasting HDL cholesterol of 4.5 mg/dL. Table 5 shows categorical changes in fasting lipids values in adolescents.

[See table 5 above]

5.8 Weight Gain

Potential consequences of weight gain should be considered prior to starting olanzapine. Patients receiving olanzapine should receive regular monitoring of weight [see Patient Counseling Information (17.7)].

Olanzapine Monotherapy in Adults—In an analysis of 13 placebo-controlled olanzapine monotherapy studies, olanzapine-treated patients gained an average of 2.6 kg (5.7 lb) compared to an average 0.3 kg (0.6 lb) weight loss in placebo-treated patients with a median exposure of 6 weeks; 22.2% of olanzapine-treated patients gained at least 7% of their baseline weight, compared to 3% of placebo-treated patients, with a median exposure to event of 8 weeks; 4.2% of olanzapine-treated patients gained at least 15% of their baseline weight, compared to 0.3% of placebo-treated patients, with a median exposure to event of 12 weeks. Clinically significant weight gain was observed across all baseline Body Mass Index (BMI) categories. Discontinuation due to weight gain occurred in 0.2% of olanzapine-treated patients and in 0% of placebo-treated patients.

In long-term studies (at least 48 weeks), the mean weight gain was 5.6 kg (12.3 lb) (median exposure of 573 days, N=2021). The percentages of patients who gained at least 7%, 15%, or 25% of their baseline body weight with long-term exposure were 64%, 32%, and 12%, respectively. Discontinuation due to weight gain occurred in 0.4% of olanzapine-treated patients following at least 48 weeks of exposure.

Table 6 includes data on adult weight gain with olanzapine pooled from 86 clinical trials. The data in each column represent data for those patients who completed treatment periods of the durations specified.

[See table 6 at left]

Olanzapine Monotherapy in Adolescents—The safety and efficacy of ZYPREXA RELPREVV have not been established in patients under the age of 18 years.

Mean increase in weight in adolescents was greater than in adults. In 4 placebo-controlled trials, discontinuation due to weight gain occurred in 1% of olanzapine-treated patients, compared to 0% of placebo-treated patients.

[See table 7 at left]

In long-term studies (at least 24 weeks), the mean weight gain was 11.2 kg (24.6 lb); (median exposure of 201 days, N=179). The percentages of adolescents who gained at least 7%, 15%, or 25% of their baseline body weight with long-term exposure were 89%, 55%, and 29%, respectively. Among adolescent patients, mean weight gain by baseline BMI category was 11.5 kg (25.3 lb), 12.1 kg (26.6 lb), and 12.7 kg (27.9 lb), respectively, for normal (N=106), overweight (N=26) and obese (N=17). Discontinuation due to weight gain occurred in 2.2% of olanzapine-treated patients following at least 24 weeks of exposure.

Table 8 shows data on adolescent weight gain with olanzapine pooled from 6 clinical trials. The data in each column represent data for those patients who completed treatment periods of the durations specified. Little clinical trial data is available on weight gain in adolescents with olanzapine beyond 6 months of treatment.

Table 8: Weight Gain with Olanzapine Use in Adolescents

Amount Gained kg (lb)	6 Weeks (N=243) (%)	6 Months (N=191) (%)
≤0	2.9	2.1
0 to ≤5 (0-11 lb)	47.3	24.6
>5 to ≤10 (11-22 lb)	42.4	26.7
>10 to ≤15 (22-33 lb)	5.8	22.0
>15 to ≤20 (33-44 lb)	0.8	12.6
>20 to ≤25 (44-55 lb)	0.8	9.4
>25 to ≤30 (55-66 lb)	0	2.1
>30 to ≤35 (66-77 lb)	0	0
>35 to ≤40 (77-88 lb)	0	0
>40 (>88 lb)	0	0.5

5.9 Tardive Dyskinesia

A syndrome of potentially irreversible, involuntary, dyskinetic movements may develop in patients treated with antipsychotic drugs. Although the prevalence of the syndrome appears to be highest among the elderly, especially elderly women, it is impossible to rely upon prevalence estimates to predict, at the inception of antipsychotic treatment, which patients are likely to develop the syndrome. Whether antipsychotic drug products differ in their potential to cause tardive dyskinesia is unknown.

The risk of developing tardive dyskinesia and the likelihood that it will become irreversible are believed to increase as the duration of treatment and the total cumulative dose of antipsychotic drugs administered to the patient increase. However, the syndrome can develop, although much less commonly, after relatively brief treatment periods at low doses or may even arise after discontinuation of treatment.

There is no known treatment for established cases of tardive dyskinesia, although the syndrome may remit, partially or completely, if antipsychotic treatment is withdrawn. Antipsychotic treatment, itself, however, may suppress (or partially suppress) the signs and symptoms of the syndrome and thereby may possibly mask the underlying process. The effect that symptomatic suppression has upon the long-term course of the syndrome is unknown.

Given these considerations, olanzapine should be prescribed in a manner that is most likely to minimize the occurrence of tardive dyskinesia. Chronic antipsychotic treatment should generally be reserved for patients (1) who suffer from a chronic illness that is known to respond to antipsychotic drugs, and (2) for whom alternative, equally effective, but potentially less harmful treatments are not available or appropriate. In patients who do require chronic treatment, the smallest dose and the shortest duration of treatment producing a satisfactory clinical response should be sought. The need for continued treatment should be reassessed periodically.

If signs and symptoms of tardive dyskinesia appear in a patient on olanzapine, drug discontinuation should be considered. However, some patients may require treatment with olanzapine despite the presence of the syndrome.

5.10 Orthostatic Hypotension

ZYPREXA RELPREVV may induce orthostatic hypotension associated with dizziness, tachycardia, bradycardia and, in some patients, syncope, probably reflecting its α_1-adrenergic antagonistic properties *[see Patient Counseling Information (17.8)]*. Syncope-related adverse reactions were reported in 0.1% of patients treated with ZYPREXA RELPREVV in clinical studies.

Olanzapine should be used with particular caution in patients with known cardiovascular disease (history of myocardial infarction or ischemia, heart failure, or conduction abnormalities), cerebrovascular disease, and conditions which would predispose patients to hypotension (dehydration, hypovolemia, and treatment with antihypertensive medications) where the occurrence of syncope, or hypotension and/or bradycardia might put the patient at increased medical risk. For patients in this population who have never taken oral olanzapine, tolerability should be established with oral olanzapine prior to initiating treatment with ZYPREXA RELPREVV *[see Dosage and Administration (2.1)]*.

Caution is necessary in patients who receive treatment with other drugs having effects that can induce hypotension, bradycardia, respiratory or central nervous system depression *[see Drug Interactions (7)]*.

5.11 Leukopenia, Neutropenia, and Agranulocytosis

Class Effect—In clinical trial and/or postmarketing experience, events of leukopenia/neutropenia have been reported temporally related to antipsychotic agents, including ZYPREXA. Agranulocytosis has also been reported.

Possible risk factors for leukopenia/neutropenia include pre-existing low white blood cell count (WBC) and history of drug-induced leukopenia/neutropenia. Patients with a history of a clinically significant low WBC or drug induced leukopenia/neutropenia should have their complete blood count (CBC) monitored frequently during the first few months of therapy and discontinuation of ZYPREXA RELPREVV should be considered at the first sign of a clinically significant decline in WBC in the absence of other causative factors.

Patients with clinically significant neutropenia should be carefully monitored for fever or other symptoms or signs of infection and treated promptly if such symptoms or signs occur. Patients with severe neutropenia (absolute neutrophil count $<1000/mm^3$ should discontinue ZYPREXA RELPREVV and have their WBC followed until recovery.

5.12 Dysphagia

Esophageal dysmotility and aspiration have been associated with antipsychotic drug use. Aspiration pneumonia is a common cause of morbidity and mortality in patients with advanced Alzheimer's disease. Olanzapine is not approved for the treatment of patients with Alzheimer's disease.

5.13 Seizures

During premarketing testing of ZYPREXA RELPREVV, seizures occurred in 0.15% of patients. During premarketing testing of oral olanzapine, seizures occurred in 0.9% of olanzapine-treated patients. There were confounding factors that may have contributed to the occurrence of seizures in many of these cases.

Olanzapine should be used cautiously in patients with a history of seizures or with conditions that potentially lower the seizure threshold, e.g., Alzheimer's dementia. Olanzapine is not approved for the treatment of patients with Alzheimer's disease. Conditions that lower the seizure threshold may be more prevalent in a population of 65 years or older.

5.14 Potential for Cognitive and Motor Impairment

Sedation was a commonly reported adverse reaction associated with ZYPREXA RELPREVV treatment, occurring at an incidence of 8% in ZYPREXA RELPREVV patients compared to 2% in placebo patients. Somnolence and sedation adverse reactions led to discontinuation in 0.6% of patients in the premarketing ZYPREXA RELPREVV database.

Since olanzapine has the potential to impair judgment, thinking, or motor skills, patients should be cautioned about operating hazardous machinery, including automobiles, until they are reasonably certain that olanzapine therapy does not affect them adversely. However, due to the risk of post-injection delirium/sedation syndrome after each injection, patients should not drive or operate heavy machinery for the remainder of the day of each injection *[see Dosage and Administration (2.1), Warnings and Precautions (5.1), and Patient Counseling Information (17.9)]*.

5.15 Body Temperature Regulation

Disruption of the body's ability to reduce core body temperature has been attributed to antipsychotic agents. Appropriate care is advised when prescribing ZYPREXA RELPREVV for patients who will be experiencing conditions which may contribute to an elevation in core body temperature, e.g., exercising strenuously, exposure to extreme heat, receiving concomitant medication with anticholinergic activity, or being subject to dehydration *[see Patient Counseling Information (17.10)]*.

5.16 Use in Patients with Concomitant Illness

Experience with ZYPREXA RELPREVV in patients with concomitant systemic illnesses is limited *[see Clinical Pharmacology (12.3)]*.

Olanzapine exhibits in vitro muscarinic receptor affinity. In premarketing clinical trials with oral olanzapine, olanzapine was associated with constipation, dry mouth, and tachycardia, all adverse reactions possibly related to cholinergic antagonism. Such adverse reactions were not often the basis for discontinuations from olanzapine, but olanzapine should be used with caution in patients with clinically significant prostatic hypertrophy, narrow angle glaucoma, or a history of paralytic ileus or related conditions.

In 5 placebo-controlled studies of oral olanzapine in elderly patients with dementia-related psychosis (n=1184), the following treatment-emergent adverse reactions were reported in olanzapine-treated patients at an incidence of at least 2% and significantly greater than placebo-treated patients: falls, somnolence, peripheral edema, abnormal gait, urinary incontinence, lethargy, increased weight, asthenia, pyrexia, pneumonia, dry mouth and visual hallucinations. The rate of discontinuation due to adverse reactions was significantly greater with oral olanzapine than placebo (13% vs 7%). Elderly patients with dementia-related psychosis treated with olanzapine are at an increased risk of death compared to placebo. Olanzapine is not approved for the treatment of patients with dementia-related psychosis *[see Boxed Warning, Warnings and Precautions (5.3), and Patient Counseling Information (17.11)]*.

Olanzapine has not been evaluated or used to any appreciable extent in patients with a recent history of myocardial infarction or unstable heart disease. Patients with these diagnoses were excluded from premarketing clinical studies. Because of the risk of orthostatic hypotension with olanzapine, caution should be observed in cardiac patients *[see Warnings and Precautions (5.10)]*.

5.17 Hyperprolactinemia

As with other drugs that antagonize dopamine D_2 receptors, olanzapine elevates prolactin levels, and the elevation persists during chronic administration. Hyperprolactinemia may suppress hypothalamic GnRH, resulting in reduced pituitary gonadotropin secretion. This, in turn, may inhibit reproductive function by impairing gonadal steroidogenesis in both female and male patients. Galactorrhea, amenorrhea, gynecomastia, and impotence have been reported in patients receiving prolactin-elevating compounds. Long-standing hyperprolactinemia when associated with hypogonadism may lead to decreased bone density in both female and male subjects.

Tissue culture experiments indicate that approximately one-third of human breast cancers are prolactin dependent in vitro, a factor of potential importance if the prescription of these drugs is contemplated in a patient with previously detected breast cancer. As is common with compounds which increase prolactin release, an increase in mammary gland neoplasia was observed in the oral olanzapine carcinogenicity studies conducted in mice and rats *[see Nonclinical Toxicology (13.1)]*. Neither clinical studies nor epidemiologic studies conducted to date have shown an association between chronic administration of this class of drugs and tumorigenesis in humans; the available evidence is considered too limited to be conclusive at this time. In premarketing studies with ZYPREXA RELPREVV, statistically significant differences among dose groups have been observed for prolactin levels *[see Adverse Reactions (6.1)]*.

In placebo-controlled olanzapine clinical studies (up to 12 weeks), changes from normal to high in prolactin concentrations were observed in 30% of adults treated with olanzapine as compared to 10.5% of adults treated with placebo. In a pooled analysis from clinical studies including 8136 adults treated with olanzapine, potentially associated clinical manifestations included menstrual-related events[1] (2% [49/3240] of females), sexual function-related events[2] (2% [150/8136] of females and males), and breast-related events[3] (0.7% [23/3240] of females, 0.2% [9/4896] of males).

In placebo-controlled olanzapine monotherapy studies in adolescent patients (up to 6 weeks) with schizophrenia or bipolar I disorder (manic or mixed episodes), changes from normal to high in prolactin concentrations were observed in 47% of olanzapine-treated patients compared to 7% of placebo-treated patients. In a pooled analysis from clinical trials including 454 adolescents treated with olanzapine, potentially associated clinical manifestations included menstrual-related events[1] (1% [2/168] of females), sexual function-related events[2] (0.7% [3/454] of females and males), and breast-related events[3] (2% [3/168] of females, 2% [7/286] of males) *[see Use in Specific Populations (8.4)]*.

[1] Based on a search of the following terms: amenorrhea, hypomenorrhea, menstruation delayed, and oligomenorrhea.

[2] Based on a search of the following terms: anorgasmia, delayed ejaculation, erectile dysfunction, decreased libido, loss of libido, abnormal orgasm, and sexual dysfunction.

[3] Based on a search of the following terms: breast discharge, enlargement or swelling, galactorrhea, gynecomastia, and lactation disorder.

5.18 Laboratory Tests

Fasting blood glucose testing and lipid profile at the beginning of, and periodically during, treatment is recommended *[see Warnings and Precautions (5.6, 5.7) and Patient Counseling Information (17.4, 17.5)]*.

6 ADVERSE REACTIONS

6.1 Clinical Trials Experience

The information below for ZYPREXA RELPREVV is derived primarily from a clinical trial database consisting of 2058 patients with approximately 1948 patient years of exposure to ZYPREXA RELPREVV. This database includes safety data from 6 open-label studies and 2 double-blind comparator studies, conducted in patients with schizophrenia or schizoaffective disorder. Additionally, data obtained from patients treated with oral olanzapine are also presented below. Adverse reactions were assessed by the collection of adverse reactions, vital signs, weights, laboratory analytes, ECGs, and the results of physical and ophthalmologic examinations. In the tables and tabulations that follow for ZYPREXA RELPREVV, the MedDRA terminology has been used to classify reported adverse reactions. Data obtained from oral olanzapine studies was reported using the COSTART dictionary.

The stated frequencies of adverse reactions represent the proportion of individuals who experienced, at least once, a treatment-emergent adverse reaction of the type listed. A reaction was considered treatment emergent if it occurred for the first time or worsened while receiving therapy following baseline evaluation. Reactions listed elsewhere in labeling may not be repeated below. The entire label should be read to gain a complete understanding of the safety profile of ZYPREXA RELPREVV.

The prescriber should be aware that the figures in the tables and tabulations cannot be used to predict the incidence of side effects in the course of usual medical practice where patient characteristics and other factors differ from those that prevailed in the clinical trials. Similarly, the cited frequencies cannot be compared with figures obtained from other clinical investigations involving different treatments, uses, and investigators. The cited figures, however, do provide the prescribing physician with some basis for estimating the relative contribution of drug and nondrug factors to the adverse reaction incidence in the population studied.

Adverse Reactions Associated with Discontinuation of Treatment in a Short-Term, Placebo-Controlled Trial

Overall, there was no difference in the incidence of discontinuation due to adverse reactions between ZYPREXA RELPREVV (4%; 13/306 patients) and placebo (5%; 5/98 patients) in an 8-week trial.

Commonly Observed Adverse Reactions in a Short-Term, Placebo-Controlled Trial

In an 8-week trial, treatment-emergent adverse reactions with an incidence of 5% or greater in at least one of the ZYPREXA RELPREVV treatment groups (210 mg/2 weeks, 405 mg/4 weeks, or 300 mg/2 weeks) and greater than placebo were: headache, sedation, weight gain, cough, diarrhea, back pain, nausea, somnolence, dry mouth, nasopharyngitis, increased appetite, and vomiting.

Adverse Reactions Occurring at an Incidence of 2% or More among ZYPREXA RELPREVV-Treated Patients in a Short-Term, Placebo-Controlled Trial

Table 9 enumerates the incidence, rounded to the nearest percent, of treatment-emergent adverse reactions that occurred in 2% or more of patients treated with ZYPREXA RELPREVV and with incidence greater than placebo who participated in the 8-week, placebo-controlled trial.

[See table 9 at top right]

Summary of Statistically Significant Changes by Dose

In a 24-week randomized, double-blind, fixed-dose study comparing 3 doses of ZYPREXA RELPREVV in patients with schizophrenia, statistically significant differences among dose groups were observed for the below safety outcomes (Table 10) [see Warnings and Precautions (5.8, 5.17)].

[See table 10 at top of next page]

Dose Dependency of Adverse Reactions in Short-Term, Placebo-Controlled Trials

Extrapyramidal Symptoms: The following table enumerates the percentage of patients with treatment-emergent extrapyramidal symptoms as assessed by categorical analyses of formal rating scales during acute therapy in a controlled clinical trial comparing oral olanzapine at 3 fixed doses with placebo in the treatment of schizophrenia in a 6-week trial.

[See table 11 on next page]

The following table enumerates the percentage of patients with treatment-emergent extrapyramidal symptoms as assessed by spontaneously reported adverse reactions during acute therapy in the same controlled clinical trial comparing olanzapine at 3 fixed doses with placebo in the treatment of schizophrenia in a 6-week trial.

[See table 12 on next page]

Dystonia, Class Effect: Symptoms of dystonia, prolonged abnormal contractions of muscle groups, may occur in susceptible individuals during the first few days of treatment. Dystonic symptoms include: spasm of the neck muscles, sometimes progressing to tightness of the throat, swallowing difficulty, difficulty breathing, and/or protrusion of the tongue. While these symptoms can occur at low doses, the frequency and severity are greater with high potency and at higher doses of first generation antipsychotic drugs. In general, an elevated risk of acute dystonia may be observed in males and younger age groups receiving antipsychotics; however, events of dystonia have been reported infrequently (<1%) with olanzapine use.

Differences among Fixed-Dose Groups Observed in Oral Olanzapine Clinical Trials

In a single 8-week randomized, double-blind, fixed-dose study comparing 10 (N=199), 20 (N=200) and 40 (N=200) mg/day of oral olanzapine in patients with schizophrenia or schizoaffective disorder, differences among 3 dose groups were observed for the following safety outcomes: weight gain, prolactin elevation, fatigue and dizziness. Mean baseline to endpoint increase in weight (10 mg/day: 1.9 kg; 20 mg/day: 2.3 kg; 40 mg/day: 3 kg) was observed with significant differences between 10 vs 40 mg/day. Incidence of treatment-emergent prolactin elevation >24.2 ng/mL (female) or >18.77 ng/mL (male) at any time during the trial (10 mg/day: 31.2%; 20 mg/day: 42.7%; 40 mg/day: 61.1%) with significant differences between 10 vs 40 mg/day and 20 vs 40 mg/day; fatigue (10 mg/day: 1.5%; 20 mg/day: 2.1%; 40 mg/day: 6.6%) with significant differences between 10 vs 40 and 20 vs 40 mg/day; and dizziness (10 mg/day: 2.6%; 20 mg/day: 1.6%; 40 mg/day: 6.6%) with significant differences between 20 vs 40 mg, was observed.

Local Injection Site Reactions

Eleven ZYPREXA RELPREVV-treated patients (3.6%) and 0 placebo-treated patients experienced treatment-emergent injection-related adverse reactions (injection site pain, buttock pain, injection site mass, induration, injection site induration) in the placebo-controlled database. The most frequently occurring treatment-emergent adverse reaction was injection site pain (2.3% ZYPREXA RELPREVV-treated; 0% placebo-treated).

Commonly Observed Adverse Reactions During the Clinical Trial Evaluation of Oral Olanzapine

In clinical trials of oral olanzapine monotherapy for the treatment of schizophrenia in adult patients, treatment-emergent adverse reactions with an incidence of 5% or greater in the olanzapine treatment arm and at least twice that of placebo were: postural hypotension, constipation, weight gain, dizziness, personality disorder, and akathisia.

Other Adverse Reactions Observed During the Clinical Trial Evaluation of Oral Olanzapine

Following is a list of treatment-emergent adverse reactions reported by patients treated with oral olanzapine (at multiple doses ≥1 mg/day) in clinical trials. This listing is not intended to include reactions (1) already listed in previous tables or elsewhere in labeling, (2) for which a drug cause was remote, (3) which were so general as to be uninformative, (4) which were not considered to have significant clinical implications, or (5) which occurred at a rate equal to or less than placebo. Reactions are classified by body system using the following definitions: frequent adverse reactions are those occurring in at least 1/100 patients; infrequent adverse reactions are those occurring in 1/100 to 1/1000 patients; rare adverse reactions are those occurring in fewer than 1/1000 patients.

Body as a Whole—*Infrequent:* chills, face edema, photosensitivity reaction, suicide attempt[1]; *Rare:* chills and fever, hangover effect, sudden death[1].

Table 9: Treatment-Emergent Adverse Reactions: Incidence in a Short-Term, Placebo-Controlled Clinical Trial with ZYPREXA RELPREVV

Body System/Adverse Reaction	Placebo (N=98)	ZYPREXA RELPREVV 405 mg/4 wks (N=100)	ZYPREXA RELPREVV 210 mg/2 wks (N=106)	ZYPREXA RELPREVV 300 mg/2 wks (N=100)
Ear and Labyrinth Disorders				
Ear pain	2	1	1	4
Gastrointestinal Disorders				
Abdominal pain[a]	2	3	3	3
Diarrhea	4	2	7	5
Dry mouth	1	2	6	4
Flatulence	0	2	2	1
Nausea	2	5	5	4
Toothache	0	3	4	3
Vomiting	2	6	1	2
General Disorders and Administration Site Conditions				
Fatigue	2	4	2	3
Injection site pain	0	2	3	2
Pain	0	0	2	3
Pyrexia	0	2	0	0
Infections and Infestations				
Nasopharyngitis	2	3	6	1
Tooth infection[b]	0	4	0	0
Upper respiratory tract infection	2	3	1	4
Viral infection	0	0	0	2
Injury, Poisoning and Procedural Complications				
Procedural pain	0	2	0	0
Investigations				
Electrocardiogram QT-corrected interval prolonged	1	0	0	2
Hepatic enzyme increased[c]	1	4	1	3
Weight increased	5	5	6	7
Metabolism and Nutrition Disorders				
Increased appetite	0	1	4	6
Musculoskeletal and Connective Tissue Disorders				
Arthralgia	0	3	3	3
Back pain	4	4	3	5
Muscle spasms	0	3	1	2
Musculoskeletal stiffness	1	1	4	4
Nervous System Disorders				
Dizziness	2	4	4	1
Dysarthria	0	0	1	2
Headache[d]	8	13	15	18
Sedation[e]	7	13	8	13
Tremor	1	3	0	1
Psychiatric Disorders				
Abnormal dreams	0	0	0	2
Hallucination, auditory	2	3	1	0
Restlessness	2	2	3	1
Sleep disorder	1	0	3	2
Thinking abnormal	1	3	0	0
Reproductive System and Breast Disorders				
Vaginal discharge	0	0	4	4
Respiratory, Thoracic and Mediastinal Disorders				
Cough	5	3	5	9
Nasal congestion[f]	3	2	1	7
Pharyngolaryngeal pain	2	2	3	3
Sneezing	0	0	0	2
Skin and Subcutaneous Tissue Disorders				
Acne	0	2	0	2
Vascular Disorders				
Hypertension	0	3	2	0

[a] The term abdominal pain upper was combined under abdominal pain.
[b] The term tooth abscess was combined under tooth infection.
[c] The terms alanine aminotransferase increased, aspartate aminotransferase increased, and gamma-glutamyltransferase increased were combined under hepatic enzyme increased.
[d] The term tension headache was combined under headache.
[e] The term somnolence was combined under sedation.
[f] The term sinus congestion was combined under nasal congestion.

Table 10: Summary of Statistically Significant Changes by Dose in a Double-Blind, Fixed-Dose Study for ZYPREXA RELPREVV[a]

	ZYPREXA RELPREVV Dose		
	150 mg/2 weeks	405 mg/4 weeks	300 mg/2 weeks
Weight: mean change in kg (N[1])	0.67 (140)	0.89 (315)	1.70[b] (140)
Prolactin: mean change in µg/L (N[1])	-5.61 (109)	-2.76 (259)	3.57[b,c] (115)
Fasting triglycerides: patients who met the criteria[d] for change from normal at baseline to high at anytime n/N[2] (%)	4/62 (6.5)	13/133 (9.8)	13/53[b,c] (24.5)

[a] Abbreviations: N[1]=Number of patients who have both baseline and post-baseline measurement; n=number of patients with an abnormal post-baseline measurement at any time; N[2]=Number of patients with a normal baseline and at least one post-baseline measurement.
[b] p<0.05 versus 150 mg/2 weeks ZYPREXA RELPREVV; pairwise p-values.
[c] p<0.05 versus 405 mg/4 weeks ZYPREXA RELPREVV; pairwise p-values.
[d] Triglycerides normal to high limits are <150 mg/dL to 200 mg/dL ≤X <500 mg/dL.

Table 11: Treatment-Emergent Extrapyramidal Symptoms Assessed by Rating Scales Incidence in a Fixed Dosage Range, Placebo-Controlled Clinical Trial of Oral Olanzapine in Schizophrenia — Acute Phase

	Percentage of Patients Reporting Event			
	Placebo	Olanzapine 5 ± 2.5 mg/day	Olanzapine 10 ± 2.5 mg/day	Olanzapine 15 ± 2.5 mg/day
Parkinsonism[a]	15	14	12	14
Akathisia[b]	23	16	19	27

[a] Percentage of patients with a Simpson-Angus Scale total score >3.
[b] Percentage of patients with a Barnes Akathisia Scale global score ≥2.

Table 12: Treatment-Emergent Extrapyramidal Symptoms Assessed by Adverse Reactions Incidence in a Fixed Dosage Range, Placebo-Controlled Clinical Trial of Oral Olanzapine in Schizophrenia — Acute Phase

	Percentage of Patients Reporting Event			
	Placebo (N=68)	Olanzapine 5 ± 2.5 mg/day (N=65)	Olanzapine 10 ± 2.5 mg/day (N=64)	Olanzapine 15 ± 2.5 mg/day (N=69)
Dystonic events[a]	1	3	2	3
Parkinsonism events[b]	10	8	14	20
Akathisia events[c]	1	5	11	10
Dyskinetic events[d]	4	0	2	1
Residual events[e]	1	2	5	1
Any extrapyramidal event	16	15	25	32

[a] Patients with the following COSTART terms were counted in this category: dystonia, generalized spasm, neck rigidity, oculogyric crisis, opisthotonos, torticollis.
[b] Patients with the following COSTART terms were counted in this category: akinesia, cogwheel rigidity, extrapyramidal syndrome, hypertonia, hypokinesia, masked facies, tremor.
[c] Patients with the following COSTART terms were counted in this category: akathisia, hyperkinesia.
[d] Patients with the following COSTART terms were counted in this category: buccoglossal syndrome, choreoathetosis, dyskinesia, tardive dyskinesia.
[e] Patients with the following COSTART terms were counted in this category: movement disorder, myoclonus, twitching.

Cardiovascular System—*Infrequent:* cerebrovascular accident, vasodilatation.
Digestive System—*Infrequent:* nausea and vomiting, tongue edema; *Rare:* ileus, intestinal obstruction, liver fatty deposit.
Hemic and Lymphatic System—*Infrequent:* leukopenia, thrombocytopenia.
Metabolic and Nutritional Disorders—*Infrequent:* alkaline phosphatase increased, bilirubinemia, hypoproteinemia.
Musculoskeletal System—*Rare:* osteoporosis.
Nervous System—*Infrequent:* ataxia, dysarthria, libido decreased, stupor; *Rare:* coma.
Respiratory System—*Infrequent:* epistaxis; *Rare:* lung edema.
Skin and Appendages—*Infrequent:* alopecia.
Special Senses—*Infrequent:* abnormality of accommodation, dry eyes; *Rare:* mydriasis.
Urogenital System—*Infrequent:* amenorrhea[2], breast pain, decreased menstruation, impotence[2], increased menstruation[2], menorrhagia[2], metrorrhagia[2], polyuria[2], urinary frequency, urinary retention, urinary urgency, urination impaired.
[1] These terms represent serious adverse events but do not meet the definition for adverse drug reactions. They are included here because of their seriousness.

[2] Adjusted for gender.

6.2 Vital Signs and Laboratory Studies
Laboratory Changes
ZYPREXA RELPREVV in Adults: Statistically significant within group mean changes for ZYPREXA RELPREVV, which were also significantly different from placebo, were observed for the following: eosinophils, monocytes, cholesterol, low-density lipoprotein (LDL), triglycerides, and direct bilirubin. There were no statistically significant differences between ZYPREXA RELPREVV and placebo in the incidence of potentially clinically significant changes in any of the laboratory values studied.
Statistically significant within group mean changes for ZYPREXA RELPREVV, which were also significantly different from oral olanzapine (in a 24-week double-blind study), were observed for the following: gamma-glutamyltranseferase (GGT) and sodium. Statistically significant differences were observed between ZYPREXA RELPREVV and oral olanzapine for the incidence of treatment-emergent low platelet count (0% ZYPREXA RELPREVV vs 1% oral olanzapine); and low total bilirubin (2.8% ZYPREXA RELPREVV vs 0.7% for oral olanzapine). There was a statistically significant difference between ZYPREXA RELPREVV and oral olanzapine in potentially clinically significant changes for high leukocyte count (0% ZYPREXA RELPREVV vs 1% oral olanzapine).

Changes in aminotransferases observed with ZYPREXA RELPREVV treatment were similar to those reported with ZYPREXA treatment. In placebo-controlled ZYPREXA RELPREVV studies, clinically significant ALT elevations (≥3 times the upper limit of the normal range) were observed in 2.7% (8/291) of patients exposed to olanzapine compared to 3.2% (3/94) of the placebo patients. None of these patients experienced jaundice. In 3 of these patients, liver enzymes reverted to the normal range despite continued treatment, and in 5 cases enzymes values decreased, but were still above the normal range at the end of therapy. Within the larger premarketing ZYPREXA RELPREVV database of 1886 patients with baseline ALT ≤90 IU/L, the incidence of ALT elevation to >200 IU/L was 0.8%. None of these patients experienced jaundice or other symptoms attributable to liver impairment and most had transient changes that tended to normalize while ZYPREXA RELPREVV treatment was continued.
Olanzapine Monotherapy in Adults: An assessment of the premarketing experience for oral olanzapine revealed an association with asymptomatic increases in ALT, AST, and GGT. Within the original premarketing database of about 2400 adult patients with baseline ALT ≤90 IU/L, the incidence of ALT elevations to >200 IU/L was 2% (50/2381). None of these patients experienced jaundice or other symptoms attributable to liver impairment and most had transient changes that tended to normalize while olanzapine treatment was continued.
In placebo-controlled oral olanzapine monotherapy studies in adults, clinically significant ALT elevations (change from <3 times the upper limit of normal [ULN] at baseline to ≥3 times ULN) were observed in 5% (77/1426) of patients exposed to olanzapine compared to 1% (10/1187) of patients exposed to placebo. ALT elevations ≥5 times ULN were observed in 2% (29/1438) of olanzapine-treated patients, compared to 0.3% (4/1196) of placebo-treated patients. ALT values returned to normal, or were decreasing, at last follow-up in the majority of patients who either continued treatment with olanzapine or discontinued olanzapine. No patient with elevated ALT values experienced jaundice, liver failure, or met the criteria for Hy's Rule.
Rare postmarketing reports of hepatitis have been received for patients taking different formulations of olanzapine. Very rare cases of cholestatic or mixed liver injury have also been reported in the postmarketing period.
Caution should be exercised in patients with signs and symptoms of hepatic impairment, in patients with pre-existing conditions associated with limited hepatic functional reserve, and in patients who are being treated with potentially hepatotoxic drugs.
Oral olanzapine administration was also associated with increases in serum prolactin [see Warnings and Precautions (5.17)], with an asymptomatic elevation of the eosinophil count in 0.3% of patients, and with an increase in CPK.
ECG Changes—Comparison of ZYPREXA RELPREVV and oral olanzapine, in a 24 week study, revealed no significant differences on ECG changes. Between-group comparisons for pooled placebo-controlled trials revealed no significant oral olanzapine/placebo differences in the proportions of patients experiencing potentially important changes in ECG parameters, including QT, QTc, and PR intervals. Oral olanzapine use was associated with a mean increase in heart rate of 2.4 beats per minute compared to no change among placebo patients. This slight tendency to tachycardia may be related to olanzapine's potential for inducing orthostatic changes [see Warnings and Precautions (5.11)].
6.3 Postmarketing Experience
Adverse reactions reported since market introduction that were temporally (but not necessarily causally) related to ZYPREXA therapy include the following: allergic reaction (e.g., anaphylactoid reaction, angioedema, pruritus or urticaria), diabetic coma, diabetic ketoacidosis, discontinuation reaction (diaphoresis, nausea, or vomiting), jaundice, neutropenia, pancreatitis, priapism, rash, rhabdomyolysis, and venous thromboembolic events (including pulmonary embolism and deep venous thrombosis). Random cholesterol levels of ≥240 mg/dL and random triglyceride levels of ≥1000 mg/dL have been reported.

7 DRUG INTERACTIONS
7.1 Potential for Other Drugs to Affect Olanzapine
Diazepam—The co-administration of diazepam with olanzapine potentiated the orthostatic hypotension observed with olanzapine [see Drug Interactions (7.2)].
Inducers of CYP1A2—Carbamazepine therapy (200 mg bid) causes an approximately 50% increase in the clearance of olanzapine. This increase is likely due to the fact that carbamazepine is a potent inducer of CYP1A2 activity. Higher daily doses of carbamazepine may cause an even greater increase in olanzapine clearance.
Alcohol—Ethanol (45 mg/70 kg single dose) did not have an effect on olanzapine pharmacokinetics. The co-administration of alcohol (i.e., ethanol) with olanzapine potentiated the orthostatic hypotension observed with olanzapine [see Drug Interactions (7.2)].

Inhibitors of CYP1A2—Fluvoxamine, a CYP1A2 inhibitor, decreases the clearance of olanzapine. This results in a mean increase in olanzapine Cmax following fluvoxamine of 54% in female nonsmokers and 77% in male smokers. The mean increase in olanzapine AUC is 52% and 108%, respectively. Lower doses of olanzapine should be considered in patients receiving concomitant treatment with fluvoxamine.
Inhibitors of CYP2D6—Fluoxetine caused a small decrease in olanzapine clearance leading to a minimal change in olanzapine steady-state concentrations and, therefore dose modification is not routinely recommended.
Warfarin—Warfarin (20 mg single dose) did not affect olanzapine pharmacokinetics *[see Drug Interactions (7.2)]*.
Inducers of CYP1A2 or Glucuronyl Transferase Enzymes—Omeprazole and rifampin may cause an increase in olanzapine clearance.

7.2 Potential for Olanzapine to Affect Other Drugs

CNS Acting Drugs—Given the primary CNS effects of olanzapine, caution should be used when olanzapine is taken in combination with other centrally acting drugs and alcohol.
Antihypertensive Agents—Olanzapine, because of its potential for inducing hypotension, may enhance the effects of certain antihypertensive agents.
Levodopa and Dopamine Agonists—Olanzapine may antagonize the effects of levodopa and dopamine agonists.
Lorazepam (IM)—Co-administration of lorazepam does not significantly affect the pharmacokinetics of olanzapine, unconjugated lorazepam, or total lorazepam. However, this co-administration of lorazepam with olanzapine potentiated the somnolence observed with either drug alone.
Lithium—Multiple doses of olanzapine (10 mg for 8 days) did not influence the kinetics of lithium. Therefore, concomitant olanzapine administration does not require dosage adjustment of lithium.
Valproate—Olanzapine (10 mg daily for 2 weeks) did not affect the steady-state plasma concentrations of valproate. Therefore, concomitant olanzapine administration does not require dosage adjustment of valproate.
Effect of Olanzapine on Drug Metabolizing Enzymes—In vitro studies utilizing human liver microsomes suggest that olanzapine has little potential to inhibit CYP1A2, CYP2C9, CYP2C19, CYP2D6, and CYP3A. Thus, olanzapine is unlikely to cause clinically important drug interactions mediated by these enzymes.
Imipramine—Single doses of olanzapine did not affect the pharmacokinetics of imipramine or its active metabolite desipramine.
Warfarin—Single doses of olanzapine did not affect the pharmacokinetics of warfarin *[see Drug Interactions (7.1)]*.
Diazepam—Olanzapine did not influence the pharmacokinetics of diazepam or its active metabolite N-desmethyldiazepam. However, diazepam co-administered with olanzapine increased the orthostatic hypotension observed with either drug given alone *[see Drug Interactions (7.1)]*.
Alcohol—Multiple doses of olanzapine did not influence the kinetics of ethanol *[see Drug Interactions (7.1)]*.
Biperiden—Multiple dosed of olanzapine did not influence the kinetics of biperiden.
Theophylline—Multiple doses of olanzapine did not affect the pharmacokinetics of theophylline or its metabolites.

8 USE IN SPECIFIC POPULATIONS

8.1 Pregnancy

Teratogenic Effects, Pregnancy Category C—In oral reproduction studies in rats at doses up to 18 mg/kg/day and in rabbits at doses up to 30 mg/kg/day (9 and 30 times the maximum recommended human daily oral dose on a mg/m^2 basis, respectively) no evidence of teratogenicity was observed. In an oral rat teratology study, early resorptions and increased numbers of nonviable fetuses were observed at a dose of 18 mg/kg/day (9 times the maximum recommended human daily oral dose on a mg/m^2 basis). Gestation was prolonged at 10 mg/kg/day (5 times the maximum recommended human daily oral dose on a mg/m^2 basis). In an oral rabbit teratology study, fetal toxicity (manifested as increased resorptions and decreased fetal weight) occurred at a maternally toxic dose of 30 mg/kg/day (30 times the maximum recommended human daily oral dose on a mg/m^2 basis). No evidence of teratogenicity or embryo-fetal toxicity was observed in rats or rabbits with ZYPREXA RELPREVV at intramuscular doses up to 75 mg/kg (1 and 2 times the maximum recommended human dose of 300 mg every 2 weeks, respectively, on a mg/m^2 basis). Placental transfer of olanzapine occurred in rat pups.
There are no adequate and well-controlled trials with olanzapine in pregnant females. Four pregnancies were observed during clinical trials with ZYPREXA RELPREVV, including 1 resulting in a normal birth and 3 therapeutic abortions. Because animal reproduction studies are not always predictive of human response, this drug should be used during pregnancy only if the potential benefit justifies the potential risk to the fetus.

8.2 Labor and Delivery

The effect of olanzapine on labor and delivery in humans is unknown. Parturition in rats was not affected by olanzapine.

8.3 Nursing Mothers

In an oral olanzapine study in lactating, healthy women, olanzapine was excreted in breast milk. Mean infant dose at steady state was estimated to be 1.8% of the maternal olanzapine dose. It is recommended that women receiving ZYPREXA RELPREVV should not breast-feed.

8.4 Pediatric Use

Safety and effectiveness of ZYPREXA RELPREVV in children and adolescent patients have not been established *[see Warnings and Precautions (5.6, 5.7, 5.8)]*.
Compared to patients from adult clinical trials, adolescents treated with oral ZYPREXA were likely to gain more weight, experience increased sedation, and have greater increases in total cholesterol, triglycerides, LDL cholesterol, prolactin and hepatic aminotransferase levels.

8.5 Geriatric Use

Clinical studies of ZYPREXA RELPREVV did not include sufficient numbers of subjects aged 65 and over to determine whether they respond differently from younger subjects. In the premarketing clinical studies with oral olanzapine, there was no indication of any different tolerability of olanzapine in elderly patients compared to younger patients with schizophrenia. Oral olanzapine studies in elderly patients with dementia-related psychosis have suggested that there may be a different tolerability profile in this population compared to younger patients with schizophrenia. Elderly patients with dementia-related psychosis treated with olanzapine are at an increased risk of death compared to placebo. In placebo-controlled studies of olanzapine in elderly patients with dementia-related psychosis, there was a higher incidence of cerebrovascular adverse events (e.g., stroke, transient ischemic attack) in patients treated with olanzapine compared to patients treated with placebo. Olanzapine is not approved for the treatment of patients with dementia-related psychosis. Also, the presence of factors that might decrease pharmacokinetic clearance or increase the pharmacodynamic response to olanzapine should lead to consideration of a lower starting dose for any geriatric patient *[see Boxed Warning, Warnings and Precautions (5.3), and Dosage and Administration (2.1)]*.

9 DRUG ABUSE AND DEPENDENCE

9.3 Dependence

In studies prospectively designed to assess abuse and dependence potential, olanzapine was shown to have acute depressive CNS effects but little or no potential of abuse or physical dependence in rats administered oral doses up to 15 times the maximum recommended human daily oral dose (20 mg) and rhesus monkeys administered oral doses up to 8 times the maximum recommended human daily oral dose on a mg/m^2 basis.
Olanzapine has not been systematically studied in humans for its potential for abuse, tolerance, or physical dependence. Because ZYPREXA RELPREVV is to be administered by healthcare professionals, the potential for misuse or abuse by patients is low.

10 OVERDOSAGE

10.1 Human Experience

During premarketing clinical studies of ZYPREXA RELPREVV, adverse reactions that presented with signs and symptoms consistent with olanzapine overdose, in particular, sedation (including coma) and/or delirium, were reported in patients following an injection of ZYPREXA RELPREVV *[see Boxed Warning and Dosage and Administration (2.1)]*. These reactions occurred in <0.1% of injections and in approximately 2% of patients who received injections for up to 46 months. These reactions were correlated with an unintentional rapid increase in serum olanzapine concentrations to supra-therapeutic ranges in some cases. While a rapid and greater than expected increase in serum olanzapine concentration has been observed in some patients with these reactions, the exact mechanism by which the drug was unintentionally introduced into the blood stream is not known. Clinical signs and symptoms included dizziness, confusion, disorientation, slurred speech, altered gait, difficulty ambulating, weakness, agitation, extrapyramidal symptoms, hypertension, convulsion, and reduced level of consciousness ranging from mild sedation to coma. Time after injection to event ranged from soon after injection to greater than 3 hours after injection. The majority of patients were hospitalized and some required supportive care, including intubation, in several cases. All patients had largely recovered by 72 hours. The risk of an event is the same at each injection, so the risk per patient is cumulative (i.e., increases with the number of injections) *[see Warnings and Precautions (5.1)]*.
In postmarketing reports of overdose with oral olanzapine alone, symptoms have been reported in the majority of cases. In symptomatic patients, symptoms with ≥10% incidence included agitation/aggressiveness, dysarthria, tachycardia, various extrapyramidal symptoms, and reduced level of consciousness ranging from sedation to coma. Among less commonly reported symptoms were the following potentially medically serious reactions: aspiration, cardiopulmonary arrest, cardiac arrhythmias (such as supraventricular tachycardia and 1 patient experiencing sinus pause with spontaneous resumption of normal rhythm), delirium, possible neuroleptic malignant syndrome, respiratory depression/arrest, convulsion, hypertension, and hypotension. Eli Lilly and Company has received reports of fatality in association with overdose of oral olanzapine alone. In 1 case of death, the amount of acutely ingested oral olanzapine was reported to be possibly as low as 450 mg of oral olanzapine; however, in another case, a patient was reported to survive an acute olanzapine ingestion of approximately 2 g of oral olanzapine.

10.2 Management of Overdose

Post-injection delirium/sedation syndrome may occur with each injection of ZYPREXA RELPREVV. Signs and symptoms consistent with olanzapine overdose have been observed, and access to emergency response services must be readily available for safe use *[see Boxed Warning and Warnings and Precautions (5.1)]*.
There is no specific antidote to olanzapine. Therefore, appropriate supportive measures should be initiated. Hypotension and circulatory collapse should be treated with appropriate measures such as intravenous fluids and/or sympathomimetic agents. (Do not use epinephrine, dopamine, or other sympathomimetics with beta-agonist activity, since beta stimulation may worsen hypotension in the setting of olanzapine-induced alpha blockade.) Respiratory support, including ventilation, may be required. Close medical supervision and monitoring should continue until the patient recovers.
The possibility of multiple drug involvement should be considered. In case of acute overdosage, establish and maintain an airway and ensure adequate oxygenation and ventilation, which may include intubation. The possibility of obtundation, seizures, or dystonic reaction of the head and neck following overdose may create a risk of aspiration with induced emesis. Cardiovascular monitoring should commence immediately and should include continuous electrocardiographic monitoring to detect possible arrhythmias.

11 DESCRIPTION

ZYPREXA RELPREVV is an atypical antipsychotic that belongs to the thienobenzodiazepine class. The chemical designation is 10H-thieno[2,3-b][1,5]benzodiazepine, 2-methyl-4-(4-methyl-1-piperazinyl)-,4,4′-methylenebis[3-hydroxy-2-naphthalenecarboxylate] (1:1), monohydrate. The formula is $C_{17}H_{22}N_4S \cdot C_{23}H_{14}O_6 \cdot H_2O$, which corresponds to a molecular weight of 718.8. The chemical structure is:

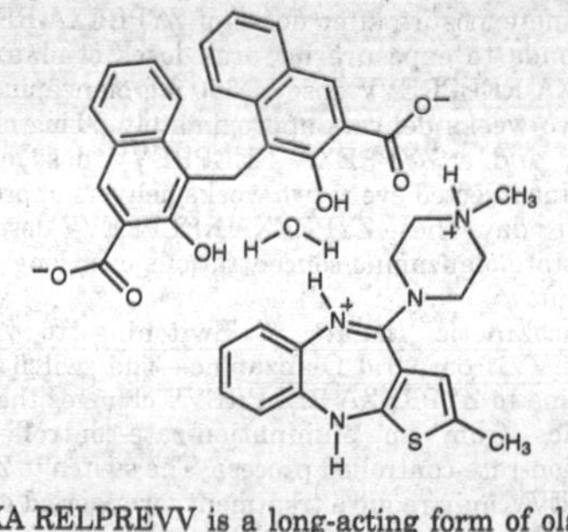

ZYPREXA RELPREVV is a long-acting form of olanzapine and is intended for deep intramuscular gluteal injection only.
ZYPREXA RELPREVV includes a vial of the drug product and a vial of the sterile diluent for ZYPREXA RELPREVV. The drug product is olanzapine pamoate monohydrate, present as a yellow solid in a glass vial equivalent to 210, 300, or 405 mg olanzapine base per vial. The diluent for ZYPREXA RELPREVV is a clear, colorless to slightly yellow solution in a glass vial and is composed of carboxymethylcellulose sodium, mannitol, polysorbate 80, sodium hydroxide and/or hydrochloric acid for pH adjustment, and water for injection. The drug product is suspended in the diluent for ZYPREXA RELPREVV to a target concentration of 150 mg olanzapine per mL prior to intramuscular injection.

12 CLINICAL PHARMACOLOGY

12.1 Mechanism of Action

The mechanism of action of olanzapine, as with other drugs having efficacy in schizophrenia, is unknown. However, it has been proposed that this drug's efficacy in schizophrenia is mediated through a combination of dopamine and serotonin type 2 ($5HT_2$) antagonism.

12.2 Pharmacodynamics

Olanzapine binds with high affinity to the following receptors: serotonin $5HT_{2A/2C}$, $5HT_6$ (K_i=4, 11, and 5 nM, respectively), dopamine $D_{1\text{-}4}$ (K_i=11-31 nM), histamine H_1 (K_i=7 nM), and adrenergic α_1 receptors (K_i=19 nM). Olanzapine is an antagonist with moderate affinity binding for serotonin $5HT_3$ (K_i=57 nM) and muscarinic $M_{1\text{-}5}$ (K_i=73, 96, 132, 32, and 48 nM, respectively). Olanzapine binds weakly to $GABA_A$, BZD, and β-adrenergic receptors (K_i>10 μM).

Antagonism at receptors other than dopamine and $5HT_2$ may explain some of the other therapeutic and side effects of olanzapine. Olanzapine's antagonism of muscarinic $M_{1\text{-}5}$ receptors may explain its anticholinergic-like effects. Olanzapine's antagonism of histamine H_1 receptors may explain the somnolence observed with this drug. Olanzapine's antagonism of adrenergic α_1 receptors may explain the orthostatic hypotension observed with this drug.

12.3 Pharmacokinetics

The fundamental pharmacokinetic properties of olanzapine are similar for ZYPREXA RELPREVV and orally administered olanzapine. Refer to the section below describing the pharmacokinetics of orally administered olanzapine for details.

Slow dissolution of ZYPREXA RELPREVV, a practically insoluble salt, after a deep intramuscular gluteal injection of a dose of ZYPREXA RELPREVV results in prolonged systemic olanzapine plasma concentrations that are sustained over a period of weeks to months. An injection every 2 or 4 weeks provides olanzapine plasma concentrations that are similar to those achieved by daily doses of oral olanzapine. The steady-state plasma concentrations for ZYPREXA RELPREVV for doses of 150 mg to 405 mg every 2 or 4 weeks are within the range of steady-state olanzapine plasma concentration known to have been associated with oral doses of 5 mg to 20 mg olanzapine once daily. The change to a slow release, rate-controlled absorption process is the only fundamental pharmacokinetic difference between the administration of ZYPREXA RELPREVV and orally administered olanzapine. The effective half-life for olanzapine after intramuscular ZYPREXA RELPREVV administration is approximately 30 days as compared to a half-life after oral administration of approximately 30 hours. Exposure to olanzapine may persist for a period of months after a ZYPREXA RELPREVV injection. The long persistence of systemic concentrations of olanzapine may be an important consideration for the long-term clinical management of the patient. Typical systemic olanzapine plasma concentrations reach a peak within the first week after injection and are at trough level immediately prior to the next injection. The olanzapine plasma concentration fluctuation between the peak and trough is comparable to the peak and trough fluctuations associated with once daily oral dosing.

Dose Proportionality and Oral Dose Correspondence—ZYPREXA RELPREVV provides a dose of 150, 210, 300, or 405 mg olanzapine. An injection of a larger dose produces a dose-proportional increase in the systemic exposure. The olanzapine exposure after doses of ZYPREXA RELPREVV corresponds to exposure for oral doses of olanzapine. A ZYPREXA RELPREVV dose of 300 mg olanzapine injected every two weeks delivers approximately 20 mg olanzapine per day and a ZYPREXA RELPREVV dose of 150 mg olanzapine injected every two weeks delivers approximately 10 mg per day. These ZYPREXA RELPREVV doses sustain steady-state olanzapine concentrations over long periods of treatment.

Pharmacokinetic Impact of Switching to ZYPREXA RELPREVV from Oral Olanzapine—The switch from oral olanzapine to ZYPREXA RELPREVV changes the pharmacokinetics from an elimination-rate-controlled to an absorption-rate-controlled process. The switch to ZYPREXA RELPREVV may require treatment for a period of approximately 3 months to re-establish steady-state conditions. Initial treatment with ZYPREXA RELPREVV is recommended at a dose corresponding to the mg/day oral dose *[see Dosage and Administration (2.1)]*. Plasma concentrations of olanzapine during the first injection interval may be lower than those maintained by a corresponding oral dose. Even though the concentrations are lower, the olanzapine concentrations remained within a therapeutically effective range and supplementation with orally administered olanzapine was generally not necessary in clinical trials.

Olanzapine is extensively distributed throughout the body, with a volume of distribution of approximately 1000 L. It is 93% bound to plasma proteins over the concentration range of 7 to 1100 ng/mL, binding primarily to albumin and α_1-acid glycoprotein.

Metabolism and Elimination—Following a single oral dose of ^{14}C labeled olanzapine, 7% of the dose of olanzapine was recovered in the urine as unchanged drug, indicating that olanzapine is highly metabolized. Approximately 57% and 30% of the dose was recovered in the urine and feces, respectively. In the plasma, olanzapine accounted for only 12% of the AUC for total radioactivity, indicating significant exposure to metabolites. After multiple dosing, the major circulating metabolites were the 10-N-glucuronide, present at steady state at 44% of the concentration of olanzapine, and 4'-N-desmethyl olanzapine, present at steady state at 31% of the concentration of olanzapine. Both metabolites lack pharmacological activity at the concentrations observed.

Direct glucuronidation and cytochrome P450 (CYP) mediated oxidation are the primary metabolic pathways for olanzapine. In vitro studies suggest that CYPs 1A2 and 2D6, and the flavin-containing monooxygenase system are involved in olanzapine oxidation. CYP2D6 mediated oxidation appears to be a minor metabolic pathway in vivo, because the clearance of olanzapine is not reduced in subjects who are deficient in this enzyme.

Intramuscular Formulations—There are two formulations of ZYPREXA which are available for intramuscular injection. One form (ZYPREXA RELPREVV) is described in this package insert. The other formulation (ZYPREXA IntraMuscular) is a solution of olanzapine. When ZYPREXA IntraMuscular is injected intramuscularly, olanzapine (as the free base) is rapidly absorbed and peak plasma concentrations occur within 15 to 45 minutes. With the exception of higher maximum plasma concentrations, the pharmacokinetics of olanzapine after ZYPREXA IntraMuscular are similar to those for orally administered olanzapine. Refer to the package insert for ZYPREXA IntraMuscular for additional information.

Specific Populations—In general, the decision to use ZYPREXA RELPREVV in specific populations should be thoughtfully considered. For patients who have never taken oral olanzapine, tolerability should be established with oral olanzapine prior to initiating treatment with ZYPREXA RELPREVV. The recommended starting dose is ZYPREXA RELPREVV 150 mg/4 wks, in patients who are debilitated, who have a predisposition to hypotensive reactions, who otherwise exhibit a combination of factors that may result in slower metabolism of olanzapine (e.g., nonsmoking female patients >65 years of age), or who may be more pharmacodynamically sensitive to olanzapine. When indicated, dose escalation should be performed with caution in these patients *[see Dosage and Administration (2.1)]*. Precautions noted below need to be carefully weighed.

Renal Impairment—Because olanzapine is highly metabolized before excretion and only 7% of the drug is excreted unchanged, renal dysfunction alone is unlikely to have a major impact on the pharmacokinetics of olanzapine. The pharmacokinetic characteristics of orally administered olanzapine were similar in patients with severe renal impairment and normal subjects, indicating that dosage adjustment based upon the degree of renal impairment is not required. In addition, olanzapine is not removed by dialysis. The effect of renal impairment on metabolite elimination has not been studied.

Hepatic Impairment—Although the presence of hepatic impairment may be expected to reduce the clearance of olanzapine, a study of the effect of impaired liver function in subjects (n=6) with clinically significant (Childs Pugh Classification A and B) cirrhosis revealed little effect on the pharmacokinetics of orally administered olanzapine.

Geriatric—In a study involving 24 healthy subjects, the mean elimination half-life of orally administered olanzapine was about 1.5 times greater in elderly (≥65 years) than in nonelderly subjects (<65 years). Caution should be used in dosing the elderly, especially if there are other factors that might additively influence drug metabolism and/or pharmacodynamic sensitivity *[see Dosage and Administration (2.1)]*.

Gender—For both oral ZYPREXA and ZYPREXA RELPREVV higher average plasma concentrations of olanzapine were observed in women than in men. There were, however, no apparent differences between men and women in effectiveness or adverse effects. Dosage modifications based on gender should not be needed.

Smoking Status—For both oral ZYPREXA and ZYPREXA RELPREVV, studies have demonstrated that the clearance of olanzapine is higher in smokers than in nonsmokers, although dosage modifications are not routinely recommended.

Race—In vivo studies of orally administered olanzapine have shown that exposures are similar among Japanese, Chinese and Caucasians, especially after normalization for body weight differences. Dosage modifications for race are, therefore, not recommended.

Combined Effects—The combined effects of age, smoking, and gender could lead to substantial pharmacokinetic differences in populations. The clearance in young smoking males, for example, may be 3 times higher than that in elderly nonsmoking females. Dosing modification may be necessary in patients who exhibit a combination of factors that may result in slower metabolism of olanzapine *[see Dosage and Administration (2.1)]*.

13 NONCLINICAL TOXICOLOGY

13.1 Carcinogenesis, Mutagenesis, Impairment of Fertility

Carcinogenesis—Oral carcinogenicity studies were conducted in mice and rats. Olanzapine was administered to mice in two 78-week studies at doses of 3, 10, 30/20 mg/kg/day (equivalent to 0.8-5 times the maximum recommended human daily oral dose on a mg/m^2 basis) and 0.25, 2, 8 mg/kg/day (equivalent to 0.06-2 times the maximum recommended human daily oral dose on a mg/m^2 basis). Rats were dosed for 2 years at doses of 0.25, 1, 2.5, 4 mg/kg/day (males) and 0.25, 1, 4, 8 mg/kg/day (females) (equivalent to 0.13-2 and 0.13-4 times the maximum recommended human daily oral dose on a mg/m^2 basis, respectively). The incidence of liver hemangiomas and hemangiosarcomas was significantly increased in 1 mouse study in female mice dosed at 8 mg/kg/day (2 times the maximum recommended human daily oral dose on a mg/m^2 basis). These tumors were not increased in another mouse study in females dosed at 10 or 30/20 mg/kg/day (2-5 times the maximum recommended human daily oral dose on a mg/m^2 basis); in this study, there was a high incidence of early mortalities in males of the 30/20 mg/kg/day group. The incidence of mammary gland adenomas and adenocarcinomas was significantly increased in female mice dosed at ≥2 mg/kg/day and in female rats dosed at ≥4 mg/kg/day (0.5 and 2 times the maximum recommended human daily oral dose on a mg/m^2 basis, respectively). Rats were also treated intramuscularly with ZYPREXA RELPREVV once a month for 2 years at doses of 5, 10, 20 mg/kg (males) and 10, 25, 50 mg/kg (females) (equivalent to 0.08-0.8 times the maximum recommended human dose of 300 mg every 2 weeks on a mg/m^2 basis; dosing was limited due to local reactions at the IM injection site). The incidence of tumors in this study was not altered when compared to solution for ZYPREXA RELPREVV control or pamoic acid treated animals. Antipsychotic drugs have been shown to chronically elevate prolactin levels in rodents. Serum prolactin levels were not measured during the olanzapine carcinogenicity studies; however, measurements during subchronic toxicity studies showed that olanzapine elevated serum prolactin levels up to 4-fold in rats at the same doses used in the carcinogenicity study. An increase in mammary gland neoplasms has been found in rodents after chronic administration of other antipsychotic drugs and is considered to be prolactin mediated. The relevance for human risk of the finding of prolactin mediated endocrine tumors in rodents is unknown *[see Warnings and Precautions (5.17)]*.

Mutagenesis—No evidence of genotoxic potential for olanzapine was found in the Ames reverse mutation test, in vivo micronucleus test in mice, the chromosomal aberration test in Chinese hamster ovary cells, unscheduled DNA synthesis test in rat hepatocytes, induction of forward mutation test in mouse lymphoma cells, or in vivo sister chromatid exchange test in bone marrow of Chinese hamsters.

Impairment of Fertility—In an oral fertility and reproductive performance study in rats, male mating performance, but not fertility, was impaired at a dose of 22.4 mg/kg/day and female fertility was decreased at a dose of 3 mg/kg/day (11 and 1.5 times the maximum recommended human daily oral dose on a mg/m^2 basis, respectively). Discontinuance of olanzapine treatment reversed the effects on male mating performance. In female rats, the precoital period was increased and the mating index reduced at 5 mg/kg/day (2.5 times the maximum recommended human daily oral dose on a mg/m^2 basis). Diestrous was prolonged and estrous delayed at 1.1 mg/kg/day (0.6 times the maximum recommended human daily oral dose on a mg/m^2 basis); therefore olanzapine may produce a delay in ovulation.

13.2 Animal Toxicology and/or Pharmacology

In animal studies with olanzapine, the principal hematologic findings were reversible peripheral cytopenias in individual dogs dosed at 10 mg/kg (17 times the maximum recommended human daily oral dose on a mg/m^2 basis), dose-related decreases in lymphocytes and neutrophils in mice, and lymphopenia in rats. A few dogs treated with 10 mg/kg developed reversible neutropenia and/or reversible hemolytic anemia between 1 and 10 months of treatment. Dose-related decreases in lymphocytes and neutrophils were seen in mice given doses of 10 mg/kg (equal to 2 times the maximum recommended human daily oral dose on a mg/m^2 basis) in studies of 3 months' duration. Nonspecific lymphopenia, consistent with decreased body weight gain, occurred in rats receiving 22.5 mg/kg (11 times the maximum recommended human daily oral dose on a mg/m^2 basis) for 3 months or 16 mg/kg (8 times the maximum recommended human daily oral dose on a mg/m^2 basis) for 6 or 12 months. No evidence of bone marrow cytotoxicity was found in any of the species examined. Bone marrows were normocellular or hypercellular, indicating that the reductions in circulating blood cells were probably due to peripheral (non-marrow) factors.

14 CLINICAL STUDIES

14.1 Schizophrenia

The short-term effectiveness of ZYPREXA RELPREVV was established in an 8-week, placebo-controlled trial in adult patients (n=404) who were experiencing psychotic symptoms and met DSM-IV or DSM-IV-TR criteria for schizophrenia. Patients were randomized to receive injections of ZYPREXA RELPREVV 210 mg every 2 weeks, ZYPREXA RELPREVV 405 mg every 4 weeks, ZYPREXA RELPREVV 300 mg every 2 weeks, or placebo every 2 weeks. Patients were discontinued from their previous antipsychotics and underwent a 2-7 day washout period. No oral antipsychotic supplementation was allowed throughout the trial. The primary efficacy measure was change from baseline to endpoint in total Positive and Negative Syndrome Scale (PANSS) score (mean baseline total PANSS score 101). Total PANSS scores showed statistically significant improvement from baseline to endpoint with each dose of ZYPREXA RELPREVV (210 mg every 2 weeks, 405 mg every 4 weeks, and 300 mg every 2 weeks) as compared to placebo. The effectiveness of ZYPREXA RELPREVV in the treatment of schizophrenia is further supported by the established effectiveness of the oral formulation of olanzapine.

A longer-term trial enrolled patients with schizophrenia (n=1065) who had remained stable for 4 to 8 weeks on open-label treatment with oral olanzapine (mean baseline total PANSS score 56) and were then randomized to continue their current oral olanzapine dose (10, 15, or 20 mg/day); or to ZYPREXA RELPREVV 150 mg every 2 weeks (405 mg every 4 weeks, 300 mg every 2 weeks, or 45 mg every 4 weeks). No oral antipsychotic supplementation was allowed throughout the trial. The primary efficacy measure was time to exacerbation of symptoms of schizophrenia defined in terms of increases in Brief Psychiatric Rating Scale (BPRS) positive symptoms or hospitalization. ZYPREXA RELPREVV doses of 150 mg every 2 weeks, 405 mg every 4 weeks, and 300 mg every 2 weeks were each statistically significantly superior to low dose ZYPREXA RELPREVV (45 mg every 4 weeks).

16 HOW SUPPLIED/STORAGE AND HANDLING
16.1 How Supplied
ZYPREXA RELPREVV convenience kit is supplied in single-use cartons. Each carton includes one vial of olanzapine pamoate monohydrate in dosage strengths that are equivalent to 210 mg olanzapine (483 mg olanzapine pamoate monohydrate), 300 mg olanzapine (690 mg olanzapine pamoate monohydrate), and 405 mg olanzapine (931 mg olanzapine pamoate monohydrate) per vial; one vial of approximately 3 mL of diluent for ZYPREXA RELPREVV used to suspend the drug product; one 3-mL syringe with pre-attached 19-gauge, 1.5-inch (38 mm) Hypodermic Needle-Pro needle with needle protection device; and two 19-gauge, 1.5-inch (38 mm) Hypodermic Needle-Pro needles with needle protection device.

Needle-Pro® is a registered trademark of Smiths Medical. NDC 0002-7635-11—single-use convenience kit: 210 mg vial (VL7635) with rust flip-off cap and 3-mL vial of sterile diluent (VL7622) with gray flip-off cap

NDC 0002-7636-11—single-use convenience kit: 300 mg vial (VL7636) with olive flip-off cap and 3-mL vial of sterile diluent (VL7622) with gray flip-off cap

NDC 0002-7637-11—single-use convenience kit: 405 mg vial (VL7637) with steel blue flip-off cap and 3-mL vial of sterile diluent (VL7622) with gray flip-off cap

16.2 Storage and Handling
ZYPREXA RELPREVV should be stored at room temperature not to exceed 30°C (86°F).

When the drug product is suspended in the solution for ZYPREXA RELPREVV, it may be held at room temperature for 24 hours. The vial should be agitated immediately prior to product withdrawal. Once the suspension is withdrawn into the syringe, it should be used immediately [see Dosage and Administration (2.2)].

17 PATIENT COUNSELING INFORMATION
See FDA-approved Medication Guide.
Patients should be advised of the following issues and asked to alert their prescriber if these occur while taking ZYPREXA RELPREVV. Patients should be advised to call their doctor if they do not think they are getting better or have concerns about their condition.

17.1 Information on Medication Guide
Prescribers or other health professionals should inform patients, their families, and their caregivers about the potential benefits and potential risks associated with treatment with ZYPREXA RELPREVV, and should counsel them in its appropriate use. A patient Medication Guide is available for ZYPREXA RELPREVV. Prescribers or other health professionals should instruct patients, their families, and their caregivers to read the Medication Guide and should assist them in understanding its contents. Patients should be given the opportunity to discuss the contents of the Medication Guide and to obtain answers to any questions they may have.

17.2 Post-Injection Delirium/Sedation Syndrome
During premarketing clinical studies, reactions that presented with signs and symptoms consistent with olanzapine overdose have been reported in patients following an injection of ZYPREXA RELPREVV. It is mandatory that patients be enrolled in the ZYPREXA RELPREVV Patient Care Pro-

gram to receive ZYPREXA RELPREVV treatment. Patients should be advised of the risk of post-injection delirium/ sedation syndrome each time they receive an injection [see Warnings and Precautions (5.1, 5.2)]. Patient and caregivers should be advised that after each ZYPREXA RELPREVV injection, patients must be observed at the healthcare facility for at least 3 hours and must be accompanied to their destination upon leaving the facility. The Medication Guide should be distributed each time patients receive an injection.

17.3 Elderly Patients with Dementia-Related Psychosis: Increased Mortality and Cerebrovascular Adverse Events (CVAE), Including Stroke
Patients and caregivers should be advised that elderly patients with dementia-related psychosis treated with antipsychotic drugs are at an increased risk of death. Patients and caregivers should be advised that elderly patients with dementia-related psychosis treated with ZYPREXA had a significantly higher incidence of cerebrovascular adverse events (e.g., stroke, transient ischemic attack) compared with placebo.

ZYPREXA RELPREVV is not approved for elderly patients with dementia-related psychosis [see Boxed Warning and Warnings and Precautions (5.3)].

17.4 Neuroleptic Malignant Syndrome (NMS)
Patients and caregivers should be counseled that a potentially fatal symptom complex sometimes referred to as NMS has been reported in association with administration of antipsychotic drugs, including ZYPREXA. Signs and symptoms of NMS include hyperpyrexia, muscle rigidity, altered mental status, and evidence of autonomic instability (irregular pulse or blood pressure, tachycardia, diaphoresis, and cardiac dysrhythmia) [see Warnings and Precautions (5.5)].

17.5 Hyperglycemia
Patients should be advised of the potential risk of hyperglycemia-related adverse reactions related to ZYPREXA RELPREVV. Patients should be monitored regularly for worsening of glucose control. Patients who have diabetes should follow their doctor's instructions about how often to check their blood sugar while taking ZYPREXA RELPREVV [see Warnings and Precautions (5.6)].

17.6 Hyperlipidemia
Patients should be counseled that hyperlipidemia has occurred during treatment with ZYPREXA RELPREVV. Patients should have their lipid profile monitored regularly [see Warnings and Precautions (5.7)].

17.7 Weight Gain
Patients should be counseled that weight gain has occurred during treatment with ZYPREXA RELPREVV. Patients should have their weight monitored regularly [see Warnings and Precautions (5.8)].

17.8 Orthostatic Hypotension
Patients should be advised of the risk of orthostatic hypotension, and in association with the use of concomitant drugs that may potentiate the orthostatic effect of ZYPREXA RELPREVV, e.g., diazepam or alcohol [see Warnings and Precautions (5.10) and Drug Interactions (7)]. Patients should be advised to change positions carefully to help prevent orthostatic hypotension, and to lie down if they feel dizzy or faint, until they feel better. Patients should be advised to call their doctor if they experience any of the following signs and symptoms associated with orthostatic hypotension: dizziness, fast or slow heart beat, or fainting.

17.9 Potential for Cognitive and Motor Impairment
Because ZYPREXA RELPREVV has the potential to impair judgment, thinking, or motor skills, patients should be cautioned about operating hazardous machinery, including automobiles, until they are reasonably certain that ZYPREXA RELPREVV therapy does not affect them adversely. Additionally, due to the risk of post-injection delirium/sedation syndrome, patients should not drive or operate heavy machinery for the remainder of the day of each injection [see Dosage and Administration (2.1) and Warnings and Precautions (5.1, 5.14)].

17.10 Body Temperature Regulation
Patients should be advised regarding appropriate care in avoiding overheating and dehydration. Patients should be advised to call their doctor right away if they become severely ill and have some or all of these symptoms of dehydration: sweating too much or not at all, dry mouth, feeling very hot, feeling thirsty, not able to produce urine [see Warnings and Precautions (5.15)].

17.11 Concomitant Medication
Patients should be advised to inform their physicians if they are taking, or plan to take, ZYPREXA or Symbyax® (olanzapine/fluoxetine combination). Patients should also be advised to inform their physicians if they are taking, plan to take, or have stopped taking any prescription or over-the-counter drugs, including herbal supplements, since there is a potential for interactions [see Drug Interactions (7)].

17.12 Alcohol
Patients should be advised to avoid alcohol while taking ZYPREXA RELPREVV [see Drug Interactions (7.1)].

17.13 Use in Specific Populations
Pregnancy—Patients should be advised to notify their physician if they become pregnant or intend to become pregnant during therapy with ZYPREXA RELPREVV [see Use in Specific Populations (8.1)].

Nursing Mothers—Patients should be advised not to breastfeed an infant if they are taking ZYPREXA RELPREVV [see Use in Specific Populations (8.3)].

Pediatric Use—Safety and effectiveness of ZYPREXA RELPREVV in patients under 18 years have not been established [see Use in Specific Populations (8.4)].

Literature revised May 27, 2010

Eli Lilly and Company
Indianapolis, IN 46285, USA
Copyright © 2009, 2010, Eli Lilly and Company. All rights reserved.
PV 5922 AMP

Medication Guide
ZYPREXA® RELPREVV™ (zy-PREX-a REL-prev)
(olanzapine)
For Extended Release Injectable Suspension
Read the Medication Guide that comes with ZYPREXA RELPREVV before you start taking it and each time before you get an injection. There may be new information. This Medication Guide does not take the place of talking to your doctor about your medical condition or treatment. Talk with your doctor if there is something you do not understand or you want to learn more about ZYPREXA RELPREVV.

What is the most important information I should know about ZYPREXA RELPREVV?
To receive ZYPREXA RELPREVV you have to:
• talk to your doctor to understand the benefits and risks of ZYPREXA RELPREVV
• register in and agree to the rules of the ZYPREXA RELPREVV Patient Care Program

Serious side effects may happen when you take ZYPREXA RELPREVV, including:
Post-injection Delirium Sedation Syndrome (PDSS): PDSS is a serious reaction that can happen after you get a ZYPREXA RELPREVV injection if the medicine gets in your blood too fast. If this happens, you may have some of these symptoms:
• feel more sleepy than usual
• feel dizzy
• feel confused or disoriented
• trouble talking or walking
• muscles feel stiff or shaking
• feel weak
• feel grouchy or angry
• feel nervous or anxious
• higher blood pressure
• seizures
• pass out (become unconscious or coma)

If you have symptoms of PDSS, you need to get medical help or be taken to an emergency room right away.

Increased risk of death in elderly patients with dementia-related psychosis: Medicines like ZYPREXA RELPREVV can raise the risk of death in elderly people who have lost touch with reality (psychosis) due to confusion and memory loss (dementia). ZYPREXA RELPREVV is not approved for treating psychosis in the elderly with dementia.

High blood sugar (hyperglycemia): High blood sugar can happen if you have diabetes already or even if you have never had diabetes. In rare cases, this could lead to ketoacidosis (build up of acid in the blood due to ketones), coma, or death. Your doctor should do lab tests to check your blood sugar before you start taking ZYPREXA RELPREVV and during treatment. In people who do not have diabetes, sometimes high blood sugar goes away when ZYPREXA RELPREVV is stopped. People with diabetes and some people who did not have diabetes before taking ZYPREXA RELPREVV need to take medicine for high blood sugar even after they stop taking ZYPREXA RELPREVV.

If you have diabetes, follow your doctor's instructions about how often to check your blood sugar while taking ZYPREXA RELPREVV.

Call your doctor if you have any of these symptoms of high blood sugar (hyperglycemia) while taking ZYPREXA RELPREVV:
• feel very thirsty
• need to urinate more than usual
• feel very hungry
• feel weak or tired
• feel sick to your stomach
• feel confused, or your breath smells fruity.

High cholesterol and triglyceride levels in the blood (fat in the blood) may happen in people treated with ZYPREXA RELPREVV, especially in teenagers (13-17 years old). ZYPREXA RELPREVV is not approved in patients less than 18 years old. You may not have any symptoms, so your doctor should do blood tests to check your cholesterol and triglyceride levels before you start taking ZYPREXA RELPREVV and during treatment.

Increase in weight (weight gain): Weight gain is very common in people who take ZYPREXA RELPREVV. Teenagers (13-17 years old) are more likely to gain weight and to gain more weight than adults. ZYPREXA RELPREVV is not approved in patients less than 18 years old. Some people may gain a lot of weight while taking ZYPREXA RELPREVV, so you and your doctor should check your weight regularly. Talk to your doctor about ways to control weight gain, such as eating a healthy, balanced diet, and exercising.

Increased risk in teenagers (13-17 years old): ZYPREXA RELPREVV is not approved in patients less than 18 years old. Possible serious risks of weight gain and increases in cholesterol and triglycerides are more common in teenagers than in adults. You and your doctor should decide if other available treatments should be used first. Before your teenager takes ZYPREXA RELPREVV, talk with your doctor about the possible long-term risks of teenagers taking ZYPREXA RELPREVV.

What is ZYPREXA RELPREVV?

ZYPREXA RELPREVV is a long-acting prescription medicine given by injection used to treat schizophrenia in adults. The symptoms of schizophrenia include hearing voices, seeing things that are not there, having beliefs that are not true, and being suspicious or withdrawn. Treatment with ZYPREXA RELPREVV may lessen some of your symptoms of schizophrenia. If you do not think you are getting better, call your doctor.

It is not known if ZYPREXA RELPREVV is safe and works in children younger than 18 years old.

What should I tell my doctor before taking ZYPREXA RELPREVV?

ZYPREXA RELPREVV may not be right for you. Before starting ZYPREXA RELPREVV, tell your doctor if you have or had:

• heart problems
• seizures
• diabetes or high blood sugar levels (hyperglycemia)
• high cholesterol or triglyceride levels in your blood
• liver problems
• low or high blood pressure
• strokes or "mini-strokes" also called transient ischemic attacks (TIAs)
• Alzheimer's disease
• narrow-angle glaucoma
• enlarged prostate in men
• bowel obstruction
• breast cancer
• thoughts of suicide or hurting yourself
• any other medical condition
• are pregnant or plan to become pregnant. It is not known if ZYPREXA RELPREVV will harm your unborn baby.
• are breast-feeding or plan to breast-feed. ZYPREXA RELPREVV can pass into your breast milk and may harm your baby. You should not breast-feed while taking ZYPREXA RELPREVV. Talk to your doctor about the best way to feed your baby if you take ZYPREXA RELPREVV.

Tell your doctor if you exercise a lot or are in hot places often.

The symptoms of schizophrenia may include **thoughts of suicide** or of hurting yourself or others. If you have these thoughts at any time, tell your doctor or go to an emergency room right away.

Tell your doctor about all the medicines that you take, including prescription and nonprescription medicines, vitamins, and herbal supplements. ZYPREXA RELPREVV and some medicines may interact with each other and may not work as well, or cause possible serious side effects. Your doctor can tell you if it is safe to take ZYPREXA RELPREVV with your other medicines. Do not start or stop any medicine while taking ZYPREXA RELPREVV without talking to your doctor first.

How will I receive ZYPREXA RELPREVV?

• ZYPREXA RELPREVV will be injected into the muscle in your buttock (gluteus) by your doctor or nurse at the clinic.
• After receiving ZYPREXA RELPREVV, you will need to stay at the clinic for at least 3 hours.
• When you leave the clinic, someone must be with you.
• You should not drive or use heavy machinery for the rest of the day after receiving ZYPREXA RELPREVV.
• Call your doctor if you do not think you are getting better or have any concerns about your condition while taking ZYPREXA RELPREVV.

What should I avoid while taking ZYPREXA RELPREVV?

• ZYPREXA RELPREVV can cause sleepiness and may affect your ability to make decisions, think clearly, or react quickly. You should not drive, operate heavy machinery, or do other dangerous activities until you know how ZYPREXA RELPREVV affects you. You should not drive or operate heavy machinery for the rest of the day after each injection.
• Avoid drinking alcohol while taking ZYPREXA RELPREVV. Drinking alcohol while you take ZYPREXA

RELPREVV may make you sleepier than if you take ZYPREXA RELPREVV alone.

What are the possible side effects of ZYPREXA RELPREVV? Serious side effects may happen when you take ZYPREXA RELPREVV, including:

• See "What is the most important information I should know about ZYPREXA RELPREVV?", which describes the risk of post-injection delirium sedation syndrome (PDSS), increased risk of death in elderly people with dementia-related psychosis and the risks of high blood sugar, high cholesterol and triglyceride levels, and weight gain.
• Increased incidence of stroke or "mini-strokes" called transient ischemic attacks (TIAs) in elderly people with dementia-related psychosis (elderly people who have lost touch with reality due to confusion and memory loss). ZYPREXA RELPREVV is not approved for these patients.
• Neuroleptic Malignant Syndrome (NMS): NMS is a rare but very serious condition that can happen in people who take antipsychotic medicines, including ZYPREXA RELPREVV. NMS can cause death and must be treated in a hospital. Call your doctor right away if you become severely ill and have any of these symptoms:
  • high fever
  • excessive sweating
  • rigid muscles
  • confusion
  • changes in your breathing, heartbeat, and blood pressure.
• Tardive Dyskinesia: This condition causes body movements that keep happening and that you can not control. These movements usually affect the face and tongue. Tardive dyskinesia may not go away, even if you stop taking ZYPREXA RELPREVV. It may also start after you stop taking ZYPREXA RELPREVV. Tell your doctor if you get any body movements that you can not control.
• Decreased blood pressure when you change positions, with symptoms of dizziness, fast or slow heart beat, or fainting.
• Difficulty swallowing, that can cause food or liquid to get into your lungs.
• Seizures: Tell your doctor if you have a seizure during treatment with ZYPREXA RELPREVV.
• Problems with control of body temperature: You could become very hot, for instance when you exercise a lot or stay in an area that is very hot. It is important for you to drink water to avoid dehydration. Call your doctor right away if you become severely ill and have any of these symptoms of dehydration:
  • sweating too much or not at all
  • dry mouth
  • feeling very hot
  • feeling thirsty
  • not able to produce urine.

Common side effects of ZYPREXA RELPREVV include: headache, sleepiness or drowsiness, weight gain, dry mouth, diarrhea, nausea, common cold, eating more (increased appetite), vomiting, cough, back pain, or pain at the injection site.

Tell your doctor about any side effect that bothers you or that does not go away.

These are not all the possible side effects with ZYPREXA RELPREVV. For more information, ask your doctor or pharmacist.

Call your doctor for medical advice about side effects. You may report side effects to FDA at 1-800-FDA-1088.

General information about ZYPREXA RELPREVV

Medicines are sometimes prescribed for purposes other than those listed in a Medication Guide.

This Medication Guide summarizes the most important information about ZYPREXA RELPREVV. If you would like more information, talk with your doctor. You can ask your doctor or pharmacist for information about ZYPREXA RELPREVV that was written for healthcare professionals. For more information about ZYPREXA RELPREVV call 1-800-Lilly-Rx (1-800-545-5979) or visit www.zyprexarelprevv.com.

What are the ingredients in ZYPREXA RELPREVV?

Active ingredient: olanzapine

Inactive ingredients: carboxymethylcellulose sodium, mannitol, polysorbate 80, sodium hydroxide and/or hydrochloric acid for pH adjustment, and water for injection.

This Medication Guide has been approved by the U.S. Food and Drug Administration.

Medication Guide issued December 11, 2009

Eli Lilly and Company
Indianapolis, IN 46285, USA
www.zyprexarelprevv.com

PV 5940 AMP

Shown in Product Identification Guide, page 311

Lundbeck Inc.
FOUR PARKWAY NORTH
DEERFIELD, IL 60015

Medical Information:
Phone: 866-402-8520
Email: luinc_druginfo@lundbeck.com
To Report Adverse Events:
Phone: 800-455-1141
Email: luinc_safety@lundbeck.com
Corporate Offices:
Phone: 847-282-1000
Fax: 847-282-1001
Email: info@lundbeck.com
www.lundbeckinc.com

NEOPROFEN® ℞
[nē-ō-prō'fĕn]
(ibuprofen lysine)
Injection for intravenous use

HIGHLIGHTS OF PRESCRIBING INFORMATION
These highlights do not include all the information needed to use NeoProfen safely and effectively. See full prescribing information for NeoProfen.
NeoProfen (ibuprofen lysine)
Injection for intravenous use
Initial U.S. Approval: 2006

——RECENT MAJOR CHANGES——
Adverse Reactions, Post-marketing Experience - June 2008 Added the terms gastrointestinal perforation and necrotizing enterocolitis.

——INDICATIONS AND USAGE——
NeoProfen is indicated to close a clinically significant patent ductus arteriosus (PDA) in premature infants weighing between 500 and 1500 g, who are no more than 32 weeks gestational age when usual medical management is ineffective. The clinical trial was conducted among infants with an asymptomatic PDA. However, the consequences beyond 8 weeks after treatment have not been evaluated; therefore, treatment should be reserved for infants with clear evidence of a clinically significant PDA.

——DOSAGE AND ADMINISTRATION——
• A course of therapy is three doses administered I.V.
• An initial dose of 10 mg/kg is followed by two doses of 5 mg/kg each, after 24 and 48 hours
• All doses should be based on birth weight
• If anuria or marked oliguria (<0.6 mL/kg/hr) is evident at the scheduled time of the second or third dose, no additional dosage should be given until laboratory studies indicate that renal function has returned to normal
• If the ductus arteriosus closes or is significantly reduced in size after completion of the first course, no further doses are necessary
• If the ductus arteriosus fails to close, then a second course of NeoProfen, alternative pharmacological therapy, or surgery may be needed

——DOSAGE FORMS AND STRENGTHS——
• 10 mg/mL as a clear sterile preservative-free solution of the l-lysine salt of ibuprofen in a 2 mL single-use vial

——CONTRAINDICATIONS——
NeoProfen is contraindicated in preterm infants:
• With proven or suspected infection that is untreated
• With congenital heart disease in whom patency of the PDA is necessary for satisfactory pulmonary or systemic blood flow
• With impaired renal function
• With thrombocytopenia, coagulation defects or who are bleeding
• With or who are suspected of having necrotizing enterocolitis

——WARNINGS AND PRECAUTIONS——
• NeoProfen has not been assessed for neurodevelopmental outcome and growth
• NeoProfen may alter the usual signs of infection.
• NeoProfen can inhibit platelet aggregation, and has been shown to prolong bleeding time in normal adult subjects
• Ibuprofen has been shown to displace bilirubin from albumin binding-sites
• NeoProfen should be administered carefully to avoid extravascular injection or leakage

——ADVERSE REACTIONS——
Most common adverse reactions (≥10%) are sepsis, anemia, intraventricular bleeding, apnea, gastrointestinal disorders, impaired renal function, respiratory infection, skin lesions, hypoglycemia, hypocalcemia, respiratory failure. (6)
To report SUSPECTED ADVERSE REACTIONS, contact Lundbeck Inc. at 1-800-455-1141 or FDA at 1-800-FDA-1088 or www.fda.gov/medwatch.

—————DRUG INTERACTIONS—————
Drug interactions in neonates have not been assessed.
See 17 for PATIENT COUNSELING INFORMATION

Revised: 01/2010

FULL PRESCRIBING INFORMATION: CONTENTS*

FULL PRESCRIBING INFORMATION

1 INDICATIONS AND USAGE

NeoProfen is indicated to close a clinically significant patent ductus arteriosus (PDA) in premature infants weighing between 500 and 1500 g, who are no more than 32 weeks gestational age when usual medical management (e.g., fluid restriction, diuretics, respiratory support, etc.) is ineffective. The clinical trial was conducted among infants with an asymptomatic PDA. However, the consequences beyond 8 weeks after treatment have not been evaluated; therefore, treatment should be reserved for infants with clear evidence of a clinically significant PDA.

2 DOSAGE AND ADMINISTRATION

2.1 Recommended Dose

A course of therapy is three doses of NeoProfen administered intravenously (administration via an umbilical arterial line has not been evaluated). An initial dose of 10 mg per kilogram is followed by two doses of 5 mg per kilogram each, after 24 and 48 hours. All doses should be based on birth weight. If anuria or marked oliguria (urinary output 0.6 mL/kg/hr) is evident at the scheduled time of the second or third dose of NeoProfen, no additional dosage should be given until laboratory studies indicate that renal function has returned to normal. If the ductus arteriosus closes or is significantly reduced in size after completion of the first course of NeoProfen, no further doses are necessary. If during continued medical management the ductus arteriosus fails to close or reopens, then a second course of NeoProfen, alternative pharmacological therapy, or surgery may be necessary.

2.2 Directions for Use

For intravenous administration only. Parenteral drug products should be inspected visually for particulate matter and discoloration prior to administration whenever solution and container permit.

For administration, NeoProfen should be diluted to an appropriate volume with dextrose or saline. NeoProfen should be prepared for infusion and administered within 30 minutes of preparation and infused continuously over a period of 15 minutes. The drug should be administered via the IV port that is nearest the insertion site. After the first withdrawal from the vial, any solution remaining must be discarded because NeoProfen contains no preservative.

Since NeoProfen is potentially irritating to tissues, it should be administered carefully to avoid extravasation.

NeoProfen should not be simultaneously administered in the same intravenous line with Total Parenteral Nutrition (TPN). If necessary, TPN should be interrupted for a 15-minute period prior to and after drug administration. Line patency should be maintained by using dextrose or saline.

3 DOSAGE FORMS AND STRENGTHS

10 mg/mL as a clear sterile preservative-free solution of the L-lysine salt of ibuprofen in a 2 mL single-use vial

4 CONTRAINDICATIONS

NeoProfen is contraindicated in:
- Preterm infants with proven or suspected infection that is untreated;
- Preterm infants with congenital heart disease in whom patency of the PDA is necessary for satisfactory pulmonary or systemic blood flow (e.g., pulmonary atresia, severe tetralogy of Fallot, severe coarctation of the aorta);
- Preterm infants who are bleeding, especially those with active intracranial hemorrhage or gastrointestinal bleeding;
- Preterm infants with thrombocytopenia;
- Preterm infants with coagulation defects;
- Preterm infants with or who are suspected of having necrotizing enterocolitis;
- Preterm infants with significant impairment of renal function.

5 WARNINGS AND PRECAUTIONS

5.1 General

There are no long-term evaluations of the infants treated with ibuprofen at durations greater than the 36 weeks postconceptual age observation period. Ibuprofen's effects on neurodevelopmental outcome and growth as well as disease processes associated with prematurity (such as retinopathy of prematurity and chronic lung disease) have not been assessed.

5.2 Infection

NeoProfen may alter the usual signs of infection. The physician must be continually on the alert and should use the drug with extra care in the presence of controlled infection and in infants at risk of infection.

5.3 Platelet Aggregation

NeoProfen, like other non-steroidal anti-inflammatory agents, can inhibit platelet aggregation. Preterm infants should be observed for signs of bleeding. Ibuprofen has been shown to prolong bleeding time (but within the normal range) in normal adult subjects. This effect may be exaggerated in patients with underlying hemostatic defects (see CONTRAINDICATIONS).

5.4 Bilirubin Displacement

Ibuprofen has been shown to displace bilirubin from albumin binding-sites; therefore, it should be used with caution in patients with elevated total bilirubin.

5.5 Administration

NeoProfen should be administered carefully to avoid extravascular injection or leakage, as solution may be irritating to tissue.

6 ADVERSE REACTIONS

6.1 Clinical Trials Experience

The most frequently reported adverse events with NeoProfen were as shown in Table 1.

Table 1. Adverse Events within 30 Days of Therapy in the Multicenter Study*

Adverse Event	% Incidence	
	NeoProfen	Placebo
Sepsis	43	37
Anemia	32	25
Total Bleeding**	32	29
Intraventricular Hemorrhage, Grades 1/2	15	13
Intraventricular Hemorrhage, Grades 3/4	15	10
Other Bleeding	6	13
Intraventricular Hemorrhage, All Grades	29	24
Apnea	28	26
Gastrointestinal Disorders non-Necrotizing Enterocolitis	22	18
Total Renal Events**	21	15
Renal Failure	1	3
Renal Insufficiency, Impairment	6	4
Urine Output Reduced	3	1
Blood Creatinine Increased	3	1
Blood Urea Increased with Hematuria	1	1
Blood Urea Increased	7	4
Respiratory Infection	19	13
Skin Lesion/Irritation	16	6
Hypoglycemia	12	6
Hypocalcemia	12	9
Respiratory Failure	10	4
Urinary Tract Infection	9	4
Adrenal Insufficiency	7	1
Hypernatremia	7	4
Edema	4	0
Atelectasis	4	1

* Within 30 days of therapy, with an event rate greater on NeoProfen than on placebo, and greater than 2 events on NeoProfen.

** A given subject may have experienced more than one specific event within these adverse event categories. Only the most severe grade of IVH counted for a given subject.

6.2 Renal Function

Compared to placebo, there was a small decrease in urinary output in the ibuprofen group on days 2-6 of life, with a compensatory increase in urine output on day 9. In other studies, adverse events classified as renal insufficiency including oliguria, elevated BUN, elevated creatinine, or renal failure were reported in ibuprofen treated infants.

6.3 Additional Adverse Events

The adverse events reported in the multicenter study and of unknown association include tachycardia, cardiac failure, abdominal distension, gastroesophageal reflux, gastritis, ileus, inguinal hernia, injection site reactions, cholestasis, various infections, feeding problems, convulsions, jaundice, hypotension, and various laboratory abnormalities including neutropenia, thrombocytopenia, and hyperglycemia.

6.4 Post-marketing Experience

The following adverse reactions have been identified from spontaneous post-marketing reports or published literature: gastrointestinal perforation and necrotizing enterocolitis. Because these reactions are reported voluntarily from a population of uncertain size, it is not always possible to reliably estimate their frequency, or establish a causal relationship to drug exposure.

7 DRUG INTERACTIONS

Drug interactions of NeoProfen in neonates have not been assessed.

10 OVERDOSAGE

The following signs and symptoms have occurred in individuals (not necessarily in premature infants) following an overdose of oral ibuprofen: breathing difficulties, coma, drowsiness, irregular heartbeat, kidney failure, low blood pressure, seizures, and vomiting. There are no specific measures to treat acute overdosage with NeoProfen. The patient should be followed for several days because gastrointestinal ulceration and hemorrhage may occur.

11 DESCRIPTION

NeoProfen® is a clear sterile preservative-free solution of the l-lysine salt of (±)-ibuprofen which is the active ingredient. (±)-Ibuprofen is a nonsteroidal anti-inflammatory agent (NSAID). L-lysine is used to create a water-soluble drug product salt suitable for intravenous administration. Each mL of NeoProfen contains 17.1 mg of ibuprofen lysine (equivalent to 10 mg of (±)-ibuprofen) in Water for Injection, USP. The pH is adjusted to 7.0 with sodium hydroxide or hydrochloric acid.

The structural formula is:

$(CH_3)_2 CHCH_2$———$CHCOOH$ (CH_3) $H_2N (CH_2)_4 CHCOOH$ (NH_2)

NeoProfen is designated chemically as α-methyl-4-(2-methyl propyl) benzeneacetic acid lysine salt. Its molecular weight is 352.48. Its empirical formula is $C_{19}H_{32}N_2O_4$. It occurs as a white crystalline solid which is soluble in water and slightly soluble in ethanol.

12 CLINICAL PHARMACOLOGY

12.1 Mechanism of Action

The mechanism of action through which ibuprofen causes closure of a patent ductus arteriosus (PDA) in neonates is not known. In adults, ibuprofen is an inhibitor of prostaglandin synthesis.

12.2 Pharmacokinetics and Bioavailability Studies

The pharmacokinetic data were obtained from 54 NeoProfen-treated premature infants included in a double-blind, placebo-controlled, randomized, multicenter study. Infants were less than 30 weeks gestational age, weighed between 500 and 1000 g, and exhibited asymptomatic PDA with evidence of echocardiographic documentation of ductal shunting. Dosing was initially 10 mg/kg followed by 5 mg/kg at 24 and 48 hours.

The population average clearance and volume of distribution values of racemic ibuprofen for premature infants at birth were 3 mL/kg/h and 320 mL/kg, respectively. Clearance increased rapidly with post-natal age (an average increase of approximately 0.5 mL/kg/h per day). Inter-individual variability in clearance and volume of distribution were 55% and 14%, respectively. In general, the half-life in infants is more than 10 times longer than in adults.

The metabolism and excretion of ibuprofen in premature infants have not been studied.

In adults, renal elimination of unchanged ibuprofen accounts for only 10-15% of the dose. The excretion of ibuprofen and metabolites occurs rapidly in both urine and feces. Approximately 80% of the dose administered orally is recovered in urine as hydroxyl and carboxyl metabolites, respectively, as a mixture of conjugated and unconjugated forms. Ibuprofen is eliminated primarily by metabolism in the liver where CYP2C9 mediates the 2- and 3-hydroxylations of R- and S-ibuprofen. Ibuprofen and its metabolites are further conjugated to acyl glucuronides.

In neonates, renal function and the enzymes associated with drug metabolism are underdeveloped at birth and substantially increase in the days after birth.

14 CLINICAL STUDIES

In a double-blind, multicenter clinical study premature infants of birth weight between 500 and 1000 g, less than 30 weeks post- conceptional age, and with echocardiographic evidence of a PDA were randomized to placebo or NeoProfen. These infants were asymptomatic from their PDA at the time of enrollment. The primary efficacy parameter was the need for rescue therapy (indomethacin, open-label ibuprofen, or surgery) to treat a hemodynamically significant PDA by study day 14. An infant was rescued if there was clinical evidence of a hemodynamically significant PDA that was echocardiographically confirmed. A hemodynamically significant PDA was defined by three of the following five criteria - bounding pulse, hyperdynamic precordium, pulmonary edema, increased cardiac silhouette, or systolic murmur - or hemodynamically significant ductus as determined by a neonatologist.

One hundred and thirty-six premature infants received either placebo or NeoProfen (10 mg/kg on the first dose and 5 mg/kg at 24 and 48 hours). Mean birth age was 1.5 days (range: 4.6-73.0 hours), mean gestational age was 26 weeks (range: 23-30 weeks), and mean weight was 798 g (range: 530-1015 g). All infants had a documented PDA with evidence of ductal shunting. As shown in Table 2, 25% of infants on NeoProfen required rescue therapy versus 48% of infants on placebo (p=0.003 from logistic regression controlling for site).

Table 2. Summary of Efficacy Results, n (%)

	NeoProfen N=68	Placebo N=68
Required rescue through study day 14		
Total	17 (25)	33 (48)
By age at treatment		
Birth to < 24 hours	3/14 (21)	8/16 (50)
24-48 hours	9/32 (28)	16/37 (43)
> 48 hours	5/22 (23)	9/15 (60)
Echocardiographically proven PDA prior to rescue	17 (100)	32 (97)
Reasons for Rescue		
Hemodynamically significant PDA per neonatologist	14 (82)	25 (76)
Bounding pulse	6 (35)	12 (36)
Systolic murmur	6 (35)	15 (45)
Pulmonary Edema	3 (18)	5 (15)
Hyperdynamic precordium	2 (12)	3 (9)
Increased cardiac silhouette	1 (6)	5 (15)

Of the infants requiring rescue within the first 14 days after the first dose of study drug, no statistically significant difference was observed between the NeoProfen and placebo groups for mean age at start of first rescue treatment (8.7 days, range 4-15 days, for the NeoProfen group and 6.9 days, range 2-15 days, for the placebo group).

The groups were similar in the number of deaths by day 14, the number of patients on a ventilator or requiring oxygenation at day 1, 4 and 14, the number of patients requiring surgical ligation of their PDA (12%), the number of cases of Pulmonary Hemorrhage and Pulmonary Hypertension by day 14, and Bronchopulmonary Dysplasia at day 28. In addition, no significant differences were noted in the incidences of Stage 2 and 3 Necrotizing Enterocolitis, Grades 3 and 4 Intraventricular Hemorrhage, Periventricular Leukomalacia and Retinopathy of Prematurity between groups as determined at 36±1 weeks adjusted gestational age.

Two supportive studies also determined that ibuprofen, either prophylactically (n=433, weight range: 400-2165 g) or as treatment (n=210, weight range: 400-2370 g), was superior to placebo (or no treatment) in preventing the need for rescue therapy for a symptomatic PDA.

16 HOW SUPPLIED/STORAGE AND HANDLING

How Supplied

NeoProfen (ibuprofen lysine) Injection is dispensed in clear glass single-use vials, each containing 2 mL of sterile solution (NDC 67386-122-52). The solution is not buffered and contains no preservatives. Each milliliter contains 17.1 mg/mL (±)-ibuprofen L-lysine [equivalent to 10 mg/mL (±)-ibuprofen] dissolved in Water for Injection, USP. NeoProfen is supplied in a carton containing 3 single-use vials.

Storage and Handling

Store at 20-25°C (68-77°F); excursions permitted 15-30°C (59-86°F) [see USP Controlled Room Temperature]. Protect from light. Store vials in carton until contents have been used.

17 PATIENT COUNSELING INFORMATION

17.1 General

Patients' caregivers should be informed that the effects of ibuprofen on infants' neurodevelopmental outcome, growth and disease process with prematurity have not been assessed in long-term studies.

17.2 Infection

NeoProfen may alter signs of infection. Patients' caregivers should be informed that the infant will be carefully monitored for any signs of infection.

17.3 Platelet Aggregation

Patients' caregivers should be informed that like other NSAIDS, NeoProfen can inhibit clot formation therefore their infant will be monitored for any signs of bleeding.

17.4 Bilirubin Displacement

Patients' caregivers should be informed that the infants' blood will be tested for increased levels of total bilirubin.

17.5 Administration

Patients' caregivers should be informed that the infants' skin and tissues will be monitored as leakage from administration may be irritating to tissue.

Manufactured for: Lundbeck Inc., Deerfield, IL 60015, U.S.A.

®Trademark of Lundbeck Inc.

Revised: January 2010

PANHEMATIN® ℞

[păn-hē′ma-tin]

Hemin For Injection

Rx only

For intravenous infusion only.

> PANHEMATIN (hemin for injection) should only be used by physicians experienced in the management of porphyrias in hospitals where the recommended clinical and laboratory diagnostic and monitoring techniques are available.
>
> PANHEMATIN therapy should be considered after an appropriate period of alternate therapy (i.e., 400 g glucose/day for 1 to 2 days). (See "WARNINGS", "PRECAUTIONS" and "DOSAGE AND ADMINISTRATION" sections.)

DESCRIPTION

PANHEMATIN (hemin for injection) is an enzyme inhibitor derived from processed red blood cells. Hemin for injection was known previously as hematin. The term hematin has been used to describe the chemical reaction product of hemin and sodium carbonate solution. Hemin is an iron containing metalloporphyrin. Chemically hemin is represented as chloro [7,12-diethenyl-3,8,13,17-tetramethyl-21H,23H-porphine-2,18-dipropanoato(2-)-N^{21},N^{22},N^{23},N^{24}] iron. The structural formula for hemin is:

PANHEMATIN is a sterile, lyophilized powder suitable for intravenous administration after reconstitution. Each dispensing vial of PANHEMATIN contains the equivalent of 313 mg hemin, 215 mg sodium carbonate and 300 mg of sorbitol. The pH may have been adjusted with hydrochloric acid; the product contains no preservatives. When mixed as directed with Sterile Water for Injection, USP, each 43 mL provides the equivalent of approximately 301 mg hemin (7 mg/mL).

CLINICAL PHARMACOLOGY

Heme acts to limit the hepatic and/or marrow synthesis of porphyrin. This action is likely due to the inhibition of δ-aminolevulinic acid synthetase, the enzyme which limits the rate of the porphyrin/heme biosynthetic pathway. The exact mechanism by which hematin produces symptomatic improvement in patients with acute episodes of the hepatic porphyrias has not been elucidated.[1,9]

Following intravenous administration of hematin in nonjaundiced human patients, an increase in fecal urobilinogen can be observed which is roughly proportional to the amount of hematin administered. This suggests an enterohepatic pathway as at least one route of elimination. Bilirubin metabolites are also excreted in the urine following hematin injections.[9]

PANHEMATIN (hemin for injection) therapy for the acute porphyrias is not curative. After discontinuation of PANHEMATIN treatment, symptoms generally return although in some cases remission is prolonged. Some neurological symptoms have improved weeks to months after therapy although little or no response was noted at the time of treatment.

Other aspects of human pharmacokinetics have not been defined.

INDICATIONS AND USAGE

PANHEMATIN (hemin for injection) is indicated for the amelioration of recurrent attacks of acute intermittent porphyria temporally related to the menstrual cycle in susceptible women.

Manifestations such as pain, hypertension, tachycardia, abnormal mental status and mild to progressive neurologic signs may be controlled in selected patients with this disorder.

Similar findings have been reported in other patients with acute intermittent porphyria, porphyria variegata and hereditary coproporphyria. PANHEMATIN is not indicated in porphyria cutanea tarda.

CONTRAINDICATIONS

PANHEMATIN is contraindicated in patients with known hypersensitivity to this drug.

WARNINGS

PANHEMATIN is made from human blood. Products made from human blood may contain infectious agents, such as viruses, that can cause disease. The risk that such products will transmit an infectious agent has been reduced by screening blood donors for prior exposure to certain viruses, by testing for the presence of certain current virus infections, and by inactivating certain viruses. Despite these measures, such products can still potentially transmit disease. There is also the possibility that unknown infectious agents may be present in such products. ALL infections thought by a physician possibly to have been transmitted by this product should be reported by the physician or other healthcare provider to Lundbeck Inc., (1-800-455-1141). The physician should discuss the risks and benefits of this product with the patient.

Because this product is made from human blood, it may carry a risk of transmitting infectious agents, e.g., viruses, and theoretically, the Creutzfeldt-Jakob disease (CJD) agent.

PANHEMATIN therapy is intended to limit the rate of porphyria/heme biosynthesis possibly by inhibiting the enzyme δ-aminolevulinic acid synthetase. For this reason, drugs such as estrogens, barbituric acid derivatives and steroid metabolites which increase the activity of δ-aminolevulinic acid synthetase should be avoided.

Also, because hemin for injection has exhibited transient, mild anticoagulant effects during clinical studies, concurrent anticoagulant therapy should be avoided.[9] The extent and duration of the hypocoagulable state induced by PANHEMATIN has not been established.

PRECAUTIONS

General

Clinical benefit from PANHEMATIN depends on prompt administration. Attacks of porphyria may progress to a point where irreversible neuronal damage has occurred. PANHEMATIN therapy is intended to prevent an attack from reaching the critical stage of neuronal degeneration. PANHEMATIN is not effective in repairing neuronal damage.[9]

Recommended dosage guidelines should be strictly followed. Reversible renal shutdown has been observed in a case where an excessive hematin dose (12.2 mg/kg) was administered in a single infusion. Oliguria and increased nitrogen retention occurred although the patient remained asymptomatic.[4] No worsening of renal function has been seen with administration of recommended dosages of hematin.[9]

A large arm vein or a central venous catheter should be utilized for the administration of PANHEMATIN to avoid the possibility of phlebitis.

Since reconstituted PANHEMATIN is not transparent, any undissolved particulate matter is difficult to see when inspected visually. Therefore, terminal filtration through a sterile 0.45 micron or smaller filter is recommended.

Tests for Diagnosis and Monitoring of Therapy

Before PANHEMATIN therapy is begun, the presence of acute porphyria must be diagnosed using the following criteria:[9]

1. Presence of clinical symptoms.
2. Positive Watson-Schwartz or Hoesch test. (A negative Watson-Schwartz or Hoesch test indicates a porphyric attack is highly unlikely. When in doubt quantitative measures of δ-aminolevulinic acid and porphobilinogen in serum or urine may aid in diagnosis.)

Urinary concentrations of the following compounds may be *monitored* during PANHEMATIN therapy. Drug effect will be demonstrated by a decrease in one or more of the following compounds.[3-6]

ALA - δ-aminolevulinic acid
UPG - uroporphyrinogen
PBG - porphobilinogen
coproporphyrin

CARCINOGENESIS, MUTAGENESIS, IMPAIRMENT OF FERTILITY

PANHEMATIN was not mutagenic in bacteria systems *in vitro* and was not clastogenic in mammalian systems *in vitro* and *in vivo*. No data are available on potential for carcinogenicity or impairment of fertility in animals or humans.

Pregnancy

Teratogenic effects-Pregnancy Category C: Animal reproduction studies have not been conducted with hematin. It is also not known whether hematin can cause fetal harm when administered to a pregnant woman or can affect reproduction capacity. For this reason PANHEMATIN should not be given to a pregnant woman unless the expected benefits are sufficiently important to the health and welfare of the patient to outweigh the unknown hazard to the fetus.

Nursing Mothers

It is not known whether this drug is excreted in human milk. Because many drugs are excreted in human milk, caution should be exercised when PANHEMATIN is administered to a nursing woman.

Pediatric Use

Safety and effectiveness in pediatric patients under 16 years of age have not been established.

Geriatric Use

Clinical studies in PANHEMATIN did not include sufficient numbers of subjects aged 65 and over to determine whether they respond differently from younger subjects. Other reported clinical experience has not identified differences in response between the elderly and younger patients. In general, dose selection for an elderly patient should be cautious, usually starting at the low end of the dosing range, reflecting the greater frequency of decreased hepatic, renal, or cardiac function, and of concomitant disease or other drug therapy.

ADVERSE REACTIONS

Reversible renal shutdown has occurred with administration of excessive doses (See "PRECAUTIONS" section). Phlebitis with or without leucocytosis and with or without mild pyrexia has occurred after administration of hematin through small arm veins.

There have been post-marketing and literature reports of thrombocytopenia and coagulopathy (including prolonged prothrombin time and prolonged partial thromboplastin time) in patients receiving PANHEMATIN. The initial literature report[8] described coagulopathy occurring in a patient receiving hematin therapy. This patient exhibited prolonged prothrombin time and partial thromboplastin time, thrombocytopenia, mild hypofibrogenemia, mild elevation of fibrin split products, and a 10% fall in hematocrit. Iron overload and serum ferritin increased have also been reported. Because these reactions are reported voluntarily from a population of uncertain size, it is not always possible to reliably estimate their frequency, or establish a causal relationship to drug exposure.

To report SUSPECTED ADVERSE REACTIONS, contact Lundbeck Inc. at 1-800-455-1141 or FDA at 1-800-FDA-1088 or *www.fda.gov/medwatch.*

OVERDOSAGE

Reversible renal shutdown has been observed in a case where an excessive hematin dose (12.2 mg/kg) was administered in a single infusion. Treatment of this case consisted of ethacrynic acid and mannitol.[7]

DOSAGE AND ADMINISTRATION

Before administering PANHEMATIN, an appropriate period of alternate therapy (i.e., 400 g glucose/day for 1 to 2 days) must be considered. If improvement is unsatisfactory for the treatment of acute attacks of porphyria, an intravenous infusion of PANHEMATIN containing a dose of 1 to 4 mg/kg/day of hematin should be given over a period of 10 to 15 minutes for 3 to 14 days based on the clinical signs. In more severe cases this dose may be repeated no earlier than every 12 hours. No more than 6 mg/kg of hematin should be given in any 24 hour period.

After reconstitution each mL of PANHEMATIN contains the equivalent of approximately 7 mg of hematin. The drug may be administered directly from the vial.

Dosage Calculation Table
1 mg hematin equivalent = 0.14 mL PANHEMATIN
2 mg hematin equivalent = 0.28 mL PANHEMATIN
3 mg hematin equivalent = 0.42 mL PANHEMATIN
4 mg hematin equivalent = 0.56 mL PANHEMATIN

Since reconstituted PANHEMATIN is not transparent, any undissolved particulate matter is difficult to see when inspected visually. Therefore, terminal filtration through a sterile 0.45 micron or smaller filter is recommended.

Preparation of Solution:

Reconstitute PANHEMATIN by aseptically adding 43 mL of Sterile Water for Injection, USP, to the dispensing vial. Immediately after adding diluent, the product should be shaken well for a period of 2 to 3 minutes to aid dissolution.

NOTE: Because PANHEMATIN contains no preservative and because PANHEMATIN undergoes rapid chemical decomposition in solution, it should not be reconstituted until immediately before use. After the first withdrawal from the vial, any solution remaining must be discarded.

No drug or chemical agent should be added to a PANHEMATIN fluid admixture unless its effect on the chemical and physical stability has first been determined.

HOW SUPPLIED

PANHEMATIN is supplied as a sterile, lyophilized black powder in single dose dispensing vials (NDC 67386-701-54). When mixed as directed with Sterile Water for Injection, USP, each 43 mL provides the equivalent of approximately 301 mg hematin (7 mg/mL). Store lyophilized powder in refrigerator at 2-8°C (36-46°F) until time of use.

Caution: The packaging (vial stopper) of this product contains natural rubber latex which may cause allergic reactions.

REFERENCES

1. Bickers, D., Treatment of the Porphyrias: Mechanisms of Action, J Invest Dermatol 77(1):107-113, 1981.
2. Watson, C. J., Hematin and Porphyria, editorial, N Engl J Med 293(12):605-607, September 18, 1975.
3. Lamon, J. M., Hematin Therapy for Acute Porphyria, Medicine 58(3):252-269, 1979.
4. Dhar, G J., et al., Effects of Hematin in Hepatic Porphyria, Ann Intern Med 83:20-30, 1975.
5. Watson, C. J., et al., Use of Hematin in the Acute Attack of the "Inducible" Hepatic Porphyrias, Adv Intern Med 23:265-286, 1978.
6. McColl, K. E., et al., Treatment with Haematin in Acute Hepatic Porphyria, Q J Med, New Series L (198):161-174, Spring, 1981.
7. Dhar, G. J., et al., Transitory Renal Failure Following Rapid Administration of a Relatively Large Amount of Hematin in a Patient with Acute Intermittent Porphyria in Clinical Remission, Acta Med Scand 203:437-443, 1978.
8. Morris, D.L., et al., Coagulopathy Associated with Hematin Treatment for Acute Intermittent Porphyria, Ann Intern Med 95:700-701, 1981.
9. Pierach, C. A., Hematin Therapy for the Porphyric Attack, Semin Liver Dis 2(2):125-131, May, 1982.

Manufactured by: APP Pharmaceuticals, Raleigh, NC 27616, U.S.A.
For: Lundbeck Inc., Deerfield, IL 60015, U.S.A.
U.S. Lic. No. 1822
® Trademark of Lundbeck Inc.
Revised: September 2010
Shown in Product Identification Guide, page 311

SABRIL®   ℞

[*SAY-bril*]
(vigabatrin)
for Oral Solution
For Oral Administration Only
Rx Only

HIGHLIGHTS OF PRESCRIBING INFORMATION
These highlights do not include all the information needed to use SABRIL safely and effectively. See full prescribing information for SABRIL.
Sabril® (vigabatrin) for Oral Solution
For Oral Administration Only   Rx Only
Initial U.S. Approval: 2009

> **WARNING: VISION LOSS**
> *See full prescribing information for complete boxed warning*
> * SABRIL causes progressive and permanent bilateral concentric visual field constriction in a high percentage of patients. In some cases, SABRIL may also reduce visual acuity.
> * Risk increases with total dose and duration of use, but no exposure to SABRIL is known that is free of risk of vision loss
> * Risk of new and worsening vision loss continues as long as SABRIL is used, and possibly after discontinuing SABRIL
> * Periodic vision testing is required for patients on SABRIL, but cannot reliably prevent vision damage
> * Because of the risk of permanent vision loss, SABRIL is available only through a special restricted distribution program

———INDICATIONS AND USAGE———
SABRIL is an antiepileptic drug (AED) indicated for:
* **Infantile Spasms (IS) - 1 Month to 2 Years of Age** (1.1)

———DOSAGE AND ADMINISTRATION———
* Infantile Spasms: Initiate therapy at 50 mg/kg/day twice daily increasing total daily dose per instructions to a maximum of 150 mg/kg/day (2.1)
* Dose adjustment recommended in renally impaired patients (2.2)
* Reduce dose gradually upon discontinuation (2.3)

———DOSAGE FORMS AND STRENGTHS———
Powder for Oral Solution: 500 mg (3.1)

———CONTRAINDICATIONS———
None (4)

———WARNINGS AND PRECAUTIONS———
* SABRIL causes permanent vision loss (5.1)
* Abnormal MRI signal changes have been reported in some infants with IS receiving SABRIL (5.3)
* Antiepileptic drugs, including SABRIL, increase the risk of suicidal thoughts and behavior (5.5)
* Dose should be tapered gradually to avoid withdrawal seizures (5.6)
* SABRIL causes anemia (5.7)
* SABRIL causes somnolence and fatigue (5.8)
* SABRIL causes peripheral neuropathy (5.9)
* SABRIL causes weight gain (5.10)
* SABRIL causes edema (5.11)

———ADVERSE REACTIONS———
Most common adverse reactions described in adults (change of ≥5% over placebo) in addition to permanent vision loss in adult controlled trials with vigabatrin were fatigue, somnolence, nystagmus, tremor, vision blurred, memory impairment, weight gain, arthralgia, abnormal coordination, and confusional state (6.1)
To report SUSPECTED ADVERSE REACTIONS, contact Lundbeck Inc. at 1-800-455-1141 or www.lundbeckinc.com or FDA at 1-800-FDA-1088 or www.fda.gov/medwatch.

———DRUG INTERACTIONS———
* Decreased phenytoin plasma levels have been reported (7.1)

———USE IN SPECIFIC POPULATIONS———
* Pregnancy: Based on animal data, may cause fetal harm. Pregnancy registry available (8.1)

- Nursing Mothers: SABRIL is excreted in human milk (8.3)
- Renal Impairment: Dose adjustment recommended (2.2, 8.5, 8.6)

See 17 for PATIENT COUNSELING INFORMATION and Medication Guide

Revised: 04/2010

FULL PRESCRIBING INFORMATION: CONTENTS*

* Sections or subsections omitted from the full prescribing information are not listed

FULL PRESCRIBING INFORMATION

WARNING: VISION LOSS
- SABRIL causes permanent vision loss in infants, children and adults. Because assessing vision loss is difficult in children, the frequency and extent of vision loss in infants and children is poorly characterized. For this reason, the data described below is primarily based on the adult experience.
- In adults, SABRIL causes permanent bilateral concentric visual field constriction in 30 percent or more of patients that ranges in severity from mild to severe, including tunnel vision to within 10 degrees of visual

---

fixation, and can result in disability. In some cases, SABRIL also can damage the central retina and may decrease visual acuity.
- The onset of vision loss from SABRIL is unpredictable, and can occur within weeks of starting treatment or sooner, or at any time during treatment, even after months or years.
- The risk of vision loss increases with increasing dose and cumulative exposure, but there is no dose or exposure known to be free of risk of vision loss.
- It is possible that vision loss can worsen despite discontinuing SABRIL.
- Because of the risk of vision loss, SABRIL should be withdrawn from patients with infantile spasms who fail to show substantial clinical benefit within 2 to 4 weeks of initiation, or sooner if treatment failure becomes obvious. Patient response to and continued need for SABRIL should be periodically reassessed.
- In infants and children, vision loss may not be detected until it is severe. Nonetheless, vision should be assessed to the extent possible at baseline (no later than 4 weeks after starting SABRIL) and at least every 3 months during therapy. Once detected, vision loss due to SABRIL is not reversible. Vision testing is also required about 3 to 6 months after the discontinuation of SABRIL therapy.
- Symptoms of vision loss from SABRIL are unlikely to be recognized by the parent or caregiver before vision loss is severe. Vision loss of milder severity, although unrecognized by the caregiver, may still adversely affect function.
- SABRIL should not be used in patients with, or at high risk of, other types of irreversible vision loss unless the benefits of treatment clearly outweigh the risks. The interaction of other types of irreversible vision damage with vision damage from SABRIL has not been well-characterized, but is likely adverse.
- SABRIL should not be used with other drugs associated with serious adverse ophthalmic effects such as retinopathy or glaucoma unless the benefits clearly outweigh the risks
- The lowest dose and shortest exposure to SABRIL should be used that is consistent with clinical objectives
- The possibility that vision loss from SABRIL may be more common, more severe or have more severe functional consequences in infants and children than in adults cannot be excluded.

Because of the risk of permanent vision loss, SABRIL is available only through a special restricted distribution program called SHARE, by calling 1-888-45-SHARE. Only prescribers and pharmacies registered with SHARE may prescribe and distribute SABRIL. In addition, SABRIL may be dispensed only to patients who are enrolled in and meet all conditions of SHARE [see WARNINGS AND PRECAUTIONS, Distribution Program for SABRIL (5.2)].

1 INDICATIONS AND USAGE

1.1 Infantile Spasms (1 Month to 2 Years of Age)
SABRIL® is indicated as monotherapy for pediatric patients with infantile spasms (IS) for whom the potential benefits outweigh the potential risk of vision loss [see WARNINGS AND PRECAUTIONS, Vision Loss (5.1)].

2 DOSAGE AND ADMINISTRATION

2.1 Infantile Spasms (1 Month to 2 Years of Age)
Physicians should review and discuss the Medication Guide with the caregiver(s) prior to preparation and administration of SABRIL. Physicians should confirm that caregiver(s) understand how to reconstitute SABRIL and to administer the correct dose to their infants.
SABRIL should be given as twice daily oral administration with or without food. The initial dosing is 50 mg/kg/day given in two divided doses and can be titrated by 25-50 mg/kg/day increments every 3 days up to a maximum of 150 mg/kg/day [see USE IN SPECIFIC POPULATIONS, Pediatric Use (8.4)].
The entire contents of the appropriate number of packets (500 mg/packet) of powder should be emptied into an empty cup, and should be dissolved in 10 mL of cold or room temperature water per packet using the 10 mL oral syringe supplied with the medication. The concentration of the final solution is 50 mg/mL. Table 1 below describes how many packets and how many mL of water will be needed to prepare each individual dose. Each individual dose should be prepared immediately before use and administered cold or at room temperature.

Table 1. Number of Packages and mL of Water used for Each Individual Dose

Each Individual Dose (Prepared and Given Twice Daily)	Number of Packets	Number of mL of Water for Dissolving
0 to 500 mg	1 packet	10 mL
501 to 1000 mg	2 packets	20 mL
1001 to 1500 mg	3 packets	30 mL

Table 2 provides the volume that should be administered as individual doses in infants of various weights is presented below:

Table 2. Infant Dosing Table

Weight (kg)	Starting Dose 50 mg/kg/day	Maximum Dose 150 mg/kg/day
3	1.5 mL twice daily	4.5 mL twice daily
4	2 mL twice daily	6 mL twice daily
5	2.5 mL twice daily	7.5 mL twice daily
6	3 mL twice daily	9 mL twice daily
7	3.5 mL twice daily	10.5 mL twice daily
8	4 mL twice daily	12 mL twice daily
9	4.5 mL twice daily	13.5 mL twice daily
10	5 mL twice daily	15 mL twice daily
11	5.5 mL twice daily	16.5 mL twice daily
12	6 mL twice daily	18 mL twice daily
13	6.5 mL twice daily	19.5 mL twice daily
14	7 mL twice daily	21 mL twice daily
15	7.5 mL twice daily	22.5 mL twice daily
16	8 mL twice daily	24 mL twice daily

2.2 Patients with Renal Impairment
SABRIL is primarily eliminated through the kidney. Information about how to adjust the dose in pediatric patients with renal impairment is unavailable.
The following dose adjustments are pertinent to the possible use of this dosage form in adults with renal impairment:
In patients with mild renal impairment (CLcr >50 to 80 mL/min), the dose should be decreased by 25%; in patients with moderate renal impairment (CLcr >30 to 50 mL/min), the dose should be decreased by 50%; and in patients with severe renal impairment (CLcr >10 to <30 mL/min), the dose should be decreased by 75%.
CLcr in mL/min may be estimated from a serum creatinine (mg/dL) determination using the following formula:
$CLcr * = [140\text{-}age\ (years)] \times weight\ (kg)/72 \times serum\ creatinine\ (mg/dL)$
$*[\times 0.85\ for\ female\ patients]$
The effect of dialysis on SABRIL clearance has not been adequately studied.
[see CLINICAL PHARMACOLOGY, Pharmacokinetics, Renal Impairment (12.3) and USE IN SPECIFIC POPULATIONS, Renal Impairment (8.6)].

2.3 General Dosing Considerations
Monitoring of SABRIL plasma concentrations to optimize therapy is not helpful. If a decision is made to discontinue SABRIL, the dose should be gradually reduced. In a controlled clinical study in patients with IS, vigabatrin was tapered by decreasing the dose at a rate of 25-50 mg/kg every 3-4 days [see WARNINGS AND PRECAUTIONS, Withdrawal of Antiepileptic Drugs (AEDs) (5.6)].

3 DOSAGE FORMS AND STRENGTHS
3.1 Powder for Oral Solution
500 mg Packet.

4 CONTRAINDICATIONS
None.

5 WARNINGS AND PRECAUTIONS
5.1 Vision Loss (see BOXED WARNING)
Because of the risk of vision loss and because SABRIL, when it is effective, provides an observable symptomatic benefit, the patient who fails to show substantial clinical benefit within 2 to 4 weeks of initiation of treatment,

should be withdrawn from SABRIL. If in the clinical judgment of the prescriber evidence of treatment failure becomes obvious earlier than 2 to 4 weeks, treatment with SABRIL should be discontinued at that time. Patient response to and continued need for treatment should be periodically assessed.

Monitoring of Vision
Because vision testing in infants and children is difficult, vision loss may not be detected until it is severe. However, monitoring of vision by an ophthalmic professional with expertise in visual field interpretation and the ability to perform dilated indirect ophthalmoscopy of the retina, must be performed at baseline (no later than 4 weeks after starting SABRIL) and at least every 3 months while on therapy. Vision testing is also required about 3 to 6 months after the discontinuation of SABRIL therapy. This assessment should include visual acuity and visual field whenever possible.

The diagnostic approach should be individualized for the patient and clinical situation, but for all patients attempts to monitor vision periodically must be documented under the SHARE program. In patients in whom vision testing is not possible, treatment may continue according to clinical judgment, with appropriate caregiver(s) counseling, and with documentation in the SHARE program of the inability to test vision. Because of variability, results from ophthalmic monitoring must be interpreted with caution, and repeat testing is recommended if results are abnormal or uninterpretable.

The onset and progression of vision loss from SABRIL is unpredictable, and may occur or worsen precipitously. Once detected, vision loss due to SABRIL is not reversible.

5.2   Distribution Program for SABRIL
SABRIL is available only under a special restricted distribution program called the SHARE program. Under the SHARE program, only prescribers and pharmacies registered with the program are able to prescribe and distribute SABRIL. In addition, SABRIL may be dispensed only to patients who are enrolled in and meet all conditions of SHARE. Contact the SHARE program at 1-888-45-SHARE. To enroll in SHARE, prescribers must understand the risks of SABRIL and complete the SHARE Prescriber Enrollment and Agreement Form indicating agreement to:
• Enroll all patients in SHARE
• Review the SABRIL Medication Guide with every caregiver
• Educate caregiver(s) on the risks of SABRIL, including the risk of vision loss [see BOXED WARNING: VISION LOSS]
• Arrange for visual field and retinal exam by an expert examiner and review visual evaluation prior to initiation of SABRIL treatment and every 3 months during therapy
• Remove patients from SABRIL therapy if the patients do not experience a meaningful reduction in seizures
• Counsel caregiver(s) who fail to comply with the program requirements
• Remove patients from SABRIL therapy whose caregiver(s) fail to comply with the program requirements after appropriate counseling

5.3   Magnetic Resonance Imaging (MRI) Abnormalities
Abnormal MRI signal changes characterized by increased T2 signal and restricted diffusion in a symmetric pattern involving the thalamus, basal ganglia, brain stem, and cerebellum have been observed in some infants treated for IS with SABRIL. In a retrospective epidemiologic study in infants with IS (N=205), the prevalence of these changes was 21.5% in SABRIL treated patients versus 4.1% in patients treated with other therapies.

In the study above, in post marketing experience, and in published literature reports, these changes generally resolved with discontinuation of treatment. In a few patients, the lesion resolved despite continued use. It has been reported that some infants exhibited coincident motor abnormalities, but no causal relationship has been established and the potential for long-term clinical sequelae has not been adequately studied.

Neurotoxicity (including convulsions and hypomyelination) was observed in rats exposed to vigabatrin during late gestation and the neonatal and juvenile periods of development. The relationship between these findings and the abnormal MRI findings in infants treated for IS with vigabatrin is unknown [see WARNINGS AND PRECAUTIONS, Neurotoxicity (5.4) and USE IN SPECIFIC POPULATIONS, Pregnancy (8.1)].

The specific pattern of signal changes observed in IS patients was not observed in older children and adult patients treated with vigabatrin for refractory complex partial seizures (CPS). In a blinded review of MRI images obtained in prospective clinical trials in patients with refractory CPS 3 years and older (N=656), no difference was observed in anatomic distribution or prevalence of MRI signal changes between vigabatrin treated and placebo patients.

5.4   Neurotoxicity
Vacuolization, characterized by fluid accumulation and separation of the outer layers of myelin, has been observed in

brain white matter tracts in adult and juvenile rats and adult mice, dogs, and possibly monkeys following administration of vigabatrin. This lesion, referred to as intramyelinic edema (IME), was seen in animals at doses within the human therapeutic range. A no-effect dose was not established in rodents or dogs. In the rat and dog, vacuolization was reversible following discontinuation of vigabatrin treatment, but, in the rat, pathologic changes consisting of swollen or degenerating axons, mineralization, and gliosis were seen in brain areas in which vacuolation had been previously observed. Vacuolization in adult animals was correlated with alterations in MRI and changes in visual and somatosensory evoked potentials (EP).

Administration of vigabatrin to rats during the neonatal and juvenile periods of development produced vacuolar changes in the gray matter (areas including the thalamus, midbrain, deep cerebellar nuclei, substantia nigra, hippocampus, and forebrain) which are considered distinct from the IME observed in vigabatrin treated adult animals. Decreased myelination, retinal dysplasia, and neurobehavioral abnormalities (convulsions, neuromotor impairment, learning deficits) were also observed following vigabatrin treatment of young rats. These effects occurred at doses associated with plasma vigabatrin levels substantially lower than those achieved clinically in infants and children.

IME has been reported in a vigabatrin treated infant on postmortem examination. The infant had hypoxic ischemic brain injury and abnormalities of myelin prior to vigabatrin treatment.

In a published study, vigabatrin (200, 400 mg/kg/day) induced apoptotic neurodegeneration in the brain of young rats when administered by intraperitoneal injection on postnatal days 5-7.

Administration of vigabatrin to female rats during pregnancy and lactation at doses below those used clinically resulted in hippocampal vacuolation and convulsions in the mature offspring.

Abnormal MRI signal changes characterized by increased T2 signal and restricted diffusion in a symmetric pattern involving the thalamus, basal ganglia, brain stem, and cerebellum have been observed in some infants treated for IS with vigabatrin. Studies of the effects of vigabatrin on MRI and EP in adult epilepsy patients have demonstrated no clear-cut abnormalities [see WARNINGS AND PRECAUTIONS, MRI Abnormalities (5.3)].

5.5   Suicidal Behavior and Ideation
The following information is pertinent to the possible use of this dosage form in adults. Antiepileptic drugs (AEDs), including SABRIL, increase the risk of suicidal thoughts or behavior in patients taking these drugs for any indication. Patients treated with any AED for any indication should be monitored for the emergence or worsening of depression, suicidal thoughts or behavior, and/or any unusual changes in mood or behavior.

Pooled analyses of 199 placebo-controlled clinical trials (mono- and adjunctive therapy) of 11 different AEDs showed that patients randomized to one of the AEDs had approximately twice the risk (adjusted Relative Risk 1.8, 95% CI: 1.2, 2.7) of suicidal thinking or behavior compared to patients randomized to placebo. In these trials, which had a median treatment duration of 12 weeks, the estimated incidence rate of suicidal behavior or ideation among 27,863 AED treated patients was 0.43%, compared to 0.24% among 16,029 placebo treated patients, representing an increase of approximately one case of suicidal thinking or behavior for every 530 patients treated. There were four suicides in drug treated patients in the trials and none in placebo treated patients, but the number is too small to allow any conclusion about drug effect on suicide.

The increased risk of suicidal thoughts or behavior with AEDs was observed as early as one week after starting drug treatment with AEDs and persisted for the duration of treatment assessed. Because most trials included in the analysis did not extend beyond 24 weeks, the risk of suicidal thoughts or behavior beyond 24 weeks could not be assessed.

The risk of suicidal thoughts or behavior was generally consistent among drugs in the data analyzed. The finding of

increased risk with AEDs of varying mechanisms of action and across a range of indications suggests that the risk applies to all AEDs used for any indication. The risk did not vary substantially by age (5-100 years) in the clinical trials analyzed. Table 3 shows absolute and relative risk by indication for all evaluated AEDs.

[See table 3 above]

The relative risk for suicidal thoughts or behavior was higher in clinical trials for epilepsy than in clinical trials for psychiatric or other conditions, but the absolute risk differences were similar for the epilepsy and psychiatric indications.

Anyone considering prescribing SABRIL or any other AED must balance the risk of suicidal thoughts or behavior with the risk of untreated illness. Epilepsy and many other illnesses for which AEDs are prescribed are themselves associated with morbidity and mortality and an increased risk of suicidal thoughts and behavior. Should suicidal thoughts and behavior emerge during treatment, the prescriber needs to consider whether the emergence of these symptoms in any given patient may be related to the illness being treated.

Patients, their caregiver(s), and families should be informed that AEDs increase the risk of suicidal thoughts and behavior and should be advised of the need to be alert for the emergence or worsening of the signs and symptoms of depression, any unusual changes in mood or behavior, or the emergence of suicidal thoughts, behavior, or thoughts about self-harm. Behaviors of concern should be reported immediately to healthcare providers.

5.6   Withdrawal of Antiepileptic Drugs (AEDs)
As with all AEDs, SABRIL should be withdrawn gradually. Caregivers should be told not to suddenly discontinue SABRIL therapy. In a controlled clinical study in patients with IS, vigabatrin was tapered by decreasing the daily dose at a rate of 25-50 mg/kg every 3-4 days [see DOSAGE AND ADMINISTRATION, General Dosing Considerations (2.3), PATIENT COUNSELING INFORMATION, Withdrawal of SABRIL Therapy (17.5)].

5.7   Anemia
In North American controlled trials in adults, 5.7% of patients (16/280) receiving SABRIL and 1.6% of patients (3/188) receiving placebo had adverse events of anemia and/or met criteria for potentially clinically important hematology changes involving hemoglobin, hematocrit, and/or RBC indices. Across U.S. controlled trials, there were mean decreases in hemoglobin of about 3% and 0% in SABRIL and placebo-treated patients, respectively, and in hematocrit of about 1% in Sabril treated patients compared to a gain of about 1% in patients treated with placebo.

In controlled and open label epilepsy trials in adults and pediatric patients, 3 SABRIL patients (0.06%, 3/4855) discontinued for anemia and 2 SABRIL patients experienced unexplained declines in hemoglobin to below 8 g/dL and/or hematocrit below 24%.

5.8   Somnolence and Fatigue
SABRIL causes somnolence and fatigue. Patients should be advised not to drive a car or operate other complex machinery until they are familiar with the effects of SABRIL on their ability to perform such activities.

Pooled data from two SABRIL controlled trials in adults demonstrated that 24% (54/222) of SABRIL patients experienced somnolence compared to 10% (14/135) of placebo patients. In those same studies, 28% of SABRIL patients experienced fatigue compared to 15% (20/135) of placebo patients. Almost 1% of SABRIL patients discontinued from clinical trials for somnolence and almost 1% discontinued for fatigue.

5.9   Peripheral Neuropathy
SABRIL has been shown to cause symptoms of peripheral neuropathy in adults. The clinical trials in pediatric patients were not adequately designed to assess whether or not these symptoms occur in the pediatric population.

In a pool of North American controlled and uncontrolled epilepsy studies, 4.2% (19/457) of SABRIL treated patients developed signs and/or symptoms of peripheral neuropathy. In the subset of North American placebo controlled epilepsy trials, 1.4% (4/280) of SABRIL treated patients and no

Table 3. Risk by Indication for Antiepileptic Drugs in the Pooled Analysis

Indication	Placebo Patients with Events per 1000 Patients	Drug Patients with Events per 1000 Patients	Relative Risk: Incidence of Drug Events in Drug Patients/Incidence in Placebo Patients	Risk Difference: Additional Drug Patients with Events per 1000 Patients
Epilepsy	1.0	3.4	3.5	2.4
Psychiatric	5.7	8.5	1.5	2.9
Other	1.0	1.8	1.9	0.9
Total	2.4	4.3	1.8	1.9

(0/188) placebo patients developed signs and/or symptoms of peripheral neuropathy. Initial manifestations of peripheral neuropathy in these trials included, in some combination, symptoms of numbness or tingling in the toes or feet, signs of reduced distal lower limb vibration or position sensation, or progressive loss of reflexes, starting at the ankles. Clinical studies in the development program were not designed to investigate peripheral neuropathy systematically and did not include nerve conduction studies, quantitative sensory testing, or skin or nerve biopsy. There is insufficient evidence to determine if development of these signs and symptoms were related to duration of SABRIL treatment, cumulative dose, or if the findings of peripheral neuropathy were completely reversible upon discontinuation of SABRIL.

5.10   Weight Gain

SABRIL has been shown to cause weight gain in adults. The clinical trials in pediatric patients were not adequately designed to assess whether or not weight gain occurs in the pediatric population.

Data pooled from randomized controlled trials found that 17% (77/443) of SABRIL patients gained ≥ 7% of baseline body weight versus 8% (22/275) of placebo patients. In these same trials, the mean weight change among SABRIL patients was 3.5 kg compared to 1.6 kg for placebo patients. In all epilepsy trials, 0.6% (31/4855) of SABRIL patients discontinued for weight gain. The long term effects of SABRIL related weight gain are not known. Weight gain was not related to the occurrence of edema.

5.11   Edema

SABRIL has been shown to cause edema in adults. The clinical trials in pediatric patients were not adequately designed to assess whether or not edema occurs in the pediatric population.

Pooled data from controlled trials demonstrated increased risk among SABRIL patients compared to placebo patients for peripheral edema (SABRIL 2%, placebo 1%), and edema (SABRIL 1%, placebo 0%). In these studies, one SABRIL and no placebo patients discontinued for an edema related AE. There was no apparent association between edema and cardiovascular adverse events such as hypertension or congestive heart failure. Edema was not associated with laboratory changes suggestive of deterioration in renal or hepatic function.

6   ADVERSE REACTIONS

SABRIL causes permanent damage to vision in a high percentage of patients [see BOXED WARNING: VISION LOSS and WARNINGS AND PRECAUTIONS, Vision Loss (5.1)].

6.1   Adverse Reactions in Clinical Trials

Because clinical trials are conducted under widely varying conditions, adverse reaction rates observed in the clinical trials of a drug cannot be directly compared to rates in the clinical trials of another drug and may not reflect the rates observed in practice.

Adverse Events in U.S. and Primary Non-U.S. Clinical Studies

In U.S. and primary non-U.S. clinical studies of 3139 adult and 999 pediatric patients treated with SABRIL, the most commonly observed (≥ 5%) adverse events associated with the use of SABRIL in combination with other AEDs were headache (18%), somnolence (17%), fatigue (16%), dizziness (15%), convulsion (11%), nasopharyngitis (10%), weight increased (10%), upper respiratory tract infection (10%), visual field defect (9%), depression (8%), tremor (7%), nystagmus (7%), nausea (7%), diarrhea (7%), memory impairment (7%), insomnia (7%), irritability (7%), coordination abnormal (7%), vision blurred (6%), diplopia (6%), vomiting (6%), influenza (6%), pyrexia (6%), and rash (6%).

The adverse reactions most commonly associated with SABRIL treatment discontinuation in ≥ 1% of IS patients were infections (1.5%), status epilepticus (1.2%), developmental coordination disorder (1.2%), dystonia (1.2%), hypotonia (1.2%), hypertonia (1.2%), weight increased (1.2%), and insomnia (1.2%).

Most Common Adverse Reactions in Controlled Clinical Trials

Infantile Spasms

In a randomized, placebo-controlled IS study with a 5 day double-blind treatment phase (n=40), the adverse events reported by >5% of SABRIL patients and that occurred more frequently than in placebo patients were somnolence (SABRIL 45%, placebo 30%), bronchitis (SABRIL 30%, placebo 15%), ear infection (SABRIL 10%, placebo 5%), and otitis media acute (SABRIL 10%, placebo 0).

In a dose response study of low-dose (18-36 mg/kg/day) versus high-dose (100-148 mg/kg/day) vigabatrin, no clear correlation between dose and incidence of adverse events was observed. The treatment emergent adverse reactions (≥ 5% in either dose group) are summarized in Table 4.

Table 4. Treatment Emergent Adverse Events Occurring in ≥5% of Patients (Study 1A)

Body System Event	SABRIL Low Dose [N = 114] %	SABRIL High Dose [N = 108] %
Eye Disorders (other than field or acuity changes)		
Strabismus	5	5
Conjunctivitis	5	2
Gastrointestinal Disorders		
Vomiting	14	20
Constipation	14	12
Diarrhea	13	12
General Disorders		
Fever	29	19
Infections		
Upper respiratory tract infection	51	46
Otitis media	44	30
Viral infection	20	19
Pneumonia	13	11
Candidiasis	8	3
Ear infection	7	14
Gastroenteritis viral	6	5
Sinusitis	5	9
Urinary tract infection	5	6
Influenza	5	3
Croup infectious	5	1
Metabolism & Nutrition Disorders		
Decreased appetite	9	7
Nervous System Disorders		
Sedation	19	17
Somnolence	17	19
Status epilepticus	6	4
Lethargy	5	7
Convulsion	4	7
Hypotonia	4	6
Psychiatric Disorders		
Irritability	16	23
Insomnia	10	12
Respiratory Disorders		
Nasal congestion	13	4
Cough	3	8
Skin & Subcutaneous Tissue Disorders		
Rash	8	11

Refractory Complex Partial Seizures in Adults

Because controlled trials in infants were of short duration and enrolled few patients, the adverse events from clinical trials in adults are presented. Table 5 lists the treatment emergent adverse reactions that occurred in ≥2% of SABRIL patients and that occurred more frequently than in placebo patients from 2 U.S. add-on clinical studies of refractory complex partial seizures in adults.

Table 5. Treatment Emergent Adverse Reactions Occurring in ≥ 2% of SABRIL Patients and More Frequently than in Placebo Patients (Studies 024 and 025)

Body System Preferred Term	SABRIL [N=222] %	Placebo [N=135] %
Eye Disorders		
Vision blurred	11	5
Diplopia	3	0
Eye disorder (other than field or acuity changes)	3	0
Asthenopia	2	0
Gastrointestinal Disorders		
Diarrhea	10	7
Nausea	9	8
Vomiting	7	6
Constipation	6	3
Abdominal pain upper	5	2
Dyspepsia	4	3
Stomach discomfort	3	1
Hemorrhoids	2	0
General Disorders		
Fatigue	27	16
Asthenia	5	2
Peripheral edema	5	1
Fever	5	3
Infections		
Nasopharyngitis	13	10
Upper respiratory tract infection	9	5
Influenza	5	4
Urinary tract infection	4	0
Injury		
Contusion	4	2
Metabolism and Nutritional Disorders		
Fluid retention	2	0
Increased appetite	2	0
Weight increased	8	3
Musculoskeletal Disorders		
Arthralgia	8	3
Back pain	6	2
Pain in extremity	5	4
Myalgia	3	2
Joint swelling	2	0
Muscle spasms	2	1
Shoulder pain	2	1
Nervous System Disorders		
Somnolence	22	13
Dizziness	21	17

Nystagmus	15	9
Tremor	14	8
Memory impairment	10	3
Coordination abnormal	9	2
Disturbance in attention	5	1
Sensory disturbance	5	2
Hyporeflexia	5	1
Parasthesia	5	1
Lethargy	4	2
Hypoaesthesia	3	2
Sedation	2	0
Status epilepticus	2	0
Dysarthria	2	1
Psychiatric Disorders		
Irritability	10	7
Depression	7	3
Confusional state	6	1
Depressed mood	4	1
Anxiety	4	3
Thinking abnormal	3	0
Abnormal behavior	3	1
Aggression	2	0
Reproductive System		
Dysmenorrhea	7	3
Respiratory, and Thoracic Disorders		
Pharyngolaryngeal pain	9	5
Dyspnea	2	0
Sinus headache	4	1

6.2 Post Marketing Experience

The following serious adverse events have been reported since approval and use of SABRIL worldwide. All serious adverse events that are not listed above as adverse events reported in clinical trials, that are not relatively common in the population and are not too vague to be useful are listed in this section. These reactions are reported voluntarily from a population of uncertain size; therefore, it is not possible to estimate their frequency or establish a causal relationship to drug exposure. Events are categorized by system organ class.

Birth Defects: Congenital cardiac defects, congenital external ear anomaly, congenital hemangioma, congenital hydronephrosis, congenital male genital malformation, congenital oral malformation, congenital vesicoureteric reflux, dentofacial anomaly, dysmorphism, fetal anticonvulsant syndrome, hamartomas, hip dysplasia, limb malformation, limb reduction defect, low set ears, renal aplasia, retinitis pigmentosa, supernumerary nipple, talipes

Ear: Deafness

Endocrine: Delayed puberty

Gastrointestinal: Gastrointestinal hemorrhage, esophagitis

General: Developmental delay, facial edema, malignant hyperthermia, multi-organ failure

Hepatobiliary: Cholestasis

Nervous System: Dystonia, encephalopathy, hypertonia, hypotonia, muscle spasticity, myoclonus, optic neuritis

Psychiatric: Acute psychosis, apathy, delirium, hypomania, neonatal agitation, psychotic disorder

Respiratory: Laryngeal edema, pulmonary embolism, respiratory failure, stridor

Skin and Subcutaneous Tissue: Angioedema, maculopapular rash, pruritus

7 DRUG INTERACTIONS

For detailed information about Drug Interactions see CLINICAL PHARMACOLOGY, Pharmacokinetics, Drug Interactions (12.3).

7.1 Phenytoin

A 16% to 20% average reduction in total phenytoin plasma levels was reported in controlled clinical studies.

7.2 Other AEDs

There are no clinically significant pharmacokinetics interactions between SABRIL and either phenobarbital or sodium valproate. Based on population pharmacokinetics, carbamazepine, clorazepate, primidone, and sodium valproate appear to have no effect on plasma concentrations of vigabatrin.

7.3 Clonazepam

In a study of 12 healthy volunteers, clonazepam (0.5 mg) co-administration had no effect on SABRIL (1.5 g twice daily) concentrations. SABRIL increases the mean C_{max} of clonazepam by 30% and decreases the mean t_{max} by 45%.

7.4 Oral Contraceptives

SABRIL is unlikely to affect the efficacy of steroid oral contraceptives.

7.5 Drug-Laboratory Test Interactions

SABRIL decreases alanine transaminase (ALT) and aspartate transaminase (AST) plasma activity in up to 90% of patients. In some patients, these enzymes become undetectable. The suppression of ALT and AST activity by SABRIL may preclude the use of these markers, especially ALT, to detect early hepatic injury.

SABRIL may increase the amount of amino acids in the urine, possibly leading to a false positive test for certain rare genetic metabolic diseases (e.g., alpha aminoadipic aciduria).

8 USE IN SPECIFIC POPULATIONS

8.1 Pregnancy

The following information is pertinent to the possible use of this dosage form in adults.

Pregnancy Category C. Vigabatrin produced developmental toxicity, including teratogenic and neurohistopathological effects, when administered to pregnant animals at clinically relevant doses. In addition, developmental neurotoxicity was observed in rats treated with vigabatrin during a period of postnatal development corresponding to the third trimester of human pregnancy. There are no adequate and well-controlled studies in pregnant women. SABRIL should be used during pregnancy only if the potential benefit justifies the potential risk to the fetus.

Administration of vigabatrin (oral doses of 50 to 200 mg/kg) to pregnant rabbits throughout the period of organogenesis was associated with an increased incidence of malformations (cleft palate) and embryo-fetal death; these findings were observed in two separate studies. The no-effect dose for teratogenicity and embryolethality in rabbits (100 mg/kg) is approximately 1/2 the maximum recommended human dose (MRHD) of 3 g/day on a body surface area (mg/m^2) basis for adults treated for refractory complex partial seizures with vigabatrin. In rats, oral administration of vigabatrin (50, 100, or 150 mg/kg) throughout organogenesis resulted in decreased fetal body weights and increased incidences of fetal anatomic variations. The no-effect dose for embryo-fetal toxicity in rats (50 mg/kg) is approximately 1/5 the MRHD in adults on a mg/m^2 basis. Oral administration of vigabatrin (50, 100, 150 mg/kg) to rats from the latter part of pregnancy through weaning produced long-term neurohistopathological (hippocampal vacuolation) and neurobehavioral (convulsions) abnormalities in the offspring. A no-effect dose for developmental neurotoxicity in rats was not established; the low-effect dose (50 mg/kg) is approximately 1/5 the MRHD in adults on a mg/m^2 basis.

In a published study, vigabatrin (300 or 450 mg/kg) was administered by intraperitoneal injection to a mutant mouse strain on a single day during organogenesis (day 7, 8, 9, 10, 11, or 12). An increase in malformations (including cleft palate) was observed at both doses.

Oral administration of vigabatrin (5, 15, or 50 mg/kg) to young rats during the neonatal and juvenile periods of development (postnatal days 4-65) produced neurobehavioral (convulsions, neuromotor impairment, learning deficits) and neurohistopathological (brain vacuolation, decreased myelination, and retinal dysplasia) abnormalities in treated animals. The early postnatal period in rats is generally thought to correspond to late pregnancy in humans in terms of brain development. The no-effect dose for developmental neurotoxicity in juvenile rats (5 mg/kg) was associated with plasma vigabatrin exposures (AUC) less than 1/30 of those measured in pediatric patients receiving an oral dose of 50 mg/kg.

Pregnancy Registry: To provide information regarding the effects of *in utero* exposure to SABRIL, physicians are advised to recommend that pregnant patients taking SABRIL enroll in the North American Antiepileptic Drug (NAAED) Pregnancy Registry. This can be done by calling the toll free number 1-888-233-2334, and must be done by patients themselves. Information on the registry can also be found at the website http://www.aedpregnancyregistry.org/.

8.3 Nursing Mothers

The following information is pertinent to the possible use of this dosage form in adults.

Vigabatrin is excreted in human milk. Because of the potential for serious adverse reactions from vigabatrin in nursing infants [see WARNINGS AND PRECAUTIONS, MRI Abnormalities (5.3) and Neurotoxicity (5.4)], a decision should be made whether to discontinue nursing or to discontinue the drug, taking into account the importance of the drug to the mother.

8.4 Pediatric Use

SABRIL is indicated as monotherapy for pediatric patients with IS (1 month to 2 years of age) for whom the potential benefits outweigh the potential risk for developing permanent vision loss.

Abnormal MRI signal changes characterized by increased T2 signal and restricted diffusion in a symmetric pattern involving the thalamus, basal ganglia, brain stem, and cerebellum have been observed in some infants treated for IS with vigabatrin. In a retrospective epidemiologic study in infants with IS (N=205), the prevalence of these changes was 21.5% in vigabatrin treated patients versus 4.1% in patients treated with other therapies. A dose-dependent relationship may exist, as children with IS who were exposed to a higher vigabatrin dose (≥125 mg/kg/day) had a prevalence of 29.5%, while those exposed to lower doses of vigabatrin had a prevalence of 12.5%; however, these differences were not statistically significant (p=0.099).

In the study above, in post marketing experience, and in published literature reports, these changes generally resolved with discontinuation of treatment, although in a few patients, the lesion resolved despite continued use. It has been reported that some infants exhibited coincident motor abnormalities, but no causal relationship has been established and the potential for long-term clinical sequelae has not been adequately studied [see WARNINGS AND PRECAUTIONS, MRI Abnormalities (5.3) and Neurotoxicity (5.4)].

The specific pattern of signal changes observed in IS patients was not observed in older children and adult patients treated with vigabatrin for refractory CPS. In a blinded review of MRI images obtained in prospective clinical trials in patients with refractory CPS 3 years and older (N=656), no difference was observed in anatomic distribution or prevalence of MRI signal changes between vigabatrin treated and placebo patients.

Oral administration of vigabatrin (5, 15, or 50 mg/kg) to young rats during the neonatal and juvenile periods of development (postnatal days 4-65) produced neurobehavioral (convulsions, neuromotor impairment, learning deficits) and neurohistopathological (brain vacuolation, decreased myelination, and retinal dysplasia) abnormalities in treated animals. The no-effect dose for developmental neurotoxicity in juvenile rats (5 mg/kg) was associated with plasma vigabatrin exposures (AUC) less than 1/30 of those measured in pediatric patients receiving an oral dose of 50 mg/kg.

8.5 Geriatric Use

The following information is pertinent to the possible use of this dosage form in adults.

Clinical studies of vigabatrin did not include sufficient numbers of patients aged 65 and over to determine whether they responded differently from younger patients.

Vigabatrin is known to be substantially excreted by the kidney, and the risk of toxic reactions to this drug may be greater in patients with impaired renal function. Because elderly patients are more likely to have decreased renal function, care should be taken in dose selection, and it may be useful to monitor renal function.

Oral administration of a single dose of 1.5 g of vigabatrin to elderly (>65 years) patients with reduced creatinine clearance (<50 mL/min) was associated with moderate to severe sedation and confusion in 4 of 5 patients, lasting up to 5 days. The renal clearance of vigabatrin was 36% lower in healthy elderly subjects (>65 years) than in young healthy males. Adjustment of dose or frequency of administration should be considered. Such patients may respond to a lower maintenance dose [see CLINICAL PHARMACOLOGY, Pharmacokinetics, Renal Impairment (12.3) and DOSAGE AND ADMINISTRATION, Patients with Renal Impairment (2.2)].

Other reported clinical experience has not identified differences in responses between the elderly and younger patients.

8.6 Renal Impairment

Information about how to adjust the dose in pediatric patients with renal impairment is unavailable.

The following dose adjustments are pertinent to the possible use of this dosage form in adults with renal impairment:

In adults, dose adjustment, including initiating treatment with a lower dose, is necessary in patients with mild (creatinine clearance >50-80 mL/min), moderate (creatinine clearance >30-50 mL/min) and severe (creatinine clearance >10-30 mL/min) renal impairment [see CLINICAL

PHARMACOLOGY, Pharmacokinetics, Renal Impairment (12.3) and DOSAGE AND ADMINISTRATION, Patients with Renal Impairment (2.2)].

9 DRUG ABUSE AND DEPENDENCE

9.1 Controlled Substance Class

Vigabatrin is not a controlled substance.

9.2 Abuse

Vigabatrin did not produce adverse events or overt behaviors associated with abuse when administered to humans or animals. It is not possible to predict the extent to which a CNS active drug will be misused, diverted, and/or abused once marketed. Consequently, physicians should carefully evaluate patients for history of drug abuse and follow such patients closely, observing them for signs of misuse or abuse of vigabatrin (e.g., incrementation of dose, drug-seeking behavior).

9.3 Dependence

Following chronic administration of vigabatrin to animals, there were no apparent withdrawal signs upon drug discontinuation. However, as with all AEDs, vigabatrin should be withdrawn gradually to minimize increased seizure frequency [see WARNINGS AND PRECAUTIONS, Withdrawal of Antiepileptic Drugs (AEDs) (5.6) and PATIENT COUNSELING INFORMATION, Withdrawal of SABRIL Therapy (17.5)].

10 OVERDOSAGE

10.1 Signs, Symptoms, and Laboratory Findings of Overdosage

Confirmed and/or suspected vigabatrin overdoses have been reported during clinical studies and in post marketing surveillance. No vigabatrin overdoses resulted in death. When reported, the vigabatrin dose ingested ranged from 3 g to 90 g, but most were between 7.5 g and 30 g. Nearly half the cases involved multiple drug ingestions including carbamazepine, barbiturates, benzodiazepines, lamotrigine, valproic acid, acetaminophen, and/or chlorpheniramine.

Coma, unconsciousness, and/or drowsiness were described in the majority of cases of vigabatrin overdose. Other less commonly reported symptoms included vertigo, psychosis, apnea or respiratory depression, bradycardia, agitation, irritability, confusion, headache, hypotension, abnormal behavior, increased seizure activity, status epilepticus, and speech disorder. These symptoms resolved with supportive care.

10.2 Treatment or Management for Overdosage

There is no specific antidote for SABRIL overdose. Standard measures to remove unabsorbed drug should be used, including elimination by emesis or gastric lavage. Supportive measures should be employed, including monitoring of vital signs and observation of the clinical status of the patients. In an *in vitro* study, activated charcoal did not significantly adsorb vigabatrin.

The effectiveness of hemodialysis in the treatment of SABRIL overdose is unknown. In isolated case reports in renal failure patients receiving therapeutic doses of vigabatrin, hemodialysis reduced vigabatrin plasma concentrations by 40% to 60%.

11 DESCRIPTION

Table 6. Description

Proprietary Name:	SABRIL®
Established Name:	Vigabatrin for Oral Solution
Dosage Form:	Packet
Route of Administration:	Oral
Pharmacologic Class of Drug:	Antiepileptic
Chemical Name:	(±) 4-amino-5-hexenoic acid
Structural Formula:	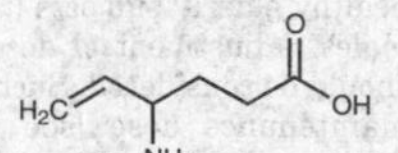

SABRIL (vigabatrin) is available as a white granular powder for oral administration. Each packet contains 500 mg vigabatrin. Each packet also contains the inactive ingredient povidone. Vigabatrin is an oral antiepileptic drug with the chemical name (±) 4-amino-5-hexenoic acid. It is a racemate consisting of two enantiomers. The molecular formula is $C_6H_{11}NO_2$ and the molecular weight is 129.16.

Vigabatrin is a white to off-white powder which is freely soluble in water, slightly soluble in methyl alcohol, very slightly soluble in ethyl alcohol and chloroform, and insoluble in toluene and hexane. The pH of a 1% aqueous solution is about 6.9. The n-octanol/water partition coefficient of vigabatrin is about 0.011 (log P=-1.96) at physiologic pH. Vigabatrin melts with decomposition in a 3-degree range within the temperature interval of 171 °C to 176 °C. The dissociation constants (pK_a) of vigabatrin are 4 and 9.7 at room temperature (25 °C).

12 CLINICAL PHARMACOLOGY

12.1 Mechanism of Action

The precise mechanism of vigabatrin's anti-seizure effect is unknown, but it is believed to be the result of its action as an irreversible inhibitor of gamma-aminobutyric acid transaminase (GABA-T), the enzyme responsible for the metabolism of the inhibitory neurotransmitter GABA. This action results in increased levels of GABA in the central nervous system.

No direct correlation between plasma concentration and efficacy has been established. The duration of drug effect is presumed to be dependent on the rate of enzyme resynthesis rather than on the rate of elimination of the drug from the systemic circulation.

12.2 Pharmacodynamics

Effects on Electrocardiogram

There is no indication of a QT/QTc prolonging effect of SABRIL in single doses up to 6.0 g. In a randomized, placebo-controlled, crossover study, 58 healthy adult subjects were administered a single oral dose of SABRIL (3 g and 6 g) and placebo. Peak concentrations for 6.0 g SABRIL were approximately 2-fold higher than the peak concentrations following the 3.0 g single oral dose.

12.3 Pharmacokinetics

Vigabatrin displayed linear pharmacokinetics after administration of single doses ranging from 0.5 g to 4 g, and after administration of repeated doses of 0.5 g to 2.0 g twice daily. Bioequivalence has been established between the oral solution and tablet formulations.

Absorption

Following oral administration, vigabatrin is essentially completely absorbed.

Time to maximum concentration (t_{max}) is approximately 2.5 hours in infants and about 1 hour in children following a single dose. There was little accumulation with multiple dosing. A food effect study involving administration of vigabatrin to healthy adult volunteers under fasting and fed conditions indicated that the C_{max} was decreased by 33%, t_{max} increased to 2 hours, and AUC was unchanged under fed conditions [see DOSAGE AND ADMINISTRATION, Infantile Spasms (2.1)].

Distribution

Vigabatrin does not bind to plasma proteins. Vigabatrin is widely distributed throughout the body; mean steady-state volume of distribution is 1.1 L/Kg (CV = 20%).

Metabolism and Elimination

Vigabatrin is not significantly metabolized; it is eliminated primarily through renal excretion. The half-life of vigabatrin in adults is about 7.5 hours and about 5.7 hours in infants. Following administration of ^{14}C-vigabatrin to healthy adult male volunteers, about 95% of total radioactivity was recovered in the urine over 72 hours with the parent drug representing about 80% of this. Vigabatrin induces CYP2C9, but does not induce other hepatic cytochrome P450 enzyme systems.

Pharmacokinetics in Special Populations

Geriatric

The renal clearance of vigabatrin in healthy elderly patients (≥ 65 years of age) was 36% less than those in healthy younger patients. A population PK analysis of patient data also confirmed these differences in age.

Pediatric

The clearance of infants and children were 2.4±0.8 and 5.7±2.5 L/h, respectively compared to 7 L/h in adults.

Gender

No gender differences were observed for the pharmacokinetic parameters of vigabatrin in patients.

Race

No specific study was conducted to investigate the effects of race on SABRIL pharmacokinetics. A cross study comparison in adults between 23 Caucasian and 7 Japanese patients who received 1, 2, and 4 g of vigabatrin indicated that the AUC, C_{max}, and half-life were similar for the two populations. However, the mean renal clearance of Caucasians (5.2 L/hr) was about 25% higher than the Japanese (4.0 L/hr). Inter-subject variability in renal clearance was 20% in Caucasians and was 30% in Japanese.

Renal Impairment

There is no information available about the pharmacokinetics of vigabatrin in pediatric patients with renal impairment.

In adult patients with mild renal impairment (CLcr from >50-80 mL/min), mean AUC increased by 30% and the terminal half-life increased by 55% (8.1 hr vs 12.5 hr) in comparison to the normal subjects. Mean AUC increased by two-fold and the terminal half-life increased by two-fold in patients with moderate renal impairment (CLcr from >30-50 mL/min) in comparison to the normal subjects. Mean AUC increased by 4.5-fold and the terminal half-life increased by 3.5-fold in patients with severe renal impairment (CLcr from >10-30 mL/min) in comparison to the normal subjects.

While dose adjustments are warranted in renally impaired pediatric patients, no data is available to guide dose adjustments in this patient population. Dosage adjustment in adults with renal impairment is recommended [see USE IN SPECIFIC POPULATIONS, Renal Impairment (8.6) and DOSAGE AND ADMINISTRATION, Patients with Renal Impairment (2.2)].

Hepatic Impairment

Vigabatrin is not significantly metabolized. The pharmacokinetics of vigabatrin in patients with impaired liver function have not been studied.

Drug Interactions

Phenytoin

A 16% to 20% average reduction in total phenytoin plasma levels was reported in controlled clinical studies. *In vitro* drug metabolism studies indicate that decreased phenytoin concentrations upon addition of vigabatrin therapy are likely due to induction of cytochrome P450 2C enzymes in some patients. Although phenytoin dose adjustments are not routinely required, dose adjustment of phenytoin should be considered if clinically indicated.

Other AEDs

When co-administered with vigabatrin, phenobarbital concentration (from phenobarbital or primidone) was reduced by an average of 8% to 16%, and sodium valproate plasma concentrations were reduced by an average of 8%. These reductions did not appear to be clinically relevant. Based on population pharmacokinetics, carbamazepine, clorazepate, primidone, and sodium valproate appear to have no effect on plasma concentrations of vigabatrin.

Clonazepam

In a study of 12 healthy volunteers, clonazepam (0.5 mg) co-administration had no effect on SABRIL (1.5 g twice daily) concentrations. SABRIL increases the mean C_{max} of clonazepam by 30% and decreases the mean t_{max} by 45%.

Alcohol

Co-administration of ethanol (0.6 g/kg) with vigabatrin (1.5 g twice daily) indicated that neither drug influences the pharmacokinetics of the other.

Oral Contraceptives

In a double-blind, placebo-controlled study using a combination oral contraceptive containing 30 µg ethinyl estradiol and 150 µg levonorgestrel, vigabatrin (3 g/day) did not interfere significantly with the cytochrome P450 isoenzyme (CYP3A)-mediated metabolism of the contraceptive tested. Based on this study, vigabatrin is unlikely to affect the efficacy of steroid oral contraceptives. Additionally, no significant difference in pharmacokinetic parameters (elimination half-life, AUC, C_{max}, apparent oral clearance, time to peak, and apparent volume of distribution) of vigabatrin were found after treatment with ethinyl estradiol and levonorgestrel.

13 NONCLINICAL TOXICOLOGY

13.1 Carcinogenesis, Mutagenesis, Impairment of Fertility

Vigabatrin showed no carcinogenic potential in mouse or rat when given in the diet at doses up to 150 mg/kg/day for 18 months (mouse) or at doses up to 150 mg/kg/day for 2 years (rat). These doses are less than the maximum recommended human dose (MRHD) for IS (150 mg/kg/day) and for refractory complex partial seizures in adults (3 g/day) on a mg/m^2 basis.

Vigabatrin was negative in *in vitro* (Ames, CHO/HGPRT mammalian cell forward gene mutation, chromosomal aberration assay in rat lymphocytes) and in *in vivo* (mouse bone marrow micronucleus) assays.

No adverse effects on male or female fertility were observed in rats at oral doses up to 150 mg/kg/day (approximately 1/2 the MRHD of 3 g/day (on a mg/m^2 basis) for adults treated for refractory complex partial seizures with vigabatrin.

14 CLINICAL STUDIES

14.1 Infantile Spasms

The effectiveness of SABRIL as monotherapy was established for IS in two multicenter controlled studies. Both studies were similar in terms of disease characteristics and prior treatments of patients and all enrolled infants had a confirmed diagnosis of IS.

Study 1

Study 1 (N=221) was a multicenter, randomized, low-dose high-dose, parallel group, partially-blinded (caregivers knew the actual dose but not whether their child was classified as low or high dose; EEG reader was blinded but investigators were not blinded) study to evaluate the safety and efficacy of vigabatrin in patients <2 years of age with new-onset Infantile Spasms. Patients with both symptomatic and cryptogenic etiologies were studied. The study was comprised of two phases. The first phase was a 14 to 21 day partially-blind phase in which patients were randomized to receive either low-dose (18-36 mg/kg/day) or high-dose (100-148 mg/kg/day) vigabatrin. Study drug was titrated over 7 days, followed by a constant dose for 7 days. If the patient became spasm-free on or before day 14, another 7 days of constant dose was administered. The primary efficacy endpoint of this study was the proportion of patients who were spasm-free for 7 consecutive days beginning within the first 14 days of vigabatrin therapy. Patients considered spasm-free were defined as those patients who remained free of spasms (evaluated according to caregiver response to direct questioning regarding spasm frequency) and who had no indication of spasms or hypsarrhythmia during 8 hours of CCTV EEG recording (including at least one sleep-wake-sleep cycle) performed within 3 days of the seventh day of spasm freedom and interpreted by a blinded EEG reader. Seventeen patients in the high dose group achieved spasm freedom compared with 8 patients in the low dose group. This difference was statistically significant (p=0.0375). Primary efficacy results are shown in Table 7.

Table 7. Spasm Freedom by Primary Criteria (Study 1A)

	SABRIL Treatment Group	
	18-36 mg/kg/day [N=114] n (%)	100-148 mg/kg/day [N=107] n (%)
Patients who Achieved Spasm Freedom	8 (7.0)	17 (15.9)

p=0.0375
Note: Primary criteria were evaluated based on caregiver assessment plus CCTV EEG confirmation within 3 days of the seventh day of spasm freedom.

Study 2

Study 2 (N=40) was a multicenter, randomized, double-blind, placebo-controlled, parallel group study consisting of a pre-treatment (baseline) period of 2-3 days, followed by a 5-day double-blind treatment phase during which patients were treated with vigabatrin (initial dose of 50 mg/kg/day with titration allowed to 150 mg/kg/day) or placebo. The primary efficacy endpoint in this study was the average percent change in daily spasm frequency, assessed during a pre-defined and consistent 2-hour window of evaluation, comparing baseline to the final 2 days of the 5-day double-blind treatment phase. No statistically significant differences were observed in the average frequency of spasms using the 2-hour evaluation window. However, a post-hoc alternative efficacy analysis, using a 24-hour clinical evaluation window found a statistically significant difference in the overall percentage of reductions in spasms between the vigabatrin group (68.9%) and the placebo group (17.0%) (p=0.030).

15 REFERENCES

None

16 HOW SUPPLIED/STORAGE AND HANDLING

16.1 SABRIL Packet

Each SABRIL packet contains 500 mg vigabatrin as a white to off-white granular powder.

NDC 67386-211-65: Packages of 50.

Store at 20-25 °C (68-77 °F). See USP controlled room temperature.

17 PATIENT COUNSELING INFORMATION

See FDA-Approved Patient Labeling (17.6)

Caregivers must be informed of the availability of a Medication Guide. They must be instructed to read the Medication Guide prior to initiating treatment with SABRIL and with each prescription refill. Doctors must review the SABRIL Medication Guide with every caregiver prior to initiation of treatment. Caregivers should be instructed to administer SABRIL only as prescribed.

Physicians should confirm that caregiver(s) understand how to reconstitute SABRIL for Oral Solution and to administer the correct dose to their infants.

17.1 Vision Loss

Caregiver(s) should be informed of the risk of permanent vision loss, particularly loss of peripheral vision from SABRIL, and the need for monitoring vision [see WARNINGS AND PRECAUTIONS, Vision Loss (5.1)].

Although vision testing in infants is insensitive, vision must be assessed to the extent possible at baseline (no later than 4 weeks after starting SABRIL) and at least every 3 months during therapy. Caregiver(s) should understand that vision testing is insensitive in infants and may not detect vision loss before it is severe. Caregiver(s) should also understand that if vision loss is documented, such loss is irreversible [see WARNINGS AND PRECAUTIONS, Vision Loss (5.1)]. Caregiver(s) should be informed that if changes in vision are suspected, they should notify their physician immediately.

17.2 MRI Abnormalities

Caregiver should be informed of the possibility of developing abnormal MRI signal changes of unknown clinical significance.

17.3 Suicidal Thinking and Behavior

The following information is pertinent to the possible use of this dosage form in adults.

Patients, their caregiver(s), and families should be counseled that AEDs, including SABRIL, may increase the risk of suicidal thoughts and behavior and should be advised of the need to be alert for the emergence or worsening of symptoms of depression, any unusual changes in mood or behavior, or the emergence of suicidal thoughts, behavior, or thoughts of self-harm. Behaviors of concern should be reported immediately to healthcare providers [see WARNINGS AND PRECAUTIONS, Suicidal Behavior and Ideation (5.5)].

17.4 Use in Pregnancy

The following information is pertinent to the possible use of this dosage form in adults.

Patients should be instructed to notify their physician if they become pregnant or intend to become pregnant during therapy, and to notify their physician if they are breast feeding or intend to breast feed during therapy [see USE IN SPECIFIC POPULATIONS, Pregnancy (8.1), Nursing Mothers (8.3)].

Patients should be encouraged to enroll in the NAAED Pregnancy Registry if they become pregnant. This registry is collecting information about the safety of antiepileptic drugs during pregnancy. To enroll, patients can call the toll free number 1-888-233-2334 [see USE IN SPECIFIC POPULATIONS, Pregnancy (8.1)]. Information on the registry can also be found at the website http://www.aedpregnancyregistry.org/.

17.5 Withdrawal of SABRIL Therapy

Caregiver(s) should be told not to suddenly discontinue SABRIL therapy in their infant. As with all AEDs, withdrawal should be gradual. In a controlled clinical study in patients with IS, vigabatrin was tapered by decreasing the daily dose at a rate of 25-50 mg/kg every 3-4 days.

17.6 FDA-Approved Medication Guide

Manufactured by: Patheon
Cincinnati, OH 45237, U.S.A.
For: Lundbeck Inc.
Deerfield, IL 60015, U.S.A.
® Trademark of Lundbeck Inc.
Issued: February 2010 30142/1

MEDICATION GUIDE

Sabril® (SAY-bril) (vigabatrin) Tablet
Sabril® (SAY-bril) (vigabatrin) for Oral Solution

Read the Medication Guide that comes with SABRIL before you or your baby starts taking SABRIL and each time you get a refill. There may be new information. This Medication Guide does not take the place of talking with your doctor about your or your baby's medical condition or treatment.

What is the most important information I should know about SABRIL?

SABRIL can cause serious side effects, including:

- **Permanent vision damage:** SABRIL can damage the vision of anyone who takes it. The most noticeable loss is in your ability to see to the side when you look straight ahead (peripheral vision). If this happens, it will not get better. People who take SABRIL do not lose all of their vision, but some people can have severe loss particularly to their peripheral vision. With severe vision loss you may only be able to see things straight in front of you (sometimes called 'tunnel vision'). You may also have blurry vision.
- **Vision loss and use of SABRIL in adults:** Because of the risk of vision loss, SABRIL is used to treat complex partial seizures (CPS) only in people who do not respond well enough to several other medicines.

Tell your doctor right away if you:

- think you are not seeing as well as before you started taking SABRIL
- start to trip, bump into things, or are more clumsy than usual
- are surprised by people or things coming in front of you that seem to come out of nowhere

These changes can mean that you have damage to your vision. Your doctor will test your visual fields (including peripheral vision) and visual acuity (ability to read an eye chart) before you start SABRIL or within 4 weeks after starting SABRIL, and at least every 3 months after that until SABRIL is stopped. Even if your vision seems fine, it is important that you get these regular vision tests because damage can happen to your vision before you notice any changes. These vision tests cannot prevent the vision damage that can happen with SABRIL, but they do allow you to stop SABRIL if vision has gotten worse, which usually will lessen further damage. If you do not have these vision tests regularly, your doctor may stop prescribing SABRIL for you. You should also have a vision test after SABRIL is stopped. If you drive and your vision is damaged by SABRIL, driving might be more dangerous, or you may not be able to drive safely at all. You should discuss this with your doctor.

- **Vision loss in babies:** Because of the risk of vision loss, SABRIL is used in babies (1 month to 2 years old) with infantile spasms (IS) only when you and your doctor decide that the possible benefits of SABRIL are more important than the risks. Parents or caregivers are not likely to recognize the symptoms of vision loss in babies until it is severe. Doctors may not find vision loss in babies until it is severe. It is difficult to test vision in babies, but all babies should have a vision test before starting SABRIL or within 4 weeks after starting SABRIL, and every 3 months after that until SABRIL is stopped. You should have a vision test for your baby after SABRIL is stopped.

Tell your doctor right away if you think that your baby is:

- not seeing as well as before taking SABRIL
- acting differently than normal

Even if your baby's vision seems fine, it is important to get regular vision tests because damage can happen before your baby acts differently. Even these regular vision exams may not show the damage to your baby's vision before it is serious and permanent. If your baby does not have these vision tests regularly, your doctor may stop prescribing SABRIL for your baby. If your baby is not able to complete vision testing, your doctor may continue prescribing SABRIL for your baby. But, your doctor will not be able to watch for vision loss in your baby.

In all people who take SABRIL:

- You are at risk for vision loss with any amount of SABRIL
- Your risk of vision loss may be higher the more SABRIL you take daily and the longer you take it
- It is not possible for your doctor to know when vision loss will happen. It could happen soon after starting SABRIL or any time during treatment. It may even happen after treatment has stopped.

Because SABRIL might cause vision loss, it is available to doctors and patients only under a special program called SHARE. As part of the SHARE program, among other things, your doctor will have to test your or your baby's vision frequently while you or your baby are being treated with SABRIL, and even after you or your baby stops treatment. You also have to agree to be in the SHARE program, and agree to have your or your baby's vision tested regularly. Your doctor will explain the details of the SHARE program to you.

MRI changes. Brain pictures taken by magnetic resonance imaging (MRI) show changes in some babies after they are given SABRIL. It is not known if these changes are harmful.

Risk of suicidal thoughts or actions. Like other antiepileptic drugs, SABRIL may cause suicidal thoughts or actions in a very small number of people, about 1 in 500 people taking it.

Call a doctor right away if you have any of these symptoms, especially if they are new, worse, or worry you:

- thoughts about suicide or dying
- attempts to commit suicide
- new or worse depression
- new or worse anxiety
- feeling agitated or restless
- panic attacks
- trouble sleeping (insomnia)
- new or worse irritability
- acting aggressive, being angry, or violent
- acting on dangerous impulses
- an extreme increase in activity and talking (mania)
- other unusual changes in behavior or mood

Suicidal thoughts or actions can be caused by things other than medicines. If you have suicidal thoughts or actions, your healthcare provider may check for other causes.

How can I watch for early symptoms of suicidal thoughts and actions?

- Pay attention to any changes, especially sudden changes, in mood, behaviors, thoughts, or feelings.
- Keep all follow-up visits with your doctor as scheduled.
- Call your doctor between visits as needed, especially if you are worried about symptoms.

Do not stop SABRIL without first talking to a healthcare provider.

- Stopping SABRIL suddenly can cause serious problems. Stopping a seizure medicine suddenly can cause seizures that will not stop (status epilepticus) in people who are being treated for seizures.

SABRIL can be prescribed only to people who are enrolled in a program called SHARE. Before you or your baby can begin taking SABRIL, you must read and agree to all of the instructions in the SHARE program.

What is SABRIL?

SABRIL Tablets is a prescription medicine used along with other treatments to treat adults with CPS if:

- The CPS does not respond well enough to several other treatments, and
- You and your doctor decide the possible benefit of taking SABRIL is more important than the risk of vision loss.

SABRIL should not be the first medicine used to treat your CPS.

SABRIL for Oral Solution is a prescription medicine used to treat babies, one month to two years old who have IS, if you and your doctor decide the possible benefits of taking SABRIL are more important than the possible risk of vision loss.

If you are an adult with CPS, you must sign an agreement form before you can receive SABRIL.

If you are the parent or caregiver of a baby with IS, you must sign an agreement form before your baby can receive SABRIL.

What should I tell my doctor before starting SABRIL?

If you are an adult with CPS, before taking SABRIL tell your doctor if you have or had:

- depression, mood problems or suicidal thoughts or behavior
- an allergic reaction to SABRIL, such as hives, itching, or trouble breathing
- any vision problems
- any kidney problems
- low red blood cell counts (anemia)
- any nervous or mental illnesses, such as depression, thoughts of suicide, or attempts at suicide
- any other medical conditions
- are breastfeeding or planning to breastfeed. SABRIL can pass into breast milk and may harm your baby. Talk to your healthcare provider about the best way to feed your baby if you take SABRIL.
- are pregnant or plan to become pregnant. It is not known if SABRIL will harm your unborn baby. You and your healthcare provider will have to decide if you should take SABRIL while you are pregnant.

Pregnancy Registry:

If you become pregnant while taking SABRIL, talk to your healthcare provider about registering with the North American Antiepileptic Drug Pregnancy Registry. You can enroll in this registry by calling 1-888-233-2334. The purpose of this registry is to collect information about the safety of antiepileptic medicine during pregnancy.

Before giving SABRIL to your baby, tell the doctor about all of your baby's medical conditions, including if your baby has or ever had:

- an allergic reaction to SABRIL, such as hives, itching, or trouble breathing
- any vision problems
- any kidney problems

Tell your doctor about all the medicines you or your baby take, including prescription and non-prescription medicines, vitamins, and herbal supplements. SABRIL and other medicines may affect each other causing side effects.

How should I take SABRIL?

If you are an adult with CPS:

- Your doctor will explain the SHARE Program to you
- You will receive SABRIL from a specialty pharmacy
- Take SABRIL tablets exactly as prescribed by your doctor. SABRIL tablets are usually taken two times each day.
- You may take SABRIL tablets with or without food
- Before you start taking SABRIL, talk to your doctor about what you should do if you miss a dose of SABRIL
- **Do not stop taking SABRIL suddenly.** This can cause serious problems. Stopping SABRIL or any seizure medicine suddenly can cause seizures that will not stop (status epilepticus) in people who are being treated for seizures. You should follow your doctor's instructions on how to stop taking SABRIL.
- Tell your doctor right away about any increase in seizures while you are stopping SABRIL
- If SABRIL does not improve your seizures enough within 3 months, your doctor will stop prescribing SABRIL for you
- **Do not stop taking SABRIL without talking to your doctor.** If SABRIL improves your seizures, you and your doctor should talk about whether the benefit of taking SABRIL is more important than the risk of vision loss, and decide if you will continue to take SABRIL.

If you are giving SABRIL to your baby for IS:

- Your doctor will explain the SHARE program to you
- You will receive SABRIL for oral solution from a specialty pharmacy
- Mix SABRIL for oral solution and give it to your baby exactly as prescribed by your doctor. Do not stop giving SABRIL for oral solution to your baby unless your doctor tells you to.
- SABRIL for oral solution is usually given two times each day

- SABRIL for oral solution can be given to your baby at the same time as their food, but the powder should not be mixed with their food. SABRIL for oral solution powder should be mixed with water only.
- See the end of this Medication Guide for detailed instructions for how to mix SABRIL for oral solution and give the medicine to your baby
- Before your baby starts taking SABRIL, speak to your baby's doctor about what to do if your baby misses a dose, vomits, spits up, or only takes part of the dose of SABRIL
- **Stopping SABRIL suddenly can cause serious problems.** Stopping SABRIL or any seizure medicine suddenly can cause seizures that will not stop. You should follow your doctor's instructions on how to stop giving SABRIL to your baby. SABRIL does not work in all babies. If your baby's seizures do not improve enough within 2 to 4 weeks, the doctor will stop SABRIL.
- **Tell your doctor right away about any increase in your baby's seizures while stopping SABRIL**

What should I avoid while taking SABRIL?

SABRIL causes sleepiness and tiredness. Adults taking SABRIL should not drive, operate machinery, or perform any hazardous task, unless you and your doctor have decided that you can do these things safely.

What are the possible side effects of SABRIL?

SABRIL can cause serious side effects. See "What is the most important information I should know about SABRIL?"

These other serious side effects happen in **adults**. It is not known if these side effects also happen in babies who take SABRIL.

- Low red blood cell counts (anemia)
- Sleepiness and tiredness. See "What should I avoid while taking SABRIL?"
- Nerve problems. Symptoms of a nerve problem can include numbness and tingling in your toes or feet. It is not known if nerve problems will go away after you stop taking SABRIL.
- Weight gain that happens without swelling
- Swelling

If you are an adult with CPS, SABRIL may make certain types of seizures worse. Tell your doctor right away if your seizures get worse.

The most common side effects of SABRIL in adults include:

- problems walking or feel uncoordinated
- feel dizzy
- shaking (tremor)
- joint pain
- memory problems and not thinking clearly
- eye problems: blurry vision, double vision and eye movements that you cannot control

If you are giving SABRIL to your baby for IS

SABRIL may make certain types of seizures worse. You should tell your baby's doctor right away if your baby's seizures get worse. Tell your baby's doctor if you see any changes in your baby's behavior.

The most common side effects of SABRIL in **babies and young children** include:

- sleepiness - SABRIL may cause your baby to be sleepy. Sleepy babies may have a harder time suckling and feeding, or may be irritable.
- ear infection
- irritability

Tell your doctor if you or your baby have any side effect that bother you or that does not go away. These are not all the possible side effects of SABRIL. For more information, ask your doctor or pharmacist.

Call your doctor for medical advice about side effects. You may report side effects to FDA at 1-800-FDA-1088.

How should I store SABRIL?

Store SABRIL tablets and SABRIL packets at room temperature, between 68 °F to 77 °F (20 °C to 25 °C).

Keep SABRIL tablets and SABRIL powder in the container they come in.

Keep SABRIL and all medicines out of the reach of children.

General information about SABRIL

Medicines are sometimes prescribed for purposes other than those listed in a Medication Guide. Do not use SABRIL for a condition for which it was not prescribed. Do not give SABRIL to other people, even if they have the same symptoms that you have. It may harm them.

This Medication Guide summarizes the most important information about SABRIL. If you would like more information about SABRIL, talk with your doctor. You can ask your pharmacist or doctor for information about SABRIL that is written for health professionals. For more information, go to **www.SABRIL.net** or call **1-800-455-1141.**

What are the ingredients in SABRIL?

Active Ingredient: vigabatrin.
Inactive Ingredients in **SABRIL tablets**: hydroxypropyl methylcellulose, magnesium stearate, microcrystalline cellulose, polyethylene glycols, povidone, sodium starch glycolate, and titanium dioxide.
Inactive Ingredient in **SABRIL powder**: povidone.

This Medication Guide has been approved by the U.S. Food and Drug Administration.
Marketed by: Lundbeck Inc., Deerfield, IL 60015, U.S.A.
® Trademark of Lundbeck Inc.
Issued: August 2009
Shown in Product Identification Guide, page 311

SABRIL®

[SAY- bril]
(vigabatrin)
Tablets
For Oral Administration Only
Rx Only

℞

HIGHLIGHTS OF PRESCRIBING INFORMATION

These highlights do not include all the information needed to use SABRIL safely and effectively. See full prescribing information for SABRIL.
Sabril® (vigabatrin) Tablets
For Oral Administration Only
Rx Only
Initial U.S. Approval: 2009

> **WARNING: VISION LOSS**
> *See full prescribing information for complete boxed warning*
> - SABRIL causes progressive and permanent bilateral concentric visual field constriction in a high percentage of patients. In some cases, SABRIL may also reduce visual acuity.
> - Risk increases with total dose and duration of use, but no exposure to SABRIL is known that is free of risk of vision loss
> - Risk of new and worsening vision loss continues as long as SABRIL is used, and possibly after discontinuing SABRIL
> - Periodic vision testing is required for patients on SABRIL, but cannot reliably prevent vision damage
> - Because of the risk of permanent vision loss, SABRIL is available only through a special restricted distribution program

INDICATIONS AND USAGE

SABRIL is an antiepileptic drug (AED) indicated for:
- **Refractory Complex Partial Seizures in Adults** (1.1). It should be used as adjunctive therapy in patients who have responded inadequately to several alternative treatments.

DOSAGE AND ADMINISTRATION

- Refractory Complex Partial Seizures in Adults: Initiate therapy at 500 mg twice daily, increasing total daily dose per instructions. The recommended dose is 1.5 grams twice daily (2.1).
- Dose adjustment recommended in renally impaired patients (2.2)
- Reduce dose gradually upon discontinuation (2.3)

DOSAGE FORMS AND STRENGTHS

Tablet: 500 mg (3.1)

CONTRAINDICATIONS

None (4)

WARNINGS AND PRECAUTIONS

- SABRIL causes permanent vision loss (5.1)
- Abnormal MRI signal changes have been reported in some infants with IS receiving SABRIL (5.3)
- Antiepileptic drugs, including SABRIL, increase the risk of suicidal thoughts and behavior (5.5)
- Dose should be tapered gradually to avoid withdrawal seizures (5.6)
- SABRIL causes anemia (5.7)
- SABRIL causes somnolence and fatigue (5.8)
- SABRIL causes peripheral neuropathy (5.9)
- SABRIL causes weight gain (5.10)
- SABRIL causes edema (5.11)

ADVERSE REACTIONS

Most common adverse reactions (change of ≥ 5% over placebo) in addition to permanent vision loss in adult controlled trials with vigabatrin were fatigue, somnolence, nystagmus, tremor, vision blurred, memory impairment, weight gain, arthralgia, abnormal coordination, and confusional state (6.1).
To report SUSPECTED ADVERSE REACTIONS, contact Lundbeck Inc. at 1-800-455-1141 or www.lundbeckinc.com or FDA at 1-800-FDA-1088 or www.fda.gov/medwatch.

DRUG INTERACTIONS

- Decreased phenytoin plasma levels have been reported (7.1)

USE IN SPECIFIC POPULATIONS

- Pregnancy: Based on animal data, may cause fetal harm. Pregnancy registry available (8.1)
- Nursing Mothers: SABRIL is excreted in human milk (8.3)
- Renal Impairment: Dose adjustment recommended (2.2, 8.5, 8.6)

See 17 for PATIENT COUNSELING INFORMATION and Medication Guide

Revised: 04/2010

FULL PRESCRIBING INFORMATION: CONTENTS *

MEDICATION GUIDE
NDC 67386-111-01
* Sections or subsections omitted from the full prescribing information are not listed

FULL PRESCRIBING INFORMATION

WARNING: VISION LOSS

- **SABRIL causes permanent bilateral concentric visual field constriction in 30 percent or more of patients that ranges in severity from mild to severe, including tunnel vision to within 10 degrees of visual fixation, and can result in disability. In some cases, SABRIL also can damage the central retina and may decrease visual acuity.**
- **The onset of vision loss from SABRIL is unpredictable, and can occur within weeks of starting treatment or sooner, or at any time during treatment, even after months or years**
- **The risk of vision loss increases with increasing dose and cumulative exposure, but there is no dose or exposure known to be free of risk of vision loss**

- **Vision testing at baseline (no later than 4 weeks after starting SABRIL) and at least every 3 months during therapy is required for adults on SABRIL. Vision testing is also required about 3 to 6 months after the discontinuation of SABRIL therapy. Once detected, vision loss due to SABRIL is not reversible. It is expected that, even with frequent monitoring, some patients will develop severe vision loss.**
- **It is possible that vision loss can worsen despite discontinuation of SABRIL**
- **Because of the risk of vision loss, SABRIL should be withdrawn from patients who fail to show substantial clinical benefit within 3 months of initiation, or sooner if treatment failure becomes obvious. Patient response to and continued need for SABRIL should be periodically reassessed.**
- **Symptoms of vision loss from SABRIL are unlikely to be recognized by patients or caregivers before vision loss is severe. Vision loss of milder severity, while often unrecognized by the patient, can still adversely affect function.**
- **SABRIL should not be used in patients with, or at high risk of, other types of irreversible vision loss unless the benefits of treatment clearly outweigh the risks. The interaction of other types of irreversible vision damage with vision damage from SABRIL has not been well-characterized, but is likely adverse.**
- **SABRIL should not be used with other drugs associated with serious adverse ophthalmic effects such as retinopathy or glaucoma unless the benefits clearly outweigh the risks**
- **The lowest dose and shortest exposure to SABRIL should be used that is consistent with clinical objectives**

Because of the risk of permanent vision loss, SABRIL is available only through a special restricted distribution program called SHARE, by calling 1-888-45-SHARE. Only prescribers and pharmacies registered with SHARE may prescribe and distribute SABRIL. In addition, SABRIL may be dispensed only to patients who are enrolled in and meet all conditions of SHARE [see WARNINGS AND PRECAUTIONS, Distribution Program for SABRIL (5.2)].

1 INDICATIONS AND USAGE

1.1 Refractory Complex Partial Seizures in Adults

SABRIL® is indicated as adjunctive therapy for adult patients with refractory complex partial seizures (CPS) who have inadequately responded to several alternative treatments and for whom the potential benefits outweigh the risk of vision loss [see WARNINGS AND PRECAUTIONS, Vision Loss (5.1)]. SABRIL is not indicated as a first line agent for complex partial seizures.

2 DOSAGE AND ADMINISTRATION

2.1 Refractory Complex Partial Seizures in Adults

SABRIL 500 mg tablets should be given as twice daily oral administration with or without food. Therapy should be initiated at 1 g/day (500 mg twice daily). Total daily dose may be increased in 500 mg increments at weekly intervals depending on response. The recommended dose of SABRIL in adults is 3 g/day (1.5 g twice daily). A 6 g/day dose has not been shown to confer additional benefit compared to the 3 g/day dose and is associated with an increased incidence of adverse events.

2.2 Patients with Renal Impairment

SABRIL is primarily eliminated through the kidney. In patients with renal impairment, dose adjustments should be made as follows:

In patients with mild renal impairment (CLcr >50 to 80 mL/min), the dose should be decreased by 25%; in patients with moderate renal impairment (CLcr >30 to 50 mL/min), the dose should be decreased by 50%; and in patients with severe renal impairment (CLcr >10 to <30 mL/min), the dose should be decreased by 75%.

CLcr in mL/min may be estimated from a serum creatinine (mg/dL) determination using the following formula:

$CLcr * = [140 - age\ (years)] \times weight\ (kg)/72 \times serum\ creatinine\ (mg/dL)]$

*[$\times$ 0.85 for female patients]

The effect of dialysis on SABRIL clearance has not been adequately studied.

[see CLINICAL PHARMACOLOGY, Pharmacokinetics, Renal Impairment (12.3) and USE IN SPECIFIC POPULATIONS, Renal Impairment (8.6)].

2.3 General Dosing Considerations

SABRIL should be withdrawn gradually. In controlled clinical studies in adults with CPS, vigabatrin was tapered by decreasing the daily dose 1 g/day on a weekly basis until

---

discontinued [see WARNINGS AND PRECAUTIONS, Withdrawal of Antiepileptic Drugs (AEDs) (5.6)].

3 DOSAGE FORMS AND STRENGTHS

3.1 Tablet

500 mg Tablet.

4 CONTRAINDICATIONS

None.

5 WARNINGS AND PRECAUTIONS

5.1 Vision Loss (see BOXED WARNING)

Because of the risk of vision loss and because SABRIL, when it is effective, provides an observable symptomatic benefit, a patient who fails to show substantial clinical benefit within 3 months of initiation of treatment, should be withdrawn from SABRIL. If in the clinical judgment of the prescriber evidence of treatment failure becomes obvious earlier than 3 months, treatment with SABRIL should be discontinued at that time. Patient response to and continued need for treatment should be periodically assessed.

Monitoring of Vision

Monitoring of vision by an ophthalmic professional with expertise in visual field interpretation and the ability to perform dilated indirect ophthalmoscopy of the retina is required. Vision testing at baseline (no later than 4 weeks after starting SABRIL) and at least every 3 months is required for adults on SABRIL. Vision testing is also required about 3 to 6 months after the discontinuation of SABRIL therapy.

The diagnostic approach should be individualized for the patient and clinical situation, but for all patients attempts to monitor vision periodically must be documented under the SHARE program. Perimetry is recommended, preferably by automated threshold visual field testing. Additional testing may also include electrophysiology (e.g., electroretinography [ERG]), retinal imaging (e.g., optical coherence tomography [OCT]), and/or other methods appropriate for the patient. In patients in whom vision testing is not possible, treatment may continue according to clinical judgment, with appropriate patient counseling and with documentation in the SHARE program of the inability to test vision. Because of variability, results from ophthalmic monitoring must be interpreted with caution, and repeat testing is recommended if results are abnormal or uninterpretable. Repeat testing in the first few weeks of treatment is recommended to establish if, and to what degree, reproducible results can be obtained, and to guide selection of appropriate ongoing monitoring for the patient.

The onset and progression of vision loss from SABRIL is unpredictable, and it may occur or worsen precipitously between tests. Once detected, vision loss due to SABRIL is not reversible. It is expected that even with frequent monitoring, some SABRIL patients will develop severe vision loss.

5.2 Distribution Program for SABRIL

SABRIL is available only under a special restricted distribution program called the SHARE program. Under the SHARE program, only prescribers and pharmacies registered with the program are able to prescribe and distribute SABRIL. In addition, SABRIL may be dispensed only to patients who are enrolled in and meet all conditions of SHARE. Contact the SHARE program at 1-888-45-SHARE. To enroll in SHARE, prescribers must understand the risks of SABRIL and complete the SHARE Prescriber Enrollment and Agreement Form indicating agreement to:

- Enroll all patients in SHARE
- Review the SABRIL Medication Guide with every patient
- Educate patients on the risks of SABRIL, including the risk of vision loss [see BOXED WARNING: VISION LOSS]
- Order and review vision assessments at initiation of SABRIL treatment and every 3 months during therapy
- Remove patients from SABRIL therapy if the patients do not experience meaningful reduction in seizures
- Counsel patients who fail to comply with the program requirements
- Remove patients from SABRIL therapy who fail to comply with the program requirements after appropriate counseling

5.3 Magnetic Resonance Imaging (MRI) Abnormalities

Abnormal MRI signal changes characterized by increased T2 signal and restricted diffusion in a symmetric pattern involving the thalamus, basal ganglia, brain stem, and cerebellum have been observed in some infants treated for Infantile Spasms (IS) with vigabatrin. In a retrospective epidemiologic study in infants with IS (N=205), the prevalence of these changes was 21.5% in vigabatrin-treated patients versus 4.1% in patients treated with other therapies.

In the study above, in post marketing experience, and in published literature reports, these changes generally re-

Table 1. Risk by Indication for Antiepileptic Drugs in the Pooled Analysis

Indication	Placebo Patients with Events per 1000 Patients	Drug Patients with Events per 1000 Patients	Relative Risk: Incidence of Drug Events in Drug Patients/Incidence in Placebo Patients	Risk Difference: Additional Drug Patients with Events per 1000 Patients
Epilepsy	1.0	3.4	3.5	2.4
Psychiatric	5.7	8.5	1.5	2.9
Other	1.0	1.8	1.9	0.9
Total	2.4	4.3	1.8	1.9

solved with discontinuation of treatment. In a few patients, the lesion resolved despite continued use. It has been reported that some infants exhibited coincident motor abnormalities, but no causal relationship has been established and the potential for long-term clinical sequelae has not been adequately studied.

Neurotoxicity (including convulsions and hypomyelination) was observed in rats exposed to vigabatrin during late gestation and the neonatal and juvenile periods of development. The relationship between these findings and the abnormal MRI findings in infants treated for IS with vigabatrin is unknown [see WARNINGS AND PRECAUTIONS, Neurotoxicity (5.4) and USE IN SPECIFIC POPULATIONS, Pregnancy (8.1)].

The specific pattern of signal changes observed in IS patients was not observed in older children and adult patients treated with vigabatrin for CPS. In a blinded review of MRI images obtained in prospective clinical trials in patients with CPS 3 years and older (N=656), no difference was observed in anatomic distribution or prevalence of MRI signal changes between vigabatrin treated and placebo patients.

For adults treated with SABRIL, routine MRI surveillance is unnecessary as there is no evidence that vigabatrin causes MRI changes in this population.

5.4 Neurotoxicity

Vacuolization, characterized by fluid accumulation and separation of the outer layers of myelin, has been observed in brain white matter tracts in adult and juvenile rats and adult mice, dogs, and possibly monkeys following administration of vigabatrin. This lesion, referred to as intramyelinic edema (IME), was seen in animals at doses within the human therapeutic range. A no-effect dose was not established in rodents or dogs. In the rat and dog, vacuolization was reversible following discontinuation of vigabatrin treatment, but, in the rat, pathologic changes consisting of swollen or degenerating axons, mineralization, and gliosis were seen in brain areas in which vacuolation had been previously observed. Vacuolization in adult animals was correlated with alterations in MRI and changes in visual and somatosensory evoked potentials (EP).

Administration of vigabatrin to rats during the neonatal and juvenile periods of development produced vacuolar changes in the gray matter (areas including the thalamus, midbrain, deep cerebellar nuclei, substantia nigra, hippocampus, and forebrain) which are considered distinct from the IME observed in vigabatrin treated adult animals. Decreased myelination, retinal dysplasia, and neurobehavioral abnormalities (convulsions, neuromotor impairment, learning deficits) were also observed following vigabatrin treatment of young rats. These effects occurred at doses associated with plasma vigabatrin levels substantially lower than those achieved clinically in infants and children.

IME has been reported in a vigabatrin treated infant on postmortem examination. The infant had hypoxic ischemic brain injury and abnormalities of myelin prior to vigabatrin treatment.

In a published study, vigabatrin (200, 400 mg/kg/day) induced apoptotic neurodegeneration in the brain of young rats when administered by intraperitoneal injection on postnatal days 5-7.

Administration of vigabatrin to female rats during pregnancy and lactation at doses below those used clinically resulted in hippocampal vacuolation and convulsions in the mature offspring.

Abnormal MRI signal changes characterized by increased T2 signal and restricted diffusion in a symmetric pattern involving the thalamus, basal ganglia, brain stem, and cerebellum have been observed in some infants treated for IS with vigabatrin. Studies of the effects of vigabatrin on MRI and EP in adult epilepsy patients have demonstrated no clear-cut abnormalities [see WARNINGS AND PRECAUTIONS, MRI Abnormalities (5.3)].

5.5 Suicidal Behavior and Ideation

Antiepileptic drugs (AEDs), including SABRIL, increase the risk of suicidal thoughts or behavior in patients taking these drugs for any indication. Patients treated with any AED for any indication should be monitored for the emergence or worsening of depression, suicidal thoughts or behavior, and/or any unusual changes in mood or behavior.

Pooled analyses of 199 placebo-controlled clinical trials (mono- and adjunctive therapy) of 11 different AEDs showed that patients randomized to one of the AEDs had approximately twice the risk (adjusted Relative Risk 1.8, 95% CI: 1.2, 2.7) of suicidal thinking or behavior compared to patients randomized to placebo. In these trials, which had a median treatment duration of 12 weeks, the estimated incidence rate of suicidal behavior or ideation among 27,863 AED treated patients was 0.43%, compared to 0.24% among 16,029 placebo treated patients, representing an increase of approximately one case of suicidal thinking or behavior for every 530 patients treated. There were four suicides in drug treated patients in the trials and none in placebo treated patients, but the number is too small to allow any conclusion about drug effect on suicide.

The increased risk of suicidal thoughts or behavior with AEDs was observed as early as one week after starting drug treatment with AEDs and persisted for the duration of treatment assessed. Because most trials included in the analysis did not extend beyond 24 weeks, the risk of suicidal thoughts or behavior beyond 24 weeks could not be assessed.

The risk of suicidal thoughts or behavior was generally consistent among drugs in the data analyzed. The finding of increased risk with AEDs of varying mechanisms of action and across a range of indications suggests that the risk applies to all AEDs used for any indication. The risk did not vary substantially by age (5-100 years) in the clinical trials analyzed. Table 1 shows absolute and relative risk by indication for all evaluated AEDs.

[See table 1 above]

The relative risk for suicidal thoughts or behavior was higher in clinical trials for epilepsy than in clinical trials for psychiatric or other conditions, but the absolute risk differences were similar for the epilepsy and psychiatric indications.

Anyone considering prescribing SABRIL or any other AED must balance the risk of suicidal thoughts or behavior with the risk of untreated illness. Epilepsy and many other illnesses for which AEDs are prescribed are themselves associated with morbidity and mortality and an increased risk of suicidal thoughts and behavior. Should suicidal thoughts and behavior emerge during treatment, the prescriber needs to consider whether the emergence of these symptoms in any given patient may be related to the illness being treated.

Patients, their caregivers, and families should be informed that AEDs increase the risk of suicidal thoughts and behavior and should be advised of the need to be alert for the emergence or worsening of the signs and symptoms of depression, any unusual changes in mood or behavior, or the emergence of suicidal thoughts, behavior, or thoughts about self-harm. Behaviors of concern should be reported immediately to healthcare providers.

5.6 Withdrawal of Antiepileptic Drugs (AEDs)

As with all AEDs, SABRIL should be withdrawn gradually. In controlled clinical studies in adults with CPS, SABRIL was tapered by decreasing the daily dose 1 g/day on a weekly basis until discontinued [see DOSAGE AND ADMINISTRATION, General Dosing Considerations (2.3), PATIENT COUNSELING INFORMATION, Withdrawal of SABRIL Therapy (17.4)].

5.7 Anemia

In North American controlled trials, 5.7% of patients (16/280) receiving SABRIL and 1.6% of patients (3/188) receiving placebo had adverse events of anemia and/or met criteria for potentially clinically important hematology changes involving hemoglobin, hematocrit, and/or RBC indices. Across U.S. controlled trials, there were mean decreases in hemoglobin of about 3% and 0% in SABRIL and placebo-treated patients, respectively, and in hematocrit of about 1% in Sabril treated patients compared to a gain of about 1% in patients treated with placebo.

In controlled and open label epilepsy trials, 3 SABRIL patients (0.06%, 3/4855) discontinued for anemia and 2 SABRIL patients experienced unexplained declines in hemoglobin to below 8 g/dL and/or hematocrit below 24%.

5.8 Somnolence and Fatigue

SABRIL causes somnolence and fatigue. Patients should be advised not to drive a car or operate other complex machinery until they are familiar with the effects of SABRIL on their ability to perform such activities.

Pooled data from two SABRIL controlled trials demonstrated that 24% (54/222) of SABRIL patients experienced somnolence compared to 10% (14/135) of placebo patients. In those same studies, 28% of SABRIL patients experienced fatigue compared to 15% (20/135) of placebo patients. Almost 1% of SABRIL patients discontinued from clinical trials for somnolence and almost 1% discontinued for fatigue.

5.9 Peripheral Neuropathy

SABRIL causes symptoms of peripheral neuropathy. In a pool of North American controlled and uncontrolled epilepsy studies, 4.2% (19/457) of SABRIL patients developed signs and/or symptoms of peripheral neuropathy. In the subset of North American placebo-controlled epilepsy trials, 1.4% (4/280) of SABRIL treated patients and no (0/188) placebo patients developed signs and/or symptoms of peripheral neuropathy. Initial manifestations of peripheral neuropathy in these trials included, in some combination, symptoms of numbness or tingling in the toes or feet, signs of reduced distal lower limb vibration or position sensation, or progressive loss of reflexes, starting at the ankles. Clinical studies in the development program were not designed to investigate peripheral neuropathy systematically and did not include nerve conduction studies, quantitative sensory testing, or skin or nerve biopsy. There is insufficient evidence to determine if development of these signs and symptoms were related to duration of SABRIL treatment, cumulative dose, or if the findings of peripheral neuropathy were completely reversible upon discontinuation of SABRIL.

5.10 Weight Gain

SABRIL causes weight gain. Data pooled from randomized controlled trials found that 17% (77/443) of SABRIL patients versus 8% (22/275) of placebo patients gained ≥ 7% of baseline body weight. In these same trials, the mean weight change among SABRIL patients was 3.5 kg compared to 1.6 kg for placebo patients. In all epilepsy trials, 0.6% (31/4855) of SABRIL patients discontinued for weight gain. The long term effects of SABRIL related weight gain are not known. Weight gain was not related to the occurrence of edema.

5.11 Edema

SABRIL causes edema. Pooled data from controlled trials demonstrated increased risk among SABRIL patients compared to placebo patients for peripheral edema (SABRIL 2%, placebo 1%), and edema (SABRIL 1%, placebo 0%). In these studies, one SABRIL and no placebo patients discontinued for an edema related AE. There was no apparent association between edema and cardiovascular adverse events such as hypertension or congestive heart failure. Edema was not associated with laboratory changes suggestive of deterioration in renal or hepatic function.

6 ADVERSE REACTIONS

SABRIL causes permanent damage to vision in a high percentage of patients [see BOXED WARNING: VISION LOSS and WARNINGS AND PRECAUTIONS, Vision Loss (5.1)].

6.1 Adverse Reactions in Clinical Trials

Because clinical trials are conducted under widely varying conditions, adverse reaction rates observed in the clinical trials of a drug cannot be directly compared to rates in the clinical trials of another drug and may not reflect the rates observed in practice.

Adverse Reactions in U.S. and Primary Non-U.S. Clinical Studies

In U.S. and primary non-U.S. clinical studies of 4,079 SABRIL treated patients, the most commonly observed (≥ 5%) adverse reactions associated with the use of SABRIL in combination with other AEDs were headache (18%), somnolence (17%), fatigue (16%), dizziness (15%), convulsion (11%), nasopharyngitis (10%), weight increased (10%), upper respiratory tract infection (10%), visual field defect (9%), depression (8%), tremor (7%), nystagmus (7%), nausea (7%), diarrhea (7%), memory impairment (7%), insomnia (7%), irritability (7%), coordination abnormal (7%), vision blurred (6%), diplopia (6%), vomiting (6%), influenza (6%), pyrexia (6%), and rash (6%).

The adverse reactions most commonly associated with SABRIL treatment discontinuation in ≥ 1% of patients were convulsion (1.4%) and depression (1.5%).

Most Common Adverse Reactions in Controlled Clinical Trials

Refractory Complex Partial Seizures in Adults

Table 2 lists the treatment emergent adverse reactions that occurred in ≥ 2% and more than one patient per SABRIL-treated group and that occurred more frequently than in placebo patients from 2 U.S. add-on clinical studies of refractory CPS in adults.

Table 2. Treatment Emergent Adverse Reactions Occurring in ≥ 2% and More than One Patient per SABRIL-Treated Group and More Frequently than in Placebo Patients (Studies 024 and 025)

Body System Preferred Term	SABRIL 3 g/day (N=134) n(%)	SABRIL 6 g/day (N=43) n(%)	Placebo (N=135) n(%)
Ear Disorders			
Tinnitus	3 (2)	0 (0)	2 (1)
Vertigo	3 (2)	2 (5)	2 (1)
Eye Disorders			
Vision blurred	18 (13)	7 (16)	7 (5)
Diplopia	9 (7)	7 (16)	4 (3)
Asthenopia	3 (2)	1 (2)	0 (0)
Eye pain	0 (0)	2 (5)	0 (0)
Gastrointestinal Disorders			
Diarrhoea	14 (10)	7 (16)	10 (7)
Nausea	13 (10)	1 (2)	11 (8)
Vomiting	9 (7)	4 (9)	8 (6)
Constipation	11 (8)	2 (5)	4 (3)
Abdominal pain upper	7 (5)	2 (5)	2 (1)
Dyspepsia	6 (4)	2 (5)	4 (3)
Stomach discomfort	5 (4)	1 (2)	1 (1)
Abdominal pain	4 (3)	1 (2)	2 (1)
Toothache	3 (2)	2 (5)	3 (2)
Abdominal distension	3 (2)	0 (0)	1 (1)
General Disorders			
Fatigue	31 (23)	17 (40)	21 (16)
Gait disturbance	8 (6)	5 (12)	9 (7)
Asthenia	7 (5)	3 (7)	2 (1)
Oedema peripheral	7 (5)	3 (7)	1 (1)
Fever	6 (4)	3 (7)	4 (3)
Chest pain	2 (1)	2 (5)	2 (1)
Thirst	3 (2)	0 (0)	0 (0)
Malaise	0 (0)	2 (5)	0 (0)
Infections			
Nasopharyngitis	19 (14)	4 (9)	14 (10)
Upper respiratory tract infection	10 (7)	4 (9)	8 (6)
Influenza	7 (5)	3 (7)	5 (4)
Urinary tract infection	5 (4)	2 (5)	0 (0)
Bronchitis	0 (0)	2 (5)	2 (1)
Injury			
Contusion	4 (3)	2 (5)	3 (2)
Joint sprain	2 (1)	1 (2)	1 (1)
Muscle strain	1 (1)	1 (2)	2 (1)
Wound secretion	0 (0)	1 (2)	0 (0)
Metabolism and Nutrition Disorders			
Increased appetite	2 (1)	2 (5)	1 (1)
Weight increased	8 (6)	6 (14)	4 (3)
Musculoskeletal Disorders			
Arthralgia	14 (10)	2 (5)	4 (3)
Back pain	6 (4)	3 (7)	3 (2)
Pain in extremity	8 (6)	1 (2)	5 (4)
Myalgia	4 (3)	2 (5)	2 (1)
Muscle twitching	1 (1)	4 (9)	2 (1)
Muscle spasms	4 (3)	0 (0)	1 (1)
Nervous System Disorders			
Headache	44 (33)	11 (26)	42 (31)
Somnolence	29 (22)	11 (26)	18 (13)
Dizziness	32 (24)	11 (26)	23 (17)
Nystagmus	17 (13)	8 (19)	12 (9)
Tremor	20 (15)	7 (16)	11 (8)
Memory impairment	9 (7)	7 (16)	4 (3)
Coordination abnormal	10 (7)	7 (16)	3 (2)
Disturbance in attention	12 (9)	0 (0)	1 (1)
Sensory disturbance	6 (4)	3 (7)	3 (2)
Hyporeflexia	6 (4)	2 (5)	1 (1)
Paraesthesia	9 (7)	1 (2)	1 (1)
Lethargy	6 (4)	3 (7)	3 (2)
Hyperreflexia	5 (4)	1 (2)	4 (3)
Hypoaesthesia	5 (4)	2 (5)	2 (1)
Sedation	5 (4)	0 (0)	0 (0)
Status epilepticus	3 (2)	2 (5)	0 (0)
Dysarthria	3 (2)	1 (2)	1 (1)
Postictal state	3 (2)	0 (0)	1 (1)
Sensory loss	0 (0)	2 (5)	0 (0)
Psychiatric Disorders			
Irritability	10 (7)	10 (23)	10 (7)
Depression	8 (6)	6 (14)	4 (3)
Confusional state	5 (4)	6 (14)	1 (1)
Anxiety	6 (4)	0 (0)	4 (3)
Depressed mood	7 (5)	0 (0)	1 (1)
Thinking abnormal	4 (3)	3 (7)	0 (0)
Abnormal behaviour	4 (3)	2 (5)	1 (1)
Expressive language disorder	2 (1)	3 (7)	1 (1)
Nervousness	3 (2)	2 (5)	3 (2)
Abnormal dreams	2 (1)	2 (5)	1 (1)
Reproductive System			
Dysmenorrhoea	12 (9)	2 (5)	4 (3)
Erectile dysfunction	0 (0)	2 (5)	0 (0)
Respiratory and Thoracic Disorders			
Pharyngolaryngeal pain	10 (7)	6 (14)	7 (5)
Cough	3 (2)	6 (14)	9 (7)
Pulmonary congestion	0 (0)	2 (5)	1 (1)
Sinus headache	8 (6)	1 (2)	1 (1)
Skin and Subcutaneous Tissue Disorders			
Rash	6 (4)	2 (5)	6 (4)

6.2   Post Marketing Experience

The following serious adverse events have been reported since approval and use of SABRIL worldwide. All serious adverse events that are not listed above as adverse events reported in clinical trials, that are not relatively common in the population and are not too vague to be useful are listed in this section. These reactions are reported voluntarily from a population of uncertain size; therefore, it is not possible to estimate their frequency or establish a causal relationship to drug exposure. Events are categorized by system organ class.

Birth Defects: Congenital cardiac defects, congenital external ear anomaly, congenital hemangioma, congenital hydronephrosis, congenital male genital malformation, congenital oral malformation, congenital vesicoureteric reflux, dentofacial anomaly, dysmorphism, fetal anticonvulsant syndrome, hamartomas, hip dysplasia, limb malformation, limb reduction defect, low set ears, renal aplasia, retinitis pigmentosa, supernumerary nipple, talipes

Ear: Deafness

Endocrine: Delayed puberty

Gastrointestinal: Gastrointestinal hemorrhage, esophagitis

General: Developmental delay, facial edema, malignant hyperthermia, multi-organ failure

Hepatobiliary: Cholestasis

Nervous System: Dystonia, encephalopathy, hypertonia, hypotonia, muscle spasticity, myoclonus, optic neuritis

Psychiatric: Acute psychosis, apathy, delirium, hypomania, neonatal agitation, psychotic disorder

Respiratory: Laryngeal edema, pulmonary embolism, respiratory failure, stridor

Skin and Subcutaneous Tissue: Angioedema, maculopapular rash, pruritus

7   DRUG INTERACTIONS

For detailed information about Drug Interactions see CLINICAL PHARMACOLOGY, Pharmacokinetics, Drug Interactions (12.3).

7.1   Phenytoin

A 16% to 20% average reduction in total phenytoin plasma levels was reported in controlled clinical studies.

7.2   Other AEDs

There are no clinically significant pharmacokinetic interactions between SABRIL and either phenobarbital or sodium valproate. Based on population pharmacokinetics, carbamazepine, clorazepate, primidone, and sodium valproate appear to have no effect on plasma concentrations of vigabatrin.

7.3   Clonazepam

In a study of 12 healthy volunteers, clonazepam (0.5 mg) co-administration had no effect on SABRIL (1.5 g twice daily) concentrations. SABRIL increases the mean C_{max} of clonazepam by 30% and decreases the mean t_{max} by 45%.

7.4   Oral Contraceptives

SABRIL is unlikely to affect the efficacy of steroid oral contraceptives.

7.5   Drug-Laboratory Test Interactions

SABRIL decreases alanine transaminase (ALT) and aspartate transaminase (AST) plasma activity in up to 90% of patients. In some patients, these enzymes become undetectable. The suppression of ALT and AST activity by SABRIL may preclude the use of these markers, especially ALT, to detect early hepatic injury.

SABRIL may increase the amount of amino acids in the urine, possibly leading to a false positive test for certain rare genetic metabolic diseases (e.g., alpha aminoadipic aciduria).

8   USE IN SPECIFIC POPULATIONS

8.1   Pregnancy

Pregnancy Category C. Vigabatrin produced developmental toxicity, including teratogenic and neurohistopathological effects, when administered to pregnant animals at clinically relevant doses. In addition, developmental neurotoxicity was observed in rats treated with vigabatrin during a period of postnatal development corresponding to the third trimester of human pregnancy. There are no adequate and well-controlled studies in pregnant women. SABRIL should be used during pregnancy only if the potential benefit justifies the potential risk to the fetus.

Table 3. Description

Proprietary Name:	SABRIL®
Established Name:	Vigabatrin Tablet
Dosage Form:	White, film-coated tablet
Route of Administration:	Oral
Pharmacologic Class of Drug:	Antiepileptic
Chemical Name:	(±) 4-amino-5-hexenoic acid
Structural Formula:	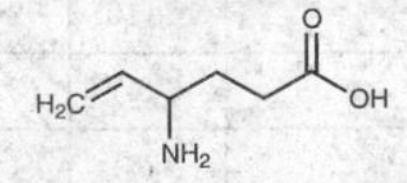

Administration of vigabatrin (oral doses of 50 to 200 mg/kg) to pregnant rabbits throughout the period of organogenesis was associated with an increased incidence of malformations (cleft palate) and embryo-fetal death; these findings were observed in two separate studies. The no-effect dose for teratogenicity and embryolethality in rabbits (100 mg/kg) is approximately 1/2 the maximum recommended human dose (MRHD) of 3 g/day on a body surface area (mg/m^2) basis. In rats, oral administration of vigabatrin (50, 100, or 150 mg/kg) throughout organogenesis resulted in decreased fetal body weights and increased incidences of fetal anatomic variations. The no-effect dose for embryo-fetal toxicity in rats (50 mg/kg) is approximately 1/5 the MRHD on a mg/m^2 basis. Oral administration of vigabatrin (50, 100, 150 mg/kg) to rats from the latter part of pregnancy through weaning produced long-term neurohistopathological (hippocampal vacuolation) and neurobehavioral (convulsions) abnormalities in the offspring. A no-effect dose for developmental neurotoxicity in rats was not established; the low-effect dose (50 mg/kg) is approximately 1/5 the MRHD on a mg/m^2 basis.

In a published study, vigabatrin (300 or 450 mg/kg) was administered by intraperitoneal injection to a mutant mouse strain on a single day during organogenesis (day 7, 8, 9, 10, 11, or 12). An increase in malformations (including cleft palate) was observed at both doses.

Oral administration of vigabatrin (5, 15, or 50 mg/kg) to young rats during the neonatal and juvenile periods of development (postnatal days 4-65) produced neurobehavioral (convulsions, neuromotor impairment, learning deficits) and neurohistopathological (brain vacuolation, decreased myelination, and retinal dysplasia) abnormalities in treated animals. The early postnatal period in rats is generally thought to correspond to late pregnancy in humans in terms of brain development. The no-effect dose for developmental neurotoxicity in juvenile rats (5 mg/kg) was associated with plasma vigabatrin exposures (AUC) less than 1/30 of those measured in pediatric patients receiving an oral dose of 50 mg/kg.

Pregnancy Registry: To provide information regarding the effects of *in utero* exposure to SABRIL, physicians are advised to recommend that pregnant patients taking SABRIL enroll in the North American Antiepileptic Drug (NAAED) Pregnancy Registry. This can be done by calling the toll free number 1-888-233-2334, and must be done by patients themselves. Information on the registry can also be found at the website http://www.aedpregnancyregistry.org/.

8.3 Nursing Mothers

Vigabatrin is excreted in human milk. Because of the potential for serious adverse reactions from vigabatrin in nursing infants [see WARNINGS AND PRECAUTIONS, MRI Abnormalities (5.3) and Neurotoxicity (5.4)], a decision should be made whether to discontinue nursing or to discontinue the drug, taking into account the importance of the drug to the mother.

8.4 Pediatric Use

The safety and efficacy of SABRIL in pediatric patients (<16 years of age) with CPS has not been established.

Abnormal MRI signal changes were observed in infants [see WARNINGS AND PRECAUTIONS, MRI Abnormalities (5.3) and Neurotoxicity (5.4)].

Oral administration of vigabatrin (5, 15, or 50 mg/kg) to young rats during the neonatal and juvenile periods of development (postnatal days 4-65) produced neurobehavioral (convulsions, neuromotor impairment, learning deficits) and neurohistopathological (brain vacuolation, decreased myelination, and retinal dysplasia) abnormalities in treated animals. The no-effect dose for developmental neurotoxicity in juvenile rats (5 mg/kg) was associated with plasma vigabatrin exposures (AUC) less than 1/30 of those measured in pediatric patients receiving an oral dose of 50 mg/kg.

8.5 Geriatric Use

Clinical studies of vigabatrin did not include sufficient numbers of patients aged 65 and over to determine whether they responded differently from younger patients.

Vigabatrin is known to be substantially excreted by the kidney, and the risk of toxic reactions to this drug may be greater in patients with impaired renal function. Because elderly patients are more likely to have decreased renal function, care should be taken in dose selection, and it may be useful to monitor renal function.

Oral administration of a single dose of 1.5 g of vigabatrin to elderly (>65 years) patients with reduced creatinine clearance (<50 mL/min) was associated with moderate to severe sedation and confusion in 4 of 5 patients, lasting up to 5 days. The renal clearance of vigabatrin was 36% lower in healthy elderly subjects (>65 years) than in young healthy males. Adjustment of dose or frequency of administration should be considered. Such patients may respond to a lower maintenance dose [see CLINICAL PHARMACOLOGY, Pharmacokinetics, Renal Impairment (12.3) and DOSAGE AND ADMINISTRATION, Patients with Renal Impairment (2.2)].

Other reported clinical experience has not identified differences in responses between the elderly and younger patients.

8.6 Renal Impairment

Dose adjustment, including initiating treatment with a lower dose, is necessary in patients with mild (creatinine clearance >50-80 mL/min), moderate (creatinine clearance >30-50 mL/min) and severe (creatinine clearance >10-30 mL/min) renal impairment [see CLINICAL PHARMACOLOGY, Pharmacokinetics, Renal Impairment (12.3) and DOSAGE AND ADMINISTRATION, Patients with Renal Impairment (2.2)].

9 DRUG ABUSE AND DEPENDENCE

9.1 Controlled Substance Class

Vigabatrin is not a controlled substance.

9.2 Abuse

Vigabatrin did not produce adverse events or overt behaviors associated with abuse when administered to humans or animals. It is not possible to predict the extent to which a CNS active drug will be misused, diverted, and/or abused once marketed. Consequently, physicians should carefully evaluate patients for history of drug abuse and follow such patients closely, observing them for signs of misuse or abuse of vigabatrin (e.g., incrementation of dose, drug-seeking behavior).

9.3 Dependence

Following chronic administration of vigabatrin to animals, there were no apparent withdrawal signs upon drug discontinuation. However, as with all AEDs, vigabatrin should be withdrawn gradually to minimize increased seizure frequency [see WARNINGS AND PRECAUTIONS, Withdrawal of Antiepileptic Drugs (AEDs) (5.6) and PATIENT COUNSELING INFORMATION, Withdrawal of SABRIL Therapy (17.4)].

10 OVERDOSAGE

10.1 Signs, Symptoms, and Laboratory Findings of Overdosage

Confirmed and/or suspected vigabatrin overdoses have been reported during clinical trials and in post marketing surveillance. No vigabatrin overdoses resulted in death. When reported, the vigabatrin dose ingested ranged from 3 g to 90 g, but most were between 7.5 g and 30 g. Nearly half the cases involved multiple drug ingestions including carbamazepine, barbiturates, benzodiazepines, lamotrigine, valproic acid, acetaminophen, and/or chlorpheniramine.

Coma, unconsciousness, and/or drowsiness were described in the majority of cases of vigabatrin overdose. Other less commonly reported symptoms included vertigo, psychosis, apnea or respiratory depression, bradycardia, agitation, irritability, confusion, headache, hypotension, abnormal behavior, increased seizure activity, status epilepticus, and speech disorder. These symptoms resolved with supportive care.

10.2 Treatment or Management for Overdosage

There is no specific antidote for SABRIL overdose. Standard measures to remove unabsorbed drug should be used, including elimination by emesis or gastric lavage. Supportive measures should be employed, including monitoring of vital signs and observation of the clinical status of the patients. In an *in vitro* study, activated charcoal did not significantly adsorb vigabatrin.

The effectiveness of hemodialysis in the treatment of SABRIL overdose is unknown. In isolated case reports in renal failure patients receiving therapeutic doses of vigabatrin, hemodialysis reduced vigabatrin plasma concentrations by 40% to 60%.

11 DESCRIPTION

[See table 3 at top left]

SABRIL (vigabatrin) is available as a white, film-coated tablet for oral administration. Each tablet contains 500 mg vigabatrin. Tablets also contain as inactive ingredients: hydroxypropyl methylcellulose, magnesium stearate, microcrystalline cellulose, polyethylene glycols, povidone, sodium starch glycolate, and titanium dioxide. Vigabatrin is an oral antiepileptic drug with the chemical name (±) 4-amino-5-hexenoic acid. It is a racemate consisting of two enantiomers. The molecular formula is $C_6H_{11}NO_2$ and the molecular weight is 129.16.

Vigabatrin is a white to off-white powder which is freely soluble in water, slightly soluble in methyl alcohol, very slightly soluble in ethyl alcohol and chloroform, and insoluble in toluene and hexane. The pH of a 1% aqueous solution is about 6.9. The n-octanol/water partition coefficient of vigabatrin is about 0.011 (log P=-1.96) at physiologic pH. Vigabatrin melts with decomposition in a 3-degree range within the temperature interval of 171 °C to 176 °C. The dissociation constants (pK_a) of vigabatrin are 4 and 9.7 at room temperature (25 °C).

12 CLINICAL PHARMACOLOGY

12.1 Mechanism of Action

The precise mechanism of vigabatrin's anti-seizure effect is unknown, but it is believed to be the result of its action as an irreversible inhibitor of γ-aminobutyric acid transaminase (GABA-T), the enzyme responsible for the metabolism of the inhibitory neurotransmitter GABA. This action results in increased levels of GABA in the central nervous system.

No direct correlation between plasma concentration and efficacy has been established. The duration of drug effect is presumed to be dependent on the rate of enzyme resynthesis rather than on the rate of elimination of the drug from the systemic circulation.

12.2 Pharmacodynamics

Effects on Electrocardiogram

There is no indication of a QT/QTc prolonging effect of SABRIL in single doses up to 6.0 g. In a randomized, placebo-controlled, crossover study, 58 healthy subjects were administered a single oral dose of SABRIL (3 g and 6 g) and placebo. Peak concentrations for 6.0 g SABRIL were approximately 2-fold higher than the peak concentrations following the 3.0 g single oral dose.

12.3 Pharmacokinetics

Vigabatrin displayed linear pharmacokinetics after administration of single doses ranging from 0.5 g to 4 g, and after administration of repeated doses of 0.5 g and 2.0 g twice daily with a half-life of about 7.5 hours. Bioequivalence has been established between the oral solution and tablet formulations.

Absorption

Following oral administration, vigabatrin is essentially completely absorbed. Time to maximum concentration (t_{max}) is approximately 1 hour following single and multiple doses. There was little accumulation with multiple dosing. A food effect study involving administration of vigabatrin to healthy volunteers under fasting and fed conditions indicated that the C_{max} was decreased by 33%, t_{max} was increased to 2 hours, and AUC was unchanged under fed conditions [see DOSAGE AND ADMINISTRATION (2)].

Distribution

Vigabatrin does not bind to plasma proteins. Vigabatrin is widely distributed throughout the body; mean steady-state volume of distribution is 1.1 L/Kg (CV = 20%).

Metabolism and Elimination

Vigabatrin is not significantly metabolized; it is eliminated primarily through renal excretion. The half-life of vigabatrin is about 7.5 hours. Following administration of $^{[14]}$C-vigabatrin to healthy male volunteers, about 95% of total radioactivity was recovered in the urine over 72 hours with the parent drug representing about 80% of this. Vigabatrin induces CYP2C9, but does not induce other hepatic cytochrome P450 enzyme systems.

Pharmacokinetics in Special Populations

Geriatric

The renal clearance of vigabatrin in healthy elderly patients (≥ 65 years of age) was 36% less than those in healthy younger patients. This finding is confirmed by an analysis of data from a controlled clinical trial.

Gender

No gender differences were observed for the pharmacokinetic parameters of vigabatrin in patients.

Race

No specific study was conducted to investigate the effects of race on SABRIL pharmacokinetics. A cross study comparison between 23 Caucasian and 7 Japanese patients who received 1, 2, and 4 g of vigabatrin indicated that the AUC, C_{max}, and half-life were similar for the two populations. However, the mean renal clearance of Caucasians (5.2 L/hr) was about 25% higher than the Japanese (4.0 L/hr). Inter-subject variability in renal clearance was 20% in Caucasians and was 30% in Japanese.

Renal Impairment

Mean AUC increased by 30% and the terminal half-life increased by 55% (8.1 hr vs 12.5 hr) in patients with mild renal impairment (CLcr from >50-80 mL/min) in comparison to normal subjects.

Mean AUC increased by two-fold and the terminal half-life increased by two-fold in patients with moderate renal impairment (CLcr from >30-50 mL/min) in comparison to normal subjects.

Mean AUC increased by 4.5-fold and the terminal half-life increased by 3.5-fold in patients with severe renal impairment (CLcr from >10-30 mL/min) in comparison to normal subjects.

Dosage adjustment, including starting at a lower dose, is recommended for patients with any degree of renal impairment [see USE IN SPECIFIC POPULATIONS, Renal Impairment (8.6) and DOSAGE AND ADMINISTRATION, Patients with Renal Impairment (2.2)].

Hepatic Impairment

Vigabatrin is not significantly metabolized. The pharmacokinetics of vigabatrin in patients with impaired liver function have not been studied.

Drug Interactions

Phenytoin

A 16% to 20% average reduction in total phenytoin plasma levels was reported in controlled clinical studies. *In vitro* drug metabolism studies indicate that decreased phenytoin concentrations upon addition of vigabatrin therapy are likely to be the result of induction of cytochrome P450 2C enzymes in some patients. Although phenytoin dose adjustments are not routinely required, dose adjustment of phenytoin should be considered if clinically indicated.

Other AEDs

When co-administered with vigabatrin, phenobarbital concentration (from phenobarbital or primidone) was reduced by an average of 8% to 16%, and sodium valproate plasma concentrations were reduced by an average of 8%. These reductions did not appear to be clinically relevant. Based on population pharmacokinetics, carbamazepine, clorazepate, primidone, and sodium valproate appear to have no effect on plasma concentrations of vigabatrin.

Clonazepam

In a study of 12 healthy volunteers, clonazepam (0.5 mg) co-administration had no effect on SABRIL (1.5 g twice daily) concentrations. SABRIL increases the mean C_{max} of clonazepam by 30% and decreases the mean t_{max} by 45%.

Alcohol

Co-administration of ethanol (0.6 g/kg) with vigabatrin (1.5 g twice daily) indicated that neither drug influences the pharmacokinetics of the other.

Oral Contraceptives

In a double-blind, placebo-controlled study using a combination oral contraceptive containing 30 μg ethinyl estradiol and 150 μg levonorgestrel, vigabatrin (3 g/day) did not interfere significantly with the cytochrome P450 isoenzyme (CYP3A)-mediated metabolism of the contraceptive tested. Based on this study, vigabatrin is unlikely to affect the efficacy of steroid oral contraceptives. Additionally, no significant difference in pharmacokinetic parameters (elimination half-life, AUC, C_{max}, apparent oral clearance, time to peak, and apparent volume of distribution) of vigabatrin were found after treatment with ethinyl estradiol and levonorgestrel.

13 NONCLINICAL TOXICOLOGY

13.1 Carcinogenesis, Mutagenesis, Impairment of Fertility

Vigabatrin showed no carcinogenic potential in mouse or rat when given in the diet at doses up to 150 mg/kg/day for 18 months (mouse) or at doses up to 150 mg/kg/day for 2 years (rat). These doses are less than the maximum recommended human dose (MRHD) of 3 g/day on a mg/m² basis.

Vigabatrin was negative in *in vitro* (Ames, CHO/HGPRT mammalian cell forward gene mutation, chromosomal aberration in rat lymphocytes) and in *in vivo* (mouse bone marrow micronucleus) assays.

No adverse effects on male or female fertility were observed in rats at oral doses up to 150 mg/kg/day (approximately 1/2 the MRHD on a mg/m² basis).

14 CLINICAL STUDIES

14.1 Complex Partial Seizures in Adults

The effectiveness of SABRIL as adjunctive therapy in adult patients with CPS was established in two U.S. multicenter, double-blind, placebo-controlled, parallel-group clinical studies. A total of 357 adults (age 18 to 60 years) with CPS, with or without secondary generalization were enrolled (Studies 1 and 2). Patients were required to be on an adequate and stable dose of an anticonvulsant, and have a history of failure on an adequate regimen of carbamazepine or phenytoin. Patients had a history of about 8 seizures per month (median) for about 20 years (median) prior to entrance into the study. These studies were not capable by design of demonstrating direct superiority of SABRIL over any other anticonvulsant added to a regimen to which the patient had not adequately responded. Further, in these studies patients had previously been treated with a limited range of anticonvulsants.

The primary measure of efficacy was the patient's reduction in mean monthly frequency of complex partial seizures plus partial seizures secondarily generalized at end of study compared to baseline.

Study 1

Study 1 (N=174) was a randomized, double-blind, placebo-controlled, dose-response study consisting of an 8-week baseline period followed by an 18-week treatment period. Patients were randomized to receive placebo or 1, 3, or 6 g/day vigabatrin administered twice daily. During the first 6 weeks following randomization, the dose was titrated upward beginning with 1 g/day and increasing by 0.5 g/day on days 1 and 5 of each subsequent week in the 3 g/day and 6 g/day groups, until the assigned dose was reached.

Results for the primary measure of effectiveness, reduction in mean monthly frequency of Complex Partial Seizures, are shown in Table 4. The 3 g/day and 6 g/day dose groups were statistically significantly superior to placebo, but the 6 g/day dose was not superior to the 3 g/day dose.

Table 4. Median Monthly Frequency of Complex Partial Seizures+

	N	Baseline	Endstudy
Placebo	45	9.0	8.8
1 g/day SABRIL	45	8.5	7.7
3 g/day SABRIL	41	8.5	3.7*
6 g/day SABRIL	43	8.5	4.5*

* P<0.05 compared to placebo

+ Including one patient with simple partial seizures with secondary generalization only

Figure 1 presents the percentage of patients (X-axis) with a percent reduction in seizure frequency (responder rate) from baseline to the maintenance phase at least as great as that represented on the Y-axis. A positive value on the Y-axis indicates an improvement from baseline (i.e., a decrease in complex partial seizure frequency), while a negative value indicates a worsening from baseline (i.e., an increase in complex partial seizure frequency). Thus, in a display of this type, a curve for an effective treatment is shifted to the left of the curve for placebo. The proportion of patients achieving any particular level of reduction in complex partial seizure frequency was consistently higher for the SABRIL 3 and 6 g/day groups compared to the placebo group. For example, 51% of patients randomized to SABRIL 3 g/day and 53% of patients randomized to Sabril 6 g/day experienced a 50% or greater reduction in seizure frequency, compared to 9% of patients randomized to placebo. Patients with an increase in seizure frequency >100% are represented on the Y-axis as equal to or greater than -100%.

Figure 1. Percent Reduction from Baseline in Seizure Frequency

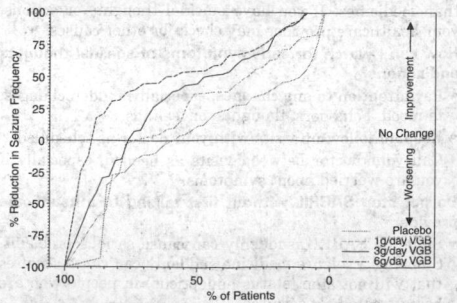

Study 2

Study 2 (N=183 randomized, 182 evaluated for efficacy) was a randomized, double-blind, placebo-controlled, parallel study consisting of an 8-week baseline period and a 16-week treatment period. During the first 4 weeks following randomization, the dose of vigabatrin was titrated upward beginning with 1 g/day and increased by 0.5 g/day on a weekly basis to the maintenance dose of 3 g/day.

Table 5. Median Monthly Frequency of Complex Partial Seizures

	N	Baseline	Endstudy
Placebo	90	9.0	7.5
3 g/day SABRIL	92	8.3	5.5*

* P<0.05 compared to placebo

Results for the primary measure of effectiveness, reduction in mean monthly complex partial seizure frequency, are shown in Table 5. Vigabatrin 3 g/day was statistically significantly superior to placebo in reducing seizure frequency. Figure 2 presents the percentage of patients (X-axis) with a percent reduction in seizure frequency (responder rate) from baseline to the maintenance phase at least as great as that represented on the Y-axis. A positive value on the Y-axis indicates an improvement from baseline (i.e., a decrease in complex partial seizure frequency), while a negative value indicates a worsening from baseline (i.e., an increase in complex partial seizure frequency). Thus, in a display of this type, a curve for an effective treatment is shifted to the left of the curve for placebo. The proportion of patients achieving any particular level of reduction in seizure frequency was consistently higher for the SABRIL 3 g/day group compared to the placebo group. For example, 39% of patients randomized to SABRIL (3 g/day) experienced a 50% or greater reduction in complex partial seizure frequency, compared to 21% of patients randomized to placebo. Patients with an increase in seizure frequency >100% are represented on the Y-axis as equal to or greater than -100%.

Figure 2. Percent Reduction from Baseline in Seizure Frequency

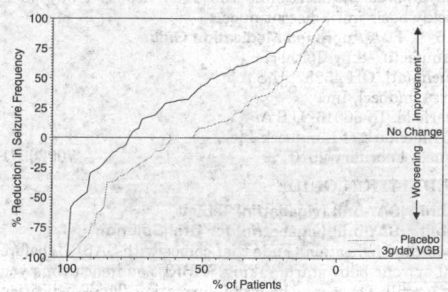

For both studies, there was no difference in the effectiveness of vigabatrin between male and female patients. Analyses of age and race were not possible as nearly all patients were between the ages of 18 to 65 and Caucasian.

15 REFERENCES

None

16 HOW SUPPLIED/STORAGE AND HANDLING

16.1 SABRIL Tablet

Each SABRIL film-coated tablet contains 500 mg vigabatrin and is white, film-coated, oval, biconvex, scored on one side, and debossed with OV 111 on the other.

NDC 67386-111-01: Bottles of 100.

Store at 20-25 °C (68-77 °F). See USP controlled room temperature.

17 PATIENT COUNSELING INFORMATION

See FDA-Approved Patient Labeling (17.5)

Patients must be informed of the availability of a Medication Guide. Patients must be instructed to read the Medication Guide prior to initiating treatment with SABRIL and with each prescription refill. Doctors must review the SABRIL Medication Guide with every patient prior to initiation of treatment. Patients should be instructed to take SABRIL only as prescribed.

17.1 Vision Loss

Patients should be informed of the risk of permanent vision loss, particularly loss of peripheral vision, from SABRIL, and the need for monitoring vision [see WARNINGS AND PRECAUTIONS, Vision Loss (5.1)].

Monitoring of vision, including assessment of visual fields and visual acuity, is required for adults at baseline (no later than 4 weeks after starting SABRIL) and at least every 3 months while on therapy unless after repeated attempts it is not possible. In those patients in whom vision testing is not possible, treatment may continue according to clinical judgment with appropriate patient counseling and with documentation in the SHARE program of the inability to test vision. Patients should be informed that if baseline or subsequent vision is not normal, SABRIL should only be used if the benefits of SABRIL treatment clearly outweigh the risks of additional vision loss.

Patients should understand that vision testing may be insensitive and may not detect vision loss before it is severe. Patients should also understand that if vision loss is documented, such loss is irreversible.

Patients should be informed that if changes in vision are suspected, they should notify their physician immediately.

17.2 Suicidal Thinking and Behavior

Patients, their caregiver(s), and families should be counseled that AEDs, including SABRIL, may increase the risk of suicidal thoughts and behavior and should be advised of the need to be alert for the emergence or worsening of symptoms of depression, any unusual changes in mood or behavior, or the emergence of suicidal thoughts, behavior, or thoughts of self-harm. Behaviors of concern should be reported immediately to healthcare providers [see WARNINGS AND PRECAUTIONS, Suicidal Behavior and Ideation (5.5)].

17.3 Use in Pregnancy

Patients should be instructed to notify their physician if they become pregnant or intend to become pregnant during therapy, and to notify their physician if they are breast feeding or intend to breast feed during therapy [see USE IN SPECIFIC POPULATIONS, Pregnancy (8.1), and Nursing Mothers (8.3)].

Patients should be encouraged to enroll in the NAAED Pregnancy Registry if they become pregnant. This registry is collecting information about the safety of antiepileptic drugs during pregnancy. To enroll, patients can call the toll free number 1-888-233-2334 [see USE IN SPECIFIC POPULATIONS, Pregnancy (8.1)]. Information on the registry can also be found at the website http://www.aedpregnancyregistry.org/.

17.4 Withdrawal of SABRIL Therapy

Patients should be told not to suddenly discontinue SABRIL therapy. As with all AEDs, withdrawal should be gradual. In controlled clinical studies in adults with CPS, vigabatrin was tapered by decreasing the daily dose 1 g/day on a weekly basis until discontinued.

17.5 FDA-Approved Medication Guide

Manufactured by: Patheon
Cincinnati, OH 45237, U.S.A.
For: Lundbeck Inc.
Deerfield, IL 60015, U.S.A.
® Trademark of Lundbeck Inc.
Issued: February 2010   70020971

MEDICATION GUIDE

Sabril® (SAY-bril) (vigabatrin) Tablet
Sabril® (SAY-bril) (vigabatrin) for Oral Solution
Read the Medication Guide that comes with SABRIL before you or your baby starts taking SABRIL and each time you get a refill. There may be new information. This Medication Guide does not take the place of talking with your doctor about your or your baby's medical condition or treatment.

What is the most important information I should know about SABRIL?

SABRIL can cause serious side effects, including:

- **Permanent vision damage:** SABRIL can damage the vision of anyone who takes it. The most noticeable loss is in your ability to see to the side when you look straight ahead (peripheral vision). If this happens, it will not get better. People who take SABRIL do not lose all of their vision, but some people can have severe loss particularly to their peripheral vision. With severe vision loss you may only be able to see things straight in front of you (sometimes called 'tunnel vision'). You may also have blurry vision.

- **Vision loss and use of SABRIL in adults:** Because of the risk of vision loss, SABRIL is used to treat complex partial seizures (CPS) only in people who do not respond well enough to several other medicines.

Tell your doctor right away if you:

- think you are not seeing as well as before you started taking SABRIL
- start to trip, bump into things, or are more clumsy than usual
- are surprised by people or things coming in front of you that seem to come out of nowhere

These changes can mean that you have damage to your vision. Your doctor will test your visual fields (including peripheral vision) and visual acuity (ability to read an eye chart) before you start SABRIL or within 4 weeks after starting SABRIL, and at least every 3 months after that until SABRIL is stopped. Even if your vision seems fine, it is important that you get these regular vision tests because damage can happen to your vision before you notice any changes. These vision tests cannot prevent the vision dam-

age that can happen with SABRIL, but they do allow you to stop SABRIL if vision has gotten worse, which usually will lessen further damage. If you do not have these vision tests regularly, your doctor may stop prescribing SABRIL for you. You should also have a vision test after SABRIL is stopped. If you drive and your vision is damaged by SABRIL, driving might be more dangerous, or you may not be able to drive safely at all. You should discuss this with your doctor.

- **Vision loss in babies:** Because of the risk of vision loss, SABRIL is used in babies (1 month to 2 years old) with infantile spasms (IS) only when you and your doctor decide that the possible benefits of SABRIL are more important than the risks. Parents or caregivers are not likely to recognize the symptoms of vision loss in babies until it is severe. Doctors may not find vision loss in babies until it is severe. It is difficult to test vision in babies, but all babies should have a vision test before starting SABRIL or within 4 weeks after starting SABRIL, and every 3 months after that until SABRIL is stopped. You should have a vision test for your baby after SABRIL is stopped.

Tell your doctor right away if you think that your baby is:

- not seeing as well as before taking SABRIL
- acting differently than normal

Even if your baby's vision seems fine, it is important to get regular vision tests because damage can happen before your baby acts differently. Even these regular vision exams may not show the damage to your baby's vision before it is serious and permanent. If your baby does not have these vision tests regularly, your doctor may stop prescribing SABRIL for your baby. If your baby is not able to complete vision testing, your doctor may continue prescribing SABRIL for your baby. But, your doctor will not be able to watch for vision loss in your baby.

> In all people who take SABRIL:
> - You are at risk for vision loss with any amount of SABRIL
> - Your risk of vision loss may be higher the more SABRIL you take daily and the longer you take it
> - It is not possible for your doctor to know when vision loss will happen. It could happen soon after starting SABRIL or any time during treatment. It may even happen after treatment has stopped.

Because SABRIL might cause vision loss, it is available to doctors and patients only under a special program called SHARE. As part of the SHARE program, among other things, your doctor will have to test your or your baby's vision frequently while you or your baby are being treated with SABRIL, and even after you or your baby stops treatment. You also have to agree to be in the SHARE program, and agree to have your or your baby's vision tested regularly. Your doctor will explain the details of the SHARE program to you.

MRI changes. Brain pictures taken by magnetic resonance imaging (MRI) show changes in some babies after they are given SABRIL. It is not known if these changes are harmful.

Risk of suicidal thoughts or actions. Like other antiepileptic drugs, SABRIL may cause suicidal thoughts or actions in a very small number of people, about 1 in 500 people taking it. Call a doctor right away if you have any of these symptoms, especially if they are new, worse, or worry you:

- thoughts about suicide or dying
- attempts to commit suicide
- new or worse depression
- new or worse anxiety
- feeling agitated or restless
- panic attacks
- trouble sleeping (insomnia)
- new or worse irritability
- acting aggressive, being angry, or violent
- acting on dangerous impulses
- an extreme increase in activity and talking (mania)
- other unusual changes in behavior or mood

Suicidal thoughts or actions can be caused by things other than medicines. If you have suicidal thoughts or actions, your healthcare provider may check for other causes.

How can I watch for early symptoms of suicidal thoughts and actions?

- Pay attention to any changes, especially sudden changes, in mood, behaviors, thoughts, or feelings.
- Keep all follow-up visits with your doctor as scheduled.
- Call your doctor between visits as needed, especially if you are worried about symptoms.

Do not stop SABRIL without first talking to a healthcare provider.

- Stopping SABRIL suddenly can cause serious problems. Stopping a seizure medicine suddenly can cause seizures that will not stop (status epilepticus) in people who are being treated for seizures.

SABRIL can be prescribed only to people who are enrolled in a program called SHARE. Before you or your baby can begin taking SABRIL, you must read and agree to all of the instructions in the SHARE program.

What is SABRIL?

SABRIL Tablets is a prescription medicine used along with other treatments to treat adults with CPS if:

- The CPS does not respond well enough to several other treatments, and
- You and your doctor decide the possible benefit of taking SABRIL is more important than the risk of vision loss.

SABRIL should not be the first medicine used to treat your CPS.

SABRIL for Oral Solution is a prescription medicine used to treat babies, one month to two years old who have IS, if you and your doctor decide the possible benefits of taking SABRIL are more important than the possible risk of vision loss.

If you are an adult with CPS, you must sign an agreement form before you can receive SABRIL.

If you are the parent or caregiver of a baby with IS, you must sign an agreement form before your baby can receive SABRIL.

What should I tell my doctor before starting SABRIL?

If you are an adult with CPS, before taking SABRIL tell your doctor if you have or had:

- depression, mood problems or suicidal thoughts or behavior
- an allergic reaction to SABRIL, such as hives, itching, or trouble breathing
- any vision problems
- any kidney problems
- low red blood cell counts (anemia)
- any nervous or mental illnesses, such as depression, thoughts of suicide, or attempts at suicide
- any other medical conditions
- are breastfeeding or planning to breastfeed. SABRIL can pass into breast milk and may harm your baby. Talk to your healthcare provider about the best way to feed your baby if you take SABRIL.
- are pregnant or plan to become pregnant. It is not known if SABRIL will harm your unborn baby. You and your healthcare provider will have to decide if you should take SABRIL while you are pregnant.

Pregnancy Registry:

If you become pregnant while taking SABRIL, talk to your healthcare provider about registering with the North American Antiepileptic Drug Pregnancy Registry. You can enroll in this registry by calling 1-888-233-2334. The purpose of this registry is to collect information about the safety of antiepileptic medicine during pregnancy.

Before giving SABRIL to your baby, tell the doctor about all of your baby's medical conditions, including if your baby has or ever had:

- an allergic reaction to SABRIL, such as hives, itching, or trouble breathing
- any vision problems
- any kidney problems

Tell your doctor about all the medicines you or your baby take, including prescription and non-prescription medicines, vitamins, and herbal supplements. SABRIL and other medicines may affect each other causing side effects.

How should I take SABRIL?

If you are an adult with CPS:

- Your doctor will explain the SHARE Program to you
- You will receive SABRIL from a specialty pharmacy
- Take SABRIL tablets exactly as prescribed by your doctor. SABRIL tablets are usually taken two times each day.
- You may take SABRIL tablets with or without food
- Before you start taking SABRIL, talk to your doctor about what you should do if you miss a dose of SABRIL
- **Do not stop taking SABRIL suddenly.** This can cause serious problems. Stopping SABRIL or any seizure medicine suddenly can cause seizures that will not stop (status epilepticus) in people who are being treated for seizures. You should follow your doctor's instructions on how to stop taking SABRIL.
- Tell your doctor right away about any increase in seizures while you are stopping SABRIL
- If SABRIL does not improve your seizures enough within 3 months, your doctor will stop prescribing SABRIL for you
- **Do not stop taking SABRIL without talking to your doctor.** If SABRIL improves your seizures, you and your doctor should talk about whether the benefit of taking SABRIL is more important than the risk of vision loss, and decide if you will continue to take SABRIL.

If you are giving SABRIL to your baby for IS:

- Your doctor will explain the SHARE program to you
- You will receive SABRIL for oral solution from a specialty pharmacy

- Mix SABRIL for oral solution and give it to your baby exactly as prescribed by your doctor. Do not stop giving SABRIL for oral solution to your baby unless your doctor tells you to.
- SABRIL for oral solution is usually given two times each day
- SABRIL for oral solution can be given to your baby at the same time as their food, but the powder should not be mixed with their food. SABRIL for oral solution powder should be mixed with water only.
- See the end of this Medication Guide for detailed instructions for how to mix SABRIL for oral solution and give the medicine to your baby
- Before your baby starts taking SABRIL, speak to your baby's doctor about what to do if your baby misses a dose, vomits, spits up, or only takes part of the dose of SABRIL
- **Stopping SABRIL suddenly can cause serious problems.** Stopping SABRIL or any seizure medicine suddenly can cause seizures that will not stop. You should follow your doctor's instructions on how to stop giving SABRIL to your baby. SABRIL does not work in all babies. If your baby's seizures do not improve enough within 2 to 4 weeks, the doctor will stop SABRIL.
- **Tell your doctor right away about any increase in your baby's seizures while stopping SABRIL**

What should I avoid while taking SABRIL?
SABRIL causes sleepiness and tiredness. Adults taking SABRIL should not drive, operate machinery, or perform any hazardous task, unless you and your doctor have decided that you can do these things safely.

What are the possible side effects of SABRIL?
SABRIL can cause serious side effects. See "What is the most important information I should know about SABRIL?"
These other serious side effects happen in **adults**. It is not known if these side effects also happen in babies who take SABRIL.

- Low red blood cell counts (anemia)
- Sleepiness and tiredness. See "What should I avoid while taking SABRIL?"
- Nerve problems. Symptoms of a nerve problem can include numbness and tingling in your toes or feet. It is not known if nerve problems will go away after you stop taking SABRIL.
- Weight gain that happens without swelling
- Swelling

If you are an adult with CPS, SABRIL may make certain types of seizures worse. Tell your doctor right away if your seizures get worse.
The most common side effects of SABRIL in adults include:

- problems walking or feel uncoordinated
- feel dizzy
- shaking (tremor)
- joint pain
- memory problems and not thinking clearly
- eye problems: blurry vision, double vision and eye movements that you cannot control

If you are giving SABRIL to your baby for IS
SABRIL may make certain types of seizures worse. You should tell your baby's doctor right away if your baby's seizures get worse. Tell your baby's doctor if you see any changes in your baby's behavior.
The most common side effects of SABRIL in **babies and young children** include:

- sleepiness - SABRIL may cause your baby to be sleepy. Sleepy babies may have a harder time suckling and feeding, or may be irritable.
- ear infection
- irritability

Tell your doctor if you or your baby have any side effect that bother you or that does not go away. These are not all the possible side effects of SABRIL. For more information, ask your doctor or pharmacist.
Call your doctor for medical advice about side effects. You may report side effects to FDA at 1-800-FDA-1088.

How should I store SABRIL?
Store SABRIL tablets and SABRIL packets at room temperature, between 68 °F to 77 °F (20 °C to 25 °C).
Keep SABRIL tablets and SABRIL powder in the container they come in.
Keep SABRIL and all medicines out of the reach of children.

General information about SABRIL
Medicines are sometimes prescribed for purposes other than those listed in a Medication Guide. Do not use SABRIL for a condition for which it was not prescribed. Do not give SABRIL to other people, even if they have the same symptoms that you have. It may harm them.
This Medication Guide summarizes the most important information about SABRIL. If you would like more information about SABRIL, talk with your doctor. You can ask your pharmacist or doctor for information about SABRIL that is written for health professionals. For more information, go to **www.SABRIL.net** or call **1-800-455-1141**.

What are the ingredients in SABRIL?
Active Ingredient: vigabatrin.
Inactive Ingredients in **SABRIL tablets**: hydroxypropyl methylcellulose, magnesium stearate, microcrystalline cellulose, polyethylene glycols, povidone, sodium starch glycolate, and titanium dioxide.
Inactive Ingredient in **SABRIL powder**: povidone.
This Medication Guide has been approved by the U.S. Food and Drug Administration.
Marketed by: Lundbeck Inc., Deerfield, IL 60015, U.S.A.
® Trademark of Lundbeck Inc.
Issued: August 2009
NDC 67386-111-01
Shown in Product Identification Guide, page 311

XENAZINE® ℞
[ZEN-uh-zeen]
(tetrabenazine)
Tablets
Rx only

DEPRESSION AND SUICIDALITY
XENAZINE can increase the risk of depression and suicidal thoughts and behavior (suicidality) in patients with Huntington's disease. Anyone considering the use of XENAZINE must balance the risks of depression and suicidality with the clinical need for control of choreiform movements. Close observation of patients for the emergence or worsening of depression, suicidality, or unusual changes in behavior should accompany therapy. Patients, their caregivers, and families should be informed of the risk of depression and suicidality and should be instructed to report behaviors of concern promptly to the treating physician.
Particular caution should be exercised in treating patients with a history of depression or prior suicide attempts or ideation, which are increased in frequency in Huntington's disease. XENAZINE is contraindicated in patients who are actively suicidal, and in patients with untreated or inadequately treated depression (see CONTRAINDICATIONS; WARNINGS - Risk of Depression and Suicidality; and PRECAUTIONS - Information for Patients).

DESCRIPTION

XENAZINE (tetrabenazine) is a monoamine depletor for oral administration. The molecular weight of tetrabenazine is 317.43, the pKa is 6.51. Tetrabenazine is a hexahydro-dimethoxy-benzoquinolizine derivative and has the following chemical name: cis rac –1,3,4,6,7,11b-hexahydro-9,10-dimethoxy-3-(2-methylpropyl)-2H-benzo[a]quinolizin-2-one. The empirical formula $C_{19}H_{27}NO_3$ is represented by the following structural formula:

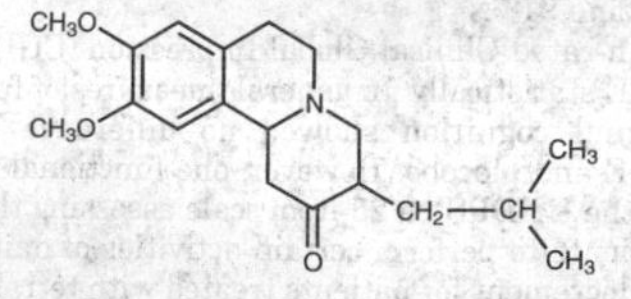

Tetrabenazine is a white to slightly yellow crystalline powder that is sparingly soluble in water and soluble in ethanol. Each XENAZINE (tetrabenazine) Tablet contains either 12.5 or 25 mg of tetrabenazine as the active ingredient. XENAZINE (tetrabenazine) Tablets contain tetrabenazine as the active ingredient and the following inactive ingredients: lactose, maize starch, talc, and magnesium stearate. The 25 mg strength tablet also contains yellow iron oxide as an inactive ingredient. XENAZINE (tetrabenazine) is supplied as a yellowish-buff scored tablet containing 25 mg of tetrabenazine, or as a white non-scored tablet containing 12.5 mg of tetrabenazine.

CLINICAL PHARMACOLOGY

Pharmacodynamics
The precise mechanism by which tetrabenazine exerts its anti-chorea effects is unknown, but is believed to be related to its effect as a reversible depletor of monoamines (such as dopamine, serotonin, norepinephrine, and histamine) from nerve terminals. Tetrabenazine reversibly inhibits the human vesicular monoamine transporter type 2 (VMAT2) ($K_i \approx 100$ nM), resulting in decreased uptake of monoamines into synaptic vesicles and depletion of monoamine stores. Human VMAT2 is also inhibited by dihydrotetrabenazine (HTBZ), a mixture of α-HTBZ and β-HTBZ. α- and β-HTBZ, major circulating metabolites in humans, exhibit high *in vitro* binding affinity to bovine VMAT2. Tetrabenazine exhibits weak *in vitro* binding affinity at the dopamine D2 receptor ($K_i = 2100$ nM).
QTc Prolongation: The effect of a single 25 or 50 mg dose of tetrabenazine on the QT interval was studied in a randomized, double-blind, placebo controlled crossover study in healthy male and female subjects with moxifloxacin as a positive control. At 50 mg, tetrabenazine caused an approximately 8 msec mean increase in QTc (90% CI: 5.0, 10.4 msec). Additional data suggest that inhibition of CYP2D6 in healthy subjects given a single 50 mg dose of tetrabenazine does not further increase the effect on the QTc interval. Effects at higher exposures to either tetrabenazine or its metabolites have not been evaluated (see PRECAUTIONS - QTc Prolongation).
Melanin Binding: Tetrabenazine or its metabolites bind to melanin-containing tissues (i.e., eye, skin, fur) in pigmented rats. After a single oral dose of radiolabeled tetrabenazine, radioactivity was still detected in eye and fur at 21 days post dosing.

Pharmacokinetics
Absorption and Distribution: Following oral administration of tetrabenazine, the extent of absorption is at least 75%. After single oral doses ranging from 12.5 to 50 mg, plasma concentrations of tetrabenazine are generally below the limit of detection because of the rapid and extensive hepatic metabolism of tetrabenazine to α-HTBZ and β-HTBZ. α-HTBZ and β-HTBZ are metabolized principally by CYP2D6. Peak plasma concentrations (C_{max}) of α-HTBZ and β-HTBZ are reached within 1 to 1½ hours post-dosing. α-HTBZ and β-HTBZ are subsequently metabolized to another major circulating metabolite, O-dealkylated-HTBZ, for which C_{max} is reached approximately 2 hours post-dosing.
The effects of food on the bioavailability of tetrabenazine were studied in subjects administered a single dose with and without food. Food had no effect on mean plasma concentrations, C_{max}, or the area under the concentration time course (AUC) of α-HTBZ or β-HTBZ. XENAZINE can therefore be administered without regard to meals.
Results of PET-scan studies in humans show that radioactivity is rapidly distributed to the brain following intravenous injection of ^{11}C-labeled tetrabenazine or α-HTBZ, with the highest binding in the striatum and lowest binding in the cortex.
The *in vitro* protein binding of tetrabenazine, α-HTBZ, and β-HTBZ was examined in human plasma for concentrations ranging from 50 to 200 ng/mL. Tetrabenazine binding ranged from 82% to 85%, α-HTBZ binding ranged from 60% to 68%, and β-HTBZ binding ranged from 59% to 63%.
Metabolism and Excretion: α-HTBZ and β-HTBZ, major circulating metabolites, have half-lives of 4-8 hours and 2-4 hours, respectively. α-HTBZ and β-HTBZ are formed by carbonyl reductase that occurs mainly in the liver. α-HTBZ is O-dealkylated by CYP450 enzymes, principally CYP2D6, with some contribution of CYP1A2. β-HTBZ is O-dealkylated principally by CYP2D6.
After oral administration in humans, at least 19 metabolites of tetrabenazine have been identified. O-dealkylated HTBZ, α-HTBZ, and β-HTBZ are the major circulating metabolites, and they are subsequently metabolized to sulfate or glucuronide conjugates. CYP1A2, CYP2A6, CYP2C9, CYP2C19, and CYP2E1 do not play a major role in metabolism of α-HTBZ or β-HTBZ based on *in vitro* studies.
The results of *in vitro* studies do not suggest that tetrabenazine, α-HTBZ, or β-HTBZ are likely to result in clinically significant inhibition of CYP2D6, CYP1A2, CYP2C8, CYP2C9, CYP2C19, CYP2E1, or CYP3A. Their effect on CYP2B6 has not been evaluated. *In vitro* studies suggest that neither tetrabenazine nor its α- or β-HTBZ metabolites is likely to result in clinically significant induction of CYP1A2, CYP3A4, CYP2B6, CYP2C8, CYP2C9, or CYP2C19.
Neither tetrabenazine nor its α- or β-HTBZ metabolites is likely to be a substrate or inhibitor of P-glycoprotein at clinically relevant concentrations *in vivo*.
Excretion: After oral administration, tetrabenazine is extensively hepatically metabolized, and the metabolites are primarily renally eliminated. In a mass balance study in 6 healthy volunteers, approximately 75% of the dose was excreted in the urine and fecal recovery accounted for approximately 7-16% of the dose. Unchanged tetrabenazine has not been found in human urine. Urinary excretion of α-HTBZ or β-HTBZ accounted for less than 10% of the administered dose. Circulating metabolites, including sulfate and glucuronide conjugates of HTBZ metabolites as well as products of oxidative metabolism, account for the majority of metabolites in the urine.

Special Populations
Pediatrics:
The pharmacokinetics of tetrabenazine and its primary metabolites have not been studied in pediatric subjects.
Geriatrics:
The pharmacokinetics of tetrabenazine and its primary metabolites have not been formally studied in geriatric subjects.

Gender:
There is no apparent effect of gender on the pharmacokinetics of α-HTBZ or β-HTBZ.

Race:
Racial differences in the pharmacokinetics of tetrabenazine and its primary metabolites have not been formally studied.

Renal Disease:
The effect of renal insufficiency on the pharmacokinetics of tetrabenazine and its primary metabolites has not been studied.

Liver Disease:
The disposition of tetrabenazine was compared in 12 patients with mild to moderate chronic liver impairment (Child-Pugh scores of 5-9) and 12 age- and gender-matched subjects with normal hepatic function who received a single 25 mg dose of tetrabenazine. In patients with hepatic impairment, tetrabenazine plasma concentrations were similar to or higher than concentrations of α-HTBZ, reflecting the markedly decreased metabolism of tetrabenazine to α-HTBZ. The mean tetrabenazine C_{max} in hepatically impaired subjects was approximately 7- to 190-fold higher than the detectable peak concentrations in healthy subjects. The elimination half-life of tetrabenazine in subjects with hepatic impairment was approximately 17.5 hours. The time to peak concentrations (t_{max}) of α-HTBZ and β-HTBZ was slightly delayed in subjects with hepatic impairment compared to age-matched controls (1.75 hrs vs. 1.0 hrs), and the elimination half lives of the α-HTBZ and β-HTBZ were prolonged to approximately 10 and 8 hours, respectively. The exposure to α-HTBZ and β-HTBZ was approximately 30-39% greater in patients with liver impairment than in age-matched controls. The safety and efficacy of this increased exposure to tetrabenazine and other circulating metabolites are unknown so that it is not possible to adjust the dosage of tetrabenazine in hepatic impairment to ensure safe use. Therefore, tetrabenazine is contraindicated in patients with hepatic impairment (see CONTRAINDICATIONS; PRECAUTIONS - Use in Patients with Concomitant Illness; and DOSAGE AND ADMINISTRATION).

CYP2D6 Poor Metabolizers
Although the pharmacokinetics of tetrabenazine and its metabolites in subjects who do not express the drug metabolizing enzyme CYP2D6 (poor metabolizers, PMs) have not been systematically evaluated, it is likely that the exposure to α-HTBZ and β-HTBZ would be increased compared to subjects who express the enzyme (extensive metabolizers, EMs), with an increase similar to that observed in patients taking strong CYP2D6 inhibitors (3- and 9-fold, respectively) (see PRECAUTIONS - Drug Interactions and DOSAGE AND ADMINISTRATION). Patients should be genotyped for CYP2D6 prior to treatment with daily doses of tetrabenazine over 50 mg (see WARNINGS - Laboratory Tests). Patients who are PMs should not be given daily doses greater than 50 mg (see DOSAGE AND ADMINISTRATION).

Drug Interactions
α-HTBZ and β-HTBZ are metabolized principally by CYP2D6. A strong CYP2D6 inhibitor (paroxetine) markedly increases exposure to these metabolites (see PRECAUTIONS - Drug Interactions).

Digoxin: Digoxin is a substrate for P-glycoprotein. A study in healthy volunteers showed that tetrabenazine (25 mg twice daily for 3 days) did not affect the bioavailability of digoxin, suggesting that at this dose, tetrabenazine does not affect P-glycoprotein in the intestinal tract. *In vitro* studies also do not suggest that tetrabenazine or its metabolites are P-glycoprotein inhibitors.

CLINICAL STUDIES

Study 1
The efficacy of XENAZINE as a treatment for the chorea of Huntington's disease was established primarily in a randomized, double-blind, placebo-controlled multi-center trial (Study 1) conducted in ambulatory patients with a diagnosis of Huntington's disease (HD). The diagnosis of HD was based on family history, neurological exam, and genetic testing. Treatment duration was 12 weeks, including a 7-week dose titration period and a 5-week maintenance period followed by a 1-week washout. The dose of XENAZINE was started at 12.5 mg/day and titrated upward at weekly intervals in 12.5 mg increments until satisfactory control of chorea was achieved, until intolerable side effects occurred, or until a maximal dose of 100 mg per day was reached.

The primary efficacy endpoint was the Total Chorea Score, an item of the Unified Huntington's Disease Rating Scale (UHDRS). On this scale, chorea is rated from 0 to 4 (with 0 representing no chorea) for 7 different parts of the body. The total score ranges from 0 to 28.

As shown in Figure 1, Total Chorea Scores for subjects in the drug group declined by an estimated 5.0 units during maintenance therapy (average of Week 9 and Week 12 scores versus baseline), compared to an estimated 1.5 units in the placebo group. The treatment effect of 3.5 units was highly statistically significant. At the Week 13 follow-up in Study 1 (1 week after discontinuation of the study medication), the Total Chorea Scores of subjects receiving XENAZINE returned to baseline.

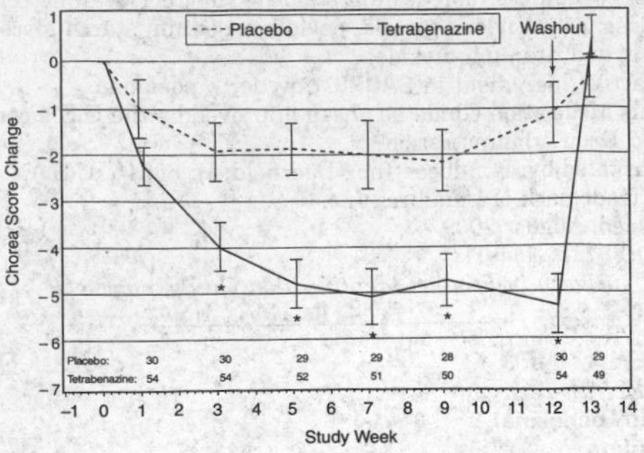

(error bars are ± s.e.m.)
*p<0.05

Figure 1. Mean ± s.e.m. Changes from Baseline in Total Chorea Score in 84 HD Subjects Treated with Tetrabenazine (n=54) or Placebo (n=30)

Figure 2 illustrates the cumulative percentages of patients from the XENAZINE and placebo treatment groups who achieved the level of reduction in the Total Chorea Score shown on the X axis. The left-ward shift of the curve (toward greater improvement) for tetrabenazine-treated patients indicates that these patients were more likely to have any given degree of improvement in chorea score. Thus, for example, about 7% of placebo patients had a 6-point or greater improvement compared to 50% of tetrabenazine-treated patients. The percentage of patients achieving reductions of at least 10, 6, and 3-points from baseline to Week 12 are shown in the inset table.

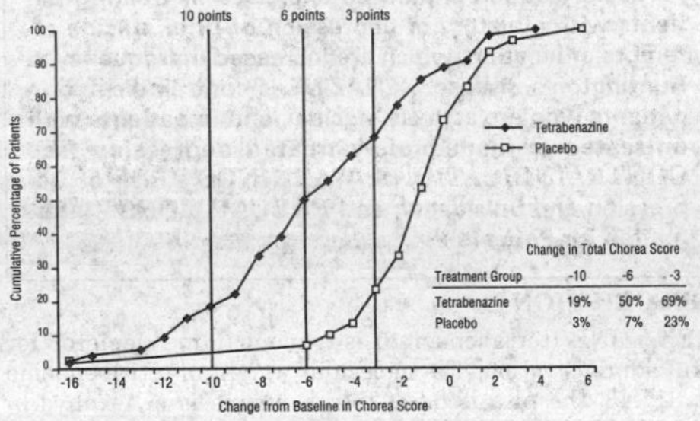

Figure 2. Cumulative Percentage of Patients with Specified Changes from Baseline in Total Chorea Score.

The Percentages of Randomized Patients within each treatment group who completed Study 1 were: Placebo 97%, Tetrabenazine 91%.

A Physician-rated Clinical Global Impression (CGI) favored XENAZINE statistically. In general, measures of functional capacity and cognition showed no difference between XENAZINE and placebo. However, one functional measure (Part 4 of the UHDRS), a 25-item scale assessing the capacity for patients to perform certain activities of daily living, showed a decrement for patients treated with tetrabenazine compared to placebo, a difference that was nominally statistically significant. A 3-item cognitive battery specifically developed to assess cognitive function in patients with HD (Part 2 of the UHDRS) also showed a decrement for patients treated with XENAZINE compared to placebo, but the difference was not statistically significant.

Study 2
A second controlled study was performed in patients who had been treated with open-label XENAZINE for at least 2 months (mean duration of treatment was 2 years). They were randomized to continuation of tetrabenazine at the same dose (n=12) or to placebo (n=6) for three days, at which time their chorea scores were compared. Although the comparison did not reach statistical significance (p=0.1), the estimate of the treatment effect was similar to that seen in Study 1 (about 3.5 units).

INDICATIONS AND USAGE

XENAZINE is indicated for the treatment of chorea associated with Huntington's disease.

CONTRAINDICATIONS

XENAZINE is contraindicated in patients who are actively suicidal, or in patients with untreated or inadequately treated depression. XENAZINE is contraindicated in patients with impaired hepatic function. XENAZINE is contraindicated in patients taking monoamine oxidase inhibitors. XENAZINE is contraindicated in patients taking reserpine. At least 20 days should elapse after stopping reserpine before starting XENAZINE (see PRECAUTIONS - Drug Interactions).

WARNINGS

Huntington's disease is a progressive disorder characterized by changes in mood, cognition, chorea, rigidity, and functional capacity over time. Although XENAZINE has been shown to decrease the chorea of HD in a 12-week controlled trial, it was also shown to cause slight worsening in mood, cognition, rigidity, and functional capacity. Whether these effects persist, resolve, or worsen with continued treatment is unknown. Therefore, proper use of the drug requires attention to all facets of the underlying disease process over time. Prescribers should periodically re-evaluate the need for XENAZINE in their patients by assessing the beneficial effect on choreiform movements and possible adverse effects, including depression, cognitive decline, parkinsonism, dysphagia, sedation/somnolence, akathisia, restlessness and disability. It may be difficult to distinguish between drug-induced side-effects and progression of the underlying disease; decreasing the dose or stopping the drug may help the clinician distinguish between the two possibilities. In some patients, underlying chorea itself may improve over time, decreasing the need for XENAZINE.

Need for Careful Dosing of XENAZINE
Proper dosing of XENAZINE involves careful titration of therapy to determine an individualized dose for each patient. When first prescribed, XENAZINE therapy should be titrated slowly over several weeks to allow the identification of a dose that both reduces chorea and is well tolerated (see DOSAGE AND ADMINISTRATION). Some adverse effects such as depression, fatigue, insomnia, sedation/somnolence, parkinsonism and akathisia may be dose-dependent and may resolve or lessen with dosage adjustment or specific treatment. If the adverse effect does not resolve or decrease, consideration should be given to discontinuing tetrabenazine.

Doses above 50 mg should not be given without CYP2D6 genotyping (see WARNINGS – Laboratory Tests and PRECAUTIONS – Drug Interactions).

Risk of Depression and Suicidality
Patients with Huntington's disease are at increased risk for depression and suicidal ideation and behavior (suicidality). Tetrabenazine increases these risks. All patients treated with tetrabenazine should be observed closely for new or worsening depression or suicidality.

In a 12-week, double-blind placebo-controlled study in patients with chorea associated with Huntington's disease, 10 of 54 patients (19%) treated with tetrabenazine were reported to have an adverse event of depression or worsening depression compared to none of the 30 placebo-treated patients. In two open-label studies (in one study, 29 patients received XENAZINE for up to 48 weeks; in the second study, 75 patients received XENAZINE for up to 80 weeks), the rate of depression/worsening depression was 35%.

In all of the HD chorea studies of tetrabenazine (n=187), one patient committed suicide, one attempted suicide, and six had suicidal ideation.

Clinicians should be alert to the heightened risk of suicide in patients with Huntington's disease regardless of depression indices. Reported rates of completed suicide among individuals with Huntington's disease range from 3-13%; over 25% of patients attempt suicide at some point in the illness.

Patients, their caregivers, and families should be informed of the risks of depression, worsening depression, and suicidality associated with XENAZINE and should be instructed to report behaviors of concern promptly to the treating physician. Patients with HD who express suicidal ideation should be evaluated immediately (see PRECAUTIONS - Information for Patients).

If depression or suicidality occurs, the dose of XENAZINE should be reduced. Initiating treatment with, or increasing the dose of, a concomitant antidepressant may also be useful. In patients with new onset depression who require antidepressants that are strong CYP2D6 inhibitors (such as paroxetine and fluoxetine), the total dose of XENAZINE should be halved (see PRECAUTIONS and DOSAGE AND ADMINISTRATION). If depression or suicidality does not resolve, consideration should be given to discontinuing treatment with tetrabenazine.

Caution should be exercised in treating patients with XENAZINE who have a history of depression or prior suicide attempts or ideation, as these patients may be at increased risk for suicidal behavior (see PRECAUTIONS - Information for Patients). Patients who are actively suicidal or with untreated or inadequately treated depression should not be treated with tetrabenazine (see CONTRAINDICATIONS).

Antidepressants that are strong CYP2D6 inhibitors significantly increase exposure to α- and β-HTBZ (see PRECAUTIONS - Drug Interactions).

Laboratory Tests
Before patients are given a daily dose of greater than 50 mg, they should be tested for the CYP2D6 gene to determine whether they are poor metabolizers (PMs) or extensive or intermediate metabolizers (EMs or IMs). When a dose of tetrabenazine is given to PMs, exposure will be substantially higher (about 3-fold for α-HTBZ and 9-fold for β-HTBZ) than it would be in EMs. The dosage should there-

fore be adjusted according to a patient's CYP2D6 metabolizer status by limiting the dose to 50 mg in patients who are CYP2D6 poor metabolizers (see CLINICAL PHARMACOLOGY and DOSAGE AND ADMINISTRATION).

Neuroleptic Malignant Syndrome (NMS)

A potentially fatal symptom complex sometimes referred to as Neuroleptic Malignant Syndrome (NMS) has been reported in association with tetrabenazine and other drugs that reduce dopaminergic transmission. Clinical manifestations of NMS are hyperpyrexia, muscle rigidity, altered mental status and evidence of autonomic instability (irregular pulse or blood pressure, tachycardia, diaphoresis, and cardiac dysrhythmia). Additional signs may include elevated creatinine phosphokinase, myoglobinuria, rhabdomyolysis, and acute renal failure. The diagnostic evaluation of patients with this syndrome is complicated. In arriving at the diagnosis, it is important to exclude cases where the clinical presentation includes both serious medical illness (e.g., pneumonia, systemic infection) and untreated or inadequately treated extrapyramidal signs and symptoms (EPS). Other important considerations in the differential diagnosis include central anticholinergic toxicity, heat stroke, drug fever, and primary central nervous system pathology. The management of NMS should include (1) immediate discontinuation of tetrabenazine and other drugs not essential to concurrent therapy; (2) intensive symptomatic treatment and medical monitoring; and (3) treatment of any concomitant serious medical problems for which specific treatments are available. There is no general agreement about specific pharmacological treatment regimens for NMS.

If the patient requires treatment with tetrabenazine after recovery from NMS, the potential reintroduction of therapy should be carefully considered. The patient should be carefully monitored, since recurrences of NMS have been reported.

PRECAUTIONS

Akathisia, Restlessness, and Agitation

In a 12-week, double-blind, placebo-controlled study in patients with chorea associated with HD, akathisia was observed in 10 (19%) of XENAZINE-treated patients and 0% of placebo-treated patients. In an 80-week open-label study, akathisia was observed in 20% of XENAZINE-treated patients. Akathisia was not observed in a 48-week open-label study. Patients receiving XENAZINE should be monitored for the presence of akathisia. Patients receiving XENAZINE should also be monitored for signs and symptoms of restlessness and agitation, as these may be indicators of developing akathisia. If a patient develops akathisia, the XENAZINE dose should be reduced; however, some patients may require discontinuation of therapy.

Parkinsonism

XENAZINE can cause parkinsonism. In a 12-week double-blind, placebo-controlled study in patients with chorea associated with HD, symptoms suggestive of parkinsonism (i.e., bradykinesia, hypertonia and rigidity) were observed in 15% of XENAZINE-treated patients compared to 0% of placebo-treated patients. In 48-week and 80-week open-label studies, symptoms suggestive of parkinsonism were observed in 10% and 3% of XENAZINE-treated patients, respectively. Because rigidity can develop as part of the underlying disease process in Huntington's disease, it may be difficult to distinguish between this drug-induced side-effect and progression of the underlying disease process. Drug-induced parkinsonism has the potential to cause more functional disability than untreated chorea for some patients with Huntington's disease. If a patient develops parkinsonism during treatment with tetrabenazine, dose reduction should be considered; in some patients, discontinuation of therapy may be necessary.

Dysphagia

Dysphagia is a component of HD. However, drugs that reduce dopaminergic transmission have been associated with esophageal dysmotility and dysphagia. The latter symptom may be associated with aspiration pneumonia. In a 12-week, double-blind, placebo-controlled study in patients with chorea associated with HD, dysphagia was observed in 4% of XENAZINE-treated patients and 3% of placebo-treated patients. In 48-week and 80-week open-label studies, dysphagia was observed in 10% and 8% of XENAZINE-treated patients, respectively. Some of the cases of dysphagia were associated with aspiration pneumonia. Whether these events were related to treatment is unknown. XENAZINE and other drugs that reduce dopaminergic transmission should be used with caution in patients with Huntington's disease at risk for aspiration pneumonia.

Sedation and Somnolence

Sedation is the most common dose-limiting adverse effect of tetrabenazine. In a 12-week, double-blind, placebo-controlled trial in patients with chorea associated with HD, sedation/somnolence was observed in 17/54 (31%) tetrabenazine-treated patients and in 1 (3%) placebo-treated patient. Sedation was the reason upward titration of tetrabenazine was stopped and/or the dose of

tetrabenazine was decreased in 15/54 (28%) patients. In all but one case, decreasing the dose of tetrabenazine resulted in decreased sedation. In 48-week and 80-week open-label studies, sedation/somnolence was observed in 17% and 57% of XENAZINE treated patients, respectively. In some patients, intolerable sedation occurred at doses that were lower than the efficacious doses.

Patients should be cautioned about performing activities requiring mental alertness, such as operating a motor vehicle or operating hazardous machinery, until they are on a maintenance dose of tetrabenazine and know how the drug affects them (see PRECAUTIONS - Information for Patients).

QTc Prolongation

XENAZINE causes a small increase (about 8 msec) in the corrected QT (QTc) interval. QT prolongation can lead to development of torsade de pointes-type ventricular tachycardia with the risk increasing as the degree of prolongation increases (see CLINICAL PHARMACOLOGY - Pharmacodynamics). The use of XENAZINE should be avoided in combination with other drugs that are known to prolong QTc, including antipsychotic medications (e.g., chlorpromazine, thioridazine, ziprasidone), antibiotics (e.g., moxifloxacin), Class 1A (e.g., quinidine, procainamide) and Class III (e.g., amiodarone, sotalol) antiarrhythmic medications, or any other medications known to prolong the QTc interval. XENAZINE should also be avoided in patients with congenital long QT syndrome and in patients with a history of cardiac arrhythmias. Certain circumstances may increase the risk of the occurrence of torsade de pointes and/or sudden death in association with the use of drugs that prolong the QTc interval, including (1) bradycardia; (2) hypokalemia or hypomagnesemia; (3) concomitant use of other drugs that prolong the QTc interval; and (4) presence of congenital prolongation of the QT interval.

Concomitant Use of Neuroleptic Drugs

Patients taking neuroleptic drugs (e.g., haloperidol, chlorpromazine, risperidone, olanzapine) were excluded from clinical studies during the tetrabenazine development program. Adverse reactions associated with tetrabenazine, such as QTc prolongation, NMS, and extrapyramidal disorders, may be exaggerated by concomitant use of dopamine antagonists.

Interaction with Alcohol

Patients should be advised that the concomitant use of alcohol or other sedating drugs may have additive effects and worsen sedation and somnolence (see PRECAUTIONS -Information for Patients).

Hypotension and Orthostatic Hypotension

XENAZINE induced postural dizziness in healthy volunteers receiving single doses of 25 or 50 mg. One subject had syncope and one subject with postural dizziness had documented orthostasis. Dizziness occurred in 4% of tetrabenazine-treated patients (vs. none on placebo) in the 12-week controlled trial; blood pressure was not measured during these events. Monitoring of vital signs on standing should be considered in patients who are vulnerable to hypotension.

Hyperprolactinemia

Tetrabenazine elevates serum prolactin concentrations in humans. Following administration of 25 mg to healthy volunteers, peak plasma prolactin levels increased 4- to 5-fold. Tissue culture experiments indicate that approximately one third of human breast cancers are prolactin-dependent *in vitro*, a factor of potential importance if tetrabenazine is being considered for a patient with previously detected breast cancer. Although amenorrhea, galactorrhea, gynecomastia and impotence can be caused by elevated serum prolactin concentrations, the clinical significance of elevated serum prolactin concentrations for most patients is unknown. Chronic increase in serum prolactin levels (although not evaluated in the tetrabenazine development program) has been associated with low levels of estrogen and increased risk of osteoporosis. If there is a clinical suspicion of symptomatic hyperprolactinemia, appropriate laboratory testing should be done and consideration should be given to discontinuation of tetrabenazine.

Tardive Dyskinesia (TD)

A potentially irreversible syndrome of involuntary, dyskinetic movements may develop in patients treated with neuroleptic drugs. In an animal model of orofacial dyskinesias, acute administration of reserpine, a monoamine depletor, has been shown to produce vacuous chewing in rats. Although the pathophysiology of tardive dyskinesia remains incompletely understood, the most commonly accepted hypothesis of the mechanism is that prolonged post-synaptic dopamine receptor blockade leads to supersensitivity to dopamine. Neither reserpine nor tetrabenazine, which are dopamine depletors, have been reported to cause clear tardive dyskinesia in humans, but as pre-synaptic dopamine depletion could theoretically lead to supersensitivity to dopamine, and tetrabenazine can cause the extrapyramidal symptoms also known to be associated with neuroleptics (e.g., parkinsonism and akathisia) physicians should be

aware of the possible risk of tardive dyskinesia. If signs and symptoms of TD appear in a patient treated with XENAZINE, drug discontinuation should be considered.

Use in Patients with Concomitant Illness

Clinical experience with tetrabenazine in patients with systemic illnesses is limited. Caution is advised in using tetrabenazine in patients with a history of depression or suicidality (see WARNINGS - Risk of Depression and Suicide). Caution is also advised in using tetrabenazine in patients with diseases, conditions, or treatments that could cause depression or increased suicidality. Tetrabenazine is contraindicated in patients with hepatic impairment (see CONTRAINDICATIONS and CLINICAL PHARMACOLOGY - Special Populations) and in patients with untreated or inadequately treated depression or who are actively suicidal.

XENAZINE has not been evaluated or used to any appreciable extent in patients with a recent history of myocardial infarction or unstable heart disease. Patients with these diagnoses were excluded from premarketing clinical trials.

Binding to Melanin-Containing Tissues

Since tetrabenazine or its metabolites bind to melanin-containing tissues, it could accumulate in these tissues over time. This raises the possibility that tetrabenazine may cause toxicity in these tissues after extended use. Neither ophthalmologic nor microscopic examination of eye was conducted in the chronic toxicity study in dogs. Ophthalmologic monitoring in humans was inadequate to exclude the possibility of injury occurring after long-term exposure.

The clinical relevance of tetrabenazine's binding to melanin-containing tissues is unknown. Although there are no specific recommendations for periodic ophthalmologic monitoring, prescribers should be aware of the possibility of long-term ophthalmologic effects.

Information for Patients

Physicians are advised to discuss the following issues with patients and their families:

Patients and their families should be told that XENAZINE may increase the risk of patients considering or attempting suicide. Patients and their families should be encouraged to be alert to the emergence of suicidal ideation and should report it immediately to the patient's physician.

Patients and their families should be told that XENAZINE may cause depression or may worsen pre-existing depression. They should be encouraged to be alert to the emergence of sadness, worsening of depression, withdrawal, insomnia, irritability, hostility (aggressiveness), akathisia (psychomotor restlessness), anxiety, agitation, or panic attacks and should report such symptoms promptly to the patient's physician.

Patients and their families should be told that the dose of XENAZINE will be titrated up slowly to the dose that is best for each patient. Sedation, akathisia, parkinsonism, depression, and difficulty swallowing may occur. Such symptoms should be promptly reported to the physician and may require dose reduction or tetrabenazine discontinuation.

Patients should be told that XENAZINE may induce sedation and somnolence and may impair the ability to perform tasks that require complex motor and mental skills. Patients should be advised that until they learn how they respond to XENAZINE they should be careful doing activities that require them to be alert, such as driving a car or operating machinery.

Patients and their families should be advised that alcohol may potentiate the sedation induced by XENAZINE.

Patients and their families should be advised to notify the physician if the patient becomes pregnant or intends to become pregnant during XENAZINE therapy, or is breastfeeding or intending to breast-feed an infant during therapy. Patients and their families should be advised to notify the physician of all medications the patient is taking and to consult with the physician before starting any new medications.

Drug Interactions

CYP2D6 inhibitors: *In vitro* studies indicate that α-HTBZ and β-HTBZ are substrates for CYP2D6. The effect of CYP2D6 inhibition on the pharmacokinetics of tetrabenazine and its metabolites was studied in 25 healthy subjects following a single 50 mg dose of tetrabenazine given after 10 days of administration of the strong CYP2D6 inhibitor paroxetine 20 mg daily. There was an approximately 30% increase in C_{max} and an approximately 3-fold increase in AUC for α-HTBZ in subjects given paroxetine prior to tetrabenazine compared to tetrabenazine given alone. For β-HTBZ, the C_{max} and AUC were increased 2.4- and 9-fold, respectively, in subjects given paroxetine prior to tetrabenazine given alone. The elimination half-life of α-HTBZ and β-HTBZ was approximately 14 hours when tetrabenazine was given with paroxetine. Caution should be used when giving any strong CYP2D6 inhibitor (such as fluoxetine, paroxetine, quinidine) to a patient already receiving a stable dose of tetrabenazine, and the daily dose of tetrabenazine should be halved (see DOSAGE AND ADMINISTRATION). The effect of moderate or weak CYP2D6 inhibitors such as duloxetine, terbinafine, amiodarone, or sertraline has not been evaluated (see DOSAGE AND ADMINISTRATION).

Other Cytochrome P450 inhibitors: Based on *in vitro* studies, a clinically significant interaction between tetrabenazine and other P450 inhibitors (other than CYP2D6 inhibitors) is not likely (see CLINICAL PHARMACOLOGY).

Reserpine: Reserpine binds irreversibly to VMAT2 and the duration of its effect is several days. Caution should therefore be used when switching a patient from reserpine to XENAZINE. The physician should wait for chorea to re-emerge before administering XENAZINE to avoid overdosage and major depletion of serotonin and norepinephrine in the CNS. At least 20 days should elapse after stopping reserpine before starting XENAZINE. XENAZINE and reserpine should not be used concomitantly (see CONTRAINDICATIONS).

Carcinogenesis, Mutagenesis, Impairment of Fertility

Carcinogenesis: Lifetime carcinogenicity studies have not been conducted with tetrabenazine.

Mutagenesis: Tetrabenazine and metabolites α-HTBZ and β-HTBZ were negative in the *in vitro* bacterial reverse mutation assay. Tetrabenazine was clastogenic in the *in vitro* chromosome aberration assay in Chinese hamster ovary cells in the presence of metabolic activation. α-HTBZ and β-HTBZ were clastogenic in the *in vitro* chromosome aberration assay in Chinese hamster lung cells in the presence and absence of metabolic activation. *In vivo* micronucleus tests were conducted in male and female rats and male mice. Tetrabenazine was negative in male mice and rats but produced an equivocal response in female rats.

Impairment of Fertility: Fertility and early embryonic development studies have not been conducted with tetrabenazine.

Pregnancy: **Pregnancy Category C**

Tetrabenazine had no clear effects on embryo-fetal development when administered to pregnant rats throughout the period of organogenesis at oral doses up to 30 mg/kg/day (or 3 times the maximum recommended human dose [MRHD]

of 100 mg/day on a mg/m^2 basis). Tetrabenazine had no effects on embryo-fetal development when administered to pregnant rabbits during the period of organogenesis at oral doses up to 60 mg/kg/day (or 12 times the MRHD on a mg/m^2 basis).

When tetrabenazine was administered to female rats (doses of 5, 15, and 30 mg/kg/day) from the beginning of organogenesis through the lactation period, an increase in stillbirths and offspring postnatal mortality was observed at 15 and 30 mg/kg/day and delayed pup maturation was observed at all doses. The no-effect dose for stillbirths and postnatal mortality was 0.5 times the MRHD on a mg/m^2 basis.

There are no adequate and well-controlled studies in pregnant women. XENAZINE should be used during pregnancy only if the potential benefit justifies the potential risk to the fetus (see PRECAUTIONS - Information for Patients).

Labor and Delivery

The effect of tetrabenazine on labor and delivery in humans is unknown.

Nursing Mothers

It is not known whether tetrabenazine or its metabolites are excreted in human milk.

Since many drugs are excreted into human milk and because of the potential for serious adverse reactions in nursing infants from tetrabenazine, a decision should be made whether to discontinue nursing or to discontinue tetrabenazine, taking into account the importance of the drug to the mother.

Pediatric Use

The safety and efficacy of tetrabenazine in children have not been established.

ADVERSE REACTIONS

During its development, tetrabenazine was administered to 773 unique subjects and patients. The conditions and duration of exposure to tetrabenazine varied greatly, and included single and multiple dose clinical pharmacology studies in healthy volunteers (n=259) and open-label (n=529) and double-blind studies (n=84) in patients.

The prescriber should be aware that the figures in the tables and tabulations cannot be used to predict the incidence of adverse effects in the course of usual medical practice where patient characteristics and other factors differ from those that prevailed in the clinical trials. Similarly, the cited frequencies cannot be compared with figures obtained from other clinical investigations involving different treatments, uses, and investigators. The cited figures, however, do provide the prescribing physician with some basis for estimating the relative contribution of drug and non-drug factors to the adverse event incidence rate in the population studied. In a randomized, 12-week, placebo-controlled clinical trial of HD subjects, adverse events (AEs) were more common in the tetrabenazine group than in the placebo group. Forty-nine of 54 (91%) patients who received XENAZINE experienced one or more AEs at any time during the study. The AEs most commonly reported (over 10%, and at least 5% greater than placebo) were sedation/somnolence (31% vs. 3% on placebo), fatigue (22% vs. 13% on placebo), insomnia (22% vs. 0% on placebo), depression (19% vs. 0% on placebo), akathisia (19% vs. 0% on placebo), and nausea (13% vs. 7% on placebo). The number and percentage of the most commonly reported AEs that occurred at any time during the study in ≥4% of tetrabenazine-treated patients, and with a greater frequency than in placebo-treated patients, are presented in Table 1 in decreasing order of frequency within body systems for the tetrabenazine group.

[See table 1 at bottom left]

Dose titration was discontinued or dosage of study drug was reduced because of one or more AEs in 28 of 54 (52%) patients randomized to tetrabenazine. These AEs consisted of sedation (15), akathisia (7), parkinsonism (4), depression (3), anxiety (2), fatigue (1) and diarrhea (1). Some patients had more than one AE and are therefore counted more than once.

The following table describes the incidence of events considered to be extrapyramidal adverse reactions.

Table 2. Treatment Emergent Extrapyramidal Symptoms in Patients Treated with Tetrabenazine and with a Greater Frequency than Placebo in the 12-Week, Double-Blind, Placebo-Controlled Trial of XENAZINE

Event	Patients (%) reporting event	
	XENAZINE n = 54	Placebo n = 30
Akathisia[1]	10 (19%)	0
Extrapyramidal event[2]	8 (15%)	0
Any extrapyramidal event	18 (33%)	0

[1] Patients with the following adverse event preferred terms were counted in this category: akathisia, hyperkinesia, restlessness.
[2] Patients with the following adverse event preferred terms were counted in this category: bradykinesia, parkinsonism, extrapyramidal disorder, hypertonia.

Patients may have had events in more than one category.

Laboratory Tests

No clinically significant changes in laboratory parameters were reported in clinical trials with XENAZINE. In controlled clinical trials, XENAZINE caused a small mean increase in ALT and AST laboratory values as compared to placebo.

Vital Signs

In controlled clinical trials, tetrabenazine did not affect blood pressure, pulse, and body weight. Orthostatic blood pressure was not consistently measured in the XENAZINE clinical trials.

To report SUSPECTED ADVERSE REACTIONS, contact the XENAZINE Information Center at 1-888-882-6013 or FDA at 1-800-FDA-1088 or www.fda.gov/medwatch.

DRUG ABUSE AND DEPENDENCE

Controlled Substance Class

Tetrabenazine is not a controlled substance.

Physical and Psychological Dependence

Clinical trials did not reveal any tendency for drug seeking behavior, though these observations were not systematic. Abuse has not been reported from the postmarketing experience in countries where tetrabenazine has been marketed. Abrupt discontinuation of tetrabenazine from patients did not produce symptoms of withdrawal or a discontinuation syndrome; only symptoms of the original disease were observed to re-emerge. As with any CNS-active drug, physicians should carefully evaluate patients for a history of drug abuse and follow such patients closely, observing them for signs of tetrabenazine misuse or abuse (such as development of tolerance, incrementation of dose, drug-seeking behavior).

Table 1. Treatment Emergent Adverse Events in Patients Treated with Tetrabenazine and with a Greater Frequency than Placebo in the 12-Week, Double-Blind, Placebo-Controlled Trial of XENAZINE

Body System	AE Term	Tetrabenazine n = 54 n (%)	Placebo n = 30 n (%)
PSYCHIATRIC DISORDERS	Sedation/somnolence	17 (31%)	1 (3%)
	Insomnia	12 (22%)	-
	Depression	10 (19%)	-
	Anxiety/anxiety aggravated	8 (15%)	1 (3%)
	Irritability	5 (9%)	1 (3%)
	Appetite decreased	2 (4%)	-
	Obsessive reaction	2 (4%)	-
CENTRAL & PERIPHERAL NERVOUS SYSTEM	Akathisia	10 (19%)	-
	Balance difficulty	5 (9%)	-
	Parkinsonism/bradykinesia	5 (9%)	-
	Dizziness	2 (4%)	-
	Dysarthria	2 (4%)	-
	Gait unsteady	2 (4%)	-
	Headache	2 (4%)	1 (3%)
GASTROINTESTINAL SYSTEM DISORDERS	Nausea	7 (13%)	2 (7%)
	Vomiting	3 (6%)	1 (3%)
BODY AS A WHOLE – GENERAL	Fatigue	12 (22%)	4 (13%)
	Fall	8 (15%)	4 (13%)
	Laceration (head)	3 (6%)	-
	Ecchymosis	3 (6%)	-
RESPIRATORY SYSTEM DISORDERS	Upper respiratory tract infection	6 (11%)	2 (7%)
	Shortness of breath	2 (4%)	-
	Bronchitis	2 (4%)	-
URINARY SYSTEM DISORDERS	Dysuria	2 (4%)	-

OVERDOSAGE

Three episodes of overdose occurred in the open-label trials performed in support of registration. Eight cases of overdose with tetrabenazine have been reported in the literature. The dose of tetrabenazine in these patients ranged from 100 mg to 1g. AEs associated with tetrabenazine overdose included acute dystonia, oculogryic crisis, nausea and vomiting, sweating, sedation, hypotension, confusion, diarrhea, hallucinations, rubor, and tremor.

Overdose Management

Treatment should consist of those general measures employed in the management of overdosage with any CNS-active drug. General supportive and symptomatic measures are recommended. Cardiac rhythm and vital signs should be monitored. In managing overdosage, the possibility of multiple drug involvement should always be considered. The physician should consider contacting a poison control center on the treatment of any overdose. Telephone numbers for certified poison control centers are listed in the *Physicians' Desk Reference®* (PDR®).

DOSAGE AND ADMINISTRATION

In patients with chorea associated with Huntington's disease, proper dosing of XENAZINE involves careful titration of therapy to determine an individualized dose for each patient. When first prescribed, XENAZINE therapy should be titrated slowly over several weeks to allow the identification of a dose for chronic use that reduces chorea and is well tolerated. Doses above 100 mg/day are not recommended for any patient.

Dosing Recommendations up to 50 mg per day

The dose of XENAZINE should be individualized. The starting dose should be 12.5 mg per day given once in the morning. After one week, the dose should be increased to 25 mg per day given as 12.5 mg twice a day. XENAZINE should be titrated up slowly at weekly intervals by 12.5 mg, to allow the identification of a dose that reduces chorea and is well tolerated. If a dose of 37.5 to 50 mg per day is needed, it should be given in a three times a day regimen. The maximum recommended single dose is 25 mg. If adverse events such as akathisia, restlessness, parkinsonism, depression, insomnia, anxiety or intolerable sedation occur, titration should be stopped and the dose should be reduced. If the adverse event does not resolve, consideration should be given to withdrawing XENAZINE treatment or initiating other specific treatment (e.g., antidepressants).

Dosing Recommendations above 50 mg per day

Patients who appear to require doses greater than 50 mg per day should be genotyped for CYP2D6.
The dose of XENAZINE should be individualized.

For CYP2D6 Extensive and Intermediate Metabolizers (patients who express CYP2D6)

At doses above 50 mg per day, XENAZINE should be titrated up slowly at weekly intervals by 12.5 mg, to allow the identification of a dose that reduces chorea and is well tolerated. Doses above 50 mg per day should be given in a three times a day regimen. The maximum recommended daily dose is 100 mg and the maximum recommended single dose is 37.5 mg. If adverse events such as akathisia, parkinsonism, depression, insomnia, anxiety or intolerable sedation occur, titration should be stopped and the dose should be reduced. If the adverse event does not resolve, consideration should be given to withdrawing XENAZINE treatment or initiating other specific treatment (e.g., antidepressants).

For CYP2D6 Poor Metabolizers (patients who do not express CYP2D6)

In patients who are CYP2D6 poor metabolizers, dosing is similar to EMs except that the recommended maximum single dose is 25 mg, and the maximum recommended daily dose is 50 mg.

Discontinuation of Treatment with XENAZINE

Treatment with XENAZINE can be discontinued without tapering. Re-emergence of chorea may occur within 12 to 18 hours after the last dose of tetrabenazine.

Resumption of Treatment

Following treatment interruption of greater than five (5) days or a treatment interruption occurring due to a change in the patient's medical condition or concomitant medications, XENAZINE therapy should be retitrated when resumed. For short-term treatment interruption of less than five (5) days, treatment can be resumed at the previous maintenance dose without titration.

SPECIAL POPULATIONS

Hepatically Impaired Patients: The use of XENAZINE in patients with liver disease is contraindicated (see CLINICAL PHARMACOLOGY – Liver Disease under Special Populations; CONTRAINDICATIONS; and PRECAUTIONS - Use in Patients with Concomitant Illness).

Patients taking CYP2D6 Inhibitors

Caution should be used when adding a strong CYP2D6 inhibitor (such as fluoxetine, paroxetine, quinidine), to a patient already receiving a stable dose of tetrabenazine. In patients receiving co-administered strong CYP2D6 inhibitors,

the daily dose of tetrabenazine should be halved. To initiate treatment with XENAZINE in patients on a stable dose of a strong CYP2D6 inhibitor, the dosing recommendations for the CYP2D6 poor metabolizers should be followed. The effect of moderate or weak CYP2D6 inhibitors such as duloxetine, terbinafine, amiodarone, or sertraline has not been evaluated (see CLINICAL PHARMACOLOGY and PRECAUTIONS).

HOW SUPPLIED

XENAZINE (tetrabenazine) tablets are available in the following strengths and packages:
The 12.5 mg XENAZINE tablets are white, cylindrical biplanar tablets with beveled edges, non-scored, embossed on one side with "CL" and "12.5".
Bottles of 112   NDC 67386-421-01.
The 25 mg XENAZINE tablets are yellowish-buff, cylindrical biplanar tablets with beveled edges, scored, embossed on one side with "CL" and "25".
Bottles of 112   NDC 67386-422-01.

STORAGE

Store at 25° C (77° F); excursions permitted to 15-30°C (59-86° F) [see USP Controlled Room Temperature].
Manufactured by:
Recipharm Fontaine SAS
Rue des Prés Potets
21121 Fontaine-les-Dijon
France
Or:
Hamol Limited
Nottingham, NG90 2DB, England
For: Biovail Corporation
Mississauga, ON L5N 8M5, Canada
Marketed by:
Lundbeck Inc.
Deerfield, IL 60015, U.S.A.
® Xenazine is a registered trademark of Cambridge Laboratories (Ireland) Limited.
Revised: July 2009
2201665 07/2009

MEDICATION GUIDE

Xenazine® *(ZEN-uh-zeen)*
(tetrabenazine) Tablets

Read the Medication Guide that comes with XENAZINE before you start taking it and each time you refill the prescription. There may be new information. This information does not take the place of talking with your doctor about your medical condition or your treatment. You should share this information with your family members and caregivers.

What is the most important information I should know about XENAZINE?

- **XENAZINE may increase the chance of depression, suicidal thoughts, or suicidal actions in some patients.**
- You should not start taking XENAZINE if you are depressed (have untreated depression or depression that is not well controlled by medicine) **or** have suicidal thoughts.
- Pay close attention to any changes, especially sudden changes, in mood, behaviors, thoughts or feelings. This is especially important when XENAZINE is started and when the dose is changed.

Call the doctor right away if you become depressed or have any of the following symptoms, especially if they are new, worse, or worry you:

- You feel sad or have crying spells.
- You are no longer interested in seeing your friends or doing things you used to enjoy.
- You are sleeping a lot *more* or a lot *less* than usual.
- You feel unimportant.
- You feel guilty.
- You feel hopeless or helpless.
- You are more irritable, angry or aggressive than usual.
- You are more or less hungry than usual or notice a big change in your body weight.
- You have trouble paying attention.
- You feel tired or sleepy all the time.
- You have thoughts about hurting yourself or ending your life.

What is XENAZINE?

XENAZINE is a medicine that is used to treat the involuntary movements (chorea) of Huntington's disease. XENAZINE does not cure the cause of the involuntary movements, and it does not treat other symptoms of Huntington's disease, such as problems with thinking or emotions.
It is not known whether XENAZINE is safe and effective in children.

Who should not take XENAZINE?

Do not take XENAZINE if you:

- are depressed or have thoughts of suicide. See "What is the most important information I should know about XENAZINE?"
- have liver problems.

- are taking a monoamine oxidase inhibitor (MAOI) medicine. Ask your doctor or pharmacist if you are not sure.
- are taking reserpine. **Do not take medicines that contain reserpine (such as Serpalan® and Renese®-R) with XENAZINE. If your doctor plans to switch you from taking reserpine to XENAZINE, you must wait at least 20 days after your last dose of reserpine before you start taking XENAZINE.**

What should I tell my doctor before taking XENAZINE?
Tell your doctor about all your medical conditions, including if you:

- have emotional or mental problems (for example, depression, nervousness, anxiety, anger, agitation, psychosis, previous suicidal thoughts or suicide attempts).
- have liver disease.
- have any allergies. See the end of this Medication Guide for a complete list of the ingredients in XENAZINE.
- have breast cancer or a history of breast cancer.
- have heart disease that is not stable, have heart failure or recently had a heart attack.
- have an irregular heart beat (cardiac arrhythmia).
- are pregnant or plan to become pregnant. It is not known if XENAZINE can harm your unborn baby.
- are breast-feeding. It is not known if XENAZINE passes into breast milk.

Tell your doctor about all the medicines you take, including prescription medicines and nonprescription medicines, vitamins and herbal products. Using XENAZINE with certain other medicines may cause serious side effects. **Do not start any new medicines while taking XENAZINE without talking to your doctor first.**

How should I take XENAZINE?

- XENAZINE is a tablet that you take by mouth.
- **Take XENAZINE exactly as prescribed by your doctor.**
- You may take XENAZINE with or without food.
- Your doctor will increase your dose of XENAZINE each week for several weeks, until you and your doctor find the best dose for you.
- If you stop taking XENAZINE or miss a dose, your involuntary movements may return or worsen in 12 to 18 hours after the last dose.
- Before starting XENAZINE, you should talk to your health care provider about what to do if you miss a dose. If you miss a dose and it is time for your next dose, do not double the dose.
- Tell your doctor if you stop taking XENAZINE for more than 5 days. **Do not take another dose until you talk to your doctor.**
- **If your doctor thinks you need to take more than 50 mg of XENAZINE each day, you will need to have a blood test to see if it is safe for you.**

What should I avoid while taking XENAZINE?
Sleepiness (sedation) is a common side effect of XENAZINE. While taking XENAZINE **do not drive a car or operate dangerous machinery until you know how XENAZINE affects you.** Drinking alcohol and taking other drugs that may also cause sleepiness while you are taking XENAZINE may increase any sleepiness caused by XENAZINE.

What are the possible side effects of XENAZINE?
XENAZINE can cause serious side effects, including:

- **Depression, suicidal thoughts, or actions.** See "What is the most important information I should know about XENAZINE?"
- **Neuroleptic Malignant Syndrome (NMS).** Call your doctor right away and go to the nearest emergency room if you develop these signs and symptoms that do not have another obvious cause:
  - - high fever
  - - stiff muscles
  - - problems thinking
  - - very fast or uneven heartbeat
  - - increased sweating
- **Parkinsonism.** Symptoms of Parkinsonism include: slight shaking, body stiffness, trouble moving or keeping your balance.
- **Restlessness.** You may get a condition where you feel a strong urge to move. This is called akathisia.
- **Trouble swallowing.** XENAZINE may increase the chance that you will have trouble swallowing. Increased coughing may be the first sign that you are having trouble swallowing. Trouble swallowing increases your risk of pneumonia.
- **Irregular heartbeat.** XENAZINE increases your chance of having certain changes in the electrical activity in your heart which can be seen on an electrocardiogram (EKG). These changes can lead to a dangerous abnormal heartbeat. Taking XENAZINE with certain medicines may increase this chance.
- **Dizziness due to blood pressure changes when you change position (orthostatic hypotension).** Change positions slowly from lying down to sitting up and from sitting up to standing when taking XENAZINE. Tell your doctor right away if you get dizzy or faint while taking XENAZINE. Your doctor may need to watch your blood pressure closely.

- **Tardive dyskinesia (TD).** TD is a condition where there is repeated facial grimacing that cannot be controlled, sticking out of the tongue, smacking of the lips, puckering and pursing of the lips, and rapid eye blinking. XENAZINE works like other drugs that can cause TD. If you get TD with XENAZINE, it is possible that the TD will not go away.

Common side effects with XENAZINE include:
- sleepiness (sedation)
- trouble sleeping
- depression
- tiredness (fatigue)
- anxiety
- restlessness
- agitation
- nausea

Tell your doctor if you have any side effects. Do not stop taking XENAZINE without talking to your doctor first.

Call your doctor for medical advice about side effects. You may report side effects to the Food and Drug Administration (FDA) at 1–800–FDA–1088.

General information about XENAZINE

XENAZINE contains the active ingredient tetrabenazine. It also contains these inactive ingredients: lactose, maize starch, talc, and magnesium stearate. The 25 mg tablet, which is pale yellow, also contains yellow iron oxide.

Medicines are sometimes prescribed for conditions that are not listed in a Medication Guide. Do not use XENAZINE for a condition for which it was not prescribed. Do not give XENAZINE to other people, even if they have the same symptoms that you have. It may harm them.

This Medication Guide summarizes the most important information about XENAZINE. If you would like more information, talk with your doctor. You can ask your doctor or pharmacist for information about XENAZINE that is written for healthcare professionals. You can also call the XENAZINE Information Center at 1-888-882-6013 or visit www.xenazineusa.com.

This Medication Guide has been approved by the U.S. Food and Drug Administration.

Manufactured by:
Recipharm Fontaine SAS
Rue des Prés Potets
21121 Fontaine-les-Dijon
France
Or:
Hamol Limited
Nottingham, NG90 2DB, England
For: Biovail Corporation
Mississauga, ON L5N 8M5, Canada
Marketed by:
Lundbeck Inc.
Deerfield, IL 60015, U.S.A.
® Xenazine is a registered trademark of Cambridge Laboratories (Ireland) Limited.
Revised: July 2009
2201665 07/2009
Shown in Product Identification Guide, page 311

Lupin Pharmaceuticals, Inc.

HARBOR PLACE TOWER
111 SOUTH CALVERT STREET, 21ST FLOOR
BALTIMORE, MD 21202

Direct Inquiries to:
Phone (410) 576-2000

SUPRAX®   ℞
[sū-praks]
(cefixime)
CEFIXIME TABLETS USP, 400 mg
Cefixime For Oral Suspension USP, 100 mg/5 mL
Cefixime For Oral Suspension USP, 200 mg/5 mL
Rx only

To reduce the development of drug-resistant bacteria and maintain the effectiveness of Suprax (cefixime) and other antibacterial drugs, Suprax should be used only to treat or prevent infections that are proven or strongly suspected to be caused by bacteria.

DESCRIPTION

Suprax (cefixime) is a semisynthetic, cephalosporin antibiotic for oral administration. Chemically, it is (6R, 7R)-7-[2-(2-Amino-4-thiazolyl)glyoxylamido]-8-oxo-3-vinyl-5-thia-1-azabicyclo[4.2.0]oct-2-ene-2-carboxylic acid, 7^2-(Z)-[O-(carboxymethyl) oxime] trihydrate.
Molecular weight = 507.50 as the trihydrate. Chemical Formula is $C_{16}H_{15}N_5O_7S_2.3H_2O$

The structural formula for cefixime is:

Suprax is available for oral administration as 400 mg film coated tablets and as powder for oral suspension which when reconstituted provides either 100 mg/5 mL or 200 mg/5 mL of cefixime as trihydrate.

Inactive ingredients contained in the 400 mg tablets are: dibasic calcium phosphate, hypromellose, titanium dioxide, lactose monohydrate, polyethylene glycol, triacetin, magnesium stearate, microcrystalline cellulose and pregelatinized starch.

The powder for oral suspension contains the following inactive ingredients: strawberry flavor, sodium benzoate, sucrose, colloidal silicon dioxide and xanthan gum.

CLINICAL PHARMACOLOGY

Suprax, given orally, is about 40%-50% absorbed whether administered with or without food; however, time to maximal absorption is increased approximately 0.8 hours when administered with food. A single 200 mg tablet of cefixime produces an average peak serum concentration of approximately 2 mcg/mL (range 1 to 4 mcg/mL); a single 400 mg tablet produces an average peak concentration of approximately 3.7 mcg/mL (range 1.3 to 7.7 mcg/mL). The oral suspension produces average peak concentrations approximately 25%-50% higher than the tablets, when tested in normal *adult* volunteers. Two hundred and 400 mg doses of oral suspension produce average peak concentrations of 3 mcg/mL (range 1 to 4.5 mcg/mL) and 4.6 mcg/mL (range 1.9 to 7.7 mcg/mL), respectively, when tested in normal *adult* volunteers. The area under the time versus concentration curve is greater by approximately 10%-25% with the oral suspension than with the tablet after doses of 100 to 400 mg, when tested in normal *adult* volunteers. This increased absorption should be taken into consideration if the oral suspension is to be substituted for the tablet. Because of the lack of bioequivalence, tablets should not be substituted for oral suspension in the treatment of otitis media. (See **DOSAGE AND ADMINISTRATION**). Cross-over studies of tablet versus suspension have not been performed in children.

Peak serum concentrations occur between 2 and 6 hours following oral administration of a single 200 mg tablet, a single 400 mg tablet or 400 mg of cefixime suspension. Peak serum concentrations occur between 2 and 5 hours following a single administration of 200 mg of suspension.

TABLE

Serum Levels of Cefixime after Administration of Tablets (mcg/mL)

DOSE	1h	2h	4h	6h	8h	12h	24h
100 mg	0.3	0.8	1	0.7	0.4	0.2	0.02
200 mg	0.7	1.4	2	1.5	1	0.4	0.03
400 mg	1.2	2.5	3.5	2.7	1.7	0.6	0.04

Serum Levels of Cefixime after Administration of Oral Suspension (mcg/mL)

DOSE	1h	2h	4h	6h	8h	12h	24h
100 mg	0.7	1.1	1.3	0.9	0.6	0.2	0.02
200 mg	1.2	2.1	2.8	2	1.3	0.5	0.07
400 mg	1.8	3.3	4.4	3.3	2.2	0.8	0.07

Approximately 50% of the absorbed dose is excreted unchanged in the urine in 24 hours. In animal studies, it was noted that cefixime is also excreted in the bile in excess of 10% of the administered dose. Serum protein binding is concentration independent with a bound fraction of approximately 65%. In a multiple dose study conducted with a research formulation which is less bioavailable than the tablet or suspension, there was little accumulation of drug in serum or urine after dosing for 14 days. The serum half-life of cefixime in healthy subjects is independent of dosage form and averages 3-4 hours but may range up to 9 hours in some normal volunteers. Average AUCs at steady state in elderly patients are approximately 40% higher than average AUCs in other healthy adults.

In subjects with moderate impairment of renal function (20 to 40 mL/min creatinine clearance), the average serum half-life of cefixime is prolonged to 6.4 hours. In severe renal impairment (5 to 20 mL/min creatinine clearance), the half-life increased to an average of 11.5 hours. The drug is not cleared significantly from the blood by hemodialysis or peritoneal dialysis. However, a study indicated that with doses of 400 mg, patients undergoing hemodialysis have similar blood profiles as subjects with creatinine clearances of 21-60 mL/min. There is no evidence of metabolism of cefixime *in vivo*.

Adequate data on CSF levels of cefixime are not available.

Microbiology

As with other cephalosporins, bactericidal action of cefixime results from inhibition of cell-wall synthesis. Cefixime is highly stable in the presence of beta-lactamase enzymes. As a result, many organisms resistant to penicillins and some cephalosporins due to the presence of beta-lactamases, may be susceptible to cefixime. Cefixime has been shown to be active against most strains of the following organisms both *in vitro* and in clinical infections (see **INDICATIONS AND USAGE**):

Gram-positive Organisms.
Streptococcus pneumoniae,
Streptococcus pyogenes.
Gram-negative Organisms.
Haemophilus influenzae
(beta-lactamase positive and negative strains),
Moraxella (Branhamella) catarrhalis
(most of which are beta-lactamase positive),
Escherichia coli,
Proteus mirabilis,
Neisseria gonorrhoeae
(including penicillinase- and non-penicillinase-producing strains).

Cefixime has been shown to be active *in vitro* against most strains of the following organisms; however, clinical efficacy has not been established.

Gram-positive Organisms.
Streptococcus agalactiae.
Gram-negative Organisms.
Haemophilus parainfluenzae
(beta-lactamase positive and negative strains),
Proteus vulgaris,
Klebsiella pneumoniae,
Klebsiella oxytoca,
Pasteurella multocida,
Providencia species,
Salmonella species,
Shigella species,
Citrobacter amalonaticus,
Citrobacter diversus,
Serratia marcescens.

Note: *Pseudomonas* species, strains of group D streptococci (including enterococci), *Listeria monocytogenes,* most strains of staphylococci (including methicillin-resistant strains) and most strains of *Enterobacter* are resistant to cefixime. In addition, most strains of *Bacteroides fragilis* and *Clostridia* are resistant to cefixime.

Susceptibility Testing
Susceptibility Tests:
Diffusion Techniques

Quantitative methods that require measurement of zone diameters give an estimate of antibiotic susceptibility. One such procedure[1-3] has been recommended for use with disks to test susceptibility to cefixime. Interpretation involves correlation of the diameters obtained in the disk test with minimum inhibitory concentration (MIC) for cefixime.

Reports from the laboratory giving results of the standard single-disk susceptibility test with a 5-mcg cefixime disk should be interpreted according to the following criteria:

Recommended Susceptibility Ranges: Agar Disk Diffusion

Organisms	Resistant	Moderately Susceptible	Susceptible
Neisseria gonorrhoeae[a]	—	—	≥ 31 mm
All other organisms	≤ 15 mm	16-18 mm	≥ 19 mm

[a] Using GC Agar Base with a defined 1% supplement without cysteine.

A report of "Susceptible" indicates that the pathogen is likely to be inhibited by generally achievable blood levels. A report of "Moderately Susceptible" indicates that inhibitory concentrations of the antibiotic may well be achieved if high dosage is used or if the infection is confined to tissues and fluids (e.g., urine) in which high antibiotic levels are attained. A report of "Resistant" indicates that achievable concentrations of the antibiotic are unlikely to be inhibitory and other therapy should be selected.

Standardized procedures require the use of laboratory control organisms. The 5-mcg disk should give the following zone diameter:

Organism	Zone diameter (mm)
E. coli ATCC 25922	23-27
N. gonorrhoeae ATCC 49226[a]	37-45

[a] Using GC Agar Base with a defined 1% supplement without cysteine.

The class disk for cephalosporin susceptibility testing (the cephalothin disk) is not appropriate because of spectrum differences with cefixime. The 5-mcg cefixime disk should be used for all *in vitro* testing of isolates.

Dilution Techniques

Broth or agar dilution methods can be used to determine the minimum inhibitory concentration (MIC) value for susceptibility of bacterial isolates to cefixime. The recommended susceptibility breakpoints are as follows:

MIC Interpretive Standards (mcg/mL)

Organisms	Resistant	Moderately Susceptible	Susceptible
Neisseria gonorrhoeae[a]	—	—	≤ 0.25
All other organisms	≥ 4	2	≤ 1

As with standard diffusion methods, dilution procedures require the use of laboratory control organisms. Standard cefixime powder should give the following MIC ranges in daily testing of quality control organisms:

Organism	MIC range (mcg/mL)
E. coli ATCC 25922	0.25-1
S. aureus ATCC 29213	8-32
N. gonorrhoeae ATCC 49226[a]	0.008-0.03

[a] Using GC Agar Base with a defined 1% supplement without cysteine.

INDICATIONS AND USAGE

To reduce the development of drug resistant bacteria and maintain the effectiveness of Suprax (cefixime) and other antibacterial drugs, Suprax should be used only to treat or prevent infections that are proven or strongly suspected to be caused by susceptible bacteria. When culture and susceptibility information are available, they should be considered in selecting or modifying antimicrobial therapy. In the absence of such data, local epidemiology and susceptibility patterns may contribute to the empiric selection of therapy. Suprax is indicated in the treatment of the following infections when caused by susceptible strains of the designated microorganisms:

Uncomplicated Urinary Tract Infections caused by *Escherichia coli* and *Proteus mirabilis.*
Otitis Media caused by *Haemophilus influenzae* (beta-lactamase positive and negative strains), *Moraxella (Branhamella) catarrhalis* (most of which are beta-lactamase positive) and *S. pyogenes**.
Note: For information on *otitis media* caused by *Streptococcus pneumoniae*, see **CLINICAL STUDIES** section.
Pharyngitis and *Tonsillitis*, caused by *S. pyogenes.*
Note: Penicillin is the usual drug of choice in the treatment of *S. pyogenes* infections, including the prophylaxis of rheumatic fever. Suprax is generally effective in the eradication of *S. pyogenes* from the nasopharynx; however, data establishing the efficacy of Suprax in the subsequent prevention of rheumatic fever are not available.
Acute Bronchitis and *Acute Exacerbations of Chronic Bronchitis*, caused by *Streptococcus pneumoniae* and *Haemophilus influenzae* (beta-lactamase positive and negative strains).
Uncomplicated gonorrhea (cervical/urethral), caused by *Neisseria gonorrhoeae* (penicillinase- and non-penicillinase-producing strains).
Appropriate cultures and susceptibility studies should be performed to determine the causative organism and its susceptibility to cefixime; however, therapy may be started while awaiting the results of these studies. Therapy should be adjusted, if necessary, once these results are known.
* Efficacy for this organism in this organ system was studied in fewer than 10 infections.

Bacteriological Outcome of Otitis Media at Two to Four Weeks Post-Therapy Based on Repeat Middle Ear Fluid Culture or Extrapolation from Clinical Outcome

Organism	Cefixime(a) 4 mg/kg BID	Cefixime(a) 8 mg/kg QD	Control(a) drugs
Streptococcus pneumoniae	48/70 (69%)	18/22 (82%)	82/100 (82%)
Haemophilus influenzae beta-lactamase negative	24/34 (71%)	13/17 (76%)	23/34 (68%)
Haemophilus influenzae beta-lactamase positive	17/22 (77%)	9/12 (75%)	1/1 (b)
Moraxella (Branhamella) catarrhalis	26/31 (84%)	5/5	18/24 (75%)
S. pyogenes	5/5	3/3	6/7
All Isolates	120/162 (74%)	48/59 (81%)	130/166 (78%)

(a) Number eradicated/number isolated.
(b) An additional 20 beta-lactamase positive strains of *Haemophilus influenzae* were isolated, but were excluded from this analysis because they were resistant to the control antibiotic. In nineteen of these, the clinical course could be assessed and a favorable outcome occurred in 10. When these cases are included in the overall bacteriological evaluation of therapy with the control drugs, 140/185 (76%) of pathogens were considered to be eradicated.

CLINICAL STUDIES

In clinical trials of otitis media in nearly 400 children between the ages of 6 months to 10 years, *Streptococcus pneumoniae* was isolated from 47% of the patients, *Haemophilus influenzae* from 34%, *Moraxella (Branhamella) catarrhalis* from 15% and *S. pyogenes* from 4%.

The overall response rate of *Streptococcus pneumoniae* to cefixime was approximately 10% lower and that of *Haemophilus influenzae* or *Moraxella (Branhamella) catarrhalis* approximately 7% higher (12% when beta-lactamase positive strains of *H. influenzae* are included) than the response rates of these organisms to the active control drugs.

In these studies, patients were randomized and treated with either cefixime at dose regimens of 4 mg/kg BID or 8 mg/kg QD, or with a standard antibiotic regimen. Sixty-nine to 70% of the patients in each group had resolution of signs and symptoms of otitis media when evaluated 2 to 4 weeks post-treatment, but persistent effusion was found in 15% of the patients. When evaluated at the completion of therapy, 17% of patients receiving cefixime and 14% of patients receiving effective comparative drugs (18% including those patients who had *Haemophilus influenzae* resistant to the control drug and who received the control antibiotic) were considered to be treatment failures. By the 2 to 4 week follow-up, a total of 30%-31% of patients had evidence of either treatment failure or recurrent disease.
[See table above]

CONTRAINDICATIONS

Suprax is contraindicated in patients with known allergy to the cephalosporin group of antibiotics.

WARNINGS

BEFORE THERAPY WITH SUPRAX IS INSTITUTED, CAREFUL INQUIRY SHOULD BE MADE TO DETERMINE WHETHER THE PATIENT HAS HAD PREVIOUS HYPERSENSITIVITY REACTIONS TO CEPHALOSPORINS, PENICILLINS, OR OTHER DRUGS. IF THIS PRODUCT IS TO BE GIVEN TO PENICILLIN-SENSITIVE PATIENTS, CAUTION SHOULD BE EXERCISED BECAUSE CROSS HYPERSENSITIVITY AMONG BETA-LACTAM ANTIBIOTICS HAS BEEN CLEARLY DOCUMENTED AND MAY OCCUR IN UP TO 10% OF PATIENTS WITH A HISTORY OF PENICILLIN ALLERGY. IF AN ALLERGIC REACTION TO SUPRAX OCCURS, DISCONTINUE THE DRUG. SERIOUS ACUTE HYPERSENSITIVITY REACTIONS MAY REQUIRE TREATMENT WITH EPINEPHRINE AND OTHER EMERGENCY MEASURES, INCLUDING OXYGEN, INTRAVENOUS FLUIDS, INTRAVENOUS ANTIHISTAMINES, CORTICOSTEROIDS, PRESSOR AMINES AND AIRWAY MANAGEMENT, AS CLINICALLY INDICATED.

Anaphylactic/anaphylactoid reactions (including shock and fatalities) have been reported with the use of cefixime.
Antibiotics, including Suprax, should be administered cautiously to any patient who has demonstrated some form of allergy, particularly to drugs.
Treatment with broad spectrum antibiotics, including Suprax, alters the normal flora of the colon and may permit overgrowth of clostridia. Studies indicate that a toxin produced by *Clostridium difficile* is a primary cause of severe antibiotic-associated diarrhea including pseudomembranous colitis.
Pseudomembranous colitis has been reported with the use of Suprax and other broad-spectrum antibiotics (including macrolides, semisynthetic penicillins, and cephalosporins); therefore, it is important to consider this diagnosis in patients who develop diarrhea in association with the use of antibiotics. Symptoms of pseudomembranous colitis may occur during or after antibiotic treatment and may range in severity from mild to life-threatening. Mild cases of pseudomembranous colitis usually respond to drug discontinuation alone. In moderate to severe cases, management should include fluids, electrolytes, and protein supplementation. If the colitis does not improve after the drug has been discontinued, or if the symptoms are severe, oral vancomycin is the drug of choice for antibiotic-associated pseudomembranous colitis produced by *C. difficile*. Other causes of colitis should be excluded.

PRECAUTIONS
General

Prescribing Suprax (Cefixime) in the absence of a proven or strongly suspected bacterial infection of a prophylactic indication is unlikely to provide benefit to the patient and increases the risk of the development of drug-resistant bacteria.

The possibility of the emergence of resistant organisms which might result in overgrowth should be kept in mind, particularly during prolonged treatment. In such use, careful observation of the patient is essential. If superinfection occurs during therapy, appropriate measures should be taken.

The dose of Suprax should be adjusted in patients with renal impairment as well as those undergoing continuous ambulatory peritoneal dialysis (CAPD) and hemodialysis (HD). Patients on dialysis should be monitored carefully. (See **DOSAGE AND ADMINISTRATION**.) Suprax should be prescribed with caution in individuals with a history of gastrointestinal disease, particularly colitis.

Cephalosporins may be associated with a fall in prothrombin activity. Those at risk include patients with renal or hepatic impairment, or poor nutritional state, as well as patients receiving a protracted course of antimicrobial therapy, and patients previously stabilized on anticoagulant therapy. Prothrombin time should be monitored in patients at risk and exogenous vitamin K administered as indicated.

Information for Patients

Patients should be counseled that antibacterial drugs, including Suprax, should only be used to treat bacterial infections. They do not treat viral infections (e.g., the common cold). When Suprax is prescribed to treat a bacterial infection, patients should be told that although it is common to feel better early in the course of therapy, the medication should be taken exactly as directed. Skipping doses or not completing the full course of therapy may: (1) decrease the effectiveness of the immediate treatment and (2) increase the likelihood that bacteria will develop resistance and will not be treatable by Suprax or other antibacterial drugs in the future.

Drug Interactions

Carbamazepine: Elevated carbamazepine levels have been reported in postmarketing experience when cefixime is administered concomitantly. Drug monitoring may be of assistance in detecting alterations in carbamazepine plasma concentrations.

Warfarin and Anticoagulants: Increased prothrombin time, with or without clinical bleeding, has been reported when cefixime is administered concomitantly.

Drug/Laboratory Test Interactions

A false-positive reaction for ketones in the urine may occur with tests using nitroprusside but not with those using nitroferricyanide.

The administration of cefixime may result in a false-positive reaction for glucose in the urine using Clinitest®**, Benedict's solution, or Fehling's solution. It is recommended that glucose tests based on enzymatic glucose oxidase reactions

PEDIATRIC DOSAGE CHART

Patient Weight (kg)	Dose/Day mg	100 mg/5 mL		200 mg/5 mL	
		Dose/Day mL	Dose/Day tsp of Suspension	Dose/Day mL	Dose/Day tsp of Suspension
6.25	50	2.5	½	1.25	¼
12.5	100	5	1	2.5	½
18.75	150	7.5	1½	3.75	¾
25	200	10	2	5	1
31.25	250	12.5	2½	6.25	1¼
37.5	300	15	3	7.5	1½

Reconstitution Directions For Oral Suspension

Strength	Bottle Size	Reconstitution Directions
100 mg/5 mL and 200 mg/5 mL	100 mL	To reconstitute, suspend with **68 mL water**. Method: Tap the bottle several times to loosen powder contents prior to reconstitution. Add approximately half the total amount of water for reconstitution and shake well. Add the remainder of water and shake well.
100 mg/5 mL and 200 mg/5 mL	75 mL	To reconstitute, suspend with **51 mL water**. Method: Tap the bottle several times to loosen powder contents prior to reconstitution. Add approximately half the total amount of water for reconstitution and shake well. Add the remainder of water and shake well.
100 mg/5 mL and 200 mg/5 mL	50 mL	To reconstitute, suspend with **34 mL water**. Method: Tap the bottle several times to loosen powder contents prior to reconstitution. Add approximately half the total amount of water for reconstitution and shake well. Add the remainder of water and shake well.
200 mg/5 mL	37.5 mL	To reconstitute, suspend with **26 mL water**. Method: Tap the bottle several times to loosen powder contents prior to reconstitution. Add approximately half the total amount of water for reconstitution and shake well. Add the remainder of water and shake well.
200 mg/5 mL	25 mL	To reconstitute, suspend with **17 mL water**. Method: Tap the bottle several times to loosen powder contents prior to reconstitution. Add approximately half the total amount of water for reconstitution and shake well. Add the remainder of water and shake well.

(such as Clinistix®** or TesTape®**) be used. A false-positive direct Coombs test has been reported during treatment with other cephalosporin antibiotics; therefore, it should be recognized that a positive Coombs test may be due to the drug.

Carcinogenesis, Mutagenesis, Impairment of Fertility
Lifetime studies in animals to evaluate carcinogenic potential have not been conducted. Cefixime did not cause point mutations in bacteria or mammalian cells, DNA damage, or chromosome damage *in vitro* and did not exhibit clastogenic potential *in vivo* in the mouse micronucleus test. In rats, fertility and reproductive performance were not affected by cefixime at doses up to 125 times the adult therapeutic dose.

Usage in Pregnancy
Pregnancy Category B. Reproduction studies have been performed in mice and rats at doses up to 400 times the human dose and have revealed no evidence of harm to the fetus due to cefixime. There are no adequate and well-controlled studies in pregnant women. Because animal reproduction studies are not always predictive of human response, this drug should be used during pregnancy only if clearly needed.

Labor and Delivery
Cefixime has not been studied for use during labor and delivery. Treatment should only be given if clearly needed.

Nursing Mothers
It is not known whether cefixime is excreted in human milk. Consideration should be given to discontinuing nursing temporarily during treatment with this drug.

Pediatric Use
Safety and effectiveness of cefixime in children aged less than six months old have not been established.
The incidence of gastrointestinal adverse reactions, including diarrhea and loose stools, in the pediatric patients receiving the suspension, was comparable to the incidence seen in adult patients receiving tablets.

ADVERSE REACTIONS

Most of adverse reactions observed in clinical trials were of a mild and transient nature. Five percent (5%) of patients in the U.S. trials discontinued therapy because of drug-related adverse reactions. The most commonly seen adverse reactions in U.S. trials of the tablet formulation were gastrointestinal events, which were reported in 30% of adult patients on either the BID or the QD regimen. Clinically mild gastrointestinal side effects occurred in 20% of all patients, moderate events occurred in 9% of all patients and severe adverse reactions occurred in 2% of all patients. Individual event rates included diarrhea 16%, loose or frequent stools 6%, abdominal pain 3%, nausea 7%, dyspepsia 3%, and flatulence 4%. The incidence of gastrointestinal adverse reactions, including diarrhea and loose stools, in pediatric patients receiving the suspension was comparable to the incidence seen in adult patients receiving tablets.
These symptoms usually responded to symptomatic therapy or ceased when cefixime was discontinued.
Several patients developed severe diarrhea and/or documented pseudomembranous colitis, and a few required hospitalization.
The following adverse reactions have been reported following the use of cefixime. Incidence rates were less than 1 in 50 (less than 2%), except as noted above for gastrointestinal events.
Gastrointestinal (see above): Diarrhea, loose stools, abdominal pain, dyspepsia, nausea, and vomiting. Several cases of documented pseudomembranous colitis were identified during the studies. The onset of pseudomembranous colitis symptoms may occur during or after therapy.
Hypersensitivity Reactions: Anaphylactic/anaphylactoid reactions (including shock and fatalities), skin rashes, urticaria, drug fever, pruritus, angioedema, and facial edema. Erythema multiforme, Stevens-Johnson syndrome, and serum sickness-like reactions have been reported.
Hepatic: Transient elevations in SGPT, SGOT, alkaline phosphatase, hepatitis, jaundice.
Renal: Transient elevations in BUN or creatinine, acute renal failure.
Central Nervous System: Headaches, dizziness, seizures.
Hemic and Lymphatic Systems: Transient thrombocytopenia, leukopenia, neutropenia, and eosinophilia. Prolongation in prothrombin time was seen rarely.
Abnormal Laboratory Tests: Hyperbilirubinemia.
Other: Genital pruritus, vaginitis, candidiasis, toxic epidermal necrolysis.
In addition to the adverse reactions listed above which have been observed in patients treated with cefixime, the following adverse reactions and altered laboratory tests have been reported for cephalosporin-class antibiotics:

Adverse reactions: Allergic reactions, superinfection, renal dysfunction, toxic nephropathy, hepatic dysfunction including cholestasis, aplastic anemia, hemolytic anemia, hemorrhage, and colitis.
Several cephalosporins have been implicated in triggering seizures, particularly in patients with renal impairment when the dosage was not reduced. (See **DOSAGE AND ADMINISTRATION** and **OVERDOSAGE**.) If seizures associated with drug therapy occur, the drug should be discontinued. Anticonvulsant therapy can be given if clinically indicated.
Abnormal Laboratory Tests: Positive direct Coombs test, elevated LDH, pancytopenia, agranulocytosis.

OVERDOSAGE

Gastric lavage may be indicated; otherwise, no specific antidote exists. Cefixime is not removed in significant quantities from the circulation by hemodialysis or peritoneal dialysis. Adverse reactions in small numbers of healthy adult volunteers receiving single doses up to 2 g of cefixime did not differ from the profile seen in patients treated at the recommended doses.

DOSAGE AND ADMINISTRATION

Adults: The recommended dose of cefixime is 400 mg daily. This may be given as a 400 mg tablet daily or as 200 mg tablet every 12 hours. For the treatment of uncomplicated cervical/urethral gonococcal infections, a single oral dose of 400 mg is recommended.
Children: The recommended dose is 8 mg/kg/day of the suspension. This may be administered as a single daily dose or may be given in two divided doses, as 4 mg/kg every 12 hours.
[See first table at top left]
Children weighing more than 50 kg or older than 12 years should be treated with the recommended adult dose.
Otitis media should be treated with the suspension. Clinical studies of otitis media were conducted with the suspension, and the suspension results in higher peak blood levels than the tablet when administered at the same dose. Therefore, the tablet should not be substituted for the suspension in the treatment of otitis media. (See **CLINICAL PHARMACOLOGY**.)
Efficacy and safety in infants aged less than six months have not been established.
In the treatment of infections due to *S. pyogenes*, a therapeutic dosage of Suprax should be administered for at least 10 days.

Renal Impairment
Suprax may be administered in the presence of impaired renal function. Normal dose and schedule may be employed in patients with creatinine clearances of 60 mL/min or greater. Patients whose clearance is between 21 and 60 mL/min or patients who are on renal hemodialysis may be given 75% of the standard dosage at the standard dosing interval (i.e., 300 mg daily). Patients whose clearance is < 20 mL/min, or patients who are on continuous ambulatory peritoneal dialysis may be given half the standard dosage at the standard dosing interval (i.e., 200 mg daily). Neither hemodialysis nor peritoneal dialysis remove significant amounts of drug from the body.
[See second table above]
After reconstitution the suspension may be kept for 14 days either at room temperature, or under refrigeration, without significant loss of potency. Keep tightly closed. Shake well before using. Discard unused portion after 14 days.

HOW SUPPLIED

Suprax®, Cefixime Tablets USP, 400 mg are white to off-white film coated capsule shaped tablets with beveled edges and a divided score line on each side, debossed with "SUPRAX" across one side and "LUPIN" across other side containing 400 mg of cefixime as the trihydrate and are supplied as follows:
NDC 27437-201-01—Bottle of 100 tablets
NDC 27437-201-08—Bottle of 50 tablets
NDC 27437-201-10—Bottle of 10 tablets with CRC
Store at 20-25°C (68-77°F) [See USP Controlled Room Temperature].
Suprax®, Cefixime for Oral Suspension USP, 100 mg/5 mL is an off-white to pale yellow colored powder. After reconstituted as directed, each 5 mL of reconstituted suspension contains 100 mg of cefixime as the trihydrate and is supplied as follows:
NDC 68180-202-03 - 50 mL Bottle
NDC 68180-202-02 - 75 mL Bottle
NDC 68180-202-01 - 100 mL Bottle
Prior to reconstitution: Store drug powder at 20-25°C (68-77°F) [See USP Controlled Room Temperature].
After reconstitution: Store at room temperature or under refrigeration.
Keep tightly closed.
Suprax®, Cefixime for Oral Suspension USP, 200 mg/5mL is an off-white to pale yellow colored powder. After reconsti-

tuted as directed, each 5 mL of reconstituted suspension contains 200 mg of cefixime as the trihydrate and is supplied as follows:
NDC 27437-206-05 - 25 mL Bottle
NDC 27437-206-06 - 37.5 mL Bottle
NDC 27437-206-03 - 50 mL Bottle
NDC 27437-206-02 - 75 mL Bottle
NDC 27437-206-01 - 100 mL Bottle
Prior to reconstitution: Store drug powder at 20-25°C (68-77°F) [See USP Controlled Room Temperature].
After reconstitution: Store at room temperature or under refrigeration.
Keep tightly closed.

REFERENCES
1. Bauer AW, Kirby WMM, Sherris JC, et al.: Antibiotic susceptibility testing by a standard single disk method. *Am J Clin Pathol* 1966; 45:493.
2. National Committee for Clinical Laboratory Standards, Approved Standard: Performance Standards for Antimicrobial Disk Susceptibility Tests (M2-A3), December 1984.
3. Standardized disk susceptibility test. Federal Register 1974; 39 (May.30): 19182–19184.
**Clinitest® and Clinistix® are registered trademarks of Ames Division, Miles Laboratories, Inc. Tes-Tape® is a registered trademark of Eli Lilly and Company.
Manufactured by:
Lupin Limited
Mumbai 400 098
INDIA
Manufactured for:
Suprax®, Cefixime Tablets USP, 400 mg
and Suprax®, Cefixime for Oral Suspension USP, 200 mg/5 mL
Lupin Pharma
Baltimore, Maryland 21202
United States
Suprax®, Cefixime for Oral Suspension USP, 100 mg/5 mL
Lupin Pharmaceuticals Inc.
Baltimore, Maryland 21202
United States
Revised: October 2008   (ID: 216394)

McNeil Consumer Healthcare
Division of McNeil-PPC, Inc.
FORT WASHINGTON, PA 19034

Direct Inquiries to:
Consumer Relationship Center
Fort Washington, PA 19034
800-962-5357

BENADRYL® ALLERGY   OTC
ULTRATAB TABLETS

Active ingredient (in each tablet)   Purpose
Diphenhydramine HCl 25 mg .... Antihistamine

Uses
• temporarily relieves these symptoms due to hay fever or other upper respiratory allergies:
  • runny nose • sneezing • itchy, watery eyes • itching of the nose or throat
• temporarily relieves these symptoms due to the common cold:
  • runny nose • sneezing

Warnings
Do not use
• to make a child sleepy
• with any other product containing diphenhydramine, even one used on skin
Ask a doctor before use if you have
• a breathing problem such as emphysema or chronic bronchitis
• glaucoma
• trouble urinating due to an enlarged prostate gland
Ask a doctor or pharmacist before use if you are taking sedatives or tranquilizers
When using this product
• marked drowsiness may occur
• avoid alcoholic drinks
• alcohol, sedatives, and tranquilizers may increase drowsiness
• be careful when driving a motor vehicle or operating machinery
• excitability may occur, especially in children
If pregnant or breast-feeding, ask a health professional before use.

Keep out of reach of children. In case of overdose, get medical help or contact a Poison Control Center right away. (1-800-222-1222)

Directions
• take every 4 to 6 hours
• do not take more than 6 times in 24 hours

adults and children 12 years and over	1 to 2 tablets
children 6 to under 12 years	1 tablet
children under 6 years	do not use this product in children under 6 years of age

Other information
• each tablet contains: **calcium 15 mg**
• store between 20–25°C (68–77°). Avoid high humidity. Protect from light.
Inactive ingredients carnauba wax, crospovidone, D&C red # 27 aluminum lake, dibasic calcium phosphate dihydrate, hypromellose, magnesium stearate, microcrystalline cellulose, polyethylene glycol, polysorbate 80, pregelatinized starch, stearic acid, titanium dioxide

---

CHILDREN'S BENADRYL® ALLERGY   OTC
LIQUID

Active ingredient (in each 5 mL)*   **Purpose**
Diphenhydramine HCl 12.5 mg .... Antihistamine
*5 mL = one teaspoon (tsp)

Uses
• temporarily relieves these symptoms due to hay fever or other upper respiratory allergies:
  • runny nose • sneezing • itchy, watery eyes • itching of the nose or throat

Warnings
Do not use
• to make a child sleepy
• with any other product containing diphenhydramine, even one used on skin
Ask a doctor before use if the child has
• a breathing problem such as chronic bronchitis
• glaucoma
• a sodium-restricted diet
Ask a doctor or pharmacist before use if the child is taking sedatives or tranquilizers
When using this product
• marked drowsiness may occur
• sedatives and tranquilizers may increase drowsiness
• excitability may occur, especially in children
Keep out of reach of children. In case of overdose, get medical help or contact a Poison Control Center right away. (1-800-222-1222)

Directions
• find right dose on chart
• use only enclosed dosing cup designed for use with this product. Do not use any other dosing device.
• take every 4 to 6 hours
• do not take more than 6 doses in 24 hours

Age (yr)	Dose
children under 2 years	do not use
children 2 to 5 years	do not use unless directed by a doctor
children 6 to 11 years	5 to 10 mL (1 to 2 tsp)

Attention: use only enclosed dosing cup designed for use with this product. Do not use any other dosing device.
Other information
• each teaspoon contains: **sodium 14 mg**
• store between 20–25°C (68–77°F). Protect from light. Store in outer carton until contents used.
Inactive ingredients anhydrous citric acid, D&C red # 33, FD&C red # 40, flavors, glycerin, monoammonium glycyrrhizinate, poloxamer 407, purified water, sodium benzoate, sodium chloride, sodium citrate, sucrose

---

IMODIUM® A-D LIQUID, CAPLETS,   OTC
AND EZ CHEWS
(loperamide hydrochloride)

Description
Each 7.5 mL (1½ teaspoonful) of *IMODIUM® A-D* liquid contains 1 mg loperamide hydrochloride. *IMODIUM® A-D* liquid has a mint flavor.
Each caplet of *IMODIUM® A-D* contains 2 mg of loperamide hydrochloride.
Each EZ Chew tablet of *IMODIUM® A-D* contains 2mg of loperamide hydrochloride.

Actions
IMODIUM® A-D contains a clinically proven antidiarrheal medication. Loperamide HCl acts by slowing intestinal motility and by affecting water and electrolyte movement through the bowel.

Use
controls symptoms of diarrhea, including Travelers' Diarrhea.

Warnings
Allergy alert: Do not use if you have ever had a rash or other allergic reaction to loperamide HCl
Do not use if you have bloody or black stool
Ask a doctor before use if you have
• fever • mucus in the stool • a history of liver disease
Ask a doctor or pharmacist before use if you are taking antibiotics
When using this product tiredness, drowsiness or dizziness may occur. Be careful when driving or operating machinery.
Stop use and ask a doctor if
• symptoms get worse • diarrhea lasts for more than 2 days
• you get abdominal swelling or bulging
These may be signs of a serious condition.
If pregnant or breast feeding, ask a health professional before use.
Keep out of reach of children. In case of overdose, get medical help or contact a Poison Control Center right away. (1-800-222-1222)

Directions
Imodium A-D Caplets and EZ Chews
• **drink plenty of clear fluids to help prevent dehydration caused by diarrhea**
• take only on an empty stomach (1 hour before or 2 hours after a meal) (EZ Chews only)
• find right dose on chart. If possible, use weight to dose; otherwise, use age.

adults and children 12 years and over	2 caplets or chew 2 tablets after the first loose stool; 1 caplet or chew 1 tablet after each subsequent loose stool; but no more than 4 caplets or chewable tablets in 24 hours
children 9–11 years (60–95 lbs)	1 caplet or chew 1 tablet after the first loose stool; ½ caplet or chew ½ tablet after each subsequent loose stool; but no more than 3 caplets or chewable tablets in 24 hours
children 6–8 years (48–59 lbs)	1 caplet or chew 1 tablet after the first loose stool; ½ caplet or chew ½ tablet after each subsequent loose stool; but no more than 2 caplets or chewable tablets in 24 hours
children under 6 years (up to 47 lbs)	ask a doctor

Imodium A-D Liquid
• **drink plenty of clear fluids to help prevent dehydration caused by diarrhea**
• find right dose on chart. If possible, use weight to dose; otherwise use age.
• shake well before using
• only use attached measuring cup to dose product

adults and children 12 years and over	30 mL (6 tsp) after the first loose stool; 15 mL (3 tsp) after each subsequent loose stool; but no more than 60 mL (12 tsp) in 24 hours

children 9–11 years (60–95 lbs)	15 mL (3 tsp) after first loose stool; 7.5 mL (1½ tsp) after each subsequent loose stool; but no more than 45 mL (9 tsp) in 24 hours
children 6–8 years (48–59 lbs)	15 mL (3 tsp) after first loose stool; 7.5 mL (1½ tsp) after each subsequent loose stool; but no more than 30 mL (6 tsp) in 24 hours
children under 6 years (up to 47 lbs)	ask a doctor

Imodium A-D Liquid Professional Dosage Schedule for children 2–5 years old (24–47 lbs): 1½ teaspoonful after first loose bowel movement, followed by 1½ teaspoonful after each subsequent loose bowel movement. Do not exceed 4½ teaspoonsful a day.

Other information:

Liquid:
- each 30 mL (6 tsp) contains: **sodium 16 mg**
- store between 20–25°C (68–77°F)

Caplets:
- each caplet contains: **calcium 10 mg**
- store between 20–25°C (68–77°F)

EZ Chews:
- **contains milk**
- store between 20–25°C (68–77°F)

Professional Information:
Overdosage information
Overdosage of loperamide HCl in man may result in constipation, CNS depression and nausea. A slurry of activated charcoal administered promptly after ingestion of loperamide hydrochloride can reduce the amount of drug that is absorbed. If vomiting occurs spontaneously upon ingestion, a slurry of 100 grams of activated charcoal should be administered orally as soon as fluids can be retained. If vomiting has not occurred, and CNS depression is evident, gastric lavage should be performed, followed by administration of 100 grams of activated charcoal slurry through the gastric tube. In the event of overdosage, patients should be monitored for signs of CNS depression for at least 24 hours. (Children may be more sensitive to CNS effects than adults.) Because children may be more sensitive to CNS effects than adults, naloxone may be administered if CNS depression is observed. If responsive to naloxone, vital signs must be monitored carefully for recurrence of symptoms of drug overdose for at least 24 hours after the last dose of naloxone.

Inactive ingredients:
Liquid: carboxymethylcellulose sodium, citric acid, D&C yellow #10, FD&C blue #1, glycerin, flavor, microcrystalline cellulose, propylene glycol, purified water, simethicone emulsion, sodium benzoate, sucralose, titanium dioxide, xanthan gum
Caplets: colloidal silicon dioxide, dibasic calcium phosphate, D&C yellow # 10 aluminum lake, FD&C blue # 1 aluminum lake, magnesium stearate, microcrystalline cellulose
EZ Chews: acesulfame potassium, basic polymethacrylate, cellulose acetate, confectioner's sugar, crospovidone, D&C yellow #10 aluminum lake, dextrose excipient, FD&C blue #1 aluminum lake, flavors, magnesium stearate, microcrystalline cellulose, milk powder, sucralose

How Supplied:
Liquid: Mint flavored liquid 4 fl. oz. and 8 fl. oz. tamper evident bottles with child resistant safety caps and special dosage cups. Mint flavored liquid 4 fl. oz. for children.
Caplets: Green scored caplets in 6s, 12s, 18, 24s, 48s and 72s blister packaging which is tamper evident and child resistant, 2s in a tamper resistant pouch.
EZ Chews: Chewable Coolmint Flavored Tablets of 20, 40 and 60.

IMODIUM® MULTI-SYMPTOM RELIEF   OTC
Caplets & Chewable Tablets

Description
Each easy to swallow caplet and mint-flavored chewable tablet of *Imodium® Multi-Symptom Relief* contains loperamide hydrochloride HCl 2 mg/simethicone 125 mg.
loperamide HCl 2mg = Anti-diarrheal
simethicone 125 mg = Anti-gas.

Actions
Imodium® Multi-Symptom Relief combines original prescription strength Imodium® to control the symptoms of diarrhea plus simethicone to relieve bloating, pressure and cramps commonly referred to as gas. Loperamide HCl acts by slowing intestinal motility and by affecting water and electrolyte movement through the bowel. Simethicone acts in the stomach and intestines by altering the surface tension of gas bubbles enabling them to coalesce, thereby freeing and eliminating the gas more easily by belching or passing flatus.

Use Relieves symptoms of diarrhea plus bloating, pressure, and cramps commonly referred to as gas

Warnings
Allergy alert: Do not use if you have ever had a rash or other allergic reaction to loperamide HCl
Do not use if you have bloody or black stool
Ask a doctor before use if you have
• fever • mucus in the stool • a history of liver disease
Ask a doctor or pharmacist before use if you are taking antibiotics
When using this product tiredness, drowsiness or dizziness may occur. Be careful when driving or operating machinery.
Stop use and ask a doctor if
• symptoms get worse • diarrhea lasts for more than 2 days • you get abdominal swelling or bulging.
These may be signs of a serious condition.
If pregnant or breast-feeding, ask a health professional before use.
Keep out of reach of children. In case of overdose, get medical help or contact a Poison Control Center right away. (1-800-222-1222)

Directions
• drink plenty of clear fluids to help prevent dehydration caused by diarrhea
• take only on an empty stomach (1 hour before or 2 hours after a meal) (caplets only)
• find right dose on chart. If possible, use weight to dose; otherwise, use age

adults and children 12 years and over	2 caplets or chew 2 tablets and take with water (for chewables) after the first loose stool; 1 caplet or chew 1 tablet and take with water (for chewables) after each subsequent loose stool; but no more than 4 caplets or chewable tablets in 24 hours
children 9–11 years (60–95 lbs)	1 caplet or chew 1 tablet and take with water (for chewables) after the first loose stool; ½ caplet or chew ½ tablet and take with water (for chewables) after each subsequent loose stool; but no more than 3 caplets/tablets in 24 hours
children 6–8 years (48–59 lbs)	1 caplet or chew 1 tablet and take with water (for chewables) after the first loose stool; ½ caplet or chew ½ tablet and take with water (for chewables) after each subsequent loose stool; but no more than 2 caplets/tablets in 24 hours
children under 6 years (up to 47 lbs)	ask a doctor

Other information:
Caplets:
• each caplet contains: **calcium 165 mg, sodium 4 mg**
• store between 20–25°C (68–77°F). Protect from light.
Chewable Tablets:
• each tablet contains: **calcium 50 mg**
• **contains milk**
• store between 20–25°C (68–77°F)

Professional Information:
Overdosage Information
Overdosage of loperamide HCl in man may result in constipation, CNS depression and nausea. A slurry of activated charcoal administered promptly after ingestion of loperamide hydrochloride can reduce the amount of drug that is absorbed. If vomiting occurs spontaneously upon ingestion, a slurry of 100 grams of activated charcoal should be administered orally as soon as fluids can be retained. If vomiting has not occurred, and CNS depression is evident, gastric lavage should be performed, followed by administration of 100 grams of activated charcoal slurry through the gastric tube. In the event of overdosage, patients should be monitored for signs of CNS depression for at least 24 hours. (Children may be more sensitive to central nervous system effects than adults.) Because children may be more sensitive to CNS effects than adults, naloxone may be administered if CNS depression is observed. If responsive to naloxone, vital signs must be monitored carefully for recurrence of symptoms of drug overdose for at least 24 hours after the last dose of naloxone. No treatment is necessary for the simethicone ingestion in this circumstance.

Inactive ingredients:
Caplets: acesulfame potassium, croscarmellose sodium, dibasic calcium phosphate, flavor, microcrystalline cellulose, stearic acid
Chewable Tablets: cellulose acetate, confectioner's sugar, D&C Yellow # 10 aluminum lake, dextrates, FD&C Blue # 1 aluminum lake, flavors, microcrystalline cellulose, milk powder, polymethacrylates, saccharin sodium, sorbitol, stearic acid, tribasic calcium phosphate

How Supplied
Mint Chewable Tablets in 18's, and blister packaging which is tamper evident and child resistant. Each Imodium® Multi-Symptom Relief tablet is round, light green in color and has "IMODIUM" embossed on one side and "2/125" on the other side. Imodium® Multi-Symptom Relief Caplets are available in blister packs of 12's and 18's and bottles of 30's, 42's. Each Imodium® Multi-Symptom Relief Caplet is oval, white color and has "IMO" embossed on one side and "2/125" on the other side.

CHILDREN'S MOTRIN® Dosing Chart

[See table 2 at top of next page]

MOTRIN® IB   OTC
(Ibuprofen)
Tablets and Caplets

Description
purpose: pain reliver/fever reducer
Active ingredient (in each caplet)
Ibuprofen 200 mg (NSAID)* .... Pain reliever/fever reducer
*nonsteroidal anti-inflammatory drug

Uses
• temporarily relieves minor aches and pains due to:
  • headache • muscular aches • minor pain of arthritis
  • toothache • backache • the common cold • menstrual cramps
• temporarily reduces fever

Warnings
Allergy alert: Ibuprofen may cause a severe allergic reaction, especially in people allergic to aspirin. Symptoms may include:
• hives • facial swelling • asthma (wheezing) • shock • skin reddening • rash • blisters
If an allergic reaction occurs, stop use and seek medical help right away.
Stomach bleeding warning: This product contains an NSAID, which may cause severe stomach bleeding. The chance is higher if you:
• are age 60 or older
• have had stomach ulcers or bleeding problems
• take a blood thinning (anticoagulant) or steroid drug
• take other drugs containing prescription or nonprescription NSAID (aspirin, ibuprofen, naproxen, or others)
• have 3 or more alcoholic drinks every day while using this product
• take more or for a longer time than directed
Do not use
• if you have ever had an allergic reaction to any other pain reliever/fever reducer
• right before or after heart surgery
Ask a doctor before use if
• you have problems or serious side effects from taking pain relievers or fever reducers
• the stomach bleeding warning applies to you
• you have a history of stomach problems, such as heartburn
• you have high blood pressure, heart disease, liver cirrhosis, or kidney disease
• you have asthma
• you are taking a diuretic
Ask a doctor or pharmacist before use if you are
• taking aspirin for heart attack or stroke, because ibuprofen may decrease this benefit of aspirin
• under a doctor's care for any serious condition
• taking any other drug
When using this product
• take with food or milk if stomach upset occurs
• the risk of heart attack or stroke may increase if you use more than directed or for longer than directed
Stop use and ask a doctor if
• you experience any of the following signs of stomach bleeding

Table 2. Children's Motrin Dosing Chart

AGE GROUP*		0-5 mos*	6-11 mos	12-23 mos	2-3 yrs	4-5 yrs	6-8 yrs	9-10 yrs	11 yrs
WEIGHT	(if possible use weight to dose; otherwise use age)	6-11 lbs	12-17 lbs	18-23 lbs	24-35 lbs	36-47 lbs	48-59 lbs	60-71 lbs	72-95 lbs
PRODUCT FORM	INGREDIENTS	Dose to be administered based on weight or age† Please advise caregivers to use the enclosed dosage device when administering medication							Maximum doses/ 24 hrs
Infants' Drops	Per 1.25 mL								
Infants' Motrin Concentrated Drops	Ibuprofen 50 mg	—	1.25 mL	1.875 mL	—	—	—	—	—	4 times in 24 hrs
Children's Liquid	Per 5 mL = 1 teaspoonful (tsp)								
Children's Motrin Suspension	Ibuprofen 100 mg	—	—	—	5 mL (1 tsp)	7.5 mL (1 ½ tsp)	10 mL (2 tsp)	12.5 mL (2 ½ tsp)	15 mL (3 tsp)	4 times in 24 hrs
Junior Strength Tablets & Caplets	Per tablet/ caplet								
Junior Strength Motrin Chewable Tablets	Ibuprofen 100 mg	—	—	—	1 tablet	1 ½ tablets	2 tablets	2 ½ tablets	3 tablets	4 times in 24 hrs
Junior Strength Motrin Caplets	Ibuprofen 100 mg	—	—	—	—	—	2 caplets	2 ½ caplets	3 caplets	4 times in 24 hrs

These products do not contain directions or complete warnings for adult use.
† Do not give more than directed. If needed, repeat dose every 6-8 hours; except for Children's Motrin Cold which is every 6 hours.
* Under 6 mos, ask a doctor.
• Do not use more than 4 times a day.
• Do not give longer than 10 days, unless directed by a doctor (see WARNINGS).
• Infants' drops: Shake well before using. Dispense liquid slowly into the child's mouth, toward the inner cheek.
• Infants' Motrin Drops are more concentrated than Children's Motrin Liquids. The Infants' Concentrated Drops have been specifically designed for use only with enclosed dosing device. Do not use any other dosing device with this product.
• Children's Motrin Liquids are less concentrated than Infants' Motrin Drops. The Children's Motrin Liquids have been specifically designed for use with the enclosed measuring cup. Use only enclosed measuring cup to dose this product. Shake well before using.
• Children's Motrin Suspensions (including cold)—replace original bottle cap to maintain child resistance

---

• feel faint, vomit blood, or have bloody or black stools.
• have stomach pain that does not get better
• pain gets worse or lasts more than 10 days
• fever gets worse or lasts more than 3 days
• redness or swelling is present in the painful area
• any new symptoms appear
If pregnant or breast-feeding, ask a health professional before use. It is especially important not to use ibuprofen during the last 3 months of pregnancy unless definitely directed to do so by a doctor because it may cause problems in the unborn child or complications during delivery.
Keep out of reach of children. In case of overdose, get medical help or contact a Poison Control Center right away. (1-800-222-1222)
Directions
• do not take more than directed
• the smallest effective dose should be used

adults and children 12 years and older	• take 1 tablet or caplet every 4 to 6 hours while symptoms persist • if pain or fever does not respond to 1 tablet or caplet, 2 tablets or caplets may be used • do not exceed 6 tablets or caplets in 24 hours, unless directed by a doctor
children under 12 years	• ask a doctor

Other information:
• store between 20–25°C (68–77°F)

Professional Information:
Overdosage information FOR ADULT MOTRIN®
IBUPROFEN
The *toxicity of ibuprofen* overdose is dependent upon the amount of drug ingested and the time elapsed since ingestion, though individual response may vary, which makes it necessary to evaluate each case individually. Although uncommon, serious toxicity and death have been reported in the medical literature with ibuprofen overdosage. The most frequently reported symptoms of ibuprofen overdose include abdominal pain, nausea, vomiting, lethargy and drowsiness. Other central nervous system symptoms include headache, tinnitus, CNS depression and seizures. Metabolic acidosis, coma, acute renal failure and apnea (primarily in very young children) may rarely occur. Cardiovascular toxicity, including hypotension, bradycardia, tachycardia and atrial fibrillation, also have been reported. The *treatment of acute ibuprofen overdose* is primarily supportive. Management of hypotension, acidosis and gastrointestinal bleeding may be necessary. In cases of acute overdose, the stomach should be emptied through ipecac-induced emesis or lavage. Emesis is most effective if initiated within 30 minutes of ingestion. Orally administered activated charcoal may help in reducing the absorption and reabsorption of ibuprofen. In children, the estimated amount of ibuprofen ingested per body weight may be helpful to predict the potential for development of toxicity although each case must be evaluated. Ingestion of less than 100 mg/kg is unlikely to produce toxicity. Children ingesting 100 to 200 mg/kg may be managed with induced emesis and a minimal observation time of four hours. Children ingesting 200 to 400 mg/kg of ibuprofen should have immediate gastric emptying and at least four hours observation in a health care facility. Children ingesting greater than 400 mg/kg require immediate medical referral, careful observation and appropriate supportive therapy. Ipecac-induced emesis is not recommended in overdoses greater than 400 mg/kg because of the risk of convulsions and the potential for aspiration of gastric contents. In adult patients the history of the dose reportedly ingested does not appear to be predictive of toxicity. The need for referral and follow-up must be judged by the circumstances at the time of the overdose ingestion. Symptomatic adults should be admitted to a health care facility for observation.

Inactive ingredients:
Tablets and Caplets: carnauba wax, colloidal silicon dioxide, corn starch, FD&C yellow #6, hypromellose, iron oxide, magnesium stearate, polydextrose, polyethylene glycol, pregelatinized starch, propylene glycol, shellac, stearic acid, titanium dioxide

How Supplied
Tablets: (orange, printed "MOTRIN IB" in black) in tamper evident packaging of 24, 50, 100, and 165.
Caplets: (orange, printed "MOTRIN IB" in black) in tamper evident packaging of 6 ct, 8 ct and 24, 50, 100, 165, 225, and 300

INFANTS' MOTRIN® ibuprofen   OTC
Concentrated Drops
CHILDREN'S MOTRIN® ibuprofen
Oral Suspension
JUNIOR STRENGTH MOTRIN® ibuprofen
Caplets and Chewable Tablets
Product information for all dosages of Children's MOTRIN have been combined under this heading

Description
Infants' MOTRIN® Concentrated Drops are available in an alcohol-free, berry-flavored suspension and a non-staining, dye-free, berry-flavored suspension. Each 1.25 mL contains ibuprofen 50 mg. *Children's MOTRIN® Oral Suspension* is available as an alcohol-free, berry, dye-free berry, bubble-gum, grape or tropical punch flavored suspension. Each 5 mL (teaspoon) of *Children's MOTRIN® Oral Suspension* contains ibuprofen 100 mg. *Junior Strength MOTRIN® Chewable Tablets* and *Junior Strength MOTRIN® Caplets* contain ibuprofen 100 mg. *Junior Strength MOTRIN® Chewable Tablets* are available in orange or grape flavors. *Junior Strength MOTRIN® Caplets* are available as easy-to-swallow caplets (capsule-shaped tablet).

Uses temporarily:
• reduces fever
• relieves minor aches and pains due to the common cold, flu, sore throat, headaches and toothaches

Directions See Table 2: Children's Motrin Dosing Chart above

Warnings
Allergy alert: Ibuprofen may cause a severe allergic reaction, especially in people allergic to aspirin. Symptoms may include:
• hives • facial swelling • asthma (wheezing) • shock • skin reddening • rash • blisters
If an allergic reaction occurs, stop use and seek medical help right away.
Stomach bleeding warning: This product contains a non-steroidal anti-inflammatory drug (NSAID), which may cause severe stomach bleeding. The chance is higher if the child:
• has had stomach ulcers or bleeding problems
• takes a blood thinning (anticoagulant) or steroid drug
• takes other drugs containing prescription or nonprescription NSAIDs (aspirin, ibuprofen, naproxen, or others)

• takes more or for a longer time than directed

Sore throat warning: Severe or persistent sore throat or sore throat accompanied by high fever, headache, nausea, and vomiting may be serious. Consult doctor promptly. Do not use more than 2 days or administer to children under 3 years of age unless directed by doctor.

Do not use
• if the child has ever had an allergic reaction to any other pain reliever/fever reducer
• right before or after heart surgery

Ask a doctor before use if
• stomach bleeding warnings applies to your child
• child has a history of stomach problems, such as heartburn
• child has problems or serious side effects from taking pain relievers or fever reducers
• child has not been drinking fluids
• child has lost a lot of fluid due to vomiting or diarrhea
• child has high blood pressure, heart disease, liver cirrhosis, or kidney disease
• child has asthma
• child is taking a diuretic

Ask a doctor or pharmacist before use if the child is
• under a doctor's care for any serious condition
• taking any other drug

When using this product
• mouth or throat burning may occur; give with food or water (*Junior Strength MOTRIN® Chewable Tablets* only)
• take with food or milk if stomach upset occurs
• the risk of heart attack or stroke may increase if you use more than directed or for longer than directed

Stop use and ask a doctor if
• child experiences any of the following signs of stomach bleeding
  • feels faint • vomits blood • has bloody or black stools
  • has stomach pain that does not get better
• stomach pain or upset gets worse or lasts
• the child does not get any relief within first day (24 hours) of treatment
• fever or pain gets worse or lasts more than 3 days
• redness or swelling is present in the painful area
• any new symptoms appear

Keep out of reach of children. In case of overdose, get medical help or contact a Poison Control Center right away (1-800-222-1222).

Other information: Infants', Children's and Junior Strength MOTRIN® products:
• store between 20–25°C (68–77°F)
Children's MOTRIN® Suspension Liquid:
• each teaspoon contains: **sodium 2 mg**
Junior Strength MOTRIN® Chewable Tablets:
• phenylketonurics: contains phenylalanine 2.8 mg per tablet

Professional Information:
Overdosage information for all infants', children's & junior strength MOTRIN® products
Ibuprofen: The *toxicity of ibuprofen* overdose is dependent upon the amount of drug ingested and the time elapsed since ingestion, though individual response may vary, which makes it necessary to evaluate each case individually. Although uncommon, serious toxicity and death have been reported in the medical literature with ibuprofen overdosage. The most frequently reported symptoms of ibuprofen overdose include abdominal pain, nausea, vomiting, lethargy and drowsiness. Other central nervous system symptoms include headache, tinnitus, CNS depression and seizures. Metabolic acidosis, coma, acute renal failure and apnea (primarily in very young children) may rarely occur. Cardiovascular toxicity, including hypotension, bradycardia, tachycardia and atrial fibrillation, also have been reported.

The *treatment of acute ibuprofen overdose* is primarily supportive. Management of hypotension, acidosis and gastrointestinal bleeding may be necessary. In cases of acute overdose, the stomach should be emptied through ipecac-induced emesis or lavage. Emesis is most effective if initiated within 30 minutes of ingestion. Orally administered activated charcoal may help in reducing the absorption and reabsorption of ibuprofen. In children, the estimated amount of ibuprofen ingested per body weight may be helpful to predict the potential for development of toxicity although each case must be evaluated. Ingestion of less than 100 mg/kg is unlikely to produce toxicity. Children ingesting 100 to 200 mg/kg may be managed with induced emesis and a minimal observation time of four hours. Children ingesting 200 to 400 mg/kg of ibuprofen should have immediate gastric emptying and at least four hours observation in a health care facility. Children ingesting greater than 400 mg/kg require immediate medical referral, careful observation and appropriate supportive therapy. Ipecac-induced emesis is not recommended in overdoses greater than 400 mg/kg because of the risk of convulsions and the potential for aspiration of gastric contents.

In adult patients the history of the dose reportedly ingested does not appear to be predictive of toxicity. The need for referral and follow-up must be judged by the circumstances at the time of the overdose ingestion. Symptomatic adults should be admitted to a health care facility for observation. **For additional emergency information, please contact your local poison control center.**

Inactive ingredients

Infants' MOTRIN® Concentrated Drops: Berry-Flavored: anhydrous citric acid, caramel, ethyl alcohol, FD&C Red #40, flavors, glycerin, polysorbate 80, pregelatinized starch, purified water, sodium benzoate, sorbitol solution, sucrose, xanthan gum. **Dye-Free Berry-Flavored:** anhydrous citric acid, caramel, ethyl alcohol, flavors, glycerin, polysorbate 80, pregelatinized starch, purified water, sodium benzoate, sorbitol solution, sucrose, xanthan gum.
Children's MOTRIN® Oral Suspension: Berry-Flavored: acesulfame potassium, anhydrous citric acid, D&C Yellow #10, FD&C Red #40, flavors, glycerin, polysorbate 80, pregelatinized starch, purified water, sodium benzoate, sucrose, xanthan gum. **Dye-Free Berry-Flavored:** acesulfame potassium, anhydrous citric acid, flavors, glycerin, polysorbate 80, pregelatinized starch, purified water, sodium benzoate, sucrose, xanthan gum. **Bubble Gum-Flavored:** acesulfame potassium, anhydrous citric acid, FD&C Red #40, flavors, glycerin, polysorbate 80, pregelatinized starch, purified water, sodium benzoate, sucrose, xanthan gum. **Grape-Flavored:** acesulfame potassium, anhydrous citric acid, D&C Red #33, FD&C Blue #1, FD&C Red #40, flavors, glycerin, polysorbate 80, pregelatinized starch, purified water, sodium benzoate, sucrose, xanthan gum. **Tropical Punch Flavored:** acesulfame potassium, anhydrous citric acid, FD&C Red #40, flavors, glycerin, polysorbate 80, pregelatinized starch, purified water, sodium benzoate, sucralose, sucrose, xanthan gum.
Junior Strength MOTRIN® Chewable Tablets: **Orange-Flavored:** acesulfame potassium, anhydrous citric acid, aspartame, FD&C Yellow #6 aluminum lake, flavor, fumaric acid, hydroxyethyl cellulose, hypromellose, magnesium stearate, mannitol, microcrystalline cellulose, povidone, sodium lauryl sulfate, sodium starch glycolate. **Grape-Flavored:** acesulfame potassium, anhydrous citric acid, aspartame, cellulose, citric acid D&C red #7 aluminum lake, D&C red #30 aluminum lake, FD&C blue #1 aluminum lake, flavor, fumaric acid, hydroxyethyl cellulose, hypromellose, magnesium stearate, mannitol, microcrystalline cellulose, povidone, sodium lauryl sulfate, sodium starch glycolate.
Easy-To-Swallow Caplets: carnauba wax, cellulose, corn starch, D&C Yellow #10 aluminum lake, FD&C Yellow #6 aluminum lake, hypromellose, polydextrose, polyethylene glycol, propylene glycol, Microcrystalline cellulose, Pregelatinized starch, shellac, sodium starch glycolate, Titanium dioxide, triacetin.

How Supplied

Infants' MOTRIN® Concentrated Drops: Berry-flavored, pink-colored liquid and Berry-Flavored, Dye-Free, white-colored liquid in ½ fl. oz. bottles w/calibrated plastic syringe. Dye-Free Berry also available in 1 oz. size.
Children's MOTRIN® Oral Suspension: Berry-flavored, pink-colored; (2 and 4 fl. oz) Berry-Flavored, Dye-Free white-colored, Bubble Gum-flavored, pink-colored, Grape-flavored, purple-colored, and Tropical Punch flavored liquid in tamper evident bottles (4 fl. oz.)
Junior Strength MOTRIN® Chewable Tablets: Orange-flavored, orange-colored chewable tablets or Grape-flavored, purple-colored chewable tablets in 24 count bottles.
Junior Strength MOTRIN® Caplets: Easy-to-swallow caplets (capsule shaped tablets) in 24 count bottles.

MOTRIN PM

Drug Facts
Active ingredients (in each caplet) Purposes
Diphenhydramine citrate 38 mg .... Nighttime sleep-aid
Ibuprofen 200 mg (NSAID)* .... Pain reliever
*nonsteroidal anti-inflammatory drug

Uses
• for relief of occasional sleeplessness when associated with minor aches and pains
• helps you fall asleep and stay asleep

Warnings
Allergy alert: Ibuprofen may cause a severe allergic reaction, especially in people allergic to aspirin. Symptoms may include:
• hives • facial swelling • asthma (wheezing) • shock • skin reddening • rash • blisters
If an allergic reaction occurs, stop use and seek medical help right away.

Stomach bleeding warning: This product contains an NSAID, which may cause severe stomach bleeding. The chance is higher if you:
• are age 60 or older
• have had stomach ulcers or bleeding problems
• take a blood thinning (anticoagulant) or steroid drug
• take other drugs containing prescription or nonprescription NSAIDs (aspirin, ibuprofen, naproxen, or others)
• have 3 or more alcoholic drinks every day while using this product
• take more or for a longer time than directed

Do not use
• if you have ever had an allergic reaction to any other pain reliever/fever reducer
• unless you have time for a full night's sleep
• in children under 12 years of age
• right before or after heart surgery
• with any other product containing diphenhydramine, even one used on skin
• if you have sleeplessness without pain

Ask a doctor before use if
• the stomach bleeding warning applies to you
• you have a history of stomach problems, such as heartburn
• you have high blood pressure, heart disease, liver cirrhosis, or kidney disease
• you are taking a diuretic
• you have a breathing problem such as emphysema or chronic bronchitis
• you have asthma
• you have glaucoma
• you have trouble urinating due to an enlarged prostate gland

Ask a doctor or pharmacist before use if you are
• taking sedatives or tranquilizers, or any other sleep-aid
• under a doctor's care for any continuing medical illness
• taking any other antihistamines
• taking aspirin for heart attack or stroke, because ibuprofen may decrease this benefit of aspirin
• taking any other drug

When using this product
• drowsiness will occur
• avoid alcoholic drinks
• do not drive a motor vehicle or operate machinery
• take with food or milk if stomach upset occurs
• the risk of heart attack or stroke may increase if you use more than directed or for longer than directed

Stop use and ask a doctor if
• you experience any of the following signs of stomach bleeding:
• feel faint • vomit blood • have bloody or black stools
• have stomach pain that does not get better
• sleeplessness persists continuously for more than 2 weeks. Insomnia may be a symptom of a serious underlying medical illness.
• redness or swelling is present in the painful area
• any new symptoms appear

If pregnant or breast-feeding, ask a health professional before use. It is especially important not to use ibuprofen during the last 3 months of pregnancy unless definitely directed to do so by a doctor because it may cause problems in the unborn child or complications during delivery.
Keep out of reach of children. In case of overdose, get medical help or contact a Poison Control Center right away. (1-800-222-1222)

Directions
• **do not take more than directed**
• **do not take longer than 10 days, unless directed by a doctor (see Warnings)**
• adults and children 12 years and over: take 2 caplets at bedtime
• do not take more than 2 caplets in 24 hours

Other information
• read all warnings and directions before use. Keep carton.
• store at 20°-25°C (68°-77°F)
• avoid excessive heat above 40°C (104°F)

Inactive ingredients colloidal silicon dioxide, croscarmellose sodium, glyceryl behenate, hydroxypropyl cellulose, lactose monohydrate, magnesium stearate, microcrystalline cellulose, polyethylene glycol, polyvinyl alcohol, pregelatinized starch, talc, titanium dioxide

---

PRECISE™ PAIN RELIEVING CREAM - REGULAR STRENGTH

Drug Facts
Active ingredients .... **Purpose**
Menthol 10% .... Topical analgesic
Methyl salicylate 10% .... Topical analgesic

---

Uses

temporarily relieves the minor aches and pains of muscles and joints associated with: • simple backache • arthritis • sprains • bruises • strains

Warnings

For external use only.

Do not use: • on wounds or damaged skin • with a heating pad • on a child under 12 years of age with arthritis-like conditions.

Ask a doctor before use if • you have redness over the affected area.

When using this product • avoid contact with eyes or mucous membranes • do not bandage tightly.

Stop use and ask a doctor if: • condition worsens or symptoms persist for more than 7 days • symptoms clear up and occur again within a few days • excessive skin irritation occurs.

Keep out of reach of children to avoid accidental ingestion. If swallowed, get medical help or contact a Poison Control Center right away. (1-800-222-1222)

Directions

• **use only as directed** • adults and children 12 years of age and older: apply to affected area not more than 3 to 4 times daily • children under 12 years of age: ask a doctor
Other Information • store at 20-25° C (68-77° F) Protect from freezing

Inactive ingredients

C12-15 alkyl benzoate, carbomer, cocoglycerides, dimethicone, distearyl ether, edetate disodium, ethylparaben, fragrance, glyceryl laurate, glyceryl stearate, methylparaben, myristyl alcohol, phenoxyethanol, propylparaben, sodium hydroxide, steareth-2, steareth-21, stearyl alcohol, water

PRECISE™ PAIN RELIEVING PATCH - EXTRA STRENGTH

Drug Facts

Active ingredients .... **Purpose**
Menthol 5% .... Topical analgesic

Uses

PRECISE™ Pain Relieving Heat Patch provide temporary relief of minor muscular and joint aches and pains associated with overexertion, strains, sprains, and arthritis.

Directions

Tear open pouch when ready to use. Peel away liner to reveal adhesive side. Place on area of pain with adhesive side toward your skin. Apply firmly. For maximum effectiveness, wear the heat patch for 8 hours. Do not use for more than 8 hours in a 24-hour period. It may take up to 30 minutes for the patch to reach its' therapeutic temperature.

Do not use:
If the heat patch is damaged or torn
With medicated lotions, creams, or ointments
On damaged, broken, or sensitive skin
On areas of bruising or swelling that has occurred within 48 hours
On people who are not capable of applying and removing the heat patch themselves, including infants, children 12 and under, and some elderly
On areas of the body where heat cannot be felt
With other forms of heat

Ask a doctor before use if you have diabetes, poor circulation, heart disease, rheumatoid arthritis, or are pregnant.

When using this product:
Check skin frequently for signs of irritation, burns or blistering – if found, stop use immediately. It is normal to experience slight skin redness after removing the heat patch. If your skin is still red after a few hours, stop using heat patch until the redness goes away completely. If product feels too hot, stop use or wear over clothing. Do not place extra pressure or tight clothing over this product. Do not use for more than 8 hours in a 24-hour period.

Stop use and call a doctor if:
You experience any discomfort, burning, swelling, rash, or other changes in your skin that persist where the heat patch is worn. After 7 days, your pain gets worse or remains unchanged, as this may be a sign of a more serious condition.

Warnings

Do not use this product while sleeping. Check skin frequently during use. This product has the potential to cause skin irritation or burns. If you find irritation or a burn, remove product immediately. IF YOU ARE 55 OR OLDER, wear the patch over a layer of clothing and not directly against your skin, as your risk of burns increase with age.
Additional Warnings The heat patch contains iron that can be harmful if ingested. If swallowed, rinse mouth with water and call a Poison Control Center immediately. If heat patch contents come in contact with your skin or eyes, rinse with water immediately. To avoid the risk of fire, DO NOT MICROWAVE THIS PRODUCT OR ATTEMPT TO RE-

HEAT. KEEP OUT OF REACH OF CHILDREN AND PETS. FOR EXTERNAL USE ONLY. KEEP AWAY FROM HEAT.

Other Information
• store between 20-25° C (68-77° F)
Inactive ingredients carboxymethylcellulose sodium, colloidal silicone dioxide, fragrance, glycerin, kaolin, methyl acrylate/2 - ethylhexyl acrylate copolymer, methylparaben, polyacrylate acid, polysorbate 80, propylparaben, sodium polyacrylate, sodium polyacrylate starch, sorbitan monooleate, sorbitol, tartaric acid, titanium dioxide, water

---

ST. JOSEPH 81 mg Aspirin   OTC
ST. JOSEPH 81 mg Adult Low Strength Aspirin Chewable & Enteric Coated Tablets

Description

Active ingredient (in each tablet)   Purpose
Aspirin 81 mg (NSAID)* .... pain reliever
*nonsteroidal anti-inflammatory drug

Uses

temporarily relieves minor aches and pains

Directions

• drink a full glass of water with each dose

adults and children 12 years and over	• take 4 to 8 tablets every 4 hours while symptoms last • do not exceed 48 tablets in 24 hours or as directed by a doctor
children under 12 years	do not use unless directed by a doctor

Warnings

Reye's syndrome: Children and teenagers who have or are recovering from chicken pox or flu-like symptoms should not use this product. When using this product, if changes in behavior with nausea and vomiting occur, consult a doctor because these symptoms could be an early sign of Reye's syndrome, a rare but serious illness.

Allergy alert: Aspirin may cause a severe allergic reaction which may include:
• hives • facial swelling • asthma (wheezing) • shock
Stomach bleeding warning: This product contains an NSAID, which may cause severe stomach bleeding. The chance is higher if you
• are age 60 or older
• have had stomach ulcers or bleeding problems
• take a blood thinning (anticoagulant) or steroid drug
• take other drugs containing prescription or nonprescription NSAIDs (aspirin, ibuprofen, naproxen, or others)
• have 3 or more alcoholic drinks every day while using this product
• take more or for a longer time than directed

Do not use
• if you have ever had an allergic reaction to any pain reliever or fever reducer
• for at least 7 days after tonsillectomy or oral surgery unless directed by a doctor (chewable tablet only)

Ask a doctor before use if
• the stomach bleeding warning applies to you
• you have a history of stomach problems such as heartburn
• you have high blood pressure, heart disease, liver cirrhosis, or kidney disease
• you have asthma
• you are taking a diuretic

Ask a doctor or pharmacist before use if you are taking a prescription drug for:
• gout • diabetes • arthritis

Stop use and ask a doctor if
• you experience any of the following signs of stomach bleeding
• feel faint • vomit blood • have bloody or black stools
• have stomach pain that does not get better
• allergic reaction occurs
• ringing in the ears or loss of hearing occurs
• pain gets worse or lasts more than 10 days
• new symptoms occur
• redness or swelling is present
This could be signs of a serious condition.

If pregnant or breast-feeding, ask a health professional before use. It is especially important not to use ibuprofen during the last 3 months of pregnancy unless definitely directed to do so by a doctor because it may cause problems in the unborn child or complications during delivery.

Keep out of reach of children. In case of overdose, get medical help or contact a Poison Control Center right away. (1-800-222-1222)

Other information:
• store between 20–25°C (68–77°F). Avoid high humidity.

Inactive ingredients: St. Joseph 81 mg Adult Low Strength Aspirin Chewable Tablets: corn starch, FD&C yellow #6 aluminum lake, flavor, mannitol, pregelatinized starch, saccharin, silicon dioxide, stearic acid.
Enteric Coated Tablets: colloidal silicon dioxide, FD&C red #40 dye, FD&C yellow #6 dye, glyceryl monostearate, iron oxide, magnesium stearate, methacrylic acid copolymer, microcrystalline cellulose, pregelatinized starch, propylene glycol, shellac, simethicone, stearic acid, triethyl citrate.

How Supplied

St. Joseph Adult Low Strength Aspirin Chewable Tablets are round, orange flavored, orange colored tablets that are debossed with the "SJ" logo. Available in: tamper evident bottles of 38 and 108 (Tri-Pack).
St. Joseph Adult Low Strength Aspirin Enteric Coated Tablets are round, pink-coated tablets that are printed with the "StJ" logo. Available in: tamper evident bottles of 36, 100, 180 and 300.

Comprehensive Prescribing Information
Description

St. Joseph Adult Low Strength Aspirin Chewable & Enteric Coated Tablets (acetylsalicylic acid) are available in 81 mg for oral administration. Aspirin is an odorless white, needle-like crystalline or powdery substance. When exposed to moisture, aspirin hydrolyzes into salicylic and acetic acids, and gives off a vinegary-odor. It is highly lipid soluble and slightly soluble in water.

Clinical Pharmacology

Mechanism of Action: Aspirin is a more potent inhibitor of both prostaglandin synthesis and platelet aggregation than other salicylic acid derivatives. The differences in activity between aspirin and salicylic acid are thought to be due to the acetyl group on the aspirin molecule. This acetyl group is responsible for the inactivation of cyclo-oxygenase via acetylation.

Pharmacokinetics: Absorption: In general, immediate release aspirin is well and completely absorbed from the gastrointestinal (GI) tract. Following absorption, aspirin is hydrolyzed to salicylic acid with peak plasma levels of salicylic acid occurring within 1–2 hours of dosing (see Pharmacokinetics—Metabolism). The rate of absorption from the GI tract is dependent upon the dosage form, the presence or absence of food, gastric pH (the presence or absence of GI antacids or buffering agents), and other physiologic factors. Enteric coated aspirin products are erratically absorbed from the GI tract.

Distribution: Salicylic acid is widely distributed to all tissues and fluids in the body including the central nervous system (CNS), breast milk, and fetal tissues. The highest concentrations are found in the plasma, liver, renal cortex, heart, and lungs. The protein binding of salicylate is concentration-dependent, i.e., nonlinear. At low concentrations (<100 micrograms/milliliter μg/mL), approximately 90 percent of plasma salicylate is bound to albumin while at higher concentrations (400 μg/mL), only about 75 percent is bound. The early signs of salicylic overdose (salicylism), including tinnitus (ringing in the ears), occur at plasma concentrations approximating 200 μg/mL. Severe toxic effects are associated with levels 400 μg/mL. (See Adverse Reactions and Overdosage.)

Metabolism: Aspirin is rapidly hydrolyzed in the plasma to salicylic acid such that plasma levels of aspirin are essentially undetectable 1–2 hours after dosing. Salicylic acid is primarily conjugated in the liver to form salicyluric acid, a phenolic glucuronide, an acyl glucuronide, and a number of minor metabolites. Salicylic acid has a plasma half-life of approximately 6 hours. Salicylate metabolism is saturable and total body clearance decreases at higher serum concentrations due to the limited ability of the liver to form both salicyluric acid and phenolic glucuronide. Following toxic doses (10–20 grams (g)), the plasma half-life may be increased to over 20 hours.

Elimination: The elimination of salicylic acid follows zero order pharmacokinetics; (i.e., the rate of drug elimination is constant in relation to plasma concentration). Renal excretion of unchanged drug depends upon urine pH. As urinary pH rises above 6.5, the renal clearance of free salicylate increases from <5 percent to 80 percent. Alkalinization of the urine is a key concept in the management of salicylate overdose. (See Overdosage.) Following therapeutic doses, approximately 10 percent is found excreted in the urine as salicylic acid, 75 percent as salicyluric acid, and 10 percent phenolic and 5 percent acyl glucuronides of salicylic acid.

Pharmacodynamics: Aspirin affects platelet aggregation by irreversibly inhibiting prostaglandin cyclo-oxygenase. The effect lasts for the life of the platelet and prevents the formation of the platelet aggregating factor thromboxane A2. Nonacetylated salicylates do not inhibit this enzyme and have no effect on platelet aggregation. At somewhat higher doses, aspirin reversibly inhibits the formation of prostaglandin I2 (prostacyclin), which is an arterial vasodilator and inhibits platelet aggregation.

At higher doses, aspirin is an effective anti-inflammatory agent, partially due to inhibition of inflammatory mediators via cyclo-oxygenase inhibition in peripheral tissues. In vitro studies suggest that other mediators of inflammation may also be suppressed by aspirin administration, although the precise mechanism of action has not been elucidated. It is this nonspecific suppression of cyclo-oxygenase activity in peripheral tissues following large doses that leads to its primary side effect of gastric irritation. (See Adverse Reactions.)

Clinical Studies

Ischemic Stroke and Transient Ischemic Attack (TIA): In clinical trials of subjects with TIA's due to fibrin platelet emboli or ischemic stroke, aspirin has been shown to significantly reduce the risk of the combined endpoint of stroke or death and the combined endpoint of TIA, stroke, or death by about 13–18 percent.

Suspected Acute Myocardial Infarction (MI): In a large, multi-center study of aspirin, streptokinase, and the combination of aspirin and streptokinase in 17,187 patients with suspected acute MI, aspirin treatment produced a 23-percent reduction in the risk of vascular mortality. Aspirin was also shown to have an additional benefit in patients given a thrombolytic agent.

Prevention of Recurrent MI and Unstable Angina Pectoris: These indications are supported by the results of six large, randomized, multi-center, placebo-controlled trials of predominantly male post-MI subjects and one randomized placebo-controlled study of men with unstable angina pectoris. Aspirin therapy in MI subjects was associated with a significant reduction (about 20 percent) in the risk of the combined endpoint of subsequent death and/or nonfatal reinfarction in these patients. In aspirin-treated unstable angina patients, the event rate was reduced to 5 percent from the 10 percent rate in the placebo group.

Chronic Stable Angina Pectoris: In a randomized, multi-center, double-blind trial designed to assess the role of aspirin for prevention of MI in patients with chronic stable angina pectoris, aspirin significantly reduced the primary combined endpoint of nonfatal MI, fatal MI, and sudden death by 34 percent. The secondary endpoint for vascular events (first occurrence of MI, stroke, or vascular death) was also significantly reduced (32 percent).

Revascularization Procedures: Most patients who undergo coronary artery revascularization procedures have already had symptomatic coronary artery disease for which aspirin is indicated. Similarly, patients with lesions of the carotid bifurcation sufficient to require carotid endarterectomy are likely to have had a precedent event. Aspirin is recommended for patients who undergo revascularization procedures if there is a preexisting condition for which aspirin is already indicated.

Rheumatologic Diseases: In clinical studies in patients with rheumatoid arthritis, juvenile rheumatoid arthritis, ankylosing spondylitis and osteoarthritis, aspirin has been shown to be effective in controlling various indices of clinical disease activity.

Animal Toxicology

The acute oral 50 percent lethal dose in rats is about 1.5 g/kilogram (kg) and in mice 1.1 g/kg. Renal papillary necrosis and decreased urinary concentrating ability occur in rodents chronically administered high doses. Dose-dependent gastric mucosal injury occurs in rats and humans. Mammals may develop aspirin toxicosis associated with GI symptoms, circulatory effects, and central nervous system depression. (See Overdosage.)

Indications and Usage

Vascular Indications (Ischemic Stroke, TIA, Acute MI, Prevention of Recurrent MI, Unstable Angina Pectoris, and Chronic Stable Angina Pectoris): Aspirin is indicated to: (1) Reduce the combined risk of death and nonfatal stroke in patients who have had ischemic stroke or transient ischemia of the brain due to fibrin platelet emboli, (2) reduce the risk of vascular mortality in patients with a suspected acute MI, (3) reduce the combined risk of death and nonfatal MI in patients with a previous MI or unstable angina pectoris, and (4) reduce the combined risk of MI and sudden death in patients with chronic stable angina pectoris.

Revascularization Procedures (Coronary Artery Bypass Graft (CABG), Percutaneous Transminase Coronary Angioplasty (PTCA), and Carotid Endarterectomy): Aspirin is indicated in patients who have undergone revascularization procedures (i.e., CABG, PTCA, or carotid endarterectomy) when there is a preexisting condition for which aspirin is already indicated.

Rheumatologic Disease Indications (Rheumatoid Arthritis, Juvenile Rheumatoid Arthritis, Spondyloarthropathies, Osteoarthritis, and the Arthritis and Pleurisy of Systemic Lupus Erythematosus (SLE)): Aspirin is indicated for the relief of the signs and symptoms of rheumatoid arthritis, juvenile rheumatoid arthritis, osteoarthritis, spondyloarthopathies, and arthritis and pleurisy associated with SLE.

Contraindications

Allergy: Aspirin is contraindicated in patients with known allergy to nonsteroidal anti-inflammatory drug products and in patients with the syndrome of asthma, rhinitis, and nasal polyps. Aspirin may cause severe urticaria, angioedema, or bronchospasm (asthma).

Reye's Syndrome: Aspirin should not be used in children or teenagers for viral infections, with or without fever, because of the risk of Reye's syndrome with concomitant use of aspirin in certain viral illnesses.

Warnings

Alcohol Warning: Patients who consume three or more alcoholic drinks every day should be counseled about the bleeding risks involved with chronic, heavy alcohol use while taking aspirin.

Coagulation Abnormalities: Even low doses of aspirin can inhibit platelet function leading to an increase in bleeding time. This can adversely affect patients with inherited (hemophilia) or acquired (liver disease or vitamin K deficiency) bleeding disorders.

GI Side Effects: GI side effects include stomach pain, heartburn, nausea, vomiting, and gross GI bleeding. Although minor upper GI symptoms, such as dyspepsia, are common and can occur anytime during therapy, physicians should remain alert for signs of ulceration and bleeding, even in the absence of previous GI symptoms. Physicians should inform patients about the signs and symptoms of GI side effects and what steps to take if they occur.

Peptic Ulcer Disease: Patients with a history of active peptic ulcer disease should avoid using aspirin, which can cause gastric mucosal irritation and bleeding.

Precautions

General: Renal Failure: Avoid aspirin in patients with severe renal failure (glomerular filtration rate less than 10 mL/minute)

Hepatic Insufficiency: Avoid aspirin in patients with severe hepatic insufficiency.

Sodium Restricted Diets: Patients with sodium-retaining states, such as congestive heart failure or renal failure, should avoid sodium-containing buffered aspirin preparations because of their high sodium content.

Laboratory Tests: Aspirin has been associated with elevated hepatic enzymes, blood urea nitrogen, serum creatinine, hyperkalemia, proteinuria, and prolonged bleeding time.

Drug Interactions: Angiotensin Converting Enzyme (ACE) Inhibitors: The hyponatremic and hypotensive effects of ACE inhibitors may be diminished by the concomitant administration of aspirin due to its indirect effect on the renin-angiotensin conversion pathway.

Acetazolamide: Concurrent use of aspirin and acetazolamide can lead to high serum concentrations of acetazolamide (and toxicity) due to competition at the renal tubule for secretion.

Anticoagulant Therapy (Heparin and Warfarin): Patients on anticoagulation therapy are at increased risk for bleeding because of drug-drug interactions and the effect on platelets. Aspirin can displace warfarin from protein binding sites, leading to prolongation of both the prothrombin time and the bleeding time. Aspirin can increase the anticoagulant activity of heparin, increasing bleeding risk.

Anticonvulsants: Salicylate can displace protein-bound phenytoin and valproic acid, leading to a decrease in the total concentration of phenytoin and an increase in serum valproic acid levels.

Beta Blockers: The hypotensive effects of beta blockers may be diminished by the concomitant administration of aspirin due to inhibition of renal prostaglandins, leading to decreased renal blood flow, and salt and fluid retention.

Diuretics: The effectiveness of diuretics in patients with underlying renal or cardiovascular disease may be diminished by the concomitant administration of aspirin due to inhibition of renal prostaglandins, leading to decreased renal blood flow and salt and fluid retention.

Methotrexate: Salicylate can inhibit renal clearance of methotrexate, leading to bone marrow toxicity, especially in the elderly or renal impaired.

Nonsteroidal Anti-Inflammatory Drugs (NSAID's): The concurrent use of aspirin with other NSAID's should be avoided because this may increase bleeding or lead to decreased renal function.

Oral Hypoglycemics: Moderate doses of aspirin may increase the effectiveness of oral hypoglycemic drugs, leading to hypoglycemia.

Uricosuric Agents (Probenecid and Sulfinpyrazone): Salicylates antagonize the uricosuric action of uricosuric agents.

Carcinogenesis, Mutagenesis, Impairment of Fertility: Administration of aspirin for 68 weeks at 0.5 percent in the feed of rats was not carcinogenic. In the Ames Salmonella assay, aspirin was not mutagenic; however, aspirin did induce chromosome aberrations in cultured human fibroblasts. Aspirin inhibits ovulation in rats. (See Pregnancy.)

Pregnancy: Pregnant women should only take aspirin if clearly needed. Because of the known effects of NSAID's on the fetal cardiovascular system (closure of the ductus arteriosus), use during the third trimester of pregnancy should be avoided. Salicylate products have also been associated with alterations in maternal and neonatal hemostasis mechanisms, decreased birth weight, and with perinatal mortality.

Labor and Delivery: Aspirin should be avoided 1 week prior to and during labor and delivery because it can result in excessive blood loss at delivery. Prolonged gestation and labor due to prostaglandin inhibition have been reported.

Nursing Mothers: Nursing mothers should avoid using aspirin because salicylate is excreted in breast milk. Use of high doses may lead to rashes, platelet abnormalities, and bleeding in nursing infants.

Pediatric Use: Pediatric dosing recommendations for juvenile rheumatoid arthritis are based on well-controlled clinical studies. An initial dose of 90–130 mg/kg/day in divided doses, with an increase as needed for anti-inflammatory efficacy (target plasma salicylate levels of 150–300 µg/mL) are effective. At high doses (i.e., plasma levels of greater than 200 µg/mL), the incidence of toxicity increases.

Adverse Reactions

Many adverse reactions due to aspirin ingestion are dose-related. The following is a list of adverse reactions that have been reported in the literature. (See Warnings.)

Body as a Whole: Fever, hypothermia, thirst.

Cardiovascular: Dysrhythmias, hypotension, tachycardia.

Central Nervous System: Agitation, cerebral edema, coma, confusion, dizziness, headache, subdural or intracranial hemorrhage, lethargy, seizures.

Fluid and Electrolyte: Dehydration, hyperkalemia, metabolic acidosis, respiratory alkalosis.

Gastrointestinal: Dyspepsia, GI bleeding, ulceration and perforation, nausea, vomiting, transient elevations of hepatic enzymes, hepatitis, Reye's Syndrome, pancreatitis.

Hematologic: Prolonged prothrombin time, disseminated intravascular coagulation, coagulopathy, thrombocytopenia.

Hypersensitivity: Acute anaphylaxis, angioedema, asthma, bronchospasm, laryngeal edema, urticaria.

Musculoskeletal: Rhabdomyolysis.

Metabolism: Hypoglycemia (in children), hyperglycemia.

Reproductive: Prolonged pregnancy and labor, stillbirths, lower birth weight infants, antepartum and postpartum bleeding.

Special Senses: Hearing loss, tinnitus. Patients with high frequency hearing loss may have difficulty perceiving tinnitus. In these patients, tinnitus cannot be used as a clinical indicator of salicylism.

Urogenital: Interstitial nephritis, papillary necrosis, proteinuria, renal insufficiency and failure.

Drug Abuse and Dependence

Aspirin is nonnarcotic. There is no known potential for addiction associated with the use of aspirin.

Overdosage

Salicylate toxicity may result from acute ingestion (overdose) or chronic intoxication. The early signs of salicylic overdose (salicylism), including tinnitus (ringing in the ears), occur at plasma concentrations approaching 200 µg/mL. Plasma concentrations of aspirin above 300 µg/mL are clearly toxic. Severe toxic effects are associated with levels above 400 µg/mL (See Clinical Pharmacology.) A single lethal dose of aspirin in adults is not known with certainty but death may be expected at 30 g. For real or suspected overdose, a Poison Control Center should be contacted immediately. Careful medical management is essential.

Signs and Symptoms: In acute overdose, severe acid-base and electrolyte disturbances may occur and are complicated by hyperthermia and dehydration. Respiratory alkalosis occurs early while hyperventilation is present, but is quickly followed by metabolic acidosis.

Treatment: Treatment consists primarily of supporting vital functions, increasing salicylate elimination, and correcting the acid-base disturbance. Gastric emptying and/or lavage is recommended as soon as possible after ingestion, even if the patient has vomited spontaneously. After lavage and/or emesis, administration of activated charcoal, as a slurry, is beneficial, if less than 3 hours have passed since ingestion. Charcoal adsorption should not be employed prior to emesis and lavage. Severity of aspirin intoxication is determined by measuring the blood salicylate level. Acid-base status should be closely followed with serial blood gas and serum pH measurements. Fluid and electrolyte balance should also be maintained. In severe cases, hyperthermia and hypovolemia are the major immediate threats to life. Children should be sponged with tepid water. Replacement fluids should be administered intravenously and augmented with correction of acidosis. Plasma electrolytes and pH should be monitored to promote alkaline diuresis of salicylate if renal function is normal. Infusion of glucose may be required to control hypoglycemia. Hemodialysis and peritoneal dialysis can be performed to reduce the body drug content. In patients with renal insufficiency or in cases of life-threatening intoxication, dialysis is usually required. Exchange transfusion may be indicated in infants and young children.

Dosage and Administration

Each dose of aspirin should be taken with a full glass of water unless the patient is fluid restricted. Anti-inflammatory and analgesic dosages should be individualized.

Ischemic Stroke and TIA: 50–325 mg once a day. Continue therapy indefinitely

Suspected Acute MI: The initial dose of 160–162.5 mg is administered as soon as an MI is suspected. The maintenance dose of 160–162.5 mg a day is continued for 30 days post-infarction. After 30 days, consider further therapy based on dosage and administration for prevention of recurrent MI.

Prevention of Recurrent MI: 75–325 mg once a day. Continue therapy indefinitely.

Unstable Angina Pectoris: 75–325 mg once a day. Continue therapy indefinitely.

Chronic Stable Angina Pectoris: 75–325 mg once a day. Continue therapy indefinitely.

CABG: 325 mg daily starting 6 hours post-procedure. Continue therapy for 1 year post-procedure.

PTCA: The initial dose of 325 mg daily should be given 2 hours pre-surgery. Maintenance dose is 160–325 mg daily. Continue therapy indefinitely.

Carotid Endarterectomy: Doses of 80 mg once daily to 650 mg twice daily, started presurgery, are recommended. Continue therapy indefinitely.

Rheumatoid Arthritis: The initial dose is 3 g a day in divided doses. Increase as needed for anti-inflammatory efficacy with target plasma salicylate levels of 150–300 µg/mL. At high doses (i.e., plasma levels of greater than 200 µg/mL), the incidence of toxicity increases.

Juvenile Rheumatoid Arthritis: Initial dose is 90–130 mg/kg/day in divided doses. Increase as needed for anti-inflammatory efficacy with target plasma salicylate levels of 150–300 µg/mL. At high doses (i.e., plasma levels of greater than 200 µg/mL), the incidence of toxicity increases.

Spondyloarthropathies: Up to 4 g per day in divided doses.

Osteoarthritis: Up to 3 g per day in divided doses.

Arthritis and Pleurisy of SLE: The initial dose is 3 g a day in divided doses. Increase as needed for anti-inflammatory efficacy with target plasma salicylate levels of 150–300 µg/mL. At high doses (i.e., plasma levels of greater than 200 µg/mL), the incidence of toxicity increases.

CHILDREN'S SUDAFED® NON-DROWSY NASAL DECONGESTANT LIQUID   OTC

Active ingredient   **Purpose**
(in each 5 mL*)
Pseudoephedrine HCl 15 mg .... Nasal decongestant

*5 mL = one tspful

Uses
- temporarily relieves nasal congestion due to the common cold, hay fever or other upper respiratory allergies
- temporarily relieves sinus congestion and pressure
- promotes nasal and/or sinus drainage

Warnings

Do not use in a child who is taking a prescription monoamine oxidase inhibitor (MAOI) (certain drugs for depression, psychiatric or emotional conditions, or Parkinson's disease), or for 2 weeks after stopping the MAOI drug. If you do not know if your child's prescription drug contains an MAOI, ask a doctor or pharmacist before giving this product.

Ask a doctor before use if the child has
- heart disease • high blood pressure • thyroid disease
- diabetes

When using this product do not exceed recommended dose

Stop use and ask a doctor if
- nervousness, dizziness, or sleeplessness occur
- symptoms do not improve within 7 days or occur with a fever

Keep out of reach of children. In case of overdose, get medical help or contact a Poison Control Center right away. (1-800-222-1222)

Directions
- find right dose on chart
- use only enclosed dosing cup designed for use with this product. Do not use any other dosing device.
- if needed, repeat dose every 4 to 6 hours
- do not use more than 4 times in 24 hours

Age (yr)	Dose (tsp or 5 mL)
under 4 years	do not use
4 to 5 years	1 teaspoonful (5 mL)
6 to 11 years	2 teaspoonfuls (10 mL)

Attention: use only enclosed dosing cup designed for use with this product. Do not use any other dosing device.

Other information
- each teaspoonful contains: **sodium 5 mg**
- store between 20–25°C (68–77°F)

Inactive ingredients anhydrous citric acid, edetate disodium, FD&C blue # 1, FD&C red # 40, flavor, glycerin, menthol, poloxamer 407, polyethylene glycol, povidone K-90, purified water, saccharin sodium, sodium benzoate, sodium citrate, sorbitol solution

---

CHILDREN'S SUDAFED PE® NASAL DECONGESTANT LIQUID   OTC

Active ingredient (in each 5 mL*)   **Purpose**
Phenylephrine HCl 2.5 mg .... Nasal decongestant
*5 mL = one teaspoonful

Use temporarily relieves nasal congestion due to the common cold, hay fever or other upper respiratory allergies

Warnings

Do not use in a child who is taking a prescription monoamine oxidase inhibitor (MAOI) (certain drugs for depression, psychiatric, or emotional conditions, or Parkinson's disease), or for 2 weeks after stopping the MAOI drug. If you do not know if your child's prescription drug contains an MAOI, ask a doctor or pharmacist before giving this product.

Ask a doctor before use if the child has
- heart disease
- high blood pressure
- thyroid disease
- diabetes
- a sodium-restricted diet

When using this product do not exceed recommended dose

Stop use and ask a doctor if
- nervousness, dizziness, or sleeplessness occur
- symptoms do not improve within 7 days or occur with a fever

Keep out of reach of children. In case of overdose, get medical help or contact a Poison Control Center right away. (1-800-222-1222)

Directions
- find right dose on chart
- use only enclosed dosing cup designed for use with this product. Do not use any other dosing device.
- if needed, repeat every 4 hours
- do not use more than 6 times in 24 hours

Age (yr)	Dose (tsp or mL)
under 4 years	do not use
4 to 5 years	1 teaspoonful (5 mL)
6 to 11 years	2 teaspoonfuls (10 mL)

Attention: use only enclosed dosing cup designed for use with this product. Do not use any other dosing device.

Other information
- each teaspoonful contains: **sodium 14 mg**
- store between 20°-25°C (68°-77°F). Protect from light. Store in outer container until contents are used.

Inactive ingredients carboxymethylcellulose sodium, citric acid, edetate disodium, FD&C red # 40, flavors, glycerin, sodium benzoate, sodium citrate, sorbitol, sucralose, water

---

SUDAFED® CONGESTION TABLETS   OTC

Active ingredient (in each tablet)   **Purpose**
Pseudoephedrine HCl 30 mg .... Nasal decongestant

Uses
- temporarily relieves sinus congestion and pressure
- temporarily relieves nasal congestion due to the common cold, hay fever or other upper respiratory allergies

Warnings

Do not use if you are now taking a prescription monoamine oxidase inhibitor (MAOI) (certain drugs for depression, psychiatric or emotional conditions, or Parkinson's disease), or for 2 weeks after stopping the MAOI drug. If you do not know if your prescription drug contains an MAOI, ask a doctor or pharmacist before taking this product.

Ask a doctor before use if you have
- heart disease
- high blood pressure
- thyroid disease
- diabetes
- trouble urinating due to an enlarged prostate gland

When using this product do not exceed recommended dose

Stop use and ask a doctor if
- nervousness, dizziness, or sleeplessness occur
- symptoms do not improve within 7 days or occur with a fever

If pregnant or breast-feeding, ask a health professional before use.

Keep out of reach of children. In case of overdose, get medical help or contact a Poison Control Center right away. (1-800-222-1222)

Directions

adults and children 12 years and over	• take 2 tablets every 4 to 6 hours • do not take more than 8 tablets in 24 hours
children ages 6 to 11 years	• take 1 tablet every 4 to 6 hours • do not take more than 4 tablets in 24 hours
children under 6 years	do not use this product in children under 6 years of age

Other information
- store between 20–25°C (68–77°F)

Inactive ingredients carnauba wax, colloidal silicon dioxide, D&C yellow #10 aluminum lake, FD&C red #40 aluminum lake, FD&C yellow #6 aluminum lake, iron oxide, magnesium stearate, microcrystalline cellulose, polyethylene glycol, polyvinyl alcohol, pregelatinized starch, shellac, sodium starch glycolate, talc, titanium dioxide

---

SUDAFED PE® CONGESTION   OTC

Drug Facts

Active ingredient (in each tablet)   **Purpose**
Phenylephrine HCl 10 mg .... Nasal decongestant

Uses
- temporarily relieves sinus congestion and pressure
- temporarily relieves nasal congestion due to the common cold, hay fever or other upper respiratory allergies

Warnings

Do not use if you are now taking a prescription monoamine oxidase inhibitor (MAOI) (certain drugs for depression, psychiatric or emotional conditions, or Parkinson's disease), or for 2 weeks after stopping the MAOI drug. If you do not know if your prescription drug contains an MAOI, ask a doctor or pharmacist before taking this product.

Ask a doctor before use if you have
- heart disease
- high blood pressure
- thyroid disease
- diabetes
- trouble urinating due to an enlarged prostate gland

When using this product do not exceed recommended dose

Stop use and ask a doctor if
- nervousness, dizziness, or sleeplessness occur
- symptoms do not improve within 7 days or occur with a fever

If pregnant or breast-feeding, ask a health professional before use.

Keep out of reach of children. In case of overdose, get medical help or contact a Poison Control Center right away. (1-800-222-1222)

Directions

adults and children 12 years of age and over	• take 1 tablet every 4 hours • do not take more than 6 tablets in 24 hours
children under 12 years	• do not use this product in children under 12 years of age

Other information
- store between 20-25° C (68-77° F)

Inactive ingredients carnauba wax, corn starch, D & C yellow # 10 aluminum lake, FD&C red # 40 aluminum lake, FD&C yellow # 6 aluminum lake, magnesium stearate, microcrystalline cellulose, polyethylene glycol, polyvinyl alcohol, powdered cellulose, pregelatinized starch, sodium starch glycolate, talc, titanium dioxide

Children's Tylenol® Dosing Chart

Attention: use only enclosed dosing device specifically designed for use with this product. Do not use any other dosing device.

AGE GROUP		0–3 mos*	4–11 mos*	12–23 mos*	2–3 yrs	4–5 yrs	6–8 yrs	9–10 yrs	11 yrs	12 yrs	
WEIGHT		6–11 lbs*	12–17 lbs*	18–23 lbs*	24–35 lbs	36–47 lbs	48–59 lbs	60–71 lbs	72–95 lbs	96 lbs and over	
PRODUCT FORM	INGREDIENTS	• shake well before using • find right dose on chart below. If possible, use weight to dose; otherwise, use age. • Dose to be administered based on weight or age • If needed, repeat dose every 4 hours mL = milliliter; tsp = teaspoonful									Maximum Doses/24 hrs
Infants' Drops	Per dropperful (0.8 mL)										
Concentrated Tylenol Infants' Drops	Acetaminophen 80 mg (in each 0.8 mL)	0.4 mL	0.8 mL	1.2 mL (0.8 + 0.4 mL)	1.6 mL) (0.8 + 0.8 mL)	—	—	—	—	—	5 times in 24 hrs
Children's Liquids	Per 5 mL = 1 teaspoonful (tsp)										
Children's Tylenol Suspension	Acetaminophen 160 mg (in each 5 mL or 1 tsp)	—	2.5 mL (½ tsp)	3.75 mL (¾ tsp)	5 mL (1 tsp)	7.5 mL (1½ tsp)	10 mL (2 tsp)	12.5 mL (2½ tsp)	15 mL (3 tsp)	—	5 times in 24 hrs
Children's Tylenol Plus Cold & Allergy Suspension	Acetaminophen 160 mg Diphenhydramine HCl 12.5 mg Phenylephrine HCl 2.5 mg	Do not use				Do not use unless directed by a doctor	10 mL (2 tsp)	10 mL (2 tsp)	10 mL (2 tsp)	—	5 times in 24 hrs
Children's Tylenol Plus Cold & Stuffy Nose Suspension	Acetaminophen 160 mg Phenylephrine Hcl 2.5 mg	Do not use				5 mL (1 tsp)	10 mL (2 tsp)	10 mL (2 tsp)	10 mL (2 tsp)	—	5 times in 24 hrs
Children's Tylenol Plus Cough and Runny Nose Suspension	Acetaminophen 160 mg Chlorpheniramine maleate 1 mg Dextromethorphan HBr 5 mg	Do not use				Do not use unless directed by a doctor	10 mL (2 tsp)	10 mL (2 tsp)	10 mL (2 tsp)	—	5 times in 24 hrs
Children's Tylenol Plus Cough and Sore Throat Suspension	Acetaminophen 160 mg Dextromethorphan HBr 5 mg	Do not use				5 mL (1 tsp)	10 mL (2 tsp)	10 mL (2 tsp)	10 mL (2 tsp)	—	5 times in 24 hrs
Children's Tylenol Plus Multi-Symptom Cold Suspension	Acetaminophen 160 mg Chlorpheniramine maleate 1 mg Dextromethorphan HBr 5 mg Phenylephrine HCl 2.5 mg	Do not use				Do not use unless directed by a doctor	10 mL (2 tsp)	10 mL (2 tsp)	10 mL (2 tsp)	—	5 times in 24 hrs
Children's Tylenol Plus Cold & Cough Suspension	Acetaminophen 160 mg Dextromethorphan HBr 5 mg Phenylephrine HCl 2.5 mg	Do not use				5 mL (1 tsp)	10 mL (2 tsp)	10 mL (2 tsp)	10 mL (2 tsp)	—	5 times in 24 hrs
Children's Tylenol Plus Flu	Acetaminophen 160 mg Chlorpheniramine maleate 1 mg Dextromethorphan HBr 5 mg Phenylephrine HCl 2.5 mg	Do not use				Do not use unless directed by a doctor	10 mL (2 tsp)	10 mL (2 tsp)	10 mL (2 tsp)	—	5 times in 24 hrs

(Table continued on next page)

CONCENTRATED TYLENOL®
acetaminophen Infants' Drops   **OTC**

CHILDREN'S TYLENOL®
acetaminophen Suspension Liquid and Meltaways

JR. TYLENOL®
acetaminophen Meltaways

Product information for all dosages of Children's TYLENOL have been combined under this heading

Description

Concentrated TYLENOL® Infants' Drops are stable, alcohol-free, grape-flavored and purple in color, cherry-flavored and red in color or dye-free cherry flavored. Each 0.8 mL contains 80 mg acetaminophen. *Concentrated TYLENOL® Infants' Drops* features the SAFE-TY-LOCK™ Bottle. The SAFE-TY-LOCK™ Bottle has a unique safety barrier inside the bottle which helps make administration easier. The integrated dropper promotes proper administration. The innovative design eliminates excess product on dropper. The star-shaped barrier inside the bottle minimizes spills and discourages pouring into a spoon. *Children's TYLENOL® Suspension Liquid* is stable, alcohol-free, cherry blast-flavored and red in color, bubble-gum yum-flavored and pink in color, grape splash-flavored and purple in color, or very berry strawberry-flavored and red in color. Each 5 mL (one teaspoonful) contains 160 mg

acetaminophen. Each *Children's TYLENOL® Meltaways* contains 80 mg acetaminophen in a grape punch or bubble-gum burst flavor. Each *Jr. TYLENOL® Meltaways* contains 160 mg acetaminophen in grape punch or bubblegum burst flavor.

Actions

Acetaminophen is a clinically proven analgesic/antipyretic. Acetaminophen is thought to produce analgesia by elevation of the pain threshold and antipyresis through action on the hypothalamic heat-regulating center. Acetaminophen is equal to aspirin in analgesic and antipyretic effectiveness and it is unlikely to produce many of the side effects associated with aspirin and aspirin-containing products.

IMPORTANT NOTICE: Updated drug information is sent bi-monthly via the PDR® Update Insert. For *monthly* email updates, register at PDR.net.

Children's Tylenol® Dosing Chart (continued)

Attention: use only enclosed dosing device specifically designed for use with this product. Do not use any other dosing device.

AGE GROUP		0–3 mos*	4–11 mos*	12–23 mos*	2–3 yrs	4–5 yrs	6–8 yrs	9–10 yrs	11 yrs	12 yrs	
WEIGHT		6–11 lbs*	12–17 lbs*	18–23 lbs*	24–35 lbs	36–47 lbs	48–59 lbs	60–71 lbs	72–95 lbs	96 lbs and over	
PRODUCT FORM	**INGREDIENTS**	• shake well before using • find right dose on chart below. If possible, use weight to dose; otherwise, use age. • Dose to be administered based on weight or age • If needed, repeat dose every 4 hours								Maximum Doses/24 hrs
							mL = milliliter; tsp = teaspoonful				
Children's Tylenol Plus Cold Suspension	Acetaminophen 160 mg Chlorpheniramine maleate 1 mg Phenylephrine HCl 2.5 mg	Do not use			Do not use unless directed by a doctor		10 mL (2 tsp)	10 mL (2 tsp)	10 mL (2 tsp)	—	5 times in 24 hrs
Children's Tablets	**Per tablet**										
Children's Tylenol Meltaway Tablets	Acetaminophen 80 mg (in each tablet)	Ask a doctor			2 tablets	3 tablets	4 tablets	5 tablets	6 tablets	—	5 times in 24 hrs
Junior Tylenol Meltaway Tablets	Acetaminophen 160 mg (in each tablet)	Ask a doctor			1 tablets**	1½ tablets**	2 tablets	2½ tablets	3 tablets	4 tablets	5 times in 24 hrs

* Ask a doctor for children under 2 years or under 24 lb.
**Ask a doctor for children under 6 years or under 48 lb.

Uses
Concentrated TYLENOL® Infants' Drops: temporarily:
• reduces fever
• relieves minor aches and pains due to: • the common cold • flu • headache • sore throat • toothache
Children's TYLENOL® Suspension Liquid and Children's TYLENOL® Meltaways: temporarily relieves minor aches and pains due to: • the common cold • flu • headache • sore throat • toothache • temporarily reduces fever
Jr. TYLENOL® Meltaways: temporarily relieves minor aches and pains due to:
• the common cold • flu • headache
• temporarily reduces fever

Directions
• this product does not contain directions or complete warnings for adult use
See Table 1: Children's Tylenol Dosing Chart on pg. 1908

Warnings
Liver warning: This product contains acetaminophen. Severe liver damage may occur if your child takes
• more than 5 doses in 24 hours, which is the maximum daily amount
• with other drugs containing acetaminophen
Sore throat warning: if sore throat is severe, persists for more than 2 days, is accompanied or followed by fever, headache, rash, nausea, or vomiting, consult a doctor promptly (excluding *Jr. TYLENOL® Meltaways*).
Ask a doctor before use if your child has liver disease
Ask a doctor or pharmacist before use if you child is taking the blood thinning drug warfarin
When using this product do not exceed recommended dose (see overdose warning)
Stop use and ask a doctor if
• pain gets worse or lasts more than 5 days
• fever gets worse or lasts more than 3 days
• new symptoms occur
• redness or swelling is present
These could be signs of a serious condition
Keep out of reach of children.
Do not use
• with any other drug containing acetaminophen (prescription or nonprescription). If you are not sure whether a drug contains acetaminophen, ask a doctor or pharmacist.
• if your child is allergic to acetaminophen or any of the inactive ingredients in this product.
Overdose warning: Taking more than the recommended dose (overdose) may cause liver damage. In case of overdose, get medical help or contact a Poison Control Center right away. (1-800-222-1222) Quick medical attention is critical for adults as well as for children even if you do not notice any signs or symptoms.
Other Information:
Concentrated TYLENOL® Infants' Drops:
• store between 20–25°C (68–77°F)

Children's TYLENOL® Suspension Liquid:
• each teaspoon contains: **sodium 2mg** (excludes Dye-Free Cherry)
• store between 20–25°C (68–77°F)
Children's TYLENOL® Meltaways:
• store between 20–25°C (68–77°F). Avoid high humidity. (Grape Punch: Protect from light.)
Jr. TYLENOL® Meltaways:
• store between 20–25°C (68–77°F). Avoid high humidity. (Grape Punch: Protect from light.)

PROFESSIONAL INFORMATION:
OVERDOSAGE INFORMATION for all Infants', Children's & Jr. Tylenol® Products
Acetaminophen:
Acetaminophen in massive overdosage may cause hepatic toxicity in some patients. In adults and adolescents (≥ 12 years of age), hepatic toxicity may occur following ingestion of greater than 7.5 to 10 grams over a period of 8 hours or less. Fatalities are infrequent (less than 3–4% of untreated cases) and have rarely been reported with overdoses of less than 15 grams. In children (<12 years of age), an acute overdosage of less than 150 mg/kg has not been associated with hepatic toxicity. Early symptoms following a potentially hepatotoxic overdose may include: nausea, vomiting, diaphoresis and general malaise. Clinical and laboratory evidence of hepatic toxicity may not be apparent until 48 to 72 hours postingestion. In adults and adolescents, any individual presenting with an unknown amount of acetaminophen ingested or with a questionable or unreliable history about the time of ingestion should have a plasma acetaminophen level drawn and be treated with N-acetylcysteine. For full prescribing information, refer to the N-acetylcysteine package insert. Do not await results of assays for plasma acetaminophen levels before initiating treatment with N-acetylcysteine. The following additional procedures are recommended: Promptly initiate gastric decontamination of the stomach. A plasma acetaminophen assay should be obtained as early as possible, but no sooner than four hours following ingestion. If an acetaminophen *extended release* product is involved, it may be appropriate to obtain an additional plasma acetaminophen level 4–6 hours following the initial acetaminophen level. If either acetaminophen level plots above the treatment line on the acetaminophen overdose nomogram, N-acetylcysteine treatment should be initiated and continued for a full course of therapy. Liver function studies should be obtained initially and repeated at 24-hour intervals. Serious toxicity or fatalities have been extremely infrequent following an acute acetaminophen overdose in young children, possibly because of differences in the way they metabolize acetaminophen. In children, the maximum potential amount ingested can be more easily estimated. If more than 150 mg/kg or an unknown amount was ingested, obtain a plasma acetaminophen level as soon as possible, but no sooner than 4 hours following ingestion. If an acetaminophen *extended release* product is involved, it may be appropriate to obtain an additional plasma acetaminophen

level 4–6 hours following the initial acetaminophen level. If either acetaminophen level plots above the treatment line on the acetaminophen overdose nomogram, N-acetylcysteine treatment should be initiated and continued for a full course of therapy. If an assay cannot be obtained and the estimated acetaminophen ingestion exceeds 150 mg/kg, dosing with N-acetylcysteine should be initiated and continued for a full course of therapy. For additional emergency information, call your regional poison center or call the Rocky Mountain Poison Center toll-free, (1-800-525-6115).
Our pediatric Tylenol® combination products contain active ingredients in addition to acetaminophen. The following is basic overdose information regarding those ingredients.
Chlorpheniramine: Chlorpheniramine toxicity should be treated as you would an antihistamine/anticholinergic overdose and is likely to be present within a few hours after acute ingestion.
Dextromethorphan: Acute dextromethorphan overdose usually does not result in serious signs and symptoms unless massive amounts have been ingested. Signs and symptoms of a substantial overdose may include nausea and vomiting, visual disturbances, CNS disturbances and urinary retention.
Diphenhydramine: Diphenhydramine toxicity should be treated as you would an antihistamine/anticholinergic overdose and is likely to be present within a few hours after acute ingestion.
Phenylephrine: Symptoms from phenylephrine overdose most often consist of hypertension, anxiety, nervousness, restlessness, tachycardia, bradycardia, headache, dizziness and/or palpitations. Symptoms usually are transient and typically require no treatment.
For additional emergency information, please contact your local poison control center.

Inactive Ingredients:
Concentrated TYLENOL® Infants' Drops: Cherry-anhydrous citric acid, FD&C red #40, flavors, glycerin, high fructose corn syrup, microcrystalline cellulose and carboxymethylcellulose sodium, purified water, sodium benzoate, sorbitol solution, xanthan gum Grape-anhydrous citric acid, D&C red #33, FD&C blue #1, flavors, glycerin, high fructose corn syrup, microcrystalline cellulose and carboxymethylcellulose sodium, purified water, sodium benzoate, sorbitol solution, xanthan gum
Cherry (Dye-Free) Flavored: anhydrous citric acid, butylparaben, flavors, glycerin, microcrystalline cellulose and carboxymethylcellulose sodium, propylene glycol, propylparaben, purified water, sorbitol solution, sucralose, xanthan gum
Children's TYLENOL® Suspension Liquids
Cherry Blast-anhydrous citric acid, butylparaben, FD&C red #40, flavors, glycerin, high fructose corn syrup, microcrystalline cellulose and carboxymethylcellulose sodium, propylene glycol, purified water, sodium benzoate, sorbitol solution, sucralose, xanthan gum

Bubble Gum-anhydrous citric acid, butylparaben, D&C Red #33, FD&C Red #40, flavors, glycerin, high fructose corn syrup, microcrystalline cellulose and carboxymethyl cellulose sodium, propylene glycol, purified water, sodium benzoate, sorbitol solution, sucralose, xanthan gum

Grape-anhydrous citric acid, butylparaben, D&C Red #33, FD&C Blue #1, flavors, glycerin, high fructose corn syrup, microcrystalline cellulose and carboxymethyl cellulose sodium, propylene glycol, purified water, sodium benzoate, sorbitol solution, sucralose, xanthan gum

Strawberry-anhydrous citric acid, butylparaben, FD&C red #40, flavors, glycerin, high fructose corn syrup, microcrystalline cellulose and carboxymethylcellulose sodium, propylene glycol, purified water, sodium benzoate, sorbitol solution, sucralose, xanthan gum

Cherry (Dye-Free) Flavored: anhydrous citric syrup, butylparaben, flavors, glycerin, microcrystalline cellulose and carboxymethylcellulose sodium, propylene glycol, propylparaben, purified water, sorbitol solution, sucralose, sucrose xanthan gum

Children's Tylenol Meltaways
Grape-Punch-Flavored: cellulose acetate, citric acid, crospovidone, dextrose, D&C red #7, D&C red #30, FD&C blue #1, flavors, magnesium stearate, povidone, sucralose.
Ch. Ty. Meltaway BB Burst-anhydrous citric acid, cellulose acetate, crospovidone, D&C red #7 calcium lake, dextrose excipient, flavor, magnesium stearate povidone, sucralose
Jr. TYLENOL® Meltaways Bubblegum Burst Flavored: anhydrous citric acid, cellulose acetate, crospovidone, D&C red #7 calcium lake, dextrose, flavors, magnesium stearate, povidone, sucralose.

How Supplied
Concentrated TYLENOL® Infants' Drops: (purple-colored grape): bottles of ½ oz (15 mL) and 1 oz (30 mL); (red-colored cherry): bottles of ½ oz and 1 oz, and dye-free cherry each with calibrated plastic dropper.
Children's TYLENOL® Suspension Liquid: (red-colored cherry blast): bottles of 2 and 4 fl oz. (pink-colored bubblegum yum, purple-colored grape splash, red-colored very berry strawberry and dye-free cherry): bottles of 4 fl. oz.
Children's TYLENOL® Meltaways: (purple-colored grape punch, pink-colored bubblegum burst, scored, imprinted "TY80"). Bottles of 30 and also blister packaged 48's and 64's.
Jr. TYLENOL® Meltaways: (pink-colored bubblegum burst, imprinted "TY 160"). Blister packaged 24's and 48's. All packages listed above are safety sealed and use child-resistant safety caps or blisters.

CHILDREN'S TYLENOL® Dosing Chart   OTC

[Note:] If possible, use weight to dose, otherwise use age. To arrive at the correct dose, weigh your child before giving TYLENOL®.
[A healthcare professional should be consulted for dosing in children under the age of two years.]
[See table on pages 1908 and 1909]
• Keep all medicines out of the reach of children
• Do NOT administer adult medicines to children
Important Instructions for Proper Use
• **Read and follow the label instructions on all TYLENOL® products**
  —Take every 4 hours as needed
  —Do not exceed more than 5 doses in 24 hours
  —Do not administer for longer than 5 days unless directed by doctor
• **Do NOT use with any other product containing acetaminophen**
• **Use only the dosing device that comes with a specific product**
• Concentrated TYLENOL® Infants' Drops are more concentrated than Children's TYLENOL® Liquids. The Concentrated Infants' Drops have been specifically designed for use with the enclosed dropper.
• Children's TYLENOL® Liquids are less concentrated than Concentrated TYLENOL® Infants' Drops. The Children's TYLENOL® Liquids have been specifically designed for use with enclosed measuring cup.
• Children's TYLENOL® Meltaway Tablets are not the same concentration as Jr. Strength TYLENOL® Meltaway Tablets. Jr. TYLENOL® Meltaway Tablets contain 160 mg of acetaminophen while Children's TYLENOL® Meltaway Tablets contain 80 mg of acetaminophen
• **If you have any questions, contact your healthcare professional or call 1-877-895-3665**

EXTRA STRENGTH TYLENOL® PM   OTC
Acetaminophen, Diphenhydramine HCl
Pain Reliever Nighttime Sleep Aid
Caplets

Drug Facts

Active ingredients (in each caplet)   **Purpose**
Acetaminophen 500 mg .... Pain reliever
Diphenhydramine HCl 25 mg .... Nighttime sleep aid

Uses
temporary relief of occasional headaches and minor aches and pains with accompanying sleeplessness

Warnings
Liver warning: This product contains acetaminophen. Severe liver damage may occur if you take
• more than 4,000 mg of acetaminophen in 24 hours
• with other drugs containing acetaminophen
• 3 or more alcoholic drinks every day while using this product
Do not use
• with any other drug containing acetaminophen (prescription or nonprescription). If you are not sure whether a drug contains acetaminophen, ask a doctor or pharmacist.
• with any product containing diphenhydramine, even one used on skin
• in children under 12 years of age
• if you have ever had an allergic reaction to this product or any of its ingredients
Ask a doctor before use if you have
• liver disease
• a breathing problem such as emphysema or chronic bronchitis
• trouble urinating due to an enlarged prostate gland
• glaucoma
Ask a doctor or pharmacist before use if you are
• taking the blood thinning drug warfarin
• taking sedatives or tranquilizers
When using this product
• drowsiness will occur
• avoid alcoholic drinks
• do not drive a motor vehicle or operate machinery
Stop use and ask a doctor if
• sleeplessness persists continuously for more than 2 weeks.
  Insomnia may be a symptom of serious underlying medical illness.
• pain gets worse or lasts more than 10 days
• fever gets worse or lasts more than 3 days
• redness or swelling is present
• new symptoms occur
These could be signs of a serious condition.
If pregnant or breast-feeding, ask a health professional before use.
Keep out of reach of children.
Overdose warning: Taking more than the recommended dose (overdose) may cause liver damage. In case of overdose, get medical help or contact a Poison Control Center right away. (1-800-222-1222) Quick medical attention is critical for adults as well as for children even if you do not notice any signs or symptoms.

Directions
• do not take more than directed (see overdose warning)

adults and children 12 years and over	• take 2 caplets at bedtime • do not take more than 2 caplets of this product in 24 hours
children under 12 years	do not use this adult product in children under 12 years of age, this will provide more than the recommended dose (overdose) and may cause liver damage

Other information
• store between 20-25°C (68-77°F)
• **do not use if carton is opened or neck wrap or foil inner seal imprinted with "SafetySeal®" is broken**
• see end panel for lot number and expiration date
Inactive ingredients
carnauba wax, FD&C blue #1 aluminum lake, FD&C blue #2 aluminum lake, hypromellose, magnesium stearate, polyethylene glycol, polysorbate 80, powdered cellulose, pregelatinized starch, propylene glycol, shellac, sodium citrate, sodium starch glycolate, titanium dioxide
Questions or comments? call 1-877-895-3665

You can feel good knowing TYLENOL PM is a pain reliever & nighttime sleep aid that is non-habit forming when used as directed.
For more information or questions, visit our website www.tylenol.com.

REGULAR STRENGTH TYLENOL®   OTC
acetaminophen Tablets
EXTRA STRENGTH TYLENOL®
acetaminophen Caplets and EZ Tabs
EXTRA STRENGTH TYLENOL®
acetaminophen Rapid Release Gels
EXTRA STRENGTH TYLENOL®
acetaminophen Adult Rapid Blast Liquid
TYLENOL® Arthritis Pain Acetaminophen
extended release Gelcaps/Caplets
TYLENOL® 8 Hour Acetaminophen
extended release Caplets

Product information for all dosage forms of Adult TYLENOL acetaminophen have been combined under this heading.

Description
Each Regular Strength TYLENOL® Tablet contains acetaminophen 325 mg. Each Extra Strength TYLENOL® Caplet, EZ Tab, or Rapid Release Gel contains acetaminophen 500 mg. Extra Strength TYLENOL® Adult Liquid is alcohol-free and each 15 mL (1 tablespoonful) contains 500 mg acetaminophen. Each TYLENOL® Arthritis Pain extended release Gelcaps/Caplet and each TYLENOL® 8 Hour extended release Caplet contains acetaminophen 650 mg.

Actions
Acetaminophen is a clinically proven analgesic/antipyretic. Acetaminophen is thought to produce analgesia by elevation of the pain threshold and antipyresis through action on the hypothalamic heat-regulating center. Acetaminophen is equal to aspirin in analgesic and antipyretic effectiveness and it is unlikely to produce many of the side effects associated with aspirin and aspirin-containing products. *Tylenol Arthritis Pain extended release* and *TYLENOL 8 Hour extended release* use a bilayer geltab/caplet. The first layer dissolves quickly while the second layer is time released to provide up to 8 hours of relief.

Uses
Regular Strength Tylenol Tablets; Extra Strength Tylenol Caplets, Rapid Release Gels, Cool Caplets, EZ tabs; Tylenol Adult Liquid; Tylenol 8 Hour extended release Caplets: temporarily relieves minor aches and pains due to:
• the common cold • headache • backache
• minor pain of arthritis • toothache
• muscular aches • premenstrual and menstrual cramps
• temporarily reduces fever
TYLENOL® Arthritis Pain extended release Caplets: temporarily relieves minor aches and pains due to:
• arthritis • the common cold • headache • toothache
• muscular aches • backache • menstrual cramps
• temporarily reduces fever
TYLENOL® Arthritis Pain extended release Gelcaps: temporarily relieves minor aches and pains due to:
• minor pain of arthritis • muscular aches • backache
• premenstrual and menstrual cramps • the common cold • headache • toothache
• temporarily reduces fever

Directions
Regular Strength TYLENOL® Tablets:
• do not take more than directed (see overdose warning)

adults and children 12 years and over	• take 2 tablets every 4 to 6 hours while symptoms last • do not take more than 12 tablets in 24 hours • do not use for more than 10 days unless directed by a doctor
children 6–11 years	• take 1 tablet every 4 to 6 hours while symptoms last • do not take more than 5 tablets in 24 hours • do not use for more than 5 days unless directed by a doctor
children under 6 years	• do not use this adult product in children under 6 years of age; this will provide more than the recommended dose (overdose) and may cause liver damage

Extra Strength TYLENOL® Caplets, EZ Tabs, or Rapid Release Gels:
• do not take more than directed (see overdose warning)

adults and children 12 years and over	• take 2 tablets, gelcaps, or caplets every 4 to 6 hours while symptoms last • do not take more than 8 tablets, gelcaps, or caplets in 24 hours • do not use for more than 10 days unless directed by a doctor
children under 12 years	do not use this adult product in children under 12 years of age; this will provide more than the recommended dose (overdose) and may cause liver damage

Extra Strength TYLENOL® Adult Liquid:
• do not take more than directed (see overdose warning)
• use only enclosed dosing cup designed for use with this product. Do not use any other dosing device.

adults and children 12 years and over	• take 2 tablespoons (tbsp.) or 1 oz in dose cup provided every 4 to 6 hours while symptoms last • do not take more than 8 tablespoons (tbsp) or 4 oz in 24 hours • do not take for more than 10 days unless directed by a doctor
children under 12 years	do not use this adult product in children under 12 years of age; this will provide more than the recommended dose (overdose) and may cause liver damage

TYLENOL® 8 Hour extended release Caplets
• do not take more than directed (see overdose warning)

adults and children 12 years and over	• take 2 caplets every 8 hours with water • swallow whole – do not crush, chew split or dissolve • do not take more than 6 caplets in 24 hours • do not use for more than 10 days unless directed by a doctor
children under 12 years	• do not use

TYLENOL® Arthritis Pain extended release Gelcaps/Caplets
• do not take more than directed (see overdose warning)

adults	• take 2 gelcaps or caplets every 8 hours with water. • Swallow only one gelcap at a time. (Gelcaps only) • take a sip of water before swallowing each geltab and wash each geltab down with water (up to a full 8 oz glass) (gelcaps only) • swallow whole – do not crush, chew split or dissolve • do not take more than 6 gelcaps or caplets in 24 hours • do not use for more than 10 days unless directed by a doctor
under 18 years of age	• ask a doctor

Warnings
Regular Strength Tylenol
Liver warning: This product contains acetaminophen. Severe liver damage may occur if
• adult takes more than 12 tablets in 24 hours, which is the maximum daily amount

• child takes more than 5 doses in 24 hours, which is the maximum daily amount
• taken with other drugs containing acetaminophen
• adult has 3 or more alcoholic drinks every day while using this product
Do not use
• with any other drug containing acetaminophen (prescription or nonprescription). If you are not sure whether a drug contains acetaminophen, ask a doctor or pharmacist.
• if you are allergic to acetaminophen or any of the inactive ingredients in this product.
Ask a doctor before use if the user has liver disease
Ask a doctor or pharmacist before use if the user is taking the blood thinning drug warfarin
Extra Strength Tylenol
Liver warning: This product contains acetaminophen. Severe liver damage may occur if you take
• more than 8 tablets, caplets, gelcaps or tablespoons in 24 hours, which is the maximum daily amount
• with other drugs containing acetaminophen
• 3 or more alcoholic drinks every day while using this product
Do not use
• with any other drug containing acetaminophen (prescription or nonprescription). If you are not sure whether a drug contains acetaminophen, ask a doctor or pharmacist.
• if you are allergic to acetaminophen or any of the inactive ingredients in this product.
Ask a doctor before use if you have liver disease
Ask a doctor or pharmacist before use if you are taking the blood thinning drug warfarin
Tylenol Arthritis Pain and Tylenol 8 Hour
Liver warning: This product contains acetaminophen. Severe liver damage may occur if you take
• more than 6 caplets or gelcaps in 24 hours, which is the maximum daily amount
• with other drugs containing acetaminophen
• 3 or more alcoholic drinks every day while using this product
Do not use
• with any other drug containing acetaminophen (prescription or nonprescription). If you are not sure whether a drug contains acetaminophen, ask a doctor or pharmacist.
• if you have difficulty swallowing large tablets or capsules. People over 65 may have difficulty swallowing these tablets.
• if you are allergic to acetaminophen or any of the inactive ingredients in this product.
Ask a doctor before use if you have liver disease
Ask a doctor or pharmacist before use if you are taking the blood thinning drug warfarin
Stop use and ask a doctor if:
• the tablet got stuck in your throat (Gelcaps only)
• pain gets worse or lasts more than 10 days
• fever gets worse or lasts more than 3 days
• new symptoms occur
• redness or swelling is present
These could be signs of a serious condition.
If pregnant or breast-feeding, ask a health professional before use.
Keep out of reach of children.
Overdose warning: Taking more than the recommended dose (overdose) may cause liver damage. In case of overdose, get medical help or contact a Poison Control Center right away. (1-800-222-1222) Quick medical attention is critical for adults as well as for children even if you do not notice any signs or symptoms.
Other information:
Regular Strength TYLENOL® Tablets
• store between 20–25°C (68–77°F)
Extra Strength TYLENOL® Caplets, EZ Tabs, or Rapid Release Gels:
• store between 20–25°C (68–77°F) (Caplet and EZ Tabs)
• store between 20–25°C (68–77°F). Avoid high humidity. (Rapid Release Gel)
Extra Strength TYLENOL® Adult Liquid
• each tablespoon contains: **sodium 9 mg**
• store between 20–25°C (68–77°F)
TYLENOL® Arthritis Pain extended release Gelcaps/Caplets and TYLENOL® 8 Hour extended release Caplets
• store at 20–25°C (68–77°F)
• avoid excessive heat 40°C (104°F)

Professional Information:
Overdosage information for all adult TYLENOL products
Acetaminophen: Acetaminophen in massive overdosage may cause hepatic toxicity in some patients. In adults and adolescents (≥ 12 years of age), hepatic toxicity may occur following ingestion of greater than 7.5 to 10 grams over a period of 8 hours or less. Fatalities are infrequent (less than 3–4% of untreated cases) and have rarely been reported

with overdoses of less than 15 grams. In children (<12 years of age), an acute overdosage of less than 150 mg/kg has not been associated with hepatic toxicity. Early symptoms following a potentially hepatotoxic overdose may include: nausea, vomiting, diaphoresis and general malaise. Clinical and laboratory evidence of hepatic toxicity may not be apparent until 48 to 72 hours postingestion. In adults and adolescents, any individual presenting with an unknown amount of acetaminophen ingested or with a questionable or unreliable history about the time of ingestion should have a plasma acetaminophen level drawn and be treated with N-acetylcysteine. For full prescribing information, refer to the N-acetylcysteine package insert. Do not await results of assays for plasma acetaminophen levels before initiating treatment with N-acetylcysteine. The following additional procedures are recommended: Promptly initiate gastric decontamination of the stomach. A plasma acetaminophen assay should be obtained as early as possible, but no sooner than four hours following ingestion. If an acetaminophen *extended release* product is involved, it may be appropriate to obtain an additional plasma acetaminophen level 4–6 hours following the initial acetaminophen level. If either acetaminophen level plots above the treatment line on the acetaminophen overdose nomogram, N-acetylcysteine treatment should be continued for a full course of therapy. Liver function studies should be obtained initially and repeated at 24-hour intervals. Serious toxicity or fatalities have been extremely infrequent following an acute acetaminophen overdose in young children, possibly because of differences in the way they metabolize acetaminophen. In children, the maximum potential amount ingested can be more easily estimated. If more than 150 mg/kg or an unknown amount was ingested, obtain a plasma acetaminophen level as soon as possible, but no sooner than 4 hours following ingestion. If an acetaminophen *extended release* product is involved, it may be appropriate to obtain an additional plasma acetaminophen level 4–6 hours following the initial acetaminophen level. If either acetaminophen level plots above the treatment line on the acetaminophen overdose nomogram, N-acetylcysteine treatment should be initiated and continued for a full course of therapy. If an assay cannot be obtained and the estimated acetaminophen ingestion exceeds 150 mg/kg, dosing with N-acetylcysteine should be initiated and continued for a full course of therapy. For additional emergency information, call your regional poison center or call the Rocky Mountain Poison Center toll-free, (1-800-525-6115).
Our adult Tylenol® combination products contain active ingredients in addition to acetaminophen. The following is basic overdose information regarding those ingredients.
Chlorpheniramine: Chlorpheniramine toxicity should be treated as you would an antihistamine/anticholinergic overdose and is likely to be present within a few hours after acute ingestion.
Dextromethorphan: Acute dextromethorphan overdose usually does not result in serious signs and symptoms unless massive amounts have been ingested. Signs and symptoms of a substantial overdose may include nausea and vomiting, visual disturbances, CNS disturbances and urinary retention.
Diphenhydramine: Diphenhydramine toxicity should be treated as you would an antihistamine/anticholinergic overdose and is likely to be present within a few hours after acute ingestion.
Doxylamine: Doxylamine toxicity should be treated as you would an antihistamine/anticholinergic overdose and is likely to be present within a few hours after acute ingestion.
Guaifenesin: Guaifenesin should be treated as a nontoxic ingestion.
Phenylephrine: Symptoms from phenylephrine overdose most often consist of hypertension, anxiety, nervousness, restlessness, tachycardia, bradycardia, headache, dizziness, and/or palpitations. Symptoms usually are transient and typically require no treatment.
Pseudoephedrine: Symptoms from pseudoephedrine overdose consist most often of mild anxiety, tachycardia and/or mild hypertension. Symptoms usually appear within 4 to 8 hours of ingestion and are transient, usually requiring no treatment.
For additional emergency information, please contact your local poison control center.
Alcohol Information: Chronic heavy alcohol abusers may be at increased risk of liver toxicity from excessive acetaminophen use, although reports of this event are rare. Reports usually involve cases of severe chronic alcoholics and the dosages of acetaminophen most often exceed recommended doses and often involve substantial overdose. Healthcare professionals should alert their patients who regularly consume large amounts of alcohol not to exceed recommended doses of acetaminophen.

Inactive ingredients:

Regular Strength TYLENOL® Tablets: cellulose, corn starch, magnesium stearate, sodium starch glycolate.

Extra Strength TYLENOL® Caplets: carnauba wax*, castor oil*, corn starch, FD&C red #40 aluminum lake, hypromellose, magnesium stearate, polyethylene glycol*, powdered cellulose, pregelatinized starch, propylene glycol, shellac, sodium starch glycolate, titanium dioxide. *contains one or more of these ingredients. **Cool Caplets:** castor oil, cellulose, corn starch, FD&C red #40, flavors, hypromellose, magnesium stearate, sodium starch glycolate, sucralose, titanium dioxide. **EZ Tabs:** anhydrous citric acid, carnauba wax, corn starch, D&C yellow #10 aluminum lake, FD&C red #40 aluminium lake, FD&C yellow #6 aluminum lake, iron oxide, magnesium stearate polyethylene glycol, polyvinyl alcohol, potassium sorbate, powdered cellulose, pregelatinized starch, propylene glycol, shellac, sodium benzoate, sodium citrate, sodium starch glycolate, sucralose, talc, titanium dioxide. **Rapid Release Gels:** benzyl alcohol, butylparaben, carboxymethylcellulose sodium, corn starch, D&C yellow #10, edetate calcium disodium, FD&C blue #1, FD&C red #40, gelatin, hypromellose, iron oxide, magnesium stearate, methylparaben, polyethylene glycol, polysorbate 80, powdered cellulose, pregelatinized starch, propylene glycol propylparaben, red iron oxide, sodium lauryl sulfate, sodium propionate, sodium starch glycolate, titanium dioxide, yellow iron oxide.

Extra Strength TYLENOL® Adult Liquid: citric acid, corn syrup, D&C red #33, FD&C red #40, flavor, polyethylene glycol, propylene glycol, purified water, saccharin sodium, sodium benzoate, sorbitol

TYLENOL® Arthritis Pain extended release **Caplets:** carnauba wax, corn starch, hydroxyethyl cellulose, hypromellose, magnesium stearate, microcrystalline cellulose, povidone, powdered cellulose, pregelatinized starch, sodium starch glycolate, titanium dioxide, triacetin. **Gelcaps:** benzyl alcohol butylparaben, castor oil, corn starch, edetate calcium disodium, FD&C blue #1 aluminum lake, FD&C blue #2 aluminum lake, gelatin, hydroxyethyl cellulose, hypromellose, magnesium stearate, microcrystalline cellulose, povidone, powdered cellulose, pregelatinized starch, shellac, sodium lauryl sulfate, sodium propionate, sodium starch glycolate, titanium dioxide.

Tylenol 8 Hour extended release **Caplets:** corn starch, D&C yellow #10 aluminum lake, FD&C red #40 aluminum lake, FD&C yellow #6 aluminum lake, hydroxyethyl cellulose, magnesium stearate, microcrystalline cellulose, polyethylene glycol, polyvinyl alcohol, povidone, powdered cellulose, pregelantinized starch, sodium starch glycolate, sucralose, talc, titanium dioxide.

How Supplied

Regular Strength TYLENOL® Tablets: (colored white, scored, imprinted "TYLENOL" and "325")—tamper-evident bottles of 100.

Extra Strength TYLENOL® Caplets: (colored white, imprinted "TYLENOL 500 mg")—vials of 10, and tamper-evident bottles of 24, 50, 100, 150, 225, and 325. *Cool Caplets* 8, 24, 50, 100, 150. *Rapid Release Gels* (colored red and light blue with an exposed grey band; gelcaps are imprinted with "TY 500") tamper-evident bottles of 8, 24, 50, 100, 150, 225, and 290. *EZ Tabs* (colored red, imprinted "tylenol EZ Tabs") tamper-evident bottles of 24, 50, 100, and 225.

Extra Strength TYLENOL® Adult Rapid Blast Liquid: Cherry-flavored liquid (colored red) 8 fl. oz. tamper-evident bottle with child resistant safety cap and special dosage cup.

TYLENOL® Arthritis Pain extended release Caplets: (colored white, engraved "TYLENOL ER") tamper-evident bottles of 24, 50, 100, 150, 225 and 290

Gelcaps: available in bottles of 20, 40 and 80

TYLENOL® 8 Hour extended release Caplets: (colored red, imprinted "8 HOUR") available in 24's, 50's, 100's, and 150's.

ZYRTEC® ALLERGY Tablets and Liquid Gels   OTC

Active ingredient (in each tablet/capsule)	Purpose
Cetirizine HCl 10 mg	Antihistamine

Uses

temporarily relieves these symptoms due to hay fever or other upper respiratory allergies:
• runny nose • sneezing • itchy, watery eyes • itching of the nose or throat

Warnings

Do not use if you have ever had an allergic reaction to this product or any of its ingredients or to an antihistamine containing hydroxyzine.

Ask a doctor before use if you have liver or kidney disease. Your doctor should determine if you need a different dose.

Ask a doctor or pharmacist before use if you are taking tranquilizers or sedatives.

When using this product
• drowsiness may occur
• avoid alcoholic drinks
• alcohol, sedatives, and tranquilizers may increase drowsiness
• be careful when driving a motor vehicle or operating machinery

Stop use and ask a doctor if an allergic reaction to this product occurs. Seek medical help right away.

If pregnant or breast-feeding:
• if breast-feeding: not recommended
• if pregnant: ask a health professional before use.

Keep out of reach of children. In case of overdose, get medical help or contact a Poison Control Center right away. (1-800-222-1222)

Directions

adults and children 6 years and over	one 10 mg tablet/capsule once daily; do not take more than one 10 mg tablet/capsule in 24 hours. A 5 mg product may be appropriate for less severe symptoms.
adults 65 years and over	ask a doctor
children under 6 years of age	ask a doctor
consumers with liver or kidney disease	ask a doctor

Other information
• store between 20° to 25°C (68° to 77°F)
Liquid gels only
• avoid high humidity and excessive heat above 40°C (104°F)
• protect from light

Zyrtec tablet Inactive Ingredients colloidal silicon dioxide, croscarmellose sodium, hypromellose, lactose monohydrate, magnesium stearate, microcrystalline cellulose, polyethylene glycol, titanium dioxide or carnauba wax, corn starch, hypromellose, lactose monohydrate, magnesium stearate, polyethylene glycol, povidone, titanium dioxide.

Zyrtec liquid gel Inactive Ingredients gelatin, glycerin, mannitol, pharmaceutical ink, polyethylene glycol 400, purified water, sodium hydroxide, sorbitan, sorbitol

How Supplied

Zyrtec® Allergy Tablets are white, film-coated, rounded off rectangular shaped tablets—bottles of 5, 14, 30, 45, 75. Zyrtec® Liquid Gels—bottles of 12, 25, 40, 60.

CHILDREN'S ZYRTEC® ALLERGY SYRUP   OTC
1 mg/mL oral solution

Active ingredient (in each 5 mL teaspoonful)	Purpose
Cetirizine HCl 5 mg	Antihistamine

Uses

temporarily relieves these symptoms due to hay fever or other upper respiratory allergies:
■ runny nose ■ sneezing ■ itchy, watery eyes ■ itching of the nose or throat

Warnings

Do not use if you have ever had an allergic reaction to this product or any of its ingredients or to an antihistamine containing hydroxyzine.

Ask a doctor before use if you have liver or kidney disease. Your doctor should determine if you need a different dose.

Ask a doctor or pharmacist before use if you are taking tranquilizers or sedatives.

When using this product
■ drowsiness may occur
■ avoid alcoholic drinks
■ alcohol, sedatives, and tranquilizers may increase drowsiness
■ be careful when driving a motor vehicle or operating machinery

Stop use and ask a doctor if an allergic reaction to this product occurs. Seek medical help right away.

If pregnant or breast-feeding:
■ if breast-feeding: not recommended
■ if pregnant: ask a health professional before use.

Keep out of reach of children. In case of overdose, get medical help or contact a Poison Control Center right away. (1-800-222-1222)

Directions
■ use only with enclosed dosing cup

adults and children 6 years and over	1 teaspoonful (5 mL) or 2 teaspoonfuls (10 mL) once daily depending upon severity of symptoms; do not take more than 2 teaspoonfuls (10 mL) in 24 hours.
adults 65 years and over	1 teaspoonful (5 mL) once daily; do not take more than 1 teaspoonful (5 mL) in 24 hours.
children 2 to under 6 years of age	1/2 teaspoonful (2.5 mL) once daily. If needed, dose can be increased to a maximum of 1 teaspoonful (5 mL) once daily or 1/2 teaspoonful (2.5 mL) every 12 hours. Do not give more than 1 teaspoonful (5 mL) in 24 hours.
children under 2 years of age	ask a doctor
consumers with liver or kidney disease	ask a doctor

Other information
■ store between 20° to 25°C (68° to 77°F)
Inactive ingredients
Bubble Gum flavor (dye-free, sugar-free) — anhydrous citric acid, flavors, propylene glycol, purified water, sodium benzoate, sorbitol solution, sucralose
Grape flavor (dye-free, sugar-free) — anhydrous citric acid, flavors, propylene glycol, purified water, sodium benzoate, sorbitol solution, sucralose
Grape flavor — flavors, glacial acetic acid, glycerin, methylparaben, propylene glycol, propylparaben, purified water, sodium acetate, sodium hydroxide, sugar

HOW SUPPLIED

Children's Zyrtec Allergy Syrup: grape flavored bottles of 4 Fl oz (118mL)

ZYRTEC® ITCHY EYE DROPS   OTC

The ingredients and uses of this product are different than other ZYRTEC® products.

Active ingredient	Purpose
Ketotifen (0.025%)	Antihistamine
(equivalent to ketotifen fumarate 0.035%)	

Use

Temporarily relieves itchy eyes due to pollen, ragweed, grass, animal hair and dander.

Warnings

Do not use
• if solution changes color or becomes cloudy
• if you are sensitive to any ingredient in this product
• to treat contact lens related irritation

When using this product
• do not touch tip of container to any surface to avoid contamination
• remove contact lenses before use
• wait at least 10 minutes before reinserting contact lenses after use
• replace cap after each use

Stop use and ask a doctor if you experience any of the following:
• eye pain
• changes in vision
• redness of the eye
• itching worsens or lasts for more than 72 hours

Keep out of reach of children
If swallowed, get medical help or contact a Poison Control Center right away. (1-800-222-1222)

Directions
• **Adults and children 3 years of age and older:** Put 1 drop in the affected eye(s) twice daily, every 8-12 hours, no more than twice per day.
• **Children under 3 years of age:** Consult a doctor.

Other information
- Only for use in the eye.
- Store at 20°–25°C (68°–77°F) [See USP Controlled Room Temperature].

Inactive ingredients benzalkonium chloride 0.01%, glycerol, sodium hydroxide and/or hydrochloric acid and water for injection.

ZYRTEC-D® Allergy & Congestion   OTC
Extended Release Tablets

Active ingredients   **Purpose**
(in each extended release tablet)
Cetirizine HCl 5 mg .... Antihistamine
Pseudoephedrine HCl 120 mg .... Nasal decongestant

Uses
■ temporarily relieves these symptoms due to hay fever or other upper respiratory allergies:
  ■ runny nose ■ sneezing
  ■ itchy, watery eyes ■ itching of the nose or throat
  ■ nasal congestion
■ reduces swelling of nasal passages
■ temporarily relieves sinus congestion and pressure
■ temporarily restores freer breathing through the nose

Warnings
Do not use
■ if you have ever had an allergic reaction to this product or any of its ingredients or to an antihistamine containing hydroxyzine.
■ if you are now taking a prescription monoamine oxidase inhibitor (MAOI) (certain drugs for depression, psychiatric or emotional conditions, or Parkinson's disease), or for 2 weeks after stopping the MAOI drug. If you do not know if your prescription drug contains an MAOI, ask a doctor or pharmacist before taking this product.
Ask a doctor before use if you have
■ heart disease
■ thyroid disease
■ diabetes
■ glaucoma
■ high blood pressure
■ trouble urinating due to an enlarged prostate gland
■ liver or kidney disease. Your doctor should determine if you need a different dose.
Ask a doctor or pharmacist before use if you are taking tranquilizers or sedatives.
When using this product
■ **do not use more than directed**
■ drowsiness may occur
■ avoid alcoholic drinks
■ alcohol, sedatives, and tranquilizers may increase drowsiness
■ be careful when driving a motor vehicle or operating machinery
Stop use and ask a doctor if
■ an allergic reaction to this product occurs. Seek medical help right away.
■ you get nervous, dizzy, or sleepless
■ symptoms do not improve within 7 days or are accompanied by fever
If pregnant or breast-feeding:
■ if breast-feeding: not recommended
■ if pregnant: ask a health professional before use.
Keep out of reach of children. In case of overdose, get medical help or contact a Poison Control Center right away. (1-800-222-1222)

Directions
■ do not break or chew tablet; swallow tablet whole

adults and children 12 years and over	take 1 tablet every 12 hours; do not take more than 2 tablets in 24 hours
adults 65 years and over	ask a doctor
children under 12 years of age	ask a doctor
consumers with liver or kidney disease	ask a doctor

Other information
■ store between 20° to 25°C (68° to 77°F)
Inactive ingredients
colloidal silicon dioxide, croscarmellose sodium, hypromellose, lactose monohydrate, magnesium stearate, microcrystalline cellulose, polyethylene glycol, titanium dioxide

How Supplied
Zyrtec D® Allergy & Congestion Tablets are white, round, bilayer tablets - in blister packs of 12 and 24

Medicis Pharmaceutical Corporation
**7720 N. DOBSON ROAD
SCOTTSDALE, AZ 85256**

For updates to the product information listed, please visit: www.Medicis.com
For Medical Information Contact:
Phone: (602) 808-8800
FAX: (602) 808-0822

DYSPORT™   ℞
[*DIS-port*]
**(abobotulinumtoxinA)
For Injection**

HIGHLIGHTS OF PRESCRIBING INFORMATION
These highlights do not include all the information needed to use DYSPORT™ for Injection safely and effectively. See full prescribing information for DYSPORT™ for Injection.
**DYSPORT™ for Injection
(abobotulinumtoxinA)
Initial U.S. Approval: April 2009**

> **Distant Spread of Toxin Effect**
> **The effects of DYSPORT™ and all botulinum toxin products may spread from the area of injection to produce symptoms consistent with botulinum toxin effects. These symptoms have been reported hours to weeks after injection. Swallowing and breathing difficulties can be life threatening and there have been reports of death. The risk of symptoms is probably greatest in children treated for spasticity but symptoms can also occur in adults, particularly in those patients who have underlying conditions that would predispose them to these symptoms.**

——INDICATIONS AND USAGE——
DYSPORT™ is an acetylcholine release inhibitor and a neuromuscular blocking agent indicated for:
- the treatment of adults with cervical dystonia to reduce the severity of abnormal head position and neck pain in both toxin-naïve and previously treated patients (1.1)
- the temporary improvement in the appearance of moderate to severe glabellar lines associated with procerus and corrugator muscle activity in adult patients <65 years of age (1.2)

——DOSAGE AND ADMINISTRATION——
- Once reconstituted, DYSPORT™ should be stored in the original container in a refrigerator (2–8°C) and used within four hours (16)
- ~~Do not freeze after reconstitution (2), (16)~~
- Protect from light (16)
- Reconstitution instructions are specific for the 300 Unit and 500 Unit vials

Cervical Dystonia (2.1)
- Initial dose of DYSPORT™ is 500 Units given intramuscularly as a divided dose among the affected muscles
- Re-treatment every 12 to 16 weeks or longer, as necessary, based on return of clinical symptoms with doses administered between 250 and 1000 Units to optimize clinical benefit
- Re-treatment should not occur in intervals of less than 12 weeks
- Titration should occur in 250 Unit steps according to the patient's response

Glabellar Lines (2.2)
- A total dose of 50 Units of DYSPORT,™ divided in five equal aliquots of 10 Units each, should be administered to affected muscles to achieve clinical effect
- Re-treatment with DYSPORT™ should be administered no more frequently than every 3 months

——DOSAGE FORMS AND STRENGTHS——
- Cervical dystonia: Single-use, sterile 500 Unit vial for reconstitution with 1 mL of 0.9 % Sodium Chloride Injection USP (without preservative) and a single-use, sterile 300 Unit vial for reconstitution with 0.6 mL of 0.9% Sodium Chloride Injection USP (without preservative) (3.1)
- Glabellar lines: Single-use, sterile 300 Unit vial for reconstitution with 2.5 mL or 1.5 mL of 0.9% Sodium Chloride Injection USP (without preservative) (3.2)

——CONTRAINDICATIONS——
- Hypersensitivity to any botulinum toxin product or excipients (4), (6.1), (6.2)
- Allergy to cow's milk protein (4)
- Infection at the proposed injection site(s) (4)

——WARNINGS AND PRECAUTIONS——
- **The potency Units of DYSPORT™ are not interchangeable with other preparations of botulinum toxin products**

and, therefore, units of biological activity of DYSPORT™ cannot be compared to or converted into units of any other botulinum toxin products (11)
- Recommended dose and frequency of administration should not be exceeded (5.1)
- Immediate medical attention may be required in cases of respiratory, speech or swallowing difficulties (5.3)
- Caution should be exercised when administering DYSPORT™ to patients with surgical alterations to the facial anatomy, marked facial asymmetry, inflammation at the injection site(s), ptosis, excessive dermatochalasis, deep dermal scarring, or thick sebaceous skin (5.4)
- Concomitant neuromuscular disorder may exacerbate clinical effects of treatment (5.5)
- DYSPORT™ contains human albumin. Based on effective donor screening and product manufacturing processes, DYSPORT™ carries an extremely remote risk for transmission of viral diseases. A theoretical risk for transmission of Creutzfeldt-Jakob disease (CJD) also is considered extremely remote. No cases of transmission of viral diseases or CJD have ever been identified for albumin (5.6)
- The possibility of an immune reaction when injected intradermally is unknown. The safety of DYSPORT™ for the treatment of hyperhidrosis has not been established (5.7)

——ADVERSE REACTIONS——
Cervical Dystonia
Most commonly observed adverse reactions (>5% of patients) are: muscular weakness, dysphagia, dry mouth, injection site discomfort, fatigue, headache, neck pain, musculoskeletal pain, dysphonia, injection site pain, and eye disorders. (6)
Glabellar Lines
The most frequently reported adverse events (≥2%) are nasopharyngitis, headache, injection site pain, injection site reaction, upper respiratory tract infection, eyelid edema, eyelid ptosis, sinusitis and nausea. (6)
To report SUSPECTED ADVERSE REACTIONS, contact 877-397-7671 or FDA at 1-800-FDA-1088 or www.fda.gov/medwatch

——DRUG INTERACTIONS——
- Patients receiving concomitant treatment of DYSPORT™ and aminoglycosides or other agents interfering with neuromuscular transmission (e.g., curare-like agents), or muscle relaxants, should be observed closely because the effect of botulinum toxin may be potentiated (7)
- Use of anticholinergic drugs may potentiate systemic anticholinergic effects (7)
- The effect of administering different botulinum neurotoxins during the course of treatment with DYSPORT™ is unknown (7)

——USE IN SPECIFIC POPULATIONS——
- Pregnancy: Based on animal data, may cause fetal harm (8.1)
- Care should be exercised when administering DYSPORT™ in elderly patients, reflecting the greater frequency of concomitant disease and other drug therapy (8.5)

See 17 for PATIENT COUNSELING INFORMATION and Medication Guide

Revised: 05/2009

*** Sections or subsections omitted from the full prescribing information are not listed**

FULL PRESCRIBING INFORMATION

DISTANT SPREAD OF TOXIN EFFECT

Postmarketing reports indicate that the effects of DYSPORT™ and all botulinum toxin products may spread from the area of injection to produce symptoms consistent with botulinum toxin effects. These may include asthenia, generalized muscle weakness, diplopia, blurred vision, ptosis, dysphagia, dysphonia, dysarthria, urinary incontinence and breathing difficulties. These symptoms have been reported hours to weeks after injection. Swallowing and breathing difficulties can be life threatening and there have been reports of death. The risk of symptoms is probably greatest in children treated for spasticity but symptoms can also occur in adults treated for spasticity and other conditions, particularly in those patients who have underlying conditions that would predispose them to these symptoms. In unapproved uses, including spasticity in children and adults, and in approved indications, cases of spread of effect have been reported at doses comparable to those used to treat cervical dystonia and at lower doses.

1 INDICATIONS AND USAGE

1.1 Cervical Dystonia

DYSPORT™ (abobotulinumtoxinA) is an acetylcholine release inhibitor and a neuromuscular blocking agent indicated for the treatment of adults with cervical dystonia to reduce the severity of abnormal head position and neck pain in both toxin-naïve and previously treated patients.

1.2 Glabellar Lines

DYSPORT™ (abobotulinumtoxinA) is an acetylcholine release inhibitor and a neuromuscular blocking agent indicated for the temporary improvement in the appearance of moderate to severe glabellar lines associated with procerus and corrugator muscle activity in adult patients <65 years of age.

2 DOSAGE AND ADMINISTRATION

The potency Units of DYSPORT™ are specific to the preparation and assay method utilized. They are not interchangeable with other preparations of botulinum toxin products and, therefore, units of biological activity of DYSPORT™ cannot be compared to or converted into units of any other botulinum toxin products assessed with any other specific assay method [*see Description (11)*].

Reconstitution instructions are specific for each of the 300 Unit vial and the 500 Unit vial. These volumes yield concentrations specific for the use for each indication.

2.1 Cervical Dystonia

The recommended initial dose of DYSPORT™ for the treatment of cervical dystonia is 500 Units given intramuscularly as a divided dose among affected muscles in patients with or without a history of prior treatment with botulinum toxin. (A description of the average DYSPORT™ dose and percentage of total dose injected into specific muscles in the pivotal clinical trials can be found in Table 5 of Section 14.1, Clinical Studies—Cervical Dystonia.) Limiting the dose injected into the sternocleidomastoid muscle may reduce the occurrence of dysphagia. Clinical studies with DYSPORT™ in cervical dystonia suggest that the peak effect occurs between two and four weeks after injection. Simultaneous EMG-guided application of DYSPORT™ may be helpful in locating active muscles not identified by physical examination alone.

Dose Modification

Where dose modification is necessary for the treatment of cervical dystonia, uncontrolled open-label studies suggest that dose adjustment can be made in 250 Unit steps according to the individual patient's response, with re-treatment every 12 weeks or longer, as necessary, based on return of clinical symptoms. Uncontrolled open-label studies also suggest that the total dose administered in a single treatment should be between 250 Units and 1000 Units. Re-treatment, if needed, should not occur in intervals of less than 12 weeks. Doses above 1000 Units have not been systematically evaluated.

2.1.1 Special Populations

Adults and elderly

The starting dose of 500 Units recommended for cervical dystonia is applicable to adults of all ages [*see Use in Specific Populations (8.5)*].

Children

The safety and effectiveness of DYSPORT™ in the treatment of cervical dystonia in children below 18 years of age has not been assessed [*see Warnings and Precautions (5.2)*].

2.1.2 Instructions for Preparation and Administration

DYSPORT™ is supplied as a single-use vial. Each 500 Unit vial of DYSPORT™ is to be reconstituted with 1 mL of 0.9% Sodium Chloride Injection USP (without preservative) to yield a solution of 500 Units per mL. Each 300 Unit vial of DYSPORT™ is to be reconstituted with 0.6 mL of 0.9% Sodium Chloride Injection USP (without preservative) to yield a solution equivalent to 250 Units per 0.5 mL. Swirl gently to dissolve.

Parenteral drug products should be inspected visually for particulate matter and discoloration prior to administration, whenever solution and container permit. Reconstituted DYSPORT™ should be clear, colorless, and free of particulate matter, otherwise it must not be injected.

A sterile 23 or 25 gauge needle should be used for administration. Administer DYSPORT™ within 4 hours of reconstitution; during this period reconstituted DYSPORT™ should be stored under refrigeration at 2–8°C (36–46°F) and protected from light. Do not freeze after reconstitution. Discard any remaining solution after injection.

2.2 Glabellar Lines

The dose of DYSPORT™ for the treatment of glabellar lines is a total of 50 Units given intramuscularly in five equal aliquots of 10 Units each to achieve clinical effect *(see Figure 1)*.

2.2.1 Special Populations

Adults

A total dose of 50 Units of DYSPORT,™ in five equal aliquots, should be administered to achieve clinical effect.

The clinical effect of DYSPORT™ may last up to four months. Repeat dose clinical studies demonstrated continued efficacy with up to four repeated administrations. It should be administered no more frequently than every three months. When used for re-treatment, DYSPORT™ should be reconstituted and injected using the same techniques as the initial treatment.

Children

DYSPORT™ for glabellar lines is not recommended for use in pediatric patients less than 18 years of age [*see Warnings and Precautions (5.2)*].

2.2.2 Instructions for Preparation and Administration

DYSPORT™ is supplied as a single-use vial. Each 300 Unit vial of DYSPORT™ is to be reconstituted with 2.5 mL of 0.9% sterile, preservative-free, saline prior to injection. The concentration of the resulting solution will be 10 Units per 0.08 mL to be delivered in five equally divided aliquots of 0.08 mL each. DYSPORT™ may also be reconstituted with 1.5 mL 0.9% sterile, preservative-free, saline for a solution of 10 Units per 0.05 mL to be delivered in five equally divided aliquots of 0.05 mL each.

Using a 21 gauge needle and aseptic technique, draw up 2.5 mL or 1.5 mL of sterile, preservative-free 0.9% saline. Insert the needle into the DYSPORT™ vial at a 45° angle and allow the saline diluent to be pulled into the vial by partial vacuum. Discard the vial if the partial vacuum has been lost. Gently rotate the vial (do not shake), until the white substance is fully dissolved. Reconstituted DYSPORT™ should be a clear, colorless solution, free of particulate matter.

Draw a single patient dose of DYSPORT™ into a sterile syringe. Expel any air bubbles in the syringe barrel. Remove the needle used to reconstitute the product and attach a 30 gauge needle.

Once reconstituted, DYSPORT™ should be stored in a refrigerator at 2–8°C (36–46°F) protected from light and used within four hours. Do not freeze reconstituted DYSPORT.™ Discard the vial and needle in accordance with local regulations.

2.2.3 Injection Technique

Glabellar facial lines arise from the activity of the lateral corrugator and vertical procerus muscles. These can be readily identified by palpating the tensed muscle mass while having the patient frown. The corrugator depresses the skin creating a "furrowed" vertical line surrounded by tensed muscle (i.e., frown lines). The location, size, and use of the muscles vary markedly among individuals. Physicians administering DYSPORT™ must understand the relevant neuromuscular and/or orbital anatomy of the area involved and any alterations to the anatomy due to prior surgical procedures.

Risk of ptosis can be mitigated by careful examination of the upper lid for separation or weakness of the levator palpebrae muscle (true ptosis), identification of lash ptosis, and evaluation of the range of lid excursion while manually depressing the frontalis to assess compensation.

In order to reduce the complication of ptosis, the following steps should be taken:

- Avoid injection near the levator palpebrae superioris, particularly in patients with larger brow depressor complexes.
- Medial corrugator injections should be placed at least 1 centimeter above the bony supraorbital ridge.
- Ensure the injected volume/dose is accurate and where feasible kept to a minimum.
- Do not inject toxin closer than 1 centimeter above the central eyebrow.

To inject DYSPORT,™ advance the needle through the skin into the underlying muscle while applying finger pressure on the superior medial orbital rim. Inject patients with a total of 50 Units in five equally divided aliquots. Using a 30 gauge needle, inject 10 Units of DYSPORT™ into each of five sites, two in each corrugator muscle, and one in the procerus muscle *(see Figure 1)*.

Figure 1

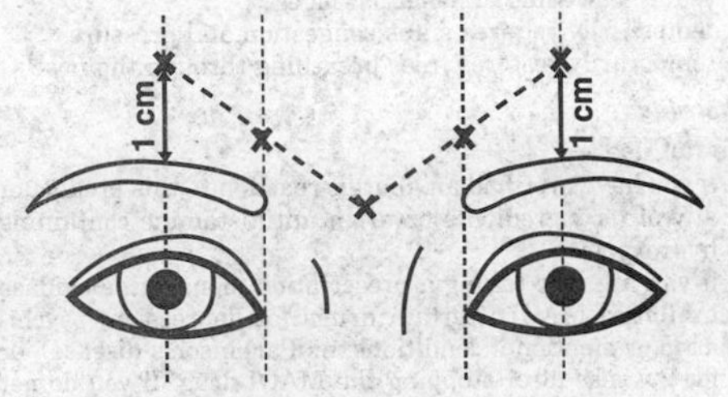

3 DOSAGE FORMS AND STRENGTHS

3.1 Cervical Dystonia

DYSPORT™ is supplied as:

- a single-use, sterile 500 Unit vial for reconstitution with 1 mL of 0.9% Sodium Chloride Injection USP (without preservative) to yield a solution of 500 Units per mL.
- a single-use, sterile 300 Unit vial for reconstitution with 0.6 mL of 0.9% Sodium Chloride Injection USP (without preservative) to yield a solution equivalent to 250 Units per 0.5 mL.

3.2 Glabellar Lines

DYSPORT™ is supplied in a single-use, sterile 300 Unit vial for reconstitution with 0.9% Sodium Chloride Injection USP (without preservative). DYSPORT™ may be reconstituted with either 2.5 mL to yield a solution of 10 Units per 0.08 mL or with 1.5 mL to yield a solution of 10 Units per 0.05 mL.

4 CONTRAINDICATIONS

DYSPORT™ is contraindicated in patients with known hypersensitivity to any botulinum toxin preparation or to any of the components in the formulation [*see Adverse Reactions (6.1), Description (11)*].

This product may contain trace amounts of cow's milk protein. Patients known to be allergic to cow's milk protein should not be treated with DYSPORT.™

DYSPORT™ is contraindicated for use in patients with infection at the proposed injection site(s).

5 WARNINGS AND PRECAUTIONS

5.1 Lack of Interchangeability between Botulinum Toxin Products

The potency Units of DYSPORT™ are specific to the preparation and assay method utilized. They are not interchangeable with other preparations of botulinum toxin products and, therefore, units of biological activity of DYSPORT™ cannot be compared to or converted into units of any other botulinum toxin products assessed with any other specific assay method [*see Description (11)*].

5.2 Spread of Toxin Effect

Post-marketing safety data from DYSPORT™ and other approved botulinum toxins suggest that botulinum toxin effects may, in some cases, be observed beyond the site of local injection. The symptoms are consistent with the mechanism of action of botulinum toxin and may include asthenia, generalized muscle weakness, diplopia, blurred vision, ptosis, dysphagia, dysphonia, dysarthria, urinary incontinence and breathing difficulties. These symptoms have been reported hours to weeks after injection. Swallowing and breathing difficulties can be life threatening and there have been reports of death related to spread of toxin effects. The risk of the symptoms is probably greatest in children treated for spasticity but symptoms can also occur in adults treated for spasticity and other conditions, and particularly in those patients who have underlying conditions that would predispose them to these symptoms. In unapproved uses, including spasticity in children and adults, and in approved indications, symptoms consistent with spread of toxin effect have been reported at doses comparable to or lower than doses used to treat cervical dystonia.

5.3 Dysphagia and Breathing Difficulties in Treatment of Cervical Dystonia

Treatment with DYSPORT™ and other botulinum toxin products can result in swallowing or breathing difficulties. Patients with pre-existing swallowing or breathing difficulties may be more susceptible to these complications. In most cases, this is a consequence of weakening of muscles in the area of injection that are involved in breathing or swallowing. When distant effects occur, additional respiratory muscles may be involved [see Warnings and Precautions (5.2)].

Deaths as a complication of severe dysphagia have been reported after treatment with botulinum toxin. Dysphagia may persist for several weeks, and require use of a feeding tube to maintain adequate nutrition and hydration. Aspiration may result from severe dysphagia and is a particular risk when treating patients in whom swallowing or respiratory function is already compromised.

Treatment of cervical dystonia with botulinum toxins may weaken neck muscles that serve as accessory muscles of ventilation. This may result in a critical loss of breathing capacity in patients with respiratory disorders who may have become dependent upon these accessory muscles. There have been post-marketing reports of serious breathing difficulties, including respiratory failure, in cervical dystonia patients.

Patients treated with botulinum toxin may require immediate medical attention should they develop problems with swallowing, speech or respiratory disorders. These reactions can occur within hours to weeks after injection with botulinum toxin [see Warnings and Precautions (5.2), Adverse Reactions (6.1), Clinical Pharmacology (12.2)].

5.4 Facial Anatomy in the Treatment of Glabellar Lines

Caution should be exercised when administering DYSPORT™ to patients with surgical alterations to the facial anatomy, excessive weakness or atrophy in the target muscle(s), marked facial asymmetry, inflammation at the injection site(s), ptosis, excessive dermatochalasis, deep dermal scarring, thick sebaceous skin [see Dosage and Administration (2.2.3)] or the inability to substantially lessen glabellar lines by physically spreading them apart [see Clinical Studies (14.2)].

Do not exceed the recommended dosage and frequency of administration of DYSPORT.™ In clinical trials, subjects who received a higher dose of DYSPORT™ had an increased incidence of eyelid ptosis.

5.5 Pre-existing Neuromuscular Disorders

Individuals with peripheral motor neuropathic diseases, amyotrophic lateral sclerosis or neuromuscular junction disorders (e.g., myasthenia gravis or Lambert-Eaton syndrome) should be monitored particularly closely when given botulinum toxin. Patients with neuromuscular disorders may be at increased risk of clinically significant effects including severe dysphagia and respiratory compromise from typical doses of DYSPORT™ [see Adverse Reactions (6.1)].

5.6 Human Albumin

This product contains albumin, a derivative of human blood. Based on effective donor screening and product manufacturing processes, it carries an extremely remote risk for transmission of viral diseases. A theoretical risk for transmission of Creutzfeldt-Jakob disease (CJD) is also considered extremely remote. No cases of transmission of viral diseases or CJD have ever been reported for albumin.

5.7 Intradermal Immune Reaction

The possibility of an immune reaction when injected intradermally is unknown. The safety of DYSPORT™ for the treatment of hyperhidrosis has not been established.

6 ADVERSE REACTIONS

The following adverse reactions to DYSPORT™ are discussed in greater detail in other sections of the labeling.

- Hypersensitivity [see Contraindications (4)]
- Dysphagia and Breathing Difficulties in Treatment of Cervical Dystonia [see Warnings and Precautions (5.3)]
- Spread of Effects from Toxin [see Warnings and Precautions (5.2)]

6.1 Clinical Studies Experience

Because clinical trials are conducted under widely varying conditions, the adverse reaction rates observed cannot be directly compared to rates in other trials and may not reflect the rates observed in clinical practice. The adverse reaction information from clinical trials does, however, provide a basis for identifying the adverse events that appear to be related to drug use and for approximating incidence rates.

Cervical Dystonia

The data described below reflect exposure to DYSPORT™ in 357 cervical dystonia patients in 6 studies. Of these, two studies were randomized, double-blind, single treatment, placebo controlled studies with subsequent optional open label treatment in which dose optimization (250 to 1000 Units per treatment) over the course of 5 treatment cycles was allowed.

Table 2: Common TEAEs by Dose in Fixed-dose Study

System Organ Class Preferred Term	DYSPORT™ Dose			
	Placebo	250 Units	500 Units	1000 Units
Any Adverse Event	30%	37%	65%	83%
Dysphagia	5%	21%	29%	39%
Dry Mouth	10%	21%	18%	39%
Muscular Weakness	0%	11%	12%	56%
Injection Site Discomfort	10%	5%	18%	22%
Dysphonia	0%	0%	18%	28%
Facial Paresis	0%	5%	0%	11%
Eye Disorders	0%	0%	6%	17%

The population was almost entirely Caucasian (99.2%) with a median age of 51 years (range 18–82 years). Most patients (86.6%) were less than 65 years of age; 58.4% were women.

Common Adverse Events

The most commonly reported adverse events (occurring in more than 5% of patients who received 500 Units of DYSPORT™ in the placebo controlled clinical trials) in cervical dystonia patients were muscular weakness, dysphagia, dry mouth, injection site discomfort, fatigue, headache, neck pain, musculoskeletal pain, dysphonia, injection site pain, and eye disorders (consisting of blurred vision, diplopia, and reduced visual acuity and accommodation). Most adverse events were reported as mild or moderate in severity. Other than injection site reactions, most adverse events became noticeable about one week after treatment and lasted several weeks.

The rates of adverse events were higher in the combined controlled and open-label experience than in the placebo-controlled trials.

During the clinical studies, two patients (<1%) experienced adverse events leading to withdrawal. One patient experienced disturbance in attention, eyelid disorder, feeling abnormal and headache, and one patient experienced dysphagia.

Table 1 compares the incidence of the most frequent treatment-emergent adverse events (TEAEs) from a single treatment cycle of 500 Units of DYSPORT™ compared to placebo [see Clinical Studies (14.1)].

Table 1: Most Common TEAEs (>5%) and Greater than Placebo: Double-blind Phase of Clinical Trials

System Organ Class Preferred Term	Double-blind Phase	
	DYSPORT™ 500 Units (N=173)	Placebo (N=182)
	%	%
Any TEAE	61	51
General disorders and administration site conditions	30	23
Injection site discomfort	13	8
Fatigue	12	10
Injection site pain	5	4
Musculoskeletal and connective tissue disorders	30	18
Muscular weakness	16	4
Musculoskeletal pain	7	3
Gastrointestinal disorders	28	15
Dysphagia	15	4
Dry mouth	13	7
Nervous system disorders	16	13
Headache	11	9
Infections and infestations	13	9
Respiratory, thoracic and mediastinal disorders	12	8

Dysphonia	6	2
Eye Disorders*	7	2

* The following preferred terms were reported: vision blurred, diplopia, visual acuity reduced, eye pain, eyelid disorder, accommodation disorder, dry eye, eye pruritus.

Dose-response relationships for common adverse events in a randomized multiple fixed-dose study in which the total dose was divided between two muscles (the sternocleidomastoid and splenius capitis) are shown in Table 2.

[See table 2 above]

Injection Site Reactions

Injection site discomfort and injection site pain were common adverse events following DYSPORT™ administration. These events were mainly of mild or moderate intensity.

Less Common Adverse Events

The following selected adverse events were reported less frequently (<5%).

Breathing Difficulties

Breathing difficulties were reported by approximately 3% of patients following DYSPORT™ administration and in 1% of placebo patients in clinical trials during the double-blind phase. These consisted mainly of dyspnea and were generally mild in intensity. The median time to onset from last dose of DYSPORT™ was approximately one week, and the median duration was approximately three weeks.

Other selected adverse events with incidences of less than 5% in the DYSPORT™ 500 Units group in the double-blind phase of clinical trials included dizziness in 3.5% of DYSPORT™-treated subjects and 1% of placebo-treated subjects, and muscle atrophy in 1% of DYSPORT™-treated subjects and in none of the placebo-treated subjects.

Laboratory Findings

Subjects treated with DYSPORT™ exhibited a small increase from baseline (0.23 mol/L) in mean blood glucose relative to placebo-treated subjects. This was not clinically significant among subjects in the development program but could be a factor in patients whose diabetes is difficult to control.

Electrocardiographic Findings

ECG measurements were only recorded in a limited number of subjects in an open-label study without a placebo or active control. This study showed a statistically significant reduction in heart rate compared to baseline, averaging about three beats per minute, observed thirty minutes after injection.

Glabellar Lines

Because clinical trials are conducted under widely varying conditions, adverse reaction rates observed in the clinical trials of a drug cannot be directly compared to rates in the clinical trials of another drug and may not be predictive of rates observed in practice.

In placebo-controlled clinical trials of DYSPORT,™ the most frequently reported adverse events (≥2%) following injection of DYSPORT™ were nasopharyngitis, headache, injection site pain, injection site reaction, upper respiratory tract infection, eyelid edema, eyelid ptosis, sinusitis and nausea. Table 3 reflects exposure to DYSPORT™ in 398 subjects aged 19 to 75 who were evaluated in the randomized, placebo-controlled clinical studies that assessed the use of DYSPORT™ for the temporary improvement in the appearance of glabellar lines [see Clinical Studies (14)]. Adverse events of any cause were reported for 48% of the DYSPORT™-treated subjects and 33% of the placebo-treated subjects. Treatment-emergent adverse events were generally mild to moderate in severity.

Table 3: Treatment-emergent Adverse Events with >1% incidence

Adverse Events by Body System	DYSPORT™ n=398 (%)*	Placebo n=496 (%)*
Any Treatment-emergent Adverse Event	191 (48)	163 (33)
Eye Disorders		
Eyelid Edema	8 (2)	0
Eyelid Ptosis	6 (2)	1 (<1)
Gastrointestinal Disorders		
Nausea	6 (2)	5 (1)
General Disorders and Administration Site Conditions		
Injection Site Pain	11 (3)	8 (2)
Injection Site Reaction	12 (3)	2 (<1)
Infections and Infestations		
Nasopharyngitis	38 (10)	21 (4)
Upper Respiratory Tract Infection	12 (3)	9 (2)
Sinusitis	8 (2)	6 (1)
Investigations		
Blood Urine Present	6 (2)	1 (<1)
Nervous System Disorders		
Headache	37 (9)	23 (5)

* Subjects who received treatment with placebo and DYSPORT™ are counted in both treatment columns.

In the overall safety database, where some subjects received up to twelve treatments with DYSPORT,™ adverse events were reported for 57% (1425/2491) of subjects. The most frequently reported of these adverse events were headache, nasopharyngitis, injection site pain, sinusitis, URI, injection site bruising, and injection site reaction (numbness, discomfort, erythema, tenderness, tingling, itching, stinging, warmth, irritation, tightness, swelling).

Adverse events that emerged after repeated injections in 2–3% of the population included bronchitis, influenza, pharyngolaryngeal pain, cough, contact dermatitis, injection site swelling, and injection site discomfort.

The incidence of eyelid ptosis did not increase in the long-term safety studies with multiple re-treatments at intervals ≥ three months. The majority of eyelid ptosis events were mild to moderate in severity and resolved over several weeks. [*see Injection Technique (2.2.3)*].

6.2 Post-marketing Spontaneous Reports

There is extensive post-marketing experience outside the U.S. for the treatment of glabellar lines. Adverse reactions are reported voluntarily from a population of uncertain size; thus, it is not always possible to estimate their frequency reliably or to establish a causal relationship to drug exposure. The following adverse reactions have been identified during post-marketing use: vertigo, eyelid ptosis, diplopia, vision blurred, photophobia, dysphagia, nausea, injection site reaction, malaise, influenza-like illness, hypersensitivity, sinusitis, amyotrophy, burning sensation, facial paresis, dizziness, headache, hypoesthesia, erythema, and excessive granulation tissue.

6.3 Immunogenicity

As with all therapeutic proteins, there is a potential for immunogenicity.

The incidence of antibody formation is highly dependent on the sensitivity and specificity of the assay. In addition, the observed incidence of antibody positivity in an assay may be influenced by several factors including assay methodology, sample handling, timing of sample collection, concomitant medications, and underlying disease. For these reasons, comparison of the incidence of antibodies across products in this class may be misleading.

Cervical Dystonia

About 3% of subjects developed antibodies (binding or neutralizing) over time with DYSPORT™ treatment. The significance of these antibodies is unknown since in the presence of binding and neutralizing antibodies some patients may continue to experience clinical benefit.

Glabellar Lines

Testing for antibodies to DYSPORT™ was performed for 1554 subjects who had up to nine cycles of treatment. Two subjects (0.13%) tested positive for binding antibodies at baseline. Three additional subjects tested positive for binding antibodies after receiving DYSPORT™ treatment. None of the subjects tested positive for neutralizing antibodies.

7 DRUG INTERACTIONS

No formal drug interaction studies have been conducted with DYSPORT.™

Patients treated concomitantly with botulinum toxins and aminoglycosides or other agents interfering with neuromuscular transmission (e.g., curare-like agents) should be observed closely because the effect of the botulinum toxin may be potentiated. Use of anticholinergic drugs after administration of DYSPORT™ may potentiate systemic anticholinergic effects such as blurred vision.

The effect of administering different botulinum neurotoxin products at the same time or within several months of each other is unknown. Excessive weakness may be exacerbated by another administration of botulinum toxin prior to the resolution of the effects of a previously administered botulinum toxin.

Excessive weakness may also be exaggerated by administration of a muscle relaxant before or after administration of DYSPORT.™

8 USE IN SPECIFIC POPULATIONS

8.1 Pregnancy

Pregnancy Category C

DYSPORT™ produced embryo-fetal toxicity when given to pregnant rats at doses similar to or greater than the maximum recommended human dose (MRHD) of 1000 Units on a body weight (Units/kg) basis.

In an embryo-fetal development study in which pregnant rats received intramuscular injections daily (2.2, 6.6, or 22 Units/kg on gestation days 6 through 17) or intermittently (44 Units/kg on gestation days 6 and 12 only) during organogenesis, increased early embryonic death was observed with both dosing schedules. The no-effect dose for embryo-fetal developmental toxicity was 2.2 Units/kg (one-tenth the MRHD on a body weight basis). Maternal toxicity was seen at 22 and 44 Units/kg. In a pre- and post-natal development study in which female rats received 6 weekly intramuscular injections (4.4, 11.1, 22.2, or 44 Units/kg) beginning on day 6 of gestation and continuing through parturition to weaning, an increase in stillbirths was observed at the highest dose, which was maternally toxic. The no-effect dose for pre- and post-natal developmental toxicity was 22.2 Units/kg (approximately equal to the MRHD on a body weight basis).

There are no adequate and well-controlled studies in pregnant women. DYSPORT™ should be used during pregnancy only if the potential benefit justifies the potential risk to the fetus.

8.3 Nursing Mothers

It is not known whether DYSPORT™ is excreted in human milk.

8.4 Pediatric Use

Cervical Dystonia

Safety and effectiveness in pediatric patients have not been established [*see Warnings and Precautions (5.2)*].

Glabellar Lines

DYSPORT™ is not recommended for use in pediatric patients less than 18 years of age.

8.5 Geriatric Use

Cervical Dystonia

There were insufficient numbers of patients aged 65 and over in the clinical studies to determine whether they respond differently than younger patients. In general, elderly patients should be observed to evaluate their tolerability of DYSPORT,™ due to the greater frequency of concomitant disease and other drug therapy [*see Dosage and Administration (2.1.1)*].

Glabellar Lines

Of the total number of subjects in the placebo-controlled clinical studies of DYSPORT,™ 8 (1%) were 65 and over. Efficacy was not observed in subjects 65 years and over [*see Clinical Studies (14.2)*]. For the entire safety database of geriatric subjects, although there was no increase in the incidence of eyelid ptosis, geriatric subjects did have an increase in the number of ocular adverse events compared to younger subjects (11% vs. 5%) [*see Dosage and Administration (2.2)*].

8.6 Ethnic Groups

Exploratory analyses in trials for glabellar lines in African-American subjects with Fitzpatrick skin types IV, V, or VI and in Hispanic subjects suggested that response rates at Day 30 were comparable to and no worse than the overall population.

10 OVERDOSAGE

Excessive doses of DYSPORT™ may be expected to produce neuromuscular weakness with a variety of symptoms. Respiratory support may be required where excessive doses cause paralysis of respiratory muscles. In the event of overdose, the patient should be medically monitored for symptoms of excessive muscle weakness or muscle paralysis [*see Warnings and Precautions (5.2)*]. Symptomatic treatment may be necessary.

Symptoms of overdose are likely not to be present immediately following injection. Should accidental injection or oral ingestion occur, the person should be medically supervised for several weeks for signs and symptoms of excessive muscle weakness or paralysis.

There is no significant information regarding overdose from clinical studies in cervical dystonia. Doses exceeding 1000 Units of DYSPORT™ were rarely studied in clinical settings for any indication.

In the event of overdose, antitoxin raised against botulinum toxin is available from the Centers for Disease Control and Prevention (CDC) in Atlanta, GA. However, the antitoxin will not reverse any botulinum toxin-induced effects already apparent by the time of antitoxin administration. In the event of suspected or actual cases of botulinum toxin poisoning, please contact your local or state Health Department to process a request for antitoxin through the CDC. If you do not receive a response within 30 minutes, please contact the CDC directly at 770-488-7100. More information can be obtained at http://www.cdc.gov/ncidod/srp/drugs/drug-service.html.

11 DESCRIPTION

Botulinum toxin type A, the active ingredient in DYSPORT™ (abobotulinumtoxinA), is a purified neurotoxin type A complex produced by fermentation of the bacterium *Clostridium botulinum* type A, Hall Strain. It is purified from the culture supernatant by a series of precipitation, dialysis, and chromatography steps. The neurotoxin complex is composed of the neurotoxin, hemagglutinin proteins and non-toxin non-hemagglutinin protein.

DYSPORT™ is supplied in a single-use, sterile vial for reconstitution intended for intramuscular injection. Each vial contains 500 or 300 Units of lyophilized abobotulinumtoxinA, 125 micrograms human serum albumin and 2.5 mg lactose. DYSPORT™ may contain trace amounts of cow's milk proteins [*see Contraindications (4)*].

One unit of DYSPORT™ corresponds to the calculated median lethal intraperitoneal dose (LD50) in mice. The method for performing the assay is specific to Ipsen's product DYSPORT.™ Due to differences in specific details such as vehicle, dilution scheme and laboratory protocols for various mouse LD50 assays, Units of biological activity of DYSPORT™ are not interchangeable with Units of any other botulinum toxin or any toxin assessed with any other specific assay method [*see Dosage Forms and Strengths (3)*].

12 CLINICAL PHARMACOLOGY

12.1 Mechanism of Action

DYSPORT™ inhibits release of the neurotransmitter, acetylcholine, from peripheral cholinergic nerve endings. Toxin activity occurs in the following sequence: Toxin heavy chain mediated binding to specific surface receptors on nerve endings, internalization of the toxin by receptor mediated endocytosis, pH-induced translocation of the toxin light chain to the cell cytosol and cleavage of SNAP25 leading to intracellular blockage of neurotransmitter exocytosis into the neuromuscular junction. This accounts for the therapeutic utility of the toxin in diseases characterized by excessive efferent activity in motor nerves.

Recovery of transmission occurs gradually as the neuromuscular junction recovers from SNAP25 cleavage and as new nerve endings are formed.

12.2 Pharmacodynamics

The primary pharmacodynamic effect of DYSPORT™ is due to chemical denervation of the treated muscle resulting in a measurable decrease of the compound muscle action potential, causing a localized reduction of muscle activity.

12.3 Pharmacokinetics

Using currently available analytical technology, it is not possible to detect DYSPORT™ in the peripheral blood following intramuscular injection at the recommended doses.

13 NONCLINICAL TOXICOLOGY

13.1 Carcinogenicity, Mutagenicity, Impairment of Fertility

Carcinogenicity

Studies to evaluate the carcinogenic potential of DYSPORT™ have not been conducted.

Mutagenicity

Genotoxicity studies have not been conducted for DYSPORT.™

Impairment of Fertility

In a fertility and early embryonic development study in rats in which either males (2.9, 7.2, 14.5 or 29 Units/kg) or females (7.4, 19.7, 39.4 or 78.8 Units/kg) received weekly intramuscular injections prior to and after mating, dose-related increases in pre-implantation loss and reduced numbers of corpora lutea were noted in treated females. Failure to mate was observed in males that received the high dose. The no-effect dose for effects on fertility was 7.4 Units/kg in females and 14.5 Units/kg in males (approximately one-half and equal to, respectively, the maximum recommended human dose of 1000 Units on a body weight basis).

Table 4: TWSTRS Total Score Efficacy Outcome from the Phase 3 Cervical Dystonia Studies Intent to Treat Population

	Study 1		Study 2	
	DYSPORT™ 500 Units N=55	Placebo N=61	DYSPORT™ 500 Units N=37	Placebo N=43
Baseline (week 0) Mean (SD)	43.8 (8.0)	45.8 (8.9)	45.1 (8.7)	46.2 (9.4)
Week 4 Mean (SD) Change from Baseline*	30.0 (12.7) -15.6 (2.0)	40.2 (11.8) -6.7 (2.0)	35.2 (13.8) -9.6 (2.0)	42.4 (12.2) -3.7 (1.8)
Treatment difference 95% confidence interval	-8.9† [-12.9 to -4.7]		-5.9† [-10.6 to -1.3]	
Week 8 Mean (SD) Change from Baseline*	29.3 (11.0) -14.7 (2.0)	39.6 (13.5) -5.9 (2.0)		
Treatment difference 95% confidence interval	-8.8† [-12.9 to -4.7]			

* Change from baseline is expressed as adjusted least squares mean (SE)
† Significant at *p*-value<0.05

Table 5: DYSPORT™ 500 Unit starting dose (units and % of the total dose) by Unilateral Muscle Injected During Double-blind Pivotal Phase 3 studies 2 and 1 Combined

Number of patients injected per muscle*		DYSPORT™ Dose Injected		Percentage of the total DYSPORT™ Dose Injected	
		Median [DYSPORT™ Units] (min, max)	75th percentile [DYSPORT™ Units]	Median [%] (min, max)	75th percentile [%]
Sternocleidomastoid	90	125 Units (50, 350)	150 Units	26.5% (10, 70)	30.0%
Splenius capitis	85	200 Units (75, 450)	250 Units	40.0% (15, 90)	50.0%
Trapezius	50	102.6 Units (50, 300)	150 Units	20.6% (10, 60)	30.0%
Levator scapulae	35	105.3 Units (50, 200)	125 Units	21.1% (10, 40)	25.0%
Scalenus (medius and anterior)	26	115.5 Units (50, 300)	150 Units	23.1% (10, 60)	30.0%
Semispinalis capitis	21	131.6 Units (50, 250)	175 Units	29.4% (10, 50)	35.0%
Longissimus	3	150 Units (100, 200)	200 Units	30.0% (20, 40)	40.0%

* Total number of patients in combined studies 2 and 1 who received initial treatment=121.

14 CLINICAL STUDIES

14.1 Cervical Dystonia

The efficacy of DYSPORT™ was evaluated in two well-controlled, randomized, double-blind, placebo-controlled, single dose, parallel group studies in treatment-naïve cervical dystonia patients. The principal analyses from these trials provide the primary demonstration of efficacy involving 252 patients (121 on DYSPORT,™ 131 on placebo) with 36% male and 64% female. Ninety-nine percent of the patients were Caucasian.

In both placebo controlled studies (Study 1 and Study 2), a dose of 500 Units DYSPORT™ was given by intramuscular injection divided among two to four affected muscles. These studies were followed by long-term open label extensions that allowed titration in 250 Unit steps to doses in a range of 250 to 1000 Units, after the initial dose of 500 Units. In the extension studies, re-treatment was determined by clinical need after a minimum of 12 weeks. The median time to re-treatment was 14 weeks and 18 weeks for the 75th percentile.

The primary assessment of efficacy was based on the total Toronto Western Spasmodic Torticollis Rating Scale (TWSTRS) change from baseline at Week 4 for both studies. The scale evaluates the severity of dystonia, patient perceived disability from dystonia, and pain. The adjusted mean change from baseline in the TWSTRS total score was statistically significantly greater for the DYSPORT™ group than the placebo group at Weeks 4 in both studies (see Table 4).
[See table 4 above]

Analyses by gender, weight, geographic region, underlying pain, cervical dystonia severity at baseline and history of treatment with botulinum toxin did not show any meaningful differences between groups.
Table 5 indicates the average DYSPORT™ dose, and percentage of total dose, injected into specific muscles in the pivotal clinical trials.
[See table 5 above]

14.2 Glabellar Lines

Three double-blind, randomized, placebo-controlled, clinical studies evaluated the efficacy of DYSPORT™ for use in the temporary improvement of the appearance of moderate to severe glabellar lines. These three studies enrolled healthy adults (ages 19–75) with glabellar lines of at least moderate severity at maximum frown. Subjects were excluded if they had marked ptosis, deep dermal scarring, or a substantial inability to lessen glabellar lines, even by physically spreading them apart. The subjects in these studies received either DYSPORT™ or placebo. The total dose was delivered in equally divided aliquots to specified injection sites (see Figure 1).
Investigators and subjects assessed efficacy at maximum frown by using a 4-point scale (none, mild, moderate, severe).
Overall treatment success was defined as post-treatment glabellar line severity of none or mild with at least 2 grade improvement from Baseline for the combined investigator and subject assessments (composite assessment) on Day 30 (see Table 6). Additional endpoints for each of the studies were post-treatment glabellar line severity of none or mild

with at least a 1 grade improvement from Baseline for the separate investigator and subject assessments on Day 30. After completion of the randomized studies, subjects were offered participation in a two-year, open-label retreatment study to assess the safety of multiple treatments.

Table 6. Treatment Success at Day 30 (None or Mild with at least 2 Grade Improvement from Baseline at Maximum Frown for the combined Investigator and Subject Assessments (Composite))

	2 Grade Improvement	
Study	DYSPORT™ n/N (%)	Placebo n/N (%)
GL-1	58/105 (55%)	0/53 (0%)
GL-2	37/71 (52%)	0/71 (0%)
GL-3	120/200 (60%)	0/100 (0%)

Treatment with DYSPORT™ reduced the severity of glabellar lines for up to four months.

Study GL-1

Study GL-1 was a single dose, double-blind, multi-center, randomized, placebo-controlled study in which 158 previously untreated subjects received either placebo or 50 Units of DYSPORT,™ administered in five aliquots of 10 Units (see Figure 1). Subjects were followed for 180 days. The mean age was 43 years; most of the subjects were women (85%), and predominantly Caucasian (49%) or Hispanic (47%). At Day 30, 55% of DYSPORT™-treated subjects achieved treatment success: a composite 2 grade improvement of glabellar line severity at maximum frown (see Table 6).

In study GL-1, the reduction of glabellar line severity at maximum frown was greater at Day 30 in the DYSPORT™ group compared to the placebo group as assessed by both Investigators and subjects (see Table 7).

Table 7. GL-1: Investigator's and Subject's Assessment of Glabellar Line Severity at Maximum Frown Using a 4-point Scale (% and Number of Subjects with Severity of None or Mild)

	Investigator's Assessment		Subject's Assessment	
Day	DYSPORT™ N=105	Placebo N=53	DYSPORT™ N=105	Placebo N=53
14	90% 95	17% 9	77% 81	9% 5
30	88% 92	4% 2	74% 78	9% 5
60	64% 67	2% 1	60% 63	6% 3
90	43% 45	6% 3	36% 38	6% 3
120	23% 24	4% 2	19% 20	6% 3
150	9% 9	2% 1	8% 8	4% 2
180	6% 6	0% 0	7% 7	8% 4

Study GL-2

Study GL-2 was a repeat dose, double-blind, multi-center, placebo-controlled, randomized study. The study was initiated with two or three open-label treatment cycles of 50 Units of DYSPORT™ administered in five aliquots of 10 Units DYSPORT™ (see Figure 1). After the open-label treatments, subjects were randomized to receive either placebo or 50 Units of DYSPORT.™ Subjects could have received up to four treatments through the course of the study. Efficacy was assessed in the final randomized treatment cycle. The study enrolled 311 subjects into the first treatment cycle and 142 subjects were randomized into the final treatment cycle. Overall, the mean age was 47 years; most of the subjects were women (86%), and predominantly Caucasian (80%).
At Day 30, 52% of DYSPORT™-treated subjects achieved treatment success: a composite 2 grade improvement of glabellar line severity at maximum frown (see Table 6).

The proportion of responders in the final treatment cycle was comparable to the proportion of responders in all prior treatment cycles.

After the final repeat treatment with DYSPORT,™ the reduction of glabellar line severity at maximum frown was greater in the DYSPORT™ group compared to the placebo group as assessed by both Investigators and subjects (see Table 8).

Table 8. GL-2: Investigator's and Subject's Assessments of Glabellar Line Severity at Maximum Frown Using a 4-point Scale (% and Number of Subjects with Severity of None or Mild)

Day	Investigator's Assessment		Subject's Assessment	
	DYSPORT™ N=71	Placebo N=71	DYSPORT™ N=71	Placebo N=71
30	85% 60	4% 3	79% 56	1% 1

Study GL-3

Study GL-3 was a single dose, double-blind, multi-center, randomized, placebo-controlled study in which 300 previously untreated subjects received either placebo or 50 Units of DYSPORT,™ administered in five aliquots of 10 Units (see Figure 1). Subjects were followed for 150 days. The mean age was 44 years; most of the subjects were women (87%), and predominantly Caucasian (75%) or Hispanic (18%).

At Day 30, 60% of DYSPORT™-treated subjects achieved treatment success: a composite 2 grade improvement of glabellar line severity at maximum frown (see Table 6).

In study GL-3, the reduction of glabellar line severity at maximum frown was greater at Day 30 in the DYSPORT™ group compared to the placebo group as assessed by both Investigators and subjects (see Table 9).

Table 9. GL-3: Investigator's and Subject's Assessment of Glabellar Line Severity at Maximum Frown Using a 4-point Scale (% and Number of Subjects with Severity of None or Mild)

Day	Investigator's Assessment		Subject's Assessment	
	DYSPORT™ N=200	Placebo N=100	DYSPORT™ N=200	Placebo N=100
14	83% 166	5% 5	83% 165	2% 2
30	86% 171	0% 0	82% 163	2% 2
60	75% 150	1% 1	65% 130	4% 4
90	51% 102	1% 1	46% 91	2% 2
120	29% 58	1% 1	31% 61	3% 3
150	16% 32	1% 1	16% 31	3% 3

Geriatric Subjects

In GL1, GL2, and GL3, there were 8 subjects aged 65 and older who were randomized to DYSPORT™ 50 Units in 5 equal aliquots of 10 Units (4) or placebo (4). None of the geriatric DYSPORT™ subjects were a treatment success at maximum frown at Day 30.

16   HOW SUPPLIED/STORAGE AND HANDLING

DYSPORT™ for Injection is supplied in a sterile, single-use, 3 mL glass vial. DYSPORT™ must be stored under refrigeration at 2–8°C (36–46°F). Protect from light.

Administer DYSPORT™ within 4 hours of reconstitution; during this period reconstituted DYSPORT™ should be stored under refrigeration at 2–8°C (36–46°F). Do not freeze after reconstitution.

Do not use after the expiration date on the vial. All vials, including expired vials, or equipment used with DYSPORT™ should be disposed of carefully as is done with all medical waste.

Cervical Dystonia
• Each vial contains 500 Units of freeze-dried abobotulinumtoxinA.
• Box containing 1 vial—NDC 15054-0500-1
• Box containing 2 vials—NDC 15054-0500-2

Glabellar Lines
• Each vial contains 300 Units of freeze-dried abobotulinumtoxinA.
• Box containing 1 vial—NDC 99207-500-30

DYSPORT™ contains a unique hologram on the vial label and carton. If you do not see the hologram, do not use the product. Instead contact 877-397-7671 between 7:00 a.m. and 5:00 p.m. Mountain Standard Time, Monday through Friday.

17   PATIENT COUNSELING INFORMATION

The physician should provide a copy of the FDA-Approved Patient Medication Guide and review the contents with the patient. Patients should be advised to inform their doctor or pharmacist if they develop any unusual symptoms (including difficulty with swallowing, speaking or breathing), or if any known symptom persists or worsens.

Patients should be counseled that if loss of strength, muscle weakness, blurred vision or drooping eyelids occur, they should avoid driving a car or engaging in other potentially hazardous activities.

Manufactured by:
Ipsen Biopharm Ltd.
Wrexham, LL13 9UF, UK
Distributed by:
Tercica, Inc.
a subsidiary of the Ipsen Group
Brisbane, CA 94005
and
Medicis Aesthetics Inc.
a wholly owned subsidiary of Medicis Pharmaceutical Corporation
Scottsdale, AZ 85256

MEDICATION GUIDE
DYSPORT™ (DIS-port)
(abobotulinumtoxinA)
Injection

Read the Medication Guide that comes with DYSPORT™ before you start using it and each time DYSPORT™ is given to you. There may be new information. This information does not take the place of talking with your doctor about your medical condition or your treatment. You should share this information with your family members and caregivers.

What is the most important information I should know about DYSPORT™?

DYSPORT™ may cause serious side effects that can be life threatening. Call your doctor or get medical help right away if you have any of these problems after treatment with DYSPORT™:

• **Problems swallowing, speaking, or breathing.** These problems can happen hours to weeks after an injection of DYSPORT™ usually because the muscles that you use to breathe and swallow can become weak after the injection. Death can happen as a complication if you have severe problems with swallowing or breathing after treatment with DYSPORT.™

• People with certain breathing problems may need to use muscles in their neck to help them breathe. These patients may be at greater risk for serious breathing problems with DYSPORT.™

• Swallowing problems may last for several weeks. People who can not swallow well may need a feeding tube to receive food and water. If swallowing problems are severe, food or liquids may go into your lungs. People who already have swallowing or breathing problems before receiving DYSPORT™ have the highest risk of getting these problems.

• **Spread of toxin effects.** In some cases, the effect of botulinum toxin may affect areas of the body away from the injection site and cause symptoms of a serious condition called botulism. The symptoms of botulism include:
• loss of strength and muscle weakness all over the body
• double vision
• blurred vision and drooping eyelids
• hoarseness or change or loss of voice (dysphonia)
• trouble saying words clearly (dysarthria)
• loss of bladder control
• trouble breathing
• trouble swallowing

These symptoms can happen hours to weeks after you receive an injection of DYSPORT.™ These problems could make it unsafe for you to drive a car or do other dangerous activities. See "What should I avoid while receiving DYSPORT™?"

What is DYSPORT™?

DYSPORT™ is a prescription medicine that is injected into muscles and used:
• to treat the abnormal head position and neck pain that happens with cervical dystonia (CD) in adults
• to improve the look of moderate to severe frown lines between the eyebrows (glabellar lines) in adults younger than 65 years of age for a short period of time (temporary)

CD is caused by muscle spasms in the neck. These spasms cause abnormal position of the head and often neck pain. After DYSPORT™ is injected into muscles, those muscles are weakened for up to 12 to 16 weeks or longer. This may help lessen your symptoms.

Frown lines (wrinkles) happen because the muscles that control facial expression are used often (muscle tightening over and over). After DYSPORT™ is injected into the muscles that control facial expression, the medicine stops the tightening of these muscles for up to 4 months.

It is not known whether DYSPORT™ is safe or effective in children under 18 years of age.

It is not known whether DYSPORT™ is safe or effective for the treatment of other types of muscle spasms. It is not known whether DYSPORT™ is safe or effective for the treatment of other wrinkles.

Who should not take DYSPORT™?

Do not take DYSPORT™ if you:
• are allergic to DYSPORT™ or any of the ingredients in DYSPORT.™ See the end of this Medication Guide for a list of ingredients in DYSPORT™
• are allergic to cow's milk protein
• had an allergic reaction to any other botulinum toxin product such as Myobloc®[1] or Botox®[1]
• have a skin infection at the planned injection site

What should I tell my doctor before taking DYSPORT™?

Tell your doctor about all your medical conditions, including if you have:
• a disease that affects your muscles and nerves (such as amyotrophic lateral sclerosis [ALS or Lou Gehrig's disease], myasthenia gravis or Lambert-Eaton syndrome). See "What is the most important information I should know about DYSPORT™?"
• allergies to any botulinum toxin product
• had any side effect from any botulinum toxin product in the past
• a breathing problem, such as asthma or emphysema
• swallowing problems
• bleeding problems
• diabetes
• a slow heart beat or other problem with your heart rate or rhythm
• plans to have surgery
• had surgery on your face
• weakness of your forehead muscles (such as trouble raising your eyebrows)
• drooping eyelids
• any other change in the way your face normally looks

Tell your doctor if you:
• are pregnant or plan to become pregnant. It is not known if DYSPORT™ can harm your unborn baby
• are breast-feeding or planning to breast-feed. It is not known if DYSPORT™ passes into breast milk

Tell your doctor about all the medicines you take, including prescription and nonprescription medicines, vitamins and herbal and other natural products. Using DYSPORT™ with certain other medicines may cause serious side effects. **Do not start any new medicines while taking DYSPORT™ without talking to your doctor first.**

Especially tell your doctor if you:
• have received any other botulinum toxin product in the last four months
• have received injections of botulinum toxin, such as Myobloc® (Botulinum Toxin Type B)[1] or Botox® (Botulinum Toxin Type A)[1] in the past; be sure your doctor knows exactly which product you received
• have recently received an antibiotic by injection
• take muscle relaxants
• take an allergy or cold medicine
• take a sleep medicine

Ask your doctor if you are not sure if your medicine is one that is listed above.

Know the medicines you take. Keep a list of your medicines with you to show your doctor and pharmacist each time you get a new medicine.

How should I take DYSPORT™?
• DYSPORT™ is an injection that your doctor will give you
• DYSPORT™ is injected into the affected muscles
• Your doctor may give you another dose of DYSPORT™ after 12 weeks or longer, if it is needed
• If you are being treated for CD, your doctor may change your dose of DYSPORT,™ until you and your doctor find the best dose for you
• The dose of DYSPORT™ is not the same as the dose of any other botulinum toxin product

What should I avoid while taking DYSPORT™?

DYSPORT™ may cause loss of strength or general muscle weakness, blurred vision, or drooping eyelids within hours to weeks of taking DYSPORT.™ **If this happens, do not** drive a car, operate machinery, or do other dangerous activities. See "What is the most important information I should know about DYSPORT™?"

What are the possible side effects of DYSPORT™?
DYSPORT™ can cause serious side effects. See "What is the most important information I should know about DYSPORT™?"

Other side effects of DYSPORT™ include:
- dry mouth
- injection site discomfort or pain
- tiredness
- headache
- neck pain
- muscle pain
- eye problems: double vision, blurred vision, decreased eyesight, problems with focusing the eyes (accommodation), drooping eyelids, swelling of the eyelids
- allergic reactions. Symptoms of an allergic reaction to DYSPORT™ may include: itching, rash, red itchy welts, wheezing, asthma symptoms, or dizziness or feeling faint. Tell your doctor or get medical help right away if you get wheezing or asthma symptoms, or if you get dizzy or faint

Tell your doctor if you have any side effect that bothers you or that does not go away. These are not all the possible side effects of DYSPORT.™ For more information, ask your doctor or pharmacist.

Call your doctor for medical advice about side effects. You may report side effects to FDA at 1-800-FDA-1088.

General information about DYSPORT™:
Medicines are sometimes prescribed for purposes other than those listed in a Medication Guide.

This Medication Guide summarizes the most important information about DYSPORT.™ If you would like more information, talk with your doctor. You can ask your doctor or pharmacist for information about DYSPORT™ that is written for healthcare professionals. For more information about DYSPORT™ call 877-397-7671 or go to www.dysport.com or www.DysportUSA.com.

What are the ingredients in DYSPORT™?
Active ingredient: (botulinum toxin Type A)
Inactive ingredients: human albumin, and lactose. DYSPORT™ may contain cow's milk protein.

Issued May 2009
This Medication Guide has been approved by the U.S. Food and Drug Administration.
Distributed by:
Tercica, Inc.
a subsidiary of the Ipsen Group
Brisbane, CA 94005
and
Medicis Aesthetics Inc.,
a wholly owned subsidiary of Medicis Pharmaceutical Corporation
Scottsdale, AZ 85256
07100055

1All trademarks are the property of their respective owners

SOLODYN®   ℞
[SO-lo-dīn]
(minocycline HCl)
Extended Release Tablets for oral use

HIGHLIGHTS OF PRESCRIBING INFORMATION
These highlights do not include all the information needed to use SOLODYN safely and effectively. See full prescribing information for SOLODYN.
SOLODYN®
(minocycline HCl) Extended Release Tablets for oral use
Initial U.S. Approval: 1971

─────────INDICATIONS AND USAGE─────────
SOLODYN is a tetracycline-class drug indicated to treat only inflammatory lesions of non-nodular moderate to severe acne vulgaris in patients 12 years of age and older. (1)

─────────DOSAGE AND ADMINISTRATION─────────
The recommended dosage of SOLODYN is approximately 1 mg/kg once daily for 12 weeks. (2)

─────────DOSAGE FORMS AND STRENGTHS─────────
Extended release tablets: 45, 55, 65, 80, 90, 105, 115, and 135 mg (3)

─────────CONTRAINDICATIONS─────────
This drug is contraindicated in persons who have shown hypersensitivity to any of the tetracyclines. (4)

─────────WARNINGS AND PRECAUTIONS─────────
- The use of SOLODYN during tooth development (last half of pregnancy, infancy, and childhood up to the age of 8 years) may cause permanent discoloration of the teeth (yellow-gray-brown). (5.1)
- If pseudomembranous colitis occurs, discontinue SOLODYN. (5.2)
- If liver injury is suspected, discontinue SOLODYN. (5.3)
- If renal impairment exists, SOLODYN doses may need to be adjusted to avoid excessive systemic accumulations of the drug and possible liver toxicity. (5.4)
- Minocycline may cause central nervous system side effects including light-headedness, dizziness, or vertigo. Advise patients. (5.5)
- Minocycline may cause pseudotumor cerebri (benign intracranial hypertension) in adults and adolescents. Discontinue SOLODYN if symptoms occur. (5.6)
- Minocycline has been associated with autoimmune syndromes; discontinue SOLODYN immediately if symptoms occur. (5.7)

─────────ADVERSE REACTIONS─────────
The most commonly observed adverse reactions (incidence ≥ 5%) are headache, fatigue, dizziness, and pruritus. (6.1)
To report SUSPECTED ADVERSE REACTIONS, contact Medicis, The Dermatology Company at 1-800-900-6389 or FDA at 1-800-FDA-1088 or www.fda.gov/medwatch.
─────────DRUG INTERACTIONS─────────
- Patients who are on anticoagulant therapy may require downward adjustment of their anticoagulant dosage. (7.1)
- The concurrent use of tetracycline and methoxyflurane has been reported to result in fatal renal toxicity. (7.3)
- To avoid contraceptive failure, female patients are advised to use a second form of contraceptive during treatment with minocycline. (7.5)
─────────USE IN SPECIFIC POPULATIONS─────────
- Minocycline like other tetracycline-class drugs can cause fetal harm when administered to a pregnant woman (5.1, 8.1)
- The use of drugs of the tetracycline-class during tooth development may cause permanent discoloration of teeth (5.1, 8.4)

See 17 for PATIENT COUNSELING INFORMATION and FDA-approved patient labeling
                                     Revised: 09/2010

FULL PRESCRIBING INFORMATION: CONTENTS*
* Sections or subsections omitted from the full prescribing information are not listed

---

FULL PRESCRIBING INFORMATION
1   INDICATIONS AND USAGE
1.1   Indication
SOLODYN is indicated to treat only inflammatory lesions of non-nodular moderate to severe acne vulgaris in patients 12 years of age and older.
1.2   Limitations of Use
SOLODYN did not demonstrate any effect on non-inflammatory acne lesions. Safety of SOLODYN has not been established beyond 12 weeks of use. This formulation of minocycline has not been evaluated in the treatment of infections [see Clinical Studies (14)].
To reduce the development of drug-resistant bacteria as well as to maintain the effectiveness of other antibacterial drugs, SOLODYN should be used only as indicated [see Warnings and Precautions (5.11)].

2   DOSAGE AND ADMINISTRATION
The recommended dosage of SOLODYN is approximately 1 mg/kg once daily for 12 weeks. Higher doses have not shown to be of additional benefit in the treatment of inflammatory lesions of acne, and may be associated with more acute vestibular side effects.
The following table shows tablet strength and body weight to achieve approximately 1 mg/kg.

Table 1: Dosing Table for SOLODYN

Patient's Weight (lbs.)	Patient's Weight (kg)	Tablet Strength (mg)	Actual mg/kg Dose
99–109	45–49	45	1–0.92
110–131	50–59	55	1.10–0.93
132–157	60–71	65	1.08–0.92
158–186	72–84	80	1.11–0.95
187–212	85–96	90	1.06–0.94
213–243	97–110	105	1.08–0.95
244–276	111–125	115	1.04–0.92
277–300	126–136	135	1.07–0.99

SOLODYN Tablets may be taken with or without food [see Clinical Pharmacology (12)]. Ingestion of food along with SOLODYN may help reduce the risk of esophageal irritation and ulceration.
In patients with renal impairment [see Warnings and Precautions (5.3)], the total dosage should be decreased by either reducing the recommended individual doses and/or by extending the time intervals between doses.

3   DOSAGE FORMS AND STRENGTHS
- 45 mg extended release tablets: gray, unscored, coated, and debossed with "DYN-045" on one side.
- 55 mg extended release tablets: pink, unscored, coated, and debossed with "DYN-055" on one side.
- 65 mg extended release tablets: blue, unscored, coated, and debossed with "DYN-065" on one side.
- 80 mg extended release tablets: gray, unscored, coated, and debossed with "DYN-080" on one side.
- 90 mg extended release tablets: yellow, unscored, coated, and debossed with "DYN-090" on one side.
- 105 mg extended release tablets: purple, unscored, coated, and debossed with "DYN-105" on one side.
- 115 mg extended release tablets: green, unscored, coated, and debossed with "DYN-115" on one side.
- 135 mg extended release tablets: pink (orange-brown), unscored, coated, and debossed with "DYN-135" on one side.

4   CONTRAINDICATIONS
This drug is contraindicated in persons who have shown hypersensitivity to any of the tetracyclines.

5   WARNINGS AND PRECAUTIONS
5.1   Teratogenic Effects
1. MINOCYCLINE, LIKE OTHER TETRACYCLINE-CLASS ANTIBIOTICS, CAN CAUSE FETAL HARM WHEN ADMINISTERED TO A PREGNANT WOMAN. IF ANY TETRACYCLINE IS USED DURING PREGNANCY OR IF THE PATIENT BECOMES PREGNANT WHILE TAKING THESE DRUGS, THE PATIENT SHOULD BE APPRISED OF THE POTENTIAL HAZARD TO THE FETUS.
SOLODYN should not be used during pregnancy or by individuals of either gender who are attempting to conceive a child [see Nonclinical Toxicology (13.1) & Use in Specific Populations 8.1)].
2. THE USE OF DRUGS OF THE TETRACYCLINE CLASS DURING TOOTH DEVELOPMENT (LAST HALF OF PREGNANCY, INFANCY, AND CHILDHOOD

UP TO THE AGE OF 8 YEARS) MAY CAUSE PERMANENT DISCOLORATION OF THE TEETH (YELLOW-GRAY-BROWN).

This adverse reaction is more common during long-term use of the drug but has been observed following repeated short-term courses. Enamel hypoplasia has also been reported. TETRACYCLINE DRUGS, THEREFORE, SHOULD NOT BE USED DURING TOOTH DEVELOPMENT.

3. All tetracyclines form a stable calcium complex in any bone-forming tissue. A decrease in fibula growth rate has been observed in premature human infants given oral tetracycline in doses of 25 mg/kg every 6 hours. This reaction was shown to be reversible when the drug was discontinued.

Results of animal studies indicate that tetracyclines cross the placenta, are found in fetal tissues, and can cause retardation of skeletal development on the developing fetus. Evidence of embryotoxicity has been noted in animals treated early in pregnancy [see Use in Specific Populations (8.1)].

5.2   Pseudomembranous Colitis
Pseudomembranous colitis has been reported with nearly all antibacterial agents and may range from mild to life-threatening. Therefore, it is important to consider this diagnosis in patients who present with diarrhea subsequent to the administration of antibacterial agents.

Treatment with antibacterial agents alters the normal flora of the colon and may permit overgrowth of clostridia. Studies indicate that a toxin produced by Clostridium difficile is a primary cause of "antibiotic-associated colitis".

After the diagnosis of pseudomembranous colitis has been established, therapeutic measures should be initiated. Mild cases of pseudomembranous colitis usually respond to discontinuation of the drug alone. In moderate to severe cases, consideration should be given to management with fluids and electrolytes, protein supplementation, and treatment with an antibacterial drug clinically effective against Clostridium difficile colitis.

5.3   Hepatotoxicity
Post-marketing cases of serious liver injury, including irreversible drug-induced hepatitis and fulminant hepatic failure (sometimes fatal) have been reported with minocycline use in the treatment of acne.

5.4   Metabolic Effects
The anti-anabolic action of the tetracyclines may cause an increase in BUN. While this is not a problem in those with normal renal function, in patients with significantly impaired function, higher serum levels of tetracycline-class antibiotics may lead to azotemia, hyperphosphatemia, and acidosis. If renal impairment exists, even usual oral or parenteral doses may lead to excessive systemic accumulations of the drug and possible liver toxicity. Under such conditions, lower than usual total doses are indicated, and if therapy is prolonged, serum level determinations of the drug may be advisable.

5.5   Central Nervous System Effects
Central nervous system side effects including light-headedness, dizziness or vertigo have been reported with minocycline therapy. Patients who experience these symptoms should be cautioned about driving vehicles or using hazardous machinery while on minocycline therapy. These symptoms may disappear during therapy and usually rapidly disappear when the drug is discontinued.

5.6   Benign Intracranial Hypertension
Pseudotumor cerebri (benign intracranial hypertension) in adults and adolescents has been associated with the use of tetracyclines. Minocycline has been reported to cause or precipitate pseudotumor cerebri, the hallmark of which is papilledema. Clinical manifestations include headache and blurred vision. Bulging fontanels have been associated with the use of tetracyclines in infants. Although signs and symptoms of pseudotumor cerebri resolve after discontinuation of treatment, the possibility for permanent sequelae such as visual loss that may be permanent or severe exists. Patients should be questioned for visual disturbances prior to initiation of treatment with tetracyclines and should be routinely checked for papilledema while on treatment. Concomitant use of isotretinoin and minocycline should be avoided because isotretinoin, a systemic retinoid, is also known to cause pseudotumor cerebri.

5.7   Autoimmune Syndromes
Tetracyclines have been associated with the development of autoimmune syndromes. The long-term use of minocycline in the treatment of acne has been associated with drug-induced lupus-like syndrome, autoimmune hepatitis and vasculitis. Sporadic cases of serum sickness have presented shortly after minocycline use. Symptoms may be manifested by fever, rash, arthralgia, and malaise. In symptomatic patients, liver function tests, ANA, CBC, and other appropriate tests should be performed to evaluate the patients. Use of all tetracycline-class drugs should be discontinued immediately.

5.8   Photosensitivity
Photosensitivity manifested by an exaggerated sunburn reaction has been observed in some individuals taking tetracyclines. This has been reported rarely with minocycline. Patients should minimize or avoid exposure to natural or artificial sunlight (tanning beds or UVA/B treatment) while using minocycline. If patients need to be outdoors while using minocycline, they should wear loose-fitting clothes that protect skin from sun exposure and discuss other sun protection measures with their physician.

5.9   Serious Skin/Hypersensitivity Reaction
Post-marketing cases of anaphylaxis and serious skin reactions such as Stevens-Johnson syndrome and erythema multiforme have been reported with minocycline use in treatment of acne.

5.10   Tissue Hyperpigmentation
Tetracycline-class antibiotics are known to cause hyperpigmentation. Tetracycline therapy may induce hyperpigmentation in many organs, including nails, bone, skin, eyes, thyroid, visceral tissue, oral cavity (teeth, mucosa, alveolar bone), sclerae and heart valves. Skin and oral pigmentation has been reported to occur independently of time or amount of drug administration, whereas other tissue pigmentation has been reported to occur upon prolonged administration. Skin pigmentation includes diffuse pigmentation as well as over sites of scars or injury.

5.11   Development of Drug Resistant Bacteria
Bacterial resistance to the tetracyclines may develop in patients using SOLODYN, therefore, the susceptibility of bacteria associated with infection should be considered in selecting antimicrobial therapy. Because of the potential for drug-resistant bacteria to develop during the use of SOLODYN, it should be used only as indicated.

5.12   Superinfection
As with other antibiotic preparations, use of SOLODYN may result in overgrowth of nonsusceptible organisms, including fungi. If superinfection occurs, the antibiotic should be discontinued and appropriate therapy instituted.

5.13   Laboratory Monitoring
Periodic laboratory evaluations of organ systems, including hematopoietic renal and hepatic studies should be performed. Appropriate tests for autoimmune syndromes should be performed as indicated.

6   ADVERSE REACTIONS
6.1   Clinical Trial Experience
Because clinical trials are conducted under prescribed conditions, adverse reaction rates observed in the clinical trial may not reflect the rates observed in practice.

The following table summarizes selected adverse reactions reported in clinical trials at a rate of ≥1% for SOLODYN.

Table 2: Selected Treatment-Emergent Adverse Reactions in at least 1% of Clinical Trial Subjects

Adverse Reactions	SOLODYN (1 mg/kg) N = 674 (%)	PLACEBO N = 364 (%)
At least one treatment-emergent event	379 (56)	197 (54)
Headache	152 (23)	83 (23)
Fatigue	62 (9)	24 (7)
Dizziness	59 (9)	17 (5)
Pruritus	31 (5)	16 (4)
Malaise	26 (4)	9 (3)
Mood alteration	17 (3)	9 (3)
Somnolence	13 (2)	3 (1)
Urticaria	10 (2)	1 (0)
Tinnitus	10 (2)	5 (1)
Arthralgia	9 (1)	2 (0)
Vertigo	8 (1)	3 (1)
Dry mouth	7 (1)	5 (1)
Myalgia	7 (1)	4 (1)

6.2   Postmarketing Experience
Adverse reactions that have been reported with minocycline hydrochloride use in a variety of indications include:

- *Skin and hypersensitivity reactions:* fixed drug eruptions, balanitis, erythema multiforme, Stevens-Johnson syndrome, anaphylactoid purpura, photosensitivity, pigmentation of skin and mucous membranes, hypersensitivity reactions, angioneurotic edema, anaphylaxis.
- *Autoimmune conditions:* polyarthralgia, pericarditis, exacerbation of systemic lupus, pulmonary infiltrates with eosinophilia, transient lupus-like syndrome.
- *Central nervous system:* pseudotumor cerebri, bulging fontanels in infants, decreased hearing.
- *Endocrine:* thyroid discoloration, abnormal thyroid function.
- *Oncology:* papillary thyroid cancer.
- *Oral:* glossitis, dysphagia, tooth discoloration.

- *Gastrointestinal:* enterocolitis, pancreatitis, hepatitis, liver failure.
- *Renal:* reversible acute renal failure.
- *Hematology:* hemolytic anemia, thrombocytopenia, eosinophilia.

Preliminary studies suggest that use of minocycline may have deleterious effects on human spermatogenesis [see Nonclinical Toxicology (13.1)].

7   DRUG INTERACTIONS
7.1   Anticoagulants
Because tetracyclines have been shown to depress plasma prothrombin activity, patients who are on anticoagulant therapy may require downward adjustment of their anticoagulant dosage.

7.2   Penicillin
Since bacteriostatic drugs may interfere with the bactericidal action of penicillin, it is advisable to avoid giving tetracycline-class drugs in conjunction with penicillin.

7.3   Methoxyflurane
The concurrent use of tetracycline and methoxyflurane has been reported to result in fatal renal toxicity.

7.4   Antacids and Iron Preparations
Absorption of tetracyclines is impaired by antacids containing aluminum, calcium or magnesium and iron-containing preparations.

7.5   Low Dose Oral Contraceptives
In a multi-center study to evaluate the effect of SOLODYN on low dose oral contraceptives, hormone levels over one menstrual cycle with and without SOLODYN 1 mg/kg once-daily were measured. Based on the results of this trial, minocycline-related changes in estradiol, progestinic hormone, FSH and LH plasma levels, of breakthrough bleeding, or of contraceptive failure, can not be ruled out. To avoid contraceptive failure, female patients are advised to use a second form of contraceptive during treatment with minocycline.

7.6   Drug/Laboratory Test Interactions
False elevations of urinary catecholamine levels may occur due to interference with the fluorescence test.

8   USE IN SPECIFIC POPULATIONS
8.1   Pregnancy
Teratogenic Effects: Pregnancy category D [see Warnings and Precautions (5.1)]

SOLODYN should not be used during pregnancy. If the patient becomes pregnant while taking this drug, the patient should be apprised of the potential hazard to the fetus and stop treatment immediately.

There are no adequate and well-controlled studies on the use of minocycline in pregnant women. Minocycline, like other tetracycline-class drugs, crosses the placenta and may cause fetal harm when administered to a pregnant woman. Rare spontaneous reports of congenital anomalies including limb reduction have been reported with minocycline use in pregnancy in post-marketing experience. Only limited information is available regarding these reports; therefore, no conclusion on causal association can be established.

Minocycline induced skeletal malformations (bent limb bones) in fetuses when administered to pregnant rats and rabbits in doses of 30 mg/kg/day and 100 mg/kg/day, respectively, (resulting in approximately 3 times and 2 times, respectively, the systemic exposure to minocycline observed in patients as a result of use of SOLODYN). Reduced mean fetal body weight was observed in studies in which minocycline was administered to pregnant rats at a dose of 10 mg/kg/day (which resulted in approximately the same level of systemic exposure to minocycline as that observed in patients who use SOLODYN).

Minocycline was assessed for effects on peri- and post-natal development of rats in a study that involved oral administration to pregnant rats from day 6 of gestation through the period of lactation (postpartum day 20), at dosages of 5, 10, or 50 mg/kg/day. In this study, body weight gain was significantly reduced in pregnant females that received 50 mg/kg/day (resulting in approximately 2.5 times the systemic exposure to minocycline observed in patients as a result of use of SOLODYN). No effects of treatment on the duration of the gestation period or the number of live pups born per litter were observed. Gross external anomalies observed in F1 pups (offspring of animals that received minocycline) included reduced body size, improperly rotated forelimbs, and reduced size of extremities. No effects were observed on the physical development, behavior, learning ability, or reproduction of F1 pups, and there was no effect on gross appearance of F2 pups (offspring of F1 animals).

8.3   Nursing Mothers
Tetracycline-class antibiotics are excreted in human milk. Because of the potential for serious adverse effects on bone and tooth development in nursing infants from the tetracycline-class antibiotics, a decision should be made whether to discontinue nursing or discontinue the drug, taking into account the importance of the drug to the mother [see Warnings and Precautions (5.1)].

8.4　Pediatric Use

SOLODYN is indicated to treat only inflammatory lesions of non-nodular moderate to severe acne vulgaris in patients 12 years and older. Safety and effectiveness in pediatric patients below the age of 12 has not been established. Use of tetracycline-class antibiotics below the age of 8 is not recommended due to the potential for tooth discoloration [see Warnings and Precautions (5.1)].

8.5　Geriatric Use

Clinical studies of SOLODYN did not include sufficient numbers of subjects aged 65 and over to determine whether they respond differently from younger subjects. Other reported clinical experience has not identified differences in responses between the elderly and younger patients. In general, dose selection for an elderly patient should be cautious, usually starting at the low end of the dosing range, reflecting the greater frequency of decreased hepatic, renal, or cardiac function, and concomitant disease or other drug therapy.

10　OVERDOSAGE

In case of overdosage, discontinue medication, treat symptomatically and institute supportive measures. Minocycline is not removed in significant quantities by hemodialysis or peritoneal dialysis.

11　DESCRIPTION

Minocycline hydrochloride, a semi synthetic derivative of tetracycline, is [4S-(4α,4aα,5aα,12aα)]-4,7-Bis(dimethylamino)-1,4,4a,5,5a,6,11,12a-octahydro-3,10,12,12a-tetrahydroxy-1,11-dioxo-2-naphthacenecarboxamide mono hydrochloride. The structural formula is represented below:

$C_{23}H_{27}N_3O_7 \cdot HCl$　　M. W. 493.95

SOLODYN Tablets for oral administration contain minocycline hydrochloride USP equivalent to 45 mg, 55 mg, 65 mg, 80 mg, 90 mg, 105 mg, 115 mg or 135 mg of minocycline. In addition, 45 mg, 55 mg, 65 mg, 80 mg, 90 mg, 105 mg, 115 mg, and 135 mg tablets contain the following inactive ingredients: lactose monohydrate NF, hypromellose type 2910 USP, magnesium stearate NF, colloidal silicon dioxide NF, and carnauba wax NF. The 45 mg tablets also contain Opadry II Gray which contains: lactose monohydrate NF, hypromellose type 2910 USP, titanium dioxide USP, triacetin USP, and iron oxide black JPE. The 55 mg tablets also contain Opadry II Pink which contains: hypromellose type 2910 USP, titanium dioxide USP, lactose monohydrate NF, polyethylene glycol 3350 NF, triacetin USP, and FD&C Red #40. The 65 mg tablets also contain Opadry II Blue which contains: hypromellose type 2910 USP, lactose monohydrate NF, FD&C Blue #1, polyethylene glycol 3350 NF, FD&C Blue #2, titanium dioxide USP, triacetin USP, and D&C Yellow #10. The 80 mg tablets also contain Opadry II Gray which contains: hypromellose type 2910 USP, lactose monohydrate NF, polyethylene glycol 3350 NF, FD&C Blue #2, FD&C Red #40, titanium dioxide USP, triacetin USP, and FD&C Yellow #6. The 90 mg tablets also contain Opadry II Yellow which contains: hypromellose type 2910 USP, lactose monohydrate NF, titanium dioxide USP, iron oxide yellow NF, polyethylene glycol 3350 NF, and triacetin USP. The 105 mg tablets also contain Opadry II Purple which contains: hypromellose type 2910 USP, lactose monohydrate NF, titanium dioxide USP, D&C Red #27, polyethylene glycol 3350 NF, triacetin USP, and FD&C Blue #1. The 115 mg tablets also contain Opadry II Green which contains: hypromellose type 2910 USP, lactose monohydrate NF, D&C Yellow #10, triacetin USP, FD&C Blue #1, titanium dioxide USP, and FD&C Blue #2. The 135 mg tablets also contain Opadry II Pink which contains: hypromellose type 2910 USP, lactose monohydrate NF, titanium dioxide USP, polyethylene glycol 3350 NF, iron oxide red NF, and triacetin USP.

12　CLINICAL PHARMACOLOGY

12.1　Mechanism of Action

The mechanism of action of SOLODYN for the treatment of acne is unknown.

12.2　Pharmacodynamics

The pharmacodynamics of SOLODYN for the treatment of acne are unknown.

12.3　Pharmacokinetics

SOLODYN Tablets are not bioequivalent to non-modified release minocycline products. Based on pharmacokinetic studies in healthy adults, SOLODYN Tablets produce a delayed T_{max} at 3.5–4.0 hours as compared to a non-modified release reference minocycline product (T_{max} at 2.25–3 hours). At steady-state (Day 6), the mean AUC(0–24) and C_{max} were 33.32 μg×hr/mL and 2.63 μg/mL for SOLODYN

Table 4: Efficacy Results at Week 12

	Study 1		Study 2	
	SOLODYN (1 mg/kg) N = 300	Placebo N = 151	SOLODYN (1 mg/kg) N = 315	Placebo N = 158
Mean Percent Improvement in Inflammatory Lesions	43.1%	31.7%	45.8%	30.8%
No. (%) of Subjects Clear or Almost Clear on the EGSA*	52 (17.3%)	12 (7.9%)	50 (15.9%)	15 (9.5%)

*Evaluator's Global Severity Assessment

Tablets and 46.35 μg×hr/mL and 2.92 μg/mL for Minocin® capsules, respectively. These parameters are based on dose adjusted to 135 mg per day for both products.

A single-dose, four-way crossover study demonstrated that SOLODYN Tablets used in the study (45 mg, 90 mg, 135 mg) exhibited dose-proportional pharmacokinetics. In another single-dose, five-way crossover pharmacokinetic study, SOLODYN Tablets 55 mg, 80 mg, and 105 mg were shown to be dose-proportional to SOLODYN Tablets 90 mg and 135 mg.

When SOLODYN Tablets were administered concomitantly with a meal that included dairy products, the extent and timing of absorption of minocycline did not differ from that of administration under fasting conditions.

Minocycline is lipid soluble and distributes into the skin and sebum.

13　NONCLINICAL TOXICOLOGY

13.1　Carcinogenesis, Mutagenesis, Impairment of Fertility

Carcinogenesis—Long-term animal studies have not been performed to evaluate the carcinogenic potential of minocycline. A structurally related compound, oxytetracycline, was found to produce adrenal and pituitary tumors in rats.

Mutagenesis—Minocycline was not mutagenic in vitro in a bacterial reverse mutation assay (Ames test) or CHO/HGPRT mammalian cell assay in the presence or absence of metabolic activation. Minocycline was not clastogenic in vitro using human peripheral blood lymphocytes or in vivo in a mouse micronucleus test.

Impairment of Fertility—Male and female reproductive performance in rats was unaffected by oral doses of minocycline of up to 300 mg/kg/day (which resulted in up to approximately 40 times the level of systemic exposure to minocycline observed in patients as a result of use of SOLODYN). However, oral administration of 100 or 300 mg/kg/day of minocycline to male rats (resulting in approximately 15 to 40 times the level of systemic exposure to minocycline observed in patients as a result of use of SOLODYN) adversely affected spermatogenesis. Effects observed at 300 mg/kg/day included a reduced number of sperm cells per gram of epididymis, an apparent reduction in the percentage of sperm that were motile, and (at 100 and 300 mg/kg/day) increased numbers of morphologically abnormal sperm cells. Morphological abnormalities observed in sperm samples included absent heads, misshapen heads, and abnormal flagella.

Limited human studies suggest that minocycline may have a deleterious effect on spermatogenesis.

SOLODYN should not be used by individuals of either gender who are attempting to conceive a child.

14　CLINICAL STUDIES

The safety and efficacy of SOLODYN in the treatment of inflammatory lesions of non-nodular moderate to severe acne vulgaris was assessed in two 12-week, multi-center, randomized, double-blind, placebo-controlled, studies in subjects ≥ 12 years. The mean age of subjects was 20 years and subjects were from the following racial groups: White (73%), Hispanic (13%), Black (11%), Asian/Pacific Islander (2%), and Other (2%).

In two efficacy and safety trials, a total of 924 subjects with non-nodular moderate to severe acne vulgaris received SOLODYN or placebo for a total of 12 weeks, according to the following dose assignments.

Table 3: Clinical Studies Dosing Table

Subject's Weight (lbs)	Subject's Weight (kg)	Available Caplet Strength (mg)	Actual mg/kg Dose
99–131	45–59	45	1–0.76
132–199	60–90	90	1.5–1
200–300	91–136	135	1.48–0.99

The two primary efficacy endpoints were:
- 1) Mean percent change in inflammatory lesion counts from Baseline to 12 weeks.

- 2) Percentage of subjects with an Evaluator's Global Severity Assessment (EGSA) of clear or almost clear at 12 weeks.

Efficacy results are presented in Table 4.

[See table above]

SOLODYN did not demonstrate any effect on non-inflammatory lesions (benefit or worsening).

16　HOW SUPPLIED/STORAGE AND HANDLING

16.1　How Supplied

SOLODYN (minocycline HCl, USP) Extended Release Tablets are supplied as aqueous film coated tablets containing minocycline hydrochloride equivalent to 45 mg, 55 mg, 65 mg, 80 mg, 90 mg, 105 mg, 115 mg or 135 mg minocycline, are supplied as follows:

The 45 mg extended release tablets are gray, unscored, coated, and debossed with "DYN-045" on one side. Each tablet contains minocycline hydrochloride equivalent to 45 mg minocycline, supplied as follows:

NDC 99207-460-30	Bottle of 30
NDC 99207-460-10	Bottle of 100

The 55 mg extended release tablets are pink, unscored, coated, and debossed with "DYN-055" on one side. Each tablet contains minocycline hydrochloride equivalent to 55 mg minocycline, supplied as follows:

NDC 99207-465-30	Bottle of 30

The 65 mg extended release tablets are blue, unscored, coated, and debossed with "DYN-065" on one side. Each tablet contains minocycline hydrochloride equivalent to 65 mg minocycline, supplied as follows:

NDC 99207-463-30	Bottle of 30

The 80 mg extended release tablets are gray, unscored, coated, and debossed with "DYN-080" on one side. Each tablet contains minocycline hydrochloride equivalent to 80 mg minocycline, supplied as follows:

NDC 99207-466-30	Bottle of 30

The 90 mg extended release tablets are yellow, unscored, coated, and debossed with "DYN-090" on one side. Each tablet contains minocycline hydrochloride equivalent to 90 mg minocycline, supplied as follows:

NDC 99207-461-30	Bottle of 30
NDC 99207-461-10	Bottle of 100

The 105 mg extended release tablets are purple, unscored, coated, and debossed with "DYN-105" on one side. Each tablet contains minocycline hydrochloride equivalent to 105 mg minocycline, supplied as follows:

NDC 99207-467-30	Bottle of 30

The 115 mg extended release tablets are green, unscored, coated, and debossed with "DYN-115" on one side. Each tablet contains minocycline hydrochloride equivalent to 115 mg minocycline, supplied as follows:

NDC 99207-464-30	Bottle of 30

The 135 mg extended release tablets are pink (orange-brown), unscored, coated, and debossed with "DYN-135" on one side. Each tablet contains minocycline hydrochloride equivalent to 135 mg minocycline, supplied as follows:

NDC 99207-462-30	Bottle of 30
NDC 99207-462-10	Bottle of 100

16.2 Storage

Store at 25°C (77°F); excursions are permitted to 15°–30°C (59°–86°F) [See USP Controlled Room Temperature].

16.3 Handling

Keep out of reach of children.

Protect from light, moisture, and excessive heat.

Dispense in tight, light-resistant container with child-resistant closure.

17 PATIENT COUNSELING INFORMATION

[See FDA-Approved Patient Labeling]

Patients taking SOLODYN (minocycline HCl, USP) Extended Release Tablets should receive the following information and instructions:

- SOLODYN should not be used by pregnant women or women attempting to conceive a child *[see Use in Specific Populations (8.1), Nonclinical Toxicology (13.1)]*.
- It is recommended that SOLODYN not be used by men who are attempting to father a child *[see Nonclinical Toxicology (13.1)]*.
- Patients should be advised that pseudomembranous colitis can occur with minocycline therapy. If patients develop watery or bloody stools, they should seek medical attention
- Patients should be counseled about the possibility of hepatotoxicity. Patients should seek medical advice if they experience symptoms which can include loss of appetite, tiredness, diarrhea, skin turning yellow, bleeding easily, confusion, and sleepiness.
- Patients who experience central nervous system symptoms *[see Warnings and Precautions (5.4)]* should be cautioned about driving vehicles or using hazardous machinery while on minocycline therapy. Patients should seek medical help for persistent headaches or blurred vision.
- Concurrent use of tetracycline may render oral contraceptives less effective *[see Drug Interactions (7.1)]*.
- Autoimmune syndromes, including drug-induced lupus-like syndrome, autoimmune hepatitis, vasculitis and serum sickness have been observed with tetracycline-class drugs, including minocycline. Symptoms may be manifested by arthralgia, fever, rash and malaise. Patients who experience such symptoms should be cautioned to stop the drug immediately and seek medical help.
- Patients should be counseled about discoloration of skin, scars, teeth or gums that can arise from minocycline therapy.
- Photosensitivity manifested by an exaggerated sunburn reaction has been observed in some individuals taking tetracyclines, including minocycline. Patients should minimize or avoid exposure to natural or artificial sunlight (tanning beds or UVA/B treatment) while using minocycline. If patients need to be outdoors while using minocycline, they should wear loose-fitting clothes that protect skin from sun exposure and discuss other sun protection measures with their physician. Treatment should be discontinued at the first evidence of skin erythema.
- SOLODYN should be taken exactly as directed. Skipping doses or not completing the full course of therapy may decrease the effectiveness of the current treatment course and increase the likelihood that bacteria will develop resistance and will not be treatable by other antibacterial drugs in the future.
- Patients should be advised to swallow SOLODYN tablets whole and not to chew, crush, or split the tablets.

FDA-Approved Patient Labeling

Patient Information

SOLODYN (SO-lo-dīn) Extended Release Tablets

(minocycline HCl, USP)

Rx only

Read all patient information that comes with SOLODYN before you start taking it and each time you get a refill. There may be new information. This leaflet does not take the place of speaking with your doctor about your condition or treatment.

What is SOLODYN?

SOLODYN is a tetracycline-class drug that contains minocycline. SOLODYN is only for the treatment of pimples and red bumps (non-nodular inflammatory lesions) that happen with moderate to severe acne in patients 12 years and older. SOLODYN did not show any effect on acne spots that were not red-looking.

SOLODYN has not been studied for use longer than 12 weeks.

SOLODYN has not been studied for the treatment of infections.

Who should not take SOLODYN?

Do not take SOLODYN if you are allergic to minocycline or any other tetracycline antibiotics. Ask your doctor or pharmacist for a list of these medicines if you are not sure. See the end of this leaflet for a complete list of ingredients in SOLODYN.

SOLODYN should not be used by pregnant women, women attempting to have a child, or children up to 8 years old because:

1. **SOLODYN may harm an unborn baby**
2. **SOLODYN may permanently turn a baby or child's teeth yellow-grey-brown during tooth development.** SOLODYN should not be used during tooth development. Tooth development happens in the last half of pregnancy and birth to age 8 years.

It is recommended that SOLODYN not be used by men who are attempting to father a child.

What should I tell my doctor before taking SOLODYN?

Tell your doctor about all of your medical conditions including if you:

- **have kidney problems.** Your doctor may prescribe a lower dose of medicine for you.
- **have any vision problems such as blurred vision.**
- **are pregnant or attempting to conceive a child.** SOLODYN may harm your unborn baby. **Stop taking SOLODYN and call your doctor if you become pregnant while taking it.**
- **are breastfeeding.** SOLODYN passes into your milk and may harm your baby. You should decide whether to use SOLODYN or breastfeed, but not both.

Tell your doctor about all the other medicines you take including prescription and nonprescription medicines, vitamins and herbal supplements. SOLODYN and other medicines may interact. Especially tell your doctor if you take:

- **birth control pills.** SOLODYN may make your birth control pills less effective. You should use a second form of birth control while taking SOLODYN.
- **a blood thinner medicine.** The dose of your blood thinner may be lowered.
- **a penicillin antibiotic medicine.** SOLODYN and penicillins should not be used together.
- **antacids that contain aluminum, calcium, or magnesium or iron-containing products.** These can affect how much SOLODYN passes into your body.
- **An acne medication that contains isotretinoin.** SOLODYN and isotretinoin should not be used together.

Know the medicines you take. Keep a list of them to show your doctor and pharmacist.

How should I take SOLODYN?

- **SOLODYN comes in 8 strengths. Your doctor will prescribe the strength that is best for your body weight. The usual dose of SOLODYN is 1 tablet each day for 12 weeks.**
- **Take SOLODYN at the same time each day, with or without food.** Taking SOLODYN with food may lower your chances of getting irritation or ulcers in your esophagus. Your esophagus is the tube that connects your mouth to your stomach.
- **Swallow SOLODYN Tablets whole. Do not chew, crush, or split the tablets.**
- **If you forget to take SOLODYN, take it as soon as you remember. Do not take more than one tablet of SOLODYN in one day.**
- **If you take too much SOLODYN at a time, call your doctor.**
- **If you do not notice an improvement in your acne after 12 weeks of treatment with SOLODYN, call your doctor.**

What are possible side effects of SOLODYN?

SOLODYN may cause serious side effects. Stop SOLODYN and call your doctor if you have:

- watery diarrhea
- bloody stools
- stomach cramps
- unusual headaches
- blurred vision
- fever
- rash
- joint pain
- feeling very tired

SOLODYN may also cause:

- **serious effects on the liver.** Symptoms can include loss of appetite, tiredness, diarrhea, skin turning yellow, bleeding easily, confusion, and sleepiness. If you have these symptoms, stop SOLODYN and call your doctor.
- **central nervous system effects.** Symptoms include light-headedness, dizziness, and a spinning feeling (vertigo). You should not drive or operate dangerous machines if you have these symptoms.
- **sun sensitivity (photosensitivity).** You may get a worse sunburn with SOLODYN. Avoid sun exposure and the use of sunlamps or tanning beds. Protect your skin while out in sunlight. Stop SOLODYN and call your doctor at the first sign of redness or sunburn.
- **darkening of skin, scars, teeth, and gums.**

The most common side effects with SOLODYN include:

- headache
- tiredness
- dizziness or spinning feeling
- itching

Call your doctor if you have a side effect that bothers you or that does not go away.

These are not all the side effects with SOLODYN. Ask your doctor or pharmacist for more information.

You may report side effects to FDA at 1-800-FDA-1088 or to Medicis at 1-800-900-6389.

How should I store SOLODYN?

- Store SOLODYN at room temperature. Keep SOLODYN Tablets in the bottle you received from the pharmacy and store away from moisture and light.
- **Keep SOLODYN and all medicines out of the reach of children.**

General Information about SOLODYN

Medicines are sometimes prescribed for conditions that are not mentioned in patient information leaflets. Do not use SOLODYN for a condition for which it was not prescribed. Do not give SOLODYN to other people, even if they have the same symptoms you have. It may harm them.

This leaflet summarizes the most important information about SOLODYN. If you would like more information, talk to your doctor. You can ask your doctor or pharmacist for information about SOLODYN that is written for health professionals.

What are the Ingredients in SOLODYN?

Active Ingredient: minocycline HCl USP equivalent to 45 mg, 55 mg, 65 mg, 80 mg, 90 mg, 105 mg, 115 mg or 135 mg of minocycline.

Inactive Ingredients: lactose monohydrate NF, hypromellose type 2910 USP, magnesium stearate NF, colloidal silicon dioxide NF, and carnauba wax NF. The 45 mg tablets also contain Opadry II Gray which contains: lactose monohydrate NF, hypromellose type 2910 USP, titanium dioxide USP, triacetin USP, and iron oxide black JPE. The 55 mg tablets also contain Opadry II Pink which contains: hypromellose type 2910 USP, titanium dioxide USP, lactose monohydrate NF, polyethylene glycol 3350 NF, triacetin USP, and FD&C Red #40. The 65 mg tablets also contain Opadry II Blue which contains: hypromellose type 2910 USP, lactose monohydrate NF, FD&C Blue #1, polyethylene glycol 3350 NF, FD&C Blue #2, titanium dioxide USP, triacetin USP, and D&C Yellow #10. The 80 mg tablets also contain Opadry II Gray which contains: hypromellose type 2910 USP, lactose monohydrate NF, polyethylene glycol 3350 NF, FD&C Blue #2, FD&C Red #40, titanium dioxide USP, triacetin USP, and FD&C Yellow #6. The 90 mg tablets also contain Opadry II Yellow which contains: hypromellose type 2910 USP, lactose monohydrate NF, titanium dioxide USP, iron oxide yellow NF, polyethylene glycol 3350 NF, and triacetin USP. The 105 mg tablets also contain Opadry II Purple which contains: hypromellose type 2910 USP, lactose monohydrate NF, titanium dioxide USP, D&C Red #27, polyethylene glycol 3350 NF, triacetin USP, and FD&C Blue #1. The 115 mg tablets also contain Opadry II Green which contains: hypromellose type 2910 USP, lactose monohydrate NF, D&C Yellow #10, triacetin USP, FD&C Blue #1, titanium dioxide USP, FD&C Blue #2. The 135 mg tablets also contain Opadry II Pink which contains: hypromellose type 2910 USP, lactose monohydrate NF, titanium dioxide USP, polyethylene glycol 3350 NF, iron oxide red NF, and triacetin USP.

SOLODYN is manufactured by WellSpring Pharmaceutical Canada Corp. for Medicis Pharmaceutical Corporation, Scottsdale, Arizona, 85256.

U.S. Patent 5,908,838[1] and Patents Pending

© 2010 Medicis Pharmaceutical Corporation

SOLODYN is a registered trademark of Medicis Pharmaceutical Corporation.

All other trademarks are the properties of their respective owners.

Manufactured for:

Medicis, The Dermatology Company

Scottsdale, AZ 85256

Manufactured by:

WellSpring Pharmaceutical Canada Corp.

Oakville, Ontario, CANADA L6H 1M5

N4605C

[1]90 mg is also covered by U.S. Patents 7,541,347 and 7,544,373

VANOS®
[vă-nōs]
(fluocinonide)
Cream, 0.1%
Rx Only

℞

For Topical Use Only
Not For Ophthalmic, Oral, Or Intravaginal Use

DESCRIPTION

VANOS (fluocinonide) Cream, 0.1% contains fluocinonide, a synthetic corticosteroid for topical dermatologic use. The corticosteroids constitute a class of primarily synthetic steroids used topically as anti-inflammatory and antipruritic agents. Fluocinonide has the chemical name 6 alpha, 9 alpha-difluoro-11 beta, 21-dihydroxy-16 alpha, 17 alpha-isopropylidenedioxypregna-1, 4-diene-3,20-dione 21-acetate. Its chemical formula is $C_{26}H_{32}F_2O_7$ and it has a molecular weight of 494.58.
It has the following chemical structure:

Fluocinonide is an almost odorless white to creamy white crystalline powder. It is practically insoluble in water and slightly soluble in ethanol.
Each gram of VANOS Cream contains 1 mg micronized fluocinonide in a cream base of propylene glycol USP, dimethyl isosorbide, glyceryl stearate (and) PEG-100 stearate, glyceryl monostearate NF, purified water USP, carbopol 980 NF, diisopropanolamine, and citric acid USP.

CLINICAL PHARMACOLOGY

Like other topical corticosteroids, VANOS (fluocinonide) Cream, has anti-inflammatory, antipruritic, and vasoconstrictive properties. The mechanism of the anti-inflammatory activity of topical corticosteroids, in general, is unclear. However, corticosteroids are thought to act by induction of phospholipase A_2 inhibitory proteins, collectively called lipocortins. It is postulated that these proteins control the biosynthesis of potent mediators of inflammation such as prostaglandins and leukotrienes by inhibiting the release of their common precursor, arachadonic acid. Arachadonic acid is released from membrane phospholipids by phospholipase A_2.

Pharmacokinetics

The extent of percutaneous absorption of topical corticosteroids is determined by many factors including the vehicle and the integrity of the epidermal barrier. Topical corticosteroids can be absorbed from normal intact skin. Inflammation and/or other disease processes in the skin may increase percutaneous absorption.
Vasoconstrictor studies performed with VANOS Cream, 0.1% in healthy subjects indicate that it is in the super-high range of potency as compared with other topical corticosteroids; however, similar blanching scores do not necessarily imply therapeutic equivalence.
Application of VANOS Cream, 0.1% twice daily for 14 days in 18 adult patients with plaque-type psoriasis (10–50% BSA, mean 19.6% BSA) showed demonstrable HPA-axis suppression in 2 patients (with 12% and 25% BSA) where the criterion for HPA-axis suppression is a serum cortisol level of less than or equal to 18 micrograms per deciliter 30 minutes after stimulation with cosyntropin ($ACTH_{1-24}$) (See **PRECAUTIONS: General** and **Pediatric Use**).
HPA-axis suppression has not been evaluated in psoriasis patients who are less than 18 years of age. HPA-axis suppression has been evaluated in pediatric patients with atopic dermatitis 12 to 18 years of age (See **PRECAUTIONS: Pediatric Use**).

CLINICAL STUDIES

Two adequate and well-controlled efficacy and safety studies of VANOS Cream have been completed, one in adult patients with plaque-type psoriasis (Table 1), and one in adult patients with atopic dermatitis (Table 2). In each of these studies, patients with between 2% and 10% body surface area involvement at Baseline treated all affected areas either once daily or twice daily with VANOS Cream for 14 consecutive days. The primary measure of efficacy was the proportion of patients whose condition was cleared or almost cleared at the end of treatment. The results of these studies are presented in the tables below as percent and number of patients achieving treatment success at Week 2.
[See table 1 above]
[See table 2 above]

Table 1: Plaque-Type Psoriasis in Adults

	VANOS Cream, once daily (n=107)	Vehicle, once daily (n=54)	VANOS Cream, twice daily (n=107)	Vehicle, twice daily (n=55)
Patients cleared	0 (0)	0 (0)	6 (6%)	0 (0)
Patients achieving treatment success*	19 (18%)	4 (7%)	33 (31%)	3 (5%)

*Cleared or almost cleared

Table 2: Atopic Dermatitis in Adults

	VANOS Cream, once daily (n=109)	Vehicle, once daily (n=50)	VANOS Cream, twice daily (n=102)	Vehicle, twice daily (n=52)
Patients cleared	11 (10%)	0 (0)	17 (17%)	0 (0)
Patients achieving treatment success*	64 (59%)	6 (12%)	58 (57%)	10 (19%)

*Cleared or almost cleared

No efficacy studies have been conducted to compare VANOS (fluocinonide) Cream, 0.1% with any other topical corticosteroid product, including fluocinonide cream 0.05%.

INDICATIONS AND USAGE

VANOS (fluocinonide) Cream, 0.1%, is a corticosteroid indicated for the relief of the inflammatory and pruritic manifestations of corticosteroid responsive dermatoses in patients 12 years of age or older (See **PRECAUTIONS: Pediatric Use**).
Treatment beyond 2 consecutive weeks is not recommended and the total dosage should not exceed 60 g/week because the safety of VANOS Cream for longer than 2 weeks has not been established and because of the potential for the drug to suppress the hypothalamic-pituitary-adrenal (HPA) axis. Therapy should be discontinued when control of the disease is achieved. If no improvement is seen within 2 weeks, reassessment of the diagnosis may be necessary. Do not use more than half of the 120 g tube per week.

CONTRAINDICATIONS

VANOS Cream is contraindicated in those patients with a history of hypersensitivity to any of the components of the preparation.

PRECAUTIONS

General

Systemic absorption of topical corticosteroids can produce reversible hypothalamic-pituitary-adrenal (HPA) axis suppression with the potential for glucocorticosteroid insufficiency after withdrawal of treatment. Manifestations of Cushing's syndrome, hyperglycemia, and glucosuria can also be produced in some patients by systemic absorption of topical corticosteroids while on treatment. Use of more than one corticosteroid-containing product at the same time may increase total systemic glucocorticoid exposure. In addition, use of VANOS Cream for longer than 2 weeks may also suppress the immune system (see **PRECAUTIONS: Carcinogenesis, Mutagenesis, and Impairment of Fertility**).
Patients applying a topical steroid to a large surface area or to areas under occlusion should be evaluated periodically for evidence of HPA-axis suppression. This may be done by using cosyntropin ($ACTH_{1-24}$) stimulation testing. Patients should not be treated with VANOS Cream for more than 2 weeks at a time and only small areas should be treated at any time due to the increased risk of HPA-axis suppression.
If HPA-axis suppression is noted, an attempt should be made to withdraw the drug, to reduce the frequency of application, or to substitute a less potent corticosteroid. Recovery of HPA-axis function is generally prompt upon discontinuation of topical corticosteroids. Infrequently, signs and symptoms of glucocorticosteroid insufficiency may occur requiring supplemental systemic corticosteroids. For information on systemic supplementation, see prescribing information for those products.
Application of VANOS Cream, 0.1% twice daily for 14 days in 18 adult patients with plaque-type psoriasis (10–50% BSA, mean 19.6% BSA) and 31 adult patients (17 treated once daily; 14 treated twice daily) with atopic dermatitis (2–10% BSA, mean 5% BSA) showed demonstrable HPA-axis suppression in 2 patients with psoriasis (with 12% and 25% BSA) and 1 patient with atopic dermatitis (treated once daily, 4% BSA) where the criterion for HPA-axis suppression is a serum cortisol level of less than or equal to 18 micrograms per deciliter 30 minutes after stimulation with cosyntropin ($ACTH_{1-24}$) (See **CLINICAL PHARMACOLOGY**).
Controlled clinical efficacy studies of VANOS Cream in pediatric patients younger than 17 years of age have not been conducted; (See **PRECAUTIONS: Pediatric Use**).

HPA-axis suppression has not been evaluated in psoriasis patients who are less than 18 years of age.
Pediatric patients may be more susceptible to systemic toxicity from equivalent doses due to their larger skin surface to body mass ratios. (See **PRECAUTIONS: Pediatric Use**).
If irritation develops, VANOS Cream should be discontinued and appropriate therapy instituted. Allergic contact dermatitis with corticosteroids is usually diagnosed by observing failure to heal rather than noting a clinical exacerbation as with most topical products not containing corticosteroids. Such an observation should be corroborated with appropriate diagnostic patch testing.
If concomitant skin infections are present or develop, an appropriate antifungal or antibacterial agent should be used. If a favorable response does not occur promptly, use of VANOS Cream should be discontinued until the infection has been adequately controlled.
VANOS Cream should not be used in the treatment of rosacea or perioral dermatitis, and should not be used on the face, groin, or axillae.

Information for the Patient

Patients using VANOS Cream should receive the following information and instructions. This information is intended to aid in the safe and effective use of this medication. It is not a disclosure of all possible adverse or unintended effects:

- 1) VANOS Cream is to be used as directed by the physician. It is for external use only. Avoid contact with the eyes. It should not be used on the face, groin, and underarms.
- 2) VANOS Cream should not be used for any disorder other than that for which it was prescribed.
- 3) The treated skin area should not be bandaged or otherwise covered or wrapped, so as to be occlusive unless directed by the physician.
- 4) Patients should report to their physician any signs of local adverse reactions.
- 5) Other corticosteroid-containing products should not be used with VANOS Cream without first talking to the physician.
- 6) As with other corticosteroids, therapy should be discontinued when control is achieved. If no improvement is seen in 2 weeks, the patient should be instructed to contact a physician. The safety of the use of VANOS Cream for longer than 2 weeks has not been established.
- 7) Patients should be informed to not use more than 60 g per week of VANOS Cream. Do not use more than half of the 120 g tube per week.
- 8) Patients should inform their physicians that they are using VANOS Cream if surgery is contemplated.
- 9) Patients should wash their hands after applying medication.

Laboratory Tests

The cosyntropin ($ACTH_{1-24}$) stimulation test may be helpful in evaluating patients for HPA-axis suppression.

Carcinogenesis, Mutagenesis, and Impairment of Fertility

Long-term animal studies have not been performed to evaluate the carcinogenic potential of VANOS Cream because of severe immunosuppression induced in a 13-week dermal rat study. The effects of fluocinonide on fertility have not been evaluated.
Fluocinonide revealed no evidence of mutagenic or clastogenic potential based on the results of two *in vitro* genotoxicity tests (Ames test and chromosomal aberration assay using human lymphocytes). However, fluocinonide was positive for clastogenic potential when tested in the *in vivo* mouse micronucleus assay.
Topical (dermal) application of 0.0003%–0.03% fluocinonide cream to rats once daily for 13 weeks resulted in a toxicity

profile generally associated with long-term exposure to corticosteroids including decreased skin thickness, adrenal atrophy, and severe immunosuppression. A NOAEL could not be determined in this study. In addition, topical (dermal) application of 0.1% fluocinonide cream plus UVR exposure to hairless mice for 13 weeks and 150–900 mg/kg/day of 0.1% fluocinonide cream to minipigs (a model which more closely approximates human skin) for 13 weeks produced glucocorticoid-related suppression of the HPA axis, with some signs of immunosuppression noted in the dermal minipig study. Although the clinical relevance of the findings in animals to humans is not clear, sustained glucocorticoid-related immune suppression may increase the risk of infection and possibly the risk for carcinogenesis.

Pregnancy Category C
Teratogenic Effects
Corticosteroids have been shown to be teratogenic in laboratory animals when administered systemically at relatively low dosage levels. Some corticosteroids have been shown to be teratogenic after dermal application in laboratory animals.

There are no adequate and well-controlled studies in pregnant women. Therefore, VANOS Cream should be used during pregnancy only if the potential benefit justifies the potential risk to the fetus.

Nursing Mothers
Systemically administered corticosteroids appear in human milk and could suppress growth, interfere with endogenous corticosteroid production, or cause other untoward effects. It is not known whether topical administration of corticosteroids could result in sufficient systemic absorption to produce detectable quantities in breast milk. Nevertheless, a decision should be made whether to discontinue nursing or to discontinue the drug, taking into account the importance of the drug to the mother.

Pediatric Use
Safety and efficacy of VANOS Cream in pediatric patients younger than 12 years of age have not been established; therefore use in pediatric patients younger than 12 years of age is not recommended.

HPA-axis suppression was studied in 4 sequential cohorts of pediatric patients with atopic dermatitis covering at least 20% of the body surface area, treated once daily or twice daily with VANOS Cream. The first cohort of 31 patients (mean 36.3% BSA) 12 to < 18 years old; the second cohort included 31 patients (mean 39.0% BSA) 6 to < 12 years old; the third cohort included 30 patients (mean 34.6% BSA) 2 to < 6 years old; the fourth cohort included 31 patients (mean 40.0% BSA) 3 months to < 2 years old. VANOS Cream caused HPA-axis suppression in 1 patient in the twice daily group in Cohort 1, 2 patients in the twice daily group in Cohort 2, and 1 patient in the twice daily group in Cohort 3. Follow-up testing 14 days after treatment discontinuation, available for all 4 suppressed patients, demonstrated a normally responsive HPA-axis. Signs of skin atrophy were present at baseline and severity was not determined making it difficult to assess local skin safety. Therefore, the safety of VANOS Cream in patients younger than 12 years of age has not been demonstrated.

Because of a higher ratio of skin surface area to body mass, pediatric patients are at a greater risk than adults of HPA-axis suppression and Cushing's syndrome when they are treated with topical corticosteroids. They are therefore also at greater risk of adrenal insufficiency during or after withdrawal of treatment. Adverse effects including striae have been reported with inappropriate use of topical corticosteroids in infants and children.

HPA-axis suppression, Cushing's syndrome, linear growth retardation, delayed weight gain, and intracranial hypertension have been reported in children receiving topical corticosteroids. Manifestations of adrenal suppression in children include low plasma cortisol levels and absence of response to cosyntropin (ACTH$_{1-24}$) stimulation. Manifestations of intracranial hypertension include bulging fontanelles, headaches, and bilateral papilledema.

Geriatric Use
Clinical studies of VANOS Cream did not include sufficient numbers of subjects aged 65 and over to determine whether they respond differently from younger subjects. In general, dose selection for an elderly patient should be cautious.

ADVERSE REACTIONS
In clinical trials, a total of 443 adult patients with atopic dermatitis or plaque-type psoriasis were treated once daily or twice daily with VANOS Cream for 2 weeks. The most commonly observed adverse events in these clinical trials were as follows:
[See table 3 below]
No other adverse events were reported by more than 1 subject receiving active treatment. The incidence of all adverse events was similar between the active treatment groups and the vehicle control groups. Safety in patients 12 to 17 years of age was similar to that observed in adults.

The following additional local adverse reactions have been reported with topical corticosteroids, and they may occur more frequently with the use of occlusive dressings and higher potency corticosteroids. These reactions are listed in an approximate decreasing order of occurrence: burning, itching, irritation, dryness, folliculitis, hypertrichosis, acneiform eruptions, hypopigmentation, perioral dermatitis, allergic contact dermatitis, maceration of the skin, secondary infection, skin atrophy, striae, and miliaria. Systemic absorption of topical corticosteroids has produced hypothalamic-pituitary-adrenal (HPA) axis suppression manifestations of Cushing's syndrome, hyperglycemia, and glucosuria in some patients.

OVERDOSAGE
Topically applied VANOS Cream can be absorbed in sufficient amounts to produce systemic effects (see PRECAUTIONS).

DOSAGE AND ADMINISTRATION
For psoriasis, apply a thin layer of VANOS Cream once or twice daily to the affected skin areas as directed by a physician. Twice daily application for the treatment of psoriasis has been shown to be more effective in achieving treatment success during 2 weeks of treatment.

For atopic dermatitis, apply a thin layer of VANOS Cream once daily to the affected skin areas as directed by a physician. Once daily application for the treatment of atopic dermatitis has been shown to be as effective as twice daily treatment in achieving treatment success during 2 weeks of treatment (See CLINICAL STUDIES).

For corticosteroid responsive dermatoses, other than psoriasis or atopic dermatitis, apply a thin layer of VANOS Cream once or twice daily to the affected areas as directed by a physician.

Treatment with VANOS Cream should be limited to 2 consecutive weeks, and no more than 60 g/week should be used. Do not use more than half of the 120 g tube per week.

Therapy should be discontinued when control has been achieved. If no improvement is seen within 2 weeks, reassessment of diagnosis may be necessary.

HOW SUPPLIED
VANOS (fluocinonide) Cream 0.1% is supplied in tubes as follows:
30 g (NDC 99207-525-30)
60 g (NDC 99207-525-60)
120 g (NDC 99207-525-10)
Store at controlled room temperature: 15° to 30°C (59° to 86°F).
Manufactured for:
Medicis, The Dermatology Company
Scottsdale, AZ 85256
Manufactured by:
Contract Pharmaceuticals Ltd.
Mississauga, Ontario
Canada L5N 6L6
Made in Canada

U.S. Patents 6,765,001; 7,217,422; 7,220,424 and Patents Pending
VANOS is a registered trademark of Medicis Pharmaceutical Corporation.
Prescribing information as of February 2010.
05100002

MedImmune, LLC
ONE MEDIMMUNE WAY
GAITHERSBURG, MD 20878

For all inquiries, including emergencies (24 hours), medical information, adverse drug experiences, product sales and ordering, and customer service, please contact:
(877) 633-4411
www.medimmune.com

FLUMIST®   ℞
[FLEW-mĭst]
Influenza Vaccine Live, Intranasal
Intranasal Spray

HIGHLIGHTS OF PRESCRIBING INFORMATION
These highlights do not include all the information needed to use FluMist safely and effectively. See full prescribing information for FluMist.
FluMist® Influenza Vaccine Live, Intranasal
Intranasal Spray
2010-2011 Formula
Initial U.S. Approval: 2003

INDICATIONS AND USAGE
FluMist is a vaccine indicated for the active immunization of individuals 2-49 years of age against influenza disease caused by influenza virus subtypes A and type B contained in the vaccine. (1)

DOSAGE AND ADMINISTRATION
For intranasal administration by a health care provider.

Age Group	Vaccination Status	Dosage Schedule
Children (2-8 years)	Not previously vaccinated with influenza vaccine	2 doses (0.2 mL* each, at least 1 month apart) (2.1)
Children (2-8 years)	Previously vaccinated with influenza vaccine	1 dose (0.2 mL*) (2.1)
Children, adolescents and adults (9-49 years)	Not applicable	1 dose (0.2 mL*) (2.1)

*Administer as 0.1 mL per nostril.

DOSAGE FORMS AND STRENGTHS
0.2 mL pre-filled, single-use intranasal spray (3)
Each 0.2 mL dose contains $10^{6.5-7.5}$ FFU (fluorescent focus units) of live attenuated influenza virus reassortants of each of the three strains for the 2010-2011 season: A/California/7/2009 (H1N1), A/Perth/16/2009 (H3N2), and B/Brisbane/60/2008. (3)

CONTRAINDICATIONS
• Hypersensitivity to eggs, egg proteins, gentamicin, gelatin, or arginine, or life-threatening reactions to previous influenza vaccination. (4.1)
• Concomitant aspirin therapy in children and adolescents. (4.2)

WARNINGS AND PRECAUTIONS
• Do not administer FluMist to children <24 months of age because of increased risk of hospitalization and wheezing observed in clinical trials. (5.1)
• FluMist should not be administered to any individuals with asthma or children < 5 years of age with recurrent wheezing because of the potential for increased risk of wheezing post vaccination. (5.2)
• If Guillain-Barré syndrome has occurred with any prior influenza vaccination, the decision to give FluMist should be based on careful consideration of the potential benefits and risks. (5.3)
• Administration of FluMist, a live virus vaccine, to immunocompromised persons should be based on careful consideration of the potential benefits and risks. (5.4)
• Safety has not been established in individuals with underlying medical conditions predisposing them to wild-type influenza infection complications. (5.5)

Table 3: Most Commonly Observed Adverse Events in Adult Clinical Trials

Adverse Event	VANOS Cream, once daily (n=216)	VANOS Cream, twice daily (n=227)	Vehicle Cream, once or twice daily (n=211)
Headache	8/216 (3.7%)	9/227 (4.0%)	6/211 (2.8%)
Application Site Burning	5/216 (2.3%)	4/227 (1.8%)	14/211 (6.6%)
Nasopharyngitis	2/216 (0.9%)	3/227 (1.3%)	3/211 (1.4%)
Nasal Congestion	3/216 (1.4%)	1/227 (0.4%)	0
Unspecified Application Site Reaction	1/216 (0.4%)	1/227 (0.4%)	3/211 (1.4%)

ADVERSE REACTIONS

Most common adverse reactions (≥ 10% in FluMist and at least 5% greater than in control) are runny nose or nasal congestion in all ages, fever >100°F in children 2-6 years of age, and sore throat in adults. (6.1)

To report SUSPECTED ADVERSE REACTIONS, contact MedImmune at 1-877-633-4411 or VAERS at 1-800-822-7967 or http://vaers.hhs.gov.

DRUG INTERACTIONS

• Antiviral agents active against influenza A and/or B: Do not administer FluMist until 48 hours after antiviral cessation. Antiviral agents should not be administered until 2 weeks after FluMist administration unless medically necessary. (7.2)

USE IN SPECIFIC POPULATIONS

• Safety and effectiveness of FluMist have not been studied in pregnant women or nursing mothers. (8.1, 8.3)

See 17 for PATIENT COUNSELING INFORMATION and FDA-approved patient labeling

Revised: 07/2010

FULL PRESCRIBING INFORMATION: CONTENTS*

* Sections or subsections omitted from the full prescribing information are not listed

FULL PRESCRIBING INFORMATION

1 INDICATIONS AND USAGE

FluMist is a vaccine indicated for the active immunization of individuals 2-49 years of age against influenza disease caused by influenza virus subtypes A and type B contained in the vaccine.

2 DOSAGE AND ADMINISTRATION

FOR INTRANASAL ADMINISTRATION BY A HEALTH CARE PROVIDER.

2.1 Dosing Information

FluMist should be administered according to the following schedule:

Age Group	Vaccination Status	Dosage Schedule
Children age 2 years through 8 years	Not previously vaccinated with influenza vaccine	2 doses (0.2 mL* each, at least 1 month apart)
Children age 2 years through 8 years	Previously vaccinated with influenza vaccine	1 dose (0.2 mL*)
Children, adolescents and adults age 9 through 49 years	Not applicable	1 dose (0.2 mL*)

* Administer as 0.1 mL per nostril.

For children age 2 years through 8 years who have not previously received influenza vaccine, the recommended dosage schedule for nasal administration is one 0.2 mL dose (0.1 mL per nostril), followed by a second 0.2 mL dose (0.1 mL per nostril) given at least 1 month later.

For all other individuals, including children age 2-8 years who have previously received influenza vaccine, the recommended schedule is one 0.2 mL dose (0.1 mL per nostril).

FluMist should be administered prior to exposure to influenza. Annual revaccination with influenza vaccine is recommended.

2.2 Administration Instructions

Each sprayer contains a single dose of FluMist; approximately one-half of the contents should be administered into each nostril. Refer to the administration diagram (Figure 1) for step-by-step administration instructions. Once FluMist has been administered, the sprayer should be disposed of according to the standard procedures for medical waste (e.g., sharps container or biohazard container).

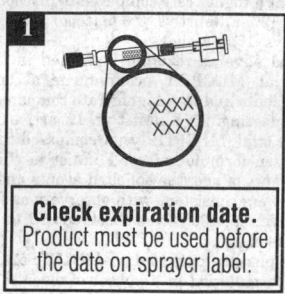

1 Check expiration date. Product must be used before the date on sprayer label.

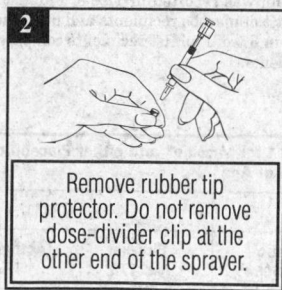

2 Remove rubber tip protector. Do not remove dose-divider clip at the other end of the sprayer.

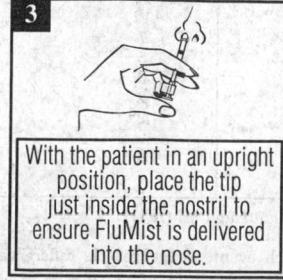

3 With the patient in an upright position, place the tip just inside the nostril to ensure FluMist is delivered into the nose.

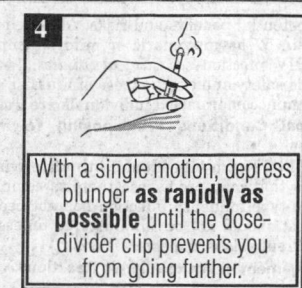

4 With a single motion, depress plunger **as rapidly as possible** until the dose-divider clip prevents you from going further.

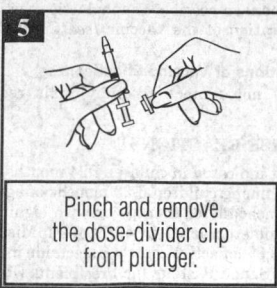

5 Pinch and remove the dose-divider clip from plunger.

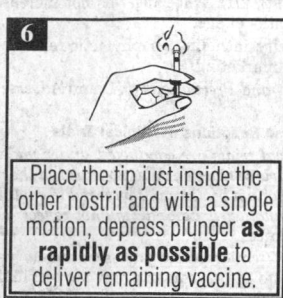

6 Place the tip just inside the other nostril and with a single motion, depress plunger **as rapidly as possible** to deliver remaining vaccine.

DO NOT INJECT. DO NOT USE A NEEDLE.

Note: Active inhalation (i.e., sniffing) is not required by the patient during FluMist administration

Figure 1

3 DOSAGE FORMS AND STRENGTHS

0.2 mL pre-filled, single-use intranasal spray.
Each 0.2 mL dose of FluMist is formulated to contain $10^{6.5-7.5}$ FFU (fluorescent focus units) of each of three live attenuated influenza virus reassortants: A/California/7/2009 (H1N1), A/Perth/16/2009 (H3N2), and B/Brisbane/60/2008.

4 CONTRAINDICATIONS

4.1 Hypersensitivity

FluMist is contraindicated in individuals with a history of hypersensitivity, especially anaphylactic reactions, to eggs, egg proteins, gentamicin, gelatin, or arginine, or with life-threatening reactions to previous influenza vaccinations.

4.2 Concomitant Pediatric and Adolescent Aspirin Therapy and Reye's Syndrome

FluMist is contraindicated in children and adolescents (2-17 years of age) receiving aspirin therapy or aspirin-containing therapy, because of the association of Reye's syndrome with aspirin and wild-type influenza infection.

5 WARNINGS AND PRECAUTIONS

5.1 Risks in Children <24 Months of Age

Do not administer FluMist to children <24 months of age. In clinical trials, an increased risk of wheezing post-vaccination was observed in FluMist recipients <24 months of age. An increase in hospitalizations was observed in children <24 months of age after vaccination with FluMist. [See Adverse Reactions (6.1).]

5.2 Asthma/Recurrent Wheezing

FluMist should not be administered to any individuals with asthma or children < 5 years of age with recurrent wheezing because of the potential for increased risk of wheezing post vaccination unless the potential benefit outweighs the potential risk.

Do not administer FluMist to individuals with severe asthma or active wheezing because these individuals have not been studied in clinical trials.

5.3 Guillain-Barré Syndrome

If Guillain-Barré syndrome has occurred within 6 weeks of any prior influenza vaccination, the decision to give FluMist should be based on careful consideration of the potential benefits and potential risks [see also Adverse Reactions (6.2)].

5.4 Altered Immunocompetence

Administration of FluMist, a live virus vaccine, to immuno-compromised persons should be based on careful consideration of the potential benefits and risks. Although FluMist was studied in 57 asymptomatic or mildly symptomatic adults with HIV infection *[see Clinical Studies (14.3)]*, data supporting the safety and effectiveness of FluMist administration in immunocompromised individuals are limited.

5.5 Medical Conditions Predisposing to Influenza Complications

The safety of FluMist in individuals with underlying medical conditions that may predispose them to complications following wild-type influenza infection has not been established. FluMist should not be administered unless the potential benefit outweighs the potential risk.

5.6 Management of Acute Allergic Reactions

Appropriate medical treatment and supervision must be available to manage possible anaphylactic reactions following administration of the vaccine *[see Contraindications (4.1)]*.

5.7 Limitations of Vaccine Effectiveness

FluMist may not protect all individuals receiving the vaccine.

6 ADVERSE REACTIONS

FluMist is not indicated in children <24 months of age. In a clinical trial, among children 6-23 months of age, wheezing requiring bronchodilator therapy or with significant respiratory symptoms occurred in 5.9% of FluMist recipients compared to 3.8% of active control (injectable influenza vaccine made by Sanofi Pasteur Inc.) recipients (Relative Risk 1.5, 95% CI: 1.2, 2.1). Wheezing was not increased in children ≥24 months of age.

Hypersensitivity, including anaphylactic reaction, has been reported post-marketing.

[See Warnings and Precautions (5.1) and Adverse Reactions (6.1, 6.2).]

6.1 Adverse Reactions in Clinical Trials

Because clinical trials are conducted under widely varying conditions, adverse reaction rates observed in the clinical trials of a drug cannot be directly compared to rates in the clinical trials of another drug and may not reflect the rates observed in practice.

A total of 9537 children and adolescents 1-17 years of age and 3041 adults 18-64 years of age received FluMist in randomized, placebo-controlled Studies D153-P501, AV006, D153-P526, AV019, and AV009 described below. In addition, 4179 children 6-59 months of age received FluMist in Study MI-CP111, a randomized, active-controlled trial. Among pediatric FluMist recipients 6 months-17 years of age, 50% were female; in the study of adults, 55% were female. In MI-CP111, AV006, D153-P526, AV019, and AV009, subjects were White (71%), Hispanic (11%), Asian (7%), Black (6%), and Other (5%), while in D153-P501, 99% of subjects were Asian.

Adverse Reactions in Children and Adolescents

In a placebo-controlled safety study (AV019) conducted in a large Health Maintenance Organization (HMO) in children 1-17 years of age (n = 9689), an increase in asthma events, captured by review of diagnostic codes, was observed in children <5 years of age (Relative Risk 3.53, 90% CI: 1.1, 15.7). This observation was prospectively evaluated in Study MI-CP111.

In MI-CP111, an active-controlled study, increases in wheezing and hospitalization (for any cause) were observed in children <24 months of age, as shown in Table 1.

Table 1 Percentages of Children with Hospitalizations and Wheezing from MI-CP111

Adverse Reaction	Age Group	FluMist	Active Control*
Hospitalizations†	6-23 months (n = 3967)	4.2%	3.2%
	24-59 months (n = 4385)	2.1%	2.5%
Wheezing‡	6-23 months (n = 3967)	5.9%	3.8%
	24-59 months (n = 4385)	2.1%	2.5%

* Injectable influenza vaccine made by Sanofi Pasteur Inc.
† From randomization through 180 days post last vaccination.
‡ Wheezing requiring bronchodilator therapy or with significant respiratory symptoms evaluated from randomization through 42 days post last vaccination.

Most hospitalizations observed were gastrointestinal and respiratory tract infections and occurred more than 6 weeks post vaccination. In post-hoc analysis, rates of hospitalization in children 6-11 months of age (n = 1376) were 6.1% in FluMist recipients and 2.6% in active control recipients.

Table 2 shows an analysis of pooled solicited events, occurring in at least 1% of FluMist recipients and at a higher rate compared to placebo, post Dose 1 for Study D153-P501 and AV006 and solicited events post Dose 1 for Study MI-CP111. Solicited events were those about which parents/guardians were specifically queried after vaccination with FluMist. In these studies, solicited events were documented for 10 days post vaccination. Solicited events post Dose 2 for FluMist were similar to those post Dose 1 and were generally observed at a lower frequency.

[See table 2 below]

In clinical studies D153-P501 and AV006, other adverse reactions in children occurring in at least 1% of FluMist recipients and at a higher rate compared to placebo were: abdominal pain (2% FluMist vs. 0% placebo) and otitis media (3% FluMist vs. 1% placebo).

An additional adverse reaction identified in the active-controlled trial, MI-CP111, occurring in at least 1% of FluMist recipients and at a higher rate compared to active control was sneezing (2% FluMist vs. 1% active control).

In a separate trial (MI-CP112) that compared the refrigerated and frozen formulations of FluMist in children and adults 5-49 years of age, the solicited events and other adverse events were consistent with observations from previous trials. Fever of >103°F was observed in 1 to 2% of children 5-8 years of age.

In a separate placebo-controlled trial (D153-P526) using the refrigerated formulation in a subset of older children and adolescents 9-17 years of age who received one dose of FluMist, the solicited events and other adverse events were generally consistent with observations from previous trials. Abdominal pain was reported in 12% of FluMist recipients compared to 4% of placebo recipients and decreased activity was reported in 6% of FluMist recipients compared to 0% of placebo recipients.

Adverse Reactions in Adults

In adults 18-49 years of age in Study AV009, summary of solicited adverse events occurring in at least 1% of FluMist recipients and at a higher rate compared to placebo include runny nose (44% FluMist vs. 27% placebo), headache (40% FluMist vs. 38% placebo), sore throat (28% FluMist vs. 17% placebo), tiredness/weakness (26% FluMist vs. 22% placebo), muscle aches (17% FluMist vs. 15% placebo), cough (14% FluMist vs. 11% placebo), and chills (9% FluMist vs. 6% placebo).

In addition to the solicited events, other adverse reactions from Study AV009 occurring in at least 1% of FluMist recipients and at a higher rate compared to placebo were: nasal congestion (9% FluMist vs. 2% placebo) and sinusitis (4% FluMist vs. 2% placebo).

6.2 Postmarketing Experience

The following adverse reactions have been identified during postapproval use of FluMist. Because these reactions are reported voluntarily from a population of uncertain size, it is not always possible to reliably estimate their frequency or establish a causal relationship to vaccine exposure.

Cardiac disorders: Pericarditis
Congenital, familial, and genetic disorders: Exacerbation of symptoms of mitochondrial encephalomyopathy (Leigh syndrome)
Gastrointestinal disorders: Nausea, vomiting, diarrhea
Immune system disorders: Hypersensitivity reactions (including anaphylactic reaction, facial edema, and urticaria)
Nervous system disorders: Guillain-Barré syndrome, Bell's Palsy, meningitis, eosinophilic meningitis, vaccine-associated encephalitis
Respiratory, thoracic, and mediastinal disorders: Epistaxis
Skin and subcutaneous tissue disorders: Rash

7 DRUG INTERACTIONS

7.1 Aspirin Therapy

Do not administer FluMist to children or adolescents who are receiving aspirin therapy or aspirin-containing therapy *[see Contraindications (4.2)]*.

7.2 Antiviral Agents Against Influenza A and/or B

The concurrent use of FluMist with antiviral agents that are active against influenza A and/or B viruses has not been evaluated. However, based upon the potential for antiviral agents to reduce the effectiveness of FluMist, do not administer FluMist until 48 hours after the cessation of antiviral therapy, and antiviral agents should not be administered until two weeks after administration of FluMist unless medically indicated. If antiviral agents and FluMist are administered concomitantly, revaccination should be considered when appropriate.

7.3 Concomitant Inactivated Vaccines

The safety and immunogenicity of FluMist when administered concurrently with inactivated vaccines have not been determined. Studies of FluMist excluded subjects who received any inactivated or subunit vaccine within two weeks of enrollment. Therefore, healthcare providers should consider the risks and benefits of concurrent administration of FluMist with inactivated vaccines.

7.4 Concomitant Live Vaccines

Concurrent administration of FluMist with the measles, mumps, and rubella vaccine and the varicella vaccine was studied in 1245 children 12-15 months of age. Adverse events were similar to those seen in other clinical trials with FluMist *[see Adverse Reactions (6.1)]*. No evidence of interference with immune responses to measles, mumps, rubella, varicella, and FluMist vaccines was observed. Concurrent administration of FluMist with the measles, mumps, and rubella vaccine and the varicella vaccine in children >15 months of age has not been studied.

7.5 Intranasal Products

There are no data regarding co-administration of FluMist with other intranasal preparations.

8 USE IN SPECIFIC POPULATIONS

8.1 Pregnancy

Pregnancy Category C

Animal reproduction studies have not been conducted with FluMist. It is not known whether FluMist can cause fetal harm when administered to a pregnant woman or can affect reproduction capacity. FluMist should be given to a pregnant woman only if clearly needed.

The effect of the vaccine on embryo-fetal and pre-weaning development was evaluated in a developmental toxicity study using pregnant rats receiving the frozen formulation. Groups of animals were administered the vaccine either once (during the period of organogenesis on gestation day 6) or twice (prior to gestation and during the period of organogenesis on gestation day 6), 250 microliter/rat/occasion (approximately 110-140 human dose equivalents), by intranasal instillation. No adverse effects on pregnancy, parturition, lactation, embryo-fetal or pre-weaning development were observed. There were no vaccine-related fetal malformations or other evidence of teratogenesis noted in this study.

Table 2 Summary of Solicited Events Observed within 10 Days after Dose 1 for Vaccine* and either Placebo or Active Control Recipients; Children 2-6 Years of Age

	D153-P501 & AV006		MI-CP111	
	FluMist N=876-1759‡	Placebo N=424-1034‡	FluMist N=2170‡	Active Control† N=2165‡
Event	%	%	%	%
Runny Nose/Nasal Congestion	58	50	51	42
Decreased Appetite	21	17	13	12
Irritability	21	19	12	11
Decreased Activity (Lethargy)	14	11	7	6
Sore Throat	11	9	5	6
Headache	9	7	3	3
Muscle Aches	6	3	2	2
Chills	4	3	2	2
Fever				
100-101°F Oral	9	6	6	4
101-102°F Oral	4	3	4	3

* Frozen formulation used in AV006; Refrigerated formulation used in D153-P501 and MI-CP111.
† Injectable influenza vaccine made by Sanofi Pasteur Inc.
‡ Number of evaluable subjects (those who returned diary cards) for each event. Range reflects differences in data collection between the 2 pooled studies.

8.3 Nursing Mothers

It is not known whether FluMist is excreted in human milk. Therefore, as some viruses are excreted in human milk, caution should be exercised if FluMist is administered to nursing mothers.

8.4 Pediatric Use

Safety and effectiveness of the vaccine has been demonstrated for children 2 years of age and older with reduction in culture-confirmed influenza rates compared to active control (injectable influenza vaccine made by Sanofi Pasteur Inc.) and placebo *[see Clinical Studies (14.1)]*. FluMist is not indicated for use in children <24 months of age. FluMist use in children <24 months has been associated with increased risk of hospitalization and wheezing in clinical trials *[see Warnings and Precautions (5.1) and Adverse Reactions (6.1)]*.

8.5 Geriatric Use

FluMist is not indicated for use in individuals ≥65 years of age. Subjects with underlying high-risk medical conditions (n = 200) were studied for safety. Compared to controls, FluMist recipients had a higher rate of sore throat.

8.6 Use in Individuals 50-64 Years of Age

FluMist is not indicated for use in individuals 50-64 years of age. In Study AV009, effectiveness was not demonstrated in individuals 50-64 years of age (n = 641). Solicited adverse events were similar in type and frequency to those reported in younger adults.

11 DESCRIPTION

FluMist (Influenza Vaccine Live, Intranasal) is a live trivalent vaccine for administration by intranasal spray. The influenza virus strains in FluMist are (a) *cold-adapted (ca)* (i.e., they replicate efficiently at 25°C, a temperature that is restrictive for replication of many wild-type influenza viruses); (b) *temperature-sensitive (ts)* (i.e., they are restricted in replication at 37°C (Type B strains) or 39°C (Type A strains), temperatures at which many wild-type influenza viruses grow efficiently); and (c) *attenuated (att)* (they do not produce classic influenza-like illness in the ferret model of human influenza infection). The cumulative effect of the antigenic properties and the *ca, ts,* and *att* phenotypes is that the attenuated vaccine viruses replicate in the nasopharynx to induce protective immunity.

No evidence of reversion has been observed in the recovered vaccine strains that have been tested (135 of possible 250 recovered isolates) *[see Clinical Studies (14.5)]*. For each of the three reassortant strains in FluMist, the six internal gene segments responsible for *ca, ts,* and *att* phenotypes are derived from a master donor virus (MDV), and the two segments that encode the two surface glycoproteins, hemagglutinin (HA) and neuraminidase (NA), are derived from the corresponding antigenically relevant wild-type influenza viruses that have been recommended by the USPHS for inclusion in the annual vaccine formulation. Thus, the three viruses contained in FluMist maintain the replication characteristics and phenotypic properties of the MDV and express the HA and NA of wild-type viruses that are related to strains expected to circulate during the 2010-2011 influenza season. For the Type A MDV, at least five genetic loci in three different internal gene segments contribute to the *ts* and *att* phenotypes. For the Type B MDV, at least three genetic loci in two different internal gene segments contribute to both the *ts* and *att* properties; five genetic loci in three gene segments control the *ca* property.

Specific pathogen-free (SPF) eggs are inoculated with each of the reassortant strains and incubated to allow vaccine virus replication. The allantoic fluid of these eggs is harvested, pooled and then clarified by filtration. The virus is concentrated by ultracentrifugation and diluted with stabilizing buffer to obtain the final sucrose and potassium phosphate concentrations. Ethylene diamine tetracetic acid (EDTA) is added to the dilution buffer for H3N2 strains. The viral harvests are then sterile filtered to produce the monovalent bulks. Each lot is tested for *ca, ts,* and *att* phenotypes and is also tested extensively by *in vitro* and *in vivo* methods to detect adventitious agents. Monovalent bulks from the three strains are subsequently blended and diluted as required to attain the desired potency with stabilizing buffers to produce the trivalent bulk vaccine. The bulk vaccine is then filled directly into individual sprayers for nasal administration.

Each pre-filled refrigerated FluMist sprayer contains a single 0.2 mL dose. Each 0.2 mL dose contains $10^{6.5-7.5}$ FFU of live attenuated influenza virus reassortants of each of the three strains: A/California/7/2009 (H1N1), A/Perth/16/2009 (H3N2), and B/Brisbane/60/2008. Each 0.2 mL dose also contains 0.188 mg/dose monosodium glutamate, 2.00 mg/dose hydrolyzed porcine gelatin, 2.42 mg/dose arginine, 13.68 mg/dose sucrose, 2.26 mg/dose dibasic potassium phosphate, 0.96 mg/dose monobasic potassium phosphate, and <0.015 mcg/mL gentamicin sulfate. FluMist contains no preservatives.

The tip attached to the sprayer is equipped with a nozzle that produces a fine mist that is primarily deposited in the nose and nasopharynx. FluMist is a colorless to pale yellow liquid and is clear to slightly cloudy.

Table 3 Comparative Efficacy against Culture-Confirmed Modified CDC-ILI* Caused by Wild-Type Strains in Children <5 Years of Age

	FluMist			Active Control†				
	N	# of Cases	Rate (cases/N)	N	# of Cases	Rate (cases/N)	% Reduction in Rate for FluMist‡	95% CI
Matched Strains								
All strains	3916	53	1.4%	3936	93	2.4%	44.5%	22.4, 60.6
A/H1N1	3916	3	0.1%	3936	27	0.7%	89.2%	67.7, 97.4
A/H3N2	3916	0	0.0%	3936	0	0.0%	–	–
B	3916	50	1.3%	3936	67	1.7%	27.3%	-4.8, 49.9
Mismatched Strains								
All strains	3916	102	2.6%	3936	245	6.2%	58.2%	47.4, 67.0
A/H1N1	3916	0	0.0%	3936	0	0.0%	–	–
A/H3N2	3916	37	0.9%	3936	178	4.5%	79.2%	70.6, 85.7
B	3916	66	1.7%	3936	71	1.8%	6.3%	-31.6, 33.3
Regardless of Match								
All strains	3916	153	3.9%	3936	338	8.6%	54.9%	45.4, 62.9
A/H1N1	3916	3	0.1%	3936	27	0.7%	89.2%	67.7, 97.4
A/H3N2	3916	37	0.9%	3936	178	4.5%	79.2%	70.6, 85.7
B	3916	115	2.9%	3936	136	3.5%	16.1%	-7.7, 34.7

ATP Population.

* Modified CDC-ILI was defined as fever (temperature ≥100°F oral or equivalent) plus cough, sore throat, or runny nose/nasal congestion on the same or consecutive days.

† Injectable influenza vaccine made by Sanofi Pasteur Inc.

‡ Reduction in rate was adjusted for country, age, prior influenza vaccination status, and wheezing history status.

12 CLINICAL PHARMACOLOGY

12.1 Mechanism of Action

Immune mechanisms conferring protection against influenza following receipt of FluMist vaccine are not fully understood. Likewise, naturally acquired immunity to wild-type influenza has not been completely elucidated. Serum antibodies, mucosal antibodies and influenza-specific T cells may play a role in prevention and recovery from infection. Influenza illness and its complications follow infection with influenza viruses. Global surveillance of influenza identifies yearly antigenic variants. For example, since 1977, antigenic variants of influenza A (H1N1 and H3N2) viruses and influenza B viruses have been in global circulation. Antibody against one influenza virus type or subtype confers limited or no protection against another. Furthermore, antibody to one antigenic variant of influenza virus might not protect against a new antigenic variant of the same type or subtype. Frequent development of antigenic variants through antigenic drift is the virologic basis for seasonal epidemics and the reason for the usual change of one or more new strains in each year's influenza vaccine. Therefore, influenza vaccines are standardized to contain the strains (i.e., typically two type A and one type B), representing the influenza viruses likely to be circulating in the United States in the upcoming winter.

Annual revaccination with the current vaccine is recommended because immunity declines during the year after vaccination, and because circulating strains of influenza virus change from year to year [1].

12.3 Pharmacokinetics

Biodistribution

A biodistribution study of intranasally administered radiolabeled placebo was conducted in 7 healthy adult volunteers. The mean percentage of the delivered doses detected were as follows: nasal cavity 89.7%, stomach 2.6%, brain 2.4%, and lung 0.4%. The clinical significance of these findings is unknown.

13 NONCLINICAL TOXICOLOGY

13.1 Carcinogenesis, Mutagenesis, Impairment of Fertility

FluMist has not been evaluated for its carcinogenic or mutagenic potential or its potential to impair fertility.

14 CLINICAL STUDIES

FluMist, in refrigerated and frozen formulations, was administered to approximately 35,000 subjects in controlled clinical studies. FluMist has been studied in placebo-controlled trials over multiple years, using different vaccine strains. Comparative efficacy has been studied where FluMist was compared to an inactivated influenza vaccine made by Sanofi Pasteur Inc.

14.1 Studies in Children and Adolescents

Study MI-CP111: Pediatric Comparative Study

A multinational, randomized, double-blind, active-controlled trial (MI-CP111) was performed to assess the efficacy and safety of FluMist compared to an injectable influenza vaccine made by Sanofi Pasteur Inc. (active control) in children <5 years of age, using the refrigerated formulation. During the 2004-2005 influenza season, a total number of 3916 children <5 years of age and without severe asthma, without use of bronchodilator or steroids and without wheezing within the prior 6 weeks were randomized to FluMist and 3936 were randomized to active control. Participants were then followed through the influenza season to identify illness caused by influenza virus. As the primary endpoint, culture-confirmed modified CDC-ILI (CDC-defined influenza-like illness) was defined as a positive culture for a wild-type influenza virus associated within ±7 days of modified CDC-ILI. Modified CDC-ILI was defined as fever (temperature ≥100°F oral or equivalent) plus cough, sore throat, or runny nose/nasal congestion on the same or consecutive days.

In the primary efficacy analysis, FluMist demonstrated a 44.5% (95% CI: 22.4, 60.6) reduction in influenza rate compared to active control as measured by culture-confirmed modified CDC-ILI caused by wild-type strains antigenically similar to those contained in the vaccine. See Table 3 for a description of the results by strain and antigenic similarity.

[See table 3 above]

Study D153-P501: Pediatric Study

A randomized, double-blind, placebo-controlled trial (D153-P501) was performed to evaluate the efficacy of FluMist in children 12 to 35 months of age without high-risk medical conditions against culture-confirmed influenza illness, using the refrigerated formulation. A total of 3174 children were randomized 3:2 (vaccine: placebo) to receive 2 doses of study vaccine or placebo at least 28 days apart in Year 1. See Table 4 for a description of the results.

Study AV006: Pediatric Study

AV006 was a multi-center, randomized, double-blind, placebo-controlled trial performed in U.S. children without high-risk medical conditions to evaluate the efficacy of FluMist against culture-confirmed influenza over two successive seasons using the frozen formulation. The primary endpoint of the trial was the prevention of culture-confirmed influenza illness due to antigenically matched wild-type influenza in children, who received two doses of vaccine in the first year and a single revaccination dose in the second year. During the first year of the study 1602 children 15-71 months of age were randomized 2:1 (vaccine: placebo). Approximately 85% of the participants in the first year returned for the second year of the study. In Year 2, children remained in the same treatment group as in year one and received a single dose of FluMist or placebo. See Table 4 for a description of the results.

[See table 4 at top of next page]

During the second year of Study AV006, the primary circulating strain was the A/Sydney/05/97 H3N2 strain, which was antigenically dissimilar from the H3N2 strain represented in the vaccine, A/Wuhan/359/95; FluMist demonstrated 87.0% (95% CI: 77.0, 92.6) efficacy against culture-confirmed influenza illness.

14.2 Study in Adults

AV009 was a multi-center, randomized, double-blind, placebo-controlled trial to evaluate effectiveness in adults 18-64 years of age without high-risk medical conditions.

Table 4 Efficacy* of FluMist vs. Placebo against Culture-Confirmed Influenza Illness due to Antigenically Matched Wild-Type Strains (D153-P501 & AV006, Year 1)

	D153-P501			AV006		
	FluMist n[†] (%)	Placebo n[†] (%)	% Efficacy (95% CI)	FluMist n[†] (%)	Placebo n[†] (%)	% Efficacy (95% CI)
	N[‡]=1653	N[‡]=1111		N[‡]=849	N[‡]=410	
Any strain	56 (3.4%)	139 (12.5%)	72.9%[§] (62.8, 80.5)	10 (1%)	73 (18%)	93.4% (87.5, 96.5)
A/H1N1	23 (1.4%)	81 (7.3%)	80.9% (69.4, 88.5)[¶]	0	0	–
A/H3N2	4 (0.2%)	27 (2.4%)	90.0% (71.4, 97.5)	4 (0.5%)	48 (12%)	96.0% (89.4, 98.5)
B	29 (1.8%)	35 (3.2%)	44.3% (6.2, 67.2)	6 (0.7%)	31 (7%)	90.5% (78.0, 95.9)

* D153-P501 and AV006 data are for subjects who received two doses of study vaccine.
† Number and percent of subjects in per-protocol efficacy analysis population with culture-confirmed influenza illness.
‡ Number of subjects in per-protocol efficacy analysis population of each treatment group of each study for the "any strain" analysis.
§ For D153-P501, influenza circulated through 12 months following vaccination.
¶ Estimate includes A/H1N1 and A/H1N2 strains. Both were considered antigenically similar to the vaccine.

Table 5 Effectiveness of FluMist* in Adults 18–49 Years of Age During the 7-week Site-Specific Outbreak Period

Endpoint	FluMist N=2411[†] n (%)	Placebo N=1226[†] n (%)	Percent Reduction	(95% CI)
Participants with one or more events of:[‡]				
Primary Endpoint:				
Any febrile illness	331 (13.73)	189 (15.42)	10.9	(-5.1, 24.4)
Secondary Endpoints:				
Severe febrile illness	250 (10.37)	158 (12.89)	19.5	(3.0, 33.2)
Febrile upper respiratory illness	213 (8.83)	142 (11.58)	23.7	(6.7, 37.5)

* Frozen formulation used.
† Number of evaluable subjects (92.7% and 93.0% of FluMist and placebo recipients, respectively).
‡ The predominantly circulating virus during the trial period was A/Sydney/05/97 (H3N2), an antigenic variant not included in the vaccine.

Participants were randomized 2:1 (vaccine: placebo). Cultures for influenza virus were not obtained from subjects in the trial, so that the efficacy against culture-confirmed influenza was not assessed. The A/Wuhan/359/95 (H3N2) strain, which was contained in FluMist, was antigenically distinct from the predominant circulating strain of influenza virus during the trial period, A/Sydney/05/97 (H3N2). Type A/Wuhan (H3N2) and Type B strains also circulated in the U.S. during the study period. The primary endpoint of the trial was the reduction in the proportion of participants with one or more episodes of any febrile illness, and prospective secondary endpoints were severe febrile illness and febrile upper respiratory illness. Effectiveness for any of the three endpoints was not demonstrated in a subgroup of adults 50-64 years of age. Primary and secondary effectiveness endpoints from the age group 18-49 years of age are presented in Table 5. Effectiveness was not demonstrated for the primary endpoint in adults 18-49 years of age.
[See table 5 above]
Effectiveness was shown in a post-hoc analysis using CDC-ILI in the age group 18-49 years.

14.3 Study in Adults with Human Immunodeficiency Virus (HIV) Infection

Safety and shedding of vaccine virus following FluMist administration were evaluated in 57 HIV-infected [median CD4 cell count of 541 cells/mm³] and 54 HIV-negative adults 18-58 years of age in a randomized, double-blind, placebo-controlled trial using the frozen formulation. No serious adverse events were reported during the one-month follow-up period. Vaccine strain (type B) virus was detected in 1 of 28 HIV-infected subjects on Day 5 and none of the HIV-negative FluMist recipients. No adverse effects on HIV viral load or CD4 counts were identified following FluMist. The effectiveness of FluMist in preventing influenza illness in HIV-infected individuals has not been evaluated.

14.4 Refrigerated Formulation Study

A double-blind, randomized, multi-center trial was conducted to evaluate the comparative immunogenicity and safety of refrigerated and frozen formulations of FluMist in individuals 5 to 49 years of age without high-risk medical conditions. Nine hundred and eighty-one subjects were randomized at a 1:1 ratio to receive either vaccine formulation. Subjects 5-8 years of age received two doses of study vaccine 46-60 days apart; subjects 9-49 years of age received one dose of study vaccine. The study met its primary endpoint. The GMT ratios of refrigerated and frozen formulations (adjusted for baseline serostatus) for H1N1, H3N2, and B

strains, respectively, were 1.24, 1.02, and 1.00 in the two dose group and 1.14, 1.12, and 0.96 in the one dose group.

14.5 Transmission Study

FluMist contains live attenuated influenza viruses that must infect and replicate in cells lining the nasopharynx of the recipient to induce immunity. Vaccine viruses capable of infection and replication can be cultured from nasal secretions obtained from vaccine recipients.
The relationship of viral replication in a vaccine recipient and transmission of vaccine viruses to other individuals has not been established.
Using the frozen formulation, a prospective, randomized, double-blind, placebo-controlled trial was performed in a daycare setting in children <3 years of age to assess the transmission of vaccine viruses from a vaccinated individual to a non-vaccinated individual. A total of 197 children 8-36 months of age were randomized to receive one dose of FluMist (n = 98) or placebo (n = 99). Virus shedding was evaluated for 21 days by culture of nasal swab specimens. Wild-type A (H3N2) influenza virus was documented to have circulated in the community and in the study population during the trial, whereas Type A (H1N1) and Type B strains did not.
At least one vaccine strain was isolated from 80% of FluMist recipients; strains were recovered from 1-21 days post vaccination (mean duration of 7.6 days ± 3.4 days). The cold-adapted (ca) and temperature-sensitive (ts) phenotypes were preserved in 135 tested of 250 strains isolated at the local laboratory. Ten influenza isolates (9 influenza A, 1 influenza B) were cultured from a total of seven placebo subjects. One placebo subject had mild symptomatic Type B virus infection confirmed as a transmitted vaccine virus by a FluMist recipient in the same playgroup. This Type B isolate retained the ca, ts, and att phenotypes of the vaccine strain, and had the same genetic sequence when compared to a Type B virus cultured from a vaccine recipient within the same playgroup. Four of the influenza Type A isolates were confirmed as wild-type A/Panama (H3N2). The remaining isolates could not be further characterized.
Assuming a single transmission event (isolation of the Type B vaccine strain), the probability of a young child acquiring vaccine virus following close contact with a single FluMist vaccinee in this daycare setting was 0.58% (95% CI: 0, 1.7) based on the Reed-Frost model. With documented transmission of one Type B in one placebo subject and possible transmission of Type A viruses in four placebo subjects, the probability of acquiring a transmitted vaccine virus was estimated to be 2.4% (95% CI: 0.13, 4.6), using the Reed-Frost model.

15 REFERENCES

1. Centers for Disease Control and Prevention. Prevention and Control of Influenza: Recommendations of the Advisory Committee on Immunization Practices (ACIP). MMWR 2009; 58(RR-8): 1-52.

16 HOW SUPPLIED/STORAGE AND HANDLING

FluMist is supplied for intranasal delivery in a package of 10 pre-filled, single-use sprayers. The single-use intranasal sprayer contains no latex.
NDC 66019-108-10
Storage and Handling
Once FluMist has been administered, the sprayer should be disposed of according to the standard procedures for medical waste (e.g., sharps container or biohazard container).
**FLUMIST SHOULD BE STORED IN A REFRIGERATOR BETWEEN 2-8°C (35-46°F) UPON RECEIPT AND UNTIL USE. THE PRODUCT MUST BE USED BEFORE THE EXPIRATION DATE ON THE SPRAYER LABEL.
DO NOT FREEZE.**
The cold chain (2 to 8°C) must be maintained when transporting FluMist.

17 PATIENT COUNSELING INFORMATION

See FDA-approved patient labeling (Information for Patients and Their Caregivers).
Vaccine recipients or their parents/guardians should be informed by the health care provider of the potential benefits and risks of FluMist, and the need for two doses at least 1 month apart in children 2-8 years old who have not previously received influenza vaccine.

17.1 Asthma and Recurrent Wheezing

Ask the vaccinee or their parent/guardian if the vaccinee has asthma. For children <5 years of age, also ask if the vaccinee has recurrent wheezing since this may be an asthma equivalent in this age group.

17.2 Vaccination with a Live Virus Vaccine

Vaccine recipients or their parents/guardians should be informed by the health care provider that FluMist is an attenuated live virus vaccine and has the potential for transmission to immunocompromised household contacts.

17.3 Adverse Event Reporting

The vaccine recipient or the parent/guardian accompanying the vaccine recipient should be told to report any suspected adverse events to the physician or clinic where the vaccine was administered.
FluMist® is a registered trademark of MedImmune, LLC.
Manufactured by:
MedImmune, LLC
Gaithersburg, MD 20878
1-877-633-4411
U.S. Government License No. 1799
Issue Date: July 2010 RAL-FLUV10

INFORMATION FOR PATIENTS AND THEIR CAREGIVERS

FluMist® (pronounced FLEW-mĭst)
(Influenza Vaccine Live, Intranasal)
Please read this Patient Information carefully before you or your child is vaccinated with FluMist.
This is a summary of information about FluMist. It does not take the place of talking with your healthcare provider about influenza vaccination. If you have questions or would like more information, please talk with your healthcare provider.
What is FluMist?
FluMist is a vaccine that is sprayed into the nose to help protect against influenza. It can be used in children, adolescents, and adults ages 2 through 49. FluMist may not prevent influenza in everyone who gets vaccinated.
Who should not get FluMist?
You should not get FluMist if you:
• are allergic to eggs, gentamicin, gelatin, or arginine
• have ever had a life-threatening reaction to influenza vaccinations
• are 2 through 17 years old and take aspirin or medicines containing aspirin

Please talk to your healthcare provider if you are not sure if the items listed above apply to you or your child.

Children under 2 years of age should not get FluMist because there is a chance they may wheeze (difficulty with breathing) after getting FluMist.
Who may not be able to get FluMist?
Tell your healthcare provider if you:
• are currently wheezing
• have a history of wheezing if under 5 years old
• have had Guillain-Barré syndrome
• have a weakened immune system or live with someone who has a severely weakened immune system
• have problems with your heart, kidneys, or lungs
• have diabetes
• are pregnant or nursing
• are taking Tamiflu®, Relenza®, amantadine, or rimantadine

If you or your child cannot take FluMist you may still be able to get an influenza shot. Talk to your healthcare provider about this.

How is FluMist given?

- FluMist is a liquid that is sprayed into the nose.
- You can breathe normally while getting FluMist. There is no need to inhale or "sniff" it.
- People over 8 years old need one dose of FluMist each year.
- Children 2 through 8 years old may need 2 doses of FluMist if they have not been vaccinated against influenza before. Your healthcare provider will decide if your child needs to come back for a second dose.

What are the possible side effects of FluMist?

The most common side effects of FluMist are:

- runny or stuffy nose
- sore throat
- fever over 100°

Other possible side effects include:

- decreased appetite
- irritability
- tiredness
- cough
- headache
- muscle ache
- chills

Call your healthcare provider or go to the emergency department right away if you or your child experience:

- hives or a bad rash
- trouble breathing
- swelling of the face, tongue, or throat

These are not all the possible side effects of FluMist. You can ask your healthcare provider for a complete list of side effects that is available to healthcare professionals.

Call your healthcare provider for medical advice about side effects. You may report side effects to VAERS at 1-800-822-7967 or *http://vaers.hhs.gov*.

What are the ingredients in FluMist?

Active Ingredient: FluMist contains 3 influenza virus strains that are weakened (A(H1N1), A(H3N2), and B).

Inactive Ingredients: monosodium glutamate, gelatin, arginine, sucrose, dibasic potassium phosphate, monobasic potassium phosphate, and gentamicin

FluMist does not contain preservatives.

If you would like more information, talk to your healthcare provider or visit *www.FluMist.com* or call 1-877-633-4411.

FluMist® is a registered trademark of MedImmune, LLC.

Other brands listed are registered trademarks of their respective owners and are not trademarks of MedImmune, LLC.

Manufactured by:
MedImmune, LLC
Gaithersburg, MD 20878

Issue date: July 2010 RAL-FLUV10

Shown in Product Identification Guide, page 311

SYNAGIS® ℞

[SĪ-nă-jĭs]

(palivizumab)
for Intramuscular Administration
Rx only

DESCRIPTION

Synagis (palivizumab) is a humanized monoclonal antibody (IgG1κ) produced by recombinant DNA technology, directed to an epitope in the A antigenic site of the F protein of respiratory syncytial virus (RSV). Synagis is a composite of human (95%) and murine (5%) antibody sequences. The human heavy chain sequence was derived from the constant domains of human IgG1 and the variable framework regions of the V_H genes Cor (1) and Cess (2). The human light chain sequence was derived from the constant domain of Cκ and the variable framework regions of the V_L gene K104 with Jκ-4 (3). The murine sequences were derived from a murine monoclonal antibody, Mab 1129 (4), in a process that involved the grafting of the murine complementarity determining regions into the human antibody frameworks. Synagis is composed of two heavy chains and two light chains and has a molecular weight of approximately 148,000 Daltons.

Synagis is supplied as a sterile, preservative-free liquid solution at 100 mg/mL to be administered by intramuscular injection (IM). Thimerosal or other mercury containing salts are not used in the production of Synagis. The solution has a pH of 6.0 and should appear clear or slightly opalescent.

Each 100 mg single-dose vial of Synagis liquid solution contains 100 mg of Synagis, 3.9 mg of histidine, 0.1 mg of glycine, and 0.5 mg of chloride in a volume of 1 mL.

Each 50 mg single-dose vial of Synagis liquid solution contains 50 mg of Synagis, 1.9 mg of histidine, 0.06 mg of glycine, and 0.2 mg of chloride in a volume of 0.5 mL.

Table 1: Incidence of RSV Hospitalization by Treatment Group

Trial		Placebo	Synagis	Difference Between Groups	Relative Reduction	p-Value
Trial 1 Impact-RSV	N	500	1002			
	Hospitalization	53 (10.6%)	48 (4.8%)	5.8%	55%	<0.001
Trial 2 CHD	N	648	639			
	Hospitalization	63 (9.7%)	34 (5.3%)	4.4%	45%	0.003

CLINICAL PHARMACOLOGY

Mechanism of Action: Synagis exhibits neutralizing and fusion-inhibitory activity against RSV. These activities inhibit RSV replication in laboratory experiments. Although resistant RSV strains may be isolated in laboratory studies, a panel of 57 clinical RSV isolates were all neutralized by Synagis (5). Synagis serum concentrations of ≥ 40 mcg/mL have been shown to reduce pulmonary RSV replication in the cotton rat model of RSV infection by 100-fold (5). The *in vivo* neutralizing activity of the active ingredient in Synagis was assessed in a randomized, placebo-controlled study of 35 pediatric patients tracheally intubated because of RSV disease. In these patients, Synagis significantly reduced the quantity of RSV in the lower respiratory tract compared to control patients (6).

Pharmacokinetics: In pediatric patients < 24 months of age without congenital heart disease (CHD), the mean half-life of Synagis was 20 days and monthly intramuscular doses of 15 mg/kg achieved mean ±SD 30 day trough serum drug concentrations of 37 ± 21 mcg/mL after the first injection, 57 ± 41 mcg/mL after the second injection, 68 ± 51 mcg/mL after the third injection and 72 ± 50 mcg/mL after the fourth injection (7). Trough concentrations following the first and fourth Synagis dose were similar in children with CHD and in non-cardiac patients. In pediatric patients given Synagis for a second season, the mean ±SD serum concentrations following the first and fourth injections were 61 ± 17 mcg/mL and 86 ± 31mcg/mL, respectively.

In 139 pediatric patients ≤ 24 months of age with hemodynamically significant CHD who received Synagis and underwent cardio-pulmonary bypass for open-heart surgery, the mean ±SD serum Synagis concentration was 98 ± 52 mcg/mL before bypass and declined to 41 ± 33 mcg/mL after bypass, a reduction of 58% (see *DOSAGE AND ADMINISTRATION*). The clinical significance of this reduction is unknown.

Specific studies were not conducted to evaluate the effects of demographic parameters on Synagis systemic exposure. However, no effects of gender, age, body weight or race on Synagis serum trough concentrations were observed in a clinical study with 639 pediatric patients with CHD (≤24 months of age) receiving five monthly intramuscular injections of 15 mg/kg of Synagis.

The pharmacokinetics and safety of Synagis liquid solution and Synagis lyophilized formulation administered IM at 15 mg/kg were studied in a cross-over trial of 153 pediatric patients ≤6 months of age with a history of prematurity. The results of this trial indicated that the trough serum concentrations of palivizumab were comparable between the liquid solution and the lyophilized formulation, which was the formulation used in the clinical studies described below.

CLINICAL STUDIES

The safety and efficacy of Synagis were assessed in two randomized, double-blind, placebo-controlled trials of prophylaxis against RSV infection in pediatric patients at high risk of an RSV-related hospitalization. Trial 1 was conducted during a single RSV season and studied a total of 1,502 patients ≤ 24 months of age with bronchopulmonary dysplasia (BPD) or infants with premature birth (≤ 35 weeks gestation) who were ≤ 6 months of age at study entry (7). Trial 2 was conducted over four consecutive seasons among a total of 1287 patients ≤ 24 months of age with hemodynamically significant congenital heart disease. In both trials participants received 15 mg/kg Synagis or an equivalent volume of placebo IM monthly for five injections and were followed for 150 days from randomization. In Trial 1, 99% of all subjects completed the study and 93% completed all five injections. In Trial 2, 96% of all subjects completed the study and 92% completed all five injections. The incidence of RSV hospitalization is shown in Table 1.

[See table 1 above]

In Trial 1, the reduction of RSV hospitalization was observed both in patients with BPD (34/266 [12.8%] placebo vs. 39/496 [7.9%] Synagis), and in premature infants without BPD (19/234 [8.1%] placebo vs. 9/506 [1.8%] Synagis). In Trial 2, reductions were observed in acyanotic (36/305 [11.8%] placebo versus 15/300 [5.0%] Synagis) and cyanotic children (27/343 [7.9%] placebo versus 19/339 [5.6%] Synagis).

The clinical studies do not suggest that RSV infection was less severe among RSV hospitalized patients who received Synagis compared to those who received placebo.

INDICATIONS AND USAGE

Synagis is indicated for the prevention of serious lower respiratory tract disease caused by respiratory syncytial virus (RSV) in pediatric patients at high risk of RSV disease. Safety and efficacy were established in infants with bronchopulmonary dysplasia (BPD), infants with a history of premature birth (≤ 35 weeks gestational age), and children with hemodynamically significant congenital heart disease (CHD) (see *CLINICAL STUDIES*).

CONTRAINDICATIONS

Synagis should not be used in pediatric patients with a history of a severe prior reaction to Synagis or other components of this product.

WARNINGS

Very rare cases of anaphylaxis including anaphylactic shock (<1 case per 100,000 patients) have been reported following initial exposure or re-exposure to Synagis (see *ADVERSE REACTIONS, Post-Marketing Experience*). Severe acute hypersensitivity reactions, estimated to be rare, (<1 case per 1,000 patients) have also been reported on initial exposure or re-exposure to Synagis (see *ADVERSE REACTIONS, Post-Marketing Experience*). If a severe hypersensitivity reaction occurs, therapy with Synagis should be permanently discontinued. If milder hypersensitivity reactions occur, caution should be used on readministration of Synagis. **If anaphylaxis or severe allergic reactions occur, administer appropriate medications (e.g., epinephrine) and provide supportive care as required.**

PRECAUTIONS

General: Synagis is for intramuscular use only. As with any intramuscular injection, Synagis should be given with caution to patients with thrombocytopenia or any coagulation disorder.

The safety and efficacy of Synagis have not been demonstrated for treatment of established RSV disease.

The single-dose vial of Synagis does not contain a preservative. Administration of Synagis should occur immediately after dose withdrawal from the vial. The vial should not be re-entered. Discard any unused portion.

Drug Interactions: No formal drug-drug interaction studies were conducted. In Trial 1, the proportions of patients in the placebo and Synagis groups who received routine childhood vaccines, influenza vaccine, bronchodilators or corticosteroids were similar and no incremental increase in adverse reactions was observed among patients receiving these agents.

Carcinogenesis, Mutagenesis, Impairment of Fertility: Carcinogenesis, mutagenesis and reproductive toxicity studies have not been performed.

Pregnancy: Pregnancy Category C: Synagis is not indicated for adult usage and animal reproduction studies have not been conducted. It is also not known whether Synagis can cause fetal harm when administered to a pregnant woman or could affect reproductive capacity.

ADVERSE REACTIONS

The most serious adverse reactions occurring with Synagis treatment are anaphylaxis and other acute hypersensitivity reactions (see *WARNINGS*). The adverse reactions most commonly observed in Synagis-treated patients were upper respiratory tract infection, otitis media, fever, rhinitis, rash, diarrhea, cough, vomiting, gastroenteritis, and wheezing. Upper respiratory tract infection, otitis media, fever, and rhinitis occurred at a rate of 1% or greater in the Synagis group compared to placebo (Table 2).

Because clinical trials are conducted under widely varying conditions, adverse event rates observed in the clinical tri-

Table 2 - Adverse Events Occurring at a Rate of 1% or Greater More Frequently in Patients[†] Receiving Synagis

Event	Synagis (n=1641) n (%)	Placebo (n=1148) n (%)
Upper respiratory infection	830 (50.6)	544 (47.4)
Otitis media	597 (36.4)	397 (34.6)
Fever	446 (27.1)	289 (25.2)
Rhinitis	439 (26.8)	282 (24.6)
Hernia	68 (4.1)	30 (2.6)
SGOT Increase	49 (3.0)	20 (1.7)

[†]Cyanosis (Synagis [9.1%]/placebo [6.9%]) and arrhythmia (Synagis [3.1%]/placebo [1.7%]) were reported during Trial 2 in CHD patients.

als of a drug cannot be directly compared to rates in the clinical trials of another drug and may not reflect the rates observed in practice. The adverse reaction information does, however, provide a basis for identifying the adverse events that appear to be related to drug use and a basis for approximating rates.

The data described reflect Synagis exposure for 1641 pediatric patients of age 3 days to 24.1 months in Trials 1 and 2. Among these patients, 496 had bronchopulmonary dysplasia, 506 were premature birth infants less than 6 months of age, and 639 had congenital heart disease. Adverse events observed in the 153 patient crossover study comparing the liquid and lyophilized formulations were similar between the two formulations, and similar to the adverse events observed with Synagis in Trials 1 and 2.

[See table 2 above]

Immunogenicity

In Trial 1, the incidence of anti-Synagis antibody following the fourth injection was 1.1% in the placebo group and 0.7% in the Synagis group. In pediatric patients receiving Synagis for a second season, one of the fifty-six patients had transient, low titer reactivity. This reactivity was not associated with adverse events or alteration in serum concentrations. Immunogenicity was not assessed in Trial 2.

These data reflect the percentage of patients whose test results were considered positive for antibodies to Synagis in an ELISA assay, and are highly dependent on the sensitivity and specificity of the assay. Additionally, the observed incidence of antibody positivity in an assay may be influenced by several factors including sample handling, concomitant medications, and underlying disease. For these reasons, comparison of the incidence of antibodies to Synagis with the incidence of antibodies to other products may be misleading.

With any monoclonal antibody, the possibility exists that a liquid solution may be more immunogenic than a lyophilized formulation. The relative immunogenicity rates between the lyophilized formulation, used in Trials 1 and 2 above, and the liquid solution have not yet been established.

Post-Marketing Experience

The following adverse reactions have been identified and reported during post-approval use of Synagis. Because the reports of these reactions are voluntary and the population is of uncertain size, it is not always possible to reliably estimate the frequency of the reaction or establish a causal relationship to drug exposure.

Blood and Lymphatic System Disorders: severe thrombocytopenia (platelet count < 50,000/microliter)

General Disorders and Administration Site Conditions: injection site reactions

Immune System Disorders: severe acute hypersensitivity reactions and anaphylaxis (including dyspnea, cyanosis, respiratory failure, urticaria, pruritus, angioedema, hypotonia, hypotension and unresponsiveness) have been reported (see *WARNINGS*). None of the reported hypersensitivity reactions were fatal. The relationship between these reactions and the development of antibodies to Synagis is unknown. Limited information from post-marketing reports suggests that, within a single RSV season, adverse events after a sixth or greater dose of Synagis are similar in character and frequency to those after the initial five doses.

OVERDOSAGE

No data from clinical studies are available on overdosage. No toxicity was observed in rabbits administered a single intramuscular or subcutaneous injection of Synagis at a dose of 50 mg/kg.

DOSAGE AND ADMINISTRATION

The recommended dose of Synagis is 15 mg/kg of body weight. Patients, including those who develop an RSV infection, should continue to receive monthly doses throughout the RSV season. The first dose should be administered prior to commencement of the RSV season. In the northern hemisphere, the RSV season typically commences in November and lasts through April, but it may begin earlier or persist later in certain communities.

Synagis serum levels are decreased after cardio-pulmonary bypass (see *CLINICAL PHARMACOLOGY*). Patients undergoing cardio-pulmonary bypass should receive a dose of Synagis as soon as possible after the cardio-pulmonary bypass procedure (even if sooner than a month from the previous dose). Thereafter, doses should be administered monthly.

Synagis should be administered in a dose of 15 mg/kg intramuscularly using aseptic technique, preferably in the anterolateral aspect of the thigh. The gluteal muscle should not be used routinely as an injection site because of the risk of damage to the sciatic nerve. The dose per month = patient weight (kg) × 15 mg/kg ÷ 100 mg/mL of Synagis. Injection volumes over 1 mL should be given as a divided dose.

Administration of Synagis

- **DO NOT DILUTE THE PRODUCT**
- **DO NOT SHAKE OR VIGOROUSLY AGITATE THE VIAL**
- Parenteral drug products should be inspected visually for particulate matter and discoloration prior to administration. Do not use any vials exhibiting particulate matter or discoloration.
- Using aseptic techniques, attach a sterile needle to a sterile syringe. Remove the flip top from the Synagis vial, and wipe the rubber stopper with a disinfectant (e.g., 70% isopropyl alcohol). Insert the needle into the vial, and withdraw into the syringe an appropriate volume of solution. Administer immediately after drawing the dose into the syringe.
- Synagis is supplied as a single-dose vial and does not contain preservatives. Do not re-enter the vial after withdrawal of drug; discard unused portion. Only administer one dose per vial.
- To prevent the transmission of hepatitis viruses or other infectious agents from one person to another, sterile disposable syringes and needles should be used. DO NOT reuse syringes and needles.

HOW SUPPLIED

Synagis is supplied in single-dose vials as a preservative-free, sterile liquid solution at 100 mg/mL for IM injection.
50 mg vial NDC 60574-4114-1
The 50 mg vial contains 50 mg Synagis in 0.5 mL.
100 mg vial NDC 60574-4113-1
The 100 mg vial contains 100 mg Synagis in 1 mL.
There is no latex in the rubber stopper used for sealing vials of Synagis. Upon receipt and until use, Synagis should be stored between 2°C and 8°C (35.6°F and 46.4°F) in its original container. DO NOT freeze. DO NOT use beyond the expiration date.

REFERENCES

1. Press E, and Hogg N. The Amino Acid Sequences of the Fd Fragments of Two Human Gamma-1 Heavy Chains. Biochem. J. 1970; 117:641-660.
2. Takahashi N, Noma T, and Honjo T. Rearranged Immunoglobulin Heavy Chain Variable Region (V_H) Pseudogene that Deletes the Second Complementarity-Determining Region. Proc. Nat. Acad. Sci. USA 1984; 81: 5194-5198.
3. Bentley D, and Rabbitts T. Human Immunoglobulin Variable Region Genes - DNA Sequences of Two V_K Genes and a Pseudogene. Nature 1980; 288:730-733.
4. Beeler JA, and Van Wyke Coelingh K. Neutralization Epitopes of the F Protein of Respiratory Syncytial Virus: Effect of Mutation Upon Fusion Function. J. Virology 1989; 63:2941-2950.
5. Johnson S, Oliver C, Prince GA, et al. Development of a Humanized Monoclonal Antibody (MEDI-493) with Potent In Vitro and In Vivo Activity Against Respiratory Syncytial Virus. J. Infect. Dis. 1997; 176:1215-1224.
6. Malley R, DeVincenzo J, Ramilo O, et al. Reduction of Respiratory Syncytial Virus (RSV) in Tracheal Aspirates in Intubated Infants by Use of Humanized Monoclonal Antibody to RSV F Protein. J. Infect. Dis. 1998; 178:1555-1561.
7. The IMpact RSV Study Group. Palivizumab, a Humanized Respiratory Syncytial Virus Monoclonal Antibody, Reduces Hospitalization From Respiratory Syncytial Virus Infection in High-Risk Infants. Pediatrics 1998; 102: 531-537.

Synagis® is a registered trademark of MedImmune, LLC
Manufactured by:
MedImmune, LLC
Gaithersburg, MD 20878
U.S. Gov't. License No. 1799
(1-877-633-4411)
Revision Date: July 2010   RAL-SYNV13

INFORMATION FOR PATIENTS AND THEIR CAREGIVERS

SYNAGIS® (SĬ-nă-jĭs)
(palivizumab)
Read this Patient Information before your child starts receiving SYNAGIS and before each injection. The information may have changed. This leaflet does not take the place of talking with your child's healthcare provider about your child's condition or treatment.

What is SYNAGIS?
SYNAGIS is a prescription medication that is used to help prevent a serious lung disease caused by Respiratory Syncytial Virus (RSV). Your child is prescribed SYNAGIS because he or she is at high risk for severe lung disease from RSV.

SYNAGIS contains man-made, disease-fighting proteins called antibodies. These antibodies help prevent RSV disease. Children at high risk for severe RSV disease often do not have enough of their own antibodies. SYNAGIS is used in certain groups of children to help prevent severe RSV disease by increasing protective RSV antibodies.

SYNAGIS is not used to treat the symptoms of RSV disease, once a child already has it. It is only used to prevent RSV disease.
SYNAGIS is not for adults.

Who should not receive SYNAGIS?
Your child should not receive SYNAGIS if they have ever had a severe allergic reaction to it or any of its ingredients. Signs and symptoms of a severe allergic reaction could include:
- a drop in blood pressure
- severe rash, hives or itching skin
- difficult, rapid or irregular breathing
- closing of the throat, difficulty swallowing
- swelling of the lips, tongue, or face
- bluish color of skin, lips or under fingernails
- muscle weakness or floppiness
- unresponsiveness

See the end of this leaflet for a list of ingredients in SYNAGIS.

What should I tell my child's healthcare provider before my child receives SYNAGIS?
Tell your child's healthcare provider about:
- **Any reactions** you believe your child has ever had to SYNAGIS.
- All your child's medical problems, including **any bleeding or bruising problems**. SYNAGIS is given by injection. If your child has a problem with bleeding or bruises easily, an injection could cause a problem.
- **All the medicines your child takes, including prescription and non-prescription medicines, vitamins, and herbal supplements**. Especially tell your child's healthcare provider if your child takes a blood thinner medicine.

How is SYNAGIS given?
- SYNAGIS is given as a monthly injection, usually in the thigh (leg) muscle, by your child's healthcare provider. Your child's healthcare provider will prescribe the amount of SYNAGIS that is right for your child (based on their weight).
- Your child's healthcare provider will give you detailed instructions on when SYNAGIS will be given.
  - "RSV season" is a term used to describe the time of year when RSV infections most commonly occur (usually fall through spring). During this time, when RSV is most active, your child will need to receive SYNAGIS shots. Your child's healthcare provider can tell you when the RSV season starts in your area.

- Your child should receive their **first SYNAGIS shot before the RSV season starts** to help protect them before RSV becomes active. If the season has already started, your child should receive their first SYNAGIS shot as soon as possible to help protect them when exposure to the virus is more likely.
- **SYNAGIS is needed every 28-30 days during the RSV season.** Each dose of SYNAGIS helps protect your child from severe RSV disease for about a month. **Keep all appointments with your child's healthcare provider.**
- If your child misses an injection, talk to your healthcare provider and schedule another injection as soon as possible.
- Your child may still get severe RSV disease after receiving SYNAGIS. Talk to your child's healthcare provider about what symptoms to look for.
- If your child already has an RSV infection and is sick, they still need to get their scheduled SYNAGIS injections to help prevent severe disease from new RSV infections.
- If your child has certain types of heart disease and has corrective surgery, your healthcare provider may need to give your child an additional SYNAGIS injection soon after surgery.

What are the possible side effects of SYNAGIS?

Over one million babies have been given SYNAGIS. Like all medicines, SYNAGIS has been associated with side effects in some patients. Most of the time, the side effects are not serious. If side effects do occur, your child may need medical attention.

Possible, serious side effects include:

- Severe allergic reactions (may occur after any dose of SYNAGIS). See "Who should not take SYNAGIS?" for a list of signs and symptoms.
- Unusual bruising and/or groups of tiny red spots on the skin.

Call your child's healthcare provider or get medical help right away if your child has any of the serious side effects listed above after any dose of SYNAGIS.

Common side effects of SYNAGIS include:

- fever
- cold-like symptoms (upper respiratory infection), including runny nose and ear infection
- rash

Other possible side effects include skin reactions around the area where the shot was given (like redness, swelling, warmth, or discomfort).

In children born with certain types of heart disease, other possible side effects include bluish color of the skin, lips or under fingernails and abnormal heart rhythms.

These are not all the possible side effects of SYNAGIS. Tell your child's healthcare provider about any side effect that bothers your child or that does not go away.

Call your healthcare provider for medical advice about side effects. You may report side effects to FDA at 1-800-FDA-1088 or call MedImmune at 1-877-633-4411.

General Information about SYNAGIS

Medicines are sometimes prescribed for purposes other than those listed in Patient Information leaflets.

This leaflet summarizes important information about SYNAGIS. If you would like more information, talk with your healthcare provider. You can ask your pharmacist or healthcare provider for information about SYNAGIS that is written for health professionals.

For more information, go to www.synagis.com or call 1-877-633-4411.

What are the ingredients in SYNAGIS?

Active Ingredient: palivizumab

Inactive Ingredients: histidine, glycine, and chloride

What is RSV?

Respiratory Syncytial Virus (RSV) is a common virus that is easily spread from person to person. RSV infects nearly all children by their second birthday. In most children, RSV infection is usually no worse than a bad cold. For some children, RSV infection can cause serious lung disease (like pneumonia and bronchiolitis) or breathing problems, and affected children may need to be admitted to the hospital or need emergency care.

Children who are more likely to get severe RSV disease (high risk children) include babies born prematurely (35 weeks or less), or babies born with certain heart or lung problems.

Issued July 2010 RAL-SYNV13

Synagis® is a registered trademark of MedImmune, LLC.

Manufactured by: MedImmune, LLC

Gaithersburg, MD 20878

Shown in Product Identification Guide, page 311

Merck

ONE MERCK DRIVE
P.O. BOX 100
WHITEHOUSE STATION, NJ 08889

For updates to the product information listed below, please check the Merck Web site, http://www.merck.com, or call 1-866-342-5683. For complete product listing, please see the Manufacturers' Index.

Direct inquiries, including 24-hour emergency information to healthcare professionals, to:

The Merck National Service Center at

(800) NSC-MERCK

(800) 672-6372

Merck U.S. operating companies include:

Merck, Sharp & Dohme Corp.

Schering Corporation

Product Identification Codes

To provide quick and positive identification of Schering products, we have imprinted the product identification number of the National Drug Code on most tablets and capsules. In some cases, identification letters also appear. Additionally, the following telephone number is provided for inquiries:

Global Medical Information
1-800-526-4099

AMINOHIPPURATE SODIUM "PAH" ℞

[am-ino-hip-pur-ate]
Injection

DESCRIPTION

Aminohippurate sodium[1] is an agent to measure effective renal plasma flow (ERPF). It is the sodium salt of para-aminohippuric acid, commonly abbreviated "PAH". It is water soluble, lipid-insoluble, and has a pKa of 3.83. The empirical formula of the anhydrous salt is $C_9H_9N_2NaO_3$ and its structural formula is:

$$H_2N-\!\!\!\left\langle\,\right\rangle\!\!\!-CONHCH_2COONa$$

It is provided as a sterile, non-preserved 20 percent aqueous solution for injection, with a pH of 6.7 to 7.6. Each 10 mL contains: Aminohippurate sodium 2 g. Inactive ingredients: Sodium hydroxide to adjust pH, water for injection, q.s.

[1] Formerly referred to as Sodium para-Aminohippurate.
Copyright © 1983 Merck Sharp & Dohme Corp., a subsidiary of **Merck & Co., Inc.**
All rights reserved

CLINICAL PHARMACOLOGY

PAH is filtered by the glomeruli and is actively secreted by the proximal tubules. At low plasma concentrations (1.0 to 2.0 mg/100 mL), an average of 90 percent of PAH is cleared by the kidneys from the renal blood stream in a single circulation. It is ideally suited for measurement of ERPF since it has a high clearance, is essentially nontoxic at the plasma concentrations reached with recommended doses, and its analytical determination is relatively simple and accurate. PAH is also used to measure the functional capacity of the renal tubular secretory mechanism or transport maximum (Tm_{PAH}). This is accomplished by elevating the plasma concentration to levels (40-60 mg/100 mL) sufficient to saturate the maximal capacity of the tubular cells to secrete PAH. Inulin clearance is generally measured during Tm_{PAH} determinations since glomerular filtration rate (GFR) must be known before calculations of secretory Tm measurements can be done (see DOSAGE AND ADMINISTRATION, Calculations).

INDICATIONS AND USAGE

Estimation of effective renal plasma flow.
Measurement of the functional capacity of the renal tubular secretory mechanism.

CONTRAINDICATIONS

Hypersensitivity to this product or to its components.

PRECAUTIONS

General

Intravenous solutions must be given with caution to patients with low cardiac reserve, since a rapid increase in plasma volume can precipitate congestive heart failure. For measurement of ERPF, small doses of PAH are used. However, in research procedures to measure Tm_{PAH}, high plasma levels are required to saturate the capacity of the tubular cells. During these procedures, the intravenous ad-

---

ministration of PAH solutions should be carried out slowly and with caution. The patient should be continuously observed for any adverse reactions.

Drug Interactions

Renal clearance measurements of PAH cannot be made with any significant accuracy in patients receiving sulfonamides, procaine, or thiazolesulfone. These compounds interfere with chemical color development essential to the analytical procedures.

Probenecid depresses tubular secretion of certain weak acids such as PAH. Therefore, patients receiving probenecid will have erroneously low ERPF and Tm_{PAH} values.

Carcinogenesis, Mutagenesis, Impairment of Fertility

Long-term studies in animals have not been done to evaluate any effects upon fertility or carcinogenic potential of PAH.

Pregnancy

Pregnancy Category C

Animal reproduction studies have not been done with PAH. It is also not known whether PAH can cause fetal harm when given to a pregnant woman or can affect reproduction capacity. PAH should be given to a pregnant woman only if clearly needed.

Nursing Mothers

It is not known whether this drug is excreted in human milk. Because many drugs are excreted in human milk, caution should be exercised when PAH is administered to a nursing woman.

Pediatric Use

Safety and effectiveness in pediatric patients have not been established.

Geriatric Use

Clinical studies of PAH did not include sufficient numbers of subjects aged 65 and over to determine whether they respond differently from younger subjects. Other reported clinical experience has not identified differences in responses between the elderly and younger patients.

ADVERSE REACTIONS

Hypersensitivity reactions including anaphylaxis, angioedema, urticaria, vasomotor disturbances, flushing, tingling, nausea, vomiting, and cramps may occur.

Patients may have a sensation of warmth or the desire to defecate or urinate during or shortly following initiation of infusion.

OVERDOSE

The intravenous LD_{50} in female mice is 7.22 g/kg.

DOSAGE AND ADMINISTRATION

For intravenous use only

Clearance measurements using single injection techniques are generally inaccurate, particularly in the measurement of ERPF. For this reason, intravenous infusions at fixed rates are used to sustain the plasma PAH concentration at the desired level.

To measure ERPF, the concentration of PAH in the plasma should be maintained at 2 mg per 100 mL, which can be achieved with a priming dose of 6 to 10 mg/kg and an infusion dose of 10 to 24 mg/min.

As a research procedure for the measurement of Tm_{PAH}, the plasma level of PAH must be sufficient to saturate the capacity of the tubular secretory cells. Concentrations from 40 to 60 mg per 100 mL are usually necessary.

Technical details of these tests may be found in Smith {1}; Wesson {2}; Bauer {3}; Pitts{4}; and Schnurr {5}.

Parenteral drug products should be inspected visually for particulate matter and discoloration prior to use, whenever solution and container permit. NOTE: The normal color range for this product is a colorless to yellow/brown solution. The efficacy is not affected by color changes within this range.

Calculations

Effective Renal Plasma Flow (ERPF)

The clearance of PAH, which is extracted almost completely from the plasma during its passage through the renal circulation, constitutes a measure of ERPF. Hence:

$ERPF = U_{PAH}V/P_{PAH}$

Where U_{PAH} = concentration of PAH (mg/mL) in the urine

V = rate of urine excretion (mL/min), and

P_{PAH} = plasma concentration of PAH (mg/mL).

Example:

U_{PAH} = 8.0 mg/mL

V = 1.5 mL/min

P_{PAH} = 0.02 mg/mL

$ERPF = 8.0 \times 1.5/0.02 = 600$ mL/min

Based on PAH clearance studies, the normal values for ERPF are:

men 675 ± 150 mL/min

women 595 ± 125 mL/min

Maximum Tubular Secretory (Tm_{PAH}) Mechanism

The quantity of PAH secreted by the tubules (Tm_{PAH}) is given by the difference between the total rate of excretion ($U_{PAH}V$) and the quantity filtered by the glomeruli (GFR × P_{PAH}). Hence:

$Tm_{PAH} = U_{PAH}V - (GFR \times P_{PAH} \times 0.83)$
The factor, 0.83, corrects for that portion of PAH which is bound to plasma protein and hence is unfilterable.
Example:
U_{PAH} = 9.55 mg/mL
V = 16.68 mL/min
GFR = 120 mL/min
P_{PAH} = 0.60 mg/mL
Then $Tm_{PAH} = 9.55 \times 16.68 - (120 \times 0.60 \times 0.83) = 100$ mg/min.
Average normal values of Tm_{PAH} are 80-90 mg/min.
The value of the expression $U_{PAH}V$, used in calculations of ERPF and Tm_{PAH}, may be found by determining the amount of PAH in a measured volume of urine excreted within a specific period of time.
These calculations are based on a body surface area of 1.73 m^2. Corrections for variations in surface area are made by multiplying the values obtained for ERPF and Tm_{PAH} by 1.73/A, where A is the subject surface area.

HOW SUPPLIED

No. 95—Aminohippurate Sodium, 20 percent sterile solution for intravenous injection, is supplied as follows:
NDC 0006-3395-11 in 10 mL vials.
Storage
Store at 25°C (77°F); excursions permitted to 15-30°C (59-86°F) [see USP Controlled Room Temperature].

REFERENCES

1. Smith, H.W.: Lectures on the kidney, University Extension Division, University of Kansas, Lawrence, Kansas, 1943.
2. Wesson, L.G., Jr.: "Physiology of the Human Kidney," New York, Grune & Stratton, 1969, pp. 632-655.
3. Bauer, J.D.; Ackermann, P.G.; Toro, G.: "Brays Clinical Laboratory Methods," ed. 7, St. Louis, Mosby, 1968.
4. Pitts, R.F.: "Physiology of the Kidney and Body Fluids," ed. 2, Chicago, Year Book Medical Publishers, 1968.
5. Schnurr, E.; Lahme, W.; Kuppers, H.: Measurement of renal clearance of inulin and PAH in the steady state without urine collection; Clinical Nephrology, *13*(1): (26-29), 1980.

Merck Sharp & Dohme Corp., a subsidiary of
MERCK & CO., INC., Whitehouse Station, NJ 08889, USA
Issued March 2010
Printed in USA
9051025

ANTIVENIN ℞

[*an-tiv-en-in*]
(Latrodectus mactans)
(Black Widow Spider Antivenin)
Equine Origin

DESCRIPTION

Antivenin (Latrodectus mactans), is a sterile, non-pyrogenic preparation derived by drying a frozen solution of specific venom-neutralizing globulins obtained from the blood serum of healthy horses immunized against venom of black widow spiders (Latrodectus mactans). It is standardized by biological assay on mice, in terms of one dose of Antivenin neutralizing the venom in not less than 6000 mouse LD_{50} of Latrodectus mactans. Thimerosal (mercury derivative) 1:10,000 is added as a preservative. When constituted as specified, it is opalescent, ranging in color from light (straw) to very dark (iced tea), and contains not more than 20.0 percent of solids.
Each vial contains not less than 6000 Antivenin units. One unit of Antivenin will neutralize one average mouse lethal dose of black widow spider venom when the Antivenin and the venom are injected simultaneously in mice under suitable conditions.

CLINICAL PHARMACOLOGY

The pharmacological mode of action is unknown and metabolic and pharmacokinetic data in humans are unavailable.

INDICATIONS AND USAGE

Antivenin (Latrodectus mactans), is used to treat patients with symptoms due to bites by the black widow spider (Latrodectus mactans). Early use of the Antivenin is emphasized for prompt relief.
Local muscular cramps begin from 15 minutes to several hours after the bite which usually produces a sharp pain similar to that caused by puncture with a needle. The exact sequence of symptoms depends somewhat on the location of the bite. The venom acts on the myoneural junctions or on the nerve endings, causing an ascending motor paralysis or destruction of the peripheral nerve endings. The groups of muscles most frequently affected at first are those of the thigh, shoulder, and back. After a varying length of time, the pain becomes more severe, spreading to the abdomen, and weakness and tremor usually develop. The abdominal muscles assume a boardlike rigidity, but tenderness is slight. Respiration is thoracic. The patient is restless and anxious. Feeble pulse, cold, clammy skin, labored breathing and speech, light stupor, and delirium may occur. Convulsions also may occur, particularly in small children. The temperature may be normal or slightly elevated. Urinary retention, shock, cyanosis, nausea and vomiting, insomnia, and cold sweats also have been reported. The syndrome following the bite of the black widow spider may be confused easily with any medical or surgical condition with acute abdominal symptoms.
The symptoms of black widow spider bite increase in severity for several hours, perhaps a day, and then very slowly become less severe, gradually passing off in the course of two or three days except in fatal cases. Residual symptoms such as general weakness, tingling, nervousness, and transient muscle spasm may persist for weeks or months after recovery from the acute stage.
If possible, the patient should be hospitalized. Other additional measures giving greatest relief are prolonged warm baths and intravenous injection of 10 mL of 10 percent solution of calcium gluconate repeated as necessary to control muscle pain. Morphine also may be required to control pain. Barbiturates may be used for extreme restlessness. However, as the venom is a neurotoxin, it can cause respiratory paralysis. This must be borne in mind when considering use of morphine or a barbiturate. Adrenocorticosteroids have been used with varying degrees of success. Supportive therapy is indicated by the condition of the patient. Local treatment of the site of the bite is of no value. Nothing is gained by applying a tourniquet or by attempting to remove venom from the site of the bite by incision and suction.
In otherwise healthy individuals between the ages of 16 and 60, the use of Antivenin may be deferred and treatment with muscle relaxants may be considered.

WARNINGS

Prior to treatment with any product prepared from horse serum, a careful review of the patient's history should be taken emphasizing prior exposure to horse serum or any allergies. Serious sickness and even death could result from the use of horse serum in a sensitive patient. A skin or conjunctival test should be performed prior to administration of Antivenin.
Skin test: Inject into (not under) the skin not more than 0.02 mL of the test material (1:10 dilution of normal horse serum in physiologic saline). Evaluate result in 10 minutes. A positive reaction is an urticarial wheal surrounded by a zone of erythema. A control test using Sodium Chloride Injection facilitates interpretation of the results.
Conjunctival test: For adults instill into the conjunctival sac one drop of a 1:10 dilution of horse serum and for children one drop of 1:100 dilution. Itching of the eye and reddening of the conjunctiva indicate a positive reaction, usually within 10 minutes.
Patients should be observed for serum sickness for an average of 8 to 12 days following administration of Antivenin.
Desensitization should be attempted only when the administration of Antivenin is considered necessary to save life. Epinephrine must be available in case of untoward reaction.
Desensitization: If the history is positive or the results of the sensitivity tests are mildly or questionably positive, Antivenin should be administered as follows to reduce the risk of an immediate severe allergic reaction:
1. In separate sterile vials or syringes prepare 1:10 or 1:100 dilutions of Antivenin in Sodium Chloride for Injection.
2. Allow at least 15 but preferably 30 minutes between injections and only proceed with the next dose if no reactions occurred following the previous dose.
3. Using a tuberculin syringe, inject subcutaneously 0.1, 0.2 and 0.5 mL of the 1:100 dilution at 15 or 30 minute intervals; repeat with the 1:10 dilution, and finally the undiluted Antivenin.
4. If there is a reaction after any of the injections, place a tourniquet proximal to the sites of injection and administer epinephrine, 1:1000 (0.3 to 1.0 mL subcutaneously, 0.05 to 0.1 mL intravenously), proximal to the tourniquet or into another extremity. Wait at least 30 minutes before giving another injection of Antivenin, the amount of which should be the same as the last one not evoking a reaction.
5. If no reaction has occurred after 0.5 mL of undiluted Antivenin has been given, it is probably safe to continue the dose at 15 minute intervals until the entire dose has been injected.

PRECAUTIONS

Carcinogenesis, Mutagenesis, Impairment of Fertility
No long term studies in animals have been performed to evaluate the potential for carcinogenesis, mutagenesis, or impairment of fertility.
Pregnancy
Pregnancy Category C. Animal reproduction studies have not been conducted with Black Widow Spider Antivenin. It is also not known whether Black Widow Spider Antivenin can cause fetal harm when administered to a pregnant woman or can affect reproduction capacity. Black Widow Spider Antivenin should be given to a pregnant woman only if clearly needed.
Nursing Mothers
It is not known whether this drug is excreted in human milk. Because many drugs are excreted in human milk, caution should be exercised when Black Widow Spider Antivenin is administered to a nursing woman.
Pediatric Use
Controlled clinical studies for safety and effectiveness in children have not been conducted.
Geriatric Use
Reported clinical experience has not identified differences in responses between the elderly and younger patients. Because of the increased risk of complications from envenomation in elderly patients, the standard of care described in the literature suggests that patients older than 60 years of age should be given Antivenin as a preferred initial therapy (see INDICATIONS AND USAGE).

ADVERSE REACTIONS

The following adverse reactions have been reported following the use of ANTIVENIN: Hypersensitivity reactions including anaphylaxis and serum sickness. Muscle cramps have also been reported.

DOSAGE AND ADMINISTRATION

Using a sterile syringe, remove from the accompanying vial 2.5 mL of Sterile Diluent for Antivenin and inject into the vial of Antivenin. With the needle still in the rubber stopper, shake the vial to dissolve the contents completely.
Parenteral drug products should be inspected visually for particulate matter prior to administration, whenever solution and container permit (see DESCRIPTION).
The dose for adults and children is the entire contents of a restored vial (2.5 mL) of Antivenin. It may be given intramuscularly, preferably in the region of the anterolateral thigh so that a tourniquet may be applied in the event of a systemic reaction. Symptoms usually subside in 1 to 3 hours. Although one dose of Antivenin usually is adequate, a second dose may be necessary in some cases.
Antivenin also may be given intravenously in 10 to 50 mL of saline solution over a 15 minute period. It is the preferred route in severe cases, or when the patient is under 12, or in shock. One restored vial usually is enough.

HOW SUPPLIED

No. 4084—Antivenin (Latrodectus mactans), equine origin is a white to gray crystalline powder, each vial containing not less than 6000 Antivenin units. Thimerosal (mercury derivative) 1:10,000 is added as preservative, **NDC** 0006-4084-00. A 2.5 mL vial of Sterile Diluent for Antivenin is included. Also supplied is a 1 mL vial of normal horse serum (1:10 dilution) for sensitivity testing. Thimerosal (mercury derivative) 1:10,000 is added as preservative.
Storage
Antivenin must be stored and shipped at 28°C (36-46°F). When reconstituted as directed, the color of Antivenin ranges from light (straw) to very dark (iced tea), but the color has no effect on potency. *Do not freeze.*

REFERENCES

Barron, W. E.: Spider Bites, J. Med. Ass. Georgia *49:* 511-512, Oct. 1960.
Micks, D. W.: Insects and Other Arthropods of Medical Importance in Texas, Tex. Rep. Biol. & Med. *18:* 624-635, Winter 1960.
Prince, G. E.: Arachnidism in Children, J. Pediat. *49:* 101-108, July 1956.
Russell, F. E.: Injuries by Venomous Animals in the United States, J. Amer. Med. Ass. *177:* 903-907, Sept. 30, 1961.
Russell, F. E.: Muscle Relaxants in Black Widow Spider (Latrodectus mactans) Poisoning, Amer. J. Med. Sci. *243:* 159-162, Feb. 1962.
Russell, F. E.: Venom Poisoning, Rational Drug Therap. *5:* 5-6, Aug. 1971.

MERCK & CO., INC., Whitehouse Station, NJ 08889, USA
Issued February 2005
Printed in USA
7972116

ASMANEX® TWISTHALER® ℞

[*ăs-măn-ĕcks*]
110 mcg, 220 mcg
(mometasone furoate inhalation powder)

HIGHLIGHTS OF PRESCRIBING INFORMATION
These highlights do not include all the information needed to use ASMANEX TWISTHALER safely and effectively. See full prescribing information for ASMANEX TWISTHALER.
ASMANEX TWISTHALER 110 mcg, 220 mcg (mometasone furoate inhalation powder)
Initial U.S. Approval: 1987

INDICATIONS AND USAGE

ASMANEX TWISTHALER is a corticosteroid indicated for:
- Maintenance treatment of asthma as prophylactic therapy in patients 4 years of age and older. (1.1)

ASMANEX TWISTHALER is NOT indicated for the relief of acute bronchospasm (1.1, 5.2) or in children less than 4 years of age (1.1, 8.4).

DOSAGE AND ADMINISTRATION

- FOR ORAL INHALATION ONLY. (2)
- Instruct patients to inhale rapidly and deeply and to rinse mouth after inhalation. (2)

[See first table at right]

DOSAGE FORMS AND STRENGTHS

- 220 mcg TWISTHALER: delivers 200 mcg mometasone furoate per actuation. (3)
- 110 mcg TWISTHALER: delivers 100 mcg mometasone furoate per actuation. (3)

CONTRAINDICATIONS

- Patients with status asthmaticus or other acute episodes of asthma where intensive measures are required. (4.1)
- Patients with a known hypersensitivity to mometasone or any of the ingredients in ASMANEX TWISTHALER. (4.2)

WARNINGS AND PRECAUTIONS

- *Candida albicans* infection of the mouth and pharynx. Monitor patients periodically for signs of adverse effects in the mouth and pharynx. Advise patients to rinse mouth after inhalation. (5.1)
- Potential worsening of existing tuberculosis, fungal, bacterial, viral, or parasitic infection, or ocular herpes simplex. More serious or even fatal course of chickenpox or measles in susceptible patients. Use caution in patients with the above because of the potential for worsening of these infections. (5.3)
- Risk of impaired adrenal function when transferring from oral steroids to inhaled corticosteroids. Taper patients slowly from systemic corticosteroids if transferring to ASMANEX TWISTHALER. (5.4)
- Hypercorticism, suppression of hypothalamic-pituitary-adrenal (HPA) function with very high dosages or at the regular dosage in susceptible individuals. If such changes occur discontinue ASMANEX TWISTHALER slowly. (5.5)
- Reduction in bone mineral density with long-term administration. Monitor patients with major risk factors for decreased bone mineral content. (5.6)
- Suppression of growth in children. Monitor growth routinely in pediatric patients receiving ASMANEX TWISTHALER. (5.7)
- Development of glaucoma, increased intraocular pressure and posterior subcapsular cataracts. Monitor patients with a change in vision or with a history of increased intraocular pressure, glaucoma, and/or cataracts closely. (5.8)

ADVERSE REACTIONS

The most common adverse reactions (incidence ≥5%) are headache, allergic rhinitis, pharyngitis, upper respiratory tract infection, sinusitis, oral candidiasis, dysmenorrhea, musculoskeletal pain, back pain, and dyspepsia. (6.1).

To report SUSPECTED ADVERSE REACTIONS, contact Schering-Plough at 1-800-526-4099 or FDA at 1-800-FDA-1088 or *www.fda.gov/medwatch*.

See 17 for PATIENT COUNSELING INFORMATION and FDA-approved patient labeling

Revised: 08/2009

FULL PRESCRIBING INFORMATION: CONTENTS*

* Sections or subsections omitted from the full prescribing information are not listed

FULL PRESCRIBING INFORMATION

1 INDICATIONS AND USAGE

1.1 Treatment of Asthma

ASMANEX® TWISTHALER® is indicated for the maintenance treatment of asthma as prophylactic therapy in patients 4 years of age and older.

Important Limitations of Use

ASMANEX TWISTHALER is NOT indicated for the relief of acute bronchospasm.

ASMANEX TWISTHALER is NOT indicated in children less than 4 years of age.

2 DOSAGE AND ADMINISTRATION

Administer ASMANEX TWISTHALER by the orally inhaled route only. Instruct patients to inhale rapidly and deeply. Advise patients to rinse the mouth after inhalation. Individual patients will experience a variable time to onset and degree of symptom relief. Maximum benefit may not be achieved for 1 to 2 weeks or longer after initiation of treatment. After asthma stability has been achieved, it is desirable to titrate to the lowest effective dosage to reduce the possibility of side effects. For patients ≥12 years of age who do not respond adequately to the starting dose after 2 weeks of therapy, higher doses may provide additional asthma control. The safety and efficacy of ASMANEX TWISTHALER when administered in excess of recommended doses have not been established.

Recommended Dosages for ASMANEX TWISTHALER Treatment

Previous Therapy	Recommended Starting Dose	Highest Recommended Daily Dose
Patients ≥12 years who received bronchodilators alone	220 mcg once daily in the evening*	440 mcg†
Patients ≥12 years who received inhaled corticosteroids	220 mcg once daily in the evening*	440 mcg†
Patients ≥12 years who received oral corticosteroids‡	440 mcg twice daily	880 mcg
Children 4–11 years of age§	110 mcg once daily in the evening*	110 mcg*

*†‡§Please refer to subsection 2.1 for full dosage recommendations and details.

Table 1: Recommended Dosages for ASMANEX TWISTHALER Treatment

Previous Therapy	Recommended Starting Dose	Highest Recommended Daily Dose
Patients ≥12 years who received bronchodilators alone	220 mcg once daily in the evening*	440 mcg†
Patients ≥12 years who received inhaled corticosteroids	220 mcg once daily in the evening*	440 mcg†
Patients ≥12 years who received oral corticosteroids‡	440 mcg twice daily	880 mcg
Children 4–11 years of age§	110 mcg once daily in the evening*	110 mcg*

* When administered once daily, ASMANEX TWISTHALER should be taken only in the evening.
† The 440 mcg daily dose may be administered in divided doses of 220 mcg twice daily or as 440 mcg once daily.
‡ **For Patients Currently Receiving Chronic Oral Corticosteroid Therapy:** Prednisone should be reduced no faster than 2.5 mg/day on a weekly basis, beginning after at least 1 week of ASMANEX TWISTHALER therapy. Monitor patients carefully for signs of asthma instability, including serial objective measures of airflow, and for signs of adrenal insufficiency during steroid taper and following discontinuation of oral corticosteroid therapy *[see Warnings and Precautions (5.4)]*.
§ Recommended pediatric dosage is 110 mcg once daily in the evening regardless of prior therapy.

2.1 Recommended Dosages in Patients 4 Years of Age and Older

The recommended starting doses and highest recommended daily dose for ASMANEX TWISTHALER treatment based on prior asthma therapy are provided in **Table 1**.

[See table 1 above]

3 DOSAGE FORMS AND STRENGTHS

ASMANEX TWISTHALER is a dry powder for inhalation that is available in two strengths.

ASMANEX TWISTHALER 220 mcg delivers 200 mcg mometasone furoate per actuation from the mouthpiece.

ASMANEX TWISTHALER 110 mcg delivers 100 mcg mometasone furoate per actuation from the mouthpiece.

4 CONTRAINDICATIONS

4.1 Status Asthmaticus

ASMANEX TWISTHALER therapy is contraindicated in the primary treatment of status asthmaticus or other acute episodes of asthma where intensive measures are required.

4.2 Hypersensitivity

ASMANEX TWISTHALER is contraindicated in patients with known hypersensitivity to mometasone or any of the ingredients in ASMANEX TWISTHALER. In the clinical trials and postmarketing experience with ASMANEX TWISTHALER, cases of allergic reaction, facial edema, urticaria, hypersensitivity, and throat tightness have been reported.

5 WARNINGS AND PRECAUTIONS

5.1 Local Effects

In clinical trials, the development of localized infections of the mouth and pharynx with *Candida albicans* occurred in 195 of 3007 patients treated with ASMANEX TWISTHALER. If oropharyngeal candidiasis develops, it should be treated with appropriate local or systemic (i.e., oral) antifungal therapy while remaining on treatment with ASMANEX TWISTHALER therapy, but at times therapy with the ASMANEX TWISTHALER may need to be interrupted. Advise patients to rinse the mouth after inhalation of ASMANEX TWISTHALER.

5.2 Acute Asthma Episodes

ASMANEX TWISTHALER is not a bronchodilator and is not indicated for rapid relief of bronchospasm or other acute episodes of asthma. Instruct patients to contact their physician immediately if episodes of asthma that are not responsive to bronchodilators occur during the course of treatment with ASMANEX TWISTHALER. During such episodes, patients may require therapy with oral corticosteroids.

5.3 Immunosuppression

Persons who are using drugs that suppress the immune system are more susceptible to infections than healthy individuals. Chickenpox and measles, for example, can have a more serious or even fatal course in susceptible children or adults using corticosteroids. In such children or adults who have not had these diseases or who are not properly immunized, particular care should be taken to avoid exposure. How the dose, route, and duration of corticosteroid administration affect the risk of developing a disseminated infection is not known. The contribution of the underlying disease and/or prior corticosteroid treatment to the risk is also not known. If exposed to chickenpox, prophylaxis with varicella zoster immune globulin (VZIG) may be indicated. If exposed to measles, prophylaxis with pooled intramuscular immunoglobulin (IG) may be indicated. (See the respective package inserts for complete VZIG and IG prescribing information.) If chickenpox develops, treatment with antiviral agents may be considered.

Inhaled corticosteroids should be used with caution, if at all, in patients with active or quiescent tuberculosis infection of the respiratory tract, untreated systemic fungal, bacterial, viral, or parasitic infections; or ocular herpes simplex.

5.4 Transferring Patients from Systemic Corticosteroid Therapy

Particular care is needed for patients who are transferred from systemically active corticosteroids to ASMANEX TWISTHALER because deaths due to adrenal insufficiency have occurred in asthmatic patients during and after transfer from systemic corticosteroids to less systemically available inhaled corticosteroids. After withdrawal from systemic corticosteroids, a number of months are required for recovery of hypothalamic-pituitary-adrenal (HPA) function. Patients who have been previously maintained on 20 mg or more per day of prednisone (or its equivalent) may be most susceptible, particularly when their systemic corticosteroids have been almost completely withdrawn. During this period of HPA suppression, patients may exhibit signs and symptoms of adrenal insufficiency when exposed to trauma, surgery, or infection (particularly gastroenteritis) or other conditions associated with severe electrolyte loss. Although ASMANEX TWISTHALER may improve control of asthma symptoms during these episodes, in recommended doses it supplies less than normal physiological amounts of corticosteroid systemically and does NOT provide the mineralocorticoid activity necessary for coping with these emergencies. During periods of stress or severe asthma attack, patients who have been withdrawn from systemic corticosteroids should be instructed to resume oral corticosteroids (in large doses) immediately and to contact their physicians for further instruction. These patients should also be instructed to carry a medical identification card indicating that they may need supplementary systemic corticosteroids during periods of stress or severe asthma attack.

Patients requiring oral corticosteroids should be weaned slowly from systemic corticosteroid use after transferring to ASMANEX TWISTHALER. Prednisone reduction can be accomplished by reducing the daily prednisone dose by 2.5 mg on a weekly basis during treatment with ASMANEX TWISTHALER [see Dosage and Administration (2)]. Lung function (FEV$_1$ or PEFR), beta-agonist use, and asthma symptoms should be carefully monitored during withdrawal of oral corticosteroids. In addition to monitoring asthma signs and symptoms, patients should be observed for signs and symptoms of adrenal insufficiency such as fatigue, lassitude, weakness, nausea and vomiting, and hypotension.

Transfer of patients from systemic corticosteroid therapy to ASMANEX TWISTHALER may unmask allergic conditions previously suppressed by the systemic corticosteroid therapy, e.g., rhinitis, conjunctivitis, eczema, arthritis, and eosinophilic conditions.

During withdrawal from oral corticosteroids, some patients may experience symptoms of systemically active corticosteroid withdrawal, e.g., joint and/or muscular pain, lassitude, and depression, despite maintenance or even improvement of respiratory function.

5.5 Hypercorticism and Adrenal Suppression

ASMANEX TWISTHALER will often help control asthma symptoms with less suppression of HPA function than therapeutically similar oral doses of prednisone. Since individual sensitivity to effects on cortisol production exists, physicians should consider this information when prescribing ASMANEX TWISTHALER. Particular care should be taken in observing patients postoperatively or during periods of stress for evidence of inadequate adrenal response. It is possible that systemic corticosteroid effects such as hypercorticism and adrenal suppression may appear in a small number of patients, particularly when ASMANEX TWISTHALER is administered at higher than recommended doses over prolonged periods of time. If such effects occur, the dosage of ASMANEX TWISTHALER should be reduced slowly, consistent with accepted procedures for reducing systemic corticosteroids and for management of asthma.

Table 2: Adverse Reactions with ≥3% Incidence in 10 Controlled Clinical Trials with ASMANEX TWISTHALER in Patients 12 Years of Age and Older Previously on Bronchodilators and/or Inhaled Corticosteroids

Adverse Reaction	(%) of Patients ASMANEX TWISTHALER 220 mcg twice daily (n=433)	440 mcg once daily (n=497)	220 mcg once daily in the evening (n=232)	Placebo (n=720)
Headache	22	17	20	20
Allergic Rhinitis	15	11	14	13
Pharyngitis	11	8	13	7
Upper Respiratory Infection	10	8	15	7
Sinusitis	6	6	5	5
Candidiasis, oral	6	4	4	2
Dysmenorrhea*	9	4	4	4
Musculoskeletal Pain	8	4	4	5
Back Pain	6	3	3	4
Dyspepsia	5	3	3	3
Myalgia	3	2	3	2
Abdominal Pain	3	2	3	2
Nausea	3	1	3	2
Average Duration of Exposure (Days)	81	70	80	62

* Percentages are based on the number of female patients.

5.6 Reduction in Bone Mineral Density

Decreases in bone mineral density (BMD) have been observed with long-term administration of products containing inhaled corticosteroids, including mometasone furoate. The clinical significance of small changes in BMD with regard to long-term outcomes is unknown. Patients with major risk factors for decreased bone mineral content, such as prolonged immobilization, family history of osteoporosis, or chronic use of drugs that can reduce bone mass (e.g., anticonvulsants and corticosteroids) should be monitored and treated with established standards of care.

In a 2-year double-blind study in 103 male and female asthma patients 18 to 50 years of age previously maintained on bronchodilator therapy (baseline FEV$_1$ 85%–88% predicted), treatment with ASMANEX TWISTHALER 220 mcg twice daily resulted in significant reductions in lumbar spine (LS) BMD at the end of the treatment period compared to placebo. The mean change from baseline to endpoint in the lumbar spine BMD was -0.015 (-1.43%) for the ASMANEX TWISTHALER group compared to 0.002 (0.25%) for the placebo group. In another 2-year double-blind study in 87 male and female asthma patients 18 to 50 years of age previously maintained on bronchodilator therapy (baseline FEV$_1$ 82%–83% predicted), treatment with ASMANEX TWISTHALER 440 mcg twice daily demonstrated no statistically significant changes in lumbar spine BMD at the end of the treatment period compared to placebo. The mean change from baseline to endpoint in the lumbar spine BMD was -0.018 (-1.57%) for the ASMANEX TWISTHALER group compared to -0.006 (-0.43%) for the placebo group.

5.7 Effect on Growth

Orally inhaled corticosteroids, including ASMANEX TWISTHALER, may cause a reduction in growth velocity when administered to pediatric patients. Monitor the growth of pediatric patients receiving ASMANEX TWISTHALER routinely (e.g., via stadiometry). To minimize the systemic effects of orally inhaled corticosteroids, including ASMANEX TWISTHALER, titrate each patient's dose to the lowest dosage that effectively controls his/her symptoms [see Use in Specific Populations (8.4)].

5.8 Glaucoma and Cataracts

In clinical trials glaucoma, increased intraocular pressure, and cataracts have been reported in 8 of 3007 patients following the administration of ASMANEX TWISTHALER. Close monitoring is warranted in patients with a change in vision or with a history of increased intraocular pressure, glaucoma, and/or cataracts.

5.9 Bronchospasm

As with other inhaled asthma medications, bronchospasm may occur with an immediate increase in wheezing after dosing. If bronchospasm occurs following dosing with ASMANEX TWISTHALER, it should be treated immediately with a fast-acting inhaled bronchodilator. Treatment with ASMANEX TWISTHALER should be discontinued and alternative therapy instituted.

6 ADVERSE REACTIONS

Systemic and local corticosteroid use may result in the following:

- *Candida albicans* infection [see Warnings and Precautions (5.1)]
- Immunosuppression [see Warnings and Precautions (5.3)]
- Hypercorticism and adrenal suppression [see Warnings and Precautions (5.5)]
- Growth effects [see Warnings and Precautions (5.7) and Use in Specific Populations (8.4)]
- Glaucoma and cataracts [see Warnings and Precautions (5.8)]

6.1 Clinical Studies Experience

The safety data described below reflect exposure to ASMANEX TWISTHALER in 2380 patients with asthma exposed for 8 to 12 weeks and 627 patients with asthma exposed for 1 year in a total of 17 clinical trials.

In adult and adolescent patients 12 years of age and older, ASMANEX TWISTHALER was studied in 10 placebo-controlled clinical trials of 8 to 12 weeks duration with a total of 1750 patients receiving ASMANEX TWISTHALER. There were also 3 trials with a total of 475 patients receiving ASMANEX TWISTHALER for 1 year. In the 8- to 12-week clinical trials, the population was 12 to 83 years of age, 38% males and 62% females, and 83% Caucasian, 8% black, 6% Hispanic, and 3% other race/ethnicity. Patients received ASMANEX TWISTHALER 110 mcg twice daily (n=133), 220 mcg once daily in the morning (n=209), 220 mcg once daily in the evening (n=232), 220 mcg twice daily (n=433), 440 mcg once daily in the morning (n=419), 440 mcg once daily in the evening (n=250), or 440 mcg twice daily (n=74). In 3 long-term safety trials (two 9-month extensions of efficacy trials and one 52-week active-controlled safety trial), 475 patients with asthma (12–83 years of age, 44% males, 56% females, 87% Caucasian, 8% black, 4% Hispanic, and 1% other race/ethnicity) received various doses of ASMANEX TWISTHALER for 1 year.

In pediatric patients 4 to 11 years of age, ASMANEX TWISTHALER was studied in 3 placebo-controlled clinical trials of 12 weeks duration with a total of 630 patients receiving ASMANEX TWISTHALER and a 52-week, active-controlled safety trial with a total of 152 patients receiving ASMANEX TWISTHALER. In the 12-week clinical trials, the population was 4 to 11 years of age, 63% males and 37% females, and 67% Caucasian, 13% black, 17% Hispanic, and

3% other race/ethnicity. Patients received ASMANEX TWISTHALER 110 mcg once daily in the evening (n=98), 110 mcg once daily in the morning (n=181), 110 mcg twice daily (n=179), or 220 mcg once daily in the morning (n=172). In the long-term active-controlled safety trial (n=152), patients with asthma (4 to 11 years of age, 60% males and 40% females, 84% Caucasian, 11% Black, and 5% Hispanic) received ASMANEX TWISTHALER 110 mcg twice daily or 220 mcg once daily in the morning for 52 weeks.

Because clinical trials are conducted under widely varying conditions, adverse reaction rates observed in the clinical trials of a drug cannot be directly compared to rates in the clinical trials of another drug and may not reflect the rates observed in practice.

Adults and Adolescents 12 Years of Age and Older: The safety results of the 10 trials that were 8 to 12 weeks in duration were pooled because patients with asthma in these studies were previously maintained on bronchodilators and/or inhaled corticosteroids. The safety results of the one 12-week clinical trial in patients with asthma previously treated with oral corticosteroids are presented separately.

In the pooled 8- to 12-week clinical trials, adverse reactions were reported in 70% of patients treated with ASMANEX TWISTHALER (n=1750) compared to 65% of patients taking placebo (n=720). **Table 2** displays the common adverse reactions (≥3% in any patient group receiving ASMANEX TWISTHALER) that occurred more frequently in patients treated with ASMANEX TWISTHALER compared to patients treated with placebo.

[See table 2 at top of previous page]

The following other adverse reactions occurred in these clinical trials with an incidence of at least 1% but less than 3% and were more common on ASMANEX TWISTHALER therapy than on placebo:

Body as a Whole: fatigue, flu-like symptoms, pain
Gastrointestinal: gastroenteritis, vomiting, anorexia
Hearing, Vestibular: earache
Resistance Mechanism: infection
Respiratory: dysphonia, epistaxis, nasal irritation, respiratory disorder, throat dry

In the 12-week trial in adult asthmatics who previously required oral corticosteroids, the effects of ASMANEX TWISTHALER therapy administered as two 220-mcg inhalations twice daily (n=46) were compared with those of placebo (n=43). Adverse reactions, whether considered drug-related or not by the investigators, reported in more than 3 patients in the ASMANEX TWISTHALER treatment group, and which occurred more frequently than in placebo were (ASMANEX TWISTHALER % vs. placebo %): musculoskeletal pain (22% vs. 14%), oral candidiasis (22% vs. 9%), sinusitis (22% vs. 19%), allergic rhinitis (20% vs. 5%), upper respiratory infection (15% vs. 14%), arthralgia (13% vs. 7%), fatigue (13% vs. 2%), depression (11% vs. 0%), and sinus congestion (9% vs. 0%). In considering these data, an increased duration of exposure for patients on ASMANEX TWISTHALER treatment (77 days vs. 58 days on placebo) should be taken into account.

Long-Term Clinical Trials Experience – 12 Years of Age and Older: In 3 long-term safety trials, 475 patients with asthma 12 years of age and older were treated with ASMANEX TWISTHALER 220 mcg twice daily (n=60), 220 mcg once daily in the morning (n=41), 220 mcg once daily in the evening (n=40), 440 mcg once daily in the morning (n=44), 440 once daily in the evening (n=41), 440 mcg twice daily (n=62), 880 mcg once daily (n=59), or at variable doses (n=128) for 52 weeks. The safety profile of ASMANEX TWISTHALER in the 52-week trials was similar to the findings in the 8- to 12-week clinical trials. In patients previously on inhaled corticosteroids, cataracts were reported in 3 patients (0.9%) treated with ASMANEX TWISTHALER, compared to 1 patient (1.7%) treated with the active comparator medication. Increased ocular pressure at the end of the study was observed in 2 patients, both on ASMANEX TWISTHALER 880 mcg once daily in the morning. Oral candidiasis, dysphonia, and dysmenorrhea were seen at a higher frequency with long-term administration than in the 8- to 12-week trials.

Pediatric Patients 4 to 11 Years of Age: In the three 12-week clinical trials in pediatric patients 4 to 11 years of age, patients with asthma were previously maintained on bronchodilators and/or inhaled corticosteroids. The safety results from 1 trial are described in **Table 3** for ASMANEX TWISTHALER 110 mcg once daily in the evening. The safety results from the other 2 trials showed similar findings.

Overall adverse reactions were reported with approximately the same frequency by patients treated with ASMANEX TWISTHALER and those receiving placebo. **Table 3** displays the common adverse reactions (≥2% in any patient group receiving ASMANEX TWISTHALER) that occurred more frequently in patients 4 to 11 years of age treated with ASMANEX TWISTHALER compared with placebo-treated patients.

Table 3: Adverse Reactions with ≥2% Incidence in a 12-Week Study with ASMANEX TWISTHALER in Patients 4 to 11 Years of Age Previously on Bronchodilators and/or Inhaled Corticosteroids

	(%) of Patients	
	ASMANEX TWISTHALER	
Adverse Reaction	110 mcg once daily in the evening (n=98)	Placebo (n=99)
Fever	7	5
Allergic Rhinitis	4	3
Abdominal Pain	6	2
Vomiting	3	2
Urinary Tract Infection	2	1
Bruise	2	0
Average Duration of Exposure (Days)	72	68

Long-Term Clinical Trials Experience in Children 4 to 11 Years of Age: In a 52-week, active-controlled, long-term safety trial, 152 patients with asthma 4 to 11 years of age were treated with ASMANEX TWISTHALER 110 mcg twice daily (n=74) or 220 mcg once daily (n=78). The safety profile for ASMANEX TWISTHALER in the 52-week trial was similar to the findings in the 12-week clinical trials.

7 DRUG INTERACTIONS

In clinical studies, the concurrent administration of ASMANEX TWISTHALER and other drugs commonly used in the treatment of asthma was not associated with any unusual adverse reactions.

7.1 Inhibitors of Cytochrome P450 3A4

Ketoconazole, a strong inhibitor of cytochrome P450 3A4, may increase plasma levels of mometasone furoate during concomitant dosing *[see Clinical Pharmacology (12.3)]*.

8 USE IN SPECIFIC POPULATIONS

8.1 Pregnancy

Pregnancy Category C: There are no adequate and well-controlled studies of ASMANEX TWISTHALER use in pregnant women. Animal reproduction studies in mice, rats, and rabbits revealed evidence of teratogenicity. Asthma is a serious and potentially life-threatening condition. Poorly controlled asthma during pregnancy is associated with adverse outcomes for mother and fetus. ASMANEX TWISTHALER should be used during pregnancy only if the potential benefit justifies the potential risk to the fetus.

There is a natural increase in corticosteroid production during pregnancy; therefore most women require a lower exogenous corticosteroid dose and may not need corticosteroid treatment during pregnancy. Infants born to mothers taking substantial oral corticosteroid doses during pregnancy should be monitored for signs of hypoadrenalism.

When administered to pregnant mice, rats, and rabbits, mometasone furoate increased fetal malformations and decreased fetal growth (measured by lower fetal weights and/or delayed ossification). Dystocia and related complications were also observed when mometasone furoate was administered to rats late in gestation. However, experience with oral corticosteroids suggests that rodents are more prone to teratogenic effects from corticosteroid exposure than humans.

In a mouse reproduction study, subcutaneous mometasone furoate produced cleft palate at approximately one-third of the maximum recommended daily human dose (MRHD) for adults on an mcg/m^2 basis and decreased fetal survival at approximately 1 time the MRHD. No toxicity was observed at approximately one-tenth of the MRHD.

In a rat reproduction study, mometasone furoate produced umbilical hernia at topical dermal doses approximately 6 times the MRHD and delays in ossification at approximately 3 times the MRHD.

In another study, rats received subcutaneous doses of mometasone throughout pregnancy or late in gestation. Treated animals had prolonged and difficult labor, fewer live births, lower birth weight, and reduced early pup survival at a dose that was approximately 6 times the MRHD for adults on an area under the curve (AUC) basis. Similar effects were not observed at approximately 3 times the MRHD.

In rabbits, mometasone furoate caused multiple malformations (e.g., flexed front paws, gallbladder agenesis, umbilical hernia, hydrocephaly) at topical dermal doses approximately 3 times the maximum recommended daily inhalation dose in adults on an mcg/m^2 basis. In an oral study, mometasone furoate increased resorptions and caused cleft palate and/or head malformations (hydrocephaly and domed head) at a dose less than the MRHD for adults based on AUC. At a dose approximately 2 times the MRHD in adults based on AUC, most litters were aborted or resorbed *[see Nonclinical Toxicology (13.2)]*.

8.3 Nursing Mothers

Systemic absorption of a single inhaled 400 mcg mometasone dose was less than 1%. It is not known if mometasone furoate is excreted in human milk. Because other corticosteroids are excreted in human milk, caution should be used when ASMANEX TWISTHALER is administered to nursing women.

8.4 Pediatric Use

The safety and effectiveness of ASMANEX TWISTHALER have been established in children 4 years of age and older. Use of ASMANEX TWISTHALER in children 12 years of age and older is supported by evidence from adequate and well-controlled clinical trials in this patient population *[see Clinical Studies (14.1) and Adverse Reactions (6.1)]*.

Use of ASMANEX TWISTHALER in pediatric patients 4 to 11 years of age is supported by evidence from adequate and well-controlled clinical trials of 12 weeks duration in 630 patients 4 to 11 years of age receiving ASMANEX TWISTHALER and one 52-week safety trial in 152 patients *[see Clinical Studies (14.1) and Adverse Reactions (6.1)]*.

Controlled clinical studies have shown that inhaled corticosteroids may cause a reduction in growth in pediatric patients. In these studies, the mean reduction in growth velocity was approximately 1 cm per year (range: 0.3–1.8 per year) and appears to depend upon dose and duration of exposure. This effect was observed in the absence of laboratory evidence of HPA axis suppression, suggesting that growth velocity is a more sensitive indicator of systemic corticosteroid exposure in pediatric patients than some commonly used tests of HPA axis function. The long-term effects of this reduction in growth velocity associated with orally inhaled corticosteroids, including the impact on final adult height, are unknown. The potential for "catch-up" growth following discontinuation of treatment with orally inhaled corticosteroids has not been adequately studied. The growth of children and adolescents (4 years of age and older) receiving orally inhaled corticosteroids, including ASMANEX TWISTHALER, should be monitored routinely (e.g., via stadiometry).

A 52-week, placebo-controlled, parallel-group study was conducted to assess the potential growth effects of ASMANEX TWISTHALER in 187 prepubescent children (131 males and 56 females) 4 to 9 years of age with asthma who were previously maintained on an inhaled beta-agonist. Treatment groups included ASMANEX TWISTHALER 110 mcg twice daily (n=44), 220 mcg once daily in the morning (n=50), 110 mcg once daily in the morning (n=48), and placebo (n=45). For each patient, an average growth rate was determined using an individual regression approach. The mean growth rates, expressed as least-squares mean in cm per year, for ASMANEX TWISTHALER 110 mcg twice daily, 220 mcg once daily in the morning, 110 mcg once daily in the morning, and placebo were 5.34, 5.93, 6.15, and 6.44, respectively. The differences from placebo and the corresponding 2-sided 95% CI of growth rates for ASMANEX TWISTHALER 110 mcg twice daily, 220 mcg once daily in the morning, and 110 mcg once daily in the morning were -1.11 (95% CI: -2.34, 0.12), -0.51 (95% CI: -1.69, 0.67), and -0.30 (95% CI: -1.48, 0.89), respectively.

The potential growth effects of prolonged treatment with orally inhaled corticosteroids should be weighed against clinical benefits obtained and the availability of safe and effective noncorticosteroid treatment alternatives. To minimize the systemic effects of orally inhaled corticosteroids, including ASMANEX TWISTHALER, each patient should be titrated to his/her lowest effective dose.

8.5 Geriatric Use

A total of 175 patients 65 years of age and over (23 of whom were 75 years of age and older) have been treated with ASMANEX TWISTHALER in controlled clinical trials. No overall differences in safety or effectiveness were observed between these and younger patients, and other reported clinical experience has not identified differences in responses between the elderly and younger patients, but greater sensitivity of some older individuals cannot be ruled out.

8.6 Hepatic Impairment

Concentrations of mometasone furoate appear to increase with severity of hepatic impairment *[see Clinical Pharmacology (12.3)]*.

10 OVERDOSAGE

Chronic overdosage may result in signs/symptoms of hypercorticism *[see Warnings and Precautions (5.5)]*. Because of low systemic bioavailability and an absence of acute drug-related systemic findings in clinical studies, acute overdose is unlikely to require any treatment other than observation. Single daily doses as high as 1200 mcg per day for 28 days were well tolerated and did not cause a significant reduction in plasma cortisol AUC (94% of placebo AUC). Single oral doses up to 8000 mcg have been studied on human volunteers with no adverse reactions reported.

11 DESCRIPTION

Mometasone furoate, the active component of the ASMANEX TWISTHALER product, is a corticosteroid with the chemical name 9,21-dichloro-11(Beta),17-dihydroxy-16(alpha)-methylpregna-1,4-diene-3,20-dione 17-(2-furoate) and the following chemical structure:

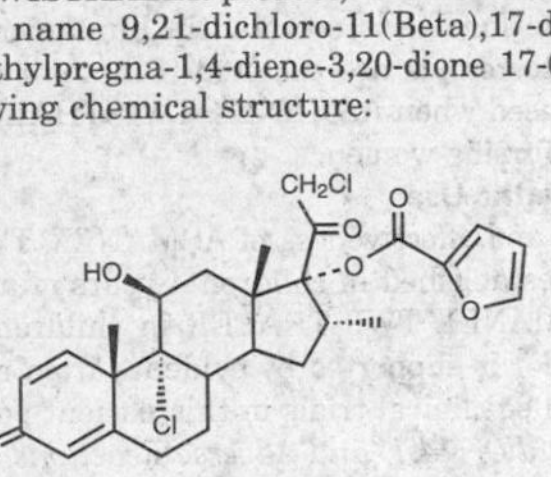

Mometasone furoate is a white powder with an empirical formula of $C_{27}H_{30}Cl_2O_6$, and molecular weight of 521.44 Daltons.

The ASMANEX TWISTHALER 110 mcg and 220 mcg products are cap-activated, inhalation-driven, multidose dry powder inhalers containing mometasone furoate and anhydrous lactose (which contains milk proteins).

Each actuation of the ASMANEX TWISTHALER 110 mcg or 220 mcg inhaler provides a measured dose of approximately 0.75 or 1.5 mg mometasone furoate inhalation powder, containing 110 or 220 mcg of mometasone furoate, respectively. This results in delivery of 100 or 200 mcg mometasone furoate from the mouthpiece, respectively, based on *in vitro* testing at flow rates of 30 L/min and 60 L/min with constant volume of 2 L. The amount of mometasone furoate emitted from the inhaler *in vitro* does not differ significantly for flow rates ranging from 28.3 L/min to 70 L/min at a constant volume of 2 L. However, the amount of drug delivered to the lung will depend on patient factors such as inspiratory flow and peak inspiratory flow through the device. In adult and adolescent patients (aged ≥12 years) with varied asthma severity, mean peak inspiratory flow rate through the device was 69 L/min (range: 54–77 L/min). In pediatric patients (aged 5–12 years) diagnosed with asthma, mean peak inspiratory flow rate in the 5- to 8-year-old subgroup was >50 L/min (minimum of 46 L/min) and for the 9- to 12-year-old subgroup was >60 L/min (minimum of 48 L/min).

12 CLINICAL PHARMACOLOGY

12.1 Mechanism of Action

Mometasone furoate is a corticosteroid demonstrating potent anti-inflammatory activity. The precise mechanism of corticosteroid action on asthma is not known. Inflammation is an important component in the pathogenesis of asthma. Corticosteroids have been shown to have a wide range of inhibitory effects on multiple cell types (e.g., mast cells, eosinophils, neutrophils, macrophages, and lymphocytes) and mediators (e.g., histamine, eicosanoids, leukotrienes, and cytokines) involved in inflammation and in the asthmatic response. These anti-inflammatory actions of corticosteroids may contribute to their efficacy in asthma.

Mometasone furoate has been shown *in vitro* to exhibit a binding affinity for the human glucocorticoid receptor, which is approximately 12 times that of dexamethasone, 7 times that of triamcinolone acetonide, 5 times that of budesonide, and 1.5 times that of fluticasone. The clinical significance of these findings is unknown.

Though effective for the treatment of asthma, corticosteroids do not affect asthma symptoms immediately. Maximum improvement in symptoms following inhaled administration of mometasone furoate may not be achieved for 1 to 2 weeks or longer after starting treatment. When corticosteroids are discontinued, asthma stability may persist for several days or longer.

12.2 Pharmacodynamics

Adrenal Function: The effects of ASMANEX TWISTHALER on adrenal function have been evaluated in 2 clinical studies: 1 in adults 18 years of age and older and 1 in pediatric patients 6 to 11 years of age. Both clinical studies were specifically designed to assess the effect of ASMANEX TWISTHALER on adrenal function.

In a 29-day, randomized, double-blind, placebo-controlled study in 64 adult and adolescent patients 18 years of age and older with asthma, ASMANEX TWISTHALER 440 mcg twice daily and 880 mcg twice daily (twice the highest recommended daily dose) were compared to both placebo and prednisone 10 mg once daily as a positive control. The 30-minute post-Cosyntropin stimulation serum cortisol concentration on Day 29 was 23.2 mcg/dL for the ASMANEX 440 mcg twice daily group (n=16) and 20.8 mcg/dL for the ASMANEX 880 mcg twice daily group (n=16), compared to 14.5 mcg/dL for the oral prednisone 10 mg group (n=16) and 25 mcg/dL for the placebo group (n=16). The difference between ASMANEX 880 mcg twice daily (twice the maximum recommended dose) and placebo was statistically significant.

In a 29-day, randomized, double-blind, placebo-controlled, parallel-group clinical trial in 50 pediatric patients 6 to 11 years of age with asthma, ASMANEX TWISTHALER 110 mcg twice daily, 220 mcg twice daily, and 440 mcg twice daily (2–8 times the highest pediatric daily recommended daily dose) were compared to placebo. HPA-axis function was assessed by 12-hour plasma cortisol AUC and 24-hour urinary-free cortisol concentrations. After 29 days of treatment, the mean changes in plasma cortisol AUC_{0-12h} from baseline were -0.11, -19.5, -21.3, and -3.47 mcg.hr/dL for the treatment groups of ASMANEX TWISTHALER 110 mcg twice daily (n=12), 220 mcg twice daily (n=12), 440 mcg twice daily (n=11), and placebo (n=7), respectively. The mean differences from placebo in the groups treated with ASMANEX TWISTHALER 110 mcg twice daily, 220 mcg twice daily, and 440 mcg twice daily were 3.4 mcg.hr/dL (95% CI: -14.0, 20.7), -16.0 mcg.hr/dL (95% CI: -33.9, 1.9), and -17.9 mcg.hr/dL (95% CI: -35.8, 0.0), respectively. For 24-hour urinary-free cortisol, after 29 days of treatment, the mean changes from baseline were -1.53, -1.33, -6.70, and -4.68 mcg/day for the groups treated with ASMANEX TWISTHALER 110 mcg twice daily (n=12), 220 mcg twice daily (n=12), 440 mcg twice daily (n=12), and placebo (n=10), respectively. The mean differences in urinary-free cortisol changes from baseline compared to placebo were 3.1 mcg/day (95% CI: -3.3, 9.6), 3.3 mcg/day (95% CI: -3.0, 9.7), and -2.0 mcg/day (95% CI: -8.6, 4.6) for the groups treated with 110 mcg twice daily, 220 mcg twice daily, and 440 mcg twice daily, respectively.

12.3 Pharmacokinetics

Absorption: Following a 1000 mcg inhaled dose of tritiated mometasone furoate inhalation powder to 6 healthy human subjects, plasma concentrations of unchanged mometasone furoate were shown to be very low compared to the total radioactivity in plasma. Following an inhaled single 400 mcg dose of ASMANEX TWISTHALER treatment to 24 healthy subjects, plasma concentrations for most subjects were near or below the lower limit of quantitation for the assay (50 pcg/mL). The mean absolute systemic bioavailability of the above single inhaled 400 mcg dose, compared to an intravenous 400 mcg dose of mometasone furoate, was determined to be less than 1%. Following administration of the recommended highest inhaled dose (400 mcg twice daily) to 64 patients for 28 days, concentration-time profiles were discernible, but with large intersubject variability. The coefficient of variation for C_{max} and AUC ranged from approximately 50% to 100%. The mean peak plasma concentrations at steady state ranged from approximately 94 to 114 pcg/mL and the mean time to peak levels ranged from approximately 1.0 to 2.5 hours.

Distribution: Based on the study employing a 1000 mcg inhaled dose of tritiated mometasone furoate inhalation powder in humans, no appreciable accumulation of mometasone furoate in the red blood cells was found. Following an intravenous 400 mcg dose of mometasone furoate, the plasma concentrations showed a biphasic decline, with a mean terminal half-life of about 5 hours and the mean steady-state volume of distribution of 152 L. The *in vitro* protein binding for mometasone furoate was reported to be 98% to 99% (in a concentration range of 5–500 ng/mL).

Metabolism: Studies have shown that mometasone furoate is primarily and extensively metabolized in the liver of all species investigated and undergoes extensive metabolism to multiple metabolites. *In vitro* studies have confirmed the primary role of CYP 3A4 in the metabolism of this compound; however, no major metabolites were identified.

Excretion: Following an intravenous dosing, the terminal half-life was reported to be about 5 hours. Following the inhaled dose of tritiated 1000 mcg mometasone furoate, the radioactivity is excreted mainly in the feces (a mean of 74%), and to a small extent in the urine (a mean of 8%) up to 7 days. No radioactivity was associated with unchanged mometasone furoate in the urine.

Special Populations: *Hepatic Impairment:* Administration of a single inhaled dose of 400 mcg mometasone furoate to subjects with mild (n=4), moderate (n=4), and severe (n=4) hepatic impairment resulted in only 1 or 2 subjects in each group having detectable peak plasma concentrations of mometasone furoate (ranging from 50–105 pcg/mL). The observed peak plasma concentrations appear to increase with severity of hepatic impairment; however, the numbers of detectable levels were few.

Renal Impairment: The effects of renal impairment on mometasone furoate pharmacokinetics have not been adequately investigated.

Pediatric: Mometasone furoate pharmacokinetics have not been investigated in the pediatric population *[see Use in Specific Populations (8.4)]*.

Gender: The effects of gender on mometasone furoate pharmacokinetics have not been adequately investigated.

Race: The effects of race on mometasone furoate pharmacokinetics have not been adequately investigated.

Drug-Drug Interaction: *Inhibitors of Cytochrome P450 3A4:* In a drug interaction study, an inhaled dose of mometasone furoate 400 mcg was given to 24 healthy subjects twice daily for 9 days and ketoconazole 200 mg (as well as placebo) were given twice daily concomitantly on Days 4 to 9. Mometasone furoate plasma concentrations were <150 pcg/mL on Day 3 prior to coadministration of ketoconazole or placebo. Following concomitant administration of ketoconazole, 4 out of 12 subjects in the ketoconazole treatment group (n=12) had peak plasma concentrations of mometasone furoate >200 pcg/mL on Day 9 (211–324 pcg/mL).

13 NONCLINICAL TOXICOLOGY

13.1 Carcinogenesis, Mutagenesis, Impairment of Fertility

In a 2-year carcinogenicity study in Sprague Dawley® rats, mometasone furoate demonstrated no statistically significant increase in the incidence of tumors at inhalation doses up to 67 mcg/kg (approximately 8 times the maximum recommended daily inhalation dose in adults on an AUC basis and 2 times the maximum recommended daily inhalation dose in pediatric patients based on an mcg/m^2 basis). In a 19-month carcinogenicity study in Swiss CD-1 mice, mometasone furoate demonstrated no statistically significant increase in the incidence of tumors at inhalation doses up to 160 mcg/kg (approximately 10 times the maximum recommended daily inhalation dose in adults on an AUC basis and 2 times the maximum recommended daily inhalation dose in pediatric patients based on an mcg/m^2 basis).

Mometasone furoate increased chromosomal aberrations in an *in vitro* Chinese hamster ovary cell assay, but did not have this effect in an *in vitro* Chinese hamster lung cell assay. Mometasone furoate was not mutagenic in the Ames test or mouse lymphoma assay, and was not clastogenic in an *in vivo* mouse micronucleus assay, a rat bone marrow chromosomal aberration assay, or a mouse male germ-cell chromosomal aberration assay. Mometasone furoate also did not induce unscheduled DNA synthesis *in vivo* in rat hepatocytes.

In reproductive studies in rats, impairment of fertility was not produced by subcutaneous doses up to 15 mcg/kg (approximately 6 times the maximum recommended daily inhalation dose in adults on an AUC basis).

13.2 Animal Toxicology and/or Pharmacology

Reproductive Toxicology Studies: In mice, mometasone furoate caused cleft palate at subcutaneous doses of 60 mcg/kg and above (less than the maximum recommended daily inhalation dose in adults on an mcg/m^2 basis). Fetal survival was reduced at 180 mcg/kg (approximately equal to the maximum recommended daily inhalation dose in adults on an mcg/m^2 basis). No toxicity was observed at 20 mcg/kg (less than the maximum recommended daily inhalation dose in adults on an mcg/m^2 basis).

In rats, mometasone furoate produced umbilical hernia at topical dermal doses of 600 mcg/kg and above (approximately 6 times the maximum recommended daily inhalation dose in adults on an mcg/m^2 basis). A dose of 300 mcg/kg (approximately 3 times the maximum recommended daily inhalation dose in adults on an mcg/m^2 basis) produced delays in ossification but no malformations.

When rats received subcutaneous doses of mometasone furoate throughout pregnancy or during the later stages of pregnancy, 15 mcg/kg (approximately 6 times the maximum recommended daily inhalation dose in adults on an AUC basis) caused prolonged and difficult labor and reduced the number of live births, birth weight, and early pup survival. Similar effects were not observed at 7.5 mcg/kg (approximately 3 times the maximum recommended daily inhalation dose in adults on an AUC basis).

In rabbits, mometasone furoate caused multiple malformations (e.g., flexed front paws, gallbladder agenesis, umbilical hernia, hydrocephaly) at topical dermal doses of 150 mcg/kg and above (approximately 3 times the maximum recommended daily inhalation dose in adults on an mcg/m^2 basis). In an oral study, mometasone furoate increased resorptions and caused cleft palate and/or head malformations (hydrocephaly and domed head) at 700 mcg/kg (less than the maximum recommended daily inhalation dose in adults on an area under the curve [AUC] basis). At 2800 mcg/kg (approximately 2 times the maximum recommended daily inhalation dose in adults on an AUC basis) most litters were aborted or resorbed. No toxicity was observed at 140 mcg/kg (less than the maximum recommended daily inhalation dose in adults on an AUC basis).

14 CLINICAL STUDIES

14.1 Asthma

Adults and Adolescents 12 Years of Age and Older: The efficacy of ASMANEX TWISTHALER in patients with asthma 12 years and older was evaluated in ten 8- to 12-week, randomized, double-blind, placebo-controlled, parallel-group clinical trials. These trials included 1750 patients ranging from 12 to 83 years of age, 38% male and 62% female, and 83% Caucasian, 8% black, 6% Hispanic, and 3% other race/ethnicity. Patients received ASMANEX TWISTHALER 110 mcg twice daily (n=133), 220 mcg once daily in the morning (n=209), 220 mcg once daily in the evening (n=232), 220 mcg twice daily (n=433), 440 mcg once daily in the morning (n=419), 440 mcg once daily in the evening (n=250), or 440 mcg twice daily (n=74). The results of the clinical trials are presented based upon previous asthma therapy.

Patients ≥ 12 Years of Age Previously Maintained on Bronchodilators Alone: ASMANEX TWISTHALER was studied in three 12-week, double-blind trials in 737 patients with mild to moderate asthma (mean baseline FEV_1 ≅ 2.6 L, 72% of predicted normal) who were maintained on short-acting beta$_2$-agonists alone. The first 2 trials evaluated doses of 440 mcg administered as 2 inhalations once daily in the morning and 1 of these studies also evaluated 220 mcg twice daily. In both trials, AM predose FEV_1 was significantly improved at endpoint (last observation) following treatment with 440 mcg ASMANEX TWISTHALER once daily in the morning as compared to placebo (14% vs. 2.5%, respectively, in 1 trial and 16% vs. 5.5% in the other). There was also a significant improvement in AM predose FEV_1 at endpoint following treatment with ASMANEX TWISTHALER 220 mcg twice daily. Other measures of lung function (AM and PM PEFR) also showed improvement compared to placebo. Patients receiving ASMANEX TWISTHALER treatment had reduced frequency of beta$_2$-agonist rescue medication use compared to those on placebo (mean reductions at endpoint 2.2 and 0.5 puffs per day, respectively, from a baseline of 4.1 puffs/day). Additionally, fewer patients receiving ASMANEX TWISTHALER 440 mcg once daily experienced asthma worsening than did patients receiving placebo.

In the third trial, 195 asthmatic patients were treated with ASMANEX TWISTHALER 220 mcg once daily in the evening or placebo. The AM FEV_1 at endpoint was significantly improved compared to placebo (mean change at endpoint 0.43 L or 16.8% vs. 0.16 L or 6%, respectively, see **Figure 1**). Evening PEF increased 24.96 L/min (7%) from baseline in the ASMANEX TWISTHALER group compared to 8.67 L/min (4%) in placebo.

FIGURE 1: A 12-Week Trial in Patients Previously Maintained on Inhaled Beta$_2$-agonists

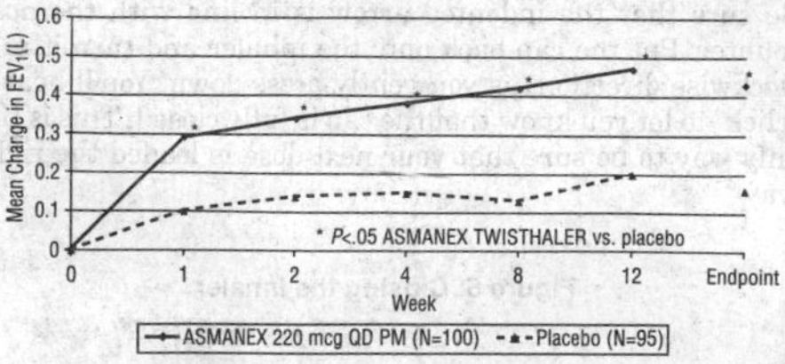
Mean Change in FEV1(L)
0.6
0.5
0.4
0.3
0.2
0.1
0
* P<.05 ASMANEX TWISTHALER vs. placebo
0
1
2
4
8
12
Endpoint
Week
ASMANEX 220 mcg QD PM (N=100)
Placebo (N=95)

Patients ≥ 12 Years of Age Previously Maintained on Inhaled Corticosteroids: The efficacy and safety of ASMANEX TWISTHALER in doses ranging from 110 mcg twice daily to 440 mcg twice daily was evaluated in 3 trials in 1072 patients previously maintained on inhaled corticosteroids. In the first 2 trials, asthmatic patients (mean baseline FEV_1 ~2.6 L, 76% predicted) were previously on either beclomethasone dipropionate [84–1200 mcg/day], flunisolide [100–2000 mcg/day], fluticasone propionate [110–880 mcg/day], or triamcinolone acetonide [300–2400 mcg/day]. The first trial included 307 patients who were treated in an open-label fashion with ASMANEX TWISTHALER 220 mcg (110 mcg × 2 inhalations) twice daily for 2 weeks followed by 12 weeks of double-blind treatment with ASMANEX TWISTHALER 440 mcg once daily in the morning or placebo. The second trial involved 365 patients who continued on their previous dose of inhaled corticosteroids during a 2-week screening period before being switched to ASMANEX TWISTHALER 440 mcg twice daily, 220 mcg twice daily, 110 mcg twice daily, beclomethasone dipropionate 168 mcg twice daily, or placebo for 12 weeks. In the first trial, AM predose FEV_1 was effectively maintained (-1.4% change from baseline to endpoint) over the 12 weeks in the patients who were randomized to ASMANEX TWISTHALER 440 mcg once daily in the morning, while decreasing 10% at endpoint in those switched to placebo. In addition, fewer patients treated with ASMANEX TWISTHALER experienced worsening of asthma compared to placebo.

In the second trial, AM predose FEV_1 was significantly increased at endpoint when patients were switched to ASMANEX TWISTHALER 220 mcg twice daily (7% increase) or 440 mcg twice daily (6.2% increase) as compared to a decrease of 7% when switched to placebo. Additionally, beta$_2$-agonist rescue medication use was decreased for patients who received ASMANEX TWISTHALER treatment relative to those on placebo (mean reduction from baseline to endpoint 1.1 puffs/day vs. increase of 0.7 puffs/day). Fewer patients receiving ASMANEX TWISTHALER treatment experienced asthma worsening than did patients receiving placebo.

The third trial evaluated the efficacy and safety of ASMANEX TWISTHALER compared to placebo in 400 asthmatic patients (mean FEV_1 67% predicted at baseline) previously maintained on beclomethasone dipropionate (hydrofluoroalkane [HFA] or chlorofluorocarbon [CFC]) 168–600 mcg/day, budesonide 200–1200 mcg/day, flunisolide 500–2000 mcg/day, fluticasone propionate 88–880 mcg/day, or triamcinolone acetonide 400–1600 mcg/day. Following a 28-day inhaled corticosteroid dose-reduction phase, patients were randomized to ASMANEX TWISTHALER 440 mcg once daily in the evening, 220 mcg once daily in the evening, 220 mcg twice daily, or placebo. At endpoint, patients who received ASMANEX TWISTHALER 220 mcg once daily in the evening, 440 mcg once daily in the evening, or 220 mcg twice daily had a significant improvement in AM FEV_1 [0.41 L (19%), 0.49 L (22%), and 0.51 L (24%) in the 220 mcg once daily in the evening, 440 mcg once daily in the evening, and 220 mcg twice daily treatment group, respectively] compared to placebo [0.16 L (8%)] (see Figure 2). Evening PEF increased 15.65 L/min (4.1%) with the 220 mcg once daily in the evening dose, 39.26 L/min (10.7%) with the 440 mcg once daily in the evening dose, and 36.7 L/min (10.8%) with the 220 mcg twice daily dose, respectively, compared to a 1.4 L/min (1%) increase with placebo. Patients receiving all doses of ASMANEX TWISTHALER treatment had reduced frequency of beta-agonist rescue medication use compared to those on placebo (mean reductions at endpoint of 1.4–1.8 puffs/day from a baseline of more than 3 puffs/day compared to an increase in use by 0.5 puffs/day for placebo). In addition, fewer patients receiving ASMANEX TWISTHALER experienced asthma worsening than did those on placebo.

FIGURE 2: A 12-Week Trial in Patients Previously Maintained on Inhaled Corticosteroids

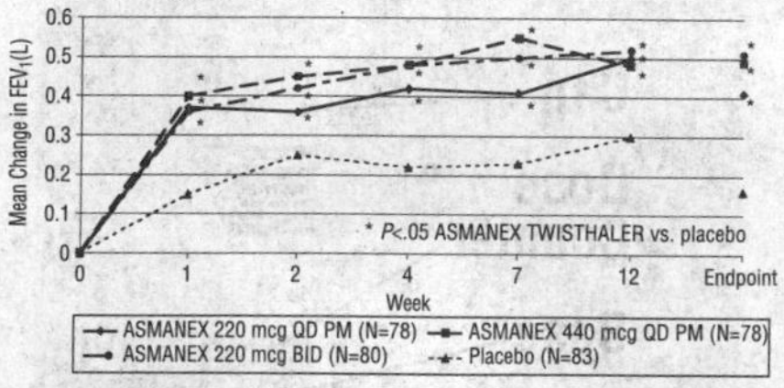
Mean Change in FEV1(L)
0.6
0.5
0.4
0.3
0.2
0.1
0
* P<.05 ASMANEX TWISTHALER vs. placebo
0
1
2
4
7
12
Endpoint
Week
ASMANEX 220 mcg QD PM (N=78)
ASMANEX 440 mcg QD PM (N=78)
ASMANEX 220 mcg BID (N=80)
Placebo (N=83)

Patients ≥ 12 Years of Age Previously Maintained on Oral Corticosteroids: The efficacy of ASMANEX TWISTHALER 440 mcg and 880 mcg twice daily was evaluated in one 12-week, double-blind trial in patients previously maintained on oral corticosteroids. A total of 132 patients requiring oral prednisone (baseline mean daily oral prednisone requirement approximately 12 mg; baseline FEV_1 of 1.8 L, 59% of predicted normal), most of whom were also on inhaled corticosteroids (baseline inhaled steroid: beclomethasone dipropionate [168–840 mcg/day], budesonide [800–1600 mcg/day], flunisolide [1000–2000 mcg/day], fluticasone propionate [440–1760 mcg/day], or triamcinolone acetonide [400–2400 mcg/day]) were studied. Patients who received ASMANEX TWISTHALER 440 mcg twice daily had a significant reduction in their oral prednisone (46%) as compared to placebo (164% increase in oral prednisone dose). Additionally, 40% of patients on ASMANEX TWISTHALER 440 mcg twice daily were able to completely discontinue their use of prednisone, whereas 60% of patients on placebo had an increase in daily prednisone use. Patients on ASMANEX TWISTHALER had significant improvement in lung function (14% increase) compared to a 12% decrease in FEV_1 in the placebo group. Additionally, mean rescue beta$_2$-agonist use was reduced to approximately 3 puffs/day from a baseline of 4–5 puffs/day with ASMANEX TWISTHALER treatment, compared to an increase of 0.3 puffs/day on placebo. Patients who received ASMANEX TWISTHALER 880 mcg twice daily experienced no additional benefit beyond that seen with 440 mcg twice daily.

Pediatric Patients 4 to 11 Years of Age: The efficacy of ASMANEX TWISTHALER in patients with asthma 4 to 11 years of age was evaluated in three 12-week, randomized, double-blind, placebo-controlled, parallel-group clinical trials. These trials included 630 patients receiving ASMANEX TWISTHALER, ranging from 4 to 11 years of age, 63% male and 37% female, and 67% Caucasian, 13% black, 17% Hispanic, and 3% other race/ethnicity. Patients received ASMANEX TWISTHALER 110 mcg once daily in the evening (n=98), 110 mcg once daily in the morning (n=181), 110 mcg twice daily (n=179), or 220 mcg once daily in the morning (n=172). The results for 1 clinical trial are described below. The other 2 clinical trials support the efficacy of ASMANEX TWISTHALER.

A 12-week, placebo-controlled trial of 296 patients 4 to 11 years of age with asthma of at least 6 months duration (mean % predicted FEV_1 at baseline ranging from 77.3%–79.7%) was conducted to demonstrate the efficacy of the ASMANEX TWISTHALER in the treatment of asthma. Patients were treated with ASMANEX TWISTHALER 110 mcg once daily in the evening (n=98) or placebo (n=99) for 12 weeks. Assessment of efficacy was based upon morning predose FEV_1. The primary endpoint was the mean change from baseline to endpoint in percent-predicted FEV_1. For the primary endpoint, improvement in the ASMANEX TWISTHALER 110 mcg once daily in the evening treatment group (4.73) was statistically significant compared to placebo (-1.77). **Figure 3** displays the results for % predicted FEV_1 change from baseline at endpoint.

In this study, secondary endpoints of morning and evening peak expiratory flow and rescue medication use were supportive of efficacy of ASMANEX TWISTHALER.

FIGURE 3: A 12-Week Trial in Children 4 to 11 Years of Age: % Predicted FEV_1 Change from Baseline Over Time and at Endpoint by Treatment Group

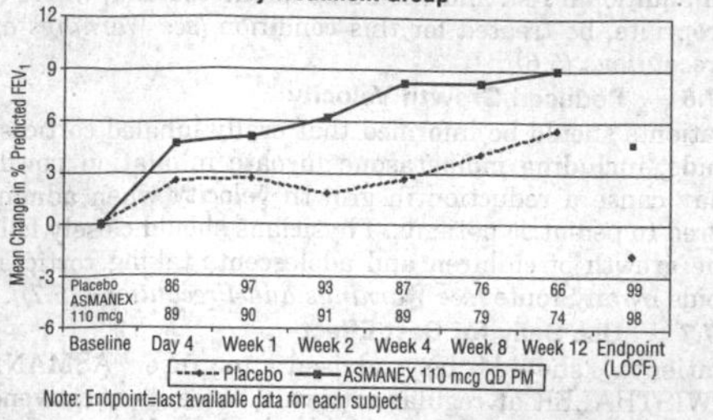
Mean Change in % Predicted FEV1
12
9
6
3
0
-3
-6
Placebo 86 97 93 87 76 66 99
ASMANEX 110 mcg 89 90 91 89 79 74 98
Baseline
Day 4
Week 1
Week 2
Week 4
Week 8
Week 12
Endpoint (LOCF)
Placebo
ASMANEX 110 mcg QD PM
Note: Endpoint=last available data for each subject

16 HOW SUPPLIED/STORAGE AND HANDLING

The ASMANEX TWISTHALER 220 mcg product is comprised of an assembled plastic cap–activated dosing mechanism with dose counter, drug-product storage unit, drug-product formulation (240 mg), and mouthpiece, covered by a white screw cap that bears the product label. The body of the inhaler is white and the turning grip is pink with a clear plastic window indicating the number of doses remaining. The inhaler will not deliver subsequent doses once the counter reaches zero ("00").

The ASMANEX TWISTHALER 110 mcg product is comprised of an assembled plastic cap–activated dosing mechanism with dose counter, drug-product storage unit, drug-product formulation (135 mg), and mouthpiece, covered by a white screw cap that bears the product label. The body of the inhaler is white and the turning grip is gray with a clear plastic window indicating the number of doses remaining. The inhaler will not deliver subsequent doses once the counter reaches zero ("00").

The ASMANEX TWISTHALER product is available as:

ASMANEX TWISTHALER 220 mcg, which delivers 200 mcg mometasone furoate from the mouthpiece: 14 inhalation units (Institutional Use Only; NDC# 0085-1341-04); 30 inhalation units (NDC# 0085-1341-03); 60 inhalation units (for more than 1 inhalation daily; NDC# 0085-1341-02); or 120 inhalation units (for more than 2 inhalations daily; NDC# 0085-1341-01).

ASMANEX TWISTHALER 110 mcg, which delivers 100 mcg mometasone furoate from the mouthpiece: 7 inhalation units (Institutional Use Only; NDC# 0085-1461-07); 30 inhalation units (NDC# 0085-1461-02).

Each inhaler is supplied in a protective foil pouch with Patient's Instructions for Use.

Store in a dry place at 25°C (77°F); excursions permitted to 15°–30°C (59°–86°F) [see USP Controlled Room Temperature].

Discard the inhaler 45 days after opening the foil pouch or when dose counter reads "00", whichever comes first.

17 PATIENT COUNSELING INFORMATION

See FDA-Approved Patient Labeling (17.9)

17.1 Oral Candidiasis

Patients should be advised that localized infections with *Candida albicans* occurred in the mouth and pharynx in some patients. If oropharyngeal candidiasis develops, it should be treated with appropriate local or systemic (i.e., oral) antifungal therapy while still continuing with ASMANEX TWISTHALER therapy, but at times therapy with ASMANEX TWISTHALER may need to be temporarily interrupted under close medical supervision. Rinsing the mouth after inhalation is advised *[see Warnings and Precautions (5.1)]*.

17.2 Acute Asthma Episodes

Patients should be advised that ASMANEX TWISTHALER is not a bronchodilator and should not be used to treat status asthmaticus or to relieve acute asthma symptoms. Acute asthma symptoms should be treated with an inhaled, short-acting beta$_2$-agonist such as albuterol [see Warnings and Precautions (5.2)].

17.3   Immunosuppression

Patients who are on immunosuppressant doses of corticosteroids should be warned to avoid exposure to chickenpox or measles and, if exposed, to consult their physician without delay. Patients should be informed of potential worsening of existing tuberculosis, fungal, bacterial, viral, or parasitic infections, or ocular herpes simplex [see Warnings and Precautions (5.3)].

17.4   Hypercorticism and Adrenal Suppression

Patients should be advised that ASMANEX TWISTHALER may cause systemic corticosteroid effects of hypercorticism and adrenal suppression. Additionally, patients should be instructed that deaths due to adrenal insufficiency have occurred during and after transfer from systemic corticosteroids. Patients should taper slowly from systemic corticosteroids if transferring to ASMANEX TWISTHALER [see Warnings and Precautions (5.5)].

17.5   Reduction in Bone Mineral Density

Patients who are at an increased risk for decreased BMD should be advised that the use of corticosteroids may pose an additional risk and should be monitored and, where appropriate, be treated for this condition [see Warnings and Precautions (5.6)].

17.6   Reduced Growth Velocity

Patients should be informed that orally inhaled corticosteroids, including mometasone furoate inhalation powder, may cause a reduction in growth velocity when administered to pediatric patients. Physicians should closely follow the growth of children and adolescents taking corticosteroids by any route [see Warnings and Precautions (5.7)].

17.7   Use Daily for Best Effect

Patients should be advised to use ASMANEX TWISTHALER at regular intervals, since its effectiveness depends on regular use. Maximum benefit may not be achieved for 1 to 2 weeks or longer after starting treatment. If symptoms do not improve in that time frame or if the condition worsens, patients should be instructed to contact their physician.

17.8   Instructions for Use

Patients should be instructed to record the date of pouch opening on the cap label, and discard the inhaler 45 days after opening the foil pouch or when the dose counter reads "00", and the final dose has been inhaled, whichever comes first. The inhaler should be held upright while removing the cap. The medication should be taken as directed, breathing rapidly and deeply, and patients should not breathe out through the inhaler. The mouthpiece should be wiped dry and the cap replaced immediately following each inhalation, rotated fully until the click is heard. Rinsing of mouth after inhalation is advised. Patients should store the unit as instructed. The dose counter displays the doses remaining. When the dose counter indicates zero, the cap will lock and the unit must be discarded. Patients should be advised that if the dose counter is not working correctly, the unit should not be used and it should be brought to their physician or pharmacist [see FDA-Approved Patient Labeling-Patient's Instructions for Use (17.9)].

17.9   FDA-Approved Patient Labeling

See accompanying Patient's Instruction for Use.
Manufactured by Schering Corporation, a subsidiary of Schering-Plough Corporation, Kenilworth, NJ 07033 USA. © 2008, Schering Corporation. All rights reserved.
U.S. Patent Nos. 5,394,868; 5,687,710; 5,740,792; 5,829,434; 5,889,015; 6,057,307; 6,240,918; 6,365,581; 6,503,537; 6,677,322; 6,949,532; and D348928.
Rev. 10/08 31340519T

The trademarks depicted in this piece are owned by their respective companies.

PATIENT'S INSTRUCTIONS FOR USE

ASMANEX® TWISTHALER® 220 mcg
(mometasone furoate inhalation powder)
ASMANEX® TWISTHALER® 110 mcg
(mometasone furoate inhalation powder)
FOR ORAL INHALATION ONLY

Please read this leaflet carefully before taking ASMANEX® TWISTHALER®.
This leaflet does not contain the complete information about this medication. If you have any questions about ASMANEX TWISTHALER, ask your health care provider or pharmacist.

IMPORTANT POINTS TO REMEMBER ABOUT ASMANEX TWISTHALER

• Your health care provider has prescribed ASMANEX TWISTHALER for you or your child. It contains a medicine called mometasone furoate. This medicine is used as maintenance treatment that helps prevent and control asthma symptoms.
• ASMANEX TWISTHALER is not a bronchodilator and should not be used for sudden symptoms of shortness of

breath. Use an inhaled short-acting bronchodilator such as albuterol to relieve sudden symptoms of shortness of breath.
• Your health care provider may prescribe bronchodilators such as albuterol for emergency relief if an acute asthma attack occurs.
• Use your ASMANEX TWISTHALER regularly and at the same time each day, as prescribed by your health care provider. You or your child may not get the most benefit for 1 to 2 weeks or longer after starting ASMANEX. If you or your child's symptoms do not improve in that time frame or if your condition gets worse, contact your health care provider.
• The cap is needed to use the ASMANEX TWISTHALER. Do not twist the mouthpiece with your hand. When the cap is removed from the TWISTHALER, the dose counter will count down by one, and show the number of doses available after this use.
• The inhaler delivers your medicine as a very fine powder that **you or your child may not taste, smell, or feel.** Do not take or give extra doses unless your health care provider has told you to.
• It is important to replace the cap after each inhalation to protect the inhaler from moisture.
• Do not use the inhaler if you notice that it is not working correctly. Take it to your health care provider or pharmacist.

HOW TO USE ASMANEX TWISTHALER OR GIVE TO YOUR CHILD

• Remove the ASMANEX TWISTHALER from its foil pouch and write the date on the cap label.
• Throw away the inhaler 45 days after this date or when the dose counter reads "00", indicating the final dose has been inhaled, whichever comes first.
• **Follow steps 1 and 2 below each time you inhale a dose from your ASMANEX TWISTHALER.**

Inhaler Parts:
See Figures 1 and 2 below to become familiar with the inhaler parts.

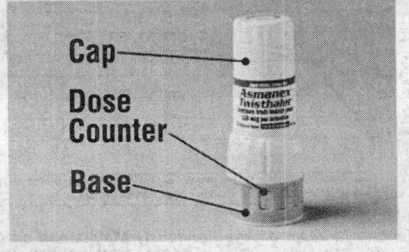
Figure 1: Inhaler (upright position)

Cap
Dose Counter
Base

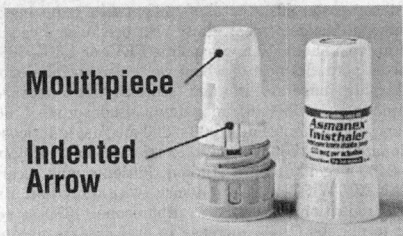
Figure 2: Inhaler with Cap Removed

Mouthpiece
Indented Arrow

Step 1:   Open inhaler
Hold the inhaler straight up (upright position) with the colored portion (the base) on the bottom (see Figure 3 below). It is important that you remove the cap of the TWISTHALER while it is in this upright position to make sure that you get the right amount of medicine with each dose.
Holding the colored base, twist the cap in a counterclockwise direction to remove it (see Figure 3 below). As you lift off the cap, the dose counter on the base will count down by one. Removing the cap loads the TWISTHALER with the medicine that you are now ready to inhale.
[See figure 3 at top of next column]
IT IS IMPORTANT TO NOTE that the indented arrow (located on the white portion of the TWISTHALER, directly above the colored base) is pointing to the dose counter (see Figure 2).

Step 2:   Inhale dose
Breathe out fully. Then bring the TWISTHALER up to your mouth or your child's mouth with the mouthpiece facing toward you or your child. Place the mouthpiece in your mouth or your child's mouth, holding it in a horizontal (on its side) position as shown below (see Figure 4). Firmly close your lips around the mouthpiece and take in a fast, deep breath. Since the medicine is a very fine powder, you may not be

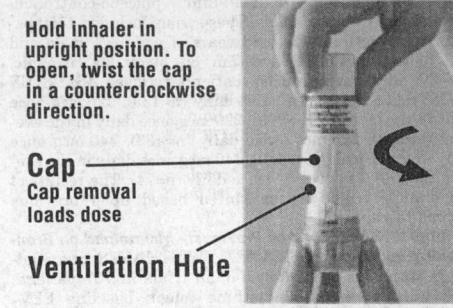
Figure 3: Cap Removal Loads Dose

Hold inhaler in upright position. To open, twist the cap in a counterclockwise direction.

Cap
Cap removal loads dose

Ventilation Hole

able to taste, smell, or feel it after inhalation. Do not cover the ventilation holes while inhaling the dose.

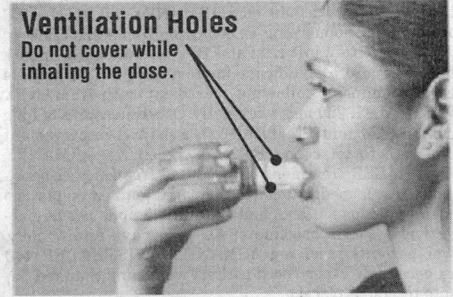
Figure 4: Inhalation

Ventilation Holes
Do not cover while inhaling the dose.

Remove the TWISTHALER from your mouth and hold your breath for about 10 seconds, or as long as you comfortably can.
IMPORTANT: DO NOT BREATHE OUT (EXHALE) INTO THE INHALER.
After you take your medicine, it is important that you wipe the mouthpiece dry, if needed, and then **REPLACE THE CAP**, firmly closing the TWISTHALER right away (see Figures 5 and 6 below).
Be sure that the indented arrow is in line with the dose counter. Put the cap back onto the inhaler and turn it in a clockwise direction, as you gently press down. You'll hear a "click" to let you know that the cap is fully closed. This is the only way to be sure that your next dose is loaded the right way.

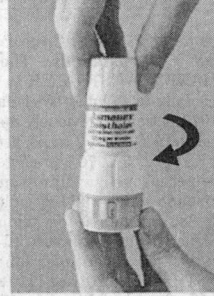
Figure 5: Closing the Inhaler

You'll hear a "click" to let you know that the cap is fully closed.

This is the only way to be sure that your next dose is properly loaded.

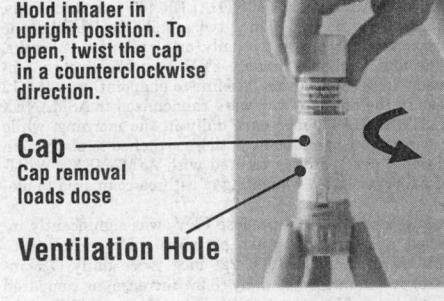
Figure 6: Closed Inhaler

Hold inhaler in upright position. To open, twist the cap in a counterclockwise direction.

Cap
Cap removal loads dose

Ventilation Hole

IT IS IMPORTANT TO REPEAT STEPS 1 AND 2 EACH TIME YOU INHALE.
Rinse your mouth after using.

STORING YOUR INHALER
- Keep your inhaler clean and dry at all times. If the mouthpiece needs cleaning, gently wipe the mouthpiece with a dry cloth or tissue as needed. Do not wash the inhaler. Avoid contact with any liquids.
- Store in a dry place at 25°C (77°F) [may range between 15°–30°C (59°–86°F)]
- Keep your inhaler out of the reach of children.

HOW TO KNOW WHEN YOUR INHALER IS EMPTY
The inhaler has a dose counter on the colored base, which shows the number of doses left to use. As you lift off the cap to take your dose, the dose counter on the base will count down by one (if you began with the dose counter reading "30" this will cause the dose counter to now read "29"). Read the numbers from top to bottom.

When the unit reads "01" this indicates the last remaining dose. After dose "01" the counter will read "00". When you replace the cap, the unit will lock and then must be thrown away. Start using a new ASMANEX TWISTHALER as instructed by your health care provider.

POSSIBLE SIDE EFFECTS WITH ASMANEX TWISTHALER
Serious Side Effects may include:
- **Fungal infections in the mouth and throat.** Patients who use inhaled steroid medicines for asthma may develop a fungal infection of the mouth. Rinse your mouth after using ASMANEX TWISTHALER.
- **Possible increased risk of infection due to a weakened immune system with using steroid medicines.** Tell your health care provider if you or your child have or had TB, are exposed to anyone with chickenpox or measles, or about any other infections you or your child had before or while using ASMANEX TWISTHALER.
- **Adrenal insufficiency (your adrenal gland cannot produce enough steroids since you were on oral steroid medicine).** If you or your child took steroids by mouth and are having them decreased (tapered) or you are being switched to ASMANEX TWISTHALER, you should be followed closely by your health care professional.
Death can occur. Tell your health care professional right away about any symptoms such as feeling tired or exhausted, weakness, nausea, vomiting, or symptoms of low blood pressure (such as dizziness or faintness). If you or your child is under stress, such as with surgery, after surgery or trauma, you may need steroids by mouth again.
- **Decreased bone mass (bone mineral density).** Patients who use inhaled steroid medicines for a long time may have an increased risk of decreased bone mass, which can affect bone strength. Talk with your health care provider about any questions about bone health.

The most common side effects with ASMANEX TWISTHALER include: headache, nasal allergy symptoms, sore throat, upper respiratory tract infection, sinus infection, fungal infections in the mouth, painful menstrual periods, muscle and bone pain, back pain, and upset stomach. Tell your health care professional about any side effects that bother you or do not go away. These are not all of the possible side effects with ASMANEX TWISTHALER. For more information, ask your health care professional.

Manufactured by Schering Corporation, a subsidiary of Schering-Plough Corporation, Kenilworth, NJ 07033 USA.
© 2008, Schering Corporation. All rights reserved.
U.S. Patent Nos. 5,394,868; 5,687,710; 5,740,792; 5,829,434; 5,889,015; 6,057,307; 6,240,918; 6,365,581; 6,503,537; 6,677,322; 6,949,532; and D348928.
Rev. 10/08
31340616T
Shown in Product Identification Guide, page 311

AVELOX®
[ă'vĕ-lŏks]
(moxifloxacin hydrochloride) Tablets
AVELOX® I.V.
(moxifloxacin hydrochloride in sodium chloride injection)

℞

WARNING:
Fluoroquinolones, including AVELOX®, are associated with an increased risk of tendinitis and tendon rupture in all ages. This risk is further increased in older patients usually over 60 years of age, in patients taking corticosteroid drugs, and in patients with kidney, heart or lung transplants (see WARNINGS).

To reduce the development of drug-resistant bacteria and maintain the effectiveness of AVELOX and other antibacterial drugs, AVELOX should be used only to treat or prevent infections that are proven or strongly suspected to be caused by bacteria.

	C_{max} (mg/L)	AUC (mg•h/L)	Half-life (hr)
Single Dose Oral			
Healthy (n = 372)	3.1 ± 1	36.1 ± 9.1	11.5-15.6*
Multiple Dose Oral			
Healthy young male/female (n = 15)	4.5 ± 0.5	48 ± 2.7	12.7 ± 1.9
Healthy elderly male (n = °)	3.8 ± 0.3	51.8 ± 6.7	
Healthy elderly female (n = 8)	4.6 ± 0.6	54.6 ± 6.7	
Healthy young male (n = 8)	3.6 ± 0.5	48.2 ± 9	
Healthy young female (n = 9)	4.2 ± 0.5	49.3 ± 9.5	

*Range of means from different studies

	C_{max} (mg/L)	AUC (mg•h/L)	Half-life (hr)
Single Dose I.V.			
Healthy young male/female (n = 56)	3.9 ± 0.9	39.3 ± 8.6	8.2-15.4*
Patients (n = 118)			
Male (n = 64)	4.4 ± 3.7		
Female (n = 54)	4.5 ± 2		
< 65 years (n = 58)	4.6 ± 4.2		
≥ 65 years (n = 60)	4.3 ± 1.3		
Multiple Dose I.V.			
Healthy young male (n = 8)	4.2 ± 0.8	38 ± 4.7	14.8 ± 2.2
Healthy elderly (n = 12; 8 male, 4 female)	6.1 ± 1.3	48.2 ± 0.9	10.1 ± 1.6
Patients† (n = 107)			
Male (n = 58)	4.2 ± 2.6		
Female (n = 49)	4.6 ± 1.5		
< 65 years (n = 52)	4.1 ± 1.4		
≥ 65 years (n = 55)	4.7 ± 2.7		

Plasma concentrations increase proportionally with dose up to the highest dose tested (1200 mg single oral dose). The mean (± SD) elimination half-life from plasma is 12 ± 1.3 hours; steady-state is achieved after at least three days with a 400 mg once daily regimen.

*Range of means from different studies
†Expected C_{max} (concentration obtained around the time of the end of the infusion)

DESCRIPTION
AVELOX (moxifloxacin hydrochloride) is a synthetic broad spectrum antibacterial agent and is available as AVELOX Tablets for oral administration and as AVELOX I.V. for intravenous administration. Moxifloxacin, a fluoroquinolone, is available as the monohydrochloride salt of 1-cyclopropyl-7-[(S,S)-2,8-diazabicyclo[4.3.0]non-8-yl]-6-fluoro-8-methoxy-1,4-dihydro-4-oxo-3 quinoline carboxylic acid. It is a slightly yellow to yellow crystalline substance with a molecular weight of 437.9. Its empirical formula is $C_{21}H_{24}FN_3O_4$*HCl and its chemical structure is as follows:

AVELOX Tablets are available as film-coated tablets containing moxifloxacin hydrochloride (equivalent to 400 mg moxifloxacin). The inactive ingredients are microcrystalline cellulose, lactose monohydrate, croscarmellose sodium, magnesium stearate, hypromellose, titanium dioxide, polyethylene glycol and ferric oxide.
AVELOX I.V. is available in ready-to-use 250 mL latex-free flexibags as a sterile, preservative free, 0.8% sodium chloride aqueous solution of moxifloxacin hydrochloride (containing 400 mg moxifloxacin) with pH ranging from 4.1 to 4.6. The appearance of the intravenous solution is yellow. The color does not affect, nor is it indicative of, product stability. The inactive ingredients are sodium chloride, USP, Water for Injection, USP, and may include hydrochloric acid and/or sodium hydroxide for pH adjustment. AVELOX I.V. contains approximately 34.2 mEq (787 mg) of sodium in 250 mL.

CLINICAL PHARMACOLOGY
Absorption
Moxifloxacin, given as an oral tablet, is well absorbed from the gastrointestinal tract. The absolute bioavailability of moxifloxacin is approximately 90 percent. Co-administration with a high fat meal (i.e., 500 calories from fat) does not affect the absorption of moxifloxacin.
Consumption of 1 cup of yogurt with moxifloxacin does not significantly affect the extent or rate of systemic absorption (AUC).
The mean (± SD) C_{max} and AUC values following single and multiple doses of 400 mg moxifloxacin given orally are summarized below.

[See first table above]
The mean (± SD) C_{max} and AUC values following single and multiple doses of 400 mg moxifloxacin given by 1 hour I.V. infusion are summarized below.
[See second table above]

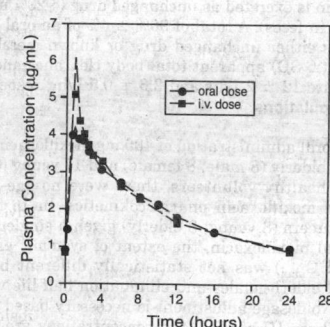

Mean Steady-State Plasma Concentrations of Moxifloxacin Obtained With Once Daily Dosing of 400 mg Either Orally (n=10) or by I.V. Infusion (n=12)

Distribution
Moxifloxacin is approximately 30-50% bound to serum proteins, independent of drug concentration. The volume of distribution of moxifloxacin ranges from 1.7 to 2.7 L/kg. Moxifloxacin is widely distributed throughout the body, with tissue concentrations often exceeding plasma concentrations. Moxifloxacin has been detected in the saliva, nasal and bronchial secretions, mucosa of the sinuses, skin blister fluid, subcutaneous tissue, skeletal muscle, and abdominal tissues and fluids following oral or intravenous administration of 400 mg. Moxifloxacin concentrations measured postdose in various tissues and fluids following a 400 mg oral and I.V. dose are summarized in the following table. The rates of elimination of moxifloxacin from tissues generally parallel the elimination from plasma.
[See table at top of next page]
Metabolism
Approximately 52% of an oral or intravenous dose of moxifloxacin is metabolized via glucuronide and sulfate conjugation. The cytochrome P450 system is not involved in moxifloxacin metabolism, and is not affected by moxifloxacin. The sulfate conjugate (M1) accounts for approximately 38% of the dose, and is eliminated primarily in the feces. Approximately 14% of an oral or intravenous dose is converted to a glucuronide conjugate (M2), which is excreted exclusively in the urine. Peak plasma concentrations

Moxifloxacin Concentrations (mean ± SD) in Tissues and the Corresponding Plasma Concentrations After a Single 400 mg Oral or Intravenous Dose*

Tissue or Fluid	N	Plasma Concentration (μg/mL)	Tissue or Fluid Concentration (μg/mL or μg/g)	Tissue Plasma Ratio
Respiratory				
Alveolar Macrophages	5	3.3 ± 0.7	61.8 ± 27.3	21.2 ± 10
Bronchial Mucosa	8	3.3 ± 0.7	5.5 ± 1.3	1.7 ± 0.3
Epithelial Lining Fluid	5	3.3 ± 0.7	24.4 ± 14.7	8.7 ± 6.1
Sinus				
Maxillary Sinus Mucosa	4	3.7 ± 1.1†	7.6 ± 1.7	2 ± 0.3
Anterior Ethmoid Mucosa	3	3.7 ± 1.1†	8.8 ± 4.3	2.2 ± 0.6
Nasal Polyps	4	3.7 ± 1.1†	9.8 ± 4.5	2.6 ± 0.6
Skin, Musculoskeletal				
Blister Fluid	5	3 ± 0.5‡	2.6 ± 0.9	0.9 ± 0.2
Subcutaneous Tissue	6	2.3 ± 0.4§	0.9 ± 0.3¶	0.4 ± 0.6
Skeletal Muscle	6	2.3 ± 0.4§	0.9 ± 0.2¶	0.4 ± 0.1
Intra-Abdominal				
Abdominal tissue	8	2.9 ± 0.5	7.6 ± 2	2.7 ± 0.8
Abdominal exudate	10	2.3 ± 0.5	3.5 ± 1.2	1.6 ± 0.7
Abscess fluid	6	2.7 ± 0.7	2.3 ± 1.5	0.8 ± 0.4

*all moxifloxacin concentrations were measured 3 hours after a single 400 mg dose, except the abdominal tissue and exudate concentrations which were measured at 2 hours post-dose and the sinus concentrations which were measured 3 hours post-dose after 5 days of dosing.
†N = 5
‡N = 7
§N = 12
¶Reflects only non-protein bound concentrations of drug.

of M2 are approximately 40% those of the parent drug, while plasma concentrations of M1 are generally less than 10% those of moxifloxacin.

In vitro studies with cytochrome (CYP) P450 enzymes indicate that moxifloxacin does not inhibit CYP3A4, CYP2D6, CYP2C9, CYP2C19, or CYP1A2, suggesting that moxifloxacin is unlikely to alter the pharmacokinetics of drugs metabolized by these enzymes.

Excretion

Approximately 45% of an oral or intravenous dose of moxifloxacin is excreted as unchanged drug (~20% in urine and ~25% in feces). A total of 96% ± 4% of an oral dose is excreted as either unchanged drug or known metabolites. The mean (± SD) apparent total body clearance and renal clearance are 12 ± 2 L/hr and 2.6 ± 0.5 L/hr, respectively.

Special Populations

Geriatric

Following oral administration of 400 mg moxifloxacin for 10 days in 16 elderly (8 male; 8 female) and 17 young (8 male; 9 female) healthy volunteers, there were no age-related changes in moxifloxacin pharmacokinetics. In 16 healthy male volunteers (8 young; 8 elderly) given a single 200 mg dose of oral moxifloxacin, the extent of systemic exposure (AUC and C_{max}) was not statistically different between young and elderly males and elimination half-life was unchanged. No dosage adjustment is necessary based on age. In large phase III studies, the concentrations around the time of the end of the infusion in elderly patients following intravenous infusion of 400 mg were similar to those observed in young patients.

Pediatric

The pharmacokinetics of moxifloxacin in pediatric subjects have not been studied.

Gender

Following oral administration of 400 mg moxifloxacin daily for 10 days to 23 healthy males (19-75 years) and 24 healthy females (19-70 years), the mean AUC and C_{max} were 8% and 16% higher, respectively, in females compared to males. There are no significant differences in moxifloxacin pharmacokinetics between male and female subjects when differences in body weight are taken into consideration.

A 400 mg single dose study was conducted in 18 young males and females. The comparison of moxifloxacin pharmacokinetics in this study (9 young females and 9 young males) showed no differences in AUC or C_{max} due to gender. Dosage adjustments based on gender are not necessary.

Race

Steady-state moxifloxacin pharmacokinetics in male Japanese subjects were similar to those determined in Caucasians, with a mean C_{max} of 4.1 μg/mL, an AUC_{24} of 47 μg•h/mL, and an elimination half-life of 14 hours, following 400 mg p.o. daily.

Renal Insufficiency

The pharmacokinetic parameters of moxifloxacin are not significantly altered in mild, moderate, severe, or end-stage renal disease. No dosage adjustment is necessary in patients with renal impairment, including those patients requiring hemodialysis (HD) or continuous ambulatory peritoneal dialysis (CAPD).

In a single oral dose study of 24 patients with varying degrees of renal function from normal to severely impaired, the mean peak concentrations (C_{max}) of moxifloxacin were reduced by 21% and 28% in the patients with moderate ($CL_{CR} \geq 30$ and ≤ 60 mL/min) and severe ($CL_{CR} < 30$ mL/min) renal impairment, respectively. The mean systemic exposure (AUC) in these patients was increased by 13%. In the moderate and severe renally impaired patients, the mean AUC for the sulfate conjugate (M1) increased by 1.7-fold (ranging up to 2.8-fold) and mean AUC and C_{max} for the glucuronide conjugate (M2) increased by 2.8-fold (ranging up to 4.8-fold) and 1.4-fold (ranging up to 2.5-fold), respectively.

The pharmacokinetics of single dose and multiple dose moxifloxacin were studied in patients with $CL_{CR} < 20$ mL/min on either hemodialysis or continuous ambulatory peritoneal dialysis (8 HD, 8 CAPD). Following a single 400 mg oral dose, the AUC of moxifloxacin in these HD and CAPD patients did not vary significantly from the AUC generally found in healthy volunteers. C_{max} values of moxifloxacin were reduced by about 45% and 33% in HD and CAPD patients, respectively, compared to healthy, historical controls. The exposure (AUC) to the sulfate conjugate (M1) increased by 1.4- to 1.5-fold in these patients. The mean AUC of the glucuronide conjugate (M2) increased by a factor of 7.5, whereas the mean C_{max} values of the glucuronide conjugate (M2) increased by a factor of 2.5 to 3, compared to healthy subjects. The sulfate and the glucuronide conjugates of moxifloxacin are not microbiologically active, and the clinical implication of increased exposure to these metabolites in patients with renal disease including those undergoing HD and CAPD has not been studied.

Oral administration of 400 mg QD moxifloxacin for 7 days to patients on HD or CAPD produced mean systemic exposure (AUC_{ss}) to moxifloxacin similar to that generally seen in healthy volunteers. Steady-state C_{max} values were about 22% lower in HD patients but were comparable between CAPD patients and healthy volunteers. Both HD and CAPD removed only small amounts of moxifloxacin from the body (approximately 9% by HD, and 3% by CAPD). HD and CAPD also removed about 4% and 2% of the glucuronide metabolite (M2), respectively.

Hepatic Insufficiency

No dosage adjustment is recommended for mild, moderate, or severe hepatic insufficiency (Child-Pugh Classes A, B, or C). However, due to metabolic disturbances associated with hepatic insufficiency, which may lead to QT prolongation, moxifloxacin should be used with caution in these patients. (See WARNINGS and DOSAGE AND ADMINISTRATION.)

In 400 mg single oral dose studies in 6 patients with mild (Child-Pugh Class A) and 10 patients with moderate (Child-Pugh Class B) hepatic insufficiency, moxifloxacin mean systemic exposure (AUC) was 78% and 102%, respectively, of 18 healthy controls and mean peak concentration (C_{max}) was 79% and 84% of controls.

The mean AUC of the sulfate conjugate of moxifloxacin (M1) increased by 3.9-fold (ranging up to 5.9-fold) and 5.7-fold (ranging up to 8-fold) in the mild and moderate groups, respectively. The mean C_{max} of M1 increased by approximately 3-fold in both groups (ranging up to 4.7- and 3.9-fold). The mean AUC of the glucuronide conjugate of moxifloxacin (M2) increased by 1.5-fold (ranging up to 2.5-fold) in both groups. The mean C_{max} of M2 increased by 1.6- and 1.3-fold (ranging up to 2.7- and 2.1-fold), respectively. The clinical significance of increased exposure to the sulfate and glucuronide conjugates has not been studied. In a subset of patients participating in a clinical trial, the plasma concentrations of moxifloxacin and metabolites determined approximately at the moxifloxacin T_{max} following the first intravenous or oral moxifloxacin dose in the Child-Pugh Class C patients (n=10) were similar to those in the Child-Pugh Class A/B patients (n=5), and also similar to those observed in healthy volunteer studies.

Photosensitivity Potential

A study of the skin response to ultraviolet (UVA and UVB) and visible radiation conducted in 32 healthy volunteers (8 per group) demonstrated that moxifloxacin does not show phototoxicity in comparison to placebo. The minimum erythematous dose (MED) was measured before and after treatment with moxifloxacin (200 mg or 400 mg once daily), lomefloxacin (400 mg once daily), or placebo. In this study, the MED measured for both doses of moxifloxacin were not significantly different from placebo, while lomefloxacin significantly lowered the MED. (See PRECAUTIONS, Information for Patients.)

It is difficult to ascribe relative photosensitivity/phototoxicity among various fluoroquinolones during actual patient use because other factors play a role in determining a subject's susceptibility to this adverse event such as: a patient's skin pigmentation, frequency and duration of sun and artificial ultraviolet light (UV) exposure, wearing of sunscreen and protective clothing, the use of other concomitant drugs and the dosage and duration of fluoroquinolone therapy (See ADVERSE REACTIONS and ADVERSE REACTIONS/Post-Marketing Adverse Event Reports).

Drug-drug Interactions

The potential for pharmacokinetic drug interactions between moxifloxacin and itraconazole, theophylline, warfarin, digoxin, atenolol, probenecid, morphine, oral contraceptives, ranitidine, glyburide, calcium, iron, and antacids has been evaluated. There was no clinically significant effect of moxifloxacin on itraconazole, theophylline, warfarin, digoxin, atenolol, oral contraceptives, or glyburide kinetics. Itraconazole, theophylline, warfarin, digoxin, probenecid, morphine, ranitidine, and calcium did not significantly affect the pharmacokinetics of moxifloxacin. These results and the data from *in vitro* studies suggest that moxifloxacin is unlikely to significantly alter the metabolic clearance of drugs metabolized by CYP3A4, CYP2D6, CYP2C9, CYP2C19, or CYP1A2 enzymes.

As with all other quinolones, iron and antacids significantly reduced bioavailability of moxifloxacin.

Itraconazole:

In a study involving 11 healthy volunteers, there was no significant effect of itraconazole (200 mg once daily for 9 days), a potent inhibitor of cytochrome P4503A4, on the pharmacokinetics of moxifloxacin (a single 400 mg dose given on the 7th day of itraconazole dosing). In addition, moxifloxacin was shown not to affect the pharmacokinetics of itraconazole.

Theophylline:

No significant effect of moxifloxacin (200 mg every twelve hours for 3 days) on the pharmacokinetics of theophylline (400 mg every twelve hours for 3 days) was detected in a study involving 12 healthy volunteers. In addition, theophylline was not shown to affect the pharmacokinetics of moxifloxacin. The effect of co-administration of a 400 mg dose of moxifloxacin with theophylline has not been studied, but it is not expected to be clinically significant based on *in vitro* metabolic data showing that moxifloxacin does not inhibit the CYP1A2 isoenzyme.

Warfarin:

No significant effect of moxifloxacin (400 mg once daily for eight days) on the pharmacokinetics of R- and S-warfarin (25 mg single dose of warfarin sodium on the fifth day) was detected in a study involving 24 healthy volunteers. No significant change in prothrombin time was observed. (See PRECAUTIONS, Drug Interactions.)

Digoxin:

No significant effect of moxifloxacin (400 mg once daily for two days) on digoxin (0.6 mg as a single dose) AUC was detected in a study involving 12 healthy volunteers. The mean digoxin C_{max} increased by about 50% during the distribution phase of digoxin. This transient increase in digoxin C_{max} is not viewed to be clinically significant. Moxifloxacin pharmacokinetics were similar in the presence or absence of digoxin. No dosage adjustment for moxifloxacin or digoxin is required when these drugs are administered concomitantly.

Atenolol:
In a crossover study involving 24 healthy volunteers (12 male; 12 female), the mean atenolol AUC following a single oral dose of 50 mg atenolol with placebo was similar to that observed when atenolol was given concomitantly with a single 400 mg oral dose of moxifloxacin. The mean C_{max} of single dose atenolol decreased by about 10% following co-administration with a single dose of moxifloxacin.

Morphine:
No significant effect of morphine sulfate (a single 10 mg intramuscular dose) on the mean AUC and C_{max} of moxifloxacin (400 mg single dose) was observed in a study of 20 healthy male and female volunteers.

Oral Contraceptives:
A placebo-controlled study in 29 healthy female subjects showed that moxifloxacin 400 mg daily for 7 days did not interfere with the hormonal suppression of oral contraception with 0.15 mg levonorgestrel/0.03 mg ethinylestradiol (as measured by serum progesterone, FSH, estradiol, and LH), or with the pharmacokinetics of the administered contraceptive agents.

Probenecid:
Probenecid (500 mg twice daily for two days) did not alter the renal clearance and total amount of moxifloxacin (400 mg single dose) excreted renally in a study of 12 healthy volunteers.

Ranitidine:
No significant effect of ranitidine (150 mg twice daily for three days as pretreatment) on the pharmacokinetics of moxifloxacin (400 mg single dose) was detected in a study involving 10 healthy volunteers.

Antidiabetic agents:
In diabetics, glyburide (2.5 mg once daily for two weeks pretreatment and for five days concurrently) mean AUC and C_{max} were 12% and 21% lower, respectively, when taken with moxifloxacin (400 mg once daily for five days) in comparison to placebo. Nonetheless, blood glucose levels were decreased slightly in patients taking glyburide and moxifloxacin in comparison to those taking glyburide alone, suggesting no interference by moxifloxacin on the activity of glyburide. These interaction results are not viewed as clinically significant.

Calcium:
Twelve healthy volunteers were administered concomitant moxifloxacin (single 400 mg dose) and calcium (single dose of 500 mg Ca^{++} dietary supplement) followed by an additional two doses of calcium 12 and 24 hours after moxifloxacin administration. Calcium had no significant effect on the mean AUC of moxifloxacin. The mean C_{max} was slightly reduced and the time to maximum plasma concentration was prolonged when moxifloxacin was given with calcium compared to when moxifloxacin was given alone (2.5 hours versus 0.9 hours). These differences are not considered to be clinically significant.

Antacids:
When moxifloxacin (single 400 mg tablet dose) was administered two hours before, concomitantly, or 4 hours after an aluminum/magnesium-containing antacid (900 mg aluminum hydroxide and 600 mg magnesium hydroxide as a single oral dose) to 12 healthy volunteers there was a 26%, 60% and 23% reduction in the mean AUC of moxifloxacin, respectively. Moxifloxacin should be taken at least 4 hours before or 8 hours after antacids containing magnesium or aluminum, as well as sucralfate, metal cations such as iron, and multivitamin preparations with zinc, or VIDEX® (didanosine) chewable/buffered tablets or the pediatric powder for oral solution. (See PRECAUTIONS, Drug Interactions and DOSAGE AND ADMINISTRATION.)

Iron: When moxifloxacin tablets were administered concomitantly with iron (ferrous sulfate 100 mg once daily for two days), the mean AUC and C_{max} of moxifloxacin was reduced by 39% and 59%, respectively. Moxifloxacin should only be taken more than 4 hours before or 8 hours after iron products. (See PRECAUTIONS, Drug Interactions and DOSAGE AND ADMINISTRATION.)

Electrocardiogram:
Prolongation of the QT interval in the ECG has been observed in some patients receiving moxifloxacin. Following oral dosing with 400 mg of moxifloxacin the mean (± SD) change in QTc from the pre-dose value at the time of maximum drug concentration was 6 msec (± 26) (n = 787). Following a course of daily intravenous dosing (400 mg; 1 hour infusion each day) the mean change in QTc from the Day 1 pre-dose value was 10 msec (±22) on Day 1 (n = 667) and 7 msec (± 24) on Day 3 (n = 667). (See WARNINGS.)

There is limited information available on the potential for a pharmacodynamic interaction in humans between moxifloxacin and other drugs that prolong the QTc interval of the electrocardiogram. Sotalol, a Class III antiarrhythmic, has been shown to further increase the QTc interval when combined with high doses of intravenous (I.V.) moxifloxacin in dogs. Therefore, moxifloxacin should be avoided with Class IA and Class III antiarrhythmics. (See ANIMAL PHARMACOLOGY, WARNINGS, and PRECAUTIONS.)

MICROBIOLOGY

Moxifloxacin has *in vitro* activity against a wide range of Gram-positive and Gram-negative microorganisms. The bactericidal action of moxifloxacin results from inhibition of the topoisomerase II (DNA gyrase) and topoisomerase IV required for bacterial DNA replication, transcription, repair, and recombination. It appears that the C8-methoxy moiety contributes to enhanced activity and lower selection of resistant mutants of Gram-positive bacteria compared to the C8-H moiety. The presence of the bulky bicycloamine substituent at the C-7 position prevents active efflux, associated with the *NorA* or *pmrA* genes seen in certain Gram-positive bacteria.

The mechanism of action for quinolones, including moxifloxacin, is different from that of macrolides, beta-lactams, aminoglycosides, or tetracyclines; therefore, microorganisms resistant to these classes of drugs may be susceptible to moxifloxacin and other quinolones. There is no known cross-resistance between moxifloxacin and other classes of antimicrobials.

In vitro resistance to moxifloxacin develops slowly via multiple-step mutations. Resistance to moxifloxacin occurs *in vitro* at a general frequency of between 1.8×10^{-9} to $< 1 \times 10^{-11}$ for Gram-positive bacteria.

Cross-resistance has been observed between moxifloxacin and other fluoroquinolones against Gram-negative bacteria. Gram-positive bacteria resistant to other fluoroquinolones may, however, still be susceptible to moxifloxacin.

Moxifloxacin has been shown to be active against most strains of the following microorganisms, both *in vitro* and in clinical infections as described in the INDICATIONS AND USAGE section.

Aerobic Gram-positive microorganisms
Enterococcus faecalis (many strains are only moderately susceptible)
Staphylococcus aureus (methicillin-susceptible strains only)
Streptococcus anginosus
Streptococcus constellatus
Streptococcus pneumoniae (including multi-drug resistant strains [MDRSP]*)
Streptococcus pyogenes

* MDRSP, Multi-drug resistant *Streptococcus pneumoniae* includes isolates previously known as PRSP (Penicillin-resistant *S. pneumoniae*), and are strains resistant to two or more of the following antibiotics: penicillin (MIC ≥ 2 μg/mL), 2nd generation cephalosporins (e.g., cefuroxime), macrolides, tetracyclines, and trimethoprim/sulfamethoxazole.

Aerobic Gram-negative microorganisms
Enterobacter cloacae
Escherichia coli
Haemophilus influenzae
Haemophilus parainfluenzae
Klebsiella pneumoniae
Moraxella catarrhalis
Proteus mirabilis

Anaerobic microorganisms
Bacteroides fragilis
Bacteroides thetaiotaomicron
Clostridium perfringens
Peptostreptococcus species

Other microorganisms
Chlamydia pneumoniae
Mycoplasma pneumoniae

The following *in vitro* data are available, **but their clinical significance is unknown.**

Moxifloxacin exhibits *in vitro* minimum inhibitory concentrations (MICs) of 2 μg/mL or less against most (≥ 90%) strains of the following microorganisms; however, the safety and effectiveness of moxifloxacin in treating clinical infections due to these microorganisms have not been established in adequate and well-controlled clinical trials.

Aerobic Gram-positive microorganisms
Staphylococcus epidermidis (methicillin-susceptible strains only)
Streptococcus agalactiae
Streptococcus viridans group

Aerobic Gram-negative microorganisms
Citrobacter freundii
Klebsiella oxytoca
Legionella pneumophila

Anaerobic microorganisms
Fusobacterium species
Prevotella species

Susceptibility Tests

Dilution Techniques: Quantitative methods are used to determine antimicrobial minimum inhibitory concentrations (MICs). These MICs provide estimates of the susceptibility of bacteria to antimicrobial compounds. The MICs should be determined using a standardized procedure. Standardized procedures are based on a dilution method[1] (broth or agar) or equivalent with standardized inoculum concentrations and standardized concentrations of moxifloxacin powder. The MIC values should be interpreted according to the following criteria:

For testing Enterobacteriaceae and methicillin-susceptible *Staphylococcus aureus:*

MIC (μg/mL)	Interpretation
≤ 2	Susceptible (S)
4	Intermediate (I)
≥ 8	Resistant (R)

For testing *Haemophilus influenzae* and *Haemophilus parainfluenzae*[a]:

MIC (μg/mL)	Interpretation
≤ 1	Susceptible (S)

[a] This interpretive standard is applicable only to broth microdilution susceptibility tests with *Haemophilus influenzae* and *Haemophilus parainfluenzae* using *Haemophilus* Test Medium[1].

The current absence of data on resistant strains precludes defining any results other than "Susceptible". Strains yielding MIC results suggestive of a "nonsusceptible" category should be submitted to a reference laboratory for further testing.

For testing *Streptococcus* species including *Streptococcus pneumoniae*[b] and *Enterococcus faecalis*:

MIC (μg/mL)	Interpretation
≤ 1	Susceptible (S)
2	Intermediate (I)
≥ 4	Resistant (R)

[b] These interpretive standards are applicable only to broth microdilution susceptibility tests using cation-adjusted Mueller-Hinton broth with 2-5% lysed horse blood.

A report of "Susceptible" indicates that the pathogen is likely to be inhibited if the antimicrobial compound in the blood reaches the concentrations usually achievable. A report of "Intermediate" indicates that the result should be considered equivocal, and, if the microorganism is not fully susceptible to alternative, clinically feasible drugs, the test should be repeated. This category implies possible clinical applicability in body sites where the drug is physiologically concentrated or in situations where a high dosage of drug can be used. This category also provides a buffer zone which prevents small uncontrolled technical factors from causing major discrepancies in interpretation. A report of "Resistant" indicates that the pathogen is not likely to be inhibited if the antimicrobial compound in the blood reaches the concentrations usually achievable; other therapy should be selected.

Standardized susceptibility test procedures require the use of laboratory control microorganisms to control the technical aspects of the laboratory procedures. Standard moxifloxacin powder should provide the following MIC values:

Microorganism		MIC (μg/mL)
Enterococcus faecalis	ATCC 29212	0.06-0.5
Escherichia coli	ATCC 25922	0.008-0.06
Haemophilus influenzae	ATCC 49247[c]	0.008-0.03
Staphylococcus aureus	ATCC 29213	0.015-0.06
Streptococcus pneumoniae	ATCC 49619[d]	0.06-0.25

[c] This quality control range is applicable to only *H. influenzae* ATCC 49247 tested by a broth microdilution procedure using *Haemophilus* Test Medium (HTM)[1].
[d] This quality control range is applicable to only *S. pneumoniae* ATCC 49619 tested by a broth microdilution procedure using cation-adjusted Mueller-Hinton broth with 2-5% lysed horse blood.

Diffusion Techniques: Quantitative methods that require measurement of zone diameters also provide reproducible estimates of the susceptibility of bacteria to antimicrobial compounds. One such standardized procedure[2] requires the use of standardized inoculum concentrations. This procedure uses paper disks impregnated with 5-μg moxifloxacin to test the susceptibility of microorganisms to moxifloxacin.

Reports from the laboratory providing results of the standard single-disk susceptibility test with a 5-μg moxifloxacin disk should be interpreted according to the following criteria:
The following zone diameter interpretive criteria should be used for testing Enterobacteriaceae and methicillin-susceptible *Staphylococcus aureus*:

Zone Diameter (mm)	Interpretation
≥ 19	Susceptible (S)
16–18	Intermediate (I)
≤ 15	Resistant (R)

For testing *Haemophilus influenzae* and *Haemophilus parainfluenzae*[e]:

Zone Diameter (mm)	Interpretation
≥ 18	Susceptible (S)

[e]This zone diameter standard is applicable only to tests with *Haemophilus influenzae* and *Haemophilus parainfluenzae* using *Haemophilus* Test Medium (HTM)[2].

The current absence of data on resistant strains precludes defining any results other than "Susceptible". Strains yielding zone diameter results suggestive of a "nonsusceptible" category should be submitted to a reference laboratory for further testing.
For testing *Streptococcus* species including *Streptococcus pneumoniae*[f] and *Enterococcus faecalis:*

Zone Diameter (mm)	Interpretation
≥ 18	Susceptible (S)
15–17	Intermediate (I)
≤ 14	Resistant (R)

[f] These interpretive standards are applicable only to disk diffusion tests using Mueller-Hinton agar supplemented with 5% sheep blood incubated in 5% CO_2.

Interpretation should be as stated above for results using dilution techniques. Interpretation involves correlation of the diameter obtained in the disk test with the MIC for moxifloxacin.
As with standardized dilution techniques, diffusion methods require the use of laboratory control microorganisms that are used to control the technical aspects of the laboratory procedures. For the diffusion technique, the 5-μg moxifloxacin disk should provide the following zone diameters in these laboratory test quality control strains:

Microorganism		Zone Diameter (mm)
Escherichia coli	ATCC 25922	28–35
Haemophilus influenzae	ATCC 49247[g]	31–39
Staphylococcus aureus	ATCC 25923	28–35
Streptococcus pneumoniae	ATCC 49619[h]	25–31

[g]These quality control limits are applicable to only *H. influenzae* ATCC 49247 testing using *Haemophilus* Test Medium (HTM)[2].
[h] These quality control limits are applicable only to tests conducted with *S. pneumoniae* ATCC 49619 tested by a disk diffusion procedure using Mueller-Hinton agar supplemented with 5% sheep blood and incubated in 5% CO_2.

Anaerobic Techniques: For anaerobic bacteria, the susceptibility to moxifloxacin as MICs can be determined by standardized procedures[3] such as reference agar dilution methods[i]. The MICs obtained should be interpreted according to the following criteria:

MIC (ug/mL)	Interpretation
≤ 2	Susceptible (S)
4	Intermediate (I)
≥ 8	Resistant (R)

[i] This interpretive standard is applicable to reference agar dilution susceptibility tests using *Brucella* agar supplemented with hemin, vitamin K_1 and 5% laked sheep blood.

Acceptable ranges of MICs (ug/mL) for control strains for reference agar dilution testing[j]:

Microorganism		MIC (ug/mL)
Bacteroides fragilis	ATCC 25285	0.12-0.5
Bacteroides thetaiotaomicron	ATCC 29741	1-4
Eubacterium lentum	ATCC 43055	0.12-0.5

[j]These quality control ranges are applicable to reference agar dilution tests using Brucella agar supplemented with hemin, vitamin K_1 and 5% laked sheep blood.

INDICATIONS AND USAGE

AVELOX Tablets and I.V. are indicated for the treatment of adults (≥ 18 years of age) with infections caused by susceptible strains of the designated microorganisms in the conditions listed below. (See DOSAGE AND ADMINISTRATION for specific recommendations. In addition, for I.V. use, see PRECAUTIONS, Geriatric Use.)
Acute Bacterial Sinusitis caused by *Streptococcus pneumoniae, Haemophilus influenzae,* or *Moraxella catarrhalis.*
Acute Bacterial Exacerbation of Chronic Bronchitis caused by *Streptococcus pneumoniae, Haemophilus influenzae, Haemophilus parainfluenzae, Klebsiella pneumoniae,* methicillin-susceptible *Staphylococcus aureus,* or *Moraxella catarrhalis.*
Community Acquired Pneumonia caused by *Streptococcus pneumoniae* (including multi-drug resistant strains*), *Haemophilus influenzae, Moraxella catarrhalis,* methicillin-susceptible *Staphylococcus aureus, Klebsiella pneumoniae, Mycoplasma pneumoniae,* or *Chlamydia pneumoniae.*
* MDRSP, Multi-drug resistant *Streptococcus pneumoniae* includes isolates previously known as PRSP (Penicillin-resistant *S. pneumoniae*), and are strains resistant to two or more of the following antibiotics: penicillin (MIC ≥ 2 μg/mL), 2nd generation cephalosporins (e.g., cefuroxime), macrolides, tetracyclines, and trimethoprim/sulfamethoxazole.
Uncomplicated Skin and Skin Structure Infections caused by methicillin-susceptible *Staphylococcus aureus* or *Streptococcus pyogenes.*
Complicated Intra-Abdominal Infections including polymicrobial infections such as abscess caused by *Escherichia coli, Bacteroides fragilis, Streptococcus anginosus, Streptococcus constellatus, Enterococcus faecalis, Proteus mirabilis, Clostridium perfringens, Bacteroides thetaiotaomicron,* or *Peptostreptococcus species.*
Complicated Skin and Skin Structure Infections caused by methicillin-susceptible *Staphylococcus aureus, Escherichia coli, Klebsiella pneumoniae,* or *Enterobacter cloacae* (See Clinical Studies).
Appropriate culture and susceptibility tests should be performed before treatment in order to isolate and identify organisms causing infection and to determine their susceptibility to moxifloxacin. Therapy with AVELOX may be initiated before results of these tests are known; once results become available, appropriate therapy should be continued.
To reduce the development of drug-resistant bacteria and maintain the effectiveness of AVELOX and other antibacterial drugs, AVELOX should be used only to treat or prevent infections that are proven or strongly suspected to be caused by susceptible bacteria. When culture and susceptibility information are available, they should be considered in selecting or modifying antibacterial therapy. In the absence of such data, local epidemiology and susceptibility patterns may contribute to the empiric selection of therapy.

CONTRAINDICATIONS

Moxifloxacin is contraindicated in persons with a history of hypersensitivity to moxifloxacin or any member of the quinolone class of antimicrobial agents.

WARNINGS

Tendinopathy and Tendon Rupture: Fluoroquinolones, including AVELOX, are associated with an increased risk of tendinitis and tendon rupture in all ages. This adverse reaction most frequently involves the Achilles tendon, and rupture of the Achilles tendon may require surgical repair. Tendinitis and tendon rupture in the rotator cuff (the shoulder), the hand, the biceps, the thumb, and other tendon sites have also been reported. The risk of developing fluoroquinolone-associated tendinitis and tendon rupture is further increased in older patients usually over 60 years of age, in patients taking corticosteroid drugs, and in patients with kidney, heart or lung transplants. Factors, in addition to age and corticosteroid use, that may independently increase the risk of tendon rupture include strenuous physical activity, renal failure, and previous tendon disorders such as rheumatoid arthritis. Tendinitis and tendon rupture have also occurred in patients taking fluoroquinolones who do not have the above risk factors. Tendon rupture can occur during or after completion of therapy; cases occurring up to several months after completion of therapy have been reported. AVELOX should be discontinued if the patient experiences pain, swelling, inflammation or rupture of a tendon. Patients should be advised to rest at the first sign of tendinitis or tendon rupture, and to contact their healthcare provider regarding changing to a non-quinolone antimicrobial drug.

THE SAFETY AND EFFECTIVENESS OF MOXIFLOXACIN IN PEDIATRIC PATIENTS, ADOLESCENTS (LESS THAN 18 YEARS OF AGE), PREGNANT WOMEN, AND LACTATING WOMEN HAVE NOT BEEN ESTABLISHED. (SEE PRECAUTIONS-PEDIATRIC USE, PREGNANCY AND NURSING MOTHERS SUBSECTIONS.)

QT prolongation: Moxifloxacin has been shown to prolong the QT interval of the electrocardiogram in some patients. The drug should be avoided in patients with known prolongation of the QT interval, patients with uncorrected hypokalemia and patients receiving Class IA (e.g., quinidine, procainamide) or Class III (e.g., amiodarone, sotalol) antiarrhythmic agents, due to the lack of clinical experience with the drug in these patient populations.
Pharmacokinetic studies between moxifloxacin and other drugs that prolong the QT interval such as cisapride, erythromycin, antipsychotics, and tricyclic antidepressants have not been performed. An additive effect of moxifloxacin and these drugs cannot be excluded; therefore caution should be exercised when moxifloxacin is given concurrently with these drugs. In premarketing clinical trials, the rate of cardiovascular adverse events was similar in 798 moxifloxacin and 702 comparator treated patients who received concomitant therapy with drugs known to prolong the QTc interval.
Moxifloxacin should be used with caution in patients with ongoing proarrhythmic conditions, such as clinically significant bradycardia, acute myocardial ischemia. The magnitude of QT prolongation may increase with increasing concentrations of the drug or increasing rates of infusion of the intravenous formulation. Therefore the recommended dose or infusion rate should not be exceeded. QT prolongation may lead to an increased risk for ventricular arrhythmias including torsade de pointes. No excess in cardiovascular morbidity or mortality attributable to QTc prolongation occurred with moxifloxacin treatment in over 15,500 patients in controlled clinical studies, including 759 patients who were hypokalemic at the start of treatment, and there was no increase in mortality in over 18,000 moxifloxacin tablet treated patients in a post-marketing observational study in which ECGs were not performed (See CLINICAL PHARMACOLOGY, Electrocardiogram. For I.V. use, see DOSAGE AND ADMINISTRATION and PRECAUTIONS, Geriatric Use.) In addition, moxifloxacin should be used with caution in patients with mild, moderate, or severe liver cirrhosis. (See CLINICAL PHARMACOLOGY, Hepatic Insufficiency.)
The oral administration of moxifloxacin caused lameness in immature dogs. Histopathological examination of the weight-bearing joints of these dogs revealed permanent lesions of the cartilage. Related quinolone-class drugs also produce erosions of cartilage of weight-bearing joints and other signs of arthropathy in immature animals of various species. (See **ANIMAL PHARMACOLOGY**.)
Convulsions have been reported in patients receiving quinolones. Quinolones may also cause central nervous system (CNS) events including: dizziness, confusion, tremors, hallucinations, depression, and, rarely, suicidal thoughts or acts. These reactions may occur following the first dose. If these reactions occur in patients receiving moxifloxacin, the drug should be discontinued and appropriate measures instituted. As with all quinolones, moxifloxacin should be used with caution in patients with known or suspected CNS disorders (e.g. severe cerebral arteriosclerosis, epilepsy) or in the presence of other risk factors that may predispose to seizures or lower the seizure threshold. (See PRECAUTIONS: General, Information for Patients, and ADVERSE REACTIONS.)

Hypersensitivity reactions: Serious anaphylactic reactions, some following the first dose, have been reported in patients receiving quinolone therapy, including moxifloxacin. Some reactions were accompanied by cardiovascular collapse, loss of consciousness, tingling, pharyngeal or facial edema, dyspnea, urticaria, and itching. Serious anaphylactic reactions require immediate emergency treatment with epinephrine. Moxifloxacin should be discontinued at the first appearance of a skin rash or any other sign of hypersensitivity. Oxygen, intravenous steroids, and airway management, including intubation, may be administered as indicated.
Other serious and sometimes fatal events, some due to hypersensitivity, and some due to uncertain etiology, have been reported rarely in patients receiving therapy with quinolones, including AVELOX. These events may be severe and generally occur following the administration of multiple doses. Clinical manifestations may include one or more of the following:

- fever, rash, or severe dermatologic reactions (e.g., toxic epidermal necrolysis, Stevens-Johnson syndrome);
- vasculitis; arthralgia; myalgia; serum sickness;
- allergic pneumonitis;
- interstitial nephritis; acute renal insufficiency or failure;
- hepatitis; jaundice; acute hepatic necrosis or failure;
- anemia, including hemolytic and aplastic; thrombocytopenia, including thrombotic thrombocytopenic purpura; leukopenia; agranulocytosis; pancytopenia; and/or other hematologic abnormalities.

The drug should be discontinued immediately at the first appearance of a skin rash, jaundice, or any other sign of hypersensitivity and supportive measures instituted (See PRECAUTIONS: Information for Patients and ADVERSE REACTIONS).

Clostridium difficile associated diarrhea (CDAD) has been reported with use of nearly all antibacterial agents, including AVELOX, and may range in severity from mild diarrhea to fatal colitis. Treatment with antibacterial agents alters the normal flora of the colon leading to overgrowth of *C. difficile*.

C. difficile produces toxins A and B which contribute to the development of CDAD. Hypertoxin producing strains of *C. difficile* cause increased morbidity and mortality, as these infections can be refractory to antimicrobial therapy and may require colectomy. CDAD must be considered in all patients who present with diarrhea following antibiotic use. Careful medical history is necessary since CDAD has been reported to occur over two months after the administration of antibacterial agents.

If CDAD is suspected or confirmed, ongoing antibiotic use not directed against *C. difficile* may need to be discontinued. Appropriate fluid and electrolyte management, protein supplementation, antibiotic treatment of *C. difficile*, and surgical evaluation should be instituted as clinically indicated.

Peripheral neuropathy: Rare cases of sensory or sensorimotor axonal polyneuropathy affecting small and/or large axons resulting in paresthesias, hypoesthesias, dysesthesias and weakness have been reported in patients receiving quinolones.

PRECAUTIONS

General:
Quinolones may cause central nervous system (CNS) events, including: nervousness, agitation, insomnia, anxiety, nightmares or paranoia. (See WARNINGS and Information for Patients.)

Moderate to severe photosensitivity/phototoxicity reactions, the latter of which may manifest as exaggerated sunburn reactions (e.g., burning, erythema, exudation, vesicles, blistering, edema) involving areas exposed to light (typically the face, "V" area of the neck, extensor surfaces of the forearms, dorsa of the hands), can be associated with the use of quinolone antibiotics after sun or UV light exposure. Therefore, excessive exposure to these sources of light should be avoided. Drug therapy should be discontinued if phototoxicity occurs (See ADVERSE REACTIONS and ADVERSE REACTIONS/Post-Marketing Adverse Event Reports).

Prescribing AVELOX in the absence of a proven or strongly suspected bacterial infection or a prophylactic indication is unlikely to provide benefit to the patient and increases the risk of the development of drug-resistant bacteria.

Information for Patients:
To assure safe and effective use of moxifloxacin, the following information and instructions should be communicated to the patient when appropriate:

Patients should be advised:

- to contact their healthcare provider if they experience pain, swelling, or inflammation of a tendon, or weakness or inability to use one of their joints; rest and refrain from exercise; and discontinue AVELOX treatment. The risk of severe tendon disorder with fluoroquinolones is higher in older patients usually over 60 years of age, in patients taking corticosteroid drugs, and in patients with kidney, heart or lung transplants.
- that antibacterial drugs including AVELOX should only be used to treat bacterial infections. They do not treat viral infections (e.g., the common cold). When AVELOX is prescribed to treat a bacterial infection, patients should be told that although it is common to feel better early in the course of therapy, the medication should be taken exactly as directed. Skipping doses or not completing the full course of therapy may (1) decrease the effectiveness of the immediate treatment and (2) increase the likelihood that bacteria will develop resistance and will not be treatable by AVELOX or other antibacterial drugs in the future.
- that moxifloxacin may produce changes in the electrocardiogram (QTc interval prolongation).
- that moxifloxacin should be avoided in patients receiving Class IA (e.g. quinidine, procainamide) or Class III (e.g. amiodarone, sotalol) antiarrhythmic agents.

- that moxifloxacin may add to the QTc prolonging effects of other drugs such as cisapride, erythromycin, antipsychotics, and tricyclic antidepressants.
- to inform their physician of any personal or family history of QTc prolongation or proarrhythmic conditions such as recent hypokalemia, significant bradycardia, acute myocardial ischemia.
- to inform their physician of any other medications when taken concurrently with moxifloxacin, including over-the-counter medications.
- to contact their physician if they experience palpitations or fainting spells while taking moxifloxacin.
- that moxifloxacin tablets may be taken with or without meals, and to drink fluids liberally.
- that moxifloxacin tablets should be taken at least 4 hours before or 8 hours after multivitamins (containing iron or zinc), antacids (containing magnesium or aluminum), sucralfate, or VIDEX® (didanosine) chewable/buffered tablets or the pediatric powder for oral solution. (See CLINICAL PHARMACOLOGY, Drug Interactions and PRECAUTIONS, Drug Interactions.)
- that moxifloxacin may be associated with hypersensitivity reactions, including anaphylactic reactions, even following a single dose, and to discontinue the drug at the first sign of a skin rash or other signs of an allergic reaction.
- that moxifloxacin may cause dizziness and lightheadedness; therefore, patients should know how they react to this drug before they operate an automobile or machinery or engage in activities requiring mental alertness or coordination.
- that photosensitivity/phototoxicity has been reported in patients receiving quinolones. Patients should minimize or avoid exposure to natural or artificial sunlight (tanning beds or UVA/B treatment) while taking quinolones. If patients need to be outdoors while using quinolones, they should wear loose-fitting clothes that protect skin from sun exposure and discuss other sun protection measures with their physician. If a sunburn-like reaction or skin eruption occurs, patients should contact their physician (see CLINICAL PHARMACOLOGY/Photosensitivity Potential).
- that convulsions have been reported in patients receiving quinolones, and they should notify their physician before taking this drug if there is a history of this condition.
- that diarrhea is a common problem caused by antibiotics which usually ends when the antibiotic is discontinued. Sometimes after starting treatment with antibiotics, patients can develop watery and bloody stools (with or without stomach cramps and fever) even as late as two or more months after having taken the last dose of the antibiotic. If this occurs, patients should contact their physician as soon as possible.

Drug Interactions:
Antacids, Sucralfate, Metal Cations, Multivitamins: Quinolones form chelates with alkaline earth and transition metal cations. Oral administration of quinolones with antacids containing aluminum or magnesium, with sucralfate, with metal cations such as iron, or with multivitamins containing iron or zinc, or with formulations containing divalent and trivalent cations such as VIDEX® (didanosine) chewable/buffered tablets or the pediatric powder for oral solution, may substantially interfere with the absorption of quinolones, resulting in systemic concentrations considerably lower than desired. Therefore, moxifloxacin should be taken at least 4 hours before or 8 hours after these agents. (See CLINICAL PHARMACOLOGY, Drug Interactions and DOSAGE AND ADMINISTRATION.)

No clinically significant drug-drug interactions between itraconazole, theophylline, warfarin, digoxin, atenolol, oral contraceptives or glyburide have been observed with moxifloxacin. Itraconazole, theophylline, digoxin, probenecid, morphine, ranitidine, and calcium have been shown not to significantly alter the pharmacokinetics of moxifloxacin. (See CLINICAL PHARMACOLOGY.)

Warfarin: No significant effect of moxifloxacin on R- and S-warfarin was detected in a clinical study involving 24 healthy volunteers. No significant changes in prothrombin time were noted in the presence of moxifloxacin. Quinolones, including moxifloxacin, have been reported to enhance the anticoagulant effects of warfarin or its derivatives in the patient population. In addition, infectious disease and its accompanying inflammatory process, age, and general status of the patient are risk factors for increased anticoagulant activity. Therefore the prothrombin time, International Normalized Ratio (INR), or other suitable anticoagulation tests should be closely monitored if a quinolone is administered concomitantly with warfarin or its derivatives.

Drugs metabolized by Cytochrome P450 enzymes: *In vitro* studies with cytochrome P450 isoenzymes (CYP) indicate that moxifloxacin does not inhibit CYP3A4, CYP2D6, CYP2C9, CYP2C19, or CYP1A2, suggesting that moxifloxacin is unlikely to alter the pharmacokinetics of

drugs metabolized by these enzymes (e.g. midazolam, cyclosporine, warfarin, theophylline).

Nonsteroidal anti-inflammatory drugs (NSAIDs): Although not observed with moxifloxacin in preclinical and clinical trials, the concomitant administration of a nonsteroidal anti-inflammatory drug with a quinolone may increase the risks of CNS stimulation and convulsions. (See WARNINGS.)

Carcinogenesis, Mutagenesis, Impairment of Fertility:
Long term studies in animals to determine the carcinogenic potential of moxifloxacin have not been performed.

Moxifloxacin was not mutagenic in 4 bacterial strains (TA 98, TA 100, TA 1535, TA 1537) used in the Ames *Salmonella* reversion assay. As with other quinolones, the positive response observed with moxifloxacin in strain TA 102 using the same assay may be due to the inhibition of DNA gyrase. Moxifloxacin was not mutagenic in the CHO/HGPRT mammalian cell gene mutation assay. An equivocal result was obtained in the same assay when v79 cells were used. Moxifloxacin was clastogenic in the v79 chromosome aberration assay, but it did not induce unscheduled DNA synthesis in cultured rat hepatocytes. There was no evidence of genotoxicity *in vivo* in a micronucleus test or a dominant lethal test in mice.

Moxifloxacin had no effect on fertility in male and female rats at oral doses as high as 500 mg/kg/day, approximately 12 times the maximum recommended human dose based on body surface area (mg/m^2), or at intravenous doses as high as 45 mg/kg/day, approximately equal to the maximum recommended human dose based on body surface area (mg/m^2). At 500 mg/kg orally there were slight effects on sperm morphology (head-tail separation) in male rats and on the estrous cycle in female rats.

Pregnancy:
Teratogenic Effects.
Pregnancy Category C:
Moxifloxacin was not teratogenic when administered to pregnant rats during organogenesis at oral doses as high as 500 mg/kg/day or 0.24 times the maximum recommended human dose based on systemic exposure (AUC), but decreased fetal body weights and slightly delayed fetal skeletal development (indicative of fetotoxicity) were observed. Intravenous administration of 80 mg/kg/day (approximately 2 times the maximum recommended human dose based on body surface area (mg/m^2)) to pregnant rats resulted in maternal toxicity and a marginal effect on fetal and placental weights and the appearance of the placenta. There was no evidence of teratogenicity at intravenous doses as high as 80 mg/kg/day. Intravenous administration of 20 mg/kg/day (approximately equal to the maximum recommended human oral dose based upon systemic exposure) to pregnant rabbits during organogenesis resulted in decreased fetal body weights and delayed fetal skeletal ossification. When rib and vertebral malformations were combined, there was an increased fetal and litter incidence of these effects. Signs of maternal toxicity in rabbits at this dose included mortality, abortions, marked reduction of food consumption, decreased water intake, body weight loss and hypoactivity. There was no evidence of teratogenicity when pregnant cynomolgus monkeys were given oral doses as high as 100 mg/kg/day (2.5 times the maximum recommended human dose based upon systemic exposure). An increased incidence of smaller fetuses was observed at 100 mg/kg/day. In an oral pre- and postnatal development study conducted in rats, effects observed at 500 mg/kg/day included slight increases in duration of pregnancy and prenatal loss, reduced pup birth weight and decreased neonatal survival. Treatment-related maternal mortality occurred during gestation at 500 mg/kg/day in this study.

Since there are no adequate or well-controlled studies in pregnant women, moxifloxacin should be used during pregnancy only if the potential benefit justifies the potential risk to the fetus.

Nursing Mothers:
Moxifloxacin is excreted in the breast milk of rats. Moxifloxacin may also be excreted in human milk. Because of the potential for serious adverse reactions in infants who are nursing from mothers taking moxifloxacin, a decision should be made whether to discontinue nursing or to discontinue the drug, taking into account the importance of the drug to the mother.

Pediatric Use:
Safety and effectiveness in pediatric patients and adolescents less than 18 years of age have not been established. Moxifloxacin causes arthropathy in juvenile animals. (See WARNINGS.)

Geriatric Use:
Geriatric patients are at increased risk for developing severe tendon disorders including tendon rupture when being treated with a fluoroquinolone such as AVELOX. This risk is further increased in patients receiving concomitant corticosteroid therapy. Tendinitis or tendon rupture can involve the Achilles, hand, shoulder, or other tendon sites and can occur during or after completion of therapy; cases occurring

up to several months after fluoroquinolone treatment have been reported. Caution should be used when prescribing AVELOX to elderly patients especially those on corticosteroids. Patients should be informed of this potential side effect and advised to discontinue AVELOX and contact their healthcare provider if any symptoms of tendinitis or tendon rupture occur (See BOXED WARNING, WARNINGS, and ADVERSE REACTIONS/Post-Marketing Adverse Event Reports).

In controlled multiple-dose clinical trials, 23% of patients receiving oral moxifloxacin were greater than or equal to 65 years of age and 9% were greater than or equal to 75 years of age. The clinical trial data demonstrate that there is no difference in the safety and efficacy of oral moxifloxacin in patients aged 65 or older compared to younger adults.

In trials of intravenous use, 42% of moxifloxacin patients were greater than or equal to 65 years of age, and 23% were greater than or equal to 75 years of age. The clinical trial data demonstrate that the safety of intravenous moxifloxacin in patients aged 65 or older was similar to that of comparator-treated patients. In general, elderly patients may be more susceptible to drug-associated effects of the QT interval. Therefore, AVELOX should be avoided in patients taking drugs that can result in prolongation of the QT interval (e.g., class IA or class III antiarrhythmics) or in patients with risk factors for torsade de pointes (e.g., known QT prolongation, uncorrected hypokalemia).

ADVERSE REACTIONS

Clinical efficacy trials enrolled over 15,500 moxifloxacin orally and intravenously treated patients, of whom over 14,900 patients received the 400 mg dose. Most adverse events reported in moxifloxacin trials were described as mild to moderate in severity and required no treatment. Moxifloxacin was discontinued due to adverse reactions thought to be drug-related in 2.9% of orally treated patients and 6.3% of sequentially (intravenous followed by oral) treated patients. The latter studies were conducted in community acquired pneumonia and complicated skin and skin structure infections and complicated intra-abdominal infections with, in general, a sicker patient population compared to the tablet studies.

Adverse reactions, judged by investigators to be at least possibly drug-related, occurring in greater than or equal to 2% of moxifloxacin treated patients were: nausea (6%), diarrhea (5%), dizziness (2%).

Additional clinically relevant uncommon events, judged by investigators to be at least possibly drug-related, that occurred in greater than or equal to 0.1% and less than 2% of moxifloxacin treated patients were:

BODY AS A WHOLE: abdominal pain, headache, asthenia, dehydration (secondary to diarrhea or reduced fluid intake), injection site reaction (including phlebitis), malaise, moniliasis, pain, allergic reaction

CARDIOVASCULAR: cardiac arrhythmia (not otherwise specified), tachycardia, palpitation, vasodilation, QT interval prolonged

DIGESTIVE: vomiting, abnormal liver function test (increased transaminases, increased bilirubin), dyspepsia, dry mouth, flatulence, oral moniliasis, constipation, GGTP increased, anorexia, stomatitis, glossitis

HEMIC AND LYMPHATIC: leukopenia, eosinophilia, prothrombin decrease (prothrombin time prolonged/International Normalized Ratio (INR) increased), thrombocythemia

METABOLIC AND NUTRITIONAL: lactic dehydrogenase increased, amylase increased

MUSCULOSKELETAL: arthralgia, myalgia

NERVOUS SYSTEM: insomnia, nervousness, vertigo, somnolence, anxiety, tremor

SKIN/APPENDAGES: rash (maculopapular, purpuric, pustular), pruritus, sweating, urticaria

SPECIAL SENSES: taste perversion

UROGENITAL: vaginal moniliasis, vaginitis

Additional clinically relevant rare events, judged by investigators to be at least possibly drug-related, that occurred in less than 0.1% of moxifloxacin treated patients were:

abnormal dreams, abnormal vision (visual disturbances temporally associated with CNS symptoms), agitation, amblyopia, amnesia, anemia, aphasia, arthritis, asthma, atrial fibrillation, back pain, chest pain, confusion, convulsions of various clinical manifestations (including grand mal convulsions), depersonalization, depression (potentially culminating in self-endangering behavior), dysphagia, dyspnea, ECG abnormal, emotional lability, face edema, gastritis, gastrointestinal disorder, hallucinations, hyperglycemia, hyperlipidemia, hypertension, hypertonia, hyperuricemia, hypesthesia, hypotension, incoordination, jaundice (predominantly cholestatic), kidney function abnormal, lab test abnormal (not specified), leg pain, paraesthesia, parosmia, pelvic pain, peripheral edema, photosensitivity/phototoxicity reactions, pseudomembranous colitis, prothrombin increase (prothrombin time decreased/International Normalized Ratio (INR) decreased), sleep disorders, speech disorders, supraventricular tachycardia, syncope, taste loss, tendon dis-

order, thinking abnormal, thrombocytopenia, thromboplastin decrease, tinnitus, tongue discoloration, ventricular tachycardia

Post-Marketing Adverse Event Reports:

Additional adverse events have been reported from worldwide post-marketing experience with moxifloxacin. Because these events are reported voluntarily from a population of uncertain size, it is not always possible to reliably estimate their frequency or establish a causal relationship to drug exposure. These events, some of them life-threatening, include anaphylactic reaction, anaphylactic shock, angioedema (including laryngeal edema), hepatic failure, including fatal cases, hepatitis (predominantly cholestatic), photosensitivity/phototoxicity reaction (see PRECAUTIONS), psychotic reaction (very rarely culminating in self-endangering behavior), renal dysfunction or renal failure, Stevens-Johnson syndrome, tendon rupture, toxic epidermal necrolysis, and ventricular tachyarrhythmias (including in very rare cases cardiac arrest and torsade de pointes, and usually in patients with concurrent severe underlying proarrhythmic conditions). Cases of altered coordination and abnormal gait as well as exacerbation of myasthenia gravis have also been reported.

LABORATORY CHANGES

Changes in laboratory parameters, without regard to drug relationship, which are not listed above and which occurred in $\geq$ 2% of patients and at an incidence greater than in controls included: increases in MCH, neutrophils, WBCs, PT ratio, ionized calcium, chloride, albumin, globulin, bilirubin; decreases in hemoglobin, RBCs, neutrophils, eosinophils, basophils, PT ratio, glucose, pO_2, bilirubin and amylase. It cannot be determined if any of the above laboratory abnormalities were caused by the drug or the underlying condition being treated.

OVERDOSAGE

Single oral overdoses up to 2.8 g were not associated with any serious adverse events. In the event of acute overdose, the stomach should be emptied and adequate hydration maintained. ECG monitoring is recommended due to the possibility of QT interval prolongation. The patient should be carefully observed and given supportive treatment. The administration of activated charcoal as soon as possible after oral overdose may prevent excessive increase of systemic moxifloxacin exposure. About 3% and 9% of the dose of moxifloxacin, as well as about 2% and 4.5% of its glucuronide metabolite are removed by continuous ambulatory peritoneal dialysis and hemodialysis, respectively.

Single oral moxifloxacin doses of 2000, 500, and 1500 mg/kg were lethal to rats, mice, and cynomolgus monkeys, respectively. The minimum lethal intravenous dose in mice and rats was 100 mg/kg. Toxic signs after administration of a single high dose of moxifloxacin to these animals included CNS and gastrointestinal effects such as decreased activity, somnolence, tremor, convulsions, vomiting and diarrhea.

DOSAGE AND ADMINISTRATION

The dose of AVELOX is 400 mg (orally or as an intravenous infusion) once every 24 hours. The duration of therapy depends on the type of infection as described below.

Infection*	Daily Dose	Duration
Acute Bacterial Sinusitis	400 mg	10 days
Acute Bacterial Exacerbation of Chronic Bronchitis	400 mg	5 days
Community Acquired Pneumonia	400 mg	7-14 days
Uncomplicated Skin and Skin Structure Infections	400 mg	7 days
Complicated Skin and Skin Structure Infections	400 mg	7-21 days
Complicated Intra-Abdominal Infections	400 mg	5-14 days

*due to the designated pathogens (See INDICATIONS AND USAGE.). For I.V. use, see Precautions, Geriatric Use.

For Complicated Intra-Abdominal Infections, therapy should usually be initiated with the intravenous formulation.

When switching from intravenous to oral dosage administration, no dosage adjustment is necessary. Patients whose therapy is started with AVELOX I.V. may be switched to AVELOX Tablets when clinically indicated at the discretion of the physician.

Oral doses of moxifloxacin should be administered at least 4 hours before or 8 hours after antacids containing magne-

sium or aluminum, as well as sucralfate, metal cations such as iron, and multivitamin preparations with zinc, or VIDEX® (didanosine) chewable/buffered tablets or the pediatric powder for oral solution. (See CLINICAL PHARMACOLOGY, Drug Interactions and PRECAUTIONS, Drug Interactions.)

Impaired Renal Function

No dosage adjustment is required in renally impaired patients, including those on either hemodialysis or continuous ambulatory peritoneal dialysis.

Impaired Hepatic Function

No dosage adjustment is recommended for mild, moderate, or severe hepatic insufficiency (Child-Pugh Classes A, B, or C). (See CLINICAL PHARMACOLOGY, Hepatic Insufficiency.)

AVELOX I.V. should be administered by INTRAVENOUS infusion only. It is not intended for intra-arterial, intramuscular, intrathecal, intraperitoneal, or subcutaneous administration.

AVELOX I.V. should be administered by intravenous infusion over a period of 60 minutes by direct infusion or through a Y-type intravenous infusion set which may already be in place. CAUTION: RAPID OR BOLUS INTRAVENOUS INFUSION MUST BE AVOIDED.

Since only limited data are available on the compatibility of moxifloxacin intravenous injection with other intravenous substances, additives or other medications should not be added to AVELOX I.V. or infused simultaneously through the same intravenous line. If the same intravenous line or a Y-type line is used for sequential infusion of other drugs, or if the "piggyback" method of administration is used, the line should be flushed before and after infusion of AVELOX I.V. with an infusion solution compatible with AVELOX I.V. as well as with other drug(s) administered via this common line.

AVELOX I.V. is compatible with the following intravenous solutions at ratios from 1:10 to 10:1:

0.9% Sodium Chloride Injection, USP	Sterile Water for Injection, USP
1M Sodium Chloride Injection	10% Dextrose for Injection, USP
5% Dextrose Injection, USP	Lactated Ringer's for Injection

Preparation for administration of AVELOX I.V. injection premix in flexible containers:

1. Close flow control clamp of administration set.
2. Remove cover from port at bottom of container.
3. Insert piercing pin from an appropriate transfer set (e.g. one that does not require excessive force, such as ISO compatible administration set) into port with a gentle twisting motion until pin is firmly seated.

NOTE: Refer to complete directions that have been provided with the administration set.

HOW SUPPLIED

Tablets

AVELOX (moxifloxacin hydrochloride) Tablets are available as oblong, dull red film-coated tablets containing 400 mg moxifloxacin.

The tablet is coded with the word "BAYER" on one side and "M400" on the reverse side.

Package	NDC Code
Bottles of 30:	0085-1733-01
Unit Dose Pack of 50:	0085-1733-02
ABC Pack of 5:	0085-1733-03

Store at 25°C (77°F); excursions permitted to 15-30°C (59-86°F) [see USP Controlled Room Temperature]. Avoid high humidity.

Intravenous Solution – Premix Bags

AVELOX I.V. (moxifloxacin hydrochloride in sodium chloride injection) is available in ready-to-use 250 mL latex-free flexible bags containing 400 mg of moxifloxacin in 0.8% saline. NO FURTHER DILUTION OF THIS PREPARATION IS NECESSARY.

Package	NDC Code
250 mL flexible container	0085-1737-01

Parenteral drug products should be inspected visually for particulate matter prior to administration. Samples containing visible particulates should not be used.

Since the premix flexible containers are for single-use only, any unused portion should be discarded.

Store at 25°C (77°F); excursions permitted to 15-30°C (59-86°F) [see USP Controlled Room Temperature].

DO NOT REFRIGERATE – PRODUCT PRECIPITATES UPON REFRIGERATION.

ANIMAL PHARMACOLOGY

Quinolones have been shown to cause arthropathy in immature animals. In studies in juvenile dogs oral doses of moxifloxacin ≥ 30 mg/kg/day (approximately 1.5 times the maximum recommended human dose based upon systemic exposure) for 28 days resulted in arthropathy. There was no evidence of arthropathy in mature monkeys and rats at oral doses up to 135 and 500 mg/kg/day, respectively.

Unlike some other members of the quinolone class, crystalluria was not observed in 6 month repeat dose studies in rats and monkeys with moxifloxacin.

No ocular toxicity was observed in a 13 week oral repeat dose study in dogs with a moxifloxacin dose of 60 mg/kg/day. Ocular toxicity was not observed in 6 month repeat dose studies in rats and monkeys (daily oral doses up to 500 mg/kg and 135 mg/kg, respectively). In beagle dogs, electroretinographic (ERG) changes were observed in a 2 week study at oral doses of 60 and 90 mg/kg/day. Histopathological changes were observed in the retina from one of four dogs at 90 mg/kg/day, a dose associated with mortality in this study.

Some quinolones have been reported to have proconvulsant activity that is exacerbated with concomitant use of non-steroidal anti-inflammatory drugs (NSAIDs). Moxifloxacin at an oral dose of 300 mg/kg did not show an increase in acute toxicity or potential for CNS toxicity (e.g., seizures) in mice when used in combination with NSAIDs such as diclofenac, ibuprofen, or fenbufen.

In dog studies, at plasma concentrations about five times the human therapeutic level, a QT-prolonging effect of moxifloxacin was found. Electrophysiological *in vitro* studies suggested an inhibition of the rapid activating component of the delayed rectifier potassium current (I_{Kr}) as an underlying mechanism. In dogs, the combined infusion of sotalol, a Class III antiarrhythmic agent, with moxifloxacin induced a higher degree of QTc prolongation than that induced by the same dose (30 mg/kg) of moxifloxacin alone.

In a local tolerability study performed in dogs, no signs of local intolerability were seen when moxifloxacin was administered intravenously. After intra-arterial injection, inflammatory changes involving the peri-arterial soft tissue were observed suggesting that intra-arterial administration of moxifloxacin should be avoided.

CLINICAL STUDIES

Acute Bacterial Exacerbation of Chronic Bronchitis

AVELOX Tablets (400 mg once daily for five days) were evaluated for the treatment of acute bacterial exacerbation of chronic bronchitis in a large, randomized, double-blind, controlled clinical trial conducted in the US. This study compared AVELOX with clarithromycin (500 mg twice daily for 10 days) and enrolled 629 patients. The primary endpoint for this trial was clinical success at 7-17 days post-therapy. The clinical success for AVELOX was 89% (222/250) compared to 89% (224/251) for clarithromycin.

The following outcomes are the clinical success rates at the follow-up visit for the clinically evaluable patient groups by pathogen:

PATHOGEN	AVELOX	Clarithromycin
Streptococcus pneumoniae	16/16 (100%)	20/23 (87%)
Haemophilus influenzae	33/37 (89%)	36/41 (88%)
Haemophilus parainfluenzae	16/16 (100%)	14/14 (100%)
Moraxella catarrhalis	29/34 (85%)	24/24 (100%)
Staphylococcus aureus	15/16 (94%)	6/8 (75%)
Klebsiella pneumoniae	18/20 (90%)	10/11 (91%)

The microbiological eradication rates (eradication plus presumed eradication) in AVELOX treated patients were *Streptococcus pneumoniae* 100%, *Haemophilus influenzae* 89%, *Haemophilus parainfluenzae* 100%, *Moraxella catarrhalis* 85%, *Staphylococcus aureus* 94%, and *Klebsiella pneumoniae* 85%.

Community Acquired Pneumonia

A large, randomized, double-blind, controlled clinical trial was conducted in the US to compare the efficacy of AVELOX Tablets (400 mg once daily) to that of high-dose clarithromycin (500 mg twice daily) in the treatment of patients with clinically and radiologically documented community acquired pneumonia. This study enrolled 474 patients (382 of whom were valid for the primary efficacy analysis conducted at the 14-35 day follow-up visit). Clinical success for clinically evaluable patients was 95% (184/194) for AVELOX and 95% (178/188) for high dose clarithromycin.

A large, randomized, double-blind, controlled trial was conducted in the US and Canada to compare the efficacy of sequential IV/PO AVELOX 400 mg QD for 7-14 days to an IV/PO fluoroquinolone control (trovafloxacin or levofloxacin) in the treatment of patients with clinically and radiologically documented community acquired pneumonia. This study enrolled 516 patients, 362 of whom were valid for the primary efficacy analysis conducted at the 7-30 day post-therapy visit. The clinical success rate was 86% (157/182) for AVELOX therapy and 89% (161/180) for the fluoroquinolone comparators.

An open-label ex-US study that enrolled 628 patients compared AVELOX to sequential IV/PO amoxicillin/clavulanate (1.2 g IV q8h/625 mg PO q8h) with or without high-dose IV/PO clarithromycin (500 mg BID). The intravenous formulations of the comparators are not FDA approved. The clinical success rate at Day 5-7 (the primary efficacy timepoint) for AVELOX therapy was 93% (241/258) and demonstrated superiority to amoxicillin/clavulanate ± clarithromycin (85%, 239/280) [95% C.I. 2.9%, 13.2%]. The clinical success rate at the 21-28 days post-therapy visit for AVELOX was 84% (216/258), which also demonstrated superiority to the comparators (74%, 208/280) [95% C.I. 2.6%, 16.3%].

The clinical success rates by pathogen across four CAP studies are presented below:

Clinical Success Rates By Pathogen (Pooled CAP Studies)

PATHOGEN	AVELOX	
Streptococcus pneumoniae	80/85	(94%)
Staphylococcus aureus	17/20	(85%)
Klebsiella pneumoniae	11/12	(92%)
Haemophilus influenzae	56/61	(92%)
Chlamydia pneumoniae	119/128	(93%)
Mycoplasma pneumoniae	73/76	(96%)
Moraxella catarrhalis	11/12	(92%)

Community Acquired Pneumonia caused by Multi-Drug Resistant *Streptococcus pneumoniae* (MDRSP)*

Avelox was effective in the treatment of community acquired pneumonia (CAP) caused by multi-drug resistant *Streptococcus pneumoniae* MDRSP* isolates. Of 37 microbiologically evaluable patients with MDRSP isolates, 35 patients (95%) achieved clinical and bacteriological success post-therapy. The clinical and bacteriological success rates based on the number of patients treated are shown in the table below.

* MDRSP, Multi-drug resistant *Streptococcus pneumoniae* includes isolates previously known as PRSP (Penicillin-resistant *S. pneumoniae*), and are strains resistant to two or more of the following antibiotics: penicillin (MIC ≥ 2 µg/mL), 2nd generation cephalosporins (e.g., cefuroxime), macrolides, tetracyclines, and trimethoprim/sulfamethoxazole.

[See first table above]

Not all isolates were resistant to all antimicrobial classes tested. Success and eradication rates are summarized in the table below:

[See second table above]

Clinical and Bacteriological Success Rates for Moxifloxacin-Treated MDRSP CAP Patients (Population: Valid for Efficacy):

Screening Susceptibility	Clinical Success		Bacteriological Success	
	n/N*	%	n/N†	%
Penicillin-resistant	21/21	100%‡	21/21	100%‡
2nd generation cephalosporin-resistant	25/26	96%‡	25/26	96%‡
Macrolide-resistant§	22/23	96%	22/23	96%
Trimethoprim/sulfamethoxazole-resistant	28/30	93%	28/30	93%
Tetracycline-resistant	17/18	94%	17/18	94%

*n = number of patients successfully treated; N = number of patients with MDRSP (from a total of 37 patients)

†n = number of patients successfully treated (presumed eradication or eradication); N = number of patients with MDRSP (from a total of 37 patients)

‡One patient had a respiratory isolate that was resistant to penicillin and cefuroxime but a blood isolate that was intermediate to penicillin and cefuroxime. The patient is included in the database based on the respiratory isolate.

§Azithromycin, clarithromycin, and erythromycin were the macrolide antimicrobials tested.

S. pneumoniae with MDRSP	Clinical Success	Bacteriological Eradication Rate
Resistant to 2 antimicrobials	12/13 (92.3%)	12/13 (92.3%)
Resistant to 3 antimicrobials	10/11 (90.9%)*	10/11 (90.9%)*
Resistant to 4 antimicrobials	6/6 (100%)	6/6 (100%)
Resistant to 5 antimicrobials	7/7 (100%)*	7/7 (100%)*
Bacteremia with MDRSP	9/9 (100%)	9/9 (100%)

*One patient had a respiratory isolate resistant to 5 antimicrobials and a blood isolate resistant to 3 antimicrobials. The patient was included in the category resistant to 5 antimicrobials.

Acute Bacterial Sinusitis

In a large, controlled double-blind study conducted in the US, AVELOX Tablets (400 mg once daily for ten days) were compared with cefuroxime axetil (250 mg twice daily for ten days) for the treatment of acute bacterial sinusitis. The trial included 457 patients valid for the primary efficacy determination. Clinical success (cure plus improvement) at the 7 to 21 day post-therapy test of cure visit was 90% for AVELOX and 89% for cefuroxime.

An additional non-comparative study was conducted to gather bacteriological data and to evaluate microbiological eradication in adult patients treated with AVELOX 400 mg once daily for seven days. All patients (n = 336) underwent antral puncture in this study. Clinical success rates and eradication/presumed eradication rates at the 21 to 37 day follow-up visit were 97% (29 out of 30) for *Streptococcus pneumoniae*, 83% (15 out of 18) for *Moraxella catarrhalis*, and 80% (24 out of 30) for *Haemophilus influenzae*.

Uncomplicated Skin and Skin Structure Infections

A randomized, double-blind, controlled clinical trial conducted in the US compared the efficacy of AVELOX 400 mg once daily for seven days with cephalexin HCl 500 mg three times daily for seven days. The percentage of patients treated for uncomplicated abscesses was 30%, furuncles 8%, cellulitis 16%, impetigo 20%, and other skin infections 26%. Adjunctive procedures (incision and drainage or debridement) were performed on 17% of the AVELOX treated patients and 14% of the comparator treated patients. Clinical success rates in evaluable patients were 89% (108/122) for AVELOX and 91% (110/121) for cephalexin HCl.

Complicated Skin and Skin Structure Infections

Two randomized, active controlled trials of cSSSI were performed. A double-blind trial was conducted primarily in North America to compare the efficacy of sequential IV/PO AVELOX 400 mg QD for 7-14 days to an IV/PO beta-lactam/beta-lactamase inhibitor control in the treatment of patients with cSSSI. This study enrolled 617 patients, 335 of which were valid for the primary efficacy analysis. A second open-label International study compared AVELOX 400 mg QD for 7-21 days to sequential IV/PO beta-lactam/beta-lactamase inhibitor control in the treatment of patients with cSSSI. This study enrolled 804 patients, 632 of which were valid for the primary efficacy analysis. Surgical incision and drainage or debridement was performed on 55% of the moxifloxacin treated and 53% of the comparator treated patients in these studies and formed an integral part of therapy for this indication. Success rates varied with the type of diagnosis ranging from 61% in patients with infected ulcers to 90% in patients with complicated erysipelas. These rates were similar to those seen with comparator drugs. The overall success rates in the evaluable patients and the clinical success by pathogen are shown below:

[See first table at top of next page]

[See second table on next page]

Complicated Intra-Abdominal Infections

Two randomized, active controlled trials of cIAI were performed. A double-blind trial was conducted primarily in North America to compare the efficacy of sequential IV/PO AVELOX 400 mg QD for 5-14 days to IV/piperacillin/tazobactam followed by PO amoxicillin/clavulanic acid in the treatment of patients with cIAI, including peritonitis, ab-

Overall Clinical Success Rates in Patients with Complicated Skin and Skin Structure Infections

Study	Moxifloxacin n/N (%)	Comparator n/N (%)	95% Confidence Interval
North America	125/162 (77.2%)	141/173 (81.5%)	-14.4%, 2%
International	254/315 (80.6%)	268/317 (84.5%)	-9.4%, 2.2%

Clinical Success Rates by Pathogen in Patients with Complicated Skin and Skin Structure Infections

Pathogen	Moxifloxacin n/N (%)	Comparator n/N (%)
Staphylococcus aureus (methicillin-susceptible strains)*	106/129 (82.2%)	120/137 (87.6%)
Escherichia coli	31/38 (81.6%)	28/33 (84.8%)
Klebsiella pneumoniae	11/12 (91.7%)	7/10 (70%)
Enterobacter cloacae	9/11 (81.8%)	4/7 (57.1%)

*methicillin susceptibility was only determined in the North American Study

Clinical Success Rates in Patients with Complicated Intra-Abdominal Infections

Study	Moxifloxacin n/N (%)	Comparator n/N (%)	95% Confidence Interval
North America (overall)	146/183 (79.8%)	153/196 (78.1%)	-7.4%,9.3%
Abscess	40/57 (70.2%)	49/63 (77.8%)*	NA†
Non-abscess	106/126 (84.1%)	104/133 (78.2%)	NA
International (overall)	199/246 (80.9%)	218/265 (82.3%)	-8.9%,4.2%
Abscess	73/93 (78.5%)	86/99 (86.9%)	NA
Non-abscess	126/153 (82.4%)	132/166 (79.5%)	NA

*excludes 2 patients who required additional surgery within the first 48 hours.
†NA - not applicable

scesses, appendicitis with perforation, and bowel perforation. This study enrolled 681 patients, 379 of which were considered clinically evaluable. A second open-label international study compared AVELOX 400 mg QD for 5-14 days to IV ceftriaxone plus IV metronidazole followed by PO amoxicillin/clavulanic acid in the treatment of patients with cIAI. This study enrolled 595 patients, 511 of which were considered clinically evaluable. The clinically evaluable population consisted of subjects with a surgically confirmed complicated infection, at least 5 days of treatment and a 25-50 day follow-up assessment for patients at the Test of Cure visit. The overall clinical success rates in the clinically evaluable patients are shown below:
[See third table above]

REFERENCES

1. Clinical and Laboratory Standards Institute, Methods for Dilution Antimicrobial Susceptibility Tests for Bacteria That Grow Aerobically-Sixth Edition. Approved Standard CLSI Document M7-A6, Vol. 23, No. 2, CLSI, Wayne, PA, January, 2003.
2. Clinical and Laboratory Standards Institute, Performance Standards for Antimicrobial Disk Susceptibility Tests-Eighth Edition. Approved Standard CLSI Document M2-A8, Vol. 23, No. 1, CLSI, Wayne, PA, January, 2003.
3. Clinical and Laboratory Standards Institute, Methods for Antimicrobial Susceptibility Testing of Anaerobic Bacteria; Approved Standard CLSI Document M11-A6, Vol. 24, No. 2, CLSI, Wayne, PA, 2004.

MEDICATION GUIDE

AVELOX® (AV-eh-locks)
(moxifloxacin hydrochloride)
Tablets
AVELOX® I.V. (AV-eh-locks)
(moxifloxacin hydrochloride in sodium chloride injection)
Read the Medication Guide that comes with AVELOX® before you start taking it and each time you get a refill. There may be new information. This Medication Guide does not take the place of talking to your healthcare provider about your medical condition or your treatment.
What is the most important information I should know about AVELOX?
AVELOX belongs to a class of antibiotics called fluoroquinolones. AVELOX can cause side effects that may be serious or even cause death. If you get any of the following serious side effects, get medical help right away. Talk with your healthcare provider about whether you should continue to take AVELOX.
• **Tendon rupture or swelling of the tendon (tendinitis)**
  • Tendons are tough cords of tissue that connect muscles to bones.
  • Pain, swelling, tears and inflammation of tendons including the back of the ankle (Achilles), shoulder, hand,

or other tendon sites can happen in people of all ages who take fluoroquinolone antibiotics, including AVELOX. The risk of getting tendon problems is higher if you:
  • are over 60 years of age
  • are taking steroids (corticosteroids)
  • have had a kidney, heart or lung transplant
• Swelling of the tendon (tendinitis) and tendon rupture (breakage) have also happened in patients who take fluoroquinolones who do not have the above risk factors.
• Other reasons for tendon ruptures can include:
  • physical activity or exercise
  • kidney failure
  • tendon problems in the past, such as in people with rheumatoid arthritis (RA)
• Call your healthcare provider right away at the first sign of tendon pain, swelling or inflammation. Stop taking AVELOX until tendinitis or tendon rupture has been ruled out by your healthcare provider. Avoid exercise and using the affected area. The most common area of pain and swelling is in the Achilles tendon at the back of your ankle. This can also happen with other tendons. Talk to your healthcare provider about the risk of tendon rupture with continued use of AVELOX. You may need a different antibiotic that is not a fluoroquinolone to treat your infection.
• Tendon rupture can happen while you are taking or after you have finished taking AVELOX. Tendon ruptures have happened up to several months after patients have finished taking their fluoroquinolone.
• Get medical help right away if you get any of the following signs or symptoms of a tendon rupture:
  • hear or feel a snap or pop in a tendon area
  • bruising right after an injury in a tendon area
  • unable to move the affected area or bear weight
• See the section **"What are the possible side effects of AVELOX?"** for more information about side effects.
What is AVELOX?
AVELOX is a fluoroquinolone antibiotic medicine used to treat certain types of infections caused by certain germs called bacteria in adults 18 years or older. It is not known if AVELOX is safe and works in people under 18 years of age. Children have a higher chance of getting bone, joint, and tendon (musculoskeletal) problems while taking fluoroquinolone antibiotic medicines.
Sometimes infections are caused by viruses rather than by bacteria. Examples include viral infections in the sinuses and lungs, such as the common cold or flu. Antibiotics, including AVELOX, do not kill viruses.
Call your healthcare provider if you think your condition is not getting better while you are taking AVELOX.
Who should not take AVELOX?
Do not take AVELOX if you have ever had a severe allergic reaction to an antibiotic known as a fluoroquinolone, or if

you are allergic to any of the ingredients in AVELOX. Ask your healthcare provider if you are not sure. See the list of ingredients in AVELOX at the end of this Medication Guide.
What should I tell my healthcare provider before taking AVELOX?
See **"What is the most important information I should know about AVELOX?"**
Tell your healthcare provider about all your medical conditions, including if you:
• have tendon problems
• have central nervous system problems (such as epilepsy)
• have nerve problems
• have or anyone in your family has an irregular heartbeat, especially a condition called "QT prolongation"
• have low blood potassium (hypokalemia)
• have a slow heartbeat (bradycardia)
• have a history of seizures
• have kidney problems
• have rheumatoid arthritis (RA) or other history of joint problems
• are pregnant or planning to become pregnant. It is not known if AVELOX will harm your unborn child.
• are breast-feeding or planning to breast-feed. It is not known if AVELOX passes into breast milk. You and your healthcare provider should decide whether you will take AVELOX or breast-feed.
Tell your healthcare provider about all the medicines you take, including prescription and non-prescription medicines, vitamins and herbal and dietary supplements. AVELOX and other medicines can affect each other causing side effects. Especially tell your healthcare provider if you take:
• an NSAID (Non-Steroidal Anti-Inflammatory Drug). Many common medicines for pain relief are NSAIDs. Taking an NSAID while you take AVELOX or other fluoroquinolones may increase your risk of central nervous system effects and seizures. See **"What are the possible side effects of AVELOX?"**
• a blood thinner (warfarin, Coumadin, Jantoven)
• a medicine to control your heart rate or rhythm (antiarrhythmic) See **"What are the possible side effects of AVELOX?"**
• an anti-psychotic medicine
• a tricyclic antidepressant
• erythromycin
• a water pill (diuretic)
• a steroid medicine. Corticosteroids taken by mouth or by injection may increase the chance of tendon injury. See **"What is the most important information I should know about AVELOX?"**
• Certain medicines may keep AVELOX from working correctly. Take AVELOX either 4 hours before or 8 hours after taking these products:
• an antacid, multivitamin, or other product that has magnesium, aluminum, iron, or zinc
• sucralfate (Carafate)
• didanosine (Videx®, Videx EC®)
Ask your healthcare provider if you are not sure if any of your medicines are listed above.
Know the medicines you take. Keep a list of your medicines and show it to your healthcare provider and pharmacist when you get a new medicine.
How should I take AVELOX?
• **Take AVELOX once a day exactly as prescribed by your healthcare provider.**
• **Take AVELOX at about the same time each day.**
• **AVELOX Tablets should be swallowed.**
• **AVELOX can be taken with or without food.**
• **Drink plenty of fluids while taking AVELOX.**
• **AVELOX I.V. is given to you by intravenous (I.V.) infusion into your vein slowly, over 60 minutes, as prescribed by your healthcare provider.**
• **Do not skip any doses, or stop taking AVELOX even if you begin to feel better, until you finish your prescribed treatment, unless:**
  • you have tendon effects (see **"What is the most important information I should know about AVELOX?"**)
  • you have a serious allergic reaction (see **"What are the possible side effects of AVELOX?"**), or your healthcare provider tells you to stop.
  • This will help make sure that all of the bacteria are killed and lower the chance that the bacteria will become resistant to AVELOX. If this happens, AVELOX and other antibiotic medicines may not work in the future.
• **If you miss a dose of AVELOX, take it as soon as you remember. Do not take more than 1 dose of AVELOX in one day.**
• **If you take too much, call your healthcare provider or get medical help immediately.**
What should I avoid while taking AVELOX?
• AVELOX can make you feel dizzy and lightheaded. Do not drive, operate machinery, or do other activities that require mental alertness or coordination until you know how AVELOX affects you.

IMPORTANT NOTICE: Updated drug information is sent bi-monthly via the PDR® Update Insert. For *monthly* email updates, register at PDR.net.

- Avoid sunlamps, tanning beds, and try to limit your time in the sun. AVELOX can make your skin sensitive to the sun (photosensitivity) and the light from sunlamps and tanning beds. You could get severe sunburn, blisters or swelling of your skin. If you get any of these symptoms while taking AVELOX, call your healthcare provider right away. You should use a sunscreen and wear a hat and clothes that cover your skin if you have to be in sunlight.

What are the possible side effects of AVELOX?

AVELOX can cause side effects that may be serious or even cause death. See **"What is the most important information I should know about AVELOX?"**

Other serious side effects of AVELOX include:

- **Central Nervous System effects**

Seizures have been reported in people who take fluoroquinolone antibiotics including AVELOX. Tell your healthcare provider if you have a history of seizures. Ask your healthcare provider whether taking AVELOX will change your risk of having a seizure.

Central Nervous System (CNS) side effects may happen as soon as after taking the first dose of AVELOX. Talk to your healthcare provider right away if you have any of these side effects, or other changes in mood or behavior:

- feeling dizzy
- seizures
- hear voices, see things, or sense things that are not there (hallucinations)
- feel restless
- tremors
- feel anxious or nervous
- confusion
- depression
- trouble sleeping
- feel more suspicious (paranoia)
- suicidal thoughts or acts
- nightmares
- **Serious allergic reactions**

Allergic reactions can happen in people taking fluoroquinolones, including AVELOX, even after only one dose. Stop taking AVELOX and get emergency medical help right away if you get any of the following symptoms of a severe allergic reaction:

- hives
- trouble breathing or swallowing
- swelling of the lips, tongue, face
- throat tightness, hoarseness
- rapid heartbeat
- faint
- yellowing of the skin or eyes. Stop taking AVELOX and tell your healthcare provider right away if you get yellowing of your skin or white part of your eyes, or if you have dark urine. These can be signs of a serious reaction to AVELOX (a liver problem).
- **Skin rash**

Skin rash may happen in people taking AVELOX even after only one dose. Stop taking AVELOX at the first sign of a skin rash and call your healthcare provider. Skin rash may be a sign of a more serious reaction to AVELOX.

- **Serious heart rhythm changes** (QT prolongation and torsade de pointes)

Tell your healthcare provider right away if you have a change in your heart beat (a fast or irregular heartbeat), or if you faint. AVELOX may cause a rare heart problem known as prolongation of the QT interval. This condition can cause an abnormal heartbeat and can be very dangerous. The chances of this event are higher in people:

- who are elderly
- with a family history of prolonged QT interval
- with low blood potassium (hypokalemia)
- who take certain medicines to control heart rhythm (antiarrhythmics)
- **Intestine (Pseudomembranous colitis)**

Pseudomembranous colitis can happen with most antibiotics, including AVELOX. Call your healthcare provider right away if you get watery diarrhea, diarrhea that does not go away, or bloody stools. You may have stomach cramps and a fever. Pseudomembranous colitis can happen 2 or more months after you have finished your antibiotic.

- **Changes in sensation and possible nerve damage (Peripheral Neuropathy)**

Damage to the nerves in arms, hands, legs, or feet can happen in people taking fluoroquinolones, including AVELOX. Talk with your healthcare provider right away if you get any of the following symptoms of peripheral neuropathy in your arms, hands, legs, or feet:

- pain
- burning
- tingling
- numbness
- weakness

AVELOX may need to be stopped to prevent permanent nerve damage.

- **Sensitivity to sunlight** (photosensitivity)
- See **"What should I avoid while taking AVELOX?"**

The most common side effects of AVELOX include nausea and diarrhea.

These are not all the possible side effects of AVELOX. Tell your healthcare provider about any side effect that bothers you or that does not go away.

Call your doctor for medical advice about side effects. You may report side effects to FDA at 1-800-FDA-1088.

How should I store AVELOX?

AVELOX Tablets

- Store AVELOX 59–86°F (15–30°C)
- Keep AVELOX away from moisture (humidity)

Keep AVELOX and all medicines out of the reach of children.

General Information about AVELOX

Medicines are sometimes prescribed for purposes other than those listed in a Medication Guide. Do not use AVELOX for a condition for which it is not prescribed. Do not give AVELOX to other people, even if they have the same symptoms that you have. It may harm them.

This Medication Guide summarizes the most important information about AVELOX. If you would like more information about AVELOX, talk with your healthcare provider. You can ask your healthcare provider or pharmacist for information about AVELOX that is written for healthcare professionals. For more information go to www.AVELOX.com or call 1-800-526-4099.

What are the ingredients in AVELOX?

- **AVELOX Tablets:**
  - Active ingredient: moxifloxacin hydrochloride
  - Inactive ingredients: microcrystalline cellulose, lactose monohydrate, croscarmellose sodium, magnesium stearate, hypromellose, titanium dioxide, polyethylene glycol, and ferric oxide
- **AVELOX I.V.:**
  - Active ingredient: moxifloxacin hydrochloride
  - Inactive ingredients: sodium chloride, USP, water for injection, USP, and may include hydrochloric acid and/or sodium hydroxide for pH adjustment

Revised October 2008

This Medication Guide has been approved by the U.S. Food and Drug Administration.

Shown in Product Identification Guide, page 311

CANCIDAS   ℞

[kan-si-das]

(caspofungin acetate)

for injection, for intravenous use

HIGHLIGHTS OF PRESCRIBING INFORMATION

These highlights do not include all the information needed to use CANCIDAS safely and effectively. See full prescribing information for CANCIDAS.

CANCIDAS (caspofungin acetate) for injection, for intravenous use

Initial U.S. Approval: 2001

INDICATIONS AND USAGE

CANCIDAS is an echinocandin antifungal drug indicated in adults and pediatric patients (3 months and older) for:

- Empirical therapy for presumed fungal infections in febrile, neutropenic patients. (1)
- Treatment of candidemia and the following *Candida* infections: intra-abdominal abscesses, peritonitis and pleural space infections. (1)
- Treatment of esophageal candidiasis. (1)
- Treatment of invasive aspergillosis in patients who are refractory to or intolerant of other therapies (e.g., amphotericin B, lipid formulations of amphotericin B, itraconazole). (1)

DOSAGE AND ADMINISTRATION

For All Patients (2.1):

- Administer by slow intravenous (IV) infusion over approximately 1 hour. Not for IV bolus administration.

- Do not mix or co-infuse CANCIDAS with other medications. Do not use diluents containing dextrose (α–D-glucose).

Adults [≥18 years of age] (2.2):

- Administer a single 70-mg loading dose on Day 1, followed by 50 mg once daily for all indications except esophageal candidiasis.
- For esophageal candidiasis, use 50 mg once daily with no loading dose.

Pediatric Patients [3 months to 17 years of age] (2.3):

- Dosing should be based on the patient's body surface area.
- For all indications, administer a single 70-mg/m² loading dose on Day 1, followed by 50 mg/m² once daily thereafter.
- **Maximum loading dose and daily maintenance dose should not exceed 70 mg, regardless of the patient's calculated dose.**

Dosing With Rifampin and Other Inducers of Drug Clearance (2.5):

- Use 70-mg once daily dose for adult patients on rifampin.
- Consider dose increase to 70 mg once daily for adult patients on nevirapine, efavirenz, carbamazepine, dexamethasone, or phenytoin.
- Pediatric patients receiving these same concomitant medications may also require an increase in dose to 70 mg/m² once daily (maximum daily dose not to exceed 70 mg).

DOSAGE FORMS AND STRENGTHS

- Vials: 50 or 70 mg lyophilized powder (plus allowance for overfill). (3)

CONTRAINDICATIONS

- CANCIDAS is contraindicated in patients with hypersensitivity to any component of this product. (4)

WARNINGS AND PRECAUTIONS

- Use with cyclosporine: Limit use to patients for whom potential benefit outweighs potential risk. Monitor patients who develop abnormal liver function tests (LFTs) during concomitant therapy and evaluate risk/benefit of continuing CANCIDAS. (5.1)
- Hepatic effects: Can cause abnormalities in LFTs and isolated cases of clinically significant hepatic dysfunction, hepatitis, or hepatic failure. Monitor patients who develop abnormal LFTs for evidence of worsening hepatic function, and evaluate risk/benefit of continuing CANCIDAS. (5.2)

ADVERSE REACTIONS

- *Adults:* Most common adverse reactions (incidence ≥10%) are diarrhea, pyrexia, ALT/AST increased, blood alkaline phosphatase increased, and blood potassium decreased. (6.1)
- *Pediatric patients:* Most common adverse reactions (incidence ≥10%) are pyrexia, diarrhea, rash, ALT/AST increased, blood potassium decreased, hypotension, and chills. (6.2)

To report SUSPECTED ADVERSE REACTIONS, contact Merck Sharp & Dohme Corp., a subsidiary of Merck & Co., Inc., at 1-877-888-4231 or FDA at 1-800-FDA-1088 or www.fda.gov/medwatch.

USE IN SPECIFIC POPULATIONS

- Pregnancy: Based on animal data, may cause fetal harm. (8.1)
- Pediatric use: Safety and efficacy in neonates and infants less than 3 months old have not been established. (8.4)
- Hepatic impairment: Reduce dose for adult patients with moderate hepatic impairment (35 mg once daily, with a 70-mg loading dose on Day 1 where appropriate). No data are available in adults with severe impairment or in pediatric patients with any degree of impairment. (8.6, 12.3)

See 17 for PATIENT COUNSELING INFORMATION

Revised: 06/2010

FULL PRESCRIBING INFORMATION: CONTENTS*

6 ADVERSE REACTIONS

FULL PRESCRIBING INFORMATION

1 INDICATIONS AND USAGE

CANCIDAS[1] is indicated in adults and pediatric patients (3 months and older) for:

- Empirical therapy for presumed fungal infections in febrile, neutropenic patients
- Treatment of candidemia and the following *Candida* infections: intra-abdominal abscesses, peritonitis and pleural space infections. CANCIDAS has not been studied in endocarditis, osteomyelitis, and meningitis due to *Candida*.
- Treatment of esophageal candidiasis *[see Clinical Studies (14.3)]*
- Treatment of invasive aspergillosis in patients who are refractory to or intolerant of other therapies (e.g., amphotericin B, lipid formulations of amphotericin B, itraconazole). CANCIDAS has not been studied as initial therapy for invasive aspergillosis.

---

2 DOSAGE AND ADMINISTRATION

2.1 Instructions for Use in All Patients

CANCIDAS should be administered by slow intravenous (IV) infusion over approximately 1 hour. CANCIDAS should not be administered by IV bolus administration.

Do not mix or co-infuse CANCIDAS with other medications, as there are no data available on the compatibility of CANCIDAS with other intravenous substances, additives, or medications. DO NOT USE DILUENTS CONTAINING DEXTROSE (α-D-GLUCOSE), as CANCIDAS is not stable in diluents containing dextrose.

2.2 Recommended Dosing in Adult Patients [≥18 years of age]

The usual dose is 50 mg once daily (following a 70-mg loading dose for most indications). The safety and efficacy of a dose of 150 mg daily (range: 1 to 51 days; median: 14 days) have been studied in 100 adult patients with candidemia and other *Candida* infections. The efficacy of CANCIDAS at this higher dose was not significantly better than the efficacy of the 50-mg daily dose of CANCIDAS. The efficacy of doses higher than 50 mg daily in the other adult patients for whom CANCIDAS is indicated is not known *[see Clinical Studies (14.2)]*.

Empirical Therapy

A single 70-mg loading dose should be administered on Day 1, followed by 50 mg once daily thereafter. Duration of treatment should be based on the patient's clinical response. Empirical therapy should be continued until resolution of neutropenia. Patients found to have a fungal infection should be treated for a minimum of 14 days; treatment should continue for at least 7 days after both neutropenia and clinical symptoms are resolved. If the 50-mg dose is well tolerated but does not provide an adequate clinical response, the daily dose can be increased to 70 mg.

Candidemia and Other Candida Infections [see Clinical Studies (14.2)]

A single 70-mg loading dose should be administered on Day 1, followed by 50 mg once daily thereafter. Duration of treatment should be dictated by the patient's clinical and microbiological response. In general, antifungal therapy should continue for at least 14 days after the last positive culture. Patients who remain persistently neutropenic may warrant a longer course of therapy pending resolution of the neutropenia.

Esophageal Candidiasis

The dose is 50 mg once daily for 7 to 14 days after symptom resolution. A 70-mg loading dose has not been studied for this indication. Because of the risk of relapse of oropharyngeal candidiasis in patients with HIV infections, suppressive oral therapy could be considered *[see Clinical Studies (14.3)]*.

Invasive Aspergillosis

A single 70-mg loading dose should be administered on Day 1, followed by 50 mg once daily thereafter. Duration of treatment should be based upon the severity of the patient's underlying disease, recovery from immunosuppression, and clinical response.

2.3 Recommended Dosing in Pediatric Patients [3 months to 17 years of age]

For all indications, a single 70-mg/m[2] loading dose should be administered on Day 1, followed by 50 mg/m[2] once daily thereafter. **The maximum loading dose and the daily maintenance dose should not exceed 70 mg, regardless of the patient's calculated dose.** Dosing in pediatric patients (3 months to 17 years of age) should be based on the patient's body surface area (BSA) as calculated by the Mosteller Formula *[see References (15)]*:

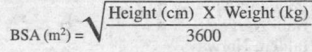

$$\text{BSA (m}^2) = \sqrt{\frac{\text{Height (cm)} \times \text{Weight (kg)}}{3600}}$$

Following calculation of the patient's BSA, the loading dose in milligrams should be calculated as BSA $(\text{m}^2) \times 70$ mg/m[2]. The maintenance dose in milligrams should be calculated as BSA $(\text{m}^2) \times 50$ mg/m[2].

Duration of treatment should be individualized to the indication, as described for each indication in adults *[see Dosage and Administration (2.2)]*. If the 50-mg/m[2] daily dose is well tolerated but does not provide an adequate clinical response, the daily dose can be increased to 70 mg/m[2] daily (not to exceed 70 mg).

2.4 Patients with Hepatic Impairment

Adult patients with mild hepatic impairment (Child-Pugh score 5 to 6) do not need a dosage adjustment. For adult patients with moderate hepatic impairment (Child-Pugh score 7 to 9), CANCIDAS 35 mg once daily is recommended based upon pharmacokinetic data *[see Clinical Pharmacology (12.3)]*. However, where recommended, a 70-mg loading dose should still be administered on Day 1. There is no clinical experience in adult patients with severe hepatic impairment (Child-Pugh score >9) and in pediatric patients with any degree of hepatic impairment.

2.5 Patients Receiving Concomitant Inducers of Drug Clearance

Adult patients on rifampin should receive 70 mg of CANCIDAS once daily. Adult patients on nevirapine, efavirenz, carbamazepine, dexamethasone, or phenytoin may require an increase in dose to 70 mg of CANCIDAS once daily *[see Drug Interactions (7)]*.

When CANCIDAS is co-administered to pediatric patients with inducers of drug clearance, such as rifampin, efavirenz, nevirapine, phenytoin, dexamethasone, or carbamazepine, a CANCIDAS dose of 70 mg/m[2] once daily (not to exceed 70 mg) should be considered *[see Drug Interactions (7)]*.

2.6 Preparation and Reconstitution for Administration

Do not mix or co-infuse CANCIDAS with other medications, as there are no data available on the compatibility of CANCIDAS with other intravenous substances, additives, or medications. DO NOT USE DILUENTS CONTAINING DEXTROSE (α-D-GLUCOSE), as CANCIDAS is not stable in diluents containing dextrose.

Preparation of CANCIDAS for Infusion

A. Equilibrate the refrigerated vial of CANCIDAS to room temperature.

B. Aseptically add 10.8 mL of 0.9% Sodium Chloride Injection, Sterile Water for Injection, Bacteriostatic Water for Injection with methylparaben and propylparaben, or Bacteriostatic Water for Injection with 0.9% benzyl alcohol to the vial.

Each vial of CANCIDAS contains an intentional overfill of CANCIDAS. Thus, the drug concentration of the resulting solution is listed in Table 1 below.

TABLE 1: Information for Preparation of CANCIDAS

CANCIDAS vial	Total Drug Content (including overfill)	Reconstitution Volume to be added	Resulting Concentration following Reconstitution
50 mg	54.6 mg	10.8 mL	5 mg/mL
70 mg	75.6 mg	10.8 mL	7 mg/mL

The white to off-white cake will dissolve completely. Mix gently until a clear solution is obtained. Visually inspect the reconstituted solution for particulate matter or discoloration during reconstitution and prior to infusion. Do not use if the solution is cloudy or has precipitated.

The reconstituted solution may be stored for up to one hour at ≤25°C (≤77°F).

CANCIDAS vials are for single use only; the remaining solution should be discarded.

C. Aseptically transfer the appropriate volume (mL) of reconstituted CANCIDAS to an IV bag (or bottle) containing 250 mL of 0.9%, 0.45%, or 0.225% Sodium Chloride Injection or Lactated Ringers Injection. Alternatively, the volume (mL) of reconstituted CANCIDAS can be added to a reduced volume of 0.9%, 0.45%, or 0.225% Sodium Chloride Injection or Lactated Ringers Injection, not to exceed a final concentration of 0.5 mg/mL.

This infusion solution must be used within 24 hours if stored at ≤25°C (≤77°F) or within 48 hours if stored refrigerated at 2 to 8°C (36 to 46°F).

Special Considerations for Pediatric Patients >3 Months of Age

Follow the reconstitution procedures described above using either the 70-mg or 50-mg vial to create the reconstituted solution *[see Dosage and Administration (2.3)]*. From the reconstituted solution in the vial, remove the volume of drug equal to the calculated loading dose or calculated maintenance dose based on a concentration of 7 mg/mL (if reconstituted from the 70-mg vial) or a concentration of 5 mg/mL (if reconstituted from the 50-mg vial).

The choice of vial should be based on total milligram dose of drug to be administered to the pediatric patient. To help ensure accurate dosing, it is recommended for pediatric doses less than 50 mg that 50-mg vials (with a concentration of 5 mg/mL) be used if available. The 70-mg vial should be reserved for pediatric patients requiring doses greater than 50 mg.

The maximum loading dose and the daily maintenance dose should not exceed 70 mg, regardless of the patient's calculated dose.

3 DOSAGE FORMS AND STRENGTHS

CANCIDAS 50 mg is a white to off-white powder/cake for infusion in a vial with a red aluminum band and a plastic cap. CANCIDAS 50-mg vial contains 54.6 mg of caspofungin.

CANCIDAS 70 mg is a white to off-white powder/cake for infusion in a vial with a yellow/orange aluminum band and a plastic cap. CANCIDAS 70-mg vial contains 75.6 mg of caspofungin.

4 CONTRAINDICATIONS

CANCIDAS is contraindicated in patients with hypersensitivity (e.g., anaphylaxis) to any component of this product *[see Adverse Reactions (6)]*.

5 WARNINGS AND PRECAUTIONS

5.1 Concomitant Use with Cyclosporine

Concomitant use of CANCIDAS with cyclosporine should be limited to patients for whom the potential benefit outweighs the potential risk. In one clinical study, 3 of 4 healthy adult subjects who received CANCIDAS 70 mg on Days 1 through 10, and also received two 3 mg/kg doses of cyclosporine 12 hours apart on Day 10, developed transient elevations of alanine transaminase (ALT) on Day 11 that were 2 to 3 times the upper limit of normal (ULN). In a separate panel of adult subjects in the same study, 2 of 8 who received CANCIDAS 35 mg daily for 3 days and cyclosporine (two 3 mg/kg doses administered 12 hours apart) on Day 1 had small increases in ALT (slightly above the ULN) on Day 2. In both groups, elevations in aspartate transaminase (AST) paralleled ALT elevations, but were of lesser magnitude. In another clinical study, 2 of 8 healthy men developed transient ALT elevations of less than 2× ULN. In this study, cyclosporine (4 mg/kg) was administered on Days 1 and 12, and CANCIDAS was administered (70 mg) daily on Days 3 through 13. In one subject, the ALT elevation occurred on Days 7 and 9 and, in the other subject, the ALT elevation occurred on Day 19. These elevations returned to normal by Day 27. In all groups, elevations in AST paralleled ALT elevations but were of lesser magnitude. In these clinical studies, cyclosporine (one 4 mg/kg dose or two 3 mg/kg doses) increased the AUC of caspofungin by approximately 35%.

In a retrospective postmarketing study, 40 immunocompromised patients, including 37 transplant recipients, were treated with CANCIDAS and cyclosporine for 1 to 290 days (median 17.5 days). Fourteen patients (35%) developed transaminase elevations >5× upper limit of normal or >3× baseline during concomitant therapy or the 14-day follow-up period; five were considered possibly related to concomitant therapy. One patient had elevated bilirubin considered possibly related to concomitant therapy. No patient developed clinical evidence of hepatotoxicity or serious hepatic events. Discontinuations due to laboratory abnormalities in hepatic enzymes from any cause occurred in four patients. Of these, 2 were considered possibly related to therapy with CANCIDAS and/or cyclosporine as well as to other possible causes.

In the prospective invasive aspergillosis and compassionate use studies, there were 4 adult patients treated with CANCIDAS (50 mg/day) and cyclosporine for 2 to 56 days. None of these patients experienced increases in hepatic enzymes.

Given the limitations of these data, CANCIDAS and cyclosporine should only be used concomitantly in those patients for whom the potential benefit outweighs the potential risk. Patients who develop abnormal liver function tests during concomitant therapy should be monitored and the risk/benefit of continuing therapy should be evaluated.

5.2 Hepatic Effects

Laboratory abnormalities in liver function tests have been seen in healthy volunteers and in adult and pediatric patients treated with CANCIDAS. In some adult and pediatric patients with serious underlying conditions who were receiving multiple concomitant medications with CANCIDAS, isolated cases of clinically significant hepatic dysfunction, hepatitis, and hepatic failure have been reported; a causal relationship to CANCIDAS has not been established. Patients who develop abnormal liver function tests during CANCIDAS therapy should be monitored for evidence of worsening hepatic function and evaluated for risk/benefit of continuing CANCIDAS therapy.

6 ADVERSE REACTIONS

The following serious adverse reactions are discussed in detail in another section of the labeling:
• Hepatic effects *[see Warnings and Precautions (5.2)]*
Anaphylaxis has been reported during administration of CANCIDAS. Possible histamine-mediated symptoms have been reported including reports of rash, facial swelling, angioedema, pruritus, sensation of warmth, or bronchospasm. Because clinical trials are conducted under widely varying conditions, adverse reaction rates observed in clinical trials of CANCIDAS cannot be directly compared to rates in clinical trials of another drug and may not reflect the rates observed in practice. The adverse reaction information from clinical trials does provide a basis for identifying adverse reactions that appear to be related to drug use and for approximating rates.

6.1 Clinical Trials Experience in Adults

The overall safety of CANCIDAS was assessed in 1865 adult individuals who received single or multiple doses of CANCIDAS: 564 febrile, neutropenic patients (empirical therapy study); 382 patients with candidemia and/or intra-abdominal abscesses, peritonitis, or pleural space infections (including 4 patients with chronic disseminated candidiasis); 297 patients with esophageal and/or oropharyngeal candidiasis; 228 patients with invasive aspergillosis; and 394 individuals in phase I studies. In the empirical therapy study patients had undergone hematopoietic stem-cell transplantation or chemotherapy. In the studies involving patients with documented *Candida* infections, the majority of the patients had serious underlying medical conditions (e.g., hematologic or other malignancy, recent major surgery, HIV) requiring multiple concomitant medications. Patients in the noncomparative *Aspergillus* studies often had serious predisposing medical conditions (e.g., bone marrow or peripheral stem cell transplants, hematologic malignancy, solid tumors or organ transplants) requiring multiple concomitant medications.

TABLE 2: Adverse Reactions Among Patients with Persistent Fever and Neutropenia* — Incidence ≥7.5% for at Least One Treatment Group by System Organ Class or Preferred Term

Adverse Reaction (MedDRA v10.1 System Organ Class and Preferred Term)	CANCIDAS[†] N=564 (percent)	AmBisome[‡] N=547 (percent)
All Systems, Any Adverse Reaction	**95**	**97**
Investigations	**58**	**63**
Alanine Aminotransferase Increased	18	20
Blood Alkaline Phosphatase Increased	15	23
Blood Potassium Decreased	15	23
Aspartate Aminotransferase Increased	14	17
Blood Bilirubin Increased	10	14
Blood Albumin Decreased	7	8
Blood Magnesium Decreased	7	9
Blood Glucose Increased	6	9
Bilirubin Conjugated Increased	5	9
Blood Urea Increased	4	8
Blood Creatinine Increased	3	11
General Disorders and Administration Site Conditions	**57**	**63**
Pyrexia	27	29
Chills	23	31
Edema Peripheral	11	12
Mucosal Inflammation	6	8
Gastrointestinal Disorders	**50**	**55**
Diarrhea	20	16
Nausea	11	20
Abdominal Pain	9	11
Vomiting	9	17
Respiratory, Thoracic and Mediastinal Disorders	**47**	**49**
Cough	11	10
Dyspnea	9	10
Rales	7	8
Infections and Infestations	**45**	**42**
Pneumonia	11	10
Skin and Subcutaneous Tissue Disorders	**42**	**37**
Rash	16	14
Nervous System Disorders	**25**	**27**
Headache	11	12
Metabolism and Nutrition Disorders	**21**	**24**
Hypokalemia	6	8
Vascular Disorders	**20**	**23**
Hypotension	6	10
Cardiac Disorders	**16**	**19**
Tachycardia	7	9

Within any system organ class, individuals may experience more than 1 adverse reaction.
* Regardless of causality
† 70 mg on Day 1, then 50 mg once daily for the remainder of treatment; daily dose was increased to 70 mg for 73 patients.
‡ 3 mg/kg/day; daily dose was increased to 5 mg/kg for 74 patients.

Empirical Therapy
In the randomized, double-blinded empirical therapy study, patients received either CANCIDAS 50 mg/day (following a 70-mg loading dose) or AmBisome[2] (amphotericin B liposome for injection, 3 mg/kg/day). In this study clinical or laboratory hepatic adverse reactions were reported in 39% and 45% of patients in the CANCIDAS and AmBisome groups, respectively. Also reported was an isolated, serious adverse reaction of hyperbilirubinemia considered possibly related to CANCIDAS. Adverse reactions occurring in ≥7.5% of the patients in either treatment group are presented in Table 2.
[See table 2 above]
The proportion of patients who experienced an infusion-related adverse reaction (defined as a systemic event, such as pyrexia, chills, flushing, hypotension, hypertension, tachycardia, dyspnea, tachypnea, rash, or anaphylaxis, that developed during the study therapy infusion and one hour following infusion) was significantly lower in the group treated with CANCIDAS (35%) than in the group treated with AmBisome (52%).

To evaluate the effect of CANCIDAS and AmBisome on renal function, nephrotoxicity was defined as doubling of serum creatinine relative to baseline or an increase of ≥1 mg/dL in serum creatinine if baseline serum creatinine was above the upper limit of the normal range. Among patients whose baseline creatinine clearance was >30 mL/min, the incidence of nephrotoxicity was significantly lower in the group treated with CANCIDAS (3%) than in the group treated with AmBisome (12%). Clinical renal events, regardless of causality, were similar between CANCIDAS (75/564, 13%) and AmBisome (85/547, 16%).

[2] Registered trademark of Gilead Sciences, Inc.

Candidemia and Other Candida Infections
In the randomized, double-blinded invasive candidiasis study, patients received either CANCIDAS 50 mg/day (following a 70-mg loading dose) or amphotericin B 0.6 to 1 mg/kg/day. Adverse reactions occurring in ≥10% of the patients in either treatment group are presented in Table 3.
[See table 3 at top of next page]

TABLE 3: Adverse Reactions Among Patients with Candidemia or other *Candida* Infections*,† — Incidence ≥10% for at Least One Treatment Group by System Organ Class or Preferred Term

Adverse Reaction (MedDRA v10.1 System Organ Class and Preferred Term)	CANCIDAS 50 mg‡ N=114 (percent)	Amphotericin B N=125 (percent)
All Systems, Any Adverse Reaction	96	99
Investigations	67	82
Blood Potassium Decreased	23	32
Blood Alkaline Phosphatase Increased	21	32
Hemoglobin Decreased	18	23
Alanine Aminotransferase Increased	16	15
Aspartate Aminotransferase Increased	16	14
Blood Bilirubin Increased	13	17
Hematocrit Decreased	13	18
Blood Creatinine Increased	11	28
Red Blood Cells Urine Positive	10	10
Blood Urea Increased	9	23
Bilirubin Conjugated Increased	8	14
Gastrointestinal Disorders	49	53
Vomiting	17	16
Diarrhea	14	10
Nausea	9	17
Infections and Infestations	48	54
Septic Shock	11	9
Pneumonia	4	10
General Disorders and Administration Site Conditions	47	63
Pyrexia	13	33
Edema Peripheral	11	12
Chills	9	30
Respiratory, Thoracic and Mediastinal Disorders	40	54
Respiratory Failure	11	12
Pleural Effusion	9	14
Tachypnea	1	11
Cardiac Disorders	26	34
Tachycardia	8	12
Skin and Subcutaneous Tissue Disorders	25	28
Rash	4	10
Vascular Disorders	25	38
Hypotension	10	16
Blood and Lymphatic System Disorders	15	13
Anemia	11	9

Within any system organ class, individuals may experience more than 1 adverse reaction.
* Intra-abdominal abscesses, peritonitis and pleural space infections.
† Regardless of causality
‡ Patients received CANCIDAS 70 mg on Day 1, then 50 mg once daily for the remainder of their treatment.

The proportion of patients who experienced an infusion-related adverse reaction (defined as a systemic event, such as pyrexia, chills, flushing, hypotension, hypertension, tachycardia, dyspnea, tachypnea, rash, or anaphylaxis, that developed during the study therapy infusion and one hour following infusion) was significantly lower in the group treated with CANCIDAS (20%) than in the group treated with amphotericin B (49%).

To evaluate the effect of CANCIDAS and amphotericin B on renal function, nephrotoxicity was defined as doubling of serum creatinine relative to baseline or an increase of ≥1 mg/dL in serum creatinine if baseline serum creatinine was above the upper limit of the normal range. In a subgroup of patients whose baseline creatinine clearance was >30 mL/min, the incidence of nephrotoxicity was significantly lower in the group treated with CANCIDAS than in the group treated with amphotericin B.

In a second randomized, double-blinded invasive candidiasis study, patients received either CANCIDAS 50 mg/day (following a 70-mg loading dose) or CANCIDAS 150 mg/day. The proportion of patients who experienced any adverse reaction was similar in the 2 treatment groups; however, this study was not large enough to detect differences in rare or unexpected adverse events. Adverse reactions occurring in ≥5% of the patients in either treatment group are presented in Table 4.
[See table 4 at top of next page]

Esophageal Candidiasis and Oropharyngeal Candidiasis
Adverse reactions occurring in ≥10% of patients with esophageal and/or oropharyngeal candidiasis are presented in Table 5.
[See table 5 on next page]

Invasive Aspergillosis
In an open-label, noncomparative aspergillosis study, in which 69 patients received CANCIDAS (70-mg loading dose on Day 1 followed by 50 mg daily), the following treatment-emergent adverse reactions were observed with an incidence of ≥12.5%: blood alkaline phosphatase increased (22%), hypotension (20%), respiratory failure (20%), pyrexia (17%), diarrhea (15%), nausea (15%), headache (15%), rash (13%), aspergillosis (13%), alanine aminotransferase increased (13%), aspartate aminotransferase increased (13%), blood bilirubin increased (13%), and blood potassium decreased (13%). Also reported infrequently in this patient population were pulmonary edema, ARDS (adult respiratory distress syndrome), and radiographic infiltrates.

6.2 Clinical Trials Experience in Pediatric Patients (3 months to 17 years of age)
The overall safety of CANCIDAS was assessed in 171 pediatric patients who received single or multiple doses of CANCIDAS. The distribution among the 153 pediatric patients who were over the age of 3 months was as follows: 104 febrile, neutropenic patients; 38 patients with candidemia and/or intra-abdominal abscesses, peritonitis, or pleural space infections; 1 patient with esophageal candidiasis; and 10 patients with invasive aspergillosis. The overall safety profile of CANCIDAS in pediatric patients is comparable to that in adult patients. Table 6 shows the incidence of adverse reactions reported in ≥7.5% of pediatric patients in clinical studies.

One patient (0.6%) receiving CANCIDAS, and three patients (12%) receiving AmBisome developed a serious drug-related adverse reaction. Two patients (1%) were discontinued from CANCIDAS and three patients (12%) were discontinued from AmBisome due to a drug-related adverse reaction. The proportion of patients who experienced an infusion-related adverse reaction (defined as a systemic event, such as pyrexia, chills, flushing, hypotension, hypertension, tachycardia, dyspnea, tachypnea, rash, or anaphylaxis, that developed during the study therapy infusion and one hour following infusion) was 22% in the group treated with CANCIDAS and 35% in the group treated with AmBisome.
[See table 6 at top of page 1952]

6.3 Overall Safety Experience of CANCIDAS in Clinical Trials
The overall safety of CANCIDAS was assessed in 2036 individuals (including 1642 adult or pediatric patients and 394 volunteers) from 34 clinical studies. These individuals received single or multiple (once daily) doses of CANCIDAS, ranging from 5 mg to 210 mg. Full safety data is available from 1951 individuals, as the safety data from 85 patients enrolled in 2 compassionate use studies was limited solely to serious adverse reactions. Treatment emergent adverse reactions, regardless of causality, which occurred in ≥5% of all individuals who received CANCIDAS in these trials, are shown in Table 7.
Overall, 1665 of the 1951 (85%) patients/volunteers who received CANCIDAS experienced an adverse reaction.

TABLE 7: Treatment-Emergent* Adverse Reactions in Patients Who Received CANCIDAS in Clinical Trials† — Incidence ≥5% for at Least One Treatment Group by System Organ Class or Preferred Term

Adverse Reaction‡ (MedDRA v10 System Organ Class and Preferred Term)	CANCIDAS (N = 1951) n	(%)
All Systems, Any Adverse Reaction	1665	(85)
Investigations	901	(46)
Alanine Aminotransferase Increased	258	(13)
Aspartate Aminotransferase Increased	233	(12)
Blood Alkaline Phosphatase Increased	232	(12)
Blood Potassium Decreased	220	(11)
Blood Bilirubin Increased	117	(6)
General Disorders and Administration Site Conditions	843	(43)
Pyrexia	381	(20)
Chills	192	(10)
Edema Peripheral	110	(6)
Gastrointestinal Disorders	754	(39)
Diarrhea	273	(14)
Nausea	166	(9)
Vomiting	146	(8)
Abdominal Pain	112	(6)
Infections and Infestations	730	(37)
Pneumonia	115	(6)
Respiratory, Thoracic, and Mediastinal Disorders	613	(31)
Cough	111	(6)
Skin and Subcutaneous Tissue Disorders	520	(27)
Rash	159	(8)
Erythema	98	(5)
Nervous System Disorders	412	(21)
Headache	193	(10)

Vascular Disorders	344	(18)
Hypotension	118	(6)

* Defined as an adverse reaction, regardless of causality, while on CANCIDAS or during the 14-day post-CANCIDAS follow-up period.
† Incidence for each preferred term is ≥5% among individuals who received at least 1 dose of CANCIDAS.
‡ Within any system organ class, individuals may experience more than 1 adverse event.

Clinically significant adverse reactions, regardless of causality or incidence which occurred in less than 5% of patients, are listed below.

- **Blood and lymphatic system disorders:** anemia, coagulopathy, febrile neutropenia, neutropenia, thrombocytopenia
- **Cardiac disorders:** arrhythmia, atrial fibrillation, bradycardia, cardiac arrest, myocardial infarction, tachycardia
- **Gastrointestinal disorders:** abdominal distension, abdominal pain upper, constipation, dyspepsia
- **General disorders and administration site conditions:** asthenia, fatigue, infusion site pain/pruritus/swelling, mucosal inflammation, edema
- **Hepatobiliary disorders:** hepatic failure, hepatomegaly, hepatotoxicity, hyperbilirubinemia, jaundice
- **Infections and infestations:** bacteremia, sepsis, urinary tract infection
- **Metabolic and nutrition disorders:** anorexia, decreased appetite, fluid overload, hypomagnesemia, hypercalcemia, hyperglycemia, hypokalemia
- **Musculoskeletal, connective tissue, and bone disorders:** arthralgia, back pain, pain in extremity
- **Nervous system disorders:** convulsion, dizziness, somnolence, tremor
- **Psychiatric disorders:** anxiety, confusional state, depression, insomnia
- **Renal and urinary disorders:** hematuria, renal failure
- **Respiratory, thoracic, and mediastinal disorders:** dyspnea, epistaxis, hypoxia, tachypnea
- **Skin and subcutaneous tissue disorders:** erythema, petechiae, skin lesion, urticaria
- **Vascular disorders:** flushing, hypertension, phlebitis

6.4 Postmarketing Experience
The following additional adverse reactions have been identified during the post-approval use of CANCIDAS. Because these reactions are reported voluntarily from a population of uncertain size, it is not always possible to reliably estimate their frequency or establish a causal relationship to drug exposure.

- **Gastrointestinal disorders:** pancreatitis
- **Hepatobiliary disorders:** hepatic necrosis
- **Skin and subcutaneous tissue disorders:** erythema multiforme, Stevens-Johnson, skin exfoliation
- **Renal and urinary disorders:** clinically significant renal dysfunction
- **General disorders and administration site conditions:** swelling and peripheral edema

7 DRUG INTERACTIONS
[See Clinical Pharmacology (12.3).]
In clinical studies, caspofungin did not induce the CYP3A4 metabolism of other drugs. Caspofungin is not a substrate for P-glycoprotein and is a poor substrate for cytochrome P450 enzymes.
Clinical studies in adult healthy volunteers show that the pharmacokinetics of CANCIDAS are not altered by itraconazole, amphotericin B, mycophenolate, nelfinavir, or tacrolimus. CANCIDAS has no effect on the pharmacokinetics of itraconazole, amphotericin B, or the active metabolite of mycophenolate.
Cyclosporine: In two adult clinical studies, cyclosporine (one 4 mg/kg dose or two 3 mg/kg doses) increased the AUC of caspofungin by approximately 35%. CANCIDAS did not increase the plasma levels of cyclosporine. There were transient increases in liver ALT and AST when CANCIDAS and cyclosporine were co-administered *[see Warnings and Precautions (5.1)]*.
Tacrolimus: For patients receiving CANCIDAS and tacrolimus, standard monitoring of tacrolimus blood concentrations and appropriate tacrolimus dosage adjustments are recommended.
Rifampin: Adult patients on rifampin should receive 70 mg of CANCIDAS daily.
Other inducers of drug clearance:
Adults: When CANCIDAS is co-administered to adult patients with inducers of drug clearance, such as efavirenz, nevirapine, phenytoin, dexamethasone, or carbamazepine, use of a daily dose of 70 mg of CANCIDAS should be considered.

TABLE 4: Adverse Reactions Among Patients with Candidemia or other *Candida* Infections*,† — Incidence ≥5% for at Least One Treatment Group by System Organ Class or Preferred Term

Adverse Reaction (MedDRA v11.0 System Organ Class and Preferred Term)	CANCIDAS 50 mg‡ N=104 (percent)	CANCIDAS 150 mg N=100 (percent)
All Systems, Any Adverse Reaction	83	83
Infections and Infestations	44	43
Septic Shock	13	14
Pneumonia	5	7
Sepsis	5	7
General Disorders and Administration Site Conditions	33	27
Pyrexia	6	6
Gastrointestinal Disorders	30	33
Vomiting	11	6
Diarrhea	6	7
Nausea	5	7
Investigations	28	35
Alkaline Phosphatase Increased	12	9
Aspartate Aminotransferase Increased	6	9
Blood potassium decreased	6	8
Alanine Aminotransferase Increased	4	7
Respiratory, Thoracic and Mediastinal Disorders	23	26
Respiratory Failure	6	2
Vascular Disorders	19	18
Hypotension	7	3
Hypertension	5	6
Skin and Subcutaneous Tissue Disorders	15	15
Decubitus Ulcer	3	5

Within any system organ class, individuals may experience more than 1 adverse event
* Intra-abdominal abscesses, peritonitis and pleural space infections.
† Regardless of causality
‡ Patients received CANCIDAS 70 mg on Day 1, then 50 mg once daily for the remainder of their treatment.

TABLE 5: Adverse Reactions Among Patients with Esophageal and/or Oropharyngeal Candidiasis* — Incidence ≥10% for at Least One Treatment Group by System Organ Class or Preferred Term

Adverse Reaction (MedDRA v10.1 System Organ Class and Preferred Term)	CANCIDAS 50 mg† N=83 (percent)	Fluconazole IV 200 mg† N=94 (percent)
All Systems, Any Adverse Reaction	90	93
Gastrointestinal Disorders	58	50
Diarrhea	27	18
Nausea	15	15
Investigations	53	61
Hemoglobin Decreased	21	16
Hematocrit Decreased	18	16
Aspartate Aminotransferase Increased	13	19
Blood Alkaline Phosphatase Increased	13	17
Alanine Aminotransferase Increased	12	17
White Blood Cell Count Decreased	12	19
General Disorders and Administration Site Conditions	31	36
Pyrexia	21	21
Vascular Disorders	19	15
Phlebitis	18	11
Nervous System Disorders	18	17
Headache	15	9

Within any system organ class, individuals may experience more than 1 adverse reaction.
* Regardless of causality
† Derived from a comparator-controlled clinical study.

Pediatric Patients: When CANCIDAS is co-administered to pediatric patients with inducers of drug clearance, such as rifampin, efavirenz, nevirapine, phenytoin, dexamethasone, or carbamazepine, a CANCIDAS dose of 70 mg/m^2 daily (not to exceed an actual daily dose of 70 mg) should be considered.

TABLE 6: Adverse Reactions Among Pediatric Patients (0 months to 17 years of age)* — Incidence ≥7.5% for at Least One Treatment Group by System Organ Class or Preferred Term

Adverse Reaction (MedDRA v10.0 System Organ Class and Preferred Term)	Noncomparative Clinical Studies CANCIDAS Any Dose N=115 (percent)	Comparator-Controlled Clinical Study of Empirical Therapy CANCIDAS 50 mg/m²† N=56 (percent)	AmBisome 3 mg/kg N=26 (percent)
All Systems, Any Adverse Reaction	95	96	89
Investigations	55	41	50
Blood Potassium Decreased	18	9	27
Aspartate Aminotransferase Increased	17	2	12
Alanine Aminotransferase Increased	14	5	12
Blood Potassium Increased	3	0	8
Protein Total Decreased	0	0	8
General Disorders and Administration Site Conditions	47	59	42
Pyrexia	29	30	23
Chills	10	13	8
Mucosal Inflammation	10	4	4
Edema	3	4	8
Respiratory, Thoracic and Mediastinal Disorders	43	32	27
Respiratory Distress	8	0	4
Cough	6	9	8
Gastrointestinal Disorders	42	41	35
Diarrhea	17	7	15
Vomiting	8	11	12
Abdominal Pain	7	4	12
Nausea	4	4	8
Infections and Infestations	40	30	35
Central Line Infection	1	9	0
Skin and Subcutaneous Tissue Disorders	33	41	39
Pruritus	7	6	8
Rash	6	23	8
Erythema	4	9	0
Vascular Disorders	24	21	19
Hypotension	12	9	8
Hypertension	10	9	4
Metabolism and Nutrition Disorders	22	11	23
Hypokalemia	8	5	4
Cardiac Disorders	17	13	19
Tachycardia	4	11	19
Nervous System Disorders	13	16	8
Headache	5	9	4
Musculoskeletal and Connective Tissue Disorders	11	14	12
Back Pain	4	0	8
Blood and Lymphatic System Disorders	10	2	15
Anemia	2	0	8
Immune System Disorders	7	7	12
Graft Versus Host Disease	1	4	8

Within any system organ class, individuals may experience more than 1 adverse reaction.
* Regardless of causality
† 70 mg/m² on Day 1, then 50 mg/m² once daily for the remainder of the treatment.

8 USE IN SPECIFIC POPULATIONS

8.1 Pregnancy
Pregnancy Category C
There are no adequate and well-controlled studies with the use of CANCIDAS in pregnant women. In animal studies, caspofungin caused embryofetal toxicity, including increased resorptions, increased peri-implantation loss, and incomplete ossification at multiple fetal sites. CANCIDAS should be used during pregnancy only if the potential benefit justifies the potential risk to the fetus.

In offspring born to pregnant rats treated with caspofungin at doses comparable to the human dose based on body surface area comparisons, there was incomplete ossification of the skull and torso and increased incidences of cervical rib. There was also an increase in resorptions and peri-implantation losses. In pregnant rabbits treated with caspofungin at doses comparable to 2 times the human dose based on body surface area comparisons, there was an increased incidence of incomplete ossification of the talus/calcaneus in offspring and increases in fetal resorptions.

Caspofungin crossed the placenta in rats and rabbits and was detectable in fetal plasma.

8.3 Nursing Mothers
It is not known whether caspofungin is present in human milk. Caspofungin was found in the milk of lactating, drug-treated rats. Because many drugs are excreted in human milk, caution should be exercised when caspofungin is administered to a nursing woman.

8.4 Pediatric Use
The safety and effectiveness of CANCIDAS in pediatric patients 3 months to 17 years of age are supported by evidence from adequate and well-controlled studies in adults, pharmacokinetic data in pediatric patients, and additional data from prospective studies in pediatric patients 3 months to 17 years of age for the following indications *[see Indications and Usage (1)]*:
- Empirical therapy for presumed fungal infections in febrile, neutropenic patients.
- Treatment of candidemia and the following *Candida* infections: intra-abdominal abscesses, peritonitis, and pleural space infections.
- Treatment of esophageal candidiasis.
- Treatment of invasive aspergillosis in patients who are refractory to or intolerant of other therapies (e.g., amphotericin B, lipid formulations of amphotericin B, itraconazole).

The efficacy and safety of CANCIDAS has not been adequately studied in prospective clinical trials involving neonates and infants under 3 months of age. Although limited pharmacokinetic data were collected in neonates and infants below 3 months of age, these data are insufficient to establish a safe and effective dose of caspofungin in the treatment of neonatal candidiasis. Invasive candidiasis in neonates has a higher rate of CNS and multi-organ involvement than in older patients; the ability of CANCIDAS to penetrate the blood-brain barrier and to treat patients with meningitis and endocarditis is unknown.

CANCIDAS has not been studied in pediatric patients with endocarditis, osteomyelitis, and meningitis due to *Candida*. CANCIDAS has also not been studied as initial therapy for invasive aspergillosis in pediatric patients.

In clinical trials, 171 pediatric patients (0 months to 17 years of age), including 18 patients who were less than 3 months of age, were given intravenous CANCIDAS. Pharmacokinetic studies enrolled a total of 66 pediatric patients, and an additional 105 pediatric patients received CANCIDAS in safety and efficacy studies *[see Clinical Pharmacology (12.3) and Clinical Studies (14.5)]*. The majority of the pediatric patients received CANCIDAS at a once-daily maintenance dose of 50 mg/m² for a mean duration of 12 days (median 9, range 1-87 days). In all studies, safety was assessed by the investigator throughout study therapy and for 14 days following cessation of study therapy. The most common adverse reactions in pediatric patients treated with CANCIDAS were pyrexia (29%), blood potassium decreased (15%), diarrhea (14%), increased aspartate aminotransferase (12%), rash (12%), increased alanine aminotransferase (11%), hypotension (11%), and chills (11%) *[see Adverse Reactions (6.2)]*.

Postmarketing hepatobiliary adverse reactions have been reported in pediatric patients with serious underlying medical conditions *[see Warnings and Precautions (5.2)]*.

8.5 Geriatric Use
Clinical studies of CANCIDAS did not include sufficient numbers of patients aged 65 and over to determine whether they respond differently from younger patients. Although the number of elderly patients was not large enough for a statistical analysis, no overall differences in safety or efficacy were observed between these and younger patients. Plasma concentrations of caspofungin in healthy older men and women (≥65 years of age) were increased slightly (approximately 28% in AUC) compared to young healthy men. A similar effect of age on pharmacokinetics was seen in patients with candidemia or other *Candida* infections (intra-abdominal abscesses, peritonitis, or pleural space infections). No dose adjustment is recommended for the elderly; however, greater sensitivity of some older individuals cannot be ruled out.

8.6 Patients with Hepatic Impairment
Adult patients with mild hepatic impairment (Child-Pugh score 5 to 6) do not need a dosage adjustment. For adult patients with moderate hepatic impairment (Child-Pugh score 7 to 9), CANCIDAS 35 mg once daily is recommended based upon pharmacokinetic data *[see Clinical Pharmacology (12.3)]*. However, where recommended, a 70-mg loading dose should still be administered on Day 1 *[see Dosage and Administration (2.4) and Clinical Pharmacology (12.3)]*. There is no clinical experience in adult patients with severe hepatic impairment (Child-Pugh score >9) and in pediatric patients 3 months to 17 years of age with any degree of hepatic impairment.

8.7 Patients with Renal Impairment
No dosage adjustment is necessary for patients with renal impairment. Caspofungin is not dialyzable; thus, supplementary dosing is not required following hemodialysis *[see Clinical Pharmacology (12.3)]*.

10 OVERDOSAGE

In 6 healthy subjects who received a single 210-mg dose, no significant adverse reactions were reported. Multiple doses above 150 mg daily have not been studied. Caspofungin is not dialyzable. The minimum lethal dose of caspofungin in rats was 50 mg/kg, a dose which is equivalent to 10 times the recommended daily dose based on relative body surface area comparison.

In clinical trials, one pediatric patient (16 years of age) unintentionally received a single dose of caspofungin of 113 mg (on Day 1), followed by 80 mg daily for an additional 7 days. No clinically significant adverse reactions were reported.

11 DESCRIPTION

CANCIDAS is a sterile, lyophilized product for intravenous (IV) infusion that contains a semisynthetic lipopeptide (echinocandin) compound synthesized from a fermentation product of *Glarea lozoyensis*. CANCIDAS is an echinocandin that inhibits the synthesis of β (1,3)-D-glucan, an integral component of the fungal cell wall.

CANCIDAS (caspofungin acetate) is 1-[(4R,5S)-5-[(2-aminoethyl)amino]-N^2-(10,12-dimethyl-1-oxotetradecyl)-4-hydroxy-L-ornithine]-5-[(3R)-3-hydroxy-L-ornithine] pneumocandin B_0 diacetate (salt). CANCIDAS 50 mg also contains: 39 mg sucrose, 26 mg mannitol, glacial acetic acid, and sodium hydroxide. CANCIDAS 70 mg also contains 54 mg sucrose, 36 mg mannitol, glacial acetic acid, and sodium hydroxide. Caspofungin acetate is a hygroscopic, white to off-white powder. It is freely soluble in water and methanol, and slightly soluble in ethanol. The pH of a saturated aqueous solution of caspofungin acetate is approximately 6.6. The empirical formula is $C_{52}H_{88}N_{10}O_{15} \cdot 2C_2H_4O_2$ and the formula weight is 1213.42. The structural formula is:

12 CLINICAL PHARMACOLOGY

12.1 Mechanism of Action

Caspofungin is an antifungal drug *[see Clinical Pharmacology (12.4)]*.

12.3 Pharmacokinetics

Adult and pediatric pharmacokinetic parameters are presented in Table 8.

Distribution

Plasma concentrations of caspofungin decline in a polyphasic manner following single 1-hour IV infusions. A short α-phase occurs immediately postinfusion, followed by a β-phase (half-life of 9 to 11 hours) that characterizes much of the profile and exhibits clear log-linear behavior from 6 to 48 hours postdose during which the plasma concentration decreases 10-fold. An additional, longer half-life phase, γ-phase, (half-life of 40-50 hours), also occurs. Distribution, rather than excretion or biotransformation, is the dominant mechanism influencing plasma clearance. Caspofungin is extensively bound to albumin (~97%), and distribution into red blood cells is minimal. Mass balance results showed that approximately 92% of the administered radioactivity was distributed to tissues by 36 to 48 hours after a single 70-mg dose of [³H] caspofungin acetate. There is little excretion or biotransformation of caspofungin during the first 30 hours after administration.

Metabolism

Caspofungin is slowly metabolized by hydrolysis and N-acetylation. Caspofungin also undergoes spontaneous chemical degradation to an open-ring peptide compound, L-747969. At later time points (≥5 days postdose), there is a low level (≤7 picomoles/mg protein, or ≤1.3% of administered dose) of covalent binding of radiolabel in plasma following single-dose administration of [³H] caspofungin acetate, which may be due to two reactive intermediates formed during the chemical degradation of caspofungin to L-747969. Additional metabolism involves hydrolysis into constitutive amino acids and their degradates, including dihydroxyhomotyrosine and N-acetyldihydroxyhomotyrosine. These two tyrosine derivatives are found only in urine, suggesting rapid clearance of these derivatives by the kidneys.

Excretion

Two single-dose radiolabeled pharmacokinetic studies were conducted. In one study, plasma, urine, and feces were collected over 27 days, and in the second study plasma was collected over 6 months. Plasma concentrations of radioactivity and of caspofungin were similar during the first 24 to 48 hours postdose; thereafter drug levels fell more rapidly. In plasma, caspofungin concentrations fell below the limit of quantitation after 6 to 8 days postdose, while radiolabel fell below the limit of quantitation at 22.3 weeks postdose. After single intravenous administration of [³H] caspofungin acetate, excretion of caspofungin and its metabolites in humans was 35% of dose in feces and 41% of dose in urine. A small amount of caspofungin is excreted unchanged in urine (~1.4% of dose). Renal clearance of parent drug is low (~0.15 mL/min) and total clearance of caspofungin is 12 mL/min.

Special Populations

Renal Impairment

In a clinical study of single 70-mg doses, caspofungin pharmacokinetics were similar in healthy adult volunteers with mild renal impairment (creatinine clearance 50 to 80 mL/min) and control subjects. Moderate (creatinine clearance 31 to 49 mL/min), severe (creatinine clearance 5 to 30 mL/min), and end-stage (creatinine clearance <10 mL/min and dialysis dependent) renal impairment moderately increased caspofungin plasma concentrations after single-dose administration (range: 30 to 49% for AUC). However, in adult patients with invasive aspergillosis, candidemia, or other *Candida* infections (intra-abdominal abscesses, peritonitis, or pleural space infections) who received multiple daily doses of CANCIDAS 50 mg, there was no significant effect of mild to end-stage renal impairment on caspofungin concentrations. No dosage adjustment is necessary for patients with renal impairment. Caspofungin is not dialyzable, thus supplementary dosing is not required following hemodialysis.

Hepatic Impairment

Plasma concentrations of caspofungin after a single 70-mg dose in adult patients with mild hepatic impairment (Child-Pugh score 5 to 6) were increased by approximately 55% in AUC compared to healthy control subjects. In a 14-day multiple-dose study (70 mg on Day 1 followed by 50 mg daily thereafter), plasma concentrations in adult patients with mild hepatic impairment were increased modestly (19 to 25% in AUC) on Days 7 and 14 relative to healthy control subjects. No dosage adjustment is recommended for patients with mild hepatic impairment.

Adult patients with moderate hepatic impairment (Child-Pugh score 7 to 9) who received a single 70-mg dose of CANCIDAS had an average plasma caspofungin increase of 76% in AUC compared to control subjects. A dosage reduction is recommended for adult patients with moderate hepatic impairment based upon these pharmacokinetic data *[see Dosage and Administration (2.4)]*.

There is no clinical experience in adult patients with severe hepatic impairment (Child-Pugh score >9) or in pediatric patients with any degree of hepatic impairment.

Gender

Plasma concentrations of caspofungin in healthy adult men and women were similar following a single 70-mg dose. After 13 daily 50-mg doses, caspofungin plasma concentrations in women were elevated slightly (approximately 22% in area under the curve [AUC]) relative to men. No dosage adjustment is necessary based on gender.

Race

Regression analyses of patient pharmacokinetic data indicated that no clinically significant differences in the pharmacokinetics of caspofungin were seen among Caucasians, Blacks, and Hispanics. No dosage adjustment is necessary on the basis of race.

Geriatric Patients

Plasma concentrations of caspofungin in healthy older men and women (≥65 years of age) were increased slightly (approximately 28% AUC) compared to young healthy men after a single 70-mg dose of caspofungin. In patients who were treated empirically or who had candidemia or other *Candida* infections (intra-abdominal abscesses, peritonitis, or pleural space infections), a similar modest effect of age was seen in older patients relative to younger patients. No dosage adjustment is necessary for the elderly *[see Use in Specific Populations (8.5)]*.

Pediatric Patients

CANCIDAS has been studied in five prospective studies involving pediatric patients under 18 years of age, including three pediatric pharmacokinetic studies [initial study in adolescents (12-17 years of age) and children (2-11 years of age) followed by a study in younger patients (3-23 months of age) and then followed by a study in neonates and infants (<3 months)] *[see Use in Specific Populations (8.4)]*. Pharmacokinetic parameters following multiple doses of CANCIDAS in pediatric and adult patients are presented in Table 8.

[See table 8 above]

Drug Interactions [see Drug Interactions (7)]

Studies *in vitro* show that caspofungin acetate is not an inhibitor of any enzyme in the cytochrome P450 (CYP) system. In clinical studies, caspofungin did not induce the CYP3A4 metabolism of other drugs. Caspofungin is not a substrate for P-glycoprotein and is a poor substrate for cytochrome P450 enzymes.

Clinical studies in adult healthy volunteers show that the pharmacokinetics of CANCIDAS are not altered by itraconazole, amphotericin B, mycophenolate, nelfinavir, or tacrolimus. CANCIDAS has no effect on the pharmacokinetics of itraconazole, amphotericin B, or the active metabolite of mycophenolate.

Cyclosporine: In two adult clinical studies, cyclosporine (one 4 mg/kg dose or two 3 mg/kg doses) increased the AUC of caspofungin by approximately 35%. CANCIDAS did not increase the plasma levels of cyclosporine. There were transient increases in liver ALT and AST when CANCIDAS and cyclosporine were co-administered *[see Warnings and Precautions (5.1)]*.

Tacrolimus: CANCIDAS reduced the blood AUC_{0-12} of tacrolimus (FK-506, Prograf) by approximately 20%, peak blood concentration (C_{max}) by 16%, and 12-hour blood concentration (C_{12hr}) by 26% in healthy adult subjects when tacrolimus (2 doses of 0.1 mg/kg 12 hours apart) was administered on the 10th day of CANCIDAS 70 mg daily, as compared to results from a control period in which tacrolimus was administered alone. For patients receiving both therapies, standard monitoring of tacrolimus blood concentrations and appropriate tacrolimus dosage adjustments are recommended.

Rifampin: A drug-drug interaction study with rifampin in adult healthy volunteers has shown a 30% decrease in caspofungin trough concentrations. Adult patients on rifampin should receive 70 mg of CANCIDAS daily.

Other inducers of drug clearance

Adults: In addition, results from regression analyses of adult patient pharmacokinetic data suggest that co-administration of other inducers of drug clearance (efavirenz, nevirapine, phenytoin, dexamethasone, or carbamazepine) with CANCIDAS may result in clinically meaningful reductions in caspofungin concentrations. It is

TABLE 8: Pharmacokinetic Parameters Following Multiple Doses of CANCIDAS in Pediatric (3 months to 17 years) and Adult Patients

Population	N	Daily Dose	AUC_{0-24hr} ($\mu g \cdot hr/mL$)	C_{1hr} ($\mu g/mL$)	C_{24hr} ($\mu g/mL$)	$t_{1/2}$ (hr)*	Cl (mL/min)
PEDIATRIC PATIENTS							
Adolescents, Aged 12-17 years	8	50 mg/m²	124.9 ± 50.4	14.0 ± 6.9	2.4 ± 1.0	11.2 ± 1.7	12.6 ± 5.5
Children, Aged 2-11 years	9	50 mg/m²	120.0 ± 33.4	16.1 ± 4.2	1.7 ± 0.8	8.2 ± 2.4	6.4 ± 2.6
Young Children, Aged 3-23 months	8	50 mg/m²	131.2 ± 17.7	17.6 ± 3.9	1.7 ± 0.7	8.8 ± 2.1	3.2 ± 0.4
ADULT PATIENTS							
Adults with Esophageal Candidiasis	6†	50 mg	87.3 ± 30.0	8.7 ± 2.1	1.7 ± 0.7	13.0 ± 1.9	10.6 ± 3.8
Adults receiving Empirical Therapy	119‡	50 mg§	–	8.0 ± 3.4	1.6 ± 0.7	–	–

* Harmonic Mean ± jackknife standard deviation
† N=5 for C_{1hr} and AUC_{0-24hr}; N=6 for C_{24hr}
‡ N=117 for C_{24hr}; N=119 for C_{1hr}
§ Following an initial 70-mg loading dose on day 1

not known which drug clearance mechanism involved in caspofungin disposition may be inducible. When CANCIDAS is co-administered to adult patients with inducers of drug clearance, such as efavirenz, nevirapine, phenytoin, dexamethasone, or carbamazepine, use of a daily dose of 70 mg of CANCIDAS should be considered.

Pediatric patients: In pediatric patients, results from regression analyses of pharmacokinetic data suggest that co-administration of dexamethasone with CANCIDAS may result in clinically meaningful reductions in caspofungin trough concentrations. This finding may indicate that pediatric patients will have similar reductions with inducers as seen in adults. When CANCIDAS is co-administered to pediatric patients with inducers of drug clearance, such as rifampin, efavirenz, nevirapine, phenytoin, dexamethasone, or carbamazepine, a CANCIDAS dose of 70 mg/m^2 daily (not to exceed an actual daily dose of 70 mg) should be considered.

[3] Registered trademark of Astellas Pharma, Inc.

12.4 Microbiology
Mechanism of Action
Caspofungin an echinocandin, inhibits the synthesis of β (1,3)-D-glucan, an essential component of the cell wall of susceptible *Aspergillus* species and *Candida* species. β (1,3)-D-glucan is not present in mammalian cells. Caspofungin has shown activity against *Candida* species and in regions of active cell growth of the hyphae of *Aspergillus fumigatus*.

Activity in vitro
Caspofungin has been shown to be active **both in vitro and in clinical infections** against most strains of the following microorganisms:
Aspergillus fumigatus
Aspergillus flavus
Aspergillus terreus
Candida albicans
Candida glabrata
Candida guilliermondii
Candida krusei
Candida parapsilosis
Candida tropicalis
Susceptibility Testing Methods [see References (15)]
Aspergillus Species and Other Filamentous fungi
No interpretive criteria have been established for *Aspergillus* species and other filamentous fungi.
Candida Species
The interpretive standards for caspofungin against *Candida* species are applicable only to tests performed using Clinical Laboratory and Standards Institute (CLSI) microbroth dilution reference method M27A for MIC (partial inhibition endpoint) read at 24 hours.
Broth Microdilution Techniques: Quantitative methods are used to determine antifungal minimum inhibitory concentrations (MICs). These MICs provide estimates of the susceptibility of *Candida* spp. to antifungal agents. MICs should be determined using a standardized procedure at 24 hours *[see References (15)]*. Standardized procedures are based on a microdilution method (broth) with standardized inoculum concentrations and standardized concentrations of caspofungin powder. The MIC values should be interpreted according to the criteria provided in Table 9.

TABLE 9: Susceptibility Interpretive Criteria for Caspofungin

Pathogen	Broth Microdilution MIC* (µg/mL) at 24 hours		
	S	I	R
Candida species	≤2	(†)	(†)

* A report of "Susceptible" indicates that the pathogen is likely to be inhibited if the antimicrobial compound in the blood reaches the concentrations usually achievable.
† The current absence of data on caspofungin-resistant isolates precludes defining any categories other than "Susceptible." Isolates yielding test results suggestive of a "Non-Susceptible" category should be retested, and if the result is confirmed, the isolate should be submitted to a reference laboratory for further testing.

Quality Control
Standardized susceptibility test procedures require the use of quality control organisms to control the technical aspects of the test procedures. Standard caspofungin powder should provide the following range of values noted in Table 10.
NOTE: Quality control microorganisms are specific strains of organisms with intrinsic biological properties relating to resistance mechanisms and their genetic expression within fungi; the specific strains used for microbiological control are not clinically significant.

TABLE 11: Favorable Response of Patients with Persistent Fever and Neutropenia

	CANCIDAS*	AmBisome*	% Difference (Confidence Interval)[†]
Number of Patients[‡]	556	539	
Overall Favorable Response	190 (33.9%)	181 (33.7%)	0.2 (-5.6, 6.0)
No documented breakthrough fungal infection	527 (94.8%)	515 (95.5%)	-0.8
Survival 7 days after end of treatment	515 (92.6%)	481 (89.2%)	3.4
No discontinuation due to toxicity or lack of efficacy	499 (89.7%)	461 (85.5%)	4.2
Resolution of fever during neutropenia	229 (41.2%)	223 (41.4%)	-0.2

* CANCIDAS: 70 mg on Day 1, then 50 mg once daily for the remainder of treatment (daily dose increased to 70 mg for 73 patients); AmBisome: 3 mg/kg/day (daily dose increased to 5 mg/kg for 74 patients).
† Overall Response: estimated % difference adjusted for strata and expressed as CANCIDAS – AmBisome (95.2% CI); Individual criteria presented above are not mutually exclusive. The percent difference calculated as CANCIDAS – AmBisome.
‡ Analysis population excluded subjects who did not have fever or neutropenia at study entry.

TABLE 10: Acceptable Quality Control Ranges* for Caspofungin to be used in Validation of Susceptibility Test Results

QC strain	Broth microdilution (MIC in µg/mL) at 24-hour
Candida parapsilosis ATCC[†] 22019	0.25–1.0
Candida krusei ATCC 6258	0.12–1.0

* Quality control ranges have not been established for this strain/antifungal agent combination due to their extensive interlaboratory variation during initial quality control studies.
† ATCC is a registered trademark of the American Type Culture Collection.

Activity in vivo
Caspofungin was active when parenterally administered to immunocompetent and immunosuppressed mice as long as 24 hours after disseminated infections with *C. albicans*, in which the endpoints were prolonged survival of infected mice and reduction of *C. albicans* from target organs. Caspofungin, administered parenterally to immunocompetent and immunosuppressed rodents, as long as 24 hours after disseminated or pulmonary infection with *Aspergillus fumigatus*, has shown prolonged survival, which has not been consistently associated with a reduction in mycological burden.

Drug Resistance
A caspofungin MIC of ≤2 µg/mL (Susceptible) indicates that the *Candida* isolate is likely to be inhibited if caspofungin therapeutic concentrations are achieved; there is insufficient treatment outcome information on isolates with reduced caspofungin susceptibility to define categories other than susceptible. Breakthrough infections with *Candida* isolates requiring caspofungin concentrations >2 µg/mL for growth inhibition have developed in a mouse model of *C. albicans* infection and in some patients with *Candida* infections. Some of these isolates had mutations in the FKS1 gene. The incidence of drug resistance by various clinical isolates of *Candida* and *Aspergillus* species is unknown.

Drug Interactions
Studies *in vitro* and *in vivo* of caspofungin, in combination with amphotericin B, suggest no antagonism of antifungal activity against either *A. fumigatus* or *C. albicans*. The clinical significance of these results is unknown.

13 NONCLINICAL TOXICOLOGY
13.1 Carcinogenesis, Mutagenesis, Impairment of Fertility
No long-term studies in animals have been performed to evaluate the carcinogenic potential of caspofungin.
Caspofungin did not show evidence of mutagenic or genotoxic potential when evaluated in the following *in vitro* assays: bacterial (Ames) and mammalian cell (V79 Chinese hamster lung fibroblasts) mutagenesis assays, the alkaline elution/rat hepatocyte DNA strand break test, and the chromosome aberration assay in Chinese hamster ovary cells. Caspofungin was not genotoxic when assessed in the mouse bone marrow chromosomal test at doses up to 12.5 mg/kg (equivalent to a human dose of 1 mg/kg based on body surface area comparisons), administered intravenously.
Fertility and reproductive performance were not affected by the intravenous administration of caspofungin to rats at doses up to 5 mg/kg. At 5 mg/kg exposures were similar to those seen in patients treated with the 70-mg dose.

13.2 Animal Toxicology and/or Pharmacology
In one 5-week study in monkeys at doses which produced exposures approximately 4 to 6 times those seen in adult patients treated with a 70-mg dose, scattered small foci of subcapsular necrosis were observed microscopically in the livers of some animals (2/8 monkeys at 5 mg/kg and 4/8 monkeys at 8 mg/kg); however, this histopathological finding was not seen in another study of 27 weeks duration at similar doses.
No treatment-related findings were seen in a 5-week study in infant monkeys at doses which produced exposures approximately 3 times those achieved in pediatric patients receiving a maintenance dose of 50 mg/m^2 daily.

14 CLINICAL STUDIES
The results of the adult clinical studies are presented by indications in Section 14.1 to 14.4. Results of pediatric clinical trials are in Section 14.5.
14.1 Empirical Therapy in Febrile, Neutropenic Patients
A double-blind study enrolled 1111 febrile, neutropenic (<500 cells/mm^3) patients who were randomized to treatment with daily doses of CANCIDAS (50 mg/day following a 70-mg loading dose on Day 1) or AmBisome (3 mg/kg/day). Patients were stratified based on risk category (high-risk patients had undergone allogeneic stem cell transplantation or had relapsed acute leukemia) and on receipt of prior antifungal prophylaxis. Twenty-four percent of patients were high risk and 56% had received prior antifungal prophylaxis. Patients who remained febrile or clinically deteriorated following 5 days of therapy could receive 70 mg/day of CANCIDAS or 5 mg/kg/day of AmBisome. Treatment was continued to resolution of neutropenia (but not beyond 28 days unless a fungal infection was documented).
An overall favorable response required meeting each of the following criteria: no documented breakthrough fungal infections up to 7 days after completion of treatment, survival for 7 days after completion of study therapy, no discontinuation of the study drug because of drug-related toxicity or lack of efficacy, resolution of fever during the period of neutropenia, and successful treatment of any documented baseline fungal infection.
Based on the composite response rates, CANCIDAS was as effective as AmBisome in empirical therapy of persistent febrile neutropenia (see Table 11).
[See table 11 above]
The rate of successful treatment of documented baseline infections, a component of the primary endpoint, was not statistically different between treatment groups.
The response rates did not differ between treatment groups based on either of the stratification variables: risk category or prior antifungal prophylaxis.
14.2 Candidemia and the Following other *Candida* Infections: Intra-Abdominal Abscesses, Peritonitis and Pleural Space Infections
In a randomized, double-blind study, patients with a proven diagnosis of invasive candidiasis received daily doses of CANCIDAS (50 mg/day following a 70-mg loading dose on Day 1) or amphotericin B deoxycholate (0.6 to 0.7 mg/kg/day for non-neutropenic patients and 0.7 to 1 mg/kg/day for neutropenic patients). Patients were stratified by both neutropenic status and APACHE II score. Patients with *Candida* endocarditis, meningitis, or osteomyelitis were excluded from this study.
Patients who met the entry criteria and received one or more doses of IV study therapy were included in the modified intention-to-treat [MITT] analysis of response at the end of IV study therapy. A favorable response at this time point required both symptom/sign resolution/improvement and microbiological clearance of the *Candida* infection.
Two hundred thirty-nine patients were enrolled. Patient disposition is shown in Table 12.
[See table 12 at top of next page]
Of the 239 patients enrolled, 224 met the criteria for inclusion in the MITT population (109 treated with CANCIDAS and 115 treated with amphotericin B). Of these 224 patients, 186 patients had candidemia (92 treated with CANCIDAS and 94 treated with amphotericin B). The majority of the patients with candidemia were non-neutropenic (87%) and had an APACHE II score less than or equal to 20 (77%) in both arms. Most candidemia infec-

tions were caused by *C. albicans* (39%), followed by *C. parapsilosis* (20%), *C. tropicalis* (17%), *C. glabrata* (8%), and *C. krusei* (3%).

At the end of IV study therapy, CANCIDAS was comparable to amphotericin B in the treatment of candidemia in the MITT population. For the other efficacy time points (Day 10 of IV study therapy, end of all antifungal therapy, 2-week post-therapy follow-up, and 6- to 8-week post-therapy follow-up), CANCIDAS was as effective as amphotericin B. Outcome, relapse and mortality data are shown in Table 13. [See table 13 below]

In this study, the efficacy of CANCIDAS in patients with intra-abdominal abscesses, peritonitis and pleural space *Candida* infections was evaluated in 19 non-neutropenic patients. Two of these patients had concurrent candidemia. *Candida* was part of a polymicrobial infection that required adjunctive surgical drainage in 11 of these 19 patients. A favorable response was seen in 9 of 9 patients with peritonitis, 3 of 4 with abscesses (liver, parasplenic, and urinary bladder abscesses), 2 of 2 with pleural space infections, 1 of 2 with mixed peritoneal and pleural infection, 1 of 1 with mixed abdominal abscess and peritonitis, and 0 of 1 with *Candida* pneumonia.

Overall, across all sites of infection included in the study, the efficacy of CANCIDAS was comparable to that of amphotericin B for the primary endpoint.

In this study, the efficacy data for CANCIDAS in neutropenic patients with candidemia were limited. In a separate compassionate use study, 4 patients with hepatosplenic candidiasis received prolonged therapy with CANCIDAS following other long-term antifungal therapy; three of these patients had a favorable response.

In a second randomized, double-blind study, 197 patients with proven invasive candidiasis received CANCIDAS 50 mg/day (following a 70-mg loading dose on Day 1) or CANCIDAS 150 mg/day. The diagnostic criteria, evaluation time points, and efficacy endpoints were similar to those employed in the prior study. Patients with *Candida* endocarditis, meningitis, or osteomyelitis were excluded. Although this study was designed to compare the safety of the two doses, it was not large enough to detect differences in rare or unexpected adverse events *[see Adverse Reactions (6.1)]*. A significant improvement in efficacy with the 150-mg daily dose was not seen when compared to the 50-mg dose.

14.3   Esophageal Candidiasis (and information on oropharyngeal candidiasis)

The safety and efficacy of CANCIDAS in the treatment of esophageal candidiasis was evaluated in one large, controlled, noninferiority, clinical trial and two smaller dose-response studies.

In all 3 studies, patients were required to have symptoms and microbiological documentation of esophageal candidiasis; most patients had advanced AIDS (with CD4 counts <50/mm³).

Of the 166 patients in the large study who had culture-confirmed esophageal candidiasis at baseline, 120 had *Candida albicans* and 2 had *Candida tropicalis* as the sole baseline pathogen whereas 44 had mixed baseline cultures containing *C. albicans* and one or more additional *Candida* species.

In the large, randomized, double-blind study comparing CANCIDAS 50 mg/day versus intravenous fluconazole 200 mg/day for the treatment of esophageal candidiasis, patients were treated for an average of 9 days (range 7-21 days). Favorable overall response at 5 to 7 days following discontinuation of study therapy required both complete resolution of symptoms and significant endoscopic improvement. The definition of endoscopic response was based on severity of disease at baseline using a 4-grade scale and required at least a two-grade reduction from baseline endoscopic score or reduction to grade 0 for patients with a baseline score of 2 or less.

The proportion of patients with a favorable overall response was comparable for CANCIDAS and fluconazole as shown in Table 14.
[See table 14 at top of next page]

The proportion of patients with a favorable symptom response was also comparable (90.1% and 89.4% for CANCIDAS and fluconazole, respectively). In addition, the proportion of patients with a favorable endoscopic response was comparable (85.2% and 86.2% for CANCIDAS and fluconazole, respectively).

As shown in Table 15, the esophageal candidiasis relapse rates at the Day 14 post-treatment visit were similar for the two groups. At the Day 28 post-treatment visit, the group treated with CANCIDAS had a numerically higher incidence of relapse; however, the difference was not statistically significant.
[See table 15 on next page]

In this trial, which was designed to establish noninferiority of CANCIDAS to fluconazole for the treatment of esophageal candidiasis, 122 (70%) patients also had oropharyngeal candidiasis. A favorable response was defined as complete resolution of all symptoms of oropharyngeal disease and all visible oropharyngeal lesions. The proportion of patients with a favorable oropharyngeal response at the 5- to 7-day

post-treatment visit was numerically lower for CANCIDAS; however, the difference was not statistically significant. Oropharyngeal candidiasis relapse rates at Day 14 and Day 28 post-treatment visits were statistically significantly higher for CANCIDAS than for fluconazole. The results are shown in Table 16.
[See table 16 on next page]

The results from the two smaller dose-ranging studies corroborate the efficacy of CANCIDAS for esophageal candidiasis that was demonstrated in the larger study.

CANCIDAS was associated with favorable outcomes in 7 of 10 esophageal *C. albicans* infections refractory to at least 200 mg of fluconazole given for 7 days, although the *in vitro* susceptibility of the infecting isolates to fluconazole was not known.

14.4   Invasive Aspergillosis

Sixty-nine patients between the ages of 18 and 80 with invasive aspergillosis were enrolled in an open-label, noncomparative study to evaluate the safety, tolerability, and efficacy of CANCIDAS. Enrolled patients had previously been refractory to or intolerant of other antifungal therapy(ies). Refractory patients were classified as those who had disease progression or failed to improve despite therapy for at least 7 days with amphotericin B, lipid formulations of amphotericin B, itraconazole, or an investigational azole with reported activity against *Aspergillus*. Intolerance to previous

therapy was defined as a doubling of creatinine (or creatinine ≥2.5 mg/dL while on therapy), other acute reactions, or infusion-related toxicity. To be included in the study, patients with pulmonary disease must have had definite (positive tissue histopathology or positive culture from tissue obtained by an invasive procedure) or probable (positive radiographic or computed tomography evidence with supporting culture from bronchoalveolar lavage or sputum, galactomannan enzyme-linked immunosorbent assay, and/or polymerase chain reaction) invasive aspergillosis. Patients with extrapulmonary disease had to have definite invasive aspergillosis. The definitions were modeled after the Mycoses Study Group Criteria *[see References (15)]*. Patients were administered a single 70-mg loading dose of CANCIDAS and subsequently dosed with 50 mg daily. The mean duration of therapy was 33.7 days, with a range of 1 to 162 days.

An independent expert panel evaluated patient data, including diagnosis of invasive aspergillosis, response and tolerability to previous antifungal therapy, treatment course on CANCIDAS, and clinical outcome.

A favorable response was defined as either complete resolution (complete response) or clinically meaningful improvement (partial response) of all signs and symptoms and attributable radiographic findings. Stable, nonprogressive disease was considered to be an unfavorable response.

TABLE 12: Disposition in Candidemia and Other *Candida* Infections (Intra-abdominal abscesses, peritonitis, and pleural space infections)

	CANCIDAS*	Amphotericin B
Randomized patients	114	125
Patients completing study†	63 (55.3%)	69 (55.2%)
DISCONTINUATIONS OF STUDY†		
All Study Discontinuations	51 (44.7%)	56 (44.8%)
Study Discontinuations due to clinical adverse events	39 (34.2%)	43 (34.4%)
Study Discontinuations due to laboratory adverse events	0 (0%)	1 (0.8%)
DISCONTINUATIONS OF STUDY THERAPY		
All Study Therapy Discontinuations	48 (42.1%)	58 (46.4%)
Study Therapy Discontinuations due to clinical adverse events	30 (26.3%)	37 (29.6%)
Study Therapy Discontinuations due to laboratory adverse events	1 (0.9%)	7 (5.6%)
Study Therapy Discontinuations due to all drug-related‡ adverse events	3 (2.6%)	29 (23.2%)

* Patients received CANCIDAS 70 mg on Day 1, then 50 mg once daily for the remainder of their treatment.
† Study defined as study treatment period and 6-8 week follow-up period.
‡ Determined by the investigator to be possibly, probably, or definitely drug-related.

TABLE 13: Outcomes, Relapse, & Mortality in Candidemia and Other *Candida* Infections (Intra-abdominal abscesses, peritonitis, and pleural space infections)

	CANCIDAS*	Amphotericin B	% Difference† after adjusting for strata (Confidence Interval)‡
Number of MITT§ patients	109	115	
FAVORABLE OUTCOMES (MITT) AT THE END OF IV STUDY THERAPY			
All MITT patients	81/109 (74.3%)	78/115 (67.8%)	7.5 (-5.4, 20.3)
Candidemia	67/92 (72.8%)	63/94 (67.0%)	7.0 (-7.0, 21.1)
Neutropenic	6/14 (43%)	5/10 (50%)	
Non-neutropenic	61/78 (78%)	58/84 (69%)	
Endophthalmitis	0/1	2/3	
Multiple Sites	4/5	4/4	
Blood/Pleural	1/1	1/1	
Blood/Peritoneal	1/1	1/1	
Blood/Urine	-	1/1	
Peritoneal/Pleural	1/2	-	
Abdominal/Peritoneal	-	1/1	
Subphrenic/Peritoneal	1/1	-	
DISSEMINATED INFECTIONS, RELAPSES AND MORTALITY			
Disseminated Infections in neutropenic patients	4/14 (28.6%)	3/10 (30.0%)	
All relapses¶	7/81 (8.6%)	8/78 (10.3%)	
Culture-confirmed relapse	5/81 (6%)	2/78 (3%)	
Overall study# mortality in MITT	36/109 (33.0%)	35/115 (30.4%)	
Mortality during study therapy	18/109 (17%)	13/115 (11%)	
Mortality attributed to *Candida*	4/109 (4%)	7/115 (6%)	

* Patients received CANCIDAS 70 mg on Day 1, then 50 mg once daily for the remainder of their treatment.
† Calculated as CANCIDAS – amphotericin B
‡ 95% CI for candidemia, 95.6% for all patients
§ Modified intention-to-treat
¶ Includes all patients who either developed a culture-confirmed recurrence of *Candida* infection or required antifungal therapy for the treatment of a proven or suspected *Candida* infection in the follow-up period.
# Study defined as study treatment period and 6-8 week follow-up period.

TABLE 14: Favorable Response Rates for Patients with Esophageal Candidiasis*

	CANCIDAS	Fluconazole	% Difference[†] (95% CI)
Day 5-7 post-treatment	66/81 (81.5%)	80/94 (85.1%)	-3.6 (-14.7, 7.5)

* Analysis excluded patients without documented esophageal candidiasis or patients not receiving at least 1 day of study therapy.
† Calculated as CANCIDAS – fluconazole

TABLE 15: Relapse Rates at 14 and 28 Days Post-Therapy in Patients with Esophageal Candidiasis at Baseline

	CANCIDAS	Fluconazole	% Difference* (95% CI)
Day 14 post-treatment	7/66 (10.6%)	6/76 (7.9%)	2.7 (-6.9, 12.3)
Day 28 post-treatment	18/64 (28.1%)	12/72 (16.7%)	11.5 (-2.5, 25.4)

* Calculated as CANCIDAS – fluconazole

TABLE 16: Oropharyngeal Candidiasis Response Rates at 5 to 7 Days Post-Therapy and Relapse Rates at 14 and 28 Days Post-Therapy in Patients with Oropharyngeal and Esophageal Candidiasis at Baseline

	CANCIDAS	Fluconazole	% Difference* (95% CI)
Response Rate Day 5-7 post-treatment	40/56 (71.4%)	55/66 (83.3%)	-11.9 (-26.8, 3.0)
Relapse Rate Day 14 post-treatment	17/40 (42.5%)	7/53 (13.2%)	29.3 (11.5, 47.1)
Relapse Rate Day 28 post-treatment	23/39 (59.0%)	18/51 (35.3%)	23.7 (3.4, 43.9)

* Calculated as CANCIDAS – fluconazole

Among the 69 patients enrolled in the study, 63 met entry diagnostic criteria and had outcome data; and of these, 52 patients received treatment for >7 days. Fifty-three (84%) were refractory to previous antifungal therapy and 10 (16%) were intolerant. Forty-five patients had pulmonary disease and 18 had extrapulmonary disease. Underlying conditions were hematologic malignancy (N=24), allogeneic bone marrow transplant or stem cell transplant (N=18), organ transplant (N=8), solid tumor (N=3), or other conditions (N=10). All patients in the study received concomitant therapies for their other underlying conditions. Eighteen patients received tacrolimus and CANCIDAS concomitantly, of whom 8 also received mycophenolate mofetil.

Overall, the expert panel determined that 41% (26/63) of patients receiving at least one dose of CANCIDAS had a favorable response. For those patients who received >7 days of therapy with CANCIDAS, 50% (26/52) had a favorable response. The favorable response rates for patients who were either refractory to or intolerant of previous therapies were 36% (19/53) and 70% (7/10), respectively. The response rates among patients with pulmonary disease and extrapulmonary disease were 47% (21/45) and 28% (5/18), respectively. Among patients with extrapulmonary disease, 2 of 8 patients who also had definite, probable, or possible CNS involvement had a favorable response. Two of these 8 patients had progression of disease and manifested CNS involvement while on therapy.

CANCIDAS is effective for the treatment of invasive aspergillosis in patients who are refractory to or intolerant of itraconazole, amphotericin B, and/or lipid formulations of amphotericin B. However, the efficacy of CANCIDAS for initial treatment of invasive aspergillosis has not been evaluated in comparator-controlled clinical studies.

14.5   Pediatric Patients
The safety and efficacy of CANCIDAS were evaluated in pediatric patients 3 months to 17 years of age in two prospective, multicenter clinical trials.

The first study, which enrolled 82 patients between 2 to 17 years of age, was a randomized, double-blind study comparing CANCIDAS (50 mg/m² IV once daily following a 70-mg/m² loading dose on Day 1 [not to exceed 70 mg daily]) to AmBisome (3 mg/kg IV daily) in a 2:1 treatment fashion (56 on caspofungin, 26 on AmBisome) as empirical therapy in pediatric patients with persistent fever and neutropenia. The study design and criteria for efficacy assessment were similar to the study in adult patients [see Clinical Studies (14.1)]. Patients were stratified based on risk category (high-risk patients had undergone allogeneic stem cell transplantation or had relapsed acute leukemia). Twenty-seven percent of patients in both treatment groups were high risk. Favorable overall response rates of pediatric patients with persistent fever and neutropenia are presented in Table 17.

TABLE 17: Favorable Overall Response Rates of Pediatric Patients with Persistent Fever and Neutropenia

	CANCIDAS	AmBisome*
Number of Patients	56	25
Overall Favorable Response	26/56 (46.4%)	8/25 (32.0%)
High risk	9/15 (60.0%)	0/7 (0.0%)
Low risk	17/41 (41.5%)	8/18 (44.4%)

* One patient excluded from analysis due to no fever at study entry.

The second study was a prospective, open-label, non-comparative study estimating the safety and efficacy of caspofungin in pediatric patients (ages 3 months to 17 years) with candidemia and other Candida infections, esophageal candidiasis, and invasive aspergillosis (as salvage therapy). The study employed diagnostic criteria which were based on established EORTC/MSG criteria of proven or probable infection; these criteria were similar to those criteria employed in the adult studies for these various indications. Similarly, the efficacy time points and endpoints used in this study were similar to those employed in the corresponding adult studies [see Clinical Studies (14.2, 14.3, and 14.4)]. All patients received CANCIDAS at 50 mg/m² IV once daily following a 70-mg/m² loading dose on Day 1 (not to exceed 70 mg daily). Among the 49 enrolled patients who received CANCIDAS, 48 were included in the efficacy analysis (one patient excluded due to not having a baseline Aspergillus or Candida infection). Of these 48 patients, 37 had candidemia or other Candida infections, 10 had invasive aspergillosis, and 1 patient had esophageal candidiasis. Most candidemia and other Candida infections were caused by C. albicans (35%), followed by C. parapsilosis (22%), C. tropicalis (14%), and C. glabrata (11%). The favorable response rate, by indication, at the end of caspofungin therapy was as follows: 30/37 (81%) in candidemia or other Candida infections, 5/10 (50%) in invasive aspergillosis, and 1/1 in esophageal candidiasis.

15   REFERENCES
1. Mosteller RD: Simplified Calculation of Body Surface Area. N Engl J Med 1987 Oct 22;317(17): 1098 (letter).
2. Reference Method for Broth Dilution Antifungal Susceptibility Testing of Filamentous Fungi; Approved Standard M38-A2 Clinical and Laboratory Standards Institute, Wayne, PA, USA.
3. Reference Method for Broth Dilution Antifungal Susceptibility Testing of Yeasts; Approved Standard M27-A3 Clinical and Laboratory Standards Institute, Wayne, PA, USA.
4. Denning DW, Lee JY, Hostetler JS, et al. NIAID Mycoses Study Group multicenter trial of oral itraconazole therapy for invasive aspergillosis. Am J Med 1994; 97: 135-144.

16   HOW SUPPLIED/STORAGE AND HANDLING
How Supplied
CANCIDAS 50 mg is a white to off-white powder/cake for infusion in a vial with a red aluminum band and a plastic cap.
NDC 0006-3822-10 supplied as one single-use vial.
CANCIDAS 70 mg is a white to off-white powder/cake for infusion in a vial with a yellow/orange aluminum band and a plastic cap.
NDC 0006-3823-10 supplied as one single-use vial.
Storage and Handling
Vials
The lyophilized vials should be stored refrigerated at 2° to 8°C (36° to 46°F).
Reconstituted Concentrate
Reconstituted CANCIDAS in the vial may be stored at ≤25°C (≤77°F) for one hour prior to the preparation of the patient infusion solution.
Diluted Product
The final patient infusion solution in the IV bag or bottle can be stored at ≤25°C (≤77°F) for 24 hours or at 2 to 8°C (36 to 46°F) for 48 hours.

17   PATIENT COUNSELING INFORMATION
• Inform patients that there have been isolated reports of serious hepatic effects from CANCIDAS therapy. Physicians will assess the risk/benefit of continuing CANCIDAS therapy if abnormal liver function tests occur during treatment.
• Inform patients that CANCIDAS can cause hypersensitivity reactions, including rash, facial swelling, pruritus, sensation of warmth, or bronchospasm.
Dist. by: Merck Sharp & Dohme Corp., a subsidiary of **MERCK & CO., INC.**, Whitehouse Station, NJ 08889, USA
Issued June 2010
9915001
516198Z 055A-06/10 3822/3823

CIPRO®   ℞
[sĭ'prō]
**(ciprofloxacin hydrochloride)
Tablets**

**CIPRO®
(ciprofloxacin)
Oral Suspension**

> **WARNING:**
> Fluoroquinolones, including CIPRO®, are associated with an increased risk of tendinitis and tendon rupture in all ages. This risk is further increased in older patients usually over 60 years of age, in patients taking corticosteroid drugs, and in patients with kidney, heart or lung transplants (See WARNINGS).

To reduce the development of drug-resistant bacteria and maintain the effectiveness of CIPRO Tablets and CIPRO Oral Suspension and other antibacterial drugs, CIPRO Tablets and CIPRO Oral Suspension should be used only to treat or prevent infections that are proven or strongly suspected to be caused by bacteria.

DESCRIPTION
CIPRO (ciprofloxacin hydrochloride) Tablets and CIPRO (ciprofloxacin*) Oral Suspension are synthetic broad spectrum antimicrobial agents for oral administration. Ciprofloxacin hydrochloride, USP, a fluoroquinolone, is the monohydrochloride monohydrate salt of 1-cyclopropyl-6-fluoro-1, 4-dihydro-4-oxo-7-(1-piperazinyl)-3-quinolinecarboxylic acid. It is a faintly yellowish to light yellow crystalline substance with a molecular weight of 385.8. Its empirical formula is $C_{17}H_{18}FN_3O_3 \cdot HCl \cdot H_2O$ and its chemical structure is as follows:

Ciprofloxacin is 1-cyclopropyl-6-fluoro-1,4-dihydro-4-oxo-7-(1-piperazinyl)-3-quinolinecarboxylic acid. Its empirical formula is $C_{17}H_{18}FN_3O_3$ and its molecular weight is 331.4. It is a faintly yellowish to light yellow crystalline substance and its chemical structure is as follows:

CIPRO film-coated tablets are available in 250 mg, 500 mg and 750 mg (ciprofloxacin equivalent) strengths. Ciprofloxacin tablets are white to slightly yellowish. The inactive ingredients are cornstarch, microcrystalline cellulose, silicon dioxide, crospovidone, magnesium stearate, hypromellose, titanium dioxide, and polyethylene glycol.

Ciprofloxacin Oral Suspension is available in 5% (5 g ciprofloxacin in 100 mL) and 10% (10 g ciprofloxacin in 100 mL) strengths. Ciprofloxacin Oral Suspension is a white to slightly yellowish suspension with strawberry flavor which may contain yellow-orange droplets. It is composed of ciprofloxacin microcapsules and diluent which are mixed prior to dispensing (See Instructions for Use/Handling). The components of the suspension have the following compositions:

Microcapsules - ciprofloxacin, povidone, methacrylic acid copolymer, hypromellose, magnesium stearate, and Polysorbate 20.

Diluent - medium-chain triglycerides, sucrose, lecithin, water, and strawberry flavor.

*Does not comply with USP with regard to "loss on drying" and "residue on ignition".

CLINICAL PHARMACOLOGY

Absorption:

Ciprofloxacin given as an oral tablet is rapidly and well absorbed from the gastrointestinal tract after oral administration. The absolute bioavailability is approximately 70% with no substantial loss by first pass metabolism. Ciprofloxacin maximum serum concentrations and area under the curve are shown in the chart for the 250 mg to 1000 mg dose range.

Dose (mg)	Maximum Serum Concentration (µg/mL)	Area Under Curve (AUC) (µg•hr/mL)
250	1.2	4.8
500	2.4	11.6
750	4.3	20.2
1000	5.4	30.8

Maximum serum concentrations are attained 1 to 2 hours after oral dosing. Mean concentrations 12 hours after dosing with 250, 500, or 750 mg are 0.1, 0.2, and 0.4 µg/mL, respectively. The serum elimination half-life in subjects with normal renal function is approximately 4 hours. Serum concentrations increase proportionately with doses up to 1000 mg. A 500 mg oral dose given every 12 hours has been shown to produce an area under the serum concentration time curve (AUC) equivalent to that produced by an intravenous infusion of 400 mg ciprofloxacin given over 60 minutes every 12 hours. A 750 mg oral dose given every 12 hours has been shown to produce an AUC at steady-state equivalent to that produced by an intravenous infusion of 400 mg given over 60 minutes every 8 hours. A 750 mg oral dose results in a C_{max} similar to that observed with a 400 mg I.V. dose. A 250 mg oral dose given every 12 hours produces an AUC equivalent to that produced by an infusion of 200 mg ciprofloxacin given every 12 hours.

Steady-state Pharmacokinetic Parameters Following Multiple Oral and I.V. Doses

Parameters	500 mg q12h, P.O.	400 mg q12h, I.V.	750 mg q12h, P.O.	400 mg q8h, I.V.
AUC (µg•hr/mL)	13.7[a]	12.7[a]	31.6[b]	32.9[c]
C_{max} (µg/mL)	2.97	4.56	3.59	4.07

[a]AUC_{0-12h}
[b]AUC 24h=$AUC_{0-12h} \times 2$
[c]AUC 24h=$AUC_{0-8h} \times 3$

Distribution:

The binding of ciprofloxacin to serum proteins is 20 to 40% which is not likely to be high enough to cause significant protein binding interactions with other drugs.

After oral administration, ciprofloxacin is widely distributed throughout the body. Tissue concentrations often exceed serum concentrations in both men and women, particularly in genital tissue including the prostate. Ciprofloxacin is present in active form in the saliva, nasal and bronchial secretions, mucosa of the sinuses, sputum, skin blister fluid, lymph, peritoneal fluid, bile, and prostatic secretions. Ciprofloxacin has also been detected in lung, skin, fat, muscle, cartilage, and bone. The drug diffuses into the cerebrospinal fluid (CSF); however, CSF concentrations are generally less than 10% of peak serum concentrations. Low levels of the drug have been detected in the aqueous and vitreous humors of the eye.

Metabolism:

Four metabolites have been identified in human urine which together account for approximately 15% of an oral dose. The metabolites have antimicrobial activity, but are less active than unchanged ciprofloxacin. Ciprofloxacin is an inhibitor of human cytochrome P450 1A2 (CYP1A2) mediated metabolism. Coadministration of ciprofloxacin with other drugs primarily metabolized by CYP1A2 results in increased plasma concentrations of these drugs and could lead to clinically significant adverse events of the coadministered drug (see **CONTRAINDICATIONS; WARNINGS; PRECAUTIONS: Drug Interactions**).

Excretion:

The serum elimination half-life in subjects with normal renal function is approximately 4 hours. Approximately 40 to 50% of an orally administered dose is excreted in the urine as unchanged drug. After a 250 mg oral dose, urine concentrations of ciprofloxacin usually exceed 200 µg/mL during the first two hours and are approximately 30 µg/mL at 8 to 12 hours after dosing. The urinary excretion of ciprofloxacin is virtually complete within 24 hours after dosing. The renal clearance of ciprofloxacin, which is approximately 300 mL/minute, exceeds the normal glomerular filtration rate of 120 mL/minute. Thus, active tubular secretion would seem to play a significant role in its elimination. Coadministration of probenecid with ciprofloxacin results in about a 50% reduction in the ciprofloxacin renal clearance and a 50% increase in its concentration in the systemic circulation. Although bile concentrations of ciprofloxacin are several fold higher than serum concentrations after oral dosing, only a small amount of the dose administered is recovered from the bile as unchanged drug. An additional 1 to 2% of the dose is recovered from the bile in the form of metabolites. Approximately 20 to 35% of an oral dose is recovered from the feces within 5 days after dosing. This may arise from either biliary clearance or transintestinal elimination.

With oral administration, a 500 mg dose, given as 10 mL of the 5% CIPRO Suspension (containing 250 mg ciprofloxacin/5mL) is bioequivalent to the 500 mg tablet. A 10 mL volume of the 5% CIPRO Suspension (containing 250 mg ciprofloxacin/5mL) is bioequivalent to a 5 mL volume of the 10% CIPRO Suspension (containing 500 mg ciprofloxacin/5mL).

Drug-drug Interactions:

When CIPRO Tablet is given concomitantly with food, there is a delay in the absorption of the drug, resulting in peak concentrations that occur closer to 2 hours after dosing rather than 1 hour whereas there is no delay observed when CIPRO Suspension is given with food. The overall absorption of CIPRO Tablet or CIPRO Suspension, however, is not substantially affected. The pharmacokinetics of ciprofloxacin given as the suspension are also not affected by food. Concurrent administration of antacids containing magnesium hydroxide or aluminum hydroxide may reduce the bioavailability of ciprofloxacin by as much as 90%. (See **PRECAUTIONS**.)

The serum concentrations of ciprofloxacin and metronidazole were not altered when these two drugs were given concomitantly.

Concomitant administration with tizanidine is contraindicated. (See **CONTRAINDICATIONS**.) Concomitant administration of ciprofloxacin with theophylline decreases the clearance of theophylline resulting in elevated serum theophylline levels and increased risk of a patient developing CNS or other adverse reactions. Ciprofloxacin also decreases caffeine clearance and inhibits the formation of paraxanthine after caffeine administration. (See **WARNINGS: PRECAUTIONS**.)

Special Populations:

Pharmacokinetic studies of the oral (single dose) and intravenous (single and multiple dose) forms of ciprofloxacin indicate that plasma concentrations of ciprofloxacin are higher in elderly subjects (> 65 years) as compared to young adults. Although the C_{max} is increased 16-40%, the increase in mean AUC is approximately 30%, and can be at least partially attributed to decreased renal clearance in the elderly. Elimination half-life is only slightly (~20%) prolonged in the elderly. These differences are not considered clinically significant. (See **PRECAUTIONS: Geriatric Use**.)

In patients with reduced renal function, the half-life of ciprofloxacin is slightly prolonged. Dosage adjustments may be required. (See **DOSAGE AND ADMINISTRATION**.)

In preliminary studies in patients with stable chronic liver cirrhosis, no significant changes in ciprofloxacin pharmacokinetics have been observed. The kinetics of ciprofloxacin in patients with acute hepatic insufficiency, however, have not been fully elucidated.

Following a single oral dose of 10 mg/kg ciprofloxacin suspension to 16 children ranging in age from 4 months to 7 years, the mean C_{max} was 2.4 µg/mL (range: 1.5–3.4 µg/mL) and the mean AUC was 9.2 µg*h/mL (range: 5.8–14.9 µg*h/mL). There was no apparent age-dependence, and no notable increase in C_{max} or AUC upon multiple dosing (10 mg/kg TID). In children with severe sepsis who were given intravenous ciprofloxacin (10 mg/kg as a 1-hour infusion), the mean C_{max} was 6.1 µg/mL (range: 4.6–8.3 µg/mL) in 10 children less than 1 year of age; and 7.2 µg/mL (range: 4.7–11.8 µg/mL) in 10 children between 1 and 5 years of age. The AUC values were 17.4 µg*h/mL (range: 11.8–32 µg*h/mL) and 16.5 µg*h/mL (range: 11–23.8 µg*h/mL) in the respective age groups. These values are within the range reported for adults at therapeutic doses. Based on population pharmacokinetic analysis of pediatric patients with various infections, the predicted mean half-life in children is approximately 4–5 hours, and the bioavailability of the oral suspension is approximately 60%.

MICROBIOLOGY

Ciprofloxacin has *in vitro* activity against a wide range of gram-negative and gram-positive microorganisms. The bactericidal action of ciprofloxacin results from inhibition of the enzymes topoisomerase II (DNA gyrase) and topoisomerase IV, which are required for bacterial DNA replication, transcription, repair, and recombination. The mechanism of action of fluoroquinolones, including ciprofloxacin, is different from that of penicillins, cephalosporins, aminoglycosides, macrolides, and tetracyclines; therefore, microorganisms resistant to these classes of drugs may be susceptible to ciprofloxacin and other quinolones. There is no known cross-resistance between ciprofloxacin and other classes of antimicrobials. *In vitro* resistance to ciprofloxacin develops slowly by multiple step mutations.

Ciprofloxacin is slightly less active when tested at acidic pH. The inoculum size has little effect when tested *in vitro*. The minimal bactericidal concentration (MBC) generally does not exceed the minimal inhibitory concentration (MIC) by more than a factor of 2.

Ciprofloxacin has been shown to be active against most strains of the following microorganisms, both *in vitro* and in clinical infections as described in the **INDICATIONS AND USAGE** section of the package insert for CIPRO (ciprofloxacin hydrochloride) Tablets and CIPRO (ciprofloxacin*) 5% and 10% Oral Suspension.

Aerobic gram-positive microorganisms

Enterococcus faecalis (Many strains are only moderately susceptible.)
Staphylococcus aureus (methicillin-susceptible strains only)
Staphylococcus epidermidis (methicillin-susceptible strains only)
Staphylococcus saprophyticus
Streptococcus pneumoniae (penicillin-susceptible strains only)
Streptococcus pyogenes

Aerobic gram-negative microorganisms

Campylobacter jejuni	*Proteus mirabilis*
Citrobacter diversus	*Proteus vulgaris*
Citrobacter freundii	*Providencia rettgeri*
Enterobacter cloacae	*Providencia stuartii*
Escherichia coli	*Pseudomonas aeruginosa*
Haemophilus influenzae	*Salmonella typhi*
Haemophilus parainfluenzae	*Serratia marcescens*
Klebsiella pneumoniae	*Shigella boydii*
Moraxella catarrhalis	*Shigella dysenteriae*
Morganella morganii	*Shigella flexneri*
Neisseria gonorrhoeae	*Shigella sonnei*

Ciprofloxacin has been shown to be active against *Bacillus anthracis* both *in vitro* and by use of serum levels as a surrogate marker (see **INDICATIONS AND USAGE** and **INHALATIONAL ANTHRAX - ADDITIONAL INFORMATION**).

The following *in vitro* data are available, **but their clinical significance is unknown.**

Ciprofloxacin exhibits *in vitro* minimum inhibitory concentrations (MICs) of 1 µg/mL or less against most (≥90%) strains of the following microorganisms; however, the safety and effectiveness of ciprofloxacin in treating clinical infections due to these microorganisms have not been established in adequate and well-controlled clinical trials.

Aerobic gram-positive microorganisms

Staphylococcus haemolyticus
Staphylococcus hominis
Streptococcus pneumoniae (penicillin-resistant strains only)

Aerobic gram-negative microorganisms

Acinetobacter lwoffi	*Pasteurella multocida*
Aeromonas hydrophila	*Salmonella enteritidis*
Edwardsiella tarda	*Vibrio cholerae*
Enterobacter aerogenes	*Vibrio parahaemolyticus*
Klebsiella oxytoca	*Vibrio vulnificus*
Legionella pneumophila	*Yersinia enterocolitica*

Most strains of *Burkholderia cepacia* and some strains of *Stenotrophomonas maltophilia* are resistant to ciprofloxacin as are most anaerobic bacteria, including *Bacteroides fragilis* and *Clostridium difficile*.

Susceptibility Tests

Dilution Techniques:
Quantitative methods are used to determine antimicrobial minimum inhibitory concentrations (MICs). These MICs provide estimates of the susceptibility of bacteria to antimicrobial compounds. The MICs should be determined using a standardized procedure. Standardized procedures are based on a dilution method[1] (broth or agar) or equivalent with standardized inoculum concentrations and standardized concentrations of ciprofloxacin powder. The MIC values should be interpreted according to the following criteria:
For testing *Enterobacteriaceae*, *Enterococcus faecalis*, methicillin-susceptible *Staphylococcus* species, penicillin-susceptible *Streptococcus pneumoniae*, *Streptococcus pyogenes*, and *Pseudomonas aeruginosa*[a]:

MIC (μg/mL)	Interpretation	
≤1	Susceptible	(S)
2	Intermediate	(I)
≥4	Resistant	(R)

[a]These interpretive standards are applicable only to broth microdilution susceptibility tests with streptococci using cation-adjusted Mueller-Hinton broth with 2-5% lysed horse blood.

For testing *Haemophilus influenzae* and *Haemophilus parainfluenzae*[b]:

MIC (μg/mL)	Interpretation	
≤1	Susceptible	(S)

[b] This interpretive standard is applicable only to broth microdilution susceptibility tests with *Haemophilus influenzae* and *Haemophilus parainfluenzae* using *Haemophilus* Test Medium[1].

The current absence of data on resistant strains precludes defining any results other than "Susceptible". Strains yielding MIC results suggestive of a "nonsusceptible" category should be submitted to a reference laboratory for further testing.
For testing *Neisseria gonorrhoeae*[c]:

MIC (μg/mL)	Interpretation
≤ 0.06	Susceptible (S)
0.12-0.5	Intermediate (I)
≥1	Resistant (R)

[c] This interpretive standard is applicable only to agar dilution test with GC agar base and 1% defined growth supplement.

A report of "Susceptible" indicates that the pathogen is likely to be inhibited if the antimicrobial compound in the blood reaches the concentrations usually achievable. A report of "Intermediate" indicates that the result should be considered equivocal, and, if the microorganism is not fully susceptible to alternative, clinically feasible drugs, the test should be repeated. This category implies possible clinical applicability in body sites where the drug is physiologically concentrated or in situations where high dosage of drug can be used. This category also provides a buffer zone, which prevents small uncontrolled technical factors from causing major discrepancies in interpretation. A report of "Resistant" indicates that the pathogen is not likely to be inhibited if the antimicrobial compound in the blood reaches the concentrations usually achievable; other therapy should be selected.
Standardized susceptibility test procedures require the use of laboratory control microorganisms to control the technical aspects of the laboratory procedures. Standard ciprofloxacin powder should provide the following MIC values:

Organism		MIC (μg/mL)
E. faecalis	ATCC 29212	0.25-2
E. coli	ATCC 25922	0.004-0.015
H. influenzae[a]	ATCC 49247	0.004-0.03
N. gonorrhoeae[b]	ATCC 49226	0.001-0.008
P. aeruginosa	ATCC 27853	0.25-1
S. aureus	ATCC 29213	0.12-0.5

[a]This quality control range is applicable to only *H. influenzae* ATCC 49247 tested by a broth microdilution procedure using *Haemophilus* Test Medium (HTM)[1].
[b]This quality control range is applicable to only *N. gonorrhoeae* ATCC 49226 tested by an agar dilution procedure using GC agar base and 1% defined growth supplement.

Diffusion Techniques:
Quantitative methods that require measurement of zone diameters also provide reproducible estimates of the susceptibility of bacteria to antimicrobial compounds. One such standardized procedure[2] requires the use of standardized inoculum concentrations. This procedure uses paper disks impregnated with 5-μg ciprofloxacin to test the susceptibility of microorganisms to ciprofloxacin.
Reports from the laboratory providing results of the standard single-disk susceptibility test with a 5-μg ciprofloxacin disk should be interpreted according to the following criteria:
For testing *Enterobacteriaceae*, *Enterococcus faecalis*, methicillin-susceptible *Staphylococcus* species, penicillin-susceptible *Streptococcus pneumoniae*, *Streptococcus pyogenes*, and *Pseudomonas aeruginosa*[a]:

Zone Diameter (mm)	Interpretation	
≥ 21	Susceptible	(S)
16-20	Intermediate	(I)
≤ 15	Resistant	(R)

[a]These zone diameter standards are applicable only to tests performed for streptococci using Mueller-Hinton agar supplemented with 5% sheep blood incubated in 5% CO_2.

For testing *Haemophilus influenzae* and *Haemophilus parainfluenzae*[b]:

Zone Diameter (mm)	Interpretation
≥ 21	Susceptible (S)

[b]This zone diameter standard is applicable only to tests with *Haemophilus influenzae* and *Haemophilus parainfluenzae* using *Haemophilus* Test Medium (HTM)[2].

The current absence of data on resistant strains precludes defining any results other than "Susceptible". Strains yielding zone diameter results suggestive of a "nonsusceptible" category should be submitted to a reference laboratory for further testing.
For testing *Neisseria gonorrhoeae*[c]:

Zone Diameter (mm)	Interpretation
≥ 41	Susceptible (S)
28-40	Intermediate (I)
≤ 27	Resistant (R)

[c]This zone diameter standard is applicable only to disk diffusion tests with GC agar base and 1% defined growth supplement.

Interpretation should be as stated above for results using dilution techniques. Interpretation involves correlation of the diameter obtained in the disk test with the MIC for ciprofloxacin.
As with standardized dilution techniques, diffusion methods require the use of laboratory control microorganisms that are used to control the technical aspects of the laboratory procedures. For the diffusion technique, the 5-μg ciprofloxacin disk should provide the following zone diameters in these laboratory test quality control strains:

Organism		Zone Diameter (mm)
E. coli	ATCC 25922	30-40
H. influenzae[a]	ATCC 49247	34-42
N. gonorrhoeae[b]	ATCC 49226	48-58
P. aeruginosa	ATCC 27853	25-33
S. aureus	ATCC 25923	22-30

[a] These quality control limits are applicable to only *H. influenzae* ATCC 49247 testing using *Haemophilus* Test Medium (HTM)[2].
[b] These quality control limits are applicable only to tests conducted with *N. gonorrhoeae* ATCC 49226 performed by disk diffusion using GC agar base and 1% defined growth supplement.

INDICATIONS AND USAGE

CIPRO is indicated for the treatment of infections caused by susceptible strains of the designated microorganisms in the conditions and patient populations listed below. Please see **DOSAGE AND ADMINISTRATION** for specific recommendations.

Adult Patients:
Urinary Tract Infections caused by *Escherichia coli*, *Klebsiella pneumoniae*, *Enterobacter cloacae*, *Serratia marcescens*, *Proteus mirabilis*, *Providencia rettgeri*, *Morganella morganii*, *Citrobacter diversus*, *Citrobacter freundii*, *Pseudomonas aeruginosa*, methicillin-susceptible *Staphylococcus epidermidis*, *Staphylococcus saprophyticus*, or *Enterococcus faecalis*.
Acute Uncomplicated Cystitis in females caused by *Escherichia coli* or *Staphylococcus saprophyticus*.
Chronic Bacterial Prostatitis caused by *Escherichia coli* or *Proteus mirabilis*.
Lower Respiratory Tract Infections caused by *Escherichia coli*, *Klebsiella pneumoniae*, *Enterobacter cloacae*, *Proteus mirabilis*, *Pseudomonas aeruginosa*, *Haemophilus influenzae*, *Haemophilus parainfluenzae*, or penicillin-susceptible *Streptococcus pneumoniae*. Also, *Moraxella catarrhalis* for the treatment of acute exacerbations of chronic bronchitis.
NOTE: Although effective in clinical trials, ciprofloxacin is not a drug of first choice in the treatment of presumed or confirmed pneumonia secondary to *Streptococcus pneumoniae*.
Acute Sinusitis caused by *Haemophilus influenzae*, penicillin-susceptible *Streptococcus pneumoniae*, or *Moraxella catarrhalis*.
Skin and Skin Structure Infections caused by *Escherichia coli*, *Klebsiella pneumoniae*, *Enterobacter cloacae*, *Proteus mirabilis*, *Proteus vulgaris*, *Providencia stuartii*, *Morganella morganii*, *Citrobacter freundii*, *Pseudomonas aeruginosa*, methicillin-susceptible *Staphylococcus aureus*, methicillin-susceptible *Staphylococcus epidermidis*, or *Streptococcus pyogenes*.
Bone and Joint Infections caused by *Enterobacter cloacae*, *Serratia marcescens*, or *Pseudomonas aeruginosa*.
Complicated Intra-Abdominal Infections (used in combination with metronidazole) caused by *Escherichia coli*, *Pseudomonas aeruginosa*, *Proteus mirabilis*, *Klebsiella pneumoniae*, or *Bacteroides fragilis*.
Infectious Diarrhea caused by *Escherichia coli* (enterotoxigenic strains), *Campylobacter jejuni*, *Shigella boydii*[†], *Shigella dysenteriae*, *Shigella flexneri* or *Shigella sonnei*[†] when antibacterial therapy is indicated.
Typhoid Fever (Enteric Fever) caused by *Salmonella typhi*.
NOTE: The efficacy of ciprofloxacin in the eradication of the chronic typhoid carrier state has not been demonstrated.
Uncomplicated cervical and urethral gonorrhea due to *Neisseria gonorrhoeae*.
Pediatric patients (1 to 17 years of age):
Complicated Urinary Tract Infections and Pyelonephritis due to *Escherichia coli*.
NOTE: Although effective in clinical trials, ciprofloxacin is not a drug of first choice in the pediatric population due to an increased incidence of adverse events compared to controls, including events related to joints and/or surrounding tissues. (See **WARNINGS, PRECAUTIONS, Pediatric Use, ADVERSE REACTIONS** and **CLINICAL STUDIES**.) Ciprofloxacin, like other fluoroquinolones, is associated with arthropathy and histopathological changes in weight-bearing joints of juvenile animals. (See **ANIMAL PHARMACOLOGY**.)
Adult and Pediatric Patients:
Inhalational anthrax (post-exposure): To reduce the incidence or progression of disease following exposure to aerosolized *Bacillus anthracis*.
Ciprofloxacin serum concentrations achieved in humans served as a surrogate endpoint reasonably likely to predict clinical benefit and provided the initial basis for approval of this indication.[4] Supportive clinical information for ciprofloxacin for anthrax post-exposure prophylaxis was obtained during the anthrax bioterror attacks of October 2001. (See also, **INHALATIONAL ANTHRAX – ADDITIONAL INFORMATION**.)
[†]Although treatment of infections due to this organism in this organ system demonstrated a clinically significant outcome, efficacy was studied in fewer than 10 patients.
If anaerobic organisms are suspected of contributing to the infection, appropriate therapy should be administered. Ap-

propriate culture and susceptibility tests should be performed before treatment in order to isolate and identify organisms causing infection and to determine their susceptibility to ciprofloxacin. Therapy with CIPRO may be initiated before results of these tests are known; once results become available appropriate therapy should be continued. As with other drugs, some strains of *Pseudomonas aeruginosa* may develop resistance fairly rapidly during treatment with ciprofloxacin. Culture and susceptibility testing performed periodically during therapy will provide information not only on the therapeutic effect of the antimicrobial agent but also on the possible emergence of bacterial resistance.

To reduce the development of drug-resistant bacteria and maintain the effectiveness of CIPRO Tablets and CIPRO Oral Suspension and other antibacterial drugs, CIPRO Tablets and CIPRO Oral Suspension should be used only to treat or prevent infections that are proven or strongly suspected to be caused by susceptible bacteria. When culture and susceptibility information are available, they should be considered in selecting or modifying antibacterial therapy. In the absence of such data, local epidemiology and susceptibility patterns may contribute to the empiric selection of therapy.

CONTRAINDICATIONS

Ciprofloxacin is contraindicated in persons with a history of hypersensitivity to ciprofloxacin, any member of the quinolone class of antimicrobial agents, or any of the product components.

Concomitant administration with tizanidine is contraindicated. (See **PRECAUTIONS: Drug Interactions.**)

WARNINGS

Tendinopathy and Tendon Rupture:

Fluoroquinolones, including CIPRO, are associated with an increased risk of tendinitis and tendon rupture in all ages. This adverse reaction most frequently involves the Achilles tendon, and rupture of the Achilles tendon may require surgical repair. Tendinitis and tendon rupture in the rotator cuff (the shoulder), the hand, the biceps, the thumb, and other tendon sites have also been reported. The risk of developing fluoroquinolone-associated tendinitis and tendon rupture is further increased in older patients usually over 60 years of age, in patients taking corticosteroid drugs, and in patients with kidney, heart or lung transplants. Factors, in addition to age and corticosteroid use, that may independently increase the risk of tendon rupture include strenuous physical activity, renal failure, and previous tendon disorders such as rheumatoid arthritis. Tendinitis and tendon rupture have also occurred in patients taking fluoroquinolones who do not have the above risk factors. Tendon rupture can occur during or after completion of therapy; cases occurring up to several months after completion of therapy have been reported. CIPRO should be discontinued if the patient experiences pain, swelling, inflammation or rupture of a tendon. Patients should be advised to rest at the first sign of tendinitis or tendon rupture, and to contact their healthcare provider regarding changing to a non-quinolone antimicrobial drug.

Pregnant Women:

THE SAFETY AND EFFECTIVENESS OF CIPROFLOXACIN IN PREGNANT AND LACTATING WOMEN HAVE NOT BEEN ESTABLISHED. (See **PRECUATIONS: Pregnancy** and **Nursing Mothers** subsections.)

Pediatrics:

Ciprofloxacin should be used in pediatric patients (less than 18 years of age) only for infections listed in the **INDICATIONS AND USAGE** section. An increased incidence of adverse events compared to controls, including events related to joints and/or surrounding tissues, has been observed. (See **ADVERSE REACTIONS.**)

In pre-clinical studies, oral administration of ciprofloxacin caused lameness in immature dogs. Histopathological examination of the weight-bearing joints of these dogs revealed permanent lesions of the cartilage. Related quinolone-class drugs also produce erosions of cartilage of weight-bearing joints and other signs of arthropathy in immature animals of various species. (See **ANIMAL PHARMACOLOGY.**)

Cytochrome P450 (CYP450):

Ciprofloxacin is an inhibitor of the hepatic CYP1A2 enzyme pathway. Coadministration of ciprofloxacin and other drugs primarily metabolized by CYP1A2 (e.g. theophylline, methylxanthines, tizanidine) results in increased plasma concentrations of the coadministered drug and could lead to clinically significant pharmacodynamic side effects of the coadministered drug.

Central Nervous System Disorders:

Convulsions, increased intracranial pressure, and toxic psychosis have been reported in patients receiving quinolones, including ciprofloxacin. Ciprofloxacin may also cause central nervous system (CNS) events including: dizziness, confusion, tremors, hallucinations, depression, and, rarely, suicidal thoughts or acts. These reactions may occur following the first dose. If these reactions occur in patients receiving ciprofloxacin, the drug should be discontinued and appropriate measures instituted. As with all quinolones, ciprofloxacin should be used with caution in patients with known or suspected CNS disorders that may predispose to seizures or lower the seizure threshold (e.g. severe cerebral arteriosclerosis, epilepsy), or in the presence of other risk factors that may predispose to seizures or lower the seizure threshold (e.g. certain drug therapy, renal dysfunction). (See **PRECAUTIONS: General, Information for Patients, Drug Interactions** and **ADVERSE REACTIONS.**)

Theophylline:

SERIOUS AND FATAL REACTIONS HAVE BEEN REPORTED IN PATIENTS RECEIVING CONCURRENT ADMINISTRATION OF CIPROFLOXACIN AND THEOPHYLLINE. These reactions have included cardiac arrest, seizure, status epilepticus, and respiratory failure. Although similar serious adverse effects have been reported in patients receiving theophylline alone, the possibility that these reactions may be potentiated by ciprofloxacin cannot be eliminated. If concomitant use cannot be avoided, serum levels of theophylline should be monitored and dosage adjustments made as appropriate.

Hypersensitivity Reactions:

Serious and occasionally fatal hypersensitivity (anaphylactic) reactions, some following the first dose, have been reported in patients receiving quinolone therapy. Some reactions were accompanied by cardiovascular collapse, loss of consciousness, tingling, pharyngeal or facial edema, dyspnea, urticaria, and itching. Only a few patients had a history of hypersensitivity reactions. Serious anaphylactic reactions require immediate emergency treatment with epinephrine. Oxygen, intravenous steroids, and airway management, including intubation, should be administered as indicated.

Other serious and sometimes fatal events, some due to hypersensitivity, and some due to uncertain etiology, have been reported rarely in patients receiving therapy with quinolones, including ciprofloxacin. These events may be severe and generally occur following the administration of multiple doses. Clinical manifestations may include one or more of the following:

- fever, rash, or severe dermatologic reactions (e.g., toxic epidermal necrolysis, Stevens-Johnson syndrome);
- vasculitis; arthralgia; myalgia; serum sickness;
- allergic pneumonitis;
- interstitial nephritis; acute renal insufficiency or failure;
- hepatitis; jaundice; acute hepatic necrosis or failure;
- anemia, including hemolytic and aplastic; thrombocytopenia, including thrombotic thrombocytopenic purpura; leukopenia; agranulocytosis; pancytopenia; and/or other hematologic abnormalities.

The drug should be discontinued immediately at the first appearance of a skin rash, jaundice, or any other sign of hypersensitivity and supportive measures instituted (See **PRECAUTIONS: Information for Patients** and **ADVERSE REACTIONS**).

Pseudomembranous Colitis:

Clostridium difficile associated diarrhea (CDAD) has been reported with use of nearly all antibacterial agents, including CIPRO, and may range in severity from mild diarrhea to fatal colitis. Treatment with antibacterial agents alters the normal flora of the colon leading to overgrowth of *C. difficile*.

C. difficile produces toxins A and B which contribute to the development of CDAD. Hypertoxin producing strains of *C. difficile* cause increased morbidity and mortality, as these infections can be refractory to antimicrobial therapy and may require colectomy. CDAD must be considered in all patients who present with diarrhea following antibiotic use. Careful medical history is necessary since CDAD has been reported to occur over two months after the administration of antibacterial agents.

If CDAD is suspected or confirmed, ongoing antibiotic use not directed against *C. difficile* may need to be discontinued. Appropriate fluid and electrolyte management, protein supplementation, antibiotic treatment of *C. difficile*, and surgical evaluation should be instituted as clinically indicated.

Peripheral neuropathy:

Rare cases of sensory or sensorimotor axonal polyneuropathy affecting small and/or large axons resulting in paresthesias, hypoesthesias, dysesthesias and weakness have been reported in patients receiving quinolones, including ciprofloxacin. Ciprofloxacin should be discontinued if the patient experiences symptoms of neuropathy including pain, burning, tingling, numbness, and/or weakness, or is found to have deficits in light touch, pain, temperature, position sense, vibratory sensation, and/or motor strength in order to prevent the development of an irreversible condition.

Syphilis:

Ciprofloxacin has not been shown to be effective in the treatment of syphilis. Antimicrobial agents used in high dose for short periods of time to treat gonorrhea may mask or delay the symptoms of incubating syphilis. All patients with gonorrhea should have a serologic test for syphilis at the time of diagnosis. Patients treated with ciprofloxacin should have a follow-up serologic test for syphilis after three months.

PRECAUTIONS

General:

Crystals of ciprofloxacin have been observed rarely in the urine of human subjects but more frequently in the urine of laboratory animals, which is usually alkaline. (See **ANIMAL PHARMACOLOGY.**) Crystalluria related to ciprofloxacin has been reported only rarely in humans because human urine is usually acidic. Alkalinity of the urine should be avoided in patients receiving ciprofloxacin. Patients should be well hydrated to prevent the formation of highly concentrated urine.

Central Nervous System:

Quinolones, including ciprofloxacin, may also cause central nervous system (CNS) events, including: nervousness, agitation, insomnia, anxiety, nightmares or paranoia. (See **WARNINGS, Information for Patients,** and **Drug Interactions.**)

Renal Impairment:

Alteration of the dosage regimen is necessary for patients with impairment of renal function. (See **DOSAGE AND ADMINISTRATION.**)

Photosensitivity/Phototoxicity: Moderate to severe photosensitivity/phototoxicity reactions, the latter of which may manifest as exaggerated sunburn reactions (e.g., burning, erythema, exudation, vesicles, blistering, edema) involving areas exposed to light (typically the face, "V" area of the neck, extensor surfaces of the forearms, dorsa of the hands), can be associated with the use of quinolones after sun or UV light exposure. Therefore, excessive exposure to these sources of light should be avoided. Drug therapy should be discontinued if phototoxicity occurs (See **ADVERSE REACTIONS/Post-Marketing Adverse Events**).

As with any potent drug, periodic assessment of organ system functions, including renal, hepatic, and hematopoietic function, is advisable during prolonged therapy.

Prescribing CIPRO Tablets and CIPRO Oral Suspension in the absence of a proven or strongly suspected bacterial infection or a prophylactic indication is unlikely to provide benefit to the patient and increases the risk of the development of drug-resistant bacteria.

Information for Patients:

Patients should be advised:

- to contact their healthcare provider if they experience pain, swelling, or inflammation of a tendon, or weakness or inability to use one of their joints; rest and refrain from exercise; and discontinue CIPRO treatment. The risk of severe tendon disorder with fluoroquinolones is higher in older patients usually over 60 years of age, in patients taking corticosteroid drugs, and in patients with kidney, heart or lung transplants.
- that antibacterial drugs including CIPRO Tablets and CIPRO Oral Suspension should only be used to treat bacterial infections. They do not treat viral infections (e.g., the common cold). When CIPRO Tablets and CIPRO Oral Suspension is prescribed to treat a bacterial infection, patients should be told that although it is common to feel better early in the course of therapy, the medication should be taken exactly as directed. Skipping doses or not completing the full course of therapy may (1) decrease the effectiveness of the immediate treatment and (2) increase the likelihood that bacteria will develop resistance and will not be treatable by CIPRO Tablets and CIPRO Oral Suspension or other antibacterial drugs in the future.
- that ciprofloxacin may be taken with or without meals and to drink fluids liberally. As with other quinolones, concurrent administration of ciprofloxacin with magnesium/aluminum antacids, or sucralfate, Videx® (didanosine) chewable/buffered tablets or pediatric powder, other highly buffered drugs, or with other products containing calcium, iron or zinc should be avoided. Ciprofloxacin may be taken two hours before or six hours after taking these products. Ciprofloxacin should not be taken with dairy products (like milk or yogurt) or calcium-fortified juices alone since absorption of ciprofloxacin may be significantly reduced; however, ciprofloxacin may be taken with a meal that contains these products.
- that ciprofloxacin may be associated with hypersensitivity reactions, even following a single dose, and to discontinue the drug at the first sign of a skin rash or other allergic reaction.
- that photosensitivity/phototoxicity has been reported in patients receiving quinolones. Patients should minimize or avoid exposure to natural or artificial sunlight (tanning beds or UVA/B treatment) while taking quinolones. If patients need to be outdoors while using quinolones, they should wear loose-fitting clothes that protect skin from sun exposure and discuss other sun protection measures with their physician. If a sunburn-like reaction or skin eruption occurs, patients should contact their physician.
- that peripheral neuropathies have been associated with ciprofloxacin use. If symptoms of peripheral neuropathy

including pain, burning, tingling, numbness and/or weakness develop, they should discontinue treatment and contact their physicians.

- that ciprofloxacin may cause dizziness and lightheadedness; therefore, patients should know how they react to this drug before they operate an automobile or machinery or engage in activities requiring mental alertness or coordination.
- that ciprofloxacin increases the effects of tizanidine (Zanaflex®). Patients should not use ciprofloxacin if they are already taking tizanidine.
- that ciprofloxacin may increase the effects of theophylline and caffeine. There is a possibility of caffeine accumulation when products containing caffeine are consumed while taking quinolones.
- that convulsions have been reported in patients receiving quinolones, including ciprofloxacin, and to notify their physician before taking this drug if there is a history of this condition.
- that ciprofloxacin has been associated with an increased rate of adverse events involving joints and surrounding tissue structures (like tendons) in pediatric patients (less than 18 years of age). Parents should inform their child's physician if the child has a history of joint-related problems before taking this drug. Parents of pediatric patients should also notify their child's physician of any joint-related problems that occur during or following ciprofloxacin therapy. (See **WARNINGS, PRECAUTIONS, Pediatric Use** and **ADVERSE REACTIONS**.)
- that diarrhea is a common problem caused by antibiotics which usually ends when the antibiotic is discontinued. Sometimes after starting treatment with antibiotics, patients can develop watery and bloody stools (with or without stomach cramps and fever) even as late as two or more months after having taken the last dose of the antibiotic. If this occurs, patients should contact their physician as soon as possible.

Drug Interactions:

In a pharmacokinetic study, systemic exposure of tizanidine (4 mg single dose) was significantly increased (Cmax 7-fold, AUC 10-fold) when the drug was given concomitantly with ciprofloxacin (500 mg bid for 3 days). The hypotensive and sedative effects of tizanidine were also potentiated. Concomitant administration of tizanidine and ciprofloxacin is contraindicated.

As with some other quinolones, concurrent administration of ciprofloxacin with theophylline may lead to elevated serum concentrations of theophylline and prolongation of its elimination half-life. This may result in increased risk of theophylline-related adverse reactions. (See **WARNINGS**.) If concomitant use cannot be avoided, serum levels of theophylline should be monitored and dosage adjustments made as appropriate.

Some quinolones, including ciprofloxacin, have also been shown to interfere with the metabolism of caffeine. This may lead to reduced clearance of caffeine and a prolongation of its serum half-life.

Concurrent administration of a quinolone, including ciprofloxacin, with multivalent cation-containing products such as magnesium/aluminum antacids, sucralfate, Videx® (didanosine) chewable/buffered tablets or pediatric powder, other highly buffered drugs, or products containing calcium, iron, or zinc may substantially decrease its absorption, resulting in serum and urine levels considerably lower than desired. (See **DOSAGE AND ADMINISTRATION** for concurrent administration of these agents with ciprofloxacin.) Histamine H$_2$-receptor antagonists appear to have no significant effect on the bioavailability of ciprofloxacin.

Altered serum levels of phenytoin (increased and decreased) have been reported in patients receiving concomitant ciprofloxacin.

The concomitant administration of ciprofloxacin with the sulfonylurea glyburide has, on rare occasions, resulted in severe hypoglycemia.

Some quinolones, including ciprofloxacin, have been associated with transient elevations in serum creatinine in patients receiving cyclosporine concomitantly.

Quinolones, including ciprofloxacin, have been reported to enhance the effects of the oral anticoagulant warfarin or its derivatives. When these products are administered concomitantly, prothrombin time or other suitable coagulation tests should be closely monitored.

Probenecid interferes with renal tubular secretion of ciprofloxacin and produces an increase in the level of ciprofloxacin in the serum. This should be considered if patients are receiving both drugs concomitantly.

Renal tubular transport of methotrexate may be inhibited by concomitant administration of ciprofloxacin potentially leading to increased plasma levels of methotrexate. This might increase the risk of methotrexate associated toxic reactions. Therefore, patients under methotrexate therapy should be carefully monitored when concomitant ciprofloxacin therapy is indicated.

Metoclopramide significantly accelerates the absorption of oral ciprofloxacin resulting in shorter time to reach maximum plasma concentrations. No significant effect was observed on the bioavailability of ciprofloxacin.

Non-steroidal anti-inflammatory drugs (but not acetyl salicylic acid) in combination of very high doses of quinolones have been shown to provoke convulsions in pre-clinical studies.

Carcinogenesis, Mutagenesis, Impairment of Fertility:

Eight *in vitro* mutagenicity tests have been conducted with ciprofloxacin, and the test results are listed below:
Salmonella/Microsome Test (Negative)
E. coli DNA Repair Assay (Negative)
Mouse Lymphoma Cell Forward Mutation Assay (Positive)
Chinese Hamster V$_{79}$ Cell HGPRT Test (Negative)
Syrian Hamster Embryo Cell Transformation Assay (Negative)
Saccharomyces cerevisiae Point Mutation Assay (Negative)
Saccharomyces cerevisiae Mitotic Crossover and Gene Conversion Assay (Negative)
Rat Hepatocyte DNA Repair Assay (Positive)
Thus, 2 of the 8 tests were positive, but results of the following 3 *in vivo* test systems gave negative results:
Rat Hepatocyte DNA Repair Assay
Micronucleus Test (Mice)
Dominant Lethal Test (Mice)
Long-term carcinogenicity studies in rats and mice resulted in no carcinogenic or tumorigenic effects due to ciprofloxacin at daily oral dose levels up to 250 and 750 mg/kg to rats and mice, respectively (approximately 1.7- and 2.5-times the highest recommended therapeutic dose based upon mg/m^2). Results from photo co-carcinogenicity testing indicate that ciprofloxacin does not reduce the time to appearance of UV-induced skin tumors as compared to vehicle control. Hairless (Skh-1) mice were exposed to UVA light for 3.5 hours five times every two weeks for up to 78 weeks while concurrently being administered ciprofloxacin. The time to development of the first skin tumors was 50 weeks in mice treated concomitantly with UVA and ciprofloxacin (mouse dose approximately equal to maximum recommended human dose based upon mg/m^2), as opposed to 34 weeks when animals were treated with both UVA and vehicle. The times to development of skin tumors ranged from 16-32 weeks in mice treated concomitantly with UVA and other quinolones.[3]

In this model, mice treated with ciprofloxacin alone did not develop skin or systemic tumors. There are no data from similar models using pigmented mice and/or fully haired mice. The clinical significance of these findings to humans is unknown.

Fertility studies performed in rats at oral doses of ciprofloxacin up to 100 mg/kg (approximately 0.7-times the highest recommended therapeutic dose based upon mg/m^2) revealed no evidence of impairment.

Pregnancy

Teratogenic Effects

Pregnancy Category C:

There are no adequate and well-controlled studies in pregnant women. An expert review of published data on experiences with ciprofloxacin use during pregnancy by TERIS – the Teratogen Information System – concluded that therapeutic doses during pregnancy are unlikely to pose a substantial teratogenic risk (quantity and quality of data=fair), but the data are insufficient to state that there is no risk.[7]

A controlled prospective observational study followed 200 women exposed to fluoroquinolones (52.5% exposed to ciprofloxacin and 68% first trimester exposures) during gestation.[8] In utero exposure to fluoroquinolones during embryogenesis was not associated with increased risk of major malformations. The reported rates of major congenital malformations were 2.2% for the fluoroquinolone group and 2.6% for the control group (background incidence of major malformations is 1-5%). Rates of spontaneous abortions, prematurity and low birth weight did not differ between the groups and there were no clinically significant musculoskeletal dysfunctions up to one year of age in the ciprofloxacin exposed children.

Another prospective follow-up study reported on 549 pregnancies with fluoroquinolone exposure (93% first trimester exposures).[9] There were 70 ciprofloxacin exposures, all within the first trimester. The malformation rates among live-born babies exposed to ciprofloxacin and to fluoroquinolones overall were both within background incidence ranges. No specific patterns of congenital abnormalities were found. The study did not reveal any clear adverse reactions due to in utero exposure to ciprofloxacin.

No differences in the rates of prematurity, spontaneous abortions, or birth weight were seen in women exposed to ciprofloxacin during pregnancy.[7,8] However, these small postmarketing epidemiology studies, of which most experience is from short term, first trimester exposure, are insufficient to evaluate the risk for less common defects or to permit reliable and definitive conclusions regarding the

safety of ciprofloxacin in pregnant women and their developing fetuses. Ciprofloxacin should not be used during pregnancy unless the potential benefit justifies the potential risk to both fetus and mother (see **WARNINGS**).

Reproduction studies have been performed in rats and mice using oral doses up to 100 mg/kg (0.6 and 0.3 times the maximum daily human dose based upon body surface area, respectively) and have revealed no evidence of harm to the fetus due to ciprofloxacin. In rabbits, oral ciprofloxacin dose levels of 30 and 100 mg/kg (approximately 0.4- and 1.3-times the highest recommended therapeutic dose based upon mg/m^2) produced gastrointestinal toxicity resulting in maternal weight loss and an increased incidence of abortion, but no teratogenicity was observed at either dose level. After intravenous administration of doses up to 20 mg/kg (approximately 0.3-times the highest recommended therapeutic dose based upon mg/m^2) no maternal toxicity was produced and no embryotoxicity or teratogenicity was observed. (See **WARNINGS**.)

Nursing Mothers:

Ciprofloxacin is excreted in human milk. The amount of ciprofloxacin absorbed by the nursing infant is unknown. Because of the potential for serious adverse reactions in infants nursing from mothers taking ciprofloxacin, a decision should be made whether to discontinue nursing or to discontinue the drug, taking into account the importance of the drug to the mother.

Pediatric Use:

Ciprofloxacin, like other quinolones, causes arthropathy and histological changes in weight-bearing joints of juvenile animals resulting in lameness. (See **ANIMAL PHARMACOLOGY**.)

Inhalational Anthrax (Post-Exposure)

Ciprofloxacin is indicated in pediatric patients for inhalational anthrax (post-exposure). The risk-benefit assessment indicates that administration of ciprofloxacin to pediatric patients is appropriate. For information regarding pediatric dosing in inhalational anthrax (post-exposure), see **DOSAGE AND ADMINISTRATION** and **INHALATIONAL ANTHRAX – ADDITIONAL INFORMATION**).

Complicated Urinary Tract Infection and Pyelonephritis

Ciprofloxacin is indicated for the treatment of complicated urinary tract infections and pyelonephritis due to *Escherichia coli*. Although effective in clinical trials, ciprofloxacin is not a drug of first choice in the pediatric population due to an increased incidence of adverse events compared to the controls, including events related to joints and/or surrounding tissues. The rates of these events in pediatric patients with complicated urinary tract infection and pyelonephritis within six weeks of follow-up were 9.3% (31/335) versus 6% (21/349) for control agents. The rates of these events occurring at any time up to the one year follow-up were 13.7% (46/335) and 9.5% (33/349), respectively. The rate of all adverse events regardless of drug relationship at six weeks was 41% (138/335) in the ciprofloxacin arm compared to 31% (109/349) in the control arm. (See **ADVERSE REACTIONS** and **CLINICAL STUDIES**.)

Cystic Fibrosis

Short-term safety data from a single trial in pediatric cystic fibrosis patients are available. In a randomized, double-blind clinical trial for the treatment of acute pulmonary exacerbations in cystic fibrosis patients (ages 5-17 years), 67 patients received ciprofloxacin I.V. 10 mg/kg/dose q8h for one week followed by ciprofloxacin tablets 20 mg/kg/dose q12h to complete 10-21 days treatment and 62 patients received the combination of ceftazidime I.V. 50 mg/kg/dose q8h and tobramycin I.V. 3 mg/kg/dose q8h for a total of 10-21 days. Patients less than 5 years of age were not studied. Safety monitoring in the study included periodic range of motion examinations and gait assessments by treatment-blinded examiners. Patients were followed for an average of 23 days after completing treatment (range 0-93 days). This study was not designed to determine long term effects and the safety of repeated exposure to ciprofloxacin.

Musculoskeletal adverse events in patients with cystic fibrosis were reported in 22% of the patients in the ciprofloxacin group and 21% in the comparison group. Decreased range of motion was reported in 12% of the subjects in the ciprofloxacin group and 16% in the comparison group. Arthralgia was reported in 10% of the patients in the ciprofloxacin group and 11% in the comparison group. Other adverse events were similar in nature and frequency between treatment arms. One of sixty-seven patients developed arthritis of the knee nine days after a ten day course of treatment with ciprofloxacin. Clinical symptoms resolved, but an MRI showed knee effusion without other abnormalities eight months after treatment. However, the relationship of this event to the patient's course of ciprofloxacin can not be definitively determined, particularly since patients with cystic fibrosis may develop arthralgias/arthritis as part of their underlying disease process.

Geriatric Use:

Geriatric patients are at increased risk for developing severe tendon disorders including tendon rupture when being treated with a fluoroquinolone such as CIPRO. This risk is further increased in patients receiving concomitant corticosteroid therapy. Tendinitis or tendon rupture can involve the Achilles, hand, shoulder, or other tendon sites and can occur during or after completion of therapy; cases occurring up to several months after fluoroquinolone treatment have been reported. Caution should be used when prescribing CIPRO to elderly patients especially those on corticosteroids. Patients should be informed of this potential side effect and advised to discontinue CIPRO and contact their healthcare provider if any symptoms of tendinitis or tendon rupture occur (See BOXED WARNING, WARNINGS, and ADVERSE REACTIONS/Post-Marketing Adverse Event Reports).

In a retrospective analysis of 23 multiple-dose controlled clinical trials of ciprofloxacin encompassing over 3500 ciprofloxacin treated patients, 25% of patients were greater than or equal to 65 years of age and 10% were greater than or equal to 75 years of age. No overall differences in safety or effectiveness were observed between these subjects and younger subjects, and other reported clinical experience has not identified differences in responses between the elderly and younger patients, but greater sensitivity of some older individuals on any drug therapy cannot be ruled out. Ciprofloxacin is known to be substantially excreted by the kidney, and the risk of adverse reactions may be greater in patients with impaired renal function. No alteration of dosage is necessary for patients greater than 65 years of age with normal renal function. However, since some older individuals experience reduced renal function by virtue of their advanced age, care should be taken in dose selection for elderly patients, and renal function monitoring may be useful in these patients. (See CLINICAL PHARMACOLOGY and DOSAGE AND ADMINISTRATION.)

In general, elderly patients may be more susceptible to drug-associated effects on the QT interval. Therefore, precaution should be taken when using CIPRO with concomitant drugs that can result in prolongation of the QT interval (e.g., class IA or class III antiarrhythmics) or in patients with risk factors for torsade de pointes (e.g., known QT prolongation, uncorrected hypokalemia).

ADVERSE REACTIONS

Adverse Reactions in Adult Patients:

During clinical investigations with oral and parenteral ciprofloxacin, 49,038 patients received courses of the drug. Most of the adverse events reported were described as only mild or moderate in severity, abated soon after the drug was discontinued, and required no treatment. Ciprofloxacin was discontinued because of an adverse event in 1% of orally treated patients.

The most frequently reported drug related events, from clinical trials of all formulations, all dosages, all drug-therapy durations, and for all indications of ciprofloxacin therapy were nausea (2.5%), diarrhea (1.6%), liver function tests abnormal (1.3%), vomiting (1%), and rash (1%).

Additional medically important events that occurred in less than 1% of ciprofloxacin patients are listed below.
BODY AS A WHOLE: headache, abdominal pain/discomfort, foot pain, pain, pain in extremities, injection site reaction (ciprofloxacin intravenous)
CARDIOVASCULAR: palpitation, atrial flutter, ventricular ectopy, syncope, hypertension, angina pectoris, myocardial infarction, cardiopulmonary arrest, cerebral thrombosis, phlebitis, tachycardia, migraine, hypotension
CENTRAL NERVOUS SYSTEM: restlessness, dizziness, lightheadedness, insomnia, nightmares, hallucinations, manic reaction, irritability, tremor, ataxia, convulsive seizures, lethargy, drowsiness, weakness, malaise, anorexia, phobia, depersonalization, depression, paresthesia, abnormal gait, grand mal convulsion
GASTROINTESTINAL: painful oral mucosa, oral candidiasis, dysphagia, intestinal perforation, gastrointestinal bleeding, cholestatic jaundice, hepatitis
HEMIC/LYMPHATIC: lymphadenopathy, petechia
METABOLIC/NUTRITIONAL: amylase increase, lipase increase
MUSCULOSKELETAL: arthralgia or back pain, joint stiffness, achiness, neck or chest pain, flare up of gout
RENAL/UROGENITAL: interstitial nephritis, nephritis, renal failure, polyuria, urinary retention, urethral bleeding, vaginitis, acidosis, breast pain
RESPIRATORY: dyspnea, epistaxis, laryngeal or pulmonary edema, hiccough, hemoptysis, bronchospasm, pulmonary embolism
SKIN/HYPERSENSITIVITY: allergic reaction, pruritus, urticaria, photosensitivity/phototoxicity reaction, flushing, fever, chills, angioedema, edema of the face, neck, lips, conjunctivae or hands, cutaneous candidiasis, hyperpigmentation, erythema nodosum, sweating
SPECIAL SENSES: blurred vision, disturbed vision (change in color perception, overbrightness of lights), decreased visual acuity, diplopia, eye pain, tinnitus, hearing loss, bad taste, chromatopsia

In several instances nausea, vomiting, tremor, irritability, or palpitation were judged by investigators to be related to elevated serum levels of theophylline possibly as a result of drug interaction with ciprofloxacin.

In randomized, double-blind controlled clinical trials comparing ciprofloxacin tablets (500 mg BID) to cefuroxime axetil (250 mg-500 mg BID) and to clarithromycin (500 mg BID) in patients with respiratory tract infections, ciprofloxacin demonstrated a CNS adverse event profile comparable to the control drugs.

Adverse Reactions in Pediatric Patients:

Ciprofloxacin, administered I.V. and/or orally, was compared to a cephalosporin for treatment of complicated urinary tract infections (cUTI) or pyelonephritis in pediatric patients 1 to 17 years of age (mean age of 6 ± 4 years). The trial was conducted in the US, Canada, Argentina, Peru, Costa Rica, Mexico, South Africa, and Germany. The duration of therapy was 10 to 21 days (mean duration of treatment was 11 days with a range of 1 to 88 days). The primary objective of the study was to assess musculoskeletal and neurological safety within 6 weeks of therapy and through one year of follow-up in the 335 ciprofloxacin- and 349 comparator-treated patients enrolled.

An Independent Pediatric Safety Committee (IPSC) reviewed all cases of musculoskeletal adverse events as well as all patients with an abnormal gait or abnormal joint exam (baseline or treatment-emergent). These events were evaluated in a comprehensive fashion and included such conditions as arthralgia, abnormal gait, abnormal joint exam, joint sprains, leg pain, back pain, arthrosis, bone pain, pain, myalgia, arm pain, and decreased range of motion in a joint. The affected joints included: knee, elbow, ankle, hip, wrist, and shoulder. Within 6 weeks of treatment initiation, the rates of these events were 9.3% (31/335) in the ciprofloxacin-treated group versus 6% (21/349) in comparator-treated patients. The majority of these events were mild or moderate in intensity. All musculoskeletal events occurring by 6 weeks resolved (clinical resolution of signs and symptoms), usually within 30 days of end of treatment. Radiological evaluations were not routinely used to confirm resolution of the events. The events occurred more frequently in ciprofloxacin-treated patients than control patients, regardless of whether they received I.V. or oral therapy. Ciprofloxacin-treated patients were more likely to report more than one event and on more than one occasion compared to control patients. These events occurred in all age groups and the rates were consistently higher in the ciprofloxacin group compared to the control group. At the end of 1 year, the rate of these events reported at any time during that period was 13.7% (46/335) in the ciprofloxacin-treated group versus 9.5% (33/349) comparator-treated patients.

An adolescent female discontinued ciprofloxacin for wrist pain that developed during treatment. An MRI performed 4 weeks later showed a tear in the right ulnar fibrocartilage. A diagnosis of overuse syndrome secondary to sports activity was made, but a contribution from ciprofloxacin cannot be excluded. The patient recovered by 4 months without surgical intervention.

Findings Involving Joint or Peri-articular Tissues as Assessed by the IPSC

	Ciprofloxacin	Comparator
All Patients (within 6 weeks)	31/335 (9.3%)	21/349 (6%)
95% Confidence Interval*	(-0.8%, +7.2%)	
Age Group		
≥ 12 months < 24 months	1/36 (2.8%)	0/41
≥ 2 years < 6 years	5/124 (4.0%)	3/118 (2.5%)
≥ 6 years < 12 years	18/143 (12.6%)	12/153 (7.8%)
≥ 12 years to 17 years	7/32 (21.9%)	6/37 (16.2%)
All Patients (within 1 year)	46/335 (13.7%)	33/349 (9.5%)
95% Confidence Interval*	(-0.6%, + 9.1%)	

*The study was designed to demonstrate that the arthropathy rate for the ciprofloxacin group did not exceed that of the control group by more than + 6%. At both the 6 week and 1 year evaluations, the 95% confidence interval indicated that it could not be concluded that ciprofloxacin group had findings comparable to the control group.

The incidence rates of neurological events within 6 weeks of treatment initiation were 3% (9/335) in the ciprofloxacin group versus 2% (7/349) in the comparator group and included dizziness, nervousness, insomnia, and somnolence.

In this trial, the overall incidence rates of adverse events regardless of relationship to study drug and within 6 weeks of treatment initiation were 41% (138/335) in the ciprofloxacin group versus 31% (109/349) in the comparator group. The most frequent events were gastrointestinal: 15% (50/335) of ciprofloxacin patients compared to 9% (31/349) of comparator patients. Serious adverse events were seen in 7.5% (25/335) of ciprofloxacin-treated patients compared to 5.7% (20/349) of control patients. Discontinuation of drug due to an adverse event was observed in 3% (10/335) of ciprofloxacin-treated patients versus 1.4% (5/349) of comparator patients. Other adverse events that occurred in at least 1% of ciprofloxacin patients were diarrhea 4.8%, vomiting 4.8%, abdominal pain 3.3%, accidental injury 3%, rhinitis 3%, dyspepsia 2.7%, nausea 2.7%, fever 2.1%, asthma 1.8% and rash 1.8%.

In addition to the events reported in pediatric patients in clinical trials, it should be expected that events reported in adults during clinical trials or post-marketing experience may also occur in pediatric patients.

Post-Marketing Adverse Event Reports:

The following adverse events have been reported from worldwide marketing experience with quinolones, including ciprofloxacin. Because these events are reported voluntarily from a population of uncertain size, it is not always possible to reliably estimate their frequency or establish a causal relationship to drug exposure. Decisions to include these events in labeling are typically based on one or more of the following factors: (1) seriousness of the event, (2) frequency of the reporting, or (3) strength of causal connection to the drug.

Agitation, agranulocytosis, albuminuria, anaphylactic reactions (including life-threatening anaphylactic shock), anosmia, candiduria, cholesterol elevation (serum), confusion, constipation, delirium, dyspepsia, dysphagia, erythema multiforme, exfoliative dermatitis, fixed eruption, flatulence, glucose elevation (blood), hemolytic anemia, hepatic failure (including fatal cases), hepatic necrosis, hyperesthesia, hypertonia, hypesthesia, hypotension (postural), jaundice, marrow depression (life threatening), methemoglobinemia, moniliasis (oral, gastrointestinal, vaginal), myalgia, myasthenia, myasthenia gravis (possible exacerbation), myoclonus, nystagmus, pancreatitis, pancytopenia (life threatening or fatal outcome), peripheral neuropathy, phenytoin alteration (serum), photosensitivity/phototoxicity reaction, potassium elevation (serum), prothrombin time prolongation or decrease, pseudomembranous colitis (the onset of pseudomembranous colitis symptoms may occur during or after antimicrobial treatment), psychosis (toxic), renal calculi, serum sickness like reaction, Stevens-Johnson syndrome, taste loss, tendinitis, tendon rupture, torsade de pointes, toxic epidermal necrolysis (Lyell's Syndrome), triglyceride elevation (serum), twitching, vaginal candidiasis, and vasculitis. (See PRECAUTIONS.) Adverse events were also reported by persons who received ciprofloxacin for anthrax post-exposure prophylaxis following the anthrax bioterror attacks of October 2001. (See also INHALATIONAL ANTHRAX - ADDITIONAL INFORMATION.)

Adverse Laboratory Changes: Changes in laboratory parameters listed as adverse events without regard to drug relationship are listed below:

Hepatic	– Elevations of ALT (SGPT) (1.9%), AST (SGOT) (1.7%), alkaline phosphatase (0.8%), LDH (0.4%), serum bilirubin (0.3%).
Hematologic	– Eosinophilia (0.6%), leukopenia (0.4%), decreased blood platelets (0.1%), elevated blood platelets (0.1%), pancytopenia (0.1%).
Renal	– Elevations of serum creatinine (1.1%), BUN (0.9%), CRYSTALLURIA, CYLINDRURIA, AND HEMATURIA HAVE BEEN REPORTED.

Other changes occurring in less than 0.1% of courses were: elevation of serum gammaglutamyl transferase, elevation of serum amylase, reduction in blood glucose, elevated uric acid, decrease in hemoglobin, anemia, bleeding diathesis, increase in blood monocytes, leukocytosis.

OVERDOSAGE

In the event of acute overdosage, reversible renal toxicity has been reported in some cases. The stomach should be emptied by inducing vomiting or by gastric lavage. The patient should be carefully observed and given supportive treatment, including monitoring of renal function and administration of magnesium, aluminum, or calcium containing antacids which can reduce the absorption of

ADULT DOSAGE GUIDELINES

Infection	Severity	Dose	Frequency	Usual Durations*
Urinary Tract	Acute Uncomplicated	250 mg	q 12 h	3 days
	Mild/Moderate	250 mg	q 12 h	7 to 14 days
	Severe/Complicated	500 mg	q 12 h	7 to 14 days
Chronic Bacterial Prostatitis	Mild/Moderate	500 mg	q 12 h	28 days
Lower Respiratory Tract	Mild/Moderate	500 mg	q 12 h	7 to 14 days
	Severe/Complicated	750 mg	q 12 h	7 to 14 days
Acute Sinusitis	Mild/Moderate	500 mg	q 12 h	10 days
Skin and	Mild/Moderate	500 mg	q 12 h	7 to 14 days
Skin Structure	Severe/Complicated	750 mg	q 12 h	7 to 14 days
Bone and Joint	Mild/Moderate	500 mg	q 12 h	≥ 4 to 6 weeks
	Severe/Complicated	750 mg	q 12 h	≥ 4 to 6 weeks
Intra-Abdominal[†]	Complicated	500 mg	q 12 h	7 to 14 days
Infectious Diarrhea	Mild/Moderate/Severe	500 mg	q 12 h	5 to 7 days
Typhoid Fever	Mild/Moderate	500 mg	q 12 h	10 days
Urethral and Cervical Gonococcal Infections	Uncomplicated	250 mg	single dose	single dose
Inhalational anthrax (post-exposure)[‡]		500 mg	q 12 h	60 days

* Generally ciprofloxacin should be continued for at least 2 days after the signs and symptoms of infection have disappeared, except for inhalational anthrax (post-exposure).
† used in conjunction with metronidazole
‡ Drug administration should begin as soon as possible after suspected or confirmed exposure.
This indication is based on a surrogate endpoint, ciprofloxacin serum concentrations achieved in humans, reasonably likely to predict clinical benefit[4]. For a discussion of ciprofloxacin serum concentrations in various human population, see **INHALATIONAL ANTHRAX – ADDITIONAL INFORMATION.**

Men: Creatinine clearance (mL/min) $= \dfrac{\text{Weight (kg)} \times (140 - \text{age})}{72 \times \text{serum creatinine (mg/dL)}}$

Women: $0.85 \times$ the value calculated for men.

PEDIATRIC DOSAGE GUIDELINES

Infection	Route of Administration	Dose (mg/kg)	Frequency	Total Duration
Complicated Urinary Tract or Pyelonephritis (patients from 1 to 17 years of age)	Intravenous	6 to 10 mg/kg (maximum 400 mg per dose; not to be exceeded even in patients weighing > 51 kg)	Every 8 hours	10-21 days*
	Oral	10 mg/kg to 20 mg/kg (maximum 750 mg per dose; not to be exceeded even in patients weighing > 51 kg)	Every 12 hours	
Inhalational Anthrax (Post-Exposure)[†]	Intravenous	10 mg/kg (maximum 400 mg per dose)	Every 12 hours	60 days
	Oral	15 mg/kg (maximum 500 mg per dose)	Every 12 hours	

* The total duration of therapy for complicated urinary tract infection and pyelonephritis in the clinical trial was determined by the physician. The mean duration of treatment was 11 days (range 10 to 21 days).
† Drug administration should begin as soon as possible after suspected or confirmed exposure to *Bacillus anthracis* spores. This indication is based on a surrogate endpoint, ciprofloxacin serum concentrations achieved in humans, reasonably likely to predict clinical benefit[4]. For a discussion of ciprofloxacin serum concentrations in various human populations, see INHALATIONAL ANTHRAX – ADDITIONAL INFORMATION.

ciprofloxacin. Adequate hydration must be maintained. Only a small amount of ciprofloxacin (< 10%) is removed from the body after hemodialysis or peritoneal dialysis. Single doses of ciprofloxacin were relatively non-toxic via the oral route of administration in mice, rats, and dogs. No deaths occurred within a 14-day post treatment observation period at the highest oral doses tested; up to 5000 mg/kg in either rodent species, or up to 2500 mg/kg in the dog. Clinical signs observed included hypoactivity and cyanosis in both rodent species and severe vomiting in dogs. In rabbits, significant mortality was seen at doses of ciprofloxacin > 2500 mg/kg. Mortality was delayed in these animals, occurring 10-14 days after dosing.
In mice, rats, rabbits and dogs, significant toxicity including tonic/clonic convulsions was observed at intravenous doses of ciprofloxacin between 125 and 300 mg/kg.

DOSAGE AND ADMINISTRATION - ADULTS

CIPRO Tablets and Oral Suspension should be administered orally to adults as described in the Dosage Guidelines table.

The determination of dosage for any particular patient must take into consideration the severity and nature of the infection, the susceptibility of the causative organism, the integrity of the patient's host-defense mechanisms, and the status of renal function and hepatic function.
The duration of treatment depends upon the severity of infection. The usual duration is 7 to 14 days; however, for severe and complicated infections more prolonged therapy may be required. Ciprofloxacin should be administered at least 2 hours before or 6 hours after magnesium/aluminum antacids, or sucralfate, or Videx® (didanosine) chewable/buffered tablets or pediatric powder for oral solution, other highly buffered drugs, or other products containing calcium, iron or zinc.
[See first table above]
Conversion of I.V. to Oral Dosing in Adults:
Patients whose therapy is started with CIPRO I.V. may be switched to CIPRO Tablets or Oral Suspension when clinically indicated at the discretion of the physician (See **CLINICAL PHARMACOLOGY** and table below for the equivalent dosing regimens).

Equivalent AUC Dosing Regimens

Cipro Oral Dosage	Equivalent Cipro I.V. Dosage
250 mg Tablet q 12 h	200 mg I.V. q 12 h
500 mg Tablet q 12 h	400 mg I.V. q 12 h
750 mg Tablet q 12 h	400 mg I.V. q 8 h

Adults with Impaired Renal Function:
Ciprofloxacin is eliminated primarily by renal excretion; however, the drug is also metabolized and partially cleared through the biliary system of the liver and through the intestine. These alternative pathways of drug elimination appear to compensate for the reduced renal excretion in patients with renal impairment. Nonetheless, some modification of dosage is recommended, particularly for patients with severe renal dysfunction. The following table provides dosage guidelines for use in patients with renal impairment:

RECOMMENDED STARTING AND MAINTENANCE DOSES FOR PATIENTS WITH IMPAIRED RENAL FUNCTION

Creatinine Clearance (mL/min)	Dose
> 50	See Usual Dosage.
30–50	250–500 mg q 12 h
5–29	250–500 mg q 18 h
Patients on hemodialysis or Peritoneal dialysis	250–500 mg q 24 h (after dialysis)

When only the serum creatinine concentration is known, the following formula may be used to estimate creatinine clearance.
[See second table at left]
The serum creatinine should represent a steady state of renal function.
In patients with severe infections and severe renal impairment, a unit dose of 750 mg may be administered at the intervals noted above. Patients should be carefully monitored.

DOSAGE AND ADMINISTRATION - PEDIATRICS

CIPRO Tablets and Oral Suspension should be administered orally as described in the Dosage Guidelines table. An increased incidence of adverse events compared to controls, including events related to joints and/or surrounding tissues, has been observed. (See **ADVERSE REACTIONS** and **CLINICAL STUDIES**.)
Dosing and initial route of therapy (i.e., I.V. or oral) for complicated urinary tract infection or pyelonephritis should be determined by the severity of the infection. In the clinical trial, pediatric patients with moderate to severe infection were initiated on 6 to 10 mg/kg I.V. every 8 hours and allowed to switch to oral therapy (10 to 20 mg/kg every 12 hours), at the discretion of the physician.
[See third table at left]
Pediatric patients with moderate to severe renal insufficiency were excluded from the clinical trial of complicated urinary tract infection and pyelonephritis. No information is available on dosing adjustments necessary for pediatric patients with moderate to severe renal insufficiency (i.e., creatinine clearance of <50 mL/min/1.73m²).

HOW SUPPLIED

CIPRO (ciprofloxacin hydrochloride) Tablets are available as round, slightly yellowish film-coated tablets containing 250 mg ciprofloxacin. The 250 mg tablet is coded with the word "BAYER" on one side and "CIP 250" on the reverse side. CIPRO is also available as capsule shaped, slightly yellowish film-coated tablets containing 500 mg or 750 mg ciprofloxacin. The 500 mg tablet is coded with the word "BAYER" on one side and "CIP 500" on the reverse side. The 750 mg tablet is coded with the word "BAYER" on one side and "CIP 750" on the reverse side. CIPRO 250 mg, 500 mg, and 750 mg are available in bottles of 50, 100, and Unit Dose packages of 100.
[See first table at top of next page]
Store below 30°C (86°F).
CIPRO Oral Suspension is supplied in 5% and 10% strengths. The drug product is composed of two components (microcapsules containing the active ingredient and diluent) which must be mixed by the pharmacist. See Instructions To The Pharmacist For Use/Handling.
[See second table on next page]
Microcapsules and diluent should be stored below 25°C (77°F) and protected from freezing.
Reconstituted product may be stored below 30°C (86°F) for 14 days. Protect from freezing. A teaspoon is provided for the patient.

	Strength	NDC Code	Tablet Identification
Bottles of 50:	750 mg	NDC 0085-1756-01	CIPRO 750
Bottles of 100:	250 mg	NDC 0085-1758-01	CIPRO 250
	500 mg	NDC 0085-1754-01	CIPRO 500
Unit Dose Package of 100:	250 mg	NDC 0085-1758-02	CIPRO 250
	500 mg	NDC 0085-1754-02	CIPRO 500
	750 mg	NDC 0085-1756-02	CIPRO 750

Strengths	Total volume after reconstitution	Ciprofloxacin Concentration	Ciprofloxacin contents per bottle	NDC Code
5%	100 mL	250 mg/5 mL	5,000 mg	0085-1777-01
10%	100 mL	500 mg/5 mL	10,000 mg	0085-1773-01

ANIMAL PHARMACOLOGY

Ciprofloxacin and other quinolones have been shown to cause arthropathy in immature animals of most species tested. (See **WARNINGS**.) Damage of weight bearing joints was observed in juvenile dogs and rats. In young beagles, 100 mg/kg ciprofloxacin, given daily for 4 weeks, caused degenerative articular changes of the knee joint. At 30 mg/kg, the effect on the joint was minimal. In a subsequent study in young beagle dogs, oral ciprofloxacin doses of 30 mg/kg and 90 mg/kg ciprofloxacin (approximately 1.3- and 3.5-times the pediatric dose based upon comparative plasma AUCs) given daily for 2 weeks caused articular changes which were still observed by histopathology after a treatment-free period of 5 months. At 10 mg/kg (approximately 0.6-times the pediatric dose based upon comparative plasma AUCs), no effects on joints were observed. This dose was also not associated with arthrotoxicity after an additional treatment-free period of 5 months. In another study, removal of weight bearing from the joint reduced the lesions but did not totally prevent them.

Crystalluria, sometimes associated with secondary nephropathy, occurs in laboratory animals dosed with ciprofloxacin. This is primarily related to the reduced solubility of ciprofloxacin under alkaline conditions, which predominate in the urine of test animals; in man, crystalluria is rare since human urine is typically acidic. In rhesus monkeys, crystalluria without nephropathy was noted after single oral doses as low as 5 mg/kg (approximately 0.07-times the highest recommended therapeutic dose based upon mg/m^2). After 6 months of intravenous dosing at 10 mg/kg/day, no nephropathological changes were noted; however, nephropathy was observed after dosing at 20 mg/kg/day for the same duration (approximately 0.2-times the highest recommended therapeutic dose based upon mg/m^2).

In dogs, ciprofloxacin at 3 and 10 mg/kg by rapid I.V. injection (15 sec.) produces pronounced hypotensive effects. These effects are considered to be related to histamine release, since they are partially antagonized by pyrilamine, an antihistamine. In rhesus monkeys, rapid I.V. injection also produces hypotension but the effect in this species is inconsistent and less pronounced.

In mice, concomitant administration of nonsteroidal anti-inflammatory drugs such as phenylbutazone and indomethacin with quinolones has been reported to enhance the CNS stimulatory effect of quinolones.

Ocular toxicity seen with some related drugs has not been observed in ciprofloxacin-treated animals.

CLINICAL STUDIES

Complicated Urinary Tract Infection and Pyelonephritis – Efficacy in Pediatric Patients:

NOTE: Although effective in clinical trials, ciprofloxacin is not a drug of first choice in the pediatric population due to an increased incidence of adverse events compared to controls, including events related to joints and/or surrounding tissues.

Ciprofloxacin, administered I.V. and/or orally, was compared to a cephalosporin for treatment of complicated urinary tract infections (cUTI) and pyelonephritis in pediatric patients 1 to 17 years of age (mean age of 6 ± 4 years). The trial was conducted in the US, Canada, Argentina, Peru, Costa Rica, Mexico, South Africa, and Germany. The duration of therapy was 10 to 21 days (mean duration of treatment was 11 days with a range of 1 to 88 days). The primary objective of the study was to assess musculoskeletal and neurological safety.

Patients were evaluated for clinical success and bacteriological eradication of the baseline organism(s) with no new infection or superinfection at 5 to 9 days post-therapy (Test of Cure or TOC). The Per Protocol population had a causative organism(s) with protocol specified colony count(s) at baseline, no protocol violation, and no premature discontinuation or loss to follow-up (among other criteria).

The clinical success and bacteriologic eradication rates in the Per Protocol population were similar between ciprofloxacin and the comparator group as shown below.

Clinical Success and Bacteriologic Eradication at Test of Cure (5 to 9 Days Post-Therapy)

	CIPRO	Comparator
Randomized Patients	337	352
Per Protocol Patients	211	231
Clinical Response at 5 to 9 Days Post-Treatment	95.7% (202/211)	92.6% (214/231)
	95% CI [-1.3%, 7.3%]	
Bacteriologic Eradication by Patient at 5 to 9 Days Post-Treatment*	84.4% (178/211)	78.3% (181/231)
	95% CI [-1.3%, 13.1%]	
Bacteriologic Eradication of the Baseline Pathogen at 5 to 9 Days Post-Treatment		
Escherichia coli	156/178 (88%)	161/179 (90%)

*Patients with baseline pathogen(s) eradicated and no new infections or superinfections/total number of patients. There were 5.5% (6/211) ciprofloxacin and 9.5% (22/231) comparator patients with superinfections or new infections.

INHALATIONAL ANTHRAX IN ADULTS AND PEDIATRICS – ADDITIONAL INFORMATION

The mean serum concentrations of ciprofloxacin associated with a statistically significant improvement in survival in the rhesus monkey model of inhalational anthrax are reached or exceeded in adult and pediatric patients receiving oral and intravenous regimens. (See **DOSAGE AND ADMINISTRATION**.) Ciprofloxacin pharmacokinetics have been evaluated in various human populations. The mean peak serum concentration achieved at steady-state in human adults receiving 500 mg orally every 12 hours is 2.97 µg/mL, and 4.56 µg/mL following 400 mg intravenously every 12 hours. The mean trough serum concentration at steady-state for both of these regimens is 0.2 µg/mL. In a study of 10 pediatric patients between 6 and 16 years of age, the mean peak plasma concentration achieved is 8.3 µg/mL and trough concentrations range from 0.09 to 0.26 µg/mL, following two 30-minute intravenous infusions of 10 mg/kg administered 12 hours apart. After the second intravenous infusion patients switched to 15 mg/kg orally every 12 hours achieve a mean peak concentration of 3.6 µg/mL after the initial oral dose. Long-term safety data, including effects on cartilage, following the administration of ciprofloxacin to pediatric patients are limited. (For additional information, see **PRECAUTIONS, Pediatric Use**.) Ciprofloxacin serum concentrations achieved in humans serve as a surrogate endpoint reasonably likely to predict clinical benefit and provide the basis for this indication.[4]

A placebo-controlled animal study in rhesus monkeys exposed to an inhaled mean dose of 11 LD$_{50}$ ($\sim$5.5 × 10^5 spores (range 5-30 LD$_{50}$) of *B. anthracis* was conducted. The minimal inhibitory concentration (MIC) of ciprofloxacin for the anthrax strain used in this study was 0.08 µg/mL. In the animals studied, mean serum concentrations of ciprofloxacin achieved at expected T$_{max}$ (1 hour post-dose) following oral dosing to steady-state ranged from 0.98 to 1.69 µg/mL. Mean steady-state trough concentrations at 12 hours post-dose ranged from 0.12 to 0.19 µg/mL[5]. Mortality due to anthrax for animals that received a 30-day regimen

of oral ciprofloxacin beginning 24 hours post-exposure was significantly lower (1/9), compared to the placebo group (9/10) [p= 0.001]. The one ciprofloxacin-treated animal that died of anthrax did so following the 30-day drug administration period.[6]

More than 9300 persons were recommended to complete a minimum of 60 days of antibiotic prophylaxis against possible inhalational exposure to *B. anthracis* during 2001. Ciprofloxacin was recommended to most of those individuals for all or part of the prophylaxis regimen. Some persons were also given anthrax vaccine or were switched to alternative antibiotics. No one who received ciprofloxacin or other therapies as prophylactic treatment subsequently developed inhalational anthrax. The number of persons who received ciprofloxacin as all or part of their post-exposure prophylaxis regimen is unknown.

Among the persons surveyed by the Centers for Disease Control and Prevention, over 1000 reported receiving ciprofloxacin as sole post-exposure prophylaxis for inhalational anthrax. Gastrointestinal adverse events (nausea, vomiting, diarrhea, or stomach pain), neurological adverse events (problems sleeping, nightmares, headache, dizziness or lightheadedness) and musculoskeletal adverse events (muscle or tendon pain and joint swelling or pain) were more frequent than had been previously reported in controlled clinical trials. This higher incidence, in the absence of a control group, could be explained by a reporting bias, concurrent medical conditions, other concomitant medications, emotional stress or other confounding factors, and/or a longer treatment period with ciprofloxacin. Because of these factors and limitations in the data collection, it is difficult to evaluate whether the reported symptoms were drug-related.

Instructions To The Pharmacist For Use/Handling Of CIPRO Oral Suspension:

CIPRO Oral Suspension is supplied in 5% (5 g ciprofloxacin in 100 mL) and 10% (10 g ciprofloxacin in 100 mL) strengths. The drug product is composed of two components (microcapsules and diluent) which must be combined prior to dispensing.

One teaspoonful (5 mL) of 5% ciprofloxacin oral suspension = 250 mg of ciprofloxacin.

One teaspoonful (5 mL) of 10% ciprofloxacin oral suspension = 500 mg of ciprofloxacin.

Appropriate Dosing Volumes of the Oral Suspensions:

Dose	5%	10%
250 mg	5 mL	2.5 mL
500 mg	10 mL	5 mL
750 mg	15 mL	7.5 mL

Preparation of the suspension:

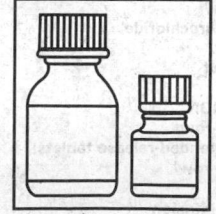

1. The small bottle contains the microcapsules, the large bottle contains the diluent.

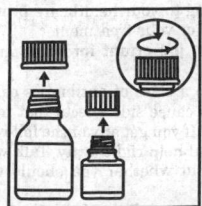

2. Open both bottles. Child-proof cap: Press down according to instructions on the cap while turning to the left.

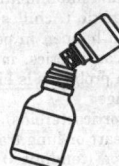

3. Pour the microcapsules completely into the larger bottle of diluent. Do not add water to the suspension.

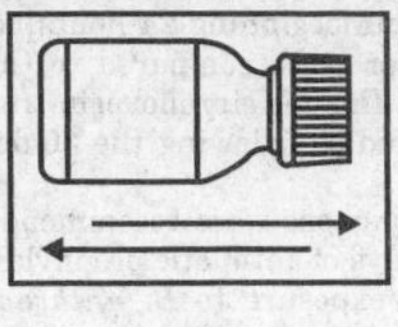

4. Remove the top layer of the diluent bottle label (to reveal the CIPRO Oral Suspension label). Close the large bottle completely according to the directions on the cap and shake vigorously for about 15 seconds. The suspension is ready for use.

CIPRO Oral Suspension should not be administered through feeding tubes due to its physical characteristics. Instruct the patient to shake CIPRO Oral Suspension vigorously each time before use for approximately 15 seconds and not to chew the microcapsules.

REFERENCES

1. National Committee for Clinical Laboratory Standards, Methods for Dilution Antimicrobial Susceptibility Tests for Bacteria That Grow Aerobically-Fifth Edition. Approved Standard NCCLS Document M7-A5, Vol. 20, No. 2, NCCLS, Wayne, PA, January, 2000.
2. National Committee for Clinical Laboratory Standards, Performance Standards for Antimicrobial Disk Susceptibility Tests-Seventh Edition. Approved Standard NCCLS Document M2-A7, Vol. 20, No. 1, NCCLS, Wayne, PA, January, 2000.
3. Report presented at the FDA's Anti-Infective Drug and Dermatological Drug Product's Advisory Committee meeting, March 31, 1993, Silver Spring, MD. Report available from FDA, CDER, Advisors and Consultants Staff, HFD-21, 1901 Chapman Avenue, Room 200, Rockville, MD 20852, USA.
4. 21 CFR 314.510 (Subpart H – Accelerated Approval of New Drugs for Life-Threatening Illnesses).
5. Kelly DJ, et al. Serum concentrations of penicillin, doxycycline, and ciprofloxacin during prolonged therapy in rhesus monkeys. J Infect Dis 1992; 166:1184-7.
6. Friedlander AM, et al. Postexposure prophylaxis against experimental inhalational anthrax. J Infect Dis 1993; 167:1239-42.
7. Friedman J, Polifka J. Teratogenic effects of drugs: a resource for clinicians (TERIS). Baltimore, Maryland: Johns Hopkins University Press, 2000:149-195.
8. Loebstein R, Addis A, Ho E, et al. Pregnancy outcome following gestational exposure to fluoroquinolones: a multicenter prospective controlled study. Antimicrob Agents Chemother. 1998;42(6):1336-1339.
9. Schaefer C, Amoura-Elefant E, Vial T, et al. Pregnancy outcome after prenatal quinolone exposure. Evaluation of a case registry of the European network of teratology information services (ENTIS). Eur J Obstet Gynecol Reprod Biol. 1996;69:83-89.

MEDICATION GUIDE

CIPRO® *(Sip-row)*
(ciprofloxacin hydrochloride)
TABLETS
CIPRO® *(Sip-row)*
(ciprofloxacin)
ORAL SUSPENSION
CIPRO® XR *(Sip-row)*
(ciprofloxacin extended-release tablets)
CIPRO® I.V. *(Sip-row)*
(ciprofloxacin)
For Intravenous Infusion

Read the Medication Guide that comes with CIPRO® before you start taking it and each time you get a refill. There may be new information. This Medication Guide does not take the place of talking to your healthcare provider about your medical condition or your treatment.

What is the most important information I should know about CIPRO?

CIPRO belongs to a class of antibiotics called fluoroquinolones. CIPRO can cause side effects that may be serious or even cause death. If you get any of the following serious side effects, get medical help right away. Talk with your healthcare provider about whether you should continue to take CIPRO.

- **Tendon rupture or swelling of the tendon (tendinitis)**
- Tendons are tough cords of tissue that connect muscles to bones.
- Pain, swelling, tears and inflammation of tendons including the back of the ankle (Achilles), shoulder, hand, or other tendon sites can happen in people of all ages who take fluoroquinolone antibiotics, including CIPRO. The risk of getting tendon problems is higher if you:
- are over 60 years of age
- are taking steroids (corticosteroids)
- have had a kidney, heart or lung transplant
- Swelling of the tendon (tendinitis) and tendon rupture (breakage) have also happened in patients who take fluoroquinolones who do not have the above risk factors.
- Other reasons for tendon ruptures can include:
- physical activity or exercise
- kidney failure
- tendon problems in the past, such as in people with rheumatoid arthritis (RA)
- Call your healthcare provider right away at the first sign of tendon pain, swelling or inflammation. Stop taking CIPRO until tendinitis or tendon rupture has been ruled out by your healthcare provider. Avoid exercise and using the affected area. The most common area of pain and swelling is the Achilles tendon at the back of your ankle. This can also happen with other tendons. Talk to your healthcare provider about the risk of tendon rupture with continued use of CIPRO. You may need a different antibiotic that is not a fluoroquinolone to treat your infection.
- Tendon rupture can happen while you are taking or after you have finished taking CIPRO. Tendon ruptures have happened up to several months after patients have finished taking their fluoroquinolone.
- Get medical help right away if you get any of the following signs or symptoms of a tendon rupture:
- hear or feel a snap or pop in a tendon area
- bruising right after an injury in a tendon area
- unable to move the affected area or bear weight
- See the section **"What are the possible side effects of CIPRO?"** for more information about side effects.

What is CIPRO?

CIPRO is a fluoroquinolone antibiotic medicine used to treat certain infections caused by certain germs called bacteria. Children less than 18 years of age have a higher chance of getting bone, joint, or tendon (musculoskeletal) problems such as pain or swelling while taking CIPRO. CIPRO should not be used as the first choice of antibiotic medicine in children under 18 years of age.

CIPRO Tablets, CIPRO Oral Suspension and CIPRO I.V. should not be used in children under 18 years old, except to treat specific serious infections, such as complicated urinary tract infections and to prevent anthrax disease after breathing the anthrax bacteria germ (inhalational exposure). It is not known if CIPRO XR is safe and works in children under 18 years of age.

Sometimes infections are caused by viruses rather than by bacteria. Examples include viral infections in the sinuses and lungs, such as the common cold or flu. Antibiotics, including CIPRO, do not kill viruses.

Call your healthcare provider if you think your condition is not getting better while you are taking CIPRO.

Who should not take CIPRO?

Do not take CIPRO if you:

- have ever had a severe allergic reaction to an antibiotic known as a fluoroquinolone, or are allergic to any of the ingredients in CIPRO. Ask your healthcare provider if you are not sure. See the list of ingredients in CIPRO at the end of this Medication Guide.
- also take a medicine called tizanidine (Zanaflex®). Serious side effects from tizanidine are likely to happen.

What should I tell my healthcare provider before taking CIPRO?

See **"What is the most important information I should know about CIPRO?"**

Tell your healthcare provider about all your medical conditions, including if you:

- have tendon problems
- have central nervous system problems (such as epilepsy)
- have nerve problems
- have or anyone in your family has an irregular heartbeat, especially a condition called "QT prolongation"
- have a history of seizures
- have kidney problems. You may need a lower dose of CIPRO if your kidneys do not work well.
- have rheumatoid arthritis (RA) or other history of joint problems
- have trouble swallowing pills
- are pregnant or planning to become pregnant. It is not known if CIPRO will harm your unborn child.
- are breast-feeding or planning to breast-feed. CIPRO passes into breast milk. You and your healthcare provider should decide whether you will take CIPRO or breast-feed.

Tell your healthcare provider about all the medicines you take, including prescription and non-prescription medicines, vitamins and herbal and dietary supplements. CIPRO and other medicines can affect each other causing side effects. Especially tell your healthcare provider if you take:

- an NSAID (Non-Steroidal Anti-Inflammatory Drug). Many common medicines for pain relief are NSAIDs. Taking an NSAID while you take CIPRO or other fluoroquinolones may increase your risk of central nervous system effects and seizures. See **"What are the possible side effects of CIPRO?"**.
- a blood thinner (warfarin, Coumadin®, Jantoven®)
- tizanidine (Zanaflex®). You should not take CIPRO if you are already taking tizanidine. See **"Who should not take CIPRO?"**
- theophylline (Theo-24®, Elixophyllin®, Theochron®, Uniphyl®, Theolair®)
- glyburide (Micronase®, Glynase®, Diabeta®, Glucovance®). See **"What are the possible side effects of CIPRO?"**
- phenytoin (Fosphenytoin Sodium®, Cerebyx®, Dilantin-125®, Dilantin®, Extended Phenytoin Sodium®, Prompt Penytoin Sodium®, Phenytek®)
- products that contain caffeine
- a medicine to control your heart rate or rhythm (antiarrhythmics) See **"What are the possible side effects of CIPRO?"**
- an anti-psychotic medicine
- a tricyclic antidepressant
- a water pill (diuretic)
- a steroid medicine. Corticosteroids taken by mouth or by injection may increase the chance of tendon injury. See **"What is the most important information I should know about CIPRO?"**
- methotrexate (Trexall®)
- Probenecid (Probalan®, Col-probenecid®)
- Metoclopromide (Reglan®, Reglan ODT®)
- Certain medicines may keep CIPRO Tablets, CIPRO Oral Suspension from working correctly. Take CIPRO Tablets and Oral Suspension either 2 hours before or 6 hours after taking these products:
- an antacid, multivitamin, or other product that has magnesium, calcium, aluminum, iron, or zinc
- sucralfate (Carafate®)
- didanosine (Videx®, Videx EC®)

Ask your healthcare provider if you are not sure if any of your medicines are listed above.

Know the medicines you take. Keep a list of your medicines and show it to your healthcare provider and pharmacist when you get a new medicine.

How should I take CIPRO?

- Take CIPRO exactly as prescribed by your healthcare provider.
- Take CIPRO Tablets in the morning and evening at about the same time each day. Swallow the tablet whole. Do not split, crush or chew the tablet. Tell your healthcare provider if you can not swallow the tablet whole.
- Take CIPRO Oral Suspension in the morning and evening at about the same time each day. Shake the CIPRO Oral Suspension bottle well each time before use for about 15 seconds to make sure the suspension is mixed well. Close the bottle completely after use.
- Take CIPRO XR one time each day at about the same time each day. Swallow the tablet whole. Do not split, crush or chew the tablet. Tell your healthcare provider if you can not swallow the tablet whole.
- CIPRO I.V. is given to you by intravenous (I.V.) infusion into your vein, slowly, over 60 minutes, as prescribed by your healthcare provider.
- CIPRO can be taken with or without food.
- CIPRO should not be taken with dairy products (like milk or yogurt) or calcium-fortified juices alone, but may be taken with a meal that contains these products.
- Drink plenty of fluids while taking CIPRO.
- Do not skip any doses, or stop taking CIPRO even if you begin to feel better, until you finish your prescribed treatment, unless:
- you have tendon effects (see **"What is the most important information I should know about CIPRO?"**),
- you have a serious allergic reaction (see **"What are the possible side effects of CIPRO?"**), or
- your healthcare provider tells you to stop.
- This will help make sure that all of the bacteria are killed and lower the chance that the bacteria will become resistant to CIPRO. If this happens, CIPRO and other antibiotic medicines may not work in the future.
- If you miss a dose of CIPRO Tablets or Oral Suspension, take it as soon as you remember. Do not take two doses at the same time, and do not take more than two doses in one day.
- If you miss a dose of CIPRO XR, take it as soon as you remember. Do not take more than one dose in one day.
- If you take too much, call your healthcare provider or get medical help immediately.

If you have been prescribed CIPRO Tablets, CIPRO Oral Suspension or CIPRO I.V. after being exposed to anthrax:

- CIPRO Tablets, Oral Suspension and I.V. has been approved to lessen the chance of getting anthrax disease or worsening of the disease after you are exposed to the anthrax bacteria germ.
- Take CIPRO exactly as prescribed by your healthcare provider. Do not stop taking CIPRO without talking with your healthcare provider. If you stop taking CIPRO too soon, it may not keep you from getting the anthrax disease.
- Side effects may happen while you are taking CIPRO Tablets, Oral Suspension or I.V. When taking your CIPRO to prevent anthrax infection, you and your healthcare provider should talk about whether the risks of stopping CIPRO too soon are more important than the risks of side effects with CIPRO.
- If you are pregnant, or plan to become pregnant while taking CIPRO, you and your healthcare provider should decide whether the benefits of taking CIPRO Tablets, Oral Suspension or I.V. for anthrax are more important than the risks.

What should I avoid while taking CIPRO?

CIPRO can make you feel dizzy and lightheaded. Do not drive, operate machinery, or do other activities that require mental alertness or coordination until you know how CIPRO affects you.

Avoid sunlamps, tanning beds, and try to limit your time in the sun. CIPRO can make your skin sensitive to the sun (photosensitivity) and the light from sunlamps and tanning beds. You could get severe sunburn, blisters or swelling of your skin. If you get any of these symptoms while taking CIPRO, call your healthcare provider right away. You should use a sunscreen and wear a hat and clothes that cover your skin if you have to be in sunlight.

What are the possible side effects of CIPRO?

CIPRO can cause side effects that may be serious or even cause death. See "What is the most important information I should know about CIPRO?"

Other serious side effects of CIPRO include:

- **Central Nervous System effects**

Seizures have been reported in people who take fluoroquinolone antibiotics including CIPRO. Tell your healthcare provider if you have a history of seizures. Ask your healthcare provider whether taking CIPRO will change your risk of having a seizure.

Central Nervous System (CNS) side effects may happen as soon as after taking the first dose of CIPRO. Talk to your healthcare provider right away if you get any of these side effects, or other changes in mood or behavior:

- feel dizzy
- seizures
- hear voices, see things, or sense things that are not there (hallucinations)
- feel restless
- tremors
- feel anxious or nervous
- confusion
- depression
- trouble sleeping
- nightmares
- feel more suspicious (paranoia)
- suicidal thoughts or acts
- **Serious allergic reactions**

Allergic reactions can happen in people taking fluoroquinolones, including CIPRO, even after only one dose. Stop taking CIPRO and get emergency medical help right away if you get any of the following symptoms of a severe allergic reaction:

- hives
- trouble breathing or swallowing
- swelling of the lips, tongue, face
- throat tightness, hoarseness
- rapid heartbeat
- faint
- yellowing of the skin or eyes. Stop taking CIPRO and tell your healthcare provider right away if you get yellowing of your skin or white part of your eyes, or if you have dark urine. These can be signs of a serious reaction to CIPRO (a liver problem).
- **Skin rash**

Skin rash may happen in people taking CIPRO even after only one dose. Stop taking CIPRO at the first sign of a skin rash and call your healthcare provider. Skin rash may be a sign of a more serious reaction to CIPRO.

- **Serious heart rhythm changes** (QT prolongation and torsade de pointes)

Tell your healthcare provider right away if you have a change in your heart beat (a fast or irregular heartbeat), or if you faint. CIPRO may cause a rare heart problem known as prolongation of the QT interval. This condition can cause an abnormal heartbeat and can be very dangerous. The chances of this event are higher in people:

- who are elderly
- with a family history of prolonged QT interval
- with low blood potassium (hypokalemia)
- who take certain medicines to control heart rhythm (antiarrhythmics)
- **Intestine infection** (Pseudomembranous colitis)

Pseudomembranous colitis can happen with most antibiotics, including CIPRO. Call your healthcare provider right away if you get watery diarrhea, diarrhea that does not go away, or bloody stools. You may have stomach cramps and a fever. Pseudomembranous colitis can happen 2 or more months after you have finished your antibiotic.

- **Changes in sensation and possible nerve damage** (Peripheral Neuropathy)

Damage to the nerves in arms, hands, legs, or feet can happen in people who take fluoroquinolones, including CIPRO. Talk with your healthcare provider right away if you get any of the following symptoms of peripheral neuropathy in your arms, hands, legs, or feet:

- pain
- burning
- tingling
- numbness
- weakness

CIPRO may need to be stopped to prevent permanent nerve damage.

- **Low blood sugar** (hypoglycemia)

People who take CIPRO and other fluoroquinolone medicines with the oral anti-diabetes medicine glyburide (Micronase, Glynase, Diabeta, Glucovance) can get low blood sugar (hypoglycemia) which can sometimes be severe. Tell your healthcare provider if you get low blood sugar with CIPRO. Your antibiotic medicine may need to be changed.

- **Sensitivity to sunlight** (photosensitivity)

See "What should I avoid while taking CIPRO?"

- **Joint Problems**

Increased chance of problems with joints and tissues around joints in children under 18 years old. Tell your child's healthcare provider if your child has any joint problems during or after treatment with CIPRO.

The most common side effects of CIPRO include:

- nausea
- headache
- diarrhea
- vomiting
- vaginal yeast infection
- changes in liver function tests
- pain or discomfort in the abdomen

These are not all the possible side effects of CIPRO. Tell your healthcare provider about any side effect that bothers you, or that does not go away.

Call your doctor for medical advice about side effects. You may report side effects to FDA at 1-800-FDA-1088.

How should I store CIPRO?

- **CIPRO Tablets**
- Store CIPRO below 86°F (30°C)
- **CIPRO Oral Suspension**
- Store CIPRO Oral Suspension below 86°F (30°C) for up to 14 days
- Do not freeze
- After treatment has been completed, any unused oral suspension should be safely thrown away
- **CIPRO XR**
- Store CIPRO XR at 59°F to 86°F (15°C to 30°C)

Keep CIPRO and all medicines out of the reach of children.

General Information about CIPRO

Medicines are sometimes prescribed for purposes other than those listed in a Medication Guide. Do not use CIPRO for a condition for which it is not prescribed. Do not give CIPRO to other people, even if they have the same symptoms that you have. It may harm them.

This Medication Guide summarizes the most important information about CIPRO. If you would like more information about CIPRO, talk with your healthcare provider. You can ask your healthcare provider or pharmacist for information about CIPRO that is written for healthcare professionals. For more information go to www.CIPRO.com or call 1-800-526-4099.

What are the ingredients in CIPRO?

- **CIPRO Tablets**
- Active ingredient: ciprofloxacin
- Inactive ingredients: cornstarch, microcrystalline cellulose, silicon dioxide, crospovidone, magnesium stearate, hypromellose, titanium dioxide, and polyethylene glycol
- **CIPRO Oral Suspension:**
- Active ingredient: ciprofloxacin
- Inactive ingredients: The components of the suspension have the following compositions: Microcapsules—ciprofloxacin, povidone, methacrylic acid copolymer, hypromellose, magnesium stearate, and Polysorbate 20. Diluent—medium-chain triglycerides, sucrose, lecithin, water, and strawberry flavor.
- **CIPRO XR:**
- Active ingredient: ciprofloxacin
- Inactive ingredients: crospovidone, hypromellose, magnesium stearate, polyethylene glycol, silica colloidal anhydrous, succinic acid, and titanium dioxide.
- **CIPRO I.V.:**
- Active ingredient: ciprofloxacin
- Inactive ingredients: lactic acid as a solubilizing agent, hydrochloric acid for pH adjustment

Revised October 2008

This Medication Guide has been approved by the U.S. Food and Drug Administration.

Manufactured by:
Bayer HealthCare Pharmaceuticals Inc.
Wayne, NJ 07470

Distributed by:
Schering-Plough
Schering Corporation
Kenilworth, NJ 07033

CIPRO is a registered trademark of Bayer Aktiengesellschaft and is used under license by Schering Corporation.

Rx Only

81532304, R.010/08 Bay o 9867 5202-2-A-U.S.-2614210
©2008 Bayer HealthCare Pharmaceuticals Inc. Printed in U.S.A.

CIPRO (ciprofloxacin*) 5% and 10% Oral Suspension Made in Italy
CIPRO (ciprofloxacin HCl) Tablets Made in Germany
Shown in Product Identification Guide, page 312

CIPRO® I.V. ℞
(ciprofloxacin)
For Intravenous Infusion

> **WARNING:**
> Fluoroquinolones, including CIPRO® I.V., are associated with an increased risk of tendinitis and tendon rupture in all ages. This risk is further increased in older patients usually over 60 years of age, in patients taking corticosteroid drugs, and in patients with kidney, heart or lung transplants (See WARNINGS).

To reduce the development of drug-resistant bacteria and maintain the effectiveness of CIPRO I.V. and other antibacterial drugs, CIPRO I.V. should be used only to treat or prevent infections that are proven or strongly suspected to be caused by bacteria.

DESCRIPTION

CIPRO® I.V. (ciprofloxacin) is a synthetic broad-spectrum antimicrobial agent for intravenous (I.V.) administration. Ciprofloxacin, a fluoroquinolone, is 1-cyclopropyl-6-fluoro-1,4-dihydro-4-oxo-7-(1piperazinyl)-3-quinolinecarboxylic acid. Its empirical formula is $C_{17}H_{18}FN_3O_3$ and its chemical structure is:

Ciprofloxacin is a faint to light yellow crystalline powder with a molecular weight of 331.4. It is soluble in dilute (0.1N) hydrochloric acid and is practically insoluble in water and ethanol. CIPRO I.V. solutions are available as sterile 1% aqueous concentrates, which are intended for dilution prior to administration, and as 0.2% ready-for-use infusion solutions in 5% Dextrose Injection. All formulas contain lactic acid as a solubilizing agent and hydrochloric acid for pH adjustment. The pH range for the 1% aqueous concentrates in vials is 3.3 to 3.9. The pH range for the 0.2% ready-for-use infusion solutions is 3.5 to 4.6.

The plastic container is latex-free and is fabricated from a specially formulated polyvinyl chloride. Solutions in contact with the plastic container can leach out certain of its chemical components in very small amounts within the expiration period, e.g., di(2-ethylhexyl) phthalate (DEHP), up to 5 parts per million. The suitability of the plastic has been confirmed in tests in animals according to USP biological tests for plastic containers as well as by tissue culture toxicity studies.

CLINICAL PHARMACOLOGY

Absorption

Following 60-minute intravenous infusions of 200 mg and 400 mg ciprofloxacin to normal volunteers, the mean maximum serum concentrations achieved were 2.1 and 4.6 μg/mL, respectively; the concentrations at 12 hours were 0.1 and 0.2 μg/mL, respectively.

Steady-state Ciprofloxacin Serum Concentrations (μg/mL) After 60-minute I.V. Infusions q 12 h.

Dose	Time after starting the infusion					
	30 min.	1 hr	3 hr	6 hr	8 hr	12 hr
200 mg	1.7	2.1	0.6	0.3	0.2	0.1
400 mg	3.7	4.6	1.3	0.7	0.5	0.2

The pharmacokinetics of ciprofloxacin are linear over the dose range of 200 to 400 mg administered intravenously. Comparison of the pharmacokinetic parameters following the 1st and 5th I.V. dose on a q 12 h regimen indicates no evidence of drug accumulation.

The absolute bioavailability of oral ciprofloxacin is within a range of 70–80% with no substantial loss by first pass metabolism. An intravenous infusion of 400-mg ciprofloxacin given over 60 minutes every 12 hours has been shown to produce an area under the serum concentration time curve (AUC) equivalent to that produced by a 500-mg oral dose given every 12 hours. An intravenous infusion of 400 mg ciprofloxacin given over 60 minutes every 8 hours has been shown to produce an AUC at steady-state equivalent to that produced by a 750-mg oral dose given every 12 hours. A 400-mg I.V. dose results in a C_{max} similar to that observed with a 750-mg oral dose. An infusion of 200 mg ciprofloxacin given every 12 hours produces an AUC equivalent to that produced by a 250-mg oral dose given every 12 hours.

Steady-state Pharmacokinetic Parameter Following Multiple Oral and I.V. Doses

Parameters	500 mg q12h, P.O.	400 mg q12h, I.V.	750 mg q12h, P.O.	400 mg q8h, I.V.
AUC (μg•hr/mL)	13.7*	12.7*	31.6†	32.9‡
C_{max} (μg/mL)	2.97	4.56	3.59	4.07

*AUC_{0-12h}
†AUC 24h=$AUC_{0-12h}\times 2$
‡AUC 24h=$AUC_{0-8h}\times 3$

Distribution

After intravenous administration, ciprofloxacin is present in saliva, nasal and bronchial secretions, sputum, skin blister fluid, lymph, peritoneal fluid, bile, and prostatic secretions. It has also been detected in the lung, skin, fat, muscle, cartilage, and bone. Although the drug diffuses into cerebrospinal fluid (CSF), CSF concentrations are generally less than 10% of peak serum concentrations. Levels of the drug in the aqueous and vitreous chambers of the eye are lower than in serum.

Metabolism

After I.V. administration, three metabolites of ciprofloxacin have been identified in human urine which together account for approximately 10% of the intravenous dose. The binding of ciprofloxacin to serum proteins is 20 to 40%. Ciprofloxacin is an inhibitor of human cytochrome P450 1A2 (CYP1A2) mediated metabolism. Coadministration of ciprofloxacin with other drugs primarily metabolized by CYP1A2 results in increased plasma concentrations of these drugs and could lead to clinically significant adverse events of the coadministered drug (see CONTRAINDICATIONS; WARNINGS; PRECAUTIONS: Drug Interactions).

Excretion

The serum elimination half-life is approximately 5–6 hours and the total clearance is around 35 L/hr. After intravenous administration, approximately 50% to 70% of the dose is excreted in the urine as unchanged drug. Following a 200-mg I.V. dose, concentrations in the urine usually exceed 200 μg/mL 0–2 hours after dosing and are generally greater than 15 μg/mL 8–12 hours after dosing. Following a 400-mg I.V. dose, urine concentrations generally exceed 400 μg/mL 0–2 hours after dosing and are usually greater than 30 μg/mL 8–12 hours after dosing. The renal clearance is approximately 22 L/hr. The urinary excretion of ciprofloxacin is virtually complete by 24 hours after dosing. Although bile concentrations of ciprofloxacin are several fold higher than serum concentrations after intravenous dosing, only a small amount of the administered dose (< 1%) is recovered from the bile as unchanged drug. Approximately 15% of an I.V. dose is recovered from the feces within 5 days after dosing.

Special Populations

Pharmacokinetic studies of the oral (single dose) and intravenous (single and multiple dose) forms of ciprofloxacin indicate that plasma concentrations of ciprofloxacin are higher in elderly subjects (> 65 years) as compared to young adults. Although the C_{max} is increased 16–40%, the increase in mean AUC is approximately 30%, and can be at least partially attributed to decreased renal clearance in the elderly. Elimination half-life is only slightly (~20%) prolonged in the elderly. These differences are not considered clinically significant. (See PRECAUTIONS: Geriatric Use.)

In patients with reduced renal function, the half-life of ciprofloxacin is slightly prolonged and dosage adjustments may be required. (See DOSAGE AND ADMINISTRATION.)

In preliminary studies in patients with stable chronic liver cirrhosis, no significant changes in ciprofloxacin pharmacokinetics have been observed. However, the kinetics of ciprofloxacin in patients with acute hepatic insufficiency have not been fully elucidated.

Following a single oral dose of 10 mg/kg ciprofloxacin suspension to 16 children ranging in age from 4 months to 7 years, the mean C_{max} was 2.4 μg/mL (range: 1.5–3.4 μg/mL) and the mean AUC was 9.2 μg*h/mL (range: 5.8–14.9 μg*h/mL). There was no apparent age-dependence, and no notable increase in C_{max} or AUC upon multiple dosing (10 mg/kg TID). In children with severe sepsis who were given intravenous ciprofloxacin (10 mg/kg as a 1-hour infusion), the mean C_{max} was 6.1 μg/mL (range: 4.6–8.3 μg/mL) in 10 children less than 1 year of age; and 7.2 μg/mL (range: 4.7–11.8 μg/mL) in 10 children between 1 and 5 years of age. The AUC values were 17.4 μg*h/mL (range: 11.8–32 μg*h/mL) and 16.5 μg*h/mL (range: 11–23.8 μg*h/mL) in the respective age groups. These values are within the range reported for adults at therapeutic doses. Based on population pharmacokinetic analysis of pediatric patients with various infections, the predicted mean half-life in children is approximately 4-5 hours, and the bioavailability of the oral suspension is approximately 60%.

Drug-drug Interactions: Concomitant administration with tizanidine is contraindicated (See CONTRAINDICATIONS). The potential for pharmacokinetic drug interactions between ciprofloxacin and theophylline, caffeine, cyclosporins, phenytoin, sulfonylurea glyburide, metronidazole, warfarin, probenecid, and piperacillin sodium has been evaluated. (See WARNINGS: PRECAUTIONS: Drug Interactions.)

MICROBIOLOGY

Ciprofloxacin has *in vitro* activity against a wide range of gram-negative and gram-positive microorganisms. The bactericidal action of ciprofloxacin results from inhibition of the enzymes topoisomerase II (DNA gyrase) and topoisomerase IV, which are required for bacterial DNA replication, transcription, repair, and recombination. The mechanism of action of fluoroquinolones, including ciprofloxacin, is different from that of penicillins, cephalosporins, aminoglycosides, macrolides, and tetracyclines; therefore, microorganisms resistant to these classes of drugs may be susceptible to ciprofloxacin and other quinolones. There is no known cross-resistance between ciprofloxacin and other classes of antimicrobials. *In vitro* resistance to ciprofloxacin develops slowly by multiple step mutations.

Ciprofloxacin is slightly less active when tested at acidic pH. The inoculum size has little effect when tested *in vitro*. The minimal bactericidal concentration (MBC) generally does not exceed the minimal inhibitory concentration (MIC) by more than a factor of 2.

Ciprofloxacin has been shown to be active against most strains of the following microorganisms, both *in vitro* and in clinical infections as described in the **INDICATIONS AND USAGE** section of the package insert for CIPRO I.V. (ciprofloxacin for intravenous infusion).

Aerobic gram-positive microorganisms
Enterococcus faecalis **(Many strains are only moderately susceptible.)**
Staphylococcus aureus **(methicillin-susceptible strains only)**
Staphylococcus epidermidis **(methicillin-susceptible strains only)**
Staphylococcus saprophyticus
Streptococcus pneumoniae **(penicillin-susceptible strains)**
Streptococcus pyogenes

Aerobic gram-negative microorganisms

Citrobacter diversus	*Morganella morganii*
Citrobacter freundii	*Proteus mirabilis*
Enterobacter cloacae	*Proteus vulgaris*
Escherichia coli	*Providencia rettgeri*
Haemophilus influenzae	*Providencia stuartii*
Haemophilus parainfluenzae	*Pseudomonas aeruginosa*
Klebsiella pneumoniae	*Serratia marcescens*
Moraxella catarrhalis	

Ciprofloxacin has been shown to be active against *Bacillus anthracis* both *in vitro* and by use of serum levels as a surrogate marker (see INDICATIONS AND USAGE and INHALATIONAL ANTHRAX - ADDITIONAL INFORMATION).

The following *in vitro* data are available, **but their clinical significance is unknown.**

Ciprofloxacin exhibits *in vitro* minimum inhibitory concentrations (MICs) of 1 μg/mL or less against most (≥ 90%) strains of the following microorganisms; however, the safety and effectiveness of ciprofloxacin intravenous formulations in treating clinical infections due to these microorganisms have not been established in adequate and well-controlled clinical trials.

Aerobic gram-positive microorganisms
Staphylococcus haemolyticus
Staphylococcus hominis
Streptococcus pneumoniae **(penicillin-resistant strains)**

Aerobic gram-negative microorganisms

Acinetobacter lwoffi	*Salmonella typhi*
Aeromonas hydrophila	*Shigella boydii*
Campylobacter jejuni	*Shigella dysenteriae*
Edwardsiella tarda	*Shigella flexneri*
Enterobacter aerogenes	*Shigella sonnei*
Klebsiella oxytoca	*Vibrio cholerae*
Legionella pneumophila	*Vibrio parahaemolyticus*
Neisseria gonorrhoeae	*Vibrio vulnificus*
Pasteurella multocida	*Yersinia enterocolitica*
Salmonella enteritidis	

Most strains of *Burkholderia cepacia* and some strains of *Stenotrophomonas maltophilia* are resistant to ciprofloxacin as are most anaerobic bacteria, including *Bacteroides fragilis* and *Clostridium difficile*.

Susceptibility Tests

Dilution Techniques:

Quantitative methods are used to determine antimicrobial minimum inhibitory concentrations (MICs). These MICs provide estimates of the susceptibility of bacteria to antimicrobial compounds. The MICs should be determined using a standardized procedure. Standardized procedures are based on a dilution method[1] (broth or agar) or equivalent with standardized inoculum concentrations and standardized concentrations of ciprofloxacin powder. The MIC values should be interpreted according to the following criteria:

For testing *Enterobacteriaceae, Enterococcus faecalis*, methicillin-susceptible *Staphylococcus* species, penicillin-susceptible *Streptococcus pneumoniae*, *Streptococcus pyogenes*, and *Pseudomonas aeruginosa*[a]:

MIC (μg/mL)	Interpretation
≤ 1	Susceptible (S)
2	Intermediate (I)
≥ 4	Resistant (R)

[a] These interpretive standards are applicable only to broth microdilution susceptibility tests with streptococci using cation-adjusted Mueller-Hinton broth with 2–5% lysed horse blood.

For testing *Haemophilus influenzae* and *Haemophilus parainfluenzae*[b]:

MIC (μg/mL)	Interpretation
≤ 1	Susceptible (S)

[b] This interpretive standard is applicable only to broth microdilution susceptibility tests with *Haemophilus influenzae* and *Haemophilus parainfluenzae* using *Haemophilus* Test Medium[1].

The current absence of data on resistant strains precludes defining any results other than "Susceptible". Strains yielding MIC results suggestive of a "nonsusceptible" category should be submitted to a reference laboratory for further testing.

A report of "Susceptible" indicates that the pathogen is likely to be inhibited if the antimicrobial compound in the blood reaches the concentrations usually achievable. A report of "Intermediate" indicates that the result should be considered equivocal, and, if the microorganism is not fully susceptible to alternative, clinically feasible drugs, the test should be repeated. This category implies possible clinical applicability in body sites where the drug is physiologically concentrated or in situations where high dosage of drug can be used. This category also provides a buffer zone, which prevents small uncontrolled technical factors from causing major discrepancies in interpretation. A report of "Resistant" indicates that the pathogen is not likely to be inhibited if the antimicrobial compound in the blood reaches the concentrations usually achievable; other therapy should be selected.

Standardized susceptibility test procedures require the use of laboratory control microorganisms to control the technical aspects of the laboratory procedures. Standard ciprofloxacin powder should provide the following MIC values:

Organism		MIC (μg/mL)
E. faecalis	ATCC 29212	0.25–2
E. coli	ATCC 25922	0.004–0.015
H. influenzae[a]	ATCC 49247	0.004–0.03
P. aeruginosa	ATCC 27853	0.25–1
S. aureus	ATCC 29213	0.12–0.5

[a] This quality control range is applicable to only *H. influenzae* ATCC 49247 tested by a broth microdilution procedure using *Haemophilus* Test Medium (HTM)[1].

Diffusion Techniques:

Quantitative methods that require measurement of zone diameters also provide reproducible estimates of the susceptibility of bacteria to antimicrobial compounds. One such standardized procedure[2] requires the use of standardized inoculum concentrations. This procedure uses paper disks impregnated with 5-μg ciprofloxacin to test the susceptibility of microorganisms to ciprofloxacin.

Reports from the laboratory providing results of the standard single-disk susceptibility test with a 5-μg ciprofloxacin disk should be interpreted according to the following criteria:

For testing *Enterobacteriaceae*, *Enterococcus faecalis*, methicillin-susceptible *Staphylococcus* species, penicillin-susceptible *Streptococcus pneumoniae*, *Streptococcus pyogenes*, and *Pseudomonas aeruginosa*[a]:

Zone Diameter (mm)	Interpretation
≥ 21	Susceptible (S)
16-20	Intermediate (I)
≤ 15	Resistant (R)

[a] These zone diameter standards are applicable only to tests performed for streptococci using Mueller-Hinton agar supplemented with 5% sheep blood incubated in 5% CO_2.

For testing *Haemophilus influenzae* and *Haemophilus parainfluenzae*[b]:

Zone Diameter (mm)	Interpretation
≥ 21	Susceptible (S)

[b] This zone diameter standard is applicable only to tests with *Haemophilus influenzae* and *Haemophilus parainfluenzae* using *Haemophilus* Test Medium (HTM)[2].

The current absence of data on resistant strains precludes defining any results other than "Susceptible". Strains yielding zone diameter results suggestive of a "nonsusceptible" category should be submitted to a reference laboratory for further testing.

Interpretation should be as stated above for results using dilution techniques. Interpretation involves correlation of the diameter obtained in the disk test with the MIC for ciprofloxacin.

As with standardized dilution techniques, diffusion methods require the use of laboratory control microorganisms that are used to control the technical aspects of the laboratory procedures. For the diffusion technique, the 5-μg ciprofloxacin disk should provide the following zone diameters in these laboratory test quality control strains:

Organism		Zone Diameter (mm)
E. coli	ATCC 25922	30-40
H. influenzae[a]	ATCC 49247	34-42
P. aeruginosa	ATCC 27853	25-33
S. aureus	ATCC 25923	22-30

[a] These quality control limits are applicable to only *H. influenzae* ATCC 49247 testing using *Haemophilus* Test Medium (HTM)[2].

INDICATIONS AND USAGE

CIPRO I.V. is indicated for the treatment of infections caused by susceptible strains of the designated microorganisms in the conditions and patient populations listed below when the intravenous administration offers a route of administration advantageous to the patient. Please see DOSAGE AND ADMINISTRATION for specific recommendations.

Adult Patients:

Urinary Tract Infections caused by *Escherichia coli* (including cases with secondary bacteremia), *Klebsiella pneumoniae* subspecies *pneumoniae*, *Enterobacter cloacae*, *Serratia marcescens*, *Proteus mirabilis*, *Providencia rettgeri*, *Morganella morganii*, *Citrobacter diversus*, *Citrobacter freundii*, *Pseudomonas aeruginosa*, methicillin-susceptible *Staphylococcus epidermidis*, *Staphylococcus saprophyticus*, or *Enterococcus faecalis*.

Lower Respiratory Infections caused by *Escherichia coli*, *Klebsiella pneumoniae* subspecies *pneumoniae*, *Enterobacter cloacae*, *Proteus mirabilis*, *Pseudomonas aeruginosa*, *Haemophilus influenzae*, *Haemophilus parainfluenzae*, or penicillin-susceptible *Streptococcus pneumoniae*. Also, *Moraxella catarrhalis* for the treatment of acute exacerbations of chronic bronchitis.

NOTE: Although effective in clinical trials, ciprofloxacin is not a drug of first choice in the treatment of presumed or confirmed pneumonia secondary to Streptococcus pneumoniae.

Nosocomial Pneumonia caused by *Haemophilus influenzae* or *Klebsiella pneumoniae*.

Skin and Skin Structure Infections caused by *Escherichia coli*, *Klebsiella pneumoniae* subspecies *pneumoniae*, *Enterobacter cloacae*, *Proteus mirabilis*, *Proteus vulgaris*, *Providencia stuartii*, *Morganella morganii*, *Citrobacter freundii*, *Pseudomonas aeruginosa*, methicillin-susceptible *Staphylococcus aureus*, methicillin-susceptible *Staphylococcus epidermidis*, or *Streptococcus pyogenes*.

Bone and Joint Infections caused by *Enterobacter cloacae*, *Serratia marcescens*, or *Pseudomonas aeruginosa*.

Complicated Intra-Abdominal Infections (used in conjunction with metronidazole) caused by *Escherichia coli*, *Pseudomonas aeruginosa*, *Proteus mirabilis*, *Klebsiella pneumoniae*, or *Bacteroides fragilis*.

Acute Sinusitis caused by *Haemophilus influenzae*, penicillin-susceptible *Streptococcus pneumoniae*, or *Moraxella catarrhalis*.

Chronic Bacterial Prostatitis caused by *Escherichia coli* or *Proteus mirabilis*.

Empirical Therapy for Febrile Neutropenic Patients in combination with piperacillin sodium. (See CLINICAL STUDIES.)

Pediatric patients (1 to 17 years of age):

Complicated Urinary Tract Infections and Pyelonephritis due to *Escherichia coli*.

NOTE: Although effective in clinical trials, ciprofloxacin is not a drug of first choice in the pediatric population due to an increased incidence of adverse events compared to controls, including events related to joints and/or surrounding tissues. (See WARNINGS, PRECAUTIONS, Pediatric Use, ADVERSE REACTIONS and CLINICAL STUDIES.)

Ciprofloxacin, like other fluoroquinolones, is associated with arthropathy and histopathological changes in weight-bearing joints of juvenile animals. (See ANIMAL PHARMACOLOGY.)

Adult and Pediatric Patients:

Inhalational anthrax (post-exposure): To reduce the incidence or progression of disease following exposure to aerosolized *Bacillus anthracis*.

Ciprofloxacin serum concentrations achieved in humans served as a surrogate endpoint reasonably likely to predict clinical benefit and provided the initial basis for approval of this indication.[4] Supportive clinical information for ciprofloxacin for anthrax post-exposure prophylaxis was obtained during the anthrax bioterror attacks of October 2001. (See also, INHALATIONAL ANTHRAX – ADDITIONAL INFORMATION).

If anaerobic organisms are suspected of contributing to the infection, appropriate therapy should be administered.

Appropriate culture and susceptibility tests should be performed before treatment in order to isolate and identify organisms causing infection and to determine their susceptibility to ciprofloxacin. Therapy with CIPRO I.V. may be initiated before results of these tests are known; once results become available, appropriate therapy should be continued.

As with other drugs, some strains of *Pseudomonas aeruginosa* may develop resistance fairly rapidly during treatment with ciprofloxacin. Culture and susceptibility testing performed periodically during therapy will provide information not only on the therapeutic effect of the antimicrobial agent but also on the possible emergence of bacterial resistance.

To reduce the development of drug-resistant bacteria and maintain the effectiveness of CIPRO I.V. and other antibacterial drugs, CIPRO I.V. should be used only to treat or prevent infections that are proven or strongly suspected to be caused by susceptible bacteria. When culture and susceptibility information are available, they should be considered in selecting or modifying antibacterial therapy. In the absence of such data, local epidemiology and susceptibility patterns may contribute to the empiric selection of therapy.

CONTRAINDICATIONS

Ciprofloxacin is contraindicated in persons with a history of hypersensitivity to ciprofloxacin, any member of the quinolone class of antimicrobial agents, or any of the product components.

Concomitant administration with tizanidine is contraindicated. (See PRECAUTIONS: Drug Interactions.)

WARNINGS

Tendinopathy and Tendon Rupture:

Fluoroquinolones, including CIPRO I.V., are associated with an increased risk of tendinitis and tendon rupture in all ages. This adverse reaction most frequently involves the Achilles tendon, and rupture of the Achilles tendon may require surgical repair. Tendinitis and tendon rupture in the rotator cuff (the shoulder), the hand, the biceps, the thumb, and other tendon sites have also been reported. The risk of developing fluoroquinolone-associated tendinitis and tendon rupture is further increased in older patients usually over 60 years of age, in patients taking corticosteroid drugs, and in patients with kidney, heart or lung transplants. Factors, in addition to age and corticosteroid use, that may independently increase the risk of tendon rupture include strenuous physical activity, renal failure, and previous tendon disorders such as rheumatoid arthritis. Tendinitis and tendon rupture have also occurred in patients taking fluoroquinolones who do not have the above risk factors. Tendon rupture can occur during or after completion of therapy; cases occurring up to several months after completion of therapy have been reported. CIPRO I.V. should be discontinued if the patient experiences pain, swelling, inflammation or rupture of a tendon. Patients should be advised to rest at the first sign of tendinitis or tendon rupture, and to contact their healthcare provider regarding changing to a non-quinolone antimicrobial drug.

Pregnant Women:

THE SAFETY AND EFFECTIVENESS OF CIPROFLOXACIN IN PREGNANT AND LACTATING WOMEN HAVE NOT BEEN ESTABLISHED. (See PRECAUTIONS: Pregnancy and Nursing Mothers subsections.)

Pediatrics:

Ciprofloxacin should be used in pediatric patients (less than 18 years of age) only for infections listed in the **INDICATIONS AND USAGE** section. An increased incidence of adverse events compared to controls, including events related to joints and/or surrounding tissues, has been observed. (See ADVERSE REACTIONS.)

In pre-clinical studies, oral administration of ciprofloxacin caused lameness in immature dogs. Histopathological examination of the weight-bearing joints of these dogs revealed permanent lesions of the cartilage. Related quinolone-class drugs also produce erosions of cartilage of weight-bearing joints and other signs of arthropathy in immature animals of various species. (See ANIMAL PHARMACOLOGY.)

Cytochrome P450 (CYP450):

Ciprofloxacin is an inhibitor of the hepatic CYP1A2 enzyme pathway. Coadministration of ciprofloxacin and other drugs primarily metabolized by CYP1A2 (e.g. theophylline, methylxanthines, tizanidine) results in increased plasma concentrations of the coadministered drug and could lead to clinically significant pharmacodynamic side effects of the coadministered drug.

Central Nervous System Disorders:

Convulsions, increased intracranial pressure and toxic psychosis have been reported in patients receiving quinolones, including ciprofloxacin. Ciprofloxacin may also cause central nervous system (CNS) events including: dizziness, confusion, tremors, hallucinations, depression, and, rarely, suicidal thoughts or acts. These reactions may occur following the first dose. If these reactions occur in patients receiving ciprofloxacin, the drug should be discontinued and appropriate measures instituted. As with all quinolones, ciprofloxacin should be used with caution in patients with known or suspected CNS disorders that may predispose to seizures or lower the seizure threshold (e.g. severe cerebral arteriosclerosis, epilepsy), or in the presence of other risk factors that may predispose to seizures or lower the seizure threshold (e.g. certain drug therapy, renal dysfunction). (See PRECAUTIONS: General, Information For Patients, Drug Interaction and ADVERSE REACTIONS.)

Theophylline:

SERIOUS AND FATAL REACTIONS HAVE BEEN REPORTED IN PATIENTS RECEIVING CONCURRENT ADMINISTRATION OF INTRAVENOUS CIPROFLOXACIN AND THEOPHYLLINE. These reactions have included cardiac arrest, seizure, status epilepticus, and respiratory failure. Although similar serious adverse events have been reported in patients receiving theophylline alone, the possibility that these reactions may be potentiated by ciprofloxacin cannot be eliminated. If concomitant use cannot be avoided, serum levels of theophylline should be monitored and dosage adjustments made as appropriate.

Hypersensitivity Reactions:

Serious and occasionally fatal hypersensitivity (anaphylactic) reactions, some following the first dose, have been reported in patients receiving quinolone therapy. Some reactions were accompanied by cardiovascular collapse, loss of consciousness, tingling, pharyngeal or facial edema, dyspnea, urticaria, and itching. Only a few patients had a history of hypersensitivity reactions. Serious anaphylactic reactions require immediate emergency treatment with epinephrine and other resuscitation measures, including oxygen, intravenous fluids, intravenous antihistamines, corticosteroids, pressor amines, and airway management, as clinically indicated.

Other serious and sometimes fatal events, some due to hypersensitivity, and some due to uncertain etiology, have been reported rarely in patients receiving therapy with quinolones, including ciprofloxacin. These events may be severe and generally occur following the administration of multiple doses. Clinical manifestations may include one or more of the following:

- fever, rash, or severe dermatologic reactions (e.g., toxic epidermal necrolysis, Stevens-Johnson syndrome);
- vasculitis; arthralgia; myalgia; serum sickness;
- allergic pneumonitis;
- interstitial nephritis; acute renal insufficiency or failure;
- hepatitis; jaundice; acute hepatic necrosis or failure;
- anemia, including hemolytic and aplastic; thrombocytopenia, including thrombotic thrombocytopenic purpura; leukopenia; agranulocytosis; pancytopenia; and/or other hematologic abnormalities.

The drug should be discontinued immediately at the first appearance of a skin rash, jaundice, or any other sign of hypersensitivity and supportive measures instituted (See PRECAUTIONS: Information for Patients and ADVERSE REACTIONS).

Pseudomembranous Colitis:

Clostridium difficile associated diarrhea (CDAD) has been reported with use of nearly all antibacterial agents, including CIPRO, and may range in severity from mild diarrhea to fatal colitis. Treatment with antibacterial agents alters the normal flora of the colon leading to overgrowth of *C. difficile*. *C. difficile* produces toxins A and B which contribute to the development of CDAD. Hypertoxin producing strains of *C. difficile* cause increased morbidity and mortality, as these infections can be refractory to antimicrobial therapy and may require colectomy. CDAD must be considered in all patients who present with diarrhea following antibiotic use. Careful medical history is necessary since CDAD has been reported to occur over two months after the administration of antibacterial agents.

If CDAD is suspected or confirmed, ongoing antibiotic use not directed against *C. difficile* may need to be discontinued. Appropriate fluid and electrolyte management, protein supplementation, antibiotic treatment of *C. difficile*, and surgical evaluation should be instituted as clinically indicated.

Peripheral neuropathy:

Rare cases of sensory or sensorimotor axonal polyneuropathy affecting small and/or large axons resulting in paresthesias, hypoesthesias, dysesthesias and weakness have been reported in patients receiving quinolones, including ciprofloxacin. Ciprofloxacin should be discontinued if the patient experiences symptoms of neuropathy including pain, burning, tingling, numbness, and/or weakness, or is found to have deficits in light touch, pain, temperature, position sense, vibratory sensation, and/or motor strength in order to prevent the development of an irreversible condition.

PRECAUTIONS

General:

INTRAVENOUS CIPROFLOXACIN SHOULD BE ADMINISTERED BY SLOW INFUSION OVER A PERIOD OF 60 MINUTES. Local I.V. site reactions have been reported with the intravenous administration of ciprofloxacin. These reactions are more frequent if infusion time is 30 minutes or less or if small veins of the hand are used. (See ADVERSE REACTIONS.)

Central Nervous System:

Quinolones, including ciprofloxacin, may also cause central nervous system (CNS) events, including: nervousness, agitation, insomnia, anxiety, nightmares or paranoia. (See WARNINGS, Information For Patients:, and Drug Interactions.)

Crystals of ciprofloxacin have been observed rarely in the urine of human subjects but more frequently in the urine of laboratory animals, which is usually alkaline. (See ANIMAL PHARMACOLOGY.) Crystalluria related to ciprofloxacin has been reported only rarely in humans because human urine is usually acidic. Alkalinity of the urine should be avoided in patients receiving ciprofloxacin. Patients should be well hydrated to prevent the formation of highly concentrated urine.

Renal Impairment:

Alteration of the dosage regimen is necessary for patients with impairment of renal function. (See DOSAGE AND ADMINISTRATION.)

Photosensitivity/Phototoxicity:

Moderate to severe photosensitivity/phototoxicity reactions, the latter of which may manifest as exaggerated sunburn reactions (e.g., burning, erythema, exudation, vesicles, blistering, edema) involving areas exposed to light (typically the face, "V" area of the neck, extensor surfaces of the forearms, dorsa of the hands), can be associated with the use of quinolones after sun or UV light exposure. Therefore, excessive exposure to these sources of light should be avoided. Drug therapy should be discontinued if phototoxicity occurs (See **ADVERSE REACTIONS**/Post-Marketing Adverse Events).

As with any potent drug, periodic assessment of organ system functions, including renal, hepatic, and hematopoietic, is advisable during prolonged therapy.

Prescribing CIPRO I.V. in the absence of a proven or strongly suspected bacterial infection or a prophylactic indication is unlikely to provide benefit to the patient and increases the risk of the development of drug-resistant bacteria.

Information For Patients:

Patients should be advised:

- to contact their healthcare provider if they experience pain, swelling, or inflammation of a tendon, or weakness or inability to use one of their joints; rest and refrain from exercise; and discontinue CIPRO I.V. treatment. The risk of severe tendon disorder with fluoroquinolones is higher in older patients usually over 60 years of age, in patients taking corticosteroid drugs, and in patients with kidney, heart or lung transplants.

- that antibacterial drugs including CIPRO I.V. should only be used to treat bacterial infections. They do not treat viral infections (e.g., the common cold). When CIPRO I.V. is prescribed to treat a bacterial infection, patients should be told that although it is common to feel better early in the course of therapy, the medication should be taken exactly as directed. Skipping doses or not completing the full course of therapy may (1) decrease the effectiveness of the immediate treatment and (2) increase the likelihood that bacteria will develop resistance and will not be treatable by CIPRO I.V. or other antibacterial drugs in the future.

- that ciprofloxacin may be associated with hypersensitivity reactions, even following a single dose, and to discontinue the drug at the first sign of a skin rash or other allergic reaction.

- that photosensitivity/phototoxicity has been reported in patients receiving quinolones. Patients should minimize or avoid exposure to natural or artificial sunlight (tanning beds or UVA/B treatment) while taking quinolones. If patients need to be outdoors while using quinolones, they should wear loose-fitting clothes that protect skin from sun exposure and discuss other sun protection measures with their physician. If a sunburn-like reaction or skin eruption occurs, patients should contact their physician.

- that ciprofloxacin may cause dizziness and lightheadedness; therefore, patients should know how they react to this drug before they operate an automobile or machinery or engage in activities requiring mental alertness or coordination.

- that ciprofloxacin increases the effects of tizanidine (Zanaflex®). Patients should not use ciprofloxacin if they are already taking tizanidine.

- that ciprofloxacin may increase the effects of theophylline and caffeine. There is a possibility of caffeine accumulation when products containing caffeine are consumed while taking ciprofloxacin.

- that peripheral neuropathies have been associated with ciprofloxacin use. If symptoms of peripheral neuropathy including pain, burning, tingling, numbness and/or weakness develop, they should discontinue treatment and contact their physicians.

- that convulsions have been reported in patients taking quinolones, including ciprofloxacin, and to notify their physician before taking this drug if there is a history of this condition.

- that ciprofloxacin has been associated with an increased rate of adverse events involving joints and surrounding tissue structures (like tendons) in pediatric patients (less than 18 years of age). Parents should inform their child's physician if the child has a history of joint-related problems before taking this drug. Parents of pediatric patients should also notify their child's physician of any joint-related problems that occur during or following ciprofloxacin therapy. (See WARNINGS, PRECAUTIONS, Pediatric Use and ADVERSE REACTIONS.)

- that diarrhea is a common problem caused by antibiotics which usually ends when the antibiotic is discontinued. Sometimes after starting treatment with antibiotics, patients can develop watery and bloody stools (with or without stomach cramps and fever) even as late as two or more months after having taken the last dose of the antibiotic. If this occurs, patients should contact their physician as soon as possible.

Drug Interactions:

In a pharmacokinetic study, systemic exposure of tizanidine (4 mg single dose) was significantly increased (C_{max} 7-fold, AUC 10-fold) when the drug was given concomitantly with ciprofloxacin (500 mg bid for 3 days). The hypotensive and sedative effects of tizanidine were also potentiated. Concomitant administration of tizanidine and ciprofloxacin is contraindicated.

As with some other quinolones, concurrent administration of ciprofloxacin with theophylline may lead to elevated serum concentrations of theophylline and prolongation of its elimination half-life. This may result in increased risk of theophylline-related adverse reactions. (See WARNINGS.) If concomitant use cannot be avoided, serum levels of theophylline should be monitored and dosage adjustments made as appropriate.

Some quinolones, including ciprofloxacin, have also been shown to interfere with the metabolism of caffeine. This may lead to reduced clearance of caffeine and prolongation of its serum half-life.

Some quinolones, including ciprofloxacin, have been associated with transient elevations in serum creatinine in patients receiving cyclosporine concomitantly.

Altered serum levels of phenytoin (increased and decreased) have been reported in patients receiving concomitant ciprofloxacin.

The concomitant administration of ciprofloxacin with the sulfonylurea glyburide has, in some patients, resulted in severe hypoglycemia. Fatalities have been reported.

The serum concentrations of ciprofloxacin and metronidazole were not altered when these two drugs were given concomitantly.

Quinolones, including ciprofloxacin, have been reported to enhance the effects of the oral anticoagulant warfarin or its derivatives. When these products are administered concomitantly, prothrombin time or other suitable coagulation tests should be closely monitored.

Probenecid interferes with renal tubular secretion of ciprofloxacin and produces an increase in the level of ciprofloxacin in the serum. This should be considered if patients are receiving both drugs concomitantly.

Renal tubular transport of methotrexate may be inhibited by concomitant administration of ciprofloxacin potentially leading to increased plasma levels of methotrexate. This might increase the risk of methotrexate associated toxic reactions. Therefore, patients under methotrexate therapy should be carefully monitored when concomitant ciprofloxacin therapy is indicated.

Non-steroidal anti-inflammatory drugs (but not acetyl salicylic acid) in combination of very high doses of quinolones have been shown to provoke convulsions in pre-clinical studies.

Following infusion of 400 mg I.V. ciprofloxacin every eight hours in combination with 50 mg/kg I.V. piperacillin sodium every four hours, mean serum ciprofloxacin concentrations were 3.02 µg/mL ½ hour and 1.18 µg/mL between 6–8 hours after the end of infusion.

Carcinogenesis, Mutagenesis, Impairment of Fertility:

Eight *in vitro* mutagenicity tests have been conducted with ciprofloxacin. Test results are listed below:

- Salmonella/Microsome Test (Negative)
- *E. coli* DNA Repair Assay (Negative)
- Mouse Lymphoma Cell Forward Mutation Assay (Positive)
- Chinese Hamster V_{79} Cell HGPRT Test (Negative)
- Syrian Hamster Embryo Cell Transformation Assay (Negative)
- *Saccharomyces cerevisiae* Point Mutation Assay (Negative)
- *Saccharomyces cerevisiae* Mitotic Crossover and Gene Conversion Assay (Negative)
- Rat Hepatocyte DNA Repair Assay (Positive)

Thus, two of the eight tests were positive, but results of the following three *in vivo* test systems gave negative results:

- Rat Hepatocyte DNA Repair Assay
- Micronucleus Test (Mice)
- Dominant Lethal Test (Mice)

Long-term carcinogenicity studies in rats and mice resulted in no carcinogenic or tumorigenic effects due to ciprofloxacin at daily oral dose levels up to 250 and 750 mg/kg to rats and mice, respectively (approximately 1.7- and 2.5-times the highest recommended therapeutic dose based upon mg/m²). Results from photo co-carcinogenicity testing indicate that ciprofloxacin does not reduce the time to appearance of UV-induced skin tumors as compared to vehicle control. Hairless (Skh-1) mice were exposed to UVA light for 3.5 hours five times every two weeks for up to 78 weeks while concurrently being administered ciprofloxacin. The time to development of the first skin tumors was 50 weeks in mice treated concomitantly with UVA and ciprofloxacin (mouse dose approximately equal to maximum recommended human dose based upon mg/m²), as opposed to 34 weeks when animals were treated with both UVA and vehicle. The times to development of skin tumors ranged from 16–32 weeks in mice treated concomitantly with UVA and other quinolones.[3]

In this model, mice treated with ciprofloxacin alone did not develop skin or systemic tumors. There are no data from similar models using pigmented mice and/or fully haired mice. The clinical significance of these findings to humans is unknown.

Fertility studies performed in rats at oral doses of ciprofloxacin up to 100 mg/kg (approximately 0.7-times the highest recommended therapeutic dose based upon mg/m²) revealed no evidence of impairment.

Pregnancy:

Teratogenic Effects

Pregnancy Category C:

There are no adequate and well-controlled studies in pregnant women. An expert review of published data on experiences with ciprofloxacin use during pregnancy by TERIS–the Teratogen Information System - concluded that therapeutic doses during pregnancy are unlikely to pose a substantial teratogenic risk (quantity and quality of data=fair), but the data are insufficient to state that there is no risk.[7]

A controlled prospective observational study followed 200 women exposed to fluoroquinolones (52.5% exposed to ciprofloxacin and 68% first trimester exposures) during gestation.[8] In utero exposure to fluoroquinolones during embryogenesis was not associated with increased risk of major malformations. The reported rates of major congenital malformations were 2.2% for the fluoroquinolone group and

2.6% for the control group (background incidence of major malformations is 1-5%). Rates of spontaneous abortions, prematurity and low birth weight did not differ between the groups and there were no clinically significant musculoskeletal dysfunctions up to one year of age in the ciprofloxacin exposed children.

Another prospective follow-up study reported on 549 pregnancies with fluoroquinolone exposure (93% first trimester exposures).[9] There were 70 ciprofloxacin exposures, all within the first trimester. The malformation rates among live-born babies exposed to ciprofloxacin and to fluoroquinolones overall were both within background incidence ranges. No specific patterns of congenital abnormalities were found. The study did not reveal any clear adverse reactions due to in utero exposure to ciprofloxacin.

No differences in the rates of prematurity, spontaneous abortions, or birth weight were seen in women exposed to ciprofloxacin during pregnancy.[7,8] However, these small postmarketing epidemiology studies, of which most experience is from short term, first trimester exposure, are insufficient to evaluate the risk for less common defects or to permit reliable and definitive conclusions regarding the safety of ciprofloxacin in pregnant women and their developing fetuses. Ciprofloxacin should not be used during pregnancy unless the potential benefit justifies the potential risk to both fetus and mother (see WARNINGS).

Reproduction studies have been performed in rats and mice using oral doses up to 100 mg/kg (0.6 and 0.3 times the maximum daily human dose based upon body surface area, respectively) and have revealed no evidence of harm to the fetus due to ciprofloxacin. In rabbits, oral ciprofloxacin dose levels of 30 and 100 mg/kg (approximately 0.4- and 1.3-times the highest recommended therapeutic dose based upon mg/m^2) produced gastrointestinal toxicity resulting in maternal weight loss and an increased incidence of abortion, but no teratogenicity was observed at either dose level. After intravenous administration of doses up to 20 mg/kg (approximately 0.3-times the highest recommended therapeutic dose based upon mg/m^2) no maternal toxicity was produced and no embryotoxicity or teratogenicity was observed. (See WARNINGS.)

Nursing Mothers:

Ciprofloxacin is excreted in human milk. The amount of ciprofloxacin absorbed by the nursing infant is unknown. Because of the potential for serious adverse reactions in infants nursing from mothers taking ciprofloxacin, a decision should be made whether to discontinue nursing or to discontinue the drug, taking into account the importance of the drug to the mother.

Pediatric Use:

Ciprofloxacin, like other quinolones, causes arthropathy and histological changes in weight-bearing joints of juvenile animals resulting in lameness. (See ANIMAL PHARMACOLOGY.)

Inhalational Anthrax (Post-Exposure)

Ciprofloxacin is indicated in pediatric patients for inhalational anthrax (post-exposure). The risk-benefit assessment indicates that administration of ciprofloxacin to pediatric patients is appropriate. For information regarding pediatric dosing in inhalational anthrax (post-exposure), see DOSAGE AND ADMINISTRATION and INHALATIONAL ANTHRAX–ADDITIONAL INFORMATION.

Complicated Urinary Tract Infection and Pyelonephritis

Ciprofloxacin is indicated for the treatment of complicated urinary tract infections and pyelonephritis due to *Escherichia coli*. Although effective in clinical trials, ciprofloxacin is not a drug of first choice in the pediatric population due to an increased incidence of adverse events compared to the controls, including those related to joints and/or surrounding tissues. The rates of these events in pediatric patients with complicated urinary tract infection and pyelonephritis within six weeks of follow-up were 9.3% (31/335) versus 6% (21/349) for control agents. The rates of these events occurring at any time up to the one year follow-up were 13.7% (46/335) and 9.5% (33/349), respectively. The rate of all adverse events regardless of drug relationship at six weeks was 41% (138/335) in the ciprofloxacin arm compared to 31% (109/349) in the control arm. (See ADVERSE REACTIONS and CLINICAL STUDIES.)

Cystic Fibrosis

Short-term safety data from a single trial in pediatric cystic fibrosis patients are available. In a randomized, double-blind clinical trial for the treatment of acute pulmonary exacerbations in cystic fibrosis patients (ages 5-17 years), 67 patients received ciprofloxacin I.V. 10 mg/kg/dose q8h for one week followed by ciprofloxacin tablets 20 mg/kg/dose q12h to complete 10-21 days treatment and 62 patients received the combination of ceftazidime I.V. 50 mg/kg/dose q8h and tobramycin I.V. 3 mg/kg/dose q8h for a total of 10-21 days. Patients less than 5 years of age were not studied. Safety monitoring in the study included periodic range of motion examinations and gait assessments by treatment-blinded examiners. Patients were followed for an average of 23 days after completing treatment (range 0-93 days). This study was not designed to determine long term effects and the safety of repeated exposure to ciprofloxacin.

Musculoskeletal adverse events in patients with cystic fibrosis were reported in 22% of the patients in the ciprofloxacin group and 21% in the comparison group. Decreased range of motion was reported in 12% of the subjects in the ciprofloxacin group and 16% in the comparison group. Arthralgia was reported in 10% of the patients in the ciprofloxacin group and 11% in the comparison group. Other adverse events were similar in nature and frequency between treatment arms. One of sixty-seven patients developed arthritis of the knee nine days after a ten day course of treatment with ciprofloxacin. Clinical symptoms resolved, but an MRI showed knee effusion without other abnormalities eight months after treatment. However, the relationship of this event to the patient's course of ciprofloxacin can not be definitively determined, particularly since patients with cystic fibrosis may develop arthralgias/arthritis as part of their underlying disease process.

Geriatric Use:

Geriatric patients are at increased risk for developing severe tendon disorders including tendon rupture when being treated with a fluoroquinolone such as CIPRO I.V. This risk is further increased in patients receiving concomitant corticosteroid therapy. Tendinitis or tendon rupture can involve the Achilles, hand, shoulder, or other tendon sites and can occur during or after completion of therapy; cases occurring up to several months after fluoroquinolone treatment have been reported. Caution should be used when prescribing CIPRO I.V. to elderly patients especially those on corticosteroids. Patients should be informed of this potential side effect and advised to discontinue CIPRO I.V. and contact their healthcare provider if any symptoms of tendinitis or tendon rupture occur (See BOXED WARNING, WARNINGS, and ADVERSE REACTIONS/Post-Marketing Adverse Event Reports).

In a retrospective analysis of 23 multiple-dose controlled clinical trials of ciprofloxacin encompassing over 3500 ciprofloxacin treated patients, 25% of patients were greater than or equal to 65 years of age and 10% were greater than or equal to 75 years of age. No overall differences in safety or effectiveness were observed between these subjects and younger subjects, and other reported clinical experience has not identified differences in responses between the elderly and younger patients, but greater sensitivity of some older individuals on any drug therapy cannot be ruled out. Ciprofloxacin is known to be substantially excreted by the kidney, and the risk of adverse reactions may be greater in patients with impaired renal function. No alteration of dosage is necessary for patients greater than 65 years of age with normal renal function. However, since some older individuals experience reduced renal function by virtue of their advanced age, care should be taken in dose selection for elderly patients, and renal function monitoring may be useful in these patients. (See CLINICAL PHARMACOLOGY and DOSAGE AND ADMINISTRATION.)

In general, elderly patients may be more susceptible to drug-associated effects on the QT interval. Therefore, precaution should be taken when using CIPRO with concomitant drugs that can result in prolongation of the QT interval (e.g., class IA or class III antiarrhythmics) or in patients with risk factors for torsade de pointes (e.g., known QT prolongation, uncorrected hypokalemia).

ADVERSE REACTIONS

Adverse Reactions in Adult Patients:

During clinical investigations with oral and parenteral ciprofloxacin, 49,038 patients received courses of the drug. Most of the adverse events reported were described as only mild or moderate in severity, abated soon after the drug was discontinued, and required no treatment. Ciprofloxacin was discontinued because of an adverse event in 1.8% of intravenously treated patients.

The most frequently reported drug related events, from clinical trials of all formulations, all dosages, all drug-therapy durations, and for all indications of ciprofloxacin therapy were nausea (2.5%), diarrhea (1.6%), liver function tests abnormal (1.3%), vomiting (1%), and rash (1%).

In clinical trials the following events were reported, regardless of drug relationship, in greater than 1% of patients treated with intravenous ciprofloxacin: nausea, diarrhea, central nervous system disturbance, local I.V. site reactions, liver function tests abnormal, eosinophilia, headache, restlessness, and rash. Many of these events were described as only mild or moderate in severity, abated soon after the drug was discontinued, and required no treatment. Local I.V. site reactions are more frequent if the infusion time is 30 minutes or less. These may appear as local skin reactions which resolve rapidly upon completion of the infusion. Subsequent intravenous administration is not contraindicated unless the reactions recur or worsen.

Additional medically important events, without regard to drug relationship or route of administration, that occurred in 1% or less of ciprofloxacin patients are listed below:

BODY AS A WHOLE: abdominal pain/discomfort, foot pain, pain, pain in extremities

CARDIOVASCULAR: cardiovascular collapse, cardiopulmonary arrest, myocardial infarction, arrhythmia, tachycardia, palpitation, cerebral thrombosis, syncope, cardiac murmur, hypertension, hypotension, angina pectoris, atrial flutter, ventricular ectopy, (thrombo)-phlebitis, vasodilation, migraine

CENTRAL NERVOUS SYSTEM: convulsive seizures, paranoia, toxic psychosis, depression, dysphasia, phobia, depersonalization, manic reaction, unresponsiveness, ataxia, confusion, hallucinations, dizziness, lightheadedness, paresthesia, anxiety, tremor, insomnia, nightmares, weakness, drowsiness, irritability, malaise, lethargy, abnormal gait, grand mal convulsion, anorexia

GASTROINTESTINAL: ileus, jaundice, gastrointestinal bleeding, *C. difficile* associated diarrhea, pseudomembranous colitis, pancreatitis, hepatic necrosis, intestinal perforation, dyspepsia, epigastric pain, constipation, oral ulceration, oral candidiasis, mouth dryness, anorexia, dysphagia, flatulence, hepatitis, painful oral mucosa

HEMIC/LYMPHATIC: agranulocytosis, prolongation of prothrombin time, lymphadenopathy, petechia

METABOLIC/NUTRITIONAL: amylase increase, lipase increase

MUSCULOSKELETAL: arthralgia, jaw, arm or back pain, joint stiffness, neck and chest pain, achiness, flare up of gout, myasthenia gravis

RENAL/UROGENITAL: renal failure, interstitial nephritis, nephritis, hemorrhagic cystitis, renal calculi, frequent urination, acidosis, urethral bleeding, polyuria, urinary retention, gynecomastia, candiduria, vaginitis, breast pain. Crystalluria, cylindruria, hematuria and albuminuria have also been reported.

RESPIRATORY: respiratory arrest, pulmonary embolism, dyspnea, laryngeal or pulmonary edema, respiratory distress, pleural effusion, hemoptysis, epistaxis, hiccough, bronchospasm

SKIN/HYPERSENSITIVITY: allergic reactions, anaphylactic reactions including life-threatening anaphylactic shock, erythema multiforme/Stevens-Johnson syndrome, exfoliative dermatitis, toxic epidermal necrolysis, vasculitis, angioedema, edema of the lips, face, neck, conjunctivae, hands or lower extremities, purpura, fever, chills, flushing, pruritus, urticaria, cutaneous candidiasis, vesicles, increased perspiration, hyperpigmentation, erythema nodosum, thrombophlebitis, burning, paresthesia, erythema, swelling, photosensitivity/phototoxicity reaction (See WARNINGS.)

SPECIAL SENSES: decreased visual acuity, blurred vision, disturbed vision (flashing lights, change in color perception, overbrightness of lights, diplopia), eye pain, anosmia, hearing loss, tinnitus, nystagmus, chromatopsia, a bad taste

In several instances, nausea, vomiting, tremor, irritability, or palpitation were judged by investigators to be related to elevated serum levels of theophylline possibly as a result of drug interaction with ciprofloxacin.

In randomized, double-blind controlled clinical trials comparing ciprofloxacin (I.V. and I.V./P.O. sequential) with intravenous beta-lactam control antibiotics, the CNS adverse event profile of ciprofloxacin was comparable to that of the control drugs.

Adverse Reactions in Pediatric Patients:

Ciprofloxacin, administered I.V. and/or orally, was compared to a cephalosporin for treatment of complicated urinary tract infections (cUTI) or pyelonephritis in pediatric patients 1 to 17 years of age (mean age of 6 ± 4 years). The trial was conducted in the US, Canada, Argentina, Peru, Costa Rica, Mexico, South Africa, and Germany. The duration of therapy was 10 to 21 days (mean duration of treatment was 11 days with a range of 1 to 88 days). The primary objective of the study was to assess musculoskeletal and neurological safety within 6 weeks of therapy and through one year of follow-up in the 335 ciprofloxacin- and 349 comparator-treated patients enrolled.

An Independent Pediatric Safety Committee (IPSC) reviewed all cases of musculoskeletal adverse events as well as all patients with an abnormal gait or abnormal joint exam (baseline or treatment-emergent). These events were evaluated in a comprehensive fashion and included such conditions as arthralgia, abnormal gait, abnormal joint exam, joint sprains, leg pain, back pain, arthrosis, bone pain, pain, myalgia, arm pain, and decreased range of motion in a joint. The affected joints included: knee, elbow, ankle, hip, wrist, and shoulder. Within 6 weeks of treatment initiation, the rates of these events were 9.3% (31/335) in the ciprofloxacin-treated group versus 6 % (21/349) in comparator-treated patients. The majority of these events were mild or moderate in intensity. All musculoskeletal events occurring by 6 weeks resolved (clinical resolution of signs and symptoms), usually within 30 days of end of treatment. Radiological evaluations were not routinely used to confirm resolution of the events. The events occurred more

Findings Involving Joint or Peri-articular Tissues as Assessed by the IPSC

	Ciprofloxacin	Comparator
All Patients (within 6 weeks)	31/335 (9.3%)	21/349 (6%)
95% Confidence Interval*	(-0.8%, +7.2%)	
Age Group		
≥ 12 months < 24 months	1/36 (2.8%)	0/41
≥ 2 years < 6 years	5/124 (4%)	3/118 (2.5%)
≥ 6 years < 12 years	18/143 (12.6%)	12/153 (7.8%)
≥ 12 years to 17 years	7/32 (21.9%)	6/37 (16.2%)
All Patients (within 1 year)	46/335 (13.7%)	33/349 (9.5%)
95% Confidence Interval*	(-0.6%, +9.1%)	

*The study was designed to demonstrate that the arthropathy rate for the ciprofloxacin group did not exceed that of the control group by more than + 6%. At both the 6 week and 1 year evaluations, the 95% confidence interval indicated that it could not be concluded that the ciprofloxacin group had findings comparable to the control group.

ADULT DOSAGE GUIDELINES

Infection*	Severity	Dose	Frequency	Usual Duration
Urinary Tract	Mild/Moderate	200 mg	q12h	7-14 Days
	Severe/Complicated	400 mg	q12h	7-14 Days
Lower	Mild/Moderate	400 mg	q12h	7-14 Days
Respiratory Tract	Severe/Complicated	400 mg	q8h	7-14 Days
Nosocomial	Mild/Moderate/Severe	400 mg	q8h	10-14 Days
Pneumonia				
Skin and	Mild/Moderate	400 mg	q12h	7-14 Days
Skin Structure	Severe/Complicated	400 mg	q8h	7-14 Days
Bone and Joint	Mild/Moderate	400 mg	q12h	≥ 4-6 Weeks
	Severe/Complicated	400 mg	q8h	≥ 4-6 Weeks
Intra-Abdominal†	Complicated	400 mg	q12h	7-14 Days
Acute Sinusitis	Mild/Moderate	400 mg	q12h	10 Days
Chronic Bacterial	Mild/Moderate	400 mg	q12h	28 Days
Prostatitis				
Empirical Therapy	Severe			
in				
Febrile Neutropenic	Ciprofloxacin	400 mg	q8h	7-14 Days
Patients	+			
	Piperacillin	50 mg/kg	q4h	
		Not to exceed		
		24 g/day		
Inhalational anthrax				
(post-exposure)‡		400 mg	q12h	60 Days

* DUE TO THE DESIGNATED PATHOGENS (See INDICATIONS AND USAGE.)
† used in conjunction with metronidazole. (See product labeling for prescribing information.)
‡ Drug administration should begin as soon as possible after suspected or confirmed exposure. This indication is based on a surrogate endpoint, ciprofloxacin serum concentrations achieved in humans, reasonably likely to predict clinical benefit.[4] For a discussion of ciprofloxacin serum concentrations in various human populations, see INHALATIONAL ANTHRAX–ADDITIONAL INFORMATION. Total duration of ciprofloxacin administration (I.V. or oral) for inhalational anthrax (post-exposure) is 60 days.

frequently in ciprofloxacin-treated patients than control patients, regardless of whether they received I.V. or oral therapy. Ciprofloxacin-treated patients were more likely to report more than one event and on more than one occasion compared to control patients. These events occurred in all age groups and the rates were consistently higher in the ciprofloxacin group compared to the control group. At the end of 1 year, the rate of these events reported at any time during that period was 13.7% (46/335) in the ciprofloxacin-treated group versus 9.5% (33/349) comparator-treated patients.

An adolescent female discontinued ciprofloxacin for wrist pain that developed during treatment. An MRI performed 4 weeks later showed a tear in the right ulnar fibrocartilage. A diagnosis of overuse syndrome secondary to sports activity was made, but a contribution from ciprofloxacin cannot be excluded. The patient recovered by 4 months without surgical intervention.
[See first table above]
The incidence rates of neurological events within 6 weeks of treatment initiation were 3% (9/335) in the ciprofloxacin group versus 2% (7/349) in the comparator group and included dizziness, nervousness, insomnia, and somnolence.
In this trial, the overall incidence rates of adverse events regardless of relationship to study drug and within 6 weeks of treatment initiation were 41% (138/335) in the ciprofloxacin group versus 31% (109/349) in the comparator group. The most frequent events were gastrointestinal: 15% (50/335) of ciprofloxacin patients compared to 9% (31/349) of comparator patients. Serious adverse events were seen in

7.5% (25/335) of ciprofloxacin-treated patients compared to 5.7% (20/349) of control patients. Discontinuation of drug due to an adverse event was observed in 3% (10/335) of ciprofloxacin-treated patients versus 1.4% (5/349) of comparator patients. Other adverse events that occurred in at least 1% of ciprofloxacin patients were diarrhea 4.8%, vomiting 4.8%, abdominal pain 3.3%, accidental injury 3%, rhinitis 3%, dyspepsia 2.7%, nausea 2.7%, fever 2.1%, asthma 1.8% and rash 1.8%.
In addition to the events reported in pediatric patients in clinical trials, it should be expected that events reported in adults during clinical trials or post-marketing experience may also occur in pediatric patients.

Post-Marketing Adverse Event Reports:
The following adverse events have been reported from worldwide marketing experience with quinolones, including ciprofloxacin. Because these events are reported voluntarily from a population of uncertain size, it is not always possible to reliably estimate their frequency or establish a causal relationship to drug exposure. Decisions to include these events in labeling are typically based on one or more of the following factors: (1) seriousness of the event, (2) frequency of the reporting, or (3) strength of causal connection to the drug.

Agitation, agranulocytosis, albuminuria, anosmia, candiduria, cholesterol elevation (serum), confusion, constipation, delirium, dyspepsia, dysphagia, erythema multiforme, exfoliative dermatitis, fixed eruption, flatulence, glucose elevation (blood), hemolytic anemia, hepatic failure (including fatal cases), hepatic necrosis, hyperesthesia, hypertonia, hypesthesia, hypotension (postural), jaundice, marrow depression (life threatening), methemoglobinemia, moniliasis (oral, gastrointestinal, vaginal), myalgia, myasthenia, myasthenia gravis (possible exacerbation), myoclonus, nystagmus, pancreatitis, pancytopenia (life threatening or fatal outcome), peripheral neuropathy, phenytoin alteration (serum), photosensitivity/phototoxicity reaction, potassium elevation (serum), prothrombin time prolongation or decrease, pseudomembranous colitis (The onset of pseudomembranous colitis symptoms may occur during or after antimicrobial treatment), psychosis (toxic), renal calculi, serum sickness like reaction, Stevens-Johnson syndrome, taste loss, tendinitis, tendon rupture, torsade de pointes, toxic epidermal necrolysis (Lyell's Syndrome), triglyceride elevation (serum), twitching, vaginal candidiasis, and vasculitis. (See **PRECAUTIONS**.)
Adverse events were also reported by persons who received ciprofloxacin for anthrax post-exposure prophylaxis following the anthrax bioterror attacks of October 2001 (See also **INHALATIONAL ANTHRAX - ADDITIONAL INFORMATION**).

Adverse Laboratory Changes:
The most frequently reported changes in laboratory parameters with intravenous ciprofloxacin therapy, without regard to drug relationship are listed below:

Hepatic	— elevations of AST (SGOT), ALT (SGPT), alkaline phosphatase, LDH, and serum bilirubin
Hematologic	— elevated eosinophil and platelet counts, decreased platelet counts, hemoglobin and/or hematocrit
Renal	— elevations of serum creatinine, BUN, and uric acid
Other	— elevations of serum creatine phosphokinase, serum theophylline (in patients receiving theophylline concomitantly), blood glucose, and triglycerides

Other changes occurring infrequently were: decreased leukocyte count, elevated atypical lymphocyte count, immature WBCs, elevated serum calcium, elevation of serum gamma-glutamyl transpeptidase (γ GT), decreased BUN, decreased uric acid, decreased total serum protein, decreased serum albumin, decreased serum potassium, elevated serum potassium, elevated serum cholesterol. Other changes occurring rarely during administration of ciprofloxacin were: elevation of serum amylase, decrease of blood glucose, pancytopenia, leukocytosis, elevated sedimentation rate, change in serum phenytoin, decreased prothrombin time, hemolytic anemia, and bleeding diathesis.

OVERDOSAGE

In the event of acute overdosage, the patient should be carefully observed and given supportive treatment, including monitoring of renal function. Adequate hydration must be maintained. Only a small amount of ciprofloxacin (< 10%) is removed from the body after hemodialysis or peritoneal dialysis.
In mice, rats, rabbits and dogs, significant toxicity including tonic/clonic convulsions was observed at intravenous doses of ciprofloxacin between 125 and 300 mg/kg.

DOSAGE AND ADMINISTRATION - ADULTS

CIPRO I.V. should be administered to adults by intravenous infusion over a period of 60 minutes at dosages described in the Dosage Guidelines table. Slow infusion of a dilute solution into a larger vein will minimize patient discomfort and reduce the risk of venous irritation. (See Preparation of CIPRO I.V. for Administration section.)

The determination of dosage for any particular patient must take into consideration the severity and nature of the infection, the susceptibility of the causative microorganism, the integrity of the patient's host-defense mechanisms, and the status of renal and hepatic function.

[See second table on previous page]

CIPRO I.V. should be administered by intravenous infusion over a period of 60 minutes.

Conversion of I.V. to Oral Dosing in Adults:

CIPRO Tablets and CIPRO Oral Suspension for oral administration are available. Parenteral therapy may be switched to oral CIPRO when the condition warrants, at the discretion of the physician. (See CLINICAL PHARMACOLOGY and table below for the equivalent dosing regimens.)

Equivalent AUC Dosing Regimens	
CIPRO Oral Dosage	Equivalent CIPRO I.V. Dosage
250 mg Tablet q 12 h	200 mg I.V. q 12 h
500 mg Tablet q 12 h	400 mg I.V. q 12 h
750 mg Tablet q 12 h	400 mg I.V. q 8 h

Parenteral drug products should be inspected visually for particulate matter and discoloration prior to administration.

Adults with Impaired Renal Function:

Ciprofloxacin is eliminated primarily by renal excretion; however, the drug is also metabolized and partially cleared through the biliary system of the liver and through the intestine. These alternative pathways of drug elimination appear to compensate for the reduced renal excretion in patients with renal impairment. Nonetheless, some modification of dosage is recommended for patients with severe renal dysfunction. The following table provides dosage guidelines for use in patients with renal impairment:

RECOMMENDED STARTING AND MAINTENANCE DOSES FOR PATIENTS WITH IMPAIRED RENAL FUNCTION

Creatinine Clearance (mL/min)	Dosage
> 30	See usual dosage.
5 - 29	200-400 mg q 18-24 hr

When only the serum creatinine concentration is known, the following formula may be used to estimate creatinine clearance:

Men:

$$\text{Creatinine clearance (mL/min)} = \frac{\text{Weight (kg)} \times (140 - \text{age})}{72 \times \text{serum creatinine (mg/dL)}}$$

Women: $0.85 \times$ the value calculated for men.

The serum creatinine should represent a steady state of renal function.

For patients with changing renal function or for patients with renal impairment and hepatic insufficiency, careful monitoring is suggested.

DOSAGE AND ADMINISTRATION - PEDIATRICS

CIPRO I.V. should be administered as described in the Dosage Guidelines table. An increased incidence of adverse events compared to controls, including events related to joints and/or surrounding tissues, has been observed. (See ADVERSE REACTIONS and CLINICAL STUDIES.)

Dosing and initial route of therapy (i.e., I.V. or oral) for complicated urinary tract infection or pyelonephritis should be determined by the severity of the infection. In the clinical trial, pediatric patients with moderate to severe infection were initiated on 6 to 10 mg/kg I.V. every 8 hours and allowed to switch to oral therapy (10 to 20 mg/kg every 12 hours), at the discretion of the physician.

[See table above]

Pediatric patients with moderate to severe renal insufficiency were excluded from the clinical trial of complicated urinary tract infection and pyelonephritis. No information is available on dosing adjustments necessary for pediatric

PEDIATRIC DOSAGE GUIDELINES

Infection	Route of Administration	Dose (mg/kg)	Frequency	Total Duration
Complicated Urinary Tract or Pyelonephritis (patients from 1 to 17 years of age)	Intravenous	6 to 10 mg/kg (maximum 400 mg per dose; not to be exceeded even in patients weighing > 51 kg)	Every 8 hours	10-21 days*
	Oral	10 mg/kg to 20 mg/kg (maximum 750 mg per dose; not to be exceeded even in patients weighing > 51 kg)	Every 12 hours	
Inhalational Anthrax (Post-Exposure)†	Intravenous	10 mg/kg (maximum 400 mg per dose)	Every 12 hours	60 days
	Oral	15 mg/kg (maximum 500 mg per dose)	Every 12 hours	

*The total duration of therapy for complicated urinary tract infection and pyelonephritis in the clinical trial was determined by the physician. The mean duration of treatment was 11 days (range 10 to 21 days).

†Drug administration should begin as soon as possible after suspected or confirmed exposure to *Bacillus anthracis* spores. This indication is based on a surrogate endpoint, ciprofloxacin serum concentrations achieved in humans, reasonably likely to predict clinical benefit.[4] For a discussion of ciprofloxacin serum concentrations in various human populations, see INHALATIONAL ANTHRAX–ADDITIONAL INFORMATION.

patients with moderate to severe renal insufficiency (i.e., creatinine clearance of < 50 mL/min/1.73m²).

Preparation of CIPRO I.V. for Administration

Vials (Injection Concentrate): THIS PREPARATION MUST BE DILUTED BEFORE USE. The intravenous dose should be prepared by aseptically withdrawing the concentrate from the vial of CIPRO I.V. This should be diluted with a suitable intravenous solution to a final concentration of 1–2mg/mL. (See COMPATIBILITY AND STABILITY.) The resulting solution should be infused over a period of 60 minutes by direct infusion or through a Y-type intravenous infusion set which may already be in place.

If the Y-type or "piggyback" method of administration is used, it is advisable to discontinue temporarily the administration of any other solutions during the infusion of CIPRO I.V. If the concomitant use of CIPRO I.V. and another drug is necessary each drug should be given separately in accordance with the recommended dosage and route of administration for each drug.

Flexible Containers: CIPRO I.V. is also available as a 0.2% premixed solution in 5% dextrose in flexible containers of 100 mL or 200 mL. The solutions in flexible containers do not need to be diluted and may be infused as described above.

COMPATIBILITY AND STABILITY

Ciprofloxacin injection 1% (10 mg/mL), when diluted with the following intravenous solutions to concentrations of 0.5 to 2 mg/mL, is stable for up to 14 days at refrigerated or room temperature storage.

- 0.9% Sodium Chloride Injection, USP
- 5% Dextrose Injection, USP
- Sterile Water for Injection
- 10% Dextrose for Injection
- 5% Dextrose and 0.225% Sodium Chloride for Injection
- 5% Dextrose and 0.45% Sodium Chloride for Injection
- Lactated Ringer's for Injection

HOW SUPPLIED

CIPRO I.V. (ciprofloxacin) is available as a clear, colorless to slightly yellowish solution. CIPRO I.V. is available in 200 mg and 400 mg strengths. The concentrate is supplied in vials while the premixed solution is supplied in latex-free flexible containers as follows:

VIAL: manufactured for Bayer HealthCare Pharmaceuticals Inc. by Bayer HealthCare LLC, Shawnee, Kansas.

SIZE	STRENGTH	NDC NUMBER
20 mL	200 mg, 1%	0085-1763-03
40 mL	400 mg, 1%	0085-1731-01

FLEXIBLE CONTAINER: Manufactured for Bayer HealthCare Pharmaceuticals Inc. by Hospira, Inc., Lake Forest, IL 60045.

SIZE	STRENGTH	NDC NUMBER
100 mL 5% Dextrose	200 mg, 0.2%	0085-1755-02
200 mL 5% Dextrose	400 mg, 0.2%	0085-1741-02

FLEXIBLE CONTAINER: Manufactured for Bayer HealthCare Pharmaceuticals Inc. by Baxter Healthcare Corporation, Deerfield, IL 60015.

SIZE	STRENGTH	NDC NUMBER
100 mL 5% Dextrose	200 mg, 0.2%	0085-1781-01
200 mL 5% Dextrose	400 mg, 0.2%	0085-1762-01

FLEXIBLE CONTAINER: Manufactured for Bayer HealthCare Pharmaceuticals Inc. Manufactured in Germany or Norway.

SIZE	STRENGTH	NDC NUMBER
100 mL 5% Dextrose	200 mg, 0.2%	0085-1759-01
200 mL 5% Dextrose	400 mg, 0.2%	0085-1782-01

STORAGE

Vial: Store between 5–30°C (41–86°F).
Flexible Container: Store between 5–25°C (41–77°F).
Protect from light, avoid excessive heat, protect from freezing.

Ciprofloxacin is also available as CIPRO (ciprofloxacin HCl) Tablets 250, 500, and 750 mg and CIPRO (ciprofloxacin*) 5% and 10% Oral Suspension.

* Does not comply with USP with regards to "loss on drying" and "residue on ignition".

ANIMAL PHARMACOLOGY

Ciprofloxacin and other quinolones have been shown to cause arthropathy in immature animals of most species tested. (See WARNINGS.) Damage of weight bearing joints was observed in juvenile dogs and rats. In young beagles, 100 mg/kg ciprofloxacin, given daily for 4 weeks, caused degenerative articular changes of the knee joint. At 30 mg/kg, the effect on the joint was minimal. In a subsequent study in young beagle dogs, oral ciprofloxacin doses of 30 mg/kg and 90 mg/kg ciprofloxacin (approximately 1.3- and 3.5-times the pediatric dose based upon comparative plasma AUCs) given daily for 2 weeks caused articular changes which were still observed by histopathology after a treatment-free period of 5 months. At 10 mg/kg (approximately 0.6-times the pediatric dose based upon comparative plasma AUCs), no effects on joints were observed. This dose was also not associated with arthrotoxicity after an additional treatment-free period of 5 months. In another study, removal of weight bearing from the joint reduced the lesions but did not totally prevent them.

Crystalluria, sometimes associated with secondary nephropathy, occurs in laboratory animals dosed with ciprofloxacin. This is primarily related to the reduced solubility of ciprofloxacin under alkaline conditions, which predominate in the urine of test animals; in man, crystalluria is rare since human urine is typically acidic. In rhesus monkeys, crystalluria without nephropathy was noted after single oral doses as low as 5 mg/kg (approximately 0.07-times the highest recommended therapeutic dose based upon mg/m²). After 6 months of intravenous dosing at 10 mg/kg/day, no nephropathological changes were noted; however, nephropathy was observed after dosing at 20 mg/kg/day for the same duration (approximately 0.2-times the highest recommended therapeutic dose based upon mg/m²).

In dogs, ciprofloxacin administered at 3 and 10 mg/kg by rapid intravenous injection (15 sec.) produces pronounced hypotensive effects. These effects are considered to be related to histamine release because they are partially antagonized by pyrilamine, an antihistamine. In rhesus monkeys, rapid intravenous injection also produces hypotension, but the effect in this species is inconsistent and less pronounced.

In mice, concomitant administration of nonsteroidal anti-inflammatory drugs, such as phenylbutazone and indomethacin, with quinolones has been reported to enhance the CNS stimulatory effect of quinolones.

Ocular toxicity, seen with some related drugs, has not been observed in ciprofloxacin-treated animals.

INHALATIONAL ANTHRAX–ADDITIONAL INFORMATION

The mean serum concentrations of ciprofloxacin associated with a statistically significant improvement in survival in the rhesus monkey model of inhalational anthrax are reached or exceeded in adult and pediatric patients receiving oral and intravenous regimens. (See DOSAGE AND ADMINISTRATION.) Ciprofloxacin pharmacokinetics have been evaluated in various human populations. The mean peak serum concentration achieved at steady-state in human adults receiving 500 mg orally every 12 hours is 2.97 μg/mL, and 4.56 μg/mL following 400 mg intravenously every 12 hours. The mean trough serum concentration at steady-state for both of these regimens is 0.2 μg/mL. In a study of 10 pediatric patients between 6 and 16 years of age, the mean peak plasma concentration achieved is 8.3 μg/mL and trough concentrations range from 0.09 to 0.26 μg/mL, following two 30-minute intravenous infusions of 10 mg/kg administered 12 hours apart. After the second intravenous infusion patients switched to 15 mg/kg orally every 12 hours achieve a mean peak concentration of 3.6 μg/mL after the initial oral dose. Long-term safety data, including effects on cartilage, following the administration of ciprofloxacin to pediatric patients are limited. (For additional information, see PRECAUTIONS, Pediatric Use.) Ciprofloxacin serum concentrations achieved in humans serve as a surrogate endpoint reasonably likely to predict clinical benefit and provide the basis for this indication.[4]

A placebo-controlled animal study in rhesus monkeys exposed to an inhaled mean dose of 11 LD_{50} ($\sim5.5 \times 10^5$) spores (range 5–30 LD_{50}) of *B. anthracis* was conducted. The minimal inhibitory concentration (MIC) of ciprofloxacin for the anthrax strain used in this study was 0.08 μg/mL. In the animals studied, mean serum concentrations of ciprofloxacin achieved at expected T_{max} (1 hour post-dose) following oral dosing to steady-state ranged from 0.98 to 1.69 μg/mL. Mean steady-state trough concentrations at 12 hours post-dose ranged from 0.12 to 0.19 μg/mL[5]. Mortality due to anthrax for animals that received a 30-day regimen of oral ciprofloxacin beginning 24 hours post-exposure was significantly lower (1/9), compared to the placebo group (9/10) [p=0.001]. The one ciprofloxacin-treated animal that died of anthrax did so following the 30-day drug administration period.[6]

More than 9300 persons were recommended to complete a minimum of 60 days of antibiotic prophylaxis against possible inhalational exposure to *B. anthracis* during 2001. Ciprofloxacin was recommended to most of those individuals for all or part of the prophylaxis regimen. Some persons were also given anthrax vaccine or were switched to alternative antibiotics. No one who received ciprofloxacin or other therapies as prophylactic treatment subsequently developed inhalational anthrax. The number of persons who received ciprofloxacin as all or part of their post-exposure prophylaxis regimen is unknown.

Among the persons surveyed by the Centers for Disease Control and Prevention, over 1000 reported receiving ciprofloxacin as sole post-exposure prophylaxis for inhalational anthrax. Gastrointestinal adverse events (nausea, vomiting, diarrhea, or stomach pain), neurological adverse events (problems sleeping, nightmares, headache, dizziness or lightheadedness) and musculoskeletal adverse events (muscle or tendon pain and joint swelling or pain) were more frequent than had been previously reported in controlled clinical trials. This higher incidence, in the absence of a control group, could be explained by a reporting bias, concurrent medical conditions, other concomitant medications, emotional stress or other confounding factors, and/or a longer treatment period with ciprofloxacin. Because of these factors and limitations in the data collection, it is difficult to evaluate whether the reported symptoms were drug-related.

CLINICAL STUDIES

EMPIRICAL THERAPY IN ADULT FEBRILE NEUTROPENIC PATIENTS

The safety and efficacy of ciprofloxacin, 400 mg I.V. q 8h, in combination with piperacillin sodium, 50 mg/kg I.V. q 4h, for the empirical therapy of febrile neutropenic patients were studied in one large pivotal multicenter, randomized trial and were compared to those of tobramycin, 2 mg/kg I.V. q 8h, in combination with piperacillin sodium, 50 mg/kg I.V. q 4h.

Clinical response rates observed in this study were as follows:

Outcomes	Ciprofloxacin/ Piperacillin N = 233 Success (%)	Tobramycin/ Piperacillin N = 237 Success (%)
Clinical Resolution of Initial Febrile Episode with No Modifications of Empirical Regimen*	63 (27%)	52 (21.9%)
Clinical Resolution of Initial Febrile Episode Including Patients with Modifications of Empirical Regimen	187 (80.3%)	185 (78.1%)
Overall Survival	224 (96.1%)	223 (94.1%)

*To be evaluated as a clinical resolution, patients had to have: (1) resolution of fever; (2) microbiological eradication of infection (if an infection was microbiologically documented); (3) resolution of signs/symptoms of infection; and (4) no modification of empirical antibiotic regimen.

Complicated Urinary Tract Infection and Pyelonephritis– Efficacy in Pediatric Patients:

NOTE: Although effective in clinical trials, ciprofloxacin is not a drug of first choice in the pediatric population due to an increased incidence of adverse events compared to controls, including events related to joints and/or surrounding tissues.

Ciprofloxacin, administered I.V. and/or orally, was compared to a cephalosporin for treatment of complicated urinary tract infections (cUTI) and pyelonephritis in pediatric patients 1 to 17 years of age (mean age of 6 ± 4 years). The trial was conducted in the US, Canada, Argentina, Peru, Costa Rica, Mexico, South Africa, and Germany. The duration of therapy was 10 to 21 days (mean duration of treatment was 11 days with a range of 1 to 88 days). The primary objective of the study was to assess musculoskeletal and neurological safety.

Patients were evaluated for clinical success and bacteriological eradication of the baseline organism(s) with no new infection or superinfection at 5 to 9 days post-therapy (Test of Cure or TOC). The Per Protocol population had a causative organism(s) with protocol specified colony count(s) at baseline, no protocol violation, and no premature discontinuation or loss to follow-up (among other criteria).

The clinical success and bacteriologic eradication rates in the Per Protocol population were similar between ciprofloxacin and the comparator group as shown below.

Clinical Success and Bacteriologic Eradication at Test of Cure (5 to 9 Days Post-Therapy)

	CIPRO	Comparator
Randomized Patients	337	352
Per Protocol Patients	211	231
Clinical Response at 5 to 9 Days Post-Treatment	95.7% (202/211)	92.6% (214/231)
		95% CI [-1.3%, 7.3%]
Bacteriologic Eradication by Patient at 5 to 9 Days Post-Treatment*	84.4% (178/211)	78.3% (181/231)
		95% CI [-1.3%, 13.1%]
Bacteriologic Eradication of the Baseline Pathogen at 5 to 9 Days Post-Treatment		
Escherichia coli	156/178 (88%)	161/179 (90%)

* Patients with baseline pathogen(s) eradicated and no new infections or superinfections/total number of patients. There were 5.5% (6/211) ciprofloxacin and 9.5% (22/231) comparator patients with superinfections or new infections.

REFERENCES

1. National Committee for Clinical Laboratory Standards, Methods for Dilution Antimicrobial Susceptibility Tests for Bacteria That Grow Aerobically - Fifth Edition. Approved Standard NCCLS Document M7-A5, Vol. 20, No. 2, NCCLS, Wayne, PA, January, 2000.
2. National Committee for Clinical Laboratory Standards, Performance Standards for Antimicrobial Disk Susceptibility Tests - Seventh Edition. Approved Standard NCCLS Document M2-A7, Vol. 20, No. 1, NCCLS, Wayne, PA, January, 2000.
3. Report presented at the FDA's Anti-Infective Drug and Dermatological Drug Products Advisory Committee Meeting, March 31, 1993, Silver Spring, MD. Report available from FDA, CDER, Advisors and Consultants Staff, HFD-21, 1901 Chapman Avenue, Room 200, Rockville, MD 20852, USA.
4. 21 CFR 314.510 (Subpart H–Accelerated Approval of New Drugs for Life-Threatening Illnesses).
5. Kelly DJ, et al. Serum concentrations of penicillin, doxycycline, and ciprofloxacin during prolonged therapy in rhesus monkeys. J Infect Dis 1992; 166: 1184-7.
6. Friedlander AM, et al. Postexposure prophylaxis against experimental inhalational anthrax. J Infect Dis 1993; 167: 1239-42.
7. Friedman J, Polifka J. Teratogenic effects of drugs: a resource for clinicians (TERIS). Baltimore, Maryland: Johns Hopkins University Press, 2000:149-195.
8. Loebstein R, Addis A, Ho E, et al. Pregnancy outcome following gestational exposure to fluoroquinolones: a multicenter prospective controlled study. Antimicrob Agents Chemother. 1998;42(6): 1336-1339.
9. Schaefer C, Amoura-Elefant E, Vial T, et al. Pregnancy outcome after prenatal quinolone exposure. Evaluation of a case registry of the European network of teratology information services (ENTIS). Eur J Obstet Gynecol Reprod Biol. 1996;69:83-89.

MEDICATION GUIDE

CIPRO® *(Sip-row)*
(ciprofloxacin hydrochloride)
TABLETS
CIPRO® *(Sip-row)*
(ciprofloxacin)
ORAL SUSPENSION
CIPRO® XR *(Sip-row)*
(ciprofloxacin extended-release tablets)
CIPRO® I.V. *(Sip-row)*
(ciprofloxacin)
For Intravenous Infusion

Read the Medication Guide that comes with CIPRO® before you start taking it and each time you get a refill. There may be new information. This Medication Guide does not take the place of talking to your healthcare provider about your medical condition or your treatment.

What is the most important information I should know about CIPRO?

CIPRO belongs to a class of antibiotics called fluoroquinolones. CIPRO can cause side effects that may be serious or even cause death. If you get any of the following serious side effects, get medical help right away. Talk with your healthcare provider about whether you should continue to take CIPRO.

• Tendon rupture or swelling of the tendon (tendinitis)
• Tendons are tough cords of tissue that connect muscles to bones.
• Pain, swelling, tears and inflammation of tendons including the back of the ankle (Achilles), shoulder, hand, or other tendon sites can happen in people of all ages who take fluoroquinolone antibiotics, including CIPRO. The risk of getting tendon problems is higher if you:
• are over 60 years of age
• are taking steroids (corticosteroids)
• have had a kidney, heart or lung transplant
• Swelling of the tendon (tendinitis) and tendon rupture (breakage) have also happened in patients who take fluoroquinolones who do not have the above risk factors.
• Other reasons for tendon ruptures can include:
• physical activity or exercise
• kidney failure
• tendon problems in the past, such as in people with rheumatoid arthritis (RA)
• Call your healthcare provider right away at the first sign of tendon pain, swelling or inflammation. Stop taking CIPRO until tendinitis or tendon rupture has been ruled out by your healthcare provider. Avoid exercise and using the affected area. The most common area of pain and swelling is the Achilles tendon at the back of your ankle. This can also happen with other tendons. Talk to your healthcare provider about the risk of tendon rupture with continued use of CIPRO. You may need a different antibiotic that is not a fluoroquinolone to treat your infection.
• Tendon rupture can happen while you are taking or after you have finished taking CIPRO. Tendon ruptures have happened up to several months after patients have finished taking their fluoroquinolone.
• Get medical help right away if you get any of the following signs or symptoms of a tendon rupture:
• hear or feel a snap or pop in a tendon area
• bruising right after an injury in a tendon area
• unable to move the affected area or bear weight
• See the section "What are the possible side effects of CIPRO?" for more information about side effects.

What is CIPRO?

CIPRO is a fluoroquinolone antibiotic medicine used to treat certain infections caused by certain germs called bacteria. Children less than 18 years of age have a higher chance of getting bone, joint, or tendon (musculoskeletal) problems such as pain or swelling while taking CIPRO. CIPRO should not be used as the first choice of antibiotic medicine in children under 18 years of age.

CIPRO Tablets, CIPRO Oral Suspension and CIPRO I.V. should not be used in children under 18 years old, except to treat specific serious infections, such as complicated urinary tract infections and to prevent anthrax disease after breathing the anthrax bacteria germ (inhalational exposure). It is not known if CIPRO XR is safe and works in children under 18 years of age.

Sometimes infections are caused by viruses rather than by bacteria. Examples include viral infections in the sinuses and lungs, such as the common cold or flu. Antibiotics, including CIPRO, do not kill viruses.

Call your healthcare provider if you think your condition is not getting better while you are taking CIPRO.

Who should not take CIPRO?

Do not take CIPRO if you:
- have ever had a severe allergic reaction to an antibiotic known as a fluoroquinolone, or are allergic to any of the ingredients in CIPRO. Ask your healthcare provider if you are not sure. See the list of ingredients in CIPRO at the end of this Medication Guide.
- also take a medicine called tizanidine (Zanaflex®). Serious side effects from tizanidine are likely to happen.

What should I tell my healthcare provider before taking CIPRO?

See "What is the most important information I should know about CIPRO?"

Tell your healthcare provider about all your medical conditions, including if you:
- have tendon problems
- have central nervous system problems (such as epilepsy)
- have nerve problems
- have or anyone in your family has an irregular heartbeat, especially a condition called "QT prolongation"
- have a history of seizures
- have kidney problems. You may need a lower dose of CIPRO if your kidneys do not work well.
- have rheumatoid arthritis (RA) or other history of joint problems
- have trouble swallowing pills
- are pregnant or planning to become pregnant. It is not known if CIPRO will harm your unborn child.
- are breast-feeding or planning to breast-feed. CIPRO passes into breast milk. You and your healthcare provider should decide whether you will take CIPRO or breast-feed.

Tell your healthcare provider about all the medicines you take, including prescription and non-prescription medicines, vitamins and herbal and dietary supplements. CIPRO and other medicines can affect each other causing side effects. Especially tell your healthcare provider if you take:
- an NSAID (Non-Steroidal Anti-Inflammatory Drug). Many common medicines for pain relief are NSAIDs. Taking an NSAID while you take CIPRO or other fluoroquinolones may increase your risk of central nervous system effects and seizures. See "What are the possible side effects of CIPRO?".
- a blood thinner (warfarin, Coumadin®, Jantoven®)
- tizanidine (Zanaflex®). You should not take CIPRO if you are already taking tizanidine. See "Who should not take CIPRO?"
- theophylline (Theo-24®, Elixophyllin®, Theochron®, Uniphyl®, Theolair®)
- glyburide (Micronase®, Glynase®, Diabeta®, Glucovance®). See "What are the possible side effects of CIPRO?"
- phenytoin (Fosphenytoin Sodium®, Cerebyx®, Dilantin-125®, Dilantin®, Extended Phenytoin Sodium®, Prompt Penytoin Sodium®, Phenytek®)
- products that contain caffeine
- a medicine to control your heart rate or rhythm (antiarrhythmics) See "What are the possible side effects of CIPRO?"
- an anti-psychotic medicine
- a tricyclic antidepressant
- a water pill (diuretic)
- a steroid medicine. Corticosteroids taken by mouth or by injection may increase the chance of tendon injury. See "What is the most important information I should know about CIPRO?"
- methotrexate (Trexall®)
- Probenecid (Probalan®, Col-probenecid®)
- Metoclopromide (Reglan®, Reglan ODT®)
- Certain medicines may keep CIPRO Tablets, CIPRO Oral Suspension from working correctly. Take CIPRO Tablets and Oral Suspension either 2 hours before or 6 hours after taking these products:
- an antacid, multivitamin, or other product that has magnesium, calcium, aluminum, iron, or zinc
- sucralfate (Carafate®)
- didanosine (Videx®, Videx EC®)

Ask your healthcare provider if you are not sure if any of your medicines are listed above.

Know the medicines you take. Keep a list of your medicines and show it to your healthcare provider and pharmacist when you get a new medicine.

How should I take CIPRO?

- Take CIPRO exactly as prescribed by your healthcare provider.
- Take CIPRO Tablets in the morning and evening at about the same time each day. Swallow the tablet whole. Do not split, crush or chew the tablet. Tell your healthcare provider if you can not swallow the tablet whole.
- Take CIPRO Oral Suspension in the morning and evening at about the same time each day. Shake the CIPRO Oral Suspension bottle well each time before use for about 15 seconds to make sure the suspension is mixed well. Close the bottle completely after use.
- Take CIPRO XR one time each day at about the same time each day. Swallow the tablet whole. Do not split, crush or chew the tablet. Tell your healthcare provider if you can not swallow the tablet whole.
- CIPRO I.V. is given to you by intravenous (I.V.) infusion into your vein, slowly, over 60 minutes, as prescribed by your healthcare provider.
- CIPRO can be taken with or without food.
- CIPRO should not be taken with dairy products (like milk or yogurt) or calcium-fortified juices alone, but may be taken with a meal that contains these products.
- Drink plenty of fluids while taking CIPRO.
- Do not skip any doses, or stop taking CIPRO even if you begin to feel better, until you finish your prescribed treatment, unless:
- you have tendon effects (see "What is the most important information I should know about CIPRO?"),
- you have a serious allergic reaction (see "What are the possible side effects of CIPRO?"), or
- your healthcare provider tells you to stop.
- This will help make sure that all of the bacteria are killed and lower the chance that the bacteria will become resistant to CIPRO. If this happens, CIPRO and other antibiotic medicines may not work in the future.
- If you miss a dose of CIPRO Tablets or Oral Suspension, take it as soon as you remember. Do not take two doses at the same time, and do not take more than two doses in one day.
- If you miss a dose of CIPRO XR, take it as soon as you remember. Do not take more than one dose in one day.
- If you take too much, call your healthcare provider or get medical help immediately.

If you have been prescribed CIPRO Tablets, CIPRO Oral Suspension or CIPRO I.V. after being exposed to anthrax:
- CIPRO Tablets, Oral Suspension and I.V. has been approved to lessen the chance of getting anthrax disease or worsening of the disease after you are exposed to the anthrax bacteria germ.
- Take CIPRO exactly as prescribed by your healthcare provider. Do not stop taking CIPRO without talking with your healthcare provider. If you stop taking CIPRO too soon, it may not keep you from getting the anthrax disease.
- Side effects may happen while you are taking CIPRO Tablets, Oral Suspension or I.V. When taking your CIPRO to prevent anthrax infection, you and your healthcare provider should talk about whether the risks of stopping CIPRO too soon are more important than the risks of side effects with CIPRO.
- If you are pregnant, or plan to become pregnant while taking CIPRO, you and your healthcare provider should decide whether the benefits of taking CIPRO Tablets, Oral Suspension or I.V. for anthrax are more important than the risks.

What should I avoid while taking CIPRO?

CIPRO can make you feel dizzy and lightheaded. Do not drive, operate machinery, or do other activities that require mental alertness or coordination until you know how CIPRO affects you.

Avoid sunlamps, tanning beds, and try to limit your time in the sun. CIPRO can make your skin sensitive to the sun (photosensitivity) and the light from sunlamps and tanning beds. You could get severe sunburn, blisters or swelling of your skin. If you get any of these symptoms while taking CIPRO, call your healthcare provider right away. You should use a sunscreen and wear a hat and clothes that cover your skin if you have to be in sunlight.

What are the possible side effects of CIPRO?

CIPRO can cause side effects that may be serious or even cause death. See "What is the most important information I should know about CIPRO?"

Other serious side effects of CIPRO include:
- Central Nervous System effects

Seizures have been reported in people who take fluoroquinolone antibiotics including CIPRO. Tell your healthcare provider if you have a history of seizures. Ask your healthcare provider whether taking CIPRO will change your risk of having a seizure.

Central Nervous System (CNS) side effects may happen as soon as after taking the first dose of CIPRO. Talk to your healthcare provider right away if you get any of these side effects, or other changes in mood or behavior:
- feel dizzy
- seizures
- hear voices, see things, or sense things that are not there (hallucinations)
- feel restless
- tremors
- feel anxious or nervous
- confusion
- depression
- trouble sleeping
- nightmares
- feel more suspicious (paranoia)
- suicidal thoughts or acts
- Serious allergic reactions

Allergic reactions can happen in people taking fluoroquinolones, including CIPRO, even after only one dose. Stop taking CIPRO and get emergency medical help right away if you get any of the following symptoms of a severe allergic reaction:
- hives
- trouble breathing or swallowing
- swelling of the lips, tongue, face
- throat tightness, hoarseness
- rapid heartbeat
- faint
- yellowing of the skin or eyes. Stop taking CIPRO and tell your healthcare provider right away if you get yellowing of your skin or white part of your eyes, or if you have dark urine. These can be signs of a serious reaction to CIPRO (a liver problem).
- Skin rash

Skin rash may happen in people taking CIPRO even after only one dose. Stop taking CIPRO at the first sign of a skin rash and call your healthcare provider. Skin rash may be a sign of a more serious reaction to CIPRO.
- Serious heart rhythm changes (QT prolongation and torsade de pointes)

Tell your healthcare provider right away if you have a change in your heart beat (a fast or irregular heartbeat), or if you faint. CIPRO may cause a rare heart problem known as prolongation of the QT interval. This condition can cause an abnormal heartbeat and can be very dangerous. The chances of this event are higher in people:
- who are elderly
- with a family history of prolonged QT interval
- with low blood potassium (hypokalemia)
- who take certain medicines to control heart rhythm (antiarrhythmics)
- Intestine infection (Pseudomembranous colitis)

Pseudomembranous colitis can happen with most antibiotics, including CIPRO. Call your healthcare provider right away if you get watery diarrhea, diarrhea that does not go away, or bloody stools. You may have stomach cramps and a fever. Pseudomembranous colitis can happen 2 or more months after you have finished your antibiotic.
- Changes in sensation and possible nerve damage (Peripheral Neuropathy)

Damage to the nerves in arms, hands, legs, or feet can happen in people who take fluoroquinolones, including CIPRO. Talk with your healthcare provider right away if you get any of the following symptoms of peripheral neuropathy in your arms, hands, legs, or feet:
- pain
- burning
- tingling
- numbness
- weakness

CIPRO may need to be stopped to prevent permanent nerve damage.
- Low blood sugar (hypoglycemia)

People who take CIPRO and other fluoroquinolone medicines with the oral anti-diabetes medicine glyburide (Micronase, Glynase, Diabeta, Glucovance) can get low blood sugar (hypoglycemia) which can sometimes be severe. Tell your healthcare provider if you get low blood sugar with CIPRO. Your antibiotic medicine may need to be changed.
- Sensitivity to sunlight (photosensitivity)

See "What should I avoid while taking CIPRO?"
- Joint Problems

Increased chance of problems with joints and tissues around joints in children under 18 years old. Tell your child's healthcare provider if your child has any joint problems during or after treatment with CIPRO.

The most common side effects of CIPRO include:
- nausea
- headache
- diarrhea
- vomiting
- vaginal yeast infection
- changes in liver function tests
- pain or discomfort in the abdomen

These are not all the possible side effects of CIPRO. Tell your healthcare provider about any side effect that bothers you, or that does not go away.

Call your doctor for medical advice about side effects. You may report side effects to FDA at 1-800-FDA-1088.

How should I store CIPRO?
- CIPRO Tablets
- Store CIPRO below 86°F (30°C)
- CIPRO Oral Suspension
- Store CIPRO Oral Suspension below 86°F (30°C) for up to 14 days
- Do not freeze
- After treatment has been completed, any unused oral suspension should be safely thrown away
- CIPRO XR
- Store CIPRO XR at 59°F to 86°F (15°C to 30°C)

Keep CIPRO and all medicines out of the reach of children.

General Information about CIPRO

Medicines are sometimes prescribed for purposes other than those listed in a Medication Guide. Do not use CIPRO for a condition for which it is not prescribed. Do not give CIPRO to other people, even if they have the same symptoms that you have. It may harm them.

This Medication Guide summarizes the most important information about CIPRO. If you would like more information about CIPRO, talk with your healthcare provider. You can ask your healthcare provider or pharmacist for information about CIPRO that is written for healthcare professionals. For more information go to www.CIPRO.com or call 1-800-526-4099.

What are the ingredients in CIPRO?
- CIPRO Tablets
- Active ingredient: ciprofloxacin
- Inactive ingredients: cornstarch, microcrystalline cellulose, silicon dioxide, crospovidone, magnesium stearate, hypromellose, titanium dioxide, and polyethylene glycol
- CIPRO Oral Suspension:
- Active ingredient: ciproflxacin
- Inactive ingredients: The components of the suspension have the following compositions: Microcapsules—ciprofloxacin, povidone, methacrylic acid copolymer, hypromellose, magnesium stearate, and Polysorbate 20. Diluent—medium-chain triglycerides, sucrose, lecithin, water, and strawberry flavor.
- CIPRO XR:
- Active ingredient: ciprofloxacin
- Inactive ingredients: crospovidone, hypromellose, magnesium stearate, polyethylene glycol, silica colloidal anhydrous, succinic acid, and titanium dioxide.
- CIPRO I.V.:
- Active ingredient: ciprofloxacin
- Inactive ingredients: lactic acid as a solubilizing agent, hydrochloric acid for pH adjustment

Revised October 2008

This Medication Guide has been approved by the U.S. Food and Drug Administration.

Manufactured for:

Bayer HealthCare Pharmaceuticals Inc.
Wayne, NJ 07470

Made in Germany or Made in Norway
By Fresenius Kabi Norge AS
NO - 1753 Halden, Norway

Distributed by:
Schering-Plough
Schering Corporation
Kenilworth, NJ 07033

CIPRO is a registered trademark of Bayer Aktiengesellschaft and is used under license by Schering Corporation.

Rx Only

81532266, R.2 09/09 ©2009 Bayer HealthCare Pharmaceuticals Inc. 14590

BAY q 3939 5202-4-A-U.S.-23 Printed In U.S.A.
Revised: 12/2009

Distributed by: Schering Plough Corporation
Shown in Product Identification Guide, page 312

CIPRO® XR ℞
[sī′prō]
(ciprofloxacin* extended-release tablets)

WARNING:
Fluoroquinolones, including CIPRO® XR, are associated with an increased risk of tendinitis and tendon rupture in all ages. This risk is further increased in older patients usually over 60 years of age, in patients taking corticosteroid drugs, and in patients with kidney, heart or lung transplants (See WARNINGS).

To reduce the development of drug-resistant bacteria and maintain the effectiveness of CIPRO XR and other antibacterial drugs, CIPRO XR should be used only to treat or prevent infections that are proven or strongly suspected to be caused by bacteria.

DESCRIPTION

CIPRO XR (ciprofloxacin* extended-release tablets) contains ciprofloxacin, a synthetic broad-spectrum antimicrobial agent for oral administration. CIPRO XR tablets are coated, bilayer tablets consisting of an immediate-release layer and an erosion-matrix type controlled-release layer. The tablets contain a combination of two types of ciprofloxacin drug substance, ciprofloxacin hydrochloride and ciprofloxacin betaine (base). Ciprofloxacin hydrochloride is 1-cyclopropyl-6-fluoro-1,4-dihydro-4-oxo-7-(1-piperazinyl)-3-quinolinecarboxylic acid hydrochloride. It is provided as a mixture of the monohydrate and the sesquihydrate. The empirical formula of the monohydrate is $C_{17}H_{18}FN_3O_3 \cdot HCl \cdot H_2O$ and its molecular weight is 385.8. The empirical formula of the sesquihydrate is $C_{17}H_{18}FN_3O_3 \cdot HCl \cdot 1.5\ H_2O$ and its molecular weight is 394.8. The drug substance is a faintly yellowish to light yellow crystalline substance. The chemical structure of the monohydrate is as follows:

Ciprofloxacin betaine is 1-cyclopropyl-6-fluoro-1, 4-dihydro-4-oxo-7-(1-piperazinyl)-3-quinolinecarboxylic acid. As a hydrate, its empirical formula is $C_{17}H_{18}FN_3O_3 \cdot 3.5\ H_2O$ and its molecular weight is 394.3. It is a pale yellowish to light yellow crystalline substance and its chemical structure is as follows:

CIPRO XR is available in 500 mg and 1000 mg (ciprofloxacin equivalent) tablet strengths. CIPRO XR tablets are nearly white to slightly yellowish, film-coated, oblong-shaped tablets. Each CIPRO XR 500 mg tablet contains 500 mg of ciprofloxacin as ciprofloxacin HCl (287.5 mg, calculated as ciprofloxacin on the dried basis) and ciprofloxacin† (212.6 mg, calculated on the dried basis). Each CIPRO XR 1000 mg tablet contains 1000 mg of ciprofloxacin as ciprofloxacin HCl (574.9 mg, calculated as ciprofloxacin on the dried basis) and ciprofloxacin† (425.2 mg, calculated on the dried basis). The inactive ingredients are crospovidone, hypromellose, magnesium stearate, polyethylene glycol, silica colloidal anhydrous, succinic acid, and titanium dioxide.

* as ciprofloxacin† and ciprofloxacin hydrochloride
† does not comply with the loss on drying test and residue on ignition test of the USP monograph.

CLINICAL PHARMACOLOGY
Absorption
CIPRO XR tablets are formulated to release drug at a slower rate compared to immediate-release tablets. Approximately 35% of the dose is contained within an immediate-release component, while the remaining 65% is contained in a slow-release matrix.

Maximum plasma ciprofloxacin concentrations are attained between 1 and 4 hours after dosing with CIPRO XR. In comparison to the 250 mg and 500 mg ciprofloxacin immediate-release BID treatment, the C_{max} of CIPRO XR 500 mg and 1000 mg once daily are higher than the corresponding BID doses, while the AUCs over 24 hours are equivalent.

The following table compares the pharmacokinetic parameters obtained at steady state for these four treatment regimens (500 mg QD CIPRO XR versus 250 mg BID ciprofloxacin immediate-release tablets and 1000 mg QD CIPRO XR versus 500 mg BID ciprofloxacin immediate-release).

[See table below]

Results of the pharmacokinetic studies demonstrate that CIPRO XR may be administered with or without food (e.g. high-fat and low-fat meals or under fasted conditions).

Distribution
The volume of distribution calculated for intravenous ciprofloxacin is approximately 2.1–2.7 L/kg. Studies with the oral and intravenous forms of ciprofloxacin have demonstrated penetration of ciprofloxacin into a variety of tissues. The binding of ciprofloxacin to serum proteins is 20% to 40%, which is not likely to be high enough to cause significant protein binding interactions with other drugs. Following administration of a single dose of CIPRO XR, ciprofloxacin concentrations in urine collected up to 4 hours after dosing averaged over 300 mg/L for both the 500 mg and 1000 mg tablets; in urine excreted from 12 to 24 hours after dosing, ciprofloxacin concentration averaged 27 mg/L for the 500 mg tablet, and 58 mg/L for the 1000 mg tablet.

Metabolism
Four metabolites of ciprofloxacin were identified in human urine. The metabolites have antimicrobial activity, but are less active than unchanged ciprofloxacin. The primary metabolites are oxociprofloxacin (M3) and sulfociprofloxacin (M2), each accounting for roughly 3% to 8% of the total dose. Other minor metabolites are desethylene ciprofloxacin (M1), and formylciprofloxacin (M4). The relative proportion of drug and metabolite in serum corresponds to the composition found in urine. Excretion of these metabolites was essentially complete by 24 hours after dosing. Ciprofloxacin is an inhibitor of human cytochrome P450 1A2 (CYP1A2) mediated metabolism. Coadministration of ciprofloxacin with other drugs primarily metabolized by CYP1A2 results in increased plasma concentrations of these drugs and could lead to clinically significant adverse events of the coadministered drug (see CONTRAINDICATIONS; WARNINGS; PRECAUTIONS: Drug Interactions).

Elimination
The elimination kinetics of ciprofloxacin are similar for the immediate-release and the CIPRO XR tablet. In studies comparing the CIPRO XR and immediate-release ciprofloxacin, approximately 35% of an orally administered dose was excreted in the urine as unchanged drug for both formulations. The urinary excretion of ciprofloxacin is virtually complete within 24 hours after dosing. The renal clearance of ciprofloxacin, which is approximately 300 mL/minute, exceeds the normal glomerular filtration rate of 120 mL/minute. Thus, active tubular secretion would seem to play a significant role in its elimination. Coadministration of probenecid with immediate-release ciprofloxacin results in about a 50% reduction in the ciprofloxacin renal clearance and a 50% increase in its concentration in the systemic circulation. Although bile concentrations of ciprofloxacin are several fold higher than serum concentrations after oral dosing with the immediate-release tablet, only a small amount of the dose administered is recovered from the bile as unchanged drug. An additional 1% to 2% of the dose is recovered from the bile in the form of metabolites. Approximately 20% to 35% of an oral dose of immediate-release ciprofloxacin is recovered from the feces within 5 days after dosing. This may arise from either biliary clearance or transintestinal elimination.

Special Populations
Pharmacokinetic studies of the immediate-release oral tablet (single dose) and intravenous (single and multiple dose) forms of ciprofloxacin indicate that plasma concentrations of ciprofloxacin are higher in elderly subjects (> 65 years) as compared to young adults. C_{max} is increased 16% to 40%, and mean AUC is increased approximately 30%, which can be at least partially attributed to decreased renal clearance in the elderly. Elimination half-life is only slightly (~20%)

Ciprofloxacin Pharmacokinetics (Mean ± SD) Following CIPRO® and CIPRO XR Administration				
	C_{max} (mg/L)	AUC_{0-24h} (mg•h/L)	$T_{1/2}$ (hr)	T_{max} (hr)*
CIPRO XR 500 mg QD	1.59 ± 0.43	7.97 ± 1.87	6.6 ± 1.4	1.5 (1.0-2.5)
CIPRO 250 mg BID	1.14 ± 0.23	8.25 ± 2.15	4.8 ± 0.6	1.0 (0.5-2.5)
CIPRO XR 1000 mg QD	3.11 ± 1.08	16.83 ± 5.65	6.31 ± 0.72	2.0 (1-4)
CIPRO 500 mg BID	2.06 ± 0.41	17.04 ± 4.79	5.66 ± 0.89	2.0 (0.5-3.5)

*median (range)

prolonged in the elderly. These differences are not considered clinically significant. (See **PRECAUTIONS, Geriatric Use.**)

In patients with reduced renal function, the half-life of ciprofloxacin is slightly prolonged. No dose adjustment is required for patients with uncomplicated urinary tract infections receiving 500 mg CIPRO XR. For complicated urinary tract infection and acute uncomplicated pyelonephritis, where 1000 mg is the appropriate dose, the dosage of CIPRO XR should be reduced to CIPRO XR 500 mg q24h in patients with creatinine clearance below 30 mL/min. (See **DOSAGE AND ADMINISTRATION.**)

In studies in patients with stable chronic cirrhosis, no significant changes in ciprofloxacin pharmacokinetics have been observed. The kinetics of ciprofloxacin in patients with acute hepatic insufficiency, however, have not been fully elucidated. (See **DOSAGE AND ADMINISTRATION.**)

Drug-drug Interactions

Concomitant administration with tizanidine is contraindicated. (See **CONTRAINDICATIONS**). Previous studies with immediate-release ciprofloxacin have shown that concomitant administration of ciprofloxacin with theophylline decreases the clearance of theophylline resulting in elevated serum theophylline levels and increased risk of a patient developing CNS or other adverse reactions. Ciprofloxacin also decreases caffeine clearance and inhibits the formation of paraxanthine after caffeine administration. Absorption of ciprofloxacin is significantly reduced by concomitant administration of multivalent cation-containing products such as magnesium/aluminum antacids, sucralfate, VIDEX® (didanosine) chewable/buffered tablets or pediatric powder, or products containing calcium, iron, or zinc. (See **WARNINGS**: **PRECAUTIONS, Drug Interactions** and **Information for Patients**, and **DOSAGE AND ADMINISTRATION.**)

Antacids: When CIPRO XR given as a single 1000 mg dose was administered two hours before, or four hours after a magnesium/aluminum-containing antacid (900 mg aluminum hydroxide and 600 mg magnesium hydroxide as a single oral dose) to 18 healthy volunteers, there was a 4% and 19% reduction, respectively, in the mean C_{max} of ciprofloxacin. The reduction in the mean AUC was 24% and 26%, respectively. CIPRO XR should be administered at least 2 hours before or 6 hours after antacids containing magnesium or aluminum, as well as sucralfate, VIDEX® (didanosine) chewable/buffered tablets or pediatric powder, other highly buffered drugs, metal cations such as iron, and multivitamin preparations with zinc. Although CIPRO XR may be taken with meals that include milk, concomitant administration with dairy products or with calcium-fortified juices alone should be avoided, since decreased absorption is possible. (See **PRECAUTIONS, Information for Patients** and **Drug Interactions**, and **DOSAGE AND ADMINISTRATION.**)

Omeprazole: When CIPRO XR was administered as a single 1000 mg dose concomitantly with omeprazole (40 mg once daily for three days) to 18 healthy volunteers, the mean AUC and C_{max} of ciprofloxacin were reduced by 20% and 23%, respectively. The clinical significance of this interaction has not been determined. (See **PRECAUTIONS, Drug Interactions.**)

MICROBIOLOGY

Ciprofloxacin has *in vitro* activity against a wide range of gram-negative and gram-positive organisms. The bactericidal action of ciprofloxacin results from inhibition of topoisomerase II (DNA gyrase) and topoisomerase IV (both Type II topoisomerases), which are required for bacterial DNA replication, transcription, repair, and recombination. The mechanism of action of quinolones, including ciprofloxacin, is different from that of other antimicrobial agents such as beta-lactams, macrolides, tetracyclines, or aminoglycosides; therefore, organisms resistant to these drugs may be susceptible to ciprofloxacin. There is no known cross-resistance between ciprofloxacin and other classes of antimicrobials. Resistance to ciprofloxacin *in vitro* develops slowly (multiple-step mutation). Resistance to ciprofloxacin due to spontaneous mutations occurs at a general frequency of between $< 10^{-9}$ to 1×10^{-6}.

Ciprofloxacin is slightly less active when tested at acidic pH. The inoculum size has little effect when tested *in vitro*. The minimal bactericidal concentration (MBC) generally does not exceed the minimal inhibitory concentration (MIC) by more than a factor of 2.

Ciprofloxacin has been shown to be active against most strains of the following microorganisms, both *in vitro* and in clinical infections as described in the **INDICATIONS AND USAGE** section.

Aerobic gram-positive microorganisms
Enterococcus faecalis (Many strains are only moderately susceptible.)
Staphylococcus saprophyticus

Aerobic gram-negative microorganisms
Escherichia coli
Klebsiella pneumoniae
Proteus mirabilis
Pseudomonas aeruginosa

The following *in vitro* data are available, but their clinical significance is unknown.

Ciprofloxacin exhibits *in vitro* minimum inhibitory concentrations (MICs) of 1 μg/mL or less against most (≥ 90%) strains of the following microorganisms; however, the safety and effectiveness of CIPRO XR in treating clinical infections due to these microorganisms have not been established in adequate and well-controlled clinical trials.

Aerobic gram-negative microorganisms

Citrobacter koseri	*Morganella morganii*
Citrobacter freundii	*Proteus vulgaris*
Edwardsiella tarda	*Providencia rettgeri*
Enterobacter aerogenes	*Providencia stuartii*
Enterobacter cloacae	*Serratia marcescens*
Klebsiella oxytoca	

Susceptibility Tests

Dilution Techniques:

Quantitative methods are used to determine antimicrobial minimal inhibitory concentrations (MICs). These MICs provide estimates of the susceptibility of bacteria to antimicrobial compounds. The MICs should be determined using a standardized procedure. Standardized procedures are based on a dilution method[1] (broth or agar) or equivalent with standardized inoculum concentrations and standardized concentrations of ciprofloxacin. The MIC values should be interpreted according to the following criteria:

For testing *Enterobacteriaceae, Enterococcus* faecalis, *Pseudomonas aeruginosa*, and *Staphylococcus* saprophyticus:

MIC (μg/mL)	Interpretation
≤ 1	Susceptible (S)
2	Intermediate (I)
≥ 4	Resistant (R)

A report of "Susceptible" indicates that the pathogen is likely to be inhibited if the antimicrobial compound in the blood reaches the concentrations usually achievable. A report of "Intermediate" indicates that the result should be considered equivocal, and, if the microorganism is not fully susceptible to alternative, clinically feasible drugs, the test should be repeated. This category implies possible clinical applicability in body sites where the drug is physiologically concentrated or in situations where high dosage of drug can be used. This category also provides a buffer zone which prevents small uncontrolled technical factors from causing major discrepancies in interpretation. A report of "Resistant" indicates that the pathogen is not likely to be inhibited if the antimicrobial compound in the blood reaches the concentrations usually achievable; other therapy should be selected.

Standardized susceptibility test procedures require the use of laboratory control microorganisms to control the technical aspects of the laboratory procedures. Standard ciprofloxacin powder should provide the following MIC values:

Microorganism		MIC Range (μg/mL)
Enterococcus faecalis	ATCC 29212	0.25-2.0
Escherichia coli	ATCC 25922	0.004-0.015
Staphylococcus aureus	ATCC 29213	0.12-0.5
Pseudomonas aeruginosa	ATCC 27853	0.25-1

Diffusion Techniques:

Quantitative methods that require measurement of zone diameters also provide reproducible estimates of the susceptibility of bacteria to antimicrobial compounds. One such standardized procedure[2] requires the use of standardized inoculum concentrations. This procedure uses paper disks impregnated with 5-μg ciprofloxacin to test the susceptibility of microorganisms to ciprofloxacin. Reports from the laboratory providing results of the standard single-disk susceptibility test with a 5-μg ciprofloxacin disk should be interpreted according to the following criteria:

For testing *Enterobacteriaceae, Enterococcus* faecalis, *Pseudomonas aeruginosa*, and *Staphylococcus* saprophyticus:

Zone Diameter (mm)	Interpretation
≥ 21	Susceptible (S)
16-20	Intermediate (I)
≤ 15	Resistant (R)

Interpretation should be as stated above for results using dilution techniques. Interpretation involves correlation of the diameter obtained in the disk test with the MIC for ciprofloxacin.

As with standardized dilution techniques, diffusion methods require the use of laboratory control microorganisms that are used to control the technical aspects of the laboratory procedures. For the diffusion technique, the 5-μg ciprofloxacin disk should provide the following zone diameters in these laboratory test quality control strains:

Microorganism		Zone Diameter (mm)
Escherichia coli	ATCC 25922	30-40
Staphylococcus aureus	ATCC 25923	22-30
Pseudomonas aeruginosa	ATCC 27853	25-33

INDICATIONS AND USAGE

CIPRO XR is indicated only for the treatment of urinary tract infections, including acute uncomplicated pyelonephritis, caused by susceptible strains of the designated microorganisms as listed below. CIPRO XR and ciprofloxacin immediate-release tablets are not interchangeable. Please see **DOSAGE AND ADMINISTRATION** for specific recommendations.

Uncomplicated Urinary Tract Infections (Acute Cystitis) caused by *Escherichia coli, Proteus mirabilis, Enterococcus faecalis*, or *Staphylococcus saprophyticus*[a].

Complicated Urinary Tract Infections caused by *Escherichia coli, Klebsiella pneumoniae, Enterococcus faecalis, Proteus mirabilis*, or *Pseudomonas aeruginosa*[a].

Acute Uncomplicated Pyelonephritis caused by *Escherichia coli.*

[a]Treatment of infections due to this organism in the organ system was studied in fewer than 10 patients.

THE SAFETY AND EFFICACY OF CIPRO XR IN TREATING INFECTIONS OTHER THAN URINARY TRACT INFECTIONS HAS NOT BEEN DEMONSTRATED. Appropriate culture and susceptibility tests should be performed before treatment in order to isolate and identify organisms causing infection and to determine their susceptibility to ciprofloxacin. Therapy with CIPRO XR may be initiated before results of these tests are known; once results become available appropriate therapy should be continued. Culture and susceptibility testing performed periodically during therapy will provide information not only on the therapeutic effect of the antimicrobial agent but also on the possible emergence of bacterial resistance.

To reduce the development of drug-resistant bacteria and maintain the effectiveness of CIPRO XR and other antibacterial drugs, CIPRO XR should be used only to treat or prevent infections that are proven or strongly suspected to be caused by susceptible bacteria. When culture and susceptibility information are available, they should be considered in selecting or modifying antibacterial therapy. In the absence of such data, local epidemiology and susceptibility patterns may contribute to the empiric selection of therapy.

CONTRAINDICATIONS

Ciprofloxacin is contraindicated in persons with a history of hypersensitivity to ciprofloxacin, any member of the quinolone class of antimicrobial agents, or any of the product components.

Concomitant administration with tizanidine is contraindicated. (See **PRECAUTIONS: Drug Interactions.**)

WARNINGS

Tendinopathy and Tendon Rupture: Fluoroquinolones, including CIPRO XR, are associated with an increased risk of tendinitis and tendon rupture in all ages. This adverse reaction most frequently involves the Achilles tendon, and rupture of the Achilles tendon may require surgical repair. Tendinitis and tendon rupture in the rotator cuff (the shoulder), the hand, the biceps, the thumb, and other tendon sites have also been reported. The risk of developing fluoroquinolone-associated tendinitis and tendon rupture is further increased in older patients usually over 60 years of age, in patients taking corticosteroid drugs, and in patients with kidney, heart or lung transplants. Factors, in addition to age and corticosteroid use, that may independently increase the risk of tendon rupture include strenuous physical activity, renal failure, and previous tendon disorders such as rheumatoid arthritis. Tendinitis and tendon rupture have also occurred in patients taking fluoroquinolones who do not have the above risk factors. Tendon rupture can occur during or after completion of therapy; cases occurring up to several months after completion of therapy have been reported. CIPRO XR should be discontinued if the patient experiences pain, swelling, inflammation or rupture of a tendon. Patients should be advised to rest at the first sign of tendinitis or tendon rupture, and to contact their healthcare provider regarding changing to a non-quinolone antimicrobial drug.

THE SAFETY AND EFFECTIVENESS OF CIPRO XR IN PEDIATRIC PATIENTS AND ADOLESCENTS (UNDER THE AGE OF 18 YEARS), PREGNANT WOMEN, AND NURSING WOMEN HAVE NOT BEEN ESTABLISHED. (See **PRECAUTIONS: Pediatric Use, Pregnancy,** and **Nursing Mothers** subsections.) The oral administration of ciprofloxacin caused lameness in immature dogs. Histopathological examination of the weight-bearing joints of these dogs revealed permanent lesions of the cartilage. Related quinolone-class drugs also produce erosions of cartilage of weight-bearing joints and other signs of arthropathy in immature animals of various species. (See **ANIMAL PHARMACOLOGY.**)

Cytochrome P450 (CYP450): Ciprofloxacin is an inhibitor of the hepatic CYP1A2 enzyme pathway. Coadministration of ciprofloxacin and other drugs primarily metabolized by CYP1A2 (e.g. theophylline, methylxanthines, tizanidine) results in increased plasma concentrations of the coadministered drug and could lead to clinically significant pharmacodynamic side effects of the coadministered drug.

Convulsions, increased intracranial pressure, and toxic psychosis have been reported in patients receiving quinolones, including ciprofloxacin. Ciprofloxacin may also cause central nervous system (CNS) events including: dizziness, confusion, tremors, hallucinations, depression, and, rarely, suicidal thoughts or acts. These reactions may occur following the first dose. If these reactions occur in patients receiving ciprofloxacin, the drug should be discontinued and appropriate measures instituted. As with all quinolones, ciprofloxacin should be used with caution in patients with known or suspected CNS disorders that may predispose to seizures or lower the seizure threshold (e.g. severe cerebral arteriosclerosis, epilepsy), or in the presence of other risk factors that may predispose to seizures or lower the seizure threshold (e.g. certain drug therapy, renal dysfunction). (See **PRECAUTIONS: General, Information for Patients, Drug Interactions** and **ADVERSE REACTIONS.**)

SERIOUS AND FATAL REACTIONS HAVE BEEN REPORTED IN PATIENTS RECEIVING CONCURRENT ADMINISTRATION OF CIPROFLOXACIN AND THEOPHYLLINE. These reactions have included cardiac arrest, seizure, status epilepticus, and respiratory failure. Although similar serious adverse effects have been reported in patients receiving theophylline alone, the possibility that these reactions may be potentiated by ciprofloxacin cannot be eliminated. If concomitant use cannot be avoided, serum levels of theophylline should be monitored and dosage adjustments made as appropriate.

Serious and occasionally fatal hypersensitivity (anaphylactic) reactions, some following the first dose, have been reported in patients receiving quinolone therapy. Some reactions were accompanied by cardiovascular collapse, loss of consciousness, tingling, pharyngeal or facial edema, dyspnea, urticaria, and itching. Only a few patients had a history of hypersensitivity reactions. Serious anaphylactic reactions require immediate emergency treatment with epinephrine. Oxygen, intravenous steroids, and airway management, including intubation, should be administered as indicated.

Other serious and sometimes fatal events, some due to hypersensitivity, and some due to uncertain etiology, have been reported rarely in patients receiving therapy with quinolones, including ciprofloxacin. These events may be severe and generally occur following the administration of multiple doses. Clinical manifestations may include one or more of the following:

- fever, rash, or severe dermatologic reactions (e.g., toxic epidermal necrolysis, Stevens-Johnson syndrome);
- vasculitis; arthralgia; myalgia; serum sickness;
- allergic pneumonitis;
- interstitial nephritis; acute renal insufficiency or failure;
- hepatitis; jaundice; acute hepatic necrosis or failure;
- anemia, including hemolytic and aplastic; thrombocytopenia, including thrombotic thrombocytopenic purpura; leukopenia; agranulocytosis; pancytopenia; and/or other hematologic abnormalities.

The drug should be discontinued immediately at the first appearance of a skin rash, jaundice, or any other sign of hypersensitivity and supportive measures instituted (See **PRECAUTIONS: Information for Patients** and **ADVERSE REACTIONS**).

Clostridium difficile associated diarrhea (CDAD) has been reported with use of nearly all antibacterial agents, including CIPRO, and may range in severity from mild diarrhea to fatal colitis. Treatment with antibacterial agents alters the normal flora of the colon leading to overgrowth of *C. difficile.* *C. difficile* produces toxins A and B which contribute to the development of CDAD. Hypertoxin producing strains of *C. difficile* cause increased morbidity and mortality, as these infections can be refractory to antimicrobial therapy and may require colectomy. CDAD must be considered in all pa-

tients who present with diarrhea following antibiotic use. Careful medical history is necessary since CDAD has been reported to occur over two months after the administration of antibacterial agents.

If CDAD is suspected or confirmed, ongoing antibiotic use not directed against *C. difficile* may need to be discontinued. Appropriate fluid and electrolyte management, protein supplementation, antibiotic treatment of *C. difficile,* and surgical evaluation should be instituted as clinically indicated.

Peripheral neuropathy: Rare cases of sensory or sensorimotor axonal polyneuropathy affecting small and/or large axons resulting in paresthesias, hypoesthesias, dysesthesias and weakness have been reported in patients receiving quinolones, including ciprofloxacin. Ciprofloxacin should be discontinued if the patient experiences symptoms of neuropathy including pain, burning, tingling, numbness, and/or weakness, or is found to have deficits in light touch, pain, temperature, position sense, vibratory sensation, and/or motor strength in order to prevent the development of an irreversible condition.

PRECAUTIONS

General:

Crystals of ciprofloxacin have been observed rarely in the urine of human subjects but more frequently in the urine of laboratory animals, which is usually alkaline. (See **ANIMAL PHARMACOLOGY.**) Crystalluria related to ciprofloxacin has been reported only rarely in humans because human urine is usually acidic. Alkalinity of the urine should be avoided in patients receiving ciprofloxacin. Patients should be well hydrated to prevent the formation of highly concentrated urine.

Quinolones, including ciprofloxacin, may also cause central nervous system (CNS) events, including: nervousness, agitation, insomnia, anxiety, nightmares or paranoia. (See **WARNINGS, Information for Patients,** and **Drug Interactions.**)

Photosensitivity/Phototoxicity:

Moderate to severe photosensitivity/phototoxicity reactions, the latter of which may manifest as exaggerated sunburn reactions (e.g., burning, erythema, exudation, vesicles, blistering, edema) involving areas exposed to light (typically the face, "V" area of the neck, extensor surfaces of the forearms, dorsa of the hands), can be associated with the use of quinolones after sun or UV light exposure. Therefore, excessive exposure to these sources of light should be avoided. Drug therapy should be discontinued if phototoxicity occurs (See **ADVERSE REACTIONS.**)

Prescribing CIPRO XR in the absence of a proven or strongly suspected bacterial infection or a prophylactic indication is unlikely to provide benefit to the patient and increases the risk of the development of drug-resistant bacteria.

Information for Patients:

Patients should be advised:

- to contact their healthcare provider if they experience pain, swelling, or inflammation of a tendon, or weakness or inability to use one of their joints; rest and refrain from exercise; and discontinue CIPRO XR treatment. The risk of severe tendon disorder with fluoroquinolones is higher in older patients usually over 60 years of age, in patients taking corticosteroid drugs, and in patients with kidney, heart or lung transplants.
- that antibacterial drugs including CIPRO XR should only be used to treat bacterial infections. They do not treat viral infections (e.g., the common cold). When CIPRO XR is prescribed to treat a bacterial infection, patients should be told that although it is common to feel better early in the course of therapy, the medication should be taken exactly as directed. Skipping doses or not completing the full course of therapy may (1) decrease the effectiveness of the immediate treatment and (2) increase the likelihood that bacteria will develop resistance and will not be treatable by CIPRO XR or other antibacterial drugs in the future.
- that CIPRO XR may be taken with or without meals and to drink fluids liberally. As with other quinolones, concurrent administration with magnesium/aluminum antacids, or sucralfate, VIDEX® (didanosine) chewable/buffered tablets or pediatric powder, other highly buffered drugs, or with other products containing calcium, iron, or zinc should be avoided. CIPRO XR may be taken two hours before or six hours after taking these products. (See **CLINICAL PHARMACOLOGY, Drug-drug Interactions, DOSAGE AND ADMINISTRATION,** and **PRECAUTIONS, Drug Interactions.**) CIPRO XR should not be taken with dairy products (like milk or yogurt) or calcium-fortified juices alone since absorption of ciprofloxacin may be significantly reduced; however, CIPRO XR may be taken with a meal that contains these products. (See **CLINICAL PHARMACOLOGY, Drug-drug Interactions, DOSAGE AND ADMINISTRATION,** and **PRECAUTIONS, Drug Interactions.**)
- if the patient should forget to take CIPRO XR at the usual time, he/she may take the dose later in the day. Do not

take more than one CIPRO XR tablet per day even if a patient misses a dose. Swallow the CIPRO XR tablet whole. **DO NOT SPLIT, CRUSH, OR CHEW THE TABLET.**

- that ciprofloxacin may be associated with hypersensitivity reactions, even following a single dose, and to discontinue CIPRO XR at the first sign of a skin rash or other allergic reaction.
- that photosensitivity/phototoxicity has been reported in patients receiving quinolones. Patients should minimize or avoid exposure to natural or artificial sunlight (tanning beds or UVA/B treatment) while taking quinolones. If patients need to be outdoors while using quinolones, they should wear loose-fitting clothes that protect skin from sun exposure and discuss other sun protection measures with their physician. If a sunburn-like reaction or skin eruption occurs, patients should contact their physician
- that peripheral neuropathies have been associated with ciprofloxacin use. If symptoms of peripheral neuropathy including pain, burning, tingling, numbness and/or weakness develop, they should discontinue treatment and contact their physicians.
- that CIPRO XR may cause dizziness and lightheadedness; therefore, patients should know how they react to this drug before they operate an automobile or machinery or engage in activities requiring mental alertness or coordination.
- that ciprofloxacin increases the effects of tizanidine (Zanaflex®). Patients should not use ciprofloxacin if they are already taking tizanidine.
- that CIPRO XR may increase the effects of theophylline and caffeine. There is a possibility of caffeine accumulation when products containing caffeine are consumed while taking quinolones.
- that convulsions have been reported in patients receiving quinolones, including ciprofloxacin, and to notify their physician before taking CIPRO XR if there is a history of this condition.
- that diarrhea is a common problem caused by antibiotics which usually ends when the antibiotic is discontinued. Sometimes after starting treatment with antibiotics, patients can develop watery and bloody stools (with or without stomach cramps and fever) even as late as two or more months after having taken the last dose of the antibiotic. If this occurs, patients should contact their physician as soon as possible.

Drug Interactions:

In a pharmacokinetic study, systemic exposure of tizanidine (4 mg single dose) was significantly increased (C_{max} 7-fold, AUC 10-fold) when the drug was given concomitantly with ciprofloxacin (500 mg bid for 3 days). The hypotensive and sedative effects of tizanidine were also potentiated. Concomitant administration of tizanidine and ciprofloxacin is contraindicated.

As with some other quinolones, concurrent administration of ciprofloxacin with theophylline may lead to elevated serum concentrations of theophylline and prolongation of its elimination half-life. This may result in increased risk of theophylline-related adverse reactions. (See **WARNINGS.**) If concomitant use cannot be avoided, serum levels of theophylline should be monitored and dosage adjustments made as appropriate.

Some quinolones, including ciprofloxacin, have also been shown to interfere with the metabolism of caffeine. This may lead to reduced clearance of caffeine and a prolongation of its serum half-life.

Concurrent administration of a quinolone, including ciprofloxacin, with multivalent cation-containing products such as magnesium/aluminum antacids, sucralfate, VIDEX® (didanosine) chewable/buffered tablets or pediatric powder, other highly buffered drugs, or products containing calcium, iron, or zinc may substantially interfere with the absorption of the quinolone, resulting in serum and urine levels considerably lower than desired. CIPRO XR should be administered at least 2 hours before or 6 hours after antacids containing magnesium or aluminum, as well as sucralfate, VIDEX® (didanosine) chewable/buffered tablets or pediatric powder, other highly buffered drugs, metal cations such as iron, and multivitamin preparations with zinc. (See **CLINICAL PHARMACOLOGY, Drug-drug Interactions, PRECAUTIONS, Information for Patients,** and **DOSAGE AND ADMINISTRATION.**)

Histamine H_2-receptor antagonists appear to have no significant effect on the bioavailability of ciprofloxacin.

Absorption of the CIPRO XR tablet was slightly diminished (20%) when given concomitantly with omeprazole. (See **CLINICAL PHARMACOLOGY, Drug-drug Interactions.**) Altered serum levels of phenytoin (increased and decreased) have been reported in patients receiving concomitant ciprofloxacin.

The concomitant administration of ciprofloxacin with the sulfonylurea glyburide has, on rare occasions, resulted in severe hypoglycemia.

Some quinolones, including ciprofloxacin, have been associated with transient elevations in serum creatinine in patients receiving cyclosporine concomitantly.

Quinolones, including ciprofloxacin, have been reported to enhance the effects of the oral anticoagulant warfarin or its derivatives. When these products are administered concomitantly, prothrombin time or other suitable coagulation tests should be closely monitored.

Probenecid interferes with renal tubular secretion of ciprofloxacin and produces an increase in the level of ciprofloxacin in the serum. This should be considered if patients are receiving both drugs concomitantly.

Renal tubular transport of methotrexate may be inhibited by concomitant administration of ciprofloxacin potentially leading to increased plasma levels of methotrexate. This might increase the risk of methotrexate associated toxic reactions. Therefore, patients under methotrexate therapy should be carefully monitored when concomitant ciprofloxacin therapy is indicated.

Metoclopramide significantly accelerates the absorption of oral ciprofloxacin resulting in a shorter time to reach maximum plasma concentrations. No significant effect was observed on the bioavailability of ciprofloxacin.

Non-steroidal anti-inflammatory drugs (but not acetyl salicylic acid) in combination of very high doses of quinolones have been shown to provoke convulsions in pre-clinical studies.

Carcinogenesis, Mutagenesis, Impairment of Fertility:
Eight *in vitro* mutagenicity tests have been conducted with ciprofloxacin, and the test results are listed below:

Salmonella/Microsome Test (Negative)
E. coli DNA Repair Assay (Negative)
Mouse Lymphoma Cell Forward Mutation Assay (Positive)
Chinese Hamster V_{79} Cell HGPRT Test (Negative)
Syrian Hamster Embryo Cell Transformation Assay (Negative)
Saccharomyces cerevisiae Point Mutation Assay (Negative)
Saccharomyces cerevisiae Mitotic Crossover and Gene Conversion Assay (Negative)
Rat Hepatocyte DNA Repair Assay (Positive)

Thus, 2 of the 8 tests were positive, but results of the following 3 *in vivo* test systems gave negative results:

Rat Hepatocyte DNA Repair Assay
Micronucleus Test (Mice)
Dominant Lethal Test (Mice)

Ciprofloxacin was not carcinogenic or tumorigenic in 2-year carcinogenicity studies with rats and mice at daily oral dose levels of 250 and 750 mg/kg, respectively (approximately 2- and 3-fold greater than the 1000 mg daily human dose based upon body surface area).

Results from photo co-carcinogenicity testing indicate that ciprofloxacin does not reduce the time to appearance of UV-induced skin tumors as compared to vehicle control. Hairless (Skh-1) mice were exposed to UVA light for 3.5 hours five times every two weeks for up to 78 weeks while concurrently being administered ciprofloxacin. The time to development of the first skin tumors was 50 weeks in mice treated concomitantly with UVA and ciprofloxacin (mouse dose approximately equal to the maximum recommended daily human dose of 1000 mg based upon mg/m²), as opposed to 34 weeks when animals were treated with both UVA and vehicle. The times to development of skin tumors ranged from 16-32 weeks in mice treated concomitantly with UVA and other quinolones.

In this model, mice treated with ciprofloxacin alone did not develop skin or systemic tumors. There are no data from similar models using pigmented mice and/or fully haired mice. The clinical significance of these findings to humans is unknown.

Fertility studies performed in rats at oral doses of ciprofloxacin up to 100 mg/kg (1.0 times the highest recommended daily human dose of 1000 mg based upon body surface area) revealed no evidence of impairment.

Pregnancy
Teratogenic Effects
Pregnancy Category C:
There are no adequate and well-controlled studies in pregnant women. An expert review of published data on experiences with ciprofloxacin use during pregnancy by TERIS – the Teratogen Information System – concluded that therapeutic doses during pregnancy are unlikely to pose a substantial teratogenic risk (quantity and quality of data=fair), but the data are insufficient to state there is no risk.

A controlled prospective observational study followed 200 women exposed to fluoroquinolones (52.5% exposed to ciprofloxacin and 68% first trimester exposures) during gestation. In utero exposure to fluoroquinolones during embryogenesis was not associated with increased risk of major malformations. The reported rates of major congenital malformations were 2.2% for the fluoroquinolone group and 2.6% for the control group (background incidence of major malformations is 1-5%). Rates of spontaneous abortions, prematurity and low birth weight did not differ between the groups and there were no clinically significant musculoskeletal dysfunctions up to one year of age in the ciprofloxacin exposed children.

Another prospective follow-up study reported on 549 pregnancies with fluoroquinolone exposure (93% first trimester exposures). There were 70 ciprofloxacin exposures, all within the first trimester. The malformation rates among live-born babies exposed to ciprofloxacin and to fluoroquinolones overall were both within background incidence ranges. No specific patterns of congenital abnormalities were found. The study did not reveal any clear adverse reactions due to in utero exposure to ciprofloxacin.

No differences in the rates of prematurity, spontaneous abortions, or birth weight were seen in women exposed to ciprofloxacin during pregnancy. However, these small post-marketing epidemiology studies, of which most experience is from short term, first trimester exposure, are insufficient to evaluate the risk for the less common defects or to permit reliable and definitive conclusions regarding the safety of ciprofloxacin in pregnant women and their developing fetuses. Ciprofloxacin should not be used during pregnancy unless potential benefit justifies the potential risk to both fetus and mother (see **WARNINGS**).

Reproduction studies have been performed in rats and mice using oral doses up to 100 mg/kg (0.7 and 0.4 times the maximum daily human dose of 1000 mg based upon body surface area, respectively) and have revealed no evidence of harm to the fetus due to ciprofloxacin. In rabbits, ciprofloxacin (30 and 100 mg/kg orally) produced gastrointestinal disturbances resulting in maternal weight loss and an increased incidence of abortion, but no teratogenicity was observed at either dose. After intravenous administration of doses up to 20 mg/kg, no maternal toxicity was produced in the rabbit, and no embryotoxicity or teratogenicity was observed.

Nursing Mothers:
Ciprofloxacin is excreted in human milk. The amount of ciprofloxacin absorbed by the nursing infant is unknown. Because of the potential for serious adverse reactions in infants nursing from mothers taking ciprofloxacin, a decision should be made whether to discontinue nursing or to discontinue the drug, taking into account the importance of the drug to the mother.

Pediatric Use:
Safety and effectiveness of CIPRO XR in pediatric patients and adolescents less than 18 years of age have not been established. Ciprofloxacin causes arthropathy in juvenile animals. (See **WARNINGS**.)

Geriatric Use:
Geriatric patients are at increased risk for developing severe tendon disorders including tendon rupture when being treated with a fluoroquinolone such as CIPRO XR. This risk is further increased in patients receiving concomitant corticosteroid therapy. Tendinitis or tendon rupture can involve the Achilles, hand, shoulder, or other tendon sites and can occur during or after completion of therapy; cases occurring up to several months after fluoroquinolone treatment have been reported. Caution should be used when prescribing CIPRO XR to elderly patients especially those on corticosteroids. Patients should be informed of this potential side effect and advised to discontinue CIPRO XR and contact their healthcare provider if any symptoms of tendinitis or tendon rupture occur (See **BOXED WARNING, WARNINGS,** and **ADVERSE REACTIONS**).

In a large, prospective, randomized CIPRO XR clinical trial in complicated urinary tract infections, 49% (509/1035) of the patients were 65 and over, while 30% (308/1035) were 75 and over. No overall differences in safety or effectiveness were observed between these subjects and younger subjects, and clinical experience with other formulations of ciprofloxacin has not identified differences in responses between the elderly and younger patients, but greater sensitivity of some older individuals cannot be ruled out. Ciprofloxacin is known to be substantially excreted by the kidney, and the risk of adverse reactions may be greater in patients with impaired renal function. No alteration of dosage is necessary for patients greater than 65 years of age with normal renal function. However, since some older individuals experience reduced renal function by virtue of their advanced age, care should be taken in dose selection for elderly patients, and renal function monitoring may be useful in these patients. (See **CLINICAL PHARMACOLOGY** and **DOSAGE AND ADMINISTRATION**.)

In general, elderly patients may be more susceptible to drug-associated effects on the QT interval. Therefore, precaution should be taken when using CIPRO XR with concomitant drugs that can result in prolongation of the QT interval (e.g., class IA or class III antiarrhythmics) or in patients with risk factors for torsade de pointes (e.g., known QT prolongation, uncorrected hypokalemia).

ADVERSE REACTIONS
Clinical trials in patients with urinary tract infections enrolled 961 patients treated with 500 mg or 1000 mg CIPRO XR. Most adverse events reported were described as mild to moderate in severity and required no treatment. The overall incidence, type and distribution of adverse events were similar in patients receiving both 500 mg and 1000 mg of CIPRO XR. Because clinical trials are conducted under widely varying conditions, adverse reaction rates observed in clinical trials of a drug cannot be directly compared to rates observed in clinical trials of another drug and may not reflect the rates observed in practice. The adverse reaction information from clinical studies does, however, provide a basis for identifying the adverse events that appear to be related to drug use and for approximating rates.

In the clinical trial of uncomplicated urinary tract infection, CIPRO XR (500 mg once daily) in 444 patients was compared to ciprofloxacin immediate-release tablets (250 mg twice daily) in 447 patients for 3 days. Discontinuations due to adverse reactions thought to be drug-related occurred in 0.2% (1/444) of patients in the CIPRO XR arm and in 0% (0/447) of patients in the control arm.

In the clinical trial of complicated urinary tract infection and acute uncomplicated pyelonephritis, CIPRO XR (1000 mg once daily) in 517 patients was compared to ciprofloxacin immediate-release tablets (500 mg twice daily) in 518 patients for 7 to 14 days. Discontinuations due to adverse reactions thought to be drug-related occurred in 3.1% (16/517) of patients in the CIPRO XR arm and in 2.3% (12/518) of patients in the control arm. The most common reasons for discontinuation in the CIPRO XR arm were nausea/vomiting (4 patients) and dizziness (3 patients). In the control arm the most common reason for discontinuation was nausea/vomiting (3 patients).

In these clinical trials, the following events occurred in ≥ 2% of all CIPRO XR patients, regardless of drug relationship: nausea (4%), headache (3%), dizziness (2%), diarrhea (2%), vomiting (2%) and vaginal moniliasis (2%).

Adverse events, judged by investigators to be at least possibly drug-related, occurring in greater than or equal to 1% of all CIPRO XR treated patients were: nausea (3%), diarrhea (2%), headache (1%), dyspepsia (1%), dizziness (1%), and vaginal moniliasis (1%). Vomiting (1%) occurred in the 1000 mg group.

Additional uncommon events, judged by investigators to be at least possibly drug-related, that occurred in less than 1% of CIPRO XR treated patients were:

BODY AS A WHOLE: abdominal pain, asthenia, malaise, photosensitivity reaction
CARDIOVASCULAR: bradycardia, migraine, syncope
DIGESTIVE: anorexia, constipation, dry mouth, flatulence, liver function tests abnormal, thirst
HEMIC/LYMPHATIC: prothrombin decrease
CENTRAL NERVOUS SYSTEM: abnormal dreams, depersonalization, depression, hypertonia, incoordination, insomnia, somnolence, tremor, vertigo
METABOLIC: hyperglycemia
SKIN/HYPERSENSIVITY: dry skin, maculopapular rash, photosensitivity/phototoxicity reactions, pruritus, rash, skin disorder, urticaria, vesiculobullous rash
SPECIAL SENSES: diplopia, taste perversion
UROGENITAL: dysmenorrhea, hematuria, kidney function abnormal, vaginitis

The following additional adverse events, some of them life threatening, regardless of incidence or relationship to drug, have been reported during clinical trials and from worldwide post-marketing experience in patients given ciprofloxacin (includes all formulations, all dosages, all drug-therapy durations, and all indications). Because these reactions have been reported voluntarily from a population of uncertain size, it is not always possible to reliably estimate their frequency or a causal relationship to drug exposure. The events in alphabetical order are:

abnormal gait, achiness, acidosis, agitation, agranulocytosis, allergic reactions (ranging from urticaria to anaphylactic reactions and including life-threatening anaphylactic shock), amylase increase, anemia, angina pectoris, angioedema, anosmia, anxiety, arrhythmia, arthralgia, ataxia, atrial flutter, bleeding diathesis, blurred vision, bronchospasm, *C. difficile* associated diarrhea, candidiasis (cutaneous, oral), candiduria, cardiac murmur, cardiopulmonary arrest, cardiovascular collapse, cerebral thrombosis, chills, cholestatic jaundice, chromatopsia, confusion, convulsion, delirium, drowsiness, dysphagia, dysphasia, dyspnea, edema (conjunctivae, face, hands, laryngeal, lips, lower extremities, neck, pulmonary), epistaxis, erythema multiforme, erythema nodosum, exfoliative dermatitis, fever, fixed eruptions, flushing, gastrointestinal bleeding, gout (flare up), grand mal convulsion, gynecomastia, hallucinations, hearing loss, hemolytic anemia, hemoptysis, hemorrhagic cystitis, hepatic failure (including fatal cases), hepatic necrosis, hepatitis, hiccup, hyperesthesia, hyperpigmentation, hypertension, hypertonia, hypesthesia, hypotension, ileus, interstitial nephritis, intestinal perforation, jaundice, joint stiffness, lethargy, lightheadedness, lipase increase, lymphadenopathy, manic reaction, marrow depression, migraine, moniliasis (oral, gastrointestinal,

DOSAGE GUIDELINES

Indication	Unit Dose	Frequency	Usual Duration
Uncomplicated Urinary Tract Infection (Acute Cystitis)	500 mg	Q24h	3 Days
Complicated Urinary Tract Infection	1000 mg	Q24h	7-14 Days
Acute Uncomplicated Pyelonephritis	1000 mg	Q24h	7-14 Days

	CIPRO XR 500 mg QD × 3 Days	CIPRO 250 mg BID × 3 Days
Randomized Patients	452	453
Per Protocol Patients*	199	223
Bacteriologic Eradication at TOC (n/N)†	188/199 (94.5%)	209/223 (93.7%)
	CI [-3.5%, 5.1%]	
Bacteriologic Eradication (by organism) at TOC (n/N)‡		
E. coli	156/160 (97.5%)	176/181 (97.2%)
E. faecalis	10/11 (90.9%)	17/21 (81.0%)
P. mirabilis	11/12 (91.7%)	7/7 (100%)
S. saprophyticus	6/7 (85.7%)	9/9 (100%)
Clinical Response at TOC (n/N)§	189/199 (95.0%)	204/223 (91.5%)
	CI [-1.1%, 8.1%]	

* The presence of a pathogen at a level of $\geq 10^5$ CFU/mL was required for microbiological evaluability criteria, except for S. saprophyticus ($\geq 10^4$ CFU/mL).
† n/N =patients with baseline organism(s) eradicated and no new infections or superinfections/total number of patients
‡ n/N =patients with specified baseline organism eradicated/patients with specified baseline organism
§ n/N = patients with clinical success/total number of patients

vaginal), myalgia, myasthenia, myasthenia gravis (possible exacerbation), myocardial infarction, myoclonus, nephritis, nightmares, nystagmus, oral ulceration, pain (arm, back, breast, chest, epigastric, eye, extremities, foot, jaw, neck, oral mucosa), palpitation, pancreatitis, pancytopenia, paranoia, paresthesia, peripheral neuropathy, perspiration (increased), petechia, phlebitis, phobia, photosensitivity/phototoxicity reaction pleural effusion, polyuria, postural hypotension, prothrombin time prolongation, pseudomembranous colitis (the onset of symptoms may occur during or after antimicrobial treatment), pulmonary embolism, purpura, renal calculi, renal failure, respiratory distress, respiratory arrest, restlessness, serum sickness-like reaction, Stevens-Johnson syndrome, sweating, tachycardia, taste loss, tendinitis, tendon rupture, tinnitus, torsade de pointes, toxic epidermal necrolysis (Lyell's syndrome), toxic psychosis, twitching, unresponsiveness, urethral bleeding, urinary retention, urination (frequent), vaginal pruritus, vasculitis, ventricular ectopy, vesicles, visual acuity (decreased), visual disturbances (flashing lights, change in color perception, overbrightness of lights).

Laboratory Changes:
The following adverse laboratory changes, in alphabetical order, regardless of incidence or relationship to drug, have been reported in patients given ciprofloxacin (includes all formulations, all dosages, all drug-therapy durations, and all indications):
Decreases in blood glucose, BUN, hematocrit, hemoglobin, leukocyte counts, platelet counts, prothrombin time, serum albumin, serum potassium, total serum protein, uric acid.
Increases in alkaline phosphatase, ALT (SGPT), AST (SGOT), atypical lymphocyte counts, blood glucose, blood monocytes, BUN, cholesterol, eosinophil counts, LDH, platelet counts, prothrombin time, sedimentation rate, serum amylase, serum bilirubin, serum calcium, serum cholesterol, serum creatine phosphokinase, serum creatinine, serum gamma-glutamyl transpeptidase (GGT), serum potassium, serum theophylline (in patients receiving theophylline concomitantly), serum triglycerides, uric acid.
Others: albuminuria, change in serum phenytoin, crystalluria, cylindruria, immature WBCs, leukocytosis, methemoglobinemia, pancytopenia.

OVERDOSAGE
In the event of acute excessive overdosage, reversible renal toxicity has been reported in some cases. The stomach should be emptied by inducing vomiting or by gastric lavage. The patient should be carefully observed and given supportive treatment, including monitoring of renal function and administration of magnesium or calcium containing antacids which can reduce the absorption of ciprofloxacin. Adequate hydration must be maintained. Only a small amount of ciprofloxacin (< 10%) is removed from the body after hemodialysis or peritoneal dialysis.
In mice, rats, rabbits and dogs, significant toxicity including tonic/clonic convulsions was observed at intravenous doses of ciprofloxacin between 125 and 300 mg/kg.
Single doses of ciprofloxacin were relatively non-toxic via the oral route of administration in mice, rats, and dogs. No deaths occurred within a 14-day post treatment observation period at the highest oral doses tested; up to 5000 mg/kg in either rodent species, or up to 2500 mg/kg in the dog. Clinical signs observed included hypoactivity and cyanosis in both rodent species and severe vomiting in dogs. In rabbits, significant mortality was seen at doses of ciprofloxacin > 2500 mg/kg. Mortality was delayed in these animals, occurring 10-14 days after dosing.

DOSAGE AND ADMINISTRATION
CIPRO XR and ciprofloxacin immediate-release tablets are not interchangeable. Cipro XR should be administered orally once daily as described in the following Dosage Guidelines table:
[See first table above]
Patients whose therapy is started with CIPRO I.V. for urinary tract infections may be switched to CIPRO XR when clinically indicated at the discretion of the physician.
CIPRO XR should be administered at least 2 hours before or 6 hours after antacids containing magnesium or aluminum, as well as sucralfate, VIDEX® (didanosine) chewable/buffered tablets or pediatric powder, other highly buffered drugs, metal cations such as iron, and multivitamin preparations with zinc. Although CIPRO XR may be taken with meals that include milk, concomitant administration with dairy products alone, or with calcium-fortified products should be avoided, since decreased absorption is possible. A 2-hour window between substantial calcium intake (> 800 mg) and dosing with CIPRO XR is recommended. CIPRO XR should be swallowed whole. DO NOT SPLIT, CRUSH, OR CHEW THE TABLET. (See CLINICAL PHARMACOLOGY, Drug-drug Interactions, PRECAUTIONS, Drug Interactions and Information for Patients.)
Impaired Renal Function:
Ciprofloxacin is eliminated primarily by renal excretion; however, the drug is also metabolized and partially cleared through the biliary system of the liver and through the intestine. These alternate pathways of drug elimination appear to compensate for the reduced renal excretion in patients with renal impairment. No dosage adjustment is required for patients with uncomplicated urinary tract infections receiving 500 mg CIPRO XR. In patients with complicated urinary tract infections and acute uncomplicated

pyelonephritis, who have a creatinine clearance of < 30 mL/min, the dose of CIPRO XR should be reduced from 1000 mg to 500 mg daily. For patients on hemodialysis or peritoneal dialysis, administer CIPRO XR after the dialysis procedure is completed. (See CLINICAL PHARMACOLOGY, Special Populations and PRECAUTIONS, Geriatric Use.)
Impaired Hepatic Function:
No dosage adjustment is required with CIPRO XR in patients with stable chronic cirrhosis. The kinetics of ciprofloxacin in patients with acute hepatic insufficiency, however, have not been fully elucidated. (See CLINICAL PHARMACOLOGY, Special Populations.)

HOW SUPPLIED
CIPRO XR is available as nearly white to slightly yellowish, film-coated, oblong-shaped tablets containing 500 mg or 1000 mg ciprofloxacin. The 500 mg tablet is coded with the word "BAYER" on one side and "C500 QD" on the reverse side. The 1000 mg tablet is coded with the word "BAYER" on one side and "C1000 QD" on the reverse side.

	Strength	NDC Code
Bottles of 50	500 mg	0085-1775-02
Bottles of 100	500 mg	0085-1775-01
Bottles of 50	1000 mg	0085-1778-03
Bottles of 100	1000 mg	0085-1778-01
Unit Dose Pack of 30	1000 mg	0085-1778-02

Store at 25°C (77°F); excursions permitted to 15-30°C (59-86°F) [see USP Controlled Room Temperature].

ANIMAL PHARMACOLOGY
Ciprofloxacin and other quinolones have been shown to cause arthropathy in immature animals of most species tested. (See WARNINGS.) Damage of weight bearing joints was observed in juvenile dogs and rats. In young beagles, 100 mg/kg ciprofloxacin, given daily for 4 weeks, caused degenerative articular changes of the knee joint. At 30 mg/kg, the effect on the joint was minimal. In a subsequent study in beagles, removal of weight bearing from the joint reduced the lesions but did not totally prevent them.
Crystalluria, sometimes associated with secondary nephropathy, occurs in laboratory animals dosed with ciprofloxacin. This is primarily related to the reduced solubility of ciprofloxacin under alkaline conditions, which predominate in the urine of test animals; in man, crystalluria is rare since human urine is typically acidic. In rhesus monkeys, crystalluria without nephropathy has been noted after single oral doses as low as 5 mg/kg. After 6 months of intravenous dosing at 10 mg/kg/day, no nephropathological changes were noted; however, nephropathy was observed after dosing at 20 mg/kg/day for the same duration.
In mice, concomitant administration of nonsteroidal anti-inflammatory drugs such as phenylbutazone and indomethacin with quinolones has been reported to enhance the CNS stimulatory effect of quinolones.
Ocular toxicity seen with some related drugs has not been observed in ciprofloxacin-treated animals.

CLINICAL STUDIES
Uncomplicated Urinary Tract Infections (acute cystitis)
CIPRO XR was evaluated for the treatment of uncomplicated urinary tract infections (acute cystitis) in a randomized, double-blind, controlled clinical trial conducted in the US. This study compared CIPRO XR (500 mg once daily for three days) with ciprofloxacin immediate-release tablets (CIPRO® 250 mg BID for three days). Of the 905 patients enrolled, 452 were randomly assigned to the CIPRO XR treatment group and 453 were randomly assigned to the control group. The primary efficacy variable was bacteriologic eradication of the baseline organism(s) with no new infection or superinfection at test-of-cure (Day 4-11 Post-therapy).
The bacteriologic eradication and clinical success rates were similar between CIPRO XR and the control group. The eradication and clinical success rates and their corresponding 95% confidence intervals for the differences between rates (CIPRO XR minus control group) are given in the following table:
[See second table above]
Complicated Urinary Tract Infections and Acute Uncomplicated Pyelonephritis
CIPRO XR was evaluated for the treatment of complicated urinary tract infections (cUTI) and acute uncomplicated pyelonephritis (AUP) in a randomized, double-blind, controlled clinical trial conducted in the US and Canada. The study enrolled 1,042 patients (521 patients per treatment arm) and compared CIPRO XR (1000 mg once daily for 7 to 14 days) with immediate-release ciprofloxacin (500 mg BID for 7 to 14 days). The primary efficacy endpoint for this trial was bacteriologic eradication of the baseline organism(s) with no new infection or superinfection at 5 to 11 days post-therapy (test-of-cure or TOC) for the Per Protocol and Modified Intent-To-Treat (MITT) populations.

The Per Protocol population was defined as patients with a diagnosis of cUTI or AUP, a causative organism(s) at baseline present at $\geq 10^5$ CFU/mL, no inclusion criteria violation, a valid test-of-cure urine culture within the TOC window, an organism susceptible to study drug, no premature discontinuation or loss to follow-up, and compliance with the dosage regimen (among other criteria). More patients in the CIPRO XR arm than in the control arm were excluded from the Per Protocol population and this should be considered in the interpretation of the study results. Reasons for exclusion with the greatest discrepancy between the two arms were no valid test-of-cure urine culture, an organism resistant to the study drug, and premature discontinuation due to adverse events.

An analysis of all patients with a causative organism(s) isolated at baseline and who received study medication, defined as the MITT population, included 342 patients in the CIPRO XR arm and 324 patients in the control arm. Patients with missing responses were counted as failures in this analysis. In the MITT analysis of cUTI patients, bacteriologic eradication was 160/271 (59.0%) versus 156/248 (62.9%) in CIPRO XR and control arm, respectively [97.5% CI* (-13.5%, 5.7%)]. Clinical cure was 184/271 (67.9%) for CIPRO XR and 182/248 (73.4%) for control arm, respectively [97.5% CI* (-14.4%, 3.5%)]. Bacterial eradication in the MITT analysis of patients with AUP at TOC was 47/71 (66.2%) and 58/76 (76.3%) for CIPRO XR and control arm, respectively [97.5% CI* (-26.8%, 6.5%)]. Clinical cure at TOC was 50/71 (70.4%) for CIPRO XR and 58/76 (76.3%) for the control arm [97.5% CI* (-22.0%, 10.4%)].
* confidence interval of the difference in rates (CIPRO XR minus control).

In the Per Protocol population, the differences between CIPRO XR and the control arm in bacteriologic eradication rates at the TOC visit were not consistent between AUP and cUTI patients. The bacteriologic eradication rate for cUTI patients was higher in the CIPRO XR arm than in the control arm. For AUP patients, the bacteriologic eradication rate was lower in the CIPRO XR arm than in the control arm. This inconsistency was not observed between the two treatment groups for clinical cure rates. Clinical cure rates were 96.1% (198/206) and 92.1% (211/229) for CIPRO XR and the control arm, respectively.

The bacterial eradication and clinical cure rates by infection type for CIPRO XR and the control arm at the TOC visit and their corresponding 97.5% confidence intervals for the differences between rates (CIPRO XR minus control arm) are given below for the Per Protocol population analysis:
[See table at right]

Of the 166 cUTI patients treated with CIPRO XR, 148 (89%) had the causative organism(s) eradicated, 8 (5%) had persistence, 5 (3%) patients developed superinfections and 5 (3%) developed new infections. Of the 177 cUTI patients treated in the control arm, 144 (81%) had the causative organism(s) eradicated, 16 (9%) patients had persistence, 3 (2%) developed superinfections and 14 (8%) developed new infections. Of the 40 patients with AUP treated with CIPRO XR, 35 (87.5%) had the causative organism(s) eradicated, 2 (5%) patients had persistence and 3 (7.5%) developed new infections. Of the 5 CIPRO XR AUP patients without eradication at TOC, 4 were considered clinical cures and did not receive alternative antibiotic therapy. Of the 52 patients with AUP treated in the control arm, 51 (98%) had the causative organism(s) eradicated. One patient (2%) had persistence.

REFERENCES

1. NCCLS, Methods for Dilution Antimicrobial Susceptibility Tests for Bacteria That Grow Aerobically-Sixth Edition. Approved Standard NCCLS Document M7-A6, Vol. 23, No. 2, NCCLS, Wayne, PA, January, 2003.
2. NCCLS, Performance Standards for Antimicrobial Disk Susceptibility Tests-Eighth Edition. Approved Standard NCCLS Document M2-A8, Vol. 23, No. 1, NCCLS, Wayne, PA, January, 2003.

MEDICATION GUIDE

CIPRO® *(Sip-row)*
(ciprofloxacin hydrochloride)
TABLETS
CIPRO® *(Sip-row)*
(ciprofloxacin)
ORAL SUSPENSION
CIPRO® XR *(Sip-row)*
(ciprofloxacin extended-release tablets)
CIPRO® I.V. *(Sip-row)*
(ciprofloxacin)
For Intravenous Infusion

Read the Medication Guide that comes with CIPRO® before you start taking it and each time you get a refill. There may be new information. This Medication Guide does not take the place of talking to your healthcare provider about your medical condition or your treatment.

What is the most important information I should know about CIPRO?

CIPRO belongs to a class of antibiotics called fluoroquinolones. CIPRO can cause side effects that may be serious or

	CIPRO XR 1000 mg QD	CIPRO 500 mg BID
Randomized Patients	521	521
Per Protocol Patients*	206	229
cUTI Patients		
Bacteriologic Eradication at TOC (n/N)†	148/166 (89.2%)	144/177 (81.4%)
	CI [-0.7%, 16.3%]	
Bacteriologic Eradication (by organism) at TOC (n/N)‡		
E. coli	91/94 (96.8%)	90/92 (97.8%)
K. pneumoniae	20/21 (95.2%)	19/23 (82.6%)
E. faecalis	17/17 (100%)	14/21 (66.7%)
P. mirabilis	11/12 (91.6%)	10/10 (100%)
P. aeruginosa	3/3 (100%)	3/3 (100%)
Clinical Cure at TOC (n/N)§	159/166 (95.8%)	161/177 (91.0%)
	CI [-1.1%, 10.8%]	
AUP Patients		
Bacteriologic Eradication at TOC (n/N)†	35/40 (87.5%)	51/52 (98.1%)
	CI [-34.8%, 6.2%]	
Bacteriologic Eradication of E. coli at TOC (n/N)‡	35/36 (97.2%)	41/41 (100%)
Clinical Cure at TOC (n/N)§	39/40 (97.5%)	50/52 (96.2%)
	CI [-15.3%, 21.1%]	

* Patients excluded from the Per Protocol population were primarily those with no causative organism(s) at baseline or no organism present at $\geq 10^5$ CFU/mL at baseline, inclusion criteria violation, no valid test-of-cure urine culture within the TOC window, an organism resistant to study drug, premature discontinuation due to an adverse event, lost to follow-up, or non-compliance with dosage regimen (among other criteria).
† n/N = patients with baseline organism(s) eradicated and no new infections or superinfections/total number of patients
‡ n/N = patients with specified baseline organism eradicated/patients with specified baseline organism
§ n/N = patients with clinical success /total number of patients

even cause death. If you get any of the following serious side effects, get medical help right away. Talk with your healthcare provider about whether you should continue to take CIPRO.

• **Tendon rupture or swelling of the tendon (tendinitis)**
• Tendons are tough cords of tissue that connect muscles to bones.
• Pain, swelling, tears and inflammation of tendons including the back of the ankle (Achilles), shoulder, hand, or other tendon sites can happen in people of all ages who take fluoroquinolone antibiotics, including CIPRO. The risk of getting tendon problems is higher if you:
• are over 60 years of age
• are taking steroids (corticosteroids)
• have had a kidney, heart or lung transplant
• Swelling of the tendon (tendinitis) and tendon rupture (breakage) have also happened in patients who take fluoroquinolones who do not have the above risk factors.
• Other reasons for tendon ruptures can include:
• physical activity or exercise
• kidney failure
• tendon problems in the past, such as in people with rheumatoid arthritis (RA)
• Call your healthcare provider right away at the first sign of tendon pain, swelling or inflammation. Stop taking CIPRO until tendinitis or tendon rupture has been ruled out by your healthcare provider. Avoid exercise and using the affected area. The most common area of pain and swelling is the Achilles tendon at the back of your ankle. This can also happen with other tendons. Talk to your healthcare provider about the risk of tendon rupture with continued use of CIPRO. You may need a different antibiotic that is not a fluoroquinolone to treat your infection.
• Tendon rupture can happen while you are taking or after you have finished taking CIPRO. Tendon ruptures have happened up to several months after patients have finished taking their fluoroquinolone.
• Get medical help right away if you get any of the following signs or symptoms of a tendon rupture:
• hear or feel a snap or pop in a tendon area
• bruising right after an injury in a tendon area
• unable to move the affected area or bear weight
• See the section "**What are the possible side effects of CIPRO?**" for more information about side effects.

What is CIPRO?
CIPRO is a fluoroquinolone antibiotic medicine used to treat certain infections caused by certain germs called bacteria.

Children less than 18 years of age have a higher chance of getting bone, joint, or tendon (musculoskeletal) problems such as pain or swelling while taking CIPRO. CIPRO should not be used as the first choice of antibiotic medicine in children under 18 years of age.
CIPRO Tablets, CIPRO Oral Suspension and CIPRO I.V. should not be used in children under 18 years old, except to treat specific serious infections, such as complicated urinary tract infections and to prevent anthrax disease after breathing the anthrax bacteria germ (inhalational exposure). It is not known if CIPRO XR is safe and works in children under 18 years of age.
Sometimes infections are caused by viruses rather than by bacteria. Examples include viral infections in the sinuses and lungs, such as the common cold or flu. Antibiotics, including CIPRO, do not kill viruses.
Call your healthcare provider if you think your condition is not getting better while you are taking CIPRO.
Who should not take CIPRO?
Do not take CIPRO if you:
• have ever had a severe allergic reaction to an antibiotic known as a fluoroquinolone, or are allergic to any of the ingredients in CIPRO. Ask your healthcare provider if you are not sure. See the list of ingredients in CIPRO at the end of this Medication Guide.
• also take a medicine called tizanidine (Zanaflex®). Serious side effects from tizanidine are likely to happen.
What should I tell my healthcare provider before taking CIPRO?
See "**What is the most important information I should know about CIPRO?**"
Tell your healthcare provider about all your medical conditions, including if you:
• have tendon problems
• have central nervous system problems (such as epilepsy)
• have nerve problems
• have or anyone in your family has an irregular heartbeat, especially a condition called "QT prolongation"
• have kidney problems. You may need a lower dose of CIPRO if your kidneys do not work well.
• have rheumatoid arthritis (RA) or other history of joint problems
• have trouble swallowing pills
• are pregnant or planning to become pregnant. It is not known if CIPRO will harm your unborn child.

- are breast-feeding or planning to breast-feed. CIPRO passes into breast milk. You and your healthcare provider should decide whether you will take CIPRO or breast-feed.

Tell your healthcare provider about all the medicines you take, including prescription and non-prescription medicines, vitamins and herbal and dietary supplements. CIPRO and other medicines can affect each other causing side effects. Especially tell your healthcare provider if you take:

- an NSAID (Non-Steroidal Anti-Inflammatory Drug). Many common medicines for pain relief are NSAIDs. Taking an NSAID while you take CIPRO or other fluoroquinolones may increase your risk of central nervous system effects and seizures. See **"What are the possible side effects of CIPRO?"**.
- a blood thinner (warfarin, Coumadin®, Jantoven®)
- tizanidine (Zanaflex®). You should not take CIPRO if you are already taking tizanidine. See **"Who should not take CIPRO?"**
- theophylline (Theo-24®, Elixophyllin®, Theochron®, Uniphyl®, Theolair®)
- glyburide (Micronase®, Glynase®, Diabeta®, Glucovance®). See **"What are the possible side effects of CIPRO?"**
- phenytoin (Fosphenytoin Sodium®, Cerebyx®, Dilantin-125®, Dilantin®, Extended Phenytoin Sodium®, Prompt Penytoin Sodium®, Phenytek®)
- products that contain caffeine
- a medicine to control your heart rate or rhythm (antiarrhythmics) See **"What are the possible side effects of CIPRO?"**
- an anti-psychotic medicine
- a tricyclic antidepressant
- a water pill (diuretic)
- a steroid medicine. Corticosteroids taken by mouth or by injection may increase the chance of tendon injury. See **"What is the most important information I should know about CIPRO?"**
- methotrexate (Trexall®)
- Probenecid (Probalan®, Col-probenecid®)
- Metoclopromide (Reglan®, Reglan ODT®)
- Certain medicines may keep CIPRO Tablets, CIPRO Oral Suspension from working correctly. Take CIPRO Tablets and Oral Suspension either 2 hours before or 6 hours after taking these products:
- an antacid, multivitamin, or other product that has magnesium, calcium, aluminum, iron, or zinc
- sucralfate (Carafate®)
- didanosine (Videx®, Videx EC®)

Ask your healthcare provider if you are not sure if any of your medicines are listed above.

Know the medicines you take. Keep a list of your medicines and show it to your healthcare provider and pharmacist when you get a new medicine.

How should I take CIPRO?

- Take CIPRO exactly as prescribed by your healthcare provider.
- Take CIPRO Tablets in the morning and evening at about the same time each day. Swallow the tablet whole. Do not split, crush or chew the tablet. Tell your healthcare provider if you can not swallow the tablet whole.
- Take CIPRO Oral Suspension in the morning and evening at about the same time each day. Shake the CIPRO Oral Suspension bottle well each time before use for about 15 seconds to make sure the suspension is mixed well. Close the bottle completely after use.
- Take CIPRO XR one time each day at about the same time each day. Swallow the tablet whole. Do not split, crush or chew the tablet. Tell your healthcare provider if you can not swallow the tablet whole.
- CIPRO I.V. is given to you by intravenous (I.V.) infusion into your vein, slowly, over 60 minutes, as prescribed by your healthcare provider.
- CIPRO can be taken with or without food.
- CIPRO should not be taken with dairy products (like milk or yogurt) or calcium-fortified juices alone, but may be taken with a meal that contains these products.
- Drink plenty of fluids while taking CIPRO.
- Do not skip any doses, or stop taking CIPRO even if you begin to feel better, until you finish your prescribed treatment, unless:
- you have tendon effects (see **"What is the most important information I should know about CIPRO?"**),
- you have a serious allergic reaction (see **"What are the possible side effects of CIPRO?"**), or
- your healthcare provider tells you to stop.
- This will help make sure that all of the bacteria are killed and lower the chance that the bacteria will become resistant to CIPRO. If this happens, CIPRO and other antibiotic medicines may not work in the future.
- If you miss a dose of CIPRO Tablets or Oral Suspension, take it as soon as you remember. Do not take two doses at the same time, and do not take more than two doses in one day.
- If you miss a dose of CIPRO XR, take it as soon as you remember. Do not take more than one dose in one day.
- If you take too much, call your healthcare provider or get medical help immediately.

If you have been prescribed CIPRO Tablets, CIPRO Oral Suspension or CIPRO I.V. after being exposed to anthrax:

- CIPRO Tablets, Oral Suspension and I.V. has been approved to lessen the chance of getting anthrax disease or worsening of the disease after you are exposed to the anthrax bacteria germ.
- Take CIPRO exactly as prescribed by your healthcare provider. Do not stop taking CIPRO without talking with your healthcare provider. If you stop taking CIPRO too soon, it may not keep you from getting the anthrax disease.
- Side effects may happen while you are taking CIPRO Tablets, Oral Suspension or I.V. When taking your CIPRO to prevent anthrax infection, you and your healthcare provider should talk about whether the risks of stopping CIPRO too soon are more important than the risks of side effects with CIPRO.
- If you are pregnant, or plan to become pregnant while taking CIPRO, you and your healthcare provider should decide whether the benefits of taking CIPRO Tablets, Oral Suspension or I.V. for anthrax are more important than the risks.

What should I avoid while taking CIPRO?

CIPRO can make you feel dizzy and lightheaded. Do not drive, operate machinery, or do other activities that require mental alertness or coordination until you know how CIPRO affects you.

Avoid sunlamps, tanning beds, and try to limit your time in the sun. CIPRO can make your skin sensitive to the sun (photosensitivity) and the light from sunlamps and tanning beds. You could get severe sunburn, blisters or swelling of your skin. If you get any of these symptoms while taking CIPRO, call your healthcare provider right away. You should use a sunscreen and wear a hat and clothes that cover your skin if you have to be in sunlight.

What are the possible side effects of CIPRO?

CIPRO can cause side effects that may be serious or even cause death. See **"What is the most important information I should know about CIPRO?"**

Other serious side effects of CIPRO include:

- **Central Nervous System effects**

Seizures have been reported in people who take fluoroquinolone antibiotics including CIPRO. Tell your healthcare provider if you have a history of seizures. Ask your healthcare provider whether taking CIPRO will change your risk of having a seizure.

Central Nervous System (CNS) side effects may happen as soon as after taking the first dose of CIPRO. Talk to your healthcare provider right away if you get any of these side effects, or other changes in mood or behavior:

- feel dizzy
- seizures
- hear voices, see things, or sense things that are not there (hallucinations)
- feel restless
- tremors
- feel anxious or nervous
- confusion
- depression
- trouble sleeping
- nightmares
- feel more suspicious (paranoia)
- suicidal thoughts or acts

- **Serious allergic reactions**

Allergic reactions can happen in people taking fluoroquinolones, including CIPRO, even after only one dose. Stop taking CIPRO and get emergency medical help right away if you get any of the following symptoms of a severe allergic reaction:

- hives
- trouble breathing or swallowing
- swelling of the lips, tongue, face
- throat tightness, hoarseness
- rapid heartbeat
- faint
- yellowing of the skin or eyes. Stop taking CIPRO and tell your healthcare provider right away if you get yellowing of your skin or white part of your eyes, or if you have dark urine. These can be signs of a serious reaction to CIPRO (a liver problem).

- **Skin rash**

Skin rash may happen in people taking CIPRO even after only one dose. Stop taking CIPRO at the first sign of a skin rash and call your healthcare provider. Skin rash may be a sign of a more serious reaction to CIPRO.

- **Serious heart rhythm changes** (QT prolongation and torsade de pointes)

Tell your healthcare provider right away if you have a change in your heart beat (a fast or irregular heartbeat), or if you faint. CIPRO may cause a rare heart problem known as prolongation of the QT interval. This condition can cause an abnormal heartbeat and can be very dangerous. The chances of this event are higher in people:

- who are elderly
- with a family history of prolonged QT interval
- with low blood potassium (hypokalemia)
- who take certain medicines to control heart rhythm (antiarrhythmics)

- **Intestine infection** (Pseudomembranous colitis)

Pseudomembranous colitis can happen with most antibiotics, including CIPRO. Call your healthcare provider right away if you get watery diarrhea, diarrhea that does not go away, or bloody stools. You may have stomach cramps and a fever. Pseudomembranous colitis can happen 2 or more months after you have finished your antibiotic.

- **Changes in sensation and possible nerve damage** (Peripheral Neuropathy)

Damage to the nerves in arms, hands, legs, or feet can happen in people who take fluoroquinolones, including CIPRO. Talk with your healthcare provider right away if you get any of the following symptoms of peripheral neuropathy in your arms, hands, legs, or feet:

- pain
- burning
- tingling
- numbness
- weakness

CIPRO may need to be stopped to prevent permanent nerve damage.

- **Low blood sugar** (hypoglycemia)

People who take CIPRO and other fluoroquinolone medicines with the oral anti-diabetes medicine glyburide (Micronase, Glynase, Diabeta, Glucovance) can get low blood sugar (hypoglycemia) which can sometimes be severe. Tell your healthcare provider if you get low blood sugar with CIPRO. Your antibiotic medicine may need to be changed.

- **Sensitivity to sunlight** (photosensitivity)

See **"What should I avoid while taking CIPRO?"**

- **Joint Problems**

Increased chance of problems with joints and tissues around joints in children under 18 years old. Tell your child's healthcare provider if your child has any joint problems during or after treatment with CIPRO.

The most common side effects of CIPRO include:

- nausea
- headache
- diarrhea
- vomiting
- vaginal yeast infection
- changes in liver function tests
- pain or discomfort in the abdomen

These are not all the possible side effects of CIPRO. Tell your healthcare provider about any side effect that bothers you, or that does not go away.

Call your doctor for medical advice about side effects. You may report side effects to FDA at 1-800-FDA-1088.

How should I store CIPRO?

- **CIPRO Tablets**
- Store CIPRO below 86°F (30°C)
- **CIPRO Oral Suspension**
- Store CIPRO Oral Suspension below 86°F (30°C) for up to 14 days
- Do not freeze
- After treatment has been completed, any unused oral suspension should be safely thrown away
- **CIPRO XR**
- Store CIPRO XR at 59°F to 86°F (15°C to 30°C)

Keep CIPRO and all medicines out of the reach of children.

General Information about CIPRO

Medicines are sometimes prescribed for purposes other than those listed in a Medication Guide. Do not use CIPRO for a condition for which it is not prescribed. Do not give CIPRO to other people, even if they have the same symptoms that you have. It may harm them.

This Medication Guide summarizes the most important information about CIPRO. If you would like more information about CIPRO, talk with your healthcare provider. You can ask your healthcare provider or pharmacist for information about CIPRO that is written for healthcare professionals. For more information go to www.CIPRO.com or call 1-800-526-4099.

What are the ingredients in CIPRO?

- **CIPRO Tablets:**
- Active ingredient: ciprofloxacin
- Inactive ingredients: cornstarch, microcrystalline cellulose, silicon dioxide, crospovidone, magnesium stearate, hypromellose, titanium dioxide, and polyethylene glycol
- **CIPRO Oral Suspension:**
- Active ingredient: ciproflxacin
- Inactive ingredients: The components of the suspension have the following compositions: Microcapsules—ciprofloxacin, povidone, methacrylic acid copolymer,

hypromellose, magnesium stearate, and Polysorbate 20. Diluent—medium-chain triglycerides, sucrose, lecithin, water, and strawberry flavor.

- **CIPRO XR:**
- Active ingredient: ciprofloxacin
- Inactive ingredients: crospovidone, hypromellose, magnesium stearate, polyethylene glycol, silica colloidal anhydrous, succinic acid, and titanium dioxide.
- **CIPRO I.V.:**
- Active ingredient: ciprofloxacin
- Inactive ingredients: lactic acid as a solubilizing agent, hydrochloric acid for pH adjustment

Revised October 2008

This Medication Guide has been approved by the U.S. Food and Drug Administration.

Manufactured by:
Bayer HealthCare Pharmaceuticals Inc.
Wayne, NJ 07470
Made in Germany
Distributed by:
Schering Plough
Schering Corporation
Kenilworth, NJ 07033
CIPRO is a registered trademark of Bayer Aktiengesellschaft and is used under license by Schering Corporation.
Rx Only
81532274, R.0Bay o 9867/q 393910/0814212
©2008 Bayer HealthCare Pharmaceuticals Inc. Printed in U.S.A.

Shown in Product Identification Guide, page 312

CLARINEX®   ℞
[klă-rĭ-nĕcks]
(desloratadine)
Tablets, Syrup, REDITABS® Tablets

PRODUCT INFORMATION

DESCRIPTION

CLARINEX (desloratadine) Tablets are light blue, round, film coated tablets containing 5 mg desloratadine, an antihistamine, to be administered orally. It also contains the following excipients: dibasic calcium phosphate dihydrate USP, microcrystalline cellulose NF, corn starch NF, talc USP, carnauba wax NF, white wax NF, coating material consisting of lactose monohydrate, hypromellose, titanium dioxide, polyethylene glycol, and FD&C Blue #2 Aluminum Lake.

CLARINEX Syrup is a clear orange colored liquid containing 0.5 mg/1 mL desloratadine. The syrup contains the following inactive ingredients: propylene glycol USP, sorbitol solution USP, citric acid (anhydrous) USP, sodium citrate dihydrate USP, sodium benzoate NF, disodium edetate USP, purified water USP. It also contains granulated sugar, natural and artificial flavor for bubble gum and FDC Yellow #6 dye.

The CLARINEX RediTabs® brand of desloratadine orally-disintegrating tablets are light red, flat-faced, round, speckled tablets with an "A" debossed on one side for the 5 mg tablets and a "K" debossed on one side for the 2.5 mg tablets. Each RediTab Tablet contains either 5 mg or 2.5 mg of desloratadine. It also contains the following inactive ingredients: mannitol USP, microcrystalline cellulose NF, pregelatinized starch, NF, sodium starch glycolate, NF, magnesium stearate NF, butylated methacrylate copolymer, crospovidone, NF, aspartame NF, citric acid USP, sodium bicarbonate USP, colloidal silicon dioxide, NF, ferric oxide red NF and tutti frutti flavoring.

Desloratadine is a white to off-white powder that is slightly soluble in water, but very soluble in ethanol and propylene glycol. It has an empirical formula: $C_{19}H_{19}ClN_2$ and a molecular weight of 310.8. The chemical name is 8-chloro-6,11-dihydro-11-(4-piperidinylidene)-5H-benzo[5,6]cyclohepta[1,2-b]pyridine and has the following structure:

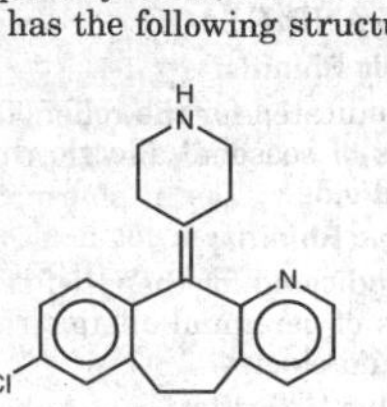

CLINICAL PHARMACOLOGY
Mechanism of Action:
Desloratadine is a long-acting tricyclic histamine antagonist with selective H_1-receptor histamine antagonist activity. Receptor binding data indicate that at a concentration of 2-3 ng/mL (7 nanomolar), desloratadine shows significant interaction with the human histamine H_1-receptor. Desloratadine inhibited histamine release from human mast cells *in vitro*.

Results of a radiolabeled tissue distribution study in rats and a radioligand H_1-receptor binding study in guinea pigs showed that desloratadine did not readily cross the blood brain barrier.

Pharmacokinetics:
Absorption:
Following oral administration of desloratadine 5 mg once daily for 10 days to normal healthy volunteers, the mean time to maximum plasma concentrations (T_{max}) occurred at approximately 3 hours post dose and mean steady state peak plasma concentrations (C_{max}) and area under the concentration-time curve (AUC) of 4 ng/mL and 56.9 ng•hr/mL were observed, respectively. Neither food nor grapefruit juice had an effect on the bioavailability (C_{max} and AUC) of desloratadine.

The pharmacokinetic profile of CLARINEX Syrup was evaluated in a three-way crossover study in 30 adult volunteers. A single dose of 10 mL of CLARINEX Syrup containing 5 mg of desloratadine was bioequivalent to a single dose of 5 mg CLARINEX Tablet. Food had no effect on the bioavailability (AUC and C_{max}) of CLARINEX Syrup.

The pharmacokinetic profile of CLARINEX RediTabs Tablets was evaluated in a three-way crossover study in 24 adult volunteers. A single CLARINEX RediTabs Tablet containing 5 mg of desloratadine was bioequivalent to a single 5 mg CLARINEX RediTabs Tablet (original formulation) for both desloratadine and 3-hydroxydesloratadine. Water had no effect on the bioavailability (AUC and C_{max}) of CLARINEX RediTabs Tablets.

Distribution:
Desloratadine and 3-hydroxydesloratadine are approximately 82% to 87% and 85% to 89%, bound to plasma proteins, respectively. Protein binding of desloratadine and 3-hydroxydesloratadine was unaltered in subjects with impaired renal function.

Metabolism:
Desloratadine (a major metabolite of loratadine) is extensively metabolized to 3-hydroxydesloratadine, an active metabolite, which is subsequently glucuronidated. The enzyme(s) responsible for the formation of 3-hydroxydesloratadine have not been identified. Data from clinical trials indicate that a subset of the general population has a decreased ability to form 3-hydroxydesloratadine, and are poor metabolizers of desloratadine. In pharmacokinetic studies (n=3748), approximately 6% of subjects were poor metabolizers of desloratadine (defined as a subject with an AUC ratio of 3-hydroxydesloratadine to desloratadine less than 0.1, or a subject with a desloratadine half-life exceeding 50 hours). These pharmacokinetic studies included subjects between the ages of 2 and 70 years, including 977 subjects aged 2-5 years, 1575 subjects aged 6-11 years, and 1196 subjects aged 12-70 years. There was no difference in the prevalence of poor metabolizers across age groups. The frequency of poor metabolizers was higher in Blacks (17%, n=988) as compared to Caucasians (2%, n=1462) and Hispanics (2%, n=1063). The median exposure (AUC) to desloratadine in the poor metabolizers was approximately 6-fold greater than in the subjects who are not poor metabolizers. Subjects who are poor metabolizers of desloratadine cannot be prospectively identified and will be exposed to higher levels of desloratadine following dosing with the recommended dose of desloratadine. In multidose clinical safety studies, where metabolizer status was identified, a total of 94 poor metabolizers and 123 normal metabolizers were enrolled and treated with CLARINEX Syrup for 15-35 days. In these studies, no overall differences in safety were observed between poor metabolizers and normal metabolizers. Although not seen in these studies, an increased risk of exposure-related adverse events in patients who are poor metabolizers cannot be ruled out.

Elimination:
The mean elimination half-life of desloratadine was 27 hours. C_{max} and AUC values increased in a dose proportional manner following single oral doses between 5 and 20 mg. The degree of accumulation after 14 days of dosing was consistent with the half-life and dosing frequency. A human mass balance study documented a recovery of approximately 87% of the ^{14}C-desloratadine dose, which was equally distributed in urine and feces as metabolic products. Analysis of plasma 3-hydroxydesloratadine showed similar T_{max} and half-life values compared to desloratadine.

Special Populations:
Geriatric:
In older subjects ($\geq$ 65 years old; n=17) following multiple-dose administration of CLARINEX Tablets, the mean C_{max} and AUC values for desloratadine were 20% greater than in younger subjects (< 65 years old). The oral total body clearance (CL/F) when normalized for body weight was similar between the two age groups. The mean plasma elimination half-life of desloratadine was 33.7 hr in subjects $\geq$ 65 years old. The pharmacokinetics for 3-hydroxydesloratadine appeared unchanged in older versus younger subjects. These

age-related differences are unlikely to be clinically relevant and no dosage adjustment is recommended in elderly subjects.

Pediatric Subjects:
In subjects 6 to 11 years old, a single dose of 5 mL of CLARINEX Syrup containing 2.5 mg of desloratadine resulted in desloratadine plasma concentrations similar to those achieved in adults administered a single 5 mg CLARINEX Tablet. In subjects 2 to 5 years old, a single dose of 2.5 mL of CLARINEX Syrup containing 1.25 mg of desloratadine resulted in desloratadine plasma concentrations similar to those achieved in adults administered a single 5 mg CLARINEX Tablet. However, the C_{max} and AUC$_t$ of the metabolite (3-OH desloratadine) were 1.27 and 1.61 times higher for the 5 mg dose of syrup administered in adults compared to the C_{max} and AUC$_t$ obtained in children 2-11 years of age receiving 1.25-2.5 mg of CLARINEX Syrup.

A single dose of either 2.5 mL or 1.25 mL of CLARINEX Syrup containing 1.25 mg or 0.625 mg, respectively, of desloratadine was administered to subjects 6 to 11 months of age and 12 to 23 months of age. The results of a population pharmacokinetic analysis indicated that a dose of 1 mg for subjects 6 to 11 months and 1.25 mg for subjects 12 to 23 months of age is required to obtain desloratadine plasma concentrations similar to those achieved in adults administered a single 5 mg dose of CLARINEX Syrup.

The CLARINEX RediTabs Tablet 2.5 mg tablet has not been evaluated in pediatric patients. Bioequivalence of the CLARINEX RediTabs Tablet and the original CLARINEX RediTabs Tablets was established in adults. In conjunction with the dose finding studies in pediatrics described, the pharmacokinetic data for CLARINEX RediTabs Tablet supports the use of the 2.5 mg dose strength in pediatric patients 6-11 years of age.

Renally Impaired:
Desloratadine pharmacokinetics following a single dose of 7.5 mg were characterized in patients with mild (n=7; creatinine clearance 51-69 mL/min/1.73 m^2), moderate (n=6; creatinine clearance 34-43 mL/min/1.73 m^2), and severe (n=6; creatinine clearance 5-29 mL/min/1.73 m^2) renal impairment or hemodialysis-dependent (n=6) patients. In patients with mild and moderate renal impairment, median C_{max} and AUC values increased by approximately 1.2- and 1.9-fold, respectively, relative to subjects with normal renal function. In patients with severe renal impairment or who were hemodialysis dependent, C_{max} and AUC values increased by approximately 1.7- and 2.5-fold, respectively. Minimal changes in 3-hydroxydesloratadine concentrations were observed. Desloratadine and 3-hydroxydesloratadine were poorly removed by hemodialysis. Plasma protein binding of desloratadine and 3-hydroxydesloratadine was unaltered by renal impairment. Dosage adjustment for patients with renal impairment is recommended (see **DOSAGE AND ADMINISTRATION** section).

Hepatically Impaired:
Desloratadine pharmacokinetics were characterized following a single oral dose in patients with mild (n=4), moderate (n=4), and severe (n=4) hepatic impairment as defined by the Child-Pugh classification of hepatic function and 8 subjects with normal hepatic function. Patients with hepatic impairment, regardless of severity, had approximately a 2.4-fold increase in AUC as compared with normal subjects. The apparent oral clearance of desloratadine in patients with mild, moderate, and severe hepatic impairment was 37%, 36%, and 28% of that in normal subjects, respectively. An increase in the mean elimination half-life of desloratadine in patients with hepatic impairment was observed. For 3-hydroxydesloratadine, the mean C_{max} and AUC values for patients with hepatic impairment were not statistically significantly different from subjects with normal hepatic function. Dosage adjustment for patients with hepatic impairment is recommended (see **DOSAGE AND ADMINISTRATION** section).

Gender:
Female subjects treated for 14 days with CLARINEX Tablets had 10% and 3% higher desloratadine C_{max} and AUC values, respectively, compared with male subjects. The 3-hydroxydesloratadine C_{max} and AUC values were also increased by 45% and 48%, respectively, in females compared with males. However, these apparent differences are not likely to be clinically relevant and therefore no dosage adjustment is recommended.

Race:
Following 14 days of treatment with CLARINEX Tablets, the C_{max} and AUC values for desloratadine were 18% and 32% higher, respectively, in Blacks compared with Caucasians. For 3-hydroxydesloratadine there was a corresponding 10% reduction in C_{max} and AUC values in Blacks compared to Caucasians. These differences are not likely to be clinically relevant and therefore no dose adjustment is recommended.

Drug Interactions:
In two controlled crossover clinical pharmacology studies in healthy male (n=12 in each study) and female (n=12 in each

Table 1
Changes in Desloratadine and 3-Hydroxydesloratadine
Pharmacokinetics in Healthy Male and Female Volunteers

	Desloratadine		3-Hydroxydesloratadine	
	C_{max}	AUC 0-24 hrs	C_{max}	AUC 0-24 hrs
Erythromycin (500 mg Q8h)	+24%	+14%	+43%	+40%
Ketoconazole (200 mg Q12h)	+45%	+39%	+43%	+72%
Azithromycin (500 mg day 1, 250 mg QD × 4 days)	+15%	+5%	+15%	+4%
Fluoxetine (20 mg QD)	+15%	+0%	+17%	+13%
Cimetidine (600 mg Q12h)	+12%	+19%	-11%	-3%

Table 2
TOTAL SYMPTOM SCORE (TSS)
Changes in a 2-Week Clinical Trial in Patients with Seasonal Allergic Rhinitis

Treatment Group (n)	Mean Baseline* (sem)	Change from Baseline** (sem)	Placebo Comparison (P-value)
CLARINEX 5.0 mg (171)	14.2 (0.3)	-4.3 (0.3)	P<0.01
Placebo (173)	13.7 (0.3)	-2.5 (0.3)	

* At baseline, a total nasal symptom score (sum of 4 individual symptoms) of at least 6 and a total non-nasal symptom score (sum of 4 individual symptoms) of at least 5 (each symptom scored 0 to 3 where 0=no symptom and 3=severe symptoms) was required for trial eligibility. TSS ranges from 0=no symptoms to 24=maximal symptoms.
**Mean reduction in TSS averaged over the 2-week treatment period.

Table 3
TOTAL SYMPTOM SCORE (TSS)
Changes in a 4-Week Clinical Trial in Patients with Perennial Allergic Rhinitis

Treatment Group (n)	Mean Baseline* (sem)	Change from Baseline** (sem)	Placebo Comparison (P-value)
CLARINEX 5.0 mg (337)	12.37 (0.18)	-4.06 (0.21)	P=0.01
Placebo (337)	12.30 (0.18)	-3.27 (0.21)	

* At baseline, average of total symptom score (sum of 5 individual nasal symptoms and 3 non-nasal symptoms, each symptom scored 0 to 3 where 0=no symptom and 3=severe symptoms) of at least 10 was required for trial eligibility. TSS ranges from 0=no symptoms to 24=maximal symptoms.
**Mean reduction in TSS averaged over the 4-week treatment period.

Table 4
PRURITUS SYMPTOM SCORE
Changes in the First Week of a Clinical Trial in Patients with Chronic Idiopathic Urticaria

Treatment Group (n)	Mean Baseline (sem)	Change from Baseline* (sem)	Placebo Comparison (P-value)
CLARINEX 5.0 mg (115)	2.19 (0.04)	-1.05 (0.07)	P<0.01
Placebo (110)	2.21 (0.04)	-0.52 (0.07)	

Pruritus scored 0 to 3 where 0=no symptom to 3=maximal symptom.
*Mean reduction in pruritus averaged over the first week of treatment.

study) volunteers, desloratadine 7.5 mg (1.5 times the daily dose) once daily was coadministered with erythromycin 500 mg every 8 hours or ketoconazole 200 mg every 12 hours for 10 days. In three separate controlled, parallel group clinical pharmacology studies, desloratadine at the clinical dose of 5 mg has been coadministered with azithromycin 500 mg followed by 250 mg once daily for 4 days (n=18) or with fluoxetine 20 mg once daily for 7 days after a 23-day pretreatment period with fluoxetine (n=18) or with cimetidine 600 mg every 12 hours for 14 days (n=18) under steady state conditions to normal healthy male and female volunteers. Although increased plasma concentrations (C_{max} and AUC 0-24 hrs) of desloratadine and 3-hydroxydesloratadine were observed (see Table 1), there were no clinically relevant changes in the safety profile of desloratadine, as assessed by electrocardiographic parameters (including the corrected QT interval), clinical laboratory tests, vital signs, and adverse events.
[See table 1 above]

Pharmacodynamics:
Wheal and Flare:
Human histamine skin wheal studies following single and repeated 5 mg doses of desloratadine have shown that the drug exhibits an antihistaminic effect by 1 hour; this activity may persist for as long as 24 hours. There was no evidence of histamine-induced skin wheal tachyphylaxis within the desloratadine 5 mg group over the 28-day treatment period. The clinical relevance of histamine wheal skin testing is unknown.

Effects on QT_c:
Single dose administration of desloratadine did not alter the corrected QT interval (QT_c) in rats (up to 12 mg/kg, oral), or guinea pigs (25 mg/kg, intravenous). Repeated oral administration at doses up to 24 mg/kg for durations up to 3 months in monkeys did not alter the QT_c at an estimated desloratadine exposure (AUC) that was approximately 955 times the mean AUC in humans at the recommended daily oral dose. See **OVERDOSAGE** section for information on human QT_c experience.

Clinical Trials:
Seasonal Allergic Rhinitis:
The clinical efficacy and safety of CLARINEX Tablets were evaluated in over 2,300 patients 12 to 75 years of age with seasonal allergic rhinitis. A total of 1,838 patients received 2.5-20 mg/day of CLARINEX in four double-blind, randomized, placebo-controlled clinical trials of 2 to 4 weeks' duration conducted in the United States. The results of these studies demonstrated the efficacy and safety of CLARINEX 5 mg in the treatment of adult and adolescent patients with seasonal allergic rhinitis. In a dose ranging trial, CLARINEX 2.5-20 mg/day was studied. Doses of 5, 7.5, 10, and 20 mg/day were superior to placebo; and no additional benefit was seen at doses above 5.0 mg. In the same study, an increase in the incidence of somnolence was observed at doses of 10 mg/day and 20 mg/day (5.2% and 7.6%, respectively), compared to placebo (2.3%).

In two 4-week studies of 924 patients (aged 15 to 75 years) with seasonal allergic rhinitis and concomitant asthma, CLARINEX Tablets 5 mg once daily improved rhinitis symptoms, with no decrease in pulmonary function. This supports the safety of administering CLARINEX Tablets to adult patients with seasonal allergic rhinitis with mild to moderate asthma.

CLARINEX Tablets 5 mg once daily significantly reduced the Total Symptom Scores (the sum of individual scores of nasal and non-nasal symptoms) in patients with seasonal allergic rhinitis. See Table 2.

[See table 2 at left]

There were no significant differences in the effectiveness of CLARINEX Tablets 5 mg across subgroups of patients defined by gender, age, or race.

Perennial Allergic Rhinitis:
The clinical efficacy and safety of CLARINEX Tablets 5 mg were evaluated in over 1,300 patients 12 to 80 years of age with perennial allergic rhinitis. A total of 685 patients received 5 mg/day of CLARINEX in two double-blind, randomized, placebo-controlled clinical trials of 4 weeks' duration conducted in the United States and internationally. In one of these studies CLARINEX Tablets 5 mg once daily was shown to significantly reduce symptoms of perennial allergic rhinitis (Table 3).

[See table 3 at left]

Chronic Idiopathic Urticaria:
The efficacy and safety of CLARINEX Tablets 5 mg once daily was studied in 416 chronic idiopathic urticaria patients 12 to 84 years of age, of whom 211 received CLARINEX. In two double-blind, placebo-controlled, randomized clinical trials of six weeks' duration, at the pre-specified one-week primary time point evaluation, CLARINEX Tablets significantly reduced the severity of pruritus when compared to placebo (Table 4). Secondary endpoints were also evaluated and during the first week of therapy CLARINEX Tablets 5 mg reduced the secondary endpoints, "Number of Hives" and the "Size of the Largest Hive," when compared to placebo.

[See table 4 at left]

The clinical safety of CLARINEX Syrup was documented in three, 15-day, double-blind, placebo-controlled safety studies in pediatric subjects with a documented history of allergic rhinitis, chronic idiopathic urticaria, or subjects who were candidates for antihistamine therapy. In the first study, 2.5 mg of CLARINEX Syrup was administered to 60 pediatric subjects 6 to 11 years of age. The second study evaluated 1.25 mg of CLARINEX Syrup administered to 55 pediatric subjects 2 to 5 years of age. In the third study, 1.25 mg of CLARINEX Syrup was administered to 65 pediatric subjects 12 to 23 months of age and 1.0 mg of CLARINEX Syrup was administered to 66 pediatric subjects 6 to 11 months of age. The results of these studies demonstrated the safety of CLARINEX Syrup in pediatric subjects 6 months to 11 years of age.

INDICATIONS AND USAGE

Seasonal Allergic Rhinitis:
CLARINEX is indicated for the relief of the nasal and non-nasal symptoms of seasonal allergic rhinitis in patients 2 years of age and older.

Perennial Allergic Rhinitis:
CLARINEX is indicated for the relief of the nasal and non-nasal symptoms of perennial allergic rhinitis in patients 6 months of age and older.

Chronic Idiopathic Urticaria:
CLARINEX is indicated for the symptomatic relief of pruritus, reduction in the number of hives, and size of hives, in patients with chronic idiopathic urticaria 6 months of age and older.

CONTRAINDICATIONS
CLARINEX Tablets 5 mg are contraindicated in patients who are hypersensitive to this medication or to any of its ingredients, or to loratadine.

PRECAUTIONS

Carcinogenesis, Mutagenesis, Impairment of Fertility:
The carcinogenic potential of desloratadine was assessed using a loratadine study in rats and a desloratadine study in mice. In a 2-year study in rats, loratadine was administered in the diet at doses up to 25 mg/kg/day (estimated desloratadine and desloratadine metabolite exposures were approximately 30 times the AUC in humans at the recommended daily oral dose). A significantly higher incidence of hepatocellular tumors (combined adenomas and carcinomas) was observed in males given 10 mg/kg/day of loratadine and in males and females given 25 mg/kg/day of loratadine. The estimated desloratadine and desloratadine metabolite exposures in rats given 10 mg/kg of loratadine were approximately 7 times the AUC in humans at the recommended daily oral dose. The clinical significance of these findings during long-term use of desloratadine is not known.

In a 2-year dietary study in mice, males and females given up to 16 mg/kg/day and 32 mg/kg/day desloratadine, respectively, did not show significant increases in the incidence of any tumors. The estimated desloratadine and metabolite exposures in mice at these doses were 12 and 27 times, respectively, the AUC in humans at the recommended daily oral dose.

In genotoxicity studies with desloratadine, there was no evidence of genotoxic potential in a reverse mutation assay (Salmonella/E. coli mammalian microsome bacterial mutagenicity assay) or in two assays for chromosomal aberrations (human peripheral blood lymphocyte clastogenicity assay and mouse bone marrow micronucleus assay).

There was no effect on female fertility in rats at desloratadine doses up to 24 mg/kg/day (estimated desloratadine and desloratadine metabolite exposures were approximately 130 times the AUC in humans at the recommended daily oral dose). A male specific decrease in fertility, demonstrated by reduced female conception rates, decreased sperm numbers and motility, and histopathologic testicular changes, occurred at an oral desloratadine dose of 12 mg/kg in rats (estimated desloratadine exposures were approximately 45 times the AUC in humans at the recommended daily oral dose). Desloratadine had no effect on fertility in rats at an oral dose of 3 mg/kg/day (estimated desloratadine and desloratadine metabolite exposures were approximately 8 times the AUC in humans at the recommended daily oral dose).

Pregnancy Category C:
Desloratadine was not teratogenic in rats at doses up to 48 mg/kg/day (estimated desloratadine and desloratadine metabolite exposures were approximately 210 times the AUC in humans at the recommended daily oral dose) or in rabbits at doses up to 60 mg/kg/day (estimated desloratadine exposures were approximately 230 times the AUC in humans at the recommended daily oral dose). In a separate study, an increase in pre-implantation loss and a decreased number of implantations and fetuses were noted in female rats at 24 mg/kg (estimated desloratadine and desloratadine metabolite exposures were approximately 120 times the AUC in humans at the recommended daily oral dose). Reduced body weight and slow righting reflex were reported in pups at doses of 9 mg/kg/day or greater (estimated desloratadine and desloratadine metabolite exposures were approximately 50 times or greater than the AUC in humans at the recommended daily oral dose). Desloratadine had no effect on pup development at an oral dose of 3 mg/kg/day (estimated desloratadine and desloratadine metabolite exposures were approximately 7 times the AUC in humans at the recommended daily oral dose). There are, however, no adequate and well-controlled studies in pregnant women. Because animal reproduction studies are not always predictive of human response, desloratadine should be used during pregnancy only if clearly needed.

Nursing Mothers:
Desloratadine passes into breast milk; therefore a decision should be made whether to discontinue nursing or to discontinue desloratadine, taking into account the importance of the drug to the mother.

Pediatric Use:
The recommended dose of CLARINEX Syrup in the pediatric population is based on cross-study comparison of the plasma concentration of CLARINEX in adults and pediatric subjects. The safety of CLARINEX Syrup has been established in 246 pediatric subjects aged 6 months to 11 years in three placebo-controlled clinical studies. Since the course of seasonal and perennial allergic rhinitis and chronic idiopathic urticaria and the effects of CLARINEX are sufficiently similar in the pediatric and adult populations, it allows extrapolation from the adult efficacy data to pediatric patients. The effectiveness of CLARINEX Syrup in these age groups is supported by evidence from adequate and well-controlled studies of CLARINEX Tablets in adults. The safety and effectiveness of CLARINEX Tablets or CLARINEX Syrup have not been demonstrated in pediatric patients less than 6 months of age.

The CLARINEX RediTabs Tablet 2.5 mg tablet has not been evaluated in pediatric patients. Bioequivalence of the CLARINEX RediTabs Tablet and the previously marketed RediTabs Tablet was established in adults. In conjunction with the dose finding studies in pediatrics described, the pharmacokinetic data for CLARINEX RediTabs Tablet supports the use of the 2.5 mg dose strength in pediatric patients 6-11 years of age.

Geriatric Use:
Clinical studies of desloratadine did not include sufficient numbers of subjects aged 65 and over to determine whether they respond differently from younger subjects. Other reported clinical experience has not identified differences between the elderly and younger patients. In general, dose selection for an elderly patient should be cautious, reflecting the greater frequency of decreased hepatic, renal, or cardiac function, and of concomitant disease or other drug therapy (see **CLINICAL PHARMACOLOGY – Special Populations**).

Information for Patients:
Patients should be instructed to use CLARINEX Tablets as directed. As there are no food effects on bioavailability, patients can be instructed that CLARINEX Tablets, Syrup, or RediTabs Tablets may be taken without regard to meals. Patients should be advised not to increase the dose or dosing frequency, as studies have not demonstrated increased effectiveness at higher doses and somnolence may occur.
Phenylketonurics: CLARINEX RediTabs Tablets contain phenylalanine 2.9 mg per 5 mg CLARINEX RediTabs Tablet or 1.4 mg per 2.5 mg CLARINEX RediTabs Tablet.

ADVERSE REACTIONS

Adults and Adolescents:
Allergic Rhinitis:
In multiple-dose placebo-controlled trials, 2,834 patients ages 12 years or older received CLARINEX Tablets at doses of 2.5 mg to 20 mg daily, of whom 1,655 patients received the recommended daily dose of 5 mg. In patients receiving 5 mg daily, the rate of adverse events was similar between CLARINEX and placebo-treated patients. The percent of patients who withdrew prematurely due to adverse events was 2.4% in the CLARINEX group and 2.6% in the placebo group. There were no serious adverse events in these trials in patients receiving desloratadine. All adverse events that were reported by greater than or equal to 2% of patients who received the recommended daily dose of CLARINEX Tablets (5.0 mg once-daily), and that were more common with CLARINEX Tablets than placebo, are listed in Table 5.

Table 5
Incidence of Adverse Events Reported by 2% or More of Adult and Adolescent Allergic Rhinitis Patients in Placebo-Controlled, Multiple-Dose Clinical Trials with the Tablet Formulation of CLARINEX

Adverse Experience	CLARINEX Tablets 5 mg (n=1,655)	Placebo (n=1,652)
Pharyngitis	4.1%	2.0%
Dry Mouth	3.0%	1.9%
Myalgia	2.1%	1.8%
Fatigue	2.1%	1.2%
Somnolence	2.1%	1.8%
Dysmenorrhea	2.1%	1.6%

The frequency and magnitude of laboratory and electrocardiographic abnormalities were similar in CLARINEX and placebo-treated patients.
There were no differences in adverse events for subgroups of patients as defined by gender, age, or race.
Chronic Idiopathic Urticaria:
In multiple-dose, placebo-controlled trials of chronic idiopathic urticaria, 211 patients ages 12 years or older received CLARINEX Tablets and 205 received placebo. Adverse events that were reported by greater than or equal to 2% of patients who received CLARINEX Tablets and that were more common with CLARINEX than placebo were (rates for CLARINEX and placebo, respectively): headache (14%, 13%), nausea (5%, 2%), fatigue (5%, 1%), dizziness (4%, 3%), pharyngitis (3%, 2%), dyspepsia (3%, 1%), and myalgia (3%, 1%).
Pediatrics:
Two hundred and forty-six pediatric subjects 6 months to 11 years of age received CLARINEX Syrup for 15 days in three placebo-controlled clinical trials. Pediatric subjects aged 6 to 11 years received 2.5 mg once a day, subjects aged 1 to 5 years received 1.25 mg once a day, and subjects 6 to 11 months of age received 1.0 mg once a day. In subjects 6 to 11 years of age, no individual adverse event was reported by 2 percent or more of the subjects. In subjects 2 to 5 years of age, adverse events reported for CLARINEX and placebo in at least 2 percent of subjects receiving CLARINEX Syrup and at a frequency greater than placebo were fever (5.5%,

5.4%), urinary tract infection (3.6%, 0%), and varicella (3.6%, 0%). In subjects 12 months to 23 months of age, adverse events reported for the CLARINEX product and placebo in at least 2 percent of subjects receiving CLARINEX Syrup and at a frequency greater than placebo were fever (16.9%, 12.9%), diarrhea (15.4%, 11.3%), upper respiratory tract infections (10.8%, 9.7%), coughing (10.8%, 6.5%), appetite increased (3.1%, 1.6%), emotional lability (3.1%, 0%), epistaxis (3.1%, 0%), parasitic infection (3.1%, 0%), pharyngitis (3.1%, 0%), rash maculopapular (3.1%, 0%). In subjects 6 months to 11 months of age, adverse events reported for CLARINEX and placebo in at least 2 percent of subjects receiving CLARINEX Syrup and at a frequency greater than placebo were upper respiratory tract infections (21.2%, 12.9%), diarrhea (19.7%, 8.1%), fever (12.1%, 1.6%), irritability (12.1%, 11.3%), coughing (10.6%, 9.7%), somnolence (9.1%, 8.1%), bronchitis (6.1%, 0%), otitis media (6.1%, 1.6%), vomiting (6.1%, 3.2%), anorexia (4.5%, 1.6%), pharyngitis (4.5%, 1.6%), insomnia (4.5%, 0%), rhinorrhea (4.5%, 3.2%), erythema (3.0%, 1.6%), and nausea (3.0%, 0%). There were no clinically meaningful changes in any electrocardiographic parameter, including the QTc interval. Only one of the 246 pediatric subjects receiving CLARINEX Syrup in the clinical trials discontinued treatment because of an adverse event.

Observed During Clinical Practice:
The following spontaneous adverse events have been reported during the marketing of desloratadine: tachycardia, palpitations, rare cases of hypersensitivity reactions (such as rash, pruritus, urticaria, edema, dyspnea, and anaphylaxis), psychomotor hyperactivity, seizures, and elevated liver enzymes including bilirubin, and very rarely, hepatitis.

DRUG ABUSE AND DEPENDENCE

There is no information to indicate that abuse or dependency occurs with CLARINEX Tablets.

OVERDOSAGE

Information regarding acute overdosage is limited to experience from clinical trials conducted during the development of the CLARINEX product. In a dose ranging trial, at doses of 10 mg and 20 mg/day somnolence was reported.
Single daily doses of 45 mg were given to normal male and female volunteers for 10 days. All ECGs obtained in this study were manually read in a blinded fashion by a cardiologist. In CLARINEX-treated subjects, there was an increase in mean heart rate of 9.2 bpm relative to placebo. The QT interval was corrected for heart rate (QTc) by both the Bazett and Fridericia methods. Using the QTc (Bazett) there was a mean increase of 8.1 msec in CLARINEX-treated subjects relative to placebo. Using QTc (Fridericia) there was a mean increase of 0.4 msec in CLARINEX-treated subjects relative to placebo. No clinically relevant adverse events were reported.
In the event of overdose, consider standard measures to remove any unabsorbed drug. Symptomatic and supportive treatment is recommended. Desloratadine and 3-hydroxydesloratadine are not eliminated by hemodialysis. Lethality occurred in rats at oral doses of 250 mg/kg or greater (estimated desloratadine and desloratadine metabolite exposures were approximately 120 times the AUC in humans at the recommended daily oral dose). The oral median lethal dose in mice was 353 mg/kg (estimated desloratadine exposures were approximately 290 times the human daily oral dose on a mg/m² basis). No deaths occurred at oral doses up to 250 mg/kg in monkeys (estimated desloratadine exposures were approximately 810 times the human daily oral dose on a mg/m² basis).

DOSAGE AND ADMINISTRATION

Adults and children 12 years of age and over:
The recommended dose of CLARINEX Tablets or CLARINEX RediTabs Tablets is one 5 mg tablet once daily or the recommended dose of CLARINEX Syrup is 2 teaspoonfuls (5 mg in 10 mL) once daily.

Children 6 to 11 years of age:
The recommended dose of CLARINEX Syrup is 1 teaspoonful (2.5 mg in 5 mL) once daily or the recommended dose of CLARINEX RediTabs Tablets is one 2.5 mg tablet once daily.

Children 12 months to 5 years of age:
The recommended dose of CLARINEX Syrup is ½ teaspoonful (1.25 mg in 2.5 mL) once daily.

Children 6 to 11 months of age:
The recommended dose of CLARINEX Syrup is 2 mL (1.0 mg) once daily.

The age-appropriate dose of CLARINEX Syrup should be administered with a commercially available measuring dropper or syringe that is calibrated to deliver 2 mL and 2.5 mL (½ teaspoon).

In adult patients with liver or renal impairment, a starting dose of one 5 mg tablet every other day is recommended based on pharmacokinetic data. Dosing recommendation for children with liver or renal impairment cannot be made due to lack of data.

Administration of CLARINEX RediTabs Tablets:
Place CLARINEX (desloratadine) RediTabs Tablets on the tongue and allow to disintegrate before swallowing. Tablet disintegration occurs rapidly. Administer with or without water. Take tablet immediately after opening the blister.

HOW SUPPLIED
CLARINEX Tablets:
Embossed "C5", light blue film coated tablets; that are packaged in high-density polyethylene plastic bottles of 100 (NDC 0085-1264-01) and 500 (NDC 0085-1264-02). Also available, CLARINEX Unit-of-Use package of 30 tablets (3 × 10; 10 blisters per card) (NDC 0085-1264-04); and Unit Dose-Hospital Pack of 100 Tablets (10 × 10; 10 blisters per card) (NDC 0085-1264-03).
Protect Unit-of-Use packaging and Unit Dose-Hospital Pack from excessive moisture.
Store at 25°C (77°F); excursions permitted to 15°-30°C (59°-86°F) [see USP Controlled Room Temperature]. Heat sensitive. Avoid exposure at or above 30°C (86°F).
CLARINEX Syrup:
Clear orange colored liquid containing 0.5 mg/1 mL desloratadine in a 16-ounce Amber glass bottle (NDC 0085-1334-01) and a 4-ounce Amber glass bottle (NDC 0085-1334-02).
Store at 25°C (77°F); excursions permitted to 15°-30°C (59°-86°F) [see USP Controlled Room Temperature]. Protect from light.
CLARINEX REDITABS (desloratadine orally-disintegrating tablets)
2.5 mg and 5 mg: Light-red, flat-faced, round, speckled tablets with an "A" debossed on one side for the 5 mg tablets and a "K" debossed on one side for the 2.5 mg tablets. One tablet per cavity in peel off foil/foil blisters. Packs of 30 tablets (containing 5 × 6's) 5 mg - NDC 0085-1384-01 and 2.5 mg - NDC 0085-1408-01.
Store at 25°C (77°F); excursions permitted to 15°-30°C (59-86°F) [see USP Controlled Room Temperature].
Schering Corporation
Kenilworth, NJ 07033 USA
Rev. 2/07   23882191T
CLARINEX REDITABS brand of desloratadine orally-disintegrating tablets are manufactured for Schering Corporation by CIMA LABS INC.®, Eden Prairie, MN 55344 USA.
U.S. Patent Nos. 4,659,716; 4,863,931; 5,178,878; 5,607,697; 6,100,274; 6,514,520; 6,709,676; and 6,979,463.
Copyright © 2004, 2005, Schering Corporation. All rights reserved.

Shown in Product Identification Guide, page 312

CLARINEX-D® 12 HOUR   ℞
[klă-rĭ-nĕks D]
(desloratadine/pseudoephedrinesulfate)
Extended Release Tablets
for oral use

HIGHLIGHTS OF PRESCRIBING INFORMATION
These highlights do not include all the information needed to use CLARINEX-D® 12 HOUR Extended Release Tablets safely and effectively. See full prescribing information for CLARINEX-D 12 HOUR Extended Release Tablets.
CLARINEX-D 12 HOUR Extended Release Tablets (desloratadine/pseudoephedrine sulfate) for oral use.
Initial U.S. Approval: 2005

──────────INDICATIONS AND USAGE──────────
CLARINEX-D 12 HOUR is a combination product containing an H1-receptor antagonist and a sympathomimetic amine indicated for:
• Relief of nasal and non-nasal symptoms of seasonal allergic rhinitis, including nasal congestion, in adults and adolescents 12 years of age and older. (1)
────────DOSAGE AND ADMINISTRATION────────
For oral use only
Adults and adolescents 12 years of age and over: The recommended dose of CLARINEX-D 12 HOUR Extended Release Tablets is one tablet twice a day. (2)
───────DOSAGE FORMS AND STRENGTHS───────
Desloratadine 2.5 mg/Pseudoephedrine sulfate 120 mg tablets. (3)
──────────CONTRAINDICATIONS──────────
• Hypersensitivity (4)
• Narrow Angle Glaucoma (4)
• Urinary Retention (4)
• Patients Receiving MAO Inhibitors or within 14 days of stopping such treatment (4)
• Severe hypertension or severe coronary artery disease (4)
──────WARNINGS AND PRECAUTIONS──────
• Cardiovascular and central nervous system effects: Use with caution in patients with cardiovascular disorders. (5.1).

• Coexisting conditions: Use with caution in patients with increased intraocular pressure, prostatic hypertrophy, diabetes mellitus, or hyperthyroidism (5.2).
──────────ADVERSE REACTIONS──────────
• The most common adverse reactions (reported in ≥2% of patients) were insomnia, headache, mouth dry, fatigue, somnolence, pharyngitis, dizziness, nausea, insomnia and anorexia. (6.1)
To report SUSPECTED ADVERSE REACTIONS, contact Schering Corporation at 800-526-4099 or FDA at 1-800-FDA-1088 or *www.fda.gov/medwatch.*
──────────DRUG INTERACTIONS──────────
Monoamine Oxidase (MAO) Inhibitors: Do not use. May potentiate the effect of pseudoephedrine on vascular system. (7.1)
──────USE IN SPECIFIC POPULATIONS──────
• Renal impairment: Avoid in patients with renal impairment (8.6)
• Hepatic impairment: Avoid in patients with hepatic impairment (8.7)
See 17 for PATIENT COUNSELING INFORMATION and FDA-approved patient labeling

Revised: 12/2009

FULL PRESCRIBING INFORMATION: CONTENTS*

FULL PRESCRIBING INFORMATION

1   INDICATIONS AND USAGE
1.1   Seasonal Allergic Rhinitis
CLARINEX-D® 12 HOUR Extended Release Tablets is indicated for the relief of the nasal and non-nasal symptoms of seasonal allergic rhinitis, including nasal congestion, in adults and adolescents 12 years of age and older.

CLARINEX-D 12 HOUR Extended Release Tablets should be administered when the antihistaminic properties of desloratadine and the nasal decongestant properties of pseudoephedrine are desired [see Clinical Pharmacology (12)].

2   DOSAGE AND ADMINISTRATION
Administer CLARINEX-D 12 HOUR Extended Release Tablet by the oral route only. Do not break, chew or crush the tablet. Swallow the tablet whole.
2.1   Adults and Adolescents 12 years of Age and Over
The recommended dose of CLARINEX-D 12 HOUR Extended Release Tablets is 1 tablet twice a day, administered approximately 12 hours apart and with or without a meal. Higher doses or increased dosing frequency of CLARINEX-D 12 HOUR Extended Release Tablets have not demonstrated increased effectiveness. Do not exceed the recommended dose as desloratadine and pseudoephedrine, the active components of CLARINEX-D 12 HOUR Extended Release Tablets have been associated with adverse effects at higher doses [see Overdosage (10.1) and (10.2)].

3   DOSAGE FORMS AND STRENGTHS
CLARINEX-D 12 HOUR Extended Release Tablets are oval shaped, blue and white bilayer tablets with "D12" embossed in the blue layer. Each tablet contains 2.5 mg desloratadine in the blue immediate-release layer and 120 mg of pseudoephedrine sulfate USP in the white extended-release layer.

4   CONTRAINDICATIONS
CLARINEX-D 12 HOUR Extended Release Tablets are contraindicated in:
• Patients with hypersensitivity to any of its ingredients, or to loratadine [see Warnings and Precautions (5.4) and Post-Marketing Experience (6.2)]
• Patients with narrow angle glaucoma
• Patients with urinary retention
• Patients receiving monoamine oxidase (MAO) inhibitor therapy or within fourteen (14) days of stopping such treatment [see Drug Interactions (7.1)].
• Patients with severe hypertension or severe coronary artery disease

5   WARNINGS AND PRECAUTIONS
5.1   Cardiovascular and Central Nervous System Effects
The pseudoephedrine sulfate contained in CLARINEX-D 12 HOUR Extended Release Tablets, like other sympathomimetic amines can produce cardiovascular and central nervous system (CNS) effects in some patients such as insomnia, dizziness, weakness, tremor, or arrhythmias. In addition central nervous system stimulation with convulsions or cardiovascular collapse with accompanying hypotension has been reported. Therefore, CLARINEX-D 12 HOUR Extended Release Tablets should be used with caution in patients with cardiovascular disorders, and should not be used in patients with severe hypertension or severe coronary artery disease.
5.2   Coexisting Conditions
CLARINEX-D 12 HOUR Extended Release Tablets contain pseudoephedrine sulfate a sympathomimetic amine and therefore should be used with caution in patients with diabetes and hyperthyroidism. Also use with caution in patients with prostatic hypertrophy or increased intraocular pressure, as urinary retention and narrow angle glaucoma may occur [see Contraindications (4)].
5.3   Co-Administration with Monoamine Oxidase (MAO) Inhibitors
CLARINEX-D 12 HOUR Extended Release Tablets should not be used in patients receiving monoamine oxidase (MAO) inhibitor therapy or within fourteen (14) days of stopping such treatment as an increase in blood pressure or hypertensive crisis, may occur [see Contraindications (4) and Drug Interactions (7.1)].
5.4   Hypersensitivity Reactions
Hypersensitivity reactions including rash, pruritus, urticaria, edema, dyspnea, and anaphylaxis have been reported after administration of desloratadine a component of CLARINEX-D 12 HOUR Extended Release Tablets. If such a reaction occurs, therapy with CLARINEX-D 12 HOUR Extended Release Tablets should be stopped and alternative treatment should be considered [see Post-marketing (6.2)].
5.5   Renal Impairment
CLARINEX-D 12 HOUR Extended Release Tablets should generally be avoided in patients with renal impairment [see Clinical Pharmacology (12)].
5.6   Hepatic Impairment
CLARINEX-D 12 HOUR Extended Release Tablets should generally be avoided in patients with hepatic impairment [see Clinical Pharmacology (12)].

6   ADVERSE REACTIONS

The following adverse reactions are discussed in greater detail in other sections of the label:
- Cardiovascular and Central Nervous System effects [see Warnings and Precautions (5.1)]
- Increased Intraocular pressure [see Warnings and Precautions (5.2)]
- Urinary retention in patients with prostatic hypertrophy [see Warnings and Precautions (5.2)]
- Hypersensitivity reactions [see Warnings and Precautions (5.4)].

6.1   Clinical Trials Experience

Because clinical trials are conducted under widely varying conditions, adverse reaction rates observed in the clinical trials of a drug cannot be directly compared to rates in the clinical trials of another drug and may not reflect the rates observed in clinical practice. The safety data described below are from 2 clinical trials with CLARINEX-D 12 HOUR Extended Release Tablets that included 1248 patients with seasonal allergic rhinitis, of which 414 patients received CLARINEX-D 12 HOUR Extended Release Tablets twice daily for up to 2 weeks. The majority of patients were between 18 and <65 years of age with a mean age of 35.8 years and were predominantly women (64%). Patient ethnicity was 82% Caucasian, 9% Black, 6 % Hispanic and 3% Asian/other ethnicity. The percentage of subjects receiving CLARINEX-D 12 HOUR Extended Release Tablets and who discontinued from the clinical trials because of an adverse event was 3.6%. Adverse reactions that were reported by ≥2% of subjects receiving CLARINEX-D 12 HOUR Extended Release Tablets are shown in Table 1.

[See table 1 at right]

There were no relevant differences in adverse reactions for subgroups of patients as defined by gender, age, or race.

6.2   Post-Marketing Experience

In addition to the adverse reactions reported during clinical trials and listed above, adverse events have been identified during post approval use of CLARINEX-D 12 HOUR Extended Release Tablets. Because these events are reported voluntarily from a population of uncertain size, it is not always possible to reliably estimate their frequency or establish a causal relationship to drug exposure. Adverse events identified from post-marketing surveillance on the use of CLARINEX-D 12 HOUR Extended Release Tablets include tachycardia, palpitations, dyspnea, rash and pruritis.

In addition to these events, the following spontaneous adverse events have been reported during the marketing of desloratadine as a single ingredient product: headache, somnolence, dizziness and rarely hypersensitivity reactions (such as urticaria, edema and anaphylaxis), and elevated liver enzymes including bilirubin and very rarely, hepatitis.

7   DRUG INTERACTIONS

No specific interaction studies have been conducted with CLARINEX-D 12 HOUR Extended Release Tablets.

7.1   Monoamine Oxidase Inhibitors

CLARINEX-D 12 HOUR Extended Release Tablets should not be used in patients receiving monoamine oxidase (MAO) inhibitor therapy or within fourteen (14) days of stopping such treatment because the action of pseudoephedrine a component of CLARINEX-D 12 HOUR Extended Release tablets on the vascular system may be potentiated by these agents. (see Contraindications (4) and Warnings and Precautions 5.3)

7.2   Beta-adrenergic blocking agents

The antihypertensive effects of beta-adrenergic blocking agents, methyldopa, and reserpine, may be reduced by sympathomimetics such as pseudoephedrine. Exercise caution when using CLARINEX-D 12 HOUR Extended Release Tablets with these agents.

7.3   Digitalis

Increased ectopic pacemaker activity can occur when pseudoephedrine is used concomitantly with digitalis. Exercise caution when using CLARINEX-D 12 HOUR Extended Release Tablets with these agents.

7.4   Inhibitors of cytochrome P450 3A4

In controlled clinical studies co-administration of desloratadine with ketoconazole, erythromycin, or azithromycin resulted in increased plasma concentrations of desloratadine and 3-hydroxydesloratadine but there were no clinically relevant changes in the safety profile of desloratadine. [see Clinical Pharmacology (12.3)]

7.5   Fluoxetine

In controlled clinical studies co-administration of desloratadine with fluoxetine, a selective serotonin reuptake inhibitor (SSRI), resulted in increased plasma concentrations of desloratadine and 3-hydroxydesloratadine but there were no clinically relevant changes in the safety profile of desloratadine [see Clinical Pharmacology (12.3)]

7.6   Cimetidine

In controlled clinical studies co-administration of desloratadine with cimetidine a histamine H2-receptor antagonist resulted in increased plasma concentrations of desloratadine and 3-hydroxydesloratadine but there were no clinically relevant changes in the safety profile of desloratadine [see Clinical Pharmacology (12.3)]

8   USE IN SPECIFIC POPULATIONS

8.1   Pregnancy

Pregnancy Category C: There are no adequate and well-controlled studies of desloratadine and pseudoephedrine in combination in pregnant women. Neither are there animal reproduction studies conducted with the combination of desloratadine and pseudoephedrine. Desloratadine was not teratogenic in rats or rabbits but affected implantation in rats. Because animal reproduction studies are not always predictive of human response, CLARINEX-D 12 HOUR Extended Release Tablets should be used during pregnancy only if clearly needed.

Desloratadine was not teratogenic in rats or rabbits at approximately 210 and 230 times, respectively, the AUC in humans at the recommended daily oral dose. An increase in pre-implantation loss and a decreased number of implantations and fetuses were noted, however, in a separate study in female rats at approximately 120 times the AUC in humans at the recommended daily oral dose. Reduced body weight and slow righting reflex were reported in pups at approximately 50 times or greater than the AUC in humans at the recommended daily oral dose. Desloratadine had no effect on pup development at approximately 7 times the AUC in humans at the recommended daily oral dose. The AUCs in comparison referred to the desloratadine exposure in rabbits and the sum of desloratadine and its metabolites exposures in rats, respectively [see Nonclinical Toxicology (13.2)]

8.3   Nursing Mothers

Desloratadine and pseudoephedrine both pass into breast milk; therefore, a decision should be made whether to discontinue nursing or to discontinue CLARINEX-D 12 HOUR Extended Release Tablets, taking into account the benefit of the drug to the nursing mother and the possible risk to the child.

8.4   Pediatric Use

CLARINEX-D 12 HOUR Extended Release Tablets are not indicated for use in pediatric patients under 12 years of age.

8.5   Geriatric Use

The number of subjects (n=10) ≥65 years old treated with CLARINEX-D 12 HOUR Extended Release Tablets was too limited to make any formal statistical comparison regarding the efficacy or safety of this drug product in this age group, or to determine whether they respond differently from younger subjects. Other reported clinical experience has not identified differences between the elderly and younger patients, although the elderly are more likely to have adverse reactions to sympathomimetic amines. In general, dose selection for an elderly patient should be cautious, reflecting the greater frequency of decreased hepatic, renal, or cardiac function, and of concomitant disease or other drug therapy [see Clinical Pharmacology (12.3)].

Pseudoephedrine, desloratadine, and their metabolites are known to be substantially excreted by the kidney, and the risk of adverse reactions may be greater in patients with renal impairment. Because elderly patients are more likely to have decreased renal function, care should be taken in dose selection, and it may be useful to monitor the patient for adverse events [see Clinical Pharmacology (12.3)].

8.6   Renal Impairment

No studies with CLARINEX-D 12 HOUR Extended Release Tablets were conducted in subjects with renal impairment. CLARINEX-D 12 HOUR Extended Release Tablets should generally be avoided in patients with renal impairment [see Warnings and Precautions (5.5) and Clinical Pharmacology (12.3)].

8.7   Hepatic Impairment

No studies with CLARINEX-D 12 HOUR Extended Release Tablets or pseudoephedrine were conducted in subjects with hepatic impairment.

CLARINEX-D 12 HOUR Extended Release Tablets should generally be avoided in patients with hepatic impairment [see Warnings and Precautions (5.6) and Clinical Pharmacology (12.3)].

8.8   Gender

No clinically significant gender-related differences were observed in the pharmacokinetic parameters of desloratadine, 3-hydroxydesloratadine or pseudoephedrine following administration of CLARINEX-D 12 HOUR Extended Release Tablets.

8.9   Race

No studies have been conducted to evaluate the effect of race on the pharmacokinetics of CLARINEX-D 12 HOUR Extended Release Tablets.

9   DRUG ABUSE AND DEPENDENCE

There is no information to indicate that abuse or dependency occurs with CLARINEX or CLARINEX-D 12 HOUR Extended Release Tablets.

10   OVERDOSAGE

In the event of overdose, consider standard measures to remove any unabsorbed drug. Symptomatic and supportive treatment is recommended. Desloratadine and 3-hydroxydesloratadine are not eliminated by hemodialysis.

10.1   Desloratadine

Information regarding acute overdosage with desloratadine is limited to experience from postmarketing adverse event reports and from clinical trials conducted during the development of the CLARINEX product. In the reported cases of overdose, there were no significant adverse events that were attributed to desloratadine. In a dose-ranging trial, at doses of 10 mg and 20 mg/day, somnolence was reported.

In another study, no clinically relevant adverse events were reported in normal male and female volunteers who were given single daily doses of CLARINEX 45 mg for 10 days [see Clinical Pharmacology (12.2)].

TABLE 1: Incidence of Adverse Reactions Reported by ≥ 2% of Patients Receiving CLARINEX-D 12 HOUR Extended Release Tablets

Adverse Reaction	CLARINEX-D® 12 HOUR BID (N = 414)	Desloratadine 5 mg QD (N = 412)	Pseudoephedrine 120 mg BID (N = 422)
Gastrointestinal Disorders			
Mouth Dry	8%	2%	8%
Nausea	2%	1%	3%
General Disorders and Administration Site Conditions			
Fatigue	4%	2%	2%
Metabolism and Nutrition Disorders			
Anorexia	2%	0%	2%
Nervous System Disorders			
Headache	8%	8%	9%
Somnolence	3%	4%	2%
Dizziness	3%	2%	2%
Psychiatric Disorders			
Insomnia	10%	3%	13%
Respiratory, Thoracic and Mediastinal Disorders			
Pharyngitis	3%	3%	3%

Lethality occurred in rats at oral doses of 250 mg/kg or greater (estimated desloratadine and desloratadine metabolite exposures were approximately 120 times the AUC in humans at the recommended daily oral dose). The oral median lethal dose in mice was 353 mg/kg (estimated desloratadine exposure was approximately 290 times the human daily oral dose on an mg/m^2 basis). No deaths occurred at oral doses up to 250 mg/kg in monkeys (estimated desloratadine exposure was approximately 810 times the human daily oral dose on an mg/m^2 basis).

10.2 Sympathomimetics

In large doses, sympathomimetics such as pseudoephedrine may give rise to giddiness, headache, nausea, vomiting, sweating, thirst, tachycardia, precordial pain, palpitations, difficulty in micturition, muscle weakness and tenseness, anxiety, restlessness, and insomnia. Many patients can present a toxic psychosis with delusions and hallucinations. Some may develop cardiac arrhythmias, circulatory collapse, convulsions, coma, and respiratory failure.

11 DESCRIPTION

CLARINEX-D 12 HOUR Extended Release Tablets are oval-shaped blue and white bilayer tablets containing 2.5 mg desloratadine in the blue immediate-release layer and 120 mg of pseudoephedrine sulfate, USP in the white extended-release layer which is released slowly, allowing for twice-daily administration.

The inactive ingredients contained in CLARINEX-D 12 HOUR Extended Release Tablets are hypromellose USP, microcrystalline cellulose NF, povidone USP, silicon dioxide NF, magnesium stearate NF, corn starch NF, edetate disodium USP, citric acid anhydrous USP, stearic acid NF and FD&C Blue No. 2 aluminum lake dye.

Desloratadine, 1 of the 2 active ingredients of CLARINEX-D 12 HOUR Extended Release Tablets, is a white to off-white powder that is slightly soluble in water, but very soluble in ethanol and propylene glycol. It has an empirical formula: $C_{19}H_{19}ClN_2$ and a molecular weight of 310.8. The chemical name is 8-chloro-6,11-dihydro-11-(4-piperdinylidene)-5*H*-benzo[5,6] cyclohepta [1,2-*b*]pyridine and has the following structure:

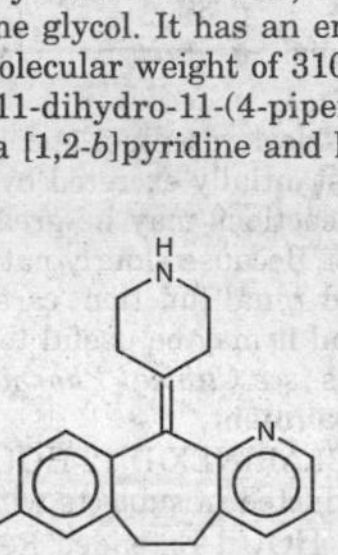

Pseudoephedrine sulfate, the other active ingredient of CLARINEX-D 12 HOUR Extended Release Tablets, is the synthetic salt of one of the naturally occurring dextrorotatory diastereomers of ephedrine and is classified as an indirect sympathomimetic amine. Pseudoephedrine sulfate is a colorless hygroscopic crystal or white, hygroscopic crystalline powder, practically odorless, with a bitter taste. It is very soluble in water, freely soluble in alcohol, and sparingly soluble in ether. The empirical formula for pseudoephedrine sulfate is $(C_{10}H_{15}NO)_2 \bullet H_2SO_4$; the chemical name is benzenemethanol, α-[1-(methylamino) ethyl]-,[*S*-(*R**,*R**)]-, sulfate (2:1)(salt); and the chemical structure is:

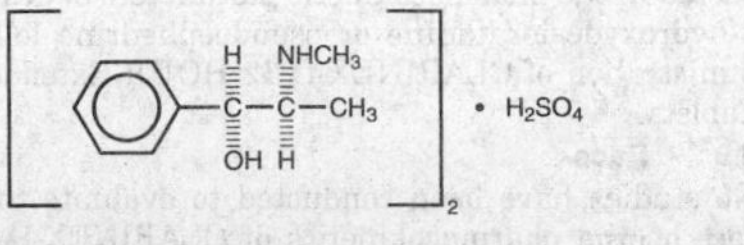

12 CLINICAL PHARMACOLOGY

12.1 Mechanism of Action

Desloratadine is a long acting tricyclic histamine antagonist with selective H_1-receptor histamine antagonist activity. Receptor binding data indicate that at a concentration of 2 to 3 ng/mL (7 nanomolar), desloratadine shows significant interaction with the human histamine H_1 receptor. Desloratadine inhibited histamine release from human mast cells *in vitro*. Results of a radiolabeled tissue distribution study in rats and a radioligand H_1-receptor-binding study in guinea pigs showed that desloratadine does not readily cross the blood brain barrier. The clinical significance of this finding is unknown.

Pseudoephedrine sulfate is an orally active sympathomimetic amine and exerts a decongestant action on the nasal mucosa. Pseudoephedrine sulfate is recognized as an effective agent for the relief of nasal congestion due to allergic rhinitis. Pseudoephedrine produces peripheral effects similar to those of ephedrine and central effects similar to, but less intense than, amphetamines. It has the potential for excitatory side effects.

12.2 Pharmacodynamics

Wheal and Flare: Human histamine skin wheal studies following single and repeated 5 mg doses of desloratadine have shown that the drug exhibits an antihistaminic effect by 1 hour; this activity may persist for as long as 24 hours. There was no evidence of histamine-induced skin wheal tachyphylaxis within the desloratadine 5mg group over the 28 day treatment period. The clinical relevance of histamine wheal skin testing is unknown.

Effects on QT_c: In clinical trials for CLARINEX-D 12 HOUR Extended Release Tablets, ECGs were recorded at baseline and endpoint within 1 to 3 hours after the last dose. The majority of ECGs were normal at both baseline and endpoint. No clinically meaningful changes were observed following treatment with CLARINEX-D 12 HOUR Extended Release Tablets for any ECG parameter, including the QTc interval. An increase in the ventricular rate of 7.1 and 6.4 bpm was observed in the CLARINEX-D 12 HOUR Extended Release Tablets and pseudoephedrine groups, respectively, compared to an increase of 3.2 bpm in subjects receiving desloratadine alone. Single daily doses of CLARINEX 45 mg were given to normal male and female volunteers for 10 days.

All ECGs obtained in this study were manually read in a blinded fashion by a cardiologist. In the CLARINEX-treated subjects, there was a mean increase in the maximum heart rate of 9.2 bpm relative to placebo. The QT interval was corrected for heart rate (QTc) by both Bazett's and Fridericia methods. Using the QTc (Bazett) there was a mean increase of 8.1 msec in the CLARINEX-treated subjects relative to placebo. Using QTc (Fridericia) there was a mean increase of 0.4 msec in CLARINEX-treated subjects relative to placebo. No clinically relevant adverse events were reported.

12.3 Pharmacokinetics

Absorption:

In a single dose pharmacokinetic study, the mean time to maximum plasma concentrations (T_{max}) for desloratadine occurred at approximately 4 to 5 hours post dose and mean peak plasma concentrations (C_{max}) and area under the concentration-time curve (AUC) of approximately 1.09 ng/mL and 31.6 ng·hr/mL, respectively, were observed. In another pharmacokinetic study, food and grapefruit juice had no effect on the bioavailability (C_{max} and AUC) of desloratadine.

For pseudoephedrine, the mean T_{max} occurred at 6 to 7 hours post dose and mean peak plasma concentrations (C_{max}) and area under the concentration-time curve (AUC) of approximately 263 ng/mL and 4588 ng·hr/mL, respectively, were observed. Food had no effect on the bioavailability (C_{max} and AUC) of pseudoephedrine.

Following oral administration of CLARINEX-D 12 HOUR Extended Release Tablets twice daily for 14 days in healthy volunteers, steady-state conditions were reached on Day 10 for desloratadine, 3-hydroxydesloratadine and pseudoephedrine. For desloratadine, mean steady-state peak plasma concentrations (C_{max}) and area under the concentration-time curve (AUC 0–12 h) of approximately 1.7 ng/mL and 16 ng·hr/mL were observed, respectively. For pseudoephedrine, mean steady state peak plasma concentrations (C_{max}) and AUC (0–12 h) of 459 ng/mL and 4658 ng•hr/mL were observed.

Distribution:

Desloratadine and 3-hydroxydesloratadine are approximately 82% to 87% and 85% to 89%, bound to plasma proteins, respectively. Protein binding of desloratadine and 3-hydroxydesloratadine was unaltered in subjects with impaired renal function.

Metabolism:

Desloratadine (a major metabolite of loratadine) is extensively metabolized to 3-hydroxydesloratadine, an active metabolite, which is subsequently glucuronidated. The enzyme(s) responsible for the formation of 3-hydroxydesloratadine have not been identified. Data from clinical trials with desloratadine indicate that a subset of the general population has a decreased ability to form 3-hydroxydesloratadine, and are poor metabolizers of desloratadine. In pharmacokinetic studies (n= 3748), approximately 6% of subjects were poor metabolizers of desloratadine (defined as a subject with an AUC ratio of 3-hydroxydesloratadine to desloratadine less than 0.1, or a subject with a desloratadine half-life exceeding 50 hours). These pharmacokinetic studies included subjects between the ages of 2 and 70 years, including 977 subjects aged 2 to 5 years, 1575 subjects aged 6 to 11 years, and 1196 subjects aged 12 to 70 years. There was no difference in the prevalence of poor metabolizers across age groups. The frequency of poor metabolizers was higher in Blacks (17%, n=988) as compared to Caucasians (2%, n=1462) and Hispanics (2%, n=1063). The median exposure (AUC) to desloratadine in the poor metabolizers was approximately 6-fold greater than in the subjects who are not poor metabolizers. Subjects who are poor metabolizers of desloratadine cannot be prospectively identified and will be exposed to higher levels of desloratadine following dosing with the recommended dose of desloratadine. In multidose clinical safety studies, where metabolizer status was prospectively identified, a total of 94 poor metabolizers and 123 normal metabolizers were enrolled and treated with CLARINEX Syrup for 15 to 35 days. In these studies, no overall differences in safety were observed between poor metabolizers and normal metabolizers. Although not seen in these studies, an increased risk of exposure-related adverse events in patients who are poor metabolizers cannot be ruled out.

Pseudoephedrine alone is incompletely metabolized (less than 1%) in the liver by N-demethylation to an inactive metabolite. The drug and its metabolite are excreted in the urine. About 55% to 96% of an administered dose of pseudoephedrine hydrochloride is excreted unchanged in the urine.

Elimination:

Following single dose administration of CLARINEX-D 12 HOUR Extended Release Tablets, the mean plasma elimination half-life of desloratadine was approximately 27 hours. In another study, following administration of single oral doses of desloratadine 5 mg, C_{max} and AUC values increased in a dose proportional manner following single oral doses between 5 and 20 mg. The degree of accumulation after 14 days of dosing was consistent with the half-life and dosing frequency. A human mass balance study documented a recovery of approximately 87% of the ^{14}C-desloratadine dose, which was equally distributed in urine and feces as metabolic products. Analysis of plasma 3-hydroxydesloratadine showed similar T_{max} and half-life values compared to desloratadine.

The mean elimination half-life of pseudoephedrine is dependent on urinary pH. The elimination half-life is approximately 3 to 6 or 9 to 16 hours when the urinary pH is 5 or 8, respectively.

Geriatric Subjects: Following multiple-dose administration of CLARINEX Tablets, the mean C_{max} and AUC values for desloratadine were 20% greater than in younger subjects (< 65 years old). The oral total body clearance (CL/F) when normalized for body weight was similar between the 2 age groups. The mean plasma elimination half-life of desloratadine was 33.7 hr in subjects ≥65 years old. The pharmacokinetics for 3-hydroxydesloratadine appeared unchanged in older vs. younger subjects. These age-related differences are unlikely to be clinically relevant and no dosage adjustment is recommended in elderly patients.

Pediatric Subjects: CLARINEX-D 12 HOUR Extended Release Tablets are not an appropriate dosage form for use in pediatric patients below 12 years of age.

Renally Impaired: Following a single dose of desloratadine 7.5 mg pharmacokinetics were characterized in subjects with mild (n=7; creatinine clearance 51–69 mL/min/1.73m^2), moderate (n=6; creatinine clearance 34–43 mL/min/1.73m^2) and severe (n=6; creatinine clearance 5–29 mL/min/1.73m^2) renal impairment or hemodialysis dependent (n=6) subjects. In subjects with mild and moderate renal impairment, median C_{max} and AUC values increased by approximately 1.2- and 1.9-fold, respectively, relative to subjects with normal renal function. In subjects with severe renal impairment or who were hemodialysis dependent, C_{max} and AUC values increased by approximately 1.7- and 2.5-fold, respectively. Minimal changes in 3-hydroxydesloratadine concentrations were observed. Desloratadine and 3-hydroxydesloratadine were poorly removed by hemodialysis. Plasma protein binding of desloratadine and 3-hydroxydesloratadine was unaltered by renal impairment.

Pseudoephedrine is primarily excreted unchanged in the urine as unchanged drug with the remainder apparently being metabolized in the liver. Therefore, pseudoephedrine may accumulate in patients with renal impairment.

Hepatically Impaired: Following a single oral dose of desloratadine, pharmacokinetics were characterized in subjects with mild (n=4), moderate (n=4) and severe (n=4) hepatic impairment as defined by the Child-Pugh classification of hepatic impairment and 8 subjects with normal hepatic function. Subjects with hepatic impairment, regardless of severity, had approximately a 2.4-fold increase in AUC as compared with normal subjects. The apparent oral clearance of desloratadine in subjects with mild, moderate, and severe hepatic impairment was 37%, 36%, and 28% of that in normal subjects, respectively. An increase in the mean elimination half-life of desloratadine in subjects with hepatic impairment was observed. For 3-hydroxydesloratadine, the mean C_{max} and AUC values for subjects with hepatic impairment combined were not statistically significantly different from subjects with normal hepatic function.

Gender: Female subjects treated for 14 days with CLARINEX Tablets had 10% and 3% higher desloratadine C_{max} and AUC values, respectively, compared with male subjects. The 3-hydroxydesloratadine C_{max} and AUC values were also increased by 45% and 48%, respectively, in females compared with males. However, these apparent differences are not considered to be clinically relevant.

Race: Following 14 days of treatment with CLARINEX Tablets, the C_{max} and AUC values for desloratadine were 18% and 32% higher, respectively in Blacks compared with

Caucasians. For 3-hydroxydesloratadine there was a corresponding 10% reduction in C_{max} and AUC values in Blacks compared to Caucasians. These differences are not considered to be clinically relevant.

Drug interaction: In 2 controlled crossover clinical pharmacology studies in healthy male (n=12 in each study) and female (n=12 in each study) subjects, desloratadine 7.5 mg (1.5 times the daily dose) once daily was co-administered with erythromycin 500 mg every 8 hours or ketoconazole 200 mg every 12 hours for 10 days. In 3 separate controlled, parallel group clinical pharmacology studies, desloratadine at the clinical dose of 5 mg has been coadministered with azithromycin 500 mg followed by 250 mg once daily for 4 days (n=18) or with fluoxetine 20 mg once daily for 7 days after a 23-day pretreatment period with fluoxetine (n=18) or with cimetidine 600 mg every 12 hours for 14 days (n=18) under steady state conditions to healthy male and female subjects. Although increased plasma concentrations (Cmax and AUC 0–24 hrs) of desloratadine and 3-hydroxydesloratadine were observed (see Table 2), there were no clinically relevant changes in the safety profile of desloratadine, as assessed by electrocardiographic parameters (including the corrected QT interval), clinical laboratory tests, vital signs and adverse events.

[See table 2 at right]

13 NONCLINICAL TOXICOLOGY

13.1 Carcinogenesis, Mutagenesis, Impairment of Fertility

There are no animal or laboratory studies on the combination product of desloratadine and pseudoephedrine sulfate to evaluate carcinogenesis, mutagenesis, or impairment of fertility.

Carcinogenicity Studies:

The carcinogenic potential of desloratadine was assessed using a loratadine study in rats and a desloratadine study in mice. In a 2-year study in rats, loratadine was administered in the diet at doses up to 25 mg/kg/day (estimated desloratadine and desloratadine metabolite exposures were approximately 30 times the AUC in humans at the recommended daily oral dose). A significantly higher incidence of hepatocellular tumors (combined adenomas and carcinomas) was observed in males given 10 mg/kg/day of loratadine and in males and females given 25 mg/kg/day of loratadine. The estimated desloratadine and desloratadine metabolite exposures in rats given 10 mg/kg of loratadine were approximately 7 times the AUC in humans at the recommended daily oral dose. The clinical significance of these findings during long-term use of desloratadine is not known.

In a 2-year dietary study in mice, males and females given up to 16 mg/kg/day and 32 mg/kg/day desloratadine, respectively, did not show significant increases in the incidence of any tumors. The estimated desloratadine and desloratadine metabolite exposures in mice at these doses were 12 and 27 times, respectively, the AUC in humans at the recommended daily oral dose.

Genotoxicity Studies:

In genotoxicity studies with desloratadine, there was no evidence of genotoxic potential in a reverse mutation assay (Salmonella/E. coli mammalian microsome bacterial mutagenicity assay) or in 2 assays for chromosomal aberrations (human peripheral blood lymphocyte clastogenicity assay and mouse bone marrow micronucleus assay).

Impairment of Fertility:

There was no effect on female fertility in rats at desloratadine doses up to 24 mg/kg/day (estimated desloratadine and desloratadine metabolite exposures were approximately 130 times the AUC in humans at the recommended daily oral dose). A male-specific decrease in fertility, demonstrated by reduced female conception rates, decreased sperm numbers and motility, and histopathologic testicular changes, occurred at an oral desloratadine dose of 12 mg/kg (estimated desloratadine and desloratadine metabolite exposures were approximately 45 times the AUC in humans at the recommended daily oral dose). Desloratadine had no effect on fertility in rats at an oral dose of 3 mg/kg/day (estimated desloratadine and desloratadine metabolite exposures were approximately 8 times the AUC in humans at the recommended daily oral dose).

13.2 Animal Toxicology and/or Pharmacology

Reproductive Toxicology Studies:

Desloratadine was not teratogenic in rats at doses up to 48 mg/kg/day (estimated desloratadine and desloratadine metabolite exposures were approximately 210 times the AUC in humans at the recommended daily oral dose) or in rabbits at doses up to 60 mg/kg/day (estimated desloratadine exposures were approximately 230 times the AUC in humans at the recommended daily oral dose). In a separate study, an increase in pre-implantation loss and a decreased number of implantations and fetuses were noted in female rats at 24 mg/kg (estimated desloratadine and desloratadine metabolite exposures were approximately 120 times the AUC in humans at the recommended daily oral

dose). Reduced body weight and slow righting reflex were reported in pups at doses of 9 mg/kg/day or greater (estimated desloratadine and desloratadine metabolite exposures were approximately 50 times or greater than the AUC in humans at the recommended daily oral dose). Desloratadine had no effect on pup development at an oral dose of 3 mg/kg/day (estimated desloratadine and desloratadine metabolite exposures were approximately 7 times the AUC in humans at the recommended daily oral dose).

14 CLINICAL STUDIES

14.1 Seasonal Allergic Rhinitis

The clinical efficacy and safety of CLARINEX-D 12 HOUR Extended Release Tablets was evaluated in two 2-week multicenter, randomized parallel group clinical trials involving 1248 subjects 12 to 78 years of age with seasonal allergic rhinitis, 414 of whom received CLARINEX-D 12 HOUR Extended Release Tablets. In the 2 trials, subjects were randomized to receive CLARINEX-D 12 HOUR Extended Release Tablets twice daily, CLARINEX Tablets 5 mg once daily, or sustained-release pseudoephedrine tablet 120 mg twice daily for 2 weeks. The majority of patients were between 18 and <65 years of age with a mean age of 35.8 years and were predominantly women (64%). Patient ethnicity was 82 % Caucasian, 9% Black, 6 % Hispanic and 3% Asian/other ethnicity. Primary efficacy variable was twice-daily reflective patient scoring of 4 nasal symptoms (rhinorrhea, nasal stuffiness/congestion, nasal itching, and sneezing) and four non-nasal symptoms (itching/burning eyes, tearing/watering eyes, redness of eyes, and itching of ears/palate) on a 4 point scale (0=none, 1=mild, 2=moderate, and 3=severe). In both trials, the antihistaminic efficacy of CLARINEX-D 12 HOUR Extended Release Tablets, as measured by total symptom score excluding nasal congestion,

was significantly greater than pseudoephedrine alone over the 2-week treatment period; and the decongestant efficacy of CLARINEX-D 12 HOUR Extended Release Tablets, as measured by nasal stuffiness/congestion, was significantly greater than CLARINEX (desloratadine alone) over the 2-week treatment period. Primary efficacy variable results from 1 of 2 trials are shown in Table 3.

[See table 3 above]

There were no significant differences in the efficacy of CLARINEX-D 12 HOUR Extended Release Tablets across subgroups of subjects defined by gender, age, or race.

16 HOW SUPPLIED/STORAGE AND HANDLING

CLARINEX-D 12 HOUR Extended Release Tablets are oval-shaped, blue and white bilayer tablets with "D12" embossed in the blue layer, containing 2.5 mg desloratadine in the blue immediate-release layer and 120 mg of pseudoephedrine sulfate USP in the white extended-release layer. CLARINEX-D 12 HOUR Extended Release Tablets are supplied in high-density polyethylene bottles of 100 (NDC 0085-1322-01).

Storage:

Store at 25°C (77°F); excursions permitted to 15–30°C (59–86°F) [see USP Controlled Room Temperature]. Avoid exposure at or above 30°C (86°F). Protect from excessive moisture. Protect from light.

17 PATIENT COUNSELING INFORMATION

[see FDA Approved Patient Labeling]

17.1 Cardiovascular and Central Nervous System Effects

Patients should be informed that pseudoephedrine, on of the active ingredients in CLARINEX-D 12 HOUR Extended Release Tablets may cause cardiovascular or central nervous system effects such as insomnia, dizziness, tremor, or arrhythmia.

TABLE 2 Changes in Desloratadine and 3-hydroxydesloratadine Pharmacokinetics in Healthy Male and Female Subjects

	Desloratadine		3-hydroxydesloratadine	
	C_{max}	AUC 0–24 hrs	C_{max}	AUC 0–24 hrs
Erythromycin (500 mg Q8h)	+24%	+14%	+43%	+40%
Ketoconazole (200 mg Q12h)	+45%	+39%	+43%	+72%
Azithromycin (500 mg day 1, 250 mg QD × 4 days)	+15%	+5%	+15%	+4%
Fluoxetine (20 mg QD)	+15%	+0%	+17%	+13%
Cimetidine (600 mg Q12h)	+12%	+19%	-11%	-3%

TABLE 3: Changes in Symptoms in a 2-Week Clinical Trial in Subjects With Seasonal Allergic Rhinitis

Treatment Group (n)	Mean Baseline* (sem)	Change (% Change) from Baseline[†] (sem)	CLARINEX-D® 12 HOUR Comparison to Components[‡] (P-value)
Total Symptom Score (Excluding Nasal Congestion)			
CLARINEX-D® 12 HOUR Extended Release Tablets BID (199)	14.18 (0.21)	-6.54 (-46.0) (0.30)	–
Pseudoephedrine tablet 120 mg BID (197)	14.06 (0.21)	-5.07 (-35.9) (0.30)	P<0.001
CLARINEX® 5 mg Tablets QD (197)	14.82 (0.21)	-5.09 (-33.5) (0.30)	P<0.001
Nasal Stuffiness/Congestion			
CLARINEX-D® 12 HOUR Extended Release Tablets BID (199)	2.47 (0.027)	-0.93 (-37.4) (0.046)	–
Pseudoephedrine tablet 120 mg BID (197)	2.46 (0.027)	-0.75 (-31.2) (0.046)	P=0.006
CLARINEX® 5 mg Tablets QD (197)	2.50 (0.027)	-0.66 (-26.7) (0.046)	**P<0.001**

Sem=Standard Error of the Mean

*To qualify at Baseline, the sum of the twice-daily diary reflective scores for the 3 days prior to Baseline and the morning of the Baseline visit were to total ≥42 for total nasal symptom score (sum of 4 nasal symptoms of rhinorrhea, nasal stuffiness/congestion, nasal itching, and sneezing) and a total of ≥35 for total non-nasal symptoms score (sum of 4 non-nasal symptoms of itching/burning eyes, tearing/watering eyes, redness of eyes, and itching of ears/palate), and a score of ≥14 for each of the individual symptoms of nasal stuffiness/congestion and rhinorrhea. Each symptom was scored on a 4-point severity scale (0=none, 1=mild, 2=moderate, 3=severe).

†Mean reduction in score averaged over the 2-week treatment period.

‡The comparison of interest is shown bolded.

17.2 Dosing
Patients should be advised not to increase the dose or dosing frequency of CLARINEX-D 12 HOUR Extended Release Tablets.

17.3 Additional Antihistamines and/or Decongestants
Patients should be advised against the concurrent use of CLARINEX-D 12 HOUR Extended Release Tablets with other antihistamines and/or decongestants.

17.4 Monoamine Oxidase (MAO) Inhibitors
Patients should be informed that due to its pseudoephedrine component, they should not use CLARINEX-D 12 HOUR with a monoamine oxidase (MAO) inhibitor or within 14 days of stopping use of an MAO inhibitor.

17.5 Coexisting Conditions
Patients with severe hypertension or severe coronary artery disease, narrow-angle glaucoma, or urinary retention should be advised not to use CLARINEX-D 12 HOUR Extended Release Tablets.

17.6 Instructions for Use
Patients should be instructed not to break, crush or chew the tablet; the tablet should be swallowed whole, and can be taken without regard to meals.

Manufactured by Schering Corporation, a subsidiary of Schering-Plough Corporation,
Kenilworth, NJ 07033 USA.
© 2006, 2009, Schering Corporation. All rights reserved.
U.S. Patent Nos. 4,659,716; 4,863,931; 5,595,997; and 6,100,274

PATIENT INFORMATION
CLARINEX-D (CLA-RI-NEX) 12 Hour Extended Release Tablets
(desloratadine and pseudoephedrine sulfate)

Read the Patient Information that comes with CLARINEX-D 12 Hour Extended Release Tablets before you start taking it and each time you get a refill. There may be new information. This leaflet is a summary of the information for patients. Your doctor or pharmacist can give you additional information. This leaflet does not take the place of talking to your doctor about your medical condition or treatment.

What is CLARINEX-D® 12 Hour Extended Release Tablets?
CLARINEX-D 12 Hour Extended Release Tablets is a prescription medicine that contains the medicines desloratadine (an antihistamine) and pseudoephedrine (a nasal decongestant). CLARINEX-D 12 Hour Extended Release Tablets is used to help control the symptoms of seasonal allergic rhinitis (sneezing, stuffy nose, runny nose and itching of the nose) in adults and children 12 years and older.
CLARINEX-D 12 Hour Extended Release Tablets is not for children under 12 years of age.

Who should not take CLARINEX-D® 12 Hour Extended Release Tablets?
Do not take CLARINEX-D 12 Hour Extended Release Tablets if you:
- are allergic to desloratadine or pseudoephedrine sulfate or any of the ingredients in CLARINEX-D 12 Hour Extended Release Tablets. See the end of this leaflet for a complete list of ingredients in CLARINEX-D 12 Hour Extended Release Tablets.
- are allergic to loratadine (Alavert, Claritin)
- have narrow angle glaucoma
- have problems with urination (urinary retention)
- take a Monoamine Oxidase Inhibitor (MAOI) medicine to treat depression, or if you stopped taking an MAOI medicine within the last 2 weeks. Ask your doctor or pharmacist if you are not sure if you take an MAOI medicine.
- have severe high blood pressure
- have severe heart disease
Talk to your doctor before taking this medicine if you have any of these conditions.

What should I tell my doctor before taking CLARINEX-D® 12 Hour Extended Release Tablets?
Before you take CLARINEX-D 12 Hour Extended Release Tablets, tell your doctor if you:
- have any of the conditions listed in the section "Who should not take CLARINEX-D 12 Hour Extended Release Tablets?"
- diabetes
- hyperthyroidism
- have prostate problems
- have liver or kidney problems
- have any other medical conditions
- are pregnant or plan to become pregnant. It is not known if CLARINEX-D 12 Hour Extended Release Tablets will harm your unborn baby. Talk to your doctor if you are pregnant or plan to become pregnant.
- are breast-feeding or plan to breast-feed. CLARINEX-D 12 Hour Extended Release Tablets **can pass into your breast milk**. Talk to your doctor about the best way to feed

your baby if you take CLARINEX-D 12 Hour Extended Release Tablets.
Tell your doctor about all the medicines your take, including prescription and non-prescription medicines, vitamins and herbal supplements. CLARINEX-D 12 Hour Extended Release Tablets may affect the way other medicines work, and other medicines may affect how CLARINEX-D 12 Hour Extended Release Tablets works. Especially tell your doctor if you take:

- Monoamine Oxidase Inhibitors (MAOI). You should not use CLARINEX-D 12 Hour Extended Release Tablets if you take a MAOI or within 2 weeks of stopping an MAOI.
- methyldopa
- reserpine (Serpalan)
- digitalis (Digoxin, Lanoxicaps, Lanoxin)
- ketoconazole (Nizoral)
- erythromycin (Ery-tab, Eryc, PCE)
- azithromycin (Zithromax, Zmax)
- antihistamines
- other decongestant medicines

Know the medicines you take. Keep a list of your medicines and show it to your doctor and pharmacist when you get a new medicine.

How should I take CLARINEX-D® 12 Hour Extended Release Tablets?
Take CLARINEX-D 12 Hour Extended Release Tablets exactly as your doctor tells you to take it.
- CLARINEX-D 12 Hour Extended Release Tablets can be taken with or without food.
- Swallow CLARINEX-D 12 Hour Extended Release Tablets whole. **Do not break, crush, or chew** CLARINEX-D 12 Hour Extended Release Tablets before swallowing. If you cannot swallow CLARINEX-D 12 Hour Extended Release Tablets whole, tell your doctor. You may need a different medicine.
- Take 1 CLARINEX-D 12 Hour Extended Release Tablet 2 times a day (every 12 hours).

What are the possible side effects of CLARINEX-D® 12 Hour Extended Release Tablets?
CLARINEX-D 12 Hour Extended Release Tablets may cause serious side effects, including:
- Cardiovascular and central nervous system effects, such as
  - unable to sleep (insomnia)
  - dizziness
  - weakness
  - tremor
  - irregular heart beat
  - seizure
  - low blood pressure
- Increased sleepiness or tiredness can happen if you take more CLARINEX-D 12 Hour Extended Release Tablets than your doctor prescribed to you.
- Allergic reactions. Stop taking CLARINEX-D 12 Hour Extended Release Tablets and call your doctor right away or get emergency help if you have any of these symptoms:
  - rash
  - itching
  - hives
  - swelling of your lips, tongue, face, and throat
  - shortness of breath or trouble breathing
The most common side effects of CLARINEX-D 12 HOUR Extended Release Tablets include:
- unable to sleep (insomnia)
- sore throat
- headache
- dizziness
- dry mouth
- nausea
- tiredness
- loss of appetite
- sleepiness
Tell your doctor if you have any side effect that bothers you or that does not go away.
These are not all of the possible side effects of CLARINEX-D 12 Hour Extended Release Tablets. For more information, ask your doctor or pharmacist.
Call your doctor for medical advice about side effects. You may report side effects to FDA at 1-800-FDA-1088.
How should I store CLARINEX-D® 12 Hour Extended Release Tablets?
- Store CLARINEX-D 12 Hour Extended Release Tablets at 59°F to 86°F (15°C to 30°C)
- Keep CLARINEX-D 12 Hour Extended Release Tablets dry and out of the light.
Keep CLARINEX-D 12 Hour Extended Release Tablets and all medicines out of the reach of children.
General information CLARINEX-D® 12 Hour Extended Release Tablets
Medicines are sometimes prescribed for purposes other than those listed in a patient information leaflet. Do not use

CLARINEX-D 12 Hour Extended Release Tablets for a condition for which it was not prescribed. Do not give CLARINEX-D 12 Hour Extended Release Tablets to other people, even if they have the same condition you have. It may harm them.
This patient information leaflet summarizes the most important information about CLARINEX-D 12 Hour Extended Release Tablets. If you would like more information, talk with your doctor. You can ask your pharmacist or doctor for information about CLARINEX-D 12 Hour Extended Release Tablets that is written for health professionals.
For more information, go to www.CLARINEX.com
What are the ingredients in CLARINEX-D® 12 Hour Extended Release Tablets?
Active ingredients: desloratadine and pseudoephedrine sulfate
Inactive ingredients: hypromellose USP, microcrystalline cellulose NF, povidone USP, silicon dioxide NF, magnesium stearate NF, corn starch NF, edetate disodium USP, citric acid anhydrous USP, stearic acid NF and FD&C Blue No. 2 aluminum lake dye.
Manufactured by Schering Corporation, a subsidiary of Schering-Plough Corporation,
Kenilworth, NJ 07033 USA.
Rev: Month/Year
© 2006, 2009, Schering Corporation. All rights reserved.
U.S. Patent Nos. 4,659,716; 4,863,931; 5,595,997; and 6,100,274
Shown in Product Identification Guide, page 312

CLARINEX-D® 24 HOUR   ℞
[klă-rĭ-nĕcks]
(desloratadine/pseudoephedrine sulfate)
Extended Release Tablets
for oral use

HIGHLIGHTS OF PRESCRIBING INFORMATION
These highlights do not include all the information needed to use CLARINEX-D® 24 HOUR Extended Release Tablets safely and effectively. See full prescribing information for CLARINEX-D 24 HOUR Extended Release Tablets.
CLARINEX-D 24 HOUR Extended Release Tablets (desloratadine/pseudoephedrine sulfate) for oral use.
Initial U.S. Approval: 2005

——————INDICATIONS AND USAGE——————
CLARINEX-D 24 HOUR is a combination product containing an H1-receptor antagonist and a sympathomimetic amine indicated for:
- Relief of nasal and non-nasal symptoms of seasonal allergic rhinitis, including nasal congestion, in adults and adolescents 12 years of age and older. (1)

————DOSAGE AND ADMINISTRATION————
For oral use only
Adults and adolescents 12 years of age and over: The recommended dose of CLARINEX-D 24 HOUR Extended Release Tablets is one tablet once daily. (2)

————DOSAGE FORMS AND STRENGTHS————
Desloratadine 5 mg/Pseudoephedrine sulfate 240 mg tablets (3)

——————CONTRAINDICATIONS——————
- Hypersensitivity (4)
- Narrow Angle Glaucoma (4)
- Urinary Retention (4)
- Patients Receiving MAO Inhibitors or within 14 days of stopping such treatment (4)
- Severe hypertension or severe coronary artery disease (4)

————WARNINGS AND PRECAUTIONS————
- Cardiovascular and central nervous system effects: Use with caution in patients with cardiovascular disorders. (5.1).
- Coexisting conditions: Use with caution in patients with increased intraocular pressure, prostatic hypertrophy, diabetes mellitus, or hyperthyroidism (5.2).

——————ADVERSE REACTIONS——————
- The most common adverse reactions (reported in ≥2% of patients) were mouth dry, headache, insomnia, fatigue, pharyngitis, somnolence, nausea, dizziness, nervousness, psychomotor hypersensitivity and anorexia. (6.1)
To report SUSPECTED ADVERSE REACTIONS, contact Schering Corporation at 800-526-4099 or FDA at 1-800-FDA-1088 or www.fda.gov/medwatch.

——————DRUG INTERACTIONS——————
Monoamine Oxidase (MAO) Inhibitors: Do not use. May potentiate the effect of pseudoephedrine on vascular system. (7.1)

————USE IN SPECIFIC POPULATIONS————
- Renal impairment: Avoid in patients with renal impairment (8.6)

• Hepatic impairment: Avoid in patients with hepatic impairment (8.7)

See 17 for PATIENT COUNSELING INFORMATION and FDA-approved patient labeling

Revised: 12/2009

FULL PRESCRIBING INFORMATION: CONTENTS*

* Sections or subsections omitted from the full prescribing information are not listed

---

FULL PRESCRIBING INFORMATION

1 INDICATIONS AND USAGE

1.1 Seasonal Allergic Rhinitis

CLARINEX-D® 24 HOUR Extended Release Tablets is indicated for the relief of the nasal and non-nasal symptoms of seasonal allergic rhinitis, including nasal congestion, in adults and adolescents 12 years of age and older. CLARINEX-D 24 HOUR Extended Release Tablets should be administered when the antihistaminic properties of desloratadine and the nasal decongestant properties of pseudoephedrine are desired [see Clinical Pharmacology (12)].

2 DOSAGE AND ADMINISTRATION

Administer CLARINEX-D 24 HOUR Extended Release Tablet by the oral route only. Do not break, chew or crush the tablet. Swallow the tablet whole.

2.1 Adults and Adolescents 12 years of Age and Over

The recommended dose of CLARINEX-D 24 HOUR Extended Release Tablets is 1 tablet once daily, administered with or without a meal. Higher doses or increased dosing frequency of CLARINEX-D 24 HOUR Extended Release Tablets have not demonstrated increased effectiveness. Do not exceed the recommended dose as desloratadine and pseudoephedrine, the active components of CLARINEX-D 24 HOUR Extended Release Tablets have been associated with adverse effects at higher doses [see Overdosage (10.1, 10.2)].

3 DOSAGE FORMS AND STRENGTHS

CLARINEX-D 24 HOUR Extended Release Tablets are oval-shaped, light blue coated tablets with "D 24" branded in black on one side. Each tablet contains 5 mg desloratadine in the tablet coating for immediate release and 240 mg pseudoephedrine sulfate, USP in an extended release core.

4 CONTRAINDICATIONS

CLARINEX-D 24 HOUR Extended Release Tablets are contraindicated in:

• Patients with hypersensitivity to any of its ingredients, or to loratadine [see Warnings and Precautions (5.4) and Post-Marketing Experience (6.2)]
• Patients with narrow angle glaucoma
• Patients with urinary retention
• Patients receiving monoamine oxidase (MAO) inhibitor therapy or within fourteen (14) days of stopping such treatment [see Drug Interactions (7.1)]
• Patients with severe hypertension or severe coronary artery disease.

5 WARNINGS AND PRECAUTIONS

5.1 Cardiovascular and Central Nervous System Effects

The pseudoephedrine sulfate contained in CLARINEX-D 24 HOUR Extended Release Tablets, like other sympathomimetic amines, can produce cardiovascular and central nervous system (CNS) effects in some patients such as insomnia, dizziness, weakness, tremor, or arrhythmias. In addition, central nervous system stimulation with convulsions or cardiovascular collapse with accompanying hypotension has been reported. Therefore, CLARINEX-D 24 HOUR Extended Release Tablets should be used with caution in patients with cardiovascular disorders, and should not be used in patients with severe hypertension or severe coronary artery disease.

5.2 Coexisting Conditions

CLARINEX-D 24 HOUR Extended Release Tablets contain pseudoephedrine sulfate, a sympathomimetic amine, and therefore should be used with caution in patients with diabetes and hyperthyroidism. Also use with caution in patients with prostatic hypertrophy or increased intraocular pressure, as urinary retention or narrow-angle glaucoma may occur [see Contraindications (4)].

5.3 Co-Administration with Monoamine Oxidase (MAO) Inhibitors

CLARINEX-D 24 HOUR Extended Release Tablets should not be used in patients receiving monoamine oxidase (MAO) inhibitor therapy or within fourteen (14) days of stopping such treatment as an increase in blood pressure or hypertensive crisis, may occur [see Contraindications (4) and Drug Interactions (7.1)].

5.4 Hypersensitivity Reactions

Hypersensitivity reactions including rash, pruritus, urticaria, edema, dyspnea, and anaphylaxis have been reported after administration of desloratadine a component of CLARINEX-D 24 HOUR Extended Release Tablets. If such a reaction occurs, therapy with CLARINEX-D 24 HOUR Extended Release Tablets should be stopped and alternative treatment should be considered [see Post-marketing (6.2)].

5.5 Renal Impairment

CLARINEX-D 24 HOUR Extended Release Tablets should generally be avoided in patients with renal impairment [see Clinical Pharmacology (12)].

5.6 Hepatic Impairment

CLARINEX-D 24 HOUR Extended Release Tablets should generally be avoided in patients with hepatic impairment [see Clinical Pharmacology (12)].

6 ADVERSE REACTIONS

The following adverse reactions are discussed in greater detail in other sections of the label:
• Cardiovascular and Central Nervous System effects [see Warnings and Precautions (5.1)]
• Increased Intraocular pressure [see Warnings and Precautions (5.2)]
• Urinary retention in patients with prostatic hypertrophy [see Warnings and Precautions (5.2)]
• Hypersensitivity reactions [see Warnings and Precautions (5.4)]

6.1 Clinical Trials Experience

Because clinical trials are conducted under widely varying conditions, adverse reaction rates observed in the clinical trials of a drug cannot be directly compared to rates in the clinical trials of another drug and may not reflect the rates observed in clinical practice. The safety data described below are from 2 clinical trials with CLARINEX-D 24 HOUR Extended Release Tablets that included 2852 patients, of which 708 patients received CLARINEX-D 24 HOUR Extended Release Tablets daily for up to 15 days. The majority of patients were between 18 and <65 years of age with a mean age of 34.3 years and were predominantly women (63%). Patient ethnicity was 79 % Caucasian, 10% Black, 8% Hispanic and 3% Asian/other ethnicity. The percentage of subjects receiving CLARINEX-D 24 HOUR Extended Release Tablets, and who discontinued from the clinical trials because of an adverse event was 3.4%. Adverse reactions that were reported by ≥ 2% of subjects receiving CLARINEX-D 24 HOUR Extended Release Tablets are shown in Table 1.

[See table 1 above]

TABLE 1: Incidence of Adverse Reactions Reported by ≥2% of Subjects Receiving CLARINEX-D 24 HOUR Extended Release Tablets

Adverse Reaction	CLARINEX-D® 24 HOUR (N =708)	Desloratadine 5 mg (N =712)	Pseudoephedrine 240 mg (N =719)
Gastrointestinal Disorders			
Mouth Dry	8%	2%	11%
Nausea	2%	1%	3%
Anorexia	2%	0%	2%
General Disorders and Administration Site Conditions			
Fatigue	3%	3%	2%
Nervous System Disorders			
Headache	6%	5%	7%
Somnolence	3%	2%	3%
Dizziness	2%	1%	2%
Psychomotor hyperactivity	2%	0%	2%
Psychiatric Disorders			
Insomnia	5%	1%	8%
Nervousness	2%	1%	1%
Respiratory, Thoracic and Mediastinal Disorders			
Pharyngitis	3%	2%	3%

There were no relevant differences in adverse reactions for subgroups of patients as defined by gender, age, or race.

6.2 Post-Marketing Experience

In addition to the adverse reactions reported during clinical trials and listed above, adverse events have been identified during post approval use of CLARINEX-D 24 HOUR Extended Release Tablets. Because these events are reported voluntarily from a population of uncertain size, it is not always possible to reliably estimate their frequency or establish a causal relationship to drug exposure. Adverse events identified from post-marketing surveillance on the use of CLARINEX-D 24 HOUR Extended Release Tablets include palpitations, pruritis and urticaria.

In addition to these events, the following spontaneous adverse events have been reported during the marketing of desloratadine as a single ingredient product: headache, somnolence, dizziness, tachycardia, and rarely hypersensitivity reactions (such as rash, edema, dyspnea, and anaphylaxis), and elevated liver enzymes including bilirubin and very rarely, hepatitis.

7 DRUG INTERACTIONS

No specific interaction studies have been conducted with CLARINEX-D 24 HOUR Extended Release Tablets.

7.1 Monoamine Oxidase Inhibitors

CLARINEX-D 24 HOUR Extended Release Tablets should not be used in patients receiving monoamine oxidase (MAO) inhibitor therapy or within fourteen (14) days of stopping such treatment because the action of pseudoephedrine a component of CLARINEX-D 24 HOUR Extended Release Tablets on the vascular system may be potentiated by these agents. *(See Contraindications (4) and Warnings and Precautions 5.4)*

7.2 Beta-adrenergic blocking agents

The antihypertensive effects of beta-adrenergic blocking agents, methyldopa, and reserpine, may be reduced by sympathomimetics such as pseudoephedrine. Exercise caution when using CLARINEX-D 24 HOUR Extended Release Tablets with these agents.

7.3 Digitalis

Increased ectopic pacemaker activity can occur when pseudoephedrine is used concomitantly with digitalis. Exercise caution when using CLARINEX-D 24 HOUR Extended Release Tablets with these agents.

7.4 Inhibitors of cytochrome P450 3A4

In controlled clinical studies co-administration of desloratadine with ketoconazole, erythromycin, or azithromycin resulted in increased plasma concentrations of desloratadine and 3-hydroxydesloratadine but there were no clinically relevant changes in the safety profile of desloratadine. *[See Clinical Pharmacology (12.3)]*

7.5 Fluoxetine

In controlled clinical studies co-administration of desloratadine with fluoxetine, a selective serotonin reuptake inhibitor (SSRI), resulted in increased plasma concentrations of desloratadine and 3-hydroxydesloratadine but there were no clinically relevant changes in the safety profile of desloratadine *[See Clinical Pharmacology (12.3)]*

7.6 Cimetidine

In controlled clinical studies co-administration of desloratadine with cimetidine a histamine H2-receptor antagonist resulted in increased plasma concentrations of desloratadine and 3-hydroxydesloratadine but there were no clinically relevant changes in the safety profile of desloratadine *[See Clinical Pharmacology (12.3)]*

8 USE IN SPECIFIC POPULATIONS

8.1 Pregnancy

Pregnancy Category C: There are no adequate and well-controlled studies of desloratadine and pseudoephedrine in combination in pregnant women. Neither are there animal reproduction studies conducted with the combination of desloratadine and pseudoephedrine. Desloratadine was not teratogenic in rats or rabbits but affected implantation in rats. Because animal reproduction studies are not always predictive of human response, CLARINEX-D 24 HOUR Extended Release Tablets should be used during pregnancy only if clearly needed.

Desloratadine was not teratogenic in rats or rabbits at approximately 210 and 230 times, respectively, the AUC in humans at the recommended daily oral dose. An increase in pre-implantation loss and a decreased number of implantations and fetuses were noted, however, in a separate study in female rats at approximately 120 times the AUC in humans at the recommended daily oral dose. Reduced body weight and slow righting reflex were reported in pups at approximately 50 times or greater than the AUC in humans at the recommended daily oral dose. Desloratadine had no effect on pup development at approximately 7 times the AUC in humans at the recommended daily oral dose. The AUCs in comparison referred to the desloratadine exposure in rabbits and the sum of desloratadine and its metabolites exposures in rats, respectively *[see Nonclinical Toxicology (13.2)]*.

8.3 Nursing Mothers

Desloratadine and pseudoephedrine both pass into breast milk; therefore, a decision should be made whether to discontinue nursing or to discontinue CLARINEX-D 24 HOUR Extended Release Tablets, taking into account the benefit of the drug to the nursing mother and the possible risk to the child.

8.4 Pediatric Use

CLARINEX-D 24 HOUR Extended Release Tablets are not indicated for use in pediatric patients under 12 years of age.

8.5 Geriatric Use

The number of subjects (n=8) ≥65 years old treated with CLARINEX-D 24 HOUR Extended Release Tablets was too limited to make any formal statistical comparison regarding the efficacy or safety of this drug product in this age group, or to determine whether they respond differently from younger subjects. Other reported clinical experience has not identified differences between the elderly and younger patients, although the elderly are more likely to have adverse reactions to sympathomimetic amines. In general, dose selection for an elderly patient should be cautious, reflecting the greater frequency of decreased hepatic, renal, or cardiac function, and of concomitant disease or other drug therapy *[see Clinical Pharmacology (12)]*.

Pseudoephedrine, desloratadine, and their metabolites are known to be substantially excreted by the kidney, and the risk of adverse reactions may be greater in patients with renal impairment. Because elderly patients are more likely to have decreased renal function, care should be taken in dose selection, and it may be useful to monitor the patient for adverse events *[see Clinical Pharmacology (12.3)]*.

8.6 Renal Impairment

No studies with CLARINEX-D 24 HOUR Extended Release Tablets were conducted in subjects with renal impairment. For CLARINEX-D 24 HOUR Extended Release Tablets should generally be avoided in patients with renal impairment *[see Warnings and Precautions (5.5) and Clinical Pharmacology (12.3)]*.

8.7 Hepatic Impairment

No studies with CLARINEX-D 24 HOUR Extended Release Tablets or pseudoephedrine have been conducted in subjects with hepatic impairment.

CLARINEX-D 24 HOUR Extended Release Tablets should generally be avoided in patients with hepatic impairment. *[see Warnings and Precautions (5.6) and Clinical Pharmacology (12.3)]*.

8.8 Gender

No clinically significant gender-related differences were observed in the pharmacokinetic parameters of desloratadine, 3-hydroxydesloratadine or pseudoephedrine following administration of CLARINEX-D 24 HOUR Extended Release Tablets.

8.9 Race

No studies have been conducted to evaluate the effect of race on the pharmacokinetics of CLARINEX-D 24 HOUR Extended Release Tablets.

9 DRUG ABUSE AND DEPENDENCE

There is no information to indicate that abuse or dependency occurs with CLARINEX or CLARINEX-D 24 HOUR Extended Release Tablets.

10 OVERDOSAGE

In the event of overdose, consider standard measures to remove any unabsorbed drug. Symptomatic and supportive treatment is recommended. Desloratadine and 3-hydroxydesloratadine are not eliminated by hemodialysis.

10.1 Desloratadine

Information regarding acute overdosage with desloratadine is limited to experience from postmarketing adverse event reports and from clinical trials conducted during the development of the CLARINEX product. In the reported cases of overdose, there were no significant adverse events that were attributed to desloratadine. In a dose ranging trial, at doses of 10 mg and 20 mg/day somnolence was reported.

In another study, no clinically relevant adverse events were reported in normal male and female volunteers who were given single daily doses of CLARINEX 45 mg for 10 days *[see Clinical Pharmacology (12.2)]*.

Lethality occurred in rats at oral doses of 250 mg/kg or greater (estimated desloratadine and desloratadine metabolite exposures were approximately 120 times the AUC in humans at the recommended daily oral dose). The oral median lethal dose in mice was 353 mg/kg (estimated desloratadine exposure was approximately 290 times the human daily oral dose on an mg/m^2 basis). No deaths occurred at oral doses up to 250 mg/kg in monkeys (estimated desloratadine exposures were approximately 810 times the human daily oral dose on an mg/m^2 basis).

10.2 Sympathomimetics

In large doses, sympathomimetics such as pseudoephedrine may give rise to giddiness, headache, nausea, vomiting, sweating, thirst, tachycardia, precordial pain, palpitations, difficulty in micturition, muscle weakness and tenseness, anxiety, restlessness, and insomnia. Many patients can present a toxic psychosis with delusions and hallucinations. Some may develop cardiac arrhythmias, circulatory collapse, convulsions, coma and respiratory failure.

11 DESCRIPTION

CLARINEX-D 24 HOUR Extended Release Tablets are light blue oval-shaped tablets containing 5 mg desloratadine in the tablet coating for immediate release and 240 mg pseudoephedrine sulfate USP in the tablet core for extended release.

The inactive ingredients contained in CLARINEX-D 24 HOUR Extended Release Tablets are hypromellose USP, ethylcellulose NF, dibasic calcium phosphate dihydrate USP, magnesium stearate NF, povidone USP, silicone dioxide NF, talc USP, polyacrylate dispersion, polyethylene glycol NF, simethicone USP, Blue Lake Blend 50726 (FD&C Blue No. 2 Lake, titanium dioxide USP and edetate disodium USP), and ink (Opacode® S-1-17746 or Opacode® S-1-4159).

Desloratadine, 1 of the 2 active ingredients of CLARINEX-D 24 HOUR Extended Release Tablets, is a white to off-white powder that is slightly soluble in water, but very soluble in ethanol and propylene glycol. It has an empirical formula: $C_{19}H_{19}ClN_2$ and a molecular weight of 310.8. The chemical name is 8-chloro-6,11-dihydro-11-(4-piperdinylidene)-5*H*-benzo[5,6]cyclohepta[1,2-*b*]pyridine and has the following structure:

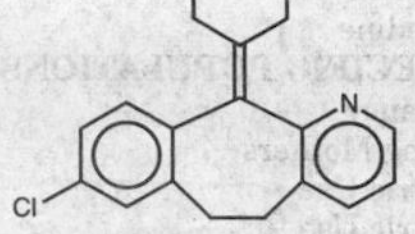

Pseudoephedrine sulfate, the other active ingredient of CLARINEX-D 24 HOUR Extended Release Tablets, is the synthetic salt of one of the naturally occurring dextrorotatory diastereomers of ephedrine and is classified as an indirect sympathomimetic amine. Pseudoephedrine sulfate is a colorless hygroscopic crystal or white, hygroscopic crystalline powder, practically odorless, with a bitter taste. It is very soluble in water, freely soluble in alcohol, and sparingly soluble in ether. The empirical formula for pseudoephedrine sulfate is $(C_{10}H_{15}NO)_2 \bullet H_2SO_4$; the chemical name is benzenemethanol, α-[1-(methylamino) ethyl]-,[*S*-(*R**,*R**)]-, sulfate (2:1)(salt); and the chemical structure is:

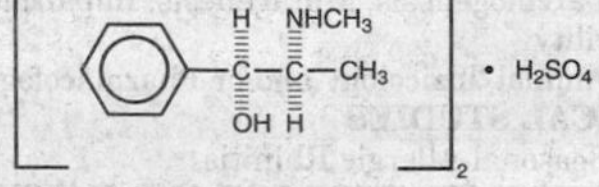

12 CLINICAL PHARMACOLOGY

12.1 Mechanism of Action

Desloratadine is a long-acting tricyclic histamine antagonist with selective H_1-receptor histamine antagonist activity. Receptor binding data indicate that at a concentration of 2 to 3 ng/mL (7 nanomolar), desloratadine shows significant interaction with the human histamine H_1-receptor. Desloratadine inhibited histamine release from human mast cells *in vitro*. Results of a radiolabeled tissue distribution study in rats and a radioligand H_1-receptor binding study in guinea pigs showed that desloratadine does not readily cross the blood brain barrier. The clinical significance of this finding is unknown.

Pseudoephedrine sulfate is an orally active sympathomimetic amine and exerts a decongestant action on the nasal mucosa.

Pseudoephedrine sulfate is recognized as an effective agent for the relief of nasal congestion due to allergic rhinitis. Pseudoephedrine produces peripheral effects similar to those of ephedrine and central effects similar to, but less intense than, amphetamines. It has the potential for excitatory side effects.

12.2 Pharmacodynamics

Wheal and Flare: Human histamine skin wheal studies following single and repeated 5 mg doses of desloratadine have shown that the drug exhibits an antihistaminic effect by 1 hour; this activity may persist for as long as 24 hours. There was no evidence of histamine-induced skin wheal tachyphylaxis within the desloratadine 5 mg group over the 28-day treatment period. The clinical relevance of histamine wheal skin testing is unknown.

Effects on QTc: In clinical trials for CLARINEX-D 24 HOUR Extended Release Tablets, ECGs were recorded at baseline and after 2 weeks of treatment within 1 to 3 hours after dosing. No clinically meaningful changes were observed following treatment with CLARINEX-D 24 HOUR Extended Release Tablets for any ECG parameter, including the QTc interval. An increase in the ventricular rate of 6.7 and 5.4 bpm was observed in the CLARINEX-D 24 HOUR Extended Release Tablets and pseudoephedrine groups, respectively, compared to an increase of 2.8 bpm in subjects receiving desloratadine alone. Single daily doses of CLARINEX 45 mg were given to normal male and female volunteers for 10 days. All ECGs obtained in this study were manually read in a blinded fashion by a cardiologist. In the CLARINEX-treated subjects, there was a mean increase in the maximum heart rate of 9.2 bpm relative to placebo. The QT interval was corrected for heart rate (QTc) by both Bazett's and Fridericia methods. Using the QTc (Bazett), there was a mean increase of 8.1 msec in the CLARINEX-treated subjects relative to placebo. Using QTc (Fridericia) there was a mean increase of 0.4 msec in CLARINEX-treated subjects relative to placebo. No clinically relevant adverse events were reported.

12.3 Pharmacokinetics

Absorption:

A bioequivalence study that compared CLARINEX-D 24 HOUR Extended Release Tablets to the monotherapy (desloratadine 5 mg, and pseudoephedrine 240 mg) showed that CLARINEX-D 24 HOUR Extended Release Tablets was not bioequivalent to the monotherapy (desloratadine 5 mg tablet). The systemic exposure to desloratadine and 3-hydroxydesloratadine was 15% to 20% lower from CLARINEX-D 24 HOUR Extended Release Tablets than those from desloratadine 5 mg tablet. Clinical trials were therefore necessary to support efficacy of CLARINEX-D 24 HOUR Extended Release Tablets *[see Clinical Studies (14)]*.

In the above single dose pharmacokinetic study the mean time to maximum plasma concentrations (T_{max}) for desloratadine occurred at approximately 6 to 7 hours post dose and mean peak plasma concentrations (C_{max}) and area under the concentration-time curve (AUC(tf)) of approximately 1.79 ng/mL and 61.1 ng•hr/mL, respectively, were observed. In another pharmacokinetic study, food and grapefruit juice had no effect on the bioavailability (C_{max} and AUC) of desloratadine.

For pseudoephedrine, the mean T_{max} occurred at 8 to 9 hours post dose and mean peak plasma concentrations (C_{max}) and AUC(tf) of 328 ng/mL and 6438 ng•hr/mL, respectively, were observed. The ingestion of food did not affect the absorption of pseudoephedrine from CLARINEX-D 24 HOUR Extended Release Tablets.

Following oral administration of CLARINEX-D 24 HOUR Extended Release Tablets once daily for 14 days in healthy volunteers, steady-state conditions were reached on Day 12 for desloratadine and 3-hydroxydesloratadine, and Day 10 for pseudoephedrine. For desloratadine, mean steady-state C_{max} and AUC (0–24h) of approximately 2.44 ng/mL and 34.8 ng•hr/mL, respectively were observed. For pseudoephedrine, mean steady-state peak plasma concentrations (C_{max}) and AUC (0–24h) of 523 ng/mL and 8795 ng•hr/mL, respectively, were observed.

Distribution:

Desloratadine and 3-hydroxydesloratadine are approximately 82% to 87% and 85% to 89%, bound to plasma proteins, respectively. Protein binding of desloratadine and 3-hydroxydesloratadine was unaltered in subjects with impaired renal function.

Metabolism

Desloratadine (a major metabolite of loratadine) is extensively metabolized to 3-hydroxydesloratadine, an active metabolite, which is subsequently glucuronidated. The enzyme(s) responsible for the formation of 3-hydroxydesloratadine have not been identified. Data from clinical trials with desloratadine indicate that a subset of the general population has a decreased ability to form 3-hydroxydesloratadine, and are poor metabolizers of desloratadine. In pharmacokinetic studies (n=3748), approximately 6% of subjects were poor metabolizers of desloratadine (defined as a subject with an AUC ratio of 3-hydroxydesloratadine to desloratadine less than 0.1, or a subject with a desloratadine half-life exceeding 50 hours). These pharmacokinetic studies included subjects between the ages of 2 and 70 years, including 977 subjects aged 2 to 5 years, 1575 subjects aged 6 to 11 years, and 1196 subjects aged 12 to 70 years. There was no difference in the prevalence of poor metabolizers across age groups. The frequency of poor metabolizers was higher in Blacks (17%, n=988) as compared to Caucasians (2%, n=1462) and Hispanics (2%, n=1063). The median exposure (AUC) to desloratadine in the poor metabolizers was approximately 6-fold greater than in the subjects who are not poor metabolizers. Subjects who are poor metabolizers of desloratadine cannot be prospectively identified and will be exposed to higher levels of desloratadine following dosing with the recommended dose of desloratadine. In multidose clinical safety studies, where metabolizer status was prospectively identified, a total of 94 poor metabolizers and 123 normal metabolizers were enrolled and treated with CLARINEX Syrup for 15 to 35 days. In these studies, no overall differences in safety were observed between poor metabolizers and normal metabolizers.

TABLE 2 Changes in Desloratadine and 3-hydroxydesloratadine Pharmacokinetics in Healthy Male and Female Subjects

	Desloratadine		3-hydroxydesloratadine	
	C_{max}	AUC 0–24 hrs	C_{max}	AUC 0–24 hrs
Erythromycin (500 mg Q8h)	+24%	+14%	+43%	+40%
Ketoconazole (200 mg Q12h)	+45%	+39%	+43%	+72%
Azithromycin (500 mg Day 1, 250 mg QD × 4 days)	+15%	+5%	+15%	+4%
Fluoxetine (20 mg QD)	+15%	+0%	+17%	+13%
Cimetidine (600 mg Q12h)	+12%	+19%	-11%	-3%

Although not seen in these studies, an increased risk of exposure-related adverse events in patients who are poor metabolizers cannot be ruled out.

Pseudoephedrine alone is incompletely metabolized (less than 1%) in the liver by N-demethylation to an inactive metabolite. The drug and its metabolite are excreted in the urine. About 55% to 96% of an administered dose of pseudoephedrine hydrochloride is excreted unchanged in the urine.

Elimination

Following single dose administration of CLARINEX-D 24 HOUR Extended Release Tablets, the mean plasma elimination half-life of desloratadine was similar to the desloratadine 5 mg tablet, approximately 24 and 27 hours, respectively. In another study, following administration of single oral doses of desloratadine 5 mg, C_{max} and AUC values increased in a dose proportional manner between 5 and 20 mg. The degree of accumulation after 14 days of dosing was consistent with the half-life and dosing frequency. A human mass balance study documented a recovery of approximately 87% of the ^{14}C-desloratadine dose, which was equally distributed in urine and feces as metabolic products. Analysis of plasma 3-hydroxydesloratadine showed similar T_{max} and half-life values compared to desloratadine.

The mean elimination half-life of pseudoephedrine is dependent on urinary pH. The elimination half-life is approximately 3 to 6 or 9 to-16 hours when the urinary pH is 5 or 8, respectively.

Geriatric Subjects: Following multiple-dose administration of CLARINEX Tablets, the mean C_{max} and AUC values for desloratadine were 20% greater than in younger subjects (<65 years old). The oral total body clearance (CL/F) when normalized for body weight was similar between the 2 age groups. The mean plasma elimination half-life of desloratadine was 33.7 hr in subjects ≥ 65 years old. The pharmacokinetics for 3-hydroxydesloratadine appeared unchanged in older vs. younger subjects. These age-related differences are unlikely to be clinically relevant and no dosage adjustment is recommended in elderly patients.

Pediatric Subjects: CLARINEX-D 24 HOUR Extended Release Tablets are not an appropriate dosage form for use in pediatric patients below 12 years of age.

Renally Impaired: Following a single dose of desloratadine 7.5 mg, pharmacokinetics were characterized in subjects with mild (n=7; creatinine clearance 51–69 mL/min/1.73 m^2), moderate (n=6; creatinine clearance 34–43 mL/min/1.73 m^2), and severe (n=6; creatinine clearance 5–29 mL/min/1.73m^2) renal impairment or hemodialysis dependent (n=6) subjects. In subjects with mild and moderate renal impairment, median C_{max} and AUC values increased by approximately 1.2- and 1.9-fold, respectively, relative to subjects with normal renal function. In subjects with severe renal impairment or who were hemodialysis dependent, C_{max} and AUC values increased by approximately 1.7- and 2.5-fold, respectively. Minimal changes in 3-hydroxydesloratadine concentrations were observed. Desloratadine and 3-hydroxydesloratadine were poorly removed by hemodialysis. Plasma protein binding of desloratadine and 3-hydroxydesloratadine was unaltered by renal impairment.

Pseudoephedrine is primarily excreted unchanged in the urine as unchanged drug; the remainder is apparently metabolized in the liver. Therefore, pseudoephedrine may accumulate in patients with renal impairment.

Hepatically Impaired: Following a single oral dose of desloratadine, pharmacokinetics were characterized in subjects with mild (n=4), moderate (n=4), and severe (n=4) hepatic impairment as defined by the Child-Pugh classification of hepatic impairment and 8 subjects with normal hepatic function. Subjects with hepatic impairment, regardless of severity, had approximately a 2.4-fold increase in AUC as compared with normal subjects. The apparent oral clearance of desloratadine in subjects with mild, moderate, and severe hepatic impairment was 37%, 36%, and 28% of that in normal subjects, respectively. An increase in the mean elimination half-life of desloratadine in subjects with hepatic impairment was observed. For 3-hydroxydesloratadine, the mean C_{max} and AUC values for subjects with hepatic impairment were not statistically significantly different from subjects with normal hepatic function.

Gender: Female subjects treated for 14 days with CLARINEX Tablets had 10% and 3% higher desloratadine C_{max} and AUC values, respectively, compared with male subjects. The 3-hydroxydesloratadine C_{max} and AUC values were also increased by 45% and 48%, respectively, in females compared with males. However, these apparent differences are not considered to be clinically relevant.

Race: Following 14 days of treatment with CLARINEX Tablets, the C_{max} and AUC values for desloratadine were 18% and 32% higher, respectively, in Blacks compared with Caucasians. For 3-hydroxydesloratadine there was a corresponding 10% reduction in C_{max} and AUC values in Blacks compared to Caucasians. These differences are not considered to be clinically relevant.

Drug interaction: In 2 controlled crossover clinical pharmacology studies in healthy male (n=12 in each study) and female (n=12 in each study) subjects, desloratadine 7.5 mg (1.5 times the daily dose) once daily was co-administered with erythromycin 500 mg every 8 hours or ketoconazole 200 mg every 12 hours for 10 days. In 3 separate controlled, parallel group clinical pharmacology studies, desloratadine at the clinical dose of 5 mg has been co-administered with azithromycin 500 mg followed by 250 mg once daily for 4 days (n=18) or with fluoxetine 20 mg once daily for 7 days after a 23-day pretreatment period with fluoxetine (n=18) or with cimetidine 600 mg every 12 hours for 14 days (n=18) under steady state conditions to healthy male and female subjects. Although increased plasma concentrations (Cmax and AUC 0–24 hrs) of desloratadine and 3-hydroxydesloratadine were observed (see Table 2), there were no clinically relevant changes in the safety profile of desloratadine, as assessed by electrocardiographic parameters (including the corrected QT interval), clinical laboratory tests, vital signs and adverse events.

[See table 2 above]

13 NONCLINICAL TOXICOLOGY

13.1 Carcinogenesis, Mutagenesis, Impairment of Fertility

There are no animal or laboratory studies on the combination product of desloratadine and pseudoephedrine sulfate to evaluate carcinogenesis, mutagenesis, or impairment of fertility.

Carcinogenicity Studies:

The carcinogenic potential of desloratadine was assessed using a loratadine study in rats and a desloratadine study in mice. In a 2-year study in rats, loratadine was administered in the diet at doses up to 25 mg/kg/day (estimated desloratadine and desloratadine metabolite exposures were approximately 30 times the AUC in humans at the recommended daily oral dose). A significantly higher incidence of hepatocellular tumors (combined adenomas and carcinomas) was observed in males given 10 mg/kg/day of loratadine and in males and females given 25 mg/kg/day of loratadine. The estimated desloratadine and desloratadine metabolite exposures in rats given 10 mg/kg of loratadine were approximately 7 times the AUC in humans at the recommended daily oral dose. The clinical significance of these findings during long-term use of desloratadine is not known.

In a 2-year dietary study in mice, males and females given up to 16 mg/kg/day and 32 mg/kg/day desloratadine, respectively, did not show significant increases in the incidence of any tumors. The estimated desloratadine and desloratadine metabolite exposures in mice at these doses were 12 and 27 times, respectively, the AUC in humans at the recommended daily oral dose.

Genotoxicity Studies:

In genotoxicity studies with desloratadine, there was no evidence of genotoxic potential in a reverse mutation assay (*Salmonella/E. coli* mammalian microsome bacterial mutagenicity assay) or in 2 assays for chromosomal aberrations (human peripheral blood lymphocyte clastogenicity assay and mouse bone marrow micronucleus assay).

Impairment of Fertility:
There was no effect on female fertility in rats at desloratadine doses up to 24 mg/kg/day (estimated desloratadine and desloratadine metabolite exposures were approximately 130 times the AUC in humans at the recommended daily oral dose). A male specific decrease in fertility, demonstrated by reduced female conception rates, decreased sperm numbers and motility, and histopathologic testicular changes, occurred at an oral desloratadine dose of 12 mg/kg in rats (estimated desloratadine and desloratadine metabolite exposures were approximately 45 times the AUC in humans at the recommended daily oral dose). Desloratadine had no effect on fertility in rats at an oral dose of 3 mg/kg/day (estimated desloratadine and desloratadine metabolite exposures were approximately 8 times the AUC in humans at the recommended daily oral dose).

13.2   Animal Toxicology and/or Pharmacology
Reproductive Toxicology Studies:
Desloratadine was not teratogenic in rats at doses up to 48 mg/kg/day (estimated desloratadine and desloratadine metabolite exposures were approximately 210 times the AUC in humans at the recommended daily oral dose) or in rabbits at doses up to 60 mg/kg/day (estimated desloratadine exposures were approximately 230 times the AUC in humans at the recommended daily oral dose). In a separate study, an increase in pre-implantation loss and a decreased number of implantations and fetuses were noted in female rats at 24 mg/kg (estimated desloratadine and desloratadine metabolite exposures were approximately 120 times the AUC in humans at the recommended daily oral dose). Reduced body weight and slow righting reflex were reported in pups at doses of 9 mg/kg/day or greater (estimated desloratadine and desloratadine metabolite exposures were approximately 50 times or greater than the AUC in humans at the recommended daily oral dose). Desloratadine had no effect on pup development at an oral dose of 3 mg/kg/day (estimated desloratadine and desloratadine metabolite exposures were approximately 7 times the AUC in humans at the recommended daily oral dose).

14   CLINICAL STUDIES
14.1   Seasonal Allergic Rhinitis
The clinical efficacy and safety of CLARINEX-D 24 HOUR Extended Release Tablets was evaluated in two 2-week multicenter, randomized parallel group clinical trials involving 2852 subjects 12 to 78 years of age with seasonal allergic rhinitis, 708 of whom received CLARINEX-D 24 HOUR Extended Release Tablets. In the 2 trials, subjects were randomized to receive CLARINEX-D 24 HOUR Extended Release Tablets once daily, CLARINEX Tablets 5 mg once daily, or sustained-release pseudoephedrine tablet 240 mg once daily for two weeks. The majority of patients were between 18 and <65 years of age with a mean age of 34.3 years and were predominantly women (63%). Patient ethnicity was 79% Caucasian, 10% Black, 8% Hispanic and 3% Asian/other ethnicity. Primary efficacy variable was twice-daily reflective patient scoring of 4 nasal symptoms (rhinorrhea, nasal stuffiness/congestion, nasal itching, and sneezing) and 4 non-nasal symptoms (itching/burning eyes, tearing/watering eyes, redness of eyes, and itching of ears/palate) on a four point scale (0=none, 1=mild, 2=moderate, and 3=severe). In both trials, the antihistaminic efficacy of CLARINEX-D 24 HOUR Extended Release Tablets, as measured by total symptom score excluding nasal congestion, was significantly greater than pseudoephedrine alone over the 2-week treatment period; and the decongestant efficacy of CLARINEX-D 24 HOUR Extended Release Tablets, as measured by nasal stuffiness/congestion, was significantly greater than CLARINEX (desloratadine alone) over the 2-week treatment period. Primary efficacy variable results from 1 of 2 trials are shown in Table 3.
[See table 3 below]
There were no significant differences in the efficacy of CLARINEX-D 24 HOUR Extended Release Tablets across subgroups of subjects defined by gender, age, or race.

16   HOW SUPPLIED/STORAGE AND HANDLING
CLARINEX-D 24 HOUR Extended Release Tablets are oval-shaped, light blue coated tablets with "D24" branded in black on one side containing 5 mg desloratadine in the tablet coating for immediate release and 240 mg pseudoephedrine sulfate USP in an extended release core. CLARINEX-D 24 HOUR Extended Release Tablets are supplied in high-density polyethylene bottles of 100 (NDC 0085-1317-01).

Storage:
Store at 25°C (77°F), excursions permitted to 15–30°C (59–86°F) [see USP Controlled Room Temperature] Heat Sensitive. Avoid exposure at or above 30°C (86°F). Protect from excessive moisture. Protect from light.

17   PATIENT COUNSELING INFORMATION
[see FDA Approved Patient Labeling]
17.1   Cardiovascular and Central Nervous System Effects
Patients should be informed that pseudoephedrine, on of the active ingredients in CLARINEX-D 24 HOUR Extended Release Tablets may cause cardiovascular or central nervous system effects such as insomnia, dizziness, tremor, or arrhythmia.
17.2   Dosing
Patients should be advised not to increase the dose or dosing frequency of CLARINEX-D 24 HOUR Extended Release Tablets.

17.3   Additional Antihistamines and/or Decongestants
Patients should be advised against the concurrent use of CLARINEX-D 24 HOUR Extended Release Tablets with other antihistamines and/or decongestants.
17.4   Monoamine Oxidase (MAO) Inhibitors
Patients should be informed that due to its pseudoephedrine component, they should not use CLARINEX-D 24 HOUR with a monoamine oxidase (MAO) inhibitor or within 14 days of stopping use of an MAO inhibitor.
17.5   Coexisting Conditions
Patients with severe hypertension or severe coronary artery disease, narrow-angle glaucoma, or urinary retention should be advised not to use CLARINEX-D 24 HOUR Extended Release Tablets.
17.6   Instructions for Use
Patients should be instructed not to break, crush or chew the tablet. The tablet should be swallowed whole, and can be taken without regard to meals.
Manufactured by Schering Corporation, a subsidiary of Schering-Plough Corporation, Kenilworth, NJ 07033 USA.
© 2005, 2009, Schering Corporation. All rights reserved.
U.S. Patent Nos. 4,659,716; 4,863,931; 5,595,997; and 6,100,274

PATIENT INFORMATION
CLARINEX-D (CLA-RI-NEX) 24 Hour Extended Release Tablets
(desloratadine and pseudoephedrine sulfate)
Read the Patient Information that comes with CLARINEX-D 24 Hour Extended Release Tablets before you start taking it and each time you get a refill. There may be new information. This leaflet is a summary of the information for patients. Your doctor or pharmacist can give you additional information. This leaflet does not take the place of talking to your doctor about your medical condition or treatment.

What is CLARINEX-D® 24 Hour Extended Release Tablets?
CLARINEX-D 24 Hour Extended Release Tablets is a prescription medicine that contains the medicines desloratadine (an antihistamine) and pseudoephedrine (a nasal decongestant). CLARINEX-D 24 Hour Extended Release Tablets is used to help control the symptoms of seasonal allergic rhinitis (sneezing, stuffy nose, runny nose and itching of the nose) in adults and children 12 years and older.
CLARINEX-D 24 Hour Extended Release Tablets is not for children under 12 years of age.

Who should not take CLARINEX-D® 24 Hour Extended Release Tablets?
Do not take CLARINEX-D 24 Hour Extended Release Tablets if you:
• are allergic to desloratadine or pseudoephedrine sulfate or any of the ingredients in CLARINEX-D 24 Hour Extended Release Tablets. See the end of this leaflet for a complete list of ingredients in CLARINEX-D 24 Hour Extended Release Tablets.
• are allergic to loratadine (Alavert, Claritin)
• have narrow angle glaucoma
• have problems with urination (urinary retention)
• take a Monoamine Oxidase Inhibitor (MAOI) medicine to treat depression, or if you stopped taking an MAOI medicine within the last 2 weeks. Ask your doctor or pharmacist if you are not sure if you take an MAOI medicine.
• have severe high blood pressure
• have severe heart disease
Talk to your doctor before taking this medicine if you have any of these conditions.

What should I tell my doctor before taking CLARINEX-D® 24 Hour Extended Release Tablets?
Before you take CLARINEX-D 24 Hour Extended Release Tablets, tell your doctor if you:
• have any of the conditions listed in the section "Who should not take CLARINEX-D 24 Hour Extended Release Tablets?"
• diabetes
• hyperthyroidism
• have prostate problems
• have liver or kidney problems
• have any other medical conditions
• are pregnant or plan to become pregnant. It is not known if CLARINEX-D 24 Hour Extended Release Tablets will harm your unborn baby. Talk to your doctor if you are pregnant or plan to become pregnant.
• are breast-feeding or plan to breast-feed. CLARINEX-D 24 Hour Extended Release Tablets **can pass into your breast milk**. Talk to your doctor about the best way to feed your baby if you take CLARINEX-D 24 Hour Extended Release Tablets.

Tell your doctor about all the medicines your take, including prescription and non-prescription medicines, vitamins and herbal supplements. CLARINEX-D 24 Hour Extended Release Tablets may affect the way other medicines work,

TABLE 3 Changes in Symptoms in a 2-Week Clinical Trial in Subjects With Seasonal Allergic Rhinitis

Treatment Group (n)	Mean Baseline* (sem)	Change (% change) from Baseline (sem)	CLARINEX-D® 24 HOUR Comparison to components‡ (P- value)
Total Symptom Score (Excluding Nasal Congestion)			
CLARINEX-D 24 HOUR Extended Release Tablets (333)	14.84 (0.15)	-5.71 (-37.4) (0.22)	-
Pseudoephedrine tablet 240 mg (337)	15.03 (0.15)	-4.95 (-32.0) (0.22)	p=0.015
CLARINEX 5 mg Tablets (337)	15.06 (0.15)	-4.78 (-30.8) (0.22)	p=0.003
Nasal Stuffiness/Congestion			
CLARINEX-D® 24 HOUR Extended Release Tablets (333)	2.56 (0.020)	-0.85 (-32.3) (0.034)	-
Pseudoephedrine tablet 240 mg (337)	2.54 (0.020)	-0.70 (-27.1) (0.034)	p=0.002
CLARINEX 5 mg Tablets (337)	2.57 (0.020)	-0.65 (-24.8) (0.034)	**p<0.001**

Sem=Standard Error of the Mean
*To qualify at Baseline, the sum of the twice-daily diary reflective scores for the 3 days prior to Baseline and the morning of the Baseline visit were to total ≥42 for total nasal symptom score (sum of 4 nasal symptoms of rhinorrhea, nasal stuffiness/congestion, nasal itching, and sneezing) and a total of ≥35 for total non-nasal symptoms score (sum of 4 non-nasal symptoms of itching/burning eyes, tearing/watering eyes, redness of eyes, and itching of ears/palate), and a score of ≥14 for each of the individual symptoms of nasal stuffiness/congestion and rhinorrhea. Each symptom was scored on a 4-point severity scale (0=none, 1=mild, 2=moderate, 3=severe).
†Mean reduction in score averaged over the 2-week treatment period.
‡The comparison of interest is shown bolded.

and other medicines may affect how CLARINEX-D 24 Hour Extended Release Tablets works. Especially tell your doctor if you take:

- Monoamine Oxidase Inhibitors (MAOI). You should not use CLARINEX-D 24 Hour Extended Release Tablets if you take a MAOI or within 2 weeks of stopping an MAOI.
- methyldopa
- reserpine (Serpalan)
- digitalis (Digoxin, Lanoxicaps, Lanoxin)
- ketoconazole (Nizoral)
- erythromycin (Ery-tab, Eryc, PCE)
- azithromycin (Zithromax, Zmax)
- antihistamines
- other decongestant medicines

Know the medicines you take. Keep a list of your medicines and show it to your doctor and pharmacist when you get a new medicine.

How should I take CLARINEX-D 24 Hour Extended Release Tablets?

- Take CLARINEX-D 24 Hour Extended Release Tablets exactly as your doctor tells you to take it.
- CLARINEX-D 24 Hour Extended Release Tablets can be taken with or without food.
- Swallow CLARINEX-D 24 Hour Extended Release Tablets whole. **Do not break, crush, or chew** CLARINEX-D 24 Hour Extended Release Tablets before swallowing. If you can not swallow CLARINEX-D 24 Hour Extended Release Tablets whole, tell your doctor. You may need a different medicine.
- Take **1** CLARINEX-D 24 Hour Extended Release Tablets every day.

What are the possible side effects of CLARINEX-D® 24 Hour Extended Release Tablets?

CLARINEX-D 24 Hour Extended Release Tablets may cause serious side effects, including:

- Cardiovascular and central nervous system effects, such as
  - unable to sleep (insomnia)
  - dizziness
  - weakness
  - tremor
  - irregular heart beat
  - seizure
  - low blood pressure
- Increased sleepiness or tiredness can happen if you take more CLARINEX-D 24 Hour Extended Release Tablets than your doctor prescribed to you.
- Allergic reactions. Stop taking CLARINEX-D 24 Hour Extended Release Tablets and call your doctor right away or get emergency help if you have any of these symptoms:
  - rash
  - itching
  - hives
  - swelling of your lips, tongue, face, and throat
  - shortness of breath or trouble breathing

The most common side effects of CLARINEX-D 24 HOUR Extended Release Tablets include:

- dry mouth
- headache
- unable to sleep (insomnia)
- tiredness
- sore throat
- sleepiness
- nausea
- dizziness
- nervousness
- restlessness
- poor appetite

Tell your doctor if you have any side effect that bothers you or that does not go away. These are not all of the possible side effects of CLARINEX-D 24 Hour Extended Release Tablets. For more information, ask your doctor or pharmacist.

Call your doctor for medical advice about side effects. You may report side effects to FDA at 1-800-FDA-1088.

How should I store CLARINEX-D® 24 Hour Extended Release Tablets?

- Store CLARINEX-D 24 Hour Extended Release Tablets at 59°F to 86°F (15°C to 30°C)
- Keep CLARINEX-D 24 Hour Extended Release Tablets dry and out of the light.

Keep CLARINEX-D 24 Hour Extended Release Tablets and all medicines out of the reach of children.

General information CLARINEX-D® 24 Hour Extended Release Tablets

Medicines are sometimes prescribed for purposes other than those listed in a patient information leaflet. Do not use CLARINEX-D 24 Hour Extended Release Tablets for a condition for which it was not prescribed. Do not give CLARINEX-D 24 Hour Extended Release Tablets to other people, even if they have the same condition you have. It may harm them.

This patient information leaflet summarizes the most important information about CLARINEX-D 24 Hour Extended Release Tablets. If you would like more information, talk with your doctor. You can ask your pharmacist or doctor for information about CLARINEX-D 24 Hour Extended Release Tablets that is written for health professionals. For more information, go to www.CLARINEX.com.

What are the ingredients in CLARINEX-D® 24 Hour Extended Release Tablets?

Active ingredients: desloratadine and pseudoephedrine sulfate

Inactive ingredients: hypromellose USP, ethylcellulose NF, dibasic calcium phosphate dihydrate USP, magnesium stearate NF, povidone USP, silicone dioxide NF, talc USP, polyacrylate dispersion, polyethylene glycol NF, simethicone USP, Blue Lake Blend 50726 (FD&C Blue No. 2 Lake, titanium dioxide USP and edetate disodium USP), and ink (Opacode® S-1-17746 or Opacode® S-1-4159).

Manufactured by Schering Corporation, a subsidiary of Schering-Plough Corporation, Kenilworth, NJ 07033 USA.

Rev: Month/Year

© 2005, 2009, Schering Corporation. All rights reserved.

U.S. Patent Nos. 4,659,716; 4,863,931; 5,595,997; and 6,100,274

CLINORIL® TABLETS   ℞

[clin-or-il]
(sulindac)

DESCRIPTION

Sulindac is a non-steroidal, anti-inflammatory indene derivative designated chemically as (Z)-5-fluoro-2-methyl-1-[[p-(methylsulfinyl)phenyl]methylene]-1H-indene-3-acetic acid. It is not a salicylate, pyrazolone or propionic acid derivative. Its empirical formula is $C_{20}H_{17}FO_3S$, with a molecular weight of 356.42. Sulindac, a yellow crystalline compound, is a weak organic acid practically insoluble in water below pH 4.5, but very soluble as the sodium salt or in buffers of pH 6 or higher.

CLINORIL[1] (Sulindac) is available in 200 mg tablets for oral administration. Each tablet contains the following inactive ingredients: cellulose, magnesium stearate, starch.

Following absorption, sulindac undergoes two major biotransformations—reversible reduction to the sulfide metabolite, and irreversible oxidation to the sulfone metabolite. Available evidence indicates that the biological activity resides with the sulfide metabolite.

The structural formulas of sulindac and its metabolites are:
[See chemical structure at top of next column]

---

[1] Registered trademark of MERCK & CO., Inc.
COPYRIGHT © 1988, 2005 MERCK & CO., Inc.
All rights reserved

CLINICAL PHARMACOLOGY

Pharmacodynamics

CLINORIL is a non-steroidal anti-inflammatory drug (NSAID) that exhibits anti-inflammatory, analgesic and antipyretic activities in animal models. The mechanism of action, like that of other NSAIDs, is not completely understood but may be related to prostaglandin synthetase inhibition.

Pharmacokinetics

Absorption

The extent of sulindac absorption from CLINORIL Tablets is similar as compared to sulindac solution.

There is no information regarding food affect on sulindac absorption. Antacids containing magnesium hydroxide 200 mg and aluminum hydroxide 225 mg per 5 ml have been shown not to significantly decrease the extent of sulindac absorption.

[See table 1 at top of next page]

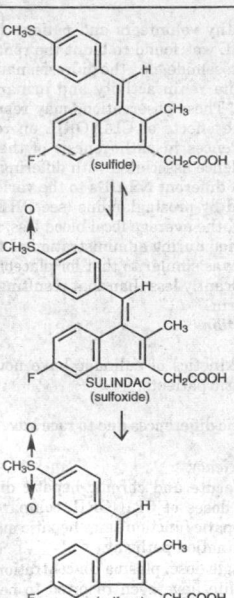

Distribution

Sulindac, and its sulfone and sulfide metabolites, are 93.1, 95.4, and 97.9% bound to plasma proteins, predominantly to albumin. Plasma protein binding measured over a concentration range (0.5-2.0 µg/mL) was constant. Following an oral, radiolabeled dose of sulindac in rats, concentrations of radiolabel in red blood cells were about 10% of those in plasma. Sulindac penetrates the blood-brain and placental barriers. Concentrations in brain did not exceed 4% of those in plasma. Plasma concentrations in the placenta and in the fetus were less than 25% and 5% respectively, of systemic plasma concentrations. Sulindac is excreted in rat milk; concentrations in milk were 10 to 20% of those levels in plasma. It is not known if sulindac is excreted in human milk.

Metabolism

Sulindac undergoes two major biotransformations of its sulfoxide moiety: oxidation to the inactive sulfone and reduction to the pharmacologically active sulfide. The latter is readily reversible in animals and in man. These metabolites are present as unchanged compounds in plasma and principally as glucuronide conjugates in human urine and bile. A dihydroxydihydro analog has also been identified as a minor metabolite in human urine.

With the twice-a-day dosage regimen, plasma concentrations of sulindac and its two metabolites accumulate: mean concentration over a dosage interval at steady state relative to the first dose averages 1.5 and 2.5 times higher, respectively, for sulindac and its active sulfide metabolite.

Sulindac and its sulfone metabolite undergo extensive enterohepatic circulation relative to the sulfide metabolite in animals. Studies in man have also demonstrated that recirculation of the parent drug sulindac and its sulfone metabolite is more extensive than that of the active sulfide metabolite. The active sulfide metabolite accounts for less than six percent of the total intestinal exposure to sulindac and its metabolites.

Biochemical as well as pharmacological evidence indicates that the activity of sulindac resides in its sulfide metabolite. An in-vitro assay for inhibition of cyclooxygenase activity exhibited an EC_{50} of 0.02 µM for sulindac sulfide. In-vivo models of inflammation indicate that activity is more highly correlated with concentrations of the metabolite than with parent drug concentrations.

Elimination

Approximately 50% of the administered dose of sulindac is excreted in the urine with the conjugated sulfone metabolite accounting for the major portion. Less than 1% of the administered dose of sulindac appears in the urine as the sulfide metabolite. Approximately 25% is found in the feces, primarily as the sulfone and sulfide metabolites.

The mean effective half-life ($T_{1/2}$) is 7.8 and 16.4 hours, respectively, for sulindac and its active sulfide metabolite.

Because CLINORIL is excreted in the urine primarily as biologically inactive forms, it may possibly affect renal function to a lesser extent than other non-steroidal anti-inflammatory drugs; however, renal adverse experiences have been reported with CLINORIL (see **ADVERSE REACTIONS**).

In a study of patients with chronic glomerular disease treated with therapeutic doses of CLINORIL, no effect was demonstrated on renal blood flow, glomerular filtration rate, or urinary excretion of prostaglandin E_2 and the primary metabolite of prostacyclin, 6-keto-$PGF_{1\alpha}$. However, in other studies in healthy volunteers and patients with liver disease, CLINORIL was found to blunt the renal responses to intravenous furosemide, i.e., the diuresis, natriuresis, increments in plasma renin activity and urinary excretion of prostaglandins. These observations may represent a differentiation of the effects of CLINORIL on renal functions based on differences in pathogenesis of the renal prostaglandin dependence associated with differing dose-response relationships of different NSAIDs to the various renal functions influenced by prostaglandins (see **PRECAUTIONS**). In healthy men, the average fecal blood loss, measured over a two-week period during administration of 400 mg per day of CLINORIL, was similar to that for placebo, and was statistically significantly less than that resulting from 4800 mg per day of aspirin.

Special Populations

Pediatric

The pharmacokinetics of sulindac have not been investigated in pediatric patients.

Race

Pharmacokinetic differences due to race have not been identified.

Hepatic Insufficiency

Patients with acute and chronic hepatic disease may require reduced doses of CLINORIL compared to patients with normal hepatic function since hepatic metabolism is an important elimination pathway.

Following a single dose, plasma concentrations of the active sulfide metabolite have been reported to be higher in patients with alcoholic liver disease compared to healthy normal subjects.

Renal Insufficiency

Sulindac pharmacokinetics have been investigated in patients with renal insufficiency. The disposition of sulindac was studied in end-stage renal disease patients requiring hemodialysis. Plasma concentrations of sulindac and it sulfone metabolite were comparable to those of normal healthy volunteers whereas concentrations of the active sulfide metabolite were significantly reduced. Plasma protein binding was reduced and the AUC of the unbound sulfide metabolite was about half that in healthy subjects.

Sulindac and its metabolites are not significantly removed from the blood in patients undergoing hemodialysis.

Since CLINORIL is eliminated primarily by the kidneys, patients with significantly impaired renal function should be closely monitored.

A lower daily dosage should be anticipated to avoid excessive drug accumulation.

In controlled clinical studies CLINORIL was evaluated in the following five conditions:

1. *Osteoarthritis*

In patients with osteoarthritis of the hip and knee, the anti-inflammatory and analgesic activity of CLINORIL was demonstrated by clinical measurements that included: assessments by both patient and investigator of overall response; decrease in disease activity as assessed by both patient and investigator; improvement in ARA Functional Class; relief of night pain; improvement in overall evaluation of pain, including pain on weight bearing and pain on active and passive motion; improvement in joint mobility, range of motion, and functional activities; decreased swelling and tenderness; and decreased duration of stiffness following prolonged inactivity.

In clinical studies in which dosages were adjusted according to patient needs, CLINORIL 200 to 400 mg daily was shown to be comparable in effectiveness to aspirin 2400 to 4800 mg daily. CLINORIL was generally well tolerated, and patients on it had a lower overall incidence of total adverse effects, of milder gastrointestinal reactions, and of tinnitus than did patients on aspirin. (See **ADVERSE REACTIONS**.)

2. *Rheumatoid arthritis*

In patients with rheumatoid arthritis, the anti-inflammatory and analgesic activity of CLINORIL was demonstrated by clinical measurements that included: assessments by both patient and investigator of overall response; decrease in disease activity as assessed by both patient and investigator; reduction in overall joint pain; reduction in duration and severity of morning stiffness; reduction in day and night pain; decrease in time required to walk 50 feet; decrease in general pain as measured on a visual analog scale; improvement in the Ritchie articular index; decrease in proximal interphalangeal joint size; improvement in ARA Functional Class; increase in grip strength; reduction in painful joint count and score; reduction in swollen joint count and score; and increased flexion and extension of the wrist.

In clinical studies in which dosages were adjusted according to patient needs, CLINORIL 300 to 400 mg daily was shown to be comparable in effectiveness to aspirin 3600 to 4800 mg daily. CLINORIL was generally well tolerated, and patients on it had a lower overall incidence of total adverse effects, of milder gastrointestinal reactions, and of tinnitus than did patients on aspirin. (See **ADVERSE REACTIONS**.)

TABLE 1

PHARMACOKINETIC PARAMETERS	NORMAL	ELDERLY
Tmax	Age 19-41 (n=24)	Age 65-87 (n=12) 400 mg qd
	(200 mg tablet)	2.54 ± 1.52 S
	3.38 ± 2.30 S	5.75 ± 2.81 SF
	4.88 ± 2.57 SP	6.83 ± 4.19 SP
	4.96 ± 2.36 SF	
	(150 mg tablet)	
	3.90 ± 2.30 S	
	5.85 ± 4.49 SP	
	6.15 ± 3.07 SF	
Renal Clearance	(200 mg tablet)	
	68.12 ± 27.56 mL/min S	
	36.58 ± 12.61 mL/min SP	
	(150 mg tablet)	
	74.39 ± 34.15 mL/min S	
	41.75 ± 13.72 mL/min SP	
Mean effective Half life (h)	7.8 S	
	16.4 SF	
	S = Sulindac	
	SF = Sulindac Sulfide	
	SP = Sulindac Sulfone	

In patients with rheumatoid arthritis, CLINORIL may be used in combination with gold salts at usual dosage levels. In clinical studies, CLINORIL added to the regimen of gold salts usually resulted in additional symptomatic relief but did not alter the course of the underlying disease.

3. *Ankylosing spondylitis*

In patients with ankylosing spondylitis, the anti-inflammatory and analgesic activity of CLINORIL was demonstrated by clinical measurements that included: assessments by both patient and investigator of overall response; decrease in disease activity as assessed by both patient and investigator; improvement in ARA Functional Class; improvement in patient and investigator evaluation of spinal pain, tenderness and/or spasm; reduction in the duration of morning stiffness; increase in the time to onset of fatigue; relief of night pain; increase in chest expansion; and increase in spinal mobility evaluated by fingers-to-floor distance, occiput to wall distance, the Schober Test, and the Wright Modification of the Schober Test. In a clinical study in which dosages were adjusted according to patient need, CLINORIL 200 to 400 mg daily was as effective as indomethacin 75 to 150 mg daily. In a second study, CLINORIL 300 to 400 mg daily was comparable in effectiveness to phenylbutazone 400 to 600 mg daily. CLINORIL was better tolerated than phenylbutazone. (See **ADVERSE REACTIONS**.)

4. *Acute painful shoulder (Acute subacromial bursitis/suprapinatus tendinitis)*

In patients with acute painful shoulder (acute subacromial bursitis/supraspinatus tendinitis), the anti-inflammatory and analgesic activity of CLINORIL was demonstrated by clinical measurements that included: assessments by both patient and investigator of overall response; relief of night pain, spontaneous pain, and pain on active motion; decrease in local tenderness; and improvement in range of motion measured by abduction, and internal and external rotation. In clinical studies in acute painful shoulder, CLINORIL 300 to 400 mg daily and oxyphenbutazone 400 to 600 mg daily were shown to be equally effective and well tolerated.

5. *Acute gouty arthritis*

In patients with acute gouty arthritis, the anti-inflammatory and analgesic activity of CLINORIL was demonstrated by clinical measurements that included: assessments by both the patient and investigator of overall response; relief of weight-bearing pain; relief of pain at rest and on active and passive motion; decrease in tenderness; reduction in warmth and swelling; increase in range of motion; and improvement in ability to function. In clinical studies, CLINORIL at 400 mg daily and phenylbutazone at 600 mg daily were shown to be equally effective. In these short-term studies in which reduction of dosage was permitted according to response, both drugs were equally well tolerated.

INDICATIONS AND USAGE

Carefully consider the potential benefits and risks of CLINORIL and other treatment options before deciding to use CLINORIL. Use the lowest effective dose for the shortest duration consistent with individual patient treatment goals (see **WARNINGS**).

CLINORIL is indicated for acute or long-term use in the relief of signs and symptoms of the following:

1. Osteoarthritis
2. Rheumatoid arthritis[2]
3. Ankylosing spondylitis
4. Acute painful shoulder (Acute subacromial bursitis/supraspinatus tendinitis)
5. Acute gouty arthritis

[2] The safety and effectiveness of CLINORIL have not been established in rheumatoid arthritis patients who are designated in the American Rheumatism Association classification as Functional Class IV (incapacitated, largely or wholly bedridden, or confined to wheelchair; little or no self-care).

CONTRAINDICATIONS

CLINORIL is contraindicated in patients with known hypersensitivity to sulindac or the excipients (see **DESCRIPTION**).

CLINORIL should not be given to patients who have experienced asthma, urticaria, or allergic-type reactions after taking aspirin or other NSAIDs. Severe, rarely fatal, anaphylactic/anaphylactoid reactions to NSAIDs have been reported in such patients (see **WARNINGS - *Anaphylactic/Anaphylactoid Reactions*, and PRECAUTIONS - *Pre-existing Asthma***).

CLINORIL is contraindicated for the treatment of perioperative pain in the setting of coronary artery bypass graft (CABG) surgery (see **WARNINGS**).

WARNINGS

CARDIOVASCULAR EFFECTS

Cardiovascular Thrombotic Events

Clinical trials of several COX-2 selective and nonselective NSAIDs of up to three years duration have shown an increased risk of serious cardiovascular (CV) thrombotic events, myocardial infarction, and stroke, which can be fatal. All NSAIDs, both COX-2 selective and nonselective, may have a similar risk. Patients with known CV disease or risk factors for CV disease may be at greater risk. To minimize the potential risk for an adverse CV event in patients treated with an NSAID, the lowest effective dose should be used for the shortest duration possible. Physicians and patients should remain alert for the development of such events, even in the absence of previous CV symptoms. Patients should be informed about the signs and/or symptoms of serious CV events and the steps to take if they occur.

There is no consistent evidence that concurrent use of aspirin mitigates the increased risk of serious CV thrombotic events associated with NSAID use. The concurrent use of aspirin and an NSAID does increase the risk of serious GI events (see **GI WARNINGS**).

Two large, controlled, clinical trials of a COX-2 selective NSAID for the treatment of pain in the first 10-14 days following CABG surgery found an increased incidence of myocardial infarction and stroke (see **CONTRAINDICATIONS**).

Hypertension

NSAIDs, including CLINORIL, can lead to onset of new hypertension or worsening of pre-existing hypertension, either of which may contribute to the increased incidence of CV events. Patients taking thiazides or loop diuretics may have impaired response to these therapies when taking NSAIDs. NSAIDs, including CLINORIL, should be used with caution in patients with hypertension. Blood pressure (BP) should be monitored closely during the initiation of NSAID treatment and throughout the course of therapy.

Congestive Heart Failure and Edema

Fluid retention and edema have been observed in some patients taking NSAIDs. CLINORIL should be used with caution in patients with fluid retention or heart failure.

Gastrointestinal Effects – Risk of Ulceration, Bleeding, and Perforation

NSAIDs, including CLINORIL, can cause serious gastrointestinal (GI) adverse events including inflammation, bleeding, ulceration, and perforation of the stomach, small intestine, or large intestine, which can be fatal. These serious adverse events can occur at any time, with or without warning symptoms, in patients treated with NSAIDs. Only one in five patients, who develop a serious upper GI adverse event on NSAID therapy is symptomatic. Upper GI ulcers, gross bleeding, or perforation caused by NSAIDs occur in approximately 1% of patients treated for 3-6 months, and in about 2-4% of patients treated for one year. These trends continue with longer duration of use, increasing the likelihood of developing a serious GI event at some time during the course of therapy. However, even short-term therapy is not without risk.

NSAIDs should be prescribed with extreme caution in those with prior history of ulcer disease or gastrointestinal bleeding. Patients with a *prior history of peptic ulcer disease and/or gastrointestinal bleeding* who use NSAIDs have a greater than 10-fold increased risk for developing a GI bleed compared to patients with neither of these risk factors. Other factors that increase the risk for GI bleeding in patients treated with NSAIDs include concomitant use of oral corticosteroids or anticoagulants, longer duration of NSAID therapy, smoking, use of alcohol, older age, and poor general health status. Most spontaneous reports of fatal GI events are in elderly or debilitated patients and therefore, special care should be taken in treating this population.

To minimize the potential risk for an adverse GI event in patients treated with an NSAID, the lowest effective dose should be used for the shortest possible duration. Patients and physicians should remain alert for signs and symptoms of GI ulceration and bleeding during NSAID therapy and promptly initiate additional evaluation and treatment if a serious GI adverse event is suspected. This should include discontinuation of the NSAID until a serious GI adverse event is ruled out. For high risk patients, alternate therapies that do not involve NSAIDs should be considered.

Hepatic Effects

In addition to hypersensitivity reactions involving the liver, in some patients the findings are consistent with those of cholestatic hepatitis (see WARNINGS, *Hypersensitivity*). As with other non-steroidal anti-inflammatory drugs, borderline elevations of one or more liver tests without any other signs and symptoms may occur in up to 15% of patients taking NSAIDs including CLINORIL. These laboratory abnormalities may progress, may remain essentially unchanged, or may be transient with continued therapy. The SGPT (ALT) test is probably the most sensitive indicator of liver dysfunction. Meaningful (3 times the upper limit of normal) elevations of SGPT or SGOT (AST) occurred in controlled clinical trials in less than 1% of patients. Notable elevations of ALT or AST (approximately three or more times the upper limit of normal) have been reported in approximately 1% of patients in clinical trials with NSAIDs. In addition, rare cases of severe hepatic reactions, including jaundice and fatal fulminant hepatitis, liver necrosis and hepatic failure, some of them with fatal outcomes have been reported.

A patient with symptoms and/or signs suggesting liver dysfunction, or in whom an abnormal liver test has occurred, should be evaluated for evidence of the development of a more severe hepatic reaction while on therapy with CLINORIL. Although such reactions as described above are rare, if abnormal liver tests persist or worsen, if clinical signs and symptoms consistent with liver disease develop, or if systemic manifestations occur (e.g., eosinophilia, rash, etc.), CLINORIL should be discontinued.

In clinical trials with CLINORIL, the use of doses of 600 mg/day has been associated with an increased incidence of mild liver test abnormalities (see DOSAGE AND ADMINISTRATION for maximum dosage recommendation).

Renal Effects

Long-term administration of NSAIDs has resulted in renal papillary necrosis and other renal injury. Renal toxicity has also been seen in patients in whom renal prostaglandins have a compensatory role in the maintenance of renal perfusion. In these patients, administration of a non-steroidal anti-inflammatory drug may cause a dose-dependent reduction in prostaglandin formation and, secondarily, in renal blood flow, which may precipitate overt renal decompensation. Patients at greatest risk of this reaction are those with impaired renal function, heart failure, liver dysfunction, those taking diuretics and ACE inhibitors, patients who are volume-depleted and the elderly. Discontinuation of NSAID therapy is usually followed by recovery to the pretreatment state.

Advanced Renal Disease

No information is available from controlled clinical studies regarding the use of CLINORIL in patients with advanced renal disease. Therefore, treatment with CLINORIL is not recommended in these patients with advanced renal disease. If CLINORIL therapy must be initiated, close monitoring of the patient's renal function is advisable.

Anaphylactic/Anaphylactoid Reactions

As with other NSAIDs, anaphylactic/anaphylactoid reactions may occur in patients without known prior exposure to CLINORIL. CLINORIL should not be given to patients with the aspirin triad. This symptom complex typically occurs in asthmatic patients who experience rhinitis with or without nasal polyps, or who exhibit severe, potentially fatal bronchospasm after taking aspirin or other NSAIDs (see CONTRAINDICATIONS and PRECAUTIONS - *Preexisting Asthma*). Emergency help should be sought in cases where an anaphylactic/anaphylactoid reaction occurs.

Skin Reactions

NSAIDs, including CLINORIL, can cause serious skin adverse events such as exfoliative dermatitis, Stevens-Johnson Syndrome (SJS), and toxic epidermal necrolysis (TEN), which can be fatal. These serious events may occur without warning. Patients should be informed about the signs and symptoms of serious skin manifestations and use of the drug should be discontinued at the first appearance of skin rash or any other sign of hypersensitivity.

Hypersensitivity

Rarely, fever and other evidence of hypersensitivity (see ADVERSE REACTIONS) including abnormalities in one or more liver function tests and severe skin reactions have occurred during therapy with CLINORIL. Fatalities have occurred in these patients. Hepatitis, jaundice, or both, with or without fever, may occur usually within the first one to three months of therapy. Determinations of liver function should be considered whenever a patient on therapy with CLINORIL develops unexplained fever, rash or other dermatologic reactions or constitutional symptoms. If unexplained fever or other evidence of hypersensitivity occurs, therapy with CLINORIL should be discontinued. The elevated temperature and abnormalities in liver function caused by CLINORIL characteristically have reverted to normal after discontinuation of therapy. Administration of CLINORIL should not be reinstituted in such patients.

Pregnancy

In late pregnancy, as with other NSAIDs, CLINORIL should be avoided because it may cause premature closure of the ductus arteriosus.

PRECAUTIONS

General

CLINORIL cannot be expected to substitute for corticosteroids or to treat corticosteroid insufficiency. Abrupt discontinuation of corticosteroids may lead to disease exacerbation. Patients on prolonged corticosteroid therapy should have their therapy tapered slowly if a decision is made to discontinue corticosteroids.

The pharmacological activity of CLINORIL in reducing fever and inflammation may diminish the utility of these diagnostic signs in detecting complications of presumed noninfectious, painful conditions.

Hematological Effects

Anemia is sometimes seen in patients receiving NSAIDs, including CLINORIL. This may be due to fluid retention, occult or gross GI blood loss, or an incompletely described effect upon erythropoiesis. Patients on long-term treatment with NSAIDs, including CLINORIL, should have their hemoglobin or hematocrit checked if they exhibit any signs or symptoms of anemia.

NSAIDs inhibit platelet aggregation and have been shown to prolong bleeding time in some patients. Unlike aspirin, their effect on platelet function is quantitatively less, of shorter duration, and reversible. Patients receiving CLINORIL who may be adversely affected by alterations in platelet function, such as those with coagulation disorders or patients receiving anticoagulants, should be carefully monitored.

Preexisting Asthma

Patients with asthma may have aspirin-sensitive asthma. The use of aspirin in patients with aspirin-sensitive asthma has been associated with severe bronchospasm which can be fatal. Since cross reactivity, including bronchospasm, between aspirin and other non-steroidal anti-inflammatory drugs has been reported in such aspirin-sensitive patients, CLINORIL should not be administered to patients with this form of aspirin sensitivity and should be used with caution in patients with preexisting asthma.

Renal Calculi

Sulindac metabolites have been reported rarely as the major or a minor component in renal stones in association with other calculus components. CLINORIL should be used with caution in patients with a history of renal lithiasis, and they should be kept well hydrated while receiving CLINORIL.

Pancreatitis

Pancreatitis has been reported in patients receiving CLINORIL (see ADVERSE REACTIONS). Should pancreatitis be suspected, the drug should be discontinued and not restarted, supportive medical therapy instituted, and the patient monitored closely with appropriate laboratory studies (e.g., serum and urine amylase, amylase/creatinine clearance ratio, electrolytes, serum calcium, glucose, lipase, etc.). A search for other causes of pancreatitis as well as those conditions which mimic pancreatitis should be conducted.

Ocular Effects

Because of reports of adverse eye findings with non-steroidal anti-inflammatory agents, it is recommended that patients who develop eye complaints during treatment with CLINORIL have ophthalmologic studies.

Hepatic Insufficiency

In patients with poor liver function, delayed, elevated and prolonged circulating levels of the sulfide and sulfone metabolites may occur. Such patients should be monitored closely; a reduction of daily dosage may be required.

SLE and Mixed Connective Tissue Disease

In patients with systemic lupus erythematosus (SLE) and mixed connective tissue disease, there may be an increased risk of aseptic meningitis (see ADVERSE REACTIONS).

Information for Patients

Patients should be informed of the following information before initiating therapy with an NSAID and periodically during the course of ongoing therapy. Patients should also be encouraged to read the NSAID Medication Guide that accompanies each prescription dispensed.

1. CLINORIL, like other NSAIDs, may cause serious CV side effects, such as MI or stroke, which may result in hospitalization and even death. Although serious CV events can occur without warning symptoms, patients should be alert for the signs and symptoms of chest pain, shortness of breath, weakness, slurring of speech, and should ask for medical advice when observing any indicative sign or symptoms. Patients should be apprised of the importance of this follow-up (see WARNINGS, *CARDIOVASCULAR EFFECTS*).

2. CLINORIL, like other NSAIDs, can cause GI discomfort and, rarely, serious GI side effects, such as ulcers and bleeding, which may result in hospitalization and even death. Although serious GI tract ulcerations and bleeding can occur without warning symptoms, patients should be alert for the signs and symptoms of ulcerations and bleeding, and should ask for medical advice when observing any indicative sign or symptoms including epigastric pain, dyspepsia, melena, and hematemesis. Patients should be apprised of the importance of this follow-up (see WARNINGS, *Gastrointestinal Effects – Risk of Ulceration, Bleeding, and Perforation*).

3. CLINORIL, like other NSAIDs, can cause serious skin side effects such as exfoliative dermatitis, SJS, and TEN, which may result in hospitalizations and even death. Although serious skin reactions may occur without warning, patients should be alert for the signs and symptoms of skin rash and blisters, fever, or other signs of hypersensitivity such as itching, and should ask for medical advice when observing any indicative signs or symptoms. Patients should be advised to stop the drug immediately if they develop any type of rash and contact their physicians as soon as possible.

4. Patients should promptly report signs or symptoms of unexplained weight gain or edema to their physicians.

5. Patients should be informed of the warning signs and symptoms of hepatotoxicity (e.g., nausea, fatigue, lethargy, pruritus, jaundice, right upper quadrant tenderness, and "flu-like" symptoms). If these occur, patients should be instructed to stop therapy and seek immediate medical therapy.

6. Patients should be informed of the signs of an anaphylactic/anaphylactoid reaction (e.g. difficulty breathing, swelling of the face or throat). If these occur, patients should be instructed to seek immediate emergency help (see WARNINGS).

7. In late pregnancy, as with other NSAIDs, CLINORIL should be avoided because it may cause premature closure of the ductus arteriosus.

Laboratory Tests

Because serious GI tract ulcerations and bleeding can occur without warning symptoms, physicians should monitor for signs or symptoms of GI bleeding. Patients on long-term treatment with NSAIDs should have their CBC and a chemistry profile checked periodically. If clinical signs and symptoms consistent with liver or renal disease develop, systemic manifestations occur (e.g., eosinophilia, rash, etc.) or if abnormal liver tests persist or worsen, CLINORIL should be discontinued.

Drug Interactions

ACE-Inhibitors and Angiotensin II Antagonists

Reports suggest that NSAIDs may diminish the antihypertensive effect of ACE-inhibitors and angiotensin II antagonists. These interactions should be given consideration in patients taking NSAIDs concomitantly with ACE-inhibitors or angiotensin II antagonists. In some patients with compromised renal function (e.g., elderly patients or patients who are volume-depleted, including those on diuretic therapy) who are being treated with non-steroidal anti-inflammatory drugs, the co-administration of an NSAID and an ACE-inhibitor or an angiotensin II antagonist may result in further deterioration of renal function, including possible acute renal failure, which is usually reversible. Therefore, monitor renal function periodically in patients receiving ACEIs or AIIAs and NSAIDS in combination therapy.

Acetaminophen
Acetaminophen had no effect on the plasma levels of sulindac or its sulfide metabolite.

Aspirin
The concomitant administration of aspirin with sulindac significantly depressed the plasma levels of the active sulfide metabolite. A double-blind study compared the safety and efficacy of CLINORIL 300 or 400 mg daily given alone or with aspirin 2.4 g/day for the treatment of osteoarthritis. The addition of aspirin did not alter the types of clinical or laboratory adverse experiences for CLINORIL; however, the combination showed an increase in the incidence of gastrointestinal adverse experiences. Since the addition of aspirin did not have a favorable effect on the therapeutic response to CLINORIL, the combination is not recommended.

Cyclosporine
Administration of non-steroidal anti-inflammatory drugs concomitantly with cyclosporine has been associated with an increase in cyclosporine-induced toxicity, possibly due to decreased synthesis of renal prostacyclin. NSAIDs should be used with caution in patients taking cyclosporine, and renal function should be carefully monitored.

Diflunisal
The concomitant administration of CLINORIL and diflunisal in normal volunteers resulted in lowering of the plasma levels of the active sulindac sulfide metabolite by approximately one-third.

Diuretics
Clinical studies, as well as post marketing observations, have shown that CLINORIL can reduce the natriuretic effect of furosemide and thiazides in some patients. This response has been attributed to inhibition of renal prostaglandin synthesis. During concomitant therapy with NSAIDs, the patient should be observed closely for signs of renal failure (see **WARNINGS**, *Renal Effects*), as well as to assure diuretic efficacy.

DMSO
DMSO should not be used with sulindac. Concomitant administration has been reported to reduce the plasma levels of the active sulfide metabolite and potentially reduce efficacy. In addition, this combination has been reported to cause peripheral neuropathy.

Lithium
NSAIDs have produced an elevation of plasma lithium levels and a reduction in renal lithium clearance. The mean minimum lithium concentration increased 15% and the renal clearance was decreased by approximately 20%. These effects have been attributed to inhibition of renal prostaglandin synthesis by the NSAID. Thus, when NSAIDs and lithium are administered concurrently, subjects should be observed carefully for signs of lithium toxicity.

Methotrexate
NSAIDs have been reported to competitively inhibit methotrexate accumulation in rabbit kidney slices. This may indicate that they could enhance the toxicity of methotrexate. Caution should be used when NSAIDs are administered concomitantly with methotrexate.

NSAIDs
The concomitant use of CLINORIL with other NSAIDs is not recommended due to the increased possibility of gastrointestinal toxicity, with little or no increase in efficacy.

Oral anticoagulants
Although sulindac and its sulfide metabolite are highly bound to protein, studies in which CLINORIL was given at a dose of 400 mg daily have shown no clinically significant interaction with oral anticoagulants. However, patients should be monitored carefully until it is certain that no change in their anticoagulant dosage is required. Special attention should be paid to patients taking higher doses than those recommended and to patients with renal impairment or other metabolic defects that might increase sulindac blood levels. The effects of warfarin and NSAIDs on GI bleeding are synergistic, such that users of both drugs together have a risk of serious GI bleeding higher than users of either drug alone.

Oral hypoglycemic agents
Although sulindac and its sulfide metabolite are highly bound to protein, studies in which CLINORIL was given at a dose of 400 mg daily, have shown no clinically significant interaction with oral hypoglycemic agents. However, patients should be monitored carefully until it is certain that no change in their hypoglycemic dosage is required. Special attention should be paid to patients taking higher doses than those recommended and to patients with renal impairment or other metabolic defects that might increase sulindac blood levels.

Probenecid
Probenecid given concomitantly with sulindac had only a slight effect on plasma sulfide levels, while plasma levels of sulindac and sulfone were increased. Sulindac was shown to produce a modest reduction in the uricosuric action of probenecid, which probably is not significant under most circumstances.

Propoxyphene hydrochloride
Propoxyphene hydrochloride had no effect on the plasma levels of sulindac or its sulfide metabolite.

Pregnancy
Teratogenic Effects. Pregnancy Category C.
Reproductive studies conducted in rats and rabbits have not demonstrated evidence of developmental abnormalities. However, animal reproduction studies are not always predictive of human response. There are no adequate and well-controlled studies in pregnant women. CLINORIL should be used in pregnancy only if the potential benefit justifies the potential risk to the fetus.

Nonteratogenic Effects
Because of the known effects of non-steroidal anti-inflammatory drugs on the fetal cardiovascular system (closure of ductus arteriosus), use during pregnancy (particularly late pregnancy) should be avoided.

The known effects of drugs of this class on the human fetus during the third trimester of pregnancy include: constriction of the ductus arteriosus prenatally, tricuspid incompetence, and pulmonary hypertension; non-closure of the ductus arteriosus postnatally which may be resistant to medical management; myocardial degenerative changes, platelet dysfunction with resultant bleeding, intracranial bleeding, renal dysfunction or failure, renal injury/dysgenesis which may result in prolonged or permanent renal failure, oligohydramnios, gastrointestinal bleeding or perforation, and increased risk of necrotizing enterocolitis.

In reproduction studies in the rat, a decrease in average fetal weight and an increase in numbers of dead pups were observed on the first day of the postpartum period at dosage levels of 20 and 40 mg/kg/day (2½ and 5 times the usual maximum daily dose in humans), although there was no adverse effect on the survival and growth during the remainder of the postpartum period. CLINORIL prolongs the duration of gestation in rats, as do other compounds of this class. Visceral and skeletal malformations observed in low incidence among rabbits in some teratology studies did not occur at the same dosage levels in repeat studies, nor at a higher dosage level in the same species.

Labor and Delivery
In rat studies with NSAIDs, as with other drugs known to inhibit prostaglandin synthesis, an increased incidence of dystocia, delayed parturition, and decreased pup survival occurred. The effects of CLINORIL on labor and delivery in pregnant women are unknown.

Nursing Mothers
It is not known whether this drug is excreted in human milk; however, it is secreted in the milk of lactating rats. Because many drugs are excreted in human milk and because of the potential for serious adverse reactions in nursing infants from CLINORIL, a decision should be made whether to discontinue nursing or to discontinue the drug, taking into account the importance of the drug to the mother.

Pediatric Use
Safety and effectiveness in pediatric patients have not been established.

Geriatric Use
As with any NSAID, caution should be exercised in treating the elderly (65 years and older) since advancing age appears to increase the possibility of adverse reactions. Elderly patients seem to tolerate ulceration or bleeding less well than other individuals and many spontaneous reports of fatal GI events are in this population (see **WARNINGS**, *Gastrointestinal Effects – Risk of Ulceration, Bleeding, and Perforation*).

CLINORIL is known to be substantially excreted by the kidney and the risk of toxic reactions to this drug may be greater in patients with impaired renal function. Because elderly patients are more likely to have decreased renal function, care should be taken in dose selection and it may be useful to monitor renal function (see **WARNINGS**, *Renal Effects*).

ADVERSE REACTIONS

The following adverse reactions were reported in clinical trials or have been reported since the drug was marketed. The probability exists of a causal relationship between CLINORIL and these adverse reactions. The adverse reactions which have been observed in clinical trials encompass observations in 1,865 patients, including 232 observed for at least 48 weeks.

Incidence Greater Than 1%
Gastrointestinal
The most frequent types of adverse reactions occurring with CLINORIL are gastrointestinal; these include gastrointestinal pain (10%), dyspepsia[3], nausea[3] with or without vomiting, diarrhea[3], constipation[3], flatulence, anorexia and gastrointestinal cramps.
Dermatologic
Rash[3], pruritus.
Central Nervous System
Dizziness[3], headache[3], nervousness.
Special Senses
Tinnitus.
Miscellaneous
Edema (see **WARNINGS**).
Incidence Less Than 1 in 100
Gastrointestinal
Gastritis, gastroenteritis or colitis. Peptic ulcer and gastrointestinal bleeding have been reported. GI perforation and intestinal strictures (diaphragms) have been reported rarely.
Liver function abnormalities; jaundice, sometimes with fever; cholestasis; hepatitis; hepatic failure.
There have been rare reports of sulindac metabolites in common bile duct "sludge" and in biliary calculi in patients with symptoms of cholecystitis who underwent a cholecystectomy.
Pancreatitis (see **PRECAUTIONS**).
Ageusia; glossitis.
Dermatologic
Stomatitis, sore or dry mucous membranes, alopecia, photosensitivity.
Erythema multiforme, toxic epidermal necrolysis, Stevens-Johnson syndrome, and exfoliative dermatitis have been reported.
Cardiovascular
Congestive heart failure, especially in patients with marginal cardiac function; palpitation; hypertension.
Hematologic
Thrombocytopenia; ecchymosis; purpura; leukopenia; agranulocytosis; neutropenia; bone marrow depression, including aplastic anemia; hemolytic anemia; increased prothrombin time in patients on oral anticoagulants (see **PRECAUTIONS**).
Genitourinary
Urine discoloration; dysuria; vaginal bleeding; hematuria; proteinuria; crystalluria; renal impairment, including renal failure; interstitial nephritis; nephrotic syndrome.
Renal calculi containing sulindac metabolites have been observed rarely.
Metabolic
Hyperkalemia.
Musculoskeletal
Muscle weakness.
Psychiatric
Depression; psychic disturbances including acute psychosis.
Nervous System
Vertigo; insomnia; somnolence; paresthesia; convulsions; syncope; aseptic meningitis (especially in patients with systemic lupus erythematosus (SLE) and mixed connective tissue disease, see **PRECAUTIONS**).
Special Senses
Blurred vision; visual disturbances; decreased hearing; metallic or bitter taste.
Respiratory
Epistaxis.
Hypersensitivity Reactions
Anaphylaxis; angioneurotic edema; urticaria; bronchial spasm; dyspnea.
Hypersensitivity vasculitis.
A potentially fatal apparent hypersensitivity syndrome has been reported. This syndrome may include constitutional symptoms (fever, chills, diaphoresis, flushing), cutaneous findings (rash or other dermatologic reactions — see above), conjunctivitis, involvement of major organs (changes in liver function including hepatic failure, jaundice, pancreatitis, pneumonitis with or without pleural effusion, leukopenia, leukocytosis, eosinophilia, disseminated intravascular coagulation, anemia, renal impairment, including renal failure), and other less specific findings (adenitis, arthralgia, arthritis, myalgia, fatigue, malaise, hypotension, chest pain, tachycardia).
Causal Relationship Unknown
A rare occurrence of fulminant necrotizing fasciitis, particularly in association with Group A β-hemolytic streptococcus, has been described in persons treated with non-steroidal anti-inflammatory agents, sometimes with fatal outcome (see also **PRECAUTIONS**, *General*).
Other reactions have been reported in clinical trials or since the drug was marketed, but occurred under circumstances where a causal relationship could not be established.

However, in these rarely reported events, that possibility cannot be excluded. Therefore, these observations are listed to serve as alerting information to physicians.
Cardiovascular
Arrhythmia.
Metabolic
Hyperglycemia.
Nervous System
Neuritis.
Special Senses
Disturbances of the retina and its vasculature.
Miscellaneous
Gynecomastia.

[3] Incidence between 3% and 9%. Those reactions occurring in 1% to 3% of patients are not marked[3].

MANAGEMENT OF OVERDOSAGE

Cases of overdosage have been reported and rarely, deaths have occurred. The following signs and symptoms may be observed following overdosage: stupor, coma, diminished urine output and hypotension.
In the event of overdosage, the stomach should be emptied by inducing vomiting or by gastric lavage, and the patient carefully observed and given symptomatic and supportive treatment.
Animal studies show that absorption is decreased by the prompt administration of activated charcoal and excretion is enhanced by alkalinization of the urine.

DOSAGE AND ADMINISTRATION

Carefully consider the potential benefits and risks of CLINORIL and other treatment options before deciding to use CLINORIL. Use the lowest effective dose for the shortest duration consistent with individual patient treatment goals (see **WARNINGS**).
After observing the response to initial therapy with CLINORIL, the dose and frequency should be adjusted to suit an individual patient's needs.
CLINORIL should be administered orally twice a day with food. The maximum dosage is 400 mg per day. Dosages above 400 mg per day are not recommended.
In osteoarthritis, rheumatoid arthritis, and ankylosing spondylitis, the recommended starting dosage is 150 mg twice a day. The dosage may be lowered or raised depending on the response.
A prompt response (within one week) can be expected in about one-half of patients with osteoarthritis, ankylosing spondylitis, and rheumatoid arthritis. Others may require longer to respond.
In acute painful shoulder (acute subacromial bursitis/supraspinatus tendinitis) and acute gouty arthritis, the recommended dosage is 200 mg twice a day. After a satisfactory response has been achieved, the dosage may be reduced according to the response. In acute painful shoulder, therapy for 7-14 days is usually adequate. In acute gouty arthritis, therapy for 7 days is usually adequate.

HOW SUPPLIED

No. 3353X—Tablets CLINORIL 200 mg are bright yellow, hexagon-shaped, compressed tablets, one side full scored, the other side half scored and debossed MSD 942. They are supplied as follows:
NDC 0006-0942-68 in bottles of 100.
Storage
Store in a well-closed container at room temperature 15-30°C (59-86°F).
Rx Only
Manufactured for:
MERCK & CO., INC., Whitehouse Station, NJ 08889, USA
By:
MERCK SHARP & DOHME Pty., Ltd.
South Granville, NSW, Australia 2142.
Issued July 2010
Printed in USA
9676108

Medication Guide For Non-Steroidal Anti-Inflammatory Drugs (Nsaids)

(See the end of this Medication Guide for a list of prescription NSAID medicines.)

What is the most important information I should know about medicines called Non-Steroidal Anti-Inflammatory Drugs (NSAIDs)?
NSAID medicines may increase the chance of a heart attack or stroke that can lead to death. This chance increases:
• with longer use of NSAID medicines
• in people who have heart disease
NSAID medicines should never be used right before or after a heart surgery called a "coronary artery bypass graft (CABG)."
NSAID medicines can cause ulcers and bleeding in the stomach and intestines at any time during treatment.

Ulcers and bleeding:
• can happen without warning symptoms
• may cause death
The chance of a person getting an ulcer or bleeding increases with:
• taking medicines called "corticosteroids" and "anticoagulants"
• longer use
• smoking
• drinking alcohol
• older age
• having poor health
NSAID medicines should only be used:
• exactly as prescribed
• at the lowest dose possible for your treatment
• for the shortest time needed

What are Non-Steroidal Anti-Inflammatory Drugs (NSAIDs)?
NSAID medicines are used to treat pain and redness, swelling, and heat (inflammation) from medical conditions such as:
• different types of arthritis
• menstrual cramps and other types of short-term pain
Who should not take a Non-Steroidal Anti-Inflammatory Drug (NSAID)?
Do not take an NSAID medicine:
• if you had an asthma attack, hives, or other allergic reaction with aspirin or any other NSAID medicine
• for pain right before or after heart bypass surgery
Tell your healthcare provider:
• about all of your medical conditions.
• about all of the medicines you take. NSAIDs and some other medicines can interact with each other and cause serious side effects. **Keep a list of your medicines to show to your healthcare provider and pharmacist.**
• if you are pregnant. **NSAID medicines should not be used by pregnant women late in their pregnancy.**
• if you are breastfeeding. **Talk to your doctor.**
What are the possible side effects of Non-Steroidal Anti-Inflammatory Drugs (NSAIDs)?

Serious side effects include:	Other side effects include:
• heart attack	• stomach pain
• stroke	• constipation
• high blood pressure	• diarrhea
• heart failure from body swelling (fluid retention)	• gas
	• heartburn
• kidney problems including kidney failure	• nausea
• bleeding and ulcers in the stomach and intestine	• vomiting
	• dizziness
• low red blood cells (anemia)	
• life-threatening skin reactions	
• life-threatening allergic reactions	
• liver problems including liver failure	
• asthma attacks in people who have asthma	

Get emergency help right away if you have any of the following symptoms:
• shortness of breath or trouble breathing
• chest pain
• weakness in one part or side of your body
• slurred speech
• swelling of the face or throat
Stop your NSAID medicine and call your healthcare provider right away if you have any of the following symptoms:
• nausea
• more tired or weaker than usual
• itching
• your skin or eyes look yellow
• stomach pain
• flu-like symptoms
• vomit blood
• there is blood in your bowel movement or it is black and sticky like tar
• unusual weight gain
• skin rash or blisters with fever
• swelling of the arms and legs, hands and feet
These are not all the side effects with NSAID medicines. Talk to your healthcare provider or pharmacist for more information about NSAID medicines.
Other information about Non-Steroidal Anti-Inflammatory Drugs (NSAIDs)
• Aspirin is an NSAID medicine but it does not increase the chance of a heart attack. Aspirin can cause bleeding in the

brain, stomach, and intestines. Aspirin can also cause ulcers in the stomach and intestines.
• Some of these NSAID medicines are sold in lower doses without a prescription (over-the-counter). Talk to your healthcare provider before using over-the-counter NSAIDs for more than 10 days.

NSAID medicines that need a prescription

Generic Name	Tradename
Celecoxib	Celebrex
Diclofenac	Cataflam, Voltaren, Arthrotec (combined with misoprostol)
Diflunisal	Dolobid
Etodolac	Lodine, Lodine XL
Fenoprofen	Nalfon, Nalfon 200
Flurbiprofen	Ansaid
Ibuprofen	Motrin, Tab-Profen, Vicoprofen* (combined with hydrocodone), Combunox (combined with oxycodone)
Indomethacin	Indocin, Indocin SR, Indo-Lemmon, Indomethegan
Ketoprofen	Oruvail
Ketorolac	Toradol
Mefenamic Acid	Ponstel
Meloxicam	Mobic
Nabumetone	Relafen
Naproxen	Naprosyn, Anaprox, Anaprox DS, EC-Naprosyn, Naprelan, Naprapac (copackaged with lansoprazole)
Oxaprozin	Daypro
Piroxicam	Feldene
Sulindac	Clinoril
Tolmetin	Tolectin, Tolectin DS, Tolectin 600

*Vicoprofen contains the same dose of ibuprofen as over-the-counter (OTC) NSAIDs, and is usually used for less than 10 days to treat pain. The OTC NSAID label warns that long term continuous use may increase the risk of heart attack or stroke.

Call your doctor for medical advice about side effects. You may report side effects to FDA at 1-800-FDA-1088.
This Medication Guide has been approved by the U.S. Food and Drug Administration.
9676108
Shown in Product Identification Guide, page 312

COMVAX® ℞
[com-vax]
[haemophilus b conjugate (meningococcal protein conjugate) and hepatitis b (recombinant) vaccine]

DESCRIPTION

COMVAX[1] [Haemophilus b Conjugate (Meningococcal Protein Conjugate) and Hepatitis B (Recombinant) Vaccine] is a sterile bivalent vaccine made of the antigenic components used in producing PedvaxHIB[1] [Haemophilus b Conjugate Vaccine (Meningococcal Protein Conjugate)] and RECOMBIVAX HB[1] [Hepatitis B Vaccine (Recombinant)]. These components are the *Haemophilus influenzae* type b capsular polysaccharide [polyribosylribitol phosphate (PRP)] that is covalently bound to an outer membrane protein complex (OMPC) of *Neisseria meningitidis* and hepatitis B surface antigen (HBsAg) from recombinant yeast cultures.
Haemophilus influenzae type b and *Neisseria meningitidis* serogroup B are grown in complex fermentation media. The primary ingredients of the phenol-inactivated fermentation medium for *Haemophilus influenzae* include an extract of yeast, nicotinamide adenine dinucleotide, hemin chloride, soy peptone, dextrose, and mineral salts and for *Neisseria meningitidis* include an extract of yeast, amino acids and mineral salts. The PRP is purified from the culture broth by

purification procedures which include ethanol fractionation, enzyme digestion, phenol extraction and diafiltration. The OMPC from *Neisseria meningitidis* is purified by detergent extraction, ultracentrifugation, diafiltration and sterile filtration.

The PRP-OMPC conjugate is prepared by the chemical coupling of the highly purified PRP (polyribosylribitol phosphate) of *Haemophilus influenzae* type b (Haemophilus b, Ross strain) to an OMPC of the B11 strain of *Neisseria meningitidis* serogroup B. The coupling of the PRP to the OMPC is necessary for enhanced immunogenicity of the PRP. This coupling is confirmed by analysis of the components of the conjugate following chemical treatment which yields a unique amino acid. After conjugation, the aqueous bulk is then adsorbed onto an amorphous aluminum hydroxyphosphate sulfate adjuvant (previously referred to as aluminum hydroxide).

HBsAg is produced in recombinant yeast cells. A portion of the hepatitis B virus gene, coding for HBsAg, is cloned into yeast, and the vaccine for hepatitis B is produced from cultures of this recombinant yeast strain according to methods developed in the Merck Research Laboratories. The antigen is harvested and purified from fermentation cultures of a recombinant strain of the yeast *Saccharomyces cerevisiae* containing the gene for the *adw* subtype of HBsAg. The fermentation process involves growth of *Saccharomyces cerevisiae* on a complex fermentation medium which consists of an extract of yeast, soy peptone, dextrose, amino acids and mineral salts.

The HBsAg protein is released from the yeast cells by mechanical cell disruption and detergent extraction, and purified by a series of physical and chemical methods, which includes ion and hydrophobic chromatography, and diafiltration. The purified protein is treated in phosphate buffer with formaldehyde and then coprecipitated with alum (potassium aluminum sulfate) to form bulk vaccine adjuvanted with amorphous aluminum hydroxyphosphate sulfate. The vaccine contains no detectable yeast DNA, and 1% or less of the protein is of yeast origin.

The individual PRP-OMPC and HBsAg adjuvanted bulks are combined to produce COMVAX. Each 0.5 mL dose of COMVAX is formulated to contain 7.5 mcg PRP conjugated to approximately 125 mcg OMPC, 5 mcg HBsAg, approximately 225 mcg aluminum as amorphous aluminum hydroxyphosphate sulfate, and 35 mcg sodium borate (decahydrate) as a pH stabilizer, in 0.9% sodium chloride. The vaccine contains not more than 0.0004% (w/v) residual formaldehyde.

The potency of the PRP-OMPC component is measured by quantitating the polysaccharide concentration by an HPLC method. The potency of the HBsAg component is measured relative to a standard by an *in vitro* immunoassay.

The product contains no preservative.

COMVAX is a sterile suspension for intramuscular injection.

CLINICAL PHARMACOLOGY

Haemophilus influenzae type b Disease

Prior to the introduction of *Haemophilus b* conjugate vaccines, *Haemophilus influenzae* type b (Hib) was the most frequent cause of bacterial meningitis and a leading cause of serious, systemic bacterial disease in young children worldwide.[1-4]

Hib disease occurred primarily in children under 5 years of age, and in the United States prior to the initiation of a vaccine program was estimated to account for nearly 20,000 cases of invasive infections annually, approximately 12,000 of which were meningitis. The mortality rate from Hib meningitis is about 5%. In addition, up to 35% of survivors develop neurologic sequelae including seizures, deafness, and mental retardation.[5,6] Other invasive diseases caused by this bacterium include cellulitis, epiglottitis, sepsis, pneumonia, septic arthritis, osteomyelitis, and pericarditis.

Prior to the introduction of the vaccine, it was estimated that 17% of all cases of Hib disease occurred in infants less than 6 months of age. The peak incidence of Hib meningitis occurred between 6 to 11 months of age. Forty-seven percent of all cases occurred by one year of age with the remaining 53% of cases occurring over the next four years.[2,20]

Among children under 5 years of age, the risk of invasive Hib disease is increased in certain populations including the following:

- Daycare attendees[7,8,9]
- Lower socio-economic groups[10]
- Blacks[11] (especially those who lack the Km(1) immunoglobulin allotype)[12]
- Caucasians who lack the G2m(23) immunoglobulin allotype[13]
- Native Americans[14-16]
- Household contacts of cases[17]

- Individuals with asplenia, sickle cell disease, or antibody deficiency syndromes.[18-19]

Prevention of Hib Disease with Vaccine

An important virulence factor of the Hib bacterium is its polysaccharide capsule (PRP). Antibody to PRP (anti-PRP) has been shown to correlate with protection against Hib disease.[3,21] While the anti-PRP level associated with protection using conjugated vaccines has not yet been determined, the level of anti-PRP associated with protection in studies using bacterial polysaccharide immune globulin or nonconjugated PRP vaccines ranged from ≥0.15 to ≥1.0 mcg/mL.[22-28]

Nonconjugated PRP vaccines are capable of stimulating B-lymphocytes to produce antibody without the help of T-lymphocytes (T-independent). The responses to many other antigens are augmented by helper T-lymphocytes (T-dependent). PedvaxHIB is a PRP-conjugate vaccine in which the PRP is covalently bound to the OMPC carrier[29] producing an antigen which is postulated to convert the T-independent antigen (PRP alone) into a T-dependent antigen resulting in both an enhanced antibody response and immunologic memory.

Clinical Trials with PedvaxHIB

The protective efficacy of the PRP-OMPC component of COMVAX was demonstrated in a randomized, double-blind, placebo-controlled study involving 3486 Native American (Navajo) infants (The Protective Efficacy Study) who completed the primary two-dose regimen for lyophilized PedvaxHIB. This population has a much higher incidence of Hib disease than the United States population as a whole and also has a lower antibody response to Haemophilus b conjugate vaccines, including PedvaxHIB.[14-16,30,31]

Each infant in this study received two doses of either placebo or lyophilized PedvaxHIB (15 mcg Haemophilus b PRP) with the first dose administered at a mean of 8 weeks of age and the second administered approximately two months later; DTP (Diphtheria and Tetanus Toxoids and whole cell Pertussis Vaccine, Adsorbed) and OPV (Poliovirus Vaccine Live Oral Trivalent) were administered concomitantly. In a subset of 416 subjects, lyophilized PedvaxHIB (15 mcg Haemophilus b PRP) induced anti-PRP levels >0.15 mcg/mL in 88% and >1.0 mcg/mL in 52% with a geometric mean titer (GMT) of 0.95 mcg/mL one to three months after the first dose; the corresponding anti-PRP levels one to three months following the second dose were 91% and 60%, respectively, with a GMT of 1.43 mcg/mL. These antibody responses were associated with a high level of protection.

Most subjects were initially followed until 15 to 18 months of age. During this time, 22 cases of invasive Hib disease occurred in the placebo group (8 cases after the first dose and 14 cases after the second dose) and only 1 case in the vaccine group (none after the first dose and 1 after the second dose). Following the primary two-dose regimen, the protective efficacy of lyophilized PedvaxHIB was calculated to be 93% with a 95% confidence interval (C.I.) of 57-98%. In the two months between the first and second doses, the difference in number of cases of disease between placebo and vaccine recipients (8 vs 0 cases, respectively) was statistically significant (p=0.008). At termination of the study, placebo recipients were offered vaccine. All original participants were then followed two years and nine months from termination of the study. During this extended follow-up, invasive Hib disease occurred in an additional 7 of the original placebo recipients prior to receiving vaccine and in 1 of the original vaccine recipients (who had received only 1 dose of vaccine). No cases of invasive Hib disease were observed in placebo recipients after they received at least one dose of vaccine. Efficacy for this follow-up period, estimated from person-days at risk, was 96.6% (95 C.I., 72.2-99.9%) in children under 18 months of age and 100% (95 C.I., 23.5-100%) in children over 18 months of age.[31] Thus, in this study, a protective efficacy of 93% was achieved with an anti-PRP level of >1.0 mcg/mL in 60% of vaccinees and a GMT of 1.43 mcg/mL one to three months after the second dose.

Hepatitis B Disease

Hepatitis B virus is an important cause of viral hepatitis. According to the Centers for Disease Control (CDC), there are an estimated 200,000-300,000 new cases of Hepatitis B infection annually in the United States.[32] There is no specific treatment for this disease. The incubation period for hepatitis B is relatively long; six weeks to six months may elapse between exposure and the onset of clinical symptoms. The prognosis following infection with hepatitis B virus is variable and dependent on at least three factors: (1) Age—infants and younger children usually experience milder initial disease than older persons but are much more likely to remain persistently infected and become at risk of developing serious chronic liver disease; (2) Dose of virus—the higher the dose, the more likely acute icteric hepatitis B will result; and, (3) Severity of associated underlying disease—underlying malignancy or pre-existing hepatic disease predisposes to increased mortality and morbidity.[34]

Hepatitis B infection fails to resolve and progresses to a chronic carrier state in 5 to 10% of older children and adults and in up to 90% of infants; chronic infection also occurs more frequently after initial anicteric hepatitis B than after initial icteric disease.[34] Consequently, carriers of HBsAg frequently give no history of having had recognized acute hepatitis. It has been estimated that more than 285 million people in the world today are persistently infected with hepatitis B virus.[35] The CDC estimates that there are approximately 1 million-1.25 million chronic carriers of hepatitis B virus in the USA.[32] Chronic carriers represent the largest human reservoir of hepatitis B virus.

A serious complication of acute hepatitis B virus infection is massive hepatic necrosis while sequelae of chronic hepatitis B include cirrhosis of the liver, chronic active hepatitis, and hepatocellular carcinoma. Chronic carriers of HBsAg appear to be at increased risk of developing hepatocellular carcinoma. Although a number of etiologic factors are associated with development of hepatocellular carcinoma, the single most important etiologic factor appears to be chronic infection with hepatitis B virus.[36] According to the CDC, hepatitis B vaccine is recognized as the first anti-cancer vaccine because it can prevent primary liver cancer.[67]

The vehicles for transmission of the virus are most often blood and blood products but the viral antigen has also been found in tears, saliva, breast milk, urine, semen, and vaginal secretions. Hepatitis B virus is capable of surviving for days on environmental surfaces exposed to body fluids containing hepatitis B virus. Infection may occur when hepatitis B virus, transmitted by infected body fluids, is implanted via mucous surfaces or percutaneously introduced through accidental or deliberate breaks in the skin. Transmission of hepatitis B virus infection is often associated with close interpersonal contact with an infected individual and with crowded living conditions.[37]

Prevention of Hepatitis B Disease with Vaccine

Hepatitis B infection and disease can be prevented through immunization with vaccines that contain viral surface antigen (HBsAg) and induce formation of protective antibody (anti-HBs).[38-39]

Multiple clinical studies have defined a protective level of anti-HBs as 1) 10 or more sample ratio units (SRU or S/N) as determined by radioimmunoassay or 2) a positive result as determined by enzyme immunoassay.[40-46] Note: 10 SRU is comparable to 10 mIU/mL of antibody.[36] The ACIP and an international group of hepatitis B experts consider an anti-HBs titer ≥10 mIU/mL an adequate response to a complete course of hepatitis B vaccine and protective against clinically significant infection (antigenemia with or without clinical disease).[36,46]

Clinical Trials with RECOMBIVAX HB

In clinical studies, 100% of 92 infants under 1 year of age born of non-carrier mothers developed a protective level of antibody (anti-HBs ≥10 mIU/mL) after receiving three 5-mcg doses of RECOMBIVAX HB at intervals of 0, 1, and 6 months.[31]

In one clinical study of RECOMBIVAX HB (2.5 mcg), which examined a different regimen of RECOMBIVAX HB, protective levels of antibody were achieved in 98% of 52 healthy infants vaccinated at 2, 4, and 12 months of age. Protective anti-HBs levels were achieved in 100% of 50 infants vaccinated at 2, 4, and 15 months of age.[47]

The protective efficacy of three 5-mcg doses of RECOMBIVAX HB, given at birth (with Hepatitis B Immune Globulin), 1, and 6 months of age, has been demonstrated in neonates born of mothers positive for both HBsAg and HBeAg (a core-associated antigenic complex which correlates with high infectivity). In this trial, after nine months of follow-up, chronic infection had not occurred in 96% of 130 infants.[48] The estimated efficacy in prevention of chronic hepatitis B infection was 95% as compared to the infection rate in untreated historical controls.[49]

Immunogenicity of COMVAX

The immunogenicity of COMVAX (7.5 mcg Haemophilus b PRP, 5 mcg HBsAg) was assessed in 1602 infants and children 6 weeks to 15 months of age in 5 clinical studies. In 2 controlled clinical trials (n=684), the immune response of COMVAX was compared with that obtained using the monovalent vaccines, PedvaxHIB (7.5 mcg Haemophilus b PRP) and RECOMBIVAX HB (5 mcg HBsAg) given at separate sites, either concurrently or one month apart. The immunogenicity of COMVAX was further assessed in 2 uncontrolled studies (n=852). In the first, a complete three-dose series of COMVAX was administered concurrently with other routine pediatric vaccines. In the second, COMVAX was administered as the third dose of Haemophilus b PRP and HBsAg concurrently with routine pediatric vaccines. COMVAX was also administered as the control arm in the evaluation of an investigational vaccine (n=66).

These studies demonstrate COMVAX to be highly immunogenic. The antibody responses are summarized below.

Antibody Responses to COMVAX in Infants Not Previously Vaccinated with Hib or Hepatitis B Vaccine

In the pivotal, controlled, multicenter, randomized, open-label study, 882 infants approximately 2 months of age, who

Table 1: Antibody Responses to COMVAX, PedvaxHIB, and RECOMBIVAX HB in Infants Not Previously Vaccinated with Hib or Hepatitis B Vaccine

Vaccine	Age (months)	Time	n	Anti-PRP % Subjects with >0.15 mcg/mL	Anti-PRP % Subjects with >1.0 mcg/mL	Anti-PRP GMT (mcg/mL)	n	Anti-HBs % Subjects ≥10 mIU/mL	Anti-HBs GMT (mIU/mL)
COMVAX		Prevaccination	633	34.4	4.7	0.1	603	10.6	0.6
(7.5 mcg PRP,	2	Dose 1*	620	88.9	51.5	1.0	595	34.3	4.2
5 mcg HBsAg)	4	Dose 2*	576	94.8	72.4†	2.5†	571	92.1	113.9
[N=661]	12/15	Dose 3‡	570	99.3	92.6	9.5	571	98.4	4467.5†
PedvaxHIB		Prevaccination	208	33.7	5.8	0.1	196	7.1	0.5
(7.5 mcg PRP)	2	Dose 1*	202	90.1	53.5	1.1	198	41.9	5.3
+	4	Dose 2*	186	95.2	76.3†	2.8†	185	98.4†	255.7
RECOMBIVAX HB	12/15	Dose 3‡	181	98.9	92.3	10.2	179	100.0†	6943.9†
(5 mcg HBsAg)									
[N=221]									

* Postvaccination responses were determined approximately two months after doses 1 and 2.
† C.I.'s of comparisons:
Dose 2 Anti-PRP: 95% C.I. on difference in % >1.0 mcg/mL (-11.2, 3.1); 95% C.I. on ratio of GMT (0.69, 1.17)
Dose 3 Anti-HBs: 95% C.I. on difference in % ≥10 mIU/mL (-2.9, -0.6); 95% C.I. on ratio of GMT (0.49, 0.91)
‡ Postvaccination responses were determined approximately one month after administration of dose 3.
More than three-quarters of the infants in the study received DTP and OPV concomitantly with the first two doses of COMVAX or PedvaxHIB plus RECOMBIVAX HB, and approximately one-third received M-M-R II[1] (Measles, Mumps, and Rubella Virus Vaccine Live) with the third dose of these vaccines at 12 or 15 months of age.

Table 2: Antibody Responses to COMVAX in Infants Previously Vaccinated with Hepatitis B Vaccine at Birth

Study	Age (months) at Vaccination	Time	n	Anti-PRP % Subjects with >0.15 mcg/mL	Anti-PRP % Subjects with >1.0 mcg/mL	Anti-PRP GMT (mcg/mL)	n	Anti-HBs % Subjects ≥10mIU/mL	Anti-HBs GMT (mIU/mL)
		Prevaccination	119	24.4	5.9	0.1	71	25.4	2.9
Study 1	2	Dose 1	Not Measured						
[N=126]	4	Dose 2*	111	94.6	81.1	3.3	111	98.2	417.2
	14/15	Dose 3*	88	100	93.2	11.0	87	98.9	3500.7
		Prevaccination	17	58.8	0	0.2	15	6.7	0.7
Study 2	2	Dose 1†	17	88.2	47.1	0.9	16	81.3	35.2
[N=19]	4	Dose 2†	17	100	76.5	2.8	16	100	281.8
	15	Dose 3†	15	100	100	8.5	16	100	3913.4

* Postvaccination responses were determined approximately 2 months after dose 2 and 1 month after dose 3.
† Postvaccination responses were determined approximately 2 months after doses 1, 2, and 3.
Infants in these studies received DTP and OPV or eIPV (enhanced inactivated poliovirus vaccine) concomitantly with the first two doses of COMVAX, while the third dose of COMVAX was given concomitantly with DTaP (diphtheria and tetanus and acellular pertussis), OPV, and M-M-R II[1] at 14-15 months of age (Study 1) or with just M-M-R II[1] at 15 months of age (Study 2).

had not previously received any Hib or hepatitis B vaccine, were assigned to receive a three-dose regimen of either COMVAX or PedvaxHIB plus RECOMBIVAX HB at approximately 2, 4, and 12-15 months of age. The proportions of evaluable vaccinees developing clinically important levels of anti-PRP (percent with >1.0 mcg/mL after the second dose, n=762) and anti-HBs (percent with ≥10 mIU/mL after the third dose, n=750) were similar in children given COMVAX or concurrent PedvaxHIB and RECOMBIVAX HB (Table 1).
The anti-PRP response after the second dose among infants given COMVAX in this study was 72.4% (C.I. 68.7, 76.0) >1.0 mcg/mL with a GMT=2.5 mcg/mL (C.I. 2.2, 2.8) and was comparable to that of infants given the PedvaxHIB and RECOMBIVAX HB controls which was 76.3% (C.I. 70.2, 82.5) with a GMT=2.8 mcg/mL (C.I. 2.2, 3.5). These responses exceed the response of Native American (Navajo) infants in a previous study of lyophilized PedvaxHIB (60% >1.0 mcg/mL; GMT=1.43 mcg/mL) that was associated with a 93% reduction in the incidence of invasive Hib disease. The efficacy of COMVAX in the prevention of invasive Hib disease is expected to be similar to that obtained with monovalent lyophilized PedvaxHIB in the Protective Efficacy Trial (see CLINICAL PHARMACOLOGY, Clinical Trials with PedvaxHIB).
The anti-HBs response after the third dose among infants given COMVAX in this study was 98.4% ≥10 mIU/mL (C.I. 97.0, 99.3) with a GMT of 4467.5 (C.I. 3786.3, 5271.3) compared to 100.0% (C.I. 97.9, 100.0) with a GMT of 6943.9 (C.I. 5555.9, 8678.7) among infants given COMVAX or concurrent PedvaxHIB and RECOMBIVAX HB.
Although the difference in anti-HBs GMT is statistically significant (p=0.011), both values are much greater than the level of 10 mIU/mL previously established as marking a protective response to hepatitis B.{42,44-46,51,52} These GMTs are higher than those observed in young infants who received the currently licensed regimen of RECOMBIVAX HB consisting of 5-mcg doses administered on the standard 0, 1, and 6-month schedule (GMT ~ 1359.9 mIU/mL).{53-55} In addition, two studies have shown that infants given 2.5-mcg doses of RECOMBIVAX HB according to the schedule used for COMVAX (2, 4, and 12-15 months of age) developed GMTs of 1245-3424 mIU/mL.{47,64} While a difference in GMT may result in differential retention of ≥10 mIU/mL of anti-HBs after a number of years, this is of no apparent clinical significance because of immunologic memory.{56,67}
Because the HBsAg component of COMVAX induces a comparable anti-HBs response to that obtained with RECOMBIVAX HB, the efficacy of COMVAX is expected to be similar (Table 1).
[See table 1 above]

Antibody Responses to COMVAX in Infants Previously Vaccinated with Hepatitis B Vaccine at Birth

Two clinical studies assessed antibody responses to a three-dose series of COMVAX in 128 evaluable infants who were previously given a birth dose of hepatitis B vaccine. Table 2 summarizes the anti-PRP and anti-HBs responses of these infants. The antibody responses were clinically comparable to those observed in the pivotal trial of COMVAX (Table 1).
[See table 2 above]

Interchangeability of COMVAX and Licensed Haemophilus b Conjugate Vaccines or Recombinant Hepatitis B Vaccines

Among 58 children previously given a primary course of PedvaxHIB, 90% (95% C.I. 78.8%, 96.1%) developed an anti-PRP response >1 mcg/mL with a GMT of 9.6 mcg/mL (95% C.I. 6.6, 14.1) in response to a dose of COMVAX at 12-15 months of age. Among 683 children previously given a primary course of another HIB or HIB-containing vaccine, 99% (95% C.I. 97.9%, 99.6%) developed an anti-PRP response >1 mcg/mL with a GMT of 14.9 mcg/mL (95% C.I. 13.7, 16.3) in response to a dose of COMVAX at 12-15 months of age.
In another study, COMVAX was administered either concomitantly or six weeks after vaccination with M-M-R[1] II and VARIVAX[1] (Varicella Virus Vaccine Live, Oka/Merck). Among 149 children who previously received 2 doses of monovalent Hepatitis B vaccine, 100% (95% C.I. 97.6%, 100.0%) developed an anti-HBs response ≥10 mIU/mL with a GMT of 2194.6 mIU/mL (95% C.I. 1667.8, 2887.8) in response to a dose of COMVAX at 12-15 months of age.

Antibody Responses to COMVAX and Concurrently Administered Vaccines

Immunogenicity results from open-labeled studies indicate that COMVAX can be administered concomitantly with DTP, DTaP, OPV, IPV (inactivated poliomyelitis vaccine), M-M-R II, and VARIVAX using separate sites and syringes for injectable vaccines.

DTP and DTaP

After a primary series of DTP (2, 4, 6 months of age) given concomitantly with COMVAX (2 and 4 months of age), 98.2% of 57 infants developed a 4-fold rise in antibody to diphtheria, 100% of 57 infants developed a 4-fold rise in antibody to tetanus, and 89.5% to 96.5% of 57 infants developed a 4-fold rise in antibody to pertussis antigens, depending on the assay used and adjusted for maternal antibody. In this trial, after 2 doses of COMVAX, 79.0% of 62 infants developed anti-PRP >1.0 mcg/mL and after 3 doses (2, 4, and 15 months of age), 100% of 59 infants developed ≥10 mIU/mL of anti-HBs.
After a primary series of DTaP and COMVAX given concomitantly at 2, 4, and 6 months of age, 100% of 18 infants had ≥0.01 antitoxin units/mL to diphtheria and tetanus and 94.4% to 100% of 18 infants developed a ≥4-fold rise in antibody to pertussis antigens, depending on the assay used and adjusted for maternal antibody. In this trial, after 2 doses of COMVAX, 85.7% of 63 infants developed anti-PRP >1.0 mcg/mL and after 3 doses administered on the compressed schedule of 2, 4, and 6 months of age, 92.9% of 56 infants developed ≥10 mIU/mL of anti-HBs.

OPV and IPV

After a primary series of OPV (2, 4, 6 months of age) given concomitantly with COMVAX (2 and 4 months of age), 98.3% of 60 infants had neutralizing antibody ≥1:4 to poliovirus type 1, 100% of 57 infants had neutralizing antibody ≥1:4 to poliovirus type 2 and 98.1% of 53 infants had neutralizing antibody ≥1:4 to poliovirus type 3. In this trial, after 2 doses of COMVAX, 79.0% of 62 infants developed anti-PRP >1.0 mcg/mL and after 3 doses, 100% of 59 infants developed ≥10 mIU/mL of anti-HBs.
After a primary series of IPV and COMVAX given concomitantly at 2, 4, and 6 months of age, 100% of 38 infants had neutralizing antibody ≥1:4 to poliovirus types 1, 2, and 3. In this trial, after 2 doses of COMVAX, 85.7% of 63 infants developed anti-PRP >1.0 mcg/mL and after 3 doses administered on the compressed schedule of 2, 4, and 6 months of age, 92.9% of 56 infants developed ≥10 mIU/mL of anti-HBs.

M M R II and VARIVAX

After concomitant vaccination of M-M-R II and VARIVAX with COMVAX (12 to 15 months of age), 99.4% of 313 children developed antibody to measles, 99.2% of 354 children developed antibody to mumps, 100% of 358 children developed antibody to rubella and 100% of 276 children developed antibody to varicella. In this trial, infants received the primary series of Hib vaccine and the first two doses of Hepatitis B vaccine in the first year of life. After the dose of COMVAX, 97.8% of 368 infants developed >1.0 mcg/mL of anti-PRP and 99.2% developed ≥10 mIU/mL of anti-HBs.

INDICATIONS AND USAGE

COMVAX is indicated for vaccination against invasive disease caused by *Haemophilus influenzae* type b and against infection caused by all known subtypes of hepatitis B virus in infants 6 weeks to 15 months of age born of HBsAg negative mothers.
Infants born to HBsAg positive mothers should receive Hepatitis B Immune Globulin and Hepatitis B Vaccine (Recombinant) at birth and should complete the hepatitis B vaccination series given according to a particular schedule (see manufacturer's circular for Hepatitis B Vaccine [Recombinant]).
Infants born to mothers of unknown HBsAg status should receive Hepatitis B Vaccine (Recombinant) at birth and should complete the hepatitis B vaccination series given according to a particular schedule (see manufacturer's circular for Hepatitis B Vaccine [Recombinant]).
Vaccination with COMVAX should ideally begin at approximately 2 months of age or as soon thereafter as possible. In order to complete the three-dose regimen of COMVAX, vaccination should be initiated no later than 10 months of age. Infants in whom vaccination with a PRP-OMPC-containing product (i.e., PedvaxHIB, COMVAX) is not initiated until 11 months of age do not require three doses of PRP-OMPC; however, three doses of an HBsAg-containing product are required for complete vaccination against hepatitis B, regardless of age. For infants and children not vaccinated according to the recommended schedule see DOSAGE AND ADMINISTRATION.
COMVAX will not protect against invasive disease caused by *Haemophilus influenzae* other than type b or against invasive disease (such as meningitis or sepsis) caused by other microorganisms. COMVAX will not prevent hepatitis caused by other viruses known to infect the liver. Because of the long incubation period for hepatitis B, it is possible for unrecognized infection to be present at the time the vaccine is given. The vaccine may not prevent hepatitis B in such patients.
As with other vaccines, COMVAX may not induce protective antibody levels immediately following vaccination and may not result in a protective antibody response in all individuals given the vaccine.

Table 3: Local Reactions and Systemic Complaints Within 5 Days After Injection Reported to Occur in ≥1.0%* of Children Given a 3-Dose Course of COMVAX Compared to These Events in Children Given Concomitant Injections of PedvaxHIB and RECOMBIVAX HB

Event	Injection 1[†] COMVAX (N=660) %	PedvaxHIB and RECOMBIVAX HB[‡] (N=221) %	Injection 2[†] COMVAX (N=645) %	PedvaxHIB and RECOMBIVAX HB[‡] (N=213) %	Injection 3 COMVAX (N=593) %	PedvaxHIB and RECOMBIVAX HB[‡] (N=193) %
Injection Site Reactions						
Pain/Soreness[§]	34.5	37.6	24.3	25.8	23.9	21.2
Erythema (>1 in.)[§]	22.4 (2.7)	25.8 (2.7)	25.7 (1.4)	23.5 (3.3)	27.2 (3.0)	24.4 (1.6)
Swelling/Induration (>1 in.)[§]	27.6 (3.0)	33.5 (4.1)	30.4 (2.9)	31.0 (3.8)	27.2 (3.2)	29.5 (4.1)
Systemic Complaints						
Irritability[§]	57.0	46.6	50.7	44.1	32.2	29.0
Somnolence[§]	49.5	47.1	37.4	31.9	21.1	22.3
Crying—						
unusual, high pitched[§]	10.6	8.6	6.7	2.3	2.9	3.6
not otherwise specified	2.3	2.3	1.4	2.3	0.7	1.6
prolonged (>4 hrs.)[§]	2.4	2.3	0.8	1.4	0.2	0
Anorexia	3.9	2.3	2.0	0.9	0.8	0.5
Vomiting	2.1	1.8	2.5	0.9	1.0	1.6
Otitis media	0.5	0	2.0	1.4	2.7	1.6
Fever (°F, rectal equiv.)[¶]						
101.0-102.9	14.2	11.9	13.8	12.2	10.5	6.4
≥103.0	0.8	0	1.6	1.4	2.7	4.3
Diarrhea	1.7	1.8	0.8	0.9	2.2	0.5
Upper respiratory infection	0.5	0.5	1.1	0.9	1.3	0.5
Rash	0.8	0	0.9	0	0.8	0.5
Rhinorrhea	0.2	0.5	1.1	0.9	1.3	2.1
Respiratory congestion	0.6	0.5	1.2	0.9	0.3	0.5
Cough	0.2	0	0.9	0.5	0.2	1.0
Candidiasis, oral	0.3	0.5	0.8	0	0.2	0
Rash, diaper	0.5	0.5	0.5	0.9	0.2	0

* Overall frequency of each event listed above is ≥1% even though the frequency after a given dose may be <1%.
† Most children received DTP and OPV concomitantly with the first two doses of COMVAX or PedvaxHIB and RECOMBIVAX HB.
‡ Injection site reactions for PedvaxHIB and RECOMBIVAX HB based on occurrence with either of the monovalent components.
§ Events prompted for on Vaccination Report Card given to parents/guardians of vaccinees.
¶ N for injections 1, 2, and 3 equals 655, 639, and 588, respectively, for COMVAX; N for injections 1, 2, and 3 equals 218, 213, and 187, respectively, for PedvaxHIB and RECOMBIVAX HB.

Use With Other Vaccines

Immunogenicity results from open-labeled studies indicate that COMVAX can be administered concomitantly with DTP, DTaP, OPV, IPV, M-M-R II, and VARIVAX using separate sites and syringes for injectable vaccines (see CLINICAL PHARMACOLOGY).

CONTRAINDICATIONS

Hypersensitivity to yeast or any component of the vaccine. The decision to administer or delay vaccination because of current or recent febrile illness depends on the severity of symptoms and on the etiology of the disease. The ACIP has recommended that immunization should be delayed during the course of an acute febrile illness.[63] All vaccines can be administered to persons with minor illnesses such as diarrhea, mild upper-respiratory infection with or without low-grade fever, or other low-grade febrile illness. Persons with moderate or severe febrile illness should be vaccinated as soon as they have recovered from the acute phase of the illness.

WARNINGS

Patients who develop symptoms suggestive of hypersensitivity after an injection should not receive further injections of the vaccine (see CONTRAINDICATIONS).

PRECAUTIONS
General

General care is to be taken by the health-care provider for the safe and effective use of this product.
As for any vaccine, adequate treatment provisions, including epinephrine, should be available for immediate use should an anaphylactic or anaphylactoid reaction occur.
As reported with Haemophilus b Polysaccharide Vaccine and another Haemophilus b Conjugate Vaccine, cases of Haemophilus b disease may occur in the week after vaccination, prior to the onset of the protective effects of the vaccines.
The packaging stopper of this product contains natural rubber latex which may cause allergic reactions.

Instructions to Health-care Provider

The health-care provider should determine the current health status and previous vaccination history of the vaccinee.
The health-care provider should question the patient, parent or guardian about reactions to a previous dose of COMVAX, PedvaxHIB or other Haemophilus b conjugate vaccines or RECOMBIVAX HB or other hepatitis B vaccines.
Injection of a blood vessel should be avoided.
COMVAX should be given with caution in infants with bleeding disorders such as hemophilia or thrombocytopenia, with steps taken to avoid the risk of hematoma following the injection.
If COMVAX is used in persons with malignancies or those receiving immunosuppressive therapy or who are otherwise immunocompromised, the expected immune response may not be obtained.
COMVAX is not contraindicated in the presence of HIV infection.[68]

Information for Vaccine Recipients and Parents/Guardians

The health-care provider should provide the vaccine information required to be given with each vaccination to the patient, parent or guardian.
The health-care provider should inform the patient, parent or guardian of the benefits and risks associated with vaccination. For risks associated with vaccination, see WARNINGS, PRECAUTIONS, and ADVERSE REACTIONS.

Laboratory Test Interactions

Sensitive tests (e.g., Latex Agglutination Kits) may detect PRP derived from the vaccine in the urine of some vaccinees for at least 30 days following vaccination with lyophilized PedvaxHIB[58]; in clinical studies with lyophilized PedvaxHIB, such children demonstrated a normal immune response to the vaccine. It is not known whether antigenuria will occur after vaccination with COMVAX.

Drug Interaction

Deferral of immunization may be considered in individuals receiving immunosuppressive therapy.

Carcinogenesis, Mutagenesis, Impairment of Fertility

COMVAX has not been evaluated for its carcinogenic or mutagenic potential, or its potential to impair fertility.

Pregnancy

Pregnancy Category C:
Animal reproduction studies have not been conducted with COMVAX. It is also not known whether COMVAX can cause fetal harm when administered to a pregnant woman or can affect reproduction capacity. COMVAX is not recommended for use in women of childbearing age.

Pediatric Use

Safety and effectiveness of COMVAX in infants below the age of 6 weeks and above the age of 15 months have not been established. However, studies have demonstrated that PedvaxHIB is safe and immunogenic when administered to infants and children up to the age of 71 months and RECOMBIVAX HB is safe and immunogenic in persons of all ages.
COMVAX should not be used in infants younger than 6 weeks of age because this will lead to a reduced anti-PRP response and may lead to immune tolerance (impaired ability to respond to subsequent exposure to the PRP antigen).[59-61]
Infants born to HBsAg-positive mothers should not receive COMVAX but instead should receive Hepatitis B Immune Globulin and Hepatitis B Vaccine (Recombinant) at birth and should complete the hepatitis B vaccination series given according to a particular schedule (see manufacturer's circular for Hepatitis B Vaccine [Recombinant]). (See DOSAGE AND ADMINISTRATION.)

Geriatric use

This vaccine is NOT recommended for use in adult populations.

ADVERSE REACTIONS

In clinical trials involving the administration of 7918 doses of COMVAX to 3561 healthy infants 6 weeks to 15 months of age, COMVAX was generally well tolerated. In these studies, infants received COMVAX with licensed pediatric vaccines (n=1745) or investigational vaccines (n=1816). Serious adverse experience data were available for all 3561 infants and non-serious adverse experience data were available for a subset of 1678 infants.

Pivotal Immunogenicity and Safety Study

In the pivotal, randomized, multicenter study, 882 infants were assigned in a 3:1 ratio to receive either COMVAX or PedvaxHIB plus RECOMBIVAX HB at separate injection sites at 2, 4, and 12-15 months of age. Children may have also received routine pediatric immunizations. The children were monitored daily for five days after each injection for injection-site and systemic adverse experiences. During this time, adverse experiences in infants who received COMVAX were generally similar in type and frequency to those observed in infants who received PedvaxHIB plus RECOMBIVAX HB.
The most frequently cited events were mild, transient signs and symptoms of inflammation at the injection site (i.e., pain/soreness, erythema, and swelling/induration), somnolence, and irritability, all of which were prompted for on report cards filled out by parents of vaccinated children. Table 3 summarizes the frequencies of injection-site and systemic adverse experiences within five days of vaccination that were reported among ≥1.0% of children in this pivotal trial. [See table 3 at left]

Infants Previously Vaccinated with Hepatitis B Vaccine

In a group of infants (N=126) given a three-dose course of COMVAX after previously receiving a dose of Hepatitis B Vaccine (Recombinant) at or shortly after birth, the type, frequency, and severity of adverse experiences did not appear to be greater than those observed in infants in the pivotal study who did not receive hepatitis B vaccine at birth.

Infants 6 Weeks to 15 Months of Age

In clinical trials, 3285 doses of COMVAX were administered to 1678 infants who were monitored for injection-site and systemic adverse experiences from Days 0 to 5 after each injection of vaccine. Of these, 855 infants had safety data following vaccination at approximately 2 months of age, 836 infants at approximately 4 months of age and 1573 infants at 12 to 15 months of age. The most frequently reported adverse experiences (≥1% of subjects for at least one injection), without regard to causality are listed in decreasing order of frequency within each body system:
Injection Site Reactions: Pain/tenderness/soreness, swelling/induration, erythema; *Body as a Whole:* Fever; *Digestive System:* Anorexia, diarrhea, vomiting; *Nervous System/Psychiatric:* Irritability, somnolence, crying; *Respiratory System:* Upper respiratory infection, rhinorrhea, cough, rhinitis; *Skin:* Rash; *Special Senses:* Otitis media.

Post-Marketing Experience

As with any vaccine, there is the possibility that broad use of COMVAX could reveal adverse experiences not observed in clinical trials. The following additional adverse reactions have been reported with the use of the marketed vaccine.
Hypersensitivity
Anaphylaxis, angioedema, urticaria, erythema multiforme
Hematologic
Thrombocytopenia
Nervous System
Seizure, febrile seizures

Potential Adverse Effects

In addition, a variety of adverse effects have been reported with marketed use of either PedvaxHIB or RECOMBIVAX HB in infants and children through 71 months of age. These adverse effects are listed below.
PedvaxHIB
Hematologic/Lymphatic
Lymphadenopathy
Skin
Sterile injection-site abscess; pain at the injection site

RECOMBIVAX HB
Hypersensitivity
Symptoms of hypersensitivity including rash, pruritus, edema, arthralgia, dyspnea, hypotension, and ecchymoses
Cardiovascular System
Tachycardia; syncope
Digestive System
Elevation of liver enzymes
Hematologic
Increased erythrocyte sedimentation rate
Musculoskeletal System
Arthritis
Nervous System
Bell's Palsy; Guillain-Barré Syndrome
Psychiatric/Behavioral
Agitation; somnolence; irritability
Skin
Stevens-Johnson Syndrome; alopecia
Special Senses
Conjunctivitis; visual disturbances

Adverse Event Reporting
Patients, parents and guardians should be instructed to report any serious adverse reactions to their health-care provider who in turn should report such events to the U.S. Department of Health and Human Services through the Vaccine Adverse Event Reporting System (VAERS), 1-800-822-7967. The health-care provider should inform the parent or guardian of the National Vaccine Injury Compensation Program (NVICP), 1-800-338-2382.

DOSAGE AND ADMINISTRATION

FOR INTRAMUSCULAR ADMINISTRATION
Do not inject intravenously, intradermally, or subcutaneously.

Recommended Schedule
Infants born to HBsAg negative mothers should be vaccinated with three 0.5 mL doses of COMVAX, ideally at 2, 4, and 12-15 months of age. If the recommended schedule cannot be followed, the interval between the first two doses should be at least six weeks and the interval between the second and third dose should be as close as possible to eight to eleven months.
Infants born to HBsAg-positive mothers should receive Hepatitis B Immune Globulin and Hepatitis B Vaccine (Recombinant) at birth and should complete the hepatitis B vaccination series given according to a particular schedule (see manufacturer's circular for Hepatitis B Vaccine [Recombinant]).
Infants born to mothers of unknown HBsAg status should receive Hepatitis B Vaccine (Recombinant) at birth and should complete the hepatitis B vaccination series given according to a particular schedule (see manufacturer's circular for Hepatitis B Vaccine [Recombinant]).
The subsequent administration of COMVAX for completion of the hepatitis B vaccination series in infants who were born to HBsAg positive mothers and received HBIG or infants born to mothers of unknown status has not been studied.
COMVAX should not be administered to any infant before the age of 6 weeks.

Modified Schedules
Children previously vaccinated with one or more doses of either hepatitis B vaccine or Haemophilus b conjugate vaccine
Children who receive one dose of hepatitis B vaccine at or shortly after birth may be administered COMVAX on the schedule of 2, 4, and 12-15 months of age. There are no data to support the use of a three-dose series of COMVAX in infants who have previously received more than one dose of hepatitis B vaccine. However, COMVAX may be administered to children otherwise scheduled to receive concurrent RECOMBIVAX HB and PedvaxHIB.
Children not vaccinated according to recommended schedule for COMVAX
Vaccination schedules for children not vaccinated according to the recommended schedule should be considered on an individual basis. The number of doses of a PRP-OMPC-containing product (i.e., COMVAX, PedvaxHIB) depends on the age that vaccination is begun. An infant 2 to 10 months of age should receive three doses of a product containing PRP-OMPC. An infant 11 to 14 months of age should receive two doses of a product containing PRP-OMPC. A child 15 to 71 months of age should receive one dose of a product containing PRP-OMPC. Infants and children, regardless of age, should receive three doses of an HBsAg-containing product.
COMVAX is for intramuscular injection. The *anterolateral thigh* is the recommended site for intramuscular injection in infants. Data suggests that injections given in the buttocks frequently are given into fatty tissue instead of into muscle. Such injections have resulted in a lower seroconversion rate (for hepatitis B vaccine) than was expected.
Injection must be accomplished with a needle long enough to ensure intramuscular deposition of the vaccine. The ACIP has recommended that for intramuscular injections, the needle should be of sufficient length to reach the muscle mass itself. In a clinical trial with COMVAX (see CLINICAL PHARMACOLOGY, Antibody Responses to COMVAX in Infants Not Previously Vaccinated with Hib or Hepatitis B Vaccine, Table 1) vaccination was accomplished with a needle length of 5/8 inches in accordance with ACIP recommendations in effect at that time.{62} ACIP currently recommends that needles of longer length (7/8 to 1 inch) be used.{63}
The vaccine should be used as supplied; no reconstitution is necessary.
Shake well before withdrawal and use. Thorough agitation is necessary to maintain suspension of the vaccine.
Parenteral drug products should be inspected visually for extraneous particulate matter and discoloration prior to administration whenever solution and container permit. After thorough agitation, COMVAX is a slightly opaque, white suspension.
It is important to use a separate sterile syringe and needle for each patient to prevent transmission of infectious agents from one person to another.

Interchangeability of COMVAX and Licensed Haemophilus b Conjugate Vaccines or Recombinant Hepatitis B Vaccines
Since 1990, the Advisory Committee on Immunization Practices (ACIP) and the Committee on Infectious Diseases of the American Academy of Pediatrics (AAP) have recommended routine immunization of infants starting at 2 months of age with a polysaccharide-protein conjugate vaccine to prevent invasive Hib disease.{32-33}
Three Hib vaccines are licensed for infant vaccination: 1) oligosaccharide conjugate Hib vaccine (HbOC) (HibTITER®[2]), 2) polyribosylribitol phosphate-tetanus toxoid conjugate (PRP-T) (ActHIB®[2] and OmniHIB®[2]and 3) Haemophilus b conjugate vaccine (meningococcal protein conjugate) (PRP-OMPC) (PedvaxHIB®). According to the ACIP, these products are now considered interchangeable for primary as well as booster vaccination.{66}
Because vaccination recommendations limited to high-risk individuals have failed to substantially lower the overall incidence of hepatitis B infection, both the Advisory Committee on Immunization Practices (ACIP) and the Committee on Infectious Diseases of the American Academy of Pediatrics (AAP) have endorsed universal infant immunization as part of a comprehensive strategy for the control of hepatitis B infection.{32,50}

[2] HibTITER is a registered trademark of Lederle Laboratories, ActHIB is a registered trademark of Aventis Pasteur Inc. and OmniHIB is a registered trademark of GlaxoSmithKline.

HOW SUPPLIED

No. 4898—COMVAX is supplied as 7.5 mcg PRP polysaccharide conjugated to approximately 125 mcg OMPC and 5 mcg HBsAg in a box of 10 single dose vials.
NDC 0006-4898-00

Storage
Store vaccine at 2-8°C (36-46°F). Storage above or below the recommended temperature may reduce potency.
DO NOT FREEZE since freezing destroys potency.

REFERENCES

1. Cochi, S.L., et al. JAMA 253: 521-529, 1985.
2. Schlech, W.F., III, et al. JAMA 253: 1749-1754, 1985.
3. Peltola, H., et al. N Engl J Med 310: 1561-1566, 1984.
4. Cardoz, M., et al. Bull WHO 59: 575-584, 1981.
5. Sell, S.H., et al. Pediatr 49: 206-217, 1972.
6. Taylor, H.G., et al. Pediatr 74: 198-205, 1984.
7. Hay, J.W., et al. Pediatr 80(3): 319-329, 1987.
8. Redmond, S.R., et al. JAMA 252: 2581-2584, 1984.
9. Istre, G.R., et al. J Pediatr 106: 190-195, 1985.
10. Fraser, D.W., et al. J Infect Dis *127:* 271-277, 1973.
11. Tarr, P.I., et al. J Pediatr *92:* 884-888, 1978.
12. Granoff, D.M., et al. J Clin Invest *74:* 1708-1714, 1984.
13. Ambrosino, D.M., et al. J Clin Invest *75:* 1935-1942, 1985.
14. Coulehan, J.L., et al. Pub Health Rep *99:* 404-409, 1984.
15. Losonsky, G.A., et al. Pediatr Infect Dis J *3:* 539-547, 1985.
16. Ward, J.I., et al. Lancet *1:* 1281-1285, 1981.
17. Ward, J.I., et al. N Engl J Med *301:* 122-126, 1979.
18. Ward, J.I., et al. J Pediatr *88:* 261-263, 1976.
19. Bartlett, A.V., et al. J Pediatr *102:* 55-58, 1983.
20. Centers for Disease Control. MMWR *34*(15): 201-205, 1985.
21. Santosham, M., et al. N Engl J Med *317:* 923-929, 1987.
22. Siber, G.R., et al. Infect Immun *45:* 248-254, 1984.
23. Smith, D.H., et al. Pediatr *52:* 637-644, 1973.
24. Robbins, J.B., et al. Pediatr Res *7:* 103-110, 1973.
25. Kaythy, H., et al. J Infect Dis *147:* 1100, 1983.
26. Peltola, H., et al. Pediatr *60:* 730-737, 1977.
27. Ward, J.I., et al. Pediatr *81:* 886-893, 1988.
28. Daum, R.S., et al. Pediatr *81:* 893-897, 1988.
29. Marburg, S., et al. J Am Chem Soc *108:* 5282-5287, 1986.
30. Letson, G.W., et al. Pediatr Infect Dis J *7*(111): 747-752, 1988.
31. Data on file at Merck Research Laboratories.
32. Centers for Disease Control. MMWR *40*(RR-1):1-25, 1991.
33. Committee on Infectious Disease. Update Pediatrics *88*(1): 169-172, 1991.
34. Robinson, W.S. "Principles and Practice of Infectious Diseases," G.L. Mandell; R.G. Douglas; J.E. Bennett (eds), vol. 2, New York, John Wiley & Sons, 1985, pp. 1002-1029.
35. Maynard, J. E., et al. "Viral Hepatitis and Liver Disease", A.J. Zuckerman (ed.), Alan R. Liss, Inc., 1988, pp. 967-969.
36. Centers for Disease Control. MMWR *39*(RR-2): 5-26, 1990.
37. Wands, J.R., et al. "Principles of Internal Medicine," G.W. Thorn, R.D. Adams, E. Braunwald, K.J. Isselbacher, R.G. Petersdorf (eds), vol. 2, McGraw-Hill, 1977, pp. 1590-1598.
38. Sitrin, R.D., Wampler, D.E., Ellis, R.W. Survey of licensed hepatitis B vaccines and their production processes. In: Ellis RW, ed. Hepatitis B vaccines in clinical practice. New York: Marcel Dekker, Inc., 1993, pp. 83-101.
39. West, D.J. Scope and design of hepatitis B vaccine clinical trials. In Ellis RW, ed. Hepatitis B vaccines in clinical practice. New York: Marcel Dekker, Inc., 1993, pp. 159-177.
40. Hadler, S.C., et al. NEJM *315*(4): 209-214, 1986.
41. Szmuness, W., et al. NEJM *303:* 833-841, 1980.
42. Francis, D.P., et al. Ann Int Med *97:* 362-366, 1982.
43. Szmuness, W., et al. NEJM *307:* 1481-1486, 1982.
44. Szmuness, W., et al. Hepatology *1:* 377-385, 1981.
45. Coutinho, R.A., et al. BMJ *286:* 1305-1308, 1983.
46. International Group: Immunisation against hepatitis B, Lancet *1*(8590): 875-876, 1988.
47. Keyserling, H.L., et al. J Pediatr *125*(1): 67-69, 1994.
48. Stevens, C.E.; Taylor, P.E.; Tong, M.J., et al. "Viral Hepatitis and Liver Diseases." A.J. Zuckerman (ed.), Alan R. Liss, Inc., 1988, pp. 982-983.
49. Stevens, C.E., et al. Pediatr *90*(1, Part 2): 170-173, 1992.
50. Universal Hepatitis B Immunization, Committee on Infectious Diseases. Pediatr *89*(4): 795-800, 1992.
51. Centers for Disease Control. MMWR *34:* 313-24, 329-35, 1985.
52. Centers for Disease Control. MMWR *36:* 353-60, 366, 1987.
53. West, D.J., et al. Pediatr Clin North Am *37:* 585-601, 1990.
54. Seto, D., et al. Pediatr Res *31*(4 Pt 2): 179A, 1992.
55. Froehlich, H. Pediatr Res *31*(4 Pt 2): 92A, 1992.
56. Jilg, W., et al. Infection *17:* 70-6, 1989.
57. West, D.J., et al. Vaccine *14:* 1019-27, 1996.
58. Goep, J.G., et al. Pediatr Infect Dis J *1*(1): 2-5, 1992.
59. Keyserling, H.L., et al. Program and Abstracts of the 30th ICAAC, 1990. (Abst. 63).
60. Ward, J.I., et al. Program and Abstracts of the 32nd ICAAC, 1992. (Abst. 984).
61. Lieberman, J.M., et al. Infect Dis, 199 (Abst.1028).
62. Centers for Disease Control. MMWR *38*(13): 205-228, 1989.
63. Centers for Disease Control. MMWR *43*(RR-1): 1994.
64. Reisenger, K.S., et al. Pediatr Res (4 pt. 2): 179A, 1993.
65. Centers for Disease Control. MMWR *46*(54): 74, 1998.
66. Centers for Disease Control. MMWR *47*(1): 9, 1998.
67. Centers for Disease Control. Federal Register, *64*(35): 9044-9045, February 23, 1999.
68. Centers for Disease Control. MMWR *42*(RR-4): 1-18, April 9, 1993.

Manuf. and Dist. by:
MERCK & CO., INC., Whitehouse Station, NJ 08889, USA
Issued August 2004
Printed in USA
9376602

COZAAR® ℞

[cō'zăr]
(losartan potassium tablets)

USE IN PREGNANCY
When used in pregnancy during the second and third trimesters, drugs that act directly on the renin-angiotensin system can cause injury and even death to the developing fetus. When pregnancy is detected, COZAAR should be discontinued as soon as possible. See WARNINGS, Fetal/Neonatal Morbidity and Mortality.

DESCRIPTION

COZAAR[1](losartan potassium) is an angiotensin II receptor (type AT_1) antagonist. Losartan potassium, a non-peptide molecule, is chemically described as 2-butyl-4-chloro-1-[p-(o-1H-tetrazol-5-ylphenyl)benzyl]imidazole-5-methanol monopotassium salt.

Its empirical formula is $C_{22}H_{22}ClKN_6O$, and its structural formula is:

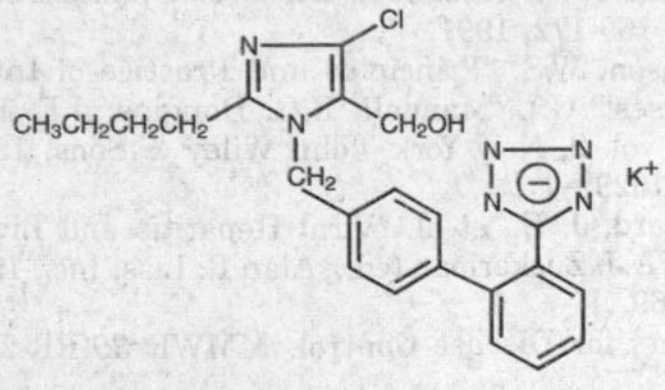

Losartan potassium is a white to off-white free-flowing crystalline powder with a molecular weight of 461.01. It is freely soluble in water, soluble in alcohols, and slightly soluble in common organic solvents, such as acetonitrile and methyl ethyl ketone. Oxidation of the 5-hydroxymethyl group on the imidazole ring results in the active metabolite of losartan.

COZAAR is available as tablets for oral administration containing either 25 mg, 50 mg or 100 mg of losartan potassium and the following inactive ingredients: microcrystalline cellulose, lactose hydrous, pregelatinized starch, magnesium stearate, hydroxypropyl cellulose, hypromellose, and titanium dioxide.

COZAAR 25 mg, 50 mg and 100 mg tablets contain potassium in the following amounts: 2.12 mg (0.054 mEq), 4.24 mg (0.108 mEq) and 8.48 mg (0.216 mEq), respectively. COZAAR 25 mg, COZAAR 50 mg, and COZAAR 100 mg may also contain carnauba wax.

[1] Registered trademark of E.I. du Pont de Nemours and Company, Wilmington, Delaware, USA

COPYRIGHT © 2003 Merck Sharp & Dohme Corp., a subsidiary of **Merck & Co., Inc.**
All rights reserved.

CLINICAL PHARMACOLOGY

Mechanism of Action

Angiotensin II [formed from angiotensin I in a reaction catalyzed by angiotensin converting enzyme (ACE, kininase II)], is a potent vasoconstrictor, the primary vasoactive hormone of the renin-angiotensin system and an important component in the pathophysiology of hypertension. It also stimulates aldosterone secretion by the adrenal cortex. Losartan and its principal active metabolite block the vasoconstrictor and aldosterone-secreting effects of angiotensin II by selectively blocking the binding of angiotensin II to the AT_1 receptor found in many tissues, (e.g., vascular smooth muscle, adrenal gland). There is also an AT_2 receptor found in many tissues but it is not known to be associated with cardiovascular homeostasis. Both losartan and its principal active metabolite do not exhibit any partial agonist activity at the AT_1 receptor and have much greater affinity (about 1000-fold) for the AT_1 receptor than for the AT_2 receptor. *In vitro* binding studies indicate that losartan is a reversible, competitive inhibitor of the AT_1 receptor. The active metabolite is 10 to 40 times more potent by weight than losartan and appears to be a reversible, non-competitive inhibitor of the AT_1 receptor.

Neither losartan nor its active metabolite inhibits ACE (kininase II, the enzyme that converts angiotensin I to angiotensin II and degrades bradykinin); nor do they bind to or block other hormone receptors or ion channels known to be important in cardiovascular regulation.

Pharmacokinetics

General

Losartan is an orally active agent that undergoes substantial first-pass metabolism by cytochrome P450 enzymes. It is converted, in part, to an active carboxylic acid metabolite that is responsible for most of the angiotensin II receptor antagonism that follows losartan treatment. Losartan metabolites have been identified in human plasma and urine. In addition to the active carboxylic acid metabolite, several inactive metabolites are formed. Following oral and intravenous administration of ^{14}C-labeled losartan potassium, circulating plasma radioactivity is primarily attributed to losartan and its active metabolite. *In vitro* studies indicate that cytochrome P450 2C9 and 3A4 are involved in the biotransformation of losartan to its metabolites. Minimal conversion of losartan to the active metabolite (less than 1% of the dose compared to 14% of the dose in normal subjects) was seen in about one percent of individuals studied.

The terminal half-life of losartan is about 2 hours and of the metabolite is about 6-9 hours.

The pharmacokinetics of losartan and its active metabolite are linear with oral losartan doses up to 200 mg and do not change over time. Neither losartan nor its metabolite accumulate in plasma upon repeated once-daily dosing.

Following oral administration, losartan is well absorbed (based on absorption of radiolabeled losartan) and undergoes substantial first-pass metabolism; the systemic bioavailability of losartan is approximately 33%. About 14% of an orally-administered dose of losartan is converted to the active metabolite. Mean peak concentrations of losartan and its active metabolite are reached in 1 hour and in 3-4 hours, respectively. While maximum plasma concentrations of losartan and its active metabolite are approximately equal, the AUC of the metabolite is about 4 times as great as that of losartan. A meal slows absorption of losartan and decreases its C_{max} but has only minor effects on losartan AUC or on the AUC of the metabolite (about 10% decreased).

The pharmacokinetics of losartan and its active metabolite were also determined after IV doses of each component separately in healthy volunteers. The volume of distribution of losartan and the active metabolite is about 34 liters and 12 liters, respectively. Total plasma clearance of losartan and the active metabolite is about 600 mL/min and 50 mL/min, respectively, with renal clearance of about 75 mL/min and 25 mL/min, respectively. After single doses of losartan administered orally, about 4% of the dose is excreted unchanged in the urine and about 6% is excreted in urine as active metabolite. Biliary excretion contributes to the elimination of losartan and its metabolites. Following oral ^{14}C-labeled losartan, about 35% of radioactivity is recovered in the urine and about 60% in the feces. Following an intravenous dose of ^{14}C-labeled losartan, about 45% of radioactivity is recovered in the urine and 50% in the feces. Both losartan and its active metabolite are highly bound to plasma proteins, primarily albumin, with plasma free fractions of 1.3% and 0.2%, respectively. Plasma protein binding is constant over the concentration range achieved with recommended doses. Studies in rats indicate that losartan crosses the blood-brain barrier poorly, if at all.

Special Populations

Pediatric: Pharmacokinetic parameters after multiple doses of losartan (average dose 0.7 mg/kg, range 0.36 to 0.97 mg/kg) as a tablet to 25 hypertensive patients aged 6 to 16 years are shown in Table 1 below. Pharmacokinetics of losartan and its active metabolite were generally similar across the studied age groups and similar to historical pharmacokinetic data in adults. The principal pharmacokinetic parameters in adults and children are shown in the table below.

[See table 1 below]

The bioavailability of the suspension formulation was compared with losartan tablets in healthy adults. The suspension and tablet are similar in their bioavailability with respect to both losartan and the active metabolite (see DOSAGE AND ADMINISTRATION, Preparation of Suspension).

Geriatric and Gender: Losartan pharmacokinetics have been investigated in the elderly (65-75 years) and in both genders. Plasma concentrations of losartan and its active metabolite are similar in elderly and young hypertensives. Plasma concentrations of losartan were about twice as high in female hypertensives as male hypertensives, but concentrations of the active metabolite were similar in males and females. No dosage adjustment is necessary (see DOSAGE AND ADMINISTRATION).

Race: Pharmacokinetic differences due to race have not been studied (see also PRECAUTIONS, Race and CLINICAL PHARMACOLOGY, Pharmacodynamics and Clinical Effects, Reduction in the Risk of Stroke, Race).

Renal Insufficiency: Following oral administration, plasma concentrations and AUCs of losartan and its active metabolite are increased by 50-90% in patients with mild (creatinine clearance of 50 to 74 mL/min) or moderate (creatinine clearance 30 to 49 mL/min) renal insufficiency. In this study, renal clearance was reduced by 55-85% for both losartan and its active metabolite in patients with mild or moderate renal insufficiency. Neither losartan nor its active metabolite can be removed by hemodialysis. No dosage adjustment is necessary for patients with renal impairment unless they are volume-depleted (see WARNINGS, Hypotension—Volume-Depleted Patients and DOSAGE AND ADMINISTRATION).

Hepatic Insufficiency: Following oral administration in patients with mild to moderate alcoholic cirrhosis of the liver, plasma concentrations of losartan and its active metabolite were, respectively, 5-times and about 1.7-times those in young male volunteers. Compared to normal subjects the total plasma clearance of losartan in patients with hepatic insufficiency was about 50% lower and the oral bioavailability was about 2-times higher. A lower starting dose is recommended for patients with a history of hepatic impairment (see DOSAGE AND ADMINISTRATION).

Drug Interactions

Losartan, administered for 12 days, did not affect the pharmacokinetics or pharmacodynamics of a single dose of warfarin. Losartan did not affect the pharmacokinetics of oral or intravenous digoxin. There is no pharmacokinetic interaction between losartan and hydrochlorothiazide. Coadministration of losartan and cimetidine led to an increase of about 18% in AUC of losartan but did not affect the pharmacokinetics of its active metabolite. Coadministration of losartan and phenobarbital led to a reduction of about 20% in the AUC of losartan and that of its active metabolite. A somewhat greater interaction (approximately 40% reduction in the AUC of active metabolite and approximately 30% reduction in the AUC of losartan) has been reported with rifampin. Fluconazole, an inhibitor of cytochrome P450 2C9, decreased the AUC of the active metabolite by approximately 40%, but increased the AUC of losartan by approximately 70% following multiple doses. Conversion of losartan to its active metabolite after intravenous administration is not affected by ketoconazole, an inhibitor of P450 3A4. The AUC of active metabolite following oral losartan was not affected by erythromycin, another inhibitor of P450 3A4, but the AUC of losartan was increased by 30%.

Pharmacodynamics and Clinical Effects

Adult Hypertension

Losartan inhibits the pressor effect of angiotensin II (as well as angiotensin I) infusions. A dose of 100 mg inhibits the pressor effect by about 85% at peak with 25-40% inhibition persisting for 24 hours. Removal of the negative feedback of angiotensin II causes a 2- to 3-fold rise in plasma renin activity and consequent rise in angiotensin II plasma concentration in hypertensive patients. Losartan does not affect the response to bradykinin, whereas ACE inhibitors increase the response to bradykinin. Aldosterone plasma concentrations fall following losartan administration. In spite of the effect of losartan on aldosterone secretion, very little effect on serum potassium was observed.

In a single-dose study in normal volunteers, losartan had no effects on glomerular filtration rate, renal plasma flow or filtration fraction. In multiple-dose studies in hypertensive patients, there were no notable effects on systemic or renal prostaglandin concentrations, fasting triglycerides, total cholesterol or HDL-cholesterol or fasting glucose concentrations. There was a small uricosuric effect leading to a minimal decrease in serum uric acid (mean decrease <0.4 mg/dL) during chronic oral administration.

The antihypertensive effects of COZAAR were demonstrated principally in 4 placebo-controlled, 6- to 12-week trials of dosages from 10 to 150 mg per day in patients with baseline diastolic blood pressures of 95-115. The studies allowed comparisons of two doses (50-100 mg/day) as once-daily or twice-daily regimens, comparisons of peak and trough effects, and comparisons of response by gender, age, and race. Three additional studies examined the antihypertensive effects of losartan and hydrochlorothiazide in combination.

The 4 studies of losartan monotherapy included a total of 1075 patients randomized to several doses of losartan and 334 to placebo. The 10- and 25-mg doses produced some effect at peak (6 hours after dosing) but small and inconsistent trough (24 hour) responses. Doses of 50, 100 and 150 mg once daily gave statistically significant systolic/diastolic mean decreases in blood pressure, compared to placebo in the range of 5.5-10.5/3.5-7.5 mmHg, with the 150-mg dose giving no greater effect than 50-100 mg.

Table 1: Pharmacokinetic Parameters in Hypertensive Adults and Children Age 6-16 Following Multiple Dosing

	Adults given 50 mg once daily for 7 days N=12		Age 6-16 given 0.7 mg/kg once daily for 7 days N=25	
	Parent	Active Metabolite	Parent	Active Metabolite
AUC_{0-24}[a] (ng•h/mL)	442 ± 173	1685 ± 452	368 ± 169	1866 ± 1076
C_{MAX} (ng/mL)[a]	224 ± 82	212 ± 73	141 ± 88	222 ± 127
$T_{1/2}$ (h)[b]	2.1 ± 0.70	7.4 ± 2.4	2.3 ± 0.8	5.6 ± 1.2
T_{PEAK} (h)[c]	0.9	3.5	2.0	4.1
CL_{REN} (mL/min)[a]	56 ± 23	20 ± 3	53 ± 33	17 ± 8

[a] Mean ± standard deviation
[b] Harmonic mean and standard deviation
[c] Median

Twice-daily dosing at 50-100 mg/day gave consistently larger trough responses than once-daily dosing at the same total dose. Peak (6 hour) effects were uniformly, but moderately, larger than trough effects, with the trough-to-peak ratio for systolic and diastolic responses 50-95% and 60-90%, respectively.

Addition of a low dose of hydrochlorothiazide (12.5 mg) to losartan 50 mg once daily resulted in placebo-adjusted blood pressure reductions of 15.5/9.2 mmHg.

Analysis of age, gender, and race subgroups of patients showed that men and women, and patients over and under 65, had generally similar responses. COZAAR was effective in reducing blood pressure regardless of race, although the effect was somewhat less in Black patients (usually a low-renin population).

The effect of losartan is substantially present within one week but in some studies the maximal effect occurred in 3-6 weeks. In long-term follow-up studies (without placebo control) the effect of losartan appeared to be maintained for up to a year. There is no apparent rebound effect after abrupt withdrawal of losartan. There was essentially no change in average heart rate in losartan-treated patients in controlled trials.

Pediatric Hypertension

The antihypertensive effect of losartan was studied in one trial enrolling 177 hypertensive pediatric patients aged 6 to 16 years old. Children who weighed <50 kg received 2.5, 25 or 50 mg of losartan daily and patients who weighed ≥50 kg received 5, 50 or 100 mg of losartan daily. Children in the lowest dose group were given losartan in a suspension formulation (see DOSAGE AND ADMINISTRATION, Preparation of Suspension). The majority of the children had hypertension associated with renal and urogenital disease. The sitting diastolic blood pressure (SiDBP) on entry into the study was higher than the 95th percentile level for the patient's age, gender, and height. At the end of three weeks, losartan reduced systolic and diastolic blood pressure, measured at trough, in a dose-dependent manner. Overall, the two higher doses (25 to 50 mg in patients <50 kg; 50 to 100 mg in patients ≥50 kg) reduced diastolic blood pressure by 5 to 6 mmHg more than the lowest dose used (2.5 mg in patients <50 kg; 5 mg in patients ≥50 kg). The lowest dose, corresponding to an average daily dose of 0.07 mg/kg, did not appear to offer consistent antihypertensive efficacy. When patients were randomized to continue losartan at the two higher doses or to placebo after 3 weeks of therapy, trough diastolic blood pressure rose in patients on placebo between 5 and 7 mmHg more than patients randomized to continuing losartan. When the low dose of losartan was randomly withdrawn, the rise in trough diastolic blood pressure was the same in patients receiving placebo and in those continuing losartan, again suggesting that the lowest dose did not have significant antihypertensive efficacy. Overall, no significant differences in the overall antihypertensive effect of losartan were detected when the patients were analyzed according to age (<, ≥12 years old) or gender. While blood pressure was reduced in all racial subgroups examined, too few non-White patients were enrolled to compare the dose-response of losartan in the non-White subgroup.

Reduction in the Risk of Stroke

The Losartan Intervention For Endpoint reduction in hypertension (LIFE) study was a multinational, double-blind study comparing COZAAR and atenolol in 9193 hypertensive patients with ECG-documented left ventricular hypertrophy. Patients with myocardial infarction or stroke within six months prior to randomization were excluded. Patients were randomized to receive once daily COZAAR 50 mg or atenolol 50 mg. If goal blood pressure (<140/90 mmHg) was not reached, hydrochlorothiazide (12.5 mg) was added first and, if needed, the dose of COZAAR or atenolol was then increased to 100 mg once daily. If necessary, other antihypertensive treatments (e.g., increase in dose of hydrochlorothiazide therapy to 25 mg or addition of other diuretic therapy, calcium-channel blockers, alpha-blockers, or centrally acting agents, but not ACE inhibitors, angiotensin II antagonists, or beta-blockers) were added to the treatment regimen to reach the goal blood pressure.

Of the randomized patients, 4963 (54%) were female and 533 (6%) were Black. The mean age was 67 with 5704 (62%) age ≥65. At baseline, 1195 (13%) had diabetes, 1326 (14%) had isolated systolic hypertension, 1469 (16%) had coronary heart disease, and 728 (8%) had cerebrovascular disease. Baseline mean blood pressure was 174/98 mmHg in both treatment groups. The mean length of follow-up was 4.8 years. At the end of study or at the last visit before a primary endpoint, 77% of the group treated with COZAAR and 73% of the group treated with atenolol were still taking study medication. Of the patients still taking study medication, the mean doses of COZAAR and atenolol were both about 80 mg/day, and 15% were taking atenolol or losartan as monotherapy, while 77% were also receiving hydrochlorothiazide (at a mean dose of 20 mg/day in each group). Blood pressure reduction measured at trough was similar

Table 2: Incidence of Primary Endpoint Events

	COZAAR		Atenolol		Risk Reduction†	95% CI	p-Value
	N (%)	Rate*	N (%)	Rate*			
Primary Composite Endpoint	508 (11)	23.8	588 (13)	27.9	13%	2% to 23%	0.021
Components of Primary Composite Endpoint (as a first event)							
Stroke (nonfatal‡)	209 (5)		286 (6)				
Myocardial infarction (nonfatal‡)	174 (4)		168 (4)				
Cardiovascular mortality	125 (3)		134 (3)				
Secondary Endpoints (any time in study)							
Stroke (fatal/nonfatal)	232 (5)	10.8	309 (7)	14.5	25%	11% to 37%	0.001
Myocardial infarction (fatal/nonfatal)	198 (4)	9.2	188 (4)	8.7	-7%	-13% to 12%	0.491
Cardiovascular mortality	204 (4)	9.2	234 (5)	10.6	11%	-7% to 27%	0.206
Due to CHD	125 (3)	5.6	124 (3)	5.6	-3%	-32% to 20%	0.839
Due to Stroke	40 (1)	1.8	62 (1)	2.8	35%	4% to 67%	0.032
Other§	39 (1)	1.8	48 (1)	2.2	16%	-28% to 45%	0.411

* Rate per 1000 patient-years of follow-up
† Adjusted for baseline Framingham risk score and level of electrocardiographic left ventricular hypertrophy
‡ First report of an event, in some cases the patient died subsequently to the event reported
§ Death due to heart failure, non-coronary vascular disease, pulmonary embolism, or a cardiovascular cause other than stroke or coronary heart disease

for both treatment groups but blood pressure was not measured at any other time of the day. At the end of study or at the last visit before a primary endpoint, the mean blood pressures were 144.1/81.3 mmHg for the group treated with COZAAR and 145.4/80.9 mmHg for the group treated with atenolol [the difference in systolic blood pressure (SBP) of 1.3 mmHg was significant (p<0.001), while the difference of 0.4 mmHg in diastolic blood pressure (DBP) was not significant (p=0.098)].

The primary endpoint was the first occurrence of cardiovascular death, nonfatal stroke, or nonfatal myocardial infarction. Patients with non-fatal events remained in the trial, so that there was also an examination of the first event of each type even if it was not the first event (e.g., a stroke following an initial myocardial infarction would be counted in the analysis of stroke). Treatment with COZAAR resulted in a 13% reduction (p=0.021) in risk of the primary endpoint compared to the atenolol group (see Figure 1 and Table 2); this difference was primarily the result of an effect on fatal and nonfatal stroke. Treatment with COZAAR reduced the risk of stroke by 25% relative to atenolol (p=0.001) (see Figure 2 and Table 2).

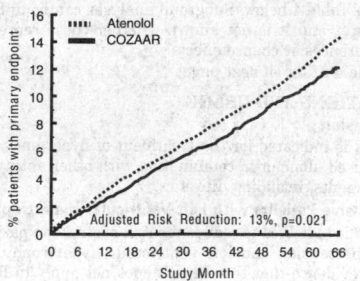

Figure 1. Kaplan-Meier estimates of the primary endpoint of time to cardiovascular death, nonfatal stroke, or nonfatal myocardial infarction in the groups treated with COZAAR and atenolol. The Risk Reduction is adjusted for baseline Framingham risk score and level of electrocardiographic left ventricular hypertrophy.

[See figure 2 at top of next column]

Table 2 shows the results for the primary composite endpoint and the individual endpoints. The primary endpoint was the first occurrence of stroke, myocardial infarction or cardiovascular death, analyzed using an intention-to-treat (ITT) approach. The table shows the number of events for each component in two different ways. The Components of Primary Endpoint (as a first event) counts only the events that define the primary endpoint, while the Secondary Endpoints count all first events of a particular type, whether or not they were preceded by a different type of event.

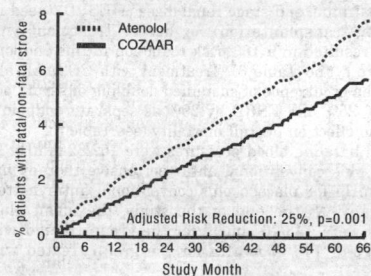

Figure 2. Kaplan-Meier estimates of the time to fatal/nonfatal stroke in the groups treated with COZAAR and atenolol. The Risk Reduction is adjusted for baseline Framingham risk score and level of electrocardiographic left ventricular hypertrophy.

[See table 2 above]

Although the LIFE study favored COZAAR over atenolol with respect to the primary endpoint (p=0.021), this result is from a single study and, therefore, is less compelling than the difference between COZAAR and placebo. Although not measured directly, the difference between COZAAR and placebo is compelling because there is evidence that atenolol is itself effective (vs. placebo) in reducing cardiovascular events, including stroke, in hypertensive patients.

Other clinical endpoints of the LIFE study were: total mortality, hospitalization for heart failure or angina pectoris, coronary or peripheral revascularization procedures, and resuscitated cardiac arrest. There were no significant differences in the rates of these endpoints between the COZAAR and atenolol groups.

For the primary endpoint and stroke, the effects of COZAAR in patient subgroups defined by age, gender, race and presence or absence of isolated systolic hypertension (ISH), diabetes, and history of cardiovascular disease (CVD) are shown in Figure 3 below. Subgroup analyses can be difficult to interpret and it is not known whether these represent true differences or chance effects.

[See figure 3 at top of next page]

Race

In the LIFE study, Black patients treated with atenolol were at lower risk of experiencing the primary composite endpoint compared with Black patients treated with COZAAR. In the subgroup of Black patients (n=533; 6% of the LIFE study patients), there were 29 primary endpoints among 263 patients on atenolol (11%, 26 per 1000 patient-years) and 46 primary endpoints among 270 patients (17%, 42 per 1000 patient-years) on COZAAR. This finding could not be explained on the basis of differences in the populations other than race or on any imbalances between treatment groups. In addition, blood pressure reductions in both treatment groups were consistent between Black and non-Black patients. Given the difficulty in interpreting subset differences in large trials, it cannot be known whether the observed difference is the result of chance. However, the LIFE study provides no evidence that the benefits of COZAAR on reducing the risk of cardiovascular events in hypertensive patients with left ventricular hypertrophy apply to Black patients.

Nephropathy in Type 2 Diabetic Patients

The Reduction of Endpoints in NIDDM with the Angiotensin II Receptor Antagonist Losartan (RENAAL) study was a randomized, placebo-controlled, double-blind, multicenter study conducted worldwide in 1513 patients with type 2 diabetes with nephropathy (defined as serum creatinine 1.3 to 3.0 mg/dl in females or males ≤60 kg and 1.5 to 3.0 mg/dl in males >60 kg and proteinuria [urinary albumin to creatinine ratio ≥300 mg/g]).

Patients were randomized to receive COZAAR 50 mg once daily or placebo on a background of conventional antihypertensive therapy excluding ACE inhibitors and angiotensin II antagonists. After one month, investigators were instructed to titrate study drug to 100 mg once daily if the trough blood pressure goal (140/90 mmHg) was not achieved. Overall, 72% of patients received the 100-mg daily dose more than 50% of the time they were on study drug. Because the study was designed to achieve equal blood pressure control in both groups, other antihypertensive agents (diuretics, calcium-channel blockers, alpha- or beta-blockers, and centrally acting agents) could be added as needed in both groups. Patients were followed for a mean duration of 3.4 years.

The study population was diverse with regard to race (Asian 16.7%, Black 15.2%, Hispanic 18.3%, White 48.6%). Overall, 63.2% of the patients were men, and 66.4% were under the age of 65 years. Almost all of the patients (96.6%) had a history of hypertension, and the patients entered the trial with a mean serum creatinine of 1.9 mg/dl and mean proteinuria (urinary albumin/creatinine) of 1808 mg/g at baseline.

The primary endpoint of the study was the time to first occurrence of any one of the following events: doubling of serum creatinine, end-stage renal disease (ESRD) (need for dialysis or transplantation), or death. Treatment with COZAAR resulted in a 16% risk reduction in this endpoint (see Figure 4 and Table 3). Treatment with COZAAR also reduced the occurrence of sustained doubling of serum creatinine by 25% and ESRD by 29% as separate endpoints, but had no effect on overall mortality (see Table 3).

The mean baseline blood pressures were 152/82 mmHg for COZAAR plus conventional antihypertensive therapy and 153/82 mmHg for placebo plus conventional antihypertensive therapy. At the end of the study, the mean blood pressures were 143/76 mmHg for the group treated with COZAAR and 146/77 mmHg for the group treated with placebo.

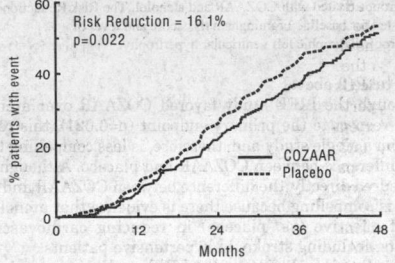

Figure 4. Kaplan-Meier curve for the primary composite endpoint of doubling of serum creatinine, end stage renal disease (need for dialysis or transplantation) or death.

[See table 3 above]

The secondary endpoints of the study were change in proteinuria, change in the rate of progression of renal disease, and the composite of morbidity and mortality from cardiovascular causes (hospitalization for heart failure, myocardial infarction, revascularization, stroke, hospitalization for unstable angina, or cardiovascular death). Compared with placebo, COZAAR significantly reduced proteinuria by an average of 34%, an effect that was evident within 3 months of starting therapy, and significantly reduced the rate of decline in glomerular filtration rate during the study by 13%, as measured by the reciprocal of the serum creatinine concentration. There was no significant difference in the incidence of the composite endpoint of cardiovascular morbidity and mortality.

The favorable effects of COZAAR were seen in patients also taking other anti-hypertensive medications (angiotensin II receptor antagonists and angiotensin converting enzyme inhibitors were not allowed), oral hypoglycemic agents and lipid-lowering agents.

For the primary endpoint and ESRD, the effects of COZAAR in patient subgroups defined by age, gender and race are

	No. of Patients	Primary Composite			Stroke (Fatal/Non-fatal)		
		COZAAR Event Rate (%)	Atenolol Event Rate (%)	Hazard Ratio (95% CI)	COZAAR Event Rate (%)	Atenolol Event Rate (%)	Hazard Ratio (95% CI)
Overall Results	9193	11	13		5	7	
Age							
<65 years	3489	7	7		3	3	
≥65 years	5704	13	16		6	9	
Gender							
Female	4963	9	11		4	6	
Male	4230	14	15		6	7	
Race							
Black	533	17	11		9	5	
White	8503	11	13		5	7	
Other*	157	9	14		5	5	
ISH							
Yes	1326	11	16		5	8	
No	7867	11	12		5	6	
Diabetes							
Yes	1195	18	23		9	11	
No	7998	10	11		5	6	
History of CVD							
Yes	2307	19	21		9	11	
No	6886	8	10		4	6	

0.3 0.5 1 2 3 ← Favors COZAAR   Favors Atenolol →
0.3 0.5 1 2 3 ← Favors COZAAR   Favors Atenolol →

Symbols are proportional to sample size.
*Other includes Asian, Hispanic, Asiatic, Multi-race, Indian, Native American, European.
†Adjusted for baseline Framingham risk score and level of electrocardiographic left ventricular hypertrophy.

Figure 3. Primary Endpoint Events†within Demographic Subgroups

Table 3: Incidence of Primary Endpoint Events

	Incidence		Risk Reduction	95% C.I.	p-Value
	Losartan	Placebo			
Primary Composite Endpoint	43.5%	47.1%	16.1%	2.3% to 27.9%	0.022
Doubling of Serum Creatinine, ESRD and Death Occurring as a First Event					
Doubling of Serum Creatinine	21.6%	26.0%			
ESRD	8.5%	8.5%			
Death	13.4%	12.6%			
Overall Incidence of Doubling of Serum Creatinine, ESRD and Death					
Doubling of Serum Creatinine	21.6%	26.0%	25.3%	7.8% to 39.4%	0.006
ESRD	19.6%	25.5%	28.6%	11.5% to 42.4%	0.002
Death	21.0%	20.3%	-1.7%	-26.9% to 18.6%	0.884

shown in Table 4 below. Subgroup analyses can be difficult to interpret and it is not known whether these represent true differences or chance effects.
[See table 4 at top of next page]

INDICATIONS AND USAGE

Hypertension

COZAAR is indicated for the treatment of hypertension. It may be used alone or in combination with other antihypertensive agents, including diuretics.

Hypertensive Patients with Left Ventricular Hypertrophy

COZAAR is indicated to reduce the risk of stroke in patients with hypertension and left ventricular hypertrophy, but there is evidence that this benefit does not apply to Black patients. (See PRECAUTIONS, Race and CLINICAL PHARMACOLOGY, Pharmacodynamics and Clinical Effects, Reduction in the Risk of Stroke, Race.)

Nephropathy in Type 2 Diabetic Patients

COZAAR is indicated for the treatment of diabetic nephropathy with an elevated serum creatinine and proteinuria (urinary albumin to creatinine ratio ≥300 mg/g) in patients with type 2 diabetes and a history of hypertension. In this population, COZAAR reduces the rate of progression of nephropathy as measured by the occurrence of doubling of serum creatinine or end stage renal disease (need for dialysis or renal transplantation) (see CLINICAL PHARMACOLOGY, Pharmacodynamics and Clinical Effects).

CONTRAINDICATIONS

COZAAR is contraindicated in patients who are hypersensitive to any component of this product.

WARNINGS

Fetal/Neonatal Morbidity and Mortality

Drugs that act directly on the renin-angiotensin system can cause fetal and neonatal morbidity and death when administered to pregnant women. Several dozen cases have been reported in the world literature in patients who were taking angiotensin converting enzyme inhibitors. When pregnancy is detected, COZAAR should be discontinued as soon as possible.

The use of drugs that act directly on the renin-angiotensin system during the second and third trimesters of pregnancy has been associated with fetal and neonatal injury, including hypotension, neonatal skull hypoplasia, anuria, reversible or irreversible renal failure, and death. Oligohydramnios has also been reported, presumably resulting from decreased fetal renal function; oligohydramnios in this setting has been associated with fetal limb contractures, craniofacial deformation, and hypoplastic lung development. Prematurity, intrauterine growth retardation, and patent ductus arteriosus have also been reported, although it is not clear whether these occurrences were due to exposure to the drug.

These adverse effects do not appear to have resulted from intrauterine drug exposure that has been limited to the first trimester.

Mothers whose embryos and fetuses are exposed to an angiotensin II receptor antagonist only during the first trimester should be so informed. Nonetheless, when patients become pregnant, physicians should have the patient discontinue the use of COZAAR as soon as possible.

Rarely (probably less often than once in every thousand pregnancies), no alternative to an angiotensin II receptor antagonist will be found. In these rare cases, the mothers should be apprised of the potential hazards to their fetuses, and serial ultrasound examinations should be performed to assess the intra-amniotic environment.

If oligohydramnios is observed, COZAAR should be discontinued unless it is considered life-saving for the mother. Contraction stress testing (CST), a non-stress test (NST), or biophysical profiling (BPP) may be appropriate, depending upon the week of pregnancy. Patients and physicians should be aware, however, that oligohydramnios may not appear until after the fetus has sustained irreversible injury.

Infants with histories of *in utero* exposure to an angiotensin II receptor antagonist should be closely observed for hypotension, oliguria, and hyperkalemia. If oliguria occurs, attention should be directed toward support of blood pressure and renal perfusion. Exchange transfusion or dialysis may be required as means of reversing hypotension and/or substituting for disordered renal function.

Losartan potassium has been shown to produce adverse effects in rat fetuses and neonates, including decreased body weight, delayed physical and behavioral development, mortality and renal toxicity. With the exception of neonatal weight gain (which was affected at doses as low as 10 mg/kg/day), doses associated with these effects exceeded 25 mg/kg/day (approximately three times the maximum recommended human dose of 100 mg on a mg/m^2 basis). These findings are attributed to drug exposure in late gestation and during lactation. Significant levels of losartan and its active metabolite were shown to be present in rat fetal plasma during late gestation and in rat milk.

Hypotension—Volume-Depleted Patients

In patients who are intravascularly volume-depleted (e.g., those treated with diuretics), symptomatic hypotension may occur after initiation of therapy with COZAAR. These conditions should be corrected prior to administration of COZAAR, or a lower starting dose should be used (see DOSAGE AND ADMINISTRATION).

Table 4: Efficacy Outcomes within Demographic Subgroups

		Primary Composite Endpoint			ESRD		
	No. of Patients	COZAAR Event Rate %	Placebo Event Rate %	Hazard Ratio (95% CI)	COZAAR Event Rate %	Placebo Event Rate %	Hazard Ratio (95% CI)
Overall Results	1513	43.5	47.1	0.839 (0.721, 0.977)	19.6	25.5	0.714 (0.576, 0.885)
Age							
<65 years	1005	44.1	49.0	0.784 (0.653, 0.941)	21.1	28.5	0.670 (0.521, 0.863)
≥65 years	508	42.3	43.5	0.978 (0.749, 1.277)	16.5	19.6	0.847 (0.560, 1.281)
Gender							
Female	557	47.8	54.1	0.762 (0.603, 0.962)	22.8	32.8	0.601 (0.436, 0.828)
Male	956	40.9	43.3	0.892 (0.733, 1.085)	17.5	21.5	0.809 (0.605, 1.081)
Race							
Asian	252	41.9	54.8	0.655 (0.453, 0.947)	18.8	27.4	0.625 (0.367, 1.066)
Black	230	40.0	39.0	0.983 (0.647, 1.495)	17.6	21.0	0.831 (0.456, 1.516)
Hispanic	277	55.0	54.0	1.003 (0.728, 1.380)	30.0	28.5	1.024 (0.661, 1.586)
White	735	40.5	43.2	0.809 (0.645, 1.013)	16.2	23.9	0.596 (0.427, 0.831)

PRECAUTIONS

General

Hypersensitivity: *Angioedema*. See ADVERSE REACTIONS, Post-Marketing Experience.

Impaired Hepatic Function

Based on pharmacokinetic data which demonstrate significantly increased plasma concentrations of losartan in cirrhotic patients, a lower dose should be considered for patients with impaired liver function (see DOSAGE AND ADMINISTRATION and CLINICAL PHARMACOLOGY, Pharmacokinetics).

Impaired Renal Function

As a consequence of inhibiting the renin-angiotensin-aldosterone system, changes in renal function have been reported in susceptible individuals treated with COZAAR; in some patients, these changes in renal function were reversible upon discontinuation of therapy.

In patients whose renal function may depend on the activity of the renin-angiotensin-aldosterone system (e.g., patients with severe congestive heart failure), treatment with angiotensin converting enzyme inhibitors has been associated with oliguria and/or progressive azotemia and (rarely) with acute renal failure and/or death. Similar outcomes have been reported with COZAAR.

In studies of ACE inhibitors in patients with unilateral or bilateral renal artery stenosis, increases in serum creatinine or blood urea nitrogen (BUN) have been reported. Similar effects have been reported with COZAAR; in some patients, these effects were reversible upon discontinuation of therapy.

Electrolyte Imbalance

Electrolyte imbalances are common in patients with renal impairment, with or without diabetes, and should be addressed. In a clinical study conducted in type 2 diabetic patients with proteinuria, the incidence of hyperkalemia was higher in the group treated with COZAAR as compared to the placebo group; however, few patients discontinued therapy due to hyperkalemia (see ADVERSE REACTIONS).

Information for Patients

Pregnancy: Female patients of childbearing age should be told about the consequences of second- and third-trimester exposure to drugs that act on the renin-angiotensin system, and they should also be told that these consequences do not appear to have resulted from intrauterine drug exposure that has been limited to the first trimester. These patients should be asked to report pregnancies to their physicians as soon as possible.

Potassium Supplements: A patient receiving COZAAR should be told not to use potassium supplements or salt substitutes containing potassium without consulting the prescribing physician (see PRECAUTIONS, Drug Interactions).

Drug Interactions

No significant drug-drug pharmacokinetic interactions have been found in interaction studies with hydrochlorothiazide, digoxin, warfarin, cimetidine and phenobarbital. Rifampin, an inducer of drug metabolism, decreased the concentrations of losartan and its active metabolite. (See CLINICAL PHARMACOLOGY, Drug Interactions.) In humans, two inhibitors of P450 3A4 have been studied. Ketoconazole did not affect the conversion of losartan to the active metabolite after intravenous administration of losartan, and erythromycin had no clinically significant effect after oral administration. Fluconazole, an inhibitor of P450 2C9, decreased active metabolite concentration and increased losartan concentration. The pharmacodynamic consequences of concomitant use of losartan and inhibitors of P450 2C9 have not been examined. Subjects who do not metabolize losartan to active metabolite have been shown to have a specific, rare defect in cytochrome P450 2C9. These data suggest that the conversion of losartan to its active metabolite is mediated primarily by P450 2C9 and not P450 3A4.

As with other drugs that block angiotensin II or its effects, concomitant use of potassium-sparing diuretics (e.g., spironolactone, triamterene, amiloride), potassium supplements, or salt substitutes containing potassium may lead to increases in serum potassium.

Lithium: As with other drugs which affect the excrction of sodium, lithium excretion may be reduced. Therefore, serum lithium levels should be monitored carefully if lithium salts are to be co-administered with angiotensin II receptor antagonists.

Non-Steroidal Anti-Inflammatory Agents including Selective Cyclooxygenase-2 Inhibitors (COX-2 Inhibitors): In patients who are elderly, volume-depleted (including those on diuretic therapy), or with compromised renal function, coadministration of NSAIDs, including selective COX-2 inhibitors, with angiotensin II receptor antagonists (including losartan) may result in deterioration of renal function, including possible acute renal failure. These effects are usually reversible. Monitor renal function periodically in patients receiving losartan and NSAID therapy.

The antihypertensive effect of angiotensin II receptor antagonists, including losartan, may be attenuated by NSAIDs, including selective COX-2 inhibitors.

Carcinogenesis, Mutagenesis, Impairment of Fertility

Losartan potassium was not carcinogenic when administered at maximally tolerated dosages to rats and mice for 105 and 92 weeks, respectively. Female rats given the highest dose (270 mg/kg/day) had a slightly higher incidence of pancreatic acinar adenoma. The maximally tolerated dosages (270 mg/kg/day in rats, 200 mg/kg/day in mice) provided systemic exposures for losartan and its pharmacologically active metabolite that were approximately 160- and 90-times (rats) and 30- and 15-times (mice) the exposure of a 50 kg human given 100 mg per day.

Losartan potassium was negative in the microbial mutagenesis and V-79 mammalian cell mutagenesis assays and in the *in vitro* alkaline elution and *in vitro* and *in vivo* chromosomal aberration assays. In addition, the active metabolite showed no evidence of genotoxicity in the microbial mutagenesis, *in vitro* alkaline elution, and *in vitro* chromosomal aberration assays.

Fertility and reproductive performance were not affected in studies with male rats given oral doses of losartan potassium up to approximately 150 mg/kg/day. The administration of toxic dosage levels in females (300/200 mg/kg/day) was associated with a significant (p<0.05) decrease in the number of corpora lutea/female, implants/female, and live fetuses/female at C-section. At 100 mg/kg/day only a decrease in the number of corpora lutea/female was observed. The relationship of these findings to drug-treatment is uncertain since there was no effect at these dosage levels on implants/pregnant female, percent post-implantation loss, or live animals/litter at parturition. In nonpregnant rats dosed at 135 mg/kg/day for 7 days, systemic exposure (AUCs) for losartan and its active metabolite were approximately 66 and 26 times the exposure achieved in man at the maximum recommended human daily dosage (100 mg).

Pregnancy

Pregnancy Categories C (first trimester) and D (second and third trimesters). See WARNINGS, Fetal/Neonatal Morbidity and Mortality.

Nursing Mothers

It is not known whether losartan is excreted in human milk, but significant levels of losartan and its active metabolite were shown to be present in rat milk. Because of the potential for adverse effects on the nursing infant, a decision should be made whether to discontinue nursing or discontinue the drug, taking into account the importance of the drug to the mother.

Pediatric Use

Antihypertensive effects of COZAAR have been established in hypertensive pediatric patients aged 6 to 16 years. There are no data on the effect of COZAAR on blood pressure in pediatric patients under the age of 6 or in pediatric patients with glomerular filtration rate <30 mL/min/1.73 m^2 (see CLINICAL PHARMACOLOGY, Pharmacokinetics, Special Populations and Pharmacodynamics and Clinical Effects, and DOSAGE AND ADMINISTRATION).

Geriatric Use

Of the total number of patients receiving COZAAR in controlled clinical studies for hypertension, 391 patients (19%) were 65 years and over, while 37 patients (2%) were 75 years and over. In a controlled clinical study for renal protection in type 2 diabetic patients with proteinuria, 248 patients (33%) were 65 years and over. In a controlled clinical study for the reduction in the combined risk of cardiovascular death, stroke and myocardial infarction in hypertensive patients with left ventricular hypertrophy, 2857 patients (62%) were 65 years and over, while 808 patients (18%) were 75 years and over. No overall differences in effectiveness or safety were observed between these patients and younger patients, but greater sensitivity of some older individuals cannot be ruled out.

Race

In the LIFE study, Black patients with hypertension and left ventricular hypertrophy had a lower risk of stroke on atenolol than on COZAAR. Given the difficulty in interpreting subset differences in large trials, it cannot be known whether the observed difference is the result of chance. However, the LIFE study does not provide evidence that the benefits of COZAAR on reducing the risk of cardiovascular events in hypertensive patients with left ventricular hypertrophy apply to Black patients. (See CLINICAL PHARMACOLOGY, Pharmacodynamics and Clinical Effects; Reduction in the Risk of Stroke.)

ADVERSE REACTIONS

Hypertension

COZAAR has been evaluated for safety in more than 3300 adult patients treated for essential hypertension and 4058 patients/subjects overall. Over 1200 patients were treated for over 6 months and more than 800 for over one year. In general, treatment with COZAAR was well-tolerated. The overall incidence of adverse experiences reported with COZAAR was similar to placebo.

In controlled clinical trials, discontinuation of therapy due to clinical adverse experiences was required in 2.3 percent of patients treated with COZAAR and 3.7 percent of patients given placebo.

The following table of adverse events is based on four 6- to 12-week, placebo-controlled trials involving over 1000 patients on various doses (10-150 mg) of losartan and over 300 patients given placebo. All doses of losartan are grouped because none of the adverse events appeared to have a dose-related frequency. The adverse experiences reported in ≥1% of patients treated with COZAAR and more commonly than placebo are shown in the table below.

	Losartan (n=1075) Incidence %	Placebo (n=334) Incidence %
Musculoskeletal		
Cramp, muscle	1	0
Pain, back	2	1
Pain, leg	1	0
Nervous System / Psychiatric		
Dizziness	3	2
Respiratory		
Congestion, nasal	2	1
Infection, upper respiratory	8	7
Sinusitis	1	0

The following adverse events were also reported at a rate of 1% or greater in patients treated with losartan, but were as, or more frequent, in the placebo group: asthenia/fatigue, edema/swelling, abdominal pain, chest pain, nausea, headache, pharyngitis, diarrhea, dyspepsia, myalgia, insomnia, cough, sinus disorder.

Adverse events occurred at about the same rates in men and women, older and younger patients, and Black and non-Black patients.

A patient with known hypersensitivity to aspirin and penicillin, when treated with COZAAR, was withdrawn from study due to swelling of the lips and eyelids and facial rash, reported as angioedema, which returned to normal 5 days after therapy was discontinued.

Superficial peeling of palms and hemolysis were reported in one subject.

In addition to the adverse events above, potentially important events that occurred in at least two patients/subjects exposed to losartan or other adverse events that occurred in <1% of patients in clinical studies are listed below. It cannot be determined whether these events were causally related to losartan: *Body as a Whole:* facial edema, fever, orthostatic effects, syncope; *Cardiovascular:* angina pectoris, second degree AV block, CVA, hypotension, myocardial infarction, arrhythmias including atrial fibrillation, palpitation, sinus bradycardia, tachycardia, ventricular tachycardia, ventricular fibrillation; *Digestive:* anorexia, constipation, dental pain, dry mouth, flatulence, gastritis, vomiting; *Hematologic:* anemia; *Metabolic:* gout; *Musculoskeletal:* arm pain, hip pain, joint swelling, knee pain, musculoskeletal pain, shoulder pain, stiffness, arthralgia, arthritis, fibromyalgia, muscle weakness; *Nervous System / Psychiatric:* anxiety, anxiety disorder, ataxia, confusion, depression, dream abnormality, hypesthesia, decreased libido, memory impairment, migraine, nervousness, paresthesia, peripheral neuropathy, panic disorder, sleep disorder, somnolence, tremor, vertigo; *Respiratory:* dyspnea, bronchitis, pharyngeal discomfort, epistaxis, rhinitis, respiratory congestion; *Skin:* alopecia, dermatitis, dry skin, ecchymosis, erythema, flushing, photosensitivity, pruritus, rash, sweating, urticaria; *Special Senses:* blurred vision, burning/stinging in the eye, conjunctivitis, taste perversion, tinnitus, decrease in visual acuity; *Urogenital:* impotence, nocturia, urinary frequency, urinary tract infection.

Persistent dry cough (with an incidence of a few percent) has been associated with ACE-inhibitor use and in practice can be a cause of discontinuation of ACE-inhibitor therapy. Two prospective, parallel-group, double-blind, randomized, controlled trials were conducted to assess the effects of losartan on the incidence of cough in hypertensive patients who had experienced cough while receiving ACE-inhibitor therapy. Patients who had typical ACE-inhibitor cough when challenged with lisinopril, whose cough disappeared on placebo, were randomized to losartan 50 mg, lisinopril 20 mg, or either placebo (one study, n=97) or 25 mg hydrochlorothiazide (n=135). The double-blind treatment period lasted up to 8 weeks. The incidence of cough is shown below.

Study 1[†]	HCTZ	Losartan	Lisinopril
Cough	25%	17%	69%
Study 2[‡]	Placebo	Losartan	Lisinopril
Cough	35%	29%	62%

[†] Demographics = (89% caucasian, 64% female)
[‡] Demographics = (90% caucasian, 51% female)

These studies demonstrate that the incidence of cough associated with losartan therapy, in a population that all had cough associated with ACE-inhibitor therapy, is similar to that associated with hydrochlorothiazide or placebo therapy.

Cases of cough, including positive re-challenges, have been reported with the use of losartan in post-marketing experience.

Pediatric Patients: No relevant differences between the adverse experience profile for pediatric patients and that previously reported for adult patients were identified.

Hypertensive Patients with Left Ventricular Hypertrophy

In the LIFE study, adverse events with COZAAR were similar to those reported previously for patients with hypertension.

Nephropathy in Type 2 Diabetic Patients

In the RENAAL study involving 1513 patients treated with COZAAR or placebo, the overall incidences of reported adverse experiences were similar for the two groups. COZAAR was generally well tolerated as evidenced by a similar incidence of discontinuations due to side effects compared to placebo (19% for COZAAR, 24% for placebo). The adverse experiences, regardless of drug relationship, reported with an incidence of ≥4% of patients treated with COZAAR and occurring more commonly than placebo, on a background of conventional antihypertensive therapy, are shown in the table below.

[See table at left]

Post-Marketing Experience

The following additional adverse reactions have been reported in post-marketing experience:

Digestive: Hepatitis (reported rarely).

General Disorders and Administration Site Conditions: Malaise.

Hemic: Thrombocytopenia (reported rarely).

Hypersensitivity: Angioedema, including swelling of the larynx and glottis, causing airway obstruction and/or swelling of the face, lips, pharynx, and/or tongue has been reported rarely in patients treated with losartan; some of these patients previously experienced angioedema with other drugs including ACE inhibitors. Vasculitis, including Henoch-Schönlein purpura, has been reported. Anaphylactic reactions have been reported.

Metabolic and Nutrition: Hyperkalemia, hyponatremia have been reported with losartan.

Musculoskeletal: Rare cases of rhabdomyolysis have been reported in patients receiving angiotensin II receptor blockers.

Nervous system disorders: Dysgeusia.

Respiratory: Dry cough (see above).

Skin: Erythroderma.

Laboratory Test Findings

In controlled clinical trials, clinically important changes in standard laboratory parameters were rarely associated with administration of COZAAR.

Creatinine, Blood Urea Nitrogen: Minor increases in blood urea nitrogen (BUN) or serum creatinine were observed in less than 0.1 percent of patients with essential hypertension treated with COZAAR alone (see PRECAUTIONS, Impaired Renal Function).

Hemoglobin and Hematocrit: Small decreases in hemoglobin and hematocrit (mean decreases of approximately 0.11 grams percent and 0.09 volume percent, respectively) occurred frequently in patients treated with COZAAR alone, but were rarely of clinical importance. No patients were discontinued due to anemia.

Liver Function Tests: Occasional elevations of liver enzymes and/or serum bilirubin have occurred. In patients with essential hypertension treated with COZAAR alone, one patient (<0.1%) was discontinued due to these laboratory adverse experiences.

	Losartan and Conventional Antihypertensive Therapy Incidence % (n=751)	Placebo and Conventional Antihypertensive Therapy Incidence % (n=762)
Body as a Whole		
Asthenia/Fatigue	14	10
Chest Pain	12	8
Fever	4	3
Infection	5	4
Influenza-like disease	10	9
Trauma	4	3
Cardiovascular		
Hypotension	7	3
Orthostatic hypotension	4	1
Digestive		
Diarrhea	15	10
Dyspepsia	4	3
Gastritis	5	4
Endocrine		
Diabetic neuropathy	4	3
Diabetic vascular disease	10	9
Eyes, Ears, Nose and Throat		
Cataract	7	5
Sinusitis	6	5
Hemic		
Anemia	14	11
Metabolic and Nutrition		
Hyperkalemia	7	3
Hypoglycemia	14	10
Weight gain	4	3
Musculoskeletal		
Back pain	12	10
Leg pain	5	4
Knee pain	5	4
Muscular weakness	7	4
Nervous System		
Hypesthesia	5	4
Respiratory		
Bronchitis	10	9
Cough	11	10
Skin		
Cellulitis	7	6
Urogenital		
Urinary tract infection	16	13

OVERDOSAGE

Significant lethality was observed in mice and rats after oral administration of 1000 mg/kg and 2000 mg/kg, respectively, about 44 and 170 times the maximum recommended human dose on a mg/m^2 basis.

Limited data are available in regard to overdosage in humans. The most likely manifestation of overdosage would be hypotension and tachycardia; bradycardia could occur from parasympathetic (vagal) stimulation. If symptomatic hypotension should occur, supportive treatment should be instituted.

Neither losartan nor its active metabolite can be removed by hemodialysis.

DOSAGE AND ADMINISTRATION

Adult Hypertensive Patients

COZAAR may be administered with other antihypertensive agents, and with or without food.

Dosing must be individualized. The usual starting dose of COZAAR is 50 mg once daily, with 25 mg used in patients with possible depletion of intravascular volume (e.g., patients treated with diuretics) (see WARNINGS, Hypotension—Volume-Depleted Patients) and patients with a history of hepatic impairment (see PRECAUTIONS, General). COZAAR can be administered once or twice daily with total daily doses ranging from 25 mg to 100 mg.

If the antihypertensive effect measured at trough using once-a-day dosing is inadequate, a twice-a-day regimen at the same total daily dose or an increase in dose may give a more satisfactory response. The effect of losartan is substantially present within one week but in some studies the maximal effect occurred in 3-6 weeks (see CLINICAL PHARMACOLOGY, Pharmacodynamics and Clinical Effects, Hypertension).

If blood pressure is not controlled by COZAAR alone, a low dose of a diuretic may be added. Hydrochlorothiazide has been shown to have an additive effect (see CLINICAL PHARMACOLOGY, Pharmacodynamics and Clinical Effects, Hypertension).

No initial dosage adjustment is necessary for elderly patients or for patients with renal impairment, including patients on dialysis.

Pediatric Hypertensive Patients ≥6 years of age

The usual recommended starting dose is 0.7 mg/kg once daily (up to 50 mg total) administered as a tablet or a suspension (see Preparation of Suspension). Dosage should be adjusted according to blood pressure response. Doses above 1.4 mg/kg (or in excess of 100 mg) daily have not been studied in pediatric patients. (See CLINICAL PHARMACOLOGY, Pharmacokinetics, Special Populations and Pharmacodynamics and Clinical Effects, and WARNINGS, Hypotension—Volume-Depleted Patients.)

COZAAR is not recommended in pediatric patients <6 years of age or in pediatric patients with glomerular filtration rate <30 mL/min/1.73 m^2 (see CLINICAL PHARMACOLOGY, Pharmacokinetics, Special Populations , Pharmacodynamics and Clinical Effects, and PRECAUTIONS).

Preparation of Suspension (for 200 mL of a 2.5 mg/mL suspension)

Add 10 mL of Purified Water USP to an 8 ounce (240 mL) amber polyethylene terephthalate (PET) bottle containing ten 50 mg COZAAR tablets. Immediately shake for at least 2 minutes. Let the concentrate stand for 1 hour and then shake for 1 minute to disperse the tablet contents. Separately prepare a 50/50 volumetric mixture of Ora-Plus™** and Ora-Sweet SF™**. Add 190 mL of the 50/50 Ora-Plus™/Ora-Sweet SF™ mixture to the tablet and water slurry in the PET bottle and shake for 1 minute to disperse the ingredients. The suspension should be refrigerated at 2-8°C (36-46°F) and can be stored for up to 4 weeks. Shake the suspension prior to each use and return promptly to the refrigerator.

** Trademark of Paddock Laboratories, Inc.

Hypertensive Patients with Left Ventricular Hypertrophy

The usual starting dose is 50 mg of COZAAR once daily. Hydrochlorothiazide 12.5 mg daily should be added and/or the dose of COZAAR should be increased to 100 mg once daily followed by an increase in hydrochlorothiazide to 25 mg once daily based on blood pressure response (see CLINICAL PHARMACOLOGY, Pharmacodynamics and Clinical Effects, Reduction in the Risk of Stroke).

Nephropathy in Type 2 Diabetic Patients

The usual starting dose is 50 mg once daily. The dose should be increased to 100 mg once daily based on blood pressure response (see CLINICAL PHARMACOLOGY, Pharmacodynamics and Clinical Effects, Nephropathy in Type 2 Diabetic Patients). COZAAR may be administered with insulin and other commonly used hypoglycemic agents (e.g., sulfonylureas, glitazones and glucosidase inhibitors).

HOW SUPPLIED

No. 8441—Tablets COZAAR, 25 mg, are white, oval, film-coated tablets with code 951 on one side and plain on the other. They are supplied as follows:

NDC 0006-0951-54 unit of use bottles of 90
NDC 0006-0951-82 bottles of 1,000.

No. 8442—Tablets COZAAR, 50 mg, are white, oval, film-coated tablets with code 952 on one side and scored on the other. They are supplied as follows:

NDC 0006-0952-31 unit of use bottles of 30
NDC 0006-0952-54 unit of use bottles of 90
NDC 0006-0952-82 bottles of 1,000

No. 3849—Tablets COZAAR, 100 mg, are white, teardrop-shaped, film-coated tablets with code 960 on one side and plain on the other. They are supplied as follows:

NDC 0006-0960-31 unit of use bottles of 30
NDC 0006-0960-54 unit of use bottles of 90
NDC 0006-0960-82 bottles of 1,000

Storage

Store at 25°C (77°F); excursions permitted to 15-30°C (59-86°F) [see USP Controlled Room Temperature]. Keep container tightly closed. Protect from light.

Manuf. for: Merck Sharp & Dohme Corp., a subsidiary of **MERCK & CO., INC.**, Whitehouse Station, NJ 08889, USA
Issued June 2010
9964202

PATIENT PACKAGE INSERT

Patient Information
COZAAR® (CO-zar)
(losartan potassium tablets)
25mg, 50mg, 100mg
Rx only
Read the Patient Information that comes with COZAAR* before you start taking it and each time you get a refill. There may be new information. This leaflet does not take the place of talking with your doctor about your condition and treatment.

---

*Registered trademark of E.I. du Pont de Nemours and Company, Wilmington, Delaware, USA
COPYRIGHT © 2006 Merck Sharp & Dohme Corp., a subsidiary of **Merck & Co., Inc.**
All rights reserved.

What is the most important information I should know about COZAAR?
Do not take COZAAR if you are pregnant or plan to become pregnant. COZAAR can harm your unborn baby causing injury and even death. Stop taking COZAAR if you become pregnant and call your doctor right away. If you plan to become pregnant, talk to your doctor about other treatment options before taking COZAAR.

What is COZAAR?
COZAAR is a prescription medicine called an angiotensin receptor blocker (ARB). It is used:
• alone or with other blood pressure medicines to lower high blood pressure (hypertension).
• to lower the chance of stroke in patients with high blood pressure and a heart problem called left ventricular hypertrophy. COZAAR may not help Black patients with this problem.
• to slow the worsening of diabetic kidney disease (nephropathy) in patients with type 2 diabetes who have or had high blood pressure.

COZAAR has not been studied in children less than 6 years old or in children with certain kidney problems.

High Blood Pressure (hypertension). Blood pressure is the force in your blood vessels when your heart beats and when your heart rests. You have high blood pressure when the force is too much. COZAAR can help your blood vessels relax so your blood pressure is lower.

Left Ventricular Hypertrophy (LVH) is an enlargement of the walls of the left chamber of the heart (the heart's main pumping chamber). LVH can happen from several things. High blood pressure is the most common cause of LVH.

Type 2 Diabetes with Nephropathy. Type 2 diabetes is a type of diabetes that happens mainly in adults. If you have diabetic nephropathy it means that your kidneys do not work properly because of damage from the diabetes.

Who should not take COZAAR?
• **Do not take COZAAR if you are allergic to any of the ingredients in COZAAR.** See the end of this leaflet for a complete list of ingredients in COZAAR.

What should I tell my doctor before taking COZAAR?
Tell your doctor about all of your medical conditions including if you:
• **are pregnant or planning to become pregnant. See "What is the most important information I should know about COZAAR?"**
• **are breast-feeding.** It is not known if COZAAR passes into your breast milk. You should choose either to take COZAAR or breast-feed, but not both.
• are vomiting a lot or having a lot of diarrhea
• have liver problems
• have kidney problems

Tell your doctor about all the medicines you take, including prescription and non-prescription medicines, vitamins, and

herbal supplements. COZAAR and certain other medicines may interact with each other. Especially tell your doctor if you are taking:
• potassium supplements
• salt substitutes containing potassium
• water pills (diuretics)
• medicines used to treat pain and arthritis, called non-steroidal anti-inflammatory drugs (NSAIDs), including COX-2 inhibitors

How should I take COZAAR?
• Take COZAAR exactly as prescribed by your doctor. Your doctor may change your dose if needed.
• COZAAR can be taken with or without food.
• If you miss a dose, take it as soon as you remember. If it is close to your next dose, do not take the missed dose. Just take the next dose at your regular time.
• If you take too much COZAAR, call your doctor or Poison Control Center, or go to the nearest hospital emergency room right away.

What are the possible side effects of COZAAR?
COZAAR may cause the following side effects that may be serious:
• **Injury or death of unborn babies. See "What is the most important information I should know about COZAAR?"**
• **Allergic reaction.** Symptoms of an allergic reaction are swelling of the face, lips, throat or tongue. Get emergency medical help right away and stop taking COZAAR.
• **Low blood pressure (hypotension).** Low blood pressure may cause you to feel faint or dizzy. Lie down if you feel faint or dizzy. Call your doctor right away.
• **For people who already have kidney problems, you may see a worsening in how well your kidneys work.** Call your doctor if you get swelling in your feet, ankles, or hands, or unexplained weight gain.

The most common side effects of COZAAR in people with high blood pressure are:
• "colds" (upper respiratory infection)
• dizziness
• stuffy nose
• back pain

The most common side effects of COZAAR in people with type 2 diabetes with diabetic kidney disease are:
• diarrhea
• tiredness
• low blood sugar
• chest pain
• high blood potassium
• low blood pressure

Tell your doctor if you get any side effect that bothers you or that won't go away.

This is **not** a complete list of side effects. For a complete list, ask your doctor or pharmacist.

How do I store COZAAR?
• Store COZAAR tablets at 59°F to 86°F (15°C to 30°C).
• Keep COZAAR in a tightly closed container that protects the medicine from light.
• **Keep COZAAR and all medicines out of the reach of children.**

General information about COZAAR
Medicines are sometimes prescribed for conditions that are not mentioned in patient information leaflets. Do not use COZAAR for a condition for which it was not prescribed. Do not give COZAAR to other people, even if they have the same symptoms that you have. It may harm them.

This leaflet summarizes the most important information about COZAAR. If you would like more information, talk with your doctor. You can ask your pharmacist or doctor for information about COZAAR that is written for health professionals.

What are the ingredients in COZAAR?
Active ingredients: losartan potassium
Inactive ingredients: microcrystalline cellulose, lactose hydrous, pregelatinized starch, magnesium stearate, hydroxypropyl cellulose, hypromellose, and titanium dioxide. COZAAR 25 mg, COZAAR 50 mg, and COZAAR 100 mg may also contain carnauba wax.
Issued December 2009
Manufactured For:
Merck Sharp & Dohme Corp., a subsidiary of
Merck & Co., Inc., Whitehouse Station, NJ 08889, USA
9964201

Shown in Product Identification Guide, page 312

CRIXIVAN®   ℞
(indinavir sulfate)
Capsules

DESCRIPTION

CRIXIVAN* (indinavir sulfate) is an inhibitor of the human immunodeficiency virus (HIV) protease. CRIXIVAN Capsules are formulated as a sulfate salt and are available for oral administration in strengths of 100, 200, and 400 mg of indinavir (corresponding to 125, 250, and 500 mg indinavir sulfate, respectively). Each capsule also contains the inactive ingredients anhydrous lactose and magnesium stearate. The capsule shell has the following inactive ingredients and dyes: gelatin, titanium dioxide, silicon dioxide, and sodium lauryl sulfate.

The chemical name for indinavir sulfate is [1(1S,2R),5(S)]-2,3,5-trideoxy-N-(2,3-dihydro-2-hydroxy-1H-inden-1-yl)-5-[2-[[(1,1-dimethylethyl)amino]carbonyl]-4-(3-pyridinylmethyl)-1-piperazinyl]-2-(phenylmethyl)-D-$erythro$-pentonamide sulfate (1:1) salt. Indinavir sulfate has the following structural formula:

Indinavir sulfate is a white to off-white, hygroscopic, crystalline powder with the molecular formula $C_{36}H_{47}N_5O_4 \cdot H_2SO_4$ and a molecular weight of 711.88. It is very soluble in water and in methanol.

MICROBIOLOGY

Mechanism of Action: HIV-1 protease is an enzyme required for the proteolytic cleavage of the viral polyprotein precursors into the individual functional proteins found in infectious HIV-1. Indinavir binds to the protease active site and inhibits the activity of the enzyme. This inhibition prevents cleavage of the viral polyproteins resulting in the formation of immature non-infectious viral particles.

Antiretroviral Activity In Vitro: The *in vitro* activity of indinavir was assessed in cell lines of lymphoblastic and monocytic origin and in peripheral blood lymphocytes. HIV-1 variants used to infect the different cell types include laboratory-adapted variants, primary clinical isolates and clinical isolates resistant to nucleoside analogue and non-nucleoside inhibitors of the HIV-1 reverse transcriptase. The IC_{95} (95% inhibitory concentration) of indinavir in these test systems was in the range of 25 to 100 nM. In drug combination studies with the nucleoside analogues zidovudine and didanosine, indinavir showed synergistic activity in cell culture. The relationship between *in vitro* susceptibility of HIV-1 to indinavir and inhibition of HIV-1 replication in humans has not been established.

Drug Resistance: Isolates of HIV-1 with reduced susceptibility to the drug have been recovered from some patients treated with indinavir. Viral resistance was correlated with the accumulation of mutations that resulted in the expression of amino acid substitutions in the viral protease. Eleven amino acid residue positions, (L10I/V/R, K20I/M/R, L24I, M46I/L, I54A/V, L63P, I64V, A71T/V, V82A/F/T, I84V, and L90M), at which substitutions are associated with resistance, have been identified. Resistance was mediated by the co-expression of multiple and variable substitutions at these positions. No single substitution was either necessary or sufficient for measurable resistance (≥4-fold increase in IC_{95}). In general, higher levels of resistance were associated with the co-expression of greater numbers of substitutions, although their individual effects varied and were not additive. At least 3 amino acid substitutions must be present for phenotypic resistance to indinavir to reach measurable levels. In addition, mutations in the p7/p1 and p1/p6 gag cleavage sites were observed in some indinavir resistant HIV-1 isolates.

In vitro phenotypic susceptibilities to indinavir were determined for 38 viral isolates from 13 patients who experienced virologic rebounds during indinavir monotherapy. Pretreatment isolates from five patients exhibited indinavir IC_{95} values of 50-100 nM. At or following viral RNA rebound (after 12-76 weeks of therapy), IC_{95} values ranged from 25 to >3000 nM, and the viruses carried 2 to 10 mutations in the protease gene relative to baseline.

Cross-Resistance to Other Antiviral Agents: Varying degrees of HIV-1 cross-resistance have been observed between indinavir and other HIV-1 protease inhibitors. In studies with ritonavir, saquinavir, and amprenavir, the extent and spectrum of cross-resistance varied with the specific mutational patterns observed. In general, the degree of cross-resistance increased with the accumulation of resistance-associated amino acid substitutions. Within a panel of 29 viral isolates from indinavir-treated patients that exhibited measurable (≥4-fold) phenotypic resistance to indinavir, all were resistant to ritonavir. Of the indinavir resistant HIV-1 isolates, 63% showed resistance to saquinavir and 81% to amprenavir.

Table 1

PK Parameter	% change in PK parameter for females relative to males	90% Confidence Interval
AUC_{0-8h} (nM•hr)	↓13%	(↓32%, ↑12%)
C_{max} (nM)	↓13%	(↓32%, ↑10%)
C_{8h} (nM)	↓22%	(↓47%, ↑15%)

↓ Indicates a decrease in the PK parameter; ↑ indicates an increase in the PK parameter.

Table 2: Drug Interactions: Pharmacokinetic Parameters for Indinavir in the Presence of the Coadministered Drug (See PRECAUTIONS, Table 9 for Recommended Alterations in Dose or Regimen)

Coadministered drug	Dose of Coadministered drug (mg)	Dose of CRIXIVAN (mg)	n	Ratio (with/without coadministered drug) of Indinavir Pharmacokinetic Parameters (90% CI); No Effect = 1.00		
				C_{max}	AUC	C_{min}
Cimetidine	600 twice daily, 6 days	400 single dose	12	1.07 (0.77, 1.49)	0.98 (0.81, 1.19)	0.82 (0.69, 0.99)
Clarithromycin	500 q12h, 7 days	800 three times daily, 7 days	10	1.08 (0.85, 1.38)	1.19 (1.00, 1.42)	1.57 (1.16, 2.12)
Delavirdine	400 three times daily	400 three times daily, 7 days	28	0.64[1] (0.48, 0.86)	No significant change[1]	2.18[1] (1.16, 4.12)
Delavirdine	400 three times daily	600 three times daily, 7 days	28	No significant change	1.53[1] (1.07, 2.20)	3.98[1] (2.04, 7.78)
Efavirenz[2]	600 once daily, 10 days	1000 three times daily, 10 days	20			
		After morning dose		No significant change[1]	0.67[1] (0.61, 0.74)	0.61[1] (0.49, 0.76)
		After afternoon dose		No significant change[1]	0.63[1] (0.54, 0.74)	0.48[1] (0.43, 0.53)
		After evening dose		0.71[1] (0.57, 0.89)	0.54[1] (0.46, 0.63)	0.43[1] (0.37, 0.50)
Fluconazole[2]	400 once daily, 8 days	1000 three times daily, 7 days	11	0.87 (0.72, 1.05)	0.76 (0.59, 0.98)	0.90 (0.72, 1.12)
Grapefruit Juice	8 oz.	400 single dose	10	0.65 (0.53, 0.79)	0.73 (0.60, 0.87)	0.90 (0.71, 1.15)
Isoniazid	300 once daily in the morning, 8 days	800 three times daily, 7 days	11	0.95 (0.88, 1.03)	0.99 (0.87, 1.13)	0.89 (0.75, 1.06)
Itraconazole	200 mg twice daily, 7 days	600 three times daily, 7 days	12	0.78[1] (0.69, 0.88)	0.99[1] (0.91, 1.06)	1.49[1] (1.28, 1.74)
Ketoconazole	400 once daily, 7 days	600 three times daily, 7 days	12	0.69[1] (0.61, 0.78)	0.80[1] (0.74, 0.87)	1.29[1] (1.11, 1.51)
	400 once daily, 7 days	400 three times daily, 7 days	12	0.42[1] (0.37, 0.47)	0.44[1] (0.41, 0.48)	0.73[1] (0.62, 0.85)
Methadone	20-60 once daily in the morning, 8 days	800 three times daily, 8 days	10	See text below for discussion of interaction.		
Quinidine	200 single dose	400 single dose	10	0.96 (0.79, 1.18)	1.07 (0.89, 1.28)	0.93 (0.73, 1.19)
Rifabutin	150 once daily in the morning, 10 days	800 three times daily, 10 days	14	0.80 (0.72, 0.89)	0.68 (0.60, 0.76)	0.60 (0.51, 0.72)
Rifabutin	300 once daily in the morning, 10 days	800 three times daily, 10 days	10	0.75 (0.61, 0.91)	0.66 (0.56, 0.77)	0.61 (0.50, 0.75)
Rifampin	600 once daily in the morning, 8 days	800 three times daily, 7 days	12	0.13 (0.08, 0.22)	0.08 (0.06, 0.11)	Not Done
Ritonavir	100 twice daily, 14 days	800 twice daily, 14 days	10, 16[3]	See text below for discussion of interaction.		
Ritonavir	200 twice daily, 14 days	800 twice daily, 14 days	9, 16[3]	See text below for discussion of interaction.		
Sildenafil	25 single dose	800 three times daily	6	See text below for discussion of interaction.		

(Table continued on next page)

CLINICAL PHARMACOLOGY

Pharmacokinetics

Absorption: Indinavir was rapidly absorbed in the fasted state with a time to peak plasma concentration (T_{max}) of 0.8 ± 0.3 hours (mean ± S.D.) (n=11). A greater than dose-proportional increase in indinavir plasma concentrations was observed over the 200-1000 mg dose range. At a dosing regimen of 800 mg every 8 hours, steady-state area under the plasma concentration time curve (AUC) was 30,691 ± 11,407 nM•hour (n=16), peak plasma concentration (C_{max}) was 12,617 ± 4037 nM (n=16), and plasma concentration eight hours post dose (trough) was 251 ± 178 nM (n=16),

Effect of Food on Oral Absorption: Administration of indinavir with a meal high in calories, fat, and protein (784 kcal, 48.6 g fat, 31.3 g protein) resulted in a 77% ± 8% reduction in AUC and an 84% ± 7% reduction in C_{max} (n=10). Administration with lighter meals (e.g., a meal of dry toast with jelly, apple juice, and coffee with skim milk and sugar or a meal of corn flakes, skim milk and sugar) resulted in little or no change in AUC, C_{max} or trough concentration.

Distribution: Indinavir was approximately 60% bound to human plasma proteins over a concentration range of 81 nM to 16,300 nM.

Metabolism: Following a 400-mg dose of ^{14}C-indinavir, 83 ± 1% (n=4) and 19 ± 3% (n=6) of the total radioactivity was recovered in feces and urine, respectively; radioactivity due to parent drug in feces and urine was 19.1% and 9.4%, respectively. Seven metabolites have been identified, one glucuronide conjugate and six oxidative metabolites. *In vitro* studies indicate that cytochrome P-450 3A4 (CYP3A4) is the major enzyme responsible for formation of the oxidative metabolites.

Elimination: Less than 20% of indinavir is excreted unchanged in the urine. Mean urinary excretion of unchanged drug was 10.4 ± 4.9% (n=10) and 12.0 ± 4.9% (n=10) following a single 700-mg and 1000-mg dose, respectively. Indinavir was rapidly eliminated with a half-life of 1.8 ± 0.4 hours (n=10). Significant accumulation was not observed after multiple dosing at 800 mg every 8 hours.

Special Populations

Hepatic Insufficiency: Patients with mild to moderate hepatic insufficiency and clinical evidence of cirrhosis had evidence of decreased metabolism of indinavir resulting in approximately 60% higher mean AUC following a single 400-mg dose (n=12). The half-life of indinavir increased to 2.8 ± 0.5 hours. Indinavir pharmacokinetics have not been studied in patients with severe hepatic insufficiency (see DOSAGE AND ADMINISTRATION, *Hepatic Insufficiency*).

Renal Insufficiency: The pharmacokinetics of indinavir have not been studied in patients with renal insufficiency.

Gender: The effect of gender on the pharmacokinetics of indinavir was evaluated in 10 HIV seropositive women who received CRIXIVAN 800 mg every 8 hours with zidovudine 200 mg every 8 hours and lamivudine 150 mg twice a day for one week. Indinavir pharmacokinetic parameters in these women were compared to those in HIV seropositive men (pooled historical control data). Differences in indinavir exposure, peak concentrations, and trough concentrations between males and females are shown in Table 1 below:
[See table 1 at top of previous page]
The clinical significance of these gender differences in the pharmacokinetics of indinavir is not known.

Race: Pharmacokinetics of indinavir appear to be comparable in Caucasians and Blacks based on pharmacokinetic studies including 42 Caucasians (26 HIV-positive) and 16 Blacks (4 HIV-positive).

Pediatric: The optimal dosing regimen for use of indinavir in pediatric patients has not been established. In HIV-infected pediatric patients (age 4-15 years), a dosage regimen of indinavir capsules, 500 mg/m^2 every 8 hours, produced AUC_{0-8hr} of 38,742 ± 24,098 nM•hour (n=34), C_{max} of 17,181 ± 9809 nM (n=34), and trough concentrations of 134 ± 91 nM (n=28). The pharmacokinetic profiles of indinavir in pediatric patients were not comparable to profiles previously observed in HIV-infected adults receiving the recommended dose of 800 mg every 8 hours. The AUC and C_{max} values were slightly higher and the trough concentrations were considerably lower in pediatric patients. Approximately 50% of the pediatric patients had trough values below 100 nM; whereas, approximately 10% of adult patients had trough levels below 100 nM. The relationship between specific trough values and inhibition of HIV replication has not been established.

Pregnant Patients: The optimal dosing regimen for use of indinavir in pregnant patients has not been established. A CRIXIVAN dose of 800 mg every 8 hours (with zidovudine 200 mg every 8 hours and lamivudine 150 mg twice a day) has been studied in 16 HIV-infected pregnant patients at 14 to 28 weeks of gestation at enrollment (study PACTG 358). The mean indinavir plasma AUC_{0-8hr} at weeks 30-32 of gestation (n=11) was 9231 nM•hr, which is 74% (95% CI: 50%, 86%) lower than that observed 6 weeks postpartum. Six of these 11 (55%) patients had mean indinavir plasma concentrations 8 hours post-dose (C_{min}) below assay threshold of reliable quantification. The pharmacokinetics of indinavir in these 11 patients at 6 weeks postpartum were generally similar to those observed in non-pregnant patients in another study (see PRECAUTIONS, *Pregnancy*).

Drug Interactions: (also see CONTRAINDICATIONS, WARNINGS, PRECAUTIONS, *Drug Interactions*)
Indinavir is an inhibitor of the cytochrome P450 isoform CYP3A4. Coadministration of CRIXIVAN and drugs primarily metabolized by CYP3A4 may result in increased plasma concentrations of the other drug, which could increase or prolong its therapeutic and adverse effects (see CONTRAINDICATIONS and WARNINGS). Based on *in vitro* data in human liver microsomes, indinavir does not in-

hibit CYP1A2, CYP2C9, CYP2E1 and CYP2B6. However, indinavir may be a weak inhibitor of CYP2D6.
Indinavir is metabolized by CYP3A4. Drugs that induce CYP3A4 activity would be expected to increase the clearance of indinavir, resulting in lowered plasma concentrations of indinavir. Coadministration of CRIXIVAN and other drugs that inhibit CYP3A4 may decrease the clearance of indinavir and may result in increased plasma concentrations of indinavir.
Drug interaction studies were performed with CRIXIVAN and other drugs likely to be coadministered and some drugs commonly used as probes for pharmacokinetic interactions. The effects of coadministration of CRIXIVAN on the AUC, C_{max} and C_{min} are summarized in Table 2 (effect of other

drugs on indinavir) and Table 3 (effect of indinavir on other drugs). For information regarding clinical recommendations, see Table 9 in PRECAUTIONS.
[See table 2 on previous page and above]
[See table 3 above and on next page]
Delaviridine: Delavirdine inhibits the metabolism of indinavir such that coadministration of 400-mg or 600-mg indinavir three times daily with 400-mg delavirdine three times daily alters indinavir AUC, C_{max} and C_{min} (see Table 2). Indinavir had no effect on delavirdine pharmacokinetics (see DOSAGE AND ADMINISTRATION, *Concomitant Therapy, Delavirdine*), based on a comparison to historical delavirdine pharmacokinetic data.

Table 2 *(cont.)*: Drug Interactions: Pharmacokinetic Parameters for Indinavir in the Presence of the Coadministered Drug (See PRECAUTIONS, Table 9 for Recommended Alterations in Dose or Regimen)

Coadministered drug	Dose of Coadministered drug (mg)	Dose of CRIXIVAN (mg)	n	Ratio (with/without coadministered drug) of Indinavir Pharmacokinetic Parameters (90% CI); No Effect = 1.00		
				C_{max}	AUC	C_{min}
St. John's wort (*Hypericum perforatum,* standardized to 0.3% hypericin)	300 three times daily with meals, 14 days	800 three times daily	8	Not Available	0.46 (0.34, 0.58)[4]	0.19 (0.06, 0.33)[4]
Stavudine (d4T)[2]	40 twice daily, 7 days	800 three times daily, 7 days	11	0.95 (0.80, 1.11)	0.95 (0.80, 1.12)	1.13 (0.83, 1.53)
Trimethoprim/ Sulfamethoxazole	800 Trimethoprim/ 160 Sulfamethoxazole q12h, 7 days	400 four times daily, 7 days	12	1.12 (0.87, 1.46)	0.98 (0.81, 1.18)	0.83 (0.72, 0.95)
Zidovudine[2]	200 three times daily, 7 days	1000 three times daily, 7 days	12	1.06 (0.91, 1.25)	1.05 (0.86, 1.28)	1.02 (0.77, 1.35)
Zidovudine/ Lamivudine (3TC)[2]	200/150 three times daily, 7 days	800 three times daily, 7 days	6, 9[5]	1.05 (0.83, 1.33)	1.04 (0.67, 1.61)	0.98 (0.56, 1.73)

All interaction studies conducted in healthy, HIV-negative adult subjects, unless otherwise indicated.
[1] Relative to indinavir 800 mg three times daily alone.
[2] Study conducted in HIV-positive subjects.
[3] Comparison to historical data on 16 subjects receiving indinavir alone.
[4] 95% CI.
[5] Parallel group design; n for indinavir + coadministered drug, n for indinavir alone.

Table 3: Drug Interactions: Pharmacokinetic Parameters for Coadministered Drug in the Presence of Indinavir (See PRECAUTIONS, Table 9 for Recommended Alterations in Dose or Regimen)

Coadministered drug	Dose of Coadministered drug (mg)	Dose of CRIXIVAN (mg)	n	Ratio (with/without CRIXIVAN) of Coadministered Drug Pharmacokinetic Parameters (90% CI); No Effect = 1.00		
				C_{max}	AUC	C_{min}
Clarithromycin	500 twice daily, 7 days	800 three times daily, 7 days	12	1.19 (1.02, 1.39)	1.47 (1.30, 1.65)	1.97 (1.58, 2.46) n=11
Efavirenz	200 once daily, 14 days	800 three times daily, 14 days	20	No significant change	No significant change	—
Ethinyl Estradiol (ORTHO-NOVUM 1/35)[1]	35 mcg, 8 days	800 three times daily, 8 days	18	1.02 (0.96, 1.09)	1.22 (1.15, 1.30)	1.37 (1.24, 1.51)
Isoniazid	300 once daily in the morning, 8 days	800 three times daily, 8 days	11	1.34 (1.12, 1.60)	1.12 (1.03, 1.22)	1.00 (0.92, 1.08)
Methadone[2]	20-60 once daily in the morning, 8 days	800 three times daily, 8 days	12	0.93 (0.84, 1.03)	0.96 (0.86, 1.06)	1.06 (0.96, 1.19)
Norethindrone (ORTHO-NOVUM 1/35)[1]	1 mcg, 8 days	800 three times daily, 8 days	18	1.05 (0.95, 1.16)	1.26 (1.20, 1.31)	1.44 (1.32, 1.57)
Rifabutin *150 mg once daily in the morning, 11 days + indinavir compared to	150 once daily in the morning, 10 days	800 three times daily, 10 days	14	1.29 (1.05, 1.59)	1.54 (1.33, 1.79)	1.99 (1.71, 2.31) n=13
300 mg once daily in the morning, 11 days alone	300 once daily in the morning, 10 days	800 three times daily, 10 days	10	2.34 (1.64, 3.35)	2.73 (1.99, 3.77)	3.44 (2.65, 4.46) n=9

(Table continued on next page)

Table 3 (cont.): Drug Interactions: Pharmacokinetic Parameters for Coadministered Drug in the Presence of Indinavir (See PRECAUTIONS, Table 9 for Recommended Alterations in Dose or Regimen)

Coadministered drug	Dose of Coadministered drug (mg)	Dose of CRIXIVAN (mg)	n	Ratio (with/without CRIXIVAN) of Coadministered Drug Pharmacokinetic Parameters (90% CI); No Effect = 1.00		
				C_{max}	AUC	C_{min}
Ritonavir	100 twice daily, 14 days	800 twice daily, 14 days	10, 4[3]	1.61 (1.13, 2.29)	1.72) (1.20, 2.48)	1.62 (0.93, 2.85)
	200 twice daily, 14 days	800 twice daily, 14 days	9, 5[3]	1.19 (0.85, 1.66)	1.96 (1.39, 2.76)	4.71 (2.66, 8.33) n=9, 4
Saquinavir						
Hard gel formulation	600 single dose	800 three times daily, 2 days	6	4.7 (2.7, 8.1)	6.0 (4.0, 9.1)	2.9 (1.7, 4.7)[4]
Soft gel formulation	800 single dose	800 three times daily, 2 days	6	6.5 (4.7, 9.1)	7.2 (4.3, 11.9)	5.5 (2.2, 14.1)[4]
Soft gel formulation	1200 single dose	800 three times daily, 2 days	6	4.0 (2.7, 5.9)	4.6 (3.2, 6.7)	5.5 (3.7, 8.3)[4]
Sildenafil	25 single dose	800 three times daily	6	See text below for discussion of interaction.		
Stavudine[5]	40 twice daily, 7 days	800 three times daily, 7 days	13	0.86 (0.73, 1.03)	1.21 (1.09, 1.33)	Not Done
Theophylline	250 single dose (on Days 1 and 7)	800 three times daily, 6 days (Days 2 to 7)	12, 4[3]	0.88 (0.76, 1.03)	1.14 (1.04, 1.24)	1.13 (0.86, 1,49) n=7, 3
Trimethoprim/ Sulfamethoxazole Trimethoprim	800 Trimethoprim/ 160 Sulfamethoxazole q12h, 7 days	400 q6h, 7 days	12	1.18 (1.05, 1.32)	1.18 (1.05, 1.33)	1.18 (1.00, 1.39)
Trimethoprim/ Sulfamethoxazole Sulfamethoxazole	800 Trimethoprim/ 160 Sulfamethoxazole q12h, 7 days	400 q6h, 7 days	12	1.01 (0.95, 1.08)	1.05 (1.01, 1.09)	1.05 (0.97, 1.14)
Vardenafil	10 single dose	800 three times daily	18	See text below for discussion of interaction.		
Zidovudine[5]	200 three times daily, 7 days	1000 three times daily, 7 days	12	0.89 (0.73, 1.09)	1.17 (1.07, 1.29)	1.51 (0.71, 3.20) n=4
Zidovudine/ Lamivudine[5] Zidovudine	200/150 three times daily, 7 days	800 three times daily, 7 days	6, 7[3]	1.23 (0.74, 2.03)	1.39 (1.02, 1.89)	1.08 (0.77, 1.50) n=5, 5
Zidovudine/ Lamivudine[5] Lamivudine	200/150 three times daily, 7 days	800 three times daily, 7 days	6, 7[3]	0.73 (0.52, 1.02)	0.91 (0.66, 1.26)	0.88 (0.59, 1.33)

All interaction studies conducted in healthy, HIV-negative adult subjects, unless otherwise indicated.
[1] Registered trademark of Ortho Pharmaceutical Corporation
[2] Study conducted in subjects on methadone maintenance.
[3] Parallel group design; n for coadministered drug + indinavir, n for coadministered drug alone.
[4] C_{6hr}
[5] Study conducted in HIV-positive subjects.

Methadone: Administration of indinavir (800 mg every 8 hours) with methadone (20 mg to 60 mg daily) for one week in subjects on methadone maintenance resulted in no change in methadone AUC. Based on a comparison to historical data, there was little or no change in indinavir AUC.
Ritonavir: Compared to historical data in patients who received indinavir 800 mg every 8 hours alone, twice-daily coadministration to volunteers of indinavir 800 mg and ritonavir with food for two weeks resulted in a 2.7-fold increase of indinavir AUC_{24h}, a 1.6-fold increase in indinavir C_{max}, and an 11-fold increase in indinavir C_{min} for a 100-mg ritonavir dose and a 3.6-fold increase of indinavir AUC_{24h}, a 1.8-fold increase in indinavir C_{max}, and a 24-fold increase in indinavir C_{min} for a 200-mg ritonavir dose. In the same study, twice-daily coadministration of indinavir (800 mg) and ritonavir (100 or 200 mg) resulted in ritonavir AUC_{24h} increases versus the same doses of ritonavir alone (see Table 3).
Sildenafil: The results of one published study in HIV-infected men (n=6) indicated that coadministration of indinavir (800 mg every 8 hours chronically) with a single 25-mg dose of sildenafil resulted in an 11% increase in average AUC_{0-8hr} of indinavir and a 48% increase in average indinavir peak concentration (C_{max}) compared to 800 mg every 8 hours alone. Average sildenafil AUC was increased by 340% following coadministration of sildenafil and indinavir compared to historical data following administration of sildenafil alone (see CONTRAINDICATIONS, WARNINGS, *Drug Interactions* and PRECAUTIONS, *Drug Interactions*).
Vardenafil: Indinavir (800 mg every 8 hours) coadministered with a single 10-mg dose of vardenafil resulted in a 16-fold increase in vardenafil AUC, a 7-fold increase in vardenafil C_{max}, and a 2-fold increase in vardenafil half-life (see WARNINGS, *Drug Interactions* and PRECAUTIONS, *Drug Interactions*).

INDICATIONS AND USAGE

CRIXIVAN in combination with antiretroviral agents is indicated for the treatment of HIV infection.
This indication is based on two clinical trials of approximately 1 year duration that demonstrated: 1) a reduction in the risk of AIDS-defining illnesses or death; 2) a prolonged suppression of HIV RNA.
Description of Studies
In all clinical studies, with the exception of ACTG 320, the AMPLICOR HIV MONITOR assay was used to determine the level of circulating HIV RNA in serum. This is an experimental use of the assay. HIV RNA results should not be directly compared to results from other trials using different HIV RNA assays or using other sample sources.

Study ACTG 320 was a multicenter, randomized, double-blind clinical endpoint trial to compare the effect of CRIXIVAN in combination with zidovudine and lamivudine with that of zidovudine plus lamivudine on the progression to an AIDS-defining illness (ADI) or death. Patients were protease inhibitor and lamivudine naive and zidovudine experienced, with CD4 cell counts of ≤200 cells/mm³. The study enrolled 1156 HIV-infected patients (17% female, 28% Black, 18% Hispanic, mean age 39 years). The mean baseline CD4 cell count was 87 cells/mm³. The mean baseline HIV RNA was 4.95 $\log_{10}$ copies/mL (89,035 copies/mL). The study was terminated after a planned interim analysis, resulting in a median follow-up of 38 weeks and a maximum follow-up of 52 weeks. Results are shown in Table 4 and Figures 1 & 2.

Table 4: ACTG 320

Endpoint	Number (%) of Patients with AIDS-defining Illness or Death	
	IDV+ZDV+L (n=577)	ZDV+L (n=579)
HIV Progression or Death	35 (6.1)	63 (10.9)
Death*	10 (1.7)	19 (3.3)

* The number of deaths is inadequate to assess the impact of Indinavir on survival.
IDV = Indinavir, ZDV = Zidovudine, L = Lamivudine

Study ACTG 320: Figure 1 - Indinavir Protocol ACTG 320 Zidovudine Experienced Plasma Viral RNA - Proportions Below 400 copies/mL

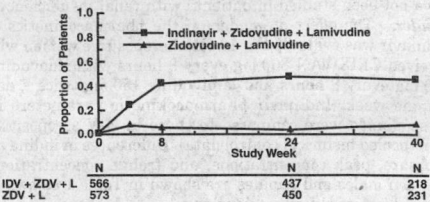

	N	N	N
IDV + ZDV + L	566	437	218
ZDV + L	573	450	231

Study ACTG 320: Figure 2 - ACTG 320 Zidovudine Experienced CD4 Cell Counts - Mean Change from Baseline

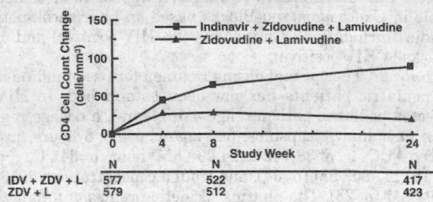

	N	N	N
IDV + ZDV + L	577	522	417
ZDV + L	579	512	423

Study 028, a double-blind, multicenter, randomized, clinical endpoint trial conducted in Brazil, compared the effects of CRIXIVAN plus zidovudine with those of CRIXIVAN alone or zidovudine alone on the progression to an ADI or death, and on surrogate marker responses. All patients were antiretroviral naive with CD4 cell counts of 50 to 250 cells/mm³. The study enrolled 996 HIV-1 seropositive patients [28% female, 11% Black, 1% Asian/Other, median age 33 years, mean baseline CD4 cell count of 152 cells/mm³, mean serum viral RNA of 4.44 $\log_{10}$ copies/mL (27,824 copies/mL)]. Treatment regimens containing zidovudine were modified in a blinded manner with the optional addition of lamivudine (median time: week 40). The median length of follow-up was 56 weeks with a maximum of 97 weeks. The study was terminated after a planned interim analysis, resulting in a median follow-up of 56 weeks and a maximum follow-up of 97 weeks. Results are shown in Table 5 and Figures 3 and 4.

Table 5: Protocol 028

Endpoint	Number (%) of Patients with AIDS-defining Illness or Death		
	IDV+ZDV (n=332)	IDV (n=332)	ZDV (n=332)
HIV Progression or Death	21 (6.3)	27 (8.1)	62 (18.7)
Death*	8 (2.4)	5 (1.5)	11 (3.3)

*The number of deaths is inadequate to assess the impact of Indinavir on survival.

Study 028: Figure 3 - Indinavir Protocol 028 Zidovudine Naive Viral RNA - Proportions Below 500 Copies/mL in Serum

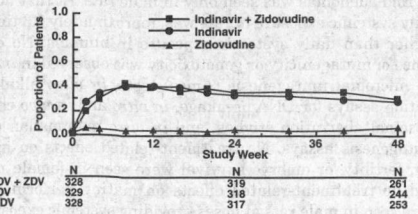

	N	N	N
IDV + ZDV	328	319	261
IDV	329	318	244
ZDV	328	317	253

Study 028: Figure 4 - Indinavir Protocol 028 Zidovudine Naive CD4 Cell Counts - Mean Change from Baseline

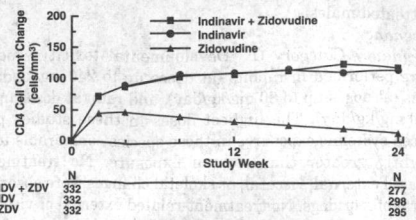

	N	N
IDV + ZDV	332	277
IDV	332	298
ZDV	332	295

Study 035 was a multicenter, randomized trial in 97 HIV-1 seropositive patients who were zidovudine-experienced (median exposure 30 months), protease-inhibitor- and lamivudine-naive, with mean baseline CD4 count 175 cells/mm³ and mean baseline serum viral RNA 4.62 log₁₀ copies/mL (41,230 copies/mL). Comparisons included CRIXIVAN plus zidovudine plus lamivudine vs. CRIXIVAN alone vs. zidovudine plus lamivudine. After at least 24 weeks of randomized, double-blind therapy, patients were switched to open-label CRIXIVAN plus lamivudine plus zidovudine. Mean changes in log₁₀ viral RNA in serum, the proportions of patients with viral RNA below 500 copies/mL in serum, and mean changes in CD4 cell counts, during 24 weeks of randomized, double-blinded therapy are summarized in Figures 5, 6, and 7, respectively. A limited number of patients remained on randomized, double-blind treatment for longer periods; based on this extended treatment experience, it appears that a greater number of subjects randomized to CRIXIVAN plus zidovudine plus lamivudine demonstrated HIV RNA levels below 500 copies/mL during one year of therapy as compared to those in other treatment groups.

Study 035: Figure 5 - Indinavir Protocol 035 Zidovudine Experienced Viral RNA - Mean Log10 Change from Baseline in Serum

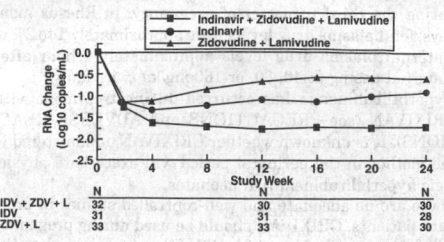

	N	N	N
IDV + ZDV + L	32	30	30
IDV	31	31	28
ZDV + L	33	33	30

Study 035: Figure 6 - Indinavir Protocol 035 Zidovudine Experienced Viral RNA - Proportions Below 500 Copies/mL in Serum

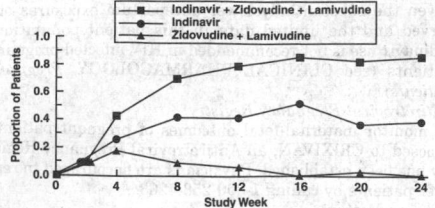

[See figure 7 at top of next column]

Genotypic Resistance in Clinical Studies

Study 006 (10/15/93-10/12/94) was a dose-ranging study in which patients were initially treated with CRIXIVAN at a dose of <2.4 g/day followed by 2.4 g/day. Study 019 (6/23/94-4/10/95) was a randomized comparison of CRIXIVAN 600 mg every 6 hours, CRIXIVAN plus zidovudine, and zidovudine alone. Table 6 shows the incidence of genotypic resistance at 24 weeks in these studies.

Study 035: Figure 7 - Indinavir Protocol 035 Zidovudine Experienced CD4 Cell Counts - Mean Change from Baseline

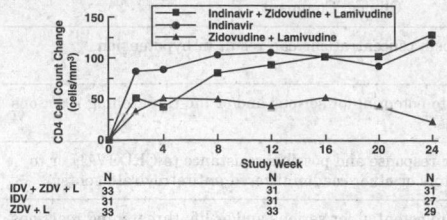

	N	N	N
IDV + ZDV + L	33	31	31
IDV	31	33	27
ZDV + L	31	33	29

Table 6: Genotypic Resistance at 24 Weeks

Treatment Group	Resistance to IDV n/N*	Resistance to ZDV n/N*
IDV		—
<2.4 g/day	31/37 (84%)	—
2.4 g/day	9/21 (43%)	1/17 (6%)
IDV/ZDV	4/22 (18%)	1/22 (5%)
ZDV	1/18 (6%)	11/17 (65%)

* N - includes patients with non-amplifiable virus at 24 weeks who had amplifiable virus at week 0.

CONTRAINDICATIONS

CRIXIVAN is contraindicated in patients with clinically significant hypersensitivity to any of its components.
Inhibition of CYP3A4 by CRIXIVAN can result in elevated plasma concentrations of the following drugs, potentially causing serious or life-threatening reactions:

Table 7: Drug Interactions With Crixivan: Contraindicated Drugs

Drug Class	Drugs Within Class That Are Contraindicated With CRIXIVAN
Alpha 1-adrenoreceptor antagonist	alfuzosin
Antiarrhythmics	amiodarone
Ergot derivatives	dihydroergotamine, ergonovine, ergotamine, methylergonovine
GI motility agents	cisapride
Neuroleptics	pimozide
PDE5 Inhibitors	Revatio[1] (sildenafil) [for treatment of pulmonary arterial hypertension]
Sedative/ hypnotics	oral midazolam, triazolam, alprazolam

[1] Registered trademark of Pfizer, Inc.

WARNINGS

ALERT: Find out about medicines that should NOT be taken with CRIXIVAN. This statement is included on the product's bottle label.
Nephrolithiasis/Urolithiasis
Nephrolithiasis/urolithiasis has occurred with CRIXIVAN therapy. The cumulative frequency of nephrolithiasis is substantially higher in pediatric patients (29%) than in adult patients (12.4%; range across individual trials: 4.7% to 34.4%). The cumulative frequency of nephrolithiasis events increases with increasing exposure to CRIXIVAN; however, the risk over time remains relatively constant. In some cases, nephrolithiasis/urolithiasis has been associated with renal insufficiency or acute renal failure, pyelonephritis with or without bacteremia. If signs or symptoms of nephrolithiasis/urolithiasis occur, (including flank pain, with or without hematuria or microscopic hematuria), temporary interruption (e.g., 1-3 days) or discontinuation of therapy may be considered. **Adequate hydration is recommended in all patients treated with CRIXIVAN. (See ADVERSE REACTIONS and DOSAGE AND ADMINISTRATION,** *Nephrolithiasis/Urolithiasis*.)
Hemolytic Anemia
Acute hemolytic anemia, including cases resulting in death, has been reported in patients treated with CRIXIVAN. Once a diagnosis is apparent, appropriate measures for the treatment of hemolytic anemia should be instituted, including discontinuation of CRIXIVAN.

Hepatitis
Hepatitis including cases resulting in hepatic failure and death has been reported in patients treated with CRIXIVAN. Because the majority of these patients had confounding medical conditions and/or were receiving concomitant therapy(ies), a causal relationship between CRIXIVAN and these events has not been established.
Hyperglycemia
New onset diabetes mellitus, exacerbation of pre-existing diabetes mellitus and hyperglycemia have been reported during post-marketing surveillance in HIV-infected patients receiving protease inhibitor therapy. Some patients required either initiation or dose adjustments of insulin or oral hypoglycemic agents for treatment of these events. In some cases, diabetic ketoacidosis has occurred. In those patients who discontinued protease inhibitor therapy, hyperglycemia persisted in some cases. Because these events have been reported voluntarily during clinical practice, estimates of frequency cannot be made and a causal relationship between protease inhibitor therapy and these events has not been established.
Drug Interactions
Concomitant use of CRIXIVAN with lovastatin, simvastatin, or rosuvastatin is not recommended. Caution should be exercised if HIV protease inhibitors, including CRIXIVAN, are used concurrently with atorvastatin. The interaction of CRIXIVAN with pravastatin and fluvastatin is not known. The risk of myopathy including rhabdomyolysis may be increased when HIV protease inhibitors, including CRIXIVAN, are used in combination with these statin drugs (see PRECAUTIONS, *Drug Interactions*).
Midazolam is extensively metabolized by CYP3A4. Coadministration with CRIXIVAN with or without ritonavir may cause a large increase in the concentration of this benzodiazepine. No drug interaction study has been performed for the co-administration of CRIXIVAN with benzodiazepines. Based on data from other CYP3A4 inhibitors, plasma concentrations of midazolam are expected to be significantly higher when midazolam is given orally. Therefore CRIXIVAN should not be co-administered with orally administered midazolam (see CONTRAINDICATIONS), whereas caution should be used with co-administration of CRIXIVAN and parenteral midazolam. Data from concomitant use of parenteral midazolam with other protease inhibitors suggest a possible 3-4 fold increase in midazolam plasma levels. If CRIXIVAN with or without ritonavir is co-administered with parenteral midazolam, it should be done in a setting which ensures close clinical monitoring and appropriate medical management in case of respiratory depression and/or prolonged sedation. Dosage reduction for midazolam should be considered, especially if more than a single dose of midazolam is administered.
Particular caution should be used when prescribing sildenafil, tadalafil, or vardenafil in patients receiving indinavir. Coadministration of CRIXIVAN with these medications is expected to substantially increase plasma concentrations of sildenafil, tadalafil, and vardenafil and may result in an increase in adverse events, including hypotension, visual changes, and priapism, which have been associated with sildenafil, tadalafil, and vardenafil (see CONTRAINDICATIONS and PRECAUTIONS, *Drug Interactions* and *Information for Patients*, and the manufacturer's complete prescribing information for sildenafil, tadalafil, or vardenafil).
Concomitant use of CRIXIVAN and St. John's wort (*Hypericum perforatum*) or products containing St. John's wort is not recommended. Coadministration of CRIXIVAN and St. John's wort has been shown to substantially decrease indinavir concentrations (see CLINICAL PHARMACOLOGY, *Drug Interactions*) and may lead to loss of virologic response and possible resistance to CRIXIVAN or to the class of protease inhibitors.

PRECAUTIONS
General
Indirect hyperbilirubinemia has occurred frequently during treatment with CRIXIVAN and has infrequently been associated with increases in serum transaminases (see also ADVERSE REACTIONS, *Clinical Trials* and *Post-Marketing Experience*). It is not known whether CRIXIVAN will exacerbate the physiologic hyperbilirubinemia seen in neonates. (See *Pregnancy*.)
Tubulointerstitial Nephritis
Reports of tubulointerstitial nephritis with medullary calcification and cortical atrophy have been observed in patients with asymptomatic severe leukocyturia (>100 cells/high power field). Patients with asymptomatic severe leukocyturia should be followed closely and monitored frequently with urinalyses. Further diagnostic evaluation may be warranted, and discontinuation of CRIXIVAN should be considered in all patients with severe leukocyturia.
Immune reconstitution syndrome has been reported in patients treated with combination antiretroviral therapy (CART), including CRIXIVAN. During the initial phase of treatment, patients responding to antiretroviral therapy

Table 8: Drugs That Should Not Be Coadministered with CRIXIVAN

Drug Class: Drug Name	Clinical Comment
Alpha 1-adrenoreceptor antagonist: alfuzosin	Potentially increased alfuzosin concentrations can result in hypotension.
Antiarrhythmics: amiodarone	CONTRAINDICATED due to potential for serious and/or life-threatening reactions such as cardiac arrhythmias.
Antimycobacterial: rifampin	May lead to loss of virologic response and possible resistance to CRIXIVAN or to the class of protease inhibitors or other coadministered antiretroviral agents.
Ergot derivatives: dihydroergotamine, ergonovine, ergotamine, methylergonovine	CONTRAINDICATED due to potential for serious and/or life-threatening reactions such as acute ergot toxicity characterized by peripheral vasospasm and ischemia of the extremitites and other tissues.
GI motility agents: cisapride	CONTRAINDICATED due to potential for serious and/or life-threatening reactions such as cardiac arrhythmias.
Herbal products: St. John's wort (*Hypericum perforatum*)	May lead to loss of virologic response and possible resistance to CRIXIVAN or to the class of protease inhibitors.
HMG-CoA Reductase inhibitors: lovastatin, simvastatin, rosuvastatin	Potential for serious reactions such as risk of myopathy including rhabdomyolysis.
Neuroleptic: pimozide	CONTRAINDICATED due to potential for serious and/or life-threatening reactions such as cardiac arrhythmias.
PDE5 inhibitor: Revatio[1] (sildenafil) [for treatment of pulmonary arterial hypertension]	A safe and effective dose has not been established when used with CRIXIVAN. There is increased potential for seldenafil-associated adverse events (which include visual disturbances, hypotension, prolonged erection, and syncope).
Protease inhibitor: atazanavir	Both CRIXIVAN and atazanavir are associated with indirect (unconjugated) hyperbilirubinemia. Combinations of these drugs have not been studied and coadministration of CRIXIVAN and atazanavir is not recommended.
Sedative/hypnotics: Oral midazolam, triazolam, alprazolam	CONTRAINDICATED due to potential for serious and/or life-threatening reactions such as prolonged or increased sedation or respiratory depression.

[1] Registered trademark of Pfizer, Inc.

whose immune system responds to CART may develop an inflammatory response to indolent or residual opportunistic infections (such as MAI, CMV, PCP, or TB), which may necessitate further evaluation and treatment.

Coexisting Conditions
Patients with hemophilia: There have been reports of spontaneous bleeding in patients with hemophilia A and B treated with protease inhibitors. In some patients, additional factor VIII was required. In many of the reported cases, treatment with protease inhibitors was continued or restarted. A causal relationship between protease inhibitor therapy and these episodes has not been established. (See ADVERSE REACTIONS, *Post-Marketing Experience*.)
Patients with hepatic insufficiency due to cirrhosis: In these patients, the dosage of CRIXIVAN should be lowered because of decreased metabolism of CRIXIVAN (see DOSAGE AND ADMINISTRATION).
Patients with renal insufficiency: Patients with renal insufficiency have not been studied.

Fat Redistribution
Redistribution/accumulation of body fat including central obesity, dorsocervical fat enlargement (buffalo hump), peripheral wasting, facial wasting, breast enlargement, and "cushingoid appearance" have been observed in patients receiving antiretroviral therapy. The mechanism and long-term consequences of these events are currently unknown. A causal relationship has not been established.

Information for Patients
A statement to patients and health care providers is included on the product's bottle label. **ALERT: Find out about medicines that should NOT be taken with CRIXIVAN.** A Patient Package Insert (PPI) for CRIXIVAN is available for patient information.
CRIXIVAN is not a cure for HIV infection and patients may continue to develop opportunistic infections and other complications associated with HIV disease. The long-term effects of CRIXIVAN are unknown at this time. CRIXIVAN has not been shown to reduce the risk of transmission of HIV to others through sexual contact or blood contamination.
Patients should be advised to remain under the care of a physician when using CRIXIVAN and should not modify or discontinue treatment without first consulting the physician. Therefore, if a dose is missed, patients should take the next dose at the regularly scheduled time and should not double this dose. Therapy with CRIXIVAN should be initiated and maintained at the recommended dosage.

CRIXIVAN may interact with some drugs; therefore, patients should be advised to report to their doctor the use of any other prescription, non-prescription medication or herbal products, particularly St. John's wort.
For optimal absorption, CRIXIVAN should be administered without food but with water 1 hour before or 2 hours after a meal. Alternatively, CRIXIVAN may be administered with other liquids such as skim milk, juice, coffee, or tea, or with a light meal, e.g., dry toast with jelly, juice, and coffee with skim milk and sugar; or corn flakes, skim milk and sugar (see CLINICAL PHARMACOLOGY, *Effect of Food on Oral Absorption* and DOSAGE AND ADMINISTRATION). Ingestion of CRIXIVAN with a meal high in calories, fat, and protein reduces the absorption of indinavir.
Patients receiving a phosphodiesterase type 5 (PDE5) inhibitor (sildenafil, tadalafil, or vardenafil) should be advised that they may be at an increased risk of PDE5 inhibitor-associated adverse events including hypotension, visual changes, and priapism, and should promptly report any symptoms to their doctors (see CONTRAINDICATIONS and WARNINGS, *Drug Interactions*).
Patients should be informed that redistribution or accumulation of body fat may occur in patients receiving antiretroviral therapy and that the cause and long-term health effects of these conditions are not known at this time.
CRIXIVAN Capsules are sensitive to moisture. Patients should be informed that CRIXIVAN should be stored and used in the original container and the desiccant should remain in the bottle.

Drug Interactions
Indinavir is an inhibitor of the cytochrome P450 isoform CYP3A4. Coadministration of CRIXIVAN and drugs primarily metabolized by CYP3A4 may result in increased plasma concentrations of the other drug, which could increase or prolong its therapeutic and adverse effects (see CONTRAINDICATIONS and WARNINGS).
Indinavir is metabolized by CYP3A4. Drugs that induce CYP3A4 activity would be expected to increase the clearance of indinavir, resulting in lowered plasma concentrations of indinavir. Coadministration of CRIXIVAN and other drugs that inhibit CYP3A4 may decrease the clearance of indinavir and may result in increased plasma concentrations of indinavir.
[See table 8 above]
[See table 9 on pages 2013 and 2014]
Carcinogenesis, Mutagenesis, Impairment of Fertility
Carcinogenicity studies were conducted in mice and rats. In mice, no increased incidence of any tumor type was ob-

served. The highest dose tested in rats was 640 mg/kg/day; at this dose a statistically significant increased incidence of thyroid adenomas was seen only in male rats. At that dose, daily systemic exposure in rats was approximately 1.3 times higher than daily systemic exposure in humans. No evidence of mutagenicity or genotoxicity was observed in *in vitro* microbial mutagenesis (Ames) tests, *in vitro* alkaline elution assays for DNA breakage, *in vitro* and *in vivo* chromosomal aberration studies, and *in vitro* mammalian cell mutagenesis assays. No treatment-related effects on mating, fertility, or embryo survival were seen in female rats and no treatment-related effects on mating performance were seen in male rats at doses providing systemic exposure comparable to or slightly higher than that with the clinical dose. In addition, no treatment-related effects were observed in fecundity or fertility of untreated females mated to treated males.

Pregnancy
Pregnancy Category C: Developmental toxicity studies were performed in rabbits (at doses up to 240 mg/kg/day), dogs (at doses up to 80 mg/kg/day), and rats (at doses up to 640 mg/kg/day). The highest doses in these studies produced systemic exposures in these species comparable to or slightly greater than human exposure. No treatment-related external, visceral, or skeletal changes were observed in rabbits or dogs. No treatment-related external or visceral changes were observed in rats. Treatment-related increases over controls in the incidence of supernumerary ribs (at exposures at or below those in humans) and of cervical ribs (at exposures comparable to or slightly greater than those in humans) were seen in rats. In all three species, no treatment-related effects on embryonic/fetal survival or fetal weights were observed.
In rabbits, at a maternal dose of 240 mg/kg/day, no drug was detected in fetal plasma 1 hour after dosing. Fetal plasma drug levels 2 hours after dosing were approximately 3% of maternal plasma drug levels. In dogs, at a maternal dose of 80 mg/kg/day, fetal plasma drug levels were approximately 50% of maternal plasma drug levels both 1 and 2 hours after dosing. In rats, at maternal doses of 40 and 640 mg/kg/day, fetal plasma drug levels were approximately 10 to 15% and 10 to 20% of maternal plasma drug levels 1 and 2 hours after dosing, respectively.
Indinavir was administered to Rhesus monkeys during the third trimester of pregnancy (at doses up to 160 mg/kg twice daily) and to neonatal Rhesus monkeys (at doses up to 160 mg/kg twice daily). When administered to neonates, indinavir caused an exacerbation of the transient physiologic hyperbilirubinemia seen in this species after birth; serum bilirubin values were approximately fourfold above controls at 160 mg/kg twice daily. A similar exacerbation did not occur in neonates after *in utero* exposure to indinavir during the third trimester of pregnancy. In Rhesus monkeys, fetal plasma drug levels were approximately 1 to 2% of maternal plasma drug levels approximately 1 hour after maternal dosing at 40, 80, or 160 mg/kg twice daily.
Hyperbilirubinemia has occurred during treatment with CRIXIVAN (see PRECAUTIONS and ADVERSE REACTIONS). It is unknown whether CRIXIVAN administered to the mother in the perinatal period will exacerbate physiologic hyperbilirubinemia in neonates.
There are no adequate and well-controlled studies in pregnant patients. CRIXIVAN should be used during pregnancy only if the potential benefit justifies the potential risk to the fetus.
A CRIXIVAN dose of 800 mg every 8 hours (with zidovudine 200 mg every 8 hours and lamivudine 150 mg twice a day) has been studied in 16 HIV-infected pregnant patients at 14 to 28 weeks of gestation at enrollment (study PACTG 358). Given the substantially lower antepartum exposures observed and the limited data in this patient population, indinavir use is not recommended in HIV-infected pregnant patients (see CLINICAL PHARMACOLOGY, *Pregnant Patients*).
Antiretroviral Pregnancy Registry
To monitor maternal-fetal outcomes of pregnant patients exposed to CRIXIVAN, an Antiretroviral Pregnancy Registry has been established. Physicians are encouraged to register patients by calling 1-800-258-4263.
Nursing Mothers
Studies in lactating rats have demonstrated that indinavir is excreted in milk. Although it is not known whether CRIXIVAN is excreted in human milk, there exists the potential for adverse effects from indinavir in nursing infants. Mothers should be instructed to discontinue nursing if they are receiving CRIXIVAN. This is consistent with the recommendation by the U.S. Public Health Service Centers for Disease Control and Prevention that HIV-infected mothers not breast-feed their infants to avoid risking postnatal transmission of HIV.

Table 9: Established and Other Potentially Significant Drug Interactions: Alteration in Dose or Regimen May Be Recommended Based on Drug Interaction Studies or Predicted Interaction (See also CLINICAL PHARMACOLOGY for magnitude of interaction, WARNINGS and DOSAGE AND ADMINISTRATION.)

Drug Name	Effect	Clinical Comment
HIV Antiviral Agents		
Delavirdine	↑ indinavir concentration	Dose reduction of CRIXIVAN to 600 mg every 8 hours should be considered when taking delavirdine 400 mg three times a day.
Didanosine		Indinavir and didanosine formulations containing buffer should be administered at least one hour apart on an empty stomach.
Efavirenz	↓ indinavir concentration	The optimal dose of indinavir, when given in combination with efavirenz, is not known. Increasing the indinavir dose to 1000 mg every 8 hours does not compensate for the increased indinavir metabolism due to efavirenz.
Nelfinavir	↑ indinavir concentration	The appropriate doses for this combination, with respect to efficacy and safety, have not been established.
Nevirapine	↓ indinavir concentration	Indinavir concentrations may be decreased in the presence of nevirapine. The appropriate doses for this combination, with respect to efficacy and safety, have not been established.
Ritonavir	↑ indinavir concentration ↑ ritonavir concentration	The appropriate doses for this combination, with respect to efficacy and safety, have not been established. Preliminary clinical data suggest that the incidence of nephrolithiasis is higher in patients receiving indinavir in combination with ritonavir than those receiving CRIXIVAN 800 mg q8h.
Saquinavir	↑ saquinavir concentration	The appropriate doses for this combination, with respect to efficacy and safety, have not been established.
Other Agents		
Antiarrhythmics: bepridil, lidocaine (systemic) and quinidine	↑ antiarrhythmic agents concentration	Caution is warranted and therapeutic concentration monitoring is recommended for antiarrhythmics when coadministered with CRIXIVAN.
Anticonvulsants: carbamazepine, phenobarbital, phenytoin	↓ indinavir concentration	Use with caution. CRIXIVAN may not be effective due to decreased indinavir concentrations in patients taking these agents concomitantly.
Antidepressant: Trazodone	↑ trazodone concentration	Concomitant use of trazodone and CRIXIVAN may increase plasma concentrations of trazodone. Adverse events of nausea, dizziness, hypotension and syncope have been observed following coadministration of trazodone and ritonavir. If trazodone is used with a CYP3A4 inhibitor such as CRIXIVAN, the combination should be used with caution and a lower dose of trazodone should be considered.
Anti-gout: Colchicine	↑ colchicine concentration	Patients with renal or hepatic impairment should not be given colchicine with CRIXIVAN. ***Treatment of gout flares:*** Co-administration of colchicine in patients on CRIXIVAN: 0.6 mg (1 tablet) × 1 dose, followed by 0.3 mg (half tablet) 1 hour later. Dose to be repeated no earlier than 3 days. ***Prophylaxis of gout flares:*** Co-administration of colchicine in patients on CRIXIVAN: If the original colchicine regimen was 0.6 mg twice a day, the regimen should be adjusted to 0.3 mg once a day. If the original colchicine regimen was 0.6 mg once a day, the regimen should be adjusted to 0.3 mg once every other day. ***Treatment of familial Mediterranean fever (FMF):*** Co-administration of colchicine in patients on CRIXIVAN: Maximum daily dose of 0.6 mg (may be given as 0.3 mg twice a day).
Calcium Channel Blockers, Dihydropyridine: e.g., felodipine, nifedipine, nicardipine	↑ dihydropyridine calcium channel blockers concentration	Caution is warranted and clinical monitoring of patients is recommended.
Clarithromycin	↑ clarithromycin concentration ↑ indinavir concentration	The appropriate doses for this combination, with respect to efficacy and safety, have not been established.
Endothelin receptor antagonist: Bosentan	↑ bosentan concentration	Co-administration of bosentan in patients on CRIXIVAN or co-administration of CRIXIVAN in patients on bosentan: Start at or adjust bosentan to 62.5 mg once daily or every other day based upon individual tolerability.

(Table continued on next page)

Pediatric Use
The optimal dosing regimen for use of indinavir in pediatric patients has not been established. A dose of 500 mg/m² every eight hours has been studied in uncontrolled studies of 70 children, 3 to 18 years of age. The pharmacokinetic profiles of indinavir at this dose were not comparable to profiles previously observed in adults receiving the recommended dose (see CLINICAL PHARMACOLOGY, *Pediatric*). Although viral suppression was observed in some of the 32 children who were followed on this regimen through 24 weeks, a substantially higher rate of nephrolithiasis was reported when compared to adult historical data (see WARNINGS, *Nephrolithiasis/Urolithiasis*). Physicians considering the use of indinavir in pediatric patients without other protease inhibitor options should be aware of the limited data available in this population and the increased risk of nephrolithiasis.

Geriatric Use
Clinical studies of CRIXIVAN did not include sufficient numbers of subjects aged 65 and over to determine whether they respond differently from younger subjects. In general, dose selection for an elderly patient should be cautious, reflecting the greater frequency of decreased hepatic, renal or cardiac function and of concomitant disease or other drug therapy.

ADVERSE REACTIONS

Clinical Trials in Adults
Nephrolithiasis/urolithiasis, including flank pain with or without hematuria (including microscopic hematuria), has been reported in approximately 12.4% (301/2429; range across individual trials: 4.7% to 34.4%) of patients receiving CRIXIVAN at the recommended dose in clinical trials with a median follow-up of 47 weeks (range: 1 day to 242 weeks; 2238 patient-years follow-up). The cumulative frequency of nephrolithiasis events increases with duration of exposure to CRIXIVAN; however, the risk over time remains relatively constant. Of the patients treated with CRIXIVAN who developed nephrolithiasis/urolithiasis in clinical trials during the double-blind phase, 2.8% (7/246) were reported to develop hydronephrosis and 4.5% (11/246) underwent stent placement. Following the acute episode, 4.9% (12/246) of patients discontinued therapy. (See WARNINGS and DOSAGE AND ADMINISTRATION, *Nephrolithiasis/Urolithiasis*.)

Asymptomatic hyperbilirubinemia (total bilirubin ≥2.5 mg/dL), reported predominantly as elevated indirect bilirubin, has occurred in approximately 14% of patients treated with CRIXIVAN. In <1% this was associated with elevations in ALT or AST.

Hyperbilirubinemia and nephrolithiasis/urolithiasis occurred more frequently at doses exceeding 2.4 g/day compared to doses ≤2.4 g/day.

Clinical adverse experiences reported in ≥2% of patients treated with CRIXIVAN alone, CRIXIVAN in combination with zidovudine or zidovudine plus lamivudine, zidovudine alone, or zidovudine plus lamivudine are presented in Table 10.

[See table 10 at top of page 2015]

In Phase I and II controlled trials, the following adverse events were reported significantly more frequently by those randomized to the arms containing CRIXIVAN than by those randomized to nucleoside analogues: rash, upper respiratory infection, dry skin, pharyngitis, taste perversion.

Selected laboratory abnormalities of severe or life-threatening intensity reported in patients treated with CRIXIVAN alone, CRIXIVAN in combination with zidovudine or zidovudine plus lamivudine, zidovudine alone, or zidovudine plus lamivudine are presented in Table 11.

[See table 11 at top of page 2016]

Post-Marketing Experience
Body As A Whole: redistribution/accumulation of body fat (see PRECAUTIONS, *Fat Redistribution*).
Cardiovascular System: cardiovascular disorders including myocardial infarction and angina pectoris; cerebrovascular disorder.
Digestive System: liver function abnormalities; hepatitis including reports of hepatic failure (see WARNINGS); pancreatitis; jaundice; abdominal distention; dyspepsia.
Hematologic: increased spontaneous bleeding in patients with hemophilia (see PRECAUTIONS); acute hemolytic anemia (see WARNINGS).
Endocrine/Metabolic: new onset diabetes mellitus, exacerbation of pre-existing diabetes mellitus, hyperglycemia (see WARNINGS).
Hypersensitivity: anaphylactoid reactions; urticaria; vasculitis.
Musculoskeletal System: arthralgia.
Nervous System/Psychiatric: oral paresthesia; depression.
Skin and Skin Appendage: rash including erythema multiforme and Stevens-Johnson syndrome; hyperpigmentation; alopecia; ingrown toenails and/or paronychia; pruritus.
Urogenital System: nephrolithiasis/urolithiasis, in some cases resulting in renal insufficiency or acute renal failure, pyelonephritis with or without bacteremia (see WARNINGS); interstitial nephritis sometimes with indinavir crystal deposits; in some patients, the interstitial nephritis did not resolve following discontinuation of CRIXIVAN; renal insufficiency; renal failure; leukocyturia (see PRECAUTIONS), crystalluria; dysuria.

Laboratory Abnormalities
Increased serum triglycerides; increased serum cholesterol.

OVERDOSAGE

There have been more than 60 reports of acute or chronic human overdosage (up to 23 times the recommended total daily dose of 2400 mg) with CRIXIVAN. The most commonly reported symptoms were renal (e.g., nephrolithiasis/urolithiasis, flank pain, hematuria) and gastrointestinal (e.g., nausea, vomiting, diarrhea).

It is not known whether CRIXIVAN is dialyzable by peritoneal or hemodialysis.

DOSAGE AND ADMINISTRATION

The recommended dosage of CRIXIVAN is 800 mg (usually two 400-mg capsules) orally every 8 hours.

CRIXIVAN must be taken at intervals of 8 hours. For optimal absorption, CRIXIVAN should be administered without food but with water 1 hour before or 2 hours after a meal. Alternatively, CRIXIVAN may be administered with other liquids such as skim milk, juice, coffee, or tea, or with a light meal, e.g., dry toast with jelly, juice, and coffee with skim milk and sugar; or corn flakes, skim milk and sugar. (See CLINICAL PHARMACOLOGY, *Effect of Food on Oral Absorption*.)

To ensure adequate hydration, it is recommended that adults drink at least 1.5 liters (approximately 48 ounces) of liquids during the course of 24 hours.

Concomitant Therapy

(See CLINICAL PHARMACOLOGY, *Drug Interactions*, and/or PRECAUTIONS, *Drug Interactions*.)

Delavirdine

Dose reduction of CRIXIVAN to 600 mg every 8 hours should be considered when administering delavirdine 400 mg three times a day.

Didanosine

If indinavir and didanosine are administered concomitantly, they should be administered at least one hour apart on an empty stomach (consult the manufacturer's product circular for didanosine).

Itraconazole

Dose reduction of CRIXIVAN to 600 mg every 8 hours is recommended when administering itraconazole 200 mg twice daily concurrently.

Ketoconazole

Dose reduction of CRIXIVAN to 600 mg every 8 hours is recommended when administering ketoconazole concurrently.

Rifabutin

Dose reduction of rifabutin to half the standard dose (consult the manufacturer's product circular for rifabutin) and a dose increase of CRIXIVAN to 1000 mg every 8 hours are recommended when rifabutin and CRIXIVAN are coadministered.

Hepatic Insufficiency

The dosage of CRIXIVAN should be reduced to 600 mg every 8 hours in patients with mild-to-moderate hepatic insufficiency due to cirrhosis.

Nephrolithiasis/Urolithiasis

In addition to adequate hydration, medical management in patients who experience nephrolithiasis/urolithiasis may include temporary interruption (e.g., 1 to 3 days) or discontinuation of therapy.

HOW SUPPLIED

CRIXIVAN Capsules are supplied as follows:

No. 3755—100 mg capsules: semi-translucent white capsules coded "CRIXIVAN™ 100 mg" in green. Available as: **NDC** 0006-0570-62 unit-of-use bottles of 180 (with desiccant).

No. 3756—200 mg capsules: semi-translucent white capsules coded "CRIXIVAN™ 200 mg" in blue. Available as: **NDC** 0006-0571-43 unit-of-use bottles of 360 (with desiccant).

No. 3758—400 mg capsules: semi-translucent white capsules coded "CRIXIVAN™ 400 mg" in green. Available as: **NDC** 0006-0573-42 unit-dose packages of 42

NDC 0006-0573-40 unit-of-use bottles of 120 (with desiccant)

NDC 0006-0573-62 unit-of-use bottles of 180 (with desiccant)

NDC 0006-0573-54 unit-of-use bottles of 90 (with desiccant)

NDC 0006-0573-18 unit-of-use bottles of 18 (with desiccant).

Storage

Bottles: Store in a tightly-closed container at room temperature, 15-30°C (59-86°F). Protect from moisture.

CRIXIVAN Capsules are sensitive to moisture. CRIXIVAN should be dispensed and stored in the original container. The desiccant should remain in the original bottle.

Unit-Dose Packages: Store at room temperature, 15-30°C (59-86°F). Protect from moisture.

Merck Sharp & Dohme Corp., a subsidiary of

MERCK & CO., INC., Whitehouse Station, NJ 08889, USA

U.S. Patent Nos.: 5,413,999; 6,645,961

Issued April 2010

Printed in USA

9640612

Table 9 *(cont.)*: Established and Other Potentially Significant Drug Interactions: Alteration in Dose or Regimen May Be Recommended Based on Drug Interaction Studies or Predicted Interaction (See also CLINICAL PHARMACOLOGY for magnitude of interaction, WARNINGS and DOSAGE AND ADMINISTRATION.)

Drug Name	Effect	Clinical Comment
Other Agents *(continued)*		
HMG-CoA Reductase Inhibitors: atorvastatin, pravastatin, fluvastatin	↑ atorvastatin concentration pravastatin, fluvastatin-interaction not studied	Use the lowest possible dose of atorvastatin with careful monitoring. If no alternative treatment is available, use with careful monitoring.
Immunosuppressants: cyclosporine, tacrolimus, sirolimus	↑ immunosuppressant agents concentration	Plasma concentrations may be increased by CRIXIVAN.
Inhaled beta agonist: Salmeterol	↑ salmeterol	Concurrent administration of salmeterol with CRIXIVAN is not recommended. The combination may result in increased risk of cardiovascular adverse events associated with salmeterol, including QT prolongation, palpitations and sinus tachycardia.
Inhaled/nasal steroid: Fluticasone	↑ fluticasone concentration	Concomitant use of fluticasone propionate and CRIXIVAN may increase plasma concentrations of fluticasone propionate. Use with caution. Consider alternatives to fluticasone propionate, particularly for long-term use. Fluticasone use is not recommended in situations where CRIXIVAN is coadministered with a potent CYP3A4 inhibitor such as ritonavir unless the potential benefit to the patient outweighs the risk of systemic corticosteroid side effects.
Itraconazole	↑ indinavir concentration	Dose reduction of CRIXIVAN to 600 mg every 8 hours is recommended when administering itraconazole concurrently.
Ketoconazole	↑ indinavir concentration	Dose reduction of CRIXIVAN to 600 mg every 8 hours should be considered.
Midazolam (parenteral administration)	↑ midazolam concentration	Concomitant use of parenteral midazolam with CRIXIVAN may increase plasma concentrations of midazolam. Coadministration should be done in a setting which ensures close clinical monitoring and appropriate medical management in case of respiratory depression and/or prolonged sedation. Dosage reduction for midazolam should be considered, especially if more than a single dose of midazolam is administered. Coadministration of oral midazolam with CRIXIVAN is CONTRAINDICATED (see Table 8).
Rifabutin	↓ indinavir concentration ↑ rifabutin concentration	Dose reduction of rifabutin to half the standard dose and a dose increase of CRIXIVAN to 1000 mg every 8 hours are recommended when rifabutin and CRIXIVAN are coadministered.
Sildenafil	↑ sildenafil concentration (only the use of sildenafil at doses used for treatment of erectile dysfunction has been studied with CRIXIVAN)	May result in an increase in PDE5 inhibitor-associated adverse events, including hypotension, syncope, visual disturbances, and priapism. *Use of sildenafil for pulmonary arterial hypertension (PAH):* Use of Revatio[1] (sildenafil) is contraindicated when used for the treatment of pulmonary arterial hypertension (PAH) [see CONTRAINDICATIONS]. *Use of sildenafil for erectile dysfunction:* Sildenafil dose should not exceed a maximum of 25 mg in a 48-hour period in patients receiving concomitant CRIXIVAN therapy. Use with increased monitoring for adverse events.
Tadalafil	↑ tadalafil concentration	May result in an increase in PDE5 inhibitor-associated adverse events, including hypotension, visual disturbances, and priapism. *Use of tadalafil for pulmonary arterial hypertension (PAH):* The following dose adjustments are recommended for use of Adcirca[2] (tadalafil) with CRIXIVAN: Co-administration of Adcirca in patients on CRIXIVAN or co-administration of CRIXIVAN in patients on Adcirca: Start at or adjust Adcirca to 20 mg once daily. Increase to 40 mg once daily based upon individual tolerability. *Use of tadalafil for erectile dysfunction:* Tadalafil dose should not exceed a maximum of 10 mg in a 72-hour period in patients receiving concomitant CRIXIVAN therapy. Use with increased monitoring for adverse events.
Vardenafil	↑ vardenafil concentration	Vardenafil dose should not exceed a maximum of 2.5 mg in a 24-hour period in patients receiving concomitant indinavir therapy.
Venlafaxine	↓ indinavir concentration	In a study of 9 healthy volunteers, venlafaxine administered under steady-state conditions at 150 mg/day resulted in a 28% decrease in the AUC of a single 800 mg oral dose of indinavir and a 36% decrease in indinavir C_{max}. Indinavir did not affect the pharmacokinetics of venlafaxine and ODV. The clinical significance of this finding is unknown.

Note: ↑ = increase; ↓ = decrease
[1] Registered trademark of Pfizer, Inc.
[2] Registered trademark of Eli Lilly and Company.

PATIENT PACKAGE INSERT

CRIXIVAN®* (indinavir sulfate) Capsules
Patient Information about
CRIXIVAN (KRIK-sih-van)
for HIV (Human Immunodeficiency Virus) Infection
Generic name: indinavir (in-DIH-nuh-veer) sulfate
ALERT: Find out about medicines that should NOT be taken with CRIXIVAN. Please also read the section "MEDICINES YOU SHOULD NOT TAKE WITH CRIXIVAN". Please read this information before you start taking CRIXIVAN. Also, read the leaflet each time you renew your prescription, just in case anything has changed. Remember, this leaflet does not take the place of careful discussions with your doctor. You and your doctor should discuss CRIXIVAN when you start taking your medication and at regular checkups. You should remain under a doctor's care when using CRIXIVAN and should not change or stop treatment without first talking with your doctor.

* Registered trademark of Merck Sharp & Dohme Corp., a subsidiary of **Merck & Co., Inc.**
Copyright © 1996, 1999 Merck Sharp & Dohme Corp., a subsidiary of **Merck & Co., Inc.**
All rights reserved

What is CRIXIVAN?
CRIXIVAN is an oral capsule used for the treatment of HIV (Human Immunodeficiency Virus). HIV is the virus that causes AIDS (acquired immune deficiency syndrome). CRIXIVAN is a type of HIV drug called a protease (PRO-tee-ase) inhibitor.

How does CRIXIVAN work?
CRIXIVAN is a protease inhibitor that fights HIV. CRIXIVAN can help reduce your chances of getting illnesses associated with HIV. CRIXIVAN can also help lower the amount of HIV in your body (called "viral load") and raise your CD4 (T) cell count. CRIXIVAN may not have these effects in all patients.
CRIXIVAN is usually prescribed with other anti-HIV drugs such as ZDV (also called AZT), 3TC, ddI, ddC, or d4T. CRIXIVAN works differently from these other anti-HIV drugs. Talk with your doctor about how you should take CRIXIVAN.

How should I take CRIXIVAN?
There are six important things you must do to help you benefit from CRIXIVAN:

1. **Take CRIXIVAN capsules every day as prescribed by your doctor.** Continue taking CRIXIVAN unless your doctor tells you to stop. Take the exact amount of CRIXIVAN that your doctor tells you to take, right from the very start. To help make sure you will benefit from CRIXIVAN, you must not skip doses or take "drug holidays". If you don't take CRIXIVAN as prescribed, the activity of CRIXIVAN may be reduced (due to resistance).

2. **Take CRIXIVAN capsules every 8 hours around the clock, every day.** It may be easier to remember to take CRIXIVAN if you take it at the same time every day. If you have questions about when to take CRIXIVAN, your doctor or health care provider can help you decide what schedule works for you.

3. **If you miss a dose by more than 2 hours, wait and then take the next dose at the regularly scheduled time.** However, if you miss a dose by less than 2 hours, take your missed dose immediately. Then take your next dose at the regularly scheduled time. Do not take more or less than your prescribed dose of CRIXIVAN at any one time.

4. **Take CRIXIVAN with water.** You can also take CRIXIVAN with other beverages such as skim or non-fat milk, juice, coffee, or tea.

5. **Ideally, take each dose of CRIXIVAN without food but with water at least one hour before or two hours after a meal.** Or you can take CRIXIVAN with a light meal. Examples of light meals include:
   dry toast with jelly, juice, and coffee (with skim or non-fat milk and sugar if you want)
   cornflakes with skim or non-fat milk and sugar
   Do not take CRIXIVAN at the same time as any meals that are high in calories, fat, and protein (for example — a bacon and egg breakfast). When taken at the same time as CRIXIVAN, these foods can interfere with CRIXIVAN being absorbed into your bloodstream and may lessen its effect.

6. **It is critical to drink plenty of fluids while taking CRIXIVAN.** Adults should drink at least six 8-ounce glasses of liquids (preferably water) throughout the day, every day. Your health care provider will give you further instructions on the amount of fluid that you should drink. **CRIXIVAN can cause kidney stones.** Having enough fluids in your body should help reduce the chances of forming a kidney stone. Call your doctor or other health care provider if you develop kidney pains (middle to lower stomach or back pain) or blood in the urine.

Table 10: Clinical Adverse Experiences Reported in ≥2% of Patients

Adverse Experience	Study 028 Considered Drug-Related and of Moderate or Severe Intensity			Study ACTG 320 of Unknown Drug Relationship and of Severe or Life-threatening Intensity	
	CRIXIVAN Percent (n=332)	CRIXIVAN plus Zidovudine Percent (n=332)	Zidovudine Percent (n=332)	CRIXIVAN plus Zidovudine plus Lamivudine Percent (n=571)	Zidovudine plus Lamivudine Percent (n=575)
Body as a Whole					
Abdominal pain	16.6	16.0	12.0	1.9	0.7
Asthenia/fatigue	2.1	4.2	3.6	2.4	4.5
Fever	1.5	1.5	2.1	3.8	3.0
Malaise	2.1	2.7	1.8	0	0
Digestive System					
Nausea	11.7	31.9	19.6	2.8	1.4
Diarrhea	3.3	3.0	2.4	0.9	1.2
Vomiting	8.4	17.8	9.0	1.4	1.4
Acid regurgitation	2.7	5.4	1.8	0.4	0
Anorexia	2.7	5.4	3.0	0.5	0.2
Appetite increase	2.1	1.5	1.2	0	0
Dyspepsia	1.5	2.7	0.9	0	0
Jaundice	1.5	2.1	0.3	0	0
Hemic and Lymphatic System					
Anemia	0.6	1.2	2.1	2.4	3.5
Musculoskeletal System					
Back pain	8.4	4.5	1.5	0.9	0.7
Nervous System / Psychiatric					
Headache	5.4	9.6	6.0	2.4	2.8
Dizziness	3.0	3.9	0.9	0.5	0.7
Somnolence	2.4	3.3	3.3	0	0
Skin and Skin Appendage					
Pruritus	4.2	2.4	1.8	0.5	0
Rash	1.2	0.6	2.4	1.1	0.5
Respiratory System					
Cough	1.5	0.3	0.6	1.6	1.0
Difficulty breathing/ dyspnea/shortness of breath	0	0.6	0.3	1.8	1.0
Urogenital System					
Nephrolithiasis/urolithiasis*	8.7	7.8	2.1	2.6	0.3
Dysuria	1.5	2.4	0.3	0.4	0.2
Special Senses					
Taste perversion	2.7	8.4	1.2	0.2	0

* Including renal colic, and flank pain with and without hematuria

Does CRIXIVAN cure HIV or AIDS?
CRIXIVAN is not a cure for HIV or AIDS. People taking CRIXIVAN may still develop infections or other conditions associated with HIV. Because of this, it is very important for you to remain under the care of a doctor. Although CRIXIVAN is not a cure for HIV or AIDS, CRIXIVAN can help reduce your chances of getting illnesses, including death, associated with HIV. CRIXIVAN may not have these effects in all patients.

Does CRIXIVAN reduce the risk of passing HIV to others?
CRIXIVAN has not been shown to reduce the risk of passing HIV to others through sexual contact or blood contamination.

Who should not take CRIXIVAN?
Do not take CRIXIVAN if you have had a serious allergic reaction to CRIXIVAN or any of its components.

What other medical problems or conditions should I discuss with my doctor?
Talk to your doctor if:
• You are pregnant or if you become pregnant while you are taking CRIXIVAN. We do not yet know how CRIXIVAN affects pregnant women or their developing babies.
• You are breast-feeding. You should stop breast-feeding if you are taking CRIXIVAN.
Also talk to your doctor if you have:
• Problems with your liver, especially if you have mild or moderate liver disease caused by cirrhosis
• Problems with your kidneys
• Diabetes
• Hemophilia
• High cholesterol and you are taking cholesterol-lowering medicines called "statins".
Tell your doctor about any medicines you are taking or plan to take, including non-prescription medicines, herbal products including St. John's wort (*Hypericum perforatum*), or dietary supplements.

Can CRIXIVAN be taken with other medications?**
MEDICINES YOU SHOULD NOT TAKE WITH CRIXIVAN

Oral VERSED® (midazolam)
ORAP® (pimozide)
PROPULSID® (cisapride)
CORDARONE® (amiodarone)
HISMANAL® (astemizole)

HALCION® (triazolam)
XANAX® (alprazolam)
REVATIO® (sildenafil for the treatment of pulmonary arterial hypertension)
UROXATRAL® (alfuzosin)
Ergot medications (e.g., Wigraine®, Cafergot®, D.H.E. 45®, Migranal®, Ergotrate®, and Methergine®)

Taking CRIXIVAN with the above medications could result in serious or life-threatening problems (such as irregular heartbeat or excessive sleepiness).
In addition, you should not take CRIXIVAN with the following:
• Rifampin, known as RIFADIN®, RIFAMATE®, RIFATER®, or RIMACTANE®.
• It is not recommended to take CRIXIVAN with the cholesterol-lowering drugs MEVACOR®* (lovastatin), ZOCOR®* (simvastatin), or CRESTOR® (rosuvastatin) because of possible drug interactions. There is also an increased risk of drug interactions between CRIXIVAN and LIPITOR® (atorvastatin); talk to your doctor before you take any of these cholesterol-reducing drugs with CRIXIVAN.
• Taking CRIXIVAN with REYATAZ® (atazanavir) is not recommended because they can both sometimes cause increased levels of bilirubin in the blood.

Table 11: Selected Laboratory Abnormalities of Severe or Life-threatening Intensity Reported in Studies 028 and ACTG 320

	CRIXIVAN	Study 028 CRIXIVAN plus Zidovudine	Zidovudine	Study ACTG 320 CRIXIVAN plus Zidovudine plus Lamivudine	Zidovudine plus Lamivudine
	Percent (n=329)	Percent (n=320)	Percent (n=330)	Percent (n=571)	Percent (n=575)
Hematology					
Decreased hemoglobin <7.0 g/dL	0.6	0.9	3.3	2.4	3.5
Decreased platelet count <50 THS/mm^3	0.9	0.9	1.8	0.2	0.9
Decreased neutrophils <0.75 THS/mm^3	2.4	2.2	6.7	5.1	14.6
Blood chemistry					
Increased ALT >500% ULN*	4.9	4.1	3.0	2.6	2.6
Increased AST >500% ULN	3.7	2.8	2.7	3.3	2.8
Total serum bilirubin >250% ULN	11.9	9.7	0.6	6.1	1.4
Increased serum amylase >200% ULN	2.1	1.9	1.8	0.9	0.3
Increased glucose >250 mg/dL	0.9	0.9	0.6	1.6	1.9
Increased creatinine >300% ULN	0	0	0.6	0.2	0

*Upper limit of the normal range.

• Taking CRIXIVAN with St. John's wort (*Hypericum perforatum*), an herbal product sold as a dietary supplement, or products containing St. John's wort is not recommended. Taking St. John's wort has been shown to decrease CRIXIVAN levels and may lead to increased viral load and possible resistance to CRIXIVAN or cross resistance to other antiretroviral drugs.

Before you take VIAGRA® (sildenafil), CIALIS® (tadalafil), or LEVITRA® (vardenafil) with CRIXIVAN, talk to your doctor about possible drug interactions and side effects. If you take any of these medicines together with CRIXIVAN, you may be at increased risk of side effects such as low blood pressure, visual changes, and penile erection lasting more than 4 hours, which have been associated with sildenafil, tadalafil, and vardenafil. If an erection lasts longer than 4 hours, you should seek immediate medical assistance to avoid permanent damage to your penis. Your doctor can explain these symptoms to you.

MEDICINES YOU CAN TAKE WITH CRIXIVAN

RETROVIR® (zidovudine, ZDV also called AZT)

EPIVIR™ (lamivudine, 3TC)

ZERIT® (stavudine, d4T)

isoniazid (INH)

BACTRIM®/SEPTRA® (trimethoprim/ sulfamethoxazole)

DIFLUCAN® (fluconazole)

BIAXIN® (clarithromycin)

ORTHO-NOVUM 1/35® (oral contraceptive)

TAGAMET® (cimetidine)

Methadone

VIDEX® (didanosine, ddI)—If you take CRIXIVAN with VIDEX, take them at least one hour apart.

MYCOBUTIN® (rifabutin)—If you take CRIXIVAN with MYCOBUTIN, your doctor may adjust both the dose of MYCOBUTIN and the dose of CRIXIVAN.

NIZORAL® (ketoconazole)—If you take CRIXIVAN with NIZORAL, your doctor may adjust the dose of CRIXIVAN.

RESCRIPTOR® (delaviridine)—If you take CRIXIVAN with RESCRIPTOR, your doctor may adjust the dose of CRIXIVAN.

SPORANOX® (itraconazole)—If you take CRIXIVAN with SPORANOX, your doctor may adjust the dose of CRIXIVAN.

SUSTIVA™ (efavirenz)—If you take CRIXIVAN with SUSTIVA, check with your doctor.

Intravenous VERSED® (midazolam)—If you take CRIXIVAN with Intravenous VERSED®, your doctor may adjust the dose of VERSED®.

Talk to your doctor about any medications you are taking.

Calcium Channel Blockers: Tell your doctor if you are taking calcium channel blockers (e.g., amlodipine, felodipine).

Antiarrhythmics: Tell your doctor if you are taking antiarrhythmics (e.g., quinidine).

Anticonvulsants: Tell your doctor if you are taking anticonvulsants (e.g., phenobarbital, phenytoin, or carbamazepine).

Steroids: Tell your doctor if you are taking steroids (e.g., dexamethasone).

** The brands listed are the registered trademarks of their respective owners and are not trademarks of Merck Sharp & Dohme Corp., a subsidiary of **Merck & Co., Inc.**

What are the possible side effects of CRIXIVAN?

Like all prescription drugs, CRIXIVAN can cause side effects. The following is **not** a complete list of side effects reported with CRIXIVAN when taken either alone or with other anti-HIV drugs. Do not rely on this leaflet alone for information about side effects. Your doctor can discuss with you a more complete list of side effects.

Some patients treated with CRIXIVAN developed kidney stones. In some of these patients this led to more severe kidney problems, including kidney failure or inflammation of the kidneys or kidney infection which sometimes spread to the blood. Drinking at least six 8-ounce glasses of liquids (preferably water) each day should help reduce the chances of forming a kidney stone (see How should I take CRIXIVAN?). Call your doctor or other health care provider if you develop kidney pains (middle to lower stomach or back pain) or blood in the urine.

Some patients treated with CRIXIVAN have had rapid breakdown of red blood cells (hemolytic anemia) which in some cases was severe or resulted in death.

Some patients treated with CRIXIVAN have had liver problems including liver failure and death. Some patients had other illnesses or were taking other drugs. It is uncertain if CRIXIVAN caused these liver problems.

Diabetes and high blood sugar (hyperglycemia) have occurred in patients taking protease inhibitors. In some of these patients, this led to ketoacidosis, a serious condition caused by poorly controlled blood sugar. Some patients had diabetes before starting protease inhibitors, others did not. Some patients required adjustments to their diabetes medication. Others needed new diabetes medication.

In some patients with hemophilia, increased bleeding has been reported.

Severe muscle pain and weakness have occurred in patients taking protease inhibitors, including CRIXIVAN, together with some of the cholesterol-lowering medicines called "statins". Call your doctor if you develop severe muscle pain or weakness.

Changes in body fat have been seen in some patients taking antiretroviral therapy. These changes may include increased amount of fat in the upper back and neck ("buffalo hump"), breast, and around the trunk. Loss of fat from the legs, arms and face may also happen. The cause and long term health effects of these conditions are not known at this time.

In some patients with advanced HIV infection (AIDS), signs and symptoms of inflammation from opportunistic infections may occur when combination antiretroviral treatment is started.

Clinical Studies

Increases in bilirubin (one laboratory test of liver function) have been reported in approximately 14% of patients. Usually, this finding has not been associated with liver problems. However, on rare occasions, a person may develop yellowing of the skin and/or eyes.

Side effects occurring in 2% or more of patients included: abdominal pain, fatigue or weakness, low red blood cell count, flank pain, painful urination, feeling unwell, nausea, upset stomach, diarrhea, vomiting, acid regurgitation, increased or decreased appetite, back pain, headache, dizziness, taste changes, rash, itchy skin, yellowing of the skin and/or eyes, upper respiratory infection, dry skin, and sore throat.

Swollen kidneys due to blocked urine flow occurred rarely.

Marketing Experience

Other side effects reported since CRIXIVAN has been marketed include: allergic reactions; severe skin reactions; yellowing of the skin and/or eyes; heart problems including heart attack; stroke; abdominal swelling; indigestion; inflammation of the kidneys; decreased kidney function; inflammation of the pancreas; joint pain; depression; itching; hives; change in skin color; hair loss; ingrown toenails with or without infection; crystals in the urine; painful urination; numbness of the mouth and increased cholesterol.

Tell your doctor promptly about these or any other unusual symptoms. If the condition persists or worsens, seek medical attention.

How should I store CRIXIVAN capsules?

• Keep CRIXIVAN capsules in the bottle they came in and at room temperature (59°-86°F).

• Keep CRIXIVAN capsules dry by leaving the small desiccant in the bottle. Keep the bottle closed.

This medication was prescribed for your particular condition. Do not use it for any other condition or give it to anybody else. Keep CRIXIVAN and all medicines out of the reach of children. If you suspect that more than the prescribed dose of this medicine has been taken, contact your local poison control center or emergency room immediately.

This leaflet provides a summary of information about CRIXIVAN. If you have any questions or concerns about either CRIXIVAN or HIV, talk to your doctor.

Merck Sharp & Dohme Corp., a subsidiary of Merck & Co., Inc.

Whitehouse Station, NJ 08889, USA

U.S. Patent Nos.: 5,413,999; 6,645,961

Issued April 2010

9640612

Shown in Product Identification Guide, page 312

DIPROLENE® AF ℞

[dĭp-rō-lēn]

brand of augmented betamethasone dipropionate*

Cream 0.05%

(potency expressed as betamethasone)

***Vehicle augments the penetration of the steroid.**

For Dermatologic Use Only — Not for Ophthalmic Use

PRODUCT INFORMATION

DESCRIPTION

DIPROLENE® AF Cream 0.05% contains betamethasone dipropionate, USP, a synthetic adrenocorticosteroid, for dermatologic use in an emollient base. Betamethasone, an analog of prednisolone, has a high degree of corticosteroid activity and a slight degree of mineralocorticoid activity. Betamethasone dipropionate is the 17,21-dipropionate ester of betamethasone.

Chemically, betamethasone dipropionate is 9-fluoro-11β, 17,21-trihydroxy-16β-methylpregna-1,4-diene-3,20-dione 17,21-dipropionate, with the empirical formula $C_{28}H_{37}FO_7$, a molecular weight of 504.6, and the following structural formula:

Betamethasone dipropionate is a white to creamy white, odorless crystalline powder, insoluble in water.

Each gram of DIPROLENE AF Cream 0.05% contains: 0.643 mg betamethasone dipropionate, USP (equivalent to 0.5 mg betamethasone) in an emollient cream base of purified water, USP; chlorocresol; propylene glycol, USP; white petrolatum, USP; white wax, NF; cyclomethicone; sorbitol solution, USP; glyceryl oleate/propylene glycol; ceteareth-30; carbomer 940, NF; and sodium hydroxide R.

CLINICAL PHARMACOLOGY

The corticosteroids are a class of compounds comprising steroid hormones secreted by the adrenal cortex and their synthetic analogs. In pharmacologic doses, corticosteroids are used primarily for their anti-inflammatory and/or immunosuppressive effects.

Topical corticosteroids, such as betamethasone dipropionate, are effective in the treatment of corticosteroid-responsive dermatoses primarily because of their anti-inflammatory, antipruritic, and vasoconstrictive actions. However, while the physiologic, pharmacologic, and clinical effects of the corticosteroids are well known, the exact mechanisms of their actions in each disease are uncertain. Betamethasone dipropionate, a corticosteroid, has been shown to have topical (dermatologic) and systemic pharmacologic and metabolic effects characteristic of this class of drugs.

Pharmacokinetics

The extent of percutaneous absorption of topical corticosteroids is determined by many factors including the vehicle, the integrity of the epidermal barrier, and the use of occlusive dressings (see **DOSAGE AND ADMINISTRATION**). Topical corticosteroids can be absorbed through normal intact skin. Inflammation and/or other disease processes in the skin may increase percutaneous absorption. Occlusive dressings substantially increase the percutaneous absorption of topical corticosteroids (see **DOSAGE AND ADMINISTRATION**).

Once absorbed through the skin, topical corticosteroids enter pharmacokinetic pathways similar to systemically administered corticosteroids. Corticosteroids are bound to plasma proteins in varying degrees, are metabolized primarily in the liver, and excreted by the kidneys. Some of the topical corticosteroids and their metabolites are also excreted into the bile.

DIPROLENE® AF Cream 0.05% was applied once daily at 7 grams per day for 1 week to diseased skin, in adult patients with psoriasis or atopic dermatitis, to study its effects on the hypothalamic-pituitary-adrenal (HPA) axis. The results suggested that the drug caused a slight lowering of adrenal corticosteroid secretion, although in no case did plasma cortisol levels go below the lower limit of the normal range.

Sixty-seven pediatric patients ages 1 to 12 years, with atopic dermatitis, were enrolled in an open-label, hypothalamic-pituitary-adrenal (HPA) axis safety study. DIPROLENE AF Cream 0.05% was applied twice daily for 2 to 3 weeks over a mean body surface area of 58% (range 35% to 95%). In 19 of 60 (32%) evaluable patients, adrenal suppression was indicated by either a ≤5 mcg/dL prestimulation cortisol, or a cosyntropin post-stimulation cortisol ≤18 mcg/dL and/or an increase of <7 mcg/dL from the baseline cortisol. Studies performed with DIPROLENE AF Cream 0.05% indicate that it is in the high range of potency as compared with other topical corticosteroids.

INDICATIONS AND USAGE

DIPROLENE® AF Cream 0.05% is a high-potency corticosteroid indicated for relief of the inflammatory and pruritic manifestations of corticosteroid-responsive dermatoses in patients 13 years and older.

CONTRAINDICATIONS

DIPROLENE® AF Cream 0.05% is contraindicated in patients who are hypersensitive to betamethasone dipropionate, to other corticosteroids, or to any ingredient in this preparation.

PRECAUTIONS

General

Systemic absorption of topical corticosteroids has produced reversible HPA axis suppression, manifestations of Cushing's syndrome, hyperglycemia, and glucosuria in some patients.

Conditions which augment systemic absorption include the application of the more potent corticosteroids, use over large surface areas, prolonged use, and the addition of occlusive dressings. Use of more than one corticosteroid-containing product at the same time may increase total systemic glucocorticoid exposure (see **DOSAGE AND ADMINISTRATION**).

Therefore, patients receiving a large dose of a potent topical steroid applied to a large surface area should be evaluated periodically for evidence of HPA axis suppression by using the urinary-free cortisol and ACTH stimulation tests. If HPA axis suppression is noted, an attempt should be made to withdraw the drug, to reduce the frequency of application, or to substitute a less potent steroid.

Recovery of HPA axis function is generally prompt and complete upon discontinuation of the drug. In an open-label pediatric study of 60 evaluable patients, of the 19 who showed evidence of suppression, 4 patients were tested 2 weeks af-

ter discontinuation of DIPROLENE® AF Cream 0.05%, and 3 of the 4 (75%) had complete recovery of HPA axis function. Infrequently, signs and symptoms of steroid withdrawal may occur, requiring supplemental systemic corticosteroids. Children may absorb proportionally larger amounts of topical corticosteroids and thus be more susceptible to systemic toxicity (see **PRECAUTIONS, Pediatric Use** section).

If irritation develops, topical corticosteroids should be discontinued and appropriate therapy instituted.

In the presence of dermatological infections, the use of an appropriate antifungal or antibacterial agent should be instituted. If a favorable response does not occur promptly, the corticosteroid should be discontinued until the infection has been adequately controlled.

Information for Patients

Patients using topical corticosteroids should receive the following information and instructions. This information is intended to aid in the safe and effective use of this medication. It is not a disclosure of all possible adverse or intended effects.

1. This medication is to be used as directed by the physician and should not be used longer than the prescribed time period. It is for external use only. Avoid contact with the eyes.
2. Patients should be advised not to use this medication for any disorder other than that for which it was prescribed.
3. The treated skin area should not be bandaged or otherwise covered or wrapped as to be occlusive (see **DOSAGE AND ADMINISTRATION**).
4. Patients should report any signs of local adverse reactions.
5. Other corticosteroid-containing products should not be used with DIPROLENE AF Cream 0.05% without first talking to your physician.

Laboratory Tests

The following tests may be helpful in evaluating HPA axis suppression:

Urinary-free cortisol test

ACTH stimulation test

Carcinogenesis, Mutagenesis, and Impairment of Fertility

Long-term animal studies have not been performed to evaluate the carcinogenic potential of betamethasone dipropionate.

Betamethasone was negative in the bacterial mutagenicity assay (*Salmonella typhimurium* and *Escherichia coli*), and in the mammalian cell mutagenicity assay (CHO/HGPRT). It was positive in the *in vitro* human lymphocyte chromosome aberration assay, and equivocal in the *in vivo* mouse bone marrow micronucleus assay. This pattern of response is similar to that of dexamethasone and hydrocortisone.

Reproductive studies with betamethasone dipropionate carried out in rabbits at doses of 1.0 mg/kg by the intramuscular route and in mice up to 33 mg/kg by the intramuscular route indicated no impairment of fertility except for dose-related increases in fetal resorption rates in both species. These doses are approximately 5- and 38-fold the human dose based on a mg/m^2 comparison, respectively.

Pregnancy

Teratogenic Effects

Pregnancy Category C

Corticosteroids are generally teratogenic in laboratory animals when administered systemically at relatively low dosage levels.

Betamethasone dipropionate has been shown to be teratogenic in rabbits when given by the intramuscular route at doses of 0.05 mg/kg. This dose is approximately 0.2-fold the maximum human dose based on a mg/m^2 comparison. The abnormalities observed included umbilical hernias, cephalocele, and cleft palates.

Some corticosteroids have been shown to be teratogenic after dermal application in laboratory animals. There are no adequate and well-controlled studies in pregnant women on teratogenic effects from topically applied corticosteroids. Therefore, topical corticosteroids should be used during pregnancy only if the potential benefit justifies the potential risk to the fetus. Drugs of this class should not be used extensively on pregnant patients, in large amounts, or for prolonged periods of time.

Nursing Mothers

It is not known whether topical administration of corticosteroids can result in sufficient systemic absorption to produce detectable quantities in breast milk. Systemically administered corticosteroids are secreted into breast milk in quantities not likely to have a deleterious effect on the infant. Nevertheless, a decision should be made whether to discontinue nursing or to discontinue the drug, taking into account the importance of the drug to the mother.

Pediatric Use

Use of DIPROLENE AF Cream 0.05% in pediatric patients 12 years of age and younger is not recommended (see **CLINICAL PHARMACOLOGY** and **ADVERSE REACTIONS**).

In an open-label study, 19 of 60 (32%) evaluable pediatric patients (aged 3 months-12 years old) using DIPROLENE AF Cream 0.05% for treatment of atopic dermatitis demon-

strated HPA axis suppression. The proportion of patients with adrenal suppression in this study was progressively greater, the younger the age group (see **CLINICAL PHARMACOLOGY, Pharmacokinetics section**).

Pediatric patients may demonstrate greater susceptibility to topical corticosteroid-induced HPA axis suppression and Cushing's syndrome than mature patients because of a larger skin surface area to body weight ratio. The study described above supports this premise, as adrenal suppression in 9-12 year olds, 6-8 year olds, 2-5 year olds, and 3 months-1 year old was 17%, 32%, 38%, and 50%, respectively.

Hypothalamic-pituitary-adrenal (HPA) axis suppression, Cushing's syndrome, and intracranial hypertension have been reported in children receiving topical corticosteroids. Manifestations of adrenal suppression in children include linear growth retardation, delayed weight gain, low plasma cortisol levels, and absence of response to ACTH stimulation. Manifestations of intracranial hypertension include bulging fontanelles, headaches, and bilateral papilledema. Chronic corticosteroid therapy may interfere with the growth and development of children.

Geriatric Use

Clinical studies of DIPROLENE AF Cream 0.05% included 104 subjects who were 65 years of age and over and 8 subjects who were 75 years of age and over. No overall differences in safety or effectiveness were observed between these subjects and younger subjects, and other reported clinical experience has not identified differences in responses between the elderly and younger patients. However, greater sensitivity of some older individuals cannot be ruled out.

ADVERSE REACTIONS

The only local adverse reaction reported to be possibly or probably related to treatment with DIPROLENE® AF Cream 0.05% during adult-controlled clinical studies was stinging. It occurred in 1 patient, 0.4%, of the 242 patients or subjects involved in the studies.

Adverse reactions reported to be possibly or probably related to treatment with DIPROLENE AF Cream 0.05% during a pediatric clinical study include signs of skin atrophy (telangiectasia, bruising, shininess). Skin atrophy occurred in 7 of 67 (10%) patients, involving all age groups from 3 months-12 years of age.

The following local adverse reactions are reported infrequently when topical corticosteroids are used as recommended. These reactions are listed in an approximate decreasing order of occurrence: burning, itching, irritation, dryness, folliculitis, hypertrichosis, acneiform eruptions, hypopigmentation, perioral dermatitis, allergic contact dermatitis, maceration of the skin, secondary infection, skin atrophy, striae, miliaria.

Systemic absorption of topical corticosteroids has produced reversible hypothalamic-pituitary-adrenal (HPA) axis suppression, manifestations of Cushing's syndrome, hyperglycemia, and glucosuria in some patients.

OVERDOSAGE

Topically applied corticosteroids can be absorbed in sufficient amounts to produce systemic effects (see **PRECAUTIONS**).

DOSAGE AND ADMINISTRATION

Apply a thin film of DIPROLENE® AF Cream 0.05% to the affected skin areas once or twice daily. <u>Treatment with DIPROLENE AF Cream 0.05% should be limited to 50 g per week.</u>

DIPROLENE AF Cream 0.05% is not to be used with occlusive dressings.

HOW SUPPLIED

DIPROLENE® AF Cream 0.05% is supplied in 15-g (NDC 0085-0517-01) and 50-g (NDC 0085-0517-04) tubes; boxes of one.

Store at 25°C (77°F); excursions permitted to 15°-30°C (59°-86°F) [see USP Controlled Room Temperature].

Schering Corporation
Kenilworth, NJ 07033 USA
Rev. 5/07   **18670356T**
Copyright © 1987, 2001, Schering Corporation. All rights reserved.

Shown in Product Identification Guide, page 312

DIPROLENE®   ℞
[dĭp-rō-lēn]
brand of augmented betamethasone dipropionate*
Lotion 0.05%
(potency expressed as betamethasone)
*Vehicle augments the penetration of the steroid.
For Dermatologic Use Only — Not for Ophthalmic Use
PRODUCT INFORMATION

DESCRIPTION

DIPROLENE® (augmented betamethasone dipropionate) Lotion contains betamethasone dipropionate, USP, a

synthetic adrenocorticosteroid, for dermatologic use. Betamethasone, an analog of prednisolone, has a high degree of corticosteroid activity and a slight degree of mineralocorticoid activity. Betamethasone dipropionate is the 17, 21-dipropionate ester of betamethasone.
Chemically, betamethasone dipropionate is 9-fluoro-11β,17,21-trihydroxy-16β-methylpregna-1,4-diene-3,20-dione 17,21-dipropionate, with the empirical formula $C_{28}H_{37}FO_7$, a molecular weight of 504.6, and the following structural formula:

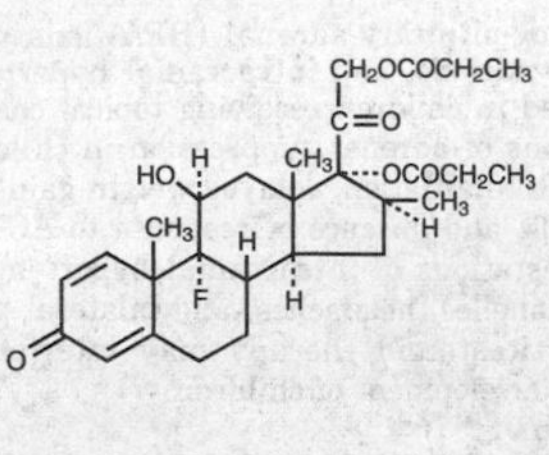

It is a white to creamy-white, odorless powder insoluble in water; freely soluble in acetone and in chloroform; sparingly soluble in alcohol.
Each gram of DIPROLENE Lotion 0.05% contains 0.643 mg betamethasone dipropionate, USP (equivalent to 0.5 mg betamethasone), in an augmented lotion base of purified water; isopropyl alcohol (30%); hydroxypropyl cellulose; propylene glycol; sodium phosphate; phosphoric acid and sodium hydroxide used to adjust the pH.

CLINICAL PHARMACOLOGY

The corticosteroids are a class of compounds comprising steroid hormones secreted by the adrenal cortex and their synthetic analogs. In pharmacologic doses, corticosteroids are used primarily for their anti-inflammatory and/or immunosuppressive effects.
Topical corticosteroids, such as betamethasone dipropionate, are effective in the treatment of corticosteroid-responsive dermatoses primarily because of their anti-inflammatory, antipruritic, and vasoconstrictive actions. However, while the physiologic, pharmacologic, and clinical effects of the corticosteroids are well known, the exact mechanisms of their actions in each disease are uncertain. Betamethasone dipropionate, a corticosteroid, has been shown to have topical (dermatologic) and systemic pharmacologic and metabolic effects characteristic of this class of drugs.

Pharmacokinetics The extent of percutaneous absorption of topical corticosteroids is determined by many factors including the vehicle, the integrity of the epidermal barrier, and the use of occlusive dressings (see **DOSAGE AND ADMINISTRATION**).
Topical corticosteroids can be absorbed through normal intact skin. Inflammation and/or other disease processes in the skin may increase percutaneous absorption. Occlusive dressings substantially increase the percutaneous absorption of topical corticosteroids (see **DOSAGE AND ADMINISTRATION**).
Once absorbed through the skin, topical corticosteroids enter pharmacokinetic pathways similar to systemically administered corticosteroids. Corticosteroids are bound to plasma proteins in varying degrees, are metabolized primarily in the liver, and excreted by the kidneys. Some of the topical corticosteroids and their metabolites are also excreted into the bile.
Studies performed with DIPROLENE® Lotion indicate that it is in the super-high range of potency as compared with other topical corticosteroids.

INDICATIONS AND USAGE

DIPROLENE® Lotion is a super-high potency corticosteroid indicated for the relief of the inflammatory and pruritic manifestations of corticosteroid-responsive dermatoses in patients 13 years of age and older. The total dose should not exceed 50 mL per week because of the potential for the drug to suppress the hypothalamic-pituitary-adrenal (HPA) axis.

CONTRAINDICATIONS

DIPROLENE® Lotion is contraindicated in patients who are hypersensitive to betamethasone dipropionate, to other corticosteroids, or to any ingredient in this preparation.

PRECAUTIONS

General Systemic absorption of topical corticosteroids has produced reversible HPA axis suppression, manifestations of Cushing's syndrome, hyperglycemia, and glucosuria in some patients.
Conditions which augment systemic absorption include the application of the more potent corticosteroids, use over large surface areas, prolonged use, and the addition of occlusive dressings. Use of more than one corticosteroid-containing product at the same time may increase total systemic glucocorticoid exposure (see **DOSAGE AND ADMINISTRATION**).
Therefore, patients receiving a large dose of a potent topical steroid applied to a large surface area should be evaluated periodically for evidence of HPA axis suppression by using the urinary-free cortisol and ACTH stimulation tests. If HPA axis suppression is noted, an attempt should be made to withdraw the drug, to reduce the frequency of application, or to substitute a less potent steroid.
Recovery of HPA axis function is generally prompt and complete upon discontinuation of the drug. Patients should not be treated with amounts of DIPROLENE® Lotion greater than 50 mL per week because of the potential for the drug to suppress HPA axis. Patients receiving super-potent corticosteroids should not be treated for more than 2 weeks at a time and only small areas should be treated at any one time due to the increased risk of HPA axis suppression.
DIPROLENE Lotion was applied once daily at 7 mL per day for 21 days to diseased scalp and body skin in patients with scalp psoriasis to study its effects on the HPA axis. In 2 out of 11 patients, the drug lowered plasma cortisol levels below normal limits. HPA axis suppression in these patients was transient and returned to normal within a week. In one of these patients, plasma cortisol levels returned to normal while treatment continued.
Infrequently, signs and symptoms of steroid withdrawal may occur, requiring supplemental systemic corticosteroids.
Pediatric patients may absorb proportionally larger amounts of topical corticosteroids and thus be more susceptible to systemic toxicity (see **PRECAUTIONS, Pediatric Use** section).
If irritation develops, topical corticosteroids should be discontinued and appropriate therapy instituted.
In the presence of dermatological infections, the use of an appropriate antifungal or antibacterial agent should be instituted. If a favorable response does not occur promptly, the corticosteroid should be discontinued until the infection has been adequately controlled.
DIPROLENE Lotion should not be used in the treatment of rosacea or perioral dermatitis, and it should not be used on the face, groin, or in the axillae.

Information for Patients Patients using topical corticosteroids should receive the following information and instructions. This information is intended to aid in the safe and effective use of this medication. It is not a disclosure of all possible adverse or intended effects.

1. This medication is to be used as directed by the physician and should not be used longer than the prescribed time period. It is for external use only. Avoid contact with the eyes.
2. This medication should not be used for any disorder other than that for which it was prescribed.
3. The treated skin area should not be bandaged, or otherwise covered or wrapped, so as to be occlusive (see **DOSAGE AND ADMINISTRATION**).
4. Patients should report to their physician any signs of local adverse reactions.
5. Patients should be advised not to use DIPROLENE® Lotion in the treatment of diaper dermatitis. DIPROLENE Lotion should not be applied in the diaper areas as diapers or plastic pants may constitute occlusive dressing (see **DOSAGE AND ADMINISTRATION**).
6. This medication should not be used on the face, underarms, or groin areas unless directed by the physician.
7. As with other corticosteroids, therapy should be discontinued when control is achieved. If no improvement is seen within 2 weeks, contact the physician.
8. Other corticosteroid-containing products should not be used with DIPROLENE Lotion.

Laboratory Tests The following tests may be helpful in evaluating patients for HPA axis suppression:
ACTH stimulation test
Urinary-free cortisol test

Carcinogenesis, Mutagenesis, and Impairment of Fertility Long-term animal studies have not been performed to evaluate the carcinogenic potential of betamethasone dipropionate. Betamethasone was negative in the bacterial mutagenicity assay (*Salmonella typhimurium* and *Escherichia coli*), and in the mammalian cell mutagenicity assay (CHO/HGPRT). It was positive in the *in vitro* human lymphocyte chromosome aberration assay, and equivocal in the *in vivo* mouse bone marrow micronucleus assay. This pattern of response is similar to that of dexamethasone and hydrocortisone. Studies in rabbits, mice, and rats using intramuscular doses up to 1, 33, and 2 mg/kg, respectively, resulted in dose-related increases in fetal resorptions in rabbits and mice.

Pregnancy ***Teratogenic Effects*** *Pregnancy Category C* Corticosteroids have been shown to be teratogenic in laboratory animals when administered systemically at relatively low dosage levels. Some corticosteroids have been shown to be teratogenic after dermal application in laboratory animals. Betamethasone dipropionate has been shown to be teratogenic in rabbits when given by the intramuscular route at doses of 0.05 mg/kg. This dose is approximately 0.2 times the human topical dose of DIPROLENE Lotion in mg/m^2 of body surface area, assuming 100% absorption and the use in a 60 kg person of 7 g per day. The abnormalities observed included umbilical hernias, cephalocele, and cleft palate. There are no adequate and well-controlled studies in pregnant women on teratogenic effects from topically applied corticosteroids. DIPROLENE Lotion should be used during pregnancy only if the potential benefit justifies the potential risk to the fetus.

Nursing Mothers Systemically administered corticosteroids appear in human milk and could suppress growth, interfere with endogenous corticosteroid production, or cause other untoward effects. It is not known whether topical administration of corticosteroids could result in sufficient systemic absorption to produce detectable quantities in human milk. Because many drugs are excreted in human milk, caution should be exercised when DIPROLENE Lotion is administered to a nursing woman.

Pediatric Use Use of DIPROLENE Lotion, 0.05%, in pediatric patients 12 years of age and younger is not recommended (see **CLINICAL PHARMACOLOGY** and **ADVERSE REACTIONS**).
Pediatric patients may demonstrate greater susceptibility to topical corticosteroid-induced HPA axis suppression and Cushing's syndrome than mature patients because of a larger skin surface area to body weight ratio.
Hypothalamic-pituitary-adrenal (HPA) axis suppression, Cushing's syndrome, and intracranial hypertension have been reported in children receiving topical corticosteroids. Manifestations of adrenal suppression in children include linear growth retardation, delayed weight gain, low plasma cortisol levels, and absence of response to ACTH stimulation. Manifestations of intracranial hypertension include bulging fontanelles, headaches, and bilateral papilledema. Chronic corticosteroid therapy may interfere with the growth and development of children.

Geriatric Use Seven clinical studies of DIPROLENE Lotion evaluated 407 subjects of which 56 subjects were 65 years of age and over and 9 subjects were 75 years of age and over. No overall differences in safety or effectiveness were observed in these clinical studies between geriatric subjects and younger subjects. There was a numerical difference for application site reactions (most frequently reported events were burning and stinging) which occurred in 15% (10/65) of geriatric subjects and 11% (38/342) of subjects less than 65 years of age. Other reported clinical experience has not identified differences in responses between the elderly and younger patients. However, greater sensitivity of some older individuals cannot be ruled out.

ADVERSE REACTIONS

The local adverse reactions which were reported with DIPROLENE® Lotion during controlled clinical trials were as follows: erythema, folliculitis, pruritus, and vesiculation each occurring in less than 1% of patients.
The following additional local adverse reactions have been reported with topical corticosteroids, and they may occur more frequently with the use of occlusive dressings and higher potency corticosteroids. These reactions are listed in an approximately decreasing order of occurrence: burning, itching, irritation, dryness, folliculitis, hypertrichosis, acneiform eruptions, hypopigmentation, perioral dermatitis, allergic contact dermatitis, secondary infection, skin atrophy, striae, and miliaria.
Systemic absorption of topical corticosteroids has produced reversible hypothalamic-pituitary-adrenal (HPA) axis suppression, manifestations of Cushing's syndrome, hyperglycemia, and glucosuria in some patients.

OVERDOSAGE

Topically applied DIPROLENE® Lotion can be absorbed in sufficient amounts to produce systemic effects (see **PRECAUTIONS**).

DOSAGE AND ADMINISTRATION

Apply a few drops of DIPROLENE® Lotion to the affected skin once or twice daily and massage lightly until the lotion disappears.
DIPROLENE Lotion is a super-high potency topical corticosteroid. **Treatment with DIPROLENE Lotion should be limited to two weeks, and amounts greater than 50 mL per week should not be used.**
As with other highly active corticosteroids, therapy should be discontinued when control is achieved. If no improvement is seen within 2 weeks, reassessment of diagnosis may be necessary.
DIPROLENE Lotion should not be used with occlusive dressings. DIPROLENE Lotion should not be applied to the diaper area if the patient requires diapers or plastic pants as these garments may constitute occlusive dressing.

HOW SUPPLIED

DIPROLENE® Lotion 0.05% is supplied in 30-mL (29 g) (NDC 0085-0962-01) and 60-mL (58 g) (NDC 0085-0962-02) plastic squeeze bottles; boxes of one.

Store at 25°C (77°F); excursions permitted to 15°-30°C (59°-86°F) [see USP Controlled Room Temperature].

Schering Corporation
Kenilworth, NJ 07033 USA
Rev. 5/07 23816431T

Shown in Product Identification Guide, page 312

DIPROLENE® ℞

[*dĭp-rō-lēn*]

brand of augmented betamethasone dipropionate*
Ointment 0.05%
(potency expressed as betamethasone)
***Vehicle augments the penetration of the steroid.**
For Dermatologic Use Only — Not for Ophthalmic Use
PRODUCT INFORMATION

DESCRIPTION

DIPROLENE® (augmented betamethasone dipropionate) Ointment contains betamethasone dipropionate, USP, a synthetic adrenocorticosteroid, for dermatologic use. Betamethasone, an analog of prednisolone, has a high degree of corticosteroid activity and a slight degree of mineralocorticoid activity. Betamethasone dipropionate is the 17, 21-dipropionate ester of betamethasone.

Chemically, betamethasone dipropionate is 9-fluoro-11β, 17,21-trihydroxy-16β-methylpregna-1,4-diene-3,20-dione 17,21-dipropionate, with the empirical formula $C_{28}H_{37}FO_7$, a molecular weight of 504.6 and the following structural formula:

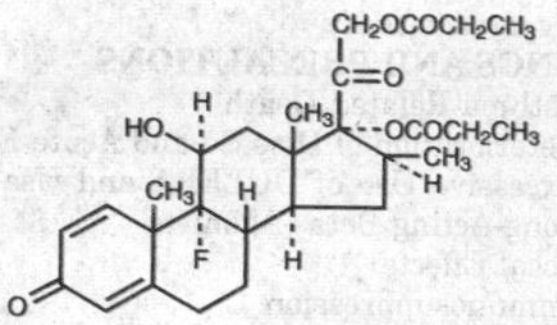

It is a white to creamy-white, odorless powder insoluble in water; freely soluble in acetone and in chloroform; sparingly soluble in alcohol.

Each gram of DIPROLENE Ointment 0.05% contains 0.643 mg betamethasone dipropionate, USP (equivalent to 0.5 mg betamethasone), in a vehicle of propylene glycol, propylene glycol stearate, white wax, and white petrolatum.

CLINICAL PHARMACOLOGY

The corticosteroids are a class of compounds comprising steroid hormones secreted by the adrenal cortex and their synthetic analogs. In pharmacologic doses, corticosteroids are used primarily for their anti-inflammatory and/or immunosuppressive effects.

Topical corticosteroids, such as betamethasone dipropionate, are effective in the treatment of corticosteroid-responsive dermatoses primarily because of their anti-inflammatory, antipruritic, and vasoconstrictive actions. However, while the physiologic, pharmacologic, and clinical effects of the corticosteroids are well known, the exact mechanisms of their actions in each disease are uncertain. Betamethasone dipropionate, a corticosteroid, has been shown to have topical (dermatologic) and systemic pharmacologic and metabolic effects characteristic of this class of drugs.

Pharmacokinetics

The extent of percutaneous absorption of topical corticosteroids is determined by many factors including the vehicle, the integrity of the epidermal barrier, and the use of occlusive dressings (see **DOSAGE AND ADMINISTRATION**).

Topical corticosteroids can be absorbed through normal intact skin. Inflammation and/or other disease processes in the skin may increase percutaneous absorption. Occlusive dressings substantially increase the percutaneous absorption of topical corticosteroids (see **DOSAGE AND ADMINISTRATION**).

Once absorbed through the skin, topical corticosteroids enter pharmacokinetic pathways similar to systemically administered corticosteroids. Corticosteroids are bound to plasma proteins in varying degrees, are metabolized primarily in the liver, and excreted by the kidneys. Some of the topical corticosteroids and their metabolites are also excreted into the bile.

Studies performed with DIPROLENE® Ointment indicate that it is in the super-high range of potency as compared with other topical corticosteroids.

INDICATIONS AND USAGE

DIPROLENE® Ointment is a super-high potency corticosteroid indicated for the relief of the inflammatory and pruritic manifestations of corticosteroid-responsive dermatoses in patients 13 years of age and older. The total dose should not exceed 50 g per week because of the potential for the drug to suppress the hypothalamic-pituitary-adrenal (HPA) axis.

CONTRAINDICATIONS

DIPROLENE® Ointment is contraindicated in patients who are hypersensitive to betamethasone dipropionate, to other corticosteroids, or to any ingredient in this preparation.

PRECAUTIONS

General

Systemic absorption of topical corticosteroids has produced reversible HPA axis suppression, manifestations of Cushing's syndrome, hyperglycemia, and glucosuria in some patients.

Conditions which augment systemic absorption include the application of the more potent corticosteroids, use over large surface areas, prolonged use, and the addition of occlusive dressings. Use of more than one corticosteroid-containing product at the same time may increase total systemic glucocorticoid exposure (see **DOSAGE AND ADMINISTRATION**).

Therefore, patients receiving a large dose of a potent topical steroid applied to a large surface area should be evaluated periodically for evidence of HPA axis suppression by using the urinary-free cortisol and ACTH stimulation tests. If HPA axis suppression is noted, an attempt should be made to withdraw the drug, to reduce the frequency of application, or to substitute a less potent steroid.

Recovery of HPA axis function is generally prompt and complete upon discontinuation of the drug. Patients should not be treated with amounts of DIPROLENE® Ointment greater than 50 g per week because of the potential for the drug to suppress HPA axis. Patients receiving super-potent corticosteroids should not be treated for more than 2 weeks at a time and only small areas should be treated at any one time due to the increased risk of HPA suppression.

At 14 g per day DIPROLENE Ointment was shown to depress the plasma levels of adrenal cortical hormones following repeated application to diseased skin in patients with psoriasis. These effects were reversible upon discontinuation of treatment. At 7 g per day DIPROLENE Ointment was shown to cause minimal inhibition of the HPA axis when applied 2 times daily for 2 to 3 weeks in healthy patients and in patients with psoriasis and eczematous disorders.

With 6 to 7 g of DIPROLENE Ointment applied once daily for 3 weeks, no significant inhibition of the HPA axis was observed in patients with psoriasis and atopic dermatitis, as measured by plasma cortisol and 24-hour urinary 17-hydroxy-corticosteroid levels. Infrequently, signs and symptoms of steroid withdrawal may occur, requiring supplemental systemic corticosteroids.

Pediatric patients may absorb proportionally larger amounts of topical corticosteroids and thus be more susceptible to systemic toxicity (see **PRECAUTIONS, Pediatric Use** section).

If irritation develops, topical corticosteroids should be discontinued and appropriate therapy instituted.

In the presence of dermatological infections, the use of an appropriate antifungal or antibacterial agent should be instituted. If a favorable response does not occur promptly, the corticosteroid should be discontinued until the infection has been adequately controlled.

DIPROLENE Ointment should not be used in the treatment of rosacea or perioral dermatitis, and it should not be used on the face, groin, or in the axillae.

Information for Patients

Patients using topical corticosteroids should receive the following information and instructions. This information is intended to aid in the safe and effective use of this medication. It is not a disclosure of all possible adverse or intended effects.

1. This medication is to be used as directed by the physician and should not be used longer than the prescribed time period. It is for external use only. Avoid contact with the eyes.
2. This medication should not be used for any disorder other than that for which it was prescribed.
3. The treated skin area should not be bandaged, otherwise covered or wrapped, so as to be occlusive (see **DOSAGE AND ADMINISTRATION**).
4. Patients should report to their physician any signs of local adverse reactions.
5. Patients should be advised not to use DIPROLENE Ointment in the treatment of diaper dermatitis. DIPROLENE Ointment should not be applied in the diaper areas as diapers or plastic pants may constitute occlusive dressing (see **DOSAGE AND ADMINISTRATION**).
6. This medication should not be used on the face, underarms, or groin areas unless directed by the physician.
7. As with other corticosteroids, therapy should be discontinued when control is achieved. If no improvement is seen within 2 weeks, contact the physician.
8. Other corticosteroid-containing products should not be used with DIPROLENE Ointment.

Laboratory Tests

The following tests may be helpful in evaluating patients for HPA axis suppression:

ACTH stimulation test
Urinary-free cortisol test

Carcinogenesis, Mutagenesis, and Impairment of Fertility

Long-term animal studies have not been performed to evaluate the carcinogenic potential of betamethasone dipropionate. Betamethasone was negative in the bacterial mutagenicity assay (*Salmonella typhimurium* and *Escherichia coli*), and in the mammalian cell mutagenicity assay (CHO/HGPRT). It was positive in the *in vitro* human lymphocyte chromosome aberration assay, and equivocal in the *in vivo* mouse bone marrow micronucleus assay. This pattern of response is similar to that of dexamethasone and hydrocortisone. Studies in rabbits, mice, and rats using intramuscular doses up to 1, 33, and 2 mg/kg, respectively, resulted in dose-related increases in fetal resorptions in rabbits and mice.

Pregnancy

Teratogenic Effects

Pregnancy Category C

Corticosteroids have been shown to be teratogenic in laboratory animals when administered systemically at relatively low dosage levels. Some corticosteroids have been shown to be teratogenic after dermal application in laboratory animals. Betamethasone dipropionate has been shown to be teratogenic in rabbits when given by the intramuscular route at doses of 0.05 mg/kg. This dose is approximately 0.2 times the human topical dose of DIPROLENE Ointment in mg/m^2 of body surface area, assuming 100% absorption and the use in a 60 kg person of 7 g per day. The abnormalities observed included umbilical hernias, cephalocele, and cleft palate. There are no adequate and well-controlled studies in pregnant women on teratogenic effects from topically applied corticosteroids. DIPROLENE Ointment should be used during pregnancy only if the potential benefit justifies the potential risk to the fetus.

Nursing Mothers

Systemically administered corticosteroids appear in human milk and could suppress growth, interfere with endogenous corticosteroid production, or cause other untoward effects. It is not known whether topical administration of corticosteroids could result in sufficient systemic absorption to produce detectable quantities in human milk. Because many drugs are excreted in human milk, caution should be exercised when DIPROLENE Ointment is administered to a nursing woman.

Pediatric Use

Use of DIPROLENE Ointment, 0.05%, in pediatric patients 12 years of age and younger is not recommended (see **CLINICAL PHARMACOLOGY** and **ADVERSE REACTIONS**).

Pediatric patients may demonstrate greater susceptibility to topical corticosteroid-induced HPA axis suppression and Cushing's syndrome than mature patients because of a larger skin surface area to body weight ratio.

Hypothalamic-pituitary-adrenal (HPA) axis suppression, Cushing's syndrome, and intracranial hypertension have been reported in children receiving topical corticosteroids. Manifestations of adrenal suppression in children include linear growth retardation, delayed weight gain, low plasma cortisol levels, and an absence of response to ACTH stimulation. Manifestations of intracranial hypertension include bulging fontanelles, headaches, and bilateral papilledema. Chronic corticosteroid therapy may interfere with the growth and development of children.

Geriatric Use

Clinical studies of DIPROLENE Ointment included 225 subjects who were 65 years of age and over and 46 subjects who were 75 years of age and over. No overall differences in safety or effectiveness were observed between these subjects and younger subjects, and other reported clinical experience has not identified differences in responses between the elderly and younger patients. However, greater sensitivity of some older individuals cannot be ruled out.

ADVERSE REACTIONS

The local adverse reactions which were reported with DIPROLENE® Ointment during controlled clinical trials were as follows: erythema, folliculitis, pruritus, and vesiculation each occurring in less than 1% of patients.

The following additional local adverse reactions have been reported with topical corticosteroids, and they may occur more frequently with the use of occlusive dressings and higher potency corticosteroids. These reactions are listed in an approximately decreasing order of occurrence: burning, itching, irritation, dryness, folliculitis, hypertrichosis, acneiform eruptions, hypopigmentation, perioral dermatitis, allergic contact dermatitis, secondary infection, skin atrophy, striae, and miliaria.

Systemic absorption of topical corticosteroids has produced reversible hypothalamic-pituitary-adrenal (HPA) axis suppression, manifestations of Cushing's syndrome, hyperglycemia, and glucosuria in some patients.

OVERDOSAGE

Topically applied DIPROLENE® Ointment can be absorbed in sufficient amounts to produce systemic effects (see **PRECAUTIONS**).

DOSAGE AND ADMINISTRATION

Apply a thin film of DIPROLENE® Ointment to the affected skin once or twice daily.

DIPROLENE® Ointment is a super-high potency topical corticosteroid. **Treatment with DIPROLENE Ointment should be limited to 50 g per week.**

As with other corticosteroids, therapy should be discontinued when control is achieved. If no improvement is seen within 2 weeks, reassessment of diagnosis may be necessary.

DIPROLENE Ointment should not be used with occlusive dressings. DIPROLENE Ointment should not be applied to the diaper area if the patient requires diapers or plastic pants as these garments may constitute occlusive dressing.

HOW SUPPLIED

DIPROLENE® Ointment 0.05% is supplied in 15-g (NDC 0085-0575-02) and 50-g (NDC 0085-0575-05) tubes; boxes of one.

Store at 25°C (77°F); excursions permitted to 15°-30°C (59°-86°F) [see USP Controlled Room Temperature].

Schering Corporation
Kenilworth, NJ 07033 USA
Rev. 5/07   18670550T
Copyright © 1983, 2004, Schering Corporation. All rights reserved.

Shown in Product Identification Guide, page 312

DULERA® 100 mcg/5 mcg   ℞
[dew-LAIR-ah]
**(mometasone furoate 100 mcg and formoterol fumarate dihydrate 5 mcg)
Inhalation Aerosol**
DULERA® 200 mcg/5 mcg
**(mometasone furoate 200 mcg and formoterol fumarate dihydrate 5 mcg)
Inhalation Aerosol
FOR ORAL INHALATION**

HIGHLIGHTS OF PRESCRIBING INFORMATION
These highlights do not include all the information needed to use DULERA safely and effectively. See full prescribing information for DULERA.

DULERA® 100 mcg/5 mcg (mometasone furoate 100 mcg and formoterol fumarate dihydrate 5 mcg) Inhalation Aerosol

DULERA® 200 mcg/5 mcg (mometasone furoate 200 mcg and formoterol fumarate dihydrate 5 mcg) Inhalation Aerosol

FOR ORAL INHALATION
Initial U.S. Approval: 2010

WARNING: ASTHMA-RELATED DEATH
See full prescribing information for complete boxed warning.
• Long-acting beta$_2$-adrenergic agonists (LABA), such as formoterol, one of the active ingredients in DULERA, increase the risk of asthma-related death. Data from a large placebo-controlled U.S. study that compared the safety of another LABA (salmeterol) or placebo added to usual asthma therapy showed an increase in asthma-related deaths in patients receiving salmeterol. This finding with salmeterol is considered a class effect of the LABA, including formoterol. Currently available data are inadequate to determine whether concurrent use of inhaled corticosteroids or other long-term asthma control drugs mitigates the increased risk of asthma-related death from LABA. Available data from controlled clinical tri-

---

als suggest that LABA increase the risk of asthma-related hospitalization in pediatric and adolescent patients.
• When treating patients with asthma, prescribe DULERA only for patients with asthma not adequately controlled on a long-term asthma control medication, such as an inhaled corticosteroid or whose disease severity clearly warrants initiation of treatment with both an inhaled corticosteroid and LABA. Once asthma control is achieved and maintained, assess the patient at regular intervals and step down therapy (e.g., discontinue DULERA) if possible without loss of asthma control, and maintain the patient on a long-term asthma control medication, such as an inhaled corticosteroid. Do not use DULERA for patients whose asthma is adequately controlled on low or medium dose inhaled corticosteroids. (1.1, 5.1)

INDICATIONS AND USAGE

DULERA is a combination product containing a corticosteroid and a long-acting beta$_2$-adrenergic agonist indicated for:
• Treatment of asthma in patients 12 years of age and older. (1.1)
Important limitations:
• Not indicated for the relief of acute bronchospasm. (1.1)

DOSAGE AND ADMINISTRATION
For oral inhalation only.
Treatment of asthma in patients ≥12 years: 2 inhalations twice daily of DULERA 100 mcg/5 mcg or 200 mcg/5 mcg. Starting dosage is based on prior asthma therapy. (2.2)

DOSAGE FORMS AND STRENGTHS
Inhalation aerosol containing a combination of mometasone furoate (100 or 200 mcg) and formoterol fumarate dihydrate (5 mcg) per actuation. (3)

CONTRAINDICATIONS
• Primary treatment of status asthmaticus or acute episodes of asthma requiring intensive measures. (4.1)
• Hypersensitivity to any of the ingredients of DULERA. (4.2)

WARNINGS AND PRECAUTIONS
• Asthma-related death: Long-acting beta$_2$-adrenergic agonists increase the risk. Prescribe only for recommended patient populations. (5.1)
• Deterioration of disease and acute episodes: Do not initiate in acutely deteriorating asthma or to treat acute symptoms. (5.2)
• Use with additional long-acting beta$_2$-agonist: Do not use in combination because of risk of overdose. (5.3)
• Localized infections: *Candida albicans* infection of the mouth and throat may occur. Monitor patients periodically for signs of adverse effects on the oral cavity. Advise patients to rinse the mouth following inhalation. (5.4)
• Immunosuppression: Potential worsening of existing tuberculosis, fungal, bacterial, viral, or parasitic infection; or ocular herpes simplex infections. More serious or even fatal course of chickenpox or measles can occur in susceptible patients. Use with caution in patients with these infections because of the potential for worsening of these infections. (5.5)
• Transferring patients from systemic corticosteroids: Risk of impaired adrenal function when transferring from oral steroids. Taper patients slowly from systemic corticosteroids if transferring to DULERA. (5.6)
• Hypercorticism and adrenal suppression: May occur with very high dosages or at the regular dosage in susceptible individuals. If such changes occur, discontinue DULERA slowly. (5.7)
• Strong cytochrome P450 3A4 inhibitors (e.g., ritonavir): Risk of increased systemic corticosteroid effects. Exercise caution when used with DULERA. (5.8)
• Paradoxical bronchospasm: Discontinue DULERA and institute alternative therapy if paradoxical bronchospasm occurs. (5.9)
• Patients with cardiovascular disorders: Use with caution because of beta-adrenergic stimulation. (5.11)
• Decreases in bone mineral density: Monitor patients with major risk factors for decreased bone mineral content. (5.12)
• Effects on growth: Monitor growth of pediatric patients. (5.13)
• Glaucoma and cataracts: Monitor patients with change in vision or with a history of increased intraocular pressure, glaucoma, and/or cataracts closely. (5.14)
• Coexisting conditions: Use with caution in patients with convulsive disorders, thyrotoxicosis, diabetes mellitus, and ketoacidosis. (5.15)
• Hypokalemia and hyperglycemia: Be alert to hypokalemia and hyperglycemia. (5.16)

ADVERSE REACTIONS
Most common adverse reactions (reported in ≥3% of patients) included:
• Nasopharyngitis, sinusitis and headache. (6.1)
To report SUSPECTED ADVERSE REACTIONS, contact Schering Corporation, a subsidiary of Merck & Co., Inc., at 1-800-526-4099 or FDA at 1-800-FDA-1088 or *www.fda.gov/medwatch*.

DRUG INTERACTIONS
• Strong cytochrome P450 3A4 inhibitors (e.g., ritonavir): Use with caution. May cause increased systemic corticosteroid effects. (7.1)
• Adrenergic agents: Use with caution. Additional adrenergic drugs may potentiate sympathetic effects. (7.2)
• Xanthine derivatives and diuretics: Use with caution. May potentiate ECG changes and/or hypokalemia. (7.3, 7.4)
• MAO inhibitors, tricyclic antidepressants, and drugs that prolong QTc interval: Use with extreme caution. May potentiate effect on the cardiovascular system. (7.5)
• Beta-blockers: Use with caution and only when medically necessary. May decrease effectiveness and produce severe bronchospasm. (7.6)

USE IN SPECIFIC POPULATIONS
• Hepatic impairment: Monitor patients for signs of increased drug exposure. (8.6)

See 17 for PATIENT COUNSELING INFORMATION and Medication Guide
                                        Revised: 06/2010

FULL PRESCRIBING INFORMATION: CONTENTS*
WARNING: ASTHMA-RELATED DEATH

* Sections or subsections omitted from the full prescribing information are not listed

FULL PRESCRIBING INFORMATION

WARNING: ASTHMA-RELATED DEATH

Long-acting beta$_2$-adrenergic agonists (LABA), such as formoterol, one of the active ingredients in DULERA, increase the risk of asthma-related death. Data from a large placebo-controlled U.S. study that compared the safety of another long-acting beta$_2$-adrenergic agonist (salmeterol) or placebo added to usual asthma therapy showed an increase in asthma-related deaths in patients receiving salmeterol. This finding with salmeterol is considered a class effect of the LABA, including formoterol. Currently available data are inadequate to determine whether concurrent use of inhaled corticosteroids or other long-term asthma control drugs mitigates the increased risk of asthma-related death from LABA. Available data from controlled clinical trials suggest that LABA increase the risk of asthma-related hospitalization in pediatric and adolescent patients. Therefore, when treating patients with asthma, DULERA should only be used for patients not adequately controlled on a long-term asthma control medication, such as an inhaled corticosteroid or whose disease severity clearly warrants initiation of treatment with both an inhaled corticosteroid and LABA. Once asthma control is achieved and maintained, assess the patient at regular intervals and step down therapy (e.g., discontinue DULERA) if possible without loss of asthma control, and maintain the patient on a long-term asthma control medication, such as an inhaled corticosteroid. Do not use DULERA for patients whose asthma is adequately controlled on low or medium dose inhaled corticosteroids. *[See Warnings and Precautions (5.1)]*

1 INDICATIONS AND USAGE

1.1 Treatment of Asthma

DULERA is indicated for the treatment of asthma in patients 12 years of age and older.

Long-acting beta$_2$-adrenergic agonists, such as formoterol, one of the active ingredients in DULERA, increase the risk of asthma-related death. Available data from controlled clinical trials suggest that LABA increase the risk of asthma-related hospitalization in pediatric and adolescent patients *[see Warnings and Precautions (5.1)]*. Therefore, when treating patients with asthma, DULERA should only be used for patients not adequately controlled on a long-term asthma control medication, such as an inhaled corticosteroid or whose disease severity clearly warrants initiation of treatment with both an inhaled corticosteroid and LABA. Once asthma control is achieved and maintained, assess the patient at regular intervals and step down therapy (e.g., discontinue DULERA) if possible without loss of asthma control, and maintain the patient on a long-term asthma control medication, such as an inhaled corticosteroid. Do not use DULERA for patients whose asthma is adequately controlled on low or medium dose inhaled corticosteroids.

Important Limitation of Use

- DULERA is NOT indicated for the relief of acute bronchospasm.

2 DOSAGE AND ADMINISTRATION

2.1 General

DULERA should be administered only by the orally inhaled route (see Instructions for Using DULERA in the Medication Guide). After each dose, the patient should be advised to rinse his/her mouth with water without swallowing.

DULERA should be primed before using for the first time by releasing 4 test sprays into the air, away from the face, shaking well before each spray. In cases where the inhaler has not been used for more than 5 days, prime the inhaler again by releasing 4 test sprays into the air, away from the face, shaking well before each spray.

The DULERA canister should only be used with the DULERA actuator. The DULERA actuator should not be used with any other inhalation drug product. Actuators from other products should not be used with the DULERA canister.

2.2 Dosing

DULERA should be administered as two inhalations twice daily every day (morning and evening) by the orally inhaled route.

Shake well prior to each inhalation.

The recommended starting dosages for DULERA treatment are based on prior asthma therapy.

Table 1: Recommended Dosages for DULERA

Previous Therapy	Recommended Dose	Maximum Recommended Daily Dose
Inhaled medium dose corticosteroids	DULERA 100 mcg/5 mcg, 2 inhalations twice daily	400 mcg/20 mcg
Inhaled high dose corticosteroids	DULERA 200 mcg/5 mcg, 2 inhalations twice daily	800 mcg/20 mcg

The maximum daily recommended dose is two inhalations of DULERA 200 mcg/5 mcg twice daily. Do not use more than two inhalations twice daily of the prescribed strength of DULERA as some patients are more likely to experience adverse effects with higher doses of formoterol. If symptoms arise between doses, an inhaled short-acting beta$_2$-agonist should be taken for immediate relief.

If a previously effective dosage regimen of DULERA fails to provide adequate control of asthma, the therapeutic regimen should be reevaluated and additional therapeutic options, e.g., replacing the current strength of DULERA with a higher strength, adding additional inhaled corticosteroid, or initiating oral corticosteroids, should be considered.

The maximum benefit may not be achieved for 1 week or longer after beginning treatment. Individual patients may experience a variable time to onset and degree of symptom relief. For patients ≥12 years of age who do not respond adequately after 2 weeks of therapy, higher strength may provide additional asthma control.

3 DOSAGE FORMS AND STRENGTHS

DULERA is a pressurized metered dose inhaler that is available in 2 strengths.

DULERA 100 mcg/5 mcg delivers 100 mcg of mometasone furoate and 5 mcg of formoterol fumarate dihydrate per actuation.

DULERA 200 mcg/5 mcg delivers 200 mcg of mometasone furoate and 5 mcg of formoterol fumarate dihydrate per actuation.

4 CONTRAINDICATIONS

4.1 Status Asthmaticus

DULERA is contraindicated in the primary treatment of status asthmaticus or other acute episodes of asthma where intensive measures are required.

4.2 Hypersensitivity

DULERA is contraindicated in patients with known hypersensitivity to mometasone furoate, formoterol fumarate, or any of the ingredients in DULERA *[see Warnings and Precautions (5.10)]*.

5 WARNINGS AND PRECAUTIONS

5.1 Asthma-Related Death

Long-acting beta$_2$-adrenergic agonists, such as formoterol, one of the active ingredients in DULERA, increase the risk of asthma-related death. Currently available data are inadequate to determine whether concurrent use of inhaled corticosteroids or other long-term asthma control drugs mitigates the increased risk of asthma-related death from LABA. Available data from controlled clinical trials suggest that LABA increase the risk of asthma-related hospitalization in pediatric and adolescent patients. Therefore, when treating patients with asthma, physicians should only prescribe DULERA for patients with asthma not adequately controlled on a long-term asthma control medication, such as an inhaled corticosteroid or whose disease severity clearly warrants initiation of treatment with both an inhaled corticosteroid and LABA. Once asthma control is achieved and maintained, assess the patient at regular intervals and step down therapy (e.g., discontinue DULERA) if possible without loss of asthma control, and maintain the patient on a long-term asthma control medication, such as an inhaled corticosteroid. Do not use DULERA for patients whose asthma is adequately controlled on low or medium dose inhaled corticosteroids.

A 28-week, placebo-controlled US study comparing the safety of salmeterol with placebo, each added to usual asthma therapy, showed an increase in asthma-related deaths in patients receiving salmeterol (13/13,176 in patients treated with salmeterol vs. 3/13,179 in patients treated with placebo; RR 4.37, 95% CI 1.25, 15.34). This finding with salmeterol is considered a class effect of the LABAs, including formoterol, one of the active ingredients in DULERA. No study adequate to determine whether the rate of asthma-related death is increased with DULERA has been conducted.

Clinical studies with formoterol suggested a higher incidence of serious asthma exacerbations in patients who received formoterol fumarate than in those who received placebo. The sizes of these studies were not adequate to precisely quantify the differences in serious asthma exacerbation rates between treatment groups.

5.2 Deterioration of Disease and Acute Episodes

DULERA should not be initiated in patients during rapidly deteriorating or potentially life-threatening episodes of asthma. DULERA has not been studied in patients with acutely deteriorating asthma. The initiation of DULERA in this setting is not appropriate.

Increasing use of inhaled, short-acting beta$_2$-agonists is a marker of deteriorating asthma. In this situation, the patient requires immediate re-evaluation with reassessment of the treatment regimen, giving special consideration to the possible need for replacing the current strength of DULERA with a higher strength, adding additional inhaled corticosteroid, or initiating systemic corticosteroids. Patients should not use more than 2 inhalations twice daily (morning and evening) of DULERA.

DULERA is not indicated for the relief of acute symptoms, i.e., as rescue therapy for the treatment of acute episodes of bronchospasm. An inhaled, short-acting beta$_2$-agonist, not DULERA, should be used to relieve acute symptoms such as shortness of breath. When prescribing DULERA, the physician must also provide the patient with an inhaled, short-acting beta$_2$-agonist (e.g., albuterol) for treatment of acute symptoms, despite regular twice-daily (morning and evening) use of DULERA.

When beginning treatment with DULERA, patients who have been taking oral or inhaled, short-acting beta$_2$-agonists on a regular basis (e.g., 4 times a day) should be instructed to discontinue the regular use of these drugs.

5.3 Excessive Use of DULERA and Use with Other Long-Acting Beta$_2$-Agonists

As with other inhaled drugs containing beta$_2$-adrenergic agents, DULERA should not be used more often than recommended, at higher doses than recommended, or in conjunction with other medications containing long-acting beta$_2$-agonists, as an overdose may result. Clinically significant cardiovascular effects and fatalities have been reported in association with excessive use of inhaled sympathomimetic drugs. Patients using DULERA should not use an additional long-acting beta$_2$-agonist (e.g., salmeterol, formoterol fumarate, arformoterol tartrate) for any reason, including prevention of exercise-induced bronchospasm (EIB) or the treatment of asthma.

5.4 Local Effects

In clinical trials, the development of localized infections of the mouth and pharynx with *Candida albicans* have occurred in patients treated with DULERA. If oropharyngeal candidiasis develops, it should be treated with appropriate local or systemic (i.e., oral) antifungal therapy while remaining on treatment with DULERA therapy, but at times therapy with DULERA may need to be interrupted. Advise patients to rinse the mouth after inhalation of DULERA.

5.5 Immunosuppression

Persons who are using drugs that suppress the immune system are more susceptible to infections than healthy individuals.

Chickenpox and measles, for example, can have a more serious or even fatal course in susceptible children or adults using corticosteroids. In such children or adults who have not had these diseases or who are not properly immunized, particular care should be taken to avoid exposure. How the dose, route, and duration of corticosteroid administration affect the risk of developing a disseminated infection is not known. The contribution of the underlying disease and/or prior corticosteroid treatment to the risk is also not known. If exposed to chickenpox, prophylaxis with varicella zoster immune globulin (VZIG) or pooled intravenous immunoglobulin (IVIG) may be indicated. If exposed to measles, prophylaxis with pooled intramuscular immunoglobulin (IG) may be indicated. (See the respective package inserts for complete VZIG and IG prescribing information.) If chickenpox develops, treatment with antiviral agents may be considered.

DULERA should be used with caution, if at all, in patients with active or quiescent tuberculosis infection of the respiratory tract, untreated systemic fungal, bacterial, viral, or parasitic infections; or ocular herpes simplex.

5.6 Transferring Patients from Systemic Corticosteroid Therapy

Particular care is needed for patients who are transferred from systemically active corticosteroids to DULERA because deaths due to adrenal insufficiency have occurred in asthmatic patients during and after transfer from systemic corticosteroids to less systemically available inhaled corticosteroids. After withdrawal from systemic corticosteroids, a number of months are required for recovery of hypothalamic-pituitary-adrenal (HPA) function.

Patients who have been previously maintained on 20 mg or more per day of prednisone (or its equivalent) may be most susceptible, particularly when their systemic corticosteroids have been almost completely withdrawn. During this period of HPA suppression, patients may exhibit signs and symptoms of adrenal insufficiency when exposed to trauma, surgery, or infection (particularly gastroenteritis) or other conditions associated with severe electrolyte loss. Although DULERA may improve control of asthma symptoms during these episodes, in recommended doses it supplies less than normal physiological amounts of corticosteroid systemically and does NOT provide the mineralocorticoid activity necessary for coping with these emergencies.

During periods of stress or severe asthma attack, patients who have been withdrawn from systemic corticosteroids should be instructed to resume oral corticosteroids (in large doses) immediately and to contact their physicians for further instruction. These patients should also be instructed to carry a medical identification card indicating that they may need supplementary systemic corticosteroids during periods of stress or severe asthma attack.

Patients requiring systemic corticosteroids should be weaned slowly from systemic corticosteroid use after transferring to DULERA. Lung function (FEV1 or PEF), beta-agonist use, and asthma symptoms should be carefully monitored during withdrawal of systemic corticosteroids. In addition to monitoring asthma signs and symptoms, patients should be observed for signs and symptoms of adrenal insufficiency such as fatigue, lassitude, weakness, nausea and vomiting, and hypotension.

Transfer of patients from systemic corticosteroid therapy to DULERA may unmask allergic conditions previously suppressed by the systemic corticosteroid therapy, e.g., rhinitis, conjunctivitis, eczema, arthritis, and eosinophilic conditions.

During withdrawal from oral corticosteroids, some patients may experience symptoms of systemically active corticosteroid withdrawal, e.g., joint and/or muscular pain, lassitude, and depression, despite maintenance or even improvement of respiratory function.

5.7 Hypercorticism and Adrenal Suppression

Mometasone furoate, a component of DULERA, will often help control asthma symptoms with less suppression of HPA function than therapeutically equivalent oral doses of prednisone. Since mometasone furoate is absorbed into the circulation and can be systemically active at higher doses, the beneficial effects of DULERA in minimizing HPA dysfunction may be expected only when recommended dosages are not exceeded and individual patients are titrated to the lowest effective dose.

Because of the possibility of systemic absorption of inhaled corticosteroids, patients treated with DULERA should be observed carefully for any evidence of systemic corticosteroid effects. Particular care should be taken in observing patients postoperatively or during periods of stress for evidence of inadequate adrenal response.

It is possible that systemic corticosteroid effects such as hypercorticism and adrenal suppression (including adrenal crisis) may appear in a small number of patients, particularly when mometasone furoate is administered at higher than recommended doses over prolonged periods of time. If such effects occur, the dosage of DULERA should be reduced slowly, consistent with accepted procedures for reducing systemic corticosteroids and for management of asthma symptoms.

5.8 Drug Interactions with Strong Cytochrome P450 3A4 Inhibitors

Caution should be exercised when considering the coadministration of DULERA with ketoconazole, and other known strong CYP3A4 inhibitors (e.g., ritonavir, atazanavir, clarithromycin, indinavir, itraconazole, nefazodone, nelfinavir, saquinavir, telithromycin) because adverse effects related to increased systemic exposure to mometasone furoate may occur [see Drug Interactions (7.1) and Clinical Pharmacology (12.3)].

5.9 Paradoxical Bronchospasm and Upper Airway Symptoms

DULERA may produce inhalation induced bronchospasm with an immediate increase in wheezing after dosing that may be life-threatening. If inhalation induced bronchospasm occurs, it should be treated immediately with an inhaled, short-acting inhaled bronchodilator. DULERA should be discontinued immediately and alternative therapy instituted.

5.10 Immediate Hypersensitivity Reactions

Immediate hypersensitivity reactions may occur after administration of DULERA, as demonstrated by cases of urticaria, flushing, allergic dermatitis, and bronchospasm.

5.11 Cardiovascular and Central Nervous System Effects

Excessive beta-adrenergic stimulation has been associated with seizures, angina, hypertension or hypotension, tachycardia with rates up to 200 beats/min, arrhythmias, nervousness, headache, tremor, palpitation, nausea, dizziness, fatigue, malaise, and insomnia. Therefore, DULERA should be used with caution in patients with cardiovascular disorders, especially coronary insufficiency, cardiac arrhythmias, and hypertension.

Formoterol fumarate, a component of DULERA, can produce a clinically significant cardiovascular effect in some patients as measured by pulse rate, blood pressure, and/or symptoms. Although such effects are uncommon after administration of DULERA at recommended doses, if they occur, the drug may need to be discontinued. In addition, beta-agonists have been reported to produce ECG changes, such as flattening of the T wave, prolongation of the QTc interval, and ST segment depression. The clinical significance of these findings is unknown. Fatalities have been reported in association with excessive use of inhaled sympathomimetic drugs.

5.12 Reduction in Bone Mineral Density

Decreases in bone mineral density (BMD) have been observed with long-term administration of products containing inhaled corticosteroids, including mometasone furoate, one of the components of DULERA. The clinical significance of small changes in BMD with regard to long-term outcomes, such as fracture, is unknown. Patients with major risk factors for decreased bone mineral content, such as prolonged immobilization, family history of osteoporosis, or chronic use of drugs that can reduce bone mass (e.g., anticonvulsants and corticosteroids) should be monitored and treated with established standards of care.

In a 2-year double-blind study in 103 male and female asthma patients 18 to 50 years of age previously maintained on bronchodilator therapy (Baseline FEV1 85%–88% predicted), treatment with mometasone furoate dry powder inhaler 200 mcg twice daily resulted in significant reductions in lumbar spine (LS) BMD at the end of the treatment period compared to placebo. The mean change from Baseline to Endpoint in the lumbar spine BMD was -0.015 (-1.43%) for the mometasone furoate group compared to 0.002 (0.25%) for the placebo group. In another 2-year double-blind study in 87 male and female asthma patients 18 to 50 years of age previously maintained on bronchodilator therapy (Baseline FEV1 82%–83% predicted), treatment with mometasone furoate 400 mcg twice daily demonstrated no statistically significant changes in lumbar spine BMD at the end of the treatment period compared to placebo. The mean change from Baseline to Endpoint in the lumbar spine BMD was -0.018 (-1.57%) for the mometasone furoate group compared to -0.006 (-0.43%) for the placebo group.

5.13 Effect on Growth

Orally inhaled corticosteroids, including DULERA, may cause a reduction in growth velocity when administered to pediatric patients. Monitor the growth of pediatric patients receiving DULERA routinely (e.g., via stadiometry). To minimize the systemic effects of orally inhaled corticosteroids, including DULERA, titrate each patient's dose to the lowest dosage that effectively controls his/her symptoms [see Use in Specific Populations (8.4)].

5.14 Glaucoma and Cataracts

Glaucoma, increased intraocular pressure, and cataracts have been reported following the use of long-term administration of inhaled corticosteroids, including mometasone furoate, a component of DULERA. Therefore, close monitoring is warranted in patients with a change in vision or with a history of increased intraocular pressure, glaucoma, and/or cataracts [see Adverse Reactions (6)].

5.15 Coexisting Conditions

DULERA, like other medications containing sympathomimetic amines, should be used with caution in patients with convulsive disorders or thyrotoxicosis; and in patients who are unusually responsive to sympathomimetic amines. Doses of the related beta₂-agonist albuterol, when administered intravenously, have been reported to aggravate preexisting diabetes mellitus and ketoacidosis.

5.16 Hypokalemia and Hyperglycemia

Beta₂-agonist medications may produce significant hypokalemia in some patients, possibly through intracellular shunting, which has the potential to produce adverse cardiovascular effects. The decrease in serum potassium is usually transient, not requiring supplementation. Clinically significant changes in blood glucose and/or serum potassium were seen infrequently during clinical studies with DULERA at recommended doses.

6 ADVERSE REACTIONS

Long-acting beta₂-adrenergic agonists, such as formoterol, one of the active ingredients in DULERA, increase the risk of asthma-related death. Currently available data are inadequate to determine whether concurrent use of inhaled corticosteroids or other long-term asthma control drugs mitigates the increased risk of asthma-related death from LABA. Available data from controlled clinical trials suggest that LABA increase the risk of asthma-related hospitalization in pediatric and adolescent patients. Data from a large placebo-controlled US trial that compared the safety of another long-acting beta₂-adrenergic agonist (salmeterol) or placebo added to usual asthma therapy showed an increase in asthma-related deaths in patients receiving salmeterol [see Warnings and Precautions (5.1)].

Systemic and local corticosteroid use may result in the following:

- Candida albicans infection [see Warnings and Precautions (5.4)]
- Immunosuppression [see Warnings and Precautions (5.5)]
- Hypercorticism and adrenal suppression [see Warnings and Precautions (5.7)]
- Growth effects in pediatrics [see Warnings and Precautions (5.13)]
- Glaucoma and cataracts [see Warnings and Precautions (5.14)]

Because clinical trials are conducted under widely varying conditions, adverse reaction rates observed in the clinical trials of a drug cannot be directly compared to rates in the clinical trials of another drug and may not reflect the rates observed in practice.

6.1 Clinical Trials Experience

The safety data described below is based on 3 clinical trials which randomized 1913 patients 12 years of age and older with asthma, including 679 patients exposed to DULERA for 12 to 26 weeks and 271 patients exposed for 1 year. DULERA was studied in two placebo- and active-controlled trials (n=781 and n=728, respectively) and in a long term 52-week safety trial (n=404). In the 12 to 26-week clinical trials, the population was 12 to 84 years of age, 41% male and 59% female, 73% Caucasians, 27% non-Caucasians. Patients received two inhalations twice daily of DULERA (100 mcg/5 mcg or 200 mcg/5 mcg), mometasone furoate MDI (100 mcg or 200 mcg), formoterol MDI (5 mcg) or placebo. In the long term 52-week active-comparator safety trial, the population was 12 years to 75 years of age with asthma, 37% male and 63% female, 47% Caucasians, 53% non-Caucasians and received two inhalations twice daily of DULERA 100 mcg/5 mcg or 200 mcg/5 mcg, or an active comparator.

The incidence of treatment emergent adverse reactions associated with DULERA in Table 2 below is based upon pooled data from 2 clinical trials 12 to 26-week in duration in patients 12 years and older treated with two inhalations twice daily of DULERA (100 mcg/5 mcg or 200 mcg/5 mcg), mometasone furoate MDI (100 mcg or 200 mcg), formoterol MDI (5mcg) or placebo.

[See table 2 at left]

Oral candidiasis has been reported in clinical trials at an incidence of 0.7% in patients using DULERA 100 mcg/5 mcg, 0.8 % in patients using DULERA 200 mcg/5 mcg and 0.5 % in the placebo group.

Table 2: Treatment-emergent adverse reactions in DULERA groups occurring at an incidence of ≥3% and more commonly than placebo

Adverse Reactions	DULERA*		Mometasone Furoate*		Formoterol*	Placebo*
	100 mcg/5 mcg n=424 n (%)	200 mcg/5 mcg n=255 n (%)	100 mcg n=192 n (%)	200 mcg n=240 n (%)	5 mcg n=202 n (%)	n=196 n (%)
Nasopharyngitis	20 (4.7)	12 (4.7)	15 (7.8)	13 (5.4)	13 (6.4)	7 (3.6)
Sinusitis	14 (3.3)	5 (2.0)	6 (3.1)	4 (1.7)	7 (3.5)	2 (1.0)
Headache	19 (4.5)	5 (2.0)	10 (5.2)	8 (3.3)	6 (3.0)	7 (3.6)
Average Duration of Exposure (days)	116	81	165	79	131	138

*All treatments were administered as two inhalations twice daily.

Long Term Clinical Trial Experience

In a long term safety trial in patients 12 years and older treated for 52 weeks with DULERA 100 mcg/5 mcg (n=141), DULERA 200 mcg/5 mcg (n=130) or an active comparator (n=133), safety outcomes in general were similar to those observed in the shorter 12 to 26 week controlled trials. No asthma-related deaths were observed. Dysphonia was observed at a higher frequency in the longer term treatment trial at a reported incidence of 7/141 (5%) patients receiving DULERA 100 mcg/5 mcg and 5/130 (3.8%) patients receiving DULERA 200 mcg/5 mcg. No clinically significant changes in blood chemistry, hematology, or ECG were observed.

7 DRUG INTERACTIONS

In clinical trials, concurrent administration of DULERA and other drugs, such as short-acting beta₂-agonist and intranasal corticosteroids have not resulted in an increased frequency of adverse drug reactions. No formal drug interaction studies have been performed with DULERA. The drug interactions of the combination are expected to reflect those of the individual components.

7.1 Inhibitors of Cytochrome P450 3A4

The main route of metabolism of corticosteroids, including mometasone furoate, a component of DULERA, is via cytochrome P450 (CYP) isoenzyme 3A4 (CYP3A4). After oral administration of ketoconazole, a strong inhibitor of CYP3A4, the mean plasma concentration of orally inhaled mometasone furoate increased. Concomitant administration of CYP3A4 inhibitors may inhibit the metabolism of, and increase the systemic exposure to, mometasone furoate. Caution should be exercised when considering the coadministration of DULERA with long-term ketoconazole and other known strong CYP3A4 inhibitors (e.g., ritonavir, atazanavir, clarithromycin, indinavir, itraconazole, nefazodone, nelfinavir, saquinavir, telithromycin) *[see Warnings and Precautions (5.8) and Clinical Pharmacology (12.3)]*.

7.2 Adrenergic agents

If additional adrenergic drugs are to be administered by any route, they should be used with caution because the pharmacologically predictable sympathetic effects of formoterol, a component of DULERA, may be potentiated.

7.3 Xanthine derivatives

Concomitant treatment with xanthine derivatives may potentiate any hypokalemic effect of formoterol, a component of DULERA.

7.4 Diuretics

Concomitant treatment with diuretics may potentiate the possible hypokalemic effect of adrenergic agonists. The ECG changes and/or hypokalemia that may result from the administration of non-potassium sparing diuretics (such as loop or thiazide diuretics) can be acutely worsened by beta-agonists, especially when the recommended dose of the beta-agonist is exceeded. Although the clinical significance of these effects is not known, caution is advised in the coadministration of DULERA with non-potassium sparing diuretics.

7.5 Monoamine oxidase inhibitors, tricyclic antidepressants, and drugs known to prolong the QTc interval

DULERA should be administered with caution to patients being treated with monoamine oxidase inhibitors, tricyclic antidepressants, or drugs known to prolong the QTc interval or within 2 weeks of discontinuation of such agents, because the action of formoterol, a component of DULERA, on the cardiovascular system may be potentiated by these agents. Drugs that are known to prolong the QTc interval have an increased risk of ventricular arrhythmias.

7.6 Beta-adrenergic receptor antagonists

Beta-adrenergic receptor antagonists (beta-blockers) and formoterol may inhibit the effect of each other when administered concurrently. Beta-blockers not only block the therapeutic effects of beta₂-agonists, such as formoterol, a component of DULERA, but may produce severe bronchospasm in patients with asthma. Therefore, patients with asthma should not normally be treated with beta-blockers. However, under certain circumstances, e.g., as prophylaxis after myocardial infarction, there may be no acceptable alternatives to the use of beta-blockers in patients with asthma. In this setting, cardioselective beta-blockers could be considered, although they should be administered with caution.

8 USE IN SPECIFIC POPULATIONS

8.1 Pregnancy

DULERA: Teratogenic Effects: Pregnancy Category C

There are no adequate and well-controlled studies of DULERA, mometasone furoate only or formoterol fumarate only in pregnant women. Animal reproduction studies of mometasone furoate and formoterol in mice, rats, and/or rabbits revealed evidence of teratogenicity as well as other developmental toxic effects. Because animal reproduction studies are not always predictive of human response, DULERA should be used during pregnancy only if the potential benefit justifies the potential risk to the fetus.

Mometasone Furoate: Teratogenic Effects

When administered to pregnant mice, rats, and rabbits, mometasone furoate increased fetal malformations and decreased fetal growth (measured by lower fetal weights and/or delayed ossification). Dystocia and related complications were also observed when mometasone furoate was administered to rats late in gestation. However, experience with oral corticosteroids suggests that rodents are more prone to teratogenic effects from corticosteroid exposure than humans.

In a mouse reproduction study, subcutaneous mometasone furoate produced cleft palate at approximately one-third of the maximum recommended daily human dose (MRHD) on a mcg/m² basis and decreased fetal survival at approximately 1 time the MRHD. No toxicity was observed at approximately one-tenth of the MRHD on a mcg/m² basis.

In a rat reproduction study, mometasone furoate produced umbilical hernia at topical dermal doses approximately 6 times the MRHD on a mcg/m² basis and delays in ossification at approximately 3 times the MRHD on a mcg/m² basis. In another study, rats received subcutaneous doses of mometasone furoate throughout pregnancy or late in gestation. Treated animals had prolonged and difficult labor, fewer live births, lower birth weight, and reduced early pup survival at a dose that was approximately 8 times the MRHD on an area under the curve (AUC) basis. Similar effects were not observed at approximately 4 times MRHD on an AUC basis.

In rabbits, mometasone furoate caused multiple malformations (e.g., flexed front paws, gallbladder agenesis, umbilical hernia, hydrocephaly) at topical dermal doses approximately 3 times the MRHD on a mcg/m² basis. In an oral study, mometasone furoate increased resorptions and caused cleft palate and/or head malformations (hydrocephaly and domed head) at a dose less than the MRHD based on AUC. At a dose approximately 2 times the MRHD based on AUC, most litters were aborted or resorbed *[see Nonclinical Toxicology (13.2)]*.

Nonteratogenic Effects:

Hypoadrenalism may occur in infants born to women receiving corticosteroids during pregnancy. Infants born to mothers taking substantial corticosteroid doses during pregnancy should be monitored for signs of hypoadrenalism.

Formoterol Fumarate: Teratogenic Effects

Formoterol fumarate administered throughout organogenesis did not cause malformations in rats or rabbits following oral administration. When given to rats throughout organogenesis, oral doses of approximately 80 times the MRHD on a mcg/m² basis and above delayed ossification of the fetus, and doses of approximately 2,400 times the MRHD on a mcg/m² basis and above decreased fetal weight. Formoterol fumarate has been shown to cause stillbirth and neonatal mortality at oral doses of approximately 2,400 times the MRHD on a mcg/m² basis and above in rats receiving the drug during the late stage of pregnancy. These effects, however, were not produced at a dose of approximately 80 times the MRHD on a mcg/m² basis.

In another testing laboratory, formoterol was shown to be teratogenic in rats and rabbits. Umbilical hernia, a malformation, was observed in rat fetuses at oral doses approximately 1,200 times and greater than the MRHD on a mcg/m² basis. Brachygnathia, a skeletal malformation, was observed in rat fetuses at an oral dose approximately 6,100 times the MRHD on a mcg/m² basis. In another study in rats, no teratogenic effects were seen at inhalation doses up to approximately 500 times the MRHD on a mcg/m² basis. Subcapsular cysts on the liver were observed in rabbit fetuses at an oral dose approximately 49,000 times the MRHD on a mcg/m² basis. No teratogenic effects were observed at oral doses up to approximately 3,000 times the MRHD on a mcg/m² basis *[see Nonclinical Toxicology (13.2)]*.

8.2 Labor and Delivery

There are no adequate and well-controlled human studies that have studied the effects of DULERA during labor and delivery.

Because beta-agonists may potentially interfere with uterine contractility, DULERA should be used during labor only if the potential benefit justifies the potential risk *[see Nonclinical Toxicology (13.2)]*.

8.3 Nursing Mothers

DULERA: It is not known whether DULERA is excreted in human milk. Because many drugs are excreted in human milk, caution should be exercised when DULERA is administered to a nursing woman.

Since there are no data from well-controlled human studies on the use of DULERA on nursing mothers, based on data for the individual components, a decision should be made whether to discontinue nursing or to discontinue DULERA, taking into account the importance of DULERA to the mother.

Mometasone Furoate: It is not known if mometasone furoate is excreted in human milk. However, other corticosteroids are excreted in human milk.

Formoterol Fumarate: In reproductive studies in rats, formoterol was excreted in the milk. It is not known whether formoterol is excreted in human milk.

8.4 Pediatric Use

The safety and effectiveness of DULERA have been established in patients 12 years of age and older in 3 clinical trials up to 52 weeks in duration. In the 3 clinical trials, 101 patients 12 to 17 years of age were treated with DULERA. Patients in this age-group demonstrated efficacy results similar to those observed in patients 18 years of age and older. There were no obvious differences in the type or frequency of adverse drug reactions reported in this age group compared to patients 18 years of age and older. Similar efficacy and safety results were observed in an additional 22 patients 12 to 17 years of age who were treated with DULERA in another clinical trial. The safety and efficacy of DULERA have not been established in children less than 12 years of age.

Controlled clinical studies have shown that inhaled corticosteroids may cause a reduction in growth velocity in pediatric patients. In these studies, the mean reduction in growth velocity was approximately 1 cm per year (range 0.3 to 1.8 per year) and appears to depend upon dose and duration of exposure. This effect was observed in the absence of laboratory evidence of hypothalamic-pituitary-adrenal (HPA) axis suppression, suggesting that growth velocity is a more sensitive indicator of systemic corticosteroid exposure in pediatric patients than some commonly used tests of HPA axis function. The long-term effects of this reduction in growth velocity associated with orally inhaled corticosteroids, including the impact on final adult height, are unknown. The potential for "catch up" growth following discontinuation of treatment with orally inhaled corticosteroids has not been adequately studied.

The growth of children and adolescents receiving orally inhaled corticosteroids, including DULERA, should be monitored routinely (e.g., via stadiometry). If a child or adolescent on any corticosteroid appears to have growth suppression, the possibility that he/she is particularly sensitive to this effect should be considered. The potential growth effects of prolonged treatment should be weighed against clinical benefits obtained and the risks associated with alternative therapies. To minimize the systemic effects of orally inhaled corticosteroids, including DULERA, each patient should be titrated to his/her lowest effective dose *[see Dosage and Administration (2.2)]*.

8.5 Geriatric Use

A total of 77 patients 65 years of age and older (of which 11 were 75 years and older) have been treated with DULERA in 3 clinical trials up to 52 weeks in duration. Similar efficacy and safety results were observed in an additional 28 patients 65 years of age and older who were treated with DULERA in another clinical trial. No overall differences in safety or effectiveness were observed between these patients and younger patients, but greater sensitivity of some older individuals cannot be ruled out. As with other products containing beta₂-agonists, special caution should be observed when using DULERA in geriatric patients who have concomitant cardiovascular disease that could be adversely affected by beta₂-agonists. Based on available data for DULERA or its active components, no adjustment of dosage of DULERA in geriatric patients is warranted.

8.6 Hepatic Impairment

Concentrations of mometasone furoate appear to increase with severity of hepatic impairment *[see Clinical Pharmacology (12.3)]*.

10 OVERDOSAGE

10.1 Signs and Symptoms

DULERA: DULERA contains both mometasone furoate and formoterol fumarate; therefore, the risks associated with overdosage for the individual components described below apply to DULERA.

Mometasone Furoate: Chronic overdosage may result in signs/symptoms of hypercorticism *[see Warnings and Precautions (5.7)]*. Single oral doses up to 8000 mcg of mometasone furoate have been studied on human volunteers with no adverse reactions reported.

Formoterol Fumarate: The expected signs and symptoms with overdosage of formoterol are those of excessive beta-adrenergic stimulation and/or occurrence or exaggeration of any of the following signs and symptoms: angina, hypertension or hypotension, tachycardia, with rates up to 200 beats/min., arrhythmias, nervousness, headache, tremor, seizures, muscle cramps, dry mouth, palpitation, nausea, dizziness, fatigue, malaise, hypokalemia, hyperglycemia, and insomnia. Metabolic acidosis may also occur. Cardiac arrest and even death may be associated with an overdose of formoterol.

The minimum acute lethal inhalation dose of formoterol fumarate in rats is 156 mg/kg (approximately 63,000 times the MRHD on a mcg/m² basis). The median lethal oral doses in Chinese hamsters, rats, and mice provide even higher multiples of the MRHD.

10.2 Treatment

DULERA: Treatment of overdosage consists of discontinuation of DULERA together with institution of appropriate symptomatic and/or supportive therapy. The judicious use of a cardioselective beta-receptor blocker may be considered, bearing in mind that such medication can produce bronchospasm. There is insufficient evidence to determine if dialysis is beneficial for overdosage of DULERA. Cardiac monitoring is recommended in cases of overdosage.

11 DESCRIPTION

DULERA 100 mcg/5 mcg and DULERA 200 mcg/5 mcg, are combinations of mometasone furoate and formoterol fumarate dihydrate for oral inhalation only.

One active component of DULERA is mometasone furoate, a corticosteroid having the chemical name 9,21-dichloro-11(Beta),17-dihydroxy-16 (alpha)-methylpregna-1,4-diene-3,20-dione 17-(2-furoate) with the following chemical structure:

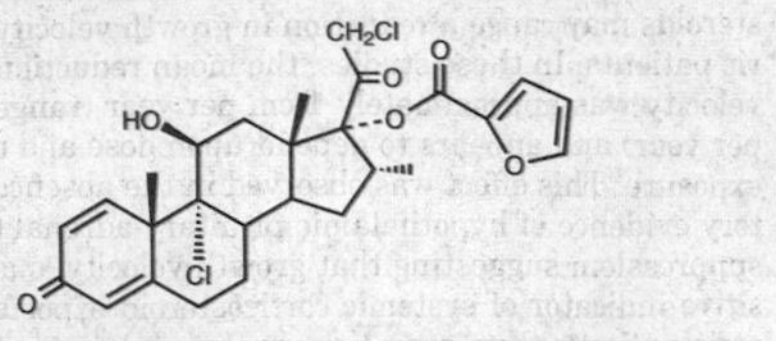

Mometasone furoate is a white powder with an empirical formula of $C_{27}H_{30}Cl_2O_6$, and molecular weight 521.44. It is practically insoluble in water; slightly soluble in methanol, ethanol, and isopropanol; soluble in acetone.

One active component of DULERA is formoterol fumarate dihydrate, a racemate. Formoterol fumarate dihydrate is a selective beta$_2$-adrenergic bronchodilator having the chemical name of (±)-2-hydroxy-5-[(1RS)-1-hydroxy-2-[[(1RS)-2-(4-methoxyphenyl)-1-methylethyl]-amino]ethyl] formanilide fumarate dihydrate with the following chemical structure:

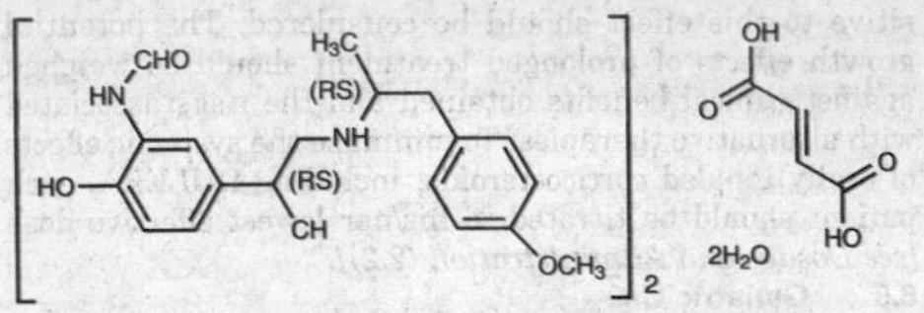

Formoterol fumarate dihydrate has a molecular weight of 840.9, and its empirical formula is $(C_{19}H_{24}N_2O_4)_2 \bullet C_4H_4O_4 \bullet 2H_2O$. Formoterol fumarate dihydrate is a white to yellowish powder, which is freely soluble in glacial acetic acid, soluble in methanol, sparingly soluble in ethanol and isopropanol, slightly soluble in water, and practically insoluble in acetone, ethyl acetate, and diethyl ether.

Each DULERA 100 mcg/5 mcg and 200 mcg/5 mcg is a hydrofluoroalkane (HFA-227) propelled pressurized metered dose inhaler containing sufficient amount of drug for 120 inhalations *[see How Supplied/Storage and Handling (16)]*. After priming, each actuation of the inhaler delivers 115 or 225 mcg of mometasone furoate and 5.5 mcg of formoterol fumarate dihydrate in 69.6 mg of suspension from the valve and delivers 100 or 200 mcg of mometasone furoate and 5 mcg of formoterol fumarate dihydrate from the actuator. The actual amount of drug delivered to the lung may depend on patient factors, such as the coordination between actuation of the device and inspiration through the delivery system. DULERA also contains anhydrous alcohol as a cosolvent and oleic acid as a surfactant.

DULERA should be primed before using for the first time by releasing 4 test sprays into the air, away from the face, shaking well before each spray. In cases where the inhaler has not been used for more than 5 days, prime the inhaler again by releasing 4 test sprays into the air, away from the face, shaking well before each spray.

12 CLINICAL PHARMACOLOGY

12.1 Mechanism of Action

DULERA: DULERA contains both mometasone furoate and formoterol fumarate; therefore, the mechanisms of actions described below for the individual components apply to DULERA. These drugs represent two different classes of medications (a synthetic corticosteroid and a selective long-acting beta$_2$-adrenergic receptor agonist) that have different effects on clinical, physiological, and inflammatory indices of asthma.

Mometasone furoate: Mometasone furoate is a corticosteroid demonstrating potent anti-inflammatory activity. The precise mechanism of corticosteroid action on asthma is not known. Inflammation is an important component in the pathogenesis of asthma. Corticosteroids have been shown to have a wide range of inhibitory effects on multiple cell types (e.g., mast cells, eosinophils, neutrophils, macrophages, and lymphocytes) and mediators (e.g., histamine, eicosanoids, leukotrienes, and cytokines) involved in inflammation and in the asthmatic response. These anti-inflammatory actions of corticosteroids may contribute to their efficacy in asthma.

Mometasone furoate has been shown *in vitro* to exhibit a binding affinity for the human glucocorticoid receptor, which is approximately 12 times that of dexamethasone, 7 times that of triamcinolone acetonide, 5 times that of budesonide, and 1.5 times that of fluticasone. The clinical significance of these findings is unknown.

Formoterol fumarate: Formoterol fumarate is a long-acting selective beta$_2$-adrenergic receptor agonist (beta$_2$-agonist). Inhaled formoterol fumarate acts locally in the lung as a bronchodilator. *In vitro* studies have shown that formoterol has more than 200-fold greater agonist activity at beta$_2$-receptors than at beta$_1$-receptors. Although beta$_2$-receptors are the predominant adrenergic receptors in bronchial smooth muscle and beta$_1$-receptors are the predominant receptors in the heart, there are also beta$_2$-receptors in the human heart comprising 10% to 50% of the total beta-adrenergic receptors. The precise function of these receptors has not been established, but they raise the possibility that even highly selective beta$_2$-agonists may have cardiac effects.

The pharmacologic effects of beta$_2$-adrenoceptor agonist drugs, including formoterol, are at least in part attributable to stimulation of intracellular adenyl cyclase, the enzyme that catalyzes the conversion of adenosine triphosphate (ATP) to cyclic-3′, 5′-adenosine monophosphate (cyclic AMP). Increased cyclic AMP levels cause relaxation of bronchial smooth muscle and inhibition of release of mediators of immediate hypersensitivity from cells, especially from mast cells.

In vitro tests show that formoterol is an inhibitor of the release of mast cell mediators, such as histamine and leukotrienes, from the human lung. Formoterol also inhibits histamine-induced plasma albumin extravasation in anesthetized guinea pigs and inhibits allergen-induced eosinophil influx in dogs with airway hyper-responsiveness. The relevance of these *in vitro* and animal findings to humans is unknown.

12.2 Pharmacodynamics

Cardiovascular Effects:

DULERA:

In a single dose, double blind placebo controlled crossover trial in 25 patients with asthma, single dose treatment of 10 mcg formoterol fumarate in combination with 400 mcg of mometasone furoate delivered via DULERA 200 mcg/5 mcg were compared to formoterol fumarate 10 mcg MDI, formoterol fumarate 12 mcg dry powder inhaler (DPI; nominal dose of formoterol fumarate delivered 10 mcg), or placebo. The degree of bronchodilation at 12 hours after dosing with DULERA was similar to formoterol fumarate delivered alone via MDI or DPI.

ECGs and blood samples for glucose and potassium were obtained prior to dosing and post dose. No downward trend in serum potassium was observed and values were within the normal range and appeared to be similar across all treatments over the 12 hour period. Mean blood glucose appeared similar across all groups for each time point. There was no evidence of significant hypokalemia or hyperglycemia in response to formoterol treatment.

No relevant changes in heart rate or changes in ECG data were observed with DULERA in the trial. No patients had a QTcB (QTc corrected by Bazett's formula) ≥500 msec during treatment.

In a single dose crossover trial involving 24 healthy subjects, single dose of formoterol fumarate 10, 20, or 40 mcg in combination with 400 mcg of mometasone furoate delivered via DULERA were evaluated for safety (ECG, blood potassium and glucose changes). ECGs and blood samples for glucose and potassium were obtained at baseline and post dose. Decrease in mean serum potassium was similar across all three treatment groups (approximately 0.3 mmol/L) and values were within the normal range. No clinically significant increases in mean blood glucose values or heart rate were observed. No subjects had a QTcB >500 msec during treatment.

Three active- and placebo-controlled trials (study duration ranging from 12, 26, and 52 weeks) evaluated 1913 patients 12 years of age and older with asthma. No clinically meaningful changes were observed in potassium and glucose values, vital signs, or ECG parameters in patients receiving DULERA.

HPA Axis Effects:

The effects of inhaled mometasone furoate administered via DULERA on adrenal function were evaluated in two clinical trials in patients with asthma. HPA-axis function was assessed by 24-hour plasma cortisol AUC. Although both these trials have open-label design and contain small number of subjects per treatment arm, results from these trials taken together demonstrated suppression of 24-hour plasma cortisol AUC for DULERA 200 mcg/5 mcg compared to placebo consistent with the known systemic effects of inhaled corticosteroid.

In a 42-day, open-label, placebo and active-controlled study 60 patients with asthma 18 years of age and older were randomized to receive two inhalations twice daily of 1 of the following treatments: DULERA 100 mcg/5 mcg, DULERA 200 mcg/5 mcg, fluticasone propionate/salmeterol xinafoate 230 mcg/21 mcg, or placebo. At Day 42, the mean change from baseline plasma cortisol AUC (0–24 hr) was 8%, 22% and 34% lower compared to placebo for the DULERA 100 mcg/5 mcg (n=13), DULERA 200 mcg/5 mcg (n=15) and fluticasone propionate/salmeterol xinafoate 230 mcg/21 mcg (n=16) treatment groups, respectively.

In a 52-week, open-label safety study, primary analysis of the plasma cortisol 24-hour AUC was performed on 57 patients with asthma who received 2 inhalations twice daily of DULERA 100 mcg/5 mcg, DULERA 200 mcg/5 mcg, fluticasone propionate/salmeterol xinafoate 250/50, or fluticasone propionate/salmeterol xinafoate 500/50. At Week 52, the mean plasma cortisol AUC (0–24 hr) was 2.2%, 29.6%, 16.7%, and 32.2% lower from baseline for the DULERA 100 mcg/5 mcg (n=18), DULERA 200 mcg/5 mcg (n=20), fluticasone propionate/salmeterol xinafoate 250/50 mcg (n=8), and fluticasone propionate/salmeterol xinafoate 500/50 mcg (n=11) treatment groups, respectively.

Other Mometasone Products

HPA Axis Effects:

The potential effect of mometasone furoate via a dry powder inhaler (DPI) on the HPA axis was assessed in a 29-day study. A total of 64 adult patients with mild to moderate asthma were randomized to one of 4 treatment groups: mometasone furoate DPI 440 mcg twice daily, mometasone furoate DPI 880 mcg twice daily, oral prednisone 10 mg once daily, or placebo. The 30-minute post-Cosyntropin stimulation serum cortisol concentration on Day 29 was 23.2 mcg/dl for the mometasone furoate DPI 440 mcg twice daily group and 20.8 mcg/dl for the mometasone furoate DPI 880 mcg twice daily group, compared to 14.5 mcg/dl for the oral prednisone 10 mg group and 25 mcg/dl for the placebo group. The difference between mometasone furoate DPI 880 mcg twice daily (twice the maximum recommended dose) and placebo was statistically significant.

12.3 Pharmacokinetics

Absorption

Mometasone furoate:

Healthy Subjects: The systemic exposures to mometasone furoate from DULERA versus mometasone furoate delivered via DPI were compared. Following oral inhalation of single and multiple doses of the DULERA, mometasone furoate was absorbed in healthy subjects with median Tmax values ranging from 0.50 to 4 hours. Following single-dose administration of higher than recommended dose of DULERA (4 inhalations of DULERA 200 mcg/5 mcg) in healthy subjects, the arithmetic mean (CV%) Cmax and AUC (0–12h) values for MF were 67.8 (49) pg/mL and 650 (51) pg•hr/mL, respectively while the corresponding estimates following 5 days of BID dosing of DULERA 800 mcg/20 mcg were 241 (36) pg/mL and 2200 (35) pg•hr/mL. Exposure to mometasone furoate increased with increasing inhaled dose of DULERA 100 mcg/5 mcg to 200 mcg/5 mcg. Studies using oral dosing of labeled and unlabeled drug have demonstrated that the oral systemic bioavailability of mometasone furoate is negligible (<1%).

The above study demonstrated that the systemic exposure to mometasone furoate (based on AUC) was approximately 52% and 25% lower on Day 1 and Day 5, respectively, following DULERA administration compared to mometasone furoate via a DPI.

Asthma Patients: Following oral inhalation of single and multiple doses of the DULERA, mometasone furoate was absorbed in asthma patients with median Tmax values ranging from 1 to 2 hours. Following single-dose administration of DULERA 400 mcg/10 mcg, the arithmetic mean (CV%) Cmax and AUC (0–12h) values for MF were 20 (88) pg/mL and 170 (94) pg•hr/mL, respectively while the corresponding estimates following BID dosing of DULERA 400 mcg/10 mcg at steady-state were 60 (36) pg/mL and 577 (40) pg•hr/mL.

Formoterol fumarate:

Healthy Subjects: When DULERA was administered to healthy subjects, formoterol was absorbed with median Tmax values ranging from 0.167 to 0.5 hour. In a single-dose study with DULERA 400 mcg/10 mcg in healthy subjects, arithmetic mean (CV%) Cmax and AUC for formoterol were 15 (50) pmol/L and 81 (51) pmol*h/L, respectively. Over the dose range of 10 to 40 mcg for formoterol from DULERA, the exposure to formoterol was dose proportional.

Asthma Patients: When DULERA was administered to patients with asthma, formoterol was absorbed with median Tmax values ranging from 0.58 to 1.97 hours. In a single-dose study with DULERA 400 mcg/10 mcg in patients with asthma, arithmetic mean (CV%) Cmax and AUC (0–12h) for formoterol were 22 (29) pmol/L and 125 (42) pmol*h/L, respectively. Following multiple-dose administration of DULERA 400 mcg/10 mcg, the steady-state arithmetic mean (CV%) Cmax and AUC (0–12h) for formoterol were 41 (59) pmol/L and 226 (54) pmol*hr/L.

Distribution

Mometasone furoate: Based on the study employing a 1000 mcg inhaled dose of tritiated mometasone furoate inhalation powder in humans, no appreciable accumulation of mometasone furoate in the red blood cells was found. Following an intravenous 400 mcg dose of mometasone furoate, the plasma concentrations showed a biphasic decline, with a mean steady-state volume of distribution of 152 liters. The *in vitro* protein binding for mometasone furoate was reported to be 98 to 99% (in a concentration range of 5 to 500 ng/mL).

Formoterol fumarate: The binding of formoterol to human plasma proteins in vitro was 61% to 64% at concentrations from 0.1 to 100 ng/mL. Binding to human serum albumin *in vitro* was 31% to 38% over a range of 5 to 500 ng/mL. The concentrations of formoterol used to assess the plasma protein binding were higher than those achieved in plasma following inhalation of a single 120 mcg dose.

Metabolism

Mometasone furoate: Studies have shown that mometasone furoate is primarily and extensively metabolized in the liver of all species investigated and undergoes extensive metabolism to multiple metabolites. In-vitro studies have confirmed the primary role of human liver cytochrome P-450 3A4 (CYP3A4) in the metabolism of this compound, however, no major metabolites were identified. Human liver CYP3A4 metabolizes mometasone furoate to 6-beta hydroxy mometasone furoate.

Formoterol fumarate: Formoterol is metabolized primarily by direct glucuronidation at either the phenolic or aliphatic hydroxyl group and O-demethylation followed by glucuronide conjugation at either phenolic hydroxyl groups. Minor pathways involve sulfate conjugation of formoterol and deformylation followed by sulfate conjugation. The most prominent pathway involves direct conjugation at the phenolic hydroxyl group. The second major pathway involves O-demethylation followed by conjugation at the phenolic 2′-hydroxyl group. Four cytochrome P450 isozymes (CYP2D6, CYP2C19, CYP2C9 and CYP2A6) are involved in the O-demethylation of formoterol. Formoterol did not inhibit CYP450 enzymes at therapeutically relevant concentrations. Some patients may be deficient in CYP2D6 or 2C19 or both. Whether a deficiency in one or both of these isozymes results in elevated systemic exposure to formoterol or systemic adverse effects has not been adequately explored.

Excretion

Mometasone furoate: Following an intravenous dosing, the terminal half-life was reported to be about 5 hours. Following the inhaled dose of tritiated 1000 mcg mometasone furoate, the radioactivity is excreted mainly in the feces (a mean of 74%), and to a small extent in the urine (a mean of 8%) up to 7 days. No radioactivity was associated with unchanged mometasone furoate in the urine. Absorbed mometasone furoate is cleared from plasma at a rate of approximately 12.5 mL/min/kg, independent of dose. The effective t½ for mometasone furoate following inhalation with DULERA was 25 hours in healthy subjects and in patients with asthma.

Formoterol fumarate: Following oral administration of 80 mcg of radiolabeled formoterol fumarate to 2 healthy subjects, 59% to 62% of the radioactivity was eliminated in the urine and 32% to 34% in the feces over a period of 104 hours. In an oral inhalation study with DULERA, renal clearance of formoterol from the blood was 217 mL/min. In single-dose studies, the mean t½ values for formoterol in plasma were 9.1 hours and 10.8 hours from the urinary excretion data. The accumulation of formoterol in plasma after multiple dose administration was consistent with the increase expected with a drug having a terminal t½ of 9 to 11 hour.

Following single inhaled doses ranging from 10 to 40 mcg to healthy subjects from the MFF MDI, 6.2% to 6.8% of the formoterol dose was excreted in urine unchanged. The (R,R) and (S,S)-enantiomers accounted, respectively, for 37% and 63% of the formoterol recovered in urine. From urinary excretion rates measured in healthy subjects, the mean terminal elimination half-lives for the (R,R)- and (S,S)-enantiomers were determined to be 13 and 9.5 hours, respectively. The relative proportion of the two enantiomers remained constant over the dose range studied.

Special Populations

Hepatic/Renal Impairment: There are no data regarding the specific use of DULERA in patients with hepatic or renal impairment.

A study evaluating the administration of a single inhaled dose of 400 mcg mometasone furoate by a dry powder inhaler to subjects with mild (n=4), moderate (n=4), and severe (n=4) hepatic impairment resulted in only 1 or 2 subjects in each group having detectable peak plasma concentrations of mometasone furoate (ranging from 50–105 pcg/mL). The observed peak plasma concentrations appear to increase with severity of hepatic impairment; however, the numbers of detectable levels were few.

Gender and Race: Specific studies to examine the effects of gender and race on the pharmacokinetics of DULERA have not been specifically studied.

Geriatrics: The pharmacokinetics of DULERA have not been specifically studied in the elderly population.

Drug-Drug Interactions

A single-dose crossover study was conducted to compare the pharmacokinetics of 4 inhalations of the following: mometasone furoate MDI, formoterol MDI, DULERA (mometasone furoate/formoterol fumarate MDI), and mometasone furoate MDI plus formoterol fumarate MDI administered concurrently. The results of the study indicated that there was no evidence of a pharmacokinetic interaction between the two components of DULERA.

Inhibitors of Cytochrome P450 Enzymes: Ketoconazole: In a drug interaction study, an inhaled dose of mometasone furoate 400 mcg delivered by a dry powder inhaler was given to 24 healthy subjects twice daily for 9 days and ketoconazole 200 mg (as well as placebo) were given twice daily concomitantly on Days 4 to 9. Mometasone furoate plasma concentrations were <150 pcg/mL on Day 3 prior to coadministration of ketoconazole or placebo. Following concomitant administration of ketoconazole, 4 out of 12 subjects in the ketoconazole treatment group (n=12) had peak plasma concentrations of mometasone furoate >200 pcg/mL on Day 9 (211–324 pcg/mL. Mometasone furoate plasma levels appeared to increase and plasma cortisol levels appeared to decrease upon concomitant administration of ketoconazole.

Specific drug-drug interaction studies with formoterol have not been performed.

13 NONCLINICAL TOXICOLOGY

13.1 Carcinogenesis, Mutagenesis, Impairment of Fertility

Mometasone furoate: In a 2-year carcinogenicity study in Sprague Dawley® rats, mometasone furoate demonstrated no statistically significant increase in the incidence of tumors at inhalation doses up to 67 mcg/kg (approximately 14 times the MRHD on an AUC basis). In a 19-month carcinogenicity study in Swiss CD-1 mice, mometasone furoate demonstrated no statistically significant increase in the incidence of tumors at inhalation doses up to 160 mcg/kg (approximately 9 times the MRHD on an AUC basis).

Mometasone furoate increased chromosomal aberrations in an *in vitro* Chinese hamster ovary cell assay, but did not have this effect in an *in vitro* Chinese hamster lung cell assay. Mometasone furoate was not mutagenic in the Ames test or mouse lymphoma assay, and was not clastogenic in an *in vivo* mouse micronucleus assay, a rat bone marrow chromosomal aberration assay, or a mouse male germ-cell chromosomal aberration assay. Mometasone furoate also did not induce unscheduled DNA synthesis *in vivo* in rat hepatocytes.

In reproductive studies in rats, impairment of fertility was not produced by subcutaneous doses up to 15 mcg/kg (approximately 8 times the MRHD on an AUC basis).

Formoterol fumarate: The carcinogenic potential of formoterol fumarate has been evaluated in 2-year drinking water and dietary studies in both rats and mice. In rats, the incidence of ovarian leiomyomas was increased at doses of 15 mg/kg and above in the drinking water study and at 20 mg/kg in the dietary study, but not at dietary doses up to 5 mg/kg (AUC exposure approximately 265 times human exposure at the MRHD). In the dietary study, the incidence of benign ovarian theca-cell tumors was increased at doses of 0.5 mg/kg and above (AUC exposure at the low dose of 0.5 mg/kg was approximately 27 times human exposure at the MRHD). This finding was not observed in the drinking water study, nor was it seen in mice (see below).

In mice, the incidence of adrenal subcapsular adenomas and carcinomas was increased in males at doses of 69 mg/kg and above in the drinking water study, but not at doses up to 50 mg/kg (AUC exposure approximately 350 times human exposure at the MRHD) in the dietary study. The incidence of hepatocarcinomas was increased in the dietary study at doses of 20 and 50 mg/kg in females and 50 mg/kg in males, but not at doses up to 5 mg/kg in either males or females (AUC exposure approximately 35 times human exposure at the MRHD). Also in the dietary study, the incidence of uterine leiomyomas and leiomyosarcomas was increased at doses of 2 mg/kg and above (AUC exposure at the low dose of 2 mg/kg was approximately 14 times human exposure at the MRHD). Increases in leiomyomas of the rodent female genital tract have been similarly demonstrated with other beta-agonist drugs.

Formoterol fumarate was not mutagenic or clastogenic in the following tests: mutagenicity tests in bacterial and mammalian cells, chromosomal analyses in mammalian cells, unscheduled DNA synthesis repair tests in rat hepatocytes and human fibroblasts, transformation assay in mammalian fibroblasts and micronucleus tests in mice and rats.

Reproduction studies in rats revealed no impairment of fertility at oral doses up to 3 mg/kg (approximately 1200 times the MRHD on a mcg/m^2 basis).

13.2 Animal Toxicology and/or Pharmacology

Animal Pharmacology

Formoterol fumarate: Studies in laboratory animals (minipigs, rodents, and dogs) have demonstrated the occurrence of cardiac arrhythmias and sudden death (with histologic evidence of myocardial necrosis) when beta-agonists and methylxanthines are administered concurrently. The clinical significance of these findings is unknown.

Reproductive Toxicology Studies

Mometasone furoate: In mice, mometasone furoate caused cleft palate at subcutaneous doses of 60 mcg/kg and above (approximately 1/3 of the maximum recommended human dose MRHD on a mcg/m^2 basis). Fetal survival was reduced at 180 mcg/kg (approximately equal to the MRHD on a mcg/m^2 basis). No toxicity was observed at 20 mcg/kg (approximately one-tenth of the MRHD on a mcg/m^2 basis). In rats, mometasone furoate produced umbilical hernia at topical dermal doses of 600 mcg/kg and above (approximately 6 times the MRHD on a mcg/m^2 basis). A dose of 300 mcg/kg (approximately 3 times the MRHD on a mcg/m^2 basis) produced delays in ossification, but no malformations.

When rats received subcutaneous doses of mometasone furoate throughout pregnancy or during the later stages of pregnancy, 15 mcg/kg (approximately 8 times the MRHD on an AUC basis) caused prolonged and difficult labor and reduced the number of live births, birth weight, and early pup survival. Similar effects were not observed at 7.5 mcg/kg (approximately 4 times the MRHD on an AUC basis).

In rabbits, mometasone furoate caused multiple malformations (e.g., flexed front paws, gallbladder agenesis, umbilical hernia, hydrocephaly) at topical dermal doses of 150 mcg/kg and above (approximately 3 times the MRHD on a mcg/m^2 basis). In an oral study, mometasone furoate increased resorptions and caused cleft palate and/or head malformations (hydrocephaly and domed head) at 700 mcg/kg (less than the MRHD on an area under the curve [AUC] basis). At 2800 mcg/kg (approximately 2 times the MRHD on an AUC basis) most litters were aborted or resorbed. No toxicity was observed at 140 mcg/kg (less than the MRHD on an AUC basis).

Formoterol fumarate: Formoterol fumarate administered throughout organogenesis did not cause malformations in rats or rabbits following oral administration. When given to rats throughout organogenesis, oral doses of 0.2 mg/kg (approximately 80 times the MRHD on a mcg/m^2 basis) and above delayed ossification of the fetus, and doses of 6 mg/kg (approximately 2400 times the MRHD on a mcg/m^2 basis) and above decreased fetal weight. Formoterol fumarate has been shown to cause stillbirth and neonatal mortality at oral doses of 6 mg/kg (approximately 2400 times the MRHD on a mcg/m^2 basis) and above in rats receiving the drug during the late stage of pregnancy. These effects, however, were not produced at a dose of 0.2 mg/kg (approximately 80 times the MRHD on a mcg/m^2 basis).

In another testing laboratory, formoterol fumarate was shown to be teratogenic in rats and rabbits. Umbilical hernia, a malformation, was observed in rat fetuses at oral doses of 3 mg/kg/day and above (approximately 1,200 times greater than the MRHD on a mcg/m^2 basis). Brachygnathia, a skeletal malformation, was observed for rat fetuses at an oral dose of 15 mg/kg/day (approximately 6,100 times the MRHD on a mcg/m^2 basis). In another study in rats, no teratogenic effects were seen at inhalation doses up to 1.2 mg/kg/day (approximately 500 times the MRHD on a mcg/m^2 basis). Subcapsular cysts on the liver were observed for rabbit fetuses at an oral dose of 60 mg/kg (approximately 49,000 times the MRHD on a mcg/m^2 basis). No teratogenic effects were observed at oral doses up to 3.5 mg/kg (approximately 3,000 times the MRHD on a mcg/m^2 basis).

14 CLINICAL STUDIES

14.1 Asthma

The safety and efficacy of DULERA were demonstrated in two randomized, double-blind, parallel group, multicenter clinical trials of 12 to 26 weeks in duration involving 1509 patients 12 years of age and older with persistent asthma uncontrolled on medium or high dose inhaled corticosteroids (baseline FEV1 means of 66% to 73% of predicted normal). These studies included a 2 to 3-week run-in period with mometasone furoate to establish a certain level of asthma control. One clinical trial compared DULERA to placebo and the individual components, mometasone furoate and formoterol (Trial 1) and one clinical trial compared two different strengths of DULERA to mometasone furoate alone (Trial 2).

Trial 1: Clinical Trial with DULERA 100 mcg/5 mcg

This 26-week, placebo controlled trial evaluated 781 patients 12 years of age and older comparing DULERA 100 mcg/5 mcg (n=191 patients), mometasone furoate 100 mcg (n=192 patients), formoterol fumarate 5 mcg

Table 3: Trial 1 - Clinically judged deterioration in asthma or reduction in lung function*

	DULERA 100 mcg/5 mcg[†] (n=191)	Mometasone furoate 100 mcg[‡] (n=192)	Formoterol 5 mcg[†] (n=202)	Placebo[†] (n=196)
Clinically judged deterioration in asthma or reduction in lung function*	58 (30%)	65 (34%)	109 (54%)	109 (56%)
Decrease in FEV1[‡]	18 (9%)	19 (10%)	31 (15%)	41 (21%)
Decrease in PEF[§]	37 (19%)	41 (21%)	62 (31%)	61 (31%)
Emergency treatment	0	1 (<1%)	4 (2%)	1 (<1%)
Hospitalization	1 (<1%)	0	0	0
Treatment with excluded asthma medication[¶]	2 (1%)	4 (2%)	17 (8%)	8 (4%)

* Includes only the first event day for each patient. Patients could have experienced more than one event criterion.
† Two inhalations, twice daily.
‡ Decrease in absolute FEV1 below the treatment period stability limit (defined as 80% of the average of the two predose FEV1 measurements taken 30 minutes and immediately prior to the first dose of randomized trial medication)
§ Decrease in AM or PM peak expiratory flow (PEF) on 2 or more consecutive days below the treatment period stability limit (defined as 70% of the AM or PM PEF obtained over the last 7 days of the run-in period)
¶ Thirty patients received glucocorticosteroids; 1 patient received formoterol via dry powder inhaler in the Formoterol 5 mcg group.

Table 4: Trial 1 – Change in trough FEV1 from baseline to Week 12

Treatment arm	N	Baseline (L)	Change from baseline at Week 12 (L)	Treatment difference from placebo (L)	P-value vs. placebo	P-value vs. formoterol
DULERA 100 mcg/5 mcg	167	2.33	0.13	0.18	<0.001	<0.001
Mometasone furoate 100 mcg	175	2.36	0.07	0.12	<0.001	0.058
Formoterol fumarate 5 mcg	141	2.29	0.00	0.05	0.170	
Placebo	145	2.30	-0.05			

LS means and p-values are from Week 12 estimates of a longitudinal analysis model.

(n=202 patients) and placebo (n=196 patients); each administered as 2 inhalations twice daily by metered dose inhalation aerosols. All other maintenance therapies were discontinued. This study included a 2 to 3-week run-in period with mometasone furoate 100 mcg, 2 inhalations twice daily. This trial included patients ranging from 12 to 76 years of age, 41% male and 59% female, and 72% Caucasian and 28% non-Caucasian. Patients had persistent asthma and were not well controlled on medium dose of inhaled corticosteroids prior to randomization. All treatment groups were balanced with regard to baseline characteristics. Mean FEV1 and mean percent predicted FEV1 were similar among all treatment groups (2.33 L, 73%). Eight (4%) patients receiving DULERA 100 mcg/5 mcg, 13 (7%) patients receiving mometasone furoate 100 mcg, 47 (23%) patients receiving formoterol fumarate 5 mcg and 46 (23%) patients receiving placebo discontinued the study early due to treatment failure.

FEV1 AUC (0–12hr) was assessed as a co-primary efficacy endpoint to evaluate the contribution of the formoterol component to DULERA. Patients receiving DULERA 100 mcg/5 mcg had significantly higher increases from baseline at Week 12 in mean FEV1 AUC (0–12 hr) compared to mometasone furoate 100 mcg (the primary treatment comparison) and vs. placebo (both p<0.001) (Figure 1). These differences were maintained through Week 26. Figure 1 shows the change from baseline post-dose serial FEV1 evaluations in Trial 1.
[See figure 1 at top of next column]
Clinically judged deteriorations in asthma or reductions in lung function were assessed as another primary endpoint to evaluate the contribution of mometasone furoate 100 mcg to DULERA 100 mcg/5 mcg (primary treatment comparison DULERA vs. formoterol). Deteriorations in asthma were defined as any of the following: a 20% decrease in FEV1; a 30% decrease in PEF on two or more consecutive days; emer-

Figure 1

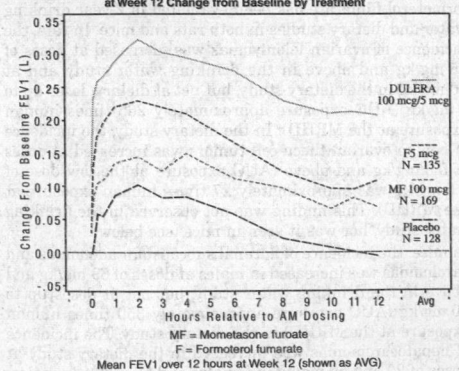

TRIAL 1 - DULERA 100 mcg/5 mcg - FEV1 Serial Evaluations for Observed Cases at Week 12 Change from Baseline by Treatment

MF = Mometasone furoate
F = Formoterol fumarate
Mean FEV1 over 12 hours at Week 12 (shown as AVG)

gency treatment, hospitalization, or treatment with systemic corticosteroids or other asthma medications not allowed per protocol. Fewer patients who received DULERA 100 mcg/5 mcg reported an event compared to patients who received formoterol 5 mcg (p<0.001).
[See table 3 above]
The change in mean trough FEV1 from baseline to Week 12 was assessed as another endpoint to evaluate the contribution of mometasone furoate 100 mcg to DULERA 100 mcg/5 mcg. A significantly greater increase in mean trough FEV1 was observed for DULERA 100 mcg/5 mcg compared to formoterol 5 mcg (the primary treatment comparison) as well as to placebo (Table 4).
[See table 4 above]

The effect of DULERA 100 mcg/5 mcg, two inhalations twice daily on selected secondary efficacy endpoints, including proportion of nights with nocturnal awakenings (-60% vs. -15%), change in total rescue medication use (-0.6 vs. +1.1 puffs/day), change in morning peak flow (+18.1 vs. -28.4 L/min) and evening peak flow (+10.8 vs. -32.1 L/min) further supports the efficacy of DULERA 100 mcg/5 mcg compared to placebo.
The subjective impact of asthma on patients' health-related quality of life was evaluated by the Asthma Quality of Life Questionnaire (AQLQ(S)) (based on a 7-point scale where 1 = maximum impairment and 7 = no impairment). A change from baseline >0.5 points is considered a clinically meaningful improvement. The mean difference in AQLQ between patients receiving DULERA 100 mcg/5 mcg and placebo was 0.5 [95% CI 0.32, 0.68].

Trial 2: Clinical Trial With DULERA 200 mcg/5 mcg
This 12-week double-blind trial evaluated 728 patients 12 years of age and older comparing DULERA 200 mcg/5 mcg (n=255 patients) with DULERA 100 mcg/5 mcg (n=233 patients) and mometasone furoate 200 mcg (n=240 patients), each administered as 2 inhalations twice daily by metered dose inhalation aerosols. All other maintenance therapies were discontinued. This trial included a 2 to 3-week run-in period with mometasone furoate 200 mcg, 2 inhalations twice daily. Patients had persistent asthma and were uncontrolled on high dose inhaled corticosteroids prior to study entry. All treatment groups were balanced with regard to baseline characteristics. This trial included patients ranging from 12 to 84 years of age, 44% male and 56% female, and 89% Caucasian and 11% non-Caucasian. Mean FEV1 and mean percent predicted FEV1 values were similar among all treatment groups (2.05 L, 66%). Eleven (5%) patients receiving DULERA 100 mcg/5 mcg, 8 (3%) patients receiving DULERA 200 mcg/5 mcg and 13 (5%) patients receiving mometasone furoate 200 mcg discontinued the trial early due to treatment failure.
The primary efficacy endpoint was the mean change in FEV1 AUC (0–12 hr) from baseline to Week 12. Patients receiving DULERA 100 mcg/5 mcg and DULERA 200 mcg/5 mcg had significantly greater increases from baseline at Day 1 in mean FEV1 AUC (0–12 hr) compared to mometasone furoate 200 mcg. The difference was maintained over 12 weeks of therapy.
Mean change in trough FEV1 from baseline to Week 12 was also assessed to evaluate the relative contribution of mometasone furoate to DULERA 100 mcg/5 mcg and DULERA 200 mcg/5 mcg (Table 5). A greater numerical increase in the mean trough FEV1 was observed for DULERA 200 mcg/5 mcg compared to DULERA 100 mcg/5 mcg and mometasone furoate 200 mcg.

Table 5: Trial 2 – Change in trough FEV1 from baseline to Week 12

Treatment arm	N	Baseline (L)	Change from baseline at Week 12 (L)
DULERA 100 mcg/5 mcg	232	2.10	0.14
DULERA 200 mcg/5 mcg	255	2.05	0.19
Mometasone furoate 200 mcg	239	2.07	0.10

Clinically judged deterioration in asthma or reduction in lung function was assessed as an additional endpoint. Fewer patients who received DULERA 200 mcg/5 mcg or DULERA 100/5 mcg compared to mometasone furoate 200 mcg alone reported an event, defined as in Trial 1 by any of the following: a 20% decrease in FEV1; a 30% decrease in PEF on two or more consecutive days; emergency treatment, hospitalization, or treatment with systemic corticosteroids or other asthma medications not allowed per protocol.
[See table 6 at top of next page]

Other Studies
In addition to Trial 1 and Trial 2, the safety and efficacy of the individual components, mometasone furoate MDI 100 mcg and 200 mcg, in comparison to placebo were demonstrated in three other, 12-week, placebo controlled trials which evaluated the mean change in FEV1 from baseline as a primary endpoint. The safety and efficacy of formoterol MDI 5 mcg alone in comparison to placebo was replicated in another 26-week trial that evaluated a lower dose of mometasone furoate MDI in combination with formoterol.

16 HOW SUPPLIED/STORAGE AND HANDLING

16.1 How Supplied

DULERA is available in two strengths (Table 7):

Table 7

Package	NDC
DULERA 100 mcg/5 mcg	0085-7206-01
DULERA 200 mcg/5 mcg	0085-4610-01

Each strength is supplied as a pressurized aluminum canister that has a blue plastic actuator integrated with a dose counter and a blue dust cap. Each 120-inhalation canister has a net fill weight of 13 grams. Each canister is placed into a carton. Each carton contains 1 canister and a Medication Guide.

Initially the dose counter will display "124" actuations. After the initial priming with 4 actuations, the dose counter will read "120" and the inhaler is now ready for use.

16.2 Storage and Handling

The DULERA canister should only be used with the DULERA actuator. The DULERA actuator should not be used with any other inhalation drug product. Actuators from other products should not be used with the DULERA canister.

The correct amount of medication in each inhalation cannot be ensured after the labeled number of actuations from the canister has been used, even though the inhaler may not feel completely empty and may continue to operate. The inhaler should be discarded when the labeled number of actuations has been used (the dose counter will read "0").

Store at controlled room temperature 20°–25°C (68°–77°F); excursions permitted to 15°–30°C (59°–86°F) [see USP Controlled Room Temperature].

For best results, the canister should be at room temperature before use. Shake well before using. Keep out of reach of children. Avoid spraying in eyes.

Contents Under Pressure: Do not puncture. Do not use or store near heat or open flame. Exposure to temperatures above 120°F may cause bursting. Never throw container into fire or incinerator.

17 PATIENT COUNSELING INFORMATION

[See Medication Guide.]

17.1 Asthma-Related Death

[See Medication Guide.]

Patients should be informed that formoterol, one of the active ingredients in DULERA, increases the risk of asthma-related death. In pediatric and adolescent patients, formoterol may increase the risk of asthma-related hospitalization. They should also be informed that data are not adequate to determine whether the concurrent use of inhaled corticosteroids, the other component of DULERA, or other long-term asthma-control therapy mitigates or eliminates this risk *[see Warnings and Precautions (5.1)]*.

17.2 Not for Acute Symptoms

DULERA is not indicated to relieve acute asthma symptoms and extra doses should not be used for that purpose. Acute symptoms should be treated with an inhaled, short-acting, beta$_2$-agonist (the health care provider should prescribe the patient with such medication and instruct the patient in how it should be used).

Patients should be instructed to seek medical attention immediately if they experience any of the following:

- If their symptoms worsen
- Significant decrease in lung function as outlined by the physician
- If they need more inhalations of a short-acting beta$_2$-agonist than usual

Patients should be advised not to increase the dose or frequency of DULERA. The daily dosage of DULERA should not exceed two inhalations twice daily. If they miss a dose, they should be instructed to take their next dose at the same time they normally do. DULERA provides bronchodilation for up to 12 hours.

Patients should not stop or reduce DULERA therapy without physician/provider guidance since symptoms may recur after discontinuation *[see Warnings and Precautions (5.2)]*.

17.3 Do Not Use Additional Long-Acting Beta$_2$-Agonists

When patients are prescribed DULERA, other long-acting beta$_2$-agonists should not be used *[see Warnings and Precautions (5.3)]*.

17.4 Risks Associated With Corticosteroid Therapy

Local Effects: Patients should be advised that localized infections with *Candida albicans* occurred in the mouth and pharynx in some patients. If oropharyngeal candidiasis develops, it should be treated with appropriate local or systemic (i.e., oral) antifungal therapy while still continuing with DULERA therapy, but at times therapy with DULERA may need to be temporarily interrupted under close medical supervision. Rinsing the mouth after inhalation is advised *[see Warnings and Precautions (5.4)]*.

Immunosuppression: Patients who are on immunosuppressant doses of corticosteroids should be warned to avoid exposure to chickenpox or measles and, if exposed, to consult their physician without delay. Patients should be informed of potential worsening of existing tuberculosis, fungal, bacterial, viral, or parasitic infections, or ocular herpes simplex *[see Warnings and Precautions (5.5)]*.

Hypercorticism and Adrenal Suppression: Patients should be advised that DULERA may cause systemic corticosteroid effects of hypercorticism and adrenal suppression. Additionally, patients should be instructed that deaths due to adrenal insufficiency have occurred during and after transfer from systemic corticosteroids. Patients should taper slowly from systemic corticosteroids if transferring to DULERA *[see Warnings and Precautions (5.7)]*.

Reduction in Bone Mineral Density: Patients who are at an increased risk for decreased BMD should be advised that the use of corticosteroids may pose an additional risk and should be monitored and, where appropriate, be treated for this condition *[see Warnings and Precautions (5.12)]*.

Reduced Growth Velocity: Patients should be informed that orally inhaled corticosteroids, a component of DULERA, may cause a reduction in growth velocity when administered to pediatric patients. Physicians should closely follow the growth of pediatric patients taking corticosteroids by any route *[see Warnings and Precautions (5.13)]*.

Glaucoma and Cataracts: Long-term use of inhaled corticosteroids may increase the risk of some eye problems (glaucoma or cataracts); regular eye examinations should be considered *[see Warnings and Precautions (5.14)]*.

17.5 Risks Associated With Beta-Agonist Therapy

Patients should be informed that treatment with beta$_2$-agonists may lead to adverse events which include palpitations, chest pain, rapid heart rate, tremor or nervousness *[see Warnings and Precautions (5.11)]*.

Manufactured by 3M Health Care Ltd., Loughborough, United Kingdom.

Manufactured for Schering Corporation, a subsidiary of Merck & Co., Inc., Whitehouse Station, NJ 08889 USA.

Copyright © 2010 Schering Corporation, a subsidiary of Merck & Co., Inc.
All rights reserved.

U.S. Patent Nos. 5889015; 6057307; 6677323; 6068832; 7067502; and 7566705.

The trademarks depicted in this piece are owned by their respective companies.

Table 6: Trial 2 - Clinically judged deterioration in asthma or reduction in lung function*

	DULERA 100 mcg/5 mcg† (n=233)	DULERA 200 mcg/5 mcg† (n=255)	Mometasone furoate 200 mcg† (n=240)
Clinically judged deterioration in asthma or reduction in lung function*	29 (12%)	31 (12%)	44 (18%)
Decrease in FEV1‡	23 (10%)	17 (7%)	33 (14%)
Decrease in PEF on two consecutive days§	2 (1%)	4 (2%)	3 (1%)
Emergency treatment	2 (1%)	1 (<1%)	1 (<1%)
Hospitalization	0	1 (<1%)	0
Treatment with excluded asthma medication¶	5 (2%)	8 (3%)	12 (5%)

* Includes only the first event day for each patient. Patients could have experienced more than one event criterion.
† Two inhalations, twice daily.
‡ Decrease in absolute FEV1 below the treatment period stability limit (defined as 80% of the average of the two predose FEV1 measurements taken 30 minutes and immediately prior to the first dose of randomized trial medication)
§ Decrease in AM or PM peak expiratory flow (PEF) below the treatment period stability limit (defined as 70% of the AM or PM PEF obtained over the last 7 days of the run-in period)
¶ Twenty four patients received glucocorticosteroids; 1 patient received albuterol in the DULERA 200 mcg / 5 mcg group.

MEDICATION GUIDE

DULERA® [dew-LAIR-ah] 100 mcg/5 mcg
(mometasone furoate 100 mcg and formoterol fumarate dihydrate 5 mcg inhalation aerosol)
DULERA® 200 mcg/5 mcg
(mometasone furoate 200 mcg and formoterol fumarate dihydrate 5 mcg inhalation aerosol)

Read the Medication Guide that comes with DULERA® before you start using it and each time you get a refill. There may be new information. This Medication Guide does not take the place of talking to your healthcare provider about your medical condition or treatment.

What is the most important information I should know about DULERA?

DULERA can cause serious side effects, including:

1. **People with asthma who take long-acting beta$_2$-adrenergic agonist (LABA) medicines such as formoterol (one of the medicines in DULERA), have an increased risk of death from asthma problems.** It is not known whether mometasone furoate, the other medicine in DULERA, reduces the risk of death from asthma problems seen with formoterol.
   - **Call your healthcare provider if breathing problems worsen over time while using DULERA. You may need different treatment.**
   - **Get emergency medical care if:**
     - breathing problems worsen quickly, and
     - you use your rescue inhaler medicine, but it does not relieve your breathing problems.
2. **DULERA should be used only if your healthcare provider decides that your asthma is not well controlled with a long-term asthma control medicine, such as an inhaled corticosteroid.**
3. When your asthma is well controlled, your healthcare provider may tell you to stop taking DULERA. Your healthcare provider will decide if you can stop DULERA without loss of asthma control. Your healthcare provider may prescribe a different long-term asthma-control medicine for you, such as an inhaled corticosteroid.
4. Children and adolescents who take LABA medicines may have an increased risk of being hospitalized for asthma problems.

What is DULERA?

DULERA combines an inhaled corticosteroid medicine, mometasone furoate (the same medicine found in ASMANEX TWISTHALER), and a long-acting beta$_2$-agonist medicine (LABA), formoterol (the same medicine found in FORADIL® AEROLIZER®).

- Inhaled corticosteroids help to decrease inflammation in the lungs. Inflammation in the lungs can lead to asthma symptoms.
- LABA medicines are used in people with asthma. LABA medicines help the muscles around the airways in your lungs stay relaxed to prevent asthma symptoms, such as wheezing and shortness of breath. These symptoms can happen when the muscles around the airways tighten. This makes it hard to breathe. In severe cases, wheezing can stop your breathing and may lead to death if not treated right away.

DULERA is used to control symptoms of asthma and prevent symptoms such as wheezing in people 12 years of age and older.

DULERA should not be used as a rescue inhaler.

DULERA contains formoterol (the same medicine found in FORADIL AEROLIZER). LABA medicines such as formoterol increase the risk of death from asthma problems.

DULERA is not for children and adults with asthma who:

- are well controlled with an asthma-control medicine, such as a low to medium dose of an inhaled corticosteroid medicine
- only need a rescue inhaler once in awhile

It is not known if DULERA is safe and effective in children less than 12 years of age.

Who should not use DULERA?

Do not use DULERA:

- to treat sudden severe symptoms of asthma
- if you are allergic to any of the ingredients in DULERA. See the end of the Medication Guide for a list of ingredients in DULERA.

What should I tell my healthcare provider before using DULERA?

Tell your healthcare provider about all of your health conditions, including if you:

- **have heart problems**
- **have high blood pressure**
- **have seizures**
- **have thyroid problems**
- **have diabetes**
- **have liver problems**
- **have osteoporosis**
- **have an immune system problem**
- **have eye problems such as increased pressure in the eye, glaucoma, or cataracts**
- **are allergic to any medicines**

- are exposed to chickenpox or measles
- **have any other medical problems**
- **are pregnant or planning to become pregnant.** It is not known if DULERA may harm your unborn baby.
- **are breastfeeding.** It is not known if DULERA passes into your milk and if it can harm your baby. You and your healthcare provider should decide if you will take DULERA while breastfeeding.

Tell your healthcare provider about all the medicines you take including prescription and non-prescription medicines, vitamins, and herbal supplements. DULERA and certain other medicines may interact with each other. This may cause serious side effects.

Especially, tell your healthcare provider if you take antifungal medicines, such as ketoconazole, or anti-HIV medicines, such as ritonavir. The anti-HIV medicines NORVIR® (ritonavir capsules) Soft Gelatin, NORVIR® (ritonavir oral solution), and KALETRA® (lopinavir/ritonavir) Tablets contain ritonavir.

Know the medicines you take. Keep a list and show it to your healthcare provider and pharmacist each time you get a new medicine.

How should I use DULERA?

See the step-by-step instructions for using DULERA at the end of this Medication Guide. Do not use DULERA unless your healthcare provider has taught you and you understand everything. Ask your healthcare provider or pharmacist if you have any questions.

- Use DULERA exactly as prescribed. **Do not use DULERA more often than prescribed.** DULERA comes in 2 strengths. Your healthcare provider has prescribed the strength that is best for you. Note the differences between DULERA and your other inhaled medications, including the differences in prescribed use and physical appearance.
- DULERA should be taken every day as 2 puffs in the morning and 2 puffs in the evening.
- If you miss a dose of DULERA, skip your missed dose and take your next dose at your regular time. Do not take DULERA more often or use more puffs than you have been prescribed.
- **While you are using DULERA 2 times each day, do not use other medicines that contain a long-acting beta₂-agonist (LABA) for any reason.** Ask your healthcare provider or pharmacist if any of your other medicines are LABA medicines.
- If you take more DULERA than your healthcare provider has prescribed, get medical help right away if you have any unusual symptoms, such as problems breathing, palpitations, chest pain, increased heart rate, nervousness or shakiness.
- Do not change or stop using DULERA or other asthma medicines used to control or treat your breathing problems unless told to do so by your healthcare provider. Your healthcare provider will change your medicines as needed.
- DULERA does not relieve sudden asthma symptoms. Always have a rescue inhaler with you to treat sudden symptoms. Use your rescue inhaler if you have breathing problems between doses of DULERA. If you do not have a rescue inhaler, call your healthcare provider to have one prescribed for you.
- Rinse your mouth with water after each dose (2 puffs) of DULERA. This will help to lessen the chance of getting a yeast infection (thrush) in the mouth and throat.
- Do not spray DULERA in your eyes. If you accidentally get DULERA in your eyes, rinse your eyes with water and if redness or irritation continues, call your healthcare provider.
- **Call your healthcare provider or get medical care right away if:**
  - your breathing problems worsen with DULERA
  - you need to use your rescue inhaler more often than usual
  - your rescue inhaler does not work as well for you at relieving symptoms
  - you use 4 or more inhalations of your rescue inhaler for 2 or more days in a row
  - you use 1 whole canister of your rescue inhaler in 8 weeks' time
  - your peak flow meter results decrease. Your healthcare provider will tell you the numbers that are right for you.
  - you have asthma and your symptoms do not improve after using DULERA regularly for 1 to 2 weeks

What are the possible side effects of DULERA?

DULERA can cause serious side effects, including:
- See "What is the most important information I should know about DULERA?"
- **Thrush in the mouth and throat.** You may develop a yeast infection (Candida albicans) in your mouth or throat. Rinse your mouth with water after using DULERA to help prevent an infection in your mouth or throat.
- **Immune system effects and a higher chance for infections.**
  - Tell your healthcare provider about any signs of infection such as:

  - fever
  - feeling tired
  - pain
  - nausea
  - body aches
  - vomiting
  - chills
- **Adrenal insufficiency.** Adrenal insufficiency is a condition in which the adrenal glands do not make enough steroid hormones. This can happen when you stop taking oral corticosteroid medicines and start inhaled corticosteroid medicines.
- **Increased wheezing right after taking DULERA.** Always have a rescue inhaler with you to treat sudden wheezing.
- **Serious allergic reactions.** Call your healthcare provider or get emergency medical care if you get any of the following symptoms of a serious allergic reaction:
  - rash
  - hives
  - swelling of the face, mouth, and tongue
  - breathing problems
- Using too much of a LABA medicine may cause:
  - **chest pain**
  - **increased or decreased blood pressure**
  - **a fast and irregular heartbeat**
  - **headache**
  - **tremor**
  - **nervousness**
  - **dizziness**
  - **weakness**
  - **seizures**
- **Lower bone mineral density.** This may be a problem for people who already have a higher chance for low bone density (osteoporosis).
- **Slowed growth in children.** A child's growth should be checked often.
- **Eye problems including glaucoma and cataracts.** You should have regular eye exams while using DULERA.
- **Decreases in blood potassium levels (hypokalemia)**
- **Increases in blood sugar levels (hyperglycemia)**

The most common side effects of DULERA include:
- inflammation of the nose and throat (nasopharyngitis)
- inflammation of the sinuses (sinusitis)
- headache

Tell your healthcare provider about any side effect that bothers you or that does not go away.

These are not all the side effects with DULERA. Ask your healthcare provider or pharmacist for more information.

Call your doctor for medical advice about side effects. You may report side effects to FDA at 1-800-FDA-1088.

You may also report side effects to Schering Corporation, a subsidiary of Merck & Co., Inc., at 1-800-526-4099.

How do I store DULERA?

- Store DULERA at room temperature between 59°F to 86°F (15°C to 30°C).
- The contents of your DULERA are under pressure. Do not puncture. Do not use or store near heat or open flame. Storage above 120°F may cause the canister to burst.
- Do not throw container into fire or incinerator.
- **Keep DULERA and all medicines out of the reach of children.**

General Information about DULERA

Medicines are sometimes prescribed for purposes other than those listed in a Medication Guide. Do not use DULERA for a condition for which it was not prescribed. Do not give your DULERA to other people, even if they have the same condition. It may harm them.

This Medication Guide summarizes the most important information about DULERA. If you would like more information, talk with your healthcare provider. You can ask your healthcare provider or pharmacist for information about DULERA that was written for healthcare professionals. For more information about DULERA, go to www.DULERA.com or call 1-800-526-4099.

What are the ingredients in DULERA?

Active ingredients: mometasone furoate and formoterol fumarate dihydrate

Inactive ingredient: hydrofluoroalkane (HFA-227), anhydrous alcohol and oleic acid

Patient Instructions for Use

DULERA®

DULERA® 100 mcg/5 mcg
(mometasone furoate 100 mcg and formoterol fumarate dihydrate 5 mcg inhalation aerosol)

DULERA® 200 mcg/5 mcg
(mometasone furoate 200 mcg and formoterol fumarate dihydrate 5 mcg inhalation aerosol)

How to use your DULERA

Before using your DULERA, read the complete instructions and use only as directed.

The parts of your DULERA:

There are 2 main parts to your DULERA inhaler – the metal canister that holds the medicine and the blue plastic actuator that sprays the medicine from the canister. The in-

haler also has a cap that covers the mouthpiece of the actuator (see Figure 1). The inhaler contains 120 actuations (puffs).

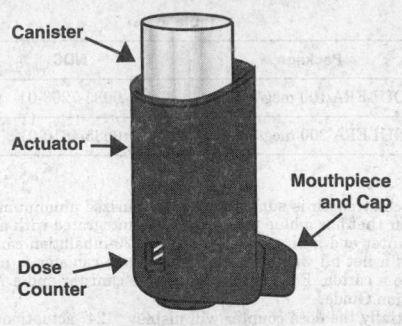

Canister
Actuator
Mouthpiece and Cap
Dose Counter

Figure 1

The inhaler comes with dose counter located on the plastic actuator. See Figure 1. The counter display will show the number of actuations (puffs) of medicine remaining. The dose counter will initially display "124" actuations remaining. Each time you press the canister, a puff of medicine is released and the counter will count down by 1. The counter will stop counting at 0.

- You should not remove the canister from the actuator because reinsertion may cause the counter to count down by 1 and discharge a puff.
- Use the DULERA canister only with the actuator supplied with the product. Do not use parts of the DULERA inhaler with parts from any other inhalation medicine.

Before using your DULERA:

Remove the cap from the mouthpiece of the actuator (see Figure 2). Check the mouthpiece for objects before use. Make sure the canister is fully inserted into the actuator.

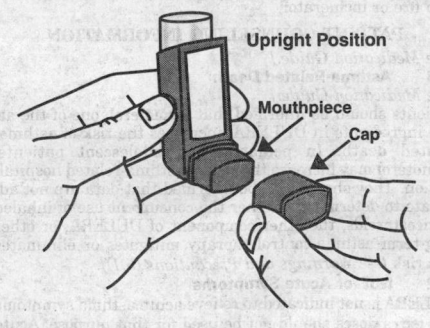

Upright Position
Mouthpiece
Cap

Figure 2

Priming your DULERA Inhaler:

Before you use DULERA for the first time, you must prime the inhaler.

1. To prime the inhaler, hold it in the upright position and release 4 actuations (puffs) into the air, away from your face.
2. Shake the inhaler well before each of the priming actuations. After priming 4 times, the dose counter should read "120".
3. **If you do not use your DULERA for more than 5 days, you will need to prime it again before use.**

Using your DULERA

4. Remove the cap from the mouthpiece of the actuator (see Figure 2). Check the mouthpiece for objects before use. Make sure the canister is fully inserted into the actuator.
5. Shake the inhaler well before each use.
6. Breathe out as fully as you comfortably can through your mouth. Push out as much air from your lungs as possible. Hold the inhaler in the upright position and place the mouthpiece into your mouth (see Figure 3). Close your lips around the mouthpiece.

[See figure 3 at top of next page]

7. Take a deep breath (inhale) in slowly through your mouth. While doing this, press down firmly and fully on the top of the canister until it stops moving in the actuator. Take your finger off the canister.
8. When you have finished breathing in, hold your breath as long as you comfortably can, up to 10 seconds. Then remove the inhaler from your mouth and breathe out through your nose, while keeping your lips closed.
9. Wait at least **30 seconds**, to take your second puff of DULERA.

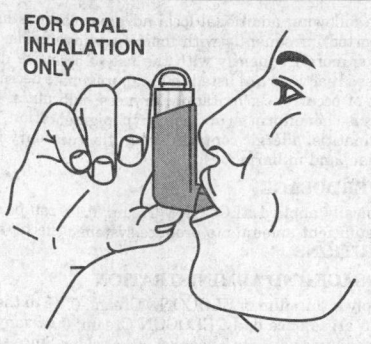

FOR ORAL INHALATION ONLY

Figure 3

10. Shake the inhaler well again and repeat steps 3 through 5 before you take your second puff of DULERA.

After using your DULERA inhaler:

11. Replace the cap over the mouthpiece right away after use.
12. After you finish taking DULERA (2 puffs), rinse your mouth with water.

Reading the counter
- The dose counter identifies the number of inhalations (puffs) left in your inhaler.
- The counter will count down each time you release a puff of medicine (either when preparing your DULERA inhaler for use or when taking the medicine).

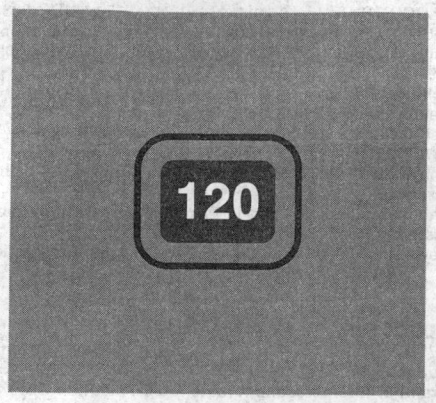

When to replace your DULERA:
- It is important that you pay attention to the number of inhalations (puffs) left in your DULERA inhaler by reading the counter.
- When the counter reads 20, you should refill your prescription or ask your healthcare provider if you need a new prescription for DULERA.
- Throw away DULERA after the counter reaches 0, indicating that you have used the number of actuations on the product label and box. Your inhaler may not feel empty and it may continue to operate, but you will not get the right amount of medicine if you keep using it.
- Never try to change the numbers on the counter or remove the counter from the actuator.
- Do not use the inhaler after the expiration date.

How do I store DULERA?
- Store DULERA at room temperature between 59°F to 86°F (15°C to 30°C).
- The contents of your DULERA canister are under pressure. Do not puncture or throw the canister into a fire or incinerator. Do not use or store it near heat or open flame. Storage above 120°F (50°C) may cause the canister to burst.
- **Keep DULERA and all medicines out of the reach of children.**

How to clean your DULERA:
The mouthpiece should be cleaned using a dry wipe after every 7 days of use.
Routine cleaning instructions:
- Remove the cap off the mouthpiece. Wipe the inside and outside surfaces of the actuator mouthpiece with a clean, dry, lint-free tissue or cloth. Put the cap back on the mouthpiece after cleaning.
- Do not attempt to unblock the actuator with a sharp object, such as a pin.
- Do not wash or put any parts of your inhaler in water.

Manufactured by 3M Health Care Ltd., Loughborough, United Kingdom.

Manufactured for Schering Corporation, a subsidiary of Merck & Co., Inc., Whitehouse Station, NJ 08889 USA.
This Medication Guide has been approved by the U.S. Food and Drug Administration. Copyright © 2010 Schering Corporation, a subsidiary of Merck & Co., Inc. All rights reserved.
The trademarks depicted in this piece are owned by their respective companies.
FORADIL is a registered trademark of Astellas Pharma Inc.
AEROLIZER is a registered trademark of Novartis AG.
NORVIR and KALETRA are registered trademarks of Abbott Laboratories.

Shown in Product Identification Guide, page 312

ELOCON® ℞
[ĕl′ ō-cŏn]
brand of (mometasone furoate cream USP)
Cream 0.1%
For Dermatologic Use Only
Not for Ophthalmic Use
PRODUCT INFORMATION

DESCRIPTION

ELOCON® Cream, 0.1% brand of (mometasone furoate cream USP) contains mometasone furoate USP for dermatologic use. Mometasone furoate is a synthetic corticosteroid with anti-inflammatory activity.

Chemically, mometasone furoate is 9α,21-dichloro-11β,17-dihydroxy-16α-methylpregna-1,4-diene-3,20-dione 17-(2-furoate), with the empirical formula $C_{27}H_{30}Cl_2O_6$, a molecular weight of 521.4 and the following structural formula:

Mometasone furoate is a white to off-white powder practically insoluble in water, slightly soluble in octanol, and moderately soluble in ethyl alcohol.

Each gram of ELOCON Cream, 0.1% contains: 1 mg mometasone furoate USP in a cream base of hexylene glycol; phosphoric acid; propylene glycol stearate (55% monoester); stearyl alcohol and ceteareth-20; titanium dioxide; aluminum starch octenylsuccinate (Gamma Irradiated); white wax; white petrolatum; and purified water.

CLINICAL PHARMACOLOGY

Like other topical corticosteroids, mometasone furoate has anti-inflammatory, antipruritic, and vasoconstrictive properties. The mechanism of the anti-inflammatory activity of the topical steroids, in general, is unclear. However, corticosteroids are thought to act by the induction of phospholipase A_2 inhibitory proteins, collectively called lipocortins. It is postulated that these proteins control the biosynthesis of potent mediators of inflammation such as prostaglandins and leukotrienes by inhibiting the release of their common precursor arachidonic acid. Arachidonic acid is released from membrane phospholipids by phospholipase A_2.

Pharmacokinetics

The extent of percutaneous absorption of topical corticosteroids is determined by many factors including the vehicle and the integrity of the epidermal barrier. Occlusive dressings with hydrocortisone for up to 24 hours have not been demonstrated to increase penetration; however, occlusion of hydrocortisone for 96 hours markedly enhances penetration. Studies in humans indicate that approximately 0.4% of the applied dose of ELOCON® Cream, 0.1% enters the circulation after 8 hours of contact on normal skin without occlusion. Inflammation and/or other disease processes in the skin may increase percutaneous absorption.

Studies performed with ELOCON Cream, 0.1% indicate that it is in the medium range of potency as compared with other topical corticosteroids.

In a study evaluating the effects of mometasone furoate cream on the hypothalamic-pituitary-adrenal (HPA) axis, 15 grams were applied twice daily for 7 days to six adult patients with psoriasis or atopic dermatitis. The cream was applied without occlusion to at least 30% of the body surface. The results show that the drug caused a slight lowering of adrenal corticosteroid secretion.

In a pediatric trial, 24 atopic dermatitis patients, of which 19 patients were age 2 to 12 years, were treated with ELOCON Cream, 0.1% once daily. The majority of patients cleared within 3 weeks.

Ninety-seven pediatric patients ages 6 to 23 months with atopic dermatitis were enrolled in an open-label, hypothalamic-pituitary-adrenal (HPA) axis safety study.

ELOCON Cream, 0.1% was applied once daily for approximately 3 weeks over a mean body surface area of 41% (range 15%–94%). In approximately 16% of patients who showed normal adrenal function by Cortrosyn test before starting treatment, adrenal suppression was observed at the end of treatment with ELOCON Cream, 0.1%. The criteria for suppression were: basal cortisol level of ≤5 mcg/dL, 30-minute post-stimulation level of ≤18 mcg/dL, or an increase of <7 mcg/dL. Follow-up testing 2 to 4 weeks after stopping treatment, available for 5 of the patients, demonstrated suppressed HPA axis function in one patient, using these same criteria.

INDICATIONS AND USAGE

ELOCON® Cream, 0.1% is a medium potency corticosteroid indicated for the relief of the inflammatory and pruritic manifestations of corticosteroid-responsive dermatoses.

ELOCON Cream, 0.1% may be used in pediatric patients 2 years of age or older, although the safety and efficacy of drug use for longer than 3 weeks have not been established (see **PRECAUTIONS, Pediatric Use** section). Since safety and efficacy of ELOCON Cream, 0.1% have not been established in pediatric patients below 2 years of age, its use in this age group is not recommended.

CONTRAINDICATIONS

ELOCON® Cream, 0.1% is contraindicated in those patients with a history of hypersensitivity to any of the components in the preparation.

PRECAUTIONS

General

Systemic absorption of topical corticosteroids can produce reversible hypothalamic-pituitary-adrenal (HPA) axis suppression with the potential for glucocorticosteroid insufficiency after withdrawal of treatment. Manifestations of Cushing's syndrome, hyperglycemia, and glucosuria can also be produced in some patients by systemic absorption of topical corticosteroids while on treatment.

Patients applying a topical steroid to a large surface area or to areas under occlusion should be evaluated periodically for evidence of HPA axis suppression. This may be done by using the ACTH stimulation, A.M. plasma cortisol, and urinary-free cortisol tests.

In a study evaluating the effects of mometasone furoate cream on the hypothalamic-pituitary-adrenal (HPA) axis, 15 grams were applied twice daily for 7 days to six adult patients with psoriasis or atopic dermatitis. The cream was applied without occlusion to at least 30% of the body surface. The results show that the drug caused a slight lowering of adrenal corticosteroid secretion.

If HPA axis suppression is noted, an attempt should be made to withdraw the drug, to reduce the frequency of application, or to substitute a less potent corticosteroid. Recovery of HPA axis function is generally prompt upon discontinuation of topical corticosteroids. Infrequently, signs and symptoms of glucocorticosteroid insufficiency may occur, requiring supplemental systemic corticosteroids. For information on systemic supplementation, see Prescribing Information for those products.

Pediatric patients may be more susceptible to systemic toxicity from equivalent doses due to their larger skin surface to body mass ratios (see **PRECAUTIONS, Pediatric Use** section).

If irritation develops, ELOCON® Cream, 0.1% should be discontinued and appropriate therapy instituted. Allergic contact dermatitis with corticosteroids is usually diagnosed by observing a failure to heal rather than noting a clinical exacerbation as with most topical products not containing corticosteroids. Such an observation should be corroborated with appropriate diagnostic patch testing.

If concomitant skin infections are present or develop, an appropriate antifungal or antibacterial agent should be used. If a favorable response does not occur promptly, use of ELOCON Cream, 0.1% should be discontinued until the infection has been adequately controlled.

Information for Patients

Patients using topical corticosteroids should receive the following information and instructions:

1. This medication is to be used as directed by the physician. It is for external use only. Avoid contact with the eyes.
2. This medication should not be used for any disorder other than that for which it was prescribed.
3. The treated skin area should not be bandaged or otherwise covered or wrapped so as to be occlusive, unless directed by the physician.
4. Patients should report to their physician any signs of local adverse reactions.
5. Parents of pediatric patients should be advised not to use ELOCON Cream, 0.1% in the treatment of diaper dermatitis. ELOCON Cream, 0.1% should not be applied in the diaper area, as diapers or plastic pants may constitute occlusive dressing (see **DOSAGE AND ADMINISTRATION**).

6. This medication should not be used on the face, underarms, or groin areas unless directed by the physician.
7. As with other corticosteroids, therapy should be discontinued when control is achieved. If no improvement is seen within 2 weeks, contact the physician.
8. Other corticosteroid-containing products should not be used with ELOCON Cream, 0.1% without first consulting with the physician.

Laboratory Tests

The following tests may be helpful in evaluating patients for HPA axis suppression:

ACTH stimulation test
A.M. plasma cortisol test
Urinary-free cortisol test

Carcinogenesis, Mutagenesis, Impairment of Fertility

Long-term animal studies have not been performed to evaluate the carcinogenic potential of ELOCON Cream, 0.1%. Long-term carcinogenicity studies of mometasone furoate were conducted by the inhalation route in rats and mice. In a 2-year carcinogenicity study in Sprague Dawley® rats, mometasone furoate demonstrated no statistically significant increase of tumors at inhalation doses up to 67 mcg/kg (approximately 0.04 times the estimated maximum clinical topical dose from ELOCON Cream, 0.1% on an mcg/m^2 basis). In a 19-month carcinogenicity study in Swiss CD-1 mice, mometasone furoate demonstrated no statistically significant increase in the incidence of tumors at inhalation doses up to 160 mcg/kg (approximately 0.05 times the estimated maximum clinical topical dose from ELOCON Cream, 0.1% on an mcg/m^2 basis).

Mometasone furoate increased chromosomal aberrations in an *in vitro* Chinese hamster ovary cell assay, but did not increase chromosomal aberrations in an *in vitro* Chinese hamster lung cell assay. Mometasone furoate was not mutagenic in the Ames test or mouse lymphoma assay, and was not clastogenic in an *in vivo* mouse micronucleus assay, a rat bone marrow chromosomal aberration assay, or a mouse male germ-cell chromosomal aberration assay. Mometasone furoate also did not induce unscheduled DNA synthesis *in vivo* in rat hepatocytes.

In reproductive studies in rats, impairment of fertility was not produced in male or female rats by subcutaneous doses up to 15 mcg/kg (approximately 0.01 times the estimated maximum clinical topical dose from ELOCON Cream, 0.1% on an mcg/m^2 basis).

Pregnancy

Teratogenic Effects

Pregnancy Category C

Corticosteroids have been shown to be teratogenic in laboratory animals when administered systemically at relatively low dosage levels. Some corticosteroids have been shown to be teratogenic after dermal application in laboratory animals.

When administered to pregnant rats, rabbits, and mice, mometasone furoate increased fetal malformations. The doses that produced malformations also decreased fetal growth, as measured by lower fetal weights and/or delayed ossification. Mometasone furoate also caused dystocia and related complications when administered to rats during the end of pregnancy.

In mice, mometasone furoate caused cleft palate at subcutaneous doses of 60 mcg/kg and above. Fetal survival was reduced at 180 mcg/kg. No toxicity was observed at 20 mcg/kg. (Doses of 20, 60, and 180 mcg/kg in the mouse are approximately 0.01, 0.02, and 0.05 times the estimated maximum clinical topical dose from ELOCON Cream, 0.1% on an mcg/m^2 basis.)

In rats, mometasone furoate produced umbilical hernias at topical doses of 600 mcg/kg and above. A dose of 300 mcg/kg produced delays in ossification, but no malformations. (Doses of 300 and 600 mcg/kg in the rat are approximately 0.2 and 0.4 times the estimated maximum clinical topical dose from ELOCON Cream, 0.1% on an mcg/m^2 basis.)

In rabbits, mometasone furoate caused multiple malformations (eg, flexed front paws, gallbladder agenesis, umbilical hernia, hydrocephaly) at topical doses of 150 mcg/kg and above (approximately 0.2 times the estimated maximum clinical topical dose from ELOCON Cream, 0.1% on an mcg/m^2 basis). In an oral study, mometasone furoate increased resorptions and caused cleft palate and/or head malformations (hydrocephaly and domed head) at 700 mcg/kg. At 2800 mcg/kg most litters were aborted or resorbed. No toxicity was observed at 140 mcg/kg. (Doses at 140, 700, and 2800 mcg/kg in the rabbit are approximately 0.2, 0.9, and 3.6 times the estimated maximum clinical topical dose from ELOCON Cream, 0.1% on an mcg/m^2 basis.)

When rats received subcutaneous doses of mometasone furoate throughout pregnancy or during the later stages of pregnancy, 15 mcg/kg caused prolonged and difficult labor and reduced the number of live births, birth weight, and early pup survival. Similar effects were not observed at 7.5 mcg/kg. (Doses of 7.5 and 15 mcg/kg in the rat are approximately 0.005 and 0.01 times the estimated maximum clinical topical dose from ELOCON Cream, 0.1% on an mcg/m^2 basis.)

There are no adequate and well-controlled studies of teratogenic effects from topically applied corticosteroids in pregnant women. Therefore, topical corticosteroids should be used during pregnancy only if the potential benefit justifies the potential risk to the fetus.

Nursing Mothers

Systemically administered corticosteroids appear in human milk and could suppress growth, interfere with endogenous corticosteroid production, or cause other untoward effects. It is not known whether topical administration of corticosteroids could result in sufficient systemic absorption to produce detectable quantities in human milk. Because many drugs are excreted in human milk, caution should be exercised when ELOCON Cream, 0.1% is administered to a nursing woman.

Pediatric Use

ELOCON Cream, 0.1% may be used with caution in pediatric patients 2 years of age or older, although the safety and efficacy of drug use for longer than 3 weeks have not been established. Use of ELOCON Cream, 0.1% is supported by results from adequate and well-controlled studies in pediatric patients with corticosteroid-responsive dermatoses. Since safety and efficacy of ELOCON Cream, 0.1% have not been established in pediatric patients below 2 years of age, its use in this age group is not recommended.

ELOCON Cream, 0.1% caused HPA axis suppression in approximately 16% of pediatric patients ages 6 to 23 months, who showed normal adrenal function by Cortrosyn test before starting treatment, and were treated for approximately 3 weeks over a mean body surface area of 41% (range 15%–94%). The criteria for suppression were: basal cortisol level of ≤5 mcg/dL, 30-minute post-stimulation level of ≤18 mcg/dL, or an increase of <7 mcg/dL. Follow-up testing 2 to 4 weeks after study completion, available for 5 of the patients, demonstrated suppressed HPA axis function in one patient, using these same criteria. Long-term use of topical corticosteroids has not been studied in this population (see **CLINICAL PHARMACOLOGY, Pharmacokinetics** section).

Because of a higher ratio of skin surface area to body mass, pediatric patients are at a greater risk than adults of HPA axis suppression and Cushing's syndrome when they are treated with topical corticosteroids. They are, therefore, also at greater risk of adrenal insufficiency during and/or after withdrawal of treatment. Pediatric patients may be more susceptible than adults to skin atrophy, including striae, when they are treated with topical corticosteroids. Pediatric patients applying topical corticosteroids to greater than 20% of body surface are at higher risk of HPA axis suppression.

HPA axis suppression, Cushing's syndrome, linear growth retardation, delayed weight gain, and intracranial hypertension have been reported in pediatric patients receiving topical corticosteroids. Manifestations of adrenal suppression in children include low plasma cortisol levels and an absence of response to ACTH stimulation. Manifestations of intracranial hypertension include bulging fontanelles, headaches, and bilateral papilledema.

ELOCON Cream, 0.1% should not be used in the treatment of diaper dermatitis.

Geriatric Use

Clinical studies of ELOCON Cream, 0.1% included 190 subjects who were 65 years of age and over and 39 subjects who were 75 years of age and over. No overall differences in safety or effectiveness were observed between these subjects and younger subjects, and other reported clinical experience has not identified differences in responses between the elderly and younger patients. However, greater sensitivity of some older individuals cannot be ruled out.

ADVERSE REACTIONS

In controlled clinical studies involving 319 patients, the incidence of adverse reactions associated with the use of ELOCON® Cream, 0.1% was 1.6%. Reported reactions included burning, pruritus, and skin atrophy. Reports of rosacea associated with the use of ELOCON Cream, 0.1% have also been received. In controlled clinical studies (n=74) involving pediatric patients 2 to 12 years of age, the incidence of adverse experiences associated with the use of ELOCON Cream, 0.1% was approximately 7%. Reported reactions included stinging, pruritus, and furunculosis.

The following adverse reactions were reported to be possibly or probably related to treatment with ELOCON Cream, 0.1% during clinical studies, in 4% of 182 pediatric patients 6 months to 2 years of age: decreased glucocorticoid levels, 2; paresthesia, 2; folliculitis, 1; moniliasis, 1; bacterial infection, 1; skin depigmentation, 1. The following signs of skin atrophy were also observed among 97 patients treated with ELOCON Cream, 0.1% in a clinical study: shininess, 4; telangiectasia, 1; loss of elasticity, 4; loss of normal skin markings, 4; thinness, 1; and bruising, 1. Striae were not observed in this study.

The following additional local adverse reactions have been reported infrequently with topical corticosteroids, but may occur more frequently with the use of occlusive dressings. These reactions are listed in an approximate decreasing order of occurrence: irritation, dryness, folliculitis, hypertrichosis, acneiform eruptions, hypopigmentation, perioral dermatitis, allergic contact dermatitis, secondary infection, striae, and miliaria.

OVERDOSAGE

Topically applied ELOCON® Cream, 0.1% can be absorbed in sufficient amounts to produce systemic effects (see **PRECAUTIONS**).

DOSAGE AND ADMINISTRATION

Apply a thin film of ELOCON® Cream, 0.1% to the affected skin areas once daily. ELOCON Cream, 0.1% may be used in pediatric patients 2 years of age or older. Since safety and efficacy of ELOCON Cream, 0.1% have not been adequately established in pediatric patients below 2 years of age, its use in this age group is not recommended (see **PRECAUTIONS, Pediatric Use** section).

As with other corticosteroids, therapy should be discontinued when control is achieved. If no improvement is seen within 2 weeks, reassessment of diagnosis may be necessary. Safety and efficacy of ELOCON Cream, 0.1% in pediatric patients for more than 3 weeks of use have not been established.

ELOCON Cream, 0.1% should not be used with occlusive dressings unless directed by a physician. ELOCON Cream, 0.1% should not be applied in the diaper area if the child still requires diapers or plastic pants, as these garments may constitute occlusive dressing.

HOW SUPPLIED

ELOCON® Cream, 0.1% is supplied in 15-g (NDC 0085-0567-01) and 45-g (NDC 0085-0567-02) tubes; boxes of one.

Store at 25°C (77°F); excursions permitted to 15°–30°C (59°–86°F) [see USP Controlled Room Temperature].

Schering-Plough
Kenilworth, NJ 07033 USA
Rev. 9/08
18724359T

Copyright © 1987, 2008, Schering Corporation. All rights reserved.
The trademarks depicted in this piece are owned by their respective companies.

Revised: 06/2009 Schering Plough Corporation

Shown in Product Identification Guide,, page 312

ELOCON® ℞
[*ĕl' ō-cŏn*]
Lotion, 0.1%
brand of (mometasone furoate topical solution USP)
For Dermatologic Use Only
Not for Ophthalmic Use

DESCRIPTION

ELOCON® Lotion, 0.1% brand of (mometasone furoate topical solution USP) contains mometasone furoate USP for dermatologic use. Mometasone furoate is a synthetic corticosteroid with anti-inflammatory activity.

Chemically, mometasone furoate is 9α,21-dichloro-11β,17-dihydroxy-16α-methylpregna-1,4-diene-3,20-dione 17-(2-furoate), with the empirical formula $C_{27}H_{30}Cl_2O_6$, a molecular weight of 521.4 and the following structural formula:

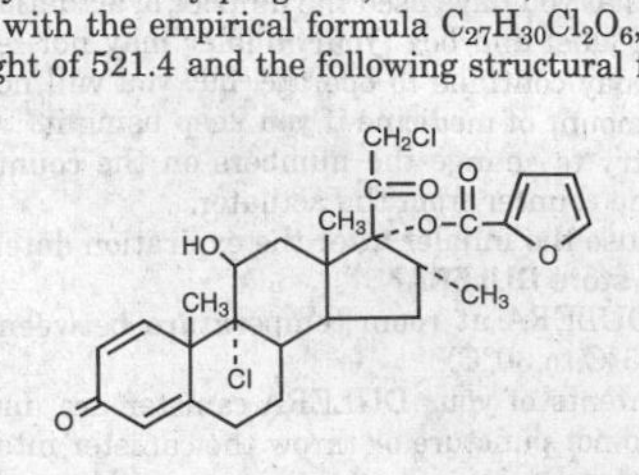

Mometasone furoate is a white to off-white powder practically insoluble in water, slightly soluble in octanol, and moderately soluble in ethyl alcohol.

Each gram of ELOCON Lotion, 0.1% contains: 1 mg mometasone furoate USP in a lotion base of isopropyl alcohol (40%); propylene glycol; hydroxypropyl cellulose; sodium phosphate monobasic monohydrate R; and purified water. May also contain phosphoric acid used to adjust the pH to approximately 4.5.

CLINICAL PHARMACOLOGY

Like other topical corticosteroids, mometasone furoate has anti-inflammatory, antipruritic, and vasoconstrictive properties. The mechanism of the anti-inflammatory activity of the topical steroids, in general, is unclear. However, corticosteroids are thought to act by the induction of phospholipase A_2 inhibitory proteins, collectively called lipocortins. It is postulated that these proteins control the biosynthesis of potent mediators of inflammation such as prostaglandins and leukotrienes by inhibiting the release of their common precursor arachidonic acid. Arachidonic acid is released from membrane phospholipids by phospholipase A_2.

Pharmacokinetics

The extent of percutaneous absorption of topical corticosteroids is determined by many factors including the vehicle and the integrity of the epidermal barrier. Occlusive dressings with hydrocortisone for up to 24 hours have not been demonstrated to increase penetration; however, occlusion of hydrocortisone for 96 hours markedly enhances penetration. Studies in humans indicate that approximately 0.7% of the applied dose of ELOCON® Ointment, 0.1% enters the circulation after 8 hours of contact on normal skin without occlusion. A similar minimal degree of absorption of the corticosteroid from the lotion formulation would be anticipated. Inflammation and/or other disease processes in the skin may increase percutaneous absorption.

Studies performed with ELOCON Lotion, 0.1% indicate that it is in the medium range of potency as compared with other topical corticosteroids.

In a study evaluating the effects of mometasone furoate lotion on the hypothalamic-pituitary-adrenal (HPA) axis, 15 mL were applied without occlusion twice daily (30 mL per day) for 7 days to four adult patients with scalp and body psoriasis. At the end of treatment, the plasma cortisol levels for each of the four patients remained within the normal range and changed little from baseline.

Sixty-five pediatric patients ages 6 to 23 months, with atopic dermatitis, were enrolled in an open-label, hypothalamic pituitary-adrenal (HPA) axis safety study. ELOCON Lotion, 0.1% was applied once daily for approximately 3 weeks over a mean body surface area of 40% (range 16%–90%). In approximately 29% of patients who showed normal adrenal function by Cortrosyn test before starting treatment, adrenal suppression was observed at the end of treatment with ELOCON Lotion, 0.1%. The criteria for suppression were: basal cortisol level of ≤5 mcg/dL, 30-minute post-stimulation level of ≤18 mcg/dL, or an increase of <7 mcg/dL. Follow-up testing 2 to 4 weeks after stopping treatment, available for 8 of the patients, demonstrated suppressed HPA axis function in one patient, using these same criteria.

INDICATIONS AND USAGE

ELOCON® Lotion, 0.1% is a medium potency corticosteroid indicated for the relief of the inflammatory and pruritic manifestations of corticosteroid-responsive dermatoses. Since safety and efficacy of ELOCON Lotion, 0.1% have not been established in pediatric patients below 12 years of age, its use in this age group is not recommended (see **PRECAUTIONS, Pediatric Use** section).

CONTRAINDICATIONS

ELOCON® Lotion, 0.1% is contraindicated in those patients with a history of hypersensitivity to any of the components in the preparation.

PRECAUTIONS

General

Systemic absorption of topical corticosteroids can produce reversible hypothalamic-pituitary-adrenal (HPA) axis suppression with the potential for glucocorticosteroid insufficiency after withdrawal of treatment. Manifestations of Cushing's syndrome, hyperglycemia, and glucosuria can also be produced in some patients by systemic absorption of topical corticosteroids while on treatment.

Patients applying a topical steroid to a large surface area or to areas under occlusion should be evaluated periodically for evidence of HPA axis suppression. This may be done by using the ACTH stimulation, A.M. plasma cortisol, and urinary-free cortisol tests.

In a study evaluating the effects of mometasone furoate lotion on the hypothalamic-pituitary-adrenal (HPA) axis, 15 mL were applied without occlusion twice daily (30 mL per day) for 7 days to four adult patients with scalp and body psoriasis. At the end of treatment, the plasma cortisol levels for each of the four patients remained within the normal range and changed little from baseline.

If HPA axis suppression is noted, an attempt should be made to withdraw the drug, to reduce the frequency of application, or to substitute a less potent corticosteroid. Recovery of HPA axis function is generally prompt upon discontinuation of topical corticosteroids. Infrequently, signs and symptoms of glucocorticosteroid insufficiency may occur, requiring supplemental systemic corticosteroids. For information on systemic supplementation, see Prescribing Information for those products.

Pediatric patients may be more susceptible to systemic toxicity from equivalent doses due to their larger skin surface to body mass ratios (see **PRECAUTIONS, Pediatric Use** section).

If irritation develops, ELOCON® Lotion, 0.1% should be discontinued and appropriate therapy instituted. Allergic

contact dermatitis with corticosteroids is usually diagnosed by observing failure to heal rather than noting a clinical exacerbation as with most topical products not containing corticosteroids. Such an observation should be corroborated with appropriate diagnostic patch testing.

If concomitant skin infections are present or develop, an appropriate antifungal or antibacterial agent should be used. If a favorable response does not occur promptly, use of ELOCON Lotion, 0.1% should be discontinued until the infection has been adequately controlled.

Information for Patients

Patients using topical corticosteroids should receive the following information and instructions:

1. This medication is to be used as directed by the physician. It is for external use only. Avoid contact with the eyes.
2. This medication should not be used for any disorder other than that for which it was prescribed.
3. The treated skin area should not be bandaged or otherwise covered or wrapped so as to be occlusive, unless directed by the physician.
4. Patients should report to their physician any signs of local adverse reactions.
5. Parents of pediatric patients should be advised not to use ELOCON Lotion, 0.1% in the treatment of diaper dermatitis. ELOCON Lotion, 0.1% should not be applied in the diaper area, as diapers or plastic pants may constitute occlusive dressing (see **DOSAGE AND ADMINISTRATION**).
6. This medication should not be used on the face, underarms, or groin areas unless directed by the physician.
7. As with other corticosteroids, therapy should be discontinued when control is achieved. If no improvement is seen within 2 weeks, contact the physician.
8. Other corticosteroid-containing products should not be used with ELOCON Lotion, 0.1% without first consulting with the physician.

Laboratory Tests

The following tests may be helpful in evaluating patients for HPA axis suppression:

ACTH stimulation test

A.M. plasma cortisol test

Urinary-free cortisol test

Carcinogenesis, Mutagenesis, Impairment of Fertility

Long-term animal studies have not been performed to evaluate the carcinogenic potential of ELOCON Lotion, 0.1%. Long-term carcinogenicity studies of mometasone furoate were conducted by the inhalation route in rats and mice. In a 2-year carcinogenicity study in Sprague Dawley® rats, mometasone furoate demonstrated no statistically significant increase of tumors at inhalation doses up to 67 mcg/kg (approximately 0.04 times the estimated maximum clinical topical dose from ELOCON Lotion, 0.1% on an mcg/m² basis). In a 19-month carcinogenicity study in Swiss CD-1 mice, mometasone furoate demonstrated no statistically significant increase in the incidence of tumors at inhalation doses up to 160 mcg/kg (approximately 0.05 times the estimated maximum clinical topical dose from ELOCON Lotion, 0.1% on an mcg/m² basis).

Mometasone furoate increased chromosomal aberrations in an *in vitro* Chinese hamster ovary cell assay, but did not increase chromosomal aberrations in an *in vitro* Chinese hamster lung cell assay. Mometasone furoate was not mutagenic in the Ames test or mouse lymphoma assay, and was not clastogenic in an *in vivo* mouse micronucleus assay, a rat bone marrow chromosomal aberration assay, or a mouse male germ-cell chromosomal aberration assay. Mometasone furoate also did not induce unscheduled DNA synthesis *in vivo* in rat hepatocytes.

In reproductive studies in rats, impairment of fertility was not produced in male or female rats by subcutaneous doses up to 15 mcg/kg (approximately 0.01 times the estimated maximum clinical topical dose from ELOCON Lotion, 0.1% on an mcg/m² basis).

Pregnancy

Teratogenic Effects

Pregnancy Category C

Corticosteroids have been shown to be teratogenic in laboratory animals when administered systemically at relatively low dosage levels. Some corticosteroids have been shown to be teratogenic after dermal application in laboratory animals.

When administered to pregnant rats, rabbits, and mice, mometasone furoate increased fetal malformations. The doses that produced malformations also decreased fetal growth, as measured by lower fetal weights and/or delayed ossification. Mometasone furoate also caused dystocia and related complications when administered to rats during the end of pregnancy.

In mice, mometasone furoate caused cleft palate at subcutaneous doses of 60 mcg/kg and above. Fetal survival was reduced at 180 mcg/kg. No toxicity was observed at 20 mcg/kg. (Doses of 20, 60, and 180 mcg/kg in the mouse are ap-

proximately 0.01, 0.02, and 0.05 times the estimated maximum clinical topical dose from ELOCON Lotion, 0.1% on an mcg/m² basis.)

In rats, mometasone furoate produced umbilical hernias at topical doses of 600 mcg/kg and above. A dose of 300 mcg/kg produced delays in ossification, but no malformations. (Doses of 300 and 600 mcg/kg in the rat are approximately 0.2 and 0.4 times the estimated maximum clinical topical dose from ELOCON Lotion, 0.1% on an mcg/m² basis.)

In rabbits, mometasone furoate caused multiple malformations (e.g., flexed front paws, gallbladder agenesis, umbilical hernia, hydrocephaly) at topical doses of 150 mcg/kg and above (approximately 0.2 times the estimated maximum clinical topical dose from ELOCON Lotion, 0.1% on an mcg/m² basis). In an oral study, mometasone furoate increased resorptions and caused cleft palate and/or head malformations (hydrocephaly and domed head) at 700 mcg/kg. At 2800 mcg/kg most litters were aborted or resorbed. No toxicity was observed at 140 mcg/kg. (Doses at 140, 700, and 2800 mcg/kg in the rabbit are approximately 0.2, 0.9, and 3.6 times the estimated maximum clinical topical dose from ELOCON Lotion, 0.1% on an mcg/m² basis.)

When rats received subcutaneous doses of mometasone furoate throughout pregnancy or during the later stages of pregnancy, 15 mcg/kg caused prolonged and difficult labor and reduced the number of live births, birth weight, and early pup survival. Similar effects were not observed at 7.5 mcg/kg. (Doses of 7.5 and 15 mcg/kg in the rat are approximately 0.005 and 0.01 times the estimated maximum clinical topical dose from ELOCON Lotion, 0.1% on an mcg/m² basis.)

There are no adequate and well-controlled studies of teratogenic effects from topically applied corticosteroids in pregnant women. Therefore, topical corticosteroids should be used during pregnancy only if the potential benefit justifies the potential risk to the fetus.

Nursing Mothers

Systemically administered corticosteroids appear in human milk and could suppress growth, interfere with endogenous corticosteroid production, or cause other untoward effects. It is not known whether topical administration of corticosteroids could result in sufficient systemic absorption to produce detectable quantities in human milk. Because many drugs are excreted in human milk, caution should be exercised when ELOCON Lotion, 0.1% is administered to a nursing woman.

Pediatric Use

Since safety and efficacy of ELOCON Lotion, 0.1% have not been established in pediatric patients below 12 years of age, its use in this age group is not recommended.

ELOCON Lotion, 0.1% caused HPA axis suppression in approximately 29% of pediatric patients ages 6 to 23 months, who showed normal adrenal function by Cortrosyn test before starting treatment, and were treated for approximately 3 weeks over a mean body surface area of 40% (range 16%–90%). The criteria for suppression were: basal cortisol level of ≤ 5 mcg/dL, 30-minute post-stimulation level of ≤18 mcg/dL, or an increase of <7 mcg/dL. Follow-up testing 2 to 4 weeks after stopping treatment, available for 8 of the patients, demonstrated suppressed HPA axis function in one patient, using these same criteria. Long-term use of topical corticosteroids has not been studied in this population (see **CLINICAL PHARMACOLOGY, Pharmacokinetics** section).

Because of a higher ratio of skin surface area to body mass, pediatric patients are at a greater risk than adults of HPA axis suppression and Cushing's syndrome when they are treated with topical corticosteroids. They are, therefore, also at greater risk of adrenal insufficiency during and/or after withdrawal of treatment. Pediatric patients may be more susceptible than adults to skin atrophy, including striae, when they are treated with topical corticosteroids. Pediatric patients applying topical corticosteroids to greater than 20% of body surface are at higher risk of HPA axis suppression.

HPA axis suppression, Cushing's syndrome, linear growth retardation, delayed weight gain, and intracranial hypertension have been reported in pediatric patients receiving topical corticosteroids. Manifestations of adrenal suppression in children include low plasma cortisol levels and absence of response to ACTH stimulation. Manifestations of intracranial hypertension include bulging fontanelles, headaches, and bilateral papilledema.

ELOCON Lotion, 0.1% should not be used in the treatment of diaper dermatitis.

Geriatric Use

Clinical studies of ELOCON Lotion, 0.1% did not include sufficient numbers of subjects aged 65 and over to determine whether they respond differently from younger subjects. Other reported clinical experience has not identified differences in responses between the elderly and younger patients. In general, dose selection for an elderly patient should be cautious.

ADVERSE REACTIONS

In clinical studies involving 209 patients, the incidence of adverse reactions associated with the use of ELOCON® Lotion, 0.1% was 3%. Reported reactions included acneiform reaction, 2; burning, 4; and itching, 1. In an irritation/sensitization study involving 156 normal subjects, the incidence of folliculitis was 3% (4 subjects).

The following adverse reactions were reported to be possibly or probably related to treatment with ELOCON Lotion, 0.1% during a clinical study, in 14% of 65 pediatric patients 6 months to 2 years of age: decreased glucocorticoid levels, 4; paresthesia, 2; dry mouth, 1; an unspecified endocrine disorder, 1; pruritus, 1; and an unspecified skin disorder, 1. The following signs of skin atrophy were also observed among 65 patients treated with ELOCON Lotion, 0.1% in a clinical study: shininess, 4; telangiectasia, 2; loss of elasticity, 2; and loss of normal skin markings, 3. Striae, thinness, and bruising were not observed in this study.

The following additional local adverse reactions have been reported infrequently with topical corticosteroids, but may occur more frequently with the use of occlusive dressings. These reactions are listed in an approximate decreasing order of occurrence: irritation, dryness, hypertrichosis, hypopigmentation, perioral dermatitis, allergic contact dermatitis, secondary infection, skin atrophy, striae, and miliaria.

OVERDOSAGE

Topically applied ELOCON® Lotion, 0.1% can be absorbed in sufficient amounts to produce systemic effects (see **PRECAUTIONS**).

DOSAGE AND ADMINISTRATION

Apply a few drops of ELOCON® Lotion, 0.1% to the affected skin areas once daily and massage lightly until it disappears. For the most effective and economical use, hold the nozzle of the bottle very close to the affected areas and gently squeeze. Since safety and efficacy of ELOCON Lotion, 0.1% have not been established in pediatric patients below 12 years of age, its use in this age group is not recommended (see **PRECAUTIONS, Pediatric Use** section).

As with other corticosteroids, therapy should be discontinued when control is achieved. If no improvement is seen within 2 weeks, reassessment of diagnosis may be necessary.

ELOCON Lotion, 0.1% should not be used with occlusive dressings unless directed by a physician. ELOCON Lotion, 0.1% should not be applied in the diaper area if the patient still requires diapers or plastic pants, as these garments may constitute occlusive dressing.

HOW SUPPLIED

ELOCON® Lotion, 0.1% is supplied in 30-mL (27.5 g) (NDC 0085-0854-01) and 60-mL (55 g) (NDC 0085-0854-02) bottles; boxes of one.

Store ELOCON Lotion, 0.1% at 25°C (77°F); excursions permitted to 15°–30°C (59°–86°F) [see USP Controlled Room Temperature].

Schering-Plough
Kenilworth, NJ 07033 USA
Rev. 9/08
32760902T

Copyright © 1989, 2008, Schering Corporation. All rights reserved.
The trademarks depicted in this piece are owned by their respective companies.

Revised: 05/2009 Schering Corporation

Shown in Product Identification Guide, page 312

ELOCON® ℞

[el' ō-cŏn]

brand of (mometasone furoate ointment USP)
Ointment, 0.1%
For Dermatologic Use Only
Not for Ophthalmic Use
PRODUCT INFORMATION

DESCRIPTION

ELOCON® Ointment, 0.1% brand of (mometasone furoate ointment USP) contains mometasone furoate USP for dermatologic use. Mometasone furoate is a synthetic corticosteroid with anti-inflammatory activity.

Chemically, mometasone furoate is 9α,21-dichloro-11β,17-dihydroxy-16α-methyl-pregna-1,4-diene-3,20-dione 17-(2-furoate), with the empirical formula $C_{27}H_{30}Cl_2O_6$, a molecular weight of 521.4 and the following structural formula:

[See chemical structure at top of next column]

Mometasone furoate is a white to off-white powder practically insoluble in water, slightly soluble in octanol, and moderately soluble in ethyl alcohol.

Each gram contains: 1 mg mometasone furoate USP in an ointment base of hexylene glycol; phosphoric acid; propylene glycol stearate (55% monoester); white wax; white petrolatum; and purified water.

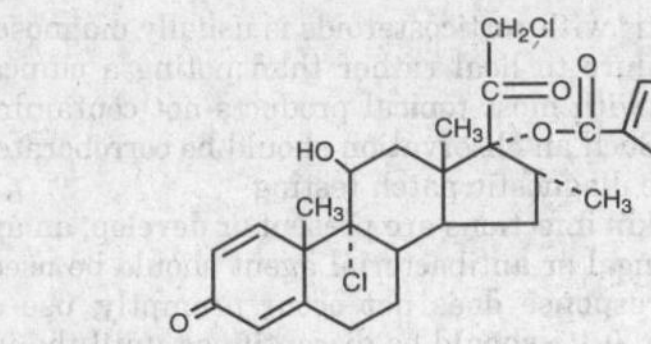

CLINICAL PHARMACOLOGY

Like other topical corticosteroids, mometasone furoate has anti-inflammatory, antipruritic, and vasoconstrictive properties. The mechanism of the anti-inflammatory activity of the topical steroids, in general, is unclear. However, corticosteroids are thought to act by the induction of phospholipase A_2 inhibitory proteins, collectively called lipocortins. It is postulated that these proteins control the biosynthesis of potent mediators of inflammation such as prostaglandins and leukotrienes by inhibiting the release of their common precursor arachidonic acid. Arachidonic acid is released from membrane phospholipids by phospholipase A_2.

Pharmacokinetics The extent of percutaneous absorption of topical corticosteroids is determined by many factors including the vehicle and the integrity of the epidermal barrier. Occlusive dressings with hydrocortisone for up to 24 hours have not been demonstrated to increase penetration; however, occlusion of hydrocortisone for 96 hours markedly enhances penetration. Studies in humans indicate that approximately 0.7% of the applied dose of ELOCON® Ointment, 0.1% enters the circulation after 8 hours of contact on normal skin without occlusion. Inflammation and/or other disease processes in the skin may increase percutaneous absorption.

Studies performed with ELOCON Ointment, 0.1% indicate that it is in the medium range of potency as compared with other topical corticosteroids.

In a study evaluating the effects of mometasone furoate ointment on the hypothalamic-pituitary-adrenal (HPA) axis, 15 grams were applied twice daily for 7 days to six adult patients with psoriasis or atopic dermatitis. The ointment was applied without occlusion to at least 30% of the body surface. The results show that the drug caused a slight lowering of adrenal corticosteroid secretion.

In a pediatric trial, 24 atopic dermatitis patients, of which 19 patients were age 2 to 12 years, were treated with ELOCON Cream, 0.1% once daily. The majority of patients cleared within 3 weeks.

Sixty-three pediatric patients ages 6 to 23 months, with atopic dermatitis, were enrolled in an open-label, hypothalamic-pituitary-adrenal (HPA) axis safety study. ELOCON Ointment, 0.1% was applied once daily for approximately 3 weeks over a mean body surface area of 39% (range 15%-99%). In approximately 27% of patients who showed normal adrenal function by Cortrosyn test before starting treatment, adrenal suppression was observed at the end of treatment with ELOCON Ointment, 0.1%. The criteria for suppression were: basal cortisol level of ≤5 mcg/dL, 30-minute post-stimulation level of ≤18 mcg/dL, or an increase of <7 mcg/dL. Follow-up testing 2 to 4 weeks after stopping treatment, available for 8 of the patients, demonstrated suppressed HPA axis function in 3 patients, using these same criteria.

INDICATIONS AND USAGE

ELOCON® Ointment, 0.1% is a medium potency corticosteroid indicated for the relief of the inflammatory and pruritic manifestations of corticosteroid-responsive dermatoses.

ELOCON Ointment, 0.1% may be used in pediatric patients 2 years of age or older, although the safety and efficacy of drug use for longer than 3 weeks have not been established (see **PRECAUTIONS, Pediatric Use** section). Since safety and efficacy of ELOCON Ointment, 0.1% have not been adequately established in pediatric patients below 2 years of age, its use in this age group is not recommended.

CONTRAINDICATIONS

ELOCON® Ointment, 0.1% is contraindicated in those patients with a history of hypersensitivity to any of the components in the preparation.

PRECAUTIONS

General Systemic absorption of topical corticosteroids can produce reversible hypothalamic-pituitary-adrenal (HPA) axis suppression with the potential for glucocorticosteroid insufficiency after withdrawal of treatment. Manifestations of Cushing's syndrome, hyperglycemia, and glucosuria can also be produced in some patients by systemic absorption of topical corticosteroids while on treatment.

Patients applying a topical steroid to a large surface area or areas under occlusion should be evaluated periodically for evidence of HPA axis suppression. This may be done by using the ACTH stimulation, A.M. plasma cortisol, and urinary-free cortisol tests.

In a study evaluating the effects of mometasone furoate ointment on the hypothalamic-pituitary-adrenal (HPA) axis, 15 grams were applied twice daily for 7 days to six adult patients with psoriasis or atopic dermatitis. The ointment was applied without occlusion to at least 30% of the body surface. The results show that the drug caused a slight lowering of adrenal corticosteroid secretion.

If HPA axis suppression is noted, an attempt should be made to withdraw the drug, to reduce the frequency of application, or to substitute a less potent corticosteroid. Recovery of HPA axis function is generally prompt upon discontinuation of topical corticosteroids. Infrequently, signs and symptoms of glucocorticosteroid insufficiency may occur, requiring supplemental systemic corticosteroids. For information on systemic supplementation, see Prescribing Information for those products.

Pediatric patients may be more susceptible to systemic toxicity from equivalent doses due to their larger skin surface to body mass ratios (see **PRECAUTIONS, Pediatric Use** section).

If irritation develops, ELOCON® Ointment, 0.1% should be discontinued and appropriate therapy instituted. Allergic contact dermatitis with corticosteroids is usually diagnosed by observing failure to heal rather than noting a clinical exacerbation as with most topical products not containing corticosteroids. Such an observation should be corroborated with appropriate diagnostic patch testing.

If concomitant skin infections are present or develop, an appropriate antifungal or antibacterial agent should be used. If a favorable response does not occur promptly, use of ELOCON Ointment, 0.1% should be discontinued until the infection has been adequately controlled.

Information for Patients Patients using topical corticosteroids should receive the following information and instructions:

1. This medication is to be used as directed by the physician. It is for external use only. Avoid contact with the eyes.
2. This medication should not be used for any disorder other than that for which it was prescribed.
3. The treated skin area should not be bandaged or otherwise covered or wrapped so as to be occlusive, unless directed by the physician.
4. Patients should report to their physician any signs of local adverse reactions.
5. Parents of pediatric patients should be advised not to use ELOCON Ointment, 0.1% in the treatment of diaper dermatitis. ELOCON Ointment, 0.1% should not be applied in the diaper area, as diapers or plastic pants may constitute occlusive dressing (see **DOSAGE AND ADMINISTRATION**).
6. This medication should not be used on the face, underarms, or groin areas unless directed by the physician.
7. As with other corticosteroids, therapy should be discontinued when control is achieved. If no improvement is seen within 2 weeks, contact the physician.
8. Other corticosteroid-containing products should not be used with ELOCON Ointment, 0.1% without first consulting with the physician.

Laboratory Tests The following tests may be helpful in evaluating patients for HPA axis suppression:

ACTH stimulation test
A.M. plasma cortisol test
Urinary-free cortisol test

Carcinogenesis, Mutagenesis, Impairment of Fertility Long-term animal studies have not been performed to evaluate the carcinogenic potential of ELOCON Ointment, 0.1%. Long-term carcinogenicity studies of mometasone furoate were conducted by the inhalation route in rats and mice. In a 2-year carcinogenicity study in Sprague Dawley® rats, mometasone furoate demonstrated no statistically significant increase of tumors at inhalation doses up to 67 mcg/kg (approximately 0.04 times the estimated maximum clinical topical dose from ELOCON Ointment, 0.1% on an mcg/m^2 basis). In a 19-month carcinogenicity study in Swiss CD-1 mice, mometasone furoate demonstrated no statistically significant increase in the incidence of tumors at inhalation doses up to 160 mcg/kg (approximately 0.05 times the estimated maximum clinical topical dose from ELOCON Ointment, 0.1% on an mcg/m^2 basis).

Mometasone furoate increased chromosomal aberrations in an *in vitro* Chinese hamster ovary cell assay, but did not increase chromosomal aberrations in an *in vitro* Chinese hamster lung cell assay. Mometasone furoate was not mutagenic in the Ames test or mouse lymphoma assay, and was not clastogenic in an *in vivo* mouse micronucleus assay, a rat bone marrow chromosomal aberration assay, or a mouse male germ-cell chromosomal aberration assay. Mometasone furoate also did not induce unscheduled DNA synthesis *in vivo* in rat hepatocytes.

In reproductive studies in rats, impairment of fertility was not produced in male or female rats by subcutaneous doses up to 15 mcg/kg (approximately 0.01 times the estimated maximum clinical topical dose from ELOCON Ointment, 0.1% on an mcg/m^2 basis).

Pregnancy ***Teratogenic Effects*** *Pregnancy Category C* Corticosteroids have been shown to be teratogenic in laboratory animals when administered systemically at relatively low dosage levels. Some corticosteroids have been shown to be teratogenic after dermal application in laboratory animals.

When administered to pregnant rats, rabbits, and mice, mometasone furoate increased fetal malformations. The doses that produced malformations also decreased fetal growth, as measured by lower fetal weights and/or delayed ossification. Mometasone furoate also caused dystocia and related complications when administered to rats during the end of pregnancy.

In mice, mometasone furoate caused cleft palate at subcutaneous doses of 60 mcg/kg and above. Fetal survival was reduced at 180 mcg/kg. No toxicity was observed at 20 mcg/kg. (Doses of 20, 60, and 180 mcg/kg in the mouse are approximately 0.01, 0.02, and 0.05 times the estimated maximum clinical topical dose from ELOCON Ointment, 0.1% on an mcg/m^2 basis.)

In rats, mometasone furoate produced umbilical hernias at topical doses of 600 mcg/kg and above. A dose of 300 mcg/kg produced delays in ossification, but no malformations. (Doses of 300 and 600 mcg/kg in the rat are approximately 0.2 and 0.4 times the estimated maximum clinical topical dose from ELOCON Ointment, 0.1% on an mcg/m^2 basis.)

In rabbits, mometasone furoate caused multiple malformations (eg, flexed front paws, gallbladder agenesis, umbilical hernia, hydrocephaly) at topical doses of 150 mcg/kg and above (approximately 0.2 times the estimated maximum clinical topical dose from ELOCON Ointment, 0.1% on an mcg/m^2 basis). In an oral study, mometasone furoate increased resorptions and caused cleft palate and/or head malformations (hydrocephaly and domed head) at 700 mcg/kg. At 2800 mcg/kg most litters were aborted or resorbed. No toxicity was observed at 140 mcg/kg. (Doses of 140, 700, and 2800 mcg/kg in the rabbit are approximately 0.2, 0.9, and 3.6 times the estimated maximum clinical topical dose from ELOCON Ointment, 0.1% on an mcg/m^2 basis.)

When rats received subcutaneous doses of mometasone furoate throughout pregnancy or during the later stages of pregnancy, 15 mcg/kg caused prolonged and difficult labor and reduced the number of live births, birth weight, and early pup survival. Similar effects were not observed at 7.5 mcg/kg. (Doses of 7.5 and 15 mcg/kg in the rat are approximately 0.005 and 0.01 times the estimated maximum clinical topical dose from ELOCON Ointment, 0.1% on an mcg/m^2 basis.)

There are no adequate and well-controlled studies of teratogenic effects from topically applied corticosteroids in pregnant women. Therefore, topical corticosteroids should be used during pregnancy only if the potential benefit justifies the potential risk to the fetus.

Nursing Mothers Systemically administered corticosteroids appear in human milk and could suppress growth, interfere with endogenous corticosteroid production, or cause other untoward effects. It is not known whether topical administration of corticosteroids could result in sufficient systemic absorption to produce detectable quantities in human milk. Because many drugs are excreted in human milk, caution should be exercised when ELOCON Ointment, 0.1% is administered to a nursing woman.

Pediatric Use ELOCON Ointment, 0.1% may be used with caution in pediatric patients 2 years of age or older, although the safety and efficacy of drug use for longer than 3 weeks have not been established. Use of ELOCON Ointment, 0.1% is supported by results from adequate and well-controlled studies in pediatric patients with corticosteroid-responsive dermatoses. Since safety and efficacy of ELOCON Ointment, 0.1% have not been adequately established in pediatric patients below 2 years of age, its use in this age group is not recommended.

ELOCON Ointment, 0.1% caused HPA axis suppression in approximately 27% of pediatric patients ages 6 to 23 months, who showed normal adrenal function by Cortrosyn test before starting treatment, and were treated for approximately 3 weeks over a mean body surface area of 39% (range 15%-99%). The criteria for suppression were: basal cortisol level of ≤5 mcg/dL, 30-minute post-stimulation level of ≤18 mcg/dL, or an increase of <7 mcg/dL. Follow-up testing 2 to 4 weeks after stopping treatment, available for 8 of the patients, demonstrated suppressed HPA axis function in 3 patients, using these same criteria. Long-term use of topical corticosteroids has not been studied in this population (see **CLINICAL PHARMACOLOGY, Pharmacokinetics** section).

Because of a higher ratio of skin surface area to body mass, pediatric patients are at a greater risk than adults of HPA axis suppression and Cushing's syndrome when they are treated with topical corticosteroids. They are, therefore, also at greater risk of glucocorticosteroid insufficiency during and/or after withdrawal of treatment. Pediatric patients may be more susceptible than adults to skin atrophy, including striae, when they are treated with topical corticosteroids. Pediatric patients applying topical corticosteroids to greater than 20% of body surface are at higher risk of HPA axis suppression.

HPA axis suppression, Cushing's syndrome, linear growth retardation, delayed weight gain, and intracranial hypertension have been reported in children receiving topical corticosteroids. Manifestations of adrenal suppression in children include low plasma cortisol levels and absence of response to ACTH stimulation. Manifestations of intracranial hypertension include bulging fontanelles, headaches, and bilateral papilledema.

ELOCON Ointment, 0.1% should not be used in the treatment of diaper dermatitis.

Geriatric Use Clinical studies of ELOCON Ointment, 0.1% included 310 subjects who were 65 years of age and over and 57 subjects who were 75 years of age and over. No overall differences in safety or effectiveness were observed between these subjects and younger subjects, and other reported clinical experience has not identified differences in responses between the elderly and younger patients. However, greater sensitivity of some older individuals cannot be ruled out.

ADVERSE REACTIONS

In controlled clinical studies involving 812 patients, the incidence of adverse reactions associated with the use of ELOCON® Ointment, 0.1% was 4.8%. Reported reactions included burning, pruritus, skin atrophy, tingling/stinging, and furunculosis. Reports of rosacea associated with the use of ELOCON Ointment, 0.1% have been received. In controlled clinical studies (n=74) involving pediatric patients 2 to 12 years of age, the incidence of adverse experiences associated with the use of ELOCON Cream is approximately 7%. Reported reactions included stinging, pruritus, and furunculosis.

The following adverse reactions were reported to be possibly or probably related to treatment with ELOCON Ointment, 0.1% during a clinical study, in 5% of 63 pediatric patients 6 months to 2 years of age: decreased glucocorticoid levels, 1; an unspecified skin disorder, 1; and a bacterial skin infection, 1. The following signs of skin atrophy were also observed among 63 patients treated with ELOCON Ointment, 0.1% in a clinical study: shininess, 4; telangiectasia, 1; loss of elasticity, 4; loss of normal skin markings, 4; and thinness, 1. Striae and bruising were not observed in this study.

The following additional local adverse reactions have been reported infrequently with topical corticosteroids, but may occur more frequently with the use of occlusive dressings. These reactions are listed in an approximate decreasing order of occurrence: irritation, dryness, folliculitis, hypertrichosis, acneiform eruptions, hypopigmentation, perioral dermatitis, allergic contact dermatitis, secondary infection, striae, and miliaria.

OVERDOSAGE

Topically applied ELOCON® Ointment, 0.1% can be absorbed in sufficient amounts to produce systemic effects (see **PRECAUTIONS**).

DOSAGE AND ADMINISTRATION

Apply a thin film of ELOCON® Ointment, 0.1% to the affected skin areas once daily. ELOCON Ointment, 0.1% may be used in pediatric patients 2 years of age or older. Since safety and efficacy of ELOCON Ointment, 0.1% have not been adequately established in pediatric patients below 2 years of age, its use in this age group is not recommended (see **PRECAUTIONS, Pediatric Use** section).

As with other corticosteroids, therapy should be discontinued when control is achieved. If no improvement is seen within 2 weeks, reassessment of diagnosis may be necessary. Safety and efficacy of ELOCON Ointment, 0.1% in pediatric patients for more than 3 weeks have not been established.

ELOCON Ointment, 0.1% should not be used with occlusive dressings unless directed by a physician.

ELOCON Ointment, 0.1% should not be applied in the diaper area if the child still requires diapers or plastic pants, as these garments may constitute occlusive dressing.

HOW SUPPLIED

ELOCON® Ointment, 0.1% is supplied in 15-g (NDC 0085-0370-01) and 45-g (NDC 0085-0370-02) tubes; boxes of one.

Store at 25°C (77°F); excursions permitted to 15-30°C (59-86°F) [see USP Controlled Room Temperature].

Schering-Plough
Kenilworth, NJ 07033 USA
Rev. 9/08 **18724243T**

Shown in Product Identification Guide, page 312

EMEND® ℞
[ē' mĕnd]
(aprepitant)
Capsules

HIGHLIGHTS OF PRESCRIBING INFORMATION
These highlights do not include all the information needed to use EMEND safely and effectively. See full prescribing information for EMEND.
EMEND (aprepitant) Capsules
Initial U.S. Approval: 2003

INDICATIONS AND USAGE

EMEND® is a substance P/neurokinin 1 (NK_1) receptor antagonist, indicated:

- in combination with other antiemetic agents for the:
  - prevention of acute and delayed nausea and vomiting associated with initial and repeat courses of highly emetogenic cancer chemotherapy (HEC) including high-dose cisplatin (1.1)
  - prevention of nausea and vomiting associated with initial and repeat courses of moderately emetogenic cancer chemotherapy (MEC) (1.1)
- for the prevention of postoperative nausea and vomiting (PONV) (1.2)

Limitations of Use (1.3)

- Not studied for the treatment of established nausea and vomiting.
- Chronic continuous administration is not recommended.

DOSAGE AND ADMINISTRATION

Prevention of Chemotherapy Induced Nausea and Vomiting (2.1)

- EMEND is given for 3 days as part of the chemotherapy induced nausea and vomiting (CINV) regimen that includes a corticosteroid and a 5-HT_3 antagonist. (2.1)
  - The recommended dose of EMEND is 125 mg orally 1 hour prior to chemotherapy treatment (Day 1) and 80 mg orally once daily in the morning on Days 2 and 3. (2.1)
  - EMEND (fosaprepitant dimeglumine) for Injection may be substituted for oral EMEND (125 mg) on Day 1 only as part of the CINV regimen. (2.1)

Prevention of Postoperative Nausea and Vomiting (2.2)

- The recommended oral dosage of EMEND for the postoperative nausea and vomiting (PONV) indication is 40 mg within 3 hours prior to induction of anesthesia. (2.2)

DOSAGE FORMS AND STRENGTHS

Capsules: 40 mg; 80 mg; 125 mg (3)

CONTRAINDICATIONS

- Hypersensitivity to any component of this medication. (4, 6.2)
- EMEND should not be used concurrently with pimozide, terfenadine, astemizole, or cisapride since inhibition of CYP3A4 by aprepitant could result in elevated plasma concentrations of these drugs, potentially causing serious or life-threatening reactions. (4)

WARNINGS AND PRECAUTIONS

- Coadministration of aprepitant with warfarin (a CYP2C9 substrate) may result in a clinically significant decrease in International Normalized Ratio (INR) of prothrombin time. (5.2)
- The efficacy of hormonal contraceptives during and for 28 days following the last dose of EMEND may be reduced. Alternative or back-up methods of contraception should be used. (5.3, 7.1)
- EMEND is a dose-dependent inhibitor of CYP3A4, and should be used with caution in patients receiving concomitant medications that are primarily metabolized through CYP3A4. (5.1)
- Caution should be exercised when administered in patients with severe hepatic impairment. (2.5, 5.4, 12.3)

ADVERSE REACTIONS

- Clinical adverse experiences for the CINV regimen in conjunction with highly and moderately emetogenic chemotherapy (incidence >10% are: alopecia, anorexia, asthenia/fatigue, constipation, diarrhea, headache, hiccups, nausea. (6.1)
- Clinical adverse experiences for the PONV regimen (incidence >5%) are: constipation, hypotension, nausea, pruritus, pyrexia. (6.1)

To report SUSPECTED ADVERSE REACTIONS, contact Merck Sharp & Dohme Corp., a subsidiary of Merck & Co., Inc., at 1-877-888-4231 or FDA at 1-800-FDA-1088 or www.fda.gov/medwatch.

DRUG INTERACTIONS

- Aprepitant is a substrate for CYP3A4; therefore, coadministration of EMEND with drugs that inhibit or induce CYP3A4 activity may result in increased or reduced plasma concentrations of aprepitant, respectively. (5.1, 7.1, 7.2).
- Aprepitant is an inducer of CYP2C9; therefore, coadministration of EMEND with drugs that are metabolized by CYP2C9 (e.g. warfarin, tolbutamide), may result in lower plasma concentrations of these drugs. (5.2, 7.1)

	Day 1	Day 2	Day 3	Day 4
EMEND*	125 mg orally	80 mg orally	80 mg orally	none
Dexamethasone[†]	12 mg orally	8 mg orally	8 mg orally	8 mg orally
Ondansetron[‡]	32 mg I.V.	none	none	none

* EMEND was administered orally 1 hour prior to chemotherapy treatment on Day 1 and in the morning on Days 2 and 3.
† Dexamethasone was administered 30 minutes prior to chemotherapy treatment on Day 1 and in the morning on Days 2 through 4. The dose of dexamethasone was chosen to account for drug interactions.
‡ Ondansetron was administered 30 minutes prior to chemotherapy treatment on Day 1.

	Day 1	Day 2	Day 3
EMEND*	125 mg orally	80 mg orally	80 mg orally
Dexamethasone[†]	12 mg orally	none	none
Ondansetron[‡]	2 × 8 mg orally	none	none

* EMEND was administered orally 1 hour prior to chemotherapy treatment on Day 1 and in the morning on Days 2 and 3.
† Dexamethasone was administered 30 minutes prior to chemotherapy treatment on Day 1. The dose of dexamethasone was chosen to account for drug interactions.
‡ Ondansetron 8-mg capsule was administered 30 to 60 minutes prior to chemotherapy treatment and one 8-mg capsule was administered 8 hours after the first dose on Day 1.

See 17 for PATIENT COUNSELING INFORMATION and FDA-approved patient labeling

Revised: 03/2010

FULL PRESCRIBING INFORMATION: CONTENTS*

FULL PRESCRIBING INFORMATION

1 INDICATIONS AND USAGE

1.1 Prevention of Chemotherapy Induced Nausea and Vomiting (CINV)

EMEND[1], in combination with other antiemetic agents, is indicated for the:
* prevention of acute and delayed nausea and vomiting associated with initial and repeat courses of highly emetogenic cancer chemotherapy (HEC) including high-dose cisplatin
* prevention of nausea and vomiting associated with initial and repeat courses of moderately emetogenic cancer chemotherapy (MEC) [see Dosage and Administration (2.1)].

[1] Registered trademark of Merck Sharp & Dohme Corp., a subsidiary of Merck & Co., Inc.
Copyright © 2003, 2005, 2006 Merck Sharp & Dohme Corp., a subsidiary of Merck & Co., Inc.
All Rights Reserved

1.2 Prevention of Postoperative Nausea and Vomiting (PONV)

EMEND is indicated for the prevention of postoperative nausea and vomiting [see Dosage and Administration (2.2)].

1.3 Limitations of Use

EMEND has not been studied for the treatment of established nausea and vomiting.
Chronic continuous administration is not recommended [see Warnings and Precautions (5.5)].

2 DOSAGE AND ADMINISTRATION

2.1 Prevention of Chemotherapy Induced Nausea and Vomiting (CINV)

Capsules of EMEND (aprepitant) are given for 3 days as part of a regimen that includes a corticosteroid and a 5-HT$_3$ antagonist. The recommended dose of EMEND is 125 mg orally 1 hour prior to chemotherapy treatment (Day 1) and 80 mg orally once daily in the morning on Days 2 and 3. EMEND may be taken with or without food.
EMEND (fosaprepitant dimeglumine) for Injection (115 mg) is a prodrug of aprepitant and may be substituted for oral EMEND (125 mg), 30 minutes prior to chemotherapy, on Day 1 only of the CINV regimen as an intravenous infusion administered over 15 minutes.
In clinical studies with EMEND, the following regimen was used for the prevention of nausea and vomiting associated with highly emetogenic cancer chemotherapy:
[See first table above]
In a clinical study with EMEND, the following regimen was used for the prevention of nausea and vomiting associated with moderately emetogenic cancer chemotherapy:
[See second table above]

2.2 Prevention of Postoperative Nausea and Vomiting (PONV)

The recommended oral dosage of EMEND is 40 mg within 3 hours prior to induction of anesthesia.
EMEND may be taken with or without food.

2.3 Geriatric Patients

No dosage adjustment is necessary for the elderly.

2.4 Patients with Renal Impairment

No dosage adjustment is necessary for patients with renal impairment or for patients with end stage renal disease (ESRD) undergoing hemodialysis.

2.5 Patients with Hepatic Impairment

No dosage adjustment is necessary for patients with mild to moderate hepatic impairment (Child-Pugh score 5 to 9). There are no clinical data in patients with severe hepatic impairment (Child-Pugh score >9).

2.6 Coadministration with Other Drugs

For additional information on dose adjustment for corticosteroids when coadministered with EMEND, see Drug Interactions (7.1).
Refer to the full prescribing information for coadministered antiemetic agents.

3 DOSAGE FORMS AND STRENGTHS

* Capsules EMEND 40 mg are opaque, hard, gelatin capsules, with white body and mustard yellow cap and "464" and "40 mg" printed radially in black ink on the body.
* Capsules EMEND 80 mg are white, opaque, hard, gelatin capsules, with "461" and "80 mg" printed radially in black ink on the body.
* Capsules EMEND 125 mg are opaque, hard, gelatin capsules, with white body and pink cap with "462" and "125 mg" printed radially in black ink on the body.

4 CONTRAINDICATIONS

EMEND is contraindicated in patients who are hypersensitive to any component of the product.
EMEND is a dose-dependent inhibitor of cytochrome P450 isoenzyme 3A4 (CYP3A4). EMEND should not be used concurrently with pimozide, terfenadine, astemizole, or cisapride. Inhibition of CYP3A4 by aprepitant could result in elevated plasma concentrations of these drugs, potentially causing serious or life-threatening reactions [see Drug Interactions (7.1)].

5 WARNINGS AND PRECAUTIONS

5.1 CYP3A4 Interactions

EMEND (aprepitant), a dose-dependent inhibitor of CYP3A4, should be used with caution in patients receiving concomitant medications that are primarily metabolized through CYP3A4. Moderate inhibition of CYP3A4 by aprepitant, 125 mg/80 mg regimen, could result in elevated plasma concentrations of these concomitant medications. Weak inhibition of CYP3A4 by a single 40 mg dose of aprepitant is not expected to alter the plasma concentrations of concomitant medications that are primarily metabolized through CYP3A4 to a clinically significant degree.
When aprepitant is used concomitantly with another CYP3A4 inhibitor, aprepitant plasma concentrations could be elevated. When EMEND is used concomitantly with medications that induce CYP3A4 activity aprepitant plasma concentrations could be reduced and this may result in decreased efficacy of EMEND [see Drug Interactions (7.1)].
Chemotherapy agents that are known to be metabolized by CYP3A4 include docetaxel, paclitaxel, etoposide, irinotecan, ifosfamide, imatinib, vinorelbine, vinblastine and vincristine. In clinical studies, EMEND (125 mg/80 mg regimen) was administered commonly with etoposide, vinorelbine, or paclitaxel. The doses of these agents were not adjusted to account for potential drug interactions.
In separate pharmacokinetic studies no clinically significant change in docetaxel or vinorelbine pharmacokinetics was observed when EMEND (125 mg/80 mg regimen) was co-administered.
Due to the small number of patients in clinical studies who received the CYP3A4 substrates vinblastine, vincristine, or ifosfamide, particular caution and careful monitoring are advised in patients receiving these agents or other chemotherapy agents metabolized primarily by CYP3A4 that were not studied [see Drug Interactions (7.1)].

5.2 Coadministration with Warfarin (a CYP2C9 substrate)

Coadministration of EMEND with warfarin may result in a clinically significant decrease in International Normalized Ratio (INR) of prothrombin time. In patients on chronic warfarin therapy, the INR should be closely monitored in the 2-week period, particularly at 7 to 10 days, following initiation of the 3-day regimen of EMEND with each chemotherapy cycle, or following administration of a single 40 mg dose of EMEND for the prevention of postoperative nausea and vomiting [see Drug Interactions (7.1)].

5.3 Coadministration with Hormonal Contraceptives

Upon coadministration with EMEND, the efficacy of hormonal contraceptives during and for 28 days following the last dose of EMEND may be reduced. Alternative or back-up methods of contraception should be used during treatment with EMEND and for 1 month following the last dose of EMEND [see Drug Interactions (7.1)].

5.4 Patients with Severe Hepatic Impairment

There are no clinical or pharmacokinetic data in patients with severe hepatic impairment (Child-Pugh score >9). Therefore, caution should be exercised when EMEND is administered in these patients [see Clinical Pharmacology (12.3) and Dosage and Administration (2.5)].

5.5 Chronic Continuous Use

Chronic continuous use of EMEND for prevention of nausea and vomiting is not recommended because it has not been studied; and because the drug interaction profile may change during chronic continuous use.

6 ADVERSE REACTIONS

The overall safety of aprepitant was evaluated in approximately 5300 individuals.

Because clinical trials are conducted under widely varying conditions, adverse reaction rates observed in the clinical trials of a drug cannot be directly compared to rates in the clinical trials of another drug and may not reflect the rates observed in clinical practice.

6.1 Clinical Trials Experience

Chemotherapy Induced Nausea and Vomiting
Highly Emetogenic Chemotherapy

In 2 well-controlled clinical trials in patients receiving highly emetogenic cancer chemotherapy, 544 patients were treated with aprepitant during Cycle 1 of chemotherapy and 413 of these patients continued in the Multiple-Cycle extension for up to 6 cycles of chemotherapy. EMEND was given in combination with ondansetron and dexamethasone.

In Cycle 1, clinical adverse experiences were reported in approximately 69% of patients treated with the aprepitant regimen compared with approximately 68% of patients treated with standard therapy. Table 1 shows the percent of patients with clinical adverse experiences reported at an incidence ≥3%.

Table 1: Percent of Patients Receiving Highly Emetogenic Chemotherapy with Clinical Adverse Experiences (Incidence ≥3%)—Cycle 1

	Aprepitant Regimen (N = 544)	Standard Therapy (N = 550)
Body as a Whole/Site Unspecified		
Asthenia/Fatigue	17.8	11.8
Dizziness	6.6	4.4
Dehydration	5.9	5.1
Abdominal Pain	4.6	3.3
Fever	2.9	3.5
Mucous Membrane Disorder	2.6	3.1
Digestive System		
Nausea	12.7	11.8
Constipation	10.3	12.2
Diarrhea	10.3	7.5
Vomiting	7.5	7.6
Heartburn	5.3	4.9
Gastritis	4.2	3.1
Epigastric Discomfort	4.0	3.1
Eyes, Ears, Nose, and Throat		
Tinnitus	3.7	3.8
Hemic and Lymphatic System		
Neutropenia	3.1	2.9
Metabolism and Nutrition		
Anorexia	10.1	9.5
Nervous System		
Headache	8.5	8.7
Insomnia	2.9	3.1
Respiratory System		
Hiccups	10.8	5.6

In addition, isolated cases of serious adverse experiences, regardless of causality, of bradycardia, disorientation, and perforating duodenal ulcer were reported in highly emetogenic CINV clinical studies.

Moderately Emetogenic Chemotherapy

During Cycle 1 of 2 moderately emetogenic chemotherapy studies, 868 patients were treated with the aprepitant regimen and 686 of these patients continued into extensions for up to 4 cycles of chemotherapy. In the combined analysis of Cycle 1 data for these 2 studies, adverse experiences were reported in approximately 69% of patients treated with the aprepitant regimen compared with approximately 72% of patients treated with standard therapy.

In the combined analysis of Cycle 1 data for these 2 studies, the adverse experience profile in both moderately emetogenic chemotherapy studies was generally comparable to the highly emetogenic chemotherapy studies. Table 2 shows the percent of patients with clinical adverse experiences reported at an incidence ≥3%.

Table 2: Percent of Patients Receiving Moderately Emetogenic Chemotherapy with Clinical Adverse Experiences (Incidence ≥3%)—Cycle 1

	Aprepitant Regimen (N = 868)	Standard Therapy (N = 846)
Blood and Lymphatic System Disorders		
Neutropenia	5.8	5.6
Metabolism and Nutrition Disorders		
Anorexia	6.2	7.2
Psychiatric Disorders		
Insomnia	2.6	3.7
Nervous System Disorders		
Headache	13.2	14.3
Dizziness	2.8	3.4
Gastrointestinal Disorders		
Constipation	10.3	15.5
Diarrhea	7.6	8.7
Dyspepsia	5.8	3.8
Nausea	5.8	5.1
Stomatitis	3.1	2.7
Skin and Subcutaneous Tissue Disorders		
Alopecia	12.4	11.9
General Disorders and General Administration Site Conditions		
Fatigue	15.4	15.6
Asthenia	4.7	4.6

In a combined analysis of these two studies, isolated cases of serious adverse experiences were similar in the two treatment groups.

Highly and Moderately Emetogenic Chemotherapy

The following additional clinical adverse experiences (incidence >0.5% and greater than standard therapy), regardless of causality, were reported in patients treated with aprepitant regimen in either HEC or MEC studies:

Infections and infestations: candidiasis, herpes simplex, lower respiratory infection, oral candidiasis, pharyngitis, septic shock, upper respiratory infection, urinary tract infection.

Neoplasms benign, malignant and unspecified (including cysts and polyps): malignant neoplasm, non-small cell lung carcinoma.

Blood and lymphatic system disorders: anemia, febrile neutropenia, thrombocytopenia.

Metabolism and nutrition disorders: appetite decreased, diabetes mellitus, hypokalemia.

Psychiatric disorders: anxiety disorder, confusion, depression.

Nervous system: peripheral neuropathy, sensory neuropathy, taste disturbance, tremor.

Eye disorders: conjunctivitis.

Cardiac disorders: myocardial infarction, palpitations, tachycardia.

Vascular disorders: deep venous thrombosis, flushing, hot flush, hypertension, hypotension.

Respiratory, thoracic and mediastinal disorders: cough, dyspnea, nasal secretion, pharyngolaryngeal pain, pneumonitis, pulmonary embolism, respiratory insufficiency, vocal disturbance.

Gastrointestinal disorders: abdominal pain upper, acid reflux, deglutition disorder, dry mouth, dysgeusia, dysphagia, eructation, flatulence, obstipation, salivation increased.

Skin and subcutaneous tissue disorders: acne, diaphoresis, pruritus, rash.

Musculoskeletal and connective tissue disorders: arthralgia, back pain, muscular weakness, musculoskeletal pain, myalgia.

Renal and urinary disorders: dysuria, renal insufficiency.

Reproductive system and breast disorders: pelvic pain.

General disorders and administrative site conditions: edema, malaise, pain, rigors.

Investigations: weight loss.

Stevens-Johnson syndrome was reported as a serious adverse experience in a patient receiving aprepitant with cancer chemotherapy in another CINV study.

Laboratory Adverse Experiences

Table 3 shows the percent of patients with laboratory adverse experiences reported at an incidence ≥3% in patients receiving highly emetogenic chemotherapy.

Table 3: Percent of Patients Receiving Highly Emetogenic Chemotherapy with Laboratory Adverse Experiences (Incidence ≥3%)—Cycle 1

	Aprepitant Regimen (N = 544)	Standard Therapy (N = 550)
Proteinuria	6.8	5.3
ALT Increased	6.0	4.3
Blood Urea Nitrogen Increased	4.7	3.5
Serum Creatinine Increased	3.7	4.3
AST Increased	3.0	1.3

The following additional laboratory adverse experiences (incidence >0.5% and greater than standard therapy), regardless of causality, were reported in patients treated with aprepitant regimen: alkaline phosphatase increased, hyperglycemia, hyponatremia, leukocytes increased, erythrocyturia, leukocyturia.

The adverse experience profiles in the Multiple-Cycle extensions of HEC and MEC studies for up to 6 cycles of chemotherapy were generally similar to that observed in Cycle 1.

Postoperative Nausea and Vomiting

In well-controlled clinical studies in patients receiving general anesthesia, 564 patients were administered 40 mg aprepitant orally and 538 patients were administered 4 mg ondansetron IV.

Clinical adverse experiences were reported in approximately 60% of patients treated with 40 mg aprepitant compared with approximately 64% of patients treated with 4 mg ondansetron IV. Table 4 shows the percent of patients with clinical adverse experiences reported at an incidence ≥3% of the combined studies.

Table 4: Percent of Patients Receiving General Anesthesia with Clinical Adverse Experiences (Incidence ≥3%)

	Aprepitant 40 mg (N = 564)	Ondansetron (N = 538)
Infections and Infestations		
Urinary Tract Infection	2.3	3.2
Blood and Lymphatic System Disorders		
Anemia	3.0	4.3
Psychiatric Disorders		
Insomnia	2.1	3.3
Nervous System Disorders		
Headache	5.0	6.5
Cardiac Disorders		
Bradycardia	4.4	3.9
Vascular Disorders		
Hypotension	5.7	4.6
Hypertension	2.1	3.2
Gastrointestinal Disorders		
Nausea	8.5	8.6
Constipation	8.5	7.6
Flatulence	4.1	5.8
Vomiting	2.5	3.9
Skin and Subcutaneous Tissue Disorders		
Pruritus	7.6	8.4
General Disorders and General Administration Site Conditions		
Pyrexia	5.9	10.6

The following additional clinical adverse experiences (incidence >0.5% and greater than ondansetron), regardless of causality, were reported in patients treated with aprepitant:
Infections and infestations: postoperative infection
Metabolism and nutrition disorders: hypokalemia, hypovolemia.
Nervous system disorders: dizziness, hypoesthesia, syncope.
Vascular disorders: hematoma
Respiratory, thoracic and mediastinal disorders: dyspnea, hypoxia, respiratory depression.
Gastrointestinal disorders: abdominal pain, abdominal pain upper, dry mouth, dyspepsia.
Skin and subcutaneous tissue disorders: urticaria
General disorders and administrative site conditions: hypothermia, pain.
Investigations: blood pressure decreased
Injury, poisoning and procedural complications: operative hemorrhage, wound dehiscence.
Other adverse experiences (incidence ≤0.5%) reported in patients treated with aprepitant 40 mg for postoperative nausea and vomiting included:
Nervous system disorders: dysarthria, sensory disturbance.
Eye disorders: miosis, visual acuity reduced.
Respiratory, thoracic and mediastinal disorders: wheezing
Gastrointestinal disorders: bowel sounds abnormal, stomach discomfort.
There were no serious adverse drug-related experiences reported in the postoperative nausea and vomiting clinical studies in patients taking 40 mg aprepitant.
Laboratory Adverse Experiences
One laboratory adverse experience, hemoglobin decreased (40 mg aprepitant 3.8%, ondansetron 4.2%), was reported at an incidence ≥3% in a patient receiving general anesthesia. The following additional laboratory adverse experiences (incidence >0.5% and greater than ondansetron), regardless of causality, were reported in patients treated with aprepitant 40 mg: blood albumin decreased, blood bilirubin increased, blood glucose increased, blood potassium decreased, glucose urine present.
The adverse experience of ALT increased occurred with similar incidence in patients treated with aprepitant 40 mg (1.1%) as in patients treated with ondansetron 4 mg (1.0%).
Other Studies
In addition, two serious adverse experiences were reported in postoperative nausea and vomiting (PONV) clinical studies in patients taking a higher dose of aprepitant: one case of constipation, and one case of sub-ileus.
Angioedema and urticaria were reported as serious adverse experiences in a patient receiving aprepitant in a non-CINV/non-PONV study.

6.2   Postmarketing Experience
The following adverse reactions have been identified during postmarketing use of aprepitant. Because these reactions are reported voluntarily from a population of uncertain size, it is generally not possible to reliably estimate their frequency or establish a causal relationship to the drug.
Skin and subcutaneous tissue disorders: pruritus, rash, urticaria.
Immune system disorders: hypersensitivity reactions including anaphylactic reactions.

7   DRUG INTERACTIONS

Aprepitant is a substrate, a weak-to-moderate (dose-dependent) inhibitor, and an inducer of CYP3A4. Aprepitant is also an inducer of CYP2C9.
7.1   Effect of Aprepitant on the Pharmacokinetics of Other Agents
CYP3A4 Substrates:
Weak inhibition of CYP3A4 by a single 40 mg dose of aprepitant is not expected to alter the plasma concentrations of concomitant medications that are primarily metabolized through CYP3A4 to a clinically significant degree. However, higher aprepitant doses or repeated dosing at any aprepitant dose may have a clinically significant effect.
As a moderate inhibitor of CYP3A4 at a dose of 125 mg/80 mg, aprepitant can increase plasma concentrations of concomitantly administered oral medications that are metabolized through CYP3A4 *[see Contraindications (4)]*. The use of fosaprepitant may increase CYP3A4 substrate plasma concentrations to a lesser degree than the use of oral aprepitant (125 mg).

5-HT₃ antagonists: In clinical drug interaction studies, aprepitant did not have clinically important effects on the pharmacokinetics of ondansetron, granisetron, or hydrodolasetron (the active metabolite of dolasetron).

Corticosteroids:
Dexamethasone: EMEND, when given as a regimen of 125 mg with dexamethasone coadministered orally as 20 mg on Day 1, and EMEND when given as 80 mg/day with dexamethasone coadministered orally as 8 mg on Days 2 through 5, increased the AUC of dexamethasone, a CYP3A4 substrate, by 2.2-fold on Days 1 and 5. The oral

dexamethasone doses should be reduced by approximately 50% when coadministered with EMEND (125 mg/80 mg regimen), to achieve exposures of dexamethasone similar to those obtained when it is given without EMEND. The daily dose of dexamethasone administered in clinical chemotherapy induced nausea and vomiting studies with EMEND reflects an approximate 50% reduction of the dose of dexamethasone *[see Dosage and Administration (2.1)]*. A single dose of EMEND (40 mg) when coadministered with a single oral dose of dexamethasone 20 mg, increased the AUC of dexamethasone by 1.45-fold. Therefore, no dose adjustment is recommended.
Methylprednisolone: EMEND, when given as a regimen of 125 mg on Day 1 and 80 mg/day on Days 2 and 3, increased the AUC of methylprednisolone, a CYP3A4 substrate, by 1.34-fold on Day 1 and by 2.5-fold on Day 3, when methylprednisolone was coadministered intravenously as 125 mg on Day 1 and orally as 40 mg on Days 2 and 3. The IV methylprednisolone dose should be reduced by approximately 25%, and the oral methylprednisolone dose should be reduced by approximately 50% when coadministered with EMEND (125 mg/80 mg regimen) to achieve exposures of methylprednisolone similar to those obtained when it is given without EMEND. Although the concomitant administration of methylprednisolone with the single 40 mg dose of aprepitant has not been studied, a single 40 mg dose of EMEND produces a weak inhibition of CYP3A4 (based on midazolam interaction study) and it is not expected to alter the plasma concentrations of methylprednisolone to a clinically significant degree. Therefore, no dose adjustment is recommended.

Chemotherapeutic agents: *[see Warnings and Precautions (5.1)]*
Docetaxel: In a pharmacokinetic study, EMEND (125 mg/80 mg regimen) did not influence the pharmacokinetics of docetaxel.
Vinorelbine: In a pharmacokinetic study, EMEND (125 mg/80 mg regimen) did not influence the pharmacokinetics of vinorelbine to a clinically significant degree.

CYP2C9 Substrates (Warfarin, Tolbutamide):
Aprepitant has been shown to induce the metabolism of S(-) warfarin and tolbutamide, which are metabolized through CYP2C9. Coadministration of EMEND with these drugs or other drugs that are known to be metabolized by CYP2C9, such as phenytoin, may result in lower plasma concentrations of these drugs.
Warfarin: A single 125-mg dose of EMEND was administered on Day 1 and 80 mg/day on Days 2 and 3 to healthy subjects who were stabilized on chronic warfarin therapy. Although there was no effect of EMEND on the plasma AUC of R(+) or S(-) warfarin determined on Day 3, there was a 34% decrease in S(-) warfarin (a CYP2C9 substrate) trough concentration accompanied by a 14% decrease in the prothrombin time (reported as International Normalized Ratio or INR) 5 days after completion of dosing with EMEND. In patients on chronic warfarin therapy, the prothrombin time (INR) should be closely monitored in the 2-week period, particularly at 7 to 10 days, following initiation of the 3-day regimen of EMEND with each chemotherapy cycle, or following administration of a single 40 mg dose of EMEND for the prevention of postoperative nausea and vomiting.
Tolbutamide: EMEND, when given as 125 mg on Day 1 and 80 mg/day on Days 2 and 3, decreased the AUC of tolbutamide (a CYP2C9 substrate) by 23% on Day 4, 28% on Day 8, and 15% on Day 15, when a single dose of tolbutamide 500 mg was administered orally prior to the administration of the 3-day regimen of EMEND and on Days 4, 8, and 15.
EMEND, when given as a 40-mg single oral dose on Day 1, decreased the AUC of tolbutamide (a CYP2C9 substrate) by 8% on Day 2, 16% on Day 4, 15% on Day 8, and 10% on Day 15, when a single dose of tolbutamide 500 mg was administered orally prior to the administration of EMEND 40 mg and on Days 2, 4, 8, and 15. This effect was not considered clinically important.

Oral contraceptives: Aprepitant, when given once daily for 14 days as a 100-mg capsule with an oral contraceptive containing 35 mcg of ethinyl estradiol and 1 mg of norethindrone, decreased the AUC of ethinyl estradiol by 43%, and decreased the AUC of norethindrone by 8%.
In another study, a daily dose of an oral contraceptive containing ethinyl estradiol and norethindrone was administered on Days 1 through 21, and EMEND was given as a 3-day regimen of 125 mg on Day 8 and 80 mg/day on Days 9 and 10 with ondansetron 32 mg IV on Day 8 and oral dexamethasone given as 12 mg on Day 8 and 8 mg/day on Days 9, 10, and 11. In the study, the AUC of ethinyl estradiol decreased by 19% on Day 10 and there was as much as a 64% decrease in ethinyl estradiol trough concentrations during Days 9 through 21. While there was no effect of EMEND on the AUC of norethindrone on Day 10, there was as much as a 60% decrease in norethindrone trough concentrations during Days 9 through 21.

In another study, a daily dose of an oral contraceptive containing ethinyl estradiol and norgestimate (which is converted to norelgestromin) was administered on Days 1 through 21, and EMEND 40 mg was given on Day 8. In the study, the AUC of ethinyl estradiol decreased by 4% and 29% on Day 8 and Day 12, respectively, while the AUC of norelgestromin increased by 18% on Day 8 and decreased by 10% on Day 12. In addition, the trough concentrations of ethinyl estradiol and norelgestromin on Days 8 through 21 were generally lower following coadministration of the oral contraceptive with EMEND 40 mg on Day 8 compared to the trough levels following administration of the oral contraceptive alone.
The coadministration of EMEND may reduce the efficacy of hormonal contraceptives (these can include birth control pills, skin patches, implants, and certain IUDs) during and for 28 days after administration of the last dose of EMEND. Alternative or back-up methods of contraception should be used during treatment with EMEND and for 1 month following the last dose of EMEND.

Midazolam: EMEND increased the AUC of midazolam, a sensitive CYP3A4 substrate, by 2.3-fold on Day 1 and 3.3-fold on Day 5, when a single oral dose of midazolam 2 mg was coadministered on Day 1 and Day 5 of a regimen of EMEND 125 mg on Day 1 and 80 mg/day on Days 2 through 5. The potential effects of increased plasma concentrations of midazolam or other benzodiazepines metabolized via CYP3A4 (alprazolam, triazolam) should be considered when coadministering these agents with EMEND (125 mg/80 mg). A single dose of EMEND (40 mg) increased the AUC of midazolam by 1.2-fold on Day 1, when a single oral dose of midazolam 2 mg was coadministered on Day 1 with EMEND 40 mg; this effect was not considered clinically important.
In another study with intravenous administration of midazolam, EMEND was given as 125 mg on Day 1 and 80 mg/day on Days 2 and 3, and midazolam 2 mg IV was given prior to the administration of the 3-day regimen of EMEND and on Days 4, 8, and 15. EMEND increased the AUC of midazolam by 25% on Day 4 and decreased the AUC of midazolam by 19% on Day 8 relative to the dosing of EMEND on Days 1 through 3. These effects were not considered clinically important. The AUC of midazolam on Day 15 was similar to that observed at baseline.
An additional study was completed with intravenous administration of midazolam and EMEND. Intravenous midazolam 2 mg was given 1 hour after oral administration of a single dose of EMEND 125 mg. The plasma AUC of midazolam was increased by 1.5-fold. Depending on clinical situations (e.g., elderly patients) and degree of monitoring available, dosage adjustment for intravenous midazolam may be necessary when it is coadministered with EMEND for the chemotherapy induced nausea and vomiting indication (125 mg on Day 1 followed by 80 mg on Days 2 and 3).
7.2   Effect of Other Agents on the Pharmacokinetics of Aprepitant
Aprepitant is a substrate for CYP3A4; therefore, coadministration of EMEND with drugs that inhibit CYP3A4 activity may result in increased plasma concentrations of aprepitant. Consequently, concomitant administration of EMEND with strong CYP3A4 inhibitors (e.g., ketoconazole, itraconazole, nefazodone, troleandomycin, clarithromycin, ritonavir, nelfinavir) should be approached with caution. Because moderate CYP3A4 inhibitors (e.g., diltiazem) result in a 2-fold increase in plasma concentrations of aprepitant, concomitant administration should also be approached with caution.
Aprepitant is a substrate for CYP3A4; therefore, coadministration of EMEND with drugs that strongly induce CYP3A4 activity (e.g., rifampin, carbamazepine, phenytoin) may result in reduced plasma concentrations of aprepitant that may result in decreased efficacy of EMEND.
Ketoconazole: When a single 125-mg dose of EMEND was administered on Day 5 of a 10-day regimen of 400 mg/day of ketoconazole, a strong CYP3A4 inhibitor, the AUC of aprepitant increased approximately 5-fold and the mean terminal half-life of aprepitant increased approximately 3-fold. Concomitant administration of EMEND with strong CYP3A4 inhibitors should be approached cautiously.
Rifampin: When a single 375-mg dose of EMEND was administered on Day 9 of a 14-day regimen of 600 mg/day of rifampin, a strong CYP3A4 inducer, the AUC of aprepitant decreased approximately 11-fold and the mean terminal half-life decreased approximately 3-fold.
Coadministration of EMEND with drugs that induce CYP3A4 activity may result in reduced plasma concentrations and decreased efficacy of EMEND.
7.3   Additional Interactions
EMEND is unlikely to interact with drugs that are substrates for the P-glycoprotein transporter, as demonstrated

by the lack of interaction of EMEND with digoxin in a clinical drug interaction study.

Diltiazem: In patients with mild to moderate hypertension, administration of aprepitant once daily, as a tablet formulation comparable to 230 mg of the capsule formulation, with diltiazem 120 mg 3 times daily for 5 days, resulted in a 2-fold increase of aprepitant AUC and a simultaneous 1.7-fold increase of diltiazem AUC. These pharmacokinetic effects did not result in clinically meaningful changes in ECG, heart rate or blood pressure beyond those changes induced by diltiazem alone.

Paroxetine: Coadministration of once daily doses of aprepitant, as a tablet formulation comparable to 85 mg or 170 mg of the capsule formulation, with paroxetine 20 mg once daily, resulted in a decrease in AUC by approximately 25% and C_{max} by approximately 20% of both aprepitant and paroxetine.

8 USE IN SPECIFIC POPULATIONS

8.1 Pregnancy
Teratogenic effects
Pregnancy Category B: Reproduction studies have been performed in rats at oral doses up to 1000 mg/kg twice daily (plasma AUC_{0-24hr} of 31.3 mcg•hr/mL, about 1.6 times the human exposure at the recommended dose) and in rabbits at oral doses up to 25 mg/kg/day (plasma AUC_{0-24hr} of 26.9 mcg•hr/mL, about 1.4 times the human exposure at the recommended dose) and have revealed no evidence of impaired fertility or harm to the fetus due to aprepitant. There are, however, no adequate and well-controlled studies in pregnant women. Because animal reproduction studies are not always predictive of human response, this drug should be used during pregnancy only if clearly needed.

8.3 Nursing Mothers
Aprepitant is excreted in the milk of rats. It is not known whether this drug is excreted in human milk. Because many drugs are excreted in human milk and because of the potential for possible serious adverse reactions in nursing infants from aprepitant and because of the potential for tumorigenicity shown for aprepitant in rodent carcinogenicity studies, a decision should be made whether to discontinue nursing or to discontinue the drug, taking into account the importance of the drug to the mother.

8.4 Pediatric Use
Safety and effectiveness of EMEND in pediatric patients have not been established.

8.5 Geriatric Use
In 2 well-controlled chemotherapy-induced nausea and vomiting clinical studies, of the total number of patients (N=544) treated with EMEND, 31% were 65 and over, while 5% were 75 and over. In well-controlled postoperative nausea and vomiting clinical studies, of the total number of patients (N=1120) treated with EMEND, 7% were 65 and over, while 2% were 75 and over. No overall differences in safety or effectiveness were observed between these subjects and younger subjects. Greater sensitivity of some older individuals cannot be ruled out. Dosage adjustment in the elderly is not necessary.

10 OVERDOSAGE

No specific information is available on the treatment of overdosage.

Drowsiness and headache were reported in one patient who ingested 1440 mg of aprepitant.

In the event of overdose, EMEND should be discontinued and general supportive treatment and monitoring should be provided. Because of the antiemetic activity of aprepitant, drug-induced emesis may not be effective.

Aprepitant cannot be removed by hemodialysis.

11 DESCRIPTION

EMEND (aprepitant) is a substance P/neurokinin 1 (NK_1) receptor antagonist, chemically described as 5-[[(2R,3S)-2-[(1R)-1-[3,5-bis(trifluoromethyl)phenyl]ethoxy]-3-(4-fluorophenyl)-4-morpholinyl]methyl]-1,2-dihydro-3H-1,2,4-triazol-3-one.

Its empirical formula is $C_{23}H_{21}F_7N_4O_3$, and its structural formula is:

Aprepitant is a white to off-white crystalline solid, with a molecular weight of 534.43. It is practically insoluble in water. Aprepitant is sparingly soluble in ethanol and isopropyl acetate and slightly soluble in acetonitrile.

Each capsule of EMEND for oral administration contains either 40 mg, 80 mg or 125 mg of aprepitant and the following inactive ingredients: sucrose, microcrystalline cellulose, hydroxypropyl cellulose and sodium lauryl sulfate. The capsule shell excipients are gelatin, titanium dioxide, and may contain sodium lauryl sulfate and silicon dioxide. The 40–mg capsule shell also contains yellow ferric oxide, and the 125–mg capsule also contains red ferric oxide and yellow ferric oxide.

12 CLINICAL PHARMACOLOGY

12.1 Mechanism of Action
Aprepitant is a selective high-affinity antagonist of human substance P/neurokinin 1 (NK_1) receptors. Aprepitant has little or no affinity for serotonin (5-HT_3), dopamine, and corticosteroid receptors, the targets of existing therapies for chemotherapy-induced nausea and vomiting (CINV) and postoperative nausea and vomiting (PONV).

Aprepitant has been shown in animal models to inhibit emesis induced by cytotoxic chemotherapeutic agents, such as cisplatin, via central actions. Animal and human Positron Emission Tomography (PET) studies with aprepitant have shown that it crosses the blood brain barrier and occupies brain NK_1 receptors. Animal and human studies show that aprepitant augments the antiemetic activity of the 5-HT_3-receptor antagonist ondansetron and the corticosteroid dexamethasone and inhibits both the acute and delayed phases of cisplatin-induced emesis.

12.2 Pharmacodynamics
NK_1 Receptor Occupancy
In two single-blind, multiple-dose, randomized, and placebo control studies, healthy young men received oral aprepitant doses of 10 mg (N=2), 30 mg (N=3), 100 mg (N=3) or 300 mg (N=5) once daily for 14 days with 2 or 3 subjects on placebo. Both plasma aprepitant concentration and NK_1 receptor occupancy in the corpus striatum by positron emission tomography were evaluated, at predose and 24 hours after the last dose. At aprepitant plasma concentrations of ~10 ng/mL and ~100 ng/mL, the NK_1 receptor occupancies were ~50% and ~90%, respectively. The oral aprepitant regimen for CINV produces mean trough plasma aprepitant concentrations >500 ng/mL, which would be expected to, based on the fitted curve with the Hill equation, result in >95% brain NK_1 receptor occupancy. However, the receptor occupancy for either CINV or PONV dosing regimen has not been determined. In addition, the relationship between NK_1 receptor occupancy and the clinical efficacy of aprepitant has not been established.

Cardiac Electrophysiology
In a randomized, double-blind, positive-controlled, thorough QTc study, a single 200-mg dose of fosaprepitant had no effect on the QTc interval. QT prolongation with the oral dosing regimens for CINV and PONV are not expected.

Table 5: Treatment Regimens in Highly Emetogenic Chemotherapy Trials

Treatment Regimen	Day 1	Days 2 to 4
Aprepitant	Aprepitant 125 mg PO Dexamethasone 12 mg PO Ondansetron 32 mg I.V.	Aprepitant 80 mg PO Daily (Days 2 and 3 only) Dexamethasone 8 mg PO Daily (morning)
Standard Therapy	Dexamethasone 20 mg PO Ondansetron 32 mg I.V.	Dexamethasone 8 mg PO Daily (morning) Dexamethasone 8 mg PO Daily (evening)

Aprepitant placebo and dexamethasone placebo were used to maintain blinding.

Table 6: Percent of Patients Receiving Highly Emetogenic Chemotherapy Responding by Treatment Group and Phase for Study 1—Cycle 1

ENDPOINTS	Aprepitant Regimen (N = 260)* %	Standard Therapy (N = 261)* %	p-Value
PRIMARY ENDPOINT			
Complete Response			
Overall[†]	73	52	<0.001
OTHER PRESPECIFIED ENDPOINTS			
Complete Response			
Acute phase[‡]	89	78	<0.001
Delayed phase[§]	75	56	<0.001
Complete Protection			
Overall	63	49	0.001
Acute phase	85	75	NS[¶]
Delayed phase	66	52	<0.001
No Emesis			
Overall	78	55	<0.001
Acute phase	90	79	0.001
Delayed phase	81	59	<0.001
No Nausea			
Overall	48	44	NS[#]
Delayed phase	51	48	NS[#]
No Significant Nausea			
Overall	73	66	NS[#]
Delayed phase	75	69	NS[#]

Visual analogue scale (VAS) score range: 0 mm = no nausea; 100 mm = nausea as bad as it could be.
* N: Number of patients (older than 18 years of age) who received cisplatin, study drug, and had at least one post-treatment efficacy evaluation.
† Overall: 0 to 120 hours post-cisplatin treatment.
‡ Acute phase: 0 to 24 hours post-cisplatin treatment.
§ Delayed phase: 25 to 120 hours post-cisplatin treatment.
¶ Not statistically significant when adjusted for multiple comparisons.
# Not statistically significant.

Table 7: Percent of Patients Receiving Highly Emetogenic Chemotherapy Responding by Treatment Group and Phase for Study 2—Cycle 1

ENDPOINTS	Aprepitant Regimen (N = 261)* %	Standard Therapy (N = 263)* %	p-Value
PRIMARY ENDPOINT			
Complete Response			
Overall[†]	63	43	<0.001
OTHER PRESPECIFIED ENDPOINTS			
Complete Response			
Acute phase[‡]	83	68	<0.001
Delayed phase[§]	68	47	<0.001
Complete Protection			
Overall	56	41	<0.001
Acute phase	80	65	<0.001
Delayed phase	61	44	<0.001
No Emesis			
Overall	66	44	<0.001
Acute phase	84	69	<0.001
Delayed phase	72	48	<0.001
No Nausea			
Overall	49	39	NS[¶]
Delayed phase	53	40	NS[¶]
No Significant Nausea			
Overall	71	64	NS[#]
Delayed phase	73	65	NS[#]

Visual analogue scale (VAS) score range: 0 mm = no nausea; 100 mm = nausea as bad as it could be.
* N: Number of patients (older than 18 years of age) who received cisplatin, study drug, and had at least one post-treatment efficacy evaluation.
† Overall: 0 to 120 hours post-cisplatin treatment.
‡ Acute phase: 0 to 24 hours post-cisplatin treatment.
§ Delayed phase: 25 to 120 hours post-cisplatin treatment.
¶ Not statistically significant when adjusted for multiple comparisons.
\# Not statistically significant.

Figure 1: Percent of Patients Receiving Highly Emetogenic Chemotherapy Who Remain Emesis Free Over Time—Cycle 1

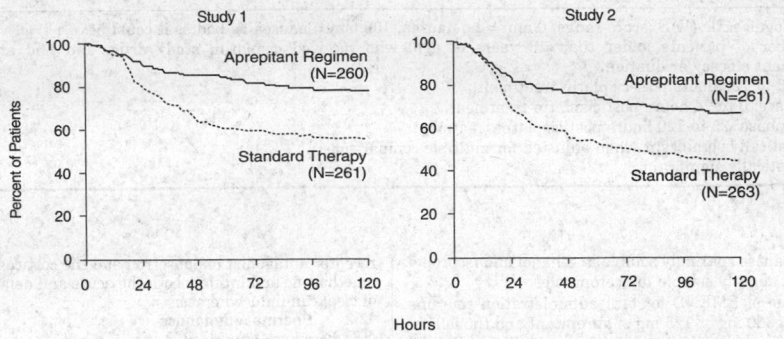

p-Value <0.001 based on a log rank test for Study 1 and Study 2; nominal p-values not adjusted for multiplicity.

12.3 Pharmacokinetics

Absorption
Following oral administration of a single 40 mg dose of EMEND in the fasted state, mean area under the plasma concentration-time curve ($AUC_{0-\infty}$) was 7.8 mcg•hr/mL and mean peak plasma concentration (C_{max}) was 0.7 mcg/mL, occurring at approximately 3 hours postdose (T_{max}). The absolute bioavailability at the 40–mg dose has not been determined.
Following oral administration of a single 125-mg dose of EMEND on Day 1 and 80 mg once daily on Days 2 and 3, the AUC_{0-24hr} was approximately 19.6 mcg•hr/mL and 21.2 mcg•hr/mL on Day 1 and Day 3, respectively. The C_{max} of 1.6 mcg/mL and 1.4 mcg/mL were reached in approximately 4 hours (T_{max}) on Day 1 and Day 3, respectively. At the dose range of 80-125 mg, the mean absolute oral bioavailability of aprepitant is approximately 60 to 65%. Oral administration of the capsule with a standard high-fat breakfast had no clinically meaningful effect on the bioavailability of aprepitant.

The pharmacokinetics of aprepitant are non-linear across the clinical dose range. In healthy young adults, the increase in $AUC_{0-\infty}$ was 26% greater than dose proportional between 80-mg and 125-mg single doses administered in the fed state.

Distribution
Aprepitant is greater than 95% bound to plasma proteins. The mean apparent volume of distribution at steady state (Vd_{ss}) is approximately 70 L in humans.
Aprepitant crosses the placenta in rats and rabbits and crosses the blood brain barrier in humans *[see Clinical Pharmacology (12.1)]*.

Metabolism
Aprepitant undergoes extensive metabolism. *In vitro* studies using human liver microsomes indicate that aprepitant is metabolized primarily by CYP3A4 with minor metabolism by CYP1A2 and CYP2C19. Metabolism is largely via oxidation at the morpholine ring and its side chains. No metabolism by CYP2D6, CYP2C9, or CYP2E1 was detected. In healthy young adults, aprepitant accounts for approxi-

mately 24% of the radioactivity in plasma over 72 hours following a single oral 300-mg dose of [^{14}C]-aprepitant, indicating a substantial presence of metabolites in the plasma. Seven metabolites of aprepitant, which are only weakly active, have been identified in human plasma.

Excretion
Following administration of a single IV 100-mg dose of [^{14}C]-aprepitant prodrug to healthy subjects, 57% of the radioactivity was recovered in urine and 45% in feces. A study was not conducted with radiolabeled capsule formulation. The results after oral administration may differ.
Aprepitant is eliminated primarily by metabolism; aprepitant is not renally excreted. The apparent plasma clearance of aprepitant ranged from approximately 62 to 90 mL/min. The apparent terminal half-life ranged from approximately 9 to 13 hours.

Special Populations
Gender
Following oral administration of a single 125-mg dose of EMEND, no difference in AUC_{0-24hr} was observed between males and females. The C_{max} for aprepitant is 16% higher in females as compared with males. The half-life of aprepitant is 25% lower in females as compared with males and T_{max} occurs at approximately the same time. These differences are not considered clinically meaningful. No dosage adjustment for EMEND is necessary based on gender.
Geriatric
Following oral administration of a single 125-mg dose of EMEND on Day 1 and 80 mg once daily on Days 2 through 5, the AUC_{0-24hr} of aprepitant was 21% higher on Day 1 and 36% higher on Day 5 in elderly (≥65 years) relative to younger adults. The C_{max} was 10% higher on Day 1 and 24% higher on Day 5 in elderly relative to younger adults. These differences are not considered clinically meaningful. No dosage adjustment for EMEND is necessary in elderly patients.
Pediatric
EMEND has not been evaluated in patients below 18 years of age.
Race
Following oral administration of a single 125-mg dose of EMEND, the AUC_{0-24hr} is approximately 25% and 29% higher in Hispanics as compared with Whites and Blacks, respectively. The C_{max} is 22% and 31% higher in Hispanics as compared with Whites and Blacks, respectively. These differences are not considered clinically meaningful. There was no difference in AUC_{0-24hr} or C_{max} between Whites and Blacks. No dosage adjustment for EMEND is necessary based on race.
Hepatic Insufficiency
Following administration of a single 125-mg dose of EMEND on Day 1 and 80 mg once daily on Days 2 and 3 to patients with mild hepatic impairment (Child-Pugh score 5 to 6), the AUC_{0-24hr} of aprepitant was 11% lower on Day 1 and 36% lower on Day 3, as compared with healthy subjects given the same regimen. In patients with moderate hepatic impairment (Child-Pugh score 7 to 9), the AUC_{0-24hr} of aprepitant was 10% higher on Day 1 and 18% higher on Day 3, as compared with healthy subjects given the same regimen. These differences in AUC_{0-24hr} are not considered clinically meaningful; therefore, no dosage adjustment for EMEND is necessary in patients with mild to moderate hepatic impairment.
There are no clinical or pharmacokinetic data in patients with severe hepatic impairment (Child-Pugh score >9) *[see Warnings and Precautions (5.4)]*.
Renal Insufficiency
A single 240-mg dose of EMEND was administered to patients with severe renal impairment (CrCl<30 mL/min) and to patients with end stage renal disease (ESRD) requiring hemodialysis.
In patients with severe renal impairment, the $AUC_{0-\infty}$ of total aprepitant (unbound and protein bound) decreased by 21% and C_{max} decreased by 32%, relative to healthy subjects. In patients with ESRD undergoing hemodialysis, the $AUC_{0-\infty}$ of total aprepitant decreased by 42% and C_{max} decreased by 32%. Due to modest decreases in protein binding of aprepitant in patients with renal disease, the AUC of pharmacologically active unbound drug was not significantly affected in patients with renal impairment compared with healthy subjects. Hemodialysis conducted 4 or 48 hours after dosing had no significant effect on the pharmacokinetics of aprepitant; less than 0.2% of the dose was recovered in the dialysate.
No dosage adjustment for EMEND is necessary for patients with renal impairment or for patients with ESRD undergoing hemodialysis.

13 NONCLINICAL TOXICOLOGY

13.1 Carcinogenesis, Mutagenesis, Impairment of Fertility
Carcinogenicity studies were conducted in Sprague-Dawley rats and in CD-1 mice for 2 years. In the rat carcinogenicity studies, animals were treated with oral doses ranging from 0.05 to 1000 mg/kg twice daily. The highest dose produced a

systemic exposure to aprepitant (plasma AUC_{0-24hr}) of 0.7 to 1.6 times the human exposure (AUC_{0-24hr} = 19.6 mcg·hr/mL) at the recommended dose of 125 mg/day. Treatment with aprepitant at doses of 5 to 1000 mg/kg twice daily caused an increase in the incidences of thyroid follicular cell adenomas and carcinomas in male rats. In female rats, it produced hepatocellular adenomas at 5 to 1000 mg/kg twice daily and hepatocellular carcinomas and thyroid follicular cell adenomas at 125 to 1000 mg/kg twice daily. In the mouse carcinogenicity studies, the animals were treated with oral doses ranging from 2.5 to 2000 mg/kg/day. The highest dose produced a systemic exposure of about 2.8 to 3.6 times the human exposure at the recommended dose. Treatment with aprepitant produced skin fibrosarcomas at 125 and 500 mg/kg/day doses in male mice.

Aprepitant was not genotoxic in the Ames test, the human lymphoblastoid cell (TK6) mutagenesis test, the rat hepatocyte DNA strand break test, the Chinese hamster ovary (CHO) cell chromosome aberration test and the mouse micronucleus test.

Aprepitant did not affect the fertility or general reproductive performance of male or female rats at doses up to the maximum feasible dose of 1000 mg/kg twice daily (providing exposure in male rats lower than the exposure at the recommended human dose and exposure in female rats at about 1.6 times the human exposure).

14 CLINICAL STUDIES

14.1 Prevention of Chemotherapy Induced Nausea and Vomiting (CINV)

Oral administration of EMEND in combination with ondansetron and dexamethasone (aprepitant regimen) has been shown to prevent acute and delayed nausea and vomiting associated with highly emetogenic chemotherapy including high-dose cisplatin, and nausea and vomiting associated with moderately emetogenic chemotherapy.

Highly Emetogenic Chemotherapy (HEC)

In 2 multicenter, randomized, parallel, double-blind, controlled clinical studies, the aprepitant regimen (see Table 6) was compared with standard therapy in patients receiving a chemotherapy regimen that included cisplatin >50 mg/m² (mean cisplatin dose = 80.2 mg/m²). Of the 550 patients who were randomized to receive the aprepitant regimen, 42% were women, 58% men, 59% White, 3% Asian, 5% Black, 12% Hispanic American, and 21% Multi-Racial. The aprepitant-treated patients in these clinical studies ranged from 14 to 84 years of age, with a mean age of 56 years. 170 patients were 65 years or older, with 29 patients being 75 years or older.

Patients (N = 1105) were randomized to either the aprepitant regimen (N = 550) or standard therapy (N = 555). The treatment regimens are defined in Table 5.

[See table 5 at top of page 2037]

During these studies 95% of the patients in the aprepitant group received a concomitant chemotherapeutic agent in addition to protocol-mandated cisplatin. The most common chemotherapeutic agents and the number of aprepitant patients exposed follows: etoposide (106), fluorouracil (100), gemcitabine (89), vinorelbine (82), paclitaxel (52), cyclophosphamide (50), doxorubicin (38), docetaxel (11).

The antiemetic activity of EMEND was evaluated during the acute phase (0 to 24 hours post-cisplatin treatment), the delayed phase (25 to 120 hours post-cisplatin treatment) and overall (0 to 120 hours post-cisplatin treatment) in Cycle 1. Efficacy was based on evaluation of the following endpoints:

Primary endpoint:

• complete response (defined as no emetic episodes and no use of rescue therapy)

Other prespecified endpoints:

• complete protection (defined as no emetic episodes, no use of rescue therapy, and a maximum nausea visual analogue scale [VAS] score <25 mm on a 0 to 100 mm scale)
• no emesis (defined as no emetic episodes regardless of use of rescue therapy)
• no nausea (maximum VAS <5 mm on a 0 to 100 mm scale)
• no significant nausea (maximum VAS <25 mm on a 0 to 100 mm scale)

A summary of the key study results from each individual study analysis is shown in Table 6 and in Table 7.

[See table 6 on page 2037]

[See table 7 at top of previous page]

In both studies, a statistically significantly higher proportion of patients receiving the aprepitant regimen in Cycle 1 had a complete response in the overall phase (primary endpoint), compared with patients receiving standard therapy. A statistically significant difference in complete response in favor of the aprepitant regimen was also observed when the acute phase and the delayed phase were analyzed separately.

In both studies, the estimated time to first emesis after initiation of cisplatin treatment was longer with the aprepitant regimen, and the incidence of first emesis was

reduced in the aprepitant regimen group compared with standard therapy group as depicted in the Kaplan-Meier curves in Figure 1.

[See figure 1 on previous page]

Patient-Reported Outcomes: The impact of nausea and vomiting on patients' daily lives was assessed in Cycle 1 of both Phase III studies using the Functional Living Index–Emesis (FLIE), a validated nausea- and vomiting-specific patient-reported outcome measure. Minimal or no impact of nausea and vomiting on patients' daily lives is defined as a FLIE total score >108. In each of the 2 studies, a higher proportion of patients receiving the aprepitant regimen reported minimal or no impact of nausea and vomiting on daily life (Study 1: 74% versus 64%; Study 2: 75% versus 64%).

Multiple-Cycle Extension: In the same 2 clinical studies, patients continued into the Multiple-Cycle extension for up to 5 additional cycles of chemotherapy. The proportion of patients with no emesis and no significant nausea by treatment group at each cycle is depicted in Figure 2. Antiemetic effectiveness for the patients receiving the aprepitant regimen is maintained throughout repeat cycles for those patients continuing in each of the multiple cycles.

[See figure 2 above]

Moderately Emetogenic Chemotherapy (MEC)

In a multicenter, randomized, double-blind, parallel-group, clinical study in breast cancer patients, the aprepitant regimen (see Table 9) was compared with a standard of care therapy in patients receiving a moderately emetogenic chemotherapy regimen that included cyclophosphamide 750-1500 mg/m²; or cyclophosphamide 500-1500 mg/m² and doxorubicin (≤60 mg/m²) or epirubicin (≤100 mg/m²).

In this study, the most common combinations were cyclophosphamide + doxorubicin (60.6%); and cyclophosphamide + epirubicin + fluorouracil (21.6%).

Of the 438 patients who were randomized to receive the aprepitant regimen, 99.5% were women. Of these, approximately 80% were White, 8% Black, 8% Asian, 4% Hispanic, and <1% Other. The aprepitant-treated patients in this clinical study ranged from 25 to 78 years of age, with a mean age of 53 years; 70 patients were 65 years or older, with 12 patients being over 74 years.

Patients (N = 866) were randomized to either the aprepitant regimen (N = 438) or standard therapy (N = 428). The treatment regimens are defined in Table 8.

[See table 8 above]

The antiemetic activity of EMEND was evaluated based on the following endpoints:

Primary endpoint:

Complete response (defined as no emetic episodes and no use of rescue therapy) in the overall phase (0 to 120 hours post-chemotherapy)

Other prespecified endpoints:

• no emesis (defined as no emetic episodes regardless of use of rescue therapy)
• no nausea (maximum VAS <5 mm on a 0 to 100 mm scale)
• no significant nausea (maximum VAS <25 mm on a 0 to 100 mm scale)
• complete protection (defined as no emetic episodes, no use of rescue therapy, and a maximum nausea visual analogue scale [VAS] score <25 mm on a 0 to 100 mm scale)
• complete response during the acute and delayed phases.

A summary of the key results from this study is shown in Table 9.

Figure 2

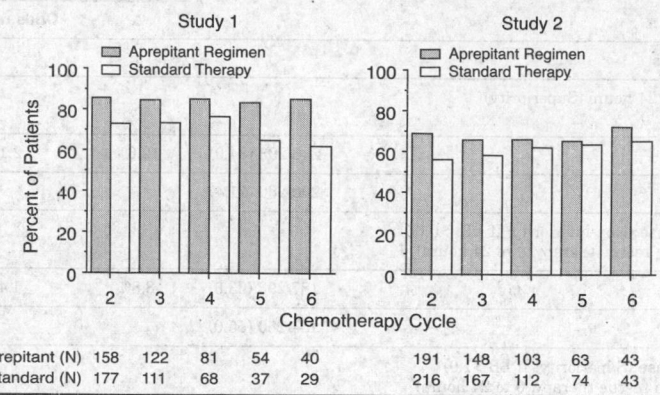

Figure 2: Proportion of Patients Receiving Highly Emetogenic Chemotherapy with No Emesis and No Significant Nausea by Treatment Group and Cycle

	2	3	4	5	6		2	3	4	5	6
Aprepitant (N)	158	122	81	54	40		191	148	103	63	43
Standard (N)	177	111	68	37	29		216	167	112	74	43

Table 8: Treatment Regimens in Moderately Emetogenic Chemotherapy Trials

Treatment Regimen	Day 1	Days 2 to 3
Aprepitant	Aprepitant 125 mg PO* Dexamethasone 12 mg PO† Ondansetron 8 mg PO × 2 doses‡	Aprepitant 80 mg PO Daily
Standard Therapy	Dexamethasone 20 mg PO Ondansetron 8 mg PO × 2 doses	Ondansetron 8 mg PO Daily (every 12 hours)

Aprepitant placebo and dexamethasone placebo were used to maintain blinding.

* 1 hour prior to chemotherapy.
† 30 minutes prior to chemotherapy.
‡ 30 to 60 minutes prior to chemotherapy and 8 hours after first ondansetron dose.

Table 9: Percent of Patients Receiving Moderately Emetogenic Chemotherapy Responding by Treatment Group and Phase—Cycle 1

ENDPOINTS	Aprepitant Regimen (N = 433)* %	Standard Therapy (N = 424)* %	p-Value
PRIMARY ENDPOINT†			
Complete Response	51	42	0.015
OTHER PRESPECIFIED ENDPOINTS†			
No Emesis	76	59	NS‡
No Nausea	33	33	NS
No Significant Nausea	61	56	NS
No Rescue Therapy	59	56	NS
Complete Protection	43	37	NS

* N: Number of patients included in the primary analysis of complete response.
† Overall: 0 to 120 hours post-chemotherapy treatment.
‡ NS when adjusted for prespecified multiple comparisons rule; unadjusted p-value <0.001.

In this study, a statistically significantly (p=0.015) higher proportion of patients receiving the aprepitant regimen

Table 11: PONV Study 1 – Response Rates for Select Efficacy Endpoints (Modified-Intention-to-Treat Population)

Treatment	n/m (%)	Aprepitant vs Ondansetron		
		Δ	Odds ratio*	Analysis
Primary Endpoints				
No Vomiting 0 to 24 hours (Superiority) (no emetic episodes)				
Aprepitant 40 mg	246/293 (84.0)	12.6%	2.1	P<0.001†
Ondansetron	200/280 (71.4)			
Complete Response (Non-inferiority: If LB‡ >0.65) (no emesis and no rescue therapy, 0 to 24 hours)				
Aprepitant 40 mg	187/293 (63.8)	8.8%	1.4	LB=1.02
Ondansetron	154/280 (55.0)			
Complete Response (Superiority: If LB >1.0) (no emesis and no rescue therapy, 0 to 24 hours)				
Aprepitant 40 mg	187/293 (63.8)	8.8%	1.4	LB=1.02§
Ondansetron	154/280 (55.0)			
Secondary Endpoint				
No Vomiting 0 to 48 (Superiority) (no emetic episodes)				
Aprepitant 40 mg	238/292 (81.5)	15.2%	2.3	P<0.001†
Ondansetron	185/279 (66.3)			

n/m = Number of responders/number of patients in analysis.
Δ Difference (%): Aprepitant 40 mg minus Ondansetron.
* Estimated odds ratio for Aprepitant versus Ondansetron. A value of >1 favors Aprepitant over Ondansetron.
† P-value of two-sided test <0.05.
‡ LB= lower bound of 1-sided 97.5% confidence interval for the odds ratio.
§ Based on the prespecified fixed sequence multiplicity strategy, Aprepitant 40 mg was not superior to Ondansetron.

(51%) in Cycle 1 had a complete response (primary endpoint) during the overall phase compared with patients receiving standard therapy (42%). The difference between treatment groups was primarily driven by the "No Emesis Endpoint", a principal component of this composite primary endpoint. In addition, a higher proportion of patients receiving the aprepitant regimen in Cycle 1 had a complete response during the acute (0-24 hours) and delayed (25-120 hours) phases compared with patients receiving standard therapy; however, the treatment group differences failed to reach statistical significance, after multiplicity adjustments.

Patient-Reported Outcomes: In a phase III study in patients receiving moderately emetogenic chemotherapy, the impact of nausea and vomiting on patients' daily lives was assessed in Cycle 1 using the FLIE. A higher proportion of patients receiving the aprepitant regimen reported minimal or no impact on daily life (64% versus 56%). This difference between treatment groups was primarily driven by the "No Vomiting Domain" of this composite endpoint.

Multiple-Cycle Extension: Patients receiving moderately emetogenic chemotherapy were permitted to continue into the Multiple-Cycle extension of the study for up to 3 additional cycles of chemotherapy. Antiemetic effect for patients receiving the aprepitant regimen is maintained during all cycles.

Postmarketing Trial: In a postmarketing, multicenter, randomized, double-blind, parallel-group, clinical study in 848 cancer patients, the aprepitant regimen (N = 430) was compared with a standard of care therapy (N = 418) in patients receiving a moderately emetogenic chemotherapy regimen that included any IV dose of oxaliplatin, carboplatin, epirubicin, idarubicin, ifosfamide, irinotecan, daunorubicin, doxorubicin; cyclophosphamide IV (<1500 mg/m²); or cytarabine IV (>1 g/m²).

Of the 430 patients who were randomized to receive the aprepitant regimen, approximately 76% were women and 24% were men. The distribution by race was 67% White, 6% Black or African American, 11% Asian, and 12% multiracial. Classified by ethnicity, 36% were Hispanic and 64% were non-Hispanic. The aprepitant-treated patients in this clinical study ranged from 22 to 85 years of age, with a mean age of 57 years; approximately 59% of the patients were 55 years or older with 32 patients being over 74 years. Patients receiving the aprepitant regimen were receiving chemotherapy for a variety of tumor types including 50% with breast cancer, 21% with gastrointestinal cancers including colorectal cancer, 13% with lung cancer and 6% with gynecological cancers.

The antiemetic activity of EMEND was evaluated based on no vomiting (with or without rescue therapy) in the overall period (0 to 120 hours post-chemotherapy) and complete response (defined as no vomiting and no use of rescue therapy) in the overall period.

A summary of the key results from this study is shown in Table 10.

Table 10: Percent of Patients Receiving Moderately Emetogenic Chemotherapy Responding by Treatment Group for Study 2—Cycle 1

ENDPOINTS	Aprepitant Regimen (N = 430)* %	Standard Therapy (N = 418)* %	p-Value
No Vomiting Overall	76	62	<0.0001
Complete Response Overall	69	56	0.0003

* N = Number of patients who received chemotherapy treatment, study drug, and had at least one post-treatment efficacy evaluation.

In this study, a statistically significantly higher proportion of patients receiving the aprepitant regimen (76%) in Cycle 1 had no vomiting during the overall phase compared with patients receiving standard therapy (62%). In addition, a higher proportion of patients receiving the aprepitant regimen (69%) in Cycle 1 had a complete response in the overall phase (0-120 hours) compared with patients receiving standard therapy (56%). In the acute phase (0 to 24 hours following initiation of chemotherapy), a higher proportion of patients receiving aprepitant compared to patients receiving standard therapy were observed to have no vomiting (92% and 84%, respectively) and complete response (89% and 80%, respectively). In the delayed phase (25 to 120 hours following initiation of chemotherapy), a higher proportion of patients receiving aprepitant compared to patients receiving standard therapy were observed to have no vomiting (78% and 67%, respectively) and complete response (71% and 61%, respectively).

In a subgroup analysis by tumor type, a numerically higher proportion of patients receiving aprepitant were observed to have no vomiting and complete response compared to patients receiving standard therapy. For gender, the difference in complete response rates between the aprepitant and

standard regimen groups was 14% in females (64.5% and 50.3%, respectively) and 4% in males (82.2% and 78.2%, respectively) during the overall phase. A similar difference for gender was observed for the no vomiting endpoint.

14.2 Prevention of Postoperative Nausea and Vomiting (PONV)

In two multicenter, randomized, double-blind, active comparator-controlled, parallel-group clinical studies (PONV Studies 1 and 2), aprepitant was compared with ondansetron for the prevention of postoperative nausea and vomiting in 1658 patients undergoing open abdominal surgery. Patients were randomized to receive 40 mg aprepitant, 125 mg aprepitant, or 4 mg ondansetron. Aprepitant was given orally with 50 mL of water 1 to 3 hours before anesthesia. Ondansetron was given intravenously immediately before induction of anesthesia. A comparison between the 125 mg dose and the 40 mg dose did not demonstrate any additional clinical benefit. The remainder of this section will focus on the results in the 40 mg aprepitant dose recommended for PONV.

Of the 564 patients who received 40 mg aprepitant, 92% were women and 8% were men; of these, 58% were White, 13% Hispanic American, 7% Multi-Racial, 14% Black, 6% Asian, and 2% Other. The age of patients treated with 40 mg aprepitant ranged from 19 to 84 years, with a mean age of 46.1 years. 46 patients were 65 years or older, with 13 patients being 75 years or older.

The antiemetic activity of EMEND was evaluated during the 0 to 48 hour period following the end of surgery. The two pivotal studies were of similar design; however, they differed in terms of study hypothesis, efficacy analyses and geographic location. PONV Study 1 was a multinational study including the U.S., whereas, PONV Study 2 was conducted entirely in the U.S.

Efficacy measures in PONV Study 1 included:
• no emesis (defined as no emetic episodes regardless of use of rescue therapy) in the 0 to 24 hours following the end of surgery (primary)
• complete response (defined as no emetic episodes and no use of rescue therapy) in the 0 to 24 hours following the end of surgery (primary)
• no emesis (defined as no emetic episodes regardless of use of rescue therapy) in the 0 to 48 hours following the end of surgery (secondary)
• time to first use of rescue medication in the 0 to 24 hours following the end of surgery (exploratory)
• time to first emesis in the 0 to 48 hours following the end of surgery (exploratory).

A closed testing procedure was applied to control the type I error for the primary endpoints.

The results of the primary and secondary endpoints for 40 mg aprepitant and 4 mg ondansetron are described in Table 11:

[See table 11 above]

The use of aprepitant did not affect the time to first use of rescue medication when compared to ondansetron. However, compared to the ondansetron group, use of aprepitant delayed the time to first vomiting, as depicted in Figure 3.

Figure 3: Percent of Patients Who Remain Emesis Free During the 48 Hours Following End of Surgery

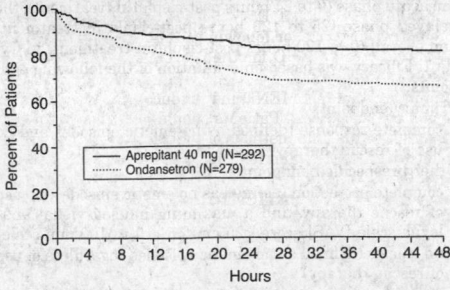

Efficacy measures in PONV Study 2 included:
• complete response (defined as no emetic episodes and no use of rescue therapy) in the 0 to 24 hours following the end of surgery (primary)
• no emesis (defined as no emetic episodes regardless of use of rescue therapy) in the 0 to 24 hours following the end of surgery (secondary)
• no use of rescue therapy in the 0 to 24 hours following the end of surgery (secondary)
• no emesis (defined as no emetic episodes regardless of use of rescue therapy) in the 0 to 48 hours following the end of surgery (secondary).

PONV Study 2 failed to satisfy its primary hypothesis that aprepitant is superior to ondansetron in the prevention of PONV as measured by the proportion of patients with complete response in the 24 hours following end of surgery. The study demonstrated that both dose levels of aprepitant had a clinically meaningful effect with respect to the

secondary endpoint "no vomiting" during the first 24 hours after surgery and showed that the use of 40 mg aprepitant was associated with a 16% improvement over ondansetron for the no vomiting endpoint.
[See table 12 at right]

16 HOW SUPPLIED/STORAGE AND HANDLING

No. 3854—80 mg capsules: White, opaque, hard gelatin capsule with "461" and "80 mg" printed radially in black ink on the body. They are supplied as follows:
NDC 0006-0461-02 unit-of-use BiPack of 2
NDC 0006-0461-06 unit-dose package of 6.
No. 3855—125 mg capsules: Opaque, hard gelatin capsule with white body and pink cap with "462" and "125 mg" printed radially in black ink on the body. They are supplied as follows:
NDC 0006-0462-06 unit-dose package of 6.
No. 3862—Unit-of-use TriPack containing one 125 mg capsule and two 80 mg capsules.
NDC 0006-3862-03.
No. 6741—40 mg capsules: Opaque, hard gelatin capsule with white body and mustard yellow cap with "464" and "40 mg" printed radially in black ink on the body. They are supplied as follows:
NDC 0006-0464-10 unit-of-use package of 1
NDC 0006-0464-05 unit-dose package of 5.
Storage
Store at 20-25°C (68-77°F) [see USP Controlled Room Temperature].

Merck Sharp & Dohme Corp., a subsidiary of
MERCK & CO., INC., Whitehouse Station, NJ 08889, USA
9985512
U.S. Patent Nos.: 5,145,684; 5,719,147; 6,048,859; 6,096,742; 6,235,735

17 PATIENT COUNSELING INFORMATION

[See FDA-Approved Patient Labeling.]
17.1 Instructions
Physicians should instruct their patients to read the patient package insert before starting therapy with EMEND and to reread it each time the prescription is renewed.
Patients should be instructed to take EMEND only as prescribed. For the prevention of chemotherapy induced nausea and vomiting (CINV), patients should be advised to take their first dose (125 mg) of EMEND 1 hour prior to chemotherapy treatment. For the prevention of postoperative nausea and vomiting (PONV), patients should receive their medication (40 mg capsule of EMEND) within 3 hours prior to induction of anesthesia.
Allergic reactions, which may be serious, and may include hives, rash and itching and cause difficulty in breathing or swallowing, have been reported in general use with EMEND. Physicians should instruct their patients to stop taking EMEND and call their doctor right away if they experience an allergic reaction.
EMEND may interact with some drugs including chemotherapy; therefore, patients should be advised to report to their doctor the use of any other prescription, nonprescription medication or herbal products.
Patients on chronic warfarin therapy should be instructed to have their clotting status closely monitored in the 2-week period, particularly at 7 to 10 days, following initiation of the 3-day regimen of EMEND 125 mg/80 mg with each chemotherapy cycle, or following administration of a single 40 mg dose of EMEND for the prevention of postoperative nausea and vomiting.
Administration of EMEND may reduce the efficacy of hormonal contraceptives. Patients should be advised to use alternative or back-up methods of contraception during treatment with EMEND and for 1 month following the last dose of EMEND.

FDA-APPROVED PATIENT LABELING
Patient Information
EMEND® (EE mend)
(aprepitant)
Capsules
Read the Patient Information that comes with EMEND before you start taking it and each time you refill your prescription. There may be new information. This leaflet does not take the place of talking with your doctor about your medical condition or treatment.
What is EMEND?
EMEND is a prescription medicine used in adults to prevent nausea and vomiting:
• caused by certain anti-cancer (chemotherapy) medicines. When used for this purpose, EMEND is always used with other medicines.
• after surgery.
EMEND is not used to treat nausea and vomiting that you already have.
EMEND should not be used continuously for a long time (chronic use).
It is not known if EMEND is safe and effective in children.

Table 12: PONV Study 2 (Modified-Intention-to-Treat Population)

Treatment	n/m (%)	Aprepitant vs Ondansetron		
		Δ	Odds ratio*	p-Value
Primary Endpoints				
Complete Response (no emesis and no rescue therapy, 0 to 24 hours)				
Aprepitant 40 mg	111/248 (44.8)	2.5%	1.1	0.61
Ondansetron	104/246 (42.3)			
Secondary Endpoints				
No Vomiting (no emetic episodes, 0 to 24 hours)				
Aprepitant 40 mg	223/248 (89.9)	16.3%	3.2	<0.001†
Ondansetron	1814/246 (73.6)			
No Use of Rescue Medication (for established emesis or nausea, 0 to 24 hours)				
Aprepitant 40 mg	112/248 (45.2)	-0.7%	1.0	0.83
Ondansetron	113/246 (45.9)			
No Vomiting 0 to 48 (Superiority) (no emetic episodes, 0 to 48 hours)				
Aprepitant 40 mg	209/247 (84.6)	17.7%	2.7	<0.001†
Ondansetron	164/245 (66.9)			

n/m = Number of responders/number of patients in analysis.
Δ Difference (%): Aprepitant 40 mg minus Ondansetron.
* Estimated odds ratio: Aprepitant 40 mg versus Ondansetron.
† Not statistically significant after pre-specified multiplicity adjustment.

Who should not take EMEND?
Do not take EMEND if you:
• are taking any of the following medicines:
  • ORAP® (pimozide)
  • SELDANE® (terfenadine)
  • HISMANAL® (astemizole)
  • PROPULSID® (cisapride)
Taking EMEND with any of these medicines could cause serious or life-threatening problems.
• are allergic to any of the ingredients in EMEND. See the end of this leaflet for a list of all the ingredients in EMEND.
What should I tell my doctor before and during treatment with EMEND?
Before you take EMEND, tell your doctor if you:
• have liver problems
• are pregnant or plan to become pregnant. It is not known if EMEND can harm your unborn baby.
  Women who use birth control medicines containing hormones to prevent pregnancy (birth control pills, skin patches, implants, and certain IUDs) should also use a back-up method of birth control during treatment with EMEND and for up to 1 month after using EMEND to prevent pregnancy.
• are breast-feeding. It is not known if EMEND passes into your milk and if it can harm your baby.
Tell your doctor about all the medicines you are taking or plan to take, including prescription and non-prescription medicines, vitamins, and herbal supplements.
EMEND may cause serious life-threatening reactions if used with certain medicines. See the section "Who should not take EMEND?"
EMEND may affect how other medicines work, and other medicines may affect how EMEND works. Ask your doctor or pharmacist before you take any new medicine. They can tell you if it is safe to take the medicine with EMEND.
Know the medicines you take. Keep a list of them to show your doctor or pharmacist when you get a new medicine.
How should I take EMEND?
• Take EMEND exactly as prescribed.
• If you take too much EMEND, call your doctor, local emergency department or poison control center right away.
• If you are receiving cancer chemotherapy, EMEND is taken as 3 doses over 3 days - starting on the day you have chemotherapy, and the two days after chemotherapy. There are two ways that your doctor may prescribe EMEND for you:
1. Capsules of EMEND by mouth for all 3 doses:
  • You should get a package that has three capsules of EMEND.

• Day 1 (Day of chemotherapy): Take one 125-mg capsule of EMEND (white and pink) by mouth 1 hour before you start your chemotherapy treatment;
• Day 2 and Day 3 (the two days after chemotherapy): Take one 80-mg capsule of EMEND (white) by mouth, each morning for the 2 days after your chemotherapy treatment.
Or
2. Intravenous (IV) injection into a vein the first day, then capsules by mouth on the two days after chemotherapy:
  • Day 1 (Day of chemotherapy): EMEND will be given to you by intravenous (IV) injection in your vein 30 minutes before you start your chemotherapy treatment.
  • You should get a package that has two capsules of EMEND.
  • Day 2 and Day 3 (the two days after chemotherapy): Take one 80-mg capsule of EMEND (white) by mouth, each morning for the 2 days after your chemotherapy treatment.
• If you are receiving chemotherapy, EMEND may be taken with or without food.
• If you are having surgery:
  • Your doctor will prescribe a 40-mg capsule of EMEND for you before surgery. You take EMEND within three hours before surgery.
  • Follow your doctor's instructions about restrictions on eating and drinking before surgery.
• If you take the blood thinner medicine warfarin sodium (COUMADIN®, JANTOVEN®), your doctor may do blood tests after you take EMEND to check your blood clotting.
What are the possible side effects of EMEND?
EMEND may cause serious side effects, including:
• **Serious allergic reactions.** Allergic reactions can happen with EMEND and may be serious. Stop taking EMEND and call your doctor right away if you have any of these signs or symptoms of an allergic reaction:
  • hives
  • rash
  • itching
  • trouble breathing or swallowing.
In people taking EMEND to prevent nausea and vomiting caused by chemotherapy, the most common side effects of EMEND include:
• tiredness
• nausea
• hiccups
• constipation
• diarrhea
• loss of appetite

- headache
- hair loss

In people taking EMEND to prevent nausea and vomiting after surgery, the most common side effects are:
- constipation
- nausea
- itch
- fever
- low blood pressure
- headache

Tell your doctor if you have any side effect that bothers you or that does not go away. These are not all of the possible side effects of EMEND. For more information ask your doctor or pharmacist.

Call your doctor for medical advice about side effects. You may report side effects to FDA at 1-800-FDA-1088.

How should I store EMEND?
- Store EMEND at room temperature, between 68°F and 77°F (20°C and 25°C).
- **Keep EMEND and all medicines out of the reach of children.**

General information about EMEND

Medicines are sometimes prescribed for conditions that are not mentioned in patient information leaflets. Do not use EMEND for a condition for which it was not prescribed. Do not give EMEND to other people, even if they have the same symptoms you have. It may harm them.

This Patient Information leaflet summarizes the most important information about EMEND. If you would like to know more information, talk with your doctor. You can ask your doctor or pharmacist for information about EMEND that is written for health professionals. For more information about EMEND call 1-800-622-4477 or go to www.emend.com.

What are the ingredients in EMEND?

Active ingredient: aprepitant

Inactive ingredients: sucrose, microcrystalline cellulose, hydroxypropyl cellulose and sodium lauryl sulfate. The capsule shell excipients are gelatin, titanium dioxide, and may contain sodium lauryl sulfate and silicon dioxide. The 125-mg capsule shell also contains red ferric oxide and yellow ferric oxide. The 40-mg capsule shell also contains yellow ferric oxide.

U.S. Patent Nos.: 5,145,684; 5,719,147; 6,048,859; 6,096,742; 6,235,735

The brands listed in the above sections "Who should not take EMEND?" and "What should I tell my doctor before and during treatment with EMEND?" are the registered trademarks of their respective owners and are not trademarks of Merck Sharp & Dohme Corp., a subsidiary of Merck & Co., Inc.

EMEND® is a registered trademark of Merck Sharp & Dohme Corp., a subsidiary of **Merck & Co., Inc.**

Copyright © 2003, 2005, 2006 Merck Sharp & Dohme Corp., a subsidiary of **Merck & Co., Inc.**

All rights reserved
Issued March 2010
Merck Sharp & Dohme Corp., a subsidiary of Merck & Co., Inc.
Whitehouse Station, NJ 08889, USA
9985410

Shown in Product Identification Guide, page 312

EMEND   ℞
[ē′mĕnd]
**(fosaprepitant dimeglumine)
For Injection**

HIGHLIGHTS OF PRESCRIBING INFORMATION
These highlights do not include all the information needed to use EMEND for Injection safely and effectively. See full prescribing information for EMEND for Injection.
EMEND (fosaprepitant dimeglumine) for Injection
Initial U.S. Approval: 2008
————INDICATIONS AND USAGE————
EMEND for Injection, in combination with other antiemetic agents, is indicated for the:
- prevention of acute and delayed nausea and vomiting associated with initial and repeat courses of highly emetogenic cancer chemotherapy (HEC) including high-dose cisplatin (1)
- prevention of nausea and vomiting associated with initial and repeat courses of moderately emetogenic cancer chemotherapy (MEC) (1)
Limitations of Use (1.1)
- Not studied for the treatment of established nausea and vomiting.
- Chronic continuous administration is not recommended.
————DOSAGE AND ADMINISTRATION————
- EMEND for Injection (115 mg) may be substituted for oral EMEND (125 mg) on Day 1 only as part of the chemotherapy induced nausea and vomiting (CINV) regimen that includes a corticosteroid and a 5-HT₃ antagonist. (2.1)

- The 3-day CINV regimen includes EMEND for Injection (115 mg) given 30 minutes prior to chemotherapy as an infusion administered over 15 minutes or EMEND (125 mg orally) on Day 1; EMEND (80 mg orally) on Days 2 and 3. (2.1)
————DOSAGE FORMS AND STRENGTHS————
One single dose per 10 mL glass vial supplied as sterile lyophilized powder for intravenous use only after reconstitution and dilution: 115 mg (3)
————CONTRAINDICATIONS————
- Hypersensitivity to any component of this medication. (4, 6.2)
- Fosaprepitant should not be used concurrently with pimozide, terfenadine, astemizole, or cisapride, since inhibition of CYP3A4 by aprepitant could result in elevated plasma concentrations of these drugs, potentially causing serious or life-threatening reactions. (4)
————WARNINGS AND PRECAUTIONS————
- Immediate hypersensitivity reactions may occur during infusion. Patients have generally responded to discontinuation. It is not recommended to reinitiate the infusion. (5.2, 6.2)
- Coadministration of aprepitant with warfarin (a CYP2C9 substrate) may result in a clinically significant decrease in International Normalized Ratio (INR) of prothrombin time. (5.3)
- The efficacy of hormonal contraceptives during and for 28 days following the last dose of fosaprepitant or aprepitant may be reduced. Alternative or back-up methods of contraception should be used. (5.4, 7.1)
- Fosaprepitant, when administered as a 3-day antiemetic regimen for CINV is a moderate inhibitor of CYP3A4, and should be used with caution in patients receiving concomitant medications that are primarily metabolized through CYP3A4. (5.1)
- Caution should be exercised when administered in patients with severe hepatic impairment. (2.5, 5.5, 12.3)
————ADVERSE REACTIONS————
- Clinical adverse experiences for the CINV regimen in conjunction with highly and moderately emetogenic chemotherapy (incidence >10%) are: alopecia, anorexia, asthenia/fatigue, constipation, diarrhea, headache, hiccups, nausea. (6.1)
- Clinical adverse experiences reported for EMEND for Injection (incidence >1%) are: infusion site pain, infusion site induration, headache. (6.1)

To report SUSPECTED ADVERSE REACTIONS, contact Merck Sharp & Dohme Corp., a subsidiary of Merck & Co., Inc., at 1-877-888-4231 or FDA at 1-800-FDA-1088 or www.fda.gov/medwatch.
————DRUG INTERACTIONS————
- Drug interactions following administration of fosaprepitant are likely to occur with drugs that interact with oral aprepitant.
- Aprepitant is a substrate for CYP3A4; therefore, coadministration of fosaprepitant or aprepitant with drugs that inhibit or induce CYP3A4 activity may result in increased or reduced plasma concentrations of aprepitant, respectively. (5.1, 7.1, 7.2)
- Aprepitant is an inducer of CYP2C9; therefore, coadministration of EMEND for Injection with drugs that are metabolized by CYP2C9 (e.g. warfarin, tolbutamide), may result in lower plasma concentrations of these drugs. (5.3, 7.1)

See 17 for PATIENT COUNSELING INFORMATION and FDA-approved patient labeling.

Revised: 03/2010

FULL PRESCRIBING INFORMATION: CONTENTS *

* Sections or subsections omitted from the full prescribing information are not listed.

FULL PRESCRIBING INFORMATION

1   INDICATIONS AND USAGE

EMEND for Injection[1] is a substance P/neurokinin-1 (NK₁) receptor antagonist indicated for use in combination with other antiemetic agents for the:
- prevention of acute and delayed nausea and vomiting associated with initial and repeat courses of highly emetogenic cancer chemotherapy (HEC) including high-dose cisplatin.
- prevention of nausea and vomiting associated with initial and repeat courses of moderately emetogenic cancer chemotherapy (MEC) *[see Dosage and Administration (2.1)]*.

[1] Registered trademark of Merck Sharp & Dohme Corp., a subsidiary of **Merck & Co., Inc.**
Copyright © 2008 Merck Sharp & Dohme Corp., a subsidiary of **Merck & Co., Inc.**
All Rights Reserved

1.1   Limitations of Use
EMEND for Injection has not been studied for the treatment of established nausea and vomiting.
Chronic continuous administration is not recommended *[see Warnings and Precautions (5.2)]*.

2   DOSAGE AND ADMINISTRATION
2.1   Prevention of Chemotherapy Induced Nausea and Vomiting (CINV)
EMEND for Injection is a sterile prodrug of aprepitant to be administered intravenously as an infusion. Aprepitant is available as capsules (EMEND[2]) for oral administration.
EMEND for Injection (115 mg) may be substituted for EMEND (125 mg) 30 minutes prior to chemotherapy, on Day 1 only of the CINV regimen as an infusion administered over 15 minutes.
EMEND for Injection should not be mixed or reconstituted with solutions for which physical and chemical compatibility have not been established. EMEND for Injection is incompatible with any solutions containing divalent cations (e.g., Ca²⁺, Mg²⁺), including Lactated Ringer's Solution and Hartmann's Solution.
EMEND for Injection may be administered with or without food.
The 3-day CINV regimen includes EMEND for Injection (115 mg) or EMEND (125 mg orally) on Day 1; EMEND (80 mg orally) on Days 2 and 3; in addition to a corticosteroid and a 5-HT₃ antagonist as specified in the tables below. In clinical studies with EMEND, the following regimen was used for the prevention of nausea and vomiting associated with highly emetogenic cancer chemotherapy:
[See first table at top of next page]
In a clinical study with EMEND, the following regimen was used for the prevention of nausea and vomiting associated with moderately emetogenic cancer chemotherapy:
[See second table on next page]

[2] Registered trademark of Merck Sharp & Dohme Corp., a subsidiary of **Merck & Co., Inc.**

2.2   Preparation of EMEND for Injection
1. Aseptically inject 5 mL 0.9% Sodium Chloride for Injection (saline) into the vial. Assure that saline is added to the vial along the vial wall in order to prevent foaming. Swirl the vial gently. Avoid shaking and jetting saline into the vial.
2. Aseptically prepare an infusion bag filled with 110 mL of saline.

3. Aseptically withdraw the entire volume from the vial and transfer it into the infusion bag containing 110 mL of saline to yield a total volume of 115 mL and a final concentration of 1 mg/1 mL.

4. Gently invert the bag 2-3 times.

The reconstituted final drug solution is stable for 24 hours at ambient room temperature (at or below 25°C).

Parenteral drug products should be inspected visually for particulate matter and discoloration before administration whenever solution and container permit.

Caution: EMEND for Injection should not be mixed or reconstituted with solutions for which physical and chemical compatibility have not been established. EMEND for Injection is incompatible with any solutions containing divalent cations (e.g., Ca^{2+}, Mg^{2+}), including Lactated Ringer's Solution and Hartmann's Solution.

2.3 Geriatric Patients
No dosage adjustment is necessary for the elderly.

2.4 Patients with Renal Impairment
No dosage adjustment is necessary for patients with renal impairment or for patients with end stage renal disease (ESRD) undergoing hemodialysis.

2.5 Patients with Hepatic Impairment
No dosage adjustment is necessary for patients with mild to moderate hepatic impairment (Child-Pugh score 5 to 9). There are no clinical data in patients with severe hepatic impairment (Child-Pugh score >9).

2.6 Coadministration with Other Drugs
For additional information on dose adjustment for corticosteroids when coadministered with EMEND for Injection, *[see Drug Interactions (7.1)]*.

Refer to the full prescribing information for coadministered antiemetic agents.

3 DOSAGE FORMS AND STRENGTHS

One 115 mg single dose per 10 mL glass vial: White to off-white lyophilized solid (Sterile lyophilized powder for intravenous use only after reconstitution and dilution).

4 CONTRAINDICATIONS

EMEND for Injection is contraindicated in patients who are hypersensitive to EMEND for Injection, aprepitant, polysorbate 80 or any other components of the product.

Aprepitant, when administered orally, is a moderate cytochrome P450 isoenzyme 3A4 (CYP3A4) inhibitor following the 3-day antiemetic dosing regimen for CINV. Since fosaprepitant is rapidly converted to aprepitant, fosaprepitant should not be used concurrently with pimozide, terfenadine, astemizole, or cisapride. Inhibition of CYP3A4 by aprepitant could result in elevated plasma concentrations of these drugs, potentially causing serious or life-threatening reactions *[see Drug Interactions (7.1)]*.

5 WARNINGS AND PRECAUTIONS

5.1 CYP3A4 Interactions
Fosaprepitant is rapidly converted to aprepitant, which is a moderate inhibitor of CYP3A4 when administered as a 3-day antiemetic dosing regimen for CINV. Fosaprepitant should be used with caution in patients receiving concomitant medications that are primarily metabolized through CYP3A4. Inhibition of CYP3A4 by aprepitant could result in elevated plasma concentrations of these concomitant medications. When fosaprepitant is used concomitantly with another CYP3A4 inhibitor, aprepitant plasma concentrations could be elevated. When aprepitant is used concomitantly with medications that induce CYP3A4 activity, aprepitant plasma concentrations could be reduced, and this may result in decreased efficacy of aprepitant *[see Drug Interactions (7.1)]*.

Chemotherapy agents that are known to be metabolized by CYP3A4 include docetaxel, paclitaxel, etoposide, irinotecan, ifosfamide, imatinib, vinorelbine, vinblastine and vincristine. In clinical studies, the oral aprepitant regimen was administered commonly with etoposide, vinorelbine, or paclitaxel. The doses of these agents were not adjusted to account for potential drug interactions.

In separate pharmacokinetic studies no clinically significant change in docetaxel or vinorelbine pharmacokinetics was observed when the oral aprepitant regimen was coadministered.

Due to the small number of patients in clinical studies who received the CYP3A4 substrates vinblastine, vincristine, or ifosfamide, particular caution and careful monitoring are advised in patients receiving these agents or other chemotherapy agents metabolized primarily by CYP3A4 that were not studied *[see Drug Interactions (7.1)]*.

5.2 Hypersensitivity Reactions
Isolated reports of immediate hypersensitivity reactions including flushing, erythema, and dyspnea have occurred during infusion of fosaprepitant. These hypersensitivity reactions have generally responded to discontinuation of the infusion and administration of appropriate therapy. It is not recommended to reinitiate the infusion in patients who experience hypersensitivity reactions.

	Day 1	Day 2	Day 3	Day 4
EMEND*	125 mg orally	80 mg orally	80 mg orally	none
Dexamethasone†	12 mg orally	8 mg orally	8 mg orally	8 mg orally
Ondansetron‡	32 mg I.V.	none	none	none

* EMEND was administered orally 1 hour prior to chemotherapy treatment on Day 1 and in the morning on Days 2 and 3.
† Dexamethasone was administered 30 minutes prior to chemotherapy treatment on Day 1 and in the morning on Days 2 through 4. The dose of dexamethasone was chosen to account for drug interactions.
‡ Ondansetron was administered 30 minutes prior to chemotherapy treatment on Day 1.

	Day 1	Day 2	Day 3
EMEND*	125 mg orally	80 mg orally	80 mg orally
Dexamethasone†	12 mg orally	none	none
Ondansetron‡	2 × 8 mg orally	none	none

* EMEND was administered orally 1 hour prior to chemotherapy treatment on Day 1 and in the morning on Days 2 and 3.
† Dexamethasone was administered 30 minutes prior to chemotherapy treatment on Day 1. The dose of dexamethasone was chosen to account for drug interactions.
‡ Ondansetron 8-mg capsule was administered 30 to 60 minutes prior to chemotherapy treatment and one 8-mg capsule was administered 8 hours after the first dose on Day 1.

5.3 Coadministration with Warfarin (a CYP2C9 substrate)
Coadministration of aprepitant with warfarin may result in a clinically significant decrease in International Normalized Ratio (INR) of prothrombin time. In patients on chronic warfarin therapy, the INR should be closely monitored in the 2-week period, particularly at 7 to 10 days, following initiation of the 3-day regimen of fosaprepitant followed by oral aprepitant with each chemotherapy cycle *[see Drug Interactions (7.1)]*.

5.4 Coadministration with Hormonal Contraceptives
Upon coadministration with aprepitant, the efficacy of hormonal contraceptives during and for 28 days following the last dose of aprepitant may be reduced. Alternative or back-up methods of contraception should be used during treatment with aprepitant and for 1 month following the last dose of aprepitant *[see Drug Interactions (7.1)]*.

5.5 Patients with Severe Hepatic Impairment
There are no clinical or pharmacokinetic data in patients with severe hepatic impairment (Child-Pugh score >9). Therefore, caution should be exercised when fosaprepitant or aprepitant is administered in these patients *[see Clinical Pharmacology (12.3) and Dosage and Administration (2.5)]*.

5.6 Chronic Continuous Use
Chronic continuous use of EMEND for Injection for prevention of nausea and vomiting is not recommended because it has not been studied; and because the drug interaction profile may change during chronic continuous use.

6 ADVERSE REACTIONS
The overall safety of aprepitant was evaluated in approximately 4900 individuals.

Since EMEND for Injection is converted to aprepitant, those adverse experiences associated with aprepitant might also be expected to occur with EMEND for Injection.

Because clinical trials are conducted under widely varying conditions, adverse reaction rates observed in the clinical trials of a drug cannot be directly compared to rates in the clinical trials of another drug and may not reflect the rates observed in clinical practice.

6.1 Clinical Trials Experience
Fosaprepitant (intravenous formulation)
In a randomized, open-label, incomplete crossover, bioequivalence study, 66 subjects were dosed with 115 mg of EMEND for Injection intravenously and 72 subjects received 125 mg of aprepitant orally. Systemic exposure of 115 mg of intravenous EMEND for Injection is equivalent to 125 mg oral aprepitant. The following clinical adverse experiences, regardless of causality, were reported in subjects dosed with EMEND for Injection: infusion site pain, 5 (7.6%); infusion site induration, 1 (1.5%); headache, 2 (3%).
Oral Aprepitant
Highly Emetogenic Chemotherapy
In 2 well-controlled clinical trials in patients receiving highly emetogenic cancer chemotherapy, 544 patients were treated with aprepitant during Cycle 1 of chemotherapy and 413 of these patients continued into the Multiple-Cycle extension for up to 6 cycles of chemotherapy. Oral aprepitant was given in combination with ondansetron and dexamethasone.
In Cycle 1, clinical adverse experiences were reported in approximately 69% of patients treated with the aprepitant regimen compared with approximately 68% of patients

treated with standard therapy. Table 1 shows the percent of patients with clinical adverse experiences reported at an incidence ≥3%.

Table 1: Percent of Patients Receiving Highly Emetogenic Chemotherapy with Clinical Adverse Experiences (Incidence ≥3%)—Cycle 1

	Aprepitant Regimen (N=544)	Standard Therapy (N=550)
Body as a Whole/Site Unspecified		
Asthenia/Fatigue	17.8	11.8
Dizziness	6.6	4.4
Dehydration	5.9	5.1
Abdominal Pain	4.6	3.3
Fever	2.9	3.5
Mucous Membrane Disorder	2.6	3.1
Digestive System		
Nausea	12.7	11.8
Constipation	10.3	12.2
Diarrhea	10.3	7.5
Vomiting	7.5	7.6
Heartburn	5.3	4.9
Gastritis	4.2	3.1
Epigastric Discomfort	4.0	3.1
Eyes, Ears, Nose, and Throat		
Tinnitus	3.7	3.8
Hemic and Lymphatic System		
Neutropenia	3.1	2.9
Metabolism and Nutrition		
Anorexia	10.1	9.5
Nervous System		
Headache	8.5	8.7
Insomnia	2.9	3.1
Respiratory System		
Hiccups	10.8	5.6

In addition, isolated cases of serious adverse experiences, regardless of causality, of bradycardia, disorientation, and perforating duodenal ulcer were reported in highly emetogenic CINV clinical studies.

Moderately Emetogenic Chemotherapy
During Cycle 1 of a moderately emetogenic chemotherapy study, 438 patients were treated with the aprepitant regimen and 385 of these patients continued into the Multiple-Cycle extension for up to 4 cycles of chemotherapy. In Cycle 1, clinical adverse experiences were reported in approximately 73% of patients treated with the aprepitant regimen compared with approximately 75% of patients treated with standard therapy. Table 2 shows the percent of patients with clinical adverse experiences reported at an incidence ≥3%.

Table 2: Percent of Patients Receiving Moderately Emetogenic Chemotherapy with Clinical Adverse Experiences (Incidence ≥3%)—Cycle 1

	Aprepitant Regimen (N=438)	Standard Therapy (N=428)
Blood and Lymphatic System Disorders		
Neutropenia	8.9	8.4
Metabolism and Nutrition Disorders		
Anorexia	4.3	5.8
Psychiatric Disorders		
Insomnia	4.1	5.6
Nervous System Disorders		
Headache	16.4	16.4
Dizziness	3.4	4.2
Vascular Disorders		
Hot Flush	3.0	1.4
Respiratory, Thoracic and Mediastinal Disorders		
Pharyngolaryngeal pain	3.0	2.3
Gastrointestinal Disorders		
Constipation	12.3	18.0
Dyspepsia	8.4	4.9
Nausea	7.1	7.5
Diarrhea	5.5	6.3
Stomatitis	5.3	4.4
Skin and Subcutaneous Tissue Disorders		
Alopecia	24.0	22.2
General Disorders and General Administration Site Conditions		
Fatigue	21.9	21.5
Asthenia	3.4	3.7
Mucosal inflammation	2.5	3.5

Isolated cases of serious adverse experiences, regardless of causality, of dehydration, enterocolitis, febrile neutropenia, hypertension, hypoesthesia, neutropenic sepsis, pneumonia, and sinus tachycardia were reported in the moderately emetogenic CINV clinical study.

Highly and Moderately Emetogenic Chemotherapy

The following additional clinical adverse experiences (incidence >0.5% and greater than standard therapy), regardless of causality, were reported in patients treated with aprepitant regimen:

Infections and infestations: candidiasis, herpes simplex, lower respiratory infection, pharyngitis, septic shock, upper respiratory infection, urinary tract infection.

Neoplasms benign, malignant and unspecified (including cysts and polyps): malignant neoplasm, non-small cell lung carcinoma.

Blood and lymphatic system disorders: anemia, febrile neutropenia, thrombocytopenia.

Metabolism and nutrition disorders: appetite decreased, diabetes mellitus, hypokalemia.

Psychiatric disorders: anxiety disorder, confusion, depression.

Nervous system: peripheral neuropathy, sensory neuropathy, taste disturbance, tremor.

Eye disorders: conjunctivitis.

Cardiac disorders: myocardial infarction, palpitations, tachycardia.

Vascular disorders: deep venous thrombosis, flushing, hypertension, hypotension.

Respiratory, thoracic and mediastinal disorders: cough, dyspnea, nasal secretion, pneumonitis, pulmonary embolism, respiratory insufficiency, vocal disturbance.

Gastrointestinal disorders: acid reflux, deglutition disorder, dry mouth, dysgeusia, dysphagia, eructation, flatulence, obstipation, salivation increased.

Skin and subcutaneous tissue disorders: acne, diaphoresis, rash.

Musculoskeletal and connective tissue disorders: arthralgia, back pain, muscular weakness, musculoskeletal pain, myalgia.

Renal and urinary disorders: dysuria, renal insufficiency.

Reproductive system and breast disorders: pelvic pain.

General disorders and administrative site conditions: edema, malaise, rigors.

Investigations: weight loss.

Laboratory Adverse Experiences

Table 3 shows the percent of patients with laboratory adverse experiences reported at an incidence ≥3% in patients receiving highly emetogenic chemotherapy.

Table 3: Percent of Patients Receiving Highly Emetogenic Chemotherapy with Laboratory Adverse Experiences (Incidence ≥3%)—Cycle 1

	Aprepitant Regimen (N=544)	Standard Therapy (N=550)
Proteinuria	6.8	5.3
ALT Increased	6.0	4.3
Blood Urea Nitrogen Increased	4.7	3.5
Serum Creatinine Increased	3.7	4.3
AST Increased	3.0	1.3

The following additional laboratory adverse experiences (incidence >0.5% and greater than standard therapy), regardless of causality, were reported in patients treated with aprepitant regimen: alkaline phosphatase increased, hyperglycemia, hyponatremia, leukocytes increased, erythrocyturia, leukocyturia.

The following laboratory adverse experiences were reported at an incidence ≥3% during Cycle 1 of the moderately emetogenic chemotherapy study in patients treated with the aprepitant regimen or standard therapy, respectively: decreased hemoglobin (2.3%, 4.7%) and decreased white blood cell count (9.3%, 9.0%).

The adverse experience profiles in the Multiple-Cycle extensions for up to 6 cycles of chemotherapy were similar to that observed in Cycle 1.

Stevens-Johnson syndrome was reported as a serious adverse experience in a patient receiving aprepitant with cancer chemotherapy in another CINV study.

Other Studies with Postoperative Nausea and Vomiting

In well-controlled clinical studies in patients receiving general anesthesia, 564 patients were administered 40 mg aprepitant orally and 538 patients were administered 4 mg ondansetron I.V. Clinical adverse experiences were reported in approximately 60% of patients treated with 40 mg aprepitant compared with approximately 64% of patients treated with 4 mg ondansetron I.V.

Additional adverse experiences were observed in patients receiving general anesthesia. In the patients treated with aprepitant (40 mg) for postoperative nausea and vomiting, the following additional adverse experiences were reported, regardless of causality, at an incidence ≥3%: anemia, bradycardia, flatulence, hypotension, pruritus, pyrexia.

The following adverse experiences were reported, regardless of causality, in patients treated with aprepitant for postoperative nausea and vomiting at an incidence of >0.5% and greater than with ondansetron: abdominal pain, abdominal pain upper, blood pressure decreased, dizziness, dyspepsia, hematoma, hypoesthesia, hypothermia, hypovolemia, hypoxia, operative hemorrhage, pain, postoperative infection, respiratory depression, syncope, urticaria, wound dehiscence.

Other adverse experiences (incidence ≤0.5%) reported, regardless of causality, in patients treated with aprepitant 40 mg for postoperative nausea and vomiting included: bowel sounds abnormal, dysarthria, miosis, sensory disturbance, stomach discomfort, visual acuity reduced, wheezing.

Laboratory Adverse Experiences with Postoperative Nausea and Vomiting

One laboratory adverse experience, hemoglobin decreased (40 mg aprepitant), was reported, regardless of causality, at an incidence ≥3% in a patient receiving general anesthesia.

The following additional laboratory adverse experiences (incidence >0.5% and greater than ondansetron), regardless of causality, were reported in patients treated with aprepitant 40 mg: blood albumin decreased, blood bilirubin increased, blood glucose increased, blood potassium decreased, glucose urine present.

The adverse experience of increased ALT occurred with similar incidence in patients treated with aprepitant as in patients treated with ondansetron.

Other Studies

In addition, two serious adverse experiences were reported in postoperative nausea and vomiting (PONV) clinical studies in patients taking a higher dose of aprepitant: one case of constipation, and one case of sub-ileus.

Angioedema and urticaria were reported as serious adverse experiences in a patient receiving aprepitant in a non-CINV/non-PONV study.

6.2 Post-marketing Experience

The following adverse reactions have been identified during post-marketing use of aprepitant. Because these reactions are reported voluntarily from a population of uncertain size, it is generally not possible to reliably estimate their frequency or establish a causal relationship to the drug.

Skin and subcutaneous tissue disorders: pruritus, rash, urticaria.

Immune system disorders: hypersensitivity reactions including anaphylactic reactions.

Immediate hypersensitivity reactions have been observed during the infusion of fosaprepitant, which may include the following: flushing, erythema, dyspnea *[see Warnings and Precautions (5.2)]*.

7 DRUG INTERACTIONS

Drug interactions following administration of fosaprepitant are likely to occur with drugs that interact with oral aprepitant. The following information was derived from data with oral aprepitant and one study conducted with fosaprepitant and oral midazolam.

Aprepitant is a substrate, a moderate inhibitor, and an inducer of CYP3A4 when administered as a 3-day antiemetic dosing regimen for CINV. Aprepitant is also an inducer of CYP2C9.

7.1 Effect of Aprepitant on the Pharmacokinetics of Other Agents

CYP3A4 Substrates:

As a moderate inhibitor of CYP3A4, aprepitant can increase plasma concentrations of concomitantly coadministered oral medications that are metabolized through CYP3A4 *[see Contraindications (4)]*.

Aprepitant has been shown to induce the metabolism of S(-) warfarin and tolbutamide, which are metabolized through CYP2C9. Coadministration of fosaprepitant or oral aprepitant with these drugs or other drugs that are known to be metabolized by CYP2C9, such as phenytoin, may result in lower plasma concentrations of these drugs.

Fosaprepitant or aprepitant is unlikely to interact with drugs that are substrates for the P-glycoprotein transporter, as demonstrated by the lack of interaction of oral aprepitant with digoxin in a clinical drug interaction study.

5-HT$_3$ antagonists: In clinical drug interaction studies, aprepitant did not have clinically important effects on the pharmacokinetics of ondansetron, granisetron or hydrodolasetron (the active metabolite of dolasetron).

Corticosteroids:

Dexamethasone: Oral aprepitant, when given as a regimen of 125 mg with dexamethasone coadministered orally as 20 mg on Day 1, and oral aprepitant when given as 80 mg/day with dexamethasone coadministered orally as 8 mg on Days 2 through 5, increased the AUC of dexamethasone, a CYP3A4 substrate, by 2.2-fold on Days 1 and 5. The oral dexamethasone doses should be reduced by approximately 50% when coadministered with a regimen of fosaprepitant followed by aprepitant, to achieve exposures of dexamethasone similar to those obtained when dexamethasone is given without aprepitant. The daily dose of dexamethasone administered in clinical CINV studies with oral aprepitant reflects an approximate 50% reduction of the dose of dexamethasone *[see Dosage and Administration (2.1)]*.

Methylprednisolone: Oral aprepitant, when given as a regimen of 125 mg on Day 1 and 80 mg/day on Days 2 and 3, increased the AUC of methylprednisolone, a CYP3A4 substrate, by 1.34-fold on Day 1 and by 2.5-fold on Day 3, when methylprednisolone was coadministered intravenously as 125 mg on Day 1 and orally as 40 mg on Days 2 and 3. The I.V. methylprednisolone dose should be reduced by approximately 25%, and the oral methylprednisolone dose should be reduced by approximately 50% when coadministered with a regimen of fosaprepitant followed by aprepitant to achieve exposures of methylprednisolone similar to those obtained when it is given without aprepitant.

Chemotherapeutic agents: *See Warnings and Precautions (5.1).*

Docetaxel: In a pharmacokinetic study, oral aprepitant (CINV regimen) did not influence the pharmacokinetics of docetaxel.

Vinorelbine: In a pharmacokinetic study, oral aprepitant (CINV regimen) did not influence the pharmacokinetics of vinorelbine to a clinically significant degree.

CYP2C9 Substrates (Warfarin, Tolbutamide):

Warfarin: A single 125-mg dose of oral aprepitant was administered on Day 1 and 80 mg/day on Days 2 and 3 to healthy subjects who were stabilized on chronic warfarin therapy. Although there was no effect of oral aprepitant on the plasma AUC of R(+) or S(-) warfarin determined on Day 3, there was a 34% decrease in S(-) warfarin (a CYP2C9 substrate) trough concentration accompanied by a 14% decrease in the prothrombin time (reported as International Normalized Ratio or INR) 5 days after completion of dosing with oral aprepitant. In patients on chronic warfarin therapy, the prothrombin time (INR) should be closely monitored in the 2-week period, particularly at 7 to 10 days, following initiation of the 3-day regimen of fosaprepitant followed by aprepitant with each chemotherapy cycle.

Tolbutamide: Oral aprepitant, when given as 125 mg on Day 1 and 80 mg/day on Days 2 and 3, decreased the AUC of tolbutamide (a CYP2C9 substrate) by 23% on Day 4, 28% on Day 8, and 15% on Day 15, when a single dose of tolbutamide 500 mg was administered orally prior to the administration of the 3-day regimen of oral aprepitant and on Days 4, 8, and 15.

Oral contraceptives: Aprepitant, when given once daily for 14 days as a 100-mg capsule with an oral contraceptive containing 35 mcg of ethinyl estradiol and 1 mg of norethindrone, decreased the AUC of ethinyl estradiol by 43%, and decreased the AUC of norethindrone by 8%.

In another study, a daily dose of an oral contraceptive containing ethinyl estradiol and norethindrone was administered on Days 1 through 21, and oral aprepitant was given as a 3-day regimen of 125 mg on Day 8 and 80 mg/day on Days 9 and 10 with ondansetron 32 mg I.V. on Day 8 and oral dexamethasone given as 12 mg on Day 8 and 8 mg/day on Days 9, 10, and 11. In the study, the AUC of ethinyl estradiol decreased by 19% on Day 10 and there was as much as a 64% decrease in ethinyl estradiol trough concentrations during Days 9 through 21. While there was no effect of oral aprepitant on the AUC of norethindrone on Day 10, there was as much as a 60% decrease in norethindrone trough concentrations during Days 9 through 21.

The coadministration of fosaprepitant or aprepitant may reduce the efficacy of hormonal contraceptives (these can include birth control pills, skin patches, implants, and certain IUDs) during and for 28 days after administration of the last dose of either. Alternative or back-up methods of contraception should be used during treatment with fosaprepitant and aprepitant and for 1 month following the last dose.

Midazolam: A study was completed with fosaprepitant and oral midazolam. Fosaprepitant was given at a dose of 100 mg over 15 minutes along with a single dose of midazolam 2 mg. The plasma AUC of midazolam was increased by 1.6-fold. This effect was not considered clinically important. Oral aprepitant increased the AUC of midazolam by 2.3-fold on Day 1 and 3.3-fold on Day 5, when a single oral dose of midazolam 2 mg was coadministered on Day 1 and Day 5 of a regimen of oral aprepitant 125 mg on Day 1 and 80 mg/day on Days 2 through 5. The potential effects of increased plasma concentrations of midazolam or other benzodiazepines metabolized via CYP3A4 (alprazolam, triazolam) should be considered when coadministering these agents with a 3-day regimen of fosaprepitant followed by aprepitant. In another study with intravenous administration of midazolam, oral aprepitant was given as 125 mg on Day 1 and 80 mg/day on Days 2 and 3, and midazolam 2 mg I.V. was given prior to the administration of the 3-day regimen of oral aprepitant and on Days 4, 8, and 15. Oral aprepitant increased the AUC of midazolam by 25% on Day 4 and decreased the AUC of midazolam by 19% on Day 8 relative to the dosing of oral aprepitant on Days 1 through 3. These effects were not considered clinically important. The AUC of midazolam on Day 15 was similar to that observed at baseline.

An additional study was completed with intravenous administration of midazolam and oral aprepitant. Intravenous midazolam 2 mg was given 1 hour after oral administration of a single dose of oral aprepitant 125 mg. The plasma AUC of midazolam was increased by 1.5-fold.

7.2 Effect of Other Agents on the Pharmacokinetics of Aprepitant

Aprepitant is a substrate for CYP3A4; therefore, coadministration of fosaprepitant or aprepitant with drugs that inhibit CYP3A4 activity may result in increased plasma concentrations of aprepitant. Consequently, concomitant administration of fosaprepitant or aprepitant with strong CYP3A4 inhibitors (e.g., ketoconazole, itraconazole, nefazodone, troleandomycin, clarithromycin, ritonavir, nelfinavir) should be approached with caution. Because moderate CYP3A4 inhibitors (e.g., diltiazem) result in a 2-fold increase in plasma concentrations of aprepitant, concomitant administration should also be approached with caution.

Aprepitant is a substrate for CYP3A4; therefore, coadministration of fosaprepitant or aprepitant with drugs that strongly induce CYP3A4 activity (e.g., rifampin, carbamazepine, phenytoin) may result in reduced plasma concentrations and decreased efficacy.

Ketoconazole: When a single 125-mg dose of oral aprepitant was administered on Day 5 of a 10-day regimen of 400 mg/day of ketoconazole, a strong CYP3A4 inhibitor, the AUC of aprepitant increased approximately 5-fold and the mean terminal half-life of aprepitant increased approximately 3-fold. Concomitant administration of fosaprepitant or aprepitant with strong CYP3A4 inhibitors should be approached cautiously.

Rifampin: When a single 375-mg dose of oral aprepitant was administered on Day 9 of a 14-day regimen of 600 mg/day of rifampin, a strong CYP3A4 inducer, the AUC of aprepitant decreased approximately 11-fold and the mean terminal half-life decreased approximately 3-fold.

Coadministration of fosaprepitant or aprepitant with drugs that induce CYP3A4 activity may result in reduced plasma concentrations and decreased efficacy.

7.3 Additional Interactions

Diltiazem: In a study in 10 patients with mild to moderate hypertension, intravenous infusion of 100 mg fosaprepitant over 15 minutes with diltiazem 120 mg 3 times daily, resulted in a 1.5-fold increase of aprepitant AUC and a 1.4-fold increase in diltiazem AUC. It also resulted in a small but clinically meaningful further maximum decrease in diastolic blood pressure [mean (SD) of 24.3 (± 10.2) mm Hg with fosaprepitant versus 15.6 (± 4.1) mm Hg without fosaprepitant] and resulted in a small further maximum decrease in systolic blood pressure [mean (SD) of 29.5 (± 7.9) mm Hg with fosaprepitant versus 23.8 (± 4.8) mm Hg without fosaprepitant], which may be clinically meaningful, but did not result in a clinically meaningful further change in heart rate or PR interval, beyond those changes induced by diltiazem alone.

In the same study, administration of aprepitant once daily, as a tablet formulation comparable to 230 mg of the capsule formulation, with diltiazem 120 mg 3 times daily for 5 days, resulted in a 2-fold increase of aprepitant AUC and a simultaneous 1.7-fold increase of diltiazem AUC. These pharmacokinetic effects did not result in clinically meaningful changes in ECG, heart rate or blood pressure beyond those changes induced by diltiazem alone.

Paroxetine: Coadministration of once daily doses of aprepitant, as a tablet formulation comparable to 85 mg or 170 mg of the capsule formulation, with paroxetine 20 mg once daily, resulted in a decrease in AUC by approximately 25% and C_{max} by approximately 20% of both aprepitant and paroxetine.

8 USE IN SPECIFIC POPULATIONS

8.1 Pregnancy

Pregnancy Category B

In the reproduction studies conducted with fosaprepitant and aprepitant, the highest systemic exposures to aprepitant were obtained following oral administration of aprepitant. Reproduction studies performed in rats at oral doses of aprepitant up to 1000 mg/kg twice daily (plasma $AUC_{0\text{-}24hr}$ of 31.3 mcg•hr/mL, about 1.6 times the human exposure at the recommended dose) and in rabbits at oral doses up to 25 mg/kg/day (plasma $AUC_{0\text{-}24hr}$ of 26.9 mcg•hr/mL, about 1.4 times the human exposure at the recommended dose) revealed no evidence of impaired fertility or harm to the fetus due to aprepitant. There are, however, no adequate and well-controlled studies in pregnant women. Because animal reproduction studies are not always predictive of human response, this drug should be used during pregnancy only if clearly needed.

8.3 Nursing Mothers

Aprepitant is excreted in the milk of rats. It is not known whether this drug is excreted in human milk. Because many drugs are excreted in human milk and because of the potential for possible serious adverse reactions in nursing infants from aprepitant and because of the potential for tumorigenicity shown for aprepitant in rodent carcinogenicity studies, a decision should be made whether to discontinue nursing or to discontinue the drug, taking into account the importance of the drug to the mother.

8.4 Pediatric Use

Safety and effectiveness in pediatric patients have not been established.

8.5 Geriatric Use

In 2 well-controlled chemotherapy-induced nausea and vomiting clinical studies, of the total number of patients (N=544) treated with oral aprepitant, 31% were 65 and over, while 5% were 75 and over. No overall differences in safety or effectiveness were observed between these subjects and younger subjects. Greater sensitivity of some older individuals cannot be ruled out. Dosage adjustment in the elderly is not necessary.

10 OVERDOSAGE

No specific information is available on the treatment of overdosage.

In the event of overdose, oral aprepitant should be discontinued and general supportive treatment and monitoring should be provided. Because of the antiemetic activity of aprepitant, drug-induced emesis may not be effective.

Aprepitant cannot be removed by hemodialysis.

11 DESCRIPTION

EMEND (fosaprepitant dimeglumine) for Injection is a sterile, lyophilized prodrug of aprepitant, a substance P/neurokinin-1 (NK_1) receptor antagonist, and is chemically described as 1-Deoxy-1-(methylamino)-D-glucitol[3-[[(2*R*, 3*S*)-2-[(1*R*)-1-[3,5-bis(trifluoromethyl)phenyl]ethoxy]-3-(4-fluorophenyl)-4-morpholinyl]methyl]-2,5-dihydro-5-oxo-1*H*-1,2,4-triazol-1-yl]phosphonate (2:1) (salt).

Its empirical formula is $C_{23}H_{22}F_7N_4O_6P \bullet 2(C_7H_{17}NO_5)$ and its structural formula is:

[See chemical structure at top of next column]

Fosaprepitant dimeglumine is a white to off-white amorphous powder with a molecular weight of 1004.83. It is freely soluble in water.

EMEND for Injection is a lyophilized prodrug of aprepitant containing polysorbate 80 (PS80), to be administered intravenously as an infusion.

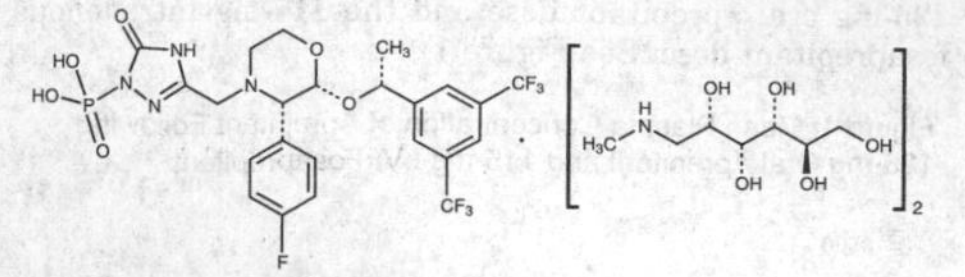

Each vial of EMEND for Injection for intravenous administration contains 188 mg of fosaprepitant dimeglumine equivalent to 115 mg of fosaprepitant and the following inactive ingredients: edetate disodium (14.4 mg), polysorbate 80 (57.5 mg), lactose anhydrous (287.5 mg), sodium hydroxide and/or hydrochloric acid (for pH adjustment). Fosaprepitant dimeglumine hereafter will be referred to as fosaprepitant.

Aprepitant is a substance P/neurokinin 1 (NK_1) receptor antagonist, chemically described as 5-[[(2*R*,3*S*)-2-[(1*R*)-1-[3,5-bis(trifluoromethyl)phenyl]ethoxy]-3-(4-fluorophenyl)-4-morpholinyl]methyl]-1,2-dihydro-3*H*-1,2,4-triazol-3-one.

Its empirical formula is $C_{23}H_{21}F_7N_4O_3$, and its structural formula is:

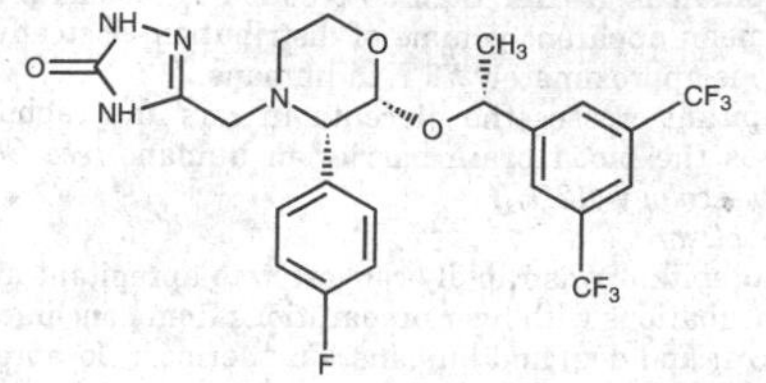

12 CLINICAL PHARMACOLOGY

Fosaprepitant, a prodrug of aprepitant, when administered intravenously is rapidly converted to aprepitant, a substance P/neurokinin 1 (NK_1) receptor antagonist. Plasma concentrations of fosaprepitant are below the limits of quantification (10 ng/mL) within 30 minutes of the completion of infusion *[see Clinical Pharmacology (12.3)]*. Upon conversion of 115 mg of fosaprepitant to aprepitant, 18.3 mg of phosphate and 73 mg of meglumine are liberated from fosaprepitant.

12.1 Mechanism of Action

Fosaprepitant is a prodrug of aprepitant and accordingly, its antiemetic effects are attributable to aprepitant.

Aprepitant is a selective high-affinity antagonist of human substance P/neurokinin 1 (NK_1) receptors. Aprepitant has little or no affinity for serotonin ($5\text{-}HT_3$), dopamine, and corticosteroid receptors, the targets of existing therapies for chemotherapy-induced nausea and vomiting (CINV). Aprepitant has been shown in animal models to inhibit emesis induced by cytotoxic chemotherapeutic agents, such as cisplatin, via central actions. Animal and human Positron Emission Tomography (PET) studies with aprepitant have shown that it crosses the blood brain barrier and occupies brain NK_1 receptors. Animal and human studies show that aprepitant augments the antiemetic activity of the $5\text{-}HT_3$-receptor antagonist ondansetron and the corticosteroid dexamethasone and inhibits both the acute and delayed phases of cisplatin-induced emesis.

12.2 Pharmacodynamics

NK_1 Receptor Occupancy

In two single-blind, multiple-dose, randomized, and placebo control studies, healthy young men received oral aprepitant doses of 10 mg (N=2), 30 mg (N=3), 100 mg (N=3) or 300 mg (N=5) once daily for 14 days with 2 or 3 subjects on placebo. Both plasma aprepitant concentration and NK-1 receptor occupancy in the corpus striatum by positron emission tomography were evaluated, at predose and 24 hours after the last dose. At aprepitant plasma concentrations of ~10 ng/mL and ~100 ng/mL, the NK-1 receptor occupancies were ~50% and ~90%, respectively. The oral aprepitant regimen for CINV produces mean trough plasma aprepitant concentrations >500 ng/mL, which would be expected to, based on the fitted curve with the Hill equation, result in >95% brain NK-1 receptor occupancy. However, the receptor occupancy for either CINV or PONV dosing regimen has not been determined. In addition, the relationship between NK-1 receptor occupancy and the clinical efficacy of aprepitant has not been established.

Cardiac Electrophysiology

In a randomized, double-blind, positive-controlled, thorough QTc study, a single 200-mg dose of fosaprepitant had no effect on the QTc interval.

12.3 Pharmacokinetics

Aprepitant after Fosaprepitant Administration

Following a single intravenous dose of fosaprepitant administered as a 15-minute infusion to healthy volunteers the mean $AUC_{0\text{-}\infty}$ of aprepitant was 31.7 (± 14.3) mcg•hr/mL and the mean maximal aprepitant concentration (C_{max}) was 3.27 (± 1.16) mcg/mL. The mean aprepitant plasma concentration at 24 hours postdose was similar between the

125-mg oral aprepitant dose and the 115-mg intravenous fosaprepitant dose (See Figure 1).

Figure 1: Mean Plasma Concentration of Aprepitant Following 125-mg Oral Aprepitant and 115-mg I.V. Fosaprepitant

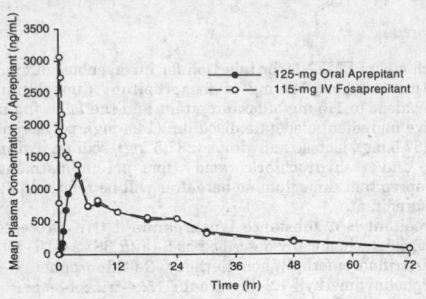

Distribution
Fosaprepitant is rapidly converted to aprepitant. Aprepitant is greater than 95% bound to plasma proteins. The mean apparent volume of distribution at steady state (Vd_{ss}) is approximately 70 L in humans.
Aprepitant crosses the placenta in rats and rabbits and crosses the blood brain barrier in humans [see Clinical Pharmacology (12.1)].
Metabolism
Fosaprepitant was rapidly converted to aprepitant in *in vitro* incubations with liver preparations from nonclinical species (rat and dog) and humans. Furthermore, fosaprepitant underwent rapid and nearly complete conversion to aprepitant in S9 preparations from multiple other human tissues including kidney, lung and ileum. Thus, it appears that the conversion of fosaprepitant to aprepitant can occur in multiple extrahepatic tissues in addition to the liver. In humans, fosaprepitant administered intravenously was rapidly converted to aprepitant within 30 minutes following the end of infusion.
Aprepitant undergoes extensive metabolism. *In vitro* studies using human liver microsomes indicate that aprepitant is metabolized primarily by CYP3A4 with minor metabolism by CYP1A2 and CYP2C19. Metabolism is largely via oxidation at the morpholine ring and its side chains. No metabolism by CYP2D6, CYP2C9, or CYP2E1 was detected. In healthy young adults, aprepitant accounts for approximately 24% of the radioactivity in plasma over 72 hours following a single oral 300-mg dose of $[^{14}C]$-aprepitant, indicating a substantial presence of metabolites in the plasma. Seven metabolites of aprepitant, which are only weakly active, have been identified in human plasma.
Excretion
Following administration of a single I.V. 100-mg dose of $[^{14}C]$-fosaprepitant to healthy subjects, 57% of the radioactivity was recovered in urine and 45% in feces.
Aprepitant is eliminated primarily by metabolism; aprepitant is not renally excreted. The apparent terminal half-life of aprepitant ranged from approximately 9 to 13 hours.
Special Populations
Fosaprepitant, a prodrug of aprepitant, when administered intravenously is rapidly converted to aprepitant.
Gender
Following oral administration of a single 125-mg dose of aprepitant, no difference in AUC_{0-24hr} was observed between males and females. The C_{max} for aprepitant is 16% higher in females as compared with males. The half-life of aprepitant is 25% lower in females as compared with males and T_{max} occurs at approximately the same time. These differences are not considered clinically meaningful. No dosage adjustment is necessary based on gender.
Geriatric
Following oral administration of a single 125-mg dose of aprepitant on Day 1 and 80 mg once daily on Days 2 through 5, the AUC_{0-24hr} of aprepitant was 21% higher on Day 1 and 36% higher on Day 5 in elderly (≥65 years) relative to younger adults. The C_{max} was 10% higher on Day 1 and 24% higher on Day 5 in elderly relative to younger adults. These differences are not considered clinically meaningful. No dosage adjustment is necessary in elderly patients.
Pediatric
Fosaprepitant has not been evaluated in patients below 18 years of age.
Race
Following oral administration of a single 125-mg dose of aprepitant, the AUC_{0-24hr} is approximately 25% and 29% higher in Hispanics as compared with Whites and Blacks, respectively. The C_{max} is 22% and 31% higher in Hispanics as compared with Whites and Blacks, respectively. These differences are not considered clinically meaningful. There was no difference in AUC_{0-24hr} or C_{max} between Whites and Blacks. No dosage adjustment is necessary based on race.

Table 4: Treatment Regimens in Highly Emetogenic Chemotherapy Trials

Treatment Regimen	Day 1	Days 2 to 4
Aprepitant	Aprepitant 125 mg PO Dexamethasone 12 mg PO Ondansetron 32 mg I.V.	Aprepitant 80 mg PO Daily (Days 2 and 3 only) Dexamethasone 8 mg PO Daily (morning)
Standard Therapy	Dexamethasone 20 mg PO Ondansetron 32 mg I.V.	Dexamethasone 8 mg PO Daily (morning) Dexamethasone 8 mg PO Daily (evening)

Aprepitant placebo and dexamethasone placebo were used to maintain blinding.

Table 5: Percent of Patients Receiving Highly Emetogenic Chemotherapy Responding by Treatment Group and Phase for Study 1 — Cycle 1

ENDPOINTS	Aprepitant Regimen (N = 260)* %	Standard Therapy (N = 261)* %	p-Value
PRIMARY ENDPOINT			
Complete Response			
Overall[†]	73	52	<0.001
OTHER PRESPECIFIED ENDPOINTS			
Complete Response			
Acute phase[‡]	89	78	<0.001
Delayed phase[§]	75	56	<0.001
Complete Protection			
Overall	63	49	0.001
Acute phase	85	75	NS[¶]
Delayed phase	66	52	<0.001
No Emesis			
Overall	78	55	<0.001
Acute phase	90	79	0.001
Delayed phase	81	59	<0.001
No Nausea			
Overall	48	44	NS[#]
Delayed phase	51	48	NS[#]
No Significant Nausea			
Overall	73	66	NS[#]
Delayed phase	75	69	NS[#]

Visual analogue scale (VAS) score range: 0 mm = no nausea; 100 mm = nausea as bad as it could be.
* N: Number of patients (older than 18 years of age) who received cisplatin, study drug, and had at least one post-treatment efficacy evaluation.
† Overall: 0 to 120 hours post-cisplatin treatment.
‡ Acute phase: 0 to 24 hours post-cisplatin treatment.
§ Delayed phase: 25 to 120 hours post-cisplatin treatment.
¶ Not statistically significant when adjusted for multiple comparisons.
# Not statistically significant.

Hepatic Insufficiency
Fosaprepitant is metabolized in various extrahepatic tissues; therefore hepatic impairment is not expected to alter the conversion of fosaprepitant to aprepitant.
Following oral administration of a single 125-mg dose of oral aprepitant on Day 1 and 80 mg once daily on Days 2 and 3 to patients with mild hepatic impairment (Child-Pugh score 5 to 6), the AUC_{0-24hr} of aprepitant was 11% lower on Day 1 and 36% lower on Day 3, as compared with healthy subjects given the same regimen. In patients with moderate hepatic impairment (Child-Pugh score 7 to 9), the AUC_{0-24hr} of aprepitant was 10% higher on Day 1 and 18% higher on Day 3, as compared with healthy subjects given the same regimen. These differences in AUC_{0-24hr} are not considered clinically meaningful; therefore, no dosage adjustment is necessary in patients with mild to moderate hepatic impairment. There are no clinical or pharmacokinetic data in patients with severe hepatic impairment (Child-Pugh score >9) [see Warnings and Precautions (5.5)].
Renal Insufficiency
A single 240-mg dose of oral aprepitant was administered to patients with severe renal impairment (CrCl<30 mL/min) and to patients with end stage renal disease (ESRD) requiring hemodialysis.
In patients with severe renal impairment, the $AUC_{0-\infty}$ of total aprepitant (unbound and protein bound) decreased by 21% and C_{max} decreased by 32%, relative to healthy sub-

jects. In patients with ESRD undergoing hemodialysis, the $AUC_{0-\infty}$ of total aprepitant decreased by 42% and C_{max} decreased by 32%. Due to modest decreases in protein binding of aprepitant in patients with renal disease, the AUC of pharmacologically active unbound drug was not significantly affected in patients with renal impairment compared with healthy subjects. Hemodialysis conducted 4 or 48 hours after dosing had no significant effect on the pharmacokinetics of aprepitant; less than 0.2% of the dose was recovered in the dialysate.
No dosage adjustment is necessary for patients with renal impairment or for patients with ESRD undergoing hemodialysis.

13 NONCLINICAL TOXICOLOGY

13.1 Carcinogenesis, Mutagenesis, Impairment of Fertility

Carcinogenicity studies were conducted in Sprague-Dawley rats and in CD-1 mice for 2 years. In the rat carcinogenicity studies, animals were treated with oral doses ranging from 0.05 to 1000 mg/kg twice daily. The highest dose produced a systemic exposure to aprepitant (plasma AUC_{0-24hr}) of 0.7 to 1.6 times the human exposure (AUC_{0-24hr} = 19.6 mcg•hr/mL) at the recommended dose of 125 mg/day. Treatment with aprepitant at doses of 5 to 1000 mg/kg twice daily caused an increase in the incidences of thyroid follicular cell adenomas and carcinomas in male rats. In female rats, it produced hepatocellular adenomas at 5 to 1000 mg/kg twice daily and hepatocellular carcinomas and thyroid follicular cell adenomas at 125 to 1000 mg/kg twice daily. In the mouse carcinogenicity studies, the animals were treated with oral doses ranging from 2.5 to 2000 mg/kg/day. The highest dose produced a systemic exposure of about 2.8 to 3.6 times the human exposure at the recommended dose. Treatment with aprepitant produced skin fibrosarcomas at 125 and 500 mg/kg/day doses in male mice. Carcinogenicity studies were not conducted with fosaprepitant.

Aprepitant and fosaprepitant were not genotoxic in the Ames test, the human lymphoblastoid cell (TK6) mutagenesis test, the rat hepatocyte DNA strand break test, the Chinese hamster ovary (CHO) cell chromosome aberration test and the mouse micronucleus test.

Fosaprepitant, when administered intravenously, is rapidly converted to aprepitant. In the fertility studies conducted with fosaprepitant and aprepitant, the highest systemic exposures to aprepitant were obtained following oral administration of aprepitant. Oral aprepitant did not affect the fertility or general reproductive performance of male or female rats at doses up to the maximum feasible dose of 1000 mg/kg twice daily (providing exposure in male rats lower than the exposure at the recommended human dose and exposure in female rats at about 1.6 times the human exposure).

14   CLINICAL STUDIES

Fosaprepitant, a prodrug of aprepitant, when administered intravenously is rapidly converted to aprepitant. Fosaprepitant 115 mg I.V. infused over 15 minutes can be substituted for 125 mg oral aprepitant on Day 1 [see Dosage and Administration (2.1)]. Pivotal efficacy studies were conducted with oral aprepitant.

Oral administration of aprepitant in combination with ondansetron and dexamethasone (aprepitant regimen) has been shown to prevent acute and delayed nausea and vomiting associated with highly emetogenic chemotherapy including high-dose cisplatin, and nausea and vomiting associated with moderately emetogenic chemotherapy.

14.1   Highly Emetogenic Chemotherapy (HEC)

In 2 multicenter, randomized, parallel, double-blind, controlled clinical studies, the aprepitant regimen (see Table 6) was compared with standard therapy in patients receiving a chemotherapy regimen that included cisplatin >50 mg/m^2 (mean cisplatin dose = 80.2 mg/m^2). Of the 550 patients who were randomized to receive the aprepitant regimen, 42% were women, 58% men, 59% White, 3% Asian, 5% Black, 12% Hispanic American, and 21% Multi-Racial. The aprepitant-treated patients in these clinical studies ranged from 14 to 84 years of age, with a mean age of 56 years. 170 patients were 65 years or older, with 29 patients being 75 years or older.

Patients (N = 1105) were randomized to either the aprepitant regimen (N = 550) or standard therapy (N = 555). The treatment regimens are defined in the Table 4.

[See table 4 at top of previous page]

During these studies 95% of the patients in the aprepitant group received a concomitant chemotherapeutic agent in addition to protocol-mandated cisplatin. The most common chemotherapeutic agents and the number of aprepitant patients exposed follow: etoposide (106), fluorouracil (100), gemcitabine (89), vinorelbine (82), paclitaxel (52), cyclophosphamide (50), doxorubicin (38), docetaxel (11).

The antiemetic activity of oral aprepitant was evaluated during the acute phase (0 to 24 hours post-cisplatin treatment), the delayed phase (25 to 120 hours post-cisplatin treatment) and overall (0 to 120 hours post-cisplatin treatment) in Cycle 1. Efficacy was based on evaluation of the following endpoints:

Primary endpoint:
• complete response (defined as no emetic episodes and no use of rescue therapy)

Other prespecified endpoints:
• complete protection (defined as no emetic episodes, no use of rescue therapy, and a maximum nausea visual analogue scale [VAS] score <25 mm on a 0 to 100 mm scale)
• no emesis (defined as no emetic episodes regardless of use of rescue therapy)
• no nausea (maximum VAS <5 mm on a 0 to 100 mm scale)
• no significant nausea (maximum VAS <25 mm on a 0 to 100 mm scale)

A summary of the key study results from each individual study analysis is shown in Table 5 and in Table 6.

[See table 5 on previous page]

[See table 6 above]

In both studies, a statistically significantly higher proportion of patients (both p<0.001) receiving the aprepitant regimen in Cycle 1 had a complete response in the overall phase (primary endpoint), compared with patients receiving standard therapy. A statistically significant difference in complete response in favor of the aprepitant regimen was also observed when the acute phase and the delayed phase were analyzed separately.

Table 6: Percent of Patients Receiving Highly Emetogenic Chemotherapy Responding by Treatment Group and Phase for Study 2 — Cycle 1

ENDPOINTS	Aprepitant Regimen (N = 261)* %	Standard Therapy (N = 263)* %	p-Value
PRIMARY ENDPOINT			
Complete Response			
Overall†	63	43	<0.001
OTHER PRESPECIFIED ENDPOINTS			
Complete Response			
Acute phase‡	83	68	<0.001
Delayed phase§	68	47	<0.001
Complete Protection			
Overall	56	41	<0.001
Acute phase	80	65	<0.001
Delayed phase	61	44	<0.001
No Emesis			
Overall	66	44	<0.001
Acute phase	84	69	<0.001
Delayed phase	72	48	<0.001
No Nausea			
Overall	49	39	NS¶
Delayed phase	53	40	NS¶
No Significant Nausea			
Overall	71	64	NS#
Delayed phase	73	65	NS#

Visual analogue scale (VAS) score range: 0 mm = no nausea; 100 mm = nausea as bad as it could be.
* N: Number of patients (older than 18 years of age) who received cisplatin, study drug, and had at least one post-treatment efficacy evaluation.
† Overall: 0 to 120 hours post-cisplatin treatment.
‡ Acute phase: 0 to 24 hours post-cisplatin treatment.
§ Delayed phase: 25 to 120 hours post-cisplatin treatment.
¶ Not statistically significant when adjusted for multiple comparisons.
# Not statistically significant.

In both studies, the estimated time to first emesis after initiation of cisplatin treatment was longer with the aprepitant regimen, and the incidence of first emesis was reduced in the aprepitant regimen group compared with standard therapy group as depicted in the Kaplan-Meier curves in Figure 2.

Figure 2: Percent of Patients Receiving Highly Emetogenic Chemotherapy Who Remain Emesis Free Over Time — Cycle 1

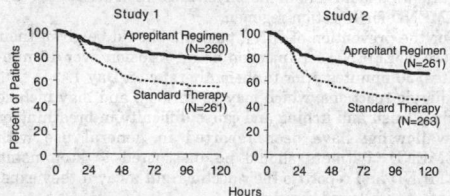

p-Value <0.001 based on a log rank test for Study 1 and Study 2; nominal p-values not adjusted for multiplicity.

Patient-Reported Outcomes: The impact of nausea and vomiting on patients' daily lives was assessed in Cycle 1 of both Phase III studies using the Functional Living Index–Emesis (FLIE), a validated nausea- and vomiting-specific patient-reported outcome measure. Minimal or no impact of nausea and vomiting on patients' daily lives is defined as a FLIE total score >108. In each of the 2 studies, a higher proportion of patients receiving the aprepitant regimen reported minimal or no impact of nausea and vomiting on daily life (Study 1: 74% versus 64%; Study 2: 75% versus 64%).

Multiple-Cycle Extension: In the same 2 clinical studies, patients continued into the Multiple-Cycle extension for up to 5 additional cycles of chemotherapy. The proportion of patients with no emesis and no significant nausea by treatment group at each cycle is depicted in Figure 3.

[See figure 3 at top of next page]

14.2   Moderately Emetogenic Chemotherapy (MEC)

In a multicenter, randomized, double-blind, parallel-group, clinical study in breast cancer patients, the aprepitant regimen (see Table 7) was compared with a standard of care

Figure 3: Proportion of Patients Receiving Highly Emetogenic Chemotherapy with No Emesis and No Significant Nausea by Treatment Group and Cycle

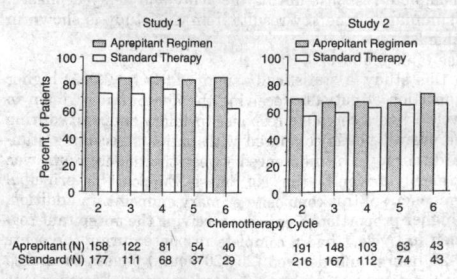

Aprepitant (N)	158	122	81	54	40	191	148	103	63	43
Standard (N)	177	111	68	37	29	216	167	112	74	43

therapy in patients receiving a moderately emetogenic chemotherapy regimen that included cyclophosphamide 750-1500 mg/m^2; or cyclophosphamide 500-1500 mg/m^2 and doxorubicin (≤60 mg/m^2) or epirubicin (≤100 mg/m^2).

In this study, the most common combinations were cyclophosphamide + doxorubicin (60.6%); and cyclophosphamide + epirubicin + fluorouracil (21.6%).

Of the 438 patients who were randomized to receive the aprepitant regimen, 99.5% were women. Of these, approximately 80% were White, 8% Black, 8% Asian, 4% Hispanic, and <1% Other. The aprepitant-treated patients in this clinical study ranged from 25 to 78 years of age, with a mean age of 53 years; 70 patients were 65 years or older, with 12 patients being over 74 years. Patients (N = 866) were randomized to either the aprepitant regimen (N = 438) or standard therapy (N = 428). The treatment regimens are defined in Table 7.

[See table 7 at top of next page]

The antiemetic activity of oral aprepitant was evaluated based on the following endpoints:

Primary endpoint:

Complete response (defined as no emetic episodes and no use of rescue therapy) in the overall phase (0 to 120 hours post-chemotherapy)

Table 7: Treatment Regimens in Moderately Emetogenic Chemotherapy Trial

Treatment Regimen	Day 1	Days 2 to 3
Aprepitant	Aprepitant 125 mg PO* Dexamethasone 12 mg PO† Ondansetron 8 mg PO × 2 doses‡	Aprepitant 80 mg PO Daily
Standard Therapy	Dexamethasone 20 mg PO Ondansetron 8 mg PO × 2 doses	Ondansetron 8 mg PO Daily (every 12 hours)

Aprepitant placebo and dexamethasone placebo were used to maintain blinding.
* 1 hour prior to chemotherapy.
† 30 minutes prior to chemotherapy.
‡ 30 to 60 minutes prior to chemotherapy and 8 hours after first ondansetron dose.

Table 8: Percent of Patients Receiving Moderately Emetogenic Chemotherapy Responding by Treatment Group and Phase — Cycle 1

ENDPOINTS	Aprepitant Regimen (N = 433)* %	Standard Therapy (N = 424)* %	p-Value
PRIMARY ENDPOINT†			
Complete Response	51	42	0.015
OTHER PRESPECIFIED ENDPOINTS†			
No Emesis	76	59	NS‡
No Nausea	33	33	NS
No Significant Nausea	61	56	NS
No Rescue Therapy	59	56	NS
Complete Protection	43	37	NS

* N: Number of patients included in the primary analysis of complete response.
† Overall: 0 to 120 hours post-chemotherapy treatment.
‡ NS when adjusted for prespecified multiple comparisons rule; unadjusted p-value <0.001.

Other prespecified endpoints:
• no emesis (defined as no emetic episodes regardless of use of rescue therapy)
• no nausea (maximum VAS <5 mm on a 0 to 100 mm scale)
• no significant nausea (maximum VAS <25 mm on a 0 to 100 mm scale)
• complete protection (defined as no emetic episodes, no use of rescue therapy, and a maximum nausea visual analogue scale [VAS] score <25 mm on a 0 to 100 mm scale)
• complete response during the acute and delayed phases.
A summary of the key results from this study is shown in Table 8.
[See table 8 above]
In this study, a statistically significantly (p=0.015) higher proportion of patients receiving the aprepitant regimen in Cycle 1 had a complete response (primary endpoint) during the overall phase compared with patients receiving standard therapy. The difference between treatment groups was primarily driven by the "No Emesis Endpoint", a principal component of this composite primary endpoint. In addition, a higher proportion of patients receiving the aprepitant regimen in Cycle 1 had a complete response during the acute (0-24 hours) and delayed (25-120 hours) phases compared with patients receiving standard therapy; however, the treatment group differences failed to reach statistical significance, after multiplicity adjustments.
Patient-Reported Outcomes: In a phase III study in patients receiving moderately emetogenic chemotherapy, the impact of nausea and vomiting on patients' daily lives was assessed in Cycle 1 using the FLIE. A higher proportion of patients receiving the aprepitant regimen reported minimal or no impact on daily life (64% versus 56%). This difference between treatment groups was primarily driven by the "No Vomiting Domain" of this composite endpoint.
Multiple-Cycle Extension: Patients receiving moderately emetogenic chemotherapy were permitted to continue into the Multiple-Cycle extension of the study for up to 3 additional cycles of chemotherapy. Antiemetic effect for patients receiving the aprepitant regimen is maintained during all cycles.

16 HOW SUPPLIED/STORAGE AND HANDLING

No. 3884—One 115 mg single dose per 10 mL glass vial: White to off-white lyophilized solid. Supplied as follows:
NDC 0006-3884-32 1 vial per carton.
Storage
Vials: Store at 2-8°C (36-46°F).
Sterile lyophilized powder for intravenous use only after reconstitution and dilution.

Manuf. for: Merck Sharp & Dohme Corp., a subsidiary of **MERCK & CO., INC.**, Whitehouse Station, NJ 08889, USA
Manufactured by:
DSM Pharmaceuticals, Inc., 5900 Martin Luther King Jr. Highway, Greenville, NC 27834
9840005
U.S. Patent Nos.: 5,512,570; 5,691,336

17 PATIENT COUNSELING INFORMATION

[See FDA-Approved Patient Labeling.]
17.1 Instructions
Physicians should instruct their patients to read the patient package insert before starting therapy with EMEND for Injection and to reread it each time the prescription is renewed.
Patients should follow the physician's instructions for the EMEND for Injection regimen.
For the prevention of CINV, patients should be given their dose of EMEND for Injection as an infusion over 15 minutes, 30 minutes prior to chemotherapy on Day 1.
Allergic reactions, which may be serious, and may include hives, rash and itching and cause difficulty in breathing or swallowing, have been reported in general use with EMEND. Patients should be instructed to stop using EMEND and report to their doctor right away if they experience an allergic reaction.
EMEND for Injection may interact with some drugs including chemotherapy; therefore, patients should be advised to report to their doctor the use of any other prescription, nonprescription medication or herbal products.
Patients on chronic warfarin therapy should be instructed to have their clotting status closely monitored in the 2-week period, particularly at 7 to 10 days, following initiation of the 3-day regimen of fosaprepitant followed by aprepitant, with each chemotherapy cycle.
Administration of EMEND for Injection may reduce the efficacy of hormonal contraceptives. Patients should be advised to use alternative or back-up methods of contraception during treatment with EMEND for Injection and for 1 month following the last dose of the 3-day aprepitant regimen.

FDA-APPROVED PATIENT LABELING

Patient Information
EMEND®
(fosaprepitant dimeglumine)
for Injection
Read the Patient Information that comes with EMEND (fosaprepitant dimeglumine) for Injection before you are given the injection each time you refill your prescription. The information may have changed. This leaflet provides only a summary of certain information about EMEND for Injection. Your doctor or pharmacist can give you an additional leaflet that is written for health professionals that contains more complete information. This leaflet does not take the place of careful discussions with your doctor. You and your doctor should discuss EMEND for Injection when you start taking your medicine.
What is EMEND for Injection?
EMEND for Injection is a prescription medicine used in adults to prevent nausea and vomiting caused by certain cancer chemotherapy medicines. EMEND for Injection is always used WITH OTHER MEDICINES. EMEND for Injection is not used to treat nausea and vomiting that you already have.
Who should not take EMEND for Injection?
Do not take EMEND for Injection if you:
• are taking any of the following medicines:
  • ORAP® (pimozide)
  • SELDANE® (terfenadine)
  • HISMANAL® (astemizole)
  • PROPULSID® (cisapride)
Taking EMEND for Injection with these medicines could cause serious or life-threatening problems.
• are allergic to fosaprepitant or any of the ingredients in EMEND for Injection. See the end of this leaflet for a list of all the ingredients in EMEND for Injection.
What should I tell my doctor before and during treatment with EMEND for Injection?
Tell your doctor about all your medical conditions, including if you:
• have liver problems.
• are pregnant or plan to become pregnant. It is not known if EMEND for Injection can harm your unborn baby.
  Women who use birth control medicines containing hormones to prevent pregnancy (these can include birth control pills, skin patches, implants, and certain IUDs) during treatment with EMEND for Injection and for up to 1 month after using EMEND for Injection should also use a back-up method of birth control to prevent pregnancy.
• are breast-feeding. It is not known if EMEND for Injection passes into your milk and if it can harm your baby.
Tell your doctor about all the medicines you are taking or plan to take, including prescription and nonprescription medicines, vitamins, and herbal supplements. EMEND for Injection may cause **serious life-threatening reactions** if used with certain medicines. (See the section "Who should not take EMEND for Injection?")
Some medicines can affect EMEND for Injection. EMEND for Injection may also affect some medicines, including chemotherapy, causing them to work differently in your body.
Your doctor may check to make sure your other medicines are working correctly while you are taking EMEND for Injection. People who take warfarin (COUMADIN®, JANTOVEN®) may need to have blood tests after each 3-day treatment to check their blood clotting.
How should I take EMEND for Injection?
EMEND for Injection is given intravenously on Day 1 only of a 3-day regimen, then EMEND capsules are taken by mouth on the two days after chemotherapy:
• **Day 1 (Day of chemotherapy):** EMEND will be given to you by intravenous (IV) injection in your vein 30 minutes before you start your chemotherapy treatment.
• You should get a package that has two capsules of EMEND.
• **Day 2 and Day 3 (the two days after chemotherapy):** Take one 80-mg capsule of EMEND (white) by mouth, each morning for the 2 days after your chemotherapy treatment.
EMEND for Injection may be given with or without food.
What are the possible side effects of EMEND for Injection?
EMEND for Injection may cause serious side effects, including:
• Allergic reactions, which may occur suddenly and may include hives, rash, itching, redness of the face or skin and may cause you to have difficult breathing or swallowing. If you have an allergic reaction, call your doctor or seek medical attention right away.
In people taking EMEND for Injection the most common side effects are:
• tiredness
• nausea
• hiccups
• constipation
• diarrhea
• loss of appetite
• headache
• hair loss
• injection site pain
• hardening of site of injection

Tell your doctor if you have any side effect that bothers you or that does not go away. These are not all of the possible side effects of EMEND for Injection. For further information ask your doctor or pharmacist.

Call your doctor for medical advice about side effects. You may report side effects to FDA at 1-800-FDA-1088.

General information about the use of EMEND for Injection
This leaflet summarizes the most important information about EMEND for Injection. If you would like to know more information, talk with your doctor. You can ask your doctor or pharmacist for information about EMEND for Injection that is written for health professionals. For more information about EMEND for Injection call 1-800-622-4477 or go to www.emend.com.

What are the ingredients in EMEND for Injection?
Active ingredient: fosaprepitant

Inactive ingredients: edetate disodium, polysorbate 80, lactose anhydrous, sodium hydroxide and/or hydrochloric acid (for pH adjustment).

U.S. Patent Nos.: 5,512,570; 5,691,336

The brands listed in the above sections **"Who should not take EMEND for Injection?"** and **"What should I tell my doctor before and during treatment with EMEND for Injection?"** are the registered trademarks of their respective owners and are not trademarks of Merck Sharp & Dohme Corp., a subsidiary of Merck & Co., Inc.

EMEND® (fosaprepitant dimeglumine) for Injection is a registered trademark of Merck Sharp & Dohme Corp., a subsidiary of **Merck & Co., Inc.**

Copyright © 2008 Merck Sharp & Dohme Corp., a subsidiary of **Merck & Co., Inc.**

All rights reserved.

Issued March 2010

Manuf. for: Merck Sharp & Dohme Corp., a subsidiary of **MERCK & CO., INC.**, Whitehouse Station, NJ 08889, USA

Manufactured by:
DSM Pharmaceuticals, Inc., 5900 Martin Luther King Jr. Highway, Greenville, NC 27834

9840005

FOLLISTIM® AQ CARTRIDGE   ℞
[*Fol-lis-tim*]
(follitropin beta injection)
For Subcutaneous Use

HIGHLIGHTS OF PRESCRIBING INFORMATION

These highlights do not include all the information needed to use FOLLISTIM® AQ Cartridge safely and effectively. See full prescribing information for FOLLISTIM® AQ Cartridge.
FOLLISTIM® AQ Cartridge (follitropin beta injection) for subcutaneous use
Initial U.S. Approval: 1997

————————RECENT MAJOR CHANGES————————
INDICATIONS AND USAGE, Induction of Spermatogenesis in Men with Primary and Secondary Hypogonadotropic Hypogonadism (HH) in Whom the Cause of Infertility Is not Due to Primary Testicular Failure (1.3) 6/2010
DOSAGE AND ADMINISTRATION, Recommended Dosing for Induction of Spermatogenesis in Men (2.4) 6/2010
WARNINGS AND PRECAUTIONS
• Ovarian Torsion (5.4) 6/2010
• Congenital Anomalies (5.6) 6/2010
• Ectopic Pregnancy (5.7) 6/2010
• Spontaneous Abortion (5.8) 6/2010
• Laboratory Tests For Men (5.10) 6/2010

————————INDICATIONS AND USAGE————————
Follistim AQ Cartridge is a gonadotropin indicated:
In Women for:
• Induction of ovulation and pregnancy in anovulatory infertile women in whom the cause of infertility is functional and not due to primary ovarian failure (1.1)
• Development of multiple follicles in ovulatory women participating in an Assisted Reproductive Technology (ART) program (1.2)
In Men for:
• Induction of spermatogenesis in men with primary and secondary hypogonadotropic hypogonadism (HH) in whom the cause of infertility is not due to primary testicular failure (1.3)

————————DOSAGE AND ADMINISTRATION————————
See Dose Conversion Table 1 for Follistim AQ Cartridge with Pen Injector (2.1)
Ovulation Induction in Women (2.2)
• Starting daily dose of 50 international units of Follistim AQ Cartridge is administered subcutaneously =for at least the first 7 days. The dose is increased by 25 or 50 international units at weekly intervals until follicular growth and/or serum estradiol levels indicate an adequate response
  • When an acceptable pre-ovulatory state is achieved, final oocyte maturation is achieved with 5000 to 10,000 international units of human chorionic gonadotropin (hCG)

• The woman and her partner should have intercourse daily, beginning on the day prior to the administration of hCG and until ovulation becomes apparent
Assisted Reproductive Technologies (ART) in Women (2.3)
• Starting dose of 125 to 175 international units of Follistim AQ Cartridge is administered subcutaneously for at least the first 4 days of treatment. Subsequent doses are adjusted based upon ovarian response as determined by ultrasound evaluation of follicular growth and serum estradiol levels
  • Final oocyte maturation is induced with a dose of 5000–10,000 international units of hCG
  • Oocyte (egg) retrieval is performed 34 to 36 hours later
Induction of Spermatogenesis in Men (2.4)
• Pretreatment with hCG alone (1500 international units twice weekly) is required. If serum testosterone levels have not normalized after 8 weeks of hCG treatment, the dose may be increased to 3000 international units twice a week
• After normalization of serum testosterone levels, administer 450 international units per week (225 international units twice weekly or 150 international units three times weekly) of Follistim AQ Cartridge subcutaneously with the same pre-treatment hCG dose used to normalize testosterone levels

————————DOSAGE FORMS AND STRENGTHS————————
Follistim AQ Cartridge 175 IU per 0.210 mL (3)
Follistim AQ Cartridge 350 IU per 0.420 mL (3)
Follistim AQ Cartridge 650 IU per 0.780 mL (3)
Follistim AQ Cartridge 975 IU per 1.170 mL (3)

————————CONTRAINDICATIONS————————
Women and men who exhibit:
• Prior hypersensitivity to recombinant hFSH products (4)
• High levels of FSH indicating primary gonadal failure (4)
• Presence of uncontrolled non-gonadal endocrinopathies (4)
• Hypersensitivity reactions related to streptomycin or neomycin (4)
• Tumor of the ovary, breast, uterus, testis, hypothalamus or pituitary gland (4)
Women who exhibit:
• Pregnancy (4, 8.1)
• Heavy or irregular vaginal bleeding of undetermined origin (4)
• Ovarian cysts or enlargement not due to polycystic ovary syndrome (PCOS) (4)

————————WARNINGS AND PRECAUTIONS————————
Treatment with Follistim AQ may result in:
• Abnormal Ovarian Enlargement (5.1)
• Ovarian Hyperstimulation Syndrome (OHSS) (5.2)
• Pulmonary and Vascular Complications (5.3)
• Ovarian Torsion (5.4)
• Multi-fetal Gestation and Birth (5.5)
• Congenital Anomalies (5.6)
• Ectopic Pregnancy (5.7)
• Spontaneous Abortion (5.8)
• Ovarian Neoplasm (5.9)

————————ADVERSE REACTIONS————————
The most common adverse reactions (≥2%) in women undergoing ovulation induction are: ovarian hyperstimulation syndrome, ovarian cyst, abdominal discomfort, abdominal pain and lower abdominal pain (6.1).

The most common adverse reactions (≥2%) in women receiving ART are ovarian hyperstimulation syndrome and abdominal pain (6.1).

The most common (≥2%) adverse reactions in men undergoing induction of spermatogenesis are headache, acne, injection site reaction, injection site pain, gynecomastia, rash and dermoid cyst (6.1)

To report SUSPECTED ADVERSE REACTIONS, contact Schering-Plough Corporation, a subsidiary of Merck & Co., Inc. at 800-526-4099 or FDA at 1-800-FDA-1088 or www.fda.gov/medwatch.

————————USE IN SPECIFIC POPULATIONS————————
• Nursing Mothers: It is not known whether this drug is excreted in human milk (8.1, 8.3)

See 17 for PATIENT COUNSELING INFORMATION and FDA-approved patient labeling

Revised: 06/2010

——
FULL PRESCRIBING INFORMATION: CONTENTS*
1   INDICATIONS AND USAGE
   1.1   Induction of ovulation and pregnancy in anovulatory infertile women in whom the cause of infertility is functional and not due to primary ovarian failure
   1.2   Development of multiple follicles in ovulatory women participating in an Assisted Reproductive Technology (ART) program
   1.3   Induction of spermatogenesis in men with primary and secondary hypogonadotropic hypogonadism (HH) in whom the cause of infertility is not due to primary testicular failure

2   DOSAGE AND ADMINISTRATION
   2.1   General Dosing Information
   2.2   Recommended Dosing for Ovulation Induction
   2.3   Recommended Dosing for ART
   2.4   Recommended Dosing for Induction of Spermatogenesis in Men
3   DOSAGE FORM AND STRENGTHS
4   CONTRAINDICATIONS
5   WARNINGS AND PRECAUTIONS
   5.1   Abnormal Ovarian Enlargement
   5.2   Ovarian Hyperstimulation Syndrome
   5.3   Pulmonary and Vascular Complications
   5.4   Ovarian Torsion
   5.5   Multi-fetal Gestation and Birth
   5.6   Congenital Anomalies
   5.7   Ectopic Pregnancy
   5.8   Spontaneous Abortion
   5.9   Ovarian Neoplasm
   5.10   Laboratory Tests
   5.11   Follistim Pen
6   ADVERSE REACTIONS
   6.1   Clinical Study Experience
   6.2   Postmarketing Experience
7   DRUG INTERACTIONS
8   USE IN SPECIFIC POPULATIONS
   8.1   Pregnancy
   8.3   Nursing Mothers
   8.4   Pediatric Use
   8.5   Geriatric Use
10   OVERDOSAGE
11   DESCRIPTION
12   CLINICAL PHARMACOLOGY
   12.1   Mechanism of Action
   12.3   Pharmacokinetics
13   NONCLINICAL TOXICOLOGY
   13.1   Carcinogenesis and Mutagenesis, Impairment of Fertility
14   CLINICAL STUDIES
   14.1   Ovulation Induction
   14.2   Assisted Reproductive Technology
   14.3   Induction of Spermatogenesis
16   HOW SUPPLIED/STORAGE AND HANDLING
17   PATIENT COUNSELING INFORMATION
   17.1   Dosing and Use of Follistim AQ Cartridge with Pen
   17.2   Therapy Duration and Necessary Monitoring in Women and Men Undergoing Treatment
   17.3   Instructions on a Missed Dose
   17.4   Ovarian Hyperstimulation Syndrome
   17.5   Multi-fetal Gestation and Birth
* Sections or subsections omitted from the full prescribing information are not listed

——

FULL PRESCRIBING INFORMATION

1   INDICATIONS AND USAGE

Follistim® AQ (follitropin beta injection) Cartridge is indicated:
In Women for:
1.1   Induction of ovulation and pregnancy in anovulatory infertile women in whom the cause of infertility is functional and not due to primary ovarian failure
Prior to initiation of treatment with Follistim AQ Cartridge:
• Women should have a complete gynecologic and endocrinologic evaluation
• Primary ovarian failure should be excluded
• The possibility of pregnancy should be excluded
• Tubal patency should be demonstrated
• The fertility status of the male partner should be evaluated

1.2   Development of multiple follicles in ovulatory women participating in an Assisted Reproductive Technology (ART) program
Prior to initiation of treatment with Follistim AQ:
• Women should have a complete gynecologic and endocrinologic evaluation and diagnosis of cause of infertility
• The possibility of pregnancy should be excluded
• The fertility status of the male partner should be evaluated

In Men for:
1.3   Induction of spermatogenesis in men with primary and secondary hypogonadotropic hypogonadism (HH) in whom the cause of infertility is not due to primary testicular failure
Prior to initiation of treatment with Follistim AQ Cartridge:
• Men should have a complete medical and endocrinologic evaluation
• Hypogonadotropic hypogonadism should be confirmed and primary testicular failure should be excluded
• Serum testosterone levels should be normalized with human chorionic gonadotropin (hCG) treatment.
• The fertility status of the female partner should be evaluated

2 DOSAGE AND ADMINISTRATION

2.1 General Dosing Information

- Parenteral drug products should be inspected visually for particulate matter and discoloration prior to administration, whenever solution and container permit. If the solution is not clear and colorless or has particles in it, the solution should not be used
- Do not add any other medicines into the Follistim AQ Cartridge
- Follistim AQ Cartridge with the pen injector device delivers on average an 18% higher amount of follitropin beta when compare to reconstituted Follistim delivered with a conventional syringe and needle. When administering Follistim AQ Cartridge, a lower starting dose and lower dose adjustments (as compared to reconstituted Follistim) should be considered. For that purpose the following Dose Conversion Table is provided:

TABLE 1: Follistim AQ Cartridge Administered Subcutaneously With the Follistim Pen Dose Conversion Table*

Lyophilized recombinant FSH dosing in ampules or vials, using conventional syringe	Follistim AQ Cartridge dosing with the Follistim Pen
75 IU	50 IU
150 IU	125 IU
225 IU	175 IU
300 IU	250 IU
375 IU	300 IU
450 IU	375 IU

*Each value represents an 18% difference rounded to the nearest 25 IU increment.

2.2 Recommended Dosing for Ovulation Induction

The dosing scheme is stepwise and is individualized for each woman [see Clinical Studies (14.1)].

- A starting daily dose of 50 international units of Follistim AQ Cartridge is administered [see Dosage and Administration (2.1)] subcutaneously daily for at least the first 7 days
- Subsequent dosage adjustments are made at weekly intervals based upon ovarian response. If an Increase in dose is indicated by the ovarian response, the increase should be made by 25 or 50 international units of Follistim AQ Cartridge at weekly intervals until follicular growth and/or serum estradiol levels indicate an adequate ovarian response

The following should be considered when planning the woman's individualized dose:

- Appropriate Follistim AQ Cartridge dose adjustment(s) should be used to prevent multiple follicular growth and cycle cancellation
- The maximum, individualized, daily dose of Follistim AQ Cartridge is 250 international units
- Treatment should continue until ultrasonic visualizations and/or serum estradiol determinations approximate the pre-ovulatory conditions seen in normal individuals
- When pre-ovulatory conditions are reached, 5000 to 10,000 international units of hCG is used to induce final oocyte maturation and ovulation.

The administration of hCG must be withheld in cases where the ovarian monitoring suggests an increased risk of OHSS on the last day of Follistim AQ Cartridge therapy [see Warnings and Precautions (5.1, 5.2, 5.10)]

- The woman and her partner should be encouraged to have intercourse daily, beginning on the day prior to the administration of hCG and until ovulation becomes apparent [see Warnings and Precautions (5.10)]
- During treatment with Follistim AQ Cartridge and during a two-week post-treatment period, woman should be assessed at least every other day for signs of excessive ovarian stimulation.

It is recommended that Follistim AQ Cartridge administration be stopped if the ovarian monitoring suggests an increased risk of OHSS or abdominal pain occurs. Most OHSS occurs after treatment has been discontinued and reaches its maximum at about seven to ten days post-ovulation

2.3 Recommended Dosing for ART

The dosing scheme follows a stepwise approach and is individualized for each woman.

- A starting dose of 125 to 175 international units of Follistim AQ Cartridge is administered [see Dosage and Administration (2.1)] subcutaneously daily for at least the first 4 days of treatment

- Subsequent dosing beyond the first 4 days of treatment is adjusted based upon the woman's ovarian response as determined by ultrasound evaluation of follicular growth and serum estradiol levels

The following should be considered when planning the woman's individualized dose:

- For most normal responding women, the daily starting dose can be continued until pre-ovulatory conditions are achieved (six to twelve days)
- For low or poor responding women, the daily dose should be increased according to the ovarian response. The maximum, individualized, daily dose of Follistim AQ Cartridge is 500 international units
- For high responding women [those at particular risk of abnormal ovarian enlargement and/or ovarian hyperstimulation syndrome (OHSS)], decrease or temporarily stop the daily dose, or discontinue the cycle according to individual response [see Warnings and Precautions (5.1, 5.2, 5.10)]
- When a sufficient number of follicles of adequate size are present, dosing of Follistim AQ Cartridge is stopped and final maturation of the oocytes is induced by administering hCG at a dose of 5000 to 10,000 international units. The administration of hCG should be withheld in cases where the ovarian monitoring suggests an increased risk of OHSS on the last day of Follistim AQ Cartridge therapy [see Warnings and Precautions (5.1, 5.2, 5.10)]
- Oocyte (egg) retrieval should be performed 34 to 36 hours following the administration of hCG

2.4 Recommended Dosing for Induction of Spermatogenesis in Men

- Pretreatment with hCG is required prior to concomitant therapy with Follistim AQ Cartridge and hCG. An initial dosage of 1500 international units of hCG should be administered at twice weekly intervals to normalize serum testosterone levels. If serum testosterone levels have not normalized after 8 weeks of hCG treatment, the hCG dose can be increased to 3000 international units twice weekly [see Clinical Studies (14.3)]
- After normal serum testosterone levels have been reached, Follistim AQ Cartridge should be administered by subcutaneous injection concomitantly with hCG treatment. Follistim is given at a dosage of 450 international units per week, as either 225 international units twice weekly or 150 international units three times per week, in combination with the same hCG dose used to normalize testosterone levels. Based on delivery of a higher dose of follitropin beta with the Follistim AQ Cartridge and pen injector [see Dosage and Administration (2.1)], a lower dose of Follistim AQ Cartridge may be considered.

The concomitant therapy should be continued for at least 3 to 4 months before any improvement in spermatogenesis can be expected. If a man has not responded after this period, the combination therapy may be continued. Treatment response has been noted at up to 12 months.

3 DOSAGE FORM AND STRENGTHS

Follistim AQ Cartridge 175 international units per 0.210 mL

Follistim AQ Cartridge 350 international units per 0.420 mL

Follistim AQ Cartridge 650 international units per 0.780 mL

Follistim AQ Cartridge 975 international units per 1.170 mL

4 CONTRAINDICATIONS

Follistim AQ Cartridge is contraindicated in women and men who exhibit:

- Prior hypersensitivity to recombinant hFSH products
- High levels of FSH indicating primary gonadal failure
- Presence of uncontrolled non-gonadal endocrinopathies (e.g., thyroid, adrenal, or pituitary disorders) [see Indications and Usage (1.1, 1.2, 1.3)]
- Hypersensitivity reactions to streptomycin or neomycin. Follistim AQ may contain traces of these antibiotics
- Tumor of the ovary, breast, uterus, testis, hypothalamus or pituitary gland

Follistim AQ Cartridge is also contraindicated in women who exhibit:

- Pregnancy [see Use in Specific Populations (8.1)]
- Heavy or irregular vaginal bleeding of undetermined origin
- Ovarian cysts or enlargement not due to polycystic ovary syndrome (PCOS)

5 WARNINGS AND PRECAUTIONS

Follistim AQ Cartridge should be used only by physicians who are experienced in infertility treatment. Follistim AQ Cartridge contains a potent gonadotropic substance capable of causing Ovarian Hyperstimulation Syndrome (OHSS) [see Warnings and Precautions (5.2)] with or without pulmonary or vascular complications [see Warnings and Precautions (5.3)] and multiple births [see Warnings and Precau-

tions (5.5)]. Gonadotropin therapy requires the availability of appropriate monitoring facilities [see Warnings and Precautions (5.10)].

Careful attention should be given to the diagnosis of infertility and in the selection of candidates for Follistim AQ Cartridge therapy [see Indications and Usage (1.1, 1.2, 1.3) and Dosage and Administration (2.2, 2.3, 2.4)].

Switching to Follistim AQ Cartridge from other brands (manufacturer), types (recombinant, urinary, etc.), and/or methods of administration (Follistim Pen, conventional syringe, etc.) may necessitate an adjustment of the dose [see Dosage and Administration (2)].

5.1 Abnormal Ovarian Enlargement

In order to minimize the hazards associated with abnormal ovarian enlargement that may occur with Follistim AQ therapy, treatment should be individualized and the lowest effective dose should be used [see Dosage and Administration (2.2, 2.3)]. Use of ultrasound monitoring of ovarian response and/or measurement of serum estradiol levels is important to minimize the risk of overstimulation [see Warnings and Precautions (5.8)].

If the ovaries are abnormally enlarged on the last day of Follistim AQ therapy, hCG should not be administered in order to reduce the chances of developing Ovarian Hyperstimulation Syndrome (OHSS). Intercourse should be prohibited in patients with significant ovarian enlargement after ovulation because of the danger of hemoperitoneum resulting from ruptured ovarian cysts [see Warnings and Precautions (5.3)].

5.2 Ovarian Hyperstimulation Syndrome

OHSS is a medical entity distinct from uncomplicated ovarian enlargement and may progress rapidly to become a serious medical condition. OHSS is characterized by a dramatic increase in vascular permeability, which can result in a rapid accumulation of fluid in the peritoneal cavity, thorax, and potentially, the pericardium. The early warning signs of OHSS developing are severe pelvic pain, nausea, vomiting, and weight gain. Abdominal pain, abdominal distension, gastrointestinal symptoms including nausea, vomiting and diarrhea, severe ovarian enlargement, weight gain, dyspnea, and oliguria have been reported with OHSS. Clinical evaluation may reveal hypovolemia, hemoconcentration, electrolyte imbalances, ascites, hemoperitoneum, pleural effusions, hydrothorax, acute pulmonary distress, and thromboembolic reactions [see Warnings and Precautions (5.3)]. Transient liver function test abnormalities suggestive of hepatic dysfunction with or without morphologic changes on liver biopsy have also been reported in association with OHSS.

OHSS occurs after gonadotropin treatment has been discontinued and it can develop rapidly, reaching its maximum about seven to ten days following treatment. Usually, OHSS resolves spontaneously with the onset of menses. If there is evidence that OHSS may be developing prior to hCG administration [see Warnings and Precautions (5.1)], the hCG must be withheld. Cases of OHSS are more common, more severe, and more protracted if pregnancy occurs; therefore, women should be assessed for the development of OHSS for at least two weeks after hCG administration.

If serious OHSS occurs, treatment should be stopped and the patient should be hospitalized. Treatment is primarily symptomatic and overall should consist of bed rest, fluid and electrolyte management, and analgesics (if needed). Because the use of diuretics can accentuate the diminished intravascular volume, diuretics should be avoided except in the late phase of resolution as described below. The management of OHSS may be divided into three phases as follows:

- *Acute Phase:*
Management should be directed at preventing hemoconcentration due to loss of intravascular volume to the third space and minimizing the risk of thromboembolic phenomena and kidney damage. Fluid intake and output, weight, hematocrit, serum and urinary electrolytes, urine specific gravity, BUN and creatinine, total proteins with albumin: globulin ratio, coagulation studies, electrocardiogram to monitor for hyperkalemia, and abdominal girth should be thoroughly assessed daily or more often based on the clinical need. Treatment, consisting of limited intravenous fluids, electrolytes, human serum albumin, is intended to normalize electrolytes while maintaining an acceptable but somewhat reduced intravascular volume. Full correction of the intravascular volume deficit may lead to an unacceptable increase in the amount of third space fluid accumulation.

- *Chronic Phase:*
After the acute phase is successfully managed as above, excessive fluid accumulation in the third space should be limited by instituting severe potassium, sodium, and fluid restriction.

- *Resolution Phase:*
As third space fluid returns to the intravascular compartment, a fall in hematocrit and increasing urinary output are observed in the absence of any increase in intake.

Peripheral and/or pulmonary edema may result if the kidneys are unable to excrete third space fluid as rapidly as it is mobilized. Diuretics may be indicated during the resolution phase, if necessary, to combat pulmonary edema. OHSS increases the risk of injury to the ovary. The ascitic, pleural, and pericardial fluid should not be removed unless there is the necessity to relieve symptoms such as pulmonary distress or cardiac tamponade. Pelvic examination may cause rupture of an ovarian cyst, which may result in hemoperitoneum, and should therefore be avoided. If bleeding occurs and requires surgical intervention, the clinical objective should be to control the bleeding and retain as much ovarian tissue as possible. During clinical trials with Follistim therapy, OHSS occurred in 7.6% of 105 women (OI) and 5.2% of 591 women (ART) treated with Follistim.

5.3 Pulmonary and Vascular Complications

Serious pulmonary conditions (e.g., atelectasis, acute respiratory distress syndrome) have been reported in women treated with gonadotropins. In addition, thromboembolic reactions both in association with, and separate from OHSS have been reported following gonadotropin therapy. Intravascular thrombosis, which may originate in venous or arterial vessels, can result in reduced blood flow to vital organs or the extremities. Women with generally recognized risk factors for thrombosis, such as a personal or family history, severe obesity, or thrombophilia, may have an increased risk of venous or arterial thrombo-embolic events, during or following treatment with gonadotropins. Sequelae of such reactions have included venous thrombophlebitis, pulmonary embolism, pulmonary infarction, cerebral vascular occlusion (stroke), and arterial occlusion resulting in loss of limb and rarely in myocardial infarction. In rare cases, pulmonary complications and/or thromboembolic reactions have resulted in death. In women with recognized risk factors, the benefits of ovulation induction or in vitro fertilization (IVF) treatment need to be weighed against the risks. It should be noted, that pregnancy itself also carries an increased risk of thrombosis.

5.4 Ovarian Torsion

Ovarian torsion has been reported after treatment with Follistim AQ and after intervention with other gonadotropins. This may be related to OHSS, pregnancy, previous abdominal surgery, past history of ovarian torsion, previous or current ovarian cyst and polycystic ovaries. Damage to the ovary due to reduced blood supply can be limited by early diagnosis and immediate detorsion.

5.5 Multi-fetal Gestation and Birth

Multi-fetal gestation and births have been reported with all gonadotopin treatments including Follistim AQ treatment. The woman and her partner should be advised of the potential risk of multi-fetal gestation and births before starting treatment.

5.6 Congenital Anomalies

The incidence of congenital malformations after ART may be slightly higher than after spontaneous conception. This slightly higher incidence is thought to be related to differences in parental characteristics (e.g., maternal age, sperm characteristics) and to the higher incidence of multi-fetal gestations after ART. There are no indications that the use of gonadotropins during ART is associated with an increased risk of congenital malformations.

5.7 Ectopic Pregnancy

Since infertile women undergoing ART, and particularly IVF, often have tubal abnormalities the incidence of ectopic pregnancies might be increased. Early confirmation of an intrauterine pregnancy should be determined by hCG testing and transvaginal ultrasound.

5.8 Spontaneous Abortion

The risk of spontaneous abortions (miscarriage) is increased with gonadotropin products. However, causality has not been established. The increased risk may be a factor of the underlying infertility.

5.9 Ovarian Neoplasm

There have been infrequent reports of ovarian neoplasms, both benign and malignant, in women who have undergone multiple drug regimens for ovulation induction; however, a causal relationship has not been established.

5.10 Laboratory Tests

For Women:
In most instances, treatment with Follistim AQ will result only in follicular growth and maturation. In order to complete the final phase of follicular maturation and to induce ovulation, hCG must be given following the administration of Follistim AQ Cartridge or when clinical assessment indicates that sufficient follicular maturation has occurred. The degree of follicular maturation and the timing of hCG administration can both be determined with the use of sonographic visualization of the ovaries and endometrial lining in conjunction with measurement of serum estradiol levels. The combination of transvaginal ultrasonography and measurement of serum estradiol levels is also useful for minimizing the risk of OHSS and multi-fetal gestation. The clinical confirmation of ovulation is obtained by the following direct or indirect indices of progesterone production as well as sonographic evidence of ovulation. Direct or indirect indices of progesterone production are:

- Urinary or serum luteinizing hormone (LH) rise
- A rise in basal body temperature
- Increase in serum progesterone
- Menstruation following the shift in basal body temperature

The following provide sonographic evidence of ovulation:
- Collapsed follicle
- Fluid in the cul-de-sac
- Features consistent with corpus luteum formation

Sonographic evaluation of the early pregnancy is also important to rule out ectopic pregnancy.

For Men:
Clinical monitoring for spermatogenesis utilizes the following indirect or direct measures:
- Serum testosterone level
- Semen analysis

5.11 Follistim Pen

The Follistim Pen is intended only for use with Follistim AQ Cartridge. The Follistim Pen is not recommended for the blind or visually impaired without the assistance of an individual with good vision who is trained in the proper use of the injection device.

6 ADVERSE REACTIONS

The following serious adverse reactions are discussed elsewhere in the labeling:
- Ovarian Hyperstimulation Syndrome [see Warnings and Precautions (5.2)]
- Atelectasis [see Warnings and Precautions (5.3)]
- Thromboembolism [see Warnings and Precautions (5.3)]
- Ovarian Torsion [see Warnings and Precautions (5.4)]
- Multi-fetal Gestation [see Warnings and Precautions (5.5)]
- Congenital Anomalies [see Warnings and Precautions (5.6)]
- Ectopic Pregnancy [see Warnings and Precautions (5.7)]
- Spontaneous Abortion [see Warnings and Precautions (5.8)]

6.1 Clinical Study Experience

Because clinical trials are conducted under widely varying conditions, adverse reactions rates observed in the clinical trials of a drug cannot be directly compared to rates in the clinical trial of another drug and may not reflect the rates observed in practice.

Ovulation Induction
In a single cycle, multi-center, assessor-blind, parallel group, comparative study, a total of 172 chronic anovulatory women who had failed to ovulate and/or conceive with clomiphene citrate therapy, were randomized and treated with Follistim (105) or a urofollitropin comparator. Adverse reactions with an incidence of greater than 2% in either treatment group are listed in Table 2.

Table 2: Common Adverse Reactions Reported at a Frequency of ≥ 2% in an Assessor Blind, Comparative Study of Women Receiving Ovulation Induction

System Organ Class/ Adverse Reactions	Treatment Number (%) of Women	
	Follistim N= 105 n (%)	Comparator N=67 n (%)
Gastrointestinal disorders		
Abdominal discomfort	3 (2.9)	1 (1.5)
Abdominal pain	3 (2.9)	2 (3.0)
Abdominal pain lower	3 (2.9)	1 (1.5)
Reproductive system and breast disorders		
Ovarian cyst	3 (2.9)	2 (3.0)
Ovarian hyperstimulation syndrome	8 (7.6)	3 (4.5)
General disorders and administration site conditions		
Pyrexia	0 (0.0)	2 (3.0)

Adverse reactions reported commonly (greater than or equal to 2 % of women treated with Follistim) in other ovulation induction clinical trials were headache, abdominal distension, constipation, diarrhea, nausea, pelvic pain, uterine enlargement, vaginal hemorrhage and injection site reaction

The following medical events have been reported subsequent to pregnancies resulting from FOLLISTIM AQ Cartridge therapy:
- Ectopic pregnancy [see Warnings and Precautions (5.7)]
- Spontaneous abortion [see Warnings and Precautions (5.8)]

ART
In a multiple cycle, multi-center, assessor-blind, parallel group, comparative study, after pituitary suppression with a gonadotropin release hormone (GnRH) agonist, a total of 989 women were randomized and treated with Follistim (N=591) or a urofollitropin comparator as part of in vitro fertilization therapy (IVF). Adverse reactions with an incidence of greater than 2% in either treatment group are listed in Table 3.

Table 3: Common Adverse Reactions Reported at a Frequency of ≥ 2% in an Assessor-Blind, Comparative Study of Women Receiving In Vitro Fertilization (IVF)

System Organ Class/ Adverse Reactions	Treatment Number (%) of Women	
	Follistim N= 591 n (%)	Comparator N=398 n (%)
Gastrointestinal disorders		
Abdominal pain	13 (2.2)	4 (1.0)
Reproductive system and breast disorders		
Ovarian hyperstimulation syndrome	31 (5.2)	17 (4.3)

Adverse reactions reported commonly (greater than or equal to 2 % of women treated with Follistim) in other IVF clinical trials were headache, abdominal distension, constipation, diarrhea, nausea, pelvic pain, breast tenderness, metrorrhagia, ovarian enlargement, vaginal hemorrhage, injection site reaction and rash.

The following medical events have been reported subsequent to pregnancies resulting from FOLLISTIM AQ Cartridge therapy:
- Ectopic pregnancy [see Warnings and Precautions (5.7)]
- Spontaneous abortion [see Warnings and Precautions (5.8)]

Induction of Spermatogenesis
In an open-label, non-comparative clinical trial, 49 men with hypogonadotropic hypogonadism were enrolled to received pretreatment with hCG, followed by combination therapy with hCG and Follistim for induction of spermatogenesis. Of the 49 men, 30 received weekly Follistim doses of 450 international units; 24 of these 30 men received a total of 48 weeks of treatment with Follistim. Adverse reactions occurring with an incidence of greater than 2% in the 30 men treated with FOLLISTIM are listed in Table 4.

Table 4: Common Adverse Reactions Reported At a Frequency of ≥ 2% in an Open-Label Clinical Trial in Men with Hypogonadotropic Hypogonadism

System Organ Class/ Adverse Reactions	Follistim Treatment N=30 n (%)
Nervous system disorders	
Headache	2 (6.7)
General disorders and administration site disorders	
Injection site reaction	2 (6.7)
Injection site pain	2 (6.7)
Skin and cutaneous tissue disorders	
Acne	2 (6.7)
Rash	1 (3.3)
Reproductive system and breast disorders	
Gynecomastia	1 (3.3)
Neoplasms benign, malignant and unspecified	
Dermoid cyst	1 (3.3)

6.2 Postmarketing Experience

The following adverse reactions have been identified during post approval use of Follistim and/or Follistim AQ Cartridge. Because these reactions are reported voluntarily from a population of uncertain size, it is not always possible to reliably estimate their frequency or establish a causal relationship to drug exposure.

Vascular disorders
Thromboembolism [see Warnings and Precautions (5.3)]

7 DRUG INTERACTIONS

No drug-drug interaction studies have been performed.

8 USE IN SPECIFIC POPULATIONS

8.1 Pregnancy

Pregnancy Category X: Follistim AQ Cartridge should not be used during pregnancy [see Contraindications (4)]

8.3 Nursing Mothers

It is not known whether this drug is excreted in human milk. Because many drugs are excreted in human milk and because of the potential for serious adverse reactions in the nursing infant from Follistim AQ Cartridge, a decision should be made whether to discontinue nursing or to discontinue the drug, taking into account the importance of the drug to the mother.

8.4 Pediatric Use

Safety and effectiveness in pediatric patients have not been established.

8.5 Geriatric Use

Clinical studies of Follistim did not include subjects aged 65 and over.

10 OVERDOSAGE

Aside from the possibility of Ovarian Hyperstimulation Syndrome *[see Warnings and Precautions (5.2, 5.3)]* and multiple gestations *[see Warnings and Precaution (5.5)]*, there is no additional information concerning the consequences of acute overdosage with Follistim AQ Cartridge.

11 DESCRIPTION

Follistim AQ Cartridge contains human follicle-stimulating hormone (hFSH), a glycoprotein hormone which is manufactured by recombinant DNA (rDNA) technology. The active drug substance, follitropin beta, has a dimeric structure containing two glycoprotein subunits (alpha and beta). Both the 92 amino acid alpha-chain and the 111 amino acid beta-chain have complex heterogeneous structures arising from two N-linked oligosaccharide chains. Follitropin beta is synthesized in a Chinese hamster ovary (CHO) cell line that has been transfected with a plasmid containing the two subunit DNA sequences encoding for hFSH. The purification process results in a highly purified preparation with a consistent hFSH isoform profile and high specific activity [as determined by the Ph. Eur. test for FSH *in vivo* bioactivity and on the basis of the molar extinction coefficient at 277 nm (ϵ_s:$mg^{-1}cm^{-1}$) = 1.066].

The biological activity is determined by measuring the increase in ovary weight in female rats. The intrinsic luteinizing hormone (LH) activity in follitropin beta is less than 1 international unit per 40,000 international units FSH. The compound is considered to contain no LH activity.

The amino acid sequence and tertiary structure of the product are indistinguishable from that of hFSH of urinary source. Also, based on available data derived from physicochemical tests and bioassay, follitropin beta and follitropin alfa, another recombinant follicle-stimulating hormone product, are indistinguishable.

Follistim AQ Cartridge is a ready for use, prefilled with solution, disposable cartridge containing either 175 IU of follitropin beta in 0.210 mL (833 IU/mL), 350 IU in 0.420 mL (833 IU/mL), 650 IU in 0.780 mL (833 IU/mL) or 975 IU in 1.170 mL (833 IU/mL) of aqueous solution for multiple dose use, with a maximal deliverable dose of either 150 IU, 300 IU, 600 IU or 900 IU, respectively. Inactive ingredients in the cartridges include: benzyl alcohol, NF 10 mg/mL; L-methionine, USP 0.5 mg/mL; polysorbate 20, NF 0.2 mg/mL; sodium citrate (dihydrate), USP 14.7 mg/mL; sucrose, NF 50 mg/mL; and water for injection, USP. Hydrochloric acid, NF and/or sodium hydroxide, NF are used to adjust the pH to 7.

Follistim AQ Cartridge is for use only with the Follistim Pen, which features an adjustable dosing system for administering the drug in a microvolume of solution. The Follistim Pen with Follistim AQ Cartridge is intended for SUBCUTANEOUS USE ONLY. .The recombinant protein in Follistim AQ Cartridge has been standardized for FSH *in vivo* bioactivity in terms of the WHO International Standard for Follicle Stimulating Hormone. (FSH) Recombinant, Human for Bioassay (code 92/642), issued by the World Health Organization Expert Committee on Biological Standardization (1995). Under current storage conditions, Follistim AQ may contain up to 11% of oxidized follitropin beta.

In clinical trials with Follistim, serum antibodies to FSH or anti-CHO cell derived proteins were not detected in any of the treated patients after exposure to Follistim for up to three cycles.

Therapeutic Class: Infertility.

12 CLINICAL PHARMACOLOGY

12.1 Mechanism of Action

Women:

Follicle-stimulating hormone (FSH), the active component in Follistim AQ Cartridge, is required for normal follicular growth, maturation, and gonadal steroid production.

In women, the level of FSH is critical for the onset and duration of follicular development, and consequently for the timing and number of follicles reaching maturity. Follistim AQ Cartridge stimulates ovarian follicular growth in women who do not have primary ovarian failure. In order to effect the final phase of follicle maturation, resumption of meiosis and rupture of the follicle in the absence of an endogenous LH surge, human chorionic gonadotropin (hCG) must be given following treatment with Follistim AQ Cartridge when patient monitoring indicates appropriate follicular development parameters have been reached.

Men:

Follistim when administered with hCG stimulates spermatogenesis in men with hypogonadotropic hypogonadism. FSH, the active component of Follistim, is the pituitary hormone responsible for spermatogenesis.

12.3 Pharmacokinetics

Pharmacokinetic parameters for Follistim AQ Cartridge were evaluated in an open-labeled, single-center, randomized study in 20 healthy women. Serum FSH values from a single subcutaneous injection of reconstituted Follistim lyophilized powder administered by conventional syringe were compared to those values following a single subcutaneous injection of Follistim AQ Cartridge administered with the Follistim Pen injector. Administration of follitropin beta with the Follistim Pen resulted an 18% increase in $AUC_{0-\infty}$ and C_{max}. The 18% difference in serum FSH concentrations resulting from administration of the two formulations was due to differences between the anticipated and actual volume delivered with the conventional syringe. The pharmacokinetic parameters for Follistim AQ Cartridge are as follows:

[See table 5 below]

Absorption:

Women:

The bioavailability of Follistim following subcutaneous and intramuscular administration was investigated in healthy, pituitary-suppressed, women given a single 300 international units dose. In these women, the area under the curve (AUC), expressed as the mean ± SD, was equivalent between the subcutaneous (455.6 ± 141.4 IU*h/L) and intramuscular (445.7 ± 135.7 IU*h/L) routes of administration. However, equivalence could not be established with respect to the peak serum FSH levels (C_{max}). The C_{max} achieved after subcutaneous administration and intramuscular administration was 5.41 ± 0.72 international units/L and 6.86 ± 2.90 international units/L, respectively. After subcutaneous or intramuscular injection the apparent dose absorbed was 77.8% and 76.4%, respectively.

The pharmacokinetics and pharmacodynamics of a single, intramuscular dose (300 international units) of Follistim were also investigated in a group (n=8) of gonadotropin-deficient, but otherwise healthy women. In these women, FSH (mean ± SD) AUC was 339 ± 105 international units*h/L, C_{max} was 4.3 ± 1.7 international units/L. C_{max} occurred at approximately 27 ± 5.4 hours after intramuscular administration.

A multiple dose, dose proportionality, pharmacokinetic study of Follistim was completed in healthy, pituitary-suppressed, female subjects given subcutaneous doses of 75, 150, or 225 international units for 7 days. Steady-state blood concentrations of FSH were reached with all doses after 5 days of treatment based on the trough concentrations of FSH just prior to dosing (C_{trough}). Peak blood concentrations with the 75, 150, and 225 international units dose were 4.30 ± 0.60 international units/L, 8.51 ± 1.16 international units/L and 13.92 ± 1.81 international units/L, respectively.

Men:

No PK studies were conducted using Follistim AQ Cartridge in men. Exposures of follitropin beta from Follistim AQ Cartridge and Follistim are expected to be equivalent after adjusting for the 18% difference in dose *[see Dosage and Administration (2)]*.

Serum levels of FSH were measured in a clinical study that compared the effects of two different dosing schedules of Follistim (150 international units three times a week or 225 international units twice a week) administered by subcutaneous injection concurrently with chorionic gonadotropin for induction of spermatogenesis in hypogonadotropic hypogonadal men. Administration of Follistim was started at week 17. Mean serum trough concentrations of FSH remained fairly constant over the treatment period. At the end of treatment (week 64), the mean serum trough concentrations of FSH were 2.09 international units/L in the 150 international units group and 3.22 international units/L in the 225 international units group. Serum trough concentrations of FSH measured prior to the first Follistim injection on the Mondays of active treatment period (weeks 17 to 64) and one week after the end of treatment period are presented in Figure 1.

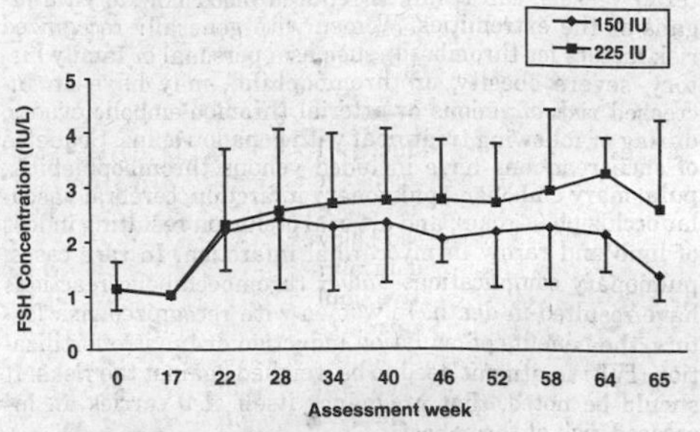

FIGURE 1: Mean (SD) Serum Trough Concentrations of FSH in Men Following Subcutaneous Administration of Follistim Using Two Different Dosing Schedules (150 International Units Three Times a Week or 225 International Units Twice a Week)

Distribution:

The volume of distribution of Follistim in healthy, pituitary-suppressed, women following intravenous administration of a 300 international units dose was approximately 8 L.

Metabolism:

The recombinant FSH in Follistim AQ Cartridge is biochemically very similar to urinary FSH and it is therefore anticipated that it is metabolized in the same manner.

Elimination:

The elimination half-life ($t_{1/2}$) following a single subcutaneous injection of 150 IU of Follistim AQ Cartridge in women was 33.4 (4.2) hours. The clearance was 0.01 (0.003) L/h/kg.

Use in Specific Populations:

Body weight: The effect of body weight on the pharmacokinetics of Follistim was evaluated in a group of European and Japanese women who were significantly different in terms of body weight. The European women had a body weight of (mean ± SD) 67.4 ± 13.5 kg and the Japanese subjects were 46.8 ± 11.6 kg. Following a single intramuscular dose of 300 international units of Follistim, the AUC was significantly smaller in European women (339 ± 105 international units*h/L) than in Japanese women (544 ± 201 international units*h/L). However, clearance per kg of body weight was essentially the same for the respective groups (0.014 and 0.013 L/hr/kg).

Geriatric Use: The pharmacokinetics of Follistim has not been studied in geriatric subjects.

Pediatric Use: The pharmacokinetics of Follistim has not been studied in pediatric subjects.

Renal Impairment: The effect of renal impairment on the pharmacokinetics of Follistim has not been studied.

Hepatic Impairment: The effect of hepatic impairment on the pharmacokinetics of Follistim has not been studied.

13 NONCLINICAL TOXICOLOGY

13.1 Carcinogenesis and Mutagenesis, Impairment of Fertility

Long-term toxicity studies in animals have not been performed with Follistim to evaluate the carcinogenic potential of the drug. Follistim was not mutagenic in the Ames test using *S. typhimurium* and *E. coli* tester strains and did not produce chromosomal aberrations in an *in vitro* assay using human lymphocytes.

14 CLINICAL STUDIES

14.1 Ovulation Induction

The efficacy of Follistim for Ovulation Induction was evaluated in a randomized, assessor-blind, parallel-group comparative, multicenter safety and efficacy study of 172 chronic anovulatory women (105 subjects on Follistim) who had previously failed to ovulate and/or conceive during clomiphene citrate treatment. The study results for ovulation rates are summarized in Table 6 and those for pregnancy rates are summarized in Table 7.

Table 5: Mean (SD) Pharmacokinetic Parameters of a Single Subcutaneous Injection of 150 IU of Follistim AQ Cartridge (n=20)

	$AUC_{0-\infty}$ (IU/L*h)	C_{max} (IU/L)	t_{max} (h)	$t_{1/2}$ (h)	CL_{app} (L/h/kg)
Follistim AQ Cartridge	215.1 (45.8)	3.4 (0.7)	12.9 (6.2)	33.4 (4.2)	0.01 (0.003)

$AUC_{0-\infty}$ Area under the curve
C_{max} Maximum concentration
t_{max} Time to maximum concentration
$t_{1/2}$ Elimination half-life
CL_{app} Clearance

Table 6: Cumulative Ovulation Rates

Cycle	Follistim (n=105)
First treatment cycle	72%
Second treatment cycle	82%
Third treatment cycle	85%

Table 7: Cumulative Ongoing*,† Pregnancy Rates

Cycle	Follistim (n=105)
First treatment cycle	14%
Second treatment cycle	19%
Third treatment cycle	23%

*All ongoing pregnancies were confirmed after at least 12 weeks after the hCG injection.
†Study was not powered to demonstrate this outcome.

14.2 Assisted Reproductive Technology

The efficacy of Follistim as part of an Assisted Reproductive Technology (ART) program was established in three studies, two of which are described below.

Follistim was evaluated in a randomized, assessor-blind, parallel-group, comparative, multicenter safety and efficacy study of 981 healthy normal ovulatory infertile women (mean age 32) treated for multiple cycles with *in vitro* fertilization and controlled ovarian stimulation with Follistim (n=585) or urofollitropin (n=396) after pituitary suppression with a GnRH agonist. The first cycle results with Follistim are summarized in Table 8.

Table 8: Results of First Cycle Treatment of Infertile Women with Follistim and In Vitro Fertilization after Pituitary Suppression With a GnRH Agonist*

Parameter	Follistim (n=585)
Total number of oocytes recovered	10.9
Ongoing† pregnancy rate/attempt‡	22.2%
Ongoing† pregnancy rate/transfer‡,§	26.0%

*All values are means.
†A single vital or multiple vital pregnancy was termed ongoing when a pregnancy, at least 12 weeks after embryo transfer (ET), was confirmed by the investigator.
‡Study was not powered to demonstrate these secondary endpoints.
§Transfers were limited to a maximum of three embryos.

Follistim was also evaluated in a randomized, assessor-blind, parallel-group, comparative, single center safety and efficacy study in 89 infertile healthy normal ovulatory women (mean age 32) treated for one cycle with *in vitro* fertilization and controlled ovarian stimulation with Follistim (n=54) or menotropins (n=35) without pituitary suppression with a GnRH agonist. The results with Follistim are summarized in Table 9.

Table 9: Results of Single Cycle Treatment of Infertile Women Treated With In Vitro Fertilization and Follistim without Pituitary Suppression*

Parameter	Follistim (n=54)
Total number of oocytes recovered	9.9
Ongoing† pregnancy rate/attempt‡	22.2%
Ongoing† pregnancy rate/transfer‡,§	30.8%

*All values are means.
†A single vital or multiple vital pregnancy was termed ongoing when a pregnancy, at least 12 weeks after embryo transfer (ET), was confirmed by the investigator.
‡Study was not powered to demonstrate these secondary endpoints.
§Transfers were limited to a maximum of three embryos.

14.3 Induction of Spermatogenesis

The safety and efficacy of Follistim administered by subcutaneous injection concomitantly chorionic gonadotropin for injection (hCG) has been examined in a multicenter, open-

Table 10: Number of Men Receiving Follistim Who Achieved a Mean Sperm Density of ≥10⁶/mL on Their Last Two Treatment Assessments

Sperm Density of $\geq 10^6$/mL	Follistim 150 international units three times a week (n=15)		Follistim 225 international units twice a week (n=15)		Overall (n=30)	
	n	%	n	%	n	%
Yes	6	40	7	47	13	43
No	9	60	8	53	17	57

label, non-comparator clinical study for induction of spermatogenesis in hypogonadotropic hypogonadal men. The study compared the effects of two different Follistim dosing schedules on semen parameters and serum levels of follicle stimulating hormone (FSH). The multicenter study involved a 16-week pretreatment phase with hCG at a dosage of 1500 international units twice a week to normalize serum testosterone levels. If serum testosterone levels did not normalize after 8 weeks of hCG treatment, the hCG dose could have been increased to 3000 international units twice a week. This phase was followed by a 48-week treatment phase. Men who were still azoospermic after the pretreatment phase were randomized to receive either 225 international units Follistim together with 1500 international units hCG twice a week or 150 international units Follistim three times a week together with 1500 international units hCG twice weekly. Men who required 3000 international units of hCG twice a week in the pretreatment phase were continued on that dosage during the treatment phase. The mean age of patients in both treatment groups was approximately 30 years (range 18 to 47 years). At baseline, mean left and right testis volumes were 4.61 ± 2.94 mL and 4.57 ± 3.00 mL, respectively, in the group receiving three weekly injections of Follistim. For the group receiving two weekly injections of Follistim, the mean left and right testis volumes were 6.54 ± 2.45 mL and 7.21 ± 2.94 mL, respectively, at baseline. The primary efficacy endpoint was the percentage of patients with a mean sperm density of $\geq 1 \times 10^6$/mL on their last two treatment assessments. The outcomes of treatment in the 30 men enrolled in the treatment phase are summarized in Table 10.
[See table 10 above]
Overall, the median time to reach a sperm concentration of 10^6 per mL was 165 days (range 25 to 327 days) in patients who demonstrated a sperm concentration of at least 10^6 per mL. The median time to reach a sperm concentration of at least 10^6 per mL was 186 days (range 25 to 327 days) for the 150 international units group and 141 days (range 43 to 204 days) for the 225 international units group. No pregnancy data were collected during the trial.
The local tolerance data were comparable between the two treatment groups. The mean percentage of days without pain calculated for all subjects in the treatment period was 91.3% for patients in the 150 international units (three times a week) and 76.0% for patients in the 225 international units (two times a week) Follistim treatment groups. In the 225 international units (twice per week) group, local symptoms judged as severe by the investigator were: itching in 1 patient (7%) , pain in 2 patients (13%), bruising in 2 patients (13%), swelling in 2 patients (13%), and redness in 1 patient (7%). In the 150 international units (three times per week) group, 1 event in 1 patient (bruising, 7%) was judged as severe. No patient discontinued treatment due to injection site reaction or injection site pain.

16 HOW SUPPLIED/STORAGE AND HANDLING

Follistim AQ Cartridge is supplied in a box containing disposable, 29 gauge, ultra-fine, ½-inch, sterile BD Micro-Fine™ Pen Needles (for use with Follistim Pen available separately) and one disposable, blister packed, prefilled 1.5 mL colorless glass cartridge, with grey rubber piston and an aluminum crimp-cap with black rubber inlay and in the following presentations:
• NDC 0052-0303-01 Follistim AQ Cartridge 175 international units per 0.210 mL (delivering 150 international units) with orange crimp-caps and 3 BD Micro-Fine Pen Needles
• NDC 0052-0313-01 Follistim AQ Cartridge 350 international units per 0.420 mL (delivering 300 international units) with silver crimp-caps and 5 BD Micro-Fine Pen Needles
• NDC 0052-0316-01 Follistim AQ Cartridge 650 international units per 0.780 mL (delivering 600 international units) with gold crimp-caps and 7 BD Micro-Fine Pen Needles
• NDC 0052-0326-01 Follistim AQ Cartridge 975 international units per 1.170 mL (delivering 900 international units) with blue crimp-caps and 10 BD Micro-Fine Pen Needles

Store refrigerated 2–8°C (36–46°F) until dispensed. Upon dispensing, the product may be stored by the patient at 2–8°C (36–46°F) until the expiration date, or at 25°C (77°F) for 3 months or until expiration date, whichever occurs first. Once the rubber inlay of the Follistim AQ Cartridge has been pierced by a needle, the product can only be stored for a maximum of 28 days at 2–25°C (36–77°F). Protect from light. Do not freeze.

17 PATIENT COUNSELING INFORMATION

See FDA-Approved Patient Labeling

17.1 Dosing and Use of Follistim AQ Cartridge with Pen
Instruct women and men on the correct usage and dosing of Follistim AQ Cartridge in conjunction with the Follistim Pen. Make sure that individuals who have used other gonadotropin products delivered by a syringe are aware of differences arising from use of the pen. Women and men should read and follow all instructions in the Follistim Pen "Instructions for Use" Manual prior to administration of Follistim AQ Cartridge.
Advise women and men of the number of doses which can be extracted from the full unused Follistim AQ Cartridge that you have prescribed.

17.2 Therapy Duration and Necessary Monitoring in Women and Men Undergoing Treatment
Prior to beginning therapy with Follistim AQ Cartridge, inform women and men about the time commitment and monitoring procedures necessary to undergo treatment [see Dosage and Administration (2), Warnings and Precautions (5.10)].

17.3 Instructions on a Missed Dose
Inform women and men that if they miss or forget to take a dose of Follistim AQ Cartridge, the next dose should not be doubled and they should call the healthcare provider for further dosing instructions.

17.4 Ovarian Hyperstimulation Syndrome
Inform women regarding the risks with use of Follistim AQ Cartridge of Ovarian Hyperstimulation Syndrome [see Warnings and Precautions (5.2)] and associated symptoms including lung and blood vessel problems [see Warnings and Precautions (5.3)] and ovarian torsion [see Warnings and Precautions (5.4)].

17.5 Multi-fetal Gestation and Birth
Inform women regarding the risk of multi-fetal gestations with the use of Follistim AQ Cartridge [see Warnings and Precautions (5.5)].

Manufactured by: Vetter Pharma-Fertigung GmbH & Co. KG, Ravensburg, Germany
Distributed by: Schering Corporation, a subsidiary of MERCK & CO., INC., Whitehouse Station, NJ 08889, USA

PATIENT INFORMATION
FOLLISTIM® (Fol-lis-tim) AQ Cartridge
(follitropin beta injection)
Read the Patient Information that comes with FOLLISTIM® AQ Cartridge before you start using it and each time you get a refill. There may be new information. This information does not take the place of talking with your healthcare provider about your medical condition or treatment.

What is Follistim AQ Cartridge?
Follistim AQ is a prescription medicine that contains follicle-stimulating hormone (FSH). The medicine is taken with the Follistim Pen.

Follistim AQ Cartridge is used:
In women:
• to help healthy ovaries to develop (mature) and release eggs
• as part of an Assisted Reproductive Technology (ART) program to help the ovaries produce more mature eggs
In men:
• to help bring about the production and development of sperm

Who should not take Follistim AQ Cartridge?
Do not take Follistim AQ Cartridge if you are a Woman or Man who:
• is allergic to recombinant human FSH products
• has a high level of FSH in your blood indicating that your ovaries (women only) or testes (men only) may be permanently damaged and do not work at all.

- has uncontrolled thyroid, pituitary, or adrenal gland problems
- is allergic to streptomycin or neomycin (types of antibiotics)
- has a tumor of the hypothalamus, pituitary gland, breast, uterus (women only), ovary (women only), or testis (men only)

Do not take Follistim AQ Cartridge if you are a Woman who:
- is pregnant or think you may be pregnant
- has heavy or irregular vaginal bleeding and the cause is not known
- has ovarian cysts or enlarged ovaries, not due to polycystic ovary syndrome (PCOS)

Talk to your healthcare provider before taking this medicine if you have any of the conditions listed above.

What should I tell my healthcare provider before taking Follistim AQ Cartridge?

Before you take Follistim AQ, tell your healthcare provider if you:
- have an increased risk of blood clots (thrombosis)
- have ever had a blood clot (thrombosis), or anyone in your immediate family has ever had a blood clot (thrombosis)
- had stomach (abdominal) surgery
- had twisting of your ovary (ovarian torsion)
- had or have a cyst in your ovary
- have polycystic ovary disease
- have any other medical conditions
- are breastfeeding or plan to breastfeed. It is not known if the medicine in Follistim AQ Cartridge passes into your breast milk. You and your healthcare provider should decide if you will take Follistim AQ Cartridge or breastfeed. You should not do both

Tell your healthcare provider about all the medicines you take, including prescription and non-prescription medicines, vitamins, and herbal supplements.

Know the medicines you take. Keep a list of them and show your healthcare provider and pharmacist when you get a new medicine.

How should I use Follistim AQ Cartridge?
- Be sure that you read, understand, and follow the "Patient Instructions for Use" that come with Follistim AQ Cartridge
- Use Follistim AQ Cartridge exactly as your healthcare provider tells you to
- Your healthcare provider will tell you how much Follistim AQ Cartridge to use, how to inject it, and how often it should be injected
- Do not inject Follistim AQ Cartridge at home until your healthcare provider has taught you the right way to put the cartridge and pen device together and to inject yourself
- Do not mix any other medicines into the Cartridge
- Do not change your dose of Follistim AQ Cartridge unless your healthcare provider tells you to
- **Call your healthcare provider immediately** if you use too much Follistim AQ Cartridge
- If you miss or forget to take a dose, do not double your next dose. Ask your healthcare provider for instructions
- Use Follistim AQ Cartridge only with the Follistim Pen
- Do not use the Follistim Pen if you are blind or visually impaired unless you have assistance from an individual with good vision who is trained in the right way to use the pen
- Do not re-use the BD Micro Fine Pen Needle
- Your healthcare provider will do blood and urine hormone tests while you are taking Follistim AQ Cartridge. Make sure you follow-up with your healthcare provider to have your blood and urine tested when told to do so

Women:
- Your healthcare provider may do ultrasound scans of your ovaries. Make sure you follow-up with your healthcare provider to have your ultrasound scans

Men:
- Your healthcare provider may test your semen while you are taking Follistim AQ Cartridge. Make sure you follow-up with your healthcare provider to give a semen sample for testing

What are the possible side effects of Follistim AQ Cartridge?

Follistim AQ Cartridge may cause serious side effects.

Serious side effects in women include:
- **Ovarian enlargement**
- **Ovarian hyperstimulation syndrome (OHSS).** OHSS is a serious medical problem that can happen when the ovaries are over stimulated. In rare cases it has caused death. OHSS causes fluid to build up suddenly in your stomach and chest areas and can cause blood clots to form. Call your healthcare provider right away if you have:
  - pain in your lower stomach area
  - nausea
  - vomiting
  - weight gain
  - diarrhea
  - decreased urine output
  - trouble breathing

- **Lung problems.** Follistim AQ Cartridge can cause you to have fluid in your lungs (atelectasis) and trouble breathing (acute respiratory distress syndrome).
- **Blood clots.** Follistim AQ Cartridge may increase your chance of having blood clots in your blood vessels. Blood clots can cause:
  - blood vessel problems (thrombophlebitis)
  - stroke
  - loss of your arm or leg
  - blood clot in your lungs (pulmonary embolus)
  - heart attack
- **Ovarian torsion.** Follistim AQ Cartridge may increase the chance of twisting of the ovaries in women with certain conditions such as OHSS, pregnancy and previous abdominal surgery. Twisting of the ovary could cause the blood flow to the ovary to be cut off
- **Pregnancy and birth of multiple babies.** Having a pregnancy with more than one baby at a time increases the health risk for you and your babies. Discuss your chances of multiple births with your healthcare provider
- **Birth defects.** A woman's age, certain sperm problems, genetic background of both parents and a pregnancy with multiple babies can increase the chance that your baby might have birth defects
- **Ectopic pregnancy (pregnancy outside of the womb).** The chance of a pregnancy outside of the womb is increased in women with damaged fallopian tubes
- **Miscarriage.** The chance of loss of an early pregnancy may be increased in women who have difficulty with becoming pregnant at all

The most common side effects of Follistim AQ Cartridge include:

In women:
- Cyst in the ovary
- stomach pain

In Men:
- headache
- pain at the injection site
- bruising, swelling or redness at the injection site
- breast enlargement
- acne

These are not all the possible side effects of Follistim AQ Cartridge. For more information, ask your healthcare provider or pharmacist.

Call your healthcare provider immediately if you get worsening or strong abdominal pain. Also, call your healthcare provider immediately if this happens some days after the last injection has been given.

Tell your healthcare provider if you have any side effect that bothers you or that does not go away

Call your doctor for medical advice about side effects. You may report side effects to FDA at 1-800-FDA-1088.

How should I store Follistim AQ Cartridge?
- Store Follistim AQ Cartridge in the refrigerator between 36°F to 46°F (2°C to 8°C) until the expiration date
- Follistim AQ can be stored at or below 77°F (25°C) for 3 months or until the expiration date, whichever comes first. Once the rubber inlay of the Follistim AQ Cartridge has been pierced by a needle, the product may be stored only for a maximum of 28 days at 36°F to 77°F (2°C to 25°C)..
- Keep Follistim AQ Cartridge away from light
- Do not freeze

Keep Follistim AQ Cartridge and all medicines out of the reach of children.

General information about Follistim AQ Cartridge

Medicines are sometimes prescribed for purposes other than those listed in the Patient Information leaflet. Do not use Follistim AQ for a condition for which it was not prescribed. Do not give Follistim AQ Cartridge to other people, even if they have the same condition that you have. It may harm them.

This Patient Information leaflet summarizes the most important information about Follistim AQ Cartridge. If you would like more information, talk with your healthcare provider. You can ask your pharmacist or healthcare provider for more information about Follistim AQ Cartridge that is written for healthcare professionals.

For more information, go to **www.follistim.com** or call 1-866-836-5633.

What are the ingredients in Follistim AQ Cartridge?

Active ingredient: follitropin beta

Inactive ingredients: sucrose, sodium citrate, benzyl alcohol, NF-10 mg/mL, L-methionine, polysorbate 20, water for injection, hydrochloric acid, or sodium hydroxide.

Manufactured by: Vetter Pharma-Fertigung GmbH & Co. KG, Ravensburg, Germany

Distributed by: Schering Corporation, a subsidiary of MERCK & CO., INC., Whitehouse Station, NJ 08889, USA

Revised 6/2010

PATIENT INSTRUCTIONS FOR USE

FOLLISTIM® (Fol-lis-tim) AQ Cartridge

(follitropin beta injection)

Read the Patient Instructions for Use that comes with FOLLISTIM® AQ Cartridge before you start using it and

each time you get a refill. There may be new information. This information does not take the place of talking with your healthcare provider about your medical condition or treatment.

A. Getting Ready
- Follistim Pen is not recommended for the blind or visually impaired user without the assistance of an individual with good vision, trained in the proper use of the injection device.
- Learn about all of the parts of the Follistim Pen (See Figure 1 and Figure 2), Follistim AQ Cartridge (Figure 3) and the BD Micro Fine™ Pen Needle (Figure 4). You will need to recognize these parts to follow the directions

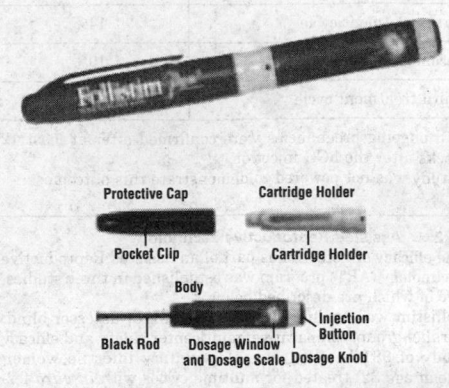

Figure 1 Follistim Pen and its Parts

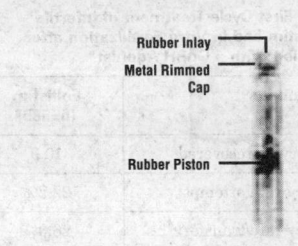

Figure 2. Parts of Follistim AQ Cartridge

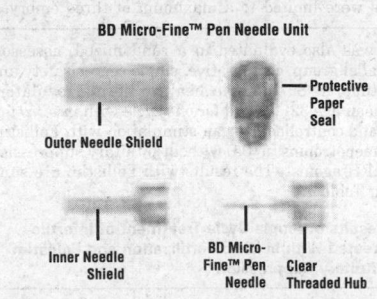

Figure 3. Parts of BD Micro-Fine Pen Needle Unit

- Remove the Cartridge out of the refrigerator
- Injecting cold drug is likely to cause discomfort. Therefore, it is recommended you allow the drug to reach room temperature before taking the injection.
- Check the liquid in the cartridge. It should appear clear and colorless. If the solution is not clear and colorless or has particles in it, **do not use it**
- **Gather the supplies you will need for your injection. You will need:**
  - a clean dry surface
  - alcohol
  - cotton balls or alcohol pads
  - sterile gauze
  - a puncture-proof container to throw away the used syringe and needle
- Wash your hands with soap and water and dry them before you use Follistim Pen or when you replace the cartridge.

B. Loading the Follistim Pen with the Follistim AQ Cartridge

• Holding the Pen Body firmly with one hand, pull off the Protective Cap with your other hand (See Figure 4). Put the cap aside on a clean, dry surface

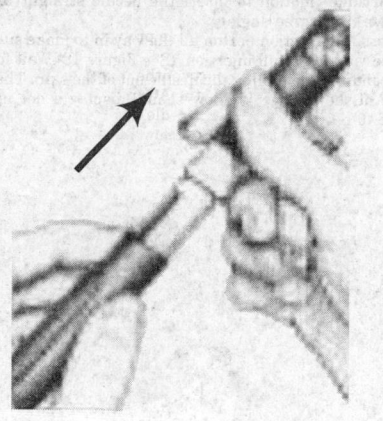

Figure 4

• Unscrew the entire Pen Body from the Cartridge Holder (See Figure 5). Place the Cartridge Holder and the Pen Body aside on a clean, dry surface

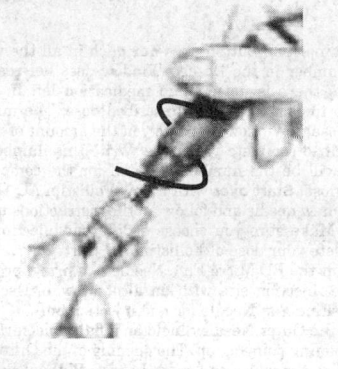

Figure 5

• Take the Follistim AQ Cartridge out of its package. Clean the rubber inlay on the cartridge with an alcohol pad. Pick up the Cartridge Holder. Put the Cartridge into the Cartridge holder (See Figure 6. The metal rimmed cap goes in first

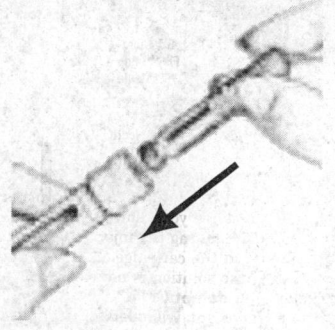

Figure 6

• Pick up the Pen Body and lower it into the Cartridge Holder. The black rod must press against the Rubber Pis-

ton on the cartridge. Screw the Pen Body fully onto the Cartridge Holder (See Figure 7). Make sure there is no gap between the Pen Body and the Cartridge Holder. The arrow (▲) on the Cartridge Holder should point to the middle of the yellow alignment mark (■) on the blue Pen Body

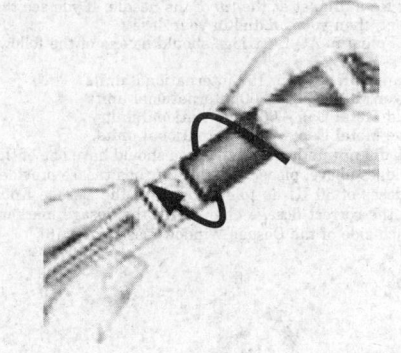

Figure 7

• Clean the open end of the Cartridge Holder with an alcohol pad (See Figure 8)

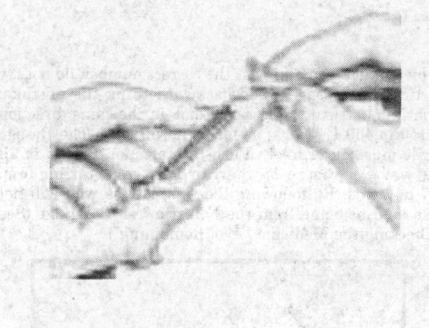

Figure 8

• Pick up a new BD Micro-Fine Pen Needle that is in its Outer Needle Shield. Peel off the protective paper seal (See Figure 9). Do **not** touch the needle. Do **not** place the open needle on any surface. **Use Only the BD Micro-Fine 0.33 mm × 12.7 mm (29G) Pen needles as supplied with the Follistim AQ Cartridge**

• You must use a new BD Micro-Fine Pen Needle with each injection. Never reuse a needle. Attach a new BD Micro-Fine Pen Needle after you make sure there is a Follistim AQ Cartridge in the Cartridge

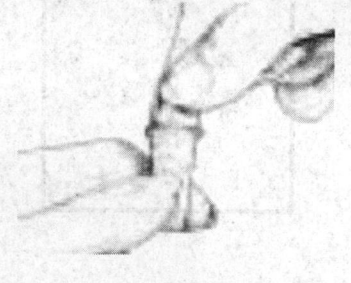

Figure 9

• Hold the Outer Needle Shield firmly in one hand while holding the Cartridge Holder firmly in the other hand. Push the end of the Cartridge Holder into the Outer Needle Shield. Screw them tightly together (See Figure 10). Place your Follistim Pen with the loaded cartridge and attached needle, flat on a clean, dry surface

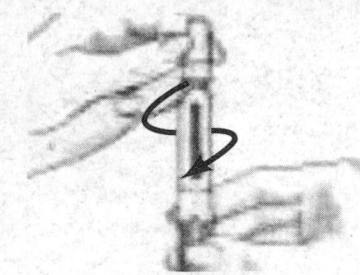

Figure 10

C. Preparing the Injection Site

• Follistim AQ Cartridge can be injected directly into a layer of fat under your skin (subcutaneously)

• When giving a subcutaneous injection, follow your healthcare provider's instructions about changing the site for each injection. This will help lower your chances of having a skin reaction

• **Do not** inject Follistim AQ Cartridge into an area that is tender, red, bruised, or hard

• The recommended site for injecting Follistim AQ Cartridge subcutaneously is:
  • just below your belly button (navel) (See Figure 11)

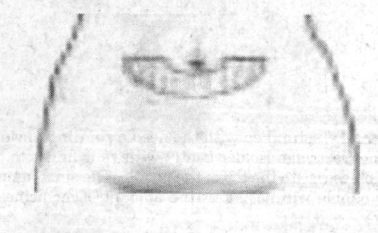

Figure 11

• The upper outer area of your thigh (See Figure 12)

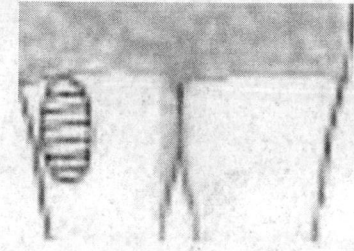

Figure 12

• Clean the skin with an alcohol wipe where the injection is to be made. Clean about two inches around the injection site where the needle will be inserted. **Do not** touch the cleaned area of skin

D. Dialing the Dose Before You Give the Injection

• Your healthcare provider will decide on the dose of Follistim AQ Cartridge to be given. This dose may be increased or decreased as your treatment progresses depending on your individual type of treatment.

• Follistim AQ Cartridge using Follistim Pen can be administered subcutaneously (beneath the skin) in prescribed doses from 50 International Units (IU) up to 450 IU, in marked 25 IU increments. The Dosage Scale on the Pen has numbers and audible clicks to help you set the correct dose

• Pull-off the outer needle shield. Leave the Inner Needle Shield-in-place over the needle attached to the Pen (See Figure 13). Do not throw the Outer Needle Shield away, you will need it later when you throw the needle away

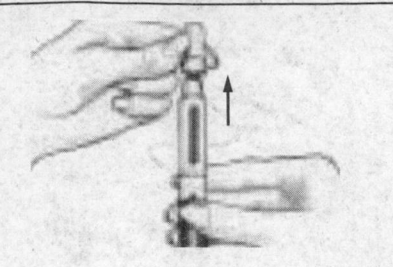

Figure 13

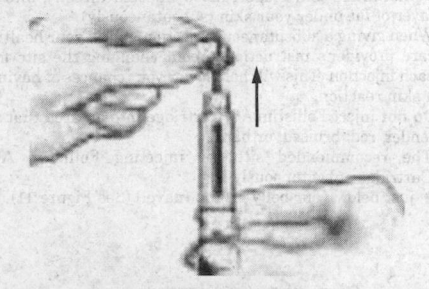

Figure 14

- Carefully remove the Inner Needle Shield and discard it (See Figure 14). Do not touch the needle or let it touch any surface while uncapped

- Hold the Follistim Pen with the needle pointing upwards. Tap the Cartridge Holder gently with your finger to help air bubbles rise to the top of the needle. The small amount of air bubble will not affect the amount of medicine you receive
- With a loaded new, unused cartridge:
1. Dial the Dosage Knob until you hear one click. With the needle pointing upwards, push in the Injection Button
2. Look for a droplet at the tip of the needle (See Figure 15). If you see the droplet, then you can dial in your dose

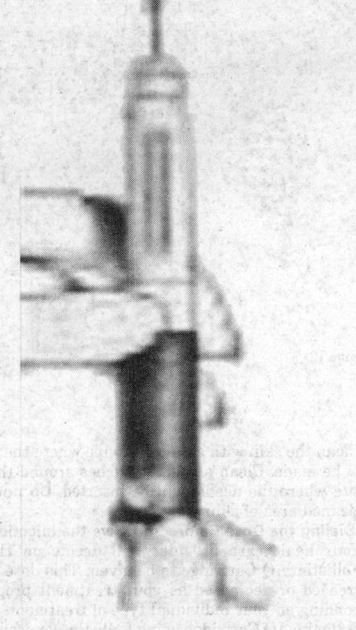

Figure 15

3. If you do **not** see a droplet, repeat Step 1 (as above) until you see droplet.
You must **make sure you see a droplet** of medicine (**check the flow of medicine**) or you may **not** inject the correct amount of medicine.

- With a partially used cartridge, to give yourself another dose of medicine you will need to attach a new BD Micro-Fine Pen Needle and look for a droplet forming at the tip of the needle (See Figure 15 above). If you see a droplet, then you can dial in your dose
If **no** droplet:
1. Dial the Dosage Knob until you hear one click. With the needle pointing upwards, push in the Injection Button
2. Look for a droplet at the tip of the needle. If you see the droplet, then you can dial in your dose
- Your Follistim AQ Cartridge should be one of the following:
  - Orange Metal Cap- 150 international units
  - Silver Metal Cap – 300 international units
  - Gold Metal Cap – 600 international units
  - Blue Metal Cap – 900 international units
If you did **not** understand that you should have one of the cartridges above, please contact your healthcare provider
- For doses of 50 IU up to 450 IU, turn the Dosage Knob until the correct dosage aligns with the dosage markers on each side of the Dosage Window (see Figure 16)

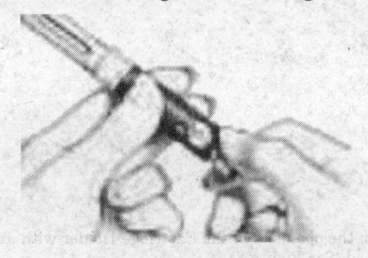

Figure 16

- If by mistake you dial past the correct number, do not try to turn the Dosage Knob backward to fix the mistake. Continue to turn the Dosage Knob in the same direction past the 450 IU mark, as far as it will turn. The Dosage Scale must move freely. Push the Injection Button in all the way. See Figure 17. Start to dial again starting from "0" upwards. By following these directions, you will not lose any medicine from the Follistim AQ Cartridge (See "Checking the Medicine Level Remaining")

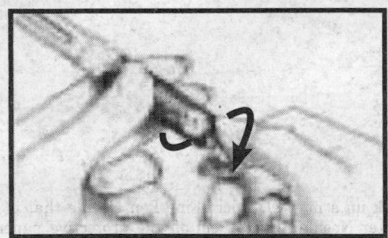

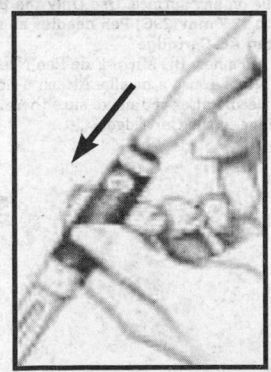

Figure 17

- **If you turn the Dosage Knob backward to correct the mistake, it will not damage the Pen, but you will lose some medication from the Follistim AQ Cartridge**
- **Never dial your dose or try to correct a dialing mistake when the needle is still in your skin as this may result in your receiving an incorrect dose.**
- **If your prescribed dose exceeds the deliverable dose of Follistim Pen or exceeds the amount remaining in the cartridge, you will need to give yourself more than one injection**

E. Giving Yourself an Injection
- Pinch a fold of skin at the cleaned injection site. **Do not** touch the cleaned area of skin
- With the other hand hold the entire Pen with Cartridge loaded and Needle on like you would a pencil. Use a quick "dart-like" motion to insert the needle straight up and down (90-degree angle)
- Press the injection button all the way in to make sure you give yourself a full injection. (See Figure 18).Wait for five seconds before pulling the needle out of the skin. The middle of the Dosage Window should display a dot next to the "0".

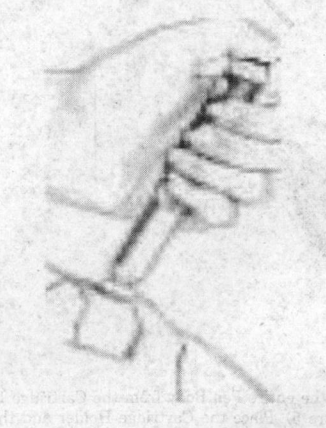

Figure 18

If the injection button does **not** push in all the way, and the number in the Dosage Window does not read "0", it means there is not enough medication left in the cartridge to complete your prescribed dose. The number in the Dosage Window will give you the amount of medicine needed to complete your dose. Write this number down. This will be the number you dial for the completion of your dose. **Start over** with a new Follistim AQ Cartridge and a new needle and follow all the instructions up to this step. Make sure you choose a different injection site to complete your dose of Follistim AQ Cartridge.
- Pull out the BD Micro-Fine Needle and firmly press down on the injection site with an alcohol swab. Use the BD Micro-Fine Pen Needle for one injection only.
- Place the Outer Needle Shield on a flat table surface with the opening pointing up. The opening of the Outer Needle Shield is the wider end with the rim. Without holding on to the Outer Needle Shield, carefully insert the needle (attached to the Follistim Pen) into the opening of the Outer Needle Shield and push down firmly. The Outer Needle Shield should now be attached to the Cartridge Holder and covering the needle (See Figure 19)

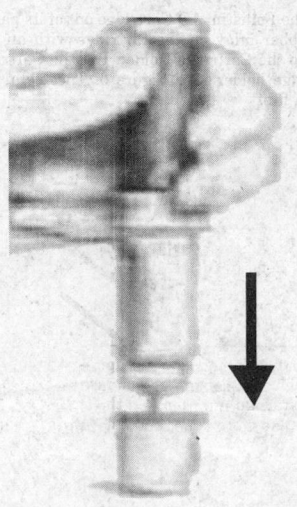

Figure 19

- Grip the Outer Needle Shield and use it to unscrew the needle from the Cartridge Holder See Figure 20). If there

heart, there are also beta$_2$-receptors in the human heart comprising 10%-50% of the total beta-adrenergic receptors. The precise function of these receptors has not been established, but they raise the possibility that even highly selective beta$_2$-agonists may have cardiac effects.

The pharmacologic effects of beta$_2$-adrenoceptor agonist drugs, including formoterol, are at least in part attributable to stimulation of intracellular adenyl cyclase, the enzyme that catalyzes the conversion of adenosine triphosphate (ATP) to cyclic-3', 5'-adenosine monophosphate (cyclic AMP). Increased cyclic AMP levels cause relaxation of bronchial smooth muscle and inhibition of release of mediators of immediate hypersensitivity from cells, especially from mast cells.

In vitro tests show that formoterol is an inhibitor of the release of mast cell mediators, such as histamine and leukotrienes, from the human lung. Formoterol also inhibits histamine-induced plasma albumin extravasation in anesthetized guinea pigs and inhibits allergen-induced eosinophil influx in dogs with airway hyper-responsiveness. The relevance of these in vitro and animal findings to humans is unknown.

Animal Pharmacology

Studies in laboratory animals (minipigs, rodents, and dogs) have demonstrated the occurrence of cardiac arrhythmias and sudden death (with histologic evidence of myocardial necrosis) when beta-agonists and methylxanthines are administered concurrently. The clinical significance of these findings is unknown.

Pharmacokinetics

Information on the pharmacokinetics of formoterol in plasma has been obtained in healthy subjects by oral inhalation of doses higher than the recommended range and in Chronic Obstructive Pulmonary Disease (COPD) patients after oral inhalation of doses at and above the therapeutic dose. Urinary excretion of unchanged formoterol was used as an indirect measure of systemic exposure. Plasma drug disposition data parallel urinary excretion, and the elimination half-lives calculated for urine and plasma are similar.

Absorption

Following inhalation of a single 120 mcg dose of formoterol fumarate by 12 healthy subjects, formoterol was rapidly absorbed into plasma, reaching a maximum drug concentration of 92 pg/mL within 5 minutes of dosing. In COPD patients treated for 12 weeks with formoterol fumarate 12 or 24 mcg b.i.d., the mean plasma concentrations of formoterol ranged between 4.0 and 8.8 pg/mL and 8.0 and 17.3 pg/mL, respectively, at 10 min, 2 h and 6 h post inhalation.

Following inhalation of 12 to 96 mcg of formoterol fumarate by 10 healthy males, urinary excretion of both (R,R)- and (S,S)-enantiomers of formoterol increased proportionally to the dose. Thus, absorption of formoterol following inhalation appeared linear over the dose range studied.

In a study in patients with asthma, when formoterol 12 or 24 mcg twice daily was given by oral inhalation for 4 weeks or 12 weeks, the accumulation index, based on the urinary excretion of unchanged formoterol ranged from 1.63 to 2.08 in comparison with the first dose. For COPD patients, when formoterol 12 or 24 mcg twice daily was given by oral inhalation for 12 weeks, the accumulation index, based on the urinary excretion of unchanged formoterol, was 1.19 - 1.38. This suggests some accumulation of formoterol in plasma with multiple dosing. The excreted amounts of formoterol at steady-state were close to those predicted based on single-dose kinetics. As with many drug products for oral inhalation, it is likely that the majority of the inhaled formoterol fumarate delivered is swallowed and then absorbed from the gastrointestinal tract.

Distribution

The binding of formoterol to human plasma proteins in vitro was 61%-64% at concentrations from 0.1 to 100 ng/mL. Binding to human serum albumin in vitro was 31%-38% over a range of 5 to 500 ng/mL. The concentrations of formoterol used to assess the plasma protein binding were higher than those achieved in plasma following inhalation of a single 120 mcg dose.

Metabolism

Formoterol is metabolized primarily by direct glucuronidation at either the phenolic or aliphatic hydroxyl group and O-demethylation followed by glucuronide conjugation at either phenolic hydroxyl groups. Minor pathways involve sulfate conjugation of formoterol and deformylation followed by sulfate conjugation. The most prominent pathway involves direct conjugation at the phenolic hydroxyl group. The second major pathway involves O-demethylation followed by conjugation at the phenolic 2'-hydroxyl group. Four cytochrome P450 isozymes (CYP2D6, CYP2C19, CYP2C9 and CYP2A6) are involved in the O-demethylation of formoterol. Formoterol did not inhibit CYP450 enzymes at therapeutically relevant concentrations. Some patients may be deficient in CYP2D6 or 2C19 or both. Whether a deficiency in one or both of these isozymes results in elevated

systemic exposure to formoterol or systemic adverse effects has not been adequately explored.

Excretion

Following oral administration of 80 mcg of radiolabeled formoterol fumarate to 2 healthy subjects, 59%-62% of the radioactivity was eliminated in the urine and 32%-34% in the feces over a period of 104 hours. Renal clearance of formoterol from blood in these subjects was about 150 mL/min. Following inhalation of a 12 mcg or 24 mcg dose by 16 patients with asthma, about 10% and 15%-18% of the total dose was excreted in the urine as unchanged formoterol and direct conjugates of formoterol, respectively. Following inhalation of 12 mcg or 24 mcg dose by 18 patients with COPD the corresponding values were 7% and 6-9% of the dose, respectively.

Based on plasma concentrations measured following inhalation of a single 120 mcg dose by 12 healthy subjects, the mean terminal elimination half-life was determined to be 10 hours. From urinary excretion rates measured in these subjects, the mean terminal elimination half-lives for the (R,R)- and (S,S)-enantiomers were determined to be 13.9 and 12.3 hours, respectively. The (R,R)- and (S,S)-enantiomers represented about 40% and 60% of unchanged drug excreted in the urine, respectively, following single inhaled doses between 12 and 120 mcg in healthy volunteers and single and repeated doses of 12 and 24 mcg in patients with asthma. Thus, the relative proportion of the two enantiomers remained constant over the dose range studied and there was no evidence of relative accumulation of one enantiomer over the other after repeated dosing.

Special Populations

Gender: After correction for body weight, formoterol pharmacokinetics did not differ significantly between males and females.

Geriatric and Pediatric: The pharmacokinetics of formoterol have not been studied in the elderly population, and limited data are available in pediatric patients.

In a study of children with asthma who were 5 to 12 years of age, when formoterol fumarate 12 or 24 mcg was given twice daily by oral inhalation for 12 weeks, the accumulation index ranged from 1.18 to 1.84 based on urinary excretion of unchanged formoterol. Hence, the accumulation in children did not exceed that in adults, where the accumulation index ranged from 1.63 to 2.08 (see above). Approximately 6% and 6.5% to 9% of the dose was recovered in the urine of the children as unchanged and conjugated formoterol, respectively.

Hepatic/Renal Impairment: The pharmacokinetics of formoterol have not been studied in subjects with hepatic or renal impairment.

Pharmacodynamics

Systemic Safety and Pharmacokinetic/Pharmacodynamic Relationships

The major adverse effects of inhaled beta$_2$-agonists occur as a result of excessive activation of the systemic beta-adrenergic receptors. The most common adverse effects in adults and adolescents include skeletal muscle tremor and cramps, insomnia, tachycardia, decreases in plasma potassium, and increases in plasma glucose.

Pharmacokinetic/pharmacodynamic (PK/PD) relationships between heart rate, ECG parameters, and serum potassium levels and the urinary excretion of formoterol were evaluated in 10 healthy male volunteers (25 to 45 years of age) following inhalation of single doses containing 12, 24, 48, or 96 mcg of formoterol fumarate. There was a linear relationship between urinary formoterol excretion and decreases in serum potassium, increases in plasma glucose, and increases in heart rate.

In a second study, PK/PD relationships between plasma formoterol levels and pulse rate, ECG parameters, and plasma potassium levels were evaluated in 12 healthy volunteers following inhalation of a single 120 mcg dose of formoterol fumarate (10 times the recommended clinical dose). Reductions of plasma potassium concentration were observed in all subjects. Maximum reductions from baseline ranged from 0.55 to 1.52 mmol/L with a median maximum reduction of 1.01 mmol/L. The formoterol plasma concentration was highly correlated with the reduction in plasma potassium concentration. Generally, the maximum effect on plasma potassium was noted 1 to 3 hours after peak formoterol plasma concentrations were achieved. A mean maximum increase of pulse rate of 26 bpm was observed 6 hours post dose. The maximum increase of mean corrected QT interval (QTc) was 25 msec when calculated using Bazett's correction and was 8 msec when calculated using Fridericia's correction. The QTc returned to baseline within 12-24 hours post-dose. Formoterol plasma concentrations were weakly correlated with pulse rate and increase of QTc duration. The effects on plasma potassium, pulse rate, and QTc interval are known pharmacological effects of this class of study drug and were not unexpected at the very high formoterol dose (120 mcg single dose, 10 times the recommended single dose) tested in this study. These effects were well-tolerated by the healthy volunteers.

The electrocardiographic and cardiovascular effects of FORADIL AEROLIZER were compared with those of albuterol and placebo in two pivotal 12-week double-blind studies of patients with asthma. A subset of patients underwent continuous electrocardiographic monitoring during three 24-hour periods. No important differences in ventricular or supraventricular ectopy between treatment groups were observed. In these two studies, the total number of patients with asthma exposed to any dose of FORADIL AEROLIZER who had continuous electrocardiographic monitoring was about 200.

Continuous electrocardiographic monitoring was not included in the clinical studies of FORADIL AEROLIZER that were performed in COPD patients. The electrocardiographic effects of FORADIL AEROLIZER were evaluated versus placebo in a 12-month pivotal double-blind study of patients with COPD. An analysis of ECG intervals was performed for patients who participated at study sites in the United States, including 46 patients treated with FORADIL AEROLIZER 12 mcg twice daily, and 50 patients treated with FORADIL AEROLIZER 24 mcg twice daily. ECGs were performed predose, and at 5-15 minutes and 2 hours postdose at study baseline and after 3, 6 and 12 months of treatment. The results showed that there was no clinically meaningful acute or chronic effect on ECG intervals, including QTc, resulting from treatment with FORADIL AEROLIZER.

Tachyphylaxis/Tolerance

In a clinical study in 19 adult patients with mild asthma, the bronchoprotective effect of formoterol, as assessed by methacholine challenge, was studied following an initial dose of 24 mcg (twice the recommended dose) and after 2 weeks of 24 mcg twice daily. Tolerance to the bronchoprotective effects of formoterol was observed as evidenced by a diminished bronchoprotective effect on FEV$_1$ after 2 weeks of dosing, with loss of protection at the end of the 12 hour dosing period.

Rebound bronchial hyper-responsiveness after cessation of chronic formoterol therapy has not been observed.

In three large clinical trials in patients with asthma, while efficacy of formoterol versus placebo was maintained, a slightly reduced bronchodilatory response (as measured by 12-hour FEV$_1$ AUC) was observed within the formoterol arms over time, particularly with the 24 mcg twice daily dose (twice the daily recommended dose). A similarly reduced FEV$_1$ AUC over time was also noted in the albuterol treatment arms (180 mcg four times daily by metered-dose inhaler).

CLINICAL TRIALS

Adolescent and Adult Asthma Trials

In a placebo-controlled, single-dose clinical trial, the onset of bronchodilation (defined as a 15% or greater increase from baseline in FEV$_1$) was similar for FORADIL AEROLIZER and albuterol 180 mcg by metered-dose inhaler.

In single-dose and multiple-dose clinical trials, the maximum improvement in FEV$_1$ for FORADIL AEROLIZER 12 mcg generally occurred within 1 to 3 hours, and an increase in FEV$_1$ above baseline was observed for 12 hours in most patients.

FORADIL AEROLIZER 12 mcg twice daily was compared to FORADIL AEROLIZER 24 mcg twice daily, albuterol 180 mcg four times daily by metered-dose inhaler, and placebo in a total of 1095 adult and adolescent patients 12 years of age and above with mild-to-moderate asthma (defined as FEV$_1$ 40%-80% of the patient's predicted normal value) who participated in two pivotal, 12-week, multicenter, randomized, double-blind, parallel group studies.

The results of both studies showed that FORADIL AEROLIZER 12 mcg twice daily resulted in significantly greater post-dose bronchodilation (as measured by serial FEV$_1$ for 12 hours post-dose) throughout the 12-week treatment period. There was no significant difference in post-dose bronchodilation between FORADIL AEROLIZER 12 mcg twice daily and FORADIL AEROLIZER 24 mcg twice daily, but serious asthma exacerbations occurred more commonly in the higher dose group (see WARNINGS and ADVERSE REACTIONS). Mean FEV$_1$ measurements from both studies are shown below for the first and last treatment days (see Figures 1 and 2).

[See figure 1a and 1b at top of next page]
[See figure 2a and 2b at top of next page]

Compared with placebo and albuterol, patients treated with FORADIL AEROLIZER 12 mcg demonstrated improvement in many secondary efficacy endpoints, including improved combined and nocturnal asthma symptom scores, fewer nighttime awakenings, fewer nights in which patients used rescue medication, and higher morning and evening peak flow rates. FORADIL AEROLIZER 24 mcg twice daily did

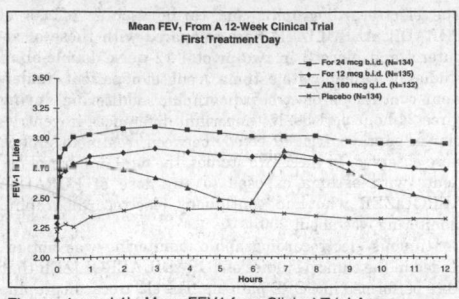

Figures 1a and 1b: Mean FEV1 from Clinical Trial A

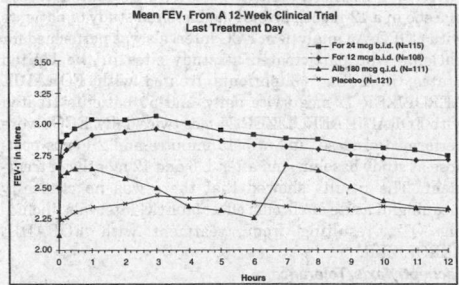

Figures 1a and 1b: Mean FEV1 from Clinical Trial A

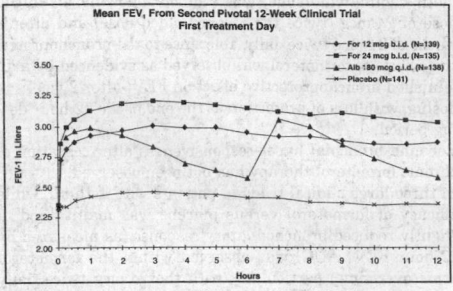

Figures 2a and 2b: Mean FEV1 from Clinical Trial B

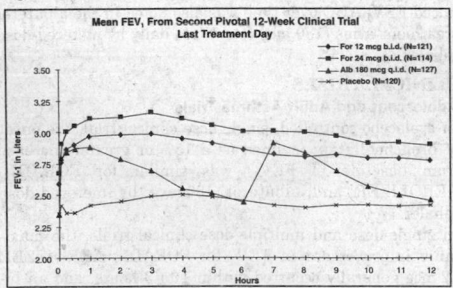

Figures 2a and 2b: Mean FEV1 from Clinical Trial B

not provide any additional improvements in these secondary endpoints compared to FORADIL AEROLIZER 12 mcg twice daily.

A 16-week, randomized, multi-center, double-blind, parallel-group study enrolled 1568 patients 12 years of age and older with mild-to-moderate asthma (defined as $FEV_1 \geq 40\%$ of the patient's predicted normal value) in three treatment groups: FORADIL AEROLIZER 12 mcg twice daily, FORADIL AEROLIZER 24 mcg twice daily, and placebo. The study's primary endpoint was the incidence of serious asthma-related adverse events. Serious asthma exacerbations occurred in 3 (0.6%) patients who received FORADIL AEROLIZER 12 mcg twice daily, 2 (0.4%) patients who received FORADIL AEROLIZER 24 mcg twice daily, and 1 (0.2%) patient who received placebo. The size of this study was not adequate to precisely quantify the differences in serious asthma exacerbation rates between treatment groups. All serious asthma exacerbations resulted in hospitalizations. While there were no deaths in the study, the duration and size of this study were not adequate to quantify the rate of asthma-related death. See WARNINGS for information about a study which compared another long-acting beta$_2$-adrenergic agonist to placebo.

Pediatric Asthma Trial
A 12-month, multi-center, randomized, double-blind, parallel-group, study compared FORADIL AEROLIZER 12 mcg twice daily and FORADIL AEROLIZER 24 mcg twice daily to placebo in a total of 518 children with asthma (ages 5-12 years) who required daily bronchodilators and

anti-inflammatory treatment. Efficacy was evaluated on the first day of treatment, at Week 12, and at the end of treatment.

FORADIL AEROLIZER 12 mcg twice daily demonstrated a greater 12-hour FEV_1 AUC compared to placebo on the first day of treatment, after twelve weeks of treatment, and after one year of treatment. FORADIL AEROLIZER 24 mcg twice daily did not result in any additional improvement in 12-hour FEV_1 AUC compared to FORADIL AEROLIZER 12 mcg twice daily.

Exercise-Induced Bronchospasm Trials
The effect of FORADIL AEROLIZER on exercise-induced bronchospasm (defined as >20% fall in FEV_1) was examined in four randomized, single-dose, double-blind, crossover studies in a total of 77 patients 4 to 41 years of age with exercise-induced bronchospasm. Exercise challenge testing was conducted 15 minutes, and 4, 8, and 12 hours following administration of a single dose of study drug (FORADIL AEROLIZER 12 mcg, albuterol 180 mcg by metered-dose inhaler, or placebo) on separate test days. FORADIL AEROLIZER 12 mcg and albuterol 180 mcg were each superior to placebo for FEV_1 measurements obtained 15 minutes after study drug administration. FORADIL AEROLIZER 12 mcg maintained superiority over placebo at 4, 8, and 12 hours after administration. Most subjects were protected from exercise-induced bronchospasm for up to 12 hours following administration of FORADIL AEROLIZER; however, some were not. The efficacy of FORADIL AEROLIZER in the prevention of exercise-induced bronchospasm when dosed on a regular twice daily regimen has not been studied.

Adult COPD Trials
In multiple-dose clinical trials in patients with COPD, FORADIL AEROLIZER 12 mcg was shown to provide onset of significant bronchodilation (defined as 15% or greater increase from baseline in FEV_1) within 5 minutes of oral inhalation after the first dose. Bronchodilation was maintained for at least 12 hours.

FORADIL AEROLIZER was studied in two pivotal, double-blind, placebo-controlled, randomized, multi-center, parallel-group trials in a total of 1634 adult patients (age range: 34-88 years; mean age: 63 years) with COPD who had a mean FEV_1 that was 46% of predicted. The diagnosis of COPD was based upon a prior clinical diagnosis of COPD, a smoking history (greater than 10 pack-years), age (at least 40 years), spirometry results (prebronchodilator baseline FEV_1 less than 70% of the predicted value, and at least 0.75 liters, with the FEV_1/VC being less than 88% for men and less than 89% for women), and symptom score (greater than zero on at least four of the seven days prior to randomization). These studies included approximately equal numbers of patients with and without baseline bronchodilator reversibility, defined as a 15% or greater increase FEV_1 after inhalation of 200 mcg of albuterol sulfate. A total of 405 patients received FORADIL AEROLIZER 12 mcg, administered twice daily. Each trial compared FORADIL AEROLIZER 12 mcg twice daily and FORADIL AEROLIZER 24 mcg twice daily with placebo and an active control drug. The active control drug was ipratropium bromide in COPD Trial A, and slow-release theophylline in COPD Trial B (the theophylline arm in this study was open-label). The treatment period was 12 weeks in COPD Trial A, and 12 months in COPD Trial B.

The results showed that FORADIL AEROLIZER 12 mcg twice daily resulted in significantly greater post-dose bronchodilation (as measured by serial FEV_1 for 12 hours post-dose; the primary efficacy analysis) compared to placebo when evaluated after 12 weeks of treatment in both trials, and after 12 months of treatment in the 12-month trial (COPD Trial B). Compared to FORADIL AEROLIZER 12 mcg twice daily, FORADIL AEROLIZER 24 mcg twice daily did not provide any additional benefit on a variety of endpoints including FEV_1.

Mean FEV_1 measurements after 12 weeks of treatment for one of the two major efficacy studies are shown in the figure below.

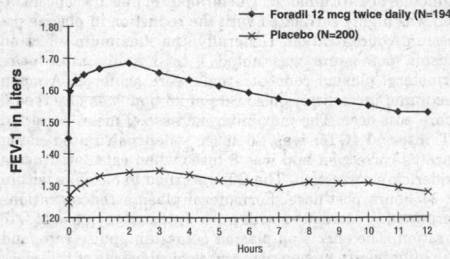

Figure 3 Mean FEV1 after 12 Weeks of treatment from COPD Trial A

FORADIL AEROLIZER 12 mcg twice daily was statistically superior to placebo at all post-dose timepoints tested (from 5

minutes to 12 hours post-dose) throughout the 12-week (COPD Trial A) and 12-month (COPD Trial B) treatment periods.

In both pivotal trials compared with placebo, patients treated with FORADIL AEROLIZER 12 mcg demonstrated improved morning pre-medication peak expiratory flow rates and took fewer puffs of rescue albuterol.

INDICATIONS AND USAGE
Asthma
FORADIL AEROLIZER is indicated for the treatment of asthma and in the prevention of bronchospasm only as concomitant therapy with a long-term asthma control medication, such as an inhaled corticosteroid, in adults and children 5 years of age and older with reversible obstructive airways disease, including patients with symptoms of nocturnal asthma.

Long acting beta$_2$ adrenergic agonists (LABA), such as formoterol, the active ingredient in FORADIL AEROLIZER, increase the risk of asthma related death (see WARNINGS). Use of FORADIL AEROLIZER for the treatment of asthma without concomitant use of a long-term asthma control medication, such as an inhaled corticosteroid, is contraindicated. Use FORADIL AEROLIZER only as additional therapy for patients with asthma who are currently taking but are inadequately controlled on a long-term asthma control medication, such as an inhaled corticosteroid. Once asthma control is achieved and maintained, assess the patient at regular intervals and step down therapy (e.g. discontinue FORADIL AEROLIZER) if possible without loss of asthma control, and maintain the patient on a long-term asthma control medication, such as an inhaled corticosteroid. Do not use FORADIL AEROLIZER for patients whose asthma is adequately controlled on low or medium dose inhaled corticosteroid.

Pediatric and Adolescent Patients
Available data from controlled clinical trials suggest that LABA increase the risk of asthma-related hospitalization in pediatric and adolescent patients (see WARNINGS). For pediatric and adolescent patients with asthma who require addition of a LABA to an inhaled corticosteroid, a fixed-dose combination product containing both an inhaled corticosteroid and LABA should ordinarily be used to ensure adherence with both drugs. In cases where use of a separate long-term asthma control medication (e.g. inhaled corticosteroid) and LABA is clinically indicated, appropriate steps must be taken to ensure adherence with both treatment components. If adherence cannot be assured, a fixed-dose combination product containing both an inhaled corticosteroid and LABA is recommended.

Exercise-Induced Bronchospasm
FORADIL AEROLIZER is also indicated for the acute prevention of exercise-induced bronchospasm (EIB) in adults and children 5 years of age and older, when administered on an occasional, as-needed basis. Use of FORADIL AEROLIZER as a single agent for the prevention of exercise-induced bronchospasm may be clinically indicated in patients who do not have persistent asthma. In patients with persistent asthma, use of FORADIL AEROLIZER for the prevention of exercise-induced bronchospasm may be clinically indicated, but the treatment of asthma should include a long-term asthma control medication, such as an inhaled corticosteroid.

Chronic Obstructive Pulmonary Disease
FORADIL AEROLIZER is indicated for the long-term, twice daily (morning and evening) administration in the maintenance treatment of bronchoconstriction in patients with Chronic Obstructive Pulmonary Disease including chronic bronchitis and emphysema.

CONTRAINDICATIONS
Because of the risk of asthma-related death and hospitalization, use of FORADIL AEROLIZER for the treatment of asthma without concomitant use of a long-term asthma control medication, such as an inhaled corticosteroid, is contraindicated (see Warnings – Asthma Related Death). FORADIL (formoterol fumarate) is contraindicated in patients with a history of hypersensitivity to formoterol fumarate or to any components of this product.

WARNINGS
ASTHMA RELATED DEATH
Long-acting beta$_2$-adrenergic agonists, such as formoterol, the active ingredient in FORADIL AEROLIZER, increase the risk of asthma-related death. Currently available data are inadequate to determine whether concurrent use of inhaled corticosteroids or other long-term asthma control drugs mitigates the increased risk of asthma-related death from LABA.

Because of this risk, use of FORADIL AEROLIZER for the treatment of asthma without concomitant use of a long-term asthma control medication, such as an inhaled corticosteroid, is contraindicated. Use FORADIL AEROLIZER only as additional therapy for patients with asthma who are currently taking but are inadequately controlled on a

NUMBER AND FREQUENCY OF SERIOUS ASTHMA EXACERBATIONS IN PATIENTS 12 YEARS OF AGE AND OLDER FROM A 16-WEEK TRIAL

	Foradil 12 mcg twice daily	Foradil 24 mcg twice daily	Placebo
Serious asthma exacerbations	3/527 (0.6%)	2/527 (0.4%)	1/514 (0.2%)

NUMBER AND FREQUENCY OF SERIOUS ASTHMA EXACERBATIONS IN PATIENTS 5-12 YEARS OF AGE FROM A 52-WEEK TRIAL

	Foradil 12 mcg twice daily	Foradil 24 mcg twice daily	Placebo
Serious asthma exacerbations	8/171 (4.7%)	11/171 (6.4%)	0/176 (0)

daily. Seven adverse events showed dose ordering among tested doses of 12 and 24 mcg administered twice daily; pharyngitis, fever, muscle cramps, increased sputum, dysphonia, myalgia, and tremor.

NUMBER AND FREQUENCY OF ADVERSE EXPERIENCES IN ADULT COPD PATIENTS TREATED IN MULTIPLE-DOSE CONTROLLED CLINICAL TRIALS

Adverse Event	FORADIL AEROLIZER 12 mcg twice daily n	(%)	Placebo n	(%)
Total patients	405	(100)	420	(100)
Upper respiratory tract infection	30	(7.4)	24	(5.7)
Pain back	17	(4.2)	17	(4.0)
Pharyngitis	14	(3.5)	10	(2.4)
Pain chest	13	(3.2)	9	(2.1)
Sinusitis	11	(2.7)	7	(1.7)
Fever	9	(2.2)	6	(1.4)
Cramps leg	7	(1.7)	2	(0.5)
Cramps muscle	7	(1.7)	0	
Anxiety	6	(1.5)	5	(1.2)
Pruritus	6	(1.5)	4	(1.0)
Sputum increased	6	(1.5)	5	(1.2)
Mouth dry	5	(1.2)	4	(1.0)

Overall, the frequency of all cardiovascular adverse events in the two pivotal studies was low and comparable to placebo (6.4% for FORADIL AEROLIZER 12 mcg twice daily, and 6.0% for placebo). There were no frequently-occurring specific cardiovascular adverse events for FORADIL AEROLIZER (frequency greater than or equal to 1% and greater than placebo).

Other adverse reactions to FORADIL AEROLIZER are similar in nature to other selective beta$_2$-adrenoceptor agonists; e.g., angina, hypertension or hypotension, tachycardia, arrhythmias, nervousness, headache, tremor, dry mouth, palpitation, muscle cramps, nausea, dizziness, fatigue, malaise, hypokalemia, hyperglycemia, metabolic acidosis and insomnia.

Post Marketing Experience

In extensive worldwide marketing experience with FORADIL, serious exacerbations of asthma, including some that have been fatal, have been reported. While most of these cases have been in patients with severe or acutely deteriorating asthma (see WARNINGS), a few have occurred in patients with less severe asthma. It is not possible to determine from these individual case reports whether FORADIL AEROLIZER contributed to the events.

Rare reports of anaphylactic reactions, including severe hypotension and angioedema, have also been received in association with the use of formoterol fumarate inhalation powder.

DRUG ABUSE AND DEPENDENCE

There was no evidence in clinical trials of drug dependence with the use of FORADIL.

OVERDOSAGE

The expected signs and symptoms with overdosage of FORADIL AEROLIZER are those of excessive beta-adrenergic stimulation and/or occurrence or exaggeration of any of the signs and symptoms listed under ADVERSE REACTIONS, e.g., angina, hypertension or hypotension, tachycardia, with rates up to 200 beats/min., arrhythmias, nervousness, headache, tremor, seizures, muscle cramps, dry mouth, palpitation, nausea, dizziness, fatigue, malaise, hypokalemia, hyperglycemia, and insomnia. Metabolic acidosis may also occur. As with all inhaled sympathomimetic medications, cardiac arrest and even death may be associated with an overdose of FORADIL AEROLIZER.

Treatment of overdosage consists of discontinuation of FORADIL AEROLIZER together with institution of appropriate symptomatic and/or supportive therapy. The judicious use of a cardioselective beta-receptor blocker may be considered, bearing in mind that such medication can produce bronchospasm. There is insufficient evidence to determine if dialysis is beneficial for overdosage of FORADIL AEROLIZER. Cardiac monitoring is recommended in cases of overdosage.

The minimum acute lethal inhalation dose of formoterol fumarate in rats is 156 mg/kg (approximately 53,000 and 25,000 times the maximum recommended daily inhalation dose in adults and children, respectively, on a mg/m^2 basis). The median lethal oral doses in Chinese hamsters, rats, and mice provide even higher multiples of the maximum recommended daily inhalation dose in humans.

DOSAGE AND ADMINISTRATION

FORADIL capsules should be administered only by the oral inhalation route and only using the AEROLIZER Inhaler (see the accompanying Medication Guide). **FORADIL capsules should not be ingested (i.e., swallowed) orally.** FORADIL capsules should always be stored in the blister, and only removed IMMEDIATELY BEFORE USE.

Treatment of Asthma

Long-acting beta$_2$-adrenergic agonists (LABA), such as formoterol, the active ingredient in FORADIL AEROLIZER, increase the risk of asthma-related death (see Warnings). **Because of this risk, use of FORADIL AEROLIZER for the treatment of asthma without concomitant use of a long-term asthma control medication, such as an inhaled corticosteroid, is contraindicated.** Use FORADIL AEROLIZER only as additional therapy for patients with asthma who are currently taking but are inadequately controlled on a long-term asthma control medication, such as an inhaled corticosteroid. Once asthma control is achieved and maintained, assess the patient at regular intervals and step down therapy (e.g. discontinue FORADIL AEROLIZER) if possible without loss of asthma control, and maintain the patient on a long-term asthma control medication, such as an inhaled corticosteroid. Do not use FORADIL AEROLIZER for patients whose asthma is adequately controlled on low or medium dose inhaled corticosteroids.

Pediatric and Adolescent Patients

Available data from controlled clinical trials suggest that LABA increase the risk of asthma-related hospitalization in pediatric and adolescent patients. For patients with asthma less than 18 years of age who require addition of a LABA to an inhaled corticosteroid, a fixed-dose combination product containing both an inhaled corticosteroid and LABA should ordinarily be used to ensure adherence with both drugs. In cases where use of a separate long-term asthma control medication (e.g. inhaled corticosteroid) and LABA is clinically indicated, appropriate steps must be taken to ensure adherence with both treatment components. If adherence cannot be assured, a fixed-dose combination product containing both an inhaled corticosteroid and LABA is recommended.

For adults and children 5 years of age and older the usual dosage is the inhalation of the contents of one 12-mcg FORADIL capsule every 12 hours using the AEROLIZER Inhaler. The patient must not exhale into the device. The total daily dose of FORADIL should not exceed one capsule twice daily (24 mcg total daily dose). More frequent administration or administration of a larger number of inhalations is not recommended. If symptoms arise between doses, an inhaled short-acting beta$_2$-agonist should be taken for immediate relief.

If a previously effective dosage regimen fails to provide the usual response, medical advice should be sought immediately as this is often a sign of destabilization of asthma. Under these circumstances, the therapeutic regimen should be re-evaluated.

For Prevention of Exercise-Induced Bronchospasm (EIB)

Use of FORADIL AEROLIZER as a single agent for the prevention of exercise-induced bronchospasm may be clinically indicated in patients who do not have persistent asthma. In patients with persistent asthma, use of FORADIL AEROLIZER for the prevention of exercise-induced bronchospasm may be clinically indicated, but the treatment of asthma should include a long-term asthma control medication, such as an inhaled corticosteroid. For adults and children 5 years of age or older, the usual dosage is the inhalation of the contents of one 12-mcg FORADIL capsule at least 15 minutes before exercise administered on an occasional as needed basis. When used intermittently as needed for prevention, protection may last up to 12 hours. Additional doses of FORADIL AEROLIZER should not be used for 12 hours after the administration of this drug. Regular, twice-daily dosing has not been studied in preventing EIB. Patients who are receiving FORADIL AEROLIZER twice daily for treatment of their asthma should not use additional doses for prevention of EIB and may require a short-acting bronchodilator.

For Maintenance Treatment of Chronic Obstructive Pulmonary Disease (COPD)

The usual dosage is the inhalation of the contents of one 12 mcg FORADIL capsule every 12 hours using the AEROLIZER inhaler.

A total daily dose of greater than 24 mcg is not recommended.

If a previously effective dosage regimen fails to provide the usual response, medical advice should be sought immediately as this is often a sign of destabilization of COPD. Under these circumstances, the therapeutic regimen should be re-evaluated and additional therapeutic options should be considered.

HOW SUPPLIED

FORADIL AEROLIZER contains: aluminum blister-packaged 12-mcg FORADIL (formoterol fumarate) clear gelatin capsules with "CG" printed on one end and "FXF" printed on the opposite end; one AEROLIZER Inhaler; and Medication Guide.

Unit Dose (blister pack)
Box of 12 (strips of 6) .... NDC 0085-1402-01
Unit Dose (blister pack)
Box of 60 (strips of 6) .... NDC 0085-1401-01

FORADIL capsules should be used with the AEROLIZER Inhaler only. The AEROLIZER Inhaler should not be used with any other capsules.

Prior to dispensing: Store in a refrigerator, 2°C-8°C (36°F-46°F)

After dispensing to patient: Store at 20°C to 25°C (68°F to 77°F) [see USP Controlled Room Temperature]. Protect from heat and moisture. CAPSULES SHOULD ALWAYS BE STORED IN THE BLISTER AND ONLY REMOVED FROM THE BLISTER IMMEDIATELY BEFORE USE.

Always discard the FORADIL capsules and AEROLIZER Inhaler by the "Use by" date and always use the new AEROLIZER Inhaler provided with each new prescription.

Keep out of the reach of children.

REV: JUNE 2010

Manufactured by:
Novartis Pharma AG, Basle, Switzerland
Distributed by:
Schering Corporation, a subsidiary of
MERCK & CO., INC.
Whitehouse Station, NJ 08889, USA
Copyright © 2010 Schering Corp.,
a subsidiary of MERCK & CO., INC.
All rights reserved.

MEDICATION GUIDE

Foradil® [FOR-a-dil] **Aerolizer®**
(formoterol fumarate inhalation powder)

Important: Do not swallow FORADIL capsules. FORADIL capsules are used only with the Aerolizer inhaler that comes with FORADIL AEROLIZER. Never place a capsule in the mouthpiece of the AEROLIZER Inhaler.

Read the Medication Guide that comes with FORADIL AEROLIZER before you start using it and each time you get a refill. There may be new information. This Medication Guide does not take the place of talking to your health care provider about your medical condition or treatment.

What is the most important information I should know about FORADIL AEROLIZER?

FORADIL AEROLIZER can cause serious side effects, including:

1. People with asthma who take long-acting beta$_2$-adrenergic agonist (LABA) medicines, such as formoterol fumarate inhalation powder (FORADIL AEROLIZER), have an increased risk of death from asthma problems.

- Call your healthcare provider if breathing problems worsen over time while using FORADIL AEROLIZER. You may need a different treatment.
- Get emergency medical care if:
  - breathing problems worsen quickly, and
  - you use your rescue inhaler medicine, but it does not relieve your breathing problems.

2. Do not use FORADIL AEROLIZER as your only asthma medicine. FORADIL AEROLIZER must only be used with a long-term asthma control medicine, such as an inhaled corticosteroid.

3. When your asthma is well controlled, your healthcare provider may tell you to stop taking FORADIL AEROLIZER. Your healthcare provider will decide if you can stop FORADIL AEROLIZER without loss of asthma control. You will continue taking your long-term asthma control medicine, such as an inhaled corticosteroid.

4. Children and adolescents who take LABA medicines may have an increased risk of being hospitalized for asthma problems.

What is FORADIL AEROLIZER?

FORADIL AEROLIZER is a long-acting beta$_2$-agonist (LABA). LABA medicines help the muscles around the airways in your lungs stay relaxed to prevent asthma symptoms, such as wheezing and shortness of breath. These symptoms can happen when the muscles around the airways tighten. This makes it hard to breathe. In severe cases, wheezing can stop your breathing and cause death if not treated right away.

FORADIL AEROLIZER is used for asthma, exercise-induced bronchospasm (EIB) and chronic obstructive pulmonary disease (COPD) as follows:

Asthma

FORADIL AEROLIZER is used with a long-term asthma control medicine, such as an inhaled corticosteroid, in adults and children ages 5 and older:
• to control symptoms of asthma, and
• to prevent symptoms such as wheezing

LABA medicines, such as FORADIL AEROLIZER, increase the risk of death from asthma problems. FORADIL AEROLIZER is not for adults and children with asthma who are well controlled with long-term asthma control medicine, such as low to medium dose of an inhaled corticosteroid medicine.

Exercise-Induced Bronchospasm (EIB)

FORADIL AEROLIZER is used to prevent wheezing caused by exercise in adults and children 5 years of age and older.
• If you have EIB only, your healthcare provider may prescribe only FORADIL AEROLIZER for your condition
• If you have EIB and asthma, your healthcare provider should also prescribe a long-term asthma control medicine, such as an inhaled corticosteroid

Chronic Obstructive Pulmonary Disease (COPD)

FORADIL AEROLIZER is used long-term, 2 times each day (morning and evening), to control symptoms of COPD and prevent wheezing in adults with COPD.

Who should not use FORADIL AEROLIZER?
• Do not take FORADIL AEROLIZER to treat your asthma without a long-term asthma control medicine, such as an inhaled corticosteroid.
• If you are allergic to formoterol fumarate or any of the ingredients in FORADIL AEROLIZER. Ask your healthcare provider if you are not sure. See the end of this Medication Guide for a complete list of ingredients in FORADIL AEROLIZER.

What should I tell my healthcare provider before using FORADIL AEROLIZER?

Tell your healthcare provider about all of your health conditions, including if you:
• have heart problems
• have high blood pressure
• have seizures
• have thyroid problems
• have diabetes
• are pregnant or planning to become pregnant. It is not known if FORADIL AEROLIZER may harm your unborn baby.
• are breastfeeding. It is not known if FORADIL AEROLIZER passes into your milk and if it can harm your baby.
• are allergic to FORADIL AEROLIZER, any other medicines, or food products.

FORADIL AEROLIZER contains lactose (milk sugar) and a small amount of milk proteins. It is possible that allergic reactions may happen in patients who have a severe milk protein allergy.

Tell your healthcare provider about all the medicines you take including prescription and non-prescription medicines, vitamins, and herbal supplements. FORADIL AEROLIZER and certain other medicines may interact with each other. This may cause serious side effects.

Know the medicines you take. Keep a list and show it to your healthcare provider and pharmacist each time you get a new medicine.

How do I use FORADIL capsules with the Aerolizer inhaler?
See the step-by-step instructions for using FORADIL Capsules with the Aerolizer inhaler at the end of this Medication Guide.

Do not use FORADIL unless your healthcare provider has taught you and you understand everything. Ask your healthcare provider or pharmacist if you have any questions.
• Children should use FORADIL AEROLIZER with an adult's help, as instructed by the child's healthcare provider.

• Use FORADIL AEROLIZER exactly as prescribed. **Do not use FORADIL AEROLIZER more often than prescribed.**
• For asthma and COPD, the usual dose is 1 FORADIL capsule inhaled through the AEROLIZER inhaler 2 times each day (morning and evening). The 2 doses should be about 12 hours apart.
• For preventing exercise-induced bronchospasm, the usual dose is 1 FORADIL capsule inhaled through the AEROLIZER inhaler at least 15 minutes before exercise, as needed. Do not use FORADIL AEROLIZER more often than every 12 hours. Do not use extra FORADIL AEROLIZER before exercise if you already use it 2 times each day.
• If you miss a dose of FORADIL AEROLIZER, just skip that dose. Take your next dose at your usual time. Never take 2 doses at one time.
• Do not use a spacer device with FORADIL AEROLIZER.
• Do not breathe into FORADIL AEROLIZER.
• While you are using FORADIL AEROLIZER 2 times each day, do not use other medicines that contain a long-acting beta$_2$-agonist (LABA) for any reason. Ask your healthcare provider or pharmacist for a list of these medicines.
• Do not stop using FORADIL AEROLIZER or any of your asthma medicines unless told to do so by your healthcare provider because your symptoms might get worse. Your healthcare provider will change your medicines as needed.
• FORADIL AEROLIZER does not relieve sudden symptoms. Always have a rescue inhaler medicine with you to treat sudden symptoms. If you do not have an inhaled, short-acting bronchodilator, contact your healthcare provider to have one prescribed for you.
• **Call your healthcare provider or get medical care right away if:**
  • your breathing problems worsen with FORADIL AEROLIZER
  • you need to use your rescue inhaler medicine more often than usual
  • your rescue inhaler medicine does not work as well for you at relieving symptoms
  • you need to use 4 or more inhalations of your rescue inhaler medicine for 2 or more days in a row
  • you use 1 whole canister of your rescue inhaler medicine in 8 weeks time
  • your peak flow meter results decrease. Your healthcare provider will tell you the numbers that are right for you.
  • you have asthma and your symptoms do not improve after using FORADIL AEROLIZER regularly for 1 week.

What are the possible side effects with FORADIL AEROLIZER?

FORADIL AEROLIZER may cause serious side effects, including:
• See "What is the most important information I should know about FORADIL AEROLIZER?"
• **Bronchospasm with wheezing or coughing and difficulty breathing**
• **Low blood potassium** (which may cause symptoms of muscle spasm, muscle weakness or abnormal heart rhythm)
• **Fast or irregular heart beat** (palpitations)
• **Serious allergic reactions including rash, hives, swelling of the face, mouth, and tongue, and breathing problems.** Call your healthcare provider or get emergency medical care if you get any symptoms of a serious allergic reaction.

Other possible side effects with FORADIL AEROLIZER include:
• chest pain
• increased blood pressure
• nervousness
• dry mouth
• muscle cramps
• nausea
• dizziness
• tiredness
• high blood sugar
• high blood acid
• trouble sleeping

Common side effects with FORADIL AEROLIZER include:
• headache
• tremor

Tell your healthcare provider about any side effect that bothers you or that does not go away.

These are not all the side effects with FORADIL AEROLIZER. Ask your healthcare provider or pharmacist for more information.

Call your doctor for medical advice about side effects. You may report side effects to FDA at 1-800-FDA-1088.

How do I store FORADIL AEROLIZER?
• Store FORADIL AEROLIZER at room temperature between 68° F and 77° F (20° C to 25° C). Protect FORADIL AEROLIZER from heat and moisture. Do not remove FORADIL capsules from their foil package until just before use.

• Always discard the old AEROLIZER inhaler by the "Use by" date and use the new one provided with each new prescription.
• Safely discard FORADIL capsules and the Aerolizer inhaler if no longer needed or is out-of-date.
• **Keep FORADIL AEROLIZER and all medicines out of the reach of children.**

General Information about FORADIL AEROLIZER

Medicines are sometimes prescribed for purposes other than those listed in a Medication Guide. Do not use FORADIL AEROLIZER for a condition for which it was not prescribed. Do not give FORADIL AEROLIZER to other people, even if they have the same condition. It may harm them.

This Medication Guide summarizes the most important information about FORADIL AEROLIZER. If you would like more information, talk with your healthcare provider. You can ask your healthcare provider or pharmacist for information about FORADIL AEROLIZER that was written for healthcare professionals. If you have any questions about the use of FORADIL AEROLIZER, call (toll-free) 1-800-526-4099 or go to www.foradil.us.

What are the ingredients in FORADIL AEROLIZER?

Active ingredient: formoterol fumarate
Inactive ingredients: lactose (contains milk proteins), gelatin (capsule shell)

Instructions for Using FORADIL AEROLIZER

Do not swallow FORADIL capsules.

Follow the instructions below for using your FORADIL AEROLIZER. **You will breathe-in (inhale) the medicine in the FORADIL capsules from the FORADIL AEROLIZER.** If you have any questions, ask your healthcare provider or pharmacist.

FORADIL AEROLIZER
• **FORADIL AEROLIZER consists of FORADIL capsules and a AEROLIZER Inhaler.**
• **FORADIL capsules come on blister cards and are wrapped in foil pouches. Do not open a foil pouch until you are ready to use FORADIL AEROLIZER.**
• **Keep your FORADIL and AEROLIZER Inhaler dry. Handle with DRY hands.**

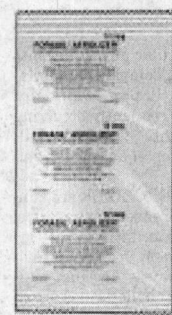

Aluminum pouch covering the foil blister cards

Foil blister card

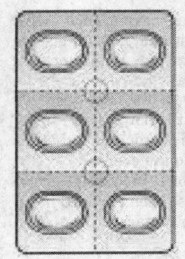

The Aerolizer consists of the following parts:
1. A cap to protect the mouthpiece of the base
2. A base that allows the proper release of medicine from the capsule. The base consists of:
3. A mouth piece
4. A capsule chamber
5. A button with "winglets" (projecting side pieces) and pins on each side
6. An air inlet channel.

With each new prescription of FORADIL AEROLIZER or refill, your pharmacist should have written the "Use by" date on the sticker on the outside of the FORADIL AEROLIZER box. Remove the "Use by" sticker on the box and place it on the AEROLIZER Inhaler cover that comes with FORADIL. If the sticker is blank, count 4 months from the date you got your FORADIL AEROLIZER from the pharmacy and write

this date on the sticker. Also, check the expiration date stamped on the box. If this date is less than 4 months from your purchase date, write this date on the sticker.
Do not use FORADIL capsules with any other capsule inhaler, and do not use the AEROLIZER inhaler to take any other capsule medicine.

Taking a dose of FORADIL AEROLIZER requires the following steps:

1. Open the foil pouch containing a blister card of FORADIL capsules. Do not remove a FORADIL capsule until you are ready for a dose.
2. Pull off the AEROLIZER Inhaler cover. (Figure 1)

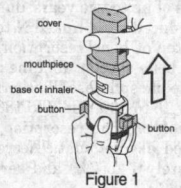

Figure 1

3. Hold the base of the AEROLIZER Inhaler firmly and twist the mouthpiece in the direction of the arrow to open. (Figure 2) Push the buttons in on each side to make sure that you can see 4 pins in the capsule well of the AEROLIZER Inhaler.

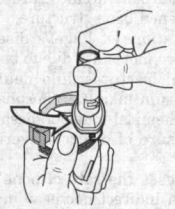

Figure 2

4. Separate one FORADIL capsule blister by tearing at the pre-cut lines. (Figure 3)

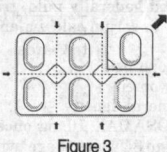

Figure 3

5. Peel the paper backing that covers one FORADIL capsule on the blister card. Push the FORADIL capsule through the foil. (Figure 4)

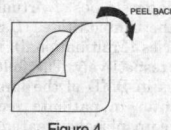

Figure 4

6. Place the FORADIL capsule in the capsule-chamber in the base of the AEROLIZER Inhaler. **Never place a capsule directly into the mouthpiece.** (Figure 5)

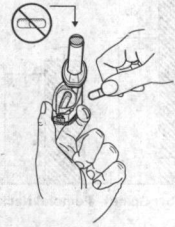

Figure 5

7. Twist the mouthpiece back to the closed position. (Figure 6)
[See figure 6 at top of next column]
8. Hold the mouthpiece of the AEROLIZER Inhaler upright and press both buttons at the same time. Only press the buttons **ONCE**. You should hear a click as the FORADIL capsule is being pierced. (Figure 7)
[See figure 7 on next column]
9. Release the buttons. If the buttons stay stuck, grasp the wings on the buttons and pull them out of the stuck position before the next step. Do not push the buttons a second time. This may cause the FORADIL capsule to break into small pieces. There is a screen built into the AEROLIZER Inhaler to hold these small pieces. It is possible that tiny pieces of a FORADIL capsule might reach your mouth or throat when

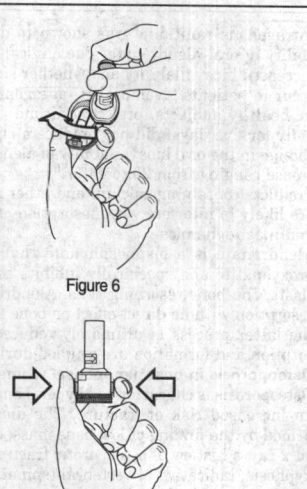

Figure 6

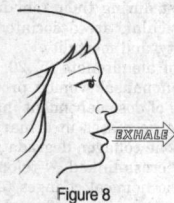

Figure 7

you inhale the medicine. This will not harm you, but to avoid this, only pierce the capsule once. The FORADIL capsules are also less likely to break into small pieces if you store them the right way (See "How do I store FORADIL AEROLIZER?").
10. Breathe out (exhale) fully. **Do not exhale into the AEROLIZER mouthpiece.** (Figure 8)

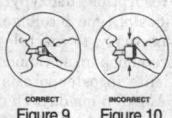

Figure 8

11. Tilt your head back slightly. Keep the AEROLIZER Inhaler level, with the blue buttons to the left and right (**not up and down**). Place the mouthpiece in your mouth and close your lips around the mouthpiece. (Figures 9 and 10)

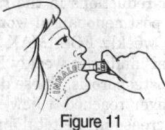

CORRECT   INCORRECT
Figure 9   Figure 10

12. Breathe in quickly and deeply (Figure 11). This will cause the FORADIL capsule to spin around in the chamber and deliver your dose of medicine. You should hear a whirring noise and experience a sweet taste in your mouth. If you do not hear the whirring noise, the capsule may be stuck. If this occurs, open the AEROLIZER Inhaler and loosen the capsule allowing it to spin freely. **Do not try to loosen the capsule by pressing the buttons again.** (You will have to repeat steps 10 to 12 again to get your dose.)

Figure 11

13. Remove the AEROLIZER Inhaler from your mouth. Continue to hold your breath as long as you can and then exhale.
14. Open the AEROLIZER Inhaler to see if any powder is still in the capsule. If any powder remains in the capsule repeat steps 10 to 13. Most people are able to empty the capsule in one or two inhalations.
15. After use, open the AEROLIZER Inhaler, remove and discard the empty capsule. Do not leave a used capsule in the chamber.
16. Close the mouthpiece and replace the cover.

Remember:
• Never breathe into the AEROLIZER Inhaler.
• Never take the AEROLIZER Inhaler apart.
• Never place a FORADIL capsule directly into the mouthpiece of the AEROLIZER Inhaler.
• Never leave a used FORADIL capsule in the AEROLIZER Inhaler chamber.
• Always use the AEROLIZER Inhaler in a level position.
• Never wash the AEROLIZER Inhaler. **Keep it dry.**

• Always keep the AEROLIZER Inhaler and FORADIL capsules in a dry place.
• Always use the new AEROLIZER Inhaler that comes with your refill.

Manufactured by:
Novartis Pharma AG, Basle, Switzerland
Distributed by:
Schering Corporation, a subsidiary of
MERCK & CO., INC.
Whitehouse Station, NJ 08889, USA
Copyright © 2010 Schering Corp., a subsidiary of MERCK & CO., INC.
All rights reserved.
FORADIL is a registered trademark of Astellas Pharma Inc.
AEROLIZER is a registered trademark of Novartis AG.
June 2010
This Medication Guide has been approved by the U.S. Food and Drug Administration.

Shown in Product Identification Guide, page 312

FOSAMAX®

[FOSS-ah-max]
(alendronate sodium)
Tablets and Oral Solution

Rx

DESCRIPTION

FOSAMAX* (alendronate sodium) is a bisphosphonate that acts as a specific inhibitor of osteoclast-mediated bone resorption. Bisphosphonates are synthetic analogs of pyrophosphate that bind to the hydroxyapatite found in bone.
Alendronate sodium is chemically described as (4-amino-1-hydroxybutylidene) bisphosphonic acid monosodium salt trihydrate.
The empirical formula of alendronate sodium is $C_4H_{12}NNaO_7P_2 \bullet 3H_2O$ and its formula weight is 325.12. The structural formula is:

$$HO-\overset{\overset{\displaystyle O}{\|}}{P}-\overset{\overset{\displaystyle CH_2}{|}\,\overset{\displaystyle CH_2}{|}\,\overset{\displaystyle CH_2}{|}\,\overset{\displaystyle NH_2}{|}}{\underset{\underset{\displaystyle OH}{}}{C}}-\overset{\overset{\displaystyle O}{\|}}{P}-ONa \cdot 3H_2O$$

Alendronate sodium is a white, crystalline, nonhygroscopic powder. It is soluble in water, very slightly soluble in alcohol, and practically insoluble in chloroform.
Tablets FOSAMAX for oral administration contain 6.53, 13.05, 45.68, 52.21 or 91.37 mg of alendronate monosodium salt trihydrate, which is the molar equivalent of 5, 10, 35, 40 and 70 mg, respectively, of free acid, and the following inactive ingredients: microcrystalline cellulose, anhydrous lactose, croscarmellose sodium, and magnesium stearate. Tablets FOSAMAX 10 mg also contain carnauba wax.
Each bottle of the oral solution contains 91.35 mg of alendronate monosodium salt trihydrate, which is the molar equivalent to 70 mg of free acid. Each bottle also contains the following inactive ingredients: sodium citrate dihydrate and citric acid anhydrous as buffering agents, sodium saccharin, artificial raspberry flavor, and purified water. Added as preservatives are sodium propylparaben 0.0225% and sodium butylparaben 0.0075%.

---

* Registered trademark of Merck Sharp & Dohme Corp., a subsidiary of **Merck & Co., Inc.**
Copyright ©1995, 1997, 2000 Merck Sharp & Dohme Corp., a subsidiary of **Merck & Co., Inc.**
All rights reserved

CLINICAL PHARMACOLOGY

Mechanism of Action
Animal studies have indicated the following mode of action. At the cellular level, alendronate shows preferential localization to sites of bone resorption, specifically under osteoclasts. The osteoclasts adhere normally to the bone surface but lack the ruffled border that is indicative of active resorption. Alendronate does not interfere with osteoclast recruitment or attachment, but it does inhibit osteoclast activity. Studies in mice on the localization of radioactive [3H]alendronate in bone showed about 10-fold higher uptake on osteoclast surfaces than on osteoblast surfaces. Bones examined 6 and 49 days after [3H]alendronate administration in rats and mice, respectively, showed that normal bone was formed on top of the alendronate, which was incorporated inside the matrix. While incorporated in bone matrix, alendronate is not pharmacologically active. Thus, alendronate must be continuously administered to suppress osteoclasts on newly formed resorption surfaces. Histomorphometry in baboons and rats showed that alendronate treatment reduces bone turnover (i.e., the number of sites at which bone is remodeled). In addition, bone formation exceeds bone resorption at these remodeling sites, leading to progressive gains in bone mass.

Pharmacokinetics

Absorption

Relative to an intravenous (IV) reference dose, the mean oral bioavailability of alendronate in women was 0.64% for doses ranging from 5 to 70 mg when administered after an overnight fast and two hours before a standardized breakfast. Oral bioavailability of the 10 mg tablet in men (0.59%) was similar to that in women when administered after an overnight fast and 2 hours before breakfast.

FOSAMAX 70 mg oral solution and FOSAMAX 70 mg tablet are equally bioavailable.

A study examining the effect of timing of a meal on the bioavailability of alendronate was performed in 49 postmenopausal women. Bioavailability was decreased (by approximately 40%) when 10 mg alendronate was administered either 0.5 or 1 hour before a standardized breakfast, when compared to dosing 2 hours before eating. In studies of treatment and prevention of osteoporosis, alendronate was effective when administered at least 30 minutes before breakfast.

Bioavailability was negligible whether alendronate was administered with or up to two hours after a standardized breakfast. Concomitant administration of alendronate with coffee or orange juice reduced bioavailability by approximately 60%.

Distribution

Preclinical studies (in male rats) show that alendronate transiently distributes to soft tissues following 1 mg/kg IV administration but is then rapidly redistributed to bone or excreted in the urine. The mean steady-state volume of distribution, exclusive of bone, is at least 28 L in humans. Concentrations of drug in plasma following therapeutic oral doses are too low (less than 5 ng/mL) for analytical detection. Protein binding in human plasma is approximately 78%.

Metabolism

There is no evidence that alendronate is metabolized in animals or humans.

Excretion

Following a single IV dose of [^{14}C]alendronate, approximately 50% of the radioactivity was excreted in the urine within 72 hours and little or no radioactivity was recovered in the feces. Following a single 10 mg IV dose, the renal clearance of alendronate was 71 mL/min (64, 78; 90% confidence interval [CI]), and systemic clearance did not exceed 200 mL/min. Plasma concentrations fell by more than 95% within 6 hours following IV administration. The terminal half-life in humans is estimated to exceed 10 years, probably reflecting release of alendronate from the skeleton. Based on the above, it is estimated that after 10 years of oral treatment with FOSAMAX (10 mg daily) the amount of alendronate released daily from the skeleton is approximately 25% of that absorbed from the gastrointestinal tract.

Special Populations

Pediatric:

The oral bioavailability in children was similar to that observed in adults; however, FOSAMAX is not indicated for use in children (see PRECAUTIONS, Pediatric Use).

Gender:

Bioavailability and the fraction of an IV dose excreted in urine were similar in men and women.

Geriatric:

Bioavailability and disposition (urinary excretion) were similar in elderly and younger patients. No dosage adjustment is necessary (see DOSAGE AND ADMINISTRATION).

Race:

Pharmacokinetic differences due to race have not been studied.

Renal Insufficiency:

Preclinical studies show that, in rats with kidney failure, increasing amounts of drug are present in plasma, kidney, spleen, and tibia. In healthy controls, drug that is not deposited in bone is rapidly excreted in the urine. No evidence of saturation of bone uptake was found after 3 weeks dosing with cumulative IV doses of 35 mg/kg in young male rats. Although no clinical information is available, it is likely that, as in animals, elimination of alendronate via the kidney will be reduced in patients with impaired renal function. Therefore, somewhat greater accumulation of alendronate in bone might be expected in patients with impaired renal function.

No dosage adjustment is necessary for patients with mild-to-moderate renal insufficiency (creatinine clearance 35 to 60 mL/min). **FOSAMAX is not recommended for patients with more severe renal insufficiency (creatinine clearance <35 mL/min) due to lack of experience with alendronate in renal failure.**

Hepatic Insufficiency:

As there is evidence that alendronate is not metabolized or excreted in the bile, no studies were conducted in patients with hepatic insufficiency. No dosage adjustment is necessary.

Drug Interactions

(also see PRECAUTIONS, Drug Interactions)

Intravenous ranitidine was shown to double the bioavailability of oral alendronate. The clinical significance of this increased bioavailability and whether similar increases will occur in patients given oral H$_2$-antagonists is unknown.

In healthy subjects, oral prednisone (20 mg three times daily for five days) did not produce a clinically meaningful change in the oral bioavailability of alendronate (a mean increase ranging from 20 to 44%).

Products containing calcium and other multivalent cations are likely to interfere with absorption of alendronate.

Pharmacodynamics

Alendronate is a bisphosphonate that binds to bone hydroxyapatite and specifically inhibits the activity of osteoclasts, the bone-resorbing cells. Alendronate reduces bone resorption with no direct effect on bone formation, although the latter process is ultimately reduced because bone resorption and formation are coupled during bone turnover.

Osteoporosis in postmenopausal women

Osteoporosis is characterized by low bone mass that leads to an increased risk of fracture. The diagnosis can be confirmed by the finding of low bone mass, evidence of fracture on x-ray, a history of osteoporotic fracture, or height loss or kyphosis, indicative of vertebral (spinal) fracture. Osteoporosis occurs in both males and females but is most common among women following the menopause, when bone turnover increases and the rate of bone resorption exceeds that of bone formation. These changes result in progressive bone loss and lead to osteoporosis in a significant proportion of women over age 50. Fractures, usually of the spine, hip, and wrist, are the common consequences. From age 50 to age 90, the risk of hip fracture in white women increases 50-fold and the risk of vertebral fracture 15- to 30-fold. It is estimated that approximately 40% of 50-year-old women will sustain one or more osteoporosis-related fractures of the spine, hip, or wrist during their remaining lifetimes. Hip fractures, in particular, are associated with substantial morbidity, disability, and mortality.

Daily oral doses of alendronate (5, 20, and 40 mg for six weeks) in postmenopausal women produced biochemical changes indicative of dose-dependent inhibition of bone resorption, including decreases in urinary calcium and urinary markers of bone collagen degradation (such as deoxypyridinoline and cross-linked N-telopeptides of type I collagen). These biochemical changes tended to return toward baseline values as early as 3 weeks following the discontinuation of therapy with alendronate and did not differ from placebo after 7 months.

Long-term treatment of osteoporosis with FOSAMAX 10 mg/day (for up to five years) reduced urinary excretion of markers of bone resorption, deoxypyridinoline and cross-linked N-telopeptides of type 1 collagen, by approximately 50% and 70%, respectively, to reach levels similar to those seen in healthy premenopausal women. Similar decreases were seen in patients in osteoporosis prevention studies who received FOSAMAX 5 mg/day. The decrease in the rate of bone resorption indicated by these markers was evident as early as one month and at three to six months reached a plateau that was maintained for the entire duration of treatment with FOSAMAX. In osteoporosis treatment studies FOSAMAX 10 mg/day decreased the markers of bone formation, osteocalcin and bone specific alkaline phosphatase by approximately 50%, and total serum alkaline phosphatase by approximately 25 to 30% to reach a plateau after 6 to 12 months. In osteoporosis prevention studies FOSAMAX 5 mg/day decreased osteocalcin and total serum alkaline phosphatase by approximately 40% and 15%, respectively. Similar reductions in the rate of bone turnover were observed in postmenopausal women during one-year studies with once weekly FOSAMAX 70 mg for the treatment of osteoporosis and once weekly FOSAMAX 35 mg for the prevention of osteoporosis. These data indicate that the rate of bone turnover reached a new steady-state, despite the progressive increase in the total amount of alendronate deposited within bone.

As a result of inhibition of bone resorption, asymptomatic reductions in serum calcium and phosphate concentrations were also observed following treatment with FOSAMAX. In the long-term studies, reductions from baseline in serum calcium (approximately 2%) and phosphate (approximately 4 to 6%) were evident the first month after the initiation of FOSAMAX 10 mg. No further decreases in serum calcium were observed for the five-year duration of treatment; however, serum phosphate returned toward prestudy levels during years three through five. Similar reductions were observed with FOSAMAX 5 mg/day. In one-year studies with once weekly FOSAMAX 35 and 70 mg, similar reductions were observed at 6 and 12 months. The reduction in serum phosphate may reflect not only the positive bone mineral balance due to FOSAMAX but also a decrease in renal phosphate reabsorption.

Osteoporosis in men

Treatment of men with osteoporosis with FOSAMAX 10 mg/day for two years reduced urinary excretion of cross-linked N-telopeptides of type I collagen by approximately 60% and

bone-specific alkaline phosphatase by approximately 40%. Similar reductions were observed in a one-year study in men with osteoporosis receiving once weekly FOSAMAX 70 mg.

Glucocorticoid-induced Osteoporosis

Sustained use of glucocorticoids is commonly associated with development of osteoporosis and resulting fractures (especially vertebral, hip, and rib). It occurs both in males and females of all ages. Osteoporosis occurs as a result of inhibited bone formation and increased bone resorption resulting in net bone loss. Alendronate decreases bone resorption without directly inhibiting bone formation.

In clinical studies of up to two years' duration, FOSAMAX 5 and 10 mg/day reduced cross-linked N-telopeptides of type I collagen (a marker of bone resorption) by approximately 60% and reduced bone-specific alkaline phosphatase and total serum alkaline phosphatase (markers of bone formation) by approximately 15 to 30% and 8 to 18%, respectively. As a result of inhibition of bone resorption, FOSAMAX 5 and 10 mg/day induced asymptomatic decreases in serum calcium (approximately 1 to 2%) and serum phosphate (approximately 1 to 8%).

Paget's disease of bone

Paget's disease of bone is a chronic, focal skeletal disorder characterized by greatly increased and disorderly bone remodeling. Excessive osteoclastic bone resorption is followed by osteoblastic new bone formation, leading to the replacement of the normal bone architecture by disorganized, enlarged, and weakened bone structure.

Clinical manifestations of Paget's disease range from no symptoms to severe morbidity due to bone pain, bone deformity, pathological fractures, and neurological and other complications. Serum alkaline phosphatase, the most frequently used biochemical index of disease activity, provides an objective measure of disease severity and response to therapy.

FOSAMAX decreases the rate of bone resorption directly, which leads to an indirect decrease in bone formation. In clinical trials, FOSAMAX 40 mg once daily for six months produced significant decreases in serum alkaline phosphatase as well as in urinary markers of bone collagen degradation. As a result of the inhibition of bone resorption, FOSAMAX induced generally mild, transient, and asymptomatic decreases in serum calcium and phosphate.

Clinical Studies

Treatment of osteoporosis

Postmenopausal women

Effect on bone mineral density

The efficacy of FOSAMAX 10 mg once daily in postmenopausal women, 44 to 84 years of age, with osteoporosis (lumbar spine bone mineral density [BMD] of at least 2 standard deviations below the premenopausal mean) was demonstrated in four double-blind, placebo-controlled clinical studies of two or three years' duration. These included two three-year, multicenter studies of virtually identical design, one performed in the United States (U.S.) and the other in 15 different countries (Multinational), which enrolled 478 and 516 patients, respectively. The following graph shows the mean increases in BMD of the lumbar spine, femoral neck, and trochanter in patients receiving FOSAMAX 10 mg/day relative to placebo-treated patients at three years for each of these studies.

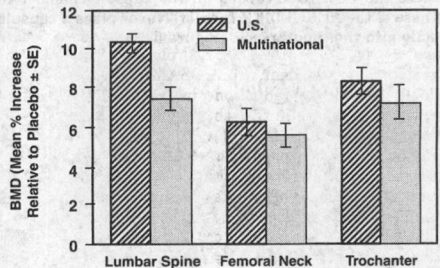

Osteoporosis Treatment Studies in Postmenopausal Women: Increase in BMD: FOSAMAX 10 mg/day at Three Years

At three years significant increases in BMD, relative both to baseline and placebo, were seen at each measurement site in each study in patients who received FOSAMAX 10 mg/day. Total body BMD also increased significantly in each study, suggesting that the increases in bone mass of the spine and hip did not occur at the expense of other skeletal sites. Increases in BMD were evident as early as three months and continued throughout the three years of treatment. (See figures below for lumbar spine results.) In the two-year extension of these studies, treatment of 147 patients with FOSAMAX 10 mg/day resulted in continued increases in BMD at the lumbar spine and trochanter (absolute additional increases between years 3 and 5: lumbar spine, 0.94%; trochanter, 0.88%). BMD at the femoral neck,

forearm and total body were maintained. FOSAMAX was similarly effective regardless of age, race, baseline rate of bone turnover, and baseline BMD in the range studied (at least 2 standard deviations below the premenopausal mean). Thus, overall FOSAMAX reverses the loss of bone mineral density, a central factor in the progression of osteoporosis.
[See figure at right]
In patients with postmenopausal osteoporosis treated with FOSAMAX 10 mg/day for one or two years, the effects of treatment withdrawal were assessed. Following discontinuation, there were no further increases in bone mass and the rates of bone loss were similar to those of the placebo groups. These data indicate that continued treatment with FOSAMAX is required to maintain the effect of the drug.
The therapeutic equivalence of once weekly FOSAMAX 70 mg (n=519) and FOSAMAX 10 mg daily (n=370) was demonstrated in a one-year, double-blind, multicenter study of postmenopausal women with osteoporosis. In the primary analysis of completers, the mean increases from baseline in lumbar spine BMD at one year were 5.1% (4.8, 5.4%; 95% CI) in the 70-mg once-weekly group (n=440) and 5.4% (5.0, 5.8%; 95% CI) in the 10-mg daily group (n=330). The two treatment groups were also similar with regard to BMD increases at other skeletal sites. The results of the intention-to-treat analysis were consistent with the primary analysis of completers.

Effect on fracture incidence
Data on the effects of FOSAMAX on fracture incidence are derived from three clinical studies: 1) U.S. and Multinational combined: a study of patients with a BMD T-score at or below minus 2.5 with or without a prior vertebral fracture, 2) Three-Year Study of the Fracture Intervention Trial (FIT): a study of patients with at least one baseline vertebral fracture, and 3) Four-Year Study of FIT: a study of patients with low bone mass but without a baseline vertebral fracture.
To assess the effects of FOSAMAX on the incidence of vertebral fractures (detected by digitized radiography; approximately one third of these were clinically symptomatic), the U.S. and Multinational studies were combined in an analysis that compared placebo to the pooled dosage groups of FOSAMAX (5 or 10 mg for three years or 20 mg for two years followed by 5 mg for one year). There was a statistically significant reduction in the proportion of patients treated with FOSAMAX experiencing one or more new vertebral fractures relative to those treated with placebo (3.2% vs. 6.2%; a 48% relative risk reduction). A reduction in the total number of new vertebral fractures (4.2 vs. 11.3 per 100 patients) was also observed. In the pooled analysis, patients who received FOSAMAX had a loss in stature that was statistically significantly less than was observed in those who received placebo (-3.0 mm vs. -4.6 mm).
The Fracture Intervention Trial (FIT) consisted of two studies in postmenopausal women: the Three-Year Study of patients who had at least one baseline radiographic vertebral fracture and the Four-Year Study of patients with low bone mass but without a baseline vertebral fracture. In both studies of FIT, 96% of randomized patients completed the studies (i.e., had a closeout visit at the scheduled end of the study); approximately 80% of patients were still taking study medication upon completion.

Fracture Intervention Trial: Three-Year Study (patients with at least one baseline radiographic vertebral fracture)
This randomized, double-blind, placebo-controlled, 2027-patient study (FOSAMAX, n=1022; placebo, n=1005) demonstrated that treatment with FOSAMAX resulted in statistically significant reductions in fracture incidence at three years as shown in the table below.
[See table above]
Furthermore, in this population of patients with baseline vertebral fracture, treatment with FOSAMAX significantly reduced the incidence of hospitalizations (25.0% vs. 30.7%).
In the Three-Year Study of FIT, fractures of the hip occurred in 22 (2.2%) of 1005 patients on placebo and 11 (1.1%) of 1022 patients on FOSAMAX, p=0.047. The figure below displays the cumulative incidence of hip fractures in this study.
[See second figure on next column]

Fracture Intervention Trial: Four-Year Study (patients with low bone mass but without a baseline radiographic vertebral fracture)
This randomized, double-blind, placebo-controlled, 4432-patient study (FOSAMAX, n=2214; placebo, n=2218) further investigated the reduction in fracture incidence due to FOSAMAX. The intent of the study was to recruit women with osteoporosis, defined as a baseline femoral neck BMD at least two standard deviations below the mean for young adult women. However, due to subsequent revisions to the normative values for femoral neck BMD, 31% of patients were found not to meet this entry criterion and thus this study included both osteoporotic and non-osteoporotic women. The results are shown in the table below for the patients with osteoporosis.
[See table at top of next page]

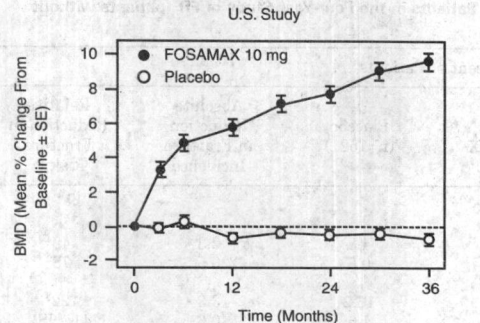

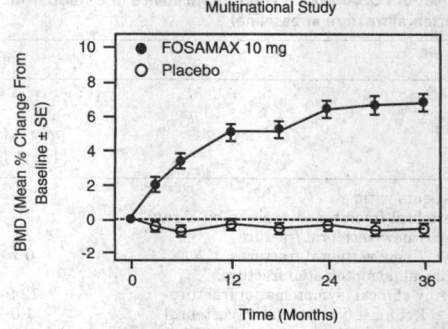

Osteoporosis Treatment Studies in Postmenopausal Women: Time Course of Effect of FOSAMAX 10 mg/day Versus Placebo: Lumbar Spine BMD Percent Change From Baseline

Effect of FOSAMAX on Fracture Incidence in the Three-Year Study of FIT (patients with vertebral fracture at baseline)

	Percent of Patients			
	FOSAMAX (n=1022)	Placebo (n=1005)	Absolute Reduction in Fracture Incidence	Relative Reduction in Fracture Risk %
Patients with:				
Vertebral fractures (diagnosed by X-ray)*				
≥ 1 new vertebral fracture	7.9	15.0	7.1	47†
≥ 2 new vertebral fractures	0.5	4.9	4.4	90†
Clinical (symptomatic) fractures				
Any clinical (symptomatic) fracture	13.8	18.1	4.3	26‡
≥ 1 clinical (symptomatic) vertebral fracture	2.3	5.0	2.7	54§
Hip fracture	1.1	2.2	1.1	51¶
Wrist (forearm) fracture	2.2	4.1	1.9	48¶

*Number evaluable for vertebral fractures: FOSAMAX, n=984; placebo, n=966
†p<0.001
‡p=0.007
§p<0.01
¶p<0.05

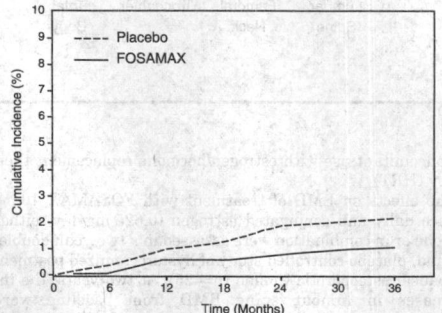

Cumulative Incidence of Hip Fractures in the Three-Year Study of FIT (patients with radiographic vertebral fracture at baseline)

Fracture results across studies
In the Three-Year Study of FIT, FOSAMAX reduced the percentage of women experiencing at least one new radiographic vertebral fracture from 15.0% to 7.9% (47% relative risk reduction, p<0.001); in the Four-Year Study of FIT, the percentage was reduced from 3.8% to 2.1% (44% relative risk reduction, p=0.001); and in the combined U.S./Multinational studies, from 6.2% to 3.2% (48% relative risk reduction, p=0.034).
FOSAMAX reduced the percentage of women experiencing multiple (two or more) new vertebral fractures from 4.2% to 0.6% (87% relative risk reduction, p<0.001) in the combined U.S./Multinational studies and from 4.9% to 0.5% (90% relative risk reduction, p<0.001) in the Three-Year Study of FIT. In the Four-Year Study of FIT, FOSAMAX reduced the percentage of osteoporotic women experiencing multiple vertebral fractures from 0.6% to 0.1% (78% relative risk reduction, p=0.035).
Thus, FOSAMAX reduced the incidence of radiographic vertebral fractures in osteoporotic women whether or not they had a previous radiographic vertebral fracture.
FOSAMAX, over a three- or four-year period, was associated with statistically significant reductions in loss of height vs. placebo in patients with and without baseline radiographic vertebral fractures. At the end of the FIT studies the between-treatment group differences were 3.2 mm in the Three-Year Study and 1.3 mm in the Four-Year Study.

Bone histology
Bone histology in 270 postmenopausal patients with osteoporosis treated with FOSAMAX at doses ranging from 1 to 20 mg/day for one, two, or three years revealed normal mineralization and structure, as well as the expected decrease in bone turnover relative to placebo. These data, together with the normal bone histology and increased bone strength observed in rats and baboons exposed to long-term alendronate treatment, support the conclusion that bone formed during therapy with FOSAMAX is of normal quality.

Men
The efficacy of FOSAMAX in men with hypogonadal or idiopathic osteoporosis was demonstrated in two clinical studies.
A two-year, double-blind, placebo-controlled, multicenter study of FOSAMAX 10 mg once daily enrolled a total of 241 men between the ages of 31 and 87 (mean, 63). All patients in the trial had either: 1) a BMD T-score ≤-2 at the femoral neck and ≤-1 at the lumbar spine, or 2) a baseline osteoporotic fracture and a BMD T-score ≤-1 at the femoral neck. At two years, the mean increases relative to placebo in BMD in men receiving FOSAMAX 10 mg/day were significant at the following sites: lumbar spine, 5.3%; femoral neck, 2.6%; trochanter, 3.1%; and total body, 1.6%. Treatment with FOSAMAX also reduced height loss (FOSAMAX, -0.6 mm vs. placebo, -2.4 mm).
A one-year, double-blind, placebo-controlled, multicenter study of once weekly FOSAMAX 70 mg enrolled a total of 167 men between the ages of 38 and 91 (mean, 66). Patients in the study had either: 1) a BMD T-score ≤-2 at the femoral neck and ≤-1 at the lumbar spine, 2) a BMD T-score ≤-2 at the lumbar spine and ≤-1 at the femoral neck, or 3) a baseline osteoporotic fracture and a BMD T-score ≤-1 at the femoral neck. At one year, the mean increases relative to placebo in BMD in men receiving FOSAMAX 70 mg once weekly were significant at the following sites: lumbar spine, 2.8%; femoral neck, 1.9%; trochanter, 2.0%; and total body, 1.2%. These increases in BMD were similar to those seen at one year in the 10 mg once-daily study.
In both studies, BMD responses were similar regardless of age (≥65 years vs. <65 years), gonadal function (baseline testosterone <9 ng/dL vs. ≥9 ng/dL), or baseline BMD (femoral neck and lumbar spine T-score ≤-2.5 vs. >-2.5).

Effect of FOSAMAX on Fracture Incidence in Osteoporotic* Patients in the Four-Year Study of FIT (patients without vertebral fracture at baseline)

	Percent of Patients			
	FOSAMAX (n=1545)	Placebo (n=1521)	Absolute Reduction in Fracture Incidence	Relative Reduction in Fracture Risk %
Patients with:				
Vertebral fractures (diagnosed by X-ray)[†]				
≥ 1 new vertebral fracture	2.5	4.8	2.3	48[‡]
≥ 2 new vertebral fractures	0.1	0.6	0.5	78[§]
Clinical (symptomatic) fractures				
Any clinical (symptomatic) fracture	12.9	16.2	3.3	22[¶]
≥ 1 clinical (symptomatic) vertebral fracture	1.0	1.6	0.6	41 (NS)[#]
Hip fracture	1.0	1.4	0.4	29 (NS)[#]
Wrist (forearm) fracture	3.9	3.8	-0.1	NS[#]

*Baseline femoral neck BMD at least 2 SD below the mean for young adult women
[†]Number evaluable for vertebral fractures: FOSAMAX, n=1426; placebo, n=1428
[‡]p<0.001
[§]p=0.035
[¶]p=0.01
[#]Not significant. This study was not powered to detect differences at these sites.

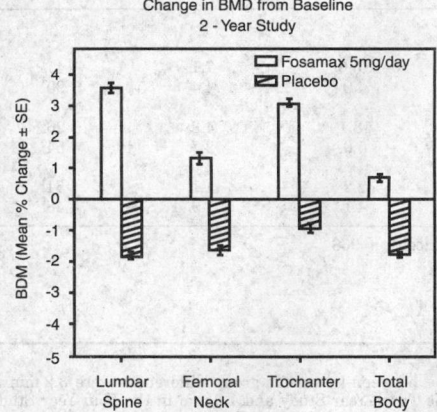

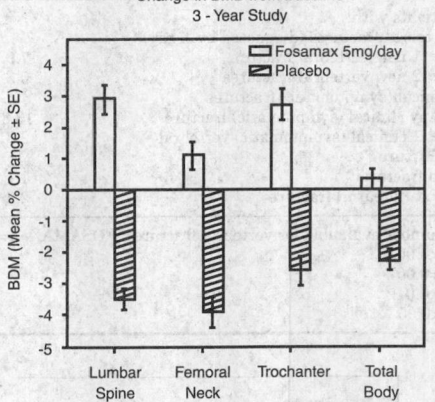

Osteoporosis Prevention Studies in Postmenopausal Women

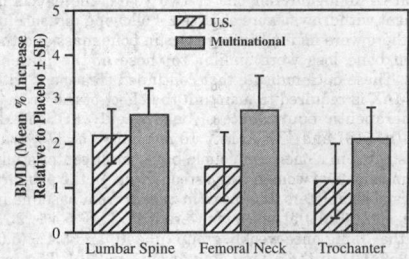

Studies in Glucocorticoid-Treated Patients: Increase in BMD: FOSAMAX 5 mg/day at One Year

Prevention of osteoporosis in postmenopausal women
Prevention of bone loss was demonstrated in two double-blind, placebo-controlled studies of postmenopausal women 40-60 years of age. One thousand six hundred nine patients (FOSAMAX 5 mg/day; n=498) who were at least six months postmenopausal were entered into a two-year study without regard to their baseline BMD. In the other study, 447 patients (FOSAMAX 5 mg/day; n=88), who were between six months and three years postmenopause, were treated for up to three years. In the placebo-treated patients BMD losses of approximately 1% per year were seen at the spine, hip (femoral neck and trochanter) and total body. In contrast, FOSAMAX 5 mg/day prevented bone loss in the majority of patients and induced significant increases in mean bone mass at each of these sites (see figures below). In addition, FOSAMAX 5 mg/day reduced the rate of bone loss at the forearm by approximately half relative to placebo. FOSAMAX 5 mg/day was similarly effective in this population regardless of age, time since menopause, race and baseline rate of bone turnover.
[See figure above]
The therapeutic equivalence of once weekly FOSAMAX 35 mg (n=362) and FOSAMAX 5 mg daily (n=361) was demonstrated in a one-year, double-blind, multicenter study of postmenopausal women without osteoporosis. In the primary analysis of completers, the mean increases from baseline in lumbar spine BMD at one year were 2.9% (2.6, 3.2%; 95% CI) in the 35-mg once-weekly group (n=307) and 3.2% (2.9, 3.5%; 95% CI) in the 5-mg daily group (n=298). The two treatment groups were also similar with regard to BMD increases at other skeletal sites. The results of the intention-to-treat analysis were consistent with the primary analysis of completers.
Bone histology
Bone histology was normal in the 28 patients biopsied at the end of three years who received FOSAMAX at doses of up to 10 mg/day.

Concomitant use with estrogen/hormone replacement therapy (HRT)
The effects on BMD of treatment with FOSAMAX 10 mg once daily and conjugated estrogen (0.625 mg/day) either alone or in combination were assessed in a two-year, double-blind, placebo-controlled study of hysterectomized postmenopausal osteoporotic women (n=425). At two years, the increases in lumbar spine BMD from baseline were significantly greater with the combination (8.3%) than with either estrogen or FOSAMAX alone (both 6.0%).
The effects on BMD when FOSAMAX was added to stable doses (for at least one year) of HRT (estrogen ± progestin) were assessed in a one-year, double-blind, placebo-controlled study in postmenopausal osteoporotic women (n=428). The addition of FOSAMAX 10 mg once daily to HRT produced, at one year, significantly greater increases in lumbar spine BMD (3.7%) vs. HRT alone (1.1%).
In these studies, significant increases or favorable trends in BMD for combined therapy compared with HRT alone were seen at the total hip, femoral neck, and trochanter. No significant effect was seen for total body BMD.
Histomorphometric studies of transiliac biopsies in 92 subjects showed normal bone architecture. Compared to placebo there was a 98% suppression of bone turnover (as assessed by mineralizing surface) after 18 months of combined treatment with FOSAMAX and HRT, 94% on FOSAMAX alone, and 78% on HRT alone. The long-term effects of combined FOSAMAX and HRT on fracture occurrence and fracture healing have not been studied.
Glucocorticoid-induced osteoporosis
The efficacy of FOSAMAX 5 and 10 mg once daily in men and women receiving glucocorticoids (at least 7.5 mg/day of prednisone or equivalent) was demonstrated in two, one-year, double-blind, randomized, placebo-controlled, multicenter studies of virtually identical design, one performed in the United States and the other in 15 different countries (Multinational [which also included FOSAMAX 2.5 mg/

day]). These studies enrolled 232 and 328 patients, respectively, between the ages of 17 and 83 with a variety of glucocorticoid-requiring diseases. Patients received supplemental calcium and vitamin D. The following figure shows the mean increases relative to placebo in BMD of the lumbar spine, femoral neck, and trochanter in patients receiving FOSAMAX 5 mg/day for each study.

After one year, significant increases relative to placebo in BMD were seen in the combined studies at each of these sites in patients who received FOSAMAX 5 mg/day. In the placebo-treated patients, a significant decrease in BMD occurred at the femoral neck (-1.2%), and smaller decreases were seen at the lumbar spine and trochanter. Total body BMD was maintained with FOSAMAX 5 mg/day. The increases in BMD with FOSAMAX 10 mg/day were similar to those with FOSAMAX 5 mg/day in all patients except for postmenopausal women not receiving estrogen therapy. In these women, the increases (relative to placebo) with FOSAMAX 10 mg/day were greater than those with FOSAMAX 5 mg/day at the lumbar spine (4.1% vs. 1.6%) and trochanter (2.8% vs. 1.7%), but not at other sites. FOSAMAX was effective regardless of dose or duration of glucocorticoid use. In addition, FOSAMAX was similarly effective regardless of age (<65 vs. ≥65 years), race (Caucasian vs. other races), gender, underlying disease, baseline BMD, baseline bone turnover, and use with a variety of common medications.
Bone histology was normal in the 49 patients biopsied at the end of one year who received FOSAMAX at doses of up to 10 mg/day.
Of the original 560 patients in these studies, 208 patients who remained on at least 7.5 mg/day of prednisone or equivalent continued into a one-year double-blind extension. After two years of treatment, spine BMD increased by 3.7% and 5.0% relative to placebo with FOSAMAX 5 and 10 mg/day, respectively. Significant increases in BMD (relative to placebo) were also observed at the femoral neck, trochanter, and total body.
After one year, 2.3% of patients treated with FOSAMAX 5 or 10 mg/day (pooled) vs. 3.7% of those treated with placebo experienced a new vertebral fracture (not significant). However, in the population studied for two years, treatment with FOSAMAX (pooled dosage groups: 5 or 10 mg for two years or 2.5 mg for one year followed by 10 mg for one year) significantly reduced the incidence of patients with a new vertebral fracture (FOSAMAX 0.7% vs. placebo 6.8%).
Paget's disease of bone
The efficacy of FOSAMAX 40 mg once daily for six months was demonstrated in two double-blind clinical studies of male and female patients with moderate to severe Paget's disease (alkaline phosphatase at least twice the upper limit of normal): a placebo-controlled, multinational study and a U.S. comparative study with etidronate disodium 400 mg/day. The following figure shows the mean percent changes from baseline in serum alkaline phosphatase for up to six months of randomized treatment.
[See figure at top of next page]
At six months the suppression in alkaline phosphatase in patients treated with FOSAMAX was significantly greater than that achieved with etidronate and contrasted with the complete lack of response in placebo-treated patients. Response (defined as either normalization of serum alkaline phosphatase or decrease from baseline ≥60%) occurred in approximately 85% of patients treated with FOSAMAX in the combined studies vs. 30% in the etidronate group and 0% in the placebo group. FOSAMAX was similarly effective regardless of age, gender, race, prior use of other bisphosphonates, or baseline alkaline phosphatase within the range studied (at least twice the upper limit of normal).
Bone histology was evaluated in 33 patients with Paget's disease treated with FOSAMAX 40 mg/day for 6 months. As in patients treated for osteoporosis (see Clinical Studies,

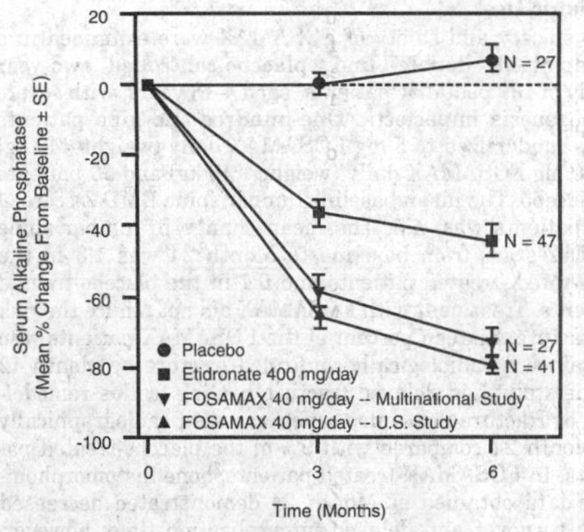

Studies in Paget's Disease of Bone: Effect on Serum Alkaline Phosphatase of FOSAMAX 40 mg/day Versus Placebo or Etidronate 400 mg/day

Treatment of osteoporosis in postmenopausal women, Bone histology), FOSAMAX did not impair mineralization, and the expected decrease in the rate of bone turnover was observed. Normal lamellar bone was produced during treatment with FOSAMAX, even where preexisting bone was woven and disorganized. Overall, bone histology data support the conclusion that bone formed during treatment with FOSAMAX is of normal quality.

ANIMAL PHARMACOLOGY

The relative inhibitory activities on bone resorption and mineralization of alendronate and etidronate were compared in the Schenk assay, which is based on histological examination of the epiphyses of growing rats. In this assay, the lowest dose of alendronate that interfered with bone mineralization (leading to osteomalacia) was 6000-fold the antiresorptive dose. The corresponding ratio for etidronate was one to one. These data suggest that alendronate administered in therapeutic doses is highly unlikely to induce osteomalacia.

INDICATIONS AND USAGE

FOSAMAX is indicated for:

- Treatment and prevention of osteoporosis in postmenopausal women
  - For the treatment of osteoporosis, FOSAMAX increases bone mass and reduces the incidence of fractures, including those of the hip and spine (vertebral compression fractures). Osteoporosis may be confirmed by the finding of low bone mass (for example, at least 2 standard deviations below the premenopausal mean) or by the presence or history of osteoporotic fracture. (See CLINICAL PHARMACOLOGY, Pharmacodynamics.)
  - For the prevention of osteoporosis, FOSAMAX may be considered in postmenopausal women who are at risk of developing osteoporosis and for whom the desired clinical outcome is to maintain bone mass and to reduce the risk of future fracture.

    Bone loss is particularly rapid in postmenopausal women younger than age 60. Risk factors often associated with the development of postmenopausal osteoporosis include early menopause; moderately low bone mass (for example, at least 1 standard deviation below the mean for healthy young adult women); thin body build; Caucasian or Asian race; and family history of osteoporosis. The presence of such risk factors may be important when considering the use of FOSAMAX for prevention of osteoporosis.
- Treatment to increase bone mass in men with osteoporosis
- Treatment of glucocorticoid-induced osteoporosis in men and women receiving glucocorticoids in a daily dosage equivalent to 7.5 mg or greater of prednisone and who have low bone mineral density (see PRECAUTIONS, Glucocorticoid-induced osteoporosis). Patients treated with glucocorticoids should receive adequate amounts of calcium and vitamin D.
- Treatment of Paget's disease of bone in men and women
  - Treatment is indicated in patients with Paget's disease of bone having alkaline phosphatase at least two times the upper limit of normal, or those who are symptomatic, or those at risk for future complications from their disease.

CONTRAINDICATIONS

- Abnormalities of the esophagus which delay esophageal emptying such as stricture or achalasia
- Inability to stand or sit upright for at least 30 minutes (see WARNINGS)
- Patients at increased risk of aspiration should not receive FOSAMAX oral solution.
- Hypersensitivity to any component of this product
- Hypocalcemia (see PRECAUTIONS, General)

WARNINGS

FOSAMAX, like other bisphosphonates administered orally, may cause local irritation of the upper gastrointestinal mucosa. Because of these possible irritant effects and a potential for worsening of the underlying disease, caution should be used when FOSAMAX is given to patients with active upper gastrointestinal problems (such as known Barrett's esophagus, dysphagia, other esophageal diseases, gastritis, duodenitis, or ulcers).

Esophageal adverse experiences, such as esophagitis, esophageal ulcers and esophageal erosions, occasionally with bleeding and rarely followed by esophageal stricture or perforation, have been reported in patients receiving treatment with oral bisphosphonates including FOSAMAX. In some cases these have been severe and required hospitalization. Physicians should therefore be alert to any signs or symptoms signaling a possible esophageal reaction and patients should be instructed to discontinue FOSAMAX and seek medical attention if they develop dysphagia, odynophagia, retrosternal pain or new or worsening heartburn.

The risk of severe esophageal adverse experiences appears to be greater in patients who lie down after taking oral bisphosphonates including FOSAMAX and/or who fail to swallow oral bisphosphonates including FOSAMAX with the recommended full glass (6-8 oz) of water, and/or who continue to take oral bisphosphonates including FOSAMAX after developing symptoms suggestive of esophageal irritation. Therefore, it is very important that the full dosing instructions are provided to, and understood by, the patient (see DOSAGE AND ADMINISTRATION). In patients who cannot comply with dosing instructions due to mental disability, therapy with FOSAMAX should be used under appropriate supervision.

There have been post-marketing reports of gastric and duodenal ulcers with oral bisphosphonate use, some severe and with complications, although no increased risk was observed in controlled clinical trials.

PRECAUTIONS

General

Causes of osteoporosis other than estrogen deficiency, aging, and glucocorticoid use should be considered.

Hypocalcemia must be corrected before initiating therapy with FOSAMAX (see CONTRAINDICATIONS). Other disorders affecting mineral metabolism (such as vitamin D deficiency) should also be effectively treated. In patients with these conditions, serum calcium and symptoms of hypocalcemia should be monitored during therapy with FOSAMAX.

Presumably due to the effects of FOSAMAX on increasing bone mineral, small, asymptomatic decreases in serum calcium and phosphate may occur, especially in patients with Paget's disease, in whom the pretreatment rate of bone turnover may be greatly elevated and in patients receiving glucocorticoids, in whom calcium absorption may be decreased.

Ensuring adequate calcium and vitamin D intake is especially important in patients with Paget's disease of bone and in patients receiving glucocorticoids.

Musculoskeletal Pain

In post marketing experience, severe and occasionally incapacitating bone, joint, and/or muscle pain has been reported in patients taking bisphosphonates that are approved for the prevention and treatment of osteoporosis (see ADVERSE REACTIONS). This category of drugs includes FOSAMAX (alendronate). Most of the patients were postmenopausal women. The time to onset of symptoms varied from one day to several months after starting the drug. Discontinue use if severe symptoms develop. Most patients had relief of symptoms after stopping. A subset had recurrence of symptoms when rechallenged with the same drug or another bisphosphonate.

In placebo-controlled clinical studies of FOSAMAX, the percentages of patients with these symptoms were similar in the FOSAMAX and placebo groups.

Dental

Osteonecrosis of the jaw (ONJ), which can occur spontaneously, is generally associated with tooth extraction and/or local infection with delayed healing, and has been reported in patients taking bisphosphonates, including FOSAMAX. Known risk factors for osteonecrosis of the jaw include invasive dental procedures (e.g., tooth extraction, dental implants, boney surgery), diagnosis of cancer, concomitant therapies (e.g., chemotherapy, corticosteroids), poor oral hygiene, and co-morbid disorders (e.g., periodontal and/or other pre-existing dental disease, anemia, coagulopathy, infection, ill-fitting dentures).

For patients requiring invasive dental procedures, discontinuation of bisphosphonate treatment may reduce the risk for ONJ. Clinical judgment of the treating physician and/or oral surgeon should guide the management plan of each patient based on individual benefit/risk assessment.

Patients who develop osteonecrosis of the jaw while on bisphosphonate therapy should receive care by an oral surgeon. In these patients, extensive dental surgery to treat ONJ may exacerbate the condition. Discontinuation of bisphosphonate therapy should be considered based on individual benefit/risk assessment.

Renal insufficency

FOSAMAX is not recommended for patients with renal insufficiency (creatinine clearance <35 mL/min). (See DOSAGE AND ADMINISTRATION.)

Glucocorticoid-induced osteoporosis

The risk versus benefit of FOSAMAX for treatment at daily dosages of glucocorticoids less than 7.5 mg of prednisone or equivalent has not been established (see INDICATIONS AND USAGE). Before initiating treatment, the hormonal status of both men and women should be ascertained and appropriate replacement considered.

A bone mineral density measurement should be made at the initiation of therapy and repeated after 6 to 12 months of combined FOSAMAX and glucocorticoid treatment.

The efficacy of FOSAMAX for the treatment of glucocorticoid-induced osteoporosis has been shown in patients with a median bone mineral density which was 1.2 standard deviations below the mean for healthy young adults.

The efficacy of FOSAMAX has been established in studies of two years' duration. The greatest increase in bone mineral density occurred in the first year with maintenance or smaller gains during the second year. Efficacy of FOSAMAX beyond two years has not been studied.

The efficacy of FOSAMAX in respect to fracture prevention has been demonstrated for vertebral fractures. However, this finding was based on very few fractures that occurred primarily in postmenopausal women. The efficacy for prevention of non-vertebral fractures has not been demonstrated.

Information for Patients

General

Physicians should instruct their patients to read the patient package insert before starting therapy with FOSAMAX and to reread it each time the prescription is renewed.

Patients should be instructed to take supplemental calcium and vitamin D, if daily dietary intake is inadequate. Weight-bearing exercise should be considered along with the modification of certain behavioral factors, such as cigarette smoking and/or excessive alcohol consumption, if these factors exist.

Dosing Instructions

Patients should be instructed that the expected benefits of FOSAMAX may only be obtained when it is taken with plain water the first thing upon arising for the day at least 30 minutes before the first food, beverage, or medication of the day. Even dosing with orange juice or coffee has been shown to markedly reduce the absorption of FOSAMAX (see CLINICAL PHARMACOLOGY, Pharmacokinetics, Absorption).

To facilitate delivery to the stomach and thus reduce the potential for esophageal irritation patients should be instructed to swallow each tablet of FOSAMAX with a full glass of water (6-8 oz). To facilitate gastric emptying patients should drink at least 2 oz (a quarter of a cup) of water after taking FOSAMAX oral solution. Patients should be instructed not to lie down for at least 30 minutes and until after their first food of the day. Patients should not chew or suck on the tablet because of a potential for oropharyngeal ulceration. Patients should be specifically instructed not to take FOSAMAX at bedtime or before arising for the day. Patients should be informed that failure to follow these instructions may increase their risk of esophageal problems. Patients should be instructed that if they develop symptoms of esophageal disease (such as difficulty or pain upon swallowing, retrosternal pain or new or worsening heartburn) they should stop taking FOSAMAX and consult their physician.

Patients should be instructed that if they miss a dose of once weekly FOSAMAX, they should take one dose on the morning after they remember. They should not take two doses on the same day but should return to taking one dose once a week, as originally scheduled on their chosen day.

Drug Interactions (also see CLINICAL PHARMACOLOGY, Pharmacokinetics, Drug Interactions)

Osteoporosis Treatment Studies in Postmenopausal Women: Adverse Experiences Considered Possibly, Probably, or Definitely Drug Related by the Investigators and Reported in ≥1% of Patients

	United States/Multinational Studies		Fracture Intervention Trial	
	FOSAMAX* % (n=196)	Placebo % (n=397)	FOSAMAX† % (n=3236)	Placebo % (n=3223)
Gastrointestinal				
abdominal pain	6.6	4.8	1.5	1.5
nausea	3.6	4.0	1.1	1.5
dyspepsia	3.6	3.5	1.1	1.2
constipation	3.1	1.8	0.0	0.2
diarrhea	3.1	1.8	0.6	0.3
flatulence	2.6	0.5	0.2	0.3
acid regurgitation	2.0	4.3	1.1	0.9
esophageal ulcer	1.5	0.0	0.1	0.1
vomiting	1.0	1.5	0.2	0.3
dysphagia	1.0	0.0	0.1	0.1
abdominal distention	1.0	0.8	0.0	0.0
gastritis	0.5	1.3	0.6	0.7
Musculoskeletal				
musculoskeletal (bone, muscle or joint) pain	4.1	2.5	0.4	0.3
muscle cramp	0.0	1.0	0.2	0.1
Nervous System / Psychiatric				
headache	2.6	1.5	0.2	0.2
dizziness	0.0	1.0	0.0	0.1
Special Senses				
taste perversion	0.5	1.0	0.1	0.0

* 10 mg/day for three years
† 5 mg/day for 2 years and 10 mg/day for either 1 or 2 additional years

Estrogen/hormone replacement therapy (HRT)
Concomitant use of HRT (estrogen ± progestin) and FOSAMAX was assessed in two clinical studies of one or two years' duration in postmenopausal osteoporotic women. In these studies, the safety and tolerability profile of the combination was consistent with those of the individual treatments; however, the degree of suppression of bone turnover (as assessed by mineralizing surface) was significantly greater with the combination than with either component alone. The long-term effects of combined FOSAMAX and HRT on fracture occurrence have not been studied (see CLINICAL PHARMACOLOGY, Clinical Studies, Concomitant use with estrogen/hormone replacement therapy (HRT) and ADVERSE REACTIONS, Clinical Studies, Concomitant use with estrogen/hormone replacement therapy).

Calcium Supplements/Antacids
It is likely that calcium supplements, antacids, and some oral medications will interfere with absorption of FOSAMAX. Therefore, patients must wait at least one-half hour after taking FOSAMAX before taking any other oral medications.

Aspirin
In clinical studies, the incidence of upper gastrointestinal adverse events was increased in patients receiving concomitant therapy with daily doses of FOSAMAX greater than 10 mg and aspirin-containing products.

Nonsteroidal Anti-inflammatory Drugs (NSAIDs)
FOSAMAX may be administered to patients taking NSAIDs. In a 3-year, controlled, clinical study (n=2027) during which a majority of patients received concomitant NSAIDs, the incidence of upper gastrointestinal adverse events was similar in patients taking FOSAMAX 5 or 10 mg/day compared to those taking placebo. However, since NSAID use is associated with gastrointestinal irritation, caution should be used during concomitant use with FOSAMAX.

Carcinogenesis, Mutagenesis, Impairment of Fertility
Harderian gland (a retro-orbital gland not present in humans) adenomas were increased in high-dose female mice (p=0.003) in a 92-week oral carcinogenicity study at doses of alendronate of 1, 3, and 10 mg/kg/day (males) or 1, 2, and 5 mg/kg/day (females). These doses are equivalent to 0.12 to 1.2 times a maximum recommended daily dose of 40 mg (Paget's disease) based on surface area, mg/m². The relevance of this finding to humans is unknown.
Parafollicular cell (thyroid) adenomas were increased in high-dose male rats (p=0.003) in a 2-year oral carcinogenicity study at doses of 1 and 3.75 mg/kg body weight. These doses are equivalent to 0.26 and 1 times a 40 mg human daily dose based on surface area, mg/m². The relevance of this finding to humans is unknown.
Alendronate was not genotoxic in the *in vitro* microbial mutagenesis assay with and without metabolic activation, in an *in vitro* mammalian cell mutagenesis assay, in an *in vitro* alkaline elution assay in rat hepatocytes, and in an *in vivo*

chromosomal aberration assay in mice. In an *in vitro* chromosomal aberration assay in Chinese hamster ovary cells, however, alendronate gave equivocal results.
Alendronate had no effect on fertility (male or female) in rats at oral doses up to 5 mg/kg/day (1.3 times a 40 mg human daily dose based on surface area, mg/m²).

Pregnancy
Pregnancy Category C:
Reproduction studies in rats showed decreased postimplantation survival at 2 mg/kg/day and decreased body weight gain in normal pups at 1 mg/kg/day. Sites of incomplete fetal ossification were statistically significantly increased in rats beginning at 10 mg/kg/day in vertebral (cervical, thoracic, and lumbar), skull, and sternebral bones. The above doses ranged from 0.26 times (1 mg/kg) to 2.6 times (10 mg/kg) a maximum recommended daily dose of 40 mg (Paget's disease) based on surface area, mg/m². No similar fetal effects were seen when pregnant rabbits were treated at doses up to 35 mg/kg/day (10.3 times a 40 mg human daily dose based on surface area, mg/m²).
Both total and ionized calcium decreased in pregnant rats at 15 mg/kg/day (3.9 times a 40 mg human daily dose based on surface area, mg/m²) resulting in delays and failures of delivery. Protracted parturition due to maternal hypocalcemia occurred in rats at doses as low as 0.5 mg/kg/day (0.13 times a 40 mg human daily dose based on surface area, mg/m²) when rats were treated from before mating through gestation. Maternotoxicity (late pregnancy deaths) occurred in the female rats treated with 15 mg/kg/day for varying periods of time ranging from treatment only during pre-mating to treatment only during early, middle, or late gestation; these deaths were lessened but not eliminated by cessation of treatment. Calcium supplementation either in the drinking water or by minipump could not ameliorate the hypocalcemia or prevent maternal and neonatal deaths due to delays in delivery; calcium supplementation IV prevented maternal, but not fetal deaths.
Bisphosphonates are incorporated into the bone matrix, from which they are gradually released over a period of years. The amount of bisphosphonate incorporated into adult bone, and hence, the amount available for release back into the systemic circulation, is directly related to the dose and duration of bisphosphonate use. There are no data on fetal risk in humans. However, there is a theoretical risk of fetal harm, predominantly skeletal, if a woman becomes pregnant after completing a course of bisphosphonate therapy. The impact of variables such as time between cessation of bisphosphonate therapy to conception, the particular bisphosphonate used, and the route of administration (intravenous versus oral) on the risk has not been studied.
There are no studies in pregnant women. FOSAMAX should be used during pregnancy only if the potential benefit justifies the potential risk to the mother and fetus.

Nursing Mothers
It is not known whether alendronate is excreted in human milk. Because many drugs are excreted in human milk, caution should be exercised when FOSAMAX is administered to nursing women.

Pediatric Use
The efficacy and safety of FOSAMAX were examined in a randomized, double-blind, placebo-controlled two-year study of 139 pediatric patients, aged 4-18 years, with severe osteogenesis imperfecta. One-hundred-and-nine patients were randomized to 5 mg FOSAMAX daily (weight <40 kg) or 10 mg FOSAMAX daily (weight ≥40 kg) and 30 patients to placebo. The mean baseline lumbar spine BMD Z-score of the patients was -4.5. The mean change in lumbar spine BMD Z-score from baseline to Month 24 was 1.3 in the FOSAMAX-treated patients and 0.1 in the placebo-treated patients. Treatment with FOSAMAX did not reduce the risk of fracture. Sixteen percent of the FOSAMAX patients who sustained a radiologically-confirmed fracture by Month 12 of the study had delayed fracture healing (callus remodeling) or fracture non-union when assessed radiographically at Month 24 compared with 9% of the placebo-treated patients. In FOSAMAX-treated patients, bone histomorphometry data obtained at Month 24 demonstrated decreased bone turnover and delayed mineralization time; however, there were no mineralization defects. There were no statistically significant differences between the FOSAMAX and placebo groups in reduction of bone pain.
FOSAMAX is not indicated for use in children.
(For clinical adverse experiences in children, see ADVERSE REACTIONS, Clinical Studies, Osteogenesis Imperfecta.)

Geriatric Use
Of the patients receiving FOSAMAX in the Fracture Intervention Trial (FIT), 71% (n=2302) were ≥65 years of age and 17% (n=550) were ≥75 years of age. Of the patients receiving FOSAMAX in the United States and Multinational osteoporosis treatment studies in women, osteoporosis studies in men, glucocorticoid-induced osteoporosis studies, and Paget's disease studies (see CLINICAL PHARMACOLOGY, Clinical Studies), 45%, 54%, 37%, and 70%, respectively, were 65 years of age or over. No overall differences in efficacy or safety were observed between these patients and younger patients, but greater sensitivity of some older individuals cannot be ruled out.

ADVERSE REACTIONS
Clinical Studies
In clinical studies of up to five years in duration adverse experiences associated with FOSAMAX usually were mild, and generally did not require discontinuation of therapy.
FOSAMAX has been evaluated for safety in approximately 8000 postmenopausal women in clinical studies.
Treatment of osteoporosis
Postmenopausal women
In two identically designed, three-year, placebo-controlled, double-blind, multicenter studies (United States and Multinational; n=994), discontinuation of therapy due to any clinical adverse experience occurred in 4.1% of 196 patients treated with FOSAMAX 10 mg/day and 6.0% of 397 patients treated with placebo. In the Fracture Intervention Trial (n=6459), discontinuation of therapy due to any clinical adverse experience occurred in 9.1% of 3236 patients treated with FOSAMAX 5 mg/day for 2 years and 10 mg/day for either one or two additional years and 10.1% of 3223 patients treated with placebo. Discontinuations due to upper gastrointestinal adverse experiences were: FOSAMAX, 3.2%; placebo, 2.7%. In these study populations, 49-54% had a history of gastrointestinal disorders at baseline and 54-89% used nonsteroidal anti-inflammatory drugs or aspirin at some time during the studies. Adverse experiences from these studies considered by the investigators as possibly, probably, or definitely drug related in ≥1% of patients treated with either FOSAMAX or placebo are presented in the following table.
[See table above]
Rarely, rash and erythema have occurred.
One patient treated with FOSAMAX (10 mg/day), who had a history of peptic ulcer disease and gastrectomy and who was taking concomitant aspirin developed an anastomotic ulcer with mild hemorrhage, which was considered drug related. Aspirin and FOSAMAX were discontinued and the patient recovered.
The adverse experience profile was similar for the 401 patients treated with either 5 or 20 mg doses of FOSAMAX in the United States and Multinational studies. The adverse experience profile for the 296 patients who received continued treatment with either 5 or 10 mg doses of FOSAMAX in the two-year extension of these studies (treatment years 4 and 5) was similar to that observed during the three-year placebo-controlled period. During the extension period, of the 151 patients treated with FOSAMAX 10 mg/day, the proportion of patients who discontinued therapy due to any clinical adverse experience was similar to that during the first three years of the study.
In a one-year, double-blind, multicenter study, the overall safety and tolerability profiles of once weekly FOSAMAX 70 mg and FOSAMAX 10 mg daily were similar. The adverse experiences considered by the investigators as

possibly, probably, or definitely drug related in ≥1% of patients in either treatment group are presented in the following table.

Osteoporosis Treatment Studies in Postmenopausal Women: Adverse Experiences Considered Possibly, Probably, or Definitely Drug Related by the Investigators and Reported in ≥1% of Patients

	Once Weekly FOSAMAX 70 mg % (n=519)	FOSAMAX 10 mg/day % (n=370)
Gastrointestinal		
abdominal pain	3.7	3.0
dyspepsia	2.7	2.2
acid regurgitation	1.9	2.4
nausea	1.9	2.4
abdominal distention	1.0	1.4
constipation	0.8	1.6
flatulence	0.4	1.6
gastritis	0.2	1.1
gastric ulcer	0.0	1.1
Musculoskeletal		
musculoskeletal (bone, muscle, joint) pain	2.9	3.2
muscle cramp	0.2	1.1

Men
In two placebo-controlled, double-blind, multicenter studies in men (a two-year study of FOSAMAX 10 mg/day and a one-year study of once weekly FOSAMAX 70 mg) the rates of discontinuation of therapy due to any clinical adverse experience were 2.7% for FOSAMAX 10 mg/day vs. 10.5% for placebo, and 6.4% for once weekly FOSAMAX 70 mg vs. 8.6% for placebo. The adverse experiences considered by the investigators as possibly, probably, or definitely drug related in ≥2% of patients treated with either FOSAMAX or placebo are presented in the following table.
[See first table above]
Prevention of osteoporosis in postmenopausal women
The safety of FOSAMAX 5 mg/day in postmenopausal women 40-60 years of age has been evaluated in three double-blind, placebo-controlled studies involving over 1,400 patients randomized to receive FOSAMAX for either two or three years. In these studies the overall safety profiles of FOSAMAX 5 mg/day and placebo were similar. Discontinuation of therapy due to any clinical adverse experience occurred in 7.5% of 642 patients treated with FOSAMAX 5 mg/day and 5.7% of 648 patients treated with placebo.
In a one-year, double-blind, multicenter study, the overall safety and tolerability profiles of once weekly FOSAMAX 35 mg and FOSAMAX 5 mg daily were similar.
The adverse experiences from these studies considered by the investigators as possibly, probably, or definitely drug related in ≥1% of patients treated with either once weekly FOSAMAX 35 mg, FOSAMAX 5 mg/day or placebo are presented in the following table.
[See second table above]
Concomitant use with estrogen/hormone replacement therapy
In two studies (of one and two years' duration) of postmenopausal osteoporotic women (total: n=853), the safety and tolerability profile of combined treatment with FOSAMAX 10 mg once daily and estrogen ± progestin (n=354) was consistent with those of the individual treatments.
Treatment of glucocorticoid-induced osteoporosis
In two, one-year, placebo-controlled, double-blind, multicenter studies in patients receiving glucocorticoid treatment, the overall safety and tolerability profiles of FOSAMAX 5 and 10 mg/day were generally similar to that of placebo. The adverse experiences considered by the investigators as possibly, probably, or definitely drug related in ≥1% of patients treated with either FOSAMAX 5 or 10 mg/day or placebo are presented in the following table.
[See third table above]
The overall safety and tolerability profile in the glucocorticoid-induced osteoporosis population that continued therapy for the second year of the studies (FOSAMAX: n=147) was consistent with that observed in the first year.
Paget's disease of bone
In clinical studies (osteoporosis and Paget's disease), adverse experiences reported in 175 patients taking FOSAMAX 40 mg/day for 3-12 months were similar to those in postmenopausal women treated with FOSAMAX 10 mg/day. However, there was an apparent increased incidence of upper gastrointestinal adverse experiences in patients taking FOSAMAX 40 mg/day (17.7% FOSAMAX vs. 10.2% placebo). One case of esophagitis and two cases of gastritis resulted in discontinuation of treatment.

Osteoporosis Studies in Men: Adverse Experiences Considered Possibly, Probably, or Definitely Drug Related by the Investigators and Reported in ≥2% of Patients

	Two-year Study		One-year Study	
	FOSAMAX 10 mg/day % (n=146)	Placebo % (n=95)	Once Weekly FOSAMAX 70 mg % (n=109)	Placebo % (n=58)
Gastrointestinal				
acid regurgitation	4.1	3.2	0.0	0.0
flatulence	4.1	1.1	0.0	0.0
gastroesophageal reflux disease	0.7	3.2	2.8	0.0
dyspepsia	3.4	0.0	2.8	1.7
diarrhea	1.4	1.1	2.8	0.0
abdominal pain	2.1	1.1	0.9	3.4
nausea	2.1	0.0	0.0	0.0

Osteoporosis Prevention Studies in Postmenopausal Women: Adverse Experiences Considered Possibly, Probably, or Definitely Drug Related by the Investigators and Reported in ≥1% of Patients

	Two/Three-Year Studies		One-Year Study	
	FOSAMAX 5 mg/day % (n=642)	Placebo % (n=648)	FOSAMAX 5 mg/day % (n=361)	Once Weekly FOSAMAX 35 mg % (n=362)
Gastrointestinal				
dyspepsia	1.9	1.4	2.2	1.7
abdominal pain	1.7	3.4	4.2	2.2
acid regurgitation	1.4	2.5	4.2	4.7
nausea	1.4	1.4	2.5	1.4
diarrhea	1.1	1.7	1.1	0.6
constipation	0.9	0.5	1.7	0.3
abdominal distention	0.2	0.3	1.4	1.1
Musculoskeletal				
musculoskeletal (bone, muscle or joint) pain	0.8	0.9	1.9	2.2

One-Year Studies in Glucocorticoid-Treated Patients: Adverse Experiences Considered Possibly, Probably, or Definitely Drug Related by the Investigators and Reported in ≥1% of Patients

	FOSAMAX 10 mg/day % (n=157)	FOSAMAX 5 mg/day % (n=161)	Placebo % (n=159)
Gastrointestinal			
abdominal pain	3.2	1.9	0.0
acid regurgitation	2.5	1.9	1.3
constipation	1.3	0.6	0.0
melena	1.3	0.0	0.0
nausea	0.6	1.2	0.6
diarrhea	0.0	0.0	1.3
Nervous System / Psychiatric			
headache	0.6	0.0	1.3

Additionally, musculoskeletal (bone, muscle or joint) pain, which has been described in patients with Paget's disease treated with other bisphosphonates, was considered by the investigators as possibly, probably, or definitely drug related in approximately 6% of patients treated with FOSAMAX 40 mg/day versus approximately 1% of patients treated with placebo, but rarely resulted in discontinuation of therapy. Discontinuation of therapy due to any clinical adverse experience occurred in 6.4% of patients with Paget's disease treated with FOSAMAX 40 mg/day and 2.4% of patients treated with placebo.
Osteogenesis Imperfecta
FOSAMAX is not indicated for use in children.
The overall safety profile of FOSAMAX in OI patients treated for up to 24 months was generally similar to that of adults with osteoporosis treated with FOSAMAX. However, there was an increased occurrence of vomiting in OI patients treated with FOSAMAX compared to placebo. During the 24-month treatment period, vomiting was observed in 32 of 109 (29.4%) patients treated with FOSAMAX and 3 of 30 (10%) patients treated with placebo.
In a pharmacokinetic study, 6 of 24 pediatric OI patients who received a single oral dose of FOSAMAX 35 or 70 mg developed fever, flu-like symptoms, and/or mild lymphocytopenia within 24 to 48 hours after administration. These events, lasting no more than 2 to 3 days and responding to acetaminophen, are consistent with an acute-phase response that has been reported in patients receiving bisphosphonates, including FOSAMAX. See ADVERSE REACTIONS, Post-Marketing Experience, Body as a Whole.

Laboratory Test Findings
In double-blind, multicenter, controlled studies, asymptomatic, mild, and transient decreases in serum calcium and phosphate were observed in approximately 18% and 10%, respectively, of patients taking FOSAMAX versus approximately 12% and 3% of those taking placebo. However, the incidences of decreases in serum calcium to <8.0 mg/dL (2.0 mM) and serum phosphate to ≤2.0 mg/dL (0.65 mM) were similar in both treatment groups.
Post-Marketing Experience
The following adverse reactions have been reported in post-marketing use:
Body as a Whole: hypersensitivity reactions including urticaria and rarely angioedema. Transient symptoms of myalgia, malaise, asthenia and rarely, fever have been reported with FOSAMAX, typically in association with initiation of treatment. Rarely, symptomatic hypocalcemia has occurred, generally in association with predisposing conditions. Rarely, peripheral edema.
Gastrointestinal: esophagitis, esophageal erosions, esophageal ulcers, rarely esophageal stricture or perforation, and oropharyngeal ulceration. Gastric or duodenal ulcers, some severe and with complications have also been reported (see WARNINGS, PRECAUTIONS, Information for Patients, and DOSAGE AND ADMINISTRATION).
Localized osteonecrosis of the jaw, generally associated with tooth extraction and/or local infection with delayed healing, has been reported rarely (see PRECAUTIONS, Dental).
Musculoskeletal: bone, joint, and/or muscle pain, occasionally severe, and rarely incapacitating (see PRECAUTIONS,

Musculoskeletal Pain); joint swelling; low-energy femoral shaft and subtrochanteric fractures.

Nervous system: dizziness and vertigo.

Skin: rash (occasionally with photosensitivity), pruritus, alopecia, rarely severe skin reactions, including Stevens-Johnson syndrome and toxic epidermal necrolysis.

Special Senses: rarely uveitis, scleritis or episcleritis.

OVERDOSAGE

Significant lethality after single oral doses was seen in female rats and mice at 552 mg/kg (3256 mg/m^2) and 966 mg/kg (2898 mg/m^2), respectively. In males, these values were slightly higher, 626 and 1280 mg/kg, respectively. There was no lethality in dogs at oral doses up to 200 mg/kg (4000 mg/m^2).

No specific information is available on the treatment of overdosage with FOSAMAX. Hypocalcemia, hypophosphatemia, and upper gastrointestinal adverse events, such as upset stomach, heartburn, esophagitis, gastritis, or ulcer, may result from oral overdosage. Milk or antacids should be given to bind alendronate. Due to the risk of esophageal irritation, vomiting should not be induced and the patient should remain fully upright.

Dialysis would not be beneficial.

DOSAGE AND ADMINISTRATION

FOSAMAX must be taken *at least* one-half hour before the first food, beverage, or medication of the day with plain water only (see PRECAUTIONS, Information for Patients). Other beverages (including mineral water), food, and some medications are likely to reduce the absorption of FOSAMAX (see PRECAUTIONS, Drug Interactions). Waiting less than 30 minutes, or taking FOSAMAX with food, beverages (other than plain water) or other medications will lessen the effect of FOSAMAX by decreasing its absorption into the body.

FOSAMAX should only be taken upon arising for the day. To facilitate delivery to the stomach and thus reduce the potential for esophageal irritation, a FOSAMAX tablet should be swallowed with a full glass of water (6-8 oz). To facilitate gastric emptying FOSAMAX oral solution should be followed by at least 2 oz (a quarter of a cup) of water. Patients should not lie down for at least 30 minutes and until after their first food of the day. FOSAMAX should not be taken at bedtime or before arising for the day. Failure to follow these instructions may increase the risk of esophageal adverse experiences (see WARNINGS, PRECAUTIONS, Information for Patients).

Patients should receive supplemental calcium and vitamin D, if dietary intake is inadequate (see PRECAUTIONS, General).

No dosage adjustment is necessary for the elderly or for patients with mild-to-moderate renal insufficiency (creatinine clearance 35 to 60 mL/min). FOSAMAX is not recommended for patients with more severe renal insufficiency (creatinine clearance <35 mL/min) due to lack of experience.

Treatment of osteoporosis in postmenopausal women (see INDICATIONS AND USAGE)

The recommended dosage is:
• one 70 mg tablet once weekly
        or
• one bottle of 70 mg oral solution once weekly
        or
• one 10 mg tablet once daily

Treatment to increase bone mass in men with osteoporosis

The recommended dosage is:
• one 70 mg tablet once weekly
        or
• one bottle of 70 mg oral solution once weekly
        or
• one 10 mg tablet once daily

Prevention of osteoporosis in postmenopausal women (see INDICATIONS AND USAGE)

The recommended dosage is:
• one 35 mg tablet once weekly
        or
• one 5 mg tablet once daily

The safety of treatment and prevention of osteoporosis with FOSAMAX has been studied for up to 7 years.

Treatment of glucocorticoid-induced osteoporosis in men and women

The recommended dosage is one 5 mg tablet once daily, except for postmenopausal women not receiving estrogen, for whom the recommended dosage is one 10 mg tablet once daily.

Paget's disease of bone in men and women

The recommended treatment regimen is 40 mg once a day for six months.

Retreatment of Paget's disease

In clinical studies in which patients were followed every six months, relapses during the 12 months following therapy occurred in 9% (3 out of 32) of patients who responded to treatment with FOSAMAX. Specific retreatment data are not available, although responses to retreatment were similar in patients who had received prior bisphosphonate therapy and those who had not. Retreatment with FOSAMAX

may be considered, following a six-month post-treatment evaluation period in patients who have relapsed, based on increases in serum alkaline phosphatase, which should be measured periodically. Retreatment may also be considered in those who failed to normalize their serum alkaline phosphatase.

HOW SUPPLIED

No. 3759—Tablets FOSAMAX, 5 mg, are white, round, uncoated tablets with an outline of a bone image on one side and code MRK 925 on the other. They are supplied as follows:

NDC 0006-0925-31 unit-of-use bottles of 30
NDC 0006-0925-58 unit-of-use bottles of 100

No. 3797—Tablets FOSAMAX, 10 mg, are white, oval, wax-polished tablets with code MRK on one side and 936 on the other. They are supplied as follows:

NDC 0006-0936-31 unit-of-use bottles of 30
NDC 0006-0936-58 unit-of-use bottles of 100
NDC 0006-0936-28 unit dose packages of 100
NDC 0006-0936-82 bottles of 1,000.

No. 3813—Tablets FOSAMAX, 35 mg, are white, oval, uncoated tablets with code 77 on one side and a bone image on the other. They are supplied as follows:

NDC 0006-0077-44 unit-of-use blister package of 4
NDC 0006-0077-21 unit dose packages of 20.

No. 8457—Tablets FOSAMAX, 40 mg, are white, triangular-shaped, uncoated tablets with code MSD 212 on one side and FOSAMAX on the other. They are supplied as follows:

NDC 0006-0212-31 unit-of-use bottles of 30.

No. 3814—Tablets FOSAMAX, 70 mg, are white, oval, uncoated tablets with code 31 on one side and an outline of a bone image on the other. They are supplied as follows:

NDC 0006-0031-44 unit-of-use blister package of 4
NDC 0006-0031-21 unit dose packages of 20.

No. 3833—Oral Solution FOSAMAX, 70 mg, is a clear, colorless solution with a raspberry flavor and is supplied as follows:

NDC 0006-3833-34 unit-of-use cartons of 4 single-dose bottles containing 75 mL each.

Storage

FOSAMAX Tablets:

Store in a well-closed container at room temperature, 15-30°C (59-86°F).

FOSAMAX Oral Solution:

Store at 25°C (77°F), excursions permitted to 15-30°C (59-86°F). [See USP Controlled Room Temperature.] Do not freeze.

Merck Sharp & Dohme Corp., a subsidiary of

MERCK & CO., INC., Whitehouse Station, NJ 08889, USA

Issued March 2010

Printed in USA

9635610

9636810

PATIENT PACKAGE INSERT

Patient Information

Once Weekly FOSAMAX® (FOSS-ah-max)

(alendronate sodium)

Tablets and Oral Solution

Read this information before you start taking FOSAMAX*. Also, read the leaflet each time you refill your prescription, just in case anything has changed. This leaflet does not take the place of discussions with your doctor. You and your doctor should discuss FOSAMAX when you start taking your medicine and at regular checkups.

---

*Registered trademark of Merck Sharp & Dohme Corp., a subsidiary of **Merck & Co., Inc.**

Copyright © 2000 Merck Sharp & Dohme Corp., a subsidiary of **Merck & Co., Inc.**

All rights reserved

What is the most important information I should know about once weekly FOSAMAX?

• **You must take once weekly FOSAMAX exactly as directed to help make sure it works and to help lower the chance of problems in your esophagus (the tube that connects your mouth and stomach). (See "How should I take once weekly FOSAMAX?").**

• **If you have chest pain, new or worsening heartburn, or have trouble or pain when you swallow, stop taking FOSAMAX and call your doctor. (See "What are the possible side effects of FOSAMAX?").**

What is FOSAMAX?

FOSAMAX is a prescription medicine for:

• The treatment or prevention of osteoporosis (thinning of bone) in women after menopause. It reduces the chance of having a hip or spinal fracture (break).

• Treatment to increase bone mass in men with osteoporosis.

• FOSAMAX tablets are for treatment and prevention of osteoporosis.

• FOSAMAX oral solution is for treatment of osteoporosis. Improvement in bone density may be observed as early as 3 months after you start taking FOSAMAX even though you won't see or feel a difference. For FOSAMAX to continue to work, you need to keep taking it.

FOSAMAX is not a hormone.

There is more information about osteoporosis at the end of this leaflet.

Who should not take FOSAMAX?

Do not take FOSAMAX (tablets or oral solution) if you:

• Have certain problems with your esophagus, the tube that connects your mouth with your stomach

• Cannot stand or sit upright for at least 30 minutes

• Have low levels of calcium in your blood

• Are allergic to FOSAMAX or any of its ingredients. A list of ingredients is at the end of this leaflet.

Do not take FOSAMAX oral solution if you have trouble swallowing liquids.

What should I tell my doctor before using FOSAMAX?

Tell your doctor about all of your medical or dental conditions, including if you:

• **have problems with swallowing**

• **have stomach or digestive problems**

• **have kidney problems**

• **are pregnant or planning to become pregnant.** It is not known if FOSAMAX can harm your unborn baby.

• **are breastfeeding.** It is not known if FOSAMAX passes into your milk and if it can harm your baby.

Tell your doctor about all medicines you take, including prescription and non-prescription medicines, vitamins, and herbal supplements.

Know the medicines you take. Keep a list of them and show it to your doctor and pharmacist each time you get a new medicine.

How should I take once weekly FOSAMAX?

• Choose the day of the week that best fits your schedule.

• Take 1 dose of FOSAMAX every week on your chosen day **after** you get up for the day and **before** taking your first food, drink, or other medicine

• Take FOSAMAX while you are sitting or standing.

• Take your FOSAMAX with plain water only as follows:

  • **TABLETS:** Swallow one tablet with a full glass (6-8 oz) of plain water.

  • **ORAL SOLUTION:** Drink one entire bottle of solution followed by at least 2 ounces (a quarter of a cup) of plain water.

Do **not** take FOSAMAX with:

Mineral water

Coffee or tea

Juice

FOSAMAX works only if it is taken on an empty stomach.

Do not chew or suck on a tablet of FOSAMAX.

After taking your FOSAMAX, wait at least 30 minutes:

• before you lie down. You may sit, stand or walk, and do normal activities like reading.

• before you take your first food or drink except for plain water.

• before you take other medicines, including antacids, calcium, and other supplements and vitamins.

Do not lie down until after your first food of the day.

• It is important that you keep taking FOSAMAX for as long as your doctor says to take it. For FOSAMAX to continue to work, you need to keep taking it.

What should I do if I miss a dose of FOSAMAX or if I take too many?

• If you miss a dose, take only 1 dose of FOSAMAX on the morning after you remember. Do not take 2 doses on the same day. Continue your usual schedule of 1 dose once a week on your chosen day.

• If you think you took more than the prescribed dose of FOSAMAX, drink a full glass of milk and call your doctor right away. Do not try to vomit. Do not lie down.

What should I avoid while taking FOSAMAX?

• Do not eat, drink, or take other medicines or supplements **before** taking FOSAMAX.

• Wait for at least 30 minutes **after** taking FOSAMAX to eat, drink, or take other medicines or supplements.

• Do not lie down for at least 30 minutes **after** taking FOSAMAX. Do not lie down until **after** your first food of the day.

What are the possible side effects of FOSAMAX?

FOSAMAX may cause problems in your esophagus (the tube that connects the mouth and stomach). (See "What is the most important information I should know about once weekly FOSAMAX?".) These problems include irritation, inflammation, or ulcers of the esophagus, which may sometimes bleed. This may occur especially if you do not drink a full glass of water with FOSAMAX or if you lie down in less than 30 minutes or before your first food of the day.

• **Stop taking FOSAMAX and call your doctor right away if you get any of these signs of possible serious problems of the esophagus:**

  • **Chest pain**

  • **New or worsening heartburn**

  • **Trouble or pain when swallowing**

• Esophagus problems may get worse if you continue to take FOSAMAX.

• Mouth sores (ulcers) may occur if the FOSAMAX tablet is chewed or dissolved in the mouth.

- You may get flu-like symptoms, typically at the start of treatment with FOSAMAX.
- You may get allergic reactions, such as hives or, in rare cases, swelling of your face, lips, tongue, or throat.
- FOSAMAX may cause jaw-bone problems in some people. Jaw-bone problems may include infection, and delayed healing after teeth are pulled.
- The most common side effect is stomach area (abdominal) pain. Less common side effects are nausea, vomiting, a full or bloated feeling in the stomach, constipation, diarrhea, black or bloody stools (bowel movements), gas, eye pain, rash that may be made worse by sunlight, hair loss, headache, dizziness, a changed sense of taste, joint swelling or swelling in the hands or legs, and bone, muscle, or joint pain.
- **Call your doctor if you develop severe bone, muscle, or joint pain.**
- Some patients have experienced fracture in a specific part of the thigh bone. Call your doctor if you develop new or unusual pain in the hip or thigh.

Tell your doctor about any side effect that bothers you or that does not go away.

These are not all the side effects with FOSAMAX. Ask your doctor or pharmacist for more information.

How do I store FOSAMAX?
- Store at room temperature, 59 to 86°F (15 to 30°C).
- Safely discard FOSAMAX that is out-of-date or no longer needed.
- **Keep FOSAMAX and all medicines out of the reach of children.**

General information about using FOSAMAX safely and effectively

Medicines are sometimes prescribed for conditions that are not mentioned in patient information leaflets. Do not use FOSAMAX for a condition for which it was not prescribed. Do not give FOSAMAX to other people, even if they have the same symptoms you have. It may harm them.

FOSAMAX is not indicated for use in children.

This leaflet is a summary of information about FOSAMAX. If you have any questions or concerns about FOSAMAX or osteoporosis, talk to your doctor, pharmacist, or other health care provider. You can ask your doctor or pharmacist for information about FOSAMAX written for health care providers. For more information, call 1-877-408-4699 (toll-free) or visit the following website: www.fosamax.com.

What are the ingredients in FOSAMAX?
Tablets

FOSAMAX tablets contain alendronate sodium as the active ingredient and the following inactive ingredients: cellulose, lactose, croscarmellose sodium and magnesium stearate.

Oral Solution

Fosamax oral solution contains alendronate sodium as the active ingredient and the following inactive ingredients: sodium citrate, citric acid, sodium saccharin, artificial raspberry flavor, purified water, sodium propylparaben and sodium butylparaben.

What should I know about osteoporosis?
Normally your bones are being rebuilt all the time. First, old bone is removed (resorbed). Then a similar amount of new bone is formed. This balanced process keeps your skeleton healthy and strong.

Osteoporosis is a thinning and weakening of the bones. It is common in women after menopause, and may also occur in men. In osteoporosis, bone is removed faster than it is formed, so overall bone mass is lost and bones become weaker. Therefore, keeping bone mass is important to keep your bones healthy. In both men and women, osteoporosis may also be caused by certain medicines called corticosteroids.

At first, osteoporosis usually has no symptoms, but it can cause fractures (broken bones). Fractures usually cause pain. Fractures of the bones of the spine may not be painful, but over time they can make you shorter. Eventually, your spine can curve and your body can become bent over. Fractures may happen during normal, everyday activity, such as lifting, or from minor injury that would normally not cause bones to break. Fractures most often occur at the hip, spine, or wrist. This can lead to pain, severe disability, or loss of ability to move around (mobility).

Who is at risk for osteoporosis?
Many things put people at risk of osteoporosis. The following people have a higher chance of getting osteoporosis:
Women who:
- Are going through or who are past menopause
Men who:
- Are elderly
People who:
- Are white (Caucasian) or oriental (Asian)
- Are thin
- Have family member with osteoporosis
- Do not get enough calcium or vitamin D
- Do not exercise
- Smoke
- Drink alcohol often
- Take bone thinning medicines (like prednisone or other corticosteroids) for a long time

What can I do to help prevent or treat osteoporosis?
In addition to FOSAMAX, your doctor may suggest one or more of the following lifestyle changes:
- **Stop smoking.** Smoking may increase your chance of getting osteoporosis.
- **Reduce the use of alcohol.** Too much alcohol may increase the risk of osteoporosis and injuries that can cause fractures.
- **Exercise regularly.** Like muscles, bones need exercise to stay strong and healthy. Exercise must be safe to prevent injuries, including fractures. Talk with your doctor before you begin any exercise program.
- **Eat a balanced diet.** Having enough calcium in your diet is important. Your doctor can advise you whether you need to change your diet or take any dietary supplements, such as calcium or vitamin D.

Rx only
Merck Sharp & Dohme Corp., a subsidiary of Merck & Co., Inc.
Whitehouse Station, NJ 08889, USA
Issued March 2010
9635610

PATIENT PACKAGE INSERT
Patient Information
FOSAMAX® (FOSS-ah-max)
(alendronate sodium) Tablets
Read this information before you start taking FOSAMAX*. Also, read the leaflet each time you refill your prescription, just in case anything has changed. This leaflet does not take the place of discussions with your doctor. You and your doctor should discuss FOSAMAX when you start taking your medicine and at regular checkups.

*Registered trademark of Merck Sharp & Dohme Corp., a subsidiary of **Merck & Co., Inc.**
Copyright ©1995, 1997, 2000 Merck Sharp & Dohme Corp., a subsidiary of **Merck & Co., Inc.**

What is the most important information I should know about FOSAMAX?
- **You must take FOSAMAX exactly as directed to help make sure it works and to help lower the chance of problems in your esophagus (the tube that connects your mouth and stomach). (See "How should I take FOSAMAX?").**
- **If you have chest pain, new or worsening heartburn, or have trouble or pain when you swallow, stop taking FOSAMAX and call your doctor. (See "What are the possible side effects of FOSAMAX?").**

What is FOSAMAX?
FOSAMAX is a prescription medicine for:
- The treatment or prevention of osteoporosis (thinning of bone) in women after menopause. It reduces the chance of having a hip or spinal fracture (break).
- Treatment to increase bone mass in men with osteoporosis.
- The treatment of osteoporosis in either men or women who are taking corticosteroid medicines (for example, prednisone).

Improvement in bone density may be observed as early as 3 months after you start taking FOSAMAX even though you won't see or feel a difference. For FOSAMAX to continue to work, you need to keep taking it.

FOSAMAX is not a hormone.

There is more information about osteoporosis at the end of this leaflet.

Who should not take FOSAMAX?
Do not take FOSAMAX if you:
- Have certain problems with your esophagus, the tube that connects your mouth with your stomach
- Cannot stand or sit upright for at least 30 minutes
- Have low levels of calcium in your blood
- Are allergic to FOSAMAX or any of its ingredients. A list of ingredients is at the end of this leaflet.

What should I tell my doctor before using FOSAMAX?
Tell your doctor about all of your medical or dental conditions, including if you:
- **have problems with swallowing**
- **have stomach or digestive problems**
- **have kidney problems**
- **are pregnant or planning to become pregnant.** It is not known if FOSAMAX can harm your unborn baby.
- **are breastfeeding.** It is not known if FOSAMAX passes into your milk and if it can harm your baby.

Tell your doctor about all medicines you take, including prescription and non-prescription medicines, vitamins, and herbal supplements.

Know the medicines you take. Keep a list of them and show it to your doctor and pharmacist each time you get a new medicine.

How should I take FOSAMAX?
- Take 1 FOSAMAX tablet once a day, every day **after** you get up for the day and **before** taking your first food, drink, or other medicine.
- Take FOSAMAX while you are sitting or standing.
- Swallow your FOSAMAX tablet with a full glass (6-8 oz) of plain water only.

Do **not** take FOSAMAX with:
Mineral water
Coffee or tea
Juice
FOSAMAX works only if taken on an empty stomach.
Do not chew or suck on a tablet of FOSAMAX.
After swallowing your FOSAMAX tablet, wait at least 30 minutes:
- before you lie down. You may sit, stand or walk, and do normal activities like reading.
- before you take your first food or drink except for plain water.
- before you take other medicines, including antacids, calcium, and other supplements and vitamins.

Do not lie down until after first food of the day.
- It is important that you keep taking FOSAMAX for as long as your doctor says to take it. For FOSAMAX to continue to work, you need to keep taking it.

What should I do if I miss a dose of FOSAMAX or if I take too many?
- If you miss a dose, do not take it later in the day. Continue your usual schedule of 1 tablet once a day the next morning.
- If you think you took more than the prescribed dose of FOSAMAX, drink a full glass of milk and call your doctor right away. Do not try to vomit. Do not lie down.

What should I avoid while taking FOSAMAX?
- Do not eat, drink, or take other medicines or supplements **before** taking FOSAMAX.
- Wait for at least 30 minutes **after** taking FOSAMAX to eat, drink, or take other medicines or supplements.
- Do not lie down for at least 30 minutes **after** taking FOSAMAX. Do not lie down until **after** your first food of the day.

What are the possible side effects of FOSAMAX?
FOSAMAX may cause problems in your esophagus (the tube that connects the mouth and stomach). (See "What is the most important information I should know about FOSAMAX?".) These problems include irritation, inflammation, or ulcers of the esophagus, which may sometimes bleed. This may occur especially if you do not drink a full glass of water with FOSAMAX or if you lie down in less than 30 minutes or before your first food of the day.
- **Stop taking FOSAMAX and call your doctor right away if you get any of these signs of possible serious problems of the esophagus:**
  - **Chest pain**
  - **New or worsening heartburn**
  - **Trouble or pain when swallowing**
- Esophagus problems may get worse if you continue to take FOSAMAX.
- Mouth sores (ulcers) may occur if the FOSAMAX tablet is chewed or dissolved in the mouth.
- You may get flu-like symptoms typically at the start of treatment with FOSAMAX.
- You may get allergic reactions, such as hives or, in rare cases, swelling of your face, lips, tongue, or throat.
- FOSAMAX may cause jaw-bone problems in some people. Jaw-bone problems include infection, and delayed healing after teeth are pulled.
- The most common side effect is stomach area (abdominal) pain. Less common side effects are nausea, vomiting, a full or bloated feeling in the stomach, constipation, diarrhea, black or bloody stools (bowel movements), gas, eye pain, rash that may be made worse by sunlight, hair loss, headache, dizziness, a changed sense of taste, joint swelling or swelling in the hands or legs, and bone, muscle, or joint pain.
- **Call your doctor if you develop severe bone, muscle, or joint pain.**
- Some patients have experienced fracture in a specific part of the thigh bone. Call your doctor if you develop new or unusual pain in the hip or thigh.

Tell your doctor about any side effect that bothers you or that does not go away.

These are not all the side effects with FOSAMAX. Ask your doctor or pharmacist for more information.

How do I store FOSAMAX?
- Store FOSAMAX at room temperature, 59 to 86°F (15 to 30°C).
- Safely discard FOSAMAX that is out-of-date or no longer needed.
- **Keep FOSAMAX and all medicines out of the reach of children.**

General information about using FOSAMAX safely and effectively

Medicines are sometimes prescribed for conditions that are not mentioned in patient information leaflets. Do not use FOSAMAX for a condition for which it was not prescribed. Do not give FOSAMAX to other people, even if they have the same symptoms you have. It may harm them.

FOSAMAX is not indicated for use in children.

This leaflet is a summary of information about FOSAMAX. If you have any questions or concerns about FOSAMAX or osteoporosis, talk to your doctor, pharmacist, or other health care provider. You can ask your doctor or pharmacist for information about FOSAMAX written for health care providers. For more information, call 1-877-408-4699 (toll-free) or visit the following website: www.fosamax.com.

What are the ingredients in FOSAMAX?

FOSAMAX contains alendronate sodium as the active ingredient and the following inactive ingredients: cellulose, lactose, croscarmellose sodium and magnesium stearate. The 10 mg tablet also contains carnauba wax.

What should I know about osteoporosis?

Normally your bones are being rebuilt all the time. First, old bone is removed (resorbed). Then a similar amount of new bone is formed. This balanced process keeps your skeleton healthy and strong.

Osteoporosis is a thinning and weakening of the bones. It is common in women after menopause, and may also occur in men. In osteoporosis, bone is removed faster than it is formed, so overall bone mass is lost and bones become weaker. Therefore, keeping bone mass is important to keep your bones healthy. In both men and women, osteoporosis may also be caused by certain medicines called corticosteroids.

At first, osteoporosis usually has no symptoms, but it can cause fractures (broken bones). Fractures usually cause pain. Fractures of the bones of the spine may not be painful, but over time they can make you shorter. Eventually, your spine can curve and your body can become bent over. Fractures may happen during normal, everyday activity, such as lifting, or from minor injury that would normally not cause bones to break. Fractures most often occur at the hip, spine, or wrist. This can lead to pain, severe disability, or loss of ability to move around (mobility).

Who is at risk for osteoporosis?

Many things put people at risk of osteoporosis. The following people have a higher chance of getting osteoporosis:
Women who:
• Are going through or who are past menopause
Men who:
• Are elderly
People who:
• Are white (Caucasian) or oriental (Asian)
• Are thin
• Have family member with osteoporosis
• Do not get enough calcium or vitamin D
• Do not exercise
• Smoke
• Drink alcohol often
• Take bone thinning medicines (like prednisone or other corticosteroids) for a long time

What can I do to help prevent or treat osteoporosis?

In addition to FOSAMAX, your doctor may suggest one or more of the following lifestyle changes:
• **Stop smoking.** Smoking may increase your chance of getting osteoporosis.
• **Reduce the use of alcohol.** Too much alcohol may increase the risk of osteoporosis and injuries that can cause fractures.
• **Exercise regularly.** Like muscles, bones need exercise to stay strong and healthy. Exercise must be safe to prevent injuries, including fractures. Talk with your doctor before you begin any exercise program.
• **Eat a balanced diet.** Having enough calcium in your diet is important. Your doctor can advise you whether you need to change your diet or take any dietary supplements, such as calcium or vitamin D.

Rx Only

Merck Sharp & Dohme Corp., a subsidiary of Merck & Co., Inc.
Whitehouse Station, NJ 08889, USA
Issued March 2010
9636810

Shown in Product Identification Guide, page 312

FOSAMAX PLUS D®   Rx

[FOSS-ah-max PLUS D]
(alendronate sodium/cholecalciferol)
Tablets

HIGHLIGHTS OF PRESCRIBING INFORMATION

These highlights do not include all the information needed to use FOSAMAX PLUS D safely and effectively. See full prescribing information for FOSAMAX PLUS D.

FOSAMAX PLUS D (alendronate sodium/cholecalciferol) tablets
Initial U.S. Approval: 2005

———RECENT MAJOR CHANGES———

Warnings and Precautions, Upper Gastrointestinal (5.1)   03/2010
Warnings and Precautions, Osteonecrosis of the Jaw (5.4)   03/2010

———INDICATIONS AND USAGE———

FOSAMAX PLUS D® is a combination of a bisphosphonate and vitamin D indicated for:
• Treatment of osteoporosis in postmenopausal women (1.1)
• Treatment to increase bone mass in men with osteoporosis (1.2)

FOSAMAX PLUS D alone should not be used to treat vitamin D deficiency. (1.3)

———DOSAGE AND ADMINISTRATION———

• 70 mg alendronate/2800 IU vitamin D_3 or 70 mg alendronate/5600 IU vitamin D_3 tablet once weekly. (2.1, 2.2, 2.3, 2.4)
• Must be taken with plain water only (6-8 oz) *at least* **30** minutes before the first food, beverage, or medication of the day. (2.3)
• Do not lie down for at least 30 minutes and until after food. (2.3)
• Do not take at bedtime or before arising. (2.3, 5.1)

———DOSAGE FORMS AND STRENGTHS———

Tablets: 70 mg/2800 IU and 70 mg/5600 IU (3)

———CONTRAINDICATIONS———

• Abnormalities of the esophagus which delay emptying such as stricture or achalasia (4, 5.1)
• Inability to stand/sit upright for at least 30 minutes (4, 5.1)
• Hypocalcemia (4, 5.2)
• Hypersensitivity to any component of this product (4, 6.2)

———WARNINGS AND PRECAUTIONS———

• Severe irritation of upper gastrointestinal mucosa can occur. Dosing instructions should be followed and caution should be used in patients with active upper GI disease. Discontinue use if new or worsening symptoms occur. (5.1)
• Hypocalcemia can worsen and must be corrected prior to use. (5.2)
• Severe bone, joint, muscle pain may occur. Discontinue use if severe symptoms develop. (5.3)
• Osteonecrosis of the jaw has been reported rarely. (5.4)

———ADVERSE REACTIONS———

The most common adverse reactions for alendronate (incidence ≥3%) are: abdominal pain, acid regurgitation, constipation, diarrhea, dyspepsia, musculoskeletal pain, nausea. (6.1)

To report SUSPECTED ADVERSE REACTIONS, contact Merck Sharp & Dohme Corp., a subsidiary of Merck & Co., Inc., at 1-877-888-4231 or FDA at 1-800-FDA-1088 or www.fda.gov/medwatch.

———DRUG INTERACTIONS———

• Calcium supplements/antacids and some medications will likely interfere with absorption of alendronate and should be taken at least 30 minutes after FOSAMAX PLUS D. (2.1, 7.1)
• Aspirin and nonsteroidal anti-inflammatory drug use may worsen gastrointestinal irritation; caution should be used. (7.2, 7.3)
• Some drugs may impair the absorption or increase the catabolism of cholecalciferol (vitamin D_3). Additional vitamin D supplementation should be considered. (7.4, 7.5, 12.3)

———USE IN SPECIFIC POPULATIONS———

• FOSAMAX PLUS D is not indicated for use in children. (8.4)
• FOSAMAX PLUS D is not recommended in patients with severe renal insufficiency (creatinine clearance <35 mL/min). (2.5, 5.5)

See 17 for PATIENT COUNSELING INFORMATION and FDA-approved patient labeling

Revised: 06/2010

FULL PRESCRIBING INFORMATION: CONTENTS*

FULL PRESCRIBING INFORMATION

1   INDICATIONS AND USAGE

FOSAMAX PLUS D[1] is indicated for:

1.1   Treatment of Osteoporosis in Postmenopausal Women

For the treatment of osteoporosis, FOSAMAX PLUS D increases bone mass and reduces the incidence of fractures, including those of the hip and spine (vertebral compression fractures).

1.2   Treatment to Increase Bone Mass in Men with Osteoporosis

1.3   Important Limitations of Use

FOSAMAX PLUS D alone should not be used to treat vitamin D deficiency.

2   DOSAGE AND ADMINISTRATION

2.1   Treatment of Osteoporosis in Postmenopausal Women

The recommended dosage is one 70 mg alendronate/2800 IU vitamin D_3 or one 70 mg alendronate/5600 IU vitamin D_3 tablet once weekly. For most osteoporotic women, the appropriate dose is FOSAMAX PLUS D (70 mg alendronate/5600 IU vitamin D_3) once weekly.

2.2   Treatment to Increase Bone Mass in Men with Osteoporosis

The recommended dosage is one 70 mg alendronate/2800 IU vitamin D_3 or one 70 mg alendronate/5600 IU vitamin D_3 tablet once weekly. For most osteoporotic men, the appropriate dose is FOSAMAX PLUS D (70 mg alendronate/5600 IU vitamin D_3) once weekly.

2.3   Dosing Instructions

FOSAMAX PLUS D must be taken *at least* one-half hour before the first food, beverage, or medication of the day with plain water only *[see Patient Counseling Information (17.3)]*. Other beverages (including mineral water), food, and some medications are likely to reduce the absorption of alendronate *[see Drug Interactions (7.1)]*. Waiting less than 30 minutes, or taking FOSAMAX PLUS D with food, beverages (other than plain water) or other medications will lessen the effect of alendronate by decreasing its absorption into the body.

To facilitate delivery to the stomach and thus reduce the potential for esophageal irritation, FOSAMAX PLUS D should only be swallowed upon arising for the day with a full glass of water (6-8 oz) and patients should not lie down for at least 30 minutes and until after their first food of the day. FOSAMAX PLUS D should not be taken at bedtime or before arising for the day. Failure to follow these instructions may increase the risk of esophageal adverse experiences *[see Warnings and Precautions (5.1); Patient Counseling Information (17.3)]*.

2.4   Recommendations for Calcium and Vitamin D Supplementation

Patients should receive supplemental calcium if dietary intake is inadequate *[see Warnings and Precautions (5.2)]*. Patients at increased risk for vitamin D insufficiency (e.g., over the age of 70 years, nursing home bound, or chronically ill) may need additional vitamin D supplementation. Patients with gastrointestinal malabsorption syndromes may require higher doses of vitamin D supplementation and measurement of 25-hydroxyvitamin D should be considered.

The recommended intake of vitamin D is 400 IU-800 IU daily. FOSAMAX PLUS D 70 mg/2800 IU and 70 mg/5600 IU are intended to provide seven days' worth of 400 and 800 IU daily vitamin D in a single, once-weekly dose, respectively.

Causes of osteoporosis other than estrogen deficiency, aging, and glucocorticoid use should be considered.

2.5 Dosing in Elderly and Renal Insufficiency

No dosage adjustment is necessary for the elderly or for patients with mild-to-moderate renal insufficiency (creatinine clearance 35 to 60 mL/min). FOSAMAX PLUS D is not recommended for patients with more severe renal insufficiency (creatinine clearance <35 mL/min) due to lack of experience.

3 DOSAGE FORMS AND STRENGTHS

- 70 mg/2800 IU tablets are white to off-white, modified capsule-shaped tablets with code 710 on one side and an outline of a bone image on the other.
- 70 mg/5600 IU tablets are white to off-white, modified rectangle-shaped tablets with code 270 on one side and an outline of a bone image on the other.

4 CONTRAINDICATIONS

- Abnormalities of the esophagus which delay esophageal emptying such as stricture or achalasia *[see Warnings and Precautions (5.1)]*
- Inability to stand or sit upright for at least 30 minutes *[see Dosage and Administration (2.3), Warnings and Precautions (5.1)]*
- Hypocalcemia *[see Warnings and Precautions (5.2)]*
- Hypersensitivity to any component of this product. Hypersensitivity reactions including urticaria and angioedema have been reported *[see Adverse Reactions (6.2)]*.

5 WARNINGS AND PRECAUTIONS

5.1 Upper Gastrointestinal Adverse Reactions

FOSAMAX PLUS D, like other bisphosphonates administered orally, may cause local irritation of the upper gastrointestinal mucosa. Because of these possible irritant effects and a potential for worsening of the underlying disease, caution should be used when FOSAMAX PLUS D is given to patients with active upper gastrointestinal problems (such as known Barrett's esophagus, dysphagia, other esophageal diseases, gastritis, duodenitis, or ulcers).

Esophageal adverse experiences, such as esophagitis, esophageal ulcers and esophageal erosions, occasionally with bleeding and rarely followed by esophageal stricture or perforation, have been reported in patients receiving treatment with oral bisphosphonates including FOSAMAX PLUS D. In some cases these have been severe and required hospitalization. Physicians should therefore be alert to any signs or symptoms signaling a possible esophageal reaction and patients should be instructed to discontinue FOSAMAX PLUS D and seek medical attention if they develop dysphagia, odynophagia, retrosternal pain or new or worsening heartburn.

The risk of severe esophageal adverse experiences appears to be greater in patients who lie down after taking oral bisphosphonates including FOSAMAX PLUS D and/or who fail to swallow oral bisphosphonates including FOSAMAX PLUS D with the recommended full glass (6-8 oz) of water, and/or who continue to take oral bisphosphonates including FOSAMAX PLUS D after developing symptoms suggestive of esophageal irritation. Therefore, it is very important that the full dosing instructions are provided to, and understood by, the patient *[see Dosage and Administration (2.3)]*. In patients who cannot comply with dosing instructions due to mental disability, therapy with FOSAMAX PLUS D should be used under appropriate supervision.

There have been post-marketing reports of gastric and duodenal ulcers with oral bisphosphonate use, some severe and with complications, although no increased risk was observed in controlled clinical trials *[see Adverse Reactions (6.2)]*.

5.2 Mineral Metabolism

Alendronate Sodium

Hypocalcemia must be corrected before initiating therapy with FOSAMAX PLUS D *[see Contraindications (4)]*. Other disorders affecting mineral metabolism (such as vitamin D deficiency) should also be effectively treated. In patients with these conditions, serum calcium and symptoms of hypocalcemia should be monitored during therapy with FOSAMAX PLUS D.

Presumably due to the effects of alendronate on increasing bone mineral, small, asymptomatic decreases in serum calcium and phosphate may occur.

Cholecalciferol

FOSAMAX PLUS D alone should not be used to treat vitamin D deficiency (commonly defined as 25-hydroxyvitamin D level below 9 ng/mL). Patients at increased risk for vitamin D insufficiency may require higher doses of vitamin D supplementation *[see Dosage and Administration (2.4)]*. Patients with gastrointestinal malabsorption syndromes may require higher doses of vitamin D supplementation and measurement of 25-hydroxyvitamin D should be considered.

Vitamin D_3 supplementation may worsen hypercalcemia and/or hypercalciuria when administered to patients with diseases associated with unregulated overproduction of 1,25 dihydroxyvitamin D (e.g., leukemia, lymphoma, sarcoidosis). Urine and serum calcium should be monitored in these patients.

5.3 Musculoskeletal Pain

In post-marketing experience, severe and occasionally incapacitating bone, joint, and/or muscle pain has been reported in patients taking bisphosphonates that are approved for the prevention and treatment of osteoporosis *[see Adverse Reactions (6.2)]*. This category of drugs includes alendronate. Most of the patients were postmenopausal women. The time to onset of symptoms varied from one day to several months after starting the drug. Discontinue use if severe symptoms develop. Most patients had relief of symptoms after stopping. A subset had recurrence of symptoms when rechallenged with the same drug or another bisphosphonate.

In placebo-controlled clinical studies of FOSAMAX, the percentages of patients with these symptoms were similar in the FOSAMAX and placebo groups.

5.4 Osteonecrosis of the Jaw

Osteonecrosis of the jaw (ONJ), which can occur spontaneously, is generally associated with tooth extraction and/or local infection with delayed healing, and has been reported in patients taking bisphosphonates, including FOSAMAX PLUS D. Known risk factors for osteonecrosis of the jaw include invasive dental procedures (e.g., tooth extraction, dental implants, bony surgery), diagnosis of cancer, concomitant therapies (e.g., chemotherapy, corticosteroids), poor oral hygiene, and co-morbid disorders (e.g., periodontal and/or other pre-existing dental disease, anemia, coagulopathy, infection, ill-fitting dentures).

For patients requiring invasive dental procedures, discontinuation of bisphosphonate treatment may reduce the risk for ONJ. Clinical judgment of the treating physician and/or oral surgeon should guide the management plan of each patient based on individual benefit/risk assessment.

Patients who develop osteonecrosis of the jaw while on bisphosphonate therapy should receive care by an oral surgeon. In these patients, extensive dental surgery to treat ONJ may exacerbate the condition. Discontinuation of bisphosphonate therapy should be considered based on individual benefit/risk assessment.

5.5 Renal Insufficiency

FOSAMAX PLUS D is not recommended for patients with renal insufficiency (creatinine clearance <35 mL/min). *[See Dosage and Administration (2.5).]*

6 ADVERSE REACTIONS

6.1 Clinical Trials Experience

Because clinical trials are conducted under widely varying conditions, adverse reaction rates observed in the clinical trials of a drug cannot be directly compared to rates in the clinical trials of another drug and may not reflect the rates observed in practice.

FOSAMAX

FOSAMAX has been evaluated for safety in approximately 8000 postmenopausal women in clinical studies.

Table 1: Osteoporosis Treatment Studies in Postmenopausal Women: Adverse Experiences Considered Possibly, Probably, or Definitely Drug Related by the Investigators and Reported in ≥1% of Patients

	United States/Multinational Studies		Fracture Intervention Trial	
	FOSAMAX* % (n=196)	Placebo % (n=397)	FOSAMAX[†] % (n=3236)	Placebo % (n=3223)
Gastrointestinal				
abdominal pain	6.6	4.8	1.5	1.5
nausea	3.6	4.0	1.1	1.5
dyspepsia	3.6	3.5	1.1	1.2
constipation	3.1	1.8	0.0	0.2
diarrhea	3.1	1.8	0.6	0.3
flatulence	2.6	0.5	0.2	0.3
acid regurgitation	2.0	4.3	1.1	0.9
esophageal ulcer	1.5	0.0	0.1	0.1
vomiting	1.0	1.5	0.2	0.3
dysphagia	1.0	0.0	0.1	0.1
abdominal distention	1.0	0.8	0.0	0.0
gastritis	0.5	1.3	0.6	0.7
Musculoskeletal				
musculoskeletal (bone, muscle or joint) pain	4.1	2.5	0.4	0.3
muscle cramp	0.0	1.0	0.2	0.1
Nervous System / Psychiatric				
headache	2.6	1.5	0.2	0.2
dizziness	0.0	1.0	0.0	0.1
Special Senses				
taste perversion	0.5	1.0	0.1	0.0

* 10 mg/day for three years
† 5 mg/day for 2 years and 10 mg/day for either 1 or 2 additional years

Postmenopausal Women
FOSAMAX daily

In two identically designed, three-year, placebo-controlled, double-blind, multicenter studies (United States and Multinational; n=994), discontinuation of therapy due to any clinical adverse experience occurred in 4.1% of 196 patients treated with FOSAMAX 10 mg/day and 6.0% of 397 patients treated with placebo. In the Fracture Intervention Trial (n=6459), discontinuation of therapy due to any clinical adverse experience occurred in 9.1% of 3236 patients treated with FOSAMAX 5 mg/day for 2 years and 10 mg/day for either one or two additional years and 10.1% of 3223 patients treated with placebo. Discontinuations due to upper gastrointestinal adverse experiences were: FOSAMAX, 3.2%; placebo, 2.7%. In these study populations, 49-54% had a history of gastrointestinal disorders at baseline and 54-89% used nonsteroidal anti-inflammatory drugs or aspirin at some time during the studies. Adverse experiences from these studies considered by the investigators as possibly, probably, or definitely drug related in ≥1% of patients treated with either FOSAMAX or placebo are presented in Table 1.

[See table 1 above]

Rarely, rash and erythema have occurred.

The adverse experience profile was similar for the 401 patients treated with either 5- or 20-mg doses of FOSAMAX in the United States and Multinational studies. The adverse experience profile for the 296 patients who received continued treatment with either 5- or 10-mg doses of FOSAMAX in the two-year extension of these studies (treatment years 4 and 5) was similar to that observed during the three-year placebo-controlled period. During the extension period, of the 151 patients treated with FOSAMAX 10 mg/day, the proportion of patients who discontinued therapy due to any clinical adverse experience was similar to that during the first three years of the study.

FOSAMAX Once-Weekly

In a one-year, double-blind, multicenter study, the overall safety and tolerability profiles of once weekly FOSAMAX 70 mg and FOSAMAX 10 mg daily were similar. The adverse experiences considered by the investigators as possibly, probably, or definitely drug related in ≥1% of patients in either treatment group are presented in Table 2.

Table 2: Osteoporosis Treatment Studies in Postmenopausal Women: Adverse Experiences Considered Possibly, Probably, or Definitely Drug Related by the Investigators and Reported in ≥1% of Patients

	Once Weekly FOSAMAX 70 mg % (n=519)	FOSAMAX 10 mg/day % (n=370)
Gastrointestinal		
abdominal pain	3.7	3.0
dyspepsia	2.7	2.2

acid regurgitation	1.9	2.4
nausea	1.9	2.4
abdominal distention	1.0	1.4
constipation	0.8	1.6
flatulence	0.4	1.6
gastritis	0.2	1.1
gastric ulcer	0.0	1.1
Musculoskeletal		
musculoskeletal (bone, muscle, joint) pain	2.9	3.2
muscle cramp	0.2	1.1

Concomitant Use With Estrogen or Estrogen/Progestin Products
In two studies (of one and two years' duration) of postmenopausal osteoporotic women (total: n=853), the safety and tolerability profile of combined treatment with FOSAMAX 10 mg once daily and estrogen ± progestin (n=354) was consistent with those of the individual treatments.
Men
In two placebo-controlled, double-blind, multicenter studies in men (a two-year study of FOSAMAX 10 mg/day and a one-year study of once weekly FOSAMAX 70 mg) the rates of discontinuation of therapy due to any clinical adverse experience were 2.7% for FOSAMAX 10 mg/day vs. 10.5% for placebo, and 6.4% for once weekly FOSAMAX 70 mg vs. 8.6% for placebo. The adverse experiences considered by the investigators as possibly, probably, or definitely drug related in ≥2% of patients treated with either FOSAMAX or placebo are presented in Table 3.
[See table 3 below]
Laboratory Test Findings
In double-blind, multicenter, controlled studies, asymptomatic, mild, and transient decreases in serum calcium and phosphate were observed in approximately 18% and 10%, respectively, of patients taking FOSAMAX versus approximately 12% and 3% of those taking placebo. However, the incidences of decreases in serum calcium to <8.0 mg/dL (2.0 mM) and serum phosphate to ≤2.0 mg/dL (0.65 mM) were similar in both treatment groups.
FOSAMAX PLUS D
In a fifteen-week double-blind, multinational study in osteoporotic postmenopausal women (n=682) and men (n=35), the safety profile of FOSAMAX PLUS D (70 mg/2800 IU) was similar to that of FOSAMAX once weekly 70 mg. In the 24-week double-blind extension study in women (n=619) and men (n=33), the safety profile of FOSAMAX PLUS D (70 mg/2800 IU) administered with an additional 2800 IU vitamin D_3 was similar to that of FOSAMAX PLUS D (70 mg/2800 IU).

6.2 Post-Marketing Experience
The following adverse reactions have been identified during post-approval use of FOSAMAX and FOSAMAX PLUS D. Because these reactions are reported voluntarily from a population of uncertain size, it is not always possible to reliably estimate their frequency or establish a causal relationship to drug exposure.
Body as a Whole: hypersensitivity reactions including urticaria and rarely angioedema. Transient symptoms of myalgia, malaise, asthenia and rarely, fever have been reported with alendronate, typically in association with initiation of treatment. Rarely, symptomatic hypocalcemia has occurred, generally in association with predisposing conditions. Rarely, peripheral edema.
Gastrointestinal: esophagitis, esophageal erosions, esophageal ulcers, rarely esophageal stricture or perforation, and oropharyngeal ulceration. Gastric or duodenal ulcers, some severe and with complications have also been reported *[see Dosage and Administration (2.3); Warnings and Precautions (5.1); Patient Counseling Information (17.3)]*.
Localized osteonecrosis of the jaw, generally associated with tooth extraction and/or local infection with delayed healing, has been reported rarely *[see Warnings and Precautions (5.4)]*.
Musculoskeletal: bone, joint, and/or muscle pain, occasionally severe, and rarely incapacitating *[see Warnings and Precautions (5.3)]*; joint swelling; low-energy femoral shaft and subtrochanteric fractures.
Nervous System: dizziness and vertigo.
Skin: rash (occasionally with photosensitivity), pruritus, alopecia, rarely severe skin reactions, including Stevens-Johnson syndrome and toxic epidermal necrolysis.
Special Senses: rarely uveitis, scleritis or episcleritis.

7 DRUG INTERACTIONS

7.1 Calcium Supplements/Antacids
It is likely that calcium supplements, antacids, and some oral medications will interfere with absorption of alendronate. Therefore, patients must wait at least one-half hour after taking FOSAMAX PLUS D before taking any other oral medications.

7.2 Aspirin
In clinical studies, the incidence of upper gastrointestinal adverse events was increased in patients receiving concomitant therapy with daily doses of FOSAMAX greater than 10 mg and aspirin-containing products.

7.3 Nonsteroidal Anti-Inflammatory Drugs (NSAIDs)
FOSAMAX PLUS D may be administered to patients taking NSAIDs. In a 3-year, controlled, clinical study (n=2027) during which a majority of patients received concomitant NSAIDs, the incidence of upper gastrointestinal adverse events was similar in patients taking FOSAMAX 5 or 10 mg/day compared to those taking placebo. However, since NSAID use is associated with gastrointestinal irritation, caution should be used during concomitant use with FOSAMAX PLUS D.

7.4 Drugs that May Impair the Absorption of Cholecalciferol
Olestra, mineral oils, orlistat, and bile acid sequestrants (e.g., cholestyramine, colestipol) may impair the absorption of vitamin D. Additional vitamin D supplementation should be considered *[see Clinical Pharmacology (12.3)]*.

7.5 Drugs that May Increase the Catabolism of Cholecalciferol
Anticonvulsants, cimetidine, and thiazides may increase the catabolism of vitamin D. Additional vitamin D supplementation should be considered *[see Clinical Pharmacology (12.3)]*.

8 USE IN SPECIFIC POPULATIONS

8.1 Pregnancy
Pregnancy Category C:
Alendronate Sodium
Reproduction studies in rats showed decreased postimplantation survival at 2 mg/kg/day and decreased body weight gain in normal pups at 1 mg/kg/day. Sites of incomplete fetal ossification were statistically significantly increased in rats beginning at 10 mg/kg/day in vertebral (cervical, thoracic, and lumbar), skull, and sternebral bones. The above doses ranged from one time (1 mg/kg) to 10 times (10 mg/kg) a maximum recommended daily dose of 10 mg/day based on surface area, mg/m^2. No similar fetal effects were seen when pregnant rabbits were treated at doses up to 35 mg/kg/day (40 times a 10 mg human daily dose based on surface area, mg/m^2).
Both total and ionized calcium decreased in pregnant rats at 15 mg/kg/day (13 times a 10-mg human daily dose based on surface area, mg/m^2) resulting in delays and failures of delivery. Protracted parturition due to maternal hypocalcemia occurred in rats at doses as low as 0.5 mg/kg/day (0.5 times a 10 mg human daily dose based on surface area, mg/m^2) when rats were treated from before mating through gestation. Maternotoxicity (late pregnancy deaths) occurred in the female rats treated with 15 mg/kg/day for varying periods of time ranging from treatment only during pre-mating to treatment only during early, middle, or late gestation; these deaths were lessened but not eliminated by cessation of treatment. Calcium supplementation either in the drinking water or by minipump could not ameliorate the hypocalcemia or prevent maternal and neonatal deaths due to delays in delivery; calcium supplementation IV prevented maternal, but not fetal deaths.
Bisphosphonates are incorporated into the bone matrix, from which they are gradually released over a period of years. The amount of bisphosphonate incorporated into adult bone, and hence, the amount available for release back into the systemic circulation, is directly related to the dose and duration of bisphosphonate use. There are no data on fetal risk in humans. However, there is a theoretical risk of fetal harm, predominantly skeletal, if a woman becomes pregnant after completing a course of bisphosphonate therapy. The impact of variables such as time between cessation of bisphosphonate therapy to conception, the particular bisphosphonate used, and the route of administration (intravenous versus oral) on the risk has not been studied.
Cholecalciferol
No data are available for cholecalciferol (vitamin D_3). Administration of high doses (≥10,000 IU/every other day) of ergocalciferol (vitamin D_2) to pregnant rabbits resulted in abortions and an increased incidence of fetal aortic stenosis. Administration of vitamin D_2 (40,000 IU/day) to pregnant rats resulted in neonatal death, decreased fetal weight, and impaired osteogenesis of long bones postnatally.
There are no studies in pregnant women. FOSAMAX PLUS D should be used during pregnancy only if the potential benefit justifies the potential risk to the mother and fetus.

8.3 Nursing Mothers
Cholecalciferol and some of its active metabolites pass into breast milk. It is not known whether alendronate is excreted in human milk. Because many drugs are excreted in human milk, caution should be exercised when FOSAMAX PLUS D is administered to nursing women.

8.4 Pediatric Use
FOSAMAX PLUS D is not indicated for use in children.
The efficacy and safety of alendronate were examined in a randomized, double-blind, placebo-controlled two-year study of 139 pediatric patients, aged 4-18 years, with severe osteogenesis imperfecta. One-hundred-and-nine patients were randomized to 5 mg alendronate daily (weight <40 kg) or 10 mg alendronate daily (weight ≥40 kg) and 30 patients to placebo. The mean baseline lumbar spine BMD Z-score of the patients was -4.5. The mean change in lumbar spine BMD Z-score from baseline to Month 24 was 1.3 in the alendronate-treated patients and 0.1 in the placebo-treated patients. Treatment with alendronate did not reduce the risk of fracture. Sixteen percent of the alendronate patients who sustained a radiologically-confirmed fracture by Month 12 of the study had delayed fracture healing (callus remodeling) or fracture non-union when assessed radiographically at Month 24 compared with 9% of the placebo-treated patients. In alendronate-treated patients, bone histomorphometry data obtained at Month 24 demonstrated decreased bone turnover and delayed mineralization time; however, there were no mineralization defects. There were no statistically significant differences between the alendronate and placebo groups in reduction of bone pain.

8.5 Geriatric Use
Of the patients receiving FOSAMAX in the Fracture Intervention Trial (FIT), 71% (n=2302) were ≥65 years of age and 17% (n=550) were ≥75 years of age. Of the patients receiving FOSAMAX in the United States and Multinational osteoporosis treatment studies in women, and osteoporosis studies in men *[see Clinical Studies (14.1)]*, 45% and 54%, respectively, were 65 years of age or over. No overall differences in efficacy or safety were observed between these patients and younger patients, but greater sensitivity of some older individuals cannot be ruled out. Dietary requirements of vitamin D_3 are increased in the elderly.

10 OVERDOSAGE

Alendronate Sodium
Significant lethality after single oral doses with alendronate was seen in female rats and mice at 552 mg/kg (3256 mg/m^2) and 966 mg/kg (2898 mg/m^2), respectively. In males, these values were slightly higher, 626 and 1280 mg/kg, respectively. There was no lethality in dogs at oral doses up to 200 mg/kg (4000 mg/m^2).
No specific information is available on the treatment of overdosage with alendronate. Hypocalcemia, hypophosphatemia, and upper gastrointestinal adverse events, such as upset stomach, heartburn, esophagitis, gastritis, or ulcer, may result from oral overdosage. Milk or antacids should be given to bind alendronate. Due to the risk of esophageal irritation, vomiting should not be induced and the patient should remain fully upright.
Dialysis would not be beneficial.
Cholecalciferol
Significant lethality occurred in mice treated with a single high oral dose of calcitriol (4 mg/kg), the hormonal metabolite of cholecalciferol.

Table 3: Osteoporosis Studies in Men: Adverse Experiences Considered Possibly, Probably, or Definitely Drug Related by the Investigators and Reported in ≥2% of Patients

	Two-year Study FOSAMAX 10 mg/day % (n=146)	Placebo % (n=95)	One-year Study Once Weekly FOSAMAX 70 mg % (n=109)	Placebo % (n=58)
Gastrointestinal				
acid regurgitation	4.1	3.2	0.0	0.0
flatulence	4.1	1.1	0.0	0.0
gastroesophageal reflux disease	0.7	3.2	2.8	0.0
dyspepsia	3.4	0.0	2.8	1.7
diarrhea	1.4	1.1	2.8	0.0
abdominal pain	2.1	1.1	0.9	3.4
nausea	2.1	0.0	0.0	0.0

There is limited information regarding doses of cholecalciferol associated with acute toxicity, although intermittent (yearly or twice yearly) single doses of ergocalciferol (vitamin D_2) as high as 600,000 IU have been given without reports of toxicity. Signs and symptoms of vitamin D toxicity include hypercalcemia, hypercalciuria, anorexia, nausea, vomiting, polyuria, polydipsia, weakness, and lethargy. Serum and urine calcium levels should be monitored in patients with suspected vitamin D toxicity. Standard therapy includes restriction of dietary calcium, hydration, and systemic glucocorticoids in patients with severe hypercalcemia.

Dialysis to remove vitamin D would not be beneficial.

11 DESCRIPTION

FOSAMAX PLUS D contains alendronate sodium, a bisphosphonate, and cholecalciferol (vitamin D_3).

Alendronate sodium is a bisphosphonate that acts as a specific inhibitor of osteoclast-mediated bone resorption. Bisphosphonates are synthetic analogs of pyrophosphate that bind to the hydroxyapatite found in bone.

Alendronate sodium is chemically described as (4-amino-1-hydroxybutylidene) bisphosphonic acid monosodium salt trihydrate.

The empirical formula of alendronate sodium is $C_4H_{12}NNaO_7P_2 \cdot 3H_2O$ and its formula weight is 325.12. The structural formula is:

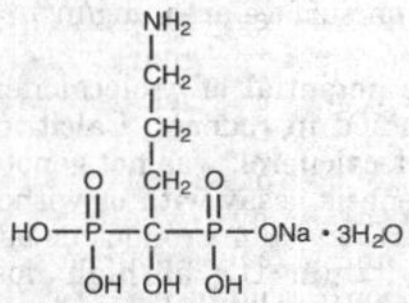

Alendronate sodium is a white, crystalline, nonhygroscopic powder. It is soluble in water, very slightly soluble in alcohol, and practically insoluble in chloroform.

Cholecalciferol (vitamin D_3) is a secosterol that is the natural precursor of the calcium-regulating hormone calcitriol (1,25 dihydroxyvitamin D_3).

The chemical name of cholecalciferol is (3β,5Z,7E)-9,10-secocholesta-5,7,10(19)-trien-3-ol. The empirical formula of cholecalciferol is $C_{27}H_{44}O$ and its molecular weight is 384.6. The structural formula is:

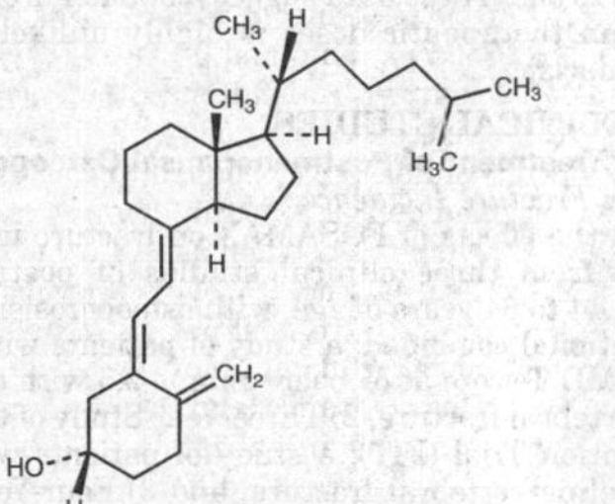

Cholecalciferol is a white, crystalline, odorless powder. Cholecalciferol is practically insoluble in water, freely soluble in usual organic solvents, and slightly soluble in vegetable oils.

FOSAMAX PLUS D for oral administration contains 91.37 mg of alendronate monosodium salt trihydrate, the molar equivalent of 70 mg of free acid, and 70 or 140 mcg of cholecalciferol, equivalent to 2800 or 5600 International Units (IU) vitamin D, respectively. Each tablet contains the following inactive ingredients: microcrystalline cellulose, lactose anhydrous, medium chain triglycerides, gelatin, croscarmellose sodium, sucrose, colloidal silicon dioxide, magnesium stearate, butylated hydroxytoluene, modified food starch, and sodium aluminum silicate.

12 CLINICAL PHARMACOLOGY

12.1 Mechanism of Action

Alendronate Sodium

Animal studies have indicated the following mode of action. At the cellular level, alendronate shows preferential localization to sites of bone resorption, specifically under osteoclasts. The osteoclasts adhere normally to the bone surface but lack the ruffled border that is indicative of active resorption. Alendronate does not interfere with osteoclast recruitment or attachment, but it does inhibit osteoclast activity. Studies in mice on the localization of radioactive [³H]alendronate in bone showed about 10–fold higher uptake on osteoclast surfaces than on osteoblast surfaces. Bones examined 6 and 49 days after [³H]alendronate administration in rats and mice, respectively, showed that normal bone was formed on top of the alendronate, which was incorporated inside the matrix. While incorporated in bone matrix, alendronate is not pharmacologically active. Thus, alendronate must be continuously administered to suppress osteoclasts on newly formed resorption surfaces. Histomorphometry in baboons and rats showed that alendronate treatment reduces bone turnover (i.e., the number of sites at which bone is remodeled). In addition, bone formation exceeds bone resorption at these remodeling sites, leading to progressive gains in bone mass.

Cholecalciferol

Vitamin D_3 is produced in the skin by photochemical conversion of 7-dehydrocholesterol to previtamin D_3 by ultraviolet light. This is followed by non-enzymatic isomerization to vitamin D_3. In the absence of adequate sunlight exposure, vitamin D_3 is an essential dietary nutrient. Vitamin D_3 in skin and dietary vitamin D_3 (absorbed into chylomicrons) is converted to 25-hydroxyvitamin D_3 in the liver. Conversion to the active calcium-mobilizing hormone 1,25-dihydroxyvitamin D_3 (calcitriol) in the kidney is stimulated by both parathyroid hormone and hypophosphatemia. The principal action of 1,25–dihydroxyvitamin D_3 is to increase intestinal absorption of both calcium and phosphate as well as regulate serum calcium, renal calcium and phosphate excretion, bone formation and bone resorption.

Vitamin D is required for normal bone formation. Vitamin D insufficiency develops when both sunlight exposure and dietary intake are inadequate. Insufficiency is associated with negative calcium balance, increased parathyroid hormone levels, bone loss, and increased risk of skeletal fracture. In severe cases, deficiency results in more severe hyperparathyroidism, hypophosphatemia, proximal muscle weakness, bone pain and osteomalacia.

12.2 Pharmacodynamics

Alendronate Sodium

Alendronate is a bisphosphonate that binds to bone hydroxyapatite and specifically inhibits the activity of osteoclasts, the bone-resorbing cells. Alendronate reduces bone resorption with no direct effect on bone formation, although the latter process is ultimately reduced because bone resorption and formation are coupled during bone turnover. Daily oral doses of alendronate (5, 20, and 40 mg for six weeks) in postmenopausal women produced biochemical changes indicative of dose-dependent inhibition of bone resorption, including decreases in urinary calcium and urinary markers of bone collagen degradation (such as deoxypyridinoline and cross-linked N–telopeptides of type I collagen). These biochemical changes tended to return toward baseline values as early as 3 weeks following the discontinuation of therapy with alendronate and did not differ from placebo after 7 months.

Long-term treatment of osteoporosis with FOSAMAX 10 mg/day (for up to five years) reduced urinary excretion of markers of bone resorption, deoxypyridinoline and cross-linked N–telopeptides of type I collagen, by approximately 50% and 70%, respectively, to reach levels similar to those seen in healthy premenopausal women. The decrease in the rate of bone resorption indicated by these markers was evident as early as one month and at three to six months reached a plateau that was maintained for the entire duration of treatment with FOSAMAX. In osteoporosis treatment studies FOSAMAX 10 mg/day decreased the markers of bone formation, osteocalcin and bone specific alkaline phosphatase by approximately 50%, and total serum alkaline phosphatase by approximately 25 to 30% to reach a plateau after 6 to 12 months. Similar reductions in the rate of bone turnover were observed in postmenopausal women during one-year studies with once weekly FOSAMAX 70 mg for the treatment of osteoporosis. These data indicate that the rate of bone turnover reached a new steady-state, despite the progressive increase in the total amount of alendronate deposited within bone.

As a result of inhibition of bone resorption, asymptomatic reductions in serum calcium and phosphate concentrations were also observed following treatment with FOSAMAX. In the long-term studies, reductions from baseline in serum calcium (approximately 2%) and phosphate (approximately 4 to 6%) were evident the first month after the initiation of FOSAMAX 10 mg. No further decreases in serum calcium were observed for the five-year duration of treatment; however, serum phosphate returned toward prestudy levels during years three through five. In one-year studies with once weekly FOSAMAX 70 mg, similar reductions were observed at 6 and 12 months. The reduction in serum phosphate may reflect not only the positive bone mineral balance due to FOSAMAX but also a decrease in renal phosphate reabsorption.

Osteoporosis in Men

Treatment of men with osteoporosis with FOSAMAX 10 mg/day for two years reduced urinary excretion of cross-linked N-telopeptides of type I collagen by approximately 60% and bone-specific alkaline phosphatase by approximately 40%. Similar reductions were observed in a one-year study in men with osteoporosis receiving once weekly FOSAMAX 70 mg.

Cholecalciferol

Vitamin D is required for normal bone formation. Vitamin D insufficiency is associated with negative calcium balance, leading to increased parathyroid hormone levels and worsening of bone loss associated with osteoporosis. When taken without vitamin D, alendronate is also associated with a reduction in serum calcium concentrations and increased parathyroid hormone levels. In a 15–week trial, 717 postmenopausal women and men, mean age 67 years, with osteoporosis (lumbar spine bone mineral density [BMD] of at least 2.5 standard deviations below the premenopausal mean) were randomized to receive either weekly FOSAMAX PLUS D 70 mg/2800 IU vitamin D or weekly FOSAMAX 70 mg alone with no vitamin D supplementation. Patients who were vitamin D deficient (25–hydroxyvitamin D <9 ng/mL) at baseline were excluded. Treatment with FOSAMAX PLUS D 70 mg/2800 IU resulted in a smaller reduction in serum calcium levels (-0.9%) when compared to FOSAMAX 70 mg alone (-1.4%). As well, treatment with FOSAMAX PLUS D 70 mg/2800 IU resulted in a significantly smaller increase in parathyroid hormone levels when compared to FOSAMAX 70 mg alone (14% and 24%, respectively).

The sufficiency of patients' vitamin D status is best assessed by measuring 25-hydroxyvitamin D levels. In the 15-week trial mentioned above, baseline 25-hydroxyvitamin D levels were 22.2 ng/mL in the FOSAMAX PLUS D group and 22.1 ng/mL in the FOSAMAX only group. After 15 weeks of treatment, the mean levels were 23.1 ng/mL and 18.4 ng/mL in the FOSAMAX PLUS D and FOSAMAX only groups, respectively. The final levels of 25-hydroxyvitamin D at Week 15 are summarized in Table 4.

[See table 4 above]

Patients (n=652) who completed the above 15-week trial continued in a 24-week extension in which all received FOSAMAX PLUS D (70 mg/2800 IU) and were randomly assigned to receive either additional once weekly vitamin D_3 2800 IU (Vitamin D_3 5600 IU group) or matching placebo (Vitamin D_3 2800 IU group). After 24 weeks of extended treatment (Week 39 from original baseline), the mean levels of 25-hydroxyvitamin D were 27.9 ng/mL and 25.6 ng/mL in the vitamin D_3 5600 IU group and vitamin D_3 2800 IU group, respectively. The percentage of patients with hypercalciuria at Week 39 was not statistically different between treatment groups.

The distribution of the final levels of 25-hydroxyvitamin D at Week 39 is summarized in Table 5.

[See table 5 at top of next page]

12.3 Pharmacokinetics

Absorption

Alendronate Sodium

Relative to an intravenous (IV) reference dose, the mean oral bioavailability of alendronate in women was 0.64% for doses ranging from 5 to 70 mg when administered after an overnight fast and two hours before a standardized breakfast. Oral bioavailability of the 10-mg tablet in men (0.59%) was similar to that in women when administered after an overnight fast and 2 hours before breakfast.

In a study, the alendronate in the FOSAMAX PLUS D (70 mg/2800 IU) tablet and the FOSAMAX (alendronate sodium) 70-mg tablet were found to be equally bioavailable. In a separate study, the alendronate in the FOSAMAX PLUS D (70 mg/5600 IU) tablet was found to be equally bioavailable to the alendronate in the FOSAMAX (alendronate sodium) 70-mg tablet.

A study examining the effect of timing of a meal on the bioavailability of alendronate was performed in 49 postmenopausal women. Bioavailability was decreased (by approximately 40%) when 10 mg alendronate was administered either 0.5 or 1 hour before a standardized breakfast, when

Table 4: 25-hydroxyvitamin D Levels after Treatment with FOSAMAX PLUS D (70 mg/2800 IU) or FOSAMAX 70 mg at Week 15*

25-hydroxyvitamin D Ranges (ng/mL)	Number (%) of Patients					
	<9	**9-14**	**15-19**	**20-24**	**25-29**	**30-62**
FOSAMAX PLUS D (70 mg/2800 IU) (N=357)	4 (1.1)	37 (10.4)	87 (24.4)	84 (23.5)	82 (23.0)	63 (17.7)
FOSAMAX 70 mg (N=351)	46 (13.1)	66 (18.8)	108 (30.8)	58 (16.5)	37 (10.5)	36 (10.3)

* Patients who were vitamin D deficient (25-hydroxyvitamin D <9 ng/mL) at baseline were excluded.

Table 5: 25-hydroxyvitamin D Levels after Treatment with FOSAMAX PLUS D at Week 39

	Number (%) of Patients					
25-hydroxyvitamin D Ranges (ng/mL)	<9	9-14	15-19	20-24	25-29	30-59
FOSAMAX PLUS D (Vitamin D_3 5600 IU group)* (N=321)	0	10 (3.1)	29 (9.0)	79 (24.6)	87 (27.1)	116 (36.1)
FOSAMAX PLUS D (Vitamin D_3 2800 IU group)† (N=320)	1 (0.3)	17 (5.3)	56 (17.5)	80 (25.0)	74 (23.1)	92 (28.8)

* Patients received FOSAMAX 70 mg or FOSAMAX PLUS D (70 mg/2800 IU) for the 15-week base study followed by FOSAMAX PLUS D (70 mg/2800 IU) and 2800 IU additional vitamin D_3 for the 24-week extension study.
† Patients received FOSAMAX 70 mg or FOSAMAX PLUS D (70 mg/2800 IU) for 15-week base study followed by FOSAMAX PLUS D (70 mg/2800 IU) and placebo for the additional vitamin D_3 for 24-week extension study.

compared to dosing 2 hours before eating. In studies of treatment and prevention of osteoporosis, alendronate was effective when administered at least 30 minutes before breakfast.
Bioavailability was negligible whether alendronate was administered with or up to two hours after a standardized breakfast. Concomitant administration of alendronate with coffee or orange juice reduced bioavailability by approximately 60%.
Cholecalciferol
Following administration of FOSAMAX PLUS D (70 mg/2800 IU) after an overnight fast and two hours before a standard meal, the baseline adjusted mean area under the serum-concentration-time curve ($AUC_{0\text{-}120\ hrs}$) for vitamin D_3 was 120.7 ng-hr/mL. The baseline adjusted mean maximal serum concentration (C_{max}) of vitamin D_3 was 4.0 ng/mL, and the baseline adjusted mean time to maximal serum concentration (T_{max}) was 10.6 hrs. The bioavailability of the 2800 IU vitamin D_3 in FOSAMAX PLUS D is similar to 2800 IU vitamin D_3 administered alone.
In a separate study, the baseline adjusted mean $AUC_{0\text{-}80\ hrs}$ and baseline adjusted mean C_{max} for vitamin D_3 were 355.6 ng-hr/mL and 10.8 ng/mL, respectively. The baseline adjusted mean T_{max} was 9.2 hrs. The bioavailability of the 5600 IU vitamin D_3 in the FOSAMAX PLUS D is similar to 5600 IU vitamin D_3 administered as two 2800 IU vitamin D_3 tablets.
Distribution
Alendronate Sodium
Preclinical studies (in male rats) show that alendronate transiently distributes to soft tissues following 1 mg/kg IV administration but is then rapidly redistributed to bone or excreted in the urine. The mean steady-state volume of distribution, exclusive of bone, is at least 28 L in humans. Concentrations of drug in plasma following therapeutic oral doses are too low (less than 5 ng/mL) for analytical detection. Protein binding in human plasma is approximately 78%.
Cholecalciferol
Following absorption, vitamin D_3 enters the blood as part of chylomicrons. Vitamin D_3 is rapidly distributed mostly to the liver where it undergoes metabolism to 25-hydroxyvitamin D_3, the major storage form. Lesser amounts are distributed to adipose tissue and stored as vitamin D_3 at these sites for later release into the circulation. Circulating vitamin D_3 is bound to vitamin D-binding protein.
Metabolism
Alendronate Sodium
There is no evidence that alendronate is metabolized in animals or humans.
Cholecalciferol
Vitamin D_3 is rapidly metabolized by hydroxylation in the liver to 25-hydroxyvitamin D_3, and subsequently metabolized in the kidney to 1,25-dihydroxyvitamin D_3, which represents the biologically active form. Further hydroxylation occurs prior to elimination. A small percentage of vitamin D_3 undergoes glucuronidation prior to elimination.
Excretion
Alendronate Sodium
Following a single IV dose of [^{14}C]alendronate, approximately 50% of the radioactivity was excreted in the urine within 72 hours and little or no radioactivity was recovered in the feces. Following a single 10-mg IV dose, the renal clearance of alendronate was 71 mL/min (64, 78; 90% confidence interval [CI]), and systemic clearance did not exceed 200 mL/min. Plasma concentrations fell by more than 95% within 6 hours following IV administration. The terminal half-life in humans is estimated to exceed 10 years, probably reflecting release of alendronate from the skeleton. Based on the above, it is estimated that after 10 years of oral treatment with FOSAMAX (10 mg daily) the amount of alendronate released daily from the skeleton is approximately 25% of that absorbed from the gastrointestinal tract.
Cholecalciferol
When radioactive vitamin D_3 was intravenously administered to healthy subjects, the mean urinary excretion of radioactivity after 48 hours was 2.4% of the administered dose, and the mean fecal excretion of radioactivity after 48 hours was 4.9% of the administered dose. In both cases, the excreted radioactivity was almost exclusively as metabolites of the parent. The mean half-life of baseline adjusted vitamin D_3 in the serum following an oral dose of FOSAMAX PLUS D is approximately 14 hours.
Special Populations
Pediatric: The oral bioavailability of alendronate in children was similar to that observed in adults; however, FOSAMAX PLUS D is not indicated for use in children *[see Use in Specific Populations (8.4)]*.
Gender: Bioavailability and the fraction of an IV dose of alendronate excreted in urine were similar in men and women.
Geriatric:
Alendronate Sodium
Bioavailability and disposition of alendronate (urinary excretion) were similar in elderly and younger patients. No dosage adjustment of alendronate is necessary *[see Dosage and Administration (2.5)]*.
Cholecalciferol
Dietary requirements of vitamin D_3 are increased in the elderly.
Race: Pharmacokinetic differences due to race have not been studied.
Renal Insufficiency:
Alendronate Sodium
Preclinical studies show that, in rats with kidney failure, increasing amounts of drug are present in plasma, kidney, spleen, and tibia. In healthy controls, drug that is not deposited in bone is rapidly excreted in the urine. No evidence of saturation of bone uptake was found after 3 weeks dosing with cumulative IV doses of 35 mg/kg in young male rats. Although no clinical information is available, it is likely that, as in animals, elimination of alendronate via the kidney will be reduced in patients with impaired renal function. Therefore, somewhat greater accumulation of alendronate in bone might be expected in patients with impaired renal function.
No dosage adjustment is necessary for patients with mild-to-moderate renal insufficiency (creatinine clearance 35 to 60 mL/min). FOSAMAX PLUS D is not recommended for patients with more severe renal insufficiency (creatinine clearance <35 mL/min) due to lack of experience with alendronate in renal failure.
Cholecalciferol
Patients with renal insufficiency will have decreased ability to form the active 1,25-dihydroxyvitamin D_3 metabolite.
Hepatic Insufficiency:
Alendronate Sodium
As there is evidence that alendronate is not metabolized or excreted in the bile, no studies were conducted in patients with hepatic insufficiency. No dosage adjustment is necessary.
Cholecalciferol
Vitamin D_3 may not be adequately absorbed in patients who have malabsorption due to inadequate bile production.
Drug Interactions
Alendronate Sodium
Intravenous ranitidine was shown to double the bioavailability of oral alendronate. The clinical significance of this increased bioavailability and whether similar increases will occur in patients given oral H_2-antagonists is unknown.
In healthy subjects, oral prednisone (20 mg three times daily for five days) did not produce a clinically meaningful change in the oral bioavailability of alendronate (a mean increase ranging from 20 to 44%).
Products containing calcium and other multivalent cations are likely to interfere with absorption of alendronate.
Cholecalciferol
Olestra, mineral oils, orlistat, and bile acid sequestrants (e.g., cholestyramine, colestipol) may impair the absorption of vitamin D. Anticonvulsants, cimetidine, and thiazides may increase the catabolism of vitamin D.

13 NONCLINICAL TOXICOLOGY

13.1 Carcinogenesis, Mutagenesis, Impairment of Fertility

The following data are based on findings for the individual components of FOSAMAX PLUS D.
Alendronate Sodium
Harderian gland (a retro-orbital gland not present in humans) adenomas were increased in high-dose female mice (p=0.003) in a 92–week oral carcinogenicity study at doses of alendronate of 1, 3, and 10 mg/kg/day (males) or 1, 2, and 5 mg/kg/day (females). These doses are equivalent to 0.5 to 4 times a maximum recommended daily dose of 10 mg based on surface area, mg/m^2. The relevance of this finding to humans is unknown.
Parafollicular cell (thyroid) adenomas were increased in high-dose male rats (p=0.003) in a 2–year oral carcinogenicity study at doses of 1 and 3.75 mg/kg body weight. These doses are equivalent to 1 and 4 times a 10-mg human daily dose based on surface area, mg/m^2. The relevance of this finding to humans is unknown.
Alendronate was not genotoxic in the *in vitro* microbial mutagenesis assay with and without metabolic activation, in an *in vitro* mammalian cell mutagenesis assay, in an *in vitro* alkaline elution assay in rat hepatocytes, and in an *in vivo* chromosomal aberration assay in mice. In an *in vitro* chromosomal aberration assay in Chinese hamster ovary cells, however, alendronate gave equivocal results.
Alendronate had no effect on fertility (male or female) in rats at oral doses up to 5 mg/kg/day (4 times a 10-mg human daily dose based on surface area, mg/m^2).
Cholecalciferol
The carcinogenic potential of cholecalciferol (vitamin D_3) has not been studied in rodents. Calcitriol, the hormonal metabolite of cholecalciferol, was not genotoxic in the Ames microbial mutagenesis assay with or without metabolic activation, and in an *in vivo* micronucleus assay in mice.
Ergocalciferol (vitamin D_2) at high doses (150,000 to 200,000 IU/kg/day) administered prior to mating resulted in altered estrous cycle and inhibition of pregnancy in rats. The potential effect of cholecalciferol on male fertility is unknown in rats.

13.2 Animal Toxicology and/or Pharmacology

The relative inhibitory activities on bone resorption and mineralization of alendronate and etidronate were compared in the Schenk assay, which is based on histological examination of the epiphyses of growing rats. In this assay, the lowest dose of alendronate that interfered with bone mineralization (leading to osteomalacia) was 6000–fold the antiresorptive dose. The corresponding ratio for etidronate was one to one. These data suggest that alendronate administered in therapeutic doses is highly unlikely to induce osteomalacia.

14 CLINICAL STUDIES

14.1 Treatment of Postmenopausal Osteoporosis

Effect on Fracture Incidence
Data on the effects of FOSAMAX on fracture incidence are derived from three clinical studies of postmenopausal women, 44 to 84 years of age, with osteoporosis: 1) U.S. and Multinational combined: a study of patients with a lumbar spine BMD T-score at or below minus 2.5 with or without a prior vertebral fracture, 2) Three-Year Study of the Fracture Intervention Trial (FIT): a study of patients with at least one baseline vertebral fracture, and 3) Four-Year Study of FIT: a study of patients with low bone mass but without a baseline vertebral fracture.
To assess the effects of FOSAMAX on the incidence of vertebral fractures (detected by digitized radiography; approximately one third of these were clinically symptomatic), the U.S. (478 patients) and Multinational (516 patients in 15 countries) studies (of virtually identical design) were combined in an analysis that compared placebo to the pooled dosage groups of FOSAMAX (5 or 10 mg for three years or 20 mg for two years followed by 5 mg for one year). There was a statistically significant reduction in the proportion of patients treated with FOSAMAX experiencing one or more new vertebral fractures relative to those treated with placebo (3.2% vs. 6.2%; a 48% relative risk reduction). A reduction in the total number of new vertebral fractures (4.2 vs. 11.3 per 100 patients) was also observed. In the pooled analysis, patients who received FOSAMAX had a loss in stature that was statistically significantly less than was observed in those who received placebo (-3.0 mm vs. -4.6 mm).
The Fracture Intervention Trial (FIT) consisted of two studies in postmenopausal women: the Three-Year Study of patients who had at least one baseline radiographic vertebral fracture and the Four-Year Study of patients with low bone mass but without a baseline vertebral fracture. In both studies of FIT, 96% of randomized patients completed the studies (i.e., had a closeout visit at the scheduled end of the study); approximately 80% of patients were still taking study medication upon completion.
Fracture Intervention Trial: Three-Year Study (patients with at least one baseline radiographic vertebral fracture)
This randomized, double-blind, placebo-controlled, 2027-patient study (FOSAMAX, n=1022; placebo, n=1005) demonstrated that treatment with FOSAMAX resulted in statistically significant reductions in fracture incidence at three years as shown in Table 6.

[See table 6 at right]

Furthermore, in this population of patients with baseline vertebral fracture, treatment with FOSAMAX significantly reduced the incidence of hospitalizations (25.0% vs. 30.7%). In the Three-Year Study of FIT, fractures of the hip occurred in 22 (2.2%) of 1005 patients on placebo and 11 (1.1%) of 1022 patients on FOSAMAX, p=0.047. Figure 1 displays the cumulative incidence of hip fractures in this study.

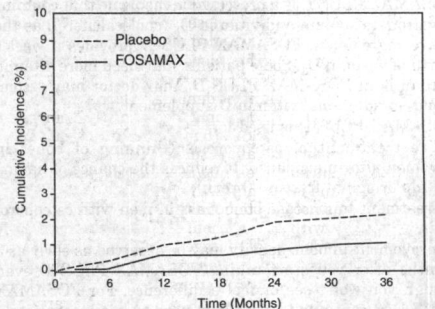

Figure 1: Cumulative Incidence of Hip Fractures in the Three-Year Study of FIT (patients with radiographic vertebral fracture at baseline)

Fracture Intervention Trial: Four-Year Study (patients with low bone mass but without a baseline radiographic vertebral fracture)

This randomized, double-blind, placebo-controlled, 4432-patient study (FOSAMAX, n=2214; placebo, n=2218) further investigated the reduction in fracture incidence due to FOSAMAX. The intent of the study was to recruit women with osteoporosis, defined as a baseline femoral neck BMD at least two standard deviations below the mean for young adult women. However, due to subsequent revisions to the normative values for femoral neck BMD, 31% of patients were found not to meet this entry criterion and thus this study included both osteoporotic and non-osteoporotic women. The results are shown in Table 7 below for the patients with osteoporosis.

[See table 7 at right]

Fracture Results Across Studies

In the Three-Year Study of FIT, FOSAMAX reduced the percentage of women experiencing at least one new radiographic vertebral fracture from 15.0% to 7.9% (47% relative risk reduction, p<0.001); in the Four-Year Study of FIT, the percentage was reduced from 3.8% to 2.1% (44% relative risk reduction, p=0.001); and in the combined U.S./Multinational studies, from 6.2% to 3.2% (48% relative risk reduction, p=0.034).

FOSAMAX reduced the percentage of women experiencing multiple (two or more) new vertebral fractures from 4.2% to 0.6% (87% relative risk reduction, p<0.001) in the combined U.S./Multinational studies and from 4.9% to 0.5% (90% relative risk reduction, p<0.001) in the Three-Year Study of FIT. In the Four-Year Study of FIT, FOSAMAX reduced the percentage of osteoporotic women experiencing multiple vertebral fractures from 0.6% to 0.1% (78% relative risk reduction, p=0.035).

Thus, FOSAMAX reduced the incidence of radiographic vertebral fractures in osteoporotic women whether or not they had a previous radiographic vertebral fracture.

FOSAMAX, over a three- or four-year period, was associated with statistically significant reductions in loss of height vs. placebo in patients with and without baseline radiographic vertebral fractures. At the end of the FIT studies the between-treatment group differences were 3.2 mm in the Three-Year Study and 1.3 mm in the Four-Year Study.

Effect on Bone Mineral Density

The efficacy of FOSAMAX 10 mg once daily in postmenopausal women with osteoporosis (lumbar spine bone mineral density [BMD] of at least 2 standard deviations below the premenopausal mean) was demonstrated in four double-blind, placebo-controlled clinical studies of two or three years' duration. These included two three-year, multicenter studies of virtually identical design, one performed in the United States (U.S.) and the other in 15 different countries (Multinational), which enrolled 478 and 516 patients, respectively. Figure 2 shows the mean increases in BMD of the lumbar spine, femoral neck, and trochanter in patients receiving FOSAMAX 10 mg/day relative to placebo-treated patients at three years for each of these studies.

[See figure 2 at top of next column]

At three years significant increases in BMD, relative both to baseline and placebo, were seen at each measurement site in each study in patients who received FOSAMAX 10 mg/day. Total body BMD also increased significantly in each study, suggesting that the increases in bone mass of the spine and hip did not occur at the expense of other skeletal sites. Increases in BMD were evident as early as three months and continued throughout the three years of treat-

Table 6: Effect of FOSAMAX on Fracture Incidence in the Three-Year Study of FIT (patients with vertebral fracture at baseline)

| | Percent of Patients | | | |
	FOSAMAX (n=1022)	Placebo (n=1005)	Absolute Reduction in Fracture Incidence	Relative Reduction in Fracture Risk %
Patients with:				
Vertebral fractures (diagnosed by X-ray)*				
≥1 new vertebral fracture	7.9	15.0	7.1	47[†]
≥2 new vertebral fractures	0.5	4.9	4.4	90[†]
Clinical (symptomatic) fractures				
Any clinical (symptomatic) fracture	13.8	18.1	4.3	26[‡]
≥1 clinical (symptomatic) vertebral fracture	2.3	5.0	2.7	54[§]
Hip fracture	1.1	2.2	1.1	51[¶]
Wrist (forearm) fracture	2.2	4.1	1.9	48[¶]

* Number evaluable for vertebral fractures: FOSAMAX, n=984; placebo, n=966
† p<0.001
‡ p=0.007
§ p<0.01
¶ p<0.05

Table 7: Effect of FOSAMAX on Fracture Incidence in Osteoporotic* Patients in the Four-Year Study of FIT (patients without vertebral fracture at baseline)

| | Percent of Patients | | | |
	FOSAMAX (n=1545)	Placebo (n=1521)	Absolute Reduction in Fracture Incidence	Relative Reduction in Fracture Risk (%)
Patients with:				
Vertebral fractures (diagnosed by X-ray)[†]				
≥1 new vertebral fracture	2.5	4.8	2.3	48[‡]
≥2 new vertebral fractures	0.1	0.6	0.5	78[§]
Clinical (symptomatic) fractures				
Any clinical (symptomatic) fracture	12.9	16.2	3.3	22[¶]
≥1 clinical (symptomatic) vertebral fracture	1.0	1.6	0.6	41 (NS)[#]
Hip fracture	1.0	1.4	0.4	29 (NS)[#]
Wrist (forearm) fracture	3.9	3.8	-0.1	NS[#]

* Baseline femoral neck BMD at least 2 SD below the mean for young adult women
† Number evaluable for vertebral fractures: FOSAMAX, n=1426; placebo, n=1428
‡ p<0.001
§ p=0.035
¶ p=0.01
\# Not significant. This study was not powered to detect differences at these sites.

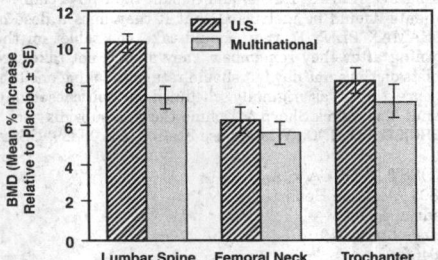

Figure 2: Osteoporosis Treatment Studies in Postmenopausal Women: Increase in BMD: FOSAMAX 10 mg/day at Three Years

ment. (See figure 3 for lumbar spine results.) In the two-year extension of these studies, treatment of 147 patients with FOSAMAX 10 mg/day resulted in continued increases in BMD at the lumbar spine and trochanter (absolute additional increases between years 3 and 5: lumbar spine, 0.94%; trochanter, 0.88%). BMD at the femoral neck, forearm and total body were maintained. FOSAMAX was similarly effective regardless of age, race, baseline rate of bone turnover, and baseline BMD in the range studied (at least 2 standard deviations below the premenopausal mean). Thus, overall FOSAMAX reverses the loss of bone mineral density, a central factor in the progression of osteoporosis.

[See figure 3 at top of next page]

In patients with postmenopausal osteoporosis treated with FOSAMAX 10 mg/day for one or two years, the effects of treatment withdrawal were assessed. Following discontinuation, there were no further increases in bone mass and the rates of bone loss were similar to those of the placebo groups. These data indicate that continued treatment with FOSAMAX is required to maintain the effect of the drug.

The therapeutic equivalence of once weekly FOSAMAX 70 mg (n=519) and FOSAMAX 10 mg daily (n=370) was demonstrated in a one-year, double-blind, multicenter study

of postmenopausal women with osteoporosis. In the primary analysis of completers, the mean increases from baseline in lumbar spine BMD at one year were 5.1% (4.8, 5.4%; 95% CI) in the 70-mg once-weekly group (n=440) and 5.4% (5.0, 5.8%; 95% CI) in the 10-mg daily group (n=330). The two treatment groups were also similar with regard to BMD increases at other skeletal sites. The results of the intention-to-treat analysis were consistent with the primary analysis of completers.

Bone Histology

Bone histology in 270 postmenopausal patients with osteoporosis treated with FOSAMAX at doses ranging from 1 to 20 mg/day for one, two, or three years revealed normal mineralization and structure, as well as the expected decrease in bone turnover relative to placebo. These data, together with the normal bone histology and increased bone strength observed in rats and baboons exposed to long-term alendronate treatment, support the conclusion that bone formed during therapy with FOSAMAX is of normal quality.

Concomitant Use with Estrogen Hormone Replacement Therapy

The effects on BMD of treatment with FOSAMAX 10 mg once daily and conjugated estrogen (0.625 mg/day) either alone or in combination were assessed in a two-year, double-blind, placebo-controlled study of hysterectomized postmenopausal osteoporotic women (n=425). At two years, the increases in lumbar spine BMD from baseline were significantly greater with the combination (8.3%) than with either estrogen or FOSAMAX alone (both 6.0%).

The effects on BMD when FOSAMAX was added to stable doses (for at least one year) of HRT (estrogen ± progestin) were assessed in a one-year, double-blind, placebo-controlled study in postmenopausal osteoporotic women (n=428). The addition of FOSAMAX 10 mg once daily to HRT produced, at one year, significantly greater increases in lumbar spine BMD (3.7%) vs. HRT alone (1.1%).

In these studies, significant increases or favorable trends in BMD for combined therapy compared with HRT alone were seen at the total hip, femoral neck, and trochanter. No significant effect was seen for total body BMD.

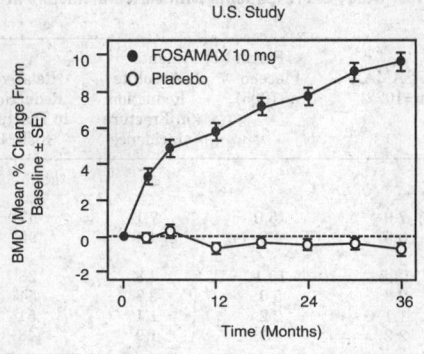

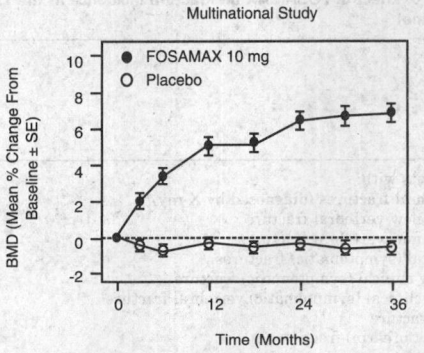

Figure 3: Osteoporosis Treatment Studies in Postmenopausal Women: Time Course of Effect of FOSAMAX 10 mg/day Versus Placebo: Lumbar Spine BMD Percent Change From Baseline

Histomorphometric studies of transiliac biopsies in 92 subjects showed normal bone architecture. Compared to placebo there was a 98% suppression of bone turnover (as assessed by mineralizing surface) after 18 months of combined treatment with FOSAMAX and HRT, 94% on FOSAMAX alone, and 78% on HRT alone. The long-term effects of combined FOSAMAX and HRT on fracture occurrence and fracture healing have not been studied.

14.2 Treatment to Increase Bone Mass in Men with Osteoporosis

The efficacy of FOSAMAX in men with hypogonadal or idiopathic osteoporosis was demonstrated in two clinical studies.

A two-year, double-blind, placebo-controlled, multicenter study of FOSAMAX 10 mg once daily enrolled a total of 241 men between the ages of 31 and 87 (mean, 63). All patients in the trial had either: 1) a BMD T-score ≤-2 at the femoral neck and ≤-1 at the lumbar spine, or 2) a baseline osteoporotic fracture and a BMD T-score ≤-1 at the femoral neck. At two years, the mean increases relative to placebo in BMD in men receiving FOSAMAX 10 mg/day were significant at the following sites: lumbar spine, 5.3%; femoral neck, 2.6%; trochanter, 3.1%; and total body, 1.6%. Treatment with FOSAMAX also reduced height loss (FOSAMAX, -0.6 mm vs. placebo, -2.4 mm).

A one-year, double-blind, placebo-controlled, multicenter study of once weekly FOSAMAX 70 mg enrolled a total of 167 men between the ages of 38 and 91 (mean, 66). Patients in the study had either: 1) a BMD T-score ≤-2 at the femoral neck and ≤-1 at the lumbar spine, 2) a BMD T-score ≤-2 at the lumbar spine and ≤-1 at the femoral neck, or 3) a baseline osteoporotic fracture and a BMD T-score ≤-1 at the femoral neck. At one year, the mean increases relative to placebo in BMD in men receiving FOSAMAX 70 mg once weekly were significant at the following sites: lumbar spine, 2.8%; femoral neck, 1.9%; trochanter, 2.0%; and total body, 1.2%. These increases in BMD were similar to those seen at one year in the 10 mg once-daily study.

In both studies, BMD responses were similar regardless of age (≥65 years vs. <65 years), gonadal function (baseline testosterone <9 ng/dL vs. ≥9 ng/dL), or baseline BMD (femoral neck and lumbar spine T-score ≤-2.5 vs. >-2.5).

16 HOW SUPPLIED/STORAGE AND HANDLING

No. 3870—Tablets FOSAMAX PLUS D 70 mg/2800 IU are white to off-white, modified capsule-shaped tablets with code 710 on one side and an outline of a bone image on the other. They are supplied as follows:
NDC 0006-0710-44 unit of use blister packages of 4.
No. 6746—Tablets FOSAMAX PLUS D 70 mg/5600 IU are white to off-white, modified rectangle-shaped tablets with code 270 on one side and an outline of a bone image on the other. They are supplied as follows:
NDC 0006-0270-44 unit of use blister packages of 4
NDC 0006-0270-21 unit dose packages of 20.
Storage
Store at 20-25°C (68-77°F), excursions between 15-30°C (59-86°F) are allowed. [See USP Controlled Room Temperature.] Protect from moisture and light. Store tablets in the original blister package until use.

17 PATIENT COUNSELING INFORMATION

[See FDA-Approved Patient Labeling (17.3).]
Physicians should instruct their patients to read the patient package insert before starting therapy with FOSAMAX PLUS D and to reread it each time the prescription is renewed.

17.1 Osteoporosis Recommendations, Including Calcium and Vitamin D Supplementation

Patients should be instructed to take supplemental calcium if intake is inadequate. Patients at increased risk for vitamin D insufficiency (e.g., over the age of 70 years, nursing home bound, or chronically ill) should be instructed to take additional vitamin D if needed *[see Dosage and Administration (2.3)]*. Patients with gastrointestinal malabsorption syndromes should be informed that they may require additional vitamin D supplementation. Weight-bearing exercise should be considered along with the modification of certain behavioral factors, such as cigarette smoking and/or excessive alcohol consumption, if these factors exist.

17.2 Dosing Instructions

Patients should be instructed that the expected benefits of FOSAMAX PLUS D may only be obtained when it is taken with plain water the first thing upon arising for the day at least 30 minutes before the first food, beverage, or medication of the day. Even dosing with orange juice or coffee has been shown to markedly reduce the absorption of alendronate *[see Clinical Pharmacology (12.3)]*.

To facilitate delivery to the stomach and thus reduce the potential for esophageal irritation, patients should be instructed to swallow each tablet of FOSAMAX PLUS D with a full glass of water (6-8 oz) and not to lie down for at least 30 minutes and until after their first food of the day. Patients should not chew or suck on the tablet because of a potential for oropharyngeal ulceration. Patients should be specifically instructed not to take FOSAMAX PLUS D at bedtime or before arising for the day. Patients should be informed that failure to follow these instructions may increase their risk of esophageal problems. Patients should be instructed that if they develop symptoms of esophageal disease (such as difficulty or pain upon swallowing, retrosternal pain or new or worsening heartburn) they should stop taking FOSAMAX PLUS D and consult their physician.

Patients should be instructed that if they miss a dose of FOSAMAX PLUS D, they should take one tablet on the morning after they remember. They should not take two tablets on the same day but should return to taking one tablet once a week, as originally scheduled on their chosen day.
Manuf. for: Merck Sharp & Dohme Corp., a subsidiary of **MERCK & CO., INC.**, Whitehouse Station, NJ 08889, USA
By:
FROSST IBERICA, S.A.
28805 Alcalá de Henares
Madrid, Spain
Issued June 2010
9664509
[1]Registered Trademark of Merck Sharp & Dohme Corp., a subsidiary of **Merck & Co., Inc.**
Copyright © 2005, 2007 Merck Sharp & Dohme Corp., a subsidiary of **Merck & Co., Inc.**
All rights reserved

17.3 FDA-Approved Patient Labeling

Patient Information
FOSAMAX PLUS D® (FOSS-ah-max PLUS D)
(alendronate sodium/cholecalciferol)
Tablets
Read the patient information before you start taking FOSAMAX PLUS D[1]. Also, read the leaflet each time you refill your prescription, just in case anything has changed. This leaflet does not take the place of discussions with your doctor about your medical condition or treatment. You and your doctor should discuss FOSAMAX PLUS D when you start taking your medicine and at regular checkups.

---

[1]Registered Trademark of Merck Sharp & Dohme Corp., a subsidiary of **Merck & Co., Inc.**
Copyright © 2005, 2007 Merck Sharp & Dohme Corp., a subsidiary of **Merck & Co., Inc.**
All rights reserved

What is the most important information I should know about FOSAMAX PLUS D?
• **You must take FOSAMAX PLUS D exactly as directed to help make sure it works and to help lower the chance** of problems in your esophagus (the tube that connects your mouth and stomach). (See "How should I take FOSAMAX PLUS D?").
• **If you have chest pain, new or worsening heartburn, or have trouble or pain when you swallow, stop taking FOSAMAX PLUS D and call your doctor.** (See "What are the possible side effects of FOSAMAX PLUS D?".)

What is FOSAMAX PLUS D?
FOSAMAX PLUS D is a prescription medicine that contains alendronate sodium and vitamin D_3 (cholecalciferol) as the active ingredients. FOSAMAX PLUS D provides a week's worth of vitamin D_3. Some patients may need more vitamin D than is in FOSAMAX PLUS D. Your doctor may recommend an additional vitamin D supplement.
FOSAMAX PLUS D is used for:
• The treatment of osteoporosis (thinning of bone) in women after menopause. It reduces the chance of having a hip or spinal fracture (break).
• Treatment to increase bone mass in men with osteoporosis.
Improvement in bone density may be observed as early as 3 months after you start taking FOSAMAX PLUS D even though you won't see or feel a difference. For FOSAMAX PLUS D to continue to work, you need to keep taking it.
FOSAMAX PLUS D should not be used to treat vitamin D deficiency.
FOSAMAX PLUS D is not a hormone.
FOSAMAX PLUS D is not for use in premenopausal women.
There is more information about osteoporosis and vitamin D at the end of this leaflet.

Who should not take FOSAMAX PLUS D?
Do not take FOSAMAX PLUS D if you:
• Have certain problems with your esophagus, the tube that connects your mouth with your stomach
• Cannot stand or sit upright for at least 30 minutes
• Have low levels of calcium in your blood
• Are allergic to FOSAMAX PLUS D or any of its ingredients. A list of ingredients is at the end of this leaflet.

What should I tell my doctor before using FOSAMAX PLUS D?

Tell your doctor about all of your medical or dental conditions, including if you:
• **have problems with swallowing**
• **have stomach or digestive problems**
• **have kidney problems**
• **have sarcoidosis, leukemia, lymphoma.** These conditions may cause changes in vitamin D.
• **are pregnant or planning to become pregnant.** It is not known if FOSAMAX PLUS D can harm your unborn baby.
• **are breastfeeding.** It is not known if FOSAMAX PLUS D passes into your milk and if it can harm your baby.
Tell your doctor about all medicines you take, including prescription and non-prescription medicines, vitamins, and herbal supplements.
Know the medicines you take. Keep a list of them and show it to your doctor and pharmacist each time you get a new medicine.

How should I take FOSAMAX PLUS D?
• Choose the day of the week that best fits your schedule.
• Take 1 tablet of FOSAMAX PLUS D every week on your chosen day **after** you get up for the day and **before** taking your first food, drink, or other medicine.
• Take FOSAMAX PLUS D while you are sitting or standing.
• Swallow your FOSAMAX PLUS D tablet with a full glass (6-8 oz) of plain water only.
Do **not** take FOSAMAX PLUS D with:
Mineral water
Coffee or tea
Juice
FOSAMAX PLUS D works only if it is taken on an empty stomach.
Do not chew or suck on a tablet of FOSAMAX PLUS D.
After swallowing your FOSAMAX PLUS D tablet, wait at least 30 minutes:
• before you lie down. You may sit, stand or walk, and do normal activities like reading.
• before you take your first food or drink except for plain water.
• before you take other medicines, including antacids, calcium, and other supplements and vitamins.
Do not lie down until after your first food of the day.
• It is important that you keep taking FOSAMAX PLUS D for as long as your doctor says to take it. For FOSAMAX PLUS D to continue to work, you need to keep taking it.

What should I do if I miss a dose of FOSAMAX PLUS D or if I take too many?
• If you miss a dose, take only 1 FOSAMAX PLUS D tablet on the morning after you remember. Do not take 2 tablets

on the same day. Continue your usual schedule of 1 FOSAMAX PLUS D tablet once a week on your chosen day.

- If you think you took more than the prescribed dose of FOSAMAX PLUS D, drink a full glass of milk and call your doctor right away. Do not try to vomit. Do not lie down.

What should I avoid while taking FOSAMAX PLUS D?

- Do not eat, drink, or take other medicines or supplements **before** taking FOSAMAX PLUS D.
- Wait for at least 30 minutes **after** taking FOSAMAX PLUS D to eat, drink, or take other medicines or supplements.
- Do not lie down for at least 30 minutes **after** taking FOSAMAX PLUS D. Do not lie down until **after** your first food of the day.

What are the possible side effects of FOSAMAX PLUS D?
FOSAMAX PLUS D may cause problems in your esophagus (the tube that connects the mouth and stomach). (See "What is the most important information I should know about FOSAMAX PLUS D?".) These problems include irritation, inflammation, or ulcers of the esophagus, which may sometimes bleed. This may occur especially if you do not drink a full glass of water with FOSAMAX PLUS D or if you lie down in less than 30 minutes or before your first food of the day.

- **Stop taking FOSAMAX PLUS D and call your doctor right away if you get any of these signs of possible serious problems of the esophagus:**
  - **Chest pain**
  - **New or worsening heartburn**
  - **Trouble or pain when swallowing**
- Esophagus problems may get worse if you continue to take FOSAMAX PLUS D.
- Mouth sores (ulcers) may occur if the FOSAMAX PLUS D tablet is chewed or dissolved in the mouth.
- You may get flu-like symptoms typically at the start of treatment with FOSAMAX PLUS D.
- You may get allergic reactions, such as hives or, in rare cases, swelling of your face, lips, tongue, or throat.
- FOSAMAX PLUS D may cause jawbone problems in some people. Jawbone problems may include infection, and delayed healing after teeth are pulled.
- The most common side effect is stomach area (abdominal) pain. Less common side effects are nausea, vomiting, a full or bloated feeling in the stomach, constipation, diarrhea, black or bloody stools (bowel movements), gas, eye pain, rash that may be made worse by sunlight, hair loss, headache, dizziness, a changed sense of taste, joint swelling or swelling in the hands or legs, and bone, muscle, or joint pain.
- **Call your doctor if you develop severe bone, muscle, or joint pain.**
- Some patients have experienced fracture in a specific part of the thigh bone. Call your doctor if you develop new or unusual pain in the hip or thigh.

Tell your doctor about any side effect that bothers you or that does not go away.

These are not all the side effects with FOSAMAX PLUS D. Ask your doctor or pharmacist for more information.

How do I store FOSAMAX PLUS D?

- Store FOSAMAX PLUS D at 68 to 77°F (20 to 25°C). Protect from moisture and light. Store tablets in the original blister package until time of use.
- Safely discard FOSAMAX PLUS D that is out-of-date or no longer needed.
- **Keep all FOSAMAX PLUS D and all medicines out of the reach of children.**

General information about using FOSAMAX PLUS D safely and effectively

Medicines are sometimes prescribed for conditions that are not mentioned in patient information leaflets. Do not use FOSAMAX PLUS D for a condition for which it was not prescribed. Do not give FOSAMAX PLUS D to other people, even if they have the same symptoms you have. It may harm them.

This leaflet is a summary of information about FOSAMAX PLUS D. If you have any questions or concerns about FOSAMAX PLUS D or osteoporosis, talk to your doctor, pharmacist, or other health care provider. You can ask your doctor or pharmacist for information about FOSAMAX PLUS D written for health care providers. For more information, call 1-877-408-4699 (toll-free) or visit the following website: www.fosamaxplusd.com.

What are the ingredients in FOSAMAX PLUS D?
Active ingredients: alendronate sodium and cholecalciferol (vitamin D₃).
Inactive ingredients: cellulose, lactose, medium chain triglycerides, gelatin, croscarmellose sodium, sucrose, colloidal silicon dioxide, magnesium stearate, butylated hydroxytoluene, modified food starch, and sodium aluminum silicate.

What should I know about vitamin D?
Vitamin D is an essential nutrient, required for calcium absorption and healthy bones. The main source is through ex-

posure to summer sunlight, which makes vitamin D in our skin. Winter sunlight in most of the United States is too weak to produce vitamin D. Even in the summer, clothing or sun block can prevent enough sunlight from getting through. In addition, as people age, their skin becomes less able to make vitamin D. Very few foods are natural sources of vitamin D. Some foods, such as milk, some brands of orange juice and breakfast cereals are fortified with vitamin D.

Too little vitamin D leads to low calcium absorption and low phosphate. These are minerals that make bones strong. Even if you are eating a diet rich in calcium or taking a calcium supplement, your body cannot absorb calcium properly unless you have enough vitamin D. Too little vitamin D may lead to bone loss and osteoporosis.

What should I know about osteoporosis?
Normally your bones are being rebuilt all the time. First, old bone is removed (resorbed). Then a similar amount of new bone is formed. This balanced process keeps your skeleton healthy and strong.

Osteoporosis is a thinning and weakening of the bones. It is common in women after menopause, and may also occur in men. In osteoporosis, bone is removed faster than it is formed, so overall bone mass is lost and bones become weaker. Therefore, keeping bone mass is important to keep your bones healthy. In both men and women, osteoporosis may also be caused by certain medicines called corticosteroids.

At first, osteoporosis usually has no symptoms, but it can cause fractures (broken bones). Fractures usually cause pain. Fractures of the bones of the spine may not be painful, but over time they can make you shorter. Eventually, your spine can curve and your body can become bent over. Fractures may happen during normal, everyday activity, such as lifting, or from minor injury that would normally not cause bones to break. Fractures most often occur at the hip, spine, or wrist. This can lead to pain, severe disability, or loss of ability to move around (mobility).

Who is at risk for osteoporosis?
Many things put people at risk of osteoporosis. The following people have a higher chance of getting osteoporosis:
Women who:
- Are going through or who are past menopause
Men who:
- Are elderly
People who:
- Are white (Caucasian) or oriental (Asian)
- Are thin
- Have family member with osteoporosis
- Do not get enough calcium or vitamin D
- Do not exercise
- Smoke
- Drink alcohol often
- Take bone thinning medicines (like prednisone or other corticosteroids) for a long time

What can I do to help treat osteoporosis?
In addition to FOSAMAX PLUS D, your doctor may suggest one or more of the following lifestyle changes:
- **Stop smoking.** Smoking may increase your chance of getting osteoporosis.
- **Reduce the use of alcohol.** Too much alcohol may increase the chance of osteoporosis and injuries that can cause fractures.
- **Exercise regularly.** Like muscles, bones need exercise to stay strong and healthy. Exercise must be safe to prevent injuries, including fractures. Talk with your doctor before you begin any exercise program.
- **Eat a balanced diet.** Having enough calcium in your diet is important. Your doctor can advise you whether you need to change your diet or take any dietary supplements, such as calcium or additional vitamin D.

Rx only
Manuf. for: Merck Sharp & Dohme Corp., a subsidiary of **MERCK & CO., INC.**, Whitehouse Station, NJ 08889, USA
By:
FROSST IBERICA, S.A.
28805 Alcalá de Henares
Madrid, Spain
Issued June 2010
9664509

Shown in Product Identification Guide, page 313

GARDASIL®　　　　　　　　　　　　　　　　　　　℞
[GARD-ah-sill]
[Human Papillomavirus Quadrivalent (Types 6, 11, 16, and 18) Vaccine, Recombinant]
Suspension for Intramuscular Injection

HIGHLIGHTS OF PRESCRIBING INFORMATION
These highlights do not include all the information needed to use GARDASIL safely and effectively. See full prescribing information for GARDASIL.
GARDASIL
[Human Papillomavirus Quadrivalent (Types 6, 11, 16, and 18) Vaccine, Recombinant]

Suspension for intramuscular injection
Initial U.S. Approval: 2006

----------RECENT MAJOR CHANGES----------
Indications and Usage (1)
　Girls and Women (1.1)　　　　　　　　　　10/2009
　Boys and Men (1.2)　　　　　　　　　　　10/2009

----------INDICATIONS AND USAGE----------
GARDASIL is a vaccine indicated in girls and women 9 through 26 years of age for the prevention of the following diseases caused by Human Papillomavirus (HPV) types included in the vaccine:
- Cervical, vulvar, and vaginal cancer caused by HPV types 16 and 18
- Genital warts (condyloma acuminata) caused by HPV types 6 and 11
And the following precancerous or dysplastic lesions caused by HPV types 6, 11, 16, and 18:
- Cervical intraepithelial neoplasia (CIN) grade 2/3 and Cervical adenocarcinoma *in situ* (AIS)
- Cervical intraepithelial neoplasia (CIN) grade 1
- Vulvar intraepithelial neoplasia (VIN) grade 2 and grade 3
- Vaginal intraepithelial neoplasia (VaIN) grade 2 and grade 3
GARDASIL is indicated in boys and men 9 through 26 years of age for the prevention of genital warts (condyloma acuminata) caused by HPV types 6 and 11. (1)
Limitations of GARDASIL Use and Effectiveness:
- GARDASIL does not eliminate the necessity for women to continue to undergo recommended cervical cancer screening. (1.3) (17)
- GARDASIL has not been demonstrated to provide protection against disease from vaccine and non-vaccine HPV types to which a person has previously been exposed through sexual activity. (1.3) (14.3) (14.4)
- GARDASIL is not intended to be used for treatment of active external genital lesions; cervical, vulvar, and vaginal cancers; CIN; VIN; or VaIN. (1.3)
- GARDASIL has not been demonstrated to protect against diseases due to HPV types not contained in the vaccine. (1.3) (14.5)
- Not all vulvar and vaginal cancers are caused by HPV, and GARDASIL protects only against those vulvar and vaginal cancers caused by HPV 16 and 18. (1.3)
- GARDASIL does not protect against genital diseases not caused by HPV. (1.3)
- Vaccination with GARDASIL may not result in protection in all vaccine recipients. (1.3)

----------DOSAGE AND ADMINISTRATION----------
0.5-mL suspension for intramuscular injection at the following schedule: 0, 2 months, 6 months. (2.1)

----------DOSAGE FORMS AND STRENGTHS----------
- 0.5-mL suspension for injection as a single-dose vial and prefilled syringe. (3) (11)

----------CONTRAINDICATIONS----------
- Hypersensitivity, including severe allergic reactions to yeast (a vaccine component), or after a previous dose of GARDASIL. (4) (11)

----------WARNINGS AND PRECAUTIONS----------
- Because vaccinees may develop syncope, sometimes resulting in falling with injury, observation for 15 minutes after administration is recommended. Syncope, sometimes associated with tonic-clonic movements and other seizure-like activity, has been reported following vaccination with GARDASIL. When syncope is associated with tonic-clonic movements, the activity is usually transient and typically responds to restoring cerebral perfusion by maintaining a supine or Trendelenburg position. (5.1)

----------ADVERSE REACTIONS----------
The most common adverse reaction was headache. Common adverse reactions (frequency of at least 1.0% and greater than AAHS control or saline placebo) are fever, nausea, dizziness; and injection-site pain, swelling, erythema, pruritus, and bruising. (6.1)
To report SUSPECTED ADVERSE REACTIONS, contact Merck & Co., Inc. at 1-877-888-4231 or VAERS at 1-800-822-7967 or www.vaers.hhs.gov.

----------DRUG INTERACTIONS----------
GARDASIL may be administered concomitantly with RECOMBIVAX HB (7.1) or with Menactra and Adacel. (7.2)

----------USE IN SPECIFIC POPULATIONS----------
Safety and effectiveness of GARDASIL have not been established in the following populations:
- Pregnant women. Physicians are encouraged to register pregnant women exposed to GARDASIL by calling 1-800-986-8999 so that Merck can monitor maternal and fetal outcomes. (8.1)
- Children below the age of 9 years. (8.4)
- Immunocompromised individuals. Response to GARDASIL may be diminished. (8.6)
- Individuals 27 years of age and older. (8.1) (14.6)

See 17 for PATIENT COUNSELING INFORMATION and FDA-approved patient labeling

Revised: 06/2010

FULL PRESCRIBING INFORMATION: CONTENTS*

* Sections or subsections omitted from the full prescribing information are not listed

---

FULL PRESCRIBING INFORMATION

1   INDICATIONS AND USAGE

1.1   Girls and Women

GARDASIL®[1] is a vaccine indicated in girls and women 9 through 26 years of age for the prevention of the following diseases caused by Human Papillomavirus (HPV) types included in the vaccine:
- Cervical, vulvar, and vaginal cancer caused by HPV types 16 and 18
- Genital warts (condyloma acuminata) caused by HPV types 6 and 11

And the following precancerous or dysplastic lesions caused by HPV types 6, 11, 16, and 18:
- Cervical intraepithelial neoplasia (CIN) grade 2/3 and Cervical adenocarcinoma *in situ* (AIS)
- Cervical intraepithelial neoplasia (CIN) grade 1
- Vulvar intraepithelial neoplasia (VIN) grade 2 and grade 3
- Vaginal intraepithelial neoplasia (VaIN) grade 2 and grade 3

1.2   Boys and Men

GARDASIL is indicated in boys and men 9 through 26 years of age for the prevention of genital warts (condyloma acuminata) caused by HPV types 6 and 11.

1.3   Limitations of GARDASIL Use and Effectiveness

The health care provider should inform the patient, parent, or guardian that vaccination does not eliminate the necessity for women to continue to undergo recommended cervical cancer screening. Women who receive GARDASIL should continue to undergo cervical cancer screening per standard of care. *[See Patient Counseling Information (17).]*

Table 1: Injection-Site Adverse Reactions in Girls and Women 9 Through 26 Years of Age*

Adverse Reaction (1 to 5 Days Postvaccination)	GARDASIL (N = 5088) %	AAHS Control[†] (N = 3470) %	Saline Placebo (N = 320) %
Injection Site			
Pain	83.9	75.4	48.6
Swelling	25.4	15.8	7.3
Erythema	24.7	18.4	12.1
Pruritus	3.2	2.8	0.6
Bruising	2.8	3.2	1.6

* The injection-site adverse reactions that were observed among recipients of GARDASIL were at a frequency of at least 1.0% and also at a greater frequency than that observed among AAHS control or saline placebo recipients.
† AAHS Control = Amorphous Aluminum Hydroxyphosphate Sulfate

GARDASIL has not been demonstrated to provide protection against disease from vaccine and non-vaccine HPV types to which a person has previously been exposed through sexual activity. *[See Clinical Studies (14.3, 14.4).]* GARDASIL is not intended to be used for treatment of active external genital lesions; cervical, vulvar, and vaginal cancers; CIN; VIN; or VaIN. GARDASIL has not been demonstrated to protect against diseases due to HPV types not contained in the vaccine. *[See Clinical Studies (14.5).]* Not all vulvar and vaginal cancers are caused by HPV, and GARDASIL protects only against those vulvar and vaginal cancers caused by HPV 16 and 18. GARDASIL does not protect against genital diseases not caused by HPV. Vaccination with GARDASIL may not result in protection in all vaccine recipients.

2   DOSAGE AND ADMINISTRATION

2.1   Dosage

GARDASIL should be administered intramuscularly as a 0.5-mL dose at the following schedule: 0, 2 months, 6 months. *[See Clinical Studies (14.7).]*

2.2   Method of Administration

For intramuscular use only.
Shake well before use. Thorough agitation immediately before administration is necessary to maintain suspension of the vaccine. GARDASIL should not be diluted or mixed with other vaccines. After thorough agitation, GARDASIL is a white, cloudy liquid. Parenteral drug products should be inspected visually for particulate matter and discoloration prior to administration. Do not use the product if particulates are present or if it appears discolored.
GARDASIL should be administered intramuscularly in the deltoid region of the upper arm or in the higher anterolateral area of the thigh.
Syncope has been reported following vaccination with GARDASIL and may result in falling with injury; observation for 15 minutes after administration is recommended. *[See Warnings and Precautions (5.1).]*
Single-Dose Vial Use
Withdraw the 0.5-mL dose of vaccine from the single-dose vial using a sterile needle and syringe and use promptly.
Prefilled Syringe Use With and Without Needle Guard (Safety) Device
Prefilled Syringe With Needle Guard (Safety) Device
Instructions for using the prefilled single-dose syringes preassembled with needle guard (safety) device

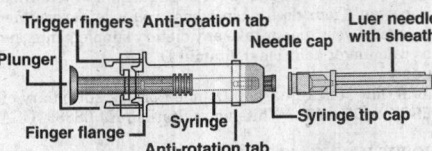

NOTE: Please use the enclosed needle for administration. If a different needle is chosen, it must fit securely on the syringe and be no longer than 1 inch to ensure proper functioning of the needle guard device. Two detachable labels are provided which can be removed after the needle is guarded.
At any of the following steps, avoid contact with the Trigger Fingers to keep from activating the safety device prematurely.
Remove Syringe Tip Cap and Needle Cap. Attach Luer Needle by pressing both Anti-Rotation Tabs to secure syringe and by twisting the Luer Needle in a clockwise direction until secured to the syringe. **Remove Needle Sheath. Administer injection** per standard protocol as stated above under DOSAGE AND ADMINISTRATION. Depress the Plunger while grasping the Finger Flange **until the entire dose has been given.** The Needle Guard Device will **NOT** activate to cover and protect the needle unless the **ENTIRE** dose has been given. While the Plunger is still depressed, remove needle from the vaccine recipient. Slowly release the Plunger and allow syringe to move up until the entire needle is guarded. For documentation of vaccination, remove detachable labels by pulling slowly on them. **Dispose in approved sharps container.**
Prefilled Syringe Without Needle Guard (Safety) Device
This package does not contain a needle guard (safety device) or a needle. Shake well before use. Attach the needle by twisting in a clockwise direction until the needle fits securely on the syringe. Administer the entire dose as per standard protocol.

3   DOSAGE FORMS AND STRENGTHS

GARDASIL is a suspension for intramuscular administration available in 0.5-mL single dose vials and prefilled syringes. See *Description (11)* for the complete listing of ingredients.

4   CONTRAINDICATIONS

Hypersensitivity, including severe allergic reactions to yeast (a vaccine component), or after a previous dose of GARDASIL. *[See Description (11).]*

5   WARNINGS AND PRECAUTIONS

5.1   Syncope

Because vaccinees may develop syncope, sometimes resulting in falling with injury, observation for 15 minutes after administration is recommended. Syncope, sometimes associated with tonic-clonic movements and other seizure-like activity, has been reported following vaccination with GARDASIL. When syncope is associated with tonic-clonic movements, the activity is usually transient and typically responds to restoring cerebral perfusion by maintaining a supine or Trendelenburg position.

5.2   Managing Allergic Reactions

Appropriate medical treatment and supervision must be readily available in case of anaphylactic reactions following the administration of GARDASIL.

6   ADVERSE REACTIONS

Overall Summary of Adverse Reactions
Headache, fever, nausea, and dizziness; and local injection site reactions (pain, swelling, erythema, pruritus, and bruising) occurred after administration with GARDASIL. Syncope, sometimes associated with tonic-clonic movements and other seizure-like activity, has been reported following vaccination with GARDASIL and may result in falling with injury; observation for 15 minutes after administration is recommended. *[See Warnings and Precautions (5.1).]*
Anaphylaxis has been reported following vaccination with GARDASIL.

6.1   Clinical Trials Experience

Because clinical trials are conducted under widely varying conditions, adverse reaction rates observed in the clinical trials of a vaccine cannot be directly compared to rates in the clinical trials of another vaccine and may not reflect the rates observed in practice.
Studies in Girls, Women, Boys, and Men 9 Through 26 Years of Age
In 6 clinical trials (4 Amorphous Aluminum Hydroxyphosphate Sulfate [AAHS]-controlled, 1 saline placebo-controlled, and 1 uncontrolled), 14,273 individuals were administered GARDASIL or AAHS control or saline placebo on the day of enrollment, and approximately 2 and 6 months thereafter, and safety was evaluated using vaccination report cards (VRC)-aided surveillance for 14 days after each injection of GARDASIL or AAHS control or saline placebo in these individuals. The individuals who were monitored using VRC-aided surveillance included 8180 individuals 9 through 26 years of age at enrollment who received GARDASIL and 6093 individuals who received AAHS control or saline placebo. Few individuals (0.2%) discontinued due to adverse reactions. The race distribution of the girls and women in the safety population was as follows: 62.3% White; 17.6% Hispanic (Black and White); 6.8% Asian; 6.7% Other; 6.4% Black; and 0.3% American Indian. The race distribution of the boys and men in the safety population was

Table 2: Injection-Site Adverse Reactions in Boys and Men 9 Through 26 Years of Age*

Adverse Reaction (1 to 5 Days Postvaccination)	GARDASIL (N = 3092) %	AAHS Control[†] (N = 2029) %	Saline Placebo (N = 274) %
Injection Site			
Pain	61.5	50.8	41.6
Erythema	16.7	14.1	14.5
Swelling	13.9	9.6	8.2

* The injection-site adverse reactions that were observed among recipients of GARDASIL were at a frequency of at least 1.0% and also at a greater frequency than that observed among AAHS control or saline placebo recipients.
† AAHS Control = Amorphous Aluminum Hydroxyphosphate Sulfate

Table 3: Postdose Evaluation of Injection-Site Adverse Reactions in Girls and Women 9 Through 26 Years of Age (1 to 5 Days Postvaccination)

Adverse Reaction	GARDASIL (% occurrence)			AAHS Control* (% occurrence)			Saline Placebo (% occurrence)		
	Post-dose 1 N[†] = 5011	Post-dose 2 N = 4924	Post-dose 3 N = 4818	Post-dose 1 N = 3410	Post-dose 2 N = 3351	Post-dose 3 N = 3295	Post-dose 1 N = 315	Post-dose 2 N = 301	Post-dose 3 N = 300
Pain	63.4	60.7	62.7	57.0	47.8	49.6	33.7	20.3	27.3
Mild/Moderate	62.5	59.7	61.2	56.6	47.3	48.9	33.3	20.3	27.0
Severe	0.9	1.0	1.5	0.4	0.5	0.6	0.3	0.0	0.3
Swelling[‡]	10.2	12.8	15.1	8.2	7.5	7.6	4.4	3.0	3.3
Mild/Moderate	9.6	11.9	14.2	8.1	7.2	7.3	4.4	3.0	3.3
Severe	0.6	0.8	0.9	0.2	0.2	0.2	0.0	0.0	0.0
Erythema[‡]	9.2	12.1	14.7	9.8	8.4	8.9	7.3	5.3	5.7
Mild/Moderate	9.0	11.7	14.3	9.5	8.4	8.8	7.3	5.3	5.7
Severe	0.2	0.3	0.4	0.3	0.1	0.1	0.0	0.0	0.0

* AAHS Control = Amorphous Aluminum Hydroxyphosphate Sulfate
† N = Number of individuals with follow-up
‡ Intensity of swelling and erythema was measured by size (inches): Mild = 0 to ≤1; Moderate = >1 to ≤2; Severe = >2.

Table 4: Postdose Evaluation of Injection-Site Adverse Reactions in Boys and Men 9 Through 26 Years of Age (1 to 5 Days Postvaccination)

Adverse Reaction	GARDASIL (% occurrence)			AAHS Control* (% occurrence)			Saline Placebo (% occurrence)		
	Post-dose 1 N[†] = 3002	Post-dose 2 N = 2897	Post-dose 3 N = 2825	Post-dose 1 N = 1950	Post-dose 2 N = 1853	Post-dose 3 N = 1799	Post-dose 1 N = 269	Post-dose 2 N = 263	Post-dose 3 N = 259
Pain	44.7	36.9	34.4	38.4	28.2	25.8	27.5	20.5	16.2
Mild/Moderate	44.5	36.5	34.1	37.9	28.2	25.5	27.5	20.2	16.2
Severe	0.2	0.5	0.3	0.4	0.1	0.3	0.0	0.4	0.0
Swelling[‡]	5.6	6.6	7.7	5.6	4.5	4.1	4.8	1.5	3.5
Mild/Moderate	5.3	6.2	7.1	5.4	4.5	4.0	4.8	1.5	3.1
Severe	0.2	0.3	0.5	0.2	0.0	0.1	0.0	0.0	0.4
Erythema[‡]	7.2	8.0	8.7	8.3	6.3	5.7	7.1	5.7	5.0
Mild/Moderate	6.8	7.7	8.3	8.0	6.2	5.6	7.1	5.7	5.0
Severe	0.3	0.2	0.3	0.2	0.1	0.1	0.0	0.0	0.0

* AAHS Control = Amorphous Aluminum Hydroxyphosphate Sulfate
† N = Number of individuals with follow-up
‡ Intensity of swelling and erythema was measured by size (inches): Mild = 0 to ≤1; Moderate = >1 to ≤2; Severe = >2.

as follows: 42.0% White; 19.7% Hispanic (Black and White); 11.0% Asian; 11.2% Other; 15.9% Black; and 0.1% American Indian.

Common Injection-Site Adverse Reactions in Girls and Women 9 Through 26 Years of Age
The injection site adverse reactions that were observed among recipients of GARDASIL at a frequency of at least 1.0% and also at a greater frequency than that observed among AAHS control or saline placebo recipients are shown in Table 1.
[See table 1 at top of previous page]
Common Injection-Site Adverse Reactions in Boys and Men 9 Through 26 Years of Age
The injection site adverse reactions that were observed among recipients of GARDASIL at a frequency of at least 1.0% and also at a greater frequency than that observed among AAHS control or saline placebo recipients are shown in Table 2.
[See table 2 above]
Evaluation of Injection-Site Adverse Reactions by Dose in Girls and Women 9 Through 26 Years of Age
An analysis of injection-site adverse reactions in girls and women by dose is shown in Table 3. Of those girls and women who reported an injection-site reaction, 94.3% judged their injection-site adverse reaction to be mild or moderate in intensity.
[See table 3 above]
Evaluation of Injection-Site Adverse Reactions by Dose in Boys and Men 9 Through 26 Years of Age
An analysis of injection-site adverse reactions in boys and men by dose is shown in Table 4. Of those boys and men who reported an injection-site reaction, 96.4% judged their injection-site adverse reaction to be mild or moderate in intensity.
[See table 4 above]
Common Systemic Adverse Reactions in Girls and Women 9 Through 26 Years of Age
Headache was the most commonly reported systemic adverse reaction in both treatment groups (GARDASIL = 28.2% and AAHS control or saline placebo = 28.4%). Fever was the next most commonly reported systemic adverse reaction in both treatment groups (GARDASIL = 13.0% and AAHS control or saline placebo = 11.2%).
Adverse reactions that were observed among recipients of GARDASIL, at a frequency of greater than or equal to 1.0% where the incidence in the GARDASIL group was greater than or equal to the incidence in the AAHS control or saline placebo group, are shown in Table 5.

Table 5: Common Systemic Adverse Reactions in Girls and Women 9 Through 26 Years of Age (GARDASIL ≥Control)*

Adverse Reactions (1 to 15 Days Postvaccination)	GARDASIL (N = 5088) %	AAHS Control[†] or Saline Placebo (N = 3790) %
Pyrexia	13.0	11.2
Nausea	6.7	6.5
Dizziness	4.0	3.7
Diarrhea	3.6	3.5
Vomiting	2.4	1.9
Cough	2.0	1.5
Toothache	1.5	1.4
Upper respiratory tract infection	1.5	1.5
Malaise	1.4	1.2
Arthralgia	1.2	0.9
Insomnia	1.2	0.9
Nasal congestion	1.1	0.9

* The adverse reactions in this table are those that were observed among recipients of GARDASIL at a frequency of at least 1.0% and greater than or equal to those observed among AAHS control or saline placebo recipients.
† AAHS Control = Amorphous Aluminum Hydroxyphosphate Sulfate

Common Systemic Adverse Reactions in Boys and Men 9 Through 26 Years of Age
Headache was the most commonly reported systemic adverse reaction in both treatment groups (GARDASIL = 12.3% and AAHS control or saline placebo = 11.2%). Fever was the next most commonly reported systemic adverse reaction in both treatment groups (GARDASIL = 8.2% and AAHS control or saline placebo = 6.5%).
Adverse reactions that were observed among recipients of GARDASIL, at a frequency of greater than or equal to 1.0% where the incidence in the group that received GARDASIL was greater than or equal to the incidence in the AAHS control or saline placebo group, are shown in Table 6.

Table 6: Common Systemic Adverse Reactions in Boys and Men 9 Through 26 Years of Age (GARDASIL ≥Control)*

Adverse Reactions (1 to 15 Days Postvaccination)	GARDASIL (N = 3092) %	AAHS Control[†] or Saline Placebo (N = 2303) %
Headache	12.3	11.2
Pyrexia	8.2	6.5
Pharyngolaryngeal pain	2.8	2.1
Diarrhea	2.7	2.2
Nasopharyngitis	2.6	2.6
Nausea	2.0	1.0
Upper respiratory tract infection	1.5	1.0
Abdominal pain upper	1.4	1.4
Myalgia	1.3	0.7
Dizziness	1.2	0.9
Vomiting	1.0	0.8

* The adverse reactions in this table are those that were observed among recipients of GARDASIL at a frequency of at least 1.0% and greater than or equal to those observed among AAHS control or saline placebo recipients.
† AAHS Control = Amorphous Aluminum Hydroxyphosphate Sulfate

Evaluation of Fever by Dose in Girls and Women 9 Through 26 Years of Age
An analysis of fever in girls and women by dose is shown in Table 7.
[See table 7 at top of next page]
Evaluation of Fever by Dose in Boys and Men 9 Through 26 Years of Age
An analysis of fever in boys and men by dose is shown in Table 8.
[See table 8 on next page]
Serious Adverse Reactions in the Entire Study Population
Across the clinical studies, 255 individuals (GARDASIL N = 126 or 0.8%; placebo N = 129 or 1.0%) out of 29,323 (GARDASIL N = 15,706; AAHS control N = 13,023; or saline placebo N = 594) individuals (9- through 45-year-old girls and women; and 9- through 26-year-old boys and men) reported a serious systemic adverse reaction.

Table 7: Postdose Evaluation of Fever in Girls and Women 9 Through 26 Years of Age (1 to 5 Days Postvaccination)

Temperature (°F)	GARDASIL (% occurrence)			AAHS Control* or Saline Placebo (% occurrence)		
	Postdose 1 N[†] = 4945	Postdose 2 N = 4804	Postdose 3 N = 4671	Postdose 1 N = 3681	Postdose 2 N = 3564	Postdose 3 N = 3467
≥100 to <102	3.7	4.1	4.4	3.1	3.8	3.6
≥102	0.3	0.5	0.5	0.2	0.4	0.5

* AAHS Control = Amorphous Aluminum Hydroxyphosphate Sulfate
† N = Number of subjects with follow-up

Table 8: Postdose Evaluation of Fever in Boys and Men 9 Through 26 Years of Age (1 to 5 Days Postvaccination)

Temperature (°F)	GARDASIL (% occurrence)			AAHS Control* or Saline Placebo (% occurrence)		
	Postdose 1 N[†] = 2971	Postdose 2 N = 2847	Postdose 3 N = 2791	Postdose 1 N = 2194	Postdose 2 N = 2079	Postdose 3 N = 2046
≥100 to <102	2.4	2.5	2.3	2.1	2.1	1.6
≥102	0.6	0.5	0.5	0.6	0.3	0.3

* AAHS Control = Amorphous Aluminum Hydroxyphosphate Sulfate
† N = Number of individuals with follow-up

Table 9: Summary of Girls and Women 9 Through 26 Years of Age Who Reported an Incident Condition Potentially Indicative of a Systemic Autoimmune Disorder After Enrollment in Clinical Trials of GARDASIL, Regardless of Causality

Conditions	GARDASIL (N = 10,706) n (%)	AAHS Control* or Saline Placebo (N = 9412) n (%)
Arthralgia/Arthritis/Arthropathy[†]	120 (1.1)	98 (1.0)
Autoimmune Thyroiditis	4 (0.0)	1 (0.0)
Celiac Disease	10 (0.1)	6 (0.1)
Diabetes Mellitus Insulin-dependent	2 (0.0)	2 (0.0)
Erythema Nodosum	2 (0.0)	4 (0.0)
Hyperthyroidism[‡]	27 (0.3)	21 (0.2)
Hypothyroidism[§]	35 (0.3)	38 (0.4)
Inflammatory Bowel Disease[¶]	7 (0.1)	10 (0.1)
Multiple Sclerosis	2 (0.0)	4 (0.0)
Nephritis[#]	2 (0.0)	5 (0.1)
Optic Neuritis	2 (0.0)	0 (0.0)
Pigmentation Disorder[Þ]	4 (0.0)	3 (0.0)
Psoriasis[ß]	13 (0.1)	15 (0.2)
Raynaud's Phenomenon	3 (0.0)	4 (0.0)
Rheumatoid Arthritis[à]	6 (0.1)	2 (0.0)
Scleroderma/Morphea	2 (0.0)	1 (0.0)
Stevens-Johnson Syndrome	1 (0.0)	0 (0.0)
Systemic Lupus Erythematosus	1 (0.0)	3 (0.0)
Uveitis	3 (0.0)	1 (0.0)
All Conditions	245 (2.3)	218 (2.3)

N = Number of individuals enrolled
n = Number of individuals with specific new Medical Conditions
NOTE: Although an individual may have had two or more new Medical Conditions, the individual is counted only once within a category. The same individual may appear in different categories.
* AAHS Control = Amorphous Aluminum Hydroxyphosphate Sulfate
† Arthralgia/Arthritis/Arthropathy includes the following terms: Arthralgia, Arthritis, Arthritis reactive, and Arthropathy
‡ Hyperthyroidism includes the following terms: Basedow's disease, Goiter, Toxic nodular goiter, and Hyperthyroidism
§ Hypothyroidism includes the following terms: Hypothyroidism and thyroiditis
¶ Inflammatory bowel disease includes the following terms: Colitis ulcerative, Crohn's disease, and Inflammatory bowel disease
# Nephritis includes the following terms: Nephritis, Glomerulonephritis minimal lesion, Glomerulonephritis proliferative
Þ Pigmentation disorder includes the following terms: Pigmentation disorder, Skin depigmentation, and Vitiligo
ß Psoriasis includes the following terms: Psoriasis, Pustular psoriasis, and Psoriatic arthropathy
à Rheumatoid arthritis includes juvenile rheumatoid arthritis. One woman counted in the rheumatoid arthritis group reported rheumatoid arthritis as an adverse experience at Day 130.

Of the entire study population (29,323 individuals), 0.04% of the reported serious systemic adverse reactions were judged to be vaccine related by the study investigator. The most frequently (frequency of 4 cases or greater with either GARDASIL, AAHS control, saline placebo, or the total of all three) reported serious systemic adverse reactions, regardless of causality, were:
Headache [0.02% GARDASIL (3 cases) vs. 0.02% AAHS control (2 cases)],
Gastroenteritis [0.02% GARDASIL (3 cases) vs. 0.02% AAHS control (2 cases)],
Appendicitis [0.03% GARDASIL (5 cases) vs. 0.01% AAHS control (1 case)],
Pelvic inflammatory disease [0.02% GARDASIL (3 cases) vs. 0.03% AAHS control (4 cases)],
Urinary tract infection [0.01% GARDASIL (2 cases) vs. 0.02% AAHS control (2 cases)],
Pneumonia [0.01% GARDASIL (2 cases) vs. 0.02% AAHS control (2 cases)],
Pyelonephritis [0.01% GARDASIL (2 cases) vs. 0.02% AAHS control (3 cases)],
Pulmonary embolism [0.01% GARDASIL (2 cases) vs. 0.02% AAHS control (2 cases)].
One case (0.006% GARDASIL; 0.0% AAHS control or saline placebo) of bronchospasm; and 2 cases (0.01% GARDASIL;

0.0% AAHS control or saline placebo) of asthma were reported as serious systemic adverse reactions that occurred following any vaccination visit.
In addition, there was 1 individual in the clinical trials, in the group that received GARDASIL, who reported two injection-site serious adverse reactions (injection-site pain and injection-site joint movement impairment).

Deaths in the Entire Study Population
Across the clinical studies, 37 deaths (GARDASIL N = 18 or 0.1%; placebo N = 19 or 0.1%) were reported in 29,323 (GARDASIL N = 15,706; AAHS control N = 13,023, saline placebo N = 594) individuals (9- through 45-year-old girls and women; and 9- through 26-year-old boys and men). The events reported were consistent with events expected in healthy adolescent and adult populations. The most common cause of death was motor vehicle accident (5 individuals who received GARDASIL and 4 individuals who received AAHS control), followed by drug overdose/suicide (2 individuals who received GARDASIL and 6 individuals who received AAHS control), gun shot wound (1 individual who received GARDASIL and 3 individuals who received AAHS control), and pulmonary embolus/deep vein thrombosis (1 individual who received GARDASIL and 1 individual who received AAHS control). In addition, there were 2 cases of sepsis, 1 case of pancreatic cancer, 1 case of arrhythmia, 1 case of pulmonary tuberculosis, 1 case of hyperthyroidism, 1 case of post-operative pulmonary embolism and acute renal failure, 1 case of traumatic brain injury/cardiac arrest, and 1 case of systemic lupus erythematosus in the group that received GARDASIL; 1 case of asphyxia, 1 case of acute lymphocytic leukemia, 1 case of chemical poisoning, and 1 case of myocardial ischemia in the AAHS control group; and 1 case of medulloblastoma in the saline placebo group.

Systemic Autoimmune Disorders in Girls and Women 9 Through 26 Years of Age
In the clinical studies, 9- through 26-year-old girls and women were evaluated for new medical conditions that occurred over the course of follow-up. New medical conditions potentially indicative of a systemic autoimmune disorder seen in the group that received GARDASIL or AAHS control or saline placebo are shown in Table 9. This population includes all girls and women who received at least one dose of GARDASIL or AAHS control or saline placebo, and had safety data available.
[See table 9 at left]

Systemic Autoimmune Disorders in Boys and Men 9 Through 26 Years of Age
In the clinical studies, 9- through 26-year-old boys and men were evaluated for new medical conditions that occurred over the course of follow-up. New medical conditions potentially indicative of a systemic autoimmune disorder seen in the group that received GARDASIL or AAHS control or saline placebo are shown in Table 10. This population includes all boys and men who received at least one dose of GARDASIL or AAHS control or saline placebo, and had safety data available.
[See table 10 at top of next page]

Safety in Concomitant Use with RECOMBIVAX HB [hepatitis B vaccine (recombinant)] in Girls and Women 16 Through 23 Years of Age
The safety of GARDASIL when administered concomitantly with RECOMBIVAX HB®[1] [hepatitis B vaccine (recombinant)] was evaluated in an AAHS-controlled study of 1871 girls and women with a mean age of 20.4 years *[see Clinical Studies (14.8)]*. The race distribution of the study individuals was as follows: 61.6% White; 23.8% Other; 11.9% Black; 1.6% Hispanic (Black and White); 0.8% Asian; and 0.3% American Indian. The rates of systemic and injection-site adverse reactions were similar among girls and women who received concomitant vaccination as compared with those who received GARDASIL or RECOMBIVAX HB [hepatitis B vaccine (recombinant)].

Safety in Concomitant Use with Menactra [Meningococcal (Groups A, C, Y and W-135) Polysaccharide Diphtheria Toxoid Conjugate Vaccine] and Adacel [Tetanus Toxoid, Reduced Diphtheria Toxoid and Acellular Pertussis Vaccine Adsorbed (Tdap)]
The safety of GARDASIL when administered concomitantly with Menactra [Meningococcal (Groups A, C, Y and W-135) Polysaccharide Diphtheria Toxoid Conjugate Vaccine] and Adacel [Tetanus Toxoid, Reduced Diphtheria Toxoid and Acellular Pertussis Vaccine Adsorbed (Tdap)] was evaluated in a randomized study of 1040 boys and girls with a mean age of 12.6 years *[see Clinical Studies (14.9)]*. The race distribution of the study subjects was as follows: 77.7% White; 1.4% Multi-racial; 12.3% Black; 6.8% Hispanic (Black and White); 1.2% Asian; 0.4% American Indian, and 0.2% Indian.
There was an increase in injection-site swelling reported at the injection site for GARDASIL (concomitant = 10.9%, non-concomitant = 6.9%) when GARDASIL was administered concomitantly with Menactra and Adacel as compared to non-concomitant (separated by 1 month) vaccination. The majority of injection-site swelling adverse experiences were reported as being mild to moderate in intensity.

6.2 Postmarketing Experience

The following adverse events have been spontaneously reported during post-approval use of GARDASIL. Because these events were reported voluntarily from a population of uncertain size, it is not possible to reliably estimate their frequency or to establish a causal relationship to vaccine exposure.

Blood and lymphatic system disorders: Autoimmune hemolytic anemia, idiopathic thrombocytopenic purpura, lymphadenopathy.

Respiratory, thoracic and mediastinal disorders: Pulmonary embolus.

Gastrointestinal disorders: Nausea, pancreatitis, vomiting.

General disorders and administration site conditions: Asthenia, chills, death, fatigue, malaise.

Immune system disorders: Autoimmune diseases, hypersensitivity reactions including anaphylactic/anaphylactoid reactions, bronchospasm, and urticaria.

Musculoskeletal and connective tissue disorders: Arthralgia, myalgia.

Nervous system disorders: Acute disseminated encephalomyelitis, dizziness, Guillain-Barré syndrome, headache, motor neuron disease, paralysis, seizures, syncope (including syncope associated with tonic-clonic movements and other seizure-like activity) sometimes resulting in falling with injury, transverse myelitis.

Vascular disorders: Deep venous thrombosis.

7 DRUG INTERACTIONS

7.1 Use with RECOMBIVAX HB

Results from clinical studies indicate that GARDASIL may be administered concomitantly (at a separate injection site) with RECOMBIVAX HB [hepatitis B vaccine (recombinant)] *[see Clinical Studies (14.8)].*

7.2 Use with Menactra and Adacel

Results from clinical studies indicate that GARDASIL may be administered concomitantly (at a separate injection site) with Menactra [Meningococcal (Groups A, C, Y and W-135) Polysaccharide Diphtheria Toxoid Conjugate Vaccine] and Adacel [Tetanus Toxoid, Reduced Diphtheria Toxoid and Acellular Pertussis Vaccine Adsorbed (Tdap)] *[see Clinical Studies (14.9)].*

7.3 Use with Hormonal Contraceptives

In clinical studies, 13,293 women (GARDASIL N = 6644; AAHS control or saline placebo N = 6649) who had post-Month 7 follow-up used hormonal contraceptives for a total of 17,597 person-years (65.1% of the total follow-up time in the studies). Use of hormonal contraceptives or lack of use of hormonal contraceptives among study participants did not alter immune response in the per protocol efficacy (PPE) population.

7.4 Use with Systemic Immunosuppressive Medications

Immunosuppressive therapies, including irradiation, antimetabolites, alkylating agents, cytotoxic drugs, and corticosteroids (used in greater than physiologic doses), may reduce the immune responses to vaccines *[see Use in Specific Populations (8.6)].*

8 USE IN SPECIFIC POPULATIONS

8.1 Pregnancy

Pregnancy Category B:

Reproduction studies have been performed in female rats at doses equivalent to the recommended human dose and have revealed no evidence of impaired female fertility or harm to the fetus due to GARDASIL. There are, however, no adequate and well-controlled studies in pregnant women. Because animal reproduction studies are not always predictive of human responses, GARDASIL should be used during pregnancy only if clearly needed.

An evaluation of the effect of GARDASIL on embryo-fetal, pre- and postweaning development was conducted using rats. One group of rats was administered GARDASIL twice prior to gestation, during the period of organogenesis (gestation Day 6) and on lactation Day 7. A second group of pregnant rats was administered GARDASIL during the period of organogenesis (gestation Day 6) and on lactation Day 7 only. GARDASIL was administered at 0.5 mL/rat/occasion (120 mcg total protein which is equivalent to the recommended human dose) by intramuscular injection. No adverse effects on mating, fertility, pregnancy, parturition, lactation, embryo-fetal or pre- and postweaning development were observed. There were no vaccine-related fetal malformations or other evidence of teratogenesis noted in this study. In addition, there were no treatment-related effects on developmental signs, behavior, reproductive performance, or fertility of the offspring.

Clinical Studies in Humans

In clinical studies, women underwent urine pregnancy testing prior to administration of each dose of GARDASIL. Women who were found to be pregnant before completion of a 3-dose regimen of GARDASIL were instructed to defer completion of their vaccination regimen until resolution of the pregnancy.

GARDASIL is not indicated for women 27 years of age or older. However, safety data in women 16 through 45 years of age was collected, and 3620 women (GARDASIL N = 1796 vs. AAHS control or saline placebo N = 1824) reported at least 1 pregnancy each.

The overall proportions of pregnancies that resulted in an adverse outcome, defined as the combined numbers of spontaneous abortion, late fetal death, and congenital anomaly cases out of the total number of pregnancy outcomes for which an outcome was known (and excluding elective terminations), were 23.3% (423/1812) in women who received GARDASIL and 24.1% (438/1820) in women who received AAHS control or saline placebo.

Overall, 54 and 63 women in the group that received GARDASIL or AAHS control or saline placebo, respectively (3.0% and 3.5% of all women who reported a pregnancy in the respective vaccination groups), experienced a serious adverse reaction during pregnancy. The most common events reported were conditions that can result in Caesarean section (e.g., failure of labor, malpresentation, cephalopelvic disproportion), premature onset of labor (e.g., threatened abortions, premature rupture of membranes), and

Table 10: Summary of Boys and Men 9 Through 26 Years of Age Who Reported an Incident Condition Potentially Indicative of a Systemic Autoimmune Disorder After Enrollment in Clinical Trials of GARDASIL, Regardless of Causality

Conditions	GARDASIL (N = 3092)	AAHS Control* or Saline Placebo (N = 2303)
	n (%)	n (%)
Alopecia Areata	1 (0.0)	0 (0.0)
Ankylosing Spondylitis	1 (0.0)	2 (0.1)
Arthralgia/Arthritis/Reactive Arthritis	30 (1.0)	17 (0.7)
Autoimmune Thrombocytopenia	1 (0.0)	0 (0.0)
Diabetes Mellitus Type 1	3 (0.1)	2 (0.1)
Hyperthyroidism	0 (0.0)	1 (0.0)
Hypothyroidism†	3 (0.1)	0 (0.0)
Inflammatory Bowel Disease‡	0 (0.0)	2 (0.1)
Myocarditis	1 (0.0)	1 (0.0)
Proteinuria	1 (0.0)	0 (0.0)
Psoriasis	0 (0.0)	2 (0.1)
Vitiligo	2 (0.1)	5 (0.2)
All Conditions	**43 (1.4)**	**32 (1.4)**

N = Number of individuals who received at least one dose of either vaccine or placebo
n = Number of individuals with specific new Medical Conditions
NOTE: Although an individual may have had two or more new Medical Conditions, the individual is counted only once within a category. The same individual may appear in different categories.
* AAHS Control = Amorphous Aluminum Hydroxyphosphate Sulfate
† Hypothyroidism includes the following terms: Hypothyroidism and Autoimmune thyroiditis
‡ Inflammatory bowel disease includes the following terms: Colitis ulcerative and Crohn's disease

Table 11: Analysis of Efficacy of GARDASIL in the PPE* Population† of 16- Through 26-Year-Old Girls and Women for Vaccine HPV Types

Population	GARDASIL		AAHS Control		% Efficacy (95% CI)
	N	Number of cases	N	Number of cases	
HPV 16- or 18-related CIN 2/3 or AIS					
Study 1‡	755	0	750	12	100.0 (65.1, 100.0)
Study 2	231	0	230	1	100.0 (-3744.9, 100.0)
Study 3	2201	0	2222	36	100.0 (89.2, 100.0)
Study 4	5306	2	5262	63	96.9 (88.2, 99.6)
Combined Protocols§	8493	2	8464	112	98.2 (93.5, 99.8)
HPV 16-related CIN 2/3 or AIS					
Combined Protocols§	7402	2	7205	93	97.9 (92.3, 99.8)
HPV 18-related CIN 2/3 or AIS					
Combined Protocols§	7382	0	7316	29	100.0 (86.6, 100.0)
HPV 16- or 18-related VIN 2/3					
Study 2	231	0	230	0	Not calculated
Study 3	2219	0	2239	6	100.0 (14.4, 100.0)
Study 4	5322	0	5275	4	100.0 (-50.3, 100.0)
Combined Protocols§	7772	0	7744	10	100.0 (55.5, 100.0)
HPV 16- or 18-related VaIN 2/3					
Study 2	231	0	230	0	Not calculated
Study 3	2219	0	2239	5	100.0 (-10.1, 100.0)
Study 4	5322	0	5275	4	100.0 (-50.3, 100.0)
Combined Protocols§	7772	0	7744	9	100.0 (49.5, 100.0)

(Table continued on next page)

Table 11 (cont.): Analysis of Efficacy of GARDASIL in the PPE* Population† of 16- Through 26-Year-Old Girls and Women for Vaccine HPV Types

Population	GARDASIL		AAHS Control		% Efficacy (95% CI)
	N	Number of cases	N	Number of cases	
HPV 6-, 11-, 16-, or 18-related CIN (CIN 1, CIN 2/3) or AIS					
Study 2	235	0	233	3	100.0 (-138.4, 100.0)
Study 3	2241	0	2258	77	100.0 (95.1, 100.0)
Study 4	5388	9	5374	145	93.8 (88.0, 97.2)
Combined Protocols§	7864	9	7865	225	96.0 (92.3, 98.2)
HPV 6-, 11-, 16-, or 18-related Genital Warts					
Study 2	235	0	233	3	100.0 (-139.5, 100.0)
Study 3	2261	0	2279	58	100.0 (93.5, 100.0)
Study 4	5404	2	5390	132	98.5 (94.5, 99.8)
Combined Protocols§	7900	2	7902	193	99.0 (96.2, 99.9)
HPV 6- and 11-related Genital Warts					
Combined Protocols§	6932	2	6856	189	99.0 (96.2, 99.9)

N = Number of individuals with at least 1 follow-up visit after Month 7
CI = Confidence Interval
Note 1: Point estimates and confidence intervals are adjusted for person-time of follow-up.
Note 2: The first analysis in the table (i.e., HPV 16- or 18-related CIN 2/3, AIS or worse) was the primary endpoint of the vaccine development plan.
Note 3: Table 11 does not include cases due to non-vaccine HPV types.
AAHS Control = Amorphous Aluminum Hydroxyphosphate Sulfate
* The PPE population consisted of individuals who received all 3 vaccinations within 1 year of enrollment, did not have major deviations from the study protocol, and were naïve (PCR negative and seronegative) to the relevant HPV type(s) (Types 6, 11, 16, and 18) prior to dose 1 and through 1 month postdose 3 (Month 7).
† See Table 13 for analysis of vaccine impact in the general population.
‡ Evaluated only the HPV 16 L1 VLP vaccine component of GARDASIL.
§ Analyses of the combined trials were prospectively planned and included the use of similar study entry criteria.

Table 12: Analysis of Efficacy of GARDASIL in the PPE Population of 16- Through 26-Year-Old Boys and Men for Vaccine HPV Types

Endpoint	GARDASIL		AAHS Control		% Efficacy (95% CI)
	N*	Number of cases	N	Number of cases	
External Genital Lesions HPV 6-, 11-, 16-, or 18-related					
External Genital Lesions	1397	3	1408	31	90.4 (69.2, 98.1)
Condyloma	1397	3	1408	28	89.4 (65.5, 97.9)
PIN 1/2/3	1397	0	1408	3	100 (-141.2, 100.0)

CI = Confidence Interval
AAHS Control = Amorphous Aluminum Hydroxyphosphate Sulfate
*N = Number of individuals with at least 1 follow-up visit after Month 7

pregnancy-related medical problems (e.g., pre-eclampsia, hyperemesis). The proportions of pregnant women who experienced such events were comparable between the groups receiving GARDASIL and AAHS control or saline placebo. There were 40 cases of congenital anomaly in pregnancies that occurred in women who received GARDASIL and 30 cases of congenital anomaly in pregnancies that occurred in women who received AAHS control or saline placebo.

Further sub-analyses were conducted to evaluate pregnancies with estimated onset within 30 days or more than 30 days from administration of a dose of GARDASIL or AAHS control or saline placebo. For pregnancies with estimated onset within 30 days of vaccination, 5 cases of congenital anomaly were observed in the group that received GARDASIL compared to 1 case of congenital anomaly in the group that received AAHS control or saline placebo. The congenital anomalies seen in pregnancies with estimated onset within 30 days of vaccination included pyloric stenosis, congenital megacolon, congenital hydronephrosis, hip dysplasia, and club foot. Conversely, in pregnancies with onset more than 30 days following vaccination, 35 cases of congenital anomaly were observed in the group that received GARDASIL compared with 29 cases of congenital anomaly in the group that received AAHS control or saline placebo.
Pregnancy Registry for GARDASIL
Merck & Co., Inc. maintains a Pregnancy Registry to monitor fetal outcomes of pregnant women exposed to GARDASIL. Patients and health care providers are encouraged to report any exposure to GARDASIL during pregnancy by calling (800) 986-8999.
8.3   Nursing Mothers
Women 16 Through 26 Years of Age
It is not known whether GARDASIL is excreted in human milk. Because many drugs are excreted in human milk, caution should be exercised when GARDASIL is administered to a nursing woman.
A total of 995 nursing mothers (vaccine N = 500, AAHS control N = 495) were given GARDASIL or AAHS control during the vaccination period of the clinical trials.
Overall, 21 and 10 infants of women who received GARDASIL or AAHS control, respectively (representing 4.2% and 2.0% of the total number of women who were breast-feeding during the period in which they received GARDASIL or AAHS control, respectively), experienced a serious adverse reaction.
In a post-hoc analysis of clinical studies, a higher number of breast-feeding infants (n = 6) whose mothers received GARDASIL had acute respiratory illnesses within 30 days post-vaccination of the mother as compared to infants (n = 2) whose mothers received AAHS control. In these studies, the rates of other adverse reactions in the mother and the nursing infant were comparable between vaccination groups.

8.4   Pediatric Use
Safety and effectiveness have not been established in pediatric patients below 9 years of age.
8.5   Geriatric Use
The safety and effectiveness of GARDASIL have not been evaluated in a geriatric population, defined as individuals aged 65 years and over.
8.6   Immunocompromised Individuals
The immunologic response to GARDASIL may be diminished in immunocompromised individuals *[see Drug Interactions (7.4)]*.
10   OVERDOSAGE
There have been reports of administration of higher than recommended doses of GARDASIL.
In general, the adverse event profile reported with overdose was comparable to recommended single doses of GARDASIL.
11   DESCRIPTION
GARDASIL, Human Papillomavirus Quadrivalent (Types 6, 11, 16, and 18) Vaccine, Recombinant, is a non-infectious recombinant quadrivalent vaccine prepared from the purified virus-like particles (VLPs) of the major capsid (L1) protein of HPV Types 6, 11, 16, and 18. The L1 proteins are produced by separate fermentations in recombinant *Saccharomyces cerevisiae* and self-assembled into VLPs. The fermentation process involves growth of *S. cerevisiae* on chemically-defined fermentation media which include vitamins, amino acids, mineral salts, and carbohydrates. The VLPs are released from the yeast cells by cell disruption and purified by a series of chemical and physical methods. The purified VLPs are adsorbed on preformed aluminum-containing adjuvant (Amorphous Aluminum Hydroxyphosphate Sulfate). The quadrivalent HPV VLP vaccine is a sterile liquid suspension that is prepared by combining the adsorbed VLPs of each HPV type and additional amounts of the aluminum-containing adjuvant and the final purification buffer.
GARDASIL is a sterile suspension for intramuscular administration. Each 0.5-mL dose contains approximately 20 mcg of HPV 6 L1 protein, 40 mcg of HPV 11 L1 protein, 40 mcg of HPV 16 L1 protein, and 20 mcg of HPV 18 L1 protein.
Each 0.5-mL dose of the vaccine contains approximately 225 mcg of aluminum (as Amorphous Aluminum Hydroxyphosphate Sulfate adjuvant), 9.56 mg of sodium chloride, 0.78 mg of L-histidine, 50 mcg of polysorbate 80, 35 mcg of sodium borate, <7 mcg yeast protein/dose, and water for injection. The product does not contain a preservative or antibiotics.
After thorough agitation, GARDASIL is a white, cloudy liquid.
12   CLINICAL PHARMACOLOGY
12.1   Mechanism of Action
HPV only infects human beings. Animal studies with analogous animal papillomaviruses suggest that the efficacy of L1 VLP vaccines may involve the development of humoral immune responses. Human beings develop a humoral immune response to the vaccine, although the exact mechanism of protection is unknown.
13   NONCLINICAL TOXICOLOGY
13.1   Carcinogenesis, Mutagenesis, Impairment of Fertility
GARDASIL has not been evaluated for the potential to cause carcinogenicity or genotoxicity.
GARDASIL administered to female rats at a dose of 120 mcg total protein, which is equivalent to the recommended human dose, had no effects on mating performance, fertility, or embryonic/fetal survival.
The effect of GARDASIL on male fertility has been studied in male rats at an intramuscular dose of 0.5 mL/rat/occasion (120 mcg total protein which is equivalent to the recommended human dose). One group of male rats was administered GARDASIL once, 3 days prior to cohabitation, and a second group of male rats was administered GARDASIL three times, at 6 weeks, 3 weeks, and 3 days prior to cohabitation. There were no treatment-related effects on reproductive performance including fertility, sperm count, and sperm motility. There were no treatment-related gross or histomorphologic and weight changes on the testes.
14   CLINICAL STUDIES
CIN 2/3 and AIS are the immediate and necessary precursors of squamous cell carcinoma and adenocarcinoma of the cervix, respectively. Their detection and removal has been shown to prevent cancer; thus, they serve as surrogate markers for prevention of cervical cancer. In the clinical studies in girls and women aged 16 through 26 years, cases of CIN 2/3 and AIS were the efficacy endpoints to assess prevention of cervical cancer. In addition, cases of VIN 2/3 and VaIN 2/3 were the efficacy endpoints to assess prevention of HPV-related vulvar and vaginal cancers, and observations

of external genital lesions were the efficacy endpoints for the prevention of genital warts.

In clinical studies in boys and men aged 16 through 26 years, efficacy was evaluated using the following endpoints: external genital warts and penile/perineal/perianal intraepithelial neoplasia (PIN) grades 1/2/3 or penile/perineal/perianal cancer.

Efficacy was assessed in 5 AAHS-controlled, double-blind, randomized Phase II and III clinical studies. The first Phase II study evaluated the HPV 16 component of GARDASIL (Study 1, N = 2391 girls and women) and the second evaluated all components of GARDASIL (Study 2, N = 551 girls and women). Two Phase III studies evaluated GARDASIL in 5442 (Study 3) and 12,157 (Study 4) girls and women. A third Phase III study, Study 5, evaluated GARDASIL in 4055 boys and men. Together, these five studies evaluated 24,596 individuals (20,541 girls and women 16 through 26 years of age at enrollment with a mean age of 20.0 years and 4055 boys and men 16 through 26 years of age at enrollment with a mean age of 20.5 years). The race distribution of the girls and women in the clinical trials was as follows: 70.4% White; 12.2% Hispanic (Black and White); 8.8% Other; 4.6% Black; 3.8% Asian; and 0.2% American Indian. The race distribution of the boys and men in the clinical trials was as follows: 35.2% White; 20.5% Hispanic (Black and White); 14.4% Other; 19.8% Black; 10.0% Asian; and 0.1% American Indian.

The median duration of follow-up was 4.0, 3.0, 3.0, 3.0, and 2.3 years for Study 1, Study 2, Study 3, Study 4, and Study 5, respectively. Individuals received vaccine or AAHS control on the day of enrollment and 2 and 6 months thereafter. Efficacy was analyzed for each study individually and for all studies in girls and women combined according to a prospective clinical plan.

Overall, 73% of 16- through 26-year-old girls and women and 83% of 16- through 26-year-old boys and men were naïve (i.e., PCR [Polymerase Chain Reaction] negative and seronegative for all 4 vaccine HPV types) to all 4 vaccine HPV types at enrollment.

A total of 27% of 16- through 26-year-old girls and women and 17% of 16- through 26-year-old boys and men had evidence of prior exposure to or ongoing infection with at least 1 of the 4 vaccine HPV types. Among these individuals, 74% of 16- through 26-year-old girls and women and 78% of 16-through 26-year-old boys and men had evidence of prior exposure to or ongoing infection with only 1 of the 4 vaccine HPV types and were naïve (PCR negative and seronegative) to the remaining 3 types.

In individuals who were naïve (PCR negative and seronegative) to all 4 vaccine HPV types, CIN, genital warts, VIN, VaIN, PIN, and persistent infection caused by any of the 4 vaccine HPV types were counted as endpoints.

Among individuals who were positive (PCR positive and/or seropositive) for a vaccine HPV type at Day 1, endpoints related to that type were not included in the analyses of prophylactic efficacy. Endpoints related to the remaining types for which the individual was naïve (PCR negative and seronegative) were counted.

For example, in individuals who were HPV 18 positive (PCR positive and/or seropositive) at Day 1, lesions caused by HPV 18 were not counted in the prophylactic efficacy evaluations. Lesions caused by HPV 6, 11, and 16 were included in the prophylactic efficacy evaluations. The same approach was used for the other types.

14.1 Prophylactic Efficacy–HPV Types 6, 11, 16, and 18 in Girls and Women 16 Through 26 Years of Age

GARDASIL was administered without prescreening for presence of HPV infection and the efficacy trials allowed enrollment of girls and women regardless of baseline HPV status (i.e., PCR status or serostatus). Girls and women with current or prior HPV infection with an HPV type contained in the vaccine were not eligible for prophylactic efficacy evaluations for that type.

The primary analyses of efficacy with respect to HPV types 6, 11, 16, and 18 were conducted in the per-protocol efficacy (PPE) population, consisting of girls and women who received all 3 vaccinations within 1 year of enrollment, did not have major deviations from the study protocol, and were naïve (PCR negative in cervicovaginal specimens and seronegative) to the relevant HPV type(s) (Types 6, 11, 16, and 18) prior to dose 1 and through 1 month Postdose 3 (Month 7). Efficacy was measured starting after the Month 7 visit. GARDASIL was efficacious in reducing the incidence of CIN (any grade including CIN 2/3); AIS; genital warts; VIN (any grade); and VaIN (any grade) related to vaccine HPV types 6, 11, 16, or 18 in those who were PCR negative and seronegative at baseline (Table 11).

In addition, girls and women who were already infected with 1 or more vaccine-related HPV types prior to vaccination were protected from precancerous cervical lesions and external genital lesions caused by the other vaccine HPV types.

[See table on pages 2085 and 2086]

Prophylactic efficacy against overall cervical and genital disease related to HPV 6, 11, 16, and 18 in an extension phase of Study 2, that included data through Month 60, was noted to be 100% (95% CI: 12.3%, 100.0%) among girls and women in the per protocol population naïve to the relevant HPV types.

GARDASIL was efficacious against HPV disease caused by HPV types 6, 11, 16, and 18 in girls and women who were naïve for those specific HPV types at baseline.

14.2 Prophylactic Efficacy–HPV Types 6, 11, 16, and 18 in Boys and Men 16 Through 26 Years of Age

The primary analyses of efficacy were conducted in the per-protocol efficacy (PPE) population. This population consisted of boys and men who received all 3 vaccinations within 1 year of enrollment, did not have major deviations from the study protocol, and were naïve (PCR negative and seronegative) to the relevant HPV type(s) (Types 6, 11, 16, and 18) prior to dose 1 and through 1 month postdose 3 (Month 7). Efficacy was measured starting after the Month 7 visit.

GARDASIL was efficacious in reducing the incidence of genital warts related to vaccine HPV types 6 and 11 in those boys and men who were PCR negative and seronegative at baseline (Table 12). Efficacy against penile/perineal/perianal intraepithelial neoplasia (PIN) grades 1/2/3 or penile/perineal/perianal cancer was not demonstrated as the number of cases was too limited to reach statistical significance. [See table 12 on previous page]

14.3 Population Impact in Girls and Women 16 Through 26 Years of Age

Effectiveness of GARDASIL in Prevention of HPV Types 6-, 11-, 16-, or 18-Related Genital Disease in Girls and Women 16 Through 26 Years of Age, Regardless of Current or Prior Exposure to Vaccine HPV Types

The clinical trials included girls and women regardless of current or prior exposure to vaccine HPV types, and additional analyses were conducted to evaluate the impact of GARDASIL with respect to HPV 6-, 11-, 16-, and 18-related cervical and genital disease in these girls and women. Here, analyses included events arising among girls and women

Table 13: Effectiveness of GARDASIL in Prevention of HPV 6, 11, 16, or 18-Related Genital Disease in Girls and Women 16 Through 26 Years of Age, Regardless of Current or Prior Exposure to Vaccine HPV Types

Endpoints	Analysis	GARDASIL or HPV 16 L1 VLP Vaccine		AAHS Control		% Reduction (95% CI)
		N	Cases	N	Cases	
HPV 16- or 18-related CIN 2/3 or AIS	Prophylactic Efficacy*	9346	4	9407	155	97.4 (93.3, 99.3)
	HPV 16 and/or HPV 18 Positive at Day 1	2870	142	2898	148†	—‡
	Girls and Women Regardless of Current or Prior Exposure to HPV 16 or 18§	9836	146	9904	303	51.8 (41.1, 60.7)¶
HPV 16- or 18-related VIN 2/3 or VaIN 2/3	Prophylactic Efficacy*	8642	1	8673	34	97.0 (82.4, 99.9)
	HPV 16 and/or HPV 18 Positive at Day 1	1880	8	1876	4	—‡
	Girls and Women Regardless of Current or Prior Exposure to HPV 16 or 18§	8955	9	8968	38	76.3 (50.0, 89.9)¶
HPV 6-, 11-, 16-, 18-related CIN (CIN 1, CIN 2/3) or AIS	Prophylactic Efficacy*	8630	16	8680	309	94.8 (91.5, 97.1)
	HPV 6, HPV 11, HPV 16, and/or HPV 18 Positive at Day 1	2466	186#	2437	213#	—‡
	Girls and Women Regardless of Current or Prior Exposure to Vaccine HPV Types§	8819	202	8854	522	61.5 (54.6, 67.4)¶
HPV 6-, 11-, 16-, or 18-related Genital Warts	Prophylactic Efficacy*	8761	10	8792	252	96.0 (92.6, 98.1)
	HPV 6, HPV 11, HPV 16, and/or HPV 18 Positive at Day 1	2501	51Þ	2475	55Þ	—‡
	Girls and Women Regardless of Current or Prior Exposure to Vaccine HPV Types§	8955	61	8968	307	80.3 (73.9, 85.3)¶
HPV 6- or 11-related Genital Warts	Prophylactic Efficacy*	7769	9	7792	246	96.4 (93.0, 98.4)
	HPV 6 and/or HPV 11 Positive at Day 1	1186	51	1176	54	—‡
	Girls and Women Regardless of Current or Prior Exposure to Vaccine HPV Types§	8955	60	8968	300	80.1 (73.7, 85.2)¶

CI = Confidence Interval
N = Number of individuals who have at least one follow-up visit after Day 1
Note 1: The 16- and 18-related CIN 2/3 or AIS composite endpoint included data from studies 1, 2, 3, and 4. All other endpoints only included data from studies 2, 3, and 4.
Note 2: Positive status at Day 1 denotes PCR positive and/or seropositive for the respective type at Day 1.
Note 3: Table 13 does not include disease due to non-vaccine HPV types.
AAHS Control = Amorphous Aluminum Hydroxyphosphate Sulfate
* Includes all individuals who received at least 1 vaccination and who were naïve (PCR negative and seronegative) to HPV 6, 11, 16, and/or 18 at Day 1. Case counting started at 1 month postdose 1.
† Out of the 148 AAHS control cases of 16/18 CIN 2/3, 2 women were missing serology or PCR results for Day 1.
‡ There is no expected efficacy since GARDASIL has not been demonstrated to provide protection against disease from vaccine HPV types to which a person has previously been exposed through sexual activity.
§ Includes all individuals who received at least 1 vaccination (regardless of baseline HPV status at Day 1). Case counting started at 1 month postdose 1.
¶ Percent reduction includes the prophylactic efficacy of GARDASIL as well as the impact of GARDASIL on the course of infections present at the start of the vaccination.
# Includes 2 AAHS control women with missing serology/PCR data at Day 1.
Þ Includes 1 woman with missing serology/PCR data at Day 1.

Table 14: Effectiveness of GARDASIL in Prevention of Any HPV Type Related Genital Disease in Girls and Women 16 Through 26 Years of Age, Regardless of Current or Prior Infection with Vaccine or Non-Vaccine HPV Types

Endpoints Caused by Vaccine or Non-vaccine HPV Types	Analysis	GARDASIL		AAHS Control		% Reduction (95% CI)
		N	Cases	N	Cases	
CIN 2/3 or AIS	Prophylactic Efficacy*	4616	77	4680	136	42.7 (23.7, 57.3)
	Girls and Women Regardless of Current or Prior Exposure to Vaccine or Non-Vaccine HPV Types†	8559	421	8592	516	18.4 (7.0, 28.4)‡
VIN 2/3 and VaIN 2/3	Prophylactic Efficacy*	4688	7	4735	31	77.1 (47.1, 91.5)
	Girls and Women Regardless of Current or Prior Exposure to Vaccine or Non-Vaccine HPV Types†	8688	30	8701	61	50.7 (22.5, 69.3)‡
CIN (Any Grade) or AIS	Prophylactic Efficacy*	4616	272	4680	390	29.7 (17.7, 40.0)
	Girls and Women Regardless of Current or Prior Exposure to Vaccine or Non-Vaccine HPV Types†	8559	967	8592	1189	19.1 (11.9, 25.8)‡
Genital Warts	Prophylactic Efficacy*	4688	29	4735	169	82.8 (74.3, 88.8)
	Girls and Women Regardless of Current or Prior Exposure to Vaccine or Non-Vaccine HPV Types†	8688	132	8701	350	62.5 (54.0, 69.5)‡

CI = Confidence Interval
AAHS Control = Amorphous Aluminum Hydroxyphosphate Sulfate
* Includes all individuals who received at least 1 vaccination and who had a Pap test that was negative for SIL [Squamous Intraepithelial Lesion] at Day 1 and were naïve to 14 common HPV types at Day 1. Case counting started at 1 month postdose 1.
† Includes all individuals who received at least 1 vaccination (regardless of baseline HPV status or Pap test result at Day 1). Case counting started at 1 month postdose 1.
‡ Percent reduction includes the prophylactic efficacy of GARDASIL as well as the impact of GARDASIL on the course of infections present at the start of the vaccination.

regardless of baseline PCR status and serostatus, including HPV infections that were present at the start of vaccination as well as events that arose from infections that were acquired after the start of vaccination.

The impact of GARDASIL in girls and women regardless of current or prior exposure to a vaccine HPV type is shown in Table 13. Impact was measured starting 1 month Postdose 1. Prophylactic efficacy denotes the vaccine's efficacy in girls and women who are naïve (PCR negative and seronegative) to the relevant HPV types at Day 1. Vaccine impact in girls and women who were positive for vaccine HPV infection, as well as vaccine impact among girls and women regardless of baseline vaccine HPV PCR status and serostatus are also presented. The majority of CIN and genital warts, VIN, and VaIN related to a vaccine HPV type detected in the group that received GARDASIL occurred as a consequence of HPV infection with the relevant HPV type that was already present at Day 1.

There was no clear evidence of protection from disease caused by HPV types for which girls and women were PCR positive regardless of serostatus at baseline.

[See table at top of previous page]

Effectiveness of GARDASIL in Prevention of Any HPV Type Related Genital Disease in Girls and Women 16 Through 26 Years of Age, Regardless of Current or Prior Infection with Vaccine or Non-Vaccine HPV Types

The impact of GARDASIL against the overall burden of HPV-related cervical, vulvar, and vaginal disease (i.e., disease caused by any HPV type) results from a combination of prophylactic efficacy against vaccine HPV types, disease contribution from vaccine HPV types present at time of vaccination, and the disease contribution from HPV types not contained in the vaccine.

Additional efficacy analyses were conducted in 2 populations: (1) a generally HPV-naïve population (negative to 14 common HPV types and had a Pap test that was negative for SIL [Squamous Intraepithelial Lesion] at Day 1), approximating a population of sexually-naïve girls and women and (2) the general study population of girls and women regardless of baseline HPV status, some of whom had HPV-related disease at Day 1.

Among generally HPV-naïve girls and women and among all girls and women in the study population (including girls and women with HPV infection at Day 1), GARDASIL reduced the overall incidence of CIN 2/3 or AIS; of VIN 2/3 or VaIN 2/3; of CIN (any grade) or AIS; and of Genital Warts (Table 14). These reductions were primarily due to reductions in lesions caused by HPV types 6, 11, 16, and 18 in girls and women naïve (seronegative and PCR negative) for

the specific relevant vaccine HPV type. Infected girls and women may already have CIN 2/3 or AIS at Day 1 and some will develop CIN 2/3 or AIS during follow-up, either related to a vaccine or non-vaccine HPV type present at the time of vaccination or related to a non-vaccine HPV type not present at the time of vaccination.

[See table 14 above]

14.4   Population Impact in Boys and Men 16 Through 26 Years of Age

Effectiveness of GARDASIL in Prevention of HPV Types 6-, 11-, 16-, or 18-Related Genital Disease in Boys and Men 16 Through 26 Years of Age, Regardless of Current or Prior Exposure to Vaccine HPV Types

Study 5 included boys and men regardless of current or prior exposure to vaccine HPV types, and additional analyses were conducted to evaluate the impact of GARDASIL with respect to HPV 6-, 11-, 16-, and 18-related genital disease in these boys and men. Here, analyses included events arising among boys and men regardless of baseline PCR status and serostatus, including HPV infections that were present at the start of vaccination as well as events that arose from infections that were acquired after the start of vaccination.

The impact of GARDASIL in boys and men regardless of current or prior exposure to a vaccine HPV type is shown in Table 15. Impact was measured starting at Day 1. Prophylactic efficacy denotes the vaccine's efficacy in boys and men who are naïve (PCR negative and seronegative) to the relevant HPV types at Day 1. Vaccine impact in boys and men who were positive for vaccine HPV infection, as well as vaccine impact among boys and men regardless of baseline vaccine HPV PCR status and serostatus are also presented. The majority of genital disease related to a vaccine HPV type detected in the group that received GARDASIL occurred as a consequence of HPV infection with the relevant HPV type that was already present at Day 1.

There was no clear evidence of protection from disease caused by HPV types for which boys and men were PCR positive regardless of serostatus at baseline.

[See table 15 at top of next page]

Effectiveness of GARDASIL in Prevention of Any HPV Type Related Genital Disease in Boys and Men 16 Through 26 Years of Age, Regardless of Current or Prior Infection with Vaccine or Non-Vaccine HPV Types

The impact of GARDASIL against the overall burden of HPV-related genital disease (i.e., disease caused by any HPV type) results from a combination of prophylactic efficacy against vaccine HPV types, disease contribution from HPV types present at time of vaccination, and the disease contribution from HPV types not contained in the vaccine.

Additional efficacy analyses from Study 5 were conducted in 2 populations: (1) a generally HPV-naïve population that consisted of boys and men who are seronegative and PCR negative to HPV 6, 11, 16, and 18 and PCR negative to HPV 31, 33, 35, 39, 45, 51, 52, 56, 58 and 59 at Day 1, approximating a population of sexually-naïve boys and men and (2) the general study population of boys and men regardless of baseline HPV status, some of whom had HPV-related disease at Day 1.

Among generally HPV-naïve boys and men and among all boys and men in Study 5 (including boys and men with HPV infection at Day 1), GARDASIL reduced the overall incidence of genital disease (Table 16). These reductions were primarily due to reductions in lesions caused by HPV types 6, 11, 16, and 18 in boys and men naïve (seronegative and PCR negative) for the specific relevant vaccine HPV type. Infected boys and men may already have genital disease at Day 1 and some will develop genital disease during follow-up, either related to a vaccine or non-vaccine HPV type present at the time of vaccination or related to a non-vaccine HPV type not present at the time of vaccination.

[See table 16 on next page]

14.5   Overall Population Impact

The subject characteristics (e.g. lifetime sex partners, geographic distribution of the subjects) influence the HPV prevalence of the population and therefore the population benefit can vary widely.

The overall efficacy of GARDASIL will vary with the baseline prevalence of HPV infection and disease, the incidence of infections against which GARDASIL has shown protection, and those infections against which GARDASIL has not been shown to protect.

The efficacy of GARDASIL for HPV types not included in the vaccine (i.e., cross-protective efficacy) is a component of the overall impact of the vaccine on rates of disease caused by HPV. Cross-protective efficacy was not demonstrated against disease caused by non-vaccine HPV types in the combined database of the Study 3 and Study 4 trials.

GARDASIL does not protect against genital disease not related to HPV. One woman who received GARDASIL in Study 3 developed an external genital well-differentiated squamous cell carcinoma at Month 24. No HPV DNA was detected in the lesion or in any other samples taken throughout the study.

In 18,150 girls and women enrolled in Study 2, Study 3, and Study 4, GARDASIL reduced definitive cervical therapy procedures by 23.9% (95% CI: 15.2%, 31.7%).

14.6   Other Studies

Data are insufficient to establish effectiveness of GARDASIL in women 27 through 45 years of age.

14.7   Immunogenicity

Assays to Measure Immune Response

The minimum anti-HPV titer that confers protective efficacy has not been determined.

Because there were few disease cases in individuals naïve (PCR negative and seronegative) to vaccine HPV types at baseline in the group that received GARDASIL, it has not been possible to establish minimum anti-HPV 6, anti-HPV 11, anti-HPV 16, and anti-HPV 18 antibody levels that protect against clinical disease caused by HPV 6, 11, 16, and/or 18.

The immunogenicity of GARDASIL was assessed in 20,132 9- through 26-year-old girls and women (GARDASIL N = 10,723; AAHS control or saline placebo N = 9409) and 5417 9- through 26-year-old boys and men (GARDASIL N = 3109; AAHS control or saline placebo N = 2308).

Type-specific immunoassays with type-specific standards were used to assess immunogenicity to each vaccine HPV type. These assays measured antibodies against neutralizing epitopes for each HPV type. The scales for these assays are unique to each HPV type; thus, comparisons across types and to other assays are not appropriate.

Immune Response to GARDASIL

The primary immunogenicity analyses were conducted in a per-protocol immunogenicity (PPI) population. This population consisted of individuals who were seronegative and PCR negative to the relevant HPV type(s) at enrollment, remained HPV PCR negative to the relevant HPV type(s) through 1 month postdose 3 (Month 7), received all 3 vaccinations, and did not deviate from the study protocol in ways that could interfere with the effects of the vaccine.

Immunogenicity was measured by (1) the percentage of individuals who were seropositive for antibodies against the relevant vaccine HPV type, and (2) the Geometric Mean Titer (GMT).

In clinical studies in girls and women, at least 99.8%, 99.8%, 99.8%, and 99.5% who received GARDASIL became anti-HPV 6, anti-HPV 11, anti-HPV 16, and anti-HPV 18 seropositive, respectively, by 1 month postdose 3 across all age groups tested.

In clinical studies in boys and men, at least 98.9%, 99.2%, 98.8%, and 97.4% who received GARDASIL became anti-HPV 6, anti-HPV 11, anti-HPV 16, and anti-HPV 18 seropositive, respectively, by 1 month postdose 3 across all age groups tested.

Across all populations, anti-HPV 6, anti-HPV 11, anti-HPV 16, and anti-HPV 18 GMTs peaked at Month 7 (Table 17 and Table 18). GMTs declined through Month 24 and then stabilized through Month 36 at levels above baseline. Table 19 displays the persistence of anti-HPV cLIA geometric mean titers by gender and age group. The duration of immunity following a complete schedule of immunization with GARDASIL has not been established.

[See table 17 at top of next page]
[See table 18 on next page]
[See table 19 at top of page 2091]

Tables 17 and 18 display the Month 7 immunogenicity data for girls and women and boys and men. Anti-HPV responses 1 month postdose 3 among 9- through 15-year-old adolescent girls were non-inferior to anti-HPV responses in 16- through 26-year-old girls and women in the combined database of immunogenicity studies for GARDASIL. Anti-HPV responses 1 month postdose 3 among 9- through 15-year-old adolescent boys were non-inferior to anti-HPV responses in 16- through 26-year-old boys and men in Study 5.

On the basis of this immunogenicity bridging, the efficacy of GARDASIL in 9- through 15-year-old adolescent girls and boys is inferred.

GMT Response to Variation in Dosing Regimen in 18- Through 26-Year-Old Women

Girls and women evaluated in the PPE population of clinical studies received all 3 vaccinations within 1 year of enrollment. An analysis of immune response data suggests that flexibility of ±1 month for Dose 2 (i.e., Month 1 to Month 3 in the vaccination regimen) and flexibility of ±2 months for Dose 3 (i.e., Month 4 to Month 8 in the vaccination regimen) do not impact the immune responses to GARDASIL.

Duration of the Immune Response to GARDASIL

The duration of immunity following a complete schedule of immunization with GARDASIL has not been established. The peak anti-HPV GMTs for HPV types 6, 11, 16, and 18 occurred at Month 7. Anti-HPV GMTs for HPV types 6, 11, 16, and 18 were similar between measurements at Month 24 and Month 60 in Study 2.

14.8   Studies with RECOMBIVAX HB [hepatitis B vaccine (recombinant)]

The safety and immunogenicity of co-administration of GARDASIL with RECOMBIVAX HB [hepatitis B vaccine (recombinant)] (same visit, injections at separate sites) were evaluated in a randomized, double-blind study of 1871 women aged 16 through 24 years at enrollment. The race distribution of the girls and women in the clinical trial was as follows: 61.6% White; 1.6% Hispanic (Black and White); 23.8% Other; 11.9% Black; 0.8% Asian; and 0.3% American Indian.

Subjects either received GARDASIL and RECOMBIVAX HB (n = 466), GARDASIL and RECOMBIVAX HB-matched placebo (n = 468), RECOMBIVAX HB and GARDASIL-matched placebo (n = 467) or RECOMBIVAX-matched placebo and GARDASIL-matched placebo (n = 470) at Day 1, Month 2 and Month 6. Immunogenicity was assessed for all vaccines 1 month post completion of the vaccination series. Concomitant administration of GARDASIL with RECOMBIVAX HB [hepatitis B vaccine (recombinant)] did not interfere with the antibody response to any of the vaccine antigens when GARDASIL was given concomitantly with RECOMBIVAX HB or separately.

14.9   Studies with Menactra [Meningococcal (Groups A, C, Y and W-135) Polysaccharide Diphtheria Toxoid Conjugate Vaccine] and Adacel [Tetanus Toxoid, Reduced Diphtheria Toxoid and Acellular Pertussis Vaccine Adsorbed (Tdap)]

The safety and immunogenicity of co-administration of GARDASIL with Menactra [Meningococcal (Groups A, C, Y and W-135) Polysaccharide Diphtheria Toxoid Conjugate Vaccine] and Adacel [Tetanus Toxoid, Reduced Diphtheria Toxoid and Acellular Pertussis Vaccine Adsorbed (Tdap)] (same visit, injections at separate sites) were evaluated in an open-labeled, randomized, controlled study of 1040 boys and girls 11 through 17 years of age at enrollment. The race distribution of the subjects in the clinical trial was as follows: 77.7% White; 6.8% Hispanic (Black and White); 1.4% Multi-racial; 12.3% Black; 1.2% Asian; 0.2% Indian; and 0.4% American Indian.

One group received GARDASIL in one limb and both Menactra and Adacel, as separate injections, in the opposite limb concomitantly on Day 1 (n = 517). The second group received the first dose of GARDASIL on Day 1 in one limb then Menactra and Adacel, as separate injections, at Month 1 in the opposite limb (n = 523). Subjects in both vaccination groups received the second dose of GARDASIL at Month 2 and the third dose at Month 6. Immunogenicity was assessed for all vaccines 1 month post completion of the vac-

cination series (1 dose for Menactra and Adacel and 3 doses for GARDASIL).

Concomitant administration of GARDASIL with Menactra [Meningococcal (Groups A, C, Y and W-135) Polysaccharide Diphtheria Toxoid Conjugate Vaccine] and Adacel [Tetanus Toxoid, Reduced Diphtheria Toxoid and Acellular Pertussis Vaccine Adsorbed (Tdap)] did not interfere with the anti-

body response to any of the vaccine antigens when GARDASIL was given concomitantly with Menactra and Adacel or separately.

16   HOW SUPPLIED/STORAGE AND HANDLING

All presentations for GARDASIL contain a suspension of 120 mcg L1 protein from HPV types 6, 11, 16, and 18 in a

Table 15: Effectiveness of GARDASIL in Prevention of HPV Types 6-, 11-, 16-, or 18-Related Genital Disease in Boys and Men 16 Through 26 Years of Age, Regardless of Current or Prior Exposure to Vaccine HPV Types

Endpoint	Analysis	GARDASIL		AAHS Control		% Reduction (95% CI)
		N	Cases	N	Cases	
External Genital Lesions	Prophylactic Efficacy*	1775	13	1770	52	75.5 (54.3, 87.7)
	HPV 6, HPV 11, HPV 16, and/or HPV 18 Positive at Day 1	168	14	167	25	—†
	Boys and Men Regardless of Current or Prior Exposure to Vaccine or Non-Vaccine HPV Types‡	1943	27	1937	77	65.5 (45.8, 78.6)§
Condyloma	Prophylactic Efficacy*	1775	10	1770	48	79.6 (59.1, 90.8)
	HPV 6, HPV 11, HPV 16, and/or HPV 18 Positive at Day 1	168	14	167	24	—†
	Boys and Men Regardless of Current or Prior Exposure to Vaccine or Non-Vaccine HPV Types‡	1943	24	1937	72	67.2 (47.3, 80.3)§
PIN 1/2/3	Prophylactic Efficacy*	1775	4	1770	4	1.2 (-430.5, 81.6)
	HPV 6, HPV 11, HPV 16, and/or HPV 18 Positive at Day 1	168	2	167	1	—†
	Boys and Men Regardless of Current or Prior Exposure to Vaccine or Non-Vaccine HPV Types‡	1943	6	1937	5	-19.2 (-393.8, 69.7)§

CI = Confidence Interval
AAHS Control = Amorphous Aluminum Hydroxyphosphate Sulfate
* Includes all individuals who received at least 1 vaccination and who were HPV-naïve (i.e., seronegative and PCR negative) at Day 1 to the vaccine HPV type being analyzed. Case counting started at Day 1.
† There is no expected efficacy since GARDASIL has not been demonstrated to provide protection against disease from vaccine HPV types to which a person has previously been exposed through sexual activity.
‡ Includes all individuals who received at least 1 vaccination. Case counting started at Day 1.
§ Percent reduction for these analyses includes the prophylactic efficacy of GARDASIL as well as the impact of GARDASIL on the course of infections present at the start of the vaccination.

Table 16: Effectiveness of GARDASIL in Prevention of Any HPV Type Related Genital Disease in Boys and Men 16 Through 26 Years of Age, Regardless of Current or Prior Infection with Vaccine or Non-Vaccine HPV Types

Endpoint	Analysis	GARDASIL		AAHS Control		% Reduction (95% CI)
		N	Cases	N	Cases	
External Genital Lesions	Generally HPV Naïve*	1275	6	1270	36	83.8 (61.2, 94.4)
	Boys and Men Regardless of Current or Prior Exposure to Vaccine or Non-Vaccine HPV Types†	1943	36	1937	89	60.2 (40.8, 73.8)‡
Condyloma	Generally HPV Naïve*	1275	5	1270	33	85.3 (62.1, 95.5)
	Boys and Men Regardless of Current or Prior Exposure to Vaccine or Non-Vaccine HPV Types†	1943	32	1937	83	62.1 (42.4, 75.6)‡
PIN 1/2/3	Generally HPV Naïve*	1275	1	1270	3	67.4 (-306.5, 99.4)
	Boys and Men Regardless of Current or Prior Exposure to Vaccine or Non-Vaccine HPV Types†	1943	7	1937	6	-15.9 (-317.5, 66.6)‡

CI = Confidence Interval
AAHS Control = Amorphous Aluminum Hydroxyphosphate Sulfate
* Includes all individuals who received at least 1 vaccination and who were seronegative and PCR negative at enrollment to HPV 6, 11, 16 and 18, and PCR negative at enrollment to HPV 31, 33, 35, 39, 45, 51, 52, 56, 58 and 59. Case counting started at Day 1.
† Includes all individuals who received at least 1 vaccination. Case counting started at Day 1.
‡ Percent reduction for these analyses includes the prophylactic efficacy of GARDASIL as well as the impact of GARDASIL on the course of infections present at the start of the vaccination.

Table 17: Summary of Month 7 Anti-HPV cLIA Geometric Mean Titers in the PPI* Population of Girls and Women

Population	N[†]	n[‡]	% Seropositive (95% CI)	GMT (95% CI) mMu[§]/mL
Anti-HPV 6				
9- through 15-year-old girls	1122	917	99.9 (99.4, 100.0)	929.2 (874.6, 987.3)
16- through 26-year-old girls and women	9862	3333	99.8 (99.6, 99.9)	545.2 (530.3, 560.6)
Anti-HPV 11				
9- through 15-year-old girls	1122	917	99.9 (99.4, 100.0)	1304.6 (1224.7, 1389.7)
16- through 26-year-old girls and women	9862	3357	99.8 (99.5, 99.9)	749.0 (726.1, 772.7)
Anti-HPV 16				
9- through 15-year-old girls	1122	915	99.9 (99.4, 100.0)	4918.5 (4556.6, 5309.1)
16- through 26-year-old girls and women	9862	3253	99.8 (99.6, 100.0)	2411.3 (2311.1, 2515.9)
Anti-HPV 18				
9- through 15-year-old girls	1122	922	99.8 (99.2, 100.0)	1042.6 (967.6, 1123.3)
16- through 26-year-old girls and women	9862	3571	99.4 (99.1, 99.7)	475.6 (459.2, 492.6)

cLIA = Competitive Luminex Immunoassay
CI = Confidence Interval
GMT = Geometric Mean Titers
* The PPI population consisted of individuals who received all 3 vaccinations within pre-defined day ranges, did not have major deviations from the study protocol, met predefined criteria for the interval between the Month 6 and Month 7 visit, and were naïve (PCR negative and seronegative) to the relevant HPV type(s) (types 6, 11, 16, and 18) prior to dose 1 and through 1 month Postdose 3 (Month 7).
† Number of individuals randomized to the respective vaccination group who received at least 1 injection.
‡ Number of individuals contributing to the analysis.
§ mMU = milli-Merck Units

Table 18: Summary of Month 7 Anti-HPV cLIA Geometric Mean Titers in the PPI* Population of Boys and Men

Population	N[†]	n[‡]	% Seropositive (95% CI)	GMT (95% CI) mMu[§]/mL
Anti-HPV 6				
9- through 15-year-old boys	1072	884	99.9 (99.4, 100.0)	1037.5 (963.5, 1117.3)
16- through 26-year-old boys and men	2026	1094	98.9 (98.1, 99.4)	447.2 (418.4, 477.9)
Anti-HPV 11				
9- through 15-year-old boys	1072	885	99.9 (99.4, 100.0)	1386.8 (1298.5, 1481.0)
16- through 26-year-old boys and men	2026	1094	99.2 (98.4, 99.6)	624.5 (588.6, 662.5)
Anti-HPV 16				
9- through 15-year-old boys	1072	882	99.8 (99.2, 100.0)	6056.5 (5601.4, 6548.6)
16- through 26-year-old boys and men	2026	1137	98.8 (97.9, 99.3)	2401.5 (2241.8, 2572.6)
Anti-HPV 18				
9- through 15-year-old boys	1072	887	99.8 (99.2, 100)	1357.4 (1249.4, 1474.7)
16- through 26-year-old boys and men	2026	1176	97.4 (96.3, 98.2)	402.6 (374.6, 432.6)

cLIA = Competitive Luminex Immunoassay
CI = Confidence Interval
GMT = Geometric Mean Titers
* The PPI population consisted of individuals who received all 3 vaccinations within pre-defined day ranges, did not have major deviations from the study protocol, met predefined criteria for the interval between the Month 6 and Month 7 visit, and were naïve (PCR negative and seronegative) to the relevant HPV type(s) (types 6, 11, 16, and 18) prior to dose 1 and through 1 month Postdose 3 (Month 7).
† Number of individuals randomized to the respective vaccination group who received at least 1 injection.
‡ Number of individuals contributing to the analysis.
§ mMU = milli-Merck Units

0.5-mL dose. GARDASIL is supplied in vials and syringes. Carton of one 0.5-mL single-dose vial. **NDC** 0006-4045-00. Carton of ten 0.5-mL single-dose vials. **NDC** 0006-4045-41. Carton of six 0.5-mL single-dose prefilled Luer Lock syringes, preassembled with UltraSafe Passive[2] delivery system. One-inch, 25-gauge needles are provided separately in the package. **NDC** 0006-4109-06. Carton of six 0.5-mL single-dose prefilled Luer Lock syringes with tip caps. **NDC** 0006-4109-09. Store refrigerated at 2 to 8°C (36 to 46°F). Do not freeze. Protect from light. GARDASIL should be administered as soon as possible after being removed from refrigeration.

GARDASIL can be out of refrigeration (at temperatures at or below 25°C/77°F), for a total time of not more than 72 hours.
[1]Registered trademark of MERCK & CO., Inc. Whitehouse Station, NJ 08889, USA
COPYRIGHT © 2006, 2009 MERCK & CO., Inc.
All rights reserved
[2]UltraSafe Passive® delivery system is a Trademark of Safety Syringes, Inc.

17   PATIENT COUNSELING INFORMATION

[See FDA-Approved Patient Labeling.]
Inform the patient, parent, or guardian:

- Vaccination does not eliminate the necessity for women to continue to undergo recommended cervical cancer screening. Women who receive GARDASIL should continue to undergo cervical cancer screening per standard of care.
- GARDASIL has not been demonstrated to provide protection against disease from vaccine and non-vaccine HPV types to which a person has previously been exposed through sexual activity.
- Since syncope has been reported following vaccination sometimes resulting in falling with injury, observation for 15 minutes after administration is recommended.
- Vaccine information is required to be given with each vaccination to the patient, parent, or guardian.
- Information regarding benefits and risks associated with vaccination.
- GARDASIL is not recommended for use in pregnant women.
- Importance of completing the immunization series unless contraindicated.
- Report any adverse reactions to their health care provider.

Manufactured and Distributed by:
MERCK & CO., INC., Whitehouse Station, NJ 08889, USA
Printed in USA
9883613

FDA-APPROVED PATIENT LABELING

USPPI
Patient Information about
GARDASIL® (pronounced "gard-Ah-sill")
Generic name: [Human Papillomavirus Quadrivalent (Types 6, 11, 16, and 18) Vaccine, Recombinant]
Read this information with care before getting GARDASIL[1]. You (the person getting GARDASIL) will need 3 doses of the vaccine. It is important to read this leaflet when you get each dose. This leaflet does not take the place of talking with your health care provider about GARDASIL.
What is GARDASIL?
GARDASIL is a vaccine (injection/shot) that is used for girls and women 9 through 26 years of age to help protect against the following diseases caused by Human Papillomavirus (HPV):
- Cervical cancer
- Vulvar and vaginal cancers
- Genital warts
- Abnormal and precancerous cervical, vaginal, and vulvar lesions
  - The diseases listed above have many causes, and GARDASIL only protects against diseases caused by certain kinds of HPV (called Type 6, Type 11, Type 16, and Type 18). Most of the time, these 4 types of HPV are responsible for the diseases listed above.
  - GARDASIL cannot protect you from a disease that is caused by other types of HPV, other viruses, or bacteria.
  - GARDASIL does not treat HPV infection.
- You cannot get HPV or any of the above diseases from GARDASIL.

GARDASIL is used for boys and men 9 through 26 years of age to help protect against genital warts.
What important information about GARDASIL should I know?
- You should continue to get routine cervical cancer screening.
- GARDASIL may not fully protect everyone who gets the vaccine.
- GARDASIL will not protect against HPV types that you already have.
Who should not get GARDASIL?
You should not get GARDASIL if you have, or have had:
- an allergic reaction after getting a dose of GARDASIL.
- a severe allergic reaction to yeast, amorphous aluminum hydroxyphosphate sulfate, polysorbate 80.
What should I tell my health care provider before getting GARDASIL?
Tell your health care provider if you:
- are pregnant or planning to get pregnant. GARDASIL is not recommended for use in pregnant women.
- have immune problems, like HIV infection, cancer, or you take medicines that affect your immune system.
- have a fever over 100°F (37.8°C).
- had an allergic reaction to another dose of GARDASIL.
- take any medicines, even those you can buy over the counter.
Your health care provider will help decide if you should get the vaccine.
How is GARDASIL given?
GARDASIL is a shot that is usually given in the arm muscle. You will need 3 shots given on the following schedule:
- Dose 1: at a date you and your health care provider choose.
- Dose 2: 2 months after Dose 1.
- Dose 3: 6 months after Dose 1.
Fainting can happen after getting GARDASIL. Sometimes people who faint can fall and hurt themselves. For this reason, your health care provider may ask you to sit or lie down

Table 19: Persistence of Anti-HPV cLIA Geometric Mean Titers by Gender and Age Group

Assay (cLIA)/ Time Point	9- to 15-year-old Boys (N* = 1072)		16- to 26-year-old Boys and Men (N* = 2026)		9- to 15-year-old Girls (N* = 1122)		16- to 26-year-old Girls and Women (N* = 9859)	
	n[†]	GMT (95% CI) mMU[‡]/mL	n[†]	GMT (95% CI) mMU[‡]/mL	n[†]	GMT (95% CI) mMU[‡]/mL	n[†]	GMT (95% CI) mMU[‡]/mL
Anti-HPV 6								
Month 07	884	1037.5 (963.5, 1117.3)	1094	447.2 (418.4, 477.9)	917	929.2 (874.6, 987.3)	3333	545.2 (530.3, 560.6)
Month 24	323	134.1 (119.5, 150.5)	907	80.3 (74.9, 86.0)	214	156.1 (135.6, 179.6)	2792	109.1 (105.2, 113.1)
Month 36[§]	342	126.6 (111.9, 143.2)	654	72.4 (68.0, 77.2)	356	129.4 (115.6, 144.8)	-	-
Month 48[¶]	-	-	-	-	-	-	2375	74.6 (71.6, 77.7)
Anti-HPV 11								
Month 07	885	1386.8 (1298.5, 1481.0)	1094	624.5 (588.6, 662.5)	917	1304.6 (1224.7, 1389.7)	3357	749.0 (726.1, 772.7)
Month 24	324	188.5 (168.4, 211.1)	907	94.6 (88.4, 101.2)	214	218.0 (188.3, 252.4)	2821	137.0 (132.0, 142.2)
Month 36[§]	342	148.8 (131.1, 169.0)	654	80.3 (75.7, 85.2)	356	148.0 (131.1, 167.1)	-	-
Month 48[¶]	-	-	-	-	-	-	2399	90.3 (86.6, 94.1)
Anti-HPV 16								
Month 07	882	6056.5 (5601.4, 6548.6)	1137	2401.5 (2241.8, 2572.6)	915	4918.5 (4556.6, 5309.1)	3253	2411.3 (2311.1, 2515.9)
Month 24	322	938.2 (825.0, 1067.0)	938	347.7 (322.5, 374.9)	211	944.2 (804.4, 1108.3)	2725	442.6 (425.0, 460.9)
Month 36[§]	341	708.8 (613.9, 818.3)	672	306.7 (287.5, 327.1)	353	642.2 (562.8, 732.8)	-	-
Month 48[¶]	-	-	-	-	-	-	2330	334.6 (319.4, 350.5)
Anti-HPV 18								
Month 07	887	1357.4 (1249.4, 1474.7)	1176	402.6 (374.6, 432.6)	922	1042.6 (967.6, 1123.3)	3571	475.6 (459.2, 492.6)
Month 24	324	131.9 (112.1, 155.3)	967	38.7 (35.2, 42.5)	214	137.7 (114.8, 165.1)	3007	50.8 (48.2, 53.5)
Month 36[§]	343	113.0 (94.7, 135.0)	690	33.4 (30.9, 36.1)	357	87.0 (74.8, 101.2)	-	-
Month 48[¶]	-	-	-	-	-	-	2536	33.8 (32.0, 35.7)

cLIA = Competitive Luminex Immunoassay
CI = Confidence Interval
GMT = Geometric Mean Titers
* N = Number of individuals randomized in the respective group who received at least 1 injection.
† n = Number of individuals in the indicated immunogenicity population.
‡ mMU = milli-Merck Units
§ Month 36 time point for 16- to 26-year-old boys and men; Month 37 for 9- to 15-year-old boys and girls. No serology samples were collected at this time point for 16- to 26-year-old girls and women.
¶ Month 48/End-of-study visits for 16- to 26-year-old girls and women were generally scheduled earlier than Month 48. Mean visit timing was Month 44. The studies in 9- to 15-year-old boys and girls and 16- to 26-year-old boys and men were planned to end prior to 48 months and therefore no serology samples were collected.

for 15 minutes after you get GARDASIL. Some people who faint might shake or become stiff. This may require evaluation or treatment by your health care provider.
Make sure that you get all 3 doses on time so that you get the best protection. If you miss a dose, talk to your health care provider.

Can other vaccines and medications be given at the same time as GARDASIL?
GARDASIL can be given at the same time as RECOMBIVAX HB®[1] [hepatitis B vaccine (recombinant)] or Menactra [Meningococcal (Groups A, C, Y and W-135) Polysaccharide Diphtheria Toxoid Conjugate Vaccine] and Adacel [Tetanus Toxoid, Reduced Diphtheria Toxoid and Acellular Pertussis Vaccine Adsorbed (Tdap)].

What are the possible side effects of GARDASIL?
The most common side effects with GARDASIL are:

• pain, swelling, itching, bruising, and redness at the injection site
• headache
• fever
• nausea
• dizziness
• vomiting
• fainting
There was no increase in side effects when GARDASIL was given at the same time as RECOMBIVAX HB [hepatitis B vaccine (recombinant)].
There was more injection-site swelling at the injection site for GARDASIL when GARDASIL was given at the same time as Menactra [Meningococcal (Groups A, C, Y and W-135) Polysaccharide Diphtheria Toxoid Conjugate Vaccine] and Adacel [Tetanus Toxoid, Reduced Diphtheria Toxoid and Acellular Pertussis Vaccine Adsorbed (Tdap)].

Tell your health care provider if you have any of the following problems because these may be signs of an allergic reaction:
• difficulty breathing
• wheezing (bronchospasm)
• hives
• rash
Tell your health care provider if you have:
• swollen glands (neck, armpit, or groin)
• joint pain
• unusual tiredness, weakness, or confusion
• chills
• generally feeling unwell
• leg pain
• shortness of breath
• chest pain
• aching muscles
• muscle weakness
• seizure
• bad stomach ache
• bleeding or bruising more easily than normal
Contact your health care provider right away if you get any symptoms that concern you, even several months after getting the vaccine.
For a more complete list of side effects, ask your health care provider.

What are the ingredients in GARDASIL?
The ingredients are proteins of HPV Types 6, 11, 16, and 18, amorphous aluminum hydroxyphosphate sulfate, yeast protein, sodium chloride, L-histidine, polysorbate 80, sodium borate, and water for injection.
This leaflet is a summary of information about GARDASIL. If you would like more information about GARDASIL or visit your health care provider or visit www.gardasil.com.
Manufactured and Distributed by:
MERCK & CO., Inc.
Whitehouse Station, NJ 08889, USA
Issued June 2010
9883613

HYZAAR® 50-12.5   ℞
(Losartan Potassium-Hydrochlorothiazide Tablets)
HYZAAR® 100-12.5
(Losartan Potassium-Hydrochlorothiazide Tablets)
HYZAAR® 100-25
(Losartan Potassium-Hydrochlorothiazide Tablets)

USE IN PREGNANCY
When used in pregnancy during the second and third trimesters, drugs that act directly on the renin-angiotensin system can cause injury and even death to the developing fetus. When pregnancy is detected, HYZAAR should be discontinued as soon as possible. See WARNINGS, *Fetal/Neonatal Morbidity and Mortality.*

DESCRIPTION
HYZAAR* 50-12.5 (losartan potassium-hydrochlorothiazide), HYZAAR* 100-12.5 (losartan potassium-hydrochlorothiazide) and HYZAAR* 100-25 (losartan potassium-hydrochlorothiazide) combine an angiotensin II receptor (type AT_1) antagonist and a diuretic, hydrochlorothiazide.
Losartan potassium, a non-peptide molecule, is chemically described as 2-butyl-4-chloro-1-[p-(o-1H-tetrazol-5-ylphenyl)benzyl]imidazole-5-methanol monopotassium salt. Its empirical formula is $C_{22}H_{22}ClKN_6O$, and its structural formula is:

Losartan potassium is a white to off-white free-flowing crystalline powder with a molecular weight of 461.01. It is freely soluble in water, soluble in alcohols, and slightly soluble in common organic solvents, such as acetonitrile and methyl ethyl ketone.
Oxidation of the 5-hydroxymethyl group on the imidazole ring results in the active metabolite of losartan.
Hydrochlorothiazide is 6-chloro-3,4-dihydro-2H-1,2,4-benzothiadiazine-7-sulfonamide 1,1-dioxide. Its empirical formula is $C_7H_8ClN_3O_4S_2$ and its structural formula is:

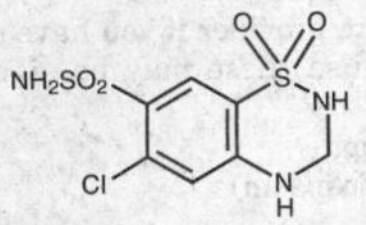

Hydrochlorothiazide is a white, or practically white, crystalline powder with a molecular weight of 297.74, which is slightly soluble in water, but freely soluble in sodium hydroxide solution.
HYZAAR is available for oral administration in three tablet combinations of losartan and hydrochlorothiazide. HYZAAR 50-12.5 contains 50 mg of losartan potassium and 12.5 mg of hydrochlorothiazide. HYZAAR 100-12.5 contains 100 mg of losartan potassium and 12.5 mg of hydrochlorothiazide. HYZAAR 100-25 contains 100 mg of losartan potassium and 25 mg of hydrochlorothiazide. Inactive ingredients are microcrystalline cellulose, lactose hydrous, pregelatinized starch, magnesium stearate, hydroxypropyl cellulose, hypromellose, and titanium dioxide. HYZAAR 50-12.5 and HYZAAR 100-25 also contain D&C yellow No. 10 aluminum lake. HYZAAR 50-12.5, HYZAAR 100-12.5, and HYZAAR 100-25 may also contain carnauba wax.
HYZAAR 50-12.5 contains 4.24 mg (0.108 mEq) of potassium, HYZAAR 100-12.5 contains 8.48 mg (0.216 mEq) of potassium, and HYZAAR 100-25 contains 8.48 mg (0.216 mEq) of potassium.

*Registered trademark of E.I. du Pont de Nemours and Company, Wilmington, Delaware, USA
Copyright © 1995, 2005 Merck Sharp & Dohme Corp., a subsidiary of **Merck & Co., Inc.**
All rights reserved.

CLINICAL PHARMACOLOGY

Mechanism of Action
Angiotensin II [formed from angiotensin I in a reaction catalyzed by angiotensin converting enzyme (ACE, kininase II)], is a potent vasoconstrictor, the primary vasoactive hormone of the renin-angiotensin system and an important component in the pathophysiology of hypertension. It also stimulates aldosterone secretion by the adrenal cortex. Losartan and its principal active metabolite block the vasoconstrictor and aldosterone-secreting effects of angiotensin II by selectively blocking the binding of angiotensin II to the AT_1 receptor found in many tissues (e.g., vascular smooth muscle, adrenal gland). There is also an AT_2 receptor found in many tissues but it is not known to be associated with cardiovascular homeostasis. Both losartan and its principal active metabolite do not exhibit any partial agonist activity at the AT_1 receptor and have much greater affinity (about 1000-fold) for the AT_1 receptor than for the AT_2 receptor. *In vitro* binding studies indicate that losartan is a reversible, competitive inhibitor of the AT_1 receptor. The active metabolite is 10 to 40 times more potent by weight than losartan and appears to be a reversible, non-competitive inhibitor of the AT_1 receptor.
Neither losartan nor its active metabolite inhibits ACE (kininase II, the enzyme that converts angiotensin I to angiotensin II and degrades bradykinin); nor do they bind to or block other hormone receptors or ion channels known to be important in cardiovascular regulation.
Hydrochlorothiazide is a thiazide diuretic. Thiazides affect the renal tubular mechanisms of electrolyte reabsorption, directly increasing excretion of sodium and chloride in approximately equivalent amounts. Indirectly, the diuretic action of hydrochlorothiazide reduces plasma volume, with consequent increases in plasma renin activity, increases in aldosterone secretion, increases in urinary potassium loss, and decreases in serum potassium. The renin-aldosterone link is mediated by angiotensin II, so coadministration of an angiotensin II receptor antagonist tends to reverse the potassium loss associated with these diuretics.
The mechanism of the antihypertensive effect of thiazides is unknown.

Pharmacokinetics
General
Losartan Potassium
Losartan is an orally active agent that undergoes substantial first-pass metabolism by cytochrome P450 enzymes. It is converted, in part, to an active carboxylic acid metabolite that is responsible for most of the angiotensin II receptor antagonism that follows losartan treatment. The terminal half-life of losartan is about 2 hours and of the metabolite is about 6-9 hours. The pharmacokinetics of losartan and its active metabolite are linear with oral losartan doses up to 200 mg and do not change over time. Neither losartan nor its metabolite accumulate in plasma upon repeated once-daily dosing.
Following oral administration, losartan is well absorbed (based on absorption of radiolabeled losartan) and undergoes substantial first-pass metabolism; the systemic bioavailability of losartan is approximately 33%. About 14% of an orally-administered dose of losartan is converted to the active metabolite. Mean peak concentrations of losartan and its active metabolite are reached in 1 hour and in 3-4 hours, respectively. While maximum plasma concentrations of losartan and its active metabolite are approximately equal, the AUC of the metabolite is about 4 times as great as that of losartan. A meal slows absorption of losartan and decreases its C_{max} but has only minor effects on losartan AUC or on the AUC of the metabolite (about 10% decreased).
Both losartan and its active metabolite are highly bound to plasma proteins, primarily albumin, with plasma free fractions of 1.3% and 0.2%, respectively. Plasma protein binding is constant over the concentration range achieved with recommended doses. Studies in rats indicate that losartan crosses the blood-brain barrier poorly, if at all.
Losartan metabolites have been identified in human plasma and urine. In addition to the active carboxylic acid metabolite, several inactive metabolites are formed. Following oral and intravenous administration of ^{14}C-labeled losartan potassium, circulating plasma radioactivity is primarily attributed to losartan and its active metabolite. *In vitro* studies indicate that cytochrome P450 2C9 and 3A4 are involved in the biotransformation of losartan to its metabolites. Minimal conversion of losartan to the active metabolite (less than 1% of the dose compared to 14% of the dose in normal subjects) was seen in about one percent of individuals studied.
The volume of distribution of losartan is about 34 liters and of the active metabolite is about 12 liters. Total plasma clearance of losartan and the active metabolite is about 600 mL/min and 50 mL/min, respectively, with renal clearance of about 75 mL/min and 25 mL/min, respectively. When losartan is administered orally, about 4% of the dose is excreted unchanged in the urine and about 6% is excreted in urine as active metabolite. Biliary excretion contributes to the elimination of losartan and its metabolites. Following oral ^{14}C-labeled losartan, about 35% of radioactivity is recovered in the urine and about 60% in the feces. Following an intravenous dose of ^{14}C-labeled losartan, about 45% of radioactivity is recovered in the urine and 50% in the feces.

Special Populations
Pediatric: Losartan pharmacokinetics have been investigated in patients 6 to 16 years (see PRECAUTIONS, *Pediatric Use*).
Geriatric and Gender: Losartan pharmacokinetics have been investigated in the elderly (65-75 years) and in both genders. Plasma concentrations of losartan and its active metabolite are similar in elderly and young hypertensives. Plasma concentrations of losartan were about twice as high in female hypertensives as male hypertensives, but concentrations of the active metabolite were similar in males and females.
Race: Pharmacokinetic differences due to race have not been studied (see also PRECAUTIONS, *Race* and CLINICAL PHARMACOLOGY, *Pharmacodynamics and Clinical Effects, Losartan Potassium, Reduction in the Risk of Stroke, Race*).
Renal Insufficiency:
Losartan: Following oral administration, plasma concentrations and AUCs of losartan and its active metabolite are increased by 50-90% in patients with mild (creatinine clearance of 50 to 74 mL/min) or moderate (creatinine clearance 30 to 49 mL/min) renal insufficiency. In this study, renal clearance was reduced by 55-85% for both losartan and its active metabolite in patients with mild or moderate renal insufficiency. Neither losartan nor its active metabolite can be removed by hemodialysis.
Hydrochlorothiazide: Following oral administration, the AUC for hydrochlorothiazide is increased by 70 and 700% for patients with mild and moderate renal insufficiency, respectively. In this study, renal clearance of hydrochlorothiazide decreased by 45 and 85% in patients with mild and moderate renal impairment, respectively.
The usual regimens of therapy with HYZAAR may be followed as long as the patient's creatinine clearance is >30 mL/min. In patients with more severe renal impairment, loop diuretics are preferred to thiazides, so HYZAAR is not recommended. (See DOSAGE AND ADMINISTRATION.)
Hepatic Insufficiency: Following oral administration in patients with mild to moderate alcoholic cirrhosis of the liver, plasma concentrations of losartan and its active metabolite were, respectively, 5 times and about 1.7 times those in young male volunteers. Compared to normal subjects, the total plasma clearance of losartan in patients with hepatic insufficiency was about 50% lower, and the oral bioavailability was about 2 times higher. The lower starting dose of losartan recommended for use in patients with hepatic impairment cannot be given using HYZAAR. Its use in such patients as a means of losartan titration is, therefore, not recommended (see DOSAGE AND ADMINISTRATION).

Drug Interactions
Losartan Potassium
Losartan, administered for 12 days, did not affect the pharmacokinetics or pharmacodynamics of a single dose of warfarin. Losartan did not affect the pharmacokinetics of oral or intravenous digoxin. There is no pharmacokinetic interaction between losartan and hydrochlorothiazide. Coadministration of losartan and cimetidine led to an increase of about 18% in AUC of losartan but did not affect the pharmacokinetics of its active metabolite. Coadministration of losartan and phenobarbital led to a reduction of about 20% in the AUC of losartan and that of its active metabolite. A somewhat greater interaction (approximately 40% reduction in the AUC of active metabolite and approximately 30% reduction in the AUC of losartan) has been reported with rifampin. Fluconazole, an inhibitor of cytochrome P450 2C9, decreased the AUC of the active metabolite by approximately 40%, but increased the AUC of losartan by approximately 70% following multiple doses. Conversion of losartan to its active metabolite after intravenous administration is not affected by ketoconazole, an inhibitor of P450 3A4. The AUC of active metabolite following oral losartan was not affected by erythromycin, another inhibitor of P450 3A4, but the AUC of losartan was increased by 30%.
Hydrochlorothiazide
After oral administration of hydrochlorothiazide, diuresis begins within 2 hours, peaks in about 4 hours and lasts about 6 to 12 hours.
Hydrochlorothiazide is not metabolized but is eliminated rapidly by the kidney. When plasma levels have been followed for at least 24 hours, the plasma half-life has been observed to vary between 5.6 and 14.8 hours. At least 61 percent of the oral dose is eliminated unchanged within 24 hours. Hydrochlorothiazide crosses the placental but not the blood-brain barrier and is excreted in breast milk.

Pharmacodynamics and Clinical Effects
Losartan Potassium
Hypertension: Losartan inhibits the pressor effect of angiotensin II (as well as angiotensin I) infusions. A dose of 100 mg inhibits the pressor effect by about 85% at peak with 25-40% inhibition persisting for 24 hours. Removal of the negative feedback of angiotensin II causes a 2- to 3-fold rise in plasma renin activity and consequent rise in angiotensin II plasma concentration in hypertensive patients. Losartan does not affect the response to bradykinin, whereas ACE inhibitors increase the response to bradykinin. Aldosterone plasma concentrations fall following losartan administration. In spite of the effect of losartan on aldosterone secretion, very little effect on serum potassium was observed.
In a single-dose study in normal volunteers, losartan had no effects on glomerular filtration rate, renal plasma flow or filtration fraction. In multiple-dose studies in hypertensive patients, there were no notable effects on systemic or renal prostaglandin concentrations, fasting triglycerides, total cholesterol or HDL-cholesterol or fasting glucose concentrations. There was a small uricosuric effect leading to a minimal decrease in serum uric acid (mean decrease <0.4 mg/dL) during chronic oral administration.
The antihypertensive effects of losartan were demonstrated principally in 4 placebo-controlled, 6- to 12-week trials of dosages from 10 to 150 mg per day in patients with baseline diastolic blood pressures of 95-115. The studies allowed comparisons of two doses (50-100 mg/day) as once-daily or twice-daily regimens, comparisons of peak and trough effects, and comparisons of response by gender, age, and race. Three additional studies examined the antihypertensive effects of losartan and hydrochlorothiazide in combination.
The 4 studies of losartan monotherapy included a total of 1075 patients randomized to several doses of losartan and 334 to placebo. The 10 and 25 mg doses produced some effect at peak (6 hours after dosing) but small and inconsistent trough (24 hour) responses. Doses of 50, 100, and 150 mg once daily gave statistically significant systolic/diastolic mean decreases in blood pressure, compared to placebo in the range of 5.5-10.5/3.5-7.5 mmHg, with the 150 mg dose giving no greater effect than 50-100 mg. Twice-daily dosing at 50-100 mg/day gave consistently larger trough responses than once-daily dosing at the same total dose. Peak (6 hour) effects were uniformly, but moderately larger than trough effects, with the trough to peak ratio for systolic and diastolic responses 50-95% and 60-90%, respectively.
Analysis of age, gender, and race subgroups of patients showed that men and women, and patients over and under 65, had generally similar responses. Losartan was effective in reducing blood pressure regardless of race, although the effect was somewhat less in Black patients (usually a low-renin population).
The effect of losartan is substantially present within one week but in some studies the maximal effect occurred in 3-6 weeks. In long-term follow-up studies (without placebo control) the effect of losartan appeared to be maintained for up to a year. There is no apparent rebound effect after abrupt withdrawal of losartan. There was essentially no change in average heart rate in losartan-treated patients in controlled trials.
Reduction in the Risk of Stroke: The Losartan Intervention For Endpoint reduction in hypertension (LIFE) study was a

multinational, double-blind study comparing losartan and atenolol in 9193 hypertensive patients with ECG-documented left ventricular hypertrophy. Patients with myocardial infarction or stroke within six months prior to randomization were excluded. Patients were randomized to receive once daily losartan 50 mg or atenolol 50 mg. If goal blood pressure (<140/90 mmHg) was not reached, hydrochlorothiazide (12.5 mg) was added first and, if needed, the dose of losartan or atenolol was then increased to 100 mg once daily. If necessary, other antihypertensive treatments (e.g., increase in dose of hydrochlorothiazide therapy to 25 mg or addition of other diuretic therapy, calcium channel blockers, alpha-blockers, or centrally acting agents, but not ACE inhibitors, angiotensin II antagonists, or beta-blockers) were added to the treatment regimen to reach the goal blood pressure.

In efforts to control blood pressure, the patients in both arms of the LIFE study were coadministered hydrochlorothiazide the majority of time they were on study drug (73.9% and 72.4% of days in the losartan and atenolol arms, respectively).

Of the randomized patients, 4963 (54%) were female and 533 (6%) were Black. The mean age was 67 with 5704 (62%) age ≥65. At baseline, 1195 (13%) had diabetes, 1326 (14%) had isolated systolic hypertension, 1469 (16%) had coronary heart disease, and 728 (8%) had cerebrovascular disease. Baseline mean blood pressure was 174/98 mmHg in both treatment groups. The mean length of follow-up was 4.8 years. At the end of study or at the last visit before a primary endpoint, 77% of the group treated with losartan and 73% of the group treated with atenolol were still taking study medication. Of the patients still taking study medication, the mean doses of losartan and atenolol were both about 80 mg/day, and 15% were taking atenolol or losartan as monotherapy, while 77% were also receiving hydrochlorothiazide (at a mean dose of 20 mg/day in each group). Blood pressure reduction measured at trough was similar for both treatment groups but blood pressure was not measured at any other time of the day. At the end of study or at the last visit before a primary endpoint, the mean blood pressures were 144.1/81.3 mmHg for the group treated with losartan and 145.4/80.9 mmHg for the group treated with atenolol [the difference in SBP of 1.3 mmHg was significant (p<0.001), while the difference of 0.4 mmHg in DBP was not significant (p=0.098)].

The primary endpoint was the first occurrence of cardiovascular death, nonfatal stroke, or nonfatal myocardial infarction. Patients with nonfatal events remained in the trial, so that there was also an examination of the first event of each type even if it was not the first event (e.g., a stroke following an initial myocardial infarction would be counted in the analysis of stroke). Treatment with losartan resulted in a 13% reduction (p=0.021) in risk of the primary endpoint compared to the atenolol group; this difference was primarily the result of an effect on fatal and nonfatal stroke. Treatment with losartan reduced the risk of stroke by 25% relative to atenolol (p=0.001).

For additional details on the LIFE study see the label for COZAAR.

Race: In the LIFE study, Black patients treated with atenolol were at lower risk of experiencing the primary composite endpoint compared with Black patients treated with losartan. In the subgroup of Black patients (n=533, 6% of the LIFE study patients), there were 29 primary endpoints among 263 patients on atenolol (11%, 26 per 1000 patient-years) and 46 primary endpoints among 270 patients (17%, 42 per 1000 patient-years) on losartan. This finding could not be explained on the basis of differences in the populations other than race or on any imbalances between treatment groups. In addition, blood pressure reductions in both treatment groups were consistent between Black and non-Black patients. Given the difficulty in interpreting subset differences in large trials, it cannot be known whether the observed difference is the result of chance. However, the LIFE study provides no evidence that the benefits of losartan on reducing the risk of cardiovascular events in hypertensive patients with left ventricular hypertrophy apply to Black patients.

Losartan Potassium-Hydrochlorothiazide
The 3 controlled studies of losartan and hydrochlorothiazide included over 1300 patients assessing the antihypertensive efficacy of various doses of losartan (25, 50 and 100 mg) and concomitant hydrochlorothiazide (6.25, 12.5 and 25 mg). A factorial study compared the combination of losartan/hydrochlorothiazide 50/12.5 mg with its components and placebo. The combination of losartan/hydrochlorothiazide 50/12.5 mg resulted in an approximately additive placebo-adjusted systolic/diastolic response (15.5/9.0 mmHg for the combination compared to 8.5/5.0 mmHg for losartan alone and 7.0/3.0 mmHg for hydrochlorothiazide alone). Another study investigated the dose-response relationship of various doses of hydrochlorothiazide (6.25, 12.5 and 25 mg) or placebo on a background of losartan (50 mg) in patients not adequately controlled (sitting diastolic blood pressure [SiDBP] 93-120 mmHg) on losartan (50 mg) alone. The third study investigated the dose-response relationship of various doses of losartan (25, 50 and 100 mg) or placebo on a background of hydrochlorothiazide (25 mg) in patients not adequately controlled (SiDBP 93-120 mmHg) on hydrochlorothiazide (25 mg) alone. These studies showed an added antihypertensive response at trough (24 hours post-dosing) of hydrochlorothiazide 12.5 or 25 mg added to losartan 50 mg of 5.5/3.5 and 10.0/6.0 mmHg, respectively. Similarly, there was an added antihypertensive response at trough when losartan 50 or 100 mg was added to hydrochlorothiazide 25 mg of 9.0/5.5 and 12.5/6.5 mmHg, respectively. There was no significant effect on heart rate.

There was no difference in response for men and women or in patients over or under 65 years of age. Black patients had a larger response to hydrochlorothiazide than non-Black patients and a smaller response to losartan. The overall response to the combination was similar for Black and non-Black patients.

Severe Hypertension (Sitting Diastolic Blood Pressure [SiDBP] ≥110 mmHg)
The safety and efficacy of HYZAAR as initial therapy for severe hypertension (defined as a mean SiDBP ≥110 mmHg confirmed on 2 separate occasions off all antihypertensive therapy) was studied in a 6-week double-blind, randomized, multicenter study. Patients were randomized to either losartan and hydrochlorothiazide (50-12.5 mg, once daily) or to losartan (50 mg, once daily) and followed for blood pressure response. Patients were titrated at 2-week intervals if their SiDBP did not reach goal (<90 mmHg). Patients on combination therapy were titrated from losartan 50 mg/hydrochlorothiazide 12.5 mg to losartan 50 mg/hydrochlorothiazide 12.5 mg (sham titration to maintain the blind) to losartan 100 mg/hydrochlorothiazide 25 mg. Patients on monotherapy were titrated from losartan 50 mg to losartan 100 mg to losartan 150 mg, as needed. The primary endpoint was a comparison at 4 weeks of patients who achieved goal diastolic blood pressure (trough SiDBP <90 mmHg).

The study enrolled 585 patients, including 264 (45%) females, 124 (21%) blacks, and 21 (4%) ≥65 years of age. The mean blood pressure at baseline for the total population was 171/113 mmHg. The mean age was 53 years. After 4 weeks of therapy, the mean SiDBP was 3.1 mmHg lower and the mean SiSBP was 5.6 mmHg lower in the group treated with HYZAAR. As a result, a greater proportion of the patients on HYZAAR reached the target diastolic blood pressure (17.6% for HYZAAR, 9.4% for losartan; p=0.006). Similar trends were seen when the patients were grouped according to gender, race or age (<, ≥ 65).

After 6 weeks of therapy, more patients who received the combination regimen reached target diastolic blood pressure than those who received the monotherapy regimen (29.8% versus 12.5%).

During the study period, there were no reported cases of syncope in either treatment group. There were 2 (0.6%) and 0 (0.0%) cases of hypotension reported in the group treated with HYZAAR and the group treated with losartan, respectively. The overall pattern of adverse events reported for patients treated with HYZAAR as initial therapy was similar to the adverse event profile for patients treated with losartan as initial therapy. For information on the specific adverse events observed during the study period, see ADVERSE REACTIONS, *Severe Hypertension*.

INDICATIONS AND USAGE
Hypertension
HYZAAR is indicated for the treatment of hypertension. This fixed dose combination is not indicated for initial therapy of hypertension, except when the hypertension is severe enough that the value of achieving prompt blood pressure control exceeds the risk of initiating combination therapy in these patients (see CLINICAL PHARMACOLOGY, *Pharmacodynamics and Clinical Effects*, and DOSAGE AND ADMINISTRATION).

Hypertensive Patients with Left Ventricular Hypertrophy
HYZAAR is indicated to reduce the risk of stroke in patients with hypertension and left ventricular hypertrophy, but there is evidence that this benefit does not apply to Black patients. (See PRECAUTIONS, *Race*, CLINICAL PHARMACOLOGY, *Pharmacodynamics and Clinical Effects*, *Losartan Potassium, Reduction in the Risk of Stroke*, *Race*, and DOSAGE AND ADMINISTRATION.)

CONTRAINDICATIONS

HYZAAR is contraindicated in patients who are hypersensitive to any component of this product.

Because of the hydrochlorothiazide component, this product is contraindicated in patients with anuria or hypersensitivity to other sulfonamide-derived drugs.

WARNINGS
Fetal/Neonatal Morbidity and Mortality
Drugs that act directly on the renin-angiotensin system can cause fetal and neonatal morbidity and death when administered to pregnant women. Several dozen cases have been reported in the world literature in patients who were taking angiotensin converting enzyme inhibitors. When pregnancy is detected, HYZAAR should be discontinued as soon as possible.

The use of drugs that act directly on the renin-angiotensin system during the second and third trimesters of pregnancy has been associated with fetal and neonatal injury, including hypotension, neonatal skull hypoplasia, anuria, reversible or irreversible renal failure, and death. Oligohydramnios has also been reported, presumably resulting from decreased fetal renal function; oligohydramnios in this setting has been associated with fetal limb contractures, craniofacial deformation, and hypoplastic lung development. Prematurity, intrauterine growth retardation, and patent ductus arteriosus have also been reported, although it is not clear whether these occurrences were due to exposure to the drug.

These adverse effects do not appear to have resulted from intrauterine drug exposure that has been limited to the first trimester.

Mothers whose embryos and fetuses are exposed to an angiotensin II receptor antagonist only during the first trimester should be so informed. Nonetheless, when patients become pregnant, physicians should have the patient discontinue the use of HYZAAR as soon as possible.

Rarely (probably less often than once in every thousand pregnancies), no alternative to an angiotensin II receptor antagonist will be found. In these rare cases, the mothers should be apprised of the potential hazards to their fetuses, and serial ultrasound examinations should be performed to assess the intra-amniotic environment.

If oligohydramnios is observed, HYZAAR should be discontinued unless it is considered life-saving for the mother. Contraction stress testing (CST), a non-stress test (NST), or biophysical profiling (BPP) may be appropriate, depending upon the week of pregnancy. Patients and physicians should be aware, however, that oligohydramnios may not appear until after the fetus has sustained irreversible injury.

Infants with histories of *in utero* exposure to an angiotensin II receptor antagonist should be closely observed for hypotension, oliguria, and hyperkalemia. If oliguria occurs, attention should be directed toward support of blood pressure and renal perfusion. Exchange transfusion or dialysis may be required as means of reversing hypotension and/or substituting for disordered renal function.

There was no evidence of teratogenicity in rats or rabbits treated with a maximum losartan potassium dose of 10 mg/kg/day in combination with 2.5 mg/kg/day of hydrochlorothiazide. At these dosages, respective exposures (AUCs) of losartan, its active metabolite, and hydrochlorothiazide in rabbits were approximately 5, 1.5, and 1.0 times those achieved in humans with 100 mg losartan in combination with 25 mg hydrochlorothiazide. AUC values for losartan, its active metabolite and hydrochlorothiazide, extrapolated from data obtained with losartan administered to rats at a dose of 50 mg/kg/day in combination with 12.5 mg/kg/day of hydrochlorothiazide, were approximately 6, 2, and 2 times greater than those achieved in humans with 100 mg of losartan in combination with 25 mg of hydrochlorothiazide. Fetal toxicity in rats, as evidenced by a slight increase in supernumerary ribs, was observed when females were treated prior to and throughout gestation with 10 mg/kg/day losartan in combination with 2.5 mg/kg/day hydrochlorothiazide. As also observed in studies with losartan alone, adverse fetal and neonatal effects, including decreased body weight, renal toxicity, and mortality, occurred when pregnant rats were treated during late gestation and/or lactation with 50 mg/kg/day losartan in combination with 12.5 mg/kg/day hydrochlorothiazide. Respective AUCs for losartan, its active metabolite and hydrochlorothiazide at these dosages in rats were approximately 35, 10 and 10 times greater than those achieved in humans with the administration of 100 mg of losartan in combination with 25 mg hydrochlorothiazide. When hydrochlorothiazide was administered without losartan to pregnant mice and rats during their respective periods of major organogenesis, at doses up to 3000 and 1000 mg/kg/day, respectively, there was no evidence of harm to the fetus. Thiazides cross the placental barrier and appear in cord blood. There is a risk of fetal or neonatal jaundice, thrombocytopenia, and possibly other adverse reactions that have occurred in adults.

Hypotension — Volume-Depleted Patients
In patients who are intravascularly volume-depleted (e.g., those treated with diuretics), symptomatic hypotension may occur after initiation of therapy with HYZAAR. This condition should be corrected prior to administration of HYZAAR (see DOSAGE AND ADMINISTRATION).

Impaired Hepatic Function
Losartan Potassium-Hydrochlorothiazide
HYZAAR is not recommended for patients with hepatic impairment who require titration with losartan. The lower

starting dose of losartan recommended for use in patients with hepatic impairment cannot be given using HYZAAR.

Hydrochlorothiazide

Thiazides should be used with caution in patients with impaired hepatic function or progressive liver disease, since minor alterations of fluid and electrolyte balance may precipitate hepatic coma.

Hypersensitivity Reaction

Hypersensitivity reactions to hydrochlorothiazide may occur in patients with or without a history of allergy or bronchial asthma, but are more likely in patients with such a history.

Systemic Lupus Erythematosus

Thiazide diuretics have been reported to cause exacerbation or activation of systemic lupus erythematosus.

Lithium Interaction

Lithium generally should not be given with thiazides (see PRECAUTIONS, *Drug Interactions, Hydrochlorothiazide, Lithium*).

PRECAUTIONS

General

Hypersensitivity: Angioedema. See ADVERSE REACTIONS, *Post-Marketing Experience*.

Losartan Potassium-Hydrochlorothiazide

In double-blind clinical trials of various doses of losartan potassium and hydrochlorothiazide, the incidence of hypertensive patients who developed hypokalemia (serum potassium <3.5 mEq/L) was 6.7% versus 3.5% for placebo; the incidence of hyperkalemia (serum potassium >5.7 mEq/L) was 0.4%. No patient discontinued due to increases or decreases in serum potassium. The mean decrease in serum potassium in patients treated with various doses of losartan and hydrochlorothiazide was 0.123 mEq/L. In patients treated with various doses of losartan and hydrochlorothiazide, there was also a dose-related decrease in the hypokalemic response to hydrochlorothiazide as the dose of losartan was increased, as well as a dose-related decrease in serum uric acid with increasing doses of losartan.

Hydrochlorothiazide

Periodic determination of serum electrolytes to detect possible electrolyte imbalance should be performed at appropriate intervals.

All patients receiving thiazide therapy should be observed for clinical signs of fluid or electrolyte imbalance: hyponatremia, hypochloremic alkalosis, and hypokalemia. Serum and urine electrolyte determinations are particularly important when the patient is vomiting excessively or receiving parenteral fluids. Warning signs or symptoms of fluid and electrolyte imbalance, irrespective of cause, include dryness of mouth, thirst, weakness, lethargy, drowsiness, restlessness, confusion, seizures, muscle pains or cramps, muscular fatigue, hypotension, oliguria, tachycardia, and gastrointestinal disturbances such as nausea and vomiting.

Hypokalemia may develop, especially with brisk diuresis, when severe cirrhosis is present, or after prolonged therapy. Interference with adequate oral electrolyte intake will also contribute to hypokalemia. Hypokalemia may cause cardiac arrhythmia and may also sensitize or exaggerate the response of the heart to the toxic effects of digitalis (e.g., increased ventricular irritability).

Although any chloride deficit is generally mild and usually does not require specific treatment except under extraordinary circumstances (as in liver disease or renal disease), chloride replacement may be required in the treatment of metabolic alkalosis.

Dilutional hyponatremia may occur in edematous patients in hot weather; appropriate therapy is water restriction, rather than administration of salt except in rare instances when the hyponatremia is life-threatening. In actual salt depletion, appropriate replacement is the therapy of choice.

Hyperuricemia may occur or frank gout may be precipitated in certain patients receiving thiazide therapy. Because losartan decreases uric acid, losartan in combination with hydrochlorothiazide attenuates the diuretic-induced hyperuricemia.

In diabetic patients, dosage adjustments of insulin or oral hypoglycemic agents may be required. Hyperglycemia may occur with thiazide diuretics. Thus latent diabetes mellitus may become manifest during thiazide therapy.

The antihypertensive effects of the drug may be enhanced in the postsympathectomy patient.

If progressive renal impairment becomes evident, consider withholding or discontinuing diuretic therapy.

Thiazides have been shown to increase the urinary excretion of magnesium; this may result in hypomagnesemia.

Thiazides may decrease urinary calcium excretion. Thiazides may cause intermittent and slight elevation of serum calcium in the absence of known disorders of calcium metabolism. Marked hypercalcemia may be evidence of hidden hyperparathyroidism. Thiazides should be discontinued before carrying out tests for parathyroid function.

Increases in cholesterol and triglyceride levels may be associated with thiazide diuretic therapy.

Impaired Renal Function

As a consequence of inhibiting the renin-angiotensin-aldosterone system, changes in renal function have been reported in susceptible individuals treated with losartan; in some patients, these changes in renal function were reversible upon discontinuation of therapy.

In patients whose renal function may depend on the activity of the renin-angiotensin-aldosterone system (e.g., patients with severe congestive heart failure), treatment with angiotensin converting enzyme inhibitors has been associated with oliguria and/or progressive azotemia and (rarely) with acute renal failure and/or death. Similar outcomes have been reported with losartan.

In studies of ACE inhibitors in patients with unilateral or bilateral renal artery stenosis, increases in serum creatinine or BUN have been reported. Similar effects have been reported with losartan; in some patients, these effects were reversible upon discontinuation of therapy.

Thiazides should be used with caution in severe renal disease. In patients with renal disease, thiazides may precipitate azotemia. Cumulative effects of the drug may develop in patients with impaired renal function.

Information for Patients

Pregnancy: Female patients of childbearing age should be told about the consequences of second- and third-trimester exposure to drugs that act on the renin-angiotensin system, and they should also be told that these consequences do not appear to have resulted from intrauterine drug exposure that has been limited to the first trimester. These patients should be asked to report pregnancies to their physicians as soon as possible.

Symptomatic Hypotension: A patient receiving HYZAAR should be cautioned that lightheadedness can occur, especially during the first days of therapy, and that it should be reported to the prescribing physician. The patients should be told that if syncope occurs, HYZAAR should be discontinued until the physician has been consulted.

All patients should be cautioned that inadequate fluid intake, excessive perspiration, diarrhea, or vomiting can lead to an excessive fall in blood pressure, with the same consequences of lightheadedness and possible syncope.

Potassium Supplements: A patient receiving HYZAAR should be told not to use potassium supplements or salt substitutes containing potassium without consulting the prescribing physician (see PRECAUTIONS, *Drug Interactions, Losartan Potassium*).

Drug Interactions

Losartan Potassium

No significant drug-drug pharmacokinetic interactions have been found in interaction studies with hydrochlorothiazide, digoxin, warfarin, cimetidine and phenobarbital. Rifampin, an inducer of drug metabolism, decreased the concentrations of losartan and its active metabolite. (See CLINICAL PHARMACOLOGY, *Drug Interactions*.) In humans, two inhibitors of P450 3A4 have been studied. Ketoconazole did not affect the conversion of losartan to the active metabolite after intravenous administration of losartan, and erythromycin had no clinically significant effect after oral administration. Fluconazole, an inhibitor of P450 2C9, decreased active metabolite concentration and increased losartan concentration. The pharmacodynamic consequences of concomitant use of losartan and inhibitors of P450 2C9 have not been examined. Subjects who do not metabolize losartan to active metabolite have been shown to have a specific, rare defect in cytochrome P450 2C9. These data suggest that the conversion of losartan to its active metabolite is mediated primarily by P450 2C9 and not P450 3A4.

As with other drugs that block angiotensin II or its effects, concomitant use of potassium-sparing diuretics (e.g., spironolactone, triamterene, amiloride), potassium supplements, or salt substitutes containing potassium may lead to increases in serum potassium (see PRECAUTIONS, *Information for Patients, Potassium Supplements*).

Lithium: As with other drugs which affect the excretion of sodium, lithium excretion may be reduced. Therefore, serum lithium levels should be monitored carefully if lithium salts are to be co-administered with angiotensin II receptor antagonists.

Non-Steroidal Anti-Inflammatory Drugs (NSAIDS) Including Selective Cyclooxygenase-2 Inhibitors (COX-2 Inhibitors): In patients who are elderly, volume-depleted (including those on diuretic therapy), or with compromised renal function, co-administration of NSAIDS, including selective COX-2 inhibitors, with angiotensin II receptor antagonists (including losartan) may result in deterioration of renal function, including possible acute renal failure. These effects are usually reversible. Monitor renal function periodically in patients receiving losartan and NSAID therapy.

The antihypertensive effect of angiotensin II receptor antagonists, including losartan, may be attenuated by NSAIDS, including selective COX-2 inhibitors.

Hydrochlorothiazide

When administered concurrently, the following drugs may interact with thiazide diuretics:

Alcohol, barbiturates, or narcotics—potentiation of orthostatic hypotension may occur.

Antidiabetic drugs (oral agents and insulin)—dosage adjustment of the antidiabetic drug may be required.

Other antihypertensive drugs—additive effect or potentiation.

Cholestyramine and colestipol resins—Absorption of hydrochlorothiazide is impaired in the presence of anionic exchange resins. Single doses of either cholestyramine or colestipol resins bind the hydrochlorothiazide and reduce its absorption from the gastrointestinal tract by up to 85 and 43 percent, respectively.

Corticosteroids, ACTH—intensified electrolyte depletion, particularly hypokalemia.

Pressor amines (e.g., norepinephrine)—possible decreased response to pressor amines but not sufficient to preclude their use.

Skeletal muscle relaxants, nondepolarizing (e.g., tubocurarine)—possible increased responsiveness to the muscle relaxant.

Lithium—should not generally be given with diuretics. Diuretic agents reduce the renal clearance of lithium and add a high risk of lithium toxicity. Refer to the package insert for lithium preparations before use of such preparations with HYZAAR.

Non-Steroidal Anti-Inflammatory Drugs (NSAIDS) Including Selective Cyclooxygenase-2 Inhibitors (COX-2 Inhibitors)—The administration of a non-steroidal anti-inflammatory agent, including a selective cyclooxygenase-2 inhibitor, can reduce the diuretic, natriuretic, and antihypertensive effects of loop, potassium-sparing and thiazide diuretics. Therefore, when HYZAAR and non-steroidal anti-inflammatory agents, including selective cyclooxygenase-2 inhibitors, are used concomitantly, the patient should be observed closely to determine if the desired effect of the diuretic is obtained.

In patients receiving diuretic therapy, co-administration of NSAIDs with angiotensin receptor blockers, including losartan, may result in deterioration of renal function, including possible acute renal failure. These effects are usuallly reversible. Monitor renal function periodically in patients receiving hydrochlorothiazide, losartan, and NSAID therapy.

Carcinogenesis, Mutagenesis, Impairment of Fertility

Losartan Potassium-Hydrochlorothiazide

No carcinogenicity studies have been conducted with the losartan potassium-hydrochlorothiazide combination.

Losartan potassium-hydrochlorothiazide when tested at a weight ratio of 4:1, was negative in the Ames microbial mutagenesis assay and the V-79 Chinese hamster lung cell mutagenesis assay. In addition, there was no evidence of direct genotoxicity in the *in vitro* alkaline elution assay in rat hepatocytes and *in vitro* chromosomal aberration assay in Chinese hamster ovary cells at noncytotoxic concentrations.

Losartan potassium, coadministered with hydrochlorothiazide, had no effect on the fertility or mating behavior of male rats at dosages up to 135 mg/kg/day of losartan and 33.75 mg/kg/day of hydrochlorothiazide. These dosages have been shown to provide respective systemic exposures (AUCs) for losartan, its active metabolite and hydrochlorothiazide that are approximately 60, 60 and 30 times greater than those achieved in humans with 100 mg of losartan potassium in combination with 25 mg of hydrochlorothiazide. In female rats, however, the coadministration of doses as low as 10 mg/kg/day of losartan and 2.5 mg/kg/day of hydrochlorothiazide was associated with slight but statistically significant decreases in fecundity and fertility indices. AUC values for losartan, its active metabolite and hydrochlorothiazide, extrapolated from data obtained with losartan administered to rats at a dose of 50 mg/kg/day in combination with 12.5 mg/kg/day of hydrochlorothiazide, were approximately 6, 2, and 2 times greater than those achieved in humans with 100 mg of losartan in combination with 25 mg of hydrochlorothiazide.

Losartan Potassium

Losartan potassium was not carcinogenic when administered at maximally tolerated dosages to rats and mice for 105 and 92 weeks, respectively. Female rats given the highest dose (270 mg/kg/day) had a slightly higher incidence of pancreatic acinar adenoma. The maximally tolerated dosages (270 mg/kg/day in rats, 200 mg/kg/day in mice) provided systemic exposures for losartan and its pharmacologically active metabolite that were approximately 160 and 90 times (rats) and 30 and 15 times (mice) the exposure of a 50 kg human given 100 mg per day.

Losartan potassium was negative in the microbial mutagenesis and V-79 mammalian cell mutagenesis assays and in the *in vitro* alkaline elution and *in vitro* and *in vivo* chromosomal aberration assays. In addition, the active metabolite showed no evidence of genotoxicity in the microbial mutagenesis, *in vitro* alkaline elution, and *in vitro* chromosomal aberration assays.

Fertility and reproductive performance were not affected in studies with male rats given oral doses of losartan potassium up to approximately 150 mg/kg/day. The administration of toxic dosage levels in females (300/200 mg/kg/day) was associated with a significant (p<0.05) decrease in the number of corpora lutea/female, implants/female, and live fetuses/female at C-section. At 100 mg/kg/day only a decrease in the number of corpora lutea/female was observed. The relationship of these findings to drug-treatment is uncertain since there was no effect at these dosage levels on implants/pregnant female, percent post-implantation loss, or live animals/litter at parturition. In nonpregnant rats dosed at 135 mg/kg/day for 7 days, systemic exposure (AUCs) for losartan and its active metabolite were approximately 66 and 26 times the exposure achieved in man at the maximum recommended human daily dosage (100 mg).

Hydrochlorothiazide

Two-year feeding studies in mice and rats conducted under the auspices of the National Toxicology Program (NTP) uncovered no evidence of a carcinogenic potential of hydrochlorothiazide in female mice (at doses of up to approximately 600 mg/kg/day) or in male and female rats (at doses of up to approximately 100 mg/kg/day). The NTP, however, found equivocal evidence for hepatocarcinogenicity in male mice.

Hydrochlorothiazide was not genotoxic *in vitro* in the Ames mutagenicity assay of *Salmonella typhimurium* strains TA 98, TA 100, TA 1535, TA 1537, and TA 1538 and in the Chinese Hamster Ovary (CHO) test for chromosomal aberrations, or *in vivo* in assays using mouse germinal cell chromosomes, Chinese hamster bone marrow chromosomes, and the *Drosophila* sex-linked recessive lethal trait gene. Positive test results were obtained only in the *in vitro* CHO Sister Chromatid Exchange (clastogenicity) and in the Mouse Lymphoma Cell (mutagenicity) assays, using concentrations of hydrochlorothiazide from 43 to 1300 μg/mL, and in the *Aspergillus nidulans* non-disjunction assay at an unspecified concentration.

Hydrochlorothiazide had no adverse effects on the fertility of mice and rats of either sex in studies wherein these species were exposed, via their diet, to doses of up to 100 and 4 mg/kg, respectively, prior to mating and throughout gestation.

Pregnancy

Pregnancy Categories C (first trimester) and D (second and third trimesters). See WARNINGS, *Fetal/Neonatal Morbidity and Mortality*.

Nursing Mothers

It is not known whether losartan is excreted in human milk, but significant levels of losartan and its active metabolite were shown to be present in rat milk. Thiazides appear in human milk. Because of the potential for adverse effects on the nursing infant, a decision should be made whether to discontinue nursing or discontinue the drug, taking into account the importance of the drug to the mother.

Pediatric Use

Safety and effectiveness of HYZAAR in pediatric patients have not been established.

Geriatric Use

In a controlled clinical study for the reduction in the combined risk of cardiovascular death, stroke and myocardial infarction in hypertensive patients with left ventricular hypertrophy, 2857 patients (62%) were 65 years and over, while 808 patients (18%) were 75 years and over. In an effort to control blood pressure in this study, patients were coadministered losartan and hydrochlorothiazide 74% of the total time they were on study drug. No overall differences in effectiveness were observed between these patients and younger patients. Adverse events were somewhat more frequent in the elderly compared to non-elderly patients for both the losartan-hydrochlorothiazide and the control groups (see CLINICAL PHARMACOLOGY, *Special Populations*).

Race

In the LIFE study, Black patients with hypertension and left ventricular hypertrophy had a lower risk of stroke on atenolol than on losartan (both cotreated with hydrochlorothiazide in the majority of patients). Given the difficulty in interpreting subset differences in large trials, it cannot be known whether the observed difference is the result of chance. However, the LIFE study does not provide evidence that the benefits of losartan on reducing the risk of cardiovascular events in hypertensive patients with left ventricular hypertrophy apply to Black patients. (See CLINICAL PHARMACOLOGY, *Pharmacodynamics and Clinical Effects; Losartan Potassium, Reduction in the Risk of Stroke*.)

ADVERSE REACTIONS

Losartan potassium-hydrochlorothiazide has been evaluated for safety in 858 patients treated for essential hypertension and 3889 patients treated for hypertension and left ventricular hypertrophy. In clinical trials with losartan potassium-hydrochlorothiazide, no adverse experiences peculiar to this combination have been observed. Adverse experiences have been limited to those that were reported previously with losartan potassium and/or hydrochlorothiazide. The overall incidence of adverse experiences reported with the combination was comparable to placebo.

In general, treatment with losartan potassium-hydrochlorothiazide was well tolerated. For the most part, adverse experiences have been mild and transient in nature and have not required discontinuation of therapy. In controlled clinical trials, discontinuation of therapy due to clinical adverse experiences was required in only 2.8% and 2.3% of patients treated with the combination and placebo, respectively.

In these double-blind controlled clinical trials, the following adverse experiences reported with losartan-hydrochlorothiazide occurred in ≥1 percent of patients, and more often on drug than placebo, regardless of drug relationship:

	Losartan Potassium-Hydrochlorothiazide (n=858)	Placebo (n=173)
Body as a Whole		
Abdominal pain	1.2	0.6
Edema/swelling	1.3	1.2
Cardiovascular		
Palpitation	1.4	0.0
Musculoskeletal		
Back pain	2.1	0.6
Nervous/Psychiatric		
Dizziness	5.7	2.9
Respiratory		
Cough	2.6	2.3
Sinusitis	1.2	0.6
Upper respiratory infection	6.1	4.6
Skin		
Rash	1.4	0.0

The following adverse events were also reported at a rate of 1% or greater, but were as, or more, common in the placebo group in studies of essential hypertension: asthenia/fatigue, diarrhea, nausea, headache, bronchitis, pharyngitis.

Adverse events occurred at about the same rates in men and women. Adverse events were somewhat more frequent in the elderly compared to non-elderly patients and somewhat more frequent in Blacks compared to non-Blacks for both the losartan-hydrochlorothiazide and the control groups.

A patient with known hypersensitivity to aspirin and penicillin, when treated with losartan potassium, was withdrawn from study due to swelling of the lips and eyelids and facial rash, reported as angioedema, which returned to normal 5 days after therapy was discontinued.

Superficial peeling of palms and hemolysis were reported in one subject treated with losartan potassium.

Losartan Potassium

Other adverse experiences that have been reported with losartan, without regard to causality, are listed below:

Body as a Whole: chest pain, facial edema, fever, orthostatic effects, syncope; *Cardiovascular:* angina pectoris, arrhythmias including atrial fibrillation, sinus bradycardia, tachycardia, ventricular tachycardia and ventricular fibrillation, CVA, hypotension, myocardial infarction, second degree AV block; *Digestive:* anorexia, constipation, dental pain, dry mouth, dyspepsia, flatulence, gastritis, vomiting; *General disorders and administration site conditions:* malaise; *Hematologic:* anemia; *Metabolic:* gout; *Musculoskeletal:* arm pain, arthralgia, arthritis, fibromyalgia, hip pain, joint swelling, knee pain, leg pain, muscle cramps, muscle weakness, musculoskeletal pain, myalgia, shoulder pain, stiffness; *Nervous System/Psychiatric:* anxiety, anxiety disorder, ataxia, confusion, depression, dream abnormality, hypesthesia, insomnia, libido decreased, memory impairment, migraine, nervousness, panic disorder, paresthesia, peripheral neuropathy, sleep disorder, somnolence, tremor, vertigo; *Respiratory:* dyspnea, epistaxis, nasal congestion, pharyngeal discomfort, respiratory congestion, rhinitis, sinus disorder; *Skin:* alopecia, dermatitis, dry skin, ecchymosis, erythema, flushing, photosensitivity, pruritus, sweating, urticaria; *Special Senses:* blurred vision, burning/stinging in the eye, conjunctivitis, decrease in visual acuity, taste perversion, tinnitus; *Urogenital:* impotence, nocturia, urinary frequency, urinary tract infection.

Hydrochlorothiazide

Other adverse experiences that have been reported with hydrochlorothiazide, without regard to causality, are listed below:

Body as a Whole: weakness; *Digestive:* pancreatitis, jaundice (intrahepatic cholestatic jaundice), sialadenitis, cramping, gastric irritation; *Hematologic:* aplastic anemia, agranulocytosis, leukopenia, hemolytic anemia, thrombocytopenia; *Hypersensitivity:* purpura, photosensitivity, urticaria, necrotizing angiitis (vasculitis and cutaneous vasculitis), fever, respiratory distress including pneumonitis and pulmonary edema; *Metabolic:* hyperglycemia, glycosuria, hyperuricemia; *Musculoskeletal:* muscle spasm; *Nervous System/Psychiatric:* restlessness; *Renal:* renal failure, renal dysfunction, interstitial nephritis; *Skin:* erythema multiforme including Stevens-Johnson syndrome, exfoliative dermatitis including toxic epidermal necrolysis; *Special Senses:* transient blurred vision, xanthopsia.

Persistent dry cough (with an incidence of a few percent) has been associated with ACE-inhibitor use and in practice can be a cause of discontinuation of ACE-inhibitor therapy. Two prospective, parallel-group, double-blind, randomized, controlled trials were conducted to assess the effects of losartan on the incidence of cough in hypertensive patients who had experienced cough while receiving ACE-inhibitor therapy. Patients who had typical ACE-inhibitor cough when challenged with lisinopril, whose cough disappeared on placebo, were randomized to losartan 50 mg, lisinopril 20 mg, or either placebo (one study, n=97) or 25 mg hydrochlorothiazide (n=135). The double-blind treatment period lasted up to 8 weeks. The incidence of cough is shown below.

Study 1[†]	HCTZ	Losartan	Lisinopril
Cough	25%	17%	69%
Study 2[††]	Placebo	Losartan	Lisinopril
Cough	35%	29%	62%

[†] Demographics = (89% caucasian, 64% female)
[††] Demographics = (90% caucasian, 51% female)

These studies demonstrate that the incidence of cough associated with losartan therapy, in a population that all had cough associated with ACE-inhibitor therapy, is similar to that associated with hydrochlorothiazide or placebo therapy.

Cases of cough, including positive re-challenges, have been reported with the use of losartan in post-marketing experience.

Severe Hypertension: In a clinical study in patients with severe hypertension (SiDBP ≥110 mmHg), the overall pattern of adverse events reported through six weeks of follow-up was similar in patients treated with HYZAAR as initial therapy and in patients treated with losartan as initial therapy. There were no reported cases of syncope in either treatment group. There were 2 (0.6%) and 0 (0.0%) cases of hypotension reported in the group treated with HYZAAR and the group treated with losartan, respectively. There were 3 (0.8%) and 2 (1.2%) cases of increased serum creatinine (>0.5 mg/dL) in the group treated with HYZAAR and the group treated with losartan, respectively, during the same time period. (See CLINICAL PHARMACOLOGY, *Pharmacodynamics and Clinical Effects, Severe Hypertension.*)

Post-Marketing Experience

The following additional adverse reactions have been reported in post-marketing experience:

Digestive: Hepatitis has been reported rarely in patients treated with losartan.

Hemic: Thrombocytopenia.

Hypersensitivity: Angioedema, including swelling of the larynx and glottis, causing airway obstruction and/or swelling of the face, lips, pharynx, and/or tongue has been reported rarely in patients treated with losartan; some of these patients previously experienced angioedema with other drugs including ACE inhibitors. Vasculitis, including Henoch-Schönlein purpura, has been reported with losartan. Anaphylactic reactions have been reported.

Metabolic and Nutrition: Hyperkalemia, hyponatremia have been reported with losartan.

Musculoskeletal: Rare cases of rhabdomyolysis have been reported in patients receiving angiotensin II receptor blockers.

Respiratory: Dry cough (see above) has been reported with losartan.

Skin: Erythroderma has been reported with losartan.

Laboratory Test Findings

In controlled clinical trials, clinically important changes in standard laboratory parameters were rarely associated with administration of HYZAAR.

Creatinine, Blood Urea Nitrogen: Minor increases in blood urea nitrogen (BUN) or serum creatinine were observed in 0.6 and 0.8 percent, respectively, of patients with essential hypertension treated with HYZAAR alone. No patient discontinued taking HYZAAR due to increased BUN. One patient discontinued taking HYZAAR due to a minor increase in serum creatinine.

Hemoglobin and Hematocrit: Small decreases in hemoglobin and hematocrit (mean decreases of approximately 0.14 grams percent and 0.72 volume percent, respectively) occurred frequently in patients treated with HYZAAR alone, but were rarely of clinical importance. No patients were discontinued due to anemia.

Liver Function Tests: Occasional elevations of liver enzymes and/or serum bilirubin have occurred. In patients with essential hypertension treated with HYZAAR alone, no patients were discontinued due to these laboratory adverse experiences.

Serum Electrolytes: See PRECAUTIONS.

OVERDOSAGE

Losartan Potassium

Significant lethality was observed in mice and rats after oral administration of 1000 mg/kg and 2000 mg/kg, respectively, about 44 and 170 times the maximum recommended human dose on a mg/m^2 basis.

Limited data are available in regard to overdosage in humans. The most likely manifestation of overdosage would be hypotension and tachycardia; bradycardia could occur from parasympathetic (vagal) stimulation. If symptomatic hypotension should occur, supportive treatment should be instituted.

Neither losartan nor its active metabolite can be removed by hemodialysis.

Hydrochlorothiazide

The oral LD$_{50}$ of hydrochlorothiazide is greater than 10 g/kg in both mice and rats. The most common signs and symptoms observed are those caused by electrolyte depletion (hypokalemia, hypochloremia, hyponatremia) and dehydration resulting from excessive diuresis. If digitalis has also been administered, hypokalemia may accentuate cardiac arrhythmias. The degree to which hydrochlorothiazide is removed by hemodialysis has not been established.

DOSAGE AND ADMINISTRATION

Hypertension

Dosing must be individualized. The usual starting dose of losartan is 50 mg once daily, with 25 mg recommended for patients with intravascular volume depletion (e.g., patients treated with diuretics) (see WARNINGS, *Hypotension — Volume-Depleted Patients*) and patients with a history of hepatic impairment (see WARNINGS, *Impaired Hepatic Function*). Losartan can be administered once or twice daily at total daily doses of 25 to 100 mg. If the antihypertensive effect measured at trough using once-a-day dosing is inadequate, a twice-a-day regimen at the same total daily dose or an increase in dose may give a more satisfactory response. Hydrochlorothiazide is effective in doses of 12.5 to 50 mg once daily and can be given at doses of 12.5 to 25 mg as HYZAAR.

To minimize dose-independent side effects, it is usually appropriate to begin combination therapy only after a patient has failed to achieve the desired effect with monotherapy. The side effects (see WARNINGS) of losartan are generally rare and apparently independent of dose; those of hydrochlorothiazide are a mixture of dose-dependent (primarily hypokalemia) and dose-independent phenomena (e.g., pancreatitis), the former much more common than the latter. Therapy with any combination of losartan and hydrochlorothiazide will be associated with both sets of dose-independent side effects.

Replacement Therapy: The combination may be substituted for the titrated components.

Dose Titration by Clinical Effect: A patient whose blood pressure is not adequately controlled with losartan monotherapy (see above) or hydrochlorothiazide alone, may be switched to HYZAAR 50-12.5 (losartan 50 mg/ hydrochlorothiazide 12.5 mg) once daily. If blood pressure remains uncontrolled after about 3 weeks of therapy, the dose may be increased to two tablets of HYZAAR 50-12.5

once daily or one tablet of HYZAAR 100-25 (losartan 100 mg/hydrochlorothiazide 25 mg) once daily. A patient whose blood pressure is not adequately controlled with losartan 100 mg monotherapy (see above) may be switched to HYZAAR 100-12.5 once daily. If blood pressure remains uncontrolled after about 3 weeks of therapy, the dose may be increased to two tablets of HYZAAR 50-12.5 once daily or one tablet of HYZAAR 100-25 (losartan 100 mg/ hydrochlorothiazide 25 mg) once daily.

A patient whose blood pressure is inadequately controlled by 25 mg once daily of hydrochlorothiazide, or is controlled but who experiences hypokalemia with this regimen, may be switched to HYZAAR 50-12.5 (losartan 50 mg/ hydrochlorothiazide 12.5 mg) once daily, reducing the dose of hydrochlorothiazide without reducing the overall expected antihypertensive response. The clinical response to HYZAAR 50-12.5 should be subsequently evaluated, and if blood pressure remains uncontrolled after about 3 weeks of therapy, the dose may be increased to two tablets of HYZAAR 50-12.5 once daily or one tablet of HYZAAR 100-25 (losartan 100 mg/hydrochlorothiazide 25 mg) once daily.

The usual dose of HYZAAR is one tablet of HYZAAR 50-12.5 once daily. More than two tablets of HYZAAR 50-12.5 once daily or more than one tablet of HYZAAR 100-25 once daily is not recommended. The maximal antihypertensive effect is attained about 3 weeks after initiation of therapy.

Use in Patients with Renal Impairment: The usual regimens of therapy with HYZAAR may be followed as long as the patient's creatinine clearance is >30 mL/min. In patients with more severe renal impairment, loop diuretics are preferred to thiazides, so HYZAAR is not recommended.

Patients with Hepatic Impairment: HYZAAR is not recommended for titration in patients with hepatic impairment (see WARNINGS, *Impaired Hepatic Function*) because the appropriate 25 mg starting dose of losartan cannot be given.

Severe Hypertension

The starting dose of HYZAAR for initial treatment of severe hypertension is one tablet of HYZAAR 50-12.5 once daily (see CLINICAL PHARMACOLOGY, *Pharmacodynamics and Clinical Effects*). For patients who do not respond adequately to HYZAAR 50-12.5 after 2 to 4 weeks of therapy, the dosage may be increased to one tablet of HYZAAR 100-25 once daily. The maximum dose is one tablet of HYZAAR 100-25 once daily. HYZAAR is not recommended as initial therapy in patients with hepatic impairment (see WARNINGS, *Impaired Hepatic Function*) because the appropriate 25 mg starting dose of losartan cannot be given. It is also not recommended for use as initial therapy in patients with intravascular volume depletion (e.g., patients treated with diuretics, see WARNINGS, *Hypotension — Volume-Depleted Patients*).

Hypertensive Patients with Left Ventricular Hypertrophy

Treatment should be initiated with COZAAR 50 mg once daily. Hydrochlorothiazide 12.5 mg should be added or HYZAAR 50-12.5 substituted if the blood pressure reduction is inadequate. If additional blood pressure reduction is needed, COZAAR 100 mg and hydrochlorothiazide 12.5 mg or HYZAAR 100-12.5 may be substituted, followed by COZAAR 100 mg and hydrochlorothiazide 25 mg or HYZAAR 100-25. For further blood pressure reduction other antihypertensives should be added (see CLINICAL PHARMACOLOGY, *Pharmacodynamics and Clinical Effects, Losartan Potassium, Reduction in the Risk of Stroke*).

HYZAAR may be administered with other antihypertensive agents.

HYZAAR may be administered with or without food.

PATIENT INFORMATION

HYZAAR®

("HY-zar")

(losartan potassium-hydrochlorothiazide tablets)

50-12.5 mg, 100-12.5 mg, 100-25 mg

Rx only

Read the Patient Information that comes with HYZAAR* before you start taking it and each time you get a refill. There may be new information. This leaflet does not take the place of talking with your doctor about your condition and treatment.

* Registered trademark of E. I. du Pont de Nemours and Company, Wilmington, Delaware, USA

What is the most important information I should know about HYZAAR?

Do not take HYZAAR if you are pregnant or plan to become pregnant. HYZAAR can harm your unborn baby causing injury and even death. Stop taking HYZAAR if you become pregnant and call your doctor right away. If you plan to become pregnant, talk to your doctor about other treatment options before taking HYZAAR.

What is HYZAAR?

HYZAAR contains 2 prescription medicines, an angiotensin receptor blocker (ARB) and a diuretic (water pill). It is used to:

• lower high blood pressure (hypertension). HYZAAR is not usually the first medicine used to treat high blood pressure.

• lower the chance of stroke in patients with high blood pressure and a heart problem called left ventricular hypertrophy (LVH). HYZAAR may not help Black patients with this problem.

HYZAAR has not been studied in children less than 18 years old.

High Blood Pressure (hypertension) Blood pressure is the force in your blood vessels when your heart beats and when your heart rests. You have high blood pressure when the force is too much. The losartan ingredient in HYZAAR can help your blood vessels relax so your blood pressure is lower. The hydrochlorothiazide ingredient in HYZAAR works by making your kidneys pass more water and salt.

Left Ventricular Hypertrophy (LVH) is an enlargement of the walls of the left chamber of the heart (the heart's main pumping chamber). LVH can happen from several things. High blood pressure is the most common cause of LVH.

Who should not take HYZAAR?

Do not take HYZAAR if you:

• are allergic to any ingredients in HYZAAR. See a complete list of ingredients in HYZAAR at the end of this leaflet.

• are allergic to any sulfonamide-containing ("sulfa") medicines. Ask your doctor if you are not sure what sulfonamide-containing ("sulfa") medicines are.

• are not passing urine.

What should I tell my doctor before taking HYZAAR?

Tell your doctor about all your medical conditions including if you:

• **are pregnant or planning to become pregnant. See "What is the most important information I should know about HYZAAR?"**

• are breast-feeding or plan to breast-feed. HYZAAR can pass into your milk and may harm your baby. You and your doctor should decide if you will take HYZAAR or breast-feed. You should not do both.

• have been vomiting (throwing up), having diarrhea, sweating a lot, or not drinking enough fluids. These could cause you to have low blood pressure.

• have liver problems

• have kidney problems

• have systemic lupus erythematosus (Lupus; SLE)

• have diabetes

• have asthma

• have gout

• have any allergies

Description	50 – 12.5 mg	100 – 12.5 mg	100 – 25 mg
Product No.	6517	6729	6596
Color	Yellow	White	Light Yellow
Shape	Oval	Oval	Oval
Obverse code	Blank	Blank	Blank
Reverse code	717	745	747
NDC			
Bottle: 30 tablets	0006-0717-31	0006-0745-31	0006-0747-31
Bottle: 90 tablets	0006-0717-54	0006-0745-54	0006-0747-54
Unit dose packs of 100	—	0006-0745-28	—
Bottle: 1000 tablets	0006-0717-82	0006-0745-82	0006-0747-82
Bottle: 4000 tablets	—	—	0006-0747-81
Bottle: 5000 tablets	—	0006-0745-86	—

Tell your doctor about all of the medicines you take, including prescription and non-prescription medicines, vitamins, and herbal supplements.

HYZAAR and certain other medicines may interact with each other. Especially tell your doctor if you are taking:

- potassium supplements
- salt substitutes containing potassium
- water pills (diuretics)
- lithium (a medicine used to treat a certain kind of depression)
- medicines used to treat pain and arthritis, called non-steroidal anti-inflammatory drugs (NSAIDs), including COX-2 inhibitors

Know the medicines you take. Keep a list of your medicines and show it to your doctor and pharmacist when you get a new medicine.

How should I take HYZAAR?

- Take HYZAAR exactly as prescribed by your doctor. Your doctor may change your dose if needed.
- HYZAAR can be taken with or without food.
- If you miss a dose, take it as soon as you remember. If it is close to your next dose, do not take the missed dose. Just take the next dose at your regular time.
- If you take too much HYZAAR, call your doctor or Poison Control Center, or go to the nearest hospital emergency room right away.
- Your doctor may do blood tests from time to time while you are taking HYZAAR.

What are the possible side effects of HYZAAR?

HYZAAR may cause the following side effects that may be serious:

- **injury or death of unborn babies.** See "What is the most important information I should know about HYZAAR?"
- **allergic reaction. Symptoms of an allergic reaction are swelling of the face, lips, throat, or tongue. Get emergency medical help right away and stop taking HYZAAR.**
- **low blood pressure (hypotension).** Low blood pressure may cause you to feel faint or dizzy. Lie down if you feel faint or dizzy. Call your doctor right away.
- **a new or worsening condition called systemic lupus erythematosus (Lupus; SLE)**
- **if you have kidney problems, you may see a worsening in how well your kidneys work.** Call your doctor if you get swelling in your feet, ankles, or hands, or unexplained weight gain.
- **If you have liver problems, you may see a worsening in how well your liver works.** Call your doctor if you get nausea, pain in the right upper stomach area (abdomen), yellow eyes or skin (which can be itchy).

The most common side effects of HYZAAR in people with high blood pressure are:

- "colds" (upper respiratory infection)
- dizziness
- stuffy nose
- back pain
- fast or irregular heartbeat (palpitations)
- rash

Tell your doctor if you get any side effect that bothers you or that won't go away. This is **not** a complete list of side effects. For a complete list, ask your doctor or pharmacist.

How should I store HYZAAR?

- Store HYZAAR at room temperature at 59°F to 86°F (15°C to 30°C).
- Keep HYZAAR in a tightly closed container, and keep HYZAAR out of the light.
- **Keep HYZAAR and all medicines out of the reach of children.**

General information about HYZAAR

Medicines are sometimes prescribed for conditions that are not mentioned in patient information leaflets. Do not use HYZAAR for a condition for which it was not prescribed. Do not give HYZAAR to other people, even if they have the same symptoms that you have. It may harm them.

This leaflet summarizes the most important information about HYZAAR. If you would like more information, talk with your doctor. You can ask your pharmacist or doctor for information that is written for health professionals.

What are the ingredients in HYZAAR?

Active ingredients: losartan potassium, hydrochlorothiazide
Inactive ingredients:
microcrystalline cellulose, lactose hydrous, pregelatinized starch, magnesium stearate, hydroxypropyl cellulose, hypromellose, titanium dioxide. HYZAAR 50-12.5 and HYZAAR 100-25 also contain D&C yellow No. 10 aluminum lake. HYZAAR 50-12.5, HYZAAR 100-12.5, and HYZAAR 100-25 may also contain carnauba wax.

Manufactured For:
Merck Sharp & Dohme Corp., a subsidiary of **Merck & Co., Inc.**
Whitehouse Station, NJ 08889, USA
Issued December 2009
Printed in USA
9964301
Shown in Product Identification Guide, page 313

IMPLANON®
(etonogestrel implant)
68 mg
For Subdermal Use Only

Rx

Women should be informed that this product does not protect against infection from HIV (the virus that causes AIDS) or other sexually transmitted diseases.

DESCRIPTION

IMPLANON® (etonogestrel implant) is an off-white, non-biodegradable, etonogestrel-containing single sterile rod implant for subdermal use. The implant is 4 cm in length with a diameter of 2 mm (see **Figure 1**). Each IMPLANON rod consists of an ethylene vinylacetate (EVA) copolymer core, containing 68 mg of the synthetic progestin etonogestrel (ENG), surrounded by an EVA copolymer skin. The release rate is 60 to 70 mcg/day in Week 5 to 6 and decreases to approximately 35 to 45 mcg/day at the end of the first year, to approximately 30 to 40 mcg/day at the end of the second year, and then to approximately 25 to 30 mcg/day at the end of the third year. IMPLANON is a progestin-only contraceptive and does not contain estrogen. IMPLANON does not contain latex and is not radio-opaque.

FIGURE 1 (Not to scale)

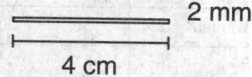

2 mm

4 cm

ENG [13-Ethyl-17-hydroxy-11-methylene-18,19-dinor-17α-pregn-4-en-20-yn-3-one], structurally derived from 19-nortestosterone, is the synthetic biologically active metabolite of the synthetic progestin desogestrel. It has a molecular weight of 324.46 and the following structural formula:

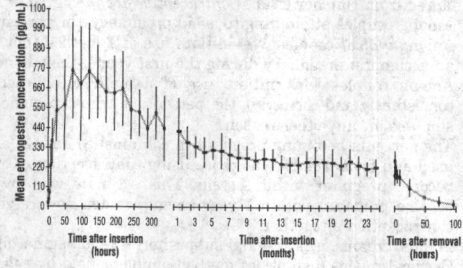

$C_{22}H_{28}O_2$

CLINICAL PHARMACOLOGY

Pharmacodynamics

The contraceptive effect of IMPLANON® (etonogestrel implant) is achieved by several mechanisms that include suppression of ovulation, increased viscosity of the cervical mucus, and alterations in the endometrium.

Pharmacokinetics

Absorption

After subdermal insertion of IMPLANON, ENG is released into the circulation and is approximately 100% bioavailable. The mean peak serum concentrations in 3 pharmacokinetic studies ranged between 781 and 894 pg/mL and were reached within the first few weeks after insertion. The mean serum ENG concentration decreases gradually over time declining to 192 to 261 pg/mL at 12 months (n=41), 154 to 194 pg/mL at 24 months (n=35), and 156 to 177 pg/mL at 36 months (n=17). The pharmacokinetic profile of IMPLANON from 1 of 3 pharmacokinetic studies is shown in **Figure 2**.

FIGURE 2: Mean Serum Concentration-time Profile of ENG During 2 Years of IMPLANON Use and After Removal in 20 Healthy Women

Distribution

The apparent volume of distribution averages about 201 L. ENG is approximately 32% bound to sex hormone binding globulin (SHBG) and 66% bound to albumin in blood.

Metabolism

In vitro data shows that ENG is metabolized in liver microsomes by the cytochrome P450 3A4 isoenzyme. The biological activity of ENG metabolites is unknown.

Excretion

The elimination half-life of ENG is approximately 25 hours. Excretion of ENG and its metabolites, either as free steroid

---

or as conjugates, is mainly in urine and to a lesser extent in feces. After removal of IMPLANON, ENG concentrations decreased below sensitivity of the assay by 1 week.

Special Populations

Overweight Women

The effectiveness of IMPLANON in overweight women has not been defined because women who weighed more than 130% of their ideal body weight were not studied. However, serum concentrations of ENG are inversely related to body weight and decrease with time after insertion. It is therefore possible that, with time, IMPLANON may be less effective in overweight women, especially in the presence of other factors that decrease etonogestrel concentrations such as concomitant use of hepatic enzyme inducers.

Race

No formal studies were conducted to evaluate the effect of race on the pharmacokinetics of IMPLANON.

Hepatic Insufficiency

No formal studies were conducted to evaluate the effect of hepatic disease on the pharmacokinetics of IMPLANON. However, ENG is metabolized by the liver and, therefore, use in patients with active liver disease is contraindicated.

Renal Insufficiency

No formal studies were conducted to evaluate the effect of renal disease on the pharmacokinetics of IMPLANON.

INDICATIONS AND USAGE

IMPLANON® (etonogestrel implant) is indicated for women for the prevention of pregnancy. IMPLANON is a long-acting (up to 3 years), reversible, contraceptive method. IMPLANON must be removed by the end of the third year and may be replaced by a new IMPLANON at the time of removal, if continued contraceptive protection is desired.

In clinical trials involving 923 subjects and 1854 women-years of IMPLANON use, the total exposure in 28-day cycles by year was

- Year 1: 10,867 cycles
- Year 2: 8595 cycles
- Year 3: 3492 cycles

The clinical trials excluded women who

- Weighed more than 130% of their ideal body weight
- Were chronically taking medications that induce liver enzymes

Among women aged 18 to 35 years of age at entry, 6 pregnancies during 20,648 cycles of use were reported. Two pregnancies occurred in each of Years 1, 2, and 3. Each conception was likely to have occurred shortly before or within 2 weeks after IMPLANON removal. With these 6 pregnancies, the cumulative Pearl Index was 0.38 pregnancies per 100 women-years of use.

The efficacy of IMPLANON does not depend on patient self-administration. IMPLANON may be less effective in women who are overweight or who are taking medications that induce liver enzymes (see **CLINICAL PHARMACOLOGY, Special Populations,** *Overweight Women,* and **PRECAUTIONS, Drug Interactions** sections).

The following table shows pregnancy rates in the first year of use for other contraceptive methods.

[See table at top of next page]

CONTRAINDICATIONS

IMPLANON® (etonogestrel implant) should not be used in women who have

- Known or suspected pregnancy
- Current or past history of thrombosis or thromboembolic disorders
- Hepatic tumors (benign or malignant), active liver disease
- Undiagnosed abnormal genital bleeding
- Known or suspected carcinoma of the breast or personal history of breast cancer
- Hypersensitivity to any of the components of IMPLANON

WARNINGS

A. WARNINGS BASED ON EXPERIENCE WITH IMPLANON® (etonogestrel implant) AND OTHER PROGESTIN-ONLY CONTRACEPTIVES

1. **Complications of Insertion and Removal**
   IMPLANON should be inserted subdermally so that it is palpable after insertion. Failure to insert IMPLANON properly may go unnoticed unless the implant is palpated immediately after insertion. Deep insertions may lead to difficult or impossible removals. Failure to remove IMPLANON may result in infertility, ectopic pregnancy, or inability to stop a drug-related adverse event. Undetected failure to insert IMPLANON may lead to an unintended pregnancy (see INSTRUCTIONS FOR INSERTION AND REMOVAL).

   In clinical trials, 1.0% of patients had complications at implant insertion and 1.7% had complications at implant removal. Complications expected of a minor surgical procedure, such as pain, paresthesias, bleeding, hematoma, scarring or infection, have been reported. Occasionally in postmarketing use, implant insertions have failed because the implant fell out of the needle or remained in the needle during insertion. Implant removals may be difficult because the implant is deep, not palpable, encased in fibrous tissue, or has migrated. Implants have broken during difficult removals.

Deep insertions may result in the need for a surgical procedure in an operating room in order to remove IMPLANON. Any of the possible complications of surgery may occur. When IMPLANON is inserted too deeply (intramuscular or in the fascia), this may cause neural or vascular damage. Too deep insertions have been associated with paraesthesia (due to neural damage), migration of the implant (due to intramuscular or fascial insertion), and in rare cases with intravascular insertion. In postmarketing use there have been cases of failure to localize and remove the implant, probably due to deep insertion. There has been 1 case of an intravascular insertion reported postmarketing which led to inability to remove the implant.

If infection develops at the insertion site, start suitable treatment. If infection persists, remove IMPLANON. Incomplete insertions or infections may lead to expulsion.

2. Ectopic Pregnancies

Be alert to the possibility of an ectopic pregnancy among patients using IMPLANON who become pregnant or complain of lower abdominal pain. Although ectopic pregnancies should be uncommon among patients using IMPLANON, a pregnancy that occurs in a patient using IMPLANON may be more likely to be ectopic than a pregnancy occurring in a patient using no contraception.

3. Bleeding Irregularities

Patients who use IMPLANON are likely to have changes in their vaginal bleeding patterns, which are often unpredictable. These may include changes in bleeding frequency or duration, or amenorrhea. Patients should be counseled regarding unpredictable bleeding irregularities so that they know what to expect. Abnormal bleeding should be evaluated as needed to exclude pathologic conditions or pregnancy. In clinical trials, bleeding changes were the single most common reason for stopping treatment with IMPLANON (11.1%, or 105 of 942 patients using IMPLANON). Most patients stopped treatment with IMPLANON because of irregular bleeding (10.8%), but some stopped because of amenorrhea (0.3%). In these studies, patients using IMPLANON had an average of 17.7 days of bleeding or spotting every 90 days (based on 3315 intervals of 90 days recorded by 780 patients). The percentages of patients having 0, 1 to 7, 8 to 21, or >21 days of spotting or bleeding over a 90-day interval while using IMPLANON is shown in the following table.

[See table at top of next page]

Bleeding patterns observed with use of IMPLANON for up to 2 years, and the proportion of 90-day intervals with these bleeding patterns, are summarized in the following table.

Bleeding Patterns Using IMPLANON During the First 2 Years of Use

Bleeding Patterns	Definitions	%
Infrequent	Less than 3 bleeding and/or spotting episodes in 90 days (excluding amenorrhea)	33.6
Amenorrhea	No bleeding and/or spotting in 90 days	22.2
Prolonged	Any bleeding and/or spotting episode lasting more than 14 days in 90 days	17.7
Frequent	More than 5 bleeding and/or spotting episodes in 90 days	6.7

% = Percentage of 90-day intervals with this pattern.
Based on 3315 recording periods of 90 day's duration in 780 women, excluding the first 90 days after implant insertion.

4. Interaction With Anti-Epileptic and Other Drugs

IMPLANON is not recommended for women who chronically take drugs that are potent hepatic enzyme inducers because etonogestrel levels may be substantially reduced in these women (see also **PRECAUTIONS, Drug Interactions** section).

Percentage of Women Experiencing an Unintended Pregnancy During the First Year of Typical and Perfect Use of Contraception and the Percentage Continuing Use at the End of the First Year: United States

Method (1)	% of Women Experiencing an Unintended Pregnancy within the First Year of Use		% of Women Continuing Use at 1 Year* (4)
	Typical Use[†] (2)	Perfect Use[‡] (3)	
Chance[§]	85	85	
Spermicides[∥]	26	6	40
Periodic abstinence	25		63
Calendar		9	
Ovulation Method		3	
Sympto-Thermal[¶]		2	
Post-Ovulation		1	
Cap[#]			
Parous Women	40	26	42
Nulliparous Women	20	9	56
Sponge			
Parous Women	40	20	42
Nulliparous Women	20	9	56
Diaphragm[#]	20	6	56
Withdrawal	19	4	
Condom**			
Female (Reality)	21	5	56
Male	14	3	61
Pill	5		71
Progestin Only		0.5	
Combined		0.1	
IUD			
Progesterone T	2.0	1.5	81
Copper T 380A	0.8	0.6	78
LNg 20	0.1	0.1	81
Depo-Provera	0.3	0.3	70
Norplant & Norplant-2	0.05	0.05	88
Female sterilization	0.5	0.5	100
Male sterilization	0.15	0.10	100

Emergency Contraceptive Pills: Treatment initiated within 72 hours after unprotected intercourse reduces the risk of pregnancy by at least 75%.[††]

Lactation Amenorrhea Method: LAM is a highly effective, temporary method of contraception.[‡‡]

Adapted from Hatcher et al., *Contraceptive Technology*, 17th Revised Edition, New York, NY: Irvington Publishers, 1998.

* Among couples attempting to avoid pregnancy, the percentage who continue to use a method for 1 year.

† Among *typical* couples who initiate use of a method (not necessarily for the first time), the percentage who experience an accidental pregnancy during the first year if they do not stop use for any other reason.

‡ Among couples who initiate use of a method (not necessarily for the first time) and who use it *perfectly* (both consistently and correctly), the percentage who experience an accidental pregnancy during the first year if they do not stop use for any other reason.

§ The percents becoming pregnant in columns (2) and (3) are based on data from populations where contraception is not used and from women who cease using contraception in order to become pregnant. Among such populations, about 89% become pregnant within 1 year. This estimate was lowered slightly (to 85%) to represent the percent who would become pregnant within 1 year among women now relying on reversible methods of contraception if they abandoned contraception altogether.

∥ Foams, creams, gels, vaginal suppositories, and vaginal film.

¶ Cervical mucus (ovulation) method supplemented by calendar in the pre-ovulatory and basal body temperature in the post-ovulation phases.

With spermicidal cream or jelly.

**Without spermicides.

†† The treatment schedule is 1 dose within 72 hours after unprotected intercourse, and a second dose 12 hours after the first dose. The FDA has declared the following brands of oral contraceptives to be safe and effective for emergency contraception: Ovral (1 dose is 2 white pills), Alesse (1 dose is 5 pink pills), Nordette or Levlen (1 dose is 4 yellow pills).

‡‡ However, to maintain effective protection against pregnancy, another method of contraception must be used as soon as menstruation resumes, the frequency or duration of breast feeds is reduced, bottle feeds are introduced, or the baby reaches 6 months of age.

Percentages of Patients with 0, 1 to 7, 8 to 21, or >21 Days of Spotting or Bleeding Over a 90-Day Interval While Using IMPLANON

Total Days of Spotting or Bleeding	Percentage of Patients		
	Treatment Days 91–180 (N=566)	Treatment Days 270–360 (N=554)	Treatment Days 640–730 (N=547)
0 days	19%	24%	17%
1–7 days	15%	13%	12%
8–21 days	30%	30%	37%
>21 days	36%	33%	35%

5. Ovarian Cysts

If follicular development occurs, atresia of the follicle is sometimes delayed, and the follicle may continue to grow beyond the size it would attain in a normal cycle. Generally, these enlarged follicles disappear spontaneously. Rarely, they can require surgery.

6. Thrombosis

There have been postmarketing reports of serious thromboembolic events, including cases of pulmonary emboli (some fatal) and strokes, in patients using IMPLANON. IMPLANON should be removed in the event of a thrombosis. Consider removal of IMPLANON in case of long-term immobilization due to surgery or illness. Women with a history of thromboembolic disorders should be made aware of the possibility of a recurrence (see also **WARNINGS**, WARNINGS BASED ON EXPERIENCE WITH COMBINATION (PROGESTIN PLUS ESTROGEN) ORAL CONTRACEPTIVES section).

B. WARNINGS BASED ON EXPERIENCE WITH COMBINATION (PROGESTIN PLUS ESTROGEN) ORAL CONTRACEPTIVES

1. Thromboembolic Disorders and Other Vascular Problems

Thromboembolism: Epidemiological investigations have associated the use of combination hormonal contraceptives with an increased incidence of venous thromboembolism (VTE, deep venous thrombosis, retinal vein thrombosis, and pulmonary embolism). The use of combination hormonal contraceptives is associated with increased risks of several serious conditions including myocardial infarction, thromboembolism, and stroke, although the risk of serious morbidity or mortality is very small in healthy women without underlying risk factors. The risk increases significantly in the presence of other underlying risk factors such as hypertension, hyperlipidemias, obesity, and diabetes.

2. Cigarette Smoking

Cigarette smoking increases the risk of serious cardiovascular side effects from the use of combination hormonal contraceptives. This risk increases with age and with heavy smoking (15 or more cigarettes per day) and is quite marked in women over 35 years old who smoke. While this is believed to be an estrogen-related effect, it is not known whether a similar risk exists with progestin-only methods. However, patients should be advised not to smoke.

3. Elevated Blood Pressure

An increase in blood pressure has been reported in women taking combination hormonal contraceptives, and this increase is more likely with continued use and with those users who are older. Studies have shown that the incidence of hypertension increases with increasing concentrations of progestins. Women with a history of hypertension-related diseases or renal disease should be discouraged from using hormonal contraceptives. If women with hypertension elect to use hormonal contraceptives, they should be monitored closely. If sustained hypertension develops during the use of hormonal contraceptives, or if a significant increase in blood pressure does not respond adequately to antihypertensive therapy, hormonal contraceptives should be discontinued. For most women, elevated blood pressure will return to normal after stopping hormonal contraceptives, and there is no difference in the occurrence of hypertension between ever- and never-users.

4. Carcinoma of the Breast and Reproductive Organs

Women with breast cancer should not use hormonal contraceptives because breast cancer may be hormonally sensitive.

The risk of having breast cancer diagnosed may be slightly increased among current and recent users of combination oral contraceptives. However, after combination oral contraceptive discontinuation, this ex-

cess risk appears to decrease over time, and within 10 years after cessation the increased risk disappears. Some studies report an increased risk with duration of use while other studies do not, and no consistent relationships have been found with dose or type of steroid. Some studies have found a small increase in risk for women who first used combination oral contraceptives before age 20. Most studies show a similar pattern of risk with combination oral contraceptive use regardless of a woman's reproductive history or her family breast cancer history.

In addition, breast cancers diagnosed in current or ever oral contraceptive users may be less clinically advanced than in never-users.

Some studies suggest that oral contraceptive use has been associated with an increase in the risk of cervical intraepithelial neoplasia in some populations of women. However, there continues to be controversy about the extent to which such findings may be due to differences in sexual behavior and other factors.

In spite of many studies on the relationship between combination oral contraceptive use and breast and cervical cancers, a cause-and-effect relationship has not been established.

5. Hepatic Neoplasia

Benign hepatic adenomas have been associated with the use of combination oral contraceptives, although the incidence of benign tumors is rare in the United States. Indirect calculations have estimated the attributable risk to be in the range of 3.3 cases/100,000 for users, a risk that increases after 4 or more years of use. Rupture of benign hepatic adenomas may cause death through intra-abdominal hemorrhage.

Studies from Britain have shown an increased risk of developing hepatocellular carcinoma in long-term (>8 years) oral contraceptive users. However, these cancers are extremely rare in the US and the attributable risk (the excess incidence) of liver cancers in oral contraceptive users approaches less than 1 per million users.

6. Gallbladder Disease

Earlier studies have reported an increased lifetime relative risk of gallbladder surgery in users of combination oral contraceptives and estrogens. More recent studies, however, have shown that the relative risk of developing gallbladder disease among combination oral contraceptive users may be minimal. The recent findings of minimal risk may be related to the use of combination oral contraceptive formulations containing lower doses of estrogens and progestins.

PRECAUTIONS

1. General

Women should be informed that this product does not protect against infection from HIV (the virus that causes AIDS) or other sexually transmitted diseases.

IMPORTANT: Pregnancy must be excluded before inserting IMPLANON® (etonogestrel implant).

2. Physical Examination and Follow-up

A complete medical evaluation, including history and physical examination and relevant laboratory tests, should be performed prior to IMPLANON insertion or reinsertion. It is good medical practice for patients using IMPLANON to have regular physical examinations. In case of undiagnosed, persistent, or recurrent abnormal vaginal bleeding, appropriate measures should be conducted to rule out malignancy. Women with a family history of breast cancer or who have breast nodules should be monitored with particular care.

3. Information for the Patient

Provide your patient with a copy of the Patient Labeling and ensure that she understands the information in the Patient Labeling before insertion and removal. A USER CARD and consent form are included in the packaging. Have the patient complete a consent form

and retain it in your records. The USER CARD should be filled out and given to the patient after IMPLANON insertion so that she will have a record of the location of IMPLANON and when IMPLANON should be removed.

4. Weight Gain

In clinical studies, mean weight gain in US IMPLANON users was 2.8 pounds after 1 year and 3.7 pounds after 2 years. How much of the weight gain was related to IMPLANON is unknown. In studies, 2.3% of IMPLANON users reported weight gain as the reason for having IMPLANON removed.

5. Carbohydrate and Lipid Metabolic Effects

IMPLANON may induce mild insulin resistance and small changes in glucose concentrations of unknown clinical significance. Women with diabetes or impaired glucose tolerance should be carefully observed while using IMPLANON.

Women who are being treated for hyperlipidemias should be followed closely if they elect to use hormonal contraceptives. Some progestins may elevate LDL levels and may render the control of hyperlipidemias more difficult.

6. Liver Function

If jaundice develops in any patient using IMPLANON, remove IMPLANON. The hormone in IMPLANON may be poorly metabolized in patients with impaired liver function.

7. Depression

Women with a history of depression should be carefully observed. Consideration should be given to removing IMPLANON in patients who become significantly depressed.

8. Contact Lenses

Contact lens wearers who develop visual changes or changes in lens tolerance should be assessed by an ophthalmologist.

9. Drug Interactions

Changes in Contraceptive Effectiveness Associated with Co-Administration of Other Drugs

a. Anti-Infective Agents and Anticonvulsants

IMPLANON is not recommended for women who require chronic use of drugs that are potent inducers of hepatic enzymes because IMPLANON is likely to be less effective for these women.

Contraceptive effectiveness may be reduced when hormonal contraceptives are coadministered with some antibiotics, antifungals, anticonvulsants, and other drugs that increase the metabolism of contraceptive steroids. This could result in an unintended pregnancy or breakthrough bleeding. Examples include: barbiturates, griseofulvin, rifampin, phenylbutazone, phenytoin, carbamazepine, felbamate, oxcarbazepine, topiramate, and modafinil. Patients should use an additional nonhormonal contraceptive method when taking medications that may decrease the efficacy of hormonal contraceptives.

b. Anti-HIV Protease Inhibitors

Several of the anti-HIV protease inhibitors have been studied with coadministration of combination oral contraceptives; significant changes (increase and decrease) in the mean area under the curve (AUC) of the estrogen and progestin have been noted in some cases. The efficacy and safety of combination oral contraceptive products may be affected with coadministration of anti-HIV protease inhibitors; it is unknown whether this applies to IMPLANON. Healthcare providers should refer to the labeling of the individual anti-HIV protease inhibitors for further drug-drug interaction information.

c. Herbal Products

Herbal products containing St. John's wort (Hypericum perforatum) may induce hepatic enzymes and p-glycoprotein transporter and may reduce the effectiveness of contraceptive steroids.

Increase in Plasma Hormone Levels Associated with Coadministered Drugs

Inhibitors of hepatic enzymes such as itraconazole or ketoconazole may increase plasma hormone levels.

10. Interactions with Laboratory Tests

Certain endocrine tests may be affected by IMPLANON use

a. Sex hormone-binding globulin concentrations may be decreased for the first 6 months after IMPLANON insertion followed by a gradual recovery.

b. Thyroxine concentrations may initially be slightly decreased followed by gradual recovery to baseline.

11. Carcinogenesis, Mutagenesis, Impairment of Fertility

In a 24-month carcinogenicity study in rats with subdermal implants releasing 10 and 20 mcg etonogestrel (ENG) per day (equal to approximately 1.8-3.6 times the systemic steady state exposure of women using IMPLANON), no drug-related carcinogenic potential was observed. ENG was not genotoxic in the *in vitro* Ames/Salmonella reverse mutation assay, the chromosomal aberration assay in Chinese hamster ovary cells or in the *in vivo* mouse micronucleus test. Fertility returned after withdrawal from treatment.

12. Pregnancy

IMPLANON is not indicated for use during pregnancy (see **CONTRAINDICATIONS**).

Teratology studies have been performed in rats and rabbits, respectively, using oral administration up to 390 and 790 times the human IMPLANON dose (based upon body surface) and revealed no evidence of fetal harm due to ENG exposure.

Studies have revealed no increased risk of birth defects in women who have used combination oral contraceptives before pregnancy or during early pregnancy. There is no evidence that the risk associated with IMPLANON is different from that of combination oral contraceptives.

IMPLANON should be removed if maintaining a pregnancy.

13. Nursing Mothers

Based on limited data, IMPLANON may be used during lactation after the fourth postpartum week. Use of IMPLANON before the fourth postpartum week has not been studied.

Small amounts of ENG are excreted in breast milk. During the first months after IMPLANON insertion, when maternal blood levels of ENG are highest, about 100 ng of ENG may be ingested by the child per day based on an average daily milk ingestion of 658 mL. Based on daily milk ingestion of 150 mL/kg, the mean daily infant ENG dose 1 month after insertion of IMPLANON is about 2.2% of the weight-adjusted maternal daily dose, or about 0.2% of the estimated absolute maternal daily dose. The health of breastfed infants whose mothers began using IMPLANON during the fourth to eighth week postpartum (n=38) was evaluated in a comparative study with infants of mothers using a nonhormonal IUD (n=33). They were breastfed for a mean duration of 14 months and followed up to 36 months of age. No significant effects and no differences between the groups were observed on the physical and psychomotor development of these infants. No differences between groups in the production or quality of breast milk were detected.

Healthcare providers should discuss both hormonal and nonhormonal contraceptive options, as steroids may not be the initial choice for these patients.

14. Return to Ovulation

In clinical trials, pregnancies occurred as early as during the first week after removal of IMPLANON. Therefore, a patient should restart contraception immediately after removal of IMPLANON if she still needs to prevent pregnancy.

15. Fluid Retention

Steroid contraceptives may cause some degree of fluid retention. They should be prescribed with caution, and only with careful monitoring, in patients with conditions which might be aggravated by fluid retention. It is unknown if IMPLANON causes fluid retention.

16. Pediatric Use

Safety and efficacy of IMPLANON have been established in women of reproductive age. Safety and efficacy are expected to be the same for postpubertal adolescents. However, no clinical studies have been conducted in women less than 18 years of age. Use of this product before menarche is not indicated.

17. Geriatric Use

This product has not been studied in women over 65 years of age and is not indicated in this population.

ADVERSE REACTIONS

See **WARNINGS** and **PRECAUTIONS** for additional important adverse events.

In clinical trials including 942 subjects, bleeding irregularities were the most common adverse event causing discontinuation of IMPLANON® (etonogestrel implant) (see following table).

Adverse Events Leading to Discontinuation of Treatment in 1% or More of Subjects in Clinical Trials

Adverse Event	All Studies N=942
Bleeding Irregularities*	11.0%
Emotional Lability†	2.3%
Weight Increase	2.3%
Headache	1.6%
Acne	1.3%
Depression‡	1.0%

* Includes "frequent", "heavy", "prolonged", "spotting", and other patterns of bleeding irregularity.
† Among US subjects, 6.1% experienced emotional lability that led to discontinuation.
‡ Among US subjects 2.4% experienced depression that led to discontinuation.

Adverse events that were reported by more than 5% of subjects in clinical trials appear in the following table.

Adverse Events Reported in More than 5% of Subjects in Clinical Trials*

Adverse Event	All Studies N=942
Headache	24.9%
Vaginitis	14.5%
Weight Increase	13.7%
Acne	13.5%
Breast Pain	12.8%
Upper Respiratory Tract Infection	12.6%
Abdominal Pain	10.9%
Pharyngitis	10.5%
Leukorrhea	9.6%
Influenza-Like Symptoms	7.6%
Dizziness	7.2%
Dysmenorrhea	7.2%
Back Pain	6.8%
Emotional Lability	6.5%
Nausea	6.4%
Pain	5.6%
Nervousness	5.6%
Sinusitis	5.6%
Depression	5.5%
Insertion Site Pain	5.2%

*List may include adverse events associated with, but unrelated to, IMPLANON use.

Other **"Less Common Adverse Events"** Reported in Less Than 5% of Subjects in Clinical Trials Include: Allergic Reaction, Alopecia, Anorexia, Anxiety, Appetite Increased, Arthralgia, Asthenia, Asthma, Breast Discharge, Breast Enlargement, Breast Fibroadenosis, Cervical Smear Test Positive, Constipation, Coughing, Crying Abnormal, Diarrhea, Dyspepsia, Dysuria, Edema, Edema Generalized, Fatigue, Fever, Flatulence, Gastritis, Hot Flushes, Hypertension, Hypoesthesia, Injection Site Reaction, Insomnia, Lactation Nonpuerperal, Libido Decreased, Migraine, Myalgia, Otitis Media, Ovarian Cyst, Pelvic Cramping, Premenstrual Tension, Pruritus, Pruritus Genital, Rash, Rhinitis, Sexual Function Abnormal, Skeletal Pain, Somnolence, Vaginal Discomfort, Vein Varicose, Vision Abnormal, Vomiting, and Weight Decrease.

Hypertrichosis has also been reported with use of progestin-only contraceptives.

Implant site complications were reported by 3.6% of subjects during any of the assessments in clinical trials. Pain was the most frequent implant site complication, reported during and/or after insertion, occurring in 2.9% of subjects. Additionally, hematoma, redness, and swelling were reported by 0.1%, 0.3%, and 0.3% of patients, respectively (see also **WARNINGS**, WARNINGS BASED ON EXPERIENCE WITH IMPLANON AND OTHER PROGESTIN-ONLY CONTRACEPTIVES, **Complications of Insertion and Removal** section).

OVERDOSAGE

Insertion of multiple rods has been reported. Overdosage may result if more than 1 IMPLANON® (etonogestrel implant) rod is in place. In case of suspected overdose, IMPLANON should be removed. It is important to remove the IMPLANON rod or other contraceptive implant(s) before inserting a new IMPLANON rod.

DOSAGE AND ADMINISTRATION

All healthcare providers performing insertions and/or removals of IMPLANON® (etonogestrel implant) must receive instruction and training and where appropriate, supervision prior to inserting or removing IMPLANON. To minimize the risk of neural or vascular damage, IMPLANON should be inserted at the inner side of the non-dominant upper arm about 8 to 10 cm (3-4 inches) above the medial epicondyle of the humerus. **IMPLANON should be inserted subdermally just under the skin to avoid the large blood vessels and nerves that lie deeper in the subcutaneous tissues in the sulcus between the triceps and biceps muscles** (see **INSTRUCTIONS FOR INSERTION AND REMOVAL**). IMPLANON must be inserted by the expiration date stated on the packaging. **Remove IMPLANON no later than 3 years after the date of insertion.**

When to Insert IMPLANON

IMPORTANT: Rule out pregnancy before inserting IMPLANON.

Timing of insertion depends on the patient's recent history, as follows

1. No preceding hormonal contraceptive use in the past month
   Counting the first day of menstruation as "Day 1", IMPLANON must be inserted between Days 1 through 5, even if the woman is still bleeding.
2. Switching from a combination hormonal contraceptive IMPLANON may be inserted
   • Anytime within 7 days after the last active (estrogen plus progestin) oral contraceptive tablet
   • Anytime during the 7-day ring-free period of NuvaRing® (etonogestrel/ethinyl estradiol vaginal ring)
   • Anytime during the 7-day patch-free period of a transdermal contraceptive system
3. Switching from a progestin-only method
   There are several types of progestin-only methods. IMPLANON insertion must be performed as follows
   • Any day of the month when switching from a progestin-only pill, do not skip any days between the last pill and insertion of IMPLANON
   • On the same day as contraceptive implant removal
   • On the same day as removal of a progestin-containing IUD
   • On the day when the next contraceptive injection would be due
4. Following first trimester abortion or miscarriage
   • IMPLANON may be inserted immediately following a complete first trimester abortion. If IMPLANON is not inserted within 5 days following a first trimester abortion, follow the instructions under "No preceding hormonal contraceptive use in the past month"
5. Following delivery or a second trimester abortion
   • IMPLANON may be inserted between 21 to 28 days postpartum if not exclusively breastfeeding or between 21 to 28 days following second trimester abortion. If more than 4 weeks have elapsed, pregnancy should be excluded and **the patient should use a nonhormonal method of birth control during the first 7 days after the insertion.** If the patient is exclusively breastfeeding, insert IMPLANON after the fourth postpartum week (see **PRECAUTIONS, Nursing Mothers** section)

If inserted as recommended above, backup contraception is not necessary. If deviating from the recommended timing of insertion, rule out pregnancy and use backup nonhormonal contraception for 7 days after IMPLANON insertion.

HOW SUPPLIED

One IMPLANON® (etonogestrel implant) package consists of a single rod implant containing 68 mg etonogestrel that is 4 cm in length and 2 mm in diameter. IMPLANON is pre-loaded in the needle of a disposable applicator. The applicator consists of acrylonitrile-butadiene-styrene body with a stainless steel needle and a polypropylene shield. The sterile applicator containing IMPLANON is packed in a blister pack.

NDC 0052-0272-01

STORAGE

Store IMPLANON® (etonogestrel implant) at 25°C (77°F); excursions permitted to 15°-30°C (59°-86°F) [see USP Controlled Room Temperature]. Protect from light. Avoid storing IMPLANON in direct sunlight or at temperatures above 30°C (86°F).

℞ only

REFERENCES FURNISHED UPON REQUEST

INSTRUCTIONS FOR INSERTION AND REMOVAL

The basis for successful use and subsequent removal of IMPLANON® (etonogestrel implant) is a correct and carefully performed subdermal insertion of the single rod implant in accordance with the instructions. If the implant is placed improperly leading to deep location or migration, it will be more difficult to remove than a correctly placed subdermal implant. All healthcare providers performing insertions and removals of IMPLANON must receive instruction and training, and where appropriate, supervision prior to inserting or removing IMPLANON.

Information concerning the insertion and removal of IMPLANON will be sent upon request free of charge [Telephone: 1-877-IMPLANON (1-877-467-5266)].

INSERTION PROCEDURE

Prior to inserting IMPLANON® (etonogestrel implant) carefully read the instructions for insertion and removal as well as the full prescribing information.

Place IMPLANON subdermally. Both you and your patient should be able to feel IMPLANON under her skin after placement.

Follow instructions carefully. All healthcare providers must receive training before inserting or removing IMPLANON. Proper IMPLANON insertion will facilitate removal. Correct timing of insertion is important (see **DOSAGE AND ADMINISTRATION, When to Insert IMPLANON** section). Perform a history and physical examination, including a gynecologic examination, before IMPLANON insertion. Ensure that the patient understands the risks and benefits of IMPLANON before insertion. Provide the patient with a copy of the Patient labeling included in packaging. Have the patient review and complete a consent form and maintain it with the patient's chart.

Exclude pregnancy before insertion.

Insert IMPLANON under aseptic conditions.

The following equipment is needed for IMPLANON insertion
- An examination table for the patient to lie on
- Sterile surgical drapes, talc-free sterile gloves, antiseptic solution, sterile marker (optional)
- Local anesthetic, needles, and syringe
- Sterile gauze, adhesive bandage, pressure bandage

An applicator and its parts are shown below (see **Figures 3a and 3b**).

FIGURE 3a: (Not to scale)

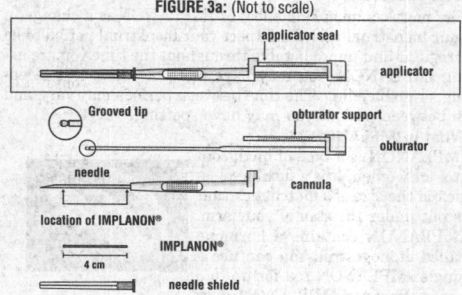

applicator seal
applicator
Grooved tip
obturator support
obturator
needle
cannula
location of IMPLANON®
IMPLANON®
4 cm
needle shield

FIGURE 3b

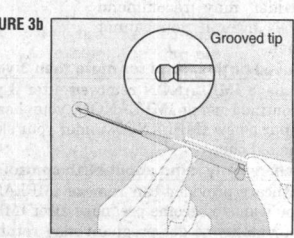

Grooved tip

Grooved tip of obturator (enlarged)

The procedure used for IMPLANON insertion is opposite from that of an injection. The obturator keeps IMPLANON in place while the cannula is retracted. The obturator must remain fixed in place while the cannula with needle is retracted from the arm. Do not push the obturator.

1. Confirm that the patient does not have allergies to IMPLANON, as well as the antiseptic and anesthetic to be used during insertion.
2. Have the patient lie on her back on the examination table with her *nondominant arm flexed at the elbow and externally rotated so that her wrist is parallel to her ear or her hand is positioned next to her head* (see **Figure 4**). [See figure 4 at top of next column]
3. Identify the insertion site, which is at the inner side of the nondominant upper arm about 8 to 10 cm (3-4 inches) above the medial epicondyle of the humerus (see **Figure 5**). **IMPLANON should be inserted subdermally just under the skin to avoid the large blood ves-**

FIGURE 4

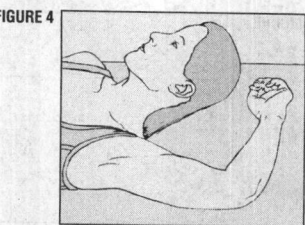

sels and nerves that lie deeper in the subcutaneous tissue of the sulcus between the biceps and triceps muscles.

4. Mark the insertion site with a sterile marker. Make 2 marks: first, mark the spot where the IMPLANON rod will be inserted, and second, mark a spot a few centimeters proximal to the first mark (see **Figure 5**). This second mark will later serve as a direction guide during IMPLANON insertion.

FIGURE 5

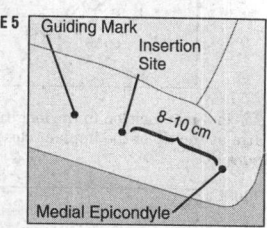

Guiding Mark
Insertion Site
8–10 cm
Medial Epicondyle

5. Clean the insertion site with an antiseptic solution.
6. Anesthetize the insertion area (for example, with anesthetic spray or by injecting 2 cc of 1% lidocaine just under the skin along the planned insertion tunnel).
7. Carefully remove the IMPLANON applicator from its blister. Keep the shield on the needle and look for the IMPLANON rod, seen as a white cylinder inside the needle tip.
8. If you don't see the IMPLANON rod, tap the top of the needle shield against a firm surface to bring the implant into the needle tip.
9. Following visual confirmation, lower the IMPLANON rod back into the needle by tapping it back into the needle tip. Then remove the needle shield, while holding the applicator upright.
10. Note that IMPLANON can fall out of the needle. Therefore, after you remove the needle shield, keep the applicator in the upright position until the moment of insertion.
11. Keep the IMPLANON needle and rod sterile. If contamination occurs, use a new package of IMPLANON with a new sterile applicator.
12. Apply counter-traction to the skin around the proposed insertion (see **Figure 6**).

FIGURE 6

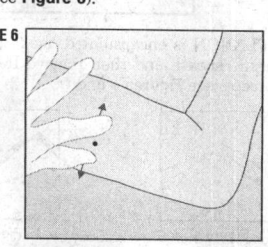

13. At a slight angle (not greater than 20°), insert **only** the tip of the needle with the beveled side up into the insertion site (see **Figure 7**).

FIGURE 7

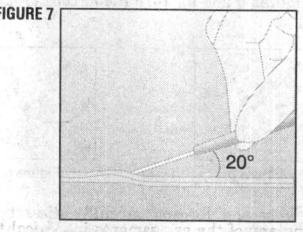

20°

14. Lower the applicator to a horizontal position. Lift the skin up with the tip of the needle, but **keep the needle in the subdermal connective tissue** (see **Figure 8**). [See figure 8 at top of next column]
15. While "tenting" (lifting) the skin, gently insert the needle to its full length. Keep the needle parallel to the surface of the skin during insertion (see **Figure 9**). [See figure 9 on next column]

FIGURE 8

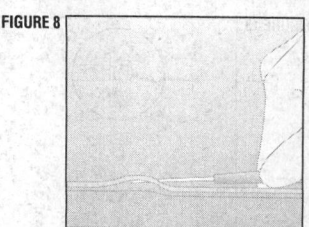

FIGURE 9

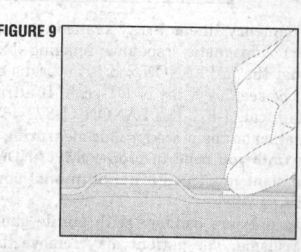

16. **If IMPLANON is placed too deeply, the removal process can be difficult or impossible. If the needle is not inserted to its full length, the implant may protrude from the insertion site and fall out.**
17. Break the seal of the applicator by pressing the obturator support (see **Figure 10**).

FIGURE 10

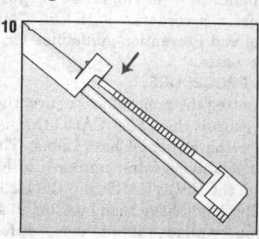

18. Turn the obturator 90° in either direction with respect to the needle (see **Figure 11**).

FIGURE 11

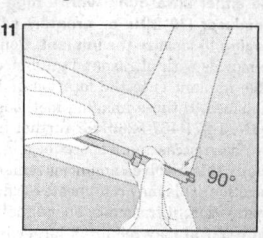

90°

19. While holding the obturator fixed in place on the arm, fully retract the cannula (see **Figure 12**). Note: This procedure is opposite from an injection. Do not push the obturator. By holding the obturator fixed in place on the arm and fully retracting the cannula, IMPLANON will be left in its correct subdermal position. Do not simultaneously retract the obturator and cannula from the patient's arm.

FIGURE 12

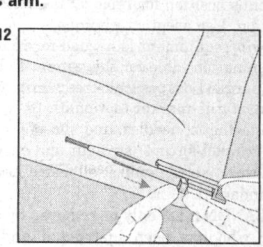

In this figure, the right hand is holding the obturator in place while the left hand is retracting the cannula.

20. Confirm that IMPLANON has been inserted by checking the tip of needle for the absence of IMPLANON. After IMPLANON insertion, the grooved tip of the obturator will be visible inside the needle (see **Figure 13**). [See figure 13 at top of next page]
21. **Always verify the presence of IMPLANON in the patient's arm immediately after insertion by palpation.** By palpating both ends of the implant, you should be able to confirm the presence of the 4-cm rod.
22. Place a small adhesive bandage over the insertion site. Request that the patient palpate IMPLANON.
23. If you cannot feel IMPLANON as a 4-cm long rod, confirm its presence using other methods. Suitable methods to locate IMPLANON are: ultrasound (US) with a

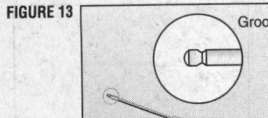

FIGURE 13

Grooved tip

high-frequency linear array transducer (10 MHz or greater) or magnetic resonance imaging (MRI). Please note that the IMPLANON rod is not radio-opaque and cannot be seen by X-ray or CT scan. If ultrasound and MRI fail, call 1-877-IMPLANON (1-877-467-5266) for information on the procedure for measuring ENG blood levels. **Until you confirm proper IMPLANON insertion, your patient must use a nonhormonal contraceptive method.**

24. Apply a pressure bandage with sterile gauze to minimize bruising. The patient may remove the pressure bandage in 24 hours and the small bandage over the insertion site in 3 to 5 days.

25. Complete the USER CARD and give it to the patient to keep. Also, complete the Patient Chart Label and affix it to the patient's medical record.

26. The applicator is for single use only. Dispose of the applicator in accordance with the Center for Disease Control and Prevention guidelines for handling of hazardous waste.

REMOVAL PROCEDURE

Before initiating the removal procedure, the healthcare provider may consult the USER CARD that is kept by the patient and/or the Patient Chart Label. The arm in which IMPLANON® (etonogestrel implant) is located should be indicated on the USER CARD and the Patient Chart Label. IMPLANON should have been inserted in the medial aspect of the upper nondominant arm. **Prior to removing IMPLANON, carefully read the instructions for removal. Find IMPLANON by palpation. If IMPLANON cannot be palpated, use either ultrasound with a high-frequency linear array transducer (10 MHz or greater) or magnetic resonance imaging to localize the implant.** Consider conducting difficult removals with ultrasound guidance. Only remove a nonpalpable implant once the location of IMPLANON has been established. If these imaging methods fail, call 1-877-IMPLANON (1-877-467-5266) for further instructions.

There have been occasional reports of migration of the implant; usually this involves minor movement relative to the original position. This may complicate localization of the implant by palpation, ultrasound, or magnetic resonance imaging, and removal may require a larger incision and more time.

Exploratory surgery without knowledge of the exact location of the implant is strongly discouraged. Removal of deeply inserted implants should be conducted with caution, in order to prevent damage to deeper neural or vascular structures in the arm, and be performed by healthcare providers familiar with the anatomy of the arm.

The patient's position for removal is similar to the position for insertion. Use aseptic technique.

The following equipment is needed for removal
- An examination table for the patient to lie on
- Sterile surgical drapes, talc-free sterile gloves, antiseptic solution, sterile marker (optional)
- Local anesthetic, needles, and syringe
- Sterile scalpel, forceps (straight and curved mosquito)
- Skin closure, sterile gauze, adhesive bandage, and pressure bandages

1. IMPLANON must only be removed by a healthcare provider who has been instructed and trained in the IMPLANON removal technique.

2. The arm in which IMPLANON is located should be indicated on the USER CARD and the Patient Chart Label. IMPLANON should be in the medial aspect of the upper nondominant arm.

3. After confirming that the patient does not have any allergies to the antiseptic, wash the patient's arm and apply an antiseptic. Locate IMPLANON by palpation and mark the end closest to the elbow, for example, with a sterile marker (see **Figure a**).

[See figure a at top of next column]

4. After determining the absence of allergies to the anesthetic agent or related drugs, anesthetize the arm, for example, with 0.5 to 1 cc 1% lidocaine at the site where the incision will be made (near the tip of IMPLANON that is closest to the elbow) (see **Figure b**). Be sure to

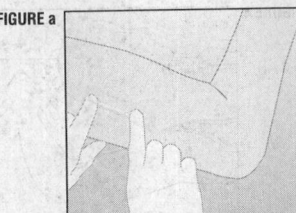

FIGURE a

inject the local anesthetic **under** IMPLANON to keep the implant close to the skin surface.

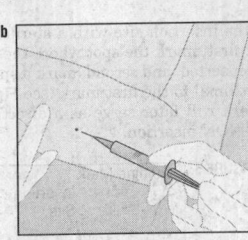

FIGURE b

5. Make a 2- to 3-mm incision in the longitudinal direction of the arm at the tip of the implant closest to the elbow (see **Figure c**).

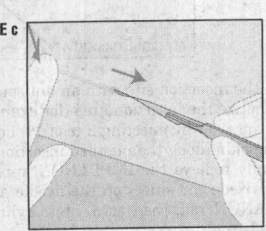

FIGURE c

6. Gently push IMPLANON toward the incision until the tip is visible. Grasp the implant with forceps (preferably curved mosquito forceps) and pull it out gently (see **Figure d**).

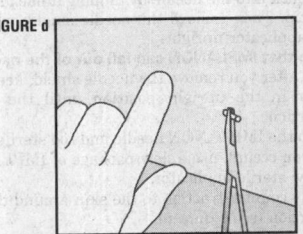

FIGURE d

7. If IMPLANON is encapsulated, make an incision into the tissue sheath and then remove IMPLANON with the forceps (see **Figures e** and **f**).

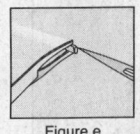 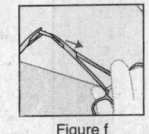

Figure e   Figure f

8. If the tip of the implant is still not visible after gently pushing it towards the incision (as in step 6), gently insert a forceps into the incision and grasp the implant (see **Figures g** and **h**). Turn the forceps around (see **Figure h**).

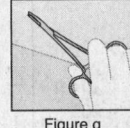 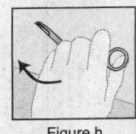

Figure g   Figure h

9. With a second forceps carefully dissect the tissue around IMPLANON and then remove IMPLANON (see **Figure i**). Be sure to remove the IMPLANON rod entirely. Confirm that the entire rod, which is 4 cm long, has been removed by measuring its length.

If the patient would like to continue using IMPLANON, insert a new IMPLANON rod immediately after the old IMPLANON rod is removed. The new IMPLANON can be inserted in the same arm, and through the same incision, or a new IMPLANON can be inserted in the

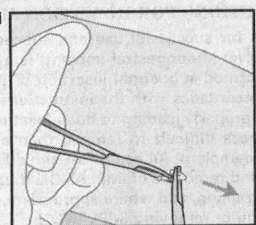

FIGURE i

other arm. If the patient does not wish to continue using IMPLANON and does not want to become pregnant, recommend another contraceptive method.

10. After removing IMPLANON, close the incision with a butterfly closure and apply an adhesive bandage.

11. Apply a pressure bandage with sterile gauze to minimize bruising.

Manufactured by N.V. Organon, Oss, The Netherlands. Distributed by Schering Corporation, a subsidiary of Schering-Plough Corporation, Kenilworth, NJ 07033 USA. © 2006, 2009, Schering Corporation. All rights reserved. Rev. 3/09   33293704T

PATIENT LABELING

IMPLANON®
(etonogestrel implant)
68 mg
For Subdermal Use Only
℞ only
IMPLANON® does not protect against infection from HIV (the virus that causes AIDS) or other sexually transmitted diseases.

Read this leaflet carefully and have your healthcare provider answer all of your questions before you decide to use IMPLANON.

What is the most important information I should know about IMPLANON®?

After you receive IMPLANON, check that it is in place by pressing your fingertips over the skin in your arm where IMPLANON was placed. You should be able to feel the IMPLANON rod. If IMPLANON is not placed properly, it may not prevent pregnancy or it may be difficult or impossible to remove.

The most common side effect of IMPLANON is a change in your menstrual periods. Expect your menstrual period to be irregular and unpredictable throughout the time you are using IMPLANON. You may have more bleeding, less bleeding, or no bleeding. The time between periods may vary, and in between periods you may have spotting.

What is IMPLANON®?

IMPLANON is a type of birth control for women. It is a flexible plastic rod the size of a matchstick that is put under the skin of your arm. IMPLANON contains a hormone called etonogestrel. You can use a single IMPLANON rod for up to 3 years. Because IMPLANON does not contain estrogen, your healthcare provider may recommend IMPLANON even if you cannot use estrogen.

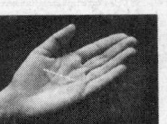

What if I need birth control for more than 3 years?

You must have IMPLANON removed after 3 years. If you want to continue using IMPLANON, your healthcare provider can put a new IMPLANON under your skin after taking out the old one.

What if I change my mind about birth control?

Your healthcare provider can remove IMPLANON at any time. If you want to become pregnant after IMPLANON removal, your ability to get pregnant may return quickly. If you don't want to get pregnant, you should start another birth control method right away.

How does IMPLANON® work?

IMPLANON prevents pregnancy in several ways. The most important way is by stopping release of an egg from your ovary. IMPLANON also changes the mucus in your cervix and this change may keep sperm from reaching the egg. Also, IMPLANON changes the lining of your uterus.

How well does IMPLANON® work?

If IMPLANON is inserted correctly, your chance of getting pregnant is very low (less than 1 pregnancy per 100 women who use IMPLANON for 1 year). It is not known if IMPLANON is as effective in very overweight women because studies did not include many overweight women.

The following chart shows the chance of getting pregnant for women who use different methods of birth control. Each box on the chart contains a list of birth control methods that are similar in effectiveness. The most effective methods are at the top of the chart. The box on the bottom of the chart shows the chance of getting pregnant for women who do not use birth control and are trying to get pregnant.

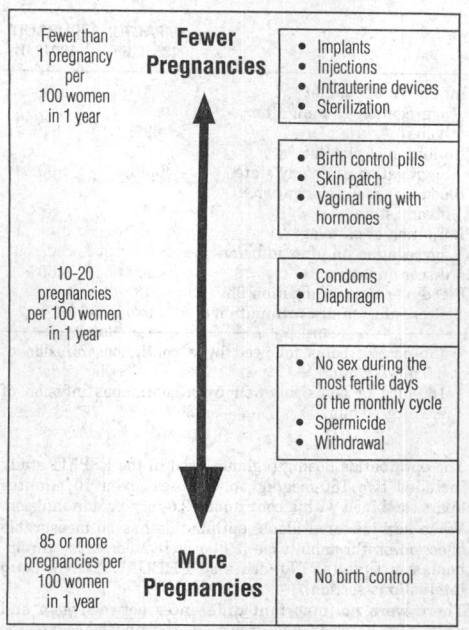

Fewer than 1 pregnancy per 100 women in 1 year	• Implants • Injections • Intrauterine devices • Sterilization
	• Birth control pills • Skin patch • Vaginal ring with hormones
10-20 pregnancies per 100 women in 1 year	• Condoms • Diaphragm
	• No sex during the most fertile days of the monthly cycle • Spermicide • Withdrawal
85 or more pregnancies per 100 women in 1 year	• No birth control

Fewer Pregnancies / **More Pregnancies**

Who should not use IMPLANON®?
Do not use IMPLANON if you
- Are pregnant or think you may be pregnant
- Have, or have had serious blood clots, such as blood clots in your legs (deep venous thrombosis), lungs (pulmonary embolism), eyes (retinal thrombosis), heart (heart attack), or head (stroke)
- Have unexplained vaginal bleeding
- Have liver disease
- Have breast cancer, now or in the past
- Are allergic to anything in IMPLANON

Tell your healthcare provider if you have ever had any of the conditions just listed. Your healthcare provider can suggest another method of birth control.

In addition, talk to your healthcare provider about using IMPLANON if you have or had
- Diabetes
- High cholesterol or triglycerides
- Headaches
- Seizures or epilepsy
- Gallbladder or kidney disease
- Depression
- High blood pressure
- Allergic reaction to anesthetics or antiseptics. These medicines will be used when IMPLANON is inserted into your arm.

If you have any of these conditions, your healthcare provider can explain what to do.

How do I use IMPLANON®?
Your healthcare provider will insert (or remove) IMPLANON in a minor surgical procedure in his or her office. IMPLANON is inserted just under the skin on the inner side of your upper arm.
The timing of insertion is important. Depending on your history, your healthcare provider may ask you to
- Have a pregnancy test before insertion
- Schedule the insertion at a specific time of your cycle (for example, within the first days of your regular menstrual bleeding)
- Use a backup method of birth control, such as condoms, for 7 days after IMPLANON insertion

Both you and your healthcare provider should check that IMPLANON is in your arm by feeling the IMPLANON implant.

If you and your healthcare provider cannot feel IMPLANON, use a nonhormonal birth control method such as condoms until your healthcare provider confirms that IMPLANON is in place. You may need special tests to check that IMPLANON is in place or to help find IMPLANON when it is time to take it out.

You will be asked to review and sign a consent form prior to inserting IMPLANON. *You will also get a USER CARD to keep at home with your health records.* Your healthcare provider will fill out the insertion and removal dates. Keep track of the removal date and schedule an appointment for removal with your healthcare provider on or before the removal date.

The insertion site is covered with 2 bandages. Leave the top bandage on for 24 hours. Keep the smaller bandage dry, clean, and in place for 3 to 5 days.

Be sure to have checkups as advised by your healthcare provider.

What are the most common side effects I can expect while using IMPLANON®?
- Irregular and Unpredictable Bleeding
The most common side effect of IMPLANON is a change in your menstrual periods. In studies, about 1 out of 10 women stopped using IMPLANON because of bleeding problems. Expect your menstrual periods to be irregular and unpredictable throughout the time you are using IMPLANON. You may have more bleeding, less bleeding, or no bleeding. The time between periods may vary, and in between periods you may have spotting.
Talk with your healthcare provider if
- You think you may be pregnant
- Your vaginal bleeding is heavy and prolonged
Besides irregular bleeding, the most frequent side effects that caused women to stop using IMPLANON in studies were
- Mood swings
- Weight gain
- Headache
- Acne
- Depression
The most common side effects reported by women using IMPLANON in clinical trials were
- Irregular bleeding
- Headache
- Vaginitis (inflammation of the vagina)
- Weight gain
- Acne
- Breast pain
- Viral infections such as colds, sore throats, sinus infections, or flu-like symptoms
- Stomach pain
- Painful periods
- Mood swings, nervousness, or depression
- Back pain
- Nausea
- Dizziness
- Pain
- Pain at the site of insertion
Rare side effects that have been reported include: extra hair on your face and body, trouble using contact lenses, and spotty darkening of the skin, especially on the face. This is not a complete list of possible side effects. Talk to your healthcare provider if you have any side effects that concern you.

What are the possible risks of using IMPLANON®?
- Complications of Insertion and Removal
Rarely, removal of IMPLANON is difficult or even impossible because IMPLANON is not where it should be. If IMPLANON cannot be removed, then the effects of IMPLANON will continue for a longer period of time.
Rarely, IMPLANON is not inserted at all due to a failed insertion, or the implant has fallen out of the needle, and then you may become pregnant. After insertion, and with direction from your healthcare provider, you should be able to feel IMPLANON under your skin. If you can't feel IMPLANON, tell your healthcare provider.
Some other problems related to insertion and removal are
- Pain, irritation, swelling, or bruising
- Scarring, including a thick scar called a keloid
- Infection
- IMPLANON breaks making it difficult to remove IMPLANON
- Thick scar tissue forming around IMPLANON making removal difficult
- Rarely, expulsion of the implant
- Rarely, need for surgery in the hospital for removal of IMPLANON
- Removals of deeply inserted implants can lead to scarring or complications such as damage to nerves or blood vessels
- Ectopic Pregnancy
If you become pregnant while using IMPLANON, you have a slightly higher chance that the pregnancy will be ectopic (occurring outside the womb) than do women who are not using birth control. Ectopic pregnancies can cause serious internal bleeding and even death.
- Interaction With Other Medicines
Certain medicines may make IMPLANON less effective and you may need to use back-up nonhormone birth control. Tell your healthcare provider about any medicines you are taking, or intend to take, including over-the-counter medicines and prescription medicines such as: barbiturates, griseofulvin, rifampin, phenylbutazone, phenytoin, carbamazepine, felbamate, oxcarbazepine, topiramate, and modafinil. Herbal remedies such as St. John's wort may also reduce the effectiveness of contraceptive drug products. This is not a complete list of drugs that may interact with IMPLANON.
When you are using IMPLANON, tell all of your healthcare providers that you have IMPLANON.

- Ovarian Cysts
Cysts on the ovaries usually go away without treatment. Sometimes surgery is needed.
- Breast Cancer
It is not known whether IMPLANON changes a woman's risk for breast cancer. If you have breast cancer now, or have had it in the past, do not use IMPLANON because some breast cancers are sensitive to hormones.
- Blood Clots (Thrombosis)
It is not known whether IMPLANON changes a woman's risk for serious blood clots called thrombosis. Thrombosis is a side effect of birth control pills and pregnancy. Because IMPLANON contains 1 of the 2 hormones that are in birth control pills, thrombosis may be a side effect of IMPLANON. There have been postmarketing reports of thrombosis among IMPLANON users.
Some examples of thrombosis are
- Legs (deep vein thrombosis)
- Lung (pulmonary embolism)
- Brain (stroke)
- Heart (heart attack)
- Eyes (blindness)
The risk of thrombosis is increased in women who smoke. If you smoke, you should quit. Your healthcare provider may be able to help.
Tell your healthcare provider at least 4 weeks before if you are going to have surgery or will need to be on bed rest. You have an increased chance of getting thrombosis during surgery or bed rest.
- Other Risks
A few women who use birth control that contains hormones may get
- High blood pressure
- Gallbladder problems
- Rare cancerous or noncancerous liver tumors

When should I call my healthcare provider?
Call your healthcare provider right away if you get any of the symptoms listed below. They may be signs of a serious problem.
- Sharp chest pain, coughing blood, or sudden shortness of breath (possible clot in the lung)
- Persistent pain in the calf (back of lower leg) (possible clot in the leg)
- Crushing chest pain or heaviness in the chest (possible heart attack)
- Sudden severe headache or vomiting, dizziness or fainting, problems with vision or speech, weakness, or numbness in an arm or leg (possible stroke)
- Sudden partial or complete blindness (possible clot in the eye)
- Yellowing of the skin or whites of the eyes (jaundice), especially with fever, tiredness, loss of appetite, dark colored urine, or light colored bowel movements (possible liver problems)
- Severe pain, swelling, or tenderness in the abdomen (possibly indicating an ectopic pregnancy, a ruptured or twisted ovarian follicle, or gallbladder or liver problems)
- Breast lumps
- Difficulty in sleeping, weakness, lack of energy, tiredness, or sadness (possible severe depression)
- Heavy vaginal bleeding

What if I become pregnant while using IMPLANON®?
You should see your healthcare provider right away. It is important to remove IMPLANON and make sure that the pregnancy is not ectopic (occurring outside the womb). Based on experience with birth control pills, IMPLANON is not likely to cause birth defects.

Can I use IMPLANON® when I am breastfeeding?
Based on a small study, you may start IMPLANON if you are breastfeeding and if you delivered your baby more than 4 weeks ago. A small amount of the active substance of IMPLANON passes into the breast milk. The health of breastfed children whose mothers were using IMPLANON has been studied up to 3 years of age in a small number of children. No effects on the growth and development of the children were seen. If you are breastfeeding and want to use IMPLANON, talk with your healthcare provider.

What if I want to become pregnant or want to stop using IMPLANON® for another reason before 3 years?
Your healthcare provider can remove IMPLANON at any time with a minor surgical procedure in the office. The information on your USER CARD may help your healthcare provider find IMPLANON.
After removal, keep the removal site clean, dry, and bandaged for 3 to 5 days to lessen the chance of infection.
If you want to become pregnant, your ability to get pregnant usually returns quickly. Some women have become pregnant within days after removal of IMPLANON. **If you do not want to become pregnant, you should start another birth control method right away.**

Additional Information
This leaflet contains important information about IMPLANON®. If you would like more information, talk

with your healthcare provider. You can ask your healthcare provider for information about IMPLANON that is written for healthcare providers. You may also call 1-877-IMPLANON (1-877-467-5266) or visit www.IMPLANON-USA.com.

Manufactured by N.V. Organon, Oss, The Netherlands. Distributed by Schering Corporation, a subsidiary of Schering-Plough Corporation, Kenilworth, NJ 07033 USA. © 2006, 2009, Schering Corporation. All rights reserved.

Rev. 3/09   33294107T

IMPLANON®
(etonogestrel implant)
68 mg

For Subdermal Use Only

PATIENT CONSENT FORM

I understand the Patient Labeling for IMPLANON®. I have discussed IMPLANON with my healthcare provider who answered all my questions. I understand that there are benefits as well as risks from using IMPLANON. I understand that there are other birth control methods and that each has its own benefits and risks.

I also understand that this Patient Consent Form is important. I understand that I need to sign this form to show that I am making an informed and careful decision to use IMPLANON, and that I have read and understand the following points.

- IMPLANON helps to keep me from getting pregnant.
- No contraceptive method is 100% effective, including IMPLANON.
- IMPLANON is made of a hormone mixed in a plastic rod.
- It is important to have IMPLANON inserted at the right time of my menstrual cycle.
- **After IMPLANON is inserted, I should check that it is in place by gently pressing my fingertips over the skin in my arm where IMPLANON was inserted. I should be able to feel the small rod.**
- IMPLANON must be removed at the end of 3 years. IMPLANON can be removed sooner if I want.
- If I have trouble finding a healthcare provider to remove IMPLANON, I can call (877) 467-5266 for help.
- IMPLANON is placed under the skin of my arm during a procedure done in my healthcare provider's office. There is a slight risk of getting a scar or an infection from this procedure.
- Removal is usually a small office procedure. However, removal may be difficult. Rarely, IMPLANON cannot be found when it is time to remove it. Special procedures, including surgery in the hospital, may be needed. Difficult removals may cause pain and scarring and may result in damage to nerves and blood vessels. If IMPLANON cannot be found, its effects may continue.
- **Most women have changes in their menstrual bleeding while using IMPLANON. I also will likely have changes in my menstrual bleeding while using IMPLANON. My bleeding may be irregular, lighter or heavier, or my bleeding may completely stop. If I think I am pregnant, I should see my healthcare provider as soon as possible.**
- I understand the warning signs for problems with IMPLANON. I should seek medical attention if any warning signs appear.
- I should tell all my healthcare providers that I am using IMPLANON.
- I need to have a medical checkup regularly and at any time I am having problems.
- IMPLANON does not protect me from HIV infection (AIDS) or any other sexually transmitted disease.

After learning about IMPLANON, I choose to use IMPLANON.

_____
(Name of Healthcare Provider)

_____
(Patient Signature)   (Date)

WITNESSED BY:
The patient above has signed this consent in my presence after I counseled her and answered her questions.

_____
(Healthcare Provider Signature)   (Date)

I have provided an accurate translation of this information to the patient whose signature appears above. She has stated that she understands the information and has had an opportunity to have her questions answered.

_____
(Signature of Translator)   (Date)

Manufactured by N.V. Organon, Oss, The Netherlands. Distributed by Schering Corporation, a subsidiary of Schering-Plough Corporation, Kenilworth, NJ 07033 USA. © 2006, 2009, Schering Corporation. All rights reserved.

Rev. 3/09   33294000T

Shown in Product Identification Guide, page 313

INTEGRILIN®   ℞
[ĭn-tĕg-rĭl-ĭn]
(eptifibatide)
INJECTION
For Intravenous Administration
PRODUCT INFORMATION

DESCRIPTION

Eptifibatide is a cyclic heptapeptide containing 6 amino acids and 1 mercaptopropionyl (des-amino cysteinyl) residue. An interchain disulfide bridge is formed between the cysteine amide and the mercaptopropionyl moieties. Chemically it is N^6-(aminoiminomethyl)-N^2-(3-mercapto-1-oxopropyl-L-lysylglycyl-L-α-aspartyl-L-tryptophyl-L-prolyl-L-cysteinamide,cyclic (1→6)-disulfide. Eptifibatide binds to the platelet receptor glycoprotein (GP) IIb/IIIa of human platelets and inhibits platelet aggregation.

The eptifibatide peptide is produced by solution-phase peptide synthesis, and is purified by preparative reverse-phase liquid chromatography and lyophilized. The structural formula is:

INTEGRILIN® (eptifibatide) Injection is a clear, colorless, sterile, non-pyrogenic solution for intravenous (IV) use with an empirical formula of $C_{35}H_{49}N_{11}O_9S_2$ and a molecular weight of 831.96. Each 10-mL vial contains 2 mg/mL of eptifibatide and each 100-mL vial contains either 0.75 mg/mL of eptifibatide or 2 mg/mL of eptifibatide. Each vial of either size also contains 5.25 mg/mL citric acid and sodium hydroxide to adjust the pH to 5.35.

CLINICAL PHARMACOLOGY
Mechanism of Action

Eptifibatide reversibly inhibits platelet aggregation by preventing the binding of fibrinogen, von Willebrand factor, and other adhesive ligands to GP IIb/IIIa. When administered intravenously, eptifibatide inhibits *ex vivo* platelet aggregation in a dose- and concentration-dependent manner. Platelet aggregation inhibition is reversible following cessation of the eptifibatide infusion; this is thought to result from dissociation of eptifibatide from the platelet.

Pharmacodynamics

Infusion of eptifibatide into baboons caused a dose-dependent inhibition of *ex vivo* platelet aggregation, with complete inhibition of aggregation achieved at infusion rates greater than 5.0 mcg/kg/min. In a baboon model that is refractory to aspirin and heparin, doses of eptifibatide that inhibit aggregation prevented acute thrombosis with only a modest prolongation (2- to 3-fold) of the bleeding time. Platelet aggregation in dogs was also inhibited by infusions of eptifibatide, with complete inhibition at 2.0 mcg/kg/min. This infusion dose completely inhibited canine coronary thrombosis induced by coronary artery injury (Folts model).

Human pharmacodynamic data were obtained in healthy subjects and in patients presenting with unstable angina (UA) or non-ST-segment elevation myocardial infarction (NSTEMI) and/or undergoing percutaneous coronary interventions. Studies in healthy subjects enrolled only males; patient studies enrolled approximately one-third women. In these studies, eptifibatide inhibited *ex vivo* platelet aggregation induced by adenosine diphosphate (ADP) and other agonists in a dose- and concentration-dependent manner. The effect of eptifibatide was observed immediately after administration of a 180-mcg/kg intravenous bolus. Table 1 shows the effects of dosing regimens of eptifibatide used in the IMPACT II and PURSUIT studies on *ex vivo* platelet aggregation induced by 20 μM ADP in PPACK-anticoagulated platelet-rich plasma and on bleeding time. The effects of the dosing regimen used in ESPRIT on platelet aggregation have not been studied.

Table 1
Platelet Inhibition and Bleeding Time

	IMPACT II 135/0.5*	PURSUIT 180/2.0†
Inhibition of platelet aggregation 15 min. after bolus	69%	84%
Inhibition of platelet aggregation at steady state	40-50%	>90%
Bleeding-time prolongation at steady state	<5×	<5×
Inhibition of platelet aggregation 4h after infusion discontinuation	<30%	<50%
Bleeding-time prolongation 6h after infusion discontinuation	1×	1.4×

* 135-mcg/kg bolus followed by a continuous infusion of 0.5 mcg/kg/min.
† 180-mcg/kg bolus followed by a continuous infusion of 2.0 mcg/kg/min.

The eptifibatide dosing regimen used in the ESPRIT study included two 180-mcg/kg bolus doses given 10 minutes apart combined with a continuous 2.0-mcg/kg/min infusion. When administered alone, eptifibatide has no measurable effect on prothrombin time (PT) or activated partial thromboplastin time (aPTT) (see also **PRECAUTIONS, Drug Interactions** section).

There were no important differences between men and women or between age groups in the pharmacodynamic properties of eptifibatide. Differences among ethnic groups have not been assessed.

Pharmacokinetics

The pharmacokinetics of eptifibatide are linear and dose-proportional for bolus doses ranging from 90 to 250 mcg/kg and infusion rates from 0.5 to 3.0 mcg/kg/min. Plasma elimination half-life is approximately 2.5 hours. Administration of a single 180-mcg/kg bolus combined with an infusion produces an early peak level, followed by a small decline prior to attaining steady state (within 4-6 hours). This decline can be prevented by administering a second 180-mcg/kg bolus 10 minutes after the first. The extent of eptifibatide binding to human plasma protein is about 25%. Clearance in patients with coronary artery disease is about 55 mL/kg/h. In healthy subjects, renal clearance accounts for approximately 50% of total body clearance, with the majority of the drug excreted in the urine as eptifibatide, deaminated eptifibatide, and other, more polar metabolites. No major metabolites have been detected in human plasma.

In patients with moderate to severe renal insufficiency (creatinine clearance <50 mL/min using the Cockcroft-Gault equation), the clearance of eptifibatide is reduced by approximately 50% and steady-state plasma levels approximately doubled (see **WARNINGS** and **DOSAGE AND ADMINISTRATION**).

Special Populations

Patients in clinical studies were older (range: 20-94 years) than those in the clinical pharmacology studies. Elderly patients with coronary artery disease demonstrated higher plasma levels and lower total body clearance of eptifibatide when given the same dose as younger patients. Limited data are available on lighter weight (<50 kg) patients over 75 years of age.

No studies have been conducted in patients with hepatic impairment.

Males and females have not demonstrated any clinically significant differences in the pharmacokinetics of eptifibatide.

CLINICAL STUDIES

Eptifibatide was studied in 3 placebo-controlled, randomized studies. PURSUIT evaluated patients with acute coronary syndromes: unstable angina (UA) or non-ST-segment elevation MI (NSTEMI). Two other studies, ESPRIT and IMPACT II, evaluated patients about to undergo a percutaneous coronary intervention (PCI). Patients underwent primarily balloon angioplasty in IMPACT II and intracoronary stent placement, with or without angioplasty, in ESPRIT.

Non-ST-segment Elevation Acute Coronary Syndrome

Non-ST-segment elevation acute coronary syndrome is defined as prolonged (≥10 minutes) symptoms of cardiac ischemia within the previous 24 hours associated with either ST-segment changes (elevations between 0.6 mm and 1 mm or depression >0.5 mm), T-wave inversion (>1 mm), or positive CK-MB. This definition includes "unstable angina" and "NSTEMI" but excludes myocardial infarction that is associated with Q waves or greater degrees of ST-segment elevation.

PURSUIT (Platelet Glycoprotein IIb/IIIa in Unstable Angina: Receptor Suppression Using INTEGRILIN® Therapy)

PURSUIT was a 726-center, 27-country, double-blind, randomized, placebo-controlled study in 10,948 patients presenting with UA or NSTEMI. Patients could be enrolled only if they had experienced cardiac ischemia at rest (≥10 minutes) within the previous 24 hours and had either ST-segment changes (elevations between 0.6 mm and 1 mm or depression >0.5 mm), T-wave inversion (>1 mm), or increased CK-MB. Important exclusion criteria included a history of bleeding diathesis, evidence of abnormal bleeding within the previous 30 days, uncontrolled hypertension, major surgery within the previous 6 weeks, stroke within the previous 30 days, any history of hemorrhagic stroke, serum creatinine >2.0 mg/dL, dependency on renal dialysis, or platelet count <100,000/mm³.

Patients were randomized to either placebo, eptifibatide 180-mcg/kg bolus followed by a 2.0-mcg/kg/min infusion (180/2.0), or eptifibatide 180-mcg/kg bolus followed by a 1.3-mcg/kg/min infusion (180/1.3). The infusion was continued for 72 hours, until hospital discharge, or until the time of coronary artery bypass grafting (CABG), whichever occurred first, except that if PCI was performed, the eptifibatide infusion was continued for 24 hours after the procedure, allowing for a duration of infusion up to 96 hours.

The lower-infusion-rate arm was stopped after the first interim analysis when the 2 active-treatment arms appeared to have the same incidence of bleeding.

Patient age ranged from 20 to 94 (mean 63) years, and 65% were male. The patients were 89% Caucasian, 6% Hispanic, and 5% Black, recruited in the United States and Canada (40%), Western Europe (39%), Eastern Europe (16%), and Latin America (5%).

This was a "real world" study; each patient was managed according to the usual standards of the investigational site; frequencies of angiography, PCI, and CABG therefore differed widely from site to site and from country to country. Of the patients in PURSUIT, 13% were managed with PCI during drug infusion, of whom 50% received intracoronary stents; 87% were managed medically (without PCI during drug infusion).

The majority of patients received aspirin (75-325 mg once daily). Heparin was administered intravenously or subcutaneously, at the physician's discretion, most commonly as an intravenous bolus of 5000 U followed by a continuous infusion of 1000 U/h. For patients weighing less than 70 kg, the recommended heparin bolus dose was 60 U/kg followed by a continuous infusion of 12 U/kg/h. A target aPTT of 50 to 70 seconds was recommended. A total of 1250 patients underwent PCI within 72 hours after randomization, in which case they received intravenous heparin to maintain an activated clotting time (ACT) of 300 to 350 seconds.

The primary endpoint of the study was the occurrence of death from any cause or new myocardial infarction (MI) (evaluated by a blinded Clinical Endpoints Committee) within 30 days of randomization.

Compared to placebo, eptifibatide administered as a 180-mcg/kg bolus followed by a 2.0-mcg/kg/min infusion significantly ($P=0.042$) reduced the incidence of endpoint events (see Table 2). The reduction in the incidence of endpoint events in patients receiving eptifibatide was evident early during treatment, and this reduction was maintained through at least 30 days (see Figure 1). Table 2 also shows the incidence of the components of the primary endpoint, death (whether or not preceded by an MI) and new MI in surviving patients at 30 days.

Table 2
Clinical Events in the PURSUIT Study

Death or MI	Placebo (n=4739) n	Eptifibatide (180/2.0) (n=4722) (%)	P-value
3 days	359 (7.6%)	279 (5.9%)	0.001
7 days	552 (11.6%)	477 (10.1%)	0.016
30 days			
Death or MI (primary endpoint)	745 (15.7%)	672 (14.2%)	0.042
Death	177 (3.7%)	165 (3.5%)	
Nonfatal MI	568 (12.0%)	507 (10.7%)	

[See figure at top of next column]

Treatment with eptifibatide prior to determination of patient management strategy reduced clinical events regardless of whether patients ultimately underwent diagnostic catheterization, revascularization (i.e., PCI or CABG surgery) or continued to receive medical management alone. Table 3 shows the incidence of death or MI within 72 hours.

Table 4
Clinical Events in the IMPACT II Study

	Placebo n (%)	Eptifibatide (135/0.5) n (%)	Eptifibatide (135/0.75) n (%)
Patients	1285	1300	1286
Abrupt Closure	65 (5.1%)	36 (2.8%)	43 (3.3%)
P-value vs. placebo		0.003	0.030
Death, MI, or Urgent Intervention			
24 hours	123 (9.6%)	86 (6.6%)	89 (6.9%)
P-value vs. placebo		0.006	0.014
48 hours	131 (10.2%)	99 (7.6%)	102 (7.9%)
P-value vs. placebo		0.021	0.045
30 days (primary endpoint)	149 (11.6%)	118 (9.1%)	128 (10.0%)
P-value vs. placebo		0.035	0.179
Death or MI			
30 days	110 (8.6%)	89 (6.8%)	95 (7.4%)
P-value vs. placebo		0.102	0.272
6 months	151 (11.9%)*	136 (10.6%)*	130 (10.3%)*
P-value vs. placebo		0.297	0.182

*Kaplan-Meier estimate of event rate.

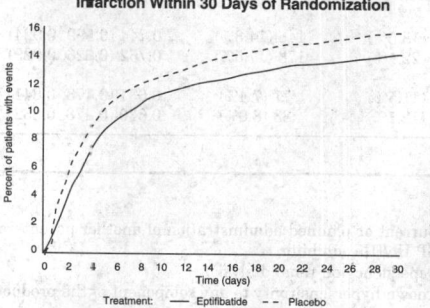

Figure 1: Kaplan-Meier Plot of Time to Death or Myocardial Infarction Within 30 Days of Randomization

Treatment: —— Eptifibatide - - - Placebo

Table 3
Clinical Events (Death or MI) in the PURSUIT Study Within 72 Hours of Randomization

	Placebo	Eptifibatide 180/2.0
Overall patient population	n=4739	n=4722
– At 72 hours	7.6%	5.9%
Patients undergoing early PCI	n=631	n=619
– Pre-procedure (nonfatal MI only)	5.5%	1.8%
– At 72 hours	14.4%	9.0%
Patients not undergoing early PCI	n=4108	n=4103
– At 72 hours	6.5%	5.4%

All of the effect of eptifibatide was established within 72 hours (during the period of drug infusion), regardless of management strategy. Moreover, for patients undergoing early PCI, a reduction in events was evident prior to the procedure.

An analysis of the results by sex suggests that women who would not routinely be expected to undergo percutaneous coronary intervention (PCI) receive less benefit from eptifibatide (95% confidence limits for relative risk of 0.94-1.28) than do men (0.72-0.90). This difference may be a true treatment difference, the effect of other differences in these subgroups, or a statistical anomaly. No differential outcomes were seen between male and female patients undergoing PCI (see results for ESPRIT).

Follow-up data were available through 165 days for 10,611 patients enrolled in the PURSUIT trial (96.9% of the initial enrollment). This follow-up included 4566 patients who received eptifibatide at the 180/2.0 dose. As reported by the investigators, the occurrence of death from any cause or new myocardial infarction for patients followed for at least 165 days was reduced from 13.6% with placebo to 12.1% with eptifibatide 180/2.0.

Percutaneous Coronary Intervention
IMPACT II (INTEGRILIN® to Minimize Platelet Aggregation and Prevent Coronary Thrombosis II)
IMPACT II was a multicenter, double-blind, randomized, placebo-controlled study conducted in the United States in 4010 patients undergoing PCI. Major exclusion criteria included a history of bleeding diathesis, major surgery within 6 weeks of treatment, gastrointestinal bleeding within 30 days, any stroke or structural CNS abnormality, uncontrolled hypertension, PT >1.2 times control, hematocrit <30%, platelet count <100,000/mm³, and pregnancy.

Patient age ranged from 24 to 89 (mean 60) years, and 75% were male. The patients were 92% Caucasian, 5% Black, and 3% Hispanic. Forty-one percent of the patients underwent PCI for ongoing ACS. Patients were randomly assigned to 1 of 3 treatment regimens, each incorporating a bolus dose initiated immediately prior to PCI followed by a continuous infusion lasting 20 to 24 hours: 1) 135-mcg/kg bolus followed by a continuous infusion of 0.5 mcg/kg/min of eptifibatide (135/0.5); 2) 135-mcg/kg bolus followed by a continuous infusion of 0.75-mcg/kg/min of eptifibatide (135/0.75); or 3) a matching placebo bolus followed by a matching placebo continuous infusion. Each patient received aspirin and an intravenous heparin bolus of 100 U/kg, with additional bolus infusions of up to 2000 additional units of heparin every 15 minutes to maintain an activated clotting time (ACT) of 300 to 350 seconds.

The primary endpoint was the composite of death, MI, or urgent revascularization, analyzed at 30 days after randomization in all patients who received at least 1 dose of study drug.

As shown in Table 4, each eptifibatide regimen reduced the rate of death, MI, or urgent intervention, although at 30 days, this finding was statistically significant only in the lower dose eptifibatide group. As in the PURSUIT study, the effects of eptifibatide were seen early and persisted throughout the 30-day period.

[See table 4 above]

ESPRIT (Enhanced Suppression of the Platelet IIb/IIIa Receptor with INTEGRILIN® Therapy)
The ESPRIT study was a multicenter, double-blind, randomized, placebo-controlled study conducted in the United States and Canada that enrolled 2064 patients undergoing elective or urgent PCI with intended intracoronary stent placement. Exclusion criteria included MI within the previous 24 hours, ongoing chest pain, administration of any oral antiplatelet or oral anticoagulant other than aspirin within 30 days of PCI (although loading doses of thienopyridine on the day of PCI were encouraged), planned PCI of a saphenous vein graft or subsequent "staged" PCI, prior stent placement in the target lesion, PCI within the previous 90 days, a history of bleeding diathesis, major surgery within 6 weeks of treatment, gastrointestinal bleeding within 30 days, any stroke or structural CNS abnormality, uncontrolled hypertension, PT >1.2 times control, hematocrit <30%, platelet count <100,000/mm³, and pregnancy.

Patient age ranged from 24 to 93 (mean 62) years and 73% of patients were male. The study enrolled 90% Caucasian, 5% African American, 2% Hispanic, and 1% Asian patients. Patients received a wide variety of stents. Patients were randomized either to placebo or eptifibatide administered as an intravenous bolus of 180 mcg/kg followed immediately by a continuous infusion of 2.0 mcg/kg/min, and a second bolus of 180 mcg/kg administered 10 minutes later (180/2.0/180). Eptifibatide infusion was continued for 18 to 24 hours after PCI or until hospital discharge, whichever came first. Each patient received at least 1 dose of aspirin (162-325 mg) and 60 U/kg of heparin as a bolus (not to exceed 6000 U) if not already receiving a heparin infusion. Additional boluses of heparin (10-40 U/kg) could be administered in order to reach a target ACT between 200 and 300 seconds.

The primary endpoint of the ESPRIT study was the composite of death, MI, urgent target vessel revascularization (UTVR), and "bailout" to open-label eptifibatide due to a thrombotic complication of PCI (TBO) (e.g., visible thrombus, "no reflow," or abrupt closure) at 48 hours. MI, UTVR, and TBO were evaluated by a blinded Clinical Events Committee.

As shown in Table 5, the incidence of the primary endpoint and selected secondary endpoints was significantly reduced

Table 5
Clinical Events in the ESPRIT Study

	Placebo (n=1024)	Eptifibatide 180/2.0/180 (n=1040)	Relative Risk (95% CI)	P-value
Death, MI, Urgent Target Vessel Revascularization, or Thrombotic "Bailout"				
48 hours (primary endpoint)	108 (10.5%)	69 (6.6%)	0.629 (0.471, 0.840)	0.0015
30 days	120 (11.7%)	78 (7.5%)	0.640 (0.488, 0.840)	0.0011
Death, MI, or Urgent Target Vessel Revascularization				
48 hours	95 (9.3%)	62 (6.0%)	0.643 (0.472, 0.875)	0.0045
30 days (key secondary endpoint)	107 (10.4%)	71 (6.8%)	0.653 (0.490, 0.871)	0.0034
Death or MI				
48 hours	94 (9.2%)	57 (5.5%)	0.597 (0.435, 0.820)	0.0013
30 days	104 (10.2%)	66 (6.3%)	0.625 (0.465, 0.840)	0.0016

Table 6
Clinical Events at 6 Months and 1 Year in the ESPRIT Study

	Placebo (n=1024)	Eptifibatide 180/2.0/180 (n=1040)	Hazard Ratio (95% CI)
Death, MI, or Target Vessel Revascularization			
6 Months	187 (18.5%)	146 (14.3%)	0.744 (0.599, 0.924)
1 Year	222 (22.1%)	178 (17.5%)	0.762 (0.626, 0.929)
Death, MI			
6 Months	117 (11.5%)	77 (7.4%)	0.631 (0.473, 0.841)
1 Year	126 (12.4%)	83 (8.0%)	0.630 (0.478, 0.832)

Percentages are Kaplan-Meier event rates.

in patients who received eptifibatide. A treatment benefit in patients who received eptifibatide was seen by 48 hours and at the end of the 30-day observation period.
[See table 5 above]
The need for thrombotic "bailout" was significantly reduced with eptifibatide at 48 hours (2.1% for placebo, 1.0% for eptifibatide; P=0.029). Consistent with previous studies of GP IIb/IIIa inhibitors, most of the benefit achieved acutely with eptifibatide was in the reduction of MI. Eptifibatide reduced the occurrence of MI at 48 hours from 9.0% for placebo to 5.4% (P=0.0015) and maintained that effect with significance at 30 days.
There was no treatment difference with respect to sex in ESPRIT. Eptifibatide reduced the incidence of the primary endpoint in both men (95% confidence limits for relative risk: 0.54, 1.07) and women (0.24, 0.72) at 48 hours.
Follow-up (12-month) mortality data were available for 2024 patients (1017 on eptifibatide) enrolled in the ESPRIT trial (98.1% of the initial enrollment). Twelve-month clinical event data were available for 1964 patients (988 on eptifibatide), representing 95.2% of the initial enrollment. As shown in Table 6, the treatment effect of eptifibatide seen at 48 hours and 30 days appeared preserved at 6 months and 1 year. Most of the benefit was in reduction of MI.
[See table 6 above]

INDICATIONS AND USAGE

INTEGRILIN® is indicated:
• For the treatment of patients with acute coronary syndrome (unstable angina/non-ST-segment elevation myocardial infarction), including patients who are to be managed medically and those undergoing percutaneous coronary intervention (PCI). In this setting, INTEGRILIN has been shown to decrease the rate of a combined endpoint of death or new myocardial infarction.
• For the treatment of patients undergoing PCI, including those undergoing intracoronary stenting. In this setting, INTEGRILIN has been shown to decrease the rate of a combined endpoint of death, new myocardial infarction, or need for urgent intervention.
In the IMPACT II, PURSUIT, and ESPRIT studies of eptifibatide, most patients received heparin and aspirin (see CLINICAL STUDIES).

CONTRAINDICATIONS

Treatment with eptifibatide is contraindicated in patients with:
• A history of bleeding diathesis, or evidence of active abnormal bleeding within the previous 30 days.
• Severe hypertension (systolic blood pressure >200 mm Hg or diastolic blood pressure >110 mm Hg) not adequately controlled on antihypertensive therapy.
• Major surgery within the preceding 6 weeks.
• History of stroke within 30 days or any history of hemorrhagic stroke.

• Current or planned administration of another parenteral GP IIb/IIIa inhibitor.
• Dependency on renal dialysis.
• Known hypersensitivity to any component of the product.

WARNINGS

Bleeding
Bleeding is the most common complication encountered during eptifibatide therapy. Administration of eptifibatide is associated with an increase in major and minor bleeding, as classified by the criteria of the Thrombolysis in Myocardial Infarction Study group (TIMI) (see ADVERSE REACTIONS). Most major bleeding associated with eptifibatide has been at the arterial access site for cardiac catheterization or from the gastrointestinal or genitourinary tract.
In patients undergoing percutaneous coronary interventions, patients receiving eptifibatide experience an increased incidence of major bleeding compared to those receiving placebo without a significant increase in transfusion requirement. Special care should be employed to minimize the risk of bleeding among these patients (see PRECAUTIONS). If bleeding cannot be controlled with pressure, infusion of eptifibatide and concomitant heparin should be stopped immediately.

Renal Insufficiency
Approximately 50% of eptifibatide is cleared by the kidney in patients with normal renal function. Total drug clearance is decreased by approximately 50% and steady-state plasma eptifibatide concentrations are doubled in patients with an estimated creatinine clearance <50 mL/min (using the Cockcroft-Gault equation). Therefore, the infusion dose should be reduced to 1 mcg/kg/min in such patients (see DOSAGE AND ADMINISTRATION). There has been no clinical experience in patients dependent on dialysis.

Platelet Count <100,000/mm³
Because it is an inhibitor of platelet aggregation, caution should be exercised when administering eptifibatide to patients with a platelet count <100,000/mm³; there has been no clinical experience with eptifibatide initiated in patients with a platelet count <100,000/mm³.

PRECAUTIONS

Bleeding Precautions
Care of the Femoral Artery Access Site in Patients Undergoing Percutaneous Coronary Intervention (PCI)
In patients undergoing PCI, treatment with eptifibatide is associated with an increase in major and minor bleeding at the site of arterial sheath placement. After PCI, eptifibatide infusion should be continued until hospital discharge or up to 18 to 24 hours, whichever comes first. Heparin use is discouraged after the PCI procedure. Early sheath removal is encouraged while eptifibatide is being infused. Prior to removing the sheath, it is recommended that heparin be discontinued for 3 to 4 hours and an aPTT of <45 seconds or ACT <150 seconds be achieved. In any case, both heparin

and eptifibatide should be discontinued and sheath hemostasis should be achieved at least 2 to 4 hours before hospital discharge.

Use of Thrombolytics, Anticoagulants, and Other Antiplatelet Agents
In the IMPACT II, PURSUIT, and ESPRIT studies, eptifibatide was used concomitantly with unfractionated heparin and aspirin (see CLINICAL STUDIES). In the ESPRIT study, clopidogrel or ticlopidine were used routinely starting the day of PCI. Because eptifibatide inhibits platelet aggregation, caution should be employed when it is used with other drugs that affect hemostasis, including thrombolytics, oral anticoagulants, nonsteroidal anti-inflammatory drugs, and dipyridamole. To avoid potentially additive pharmacologic effects, concomitant treatment with other inhibitors of platelet receptor GP IIb/IIIa should be avoided.
There is only a small experience with concomitant use of eptifibatide and thrombolytics. In a study of 180 patients with acute myocardial infarction (AMI), eptifibatide (in regimens up to a bolus of 180 mcg/kg followed by a continuous infusion of 0.75 mcg/kg/min for 24 hours) was administered concomitantly with the approved "accelerated" regimen of alteplase, a thrombolytic agent. The studied regimens of eptifibatide did not increase the incidence of major bleeding or transfusion compared to the incidence seen when alteplase was given alone.
In the IMPACT II study, 15 patients received a thrombolytic agent in conjunction with the 135/0.5 dosing regimen, 2 of whom experienced a major bleed. In the PURSUIT study, 40 patients who received eptifibatide at the 180/2.0 dosing regimen received a thrombolytic agent, 10 of whom experienced a major bleed.
In another AMI study involving 181 patients, eptifibatide (in regimens up to a bolus of 180 mcg/kg followed by a continuous infusion of up to 2.0 mcg/kg/min for up to 72 hours) was administered concomitantly with streptokinase (1.5 million U over 60 minutes), another thrombolytic agent. At the highest studied infusion rates (1.3 mcg/kg/min and 2.0 mcg/kg/min), eptifibatide was associated with an increase in the incidence of bleeding and transfusions compared to the incidence seen when streptokinase was given alone.
These limited data on the use of eptifibatide in patients receiving thrombolytic agents do not allow an estimate of the bleeding risk associated with concomitant use of thrombolytics. Systemic thrombolytic therapy should be used with caution in patients who have received eptifibatide.

Minimization of Vascular and Other Trauma
Arterial and venous punctures, intramuscular injections, and the use of urinary catheters, nasotracheal intubation, and nasogastric tubes should be minimized. When obtaining intravenous access, noncompressible sites (e.g., subclavian or jugular veins) should be avoided.

Laboratory Tests
Before infusion of eptifibatide, the following laboratory tests should be performed to identify preexisting hemostatic abnormalities: hematocrit or hemoglobin, platelet count, serum creatinine, and PT/aPTT. In patients undergoing PCI, the activated clotting time (ACT) should also be measured.

Maintaining Target aPTT and ACT
The aPTT should be maintained between 50 and 70 seconds unless PCI is to be performed. In patients treated with heparin, bleeding can be minimized by close monitoring of the aPTT. Table 7 displays the risk of major bleeding according to the maximum aPTT attained within 72 hours in the PURSUIT study.
[See table 7 at top of next page]
The ESPRIT study stipulated a target ACT of 200 to 300 seconds during PCI. Patients receiving eptifibatide 180/2.0/180 (mean ACT: 284 seconds) experienced an increased incidence of bleeding relative to placebo (mean ACT: 276 seconds), primarily at the femoral artery access site. At these lower ACTs, bleeding was less than previously reported with eptifibatide in the PURSUIT and IMPACT II studies. The aPTT or ACT should be checked prior to arterial sheath removal. The sheath should not be removed unless the aPTT is <45 seconds or the ACT is <150 seconds.

Thrombocytopenia
If the patient experiences a confirmed platelet decrease to <100,000/mm³, INTEGRILIN® and heparin should be discontinued and the condition appropriately monitored and treated.

Drug Interactions
Enoxaparin dosed as a 1.0-mg/kg subcutaneous injection q12h for 4 doses did not alter the pharmacokinetics of eptifibatide or the level of platelet aggregation in healthy adults.

Geriatric Use
The PURSUIT and IMPACT II clinical studies enrolled patients up to the age of 94 years (45% were age 65 and over; 12% were age 75 and older). There was no apparent difference in efficacy between older and younger patients treated

with eptifibatide. The incidence of bleeding complications was higher in the elderly in both placebo and eptifibatide groups, and the incremental risk of eptifibatide-associated bleeding was greater in the older patients. No dose adjustment was made for elderly patients, but patients over 75 years of age had to weigh at least 50 kg to be enrolled in the PURSUIT study; no such limitation was stipulated in the ESPRIT study (see also **ADVERSE REACTIONS**).

Carcinogenesis, Mutagenesis, Impairment of Fertility
No long-term studies in animals have been performed to evaluate the carcinogenic potential of eptifibatide. Eptifibatide was not genotoxic in the Ames test, the mouse lymphoma cell (L 5178Y, TK+/-) forward mutation test, the human lymphocyte chromosome aberration test, or the mouse micronucleus test. Administered by continuous intravenous infusion at total daily doses up to 72 mg/kg/day (about 4 times the recommended maximum daily human dose on a body surface area basis), eptifibatide had no effect on fertility and reproductive performance of male and female rats.

Pregnancy
Pregnancy Category B
Teratology studies have been performed by continuous intravenous infusion of eptifibatide in pregnant rats at total daily doses of up to 72 mg/kg/day (about 4 times the recommended maximum daily human dose on a body surface area basis) and in pregnant rabbits at total daily doses of up to 36 mg/kg/day (also about 4 times the recommended maximum daily human dose on a body surface area basis). These studies revealed no evidence of harm to the fetus due to eptifibatide. There are, however, no adequate and well-controlled studies in pregnant women with eptifibatide. Because animal reproduction studies are not always predictive of human response, eptifibatide should be used during pregnancy only if clearly needed.

Pediatric Use
Safety and effectiveness of eptifibatide in pediatric patients have not been studied.

Nursing Mothers
It is not known whether eptifibatide is excreted in human milk. Because many drugs are excreted in human milk, caution should be exercised when eptifibatide is administered to a nursing mother.

ADVERSE REACTIONS
A total of 16,782 patients were treated in the Phase III clinical trials (PURSUIT, ESPRIT, and IMPACT II). These 16,782 patients had a mean age of 62 years (range: 20-94 years). Eighty-nine percent of the patients were Caucasian, with the remainder being predominantly Black (5%) and Hispanic (5%). Sixty-eight percent were men. Because of the different regimens used in PURSUIT, IMPACT II, and ESPRIT, data from the 3 studies were not pooled.

Bleeding
The incidences of bleeding events and transfusions in the PURSUIT, IMPACT II, and ESPRIT studies are shown in Table 8. Bleeding was classified as major or minor by the criteria of the TIMI study group. Major bleeding events consisted of intracranial hemorrhage and other bleeding that led to decreases in hemoglobin greater than 5 g/dL. Minor bleeding events included spontaneous gross hematuria, spontaneous hematemesis, other observed blood loss with a hemoglobin decrease of more than 3 g/dL, and other hemoglobin decreases that were greater than 4 g/dL but less than 5 g/dL. In patients who received transfusions, the corresponding loss in hemoglobin was estimated through an adaptation of the method of Landefeld et al.

[See table 8 above]

The majority of major bleeding events in the ESPRIT study occurred at the vascular access site (1 and 8 patients, or 0.1% and 0.8% in the placebo and eptifibatide groups, respectively). Bleeding at "other" locations occurred in 0.2% and 0.4% of patients, respectively.

In the PURSUIT study, the greatest increase in major bleeding in eptifibatide-treated patients compared to placebo-treated patients was also associated with bleeding at the femoral artery access site (2.8% vs. 1.3%). Oropharyngeal (primarily gingival), genitourinary, gastrointestinal, and retroperitoneal bleeding were also seen more commonly in eptifibatide-treated patients compared to placebo-treated patients.

Among patients experiencing a major bleed in the IMPACT II study, an increase in bleeding on eptifibatide versus placebo was observed only for the femoral artery access site (3.2% vs. 2.8%).

Table 9 displays the incidence of TIMI *major* bleeding according to the cardiac procedures carried out in the PURSUIT study. The most common bleeding complications were related to cardiac revascularization (CABG-related or femoral artery access site bleeding). A corresponding table for ESPRIT is not presented, as every patient underwent PCI in the ESPRIT study and only 11 patients underwent CABG.

[See table 9 above]

Table 7
Major Bleeding by Maximal aPTT Within 72 Hours in the PURSUIT Study

	Placebo n (%)	Eptifibatide 180/1.3* n (%)	Eptifibatide 180/2.0 n (%)
Maximum aPTT (seconds)			
<50	44/721 (6.1%)	21/244 (8.6%)	44/743 (5.9%)
50 to 70 (recommended)	92/908 (10.1%)	28/259 (10.8%)	99/883 (11.2%)
>70	281/2786 (10.1%)	99/891 (11.1%)	345/2811 (12.3%)

*Administered only until the first interim analysis.

Table 8
Bleeding Events and Transfusions in the PURSUIT, ESPRIT and IMPACT II Studies

PURSUIT

	Placebo n (%)	Eptifibatide 180/1.3* n (%)	Eptifibatide 180/2.0 n (%)
Patients	4696	1472	4679
Major bleeding†	425 (9.3%)	152 (10.5%)	498 (10.8%)
Minor bleeding†	347 (7.6%)	152 (10.5%)	604 (13.1%)
Requiring transfusions‡	490 (10.4%)	188 (12.8%)	601 (12.8%)

ESPRIT

	Placebo n (%)	Eptifibatide 180/2.0/180 n (%)
Patients	1024	1040
Major bleeding†	4 (0.4%)	13 (1.3%)
Minor bleeding†	18 (2.0%)	29 (3.0%)
Requiring transfusions‡	11 (1.1%)	16 (1.5%)

IMPACT II

	Placebo n (%)	Eptifibatide 135/0.5 n (%)	Eptifibatide 135/0.75 n (%)
Patients	1285	1300	1286
Major bleeding†	55 (4.5%)	55 (4.4%)	58 (4.7%)
Minor bleeding†	115 (9.3%)	146 (11.7%)	177 (14.2%)
Requiring transfusions‡	66 (5.1%)	71 (5.5%)	74 (5.8%)

Note: Denominator is based on patients for whom data are available.
* Administered only until the first interim analysis.
† For major and minor bleeding, patients are counted only once according to the most severe classification.
‡ Includes transfusions of whole blood, packed red blood cells, fresh frozen plasma, cryoprecipitate, platelets, and autotransfusion during the initial hospitalization.

Table 9
Major Bleeding by Procedures in the PURSUIT Study

	Placebo n (%)	Eptifibatide 180/1.3* n (%)	Eptifibatide 180/2.0 n (%)
Patients	4577	1451	4604
Overall Incidence of Major Bleeding	425 (9.3%)	152 (10.5%)	498 (10.8%)
Breakdown by Procedure:			
CABG	375 (8.2%)	123 (8.5%)	377 (8.2%)
Angioplasty without CABG	27 (0.6%)	16 (1.1%)	64 (1.4%)
Angiography without Angioplasty or CABG	11 (0.2%)	7 (0.5%)	29 (0.6%)
Medical Therapy Only	12 (0.3%)	6 (0.4%)	28 (0.6%)

Note: Denominators are based on the total number of patients whose TIMI classification was resolved.
*Administered only until the first interim analysis.

In the PURSUIT and ESPRIT studies, the risk of major bleeding with eptifibatide increased as patient weight decreased. This relationship was most apparent for patients weighing less than 70 kg.

Bleeding adverse events resulting in discontinuation of study drug were more frequent among patients receiving eptifibatide than placebo (4.6% vs. 0.9% in ESPRIT, 8% vs. 1% in PURSUIT, 3.5% vs. 1.9% in IMPACT II).

Intracranial Hemorrhage and Stroke
Intracranial hemorrhage was rare in the PURSUIT, IMPACT II, and ESPRIT clinical studies. In the PURSUIT study, 3 patients in the placebo group, 1 patient in the group treated with eptifibatide 180/1.3, and 5 patients in the group treated with eptifibatide 180/2.0 experienced a hemorrhagic stroke. The overall incidence of stroke was 0.5% in patients receiving eptifibatide 180/1.3, 0.7% in patients receiving eptifibatide 180/2.0, and 0.8% in placebo patients.
In the IMPACT II study, intracranial hemorrhage was experienced by 1 patient treated with eptifibatide 135/0.5, 2 patients treated with eptifibatide 135/0.75, and 2 patients in the placebo group. The overall incidence of stroke was 0.5% in patients receiving 135/0.5 eptifibatide, 0.7% in patients receiving eptifibatide 135/0.75, and 0.7% in the placebo group.
In the ESPRIT study, there were 3 hemorrhagic strokes, 1 in the placebo group and 2 in the eptifibatide group. In addition there was 1 case of cerebral infarction in the eptifibatide group.

Thrombocytopenia
In the PURSUIT and IMPACT II studies, the incidence of thrombocytopenia (<100,000/mm³ or ≥50% reduction from baseline) and the incidence of platelet transfusions were similar between patients treated with eptifibatide and placebo. In the ESPRIT study, the incidence was 0.6% in the placebo group and 1.2% in the eptifibatide group.

Allergic Reactions
In the PURSUIT study, anaphylaxis was reported in 7 patients receiving placebo (0.15%) and 7 patients receiving eptifibatide 180/2.0 (0.16%). In the IMPACT II study, anaphylaxis was reported in 1 patient (0.08%) on placebo and in no patients on eptifibatide. In the IMPACT II study, 2 patients (1 patient [0.04%] receiving eptifibatide and 1 patient

INTEGRILIN Dosing Charts by Weight

Patient Weight		180 mcg/kg Bolus Volume	2.0 mcg/kg/min Infusion Volume		1.0 mcg/kg/min Infusion Volume	
(kg)	(lb)	(from 2-mg/mL vial)	(from 2-mg/mL 100-mL vial)	(from 0.75-mg/mL 100-mL vial)	(from 2-mg/mL 100-mL vial)	(from 0.75-mg/mL 100-mL vial)
37-41	81-91	3.4 mL	2.0 mL/h	6.0 mL/h	1.0 mL/h	3.0 mL/h
42-46	92-102	4.0 mL	2.5 mL/h	7.0 mL/h	1.3 mL/h	3.5 mL/h
47-53	103-117	4.5 mL	3.0 mL/h	8.0 mL/h	1.5 mL/h	4.0 mL/h
54-59	118-130	5.0 mL	3.5 mL/h	9.0 mL/h	1.8 mL/h	4.5 mL/h
60-65	131-143	5.6 mL	3.8 mL/h	10.0 mL/h	1.9 mL/h	5.0 mL/h
66-71	144-157	6.2 mL	4.0 mL/h	11.0 mL/h	2.0 mL/h	5.5 mL/h
72-78	158-172	6.8 mL	4.5 mL/h	12.0 mL/h	2.3 mL/h	6.0 mL/h
79-84	173-185	7.3 mL	5.0 mL/h	13.0 mL/h	2.5 mL/h	6.5 mL/h
85-90	186-198	7.9 mL	5.3 mL/h	14.0 mL/h	2.7 mL/h	7.0 mL/h
91-96	199-212	8.5 mL	5.6 mL/h	15.0 mL/h	2.8 mL/h	7.5 mL/h
97-103	213-227	9.0 mL	6.0 mL/h	16.0 mL/h	3.0 mL/h	8.0 mL/h
104-109	228-240	9.5 mL	6.4 mL/h	17.0 mL/h	3.2 mL/h	8.5 mL/h
110-115	241-253	10.2 mL	6.8 mL/h	18.0 mL/h	3.4 mL/h	9.0 mL/h
116-121	254-267	10.7 mL	7.0 mL/h	19.0 mL/h	3.5 mL/h	9.5 mL/h
>121	>267	11.3 mL	7.5 mL/h	20.0 mL/h	3.7 mL/h	10.0 mL/h

[0.08%] receiving placebo) discontinued study drug because of allergic reactions. In the ESPRIT study, there were no cases of anaphylaxis reported. There were 3 patients who suffered an allergic reaction, 1 on placebo and 2 on eptifibatide. In addition, 1 patient in the placebo group was diagnosed with urticaria.

The potential for development of antibodies to eptifibatide has been studied in 433 subjects. Eptifibatide was nonantigenic in 412 patients receiving a single administration of eptifibatide (135-mcg/kg bolus followed by a continuous infusion of either 0.5 mcg/kg/min or 0.75 mcg/kg/min), and in 21 subjects to whom eptifibatide (135-mcg/kg bolus followed by a continuous infusion of 0.75 mcg/kg/min) was administered twice, 28 days apart. In both cases, plasma for antibody detection was collected approximately 30 days after each dose. The development of antibodies to eptifibatide at higher doses has not been evaluated.

Other Adverse Reactions

In the PURSUIT and ESPRIT studies, the incidence of serious nonbleeding adverse events was similar in patients receiving placebo or eptifibatide (19% and 19%, respectively, in PURSUIT; 6% and 7%, respectively, in ESPRIT). In PURSUIT, the only serious nonbleeding adverse event that occurred at a rate of at least 1% and was more common with eptifibatide than placebo (7% vs. 6%) was hypotension. Most of the serious nonbleeding events consisted of cardiovascular events typical of an unstable angina population. In the IMPACT II study, serious nonbleeding events that occurred in greater than 1% of patients were uncommon and similar in incidence between placebo- and eptifibatide-treated patients.

Discontinuation of study drug due to adverse events other than bleeding was uncommon in the PURSUIT, IMPACT II, and ESPRIT studies, with no single event occurring in >0.5% of the study population (except for "other" in the ESPRIT study). In the PURSUIT study, nonbleeding adverse events leading to discontinuation occurred in the eptifibatide and placebo groups in the following body systems with an incidence of ≥0.1%: cardiovascular system (0.3% and 0.3%), digestive system (0.1% and 0.1%), hemic/lymphatic system (0.1% and 0.1%), nervous system (0.3% and 0.4%), urogenital system (0.1% and 0.1%), and whole body system (0.2% and 0.2%). In the ESPRIT study, the following nonbleeding adverse events leading to discontinuation occurred in the eptifibatide and placebo groups with an incidence of ≥0.1%: "other" (1.2% and 1.1%). In the IMPACT II study, nonbleeding adverse events leading to discontinuation occurred in the 135/0.5 eptifibatide and placebo groups in the following body systems with an incidence of ≥0.1%: whole body (0.3% and 0.1%), cardiovascular system (1.4% and 1.4%), digestive system (0.2% and 0%), hemic/lymphatic system (0.2% and 0%), nervous system (0.3% and 0.2%), and respiratory system (0.1% and 0.1%).

Postmarketing Experience

The following adverse events have been reported in postmarketing experience, primarily with eptifibatide in combination with heparin and aspirin: cerebral, GI, and pulmonary hemorrhage. Fatal bleeding events have been reported. Acute profound thrombocytopenia has been reported.

OVERDOSAGE

There has been only limited experience with overdosage of eptifibatide. There were 8 patients in the IMPACT II study, 9 patients in the PURSUIT study, and no patients in the ESPRIT study who received bolus doses and/or infusion doses more than double those called for in the protocols. None of these patients experienced an intracranial bleed or other major bleeding.

Eptifibatide was not lethal to rats, rabbits, or monkeys when administered by continuous intravenous infusion for 90 minutes at a total dose of 45 mg/kg (about 2-5 times the recommended maximum daily human dose on a body surface area basis). Symptoms of acute toxicity were loss of righting reflex, dyspnea, ptosis, and decreased muscle tone in rabbits and petechial hemorrhages in the femoral and abdominal areas of monkeys.

From *in vitro* studies, eptifibatide is not extensively bound to plasma proteins and thus may be cleared from plasma by dialysis.

DOSAGE AND ADMINISTRATION

The safety and efficacy of eptifibatide has been established in clinical studies that employed concomitant use of heparin and aspirin. Different dose regimens of eptifibatide were used in the major clinical studies (see **CLINICAL STUDIES**).

Acute Coronary Syndrome

The recommended adult dosage of eptifibatide in patients with acute coronary syndrome and normal renal function is an intravenous bolus of 180 mcg/kg as soon as possible following diagnosis, followed by a continuous infusion of 2.0 mcg/kg/min until hospital discharge or initiation of CABG surgery, up to 72 hours. If a patient is to undergo a percutaneous coronary intervention (PCI) while receiving eptifibatide, the infusion should be continued up to hospital discharge, or for up to 18 to 24 hours after the procedure, whichever comes first, allowing for up to 96 hours of therapy.

Patients With Creatinine Clearance Less Than 50 mL/min

The recommended adult dosage of eptifibatide in patients with acute coronary syndrome with an estimated creatinine clearance (using the Cockcroft-Gault equation)* <50 mL/min is an intravenous bolus of 180 mcg/kg as soon as possible following diagnosis, immediately followed by a continuous infusion of 1.0 mcg/kg/min.

Percutaneous Coronary Intervention (PCI)

The recommended adult dosage of eptifibatide in patients with normal renal function is an intravenous bolus of 180 mcg/kg administered immediately before the initiation of PCI followed by a continuous infusion of 2.0 mcg/kg/min and a second 180-mcg/kg bolus 10 minutes after the first bolus. Infusion should be continued until hospital discharge, or for up to 18 to 24 hours, whichever comes first. A minimum of 12 hours of infusion is recommended.

Patients With Creatinine Clearance Less Than 50 mL/min

The recommended adult dose of eptifibatide in patients with an estimated creatinine clearance (using the Cockcroft-Gault equation)* <50 mL/min is an intravenous bolus of 180 mcg/kg administered immediately before the initiation of the procedure, immediately followed by a continuous infusion of 1.0 mcg/kg/min and a second 180-mcg/kg bolus administered 10 minutes after the first.

In patients who undergo coronary artery bypass graft surgery, eptifibatide infusion should be discontinued prior to surgery.

* Use the Cockcroft-Gault equation with actual body weight to calculate creatinine clearance:

Males: $$\frac{(140 - \text{age}) \times (\text{actual body wt in kg})}{72 \times (\text{serum creatinine})}$$

Females: $$\frac{(140 - \text{age}) \times (\text{actual body wt in kg}) \times 0.85}{72 \times (\text{serum creatinine})}$$

Aspirin and Heparin Dosing Recommendations

In the clinical trials that showed eptifibatide to be effective, most patients received concomitant aspirin and heparin. The recommended aspirin and heparin doses to be used are as follows:

Acute Coronary Syndrome

Aspirin:

160 to 325 mg orally initially and daily thereafter

Heparin:

Target aPTT 50 to 70 seconds during medical management
- If weight ≥70 kg, 5000-U bolus followed by infusion of 1000 U/hr.
- If weight <70 kg, 60-U/kg bolus followed by infusion of 12 U/kg/hr.

Target ACT 200 to 300 seconds during PCI
- If heparin is initiated prior to PCI, additional boluses during PCI to maintain an ACT target of 200 to 300 seconds.
- Heparin infusion after the PCI is discouraged.

PCI

Aspirin:

160 to 325 mg orally 1 to 24 hours prior to PCI and daily thereafter

Heparin:

Target ACT 200 to 300 seconds
- 60-U/kg bolus initially in patients not treated with heparin within 6 hours prior to PCI.
- Additional boluses during PCI to maintain ACT within target.
- Heparin infusion after the PCI is strongly discouraged.

Patients requiring thrombolytic therapy should have eptifibatide infusions stopped.

Instructions for Administration

1. Like other parenteral drug products, INTEGRILIN® solutions should be inspected visually for particulate matter and discoloration prior to administration, whenever solution and container permit.
2. INTEGRILIN may be administered in the same intravenous line as alteplase, atropine, dobutamine, heparin, lidocaine, meperidine, metoprolol, midazolam, morphine, nitroglycerin, or verapamil. INTEGRILIN should not be administered through the same intravenous line as furosemide.
3. INTEGRILIN may be administered in the same IV line with 0.9% NaCl or 0.9% NaCl/5% dextrose. With either vehicle, the infusion may also contain up to 60 mEq/L of potassium chloride. No incompatibilities have been observed with intravenous administration sets. No compatibility studies have been performed with PVC bags.
4. The bolus dose(s) of INTEGRILIN should be withdrawn from the 10-mL vial into a syringe. The bolus dose(s) should be administered by IV push.
5. Immediately following the bolus dose administration, a continuous infusion of INTEGRILIN should be initiated. When using an intravenous infusion pump, INTEGRILIN should be administered undiluted directly from the 100-mL vial. The 100-mL vial should be spiked with a vented infusion set. Care should be taken to center the spike within the circle on the stopper top.

INTEGRILIN is to be administered by volume according to patient weight. Patients should receive INTEGRILIN according to the following table:

[See table above]

HOW SUPPLIED

INTEGRILIN® (eptifibatide) Injection is supplied as a sterile solution in 10-mL vials containing 20 mg of eptifibatide (NDC 0085-1177-01) and 100-mL vials containing either 75 mg of eptifibatide (NDC 0085-1136-01) or 200 mg of eptifibatide (NDC 0085-1177-02).

Vials should be stored refrigerated at 2°-8°C (36°-46°F). Vials may be transferred to room temperature storage† for a period not to exceed 2 months. Upon transfer, vial cartons must be marked by the dispensing pharmacist with a "DISCARD BY" date (2 months from the transfer date or the labeled expiration date, whichever comes first).

Do not use beyond the labeled expiration date. Protect from light until administration. Discard any unused portion left in the vial.

†Store at 25°C (77°F); excursions permitted to 15°-30°C (59°-86°F) [see USP Controlled Room Temperature].

Manufactured for Schering Corporation, a subsidiary of Schering-Plough Corporation, Kenilworth, NJ 07033 USA.

U.S. Patent Nos. 5,686,570; 5,747,447; 5,756,451; 5,807,825; and 5,968,902.

INTEGRILIN is a registered trademark of Millennium Pharmaceuticals, Inc.

Rev. 1/09 **31447119T**

Shown in Product Identification Guide, page 313

INTRON® A ℞

[*ĭn' trŏn*]

Interferon alfa-2b, recombinant

For Injection

PRODUCT INFORMATION

WARNING

Alpha interferons, including INTRON® A, cause or aggravate fatal or life-threatening neuropsychiatric, autoimmune, ischemic, and infectious disorders. Patients

should be monitored closely with periodic clinical and laboratory evaluations. Patients with persistently severe or worsening signs or symptoms of these conditions should be withdrawn from therapy. In many but not all cases these disorders resolve after stopping INTRON A therapy. See WARNINGS and ADVERSE REACTIONS.

DESCRIPTION

INTRON® A (Interferon alfa-2b) for intramuscular, subcutaneous, intralesional, or intravenous Injection is a purified sterile recombinant interferon product.

INTRON A recombinant for Injection has been classified as an alpha interferon and is a water-soluble protein with a molecular weight of 19,271 daltons produced by recombinant DNA techniques. It is obtained from the bacterial fermentation of a strain of *Escherichia coli* bearing a genetically engineered plasmid containing an interferon alfa-2b gene from human leukocytes. The fermentation is carried out in a defined nutrient medium containing the antibiotic tetracycline hydrochloride at a concentration of 5 to 10 mg/L; the presence of this antibiotic is not detectable in the final product. The specific activity of interferon alfa-2b, recombinant is approximately 2.6×10^8 IU/mg protein as measured by the HPLC assay.

[See first table above]

Prior to administration, the INTRON A Powder for Injection is to be reconstituted with the provided Diluent for INTRON A (Sterile Water for Injection USP) (see **DOSAGE AND ADMINISTRATION**). INTRON A Powder for Injection is a white to cream-colored powder.

[See second table at right]

[See third table at right]

These packages do not require reconstitution prior to administration (see **DOSAGE AND ADMINISTRATION**). INTRON A Solution for Injection is a clear, colorless solution.

CLINICAL PHARMACOLOGY

General

The interferons are a family of naturally occurring small proteins and glycoproteins with molecular weights of approximately 15,000 to 27,600 daltons produced and secreted by cells in response to viral infections and to synthetic or biological inducers.

Preclinical Pharmacology

Interferons exert their cellular activities by binding to specific membrane receptors on the cell surface. Once bound to the cell membrane, interferons initiate a complex sequence of intracellular events. *In vitro* studies demonstrated that these include the induction of certain enzymes, suppression of cell proliferation, immunomodulating activities such as enhancement of the phagocytic activity of macrophages and augmentation of the specific cytotoxicity of lymphocytes for target cells, and inhibition of virus replication in virus-infected cells.

In a study using human hepatoblastoma cell line HB 611, the *in vitro* antiviral activity of alpha interferon was demonstrated by its inhibition of hepatitis B virus (HBV) replication.

The correlation between these *in vitro* data and the clinical results is unknown. Any of these activities might contribute to interferon's therapeutic effects.

Pharmacokinetics

The pharmacokinetics of INTRON® A were studied in 12 healthy male volunteers following single doses of 5 million IU/m^2 administered intramuscularly, subcutaneously, and as a 30 minute intravenous infusion in a crossover design. The mean serum INTRON A concentrations following intramuscular and subcutaneous injections were comparable. The maximum serum concentrations obtained via these routes were approximately 18 to 116 IU/mL and occurred 3 to 12 hours after administration. The elimination half-life of INTRON A following both intramuscular and subcutaneous injections was approximately 2 to 3 hours. Serum concentrations were undetectable by 16 hours after the injections. After intravenous administration, serum INTRON A concentrations peaked (135–273 IU/mL) by the end of the 30-minute infusion, then declined at a slightly more rapid rate than after intramuscular or subcutaneous drug administration, becoming undetectable 4 hours after the infusion. The elimination half-life was approximately 2 hours.

Urine INTRON A concentrations following a single dose (5 million IU/m^2) were not detectable after any of the parenteral routes of administration. This result was expected since preliminary studies with isolated and perfused rabbit kidneys have shown that the kidney may be the main site of interferon catabolism.

There are no pharmacokinetic data available for the intralesional route of administration.

Serum Neutralizing Antibodies

In INTRON A-treated patients tested for antibody activity in clinical trials, serum anti-interferon neutralizing antibodies were detected in 0% (0/90) of patients with hairy cell

Powder for Injection

Vial Strength Million IU	mL Diluent	Final Concentration after Reconstitution million IU/mL*	mg INTRON A[†] per vial	Route of Administration
10	1	10	0.038	IM, SC, IV, IL
18	1	18	0.069	IM, SC, IV
50	1	50	0.192	IM, SC, IV

* Each mL also contains 20 mg glycine, 2.3 mg sodium phosphate dibasic, 0.55 mg sodium phosphate monobasic, and 1.0 mg human albumin.
† Based on the specific activity of approximately 2.6×10^8 IU/mg protein, as measured by HPLC assay.

Solution Vials for Injection

Vial Strength	Concentration*	mg INTRON A[†] per vial	Route of Administration
18[‡] MIU multidose	3 million IU/0.5 mL	0.088	IM, SC
25[§] MIU multidose	5 million IU/0.5 mL	0.123	IM, SC, IL

* Each mL contains 7.5 mg sodium chloride, 1.8 mg sodium phosphate dibasic, 1.3 mg sodium phosphate monobasic, 0.1 mg edetate disodium, 0.1 mg polysorbate 80, and 1.5 mg m-cresol as a preservative.
† Based on the specific activity of approximately 2.6×10^8 IU/mg protein as measured by HPLC assay.
‡ This is a multidose vial which contains a total of 22.8 million IU of interferon alfa-2b, recombinant per 3.8 mL in order to provide the delivery of six 0.5-mL doses, each containing 3 million IU of INTRON A (for a label strength of 18 million IU).
§ This is a multidose vial which contains a total of 32.0 million IU of interferon alfa-2b, recombinant per 3.2 mL in order to provide the delivery of five 0.5-mL doses, each containing 5 million IU of INTRON A (for a label strength of 25 million IU).

Solution in Multidose Pens for Injection

Pen Strength	Concentration* Million IU/1.5 ml	INTRON A Dose Delivered (6 doses, 0.2 mL each)	mg INTRON A[†] per 1.5 mL	Route of Administration
3 MIU	22.5	3 MIU/0.2 ml	0.087	SC
5 MIU	37.5	5 MIU/0.2 ml	0.144	SC
10 MIU	75	10 MIU/0.2 ml	0.288	SC

* Each mL also contains 7.5 mg sodium chloride, 1.8 mg sodium phosphate dibasic, 1.3 mg sodium phosphate monobasic, 0.1 mg edetate disodium, 0.1 mg polysorbate 80, and 1.5 mg m-cresol as a preservative.
† Based on the specific activity of approximately 2.6×10^8 IU/mg protein as measured by HPLC assay.

leukemia, 0.8% (2/260) of patients treated intralesionally for condylomata acuminata, and 4% (1/24) of patients with AIDS-Related Kaposi's Sarcoma. Serum neutralizing antibodies have been detected in <3% of patients treated with higher INTRON A doses in malignancies other than hairy cell leukemia or AIDS-Related Kaposi's Sarcoma. The clinical significance of the appearance of serum anti-interferon neutralizing activity in these indications is not known.

Serum anti-interferon neutralizing antibodies were detected in 7% (12/168) of patients either during treatment or after completing 12 to 48 weeks of treatment with 3 million IU TIW of INTRON A therapy for chronic hepatitis C and in 13% (6/48) of patients who received INTRON A therapy for chronic hepatitis B at 5 million IU QD for 4 months, and in 3% (1/33) of patients treated at 10 million IU TIW. Serum anti-interferon neutralizing antibodies were detected in 9% (5/53) of pediatric patients who received INTRON A therapy for chronic hepatitis B at 6 million IU/m^2 TIW. Among all chronic hepatitis B or C patients, pediatrics and adults with detectable serum neutralizing antibodies, the titers detected were low (22/24 with titers ≤1:40 and 2/24 with titers ≤1:160). The appearance of serum anti-interferon neutralizing activity did not appear to affect safety or efficacy.

Hairy Cell Leukemia

In clinical trials in patients with hairy cell leukemia, there was depression of hematopoiesis during the first 1 to 2 months of INTRON A treatment, resulting in reduced numbers of circulating red and white blood cells, and platelets. Subsequently, both splenectomized and nonsplenectomized patients achieved substantial and sustained improvements in granulocytes, platelets, and hemoglobin levels in 75% of treated patients and at least some improvement (minor responses) occurred in 90%. INTRON A treatment resulted in a decrease in bone marrow hypercellularity and hairy cell infiltrates. The hairy cell index (HCI), which represents the percent of bone marrow cellularity times the percent of hairy cell infiltrate, was ≥50% at the beginning of the study in 87% of patients. The percentage of patients with such an HCI decreased to 25% after 6 months and to 14% after 1 year. These results indicate that even though hematologic

improvement had occurred earlier, prolonged INTRON A treatment may be required to obtain maximal reduction in tumor cell infiltrates in the bone marrow.

The percentage of patients with hairy cell leukemia who required red blood cell or platelet transfusions decreased significantly during treatment and the percentage of patients with confirmed and serious infections declined as granulocyte counts improved. Reversal of splenomegaly and of clinically significant hypersplenism was demonstrated in some patients.

A study was conducted to assess the effects of extended INTRON A treatment on duration of response for patients who responded to initial therapy. In this study, 126 responding patients were randomized to receive additional INTRON A treatment for 6 months or observation for a comparable period, after 12 months of initial INTRON A therapy. During this 6-month period, 3% (2/66) of INTRON A-treated patients relapsed compared with 18% (11/60) who were not treated. This represents a significant difference in time to relapse in favor of continued INTRON A treatment (P=0.006/0.01, Log Rank/Wilcoxon). Since a small proportion of the total population had relapsed, median time to relapse could not be estimated in either group. A similar pattern in relapses was seen when all randomized treatment, including that beyond 6 months, and available follow-up data were assessed. The 15% (10/66) relapses among INTRON A patients occurred over a significantly longer period of time than the 40% (24/60) with observation (P=0.0002/0.0001, Log Rank/Wilcoxon). Median time to relapse was estimated, using the Kaplan-Meier method, to be 6.8 months in the observation group but could not be estimated in the INTRON A group.

Subsequent follow-up with a median time of approximately 40 months demonstrated an overall survival of 87.8%. In a comparable historical control group followed for 24 months, overall median survival was approximately 40%.

Malignant Melanoma

The safety and efficacy of INTRON A was evaluated as adjuvant to surgical treatment in patients with melanoma who were free of disease (post surgery) but at high risk for systemic recurrence. These included patients with lesions of Breslow thickness >4 mm, or patients with lesions of any Breslow thickness with primary or recurrent nodal involvement. In a randomized, controlled trial in 280 patients, 143 patients received INTRON A therapy at 20 million IU/m^2 intravenously five times per week for 4 weeks (induction phase) followed by 10 million IU/m^2 subcutaneously three times per week for 48 weeks (maintenance phase). In the clinical trial, the median daily INTRON A dose administered to patients was 19.1 million IU/m^2 during the induction phase and 9.1 million IU/m^2 during the maintenance phase. INTRON A therapy was begun ≤56 days after surgical resection. The remaining 137 patients were observed.

INTRON A therapy produced a significant increase in relapse-free and overall survival. Median time to relapse for the INTRON A-treated patients vs observation patients was 1.72 years vs 0.98 years (P<0.01, stratified Log Rank). The estimated 5-year relapse-free survival rate, using the Kaplan-Meier method, was 37% for INTRON A-treated patients vs 26% for observation patients. Median overall survival time for INTRON A-treated patients vs observation patients was 3.82 years vs 2.78 years (P=0.047, stratified Log Rank). The estimated 5-year overall survival rate, using the Kaplan-Meier method, was 46% for INTRON A-treated patients vs 37% for observation patients.

In a second study of 642 resected high-risk melanoma patients, subjects were randomized equally to one of three groups: high-dose INTRON A therapy for 1 year (same schedule as above), low-dose INTRON A therapy for 2 years (3 MU/d TIW SC), and observation. Consistent with the earlier trial, high-dose INTRON A therapy demonstrated an improvement in relapse-free survival (3-year estimated RFS 48% vs 41%; median RFS 2.4 vs 1.6 years, P=not significant). Relapse-free survival in the low-dose INTRON A arm was similar to that seen in the observation arm. Neither high-dose nor low-dose INTRON A therapy showed a benefit in overall survival as compared to observation in this study.

Follicular Lymphoma

The safety and efficacy of INTRON A in conjunction with CHVP, a combination chemotherapy regimen, was evaluated as initial treatment in patients with clinically aggressive, large tumor burden, Stage III/IV follicular Non-Hodgkin's Lymphoma. Large tumor burden was defined by the presence of any one of the following: a nodal or extranodal tumor mass with a diameter of >7 cm; involvement of at least three nodal sites (each with a diameter of >3 cm); systemic symptoms; splenomegaly; serous effusion, orbital or epidural involvement; ureteral compression; or leukemia.

In a randomized, controlled trial, 130 patients received CHVP therapy and 135 patients received CHVP therapy plus INTRON A therapy at 5 million IU subcutaneously three times weekly for the duration of 18 months. CHVP chemotherapy consisted of cyclophosphamide 600 mg/m^2, doxorubicin 25 mg/m^2, and teniposide (VM-26) 60 mg/m^2, administered intravenously on Day 1 and prednisone at a daily dose of 40 mg/m^2 given orally on Days 1 to 5. Treatment consisted of six CHVP cycles administered monthly, followed by an additional six cycles administered every 2 months for 1 year. Patients in both treatment groups received a total of 12 CHVP cycles over 18 months.

The group receiving the combination of INTRON A therapy plus CHVP had a significantly longer progression-free survival (2.9 years vs 1.5 years, P=0.0001, Log Rank test). After a median follow-up of 6.1 years, the median survival for patients treated with CHVP alone was 5.5 years while median survival for patients treated with CHVP plus INTRON A therapy had not been reached (P=0.004, Log Rank test). In three additional published, randomized, controlled studies of the addition of interferon alpha to anthracycline-containing combination chemotherapy regimens,[1-3] the addition of interferon alpha was associated with significantly prolonged progression-free survival. Differences in overall survival were not consistently observed.

Condylomata Acuminata

Condylomata acuminata (venereal or genital warts) are associated with infections of the human papilloma virus (HPV). The safety and efficacy of INTRON A in the treatment of condylomata acuminata were evaluated in three controlled double-blind clinical trials. In these studies, INTRON A doses of 1 million IU per lesion were administered intralesionally three times a week (TIW), in ≤5 lesions per patient for 3 weeks. The patients were observed for up to 16 weeks after completion of the full treatment course.

INTRON A treatment of condylomata was significantly more effective than placebo, as measured by disappearance of lesions, decreases in lesion size, and by an overall change in disease status. Of 192 INTRON A-treated patients and 206 placebo-treated patients who were evaluable for efficacy at the time of best response during the course of the study, 42% of INTRON A patients vs 17% of placebo patients experienced clearing of all treated lesions. Likewise, 24% of INTRON A patients vs 8% of placebo patients experienced marked (≥75% to <100%) reduction in lesion size, 18% vs 9% experienced moderate (≥50% to ≤75%) reduction in lesion size, 10% vs 42% had a slight (<50%) reduction in lesion size, 5% vs 24% had no change in lesion size, and 0% vs 1% experienced exacerbation (P<0.001).

In one of these studies, 43% (54/125) of patients in whom multiple (≤3) lesions were treated experienced complete clearing of all treated lesions during the course of the study. Of these patients, 81% remained cleared 16 weeks after treatment was initiated.

Patients who did not achieve total clearing of all their treated lesions had these same lesions treated with a second course of therapy. During this second course of treatment, 38% to 67% of patients had clearing of all treated lesions. The overall percentage of patients who had cleared all their treated lesions after two courses of treatment ranged from 57% to 85%.

INTRON A-treated lesions showed improvement within 2 to 4 weeks after the start of treatment in the above study; maximal response to INTRON A therapy was noted 4 to 8 weeks after initiation of treatment.

The response to INTRON A therapy was better in patients who had condylomata for shorter durations than in patients with lesions for a longer duration.

Another study involved 97 patients in whom three lesions were treated with either an intralesional injection of 1.5 million IU of INTRON A per lesion followed by a topical application of 25% podophyllin, or a topical application of 25% podophyllin alone. Treatment was given once a week for 3 weeks. The combined treatment of INTRON A and podophyllin was shown to be significantly more effective than podophyllin alone, as determined by the number of patients whose lesions cleared. This significant difference in response was evident after the second treatment (Week 3) and continued through 8 weeks posttreatment. At the time of the patient's best response, 67% (33/49) of the INTRON A- and podophyllin-treated patients had all three treated lesions clear while 42% (20/48) of the podophyllin-treated patients had all three clear (P=0.003).

AIDS-Related Kaposi's Sarcoma

The safety and efficacy of INTRON A in the treatment of Kaposi's Sarcoma (KS), a common manifestation of the Acquired Immune Deficiency Syndrome (AIDS), were evaluated in clinical trials in 144 patients.

In one study, INTRON A doses of 30 million IU/m^2 were administered subcutaneously three times per week (TIW) to patients with AIDS-Related KS. Doses were adjusted for patient tolerance. The average weekly dose delivered in the first 4 weeks was 150 million IU; at the end of 12 weeks this averaged 110 million IU/week; and by 24 weeks averaged 75 million IU/week.

Forty-four percent of asymptomatic patients responded vs 7% of symptomatic patients. The median time to response was approximately 2 months and 1 month, respectively, for asymptomatic and symptomatic patients. The median duration of response was approximately 3 months and 1 month, respectively, for the asymptomatic and symptomatic patients. Baseline T4/T8 ratios were 0.46 for responders vs 0.33 for nonresponders.

In another study, INTRON A doses of 35 million IU were administered subcutaneously, daily (QD), for 12 weeks. Maintenance treatment, with every other day dosing (QOD), was continued for up to 1 year in patients achieving antitumor and antiviral responses. The median time to response was 2 months and the median duration of response was 5 months in the asymptomatic patients.

In all studies, the likelihood of response was greatest in patients with relatively intact immune systems as assessed by baseline CD4 counts (interchangeable with T4 counts). Results at doses of 30 million IU/m^2 TIW and 35 million IU/QD were subcutaneously similar and are provided together in TABLE 1. This table demonstrates the relationship of response to baseline CD4 count in both asymptomatic and symptomatic patients in the 30 million IU/m^2 TIW and the 35 million IU/QD treatment groups.

In the 30 million IU study group, 7% (5/72) of patients were complete responders and 22% (16/72) of the patients were partial responders. The 35 million IU study had 13% (3/23 patients) complete responders and 17% (4/23) partial responders.

For patients who received 30 million IU TIW, the median survival time was longer in patients with CD4 >200 (30.7 months) than in patients with CD4 ≤200 (8.9 months). Among responders, the median survival time was 22.6 months vs 9.7 months in nonresponders.

Chronic Hepatitis C

The safety and efficacy of INTRON A in the treatment of chronic hepatitis C was evaluated in 5 randomized clinical studies in which an INTRON A dose of 3 million IU three times a week (TIW) was assessed. The initial three studies were placebo-controlled trials that evaluated a 6-month (24-week) course of therapy. In each of the three studies, INTRON A therapy resulted in a reduction in serum alanine aminotransferase (ALT) in a greater proportion of patients vs control patients at the end of 6 months of dosing. During the 6 months of follow-up, approximately 50% of the patients who responded maintained their ALT response. A combined analysis comparing pretreatment and posttreatment liver biopsies revealed histological improvement in a statistically significantly greater proportion of INTRON A-treated patients compared to controls.

Two additional studies have investigated longer treatment durations (up to 24 months).[5,6] Patients in the two studies to evaluate longer duration of treatment had hepatitis with or without cirrhosis in the absence of decompensated liver disease. Complete response to treatment was defined as normalization of the final two serum ALT levels during the treatment period. A sustained response was defined as a complete response at the end of the treatment period, with sustained normal ALT values lasting at least 6 months following discontinuation of therapy.

In Study 1, all patients were initially treated with INTRON A 3 million IU TIW subcutaneously for 24 weeks (run-in-period). Patients who completed the initial 24-week treatment period were then randomly assigned to receive no further treatment, or to receive 3 million IU TIW for an additional 48 weeks. In Study 2, patients who met the entry criteria were randomly assigned to receive INTRON A 3 million IU TIW subcutaneously for 24 weeks or to receive INTRON A 3 million IU TIW subcutaneously for 96 weeks. In both studies, patient follow-up was variable and some data collection was retrospective.

Results show that longer durations of INTRON A therapy improved the sustained response rate (see TABLE 2). In patients with complete responses (CR) to INTRON A therapy after 6 months of treatment (149/352 [42%]), responses were less often sustained if drug was discontinued (21/70 [30%]) than if it was continued for 18 to 24 months (44/79 [56%]). Of all patients randomized, the sustained response rate in the patients receiving 18 or 24 months of therapy was 22% and 26%, respectively, in the two trials. In patients who did not have a CR by 6 months, additional therapy did not result in significantly more responses, since almost all patients who responded to therapy did so within the first 16 weeks of treatment.

A subset (<50%) of patients from the combined extended dosing studies had liver biopsies performed both before and after INTRON A treatment. Improvement in necroinflammatory activity as assessed retrospectively by the Knodell (Study 1) and Scheuer (Study 2) Histology Activity Indices was observed in both studies. A higher number of patients (58%, 45/78) improved with extended therapy than with shorter (6 months) therapy (38%, 34/89) in this subset.

Combination treatment with INTRON A and REBETOL® (ribavirin, USP) provided a significant reduction in virologic load and improved histologic response in adult patients with compensated liver disease who were treatment naïve or had relapsed following therapy with alpha interferon alone; pediatric patients previously untreated with alpha interferon experienced a sustained virologic response. See REBETOL package insert for additional information.

Chronic Hepatitis B

Adults

The safety and efficacy of INTRON A in the treatment of chronic hepatitis B were evaluated in three clinical trials in which INTRON A doses of 30 to 35 million IU per week were administered subcutaneously (SC), as either 5 million IU daily (QD), or 10 million IU three times a week (TIW) for 16 weeks vs no treatment. All patients were 18 years of age or older with compensated liver disease, and had chronic hepatitis B virus (HBV) infection (serum HBsAg positive for at least 6 months) and HBV replication (serum HBeAg positive). Patients were also serum HBV-DNA positive, an additional indicator of HBV replication, as measured by a research assay.[7,8] All patients had elevated serum alanine aminotransferase (ALT) and liver biopsy findings compatible with the diagnosis of chronic hepatitis. Patients with the presence of antibody to human immunodeficiency virus (anti-HIV) or antibody to hepatitis delta virus (anti-HDV) in the serum were excluded from the studies.

Virologic response to treatment was defined in these studies as a loss of serum markers of HBV replication (HBeAg and HBV DNA). Secondary parameters of response included loss of serum HBsAg, decreases in serum ALT, and improvement in liver histology.

In each of two randomized controlled studies, a significantly greater proportion of INTRON A-treated patients exhibited a virologic response compared with untreated control patients (see TABLE 3). In a third study without a concurrent control group, a similar response rate to INTRON A therapy was observed. Pretreatment with prednisone, evaluated in two of the studies, did not improve the response rate and provided no additional benefit.

The response to INTRON A therapy was durable. No patient responding to INTRON A therapy at a dose of 5 million IU QD or 10 million IU TIW relapsed during the follow-up period, which ranged from 2 to 6 months after treatment ended. The loss of serum HBeAg and HBV DNA was maintained in 100% of 19 responding patients followed for 3.5 to 36 months after the end of therapy.

In a proportion of responding patients, loss of HBeAg was followed by the loss of HBsAg. HBsAg was lost in 27% (4/15) of patients who responded to INTRON A therapy at a dose of 5 million IU QD, and 35% (8/23) of patients who responded to 10 million IU TIW. No untreated control patient lost HBsAg in these studies.

In an ongoing study to assess the long-term durability of virologic response, 64 patients responding to INTRON A therapy have been followed for 1.1 to 6.6 years after treatment; 95% (61/64) remain serum HBeAg negative, and 49% (30/61) lost serum HBsAg.

INTRON A therapy resulted in normalization of serum ALT in a significantly greater proportion of treated patients compared to untreated patients in each of two controlled studies (see TABLE 4). In a third study without a concurrent control group, normalization of serum ALT was observed in 50% (12/24) of patients receiving INTRON A therapy.

Virologic response was associated with a reduction in serum ALT to normal or near normal ($\leq$1.5 × the upper limit of normal) in 87% (13/15) of patients responding to INTRON A therapy at 5 million IU QD, and 100% (23/23) of patients responding to 10 million IU TIW.

Improvement in liver histology was evaluated in Studies 1 and 3 by comparison of pretreatment and 6-month posttreatment liver biopsies using the semiquantitative Knodell Histology Activity Index.[9] No statistically significant difference in liver histology was observed in treated patients compared to control patients in Study 1. Although statistically significant histological improvement from baseline was observed in treated patients in Study 3 (P$\leq$0.01), there was no control group for comparison. Of those patients exhibiting a virologic response following treatment with 5 million IU QD or 10 million IU TIW, histological improvement was observed in 85% (17/20) compared to 36% (9/25) of patients who were not virologic responders. The histological improvement was due primarily to decreases in severity of necrosis, degeneration, and inflammation in the periportal, lobular, and portal regions of the liver (Knodell Categories I + II + III). Continued histological improvement was observed in four responding patients who lost serum HBsAg and were followed 2 to 4 years after the end of INTRON A therapy.[10]

Pediatrics

The safety and efficacy of INTRON A in the treatment of chronic hepatitis B was evaluated in one randomized controlled trial of 149 patients ranging from 1 year to 17 years of age. Seventy-two patients were treated with 3 million IU/m² of INTRON A therapy administered subcutaneously three times a week (TIW) for 1 week; the dose was then escalated to 6 million IU/m² TIW for a minimum of 16 weeks up to 24 weeks. The maximum weekly dosage was 10 million IU TIW. Seventy-seven patients were untreated controls. Study entry and response criteria were identical to those described in the adult patient population.

Patients treated with INTRON A therapy had a better response (loss of HBV DNA and HBeAg at 24 weeks of follow-up) compared to the untreated controls (24% [17/72] vs 10% [8/77] P=0.05). Sixteen of the 17 responders treated with INTRON A therapy remained HBV DNA and HBeAg negative and had a normal serum ALT 12 to 24 months after completion of treatment. Serum HBsAg became negative in 7 out of 17 patients who responded to INTRON A therapy. None of the control patients who had an HBV DNA and HBeAg response became HBsAg negative. At 24 weeks of follow-up, normalization of serum ALT was similar in patients treated with INTRON A therapy (17%, 12/72) and in untreated control patients (16%, 12/77). Patients with a baseline HBV DNA <100 pg/mL were more likely to respond to INTRON A therapy than were patients with a baseline HBV DNA >100 pg/mL (35% vs 9%, respectively). Patients who contracted hepatitis B through maternal vertical transmission had lower response rates than those who contracted the disease by other means (5% vs 31%, respectively). There was no evidence that the effects on HBV DNA and HBeAg were limited to specific subpopulations based on age, gender, or race.

TABLE 1 RESPONSE BY BASELINE CD4 COUNT* IN AIDS-RELATED KS PATIENTS

	30 million IU/m² TIW, SC and 35 million IU QD, SC			
	Asymptomatic		Symptomatic	
CD4<200	4/14	(29%)	0/19	(0%)
200≤CD4≤400	6/12	(50%)	0/5	(0%)
CD4>400	5/7	(71%)	0/0	(0%)

} 58%

*Data for CD4, and asymptomatic and symptomatic classification were not available for all patients.

[See table 2 above]

TABLE 2 SUSTAINED ALT RESPONSE RATE VS DURATION OF THERAPY IN CHRONIC HEPATITIS C PATIENTS INTRON A 3 Million IU TIW

	Treatment Group* - Number of Patients (%)		
Study Number	INTRON A 3 million IU 24 weeks of treatment	INTRON A 3 million IU 72 or 96 weeks of treatment[†]	Difference (Extended - 24 weeks) (95% CI)[‡]
	ALT response at the end of follow-up		
1	12/101 (12%)	23/104 (22%)	10% (-3, 24)
2	9/67 (13%)	21/80 (26%)	13% (-4, 30)
Combined Studies	21/168 (12.5%)	44/184 (24%)	11.4% (2, 21)
	ALT response at the end of treatment		
1	40/101 (40%)	51/104 (49%)	—
2	32/67 (48%)	35/80 (44%)	—

* Intent to treat groups.
† Study 1: 72 weeks of treatment; Study 2: 96 weeks of treatment.
‡ Confidence intervals adjusted for multiple comparisons due to 3 treatment arms in the study.

TABLE 3 VIROLOGIC RESPONSE* IN CHRONIC HEPATITIS B PATIENTS

	Treatment Group[†] - Number of Patients (%)						
Study Number	INTRON A 5 million IU QD		INTRON A 10 million IU TIW		Untreated Controls		P[‡] Value
1[7]	15/38	(39%)	—	—	3/42	(7%)	0.0009
2	—	—	10/24	(42%)	1/22	(5%)	0.005
3[8]	—	—	13/24[§]	(54%)	2/27	(7%)[§]	NA[§]
All Studies	15/38	(39%)	23/48	(48%)	6/91	(7%)	—

* Loss of HBeAg and HBV DNA by 6-months posttherapy.
† Patients pretreated with prednisone not shown.
‡ INTRON A treatment group vs untreated control.
§ Untreated control patients evaluated after 24-week observation period. A subgroup subsequently received INTRON A therapy. A direct comparison is not applicable (NA).

TABLE 4 ALT RESPONSES* IN CHRONIC HEPATITIS B PATIENTS

	Treatment Group - Number of Patients (%)						
Study Number	INTRON A 5 million IU QD		INTRON A 10 million IU TIW		Untreated Controls		P[†] Value
1	16/38	(42%)	—	—	8/42	(19%)	0.03
2	—	—	10/24	(42%)	1/22	(5%)	0.0034
3	—	—	12/24[‡]	(50%)	2/27	(7%)[‡]	NA[‡]
All Studies	16/38	(42%)	22/48	(46%)	11/91	(12%)	—

* Reduction in serum ALT to normal by 6-months posttherapy.
† INTRON A treatment group vs untreated control.
‡ Untreated control patients evaluated after 24-week observation period. A subgroup subsequently received INTRON A therapy. A direct comparison is not applicable (NA).

[See table 3 above]
[See table 4 above]

INDICATIONS AND USAGE

Hairy Cell Leukemia

INTRON® A is indicated for the treatment of patients 18 years of age or older with hairy cell leukemia.

Malignant Melanoma

INTRON A is indicated as adjuvant to surgical treatment in patients 18 years of age or older with malignant melanoma who are free of disease but at high risk for systemic recurrence, within 56 days of surgery.

Follicular Lymphoma

INTRON A is indicated for the initial treatment of clinically aggressive (see Clinical Experience) follicular Non-Hodgkin's Lymphoma in conjunction with anthracycline-containing combination chemotherapy in patients 18 years of age or older. Efficacy of INTRON A therapy in patients with low-grade, low-tumor burden follicular Non-Hodgkin's Lymphoma has not been demonstrated.

Condylomata Acuminata

INTRON A is indicated for intralesional treatment of selected patients 18 years of age or older with condylomata acuminata involving external surfaces of the genital and perianal areas (see DOSAGE AND ADMINISTRATION). The use of this product in adolescents has not been studied.

AIDS-Related Kaposi's Sarcoma

INTRON A is indicated for the treatment of selected patients 18 years of age or older with AIDS-Related Kaposi's Sarcoma. The likelihood of response to INTRON A therapy is greater in patients who are without systemic symptoms, who have limited lymphadenopathy and who have a relatively intact immune system as indicated by total CD4 count.

Chronic Hepatitis C

INTRON A is indicated for the treatment of chronic hepatitis C in patients 18 years of age or older with compensated liver disease who have a history of blood or blood-product exposure and/or are HCV antibody positive. Studies in these patients demonstrated that INTRON A therapy can produce clinically meaningful effects on this disease, manifested by normalization of serum alanine aminotransferase (ALT) and reduction in liver necrosis and degeneration.

A liver biopsy should be performed to establish the diagnosis of chronic hepatitis. Patients should be tested for the presence of antibody to HCV. Patients with other causes of chronic hepatitis, including autoimmune hepatitis, should be excluded. Prior to initiation of INTRON A therapy, the physician should establish that the patient has compensated liver disease. The following patient entrance criteria for compensated liver disease were used in the clinical studies and should be considered before INTRON A treatment of patients with chronic hepatitis C:

- No history of hepatic encephalopathy, variceal bleeding, ascites, or other clinical signs of decompensation
- Bilirubin   ≤2 mg/dL
- Albumin   Stable and within normal limits
- Prothrombin Time   <3 seconds prolonged
- WBC   ≥3000/mm³
- Platelets   ≥70,000/mm³

Serum creatinine should be normal or near normal.

Prior to initiation of INTRON A therapy, CBC and platelet counts should be evaluated in order to establish baselines for monitoring potential toxicity. These tests should be repeated at Weeks 1 and 2 following initiation of INTRON A therapy, and monthly thereafter. Serum ALT should be evaluated at approximately 3-month intervals to assess response to treatment (see **DOSAGE AND ADMINISTRATION**).

Patients with preexisting thyroid abnormalities may be treated if thyroid-stimulating hormone (TSH) levels can be maintained in the normal range by medication. TSH levels must be within normal limits upon initiation of INTRON A treatment and TSH testing should be repeated at 3 and 6 months (see **PRECAUTIONS, Laboratory Tests** section).

INTRON A in combination with REBETOL® is indicated for the treatment of chronic hepatitis C in patients 3 years of age and older with compensated liver disease previously untreated with alpha interferon therapy and in patients 18 years of age and older who have relapsed following alpha interferon therapy. See REBETOL package insert for additional information.

Chronic Hepatitis B

INTRON A is indicated for the treatment of chronic hepatitis B in patients 1 year of age or older with compensated liver disease. Patients who have been serum HBsAg positive for at least 6-months and have evidence of HBV replication (serum HBeAg positive) with elevated serum ALT are candidates for treatment. Studies in these patients demonstrated that INTRON A therapy can produce virologic remission of this disease (loss of serum HBeAg) and normalization of serum aminotransferases. INTRON A therapy resulted in the loss of serum HBsAg in some responding patients.

Prior to initiation of INTRON A therapy, it is recommended that a liver biopsy be performed to establish the presence of chronic hepatitis and the extent of liver damage. The physician should establish that the patient has compensated liver disease. The following patient entrance criteria for compensated liver disease were used in the clinical studies and should be considered before INTRON A treatment of patients with chronic hepatitis B:

- No history of hepatic encephalopathy, variceal bleeding, ascites, or other signs of clinical decompensation
- Bilirubin   Normal
- Albumin   Stable and within normal limits
- Prothrombin Time *Adults* <3 seconds prolonged
        Pediatrics ≤2 seconds prolonged
- WBC   ≥4000/mm^3
- Platelets   *Adults* ≥100,000/mm^3
        Pediatrics ≥150,000/mm^3

Patients with causes of chronic hepatitis other than chronic hepatitis B or chronic hepatitis C should not be treated with INTRON A. CBC and platelet counts should be evaluated prior to initiation of INTRON A therapy in order to establish baselines for monitoring potential toxicity. These tests should be repeated at treatment Weeks 1, 2, 4, 8, 12, and 16. Liver function tests, including serum ALT, albumin, and bilirubin, should be evaluated at treatment Weeks 1, 2, 4, 8, 12, and 16. HBeAg, HBsAg, and ALT should be evaluated at the end of therapy, as well as 3- and 6-months posttherapy, since patients may become virologic responders during the 6-month period following the end of treatment. In clinical studies in adults, 39% (15/38) of responding patients lost HBeAg 1 to 6 months following the end of INTRON A therapy. Of responding patients who lost HBsAg, 58% (7/12) did so 1 to 6 months posttreatment.

A transient increase in ALT ≥2 times baseline value (flare) can occur during INTRON A therapy for chronic hepatitis B. In clinical trials in adults and pediatrics, this flare generally occurred 8 to 12 weeks after initiation of therapy and was more frequent in responders (*adults* 63%, 24/38; *pediatrics* 59%, 10/17) than in nonresponders (*adults* 27%, 13/48; *pediatrics* 35%, 19/55). However, in adults and pediatrics, elevations in bilirubin ≥3 mg/dL (≥2 times ULN) occurred infrequently (*adults* 2%, 2/86; *pediatrics* 3%, 2/72) during therapy. When ALT flare occurs, in general, INTRON A therapy should be continued unless signs and symptoms of liver failure are observed. During ALT flare, clinical symptomatology and liver function tests including ALT, prothrombin time, alkaline phosphatase, albumin, and bilirubin, should be monitored at approximately 2-week intervals (see **WARNINGS**).

CONTRAINDICATIONS

INTRON® A is contraindicated in patients with:
- Hypersensitivity to interferon alpha or any component of the product.
- Autoimmune hepatitis.
- Decompensated liver disease.

INTRON A and REBETOL® combination therapy is additionally contraindicated in:
- Patients with hypersensitivity to ribavirin or any other component of the product
- Women who are pregnant
- Men whose female partners are pregnant

- Patients with hemoglobinopathies (e.g. thalassemia major, sickle cell anemia)
- Patients with creatinine clearance < 50 mL/min

See REBETOL package insert for additional information.

WARNINGS

General

Moderate to severe adverse experiences may require modification of the patient's dosage regimen, or in some cases termination of INTRON® A therapy. Because of the fever and other "flu-like" symptoms associated with INTRON A administration, it should be used cautiously in patients with debilitating medical conditions, such as those with a history of pulmonary disease (e.g., chronic obstructive pulmonary disease) or diabetes mellitus prone to ketoacidosis. Caution should also be observed in patients with coagulation disorders (eg, thrombophlebitis, pulmonary embolism) or severe myelosuppression.

Cardiovascular Disorders

INTRON A therapy should be used cautiously in patients with a history of cardiovascular disease. Those patients with a history of myocardial infarction and/or previous or current arrhythmic disorder who require INTRON A therapy should be closely monitored (see **PRECAUTIONS, Laboratory Tests** section). Cardiovascular adverse experiences, which include hypotension, arrhythmia, or tachycardia of 150 beats per minute or greater, and rarely, cardiomyopathy and myocardial infarction have been observed in some INTRON A-treated patients. Some patients with these adverse events had no history of cardiovascular disease. Transient cardiomyopathy was reported in approximately 2% of the AIDS-Related Kaposi's Sarcoma patients treated with INTRON A. Hypotension may occur during INTRON A administration, or up to 2 days posttherapy, and may require supportive therapy including fluid replacement to maintain intravascular volume.

Supraventricular arrhythmias occurred rarely and appeared to be correlated with preexisting conditions and prior therapy with cardiotoxic agents. These adverse experiences were controlled by modifying the dose or discontinuing treatment, but may require specific additional therapy.

Cerebrovascular Disorders

Ischemic and hemorrhagic cerebrovascular events have been observed in patients treated with interferon alpha-based therapies, including INTRON A. Events occurred in patients with few or no reported risk factors for stroke, including patients less than 45 years of age. Because these are spontaneous reports, estimates of frequency cannot be made and a causal relationship between interferon alpha-based therapies and these events is difficult to establish.

Neuropsychiatric Disorders

DEPRESSION AND SUICIDAL BEHAVIOR INCLUDING SUICIDAL IDEATION, SUICIDAL ATTEMPTS, AND COMPLETED SUICIDES, HOMICIDAL IDEATION, AND AGGRESSIVE BEHAVIOR SOMETIMES DIRECTED TOWARDS OTHERS, HAVE BEEN REPORTED IN ASSOCIATION WITH TREATMENT WITH ALPHA INTERFERONS, INCLUDING INTRON A THERAPY. If patients develop psychiatric problems, including clinical depression, it is recommended that the patients be carefully monitored during treatment and in the 6-month follow-up period.

Patients with a preexisting psychiatric condition, especially depression, or a history of severe psychiatric disorder should not be treated with INTRON A.[11] INTRON A therapy should be discontinued for any patient developing severe depression or other psychiatric disorder during treatment. Obtundation and coma have also been observed in some patients, usually elderly, treated at higher doses. While these effects are usually rapidly reversible upon discontinuation of therapy, full resolution of symptoms has taken up to 3 weeks in a few severe episodes. If psychiatric symptoms persist or worsen, or suicidal ideation or aggressive behavior towards others is identified, it is recommended that treatment with INTRON A be discontinued and the patient followed, with psychiatric intervention as appropriate. Narcotics, hypnotics, or sedatives may be used concurrently with caution and patients should be closely monitored until the adverse effects have resolved. Suicidal ideation or attempts occurred more frequently among pediatric patients, primarily adolescents, compared to adult patients (2.4% vs 1%) during treatment and off-therapy follow-up. Cases of encephalopathy have also been observed in some patients, usually elderly, treated with higher doses of INTRON A.

Bone marrow toxicity

INTRON A therapy suppresses bone marrow function and may result in severe cytopenias including aplastic anemia. It is advised that complete blood counts (CBC) be obtained pretreatment and monitored routinely during therapy (see **PRECAUTIONS, Laboratory Tests** section). INTRON A therapy should be discontinued in patients who develop severe decreases in neutrophil (<0.5 × 10^9/L) or platelet counts (<25 × 10^9/L) (see **DOSAGE AND ADMINISTRATION, Guidelines for Dose Modification**).

Ophthalmologic Disorders

Decrease or loss of vision, retinopathy including macular edema, retinal artery or vein thrombosis, retinal hemorrhages and cotton wool spots; optic neuritis, papilledema and serous retinal detachment may be induced or aggravated by treatment with interferon alfa-2b or other alpha interferons. All patients should receive an eye examination at baseline. Patients with preexisting ophthalmologic disorders (e.g., diabetic or hypertensive retinopathy) should receive periodic ophthalmologic exams during interferon alpha treatment. Any patient who develops ocular symptoms should receive a prompt and complete eye examination. Interferon alfa-2b treatment should be discontinued in patients who develop new or worsening ophthalmologic disorders.

Endocrine Disorders

Infrequently, patients receiving INTRON A therapy developed thyroid abnormalities, either hypothyroid or hyperthyroid. The mechanism by which INTRON A may alter thyroid status is unknown. Patients with preexisting thyroid abnormalities whose thyroid function cannot be maintained in the normal range by medication should not be treated with INTRON A. Prior to initiation of INTRON A therapy, serum TSH should be evaluated. Patients developing symptoms consistent with possible thyroid dysfunction during the course of INTRON A therapy should have their thyroid function evaluated and appropriate treatment instituted. Therapy should be discontinued for patients developing thyroid abnormalities during treatment whose thyroid function cannot be normalized by medication. Discontinuation of INTRON A therapy has not always reversed thyroid dysfunction occurring during treatment. Diabetes mellitus has been observed in patients treated with alpha interferons. Patients with these conditions who cannot be effectively treated by medication should not begin INTRON A therapy. Patients who develop these conditions during treatment and cannot be controlled with medication should not continue INTRON A therapy.

Gastrointestinal Disorders

Hepatotoxicity, including fatality, has been observed in interferon alpha-treated patients, including those treated with INTRON A. Any patient developing liver function abnormalities during treatment should be monitored closely and if appropriate, treatment should be discontinued.

Pulmonary Disorders

Dyspnea, pulmonary infiltrates, pneumonia, bronchiolitis obliterans, interstitial pneumonitis, pulmonary hypertension, and sarcoidosis, some resulting in respiratory failure and/or patient deaths, may be induced or aggravated by INTRON A or other alpha interferons. Recurrence of respiratory failure has been observed with interferon rechallenge. The etiologic explanation for these pulmonary findings has yet to be established. Any patient developing fever, cough, dyspnea, or other respiratory symptoms should have a chest X-ray taken. If the chest X-ray shows pulmonary infiltrates or there is evidence of pulmonary function impairment, the patient should be closely monitored, and, if appropriate, interferon alpha treatment should be discontinued. While this has been reported more often in patients with chronic hepatitis C treated with interferon alpha, it has also been reported in patients with oncologic diseases treated with interferon alpha.

Autoimmune Disorders

Rare cases of autoimmune diseases including thrombocytopenia, vasculitis, Raynaud's phenomenon, rheumatoid arthritis, lupus erythematosus, and rhabdomyolysis have been observed in patients treated with alpha interferons, including patients treated with INTRON A. In very rare cases the event resulted in fatality. The mechanism by which these events developed and their relationship to interferon alpha therapy is not clear. Any patient developing an autoimmune disorder during treatment should be closely monitored and, if appropriate, treatment should be discontinued.

Human Albumin

The powder formulations of this product contain albumin, a derivative of human blood. Based on effective donor screening and product manufacturing processes, it carries an extremely remote risk for transmission of viral diseases. A theoretical risk for transmission of Creutzfeldt-Jakob disease (CJD) also is considered extremely remote. No cases of transmission of viral diseases or CJD have ever been identified for albumin.

AIDS-Related Kaposi's Sarcoma

INTRON A therapy should not be used for patients with rapidly progressive visceral disease (see **CLINICAL PHARMACOLOGY**). Also of note, there may be synergistic adverse effects between INTRON A and zidovudine. Patients receiving concomitant zidovudine have had a higher incidence of neutropenia than that expected with zidovudine alone. Careful monitoring of the WBC count is indicated in all patients who are myelosuppressed and in all patients receiving other myelosuppressive medications. The effects of INTRON A when combined with other drugs used in the treatment of AIDS-related disease are unknown.

TREATMENT-RELATED ADVERSE EXPERIENCES BY INDICATION

Dosing Regimens
Percentage (%) of Patients*

ADVERSE EXPERIENCE	MALIGNANT MELANOMA 20 MIU/m² Induction (IV) 10 MIU/m² Maintenance (SC) N=143	FOLLICULAR LYMPHOMA 5 MIU TIW/SC N=135	HAIRY CELL LEUKEMIA 2 MIU/m² TIW/SC N=145	CONDYLOMATA ACUMINATA 1 MIU/lesion N=352	AIDS-RELATED KAPOSI'S SARCOMA 30 MIU/m² TIW/SC N=74	35 MIU QD/SC N=29	CHRONIC HEPATITIS C† 3 MIU TIW N=183	CHRONIC HEPATITIS B Adults 5 MIU QD N=101	10 MIU TIW N=78	CHRONIC HEPATITIS B Pediatrics 6 MIU/m² TIW N=116
Application-Site Disorders										
injection site inflammation	—	1	20	—	—	—	5	3	—	—
other (≤5%)	burning, injection site bleeding, injection site pain, injection site reaction (5% in chronic hepatitis B pediatrics), itching									
Blood Disorders (<5%)	anemia, anemia hypochromic, granulocytopenia, hemolytic anemia, leukopenia, lymphocytosis, neutropenia (9% in chronic hepatitis C, 14% in chronic hepatitis B pediatrics), thrombocytopenia (10% in chronic hepatitis C) (bleeding 8% in malignant melanoma), thrombocytopenia purpura									
Body as a Whole										
facial edema		1	—	<1	—	10	<1	3	1	<1
weight decrease	3	13	<1	<1	5	10	10	2	5	3
other (≤5%)	allergic reaction, cachexia, dehydration, earache, hernia, edema, hypercalcemia, hyperglycemia, hypothermia, inflammation nonspecific, lymphadenitis, lymphadenopathy, mastitis, periorbital edema, poor peripheral circulation, peripheral edema (6% in follicular lymphoma), phlebitis superficial, scrotal/penile edema, thirst, weakness, weight increase									
Cardiovascular System Disorders (<5%)	angina, arrhythmia, atrial fibrillation, bradycardia, cardiac failure, cardiomegaly, cardiomyopathy, coronary artery disorder, extrasystoles, heart valve disorder, hematoma, hypertension (9% in chronic hepatitis C), hypotension, palpitations, phlebitis, postural hypotension, pulmonary embolism, Raynaud's disease, tachycardia, thrombosis, varicose vein									
Endocrine System Disorders (<5%)	aggravation of diabetes mellitus, goiter, gynecomastia, hyperglycemia, hyperthyroidism, hypertriglyceridemia, hypothyroidism, virilism									
Flu-like Symptoms										
fever	81	56	68	56	47	55	34	66	86	94
headache	62	21	39	47	36	21	43	61	44	57
chills	54	—	46	45	—	—	—	—	—	—
myalgia	75	16	39	44	34	28	43	59	40	27
fatigue	96	8	61	18	84	48	23	75	69	71
increased sweating	6	13	8	2	4	21	4	1	1	3
asthenia	—	63	7	—	11	—	40	5	15	5
rigors	2	7	—	—	30	14	16	38	42	30
arthralgia	6	8	8	9	—	3	16	19	8	15
dizziness	23	—	12	9	7	24	9	13	10	8
influenza-like symptoms	10	18	37	—	45	79	26	5	—	<1
back pain	—	15	19	6	1	3	—	—	—	—
dry mouth	1	2	19	—	22	28	5	6	5	—
chest pain	2	8	<1	<1	1	28	5	4	—	—
malaise	6	—	—	14	5	—	13	9	6	3
pain (unspecified)	15	9	18	3	3	3	—	—	—	—
other (<5%)	chest pain substernal, hyperthermia, rhinitis, rhinorrhea									
Gastrointestinal System Disorders										
diarrhea	35	19	18	2	18	45	13	19	8	12
anorexia	69	21	19	1	38	41	14	43	53	43
nausea	66	24	21	17	28	21	19	50	33	18
taste alteration	24	2	13	<1	5	7	2	10	—	—
abdominal pain	2	20	<5	1	5	21	16	5	4	23
loose stools	—	1	—	<1	—	10	2	2	—	2
vomiting	‡	32	6	2	11	14	8	7	10	27
constipation	1	14	<1	—	1	10	4	5	—	2
gingivitis	2§	7§	—	—	—	14	—	1	—	—
dyspepsia	—	2	—	2	4	—	7	3	8	3
other (<5%)	abdominal ascites, abdominal distension, colitis, dysphagia, eructation, esophagitis, flatulence, gallstones, gastric ulcer, gastritis, gastroenteritis, gastrointestinal disorder (7% in follicular lymphoma), gastrointestinal hemorrhage, gastrointestinal mucosal discoloration, gingival bleeding, gum hyperplasia, halitosis, hemorrhoids, increased appetite, increased saliva, intestinal disorder, melena, mouth ulceration, mucositis, oral hemorrhage, oral leukoplakia, rectal bleeding after stool, rectal hemorrhage, stomatitis, stomatitis ulcerative, taste loss, tongue disorder, tooth disorder									
Liver and Biliary System Disorders (<5%)	abnormal hepatic function tests, biliary pain, bilirubinemia, hepatitis, increased lactate dehydrogenase, increased transaminases (SGOT/SGPT) (elevated SGOT 63% in malignant melanoma and 24% in follicular lymphoma), jaundice, right upper quadrant pain (15% in chronic hepatitis C), and very rarely, hepatic encephalopathy, hepatic failure, and death									
Musculoskeletal System Disorders										
musculoskeletal pain	—	18	—	—	—	—	21	9	1	10
Other (<5%)	arteritis, arthritis, arthritis aggravated, arthrosis, bone disorder, bone pain, carpal tunnel syndrome, hyporeflexia, leg cramps, muscle atrophy, muscle weakness, polyarteritis nodosa, tendinitis, rheumatoid arthritis, spondylitis									

(Table continued on next page)

Chronic Hepatitis C and Chronic Hepatitis B

Patients with decompensated liver disease, autoimmune hepatitis or a history of autoimmune disease, and patients who are immunosuppressed transplant recipients should not be treated with INTRON A. There are reports of worsening liver disease, including jaundice, hepatic encephalopathy, hepatic failure, and death following INTRON A therapy in such patients. Therapy should be discontinued for any patient developing signs and symptoms of liver failure.

Chronic hepatitis B patients with evidence of decreasing hepatic synthetic functions, such as decreasing albumin levels or prolongation of prothrombin time, who nevertheless meet the entry criteria to start therapy, may be at increased risk of clinical decompensation if a flare of aminotransferases occurs during INTRON A treatment. In such patients, if increases in ALT occur during INTRON A therapy for chronic hepatitis B, they should be followed carefully, including close monitoring of clinical symptomatology and liver function tests, including ALT, prothrombin time, alkaline phosphatase, albumin, and bilirubin. In considering these patients for INTRON A therapy, the potential risks must be evaluated against the potential benefits of treatment.

Peripheral Neuropathy

Peripheral neuropathy has been reported when alpha interferons were given in combination with telbivudine. In one clinical trial, an increased risk and severity of peripheral neuropathy was observed with the combination use of

TREATMENT-RELATED ADVERSE EXPERIENCES BY INDICATION (cont.)

Dosing Regimens
Percentage (%) of Patients*

ADVERSE EXPERIENCE	MALIGNANT MELANOMA 20 MIU/m² Induction (IV) 10 MIU/m² Maintenance (SC) N=143	FOLLICULAR LYMPHOMA 5 MIU TIW/SC N=135	HAIRY CELL LEUKEMIA 2 MIU/m² TIW/SC N=145	CONDYLOMATA ACUMINATA 1 MIU/lesion N=352	AIDS-RELATED KAPOSI'S SARCOMA 30 MIU/m² TIW/SC N=74	AIDS-RELATED KAPOSI'S SARCOMA 35 MIU QD/SC N=29	CHRONIC HEPATITIS C† 3 MIU TIW N=183	CHRONIC HEPATITIS B Adults 5 MIU QD N=101	CHRONIC HEPATITIS B Adults 10 MIU TIW N=78	CHRONIC HEPATITIS B Pediatrics 6 MIU/m² TIW N=116
Nervous System and Psychiatric Disorders										
depression	40	9	6	3	9	28	19	17	6	4
paresthesia	13	13	6	1	3	21	5	6	3	<1
impaired concentration	—	1	—	<1	3	14	3	8	5	3
amnesia	¶	1	<5	—	—	14	—	—	—	2
confusion	8	2	<5	4	12	10	1	—	—	—
hypoesthesia	—	1	<5	1	—	10	—	—	—	—
irritability	1	1	—	—	—	—	13	16	12	22
somnolence	1	2	<5	3	3	—	33#	14	9	5
anxiety	1	9	5	<1	1	3	5	2	—	3
insomnia	5	4	—	<1	3	3	12	11	6	8
nervousness	1	1	—	—	—	3	2	3	—	3
decreased libido	1	1	<5	—	—	—	1	5	1	—
other (<5%)	abnormal coordination, abnormal dreaming, abnormal gait, abnormal thinking, aggravated depression, aggressive reaction, agitation (7% in chronic hepatitis B pediatrics), alcohol intolerance, apathy, aphasia, ataxia, Bell's palsy, CNS dysfunction, coma, convulsions, delirium, dysphonia, emotional lability, extrapyramidal disorder, feeling of ebriety, flushing, hearing disorder, hearing impairment, hot flashes, hyperesthesia, hyperkinesia, hypertonia, hypokinesia, impaired consciousness, labyrinthine disorder, loss of consciousness, manic depression, manic reaction, migraine, neuralgia, neuritis, neuropathy, neurosis, paresis, paroniria, parosmia, personality disorder, polyneuropathy, psychosis, speech disorder, stroke, suicidal ideation, suicide attempt, syncope, tinnitus, tremor, twitching, vertigo (8% in follicular lymphoma)									
Reproduction System Disorders (<5%)	amenorrhea (12% in follicular lymphoma), dysmenorrhea, impotence, leukorrhea, menorrhagia, menstrual irregularity, pelvic pain, penis disorder, sexual dysfunction, uterine bleeding, vaginal dryness									
Resistance Mechanism Disorders										
moniliasis	—	1	—	<1	—	17	—	—	—	—
herpes simplex	1	2	—	1	—	3	1	5	—	—
other (<5%)	abscess, conjunctivitis, fungal infection, hemophilus, herpes zoster, infection, infection bacterial, infection nonspecific (7% in follicular lymphoma), infection parasitic, otitis media, sepsis, stye, trichomonas, upper respiratory tract infection, viral infection (7% in chronic hepatitis C)									
Respiratory System Disorders										
dyspnea	15	14	<1	—	1	34	3	5	—	5
coughing	6	13	<1	—	—	31	1	4	—	5
pharyngitis	2	8	<5	1	1	31	3	7	1	7
sinusitis	1	4	—	—	—	21	2	—	—	—
nonproductive coughing	2	7	—	—	1	14	0	1	—	—
nasal congestion	1	1	—	1	—	10	<1	4	—	—
other (≤5%)	asthma, bronchitis (10% in follicular lymphoma), bronchospasm, cyanosis, epistaxis (7% in chronic hepatitis B pediatrics), hemoptysis, hypoventilation, laryngitis, lung fibrosis, pleural effusion, orthopnea, pleural pain, pneumonia, pneumonitis, pneumothorax, rales, respiratory disorder, respiratory insufficiency, sneezing, tonsillitis, tracheitis, wheezing									
Skin and Appendages Disorders										
dermatitis	1	—	8	—	—	—	2	1	—	—
alopecia	29	23	8	—	12	31	28	26	38	17
pruritus	—	10	11	1	7	—	9	6	4	3
rash	19	13	25	—	9	10	5	8	1	5
dry skin	1	3	9	—	1	3	4	3	—	<1
other (<5%)	abnormal hair texture, acne, cellulitis, cyanosis of the hand, cold and clammy skin, dermatitis lichenoides, eczema, epidermal necrolysis, erythema, erythema nodosum, folliculitis, furunculosis, increased hair growth, lacrimal gland disorder, lacrimation, lipoma, maculopapular rash, melanosis, nail disorders, nonherpetic cold sores, pallor, peripheral ischemia, photosensitivity, pruritus genital, psoriasis, psoriasis aggravated, purpura (5% in chronic hepatitis C), rash erythematous, sebaceous cyst, skin depigmentation, skin discoloration, skin nodule, urticaria, vitiligo									
Urinary System Disorders (<5%)	albumin/protein in urine, cystitis, dysuria, hematuria, incontinence, increased BUN, micturition disorder, micturition frequency, nocturia, polyuria (10% in follicular lymphoma), renal insufficiency, urinary tract infection (5% in chronic hepatitis C)									
Vision Disorders (<5%)	abnormal vision, blurred vision, diplopia, dry eyes, eye pain, nystagmus, photophobia									

* Dash (—) indicates not reported
† Percentages based upon a summary of all adverse events during 18 to 24 months of treatment
‡ Vomiting was reported with nausea as a single term
§ Includes stomatitis/mucositis
¶ Amnesia was reported with confusion as a single term
# Predominantly lethargy

telbivudine and pegylated interferon alfa-2a as compared to telbivudine alone. The safety and efficacy of telbivudine in combination with interferons for the treatment of chronic hepatitis B has not been demonstrated.

Use with Ribavirin (See also REBETOL® package insert)
REBETOL may cause birth defects and/or death of the unborn child. REBETOL therapy should not be started until a report of a negative pregnancy test has been obtained immediately prior to initiation of therapy. Patients should use at least two forms of contraception and have monthly pregnancy tests (see **CONTRAINDICATIONS** and **PRECAUTIONS: Information for Patients**).

Combination treatment with INTRON A and REBETOL was associated with hemolytic anemia. Hemoglobin <10 g/dL was observed in approximately 10% of adult and pediatric patients in clinical trials. Anemia occurred within 1 to 2 weeks of initiation of ribavirin therapy. Combination treatment with INTRON A and REBETOL should **not** be used in patients with creatinine clearance <50 mL/min. See REBETOL package insert for additional information.

PRECAUTIONS
General
Acute serious hypersensitivity reactions (e.g., urticaria, angioedema, bronchoconstriction, anaphylaxis) have been ob-

served rarely in INTRON® A-treated patients; if such an acute reaction develops, the drug should be discontinued immediately and appropriate medical therapy instituted. Transient rashes have occurred in some patients following injection, but have not necessitated treatment interruption. While fever may be related to the flu-like syndrome reported commonly in patients treated with interferon, other causes of persistent fever should be ruled out.

There have been reports of interferon, including INTRON A, exacerbating preexisting psoriasis and sarcoidosis as well as development of new sarcoidosis. Therefore, INTRON A

IMPORTANT NOTICE: Updated drug information is sent bi-monthly via the PDR® Update Insert. For *monthly* email updates, register at PDR.net.

therapy should be used in these patients only if the potential benefit justifies the potential risk.

Variations in dosage, routes of administration, and adverse reactions exist among different brands of interferon. Therefore, do not use different brands of interferon in any single treatment regimen.

Triglycerides

Elevated triglyceride levels have been observed in patients treated with interferons, including INTRON A therapy. Elevated triglyceride levels should be managed as clinically appropriate. Hypertriglyceridemia may result in pancreatitis. Discontinuation of INTRON A therapy should be considered for patients with persistently elevated triglycerides (e.g., triglycerides >1000 mg/dL) associated with symptoms of potential pancreatitis, such as abdominal pain, nausea, or vomiting.

Drug Interactions

Interactions between INTRON A and other drugs have not been fully evaluated. Caution should be exercised when administering INTRON A therapy in combination with other potentially myelosuppressive agents such as zidovudine. Concomitant use of alpha interferon and theophylline decreases theophylline clearance, resulting in a 100% increase in serum theophylline levels.

Information for Patients

Patients receiving INTRON A alone or in combination with REBETOL® should be informed of the risks and benefits associated with treatment and should be instructed on proper use of the product. To supplement your discussion with a patient, you may wish to provide patients with a copy of the **MEDICATION GUIDE.**

Patients should be informed of, and advised to seek medical attention for, symptoms indicative of serious adverse reactions associated with this product. Such adverse reactions may include depression (suicidal ideation), cardiovascular (chest pain), ophthalmologic toxicity (decrease in/or loss of vision), pancreatitis or colitis (severe abdominal pain), and cytopenias (high persistent fevers, bruising, dyspnea). Patients should be advised that some side effects such as fatigue and decreased concentration might interfere with the ability to perform certain tasks. Patients who are taking INTRON A in combination with REBETOL must be thoroughly informed of the risks to a fetus. Female patients and female partners of male patients must be told to use two forms of birth control during treatment and for six months after therapy is discontinued (see **MEDICATION GUIDE**). Patients should be advised to remain well hydrated during the initial stages of treatment and that use of an antipyretic may ameliorate some of the flu-like symptoms.

If a decision is made to allow a patient to self-administer INTRON A, a puncture resistant container for the disposal of needles and syringes should be supplied. Patients self-administering INTRON A should be instructed on the proper disposal of needles and syringes and cautioned against reuse.

Dental and Periodontal Disorders

Dental and periodontal disorders have been reported in patients receiving ribavirin and interferon combination therapy. In addition, dry mouth could have a damaging effect on teeth and mucous membranes of the mouth during long-term treatment with the combination of REBETOL and interferon alfa-2b. Patients should brush their teeth thoroughly twice daily and have regular dental examinations. In addition, some patients may experience vomiting. If this reaction occurs, they should be advised to rinse out their mouth thoroughly afterwards.

Laboratory Tests

In addition to those tests normally required for monitoring patients, the following laboratory tests are recommended for all patients on INTRON A therapy, prior to beginning treatment and then periodically thereafter.

• Standard hematologic tests - including hemoglobin, complete and differential white blood cell counts, and platelet count.

• Blood chemistries - electrolytes, liver function tests, and TSH.

Those patients who have preexisting cardiac abnormalities and/or are in advanced stages of cancer should have electrocardiograms taken prior to and during the course of treatment.

Mild-to-moderate leukopenia and elevated serum liver enzyme (SGOT) levels have been reported with intralesional administration of INTRON A (see **ADVERSE REACTIONS**); therefore, the monitoring of these laboratory parameters should be considered.

Baseline chest X-rays are *suggested* and should be repeated if clinically indicated.

For malignant melanoma patients, differential WBC count and liver function tests should be monitored weekly during the induction phase of therapy and monthly during the maintenance phase of therapy.

For specific recommendations in chronic hepatitis C and chronic hepatitis B, see **INDICATIONS AND USAGE.**

Carcinogenesis, Mutagenesis, Impairment of Fertility

Studies with INTRON A have not been performed to determine carcinogenicity.

Interferon may impair fertility. In studies of interferon administration in nonhuman primates, menstrual cycle abnormalities have been observed. Decreases in serum estradiol and progesterone concentrations have been reported in women treated with human leukocyte interferon.[12] Therefore, fertile women should not receive INTRON A therapy unless they are using effective contraception during the therapy period. INTRON A therapy should be used with caution in fertile men.

Mutagenicity studies have demonstrated that INTRON A is not mutagenic.

Studies in mice (0.1, 1.0 million IU/day), rats (4, 20, 100 million IU/kg/day), and cynomolgus monkeys (1.1 million IU/kg/day; 0.25, 0.75, 2.5 million IU/kg/day) injected with INTRON A for up to 9 days, 3 months, and 1 month, respectively, have revealed no evidence of toxicity. However, in cynomolgus monkeys (4, 20, 100 million IU/kg/day) injected daily for 3 months with INTRON A, toxicity was observed at the mid and high doses and mortality was observed at the high dose.

However, due to the known species-specificity of interferon, the effects in animals are unlikely to be predictive of those in man.

INTRON A in combination with REBETOL should be used with caution in fertile men. See the REBETOL package insert for additional information.

Pregnancy Category C

INTRON A has been shown to have abortifacient effects in *Macaca mulatta* (rhesus monkeys) at 15 and 30 million IU/kg (estimated human equivalent of 5 and 10 million IU/kg, based on body surface area adjustment for a 60-kg adult). There are no adequate and well-controlled studies in pregnant women. INTRON A therapy should be used during pregnancy only if the potential benefit justifies the potential risk to the fetus.

Pregnancy Category X applies to combination treatment with INTRON A and REBETOL (see **CONTRAINDICATIONS**). See REBETOL package insert for additional information. Significant teratogenic and/or embryocidal effects have been demonstrated in all animal species exposed to ribavirin. REBETOL therapy is contraindicated in women who are pregnant and in the male partners of women who are pregnant. See **CONTRAINDICATIONS** and the REBETOL package insert.

Ribavirin Pregnancy Registry: A Ribavirin Pregnancy Registry has been established to monitor maternal-fetal outcomes of pregnancies in female patients and female partners of male patients exposed to ribavirin during treatment and for 6 months following cessation of treatment. Physicians and patients are encouraged to report such cases by calling 1-800-593-2214.

Nursing Mothers

It is not known whether this drug is excreted in human milk. However, studies in mice have shown that mouse interferons are excreted into the milk. Because of the potential for serious adverse reactions from the drug in nursing infants, a decision should be made whether to discontinue nursing or to discontinue INTRON A therapy, taking into account the importance of the drug to the mother.

Pediatric Use

General

Safety and effectiveness in pediatric patients have not been established for indications other than chronic hepatitis B and chronic hepatitis C.

Chronic Hepatitis B

Safety and effectiveness in pediatric patients ranging in age from 1 to 17 years have been established based upon one controlled clinical trial (see **CLINICAL PHARMACOLOGY, INDICATIONS AND USAGE,** and **DOSAGE AND ADMINISTRATION, Chronic Hepatitis B Pediatrics** section).

Chronic Hepatitis C

Safety and effectiveness in pediatric patients ranging in age from 3 to 16 years have been established based upon clinical studies in 118 patients. See REBETOL package insert for additional information. Suicidal ideation or attempts occurred more frequently among pediatric patients compared to adult patients (2.4% vs 1%) during treatment and off-therapy follow-up (see **WARNINGS, Neuropsychiatric Disorders** section). During a 48-week course of therapy there was a decrease in the rate of linear growth (mean percentile assignment decrease of 7%) and a decrease in the rate of weight gain (mean percentile assignment decrease of 9%). A general reversal of these trends was noted during the 24-week post-treatment period.

Geriatric Use

In all clinical studies of INTRON A, including studies as monotherapy and in combination with REBETOL (ribavirin, USP) Capsules, only a small percentage of the subjects were aged 65 and over. These numbers were too few to determine if they respond differently from younger subjects

except for the clinical trials of INTRON A in combination with REBETOL, where elderly subjects had a higher frequency of anemia (67%) than did younger patients (28%).

In a database consisting of clinical study and postmarketing reports for various indications, cardiovascular adverse events and confusion were reported more frequently in elderly patients receiving INTRON A therapy compared to younger patients.

In general, INTRON A therapy should be administered to elderly patients cautiously, reflecting the greater frequency of decreased hepatic, renal, bone marrow, and/or cardiac function and concomitant disease or other drug therapy. INTRON A is known to be substantially excreted by the kidney, and the risk of adverse reactions to INTRON A may be greater in patients with impaired renal function. Because elderly patients often have decreased renal function, patients should be carefully monitored during treatment, and dose adjustments made based on symptoms and/or laboratory abnormalities (see **CLINICAL PHARMACOLOGY** and **DOSAGE AND ADMINISTRATION**).

ADVERSE REACTIONS

General

The adverse experiences listed below were reported to be possibly or probably related to INTRON® A therapy during clinical trials. Most of these adverse reactions were mild to moderate in severity and were manageable. Some were transient and most diminished with continued therapy.

The most frequently reported adverse reactions were "flu-like" symptoms, particularly fever, headache, chills, myalgia, and fatigue. More severe toxicities are observed generally at higher doses and may be difficult for patients to tolerate.

[See table on pages 2113 and 2114]

Hairy Cell Leukemia

The adverse reactions most frequently reported during clinical trials in 145 patients with hairy cell leukemia were the "flu-like" symptoms of fever (68%), fatigue (61%), and chills (46%).

Malignant Melanoma

The INTRON A dose was modified because of adverse events in 65% (n=93) of the patients. INTRON A therapy was discontinued because of adverse events in 8% of the patients during induction and 18% of the patients during maintenance. The most frequently reported adverse reaction was fatigue, which was observed in 96% of patients. Other adverse reactions that were recorded in >20% of INTRON A-treated patients included neutropenia (92%), fever (81%), myalgia (75%), anorexia (69%), vomiting/nausea (66%), increased SGOT (63%), headache (62%), chills (54%), depression (40%), diarrhea (35%), alopecia (29%), altered taste sensation (24%), dizziness/vertigo (23%), and anemia (22%).

Adverse reactions classified as severe or life-threatening (ECOG Toxicity Criteria grade 3 or 4) were recorded in 66% and 14% of INTRON A-treated patients, respectively. Severe adverse reactions recorded in >10% of INTRON A-treated patients included neutropenia/leukopenia (26%), fatigue (23%), fever (18%), myalgia (17%), headache (17%), chills (16%), and increased SGOT (14%). Grade 4 fatigue was recorded in 4% and grade 4 depression was recorded in 2% of INTRON A-treated patients. No other grade 4 AE was reported in more than 2 INTRON A-treated patients. Lethal hepatotoxicity occurred in 2 INTRON A-treated patients early in the clinical trial. No subsequent lethal hepatotoxicities were observed with adequate monitoring of liver function tests (see **PRECAUTIONS, Laboratory Tests** section).

Follicular Lymphoma

Ninety-six percent of patients treated with CHVP plus INTRON A therapy and 91% of patients treated with CHVP alone reported an adverse event of any severity. Asthenia, fever, neutropenia, increased hepatic enzymes, alopecia, headache, anorexia, "flu-like" symptoms, myalgia, dyspnea, thrombocytopenia, paresthesia, and polyuria occurred more frequently in the CHVP plus INTRON A-treated patients than in patients treated with CHVP alone. Adverse reactions classified as severe or life threatening (World Health Organization grade 3 or 4) recorded in >5% of CHVP plus INTRON A-treated patients included neutropenia (34%), asthenia (10%), and vomiting (10%). The incidence of neutropenic infection was 6% in CHVP plus INTRON A vs 2% in CHVP alone. One patient in each treatment group required hospitalization.

Twenty-eight percent of CHVP plus INTRON A-treated patients had a temporary modification/interruption of their INTRON A therapy, but only 13 patients (10%) permanently stopped INTRON A therapy because of toxicity. There were four deaths on study; two patients committed suicide in the CHVP plus INTRON A arm and two patients in the CHVP arm had unwitnessed sudden death. Three patients with hepatitis B (one of whom also had alcoholic cirrhosis) developed hepatotoxicity leading to discontinuation of INTRON A. Other reasons for discontinuation included

Abnormal Laboratory Test Values by Indication

Dosing Regimens
Percentage (%) of Patients

LABORATORY TESTS	MALIGNANT MELANOMA 20 MIU/m² Induction (IV) 10 MIU/m² Maintenance (SC) N=143	FOLLICULAR LYMPHOMA 5 MIU TIW/SC N=135	HAIRY CELL LEUKEMIA 2 MIU/m² TIW/SC N=145	CONDYLOMATA ACUMINATA 1 MIU/lesion N=352	AIDS-RELATED KAPOSI'S SARCOMA 30 MIU/m² TIW/SC N=69–73	AIDS-RELATED KAPOSI'S SARCOMA 35 MIU QD/SC N=26–28	CHRONIC HEPATITIS C 3 MIU TIW N=140–171	CHRONIC HEPATITIS C 5 MIU QD N=96–101	CHRONIC HEPATITIS B Adults 10 MIU TIW N=75–103	CHRONIC HEPATITIS B Pediatrics 6 MIU/m² TIW N=113–115
Hemoglobin	22	8	NA	1	15		26*	32†	23†	17‡
White Blood Cell Count	§	—	NA	17	10	22	26¶	68¶	34¶	9¶
Platelet Count	15	13	NA	—	0	8	15#	12#	5#	1#
Serum Creatinine	3	2	0	—	—	—	6	3	0	3
Alkaline Phosphatase	13	—	4	—	—	—	—	8	4	0
Lactate Dehydrogenase	1	—	0	—	—	—	—	—	—	—
Serum Urea Nitrogen	12	4	0	—	—	—	—	2	0	2
SGOT	63	24	4	12	11	41	—	—	—	—
SGPT	2	—	13	—	10	15	—	—	—	—
Granulocyte Count										
• Total	92	36	NA	—	31	39	45Þ	75Þ	61Þ	70Þ
• 1000–<1500/mm³	66	—	—	—	—	—	32	30	32	43
• 750–<1000/mm³	—	21	—	—	—	—	10	24	18	18
• 500–<750/mm³	25	—	—	—	—	—	1	17	9	7
• <500/mm³	1	13	—	—	—	—	2	4	2	2

NA-Not Applicable-Patients' initial hematologic laboratory test values were abnormal due to their condition.
* Decrease of ≥2 g/dL; 20% 2–<3 g/dL; 6% ≥3 g/dL
† Decrease of ≥2 g/dL
‡ Decrease of ≥2 g/dL; 14% 2–<3 g/dL; 3% ≥3 g/dL
§ White Blood Cell Count was reported as neutropenia
¶ Decrease to <3000/mm³
# Decrease to <70,000/mm³
Þ Neutrophils plus bands

intolerable asthenia (5/135), severe flu symptoms (2/135), and one patient each with exacerbation of ankylosing spondylitis, psychosis, and decreased ejection fraction.

Condylomata Acuminata
Eighty-eight percent (311/352) of patients treated with INTRON A for condylomata acuminata who were evaluable for safety reported an adverse reaction during treatment. The incidence of the adverse reactions reported increased when the number of treated lesions increased from one to five. All 40 patients who had five warts treated reported some type of adverse reaction during treatment.
Adverse reactions and abnormal laboratory test values reported by patients who were re-treated were qualitatively and quantitatively similar to those reported during the initial INTRON A treatment period.

AIDS-Related Kaposi's Sarcoma
In patients with AIDS-Related Kaposi's Sarcoma, some type of adverse reaction occurred in 100% of the 74 patients treated with 30 million IU/m² three times a week and in 97% of the 29 patients treated with 35 million IU per day. Of these adverse reactions, those classified as severe (World Health Organization grade 3 or 4) were reported in 27% to 55% of patients. Severe adverse reactions in the 30 million IU/m² TIW study included: fatigue (20%), influenza-like symptoms (15%), anorexia (12%), dry mouth (4%), headache (4%), confusion (3%), fever (3%), myalgia (3%), and nausea and vomiting (1% each). Severe adverse reactions for patients who received the 35 million IU QD included: fever (24%), fatigue (17%), influenza-like symptoms (14%), dyspnea (14%), headache (10%), pharyngitis (7%), and ataxia, confusion, dysphagia, GI hemorrhage, abnormal hepatic function, increased SGOT, myalgia, cardiomyopathy, face edema, depression, emotional lability, suicide attempt, chest pain, and coughing (1 patient each). Overall, the incidence of severe toxicity was higher among patients who received the 35 million IU per day dose.

Chronic Hepatitis C
Two studies of extended treatment (18–24 months) with INTRON A show that approximately 95% of all patients treated experience some type of adverse event and that patients treated for extended duration continue to experience adverse events throughout treatment. Most adverse events reported are mild to moderate in severity. However, 29/152 (19%) of patients treated for 18 to 24 months experienced a serious adverse event compared to 11/163 (7%) of those treated for 6 months. Adverse events which occur or persist during extended treatment are similar in type and severity to those occurring during short-course therapy.
Of the patients achieving a complete response after 6 months of therapy, 12/79 (15%) subsequently discontinued

INTRON A treatment during extended therapy because of adverse events, and 23/79 (29%) experienced severe adverse events (WHO grade 3 or 4) during extended therapy.
In patients using combination treatment with INTRON A and REBETOL, the primary toxicity observed was hemolytic anemia. Reductions in hemoglobin levels occurred within the first 1 to 2 weeks of therapy. Cardiac and pulmonary events associated with anemia occurred in approximately 10% of patients treated with INTRON A/REBETOL therapy. See REBETOL package insert for additional information.

Chronic Hepatitis B
Adults
In patients with chronic hepatitis B, some type of adverse reaction occurred in 98% of the 101 patients treated at 5 million IU QD and 90% of the 78 patients treated at 10 million IU TIW. Most of these adverse reactions were mild to moderate in severity, were manageable, and were reversible following the end of therapy.
Adverse reactions classified as severe (causing a significant interference with normal daily activities or clinical state) were reported in 21% to 44% of patients. The severe adverse reactions reported most frequently were the "flu-like" symptoms of fever (28%), fatigue (15%), headache (5%), myalgia (4%), rigors (4%), and other severe "flu-like" symptoms, which occurred in 1% to 3% of patients. Other severe adverse reactions occurring in more than one patient were alopecia (8%), anorexia (6%), depression (3%), nausea (3%), and vomiting (2%).
To manage side effects, the dose was reduced, or INTRON A therapy was interrupted in 25% to 38% of patients. Five percent of patients discontinued treatment due to adverse experiences.
Pediatrics
In pediatric patients, the most frequently reported adverse events were those commonly associated with interferon treatment: flu-like symptoms (100%), gastrointestinal system disorders (46%), and nausea and vomiting (40%). Neutropenia (13%) and thrombocytopenia (30%) were also reported. None of the adverse events were life threatening. The majority were moderate to severe and resolved upon dose reduction or drug discontinuation.
[See table above]

Postmarketing Experience
The following adverse reactions have been identified during post-approval use of Intron A alone or in combination with Rebetol. Because these reactions are reported voluntarily from a population of uncertain size, it is not always possible to reliably estimate their frequency or establish a causal relationship to drug exposure.

Blood and Lymphatic System Disorders
pancytopenia (concurrent anemia, leukopenia, thrombocytopenia), aplastic anemia, pure red cell aplasia, thrombotic thrombocytopenic purpura, idiopathic thrombocytopenic purpura
Ear and Labyrinth Disorders
hearing loss
Eye Disorders
Vogt-Koyanagi-Harada syndrome, serous retinal detachment
Gastrointestinal Disorders
pancreatitis
General Disorders and Administration Site Conditions
asthenic conditions (including asthenia, malaise, fatigue)
Immune System Disorders
cases of acute hypersensitivity reactions, including anaphylaxis and angioedema, systemic lupus erythematosus, sarcoidosis or exacerbation of sarcoidosis
Musculoskeletal and Connective Tissue Disorders
myositis
Nervous System Disorders
peripheral neuropathy
Psychiatric Disorders
homicidal ideation, psychosis including hallucinations
Renal and Urinary Disorders
renal failure, renal insufficiency, nephrotic syndrome
Respiratory, thoracic and mediastinal disorders
pulmonary hypertension
Skin and Subcutaneous Tissue Disorders
injection site necrosis, Stevens-Johnson syndrome, toxic epidermal necrolysis, erythema multiforme, urticaria

OVERDOSAGE
There is limited experience with overdosage. Postmarketing surveillance includes reports of patients receiving a single dose as great as 10 times the recommended dose. In general, the primary effects of an overdose are consistent with the effects seen with therapeutic doses of interferon alfa-2b. Hepatic enzyme abnormalities, renal failure, hemorrhage, and myocardial infarction have been reported with single administration overdoses and/or with longer durations of treatment than prescribed (see **ADVERSE REACTIONS**). Toxic effects after ingestion of interferon alfa-2b are not expected because interferons are poorly absorbed orally. Consultation with a poison center is recommended.

Treatment
There is no specific antidote for interferon alfa-2b. Hemodialysis and peritoneal dialysis are not considered effective for treatment of overdose.

DOSAGE AND ADMINISTRATION
General

IMPORTANT: INTRON® A is supplied as 1) Powder for Injection/Reconstitution; 2) Solution for Injection in Vials; 3) Solution for Injection in Multidose Pens. **Not all dosage forms and strengths are appropriate for some indications.** It is important that you carefully read the instructions below for the indication you are treating to ensure you are using an appropriate dosage form and strength.

To enhance the tolerability of INTRON A, injections should be administered in the evening when possible.

To reduce the incidence of certain adverse reactions, acetaminophen may be administered at the time of injection.

Hairy Cell Leukemia
(see DOSAGE AND ADMINISTRATION, General section)
Dose

The recommended dose for the treatment of hairy cell leukemia is 2 million IU/m^2 administered intramuscularly or subcutaneously 3 times a week for up to 6 months. Patients with platelet counts of less than $50,000/mm^3$ should not be administered INTRON A intramuscularly, but instead by subcutaneous administration. Patients who are responding to therapy may benefit from continued treatment.
[See first table above]

NOTE: INTRON A Powder for Injection does not contain a preservative. The vial must be discarded after reconstitution and withdrawal of a single dose.

Dose adjustment

- If severe adverse reactions develop, the dosage should be modified (50% reduction) or therapy should be temporarily withheld until the adverse reactions abate and then resume at 50% (1 MIU/m^2 TIW).
- If severe adverse reactions persist or recur following dosage adjustment, INTRON A should be permanently discontinued.
- INTRON A should be discontinued for progressive disease or failure to respond after six months of treatment.

Malignant Melanoma
(see DOSAGE AND ADMINISTRATION, General section)

INTRON A adjuvant treatment of malignant melanoma is given in two phases, induction and maintenance.
Induction Recommended Dose

The recommended daily dose of INTRON A in induction is 20 million IU/m^2 as an intravenous infusion, over 20 minutes, 5 consecutive days per week, for 4 weeks (see Dose Adjustment below).

Dosage Forms for This Indication

Dosage Form	Concentration	Route
Powder 10 MIU	10 MIU/mL	IV
Powder 18 MIU	18 MIU/mL	IV
Powder 50 MIU	50 MIU/mL	IV

NOTE: INTRON A Solution for Injection in vials or Multidose Pens is NOT recommended for intravenous administration and should not be used for the induction phase of malignant melanoma.

NOTE: INTRON A Powder for Injection does not contain a preservative. The vial must be discarded after reconstitution and withdrawal of a single dose.

Dose Adjustment

NOTE: Regular laboratory testing should be performed to monitor laboratory abnormalities for the purpose of dose modifications (see **PRECAUTIONS, Laboratory Tests** section).

- INTRON A should be withheld for severe adverse reactions, including granulocyte counts >$250mm^3$ but <$500mm^3$ or SGPT/SGOT >5–10× upper limit of normal, until adverse reactions abate. INTRON A treatment should be restarted at 50% of the previous dose.
- INTRON A should be permanently discontinued for:
  - Toxicity that does not abate after withholding INTRON A
  - Severe adverse reactions which recur in patients receiving reduced doses of INTRON A
  - Granulocyte count <$250mm^3$ or SGPT/SGOT of >10× upper limit of normal

Maintenance Recommended Dose

The recommended dose of INTRON A for maintenance is 10 million IU/m^2 as a subcutaneous injection three times per week for 48 weeks (see Dose Adjustment below).
[See second table above]

NOTE: INTRON A Powder for Injection does not contain a preservative. The vial must be discarded after reconstitution and withdrawal of a single dose.

Dose Adjustment

NOTE: Regular laboratory testing should be performed to monitor laboratory abnormalities for the purpose of dose modifications (see **PRECAUTIONS, Laboratory Tests** section).

Dosage Forms for This Indication

Dosage Form	Concentration	Route	Fixed Doses
Powder 10 MIU (single-dose)	10 MIU/mL	IM, SC	N/A
Solution 18 MIU multidose	6 MIU/mL	IM, SC	N/A
Solution 25 MIU multidose	10 MIU/mL	IM, SC	N/A
Pen 3 MIU/dose multidose	15 MIU/mL	SC	1.5, 3.0, 4.5
Pen 5 MIU/dose multidose	25 MIU/mL	SC	2.5, 5.0

Dosage Forms for This Indication

Dosage Form	Concentration	Route	Fixed Doses
Powder 10 MIU (single-dose)*	10 MIU/mL	SC	N/A
Powder 18 MIU (single dose)†	18 MIU/mL	SC	N/A
Solution 18 MIU multidose	6 MIU/mL	SC	N/A
Solution 25 MIU multidose	10 MIU/mL	SC	N/A
Pen 3 MIU/dose multidose*	15 MIU/mL	SC	1.5, 3.0, 4.5, 6.0
Pen 5 MIU/dose multidose	25 MIU/mL	SC	7.5, 10.0
Pen 10 MIU/dose multidose	50 MIU/mL	SC	10.0, 15.0, 20.0

* Patients receiving 50% dose reduction only
† Patients receiving full dose only

Dosage Forms for this Indication

Dosage Form	Concentration	Route	Fixed Doses
Powder 10 MIU (single-dose)	10 MIU/mL	SC	N/A
Solution 18 MIU multidose	6 MIU/mL	SC	N/A
Solution 25 MIU multidose	10 MIU/mL	SC	N/A
Pen 5 MIU/dose multidose	25 MIU/mL	SC	2.5, 5.0
Pen 10 MIU/dose multidose	50 MIU/mL	SC	5.0

- INTRON A should be withheld for severe adverse reactions, including granulocyte counts >$250mm^3$ but <$500mm^3$ or SGPT/SGOT >5–10× upper limit of normal, until adverse reactions abate. INTRON A treatment should be restarted at 50% of the previous dose.
- INTRON A should be permanently discontinued for:
  - Toxicity that does not abate after withholding INTRON A
  - Severe adverse reactions which recur in patients receiving reduced doses of INTRON A
  - Granulocyte count <$250mm^3$ or SGPT/SGOT of >10× upper limit of normal

Follicular Lymphoma
(see DOSAGE and ADMINISTRATION, General section)
Dose

The recommended dose of INTRON A for the treatment of follicular lymphoma is 5 million IU subcutaneously three times per week for up to 18 months in conjunction with anthracycline-containing chemotherapy regimen and following completion of the chemotherapy regimen.
[See third table above]

NOTE: INTRON A Powder for Injection does not contain a preservative. The vial must be discarded after reconstitution and withdrawal of a single dose.

Dose Adjustment

- Doses of myelosuppressive drugs were reduced by 25% from a full-dose CHOP regimen, and cycle length increased by 33% (eg, from 21 to 28 days) when alpha interferon was added to the regimen.
- Delay chemotherapy cycle if neutrophil count was <$1500/mm^3$ or platelet count was <$75,000/mm^3$.
- INTRON A should be permanently discontinued if SGOT exceeds >5× the upper limit of normal or serum creatinine >2.0 mg/dL (see **WARNINGS**).
- Administration of INTRON A therapy should be withheld for a neutrophil count <$1000/mm^3$, or a platelet count <$50,000/mm^3$.
- INTRON A dose should be reduced by 50% (2.5 MIU TIW) for a neutrophil count >$1000/mm^3$, but <$1500/mm^3$. The INTRON A dose may be re-escalated to the starting dose (5 million IU TIW) after resolution of hematologic toxicity (ANC >$1500/mm^3$).

Condylomata Acuminata
(see DOSAGE and ADMINISTRATION, General section)
Dose

The recommended dose is 1.0 million IU per lesion in a maximum of 5 lesions in a single course. The lesions should be injected three times weekly on alternate days for 3 weeks. An additional course may be administered at 12 to 16 weeks.

Dosage Forms for This Indication

Dosage Form	Concentration	Route
Powder 10 MIU (single-dose)	10 MIU/mL	IL
Solution 25 MIU multidose	10 MIU/mL	IL

NOTE: INTRON A Powder for Injection does not contain a preservative. The vial must be discarded after reconstitution and withdrawal of a single dose.

NOTE: Do not use the following formulations for this indication:
- the 18 million or 50 million IU Powder for Injection
- the 18 million IU multidose INTRON A Solution for Injection
- the Multidose Pens

Dose Adjustment
None

Technique for Injection

The injection should be administered intralesionally using a Tuberculin or similar syringe and a 25- to 30-gauge needle. The needle should be directed at the center of the base of the wart and at an angle almost parallel to the plane of the skin (approximately that in the commonly used PPD test). This will deliver the interferon to the dermal core of the lesion, infiltrating the lesion and causing a small wheal. Care should be taken not to go beneath the lesion too deeply; subcutaneous injection should be avoided, since this area is below the base of the lesion. Do not inject too superficially since this will result in possible leakage, infiltrating only the keratinized layer and not the dermal core.

Dosage Forms for this Indication

Dosage Form	Concentration	Route	Fixed Doses
Solution 18 MIU multidose	6 MIU/mL	IM, SC	N/A
Pen 3 MIU/dose multidose	15 MIU/mL	SC	1.5, 3.0

Dosage Forms for this Indication

Dosage Form	Concentration	Route	Fixed Doses
Powder 10 MIU (single-dose)	10 MIU/mL	IM, SC	N/A
Solution 25 MIU multidose	10 MIU/mL	IM, SC	N/A
Pen 5 MIU/dose multidose	25 MIU/mL	SC	2.5, 5.0, 10.0
Pen 10 MIU/dose multidose	50 MIU/mL	SC	5.0, 10.0

Dosage Forms for this Indication

Dosage Form	Concentration	Route	Fixed Doses
Powder 10 MIU (single-dose)	10 MIU/mL	SC	N/A
Solution 25 MIU multidose	10 MIU/mL	SC	N/A
Pen 3 MIU/dose multidose	15 MIU/mL	SC	1.5, 3.0, 4.5, 6.0
Pen 5 MIU/dose multidose	25 MIU/mL	SC	2.5, 5.0, 7.5, 10.0
Pen 10 MIU/dose multidose	50 MIU/mL	SC	5.0, 10.0, 15.0, 20.0

INTRON A Dose	White Blood Cell Count	Granulocyte Count	Platelet Count
Reduce 50%	$<1.5 \times 10^9$/L	$<0.75 \times 10^9$/L	$<50 \times 10^9$/L
Permanently Discontinue	$<1.0 \times 10^9$/L	$<0.5 \times 10^9$/L	$<25 \times 10^9$/L

AIDS-Related Kaposi's Sarcoma
(see DOSAGE and ADMINISTRATION, General section)
Dose
The recommended dose of INTRON A for Kaposi's Sarcoma is 30 million IU/m²/dose administered subcutaneously or intramuscularly three times a week until disease progression or maximal response has been achieved after 16 weeks of treatment. Dose reduction is frequently required (see Dose Adjustment below).

Dosage Forms for this Indication

Dosage Form	Concentration	Route
Powder 50 MIU	50 MIU/mL	IM, SC

NOTE: INTRON A Solution for Injection either in vials or in Multidose Pens should NOT be used for AIDS-Related Kaposi's Sarcoma.
NOTE: INTRON A Powder for Injection does not contain a preservative. The vial must be discarded after reconstitution and withdrawal of a single dose.
Dose Adjustment
• INTRON A dose should be reduced by 50% or withheld for severe adverse reactions.
• INTRON A may be resumed at a reduced dose if severe adverse reactions abate with interruption of dosing.
• INTRON A should be permanently discontinued if severe adverse reactions persist or if they recur in patients receiving a reduced dose.

Chronic Hepatitis C
(see DOSAGE and ADMINISTRATION, General section)
Dose
The recommended dose of INTRON A for the treatment of chronic hepatitis C is 3 million IU three times a week (TIW) administered subcutaneously or intramuscularly. In patients tolerating therapy with normalization of ALT at 16 weeks of treatment, INTRON A therapy should be extended to 18 to 24 months (72 to 96 weeks) at 3 million IU TIW to improve the sustained response rate (see CLINICAL PHARMACOLOGY, Chronic Hepatitis C section). Patients who do not normalize their ALTs or have persistently high levels of HCV RNA after 16 weeks of therapy rarely achieve a sustained response with extension of treatment. Consideration should be given to discontinuing these patients from therapy.

When INTRON A is administered in combination with REBETOL®, patients with impaired renal function and/or those over the age of 50 should be carefully monitored with respect to the development of anemia. See REBETOL package insert for dosing when used in combination with REBETOL for adults and pediatric patients.
[See first table above]
Dose adjustment
If severe adverse reactions develop during INTRON A treatment, the dose should be modified (50% reduction) or therapy should be temporarily discontinued until the adverse reactions abate. If intolerance persists after dose adjustment, INTRON A therapy should be discontinued.

Chronic Hepatitis B Adults
(see DOSAGE and ADMINISTRATION, General section)
Dose
The recommended dose of INTRON A for the treatment of chronic hepatitis B is 30 to 35 million IU per week, administered subcutaneously or intramuscularly, either as 5 million IU daily (QD) or as 10 million IU three times a week (TIW) for 16 weeks.
[See second table above]
NOTE: INTRON A Powder for Injection does not contain a preservative. The vial must be discarded after reconstitution and withdrawal of a single dose.

Chronic Hepatitis B Pediatrics
(see DOSAGE and ADMINISTRATION, General section)
Dose
The recommended dose of INTRON A for the treatment of chronic hepatitis B is 3 million IU/m² three times a week (TIW) for the first week of therapy followed by dose escalation to 6 million IU/m² TIW (maximum of 10 million IU TIW) administered subcutaneously for a total duration of 16 to 24 weeks.
[See third table above]
NOTE: INTRON A Powder for Injection does not contain a preservative. The vial must be discarded after reconstitution and withdrawal of a single-dose.
Dose adjustment
If severe adverse reactions or laboratory abnormalities develop during INTRON A therapy, the dose should be modified (50% reduction) or discontinued if appropriate, until the adverse reactions abate. If intolerance persists after dose adjustment, INTRON A therapy should be discontinued.
For patients with decreases in white blood cell, granulocyte or platelet counts, the following guidelines for dose modification should be followed:

[See fourth table below]
INTRON A therapy was resumed at up to 100% of the initial dose when white blood cell, granulocyte, and/or platelet counts returned to normal or baseline values.

PREPARATION AND ADMINISTRATION
Reconstitution of INTRON® A Powder for Injection
The reconstituted solution is clear and colorless to light yellow. The INTRON A powder reconstituted with Sterile Water for Injection USP is a single-use vial and does not contain a preservative. **DO NOT RE-ENTER VIAL AFTER WITHDRAWING THE DOSE. DISCARD UNUSED PORTION** (see **DOSAGE and ADMINISTRATION**). Once the dose from the single-dose vial has been withdrawn, the sterility of any remaining product can no longer be guaranteed. Pooling of unused portions of some medications has been linked to bacterial contamination and morbidity.

• **Intramuscular, Subcutaneous, or Intralesional Administration**
Inject 1 mL Diluent (Sterile Water for Injection USP) for INTRON A into the INTRON A vial. Swirl gently to hasten complete dissolution of the powder. The appropriate INTRON A dose should then be withdrawn and injected intramuscularly, subcutaneously, or intralesionally (see **MEDICATION GUIDE** for detailed instructions).
Please refer to the **MEDICATION GUIDE** for detailed, step-by-step instructions on how to inject the INTRON A dose. After preparation and administration of the INTRON A injection, it is essential to follow the procedure for proper disposal of syringes and needles (see **MEDICATION GUIDE** for detailed instructions).
Parenteral drug products should be inspected visually for particulate matter and discoloration prior to administration.

• **Intravenous Infusion**
The infusion solution should be prepared immediately prior to use. Based on the desired dose, the appropriate vial strength(s) of INTRON A should be reconstituted with the diluent provided. Inject 1 mL Diluent (Sterile Water for Injection USP) for INTRON A into the INTRON A vial. Swirl gently to hasten complete dissolution of the powder. The appropriate INTRON A dose should then be withdrawn and injected into a 100-mL bag of 0.9% Sodium Chloride Injection USP. The final concentration of INTRON A should not be less than 10 million IU/100 mL.
Please refer to the **MEDICATION GUIDE** for detailed, step-by-step instructions on how to inject the INTRON A dose. After preparation and administration of INTRON A, it is essential to follow the procedure for proper disposal of syringes and needles.

INTRON A Solution for Injection in Vials
INTRON A Solution for Injection is supplied in two multidose vials. The solutions for injection do not require reconstitution prior to administration; the solution is clear and colorless.
The appropriate dose should be withdrawn from the vial and injected intramuscularly, subcutaneously, or intralesionally.
INTRON A Solution for Injection is not recommended for intravenous administration.
Solution for Injection in Multidose Pens
The INTRON A Solution for Injection Multidose Pens are designed to deliver 3 to 12 doses, depending on the individual dose, using a simple dial mechanism, and are for subcutaneous injections only. Only the needles provided in the packaging should be used for the INTRON A Solution for Injection Multidose Pen. A new needle is to be used each time a dose is delivered using the pen. To avoid the possible transmission of disease, each INTRON A Solution for Injection Multidose Pen is for single patient use only.
Please refer to the **MEDICATION GUIDE** for detailed, step-by-step instructions on how to inject the INTRON A dose. After preparation and administration of INTRON A, it is essential to follow the procedure for proper disposal of syringes and needles.

HOW SUPPLIED
INTRON® A Powder for Injection
INTRON A Powder for Injection, 10 million IU per vial and Diluent for INTRON A (Sterile Water for Injection USP) 1 mL per vial; boxes containing 1 INTRON A vial and 1 vial of INTRON A Diluent (NDC 0085-0571-02).
INTRON A Powder for Injection, 18 million IU per vial and Diluent for INTRON A (Sterile Water for Injection USP) 1 mL per vial; boxes containing 1 vial of INTRON A and 1 vial of INTRON A Diluent (NDC 0085-1110-01).
INTRON A Powder for Injection, 50 million IU per vial and Diluent for INTRON A (Sterile Water for Injection USP) 1 mL per vial; boxes containing 1 INTRON A vial and 1 vial of INTRON A Diluent (NDC 0085-0539-01).
INTRON A Solution for Injection in Multidose Pens
INTRON A Solution for Injection, 6 doses of 3 million IU (18 million IU) Multidose Pen (22.5 million IU per 1.5 mL per pen); boxes containing 1 INTRON A Multidose Pen, six disposable needles and alcohol swabs (NDC 0085-1242-01).
INTRON A Solution for Injection, 6 doses of 5 million IU (30 million IU) Multidose Pen (37.5 million IU per 1.5 mL per pen); boxes containing 1 INTRON A Multidose Pen, six disposable needles and alcohol swabs (NDC 0085-1235-01).

INTRON A Solution for Injection, 6 doses of 10 million IU (60 million IU) Multidose Pen (75 million IU per 1.5 mL per pen); boxes containing 1 INTRON A Multidose Pen, six disposable needles and alcohol swabs (NDC 0085-1254-01).

INTRON A Solution for Injection in Vials

INTRON A Solution for Injection, 18 million IU multidose vial (22.8 million IU per 3.8 mL per vial); boxes containing 1 vial of INTRON A Solution for Injection (NDC 0085-1168-01).

INTRON A Solution for Injection, 25 million IU multidose vial (32 million IU per 3.2 mL per vial); boxes containing 1 vial of INTRON A Solution for Injection (NDC 0085-1133-01).

Storage

• INTRON A Powder for Injection/Reconstitution

INTRON A Powder for Injection should be stored at 2° to 8°C (36°–46°F). After reconstitution, the solution should be used immediately, but may be stored up to 24 hours at 2°–8°C (36°–46°F).

• INTRON A Solution for Injection in Vials

INTRON A Solution for Injection in Vials should be stored at 2°–8°C (36°–46°F).

• INTRON A Solution for Injection in Multidose Pens

INTRON A Solution for Injection in Multidose Pens should be stored at 2°–8°C (36°–46°

REFERENCES

1. Smalley R, et al. *N Engl J Med.* 1992;327:1336–1341.
2. Aviles A, et al. *Leukemia and Lymphoma.* 1996;20: 495–499.
3. Unterhalt M, et al. *Blood.* 1996;88:(10 Suppl 1):1744A.
4. Schiller J, et al. *J. Biol Response Mod.* 1989;8:252–261.
5. Poynard T, et al. *N Engl J Med.* 1995;332:(22) 1457–1462.
6. Lin R, et al. *J Hepatol.* 1995;23:487–496.
7. Perrillo R, et al. *N Engl J Med.* 1990;323:295–301.
8. Perez V, et al. *J Hepatol.* 1990;11:S113–S117.
9. Knodell R, et al. *Hepatology.* 1981;1:431–435.
10. Perrillo R, et al. *Ann Intern Med.* 1991;115:113–115.
11. Renault P, et al. *Arch Intern Med.* 1987;147:1577–1580.
12. Kauppila A, et al. *Int J Cancer.* 1982;29:291–294.

Manufactured by Schering Corporation, a subsidiary of Schering-Plough Corporation, Kenilworth, NJ 07033 USA. Rev. 2/10

© 1986, 2008, Schering Corporation. All rights reserved.

U.S. Patent Nos. 5,935,566 and 6,610,830

MEDICATION GUIDE

INTRON® A

(Interferon alfa-2b, recombinant)

Including appendix with instructions for using INTRON A Multidose Pen for Injection

Read this Medication Guide carefully before you start to take INTRON A (In-tron aye) for Injection alone or INTRON A in combination with REBETOL® (REB-eh-tole) (ribavirin, USP) Capsules. Read the Medication Guide each time you refill your prescription because there may be new information. The information in this Medication Guide does not take the place of talking with your healthcare provider. If you are taking INTRON A and REBETOL combination therapy, also read the Medication Guide for REBETOL (ribavirin, USP) Capsules.

What is the most important information I should know about INTRON® A?

INTRON A is a treatment for some people who have hairy cell leukemia, malignant melanoma, follicular lymphoma, AIDS-related Kaposi's sarcoma, chronic hepatitis B, chronic hepatitis C, and condylomata acuminata. If you have chronic hepatitis C, your healthcare provider may prescribe INTRON A in combination with REBETOL®. INTRON A used by itself or with REBETOL can help you, but can also have serious side effects and may cause death in rare cases. Before starting treatment, you should talk to your healthcare provider about the possible benefits and possible side effects of INTRON A alone or in combination with REBETOL, to decide if this treatment is right for you. While taking INTRON A alone or in combination with REBETOL, you need to see a healthcare provider regularly for medical examinations and lab tests to make sure the treatment is working and to check for side effects.

You should call your healthcare provider immediately if you develop any of these conditions while taking INTRON A:

• you become pregnant or if you are a male and your female partner becomes pregnant
• new or worsening mental health problems such as thoughts about hurting or killing yourself or others
• decreased vision
• trouble breathing or chest pain
• severe stomach or lower back pain
• bloody diarrhea or bloody bowel movements
• high fever
• easy bruising or bleeding

The most serious possible side effects of INTRON A include:

RISK TO PREGNANCY. Combination INTRON A and

REBETOL therapy can cause death, serious birth defects or other harm to your unborn child. If you are pregnant, you or your male partner must not take INTRON A and REBETOL combination therapy. You must not become pregnant while either you or your partner are taking the combination of INTRON A and REBETOL and for 6 months after you stop taking the combination. If you are a woman of childbearing age you must have negative pregnancy tests immediately before starting treatment, during treatment, and for 6 months after you have stopped treatment. You should use two forms of birth control during and for 6 months after you have stopped treatment. If you are a man taking INTRON A/REBETOL combination therapy, one of the two forms of birth control should be a condom. You must use birth control even if you believe that you are not fertile or that your fertility is low. You should talk to your healthcare provider about birth control for you and your partner. If you or your partner becomes pregnant while either of you is being treated or within 6 months of stopping treatment, tell your healthcare provider right away. There is a Ribavirin Pregnancy Registry that collects information about pregnancy outcomes in female patients and female partners of male patients exposed to ribavirin. You or your healthcare provider are encouraged to contact the Registry at 1-800-593-2214.

Mental health problems and suicide. INTRON A may cause patients to develop mood or behavioral problems. These can include irritability (getting easily upset) and depression (feeling low, feeling bad about yourself, or feeling hopeless). Some patients may have aggressive behavior. Former drug addicts may fall back into drug addiction or overdose. Some patients think about hurting or killing themselves or other people. Some patients have killed themselves (suicide) or hurt themselves or others. You must tell your healthcare provider if you are being treated for a mental illness or had treatment in the past for any mental illness, including depression and suicidal behavior. You should also tell your healthcare provider if you have ever been addicted to drugs or alcohol.

Eye problems. Changes in vision such as a decrease or loss of vision (blindness) may happen in some patients. You should have an eye exam before you take INTRON A. If you have eye problems or have had them in the past, you may need eye exams while you are taking INTRON A. Tell your healthcare provider or eye doctor right away if you have changes in your vision while taking INTRON A.

Heart problems. Some patients taking INTRON A may develop problems with their heart, including low blood pressure, fast heart rate, and very rarely, heart attacks. Tell your healthcare provider if you have had any heart problems in the past.

Blood problems. INTRON A commonly lowers two types of blood cells (white blood cells and platelets). In some patients, these blood counts may fall to dangerously low levels. If your blood cell counts become very low, you could get infections or have bleeding problems.

If you are taking INTRON A and REBETOL combination therapy, REBETOL can cause a drop in your number of red blood cells (anemia). A very low red blood cell count can be dangerous, especially if you have heart or breathing problems.

For other possible side effects of INTRON A, see "What are the possible side effects of INTRON A?" in this Medication Guide.

Body organ problems. INTRON A may cause lung problems including: trouble breathing, pneumonia, inflammation of lung tissue, and new or worse high blood pressure in the lungs (pulmonary hypertension), which can be severe and may in some cases lead to death. Certain symptoms like severe stomach pain may mean that your internal organs are being damaged. Cases of weakness, loss of coordination, and numbness due to stroke have been reported in patients taking Intron A, including patients with few or no reported risk factors for stroke.

What is INTRON® A?

The INTRON A product contains a man-made protein called interferon. Interferon is a protein that is part of the body's immune system that "interferes" with the growth of viruses or cancer cells.

It is not known if INTRON A or INTRON A/REBETOL® combination therapy can cure hepatitis B or C (*permanently eliminate the virus*) or if it can prevent liver failure or liver cancer that is caused by hepatitis B or C infection.

It is also not known if INTRON A or INTRON A/REBETOL combination therapy will prevent one infected person from infecting another person with hepatitis B or C.

Who should not take INTRON® A?

Do not take INTRON A alone or in combination with REBETOL® if you:

• are pregnant, planning to get pregnant, or breast-feeding
• are a male patient on combination therapy and have a female sexual partner who is pregnant or plans to become

pregnant while you are being treated with REBETOL or during the 6 months after your treatment has ended

• have autoimmune hepatitis (hepatitis caused by your immune system attacking your liver) or unstable liver disease (yellowing of the skin and eyes, swelling of the abdomen)
• had an allergic reaction to another alpha interferon or ribavirin or are allergic to any of the ingredients in INTRON A or REBETOL

If you have any of the following conditions or serious medical problems, tell your healthcare provider before taking INTRON A alone or in combination with REBETOL:

• depression or anxiety
• eye problems
• sleep problems
• high blood pressure
• previous heart attack, or other heart problems
• liver problems (other than hepatitis B or C)
• any kind of autoimmune disease (where the body's immune system attacks the body's own cells), such as psoriasis, sarcoidosis, systemic lupus erythematosus, rheumatoid arthritis
• thyroid problems
• diabetes
• colitis (inflammation of the bowels)
• cancer
• hepatitis B or C infection
• HIV infection (the virus that causes AIDS)
• kidney problems
• bleeding problems
• alcoholism
• drug abuse or addiction
• body organ transplant and are taking medicine that keeps your body from rejecting your transplant (suppresses your immune system)
• high blood triglycerides (fat particles normally found in your blood)

Tell your healthcare provider about all the medicines you take, including prescription and non- prescription medicines, vitamins, and herbal supplements. INTRON A and certain other medicines may affect each other and cause side effects.

Especially tell your doctor if you take the anti-hepatitis B medicine telbivudine (Tyzeka). See "What are the possible side effects of INTRON A?"

Know the medicines you take. Keep a list of them and show it to your healthcare provider and pharmacist when you get a new medicine.

How should I take INTRON® A?

To get the most benefit from this medicine, it is important that you take INTRON A exactly as your healthcare provider tells you. Your healthcare provider will decide your dose of INTRON A and how often you will take it. Do not take more than your prescribed dose. INTRON A is given as an injection either under the skin (subcutaneous) or into a muscle (intramuscular). You should be completely comfortable with how to prepare and measure your dose of INTRON A and how to inject yourself before you use INTRON A for the first time. Your healthcare provider will train you on how to use and inject INTRON A properly.

INTRON A comes in different strengths and different forms (a powder in a vial, a solution in a vial, and a Multidose Pen). Your healthcare provider will determine which form is best for you. The instructions for giving a dose of INTRON A are at the end of this leaflet.

If you miss a dose of INTRON A, take the missed dose as soon as possible during the same day or the next day, then continue on your regular dosing schedule. If several days go by after you miss a dose, check with your healthcare provider to see what to do. **Do not double your next dose** or take more than your prescribed dose without talking to your healthcare provider. Call your healthcare provider right away if you take more than your prescribed dose. Your healthcare provider may wish to examine you more closely and take blood for testing.

If you are taking INTRON A in combination with REBETOL®, you should also read the Medication Guide for REBETOL (ribavirin, USP) for more information about side effects and how to take REBETOL. **REBETOL capsules should be taken twice a day with food.** Taking REBETOL with food helps your body take up more of the medicine. Taking REBETOL at the same time of day every day will help keep the amount of medicine in your body at a steady level. This can help your healthcare provider decide how your treatment is working and how to change the number of REBETOL capsules you take if you have side effects. If you miss a dose of REBETOL, take the missed dose as soon as possible during the same day. If an entire day has passed, check with your healthcare provider about what to do. **Do not double your next dose.**

You must see your healthcare provider on a regular basis for blood tests so your healthcare provider can check how the treatment is working for you and to check for side effects.

Tell your healthcare provider if you are taking or planning to take other prescription or nonprescription medicines, including vitamin and mineral supplements and herbal medicines.

What should I avoid while taking INTRON® A?

- Avoid becoming pregnant while taking INTRON A. INTRON A alone and INTRON A taken in combination with REBETOL® may harm your unborn child or cause you to lose your baby (miscarry). If you or your partner becomes pregnant during treatment or during the 6 months after treatment with INTRON A/REBETOL combination therapy, immediately report the pregnancy to your healthcare provider. Your healthcare provider will make decisions about your treatment. Your healthcare provider should call 1-800-593-2214. Your healthcare provider will be asked to give follow-up information about the pregnancy.
- Do not breast-feed your baby while taking INTRON A.
- Avoid taking telbivudine (Tyzeka), a drug used to treat hepatitis B. People who take INTRON A or other alpha interferon products with telbivudine (Tyzeka) can have nerve problems such as continuing numbness, tingling, or burning sensation in the arms or legs, or problems walking.

What are the possible side effects of INTRON® A?

INTRON A may cause serious side effects including:
- See "What is the most important information I should know about INTRON A?"
- **Other body organ problems.** Certain symptoms like severe pain in the middle of your body, nausea, and vomiting may mean that your liver or pancreas is being damaged. A few patients have inflammation of the kidney. If you have severe stomach or back pains or a fever, you should call your health care provider right away.
- **Thyroid problems.** Some patients develop changes in the function of their thyroid. Symptoms of thyroid changes include the inability to concentrate, feeling cold or hot all the time, a change in your weight and changes to your skin.
- **New or worsening autoimmune disease.** Some patients taking INTRON A develop autoimmune diseases (a condition where the body's immune cells attack other cells or organs in the body), including rheumatoid arthritis, systemic lupus erythematosus, sarcoidosis, and psoriasis. In some patients who already have an autoimmune disease, the disease may worsen while on INTRON A.
- **Nerve problems.** People who take INTRON A or other alpha interferon products with telbivudine (Tyzeka) can have nerve problems such as continuing numbness, tingling, or burning sensation in the arms or legs (peripheral neuropathy). Call your healthcare provider if you have any of these symptoms.

Common but less serious side effects include:
- **Flu-like symptoms.** Most patients who take INTRON A have "flu-like" symptoms (headache, muscle aches, tiredness, and fever) that usually lessen after the first few weeks of therapy. You can reduce some of these symptoms by injecting your INTRON A dose at bedtime. Over-the-counter pain and fever medications can be used to prevent or reduce the fever and headache. If your fever does not go away you should tell your healthcare provider.
- **Extreme fatigue (tiredness).** Many patients become extremely tired while on INTRON A.
- **Appetite problems.** Nausea, loss of appetite, and weight loss occur commonly.
- **Blood sugar problems.** Some patients develop problems with the way their body controls their blood sugar and may develop high blood sugar or diabetes.
- **Skin reactions.** Redness, swelling, and itching are common at the site of injection. If after several days these symptoms do not disappear, contact your healthcare provider. You may get a rash during therapy. If this occurs, your healthcare provider may recommend medicine to treat the rash.
- **Hair thinning.** Hair thinning is common during INTRON A treatment. Hair loss stops and hair growth returns after therapy is stopped.

These are not all the side effects of INTRON A or INTRON A/REBETOL® combination therapy. Your healthcare provider can give you a more complete list.
Call your doctor for medical advice about side effects. You may report side effects to FDA at 1–800–FDA–1088.

General advice about prescription medicines

Medicines are sometimes prescribed for purposes other than those listed in a Medication Guide. If you have any concerns about the INTRON A product, ask your healthcare provider. Your healthcare provider can give you additional information about INTRON A. Do not use INTRON A for a condition for which it was not prescribed. Do not share this medication with other people.

This Medication Guide has been approved by the U.S. Food and Drug Administration.

Manufactured by: Schering Corporation Kenilworth, NJ 07033 USA
Issued: August 2009
Instructional leaflet and video are available through your healthcare provider.

Rev. 8/09

Medication Guide Appendix: Instructions for Preparing and Giving a Dose of INTRON® A Multidose Pen

The INTRON A Solution for Injection Multidose Pen is a pre-filled, Multidose Pen that contains six doses of either 3, 5, or 10 million international units (MIU) of INTRON A. The Multidose Pen can also be used for different doses if your healthcare provider wants you to increase or decrease your dose.

The Multidose Pen can provide between 3 to 12 doses depending upon the dose your healthcare provider tells you to use. The Multidose Pen prescribed for you by your healthcare provider will be one of the following:
- 3 Million International Units (MIU) with a brown push button and a brown color-coding strip. The different doses that it can deliver are 1.5 MIU, 3.0 MIU, 4.5 MIU, and 6.0 MIU. Six MIU is the maximum dose that this pen can deliver at one time.
- 5 Million International Units (MIU) with a light blue push button and a light blue color-coding strip. The different doses that it can deliver are 2.5 MIU, 5.0 MIU, 7.5 MIU, and 10.0 MIU. Ten MIU is the maximum dose that this pen can deliver at one time.
- 10 Million International Units (MIU) with a pink push button and a pink color-coding strip. The different doses that it can deliver are 5.0 MIU, 10.0 MIU, 15.0 MIU, and 20.0 MIU. Twenty MIU is the maximum dose that this pen can deliver at one time.

Make sure that you have the correct INTRON A Multidose Pen as prescribed by your healthcare provider.

Description of your INTRON® A Multidose Pen

- The INTRON A Multidose Pen should **ONLY** be used with **Novofine®** needles. These are the needles that come packaged with the pen. If you use other needles the pen may not work properly and you could get the wrong dose of INTRON A.

The two diagrams below show all the different parts of the INTRON A Multidose Pen and the Novofine needle. The parts of the pen you need to become familiar with are:

INTRON A Pen   **Novofine Needle Assembly**

Cap
Cap scale
Needle
Rubber membrane
Color coded band
INTRON A reservoir
Dosage indicator
Pen barrel
Color coded label
Push button scale
Push button
Outer needle cap
Inner needle cap
Needle
Protective tab

- The **color-coded push button** and **push button scale**. These are located at the bottom of the pen when it is held with the cap side up. This tells you the dose that has been set.
- The **color-coding** band. This is located on the INTRON A reservoir. The band lets you know the dose that you are using. The 3 MIU INTRON A Multidose Pen has a brown push button, a brown color-coding band, and color-coded label. The 5 MIU INTRON A Multidose Pen has a light blue push button, a light blue color-coding band, and color-coded label. The 10 MIU INTRON A Multidose Pen has a pink push button, a pink color-coding band, and color-coded label.
- The **cap**. The cap is used for setting the dose and storing the pen. You will not be able to set the dose or completely close the pen unless you line up the **triangle** on the **cap scale** with the **dosage indicator** on the barrel.

To avoid the possible transmission of disease, do not allow anyone else to use your multidose pen.

Storing INTRON® A Solution Multidose Pen for Injection

INTRON A Solution Multidose Pen for Injection should be stored in the refrigerator between 2° and 8°C (36° and 46°F). Discard any unused INTRON A pen remaining after 4 weeks. **DO NOT FREEZE.**

How do I prepare for an injection using the INTRON® A Multidose Pen?

1. Find a well-lit, clean, flat working surface such as a table. Collect the supplies you will need for an injection:
   - the INTRON A Multidose Pen
   - two alcohol swabs
   - a cotton ball or gauze
   - a puncture-proof disposable container
2. Before removing the Multidose Pen from the carton, check the date printed on the carton to make sure that the expiration date has not passed. Do not use if the expiration date has passed.
3. Wash your hands with soap and warm water. It is important to keep your work area, your hands, and injection site clean to minimize the risk of infection.
4. Remove the Multidose Pen from the carton. Pull the cap off the pen and wipe the rubber membrane with one alcohol swab.

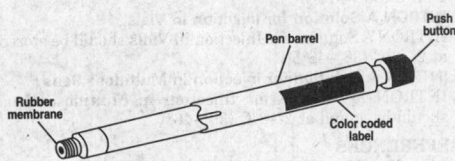

5. Check the solution inside the pen. The solution should be clear and colorless, without particles. Do not use the INTRON A if the medicine is cloudy, has particles, or is any color besides clear and colorless.
6. Remove the paper backing from the Novofine® needle by pulling the paper tab. You will see the back of the needle once the paper tab is removed.

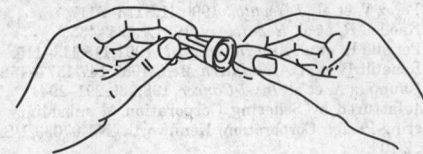

7. Keep the needle in its outer clear needle cap and gently push the Novofine needle straight into the pen's rubber membrane you just cleaned. Screw the needle onto the INTRON A Multidose Pen by turning it clockwise.

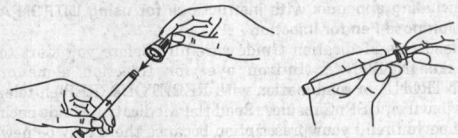

8. With the needle facing up, pull off the outer clear needle cap and set the outer needle cap down on your flat work surface for later use. Next, carefully pull off the white inner needle cap. The needle will now be exposed.

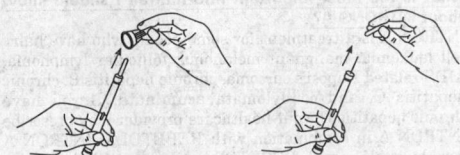

9. Keep the needle facing up and remove any air bubbles that may be in the reservoir by tapping the reservoir with your finger. If you have any air bubbles, they will rise to the top of the reservoir.

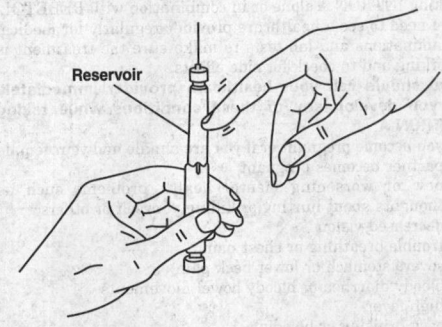

10. Hold the pen by the barrel and turn the INTRON A reservoir clockwise until you feel it click into place.

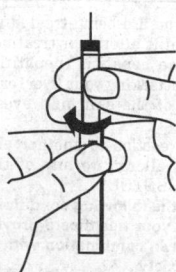

11. Keep the needle facing up and press the push button all the way up. A drop of INTRON A solution should come out of the tip of the needle.

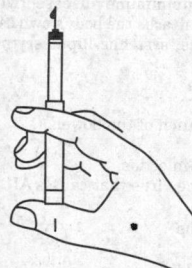

12. Place the cap back on the INTRON A multidose pen. Make sure you line up the black triangle on the pen cap with the dosage indicator on the pen barrel. The pen is now ready to set the dose.

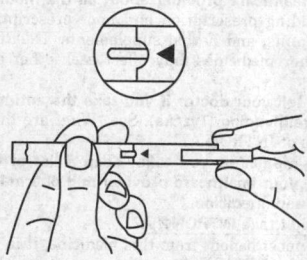

Setting the dose prescribed by your healthcare provider
13. Hold the pen horizontally in the middle of the pen barrel so the push button can move freely. With the other hand, hold the Multidose Pen cap.

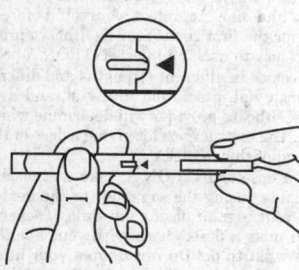

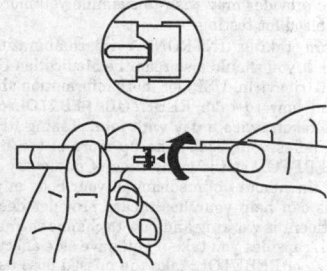

14. Set the dose prescribed by your healthcare provider by turning the cap clockwise. With each clockwise turn, the push button will start to rise and you will see the push button scale. Do not use force to turn the pen cap or you may damage the pen.

• To set a 3.0 MIU dose using the 3 MIU multidose pen, turn the cap 2 full turns (10 clicks) = 3.0 MIU.

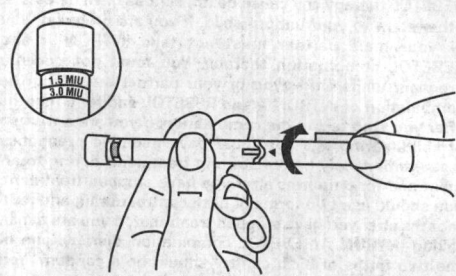

• To set a 5 MIU dose using the 5 MIU multidose pen, turn the cap 2 full turns (10 clicks) = 5.0 MIU.

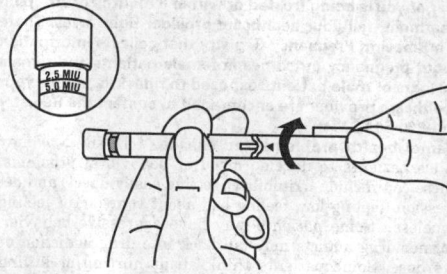

• To set a 10 MIU dose using the 10 MIU multidose pen, turn the cap 2 full turns (10 clicks) = 10.0 MIU.

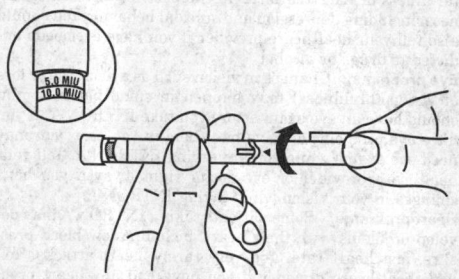

15. After each complete turn, make sure the triangle on the cap is lined up with the dosage indicator on the pen barrel.

IF YOUR HEALTHCARE PROVIDER HAS PRESCRIBED A DOSE OTHER THAN 3.0, 5.0, OR 10.0 MIU, THE DOSE CAN BE SET BY TURNING THE CAP AS MANY TIMES AS SHOWN BELOW:

A dose prescribed other than 3.0 MIU from the 3 MIU multidose pen

1 full turn (5 clicks) = 1.5 MIU
3 full turns (15 clicks) = 4.5 MIU
4 full turns (20 clicks) = 6.0 MIU

A dose prescribed other than 5.0 MIU from the 5 MIU multidose pen

1 full turn (5 clicks) = 2.5 MIU
3 full turns (15 clicks) = 7.5 MIU
4 full turns (20 clicks) = 10.0 MIU

A dose prescribed other than 10.0 MIU from the 10 MIU multidose pen

1 full turn (5 clicks) = 5.0 MIU
3 full turns (15 clicks) = 15.0 MIU
4 full turns (20 clicks) = 20.0 MIU

16. Check the push button scale to make sure you have set the correct dose.
17. If you have set a wrong dose, turn the cap back (counterclockwise) as far as you can until the push button is all the way in and the push button scale is completely covered, then begin at step 13 again.
18. Gently warm the INTRON® A Solution for Injection by slowly rolling the capped Multidose Pen in the palms of your hands for about 1 minute. DO NOT SHAKE.
19. Place the Multidose Pen on your flat work surface until you are ready to inject INTRON A.

Choosing an injection site
You should inject a dose of INTRON® A subcutaneously (under the skin). If it is too difficult for you to inject, ask someone who has been trained to give injections to help you. The best sites for injection are areas on your body with a layer of fat between skin and muscle such as:
• the front of the middle thighs
• the outer area of the upper arms

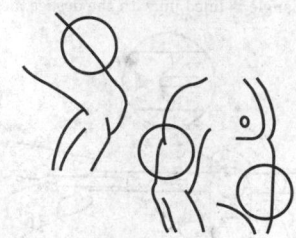

• the abdomen, except around the navel

You should use a different site each time you inject INTRON A to avoid soreness at any one site. Do not inject INTRON A into an area where the skin is irritated, red, bruised, infected or has scars, stretch marks, or lumps.

Injecting your dose of INTRON® A
1. Clean the injection site with a new alcohol swab.
2. Pick up the Multidose Pen from your flat work surface and remove the cap from the needle.
3. With one hand, pinch a fold of the skin at the cleaned injection site.
4. With the other hand, hold the Multidose Pen (like a pencil) at a **45-degree angle** to the skin. With a quick "dart-like" motion, push the needle into the skin.

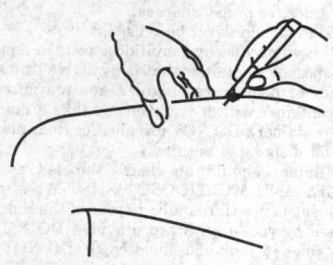

5. After the needle is in, remove the hand used to pinch the skin and use it to hold the pen barrel. If blood comes into the pen reservoir, the needle has entered a blood vessel. **Do not inject INTRON A.** Withdraw the needle and discard the used Multi-dose pen in the puncture-proof container. Contact your healthcare provider. Repeat the steps to prepare for an injection.
6. If no blood is present in the pen reservoir, inject the medicine by gently pressing the push button all the way down.
7. Leave the needle in place for a few seconds while holding down the push button.
8. Slowly release the push button and pull the needle out of the skin.
9. Place a cotton ball or gauze over the injection site and press for several seconds. Do not massage the injection site. If there is bleeding, cover the injection site with a bandage.
10. It is important to check your injection site approximately two hours after your injection for redness, swelling, or tenderness. These are signs of inflammation that you may need to talk to your healthcare provider about if they do not go away.

Removing the needle from the multidose pen
11. Using a scooping motion, carefully replace the outer clear needle cap (like capping a pen).

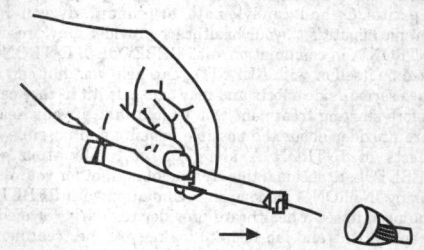

12. Once capped, remove the needle by holding the clear outer needle cap with one hand and holding the pen barrel with the other hand, turning counterclockwise.

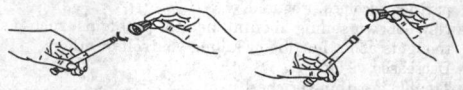

13. Carefully lift the needle off the pen and discard the capped needle. See *"How should I dispose of materials used to inject INTRON® A?"*

14. Replace the pen cap over the pen reservoir so that the black triangle is lined up with the dosage indicator.

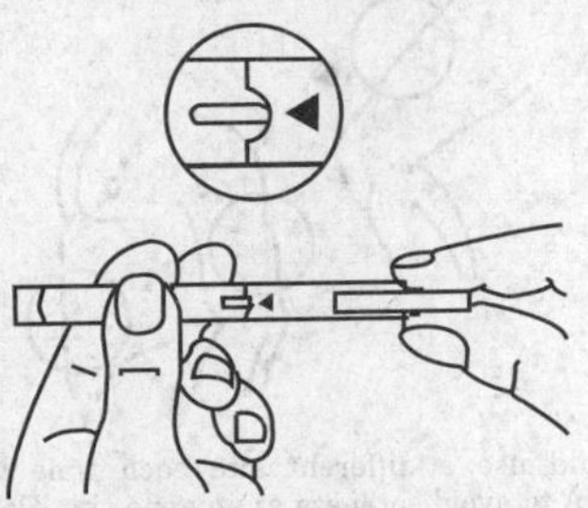

Storing INTRON A Solution Multidose Pen for Injection
INTRON A Solution Multidose Pen for Injection should be stored in the refrigerator between 2° and 8°C (36° and 46°F). **DO NOT FREEZE.** Discard any unused INTRON A pen remaining after 4 weeks.

How should I dispose of material used to inject INTRON® A?
There may be special state and local laws for disposal of used needles and multidose pens. Your healthcare provider should provide you with instructions on how to properly dispose of your used needles and multidose pens. Always follow those instructions. The instructions below should be used as a general guide for proper disposal.
- The needles should never be reused.
- Place all used needles and multidose pens in a puncture-proof disposable container that is available through your pharmacy or healthcare provider. You may use a hard plastic container with a screw-on cap (like a laundry detergent container). DO NOT use glass or clear plastic containers for disposal of needles.
- The container should be clearly labeled as "USED NEEDLES AND MULTIDOSE PENS." When the container is about two-thirds full, dispose of the container as instructed by your healthcare provider. DO NOT throw the container in your household trash. DO NOT recycle.
- **Always keep the container out of the reach of children.**

Schering Corporation Kenilworth, NJ 07033 USA
Copyright© 1996, 2001, 2006, Schering Corporation. All rights reserved.
U.S. Patent Nos. 5,935,566 and 6,610,830.
Novofine is a registered trademark of Novo Nordisk A/S.
Rev 7/09

MEDICATION GUIDE

INTRON A
(Interferon alfa-2b, recombinant)
Including appendix with instructions for using INTRON A Powder for Injection

Read this Medication Guide carefully before you start to take INTRON A (In-tron aye) for Injection alone or INTRON A in combination with REBETOL® (REB-eh-tole) (ribavirin, USP) Capsules. Read the Medication Guide each time you refill your prescription because there may be new information. The information in this Medication Guide does not take the place of talking with your healthcare provider. If you are taking INTRON A and REBETOL combination therapy, also read the Medication Guide for REBETOL (ribavirin, USP) Capsules.

What is the most important information I should know about INTRON® A?
INTRON A is a treatment for some people who have hairy cell leukemia, malignant melanoma, follicular lymphoma, AIDS-related Kaposi's sarcoma, chronic hepatitis B, chronic hepatitis C, and condylomata acuminata. If you have chronic hepatitis C, your healthcare provider may prescribe INTRON A in combination with REBETOL®. INTRON® A used by itself or with REBETOL can help you, but can also have serious side effects and may cause death in rare cases. Before starting treatment, you should talk to your healthcare provider about the possible benefits and possible side effects of INTRON A alone or in combination with REBETOL, to decide if this treatment is right for you. While taking INTRON A alone or in combination with REBETOL, you need to see a healthcare provider regularly for medical examinations and lab tests to make sure the treatment is working and to check for side effects.

You should call your healthcare provider immediately if you develop any of these conditions while taking INTRON A:
- You become pregnant or if you are a male and your female partner becomes pregnant
- New or worsening mental health problems such as thoughts about hurting or killing yourself or others
- Decreased vision
- Trouble breathing or chest pain
- Severe stomach or lower back pain
- Bloody diarrhea or bloody bowel movements
- High fever
- Easy bruising or bleeding

The most serious possible side effects of INTRON A include:
RISK TO PREGNANCY. Combination INTRON A and REBETOL therapy can cause death, serious birth defects or other harm to your unborn child. If you are pregnant, you or your male partner must not take INTRON A and REBETOL combination therapy. You must not become pregnant while either you or your partner are taking the combination of INTRON A and REBETOL and for 6 months after you stop taking the combination. If you are a woman of childbearing age you must have negative pregnancy tests immediately before starting treatment, during treatment and for 6 months after you have stopped treatment. You should use two forms of birth control during and for 6 months after you have stopped treatment. If you are a man taking INTRON A/REBETOL combination therapy, one of the two forms of birth control should be a condom. You must use birth control even if you believe that you are not fertile or that your fertility is low. You should talk to your healthcare provider about birth control for you and your partner. If you or your partner becomes pregnant while either of you is being treated or within 6 months of stopping treatment, tell your healthcare provider right away. There is a Ribavirin Pregnancy Registry that collects information about pregnancy outcomes in female patients and female partners of male patients exposed to ribavirin. You or your healthcare provider are encouraged to contact the Registry at 1-800-593-2214.

Mental health problems and suicide. INTRON A may cause patients to develop mood or behavioral problems. These can include irritability (getting easily upset) and depression (feeling low, feeling bad about yourself, or feeling hopeless). Some patients may have aggressive behavior. Former drug addicts may fall back into drug addiction or overdose. Some patients think about hurting or killing themselves or other people. Some patients have killed themselves (suicide) or hurt themselves or others. You must tell your healthcare provider if you are being treated for a mental illness or had treatment in the past for any mental illness, including depression and suicidal behavior. You should also tell your healthcare provider if you have ever been addicted to drugs or alcohol.

Eye problems. Changes in vision such as a decrease or loss of vision (blindness) may happen in some patients. You should have an eye exam before you take INTRON A. If you have eye problems or have had them in the past, you may need eye exams while you are taking INTRON A. Tell your healthcare provider or eye doctor right away if you have changes in your vision while taking INTRON A.

Heart problems. Some patients taking INTRON A may develop problems with their heart, including low blood pressure, fast heart rate, and very rarely, heart attacks. Tell your healthcare provider if you have had any heart problems in the past.

Blood problems. INTRON A commonly lowers two types of blood cells (white blood cells and platelets). In some patients, these blood counts may fall to dangerously low levels. If your blood cell counts become very low, you could get infections or have bleeding problems.

If you are taking INTRON A and REBETOL combination therapy, REBETOL can cause a drop in your number of red blood cells (anemia). A very low red blood cell count can be dangerous, especially if you have heart or breathing problems.

For other possible side effects of INTRON A, *see "What are the possible side effects of INTRON A?" in this Medication Guide.*

Body organ problems. INTRON A may cause lung problems including: trouble breathing, pneumonia, inflammation of lung tissue, and new or worse high blood pressure in the lungs (pulmonary hypertension), which can be severe and may in some cases lead to death. Certain symptoms like severe stomach pain may mean that your internal organs are being damaged. Cases of weakness, loss of coordination, and numbness due to stroke have been reported in patients taking Intron A, including patients with few or no reported risk factors for stroke.

What is INTRON® A?
The INTRON A product contains a man-made protein called interferon. Interferon is a protein that is part of the body's immune system that "interferes" with the growth of viruses or cancer cells.

It is not known if INTRON A or INTRON A/REBETOL® combination therapy can cure hepatitis B or C (permanently eliminate the virus) or if it can prevent liver failure or liver cancer that is caused by hepatitis B or C infection.

It is also not known if INTRON A or INTRON A/REBETOL combination therapy will prevent one infected person from infecting another person with hepatitis B or C.

Who should not take INTRON® A?
Do not take INTRON A alone or in combination with REBETOL® if you:
- are pregnant, planning to get pregnant, or breast-feeding
- are a male patient on combination therapy and have a female sexual partner who is pregnant or plans to become pregnant while you are being treated with REBETOL or during the 6 months after your treatment has ended
- have autoimmune hepatitis (hepatitis caused by your immune system attacking your liver) or unstable liver disease (yellowing of the skin and eyes, swelling of the abdomen)
- had an allergic reaction to another alpha interferon or ribavirin or are allergic to any of the ingredients in INTRON A or REBETOL

If you have any of the following conditions or serious medical problems, tell your healthcare provider before taking INTRON A alone or in combination with REBETOL:
- depression or anxiety
- eye problems
- sleep problems
- high blood pressure
- previous heart attack, or other heart problems
- liver problems (other than hepatitis B or C)
- any kind of autoimmune disease (where the body's immune system attacks the body's own cells), such as psoriasis, sarcoidosis, systemic lupus erythematosus, rheumatoid arthritis
- thyroid problems
- diabetes
- colitis (inflammation of the bowels)
- cancer
- hepatitis B or C infection
- HIV infection (the virus that causes AIDS)
- kidney problems
- bleeding problems
- alcoholism
- drug abuse or addiction
- body organ transplant and are taking medicine that keeps your body from rejecting your transplant (suppresses your immune system)
- high blood triglycerides (fat particles normally found in your blood)

Tell your healthcare provider about all the medicines you take, including prescription and non- prescription medicines, vitamins, and herbal supplements. INTRON A and certain other medicines may affect each other and cause side effects.

Especially tell your doctor if you take the anti-hepatitis B medicine telbivudine (Tyzeka). See "What are the possible side effects of INTRON A?"

Know the medicines you take. Keep a list of them and show it to your healthcare provider and pharmacist when you get a new medicine.

How should I take INTRON® A?
To get the most benefit from this medicine, it is important that you take INTRON A exactly as your healthcare provider tells you. Your healthcare provider will decide your dose of INTRON A and how often you will take it. Do not take more than your prescribed dose. INTRON A is given as an injection either under the skin (subcutaneous) or into a muscle (intramuscular). You should be completely comfortable with how to prepare and measure your dose of INTRON A and how to inject yourself before you use INTRON A for the first time. Your healthcare provider will train you on how to use and inject INTRON A properly.

INTRON A comes in different strengths and different forms (a powder in a vial, a solution in a vial, and a multidose pen). Your healthcare provider will determine which form is best for you. The instructions for giving a dose of INTRON A are at the end of this leaflet.

If you miss a dose of INTRON A, take the missed dose as soon as possible during the same day or the next day, then continue on your regular dosing schedule. If several days go by after you miss a dose, check with your healthcare provider to see what to do. **Do not double your next dose** or take more than your prescribed dose without talking to your healthcare provider. Call your healthcare provider right away if you take more than your prescribed dose. Your healthcare provider may wish to examine you more closely and take blood for testing.

If you are taking INTRON A in combination with REBETOL®, you should also read the Medication Guide for REBETOL (ribavirin, USP) for more information about side effects and how to take REBETOL. **REBETOL capsules should be taken twice a day with food.** Taking REBETOL with food helps your body take up more of the medicine. Taking REBETOL at the same time of day every day will help keep the amount of medicine in your body at a steady level. This can help your healthcare provider decide how your treatment is working and how to change the number of REBETOL capsules you take if you have side effects. If you miss a dose of REBETOL, take the missed dose as soon as possible during the same day. If an entire day has passed, check with your healthcare provider about what to do. **Do not double your next dose.**

You must see your healthcare provider on a regular basis for blood tests so your healthcare provider can check how the treatment is working for you and to check for side effects.

Tell your healthcare provider if you are taking or planning to take other prescription or nonprescription medicines, including vitamin and mineral supplements and herbal medicines.

What should I avoid while taking INTRON® A?

- Avoid becoming pregnant while taking INTRON A. INTRON A alone and INTRON A taken in combination with REBETOL® may harm your unborn child or cause you to lose your baby (miscarry). If you or your partner becomes pregnant during treatment or during the 6 months after treatment with INTRON A/REBETOL combination therapy, immediately report the pregnancy to your healthcare provider. Your healthcare provider will make decisions about your treatment. Your healthcare provider should call 1-800-593-2214. Your healthcare provider will be asked to give follow-up information about the pregnancy.
- Do not breast-feed your baby while taking INTRON A.
- Avoid taking telbivudine (Tyzeka), a drug used to treat hepatitis B. People who take INTRON A or other alpha interferon products with telbivudine (Tyzeka) can have nerve problems such as continuing numbness, tingling, or burning sensation in the arms or legs, or problems walking.

What are the possible side effects of INTRON® A?

INTRON A may cause serious side effects including:

- See "What is the most important information I should know about INTRON A?"
- **Other body organ problems.** Certain symptoms like severe pain in the middle of your body, nausea, and vomiting may mean that your liver or pancreas is being damaged. A few patients have inflammation of the kidney. If you have severe stomach or back pains or a fever, you should call your health care provider right away.
- **Thyroid problems.** Some patients develop changes in the function of their thyroid. Symptoms of thyroid changes include the inability to concentrate, feeling cold or hot all the time, a change in your weight and changes to your skin.
- **New or worsening autoimmune disease.** Some patients taking INTRON A develop autoimmune diseases (a condition where the body's immune cells attack other cells or organs in the body), including rheumatoid arthritis, systemic lupus erythematosus, sarcoidosis, and psoriasis. In some patients who already have an autoimmune disease, the disease may worsen while on INTRON A.
- **Nerve problems.** People who take INTRON A or other alpha interferon products with telbivudine (Tyzeka) can have nerve problems such as continuing numbness, tingling, or burning sensation in the arms or legs (peripheral neuropathy). Call your healthcare provider if you have any of these symptoms.

Common but less serious side effects include:

- **Flu-like symptoms.** Most patients who take INTRON A have "flu-like" symptoms (headache, muscle aches, tiredness, and fever) that usually lessen after the first few weeks of therapy. You can reduce some of these symptoms by injecting your INTRON A dose at bedtime. Over-the-counter pain and fever medications can be used to prevent or reduce the fever and headache. If your fever does not go away you should tell your healthcare provider.
- **Extreme fatigue (tiredness).** Many patients become extremely tired while on INTRON A.
- **Appetite problems.** Nausea, loss of appetite, and weight loss occur commonly.
- **Blood sugar problems.** Some patients develop problems with the way their body controls their blood sugar and may develop high blood sugar or diabetes.
- **Skin reactions.** Redness, swelling, and itching are common at the site of injection. If after several days these symptoms do not disappear, contact your healthcare provider. You may get a rash during therapy. If this occurs, your healthcare provider may recommend medicine to treat the rash.
- **Hair thinning.** Hair thinning is common during INTRON A treatment. Hair loss stops and hair growth returns after therapy is stopped.

These are not all the side effects of INTRON A or INTRON A/REBETOL® combination therapy. Your healthcare provider can give you a more complete list.

Call your doctor for medical advice about side effects. You may report side effects to FDA at 1-800-FDA-1088.

General advice about prescription medicines

Medicines are sometimes prescribed for purposes other than those listed in a Medication Guide. If you have any concerns about the INTRON® A product, ask your healthcare provider. Your health care provider can give you additional information about INTRON A. Do not use INTRON A for a condition for which it was not prescribed. Do not share this medication with other people.

This Medication Guide has been approved by the U.S. Food and Drug Administration.

Manufactured by: Schering Corporation Kenilworth, NJ 07033 USA

Issued: August 2009
Copyright © 1996, 2008, Schering Corporation.
All rights reserved.
Rev. 8/09

Medication Guide Appendix: Instructions for Preparing and Giving a Dose of INTRON® A Powder for Injection

- INTRON A medication has been supplied to you as a powder form that requires you to add the supplied liquid (DILUENT) to the powder. The liquid (DILUENT) is supplied to you in a vial.

The INTRON® A Powder for Injection may be supplied to you in 10 million IU, 18 million IU, or 50 million IU vials. These packages contain 1 vial of INTRON A powder and 1 vial of DILUENT (Sterile Water for Injection, USP). Syringes are not supplied to you. Talk to your healthcare provider about what syringes you should use.

Storing INTRON® A Powder for Injection

Before and after reconstitution, INTRON A Powder for Injection should be stored in the refrigerator between 2° and 8°C (36° and 46°F). **DO NOT FREEZE.**

NOTE: INTRON A Powder for Injection does not contain a preservative. The vial must be discarded after reconstitution and withdrawal of a single dose.

Preparing a dose of INTRON® A Powder for Injection

1. Find a well lit, clean, flat working surface such as a table. Collect the supplies you will need for an injection:
   - a vial of INTRON A powder
   - a vial of DILUENT (Sterile Water for Injection, USP)
   - a single-use, disposable syringe, as prescribed by your healthcare provider
   - a cotton ball or gauze
   - two alcohol swabs
   - a puncture-proof disposable container
2. Before removing the vials from the carton, check the expiration date printed on the carton to make sure that the expiration date has not passed. Do not use if the expiration date has passed.
3. Wash your hands with soap and warm water. It is important to keep your work area, your hands and injection site clean to minimize the risk of infection.
4. Gently warm the DILUENT vial by slowly rolling the vial in the palms of your hands for one minute.
5. Remove the protective caps from both vials (INTRON A powder and the supplied DILUENT). Clean the rubber stopper on the top of each vial with an alcohol swab.
6. Open the syringe package and remove the syringe.
7. Remove the needle cover from the syringe. Fill the syringe with air by pulling the plunger back to the mark on the syringe that matches the dose prescribed by your health care provider.

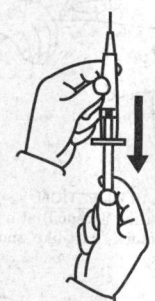

8. Hold the DILUENT vial on your flat working surface without touching the cleaned rubber stopper with your hands.
9. Insert the needle straight down through the middle of the rubber stopper of the vial containing the DILUENT. Slowly inject all the air from the syringe into the air space above the DILUENT.

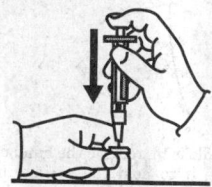

10. Keep the needle in the vial and turn the vial upside down. Make sure the tip of the needle is in the DILUENT. Slowly pull the plunger back to fill the syringe with DILUENT to the number (mL or cc) that your healthcare provider instructed you to use.

[See figure at top of next column]

11. With the needle still inserted in the vial, check the syringe for air bubbles. If there are any air bubbles, gently tap the syringe with your finger until the air bubbles rise to the top of the syringe. Slowly push the plunger up

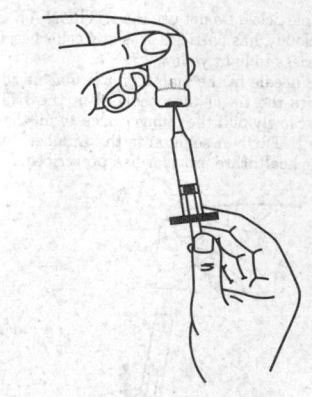

to remove the air bubbles. If you push DILUENT back into the vial, slowly pull back on the plunger to again draw the correct amount of DILUENT back into the syringe.

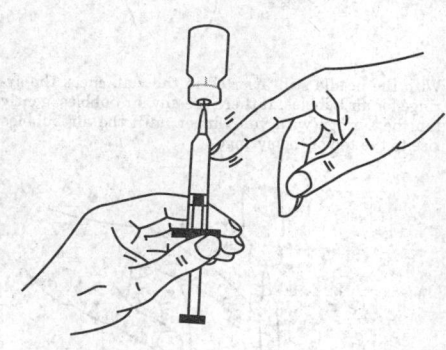

12. Remove the needle from the vial. Do not let the syringe touch anything.
13. Without touching the cleaned rubber stopper, insert the needle through the middle of the rubber stopper and gently place the needle tip, at an angle, against the side of the INTRON A powder vial.
14. Slowly push the plunger down to inject the DILUENT. The stream of liquid should run down the sides of the glass vial. **DO NOT INJECT THE DILUENT DIRECTLY AT THE WHITE POWDER.**

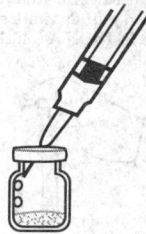

15. Do not remove the needle from the vial.
16. To dissolve the white powder, gently swirl the INTRON A vial in a circular motion until the powder is completely dissolved. **DO NOT SHAKE.** If the solution is foamy, wait a few minutes until the bubbles have settled before withdrawing your dose from the vial.

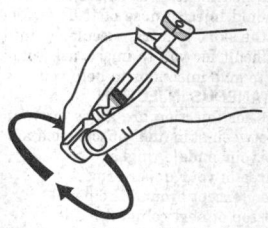

17. Check the solution inside the vial of the INTRON A. The solution should be clear and colorless to light yellow,

without particles. Do not use the INTRON A if the medicine is cloudy, has particles or is any color besides clear and colorless to light yellow.

18. With the needle in the vial, turn the vial upside down. Make sure the tip of the needle is in the INTRON A solution. Slowly pull the plunger back to fill the syringe with the INTRON A solution to the number (mL or cc) that your healthcare provider has prescribed.

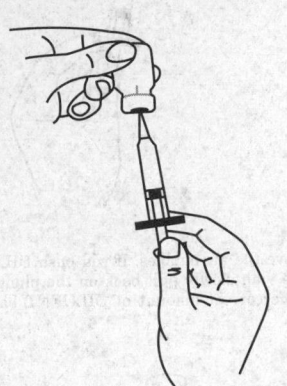

19. With the needle still inserted in the vial, check the syringe for air bubbles. If there are any air bubbles, gently tap the syringe with your finger until the air bubbles rise to the top of the syringe.

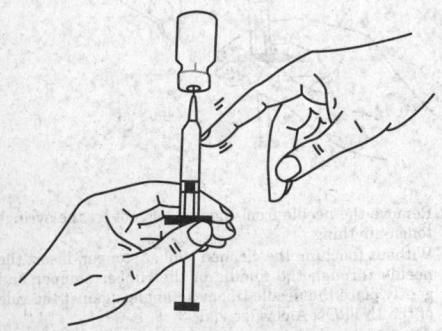

20. Slowly push the plunger up to remove the air bubbles. If you push solution back into the vial, slowly pull back on the plunger again to draw the correct amount of INTRON A solution back into the syringe.

21. Do not remove the needle from the vial. Lay the vial and syringe on its side on your flat work surface until you are ready to inject the INTRON A solution.

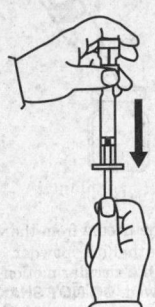

Choosing an Injection site
Based on your treatment, your health care provider will tell you if you should inject a dose of INTRON® A subcutaneously (under the skin) or intramuscularly (into the muscle). If it is too difficult for you to inject, ask someone who has been trained to give injections to help you.

FOR SUBCUTANEOUS INJECTION
The best sites for injection are areas on your body with a layer of fat between skin and muscle such as:
- the front of your middle thighs
- the outer area of your upper arms
- the abdomen, except around the navel
[See figure at top of next column]

FOR INTRAMUSCULAR INJECTION
The best sites for injection into your muscle are:
- the front of the middle thighs
- the upper arms

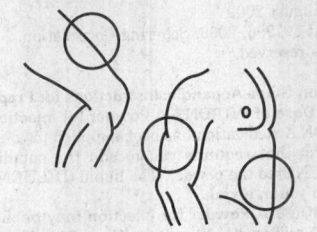

- the upper outer areas of the buttocks

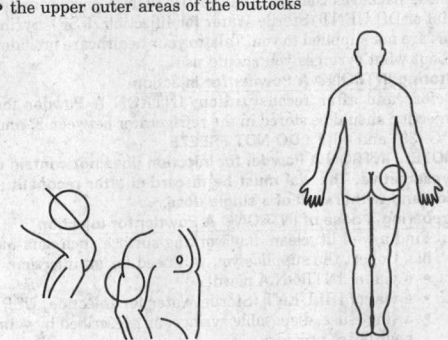

You should use a different site each time you inject INTRON A to avoid soreness at any one site. Do not inject INTRON A into an area where the skin is irritated, red, bruised, infected or has scars, stretch marks or lumps.

Injecting the dose of INTRON® A
1. Clean the injection site with a new alcohol swab.
2. Pick up the vial and syringe from your flat work surface. Remove the syringe and needle from the vial. Hold the syringe in the hand that you will use to inject INTRON A. Do not touch the needle or allow it to touch the work surface.
3. With your free hand, pinch a fold of the skin at the cleaned injection site.

FOR SUBCUTANEOUS INJECTION:
4a. Hold the syringe (like a pencil) at a **45-degree angle** to the skin. With a quick "dart-like" motion, push the needle into the skin.

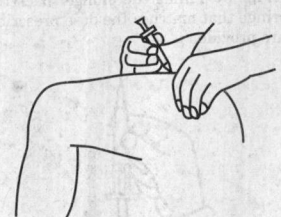

FOR INTRAMUSCULAR INJECTION:
4b. Hold the syringe (like a pencil) at a **90-degree angle** to the skin. With a quick "dart-like" motion, push the needle into the muscle.

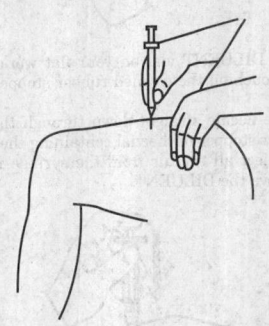

5. After the needle is in, remove the hand used to pinch the skin and use it to hold the syringe barrel. Pull the plunger back slightly. If blood comes into the syringe, the needle has entered a blood vessel. Do not inject INTRON A. Withdraw the needle and discard the syringe in the puncture-proof container. *See "How should I dispose of materials used to inject INTRON A?"* Prepare a new dose of INTRON A using a new INTRON A Powder for Injection vial and prepare a new injection site.

6. If no blood is present in the syringe, inject the medicine by gently pushing the plunger all the way down until the syringe is empty.

7. When the syringe is empty, pull the needle out of the skin and place a cotton ball or gauze over the injection site and press for several seconds. Do not massage the injection site. If there is bleeding, cover the injection site with a bandage.

8. Dispose of syringe and needle. *See "How should I dispose of materials used to inject INTRON A?"*

9. It is important to check your injection site approximately two hours after your injection for redness, swelling, or tenderness. These are signs of inflammation that you may need to talk to your healthcare provider about if they do not go away.

How should I dispose of materials used to inject INTRON A?
There may be special state and local laws for disposal of used needles and syringes. Your healthcare provider should provide you with instructions on how to properly dispose of your used syringes and needles. Always follow those instructions. The instructions below should be used as a general guide for proper disposal.
- The needles and syringes should never be reused.
- Place all used needles and syringes in a puncture-proof disposable container that is available through your pharmacy or healthcare provider. You may also use a hard plastic container with a screw-on cap (like a laundry detergent container).
- DO NOT use glass or clear plastic containers for disposal of needles and syringes.

The container should be clearly labeled as "USED SYRINGES AND NEEDLES." When the container is about two-thirds full, tighten the lid. Tape the cap or lid to make sure it does not come off. Dispose of the container as instructed by your healthcare provider. DO NOT throw the container in your household trash. DO NOT recycle.
- **Always keep the container out of reach of children.**

Schering Corporation
Kenilworth, NJ 07033 USA
Copyright © 1996, 2001, 2004, Schering Corporation. All rights reserved.
Rev. 8/09
U.S. Patent No. 5,935,566 and 6,610,830.

MEDICATION GUIDE
INTRON® A
(Interferon alfa-2b, recombinant)
Including appendix with instructions for using INTRON A Solution for Injection
Read this Medication Guide carefully before you start to take INTRON A (In-tron aye) for Injection alone or INTRON A in combination with REBETOL® (REB-eh-tole) (ribavirin, USP) Capsules. Read the Medication Guide each time you refill your prescription because there may be new information. The information in this Medication Guide does not take the place of talking with your healthcare provider. If you are taking INTRON A and REBETOL combination therapy, also read the Medication Guide for REBETOL (ribavirin, USP) Capsules.

What is the most important information I should know about INTRON® A?
INTRON A is a treatment for some people who have hairy cell leukemia, malignant melanoma, follicular lymphoma, AIDS-related Kaposi's sarcoma, chronic hepatitis B, chronic hepatitis C, and condylomata acuminata. If you have chronic hepatitis C, your healthcare provider may prescribe INTRON A in combination with REBETOL®. INTRON A used by itself or with REBETOL can help you, but can also have serious side effects and may cause death in rare cases. Before starting treatment, you should talk to your healthcare provider about the possible benefits and possible side effects of INTRON A alone or in combination with REBETOL, to decide if this treatment is right for you. While taking INTRON A alone or in combination with REBETOL, you need to see a healthcare provider regularly for medical examinations and lab tests to make sure the treatment is working and to check for side effects.

You should call your healthcare provider immediately if you develop any of these conditions while taking INTRON A:
- You become pregnant or if you are a male and your female partner becomes pregnant
- New or worsening mental health problems such as thoughts about hurting or killing yourself or others
- Decreased vision
- Trouble breathing or chest pain
- Severe stomach or lower back pain
- Bloody diarrhea or bloody bowel movements
- High fever
- Easy bruising or bleeding

The most serious possible side effects of INTRON A include:
RISK TO PREGNANCY. Combination INTRON A and REBETOL therapy can cause death, serious birth defects or other harm to your unborn child. If you are pregnant, you or your male partner must not take INTRON A and REBETOL combination therapy. You must not become pregnant while either you or your partner are taking the combination of INTRON A and REBETOL and for 6 months

after you stop taking the combination. If you are a woman of childbearing age you must have negative pregnancy tests immediately before starting treatment, during treatment and for 6 months after you have stopped treatment. You should use two forms of birth control during and for 6 months after you have stopped treatment. If you are a man taking INTRON A/REBETOL combination therapy, one of the two forms of birth control should be a condom. You must use birth control even if you believe that you are not fertile or that your fertility is low. You should talk to your healthcare provider about birth control for you and your partner. If you or your partner becomes pregnant while either of you is being treated or within 6 months of stopping treatment, tell your healthcare provider right away. There is a Ribavirin Pregnancy Registry that collects information about pregnancy outcomes in female patients and female partners of male patients exposed to ribavirin. You or your healthcare provider are encouraged to contact the Registry at 1-800-593-2214.

Mental health problems and suicide. INTRON A may cause patients to develop mood or behavioral problems. These can include irritability (getting easily upset) and depression (feeling low, feeling bad about yourself, or feeling hopeless). Some patients may have aggressive behavior. Former drug addicts may fall back into drug addiction or overdose. Some patients think about hurting or killing themselves or other people. Some patients have killed themselves (suicide) or hurt themselves or others. You must tell your healthcare provider if you are being treated for a mental illness or had treatment in the past for any mental illness, including depression and suicidal behavior. You should also tell your healthcare provider if you have ever been addicted to drugs or alcohol.

Eye problems. Changes in vision such as a decrease or loss of vision (blindness) may happen in some patients. You should have an eye exam before you take INTRON A. If you have eye problems or have had them in the past, you may need eye exams while you are taking INTRON A. Tell your healthcare provider or eye doctor right away if you have changes in your vision while taking INTRON A.

Heart problems. Some patients taking INTRON A may develop problems with their heart, including low blood pressure, fast heart rate, and very rarely, heart attacks. Tell your healthcare provider if you have had any heart problems in the past.

Blood problems. INTRON A commonly lowers two types of blood cells (white blood cells and platelets). In some patients, these blood counts may fall to dangerously low levels. If your blood cell counts become very low, you could get infections or have bleeding problems.

If you are taking INTRON A and REBETOL combination therapy, REBETOL can cause a drop in your number of red blood cells (anemia). A very low red blood cell count can be dangerous, especially if you have heart or breathing problems.

For other possible side effects of INTRON A, see "What are the possible side effects of INTRON A?" in this Medication Guide.

Body organ problems. INTRON A may cause lung problems including: trouble breathing, pneumonia, inflammation of lung tissue, and new or worse high blood pressure of the lungs (pulmonary hypertension), which can be severe and may in some cases lead to death. Certain symptoms like severe stomach pain may mean that your internal organs are being damaged. Cases of weakness, loss of coordination, and numbness due to stroke have been reported in patients taking Intron A, including patients with few or no reported risk factors for stroke.

What is INTRON® A?

The INTRON A product contains a man-made protein called interferon. Interferon is a protein that is part of the body's immune system that "interferes" with the growth of viruses or cancer cells.

It is not known if INTRON A or INTRON A/REBETOL® combination therapy can cure hepatitis B or C (permanently eliminate the virus) or if it can prevent liver failure or liver cancer that is caused by hepatitis B or C infection.

It is also not known if INTRON A or INTRON A/REBETOL combination therapy will prevent one infected person from infecting another person with hepatitis B or C.

Who should not take INTRON® A?

Do not take INTRON A alone or in combination with REBETOL® if you:

• are pregnant, planning to get pregnant, or breast-feeding
• are a male patient on combination therapy and have a female sexual partner who is pregnant or plans to become pregnant while you are being treated with REBETOL or during the 6 months after your treatment has ended
• have autoimmune hepatitis (hepatitis caused by your immune system attacking your liver) or unstable liver disease (yellowing of the skin and eyes, swelling of the abdomen)

• had an allergic reaction to another alpha interferon or ribavirin or are allergic to any of the ingredients in INTRON A or REBETOL

If you have any of the following conditions or serious medical problems, tell your healthcare provider before taking INTRON A alone or in combination with REBETOL:

• depression or anxiety
• eye problems
• sleep problems
• high blood pressure
• previous heart attack, or other heart problems
• liver problems (other than hepatitis B or C)
• any kind of autoimmune disease (where the body's immune system attacks the body's own cells), such as psoriasis, sarcoidosis, systemic lupus erythematosus, rheumatoid arthritis
• thyroid problems
• diabetes
• colitis (inflammation of the bowels)
• cancer
• hepatitis B or C infection
• HIV infection (the virus that causes AIDS)
• kidney problems
• bleeding problems
• alcoholism
• drug abuse or addiction
• body organ transplant and are taking medicine that keeps your body from rejecting your transplant (suppresses your immune system)
• high blood triglycerides (fat particles normally found in your blood)

Tell your healthcare provider about all the medicines you take, including prescription and non-prescription medicines, vitamins, and herbal supplements. INTRON A and certain other medicines may affect each other and cause side effects.

Especially tell your doctor if you take the anti-hepatitis B medicine telbivudine (Tyzeka). See "What are the possible side effects of INTRON A?"

Know the medicines you take. Keep a list of them and show it to your healthcare provider and pharmacist when you get a new medicine.

How should I take INTRON® A?

To get the most benefit from this medicine, it is important that you take INTRON A exactly as your healthcare provider tells you. Your healthcare provider will decide your dose of INTRON A and how often you will take it. Do not take more than your prescribed dose. INTRON A is given as an injection either under the skin (subcutaneous) or into a muscle (intramuscular). You should be completely comfortable with how to prepare and measure your dose of INTRON A and how to inject yourself before you use INTRON A for the first time. Your healthcare provider will train you on how to use and inject INTRON A properly.

INTRON A comes in different strengths and different forms (a powder in a vial, a solution in a vial, and a multidose pen). Your healthcare provider will determine which form is best for you. The instructions for giving a dose of INTRON A are at the end of this leaflet.

If you miss a dose of INTRON A, take the missed dose as soon as possible during the same day or the next day, then continue on your regular dosing schedule. If several days go by after you miss a dose, check with your healthcare provider to see what to do. **Do not double your next dose** or take more than your prescribed dose without talking to your healthcare provider. Call your healthcare provider right away if you take more than your prescribed dose. Your healthcare provider may wish to examine you more closely and take blood for testing.

If you are taking INTRON A in combination with REBETOL®, you should also read the Medication Guide for REBETOL (ribavirin, USP) for more information about side effects and how to take REBETOL. **REBETOL capsules should be taken twice a day with food.** Taking REBETOL with food helps your body take up more of the medicine. Taking REBETOL at the same time of day every day will help keep the amount of medicine in your body at a steady level. This can help your healthcare provider decide how your treatment is working and how to change the number of REBETOL capsules you take if you have side effects. If you miss a dose of REBETOL, take the missed dose as soon as possible during the same day. If an entire day has passed, check with your healthcare provider about what to do. **Do not double your next dose.**

You must see your healthcare provider on a regular basis for blood tests so your healthcare provider can check how the treatment is working for you and to check for side effects. Tell your healthcare provider if you are taking or planning to take other prescription or nonprescription medicines, including vitamin and mineral supplements and herbal medicines.

What should I avoid while taking INTRON® A?

• Avoid becoming pregnant while taking INTRON A. INTRON A alone and INTRON A taken in combination

with REBETOL® may harm your unborn child or cause you to lose your baby (miscarry). If you or your partner becomes pregnant during treatment or during the 6 months after treatment with INTRON A/REBETOL combination therapy, immediately report the pregnancy to your healthcare provider. Your healthcare provider will make decisions about your treatment. Your healthcare provider should call 1-800-593-2214. Your healthcare provider will be asked to give follow-up information about the pregnancy.

• Do not breast-feed your baby while taking INTRON A.
• Avoid taking telbivudine (Tyzeka), a drug used to treat hepatitis B. People who take INTRON A or other alpha interferon products with telbivudine (Tyzeka) can have nerve problems such as continuing numbness, tingling, or burning sensation in the arms or legs, or problems walking.

What are the possible side effects of INTRON® A?

INTRON A may cause serious side effects including:

• See "What is the most important information I should know about INTRON A?"
• **Other body organ problems.** Certain symptoms like severe pain in the middle of your body, nausea, and vomiting may mean that your liver or pancreas is being damaged. A few patients have inflammation of the kidney. If you have severe stomach or back pains or a fever, you should call your healthcare provider right away.
• **Thyroid problems.** Some patients develop changes in the function of their thyroid. Symptoms of thyroid changes include the inability to concentrate, feeling cold or hot all the time, a change in your weight and changes to your skin.
• **New or worsening autoimmune disease.** Some patients taking INTRON A develop autoimmune diseases (a condition where the body's immune cells attack other cells or organs in the body), including rheumatoid arthritis, systemic lupus erythematosus, sarcoidosis, and psoriasis. In some patients who already have an autoimmune disease, the disease may worsen while on INTRON A.
• **Nerve problems.** People who take INTRON A or other alpha interferon products with telbivudine (Tyzeka) can have nerve problems such as continuing numbness, tingling, or burning sensation in the arms or legs (peripheral neuropathy). Call your healthcare provider if you have any of these symptoms.

Common but less serious side effects include:

• **Flu-like symptoms.** Most patients who take INTRON A have "flu-like" symptoms (headache, muscle aches, tiredness, and fever) that usually lessen after the first few weeks of therapy. You can reduce some of these symptoms by injecting your INTRON A dose at bedtime. Over-the-counter pain and fever medications can be used to prevent or reduce the fever and headache. If your fever does not go away you should tell your healthcare provider.
• **Extreme fatigue (tiredness).** Many patients become extremely tired while on INTRON A.
• **Appetite problems.** Nausea, loss of appetite, and weight loss occur commonly.
• **Blood sugar problems.** Some patients develop problems with the way their body controls their blood sugar and may develop high blood sugar or diabetes.
• **Skin reactions.** Redness, swelling, and itching are common at the site of injection. If after several days these symptoms do not disappear, contact your healthcare provider. You may get a rash during therapy. If this occurs, your healthcare provider may recommend medicine to treat the rash.
• **Hair thinning.** Hair thinning is common during INTRON A treatment. Hair loss stops and hair growth returns after therapy is stopped.

These are not all the side effects of INTRON A or INTRON A/REBETOL® combination therapy. Your healthcare provider can give you a more complete list.

Call your doctor for medical advice about side effects. You may report side effects to FDA at 1–800–FDA–1088.

General advice about prescription medicines

Medicines are sometimes prescribed for purposes other than those listed in a Medication Guide. If you have any concerns about the INTRON A product, ask your healthcare provider. Your health care provider can give you additional information about INTRON A. Do not use INTRON A for a condition for which it was not prescribed. Do not share this medication with other people.

This Medication Guide has been approved by the U.S. Food and Drug Administration.

Manufactured by: Schering Corporation Kenilworth, NJ 07033 USA

Issued: August 2009

Rev. 8/09

Medication Guide Appendix: Instructions for Preparing and Giving a Dose of INTRON® A Solution for Injection
• INTRON A medication has been supplied to you in a liquid form in a vial.

The INTRON® A Solution for Injection may be supplied to you as:
• **INTRON A Solution 18 million IU and 25 million IU multidose vial.** These packages contain 1 vial of INTRON A solution. Syringes are not supplied to you. Talk to your healthcare provider about what syringes you should use.

Storing INTRON® A Solution for Injection
INTRON A Solution for Injection should be stored in the refrigerator between 2° and 8°C (36° and 46°F). **DO NOT FREEZE.** After using the 18 or 25 million IU multidose vials, discard any unused INTRON A solution remaining after one month.

Preparing a Dose of INTRON® A Solution for Injection
1. Find a well lit, clean, flat working surface such as a table. Collect the supplies you will need for an injection:
   • A vial of INTRON A solution
   • A syringe you have obtained for use with the multi-use vials.
   • A cotton ball or gauze
   • Two alcohol swabs
   • A puncture-proof disposable container
2. Before removing contents from the carton, check the expiration date printed on the carton to make sure that the expiration date has not passed. Do not use if the expiration date has passed.
3. Wash your hands with soap and warm water. It is important to keep your work area, your hands and injection site clean to minimize the risk of infection.
4. Remove one vial of INTRON A solution from the carton.
5. Check the vial of INTRON A. The solution should be clear and colorless, without particles. Do not use the vial of INTRON A if the medicine is cloudy, has particles or is any color besides clear and colorless.
6. Remove the protective plastic cap from the top of the INTRON A vial. Clean the rubber stopper on the top of the INTRON A vial with an alcohol swab.
7. Gently warm the INTRON A solution by slowly rolling the vial in the palms of your hands for about one minute. **DO NOT SHAKE.**

Open the package for the syringe you are using and if it does not have a needle attached, then attach one of the needles you have obtained to the syringe.

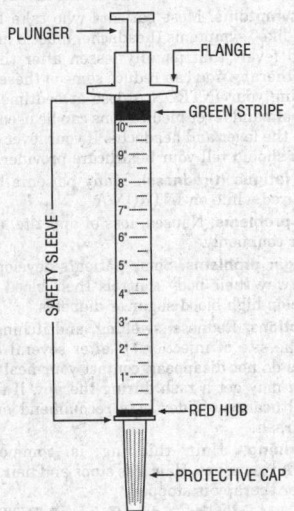

PLUNGER — FLANGE — GREEN STRIPE — SAFETY SLEEVE — RED HUB — PROTECTIVE CAP

8. Remove the protective cap from the needle of the syringe. Fill the syringe with air by pulling the plunger back to the mark on the syringe that matches the dose as prescribed by your healthcare provider.

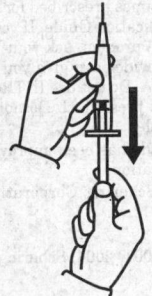

9. Hold the vial of INTRON A Solution for Injection on your flat working surface without touching the cleaned rubber stopper with your hands.

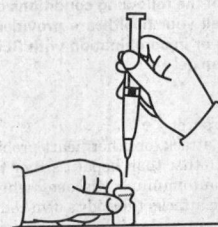

10. Insert the needle straight down through the middle of the rubber stopper of the vial containing the INTRON A solution. Slowly inject all the air from the syringe into the air space above the solution.

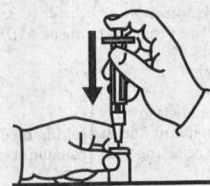

11. Keep the needle in the vial and turn the vial upside down. Make sure the tip of the needle is in the INTRON A solution. Slowly pull the plunger back to fill the syringe with INTRON A solution to the number (mL or cc) as prescribed by your healthcare provider.

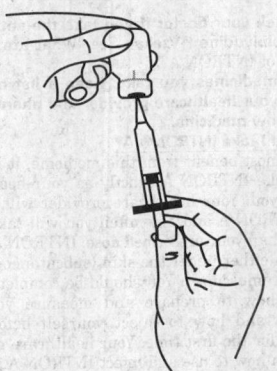

12. With the needle in the vial, check the syringe for air bubbles. If there are any air bubbles, gently tap the syringe with your finger until the air bubbles rise to the top of the syringe. Slowly push the plunger up to remove the air bubbles. If you push solution back into the vial, slowly pull back on the plunger to again draw the correct dose as prescribed by your healthcare provider.

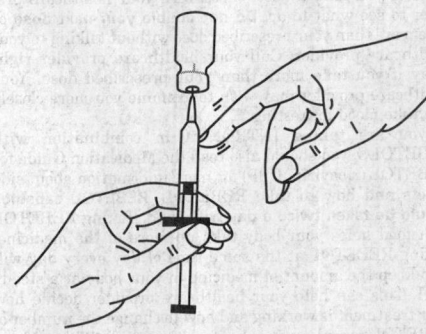

13. Do not remove the needle from the vial. Lay the vial and syringe on its side on your flat work surface until you are ready to inject the INTRON A solution.

Choosing an Injection site
Based on your treatment, your healthcare provider will tell you if you should inject a dose of INTRON® A subcutaneously (under the skin) or intramuscularly (into the muscle). If it is too difficult for you to inject, ask someone who has been trained to give injections to help you.

FOR SUBCUTANEOUS INJECTION
The best sites for injection are areas on your body with a layer of fat between skin and muscle such as:
• the front of your middle thighs
• the outer area of your upper arms

• the abdomen, except around the navel

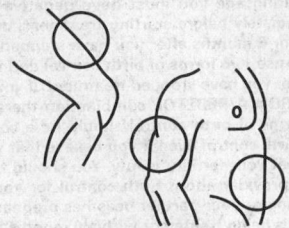

FOR INTRAMUSCULAR INJECTION
The best sites for injection into your muscle are:
• the front of the middle thighs
• the upper arms
• the upper outer areas of the buttocks

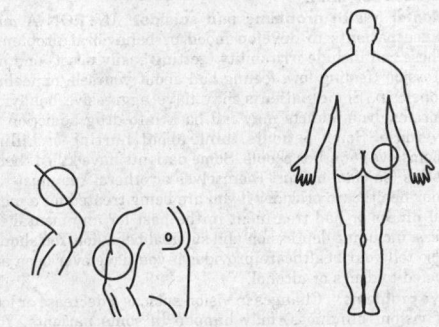

You should use a different site each time you inject INTRON® A to avoid soreness at any one site. Do not inject INTRON A into an area where the skin is irritated, red, bruised, infected or has scars, stretch marks or lumps.

Injecting the Dose of INTRON® A
1. Clean the injection site with a new alcohol swab.
2. Pick up the vial and syringe from your flat work surface. Remove the syringe and needle from the vial. Hold the syringe in the hand that you will use to inject INTRON A. Do not touch the needle or allow it to touch the work surface.
3. With your free hand, pinch a fold of the skin at the cleaned injection site.

FOR SUBCUTANEOUS INJECTION:
4a. Hold the syringe (like a pencil) at a **45-degree angle** to the skin. With a quick "dart-like" motion, push the needle into the skin.

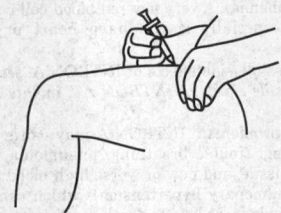

FOR INTRAMUSCULAR INJECTION:
4b. Hold the syringe (like a pencil) at a **90-degree angle** to the skin. With a quick "dart-like" motion, push the needle into the muscle.

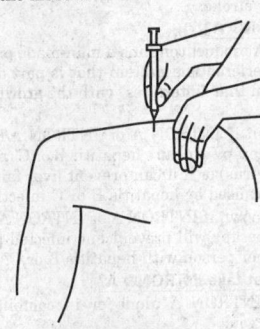

5. After the needle is in, remove the hand used to pinch the skin and use it to hold the syringe barrel. Pull the plunger back slightly. If blood comes into the syringe, the needle has entered a blood vessel. **Do not inject INTRON® A.** Withdraw the needle and discard the syringe in the puncture-proof container. See *"How should I dispose of materials used to inject INTRON A?"*) Prepare a new dose of INTRON A and prepare a new injection site.

6. If no blood is present in the syringe, inject the medicine by gently pushing the plunger all the way down until the syringe is empty.

7. When the syringe is empty, pull the needle out of the skin and place a cotton ball or gauze over the injection site and press for several seconds. Do not massage the injection site. If there is bleeding, cover the injection site with a bandage.

8. Dispose of syringe and needle. *See "How should I dispose of materials used to inject INTRON A?"*

9. If after using a multidose vial (18 million IU or 25 million IU) there is enough solution left in the vial for another dose, refrigerate the INTRON A vial after use. Discard any unused INTRON A solution remaining after 1 month.

10. It is important to check your injection site approximately two hours after your injection for redness, swelling, or tenderness. These are signs of inflammation that you may need to talk to your healthcare provider about if they do not go away.

How should I dispose of materials used to inject INTRON® A?

There may be special state and local laws for disposal of used needles and syringes. Your healthcare provider should provide you with instructions on how to properly dispose of your used syringes and needles. Always follow those instructions. The instructions below should be used as a general guide for proper disposal.

• **The needles and syringes should never be reused.**

• Place all used needles and syringes in a puncture-proof disposable container that is available through your pharmacy or healthcare provider. You may also use a hard plastic container with a screw-on cap (like a laundry detergent container).

• Do not use glass or clear plastic containers for disposal of needles and syringes.

• The container used for the disposal of syringes and needles should be clearly labeled as "USED SYRINGES AND NEEDLES." When the container is almost full, tighten the lid. Tape the cap or lid to make sure it does not come off. Dispose of the container as instructed by your healthcare provider.

DO NOT throw the container in your household trash and DO NOT recycle.

• **Always keep the container out of reach of children**

Schering Corporation Kenilworth, NJ 07033 USA

U.S. Patent No. 5,935,566 and 6,610,830.
Rev. 8/09
Shown in Product Identification Guide, page 313

INVANZ® ℞
[invanz]
(ertapenem for injection)

To reduce the development of drug-resistant bacteria and maintain the effectiveness of INVANZ and other antibacterial drugs, INVANZ should be used only to treat or prevent infections that are proven or strongly suspected to be caused by bacteria.

For Intravenous or Intramuscular Use

DESCRIPTION

INVANZ* (Ertapenem for Injection) is a sterile, synthetic, parenteral, 1-β methyl-carbapenem that is structurally related to beta-lactam antibiotics.

Chemically, INVANZ is described as [4R-[3(3S*,5S*),4α,5β,6β(R*)]]-3-[[5-[[(3-carboxyphenyl)amino]carbonyl]-3-pyrrolidinyl]thio]-6-(1-hydroxyethyl)-4-methyl-7-oxo-1-azabicyclo[3.2.0]hept-2-ene-2-carboxylic acid monosodium salt. Its molecular weight is 497.50. The empirical formula is $C_{22}H_{24}N_3O_7SNa$, and its structural formula is:

Ertapenem sodium is a white to off-white hygroscopic, weakly crystalline powder. It is soluble in water and 0.9% sodium chloride solution, practically insoluble in ethanol, and insoluble in isopropyl acetate and tetrahydrofuran. INVANZ is supplied as sterile lyophilized powder for intravenous infusion after reconstitution with appropriate diluent (see DOSAGE AND ADMINISTRATION, PREPARATION OF SOLUTION) and transfer to 50 mL 0.9% Sodium Chloride Injection or for intramuscular injection following reconstitution with 1% lidocaine hydrochloride. Each vial contains 1.046 grams ertapenem sodium, equivalent to 1 gram ertapenem. The sodium content is approximately 137 mg (approximately 6.0 mEq).

Each vial of INVANZ contains the following inactive ingredients: 175 mg sodium bicarbonate and sodium hydroxide to adjust pH to 7.5.

---

*Registered trademark of Merck Sharp & Dohme Corp., a subsidiary of **Merck & Co., Inc.**
COPYRIGHT © 2001, 2003–2007 Merck Sharp & Dohme Corp., a subsidiary of **Merck & Co., Inc.**
All rights reserved

CLINICAL PHARMACOLOGY

Pharmacokinetics

Average plasma concentrations (mcg/mL) of ertapenem following a single 30-minute infusion of a 1 g intravenous (IV) dose and administration of a single 1 g intramuscular (IM) dose in healthy young adults are presented in Table 1.

[See table 1 above]

The area under the plasma concentration-time curve (AUC) of ertapenem in adults increased less-than dose-proportional based on total ertapenem concentrations over the 0.5 to 2 g dose range, whereas the AUC increased greater-than dose proportional based on unbound ertapenem concentrations. Ertapenem exhibits non-linear pharmacokinetics due to concentration-dependent plasma protein binding at the proposed therapeutic dose. (See CLINICAL PHARMACOLOGY, *Distribution*.)

There is no accumulation of ertapenem following multiple IV or IM 1 g daily doses in healthy adults.

Average plasma concentrations (mcg/mL) of ertapenem in pediatric patients are presented in Table 2.

[See table 2 above]

Absorption

Ertapenem, reconstituted with 1% lidocaine HCl injection, USP (in saline without epinephrine), is almost completely absorbed following intramuscular (IM) administration at the recommended dose of 1 g. The mean bioavailability is approximately 90%. Following 1 g daily IM administration, mean peak plasma concentrations (C_{max}) are achieved in approximately 2.3 hours (T_{max}).

Distribution

Ertapenem is highly bound to human plasma proteins, primarily albumin. In healthy young adults, the protein binding of ertapenem decreases as plasma concentrations increase, from approximately 95% bound at an approximate plasma concentration of <100 micrograms (mcg)/mL to approximately 85% bound at an approximate plasma concentration of 300 mcg/mL.

The apparent volume of distribution at steady state (V_{ss}) of ertapenem in adults is approximately 0.12 liter/kg, approximately 0.2 liter/kg in pediatric patients 3 months to 12 years of age and approximately 0.16 liter/kg in pediatric patients 13 to 17 years of age.

The concentrations of ertapenem achieved in suction-induced skin blister fluid at each sampling point on the third day of 1 g once daily IV doses are presented in Table 3. The ratio of AUC_{0-24} in skin blister fluid/AUC_{0-24} in plasma is 0.61.

[See table 3 above]

The concentration of ertapenem in breast milk from 5 lactating women with pelvic infections (5 to 14 days postpartum) was measured at random time points daily for 5 consecutive days following the last 1 g dose of intravenous therapy (3-10 days of therapy). The concentration of ertapenem in breast milk within 24 hours of the last dose of therapy in all 5 women ranged from <0.13 (lower limit of quantitation) to 0.38 mcg/mL; peak concentrations were not assessed. By day 5 after discontinuation of therapy, the level of ertapenem was undetectable in the breast milk of 4 women and below the lower limit of quantitation (<0.13 mcg/mL) in 1 woman.

Metabolism

In healthy young adults, after infusion of 1 g IV radiolabeled ertapenem, the plasma radioactivity consists predominantly (94%) of ertapenem. The major metabolite of ertapenem is the inactive ring-opened derivative formed by hydrolysis of the beta-lactam ring.

In vitro studies in human liver microsomes indicate that ertapenem does not inhibit metabolism mediated by any of the following cytochrome p450 (CYP) isoforms: 1A2, 2C9, 2C19, 2D6, 2E1 and 3A4. (See PRECAUTIONS, *Drug Interactions*.)

Table 1
Plasma Concentrations of Ertapenem in Adults After Single Dose Administration

Dose/Route	Average Plasma Concentrations (mcg/mL)								
	0.5 hr	1 hr	2 hr	4 hr	6 hr	8 hr	12 hr	18 hr	24 hr
1 g IV*	155	115	83	48	31	20	9	3	1
1 g IM	33	53	67	57	40	27	13	4	2

* Infused at a constant rate over 30 minutes

Table 2
Plasma Concentrations of Ertapenem in Pediatric Patients After Single IV* Dose Administration

Age Group	Dose	Average Plasma Concentrations (mcg/mL)							
		0.5 hr	1 hr	2 hr	4 hr	6 hr	8 hr	12 hr	24 hr
3 to 23 months	15 mg/kg†	103.8	57.3	43.6	23.7	13.5	8.2	2.5	-
	20 mg/kg†	126.8	87.6	58.7	28.4	-	12.0	3.4	0.4
	40 mg/kg‡	199.1	144.1	95.7	58.0	-	20.2	7.7	0.6
2 to 12 years	15 mg/kg†	113.2	63.9	42.1	21.9	12.8	7.6	3.0	-
	20 mg/kg†	147.6	97.6	63.2	34.5	-	12.3	4.9	0.5
	40 mg/kg‡	241.7	152.7	96.3	55.6	-	18.8	7.2	0.6
13 to 17 years	20 mg/kg†	170.4	98.3	67.8	40.4	-	16.0	7.0	1.1
	1 g§	155.9	110.9	74.8	-	24.0	-	6.2	-
	40 mg/kg‡	255.0	188.7	127.9	76.2	-	31.0	15.3	2.1

* Infused at a constant rate over 30 minutes
† up to a maximum dose of 1 g/day
‡ up to a maximum dose of 2 g/day
§ Based on three patients receiving 1 g ertapenem who volunteered for pharmacokinetic assessment in one of the two safety and efficacy studies

Table 3
Concentrations (mcg/mL) of Ertapenem in Adult Skin Blister Fluid at each
Sampling Point on the Third Day of 1-g Once Daily IV Doses

0.5 hr	1 hr	2 hr	4 hr	8 hr	12 hr	24 hr
7	12	17	24	24	21	8

Table 4
Susceptibility Interpretive Criteria for Ertapenem

Pathogen	Minimum Inhibitory Concentrations* MIC (µg/mL)			Disk Diffusion* Zone Diameter (mm)		
	S	I	R	S	I	R
Enterobacteriaceae and *Staphylococcus* spp.	≤2.0	4.0	≥8.0	≥19	16–18	≤15
Haemophilus spp.	≤0.5	-	-	≥19	-	-
Streptococcus pneumoniae†,‡	≤1.0	-	-	≥19	-	-
Streptococcus spp. other than *Streptococcus pneumoniae*§,¶	≤1.0	-	-	≥19	-	-
Anaerobes	≤4.0	8.0	≥16.0	-	-	-

* The current absence of data in resistant isolates precludes defining any results other than "Susceptible". Isolates yielding MIC results suggestive of a "Nonsusceptible" category should be submitted to a reference laboratory for further testing.

† *Streptococcus pneumoniae* that are susceptible to penicillin (penicillin MIC ≤0.06 µg/mL) can be considered susceptible to ertapenem. Testing of ertapenem against penicillin-intermediate or penicillin-resistant isolates is not recommended since reliable interpretive criteria for ertapenem are not available.

‡ *Streptococcus pneumoniae* that are susceptible to penicillin (1-µg oxacillin disk zone diameter ≥20 mm), can be considered susceptible to ertapenem. Isolates with 1-µg oxacillin zone diameter ≤19 mm should be tested against ertapenem using an MIC method.

§ *Streptococcus* spp. other than *Streptococcus pneumoniae* that are susceptible to penicillin (MIC ≤0.12 µg/mL) can be considered susceptible to ertapenem. Testing of ertapenem against penicillin-intermediate or penicillin-resistant isolates is not recommended since reliable interpretive criteria for ertapenem are not available.

¶ *Streptococcus* spp. other than *Streptococcus pneumoniae* that are susceptible to penicillin (10-units penicillin disk zone diameter ≥24 mm), can be considered susceptible to ertapenem. Isolates with 10-units penicillin disk zone diameter <24 mm should be tested against ertapenem using an MIC method. Penicillin disk diffusion interpretive criteria are not available for viridans group streptococci and they should not be tested against ertapenem.

In vitro studies indicate that ertapenem does not inhibit P-glycoprotein-mediated transport of digoxin or vinblastine and that ertapenem is not a substrate for P-glycoprotein-mediated transport. (See PRECAUTIONS, *Drug Interactions*.)

Elimination

Ertapenem is eliminated primarily by the kidneys. The mean plasma half-life in healthy young adults is approximately 4 hours and the plasma clearance is approximately 1.8 L/hour. The mean plasma half-life in pediatric patients 13 to 17 years of age is approximately 4 hours and approximately 2.5 hours in pediatric patients 3 months to 12 years of age.

Following the administration of 1 g IV radiolabeled ertapenem to healthy young adults, approximately 80% is recovered in urine and 10% in feces. Of the 80% recovered in urine, approximately 38% is excreted as unchanged drug and approximately 37% as the ring-opened metabolite.

In healthy young adults given a 1 g IV dose, the mean percentage of the administered dose excreted in urine was 17.4% during 0-2 hours postdose, 5.4% during 4-6 hours postdose, and 2.4% during 12-24 hours postdose.

Special Populations

Renal Insufficiency

Total and unbound fractions of ertapenem pharmacokinetics were investigated in 26 adult subjects (31 to 80 years of age) with varying degrees of renal impairment. Following a single 1 g IV dose of ertapenem, the unbound AUC increased 1.5-fold and 2.3-fold in subjects with mild renal insufficiency (CL_{CR} 60-90 mL/min/1.73 m^2) and moderate renal insufficiency (CL_{CR} 31-59 mL/min/1.73 m^2), respectively, compared with healthy young subjects (25 to 45 years of age). No dosage adjustment is necessary in patients with CL_{CR} ≥31 mL/min/1.73 m^2. The unbound AUC increased 4.4-fold and 7.6-fold in subjects with advanced renal insufficiency (CL_{CR} 5-30 mL/min/1.73 m^2) and end-stage renal insufficiency (CL_{CR} <10 mL/min/1.73 m^2), respectively, compared with healthy young subjects. The effects of renal insufficiency on AUC of total drug were of smaller magnitude. The recommended dose of ertapenem in adult patients with CL_{CR} ≤30 mL/min/1.73 m^2 is 0.5 grams every 24 hours. Following a single 1 g IV dose given immediately prior to a 4 hour hemodialysis session in 5 adult patients with end-stage renal insufficiency, approximately 30% of the dose was recovered in the dialysate. A supplementary dose of 150 mg is recommended if ertapenem is administered within 6 hours prior to hemodialysis. (See DOSAGE AND ADMINISTRATION.) There are no data in pediatric patients with renal insufficiency.

Hepatic Insufficiency

The pharmacokinetics of ertapenem in patients with hepatic insufficiency have not been established. However, ertapenem does not appear to undergo hepatic metabolism based on *in vitro* studies and approximately 10% of an administered dose is recovered in the feces. (See PRECAUTIONS and DOSAGE AND ADMINISTRATION.)

Gender

The effect of gender on the pharmacokinetics of ertapenem was evaluated in healthy male (n = 8) and healthy female (n = 8) subjects. The differences observed could be attributed to body size when body weight was taken into consideration. No dose adjustment is recommended based on gender.

Geriatric Patients

The impact of age on the pharmacokinetics of ertapenem was evaluated in healthy male (n = 7) and healthy female (n = 7) subjects ≥65 years of age. The total and unbound AUC increased 37% and 67%, respectively, in elderly adults relative to young adults. These changes were attributed to age-related changes in creatinine clearance. No dosage adjustment is necessary for elderly patients with normal (for their age) renal function.

Pediatric Patients

Plasma concentrations of ertapenem are comparable in pediatric patients 13 to 17 years of age and adults following a 1 g once daily IV dose.

Following the 20 mg/kg dose (up to a maximum dose of 1 g), the pharmacokinetic parameter values in patients 13 to 17 years of age (N = 6) were generally comparable to those in healthy young adults.

Plasma concentrations at the midpoint of the dosing interval following a single 15 mg/kg IV dose of ertapenem in patients 3 months to 12 years of age are comparable to plasma concentrations at the midpoint of the dosing interval following a 1 g once daily IV dose in adults (see *Pharmacokinetics*). The plasma clearance (mL/min/kg) of ertapenem in patients 3 months to 12 years of age is approximately 2-fold higher as compared to that in adults. At the 15 mg/kg dose, the AUC value (doubled to model a twice daily dosing regimen, i.e., 30 mg/kg/day exposure) in patients 3 months to 12 years of age was comparable to the AUC value in young healthy adults receiving a 1 g IV dose of ertapenem.

Microbiology

Ertapenem has *in vitro* activity against gram-positive and gram-negative aerobic and anaerobic bacteria. The bactericidal activity of ertapenem results from the inhibition of cell wall synthesis and is mediated through ertapenem binding to penicillin binding proteins (PBPs). In *Escherichia coli*, it has strong affinity toward PBPs 1a, 1b, 2, 3, 4 and 5 with preference for PBPs 2 and 3. Ertapenem is stable against hydrolysis by a variety of beta-lactamases, including penicillinases, and cephalosporinases and extended spectrum beta-lactamases. Ertapenem is hydrolyzed by metallo-beta-lactamases.

Ertapenem has been shown to be active against most isolates of the following microorganisms *in vitro* and in clinical infections. (See INDICATIONS AND USAGE):

Aerobic and facultative gram-positive microorganisms:

Staphylococcus aureus (methicillin susceptible isolates only)
Streptococcus agalactiae
Streptococcus pneumoniae (penicillin susceptible isolates only)
Streptococcus pyogenes

Note: Methicillin-resistant staphylococci and *Enterococcus* spp. are resistant to ertapenem.

Aerobic and facultative gram-negative microorganisms:

Escherichia coli
Haemophilus influenzae (Beta-lactamase negative isolates only)
Klebsiella pneumoniae
Moraxella catarrhalis
Proteus mirabilis

Anaerobic microorganisms:

Bacteroides fragilis
Bacteroides distasonis
Bacteroides ovatus
Bacteroides thetaiotaomicron
Bacteroides uniformis
Clostridium clostridioforme
Eubacterium lentum
Peptostreptococcus species
Porphyromonas asaccharolytica
Prevotella bivia

The following *in vitro* data are available, **but their clinical significance is unknown.**

At least 90% of the following microorganisms exhibit an *in vitro* minimum inhibitory concentration (MIC) less than or equal to the susceptible breakpoint for ertapenem; however, the safety and effectiveness of ertapenem in treating clinical infections due to these microorganisms have not been established in adequate and well-controlled clinical studies:

Aerobic and facultative gram-positive microorganisms:

Staphylococcus epidermidis (methicillin susceptible isolates only)
Streptococcus pneumoniae (penicillin-intermediate isolates only)

Aerobic and facultative gram-negative microorganisms:

Citrobacter freundii
Citrobacter koseri
Enterobacter aerogenes
Enterobacter cloacae
Haemophilus influenzae (Beta-lactamase positive isolates)
Haemophilus parainfluenzae
Klebsiella oxytoca (excluding ESBL producing isolates)
Morganella morganii
Proteus vulgaris
Providencia rettgeri
Providencia stuartii
Serratia marcescens

Anaerobic microorganisms:

Bacteroides vulgatus
Clostridium perfringens
Fusobacterium spp.

Susceptibility Tests Methods:

When available, the results of *in vitro* susceptibility tests should be provided to the physician as periodic reports which describe the susceptibility profile of nosocomial and community-acquired pathogens. These reports should aid the physician in selecting the most effective antimicrobial.

Dilution Techniques:

Quantitative methods are used to determine antimicrobial minimum inhibitory concentrations (MICs). These MICs provide estimates of the susceptibility of bacteria to antimicrobial compounds. The MICs should be determined using a standardized procedure. Standardized procedures are based on a broth dilution method[1,2] or equivalent with standardized inoculum concentrations and standardized concentrations of ertapenem powder. The MIC values should be interpreted according to criteria provided in Table 4.

Diffusion Techniques:

Quantitative methods that require measurement of zone diameters also provide reproducible estimates of the susceptibility of bacteria to antimicrobial compounds. One such standardized procedure[2,3] requires the use of standardized inoculum concentrations. This procedure uses paper disks impregnated with 10-µg ertapenem to test the susceptibility of microorganisms to ertapenem. The disk diffusion interpretive criteria should be interpreted according to criteria provided in Table 4.

Anaerobic Techniques:

For anaerobic bacteria, the susceptibility to ertapenem as MICs can be determined by standardized test methods[4]. The MIC values obtained should be interpreted according to criteria provided in Table 4.

[See table 4 above]

Note: *Staphylococcus* spp. can be considered susceptible to ertapenem if the penicillin MIC is ≤0.12 µg/mL. If the penicillin MIC is >0.12 µg/mL, then test oxacillin. *Staphylococcus aureus* can be considered susceptible to ertapenem if the oxacillin MIC is ≤2.0 µg/mL and resistant to ertapenem if the oxacillin MIC is ≥4.0 µg/mL. Coagulase negative staphylococci can be considered susceptible to ertapenem if the oxacillin MIC is ≤0.25 µg/mL and resistant to ertapenem if the oxacillin MIC ≤0.5 µg/mL.

Staphylococcus spp. can be considered susceptible to ertapenem if the penicillin (10 U disk) zone is ≥29 mm. If the penicillin zone is ≤28 mm, then test oxacillin by disk diffusion (1 µg disk). *Staphylococcus aureus* can be considered susceptible to ertapenem if the oxacillin (1 μg disk) zone is ≥13 mm and resistant to ertapenem if the oxacillin zone is ≤10 mm. Coagulase negative staphylococci can be considered susceptible to ertapenem if the oxacillin zone is ≥18 mm and resistant to ertapenem if the oxacillin (1 μg disk) zone is ≤17 mm.

A report of "Susceptible" indicates that the pathogen is likely to be inhibited if the antimicrobial compound in blood reaches the concentrations usually achievable. A report of "Intermediate" indicates that the result should be considered equivocal, and, if the microorganism is not fully susceptible to alternative, clinically feasible drugs, the test should be repeated. This category implies possible clinical applicability in body sites where the drug is physiologically concentrated or in situations where high dosage of drug can be used. This category also provides a buffer zone which prevents small uncontrolled technical factors from causing major discrepancies in interpretation. A report of "Resistant" indicates that the pathogen is not likely to be inhibited if the antimicrobial compound in the blood reaches the concentrations usually achievable; other therapy should be selected.

Quality Control

Standardized susceptibility test procedures require the use of laboratory control microorganisms to control the technical aspects of the laboratory procedures[1,2,3,4]. Quality control microorganisms are specific strains of organisms with intrinsic biological properties. QC strains are very stable strains which will give a standard and repeatable susceptibility pattern. The specific strains used for microbiological quality control are not clinically significant. Standard ertapenem powder should provide the following range of values noted in Table 5.

[See table 5 at right]

Table 5
Acceptable Quality Control Ranges for Ertapenem

Microorganism	Minimum Inhibitory Concentrations MIC Range (μg/mL)	Disk Diffusion Zone Diameter (mm)
Escherichia coli ATCC 25922	0.004-0.016	29-36
Haemophilus influenzae ATCC 49766	0.016-0.06	27-33
Staphylococcus aureus ATCC 29213	0.06-0.25	
Staphylococcus aureus ATCC 25923	-	24-31
Streptococcus pneumoniae ATCC 49619	0.03-0.25	28-35
Bacteroides fragilis ATCC 25285	0.06-0.5* 0.06-0.25†	-
Bacteroides thetaiotaomicron ATCC 29741	0.5-2.0* 0.25-1.0†	-
Eubacterium lentum ATCC 43055	0.5-4.0* 0.5-2.0†	-

* Quality control ranges for broth microdilution testing
† Quality control ranges for agar microdilution testing

INDICATIONS AND USAGE

Treatment

INVANZ is indicated for the treatment of patients with the following moderate to severe infections caused by susceptible isolates of the designated microorganisms. (See DOSAGE AND ADMINISTRATION):

Complicated Intra-abdominal Infections due to *Escherichia coli*, *Clostridium clostridioforme*, *Eubacterium lentum*, *Peptostreptococcus* species, *Bacteroides fragilis*, *Bacteroides distasonis*, *Bacteroides ovatus*, *Bacteroides thetaiotaomicron*, or *Bacteroides uniformis*.

Complicated Skin and Skin Structure Infections, including diabetic foot infections without osteomyelitis due to *Staphylococcus aureus* (methicillin susceptible isolates only), *Streptococcus agalactiae*, *Streptococcus pyogenes*, *Escherichia coli*, *Klebsiella pneumoniae*, *Proteus mirabilis*, *Bacteroides fragilis*, *Peptostreptococcus* species, *Porphyromonas asaccharolytica*, or *Prevotella bivia*. INVANZ has not been studied in diabetic foot infections with concomitant osteomyelitis (see CLINICAL STUDIES).

Community Acquired Pneumonia due to *Streptococcus pneumoniae* (penicillin susceptible isolates only) including cases with concurrent bacteremia, *Haemophilus influenzae* (beta-lactamase negative isolates only), or *Moraxella catarrhalis*.

Complicated Urinary Tract Infections including pyelonephritis due to *Escherichia coli*, including cases with concurrent bacteremia, or *Klebsiella pneumoniae*.

Acute Pelvic Infections including postpartum endomyometritis, septic abortion and post surgical gynecologic infections due to *Streptococcus agalactiae*, *Escherichia coli*, *Bacteroides fragilis*, *Porphyromonas asaccharolytica*, *Peptostreptococcus* species, or *Prevotella bivia*.

Prevention

INVANZ is indicated in adults for the **prophylaxis of surgical site infection following elective colorectal surgery**.

Appropriate specimens for bacteriological examination should be obtained in order to isolate and identify the causative organisms and to determine their susceptibility to ertapenem. Therapy with INVANZ (ertapenem) may be initiated empirically before results of these tests are known; once results become available, antimicrobial therapy should be adjusted accordingly.

To reduce the development of drug-resistant bacteria and maintain the effectiveness of INVANZ and other antibacterial drugs, INVANZ should be used only to treat or prevent infections that are proven or strongly suspected to be caused by susceptible bacteria. When culture and susceptibility information are available, they should be considered in selecting or modifying antibacterial therapy. In the absence of such data, local epidemiology and susceptibility patterns may contribute to the empiric selection of therapy.

CONTRAINDICATIONS

INVANZ is contraindicated in patients with known hypersensitivity to any component of this product or to other drugs in the same class or in patients who have demonstrated anaphylactic reactions to beta-lactams.

Due to the use of lidocaine HCl as a diluent, INVANZ administered intramuscularly is contraindicated in patients with a known hypersensitivity to local anesthetics of the amide type. (Refer to the prescribing information for lidocaine HCl.)

WARNINGS

SERIOUS AND OCCASIONALLY FATAL HYPERSENSITIVITY (ANAPHYLACTIC) REACTIONS HAVE BEEN REPORTED IN PATIENTS RECEIVING THERAPY WITH BETA-LACTAMS. THESE REACTIONS ARE MORE LIKELY TO OCCUR IN INDIVIDUALS WITH A HISTORY OF SENSITIVITY TO MULTIPLE ALLERGENS. THERE HAVE BEEN REPORTS OF INDIVIDUALS WITH A HISTORY OF PENICILLIN HYPERSENSITIVITY WHO HAVE EXPERIENCED SEVERE HYPERSENSITIVITY REACTIONS WHEN TREATED WITH ANOTHER BETA-LACTAM. BEFORE INITIATING THERAPY WITH INVANZ, CAREFUL INQUIRY SHOULD BE MADE CONCERNING PREVIOUS HYPERSENSITIVITY REACTIONS TO PENICILLINS, CEPHALOSPORINS, OTHER BETA-LACTAMS AND OTHER ALLERGENS. IF AN ALLERGIC REACTION TO INVANZ OCCURS, DISCONTINUE THE DRUG IMMEDIATELY. **SERIOUS ANAPHYLACTIC REACTIONS REQUIRE IMMEDIATE EMERGENCY TREATMENT WITH EPINEPHRINE, OXYGEN, INTRAVENOUS STEROIDS, AND AIRWAY MANAGEMENT, INCLUDING INTUBATION. OTHER THERAPY MAY ALSO BE ADMINISTERED AS INDICATED.**

Seizure Potential

Seizures and other CNS adverse experiences have been reported during treatment with INVANZ. (See PRECAUTIONS and ADVERSE REACTIONS.)

Case reports in the literature have shown that co-administration of carbapenems, including ertapenem, to patients receiving valproic acid or divalproex sodium results in a reduction in valproic acid concentrations. The valproic acid concentrations may drop below the therapeutic range as a result of this interaction, therefore increasing the risk of breakthrough seizures. Increasing the dose of valproic acid or divalproex sodium may not be sufficient to overcome this interaction. The concomitant use of ertapenem and valproic acid/divalproex sodium is generally not recommended. Anti-bacterials other than carbapenems should be considered to treat infections in patients whose seizures are well controlled on valproic acid or divalproex sodium. If administration of INVANZ is necessary, supplemental anticonvulsant therapy should be considered. (See PRECAUTIONS, *Drug Interactions*.)

Clostridium difficile associated diarrhea (CDAD) has been reported with use of nearly all antibacterial agents, including ertapenem, and may range in severity from mild diarrhea to fatal colitis. Treatment with antibacterial agents alters the normal flora of the colon leading to overgrowth of *Clostridium difficile*.

Clostridium difficile produces toxins A and B which contribute to the development of CDAD. Hypertoxin producing strains of *Clostridium difficile* cause increased morbidity and mortality, as these infections can be refractory to antimicrobial therapy and may require colectomy. CDAD must be considered in all patients who present with diarrhea following antibiotic use. Careful medical history is necessary since CDAD has been reported to occur over two months after the administration of antibacterial agents.

If CDAD is suspected or confirmed, ongoing antibiotic use not directed against *Clostridium difficile* may need to be discontinued. Appropriate fluid and electrolyte management, protein supplementation, antibiotic treatment of *Clostridium difficile*, and surgical evaluation should be instituted as clinically indicated.

Lidocaine HCl is the diluent for intramuscular administration of INVANZ. Refer to the prescribing information for lidocaine HCl.

PRECAUTIONS

General

During clinical investigations in adult patients treated with INVANZ (1 g once a day), seizures, irrespective of drug relationship, occurred in 0.5% of patients during study therapy plus 14-day follow-up period. (See ADVERSE REACTIONS.) These experiences have occurred most commonly in patients with CNS disorders (e.g., brain lesions or history of seizures) and/or compromised renal function. Close adherence to the recommended dosage regimen is urged, especially in patients with known factors that predispose to convulsive activity. Anticonvulsant therapy should be continued in patients with known seizure disorders. If focal tremors, myoclonus, or seizures occur, patients should be evaluated neurologically, placed on anticonvulsant therapy if not already instituted, and the dosage of INVANZ reexamined to determine whether it should be decreased or the antibiotic discontinued. Dosage adjustment of INVANZ is recommended in patients with reduced renal function. (See DOSAGE AND ADMINISTRATION.)

As with other antibiotics, prolonged use of INVANZ may result in overgrowth of non-susceptible organisms. Repeated evaluation of the patient's condition is essential. If superinfection occurs during therapy, appropriate measures should be taken.

Prescribing INVANZ in the absence of a proven or strongly suspected bacterial infection or a prophylactic indication is unlikely to provide benefit to the patient and increases the risk of the development of drug-resistant bacteria.

Caution should be taken when administering INVANZ intramuscularly to avoid inadvertent injection into a blood vessel. (See DOSAGE AND ADMINISTRATION.)

Lidocaine HCl is the diluent for intramuscular administration of INVANZ. Refer to the prescribing information for lidocaine HCl for additional precautions.

Information for Patients

Patients should be counseled to inform their physician if they are taking valproic acid or divalproex sodium. Valproic acid concentrations in the blood may drop below the therapeutic range upon co-administration with INVANZ. If treatment with INVANZ is necessary and continued, alternative or supplemental anti-convulsant medication to prevent and/or treat seizures may be needed.

Patients should be counseled that antibacterial drugs including INVANZ should only be used to treat bacterial infections. They do not treat viral infections (e.g., the common cold). When INVANZ is prescribed to treat a bacterial infection, patients should be told that although it is common to feel better early in the course of therapy, the medication should be taken exactly as directed. Skipping doses or not completing the full course of therapy may (1) decrease the effectiveness of the immediate treatment and (2) increase the likelihood that bacteria will develop resistance and will not be treatable by INVANZ or other antibacterial drugs in the future.

Diarrhea is a common problem caused by antibiotics which usually ends when the antibiotic is discontinued. Sometimes after starting treatment with antibiotics, patients can develop watery and bloody stools (with or without stomach cramps and fever) even as late as two or more months after having taken the last dose of the antibiotic. If this occurs, patients should contact their physician as soon as possible.

Laboratory Tests
While INVANZ possesses toxicity similar to the beta-lactam group of antibiotics, periodic assessment of organ system function, including renal, hepatic, and hematopoietic, is advisable during prolonged therapy.

Drug Interactions
When ertapenem is co-administered with probenecid (500 mg p.o. every 6 hours), probenecid competes for active tubular secretion and reduces the renal clearance of ertapenem. Based on total ertapenem concentrations, probenecid increased the AUC by 25% and reduced the plasma and renal clearances by 20% and 35%, respectively. The half-life increased from 4.0 to 4.8 hours. Because of the small effect on half-life, the coadministration with probenecid to extend the half-life of ertapenem is not recommended. *In vitro* studies indicate that ertapenem does not inhibit P-glycoprotein-mediated transport of digoxin or vinblastine and that ertapenem is not a substrate for P-glycoprotein-mediated transport. *In vitro* studies in human liver microsomes indicate that ertapenem does not inhibit metabolism mediated by any of the following six cytochrome p450 (CYP) isoforms: 1A2, 2C9, 2C19, 2D6, 2E1 and 3A4. Drug interactions caused by inhibition of P-glycoprotein-mediated drug clearance or CYP-mediated drug clearance with the listed isoforms are unlikely. (See CLINICAL PHARMACOLOGY, *Distribution and Metabolism.*)
Other than with probenecid, no specific clinical drug interaction studies have been conducted.
Case reports in the literature have shown that co-administration of carbapenems, including ertapenem, to patients receiving valproic acid or divalproex sodium results in a reduction of valproic acid concentrations. The valproic acid concentrations may drop below the therapeutic range as a result of this interaction, therefore increasing the risk of breakthrough seizures. Although the mechanism of this interaction is unknown, data from *in vitro* and animal studies suggest that carbapenems may inhibit the hydrolysis of valproic acid's glucuronide metabolite (VPA-g) back to valproic acid, thus decreasing the serum concentrations of valproic acid. (See WARNINGS, *Seizure Potential*.)

Carcinogenesis, Mutagenesis, Impairment of Fertility
No long-term studies in animals have been performed to evaluate the carcinogenic potential of ertapenem.
Ertapenem was neither mutagenic nor genotoxic in the following *in vitro* assays: alkaline elution/rat hepatocyte assay, chromosomal aberration assay in Chinese hamster ovary cells, and TK6 human lymphoblastoid cell mutagenesis assay; and in the *in vivo* mouse micronucleus assay.
In mice and rats, IV doses of up to 700 mg/kg/day (for mice, approximately 3 times the recommended human dose of 1 g based on body surface area and for rats, approximately 1.2 times the human exposure at the recommended dose of 1 g based on plasma AUCs) resulted in no effects on mating performance, fecundity, fertility, or embryonic survival.

Pregnancy: Teratogenic Effects
Pregnancy Category B: In mice and rats given IV doses of up to 700 mg/kg/day (for mice, approximately 3 times the recommended human dose of 1 g based on body surface area and for rats, approximately 1.2 times the human exposure at the recommended dose of 1 g based on plasma AUCs), there was no evidence of developmental toxicity as assessed by external, visceral, and skeletal examination of the fetuses. However, in mice given 700 mg/kg/day, slight decreases in average fetal weights and an associated decrease in the average number of ossified sacrocaudal vertebrae were observed. Ertapenem crosses the placental barrier in rats.
There are, however, no adequate and well-controlled studies in pregnant women. Because animal reproduction studies are not always predictive of human response, this drug should be used during pregnancy only if clearly needed.

Nursing Mothers
Ertapenem is excreted in human breast milk. (See CLINICAL PHARMACOLOGY, *Distribution.*) Caution should be exercised when INVANZ is administered to a nursing woman. INVANZ should be administered to nursing mothers only when the expected benefit outweighs the risk.

Labor and Delivery
INVANZ has not been studied for use during labor and delivery.

Pediatric Use
Safety and effectiveness of INVANZ in pediatric patients 3 months to 17 years of age are supported by evidence from adequate and well-controlled studies in adults, pharmacokinetic data in pediatric patients, and additional data from comparator-controlled studies in pediatric patients 3 months to 17 years of age with the following infections (see INDICATIONS AND USAGE and CLINICAL STUDIES):
• Complicated Intra-abdominal Infections
• Complicated Skin and Skin Structure Infections
• Community Acquired Pneumonia
• Complicated Urinary Tract Infections
• Acute Pelvic Infections
INVANZ is not recommended in infants under 3 months of age as no data are available.
INVANZ is not recommended in the treatment of meningitis in the pediatric population due to lack of sufficient CSF penetration.

Geriatric Use
Of the 1,835 patients in Phase IIb/III studies treated with INVANZ, approximately 26 percent were 65 and over, while approximately 12 percent were 75 and over. No overall differences in safety or effectiveness were observed between these patients and younger patients. Other reported clinical experience has not identified differences in responses between the elderly and younger patients, but greater sensitivity of some older individuals cannot be ruled out.
This drug is known to be substantially excreted by the kidney, and the risk of toxic reactions to this drug may be greater in patients with impaired renal function. Because elderly patients are more likely to have decreased renal function, care should be taken in dose selection, and it may be useful to monitor renal function. (See DOSAGE AND ADMINISTRATION.)

Hepatic Insufficiency
The pharmacokinetics of ertapenem in patients with hepatic insufficiency have not been established. Of the total number of patients in clinical studies, 37 patients receiving ertapenem 1 g daily and 36 patients receiving comparator drugs were considered to have Child-Pugh Class A, B, or C liver impairment. The incidence of adverse experiences in patients with hepatic impairment was similar between the ertapenem group and the comparator groups.

ANIMAL PHARMACOLOGY

In repeat-dose studies in rats, treatment-related neutropenia occurred at every dose-level tested, including the lowest dose of 2 mg/kg (approximately 2% of the human dose on a body surface area basis).
Studies in rabbits and Rhesus monkeys were inconclusive with regard to the effect on neutrophil counts.

ADVERSE REACTIONS

Adults
Clinical studies enrolled 1954 patients treated with ertapenem; in some of the clinical studies, parenteral therapy was followed by a switch to an appropriate oral antimicrobial. (See CLINICAL STUDIES.) Most adverse experiences reported in these clinical studies were described as mild to moderate in severity. Ertapenem was discontinued due to adverse experiences in 4.7% of patients. Table 6 shows the incidence of adverse experiences reported in ≥1.0% of patients in these studies. The most common drug-related adverse experiences in patients treated with INVANZ, including those who were switched to therapy with an oral antimicrobial, were diarrhea (5.5%), infused vein complication (3.7%), nausea (3.1%), headache (2.2%), vaginitis in females (2.1%), phlebitis/thrombophlebitis (1.3%), and vomiting (1.1%).
[See table 6 at left]
In patients treated for complicated intra-abdominal infections, death occurred in 4.7% (15/316) of patients receiving ertapenem and 2.6% (8/307) of patients receiving comparator drug. These deaths occurred in patients with significant co-morbidity and/or severe baseline infections. Deaths were considered unrelated to study drugs by investigators.
In clinical studies, seizure was reported during study therapy plus 14-day follow-up period in 0.5% of patients treated with ertapenem, 0.3% of patients treated with piperacillin/tazobactam and 0% of patients treated with ceftriaxone. (See PRECAUTIONS.)
Additional adverse experiences that were reported with INVANZ with an incidence >0.1% within each body system are listed below:
Body as a whole: abdominal distention, pain, chills, septicemia, septic shock, dehydration, gout, malaise, necrosis, candidiasis, weight loss, facial edema, injection site induration, injection site pain, flank pain, and syncope;

Table 6
Incidence (%) of Adverse Experiences Reported
During Study Therapy Plus 14-Day Follow-Up in ≥1.0% of Adult Patients
Treated With INVANZ in Clinical Studies

Adverse Events	INVANZ* 1 g daily (N = 802)	Piperacillin/ Tazobactam* 3.375 g q6h (N = 774)	INVANZ† 1 g daily (N = 1152)	Ceftriaxone† 1 or 2 g daily (N = 942)
Local:				
Extravasation	1.9	1.7	0.7	1.1
Infused vein complication	7.1	7.9	5.4	6.7
Phlebitis/thrombophlebitis	1.9	2.7	1.6	2.0
Systemic:				
Asthenia/fatigue	1.2	0.9	1.2	1.1
Death	2.5	1.6	1.3	1.6
Edema/swelling	3.4	2.5	2.9	3.3
Fever	5.0	6.6	2.3	3.4
Abdominal pain	3.6	4.8	4.3	3.9
Chest pain	1.5	1.4	1.0	2.5
Hypertension	1.6	1.4	0.7	1.0
Hypotension	2.0	1.4	1.0	1.2
Tachycardia	1.6	1.3	1.3	0.7
Acid regurgitation	1.6	0.9	1.1	0.6
Oral candidiasis	0.1	1.3	1.4	1.9
Constipation	4.0	5.4	3.3	3.1
Diarrhea	10.3	12.1	9.2	9.8
Dyspepsia	1.1	0.6	1.0	1.6
Nausea	8.5	8.7	6.4	7.4
Vomiting	3.7	5.3	4.0	4.0
Leg pain	1.1	0.5	0.4	0.3
Anxiety	1.4	1.3	0.8	1.2
Altered mental status‡	5.1	3.4	3.3	2.5
Dizziness	2.1	3.0	1.5	2.1
Headache	5.6	5.4	6.8	6.9
Insomnia	3.2	5.2	3.0	4.1
Cough	1.6	1.7	1.3	0.5
Dyspnea	2.6	1.8	1.0	2.4
Pharyngitis	0.7	1.4	1.1	0.6
Rales/rhonchi	1.1	1.0	0.5	0.5
Respiratory distress	1.0	0.4	0.2	0.2
Erythema	1.6	1.7	1.2	1.2
Pruritus	2.0	2.6	1.0	1.9
Rash	2.5	3.1	2.3	1.5
Vaginitis	1.4	1.0	3.3	3.7

* Includes Phase IIb/III Complicated intra-abdominal infections, Complicated skin and skin structure infections and Acute pelvic infections studies
† Includes Phase IIb/III Community acquired pneumonia and Complicated urinary tract infections, and Phase IIa studies
‡ Includes agitation, confusion, disorientation, decreased mental acuity, changed mental status, somnolence, stupor

Cardiovascular System: heart failure, hematoma, cardiac arrest, bradycardia, arrhythmia, atrial fibrillation, heart murmur, ventricular tachycardia, asystole, and subdural hemorrhage;

Digestive System: gastrointestinal hemorrhage, anorexia, flatulence, *C. difficile* associated diarrhea, stomatitis, dysphagia, hemorrhoids, ileus, cholelithiasis, duodenitis, esophagitis, gastritis, jaundice, mouth ulcer, pancreatitis, and pyloric stenosis;

Nervous System & Psychiatric: nervousness, seizure (see WARNINGS and PRECAUTIONS), tremor, depression, hypesthesia, spasm, paresthesia, aggressive behavior, and vertigo;

Respiratory System: pleural effusion, hypoxemia, bronchoconstriction, pharyngeal discomfort, epistaxis, pleuritic pain, asthma, hemoptysis, hiccups, and voice disturbance;

Skin & Skin Appendage: sweating, dermatitis, desquamation, flushing, and urticaria;

Special Senses: taste perversion;

Urogenital System: renal insufficiency, oliguria/anuria, vaginal pruritus, hematuria, urinary retention, bladder dysfunction, vaginal candidiasis, and vulvovaginitis.

In a clinical trial for the treatment of diabetic foot infections in which 289 adult diabetic patients were treated with ertapenem, the adverse experience profile was generally similar to that seen in previous clinical trials.

In a clinical study in adults for the prophylaxis of surgical site infection following elective colorectal surgery in which 476 patients received a 1 g dose of ertapenem 1 hour prior to surgery and were then followed for safety 14 days post surgery, the overall adverse experience profile was generally comparable to that observed for ertapenem in previous clinical trials. Table 7 shows the incidence of adverse experiences other than those previously described above for ertapenem, regardless of causality, reported in ≥1.0% of patients in this study.

[See table 7 above]

Additional adverse experiences that were reported in this prophylaxis study with INVANZ, regardless of causality, with an incidence <1.0% and >0.5% within each body system are listed below:

Gastrointestinal Disorders: dry mouth, hematochezia;

General Disorders and Administration Site Condition: crepitations;

Infections and Infestations: abdominal abscess, fungal rash, pelvic abscess;

Injury, Poisoning and Procedural Complications: incision site complication, incision site hemorrhage, intestinal stoma complication;

Musculoskeletal and Connective Tissue Disorders: muscle spasms;

Nervous System Disorders: cerebrovascular accident;

Renal and Urinary Disorders: pollakiuria;

Respiratory, Thoracic and Mediastinal Disorders: crackles lung, lung infiltration, pulmonary congestion, pulmonary embolism, wheezing.

Pediatric Patients

Clinical studies enrolled 384 patients treated with ertapenem; in some of the clinical studies, parenteral therapy was followed by a switch to an appropriate oral antimicrobial. (See CLINICAL STUDIES.) The overall adverse experience profile in pediatric patients is comparable to that in adult patients. Table 8 shows the incidence of adverse experiences reported in ≥1.0% of pediatric patients in clinical studies. The most common drug-related adverse experiences in pediatric patients treated with INVANZ, including those who were switched to therapy with an oral antimicrobial, were diarrhea (6.5%), infusion site pain (5.5%), infusion site erythema (2.6%), vomiting (2.1%).

[See table 8 at right]

Additional adverse experiences that were reported with INVANZ with an incidence <1.0% and >0.5% within each body system are listed below:

General Disorders and Administration Site Condition: chest pain, infusion site pruritus;

Infections and Infestations: candidiasis, ear infection, oral candidiasis;

Metabolism and Nutrition Disorders: decreased appetite;

Musculoskeletal and Connective Tissue Disorders: arthralgia;

Nervous System Disorders: somnolence;

Psychiatric Disorders: insomnia;

Reproductive System and Breast Disorders: genital rash;

Respiratory, Thoracic and Mediastinal Disorders: pleural effusion, rhinitis, rhinorrhea;

Skin and Subcutaneous Tissue Disorders: dermatitis atopic, rash erythematous, skin lesion;

Vascular Disorders: phlebitis.

Post-Marketing Experience

The following post-marketing adverse experiences have been reported:

Immune System: anaphylaxis including anaphylactoid reactions

Psychiatric Disorders: altered mental status (including aggression, delirium, hallucinations)

Nervous System: dyskinesia, myoclonus, tremor

Skin and Subcutaneous Tissue Disorders: Drug Rash with Eosinophilia and Systemic Symptoms (DRESS syndrome)

Adverse Laboratory Changes

Adults

Laboratory adverse experiences that were reported during therapy in ≥1.0% of adult patients treated with INVANZ in clinical studies are presented in Table 9. Drug-related laboratory adverse experiences that were reported during therapy in ≥1.0% of adult patients treated with INVANZ, including those who were switched to therapy with an oral antimicrobial, in clinical studies were ALT increased (6.0%), AST increased (5.2%), serum alkaline phosphatase increased (3.4%), platelet count increased (2.8%), and eosinophils increased (1.1%). Ertapenem was discontinued due to laboratory adverse experiences in 0.3% of patients.

[See table 9 at top of next page]

Additional laboratory adverse experiences that were reported during therapy in >0.1% but <1.0% of patients treated with INVANZ in clinical studies include: increases in BUN, direct and indirect serum bilirubin, serum sodium, monocytes, PTT, urine epithelial cells; decreases in serum bicarbonate.

In a clinical trial for the treatment of diabetic foot infections in which 289 adult diabetic patients were treated with ertapenem, the laboratory adverse experience profile was generally similar to that seen in previous clinical trials.

In a clinical study in adults for the prophylaxis of surgical site infection following elective colorectal surgery in which 476 patients received a 1 g dose of ertapenem 1 hour prior to surgery and were then followed for safety 14 days post surgery, the overall laboratory adverse experience profile was generally comparable to that observed for ertapenem in previous clinical trials. Additional laboratory adverse

Table 7
Incidence (%) of Adverse Experiences Reported During Study Therapy Plus 14-Day Follow-Up in ≥1.0% of Adult Patients Treated With INVANZ for Prophylaxis of Surgical Site Infections Following Elective Colorectal Surgery

Adverse Events	INVANZ 1 g (N = 476)	Cefotetan 2 g (N = 476)
Anemia	5.7	6.9
Small intestinal obstruction	2.1	1.9
Cellulitis	1.5	1.5
C. difficile infection or colitis	1.7	0.6
Pneumonia	2.1	4.0
Postoperative infection	2.3	4.0
Urinary tract infection	3.8	5.5
Wound infection	6.5	12.4
Anastomotic leak	1.5	1.3
Seroma	1.3	1.9
Wound complication	2.9	2.3
Wound dehiscence	1.3	1.5
Wound secretion	1.9	2.1
Dysuria	1.1	1.3
Atelectasis	3.4	1.9

Table 8
Incidence (%) of Adverse Experiences Reported During Study Therapy Plus 14-Day Follow-Up in ≥1.0% of Pediatric Patients Treated With INVANZ in Clinical Studies

Adverse Events	INVANZ*† (N = 384)	Ceftriaxone* (N = 100)	Ticarcillin/ Clavulanate† (N = 24)
Local:			
Infusion Site Erythema	3.9	3.0	8.3
Infusion Site Induration	1.0	1.0	0.0
Infusion Site Pain	7.0	4.0	20.8
Infusion Site Phlebitis	1.8	3.0	0.0
Infusion Site Swelling	1.8	1.0	4.2
Infusion Site Warmth	1.3	1.0	4.2
Systemic:			
Abdominal Pain	4.7	3.0	4.2
Upper Abdominal Pain	1.0	2.0	0.0
Constipation	2.3	0.0	0.0
Diarrhea	11.7	17.0	4.2
Loose Stools	2.1	0.0	0.0
Nausea	1.6	0.0	0.0
Vomiting	10.2	11.0	8.3
Pyrexia	4.9	6.0	8.3
Abdominal Abscess	1.0	0.0	4.2
Herpes Simplex	1.0	1.0	4.2
Nasopharyngitis	1.6	6.0	0.0
Upper Respiratory Tract Infection	2.3	3.0	0.0
Viral Pharyngitis	1.0	0.0	0.0
Hypothermia	1.6	1.0	0.0
Dizziness	1.6	0.0	0.0
Headache	4.4	4.0	0.0
Cough	4.4	3.0	0.0
Wheezing	1.0	0.0	0.0
Dermatitis	1.0	1.0	0.0
Pruritus	1.6	0.0	0.0
Diaper Dermatitis	4.7	4.0	0.0
Rash	2.9	2.0	8.3

* Includes Phase IIb Complicated skin and skin structure infections. Community acquired pneumonia and Complicated urinary tract infections studies in which patients 3 months to 12 years of age received INVANZ 15 mg/kg IV twice daily up to a maximum of 1 g or ceftriaxone 50 mg/kg/day IV in two divided doses up to a maximum of 2 g, and patients 13 to 17 years of age received INVANZ 1 g IV daily or ceftriaxone 50 mg/kg/day IV in a single daily dose.

† Includes Phase IIb Acute pelvic infections and Complicated intra-abdominal infections studies in which patients 3 months to 12 years of age received INVANZ 15 mg/kg IV twice daily up to a maximum of 1 g and patients 13 to 17 years of age received INVANZ 1 g IV daily or ticarcillin/clavulanate 50 mg/kg for patients <60 kg or ticarcillin/clavulanate 3.0 g for patients >60 kg, 4 or 6 times a day.

Table 9
Incidence* (%) of Specific Laboratory Adverse Experiences Reported
During Study Therapy Plus 14-Day Follow-Up in ≥1.0% of Adult Patients Treated
With INVANZ in Clinical Studies

Adverse laboratory experiences	INVANZ‡ 1 g daily (n† = 766)	Piperacillin/ Tazobactam‡ 3.375 g q6h (n† = 755)	INVANZ§ 1 g daily (n† = 1122)	Ceftriaxone§ 1 or 2 g daily (n† = 920)
ALT increased	8.8	7.3	8.3	6.9
AST increased	8.4	8.3	7.1	6.5
Serum albumin decreased	1.7	1.5	0.9	1.6
Serum alkaline phosphatase increased	6.6	7.2	4.3	2.8
Serum creatinine increased	1.1	2.7	0.9	1.2
Serum glucose increased	1.2	2.3	1.7	2.0
Serum potassium decreased	1.7	2.8	1.8	2.4
Serum potassium increased	1.3	0.5	0.5	0.7
Total serum bilirubin increased	1.7	1.4	0.6	1.1
Eosinophils increased	1.1	1.1	2.1	1.8
Hematocrit decreased	3.0	2.9	3.4	2.4
Hemoglobin decreased	4.9	4.7	4.5	3.5
Platelet count decreased	1.1	1.2	1.1	1.0
Platelet count increased	6.5	6.3	4.3	3.5
Segmented neutrophils decreased	1.0	0.3	1.5	0.8
Prothrombin time increased	1.2	2.0	0.3	0.9
WBC decreased	0.8	0.7	1.5	1.4
Urine RBCs increased	2.5	2.9	1.1	1.0
Urine WBCs increased	2.5	3.2	1.6	1.1

* Number of patients with laboratory adverse experiences/Number of patients with the laboratory test
† Number of patients with one or more laboratory tests
‡ Includes Phase IIb/III Complicated intra-abdominal infections, Complicated skin and skin structure infections and Acute pelvic infections studies
§ Includes Phase IIb/III Community acquired pneumonia and Complicated urinary tract infections, and Phase IIa studies

Table 10
Incidence* (%) of Specific Laboratory Adverse Experiences Reported
During Study Therapy Plus 14-Day Follow-Up in ≥1.0% of Pediatric Patients Treated
With INVANZ in Clinical Studies

Adverse laboratory experiences	INVANZ (n† = 379)	Ceftriaxone (n† = 97)	Ticarcillin/ Clavulanate (n† = 24)
ALT Increased	3.8	1.1	4.3
Alkaline Phosphatase Increased	1.1	0.0	0.0
AST Increased	3.8	1.1	4.3
Eosinophil Count Increased	1.1	2.1	0.0
Neutrophil Count Decreased	5.8	3.1	0.0
Platelet Count Increased	1.3	0.0	8.7

* Number of patients with laboratory adverse experiences/Number of patients with the laboratory test; where at least 300 patients had the test
† Number of patients with one or more laboratory tests

Table 11
Treatment Guidelines for Adults and Pediatric Patients With Normal Renal Function* and Body Weight

Infection†	Daily Dose (IV or IM) Adults and Pediatric Patients 13 years of age and older	Daily Dose (IV or IM) Pediatric Patients 3 months to 12 years of age	Recommended Duration of Total Antimicrobial Treatment
Complicated intra-abdominal infections	1 g	15 mg/kg twice daily‡	5 to 14 days
Complicated skin and skin structure infections, including diabetic foot infections§	1 g	15 mg/kg twice daily‡	7 to 14 days¶
Community acquired pneumonia	1 g	15 mg/kg twice daily‡	10 to 14 days#
Complicated urinary tract infections, including pyelonephritis	1 g	15 mg/kg twice daily‡	10 to 14 days#
Acute pelvic infections including postpartum endomyometritis, septic abortion and post surgical gynecologic infections	1 g	15 mg/kg twice daily‡	3 to 10 days

* defined as creatinine clearance >90 mL/min/1.73 m²
† due to the designated pathogens (see INDICATIONS AND USAGE)
‡ not to exceed 1 g/day
§ INVANZ has not been studied in diabetic foot infections with concomitant osteomyelitis (see CLINICAL STUDIES).
¶ adult patients with diabetic foot infections received up to 28 days of treatment (parenteral or parenteral plus oral switch therapy)
# duration includes a possible switch to an appropriate oral therapy, after at least 3 days of parenteral therapy, once clinical improvement has been demonstrated.

experiences that were reported during therapy and the 14 days post surgery period in >1.0% of patients, regardless of causality, include: white blood cell count increased and urine protein present.

Pediatric Patients

Laboratory adverse experiences that were reported during therapy in ≥1.0% of pediatric patients treated with INVANZ in clinical studies are presented in Table 10. Drug-related laboratory adverse experiences that were reported during therapy in ≥2.0% of pediatric patients treated with INVANZ, including those who were switched to therapy with an oral antimicrobial, in clinical studies were neutrophil count decreased (3.0%), ALT increased (2.2%), and AST increased (2.1%).

[See table 10 below]

Additional laboratory adverse experiences that were reported during therapy in >0.5% but <1.0% of patients treated with INVANZ in clinical studies include: white blood cell count decreased and urine protein present.

OVERDOSAGE

No specific information is available on the treatment of overdosage with INVANZ. Intentional overdosing of INVANZ is unlikely. Intravenous administration of INVANZ at a dose of 2 g over 30 min or 3 g over 1-2h in healthy adult volunteers resulted in an increased incidence of nausea. In clinical studies in adults, inadvertent administration of three 1 g doses of INVANZ in a 24 hour period resulted in diarrhea and transient dizziness in one patient. In pediatric clinical studies, a single IV dose of 40 mg/kg up to a maximum of 2 g did not result in toxicity.

In the event of an overdose, INVANZ should be discontinued and general supportive treatment given until renal elimination takes place.

INVANZ can be removed by hemodialysis; the plasma clearance of the total fraction of ertapenem was increased 30% in subjects with end-stage renal insufficiency when hemodialysis (4 hour session) was performed immediately following administration. However, no information is available on the use of hemodialysis to treat overdosage.

DOSAGE AND ADMINISTRATION

The dose of INVANZ in patients 13 years of age and older is 1 gram (g) given once a day. The dose of INVANZ in patients 3 months to 12 years of age is 15 mg/kg twice daily (not to exceed 1 g/day). INVANZ may be administered by intravenous infusion for up to 14 days or intramuscular injection for up to 7 days. When administered intravenously, INVANZ should be infused over a period of 30 minutes.

Intramuscular administration of INVANZ may be used as an alternative to intravenous administration in the treatment of those infections for which intramuscular therapy is appropriate.

DO NOT MIX OR CO-INFUSE INVANZ WITH OTHER MEDICATIONS. DO NOT USE DILUENTS CONTAINING DEXTROSE (α-D-GLUCOSE).

Table 11 presents treatment guidelines for INVANZ.

[See table 11 at left]

Table 12 presents prophylaxis guidelines for INVANZ.

[See table 12 at top of next page]

Patients with Renal Insufficiency: INVANZ may be used for the treatment of infections in adult patients with renal insufficiency. In patients whose creatinine clearance is >30 mL/min/1.73 m², no dosage adjustment is necessary. Adult patients with advanced renal insufficiency (creatinine clearance ≤30 mL/min/1.73 m²) and end-stage renal insufficiency (creatinine clearance ≤10 mL/min/1.73 m²) should receive 500 mg daily. There are no data in pediatric patients with renal insufficiency.

Patients on Hemodialysis: When adult patients on hemodialysis are given the recommended daily dose of 500 mg of INVANZ within 6 hours prior to hemodialysis, a supplementary dose of 150 mg is recommended following the hemodialysis session. If INVANZ is given at least 6 hours prior to hemodialysis, no supplementary dose is needed. There are no data in patients undergoing peritoneal dialysis or hemofiltration. There are no data in pediatric patients on hemodialysis.

When only the serum creatinine is available, the following formula** may be used to estimate creatinine clearance. The serum creatinine should represent a steady state of renal function.

Males: $\dfrac{\text{(weight in kg)} \times \text{(140-age in years)}}{(72) \times \text{serum creatinine (mg/100 mL)}}$

Females: $(0.85) \times$ (value calculated for males)

Patients with Hepatic Insufficiency: No dose adjustment recommendations can be made in patients with impaired hepatic function. (See CLINICAL PHARMACOLOGY, *Special Populations, Hepatic Insufficiency* and PRECAUTIONS.)

Table 12
Prophylaxis Guidelines for Adults

Indication	Daily Dose (IV) Adults	Recommended Duration of Total Antimicrobial Treatment
Prophylaxis of surgical site infection following elective colorectal surgery	1 g	Single intravenous dose given 1 hour prior to surgical incision

No dosage adjustment is recommended based on age (13 years of age and older) or gender. (See CLINICAL PHARMACOLOGY, *Special Populations*.)

**Cockcroft and Gault equation: Cockcroft DW, Gault MH. Prediction of creatinine clearance from serum creatinine. Nephron. 1976
PREPARATION OF SOLUTION
Vials
Adults and pediatric patients 13 years of age and older
Preparation for intravenous administration:
DO NOT MIX OR CO-INFUSE INVANZ WITH OTHER MEDICATIONS. DO NOT USE DILUENTS CONTAINING DEXTROSE (α-D-GLUCOSE).
INVANZ MUST BE RECONSTITUTED AND THEN DILUTED PRIOR TO ADMINISTRATION.
1. Reconstitute the contents of a 1 g vial of INVANZ with 10 mL of one of the following: Water for Injection, 0.9% Sodium Chloride Injection or Bacteriostatic Water for Injection.
2. Shake well to dissolve and immediately transfer contents of the reconstituted vial to 50 mL of 0.9% Sodium Chloride Injection.
3. Complete the infusion within 6 hours of reconstitution.
Preparation for intramuscular administration:
INVANZ MUST BE RECONSTITUTED PRIOR TO ADMINISTRATION.
1. Reconstitute the contents of a 1 g vial of INVANZ with 3.2 mL of 1.0% lidocaine HCl injection*** (**without epinephrine**). Shake vial thoroughly to form solution.
2. Immediately withdraw the contents of the vial and administer by deep intramuscular injection into a large muscle mass (such as the gluteal muscles or lateral part of the thigh).
3. The reconstituted IM solution should be used within 1 hour after preparation. **NOTE: THE RECONSTITUTED SOLUTION SHOULD NOT BE ADMINISTERED INTRAVENOUSLY.**
Pediatric patients 3 months to 12 years of age:
Preparation for intravenous administration:
DO NOT MIX OR CO-INFUSE INVANZ WITH OTHER MEDICATIONS. DO NOT USE DILUENTS CONTAINING DEXTROSE (α-D-GLUCOSE).
INVANZ MUST BE RECONSTITUTED AND THEN DILUTED PRIOR TO ADMINISTRATION.
1. Reconstitute the contents of a 1 g vial of INVANZ with 10 mL of one of the following: Water for Injection, 0.9% Sodium Chloride Injection or Bacteriostatic Water for Injection.
2. Shake well to dissolve and immediately withdraw a volume equal to 15 mg/kg of body weight (not to exceed 1 g/day) and dilute in 0.9% Sodium Chloride Injection to a final concentration of 20 mg/mL or less.
3. Complete the infusion within 6 hours of reconstitution.
Preparation for intramuscular administration:
INVANZ MUST BE RECONSTITUTED PRIOR TO ADMINISTRATION.
1. Reconstitute the contents of a 1 g vial of INVANZ with 3.2 mL of 1.0% lidocaine HCl injection*** (**without epinephrine**). Shake vial thoroughly to form solution.
2. Immediately withdraw a volume equal to 15 mg/kg of body weight (not to exceed 1 g/day) and administer by deep intramuscular injection into a large muscle mass (such as the gluteal muscles or lateral part of the thigh).
3. The reconstituted IM solution should be used within 1 hour after preparation. **NOTE: THE RECONSTITUTED SOLUTION SHOULD NOT BE ADMINISTERED INTRAVENOUSLY.**

***Refer to the prescribing information for lidocaine HCl.
ADD-Vantage®[†] Vials
See separate INSTRUCTIONS FOR USE OF INVANZ (Ertapenem for Injection) IN ADD-Vantage® VIALS. INVANZ in ADD-Vantage® vials should be reconstituted with ADD-Vantage® diluent containers containing 50 mL or 100 mL of 0.9% Sodium Chloride Injection.
Parenteral drug products should be inspected visually for particulate matter and discoloration prior to use, whenever solution and container permit. Solutions of INVANZ range from colorless to pale yellow. Variations of color within this range do not affect the potency of the product.

[†] Registered trademark of Hospira Laboratories, Inc

STORAGE AND STABILITY
Before reconstitution
Do not store lyophilized powder above 25°C (77°F).
Reconstituted and infusion solutions
The reconstituted solution, immediately diluted in 0.9% Sodium Chloride Injection (see DOSAGE AND ADMINISTRATION, PREPARATION OF SOLUTION), **may be stored at room temperature (25°C) and used within 6 hours or stored for 24 hours under refrigeration (5°C) and used within 4 hours after removal from refrigeration. Solutions of INVANZ should not be frozen.**

HOW SUPPLIED
INVANZ is supplied as a sterile lyophilized powder in single dose vials containing ertapenem for intravenous infusion or for intramuscular injection as follows:
    No. 3843—1 g ertapenem equivalent
    NDC 0006-3843-71 in trays of 10 vials
INVANZ is supplied as a sterile lyophilized powder in single dose ADD-Vantage® vials containing ertapenem for intravenous infusion as follows:
    No. 3845—1 g ertapenem equivalent
    NDC 0006-3845-71 in trays of 10 ADD-Vantage® vials.

CLINICAL STUDIES
Adults
Complicated Intra-Abdominal Infections
Ertapenem was evaluated in adults for the treatment of complicated intra-abdominal infections in a clinical trial. This study compared ertapenem (1 g intravenously once a day) with piperacillin/tazobactam (3.375 g intravenously every 6 hours) for 5 to 14 days and enrolled 665 patients with localized complicated appendicitis, and any other complicated intra-abdominal infection including colonic, small intestinal, and biliary infections and generalized peritonitis. The combined clinical and microbiologic success rates in the microbiologically evaluable population at 4 to 6 weeks posttherapy (test-of-cure) were 83.6% (163/195) for ertapenem and 80.4% (152/189) for piperacillin/tazobactam.
Complicated Skin and Skin Structure Infections
Ertapenem was evaluated in adults for the treatment of complicated skin and skin structure infections in a clinical trial. This study compared ertapenem (1 g intravenously once a day) with piperacillin/tazobactam (3.375 g intravenously every 6 hours) for 7 to 14 days and enrolled 540 patients including patients with deep soft tissue abscess, post-traumatic wound infection and cellulitis with purulent drainage. The clinical success rates at 10 to 21 days posttherapy (test-of-cure) were 83.9% (141/168) for ertapenem and 85.3% (145/170) for piperacillin/tazobactam.
Diabetic Foot Infections
Ertapenem was evaluated in adults for the treatment of diabetic foot infections without concomitant osteomyelitis in a multicenter, randomized, double-blind clinical trial. This study compared ertapenem (1 g intravenously once a day) with piperacillin/tazobactam (3.375 g intravenously every 6 hours). Test-of-cure was defined as clinical response between treatment groups in the clinically evaluable population at the 10-day posttherapy follow-up visit. The study included 295 patients randomized to ertapenem and 291 patients to piperacillin/tazobactam. Both regimens allowed the option to switch to oral amoxicillin/clavulanate for a total of 5 to 28 days of treatment (parenteral and oral). All patients were eligible to receive appropriate adjunctive treatment methods, such as debridement, as is typically required in the treatment of diabetic foot infections, and most patients received these treatments. Patients with suspected osteomyelitis could be enrolled if all the infected bone was removed within 2 days of initiation of study therapy, and preferably within the prestudy period. Investigators had the option to add open-label vancomycin if enterococci or methicillin-resistant *Staphylococcus aureus* (MRSA) were among the pathogens isolated or if patients had a history of MRSA infection and additional therapy was indicated in the opinion of the investigator. Two hundred and four (204) patients randomized to ertapenem and 202 patients randomized to piperacillin/tazobactam were clinically evaluable. The clinical success rates at 10 days posttherapy were 75.0% (153/204) for ertapenem and 70.8% (143/202) for piperacillin/tazobactam.
Community Acquired Pneumonia
Ertapenem was evaluated in adults for the treatment of community acquired pneumonia in two clinical trials. Both studies compared ertapenem (1 g parenterally once a day) with ceftriaxone (1 g parenterally once a day) and enrolled a total of 866 patients. Both regimens allowed the option to switch to oral amoxicillin/clavulanate for a total of 10 to 14 days of treatment (parenteral and oral). In the first study the primary efficacy parameter was the clinical success rate in the clinically evaluable population and success rates were 92.3% (168/182) for ertapenem and 91.0% (183/201) for ceftriaxone at 7 to 14 days posttherapy (test-of-cure). In the second study the primary efficacy parameter was the clinical success rate in the microbiologically evaluable population and success rates were 91% (91/100) for ertapenem and 91.8% (45/49) for ceftriaxone at 7 to 14 days posttherapy (test-of-cure).
Complicated Urinary Tract Infections Including Pyelonephritis
Ertapenem was evaluated in adults for the treatment of complicated urinary tract infections including pyelonephritis in two clinical trials. Both studies compared ertapenem (1 g parenterally once a day) with ceftriaxone (1 g parenterally once a day) and enrolled a total of 850 patients. Both regimens allowed the option to switch to oral ciprofloxacin (500 mg twice daily) for a total of 10 to 14 days of treatment (parenteral and oral). The microbiological success rates (combined studies) at 5 to 9 days posttherapy (test-of-cure) were 89.5% (229/256) for ertapenem and 91.1% (204/224) for ceftriaxone.
Acute Pelvic Infections Including Endomyometritis, Septic Abortion and Post-Surgical Gynecological Infections
Ertapenem was evaluated in adults for the treatment of acute pelvic infections in a clinical trial. This study compared ertapenem (1 g intravenously once a day) with piperacillin/tazobactam (3.375 g intravenously every 6 hours) for 3 to 10 days and enrolled 412 patients including 350 patients with obstetric/postpartum infections and 45 patients with septic abortion. The clinical success rates in the clinically evaluable population at 2 to 4 weeks posttherapy (test-of-cure) were 93.9% (153/163) for ertapenem and 91.5% (140/153) for piperacillin/tazobactam.
Prophylaxis of Surgical Site Infections Following Elective Colorectal Surgery
Ertapenem was evaluated in adults for prophylaxis of surgical site infection following elective colorectal surgery in a multicenter, randomized, double-blind clinical trial. This study compared a single intravenous dose of ertapenem (1 g) versus cefotetan (2 g) administered over 30 minutes, 1 hour before elective colorectal surgery. Test-of-prophylaxis was defined as no evidence of surgical site infection, post-operative anastomotic leak, or unexplained antibiotic use in the clinically evaluable population up to and including at the 4-week posttreatment follow-up visit. The study included 500 patients randomized to ertapenem and 502 patients randomized to cefotetan. The modified intent-to-treat (MITT) population consisted of 451 ertapenem patients and 450 cefotetan patients and included all patients who were randomized, treated, and underwent elective colorectal surgery with adequate bowel preparation. The clinically evaluable population was a subset of the MITT population and consisted of patients who received a complete dose of study therapy no more than two hours prior to surgical incision and no more than six hours before surgical closure. Clinically evaluable patients had sufficient information to determine outcome at the 4-week follow-up assessment and had no confounding factors that interfered with the assessment of that outcome. Examples of confounding factors included prior or concomitant antibiotic violations, the need for a second surgical procedure during the study period, and identification of a distant site infection with concomitant antibiotic administration and no evidence of subsequent wound infection. Three-hundred forty-six (346) patients randomized to ertapenem and 339 patients randomized to cefotetan were clinically evaluable. The prophylactic success rates at 4 weeks posttreatment in the clinically evaluable population were 70.5% (244/346) for ertapenem and 57.2% (194/339) for cefotetan (difference 13.3%, [95% C.I.: 6.1, 20.4], p<0.001). Prophylaxis failure due to surgical site infections occurred in 18.2% (63/346) ertapenem patients and 31.0% (105/339) cefotetan patients. Post-operative anastomotic leak occurred in 2.9% (10/346) ertapenem patients and 4.1% (14/339) cefotetan patients. Unexplained antibiotic use occurred in 8.4% (29/346) ertapenem patients and 7.7% (26/339) cefotetan patients. Though patient numbers were small in some subgroups, in general, clinical response rates by age, gender, and race were consistent with the results found in the clinically evaluable population. In the MITT analysis, the prophylactic success rates at 4 weeks post-

treatment were 58.3% (263/451) for ertapenem and 48.9% (220/450) for cefotetan (difference 9.4%, [95% C.I.: 2.9, 15.9], p = 0.002). A statistically significant difference favoring ertapenem over cefotetan with respect to the primary endpoint has been observed at a significance level of 5% in this study. A second adequate and well-controlled study to confirm these findings has not been conducted; therefore, the clinical superiority of ertapenem over cefotetan has not been demonstrated.

Pediatric Patients
Ertapenem was evaluated in pediatric patients 3 months to 17 years of age in two randomized, multicenter clinical trials. The first study enrolled 404 patients and compared ertapenem (15 mg/kg IV every 12 hours in patients 3 months to 12 years of age, and 1 g IV once a day in patients 13 to 17 years of age) to ceftriaxone (50 mg/kg/day IV in two divided doses in patients 3 months to 12 years of age and 50 mg/kg/day IV as a single daily dose in patients 13 to 17 years of age) for the treatment of complicated urinary tract infection (UTI), skin and soft tissue infection (SSTI), or community-acquired pneumonia (CAP). Both regimens allowed the option to switch to oral amoxicillin/clavulanate for a total of up to 14 days of treatment (parenteral and oral). The microbiological success rates in the evaluable per protocol (EPP) analysis in patients treated for UTI were 87.0% (40/46) for ertapenem and 90.0% (18/20) for ceftriaxone. The clinical success rates in the EPP analysis in patients treated for SSTI were 95.5% (64/67) for ertapenem and 100% (26/26) for ceftriaxone, and in patients treated for CAP were 96.1% (74/77) for ertapenem and 96.4% (27/28) for ceftriaxone.

The second study enrolled 112 patients and compared ertapenem (15 mg/kg IV every 12 hours in patients 3 months to 12 years of age, and 1 g IV once a day in patients 13 to 17 years of age) to ticarcillin/clavulanate (50 mg/kg for patients <60 kg or 3.0 g for patients >60 kg, 4 or 6 times a day) up to 14 days for the treatment of complicated intra-abdominal infections (IAI) and acute pelvic infections (API). In patients treated for IAI (primarily patients with perforated or complicated appendicitis), the clinical success rates were 83.7% (36/43) for ertapenem and 63.6% (7/11) for ticarcillin/clavulanate in the EPP analysis. In patients treated for API (post-operative or spontaneous obstetrical endomyometritis, or septic abortion) the clinical success rates were 100% (23/23) for ertapenem and 100% (4/4) for ticarcillin/clavulanate in the EPP analysis.

REFERENCES
1. Clinical and Laboratory Standards Institute (CLSI). Methods for Dilution Antimicrobial Susceptibility Tests for Bacteria that Grow Aerobically. Seventh Edition; Approved Standard, CLSI Document M7-A7, Clinical and Laboratory Standards Institute, Wayne, PA, January 2006.
2. Clinical and Laboratory Standards Institute (CLSI). Performance Standards for Antimicrobial Disk Susceptibility Testing—Sixteenth Informational Supplement. Approved Standard, CLSI Document M100-S16. Clinical and Laboratory Standards Institute, Wayne, PA, January 2006.
3. Clinical and Laboratory Standards Institute (CLSI). Performance Standards for Antimicrobial Disk Susceptibility Tests. Ninth Edition; Approved Standard, CLSI Document M2-A9. Clinical and Laboratory Standards Institute, Wayne, PA, January 2006.
4. Clinical and Laboratory Standards Institute (CLSI). *Methods for Antimicrobial Susceptibility Testing of Anaerobic Bacteria*– Sixth Edition; Approved Standard, CLSI Document M11-A6. Clinical and Laboratory Standards Institute, Wayne, PA, January 2004.

Manuf. for:
Merck Sharp & Dohme Corp., a subsidiary of **MERCK & CO., INC.**
Whitehouse Station, NJ 08889, USA
By: Laboratories Merck Sharp & Dohme-Chibret
63963 Clermont-Ferrand Cedex 9, France
US Patent Nos.: 5,478,820; 5,952,323; 5,652,233
9709712 Issued March 2010.

INSTRUCTIONS FOR USE OF INVANZ®*
(Ertapenem for Injection)
IN ADD-Vantage®† VIALS
For I.V. Use Only.
INSTRUCTIONS FOR USE
To Open Diluent Container:
Peel overwrap from the corner and remove container. Some opacity of the plastic due to moisture absorption during the sterilization process may be observed. This is normal and does not affect the solution quality or safety. The opacity will diminish gradually.

To Assemble Vial and Flexible Diluent Container:
(Use Aseptic Technique)
1. Remove the protective covers from the top of the vial and the vial port on the diluent container as follows:
   a. To remove the breakaway vial cap, swing the pull ring over the top of the vial and pull down far enough to start the opening. (SEE FIGURE 1.) Pull the ring approximately half way around the cap and then pull straight up to remove the cap. (SEE FIGURE 2.) NOTE: DO NOT ACCESS VIAL WITH SYRINGE.

---

* Merck Sharp & Dohme Corp., a subsidiary of **Merck & Co., Inc.**
Copyright © 2006 Merck Sharp & Dohme Corp., a subsidiary of **Merck & Co., Inc.**
All rights reserved
† Registered trademark of Hospira Laboratories, Inc.

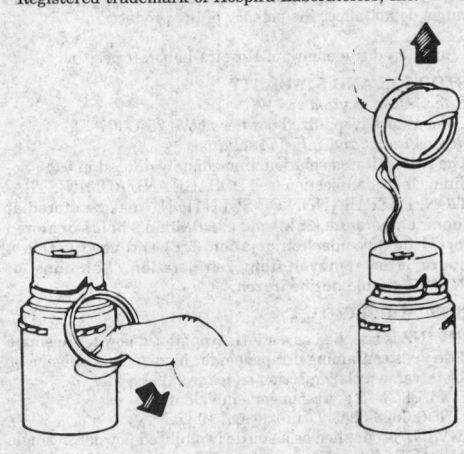

Fig. 1   Fig. 2

   b. To remove the vial port cover, grasp the tab on the pull ring, pull up to break the three tie strings, then pull back to remove the cover. (SEE FIGURE 3.)
2. Screw the vial into the vial port until it will go no further. THE VIAL MUST BE SCREWED IN TIGHTLY TO ASSURE A SEAL. This occurs approximately ½ turn (180°) after the first audible click. (SEE FIGURE 4.) The clicking sound does not assure a seal; the vial must be turned as far as it will go. NOTE: Once vial is seated, do not attempt to remove. (SEE FIGURE 4.)
3. Recheck the vial to assure that it is tight by trying to turn it further in the direction of assembly.
4. Label appropriately.

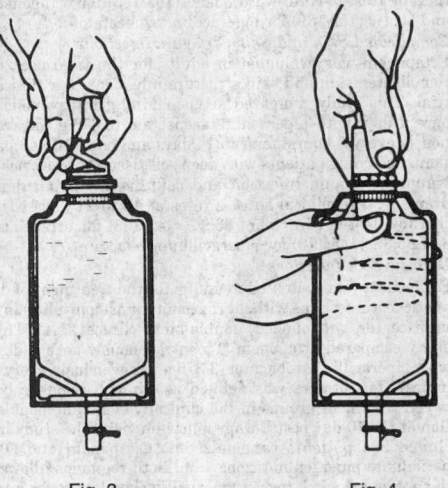

Fig. 3   Fig. 4

To Prepare Admixture:
1. Squeeze the bottom of the diluent container gently to inflate the portion of the container surrounding the end of the drug vial.
2. With the other hand, push the drug vial down into the container telescoping the walls of the container. Grasp the inner cap of the vial through the walls of the container. (SEE FIGURE 5.)
3. Pull the inner cap from the drug vial. (SEE FIGURE 6.) Verify that the rubber stopper has been pulled out, allowing the drug and diluent to mix.

4. Mix container contents thoroughly and use within the specified time.

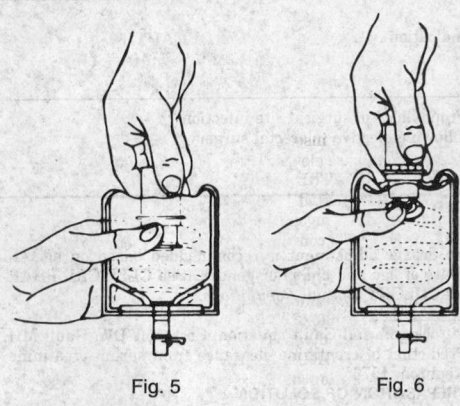

Fig. 5   Fig. 6

Preparation for Administration:
(Use Aseptic Technique)
1. Confirm the activation and admixture of vial contents.
2. Check for leaks by squeezing container firmly. If leaks are found, discard unit as sterility may be impaired.
3. Close flow control clamp of administration set.
4. Remove cover from outlet port at bottom of container.
5. Insert piercing pin of administration set into port with a twisting motion until the pin is firmly seated. NOTE: See full directions on administration set carton.
6. Lift the free end of the hanger loop on the bottom of the vial, breaking the two tie strings. Bend the loop outward to lock it in the upright position, then suspend container from hanger.
7. Squeeze and release drip chamber to establish proper fluid level in chamber.
8. Open flow control clamp and clear air from set. Close clamp.
9. Attach set to venipuncture device. If device is not indwelling, prime and make venipuncture.
10. Regulate rate of administration with flow control clamp.

WARNING: Do not use flexible container in series connections.
Storage
INVANZ (Ertapenem for Injection) 1 g single dose ADD-Vantage® vials should be prepared with ADD-Vantage® diluent containers containing 50 mL or 100 mL of 0.9% Sodium Chloride Injection. When prepared with this diluent, INVANZ (Ertapenem for Injection) maintains satisfactory potency **for 6 hours at room temperature (25°C) or for 24 hours under refrigeration (5°C) and used within 4 hours after removal from refrigeration. Solutions of INVANZ should not be frozen.**
Before administering, see accompanying package circular for INVANZ (Ertapenem for Injection).
Manuf. for:
Merck Sharp & Dohme Corp., a subsidiary of **MERCK & CO., INC.**
Whitehouse Station, NJ 08889, USA
By: Laboratories Merck Sharp & Dohme-Chibret
63963 Clermont-Ferrand Cedex 9, France
US Patent Nos.: 5,478,820; 5,952,323; 5,652,233
Issued March 2010.

ISENTRESS®   ℞
(raltegravir)
Tablets

HIGHLIGHTS OF PRESCRIBING INFORMATION
These highlights do not include all the information needed to use ISENTRESS safely and effectively. See full prescribing information for ISENTRESS.
ISENTRESS (raltegravir) Tablets
Initial U.S. Approval: 2007
————RECENT MAJOR CHANGES————
Indications And Usage (1)   06/2010
————INDICATIONS AND USAGE————
ISENTRESS® is a human immunodeficiency virus integrase strand transfer inhibitor (HIV-1 INSTI) indicated:
• In combination with other antiretroviral agents for the treatment of HIV-1 infection in adult patients (1).
The safety and efficacy of ISENTRESS have not been established in pediatric patients (1).
———— DOSAGE AND ADMINISTRATION ————
• 400 mg administered orally, twice daily with or without food (2).
• During coadministration with rifampin, 800 mg twice daily (2).

DOSAGE FORMS AND STRENGTHS

Tablets: 400 mg (3).

CONTRAINDICATIONS

None (4).

WARNINGS AND PRECAUTIONS

Monitor for Immune Reconstitution Syndrome (5.1).

ADVERSE REACTIONS

- The most common adverse reactions of moderate to severe intensity (≥2%) which occurred at a higher rate than the comparator are insomnia and headache (6.1).
- Creatine kinase elevations were observed in subjects who received ISENTRESS. Myopathy and rhabdomyolysis have been reported. Use with caution in patients at increased risk of myopathy or rhabdomyolysis, such as patients receiving concomitant medications known to cause these conditions (6.1).

To report SUSPECTED ADVERSE REACTIONS, contact Merck Sharp & Dohme Corp., a subsidiary of Merck & Co., Inc., at 1-877-888-4231 or FDA at 1-800-FDA-1088 or www.fda.gov/medwatch.

DRUG INTERACTIONS

- Coadministration of ISENTRESS with drugs that are strong inducers of UGT1A1 may result in reduced plasma concentrations of raltegravir (7.2).

USE IN SPECIFIC POPULATIONS

Pregnancy:

- ISENTRESS should be used during pregnancy only if the potential benefit justifies the potential risk to the fetus. Physicians are encouraged to register pregnant women exposed to ISENTRESS by calling 1-800-258-4263 so that Merck Sharp & Dohme Corp., a subsidiary of Merck & Co., Inc., can monitor maternal and fetal outcomes (8.1).

Nursing Mothers:

- Breast-feeding is not recommended while taking ISENTRESS (8.3).

See 17 for PATIENT COUNSELING INFORMATION and FDA-approved patient labeling

Revised: 06/2010

FULL PRESCRIBING INFORMATION: CONTENTS*

*** Sections or subsections omitted from the full prescribing information are not listed**

FULL PRESCRIBING INFORMATION

1 INDICATIONS AND USAGE

ISENTRESS[1] is indicated in combination with other antiretroviral agents for the treatment of human immunodeficiency virus (HIV-1) infection in adult patients.

This indication is based on analyses of plasma HIV-1 RNA levels through 96 weeks in three double-blind controlled studies of ISENTRESS. Two of these studies were conducted in clinically advanced, 3-class antiretroviral (NNRTI, NRTI, PI) treatment-experienced adults and one was conducted in treatment-naïve adults.

The use of other active agents with ISENTRESS is associated with a greater likelihood of treatment response *[see Clinical Studies (14)]*.

Table 2: Selected Grade 2 to 4 Laboratory Abnormalities Reported in Treatment-Naïve Subjects (96 Week Analysis)

Laboratory Parameter Preferred Term (Unit)	Limit	Randomized Study Protocol 021: ISENTRESS 400 mg Twice Daily + Emtricitabine (+) Tenofovir (N = 281)	Efavirenz 600 mg At Bedtime + Emtricitabine (+) Tenofovir (N = 282)
Hematology			
Absolute neutrophil count ($10^3/\mu L$)			
Grade 2	0.75 - 0.999	3%	4%
Grade 3	0.50 - 0.749	2%	1%
Grade 4	<0.50	<1%	<1%
Hemoglobin (gm/dL)			
Grade 2	7.5 - 8.4	1%	1%
Grade 3	6.5 - 7.4	<1%	1%
Grade 4	<6.5	<1%	0%
Platelet count ($10^3/\mu L$)			
Grade 2	50 - 99.999	2%	0%
Grade 3	25 - 49.999	<1%	<1%
Grade 4	<25	0%	0%

(Table continued on next page)

The safety and efficacy of ISENTRESS have not been established in pediatric patients.

[1] Registered trademark of Merck Sharp & Dohme Corp., a subsidiary of **Merck & Co., Inc.**

Copyright © 2007, 2009 Merck Sharp & Dohme Corp., a subsidiary of **Merck & Co., Inc.**
All rights reserved

2 DOSAGE AND ADMINISTRATION

For the treatment of patients with HIV-1 infection, the dosage of ISENTRESS is 400 mg administered orally, twice daily with or without food. During coadministration with rifampin, the recommended dosage of ISENTRESS is 800 mg twice daily with or without food.

3 DOSAGE FORMS AND STRENGTHS

400 mg pink, oval-shaped, film-coated tablets with "227" on one side.

4 CONTRAINDICATIONS

None

5 WARNINGS AND PRECAUTIONS

5.1 Immune Reconstitution Syndrome

During the initial phase of treatment, patients responding to antiretroviral therapy may develop an inflammatory response to indolent or residual opportunistic infections (such as *Mycobacterium avium* complex, cytomegalovirus, *Pneumocystis jiroveci* pneumonia, *Mycobacterium* tuberculosis, or reactivation of varicella zoster virus), which may necessitate further evaluation and treatment.

6 ADVERSE REACTIONS

6.1 Clinical Trials Experience

Because clinical trials are conducted under widely varying conditions, adverse reaction rates observed in the clinical trials of a drug cannot be directly compared to rates in the clinical trials of another drug and may not reflect the rates observed in practice.

Treatment-Naïve Studies

The following safety assessment of ISENTRESS in treatment-naïve subjects is based on the randomized double-blind active controlled study of treatment-naïve subjects, STARTMRK (Protocol 021) with ISENTRESS 400 mg twice daily in combination with a fixed dose of emtricitabine 200 mg (+) tenofovir 300 mg, (N=281) versus efavirenz (EFV) 600 mg at bedtime in combination with emtricitabine (+) tenofovir, (N=282). During double-blind treatment, the total follow-up for subjects receiving ISENTRESS 400 mg twice daily + emtricitabine (+) tenofovir was 480 patient-years and 463 patient-years for subjects receiving efavirenz 600 mg at bedtime + emtricitabine (+) tenofovir.

In Protocol 021, the rate of discontinuation of therapy due to adverse reactions was 4% in subjects receiving ISENTRESS + emtricitabine (+) tenofovir and 7% in subjects receiving efavirenz + emtricitabine (+) tenofovir.

The clinical adverse drug reactions (ADRs) listed below were considered by investigators to be causally related to ISENTRESS + emtricitabine (+) tenofovir or efavirenz + emtricitabine (+) tenofovir. Clinical ADRs of moderate to severe intensity occurring in ≥2% of treatment-naïve subjects treated with ISENTRESS and occurring at a higher rate than efavirenz are presented in Table 1.

Table 1: Adverse Reactions* of Moderate to Severe Intensity† Occurring in ≥2% of Treatment-Naïve Adult Subjects Receiving ISENTRESS and at a Higher Rate Compared to Efavirenz (96 Week Analysis)

System Organ Class, Preferred Term	Randomized Study Protocol 021: ISENTRESS 400 mg Twice Daily + Emtricitabine (+) Tenofovir (n = 281)‡ %	Efavirenz 600 mg At Bedtime + Emtricitabine (+) Tenofovir (n = 282)‡ %
Psychiatric Disorders		
Insomnia	4	3

* Includes adverse experiences considered by investigators to be at least possibly, probably, or definitely related to the drug.

† Intensities are defined as follows: Moderate (discomfort enough to cause interference with usual activity); Severe (incapacitating with inability to work or do usual activity).

‡ n = total number of subjects per treatment group

Laboratory Abnormalities

The percentages of adult subjects treated with ISENTRESS 400 mg twice daily or efavirenz in Protocol 021 with selected Grades 2 to 4 laboratory abnormalities that represent a worsening Grade from baseline are presented in Table 2.

[See table 2 above and on next page]

Lipids, Change from Baseline

Changes from baseline in fasting lipids are shown in Table 3.

[See table 3 on next page]

Treatment-Experienced Studies

The safety assessment of ISENTRESS in treatment-experienced subjects is based on the pooled safety data from the randomized, double-blind, placebo-controlled trials, BENCHMRK 1 and BENCHMRK 2 (Protocols 018 and 019) in antiretroviral treatment-experienced HIV-1 infected adult subjects. A total of 462 subjects received the recommended dose of ISENTRESS 400 mg twice daily in combination with optimized background therapy (OBT) compared to 237 subjects taking placebo in combination with OBT. The median duration of therapy in these trials was 96 weeks for subjects receiving ISENTRESS and 38 weeks for subjects receiving placebo. The total exposure to ISENTRESS was 708 patient-years versus 244 patient-years on placebo. The rates of discontinuation due to adverse events were 4% in subjects receiving ISENTRESS and 5% in subjects receiving placebo.

Clinical ADRs were considered by investigators to be causally related to ISENTRESS + OBT or placebo + OBT. Clinical ADRs of moderate to severe intensity occurring in ≥2% of subjects treated with ISENTRESS and occurring at a higher rate compared to placebo are presented in Table 4.

Table 4: Adverse Drug Reactions* of Moderate to Severe Intensity† Occurring in ≥2% of Treatment-Experienced Adult Subjects Receiving ISENTRESS and at a Higher Rate Compared to Placebo (96 Week Analysis)

System Organ Class, Adverse Reactions	Randomized Studies Protocol 018 and 019	
	ISENTRESS 400 mg Twice Daily + OBT (n = 462)‡	Placebo + OBT (n = 237)‡
Nervous System Disorders		
Headache	2	<1

* Includes adverse reactions at least possibly, probably, or definitely related to the drug.
† Intensities are defined as follows: Moderate (discomfort enough to cause interference with usual activity); Severe (incapacitating with inability to work or do usual activity).
‡ n=total number of subjects per treatment group.

Laboratory Abnormalities
The percentages of adult subjects treated with ISENTRESS 400 mg twice daily or placebo in Protocols 018 and 019 with selected Grade 2 to 4 laboratory abnormalities representing a worsening Grade from baseline are presented in Table 5. [See table 5 at top of next page]

Less Common Adverse Reactions Observed in Treatment-Naïve and Treatment-Experienced Studies
The following ADRs occurred in <2% of treatment-naïve or treatment-experienced subjects receiving ISENTRESS in a combination regimen. These events have been included because of their seriousness, increased frequency on ISENTRESS compared with efavirenz or placebo, or investigator's assessment of potential causal relationship.
Gastrointestinal Disorders: abdominal pain, gastritis, dyspepsia, vomiting, nausea
General Disorders and Administration Site Conditions: fatigue, asthenia
Hepatobiliary Disorders: hepatitis
Immune System Disorders: hypersensitivity
Infections and Infestations: genital herpes, herpes zoster
Nervous System Disorders: dizziness
Psychiatric Disorders: depression (particularly in subjects with a pre-existing history of psychiatric illness), including suicidal ideation and behaviors
Renal and Urinary Disorders: nephrolithiasis, renal failure

Selected Adverse Events
Cancers were reported in treatment-experienced subjects who initiated ISENTRESS or placebo, both with OBT, and in treatment-naïve subjects who initiated ISENTRESS or efavirenz, both with emtricitabine (+) tenofovir; several were recurrent. The types and rates of specific cancers were those expected in a highly immunodeficient population (many had CD4+ counts below 50 cells/mm³ and most had prior AIDS diagnoses). The risk of developing cancer in these studies was similar in the group receiving ISENTRESS and the group receiving the comparator.
Grade 2-4 creatine kinase laboratory abnormalities were observed in subjects treated with ISENTRESS (see Table 5). Myopathy and rhabdomyolysis have been reported. Use with caution in patients at increased risk of myopathy or rhabdomyolysis, such as patients receiving concomitant medications known to cause these conditions.
Rash occurred more commonly in treatment-experienced subjects receiving regimens containing ISENTRESS + darunavir/ritonavir compared to subjects receiving ISENTRESS without darunavir/ritonavir or darunavir/ritonavir without ISENTRESS. However, rash that was considered drug related occurred at similar rates for all three groups. These rashes were mild to moderate in severity and did not limit therapy; there were no discontinuations due to rash.

Patients with Co-existing Conditions
Patients Co-infected with Hepatitis B and/or Hepatitis C Virus
In the randomized, double-blind, placebo-controlled trials, treatment-experienced subjects (N = 114/699 or 16%) and treatment-naïve subjects (N = 34/563 or 6%) with chronic (but not acute) active hepatitis B and/or hepatitis C virus co-infection were permitted to enroll provided that baseline liver function tests did not exceed 5 times the upper limit of normal (ULN). In general the safety profile of ISENTRESS in subjects with hepatitis B and/or hepatitis C virus co-infection was similar to that in subjects without hepatitis B and/or hepatitis C virus co-infection, although the rates of AST and ALT abnormalities were higher in the subgroup with hepatitis B and/or hepatitis C virus co-infection for all treatment groups. In treatment-experienced subjects,

Table 2 (cont.): Selected Grade 2 to 4 Laboratory Abnormalities Reported in Treatment-Naïve Subjects (96 Week Analysis)

Laboratory Parameter Preferred Term (Unit)	Limit	Randomized Study Protocol 021	
		ISENTRESS 400 mg Twice Daily + Emtricitabine (+) Tenofovir (N = 281)	Efavirenz 600 mg At Bedtime + Emtricitabine (+) Tenofovir (N = 282)
Blood chemistry			
Fasting (non-random) serum glucose test (mg/dL)			
Grade 2	126 - 250	3%	4%
Grade 3	251 - 500	1%	0%
Grade 4	>500	0%	0%
Total serum bilirubin			
Grade 2	1.6 - 2.5 × ULN	4%	0%
Grade 3	2.6 - 5.0 × ULN	1%	0%
Grade 4	>5.0 × ULN	0%	0%
Serum aspartate aminotransferase			
Grade 2	2.6 - 5.0 × ULN	4%	5%
Grade 3	5.1 - 10.0 × ULN	2%	2%
Grade 4	>10.0 × ULN	1%	<1%
Serum alanine aminotransferase			
Grade 2	2.6 - 5.0 × ULN	6%	9%
Grade 3	5.1 - 10.0 × ULN	1%	2%
Grade 4	>10.0 × ULN	1%	1%
Serum alkaline phosphatase			
Grade 2	2.6 - 5.0 × ULN	1%	3%
Grade 3	5.1 - 10.0 × ULN	0%	<1%
Grade 4	>10.0 × ULN	0%	<1%

ULN = Upper limit of normal range

Table 3: Lipid Values, Mean Change from Baseline, Protocol 021

Laboratory Parameter Preferred Term	ISENTRESS 400 mg Twice Daily + Emtricitabine (+) Tenofovir N = 281			Efavirenz 600 mg At Bedtime + Emtricitabine (+) Tenofovir N = 282		
			Change from Baseline at Week 96			Change from Baseline at Week 96
	Baseline Mean (mg/dL)	Week 96 Mean (mg/dL)	Mean Change (mg/dL)	Baseline Mean (mg/dL)	Week 96 Mean (mg/dL)	Mean Change (mg/dL)
LDL-Cholesterol*	96	103	7	93	115	21
HDL-Cholesterol*	39	42	3	38	48	10
Total Cholesterol*	159	169	10	156	194	38
Triglyceride*	125	121	-4	137	177	40

* Fasting (non-random) laboratory tests.
Notes:
N = Number of subjects in the treatment group. The analysis is based on all available data.
If subjects initiated or increased serum lipid-reducing agents, the last available lipid values prior to the change in therapy were used in the analysis. If the missing data was due to other reasons, subjects were censored thereafter for the analysis. At baseline, serum lipid-reducing agents were used in 5% of subjects in the group receiving ISENTRESS and 3% in the efavirenz group. Through Week 96, serum lipid-reducing agents were used in 7% of subjects in the group receiving ISENTRESS and 9% in the efavirenz group.

Grade 2 or higher laboratory abnormalities that represent a worsening Grade from baseline of AST, ALT or total bilirubin occurred in 29%, 34% and 13%, respectively, of co-infected subjects treated with ISENTRESS as compared to 11%, 10% and 9% of all other subjects treated with ISENTRESS. In treatment-naïve subjects, Grade 2 or higher laboratory abnormalities that represent a worsening Grade from baseline of AST, ALT or total bilirubin occurred in 17%, 28% and 17%, respectively, of co-infected subjects treated with ISENTRESS as compared to 6%, 6% and 3% of all others subjects treated with ISENTRESS.

6.2 Postmarketing Experience
The following adverse reactions have been identified during postapproval use of ISENTRESS. Because these reactions are reported voluntarily from a population of uncertain size, it is not always possible to reliably estimate their frequency or establish a causal relationship to drug exposure.
Blood and Lymphatic System Disorders: thrombocytopenia
Musculoskeletal and Connective Tissue Disorders: rhabdomyolysis
Psychiatric Disorders: anxiety, paranoia
Skin and Subcutaneous Tissue Disorders: rash, Stevens-Johnson syndrome

7 DRUG INTERACTIONS
7.1 Effect of Raltegravir on the Pharmacokinetics of Other Agents
Raltegravir does not inhibit (IC_{50}>100 µM) CYP1A2, CYP2B6, CYP2C8, CYP2C9, CYP2C19, CYP2D6 or CYP3A *in vitro*. Moreover, *in vitro*, raltegravir did not induce CYP1A2, CYP2B6 or CYP3A4. A midazolam drug interaction study confirmed the low propensity of raltegravir to alter the pharmacokinetics of agents metabolized by CYP3A4 *in vivo* by demonstrating a lack of effect of raltegravir on the pharmacokinetics of midazolam, a sensitive CYP3A4 substrate. Similarly, raltegravir is not an inhibitor (IC_{50}>50 µM) of the UDP-glucuronosyltransferases (UGT) tested (UGT1A1, UGT2B7), and raltegravir does not inhibit P-glycoprotein-mediated transport. Based on these data, ISENTRESS is not expected to affect the pharmacokinetics of drugs that are substrates of these enzymes or P-glycoprotein (e.g., protease inhibitors, NNRTIs, opioid analgesics, statins, azole antifungals, proton pump inhibitors and anti-erectile dysfunction agents).
In drug interaction studies, raltegravir did not have a clinically meaningful effect on the pharmacokinetics of the following: hormonal contraceptives, methadone, lamivudine, tenofovir, etravirine, darunavir/ritonavir.

7.2 Effect of Other Agents on the Pharmacokinetics of Raltegravir

Raltegravir is not a substrate of cytochrome P450 (CYP) enzymes. Based on *in vivo* and *in vitro* studies, raltegravir is eliminated mainly by metabolism via a UGT1A1-mediated glucuronidation pathway.

Rifampin, a strong inducer of UGT1A1, reduces plasma concentrations of ISENTRESS. Therefore, the dose of ISENTRESS should be increased during coadministration with rifampin *[see Dosage and Administration (2)]*. The impact of other inducers of drug metabolizing enzymes, such as phenytoin and phenobarbital, on UGT1A1 is unknown. Coadministration of ISENTRESS with drugs that inhibit UGT1A1 may increase plasma levels of raltegravir.

Selected drug interactions are presented in Table 6 *[see Clinical Pharmacology (12.3)]*.

[See table 6 at top of next page]

8 USE IN SPECIFIC POPULATIONS

8.1 Pregnancy

Pregnancy Category C

ISENTRESS should be used during pregnancy only if the potential benefit justifies the potential risk to the fetus. There are no adequate and well-controlled studies in pregnant women. In addition, there have been no pharmacokinetic studies conducted in pregnant patients.

Developmental toxicity studies were performed in rabbits (at oral doses up to 1000 mg/kg/day) and rats (at oral doses up to 600 mg/kg/day). The reproductive toxicity study in rats was performed with pre-, peri-, and postnatal evaluation. The highest doses in these studies produced systemic exposures in these species approximately 3- to 4-fold the exposure at the recommended human dose. In both rabbits and rats, no treatment-related effects on embryonic/fetal survival or fetal weights were observed. In addition, no treatment-related external, visceral, or skeletal changes were observed in rabbits. However, treatment-related increases over controls in the incidence of supernumerary ribs were seen in rats at 600 mg/kg/day (exposures 3-fold the exposure at the recommended human dose).

Placenta transfer of drug was demonstrated in both rats and rabbits. At a maternal dose of 600 mg/kg/day in rats, mean drug concentrations in fetal plasma were approximately 1.5- to 2.5-fold greater than in maternal plasma at 1 hour and 24 hours postdose, respectively. Mean drug concentrations in fetal plasma were approximately 2% of the mean maternal concentration at both 1 and 24 hours postdose at a maternal dose of 1000 mg/kg/day in rabbits.

Antiretroviral Pregnancy Registry

To monitor maternal-fetal outcomes of pregnant patients exposed to ISENTRESS, an Antiretroviral Pregnancy Registry has been established. Physicians are encouraged to register patients by calling 1-800-258-4263.

8.3 Nursing Mothers

Breast-feeding is not recommended while taking ISENTRESS. In addition, it is recommended that HIV-1-infected mothers not breast-feed their infants to avoid risking postnatal transmission of HIV-1.

It is not known whether raltegravir is secreted in human milk. However, raltegravir is secreted in the milk of lactating rats. Mean drug concentrations in milk were approximately 3-fold greater than those in maternal plasma at a maternal dose of 600 mg/kg/day in rats. There were no effects in rat offspring attributable to exposure of ISENTRESS through the milk.

8.4 Pediatric Use

Safety and effectiveness of ISENTRESS in pediatric patients have not been established.

8.5 Geriatric Use

Clinical studies of ISENTRESS did not include sufficient numbers of subjects aged 65 and over to determine whether they respond differently from younger subjects. Other reported clinical experience has not identified differences in responses between the elderly and younger subjects. In general, dose selection for an elderly patient should be cautious, reflecting the greater frequency of decreased hepatic, renal, or cardiac function, and of concomitant disease or other drug therapy.

8.6 Use in Patients with Hepatic Impairment

No clinically important pharmacokinetic differences between subjects with moderate hepatic impairment and healthy subjects were observed. No dosage adjustment is necessary for patients with mild to moderate hepatic impairment. The effect of severe hepatic impairment on the pharmacokinetics of raltegravir has not been studied *[see Clinical Pharmacology (12.3)]*.

8.7 Use in Patients with Renal Impairment

No clinically important pharmacokinetic differences between subjects with severe renal impairment and healthy subjects were observed. No dosage adjustment is necessary *[see Clinical Pharmacology (12.3)]*.

10 OVERDOSAGE

No specific information is available on the treatment of overdosage with ISENTRESS. Doses as high as 1600-mg single dose and 800-mg twice-daily multiple doses were studied in healthy volunteers without evidence of toxicity. Occasional doses of up to 1800 mg per day were taken in the clinical studies of HIV-1 infected subjects without evidence of toxicity.

In the event of an overdose, it is reasonable to employ the standard supportive measures, e.g., remove unabsorbed material from the gastrointestinal tract, employ clinical monitoring (including obtaining an electrocardiogram), and institute supportive therapy if required. The extent to which ISENTRESS may be dialyzable is unknown.

11 DESCRIPTION

ISENTRESS contains raltegravir potassium, a human immunodeficiency virus integrase strand transfer inhibitor. The chemical name for raltegravir potassium is N-[(4-Fluorophenyl)methyl]-1,6-dihydro-5-hydroxy-1-methyl-2-[1-methyl-1-[[(5-methyl-1,3,4-oxadiazol-2-yl)carbonyl]amino]ethyl]-6-oxo-4-pyrimidinecarboxamide monopotassium salt.

The empirical formula is $C_{20}H_{20}FKN_4O_5$ and the molecular weight is 482.51. The structural formula is:

Raltegravir potassium is a white to off-white powder. It is soluble in water, slightly soluble in methanol, very slightly soluble in ethanol and acetonitrile and insoluble in isopropanol.

Each film-coated tablet of ISENTRESS for oral administration contains 434.4 mg of raltegravir potassium (as salt), equivalent to 400 mg of raltegravir (free phenol) and the following inactive ingredients: microcrystalline cellulose, lactose monohydrate, calcium phosphate dibasic anhydrous, hypromellose 2208, poloxamer 407 (contains 0.01% butylated hydroxytoluene as antioxidant), sodium stearyl fumarate, magnesium stearate. In addition, the film coating contains the following inactive ingredients: polyvinyl alcohol,

Table 5: Selected Grade 2 to 4 Laboratory Abnormalities Reported in Treatment-Experienced Subjects (96 Week Analysis)

Laboratory Parameter Preferred Term (Unit)	Limit	Randomized Studies Protocol 018 and 019	
		ISENTRESS 400 mg Twice Daily + OBT (N = 462)	Placebo + OBT (N = 237)
Hematology			
Absolute neutrophil count (10^3/µL)			
Grade 2	0.75 - 0.999	4%	5%
Grade 3	0.50 - 0.749	3%	3%
Grade 4	<0.50	1%	<1%
Hemoglobin (gm/dL)			
Grade 2	7.5 - 8.4	1%	3%
Grade 3	6.5 - 7.4	1%	1%
Grade 4	<6.5	<1%	0%
Platelet count (10^3/µL)			
Grade 2	50 - 99.999	3%	5%
Grade 3	25 - 49.999	1%	<1%
Grade 4	<25	1%	<1%
Blood chemistry			
Fasting (non-random) serum glucose test (mg/dL)			
Grade 2	126 - 250	10%	7%
Grade 3	251 - 500	3%	1%
Grade 4	>500	0%	0%
Total serum bilirubin			
Grade 2	1.6 - 2.5 × ULN	6%	3%
Grade 3	2.6 - 5.0 × ULN	3%	3%
Grade 4	>5.0 × ULN	1%	0%
Serum aspartate aminotransferase			
Grade 2	2.6 - 5.0 × ULN	9%	7%
Grade 3	5.1 - 10.0 × ULN	4%	3%
Grade 4	>10.0 × ULN	1%	1%
Serum alanine aminotransferase			
Grade 2	2.6 - 5.0 × ULN	9%	9%
Grade 3	5.1 - 10.0 × ULN	4%	2%
Grade 4	>10.0 × ULN	1%	2%
Serum alkaline phosphatase			
Grade 2	2.6 - 5.0 × ULN	2%	<1%
Grade 3	5.1 - 10.0 × ULN	<1%	1%
Grade 4	>10.0 × ULN	1%	<1%
Serum pancreatic amylase test			
Grade 2	1.6 - 2.0 × ULN	2%	1%
Grade 3	2.1 - 5.0 × ULN	4%	3%
Grade 4	>5.0 × ULN	<1%	<1%
Serum lipase test			
Grade 2	1.6 - 3.0 × ULN	5%	4%
Grade 3	3.1 - 5.0 × ULN	2%	1%
Grade 4	>5.0 × ULN	0%	0%
Serum creatine kinase			
Grade 2	6.0 - 9.9 × ULN	2%	2%
Grade 3	10.0 - 19.9 × ULN	4%	3%
Grade 4	≥20.0 × ULN	3%	1%

ULN = Upper limit of normal range

Table 6: Selected Drug Interactions

Concomitant Drug Class: Drug Name	Effect on Concentration of Raltegravir	Clinical Comment
HIV-1-Antiviral Agents		
atazanavir	↑	Atazanavir, a strong inhibitor of UGT1A1, increases plasma concentrations of raltegravir. However, since concomitant use of ISENTRESS with atazanavir/ritonavir did not result in a unique safety signal in Phase 3 studies, no dose adjustment is recommended.
atazanavir/ritonavir	↑	Atazanavir/ritonavir increases plasma concentrations of raltegravir. However, since concomitant use of ISENTRESS with atazanavir/ritonavir did not result in a unique safety signal in Phase 3 studies, no dose adjustment is recommended.
efavirenz	↓	Efavirenz reduces plasma concentrations of raltegravir. The clinical significance of this interaction has not been directly assessed.
etravirine	↓	Etravirine reduces plasma concentrations of raltegravir. The clinical significance of this interaction has not been directly assessed.
tipranavir/ritonavir	↓	Tipranavir/ritonavir reduces plasma concentrations of raltegravir. However, since comparable efficacy was observed for this combination relative to other ISENTRESS-containing regimens in Phase 3 studies 018 and 019, no dose adjustment is recommended.
Other Agents		
omeprazole	↑	Coadministration of medicinal products that increase gastric pH (e.g., omeprazole) may increase raltegravir levels based on increased raltegravir solubility at higher pH. However, since concomitant use of ISENTRESS with proton pump inhibitors and H2 blockers did not result in a unique safety signal in Phase 3 studies, no dose adjustment is recommended.
rifampin	↓	Rifampin, a strong inducer of UGT1A1, reduces plasma concentrations of raltegravir. The recommended dosage of ISENTRESS is 800 mg twice daily during coadministration with rifampin.

titanium dioxide, polyethylene glycol 3350, talc, red iron oxide and black iron oxide.

12 CLINICAL PHARMACOLOGY

12.1 Mechanism of Action

Raltegravir is an HIV-1 antiviral drug [see Clinical Pharmacology (12.4)].

12.2 Pharmacodynamics

In a monotherapy study raltegravir (400 mg twice daily) demonstrated rapid antiviral activity with mean viral load reduction of $1.66 \log_{10}$ copies/mL by Day 10.

In the randomized, double-blind, placebo-controlled, dose-ranging trial, Protocol 005, and Protocols 018 and 019, antiviral responses were similar among subjects regardless of dose.

Effects on Electrocardiogram

In a randomized, placebo-controlled, crossover study, 31 healthy subjects were administered a single oral supra-therapeutic dose of raltegravir 1600 mg and placebo. Peak raltegravir plasma concentrations were approximately 4-fold higher than the peak concentrations following a 400 mg dose. ISENTRESS did not appear to prolong the QTc interval for 12 hours postdose. After baseline and placebo adjustment, the maximum mean QTc change was -0.4 msec (1-sided 95% upper CI: 3.1 msec).

12.3 Pharmacokinetics

Absorption

Raltegravir is absorbed with a T_{max} of approximately 3 hours postdose in the fasted state. Raltegravir AUC and C_{max} increase dose proportionally over the dose range 100 mg to 1600 mg. Raltegravir C_{12hr} increases dose proportionally over the dose range of 100 to 800 mg and increases slightly less than dose proportionally over the dose range 100 mg to 1600 mg. With twice-daily dosing, pharmacokinetic steady state is achieved within approximately the first 2 days of dosing. There is little to no accumulation in AUC and C_{max}. The average accumulation ratio for C_{12hr} ranged from approximately 1.2 to 1.6.

The absolute bioavailability of raltegravir has not been established.

In subjects who received 400 mg twice daily alone, raltegravir drug exposures were characterized by a geometric mean AUC_{0-12hr} of 14.3 μM•hr and C_{12hr} of 142 nM. Considerable variability was observed in the pharmacokinetics of raltegravir. For observed C_{12hr} in Protocols 018 and

019, the coefficient of variation (CV) for inter-subject variability = 212% and the CV for intra-subject variability = 122%.

Effect of Food on Oral Absorption

ISENTRESS may be administered with or without food. Raltegravir was administered without regard to food in the pivotal safety and efficacy studies in HIV-1-infected patients. The effect of consumption of low-, moderate- and high-fat meals on steady-state raltegravir pharmacokinetics was assessed in healthy volunteers. Administration of multiple doses of raltegravir following a moderate-fat meal (600 Kcal, 21 g fat) did not affect raltegravir AUC to a clinically meaningful degree with an increase of 13% relative to fasting. Raltegravir C_{12hr} was 66% higher and C_{max} was 5% higher following a moderate-fat meal compared to fasting. Administration of raltegravir following a high-fat meal (825 Kcal, 52 g fat) increased AUC and C_{max} by approximately 2-fold and increased C_{12hr} by 4.1-fold. Administration of raltegravir following a low-fat meal (300 Kcal, 2.5 g fat) decreased AUC and C_{max} by 46% and 52%, respectively; C_{12hr} was essentially unchanged. Food appears to increase pharmacokinetic variability relative to fasting.

Distribution

Raltegravir is approximately 83% bound to human plasma protein over the concentration range of 2 to 10 μM.

Metabolism and Excretion

The apparent terminal half-life of raltegravir is approximately 9 hours, with a shorter α-phase half-life (~1 hour) accounting for much of the AUC. Following administration of an oral dose of radiolabeled raltegravir, approximately 51 and 32% of the dose was excreted in feces and urine, respectively. In feces, only raltegravir was present, most of which is likely derived from hydrolysis of raltegravir-glucuronide secreted in bile as observed in preclinical species. Two components, namely raltegravir and raltegravir-glucuronide, were detected in urine and accounted for approximately 9 and 23% of the dose, respectively. The major circulating entity was raltegravir and represented approximately 70% of the total radioactivity; the remaining radioactivity in plasma was accounted for by raltegravir-glucuronide. Studies using isoform-selective chemical inhibitors and cDNA-expressed UDP-glucuronosyltransferases (UGT) show that UGT1A1 is the main enzyme responsible for the formation of raltegravir-glucuronide. Thus, the data indicate that the major mechanism of clearance of raltegravir in humans is UGT1A1-mediated glucuronidation.

Special Populations

Pediatric

The pharmacokinetics of raltegravir in pediatric patients has not been established.

Age

The effect of age on the pharmacokinetics of raltegravir was evaluated in the composite analysis. No dosage adjustment is necessary.

Race

The effect of race on the pharmacokinetics of raltegravir was evaluated in the composite analysis. No dosage adjustment is necessary.

Gender

A study of the pharmacokinetics of raltegravir was performed in healthy adult males and females. Additionally, the effect of gender was evaluated in a composite analysis of pharmacokinetic data from 103 healthy subjects and 28 HIV-1 infected subjects receiving raltegravir monotherapy with fasted administration. No dosage adjustment is necessary.

Hepatic Impairment

Raltegravir is eliminated primarily by glucuronidation in the liver. A study of the pharmacokinetics of raltegravir was performed in subjects with moderate hepatic impairment. Additionally, hepatic impairment was evaluated in the composite pharmacokinetic analysis. There were no clinically important pharmacokinetic differences between subjects with moderate hepatic impairment and healthy subjects. No dosage adjustment is necessary for patients with mild to moderate hepatic impairment. The effect of severe hepatic impairment on the pharmacokinetics of raltegravir has not been studied.

Renal Impairment

Renal clearance of unchanged drug is a minor pathway of elimination. A study of the pharmacokinetics of raltegravir was performed in subjects with severe renal impairment. Additionally, renal impairment was evaluated in the composite pharmacokinetic analysis. There were no clinically important pharmacokinetic differences between subjects with severe renal impairment and healthy subjects. No dosage adjustment is necessary. Because the extent to which ISENTRESS may be dialyzable is unknown, dosing before a dialysis session should be avoided.

UGT1A1 Polymorphism

There is no evidence that common UGT1A1 polymorphisms alter raltegravir pharmacokinetics to a clinically meaningful extent. In a comparison of 30 subjects with *28/*28 genotype (associated with reduced activity of UGT1A1) to 27 subjects with wild-type genotype, the geometric mean ratio (90% CI) of AUC was 1.41 (0.96, 2.09).

Drug Interactions [see Drug Interactions (7)]

[See table 7 at top of next page]

12.4 Microbiology

Mechanism of Action

Raltegravir inhibits the catalytic activity of HIV-1 integrase, an HIV-1 encoded enzyme that is required for viral replication. Inhibition of integrase prevents the covalent insertion, or integration, of unintegrated linear HIV-1 DNA into the host cell genome preventing the formation of the HIV-1 provirus. The provirus is required to direct the production of progeny virus, so inhibiting integration prevents propagation of the viral infection. Raltegravir did not significantly inhibit human phosphoryltransferases including DNA polymerases α, β, and γ.

Antiviral Activity in Cell Culture

Raltegravir at concentrations of 31 ± 20 nM resulted in 95% inhibition (EC_{95}) of viral spread (relative to an untreated virus-infected culture) in human T-lymphoid cell cultures infected with the cell-line adapted HIV-1 variant H9IIIB. In addition, 5 clinical isolates of HIV-1 subtype B had EC_{95} values ranging from 9 to 19 nM in cultures of mitogen-activated human peripheral blood mononuclear cells. In a single-cycle infection assay, raltegravir inhibited infection of 23 HIV-1 isolates representing 5 non-B subtypes (A, C, D, F, and G) and 5 circulating recombinant forms (AE, AG, BF, BG, and cpx) with EC_{50} values ranging from 5 to 12 nM. Raltegravir also inhibited replication of an HIV-2 isolate when tested in CEM×174 cells (EC_{95} value = 6 nM). Additive to synergistic antiretroviral activity was observed when human T-lymphoid cells infected with the H9IIIB variant of HIV-1 were incubated with raltegravir in combination with non-nucleoside reverse transcriptase inhibitors (delavirdine, efavirenz, or nevirapine); nucleoside analog reverse transcriptase inhibitors (abacavir, didanosine, lamivudine, stavudine, tenofovir, zalcitabine, or zidovudine); protease inhibitors (amprenavir, atazanavir, indinavir, lopinavir, nelfinavir, ritonavir, or saquinavir); or the entry inhibitor enfuvirtide.

Resistance

The mutations observed in the HIV-1 integrase coding sequence that contributed to raltegravir resistance (evolved

Table 7: Effect of Other Agents on the Pharmacokinetics of Raltegravir

Coadministered Drug	Coadministered Drug Dose/Schedule	Raltegravir Dose/Schedule	n	Ratio (90% Confidence Interval) of Raltegravir Pharmacokinetic Parameters with/without Coadministered Drug; No Effect = 1.00		
				C_{max}	AUC	C_{min}
atazanavir	400 mg daily	100 mg single dose	10	1.53 (1.11, 2.12)	1.72 (1.47, 2.02)	1.95 (1.30, 2.92)
atazanavir/ ritonavir	300 mg/100 mg daily	400 mg twice daily	10	1.24 (0.87, 1.77)	1.41 (1.12, 1.78)	1.77 (1.39, 2.25)
efavirenz	600 mg daily	400 mg single dose	9	0.64 (0.41, 0.98)	0.64 (0.52, 0.80)	0.79 (0.49, 1.28)
etravirine	200 mg twice daily	400 mg twice daily	19	0.89 (0.68, 1.15)	0.90 (0.68, 1.18)	0.66 (0.34, 1.26)
omeprazole	20 mg daily	400 mg single dose	14 (10 for AUC)	4.15 (2.82, 6.10)	3.12 (2.13, 4.56)	1.46 (1.10, 1.93)
rifampin	600 mg daily	400 mg single dose	9	0.62 (0.37, 1.04)	0.60 (0.39, 0.91)	0.39 (0.30 0.51)
rifampin	600 mg daily	400 mg twice daily when administered alone; 800 mg twice daily when administered with rifampin	14	1.62 (1.12, 2.33)	1.27 (0.94 1.71)	0.47 (0.36, 0.61)
ritonavir	100 mg twice daily	400 mg single dose	10	0.76 (0.55, 1.04)	0.84 (0.70, 1.01)	0.99 (0.70, 1.40)
tenofovir	300 mg daily	400 mg twice daily	9	1.64 (1.16, 2.32)	1.49 (1.15, 1.94)	1.03 (0.73, 1.45)
tipranavir/ ritonavir	500 mg/200 mg twice daily	400 mg twice daily	15 (14 for C_{min})	0.82 (0.46, 1.46)	0.76 (0.49, 1.19)	0.45 (0.31, 0.66)

either in cell culture or in subjects treated with raltegravir) generally included an amino acid substitution at either Y143 (changed to C, H, or R) or Q148 (changed to H, K, or R) or N155 (changed to H) plus one or more additional substitutions (i.e., L74M, E92Q, T97A, E138A/K, G140A/S, V151I, G163R, H183P, Y226C/D/F/H, S230R, and D232N).

Treatment-Naïve Subjects: By Week 96 in the STARTMRK trial, the primary raltegravir resistance-associated substitutions were observed in 4 (2 with Y143H/R and 2 with Q148H/R) of the 10 virologic failure subjects with evaluable genotypic data from paired baseline and raltegravir treatment-failure isolates.

Treatment-Experienced Subjects: By Week 96 in the BENCHMRK trials, at least one of the primary raltegravir resistance-associated substitutions, Y143C/H/R, Q148H/ K/R, and N155H, was observed in 76 of the 112 virologic failure subjects with evaluable genotypic data from paired baseline and raltegravir treatment-failure isolates. The emergence of the primary raltegravir resistance-associated substitutions was observed cumulatively in 70 subjects by Week 48 and 78 subjects by Week 96, 15.2% and 17% of the raltegravir recipients, respectively. Some (n=58) of those HIV-1 isolates harboring one or more of the primary raltegravir resistance-associated substitutions were evaluated for raltegravir susceptibility yielding a median decrease of 26.3-fold (mean 48.9 ± 44.8-fold decrease, ranging from 0.8- to 159-fold) compared to the wild-type reference.

13 NONCLINICAL TOXICOLOGY

13.1 Carcinogenesis, Mutagenesis, Impairment of Fertility

Carcinogenicity studies of raltegravir in mice did not show any carcinogenic potential. At the highest dose levels, 400 mg/kg/day in females and 250 mg/kg/day in males, systemic exposure was 1.8-fold (females) or 1.2-fold (males) greater than the AUC (54 μM•hr) at the 400-mg twice daily human dose. Treatment-related squamous cell carcinoma of nose/nasopharynx was observed in female rats dosed with *600 mg/kg/day raltegravir for 104 weeks. These tumors* were possibly the result of local deposition and/or aspiration of drug in the mucosa of the nose/nasopharynx during dosing. No tumors of the nose/nasopharynx were observed in rats dosed with 150 mg/kg/day (males) and 50 mg/kg/day (females) and the systemic exposure in rats was 1.7-fold (males) to 1.4-fold (females) greater than the AUC (54 μM•hr) at the 400-mg twice daily human dose.

No evidence of mutagenicity or genotoxicity was observed in *in vitro* microbial mutagenesis (Ames) tests, *in vitro* alkaline elution assays for DNA breakage, and *in vitro* and *in vivo* chromosomal aberration studies.

No effect on fertility was seen in male and female rats at doses up to 600 mg/kg/day which resulted in a 3-fold exposure above the exposure at the recommended human dose.

14 CLINICAL STUDIES

Description of Clinical Studies

The evidence of durable efficacy of ISENTRESS is based on the analyses of 96-week data from an ongoing, randomized, double-blind, active-control trial, STARTMRK (Protocol 021) in antiretroviral treatment-naïve HIV-1 infected adult subjects and from 2 ongoing, randomized, double-blind, placebo-controlled studies, BENCHMRK 1 and BENCHMRK 2 (Protocols 018 and 019), in antiretroviral treatment-experienced HIV-1 infected adult subjects.

Treatment-Naïve Subjects

STARTMRK (Protocol 021) is a Phase 3 study to evaluate the safety and antiretroviral activity of ISENTRESS 400 mg twice daily + emtricitabine (+) tenofovir versus efavirenz 600 mg at bedtime plus emtricitabine (+) tenofovir in treatment-naïve HIV-1-infected subjects with HIV-1 RNA >5000 copies/mL. Randomization was stratified by screening HIV-1 RNA level (≤50,000 copies/mL; and >50,000 copies/mL) and by hepatitis status.

Table 8 shows the demographic characteristics of subjects in the group receiving ISENTRESS 400 mg twice daily and subjects in the comparator group.

Table 8: Baseline Characteristics

Randomized Study Protocol 021	ISENTRESS 400 mg Twice Daily (N = 281)	Efavirenz 600 mg At Bedtime (N = 282)
Gender		
Male	81%	82%
Female	19%	18%
Race		
White	41%	44%
Black	12%	8%
Asian	13%	11%
Hispanic	21%	24%
Native American	<1%	<1%
Multiracial	12%	13%
Region		
Latin America	35%	34%
Southeast Asia	12%	10%
North America	29%	32%
EU/Australia	23%	23%
Age (years)		
18-64	99%	99%
≥65	1%	1%
Mean (SD)	38 (9)	37 (10)
Median (min, max)	37 (19 to 67)	36 (19 to 71)
CD4+ Cell Count (cells/ microL)		
Mean (SD)	219 (124)	217 (134)
Median (min, max)	212 (1 to 620)	204 (4 to 807)
Plasma HIV-1 RNA (log_{10} copies/mL)		
Mean (SD)	5 (1)	5 (1)
Median (min, max)	5 (3 to 6)	5 (4 to 6)
Plasma HIV-1 RNA (copies/mL)		
Geometric Mean	103205	106215
Median (min, max)	114000 (400 to 750000)	104000 (4410 to 750000)
History of AIDS*		
Yes	19%	21%
Viral Subtype		
Clade B	78%	82%
Non-Clade B[†]	21%	17%
Baseline Plasma HIV-1 RNA		
≤100,000 copies/mL	45%	49%
>100,000 copies/mL	55%	51%
Baseline CD4+ Cell Counts		
≤50 cells/mm³	10%	11%
>50 cells/mm³ and ≤200 cells/mm³	37%	37%
>200 cells/mm³	53%	51%
Hepatitis Status		
Hepatitis B or C Positive[‡]	6%	6%

* Includes additional subjects identified as having a history of AIDS.
† Non-Clade B Subtypes (# of subjects): Clade A (4), A/C (1), A/G (2), A1 (1), AE (29), AG (12), BF (6), C (37), D (2), F (2), F1 (5), G (2), Complex (3).
‡ Evidence of hepatitis B surface antigen or evidence of HCV RNA by polymerase chain reaction (PCR) quantitative test for hepatitis C Virus.
Notes:
ISENTRESS and Efavirenz were administered with emtricitabine (+) tenofovir
N = Number of subjects in each group

Week 96 outcomes from Protocol 021 are shown in Table 9. [See table 9 at top of next page]

The mean changes in CD4 count from baseline were 217 cells/mm³ in the group receiving ISENTRESS 400 mg twice daily and 199 cells/mm³ in the group receiving Efavirenz 600 mg at bedtime.

Treatment-Experienced Subjects

BENCHMRK 1 and BENCHMRK 2 are Phase 3 studies to evaluate the safety and antiretroviral activity of ISENTRESS 400 mg twice daily in combination with an optimized background therapy (OBT), versus OBT alone, in HIV-1-infected subjects, 16 years or older, with documented resistance to at least 1 drug in each of 3 classes (NNRTIs, NRTIs, PIs) of antiretroviral therapies. Randomization was stratified by degree of resistance to PI (1PI vs. >1PI) and the use of enfuvirtide in the OBT. Prior to randomization, OBT was selected by the investigator based on genotypic/ phenotypic resistance testing and prior ART history.

Table 10 shows the demographic characteristics of subjects in the group receiving ISENTRESS 400 mg twice daily and subjects in the placebo group.
[See table 10 on next page]

Table 11 compares the characteristics of optimized background therapy at baseline in the group receiving ISENTRESS 400 mg twice daily and subjects in the control group.
[See table 11 at top of page 2141]

Table 9: Virologic Outcomes of Randomized Treatment of Protocol 021 at 96 Weeks

	ISENTRESS 400 mg Twice Daily (N = 281)	Efavirenz 600 mg At Bedtime (N = 282)	Difference (ISENTRESS–Efavirenz) (CI)
Subjects with HIV-1 RNA less than 50 copies/mL	82%	78%	3.8% (-2.8%, 10.4%)
Virologic Failure*	9%	10%	
No virologic data at Week 96 Window Reasons			
Discontinued study due to AE or death†	4%	7%	
Discontinued study for other reasons‡	5%	4%	
Missing data during window but on study	1%	1%	

* Includes subjects who discontinued prior to Week 96 for lack of efficacy, subjects changed OBT due to lack of efficacy prior to Week 96, or subjects who are ≥50 copies in the 96 week window.
† Includes subjects who discontinued due to AE or Death at any time point from Day 1 through the Week 96 window if this resulted in no virologic data on treatment during Week 96 visit window.
‡ Other includes: withdrew consent, loss to follow-up, moved etc., if the viral load at the time of discontinuation was <50 copies/mL.

Table 10: Baseline Characteristics

Randomized Studies Protocol 018 and 019	ISENTRESS 400 mg Twice Daily + OBT (N = 462)	Placebo + OBT (N = 237)
Gender		
Male	88%	89%
Female	12%	11%
Race		
White	65%	73%
Black	14%	11%
Asian	3%	3%
Hispanic	11%	8%
Others	6%	5%
Age (years)		
Median (min, max)	45 (16 to 74)	45 (17 to 70)
CD4+ Cell Count		
Median (min, max), cells/mm^3	119 (1 to 792)	123 (0 to 759)
≤50 cells/mm^3	32%	33%
>50 and ≤200 cells/mm^3	37%	36%
Plasma HIV-1 RNA		
Median (min, max), log$_{10}$ copies/mL	4.8 (2 to 6)	4.7 (2 to 6)
>100,000 copies/mL	36%	33%
History of AIDS		
Yes	92%	91%
Prior Use of ART, Median (1st Quartile, 3rd Quartile)		
Years of ART Use	10 (7 to 12)	10 (8 to 12)
Number of ART	12 (9 to 15)	12 (9 to 14)
Hepatitis Co-infection*		
No Hepatitis B or C virus	83%	84%
Hepatitis B virus only	8%	3%
Hepatitis C virus only	8%	12%
Co-infection of Hepatitis B and C virus	1%	1%
Stratum		
Enfuvirtide in OBT	38%	38%
Resistant to ≥2 PI	97%	95%

* Hepatitis B virus surface antigen positive or hepatitis C virus antibody positive.

Week 96 outcomes for the 699 subjects randomized and treated with the recommended dose of ISENTRESS 400 mg twice daily or placebo in the pooled BENCHMRK 1 and 2 studies are shown in Table 12.
[See table 12 on next page]
The mean changes in CD4 count from baseline were 118 cells/mm^3 in the group receiving ISENTRESS 400 mg twice daily and 47 cells/mm^3 for the control group.
Treatment-emergent CDC Category C events occurred in 4% of the group receiving ISENTRESS 400 mg twice daily and 5% of the control group.
Virologic responses at Week 96 by baseline genotypic and phenotypic sensitivity score are shown in Table 13.
[See table 13 on next page]

16   HOW SUPPLIED/STORAGE AND HANDLING

ISENTRESS tablets 400 mg are pink, oval-shaped, film-coated tablets with "227" on one side. They are supplied as follows:
NDC 0006-0227-61 unit-of-use bottles of 60.
No. 3894

Storage and Handling
Store at 20-25°C (68-77°F); excursions permitted to 15-30°C (59-86°F). See USP Controlled Room Temperature.
Distributed by:
Merck Sharp & Dohme Corp., a subsidiary of Merck & Co., Inc.
Whitehouse Station, NJ 08889, USA
9795110
U.S. Patent Nos. US 7,169,780

17   PATIENT COUNSELING INFORMATION

[See FDA-Approved Patient Labeling.]
Patients should be informed that ISENTRESS is not a cure for HIV infection or AIDS. They should also be told that people taking ISENTRESS may still get infections or other conditions common in people with HIV (opportunistic infections). Patients should also be told that it is very important that they stay under a physician's care during treatment with ISENTRESS.
Patients should be informed that ISENTRESS does not reduce the chance of passing HIV to others through sexual contact, sharing needles, or being exposed to blood. Patients should be advised to continue to practice safer sex and to use latex or polyurethane condoms or other barrier methods to lower the chance of sexual contact with any body fluids such as semen, vaginal secretions or blood. Patients should also be advised to never re-use or share needles.
Physicians should instruct their patients that if they miss a dose, they should take it as soon as they remember. If they do not remember until it is time for the next dose, they should be instructed to skip the missed dose and go back to the regular schedule. Patients should not take two tablets of ISENTRESS at the same time.
Physicians should instruct their patients to read the Patient Package Insert before starting ISENTRESS therapy and to reread each time the prescription is renewed. Patients should be instructed to inform their physician or pharmacist if they develop any unusual symptom, or if any known symptom persists or worsens.

FDA-Approved Patient Labeling
Patient Information
ISENTRESS® (eye sen tris)
(raltegravir)
Tablets
Read the patient information that comes with ISENTRESS[1] before you start taking it and each time you get a refill. There may be new information. This leaflet is a summary of the information for patients. Your doctor or pharmacist can give you additional information. This leaflet does not take the place of talking with your doctor about your medical condition or your treatment.

What is ISENTRESS?
- ISENTRESS is an anti-HIV (antiretroviral) medicine used for the treatment of HIV. The term HIV stands for Human Immunodeficiency Virus. It is the virus that causes AIDS (Acquired Immune Deficiency Syndrome). ISENTRESS is used along with other anti-HIV medicines. ISENTRESS will NOT cure HIV infection.
- People taking ISENTRESS may still develop infections, including opportunistic infections or other conditions that happen with HIV infection.
- Stay under the care of your doctor during treatment with ISENTRESS.
- The safety and effectiveness of ISENTRESS in children has not been studied.

ISENTRESS must be used with other anti-HIV medicines.
How does ISENTRESS work?
- ISENTRESS blocks an enzyme which the virus (HIV) needs in order to make more virus. The enzyme that ISENTRESS blocks is called HIV integrase.
- When used with other anti-HIV medicines, ISENTRESS may do two things:
  1. Reduce the amount of HIV in your blood. This is called your "viral load".
  2. Increase the number of white blood cells called CD4 (T) cells.
- ISENTRESS may not have these effects in all patients.

Does ISENTRESS lower the chance of passing HIV to other people?
No. ISENTRESS does not reduce the chance of passing HIV to others through sexual contact, sharing needles, or being exposed to your blood.
- Continue to practice safer sex.
- Use latex or polyurethane condoms or other barrier methods to lower the chance of sexual contact with any body fluids. This includes semen from a man, vaginal secretions from a woman, or blood.
- Never re-use or share needles.
Ask your doctor if you have any questions about safer sex or how to prevent passing HIV to other people.

What should I tell my doctor before and during treatment with ISENTRESS?
Tell your doctor about all of your medical conditions. Include any of the following that applies to you:
- You have any allergies.
- You are pregnant or plan to become pregnant.
  - ISENTRESS is not recommended for use during pregnancy. ISENTRESS has not been studied in pregnant women. If you take ISENTRESS while you are pregnant, talk to your doctor about how you can be included in the Antiretroviral Pregnancy Registry.
- You are breast-feeding or plan to breast-feed.
  - It is recommended that HIV-infected women should not breast-feed their infants. This is because their babies could be infected with HIV through their breast milk.
  - Talk with your doctor about the best way to feed your baby.

Tell your doctor about all the medicines you take. Include the following:
- prescription medicines, including rifampin (a medicine used to treat some infections such as tuberculosis)
- non-prescription medicines

- vitamins
- herbal supplements

Know the medicines you take.

- Keep a list of your medicines. Show the list to your doctor and pharmacist when you get a new medicine.

How should I take ISENTRESS?
Take ISENTRESS exactly as your doctor has prescribed.
The recommended dose is as follows:

- Take only one 400-mg tablet at a time.
- Take it twice a day.
- Take it by mouth.
- Take it with or without food.

Do not change your dose or stop taking ISENTRESS or your other anti-HIV medicines without first talking with your doctor.

IMPORTANT: Take ISENTRESS exactly as your doctor prescribed and at the right times of day because if you don't:

- The amount of virus (HIV) in your blood may increase if the medicine is stopped for even a short period of time.
- The virus may develop resistance to ISENTRESS and become harder to treat.
- Your medicines may stop working to fight HIV.
- The activity of ISENTRESS may be reduced (due to resistance).

If you fail to take ISENTRESS the way you should, here's what to do:

- If you miss a dose, take it as soon as you remember. If you do not remember until it is time for your next dose, skip the missed dose and go back to your regular schedule. Do NOT take two tablets of ISENTRESS at the same time. In other words, do NOT take a double dose.
- If you take too much ISENTRESS, call your doctor or local Poison Control Center.

Be sure to keep a supply of your anti-HIV medicines.

- When your ISENTRESS supply starts to run low, get more from your doctor or pharmacy.
- Do not wait until your medicine runs out to get more.

What are the possible side effects of ISENTRESS?
When ISENTRESS has been given with other anti-HIV drugs, side effects included:

- nausea
- headache
- tiredness
- weakness
- trouble sleeping
- stomach pain
- dizziness
- depression
- suicidal thoughts and actions

Other side effects include rash, severe skin reactions, feeling anxious, paranoia, low blood platelet count.

A condition called Immune Reconstitution Syndrome can happen in some patients with advanced HIV infection (AIDS) when combination antiretroviral treatment is started. Signs and symptoms of inflammation from opportunistic infections that a person has or had may occur as the medicines work to treat the HIV infection and help to strengthen the immune system. Call your doctor right away if you notice any signs or symptoms of an infection after starting ISENTRESS with other anti-HIV medicines.

Contact your doctor promptly if you experience unexplained muscle pain, tenderness, or weakness while taking ISENTRESS. This is because on rare occasions, muscle problems can be serious and can lead to kidney damage.

Rash occurred more often in patients taking ISENTRESS and darunavir together than with either drug separately, but was generally mild.

Tell your doctor if you have any side effects that bother you. These are not all the side effects of ISENTRESS. For more information, ask your doctor or pharmacist.

How should I store ISENTRESS?

- Store ISENTRESS at room temperature (68 to 77°F).
- **Keep ISENTRESS and all medicines out of the reach of children.**

General information about the use of ISENTRESS
Medicines are sometimes prescribed for conditions that are not mentioned in patient information leaflets.

- Do not use ISENTRESS for a condition for which it was not prescribed.
- Do not give ISENTRESS to other people, even if they have the same symptoms you have. It may harm them.

This leaflet gives you the most important information about ISENTRESS.

- If you would like to know more, talk with your doctor.
- You can ask your doctor or pharmacist for additional information about ISENTRESS that is written for health professionals.
- For more information go to www.ISENTRESS.com or call 1-800-622-4477.

What are the ingredients in ISENTRESS?
Active ingredient: Each film-coated tablet contains 400 mg of raltegravir.

Table 11: Characteristics of Optimized Background Therapy at Baseline

Randomized Studies Protocol 018 and 019	ISENTRESS 400 mg Twice Daily + OBT (N = 462)	Placebo + OBT (N = 237)
Number of ARTs in OBT Median (min, max)	4 (1 to 7)	4 (2 to 7)
Number of Active PI in OBT by Phenotypic Resistance Test*		
0	36%	41%
1 or more	60%	58%
Phenotypic Sensitivity Score (PSS)†		
0	15%	18%
1	31%	30%
2	31%	28%
3 or more	18%	20%
Genotypic Sensitivity Score (GSS)†		
0	25%	27%
1	38%	40%
2	24%	21%
3 or more	11%	10%

* Darunavir use in OBT in darunavir-naïve subjects was counted as one active PI.
† The Phenotypic Sensitivity Score (PSS) and the Genotypic Sensitivity Score (GSS) were defined as the total oral ARTs in OBT to which a subject's viral isolate showed phenotypic sensitivity and genotypic sensitivity, respectively, based upon phenotypic and genotypic resistance tests. Enfuvirtide use in OBT in enfuvirtide-naïve subjects was counted as one active drug in OBT in the GSS and PSS. Similarly, darunavir use in OBT in darunavir-naïve subjects was counted as one active drug in OBT.

Table 12: Virologic Outcomes of Randomized Treatment of Protocols 018 and 019 at 96 Weeks (Pooled Analysis)

	ISENTRESS 400 mg Twice Daily + OBT (N = 462)	Placebo + OBT (N = 237)
Subjects with HIV-1 RNA less than 50 copies/mL	55%	27%
Virologic Failure*	35%	66%
No virologic data at Week 96 Window Reasons		
Discontinued study due to AE or death†	3%	3%
Discontinued study for other reasons‡	4%	4%
Missing data during window but on study	4%	<1%

* Includes subjects who switched to open-label raltegravir after Week 16 due to the protocol-defined virologic failure, subjects who discontinued prior to Week 96 for lack of efficacy, subjects changed OBT due to lack of efficacy prior to Week 96, or subjects who were ≥50 copies in the 96 week window.
† Includes subjects who discontinued due to AE or Death at any time point from Day 1 through the Week 96 window if this resulted in no virologic data on treatment during the Week 96 window.
‡ Other includes: withdrew consent, loss to follow-up, moved etc., if the viral load at the time of discontinuation was <50 copies/mL.

Table 13: Virologic Response at 96 Week Window by Baseline Genotypic/Phenotypic Sensitivity Score

	Percent with HIV-1 RNA <50 copies/mL At Week 96			
	ISENTRESS 400 mg Twice Daily + OBT (N = 462)		Placebo + OBT (N = 237)	
	n		n	
Phenotypic Sensitivity Score (PSS)*				
0	67	43	43	5
1	144	58	71	23
2	142	61	66	32
3 or more	85	48	48	42
Genotypic Sensitivity Score (GSS)*				
0	116	39	65	5
1	177	62	95	26
2	111	61	49	53
3 or more	51	49	23	35

* The Phenotypic Sensitivity Score (PSS) and the Genotypic Sensitivity Score (GSS) were defined as the total oral ARTs in OBT to which a subject's viral isolate showed phenotypic sensitivity and genotypic sensitivity, respectively, based upon phenotypic and genotypic resistance tests. Enfuvirtide use in OBT in enfuvirtide-naïve subjects was counted as one active drug in OBT in the GSS and PSS. Similarly, darunavir use in OBT in darunavir-naïve subjects was counted as one active drug in OBT.

Inactive ingredients: Microcrystalline cellulose, lactose monohydrate, calcium phosphate dibasic anhydrous, hypromellose 2208, poloxamer 407 (contains 0.01% butyl- ated hydroxytoluene as antioxidant), sodium stearyl fumarate, magnesium stearate. In addition, the film coating contains the following inactive ingredients: polyvinyl alcohol, titanium dioxide, polyethylene glycol 3350, talc, red iron oxide and black iron oxide.

Distributed by:

Merck Sharp & Dohme Corp., a subsidiary of Merck & Co., Inc.

Whitehouse Station, NJ 08889, USA

Revised June 2010

9795110

U.S. Patent Nos. US 7,169,780

Shown in Product Identification Guide, page 313

JANUMET® ℞

[*JAN-you-met*]

(sitagliptin/metformin HCl)

Tablets

HIGHLIGHTS OF PRESCRIBING INFORMATION

These highlights do not include all the information needed to use JANUMET safely and effectively. See full prescribing information for JANUMET.

JANUMET® (sitagliptin/metformin HCl) tablets

Initial U.S. Approval: 2007

WARNING: LACTIC ACIDOSIS

See full prescribing information for complete boxed warning.

- Lactic acidosis can occur due to metformin accumulation. The risk increases with conditions such as sepsis, dehydration, excess alcohol intake, hepatic insufficiency, renal impairment, and acute congestive heart failure. (5.1)
- Symptoms include malaise, myalgias, respiratory distress, increasing somnolence, and nonspecific abdominal distress. Laboratory abnormalities include low pH, increased anion gap and elevated blood lactate. (5.1)
- If acidosis is suspected, discontinue JANUMET and hospitalize the patient immediately. (5.1)

———RECENT MAJOR CHANGES———

Indications and Usage (1)	02/2010
Dosage and Administration	
Recommended Dosing (2.1)	02/2010
Warnings and Precautions	
Pancreatitis (5.2)	12/2009
Use with Medications Known to Cause	
Hypoglycemia (5.9)	02/2010

———INDICATIONS AND USAGE———

JANUMET is a dipeptidyl peptidase-4 (DPP-4) inhibitor and biguanide combination product indicated as an adjunct to diet and exercise to improve glycemic control in adults with type 2 diabetes mellitus when treatment with both sitagliptin and metformin is appropriate. (1)

Important Limitations of Use:
- JANUMET should not be used in patients with type 1 diabetes or for the treatment of diabetic ketoacidosis. (1)
- JANUMET has not been studied in patients with a history of pancreatitis. (1, 5.2)

———DOSAGE AND ADMINISTRATION———

- Individualize the starting dose of JANUMET based on the patient's current regimen. (2.1)
- May adjust the dosing based on effectiveness and tolerability while not exceeding the maximum recommended daily dose of 100 mg sitagliptin and 2000 mg metformin. (2.1)
- JANUMET should be given twice daily with meals, with gradual dose escalation, to reduce the gastrointestinal (GI) side effects due to metformin. (2.1)

———DOSAGE FORMS AND STRENGTHS———

Tablets: 50 mg sitagliptin/500 mg metformin HCl and 50 mg sitagliptin/1000 mg metformin HCl (3)

———CONTRAINDICATIONS———

- Renal dysfunction, e.g., serum creatinine ≥1.5 mg/dL [males], ≥1.4 mg/dL [females] or abnormal creatinine clearance. (4, 5.1, 5.4)
- Acute or chronic metabolic acidosis, including diabetic ketoacidosis, with or without coma. (4, 5.1)
- History of a serious hypersensitivity reaction to JANUMET or sitagliptin (one of the components of JANUMET), such as anaphylaxis or angioedema. (5.14, 6.2)
- Temporarily discontinue JANUMET in patients undergoing radiologic studies involving intravascular administration of iodinated contrast materials. (4, 5.1, 5.11)

———WARNINGS AND PRECAUTIONS———

- Do not use JANUMET in patients with hepatic disease. (5.1, 5.3)
- Before initiating JANUMET and at least annually thereafter, assess renal function and verify as normal. (4, 5.1, 5.4, 5.10)
- There have been postmarketing reports of acute pancreatitis, including fatal and non-fatal hemorrhagic or necrotizing pancreatitis. If pancreatitis is suspected, promptly discontinue JANUMET. (5.2)
- Measure hematologic parameters annually. (5.5, 6.1)
- Warn patients against excessive alcohol intake. (5.1, 5.6)
- May need to discontinue JANUMET and temporarily use insulin during periods of stress and decreased intake of fluids and food as may occur with fever, trauma, infection or surgery. (5.7, 5.8, 5.12, 5.13)
- Promptly evaluate patients previously controlled on JANUMET who develop laboratory abnormalities or clinical illness for evidence of ketoacidosis or lactic acidosis. (5.1, 5.8, 5.12, 5.13)
- When used with an insulin secretagogue (e.g., sulfonylurea) or with insulin, a lower dose of the insulin secretagogue or insulin may be required to reduce the risk of hypoglycemia. (2.1, 5.9)
- There have been postmarketing reports of serious allergic and hypersensitivity reactions in patients treated with sitagliptin (one of the components of JANUMET), such as anaphylaxis, angioedema, and exfoliative skin conditions including Stevens-Johnson syndrome. In such cases, promptly stop JANUMET, assess for other potential causes, institute appropriate monitoring and treatment, and initiate alternative treatment for diabetes. (5.14, 6.2)
- There have been no clinical studies establishing conclusive evidence of macrovascular risk reduction with JANUMET or any other anti-diabetic drug. (5.15)

———ADVERSE REACTIONS———

- The most common adverse reactions reported in ≥5% of patients simultaneously started on sitagliptin and metformin and more commonly than in patients treated with placebo were diarrhea, upper respiratory tract infection, and headache. (6.1)
- Adverse reactions reported in ≥5% of patients treated with sitagliptin in combination with sulfonylurea and metformin and more commonly than in patients treated with placebo in combination with sulfonylurea and metformin were hypoglycemia and headache. (6.1)
- Hypoglycemia was the only adverse reaction reported in ≥5% of patients treated with sitagliptin in combination with insulin and metformin and more commonly than in patients treated with placebo in combination with insulin and metformin. (6.1)
- Nasopharyngitis was the only adverse reaction reported in ≥5% of patients treated with sitagliptin monotherapy and more commonly than in patients given placebo. (6.1)
- The most common (>5%) adverse reactions due to initiation of metformin therapy are diarrhea, nausea/vomiting, flatulence, abdominal discomfort, indigestion, asthenia, and headache. (6.1)

To report SUSPECTED ADVERSE REACTIONS, contact Merck Sharp & Dohme Corp., a subsidiary of Merck & Co., Inc., at 1-877-888-4231 or FDA at 1-800-FDA-1088 or www.fda.gov/medwatch.

———DRUG INTERACTIONS———

- Cationic drugs eliminated by renal tubular secretion: Use with caution. (5.10, 7.1)

———USE IN SPECIFIC POPULATIONS———

- Safety and effectiveness of JANUMET in children under 18 years have not been established. (8.4)
- There are no adequate and well-controlled studies in pregnant women. To report drug exposure during pregnancy call 1-800-986-8999. (8.1)

See 17 for PATIENT COUNSELING INFORMATION and FDA-approved Medication Guide

Revised: 02/2010

FULL PRESCRIBING INFORMATION

WARNING: LACTIC ACIDOSIS

Lactic acidosis is a rare, but serious complication that can occur due to metformin accumulation. The risk increases with conditions such as sepsis, dehydration, excess alcohol intake, hepatic insufficiency, renal impairment, and acute congestive heart failure.

The onset is often subtle, accompanied only by nonspecific symptoms such as malaise, myalgias, respiratory distress, increasing somnolence, and nonspecific abdominal distress.

Laboratory abnormalities include low pH, increased anion gap and elevated blood lactate.

If acidosis is suspected, JANUMET[1] should be discontinued and the patient hospitalized immediately. [*See Warnings and Precautions (5.1).*]

---

1 INDICATIONS AND USAGE

JANUMET is indicated as an adjunct to diet and exercise to improve glycemic control in adults with type 2 diabetes mellitus when treatment with both sitagliptin and metformin is appropriate. [*See Clinical Studies (14).*]

Important Limitations of Use

JANUMET should not be used in patients with type 1 diabetes or for the treatment of diabetic ketoacidosis, as it would not be effective in these settings.

JANUMET has not been studied in patients with a history of pancreatitis. It is unknown whether patients with a history of pancreatitis are at increased risk for the development of pancreatitis while using JANUMET. [*See Warnings and Precautions (5.2).*]

2 DOSAGE AND ADMINISTRATION

2.1 Recommended Dosing

The dosage of JANUMET should be individualized on the basis of the patient's current regimen, effectiveness, and tolerability while not exceeding the maximum recommended daily dose of 100 mg sitagliptin and 2000 mg metformin. Initial combination therapy or maintenance of combination therapy should be individualized and left to the discretion of the health care provider.

JANUMET should generally be given twice daily with meals, with gradual dose escalation, to reduce the gastrointestinal (GI) side effects due to metformin.

The starting dose of JANUMET should be based on the patient's current regimen. JANUMET should be given twice daily with meals. The following doses are available:

50 mg sitagliptin/500 mg metformin hydrochloride

50 mg sitagliptin/1000 mg metformin hydrochloride.

The recommended starting dose in patients not currently treated with metformin is 50 mg sitagliptin/500 mg metformin hydrochloride twice daily, with gradual dose escalation recommended to reduce gastrointestinal side effects associated with metformin.

The starting dose in patients already treated with metformin should provide sitagliptin dosed as 50 mg twice daily (100 mg total daily dose) and the dose of metformin already being taken. For patients taking metformin 850 mg twice daily, the recommended starting dose of JANUMET is 50 mg sitagliptin/1000 mg metformin hydrochloride twice daily.

Patients treated with an insulin secretagogue or insulin
Co-administration of JANUMET with an insulin secretagogue (e.g., sulfonylurea) or insulin may require lower doses of the insulin secretagogue or insulin to reduce the risk of hypoglycemia [see Warnings and Precautions (5.9)].

No studies have been performed specifically examining the safety and efficacy of JANUMET in patients previously treated with other oral antihyperglycemic agents and switched to JANUMET. Any change in therapy of type 2 diabetes should be undertaken with care and appropriate monitoring as changes in glycemic control can occur.

3 DOSAGE FORMS AND STRENGTHS

- 50 mg/500 mg tablets are light pink, capsule-shaped, film-coated tablets with "575" debossed on one side.
- 50 mg/1000 mg tablets are red, capsule-shaped, film-coated tablets with "577" debossed on one side.

4 CONTRAINDICATIONS

JANUMET (sitagliptin/metformin HCl) is contraindicated in patients with:

- Renal disease or renal dysfunction, e.g., as suggested by serum creatinine levels ≥1.5 mg/dL [males], ≥1.4 mg/dL [females] or abnormal creatinine clearance which may also result from conditions such as cardiovascular collapse (shock), acute myocardial infarction, and septicemia [see Warnings and Precautions (5.1)].
- Acute or chronic metabolic acidosis, including diabetic ketoacidosis, with or without coma.
- History of a serious hypersensitivity reaction to JANUMET or sitagliptin (one of the components of JANUMET), such as anaphylaxis or angioedema. [See Warnings and Precautions (5.14); Adverse Reactions (6.2).]

JANUMET should be temporarily discontinued in patients undergoing radiologic studies involving intravascular administration of iodinated contrast materials, because use of such products may result in acute alteration of renal function [see Warnings and Precautions (5.11)].

5 WARNINGS AND PRECAUTIONS

5.1 Lactic Acidosis

Metformin hydrochloride
Lactic acidosis is a rare, but serious, metabolic complication that can occur due to metformin accumulation during treatment with JANUMET; when it occurs, it is fatal in approximately 50% of cases. Lactic acidosis may also occur in association with a number of pathophysiologic conditions, including diabetes mellitus, and whenever there is significant tissue hypoperfusion and hypoxemia. Lactic acidosis is characterized by elevated blood lactate levels (>5 mmol/L), decreased blood pH, electrolyte disturbances with an increased anion gap, and an increased lactate/pyruvate ratio. When metformin is implicated as the cause of lactic acidosis, metformin plasma levels >5 µg/mL are generally found. The reported incidence of lactic acidosis in patients receiving metformin hydrochloride is very low (approximately 0.03 cases/1000 patient-years, with approximately 0.015 fatal cases/1000 patient-years). In more than 20,000 patient-years exposure to metformin in clinical trials, there were no reports of lactic acidosis. Reported cases have occurred primarily in diabetic patients with significant renal insufficiency, including both intrinsic renal disease and renal hypoperfusion, often in the setting of multiple concomitant medical/surgical problems and multiple concomitant medications. Patients with congestive heart failure requiring pharmacologic management, in particular those with unstable or acute congestive heart failure who are at risk of hypoperfusion and hypoxemia, are at increased risk of lactic acidosis. The risk of lactic acidosis increases with the degree of renal dysfunction and the patient's age. The risk of lactic acidosis may, therefore, be significantly decreased by regular monitoring of renal function in patients taking metformin and by use of the minimum effective dose of metformin. In particular, treatment of the elderly should be accompanied by careful monitoring of renal function. Metformin treatment should not be initiated in patients ≥80 years of age unless measurement of creatinine clearance demonstrates that renal function is not reduced, as these patients are more susceptible to developing lactic acidosis. In addition, metformin should be promptly withheld in the presence of any condition associated with hypoxemia, dehydration, or sepsis. Because impaired hepatic function may significantly limit the ability to clear lactate, metformin should generally be avoided in patients with clinical or laboratory evidence of hepatic disease. Patients should be cautioned against excessive alcohol intake, either *acute or chronic*, when taking metformin, since alcohol potentiates the effects of metformin hydrochloride on lactate metabolism. In addition, metformin should be temporarily discontinued prior to any intravascular radiocontrast study and for any surgical procedure [see Warnings and Precautions (5.4, 5.6, 5.7, 5.11)].

The onset of lactic acidosis often is subtle, and accompanied only by nonspecific symptoms such as malaise, myalgias, respiratory distress, increasing somnolence, and nonspecific abdominal distress. There may be associated hypothermia, hypotension, and resistant bradyarrhythmias with more marked acidosis. The patient and the patient's physician must be aware of the possible importance of such symptoms and the patient should be instructed to notify the physician immediately if they occur [see Warnings and Precautions (5.12)]. Metformin should be withdrawn until the situation is clarified. Serum electrolytes, ketones, blood glucose, and if indicated, blood pH, lactate levels, and even blood metformin levels may be useful. Once a patient is stabilized on any dose level of metformin, gastrointestinal symptoms, which are common during initiation of therapy, are unlikely to be drug related. Later occurrence of gastrointestinal symptoms could be due to lactic acidosis or other serious disease.

Levels of fasting venous plasma lactate above the upper limit of normal but less than 5 mmol/L in patients taking metformin do not necessarily indicate impending lactic acidosis and may be explainable by other mechanisms, such as poorly controlled diabetes or obesity, vigorous physical activity, or technical problems in sample handling [see Warnings and Precautions (5.8, 5.13)].

Lactic acidosis should be suspected in any diabetic patient with metabolic acidosis lacking evidence of ketoacidosis (ketonuria and ketonemia).

Lactic acidosis is a medical emergency that must be treated in a hospital setting. In a patient with lactic acidosis who is taking metformin, the drug should be discontinued immediately and general supportive measures promptly instituted. Because metformin hydrochloride is dialyzable (with a clearance of up to 170 mL/min under good hemodynamic conditions), prompt hemodialysis is recommended to correct the acidosis and remove the accumulated metformin. Such management often results in prompt reversal of symptoms and recovery [see Contraindications (4); Warnings and Precautions (5.6, 5.7, 5.10, 5.11, 5.12)].

5.2 Pancreatitis

There have been postmarketing reports of acute pancreatitis, including fatal and non-fatal hemorrhagic or necrotizing pancreatitis, in patients taking JANUMET. After initiation of JANUMET, patients should be observed carefully for signs and symptoms of pancreatitis. If pancreatitis is suspected, JANUMET should promptly be discontinued and appropriate management should be initiated. It is unknown whether patients with a history of pancreatitis are at increased risk for the development of pancreatitis while using JANUMET.

5.3 Impaired Hepatic Function

Since impaired hepatic function has been associated with some cases of lactic acidosis, JANUMET should generally be avoided in patients with clinical or laboratory evidence of hepatic disease.

5.4 Assessment of Renal Function

Metformin and sitagliptin are known to be substantially excreted by the kidney. The risk of metformin accumulation and lactic acidosis increases with the degree of impairment of renal function. Thus, patients with serum creatinine levels above the upper limit of normal for their age should not receive JANUMET. In the elderly, JANUMET should be carefully titrated to establish the minimum dose for adequate glycemic effect, because aging can be associated with reduced renal function. [See Warnings and Precautions (5.1) and Use in Specific Populations (8.5).]

Before initiation of therapy with JANUMET and at least annually thereafter, renal function should be assessed and verified as normal. In patients in whom development of renal dysfunction is anticipated, particularly in elderly patients, renal function should be assessed more frequently and JANUMET discontinued if evidence of renal impairment is present.

5.5 Vitamin B₁₂ Levels

In controlled clinical trials of metformin of 29 weeks duration, a decrease to subnormal levels of previously normal serum Vitamin B_{12} levels, without clinical manifestations, was observed in approximately 7% of patients. Such decrease, possibly due to interference with B_{12} absorption from the B_{12}-intrinsic factor complex, is, however, very rarely associated with anemia and appears to be rapidly reversible with discontinuation of metformin or Vitamin B_{12} supplementation. Measurement of hematologic parameters on an annual basis is advised in patients on JANUMET and any apparent abnormalities should be appropriately investigated and managed. [See Adverse Reactions (6.1).]

Certain individuals (those with inadequate Vitamin B_{12} or calcium intake or absorption) appear to be predisposed to developing subnormal Vitamin B_{12} levels. In these patients, routine serum Vitamin B_{12} measurements at two- to three-year intervals may be useful.

5.6 Alcohol Intake

Alcohol is known to potentiate the effect of metformin on lactate metabolism. Patients, therefore, should be warned against excessive alcohol intake, acute or chronic, while receiving JANUMET.

5.7 Surgical Procedures

Use of JANUMET should be temporarily suspended for any surgical procedure (except minor procedures not associated with restricted intake of food and fluids) and should not be restarted until the patient's oral intake has resumed and renal function has been evaluated as normal.

5.8 Change in Clinical Status of Patients with Previously Controlled Type 2 Diabetes

A patient with type 2 diabetes previously well controlled on JANUMET who develops laboratory abnormalities or clinical illness (especially vague and poorly defined illness) should be evaluated promptly for evidence of ketoacidosis or lactic acidosis. Evaluation should include serum electrolytes and ketones, blood glucose and, if indicated, blood pH, lactate, pyruvate, and metformin levels. If acidosis of either form occurs, JANUMET must be stopped immediately and other appropriate corrective measures initiated.

5.9 Use with Medications Known to Cause Hypoglycemia

Sitagliptin
When sitagliptin was used in combination with a sulfonylurea or with insulin, medications known to cause hypoglycemia, the incidence of hypoglycemia was increased over that of placebo used in combination with a sulfonylurea or with insulin [see Adverse Reactions (6)]. Therefore, patients also receiving an insulin secretagogue (e.g., sulfonylurea) or insulin may require a lower dose of the insulin secretagogue or insulin to reduce the risk of hypoglycemia [see Dosage and Administration (2.1)].

Metformin hydrochloride
Hypoglycemia does not occur in patients receiving metformin alone under usual circumstances of use, but could occur when caloric intake is deficient, when strenuous exercise is not compensated by caloric supplementation, or during concomitant use with other glucose-lowering agents (such as sulfonylureas and insulin) or ethanol. Elderly, debilitated, or malnourished patients, and those with adrenal or pituitary insufficiency or alcohol intoxication are particularly susceptible to hypoglycemic effects. Hypoglycemia may be difficult to recognize in the elderly, and in people who are taking β-adrenergic blocking drugs.

5.10 Concomitant Medications Affecting Renal Function or Metformin Disposition

Concomitant medication(s) that may affect renal function or result in significant hemodynamic change or may interfere with the disposition of metformin, such as cationic drugs that are eliminated by renal tubular secretion [see Drug Interactions (7.1)], should be used with caution.

5.11 Radiologic Studies with Intravascular Iodinated Contrast Materials

Intravascular contrast studies with iodinated materials (for example, intravenous urogram, intravenous cholangiography, angiography, and computed tomography (CT) scans with intravascular contrast materials) can lead to acute alteration of renal function and have been associated with lactic acidosis in patients receiving metformin [see Contraindications (4)]. Therefore, in patients in whom any such study is planned, JANUMET should be temporarily discontinued at the time of or prior to the procedure, and withheld for 48 hours subsequent to the procedure and reinstituted only after renal function has been re-evaluated and found to be normal.

5.12 Hypoxic States

Cardiovascular collapse (shock) from whatever cause, acute congestive heart failure, acute myocardial infarction and other conditions characterized by hypoxemia have been associated with lactic acidosis and may also cause prerenal azotemia. When such events occur in patients on JANUMET therapy, the drug should be promptly discontinued.

5.13 Loss of Control of Blood Glucose

When a patient stabilized on any diabetic regimen is exposed to stress such as fever, trauma, infection, or surgery, a temporary loss of glycemic control may occur. At such times, it may be necessary to withhold JANUMET and temporarily administer insulin. JANUMET may be reinstituted after the acute episode is resolved.

5.14 Hypersensitivity Reactions

There have been postmarketing reports of serious hypersensitivity reactions in patients treated with sitagliptin, one of the components of JANUMET. These reactions include anaphylaxis, angioedema, and exfoliative skin conditions including Stevens-Johnson syndrome. Because these reactions are reported voluntarily from a population of uncertain size, it is generally not possible to reliably estimate their frequency or establish a causal relationship to drug exposure. Onset of these reactions occurred within the first 3 months after initiation of treatment with sitagliptin, with some reports occurring after the first dose. If a hypersensitivity reaction is suspected, discontinue JANUMET, assess for other potential causes for the event, and institute

Table 1: Sitagliptin and Metformin Co-administered to Patients with Type 2 Diabetes Inadequately Controlled on Diet and Exercise: Adverse Reactions Reported (Regardless of Investigator Assessment of Causality) in ≥5% of Patients Receiving Combination Therapy (and Greater than in Patients Receiving Placebo)*

	Number of Patients (%)			
	Placebo	Sitagliptin 100 mg QD	Metformin 500 mg/ Metformin 1000 mg bid[†]	Sitagliptin 50 mg bid + Metformin 500 mg/ Metformin 1000 mg bid[†]
	N = 176	N = 179	N = 364[†]	N = 372[†]
Diarrhea	7 (4.0)	5 (2.8)	28 (7.7)	28 (7.5)
Upper Respiratory Tract Infection	9 (5.1)	8 (4.5)	19 (5.2)	23 (6.2)
Headache	5 (2.8)	2 (1.1)	14 (3.8)	22 (5.9)

* Intent-to-treat population.
† Data pooled for the patients given the lower and higher doses of metformin.

Table 2: Pre-selected Gastrointestinal Adverse Reactions (Regardless of Investigator Assessment of Causality) Reported in Patients with Type 2 Diabetes Receiving Sitagliptin and Metformin

	Number of Patients (%)					
	Study of Sitagliptin and Metformin in Patients Inadequately Controlled on Diet and Exercise				Study of Sitagliptin Add-on in Patients Inadequately Controlled on Metformin Alone	
	Placebo	Sitagliptin 100 mg QD	Metformin 500 mg/ Metformin 1000 mg bid*	Sitagliptin 50 mg bid + Metformin 500 mg/ Metformin 1000 mg bid*	Placebo and Metformin ≥1500 mg daily	Sitagliptin 100 mg QD and Metformin ≥1500 mg daily
	N = 176	N = 179	N = 364	N = 372	N = 237	N = 464
Diarrhea	7 (4.0)	5 (2.8)	28 (7.7)	28 (7.5)	6 (2.5)	11 (2.4)
Nausea	2 (1.1)	2 (1.1)	20 (5.5)	18 (4.8)	2 (0.8)	6 (1.3)
Vomiting	1 (0.6)	0 (0.0)	2 (0.5)	8 (2.2)	2 (0.8)	5 (1.1)
Abdominal Pain[†]	4 (2.3)	6 (3.4)	14 (3.8)	11 (3.0)	9 (3.8)	10 (2.2)

* Data pooled for the patients given the lower and higher doses of metformin.
† Abdominal discomfort was included in the analysis of abdominal pain in the study of initial therapy.

Table 3: Incidence and Rate of Hypoglycemia* (Regardless of Investigator Assessment of Causality) in Placebo-Controlled Clinical Studies of Sitagliptin in Combination with Metformin Co-administered with Glimepiride or Insulin

Add-On to Glimepiride + Metformin (24 weeks)	Sitagliptin 100 mg + Metformin + Glimepiride	Placebo + Metformin + Glimepiride
	N = 116	N = 113
Overall (%)	19 (16.4)	1 (0.9)
Rate (episodes/patient-year)[†]	0.82	0.02
Severe (%)[‡]	0 (0.0)	0 (0.0)

Add-On to Insulin + Metformin (24 weeks)	Sitagliptin 100 mg + Metformin + Insulin	Placebo + Metformin + Insulin
	N = 229	N = 233
Overall (%)	35 (15.3)	19 (8.2)
Rate (episodes/patient-year)[†]	0.98	0.61
Severe (%)[‡]	1 (0.4)	1 (0.4)

* Adverse reactions of hypoglycemia were based on all reports of symptomatic hypoglycemia; a concurrent glucose measurement was not required: Intent to Treat Population.
† Based on total number of events (i.e., a single patient may have had multiple events).
‡ Severe events of hypoglycemia were defined as those events requiring medical assistance or exhibiting depressed level/ loss of consciousness or seizure.

alternative treatment for diabetes. [See Adverse Reactions (6.2).]

Macrovascular Outcomes
There have been no clinical studies establishing conclusive evidence of macrovascular risk reduction with JANUMET or any other anti-diabetic drug.

6   ADVERSE REACTIONS
6.1   Clinical Trials Experience
Because clinical trials are conducted under widely varying conditions, adverse reaction rates observed in the clinical trials of a drug cannot be directly compared to rates in the clinical trials of another drug and may not reflect the rates observed in practice.

Sitagliptin and Metformin Co-administration in Patients with Type 2 Diabetes Inadequately Controlled on Diet and Exercise
Table 1 summarizes the most common (≥5% of patients) adverse reactions reported (regardless of investigator assessment of causality) in a 24-week placebo-controlled factorial study in which sitagliptin and metformin were co-administered to patients with type 2 diabetes inadequately controlled on diet and exercise.
[See table above]
Sitagliptin Add-on Therapy in Patients with Type 2 Diabetes Inadequately Controlled on Metformin Alone
In a 24-week placebo-controlled trial of sitagliptin 100 mg administered once daily added to a twice daily metformin

regimen, there were no adverse reactions reported regardless of investigator assessment of causality in ≥5% of patients and more commonly than in patients given placebo. Discontinuation of therapy due to clinical adverse reactions was similar to the placebo treatment group (sitagliptin and metformin, 1.9%; placebo and metformin, 2.5%).
Gastrointestinal Adverse Reactions
The incidences of pre-selected gastrointestinal adverse experiences in patients treated with sitagliptin and metformin were similar to those reported for patients treated with metformin alone. See Table 2.
[See table 2 below]
Sitagliptin in Combination with Metformin and Glimepiride
In a 24-week placebo-controlled study of sitagliptin 100 mg as add-on therapy in patients with type 2 diabetes inadequately controlled on metformin and glimepiride (sitagliptin, N=116; placebo, N=113), the adverse reactions reported regardless of investigator assessment of causality in ≥5% of patients treated with sitagliptin and more commonly than in patients treated with placebo were: hypoglycemia (Table 3) and headache (6.9%, 2.7%).
Sitagliptin in Combination with Metformin and Rosiglitazone
In a placebo-controlled study of sitagliptin 100 mg as add-on therapy in patients with type 2 diabetes inadequately controlled on metformin and rosiglitazone (sitagliptin, N=181; placebo, N=97), the adverse reactions reported regardless of investigator assessment of causality through Week 18 in ≥5% of patients treated with sitagliptin and more commonly than in patients treated with placebo were: upper respiratory tract infection (sitagliptin, 5.5%; placebo, 5.2%) and nasopharyngitis (6.1%, 4.1%). Through Week 54, the adverse reactions reported regardless of investigator assessment of causality in ≥5% of patients treated with sitagliptin and more commonly than in patients treated with placebo were: upper respiratory tract infection (sitagliptin, 15.5%; placebo, 6.2%), nasopharyngitis (11.0%, 9.3%), peripheral edema (8.3%, 5.2%), and headache (5.5%, 4.1%).
Sitagliptin in Combination with Metformin and Insulin
In a 24-week placebo-controlled study of sitagliptin 100 mg as add-on therapy in patients with type 2 diabetes inadequately controlled on metformin and insulin (sitagliptin, N=229; placebo, N=233), the only adverse reaction reported regardless of investigator assessment of causality in ≥5% of patients treated with sitagliptin and more commonly than in patients treated with placebo was hypoglycemia (Table 3).
Hypoglycemia
In all (N=5) studies, adverse reactions of hypoglycemia were based on all reports of symptomatic hypoglycemia; a concurrent glucose measurement was not required although most (77%) reports of hypoglycemia were accompanied by a blood glucose measurement ≤70 mg/dL. When the combination of sitagliptin and metformin was co-administered with a sulfonylurea or with insulin, the percentage of patients reporting at least one adverse reaction of hypoglycemia was higher than that observed with placebo and metformin co-administered with a sulfonylurea or with insulin (Table 3).
[See table 3 at left]
The overall incidence of reported adverse reactions of hypoglycemia in patients with type 2 diabetes inadequately controlled on diet and exercise was 0.6% in patients given placebo, 0.6% in patients given sitagliptin alone, 0.8% in patients given metformin alone, and 1.6% in patients given sitagliptin in combination with metformin. In patients with type 2 diabetes inadequately controlled on metformin alone, the overall incidence of adverse reactions of hypoglycemia was 1.3% in patients given add-on sitagliptin and 2.1% in patients given add-on placebo.
In the study of sitagliptin and add-on combination therapy with metformin and rosiglitazone, the overall incidence of hypoglycemia was 2.2% in patients given add-on sitagliptin and 0.0% in patients given add-on placebo through Week 18. Through Week 54, the overall incidence of hypoglycemia was 3.9% in patients given add-on sitagliptin and 1.0% in patients given add-on placebo.
With the combination of sitagliptin and metformin, no clinically meaningful changes in vital signs or in ECG (including in QTc interval) were observed.
The most common adverse experience in sitagliptin monotherapy reported regardless of investigator assessment of causality in ≥5% of patients and more commonly than in patients given placebo was nasopharyngitis.
The most common (>5%) established adverse reactions due to initiation of metformin therapy are diarrhea, nausea/ vomiting, flatulence, abdominal discomfort, indigestion, asthenia, and headache.
Laboratory Tests
Sitagliptin
The incidence of laboratory adverse reactions was similar in patients treated with sitagliptin and metformin (7.6%) compared to patients treated with placebo and metformin (8.7%). In most but not all studies, a small increase in white blood cell count (approximately 200 cells/microL difference

in WBC vs placebo; mean baseline WBC approximately 6600 cells/microL) was observed due to a small increase in neutrophils. This change in laboratory parameters is not considered to be clinically relevant.

Metformin hydrochloride

In controlled clinical trials of metformin of 29 weeks duration, a decrease to subnormal levels of previously normal serum Vitamin B_{12} levels, without clinical manifestations, was observed in approximately 7% of patients. Such decrease, possibly due to interference with B_{12} absorption from the B_{12}-intrinsic factor complex, is, however, very rarely associated with anemia and appears to be rapidly reversible with discontinuation of metformin or Vitamin B_{12} supplementation. *[See Warnings and Precautions (5.5).]*

6.2 Postmarketing Experience

The following additional adverse reactions have been identified during postapproval use of JANUMET or sitagliptin, one of the components of JANUMET. Because these reactions are reported voluntarily from a population of uncertain size, it is generally not possible to reliably estimate their frequency or establish a causal relationship to drug exposure.

Hypersensitivity reactions include anaphylaxis, angioedema, rash, urticaria, cutaneous vasculitis, and exfoliative skin conditions including Stevens-Johnson syndrome *[see Warnings and Precautions (5.14)]*; upper respiratory tract infection; hepatic enzyme elevations; acute pancreatitis, including fatal and non-fatal hemorrhagic and necrotizing pancreatitis *[see Limitations of Use (1); Warnings and Precautions (5.2)]*.

7 DRUG INTERACTIONS

7.1 Cationic drugs

Cationic drugs (e.g., amiloride, digoxin, morphine, procainamide, quinidine, quinine, ranitidine, triamterene, trimethoprim, or vancomycin) that are eliminated by renal tubular secretion theoretically have the potential for interaction with metformin by competing for common renal tubular transport systems. Such interaction between metformin and oral cimetidine has been observed in normal healthy volunteers in both single- and multiple-dose metformin-cimetidine drug interaction studies, with a 60% increase in peak metformin plasma and whole blood concentrations and a 40% increase in plasma and whole blood metformin AUC. There was no change in elimination half-life in the single-dose study. Metformin had no effect on cimetidine pharmacokinetics. Although such interactions remain theoretical (except for cimetidine), careful patient monitoring and dose adjustment of JANUMET and/or the interfering drug is recommended in patients who are taking cationic medications that are excreted via the proximal renal tubular secretory system.

7.2 Digoxin

There was a slight increase in the area under the curve (AUC, 11%) and mean peak drug concentration (C_{max}, 18%) of digoxin with the co-administration of 100 mg sitagliptin for 10 days. These increases are not considered likely to be clinically meaningful. Digoxin, as a cationic drug, has the potential to compete with metformin for common renal tubular transport systems, thus affecting the serum concentrations of either digoxin, metformin or both. Patients receiving digoxin should be monitored appropriately. No dosage adjustment of digoxin or JANUMET is recommended.

7.3 Glyburide

In a single-dose interaction study in type 2 diabetes patients, co-administration of metformin and glyburide did not result in any changes in either metformin pharmacokinetics or pharmacodynamics. Decreases in glyburide AUC and C_{max} were observed, but were highly variable. The single-dose nature of this study and the lack of correlation between glyburide blood levels and pharmacodynamic effects make the clinical significance of this interaction uncertain.

7.4 Furosemide

A single-dose, metformin-furosemide drug interaction study in healthy subjects demonstrated that pharmacokinetic parameters of both compounds were affected by co-administration. Furosemide increased the metformin plasma and blood C_{max} by 22% and blood AUC by 15%, without any significant change in metformin renal clearance. When administered with metformin, the C_{max} and AUC of furosemide were 31% and 12% smaller, respectively, than when administered alone, and the terminal half-life was decreased by 32%, without any significant change in furosemide renal clearance. No information is available about the interaction of metformin and furosemide when co-administered chronically.

7.5 Nifedipine

A single-dose, metformin-nifedipine drug interaction study in normal healthy volunteers demonstrated that co-administration of nifedipine increased plasma metformin C_{max} and AUC by 20% and 9%, respectively, and increased the amount excreted in the urine. T_{max} and half-life were unaffected. Nifedipine appears to enhance the absorption of metformin. Metformin had minimal effects on nifedipine.

7.6 The Use of Metformin with Other Drugs

Certain drugs tend to produce hyperglycemia and may lead to loss of glycemic control. These drugs include the thiazides and other diuretics, corticosteroids, phenothiazines, thyroid products, estrogens, oral contraceptives, phenytoin, nicotinic acid, sympathomimetics, calcium channel blocking drugs, and isoniazid. When such drugs are administered to a patient receiving JANUMET the patient should be closely observed to maintain adequate glycemic control.

In healthy volunteers, the pharmacokinetics of metformin and propranolol, and metformin and ibuprofen were not affected when co-administered in single-dose interaction studies.

Metformin is negligibly bound to plasma proteins and is, therefore, less likely to interact with highly protein-bound drugs such as salicylates, sulfonamides, chloramphenicol, and probenecid, as compared to the sulfonylureas, which are extensively bound to serum proteins.

8 USE IN SPECIFIC POPULATIONS

8.1 Pregnancy

Pregnancy Category B:

JANUMET

There are no adequate and well-controlled studies in pregnant women with JANUMET or its individual components; therefore, the safety of JANUMET in pregnant women is not known. JANUMET should be used during pregnancy only if clearly needed.

Merck Sharp & Dohme Corp., a subsidiary of Merck & Co., Inc., maintains a registry to monitor the pregnancy outcomes of women exposed to JANUMET while pregnant. Health care providers are encouraged to report any prenatal exposure to JANUMET by calling the Pregnancy Registry at (800) 986-8999.

No animal studies have been conducted with the combined products in JANUMET to evaluate effects on reproduction. The following data are based on findings in studies performed with sitagliptin or metformin individually.

Sitagliptin

Reproduction studies have been performed in rats and rabbits. Doses of sitagliptin up to 125 mg/kg (approximately 12 times the human exposure at the maximum recommended human dose) did not impair fertility or harm the fetus. There are, however, no adequate and well-controlled studies with sitagliptin in pregnant women.

Sitagliptin administered to pregnant female rats and rabbits from gestation day 6 to 20 (organogenesis) was not teratogenic at oral doses up to 250 mg/kg (rats) and 125 mg/kg (rabbits), or approximately 30 and 20 times human exposure at the maximum recommended human dose (MRHD) of 100 mg/day based on AUC comparisons. Higher doses increased the incidence of rib malformations in offspring at 1000 mg/kg, or approximately 100 times human exposure at the MRHD.

Sitagliptin administered to female rats from gestation day 6 to lactation day 21 decreased body weight in male and female offspring at 1000 mg/kg. No functional or behavioral toxicity was observed in offspring of rats.

Placental transfer of sitagliptin administered to pregnant rats was approximately 45% at 2 hours and 80% at 24 hours postdose. Placental transfer of sitagliptin administered to pregnant rabbits was approximately 66% at 2 hours and 30% at 24 hours.

Metformin hydrochloride

Metformin was not teratogenic in rats and rabbits at doses up to 600 mg/kg/day. This represents an exposure of about 2 and 6 times the maximum recommended human daily dose of 2,000 mg based on body surface area comparisons for rats and rabbits, respectively. Determination of fetal concentrations demonstrated a partial placental barrier to metformin.

8.3 Nursing Mothers

No studies in lactating animals have been conducted with the combined components of JANUMET. In studies performed with the individual components, both sitagliptin and metformin are secreted in the milk of lactating rats. It is not known whether sitagliptin is excreted in human milk. Because many drugs are excreted in human milk, caution should be exercised when JANUMET is administered to a nursing woman.

8.4 Pediatric Use

Safety and effectiveness of JANUMET in pediatric patients under 18 years have not been established.

8.5 Geriatric Use

JANUMET

Because sitagliptin and metformin are substantially excreted by the kidney, and because aging can be associated with reduced renal function, JANUMET should be used with caution as age increases. Care should be taken in dose selection and should be based on careful and regular monitoring of renal function. *[See Warnings and Precautions (5.1, 5.4); Clinical Pharmacology (12.3).]*

Sitagliptin

Of the total number of subjects (N=3884) in Phase II and III clinical studies of sitagliptin, 725 patients were 65 years and over, while 61 patients were 75 years and over. No overall differences in safety or effectiveness were observed between subjects 65 years and over and younger subjects. While this and other reported clinical experience have not identified differences in responses between the elderly and younger patients, greater sensitivity of some older individuals cannot be ruled out.

Metformin hydrochloride

Controlled clinical studies of metformin did not include sufficient numbers of elderly patients to determine whether they respond differently from younger patients, although other reported clinical experience has not identified differences in responses between the elderly and young patients. Metformin should only be used in patients with normal renal function. The initial and maintenance dosing of metformin should be conservative in patients with advanced age, due to the potential for decreased renal function in this population. Any dose adjustment should be based on a careful assessment of renal function. *[See Contraindications (4); Warnings and Precautions (5.4); and Clinical Pharmacology (12.3).]*

10 OVERDOSAGE

Sitagliptin

During controlled clinical trials in healthy subjects, single doses of up to 800 mg sitagliptin were administered. Maximal mean increases in QTc of 8.0 msec were observed in one study at a dose of 800 mg sitagliptin, a mean effect that is not considered clinically important *[see Clinical Pharmacology (12.2)]*. There is no experience with doses above 800 mg in humans. In Phase I multiple-dose studies, there were no dose-related clinical adverse reactions observed with sitagliptin with doses of up to 400 mg per day for periods of up to 28 days.

In the event of an overdose, it is reasonable to employ the usual supportive measures, e.g., remove unabsorbed material from the gastrointestinal tract, employ clinical monitoring (including obtaining an electrocardiogram), and institute supportive therapy as indicated by the patient's clinical status.

Sitagliptin is modestly dialyzable. In clinical studies, approximately 13.5% of the dose was removed over a 3- to 4-hour hemodialysis session. Prolonged hemodialysis may be considered if clinically appropriate. It is not known if sitagliptin is dialyzable by peritoneal dialysis.

Metformin hydrochloride

Overdose of metformin hydrochloride has occurred, including ingestion of amounts greater than 50 grams. Hypoglycemia was reported in approximately 10% of cases, but no causal association with metformin hydrochloride has been established. Lactic acidosis has been reported in approximately 32% of metformin overdose cases *[see Warnings and Precautions (5.1)]*. Metformin is dialyzable with a clearance of up to 170 mL/min under good hemodynamic conditions. Therefore, hemodialysis may be useful for removal of accumulated drug from patients in whom metformin overdosage is suspected.

11 DESCRIPTION

JANUMET (sitagliptin/metformin HCl) tablets contain two oral antihyperglycemic drugs used in the management of type 2 diabetes: sitagliptin and metformin hydrochloride.

Sitagliptin

Sitagliptin is an orally-active inhibitor of the dipeptidyl peptidase-4 (DPP-4) enzyme. Sitagliptin is present in JANUMET tablets in the form of sitagliptin phosphate monohydrate. Sitagliptin phosphate monohydrate is described chemically as 7-[(3*R*)-3-amino-1-oxo-4-(2,4,5-trifluorophenyl)butyl]-5,6,7,8-tetrahydro-3-(trifluoromethyl)-1,2,4-triazolo[4,3-*a*]pyrazine phosphate (1:1) monohydrate with an empirical formula of $C_{16}H_{15}F_6N_5O \bullet H_3PO_4 \bullet H_2O$ and a molecular weight of 523.32. The structural formula is:

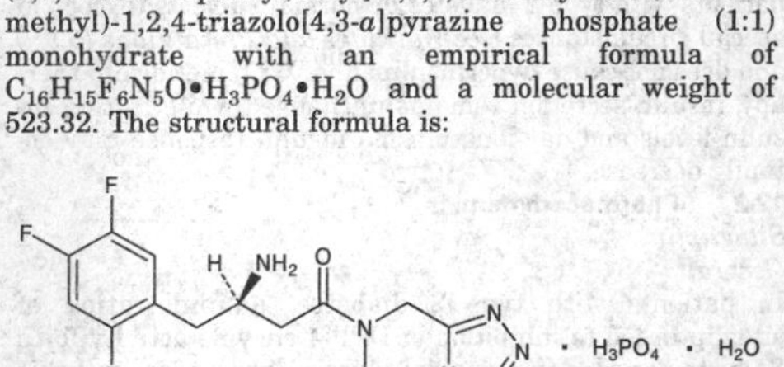

Sitagliptin phosphate monohydrate is a white to off-white, crystalline, non-hygroscopic powder. It is soluble in water and N,N-dimethyl formamide; slightly soluble in methanol; very slightly soluble in ethanol, acetone, and acetonitrile; and insoluble in isopropanol and isopropyl acetate.

Metformin hydrochloride

Metformin hydrochloride (*N,N*-dimethylimidodicarbonimidic diamide hydrochloride) is not chemically or pharmacologically related to any other classes of oral antihyperglycemic agents. Metformin hydrochloride is a white to off-white crystalline compound with a molecular formula of $C_4H_{11}N_5{\bullet}HCl$ and a molecular weight of 165.63. Metformin hydrochloride is freely soluble in water and is practically insoluble in acetone, ether, and chloroform. The pK_a of metformin is 12.4. The pH of a 1% aqueous solution of metformin hydrochloride is 6.68. The structural formula is as shown:

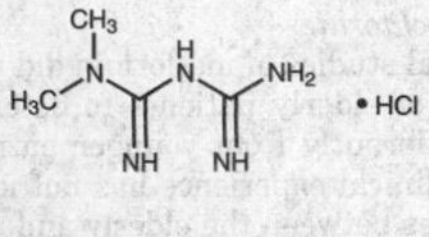

JANUMET

JANUMET is available for oral administration as tablets containing 64.25 mg sitagliptin phosphate monohydrate and metformin hydrochloride equivalent to: 50 mg sitagliptin as free base and 500 mg metformin hydrochloride (JANUMET 50 mg/500 mg) or 1000 mg metformin hydrochloride (JANUMET 50 mg/1000 mg). Each film-coated tablet of JANUMET contains the following inactive ingredients: microcrystalline cellulose, polyvinylpyrrolidone, sodium lauryl sulfate, and sodium stearyl fumarate. In addition, the film coating contains the following inactive ingredients: polyvinyl alcohol, polyethylene glycol, talc, titanium dioxide, red iron oxide, and black iron oxide.

12 CLINICAL PHARMACOLOGY

12.1 Mechanism of Action

JANUMET

JANUMET combines two antihyperglycemic agents with complementary mechanisms of action to improve glycemic control in patients with type 2 diabetes: sitagliptin, a dipeptidyl peptidase-4 (DPP-4) inhibitor, and metformin hydrochloride, a member of the biguanide class.

Sitagliptin

Sitagliptin is a DPP-4 inhibitor, which is believed to exert its actions in patients with type 2 diabetes by slowing the inactivation of incretin hormones. Concentrations of the active intact hormones are increased by sitagliptin, thereby increasing and prolonging the action of these hormones. Incretin hormones, including glucagon-like peptide-1 (GLP-1) and glucose-dependent insulinotropic polypeptide (GIP), are released by the intestine throughout the day, and levels are increased in response to a meal. These hormones are rapidly inactivated by the enzyme DPP-4. The incretins are part of an endogenous system involved in the physiologic regulation of glucose homeostasis. When blood glucose concentrations are normal or elevated, GLP-1 and GIP increase insulin synthesis and release from pancreatic beta cells by intracellular signaling pathways involving cyclic AMP. GLP-1 also lowers glucagon secretion from pancreatic alpha cells, leading to reduced hepatic glucose production. By increasing and prolonging active incretin levels, sitagliptin increases insulin release and decreases glucagon levels in the circulation in a glucose-dependent manner. Sitagliptin demonstrates selectivity for DPP-4 and does not inhibit DPP-8 or DPP-9 activity *in vitro* at concentrations approximating those from therapeutic doses.

Metformin hydrochloride

Metformin is an antihyperglycemic agent which improves glucose tolerance in patients with type 2 diabetes, lowering both basal and postprandial plasma glucose. Its pharmacologic mechanisms of action are different from other classes of oral antihyperglycemic agents. Metformin decreases hepatic glucose production, decreases intestinal absorption of glucose, and improves insulin sensitivity by increasing peripheral glucose uptake and utilization. Unlike sulfonylureas, metformin does not produce hypoglycemia in either patients with type 2 diabetes or normal subjects (except in special circumstances *[see Warnings and Precautions (5.9)]*) and does not cause hyperinsulinemia. With metformin therapy, insulin secretion remains unchanged while fasting insulin levels and day-long plasma insulin response may actually decrease.

12.2 Pharmacodynamics

Sitagliptin

General

In patients with type 2 diabetes, administration of sitagliptin led to inhibition of DPP-4 enzyme activity for a 24-hour period. After an oral glucose load or a meal, this DPP-4 inhibition resulted in a 2- to 3-fold increase in circulating levels of active GLP-1 and GIP, decreased glucagon concentrations, and increased responsiveness of insulin release to glucose, resulting in higher C-peptide and insulin concentrations. The rise in insulin with the decrease in glucagon was associated with lower fasting glucose concentrations and reduced glucose excursion following an oral glucose load or a meal.

Sitagliptin and Metformin hydrochloride Co-administration

In a two-day study in healthy subjects, sitagliptin alone increased active GLP-1 concentrations, whereas metformin alone increased active and total GLP-1 concentrations to similar extents. Co-administration of sitagliptin and metformin had an additive effect on active GLP-1 concentrations. Sitagliptin, but not metformin, increased active GIP concentrations. It is unclear what these findings mean for changes in glycemic control in patients with type 2 diabetes.

In studies with healthy subjects, sitagliptin did not lower blood glucose or cause hypoglycemia.

Cardiac Electrophysiology

In a randomized, placebo-controlled crossover study, 79 healthy subjects were administered a single oral dose of sitagliptin 100 mg, sitagliptin 800 mg (8 times the recommended dose), and placebo. At the recommended dose of 100 mg, there was no effect on the QTc interval obtained at the peak plasma concentration, or at any other time during the study. Following the 800-mg dose, the maximum increase in the placebo-corrected mean change in QTc from baseline at 3 hours postdose was 8.0 msec. This increase is not considered to be clinically significant. At the 800-mg dose, peak sitagliptin plasma concentrations were approximately 11 times higher than the peak concentrations following a 100-mg dose.

In patients with type 2 diabetes administered sitagliptin 100 mg (N=81) or sitagliptin 200 mg (N=63) daily, there were no meaningful changes in QTc interval based on ECG data obtained at the time of expected peak plasma concentration.

12.3 Pharmacokinetics

JANUMET

The results of a bioequivalence study in healthy subjects demonstrated that the JANUMET (sitagliptin/metformin HCl) 50 mg/500 mg and 50 mg/1000 mg combination tablets are bioequivalent to co-administration of corresponding doses of sitagliptin (JANUVIA®[2]) and metformin hydrochloride as individual tablets.

Absorption

Sitagliptin

The absolute bioavailability of sitagliptin is approximately 87%. Co-administration of a high-fat meal with sitagliptin had no effect on the pharmacokinetics of sitagliptin.

Metformin hydrochloride

The absolute bioavailability of a metformin hydrochloride 500-mg tablet given under fasting conditions is approximately 50-60%. Studies using single oral doses of metformin hydrochloride tablets 500 mg to 1500 mg, and 850 mg to 2550 mg, indicate that there is a lack of dose proportionality with increasing doses, which is due to decreased absorption rather than an alteration in elimination. Food decreases the extent of and slightly delays the absorption of metformin, as shown by approximately a 40% lower mean peak plasma concentration (C_{max}), a 25% lower area under the plasma concentration versus time curve (AUC), and a 35-minute prolongation of time to peak plasma concentration (T_{max}) following administration of a single 850-mg tablet of metformin with food, compared to the same tablet strength administered fasting. The clinical relevance of these decreases is unknown.

Distribution

Sitagliptin

The mean volume of distribution at steady state following a single 100-mg intravenous dose of sitagliptin to healthy subjects is approximately 198 liters. The fraction of sitagliptin reversibly bound to plasma proteins is low (38%).

Metformin hydrochloride

The apparent volume of distribution (V/F) of metformin following single oral doses of metformin hydrochloride tablets 850 mg averaged 654 ± 358 L. Metformin is negligibly bound to plasma proteins, in contrast to sulfonylureas, which are more than 90% protein bound. Metformin partitions into erythrocytes, most likely as a function of time. At usual clinical doses and dosing schedules of metformin hydrochloride tablets, steady-state plasma concentrations of metformin are reached within 24-48 hours and are generally <1 mcg/mL. During controlled clinical trials of metformin, maximum metformin plasma levels did not exceed 5 mcg/mL, even at maximum doses.

Metabolism

Sitagliptin

Approximately 79% of sitagliptin is excreted unchanged in the urine with metabolism being a minor pathway of elimination.

Following a [^{14}C]sitagliptin oral dose, approximately 16% of the radioactivity was excreted as metabolites of sitagliptin. Six metabolites were detected at trace levels and are not expected to contribute to the plasma DPP-4 inhibitory activity of sitagliptin. *In vitro* studies indicated that the primary enzyme responsible for the limited metabolism of sitagliptin was CYP3A4, with contribution from CYP2C8.

Metformin hydrochloride

Intravenous single-dose studies in normal subjects demonstrate that metformin is excreted unchanged in the urine and does not undergo hepatic metabolism (no metabolites have been identified in humans) nor biliary excretion.

Excretion

Sitagliptin

Following administration of an oral [^{14}C]sitagliptin dose to healthy subjects, approximately 100% of the administered radioactivity was eliminated in feces (13%) or urine (87%) within one week of dosing. The apparent terminal $t_{1/2}$ following a 100-mg oral dose of sitagliptin was approximately 12.4 hours and renal clearance was approximately 350 mL/min.

Elimination of sitagliptin occurs primarily via renal excretion and involves active tubular secretion. Sitagliptin is a substrate for human organic anion transporter-3 (hOAT-3), which may be involved in the renal elimination of sitagliptin. The clinical relevance of hOAT-3 in sitagliptin transport has not been established. Sitagliptin is also a substrate of p-glycoprotein, which may also be involved in mediating the renal elimination of sitagliptin. However, cyclosporine, a p-glycoprotein inhibitor, did not reduce the renal clearance of sitagliptin.

Metformin hydrochloride

Renal clearance is approximately 3.5 times greater than creatinine clearance, which indicates that tubular secretion is the major route of metformin elimination. Following oral administration, approximately 90% of the absorbed drug is eliminated via the renal route within the first 24 hours, with a plasma elimination half-life of approximately 6.2 hours. In blood, the elimination half-life is approximately 17.6 hours, suggesting that the erythrocyte mass may be a compartment of distribution.

Special Populations

Renal Insufficiency

JANUMET

JANUMET should not be used in patients with renal insufficiency *[see Contraindications (4); Warnings and Precautions (5.4)]*.

Sitagliptin

An approximately 2-fold increase in the plasma AUC of sitagliptin was observed in patients with moderate renal insufficiency, and an approximately 4-fold increase was observed in patients with severe renal insufficiency including patients with ESRD on hemodialysis, as compared to normal healthy control subjects.

Metformin hydrochloride

In patients with decreased renal function (based on measured creatinine clearance), the plasma and blood half-life of metformin is prolonged and the renal clearance is decreased in proportion to the decrease in creatinine clearance.

Hepatic Insufficiency

Sitagliptin

In patients with moderate hepatic insufficiency (Child-Pugh score 7 to 9), mean AUC and C_{max} of sitagliptin increased approximately 21% and 13%, respectively, compared to healthy matched controls following administration of a single 100-mg dose of sitagliptin. These differences are not considered to be clinically meaningful.

There is no clinical experience in patients with severe hepatic insufficiency (Child-Pugh score >9).

Metformin hydrochloride

No pharmacokinetic studies of metformin have been conducted in patients with hepatic insufficiency.

Gender

Sitagliptin

Gender had no clinically meaningful effect on the pharmacokinetics of sitagliptin based on a composite analysis of Phase I pharmacokinetic data and on a population pharmacokinetic analysis of Phase I and Phase II data.

Metformin hydrochloride

Metformin pharmacokinetic parameters did not differ significantly between normal subjects and patients with type 2 diabetes when analyzed according to gender. Similarly, in controlled clinical studies in patients with type 2 diabetes, the antihyperglycemic effect of metformin was comparable in males and females.

Geriatric

Sitagliptin

When the effects of age on renal function are taken into account, age alone did not have a clinically meaningful impact on the pharmacokinetics of sitagliptin based on a population pharmacokinetic analysis. Elderly subjects (65 to 80 years) had approximately 19% higher plasma concentrations of sitagliptin compared to younger subjects.

Metformin hydrochloride

Limited data from controlled pharmacokinetic studies of metformin in healthy elderly subjects suggest that total plasma clearance of metformin is decreased, the half life is prolonged, and C_{max} is increased, compared to healthy young subjects. From these data, it appears that the change in metformin pharmacokinetics with aging is primarily accounted for by a change in renal function (see **GLUCOPHAGE[3]** prescribing information: **CLINICAL PHARMACOLOGY**, Special Populations, Geriatrics).

JANUMET treatment should not be initiated in patients ≥80 years of age unless measurement of creatinine clearance demonstrates that renal function is not reduced [see Warnings and Precautions (5.1, 5.4)].

Pediatric
No studies with JANUMET have been performed in pediatric patients.

Race
Sitagliptin
Race had no clinically meaningful effect on the pharmacokinetics of sitagliptin based on a composite analysis of available pharmacokinetic data, including subjects of white, Hispanic, black, Asian, and other racial groups.

Metformin hydrochloride
No studies of metformin pharmacokinetic parameters according to race have been performed. In controlled clinical studies of metformin in patients with type 2 diabetes, the antihyperglycemic effect was comparable in whites (n=249), blacks (n=51), and Hispanics (n=24).

Body Mass Index (BMI)
Sitagliptin
Body mass index had no clinically meaningful effect on the pharmacokinetics of sitagliptin based on a composite analysis of Phase I pharmacokinetic data and on a population pharmacokinetic analysis of Phase I and Phase II data.

Drug Interactions
Sitagliptin and Metformin hydrochloride
Co-administration of multiple doses of sitagliptin (50 mg) and metformin (1000 mg) given twice daily did not meaningfully alter the pharmacokinetics of either sitagliptin or metformin in patients with type 2 diabetes.
Pharmacokinetic drug interaction studies with JANUMET have not been performed; however, such studies have been conducted with the individual components of JANUMET (sitagliptin and metformin hydrochloride).

Sitagliptin
In Vitro Assessment of Drug Interactions
Sitagliptin is not an inhibitor of CYP isozymes CYP3A4, 2C8, 2C9, 2D6, 1A2, 2C19 or 2B6, and is not an inducer of CYP3A4. Sitagliptin is a p-glycoprotein substrate, but does not inhibit p-glycoprotein mediated transport of digoxin. Based on these results, sitagliptin is considered unlikely to cause interactions with other drugs that utilize these pathways.
Sitagliptin is not extensively bound to plasma proteins. Therefore, the propensity of sitagliptin to be involved in clinically meaningful drug-drug interactions mediated by plasma protein binding displacement is very low.

In Vivo Assessment of Drug Interactions
Effect of Sitagliptin on Other Drugs
In clinical studies, as described below, sitagliptin did not meaningfully alter the pharmacokinetics of metformin, glyburide, simvastatin, rosiglitazone, warfarin, or oral contraceptives, providing *in vivo* evidence of a low propensity for causing drug interactions with substrates of CYP3A4, CYP2C8, CYP2C9, and organic cationic transporter (OCT).
Digoxin: Sitagliptin had a minimal effect on the pharmacokinetics of digoxin. Following administration of 0.25 mg digoxin concomitantly with 100 mg of sitagliptin daily for 10 days, the plasma AUC of digoxin was increased by 11%, and the plasma C_{max} by 18%.
Sulfonylureas: Single-dose pharmacokinetics of glyburide, a CYP2C9 substrate, was not meaningfully altered in subjects receiving multiple doses of sitagliptin. Clinically meaningful interactions would not be expected with other sulfonylureas (e.g., glipizide, tolbutamide, and glimepiride) which, like glyburide, are primarily eliminated by CYP2C9 [see Warnings and Precautions (5.9)].
Simvastatin: Single-dose pharmacokinetics of simvastatin, a CYP3A4 substrate, was not meaningfully altered in subjects receiving multiple daily doses of sitagliptin. Therefore, sitagliptin is not an inhibitor of CYP3A4-mediated metabolism.
Thiazolidinediones: Single-dose pharmacokinetics of rosiglitazone was not meaningfully altered in subjects receiving multiple daily doses of sitagliptin, indicating that sitagliptin is not an inhibitor of CYP2C8-mediated metabolism.
Warfarin: Multiple daily doses of sitagliptin did not meaningfully alter the pharmacokinetics, as assessed by measurement of S(-) or R(+) warfarin enantiomers, or pharmacodynamics (as assessed by measurement of prothrombin INR) of a single dose of warfarin. Because S(-) warfarin is primarily metabolized by CYP2C9, these data also support the conclusion that sitagliptin is not a CYP2C9 inhibitor.
Oral Contraceptives: Co-administration with sitagliptin did not meaningfully alter the steady-state pharmacokinetics of norethindrone or ethinyl estradiol.

Effect of Other Drugs on Sitagliptin
Clinical data described below suggest that sitagliptin is not susceptible to clinically meaningful interactions by co-administered medications.

Table 4: Glycemic Parameters at Final Visit (24-Week Study) for Sitagliptin and Metformin, Alone and in Combination in Patients with Type 2 Diabetes Inadequately Controlled on Diet and Exercise*

	Placebo	Sitagliptin 100 mg QD	Metformin 500 mg bid	Metformin 1000 mg bid	Sitagliptin 50 mg bid + Metformin 500 mg bid	Sitagliptin 50 mg bid + Metformin 1000 mg bid
A1C (%)	N = 165	N = 175	N = 178	N = 177	N = 183	N = 178
Baseline (mean)	8.7	8.9	8.9	8.7	8.8	8.8
Change from baseline (adjusted mean[†])	0.2	-0.7	-0.8	-1.1	-1.4	-1.9
Difference from placebo (adjusted mean[†]) (95% CI)		-0.8[‡] (-1.1, -0.6)	-1.0[‡] (-1.2, -0.8)	-1.3[‡] (-1.5, -1.1)	-1.6[‡] (-1.8, -1.3)	-2.1[‡] (-2.3, -1.8)
Patients (%) achieving A1C <7%	15 (9%)	35 (20%)	41 (23%)	68 (38%)	79 (43%)	118 (66%)
% Patients receiving rescue medication	32	21	17	12	8	2
FPG (mg/dL)	N = 169	N = 178	N = 179	N = 179	N = 183	N = 180
Baseline (mean)	196	201	205	197	204	197
Change from baseline (adjusted mean[†])	6	-17	-27	-29	-47	-64
Difference from placebo (adjusted mean[†]) (95% CI)		-23[‡] (-33, -14)	-33[‡] (-43, -24)	-35[‡] (-45, -26)	-53[‡] (-62, -43)	-70[‡] (-79, -60)
2-hour PPG (mg/dL)	N = 129	N = 136	N = 141	N = 138	N = 147	N = 152
Baseline (mean)	277	285	293	283	292	287
Change from baseline (adjusted mean[†])	0	-52	-53	-78	-93	-117
Difference from placebo (adjusted mean[†]) (95% CI)		-52[‡] (-67, -37)	-54[‡] (-69, -39)	-78[‡] (-93, -63)	-93[‡] (-107, -78)	-117[‡] (-131, -102)

* Intent to Treat Population using last observation on study prior to glyburide (glibenclamide) rescue therapy.
† Least squares means adjusted for prior antihyperglycemic therapy status and baseline value.
‡ $p < 0.001$ compared to placebo.

Cyclosporine: A study was conducted to assess the effect of cyclosporine, a potent inhibitor of p-glycoprotein, on the pharmacokinetics of sitagliptin. Co-administration of a single 100-mg oral dose of sitagliptin and a single 600-mg oral dose of cyclosporine increased the AUC and C_{max} of sitagliptin by approximately 29% and 68%, respectively. These modest changes in sitagliptin pharmacokinetics were not considered to be clinically meaningful. The renal clearance of sitagliptin was also not meaningfully altered. Therefore, meaningful interactions would not be expected with other p-glycoprotein inhibitors.
Metformin hydrochloride
[See Drug Interactions (7.1, 7.3, 7.4, 7.5, 7.6).]

13 NONCLINICAL TOXICOLOGY
13.1 Carcinogenesis, Mutagenesis, Impairment of Fertility
JANUMET
No animal studies have been conducted with the combined products in JANUMET to evaluate carcinogenesis, mutagenesis or impairment of fertility. The following data are based on the findings in studies with sitagliptin and metformin individually.
Sitagliptin
A two-year carcinogenicity study was conducted in male and female rats given oral doses of sitagliptin of 50, 150, and 500 mg/kg/day. There was an increased incidence of combined liver adenoma/carcinoma in males and females and of liver carcinoma in females at 500 mg/kg. This dose results in exposures approximately 60 times the human exposure at the maximum recommended daily adult human dose (MRHD) of 100 mg/day based on AUC comparisons. Liver tumors were not observed at 150 mg/kg, approximately 20 times the human exposure at the MRHD. A two-year carcinogenicity study was conducted in male and female mice given oral doses of sitagliptin of 50, 125, 250, and 500 mg/kg/day. There was no increase in the incidence of tumors in any organ up to 500 mg/kg, approximately 70 times human exposure at the MRHD. Sitagliptin was not mutagenic or clastogenic with or without metabolic activation in the Ames bacterial mutagenicity assay, a Chinese hamster ovary (CHO) chromosome aberration assay, an *in vitro* cytogenetics assay in CHO, an *in vitro* rat hepatocyte DNA alkaline elution assay, and an *in vivo* micronucleus assay.
In rat fertility studies with oral gavage doses of 125, 250, and 1000 mg/kg, males were treated for 4 weeks prior to mating, during mating, up to scheduled termination (approximately 8 weeks total), and females were treated 2 weeks prior to mating through gestation day 7. No adverse effect on fertility was observed at 125 mg/kg (approximately 12 times human exposure at the MRHD of 100 mg/day based on AUC comparisons). At higher doses, nondose-

related increased resorptions in females were observed (approximately 25 and 100 times human exposure at the MRHD based on AUC comparison).
Metformin hydrochloride
Long-term carcinogenicity studies have been performed in rats (dosing duration of 104 weeks) and mice (dosing duration of 91 weeks) at doses up to and including 900 mg/kg/day and 1500 mg/kg/day, respectively. These doses are both approximately four times the maximum recommended human daily dose of 2000 mg based on body surface area comparisons. No evidence of carcinogenicity with metformin was found in either male or female mice. Similarly, there was no tumorigenic potential observed with metformin in male rats. There was, however, an increased incidence of benign stromal uterine polyps in female rats treated with 900 mg/kg/day.
There was no evidence of a mutagenic potential of metformin in the following *in vitro* tests: Ames test (*S. typhimurium*), gene mutation test (mouse lymphoma cells), or chromosomal aberrations test (human lymphocytes). Results in the *in vivo* mouse micronucleus test were also negative. Fertility of male or female rats was unaffected by metformin when administered at doses as high as 600 mg/kg/day, which is approximately three times the maximum recommended human daily dose based on body surface area comparisons.

14 CLINICAL STUDIES
The co-administration of sitagliptin and metformin has been studied in patients with type 2 diabetes inadequately controlled on diet and exercise and in combination with other antihyperglycemic agents.
There have been no clinical efficacy studies conducted with JANUMET; however, bioequivalence of JANUMET with co-administered sitagliptin and metformin hydrochloride tablets was demonstrated.
Sitagliptin and Metformin Co-administration in Patients with Type 2 Diabetes Inadequately Controlled on Diet and Exercise
A total of 1091 patients with type 2 diabetes and inadequate glycemic control on diet and exercise participated in a 24-week, randomized, double-blind, placebo-controlled factorial study designed to assess the efficacy of sitagliptin and metformin co-administration. Patients on an antihyperglycemic agent (N=541) underwent a diet, exercise, and drug washout period of up to 12 weeks duration. After the washout period, patients with inadequate glycemic control (A1C 7.5% to 11%) were randomized after completing a 2-week single-blind placebo run-in period. Patients not on antihyperglycemic agents at study entry (N=550) with inadequate glycemic control (A1C 7.5% to 11%) immediately entered the 2-week single-blind placebo run-in period and then were

Table 5: Glycemic Parameters at Final Visit (24-Week Study) of Sitagliptin as Add-on Combination Therapy with Metformin*

	Sitagliptin 100 mg QD + Metformin	Placebo + Metformin
A1C (%)	**N = 453**	**N = 224**
Baseline (mean)	8.0	8.0
Change from baseline (adjusted mean†)	-0.7	-0.0
Difference from placebo + metformin (adjusted mean†)	-0.7‡	
(95% CI)	(-0.8, -0.5)	
Patients (%) achieving A1C <7%	213 (47%)	41 (18%)
FPG (mg/dL)	**N = 454**	**N = 226**
Baseline (mean)	170	174
Change from baseline (adjusted mean†)	-17	9
Difference from placebo + metformin (adjusted mean†)	-25‡	
(95% CI)	(-31, -20)	
2-hour PPG (mg/dL)	**N = 387**	**N = 182**
Baseline (mean)	275	272
Change from baseline (adjusted mean†)	-62	-11
Difference from placebo + metformin (adjusted mean†)	-51‡	
(95% CI)	(-61, -41)	

* Intent to Treat Population using last observation on study prior to pioglitazone rescue therapy.
† Least squares means adjusted for prior antihyperglycemic therapy and baseline value.
‡ p<0.001 compared to placebo + metformin.

Table 6: Glycemic Parameters at Final Visit (24-Week Study) for Sitagliptin in Combination with Metformin and Glimepiride*

	Sitagliptin 100 mg + Metformin and Glimepiride	Placebo + Metformin and Glimepiride
A1C (%)	**N = 115**	**N = 105**
Baseline (mean)	8.3	8.3
Change from baseline (adjusted mean†)	-0.6	0.3
Difference from placebo (adjusted mean†)	-0.9‡	
(95% CI)	(-1.1, -0.7)	
Patients (%) achieving A1C <7%	26 (23%)	1 (1%)
FPG (mg/dL)	**N = 115**	**N = 109**
Baseline (mean)	179	179
Change from baseline (adjusted mean†)	-8	13
Difference from placebo (adjusted mean†)	-21‡	
(95% CI)	(-32, -10)	

* Intent to Treat Population using last observation on study prior to pioglitazone rescue therapy.
† Least squares means adjusted for prior antihyperglycemic therapy status and baseline value.
‡ p<0.001 compared to placebo.

randomized. Approximately equal numbers of patients were randomized to receive placebo, 100 mg of sitagliptin once daily, 500 mg or 1000 mg of metformin twice daily, or 50 mg of sitagliptin twice daily in combination with 500 mg or 1000 mg of metformin twice daily. Patients who failed to meet specific glycemic goals during the study were treated with glyburide (glibenclamide) rescue.
Sitagliptin and metformin co-administration provided significant improvements in A1C, FPG, and 2-hour PPG compared to placebo, to metformin alone, and to sitagliptin alone (Table 4, Figure 1). Mean reductions from baseline in A1C were generally greater for patients with higher baseline A1C values. For patients not on an antihyperglycemic agent at study entry, mean reductions from baseline in A1C were: sitagliptin 100 mg once daily, -1.1%; metformin 500 mg bid, -1.1%; metformin 1000 mg bid, -1.2%; sitagliptin 50 mg bid with metformin 500 mg bid, -1.6%; sitagliptin 50 mg bid with metformin 1000 mg bid, -1.9%; and for patients receiving placebo, -0.2%. Lipid effects were generally neutral. The decrease in body weight in the groups given sitagliptin in combination with metformin was similar to that in the groups given metformin alone or placebo.
[See table 4 at top of previous page]
[See figure 1 at top of next column]
In addition, this study included patients (N=117) with more severe hyperglycemia (A1C >11% or blood glucose >280 mg/dL) who were treated with twice daily open-label sitagliptin 50 mg and metformin 1000 mg. In this group of patients, the mean baseline A1C value was 11.2%, mean FPG was 314 mg/dL, and mean 2-hour PPG was 441 mg/dL. After 24 weeks, mean decreases from baseline of -2.9% for A1C, -127 mg/dL for FPG, and -208 mg/dL for 2-hour PPG were observed.

Figure 1: Mean Change from Baseline for A1C (%) over 24 Weeks with Sitagliptin and Metformin, Alone and in Combination in Patients with Type 2 Diabetes Inadequately Controlled with Diet and Exercise†

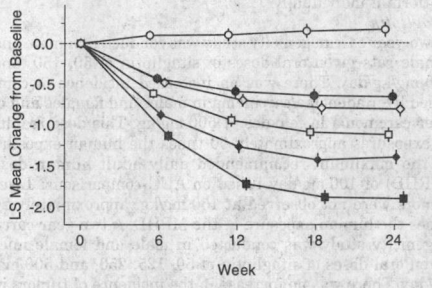

○ Placebo
● Sitagliptin 100 mg q.d.
◇ Metformin 500 mg b.i.d.
□ Metformin 1000 mg b.i.d.
◆ Sitagliptin 50 mg b.i.d. + Metformin 500 mg b.i.d.
■ Sitagliptin 50 mg b.i.d. + Metformin 1000 mg b.i.d.

† Intention to Treat Population; Least squares means adjusted for prior antihyperglycemic therapy and baseline value.

Initial combination therapy or maintenance of combination therapy should be individualized and are left to the discretion of the health care provider.

Sitagliptin Add-on Therapy in Patients with Type 2 Diabetes Inadequately Controlled on Metformin Alone
A total of 701 patients with type 2 diabetes participated in a 24-week, randomized, double-blind, placebo-controlled study designed to assess the efficacy of sitagliptin in combination with metformin. Patients already on metformin

(N=431) at a dose of at least 1500 mg per day were randomized after completing a 2-week, single-blind placebo run-in period. Patients on metformin and another antihyperglycemic agent (N=229) and patients not on any antihyperglycemic agents (off therapy for at least 8 weeks, N=41) were randomized after a run-in period of approximately 10 weeks on metformin (at a dose of at least 1500 mg per day) in monotherapy. Patients were randomized to the addition of either 100 mg of sitagliptin or placebo, administered once daily. Patients who failed to meet specific glycemic goals during the studies were treated with pioglitazone rescue.
In combination with metformin, sitagliptin provided significant improvements in A1C, FPG, and 2-hour PPG compared to placebo with metformin (Table 5). Rescue glycemic therapy was used in 5% of patients treated with sitagliptin 100 mg and 14% of patients treated with placebo. A similar decrease in body weight was observed for both treatment groups.
[See table 5 at left]

Sitagliptin Add-on Therapy in Patients with Type 2 Diabetes Inadequately Controlled on the Combination of Metformin and Glimepiride
A total of 441 patients with type 2 diabetes participated in a 24-week, randomized, double-blind, placebo-controlled study designed to assess the efficacy of sitagliptin in combination with glimepiride, with or without metformin. Patients entered a run-in treatment period on glimepiride (≥4 mg per day) alone or glimepiride in combination with metformin (≥1500 mg per day). After a dose-titration and dose-stable run-in period of up to 16 weeks and a 2-week placebo run-in period, patients with inadequate glycemic control (A1C 7.5% to 10.5%) were randomized to the addition of either 100 mg of sitagliptin or placebo, administered once daily. Patients who failed to meet specific glycemic goals during the studies were treated with pioglitazone rescue.
Patients receiving sitagliptin with metformin and glimepiride had significant improvements in A1C and FPG compared to patients receiving placebo with metformin and glimepiride (Table 6), with mean reductions from baseline relative to placebo in A1C of -0.9% and in FPG of -21 mg/dL. Rescue therapy was used in 8% of patients treated with sitagliptin 100 mg and 29% of patients treated with add-on placebo. The patients treated with add-on sitagliptin had a mean increase in body weight of 1.1 kg vs. add-on placebo (+0.4 kg vs. -0.7 kg). In addition, add-on sitagliptin resulted in an increased rate of hypoglycemia compared to add-on placebo. *[See Warnings and Precautions (5.9); Adverse Reactions (6.1).]*
[See table 6 at left]

Sitagliptin Add-on Therapy in Patients with Type 2 Diabetes Inadequately Controlled on the Combination of Metformin and Rosiglitazone
A total of 278 patients with type 2 diabetes participated in a 54-week, randomized, double-blind, placebo-controlled study designed to assess the efficacy of sitagliptin in combination with metformin and rosiglitazone. Patients on dual therapy with metformin ≥1500 mg/day and rosiglitazone ≥4 mg/day or with metformin ≥1500 mg/day and pioglitazone ≥30 mg/day (switched to rosiglitazone ≥4 mg/day) entered a dose-stable run-in period of 6 weeks. Patients on other dual therapy were switched to metformin ≥1500 mg/day and rosiglitazone ≥4 mg/day in a dose titration/stabilization run-in period of up to 20 weeks in duration. After the run-in period, patients with inadequate glycemic control (A1C 7.5% to 11%) were randomized 2:1 to the addition of either 100 mg of sitagliptin or placebo, administered once daily. Patients who failed to meet specific glycemic goals during the studies were treated with glipizide (or other sulfonylurea) rescue. The primary time point for evaluation of glycemic parameters was Week 18.
In combination with metformin and rosiglitazone, sitagliptin provided significant improvements in A1C, FPG, and 2-hour PPG compared to placebo with metformin and rosiglitazone (Table 7) at Week 18. At Week 54, mean reduction in A1C was -1.0% for patients treated with sitagliptin and -0.3% for patients treated with placebo in an analysis based on the intent to treat population. Rescue therapy was used in 18% of patients treated with sitagliptin 100 mg and 40% of patients treated with placebo. There was no significant difference between sitagliptin and placebo in body weight change.
[See table 7 at top of next page]

Sitagliptin Add-on Therapy in Patients with Type 2 Diabetes Inadequately Controlled on the Combination of Metformin and Insulin
A total of 641 patients with type 2 diabetes participated in a 24-week, randomized, double-blind, placebo-controlled study designed to assess the efficacy of sitagliptin as add-on to insulin therapy. Approximately 75% of patients were also taking metformin. Patients entered a 2-week, single-blind run-in treatment period on pre-mixed, long-acting, or intermediate-acting insulin, with or without metformin

Table 7: Glycemic Parameters at Week 18 for Sitagliptin in Add-on Combination Therapy with Metformin and Rosiglitazone*

	Week 18	
	Sitagliptin 100 mg + Metformin + Rosiglitazone	Placebo + Metformin + Rosiglitazone
A1C (%)	N =176	N = 93
Baseline (mean)	8.8	8.7
Change from baseline (adjusted mean[†])	-1.0	-0.4
Difference from placebo + rosiglitazone + metformin (adjusted mean[†]) (95% CI)	-0.7[‡] (-0.9, -0.4)	
Patients (%) achieving A1C <7%	39 (22%)	9 (10%)
FPG (mg/dL)	N = 179	N = 94
Baseline (mean)	181	182
Change from baseline (adjusted mean[†])	-30	-11
Difference from placebo + rosiglitazone + metformin (adjusted mean[†]) (95% CI)	-18[‡] (-26, -10)	
2-hour PPG (mg/dL)	N = 152	N = 80
Baseline (mean)	256	248
Change from baseline (adjusted mean[†])	-59	-21
Difference from placebo + rosiglitazone + metformin (adjusted mean[†]) (95% CI)	-39[‡] (-51, -26)	

* Intent to Treat Population using last observation on study prior to glipizide (or other sulfonylurea) rescue therapy.
† Least squares means adjusted for prior antihyperglycemic therapy status and baseline value.
‡ p<0.001 compared to placebo + metformin + rosiglitazone.

Table 8: Glycemic Parameters at Final Visit (24-Week Study) for Sitagliptin as Add-on Combination Therapy with Metformin and Insulin*

	Sitagliptin 100 mg + Metformin + Insulin	Placebo + Metformin + Insulin
A1C (%)	N = 223	N = 229
Baseline (mean)	8.7	8.6
Change from baseline (adjusted mean[†,‡])	-0.7	-0.1
Difference from placebo (adjusted mean[†]) (95% CI)	-0.5[§] (-0.7, -0.4)	
Patients (%) achieving A1C % <7%	32 (14%)	12 (5%)
FPG (mg/dL)	N = 225	N = 229
Baseline (mean)	173	176
Change from baseline (adjusted mean[†])	-22	-4
Difference from placebo (adjusted mean[†]) (95% CI)	-18[§] (-28, -8.4)	
2-hour PPG (mg/dL)	N = 182	N = 189
Baseline (mean)	281	281
Change from baseline (adjusted mean[†])	-39	1
Difference from placebo (adjusted mean[†]) (95% CI)	-40[§] (-53, -28)	

* Intent to Treat Population using last observation on study prior to rescue therapy.
† Least squares mean adjusted for insulin use at the screening visit, type of insulin used at the screening visit (pre-mixed vs. non pre-mixed [intermediate- or long-acting]), and baseline value.
‡ Treatment by insulin stratum interaction was not significant (p >0.10).
§ p<0.001 compared to placebo.

(≥1500 mg per day). Patients using short-acting insulins were excluded unless the short-acting insulin was administered as part of a pre-mixed insulin. After the run-in period, patients with inadequate glycemic control (A1C 7.5% to 11%) were randomized to the addition of either 100 mg of sitagliptin (N=229) or placebo (N=233), administered once daily. Patients were on a stable dose of insulin prior to enrollment with no changes in insulin dose permitted during the run-in period. Patients who failed to meet specific glycemic goals during the double-blind treatment period were to have uptitration of the background insulin dose as rescue therapy.

Among patients also receiving metformin, the median daily insulin (pre-mixed, intermediate or long acting) dose at baseline was 40 units in the sitagliptin-treated patients and 42 units in the placebo-treated patients. The median change from baseline in daily dose of insulin was zero for both groups at the end of the study. Patients receiving sitagliptin with metformin and insulin had significant improvements in A1C, FPG and 2-hour PPG compared to patients receiving placebo with metformin and insulin (Table 8). The adjusted mean change from baseline in body weight was -0.3 kg in patients receiving sitagliptin with metformin and insulin and -0.2 kg in patients receiving placebo with metformin and insulin. There was an increased rate of hypoglycemia in patients treated with sitagliptin. [See Warnings and Precautions (5.9); Adverse Reactions (6.1).]
[See table 8 above]

Sitagliptin Add-on Therapy vs. Glipizide Add-on Therapy in Patients with Type 2 Diabetes Inadequately Controlled on Metformin

The efficacy of sitagliptin was evaluated in a 52-week, double-blind, glipizide-controlled noninferiority trial in patients with type 2 diabetes. Patients not on treatment or on other antihyperglycemic agents entered a run-in treatment period of up to 12 weeks duration with metformin monotherapy (dose of ≥1500 mg per day) which included washout of medications other than metformin, if applicable. After the run-in period, those with inadequate glycemic control (A1C 6.5% to 10%) were randomized 1:1 to the addition of sitagliptin 100 mg once daily or glipizide for 52 weeks. Patients receiving glipizide were given an initial dosage of 5 mg/day and then electively titrated over the next 18 weeks to a maximum dosage of 20 mg/day as needed to optimize glycemic control. Thereafter, the glipizide dose was to be kept constant, except for down-titration to prevent hypoglycemia. The mean dose of glipizide after the titration period was 10 mg.

After 52 weeks, sitagliptin and glipizide had similar mean reductions from baseline in A1C in the intent-to-treat analysis (Table 9). These results were consistent with the per protocol analysis (Figure 2). A conclusion in favor of the noninferiority of sitagliptin to glipizide may be limited to patients with baseline A1C comparable to those included in the study (over 70% of patients had baseline A1C <8% and over 90% had A1C <9%).

Table 9: Glycemic Parameters in a 52-Week Study Comparing Sitagliptin to Glipizide as Add-On Therapy in Patients Inadequately Controlled on Metformin (Intent-to-Treat Population)*

	Sitagliptin 100 mg + Metformin	Glipizide + Metformin
A1C (%)	N = 576	N = 559
Baseline (mean)	7.7	7.6
Change from baseline (adjusted mean[†])	-0.5	-0.6
FPG (mg/dL)	N = 583	N = 568
Baseline (mean)	166	164
Change from baseline (adjusted mean[†])	-8	-8

* The Intent to Treat Analysis used the patients' last observation in the study prior to discontinuation.
† Least squares means adjusted for prior antihyperglycemic therapy status and baseline A1C value.

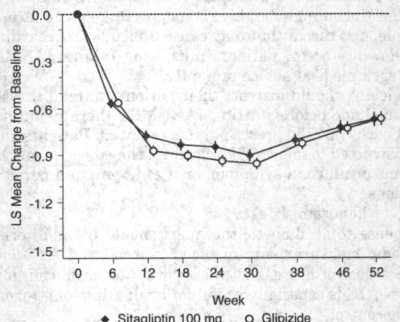

Figure 2: Mean Change from Baseline for A1C (%) Over 52 Weeks in a Study Comparing Sitagliptin to Glipizide as Add-On Therapy in Patients Inadequately Controlled on Metformin (Per Protocol Population)[†]

† The per protocol population (mean baseline A1C of 7.5%) included patients without major protocol violations who had observations at baseline and at Week 52.

The incidence of hypoglycemia in the sitagliptin group (4.9%) was significantly (p<0.001) lower than that in the glipizide group (32.0%). Patients treated with sitagliptin exhibited a significant mean decrease from baseline in body weight compared to a significant weight gain in patients administered glipizide (-1.5 kg vs. +1.1 kg).

16   HOW SUPPLIED/STORAGE AND HANDLING

No. 6747—Tablets JANUMET, 50 mg/500 mg, are light pink, capsule-shaped, film-coated tablets with "575" debossed on one side. They are supplied as follows:
NDC 0006-0575-61 unit-of-use bottles of 60
NDC 0006-0575-62 unit-of-use bottles of 180
NDC 0006-0575-52 unit dose blister packages of 50
NDC 0006-0575-82 bulk bottles of 1000.

No. 6749—Tablets JANUMET, 50 mg/1000 mg, are red, capsule-shaped, film-coated tablets with "577" debossed on one side. They are supplied as follows:
NDC 0006-0577-61 unit-of-use bottles of 60
NDC 0006-0577-62 unit-of-use bottles of 180
NDC 0006-0577-52 unit dose blister packages of 50
NDC 0006-0577-82 bulk bottles of 1000.
Store at 20-25°C (68-77°F), excursions permitted to 15-30°C (59-86°F), [See USP Controlled Room Temperature].

17 PATIENT COUNSELING INFORMATION
See FDA-approved Medication Guide.

17.1 Instructions
Patients should be informed of the potential risks and benefits of JANUMET and of alternative modes of therapy. They should also be informed about the importance of adherence to dietary instructions, regular physical activity, periodic blood glucose monitoring and A1C testing, recognition and management of hypoglycemia and hyperglycemia, and assessment for diabetes complications. During periods of stress such as fever, trauma, infection, or surgery, medication requirements may change and patients should be advised to seek medical advice promptly.

The risks of lactic acidosis due to the metformin component, its symptoms, and conditions that predispose to its development, as noted in Warnings and Precautions (5.1), should be explained to patients. Patients should be advised to discontinue JANUMET immediately and to promptly notify their health practitioner if unexplained hyperventilation, myalgia, malaise, unusual somnolence, dizziness, slow or irregular heart beat, sensation of feeling cold (especially in the extremities) or other nonspecific symptoms occur. Gastrointestinal symptoms are common during initiation of metformin treatment and may occur during initiation of JANUMET therapy; however, patients should consult their physician if they develop unexplained symptoms. Although gastrointestinal symptoms that occur after stabilization are unlikely to be drug related, such an occurrence of symptoms should be evaluated to determine if it may be due to lactic acidosis or other serious disease.

Patients should be counseled against excessive alcohol intake, either acute or chronic, while receiving JANUMET.
Patients should be informed about the importance of regular testing of renal function and hematological parameters when receiving treatment with JANUMET.
Patients should be informed that acute pancreatitis has been reported during postmarketing use of JANUMET. Patients should be informed that persistent severe abdominal pain, sometimes radiating to the back, which may or may not be accompanied by vomiting, is the hallmark symptom of acute pancreatitis. Patients should be instructed to promptly discontinue JANUMET and contact their physician if persistent severe abdominal pain occurs [see Warnings and Precautions (5.2)].
Patients should be informed that the incidence of hypoglycemia is increased when JANUMET is added to an insulin secretagogue (e.g., sulfonylurea) or insulin therapy and that a lower dose of the insulin secretagogue or insulin may be required to reduce the risk of hypoglycemia.
Patients should be informed that allergic reactions have been reported during postmarketing use of sitagliptin, one of the components of JANUMET. If symptoms of allergic reactions (including rash, hives, and swelling of the face, lips, tongue, and throat that may cause difficulty in breathing or swallowing) occur, patients must stop taking JANUMET and seek medical advice promptly.
Physicians should instruct their patients to read the Medication Guide before starting JANUMET therapy and to reread each time the prescription is renewed. Patients should be instructed to inform their doctor if they develop any bothersome or unusual symptom, or if any symptom persists or worsens.

17.2 Laboratory Tests
Response to all diabetic therapies should be monitored by periodic measurements of blood glucose and A1C levels, with a goal of decreasing these levels towards the normal range. A1C is especially useful for evaluating long-term glycemic control.
Initial and periodic monitoring of hematologic parameters (e.g., hemoglobin/hematocrit and red blood cell indices) and renal function (serum creatinine) should be performed, at least on an annual basis. While megaloblastic anemia has rarely been seen with metformin therapy, if this is suspected, Vitamin B$_{12}$ deficiency should be excluded.

Dist. by: Merck Sharp & Dohme Corp., a subsidiary of
MERCK & CO., INC., Whitehouse Station, NJ 08889, USA
9984500
US Patent No.: 6,699,871
[1,2] Registered trademark of Merck Sharp & Dohme Corp., a subsidiary of **Merck & Co., Inc.**
[3] GLUCOPHAGE® is a registered trademark of Merck Sante S.A.S., an associate of Merck KGaA of Darmstadt, Germany. Licensed to Bristol-Myers Squibb Company.
Copyright © 2007, 2008, 2009, 2010 Merck Sharp & Dohme Corp., a subsidiary of **Merck & Co., Inc.**
All rights reserved

MEDICATION GUIDE
JANUMET® (JAN-you-met)
(sitagliptin/metformin hydrochloride)
Tablets
Read this Medication Guide carefully before you start taking JANUMET and each time you get a refill. There may be new information. This information does not take the place of talking with your doctor about your medical condition or your treatment. If you have any questions about JANUMET, ask your doctor or pharmacist.

What is the most important information I should know about JANUMET?
Serious side effects can happen in people taking JANUMET, including:
1. Lactic Acidosis. Metformin, one of the medicines in JANUMET, can cause a rare but serious condition called lactic acidosis (a build-up of lactic acid in the blood) that can cause death. Lactic acidosis is a medical emergency and must be treated in the hospital.
Stop taking JANUMET and call your doctor right away if you get any of the following symptoms, which could be signs of lactic acidosis.
You:
• feel very weak or tired.
• have unusual (not normal) muscle pain.
• have trouble breathing.
• have unusual sleepiness or sleep longer than usual.
• have sudden stomach or intestinal problems with nausea and vomiting or diarrhea.
• feel cold, especially in your arms and legs.
• feel dizzy or lightheaded.
• have a slow or irregular heartbeat.
You have a higher chance of getting lactic acidosis if you:
• have kidney problems. People whose kidneys are not working properly should not take JANUMET.
• have liver problems.
• have congestive heart failure that requires treatment with medicines.
• drink alcohol very often, or drink a lot of alcohol in short-term "binge" drinking.
• get dehydrated (lose a large amount of body fluids). This can happen if you are sick with a fever, vomiting, or diarrhea. Dehydration can also happen when you sweat a lot with activity or exercise and do not drink enough fluids.
• have certain x-ray tests with dyes or contrast agents that are injected into your body.
• have surgery.
• have a heart attack, severe infection, or stroke.
• are 80 years of age or older and have not had your kidneys tested.
2. Pancreatitis (inflammation of the pancreas) which may be severe and lead to death.
Certain medical problems make you more likely to get pancreatitis.
Before you start taking JANUMET:
Tell your doctor if you have ever had
• pancreatitis
• stones in your gallbladder (gallstones)
• a history of alcoholism
• high blood triglyceride levels
Stop taking JANUMET and call your doctor right away if you have pain in your stomach area (abdomen) that is severe and will not go away. The pain may be felt going from your abdomen through to your back. The pain may happen with or without vomiting. These may be symptoms of pancreatitis.

What is JANUMET?
• JANUMET is a prescription medicine that contains two prescription diabetes medicines, sitagliptin (JANUVIA®) and metformin. JANUMET can be used along with diet and exercise to lower blood sugar in adults with type 2 diabetes.
• JANUMET is not for people with type 1 diabetes.
• JANUMET is not for people with diabetic ketoacidosis (increased ketones in your blood or urine).
• If you have had pancreatitis (inflammation of the pancreas) in the past, it is not known if you have a higher chance of getting pancreatitis while you take JANUMET.
• It is not known if JANUMET is safe and effective when used in children under 18 years of age.

Who should not take JANUMET?
Do not take JANUMET if:
• you are allergic to any of the ingredients in JANUMET. See the end of this Medication Guide for a complete list of ingredients in JANUMET.
Symptoms of a serious allergic reaction to JANUMET may include:
• rash
• raised red patches on your skin (hives)
• swelling of the face, lips, tongue, and throat that may cause difficulty in breathing or swallowing
• you have kidneys which are not working properly.
• you are going to get an injection of dye or contrast agents for an x-ray procedure, JANUMET will need to be stopped

for a short time. Talk to your doctor about when you should stop JANUMET and when you should start JANUMET again. See **"What is the most important information I should know about JANUMET?"**
What should I tell my doctor before taking JANUMET?
Before you take JANUMET, tell your doctor if you:
• have or have had inflammation of your pancreas (pancreatitis).
• have kidney problems.
• have liver problems.
• have heart problems, including congestive heart failure.
• are older than 80 years. If you are over 80 years old you should not take JANUMET unless your kidneys have been checked and they are normal.
• drink alcohol very often, or drink a lot of alcohol in short-term "binge" drinking.
• have any other medical conditions.
• are pregnant or plan to become pregnant. It is not known if JANUMET will harm your unborn baby. If you are pregnant, talk with your doctor about the best way to control your blood sugar while you are pregnant.
Pregnancy Registry: If you take JANUMET at any time during your pregnancy, talk with your doctor about how you can join the JANUMET pregnancy registry. The purpose of this registry is to collect information about the health of you and your baby. You can enroll in this registry by calling 1-800-986-8999.
• are breast-feeding or plan to breast-feed. It is not known if JANUMET will pass into your breast milk. Talk with your doctor about the best way to feed your baby if you are taking JANUMET.
Tell your doctor about all the medicines you take, including prescription and non-prescription medicines, vitamins, and herbal supplements. JANUMET may affect how well other drugs work and some drugs can affect how well JANUMET works.
Know the medicines you take. Keep a list of your medicines and show it to your doctor and pharmacist when you get a new medicine.
How should I take JANUMET?
• Take JANUMET exactly as your doctor tells you.
• Your doctor may change your dose of JANUMET if needed.
• Your doctor may tell you to take JANUMET along with certain other diabetes medicines. Low blood sugar can happen more often when JANUMET is taken with certain other diabetes medicines. See **"What are the possible side effects of JANUMET?"**
• Take JANUMET with meals to lower your chance of having an upset stomach.
• Continue to take JANUMET as long as your doctor tells you.
• If you take too much JANUMET, call your doctor or local Poison Control Center right away.
• If you miss a dose, take it with food as soon as you remember. If you do not remember until it is time for your next dose, skip the missed dose and go back to your regular schedule. Do not take two doses of JANUMET at the same time.
• You may need to stop taking JANUMET for a short time. Call your doctor for instructions if you:
• are dehydrated (have lost too much body fluid). Dehydration can occur if you are sick with severe vomiting, diarrhea or fever, or if you drink a lot less fluid than normal.
• plan to have surgery.
• are going to get an injection of dye or contrast agent for an x-ray procedure. See **"What is the most important information I should know about JANUMET?"** and **"Who should not take JANUMET?"**
• When your body is under some types of stress, such as fever, trauma (such as a car accident), infection or surgery, the amount of diabetes medicine that you need may change. Tell your doctor right away if you have any of these problems and follow your doctor's instructions.
• Check your blood sugar as your doctor tells you to.
• Stay on your prescribed diet and exercise program while taking JANUMET.
• Talk to your doctor about how to prevent, recognize and manage low blood sugar (hypoglycemia), high blood sugar (hyperglycemia), and problems you have because of your diabetes.
• Your doctor will check your diabetes with regular blood tests, including your blood sugar levels and your hemoglobin A1C.
• Your doctor will do blood tests to check how well your kidneys are working before and during your treatment with JANUMET.
What are the possible side effects of JANUMET?
Serious side effects have occurred in people taking JANUMET.
• See **"What is the most important information I should know about JANUMET?"**
• **Low blood sugar (hypoglycemia).** If you take JANUMET with another medicine that can cause low blood sugar, such as a sulfonylurea or insulin, your risk of getting low

blood sugar is higher. The dose of your sulfonylurea medicine or insulin may need to be lowered while you use JANUMET. Signs and symptoms of low blood sugar may include:

- headache
- drowsiness
- weakness
- dizziness
- confusion
- irritability
- hunger
- fast heart beat
- sweating
- feeling jittery

- **Serious allergic reactions.** If you have any symptoms of a serious allergic reaction, stop taking JANUMET and call your doctor right away. See "**Who should not take JANUMET?**". Your doctor may give you a medicine for your allergic reaction and prescribe a different medicine for your diabetes.

The most common side effects of JANUMET include:
- stuffy or runny nose and sore throat
- upper respiratory infection
- diarrhea
- nausea and vomiting
- gas, upset stomach, indigestion
- weakness
- headache

Taking JANUMET with meals can help lessen the common stomach side effects of metformin that usually happen at the beginning of treatment. If you have unusual or sudden stomach problems, talk with your doctor. Stomach problems that start later during treatment may be a sign of something more serious.

JANUMET may have other side effects, including:
- swelling of the hands or legs. Swelling of the hands and legs can happen if you take JANUMET in combination with rosiglitazone (Avandia®). Rosiglitazone is another type of diabetes medicine.

These are not all the possible side effects of JANUMET. For more information, ask your doctor or pharmacist.

Tell your doctor if you have any side effect that bothers you, is unusual, or does not go away.

Call your doctor for medical advice about side effects. You may report side effects to FDA at 1-800-FDA-1088.

How should I store JANUMET?

Store JANUMET at 68°F to 77°F (20°C to 25°C).

Keep JANUMET and all medicines out of the reach of children.

General information about the use of JANUMET

Medicines are sometimes prescribed for purposes other than those listed in Medication Guides. Do not use JANUMET for a condition for which it was not prescribed. Do not give JANUMET to other people, even if they have the same symptoms you have. It may harm them.

This Medication Guide summarizes the most important information about JANUMET. If you would like to know more information, talk with your doctor. You can ask your doctor or pharmacist for additional information about JANUMET that is written for health care professionals. For more information go to www.JANUMET.com or call 1-800-622-4477.

What are the ingredients in JANUMET?

Active ingredients: sitagliptin and metformin hydrochloride.

Inactive ingredients: microcrystalline cellulose, polyvinyl-pyrrolidone, sodium lauryl sulfate, and sodium stearyl fumarate. The tablet film coating contains the following inactive ingredients: polyvinyl alcohol, polyethylene glycol, talc, titanium dioxide, red iron oxide, and black iron oxide.

What is type 2 diabetes?

Type 2 diabetes is a condition in which your body does not make enough insulin, and the insulin that your body produces does not work as well as it should. Your body can also make too much sugar. When this happens, sugar (glucose) builds up in the blood. This can lead to serious medical problems.

High blood sugar can be lowered by diet and exercise, and by certain medicines when necessary.

JANUMET® and JANUVIA® are registered trademarks of Merck Sharp & Dohme Corp., a subsidiary of **Merck & Co., Inc.**

Avandia® is a registered trademark of GlaxoSmithKline.

Copyright © 2010 Merck Sharp & Dohme Corp., a subsidiary of **Merck & Co., Inc.**

All rights reserved

Revised February 2010

Dist. by: Merck Sharp & Dohme Corp., a subsidiary of **MERCK & CO., INC.**, Whitehouse Station, NJ 08889, USA

9984500

This Medication Guide has been approved by the US Food and Drug Administration.

Shown in Product Identification Guide, page 313

JANUVIA®

R

[ja-new'-vee-a]
(sitagliptin)
Tablets

HIGHLIGHTS OF PRESCRIBING INFORMATION

These highlights do not include all the information needed to use JANUVIA safely and effectively. See full prescribing information for JANUVIA.

JANUVIA® (sitagliptin) Tablets
Initial U.S. Approval: 2006

——RECENT MAJOR CHANGES——

Indications and Usage
  Important Limitations of Use (1.2) 02/2010
Dosage and Administration
  Concomitant Use with an Insulin Secretagogue (e.g., Sulfonylurea) or with Insulin (2.3) 02/2010
Warnings and Precautions
  Pancreatitis (5.1) 12/2009
Use with Medications Known to Cause Hypoglycemia (5.3) 02/2010

——INDICATIONS AND USAGE——

JANUVIA is a dipeptidyl peptidase-4 (DPP-4) inhibitor indicated as an adjunct to diet and exercise to improve glycemic control in adults with type 2 diabetes mellitus. (1.1)

Important Limitations of Use:
- JANUVIA should not be used in patients with type 1 diabetes or for the treatment of diabetic ketoacidosis. (1.2)
- JANUVIA has not been studied in patients with a history of pancreatitis. (1.2, 5.1)

——DOSAGE AND ADMINISTRATION——

The recommended dose of JANUVIA is 100 mg once daily. JANUVIA can be taken with or without food. (2.1)
Dosage adjustment is recommended for patients with moderate or severe renal insufficiency or end-stage renal disease. (2.2)

Dosage Adjustment in Patients With Moderate, Severe and End Stage Renal Disease (ESRD) (2.2)

50 mg once daily	25 mg once daily
Moderate CrCl ≥30 to <50 mL/min ~Serum Cr levels [mg/dL] Men: >1.7–≤3.0; Women: >1.5–≤2.5	Severe and ESRD CrCl <30 mL/min ~Serum Cr levels [mg/dL] Men: >3.0; Women: >2.5; or on dialysis

——DOSAGE FORMS AND STRENGTHS——

Tablets: 100 mg, 50 mg, and 25 mg (3)

——CONTRAINDICATIONS——

History of a serious hypersensitivity reaction to sitagliptin, such as anaphylaxis or angioedema. (5.4, 6.2)

——WARNINGS AND PRECAUTIONS——

- There have been postmarketing reports of acute pancreatitis, including fatal and non-fatal hemorrhagic or necrotizing pancreatitis. If pancreatitis is suspected, promptly discontinue JANUVIA. (5.1)
- Dosage adjustment is recommended in patients with moderate or severe renal insufficiency and in patients with ESRD. Assessment of renal function is recommended prior to initiating JANUVIA and periodically thereafter. (2.2, 5.2)
- There is an increased risk of hypoglycemia when JANUVIA is added to an insulin secretagogue (e.g., sulfonylurea) or insulin therapy. Consider lowering the dose of the sulfonylurea or insulin to reduce the risk of hypoglycemia. (2.3, 5.3)
- There have been postmarketing reports of serious allergic and hypersensitivity reactions in patients treated with JANUVIA such as anaphylaxis, angioedema, and exfoliative skin conditions including Stevens-Johnson syndrome. In such cases, promptly stop JANUVIA, assess for other potential causes, institute appropriate monitoring and treatment, and initiate alternative treatment for diabetes. (5.4, 6.2)
- There have been no clinical studies establishing conclusive evidence of macrovascular risk reduction with JANUVIA or any other anti-diabetic drug. (5.5)

——ADVERSE REACTIONS——

Adverse reactions reported in ≥5% of patients treated with JANUVIA and more commonly than in patients treated with placebo are: upper respiratory tract infection, nasopharyngitis and headache. In the add-on to sulfonylurea and add-on to insulin studies, hypoglycemia was also more commonly reported in patients treated with JANUVIA compared to placebo. (6.1)

To report SUSPECTED ADVERSE REACTIONS, contact Merck Sharp & Dohme Corp., a subsidiary of Merck & Co., Inc., at 1-877-888-4231 or FDA at 1-800-FDA-1088 or www.fda.gov/medwatch.

——USE IN SPECIFIC POPULATIONS——

- Safety and effectiveness of JANUVIA in children under 18 years have not been established. (8.4)
- There are no adequate and well-controlled studies in pregnant women. To report drug exposure during pregnancy call 1-800-986-8999. (8.1)

See 17 for PATIENT COUNSELING INFORMATION and Medication Guide

Revised: 02/2010

FULL PRESCRIBING INFORMATION: CONTENTS*

*Sections or subsections omitted from the full prescribing information are not listed

FULL PRESCRIBING INFORMATION

1 INDICATIONS AND USAGE

1.1 Monotherapy and Combination Therapy

JANUVIA[1] is indicated as an adjunct to diet and exercise to improve glycemic control in adults with type 2 diabetes mellitus. *[See Clinical Studies (14).]*

1.2 Important Limitations of Use

JANUVIA should not be used in patients with type 1 diabetes or for the treatment of diabetic ketoacidosis, as it would not be effective in these settings.

JANUVIA has not been studied in patients with a history of pancreatitis. It is unknown whether patients with a history of pancreatitis are at increased risk for the development of pancreatitis while using JANUVIA. *[See Warnings and Precautions (5.1).]*

2 DOSAGE AND ADMINISTRATION

2.1 Recommended Dosing

The recommended dose of JANUVIA is 100 mg once daily. JANUVIA can be taken with or without food.

2.2 Patients with Renal Insufficiency

For patients with mild renal insufficiency (creatinine clearance [CrCl] ≥50 mL/min, approximately corresponding to serum creatinine levels of ≤1.7 mg/dL in men and ≤1.5 mg/dL in women), no dosage adjustment for JANUVIA is required.

For patients with moderate renal insufficiency (CrCl ≥30 to <50 mL/min, approximately corresponding to serum creatinine levels of >1.7 to ≤3.0 mg/dL in men and >1.5 to ≤2.5 mg/dL in women), the dose of JANUVIA is 50 mg once daily.

For patients with severe renal insufficiency (CrCl <30 mL/min, approximately corresponding to serum creatinine levels of >3.0 mg/dL in men and >2.5 mg/dL in women) or with end-stage renal disease (ESRD) requiring hemodialysis or peritoneal dialysis, the dose of JANUVIA is 25 mg once daily. JANUVIA may be administered without regard to the timing of hemodialysis.

Because there is a need for dosage adjustment based upon renal function, assessment of renal function is recommended prior to initiation of JANUVIA and periodically thereafter. Creatinine clearance can be estimated from serum creatinine using the Cockcroft-Gault formula. *[See Clinical Pharmacology (12.3).]*

2.3   Concomitant Use with an Insulin Secretagogue (e.g., Sulfonylurea) or with Insulin
When JANUVIA is used in combination with an insulin secretagogue (e.g., sulfonylurea) or with insulin, a lower dose of the insulin secretagogue or insulin may be required to reduce the risk of hypoglycemia. *[See Warnings and Precautions (5.3).]*

3   DOSAGE FORMS AND STRENGTHS
- 100 mg tablets are beige, round, film-coated tablets with "277" on one side.
- 50 mg tablets are light beige, round, film-coated tablets with "112" on one side.
- 25 mg tablets are pink, round, film-coated tablets with "221" on one side.

4   CONTRAINDICATIONS
History of a serious hypersensitivity reaction to sitagliptin, such as anaphylaxis or angioedema. *[See Warnings and Precautions (5.4); Adverse Reactions (6.2).]*

5   WARNINGS AND PRECAUTIONS
5.1   Pancreatitis
There have been postmarketing reports of acute pancreatitis, including fatal and non-fatal hemorrhagic or necrotizing pancreatitis, in patients taking JANUVIA. After initiation of JANUVIA, patients should be observed carefully for signs and symptoms of pancreatitis. If pancreatitis is suspected, JANUVIA should promptly be discontinued and appropriate management should be initiated. It is unknown whether patients with a history of pancreatitis are at increased risk for the development of pancreatitis while using JANUVIA.

5.2   Use in Patients with Renal Insufficiency
A dosage adjustment is recommended in patients with moderate or severe renal insufficiency and in patients with ESRD requiring hemodialysis or peritoneal dialysis. *[See Dosage and Administration (2.2); Clinical Pharmacology (12.3).]*

5.3   Use with Medications Known to Cause Hypoglycemia
When JANUVIA was used in combination with a sulfonylurea or with insulin, medications known to cause hypoglycemia, the incidence of hypoglycemia was increased over that of placebo used in combination with a sulfonylurea or with insulin. *[See Adverse Reactions (6.1).]* Therefore, a lower dose of sulfonylurea or insulin may be required to reduce the risk of hypoglycemia. *[See Dosage and Administration (2.3).]*

5.4   Hypersensitivity Reactions
There have been postmarketing reports of serious hypersensitivity reactions in patients treated with JANUVIA. These reactions include anaphylaxis, angioedema, and exfoliative skin conditions including Stevens-Johnson syndrome. Because these reactions are reported voluntarily from a population of uncertain size, it is generally not possible to reliably estimate their frequency or establish a causal relationship to drug exposure. Onset of these reactions occurred within the first 3 months after initiation of treatment with JANUVIA, with some reports occurring after the first dose. If a hypersensitivity reaction is suspected, discontinue JANUVIA, assess for other potential causes for the event, and institute alternative treatment for diabetes. *[See Adverse Reactions (6.2).]*

5.5   Macrovascular Outcomes
There have been no clinical studies establishing conclusive evidence of macrovascular risk reduction with JANUVIA or any other anti-diabetic drug.

6   ADVERSE REACTIONS
6.1   Clinical Trials Experience
Because clinical trials are conducted under widely varying conditions, adverse reaction rates observed in the clinical trials of a drug cannot be directly compared to rates in the clinical trials of another drug and may not reflect the rates observed in practice.
In controlled clinical studies as both monotherapy and combination therapy with metformin, pioglitazone, or rosiglitazone and metformin, the overall incidence of adverse reactions, hypoglycemia, and discontinuation of therapy due to clinical adverse reactions with JANUVIA were similar to placebo. In combination with glimepiride, with or without metformin, the overall incidence of clinical adverse reactions with JANUVIA was higher than with placebo, in part related to a higher incidence of hypoglycemia (see Table 3); the incidence of discontinuation due to clinical adverse reactions was similar to placebo.
Two placebo-controlled monotherapy studies, one of 18- and one of 24-week duration, included patients treated with JANUVIA 100 mg daily, JANUVIA 200 mg daily, and placebo. Five placebo-controlled add-on combination therapy

studies were also conducted: one with metformin; one with pioglitazone; one with metformin and rosiglitazone; one with glimepiride (with or without metformin); and one with insulin (with or without metformin). In these studies, patients with inadequate glycemic control on a stable dose of the background therapy were randomized to add-on therapy with JANUVIA 100 mg daily or placebo. The adverse reactions, excluding hypoglycemia, reported regardless of investigator assessment of causality in ≥5% of patients treated with JANUVIA 100 mg daily and more commonly than in patients treated with placebo, are shown in Table 1 for the clinical trials of at least 18 weeks duration. Incidences of hypoglycemia are shown in Table 3.

Table 1: Placebo-Controlled Clinical Studies of JANUVIA Monotherapy or Add-on Combination Therapy with Pioglitazone, Metformin + Rosiglitazone, or Glimepiride +/- Metformin: Adverse Reactions (Excluding Hypoglycemia) Reported in ≥5% of Patients and More Commonly than in Patients Given Placebo, Regardless of Investigator Assessment of Causality*

	Number of Patients (%)	
Monotherapy (18 or 24 weeks)	JANUVIA 100 mg	Placebo
	N = 443	N = 363
Nasopharyngitis	23 (5.2)	12 (3.3)
Combination with Pioglitazone (24 weeks)	**JANUVIA 100 mg + Pioglitazone**	**Placebo + Pioglitazone**
	N = 175	N = 178
Upper Respiratory Tract Infection	11 (6.3)	6 (3.4)
Headache	9 (5.1)	7 (3.9)
Combination with Metformin + Rosiglitazone (18 weeks)	**JANUVIA 100 mg + Metformin + Rosiglitazone**	**Placebo + Metformin + Rosiglitazone**
	N = 181	N = 97
Upper Respiratory Tract Infection	10 (5.5)	5 (5.2)
Nasopharyngitis	11 (6.1)	4 (4.1)
Combination with Glimepiride (+/- Metformin) (24 weeks)	**JANUVIA 100 mg + Glimepiride (+/- Metformin)**	**Placebo + Glimepiride (+/- Metformin)**
	N = 222	N = 219
Nasopharyngitis	14 (6.3)	10 (4.6)
Headache	13 (5.9)	5 (2.3)

*Intent to treat population

In the 24-week study of patients receiving JANUVIA as add-on combination therapy with metformin, there were no adverse reactions reported regardless of investigator assessment of causality in ≥5% of patients and more commonly than in patients given placebo.
In the 24-week study of patients receiving JANUVIA as add-on therapy to insulin (with or without metformin), there were no adverse reactions reported regardless of investigator assessment of causality in ≥5% of patients and more commonly than in patients given placebo, except for hypoglycemia (see Table 3).
In the study of JANUVIA as add-on combination therapy with metformin and rosiglitazone (Table 1), through Week 54 the adverse reactions reported regardless of investigator

Table 2: Initial Therapy with Combination of Sitagliptin and Metformin: Adverse Reactions Reported (Regardless of Investigator Assessment of Causality) in ≥5% of Patients Receiving Combination Therapy (and Greater than in Patients Receiving Metformin alone, Sitagliptin alone, and Placebo)*

	Number of Patients (%)			
	Placebo	Sitagliptin (JANUVIA) 100 mg QD	Metformin 500 or 1000 mg bid†	Sitagliptin 50 mg bid + Metformin 500 or 1000 mg bid†
	N = 176	N = 179	N = 364†	N = 372†
Upper Respiratory Infection	9 (5.1)	8 (4.5)	19 (5.2)	23 (6.2)
Headache	5 (2.8)	2 (1.1)	14 (3.8)	22 (5.9)

* Intent-to-treat population.
† Data pooled for the patients given the lower and higher doses of metformin.

assessment of causality in ≥5% of patients treated with JANUVIA and more commonly than in patients treated with placebo were: upper respiratory tract infection (JANUVIA, 15.5%; placebo, 6.2%), nasopharyngitis (11.0%, 9.3%), peripheral edema (8.3%, 5.2%), and headache (5.5%, 4.1%).
In a pooled analysis of the two monotherapy studies, the add-on to metformin study, and the add-on to pioglitazone study, the incidence of selected gastrointestinal adverse reactions in patients treated with JANUVIA was as follows: abdominal pain (JANUVIA 100 mg, 2.3%; placebo, 2.1%), nausea (1.4%, 0.6%), and diarrhea (3.0%, 2.3%).
In an additional, 24-week, placebo-controlled factorial study of initial therapy with sitagliptin in combination with metformin, the adverse reactions reported (regardless of investigator assessment of causality) in ≥5% of patients are shown in Table 2.
[See table 2 above]
In a 24-week study of initial therapy with JANUVIA in combination with pioglitazone, there were no adverse reactions reported (regardless of investigator assessment of causality) in ≥5% of patients and more commonly than in patients given pioglitazone alone.
No clinically meaningful changes in vital signs or in ECG (including in QTc interval) were observed in patients treated with JANUVIA.

Hypoglycemia
In all (N=9) studies, adverse reactions of hypoglycemia were based on all reports of symptomatic hypoglycemia. A concurrent blood glucose measurement was not required although most (74%) reports of hypoglycemia were accompanied by a blood glucose measurement ≤70 mg/dL. When JANUVIA was co-administered with a sulfonylurea or with insulin, the percentage of patients with at least one adverse reaction of hypoglycemia was higher than in the corresponding placebo group (Table 3).

Table 3: Incidence and Rate of Hypoglycemia* in Placebo-Controlled Clinical Studies when JANUVIA was used as Add-On Therapy to Glimepiride (with or without Metformin) or Insulin (with or without Metformin), Regardless of Investigator Assessment of Causality

Add-On to Glimepiride (+/- Metformin) (24 weeks)	JANUVIA 100 mg + Glimepiride (+/- Metformin)	Placebo + Glimepiride (+/- Metformin)
	N = 222	N = 219
Overall (%)	27 (12.2)	4 (1.8)
Rate (episodes/patient-year)†	0.59	0.24
Severe (%)‡	0 (0.0)	0 (0.0)
Add-On to Insulin (+/- Metformin) (24 weeks)	**JANUVIA 100 mg + Insulin (+/- Metformin)**	**Placebo + Insulin (+/- Metformin)**
	N = 322	N = 319
Overall (%)	50 (15.5)	25 (7.8)
Rate (episodes/patient-year)†	1.06	0.51
Severe (%)‡	2 (0.6)	1 (0.3)

* Adverse reactions of hypoglycemia were based on all reports of symptomatic hypoglycemia; a concurrent glucose measurement was not required; intent to treat population.
†Based on total number of events (i.e., a single patient may have had multiple events).
‡ Severe events of hypoglycemia were defined as those events requiring medical assistance or exhibiting depressed level/loss of consciousness or seizure.

In a pooled analysis of the two monotherapy studies, the add-on to metformin study, and the add-on to pioglitazone study, the overall incidence of adverse reactions of hypoglycemia was 1.2% in patients treated with JANUVIA 100 mg and 0.9% in patients treated with placebo.

In the study of JANUVIA as add-on combination therapy with metformin and rosiglitazone, the overall incidence of hypoglycemia was 2.2% in patients given add-on JANUVIA and 0.0% in patients given add-on placebo through Week 18. Through Week 54, the overall incidence of hypoglycemia was 3.9% in patients given add-on JANUVIA and 1.0% in patients given add-on placebo.

In the 24-week, placebo-controlled factorial study of initial therapy with JANUVIA in combination with metformin, the incidence of hypoglycemia was 0.6% in patients given placebo, 0.6% in patients given JANUVIA alone, 0.8% in patients given metformin alone, and 1.6% in patients given JANUVIA in combination with metformin.

In the study of JANUVIA as initial therapy with pioglitazone, one patient taking JANUVIA experienced a severe episode of hypoglycemia. There were no severe hypoglycemia episodes reported in other studies except in the study involving co-administration with insulin.

Laboratory Tests

Across clinical studies, the incidence of laboratory adverse reactions was similar in patients treated with JANUVIA 100 mg compared to patients treated with placebo. A small increase in white blood cell count (WBC) was observed due to an increase in neutrophils. This increase in WBC (of approximately 200 cells/microL vs placebo, in four pooled placebo-controlled clinical studies, with a mean baseline WBC count of approximately 6600 cells/microL) is not considered to be clinically relevant. In a 12-week study of 91 patients with chronic renal insufficiency, 37 patients with moderate renal insufficiency were randomized to JANUVIA 50 mg daily, while 14 patients with the same magnitude of renal impairment were randomized to placebo. Mean (SE) increases in serum creatinine were observed in patients treated with JANUVIA [0.12 mg/dL (0.04)] and in patients treated with placebo [0.07 mg/dL (0.07)]. The clinical significance of this added increase in serum creatinine relative to placebo is not known.

6.2 Postmarketing Experience

The following additional adverse reactions have been identified during postapproval use of JANUVIA. Because these reactions are reported voluntarily from a population of uncertain size, it is generally not possible to reliably estimate their frequency or establish a causal relationship to drug exposure.

Hypersensitivity reactions include anaphylaxis, angioedema, rash, urticaria, cutaneous vasculitis, and exfoliative skin conditions including Stevens-Johnson syndrome *[see Warnings and Precautions (5.4)]*; hepatic enzyme elevations; acute pancreatitis, including fatal and non-fatal hemorrhagic and necrotizing pancreatitis *[see Limitations of Use (1.2); Warnings and Precautions (5.1)]*.

7 DRUG INTERACTIONS

7.1 Digoxin

There was a slight increase in the area under the curve (AUC, 11%) and mean peak drug concentration (C_{max}, 18%) of digoxin with the co-administration of 100 mg sitagliptin for 10 days. Patients receiving digoxin should be monitored appropriately. No dosage adjustment of digoxin or JANUVIA is recommended.

8 USE IN SPECIFIC POPULATIONS

8.1 Pregnancy

Pregnancy Category B:

Reproduction studies have been performed in rats and rabbits. Doses of sitagliptin up to 125 mg/kg (approximately 12 times the human exposure at the maximum recommended human dose) did not impair fertility or harm the fetus. There are, however, no adequate and well-controlled studies in pregnant women. Because animal reproduction studies are not always predictive of human response, this drug should be used during pregnancy only if clearly needed.

Merck Sharp & Dohme Corp., a subsidiary of Merck & Co., Inc., maintains a registry to monitor the pregnancy outcomes of women exposed to JANUVIA while pregnant. Health care providers are encouraged to report any prenatal exposure to JANUVIA by calling the Pregnancy Registry at (800) 986-8999.

Sitagliptin administered to pregnant female rats and rabbits from gestation day 6 to 20 (organogenesis) was not teratogenic at oral doses up to 250 mg/kg (rats) and 125 mg/kg (rabbits), or approximately 30- and 20-times human exposure at the maximum recommended human dose (MRHD) of 100 mg/day based on AUC comparisons. Higher doses increased the incidence of rib malformations in offspring at 1000 mg/kg, or approximately 100 times human exposure at the MRHD.

Sitagliptin administered to female rats from gestation day 6 to lactation day 21 decreased body weight in male and female offspring at 1000 mg/kg. No functional or behavioral toxicity was observed in offspring of rats.

Placental transfer of sitagliptin administered to pregnant rats was approximately 45% at 2 hours and 80% at 24 hours postdose. Placental transfer of sitagliptin administered to pregnant rabbits was approximately 66% at 2 hours and 30% at 24 hours.

8.3 Nursing Mothers

Sitagliptin is secreted in the milk of lactating rats at a milk to plasma ratio of 4:1. It is not known whether sitagliptin is excreted in human milk. Because many drugs are excreted in human milk, caution should be exercised when JANUVIA is administered to a nursing woman.

8.4 Pediatric Use

Safety and effectiveness of JANUVIA in pediatric patients under 18 years of age have not been established.

8.5 Geriatric Use

Of the total number of subjects (N=3884) in pre-approval clinical safety and efficacy studies of JANUVIA, 725 patients were 65 years and over, while 61 patients were 75 years and over. No overall differences in safety or effectiveness were observed between subjects 65 years and over and younger subjects. While this and other reported clinical experience have not identified differences in responses between the elderly and younger patients, greater sensitivity of some older individuals cannot be ruled out.

This drug is known to be substantially excreted by the kidney. Because elderly patients are more likely to have decreased renal function, care should be taken in dose selection in the elderly, and it may be useful to assess renal function in these patients prior to initiating dosing and periodically thereafter *[see Dosage and Administration (2.2); Clinical Pharmacology (12.3)]*.

10 OVERDOSAGE

During controlled clinical trials in healthy subjects, single doses of up to 800 mg JANUVIA were administered. Maximal mean increases in QTc of 8.0 msec were observed in one study at a dose of 800 mg JANUVIA, a mean effect that is not considered clinically important *[see Clinical Pharmacology (12.2)]*. There is no experience with doses above 800 mg in humans. In Phase I multiple-dose studies, there were no dose-related clinical adverse reactions observed with JANUVIA with doses of up to 600 mg per day for periods of up to 10 days and 400 mg per day for up to 28 days.

In the event of an overdose, it is reasonable to employ the usual supportive measures, e.g., remove unabsorbed material from the gastrointestinal tract, employ clinical monitoring (including obtaining an electrocardiogram), and institute supportive therapy as dictated by the patient's clinical status.

Sitagliptin is modestly dialyzable. In clinical studies, approximately 13.5% of the dose was removed over a 3- to 4-hour hemodialysis session. Prolonged hemodialysis may be considered if clinically appropriate. It is not known if sitagliptin is dialyzable by peritoneal dialysis.

11 DESCRIPTION

JANUVIA Tablets contain sitagliptin phosphate, an orally-active inhibitor of the dipeptidyl peptidase-4 (DPP-4) enzyme.

Sitagliptin phosphate monohydrate is described chemically as 7-[(3*R*)-3-amino-1-oxo-4-(2,4,5-trifluorophenyl)butyl]-5,6,7,8-tetrahydro-3-(trifluoromethyl)-1,2,4-triazolo[4,3-*a*]pyrazine phosphate (1:1) monohydrate.

The empirical formula is $C_{16}H_{15}F_6N_5O \bullet H_3PO_4 \bullet H_2O$ and the molecular weight is 523.32. The structural formula is:

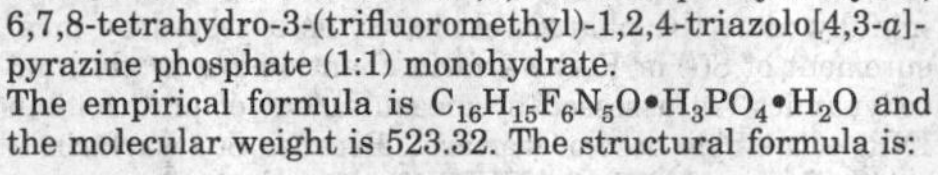

Sitagliptin phosphate monohydrate is a white to off-white, crystalline, non-hygroscopic powder. It is soluble in water and N,N-dimethyl formamide; slightly soluble in methanol; very slightly soluble in ethanol, acetone, and acetonitrile; and insoluble in isopropanol and isopropyl acetate.

Each film-coated tablet of JANUVIA contains 32.13, 64.25, or 128.5 mg of sitagliptin phosphate monohydrate, which is equivalent to 25, 50, or 100 mg, respectively, of free base and the following inactive ingredients: microcrystalline cellulose, anhydrous dibasic calcium phosphate, croscarmellose sodium, magnesium stearate, and sodium stearyl fumarate. In addition, the film coating contains the following inactive ingredients: polyvinyl alcohol, polyethylene glycol, talc, titanium dioxide, red iron oxide, and yellow iron oxide.

12 CLINICAL PHARMACOLOGY

12.1 Mechanism of Action

Sitagliptin is a DPP-4 inhibitor, which is believed to exert its actions in patients with type 2 diabetes by slowing the inactivation of incretin hormones. Concentrations of the active intact hormones are increased by JANUVIA, thereby increasing and prolonging the action of these hormones. Incretin hormones, including glucagon-like peptide-1 (GLP-1) and glucose-dependent insulinotropic polypeptide (GIP), are released by the intestine throughout the day, and levels are increased in response to a meal. These hormones are rapidly inactivated by the enzyme, DPP-4. The incretins are part of an endogenous system involved in the physiologic regulation of glucose homeostasis. When blood glucose concentrations are normal or elevated, GLP-1 and GIP increase insulin synthesis and release from pancreatic beta cells by intracellular signaling pathways involving cyclic AMP. GLP-1 also lowers glucagon secretion from pancreatic alpha cells, leading to reduced hepatic glucose production. By increasing and prolonging active incretin levels, JANUVIA increases insulin release and decreases glucagon levels in the circulation in a glucose-dependent manner. Sitagliptin demonstrates selectivity for DPP-4 and does not inhibit DPP-8 or DPP-9 activity *in vitro* at concentrations approximating those from therapeutic doses.

12.2 Pharmacodynamics

General

In patients with type 2 diabetes, administration of JANUVIA led to inhibition of DPP-4 enzyme activity for a 24-hour period. After an oral glucose load or a meal, this DPP-4 inhibition resulted in a 2- to 3-fold increase in circulating levels of active GLP-1 and GIP, decreased glucagon concentrations, and increased responsiveness of insulin release to glucose, resulting in higher C-peptide and insulin concentrations. The rise in insulin with the decrease in glucagon was associated with lower fasting glucose concentrations and reduced glucose excursion following an oral glucose load or a meal.

In a two-day study in healthy subjects, sitagliptin alone increased active GLP-1 concentrations, whereas metformin alone increased active and total GLP-1 concentrations to similar extents. Co-administration of sitagliptin and metformin had an additive effect on active GLP-1 concentrations. Sitagliptin, but not metformin, increased active GIP concentrations. It is unclear how these findings relate to changes in glycemic control in patients with type 2 diabetes.

In studies with healthy subjects, JANUVIA did not lower blood glucose or cause hypoglycemia.

Cardiac Electrophysiology

In a randomized, placebo-controlled crossover study, 79 healthy subjects were administered a single oral dose of JANUVIA 100 mg, JANUVIA 800 mg (8 times the recommended dose), and placebo. At the recommended dose of 100 mg, there was no effect on the QTc interval obtained at the peak plasma concentration, or at any other time during the study. Following the 800 mg dose, the maximum increase in the placebo-corrected mean change in QTc from baseline was observed at 3 hours postdose and was 8.0 msec. This increase is not considered to be clinically significant. At the 800 mg dose, peak sitagliptin plasma concentrations were approximately 11 times higher than the peak concentrations following a 100 mg dose.

In patients with type 2 diabetes administered JANUVIA 100 mg (N=81) or JANUVIA 200 mg (N=63) daily, there were no meaningful changes in QTc interval based on ECG data obtained at the time of expected peak plasma concentration.

12.3 Pharmacokinetics

The pharmacokinetics of sitagliptin has been extensively characterized in healthy subjects and patients with type 2 diabetes. After oral administration of a 100 mg dose to healthy subjects, sitagliptin was rapidly absorbed, with peak plasma concentrations (median T_{max}) occurring 1 to 4 hours postdose. Plasma AUC of sitagliptin increased in a dose-proportional manner. Following a single oral 100 mg dose to healthy volunteers, mean plasma AUC of sitagliptin was 8.52 μM•hr, C_{max} was 950 nM, and apparent terminal half-life ($t_{1/2}$) was 12.4 hours. Plasma AUC of sitagliptin increased approximately 14% following 100 mg doses at steady-state compared to the first dose. The intra-subject and inter-subject coefficients of variation for sitagliptin AUC were small (5.8% and 15.1%). The pharmacokinetics of sitagliptin was generally similar in healthy subjects and in patients with type 2 diabetes.

Absorption

The absolute bioavailability of sitagliptin is approximately 87%. Because coadministration of a high-fat meal with JANUVIA had no effect on the pharmacokinetics, JANUVIA may be administered with or without food.

Distribution

The mean volume of distribution at steady state following a single 100 mg intravenous dose of sitagliptin to healthy subjects is approximately 198 liters. The fraction of sitagliptin reversibly bound to plasma proteins is low (38%).

Metabolism

Approximately 79% of sitagliptin is excreted unchanged in the urine with metabolism being a minor pathway of elimination.

Following a [^{14}C]sitagliptin oral dose, approximately 16% of the radioactivity was excreted as metabolites of sitagliptin.

$$CrCl = \frac{[140 - \text{age (years)}] \times \text{weight (kg)}}{[72 \times \text{serum creatinine (mg/dL)}]} \{\times 0.85 \text{ for female patients}\}$$

Six metabolites were detected at trace levels and are not expected to contribute to the plasma DPP-4 inhibitory activity of sitagliptin. *In vitro* studies indicated that the primary enzyme responsible for the limited metabolism of sitagliptin was CYP3A4, with contribution from CYP2C8.

Excretion

Following administration of an oral [^{14}C]sitagliptin dose to healthy subjects, approximately 100% of the administered radioactivity was eliminated in feces (13%) or urine (87%) within one week of dosing. The apparent terminal $t_{1/2}$ following a 100 mg oral dose of sitagliptin was approximately 12.4 hours and renal clearance was approximately 350 mL/min.

Elimination of sitagliptin occurs primarily via renal excretion and involves active tubular secretion. Sitagliptin is a substrate for human organic anion transporter-3 (hOAT-3), which may be involved in the renal elimination of sitagliptin. The clinical relevance of hOAT-3 in sitagliptin transport has not been established. Sitagliptin is also a substrate of p-glycoprotein, which may also be involved in mediating the renal elimination of sitagliptin. However, cyclosporine, a p-glycoprotein inhibitor, did not reduce the renal clearance of sitagliptin.

Special Populations

Renal Insufficiency

A single-dose, open-label study was conducted to evaluate the pharmacokinetics of JANUVIA (50 mg dose) in patients with varying degrees of chronic renal insufficiency compared to normal healthy control subjects. The study included patients with renal insufficiency classified on the basis of creatinine clearance as mild (50 to <80 mL/min), moderate (30 to <50 mL/min), and severe (<30 mL/min), as well as patients with ESRD on hemodialysis. In addition, the effects of renal insufficiency on sitagliptin pharmacokinetics in patients with type 2 diabetes and mild or moderate renal insufficiency were assessed using population pharmacokinetic analyses. Creatinine clearance was measured by 24–hour urinary creatinine clearance measurements or estimated from serum creatinine based on the Cockcroft-Gault formula:

[See table above]

Compared to normal healthy control subjects, an approximate 1.1- to 1.6-fold increase in plasma AUC of sitagliptin was observed in patients with mild renal insufficiency. Because increases of this magnitude are not clinically relevant, dosage adjustment in patients with mild renal insufficiency is not necessary. Plasma AUC levels of sitagliptin were increased approximately 2-fold and 4-fold in patients with moderate renal insufficiency and in patients with severe renal insufficiency, including patients with ESRD on hemodialysis, respectively. Sitagliptin was modestly removed by hemodialysis (13.5% over a 3- to 4-hour hemodialysis session starting 4 hours postdose). To achieve plasma concentrations of sitagliptin similar to those in patients with normal renal function, lower dosages are recommended in patients with moderate and severe renal insufficiency, as well as in ESRD patients requiring hemodialysis. *[See Dosage and Administration (2.2).]*

Hepatic Insufficiency

In patients with moderate hepatic insufficiency (Child-Pugh score 7 to 9), mean AUC and C_{max} of sitagliptin increased approximately 21% and 13%, respectively, compared to healthy matched controls following administration of a single 100 mg dose of JANUVIA. These differences are not considered to be clinically meaningful. No dosage adjustment for JANUVIA is necessary for patients with mild or moderate hepatic insufficiency.

There is no clinical experience in patients with severe hepatic insufficiency (Child-Pugh score >9).

Body Mass Index (BMI)

No dosage adjustment is necessary based on BMI. Body mass index had no clinically meaningful effect on the pharmacokinetics of sitagliptin based on a composite analysis of Phase I pharmacokinetic data and on a population pharmacokinetic analysis of Phase I and Phase II data.

Gender

No dosage adjustment is necessary based on gender. Gender had no clinically meaningful effect on the pharmacokinetics of sitagliptin based on a composite analysis of Phase I pharmacokinetic data and on a population pharmacokinetic analysis of Phase I and Phase II data.

Geriatric

No dosage adjustment is required based solely on age. When the effects of age on renal function are taken into account, age alone did not have a clinically meaningful impact on the pharmacokinetics of sitagliptin based on a population pharmacokinetic analysis. Elderly subjects (65 to 80 years) had approximately 19% higher plasma concentrations of sitagliptin compared to younger subjects.

Pediatric

Studies characterizing the pharmacokinetics of sitagliptin in pediatric patients have not been performed.

Race

No dosage adjustment is necessary based on race. Race had no clinically meaningful effect on the pharmacokinetics of sitagliptin based on a composite analysis of available pharmacokinetic data, including subjects of white, Hispanic, black, Asian, and other racial groups.

Drug Interactions

In Vitro Assessment of Drug Interactions

Sitagliptin is not an inhibitor of CYP isozymes CYP3A4, 2C8, 2C9, 2D6, 1A2, 2C19 or 2B6, and is not an inducer of CYP3A4. Sitagliptin is a p-glycoprotein substrate, but does not inhibit p–glycoprotein mediated transport of digoxin. Based on these results, sitagliptin is considered unlikely to cause interactions with other drugs that utilize these pathways.

Sitagliptin is not extensively bound to plasma proteins. Therefore, the propensity of sitagliptin to be involved in clinically meaningful drug–drug interactions mediated by plasma protein binding displacement is very low.

In Vivo Assessment of Drug Interactions

Effects of Sitagliptin on Other Drugs

In clinical studies, as described below, sitagliptin did not meaningfully alter the pharmacokinetics of metformin, glyburide, simvastatin, rosiglitazone, warfarin, or oral contraceptives, providing *in vivo* evidence of a low propensity for causing drug interactions with substrates of CYP3A4, CYP2C8, CYP2C9, and organic cationic transporter (OCT).

Digoxin: Sitagliptin had a minimal effect on the pharmacokinetics of digoxin. Following administration of 0.25 mg digoxin concomitantly with 100 mg of JANUVIA daily for 10 days, the plasma AUC of digoxin was increased by 11%, and the plasma C_{max} by 18%.

Metformin: Co-administration of multiple twice-daily doses of sitagliptin with metformin, an OCT substrate, did not meaningfully alter the pharmacokinetics of metformin in patients with type 2 diabetes. Therefore, sitagliptin is not an inhibitor of OCT-mediated transport.

Sulfonylureas: Single-dose pharmacokinetics of glyburide, a CYP2C9 substrate, was not meaningfully altered in subjects receiving multiple doses of sitagliptin. Clinically meaningful interactions would not be expected with other sulfonylureas (e.g., glipizide, tolbutamide, and glimepiride) which, like glyburide, are primarily eliminated by CYP2C9.

Simvastatin: Single-dose pharmacokinetics of simvastatin, a CYP3A4 substrate, was not meaningfully altered in subjects receiving multiple daily doses of sitagliptin. Therefore, sitagliptin is not an inhibitor of CYP3A4-mediated metabolism.

Thiazolidinediones: Single-dose pharmacokinetics of rosiglitazone, was not meaningfully altered in subjects receiving multiple daily doses of sitagliptin, indicating that JANUVIA is not an inhibitor of CYP2C8-mediated metabolism.

Warfarin: Multiple daily doses of sitagliptin did not meaningfully alter the pharmacokinetics, as assessed by measurement of S(-) or R(+) warfarin enantiomers, or pharmacodynamics (as assessed by measurement of prothrombin INR) of a single dose of warfarin. Because S(-) warfarin is primarily metabolized by CYP2C9, these data also support the conclusion that sitagliptin is not a CYP2C9 inhibitor.

Oral Contraceptives: Co-administration with sitagliptin did not meaningfully alter the steady-state pharmacokinetics of norethindrone or ethinyl estradiol.

Effects of Other Drugs on Sitagliptin

Clinical data described below suggest that sitagliptin is not susceptible to clinically meaningful interactions by co-administered medications.

Metformin: Co-administration of multiple twice-daily doses of metformin with sitagliptin did not meaningfully alter the pharmacokinetics of sitagliptin in patients with type 2 diabetes.

Cyclosporine: A study was conducted to assess the effect of cyclosporine, a potent inhibitor of p-glycoprotein, on the pharmacokinetics of sitagliptin. Co-administration of a single 100 mg oral dose of JANUVIA and a single 600 mg oral dose of cyclosporine increased the AUC and C_{max} of sitagliptin by approximately 29% and 68%, respectively. These modest changes in sitagliptin pharmacokinetics were not considered to be clinically meaningful. The renal clearance of sitagliptin was also not meaningfully altered. Therefore, meaningful interactions would not be expected with other p-glycoprotein inhibitors.

13 NONCLINICAL TOXICOLOGY

13.1 Carcinogenesis, Mutagenesis, Impairment of Fertility

A two-year carcinogenicity study was conducted in male and female rats given oral doses of sitagliptin of 50, 150, and 500 mg/kg/day. There was an increased incidence of combined liver adenoma/carcinoma in males and females and of liver carcinoma in females at 500 mg/kg. This dose results in exposures approximately 60 times the human exposure at the maximum recommended daily adult human dose (MRHD) of 100 mg/day based on AUC comparisons. Liver tumors were not observed at 150 mg/kg, approximately 20 times the human exposure at the MRHD. A two-year carcinogenicity study was conducted in male and female mice given oral doses of sitagliptin of 50, 125, 250, and 500 mg/kg/day. There was no increase in the incidence of tumors in any organ up to 500 mg/kg, approximately 70 times human exposure at the MRHD. Sitagliptin was not mutagenic or clastogenic with or without metabolic activation in the Ames bacterial mutagenicity assay, a Chinese hamster ovary (CHO) chromosome aberration assay, an *in vitro* cytogenetics assay in CHO, an *in vitro* rat hepatocyte DNA alkaline elution assay, and an *in vivo* micronucleus assay.

In rat fertility studies with oral gavage doses of 125, 250, and 1000 mg/kg, males were treated for 4 weeks prior to mating, during mating, up to scheduled termination (approximately 8 weeks total) and females were treated 2 weeks prior to mating through gestation day 7. No adverse effect on fertility was observed at 125 mg/kg (approximately 12 times human exposure at the MRHD of 100 mg/day based on AUC comparisons). At higher doses, nondose-related increased resorptions in females were observed (approximately 25 and 100 times human exposure at the MRHD based on AUC comparison).

14 CLINICAL STUDIES

There were approximately 5200 patients with type 2 diabetes randomized in nine double-blind, placebo-controlled clinical safety and efficacy studies conducted to evaluate the effects of sitagliptin on glycemic control. In a pooled analysis of seven of these studies, the ethnic/racial distribution was approximately 59% white, 20% Hispanic, 10% Asian, 6% black, and 6% other groups. Patients had an overall mean age of approximately 55 years (range 18 to 87 years). In addition, an active (glipizide)-controlled study of 52-weeks duration was conducted in 1172 patients with type 2 diabetes who had inadequate glycemic control on metformin.

In patients with type 2 diabetes, treatment with JANUVIA produced clinically significant improvements in hemoglobin A1C, fasting plasma glucose (FPG) and 2-hour postprandial glucose (PPG) compared to placebo.

14.1 Monotherapy

A total of 1262 patients with type 2 diabetes participated in two double-blind, placebo-controlled studies, one of 18-week and another of 24-week duration, to evaluate the efficacy and safety of JANUVIA monotherapy. In both monotherapy studies, patients currently on an antihyperglycemic agent discontinued the agent, and underwent a diet, exercise, and drug wash-out period of about 7 weeks. Patients with inadequate glycemic control (A1C 7% to 10%) after the wash-out period were randomized after completing a 2-week single-blind placebo run-in period; patients not currently on antihyperglycemic agents (off therapy for at least 8 weeks) with inadequate glycemic control (A1C 7% to 10%) were randomized after completing the 2-week single-blind placebo run-in period. In the 18-week study, 521 patients were randomized to placebo, JANUVIA 100 mg, or JANUVIA 200 mg, and in the 24-week study 741 patients were randomized to placebo, JANUVIA 100 mg, or JANUVIA 200 mg. Patients who failed to meet specific glycemic goals during the studies were treated with metformin rescue, added on to placebo or JANUVIA.

Treatment with JANUVIA at 100 mg daily provided significant improvements in A1C, FPG, and 2-hour PPG compared to placebo (Table 4). In the 18-week study, 9% of patients receiving JANUVIA 100 mg and 17% who received placebo required rescue therapy. In the 24-week study, 9% of patients receiving JANUVIA 100 mg and 21% of patients receiving placebo required rescue therapy. The improvement in A1C compared to placebo was not affected by gender, age, race, prior antihyperglycemic therapy, or baseline BMI. As is typical for trials of agents to treat type 2 diabetes, the mean reduction in A1C with JANUVIA appears to be related to the degree of A1C elevation at baseline. In these 18- and 24-week studies, among patients who were not on an antihyperglycemic agent at study entry, the reductions from baseline in A1C were -0.7% and -0.8%, respectively, for those given JANUVIA, and -0.1% and -0.2%, respectively, for those given placebo. Overall, the 200 mg daily dose did not provide greater glycemic efficacy than the 100 mg daily dose. The effect of JANUVIA on lipid endpoints was similar to placebo. Body weight did not increase from baseline with JANUVIA therapy in either study, compared to a small reduction in patients given placebo.

[See table 4 at top of next page]

Additional Monotherapy Study

A multinational, randomized, double-blind, placebo-controlled study was also conducted to assess the safety and tolerability of JANUVIA in 91 patients with type 2 diabetes and chronic renal insufficiency (creatinine clearance <50 mL/min). Patients with moderate renal insufficiency received 50 mg daily of JANUVIA and those with severe renal insufficiency or with ESRD on hemodialysis or peritoneal dialysis received 25 mg daily. In this study, the safety and tolerability of JANUVIA were generally similar to placebo. A small increase in serum creatinine was reported in patients with moderate renal insufficiency treated with JANUVIA relative to those on placebo. In addition, the reductions in A1C and FPG with JANUVIA compared to placebo were generally similar to those observed in other monotherapy studies. [See Clinical Pharmacology (12.3).]

14.2 Combination Therapy

Add-on Combination Therapy with Metformin

A total of 701 patients with type 2 diabetes participated in a 24-week, randomized, double-blind, placebo-controlled study designed to assess the efficacy of JANUVIA in combination with metformin. Patients already on metformin (N=431) at a dose of at least 1500 mg per day were randomized after completing a 2-week single-blind placebo run-in period. Patients on metformin and another antihyperglycemic agent (N=229) and patients not on any antihyperglycemic agents (off therapy for at least 8 weeks, N=41) were randomized after a run-in period of approximately 10 weeks on metformin (at a dose of at least 1500 mg per day) in monotherapy. Patients with inadequate glycemic control (A1C 7% to 10%) were randomized to the addition of either 100 mg of JANUVIA or placebo, administered once daily. Patients who failed to meet specific glycemic goals during the studies were treated with pioglitazone rescue.

In combination with metformin, JANUVIA provided significant improvements in A1C, FPG, and 2-hour PPG compared to placebo with metformin (Table 5). Rescue glycemic therapy was used in 5% of patients treated with JANUVIA 100 mg and 14% of patients treated with placebo. A similar decrease in body weight was observed for both treatment groups.

Table 5: Glycemic Parameters at Final Visit (24-Week Study) for JANUVIA in Add-on Combination Therapy with Metformin*

	JANUVIA 100 mg + Metformin	Placebo + Metformin
A1C (%)	**N = 453**	**N = 224**
Baseline (mean)	8.0	8.0
Change from baseline (adjusted mean[†])	-0.7	-0.0
Difference from placebo + metformin (adjusted mean[†])	-0.7[‡]	
(95% CI)	(-0.8, -0.5)	
Patients (%) achieving A1C <7%	213 (47%)	41 (18%)
FPG (mg/dL)	**N = 454**	**N = 226**
Baseline (mean)	170	174
Change from baseline (adjusted mean[†])	-17	9
Difference from placebo + metformin (adjusted mean[†])	-25[‡]	
(95% CI)	(-31, -20)	
2-hour PPG (mg/dL)	**N = 387**	**N = 182**
Baseline (mean)	275	272
Change from baseline (adjusted mean[†])	-62	-11
Difference from placebo + metformin (adjusted mean[†])	-51[‡]	
(95% CI)	(-61, -41)	

* Intent to Treat Population using last observation on study prior to pioglitazone rescue therapy.
[†] Least squares means adjusted for prior antihyperglycemic therapy and baseline value.
[‡] p<0.001 compared to placebo + metformin.

Initial Combination Therapy with Metformin

A total of 1091 patients with type 2 diabetes and inadequate glycemic control on diet and exercise participated in a 24-week, randomized, double-blind, placebo-controlled factorial study designed to assess the efficacy of sitagliptin as initial therapy in combination with metformin. Patients on an antihyperglycemic agent (N=541) discontinued the agent, and underwent a diet, exercise, and drug washout period of up to 12 weeks duration. After the washout period, patients

Table 4: Glycemic Parameters in 18- and 24-Week Placebo-Controlled Studies of JANUVIA in Patients with Type 2 Diabetes*

	18-Week Study		24-Week Study	
	JANUVIA 100 mg	Placebo	JANUVIA 100 mg	Placebo
A1C (%)	**N = 193**	**N = 103**	**N = 229**	**N = 244**
Baseline (mean)	8.0	8.1	8.0	8.0
Change from baseline (adjusted mean[†])	-0.5	0.1	-0.6	0.2
Difference from placebo (adjusted mean[†])	-0.6[‡]		-0.8[‡]	
(95% CI)	(-0.8, -0.4)		(-1.0, -0.6)	
Patients (%) achieving A1C <7%	69 (36%)	16 (16%)	93 (41%)	41 (17%)
FPG (mg/dL)	**N = 201**	**N = 107**	**N = 234**	**N = 247**
Baseline (mean)	180	184	170	176
Change from baseline (adjusted mean[†])	-13	7	-12	5
Difference from placebo (adjusted mean[†])	-20[‡]		-17[‡]	
(95% CI)	(-31, -9)		(-24, -10)	
2-hour PPG (mg/dL)	§	§	**N = 201**	**N = 204**
Baseline (mean)			257	271
Change from baseline (adjusted mean[†])			-49	-2
Difference from placebo (adjusted mean[†])			-47[‡]	
(95% CI)			(-59, -34)	

* Intent to Treat Population using last observation on study prior to metformin rescue therapy.
[†] Least squares means adjusted for prior antihyperglycemic therapy status and baseline value.
[‡] p<0.001 compared to placebo.
§ Data not available.

Table 6: Glycemic Parameters at Final Visit (24-Week Study) for Sitagliptin and Metformin, Alone and in Combination as Initial Therapy*

	Placebo	Sitagliptin (JANUVIA) 100 mg QD	Metformin 500 mg bid	Metformin 1000 mg bid	Sitagliptin 50 mg bid + Metformin 500 mg bid	Sitagliptin 50 mg bid + Metformin 1000 mg bid
A1C (%)	**N = 165**	**N = 175**	**N = 178**	**N = 177**	**N = 183**	**N = 178**
Baseline (mean)	8.7	8.9	8.9	8.7	8.8	8.8
Change from baseline (adjusted mean[†])	0.2	-0.7	-0.8	-1.1	-1.4	-1.9
Difference from placebo (adjusted mean[†])		-0.8[‡]	-1.0[‡]	-1.3[‡]	-1.6[‡]	-2.1[‡]
(95% CI)		(-1.1, -0.6)	(-1.2, -0.8)	(-1.5, -1.1)	(-1.8, -1.3)	(-2.3, -1.8)
Patients (%) achieving A1C <7%	15 (9%)	35 (20%)	41 (23%)	68 (38%)	79 (43%)	118 (66%)
% Patients receiving rescue medication	32	21	17	12	8	2
FPG (mg/dL)	**N = 169**	**N = 178**	**N = 179**	**N = 179**	**N = 183**	**N = 180**
Baseline (mean)	196	201	205	197	204	197
Change from baseline (adjusted mean[†])	6	-17	-27	-29	-47	-64
Difference from placebo (adjusted mean[†])		-23[‡]	-33[‡]	-35[‡]	-53[‡]	-70[‡]
(95% CI)		(-33, -14)	(-43, -24)	(-45, -26)	(-62, -43)	(-79, -60)
2-hour PPG (mg/dL)	**N = 129**	**N = 136**	**N = 141**	**N = 138**	**N = 147**	**N = 152**
Baseline (mean)	277	285	293	283	292	287
Change from baseline (adjusted mean[†])	0	-52	-53	-78	-93	-117
Difference from placebo (adjusted mean[†])		-52[‡]	-54[‡]	-78[‡]	-93[‡]	-117[‡]
(95% CI)		(-67, -37)	(-69, -39)	(-93, -63)	(-107, -78)	(-131, -102)

* Intent to Treat Population using last observation on study prior to glyburide (glibenclamide) rescue therapy.
[†] Least squares means adjusted for prior antihyperglycemic therapy status and baseline value.
[‡] p<0.001 compared to placebo.

with inadequate glycemic control (A1C 7.5% to 11%) were randomized after completing a 2-week single-blind placebo run-in period. Patients not on antihyperglycemic agents at study entry (N=550) with inadequate glycemic control (A1C 7.5% to 11%) immediately entered the 2-week single-blind placebo run-in period and then were randomized. Approximately equal numbers of patients were randomized to receive initial therapy with placebo, 100 mg of JANUVIA once daily, 500 mg or 1000 mg of metformin twice daily, or 50 mg of sitagliptin twice daily in combination with 500 mg or 1000 mg of metformin twice daily. Patients who failed to meet specific glycemic goals during the study were treated with glyburide (glibenclamide) rescue.

Initial therapy with the combination of JANUVIA and metformin provided significant improvements in A1C, FPG, and 2-hour PPG compared to placebo, to metformin alone, and to

JANUVIA alone (Table 6, Figure 1). Mean reductions from baseline in A1C were generally greater for patients with higher baseline A1C values. For patients not on an antihyperglycemic agent at study entry, mean reductions from baseline in A1C were: JANUVIA 100 mg once daily, -1.1%; metformin 500 mg bid, -1.1%; metformin 1000 mg bid, -1.2%; sitagliptin 50 mg bid with metformin 500 mg bid, -1.6%; sitagliptin 50 mg bid with metformin 1000 mg bid, -1.9%; and for patients receiving placebo, -0.2%. Lipid effects were generally neutral. The decrease in body weight in the groups given sitagliptin in combination with metformin was similar to that in the groups given metformin alone or placebo.
[See table 6 above]
[See figure 1 at top of next page]
In addition, this study included patients (N=117) with more severe hyperglycemia (A1C >11% or blood glucose

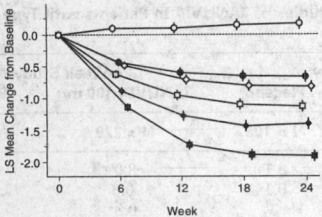

○ Placebo
● Sitagliptin 100 mg q.d.
◇ Metformin 500 mg b.i.d.
□ Metformin 1000 mg b.i.d.
◆ Sitagliptin 50 mg b.i.d. + Metformin 500 mg b.i.d.
■ Sitagliptin 50 mg b.i.d. + Metformin 1000 mg b.i.d.

† All Patients Treated Population Least squares means adjusted for prior antihyperglycemic therapy and baseline value.

Figure 1: Mean Change from Baseline for A1C (%) over 24 Weeks with Sitagliptin and Metformin, Alone and in Combination as Initial Therapy in Patients with Type 2 Diabetes†

>280 mg/dL) who were treated with twice daily open-label JANUVIA 50 mg and metformin 1000 mg. In this group of patients, the mean baseline A1C value was 11.2%, mean FPG was 314 mg/dL, and mean 2-hour PPG was 441 mg/dL. After 24 weeks, mean decreases from baseline of -2.9% for A1C, -127 mg/dL for FPG, and -208 mg/dL for 2-hour PPG were observed.

Initial combination therapy or maintenance of combination therapy may not be appropriate for all patients. These management options are left to the discretion of the health care provider.

Active-Controlled Study vs Glipizide in Combination with Metformin

The efficacy of JANUVIA was evaluated in a 52-week, double-blind, glipizide-controlled noninferiority trial in patients with type 2 diabetes. Patients not on treatment or on other antihyperglycemic agents entered a run-in treatment period of up to 12 weeks duration with metformin monotherapy (dose of ≥1500 mg per day) which included washout of medications other than metformin, if applicable. After the run-in period, those with inadequate glycemic control (A1C 6.5% to 10%) were randomized 1:1 to the addition of JANUVIA 100 mg once daily or glipizide for 52 weeks. Patients receiving glipizide were given an initial dosage of 5 mg/day and then electively titrated over the next 18 weeks to a maximum dosage of 20 mg/day as needed to optimize glycemic control. Thereafter, the glipizide dose was to be kept constant, except for down-titration to prevent hypoglycemia. The mean dose of glipizide after the titration period was 10 mg.

After 52 weeks, JANUVIA and glipizide had similar mean reductions from baseline in A1C in the intent-to-treat analysis (Table 7). These results were consistent with the per protocol analysis (Figure 2). A conclusion in favor of the noninferiority of JANUVIA to glipizide may be limited to patients with baseline A1C comparable to those included in the study (over 70% of patients had baseline A1C <8% and over 90% had A1C <9%).

Table 7: Glycemic Parameters in a 52-Week Study Comparing JANUVIA to Glipizide as Add-On Therapy in Patients Inadequately Controlled on Metformin (Intent-to-Treat Population)*

	JANUVIA 100 mg	Glipizide
A1C (%)	N = 576	N = 559
Baseline (mean)	7.7	7.6
Change from baseline (adjusted mean†)	-0.5	-0.6
FPG (mg/dL)	N = 583	N = 568
Baseline (mean)	166	164
Change from baseline (adjusted mean†)	-8	-8

* The Intent to Treat Analysis used the patients' last observation in the study prior to discontinuation.
† Least squares means adjusted for prior antihyperglycemic therapy status and baseline A1C value.

[See figure 2 at top of next column]

The incidence of hypoglycemia in the JANUVIA group (4.9%) was significantly (p<0.001) lower than that in the glipizide group (32.0%). Patients treated with JANUVIA exhibited a significant mean decrease from baseline in body weight compared to a significant weight gain in patients administered glipizide (-1.5 kg vs +1.1 kg).

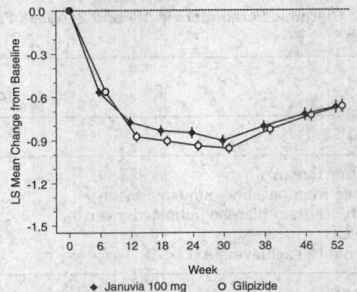

◆ Januvia 100 mg   ○ Glipizide

† The per protocol population (mean baseline A1C of 7.5%) included patients without major protocol violations who had observations at baseline and at Week 52.

Figure 2: Mean Change from Baseline for A1C (%) Over 52 Weeks in a Study Comparing JANUVIA to Glipizide as Add-On Therapy in Patients Inadequately Controlled on Metformin (Per Protocol Population)†

Add-on Combination Therapy with Pioglitazone

A total of 353 patients with type 2 diabetes participated in a 24-week, randomized, double-blind, placebo-controlled study designed to assess the efficacy of JANUVIA in combination with pioglitazone. Patients on any oral antihyperglycemic agent in monotherapy (N=212) or on a PPARγ agent in combination therapy (N=106) or not on an antihyperglycemic agent (off therapy for at least 8 weeks, N=34) were switched to monotherapy with pioglitazone (at a dose of 30-45 mg per day), and completed a run-in period of approximately 12 weeks in duration. After the run-in period on pioglitazone monotherapy, patients with inadequate glycemic control (A1C 7% to 10%) were randomized to the addition of either 100 mg of JANUVIA or placebo, administered once daily. Patients who failed to meet specific glycemic goals during the studies were treated with metformin rescue. Glycemic endpoints measured were A1C and fasting glucose.

In combination with pioglitazone, JANUVIA provided significant improvements in A1C and FPG compared to placebo with pioglitazone (Table 8). Rescue therapy was used in 7% of patients treated with JANUVIA 100 mg and 14% of patients treated with placebo. There was no significant difference between JANUVIA and placebo in body weight change.

Table 8: Glycemic Parameters at Final Visit (24-Week Study) for JANUVIA in Add-on Combination Therapy with Pioglitazone*

	JANUVIA 100 mg + Pioglitazone	Placebo + Pioglitazone
A1C (%)	N = 163	N = 174
Baseline (mean)	8.1	8.0
Change from baseline (adjusted mean†)	-0.9	-0.2
Difference from placebo + pioglitazone (adjusted mean†)	-0.7‡	
(95% CI)	(-0.9, -0.5)	
Patients (%) achieving A1C <7%	74 (45%)	40 (23%)
FPG (mg/dL)	N = 163	N = 174
Baseline (mean)	168	166
Change from baseline (adjusted mean†)	-17	1
Difference from placebo + pioglitazone (adjusted mean†)	-18‡	
(95% CI)	(-24, -11)	

* Intent to Treat Population using last observation on study prior to metformin rescue therapy.
† Least squares means adjusted for prior antihyperglycemic therapy status and baseline value.
‡ p<0.001 compared to placebo + pioglitazone.

Initial Combination Therapy with Pioglitazone

A total of 520 patients with type 2 diabetes and inadequate glycemic control on diet and exercise participated in a 24-week, randomized, double-blind study designed to assess the efficacy of JANUVIA as initial therapy in combination with pioglitazone. Patients not on antihyperglycemic agents at study entry (<4 weeks cumulative therapy over the past 2 years, and with no treatment over the prior 4 months) with inadequate glycemic control (A1C 8% to 12%) immediately entered the 2-week single-blind placebo run-in period and then were randomized. Approximately equal numbers of pa-

tients were randomized to receive initial therapy with 100 mg of JANUVIA in combination with 30 mg of pioglitazone once daily or 30 mg of pioglitazone once daily as monotherapy. There was no glycemic rescue therapy in this study. Initial therapy with the combination of JANUVIA and pioglitazone provided significant improvements in A1C, FPG, and 2-hour PPG compared to pioglitazone monotherapy (Table 9). The improvement in A1C was generally consistent across subgroups defined by gender, age, race, baseline BMI, baseline A1C, or duration of disease. In this study, patients treated with JANUVIA in combination with pioglitazone had a mean increase in body weight of 1.1 kg compared to pioglitazone alone (3.0 kg vs. 1.9 kg). Lipid effects were generally neutral.

Table 9: Glycemic Parameters at Final Visit (24-Week Study) for JANUVIA in Combination with Pioglitazone as Initial Therapy*

	JANUVIA 100 mg + Pioglitazone	Pioglitazone
A1C (%)	N = 251	N = 246
Baseline (mean)	9.5	9.4
Change from baseline (adjusted mean†)	-2.4	-1.5
Difference from placebo + pioglitazone (adjusted mean†)	-0.9‡	
(95% CI)	(-1.1, -0.7)	
Patients (%) achieving A1C <7%	151 (60%)	68 (28%)
FPG (mg/dL)	N = 256	N = 253
Baseline (mean)	203	201
Change from baseline (adjusted mean†)	-63	-40
Difference from placebo + pioglitazone (adjusted mean†)	-23‡	
(95% CI)	(-30, -15)	
2-hour PPG (mg/dL)	N = 216	N = 211
Baseline (mean)	283	284
Change from baseline (adjusted mean†)	-114	-69
Difference from placebo + pioglitazone (adjusted mean†)	-45‡	
(95% CI)	(-57, -32)	

* Intent to Treat Population using last observation on study.
† Least squares means adjusted for baseline value.
‡ p<0.001 compared to placebo + pioglitazone.

Add-on Combination Therapy with Metformin and Rosiglitazone

A total of 278 patients with type 2 diabetes participated in a 54-week, randomized, double-blind, placebo-controlled study designed to assess the efficacy of JANUVIA in combination with metformin and rosiglitazone. Patients on dual therapy with metformin ≥1500 mg/day and rosiglitazone ≥4 mg/day or with metformin ≥1500 mg/day and pioglitazone ≥30 mg/day (switched to rosiglitazone ≥4 mg/day) entered a dose-stable run-in period of 6 weeks. Patients on other dual therapy were switched to metformin ≥1500 mg/day and rosiglitazone ≥4 mg/day in a dose titration/stabilization run-in period of up to 20 weeks in duration. After the run-in period, patients with inadequate glycemic control (A1C 7.5% to 11%) were randomized 2:1 to the addition of either 100 mg of JANUVIA or placebo, administered once daily. Patients who failed to meet specific glycemic goals during the study were treated with glipizide (or other sulfonylurea) rescue. The primary time point for evaluation of glycemic parameters was Week 18.

In combination with metformin and rosiglitazone, JANUVIA provided significant improvements in A1C, FPG, and 2-hour PPG compared to placebo with metformin and rosiglitazone (Table 10) at Week 18. At Week 54, mean reduction in A1C was -1.0% for patients treated with JANUVIA and -0.3% for patients treated with placebo in an analysis based on the intent to treat population. Rescue therapy was used in 18% of patients treated with JANUVIA 100 mg and 40% of patients treated with placebo. There was no significant difference between JANUVIA and placebo in body weight change.

Table 10: Glycemic Parameters at Week 18 for JANUVIA in Add-on Combination Therapy with Metformin and Rosiglitazone*

	JANUVIA 100 mg + Metformin + Rosiglitazone	Placebo + Metformin + Rosiglitazone
A1C (%)	**N = 176**	**N = 93**
Baseline (mean)	8.8	8.7
Change from baseline (adjusted mean[†])	-1.0	-0.4
Difference from placebo + rosiglitazone + metformin (adjusted mean[†])	-0.7[‡]	
(95% CI)	(-0.9, -0.4)	
Patients (%) achieving A1C <7%	39 (22%)	9 (10%)
FPG (mg/dL)	**N = 179**	**N = 94**
Baseline (mean)	181	182
Change from baseline (adjusted mean[†])	-30	-11
Difference from placebo + rosiglitazone + metformin (adjusted mean[†])	-18[‡]	
(95% CI)	(-26, -10)	
2-hour PPG (mg/dL)	**N = 152**	**N = 80**
Baseline (mean)	256	248
Change from baseline (adjusted mean[†])	-59	-21
Difference from placebo + rosiglitazone + metformin (adjusted mean[†])	-39[‡]	
(95% CI)	(-51, -26)	

* Intent to Treat Population using last observation on study prior to glipizide (or other sulfonylurea) rescue therapy.
† Least squares means adjusted for prior antihyperglycemic therapy status and baseline value.
‡ p<0.001 compared to placebo + metformin + rosiglitazone.

Add-on Combination Therapy with Glimepiride, with or without Metformin
A total of 441 patients with type 2 diabetes participated in a 24-week, randomized, double-blind, placebo-controlled study designed to assess the efficacy of JANUVIA in combination with glimepiride, with or without metformin. Patients entered a run-in treatment period on glimepiride (≥4 mg per day) alone or glimepiride in combination with metformin (≥1500 mg per day). After a dose-titration and dose-stable run-in period of up to 16 weeks and a 2-week placebo run-in period, patients with inadequate glycemic control (A1C 7.5% to 10.5%) were randomized to the addition of either 100 mg of JANUVIA or placebo, administered once daily. Patients who failed to meet specific glycemic goals during the studies were treated with pioglitazone rescue.
In combination with glimepiride, with or without metformin, JANUVIA provided significant improvements in A1C and FPG compared to placebo (Table 11). In the entire study population (patients on JANUVIA in combination with glimepiride and patients on JANUVIA in combination with glimepiride and metformin), a mean reduction from baseline relative to placebo in A1C of -0.7% and in FPG of -20 mg/dL was seen. Rescue therapy was used in 12% of patients treated with JANUVIA 100 mg and 27% of patients treated with placebo. In this study, patients treated with JANUVIA had a mean increase in body weight of 1.1 kg vs. placebo (+0.8 kg vs. -0.4 kg). In addition, there was an increased rate of hypoglycemia. *[See Warnings and Precautions (5.3); Adverse Reactions (6.1).]*
[See table 11 above]

Add-on Combination Therapy with Insulin (with or without Metformin)
A total of 641 patients with type 2 diabetes participated in a 24-week, randomized, double-blind, placebo-controlled study designed to assess the efficacy of JANUVIA as add-on to insulin therapy (with or without metformin). The racial distribution in this study was approximately 70% white, 18% Asian, 7% black, and 5% other groups. Approximately 14% of the patients in this study were Hispanic. Patients entered a 2-week, single-blind run-in treatment period on

Table 11: Glycemic Parameters at Final Visit (24-Week Study) for JANUVIA as Add-On Combination Therapy with Glimepiride, with or without Metformin*

	JANUVIA 100 mg + Glimepiride	Placebo + Glimepiride	JANUVIA 100 mg + Glimepiride + Metformin	Placebo + Glimepiride + Metformin
A1C (%)	**N = 102**	**N = 103**	**N = 115**	**N = 105**
Baseline (mean)	8.4	8.5	8.3	8.3
Change from baseline (adjusted mean[†])	-0.3	0.3	-0.6	0.3
Difference from placebo (adjusted mean[†])	-0.6[‡]		-0.9[‡]	
(95% CI)	(-0.8, -0.3)		(-1.1, -0.7)	
Patients (%) achieving A1C <7%	11 (11%)	9 (9%)	26 (23%)	1 (1%)
FPG (mg/dL)	**N = 104**	**N = 104**	**N = 115**	**N = 109**
Baseline (mean)	183	185	179	179
Change from baseline (adjusted mean[†])	-1	18	-8	13
Difference from placebo (adjusted mean[†])	-19[§]		-21[‡]	
(95% CI)	(-32, -7)		(-32, -10)	

* Intent to Treat Population using last observation on study prior to pioglitazone rescue therapy.
† Least squares means adjusted for prior antihyperglycemic therapy status and baseline value.
‡ p<0.001 compared to placebo.
§ p<0.01 compared to placebo.

pre-mixed, long-acting, or intermediate-acting insulin, with or without metformin (≥1500 mg per day). Patients using short-acting insulins were excluded unless the short-acting insulin was administered as part of a pre-mixed insulin. After the run-in period, patients with inadequate glycemic control (A1C 7.5% to 11%) were randomized to the addition of either 100 mg of JANUVIA or placebo, administered once daily. Patients were on a stable dose of insulin prior to enrollment with no changes in insulin dose permitted during the run-in period. Patients who failed to meet specific glycemic goals during the double-blind treatment period were to have uptitration of the background insulin dose as rescue therapy.
The median daily insulin dose at baseline was 42 units in the patients treated with JANUVIA and 45 units in the placebo-treated patients.
The median change from baseline in daily dose of insulin was zero for both groups at the end of the study. In combination with insulin (with or without metformin), JANUVIA provided significant improvements in A1C, FPG, and 2-hour PPG compared to placebo (Table 12). Both treatment groups had an adjusted mean increase in body weight of 0.1 kg from baseline to Week 24. There was an increased rate of hypoglycemia in patients treated with JANUVIA. *[See Warnings and Precautions (5.3); Adverse Reactions (6.1).]*

Table 12: Glycemic Parameters at Final Visit (24-Week Study) for JANUVIA as Add-on Combination Therapy with Insulin*

	JANUVIA 100 mg + Insulin (+/- Metformin)	Placebo + Insulin (+/- Metformin)
A1C (%)	**N = 305**	**N = 312**
Baseline (mean)	8.7	8.6
Change from baseline (adjusted mean[†])	-0.6	-0.1
Difference from placebo (adjusted mean[†,‡])	-0.6[§]	
(95% CI)	(-0.7, -0.4)	
Patients (%) achieving A1C <7%	39 (12.8%)	16 (5.1%)
FPG (mg/dL)	**N = 310**	**N = 313**
Baseline (mean)	176	179
Change from baseline (adjusted mean[†])	-18	-4
Difference from placebo (adjusted mean[†])	-15[§]	
(95% CI)	(-23, -7)	
2-hour PPG (mg/dL)	**N = 240**	**N = 257**
Baseline (mean)	291	292
Change from baseline (adjusted mean[†])	-31	5
Difference from placebo (adjusted mean[†])	-36[§]	
(95% CI)	(-47, -25)	

* Intent to Treat Population using last observation on study prior to rescue therapy.

† Least squares means adjusted for metformin use at the screening visit (yes/no), type of insulin used at the screening visit (pre-mixed vs. non-pre-mixed [intermediate- or long-acting]), and baseline value.
‡ Treatment by stratum interaction was not significant (p>0.10) for metformin stratum and for insulin stratum.
§ p<0.001 compared to placebo.

16   HOW SUPPLIED/STORAGE AND HANDLING
No. 6737—Tablets JANUVIA, 25 mg, are pink, round, film-coated tablets with "221" on one side. They are supplied as follows:
NDC 0006-0221-31 unit-of-use bottles of 30
NDC 0006-0221-54 unit-of-use bottles of 90
NDC 0006-0221-28 unit dose blister packages of 100.
No. 6738—Tablets JANUVIA, 50 mg, are light beige, round, film-coated tablets with "112" on one side. They are supplied as follows:
NDC 0006-0112-31 unit-of-use bottles of 30
NDC 0006-0112-54 unit-of-use bottles of 90
NDC 0006-0112-28 unit dose blister packages of 100.
No. 6739—Tablets JANUVIA, 100 mg, are beige, round, film-coated tablets with "277" on one side. They are supplied as follows:
NDC 0006-0277-31 unit-of-use bottles of 30
NDC 0006-0277-54 unit-of-use bottles of 90
NDC 0006-0277-28 unit dose blister packages of 100
NDC 0006-0277-74 bottles of 500
NDC 0006-0277-82 bottles of 1000.
Storage
Store at 20-25°C (68-77°F), excursions permitted to 15-30°C (59-86°F), [see USP Controlled Room Temperature].

17   PATIENT COUNSELING INFORMATION
See FDA-approved Medication Guide.
17.1   Instructions
Patients should be informed of the potential risks and benefits of JANUVIA and of alternative modes of therapy. Patients should also be informed about the importance of adherence to dietary instructions, regular physical activity, periodic blood glucose monitoring and A1C testing, recognition and management of hypoglycemia and hyperglycemia, and assessment for diabetes complications. During periods of stress such as fever, trauma, infection, or surgery, medication requirements may change and patients should be advised to seek medical advice promptly.
Patients should be informed that acute pancreatitis has been reported during postmarketing use of JANUVIA. Patients should be informed that persistent severe abdominal pain, sometimes radiating to the back, which may or may not be accompanied by vomiting, is the hallmark symptom of acute pancreatitis. Patients should be instructed to promptly discontinue JANUVIA and contact their physician if persistent severe abdominal pain occurs *[see Warnings and Precautions (5.1)]*.
Patients should be informed that the incidence of hypoglycemia is increased when JANUVIA is added to a sulfonylurea or insulin and that a lower dose of the sulfonylurea or insulin may be required to reduce the risk of hypoglycemia. Patients should be informed that allergic reactions have been reported during postmarketing use of JANUVIA. If symptoms of allergic reactions (including rash, hives, and swelling of the face, lips, tongue, and throat that may cause difficulty in breathing or swallowing) occur, patients must stop taking JANUVIA and seek medical advice promptly.

Physicians should instruct their patients to read the Medication Guide before starting JANUVIA therapy and to re-read each time the prescription is renewed. Patients should be instructed to inform their doctor or pharmacist if they develop any unusual symptom, or if any known symptom persists or worsens.

17.2   Laboratory Tests
Patients should be informed that response to all diabetic therapies should be monitored by periodic measurements of blood glucose and A1C levels, with a goal of decreasing these levels towards the normal range. A1C is especially useful for evaluating long-term glycemic control. Patients should be informed of the potential need to adjust dose based on changes in renal function tests over time.
Manuf. for: Merck Sharp & Dohme Corp., a subsidiary of **MERCK & CO., INC.**, Whitehouse Station, NJ 08889, USA
Manufactured by:
Merck Sharp & Dohme (Italia) S.p.A.
Via Emilia, 21
27100 – Pavia, Italy
9984400
US Patent No.: 6,699,871
[1]Registered trademark of Merck Sharp & Dohme Corp., a subsidiary of **Merck & Co., Inc.**
Copyright © 2006, 2007, 2009, 2010 Merck Sharp & Dohme Corp., a subsidiary of **Merck & Co., Inc.**
All rights reserved

MEDICATION GUIDE
JANUVIA® (jah-NEW-vee-ah)
(sitagliptin)
Tablets

Read this Medication Guide carefully before you start taking JANUVIA and each time you get a refill. There may be new information. This information does not take the place of talking with your doctor about your medical condition or your treatment. If you have any questions about JANUVIA, ask your doctor or pharmacist.

What is the most important information I should know about JANUVIA?
Serious side effects can happen in people taking JANUVIA, including inflammation of the pancreas (pancreatitis) which may be severe and lead to death.
Certain medical problems make you more likely to get pancreatitis.

Before you start taking JANUVIA:
Tell your doctor if you have ever had
• pancreatitis
• stones in your gallbladder (gallstones)
• a history of alcoholism
• high blood triglyceride levels
Stop taking JANUVIA and call your doctor right away if you have pain in your stomach area (abdomen) that is severe and will not go away. The pain may be felt going from your abdomen through to your back. The pain may happen with or without vomiting. These may be symptoms of pancreatitis.

What is JANUVIA?
• JANUVIA is a prescription medicine used along with diet and exercise to lower blood sugar in adults with type 2 diabetes.
• JANUVIA is not for people with type 1 diabetes.
• JANUVIA is not for people with diabetic ketoacidosis (increased ketones in your blood or urine).
• If you have had pancreatitis (inflammation of the pancreas) in the past, it is not known if you have a higher chance of getting pancreatitis while you take JANUVIA.
• It is not known if JANUVIA is safe and effective when used in children under 18 years of age.

Who should not take JANUVIA?
Do not take JANUVIA if:
• you are allergic to any of the ingredients in JANUVIA. See the end of this Medication Guide for a complete list of ingredients in JANUVIA.
Symptoms of a serious allergic reaction to JANUVIA may include:
• rash
• raised red patches on your skin (hives)
• swelling of the face, lips, tongue, and throat that may cause difficulty in breathing or swallowing

What should I tell my doctor before taking JANUVIA?
Before you take JANUVIA, tell your doctor if you:
• have or have had inflammation of your pancreas (pancreatitis).
• have kidney problems.
• have any other medical conditions.
• are pregnant or plan to become pregnant. It is not known if JANUVIA will harm your unborn baby. If you are pregnant, talk with your doctor about the best way to control your blood sugar while you are pregnant.

Pregnancy Registry: If you take JANUVIA at any time during your pregnancy, talk with your doctor about how you can join the JANUVIA pregnancy registry. The purpose of this registry is to collect information about the

health of you and your baby. You can enroll in this registry by calling 1-800-986-8999.
• are breast-feeding or plan to breast-feed. It is not known if JANUVIA will pass into your breast milk. Talk with your doctor about the best way to feed your baby if you are taking JANUVIA.

Tell your doctor about all the medicines you take, including prescription and non-prescription medicines, vitamins, and herbal supplements.
Know the medicines you take. Keep a list of your medicines and show it to your doctor and pharmacist when you get a new medicine.

How should I take JANUVIA?
• Take JANUVIA 1 time each day exactly as your doctor tells you.
• You can take JANUVIA with or without food.
• Your doctor may do blood tests from time to time to see how well your kidneys are working. Your doctor may change your dose of JANUVIA based on the results of your blood tests.
• Your doctor may tell you to take JANUVIA along with other diabetes medicines. Low blood sugar can happen more often when JANUVIA is taken with certain other diabetes medicines. See "**What are the possible side effects of JANUVIA?**"
• If you miss a dose, take it as soon as you remember. If you do not remember until it is time for your next dose, skip the missed dose and go back to your regular schedule. Do not take two doses of JANUVIA at the same time.
• If you take too much JANUVIA, call your doctor or local Poison Control Center right away.
• When your body is under some types of stress, such as fever, trauma (such as a car accident), infection or surgery, the amount of diabetes medicine that you need may change. Tell your doctor right away if you have any of these conditions and follow your doctor's instructions.
• Check your blood sugar as your doctor tells you to.
• Stay on your prescribed diet and exercise program while taking JANUVIA.
• Talk to your doctor about how to prevent, recognize and manage low blood sugar (hypoglycemia), high blood sugar (hyperglycemia), and problems you have because of your diabetes.
• Your doctor will check your diabetes with regular blood tests, including your blood sugar levels and your hemoglobin A1C.

What are the possible side effects of JANUVIA?
Serious side effects have occurred in people taking JANUVIA.
• See "**What is the most important information I should know about JANUVIA?**"
• **Low blood sugar (hypoglycemia).** If you take JANUVIA with another medicine that can cause low blood sugar, such as a sulfonylurea or insulin, your risk of getting low blood sugar is higher. The dose of your sulfonylurea medicine or insulin may need to be lowered while you use JANUVIA. Signs and symptoms of low blood sugar may include:

• headache	• irritability
• drowsiness	• hunger
• weakness	• fast heart beat
• dizziness	• sweating
• confusion	• feeling jittery

• **Serious allergic reactions.** If you have any symptoms of a serious allergic reaction, stop taking JANUVIA and call your doctor right away. See "**Who should not take JANUVIA?**". Your doctor may give you a medicine for your allergic reaction and prescribe a different medicine for your diabetes.
The most common side effects of JANUVIA include:
• upper respiratory infection
• stuffy or runny nose and sore throat
• headache
JANUVIA may have other side effects, including:
• stomach upset and diarrhea
• swelling of the hands or legs, when JANUVIA is used with rosiglitazone (Avandia®). Rosiglitazone is another type of diabetes medicine.
These are not all the possible side effects of JANUVIA. For more information, ask your doctor or pharmacist.
Tell your doctor if you have any side effect that bothers you, is unusual or does not go away.
Call your doctor for medical advice about side effects. You may report side effects to FDA at 1-800-FDA-1088.

How should I store JANUVIA?
Store JANUVIA at 68°F to 77°F (20°C to 25°C).
Keep JANUVIA and all medicines out of the reach of children.

General information about the use of JANUVIA
Medicines are sometimes prescribed for purposes that are not listed in Medication Guides. Do not use JANUVIA for a condition for which it was not prescribed. Do not give JANUVIA to other people, even if they have the same symptoms you have. It may harm them.
This Medication Guide summarizes the most important information about JANUVIA. If you would like to know more information, talk with your doctor. You can ask your doctor or pharmacist for additional information about JANUVIA that is written for health professionals. For more information, go to www.JANUVIA.com or call 1-800-622-4477.

What are the ingredients in JANUVIA?
Active ingredient: sitagliptin
Inactive ingredients: microcrystalline cellulose, anhydrous dibasic calcium phosphate, croscarmellose sodium, magnesium stearate, and sodium stearyl fumarate. The tablet film coating contains the following inactive ingredients: polyvinyl alcohol, polyethylene glycol, talc, titanium dioxide, red iron oxide, and yellow iron oxide.

What is type 2 diabetes?
Type 2 diabetes is a condition in which your body does not make enough insulin, and the insulin that your body produces does not work as well as it should. Your body can also make too much sugar. When this happens, sugar (glucose) builds up in the blood. This can lead to serious medical problems.
High blood sugar can be lowered by diet and exercise, and by certain medicines when necessary.
JANUVIA® is a registered trademark of Merck Sharp & Dohme Corp., a subsidiary of **Merck & Co., Inc.**
Avandia® is a registered trademark of GlaxoSmithKline.
Copyright © 2010 Merck Sharp & Dohme Corp., a subsidiary of **Merck & Co., Inc.**
All rights reserved
Revised February 2010
Manuf. for: Merck Sharp & Dohme Corp., a subsidiary of **MERCK & CO., INC.**, Whitehouse Station, NJ 08889, USA
Manufactured by:
Merck Sharp & Dohme (Italia) S.p.A.
Via Emilia, 21
27100 – Pavia, Italy
9984400
This Medication Guide has been approved by the U.S. Food and Drug Administration.

Shown in Product Identification Guide, page 313

LEVITRA®   ℞
[lĕ-vē-trǎ]
(vardenafil HCl)
TABLETS

DESCRIPTION
LEVITRA® is an oral therapy for the treatment of erectile dysfunction. This monohydrochloride salt of vardenafil is a selective inhibitor of cyclic guanosine monophosphate (cGMP)-specific phosphodiesterase type 5 (PDE5).
Vardenafil HCl is designated chemically as piperazine, 1-[[3-(1,4-dihydro-5-methyl-4-oxo-7-propylimidazo[5,1-*f*][1,2,4]triazin-2-yl)-4-ethoxyphenyl]sulfonyl]-4-ethyl-, monohydrochloride and has the following structural formula:

Vardenafil HCl is a nearly colorless, solid substance with a molecular weight of 579.1 g/mol and a solubility of 0.11 mg/mL in water. LEVITRA is formulated as orange, round, film-coated tablets with "BAYER" cross debossed on one side and "2.5", "5", "10", and "20" on the other side corresponding to 2.5 mg, 5 mg, 10 mg, and 20 mg of vardenafil, respectively. In addition to the active ingredient, vardenafil HCl, each tablet contains microcrystalline cellulose, crospovidone, colloidal silicon dioxide, magnesium stearate, hypromellose, polyethylene glycol, titanium dioxide, yellow ferric oxide, and red ferric oxide.

CLINICAL PHARMACOLOGY
Mechanism of Action
Penile erection is a hemodynamic process initiated by the relaxation of smooth muscle in the corpus cavernosum and its associated arterioles. During sexual stimulation, nitric oxide is released from nerve endings and endothelial cells in

the corpus cavernosum. Nitric oxide activates the enzyme guanylate cyclase resulting in increased synthesis of cyclic guanosine monophosphate (cGMP) in the smooth muscle cells of the corpus cavernosum. The cGMP in turn triggers smooth muscle relaxation, allowing increased blood flow into the penis, resulting in erection. The tissue concentration of cGMP is regulated by both the rates of synthesis and degradation via phosphodiesterases (PDEs). The most abundant PDE in the human corpus cavernosum is the cGMP-specific phosphodiesterase type 5 (PDE5); therefore, the inhibition of PDE5 enhances erectile function by increasing the amount of cGMP. Because sexual stimulation is required to initiate the local release of nitric oxide, the inhibition of PDE5 has no effect in the absence of sexual stimulation.

In vitro studies have shown that vardenafil is a selective inhibitor of PDE5. The inhibitory effect of vardenafil is more selective on PDE5 than for other known phosphodiesterases (>15-fold relative to PDE6, >130-fold relative to PDE1, >300-fold relative to PDE11, and >1,000-fold relative to PDE2, 3, 4, 7, 8, 9, and 10).

Pharmacokinetics

The pharmacokinetics of vardenafil are approximately dose proportional over the recommended dose range. Vardenafil is eliminated predominantly by hepatic metabolism, mainly by CYP3A4 and to a minor extent, CYP2C isoforms. Concomitant use with potent CYP3A4 inhibitors such as ritonavir, indinavir, ketoconazole, as well as moderate CYP3A inhibitors such as erythromycin results in significant increases of plasma levels of vardenafil (see **PRECAUTIONS, WARNINGS** and **DOSAGE AND ADMINISTRATION**). Mean vardenafil plasma concentrations measured after the administration of a single oral dose of 20 mg to healthy male volunteers are depicted in Figure 1.

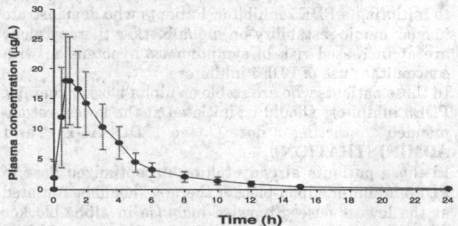

Figure 1: Plasma Vardenafil Concentration (Mean ± SD) Curve for a Single 20 mg LEVITRA Dose

Absorption:
Vardenafil is rapidly absorbed with absolute bioavailability of approximately 15%. Maximum observed plasma concentrations after a single 20 mg dose in healthy volunteers are usually reached between 30 minutes and 2 hours (median 60 minutes) after oral dosing in the fasted state. Two food-effect studies were conducted which showed that high-fat meals caused a reduction in C_{max} by 18%-50%.

Distribution:
The mean steady-state volume of distribution (Vss) for vardenafil is 208 L, indicating extensive tissue distribution. Vardenafil and its major circulating metabolite, M1, are highly bound to plasma proteins (about 95% for parent drug and M1). This protein binding is reversible and independent of total drug concentrations.
Following a single oral dose of 20 mg vardenafil in healthy volunteers, a mean of 0.00018% of the administered dose was obtained in semen 1.5 hours after dosing.

Metabolism:
Vardenafil is metabolized predominantly by the hepatic enzyme CYP3A4, with contribution from the CYP3A5 and CYP2C isoforms. The major circulating metabolite, M1, results from desethylation at the piperazine moiety of vardenafil. M1 is subject to further metabolism. The plasma concentration of M1 is approximately 26% that of the parent compound. This metabolite shows a phosphodiesterase selectivity profile similar to that of vardenafil and an *in vitro* inhibitory potency for PDE5 28% of that of vardenafil. Therefore, M1 accounts for approximately 7% of total pharmacologic activity.

Excretion:
The total body clearance of vardenafil is 56 L/h, and the terminal half-life of vardenafil and its primary metabolite (M1) is approximately 4-5 hours. After oral administration, vardenafil is excreted as metabolites predominantly in the feces (approximately 91-95% of administered oral dose) and to a lesser extent in the urine (approximately 2-6% of administered oral dose).

Pharmacokinetics in Special Populations
Pediatrics: Vardenafil trials were not conducted in the pediatric population.
Geriatrics: In a healthy volunteer study of elderly males (≥65 years) and younger males (18–45 years), mean C_{max} and AUC were 34% and 52% higher, respectively, in the elderly males (see **PRECAUTIONS, Geriatric Use** and **DOS-**

Table 1. Mean QT and QT_c changes in msec (90% CI) from baseline relative to placebo at 1 hour post-dose with different methodologies to correct for the effect of heart rate.

Drug/Dose	QT Uncorrected (msec)	Fridericia QT Correction (msec)	Individual QT Correction (msec)
Vardenafil 10 mg	-2 (-4, 0)	8 (6, 9)	4 (3, 6)
Vardenafil 80 mg	-2 (-4, 0)	10 (8, 11)	6 (4, 7)
Moxifloxacin* 400 mg	3 (1, 5)	8 (6, 9)	7 (5, 8)

*Active control (drug known to prolong QT)

AGE AND ADMINISTRATION). Consequently, a lower starting dose of LEVITRA (5 mg) in patients ≥65 years of age should be considered.
Renal Insufficiency: In volunteers with mild renal impairment (CL_{cr} = 50-80 ml/min), the pharmacokinetics of vardenafil were similar to those observed in a control group with normal renal function. In the moderate (CL_{cr} = 30-50 ml/min) or severe (CL_{cr}<30 ml/min) renal impairment groups, the AUC of vardenafil was 20–30% higher compared to that observed in a control group with normal renal function (CL_{cr}>80 ml/min). Vardenafil pharmacokinetics have not been evaluated in patients requiring renal dialysis (see **PRECAUTIONS, Renal Insufficiency,** and **DOSAGE AND ADMINISTRATION**).
Hepatic Insufficiency: In volunteers with mild hepatic impairment (Child-Pugh A), the C_{max} and AUC following a 10 mg vardenafil dose were increased by 22% and 17%, respectively, compared to healthy control subjects. In volunteers with moderate hepatic impairment (Child-Pugh B), the C_{max} and AUC following a 10 mg vardenafil dose were increased by 130% and 160%, respectively, compared to healthy control subjects. Consequently, a starting dose of 5 mg is recommended for patients with moderate hepatic impairment, and the maximum dose should not exceed 10 mg (see **PRECAUTIONS** and **DOSAGE AND ADMINISTRATION**). Vardenafil has not been evaluated in patients with severe (Child-Pugh C) hepatic impairment.

Pharmacodynamics
Effects on Blood Pressure:
In a clinical pharmacology study of patients with erectile dysfunction, single doses of vardenafil 20 mg caused a mean maximum decrease in supine blood pressure of 7 mmHg systolic and 8 mmHg diastolic (compared to placebo), accompanied by a mean maximum increase of heart rate of 4 beats per minute. The maximum decrease in blood pressure occurred between 1 and 4 hours after dosing. Following multiple dosing for 31 days, similar blood pressure responses were observed on Day 31 as on Day 1. Vardenafil may add to the blood pressure lowering effects of antihypertensive agents (see **PRECAUTIONS, Drug Interactions**).
Effects on Blood Pressure and Heart Rate when LEVITRA is Combined with Nitrates:
A study was conducted in which the blood pressure and heart rate response to 0.4 mg nitroglycerin (NTG) sublingually was evaluated in 18 healthy subjects following pretreatment with LEVITRA 20 mg at various times before NTG administration. LEVITRA 20 mg caused an additional time-related reduction in blood pressure and increase in heart rate in association with NTG administration. The blood pressure effects were observed when LEVITRA 20 mg was dosed 1 or 4 hours before NTG and the heart rate effects were observed when 20 mg was dosed 1, 4, or 8 hours before NTG. Additional blood pressure and heart rate changes were not detected when LEVITRA 20 mg was dosed 24 hours before NTG. (See Figure 2.)

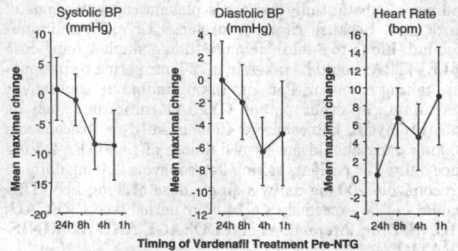

Figure 2: Placebo-subtracted point estimates (with 90% CI) of mean maximal blood pressure and heart rate effects of pre-dosing with LEVITRA 20 mg at 24, 8, 4, and 1 hour before 0.4 mg NTG sublingually.

Because the disease state of patients requiring nitrate therapy is anticipated to increase the likelihood of hypotension,

the use of vardenafil by patients on nitrate therapy or on nitric oxide donors is contraindicated (see **CONTRAINDICATIONS**).
Electrophysiology:
The effect of 10 mg and 80 mg vardenafil on QT interval was evaluated in a single-dose, double-blind, randomized, placebo- and active-controlled (moxifloxacin 400 mg) crossover study in 59 healthy males (81% White, 12% Black, 7% Hispanic) aged 45-60 years. The QT interval was measured at one hour post dose because this time point approximates the average time of peak vardenafil concentration. The 80 mg dose of LEVITRA (four times the highest recommended dose) was chosen because this dose yields plasma concentrations covering those observed upon co-administration of a low-dose of LEVITRA (5 mg) and 600 mg BID of ritonavir. Of the CYP3A4 inhibitors that have been studied, ritonavir causes the most significant drug-drug interaction with vardenafil. Table 1 summarizes the effect on mean uncorrected QT and mean corrected QT interval (QT_c) with different methods of correction (Fridericia and a linear individual correction method) at one hour post-dose. No single correction method is known to be more valid than the other. In this study, the mean increase in heart rate associated with a 10 mg dose of LEVITRA compared to placebo was 5 beats/minute and with an 80 mg dose of LEVITRA the mean increase was 6 beats/minute.
[See table 1 above]
Therapeutic and supratherapeutic doses of vardenafil and the active control moxifloxacin produced similar increases in QT_c interval. This study, however, was not designed to make direct statistical comparisons between the drug or the dose levels. The clinical impact of these QT_c changes is unknown (see **PRECAUTIONS**).
In a separate postmarketing study of 44 healthy volunteers, single doses of 10 mg LEVITRA resulted in a placebo-subtracted mean change from baseline of QTcF (Fridericia correction) of 5 msec (90% CI: 2,8). Single doses of gatifloxacin 400 mg resulted in a placebo-subtracted mean change from baseline QTcF of 4 msec (90% CI: 1,7). When LEVITRA 10 mg and gatifloxacin 400 mg were co-administered, the mean QTcF change from baseline was additive when compared to either drug alone and produced a mean QTcF change of 9 msec from baseline (90% CI: 6,11). The clinical impact of these QT changes is unknown (see **PRECAUTIONS,** Congenital or Acquired QT Prolongation).
Effects on Exercise Treadmill Test in Patients with Coronary Artery Disease (CAD):
In two independent trials that assessed 10 mg (n=41) and 20 mg (n=39) vardenafil, respectively, vardenafil did not alter the total treadmill exercise time compared to placebo. The patient population included men aged 40-80 years with stable exercise-induced angina documented by at least one of the following: 1) prior history of MI, CABG, PTCA, or stenting (not within 6 months); 2) positive coronary angiogram showing at least 60% narrowing of the diameter of at least one major coronary artery; or 3) a positive stress echocardiogram or stress nuclear perfusion study.
Results of these studies showed that LEVITRA did not alter the total treadmill exercise time compared to placebo (10 mg LEVITRA vs. placebo: 433±109 and 426±105 seconds, respectively; 20 mg LEVITRA vs. placebo: 414±111 and 411±124 seconds, respectively). The total time to angina was not altered by LEVITRA when compared to placebo (10 mg LEVITRA vs. placebo: 291±123 and 292±110 seconds; 20 mg LEVITRA vs. placebo: 354±137 and 347±143 seconds, respectively). The total time to 1 mm or greater ST-segment depression was similar to placebo in both the 10 mg and the 20 mg LEVITRA groups (10 mg LEVITRA vs. placebo: 380±108 and 334±108 seconds; 20 mg LEVITRA vs. placebo: 364±101 and 366±105 seconds, respectively).
Effects on Vision:
Single oral doses of phosphodiesterase inhibitors have demonstrated transient dose-related impairment of color

discrimination (blue/green) using the Farnsworth-Munsell 100-hue test and reductions in electroretinogram (ERG) b-wave amplitudes, with peak effects near the time of peak plasma levels. These findings are consistent with the inhibition of PDE6 in rods and cones, which is involved in phototransduction in the retina. The findings were most evident one hour after administration, diminishing but still present 6 hours after administration. In a single dose study in 25 normal males, LEVITRA 40 mg, twice the maximum daily recommended dose, did not alter visual acuity, intraocular pressure, fundoscopic and slit lamp findings.

In another double-blind, placebo controlled clinical trial, at least 15 doses of 20 mg vardenafil were administered over 8 weeks versus placebo to 52 males. Thirty-two (32) males (62%) of the patients completed the trial. Retinal function was measured by ERG and FM-100 test 2, 6 and 24 hours after dosing. The trial was designed to detect changes in retinal function that might occur in more than 10% of patients. Vardenafil did not produce clinically significant ERG or FM-100 effects in healthy men compared to placebo. Two patients on vardenafil in the trial reported episodes of transient cyanopsia (objects appear blue).

CLINICAL STUDIES

LEVITRA was evaluated in four major double-blind, randomized, placebo-controlled, fixed-dose, parallel design, multicenter trials in 2431 men aged 20-83 (mean age 57 years; 78% White, 7% Black, 2% Asian, 3% Hispanic and 10% Other/Unknown). The doses of LEVITRA in these studies were 5 mg, 10 mg, and 20 mg. Two of these trials were conducted in the general ED population and two in special ED populations (one in patients with diabetes mellitus and one in post-prostatectomy patients). LEVITRA was dosed without regard to meals on an as needed basis in men with erectile dysfunction (ED), many of whom had multiple other medical conditions. The primary endpoints were assessed at 3 months.

Primary efficacy assessment in all four major trials was by means of the Erectile Function (EF) Domain score of the validated International Index of Erectile Function (IIEF) Questionnaire and two questions from the Sexual Encounter Profile (SEP) dealing with the ability to achieve vaginal penetration (SEP2), and the ability to maintain an erection long enough for successful intercourse (SEP3).

In all four fixed-dose efficacy trials, LEVITRA showed clinically meaningful and statistically significant improvement in the EF Domain, SEP2, and SEP3 scores compared to placebo. The mean baseline EF Domain score in these trials was 11.8 (scores range from 0-30 where lower scores represent more severe disease). LEVITRA (5 mg, 10 mg, and 20 mg) was effective in all age categories (<45, 45 to <65, and ≥65 years) and was also effective regardless of race (White, Black, Other).

Trials in a General Erectile Dysfunction Population: In the major North American fixed-dose trial, 762 patients (mean age 57, range 20-83 years; 79% White, 13% Black, 4% Hispanic, 2% Asian and 2% Other) were evaluated. The mean baseline EF Domain scores were 13, 13, 13, 14 for the LEVITRA 5 mg, 10 mg, 20 mg and placebo groups, respectively. There was significant improvement (p <0.0001) at 3 months with LEVITRA (EF Domain scores of 18, 21, 21, for the 5 mg, 10 mg, and 20 mg dose groups, respectively) compared to the placebo group (EF Domain score of 15). The European trial (total N=803) confirmed these results. The improvement in mean score was maintained at all doses at 6 months in the North American trial.

In the North American trial, LEVITRA significantly improved the rates of achieving an erection sufficient for penetration (SEP2) at doses of 5 mg, 10 mg, and 20 mg compared to placebo (65%, 75%, and 80%, respectively, compared to a 52% response in the placebo group at 3 months; p <0.0001). The European trial confirmed these results.

LEVITRA demonstrated a clinically meaningful and statistically significant increase in the overall per-patient rate of maintenance of erection to successful intercourse (SEP3) (51% on 5 mg, 64% on 10 mg, and 65% on 20 mg, respectively, compared to 32% on placebo; p <0.0001) at 3 months in the North American trial. The European trial showed comparable efficacy. This improvement in mean score was maintained at all doses at 6 months in the North American trial.

Trial in Patients with ED and Diabetes Mellitus: LEVITRA demonstrated clinically meaningful and statistically significant improvement in erectile function in a prospective, fixed-dose (10 and 20 mg LEVITRA), double-blind, placebo-controlled trial of patients with diabetes mellitus (n=439; mean age 57 years, range 33-81; 80% White, 9% Black, 8% Hispanic, and 3% Other).

Significant improvements in the EF Domain were shown in this study (EF Domain scores of 17 on 10 mg LEVITRA and 19 on 20 mg LEVITRA compared to 13 on placebo; p <0.0001).

LEVITRA significantly improved the overall per-patient rate of achieving an erection sufficient for penetration (SEP2) (61% on 10 mg and 64% on 20 mg LEVITRA compared to 36% on placebo; p <0.0001).

LEVITRA demonstrated a clinically meaningful and statistically significant increase in the overall per-patient rate of maintenance of erection to successful intercourse (SEP3) (49% on 10 mg, 54% on 20 mg LEVITRA compared to 23% on placebo; p <0.0001).

Trial in Patients with ED after Radical Prostatectomy: LEVITRA demonstrated clinically meaningful and statistically significant improvement in erectile function in a prospective, fixed-dose (10 and 20 mg LEVITRA), double-blind, placebo-controlled trial in post-prostatectomy patients (n=427, mean age 60, range 44-77 years; 93% White, 5% Black, 2% Other).

Significant improvements in the EF Domain were shown in this study (EF Domain scores of 15 on 10 mg LEVITRA and 15 on 20 mg LEVITRA compared to 9 on placebo; p <0.0001).

LEVITRA significantly improved the overall per-patient rate of achieving an erection sufficient for penetration (SEP2) (47% on 10 mg and 48% on 20 mg LEVITRA compared to 22% on placebo; p <0.0001).

LEVITRA demonstrated a clinically meaningful and statistically significant increase in the overall per-patient rate of maintenance of erection to successful intercourse (SEP3) (37% on 10 mg, 34% on 20 mg LEVITRA compared to 10% on placebo; p <0.0001).

INDICATIONS AND USAGE

LEVITRA is indicated for the treatment of erectile dysfunction.

CONTRAINDICATIONS

Nitrates: Administration of LEVITRA with nitrates (either regularly and/or intermittently) and nitric oxide donors is contraindicated (see **CLINICAL PHARMACOLOGY, Pharmacodynamics, Effects on Blood Pressure and Heart Rate when LEVITRA is Combined with Nitrates**). Consistent with the effects of PDE5 inhibition on the nitric oxide/cyclic guanosine monophosphate pathway, PDE5 inhibitors may potentiate the hypotensive effects of nitrates. A suitable time interval following LEVITRA dosing for the safe administration of nitrates or nitric oxide donors has not been determined.

Hypersensitivity: LEVITRA is contraindicated for patients with a known hypersensitivity to any component of the tablet.

WARNINGS

Cardiovascular effects

General: Physicians should consider the cardiovascular status of their patients, since there is a degree of cardiac risk associated with sexual activity. In men for whom sexual activity is not recommended because of their underlying cardiovascular status, any treatment for erectile dysfunction, including LEVITRA, generally should not be used.

Left Ventricular Outflow Obstruction: Patients with left ventricular outflow obstruction, e.g., aortic stenosis and idiopathic hypertrophic subaortic stenosis, can be sensitive to the action of vasodilators including Type 5 phosphodiesterase inhibitors.

Blood Pressure Effects: LEVITRA has systemic vasodilatory properties that resulted in transient decreases in supine blood pressure in healthy volunteers (mean maximum decrease of 7 mmHg systolic and 8 mmHg diastolic) (see **CLINICAL PHARMACOLOGY, Pharmacodynamics**). While this normally would be expected to be of little consequence in most patients, prior to prescribing LEVITRA, physicians should carefully consider whether their patients with underlying cardiovascular disease could be affected adversely by such vasodilatory effects.

Effect of Co-administration of Potent CYP3A4 Inhibitors

Long-term safety information is not available on the concomitant administration of vardenafil with HIV protease inhibitors. Concomitant administration with ritonavir or indinavir substantially increases plasma concentrations of vardenafil. Because ritonavir prolongs LEVITRA elimination half-life (5 to 6-fold), no more than a single 2.5 mg dose of LEVITRA should be taken in a 72-hour period by patients also taking ritonavir. Patients taking indinavir, saquinavir, atazanavir or other potent CYP3A4 inhibitors such as clarithromycin, ketoconazole 400 mg daily, or itraconazole 400 mg daily should not exceed a dose of LEVITRA 2.5 mg once daily. For patients taking ketoconazole 200 mg daily or itraconazole 200 mg daily, a single dose of 5 mg LEVITRA should not be exceeded in a 24-hour period (see **PRECAUTIONS, Drug Interactions** and **DOSAGE AND ADMINISTRATION**).

Other Effects

There have been rare reports of prolonged erections greater than 4 hours and priapism (painful erections greater than 6 hours in duration) for this class of compounds, including vardenafil. In the event that an erection persists longer than 4 hours, the patient should seek immediate medical

assistance. If priapism is not treated immediately, penile tissue damage and permanent loss of potency may result.

Patient Subgroups Not Studied in Clinical Trials

There are no controlled clinical data on the safety or efficacy of LEVITRA in the following patients; and therefore its use is not recommended until further information is available.

• unstable angina; hypotension (resting systolic blood pressure of <90 mmHg); uncontrolled hypertension (>170/110 mmHg); recent history of stroke, life-threatening arrhythmia, or myocardial infarction (within the last 6 months); severe cardiac failure
• severe hepatic impairment (Child-Pugh C)
• end stage renal disease requiring dialysis
• known hereditary degenerative retinal disorders, including retinitis pigmentosa

PRECAUTIONS

The evaluation of erectile dysfunction should include a determination of potential underlying causes, a medical assessment, and the identification of appropriate treatment. Before prescribing LEVITRA, it is important to note the following:

Alpha-blockers:

Caution is advised when PDE5 inhibitors are co-administered with alpha-blockers. Phosphodiesterase Type 5 (PDE5) inhibitors, including LEVITRA, and alpha-adrenergic blocking agents are both vasodilators with blood-pressure lowering effects. When vasodilators are used in combination, an additive effect on blood pressure may be anticipated. In some patients, concomitant use of these two drug classes can lower blood pressure significantly (see **PRECAUTIONS, Drug Interactions**) leading to symptomatic hypotension (e.g., fainting). Consideration should be given to the following:

• Patients should be stable on alpha-blocker therapy prior to initiating a PDE5 inhibitor. Patients who demonstrate hemodynamic instability on alpha-blocker therapy alone are at increased risk of symptomatic hypotension with concomitant use of PDE5 inhibitors.
• In those patients who are stable on alpha-blocker therapy, PDE5 inhibitors should be initiated at the lowest recommended starting dose (see **DOSAGE and ADMINISTRATION**).
• In those patients already taking an optimized dose of PDE5 inhibitor, alpha-blocker therapy should be initiated at the lowest dose. Stepwise increase in alpha-blocker dose may be associated with further lowering of blood pressure in patients taking a PDE5 inhibitor.
• Safety of combined use of PDE5 inhibitors and alpha-blockers may be affected by other variables, including intravascular volume depletion and other anti-hypertensive drugs.

Hepatic Insufficiency:

In volunteers with moderate impairment (Child-Pugh B), the C_{max} and AUC following a 10 mg vardenafil dose were increased 130% and 160%, respectively, compared to healthy control subjects. Consequently, a starting dose of 5 mg is recommended for patients with moderate hepatic impairment and the maximum dose should not exceed 10 mg (see **CLINICAL PHARMACOLOGY, Pharmacokinetics in Special Populations**, and **DOSAGE AND ADMINISTRATION**). Vardenafil has not been evaluated in patients with severe hepatic impairment (Child-Pugh C).

Congenital or Acquired QT Prolongation: In a study of the effect of LEVITRA on QT interval in 59 healthy males (see **CLINICAL PHARMACOLOGY, Electrophysiology**), therapeutic (10 mg) and supratherapeutic (80 mg) doses of LEVITRA and the active control moxifloxacin (400 mg) produced similar increases in QT_c interval. A postmarketing study evaluating the effect of combining LEVITRA with another drug of comparable QT effect showed an additive QT effect when compared with either drug alone (see **CLINICAL PHARMACOLOGY, Electrophysiology**). These observations should be considered in clinical decisions when prescribing LEVITRA to patients with known history of QT prolongation or patients who are taking medications known to prolong the QT interval. Patients taking Class 1A (e.g. quinidine, procainamide) or Class III (e.g. amiodarone, sotalol) antiarrhythmic medications or those with congenital QT prolongation, should avoid using LEVITRA.

Renal Insufficiency:

In patients with moderate (CL_{cr} = 30-50 ml/min) to severe (CL_{cr} <30 ml/min) renal impairment, the AUC of vardenafil was 20–30% higher compared to that observed in a control group with normal renal function (CL_{cr} >80 ml/min) (see **CLINICAL PHARMACOLOGY, Pharmacokinetics in Special Populations**). Vardenafil pharmacokinetics have not been evaluated in patients requiring renal dialysis.

General: In humans, vardenafil alone in doses up to 20 mg does not prolong the bleeding time. There is no clinical evidence of any additive prolongation of the bleeding time when vardenafil is administered with aspirin. Vardenafil has not been administered to patients with bleeding disorders or significant active peptic ulceration. Therefore

LEVITRA should be administered to these patients after careful benefit-risk assessment.
Treatment for erectile dysfunction should generally be used with caution by patients with anatomical deformation of the penis (such as angulation, cavernosal fibrosis, or Peyronie's disease) or by patients who have conditions that may predispose them to priapism (such as sickle cell anemia, multiple myeloma, or leukemia).
The safety and efficacy of LEVITRA used in combination with other treatments for erectile dysfunction have not been studied. Therefore, the use of such combinations is not recommended.

Information for Patients

Physicians should discuss with patients the contraindication of LEVITRA with regular and/or intermittent use of organic nitrates. Patients should be counseled that concomitant use of LEVITRA with nitrates could cause blood pressure to suddenly drop to an unsafe level, resulting in dizziness, syncope, or even heart attack or stroke.
Physicians should inform their patients that in some patients concomitant use of PDE5 inhibitors, including LEVITRA, with alpha-blockers can lower blood pressure significantly leading to symptomatic hypotension (e.g., fainting). Patients prescribed LEVITRA who are taking alpha-blockers should be started on the lowest recommended starting dose of LEVITRA (see **Drug Interactions** and **DOSAGE AND ADMINISTRATION**). Patients should be advised of the possible occurrence of symptoms related to postural hypotension and appropriate countermeasures. Patients should be advised to contact the prescribing physician if other anti-hypertensive drugs or new medications that may interact with LEVITRA are prescribed by another healthcare provider.
Physicians should discuss with patients the appropriate use of LEVITRA and its anticipated benefits. It should be explained that sexual stimulation is required for an erection to occur after taking LEVITRA. LEVITRA should be taken approximately 60 minutes before sexual activity. Patients should be counseled regarding the dosing of LEVITRA. Patients should be advised to contact their healthcare provider for dose modification if they are not satisfied with the quality of their sexual performance with LEVITRA or in the case of an unwanted effect. Patients should be advised to contact the prescribing physician if new medications that may interact with LEVITRA are prescribed by another healthcare provider.
Physicians should advise patients to stop use of all PDE5 inhibitors, including LEVITRA, and seek medical attention in the event of sudden loss of vision in one or both eyes. Such an event may be a sign of non-arteritic anterior ischemic optic neuropathy (NAION), a cause of decreased vision, including permanent loss of vision, that has been reported rarely post-marketing in temporal association with the use of all PDE5 inhibitors. It is not possible to determine whether these events were related directly to the use of PDE5 inhibitors or to other factors. Physicians should also discuss with patients the increased risk of NAION in individuals who have already experienced NAION in one eye, including whether such individuals could be adversely affected by use of vasodilators such as PDE5 inhibitors (see **POST-MARKETING EXPERIENCE,** Ophthalmologic).
Physicians should advise patients to stop taking PDE5 inhibitors, including LEVITRA, and seek prompt medical attention in the event of sudden decrease or loss of hearing. These events, which may be accompanied by tinnitus and dizziness, have been reported in temporal association to the intake of PDE5 inhibitors, including LEVITRA. It is not possible to determine whether these events are related directly to the use of PDE5 inhibitors or to other factors (see **ADVERSE REACTIONS**).
Physicians should discuss with patients the potential cardiac risk of sexual activity for patients with preexisting cardiovascular risk factors.
The use of LEVITRA offers no protection against sexually transmitted diseases. Counseling of patients about protective measures necessary to guard against sexually transmitted diseases, including the Human Immunodeficiency Virus (HIV), should be considered.
Physicians should inform patients that there have been rare reports of prolonged erections greater than 4 hours and priapism (painful erections greater than 6 hours in duration) for LEVITRA and this class of compounds. In the event that an erection persists longer than 4 hours, the patient should seek immediate medical assistance. If priapism is not treated immediately, penile tissue damage and permanent loss of potency may result.

Drug Interactions

Effect of other drugs on LEVITRA
In vitro studies: Studies in human liver microsomes showed that vardenafil is metabolized primarily by cytochrome P450 (CYP) isoforms 3A4/5, and to a lesser degree by CYP2C9. Therefore, inhibitors of these enzymes are expected to reduce vardenafil clearance (see **WARNINGS** and **DOSAGE AND ADMINISTRATION**).

Table 2: Mean (95% C.I.) maximal change from baseline in systolic blood pressure (mmHg) following vardenafil 5 mg in BPH patients on stable alpha-blocker therapy (Study 1)

Alpha-Blocker		Simultaneous dosing of Vardenafil 5 mg and Alpha-Blocker, Placebo-Subtracted	Dosing of Vardenafil 5 mg and Alpha-Blocker Separated by 6 Hours, Placebo-Subtracted
Terazosin	Standing SBP	-3 (-6.7, 0.1)	-4 (-7.4, -0.5)
5 or 10 mg daily	Supine SBP	-4 (-6.7, -0.5)	-4 (-7.1, -0.7)
Tamsulosin	Standing SBP	-6 (-9.9, -2.1)	-4 (-8.3, -0.5)
0.4 mg daily	Supine SBP	-4 (-7.0, -0.8)	-5 (-7.9, -1.7)

In vivo studies: Cytochrome P450 Inhibitors
Cimetidine (400 mg b.i.d.) had no effect on vardenafil bioavailability (AUC) and maximum concentration (C_{max}) of vardenafil when co-administered with 20 mg LEVITRA in healthy volunteers.
Erythromycin (500 mg t.i.d.) produced a 4-fold increase in vardenafil AUC and a 3-fold increase in C_{max} when co-administered with LEVITRA 5 mg in healthy volunteers (see **DOSAGE AND ADMINISTRATION**). It is recommended not to exceed a single 5 mg dose of LEVITRA in a 24-hour period when used in combination with erythromycin.
Ketoconazole (200 mg once daily) produced a 10-fold increase in vardenafil AUC and a 4-fold increase in C_{max} when co-administered with LEVITRA (5 mg) in healthy volunteers. A 5-mg LEVITRA dose should not be exceeded when used in combination with 200 mg once daily ketoconazole. Since higher doses of ketoconazole (400 mg daily) may result in higher increases in C_{max} and AUC, a single 2.5 mg dose of LEVITRA should not be exceeded in a 24-hour period when used in combination with ketoconazole 400 mg daily (see **WARNINGS** and **DOSAGE AND ADMINISTRATION**).
HIV Protease Inhibitors:
Indinavir (800 mg t.i.d.) co-administered with LEVITRA 10 mg resulted in a 16-fold increase in vardenafil AUC, a 7-fold increase in vardenafil C_{max} and a 2-fold increase in vardenafil half-life. It is recommended not to exceed a single 2.5 mg LEVITRA dose in a 24-hour period when used in combination with indinavir (see **WARNINGS** and **DOSAGE AND ADMINISTRATION**).
Ritonavir (600 mg b.i.d.) co-administered with LEVITRA 5 mg resulted in a 49-fold increase in vardenafil AUC and a 13-fold increase in vardenafil C_{max}. The interaction is a consequence of blocking hepatic metabolism of vardenafil by ritonavir, a highly potent CYP3A4 inhibitor, which also inhibits CYP2C9. Ritonavir significantly prolonged the half-life of vardenafil to 26 hours. Consequently, it is recommended not to exceed a single 2.5 mg LEVITRA dose in a 72-hour period when used in combination with ritonavir (see **WARNINGS** and **DOSAGE AND ADMINISTRATION**).
Other CYP3A4 inhibitors: Although specific interactions have not been studied, other CYP3A4 inhibitors, including grapefruit juice would likely increase vardenafil exposure.
Other Drug Interactions: No pharmacokinetic interactions were observed between vardenafil and the following drugs: glyburide, warfarin, digoxin, Maalox, and ranitidine. In the warfarin study, vardenafil had no effect on the prothrombin time or other pharmacodynamic parameters.
Effects of LEVITRA on other drugs
In vitro studies:
Vardenafil and its metabolites had no effect on CYP1A2, 2A6, and 2E1 (Ki >100 µM). Weak inhibitory effects toward other isoforms (CYP2C8, 2C9, 2C19, 2D6, 3A4) were found, but Ki values were in excess of plasma concentrations achieved following dosing. The most potent inhibitory activity was observed for vardenafil metabolite M1, which had a Ki of 1.4 µM toward CYP3A4, which is about 20 times higher than the M1 C_{max} values after an 80 mg LEVITRA dose.
In vivo studies:
Nitrates: The blood pressure lowering effects of sublingual nitrates (0.4 mg) taken 1 and 4 hours after vardenafil and increases in heart rate when taken at 1, 4 and 8 hours were potentiated by a 20 mg dose of LEVITRA in healthy middle-aged subjects. These effects were not observed when LEVITRA 20 mg was taken 24 hours before the NTG. Potentiation of the hypotensive effects of nitrates for patients with ischemic heart disease has not been evaluated, and concomitant use of LEVITRA and nitrates is contraindicated (see **CLINICAL PHARMACOLOGY, Pharmacodynamics,** Effects on Blood Pressure and Heart Rate when LEVITRA is Combined with Nitrates; CONTRAINDICATIONS).
Nifedipine: Vardenafil 20 mg, when co-administered with slow-release nifedipine 30 mg or 60 mg once daily, did not affect the relative bioavailability (AUC) or maximum concentration (C_{max}) of nifedipine, a drug that is metabolized via CYP3A4. Nifedipine did not alter the plasma levels of LEVITRA when taken in combination. In these patients whose hypertension was controlled with nifedipine, LEVITRA 20 mg produced mean additional supine systolic/diastolic blood pressure reductions of 6/5 mmHg compared to placebo.
Alpha-blockers:
Blood pressure effects in patients on stable alpha-blocker treatment:
Two clinical pharmacology studies were conducted in patients with benign prostatic hyperplasia (BPH) on stable-dose alpha-blocker treatment for at least four weeks.
Study 1: This study was designed to evaluate the effect of 5 mg vardenafil compared to placebo when administered to BPH patients on chronic alpha-blocker therapy in two separate cohorts: tamsulosin 0.4 mg daily (cohort 1, n=21) and terazosin 5 or 10 mg daily (cohort 2, n=21). The design was a randomized, double blind, cross-over study with four treatments: vardenafil 5 mg or placebo administered simultaneously with the alpha-blocker and vardenafil 5 mg or placebo administered 6 hours after the alpha-blocker. Blood pressure and pulse were evaluated over the 6-hour interval after vardenafil dosing. For BP results see Table 2. One patient after simultaneous treatment with 5 mg vardenafil and 10 mg terazosin exhibited symptomatic hypotension with standing blood pressure of 80/60 mmHg occurring one hour after administration and subsequent mild dizziness and moderate lightheadedness lasting for 6 hours. For vardenafil and placebo, five and two patients, respectively, experienced a decrease in standing systolic blood pressure (SBP) of >30 mmHg following simultaneous administration of terazosin. Hypotension was not observed when vardenafil 5 mg and terazosin were administered 6 hours apart. Following simultaneous administration of vardenafil 5 mg and tamsulosin, two patients had a standing SBP of <85 mmHg; two and one patient (vardenafil and placebo, respectively) had a decrease in standing SBP of >30 mmHg. When tamsulosin and vardenafil 5 mg were separated by 6 hours, two patients had a standing SBP <85 mmHg and one patient had a decrease in SBP of >30 mmHg. There were no severe adverse events related to hypotension reported during the study. There were no cases of syncope.
[See table 2 above]
Blood pressure effects (standing SBP) in normotensive men on stable dose tamsulosin 0.4 mg following simultaneous administration of vardenafil 5 mg or placebo, or following administration of vardenafil 5 mg or placebo separated by 6 hours are shown in Figure 3. Blood pressure effects (standing SBP) in normotensive men on stable dose terazosin (5 or 10 mg) following simultaneous administration of vardenafil 5 mg or placebo, or following administration of vardenafil 5 mg or placebo separated by 6 hours, are shown in Figure 4.

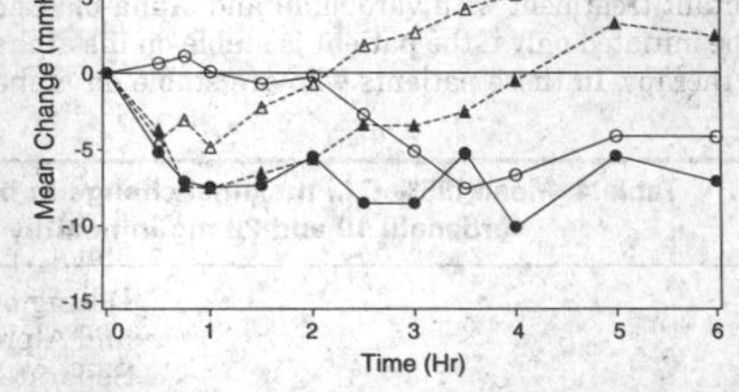

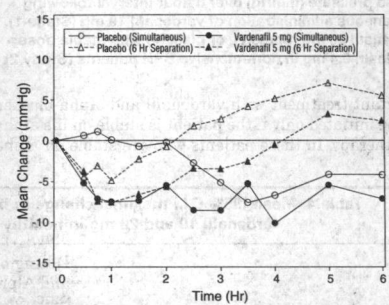

Figure 3: Mean change from baseline in standing systolic blood pressure (mmHg) over 6 hour interval following simultaneous or 6 hr separation administration of vardenafil 5 mg or placebo with stable dose tamsulosin 0.4 mg in normotensive BPH patients (Study 1)

[See figure 4 at top of next page]
Study 2: This study was designed to evaluate the effect of 10 mg vardenafil (stage 1) and 20 mg vardenafil (stage 2) compared to placebo, when administered to a single cohort of BPH patients (n=23) on stable therapy with tamsulosin 0.4 mg or 0.8 mg daily for at least four weeks. The design was a randomized, double blind, two-period cross-over

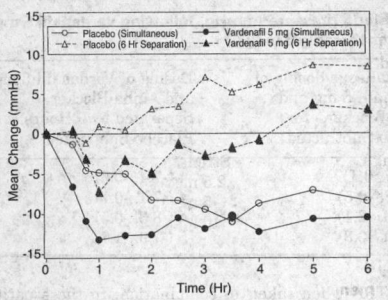

Figure 4: Mean change from baseline in standing systolic blood pressure (mmHg) over 6 hour interval following simultaneous or 6 hr separation administration of vardenafil 5 mg or placebo with stable dose terazosin (5 or 10 mg) in normotensive BPH patients (Study 1)

study. Vardenafil or placebo was given simultaneously with tamsulosin. Blood pressure and pulse were evaluated over the 6-hour interval after vardenafil dosing. For BP results see Table 3. One patient experienced a decrease from baseline in standing SBP of >30 mmHg following vardenafil 10 mg. There were no other instances of outlier blood pressure values (standing SBP <85 mmHg or decrease from baseline in standing SBP of >30 mmHg). Three patients reported dizziness following vardenafil 20 mg. There were no cases of syncope.

Table 3: Mean (95% C.I.) maximal change from baseline in systolic blood pressure (mmHg) following vardenafil 10 and 20 mg in BPH patients on stable alpha-blocker therapy with tamsulosin 0.4 or 0.8 mg daily (Study 2)

	Vardenafil 10 mg Placebo-subtracted	Vardenafil 20 mg Placebo-subtracted
Standing SBP	-4 (-6.8, -0.3)	-4 (-6.8, -1.4)
Supine SBP	-5 (-8.2, -0.8)	-4 (-6.3, -1.8)

Blood pressure effects (standing SBP) in normotensive men on stable dose tamsulosin 0.4 mg following simultaneous administration of vardenafil 20 mg or placebo, or following administration of vardenafil 20 mg or placebo separated by 6 hours are shown in Figure 5.

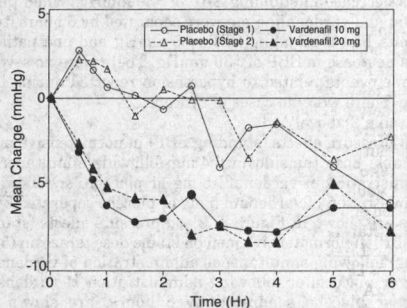

Figure 5: Mean change from baseline in standing systolic blood pressure (mmHg) over 6 hour interval following simultaneous administration of vardenafil 10 mg (Stage 1), vardenafil 20 mg (Stage 2), or placebo with stable dose tamsulosin 0.4 mg in normotensive BPH patients (Study 2)

Concomitant treatment with vardenafil and alpha-blockers should be initiated only if the patient is stable on his alpha-blocker therapy. In those patients who are stable on alpha-

blocker therapy, LEVITRA should be initiated at the lowest recommended starting dose (see **DOSAGE and ADMINISTRATION**).

Blood pressure effects in normotensive men after forced titration with alpha-blockers:
Two randomized, double blind, placebo-controlled clinical pharmacology studies with healthy normotensive volunteers (age range, 45-74 years) were performed after forced titration of the alpha-blocker terazosin to 10 mg daily over 14 days (n=29), and after initiation of tamsulosin 0.4 mg daily for five days (n=24). There were no severe adverse events related to hypotension in either study. Symptoms of hypotension were a cause for withdrawal in 2 subjects receiving terazosin and in 4 subjects receiving tamsulosin. Instances of outlier blood pressure values (defined as standing SBP <85 mmHg and/or a decrease from baseline of standing SBP >30 mmHg) were observed in 9/24 subjects receiving tamsulosin and 19/29 receiving terazosin. The incidence of subjects with standing SBP <85 mmHg given vardenafil and terazosin to achieve simultaneous T_{max} led to early termination of that arm of the study. In most (7/8) of these subjects, instances of standing SBP <85 mmHg were not associated with symptoms. Among subjects treated with terazosin, outlier values were observed more frequently when vardenafil and terazosin were given to achieve simultaneous T_{max} than when dosing was administered to separate T_{max} by 6 hours. There were 3 cases of dizziness observed with concomitant administration of terazosin and vardenafil. Seven subjects experienced dizziness mainly occurring with simultaneous T_{max} administration of tamsulosin. There were no cases of syncope.
[See table 4 below]

TERAZOSIN

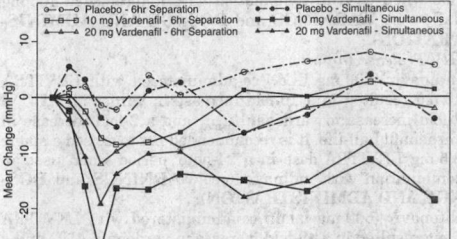

Figure 6: Mean change from baseline in standing systolic blood pressure (mmHg) over 6 hour interval following simultaneous or 6 hr separation administration of vardenafil 10 mg, vardenafil 20 mg or placebo with terazosin (10 mg) in healthy volunteers

[See figure 7 at top of next column]
Ritonavir and indinavir: Upon concomitant administration of 5 mg of LEVITRA with 600 mg BID ritonavir, the C_{max} and AUC of ritonavir were reduced by approximately 20%. Upon administration of 10 mg of LEVITRA with 800 mg TID indinavir, the C_{max} and AUC of indinavir were reduced by 40% and 30%, respectively.
Alcohol: Alcohol (0.5 g/kg body weight: approximately 40 mL of absolute alcohol in a 70 kg person) and vardenafil plasma levels were not altered when dosed simultaneously. LEVITRA (20 mg) did not potentiate the hypotensive effects of alcohol during the 4-hour observation period in healthy volunteers when administered with alcohol (0.5 g/kg body weight).
Aspirin: LEVITRA (10 mg and 20 mg) did not potentiate the increase in bleeding time caused by aspirin (two 81 mg tablets).

TAMSULOSIN

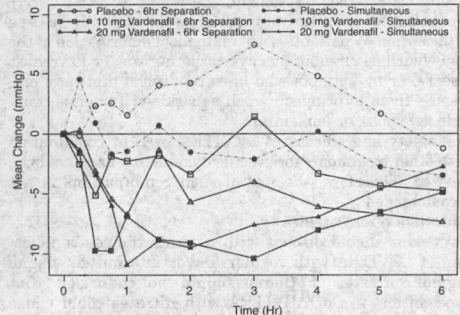

Figure 7: Mean change from baseline in standing systolic blood pressure (mmHg) over 6 hour interval following simultaneous or 6 hr separation administration of vardenafil 10 mg, vardenafil 20 mg or placebo with tamsulosin (0.4 mg) in healthy volunteers

Other interactions: LEVITRA had no effect on the pharmacodynamics of glyburide (glucose and insulin concentrations) and warfarin (prothrombin time or other pharmacological parameters).

Carcinogenesis, Mutagenesis, Impairment of Fertility
Vardenafil was not carcinogenic in rats and mice when administered daily for 24 months. In these studies systemic drug exposures (AUCs) for unbound (free) vardenafil and its major metabolite were approximately 400- and 170-fold for male and female rats, respectively, and 21- and 37-fold for male and female mice, respectively, the exposures observed in human males given the Maximum Recommended Human Dose (MRHD) of 20 mg. Vardenafil was not mutagenic as assessed in either the *in vitro* bacterial Ames assay or the forward mutation assay in Chinese hamster V_{79} cells. Vardenafil was not clastogenic as assessed in either the *in vitro* chromosomal aberration test or the *in vivo* mouse micronucleus test. Vardenafil did not impair fertility in male and female rats administered doses up to 100 mg/kg/day for 28 days prior to mating in male, and for 14 days prior to mating and through day 7 of gestation in females. In a corresponding 1-month rat toxicity study, this dose produced an AUC value for unbound vardenafil 200 fold greater than AUC in humans at the MRHD of 20 mg.
There was no effect on sperm motility or morphology after single 20 mg oral doses of vardenafil in healthy volunteers.

Pregnancy, Nursing Mothers and Pediatric Use
LEVITRA is not indicated for use in women, newborns, or children. Vardenafil was secreted into the milk of lactating rats at concentrations approximately 10-fold greater than found in the plasma. Following a single oral dose of 3 mg/kg, 3.3% of the administered dose was excreted into the milk within 24 hours. It is not known if vardenafil is excreted in human breast milk.

Pregnancy Category B:
No evidence of specific potential for teratogenicity, embryotoxicity or fetotoxicity was observed in rats and rabbits that received vardenafil at up to 18 mg/kg/day during organogenesis. This dose is approximately 100 fold (rat) and 29 fold (rabbit) greater than the AUC values for unbound vardenafil and its major metabolite in humans given the MRHD of 20 mg. In the rat pre-and postnatal development study, the NOAEL (no observed adverse effect level) for maternal toxicity was 8 mg/kg/day. Retarded physical development of pups in the absence of maternal effects was observed following maternal exposure to 1 and 8 mg/kg possibly due to vasodilatation and/or secretion of the drug into milk. The number of living pups born to rats exposed pre- and postnatally was reduced at 60 mg/kg/day. Based on the results of the pre- and postnatal study, the developmental NOAEL is less than 1 mg/kg/day. Based on plasma exposures in the rat developmental toxicity study, 1 mg/kg/day in the pregnant rat is estimated to produce total AUC values for unbound vardenafil and its major metabolite comparable to the human AUC at the MRHD of 20 mg. There are no adequate and well-controlled trials of vardenafil in pregnant women.

Geriatric Use
Elderly males age 65 years and older have higher vardenafil plasma concentrations than younger males (18–45 years), mean C_{max} and AUC were 34% and 52% higher, respectively (see **CLINICAL PHARMACOLOGY, Pharmacokinetics in Special Populations**, and **DOSAGE AND ADMINISTRATION**). Phase 3 clinical trials included more than 834 elderly patients, and no differences in safety or effectiveness of LEVITRA 5, 10, or 20 mg were noted when these elderly patients were compared to younger patients. However, due to increased vardenafil concentrations in the elderly, a starting dose of 5 mg LEVITRA should be considered in patients ≥65 years of age.

Table 4. Mean (95% C.I.) maximal change in baseline in systolic blood pressure (mmHg) following vardenafil 10 and 20 mg in healthy volunteers on daily alpha-blocker therapy

Alpha-Blocker		Dosing of Vardenafil and Alpha-Blocker Separated by 6 Hours		Simultaneous dosing of Vardenafil and Alpha-Blocker	
		Vardenafil 10 mg Placebo-Subtracted	Vardenafil 20 mg Placebo-Subtracted	Vardenafil 10 mg Placebo-Subtracted	Vardenafil 20 mg Placebo-Subtracted
Terazosin 10 mg daily	Standing SBP	-7 (-10, -3)	-11 (-14, -7)	-23 (-31, 16)*	-14 (-33, 11)*
	Supine SBP	-5 (-8, -2)	-7 (-11, -4)	-7 (-25, 19)*	-7 (-31, 22)*
Tamsulosin 0.4 mg daily	Standing SBP	-4 (-8, -1)	-8 (-11, -4)	-8 (-14, -2)	-8 (-14, -1)
	Supine SBP	-4 (-8, 0)	-7 (-11, -3)	-5 (-9, -2)	-3 (-7, 0)

*Due to the sample size, confidence intervals may not be an accurate measure for these data. These values represent the range for the difference.

ADVERSE REACTIONS

LEVITRA was administered to over 4430 men (mean age 56, range 18-89 years; 81% White, 6% Black, 2% Asian, 2% Hispanic and 9% Other) during controlled and uncontrolled clinical trials worldwide. Over 2200 patients were treated for 6 months or longer, and 880 patients were treated for at least 1 year.

In placebo-controlled clinical trials, the discontinuation rate due to adverse events was 3.4% for LEVITRA compared to 1.1% for placebo.

When LEVITRA was taken as recommended in placebo-controlled clinical trials, the following adverse events were reported (see **Table 5**).

Table 5: Adverse Events Reported By ≥2% of Patients Treated with LEVITRA and More Frequent on Drug than Placebo in Fixed and Flexible* Dose Randomized, Controlled Trials of 5 mg, 10 mg, or 20 mg Vardenafil

Adverse Event	Percentage of Patients Reporting Event	
	Placebo N = 1199	LEVITRA N = 2203
Headache	4%	15%
Flushing	1%	11%
Rhinitis	3%	9%
Dyspepsia	1%	4%
Accidental Injury†	2%	3%
Sinusitis	1%	3%
Flu Syndrome	2%	3%
Dizziness	1%	2%
Increased Creatine Kinase	1%	2%
Nausea	1%	2%

* Flexible dose studies started all patients at LEVITRA 10 mg and allowed decrease in dose to 5 mg or increase in dose to 20 mg based on side effects and efficacy.

† All the events listed in the above table were deemed to be adverse drug reactions with the exception of accidental injury.

Back pain was reported in 2.0% of patients treated with LEVITRA and 1.7% of patients on placebo.

Placebo-controlled trials suggested a dose effect in the incidence of some adverse events (headache, flushing, dyspepsia, nausea, rhinitis) over the 5 mg, 10 mg, and 20 mg doses of LEVITRA. The following section identifies additional, less frequent events (<2%) reported during the clinical development of LEVITRA. Excluded from this list are those events that are infrequent and minor, those events that may be commonly observed in the absence of drug therapy, and those events that are not reasonably associated with the drug.

BODY AS A WHOLE: anaphylactic reaction (including laryngeal edema), asthenia, face edema, pain

AUDITORY: sudden decrease or loss of hearing, tinnitus

CARDIOVASCULAR: angina pectoris, chest pain, hypertension, hypotension, myocardial ischemia, myocardial infarction, palpitation, postural hypotension, syncope, tachycardia

DIGESTIVE: abdominal pain, abnormal liver function tests, diarrhea, dry mouth, dysphagia, esophagitis, gastritis, gastroesophageal reflux, GGTP increased, vomiting

MUSCULOSKELETAL: arthralgia, back pain, myalgia, neck pain

NERVOUS: hypertonia, hypesthesia, insomnia, paresthesia, somnolence, vertigo

RESPIRATORY: dyspnea, epistaxis, pharyngitis

SKIN AND APPENDAGES: photosensitivity reaction, pruritus, rash, sweating

OPHTHALMOLOGIC: abnormal vision, blurred vision, chromatopsia, changes in color vision, conjunctivitis (increased redness of the eye), dim vision, eye pain, glaucoma, photophobia, watery eyes

UROGENITAL: abnormal ejaculation, priapism (including prolonged or painful erections)

POST-MARKETING EXPERIENCE

Ophthalmologic

Non-arteritic anterior ischemic optic neuropathy (NAION), a cause of decreased vision including permanent loss of vision, has been reported rarely post-marketing in temporal association with the use of phosphodiesterase type 5 (PDE5) inhibitors, including LEVITRA. Most, but not all, of these patients had underlying anatomic or vascular risk factors for development of NAION, including but not necessarily limited to: low cup to disc ratio ("crowded disc"), age over 50, diabetes, hypertension, coronary artery disease, hyperlipidemia and smoking. It is not possible to determine whether these events are related directly to the use of PDE5 inhibitors, to the patient's underlying vascular risk factors or anatomical defects, to a combination of these factors, or to other factors (see **PRECAUTIONS, Information for Patients**).

Visual disturbances including vision loss (temporary or permanent), such as visual field defect, retinal vein occlusion, and reduced visual acuity, have also been reported rarely in post-marketing experience. It is not possible to determine whether these events are related directly to the use of LEVITRA.

Neurologic

Seizure, seizure recurrence and transient global amnesia have been reported post-marketing in temporal association with LEVITRA.

Otologic

Cases of sudden decrease or loss of hearing have been reported post-marketing in temporal association with the use of PDE5 inhibitors, including LEVITRA. In some cases, medical conditions and other factors were reported that may have also played a role in the otologic adverse events. In many cases, medical follow-up information was limited. It is not possible to determine whether these reported events are related directly to the use of LEVITRA, to the patient's underlying risk factors for hearing loss, a combination of these factors, or to other factors (see **PRECAUTIONS, Information for Patients**).

OVERDOSAGE

The maximum dose of LEVITRA for which human data are available is a single 120 mg dose administered to eight healthy male volunteers. The majority of these subjects experienced reversible back pain/myalgia and/or "abnormal vision."

In cases of overdose, standard supportive measures should be taken as required. Renal dialysis is not expected to accelerate clearance because vardenafil is highly bound to plasma proteins and is not significantly eliminated in the urine.

DOSAGE AND ADMINISTRATION

For most patients, the recommended starting dose of LEVITRA is 10 mg, taken orally approximately 60 minutes before sexual activity. The dose may be increased to a maximum recommended dose of 20 mg or decreased to 5 mg based on efficacy and side effects. The maximum recommended dosing frequency is once per day. LEVITRA can be taken with or without food. Sexual stimulation is required for a response to treatment.

Geriatrics: A starting dose of 5 mg LEVITRA should be considered in patients ≥65 years of age (see **CLINICAL PHARMACOLOGY, Pharmacokinetics in Special Populations** and **PRECAUTIONS**).

Hepatic Impairment: For patients with mild hepatic impairment (Child-Pugh A), no dose adjustment of LEVITRA is required. Vardenafil clearance is reduced in patients with moderate hepatic impairment (Child-Pugh B), and a starting dose of 5 mg LEVITRA is recommended. The maximum dose in patients with moderate hepatic impairment should not exceed 10 mg. LEVITRA has not been evaluated in patients with severe hepatic impairment (Child-Pugh C) (see **CLINICAL PHARMACOLOGY**, Metabolism and Excretion, **WARNINGS** and **PRECAUTIONS**).

Renal Impairment: For patients with mild (CL_{cr} = 50-80 ml/min), moderate (CL_{cr} = 30-50 ml/min), or severe (CL_{cr} <30 ml/min) renal impairment, no dose adjustment is required. LEVITRA has not been evaluated in patients on renal dialysis (see **CLINICAL PHARMACOLOGY**, Metabolism and Excretion and **PRECAUTIONS**).

Concomitant Medications: The dosage of LEVITRA may require adjustment in patients receiving potent CYP3A4 inhibitors such as ketoconazole, itraconazole, ritonavir, indinavir, saquinavir, atazanavir, and clarithromycin as well as in other patients receiving moderate CYP3A4 inhibitors such as erythromycin (see **WARNINGS, PRECAUTIONS, Drug Interactions**). For ritonavir, a single dose of 2.5 mg LEVITRA should not be exceeded in a 72-hour period. For indinavir, saquinavir, atazanavir, ketoconazole 400 mg daily, itraconazole 400 mg daily, and clarithromycin, a single dose of 2.5 mg LEVITRA should not be exceeded in a 24-hour period. For ketoconazole 200 mg daily, itraconazole 200 mg daily, and erythromycin, a single dose of 5 mg LEVITRA should not be exceeded in a 24-hour period. For alpha-blockers, caution is advised when PDE5 inhibitors, including LEVITRA, are used concomitantly with alpha-blockers because of the potential for an additive effect on blood pressure. In some patients, concomitant use of these two drug classes can lower blood pressure significantly (see **PRECAUTIONS, Alpha-blockers** and **Drug Interactions**) leading to symptomatic hypotension (e.g., fainting). Concomitant treatment should be initiated only if the patient is stable on his alpha blocker therapy. In those patients who are stable on alpha-blocker therapy, LEVITRA should be initiated at a dose of 5 mg (2.5 mg when used concomitantly with certain CYP3A4 inhibitors - see **Drug Interactions**).

HOW SUPPLIED

LEVITRA (vardenafil HCl) is formulated as orange, film-coated round tablets with debossed "BAYER" cross on one side and "2.5", "5", "10", and "20" on the other side equivalent to 2.5 mg, 5 mg, 10 mg, and 20 mg of vardenafil, respectively.

Package	Strength	NDC Code
Bottles of 30	2.5 mg	0085-1923-01
	5 mg	0085-1945-01
	10 mg	0085-1901-01
	20 mg	0085-1934-01

Recommended Storage:
Store at 25°C (77°F); excursions permitted to 15-30°C (59-86°F) [see USP Controlled Room Temperature].
Manufactured by:
Bayer HealthCare Pharmaceuticals Inc.
Wayne, NJ 07470
Made in Germany
Marketed By
GlaxoSmithKline
Research Triangle Park NC 27709
Distributed and Marketed By:
Schering-Plough
Schering Corporation
Kenilworth, NJ 07033
LEVITRA is a registered trademark of Bayer Aktiengesellschaft and is used under license by GlaxoSmithKline and Schering Corporation.
Rx Only
08918646IP, R.7 12/08 14272
©2008 Bayer HealthCare Pharmaceuticals Inc.
Printed in U.S.A.

PATIENT INFORMATION

LEVITRA® (Luh-VEE-Trah)
(vardenafil HCl) Tablets
Read the Patient Information about LEVITRA before you start taking it and again each time you get a refill. There may be new information. You may also find it helpful to share this information with your partner. This leaflet does not take the place of talking with your doctor. You and your doctor should talk about LEVITRA when you start taking it and at regular checkups. If you do not understand the information, or have questions, talk with your doctor or pharmacist.

WHAT IMPORTANT INFORMATION SHOULD YOU KNOW ABOUT LEVITRA?
LEVITRA can cause your blood pressure to drop suddenly to an unsafe level if it is taken with certain other medicines. With a sudden drop in blood pressure, you could get dizzy, faint, or have a heart attack or stroke.
Do not take LEVITRA if you:
• take any medicines called "nitrates."
• use recreational drugs called "poppers" like amyl nitrate and butyl nitrate.
(See "Who Should Not Take Levitra?")
Tell all your healthcare providers that you take LEVITRA. If you need emergency medical care for a heart problem, it will be important for your healthcare provider to know when you last took LEVITRA.
WHAT IS LEVITRA?
LEVITRA is a prescription medicine taken by mouth for the treatment of erectile dysfunction (ED) in men.
ED is a condition where the penis does not harden and expand when a man is sexually excited, or when he cannot keep an erection. A man who has trouble getting or keeping an erection should see his doctor for help if the condition bothers him. LEVITRA may help a man with ED get and keep an erection when he is sexually excited.
LEVITRA does not:
• cure ED
• increase a man's sexual desire
• protect a man or his partner from sexually transmitted diseases, including HIV. Speak to your doctor about ways to guard against sexually transmitted diseases.
• serve as a male form of birth control
LEVITRA is only for men with ED. LEVITRA is not for women or children. LEVITRA must be used only under a doctor's care.
HOW DOES LEVITRA WORK?
When a man is sexually stimulated, his body's normal physical response is to increase blood flow to his penis. This results in an erection. LEVITRA helps increase blood flow to the penis and may help men with ED get and keep an erection satisfactory for sexual activity. Once a man has completed sexual activity, blood flow to his penis decreases, and his erection goes away.
WHO CAN TAKE LEVITRA?
Talk to your doctor to decide if LEVITRA is right for you. LEVITRA has been shown to be effective in men over the age of 18 years who have erectile dysfunction, including men with diabetes or who have undergone prostatectomy.

WHO SHOULD NOT TAKE LEVITRA?

Do not take LEVITRA if you:

- **take any medicines called "nitrates"** (See "What important information should you know about LEVITRA?"). Nitrates are commonly used to treat angina. Angina is a symptom of heart disease and can cause pain in your chest, jaw, or down your arm.
  Medicines called nitrates include nitroglycerin that is found in tablets, sprays, ointments, pastes, or patches. Nitrates can also be found in other medicines such as isosorbide dinitrate or isosorbide mononitrate. Some recreational drugs called "poppers" also contain nitrates, such as amyl nitrate and butyl nitrate. Do not use LEVITRA if you are using these drugs. Ask your doctor or pharmacist if you are not sure if any of your medicines are nitrates.
- **you have been told by your healthcare provider to not have sexual activity because of health problems.** Sexual activity can put an extra strain on your heart, especially if your heart is already weak from a heart attack or heart disease.
- **are allergic to LEVITRA or any of its ingredients.** The active ingredient in LEVITRA is called vardenafil. See the end of this leaflet for a complete list of ingredients.

WHAT SHOULD YOU DISCUSS WITH YOUR DOCTOR BEFORE TAKING LEVITRA?

Before taking LEVITRA, tell your doctor about all your medical problems, including if you:

- **have heart problems** such as angina, heart failure, irregular heartbeats, or have had a heart attack. Ask your doctor if it is safe for you to have sexual activity.
- **have low blood pressure or** have high blood pressure that is not controlled
- **have had a stroke**
- **have had a seizure**
- **or any family members have a rare heart condition known as prolongation of the QT interval (long QT syndrome)**
- **have liver problems**
- **have kidney problems and require dialysis**
- **have retinitis pigmentosa,** a rare genetic (runs in families) eye disease
- **have ever had severe vision loss, or if you have an eye condition called non-arteritic anterior ischemic optic neuropathy (NAION)**
- **have stomach ulcers**
- **have a bleeding problem**
- **have a deformed penis shape** or Peyronie's disease
- **have had an erection that lasted more than 4 hours**
- **have blood cell problems** such as sickle cell anemia, multiple myeloma, or leukemia

CAN OTHER MEDICATIONS AFFECT LEVITRA?

Tell your doctor about all the medicines you take including prescription and non-prescription medicines, vitamins, and herbal supplements. LEVITRA and other medicines may affect each other. Always check with your doctor before starting or stopping any medicines. Especially tell your doctor if you take any of the following:

- medicines called nitrates (See "What important information should you know about LEVITRA?")
- medicines called alpha-blockers. These include Hytrin® (terazosin HCl), Flomax® (tamsulosin HCl), Cardura® (doxazosin mesylate), Minipress® (prazosin HCl) or Uroxatral® (alfuzosin HCl). Alpha-blockers are sometimes prescribed for prostate problems or high blood pressure. In some patients the use of PDE5 inhibitor drugs, including LEVITRA, with alpha-blockers can lower blood pressure significantly leading to fainting. You should contact the prescribing physician if alpha-blockers or other drugs that lower blood pressure are prescribed by another healthcare provider.
- medicines that treat abnormal heartbeat. These include quinidine, procainamide, amiodarone and sotalol.
- ritonavir (Norvir®) or indinavir sulfate (Crixivan®) saquinavir (Fortavase® or Invirase®) or atazanavir (Reyataz®)
- ketoconazole or itraconazole (such as Nizoral® or Sporanox®)
- erythromycin or clarithromycin
- other medicines or treatments for ED

HOW SHOULD YOU TAKE LEVITRA?

Take LEVITRA exactly as your doctor prescribes. LEVITRA comes in different doses (2.5 mg, 5 mg, 10 mg, and 20 mg). For most men, the recommended starting dose is 10 mg.
Take LEVITRA no more than once a day. Doses should be taken at least 24 hours apart. Some men can only take a low dose of LEVITRA because of medical conditions or medicines they take. Your doctor will prescribe the dose that is right for you.

- If you are older than 65 or have liver problems, your doctor may start you on a lower dose of LEVITRA.
- If you have prostate problems or high blood pressure, for which you take medicines called alpha-blockers, your doctor may start you on a lower dose of LEVITRA.
- If you are taking certain other medicines your doctor may prescribe a lower starting dose and limit you to one dose of LEVITRA in a 72-hour (3 days) period.

Take 1 LEVITRA tablet about 1 hour (60 minutes) before sexual activity. Some form of sexual stimulation is needed for an erection to happen with LEVITRA. LEVITRA may be taken with or without meals.
Do not change your dose of LEVITRA without talking to your doctor. Your doctor may lower your dose or raise your dose, depending on how your body reacts to LEVITRA.
If you take too much LEVITRA, call your doctor or emergency room right away.

WHAT ARE THE POSSIBLE SIDE EFFECTS OF LEVITRA?

The most common side effects with LEVITRA are headache, flushing, stuffy or runny nose, indigestion, upset stomach, or dizziness. These side effects usually go away after a few hours. Call your doctor if you get a side effect that bothers you or one that will not go away.

LEVITRA may uncommonly cause:

- **an erection that won't go away (priapism).** If you get an erection that lasts more than 4 hours, get medical help right away. Priapism must be treated as soon as possible or lasting damage can happen to your penis including the inability to have erections.
- **color vision changes,** such as seeing a blue tinge to objects or having difficulty telling the difference between the colors blue and green.

In rare instances, men taking PDE5 inhibitors (oral erectile dysfunction medicines, including LEVITRA) reported a sudden decrease or loss of vision in one or both eyes. It is not possible to determine whether these events are related directly to these medicines, to other factors such as high blood pressure or diabetes, or to a combination of these. If you experience sudden decrease or loss of vision, stop taking PDE5 inhibitors, including LEVITRA, and call a doctor right away.
Sudden loss or decrease in hearing, sometimes with ringing in the ears and dizziness, has been rarely reported in people taking PDE5 inhibitors, including LEVITRA. It is not possible to determine whether these events are related directly to the PDE5 inhibitors, to other diseases or medications, to other factors, or to a combination of factors. If you experience these symptoms, stop taking LEVITRA and contact a doctor right away.
These are not all the side effects of LEVITRA. For more information, ask your doctor or pharmacist.

HOW SHOULD LEVITRA BE STORED?

- Store LEVITRA at room temperature between 59° and 86° F (15° to 30° C).
- **Keep LEVITRA and all medicines out of the reach of children.**

GENERAL INFORMATION ABOUT LEVITRA.

Medicines are sometimes prescribed for conditions other than those described in patient information leaflets. Do not use LEVITRA for a condition for which it was not prescribed. Do not give LEVITRA to other people, even if they have the same symptoms that you have. It may harm them. This leaflet summarizes the most important information about LEVITRA. If you would like more information, talk with your healthcare provider. You can ask your doctor or pharmacist for information about LEVITRA that is written for health professionals.
For more information you can also visit www.LEVITRA.com, or call 1-866-LEVITRA.

WHAT ARE THE INGREDIENTS OF LEVITRA?

Active Ingredient: vardenafil hydrochloride
Inactive Ingredients: microcrystalline cellulose, crospovidone, colloidal silicon dioxide, magnesium stearate, hypromellose, polyethylene glycol, titanium dioxide, yellow ferric oxide, and red ferric oxide.
Norvir (ritonavir) is a trademark of Abbott Laboratories
Crixivan (indinavir sulfate) is a trademark of Merck & Co., Inc.
Invirase or Fortavase (saquinavir mesylate) is a trademark of Roche Laboratories Inc.
Reyataz (atazanavir sulfate) is a trademark of Bristol-Myers Squibb Company
Nizoral (ketoconazole) is a trademark of Johnson & Johnson
Sporanox (itraconazole) is a trademark of Johnson & Johnson
Hytrin (terazosin HCl) is a trademark of Abbott Laboratories
Flomax (tamsulosin HCl) is a trademark of Yamanouchi Pharmaceutical Co., Ltd.
Cardura (doxazosin mesylate) is a trademark of Pfizer Inc.
Minipress (prazosin HCl) is a trademark of Pfizer Inc.
Uroxatral (alfuzosin HCl) is a trademark of Sanofi-Synthelabo
Manufactured by:
Bayer HealthCare Pharmaceuticals Inc.
Wayne, NJ 07470
Made in Germany
Marketed By:
GlaxoSmithKline Research
Triangle Park NC 27709

Distributed and Marketed By:
Schering-Plough
Schering Corporation
Kenilworth, NJ 07033
LEVITRA is a registered trademark of Bayer Aktiengesellschaft and is used under license by GlaxoSmithKline and Schering Corporation.
Rx Only
08918646IP, R.7 12/08 14272
©2008 Bayer HealthCare Pharmaceuticals Inc. Printed in U.S.A.
Revised: 11/2007 Bayer HealthCare Pharmaceuticals Inc.
Shown in Product Identification Guide, page 313

LOTRISONE® CREAM
LOTRISONE® LOTION   ℞

[lō-trĭ-sōn]
(clotrimazole and betamethasone dipropionate)

FOR TOPICAL USE ONLY. NOT FOR OPHTHALMIC, ORAL, OR INTRAVAGINAL USE. NOT RECOMMENDED FOR PATIENTS UNDER THE AGE OF 17 YEARS AND NOT RECOMMENDED FOR DIAPER DERMATITIS.

DESCRIPTION

LOTRISONE® Cream and Lotion contain combinations of clotrimazole, a synthetic antifungal agent, and betamethasone dipropionate, a synthetic corticosteroid, for dermatologic use.
Chemically, clotrimazole is 1–(o-chloro-α,α-diphenylbenzyl) imidazole, with the empirical formula $C_{22}H_{17}ClN_2$, a molecular weight of 344.84, and the following structural formula:

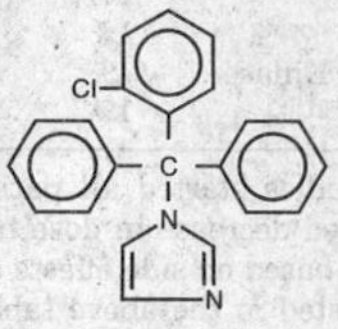

Clotrimazole is an odorless, white crystalline powder, insoluble in water and ethanol.
Betamethasone dipropionate has the chemical name 9-fluoro-11β,17,21-trihydroxy-16β-methylpregna-1,4-diene-3,20-dione 17,21-dipropionate, with the empirical formula $C_{28}H_{37}FO_7$, a molecular weight of 504.59, and the following structural formula:

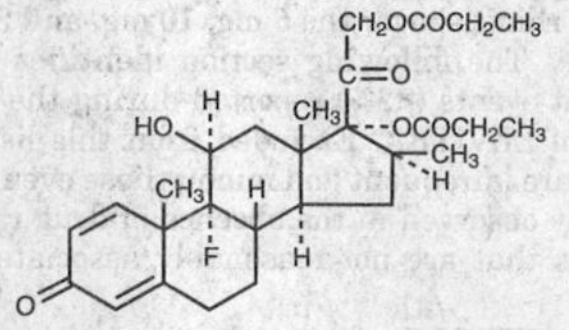

Betamethasone dipropionate is a white to creamy white, odorless crystalline powder, insoluble in water.
Each gram of **LOTRISONE Cream** contains 10 mg clotrimazole and 0.643 mg betamethasone dipropionate (equivalent to 0.5 mg betamethasone), in a hydrophilic cream consisting of purified water, mineral oil, white petrolatum, cetyl alcohol plus stearyl alcohol, ceteareth-30, propylene glycol, sodium phosphate monobasic monohydrate, and phosphoric acid; benzyl alcohol as a preservative.
LOTRISONE Cream may contain sodium hydroxide. LOTRISONE Cream is smooth, uniform, and white to off-white in color.
Each gram of **LOTRISONE Lotion** contains 10 mg clotrimazole and 0.643 mg betamethasone dipropionate (equivalent to 0.5 mg betamethasone), in a hydrophilic base of purified water, mineral oil, white petrolatum, cetyl alcohol plus stearyl alcohol, ceteareth-30, propylene glycol, sodium phosphate monobasic monohydrate, and phosphoric acid; benzyl alcohol as a preservative.
LOTRISONE Lotion may contain sodium hydroxide. LOTRISONE Lotion is opaque and white in color.

CLINICAL PHARMACOLOGY

Clotrimazole and Betamethasone Dipropionate
LOTRISONE® Cream has been shown to be at least as effective as clotrimazole alone in a different cream vehicle. No comparative studies have been conducted with LOTRISONE® Lotion and clotrimazole alone. Use of corticosteroids in the treatment of a fungal infection may lead to suppression of host inflammation leading to worsening or decreased cure rate.
Clotrimazole
Skin penetration and systemic absorption of clotrimazole following topical application of LOTRISONE Cream or Lotion have not been studied. The following information was obtained using 1% clotrimazole cream and solution formulations. Six hours after the application of radioactive clotrimazole 1% cream and 1% solution onto intact and acutely inflamed skin, the concentration of clotrimazole

varied from 100 mcg/cm³ in the stratum corneum, to 0.5 to 1 mcg/cm³ in the reticular dermis, and 0.1 mcg/cm³ in the subcutis. No measurable amount of radioactivity (<0.001 mcg/mL) was found in the serum within 48 hours after application under occlusive dressing of 0.5 mL of the solution or 0.8 g of the cream. Only 0.5% or less of the applied radioactivity was excreted in the urine.

Microbiology
Mechanism of Action: Clotrimazole is an imidazole antifungal agent. Imidazoles inhibit 14-α-demethylation of lanosterol in fungi by binding to one of the cytochrome P-450 enzymes. This leads to the accumulation of 14-α-methylsterols and reduced concentrations of ergosterol, a sterol essential for a normal fungal cytoplasmic membrane. The methylsterols may affect the electron transport system, thereby inhibiting growth of fungi.

Activity *In Vivo*: Clotrimazole has been shown to be active against most strains of the following dermatophytes, both *in vitro* and in clinical infections as described in the **INDICATIONS AND USAGE** section: *Epidermophyton floccosum*, *Trichophyton mentagrophytes*, and *Trichophyton rubrum*.

Activity *In Vitro*: *In vitro*, clotrimazole has been shown to have activity against many dermatophytes, **but the clinical significance of this information is unknown.**

Drug Resistance: Strains of dermatophytes having a natural resistance to clotrimazole have not been reported. Resistance to azoles including clotrimazole has been reported in some *Candida* species.

No single-step or multiple-step resistance to clotrimazole has developed during successive passages of *Trichophyton mentagrophytes*.

Betamethasone Dipropionate
Betamethasone dipropionate, a corticosteroid, has been shown to have topical (dermatologic) and systemic pharmacologic and metabolic effects characteristic of this class of drugs.

Pharmacokinetics
The extent of percutaneous absorption of topical corticosteroids is determined by many factors, including the vehicle, the integrity of the epidermal barrier, and the use of occlusive dressings (see **DOSAGE AND ADMINISTRATION**). Topical corticosteroids can be absorbed from normal intact skin. Inflammation and/or other disease processes in the skin may increase percutaneous absorption of topical corticosteroids. Occlusive dressings substantially increase the percutaneous absorption of topical corticosteroids (see **DOSAGE AND ADMINISTRATION**).

Once absorbed through the skin, the pharmacokinetics of topical corticosteroids are similar to systemically administered corticosteroids. Corticosteroids are bound to plasma proteins in varying degrees. Corticosteroids are metabolized primarily in the liver and are then excreted by the kidneys. Some of the topical corticosteroids and their metabolites are also excreted into the bile.

Studies performed with LOTRISONE Cream and Lotion indicate that these topical combination antifungal/corticosteroids may have vasoconstrictor potencies in a range that is comparable to high-potency topical corticosteroids. Therefore, use is not recommended in patients less than 17 years of age, in diaper dermatitis, and under occlusion.

CLINICAL STUDIES (LOTRISONE® Cream)
In clinical studies of tinea corporis, tinea cruris, and tinea pedis, patients treated with LOTRISONE Cream showed a better clinical response at the first return visit than patients treated with clotrimazole cream. In tinea corporis and tinea cruris, the patient returned 3 to 5 days after starting treatment, and in tinea pedis, after 1 week. Mycological cure rates observed in patients treated with LOTRISONE Cream were as good as or better than in those patients treated with clotrimazole cream. In these same clinical studies, patients treated with LOTRISONE Cream showed better clinical responses and mycological cure rates when compared with patients treated with betamethasone dipropionate cream.

CLINICAL STUDIES (LOTRISONE® Lotion)
In the treatment of tinea pedis twice daily for 4 weeks, LOTRISONE Lotion was shown to be superior to vehicle in relieving symptoms of erythema, scaling, pruritus, and maceration at Week 2. LOTRISONE Lotion was also shown to have a superior mycological cure rate compared to vehicle 2 weeks after discontinuation of treatment. It is unclear if the relief of symptoms at 2 weeks in this clinical study with LOTRISONE Lotion was due to the contribution of betamethasone dipropionate, clotrimazole, or both.

In the treatment of tinea cruris twice daily for 2 weeks, LOTRISONE Lotion was shown to be superior to vehicle in the relief of symptoms of erythema, scaling, and pruritus after 3 days. It is unclear if the relief of symptoms after 3 days in this clinical study with LOTRISONE Lotion was due to the contribution of betamethasone dipropionate, clotrimazole, or both.

The comparative efficacy and safety of LOTRISONE Lotion versus clotrimazole alone in a lotion vehicle have not been

studied in the treatment of tinea pedis or tinea cruris or tinea corporis. The comparative efficacy and safety of LOTRISONE Lotion and LOTRISONE® Cream have also not been studied.

INDICATIONS AND USAGE
LOTRISONE® Cream and Lotion are indicated in patients 17 years and older for the topical treatment of symptomatic inflammatory tinea pedis, tinea cruris, and tinea corporis due to *Epidermophyton floccosum*, *Trichophyton mentagrophytes*, and *Trichophyton rubrum*. Effective treatment without the risks associated with topical corticosteroid use may be obtained using a topical antifungal agent that does not contain a corticosteroid, especially for noninflammatory tinea infections. The efficacy of LOTRISONE Cream or Lotion for the treatment of infections caused by zoophilic dermatophytes (eg, *Microsporum canis*) has not been established. Several cases of treatment failure of LOTRISONE Cream in the treatment of infections caused by *Microsporum canis* have been reported.

CONTRAINDICATIONS
LOTRISONE® Cream or Lotion is contraindicated in patients who are sensitive to clotrimazole, betamethasone dipropionate, other corticosteroids or imidazoles, or to any ingredient in these preparations.

PRECAUTIONS
General
Systemic absorption of topical corticosteroids can produce reversible hypothalamic-pituitary-adrenal (HPA) axis suppression with the potential for glucocorticosteroid insufficiency after withdrawal of treatment. Manifestations of Cushing's syndrome, hyperglycemia, and glucosuria can also be produced in some patients by systemic absorption of topical corticosteroids while on treatment.

Conditions which augment systemic absorption include use over large surface areas, prolonged use, and use under occlusive dressings. Use of more than one corticosteroid-containing product at the same time may increase total systemic glucocorticoid exposure. Patients applying LOTRISONE® Cream or Lotion to a large surface area or to areas under occlusion should be evaluated periodically for evidence of HPA axis suppression. This may be done by using the ACTH stimulation, morning plasma cortisol, and urinary-free cortisol tests.

If HPA axis suppression is noted, an attempt should be made to withdraw the drug, to reduce the frequency of application, or to substitute a less potent corticosteroid. Recovery of HPA axis function is generally prompt upon discontinuation of topical corticosteroids. Infrequently, signs and symptoms of glucocorticosteroid insufficiency may occur, requiring supplemental systemic corticosteroids.

In a small study, LOTRISONE Cream was applied using large dosages, 7 g daily for 14 days (BID) to the crural area of normal adult subjects. Three of the 8 normal subjects on whom LOTRISONE Cream was applied exhibited low morning plasma cortisol levels during treatment. One of these subjects had an abnormal Cortrosyn test. The effect on morning plasma cortisol was transient and subjects recovered 1 week after discontinuing dosing. In addition, 2 separate studies in pediatric patients demonstrated adrenal suppression as determined by cosyntropin testing (see **PRECAUTIONS, Pediatric Use** section).

Pediatric patients may be more susceptible to systemic toxicity from equivalent doses due to their larger skin surface to body mass ratios (see **PRECAUTIONS, Pediatric Use** section).

If irritation develops, LOTRISONE Cream or Lotion should be discontinued and appropriate therapy instituted.

THE SAFETY OF LOTRISONE CREAM OR LOTION HAS NOT BEEN DEMONSTRATED IN THE TREATMENT OF DIAPER DERMATITIS. ADVERSE EVENTS CONSISTENT WITH CORTICOSTEROID USE HAVE BEEN OBSERVED IN PATIENTS TREATED WITH LOTRISONE CREAM FOR DIAPER DERMATITIS. THE USE OF LOTRISONE CREAM OR LOTION IN THE TREATMENT OF DIAPER DERMATITIS IS NOT RECOMMENDED.

Information for Patients
Patients using LOTRISONE Cream or Lotion should receive the following information and instructions:
1. The medication is to be used as directed by the physician and is not recommended for use longer than the prescribed time period. It is for external use only. Avoid contact with the eyes, the mouth, or intravaginally.
2. This medication is to be used for the full prescribed treatment time, even though the symptoms may have improved. Notify the physician if there is no improvement after 1 week of treatment for tinea cruris or tinea corporis, or after 2 weeks for tinea pedis.
3. This medication should only be used for the disorder for which it was prescribed.
4. Other corticosteroid-containing products should not be used with LOTRISONE without first talking with your physician.

5. The treated skin area should not be bandaged, covered, or wrapped so as to be occluded (see **DOSAGE AND ADMINISTRATION**).
6. Any signs of local adverse reactions should be reported to your physician.
7. Patients should avoid sources of infection or reinfection.
8. When using LOTRISONE Cream or Lotion in the groin area, patients should use the medication for 2 weeks only, and apply the cream or lotion sparingly. Patients should wear loose-fitting clothing. Notify the physician if the condition persists after 2 weeks.
9. The safety of LOTRISONE Cream or Lotion has not been demonstrated in the treatment of diaper dermatitis. Adverse events consistent with corticosteroid use have been observed in patients treated with LOTRISONE Cream for diaper dermatitis. The use of LOTRISONE Cream or Lotion in the treatment of diaper dermatitis is not recommended.

Laboratory Tests
If there is a lack of response to LOTRISONE Cream or Lotion, appropriate confirmation of the diagnosis, including possible mycological studies, is indicated before instituting another course of therapy.

The following tests may be helpful in evaluating HPA axis suppression due to the corticosteroid components:
   Urinary-free cortisol test
   Morning plasma cortisol test
   ACTH (cosyntropin) stimulation test

Carcinogenesis, Mutagenesis, Impairment of Fertility
There are no adequate laboratory animal studies with either the combination of clotrimazole and betamethasone dipropionate or with either component individually to evaluate carcinogenesis.

Betamethasone was negative in the bacterial mutagenicity assay (*Salmonella typhimurium* and *Escherichia coli*) and in the mammalian cell mutagenicity assay (CHO/HGPRT). It was positive in the *in vitro* human lymphocyte chromosome aberration assay, and equivocal in the *in vivo* mouse bone marrow micronucleus assay. This pattern of response is similar to that of dexamethasone and hydrocortisone.

Reproductive studies with betamethasone dipropionate carried out in rabbits at doses of 1.0 mg/kg by the intramuscular route and in mice up to 33 mg/kg by the intramuscular route indicated no impairment of fertility except for dose-related increases in fetal resorption rates in both species. These doses are approximately 5- and 38-fold the maximum human dose based on body surface areas, respectively.

In a combined study of the effects of clotrimazole on fertility, teratogenicity, and postnatal development, male and female rats were dosed orally (diet admixture) with levels of 5, 10, 25, or 50 mg/kg/day (approximately 1–8 times the maximum dose in a 60-kg adult based on body surface area) from 10 weeks prior to mating until 4 weeks postpartum. No adverse effects on the duration of estrous cycle, fertility, or duration of pregnancy were noted.

Pregnancy
Teratogenic Effects: Pregnancy Category C
There have been no teratogenic studies performed in animals or humans with the combination of clotrimazole and betamethasone dipropionate. Corticosteroids are generally teratogenic in laboratory animals when administered at relatively low dosage levels.

Studies in pregnant rats with intravaginal doses up to 100 mg/kg (15 times the maximum human dose) revealed no evidence of fetotoxicity due to clotrimazole exposure.

No increase in fetal malformations was noted in pregnant rats receiving oral (gastric tube) clotrimazole doses up to 100 mg/kg/day during gestation Days 6 to 15. However, clotrimazole dosed at 100 mg/kg/day was embryotoxic (increased resorptions), fetotoxic (reduced fetal weights), and maternally toxic (reduced body weight gain) to rats. Clotrimazole dosed at 200 mg/kg/day (30 times the maximum human dose) was maternally lethal, and therefore fetuses were not evaluated in this group. Also in this study, doses up to 50 mg/kg/day (8 times the maximum human dose) had no adverse effects on dams or fetuses. However, in the combined fertility, teratogenicity, and postnatal development study described above, 50 mg/kg clotrimazole, was associated with reduced maternal weight gain and reduced numbers of offspring reared to 4 weeks.

Oral clotrimazole doses of 25, 50, 100, and 200 mg/kg/day (2–15 times the maximum human dose) were not teratogenic in mice. No evidence of maternal toxicity or embryotoxicity was seen in pregnant rabbits dosed orally with 60, 120, or 180 mg/kg/day (18–55 times the maximum human dose).

Betamethasone dipropionate has been shown to be teratogenic in rabbits when given by the intramuscular route at doses of 0.05 mg/kg. This dose is approximately one-fifth the maximum human dose. The abnormalities observed included umbilical hernias, cephalocele, and cleft palates. Betamethasone dipropionate has not been tested for teratogenic potential by the dermal route of administration. Some corticosteroids have been shown to be teratogenic after dermal application to laboratory animals.

There are no adequate and well-controlled studies in pregnant women of the teratogenic effects of topically applied corticosteroids. Therefore, LOTRISONE Cream or Lotion should be used during pregnancy only if the potential benefit justifies the potential risk to the fetus.

Nursing Mothers

Systemically administered corticosteroids appear in human milk and could suppress growth, interfere with endogenous corticosteroid production, or cause other untoward effects. It is not known whether topical administration of corticosteroids could result in sufficient systemic absorption to produce detectable quantities in human milk. Because many drugs are excreted in human milk, caution should be exercised when LOTRISONE Cream or Lotion is administered to a nursing woman.

Pediatric Use

Adverse events consistent with corticosteroid use have been observed in patients under 12 years of age treated with LOTRISONE Cream. In open-label studies, 17 of 43 (39.5%) evaluable pediatric patients (aged 12–16 years old) using LOTRISONE Cream for treatment of tinea pedis demonstrated adrenal suppression as determined by cosyntropin testing. In another open-label study, 8 of 17 (47.1%) evaluable pediatric patients (aged 12–16 years old) using LOTRISONE Cream for treatment of tinea cruris demonstrated adrenal suppression as determined by cosyntropin testing. **THE USE OF LOTRISONE CREAM OR LOTION IN THE TREATMENT OF PATIENTS UNDER 17 YEARS OF AGE OR PATIENTS WITH DIAPER DERMATITIS IS NOT RECOMMENDED.**

Because of a higher ratio of skin surface area to body mass, pediatric patients under the age of 12 years are at a higher risk with LOTRISONE Cream or Lotion. The studies described above suggest that pediatric patients under the age of 17 years may also have this risk. They are at increased risk of developing Cushing's syndrome while on treatment and adrenal insufficiency after withdrawal of treatment. Adverse effects, including striae and growth retardation, have been reported with inappropriate use of LOTRISONE Cream in infants and children (see **PRECAUTIONS** and **ADVERSE REACTIONS**).

Hypothalamic-pituitary-adrenal (HPA) axis suppression, Cushing's syndrome, linear growth retardation, delayed weight gain, and intracranial hypertension have been reported in children receiving topical corticosteroids. Manifestations of adrenal suppression in children include low plasma cortisol levels and absence of response to ACTH stimulation. Manifestations of intracranial hypertension include bulging fontanelles, headaches, and bilateral papilledema.

Geriatric Use

Clinical studies of LOTRISONE Cream and Lotion did not include sufficient numbers of subjects aged 65 and over to determine whether they respond differently from younger subjects. Postmarket adverse event reporting for LOTRISONE Cream in patients aged 65 and above includes reports of skin atrophy and rare reports of skin ulceration. Caution should be exercised with the use of these corticosteroid-containing topical products on thinning skin. **THE USE OF LOTRISONE CREAM OR LOTION UNDER OCCLUSION, SUCH AS IN DIAPER DERMATITIS, IS NOT RECOMMENDED.**

ADVERSE REACTIONS

Adverse reactions reported for LOTRISONE® Cream in clinical trials were paresthesia in 1.9% of patients, and rash, edema, and secondary infection, each in less than 1% of patients.

Adverse reactions reported for LOTRISONE® Lotion in clinical trials were burning and dry skin in 1.6% of patients and stinging in less than 1% of patients.

The following local adverse reactions have been reported with topical corticosteroids and may occur more frequently with the use of occlusive dressings. These reactions are listed in an approximate decreasing order of occurrence: itching, irritation, dryness, folliculitis, hypertrichosis, acneiform eruptions, hypopigmentation, perioral dermatitis, allergic contact dermatitis, maceration of the skin, secondary infection, skin atrophy, striae, miliaria, capillary fragility (ecchymoses), telangiectasia, and sensitization (local reactions upon repeated application of product). In the pediatric population, reported adverse events for LOTRISONE Cream include growth retardation, benign intracranial hypertension, Cushing's syndrome (HPA axis suppression), and local cutaneous reactions, including skin atrophy.

Systemic absorption of topical corticosteroids has produced reversible hypothalamic-pituitary-adrenal (HPA) axis suppression, manifestations of Cushing's syndrome, hyperglycemia, and glucosuria in some patients.

Adverse reactions reported with the use of clotrimazole are as follows: erythema, stinging, blistering, peeling, edema, pruritus, urticaria, and general irritation of the skin.

OVERDOSAGE

Amounts greater than 45 g/week of LOTRISONE® Cream or 45 mL/week of LOTRISONE® Lotion should not be used. Acute overdosage with topical application of LOTRISONE Cream or Lotion is unlikely and would not be expected to lead to a life-threatening situation. LOTRISONE Cream or Lotion should not be used for longer than the prescribed time period.

Topically applied corticosteroids, such as the one contained in LOTRISONE Cream or Lotion can be absorbed in sufficient amounts to produce systemic effects (see **PRECAUTIONS**).

DOSAGE AND ADMINISTRATION

Gently massage sufficient LOTRISONE® Cream or Lotion into the affected skin areas twice a day, in the morning and evening.

LOTRISONE Cream or Lotion should not be used longer than 2 weeks in the treatment of tinea corporis or tinea cruris, and amounts greater than 45 g per week of LOTRISONE Cream or amounts greater than 45 mL per week of LOTRISONE Lotion should not be used. If a patient with tinea corporis or tinea cruris shows no clinical improvement after 1 week of treatment with LOTRISONE Cream or Lotion, the diagnosis should be reviewed.

LOTRISONE Cream or Lotion should not be used longer than 4 weeks in the treatment of tinea pedis and amounts greater than 45 g per week of LOTRISONE Cream or amounts greater than 45 mL per week of LOTRISONE Lotion should not be used. If a patient with tinea pedis shows no clinical improvement after 2 weeks of treatment with LOTRISONE Cream or Lotion, the diagnosis should be reviewed.

LOTRISONE Cream or Lotion should not be used with occlusive dressings.

HOW SUPPLIED

LOTRISONE® Cream is supplied in 15-g (NDC 0085-0924-01) and 45-g tubes (NDC 0085-0924-02), boxes of one. **Store at 25°C (77°F); excursions permitted to 15°–30°C (59°–86°F) [see USP Controlled Room Temperature].**

LOTRISONE® Lotion is supplied in 30-mL bottles (NDC 0085-0809-01), boxes of one. **Store at 25°C (77°F) in the upright position only; excursions permitted between 15°C and 30°C (59°F and 86°F).**

SHAKE LOTION WELL BEFORE EACH USE.

Rx only

Manufactured by Schering Corporation, a subsidiary of Schering-Plough Corporation, Kenilworth, NJ 07033 USA.

Rev. 6/09 24441962T

Copyright © 2000, 2007, Schering Corporation. All rights reserved.

LOTRISONE® Cream
LOTRISONE® Lotion

(clotrimazole and betamethasone dipropionate)

Patient's Instructions for Use

SHAKE LOTION WELL BEFORE EACH USE

Patient Information Leaflet

What is LOTRISONE® Cream or Lotion?

LOTRISONE Cream and Lotion are medications used on the skin to treat fungal infections of the feet, groin, and body, as diagnosed by your doctor. LOTRISONE Cream or Lotion should be used for fungal infections that are inflamed and have symptoms of redness and/or itching. Talk to your doctor if your fungal infection does not have these symptoms. LOTRISONE Cream and Lotion contain a corticosteroid. Notify your doctor if you notice side effects with the use of LOTRISONE Cream or Lotion (see **"What are the possible side effects of LOTRISONE Cream and Lotion?"** below). LOTRISONE Cream or Lotion is not to be used in the eyes, in the mouth, or in the vagina.

How do LOTRISONE® Cream and Lotion work?

LOTRISONE Cream and Lotion are combinations of an antifungal agent (clotrimazole) and a corticosteroid (betamethasone dipropionate). Clotrimazole works against fungus. Betamethasone dipropionate, a corticosteroid, is used to help relieve redness, swelling, itching, and other discomforts of fungal infections.

Who should NOT use LOTRISONE® Cream or Lotion?

LOTRISONE Cream and Lotion are not recommended for use in patients under the age of 17 years. LOTRISONE Cream or Lotion is not recommended for use in diaper rash. Patients who are sensitive to clotrimazole and betamethasone dipropionate, other imidazoles or corticosteroids, or any ingredients in the preparation should not use LOTRISONE Cream and Lotion.

How should I use LOTRISONE® Cream or Lotion?

Gently massage sufficient LOTRISONE Cream or Lotion into the affected and surrounding skin areas twice a day, in the morning and evening. Treatment for 2 weeks on the groin or on the body, and for 4 weeks on the feet is recommended. The use of LOTRISONE Cream or Lotion for longer than 4 weeks is not recommended for any condition. Prolonged use of LOTRISONE Cream or Lotion may lead to unwanted side effects.

What other important information should I know about LOTRISONE® Cream and Lotion?

1. This medication is to be used for the full prescribed treatment time, even though the symptoms may have improved. Notify your doctor if there is no improvement after 1 week of treatment on the groin or body or after 2 weeks on the feet.
2. This medication should only be used for the disorder for which it was prescribed.
3. The treated skin area should not be bandaged or otherwise covered or wrapped.
4. Other corticosteroid-containing products should not be used with LOTRISONE without first talking with your physician.
5. Any signs of side effects where LOTRISONE Cream or Lotion is applied should be reported to your doctor.
6. When using LOTRISONE Cream or Lotion in the groin area, it is especially important to use the medication for 2 weeks only, and to apply the cream or lotion sparingly. You should tell your doctor if your problem persists after 2 weeks. You should also wear loose-fitting clothing so as to avoid tightly covering the area where LOTRISONE Cream or Lotion is applied.
7. This medication is not recommended for use in diaper rash.

What are the possible side effects of LOTRISONE® Cream and Lotion?

The following side effects have been reported with topical corticosteroid medications: itching, irritation, dryness, infection of the hair follicles, increased hair, acne, fragile blood vessels, spider veins, sensitization (local reactions upon repeated application of product), change in skin color, allergic skin reaction, skin thinning, and stretch marks. In children, reported adverse events for LOTRISONE Cream include slower growth, Cushing's syndrome (a type of hormone imbalance that can be very serious), and local skin reactions, including thinning skin and stretch marks. Hormone imbalance (adrenal suppression) was demonstrated in clinical studies in children.

Can LOTRISONE® Cream or Lotion be used if I am pregnant or plan to become pregnant or if I am nursing?

Before using LOTRISONE Cream or Lotion, tell your doctor if you are pregnant or plan to become pregnant. Also, tell your doctor if you are nursing.

How should LOTRISONE® Cream or Lotion be stored?

LOTRISONE Cream should be stored at 25°C (77°F); excursions permitted to 15°–30°C (59°–86°F) [see USP Controlled Room Temperature].

LOTRISONE Lotion should be stored at 25°C (77°F) in the upright position only; excursions permitted between 15°C and 30°C (59°F and 86°F). Shake well before using LOTRISONE Lotion.

General advice about prescription medicines

This medicine was prescribed for your particular condition. Only use LOTRISONE® Cream or Lotion to treat the condition for which your doctor has prescribed. Do not give LOTRISONE Cream or Lotion to other people. It may harm them.

This leaflet summarizes the most important information about LOTRISONE Cream and Lotion. If you would like more information, talk with your doctor. You can ask your pharmacist or doctor for information about LOTRISONE Cream and Lotion that is written for health professionals.

Rx only

Manufactured by Schering Corporation, a subsidiary of Schering-Plough Corporation, Kenilworth, NJ 07033 USA.

Copyright © 2000, 2007, Schering Corporation. All rights reserved.

Rev. 6/09 **31642124T**

Shown in Product Identification Guide, page 313

M-M-R® II ℞

[em em ar too]

(MEASLES, MUMPS, and RUBELLA VIRUS VACCINE LIVE)

DESCRIPTION

M-M-R[1] II (Measles, Mumps, and Rubella Virus Vaccine Live) is a live virus vaccine for vaccination against measles (rubeola), mumps, and rubella (German measles).

M-M-R II is a sterile lyophilized preparation of (1) ATTENUVAX[1] (Measles Virus Vaccine Live), a more attenuated line of measles virus, derived from Enders' attenuated Edmonston strain and propagated in chick embryo cell culture; (2) MUMPSVAX[1] (Mumps Virus Vaccine Live), the Jeryl Lynn[2] (B level) strain of mumps virus propagated in chick embryo cell culture; and (3) MERUVAX[1] II (Rubella Virus Vaccine Live), the Wistar RA 27/3 strain of live attenuated rubella virus propagated in WI-38 human diploid lung fibroblasts.(1,2)

The growth medium for measles and mumps is Medium 199 (a buffered salt solution containing vitamins and amino acids and supplemented with fetal bovine serum) containing SPGA (sucrose, phosphate, glutamate, and recombinant human albumin) as stabilizer and neomycin.

The growth medium for rubella is Minimum Essential Medium (MEM) [a buffered salt solution containing vitamins and amino acids and supplemented with fetal bovine serum] containing recombinant human albumin and neomycin. Sorbitol and hydrolyzed gelatin stabilizer are added to the individual virus harvests.

The cells, virus pools, and fetal bovine serum are all screened for the absence of adventitious agents.

The reconstituted vaccine is for subcutaneous administration. Each 0.5 mL dose contains not less than 1,000 TCID$_{50}$ (tissue culture infectious doses) of measles virus; 12,500 TCID$_{50}$ of mumps virus; and 1,000 TCID$_{50}$ of rubella virus. Each dose of the vaccine is calculated to contain sorbitol (14.5 mg), sodium phosphate, sucrose (1.9 mg), sodium chloride, hydrolyzed gelatin (14.5 mg), recombinant human albumin ($\leq$0.3 mg), fetal bovine serum (<1 ppm), other buffer and media ingredients and approximately 25 mcg of neomycin. The product contains no preservative.

Before reconstitution, the lyophilized vaccine is a light yellow compact crystalline plug. M-M-R II, when reconstituted as directed, is clear yellow.

---

[1] Registered trademark of MERCK & CO., Inc.
COPYRIGHT © 2009 MERCK & CO., Inc.
All rights reserved
[2] Trademark of MERCK & CO., Inc.

CLINICAL PHARMACOLOGY

Measles, mumps, and rubella are three common childhood diseases, caused by measles virus, mumps virus (paramyxoviruses), and rubella virus (togavirus), respectively, that may be associated with serious complications and/or death. For example, pneumonia and encephalitis are caused by measles. Mumps is associated with aseptic meningitis, deafness and orchitis; and rubella during pregnancy may cause congenital rubella syndrome in the infants of infected mothers.

The impact of measles, mumps, and rubella vaccination on the natural history of each disease in the United States can be quantified by comparing the maximum number of measles, mumps, and rubella cases reported in a given year prior to vaccine use to the number of cases of each disease reported in 1995. For measles, 894,134 cases reported in 1941 compared to 288 cases reported in 1995 resulted in a 99.97% decrease in reported cases; for mumps, 152,209 cases reported in 1968 compared to 840 cases reported in 1995 resulted in a 99.45% decrease in reported cases; and for rubella, 57,686 cases reported in 1969 compared to 200 cases reported in 1995 resulted in a 99.65% decrease.[3]

Clinical studies of 284 triple seronegative children, 11 months to 7 years of age, demonstrated that M-M-R II is highly immunogenic and generally well tolerated. In these studies, a single injection of the vaccine induced measles hemagglutination-inhibition (HI) antibodies in 95%, mumps neutralizing antibodies in 96%, and rubella HI antibodies in 99% of susceptible persons. However, a small percentage (1-5%) of vaccinees may fail to seroconvert after the primary dose (see also INDICATIONS AND USAGE, Recommended Vaccination Schedule).

A study[4] of 6-month-old and 15-month-old infants born to vaccine-immunized mothers demonstrated that, following vaccination with ATTENUVAX, 74% of the 6-month-old infants developed detectable neutralizing antibody (NT) titers while 100% of the 15-month-old infants developed NT. This rate of seroconversion is higher than that previously reported for 6-month-old infants born to naturally immune mothers tested by HI assay. When the 6-month-old infants of immunized mothers were revaccinated at 15 months, they developed antibody titers equivalent to the 15-month-old vaccinees. The lower seroconversion rate in 6-month-olds has two possible explanations: 1) Due to the limit of the detection level of the assays (NT and enzyme immunoassay [EIA]), the presence of trace amounts of undetectable maternal antibody might interfere with the seroconversion of infants; or 2) The immune system of 6-month-olds is not always capable of mounting a response to measles vaccine as measured by the two antibody assays.

There is some evidence to suggest that infants who are born to mothers who had wild-type measles and who are vaccinated at less than one year of age may not develop sustained antibody levels when later revaccinated. The advantage of early protection must be weighed against the chance for failure to respond adequately on reimmunization.[5,6]

Efficacy of measles, mumps, and rubella vaccines was established in a series of double-blind controlled field trials which demonstrated a high degree of protective efficacy afforded by the individual vaccine components.[7-12] These studies also established that seroconversion in response to vaccination against measles, mumps, and rubella paralleled protection from these diseases.[13-15]

Following vaccination, antibodies associated with protection can be measured by neutralization assays, HI, or ELISA (enzyme linked immunosorbent assay) tests. Neutralizing and ELISA antibodies to measles, mumps, and rubella viruses are still detectable in most individuals 11 to 13 years after primary vaccination.[16-18] See INDICATIONS AND USAGE, Non-Pregnant Adolescent and Adult Females, for Rubella Susceptibility Testing.

The RA 27/3 rubella strain in M-M-R II elicits higher immediate post-vaccination HI, complement-fixing and neutralizing antibody levels than other strains of rubella vaccine[19-25] and has been shown to induce a broader profile of circulating antibodies including anti-theta and anti-iota precipitating antibodies.[26,27] The RA 27/3 rubella strain immunologically simulates natural infection more closely than other rubella vaccine viruses.[27-29] The increased levels and broader profile of antibodies produced by RA 27/3 strain rubella virus vaccine appear to correlate with greater resistance to subclinical reinfection with the wild virus,[27,29-31] and provide greater confidence for lasting immunity.

INDICATIONS AND USAGE

Recommended Vaccination Schedule

M-M-R II is indicated for simultaneous vaccination against measles, mumps, and rubella in individuals 12 months of age or older.

Individuals first vaccinated at 12 months of age or older should be revaccinated prior to elementary school entry. Revaccination is intended to seroconvert those who do not respond to the first dose. The Advisory Committee on Immunization Practices (ACIP) recommends administration of the first dose of M-M-R II at 12 to 15 months of age and administration of the second dose of M-M-R II at 4 to 6 years of age.[59] In addition, some public health jurisdictions mandate the age for revaccination. Consult the complete text of applicable guidelines regarding routine revaccination including that of high-risk adult populations.

Measles Outbreak Schedule

Infants Between 6 to 12 Months of Age

Local health authorities may recommend measles vaccination of infants between 6 to 12 months of age in outbreak situations. This population may fail to respond to the components of the vaccine. Safety and effectiveness of mumps and rubella vaccine in infants less than 12 months of age have not been established. The younger the infant, the lower the likelihood of seroconversion (see CLINICAL PHARMACOLOGY). Such infants should receive a second dose of M-M-R II between 12 to 15 months of age followed by revaccination at elementary school entry.[59]

Unnecessary doses of a vaccine are best avoided by ensuring that written documentation of vaccination is preserved and a copy given to each vaccinee's parent or guardian.

Other Vaccination Considerations

Non-Pregnant Adolescent and Adult Females

Immunization of susceptible non-pregnant adolescent and adult females of childbearing age with live attenuated rubella virus vaccine is indicated if certain precautions are observed (see below and PRECAUTIONS). Vaccinating susceptible postpubertal females confers individual protection against subsequently acquiring rubella infection during pregnancy, which in turn prevents infection of the fetus and consequent congenital rubella injury.[33]

Women of childbearing age should be advised not to become pregnant for 3 months after vaccination and should be informed of the reasons for this precaution.

The ACIP has stated "If it is practical and if reliable laboratory services are available, women of childbearing age who are potential candidates for vaccination can have serologic tests to determine susceptibility to rubella. However, with the exception of premarital and prenatal screening, routinely performing serologic tests for all women of childbearing age to determine susceptibility (so that vaccine is given only to proven susceptible women) can be effective but is expensive. Also, 2 visits to the health-care provider would be necessary—one for screening and one for vaccination. Accordingly, rubella vaccination of a woman who is not known to be pregnant and has no history of vaccination is justifiable without serologic testing—and may be preferable, particularly when costs of serology are high and follow-up of identified susceptible women for vaccination is not assured."[33]

Postpubertal females should be informed of the frequent occurrence of generally self-limited arthralgia and/or arthritis beginning 2 to 4 weeks after vaccination (see ADVERSE REACTIONS).

Postpartum Women

It has been found convenient in many instances to vaccinate rubella-susceptible women in the immediate postpartum period (see PRECAUTIONS, Nursing Mothers).

Other Populations

Previously unvaccinated children older than 12 months who are in contact with susceptible pregnant women should re-

ceive live attenuated rubella vaccine (such as that contained in monovalent rubella vaccine or in M-M-R II) to reduce the risk of exposure of the pregnant woman.

Individuals planning travel outside the United States, if not immune, can acquire measles, mumps, or rubella and import these diseases into the United States. Therefore, prior to international travel, individuals known to be susceptible to one or more of these diseases can either receive the indicated monovalent vaccine (measles, mumps, or rubella), or a combination vaccine as appropriate. However, M-M-R II is preferred for persons likely to be susceptible to mumps and rubella; and if monovalent measles vaccine is not readily available, travelers should receive M-M-R II regardless of their immune status to mumps or rubella.[34-36]

Vaccination is recommended for susceptible individuals in high-risk groups such as college students, health-care workers, and military personnel.[33,34,37]

According to ACIP recommendations, most persons born in 1956 or earlier are likely to have been infected with measles naturally and generally need not be considered susceptible. All children, adolescents, and adults born after 1956 are considered susceptible and should be vaccinated, if there are no contraindications. This includes persons who may be immune to measles but who lack adequate documentation of immunity such as: (1) physician-diagnosed measles, (2) laboratory evidence of measles immunity, or (3) adequate immunization with live measles vaccine on or after the first birthday.[34]

The ACIP recommends that "Persons vaccinated with inactivated vaccine followed within 3 months by live vaccine should be revaccinated with two doses of live vaccine. Revaccination is particularly important when the risk of exposure to wild-type measles virus is increased, as may occur during international travel."[34]

Post-Exposure Vaccination

Vaccination of individuals exposed to wild-type measles may provide some protection if the vaccine can be administered within 72 hours of exposure. If, however, vaccine is given a few days before exposure, substantial protection may be afforded.[34,38,39] There is no conclusive evidence that vaccination of individuals recently exposed to wild-type mumps or wild-type rubella will provide protection.[33,37]

Use With Other Vaccines

See DOSAGE AND ADMINISTRATION, Use With Other Vaccines.

CONTRAINDICATIONS

Hypersensitivity to any component of the vaccine, including gelatin.[40]

Do not give M-M-R II to pregnant females; the possible effects of the vaccine on fetal development are unknown at this time. If vaccination of postpubertal females is undertaken, pregnancy should be avoided for three months following vaccination (see INDICATIONS AND USAGE, Non-Pregnant Adolescent and Adult Females and PRECAUTIONS, Pregnancy).

Anaphylactic or anaphylactoid reactions to neomycin (each dose of reconstituted vaccine contains approximately 25 mcg of neomycin).

Febrile respiratory illness or other active febrile infection. However, the ACIP has recommended that all vaccines can be administered to persons with minor illnesses such as diarrhea, mild upper respiratory infection with or without low-grade fever, or other low-grade febrile illness.[41]

Patients receiving immunosuppressive therapy. This contraindication does not apply to patients who are receiving corticosteroids as replacement therapy, e.g., for Addison's disease.

Individuals with blood dyscrasias, leukemia, lymphomas of any type, or other malignant neoplasms affecting the bone marrow or lymphatic systems.

Primary and acquired immunodeficiency states, including patients who are immunosuppressed in association with AIDS or other clinical manifestations of infection with human immunodeficiency viruses;[41-43] cellular immune deficiencies; and hypogammaglobulinemic and dysgammaglobulinemic states. Measles inclusion body encephalitis[60] (MIBE), pneumonitis[61] and death as a direct consequence of disseminated measles vaccine virus infection have been reported in immunocompromised individuals inadvertently vaccinated with measles-containing vaccine.

Individuals with a family history of congenital or hereditary immunodeficiency, until the immune competence of the potential vaccine recipient is demonstrated.

WARNINGS

Due caution should be employed in administration of M-M-R II to persons with a history of cerebral injury, individual or family histories of convulsions, or any other condition in which stress due to fever should be avoided. The physician should be alert to the temperature elevation which may occur following vaccination (see ADVERSE REACTIONS).

Hypersensitivity to Eggs

Live measles vaccine and live mumps vaccine are produced in chick embryo cell culture. Persons with a history of anaphylactic, anaphylactoid, or other immediate reactions (e.g., hives, swelling of the mouth and throat, difficulty breathing, hypotension, or shock) subsequent to egg ingestion may be at an enhanced risk of immediate-type hypersensitivity reactions after receiving vaccines containing traces of chick embryo antigen. The potential risk to benefit ratio should be carefully evaluated before considering vaccination in such cases. Such individuals may be vaccinated with extreme caution, having adequate treatment on hand should a reaction occur (see PRECAUTIONS).{45}

However, the AAP has stated, "Most children with a history of anaphylactic reactions to eggs have no untoward reactions to measles or MMR vaccine. Persons are not at increased risk if they have egg allergies that are not anaphylactic, and they should be vaccinated in the usual manner. In addition, skin testing of egg-allergic children with vaccine has not been predictive of which children will have an immediate hypersensitivity reaction...Persons with allergies to chickens or chicken feathers are not at increased risk of reaction to the vaccine."{44}

Hypersensitivity to Neomycin

The AAP states, "Persons who have experienced anaphylactic reactions to topically or systemically administered neomycin should not receive measles vaccine. Most often, however, neomycin allergy manifests as a contact dermatitis, which is a delayed-type (cell-mediated) immune response rather than anaphylaxis. In such persons, an adverse reaction to neomycin in the vaccine would be an erythematous, pruritic nodule or papule, 48 to 96 hours after vaccination. A history of contact dermatitis to neomycin is not a contraindication to receiving measles vaccine."{44}

Thrombocytopenia

Individuals with current thrombocytopenia may develop more severe thrombocytopenia following vaccination. In addition, individuals who experienced thrombocytopenia with the first dose of M-M-R II (or its component vaccines) may develop thrombocytopenia with repeat doses. Serologic status may be evaluated to determine whether or not additional doses of vaccine are needed. The potential risk to benefit ratio should be carefully evaluated before considering vaccination in such cases (see ADVERSE REACTIONS).

PRECAUTIONS

General

Adequate treatment provisions including epinephrine injection (1:1000), should be available for immediate use should an anaphylactic or anaphylactoid reaction occur.

Special care should be taken to ensure that the injection does not enter a blood vessel.

Children and young adults who are known to be infected with human immunodeficiency viruses and are not immunosuppressed may be vaccinated. However, vaccinees who are infected with HIV should be monitored closely for vaccine-preventable diseases because immunization may be less effective than for uninfected persons (see CONTRAINDICATIONS).{42,43}

Vaccination should be deferred for 3 months or longer following blood or plasma transfusions, or administration of immune globulin (human).{44}

Excretion of small amounts of the live attenuated rubella virus from the nose or throat has occurred in the majority of susceptible individuals 7 to 28 days after vaccination. There is no confirmed evidence to indicate that such virus is transmitted to susceptible persons who are in contact with the vaccinated individuals. Consequently, transmission through close personal contact, while accepted as a theoretical possibility, is not regarded as a significant risk.{33} However, transmission of the rubella vaccine virus to infants via breast milk has been documented (see Nursing Mothers).

There are no reports of transmission of live attenuated measles or mumps viruses from vaccinees to susceptible contacts.

It has been reported that live attenuated measles, mumps and rubella virus vaccines given individually may result in a temporary depression of tuberculin skin sensitivity. Therefore, if a tuberculin test is to be done, it should be administered either before or simultaneously with M-M-R II.

Children under treatment for tuberculosis have not experienced exacerbation of the disease when immunized with live measles virus vaccine;{46} no studies have been reported to date of the effect of measles virus vaccines on untreated tuberculous children. However, individuals with active untreated tuberculosis should not be vaccinated.

As for any vaccine, vaccination with M-M-R II may not result in protection in 100% of vaccinees.

The health-care provider should determine the current health status and previous vaccination history of the vaccinee.

The health-care provider should question the patient, parent, or guardian about reactions to a previous dose of M-M-R II or other measles-, mumps-, or rubella-containing vaccines.

Information for Patients

The health-care provider should provide the vaccine information required to be given with each vaccination to the patient, parent, or guardian.

The health-care provider should inform the patient, parent, or guardian of the benefits and risks associated with vaccination. For risks associated with vaccination see WARNINGS, PRECAUTIONS, and ADVERSE REACTIONS.

Patients, parents, or guardians should be instructed to report any serious adverse reactions to their health-care provider who in turn should report such events to the U.S. Department of Health and Human Services through the Vaccine Adverse Event Reporting System (VAERS), 1-800-822-7967.{47}

Pregnancy should be avoided for 3 months following vaccination, and patients should be informed of the reasons for this precaution (see INDICATIONS AND USAGE, Non-Pregnant Adolescent and Adult Females, CONTRAINDICATIONS, and PRECAUTIONS, Pregnancy).

Laboratory Tests

See INDICATIONS AND USAGE, Non-Pregnant Adolescent and Adult Females, for Rubella Susceptibility Testing, and CLINICAL PHARMACOLOGY.

Drug Interactions

See DOSAGE AND ADMINISTRATION, Use With Other Vaccines.

Immunosuppressive Therapy

The immune status of patients about to undergo immunosuppressive therapy should be evaluated so that the physician can consider whether vaccination prior to the initiation of treatment is indicated (see CONTRAINDICATIONS and PRECAUTIONS).

The ACIP has stated that "patients with leukemia in remission who have not received chemotherapy for at least 3 months may receive live virus vaccines. Short-term (<2 weeks), low- to moderate-dose systemic corticosteroid therapy, topical steroid therapy (e.g. nasal, skin), long-term alternate-day treatment with low to moderate doses of short-acting systemic steroid, and intra-articular, bursal, or tendon injection of corticosteroids are not immunosuppressive in their usual doses and do not contraindicate the administration of [measles, mumps, or rubella vaccine]."{33,34,37}

Immune Globulin

Administration of immune globulins concurrently with M-M-R II may interfere with the expected immune response.{33,34,44}

See also PRECAUTIONS, General.

Carcinogenesis, Mutagenesis, Impairment of Fertility

M-M-R II has not been evaluated for carcinogenic or mutagenic potential, or potential to impair fertility.

Pregnancy

Pregnancy Category C

Animal reproduction studies have not been conducted with M-M-R II. It is also not known whether M-M-R II can cause fetal harm when administered to a pregnant woman or can affect reproduction capacity. Therefore, the vaccine should not be administered to pregnant females; furthermore, pregnancy should be avoided for 3 months following vaccination (see INDICATIONS AND USAGE, Non-Pregnant Adolescent and Adult Females and CONTRAINDICATIONS).

In counseling women who are inadvertently vaccinated when pregnant or who become pregnant within 3 months of vaccination, the physician should be aware of the following: (1) In a 10-year survey involving over 700 pregnant women who received rubella vaccine within 3 months before or after conception (of whom 189 received the Wistar RA 27/3 strain), none of the newborns had abnormalities compatible with congenital rubella syndrome;{48} (2) Mumps infection during the first trimester of pregnancy may increase the rate of spontaneous abortion. Although mumps vaccine virus has been shown to infect the placenta and fetus, there is no evidence that it causes congenital malformations in humans;{37} and (3) Reports have indicated that contracting wild-type measles during pregnancy enhances fetal risk. Increased rates of spontaneous abortion, stillbirth, congenital defects and prematurity have been observed subsequent to infection with wild-type measles during pregnancy.{57,58} There are no adequate studies of the attenuated (vaccine) strain of measles virus in pregnancy. However, it would be prudent to assume that the vaccine strain of virus is also capable of inducing adverse fetal effects.

Nursing Mothers

It is not known whether measles or mumps vaccine virus is secreted in human milk. Recent studies have shown that lactating postpartum women immunized with live attenuated rubella vaccine may secrete the virus in breast milk and transmit it to breast-fed infants.{49} In the infants with serological evidence of rubella infection, none exhibited severe disease; however, one exhibited mild clinical illness typical of acquired rubella.{50,51} Caution should be exercised when M-M-R II is administered to a nursing woman.

Pediatric Use

Safety and effectiveness of measles vaccine in infants below the age of 6 months have not been established (see also CLINICAL PHARMACOLOGY). Safety and effectiveness of mumps and rubella vaccine in infants less than 12 months of age have not been established.

Geriatric Use

Clinical studies of M-M-R II did not include sufficient numbers of seronegative subjects aged 65 and over to determine whether they respond differently from younger subjects. Other reported clinical experience has not identified differences in responses between the elderly and younger subjects.

ADVERSE REACTIONS

The following adverse reactions are listed in decreasing order of severity, without regard to causality, within each body system category and have been reported during clinical trials, with use of the marketed vaccine, or with use of monovalent or bivalent vaccine containing measles, mumps, or rubella:

Body as a Whole

Panniculitis; atypical measles; fever; syncope; headache; dizziness; malaise; irritability.

Cardiovascular System

Vasculitis.

Digestive System

Pancreatitis; diarrhea; vomiting; parotitis; nausea.

Endocrine System

Diabetes mellitus.

Hemic and Lymphatic System

Thrombocytopenia (see WARNINGS, Thrombocytopenia); purpura; regional lymphadenopathy; leukocytosis.

Immune System

Anaphylaxis and anaphylactoid reactions have been reported as well as related phenomena such as angioneurotic edema (including peripheral or facial edema) and bronchial spasm in individuals with or without an allergic history.

Musculoskeletal System

Arthritis; arthralgia; myalgia.

Arthralgia and/or arthritis (usually transient and rarely chronic), and polyneuritis are features of infection with wild-type rubella and vary in frequency and severity with age and sex, being greatest in adult females and least in prepubertal children. This type of involvement as well as myalgia and paresthesia, have also been reported following administration of MERUVAX II.

Chronic arthritis has been associated with wild-type rubella infection and has been related to persistent virus and/or viral antigen isolated from body tissues. Only rarely have vaccine recipients developed chronic joint symptoms.

Following vaccination in children, reactions in joints are uncommon and generally of brief duration. In women, incidence rates for arthritis and arthralgia are generally higher than those seen in children (children: 0-3%; women: 12-26%),{17,52,53} and the reactions tend to be more marked and of longer duration. Symptoms may persist for a matter of months or on rare occasions for years. In adolescent girls, the reactions appear to be intermediate in incidence between those seen in children and in adult women. Even in women older than 35 years, these reactions are generally well tolerated and rarely interfere with normal activities.

Nervous System

Encephalitis; encephalopathy; measles inclusion body encephalitis (MIBE) (see CONTRAINDICATIONS); subacute sclerosing panencephalitis (SSPE); Guillain-Barré Syndrome (GBS); febrile convulsions; afebrile convulsions or seizures; ataxia; polyneuritis; polyneuropathy; ocular palsies; paresthesia.

Experience from more than 80 million doses of all live measles vaccines given in the U.S. through 1975 indicates that significant central nervous system reactions such as encephalitis and encephalopathy, occurring within 30 days after vaccination, have been temporally associated with measles vaccine very rarely.{54} In no case has it been shown that reactions were actually caused by vaccine. The Centers for Disease Control and Prevention has pointed out that "a certain number of cases of encephalitis may be expected to occur in a large childhood population in a defined period of time even when no vaccines are administered". However, the data suggest the possibility that some of these cases may have been caused by measles vaccines. The risk of such serious neurological disorders following live measles virus vaccine administration remains far less than that for encephalitis and encephalopathy with wild-type measles (one per two thousand reported cases).

Post-marketing surveillance of the more than 200 million doses of M-M-R and M-M-R II that have been distributed worldwide over 25 years (1971 to 1996) indicates that serious adverse events such as encephalitis and encephalopathy continue to be rarely reported.{17}

There have been reports of subacute sclerosing panencephalitis (SSPE) in children who did not have a history of infection with wild-type measles but did receive measles vaccine.

Some of these cases may have resulted from unrecognized measles in the first year of life or possibly from the measles vaccination. Based on estimated nationwide measles vaccine distribution, the association of SSPE cases to measles vaccination is about one case per million vaccine doses distributed. This is far less than the association with infection with wild-type measles, 6-22 cases of SSPE per million cases of measles. The results of a retrospective case-controlled study conducted by the Centers for Disease Control and Prevention suggest that the overall effect of measles vaccine has been to protect against SSPE by preventing measles with its inherent higher risk of SSPE.(55)

Cases of aseptic meningitis have been reported to VAERS following measles, mumps, and rubella vaccination. Although a causal relationship between the Urabe strain of mumps vaccine and aseptic meningitis has been shown, there is no evidence to link Jeryl Lynn™ mumps vaccine to aseptic meningitis.

Respiratory System

Pneumonia; pneumonitis (see CONTRAINDICATIONS); sore throat; cough; rhinitis.

Skin

Stevens-Johnson syndrome; erythema multiforme; urticaria; rash; measles-like rash; pruritis.

Local reactions including burning/stinging at injection site; wheal and flare; redness (erythema); swelling; induration; tenderness; vesiculation at injection site.

Special Senses—Ear

Nerve deafness; otitis media.

Special Senses—Eye

Retinitis; optic neuritis; papillitis; retrobulbar neuritis; conjunctivitis.

Urogenital System

Epididymitis; orchitis.

Other

Death from various, and in some cases unknown, causes has been reported rarely following vaccination with measles, mumps, and rubella vaccines; however, a causal relationship has not been established in healthy individuals (see CONTRAINDICATIONS). No deaths or permanent sequelae were reported in a published post-marketing surveillance study in Finland involving 1.5 million children and adults who were vaccinated with M-M-R II during 1982 to 1993.(56)

Under the National Childhood Vaccine Injury Act of 1986, health-care providers and manufacturers are required to record and report certain suspected adverse events occurring within specific time periods after vaccination. However, the U.S. Department of Health and Human Services (DHHS) has established a Vaccine Adverse Event Reporting System (VAERS) which will accept all reports of suspected events.(47) A VAERS report form as well as information regarding reporting requirements can be obtained by calling VAERS 1-800-822-7967.

DOSAGE AND ADMINISTRATION

FOR SUBCUTANEOUS ADMINISTRATION

Do not inject intravascularly.

The dose for any age is 0.5 mL administered subcutaneously, preferably into the outer aspect of the upper arm.

The recommended age for primary vaccination is 12 to 15 months.

Revaccination with M-M-R II is recommended prior to elementary school entry. See also INDICATIONS AND USAGE, Recommended Vaccination Schedule.

Children first vaccinated when younger than 12 months of age should receive another dose between 12 to 15 months of age followed by revaccination prior to elementary school entry.(59) See also INDICATIONS AND USAGE, Measles Outbreak Schedule.

Immune Globulin (IG) is not to be given concurrently with M-M-R II (see PRECAUTIONS, General and PRECAUTIONS, Drug Interactions).

CAUTION: A sterile syringe free of preservatives, antiseptics, and detergents should be used for each injection and/or reconstitution of the vaccine because these substances may inactivate the live virus vaccine. A 25 gauge, 5/8″ needle is recommended.

To reconstitute, use only the diluent supplied, since it is free of preservatives or other antiviral substances which might inactivate the vaccine.

Single Dose Vial—First withdraw the entire volume of diluent into the syringe to be used for reconstitution. Inject all the diluent in the syringe into the vial of lyophilized vaccine, and agitate to mix thoroughly. If the lyophilized vaccine cannot be dissolved, discard. Withdraw the entire contents into a syringe and inject the total volume of restored vaccine subcutaneously.

It is important to use a separate sterile syringe and needle for each individual patient to prevent transmission of hepatitis B and other infectious agents from one person to another.

Parenteral drug products should be inspected visually for particulate matter and discoloration prior to administration whenever solution and container permit. M-M-R II, when reconstituted, is clear yellow.

Use With Other Vaccines

M-M-R II should be given one month before or after administration of other live viral vaccines.

M-M-R II has been administered concurrently with VARIVAX[1] [Varicella Virus Vaccine Live (Oka/Merck)], and PedvaxHIB[1] [*Haemophilus b* Conjugate Vaccine (Meningococcal Protein Conjugate)] using separate injection sites and syringes. No impairment of immune response to individually tested vaccine antigens was demonstrated. The type, frequency, and severity of adverse experiences observed with M-M-R II were similar to those seen when each vaccine was given alone.

Routine administration of DTP (diphtheria, tetanus, pertussis) and/or OPV (oral poliovirus vaccine) concurrently with measles, mumps and rubella vaccines is not recommended because there are limited data relating to the simultaneous administration of these antigens.

However, other schedules have been used. The ACIP has stated "Although data are limited concerning the simultaneous administration of the entire recommended vaccine series (i.e., DTaP [or DTwP], IPV [or OPV], Hib with or without Hepatitis B vaccine, and varicella vaccine), data from numerous studies have indicated no interference between routinely recommended childhood vaccines (either live, attenuated, or killed). These findings support the simultaneous use of all vaccines as recommended."(32)

HOW SUPPLIED

No. 4681—M-M-R II is supplied as follows: (1) a box of 10 single-dose vials of lyophilized vaccine (package A), **NDC** 0006-4681-00; and (2) a box of 10 vials of diluent (package B). To conserve refrigerator space, the diluent may be stored separately at room temperature.

Storage

To maintain potency, M-M-R II must be stored between -58°F and +46°F (-50°C to +8°C). Use of dry ice may subject M-M-R II to temperatures colder than -58°F (-50°C).

Protect the vaccine from light at all times, since such exposure may inactivate the viruses.

Before reconstitution, store the lyophilized vaccine at 36°F to 46°F (2°C to 8°C). The diluent may be stored in the refrigerator with the lyophilized vaccine or separately at room temperature. **Do not freeze the diluent.**

It is recommended that the vaccine be used as soon as possible after reconstitution. Store reconstituted vaccine in the vaccine vial in a dark place at 36°F to 46°F (2°C to 8°C) and discard if not used within 8 hours.

For information regarding stability under conditions other than those recommended, call 1-800-MERCK-90.

REFERENCES

1. Plotkin, S.A.; Cornfeld, D.; Ingalls, T.H.: Studies of immunization with living rubella virus: Trials in children with a strain cultured from an aborted fetus, Am. J. Dis. Child. *110:* 381-389, 1965.
2. Plotkin, S.A.; Farquhar, J.; Katz, M.; Ingalls, T.H.: A new attenuated rubella virus grown in human fibroblasts: Evidence for reduced nasopharyngeal excretion, Am. J. Epidemiol. *86:* 468-477, 1967.
3. Monthly Immunization Table, MMWR *45*(1): 24-25, January 12, 1996.
4. Johnson, C.E.; et al: Measles Vaccine Immunogenicity in 6- Versus 15-Month-Old Infants Born to Mothers in the Measles Vaccine Era, Pediatrics, *93*(6): 939-943, 1994.
5. Linneman, C.C.; et al: Measles Immunity After Vaccination: Results in Children Vaccinated Before 10 Months of Age, Pediatrics, *69*(3): 332-335, March 1982.
6. Stetler, H.C.; et al: Impact of Revaccinating Children Who Initially Received Measles Vaccine Before 10 Months of Age, Pediatrics 77(4): 471-476, April 1986.
7. Hilleman, M.R.; Buynak, E.B.; Weibel, R.E.; et al: Development and Evaluation of the Moraten Measles Virus Vaccine, JAMA *206*(3): 587-590, 1968.
8. Weibel, R.E.; Stokes, J.; Buynak, E.B.; et al: Live, Attenuated Mumps Virus Vaccine 3. Clinical and Serologic Aspects in a Field Evaluation, N. Engl. J. Med. *276:* 245-251, 1967.
9. Hilleman, M.R.; Weibel, R.E.; Buynak, E.B.; et al: Live, Attenuated Mumps Virus Vaccine 4. Protective Efficacy as Measured in a Field Evaluation, N. Engl. J. Med. *276:* 252-258, 1967.
10. Cutts, F.T.; Henderson, R.H.; Clements, C.J.; et al: Principles of measles control, Bull WHO *69*(1): 1-7, 1991.
11. Weibel, R.E.; Buynak, E.B.; Stokes, J.; et al: Evaluation Of Live Attenuated Mumps Virus Vaccine, Strain Jeryl Lynn, First International Conference on Vaccines Against Viral and Rickettsial Diseases of Man, World Health Organization, No. 147, May 1967.
12. Leibhaber, H.; Ingalls, T.H.; LeBouvier, G.L.; et al: Vaccination With RA 27/3 Rubella Vaccine, Am. J. Dis. Child. *123:* 133-136, February 1972.
13. Rosen, L.: Hemagglutination and Hemagglutination-Inhibition with Measles Virus, Virology *13:* 139-141, January 1961.
14. Brown, G.C.; et al: Fluorescent-Antibody Marker for Vaccine-Induced Rubella Antibodies, Infection and Immunity *2*(4): 360-363, 1970.
15. Buynak, E.B.; et al: Live Attenuated Mumps Virus Vaccine 1. Vaccine Development, Proceedings of the Society for Experimental Biology and Medicine, *123:* 768-775, 1966.
16. Weibel, R.E.; Carlson, A.J.; Villarejos, V.M.; Buynak, E.B.; McLean, A.A.; Hilleman, M.R.: Clinical and Laboratory Studies of Combined Live Measles, Mumps, and Rubella Vaccines Using the RA 27/3 Rubella Virus, Proc. Soc. Exp. Biol. Med. *165:* 323-326, 1980.
17. Unpublished data from the files of Merck Research Laboratories.
18. Watson, J.C.; Pearson, J.S.; Erdman, D.D.; et al: An Evaluation of Measles Revaccination Among School-Entry Age Children, 31st Interscience Conference on Antimicrobial Agents and Chemotherapy, Abstract #268, 143, 1991.
19. Fogel, A.; Moshkowitz, A.; Rannon, L.; Gerichter, Ch.B.: Comparative trials of RA 27/3 and Cendehill rubella vaccines in adult and adolescent females, Am. J. Epidemiol. *93:* 392-393, 1971.
20. Andzhaparidze, O.G.; Desyatskova, R.G.; Chervonski, G.I.; Pryanichnikova, L.V.: Immunogenicity and reactogenicity of live attenuated rubella virus vaccines, Am. J. Epidemiol. *91:* 527-530, 1970.
21. Freestone, D.S.; Reynolds, G.M.; McKinnon, J.A.; Prydie, J.: Vaccination of schoolgirls against rubella. Assessment of serological status and a comparative trial of Wistar RA 27/3 and Cendehill strain live attenuated rubella vaccines in 13-year-old schoolgirls in Dudley, Br. J. Prev. Soc. Med. *29:* 258-261, 1975.
22. Grillner, L.; Hedstrom, C.E.; Bergstrom, H.; Forssman, L.; Rigner, A.; Lycke, E.: Vaccination against rubella of newly delivered women, Scand. J. Infect. Dis. *5:* 237-241, 1973.
23. Grillner, L.: Neutralizing antibodies after rubella vaccination of newly delivered women: a comparison between three vaccines, Scand. J. Infect. Dis. *7:* 169-172, 1975.
24. Wallace, R.B.; Isacson, P.: Comparative trial of HPV-77, DE-5 and RA 27/3 live-attenuated rubella vaccines, Am. J. Dis. Child. *124:* 536-538, 1972.
25. Lalla, M.; Vesikari, T.; Virolainen, M.: Lymphoblast proliferation and humoral antibody response after rubella vaccination, Clin. Exp. Immunol. *15:* 193-202, 1973.
26. LeBouvier, G.L.; Plotkin, S.A.: Precipitin responses to rubella vaccine RA 27/3, J. Infect. Dis. *123:* 220-223, 1971.
27. Horstmann, D.M.: Rubella: The challenge of its control, J. Infect. Dis. *123:* 640-654, 1971.
28. Ogra, P.L.; Kerr-Grant, D.; Umana, G.; Dzierba, J.; Weintraub, D.: Antibody response in serum and nasopharynx after naturally acquired and vaccine-induced infection with rubella virus, N. Engl. J. Med. *285:* 1333-1339, 1971.
29. Plotkin, S.A.; Farquhar, J.D.; Ogra, P.L.: Immunologic properties of RA 27/3 rubella virus vaccine, J. Am. Med. Assoc. *225:* 585-590, 1973.
30. Liebhaber, H.; Ingalls, T.H.; LeBouvier, G.L.; Horstmann, D.M.: Vaccination with RA 27/3 rubella vaccine. Persistence of immunity and resistance to challenge after two years, Am. J. Dis. Child. *123:* 133-136, 1972.
31. Farquhar, J.D.: Follow-up on rubella vaccinations and experience with subclinical reinfection, J. Pediatr. *81:* 460-465, 1972.
32. Centers for Disease Control and Prevention. Recommended childhood immunization schedule — United States, January-June 1996, MMWR *44*(51 & 52): 940-943, January 5, 1996.
33. Rubella Prevention: Recommendation of the Immunization Practices Advisory Committee (ACIP), MMWR *39*(RR-15): 1-18, November 23, 1990.
34. Measles Prevention: Recommendations of the Immunization Practices Advisory Committee (ACIP), MMWR *38*(S-9): 5-22, December 29, 1989.
35. Jong, E.C., The Travel and Tropical Medicine Manual, W.B. Saunders Company, p. 12-16, 1987.
36. Committee on Immunization Council of Medical Societies, American College of Physicians, Phila., PA, Guide for Adult Immunization, First Edition, 1985.
37. Recommendations of the Immunization Practices Advisory Committee (ACIP), Mumps Prevention, MMWR *38*(22): 388-400, June 9, 1989.
38. King, G.E.; Markowitz, L.E.; Patriarca, P.A.; et al: Clinical Efficacy of Measles Vaccine During the 1990 Measles Epidemic, Pediatr. Infect. Dis. J. *10*(12): 883-888, December 1991.
39. Krasinski, K.; Borkowsky, W.: Measles and Measles Immunity in Children Infected With Human Immunodeficiency Virus, JAMA *261*(17): 2512-2516, 1989.

40. Kelso, J.M.; Jones, R.T.; Yunginger, J.W.: Anaphylaxis to measles, mumps, and rubella vaccine mediated by IgE to gelatin, J. Allergy Clin. Immunol. *91:* 867-872, 1993.
41. General Recommendations on Immunization, Recommendations of the Advisory Committee on Immunization Practices, MMWR *43*(RR-1): 1-38, January 28, 1994.
42. Center for Disease Control: Immunization of Children Infected with Human T-Lymphotropic Virus Type III/ Lymphadenopathy- Associated Virus, Annals of Internal Medicine, *106:* 75-78, 1987.
43. Krasinski, K.; Borkowsky, W.; Krugman, S.: Antibody following measles immunization in children infected with human T-cell lymphotropic virus-type III/lymphadenopathy associated virus (HTLV-III/LAV) [Abstract]. In: Program and abstracts of the International Conference on Acquired Immunodeficiency Syndrome, Paris, France, June 23-25, 1986.
44. Peter, G.; et al (eds): Report of the Committee on Infectious Diseases, Twenty-fourth Edition, American Academy of Pediatrics, 344-357, 1997.
45. Isaacs, D.; Menser, M.: Modern Vaccines, Measles, Mumps, Rubella, and Varicella, Lancet *335:* 1384-1387, June 9, 1990.
46. Starr, S.; Berkovich, S.: The effect of measles, gamma globulin modified measles, and attenuated measles vaccine on the course of treated tuberculosis in children, Pediatrics *35:* 97-102, January 1965.
47. Vaccine Adverse Event Reporting System — United States, MMWR *39*(41): 730-733, October 19, 1990.
48. Rubella vaccination during pregnancy — United States, 1971-1981. MMWR *31*(35): 477-481, September 10, 1982.
49. Losonsky, G.A.; Fishaut, J.M.; Strussenber, J.; Ogra, P.L.: Effect of immunization against rubella on lactation products. II. Maternal-neonatal interactions, J. Infect. Dis. *145:* 661-666, 1982.
50. Landes, R.D.; Bass, J.W.; Millunchick, E.W.; Oetgen, W.J.: Neonatal rubella following postpartum maternal immunization, J. Pediatr. *97:* 465-467, 1980.
51. Lerman, S.J.: Neonatal rubella following postpartum maternal immunization, J. Pediatr. *98:* 668, 1981. (Letter)
52. Gershon, A.; et al: Live attenuated rubella virus vaccine: comparison of responses to HPV-77-DE5 and RA 27/3 strains, Am. J. Med. Sci. *279*(2): 95-97, 1980.
53. Weibel, R.E.; et al: Clinical and laboratory studies of live attenuated RA 27/3 and HPV-77-DE rubella virus vaccines, Proc. Soc. Exp. Biol. Med. *165:* 44-49, 1980.
54. CDC. Important Information about Measles, Mumps, and Rubella, and Measles, Mumps, and Rubella Vaccines. 1980. 1983.
55. CDC, Measles Surveillance, Report No. 11, p. 14, September 1982.
56. Peltola, H.; et al: The elimination of indigenous measles, mumps, and rubella from Finland by a 12-year, two dose vaccination program. N. Engl. J. Med. *331:* 1397-1402, 1994.
57. Eberhart-Phillips, J.E.; et al: Measles in pregnancy: a descriptive study of 58 cases. Obstetrics and Gynecology, *82*(5): 797-801, November 1993.
58. Jespersen, C.S.; et al: Measles as a cause of fetal defects: A retrospective study of ten measles epidemics in Greenland. Acta Paediatr Scand. *66:* 367-372, May 1977.
59. Measles, Mumps, and Rubella—Vaccine Use and Strategies for Elimination of Measles, Rubella, and Congenital Rubella Syndrome and Control of Mumps: Recommendations of the Advisory Committee on Immunization Practices (ACIP), MMWR *47*(RR-8): May 22, 1998.
60. Bitnum, A.; et al: Measles Inclusion Body Encephalitis Caused by the Vaccine Strain of Measles Virus. Clin. Infect. Dis. *29:* 855-861, 1999.
61. Angel, J.B.; et al: Vaccine Associated Measles Pneumonitis in an Adult with AIDS. Annals of Internal Medicine, *129:* 104-106, 1998.

Dist. by:
MERCK & CO., INC., Whitehouse Station, NJ 08889, USA
Issued March 2010
Printed in USA
9912201

PATIENT PACKAGE INSERT

Patient Information about
M-M-R® II (pronounced "em em ar too")
Generic name: Measles, Mumps, and Rubella Virus Vaccine Live

This is a summary of information about M-M-R II[1] You should read it before you or your child receives the vaccine. If you have any questions about the vaccine after reading this leaflet, you should ask your health care provider. This is a summary only. It does not take the place of talking about M-M-R II with your doctor, nurse, or other health care provider. Only your health care provider can decide if M-M-R II is right for you or your child.

What is M-M-R II and how does it work?

M-M-R II is also known as Measles, Mumps, and Rubella Virus Vaccine Live. It is a live virus vaccine that is given as a shot. This vaccine is usually given to people one year old or older. It is meant to help prevent measles (rubeola), mumps, and rubella (German measles).
M-M-R II contains weakened forms of measles virus, mumps virus, and rubella virus.
M-M-R II works by helping the immune system protect you or your child from getting measles, mumps, or rubella. M-M-R II may not protect everyone who gets the vaccine. M-M-R II does not treat measles, mumps, or rubella once you or your child has them.

What do I need to know about measles, mumps, and rubella?

Measles is also known as rubeola. It is a serious illness. Measles virus can be passed to others if you have it. Measles can give you a high fever, cough, and a rash. The illness can last for 1 to 2 weeks. In rare cases, it can also cause an infection of the brain. This could lead to seizures, hearing loss, mental retardation, and even death.
Mumps can also be passed to others. This virus can cause fever and headache. It also makes the glands under your jaw swell and be painful. The illness often lasts for several days. Sometimes, mumps can make the testicles swell and be painful. In some cases, it can cause meningitis, which is a mild swelling of the coverings of the brain and spinal cord.
Rubella is also known as German measles. It is often a mild illness. Rubella virus can cause a mild fever, swollen glands in the neck, pain and swelling in the joints, and a rash that lasts for a short time. It can be very dangerous if a pregnant woman catches it. Women who catch German measles when they are pregnant can have babies who are stillborn. Also, the babies may be blind or deaf, or have heart disease or mental retardation.

Who should not get M-M-R II?

Do not get M-M-R II if you or your child:
- are allergic to any of its ingredients (This includes gelatin or neomycin. See the ingredient list at the end of this leaflet.);
- have a weakened immune system, such as an immune deficiency, an inherited immune disorder, leukemia, lymphoma, or HIV/ AIDS;
- take high doses of steroids by mouth or in a shot;
- have a fever higher than 101.3°F (38.5°C);
- are pregnant or plan to get pregnant within the next three months.

How is M-M-R II given?

M-M-R II is given as a shot to people one year old or older. The dose of the vaccine is the same for everyone. If your child gets the shot when he or she is one year old or older, a second dose is recommended. Often, the second dose is given right before the child goes to elementary school (4 to 6 years of age). If your child is less than one year old when he or she first gets the shot, a second dose should be given when they are 12 to 15 months old. Then, a third shot should be given between 4 and 6 years of age. Your doctor will decide the best time and number of shots by using official recommendations.
If a dose is missed, your health care provider will let you know when you should have it.
Non-pregnant adolescent and adult females of childbearing age who are susceptible to rubella can be vaccinated with M-M-R II (or live attenuated rubella virus vaccine) if certain precautions are taken. In many cases, it is convenient to give the vaccine to women at risk for rubella right after they give birth.

What are the possible side effects of M-M-R II?

The most common side effect of vaccination with M-M-R II is burning and/or stinging at the site of the shot for a short time. Other side effects may include:
- Fever
- Rash

Less common side effects may also include:
- Swelling of the testicles
- Joint pain and/or swelling

Some side effects are rare but may be serious. You should call your health care provider if you notice any of the following problems:
- Difficulty breathing, wheezing, hives, or a skin rash may be signs of an allergic reaction.
- Bleeding or bruising under the skin.
- Seizures, a severe headache, or a change in behavior or consciousness.

Other side effects may also occur. Your doctor has a more complete list of side effects for M-M-R II.
Contact your doctor or health care provider if you or your child have any new or unusual symptoms after receiving M-M-R II.
You may also report any adverse reactions to your doctor or your child's health care provider or submit a report directly to the Vaccine Adverse Event Reporting System (VAERS). The VAERS toll-free number is 1-800-822-7967 or you may report online to www.vaers.hhs.gov.

What are the ingredients of M-M-R II?

Active Ingredients: weakened forms of the measles, mumps, and rubella viruses.
Inactive Ingredients: sorbitol, sodium phosphate, potassium phosphate, sucrose, sodium chloride, hydrolyzed gelatin, recombinant human albumin, fetal bovine serum, other buffer and media ingredients, neomycin.

What else should I know about M-M-R II?

If you get M-M-R II while you are pregnant, please call 1-800-986-8999. Or, you can have your health care provider call.
This leaflet summarizes important information about M-M-R II.
If you would like more information, talk to your health care provider or call 1-800-622-4477.
Rx Only
Issued March 2010
9912201
Dist. by:
MERCK & CO., INC., Whitehouse Station, NJ 08889, USA

MAXALT® ℞
[max-awlt]
(rizatriptan benzoate)
Tablets

MAXALT-MLT® ℞
(rizatriptan benzoate)
Orally Disintegrating Tablets

DESCRIPTION

MAXALT[1] contains rizatriptan benzoate, a selective 5-hydroxytryptamine$_{1B/1D}$ (5-HT$_{1B/1D}$) receptor agonist.
Rizatriptan benzoate is described chemically as: *N,N*-dimethyl-5-(1*H*-1,2,4-triazol-1-ylmethyl)-1*H*-indole-3-ethanamine monobenzoate and its structural formula is:

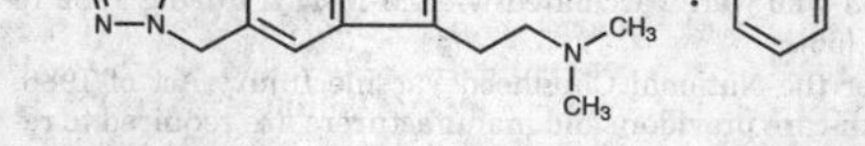

Its empirical formula is $C_{15}H_{19}N_5 \cdot C_7H_6O_2$, representing a molecular weight of the free base of 269.4. Rizatriptan benzoate is a white to off-white, crystalline solid that is soluble in water at about 42 mg per mL (expressed as free base) at 25°C.
MAXALT Tablets and MAXALT-MLT[1] Orally Disintegrating Tablets are available for oral administration in strengths of 5 and 10 mg (corresponding to 7.265 mg or 14.53 mg of the benzoate salt, respectively). Each compressed tablet contains the following inactive ingredients: lactose monohydrate, microcrystalline cellulose, pregelatinized starch, ferric oxide (red), and magnesium stearate.
Each lyophilized orally disintegrating tablet contains the following inactive ingredients: gelatin, mannitol, glycine, aspartame, and peppermint flavor.

[1] Registered trademark of Merck Sharp & Dohme Corp., a subsidiary of **Merck & Co., Inc.**
COPYRIGHT © 1998, 2006 Merck Sharp & Dohme Corp., a subsidiary of **Merck & Co., Inc.**
All rights reserved

CLINICAL PHARMACOLOGY

Mechanism of Action

Rizatriptan binds with high affinity to human cloned 5-HT$_{1B}$ and 5-HT$_{1D}$ receptors. Rizatriptan has weak affinity for other 5-HT$_1$ receptor subtypes (5-HT$_{1A}$, 5-HT$_{1E}$, 5-HT$_{1F}$) and the 5-HT$_7$ receptor, but has no significant activity at 5-HT$_2$, 5-HT$_3$, alpha- and beta-adrenergic, dopaminergic, histaminergic, muscarinic or benzodiazepine receptors.
Current theories on the etiology of migraine headache suggest that symptoms are due to local cranial vasodilatation and/or to the release of vasoactive and pro-inflammatory peptides from sensory nerve endings in an activated trigeminal system. The therapeutic activity of rizatriptan in migraine can most likely be attributed to agonist effects at 5-HT$_{1B/1D}$ receptors on the extracerebral, intracranial blood vessels that become dilated during a migraine attack and on nerve terminals in the trigeminal system. Activation of these receptors results in cranial vessel constriction, inhibition of neuropeptide release and reduced transmission in trigeminal pain pathways.

Pharmacokinetics

Rizatriptan is completely absorbed following oral administration. The mean oral absolute bioavailability of the MAXALT Tablet is about 45%, and mean peak plasma concentrations (C_{max}) are reached in approximately 1-1.5 hours

(T_{max}). The presence of a migraine headache did not appear to affect the absorption or pharmacokinetics of rizatriptan. Food has no significant effect on the bioavailability of rizatriptan but delays the time to reach peak concentration by an hour. In clinical trials, MAXALT was administered without regard to food. The plasma half-life of rizatriptan in males and females averages 2-3 hours.

The bioavailability and C_{max} of rizatriptan were similar following administration of MAXALT Tablets and MAXALT-MLT Orally Disintegrating Tablets, but the rate of absorption is somewhat slower with MAXALT-MLT, with T_{max} averaging 1.6-2.5 hours. AUC of rizatriptan is approximately 30% higher in females than in males. No accumulation occurred on multiple dosing.

The mean volume of distribution is approximately 140 liters in male subjects and 110 liters in female subjects. Rizatriptan is minimally bound (14%) to plasma proteins.

The primary route of rizatriptan metabolism is via oxidative deamination by monoamine oxidase-A (MAO-A) to the indole acetic acid metabolite, which is not active at the 5-$HT_{1B/1D}$ receptor. N-monodesmethyl-rizatriptan, a metabolite with activity similar to that of parent compound at the 5-$HT_{1B/1D}$ receptor, is formed to a minor degree. Plasma concentrations of N-monodesmethyl-rizatriptan are approximately 14% of those of parent compound, and it is eliminated at a similar rate. Other minor metabolites, the N-oxide, the 6-hydroxy compound, and the sulfate conjugate of the 6-hydroxy metabolite are not active at the 5-$HT_{1B/1D}$ receptor.

The total radioactivity of the administered dose recovered over 120 hours in urine and feces was 82% and 12%, respectively, following a single 10 mg oral administration of ^{14}C-rizatriptan. Following oral administration of ^{14}C-rizatriptan, rizatriptan accounted for about 17% of circulating plasma radioactivity. Approximately 14% of an oral dose is excreted in urine as unchanged rizatriptan while 51% is excreted as indole acetic acid metabolite, indicating substantial first pass metabolism.

Cytochrome P450 Isoforms: Rizatriptan is not an inhibitor of the activities of human liver cytochrome P450 isoforms 3A4/5, 1A2, 2C9, 2C19, or 2E1; rizatriptan is a competitive inhibitor (Ki=1400 nM) of cytochrome P450 2D6, but only at high, clinically irrelevant concentrations.

Special Populations

Age: Rizatriptan pharmacokinetics in healthy elderly non-migraineur volunteers (age 65-77 years) were similar to those in younger non-migraineur volunteers (age 18-45 years).

Gender: The mean $AUC_{0-\infty}$ and C_{max} of rizatriptan (10 mg orally) were about 30% and 11% higher in females as compared to males, respectively, while T_{max} occurred at approximately the same time.

Hepatic impairment: Following oral administration in patients with hepatic impairment caused by mild to moderate alcoholic cirrhosis of the liver, plasma concentrations of rizatriptan were similar in patients with mild hepatic insufficiency compared to a control group of healthy subjects; plasma concentrations of rizatriptan were approximately 30% greater in patients with moderate hepatic insufficiency. (See PRECAUTIONS.)

Renal impairment: In patients with renal impairment (creatinine clearance 10-60 mL/min/1.73 m^2), the $AUC_{0-\infty}$ of rizatriptan was not significantly different from that in healthy subjects. In hemodialysis patients, (creatinine clearance < 2 mL/min/1.73 m^2), however, the AUC for rizatriptan was approximately 44% greater than that in patients with normal renal function. (See PRECAUTIONS.)

Race: Pharmacokinetic data revealed no significant differences between African American and Caucasian subjects.

Drug Interactions

(See also PRECAUTIONS, Drug Interactions.)

Monoamine oxidase inhibitors: Rizatriptan is principally metabolized via monoamine oxidase, 'A' subtype (MAO-A). Plasma concentrations of rizatriptan may be increased by drugs that are selective MAO-A inhibitors (e.g., moclobemide) or nonselective MAO inhibitors [type A and B] (e.g., isocarboxazid, phenelzine, tranylcypromine, and pargyline). In a drug interaction study, when MAXALT 10 mg was administered to subjects (n=12) receiving concomitant therapy with the selective, reversible MAO-A inhibitor, moclobemide 150 mg t.i.d., there were mean increases in rizatriptan AUC and C_{max} of 119% and 41% respectively; and the AUC of the active N-monodesmethyl metabolite of rizatriptan was increased more than 400%. The interaction would be expected to be greater with irreversible MAO inhibitors. No pharmacokinetic interaction is anticipated in patients receiving selective MAO-B inhibitors. (See CONTRAINDICATIONS; PRECAUTIONS, Drug Interactions.)

Propranolol: In a study of concurrent administration of propranolol 240 mg/day and a single dose of rizatriptan 10 mg in healthy subjects (n=11), mean plasma AUC for rizatriptan was increased by 70% during propranolol administration, and a fourfold increase was observed in one subject. The AUC of the active N-monodesmethyl metabolite of rizatriptan was not affected by propranolol. (See PRECAUTIONS; DOSAGE AND ADMINISTRATION.)

Nadolol/Metoprolol: In a drug interactions study, effects of multiple doses of nadolol 80 mg or metoprolol 100 mg every 12 hours on the pharmacokinetics of a single dose of 10 mg rizatriptan were evaluated in healthy subjects (n=12). No pharmacokinetic interactions were observed.

Paroxetine: In a study of the interaction between the selective serotonin reuptake inhibitor (SSRI) paroxetine 20 mg/day for two weeks and a single dose of MAXALT 10 mg in healthy subjects (n=12), neither the plasma concentrations of rizatriptan nor its safety profile were affected by paroxetine (see WARNINGS and PRECAUTIONS, Information for Patients.)

Oral contraceptives: In a study of concurrent administration of an oral contraceptive during 6 days of administration of MAXALT (10-30 mg/day) in healthy female volunteers (n=18), rizatriptan did not affect plasma concentrations of ethinyl estradiol or norethindrone.

Clinical Studies

The efficacy of MAXALT Tablets was established in four multicenter, randomized, placebo-controlled trials. Patients enrolled in these studies were primarily female (84%) and Caucasian (88%), with a mean age of 40 years (range of 18 to 71). Patients were instructed to treat a moderate to severe headache. Headache response, defined as a reduction of moderate or severe headache pain to no or mild headache pain, was assessed for up to 2 hours (Study 1) or up to 4 hours after dosing (Studies 2, 3 and 4). Associated symptoms of nausea, photophobia, and phonophobia and maintenance of response up to 24 hours postdose were evaluated. A second dose of MAXALT Tablets was allowed 2 to 24 hours after dosing for treatment of recurrent headache in Studies 1 and 2. Additional analgesics and/or antiemetics were allowed 2 hours after initial treatment for rescue in all four studies.

In all studies, the percentage of patients achieving headache response 2 hours after treatment was significantly greater in patients who received either MAXALT 5 or 10 mg compared to those who received placebo. In a separate study, doses of 2.5 mg were not different from placebo. Doses greater than 10 mg were associated with an increased incidence of adverse effects. The results from the 4 controlled studies using the marketed formulation are summarized in Table 1.

Table 1: Response Rates 2 Hours Following Treatment of Initial Headache

Study	Placebo	MAXALT Tablets 5 mg	MAXALT Tablets 10 mg
1	35% (n=304)	62%* (n=458)	71%*,† (n=456)
2‡	37% (n=82)	—	77%* (n=320)
3	23% (n= 80)	63%* (n=352)	—
4	40% (n=159)	60%* (n=164)	67%* (n=385)

* p value < 0.05 in comparison with placebo
† p value < 0.05 in comparison with 5 mg
‡ Results for initial headache only.

Comparisons of drug performance based upon results obtained in different clinical trials are never reliable. Because studies are conducted at different times, with different samples of patients, by different investigators, employing different criteria and/or different interpretations of the same criteria, under different conditions (dose, dosing regimen, etc.), quantitative estimates of treatment response and the timing of response may be expected to vary considerably from study to study.

The estimated probability of achieving an initial headache response within 2 hours following treatment is depicted in Figure 1.

[See figure 1 at top of next column]

For patients with migraine-associated photophobia, phonophobia, and nausea at baseline, there was a decreased incidence of these symptoms following administration of MAXALT compared to placebo.

Two to 24 hours following the initial dose of study treatment, patients were allowed to use additional treatment for pain response in the form of a second dose of study treatment or other medication. The estimated probability of patients taking a second dose or other medication for migraine over the 24 hours following the initial dose of study treatment is summarized in Figure 2.

[See figure 2 on next column]

Efficacy was unaffected by the presence of aura; by the gender, or age of the patient; or by concomitant use of common migraine prophylactic drugs (e.g., beta-blockers, calcium channel blockers, tricyclic antidepressants) or oral contraceptives. In two additional similar studies, efficacy was unaffected by relationship to menses. There were insufficient data to assess the impact of race on efficacy.

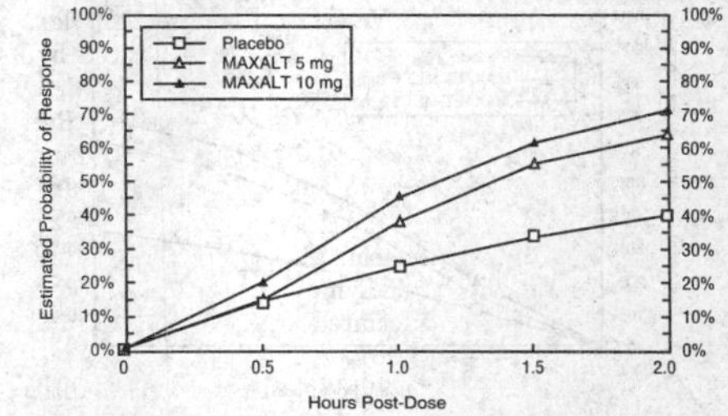

†† Figure 1 shows the Kaplan-Meier plot of the probability over time of obtaining headache response (no or mild pain) following treatment with rizatriptan or placebo. The averages displayed are based on pooled data from 4 placebo-controlled, outpatient trials providing evidence of efficacy (Studies 1, 2, 3, and 4). Patients taking additional treatment or not achieving headache response prior to 2 hours were censored at 2 hours.

Figure 1: Estimated Probability of Achieving an Initial Headache Response by 2 Hours††

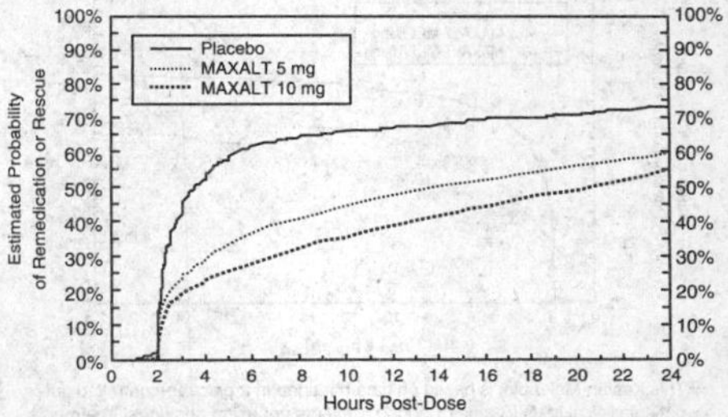

††† This Kaplan-Meier plot is based on data obtained in 4 placebo-controlled outpatient clinical trials (Studies 1, 2, 3, and 4). Patients not using additional treatment were censored at 24 hours. The plot includes both patients who had headache response at 2 hours and those who had no response to the initial dose. Remedication was not allowed within 2 hours post-dose.

Figure 2: Estimated Probability of Patients Taking a Second Dose of MAXALT Tablets or Other Medication for Migraines Over the 24 Hours Following the Initial Dose of Study Treatment†††

In a single study in adolescents (n=291), there were no statistically significant differences between treatment groups. The headache response rates at 2 hours were 66% and 56% for MAXALT 5 mg Tablets and placebo, respectively.

MAXALT-MLT Orally Disintegrating Tablets

The efficacy of MAXALT-MLT was established in two multicenter, randomized, placebo-controlled trials that were similar in design to the trials of MAXALT Tablets. Patients were instructed to treat a moderate to severe headache. Patients treated in these studies were primarily female (88%) and Caucasian (95%), with a mean age of 42 years (range 18-72).

In both studies, the percentage of patients achieving headache response 2 hours after treatment was significantly greater in patients who received either MAXALT-MLT 5 or 10 mg compared to those who received placebo. The results from the 2 controlled studies using the marketed formulation are summarized in Table 2.

Table 2: Response Rates 2 Hours Following Treatment of Initial Headache

Study	Placebo	MAXALT-MLT 5 mg	MAXALT-MLT 10 mg
1	47% (n=98)	66%* (n=100)	66%* (n=113)
2	28% (n=180)	59%* (n=181)	74%*,† (n=186)

* p value < 0.01 in comparison with placebo
† p value < 0.01 in comparison with 5 mg

The estimated probability of achieving an initial headache response by 2 hours following treatment with MAXALT-MLT is depicted in Figure 3.

[See figure 3 on next page]

For patients with migraine-associated photophobia and phonophobia at baseline, there was a decreased incidence of these symptoms following administration of MAXALT-MLT as compared to placebo.

Two to 24 hours following the initial dose of study treatment, patients were allowed to use additional treatment for pain response in the form of a second dose of study treatment or other medication. The estimated probability of patients taking a second dose or other medication for migraine over the 24 hours following the initial dose of study treatment is summarized in Figure 4.

[See figure 4 on next page]

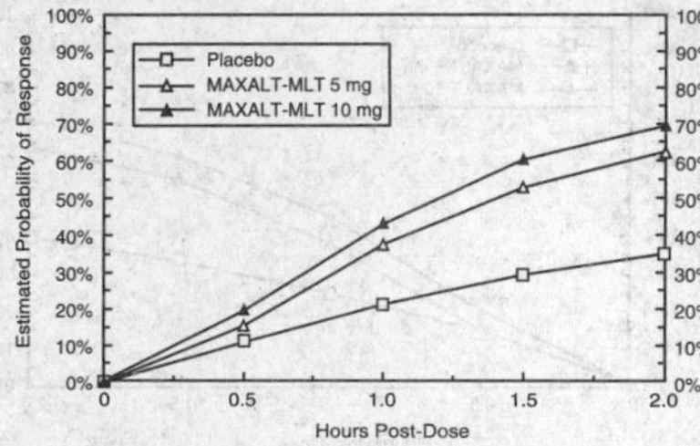

‡Figure 3 shows the Kaplan-Meier plot of the probability over time of obtaining headache response (no or mild pain) following treatment with MAXALT-MLT or placebo. The averages displayed are based on pooled data from 2 placebo-controlled, outpatient trials providing evidence of efficacy (Studies 1 and 2). Patients taking additional treatment or not achieving headache response prior to 2 hours were censored at 2 hours.

Figure 3: Estimated Probability of Achieving an Initial Headache Response with MAXALT-MLT by 2 Hours‡

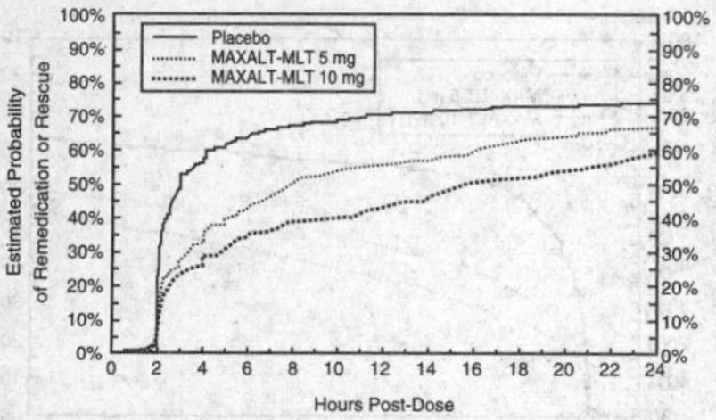

‡‡This Kaplan-Meier plot is based on data obtained in 2 placebo-controlled outpatient clinical trials (Studies 1 and 2). Patients not using additional treatments were censored at 24 hours. The plot includes both patients who had headache response at 2 hours and those who had no response to the initial dose. Remedication was not allowed within 2 hours post-dose.

Figure 4: Estimated Probability of Patients Taking a Second Dose of MAXALT-MLT or Other Medication for Migraines Over the 24 Hours Following the Initial Dose of Study Treatment‡‡

INDICATIONS AND USAGE

MAXALT is indicated for the acute treatment of migraine attacks with or without aura in adults.

MAXALT is not intended for the prophylactic therapy of migraine or for use in the management of hemiplegic or basilar migraine (see CONTRAINDICATIONS). Safety and effectiveness of MAXALT have not been established for cluster headache, which is present in an older, predominantly male population.

CONTRAINDICATIONS

MAXALT should not be given to patients with ischemic heart disease (e.g., angina pectoris, history of myocardial infarction, or documented silent ischemia) or to patients who have symptoms or findings consistent with ischemic heart disease, coronary artery vasospasm, including Prinzmetal's variant angina, or other significant underlying cardiovascular disease (see WARNINGS).

Because MAXALT may increase blood pressure, it should not be given to patients with uncontrolled hypertension (see WARNINGS).

MAXALT should not be used within 24 hours of treatment with another 5-HT$_1$ agonist, or an ergotamine-containing or ergot-type medication like dihydroergotamine or methysergide.

MAXALT should not be administered to patients with hemiplegic or basilar migraine.

Concurrent administration of MAO inhibitors or use of rizatriptan within 2 weeks of discontinuation of MAO inhibitor therapy is contraindicated (see CLINICAL PHARMACOLOGY, Drug Interactions and PRECAUTIONS, Drug Interactions).

MAXALT is contraindicated in patients who are hypersensitive to rizatriptan or any of its inactive ingredients.

WARNINGS

MAXALT should only be used where a clear diagnosis of migraine has been established.

Risk of Myocardial Ischemia and/or Infarction and Other Adverse Cardiac Events: **Because of the potential of this class of compounds (5-HT$_{1B/1D}$ agonists) to cause coronary vasospasm, MAXALT should not be given to patients with documented ischemic or vasospastic coronary artery disease (see CONTRAINDICATIONS). It is strongly recommended that rizatriptan not be given to patients in whom unrecognized coronary artery disease (CAD) is predicted by the presence of risk factors (e.g., hypertension, hypercholesterolemia, smoker, obesity, diabetes, strong family history of CAD, female with surgical or physiological menopause, or male over 40 years of age) unless a cardiovascular evaluation provides satisfactory clinical evidence that the patient is reasonably free of coronary artery and ischemic myocardial disease or other significant underlying cardiovascular disease. The sensitivity of cardiac diagnostic procedures to detect cardiovascular disease or predisposition to coronary artery vasospasm is modest, at best. If, during the cardiovascular evaluation, the patient's medical history, electrocardiographic or other investigations reveal findings indicative of, or consistent with, coronary artery vasospasm or myocardial ischemia, rizatriptan should not be administered (see CONTRAINDICATIONS).**

For patients with risk factors predictive of CAD, who are determined to have a satisfactory cardiovascular evaluation, it is strongly recommended that administration of the first dose of rizatriptan take place in the setting of a physician's office or similar medically staffed and equipped facility unless the patient has previously received rizatriptan. Because cardiac ischemia can occur in the absence of clinical symptoms, consideration should be given to obtaining on the first occasion of use an electrocardiogram (ECG) during the interval immediately following MAXALT, in these patients with risk factors.

It is recommended that patients who are intermittent long-term users of MAXALT and who have or acquire risk factors predictive of CAD, as described above, undergo periodic interval cardiovascular evaluation as they continue to use MAXALT.

The systematic approach described above is intended to reduce the likelihood that patients with unrecognized cardiovascular disease will be inadvertently exposed to rizatriptan.

Cardiac Events and Fatalities Associated with 5-HT$_1$ Agonists: Serious adverse cardiac events, including acute myocardial infarction, have been reported within a few hours following the administration of rizatriptan. Life-threatening disturbances of cardiac rhythm and death have been reported within a few hours following the administration of other 5-HT$_1$ agonists. Considering the extent of use of 5-HT$_1$ agonists in patients with migraine, the incidence of these events is extremely low. MAXALT can cause coronary vasospasm. Because of the close proximity of the events to MAXALT use, a causal relationship cannot be excluded. In the cases where there has been known underlying coronary artery disease, the relationship is uncertain.

Premarketing experience with rizatriptan: Among the 3700 patients with migraine who participated in premarketing clinical trials of MAXALT, one patient was reported to have chest pain with possible ischemic ECG changes following a single dose of 10 mg.

Postmarketing experience with rizatriptan: Serious cardiovascular events have been reported in association with the use of MAXALT. The uncontrolled nature of postmarketing surveillance, however, makes it impossible to determine definitively the proportion of the reported cases that were actually caused by rizatriptan or to reliably assess causation in individual cases.

Cerebrovascular Events and Fatalities Associated with 5-HT$_1$ Agonists: Cerebral hemorrhage, subarachnoid hemorrhage, stroke, and other cerebrovascular events have been reported in patients treated with 5-HT$_1$ agonists; and some have resulted in fatalities. In a number of cases, it appears possible that the cerebrovascular events were primary, the agonist having been administered in the incorrect belief that the symptoms experienced were a consequence of migraine, when they were not. It should be noted that patients with migraine may be at increased risk of certain cerebrovascular events (e.g., stroke, hemorrhage, transient ischemic attack).

Other Vasospasm-Related Events: 5-HT$_1$ agonists may cause vasospastic reactions other than coronary artery vasospasm. Both peripheral vascular ischemia and colonic ischemia with abdominal pain and bloody diarrhea have been reported with 5-HT$_1$ agonists.

Increase in Blood Pressure: Significant elevation in blood pressure, including hypertensive crisis, has been reported on rare occasions in patients receiving 5-HT$_1$ agonists with and without a history of hypertension. In healthy young male and female subjects who received maximal doses of MAXALT (10 mg every 2 hours for 3 doses), slight increases in blood pressure (approximately 2-3 mmHg) were observed. Rizatriptan is contraindicated in patients with uncontrolled hypertension (see CONTRAINDICATIONS).

An 18% increase in mean pulmonary artery pressure was seen following dosing with another 5-HT$_1$ agonist in a study evaluating subjects undergoing cardiac catheterization.

Serotonin Syndrome: The development of a potentially life-threatening serotonin syndrome may occur with triptans, including MAXALT treatment, particularly during combined use with selective serotonin reuptake inhibitors (SSRIs) or serotonin norepinephrine reuptake inhibitors (SNRIs). If concomitant treatment with rizatriptan and an SSRI (e.g., fluoxetine, paroxetine, sertraline, fluvoxamine, citalopram, escitalopram) or SNRI (e.g., venlafaxine, duloxetine) is clinically warranted, careful observation of the patient is advised, particularly during treatment initiation and dose increases. Serotonin syndrome symptoms may include mental status changes (e.g., agitation, hallucinations, coma), autonomic instability (e.g., tachycardia, labile blood pressure, hyperthermia), neuromuscular aberrations (e.g., hyperreflexia, incoordination) and/or gastrointestinal symptoms (e.g., nausea, vomiting, diarrhea) (see PRECAUTIONS, Drug Interactions).

PRECAUTIONS

General

As with other 5-HT$_{1B/1D}$ agonists, sensations of tightness, pain, pressure, and heaviness have been reported after treatment with MAXALT in the precordium, throat, neck and jaw. These events have not been associated with arrhythmias or definite ischemic ECG changes in clinical trials (one patient experienced chest pain with possible ischemic ECG changes). Because drugs in this class may cause coronary artery vasospasm, patients who experience signs or symptoms suggestive of angina following dosing should be evaluated for the presence of CAD or a predisposition to Prinzmetal's variant angina before receiving additional doses of medication, and should be monitored electrocardiographically if dosing is resumed and similar symptoms recur. Similarly, patients who experience other symptoms or signs suggestive of decreased arterial flow, such as ischemic bowel syndrome or Raynaud's syndrome following the use of any 5-HT$_1$ agonist are candidates for further evaluation (see WARNINGS).

Rizatriptan should also be administered with caution to patients with diseases that may alter the absorption, metabolism, or excretion of drugs (see CLINICAL PHARMACOLOGY, Special Populations).

Renally Impaired Patients: Rizatriptan should be used with caution in dialysis patients due to a decrease in the clearance of rizatriptan (see CLINICAL PHARMACOLOGY, Special Populations).

Hepatically Impaired Patients: Rizatriptan should be used with caution in patients with moderate hepatic insufficiency due to an increase in plasma concentrations of approximately 30% (see CLINICAL PHARMACOLOGY, Special Populations).

For a given attack, if a patient has no response to the first dose of rizatriptan, the diagnosis of migraine should be reconsidered before administration of a second dose.

Binding to Melanin-Containing Tissues

The propensity for rizatriptan to bind melanin has not been investigated. Based on its chemical properties, rizatriptan may bind to melanin and accumulate in melanin rich tissue (e.g., eye) over time. This raises the possibility that rizatriptan could cause toxicity in these tissues after extended use. There were, however, no adverse ophthalmologic changes related to treatment with rizatriptan in the one year dog toxicity study. Although no systematic monitoring of ophthalmologic function was undertaken in clinical trials, and no specific recommendations for ophthalmologic monitoring are offered, prescribers should be aware of the possibility of long-term ophthalmologic effects.

Phenylketonurics

Phenylketonuric patients should be informed that MAXALT-MLT Orally Disintegrating Tablets contain phenylalanine (a component of aspartame). Each 5-mg orally disintegrating tablet contains 1.05 mg phenylalanine, and each 10-mg orally disintegrating tablet contains 2.10 mg phenylalanine.

Information for Patients

Migraine or treatment with MAXALT may cause somnolence in some patients. Dizziness has also been reported in some patients receiving MAXALT. Patients should, therefore, evaluate their ability to perform complex tasks during migraine attacks and after administration of MAXALT.

Physicians should instruct their patients to read the patient package insert before taking MAXALT. See the accompanying PATIENT INFORMATION leaflet.

Patients should be cautioned about the risk of serotonin syndrome with the use of rizatriptan or other triptans, especially during combined use with selective serotonin reuptake inhibitors (SSRIs) or serotonin norepinephrine reuptake inhibitors (SNRIs) (see WARNINGS).

MAXALT-MLT Orally Disintegrating Tablets

Patients should be instructed not to remove the blister from the outer pouch until just prior to dosing. The blister pack should then be peeled open with dry hands and the orally disintegrating tablet placed on the tongue, where it will dissolve and be swallowed with the saliva.

Laboratory Tests

No specific laboratory tests are recommended for monitoring patients prior to and/or after treatment with MAXALT.

Drug Interactions

(See also CLINICAL PHARMACOLOGY, Drug Interactions.)

Propranolol: Rizatriptan 5 mg should be used in patients taking propranolol, as propranolol has been shown to increase the plasma concentrations of rizatriptan by 70% (see CLINICAL PHARMACOLOGY, Drug Interactions; DOSAGE AND ADMINISTRATION).

Ergot-containing drugs: Ergot-containing drugs have been reported to cause prolonged vasospastic reactions. *Because* there is a theoretical basis that these effects may be additive, use of ergotamine-containing or ergot-type medications (like dihydroergotamine or methysergide) and rizatriptan within 24 hours is contraindicated (see CONTRAINDICATIONS).

Other 5-HT$_1$ agonists: The administration of rizatriptan with other 5-HT$_1$ agonists has not been evaluated in migraine patients. Because their vasospastic effects may be additive, coadministration of rizatriptan and other 5-HT$_1$ agonists within 24 hours of each other is not recommended (see CONTRAINDICATIONS).

Selective Serotonin Reuptake Inhibitors/Serotonin Norepinephrine Reuptake Inhibitors and Serotonin Syndrome: Cases of life-threatening serotonin syndrome have been reported during combined use of selective serotonin reuptake inhibitors (SSRIs) or serotonin norepinephrine reuptake inhibitors (SNRIs) and triptans (see WARNINGS).

Monoamine oxidase inhibitors: Rizatriptan should not be administered to patients taking MAO-A inhibitors and nonselective MAO inhibitors; it has been shown that moclobemide (a specific MAO-A inhibitor) increased the systemic exposure of rizatriptan and its metabolite (see CLINICAL PHARMACOLOGY, Drug Interactions; CONTRAINDICATIONS).

Drug/Laboratory Test Interactions

MAXALT is not known to interfere with commonly employed clinical laboratory tests.

Carcinogenesis, Mutagenesis, Impairment of Fertility

Carcinogenesis: The lifetime carcinogenic potential of rizatriptan was evaluated in a 100-week study in mice and a 106-week study in rats at oral gavage doses of up to 125 mg/kg/day. Exposure data were not obtained in those studies, but plasma AUC's of parent drug measured in other studies after 5 and 21 weeks of oral dosing in mice and rats, respectively, indicate that the exposures to parent drug at the highest dose level in the carcinogenicity studies would have been approximately 150 times (mice) and 240 times (rats) average AUC's measured in humans after three 10 mg doses, the maximum recommended total daily dose. There was no evidence of an increase in tumor incidence related to rizatriptan in either species.

Mutagenesis: Rizatriptan, with and without metabolic activation, was neither mutagenic, nor clastogenic in a battery of *in vitro* and *in vivo* genetic toxicity studies, including: the microbial mutagenesis (Ames) assay, the *in vitro* mammalian cell mutagenesis assay in V-79 Chinese hamster lung cells, the *in vitro* alkaline elution assay in rat hepatocytes, the *in vitro* chromosomal aberration assay in Chinese hamster ovary cells and the *in vivo* chromosomal aberration assay in mouse bone marrow.

Impairment of Fertility: In a fertility study in rats, altered estrus cyclicity and delays in time to mating were observed in females treated orally with 100 mg/kg/day rizatriptan. Plasma drug exposure (AUC) at this dose was approximately 225 times the exposure in humans receiving the maximum recommended daily dose (MRDD) of 30 mg. The no-effect dose was 10 mg/kg/day (approximately 15 times the human exposure at the MRDD). There were no other fertility-related effects in the female rats. There was no impairment of fertility or reproductive performance in male rats treated with up to 250 mg/kg/day (approximately 550 times the human exposure at the MRDD).

Pregnancy:

Pregnancy Category C

In a general reproductive study in rats, birth weights and pre- and post-weaning weight gain were reduced in the offspring of females treated prior to and during mating and throughout gestation and lactation with doses of 10 and 100 mg/kg/day. Maternal drug exposures (AUC) at these doses were approximately 15 and 225 times, respectively, the exposure in humans receiving the maximum recommended daily dose (MRDD) of 30 mg. In a pre- and postnatal developmental toxicity study in rats, an increase in mortality of the offspring at birth and for the first three days after birth, a decrease in pre- and post-weaning weight gain, and decreased performance in a passive avoidance test (which indicates a decrease in learning capacity of the offspring) were observed at doses of 100 and 250 mg/kg/day. The no-effect dose for all of these effects was 5 mg/kg/day, approximately 7.5 times the exposure in humans receiving the MRDD. With doses of 100 and 250 mg/kg/day, the decreases in average weight of both the male and female offspring persisted into adulthood. All of these effects on the offspring in both reproductive toxicity studies occurred in the absence of any apparent maternal toxicity.

In embryofetal development studies, no teratogenic effects were observed when pregnant rats and rabbits were administered doses of 100 and 50 mg/kg/day, respectively, during organogenesis. Fetal weights were decreased in conjunction with decreased maternal weight gain at the highest doses (maternal exposures approximately 225 and 115 times the human exposure at the MRDD in rats and rabbits, respectively). The developmental no-effect dose in these studies was 10 mg/kg/day in both rats and rabbits (maternal exposures approximately 15 times human exposure at the MRDD). Toxicokinetic studies demonstrated placental transfer of drug in both species.

There are no adequate and well-controlled studies in pregnant women; therefore, rizatriptan should be used during pregnancy only if the potential benefit justifies the potential risk to the fetus.

Merck Sharp & Dohme Corp., a subsidiary of Merck & Co., Inc., maintains a registry to monitor the pregnancy outcomes of women exposed to MAXALT while pregnant. Healthcare providers are encouraged to report any prenatal exposure to MAXALT by calling the Pregnancy Registry at (800) 986-8999.

Nursing Mothers

It is not known whether this drug is excreted in human milk. Because many drugs are excreted in human milk, caution should be exercised when MAXALT is administered to women who are breast-feeding. Rizatriptan is extensively excreted in rat milk, at a level of 5-fold or greater than maternal plasma levels.

Pediatric Use

Safety and effectiveness of rizatriptan in pediatric patients have not been established; therefore, MAXALT is not recommended for use in patients under 18 years of age.

The efficacy of MAXALT Tablets (5 mg) in patients aged 12 to 17 years was not established in a randomized placebo-controlled trial of 291 adolescent migraineurs (see Clinical Studies). Adverse events observed were similar in nature to those reported in clinical trials in adults. Postmarketing experience with other triptans includes a limited number of reports that describe pediatric patients who have experienced clinically serious adverse events that are similar in nature to those reported rarely in adults. The long-term safety of rizatriptan in pediatric patients has not been studied.

Geriatric Use

The pharmacokinetics of rizatriptan were similar in elderly (aged ≥ 65 years) and in younger adults. Because migraine occurs infrequently in the elderly, clinical experience with MAXALT is limited in such patients. In clinical trials, there were no apparent differences in efficacy or in overall adverse experience rates between patients under 65 years of age and those 65 and above (n=17).

ADVERSE REACTIONS

Serious cardiac events, including some that have been fatal, have occurred following use of 5-HT$_1$ agonists. These events are extremely rare and most have been reported in patients with risk factors predictive of CAD. Events reported have included coronary artery vasospasm, transient myocardial ischemia, myocardial infarction, ventricular tachycardia, and ventricular fibrillation (see CONTRAINDICATIONS, WARNINGS, and PRECAUTIONS).

Incidence in Controlled Clinical Trials: Adverse experiences to rizatriptan were assessed in controlled clinical trials that included over 3700 patients who received single or multiple doses of MAXALT Tablets. The most common adverse events during treatment with MAXALT were asthenia/fatigue, somnolence, pain/pressure sensation and dizziness. These events appeared to be dose related. In long term extension studies where patients were allowed to treat multiple attacks for up to 1 year, 4% (59 out of 1525 patients) withdrew because of adverse experiences.

Table 3 lists the adverse events regardless of drug relationship (incidence ≥ 2% and greater than placebo) after a single dose of MAXALT. The events cited reflect experience gained under closely monitored conditions of clinical trials in a highly selected patient population. In actual clinical practice or in other clinical trials, these frequency estimates may not apply, as the conditions of use, reporting behavior, and the kinds of patients treated may differ.

Table 3: Incidence (≥ 2% and Greater than Placebo) of Adverse Experiences After a Single Dose of MAXALT Tablets or Placebo

	% of Patients		
Adverse Experiences	MAXALT 5 mg (N=977)	MAXALT 10 mg (N=1167)	Placebo (N=627)
Atypical Sensations	4	5	4
Paresthesia	3	4	<2
Pain and other Pressure Sensations	6	9	3
Chest Pain: tightness/pressure and/or heaviness	<2	3	1
Neck/throat/jaw: pain/tightness/ pressure	<2	2	1
Regional Pain: tightness/pressure/ heaviness	<1	2	0
Pain, location unspecified	3	3	<2
Digestive	9	13	8
Dry Mouth	3	3	1
Nausea	4	6	4
Neurological	14	20	11
Dizziness	4	9	5
Headache	<2	2	<1
Somnolence	4	8	4
Other			
Asthenia/fatigue	4	7	2

MAXALT was generally well-tolerated. Adverse experiences were typically mild in intensity and were transient. The frequencies of adverse experiences in clinical trials did not increase when up to three doses were taken within 24 hours. Adverse event frequencies were also unchanged by concomitant use of drugs commonly taken for migraine prophylaxis (including propranolol), oral contraceptives, or analgesics. The incidences of adverse experiences were not affected by age or gender. There were insufficient data to assess the impact of race on the incidence of adverse events.

Other Events Observed in Association with the Administration of MAXALT: In the section that follows, the frequencies of less commonly reported adverse clinical events are presented. Because the reports include events observed in open studies, the role of MAXALT in their causation cannot be reliably determined. Furthermore, variability associated with adverse event reporting, the terminology used to describe adverse events, etc., limit the value of the quantitative frequency estimates provided. Event frequencies are calculated as the number of patients who used MAXALT (N=3716) and reported an event divided by the total number of patients exposed to MAXALT. All reported events are included, except those already listed in the previous table, those too general to be informative, and those not reasonably associated with the use of the drug. Events are further classified within body system categories and enumerated in order of decreasing frequency using the following definitions: frequent adverse events are those defined as those occurring in at least (>)1/100 patients; infrequent adverse experiences are those occurring in 1/100 to 1/1000 patients; and rare adverse experiences are those occurring in fewer than 1/1000 patients.

General: Infrequent were chills, heat sensitivity, facial edema, hangover effect, and abdominal distention. Rare were fever, orthostatic effects, syncope and edema/swelling.

Atypical Sensations: Frequent were warm/cold sensations.

Cardiovascular: Frequent was palpitation. Infrequent were tachycardia, cold extremities, hypertension, arrhythmia, and bradycardia. Rare was angina pectoris.

Digestive: Frequent were diarrhea and vomiting. Infrequent were dyspepsia, thirst, acid regurgitation, dysphagia, constipation, flatulence, and tongue edema. Rare were anorexia, appetite increase, gastritis, paralysis (tongue), and eructation.

Metabolic: Infrequent was dehydration.

Musculoskeletal: Infrequent were muscle weakness, stiffness, myalgia, muscle cramp, musculoskeletal pain, arthralgia, and muscle spasm.

Neurological/Psychiatric: Frequent were hypesthesia, mental acuity decreased, euphoria and tremor. Infrequent were nervousness, vertigo, insomnia, anxiety, depression, disorientation, ataxia, dysarthria, confusion, dream abnormality, gait abnormality, irritability, memory impairment, agitation and hyperesthesia. Rare were: dysesthesia, depersonalization, akinesia/bradykinesia, apprehension, hyperkinesia, hypersomnia, and hyporeflexia.

Respiratory: Frequent was dyspnea. Infrequent were pharyngitis, irritation (nasal), congestion (nasal), dry throat, upper respiratory infection, yawning, respiratory congestion (nasal), dry nose, epistaxis, and sinus disorder. Rare were cough, hiccups, hoarseness, rhinorrhea, sneezing, tachypnea, and pharyngeal edema.

Special Senses: Infrequent were blurred vision, tinnitus, dry eyes, burning eye, eye pain, eye irritation, ear pain, and tearing. Rare were hyperacusis, smell perversion, photophobia, photopsia, itching eye, and eye swelling.

Skin and Skin Appendage: Frequent was flushing. Infrequent were sweating, pruritus, rash, and urticaria. Rare were erythema, acne, and photosensitivity.

Urogenital System: Frequent was hot flashes. Infrequent were urinary frequency, polyuria, and menstruation disorder. Rare was dysuria.

The adverse experience profile seen with MAXALT-MLT Orally Disintegrating Tablets was similar to that seen with MAXALT Tablets.

Postmarketing Experience

The following section enumerates potentially important adverse events that have occurred in clinical practice and which have been reported spontaneously to various surveillance systems. The events enumerated represent reports arising from both domestic and non-domestic use of rizatriptan. The events enumerated include all except those already listed in the ADVERSE REACTIONS section above or those too general to be informative. Because the reports cite events reported spontaneously from worldwide post-marketing experience, frequency of events and the role of rizatriptan in their causation cannot be reliably determined.

Cardiovascular: Myocardial ischemia, myocardial infarction, peripheral vascular ischemia (see WARNINGS).

Cerebrovascular: Stroke.

Neurological/Psychiatric: Serotonin syndrome (see WARNINGS), seizure.

Special Senses: Dysgeusia.

General: Hypersensitivity reaction, anaphylaxis/anaphylactoid reaction, angioedema (e.g., facial edema, tongue swelling, pharyngeal edema), wheezing, toxic epidermal necrolysis.

DRUG ABUSE AND DEPENDENCE

Although the abuse potential of MAXALT has not been specifically assessed, no abuse of, tolerance to, withdrawal from, or drug-seeking behavior was observed in patients who received MAXALT in clinical trials or their extensions. The 5-HT$_{1B/1D}$ agonists, as a class, have not been associated with drug abuse.

OVERDOSAGE

No overdoses of MAXALT were reported during clinical trials.

Rizatriptan 40 mg (administered as either a single dose or as two doses with a 2-hour interdose interval) was generally well tolerated in over 300 patients; dizziness and somnolence were the most common drug-related adverse effects.

In a clinical pharmacology study in which 12 subjects received rizatriptan, at total cumulative doses of 80 mg (given within four hours), two subjects experienced syncope and/or bradycardia. One subject, a female aged 29 years, developed vomiting, bradycardia, and dizziness beginning three hours after receiving a total of 80 mg rizatriptan (administered over two hours); a third degree AV block, responsive to atropine, was observed an hour after the onset of the other symptoms. The second subject, a 25 year old male, experienced transient dizziness, syncope, incontinence, and a 5-second systolic pause (on ECG monitor) immediately after a painful venipuncture. The venipuncture occurred two hours after the subject had received a total of 80 mg rizatriptan (administered over four hours).

In addition, based on the pharmacology of rizatriptan, hypertension or other more serious cardiovascular symptoms could occur after overdosage. Gastrointestinal decontamination, (i.e., gastric lavage followed by activated charcoal) should be considered in patients suspected of an overdose with MAXALT. Clinical and electrocardiographic monitoring should be continued for at least 12 hours, even if clinical symptoms are not observed.

The effects of hemo- or peritoneal dialysis on serum concentrations of rizatriptan are unknown.

DOSAGE AND ADMINISTRATION

In controlled clinical trials, single doses of 5 and 10 mg of MAXALT Tablets or MAXALT-MLT were effective for the acute treatment of migraines in adults. There is evidence that the 10-mg dose may provide a greater effect than the 5-mg dose (see CLINICAL PHARMACOLOGY, Clinical Studies). Individuals may vary in response to doses of MAXALT Tablets. The choice of dose should therefore be made on an individual basis, weighing the possible benefit of the 10-mg dose with the potential risk for increased adverse events.

Redosing: Doses should be separated by at least 2 hours; no more than 30 mg should be taken in any 24-hour period. The safety of treating, on average, more than four headaches in a 30-day period has not been established.

Patients receiving propranolol: In patients receiving propranolol, the 5-mg dose of MAXALT should be used, up to a maximum of 3 doses in any 24-hour period. (See CLINICAL PHARMACOLOGY, Drug Interactions.)

For MAXALT-MLT Orally Disintegrating Tablets, administration with liquid is not necessary. The orally disintegrating tablet is packaged in a blister within an outer aluminum pouch. Patients should be instructed not to remove the blister from the outer pouch until just prior to dosing. The blister pack should then be peeled open with dry hands and the orally disintegrating tablet placed on the tongue, where it will dissolve and be swallowed with the saliva.

HOW SUPPLIED

No. 3732—MAXALT Tablets, 5 mg, are pale pink, capsule-shaped, compressed tablets coded MRK on one side and 266 on the other. They are supplied as follows:
NDC 0006-0266-12, carton of 12 tablets.

No. 3733—MAXALT Tablets, 10 mg, are pale pink, capsule-shaped, compressed tablets coded MAXALT on one side and MRK 267 on the other. They are supplied as follows:
NDC 0006-0267-12, carton of 12 tablets.

No. 3800—MAXALT-MLT Orally Disintegrating Tablets, 5 mg, are white to off-white, round lyophilized orally disintegrating tablets debossed with a modified triangle on one side, and measuring 10.0-11.5 mm (side-to-side) with a peppermint flavor. Each orally disintegrating tablet is individually packaged in a blister inside an aluminum pouch (sachet). They are supplied as follows:
NDC 0006-3800-12, 4 × unit of use carrying case of 3 orally disintegrating tablets (12 tablets total).

No. 3801—MAXALT-MLT Orally Disintegrating Tablets, 10 mg, are white to off-white, round lyophilized orally disintegrating tablets debossed with a modified square on one side, and measuring 12.0-13.8 mm (side-to-side) with a peppermint flavor. Each orally disintegrating tablet is individually packaged in a blister inside an aluminum pouch (sachet). They are supplied as follows:
NDC 0006-3801-12, 4 × unit of use carrying case of 3 orally disintegrating tablets (12 tablets total).

Storage

Store MAXALT Tablets at room temperature, 15-30°C (59-86°F). Dispense in a tight container, if product is subdivided.

Store MAXALT-MLT Orally Disintegrating Tablets at room temperature, 15-30°C (59-86°F). The patient should be instructed not to remove the blister from the outer aluminum pouch until the patient is ready to consume the orally disintegrating tablet inside.

MAXALT Tablets are manufactured for:
Merck Sharp & Dohme Corp., a subsidiary of
MERCK & CO., INC., Whitehouse Station, NJ 08889, USA
By:
MSD, Ltd. Cramlington
Northumberland, NE23 3JU, UK

MAXALT-MLT Orally Disintegrating Tablets are manufactured for:
Merck Sharp & Dohme Corp., a subsidiary of
MERCK & CO., INC., Whitehouse Station, NJ 08889, USA
By:
Catalent UK Swindon, Zydis Ltd.
Swindon, Wiltshire, SN5 8RU, UK
US Patent No.: 5,298,520
Issued December 2009
9652507

PATIENT PACKAGE INSERT

Patient Information about
MAXALT® (max-awlt) and **MAXALT-MLT®**
for Migraine
Generic name: rizatriptan benzoate
Please read this information before you start taking MAXALT[1]. Also, read the leaflet each time you renew your prescription, just in case anything has changed. Remember, this leaflet does not take the place of careful discussions with your doctor. You and your doctor should discuss MAXALT when you start taking your medication and at regular checkups.

What is MAXALT and what is it used for?

MAXALT is a medication used for the treatment of migraine attacks in adults. MAXALT is a member of a class of drugs called selective 5-HT$_{1B/1D}$ receptor agonists.

It is available as a traditional tablet (MAXALT) and as an orally disintegrating tablet (MAXALT-MLT[1]). Unless otherwise stated, the information contained in this leaflet applies both to MAXALT Tablets and to MAXALT-MLT Orally Disintegrating Tablets.

Tell your doctor about your symptoms. Your doctor will decide if you have migraine. Use MAXALT only for a migraine attack. MAXALT should not be used to treat headaches that might be caused by other, more serious conditions.

You will find more information about migraine at the end of this leaflet.

How should I take MAXALT?

Your doctor has prescribed either a 5-mg or 10-mg dosage of MAXALT or MAXALT-MLT for your migraine attack. When you have a migraine headache, take your medication as directed by your doctor.

MAXALT Tablets

If you are using MAXALT Tablets, swallow the tablet whole with liquid.

MAXALT-MLT Orally Disintegrating Tablets

If you are using MAXALT-MLT, leave the orally disintegrating tablet in its package until you are ready to take it. Remove the blister from the foil pouch. Do not push the tablet through the blister; rather, peel open the blister pack with dry hands and place the tablet on your tongue. The tablet will dissolve rapidly and be swallowed with your saliva. No liquid is needed to take the orally disintegrating tablet.

If your headache comes back after your initial dose, a second dose may be taken anytime after 2 hours of administering the first dose. For any attack where you have no re-

sponse to the first dose, do not take a second dose without first consulting with your doctor. Do not take more than 30 mg of MAXALT in a 24-hour period (for example, do not take more than three 10-mg tablets in a 24-hour period).

If you are receiving propranolol, you should use the 5-mg dose of MAXALT or MAXALT-MLT, up to a maximum of 3 doses (15 mg total) in a 24-hour period.

If your condition worsens, seek medical attention.

Who should not take MAXALT?

Do not take MAXALT if you:

- have had a serious allergic reaction to MAXALT or any of its ingredients
- have uncontrolled high blood pressure
- have heart disease or history of heart disease
- are currently taking monoamine oxidase (MAO) inhibitors[2] such as phenelzine sulfate (NARDIL®) or tranylcypromine sulfate (PARNATE®) for mental depression, or have taken MAO inhibitors within the last two weeks.

MAXALT should not be used within 24 hours of treatment with another 5-HT$_1$ agonist[2] such as sumatriptan (IMITREX®), naratriptan (AMERGE™) or zolmitriptan (ZOMIG™); or ergotamine-type medications such as ergotamine (BELLERGAL-S®, CAFERGOT®, ERGOMAR®, WIGRAINE®), dihydro-ergotamine (D.H.E. 45®), or methysergide (SANSERT®).

[2] The brands listed are the trademarks of their respective owners and are not trademarks of Merck Sharp & Dohme Corp., a subsidiary of **Merck & Co., Inc.**

What should I tell my doctor before and during treatment with MAXALT?

Tell your doctor:

- about any past or present medical problems
- about any history of high blood pressure, chest pain, shortness of breath, heart disease, or stroke
- about any risk factors for heart disease or blood vessel disease
  - high blood pressure or diabetes
  - high cholesterol
  - obesity
  - smoking
  - family history of heart disease or blood vessel disease
  - post menopausal
  - male over 40
- about any allergies you have or have had
- if you are pregnant or plan to become pregnant
- if you are breast-feeding or plan to breast-feed
- about all drugs you are taking or plan to take, including those obtained without a prescription, and those you normally take for a migraine
- if you take selective serotonin reuptake inhibitors (SSRIs) or serotonin norepinephrine reuptake inhibitors (SNRIs), two types of drugs for depression or other disorders. Common SSRIs[2] are CELEXA® (citalopram HBr), LEXAPRO® (escitalopram oxalate), PAXIL® (paroxetine), PROZAC®/SARAFEM® (fluoxetine), SYMBYAX® (olanzapine/fluoxetine), ZOLOFT® (sertraline), and fluvoxamine. Common SNRIs[2] are CYMBALTA® (duloxetine) and EFFEXOR® (venlafaxine).

MAXALT-MLT orally disintegrating tablets contain aspartame, a source of phenylalanine.

Phenylketonurics: MAXALT-MLT 5-mg and 10-mg orally disintegrating tablets contain 1.05 and 2.10 mg phenylalanine, respectively.

What if I am pregnant?

Do not use MAXALT if you are pregnant, think you might be pregnant, are trying to become pregnant, or are not using adequate contraception, unless you have discussed this with your doctor.

Can I take MAXALT with other medications[2]?

Do not take MAXALT with any other drug in the same class within 24 hours, such as sumatriptan (IMITREX®), naratriptan (AMERGE™) or zolmitriptan (ZOMIG™).

Do not take MAXALT within 24 hours of taking ergotamine-type medications such as ergotamine (BELLERGAL-S®, CAFERGOT®, ERGOMAR®, WIGRAINE®), dihydroergotamine (D.H.E. 45®) or methysergide (SANSERT®) to treat your migraine.

Do not take MAXALT when you are taking monoamine oxidase (MAO) inhibitors, such as phenelzine sulfate (NARDIL®) or tranylcypromine sulfate (PARNATE®) for mental depression, or if it has been less than two weeks since you stopped taking an MAO inhibitor.

Ask your doctor for instructions about taking MAXALT if you are now taking propranolol (INDERAL®). (See **How should I take MAXALT?** section.)

Ask your doctor for instructions about taking MAXALT if you are now taking selective serotonin reuptake inhibitors (SSRIs) or serotonin norepinephrine reuptake inhibitors (SNRIs), two types of drugs for depression or other disorders. (See **What should I tell my doctor before and during treatment with MAXALT?** section.)

What are the possible side effects of MAXALT?
Like all prescription drugs, MAXALT can cause side effects. In studies, MAXALT was generally well-tolerated. The side effects were usually mild and temporary. The following is **not** a complete list of side effects reported with MAXALT. Do not rely on this leaflet alone for information about side effects. Ask your doctor to discuss with you the more complete list of side effects.
In studies, the **most common** side effects reported were:
- **dizziness**
- **sleepiness, tiredness, fatigue**
- **pain or pressure sensation (e.g., in the chest or throat)**

If you experience dizziness, sleepiness, tiredness or fatigue, you should evaluate your ability to perform complex tasks such as driving or operating heavy machinery.
Other, **less common** side effects reported in studies or general use were related to the:
Heart and blood vessels-Alterations in heartbeat, increased blood pressure and spasm of blood vessels of the extremities including coldness and numbness of the hands or feet.
Muscles-Muscle weakness, stiffness, and spasm; and muscle and bone pain.
Nervous system-Nervousness, decreased mental sharpness, tremor, headache, abnormal sensation, vertigo, sleep disturbance, mood and personality changes, alterations in speech and movement, memory impairment, confusion, dream abnormality and seizure.
Digestive system-Stomach upset, diarrhea, dry mouth, constipation, gas, thirst, acid reflux, difficulty swallowing, changes in appetite, burping and inability of the tongue to move.
Skin-Flushing (redness of the face lasting a short time), hot flashes, sweating, itching, rash, acne and skin reaction to sunlight.
Respiratory-Difficult or rapid breathing, dryness or discomfort of the throat or nose, nosebleed, yawning and sinus disorder, cold-like symptoms, cough, and hiccups.
Special Senses-Visual disturbances, ringing in the ears, ear pain, eye discomfort, swelling or tearing, alterations in hearing and smelling, visual intolerance to light, and bad taste.
Miscellaneous-Allergic reactions including swelling of face, lips, tongue and/or throat which may cause difficulty in breathing and/or swallowing, wheezing, hives, rash, and severe sloughing of the skin. Also chills, heat sensitivity, swelling, bloating, hangover effect, fever, fainting, dizziness on standing up, warm/cold sensations, dehydration and changes in urination and menstruation.
As with other drugs in this class, there have been very rare reports of heart attack and stroke generally occurring in patients with risk factors for heart and blood vessel disease (see **What should I tell my doctor before and during treatment with MAXALT?**).
Tell your doctor about these or any other symptoms. If the symptoms persist or worsen, seek medical attention promptly. In addition, tell your doctor if you experience any symptoms that suggest an allergic reaction (see **Miscellaneous** above) after taking MAXALT.
What should I do if I take an overdose?
If you take more medication than you have been told to take, you should contact your doctor, hospital emergency department, or nearest poison control center immediately.
What is migraine and how does it differ from other headaches?
Migraine is an intense, throbbing, typically one-sided headache that often includes nausea, vomiting, sensitivity to light, and sensitivity to sound. According to many migraine sufferers, the pain and symptoms from a migraine headache are more intense than the pain and symptoms of a common headache.
Some people may have visual symptoms before the headache, such as flashing lights or wavy lines, called an aura. Migraine attacks typically last for hours or, rarely, for more than a day, and they can return frequently. The severity and frequency of migraine attacks may vary.
Based on your symptoms, your doctor will decide whether you have migraine.
Who gets migraine?
Migraine headaches tend to occur in members of the same family. Both men and women get migraine, but it is more common in women.
What may trigger a migraine attack?
Certain things are thought to trigger migraine attacks in some people. Some of these triggers are:
- certain foods or beverages (e.g., cheese, chocolate, citrus fruit, caffeine, alcohol)
- stress
- change in a behavior (e.g., under/oversleeping; missing a meal; change in diet)
- hormonal changes in women (e.g., menstruation)

You may be able to prevent migraine attacks or diminish their frequency if you understand what specifically triggers your attacks. Keeping a headache diary may help you identify and monitor the possible migraine triggers you encounter. Once the triggers are identified, you and your doctor can modify your treatment and lifestyle appropriately.
How does MAXALT work during a migraine attack?
Treatment with MAXALT:
1. Reduces swelling of blood vessels surrounding the brain. This swelling results in the headache pain of a migraine attack.
2. Blocks the release of substances from nerve endings that cause more pain and other symptoms of migraine.
3. Interrupts the sending of specific pain signals to your brain.

It is thought that each of these actions contributes to relief of your symptoms by MAXALT.
How should I store MAXALT?
Keep your medicine in a safe place where children cannot reach it. It may be harmful to children. Store your medication away from heat, light, moisture, and at a controlled room temperature 59°-86°F (15°-30°C). If your medication has expired, throw it away as instructed. If your doctor decides to stop your treatment, do not keep any leftover medicine unless your doctor tells you to do so. Throw away your medicine as instructed. Be sure that the discarded tablets are out of the reach of children.
If you are storing MAXALT-MLT, do not remove the blister from the outer aluminum pouch until you are ready to take the medication inside.
This leaflet provides a summary of information about MAXALT. If you have any questions or concerns about either MAXALT or migraine, talk to your doctor. In addition, talk to your pharmacist or other health care provider.
MAXALT Tablets are manufactured for:
Merck Sharp & Dohme Corp., a subsidiary of
MERCK & CO., INC., Whitehouse Station, NJ 08889, USA
By:
MSD, Ltd. Cramlington
Northumberland, NE23 3JU, UK
MAXALT-MLT Orally Disintegrating Tablets are manufactured for:
Merck Sharp & Dohme Corp., a subsidiary of
MERCK & CO., INC., Whitehouse Station, NJ 08889, USA
By:
Catalent UK Swindon, Zydis Ltd.
Swindon, Wiltshire, SN5 8RU, UK
US Patent No.: 5,298,520
Issued December 2009
9652507
Shown in Product Identification Guide, page 313

MEVACOR® ℞

[mevacor]
(lovastin)
Tablets

DESCRIPTION

MEVACOR[1] (Lovastatin) is a cholesterol lowering agent isolated from a strain of *Aspergillus terreus.* After oral ingestion, lovastatin, which is an inactive lactone, is hydrolyzed to the corresponding β-hydroxyacid form. This is a principal metabolite and an inhibitor of 3-hydroxy-3-methylglutaryl-coenzyme A (HMG-CoA) reductase. This enzyme catalyzes the conversion of HMG-CoA to mevalonate, which is an early and rate limiting step in the biosynthesis of cholesterol.
Lovastatin is [1*S* -[1α(*R**),3α,7β,8β(2*S**,4*S**),8aβ]]-1,2,3,7,8,8a-hexahydro-3,7-dimethyl-8-[2-(tetrahydro-4-hydroxy-6-oxo-2*H*-pyran-2-yl)ethyl]-1-naphthalenyl 2-methylbutanoate. The empirical formula of lovastatin is $C_{24}H_{36}O_5$ and its molecular weight is 404.55. Its structural formula is:

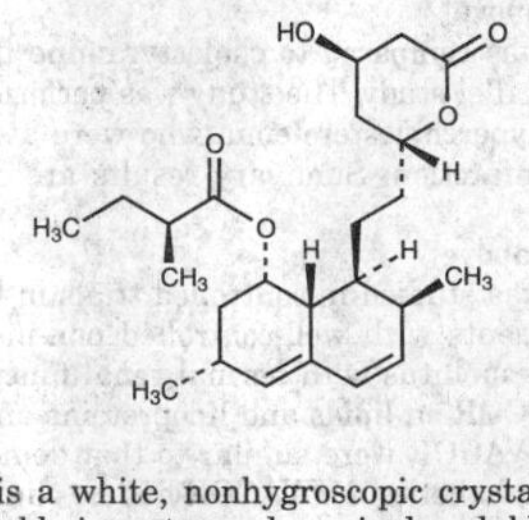

Lovastatin is a white, nonhygroscopic crystalline powder that is insoluble in water and sparingly soluble in ethanol, methanol, and acetonitrile.
Tablets MEVACOR are supplied as 20 mg and 40 mg tablets for oral administration. In addition to the active ingredient lovastatin, each tablet contains the following inactive ingredients: cellulose, lactose, magnesium stearate, and starch. Butylated hydroxyanisole (BHA) is added as a preservative. Tablets MEVACOR 20 mg also contain FD&C Blue 2 aluminum lake. Tablets MEVACOR 40 mg also contain D&C Yellow 10 aluminum lake and FD&C Blue 2 aluminum lake.

[1] Registered trademark of Merck Sharp & Dohme Corp., a subsidiary of **Merck & Co., Inc.**

CLINICAL PHARMACOLOGY

The involvement of low-density lipoprotein cholesterol (LDL–C) in atherogenesis has been well-documented in clinical and pathological studies, as well as in many animal experiments. Epidemiological and clinical studies have established that high LDL–C and low high-density lipoprotein cholesterol (HDL–C) are both associated with coronary heart disease. However, the risk of developing coronary heart disease is continuous and graded over the range of cholesterol levels and many coronary events do occur in patients with total cholesterol (total–C) and LDL–C in the lower end of this range.
MEVACOR has been shown to reduce both normal and elevated LDL–C concentrations. LDL is formed from very low-density lipoprotein (VLDL) and is catabolized predominantly by the high affinity LDL receptor. The mechanism of the LDL-lowering effect of MEVACOR may involve both reduction of VLDL–C concentration, and induction of the LDL receptor, leading to reduced production and/or increased catabolism of LDL–C. Apolipoprotein B also falls substantially during treatment with MEVACOR. Since each LDL particle contains one molecule of apolipoprotein B, and since little apolipoprotein B is found in other lipoproteins, this strongly suggests that MEVACOR does not merely cause cholesterol to be lost from LDL, but also reduces the concentration of circulating LDL particles. In addition, MEVACOR can produce increases of variable magnitude in HDL–C, and modestly reduces VLDL–C and plasma triglycerides (TG) (see Tables I-III under Clinical Studies). The effects of MEVACOR on Lp(a), fibrinogen, and certain other independent biochemical risk markers for coronary heart disease are unknown.
MEVACOR is a specific inhibitor of HMG–CoA reductase, the enzyme which catalyzes the conversion of HMG–CoA to mevalonate. The conversion of HMG–CoA to mevalonate is an early step in the biosynthetic pathway for cholesterol.
Pharmacokinetics
Lovastatin is a lactone which is readily hydrolyzed *in vivo* to the corresponding β–hydroxyacid, a potent inhibitor of HMG–CoA reductase. Inhibition of HMG–CoA reductase is the basis for an assay in pharmacokinetic studies of the β–hydroxyacid metabolites (active inhibitors) and, following base hydrolysis, active plus latent inhibitors (total inhibitors) in plasma following administration of lovastatin.
Following an oral dose of ^{14}C–labeled lovastatin in man, 10% of the dose was excreted in urine and 83% in feces. The latter represents absorbed drug equivalents excreted in bile, as well as any unabsorbed drug. Plasma concentrations of total radioactivity (lovastatin plus ^{14}C–metabolites) peaked at 2 hours and declined rapidly to about 10% of peak by 24 hours postdose. Absorption of lovastatin, estimated relative to an intravenous reference dose, in each of four animal species tested, averaged about 30% of an oral dose. In animal studies, after oral dosing, lovastatin had high selectivity for the liver, where it achieved substantially higher concentrations than in non-target tissues. Lovastatin undergoes extensive first-pass extraction in the liver, its primary site of action, with subsequent excretion of drug equivalents in the bile. As a consequence of extensive hepatic extraction of lovastatin, the availability of drug to the general circulation is low and variable. In a single dose study in four hypercholesterolemic patients, it was estimated that less than 5% of an oral dose of lovastatin reaches the general circulation as active inhibitors. Following administration of lovastatin tablets the coefficient of variation, based on between-subject variability, was approximately 40% for the area under the curve (AUC) of total inhibitory activity in the general circulation.
Both lovastatin and its β–hydroxyacid metabolite are highly bound (>95%) to human plasma proteins. Animal studies demonstrated that lovastatin crosses the blood-brain and placental barriers.
The major active metabolites present in human plasma are the β–hydroxyacid of lovastatin, its 6′–hydroxy derivative, and two additional metabolites. Peak plasma concentrations of both active and total inhibitors were attained within 2 to 4 hours of dose administration. While the recommended therapeutic dose range is 10 to 80 mg/day, linearity of inhibitory activity in the general circulation was established by a single dose study employing lovastatin tablet dosages from 60 to as high as 120 mg. With a once-a-day dosing regimen, plasma concentrations of total inhibitors over a dosing interval achieved a steady state between the second and third days of therapy and were about 1.5 times those following a single dose. When lovastatin was given under fasting conditions, plasma concentrations of

TABLE I: MEVACOR vs. Placebo (Mean Percent Change from Baseline After 6 Weeks)

DOSAGE	N	TOTAL-C	LDL-C	HDL-C	LDL-C/HDL-C	TOTAL-C/HDL-C	TG.
Placebo	33	−2	−1	−1	0	+1	+9
MEVACOR							
10 mg q.p.m.	33	−16	−21	+5	−24	−19	−10
20 mg q.p.m.	33	−19	−27	+6	−30	−23	+9
10 mg b.i.d.	32	−19	−28	+8	−33	−25	−7
40 mg q.p.m.	33	−22	−31	+5	−33	−25	−8
20 mg b.i.d.	36	−24	−32	+2	−32	−24	−6

TABLE II: MEVACOR vs. Cholestyramine (Percent Change from Baseline After 12 Weeks)

TREATMENT	N	TOTAL-C (mean)	LDL-C (mean)	HDL-C (mean)	LDL-C/HDL-C (mean)	TOTAL-C/HDL-C (mean)	VLDL-C (median)	TG. (mean)
MEVACOR								
20 mg b.i.d.	85	−27	−32	+9	−36	−31	−34	−21
40 mg b.i.d.	88	−34	−42	+8	−44	−37	−31	−27
Cholestyramine								
12 g b.i.d.	88	−17	−23	+8	−27	−21	+2	+11

TABLE III: MEVACOR vs. Placebo (Percent Change from Baseline—Average Values Between Weeks 12 and 48)

DOSAGE	N*	TOTAL-C (mean)	LDL-C (mean)	HDL-C (mean)	LDL-C/HDL-C (mean)	TOTAL-C/HDL-C (mean)	TG. (median)
Placebo	1663	+0.7	+0.4	+2.0	+0.2	+0.6	+4
MEVACOR							
20 mg q.p.m.	1642	−17	−24	+6.6	−27	−21	−10
40 mg q.p.m.	1645	−22	−30	+7.2	−34	−26	−14
20 mg b.i.d.	1646	−24	−34	+8.6	−38	−29	−16
40 mg b.i.d.	1649	−29	−40	+9.5	−44	−34	−19

*Patients enrolled.

total inhibitors were on average about two-thirds those found when lovastatin was administered immediately after a standard test meal.

In a study of patients with severe renal insufficiency (creatinine clearance 10–30 mL/min), the plasma concentrations of total inhibitors after a single dose of lovastatin were approximately two-fold higher than those in healthy volunteers.

In a study including 16 elderly patients between 70–78 years of age who received MEVACOR 80 mg/day, the mean plasma level of HMG–CoA reductase inhibitory activity was increased approximately 45% compared with 18 patients between 18–30 years of age (see PRECAUTIONS, Geriatric Use).

Although the mechanism is not fully understood, cyclosporine has been shown to increase the AUC of HMG-CoA reductase inhibitors. The increase in AUC for lovastatin and lovastatin acid is presumably due, in part, to inhibition of CYP3A4.

The risk of myopathy is increased by high levels of HMG–CoA reductase inhibitory activity in plasma. Potent inhibitors of CYP3A4 can raise the plasma levels of HMG–CoA reductase inhibitory activity and increase the risk of myopathy (see WARNINGS, Myopathy/Rhabdomyolysis and PRECAUTIONS, Drug Interactions).

Lovastatin is a substrate for cytochrome P450 isoform 3A4 (CYP3A4) (see PRECAUTIONS, Drug Interactions). Grapefruit juice contains one or more components that inhibit CYP3A4 and can increase the plasma concentrations of drugs metabolized by CYP3A4. In one study[2], 10 subjects consumed 200 mL of double-strength grapefruit juice (one can of frozen concentrate diluted with one rather than 3 cans of water) three times daily for 2 days and an additional 200 mL double-strength grapefruit juice together with and 30 and 90 minutes following a single dose of 80 mg lovastatin on the third day. This regimen of grapefruit juice resulted in a mean increase in the serum concentration of lovastatin and its β-hydroxyacid metabolite (as measured by the area under the concentration-time curve) of 15–fold and 5–fold, respectively [as measured using a chemical assay—high performance liquid chromatography]. In a second study, 15 subjects consumed one 8 oz glass of single-strength grapefruit juice (one can of frozen concentrate diluted with 3 cans of water) with breakfast for 3 consecutive days and a single dose of 40 mg lovastatin in the evening of the third day. This regimen of grapefruit juice resulted in a mean increase in the plasma concentration (as measured by the area under the concentration-time curve) of active and total HMG–CoA reductase inhibitory activity [using an enzyme inhibition assay both before (for active inhibitors) and after (for total inhibitors) base hydrolysis] of 1.34–fold and 1.36–fold, respectively, and of lovastatin and its β–hydroxy-

acid metabolite [measured using a chemical assay—liquid chromatography/tandem mass spectrometry —different from that used in the first[2] study] of 1.94–fold and 1.57–fold, respectively. The effect of amounts of grapefruit juice between those used in these two studies on lovastatin pharmacokinetics has not been studied.

[2] Kantola, T, et al., Clin Pharmacol Ther 1998; 63(4): 397–402.

Clinical Studies in Adults

MEVACOR has been shown to be highly effective in reducing total–C and LDL–C in heterozygous familial and non-familial forms of primary hypercholesterolemia and in mixed hyperlipidemia. A marked response was seen within 2 weeks, and the maximum therapeutic response occurred within 4-6 weeks. The response was maintained during continuation of therapy. Single daily doses given in the evening were more effective than the same dose given in the morning, perhaps because cholesterol is synthesized mainly at night.

In multicenter, double-blind studies in patients with familial or non-familial hypercholesterolemia, MEVACOR, administered in doses ranging from 10 mg q.p.m. to 40 mg b.i.d., was compared to placebo. MEVACOR consistently and significantly decreased plasma total–C, LDL–C, total–C/HDL–C ratio and LDL–C/HDL–C ratio. In addition, MEVACOR produced increases of variable magnitude in HDL–C, and modestly decreased VLDL–C and plasma TG (see Tables I through III for dose response results).

The results of a study in patients with primary hypercholesterolemia are presented in Table I.

[See table I above]

MEVACOR was compared to cholestyramine in a randomized open parallel study. The study was performed with patients with hypercholesterolemia who were at high risk of myocardial infarction. Summary results are presented in Table II.

[See table II above]

MEVACOR was studied in controlled trials in hypercholesterolemic patients with well-controlled non-insulin dependent diabetes mellitus with normal renal function. The effect of MEVACOR on lipids and lipoproteins and the safety profile of MEVACOR were similar to that demonstrated in studies in nondiabetics. MEVACOR had no clinically important effect on glycemic control or on the dose requirement of oral hypoglycemic agents.

Expanded Clinical Evaluation of Lovastatin (EXCEL) Study

MEVACOR was compared to placebo in 8,245 patients with hypercholesterolemia (total-C 240-300 mg/dL [6.2 mmol/L-7.6 mmol/L], LDL–C >160 mg/dL [4.1 mmol/L]) in the randomized, double-blind, parallel, 48–week EXCEL study. All changes in the lipid measurements (Table III) in

MEVACOR treated patients were dose-related and significantly different from placebo (p≤0.001). These results were sustained throughout the study.

[See table III at left]

Air Force/Texas Coronary Atherosclerosis Prevention Study (AFCAPS/TexCAPS)

The Air Force/Texas Coronary Atherosclerosis Prevention Study (AFCAPS/TexCAPS), a double-blind, randomized, placebo-controlled, primary prevention study, demonstrated that treatment with MEVACOR decreased the rate of acute major coronary events (composite endpoint of myocardial infarction, unstable angina, and sudden cardiac death) compared with placebo during a median of 5.1 years of follow-up. Participants were middle-aged and elderly men (ages 45-73) and women (ages 55-73) without symptomatic cardiovascular disease with average to moderately elevated total–C and LDL–C, below average HDL–C, and who were at high risk based on elevated total–C/HDL–C. In addition to age, 63% of the participants had at least one other risk factor (baseline HDL–C <35 mg/dL, hypertension, family history, smoking and diabetes).

AFCAPS/TexCAPS enrolled 6,605 participants (5,608 men, 997 women) based on the following lipid entry criteria: total–C range of 180-264 mg/dL, LDL–C range of 130-190 mg/dL, HDL–C of ≤45 mg/dL for men and ≤47 mg/dL for women, and TG of ≤400 mg/dL. Participants were treated with standard care, including diet, and either MEVACOR 20-40 mg daily (n=3,304) or placebo (n=3,301). Approximately 50% of the participants treated with MEVACOR were titrated to 40 mg daily when their LDL–C remained >110 mg/dL at the 20–mg starting dose.

MEVACOR reduced the risk of a first acute major coronary event, the primary efficacy endpoint, by 37% (MEVACOR 3.5%, placebo 5.5%; p<0.001; Figure 1). A first acute major coronary event was defined as myocardial infarction (54 participants on MEVACOR, 94 on placebo) or unstable angina (54 vs. 80) or sudden cardiac death (8 vs. 9). Furthermore, among the secondary endpoints, MEVACOR reduced the risk of unstable angina by 32% (1.8 vs. 2.6%; p=0.023), of myocardial infarction by 40% (1.7 vs. 2.9%; p=0.002), and of undergoing coronary revascularization procedures (e.g., coronary artery bypass grafting or percutaneous transluminal coronary angioplasty) by 33% (3.2 vs. 4.8%; p=0.001). Trends in risk reduction associated with treatment with MEVACOR were consistent across men and women, smokers and non-smokers, hypertensives and non-hypertensives, and older and younger participants. Participants with ≥2 risk factors had risk reductions (RR) in both acute major coronary events (RR 43%) and coronary revascularization procedures (RR 37%). Because there were too few events among those participants with age as their only risk factor in this study, the effect of MEVACOR on outcomes could not be adequately assessed in this subgroup.

Figure 1: Acute Major Coronary Events (Primary Endpoint)

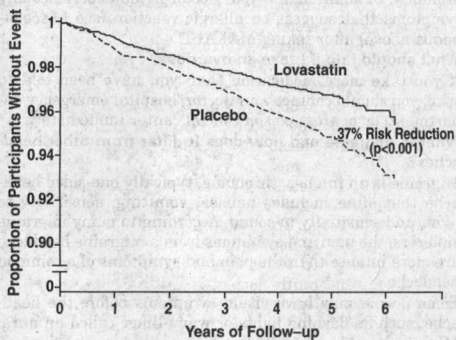

Atherosclerosis

In the Canadian Coronary Atherosclerosis Intervention Trial (CCAIT), the effect of therapy with lovastatin on coronary atherosclerosis was assessed by coronary angiography in hyperlipidemic patients. In the randomized, double-blind, controlled clinical trial, patients were treated with conventional measures (usually diet and 325 mg of aspirin every other day) and either lovastatin 20-80 mg daily or placebo. Angiograms were evaluated at baseline and at two years by computerized quantitative coronary angiography (QCA). Lovastatin significantly slowed the progression of lesions as measured by the mean change per-patient in minimum lumen diameter (the primary endpoint) and percent diameter stenosis, and decreased the proportions of patients categorized with disease progression (33% vs. 50%) and with new lesions (16% vs. 32%).

In a similarly designed trial, the Monitored Atherosclerosis Regression Study (MARS), patients were treated with diet and either lovastatin 80 mg daily or placebo. No statistically significant difference between lovastatin and placebo was seen for the primary endpoint (mean change per patient in percent diameter stenosis of all lesions), or for most secondary QCA endpoints. Visual assessment by angiographers who formed a consensus opinion of overall angiographic change (Global Change Score) was also a secondary endpoint. By this endpoint, significant slowing of disease was seen, with regression in 23% of patients treated with lovastatin compared to 11% of placebo patients.

In the Familial Atherosclerosis Treatment Study (FATS), either lovastatin or niacin in combination with a bile acid sequestrant for 2.5 years in hyperlipidemic subjects significantly reduced the frequency of progression and increased the frequency of regression of coronary atherosclerotic lesions by QCA compared to diet and, in some cases, low-dose resin.

The effect of lovastatin on the progression of atherosclerosis in the coronary arteries has been corroborated by similar findings in another vasculature. In the Asymptomatic Carotid Artery Progression Study (ACAPS), the effect of therapy with lovastatin on carotid atherosclerosis was assessed by B–mode ultrasonography in hyperlipidemic patients with early carotid lesions and without known coronary heart disease at baseline. In this double-blind, controlled clinical trial, 919 patients were randomized in a 2 × 2 factorial design to placebo, lovastatin 10-40 mg daily and/or warfarin. Ultrasonograms of the carotid walls were used to determine the change per patient from baseline to three years in mean maximum intimal-medial thickness (IMT) of 12 measured segments. There was a significant regression of carotid lesions in patients receiving lovastatin alone compared to those receiving placebo alone (p=0.001). The predictive value of changes in IMT for stroke has not yet been established. In the lovastatin group there was a significant reduction in the number of patients with major cardiovascular events relative to the placebo group (5 vs. 14) and a significant reduction in all-cause mortality (1 vs. 8).

Eye
There was a high prevalence of baseline lenticular opacities in the patient population included in the early clinical trials with lovastatin. During these trials the appearance of new opacities was noted in both the lovastatin and placebo groups. There was no clinically significant change in visual acuity in the patients who had new opacities reported nor was any patient, including those with opacities noted at baseline, discontinued from therapy because of a decrease in visual acuity.

A three–year, double-blind, placebo-controlled study in hypercholesterolemic patients to assess the effect of lovastatin on the human lens demonstrated that there were no clinically or statistically significant differences between the lovastatin and placebo groups in the incidence, type or progression of lenticular opacities. There are no controlled clinical data assessing the lens available for treatment beyond three years.

Clinical Studies in Adolescent Patients
Efficacy of Lovastatin in Adolescent Boys with Heterozygous Familial Hypercholesterolemia
In a double-blind, placebo-controlled study, 132 boys 10-17 years of age (mean age 12.7 yrs) with heterozygous familial hypercholesterolemia (heFH) were randomized to lovastatin (n=67) or placebo (n=65) for 48 weeks. Inclusion in the study required a baseline LDL–C level between 189 and 500 mg/dL and at least one parent with an LDL–C level >189 mg/dL. The mean baseline LDL–C value was 253.1 mg/dL (range: 171-379 mg/dL) in the MEVACOR group compared to 248.2 mg/dL (range: 158.5-413.5 mg/dL) in the placebo group. The dosage of lovastatin (once daily in the evening) was 10 mg for the first 8 weeks, 20 mg for the second 8 weeks, and 40 mg thereafter.

MEVACOR significantly decreased plasma levels of total–C, LDL–C and apolipoprotein B (see Table IV).

[See table IV above]

The mean achieved LDL–C value was 190.9 mg/dL (range: 108-336 mg/dL) in the MEVACOR group compared to 244.8 mg/dL (range: 135-404 mg/dL) in the placebo group.

Efficacy of Lovastatin in Post-Menarchal Girls with Heterozygous Familial Hypercholesterolemia
In a double-blind, placebo-controlled study, 54 girls 10-17 years of age who were at least 1 year post-menarche with heFH were randomized to lovastatin (n=35) or placebo (n=19) for 24 weeks. Inclusion in the study required a baseline LDL–C level of 160-400 mg/dL and a parental history of familial hypercholesterolemia. The mean baseline LDL–C value was 218.3 mg/dL (range: 136.3-363.7 mg/dL) in the MEVACOR group compared to 198.8 mg/dL (range: 151.1-283.1 mg/dL) in the placebo group. The dosage of lovastatin (once daily in the evening) was 20 mg for the first 4 weeks, and 40 mg thereafter.

MEVACOR significantly decreased plasma levels of total–C, LDL–C, and apolipoprotein B (see Table V).

[See table V above]

The mean achieved LDL–C value was 154.5 mg/dL (range: 82-286 mg/dL) in the MEVACOR group compared to 203.5 mg/dL (range: 135-304 mg/dL) in the placebo group.

TABLE IV: Lipid-lowering Effects of Lovastatin in Adolescent Boys with Heterozygous Familial Hypercholesterolemia (Mean Percent Change from Baseline at Week 48 in Intention-to-Treat Population)

DOSAGE	N	TOTAL-C	LDL-C	HDL-C	TG.*	Apolipoprotein B
Placebo	61	−1.1	−1.4	−2.2	−1.4	−4.4
MEVACOR	64	−19.3	−24.2	+1.1	−1.9	−21

*data presented as median percent changes

TABLE V: Lipid-lowering Effects of Lovastatin in Post-Menarchal Girls with Heterozygous Familial Hypercholesterolemia (Mean Percent Change from Baseline at Week 24 in Intention-to-Treat Population)

DOSAGE	N	TOTAL-C	LDL-C	HDL-C	TG.*	Apolipoprotein B
Placebo	18	+3.6	+2.5	+4.8	−3.0	+6.4
MEVACOR	35	−22.4	−29.2	+2.4	−22.7	−24.4

*data presented as median percent changes

NCEP Treatment Guidelines: LDL–C Goals and Cutpoints for Therapeutic Lifestyle Changes and Drug Therapy in Different Risk Categories

Risk Category	LDL Goal (mg/dL)	LDL Level at Which to Initiate Therapeutic Lifestyle Changes (mg/dL)	LDL Level at Which to Consider Drug Therapy (mg/dL)
CHD* or CHD risk equivalents (10-year risk >20%)	<100	≥100	≥130 (100–129: drug optional)†
2+ Risk factors (10 year-risk ≤20%)	<130	≥130	10-year risk 10–20%: ≥130 10-year risk <10%: ≥160
0–1 Risk factor‡	<160	≥160	≥190 (160–189: LDL-lowering drug optional)

*CHD, coronary heart disease
†Some authorities recommend use of LDL-lowering drugs in this category if an LDL–C level of <100 mg/dL cannot be achieved by therapeutic lifestyle changes. Others prefer use of drugs that primarily modify triglycerides and HDL–C, e.g., nicotinic acid and fibrate. Clinical judgment also may call for deferring drug therapy in this subcategory.
‡Almost all people with 0–1 risk factor have a 10-year risk <10%; thus, 10-year risk assessment in people with 0–1 risk factor is not necessary.

The safety and efficacy of doses above 40 mg daily have not been studied in children. The long-term efficacy of lovastatin therapy in childhood to reduce morbidity and mortality in adulthood has not been established.

INDICATIONS AND USAGE
Therapy with MEVACOR should be a component of multiple risk factor intervention in those individuals with dyslipidemia at risk for atherosclerotic vascular disease. MEVACOR should be used in addition to a diet restricted in saturated fat and cholesterol as part of a treatment strategy to lower total–C and LDL–C to target levels when the response to diet and other nonpharmacological measures alone has been inadequate to reduce risk.
Primary Prevention of Coronary Heart Disease
In individuals without symptomatic cardiovascular disease, average to moderately elevated total–C and LDL–C, and below average HDL–C, MEVACOR is indicated to reduce the risk of:
- Myocardial infarction
- Unstable angina
- Coronary revascularization procedures
(See CLINICAL PHARMACOLOGY, Clinical Studies.)
Coronary Heart Disease
MEVACOR is indicated to slow the progression of coronary atherosclerosis in patients with coronary heart disease as part of a treatment strategy to lower total–C and LDL–C to target levels.
Hypercholesterolemia
Therapy with lipid-altering agents should be a component of multiple risk factor intervention in those individuals at significantly increased risk for atherosclerotic vascular disease due to hypercholesterolemia. MEVACOR is indicated as an adjunct to diet for the reduction of elevated total–C and LDL–C levels in patients with primary hypercholesterolemia (Types IIa and IIb[3]), when the response to diet restricted in saturated fat and cholesterol and to other nonpharmacological measures alone has been inadequate.

---
[3] Classification of Hyperlipoproteinemias

Type	Lipoproteins elevated	Lipid Elevations major	minor
I	chylomicrons	TG	↑→C
IIa	LDL	C	—
IIb	LDL, VLDL	C	TG
III (rare)	IDL	C/TG	—
IV	VLDL	TG	↑→C
V (rare)	chylomicrons, VLDL	TG	↑→C

IDL = intermediate-density lipoprotein.

Adolescent Patients with Heterozygous Familial Hypercholesterolemia
MEVACOR is indicated as an adjunct to diet to reduce total–C, LDL–C and apolipoprotein B levels in adolescent boys and girls who are at least one year post-menarche, 10-17 years of age, with heFH if after an adequate trial of diet therapy the following findings are present:
1. LDL–C remains >189 mg/dL or
2. LDL–C remains >160 mg/dL and:
   • there is a positive family history of premature cardiovascular disease or
   • two or more other CVD risk factors are present in the adolescent patient
General Recommendations
Prior to initiating therapy with lovastatin, secondary causes for hypercholesterolemia (e.g., poorly controlled diabetes mellitus, hypothyroidism, nephrotic syndrome, dysproteinemias, obstructive liver disease, other drug therapy, alcoholism) should be excluded, and a lipid profile performed to measure total–C, HDL–C, and TG. For patients with TG less than 400 mg/dL (<4.5 mmol/L), LDL–C can be estimated using the following equation:
LDL–C = total–C − [0.2 × (TG) + HDL–C]
For TG levels >400 mg/dL (>4.5 mmol/L), this equation is less accurate and LDL–C concentrations should be determined by ultracentrifugation. In hypertriglyceridemic patients, LDL–C may be low or normal despite elevated total–C. In such cases, MEVACOR is not indicated.
The National Cholesterol Education Program (NCEP) Treatment Guidelines are summarized below:
[See third table above]
After the LDL–C goal has been achieved, if the TG is still ≥200 mg/dL, non-HDL–C (total–C minus HDL–C) becomes a secondary target of therapy. Non-HDL–C goals are set 30 mg/dL higher than LDL–C goals for each risk category. At the time of hospitalization for an acute coronary event, consideration can be given to initiating drug therapy at discharge if the LDL–C is ≥130 mg/dL (see NCEP Guidelines above).

Since the goal of treatment is to lower LDL-C, the NCEP recommends that LDL-C levels be used to initiate and assess treatment response. Only if LDL-C levels are not available, should the total-C be used to monitor therapy.

Although MEVACOR may be useful to reduce elevated LDL-C levels in patients with combined hypercholesterolemia and hypertriglyceridemia where hypercholesterolemia is the major abnormality (Type IIb hyperlipoproteinemia), it has not been studied in conditions where the major abnormality is elevation of chylomicrons, VLDL or IDL (i.e., hyperlipoproteinemia types I, III, IV, or V).[3]

The NCEP classification of cholesterol levels in pediatric patients with a familial history of hypercholesterolemia or premature cardiovascular disease is summarized below:

Category	Total-C (mg/dL)	LDL-C (mg/dL)
Acceptable	<170	<110
Borderline	170–199	110–129
High	≥200	≥130

Children treated with lovastatin in adolescence should be re-evaluated in adulthood and appropriate changes made to their cholesterol lowering regimen to achieve adult goals for LDL-C.

CONTRAINDICATIONS

Hypersensitivity to any component of this medication.

Active liver disease or unexplained persistent elevations of serum transaminases (see WARNINGS).

Pregnancy and lactation (see PRECAUTIONS, Pregnancy and Nursing Mothers). Atherosclerosis is a chronic process and the discontinuation of lipid-lowering drugs during pregnancy should have little impact on the outcome of long-term therapy of primary hypercholesterolemia. Moreover, cholesterol and other products of the cholesterol biosynthesis pathway are essential components for fetal development, including synthesis of steroids and cell membranes. Because of the ability of inhibitors of HMG–CoA reductase such as MEVACOR to decrease the synthesis of cholesterol and possibly other products of the cholesterol biosynthesis pathway, MEVACOR is contraindicated during pregnancy and in nursing mothers. **MEVACOR should be administered to women of childbearing age only when such patients are highly unlikely to conceive.** If the patient becomes pregnant while taking this drug, MEVACOR should be discontinued immediately and the patient should be apprised of the potential hazard to the fetus (see PRECAUTIONS, Pregnancy).

WARNINGS

Myopathy / Rhabdomyolysis

Lovastatin, like other inhibitors of HMG–CoA reductase, occasionally causes myopathy manifested as muscle pain, tenderness or weakness with creatine kinase (CK) above ten times the upper limit of normal (ULN). Myopathy sometimes takes the form of rhabdomyolysis with or without acute renal failure secondary to myoglobinuria, and rare fatalities have occurred. The risk of myopathy is increased by high levels of HMG–CoA reductase inhibitory activity in plasma.

As with other HMG-CoA reductase inhibitors, the risk of myopathy/rhabdomyolysis is dose related. In a clinical study (EXCEL) in which patients were carefully monitored and some interacting drugs were excluded, there was one case of myopathy among 4933 patients randomized to lovastatin 20-40 mg daily for 48 weeks, and 4 among 1649 patients randomized to 80 mg daily.

All patients starting therapy with lovastatin, or whose dose of lovastatin is being increased, should be advised of the risk of myopathy and told to report promptly any unexplained muscle pain, tenderness or weakness. Lovastatin therapy should be discontinued immediately if myopathy is diagnosed or suspected. In most cases, muscle symptoms and CK increases resolved when treatment was promptly discontinued. Periodic CK determinations may be considered in patients starting therapy with lovastatin or whose dose is being increased, but there is no assurance that such monitoring will prevent myopathy.

Many of the patients who have developed rhabdomyolysis on therapy with lovastatin have had complicated medical histories, including renal insufficiency usually as a consequence of long-standing diabetes mellitus. Such patients merit closer monitoring. Therapy with lovastatin should be temporarily stopped a few days prior to elective major surgery and when any major medical or surgical condition supervenes.

The risk of myopathy/rhabdomyolysis is increased by concomitant use of lovastatin with the following:

Potent inhibitors of CYP3A4: Lovastatin, like several other inhibitors of HMG-CoA reductase, is a substrate of cytochrome P450 3A4 (CYP3A4). When lovastatin is used with a potent inhibitor of CYP3A4, elevated plasma levels of HMG-CoA reductase inhibitory activity can increase the risk of myopathy and rhabdomyolysis, particularly with higher doses of lovastatin.

The use of lovastatin concomitantly with the potent CYP3A4 inhibitors itraconazole, ketoconazole, erythromycin, clarithromycin, telithromycin, HIV protease inhibitors, nefazodone, or large quantities of grapefruit juice (>1 quart daily) should be avoided. Concomitant use of other medicines labeled as having a potent inhibitory effect on CYP3A4 should be avoided unless the benefits of combined therapy outweigh the increased risk. If treatment with itraconazole, ketoconazole, erythromycin, clarithromycin or telithromycin is unavoidable, therapy with lovastatin should be suspended during the course of treatment.

Gemfibrozil, particularly with higher doses of lovastatin: The dose of lovastatin should not exceed 20 mg daily in patients receiving concomitant medication with gemfibrozil. The combined use of lovastatin with gemfibrozil should be avoided, unless the benefits are likely to outweigh the increased risks of this drug combination.

Other lipid-lowering drugs (other fibrates or ≥1 g/day of niacin): The dose of lovastatin should not exceed 20 mg daily in patients receiving concomitant medication with other fibrates or ≥1 g/day of niacin. Caution should be used when prescribing other fibrates or lipid-lowering doses (≥1 g/day) of niacin with lovastatin, as these agents can cause myopathy when given alone. **The benefit of further alterations in lipid levels by the combined use of lovastatin with other fibrates or niacin should be carefully weighed against the potential risks of these combinations.**

Cyclosporine or danazol, with higher doses of lovastatin: The dose of lovastatin should not exceed 20 mg daily in patients receiving concomitant medication with cyclosporine or danazol. The benefits of the use of lovastatin in patients receiving cyclosporine or danazol should be carefully weighed against the risks of these combinations.

Amiodarone or verapamil: The dose of lovastatin should not exceed 40 mg daily in patients receiving concomitant medication with amiodarone or verapamil. The combined use of lovastatin at doses higher than 40 mg daily with amiodarone or verapamil should be avoided unless the clinical benefit is likely to outweigh the increased risk of myopathy. The risk of myopathy/rhabdomyolysis is increased when either amiodarone or verapamil is used concomitantly with higher doses of a closely related member of the HMG-CoA reductase inhibitor class.

Prescribing recommendations for interacting agents are summarized in Table VI (see also CLINICAL PHARMACOLOGY, Pharmacokinetics; PRECAUTIONS, Drug Interactions; DOSAGE AND ADMINISTRATION).

TABLE VI: Drug Interactions Associated with Increased Risk of Myopathy/Rhabdomyolysis

Interacting Agents	Prescribing Recommendations
Itraconazole Ketoconazole Erythromycin Clarithromycin Telithromycin HIV protease inhibitors Nefazodone	Avoid lovastatin
Gemfibrozil Other fibrates Lipid-lowering doses (≥1 g/day) of niacin Cyclosporine Danazol	Do not exceed 20 mg lovastatin daily
Amiodarone Verapamil	Do not exceed 40 mg lovastatin daily
Grapefruit juice	Avoid large quantities of grapefruit juice (>1 quart daily)

Liver Dysfunction

Persistent increases (to more than 3 times the upper limit of normal) in serum transaminases occurred in 1.9% of adult patients who received lovastatin for at least one year in early clinical trials (see ADVERSE REACTIONS). When the drug was interrupted or discontinued in these patients, the transaminase levels usually fell slowly to pretreatment levels. The increases usually appeared 3 to 12 months after the start of therapy with lovastatin, and were not associated with jaundice or other clinical signs or symptoms. There was no evidence of hypersensitivity. In the EXCEL study (see CLINICAL PHARMACOLOGY, Clinical Studies), the incidence of persistent increases in serum transaminases over 48 weeks was 0.1% for placebo, 0.1% at 20 mg/day, 0.9% at 40 mg/day, and 1.5% at 80 mg/day in patients on lovastatin. However, in post-marketing experience with MEVACOR, symptomatic liver disease has been reported rarely at all dosages (see ADVERSE REACTIONS). In AFCAPS/TexCAPS, the number of participants with consecutive elevations of either alanine aminotransferase (ALT) or aspartate aminotransferase (AST) (>3 times the upper limit of normal), over a median of 5.1 years of follow-up, was not significantly different between the MEVACOR and placebo groups (18 [0.6%] vs. 11 [0.3%]). The starting dose of MEVACOR was 20 mg/day; 50% of the MEVACOR treated participants were titrated to 40 mg/day at Week 18. Of the 18 participants on MEVACOR with consecutive elevations of either ALT or AST, 11 (0.7%) elevations occurred in participants taking 20 mg/day, while 7 (0.4%) elevations occurred in participants titrated to 40 mg/day. Elevated transaminases resulted in discontinuation of 6 (0.2%) participants from therapy in the MEVACOR group (n=3,304) and 4 (0.1%) in the placebo group (n=3,301).

It is recommended that liver function tests be performed prior to initiation of therapy in patients with a history of liver disease, or when otherwise clinically indicated. It is recommended that liver function tests be performed in all patients prior to use of 40 mg or more daily and thereafter when clinically indicated. Patients who develop increased transaminase levels should be monitored with a second liver function evaluation to confirm the finding and be followed thereafter with frequent liver function tests until the abnormality(ies) returns to normal. Should an increase in AST or ALT of three times the upper limit of normal or greater persist, withdrawal of therapy with MEVACOR is recommended.

The drug should be used with caution in patients who consume substantial quantities of alcohol and/or have a past history of liver disease. Active liver disease or unexplained transaminase elevations are contraindications to the use of lovastatin.

As with other lipid-lowering agents, moderate (less than three times the upper limit of normal) elevations of serum transaminases have been reported following therapy with MEVACOR (see ADVERSE REACTIONS). These changes appeared soon after initiation of therapy with MEVACOR, were often transient, were not accompanied by any symptoms and interruption of treatment was not required.

PRECAUTIONS

General

Lovastatin may elevate creatine phosphokinase and transaminase levels (see WARNINGS and ADVERSE REACTIONS). This should be considered in the differential diagnosis of chest pain in a patient on therapy with lovastatin.

Homozygous Familial Hypercholesterolemia

MEVACOR is less effective in patients with the rare homozygous familial hypercholesterolemia, possibly because these patients have no functional LDL receptors. MEVACOR appears to be more likely to raise serum transaminases (see ADVERSE REACTIONS) in these homozygous patients.

Information for Patients

Patients should be advised about substances they should not take concomitantly with lovastatin and be advised to report promptly unexplained muscle pain, tenderness, or weakness (see list below and WARNINGS, Myopathy/Rhabdomyolysis). Patients should also be advised to inform other physicians prescribing a new medication that they are taking MEVACOR.

Drug Interactions

CYP3A4 Interactions

Lovastatin is metabolized by CYP3A4 but has no CYP3A4 inhibitory activity; therefore it is not expected to affect the plasma concentrations of other drugs metabolized by CYP3A4. Potent inhibitors of CYP3A4 (below) increase the risk of myopathy by reducing the elimination of lovastatin. See WARNINGS, Myopathy/Rhabdomyolysis, and CLINICAL PHARMACOLOGY, Pharmacokinetics.

Itraconazole
Ketoconazole
Erythromycin
Clarithromycin
Telithromycin
HIV protease inhibitors
Nefazodone
Large quantities of grapefruit juice (>1 quart daily)

Interactions With Lipid-Lowering Drugs That Can Cause Myopathy When Given Alone

The risk of myopathy is also increased by the following lipid-lowering drugs that are not potent CYP3A4 inhibitors, but which can cause myopathy when given alone. See WARNINGS, Myopathy/Rhabdomyolysis.

Gemfibrozil
Other fibrates
Niacin (nicotinic acid) (≥1 g/day)

Other Drug Interactions

Cyclosporine or Danazol: The risk of myopathy/rhabdomyolysis is increased by concomitant administration of cyclosporine or danazol particularly with higher doses of lovastatin (see WARNINGS, Myopathy/Rhabdomyolysis; CLINICAL PHARMACOLOGY, Pharmacokinetics).

Amiodarone or Verapamil: The risk of myopathy/rhabdomyolysis is increased when either amiodarone or verapamil is used concomitantly with a closely related member of the HMG–CoA reductase inhibitor class (see WARNINGS, Myopathy/Rhabdomyolysis).

Coumarin Anticoagulants: In a small clinical trial in which lovastatin was administered to warfarin treated patients, no effect on prothrombin time was detected. However, another HMG-CoA reductase inhibitor has been found to produce a less than two-second increase in prothrombin time in healthy volunteers receiving low doses of warfarin. Also, bleeding and/or increased prothrombin time have been reported in a few patients taking coumarin anticoagulants concomitantly with lovastatin. It is recommended that in patients taking anticoagulants, prothrombin time be determined before starting lovastatin and frequently enough during early therapy to insure that no significant alteration of prothrombin time occurs. Once a stable prothrombin time has been documented, prothrombin times can be monitored at the intervals usually recommended for patients on coumarin anticoagulants. If the dose of lovastatin is changed, the same procedure should be repeated. Lovastatin therapy has not been associated with bleeding or with changes in prothrombin time in patients not taking anticoagulants.

Propranolol: In normal volunteers, there was no clinically significant pharmacokinetic or pharmacodynamic interaction with concomitant administration of single doses of lovastatin and propranolol.

Digoxin: In patients with hypercholesterolemia, concomitant administration of lovastatin and digoxin resulted in no effect on digoxin plasma concentrations.

Oral Hypoglycemic Agents: In pharmacokinetic studies of MEVACOR in hypercholesterolemic non-insulin dependent diabetic patients, there was no drug interaction with glipizide or with chlorpropamide (see CLINICAL PHARMACOLOGY, Clinical Studies).

Endocrine Function

HMG–CoA reductase inhibitors interfere with cholesterol synthesis and as such might theoretically blunt adrenal and/or gonadal steroid production. Results of clinical trials with drugs in this class have been inconsistent with regard to drug effects on basal and reserve steroid levels. However, clinical studies have shown that lovastatin does not reduce basal plasma cortisol concentration or impair adrenal reserve, and does not reduce basal plasma testosterone concentration. Another HMG–CoA reductase inhibitor has been shown to reduce the plasma testosterone response to HCG. In the same study, the mean testosterone response to HCG was slightly but not significantly reduced after treatment with lovastatin 40 mg daily for 16 weeks in 21 men. The effects of HMG-CoA reductase inhibitors on male fertility have not been studied in adequate numbers of male patients. The effects, if any, on the pituitary-gonadal axis in pre-menopausal women are unknown. Patients treated with lovastatin who develop clinical evidence of endocrine dysfunction should be evaluated appropriately. Caution should also be exercised if an HMG–CoA reductase inhibitor or other agent used to lower cholesterol levels is administered to patients also receiving other drugs (e.g., ketoconazole, spironolactone, cimetidine) that may decrease the levels or activity of endogenous steroid hormones.

CNS Toxicity

Lovastatin produced optic nerve degeneration (Wallerian degeneration of retinogeniculate fibers) in clinically normal dogs in a dose-dependent fashion starting at 60 mg/kg/day, a dose that produced mean plasma drug levels about 30 times higher than the mean drug level in humans taking the highest recommended dose (as measured by total enzyme inhibitory activity). Vestibulocochlear Wallerian-like degeneration and retinal ganglion cell chromatolysis were also seen in dogs treated for 14 weeks at 180 mg/kg/day, a dose which resulted in a mean plasma drug level (C_{max}) similar to that seen with the 60 mg/kg/day dose.

CNS vascular lesions, characterized by perivascular hemorrhage and edema, mononuclear cell infiltration of perivascular spaces, perivascular fibrin deposits and necrosis of small vessels, were seen in dogs treated with lovastatin at a dose of 180 mg/kg/day, a dose which produced plasma drug levels (C_{max}) which were about 30 times higher than the mean values in humans taking 80 mg/day.

Similar optic nerve and CNS vascular lesions have been observed with other drugs of this class.

Cataracts were seen in dogs treated for 11 and 28 weeks at 180 mg/kg/day and 1 year at 60 mg/kg/day.

Carcinogenesis, Mutagenesis, Impairment of Fertility

In a 21-month carcinogenic study in mice, there was a statistically significant increase in the incidence of hepatocellular carcinomas and adenomas in both males and females

at 500 mg/kg/day. This dose produced a total plasma drug exposure 3 to 4 times that of humans given the highest recommended dose of lovastatin (drug exposure was measured as total HMG–CoA reductase inhibitory activity in extracted plasma). Tumor increases were not seen at 20 and 100 mg/kg/day, doses that produced drug exposures of 0.3 to 2 times that of humans at the 80 mg/day dose. A statistically significant increase in pulmonary adenomas was seen in female mice at approximately 4 times the human drug exposure. (Although mice were given 300 times the human dose [HD] on a mg/kg body weight basis, plasma levels of total inhibitory activity were only 4 times higher in mice than in humans given 80 mg of MEVACOR.)

There was an increase in incidence of papilloma in the non-glandular mucosa of the stomach of mice beginning at exposures of 1 to 2 times that of humans. The glandular mucosa was not affected. The human stomach contains only glandular mucosa.

In a 24-month carcinogenicity study in rats, there was a positive dose response relationship for hepatocellular carcinogenicity in males at drug exposures between 2-7 times that of human exposure at 80 mg/day (doses in rats were 5, 30 and 180 mg/kg/day).

An increased incidence of thyroid neoplasms in rats appears to be a response that has been seen with other HMG–CoA reductase inhibitors.

A chemically similar drug in this class was administered to mice for 72 weeks at 25, 100, and 400 mg/kg body weight, which resulted in mean serum drug levels approximately 3, 15, and 33 times higher than the mean human serum drug concentration (as total inhibitory activity) after a 40 mg oral dose. Liver carcinomas were significantly increased in high dose females and mid- and high dose males, with a maximum incidence of 90 percent in males. The incidence of adenomas of the liver was significantly increased in mid- and high dose females. Drug treatment also significantly increased the incidence of lung adenomas in mid- and high dose males and females. Adenomas of the Harderian gland (a gland of the eye of rodents) were significantly higher in high dose mice than in controls.

No evidence of mutagenicity was observed in a microbial mutagen test using mutant strains of *Salmonella typhimurium* with or without rat or mouse liver metabolic activation. In addition, no evidence of damage to genetic material was noted in an *in vitro* alkaline elution assay using rat or mouse hepatocytes, a V–79 mammalian cell forward mutation study, an *in vitro* chromosome aberration study in CHO cells, or an *in vivo* chromosomal aberration assay in mouse bone marrow.

Drug-related testicular atrophy, decreased spermatogenesis, spermatocytic degeneration and giant cell formation were seen in dogs starting at 20 mg/kg/day. Similar findings were seen with another drug in this class. No drug-related effects on fertility were found in studies with lovastatin in rats. However, in studies with a similar drug in this class, there was decreased fertility in male rats treated for 34 weeks at 25 mg/kg body weight, although this effect was not observed in a subsequent fertility study when this same dose was administered for 11 weeks (the entire cycle of spermatogenesis, including epididymal maturation). In rats treated with this same reductase inhibitor at 180 mg/kg/day, seminiferous tubule degeneration (necrosis and loss of spermatogenic epithelium) was observed. No microscopic changes were observed in the testes from rats of either study. The clinical significance of these findings is unclear.

Pregnancy

Pregnancy Category X

See CONTRAINDICATIONS.

Safety in pregnant women has not been established.

Lovastatin has been shown to produce skeletal malformations in offspring of pregnant mice and rats dosed during gestation at 80 mg/kg/day (affected mouse fetuses/total: 8/307 compared to 4/289 in the control group; affected rat fetuses/total: 6/324 compared to 2/308 in the control group). Female rats dosed before mating through gestation at 80 mg/kg/day also had fetuses with skeletal malformations (affected fetuses/total: 1/152 compared to 0/171 in the control group). The 80 mg/kg/day dose in mice is 7 times the human dose based on body surface area and in rats results in 5 times the human exposure based on AUC. In pregnant rats given doses of 2, 20, or 200 mg/kg/day and treated through lactation, the following effects were observed: neonatal mortality (4.1%, 3.5%, and 46%, respectively, compared to 0.6% in the control group), decreased pup body weights throughout lactation (up to 5%, 8%, and 38%, respectively, below control), supernumerary ribs in dead pups (affected fetuses/total: 0/7, 1/17, and 11/79, respectively, compared to 0/5 in the control group), delays in ossification in dead pups (affected fetuses/total: 0/7, 0/17, and 1/79, respectively, compared to 0/5 in the control group) and delays in pup development (delays in the appearance of an auditory startle response at 200 mg/kg/day and free-fall righting reflexes at 20 and 200 mg/kg/day).

Direct dosing of neonatal rats by subcutaneous injection with 10 mg/kg/day of the open hydroxyacid form of lovastatin resulted in delayed passive avoidance learning in female rats (mean of 8.3 trials to criterion, compared to 7.3 and 6.4 in untreated and vehicle-treated controls; no effects on retention 1 week later) at exposures 4 times the human systemic exposure at 80 mg/day based on AUC. No effect was seen in male rats. No evidence of malformations was observed when pregnant rabbits were given 5 mg/kg/day (doses equivalent to a human dose of 80 mg/day based on body surface area) or a maternally toxic dose of 15 mg/kg/day (3 times the human dose of 80 mg/day based on body surface area).

Rare clinical reports of congenital anomalies following intrauterine exposure to HMG-CoA reductase inhibitors have been received. However, in an analysis[4] of greater than 200 prospectively followed pregnancies exposed during the first trimester to MEVACOR or another closely related HMG-CoA reductase inhibitor, the incidence of congenital anomalies was comparable to that seen in the general population. This number of pregnancies was sufficient to exclude a 3-fold or greater increase in congenital anomalies over the background incidence.

Maternal treatment with MEVACOR may reduce the fetal levels of mevalonate, which is a precursor of cholesterol biosynthesis. Atherosclerosis is a chronic process, and ordinarily discontinuation of lipid-lowering drugs during pregnancy should have little impact on the long-term risk associated with primary hypercholesterolemia. For these reasons, MEVACOR should not be used in women who are pregnant, or can become pregnant (see CONTRAINDICATIONS). MEVACOR should be administered to women of child-bearing potential only when such patients are highly unlikely to conceive and have been informed of the potential hazards. Treatment should be immediately discontinued as soon as pregnancy is recognized.

[4] Manson, J.M., Freyssinges, C., Ducrocq, M.B., Stephenson, W.P., Postmarketing Surveillance of Lovastatin and Simvastatin Exposure During Pregnancy. *Reproductive Toxicology.* 10(6):439-446. 1996.

Nursing Mothers

It is not known whether lovastatin is excreted in human milk. Because a small amount of another drug in this class is excreted in human breast milk and because of the potential for serious adverse reactions in nursing infants, women taking MEVACOR should not nurse their infants (see CONTRAINDICATIONS).

Pediatric Use

Safety and effectiveness in patients 10-17 years of age with heFH have been evaluated in controlled clinical trials of 48 weeks duration in adolescent boys and controlled clinical trials of 24 weeks duration in girls who were at least 1 year post-menarche. Patients treated with lovastatin had an adverse experience profile generally similar to that of patients treated with placebo. **Doses greater than 40 mg have not been studied in this population.** In these limited controlled studies, there was no detectable effect on growth or sexual maturation in the adolescent boys or on menstrual cycle length in girls. See CLINICAL PHARMACOLOGY, Clinical Studies in Adolescent Patients; ADVERSE REACTIONS, Adolescent Patients; and DOSAGE AND ADMINISTRATION, Adolescent Patients (10-17 years of age) with Heterozygous Familial Hypercholesterolemia. Adolescent females should be counseled on appropriate contraceptive methods while on lovastatin therapy (see CONTRAINDICATIONS and PRECAUTIONS, Pregnancy). **Lovastatin has not been studied in pre-pubertal patients or patients younger than 10 years of age.**

Geriatric Use

A pharmacokinetic study with lovastatin showed the mean plasma level of HMG–CoA reductase inhibitory activity to be approximately 45% higher in elderly patients between 70-78 years of age compared with patients between 18-30 years of age; however, clinical study experience in the elderly indicates that dosage adjustment based on this age-related pharmacokinetic difference is not needed. In the two large clinical studies conducted with lovastatin (EXCEL and AFCAPS/TexCAPS), 21% (3094/14850) of patients were ≥65 years of age. Lipid-lowering efficacy with lovastatin was at least as great in elderly patients compared with younger patients, and there were no overall differences in safety over the 20 to 80 mg/day dosage range (see CLINICAL PHARMACOLOGY).

ADVERSE REACTIONS

MEVACOR is generally well tolerated; adverse reactions usually have been mild and transient.

Phase III Clinical Studies

In Phase III controlled clinical studies involving 613 patients treated with MEVACOR, the adverse experience profile was similar to that shown below for the 8,245-patient EXCEL study (see Expanded Clinical Evaluation of Lovastatin (EXCEL) Study).

	Placebo (N = 1663) %	MEVACOR 20 mg q.p.m. (N = 1642) %	MEVACOR 40 mg q.p.m. (N = 1645) %	MEVACOR 20 mg b.i.d. (N = 1646) %	MEVACOR 40 mg b.i.d. (N = 1649) %
Body As a Whole					
Asthenia	1.4	1.7	1.4	1.5	1.2
Gastrointestinal					
Abdominal pain	1.6	2.0	2.0	2.2	2.5
Constipation	1.9	2.0	3.2	3.2	3.5
Diarrhea	2.3	2.6	2.4	2.2	2.6
Dyspepsia	1.9	1.3	1.3	1.0	1.6
Flatulence	4.2	3.7	4.3	3.9	4.5
Nausea	2.5	1.9	2.5	2.2	2.2
Musculoskeletal					
Muscle cramps	0.5	0.6	0.8	1.1	1.0
Myalgia	1.7	2.6	1.8	2.2	3.0
Nervous System / Psychiatric					
Dizziness	0.7	0.7	1.2	0.5	0.5
Headache	2.7	2.6	2.8	2.1	3.2
Skin					
Rash	0.7	0.8	1.0	1.2	1.3
Special Senses					
Blurred vision	0.8	1.1	0.9	0.9	1.2

Persistent increases of serum transaminases have been noted (see WARNINGS, Liver Dysfunction). About 11% of patients had elevations of CK levels of at least twice the normal value on one or more occasions. The corresponding values for the control agent cholestyramine was 9 percent. This was attributable to the noncardiac fraction of CK. Large increases in CK have sometimes been reported (see WARNINGS, Myopathy/Rhabdomyolysis).

Expanded Clinical Evaluation of Lovastatin (EXCEL) Study
MEVACOR was compared to placebo in 8,245 patients with hypercholesterolemia (total-C 240-300 mg/dL [6.2-7.8 mmol/L]) in the randomized, double-blind, parallel, 48 week EXCEL study. Clinical adverse experiences reported as possibly, probably or definitely drug-related in ≥1% in any treatment group are shown in the table below. For no event was the incidence on drug and placebo statistically different.
[See table above]
Other clinical adverse experiences reported as possibly, probably or definitely drug-related in 0.5 to 1.0 percent of patients in any drug-treated group are listed below. In all these cases the incidence on drug and placebo was not statistically different. *Body as a Whole:* chest pain; *Gastrointestinal:* acid regurgitation, dry mouth, vomiting; *Musculoskeletal:* leg pain, shoulder pain, arthralgia; *Nervous System / Psychiatric:* insomnia, paresthesia; *Skin:* alopecia, pruritus; *Special Senses:* eye irritation.
In the EXCEL study (see CLINICAL PHARMACOLOGY, Clinical Studies), 4.6% of the patients treated up to 48 weeks were discontinued due to clinical or laboratory adverse experiences which were rated by the investigator as possibly, probably or definitely related to therapy with MEVACOR. The value for the placebo group was 2.5%.
Air Force / Texas Coronary Atherosclerosis Prevention Study (AFCAPS / TexCAPS)
In AFCAPS/TexCAPS (see CLINICAL PHARMACOLOGY, Clinical Studies) involving 6,605 participants treated with 20-40 mg/day of MEVACOR (n=3,304) or placebo (n=3,301), the safety and tolerability profile of the group treated with MEVACOR was comparable to that of the group treated with placebo during a median of 5.1 years of follow-up. The adverse experiences reported in AFCAPS/TexCAPS were similar to those reported in EXCEL (see ADVERSE REACTIONS, Expanded Clinical Evaluation of Lovastatin (EXCEL) Study).
Concomitant Therapy
In controlled clinical studies in which lovastatin was administered concomitantly with cholestyramine, no adverse reactions peculiar to this concomitant treatment were observed. The adverse reactions that occurred were limited to those reported previously with lovastatin or cholestyramine. Other lipid-lowering agents were not administered concomitantly with lovastatin during controlled clinical studies. Preliminary data suggests that the addition of gemfibrozil to therapy with lovastatin is not associated with greater reduction in LDL–C than that achieved with lovastatin alone. In uncontrolled clinical studies, most of the patients who have developed myopathy were receiving concomitant therapy with cyclosporine, gemfibrozil or niacin (nicotinic acid). The combined use of lovastatin at doses exceeding 20 mg/day with cyclosporine, gemfibrozil, other fibrates or lipid-lowering doses (≥1 g/day) of niacin should be avoided (see WARNINGS, Myopathy/Rhabdomyolysis).
The following effects have been reported with drugs in this class. Not all the effects listed below have necessarily been associated with lovastatin therapy.

Skeletal: muscle cramps, myalgia, myopathy, rhabdomyolysis, arthralgias.
Neurological: dysfunction of certain cranial nerves (including alteration of taste, impairment of extra-ocular movement, facial paresis), tremor, dizziness, vertigo, memory loss, paresthesia, peripheral neuropathy, peripheral nerve palsy, psychic disturbances, anxiety, insomnia, depression.
Hypersensitivity Reactions: An apparent hypersensitivity syndrome has been reported rarely which has included one or more of the following features: anaphylaxis, angioedema, lupus erythematous-like syndrome, polymyalgia rheumatica, dermatomyositis, vasculitis, purpura, thrombocytopenia, leukopenia, hemolytic anemia, positive ANA, ESR increase, eosinophilia, arthritis, arthralgia, urticaria, asthenia, photosensitivity, fever, chills, flushing, malaise, dyspnea, toxic epidermal necrolysis, erythema multiforme, including Stevens-Johnson syndrome.
Gastrointestinal: pancreatitis, hepatitis, including chronic active hepatitis, cholestatic jaundice, fatty change in liver; and rarely, cirrhosis, fulminant hepatic necrosis, and hepatoma; anorexia, vomiting.
Skin: alopecia, pruritus. A variety of skin changes (e.g., nodules, discoloration, dryness of skin/mucous membranes, changes to hair/nails) have been reported.
Reproductive: gynecomastia, loss of libido, erectile dysfunction.
Eye: progression of cataracts (lens opacities), ophthalmoplegia.
Laboratory Abnormalities: elevated transaminases, alkaline phosphatase, γ-glutamyl transpeptidase, and bilirubin; thyroid function abnormalities.
Adolescent Patients (ages 10–17 years)
In a 48–week controlled study in adolescent boys with heFH (n=132) and a 24–week controlled study in girls who were at least 1 year post-menarche with heFH (n=54), the safety and tolerability profile of the groups treated with MEVACOR (10 to 40 mg daily) was generally similar to that of the groups treated with placebo (see CLINICAL PHARMACOLOGY, Clinical Studies in Adolescent Patients and PRECAUTIONS, Pediatric Use).

OVERDOSAGE

After oral administration of MEVACOR to mice, the median lethal dose observed was >15 g/m². Five healthy human volunteers have received up to 200 mg of lovastatin as a single dose without clinically significant adverse experiences. A few cases of accidental overdosage have been reported; no patients had any specific symptoms, and all patients recovered without sequelae. The maximum dose taken was 5-6 g.
Until further experience is obtained, no specific treatment of overdosage with MEVACOR can be recommended.
The dialyzability of lovastatin and its metabolites in man is not known at present.

DOSAGE AND ADMINISTRATION

The patient should be placed on a standard cholesterol-lowering diet before receiving MEVACOR and should continue on this diet during treatment with MEVACOR (see NCEP Treatment Guidelines for details on dietary therapy). MEVACOR should be given with meals.
Adult Patients
The usual recommended starting dose is 20 mg once a day given with the evening meal. The recommended dosing range of lovastatin is 10-80 mg/day in single or two divided doses; the maximum recommended dose is 80 mg/day. Doses should be individualized according to the recommended goal of therapy (see NCEP Guidelines and CLINICAL PHARMACOLOGY). Patients requiring reductions in LDL–C of 20% or more to achieve their goal (see INDICATIONS AND USAGE) should be started on 20 mg/day of MEVACOR. A starting dose of 10 mg of lovastatin may be considered for patients requiring smaller reductions. Adjustments should be made at intervals of 4 weeks or more. The 10 mg dosage is provided for information purposes only. Although lovastatin tablets 10 mg are available in the marketplace, MEVACOR is no longer marketed in the 10 mg strength.
Cholesterol levels should be monitored periodically and consideration should be given to reducing the dosage of MEVACOR if cholesterol levels fall significantly below the targeted range.
Dosage in Patients taking Cyclosporine or Danazol
In patients taking cyclosporine or danazol concomitantly with lovastatin (see WARNINGS, Myopathy/Rhabdomyolysis), therapy should begin with 10 mg of lovastatin and should not exceed 20 mg/day.
Dosage in Patients taking Amiodarone or Verapamil
In patients taking amiodarone or verapamil concomitantly with MEVACOR, the dose should not exceed 40 mg/day (see WARNINGS, Myopathy/Rhabdomyolysis and PRECAUTIONS, Drug Interactions, Other drug interactions).
Adolescent Patients (10-17 years of age) with Heterozygous Familial Hypercholesterolemia
The recommended dosing range of lovastatin is 10-40 mg/day; the maximum recommended dose is 40 mg/day. Doses should be individualized according to the recommended goal of therapy (see NCEP Pediatric Panel Guidelines[5], CLINICAL PHARMACOLOGY, and INDICATIONS AND USAGE). Patients requiring reductions in LDL–C of 20% or more to achieve their goal should be started on 20 mg/day of MEVACOR. A starting dose of 10 mg of lovastatin may be considered for patients requiring smaller reductions. Adjustments should be made at intervals of 4 weeks or more.

[5] National Cholesterol Education Program (NCEP): Highlights of the Report of the Expert Panel on Blood Cholesterol Levels in Children and Adolescents. *Pediatrics.* 89(3): 495-501. 1992.
Concomitant Lipid-Lowering Therapy
MEVACOR is effective alone or when used concomitantly with bile-acid sequestrants. If MEVACOR is used in combination with gemfibrozil, other fibrates or lipid-lowering doses (≥1 g/day) of niacin, the dose of MEVACOR should not exceed 20 mg/day (see WARNINGS, Myopathy/Rhabdomyolysis and PRECAUTIONS, Drug Interactions).
Dosage in Patients with Renal Insufficiency
In patients with severe renal insufficiency (creatinine clearance <30 mL/min), dosage increases above 20 mg/day should be carefully considered and, if deemed necessary, implemented cautiously (see CLINICAL PHARMACOLOGY and WARNINGS, Myopathy/Rhabdomyolysis).

HOW SUPPLIED

No. 8123—Tablets MEVACOR 20 mg are blue, octagonal tablets, coded MSD 731 on one side and plain on the other. They are supplied as follows:
NDC 0006-0731-61 unit of use bottles of 60.
No. 8124—Tablets MEVACOR 40 mg are green, octagonal tablets, coded MSD 732 on one side and plain on the other. They are supplied as follows:
NDC 0006-0732-61 unit of use bottles of 60.
Storage
Store at 20-25°C (68-77°F). [See USP Controlled Room Temperature.] Tablets MEVACOR must be protected from light and stored in a well-closed, light-resistant container.
Manuf. for: Merck Sharp & Dohme Corp., a subsidiary of **MERCK & CO., INC.,** Whitehouse Station, NJ 08889, USA
By:
Mylan Pharmaceuticals Inc.
Morgantown, WV 26505, USA
OR
Mylan Pharmaceuticals ULC
Etobicoke, Ontario, Canada M8Z 2S6
Issued May 2010
9844661
014-874-01
Shown in Product Identification Guide, page 313

NASONEX®   ℞
[nā-sō-něks]
(mometasone furoate monohydrate)
Nasal Spray 50 mcg†

†calculated on the anhydrous basis
HIGHLIGHTS OF PRESCRIBING INFORMATION
These highlights do not include all the information needed to use NASONEX safely and effectively. See full prescribing information for NASONEX.
NASONEX ® (mometasone furoate monohydrate) Nasal Spray 50 mcg†
†calculated on the anhydrous basis
Initial U.S. Approval: 1997

INDICATIONS AND USAGE

NASONEX is a corticosteroid indicated for:
1. Treatment of Nasal Symptoms of Allergic Rhinitis (1.1)
2. Treatment of Nasal Congestion Associated with Seasonal Allergic Rhinitis (1.2)
3. Prophylaxis of Seasonal Allergic Rhinitis (1.3)
4. Treatment of Nasal Polyps (1.4)

DOSAGE AND ADMINISTRATION

For Intranasal Use Only
- Treatment of Nasal Symptoms of Allergic Rhinitis (2.1)
  Adults & Adolescents (12 yrs. and older): 2 sprays in each nostril once daily
  Children (2–11 yrs.): 1 spray in each nostril once daily
- Treatment of Nasal Congestion Associated with Seasonal Allergic Rhinitis (2.2)
  Adults & Adolescents (12 yrs. and older): 2 sprays in each nostril once daily
  Children (2–11 yrs.): 1 spray in each nostril once daily
- Prophylaxis of Seasonal Allergic Rhinitis (2.3)
  Adults & Adolescents (12 yrs. and older): 2 sprays in each nostril once daily
- Treatment of Nasal Polyps (2.4)
  Adults (18 yrs and older): 2 sprays in each nostril twice daily. 2 sprays in each nostril once daily may also be effective in some patients.

DOSAGE FORMS AND STRENGTHS

Nasal Spray: 50 mcg of mometasone furoate in each 100-microliter spray (3)

CONTRAINDICATIONS

Patients with known hypersensitivity to mometasone furoate or any of the ingredients of NASONEX. (4)

WARNINGS AND PRECAUTIONS

- Epistaxis, nasal ulceration, *Candida albicans* infection, nasal septal perforation, impaired wound healing. Monitor patients periodically for signs of adverse effects on the nasal mucosa. Avoid use in patients with recent nasal ulcers, nasal surgery, or nasal trauma. (5.1)
- Potential worsening of existing tuberculosis; fungal, bacterial, viral, or parasitic infections; or ocular herpes simplex. More serious or even fatal course of chickenpox or measles in susceptible patients. Use caution in patients with the above because of the potential for worsening of these infections. (5.4)
- Hypercorticism and adrenal suppression with higher than recommended dosages or at the regular dosage in susceptible individuals. If such changes occur, discontinue NASONEX Nasal Spray slowly. (5.5)
- Potential reduction in growth velocity in children. Monitor growth routinely in pediatric patients receiving NASONEX Nasal Spray. (5.6, 8.4)

ADVERSE REACTIONS

The most common adverse reactions (≥5%) included headache, viral infection, pharyngitis, epistaxis and cough. (6)

To report SUSPECTED ADVERSE REACTIONS, contact Schering-Plough at 800-526-4099 or FDA at 1-800-FDA-1088 or www.fda.gov/medwatch.

See 17 for PATIENT COUNSELING INFORMATION and FDA-approved patient labeling

Revised: 06/2010

FULL PRESCRIBING INFORMATION

1. INDICATIONS AND USAGE

1.1 Treatment of Allergic Rhinitis

NASONEX® Nasal Spray 50 mcg is indicated for the treatment of the nasal symptoms of seasonal allergic and perennial allergic rhinitis, in adults and pediatric patients 2 years of age and older.

1.2 Treatment of Nasal Congestion Associated with Seasonal Allergic Rhinitis

NASONEX Nasal Spray 50 mcg is indicated for the relief of nasal congestion associated with seasonal allergic rhinitis, in adults and pediatric patients 2 years of age and older.

1.3 Prophylaxis of Seasonal Allergic Rhinitis

NASONEX Nasal Spray 50 mcg is indicated for the prophylaxis of the nasal symptoms of seasonal allergic rhinitis in adult and adolescent patients 12 years and older.

1.4 Treatment of Nasal Polyps

NASONEX Nasal Spray 50 mcg is indicated for the treatment of nasal polyps in patients 18 years of age and older.

2. DOSAGE AND ADMINISTRATION

Administer NASONEX Nasal Spray 50 mcg by the intranasal route only. Prior to initial use of NASONEX Nasal Spray, 50 mcg, the pump must be primed by actuating ten times or until a fine spray appears. The pump may be stored unused for up to 1 week without repriming. If unused for more than 1 week, reprime by actuating two times, or until a fine spray appears.

2.1 Treatment of Allergic Rhinitis

Adults and Adolescents 12 Years of Age and Older:
The recommended dose for treatment of the nasal symptoms of seasonal allergic and perennial allergic rhinitis is 2 sprays (50 mcg of mometasone furoate in each spray) in each nostril once daily (total daily dose of 200 mcg).

Children 2 to 11 Years of Age:
The recommended dose for treatment of the nasal symptoms of seasonal allergic and perennial allergic rhinitis is 1 spray (50 mcg of mometasone furoate in each spray) in each nostril once daily (total daily dose of 100 mcg).

2.2 Treatment of Nasal Congestion Associated with Seasonal Allergic Rhinitis

Adults and Adolescents 12 Years of Age and Older:
The recommended dose for treatment of nasal congestion associated with seasonal allergic rhinitis is two sprays (50 mcg of mometasone furoate in each spray) in each nostril once daily (total daily dose of 200 mcg).

Children 2 to 11 Years of Age:
The recommended dose for treatment of nasal congestion associated with seasonal allergic rhinitis is one spray (50 mcg of mometasone furoate in each spray) in each nostril once daily (total daily dose of 100 mcg).

2.3 Prophylaxis of Seasonal Allergic Rhinitis

Adults and Adolescents 12 Years of Age and Older:
The recommended dose for prophylaxis treatment of nasal symptoms of seasonal allergic rhinitis is 2 sprays (50 mcg of mometasone furoate in each spray) in each nostril once daily (total daily dose of 200 mcg).

In patients with a known seasonal allergen that precipitates nasal symptoms of seasonal allergic rhinitis, prophylaxis with NASONEX Nasal Spray 50 mcg (200 mcg/day) is recommended 2 to 4 weeks prior to the anticipated start of the pollen season.

2.4 Treatment of Nasal Polyps

Adults 18 Years of Age and Older:
The recommended dose for the treatment of nasal polyps is 2 sprays (50 mcg of mometasone furoate in each spray) in each nostril twice daily (total daily dose of 400 mcg). A dose of 2 sprays (50 mcg of mometasone furoate in each spray) in each nostril once daily (total daily dose of 200 mcg) is also effective in some patients.

3. DOSAGE FORMS AND STRENGTHS

NASONEX Nasal Spray 50 mcg is a metered-dose, manual pump spray unit containing an aqueous suspension of mometasone furoate monohydrate equivalent to 0.05% w/w mometasone furoate calculated on the anhydrous basis. After initial priming (10 actuations), each actuation of the pump delivers a metered spray containing 100 mg or 100 microliter of suspension containing mometasone furoate monohydrate equivalent to 50 mcg of mometasone furoate calculated on the anhydrous basis. Each bottle of NASONEX Nasal Spray 50 mcg provides 120 sprays.

4. CONTRAINDICATIONS

NASONEX Nasal Spray is contraindicated in patients with known hypersensitivity to mometasone furoate or any of its ingredients.

5. WARNINGS AND PRECAUTIONS

5.1 Local Nasal Effects

Epistaxis
In clinical studies, epistaxis was observed more frequently in patients with allergic rhinitis with NASONEX Nasal Spray than those who received placebo *[see Adverse Reactions (6)]*.

Candida Infection
In clinical studies with NASONEX Nasal Spray 50 mcg, the development of localized infections of the nose and pharynx with *Candida albicans* has occurred. When such an infection develops, use of NASONEX Nasal Spray 50 mcg should be discontinued and appropriate local or systemic therapy instituted, if needed.

Nasal Septum Perforation
Instances of nasal septum perforation have been reported following the intranasal application of corticosteroids. As with any long-term topical treatment of the nasal cavity, patients using NASONEX Nasal Spray 50 mcg over several months or longer should be examined periodically for possible changes in the nasal mucosa.

Impaired Wound Healing
Because of the inhibitory effect of corticosteroids on wound healing, patients who have experienced recent nasal septum ulcers, nasal surgery, or nasal trauma should not use a nasal corticosteroid until healing has occurred.

5.2 Glaucoma and Cataracts

Nasal and inhaled corticosteroids may result in the development of glaucoma and/or cataracts. Therefore, close monitoring is warranted in patients with a change in vision or with a history of increased intraocular pressure, glaucoma, and/or cataracts.

Glaucoma and cataract formation was evaluated in one controlled study of 12 weeks' duration and one uncontrolled study of 12 months' duration in patients treated with NASONEX Nasal Spray, 50 mcg at 200 mcg/day, using intraocular pressure measurements and slit lamp examination. No significant change from baseline was noted in the mean intraocular pressure measurements for the 141 NASONEX-treated patients in the 12-week study, as compared with 141 placebo-treated patients. No individual NASONEX-treated patient was noted to have developed a significant elevation in intraocular pressure or cataracts in this 12-week study. Likewise, no significant change from baseline was noted in the mean intraocular pressure measurements for the 139 NASONEX-treated patients in the 12-month study and again, no cataracts were detected in these patients. Nonetheless, nasal and inhaled corticosteroids have been associated with the development of glaucoma and/or cataracts.

5.3 Hypersensitivity Reactions

Hypersensitivity reactions including instances of wheezing may occur after the intranasal administration of mometasone furoate monohydrate. Discontinue Nasonex Nasal Spray if such reactions occur *[see Contraindications (4)]*.

5.4 Immunosuppression

Persons who are on drugs which suppress the immune system are more susceptible to infections than healthy individuals. Chickenpox and measles, for example, can have a more serious or even fatal course in nonimmune children or adults on corticosteroids. In such children or adults who have not had these diseases, particular care should be taken to avoid exposure. How the dose, route, and duration of corticosteroid administration affect the risk of developing a disseminated infection is not known. The contribution of the underlying disease and/or prior corticosteroid treatment to the risk is also not known. If exposed to chickenpox, prophylaxis with varicella zoster immune globin (VZIG) may be indicated. If exposed to measles, prophylaxis with pooled intramuscular immunoglobulin (IG) may be indicated. (See the respective package inserts for complete VZIG and IG prescribing information.) If chickenpox develops, treatment with antiviral agents may be considered.

Corticosteroids should be used with caution, if at all, in patients with active or quiescent tuberculous infection of the respiratory tract, or in untreated fungal, bacterial, systemic viral infections, or ocular herpes simplex because of the potential for worsening of these infections.

5.5 Hypothalamic-Pituitary-Adrenal Axis Effect

Hypercorticism and Adrenal Suppression

When intranasal steroids are used at higher than recommended dosages or in susceptible individuals at recommended dosages, systemic corticosteroid effects such as hypercorticism and adrenal suppression may appear. If such changes occur, the dosage of Nasonex Nasal Spray should be discontinued slowly, consistent with accepted procedures for discontinuing oral corticosteroid therapy.

5.6 Effect on Growth

Corticosteroids may cause a reduction in growth velocity when administered to pediatric patients. Monitor the growth routinely of pediatric patients receiving NASONEX Nasal Spray. To minimize the systemic effects of intranasal corticosteroids, including NASONEX Nasal Spray, titrate each patient's dose to the lowest dosage that effectively controls his/her symptoms [*see Use in Specific Populations (8.4)*].

6. ADVERSE REACTIONS

Systemic and local corticosteroid use may result in the following:

- Epistaxis, ulcerations, Candida albicans infection, impaired wound healing [*see Warnings and Precautions (5.1)*].
- Cataracts and glaucoma [*see Warnings and Precautions (5.2)*]
- Immunosuppression [*see Warnings and Precautions (5.4)*]
- Hypothalamic-pituitary-adrenal (HPA) axis effects, including growth reduction [*see Warnings and Precautions (5.5, 5.6), Use in Specific Populations (8.4)*]

6.1 Clinical Trials Experience

Because clinical trials are conducted under widely varying conditions, adverse reaction rates observed in the clinical trials of a drug cannot be directly compared to rates in the clinical trials of another drug and may not reflect the rates observed in practice.

Allergic Rhinitis

Adults and adolescents 12 years of age and older

In controlled US and international clinical studies, a total of 3210 adult and adolescent patients 12 years and older with allergic rhinitis received treatment with NASONEX Nasal Spray 50 mcg at doses of 50 to 800 mcg/day. The majority of patients (n = 2103) were treated with 200 mcg/day. A total of 350 adult and adolescent patients have been treated for one year or longer. Adverse events did not differ significantly based on age, sex, or race. Four percent or less of patients in clinical trials discontinued treatment because of adverse events and the discontinuation rate was similar for the vehicle and active comparators.

All adverse events (regardless of relationship to treatment) reported by 5% or more of adult and adolescent patients ages 12 years and older who received NASONEX Nasal Spray 50 mcg, 200 mcg/day vs. placebo and that were more common with NASONEX Nasal Spray 50 mcg than placebo, are displayed in TABLE 1 below.

TABLE 1. ADULT AND ADOLESCENT PATIENTS 12 YEARS AND OLDER – ADVERSE EVENTS FROM CONTROLLED CLINICAL TRIALS IN SEASONAL ALLERGIC AND PERENNIAL ALLERGIC RHINITIS (PERCENT OF PATIENTS REPORTING)

	NASONEX 200 mcg (n = 2103)	VEHICLE PLACEBO (n = 1671)
Headache	26	22
Viral Infection	14	11
Pharyngitis	12	10
Epistaxis/Blood-Tinged Mucus	11	6
Coughing	7	6
Upper Respiratory Tract Infection	6	2
Dysmenorrhea	5	3
Musculoskeletal Pain	5	3
Sinusitis	5	3

Other adverse events which occurred in less than 5% but greater than or equal to 2% of adult and adolescent patients (ages 12 years and older) treated with NASONEX Nasal Spray 50 mcg, 200-mcg/day (regardless of relationship to treatment), and more frequently than in the placebo group included: arthralgia, asthma, bronchitis, chest pain, conjunctivitis, diarrhea, dyspepsia, earache, flu-like symptoms, myalgia, nausea, and rhinitis.

Pediatric patients < 12 years of age

In controlled US and international studies, a total of 990 pediatric patients (ages 3 to 11 years) with allergic rhinitis received treatment with NASONEX Nasal Spray 50 mcg, at doses of 25 to 200 mcg/day. The majority of pediatric patients (n = 720) were treated with 100 mcg/day. A total of 163 pediatric patients have been treated for one year or longer. Two percent or less of patients in clinical trials who received NASONEX Nasal Spray 50 mcg discontinued treatment because of adverse events and the discontinuation rate was similar for the placebo and active comparators.

Adverse events which occurred in ≥5% of pediatric patients (ages 3 to 11 years) treated with NASONEX Nasal Spray 50 mcg, 100 mcg/day vs. placebo (regardless of relationship to treatment) and more frequently than in the placebo group included upper respiratory tract infection (5% in NASONEX Nasal Spray 50 mcg group vs. 4% in placebo) and vomiting (5% in NASONEX Nasal Spray 50 mcg group vs. 4% in placebo).

Other adverse events which occurred in less than 5% but greater than or equal to 2% of pediatric patients (ages 3 to 11 years) treated NASONEX Nasal Spray 50 mcg, 100-mcg/day vs. placebo (regardless of relationship to treatment) and more frequently than in the placebo group included: diarrhea, nasal irritation, otitis media, and wheezing.

The adverse event (regardless of relationship to treatment) reported by 5% of pediatric patients ages 2 to 5 years who received NASONEX Nasal Spray, 50 mcg, 100 mcg/day in a clinical trial vs. placebo including 56 subjects (28 each NASONEX Nasal Spray, 50 mcg and placebo) and that was more common with NASONEX Nasal Spray, 50 mcg than placebo, included: upper respiratory tract infection (7% vs. 0%, respectively). The other adverse event which occurred in less than 5% but greater than or equal to 2% of mometasone furoate pediatric patients ages 2 to 5 years treated with 100-mcg doses vs. placebo (regardless of relationship to treatment) and more frequently than in the placebo group included: skin trauma.

Nasal Polyps

In controlled clinical studies, the types of adverse events observed in patients with nasal polyps were similar to those observed for patients with allergic rhinitis. A total of 594 adult patients (ages 18 to 86 years) received NASONEX Nasal Spray 50 mcg at doses of 200 mcg once or twice daily for up to 4 months for treatment of nasal polyps. The overall incidence of adverse events for patients treated with NASONEX Nasal Spray 50 mcg was comparable to patients with the placebo except for epistaxis, which was 9% for 200 mcg once daily, 13% for 200 mcg twice daily, and 5% for the placebo.

Nasal ulcers and nasal and oral candidiasis were also reported in patients treated with NASONEX Nasal Spray 50 mcg primarily in patients treated for longer than 4 weeks.

Nasal Congestion Associated with Seasonal Allergic Rhinitis

A total of 1008 patients aged 12 years and older received NASONEX Nasal Spray 50 mcg 200 mcg/day (n = 506) or placebo (n = 502) for 15 days. Adverse events that occurred more frequently in patients treated with NASONEX Nasal Spray 50 mcg than in patients with the placebo included sinus headache (1.2% in NASONEX Nasal Spray 50 mcg group vs. 0.2% in placebo) and epistaxis (1% in NASONEX Nasal Spray 50 mcg group vs. 0.2% in placebo) and the overall adverse event profile was similar to that observed in the other allergic rhinitis trials.

6.2 Post-Marketing Experience

The following adverse reactions have been identified during the post-marketing period for NASONEX Nasal Spray 50 mcg: nasal burning and irritation, anaphylaxis and angioedema, disturbances in taste and smell and nasal septal perforation. Because these reactions are reported voluntarily from a population of uncertain size, it is not always possible to reliably estimate their frequency or establish a causal relationship to drug exposure.

7. DRUG INTERACTIONS

No formal drug-drug interaction studies have been conducted with NASONEX Nasal Spray 50 mcg.

Inhibitors of Cytochrome P450 3A4: Studies have shown that mometasone furoate is primarily and extensively metabolized in the liver of all species investigated and undergoes extensive metabolism to multiple metabolites. *In vitro* studies have confirmed the primary role of cytochrome CYP 3A4 in the metabolism of this compound. Coadministration with ketoconazole, a potent CYP 3A4 inhibitor, may increase the plasma concentrations of mometasone furoate [*see Clinical Pharmacology (12.3)*].

8. USE IN SPECIFIC POPULATIONS

8.1 Pregnancy

Teratogenic Effects: Pregnancy Category C: There are no adequate and well-controlled studies in pregnant women. NASONEX Nasal Spray 50 mcg, like other corticosteroids, should be used during pregnancy only if the potential benefits justify the potential risk to the fetus. Experience with oral corticosteroids since their introduction in pharmacologic, as opposed to physiologic, doses suggests that rodents are more prone to teratogenic effects from corticosteroids than humans. In addition, because there is a natural increase in corticosteroid production during pregnancy, most women will require a lower exogenous corticosteroid dose and many will not need corticosteroid treatment during pregnancy.

In mice, mometasone furoate caused cleft palate at subcutaneous doses (less than the MRDID in adults on a mcg/m^2 basis). Fetal survival was reduced at approximately 2 times the MRDID in adults on a mcg/m^2 basis. No toxicity was observed at less than the MRDID in adults on a mcg/m^2 basis.

In rats, mometasone furoate produced umbilical hernia at topical dermal doses approximately 10 times the MRDID in adults on a mcg/m^2 basis. A topical dermal dose approximately 6 times the MRDID in adults on a mcg/m^2 basis produced delays in ossification, but no malformations.

In rabbits, mometasone furoate caused multiple malformations (e.g., flexed front paws, gallbladder agenesis, umbilical hernia, and hydrocephaly) at topical dermal doses approximately 6 times the MRDID in adults on a mcg/m^2 basis. In an oral study, mometasone furoate increased resorptions and caused cleft palate and/or head malformations (hydrocephaly or domed head) at approximately 30 times the MRDID in adults on a mcg/m^2 basis. At approximately 110 times the MRDID in adults on a mcg/m^2 basis, most litters were aborted or resorbed. No toxicity was observed at approximately 6 times the MRDID in adults on a mcg/m^2 basis.

When rats received subcutaneous doses of mometasone furoate throughout pregnancy or during the later stages of pregnancy, a dose less than the MRDID in adults on a mcg/m^2 basis caused prolonged and difficult labor and reduced the number of live births, birth weight, and early pup survival.

Nonteratogenic Effects: Hypoadrenalism may occur in infants born to women receiving corticosteroids during pregnancy. Such infants should be carefully monitored.

8.3 Nursing Mothers

It is not known if mometasone furoate is excreted in human milk. Because other corticosteroids are excreted in human milk, caution should be used when NASONEX Nasal Spray, 50 mcg is administered to nursing women.

8.4 Pediatric Use

The safety and effectiveness of NASONEX Nasal Spray 50 mcg for allergic rhinitis in children 12 years of age and older have been established [*see Adverse Reactions (6.1) and Clinical Studies (14.1)*]. Use of NASONEX Nasal Spray 50 mcg for allergic rhinitis in pediatric patients 2 to 11 years of age is supported by safety and efficacy data from clinical studies. Seven hundred and twenty (720) patients 3 to 11 years of age with allergic rhinitis were treated with mometasone furoate nasal spray 50 mcg (100 mcg total daily dose) in controlled clinical trials [*see Adverse Reactions (6.1) and Clinical Studies (14.2)*]. Twenty-eight (28) patients 2 to 5 years of age with allergic rhinitis were treated with mometasone furoate nasal spray 50 mcg (100 mcg total daily dose) in a controlled trial to evaluate safety [*see Adverse Reactions (6.1)*]. Safety and effectiveness of Nasonex Nasal Spray 50 mcg for allergic rhinitis in children less than 2 years of age have not been established. The safety and effectiveness of Nasonex Nasal Spray 50 mcg in children less than 18 years of age with nasal polyps have not been established.

Controlled clinical studies have shown intranasal corticosteroids may cause a reduction in growth velocity in pediatric patients. This effect has been observed in the absence of laboratory evidence of hypothalamic-pituitary-adrenal (HPA) axis suppression, suggesting that growth velocity is a more sensitive indicator of systemic corticosteroid exposure in pediatric patients than some commonly used tests of HPA axis function. The long-term effects of this reduction in growth velocity associated with intranasal corticosteroids, including the impact on final adult height, are unknown. The potential for "catch up" growth following discontinuation of treatment with intranasal corticosteroids has not been adequately studied. The growth of pediatric patients receiving intranasal corticosteroids, including NASONEX Nasal Spray, 50 mcg, should be monitored routinely (e.g., via stadiometry). The potential growth effects of prolonged treatment should be weighed against clinical benefits obtained and the availability of safe and effective *noncortico-*

steroid treatment alternatives. To minimize the systemic effects of intranasal corticosteroids, including NASONEX Nasal Spray, 50 mcg, each patient should be titrated to his/her lowest effective dose.

A clinical study to assess the effect of NASONEX Nasal Spray 50 mcg (100 mcg total daily dose) on growth velocity has been conducted in pediatric patients 3 to 9 years of age with allergic rhinitis. No statistically significant effect on growth velocity was observed for NASONEX Nasal Spray 50 mcg compared to placebo following one year of treatment. No evidence of clinically relevant HPA axis suppression was observed following a 30-minute cosyntropin infusion.

The potential of NASONEX Nasal Spray 50 mcg to cause growth suppression in susceptible patients or when given at higher doses cannot be ruled out.

8.5 Geriatric Use

A total of 280 patients above 64 years of age with allergic rhinitis or nasal polyps (age range 64 to 86 years) have been treated with NASONEX Nasal Spray 50 mcg for up to 3 or 4 months, respectively. The adverse reactions reported in this population were similar in type and incidence to those reported by younger patients.

8.6 Hepatic Impairment

Concentrations of mometasone furoate appear to increase with severity of hepatic impairment *[see Clinical Pharmacology (12.3)]*

10. OVERDOSAGE

There are no data available on the effects of acute or chronic overdosage with NASONEX Nasal Spray 50 mcg. Because of low systemic bioavailability, and an absence of acute drug-related systemic findings in clinical studies, overdose is unlikely to require any therapy other than observation. Intranasal administration of 1600 mcg (4 times the recommended dose of NASONEX Nasal Spray 50 mcg for the treatment of nasal polyps in patients 18 years of age and older) daily for 29 days, to healthy human volunteers, showed no increased incidence of adverse events. Single intranasal doses up to 4000 mcg and oral inhalation doses up to 8000 mcg have been studied in human volunteers with no adverse effects reported. Chronic over dosage with any corticosteroid may result in signs or symptoms of hypercorticism [*see Warnings and Precautions (5.4)*]. Acute overdosage with this dosage form is unlikely since one bottle of NASONEX Nasal Spray 50 mcg contains approximately 8500 mcg of mometasone furoate.

11. DESCRIPTION

Mometasone furoate monohydrate, the active component of NASONEX Nasal Spray, 50 mcg, is an anti-inflammatory corticosteroid having the chemical name, 9,21-Dichloro-11ß,17-dihydroxy-16α-methylpregna-1,4-diene-3,20-dione-17-(2 furoate) monohydrate, and the following chemical structure:

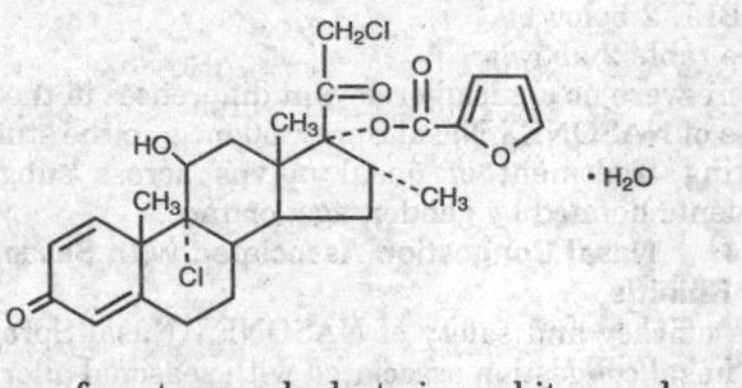

Mometasone furoate monohydrate is a white powder, with an empirical formula of $C_{27}H_{30}Cl_2O_6 \bullet H_2O$, and a molecular weight of 539.45. It is practically insoluble in water; slightly soluble in methanol, ethanol, and isopropanol; soluble in acetone and chloroform; and freely soluble in tetrahydrofuran. Its partition coefficient between octanol and water is greater than 5000.

NASONEX Nasal Spray 50 mcg is a metered-dose, manual pump spray unit containing an aqueous suspension of mometasone furoate monohydrate equivalent to 0.05% w/w mometasone furoate calculated on the anhydrous basis; in an aqueous medium containing glycerin, microcrystalline cellulose and carboxymethylcellulose sodium, sodium citrate, citric acid, benzalkonium chloride, and polysorbate 80. The pH is between 4.3 and 4.9.

12. CLINICAL PHARMACOLOGY

12.1 Mechanism of Action

NASONEX Nasal Spray 50 mcg is a corticosteroid demonstrating potent anti-inflammatory properties. The precise mechanism of corticosteroid action on allergic rhinitis is not known. Corticosteroids have been shown to have a wide range of effects on multiple cell types (e.g., mast cells, eosinophils, neutrophils, macrophages, and lymphocytes) and mediators (e.g., histamine, eicosanoids, leukotrienes, and cytokines) involved in inflammation.

In two clinical studies utilizing nasal antigen challenge, NASONEX Nasal Spray, 50 mcg decreased some markers of the early- and late-phase allergic response. These observations included decreases (vs. placebo) in histamine and eosinophil cationic protein levels, and reductions (vs. baseline) in eosinophils, neutrophils, and epithelial cell adhesion proteins. The clinical significance of these findings is not known.

The effect of NASONEX Nasal Spray, 50 mcg on nasal mucosa following 12 months of treatment was examined in 46 patients with allergic rhinitis. There was no evidence of atrophy and there was a marked reduction in intraepithelial eosinophilia and inflammatory cell infiltration (e.g., eosinophils, lymphocytes, monocytes, neutrophils, and plasma cells).

12.2 Pharmacodynamics

Adrenal Function in Adults: Four clinical pharmacology studies have been conducted in humans to assess the effect of NASONEX Nasal Spray, 50 mcg at various doses on adrenal function. In one study, daily doses of 200 and 400 mcg of NASONEX Nasal Spray, 50 mcg and 10 mg of prednisone were compared to placebo in 64 patients (22 to 44 years of age) with allergic rhinitis. Adrenal function before and after 36 consecutive days of treatment was assessed by measuring plasma cortisol levels following a 6-hour Cortrosyn (ACTH) infusion and by measuring 24-hour urinary-free cortisol levels. NASONEX Nasal Spray, 50 mcg, at both the 200- and 400-mcg dose, was not associated with a statistically significant decrease in mean plasma cortisol levels post-Cortrosyn infusion or a statistically significant decrease in the 24-hour urinary-free cortisol levels compared to placebo. A statistically significant decrease in the mean plasma cortisol levels post-Cortrosyn infusion and 24-hour urinary-free cortisol levels was detected in the prednisone treatment group compared to placebo.

A second study assessed adrenal response to NASONEX Nasal Spray, 50 mcg (400 and 1600 mcg/day), prednisone (10 mg/day), and placebo, administered for 29 days in 48 male volunteers (21 to 40 years of age). The 24-hour plasma cortisol area under the curve (AUC_{0-24}), during and after an 8-hour Cortrosyn infusion and 24-hour urinary-free cortisol levels were determined at baseline and after 29 days of treatment. No statistically significant differences in adrenal function were observed with NASONEX Nasal Spray, 50 mcg compared to placebo.

A third study evaluated single, rising doses of NASONEX Nasal Spray, 50 mcg (1000, 2000, and 4000 mcg/day), orally administered mometasone furoate (2000, 4000, and 8000 mcg/day), orally administered dexamethasone (200, 400, and 800 mcg/day), and placebo (administered at the end of each series of doses) in 24 male volunteers (22 to 39 years of age). Dose administrations were separated by at least 72 hours. Determination of serial plasma cortisol levels at 8 AM and for the 24-hour period following each treatment were used to calculate the plasma cortisol area under the curve (AUC_{0-24}). In addition, 24-hour urinary-free cortisol levels were collected prior to initial treatment administration and during the period immediately following each dose. No statistically significant decreases in the plasma cortisol AUC, 8 AM cortisol levels, or 24-hour urinary-free cortisol levels were observed in volunteers treated with either NASONEX Nasal Spray, 50 mcg or oral mometasone, as compared with placebo treatment. Conversely, nearly all volunteers treated with the three doses of dexamethasone demonstrated abnormal 8 AM cortisol levels (defined as a cortisol level <10 mcg/dL), reduced 24-hour plasma AUC values, and decreased 24-hour urinary-free cortisol levels, as compared to placebo treatment.

In a fourth study, adrenal function was assessed in 213 patients (18 to 81 years of age) with nasal polyps before and after 4 months of treatment with either NASONEX Nasal Spray, 50 mcg, (200 mcg once or twice daily) or placebo by measuring 24-hour urinary-free cortisol levels. NASONEX Nasal Spray, 50 mcg, at both doses (200 and 400 mcg/day), was not associated with statistically significant decreases in the 24-hour urinary-free cortisol levels compared to placebo.

Three clinical pharmacology studies have been conducted in pediatric patients to assess the effect of mometasone furoate nasal spray on the adrenal function at daily doses of 50, 100, and 200 mcg vs. placebo. In one study, adrenal function before and after 7 consecutive days of treatment was assessed in 48 pediatric patients with allergic rhinitis (ages 6 to 11 years) by measuring morning plasma cortisol and 24-hour urinary-free cortisol levels. Mometasone furoate nasal spray, at all three doses, was not associated with a statistically significant decrease in mean plasma cortisol levels or a statistically significant decrease in the 24-hour urinary-free cortisol levels compared to placebo. In the second study, adrenal function before and after 14 consecutive days of treatment was assessed in 48 pediatric patients (ages 3 to 5 years) with allergic rhinitis by measuring plasma cortisol levels following a 30-minute Cortrosyn infusion. Mometasone furoate nasal spray, 50 mcg, at all three doses (50, 100, and 200 mcg/day), was not associated with a statistically significant decrease in mean plasma cortisol levels post-Cortrosyn infusion compared to placebo. All patients had a normal response to Cortrosyn. In the third study, adrenal function before and after up to 42 consecutive days of once-daily treatment was assessed in 52 patients with allergic rhinitis (ages 2 to 5 years), 28 of whom received mometasone furoate nasal spray, 50 mcg per nostril (total daily dose 100 mcg), by measuring morning plasma cortisol and 24-hour urinary-free cortisol levels. Mometasone furoate nasal spray was not associated with a statistically significant decrease in mean plasma cortisol levels or a statistically significant decrease in the 24-hour urinary-free cortisol levels compared to placebo.

12.3 Pharmacokinetics

Absorption:

Mometasone furoate monohydrate administered as a nasal spray suspension has very low bioavailability (<1%) in plasma using a sensitive assay with a lower quantitation limit (LOQ) of 0.25 pcg/mL.

Distribution:

The *in vitro* protein binding for mometasone furoate was reported to be 98% to 99% in concentration range of 5 to 500 ng/mL.

Metabolism:

Studies have shown that any portion of a mometasone furoate dose which is swallowed and absorbed undergoes extensive metabolism to multiple metabolites. There are no major metabolites detectable in plasma. Upon *in vitro* incubation, one of the minor metabolites formed is 6ß-hydroxy-mometasone furoate. In human liver microsomes, the formation of the metabolite is regulated by cytochrome P-450 3A4 (CYP3A4).

Elimination:

Following intravenous administration, the effective plasma elimination half-life of mometasone furoate is 5.8 hours. Any absorbed drug is excreted as metabolites mostly via the bile, and to a limited extent, into the urine.

Specific Populations:

Hepatic Impairment: Administration of a single inhaled dose of 400 mcg mometasone furoate to subjects with mild (n=4), moderate (n=4), and severe (n=4) hepatic impairment resulted in only 1 or 2 subjects in each group having detectable peak plasma concentrations of mometasone furoate (ranging from 50 to 105 pcg/mL). The observed peak plasma concentrations appear to increase with severity of hepatic impairment, however, the numbers of detectable levels were few.

Renal Impairment: The effects of renal impairment on mometasone furoate pharmacokinetics have not been adequately investigated.

Pediatric: Mometasone furoate pharmacokinetics have not been investigated in the pediatric population [see Use in Specific Populations (8.4)].

Gender: The effects of gender on mometasone furoate pharmacokinetics have not been adequately investigated.

Race: The effects of race on mometasone furoate pharmacokinetics have not been adequately investigated.

Drug-Drug Interactions:

Inhibitors of Cytochrome P450 3A4: In a drug interaction study, an inhaled dose of mometasone furoate 400 mcg was given to 24 healthy subjects twice daily for 9 days and ketoconazole 200 mg (as well as placebo) were given twice daily concomitantly on Days 4 to 9. Mometasone furoate plasma concentrations were <150 pcg/mL on Day 3 prior to coadministration of ketoconazole or placebo. Following concomitant administration of ketoconazole, 4 out of 12 subjects in the ketoconazole treatment group (n=12) had peak plasma concentrations of mometasone furoate >200 pcg/mL on Day 9 (211–324 pcg/mL).

13. NONCLINICAL TOXICOLOGY

13.1 Carcinogenesis, Mutagenesis, Impairment of Fertility

In a 2-year carcinogenicity study in Sprague Dawley rats, mometasone furoate demonstrated no statistically significant increase in the incidence of tumors at inhalation doses up to 67 mcg/kg (approximately 1 and 2 times the maximum recommended daily intranasal dose [MRDID] in adults [400 mcg] and children [100 mcg], respectively, on a mcg/m^2 basis). In a 19-month carcinogenicity study in Swiss CD-1 mice, mometasone furoate demonstrated no statistically significant increase in the incidence of tumors at inhalation doses up to 160 mcg/kg (approximately 2 times the MRDID in adults and children, respectively, on a mcg/m^2 basis).

Mometasone furoate increased chromosomal aberrations in an *in vitro* Chinese hamster ovary-cell assay, but did not increase chromosomal aberrations in an *in vitro* Chinese hamster lung cell assay. Mometasone furoate was not mutagenic in the Ames test or mouse-lymphoma assay, and was not clastogenic in an *in vivo* mouse micronucleus assay and a rat bone marrow chromosomal aberration assay or a mouse male germ-cell chromosomal aberration assay. Mometasone furoate also did not induce unscheduled DNA synthesis *in vivo* in rat hepatocytes.

In reproductive studies in rats, impairment of fertility was not produced by subcutaneous doses up to 15 mcg/kg (less than the MRDID in adults on a mcg/m^2 basis).

TABLE 2: EFFECT OF NASONEX NASAL SPRAY IN TWO RANDOMIZED, PLACEBO-CONTROLLED TRIALS IN PATIENTS WITH NASAL POLYPS

	NASONEX 200 mcg qd	NASONEX 200 mcg bid	Placebo	P value for NASONEX 200 mcg qd vs. placebo	P value for NASONEX 200 mcg bid vs. placebo
Study 1	N = 115	N = 122	N = 117		
Baseline bilateral polyp grade*	4.21	4.27	4.25		
Mean change from baseline in bilateral polyps grade	-1.15	-0.96	-0.50	<0.001	0.01
Baseline nasal congestion†	2.29	2.35	2.28		
Mean change from baseline in nasal congestion	-0.47	-0.61	-0.24	0.001	<0.001
Study 2	N = 102	N = 102	N = 106		
Baseline bilateral polyp grade*	4.00	4.10	4.17		
Mean change from baseline in bilateral polyps grade	-0.78	-0.96	-0.62	0.33	0.04
Baseline nasal congestion†	2.23	2.20	2.18		
Mean change from baseline in nasal congestion	-0.42	-0.66	-0.23	0.01	<0.001

* polyps in each nasal fossa were graded by the investigator based on endoscopic visualization, using a scale of 0–3 where 0 = no polyps; 1 = polyps in the middle meatus, not reaching below the inferior border of the middle turbinate; 2 = polyps reaching below the inferior border of the middle turbinate but not the inferior border of the inferior turbinate; 3 = polyps reaching to or below the border of the inferior turbinate, or polyps medial to the middle turbinate (score reflects sum of left and right nasal fossa grades).

† nasal congestion/obstruction was scored daily by the patient using a 0–3 categorical scale where 0 = no symptoms, 1 = mild symptoms, 2 = moderate symptoms and 3 = severe symptoms.

TABLE 3: EFFECT OF NASONEX NASAL SPRAY IN TWO RANDOMIZED, PLACEBO-CONTROLLED TRIALS ON NASAL CONGESTION IN PATIENTS WITH SEASONAL ALLERGIC RHINITIS

Treatment (Patient Number)	Baseline * LS Mean †	Change from Baseline LS Mean †	Difference from Placebo LS Mean †	P value for NASONEX 200 mcg qd vs. placebo
Study 1				
NASONEX 200 mcg qd (N=176)	2.63	-0.64	-0.15	0.006
Placebo (N=175)	2.62	-0.49		
Study 2				
NASONEX 200 mcg qd (N=168)	2.62	-0.71	-0.31	<0.001
Placebo (N=164)	2.60	-0.40		

* nasal congestion/obstruction was scored daily by the patient using a 0–3 categorical scale where 0= no symptoms, 1=mild symptoms, 2=moderate symptoms and 3 =severe symptoms.

† LS Mean and p- value was from an ANCOVA model with treatment, baseline value, and center effects.

13.2 Animal Toxicology and/or Pharmacology Reproduction Toxicology Studies

In mice, mometasone furoate caused cleft palate at subcutaneous doses of 60 mcg/kg and above (less than the MRDID in adults on a mcg/m² basis). Fetal survival was reduced at 180 mcg/kg (approximately 2 times the MRDID in adults on a mcg/m² basis). No toxicity was observed at 20 mcg/kg (less than the MRDID in adults on a mcg/m² basis).

In rats, mometasone furoate produced umbilical hernia at topical dermal doses of 600 mcg/kg and above (approximately 10 times the MRDID in adults on a mcg/m² basis). A dose of 300 mcg/kg (approximately 6 times the MRDID in adults on a mcg/m² basis) produced delays in ossification, but no malformations. In rabbits, mometasone furoate caused multiple malformations (e.g., flexed front paws, gallbladder agenesis, umbilical hernia, hydrocephaly) at topical dermal doses of 150 mcg/kg and above (approximately 6 times the MRDID in adults on a mcg/m² basis). In an oral study, mometasone furoate increased resorptions and caused cleft palate and/or head malformations (hydrocephaly or domed head) at 700 mcg/kg (approximately 30 times the MRDID in adults on a mcg/m² basis). At 2800 mcg/kg (approximately 110 times the MRDID in adults on a mcg/m² basis), most litters were aborted or resorbed. No toxicity was observed at 140 mcg/kg (approximately 6 times the MRDID in adults on a mcg/m² basis).

When rats received subcutaneous doses of mometasone furoate throughout pregnancy or during the later stages of pregnancy, 15 mcg/kg (less than the MRDID in adults on a mcg/m² basis) caused prolonged and difficult labor and reduced the number of live births, birth weight, and early pup survival. Similar effects were not observed at 7.5 mcg/kg (less than the MRDID in adults on a mcg/m² basis).

14. CLINICAL STUDIES

14.1 Allergic Rhinitis in Adults and Adolescents

The efficacy and safety of NASONEX Nasal Spray, 50 mcg in the prophylaxis and treatment of seasonal allergic rhinitis and the treatment of perennial allergic rhinitis have been evaluated in 18 controlled trials, and one uncontrolled clinical trial, in approximately 3000 adults (ages 17 to 85 years) and adolescents (ages 12 to 16 years). Of the total number of patients, there were 1757 males and 1453 females, including a total of 283 adolescents (182 boys and 101 girls) with seasonal allergic or perennial allergic rhinitis. Patients were treated with NASONEX Nasal Spray 50 mcg at doses ranging from 50 to 800 mcg/day. The majority of patients were treated with 200 mcg/day. The allergic rhinitis trials evaluated the total nasal symptom scores that included stuffiness, rhinorrhea, itching, and sneezing. Patients treated with NASONEX Nasal Spray 50 mcg, 200 mcg/day had a significant decrease in total nasal symptom scores compared to placebo-treated patients. No additional benefit was observed for mometasone furoate doses greater than 200 mcg/day. A total of 350 patients have been treated with NASONEX Nasal Spray 50 mcg for 1 year or longer.

In patients with seasonal allergic rhinitis, NASONEX Nasal Spray 50 mcg, demonstrated improvement in nasal symptoms (vs. placebo) within 11 hours after the first dose based on one single-dose, parallel-group study of patients in an outdoor "park" setting (park study) and one environmental exposure unit (EEU) study, and within 2 days in two randomized, double-blind, placebo-controlled, parallel-group seasonal allergic rhinitis studies. Maximum benefit is usually achieved within 1 to 2 weeks after initiation of dosing.

Prophylaxis of seasonal allergic rhinitis for patients 12 years of age and older with NASONEX Nasal Spray 50 mcg, given at a dose of 200 mcg/day, was evaluated in two clinical studies in 284 patients. These studies were designed such that patients received 4 weeks of prophylaxis with NASONEX Nasal Spray 50 mcg prior to the anticipated onset of the pollen season; however, some patients received only 2 to 3 weeks of prophylaxis. Patients receiving 2 to 4 weeks of prophylaxis with NASONEX Nasal Spray 50 mcg demonstrated a statistically significantly smaller mean increase in total nasal symptom scores with onset of the pollen season as compared to placebo patients.

14.2 Allergic Rhinitis in Pediatrics

The efficacy and safety of NASONEX Nasal Spray 50 mcg in the treatment of seasonal allergic and perennial allergic rhinitis in pediatric patients (ages 3 to 11 years) have been evaluated in four controlled trials. This included approximately 990 pediatric patients ages 3 to 11 years (606 males and 384 females) with seasonal allergic or perennial allergic rhinitis treated with mometasone furoate nasal spray at doses ranging from 25 to 200 mcg/day. Pediatric patients treated with NASONEX Nasal Spray 50 mcg (100 mcg total daily dose, 374 patients) had a significant decrease in total nasal symptom (nasal congestion, rhinorrhea, itching, and sneezing) scores, compared to placebo-treated patients. No additional benefit was observed for the 200-mcg mometasone furoate total daily dose in pediatric patients (ages 3 to 11 years). A total of 163 pediatric patients have been treated for 1 year.

14.3 Nasal Polyps

Two studies were performed to evaluate the efficacy and safety of NASONEX Nasal Spray in the treatment of nasal polyps. These studies involved 664 patients with nasal polyps, 441 of whom received NASONEX Nasal Spray. These studies were randomized, double-blind, placebo-controlled, parallel-group, multicenter studies in patients 18 to 86 years of age with bilateral nasal polyps. Patients were randomized to receive NASONEX Nasal Spray 200 mcg once daily, 200 mcg twice daily or placebo for a period of 4 months. The co-primary efficacy endpoints were 1) change from baseline in nasal congestion/obstruction averaged over the first month of treatment; and 2) change from baseline to last assessment in bilateral polyp grade during the entire 4 months of treatment as assessed by endoscopy. Efficacy was demonstrated in both studies at a dose of 200 mcg twice daily and in one study at a dose of 200 mcg once a day (see TABLE 2 below).

[See table 2 above]

There were no clinically relevant differences in the effectiveness of NASONEX Nasal Spray, 50 mcg, in the studies evaluating treatment of nasal polyps across subgroups of patients defined by gender, age, or race.

14.4 Nasal Congestion Associated with Seasonal Allergic Rhinitis

The efficacy and safety of NASONEX Nasal Spray 50 mcg for nasal congestion associated with seasonal allergic rhinitis were evaluated in three randomized, placebo-controlled, double blind clinical trials of 15 days duration. The three trials included a total of 1008 patients 12 years of age and older with nasal congestion associated with seasonal allergic rhinitis, of whom 506 received NASONEX Nasal Spray 200 mcg daily and 502 received placebo. Of the 1008 patients, the majority 784 (78 %) were Caucasians. The majority of the patients were between 18 to < 65 years of age with a mean age of 38.8 years and were predominantly women (66%). The primary efficacy endpoint was the change from baseline in average morning and evening reflective nasal congestion score over treatment day 1 to day 15. The key secondary efficacy endpoint was the change from baseline in average morning and evening reflective total nasal symptom score (TNSS = rhinorrhea [nasal discharge/runny nose or postnasal drip], nasal congestion/stuffiness, nasal itching, sneezing) averaged over treatment day 1 to 15. Two out of three studies demonstrated that treatment with Nasonex Nasal Spray significantly reduced the nasal congestion symptom score and the TNSS compared to placebo in patients 12 years of age and older with seasonal allergic rhinitis (see TABLE 3 and 4 below).

[See table 3 above]

[See table 4 at top of next page]

Based on results in other studies with NASONEX Nasal Spray in pediatric patients, effects on nasal congestion associated with seasonal allergic rhinitis in patients below 12 years of age is similar to those seen in adults and adolescents [see Clinical Studies (14.2)].

16. HOW SUPPLIED/STORAGE AND HANDLING

NASONEX (mometasone furoate monohydrate) Nasal Spray, 50 mcg is supplied in a white, high-density, polyethylene bottle fitted with a white metered-dose, manual spray pump, and blue cap. It contains 17 g of product formulation, 120 sprays, each delivering 50 mcg of mometasone furoate per actuation.
(NDC 0085-1288-01).

Store at 25°C (77°F); excursions permitted to 15° to 30°C (59° to 86°F) [see USP Controlled Room Temperature]. Protect from light.

When NASONEX Nasal Spray, 50 mcg is removed from its cardboard container, prolonged exposure of the product to direct light should be avoided. Brief exposure to light, as with normal use, is acceptable.

SHAKE WELL BEFORE EACH USE.

Keep out of reach of children.

17. PATIENT COUNSELING INFORMATION

See FDA-approved labeling

17.1 Local Nasal Effect

Patients should be informed that treatment with NASONEX Nasal Spray 50 mcg may be associated with adverse reactions which include epistaxis (nose bleed) and nasal septum perforation. Candida infection may also occur. Because of the inhibitory effect of corticosteroids on wound healing, patients who have experienced recent nasal septum ulcers, nasal surgery, or nasal trauma should not use a nasal corticosteroid until healing has occurred *[see Warnings and Precautions (5.1)]*. Patients should be cautioned not to spray NASONEX Nasal Spray 50 mcg directly onto the nasal septum.

17.2 Glaucoma and Cataracts

Patients should be informed that nasal and inhaled corticosteroids may result in the development of glaucoma and/or cataracts. Therefore, close monitoring is warranted in patients with a change in vision or with a history of increased intraocular pressure, glaucoma, and/or cataracts. Patients should be cautioned not to spray NASONEX Nasal Spray 50 mcg into the eyes *[see Warnings and Precautions (5.2)]*.

17.3 Immunosuppression

Persons who are on immunosuppressant doses of corticosteroids should be warned to avoid exposure to chickenpox or measles, and patients should also be advised that if they are exposed, medical advice should be sought without delay *[see Warnings and Precautions (5.4)]*.

17.4 Use Regularly for Best Effect

Patients should use NASONEX Nasal Spray 50 mcg on a regular basis for optimal effect. Improvement in nasal symptoms of allergic rhinitis has been shown to occur within 1 to 2 days after initiation of dosing. Maximum benefit is usually achieved within 1 to 2 weeks after initiation of dosing. Patients should not increase the prescribed dosage but should contact their physician if symptoms do not improve, or if the condition worsens. Administration to young children should be aided by an adult.

If a patient missed a dose, the patient should be advised to take the dose as soon as they remember. The patient should not take more than the recommended dose for the day.

Manufactured by Schering Corporation, a subsidiary of Schering-Plough Corporation, Kenilworth, NJ 07033 USA.

Schering-Plough

© 1997, 2009 Schering Corporation. All rights reserved.

U.S. Patent Nos. D355,844; 5,837,699; 6,127,353; and 6,723,713.

PATIENT INFORMATION

NASONEX® [nā-sō-nĕks] (mometasone furoate monohydrate) **Nasal Spray, 50 mcg**

FOR INTRANASAL USE ONLY

Read the Patient Information that comes with NASONEX before you start using it and each time you get a refill. There may be new information. This Patient Information does not take the place of talking to your health-care provider about your medical condition or treatment. If you have any questions about NASONEX, ask your health-care provider.

What is NASONEX?

NASONEX Nasal Spray is a man-made (synthetic) corticosteroid medicine that is used to:

- to treat the nasal symptoms of seasonal and year-round allergic rhinitis (inflammation of the lining of the nose) in adults and children 2 years of age and older.
- to treat nasal congestion that happens with seasonal allergic rhinitis in adults and children 2 years of age and older.
- to prevent nasal symptoms of seasonal allergic rhinitis in people 12 years of age and older.
- to treat nasal polyps in people 18 years and older.

The safety and effectiveness of NASONEX has not been shown:

- In children under 2 years of age to treat allergic rhinitis.
- In children under 18 years of age to treat nasal polyps.

TABLE 4: EFFECT OF NASONEX NASAL SPRAY ON TNSS IN TWO RANDOMIZED, PLACEBO-CONTROLLED TRIALS IN PATIENTS WITH SEASONAL ALLERGIC RHINITIS

Treatment (Patient Number)	Baseline * LS Mean [†]	Change from Baseline LS Mean [†]	Difference from Placebo LS Mean [†]	P value for NASONEX 200 mcg qd vs. placebo
Study 1				
NASONEX 200 mcg qd (N=176)	9.60	-2.68	-0.83	<0.001
Placebo (N=175)	9.66	-1.85		
Study 2				
NASONEX 200 mcg qd (N=168)	9.39	-3.00	-1.27	<0.001
Placebo (N=164)	9.50	-1.73		

* TNSS was the sum of four individual symptom scores: rhinorrhea, nasal congestion/stuffiness, nasal itching and sneezing. Each symptom was to be rated on a scale of 0 = none, 1 = mild, 2 = moderate, 3 = severe.
† LS Mean and p- value was from an ANCOVA model with treatment, baseline value, and center effects.

Who should not use NASONEX?

Do not use NASONEX if you are allergic to any of the ingredients in NASONEX. See the end of this leaflet for a complete list of ingredients in NASONEX.

What should I tell my health-care provider before using NASONEX?

Before you take NASONEX, tell your health-care provider if you:

- have had recent nasal sores, nasal surgery, or nasal injury.
- have eye or vision problems, such as cataracts or glaucoma (increased pressure in your eye).
- have tuberculosis or any untreated fungal, bacterial, viral infections, or eye infections caused by herpes.
- have been near someone who has chickenpox or measles.
- are not feeling well or have any other symptoms that you do not understand.
- have any other medical conditions.
- **are pregnant or planning to become pregnant.** It is not known if NASONEX will harm your unborn baby. Talk to your doctor if you are pregnant or plan to become pregnant.
- **are breast-feeding or planning to breast-feed.** It is not known whether NASONEX passes into your breast milk.

Tell your healthcare provider about all the medicines you take including prescription and non-prescription medicines, vitamins, and herbal supplements.

NASONEX and other medicines may affect each other and cause side effects. NASONEX may affect the way other medicines work, and other medicines may affect how NASONEX works.

Know the list of medicine you take. Keep a list of your medications with you to show your healthcare provider and pharmacist when a new medication is prescribed.

How should I use NASONEX?

- Use NASONEX exactly as prescribed by your health-care provider.
- This medicine is for use in the _nose only_. Do not spray it into your mouth or eyes.
- An adult should help a young child use this medicine.
- For best results, you should keep using NASONEX regularly each day without missing a dose. If you do miss a dose of NASONEX, take it as soon as you remember. However, do not take more than the daily dose prescribed by your doctor.
- Do not use NASONEX more often than prescribed. Ask your health-care provider if you have any questions.
- For detailed instructions on how to use NASONEX Nasal Spray, see the **"Patient's Instructions for Use"** at the end of this leaflet.

See your health-care provider regularly to assess your symptoms while taking NASONEX and to check for side effects.

What should I avoid while taking NASONEX?

If you are taking other corticosteroid medicines for allergy, either by mouth or injection, your health-care provider may advise you to stop taking them once you begin using NASONEX.

What are the possible side effects of NASONEX?

NASONEX may cause serious side effects, including:

- **Thrush (candida), a fungal infection in your nose and throat.** Tell your doctor if you have any redness or white colored patches in your nose or throat.
- **Slow wound healing. Do not** use NASONEX until your nose has healed if you have a sore in your nose, if you have surgery on your nose, or if your nose has been injured.
- **Some people may have eye problems, including glaucoma and cataracts.** You should have regular eye exams.

- **Immune system problems that may increase you risk of infections.** You are more likely to get infections if you take medicines that weaken your immune system. Avoid contact with people who have contagious diseases such as chicken pox or measles while using NASONEX. Symptoms of infection may include: fever, pain, aches, chills, feeling tired, nausea and vomiting. Tell your doctor about any signs of infection while you are using NASONEX.
- **Adrenal insufficiency.** Adrenal insufficiency is a condition in which the adrenal glands do not make enough steroid hormones. Symptoms of adrenal insufficiency can include: tiredness, weakness, nausea and vomiting and low blood pressure.

The most common side effects of NASONEX include:

- Headache
- viral infection
- sore throat
- nosebleeds
- cough

Tell your health-care provider if you have any side effect that bothers you or that does not go away.

These are not all the possible side effects of NASONEX. For more information ask your health-care provider or pharmacist.

Call your doctor for medical advice about side effects. You may report side effects to FDA at 1-800-FDA-1088.

How should I store NASONEX?

- Store NASONEX at room temperature between 59°F to 86°F (15°C to 30°C).
- Avoid prolonged exposure NASONEX container to bright light.
- Shake well before each use.

Keep NASONEX and all medicines out of the reach of children.

General information about NASONEX

Medicines are sometimes prescribed for conditions that are not listed in a Patient Information leaflet. Do not use NASONEX for a condition for which it was not prescribed. Do not give NASONEX to other people even if they have the same symptoms you have. It may harm them.

This Patient Information leaflet provides a summary of the most important information about NASONEX. If you would like more information, talk with your health-care provider. You can ask your health-care provider or pharmacist for information about NASONEX that is written for health professionals.

For more information, go to www.NASONEX.com or call 1-800-526-4099.

What are the ingredients in NASONEX?

Active Ingredients: mometasone furoate monohydrate

Inactive Ingredients: glycerin, microcrystalline cellulose and carboxymethylcellulose sodium, sodium citrate, citric acid, benzalkonium chloride, and polysorbate 80.

Patient Instructions for Use

For use in your nose only.

Read the Patient Instructions for Use carefully before you start to use your NASONEX Nasal Spray. If you have any questions, ask your health-care provider.

Shake the bottle well before each use.

- 1.Remove the plastic cap (Figure 1).

[See figure 1 at top of next page]

- 2.Before you use NASONEX for the first time prime the pump by pressing downward on the shoulders of the white nasal applicator using your index finger and middle finger while holding the base of the bottle with your thumb (Figure 2). **Do Not** pierce the nasal applicator. Press down and release the pump 10 times or until a fine spray appears. **Do Not** spray into eyes. The pump is now ready to use. The pump may be stored unused for up to 1 week without

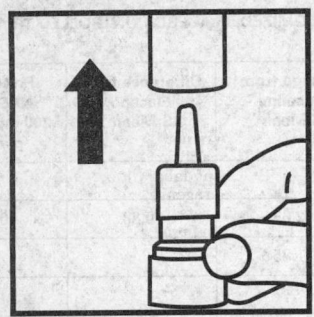

Figure 1

repriming. If unused for more than 1 week, reprime by spraying 2 times or until a fine spray appears.

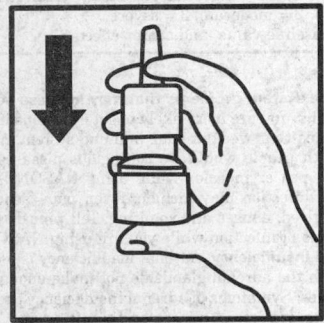

Figure 2

- 3. Gently blow your nose to clear the nostrils. Close 1 nostril. Tilt your head forward slightly, keep the bottle upright, carefully insert the nasal applicator into the other nostril (Figure 3). **Do Not** spray directly onto the nasal septum (the wall between the two nostrils).

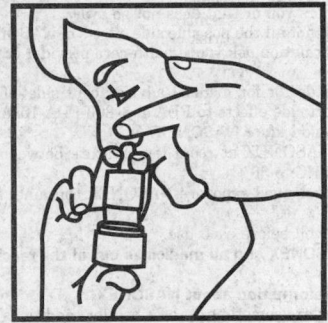

Figure 3

- 4. For each spray, hold the spray bottle upright and press firmly downward 1 time on the shoulders of the white nasal applicator using your index and middle fingers while supporting the base of the bottle with your thumb. Breathe gently inward through the nostril (Figure 4).

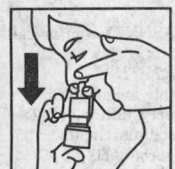

Note: It is important to keep the Nasonex unit in an upright orientation (as seen in Figure 4). Failure to do so may result in an incomplete or non-existent spray.

Figure 4

- 5. Then breathe out through the mouth.
- 6. Repeat in the other nostril.
- 7. Wipe the nasal applicator with a clean tissue and replace the plastic cap.

Each bottle of NASONEX Nasal Spray contains enough medicine for you to spray medicine from the bottle 120 times. Do not use the bottle of NASONEX Nasal Spray after 120 sprays. Additional sprays after the 120 sprays may not contain the right amount of medicine, **you should keep track of the number of sprays used from each bottle of NASONEX Nasal Spray,** and throw away the bottle even if it

has medicine still left in. **Do not count any sprays used for priming the device.** Talk with your health-care provider before your supply runs out to see if you should get a refill of your medicine.

Pediatric Use: Administration to young children should be done by an adult. Steps 1 through 7 from the **Patient Instructions for Use,** should be followed.

Cleaning: Do not try to unblock the nasal applicator with a sharp object. Please see **Applicator Cleaning Instructions.**

Patient Instruction for cleaning applicator

- 1. To clean the nasal applicator, remove the plastic cap (Figure 6).

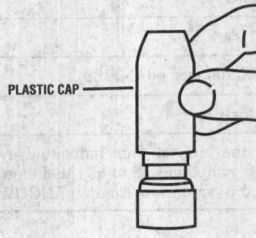

PLASTIC CAP

Figure 6

- 2. Pull gently upward on the white nasal applicator to remove (Figure 7).

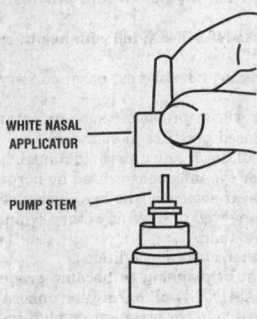

WHITE NASAL APPLICATOR

PUMP STEM

Figure 7

- 3. Soak the nasal applicator in cold tap water and rinse both ends of the nasal applicator under cold tap water and dry. (Figure 8). **Do not try to unblock the nasal applicator by inserting a pin or other sharp object as this will damage the applicator and cause you not to get the right dose of medicine.**

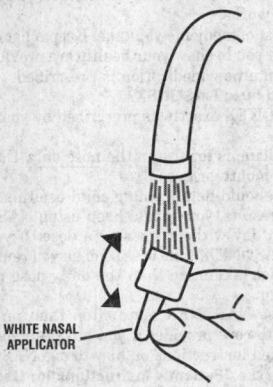

WHITE NASAL APPLICATOR

Figure 8

- 4. Rinse the plastic cap under cold water and dry (Figure 9).

[See figure 9 at top of next column]

- 5. Put the nasal applicator back together making sure the pump stem is reinserted into the applicator's center hole (Figure 10).

[See figure 10 on next column]

- 6. Reprime the pump by pressing downward on the shoulders of the white nasal applicator using your index and middle fingers while holding the base of the bottle with your thumb. Press down and release the pump 2 times or until a fine spray appears. **Do Not** spray into eyes. The pump is now ready to use. The pump may be stored unused for up to 1 week without repriming. If unused for more than 1 week, reprime by spraying 2 times or until a fine spray appears (Figure 11).

[See figure 11 on next column]

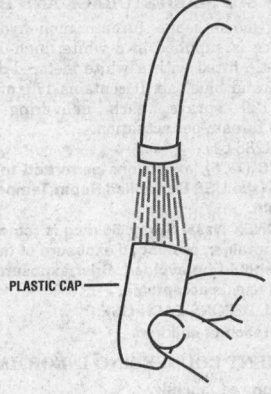

PLASTIC CAP

Figure 9

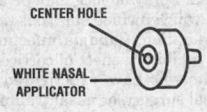

CENTER HOLE

WHITE NASAL APPLICATOR

PUMP STEM

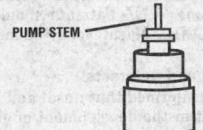

Figure 10

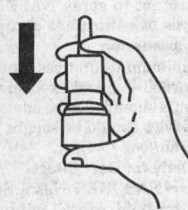

Figure 11

- 7. Replace the plastic cap (Figure 12).

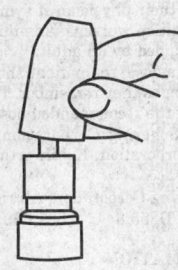

Figure 12

Manufactured by Schering Corporation, a subsidiary of Schering-Plough Corporation, Kenilworth, NJ 07033 USA.

Schering-Plough

© 1997, 2009 Schering Corporation. All rights reserved.

U.S. Patent Nos. D355,844; 5,837,699; 6,127,353; and 6,723,713.

Rev. 05/10

Shown in Product Identification Guide, page 313

NITRO-DUR®

[Nĭ-trō-Dŭr]

(nitroglycerin)

Transdermal Infusion System

PRODUCT INFORMATION

DESCRIPTION

Nitroglycerin is 1,2,3-propanetriol trinitrate, an organic nitrate whose structural formula is:

$$H_2CONO_2$$
$$|$$
$$HCONO_2$$
$$|$$
$$H_2CONO_2$$

and whose molecular weight is 227.09. The organic nitrates are vasodilators, active on both arteries and veins.
The NITRO-DUR (nitroglycerin) Transdermal Infusion System is a flat unit designed to provide continuous controlled release of nitroglycerin through intact skin. The rate of release of nitroglycerin is linearly dependent upon the area of the applied system; each cm^2 of applied system delivers approximately 0.02 mg of nitroglycerin per hour. Thus, the 5-, 10-, 15-, 20-, 30-, and 40-cm^2 systems deliver approximately 0.1, 0.2, 0.3, 0.4, 0.6, and 0.8 mg of nitroglycerin per hour, respectively.
The remainder of the nitroglycerin in each system serves as a reservoir and is not delivered in normal use. After 12 hours, for example, each system has delivered approximately 6% of its original content of nitroglycerin.
The NITRO-DUR transdermal system contains nitroglycerin in acrylic-based polymer adhesives with a resinous cross-linking agent to provide a continuous source of active ingredient. Each unit is sealed in a paper polyethylene-foil pouch.
Cross section of the system.

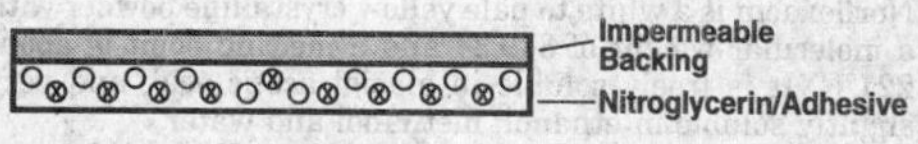

CLINICAL PHARMACOLOGY

The principal pharmacological action of nitroglycerin is relaxation of vascular smooth muscle and consequent dilatation of peripheral arteries and veins, especially the latter. Dilatation of the veins promotes peripheral pooling of blood and decreases venous return to the heart, thereby reducing left ventricular end-diastolic pressure and pulmonary capillary wedge pressure (preload). Arteriolar relaxation reduces systemic vascular resistance, systolic arterial pressure, and mean arterial pressure (afterload). Dilatation of the coronary arteries also occurs. The relative importance of preload reduction, afterload reduction, and coronary dilatation remains undefined.
Dosing regimens for most chronically used drugs are designed to provide plasma concentrations that are continuously greater than a minimally effective concentration. This strategy is inappropriate for organic nitrates. Several well-controlled clinical trials have used exercise testing to assess the antianginal efficacy of continuously delivered nitrates. In the large majority of these trials, active agents were indistinguishable from placebo after 24 hours (or less) of continuous therapy. Attempts to overcome nitrate tolerance by dose escalation, even to doses far in excess of those used acutely, have consistently failed. Only after nitrates have been absent from the body for several hours has their antianginal efficacy been restored.

Pharmacokinetics:

The volume of distribution of nitroglycerin is about 3 L/kg, and nitroglycerin is cleared from this volume at extremely rapid rates, with a resulting serum half-life of about 3 minutes. The observed clearance rates (close to 1 L/kg/min) greatly exceed hepatic blood flow; known sites of extrahepatic metabolism include red blood cells and vascular walls. The first products in the metabolism of nitroglycerin are inorganic nitrate and the 1,2- and 1,3-dinitroglycerols. The dinitrates are less effective vasodilators than nitroglycerin, but they are longer-lived in the serum, and their net contribution to the overall effect of chronic nitroglycerin regimens is not known. The dinitrates are further metabolized to (nonvasoactive) mononitrates and, ultimately, to glycerol and carbon dioxide.
To avoid development of tolerance to nitroglycerin, drug-free intervals of 10 to 12 hours are known to be sufficient; shorter intervals have not been well studied. In one well-controlled clinical trial, subjects receiving nitroglycerin appeared to exhibit a rebound or withdrawal effect, so that their exercise tolerance at the end of the daily drug-free interval was *less* than that exhibited by the parallel group receiving placebo.
In healthy volunteers, steady-state plasma concentrations of nitroglycerin are reached by about 2 hours after application of a patch and are maintained for the duration of wearing the system (observations have been limited to 24 hours). Upon removal of the patch, the plasma concentration declines with a half-life of about an hour.

Clinical Trials:

Regimens in which nitroglycerin patches were worn for 12 hours daily have been studied in well-controlled trials up to 4 weeks in duration. Starting about 2 hours after application and continuing until 10 to 12 hours after application, patches that deliver at least 0.4 mg of nitroglycerin per hour have consistently demonstrated greater antianginal activity than placebo. Lower-dose patches have not been as well studied, but in one large, well-controlled trial in which higher-dose patches were also studied, patches delivering 0.2 mg/hr had significantly *less* antianginal activity than placebo.
It is reasonable to believe that the rate of nitroglycerin absorption from patches may vary with the site of application, but this relationship has not been adequately studied.

INDICATIONS AND USAGE

Transdermal nitroglycerin is indicated for the prevention of angina pectoris due to coronary artery disease. The onset of action of transdermal nitroglycerin is not sufficiently rapid for this product to be useful in aborting an acute attack.

CONTRAINDICATIONS

Allergic reactions to organic nitrates are extremely rare, but they do occur. Nitroglycerin is contraindicated in patients who are allergic to it. Allergy to the adhesives used in nitroglycerin patches has also been reported, and it similarly constitutes a contraindication to the use of this product.

WARNINGS

Amplification of the vasodilatory effects of the NITRO-DUR patch by phosphodiesterase inhibitors, eg, sildenafil can result in severe hypotension. The time course and dose dependence of this interaction have not been studied. Appropriate supportive care has not been studied, but it seems reasonable to treat this as a nitrate overdose, with elevation of the extremities and with central volume expansion.
The benefits of transdermal nitroglycerin in patients with acute myocardial infarction or congestive heart failure have not been established. If one elects to use nitroglycerin in these conditions, careful clinical or hemodynamic monitoring must be used to avoid the hazards of hypotension and tachycardia.
A cardioverter/defibrillator should not be discharged through a paddle electrode that overlies a NITRO-DUR patch. The arcing that may be seen in this situation is harmless in itself, but it may be associated with local current concentration that can cause damage to the paddles and burns to the patient.

PRECAUTIONS

General:

Severe hypotension, particularly with upright posture, may occur with even small doses of nitroglycerin, particularly in the elderly. The NITRO-DUR Transdermal Infusion System should therefore be used with caution in elderly patients who may be volume-depleted, are on multiple medications, or who, for whatever reason, are already hypotensive. Hypotension induced by nitroglycerin may be accompanied by paradoxical bradycardia and increased angina pectoris.
Elderly patients may be more susceptible to hypotension and may be at greater risk of falling at the therapeutic doses of nitroglycerin.
Nitrate therapy may aggravate the angina caused by hypertrophic cardiomyopathy, particularly in the elderly.
In industrial workers who have had long-term exposure to unknown (presumably high) doses of organic nitrates, tolerance clearly occurs. Chest pain, acute myocardial infarction, and even sudden death have occurred during temporary withdrawal of nitrates from these workers, demonstrating the existence of true physical dependence.
Several clinical trials in patients with angina pectoris have evaluated nitroglycerin regimens which incorporated a 10- to 12-hour, nitrate-free interval. In some of these trials, an increase in the frequency of anginal attacks during the nitrate-free interval was observed in a small number of patients. In one trial, patients had decreased exercise tolerance at the end of the nitrate-free interval. Hemodynamic rebound has been observed only rarely; on the other hand, few studies were so designed that rebound, if it had occurred, would have been detected. The importance of these observations to the routine, clinical use of transdermal nitroglycerin is unknown.

Information for Patients:

Daily headaches sometimes accompany treatment with nitroglycerin. In patients who get these headaches, the headaches may be a marker of the activity of the drug. Patients should resist the temptation to avoid headaches by altering the schedule of their treatment with nitroglycerin, since loss of headache may be associated with simultaneous loss of antianginal efficacy.
Treatment with nitroglycerin may be associated with lightheadedness on standing, especially just after rising from a recumbent or seated position. This effect may be more frequent in patients who have also consumed alcohol.
After normal use, there is enough residual nitroglycerin in discarded patches that they are a potential hazard to children and pets
A patient leaflet is supplied with the systems.

Drug Interactions:

The vasodilating effects of nitroglycerin may be additive with those of other vasodilators. Alcohol, in particular, has been found to exhibit additive effects of this variety.

Carcinogenesis, Mutagenesis, Impairment of Fertility:

Animal carcinogenesis studies with topically applied nitroglycerin have not been performed.
Rats receiving up to 434 mg/kg/day of dietary nitroglycerin for 2 years developed dose-related fibrotic and neoplastic changes in liver, including carcinomas, and interstitial cell tumors in testes. At high dose, the incidences of hepatocellular carcinomas in both sexes were 52% vs 0% in controls, and incidences of testicular tumors were 52% vs 8% in controls. Lifetime dietary administration of up to 1058 mg/kg/day of nitroglycerin was not tumorigenic in mice.
Nitroglycerin was weakly mutagenic in Ames tests performed in two different laboratories. Nevertheless, there was no evidence of mutagenicity in an *in vivo* dominant lethal assay with male rats treated with doses up to about 363 mg/kg/day, po, or in *in vitro* cytogenetic tests in rat and dog tissues.
In a three-generation reproduction study, rats received dietary nitroglycerin at doses up to about 434 mg/kg/day for 6 months prior to mating of the F_0 generation with treatment continuing through successive F_1 and F_2 generations. The high dose was associated with decreased feed intake and body weight gain in both sexes at all matings. No specific effect on the fertility of the F_0 generation was seen. Infertility noted in subsequent generations, however, was attributed to increased interstitial cell tissue and aspermatogenesis in the high-dose males. In this three-generation study there was no clear evidence of teratogenicity.

Pregnancy: Pregnancy Category C:

Animal teratology studies have not been conducted with nitroglycerin transdermal systems. Teratology studies in rats and rabbits, however, were conducted with topically applied nitroglycerin ointment at doses up to 80 mg/kg/day and 240 mg/kg/day, respectively. No toxic effects on dams or fetuses were seen at any dose tested. There are no adequate and well-controlled studies in pregnant women. Nitroglycerin should be given to a pregnant woman only if clearly needed.

Nursing Mothers:

It is not known whether nitroglycerin is excreted in human milk. Because many drugs are excreted in human milk, caution should be exercised when nitroglycerin is administered to a nursing woman.

Pediatric Use:

Safety and effectiveness in pediatric patients have not been established.

Geriatric Use:

Clinical studies of NITRO-DUR Transdermal Infusion System did not include sufficient information to determine whether subjects 65 years and older respond differently from younger subjects. Additional clinical data from the published literature indicate that the elderly demonstrate increased sensitivity to nitrates, which may result in hypotension and increased risk of falling. In general, dose selection for an elderly patient should be cautious, usually starting at the low end of the dosing range, reflecting the greater frequency of the decreased hepatic, renal, or cardiac function, and of concomitant disease or other drug therapy.

ADVERSE REACTIONS

Adverse reactions to nitroglycerin are generally dose related, and almost all of these reactions are the result of nitroglycerin's activity as a vasodilator. Headache, which may be severe, is the most commonly reported side effect. Headache may be recurrent with each daily dose, especially at higher doses. Transient episodes of lightheadedness, occasionally related to blood pressure changes, may also occur. Hypotension occurs infrequently, but in some patients it may be severe enough to warrant discontinuation of therapy. Syncope, crescendo angina, and rebound hypertension have been reported but are uncommon.
Allergic reactions to nitroglycerin are also uncommon, and the great majority of those reported have been cases of contact dermatitis or fixed drug eruptions in patients receiving nitroglycerin in ointments or patches. There have been a few reports of genuine anaphylactoid reactions, and these reactions can probably occur in patients receiving nitroglycerin by any route.
Extremely rarely, ordinary doses of organic nitrates have caused methemoglobinemia in normal-seeming patients. Methemoglobinemia is so infrequent at these doses that further discussion of its diagnosis and treatment is deferred (see **OVERDOSAGE**).
Application-site irritation may occur but is rarely severe.
In two placebo-controlled trials of intermittent therapy with nitroglycerin patches at 0.2 to 0.8 mg/hr, the most frequent adverse reactions among 307 subjects were as follows:

	Placebo	Patch
Headache	18%	63%
Lightheadedness	4%	6%
Hypotension, and/or Syncope	0%	4%
Increased Angina	2%	2%

OVERDOSAGE

Hemodynamic Effects:

Nitroglycerin toxicity is generally mild. The estimated adult oral lethal dose of nitroglycerin is 200 mg to 1,200 mg. Infants may be more susceptible to toxicity from nitroglycerin. Consultation with a poison center should be considered.

NITRO-DUR System Rated Release In Vivo*	Total Nitroglycerin Content	System Size	Package Size
0.1 mg/hr	20 mg	5 cm²	Unit Dose 30 (NDC 0085-3305-30) Institutional Package 30 (NDC 0085-3305-35)
0.2 mg/hr	40 mg	10 cm²	Unit Dose 30 (NDC 0085-3310-30) Institutional Package 30 (NDC 0085-3310-35)
0.3 mg/hr	60 mg	15 cm²	Unit Dose 30 (NDC 0085-3315-30) Institutional Package 30 (NDC 0085-3315-35)
0.4 mg/hr	80 mg	20 cm²	Unit Dose 30 (NDC 0085-3320-30) Institutional Package 30 (NDC 0085-3320-35)
0.6 mg/hr	120 mg	30 cm²	Unit Dose 30 (NDC 0085-3330-30) Institutional Package 30 (NDC 0085-3330-35)
0.8 mg/hr	160 mg	40 cm²	Unit Dose 30 (NDC 0085-0819-30) Institutional Package 30 (NDC 0085-0819-35)

*Release rates were formerly described in terms of drug delivered per 24 hours. In these terms, the supplied NITRO-DUR systems would be rated at 2.5 mg/24 hours (0.1 mg/hour), 5 mg/24 hours (0.2 mg/hour), 7.5 mg/24 hours (0.3 mg/hour), 10 mg/24 hours (0.4 mg/hour), and 15 mg/24 hours (0.6 mg/hour).

Laboratory determinations of serum levels of nitroglycerin and its metabolites are not widely available, and such determinations have, in any event, no established role in the management of nitroglycerin overdose.

No data are available to suggest physiological maneuvers (eg, maneuvers to change the pH of the urine) that might accelerate elimination of nitroglycerin and its active metabolites. Similarly, it is not known which – if any – of these substances can usefully be removed from the body by hemodialysis.

No specific antagonist to the vasodilator effects of nitroglycerin is known, and no intervention has been subject to controlled study as a therapy of nitroglycerin overdose. Because the hypotension associated with nitroglycerin overdose is the result of venodilatation and arterial hypovolemia, prudent therapy in this situation should be directed toward increase in central fluid volume. Passive elevation of the patient's legs may be sufficient, but intravenous infusion of normal saline or similar fluid may also be necessary. The use of epinephrine or other arterial vasoconstrictors in this setting is likely to do more harm than good.

In patients with renal disease or congestive heart failure, therapy resulting in central volume expansion is not without hazard. Treatment of nitroglycerin overdose in these patients may be subtle and difficult, and invasive monitoring may be required.

Methemoglobinemia:

Nitrate ions liberated during metabolism of nitroglycerin can oxidize hemoglobin into methemoglobin. Even in patients totally without cytochrome b_5 reductase activity, however, and even assuming that the nitrate moieties of nitroglycerin are quantitatively applied to oxidation of hemoglobin, about 1 mg/kg of nitroglycerin should be required before any of these patients manifests clinically significant ($\geq$10%) methemoglobinemia. In patients with normal reductase function, significant production of methemoglobin should require even larger doses of nitroglycerin. In one study in which 36 patients received 2 to 4 weeks of continuous nitroglycerin therapy at 3.1 to 4.4 mg/hr, the average methemoglobin level measured was 0.2%; this was comparable to that observed in parallel patients who received placebo.

Notwithstanding these observations, there are case reports of significant methemoglobinemia in association with moderate overdoses of organic nitrates. None of the affected patients had been thought to be unusually susceptible.

Methemoglobin levels are available from most clinical laboratories. The diagnosis should be suspected in patients who exhibit signs of impaired oxygen delivery despite adequate cardiac output and adequate arterial PO_2. Classically, methemoglobinemic blood is described as chocolate brown, without color change on exposure to air.

Methemoglobinemia should be treated with methylene blue if the patient develops cardiac or CNS effects of hypoxia. The initial dose is 1 to 2 mg/kg infused intravenously over 5 minutes. Repeat methemoglobin levels should be obtained 30 minutes later and a repeat dose of 0.5 to 1.0 mg/kg may be used if the level remains elevated and the patient is still symptomatic. Relative contraindications for methylene blue include known NADH methemoglobin reductase deficiency or G-6-PD deficiency. Infants under the age of 4 months may

not respond to methylene blue due to immature NADH methemoglobin reductase. Exchange transfusion has been used successfully in critically ill patients when methemoglobinemia is refractory to treatment.

DOSAGE AND ADMINISTRATION

The suggested starting dose is between 0.2 mg/hr* and 0.4 mg/hr*. Doses between 0.4 mg/hr* and 0.8 mg/hr* have shown continued effectiveness for 10 to 12 hours daily for at least 1 month (the longest period studied) of intermittent administration. Although the minimum nitrate-free interval has not been defined, data show that a nitrate-free interval of 10 to 12 hours is sufficient (see **CLINICAL PHARMACOLOGY**). Thus, an appropriate dosing schedule for nitroglycerin patches would include a daily patch-on period of 12 to 14 hours and a daily patch-off period of 10 to 12 hours.

*Release rates were formerly described in terms of drug delivered per 24 hours. In these terms, the supplied NITRO-DUR systems would be rated at 2.5 mg/24 hours (0.1 mg/hour), 5 mg/24 hours (0.2 mg/hour), 7.5 mg/24 hours (0.3 mg/hour), 10 mg/24 hours (0.4 mg/hour), and 15 mg/24 hours (0.6 mg/hour).

Although some well-controlled clinical trials using exercise tolerance testing have shown maintenance of effectiveness when patches are worn continuously, the large majority of such controlled trials have shown the development of tolerance (ie, complete loss of effect) within the first 24 hours after therapy was initiated. Dose adjustment, even to levels much higher than generally used, did not restore efficacy.

HOW SUPPLIED

[See table above]

Store at 25°C (77°F); excursions permitted to 15-30°C (59-86°F) [see USP Controlled Room Temperature]. Do not refrigerate.

Rx only

Key Pharmaceuticals, Inc.
Kenilworth, NJ 07033 USA
Rev. 12/04   18143690
Copyright © 1987, 2002, Key Pharmaceuticals, Inc.
All rights reserved.
Shown in Product Identification Guide, page 313

NOROXIN®   ℞
[nor-AHK-sin]
(norfloxacin)
Tablets

WARNING:
Fluoroquinolones, including NOROXIN, are associated with an increased risk of tendinitis and tendon rupture in all ages. This risk is further increased in older patients usually over 60 years of age, in patients taking corticosteroid drugs, and in patients with kidney, heart or lung transplants (see WARNINGS).

To reduce the development of drug-resistant bacteria and maintain the effectiveness of NOROXIN[1] and other antibac-

terial drugs, NOROXIN should be used only to treat or prevent infections that are proven or strongly suspected to be caused by bacteria.

DESCRIPTION

NOROXIN (Norfloxacin) is a synthetic, broad-spectrum antibacterial agent for oral administration. Norfloxacin, a fluoroquinolone, is 1-ethyl-6-fluoro-1,4-dihydro-4-oxo-7-(1-piperazinyl)-3-quinolinecarboxylic acid. Its empirical formula is $C_{16}H_{18}FN_3O_3$ and the structural formula is:

Norfloxacin is a white to pale yellow crystalline powder with a molecular weight of 319.34 and a melting point of about 221°C. It is freely soluble in glacial acetic acid, and very slightly soluble in ethanol, methanol and water.

NOROXIN is available in 400-mg tablets. Each tablet contains the following inactive ingredients: cellulose, croscarmellose sodium, hydroxypropyl cellulose, hydroxypropyl methylcellulose, magnesium stearate, and titanium dioxide. Norfloxacin, a fluoroquinolone, differs from non-fluorinated quinolones by having a fluorine atom at the 6 position and a piperazine moiety at the 7 position.

CLINICAL PHARMACOLOGY

In fasting healthy volunteers, at least 30-40% of an oral dose of NOROXIN is absorbed. Absorption is rapid following single doses of 200 mg, 400 mg and 800 mg. At the respective doses, mean peak serum and plasma concentrations of 0.8, 1.5 and 2.4 µg/mL are attained approximately one hour after dosing. The presence of food and/or dairy products may decrease absorption. The effective half-life of norfloxacin in serum and plasma is 3-4 hours. Steady-state concentrations of norfloxacin will be attained within two days of dosing.

In healthy elderly volunteers (65-75 years of age with normal renal function for their age), norfloxacin is eliminated more slowly because of their slightly decreased renal function. Following a single 400-mg dose of norfloxacin, the mean ($\pm$ SD) AUC and C_{max} of 9.8 (2.83) µg•hr/mL and 2.02 (0.77) µg/mL, respectively, were observed in healthy elderly volunteers. The extent of systemic exposure was slightly higher than that seen in younger adults (AUC 6.4 µg•hr/mL and C_{max} 1.5 µg/mL). Drug absorption appears unaffected. However, the effective half-life of norfloxacin in these elderly subjects is 4 hours.

There is no information on accumulation of norfloxacin with repeated administration in elderly patients. However, no dosage adjustment is required based on age alone. In elderly patients with reduced renal function, the dosage should be adjusted as for other patients with renal impairment (see DOSAGE AND ADMINISTRATION, *Renal Impairment*).

The disposition of norfloxacin in patients with creatinine clearance rates greater than 30 mL/min/1.73 m² is similar to that in healthy volunteers. In patients with creatinine clearance rates equal to or less than 30 mL/min/1.73 m², the renal elimination of norfloxacin decreases so that the effective serum half-life is 6.5 hours. In these patients, alteration of dosage is necessary (see DOSAGE AND ADMINISTRATION). Drug absorption appears unaffected by decreasing renal function.

Norfloxacin is eliminated through metabolism, biliary excretion, and renal excretion. After a single 400-mg dose of NOROXIN, mean antimicrobial activities equivalent to 278, 773, and 82 µg of norfloxacin/g of feces were obtained at 12, 24, and 48 hours, respectively. Renal excretion occurs by both glomerular filtration and tubular secretion as evidenced by the high rate of renal clearance (approximately 275 mL/min). Within 24 hours of drug administration, 26 to 32% of the administered dose is recovered in the urine as norfloxacin with an additional 5-8% being recovered in the urine as six active metabolites of lesser antimicrobial potency. Only a small percentage (less than 1%) of the dose is recovered thereafter. Fecal recovery accounts for another 30% of the administered dose. In elderly subjects (average creatinine clearance 91 mL/min/1.73 m²) approximately 22% of the administered dose was recovered in urine and renal clearance averaged 154 mL/min.

Two to three hours after a single 400-mg dose, urinary concentrations of 200 µg/mL or more are attained in the urine. In healthy volunteers, mean urinary concentrations of norfloxacin remain above 30 µg/mL for at least 12 hours following a 400-mg dose. The urinary pH may affect the solubility of norfloxacin. Norfloxacin is least soluble at urinary pH of 7.5 with greater solubility occurring at pHs above and below this value. The serum protein binding of norfloxacin is between 10 and 15%.

The following are mean concentrations of norfloxacin in various fluids and tissues measured 1 to 4 hours post-dose after two 400-mg doses, unless otherwise indicated:

Renal Parenchyma	7.3 µg/g
Prostate	2.5 µg/g
Seminal Fluid	2.7 µg/mL
Testicle	1.6 µg/g
Uterus/Cervix	3.0 µg/g
Vagina	4.3 µg/g
Fallopian Tube	1.9 µg/g
Bile	6.9 µg/mL (after two 200-mg doses)

Microbiology

Norfloxacin has in vitro activity against a broad range of gram-positive and gram-negative aerobic bacteria. The fluorine atom at the 6 position provides increased potency against gram-negative organisms, and the piperazine moiety at the 7 position is responsible for antipseudomonal activity.

Norfloxacin inhibits bacterial deoxyribonucleic acid synthesis and is bactericidal. At the molecular level, three specific events are attributed to norfloxacin in E. coli cells:
1. inhibition of the ATP-dependent DNA supercoiling reaction catalyzed by DNA gyrase,
2. inhibition of the relaxation of supercoiled DNA,
3. promotion of double-stranded DNA breakage.

Resistance to norfloxacin due to spontaneous mutation in vitro is a rare occurrence (range: 10^{-9} to 10^{-12} cells). Resistant organisms have emerged during therapy with norfloxacin in less than 1% of patients treated. Organisms in which development of resistance is greatest are the following:

Pseudomonas aeruginosa
Klebsiella pneumoniae
Acinetobacter spp.
Enterococcus spp.

For this reason, when there is a lack of satisfactory clinical response, repeat culture and susceptibility testing should be done. Nalidixic acid-resistant organisms are generally susceptible to norfloxacin in vitro; however, these organisms may have higher minimum inhibitory concentrations (MICs) to norfloxacin than nalidixic acid-susceptible strains. There is generally no cross-resistance between norfloxacin and other classes of antibacterial agents. Therefore, norfloxacin may demonstrate activity against indicated organisms resistant to some other antimicrobial agents including the aminoglycosides, penicillins, cephalosporins, tetracyclines, macrolides, and sulfonamides, including combinations of sulfamethoxazole and trimethoprim. Antagonism has been demonstrated in vitro between norfloxacin and nitrofurantoin.

Norfloxacin has been shown to be active against most strains of the following microorganisms both in vitro and in clinical infections as described in the **INDICATIONS AND USAGE** section.

Gram-positive aerobes:
Enterococcus faecalis
Staphylococcus aureus
Staphylococcus epidermidis
Staphylococcus saprophyticus
Streptococcus agalactiae

Gram-negative aerobes:
Citrobacter freundii
Enterobacter aerogenes
Enterobacter cloacae
Escherichia coli
Klebsiella pneumoniae
Neisseria gonorrhoeae
Proteus mirabilis
Proteus vulgaris
Pseudomonas aeruginosa
Serratia marcescens

The following in vitro data are available, **but their clinical significance is unknown.**

Norfloxacin exhibits in vitro MICs of ≤4 µg/mL against most (≥90%) strains of the following microorganisms; however, the safety and effectiveness of norfloxacin in treating clinical infections due to these microorganisms have not been established in adequate and well-controlled clinical trials.

Gram-negative aerobes:
Citrobacter diversus
Edwardsiella tarda
Enterobacter agglomerans
Haemophilus ducreyi
Klebsiella oxytoca
Morganella morganii
Providencia alcalifaciens
Providencia rettgeri
Providencia stuartii
Pseudomonas fluorescens
Pseudomonas stutzeri

Other:
Ureaplasma urealyticum
NOROXIN is not generally active against obligate anaerobes.

Norfloxacin has not been shown to be active against *Treponema pallidum* (see WARNINGS).

Susceptibility Tests
Dilution Techniques:

Quantitative methods are used to determine antimicrobial MICs. These MICs provide estimates of the susceptibility of bacteria to antimicrobial compounds. The MICs should be determined using a standardized procedure. Standardized procedures are based on a dilution method[1] (broth, agar, or microdilution) or equivalent with standardized inoculum concentrations and standardized concentrations of norfloxacin powder. The MIC values should be interpreted according to the following criteria[2]:

MIC (µg/mL)	Interpretation
≤4	Susceptible (S)
8	Intermediate (I)
≥16	Resistant (R)

A report of "Susceptible" indicates that the pathogen is likely to be inhibited if the antimicrobial compound in the blood reaches the concentrations usually achievable. A report of "Intermediate" indicates that the result should be considered equivocal, and, if the microorganism is not fully susceptible to alternative, clinically feasible drugs, the test should be repeated. This category implies possible clinical applicability in body sites where the drug is physiologically concentrated or in situations where high dosage of drug can be used. This category also provides a buffer zone which prevents small uncontrolled technical factors from causing major discrepancies in interpretation. A report of "Resistant" indicates that the pathogen is not likely to be inhibited if the antimicrobial compound in the blood reaches the concentrations usually achievable; other therapy should be selected.

Standardized susceptibility test procedures require use of laboratory control microorganisms to control the technical aspects of the laboratory procedures. Standard norfloxacin powder should provide the following MIC values:

Organism	MIC range (µg/mL)
E. coli ATCC 25922	0.03-0.12
E. faecalis ATCC 29212	2-8
P. aeruginosa ATCC 27853	1-4
S. aureus ATCC 29213	0.5-2

[2] These interpretative criteria apply only to isolates from urinary tract infections. There are no established norfloxacin interpretive criteria for *Neisseria gonorrhoeae* or organisms isolated from other infection sites.

Diffusion Techniques:

Quantitative methods that require measurement of zone diameters also provide reproducible estimates of the susceptibility of bacteria to antimicrobial compounds. One such standardized procedure[2] requires the use of standardized inoculum concentrations. This procedure uses paper disks impregnated with 10-µg norfloxacin to test the susceptibility of microorganisms to norfloxacin. Reports from the laboratory providing results of the standard single-disk susceptibility test with a 10-µg norfloxacin disk should be interpreted according to the following criteria[2]:

Zone diameter (mm)	Interpretation
≥17	Susceptible (S)
13-16	Intermediate (I)
≤12	Resistant (R)

Interpretation should be as stated above for results using dilution techniques. Interpretation involves correlation of the diameter obtained in the disk test with the MIC for norfloxacin.

As with standard dilution techniques, diffusion methods require the use of laboratory control microorganisms that are used to control the technical aspects of the laboratory procedures. For the diffusion techniques, the 10-µg norfloxacin disk should provide the following zone diameters in these laboratory test quality control strains:

Organism	Zone Diameter (mm)
E. coli ATCC 25922	28-35
P. aeruginosa ATCC 27853	22-29
S. aureus ATCC 25923	17-28

INDICATIONS AND USAGE

NOROXIN is indicated for the treatment of adults with the following infections caused by susceptible strains of the designated microorganisms:

Urinary tract infections:
Uncomplicated urinary tract infections (including cystitis) due to *Enterococcus faecalis, Escherichia coli, Klebsiella pneumoniae, Proteus mirabilis, Pseudomonas aeruginosa, Staphylococcus epidermidis, Staphylococcus saprophyticus, Citrobacter freundii[3], Enterobacter aerogenes[3], Enterobacter cloacae[3], Proteus vulgaris[3], Staphylococcus aureus[3],* or *Streptococcus agalactiae[3].*

Complicated urinary tract infections due to *Enterococcus faecalis, Escherichia coli, Klebsiella pneumoniae, Proteus mirabilis, Pseudomonas aeruginosa,* or *Serratia marcescens.[3]*

[3] Efficacy for this organism in this organ system was studied in fewer than 10 infections.

Sexually transmitted diseases
(see WARNINGS):
Uncomplicated urethral and cervical gonorrhea due to *Neisseria gonorrhoeae.*

Prostatitis:
Prostatitis due to *Escherichia coli.*
(See DOSAGE AND ADMINISTRATION for appropriate dosing instructions.)
Penicillinase production should have no effect on norfloxacin activity.

Appropriate culture and susceptibility tests should be performed before treatment in order to isolate and identify organisms causing the infection and to determine their susceptibility to norfloxacin. Therapy with norfloxacin may be initiated before results of these tests are known; once results become available, appropriate therapy should be given. Repeat culture and susceptibility testing performed periodically during therapy will provide information not only on the therapeutic effect of the antimicrobial agents but also on the possible emergence of bacterial resistance. To reduce the development of drug-resistant bacteria and maintain the effectiveness of NOROXIN and other antibacterial drugs, NOROXIN should be used only to treat or prevent infections that are proven or strongly suspected to be caused by susceptible bacteria. When culture and susceptibility information are available, they should be considered in selecting or modifying antibacterial therapy. In the absence of such data, local epidemiology and susceptibility patterns may contribute to the empiric selection of therapy.

CONTRAINDICATIONS

NOROXIN (norfloxacin) is contraindicated in persons with a history of hypersensitivity, tendinitis, or tendon rupture associated with the use of norfloxacin or any member of the quinolone group of antimicrobial agents.

WARNINGS

Tendinopathy and Tendon Rupture: Fluoroquinolones, including NOROXIN, are associated with an increased risk of tendinitis and tendon rupture in all ages. This adverse reaction most frequently involves the Achilles tendon, and rupture of the Achilles tendon may require surgical repair. Tendinitis and tendon rupture in the rotator cuff (the shoulder), the hand, the biceps, the thumb, and other tendon sites have also been reported. The risk of developing fluoroquinolone-associated tendinitis and tendon rupture is further increased in older patients usually over 60 years of age, in patients taking corticosteroid drugs, and in patients with kidney, heart or lung transplants. Factors, in addition to age and corticosteroid use, that may independently increase the risk of tendon rupture include strenuous physical activity, renal failure, and previous tendon disorders such as rheumatoid arthritis. Tendinitis and tendon rupture have also occurred in patients taking fluoroquinolones who do not have the above risk factors. Tendon rupture can occur during or after completion of therapy; cases occurring up to several months after completion of therapy have been reported. NOROXIN should be discontinued if the patient experiences pain, swelling, inflammation or rupture of a tendon. Patients should be advised to rest at the first sign of tendinitis or tendon rupture, and to contact their healthcare provider regarding changing to a non-quinolone antimicrobial drug.

Safety in Children, Adolescents, Nursing mothers, and during Pregnancy: THE SAFETY AND EFFICACY OF ORAL NORFLOXACIN IN PEDIATRIC PATIENTS, ADOLESCENTS (UNDER THE AGE OF 18), PREGNANT WOMEN, AND NURSING MOTHERS HAVE NOT BEEN ESTABLISHED.

(See PRECAUTIONS, *Pediatric Use, Pregnancy, and Nursing Mothers* subsections.) The oral administration of single doses of norfloxacin, 6 times[4] the recommended human clinical dose (on a mg/kg basis), caused lameness in immature dogs. Histologic examination of the weight-bearing joints of these dogs revealed permanent lesions of the cartilage. Other quinolones also produced erosions of the cartilage in weight-bearing joints and other signs of arthropathy in immature animals of various species (see ANIMAL PHARMACOLOGY).

Seizures: Convulsions have been reported in patients receiving norfloxacin. Convulsions, increased intracranial pressure, and toxic psychoses have been reported in patients receiving drugs in this class. Quinolones may also cause central nervous system (CNS) stimulation which may lead to tremors, restlessness, lightheadedness, confusion, and hallucinations. If these reactions occur in patients receiving norfloxacin, the drug should be discontinued and appropriate measures instituted.

The effects of norfloxacin on brain function or on the electrical activity of the brain have not been tested. Therefore, until more information becomes available, norfloxacin, like all other quinolones, should be used with caution in patients with known or suspected CNS disorders, such as severe cerebral arteriosclerosis, epilepsy, and other factors which predispose to seizures (See ADVERSE REACTIONS).

Hypersensitivity Reactions: Serious and occasionally fatal hypersensitivity (anaphylactic) reactions, some following the first dose, have been reported in patients receiving quinolone therapy, including NOROXIN. Some reactions were accompanied by cardiovascular collapse, loss of consciousness, tingling, pharyngeal or facial edema, dyspnea, urticaria and itching. Only a few patients had a history of hypersensitivity reactions. If an allergic reaction to norfloxacin occurs, discontinue the drug. Serious acute hypersensitivity reactions require immediate emergency treatment with epinephrine. Oxygen, intravenous fluids, antihistamines, corticosteroids, pressor amines, and airway management, including intubation, should be administered as indicated.

Other serious and sometimes fatal events, some due to hypersensitivity, and some due to uncertain etiology, have been reported rarely in patients receiving therapy with quinolones, including NOROXIN. These events may be severe and generally occur following the administration of multiple doses. Clinical manifestations may include one or more of the following:

• fever, rash or severe dermatologic reactions (e.g., toxic epidermal necrolysis, Stevens-Johnson syndrome);
• vasculitis; arthralgia; myalgia; serum sickness;
• allergic pneumonitis;
• interstitial nephritis; acute renal insufficiency or failure;
• hepatitis; jaundice; acute hepatic necrosis or failure;
• anemia, including hemolytic and aplastic; thrombocytopenia, including thrombotic thrombocytopenic purpura; leukopenia; agranulocytosis; pancytopenia; and/or other hematologic abnormalities.

The drug should be discontinued immediately at the first appearance of a skin rash, jaundice, or any other sign of hypersensitivity, and supportive measures should be instituted (see PRECAUTIONS, *Information for Patients* and ADVERSE REACTIONS).

Clostridium difficile associated diarrhea: Clostridium difficile associated diarrhea (CDAD) has been reported with use of nearly all antibacterial agents, including NOROXIN, and may range in severity from mild diarrhea to fatal colitis. Treatment with antibacterial agents alters the normal flora of the colon leading to overgrowth of *C. difficile.*
C. difficile produces toxins A and B which contribute to the development of CDAD.

Hypertoxin producing strains of *C. difficile* cause increased morbidity and mortality, as these infections can be refractory to antimicrobial therapy and may require colectomy. CDAD must be considered in all patients who present with diarrhea following antibiotic use. Careful medical history is necessary since CDAD has been reported to occur over two months after the administration of antibacterial agents.

If CDAD is suspected or confirmed, ongoing antibiotic use not directed against *C. difficile* may need to be discontinued. Appropriate fluid and electrolyte management, protein supplementation, antibiotic treatment of *C. difficile,* and surgical evaluation should be instituted as clinically indicated.

Peripheral neuropathy: Rare cases of sensory or sensorimotor axonal polyneuropathy affecting small and/or large axons resulting in paresthesias, hypoesthesias, dysesthesias and weakness have been reported in patients receiving quinolones, including norfloxacin. Norfloxacin should be discontinued if the patient experiences symptoms of neuropathy including pain, burning, tingling, numbness, and/or weakness, or is found to have deficits in light touch, pain, temperature, position sense, vibratory sensation, and/or motor strength in order to prevent the development of an irreversible condition.

Syphilis treatment: Norfloxacin has **not** been shown to be effective in the treatment of syphilis. Antimicrobial agents used in high doses for short periods of time to treat gonorrhea may mask or delay the symptoms of incubating syphilis. All patients with gonorrhea should have a serologic test for syphilis at the time of diagnosis. Patients treated with norfloxacin should have a follow-up serologic test for syphilis after three months.

---

[4] Based on a patient weight of 50 kg.

PRECAUTIONS
General
Needle-shaped crystals were found in the urine of some volunteers who received either placebo, 800 mg norfloxacin, or 1600 mg norfloxacin (at or twice the recommended daily dose, respectively) while participating in a double-blind, crossover study comparing single doses of norfloxacin with placebo. While crystalluria is not expected to occur under usual conditions with a dosage regimen of 400 mg b.i.d., as a precaution, the daily recommended dosage should not be exceeded and the patient should drink sufficient fluids to ensure a proper state of hydration and adequate urinary output.

Alteration in dosage regimen is necessary for patients with impaired renal function (see DOSAGE AND ADMINISTRATION).

Moderate to severe photosensitivity/phototoxicity reactions, the latter of which may manifest as exaggerated sunburn reactions (e.g., burning, erythema, exudation, vesicles, blistering, edema) involving areas exposed to light (typically the face, "V" area of the neck, extensor surfaces of the forearms, dorsa of the hands), can be associated with the use of quinolone antibiotics after sun or UV light exposure. Therefore, excessive exposure to these sources of light should be avoided. Drug therapy should be discontinued if phototoxicity occurs (see ADVERSE REACTIONS, *Post-Marketing*).

Rarely, hemolytic reactions have been reported in patients with latent or actual defects in glucose-6-phosphate dehydrogenase activity who take quinolone antibacterial agents, including norfloxacin (See ADVERSE REACTIONS).

Quinolones, including norfloxacin, may exacerbate the signs of myasthenia gravis and lead to life-threatening weakness of the respiratory muscles. Caution should be exercised when using quinolones, including NOROXIN, in patients with myasthenia gravis (see ADVERSE REACTIONS).

Prescribing NOROXIN in the absence of a proven or strongly suspected bacterial infection or a prophylactic indication is unlikely to provide benefit to the patient and increases the risk of the development of drug-resistant bacteria.

Information for Patients
Patients should be advised:

— to contact their healthcare provider if they experience pain, swelling, or inflammation of a tendon, or weakness or inability to use one of their joints; rest and refrain from exercise; and discontinue NOROXIN treatment. The risk of severe tendon disorders with fluoroquinolones is higher in older patients usually over 60 years of age, in patients taking corticosteroid drugs, and in patients with kidney, heart or lung transplants.

— that norfloxacin may cause changes in the electrocardiogram (QTc interval prolongation).

— that norfloxacin should be avoided in patients receiving class IA (e.g., quinidine, procainamide) or class III (e.g., amiodarone, sotalol) antiarrhythmic agents.

— that norfloxacin should be used with caution in subjects receiving drugs that affect the QTc interval such as cisapride, erythromycin, antipsychotics, and tricyclic antidepressants.

— to inform their physicians of any personal or family history of QTc prolongation or proarrhythmic conditions such as hypokalemia, bradycardia or recent myocardial ischemia.

— that peripheral neuropathies have been associated with norfloxacin use. If symptoms of peripheral neuropathy including pain, burning, tingling, numbness, and/or weakness develop, they should discontinue treatment and contact their physicians.

— to drink fluids liberally.

— that norfloxacin should be taken at least one hour before or at least two hours after a meal or ingestion of milk and/or other dairy products.

— that multivitamins or other products containing iron or zinc, antacids or Videx[®5] (Didanosine), chewable/buffered tablets or the pediatric powder for oral solution, should not be taken within the two-hour period before or within the two-hour period after taking norfloxacin (see PRECAUTIONS, *Drug Interactions*).

— that norfloxacin can cause dizziness and lightheadedness and, therefore, patients should know how they react to norfloxacin before they operate an automobile or machinery or engage in activities requiring mental alertness and coordination.

— that norfloxacin may be associated with hypersensitivity reactions, even following the first dose, and to discontinue the drug at the first sign of a skin rash or other allergic reaction.

— that photosensitivity/phototoxicity has been reported in patients receiving quinolones. Patients should minimize or avoid exposure to natural or artificial sunlight (tanning beds or UVA/B treatment) while taking quinolones. If patients need to be outdoors while using quinolones, they should wear loose-fitting clothes that protect skin from sun exposure and discuss other sun protection measures with their physician. If a sunburn-like reaction or skin eruption occurs, patients should contact their physician.

— that some quinolones may increase the effects of theophylline and/or caffeine (see PRECAUTIONS, *Drug Interactions*).

— that convulsions have been reported in patients taking quinolones, including norfloxacin, and to notify their physician before taking this drug if there is a history of this condition.

— that diarrhea is a common problem caused by antibiotics, which usually ends when the antibiotic is discontinued. Sometimes after starting the treatment with antibiotics, patients can develop watery and bloody stools (with or without stomach cramps and fever) even as late as two or more months after having taken the last dose of the antibiotic. If this occurs, patients should contact their physician as soon as possible.

Patients should be counseled that antibacterial drugs including NOROXIN should only be used to treat bacterial infections. They do not treat viral infections (e.g., the common cold). When NOROXIN is prescribed to treat a bacterial infection, patients should be told that although it is common to feel better early in the course of therapy, the medication should be taken exactly as directed. Skipping doses or not completing the full course of therapy may (1) decrease the effectiveness of the immediate treatment and (2) increase the likelihood that bacteria will develop resistance and will not be treatable by NOROXIN or other antibacterial drugs in the future.

---

[5] Registered trademark of Bristol-Myers Squibb Company

Laboratory Tests
As with any potent antibacterial agent, periodic assessment of organ system functions, including renal, hepatic, and hematopoietic, is advisable during prolonged therapy.

Drug Interactions
Quinolones, including norfloxacin, have been shown *in vitro* to inhibit CYP1A2. Concomitant use with drugs metabolized by CYP1A2 (e.g., caffeine, clozapine, ropinirole, tacrine, theophylline, tizanidine) may result in increased substrate drug concentrations when given in usual doses. Patients taking any of these drugs concomitantly with norfloxacin should be carefully monitored.

Elevated plasma levels of theophylline have been reported with concomitant quinolone use. There have been reports of theophylline-related side effects in patients on concomitant therapy with norfloxacin and theophylline. Therefore, monitoring of theophylline plasma levels should be considered and dosage of theophylline adjusted as required.

Elevated serum levels of cyclosporine have been reported with concomitant use of cyclosporine with norfloxacin. Therefore, cyclosporine serum levels should be monitored and appropriate cyclosporine dosage adjustments made when these drugs are used concomitantly.

Quinolones, including norfloxacin, may enhance the effects of oral anticoagulants, including warfarin or its derivatives or similar agents. When these products are administered concomitantly, prothrombin time or other suitable coagulation tests should be closely monitored.

The concomitant administration of quinolones including norfloxacin with glyburide (a sulfonylurea agent) has, on rare occasions, resulted in severe hypoglycemia. Therefore, monitoring of blood glucose is recommended when these agents are co-administered.

Diminished urinary excretion of norfloxacin has been reported during the concomitant administration of probenecid and norfloxacin.

The concomitant use of nitrofurantoin is not recommended since nitrofurantoin may antagonize the antibacterial effect of NOROXIN in the urinary tract.

Multivitamins, or other products containing iron or zinc, antacids or sucralfate, should not be administered concomitantly with, or within 2 hours of, the administration of norfloxacin, because they may interfere with absorption resulting in lower serum and urine levels of norfloxacin.

Videx® (Didanosine) chewable/buffered tablets or the pediatric powder for oral solution should not be administered concomitantly with, or within 2 hours of, the administration of norfloxacin, because these products may interfere with absorption resulting in lower serum and urine levels of norfloxacin.

Some quinolones have also been shown to interfere with the metabolism of caffeine. This may lead to reduced clearance of caffeine and a prolongation of its plasma half-life that may lead to accumulation of caffeine in plasma when products containing caffeine are consumed while taking norfloxacin.

The concomitant administration of a non-steroidal anti-inflammatory drug (NSAID) with a quinolone, including norfloxacin, may increase the risk of CNS stimulation and convulsive seizures. Therefore, NOROXIN should be used with caution in individuals receiving NSAIDS concomitantly.

Carcinogenesis, Mutagenesis, Impairment of Fertility

No increase in neoplastic changes was observed with norfloxacin as compared to controls in a study in rats, lasting up to 96 weeks at doses 8-9 times[4] the usual human dose (on a mg/kg basis).

Norfloxacin was tested for mutagenic activity in a number of *in vivo* and *in vitro* tests. Norfloxacin had no mutagenic effect in the dominant lethal test in mice and did not cause chromosomal aberrations in hamsters or rats at doses 30-60 times[4] the usual human dose (on a mg/kg basis). Norfloxacin had no mutagenic activity *in vitro* in the Ames microbial mutagen test, Chinese hamster fibroblasts and V-79 mammalian cell assay. Although norfloxacin was weakly positive in the Rec-assay for DNA repair, all other mutagenic assays were negative including a more sensitive test (V-79).

Norfloxacin did not adversely affect the fertility of male and female mice at oral doses up to 30 times[4] the usual human dose (on a mg/kg basis).

Pregnancy

Teratogenic Effects

Pregnancy Category C

Norfloxacin has been shown to produce embryonic loss in monkeys when given in doses 10 times[4] the maximum daily total human dose (on a mg/kg basis). At this dose, peak plasma levels obtained in monkeys were approximately 2 times those obtained in humans. There has been no evidence of a teratogenic effect in any of the animal species tested (rat, rabbit, mouse, monkey) at 6-50 times[4] the maximum daily human dose (on a mg/kg basis). There are, however, no adequate and well-controlled studies in pregnant women. Norfloxacin should be used during pregnancy only if the potential benefit justifies the potential risk to the fetus.

Nursing Mothers

It is not known whether norfloxacin is excreted in human milk.

When a 200-mg dose of NOROXIN was administered to nursing mothers, norfloxacin was not detected in human milk. However, because the dose studied was low, because other drugs in this class are secreted in human milk, and because of the potential for serious adverse reactions from norfloxacin in nursing infants, a decision should be made to discontinue nursing or to discontinue the drug, taking into account the importance of the drug to the mother.

Pediatric Use

The safety and effectiveness of oral norfloxacin in pediatric patients and adolescents below the age of 18 years have not been established. Norfloxacin causes arthropathy in juvenile animals of several animal species (see WARNINGS and ANIMAL PHARMACOLOGY).

Geriatric Use

Geriatric patients are at increased risk for developing severe tendon disorders including tendon rupture when being treated with a fluoroquinolone such as NOROXIN. This risk is further increased in patients receiving concomitant corticosteroid therapy. Tendinitis or tendon rupture can involve the Achilles, hand, shoulder, or other tendon sites and can occur during or after completion of therapy; cases occurring up to several months after fluoroquinolone treatment have been reported. Caution should be used when prescribing NOROXIN to elderly patients, especially those on corticosteroids. Patients should be informed of this potential side effect and advised to discontinue NOROXIN and contact their healthcare provider if any symptoms of tendinitis or tendon rupture occur (see Boxed Warning; WARNINGS; and ADVERSE REACTIONS, *Post-Marketing*).

Of the 340 subjects in one large clinical study of NOROXIN for treatment of urinary tract infections, 103 patients were 65 and older, 77 of whom were 70 and older; no overall differences in safety and effectiveness were evident between these subjects and younger subjects. In clinical practice, no difference in the type of reported adverse experiences have been observed between the elderly and younger patients except for a possible increased risk of tendon rupture in elderly patients *receiving concomitant corticosteroids* (see WARNINGS). In addition, increased risk for other adverse experiences in some older individuals cannot be ruled out (see ADVERSE REACTIONS).

This drug is known to be substantially excreted by the kidney, and the risk of toxic reactions to this drug may be greater in patients with impaired renal function. Because elderly patients are more likely to have decreased renal function, care should be taken in dose selection, and it may be useful to monitor renal function (see DOSAGE AND ADMINISTRATION).

A pharmacokinetic study of NOROXIN in elderly volunteers (65 to 75 years of age with normal renal function for their age) was carried out (see CLINICAL PHARMACOLOGY).

In general, elderly patients may be more susceptible to drug-associated effects of the QTc interval. Therefore, precaution should be taken when using NOROXIN concomitantly with drugs that can result in prolongation of the QTc interval (e.g., class IA or class III antiarrhythmics) or in patients with risk factors for torsades de pointes (e.g., known QTc prolongation, uncorrected hypokalemia).

Infection	Description	Unit Dose	Frequency	Duration	Daily Dose
Urinary Tract	Uncomplicated UTI's (cystitis) due to *E. coli, K. pneumoniae,* or *P. mirabilis*	400 mg	q12h	3 days	800 mg
	Uncomplicated UTI's due to other indicated organisms	400 mg	q12h	7-10 days	800 mg
	Complicated UTI's	400 mg	q12h	10-21 days	800 mg
Sexually Transmitted Diseases	Uncomplicated Gonorrhea	800 mg	single dose	1 day	800 mg
Prostatitis	Acute or Chronic	400 mg	q12h	28 days	800 mg

ADVERSE REACTIONS

Single-Dose Studies

In clinical trials involving 82 healthy subjects and 228 patients with gonorrhea, treated with a single dose of norfloxacin, 6.5% reported drug-related adverse experiences. However, the following incidence figures were calculated without reference to drug relationship.

The most common adverse experiences (>1.0%) were: dizziness (2.6%), nausea (2.6%), headache (2.0%), and abdominal cramping (1.6%).

Additional reactions (0.3%-1.0%) were: anorexia, diarrhea, hyperhidrosis, asthenia, anal/rectal pain, constipation, dyspepsia, flatulence, tingling of the fingers, and vomiting.

Laboratory adverse changes considered drug-related were reported in 4.5% of patients/subjects. These laboratory changes were: increased AST (SGOT) (1.6%), decreased WBC (1.3%), decreased platelet count (1.0%), increased urine protein (1.0%), decreased hematocrit and hemoglobin (0.6%), and increased eosinophils (0.6%).

Multiple-Dose Studies

In clinical trials involving 52 healthy subjects and 1980 patients with urinary tract infections or prostatitis treated with multiple doses of norfloxacin, 3.6% reported drug-related adverse experiences. However, the incidence figures below were calculated without reference to drug relationship.

The most common adverse experiences (>1.0%) were: nausea (4.2%), headache (2.8%), dizziness (1.7%), and asthenia (1.3%).

Additional reactions (0.3%-1.0%) were: abdominal pain, back pain, constipation, diarrhea, dry mouth, dyspepsia/heartburn, fever, flatulence, hyperhidrosis, loose stools, pruritus, rash, somnolence, and vomiting.

Less frequent reactions (0.1%-0.2%) included: abdominal swelling, allergies, anorexia, anxiety, bitter taste, blurred vision, bursitis, chest pain, chills, depression, dysmenorrhea, edema, erythema, foot or hand swelling, insomnia, mouth ulcer, myocardial infarction, palpitation, pruritus ani, renal colic, sleep disturbances, and urticaria.

Abnormal laboratory values observed in these patients/subjects were: eosinophilia (1.5%), elevation of ALT (SGPT) (1.4%), decreased WBC and/or neutrophil count (1.4%), elevation of AST (SGOT) (1.4%), and increased alkaline phosphatase (1.1%). Those occurring less frequently included increased BUN, increased LDH, increased serum creatinine, decreased hematocrit, and glycosuria.

Post-Marketing

The most frequently reported adverse reaction in post-marketing experience is rash.

CNS effects characterized as generalized seizures, myoclonus and tremors have been reported with NOROXIN (see WARNINGS). Visual disturbances have been reported with drugs in this class.

The following additional adverse reactions have been reported since the drug was marketed:

Hypersensitivity Reactions

Hypersensitivity reactions have been reported including anaphylactoid reactions, angioedema, dyspnea, vasculitis, urticaria, arthritis, arthralgia and myalgia (see WARNINGS).

Skin

Toxic epidermal necrolysis, Stevens-Johnson syndrome and erythema multiforme, exfoliative dermatitis, photosensitivity/phototoxicity reactions (see PRECAUTIONS).

Gastrointestinal

Pseudomembranous colitis, hepatitis, jaundice including cholestatic jaundice and elevated liver function tests, pancreatitis (rare), stomatitis. The onset of pseudomembranous colitis symptoms may occur during or after antibacterial treatment (see WARNINGS).

Hepatic

Hepatic failure, including fatal cases.

Cardiovascular

On rare occasions, prolonged QTc interval and ventricular arrhythmia including torsades de pointes.

Renal

Interstitial nephritis, renal failure.

Nervous System/Psychiatric

Peripheral neuropathy, Guillain-Barré syndrome, ataxia, paresthesia, hypoesthesia, psychic disturbances including psychotic reactions and confusion.

Musculoskeletal

Tendinitis, tendon rupture; exacerbation of myasthenia gravis (see PRECAUTIONS); elevated creatine kinase (CK).

Hematologic

Neutropenia; leukopenia; agranulocytosis; hemolytic anemia, sometimes associated with glucose-6-phosphate dehydrogenase deficiency; thrombocytopenia.

Special Senses

Hearing loss, tinnitus, diplopia, dysgeusia.

Other adverse events reported with quinolones include: agranulocytosis, albuminuria, candiduria, crystalluria, cylindruria, dysphagia, elevation of blood glucose, elevation of serum cholesterol, elevation of serum potassium, elevation of serum triglycerides, hematuria, hepatic necrosis, symptomatic hypoglycemia, nystagmus, postural hypotension, prolongation of prothrombin time, and vaginal candidiasis.

OVERDOSAGE

No significant lethality was observed in male and female mice and rats at single oral doses up to 4 g/kg.

In the event of acute overdosage, the stomach should be emptied by inducing vomiting or by gastric lavage, and the patient carefully observed and given symptomatic and supportive treatment. Adequate hydration must be maintained.

DOSAGE AND ADMINISTRATION

Tablets NOROXIN should be taken at least one hour before or at least two hours after a meal or ingestion of milk and/or other dairy products. Multivitamins, other products containing iron or zinc, antacids containing magnesium and aluminum, sucralfate, or Videx® (Didanosine), chewable/buffered tablets or the pediatric powder for oral solution, should not be taken within 2 hours of administration of norfloxacin. Tablets NOROXIN should be taken with a glass of water. Patients receiving NOROXIN should be well hydrated (see PRECAUTIONS).

Normal Renal Function

The recommended daily dose of NOROXIN is as described in the following chart:

[See table above]

Renal Impairment

NOROXIN may be used for the treatment of urinary tract infections in patients with renal insufficiency. In patients with a creatinine clearance rate of 30 mL/min/1.73 m^2 or less, the recommended dosage is one 400-mg tablet once daily for the duration given above. At this dosage, the urinary concentration exceeds the MICs for most urinary pathogens susceptible to norfloxacin, even when the creatinine clearance is less than 10 mL/min/1.73 m^2.

When only the serum creatinine level is available, the following formula (based on sex, weight, and age of the patient) may be used to convert this value into creatinine clearance. The serum creatinine should represent a steady state of renal function.

$$\text{Males: } \frac{(\text{weight in kg}) \times (140 - \text{age})}{(72) \times \text{serum creatinine (mg/100 mL)}}$$

$$\text{Females: } (0.85) \times (\text{above value})$$

Elderly

Elderly patients being treated for urinary tract infections who have a creatinine clearance of greater than 30 mL/min/1.73 m^2 should receive the dosages recommended under *Normal Renal Function.*

Elderly patients being treated for urinary tract infections who have a creatinine clearance of 30 mL/min/1.73 m^2 or less should receive 400 mg once daily as recommended under *Renal Impairment*.

HOW SUPPLIED

No. 8338—Tablets NOROXIN 400 mg are white to off-white, oval shaped, film-coated tablets, coded 705 on one side and plain on the other. They are supplied as follows:

NDC 0006-0705-68 bottles of 100
NDC 0006-0705-20 unit of use bottles of 20.

Storage

Store at 25°C (77°F); excursions permitted to 15-30°C (59-86°F) [see USP Controlled Room Temperature]. Keep container tightly closed.

ANIMAL PHARMACOLOGY

Norfloxacin and related drugs have been shown to cause arthropathy in immature animals of most species tested (see WARNINGS).

Crystalluria has occurred in laboratory animals tested with norfloxacin. In dogs, needle-shaped drug crystals were seen in the urine at doses of 50 mg/kg/day. In rats, crystals were reported following doses of 200 mg/kg/day.

Embryo lethality and slight maternotoxicity (vomiting and anorexia) were observed in cynomolgus monkeys at doses of 150 mg/kg/day or higher.

Ocular toxicity, seen with some related drugs, was not observed in any norfloxacin-treated animals.

REFERENCES

1. National Committee for Clinical Laboratory Standards, Methods for dilution antimicrobial susceptibility tests for bacteria that grow aerobically - 3rd ed., Approved Standard NCCLS Document M7-A3, Vol. 13, No. 25, NCCLS, Villanova, PA, 1993.
2. National Committee for Clinical Laboratory Standards, Performance standards for antimicrobial disk susceptibility tests - 5th ed., Approved Standard NCCLS Document M2-A5, Vol. 13, No. 24, NCCLS, Villanova, PA, 1993.

Manuf. for: Merck Sharp & Dohme Corp., a subsidiary of **MERCK & CO., INC.**, Whitehouse Station, NJ 08889, USA
By: Merck Sharp & Dohme (Italia) S.p.A.
Via Emilia, 21
27100 Pavia, Italy
Issued February 2010
Printed in USA
9900802

MEDICATION GUIDE

NOROXIN® [nor-AHK-sin]
(norfloxacin)
400 mg Tablets

Read the Medication Guide that comes with NOROXIN[1] before you start taking it and each time you get a refill. There may be new information. This Medication Guide does not take the place of talking to your healthcare provider about your medical condition or your treatment.

What is the most important information I should know about NOROXIN?

NOROXIN belongs to a class of antibiotics called fluoroquinolones. NOROXIN can cause side effects that may be serious or even cause death. If you develop any of the following serious side effects, get medical help right away. Talk with your healthcare provider about whether you should continue to take NOROXIN.

Tendon rupture or swelling of the tendon (tendinitis).

- Tendons are tough cords of tissue that connect muscle to bones.
- Pain, swelling, tears and inflammation of tendons including the back of the ankle (Achilles), shoulder, hand, or other tendon sites can happen in people of all ages who take fluoroquinolone antibiotics, including NOROXIN. The risk of getting tendon problems is higher if you:
  - are over 60 years of age
  - are taking steroids (corticosteroids)
  - have had a kidney, heart or lung transplant
- Swelling of the tendon (tendinitis) and tendon rupture (breakage) have also happened in patients who take fluoroquinolones who do not have the above risk factors.
- Other reasons for tendon ruptures can include:
  - physical activity or exercise
  - kidney failure
  - tendon problems in the past, such as in people with rheumatoid arthritis (RA).
- Call your healthcare provider right away at the first sign of tendon pain, swelling or inflammation. Stop taking NOROXIN until tendinitis or tendon rupture has been ruled out by your healthcare provider. Avoid exercise and using the affected area. The most common area of pain and swelling is the Achilles tendon at the back of your ankle. This can also happen with other tendons. Talk to your healthcare provider about the risk of tendon rupture with

continued use of NOROXIN. You may need a different antibiotic that is not a fluoroquinolone to treat your infection.
- Tendon rupture can happen while you are taking or after you have finished taking NOROXIN. Tendon ruptures have happened up to several months after patients have finished taking their fluoroquinolone.
- Get medical help right away if you get any of the following signs or symptoms of a tendon rupture:
  - hear or feel a snap or pop in a tendon area
  - bruising right after an incident in a tendon area
  - unable to move the affected area or bear weight
- See the section "**What are the possible side effects of NOROXIN?**" for more information about side effects.

What is NOROXIN?

NOROXIN is a fluoroquinolone antibiotic medicine used in adults to treat certain infections caused by certain germs called bacteria. It is not known if NOROXIN is safe and works in children under 18 years of age. Children have a higher chance of getting bone and joint (musculoskeletal) problems while taking NOROXIN.

Sometimes infections are caused by viruses rather than by bacteria. Examples include viral infections in the sinuses and lungs, such as the common cold or flu. Antibiotics including NOROXIN do not kill viruses.

Call your healthcare provider if you think your condition is not getting better while you are taking NOROXIN.

Who should not take NOROXIN?

Do not take NOROXIN if you:

- have ever had a severe allergic reaction to an antibiotic known as a fluoroquinolone, or are allergic to any of the ingredients in NOROXIN. Ask your healthcare provider if you are not sure. See the list of ingredients in NOROXIN at the end of this Medication Guide.
- have had tendinitis or tendon rupture with the use of NOROXIN or another fluoroquinolone antibiotic.

What should I tell my healthcare provider before taking NOROXIN?

See "**What is the most important information I should know about NOROXIN?**"

Tell your healthcare provider about all your medical conditions, including if you:

- have tendon problems
- have central nervous system problems (such as epilepsy)
- have nerve problems
- have myasthenia gravis
- have or anyone in your family has an irregular heartbeat, especially a condition called "QTc prolongation."
- have low potassium (hypokalemia)
- have a slow heartbeat called bradycardia
- have a history of seizures
- have kidney problems. You may need a lower dose of NOROXIN if your kidneys do not work well.
- have rheumatoid arthritis (RA) or other history of joint problems
- are pregnant or planning to become pregnant. It is not known if NOROXIN will harm your unborn child.
- are breast-feeding or planning to breast-feed. It is not known if NOROXIN passes into breast milk. You and your healthcare provider should decide whether you will take NOROXIN or breast-feed.

Tell your healthcare provider about all the medicines you take, including prescription and nonprescription medicines, vitamins, and herbal and dietary supplements. NOROXIN and other medicines[6] can affect each other causing side effects. Especially tell your healthcare provider if you take:

- an NSAID (Non-Steroidal Anti-Inflammatory Drug). Many common medicines for pain relief are NSAIDs. Taking an NSAID while you take NOROXIN or other fluoroquinolones may increase your risk of central nervous system effects and seizures. See "**What are the possible side effects of NOROXIN?**"
- glyburide (Micronase, Glynase, Diabeta, Glucovance). See "**What are the possible side effects of NOROXIN?**"
- a blood thinner (warfarin, Coumadin, Jantoven)
- a medicine to control your heart rate or rhythm (antiarrhythmics). See "**What are the possible side effects of NOROXIN?**"
- an anti-psychotic medicine
- a tricyclic antidepressant
- erythromycin
- a water pill (diuretic)
- a steroid medicine. Corticosteroids taken by mouth or by injection may increase the chance of tendon injury.
- probenecid (Probalan, Col-probenecid)
- cyclosporine (Gengraf, Sandimmune, Neoral)
- products that contain caffeine
- clozapine (Fazaclo ODT, Clozaril)
- ropinirole (Requip, Requip XL)
- tacrine (Cognex)
- tizanidine (Zanaflex)
- theophylline (Theo-24, Elixophyllin, Theochron, Uniphyl, Theolair)
- cisapride (Propulsid)

certain medicines may keep NOROXIN from working correctly. Take NOROXIN either 2 hours before or 2 hours after taking these products:
  - an antacid, multivitamin or other product that has iron or zinc
  - sucralfate (Carafate)
  - didanosine (Videx, Videx EC)
- You should not take the medicine nitrofuantoin (furadantin, macrodantin, macrobid) while taking NOROXIN.

Ask your healthcare provider if you are not sure if your medicine is listed above.

Know the medicines you take. Keep a list of your medicines and show it to your healthcare provider and pharmacist when you get a new medicine.

How should I take NOROXIN?

- Take NOROXIN exactly as prescribed by your healthcare provider.
- NOROXIN is usually taken every 12 hours for patients with normal kidney function.
- Take NOROXIN with a glass of water.
- Drink plenty of fluids while taking NOROXIN.
- Take NOROXIN at least one hour before or 2 hours after a meal or having milk or other dairy products.
- Do not skip any doses, or stop taking NOROXIN even if you begin to feel better, until you finish your prescribed treatment, unless:
  - you have tendon effects (see "**What is the most important information I should know about NOROXIN?**"),
  - you have a serious allergic reaction (see "**What are the possible side effects of NOROXIN?**"), or
  - your healthcare provider tells you to stop. This will help make sure that all of the bacteria are killed and lower the chance that the bacteria will become resistant to NOROXIN. If this happens, NOROXIN and other antibiotic medicines may not work in the future.
- If you miss a dose of NOROXIN, take it as soon as you remember. Do not take two doses of NOROXIN at the same time. Do not take more than 2 doses of NOROXIN in one day.
- If you take too much, call your healthcare provider or get medical help immediately.

What should I avoid while taking NOROXIN?

- NOROXIN can make you feel dizzy and lightheaded. Do not drive, operate machinery, or do other activities that require mental alertness or coordination until you know how NOROXIN affects you.
- Avoid sunlamps and tanning beds, and try to limit your time in the sun. NOROXIN can make your skin sensitive to the sun (photosensitivity) and the light from sunlamps and tanning beds. You could get severe sunburn, blisters or swelling of your skin. If you get any of these symptoms while taking NOROXIN, call your healthcare provider right away. You should use sunscreen and wear a hat and clothes that cover your skin if you have to be in sunlight.

What are the possible side effects of NOROXIN?

NOROXIN can cause side effects that may be serious or even cause death. See "**What is the most important information I should know about NOROXIN?**"

Other serious side effects of NOROXIN include:

- **Central Nervous System Effects.** Seizures have been reported in people who take fluoroquinolone antibiotics including NOROXIN. Tell your healthcare provider if you have a history of seizures. Ask your healthcare provider whether taking NOROXIN will change your risk of having a seizure.

  Central Nervous System (CNS) side effects may happen as soon as after taking the first dose of NOROXIN. Talk to your healthcare provider right away if you get any of these side effects, or other changes in mood or behavior:
  - feel lightheaded
  - seizures
  - hear voices, see things, or sense things that are not there (hallucinations)
  - feel restless
  - tremors
  - feel anxious or nervous
  - confusion
  - feel more suspicious (paranoia)
- **Serious allergic reactions.** Allergic reactions can happen in people who take fluoroquinolones, including NOROXIN, even after only one dose. Stop taking NOROXIN and get emergency medical help right away if you get any of the following symptoms of a severe allergic reaction:
  - hives
  - trouble breathing or swallowing
  - swelling of the lips, tongue, face
  - throat tightness, hoarseness
  - rapid heartbeat
  - faint
- yellowing of the skin or eyes. Stop taking NOROXIN and tell your healthcare provider right away if you get

yellowing of your skin or white part of your eyes, or if you have dark urine. These can be signs of a serious reaction to NOROXIN (a liver problem).

- **Skin rash.** Skin rash may happen in people taking NOROXIN, even after only one dose. Stop taking NOROXIN at the first sign of a skin rash and call your healthcare provider. Skin rash may be sign of a more serious reaction to NOROXIN.
- **Serious heart rhythm changes (QTc prolongation and torsade de pointes).** Tell your healthcare provider right away if you have a change in your heart beat (a fast or irregular heartbeat), or if you faint. NOROXIN may cause a rare heart problem known as prolongation of the QTc interval. This condition can cause an abnormal heartbeat and can be very dangerous. The chances of this happening are higher in people:
  - who are elderly
  - with a family history of prolonged QTc interval
  - with low blood potassium (hypokalemia)
  - who take certain medicines to control heart rhythm (antiarrhythmics)
- **Worsening of myasthenia gravis symptoms.** Fluoroquinolones, including NOROXIN, may worsen the signs of myasthenia gravis. This may cause trouble breathing which may be life-threatening. Tell your healthcare provider right away if you get this symptom.
- **Intestine infection (Pseudomembranous colitis).** Pseudomembranous colitis can happen with most antibiotics, including NOROXIN. Call your healthcare provider right away if you get watery diarrhea, diarrhea that does not go away, or bloody stools. You may have stomach cramps and a fever. Pseudomembranous colitis can happen 2 or more months after you have finished your antibiotic.
- **Changes in sensation and possible nerve damage (Peripheral Neuropathy).** Damage to the nerves in arms, hands, legs, or feet can happen in people taking fluoroquinolones, including NOROXIN. Talk with your healthcare provider right away if you get any of the following symptoms of peripheral neuropathy in your arms, hands, legs, or feet:
  - pain
  - burning
  - tingling
  - numbness
  - weakness
NOROXIN may need to be stopped to prevent permanent nerve damage.
- **Low blood sugar (hypoglycemia).** People taking NOROXIN and other fluoroquinolone medicines with the oral anti-diabetes medicine glyburide (Micronase, Glynase, Diabeta, Glucovance) can get low blood sugar (hypoglycemia) which can sometimes be severe. Tell your healthcare provider if you get low blood sugar while taking NOROXIN. Your antibiotic medicine may need to be changed.
- **Sensitivity to sunlight (photosensitivity).** See "What should I avoid while taking NOROXIN?"

The most common side effects of NOROXIN include:
- dizziness
- nausea
- diarrhea
- heartburn
- headache
- stomach (abdominal) cramping
- weakness
- changes in certain liver function tests
These are not all the possible side effects of NOROXIN. Tell your healthcare provider about any side effect that bothers you or that does not go away.
Call your healthcare provider for medical advice about side effects. You may report side effects to FDA at 1-800-FDA-1088.

How should I store NOROXIN?
Store between 59-86°F (15-30°C).
Keep container closed tightly.
Keep NOROXIN and all medicines out of the reach of children.
General Information about NOROXIN
Medicines are sometimes prescribed for purposes other than those listed in a Medication Guide. Do not use NOROXIN for a condition for which it is not prescribed. Do not give NOROXIN to other people, even if they have the same symptoms that you have. It may harm them.
This Medication Guide summarizes the most important information about NOROXIN. If you would like more information about NOROXIN, talk with your healthcare provider. You can ask your healthcare provider or pharmacist for information about NOROXIN that is written for healthcare professionals. For more information call 1-800-622-4477.
What are the ingredients in NOROXIN?
Active ingredient: norfloxacin
Inactive ingredients: cellulose, croscarmellose sodium, hydroxypropyl cellulose, hydroxypropyl methylcellulose, magnesium stearate and titanium dioxide

Revised February 2010
Manuf. for: Merck Sharp & Dohme Corp., a subsidiary of **MERCK & CO., INC.,** Whitehouse Station, NJ 08889, USA
Manufactured by:
Merck Sharp & Dohme (Italia) S.p.A.
Via Emilia, 21
27100 Pavia, Italy
9900802
This Medication Guide has been approved by the U.S. Food and Drug Administration.

[6] Other brands listed are the trademarks of their respective owners and are not trademarks of Merck Sharp & Dohme Corp.
Revised: 02/2010
Distributed by: Merck Sharp & Dohme Corp.
Shown in Product Identification Guide, page 313

NOXAFIL®
(posaconazole)
Oral Suspension
Product Information
℞

DESCRIPTION
NOXAFIL® (posaconazole) is a triazole antifungal agent available as a suspension for oral administration.
Posaconazole is designated chemically as 4-[4-[4-[4-[[(3R,5R)-5-(2,4-difluorophenyl)tetrahydro-5-(1H-1,2,4-triazol-1-ylmethyl)-3-furanyl]methoxy]phenyl]-1-piperazinyl]phenyl]-2-[(1S 2S)-1-ethyl-2-hydroxypropyl]-2,4-dihydro-3H-1,2,4-triazol-3-one with an empirical formula of $C_{37}H_{42}F_2N_8O_4$ and a molecular weight of 700.8. The structural formula is:

Posaconazole is a white powder and is insoluble in water. NOXAFIL Oral Suspension is a white, cherry-flavored immediate-release suspension containing 40 mg of posaconazole per mL and the following inactive ingredients: polysorbate 80, simethicone, sodium benzoate, sodium citrate dihydrate, citric acid monohydrate, glycerin, xanthan gum, liquid glucose, titanium dioxide, artificial cherry flavor, and purified water.

CLINICAL PHARMACOLOGY
Pharmacokinetics *Absorption* Posaconazole is absorbed with a median T_{max} of ~3 to 5 hours. Dose proportional increases in plasma exposure (AUC) to posaconazole were observed following single oral doses from 50 mg to 800 mg and following multiple-dose administration from 50 mg BID to 400 mg BID. No further increases in exposure were observed when the dose was increased from 400 mg BID to 600 mg BID in febrile neutropenic patients or those with refractory invasive fungal infections. Steady-state plasma concentrations are attained at 7 to 10 days following multiple-dose administration.

Following single-dose administration of 200 mg, the mean AUC and C_{max} of posaconazole are approximately 3 times higher when administered with a nonfat meal and approximately 4 times higher when administered with a high-fat meal (~50 gm fat) relative to the fasted state. Following single-dose administration of 400 mg, the mean AUC and C_{max} of posaconazole are approximately 3 times higher when administered with a liquid nutritional supplement (14 gm fat) relative to the fasted state (see **Table 1**). In order to assure attainment of adequate plasma concentrations, it is recommended to administer posaconazole with food or a nutritional supplement (see **DOSAGE AND ADMINISTRATION**).
[See table 1 below]
In 12 healthy volunteers who received a single 400-mg dose of NOXAFIL® Oral Suspension in the fasted state, 5 minutes before, during, and 20 minutes after a high-fat meal in a 4-way crossover design, the coadministration of NOXAFIL with a high-fat meal significantly increased the extent of absorption of posaconazole compared to in the fasted state. However, the magnitude of the food effect varied with timing of the meals. When NOXAFIL was administered during a high-fat meal, the mean C_{max} and AUC increased by 339% and 382% compared to in the fasted state, respectively. When NOXAFIL was administered 20 minutes after a high-fat meal, the mean C_{max} and AUC also increased by 333% and 387% compared to in the fasted state, respectively. When NOXAFIL was administered 5 minutes before a high-fat meal, the mean C_{max} and AUC increased by 96% and 111% compared to in the fasted state, respectively (see **DOSAGE AND ADMINISTRATION**).
In 12 healthy volunteers who received 400 mg BID and 200 mg QID of NOXAFIL Oral Suspension for 7 days in the fasted state and with liquid nutritional supplement (BOOST® Drink) in a 4-way crossover design, the administration of NOXAFIL 400 mg BID with BOOST increased the mean C_{max} and AUC by 65% and 66%, respectively, compared to NOXAFIL 400 mg BID in the fasted state. However, when NOXAFIL 200 mg QID was administered with BOOST, the mean C_{max} and AUC were not affected compared to NOXAFIL 200 mg QID in the fasted state.
In 12 healthy volunteers who received 400 mg BID and 200 mg QID of NOXAFIL Oral Suspension for 7 days in the fasted state and with liquid nutritional supplement (BOOST Drink) in a 4-way crossover design, the absorption of posaconazole was significantly increased when NOXAFIL was administered by dividing the total daily dose from 400 mg BID to 200 mg QID regardless of under-fasted conditions or with a liquid nutritional supplement. In the fasted state, the mean C_{max} and AUC increased by 136% and 161%, respectively, when NOXAFIL was administered as 200 mg QID compared to 400 mg BID. When NOXAFIL was administered as 200 mg QID with BOOST, the mean C_{max} and AUC increased by 44% and 54%, respectively, compared to 400 mg BID with BOOST.
In 12 healthy volunteers who received a single 400-mg dose of NOXAFIL Oral Suspension alone, or with ginger ale (carbonated acidic beverage), or with esomeprazole, or both ginger ale and esomeprazole in the fasted state in a 4-way crossover design, the coadministration of NOXAFIL with ginger ale increased the mean C_{max} and AUC by 92% and

TABLE 1: The Mean (%CV) [min-max] Posaconazole Pharmacokinetic Parameters Following Single-dose Suspension Administration of 200 mg and 400 mg Under Fed and Fasted Conditions

Dose (mg)	C_{max} (ng/mL)	T_{max}* (hr)	AUC(I) (ng·hr/mL)	CL/F (L/hr)	$t_{1/2}$ (hr)
200 mg fasted (n=20)[‡]	132 (50) [45-267]	3.50 [1.5-36†]	4179 (31) [2705-7269]	51 (25) [28-74]	23.5 (25) [15.3-33.7]
200 mg nonfat (n=20)[‡]	378 (43) [131-834]	4 [3-5]	10,753 (35) [4579-17,092]	21 (39) [12-44]	22.2 (18) [17.4-28.7]
200 mg high fat (54 gm fat)† (n=20)[‡]	512 (34) [241-1016]	5 [4-5]	15,059 (26) [10,341-24,476]	14 (24) [8.2-19]	23.0 (19) [17.2-33.4]
400 mg fasted (n=23)[§]	121 (75) [27-366]	4 [2-12]	5258 (48) [2834-9567]	91 (40) [42-141]	27.3 (26) [16.8-38.9]
400 mg with liquid nutritional supplement (14 gm fat) (n=23)[§]	355 (43) [145-720]	5 [4-8]	11,295 (40) [3865-20,592]	43 (56) [19-103]	26.0 (19) [18.2-35.0]

* Median [min-max].
† The subject with T_{max} of 36 hrs had relatively constant plasma levels over 36 hrs (1.7 ng/mL difference between 4 hrs and 36 hrs).
‡ n=15 for AUC(I), CL/F and $t_{1/2}$.
§ n=10 for AUC(I), CL/F and $t_{1/2}$.

TABLE 2: The Mean (%CV) [min-max] Posaconazole Steady-state Pharmacokinetic Parameters in Patients Following Oral Administration of Posaconazole 200 mg TID and 400 mg BID

Dose*	Cav (ng/mL)	AUC‖ (ng·hr/mL)	CL/F (L/hr)	V/F (L)	t$_{1/2}$ (hr)
200 mg TID[†] (n=252)	1103 (67) [21.5-3650]	ND¶	ND¶	ND¶	ND¶
200 mg TID[‡] (n=215)	583 (65) [89.7-2200]	15,900 (62) [4100-56,100]	51.2 (54) [10.7-146]	2425 (39) [828-5702]	37.2 (39) [19.1-148]
400 mg BID[§] (n=23)	723 (86) [6.70-2256]	9093 (80) [1564-26,794]	76.1 (78) [14.9-256]	3088 (84) [407-13,140]	31.7 (42) [12.4-67.3]

Note: Cav based on observed data; other pharmacokinetic parameters based on estimates from population pharmacokinetic analyses.
* Oral suspension administration.
[†] Allogeneic hematopoietic stem cell transplant (HSCT) recipients with graft-vs.-host disease.
[‡] Neutropenic patients who were receiving cytotoxic chemotherapy for acute myelogenous leukemia or myelodysplastic syndromes.
[§] Febrile neutropenic patients or patients with refractory invasive fungal infections, Cav n=24.
‖ AUC (0-24 hr) for 200 mg TID and AUC (0-12 hr) for 400 mg BID.
¶ Not done.

TABLE 3: Summary of the Effect of Coadministered Drugs on Posaconazole in Healthy Volunteers

Coadministered Drug (Postulated Mechanism of Interaction)	Coadministered Drug Dose/ Schedule	Posaconazole Dose/Schedule	Effect on Bioavailability of Posaconazole		Recommendations
			Change in Mean C$_{max}$ (ratio estimate*; 90% CI of the ratio estimate)	Change in Mean AUC (ratio estimate*; 90% CI of the ratio estimate)	
Rifabutin (UDP-G Induction)	300 mg QD × 17 days	200 mg (tablets) QD × 10 days	↓43% (0.57; 0.43-0.75)	↓49% (0.51; 0.37-0.71)	Avoid concomitant use unless the benefit outweighs the risks.
Phenytoin (UDP-G Induction)	200 mg QD × 10 days	200 mg (tablets) QD × 10 days	↓41% (0.59; 0.44-0.79)	↓50% (0.50; 0.36-0.71)	Avoid concomitant use unless the benefit outweighs the risks.
Cimetidine (Alteration of Gastric pH)	400 mg BID × 10 days	200 mg (tablets) QD × 10 days	↓39% (0.61; 0.53-0.70)	↓39% (0.61; 0.54-0.69)	Avoid concomitant use unless the benefit outweighs the risks.
Efavirenz (UDP-G Induction)	400 mg QD × 10 and 20 days	400 mg (oral suspension) BID × 10 and 20 days	↓45% (0.55; 0.47-0.66)	↓50% (0.50; 0.43-0.60)	Avoid concomitant use unless the benefit outweighs the risks.
Esomeprazole (Increase in Gastric pH)	40 mg QAM × 3 days	400 mg (oral suspension) single dose	↓46% (0.54; 0.43-0.69)	↓32% (0.68; 0.57-0.81)	Monitor closely for breakthrough fungal infections.
Metoclopramide (Increase in Gastric motility)	10 mg TID × 2 days	400 mg (oral suspension) single dose	↓21% (0.79; 0.72-0.87)	↓19% (0.81; 0.72-0.91)	Monitor closely for breakthrough fungal infections.

*Ratio Estimate is the ratio of coadministered drug plus posaconazole to posaconazole alone for C$_{max}$ or AUC.

70% compared to NOXAFIL alone, respectively. The coadministration of NOXAFIL with esomeprazole (proton pump inhibitor) decreased the mean C$_{max}$ and AUC by 46% and 32% compared to NOXAFIL alone, respectively. The coadministration of NOXAFIL with both ginger ale and esomeprazole decreased the mean C$_{max}$ and AUC by 33% and 21% compared to NOXAFIL alone, respectively (see **CLINICAL PHARMACOLOGY, Drug Interactions; PRECAUTIONS, Drug Interactions** sections and **DOSAGE AND ADMINISTRATION**).

In 12 subjects who received single 400-mg dose of NOXAFIL Oral Suspension with BOOST, or with a prokinetic agent (metoclopramide 10 mg TID for 2 days) and BOOST, or with an antikinetic agent (loperamide 4-mg single dose) and BOOST in a 3-way crossover design, the coadministration of NOXAFIL with metoclopramide decreased the mean C$_{max}$ and AUC by 21% and 19%, respectively, compared to NOXAFIL alone. When NOXAFIL was coadministered with loperamide, the mean C$_{max}$ and AUC were decreased by 3% and increased by 11%, respectively, compared to NOXAFIL alone (see **CLINICAL PHARMACOLOGY, Drug Interactions** and **PRECAUTIONS, Drug Interactions** sections).

In 16 healthy volunteers who received a single 400-mg dose of NOXAFIL either orally or via an NG tube in a crossover design, the mean C$_{max}$ and AUC decreased by 19% and 23%, respectively, when NOXAFIL was administered via an NG tube compared to when POS was administered orally. In 5

subjects, the C$_{max}$ and AUC decreased substantially (range: -27% to -53% and -33% to -51%, respectively) when NOXAFIL was administered via an NG tube compared to when NOXAFIL was administered orally. It is recommended to closely monitor patients for breakthrough fungal infections when NOXAFIL is administered via an NG tube because a lower plasma exposure may be associated with an increased risk of treatment failure (see **CLINICAL PHARMACOLOGY, Exposure Response Relationship** section).

Distribution Posaconazole has an apparent volume of distribution of 1774 L, suggesting extensive extravascular distribution and penetration into the body tissues. Posaconazole is highly protein bound (>98%), predominantly to albumin.

Metabolism Posaconazole primarily circulates as the parent compound in plasma. Of the circulating metabolites, the majority are glucuronide conjugates formed via UDP glucuronidation (phase 2 enzymes). Posaconazole does not have any major circulating oxidative (CYP450 mediated) metabolites. The excreted metabolites in urine and feces account for ~17% of the administered radiolabeled dose.

Excretion Posaconazole is eliminated with a mean half-life (t$_{1/2}$) of 35 hours (range: 20-66 hours) and a total body clearance (CL/F) of 32 L/hr. Posaconazole is predominantly eliminated in the feces (71% of the radiolabeled dose up to 120 hours) with the major component eliminated as parent drug

(66% of the radiolabeled dose). Renal clearance is a minor elimination pathway, with 13% of the radiolabeled dose excreted in urine up to 120 hours (<0.2% of the radiolabeled dose is parent drug).

Summary of Pharmacokinetic Parameters The mean (%CV) [min-max] posaconazole average steady-state plasma concentrations (Cav) and steady-state pharmacokinetic parameters in patients following administration of 200 mg TID and 400 mg BID of the oral suspension are provided in **Table 2.**

[See table 2 at left]

The variability in average plasma posaconazole concentrations in patients was relatively higher than that in healthy subjects.

Exposure Response Relationship In clinical studies of immunocompromised patients, a wide range of plasma exposures to posaconazole was noted. A pharmacokinetic-pharmacodynamic analysis of patient data revealed an apparent association between average posaconazole concentrations (Cav) and prophylactic efficacy. A lower Cav may be associated with an increased risk of treatment failure [defined in the study as treatment discontinuation, use of empiric systemic antifungal therapy (SAF), or invasive fungal infections (IFI)].

To enhance the oral absorption of posaconazole and optimize plasma concentrations:
- Each dose of NOXAFIL Oral Suspension should be administered during or immediately (i.e., within 20 minutes) following a full meal or liquid nutritional supplement. For patients who cannot eat a full meal or tolerate an oral nutritional supplement, alternative antifungal therapy should be considered or patients should be monitored closely for breakthrough fungal infections.
- Patients who have severe diarrhea or vomiting should be monitored closely for breakthrough fungal infections.
- Coadministration of drugs that can decrease the plasma concentrations of posaconazole should generally be avoided unless the benefit outweighs the risk. If such drugs are necessary, patients should be monitored closely for breakthrough fungal infections (see **CLINICAL PHARMACOLOGY, Drug Interactions** section).

Pharmacokinetics in Special Populations *Gender* The pharmacokinetics of posaconazole are comparable in men and women. No adjustment in the dosage of NOXAFIL is necessary based on gender.

Race The pharmacokinetic profile of posaconazole is not significantly affected by race. No adjustment in the dosage of NOXAFIL is necessary based on race.

Geriatric The pharmacokinetics of posaconazole are comparable in young and elderly subjects (≥65 years of age). No adjustment in the dosage of NOXAFIL is necessary in elderly patients (≥65 years of age) based on age.

Pediatric In the prophylaxis studies, the mean steady-state posaconazole average concentration (Cav) was similar among 10 adolescents (13-17 years of age) and adults (≥18 years of age). This is consistent with pharmacokinetic data from another study in which mean steady-state posaconazole Cav from 12 adolescent patients (8-17 years of age) was similar to that in the adults (≥18 years of age).

Hepatic Insufficiency After a single oral dose of posaconazole 400 mg, the mean AUC was 43%, 27%, and 21% higher in subjects with mild (Child-Pugh Class A, N=6), moderate (Child-Pugh Class B, N=6), and severe (Child-Pugh Class C, N=6) hepatic insufficiency, respectively, compared to subjects with normal hepatic function (N=18). Compared to subjects with normal hepatic function, the mean C$_{max}$ was 1% higher, 40% higher, and 34% lower in subjects with mild, moderate, and severe hepatic insufficiency, respectively. The mean apparent oral clearance (CL/F) was reduced by 18%, 36%, and 28% in subjects with mild, moderate, and severe hepatic insufficiency, respectively, compared to subjects with normal hepatic function. The elimination half-life (t$_{1/2}$) was 27 hours, 39 hours, 27 hours, and 43 hours in subjects with normal hepatic function and mild, moderate, and severe hepatic insufficiency, respectively.

It is recommended that no dose adjustment of NOXAFIL is needed in patients with mild to severe hepatic insufficiency (Child-Pugh Class A, B, and C) (see **WARNINGS** and **DOSAGE AND ADMINISTRATION**).

Renal Insufficiency Following single-dose administration of 400 mg of the oral suspension, there was no significant effect of mild (CLcr: 50-80 mL/min/1.73m², n=6) and moderate (CLcr: 20-49 mL/min/1.73m², n=6) renal insufficiency on posaconazole pharmacokinetics; therefore, no dose adjustment is required in patients with mild to moderate renal impairment. In subjects with severe renal insufficiency (CLcr: <20 mL/min/1.73m²), the mean plasma exposure (AUC) was similar to that in patients with normal renal function (CLcr: >80 mL/min/1.73m²); however, the range of the AUC estimates was highly variable (CV=96%) in these subjects with severe renal insufficiency as compared to that in the other renal impairment groups (CV<40%). Due to the variability in exposure, patients with severe renal impairment should be monitored closely for breakthrough fungal infections (see **DOSAGE AND ADMINISTRATION**).

Electrocardiogram Evaluation Multiple, time-matched ECGs collected over a 12-hour period were recorded at baseline and steady-state from 173 healthy male and female volunteers (18-85 years of age) administered posaconazole 400 mg BID with a high-fat meal. In this pooled analysis, the mean QTc (Fridericia) interval change from baseline was -5 msec following administration of the recommended clinical dose. A decrease in the QTc(F) interval (-3 msec) was also observed in a small number of subjects (n=16) administered placebo. The placebo-adjusted mean maximum QTc(F) interval change from baseline was <0 msec (-8 msec). No healthy subject administered posaconazole had a QTc(F) interval ≥500 msec or an increase ≥60 msec in their QTc(F) interval from baseline (see **PRECAUTIONS**).

Drug Interactions *Effect of Other Drugs on Posaconazole* Posaconazole is primarily metabolized via UDP glucuronidation (phase 2 enzymes) and is a substrate for p-glycoprotein (P-gp) efflux. Therefore, inhibitors or inducers of these clearance pathways may affect posaconazole plasma concentrations. A summary of drugs studied clinically, which affect posaconazole concentrations, is provided in **Table 3** (see **PRECAUTIONS, Drug Interactions** section). [See table 3 on previous page]

Coadministration of these drugs listed in **Table 3** with posaconazole may result in lower plasma concentrations of posaconazole.

No clinically relevant effect on posaconazole bioavailability and/or plasma concentrations was observed when administered with an antacid, glipizide, ritonavir, loperamide, or H2 receptor antagonists other than cimetidine; therefore, no posaconazole dose adjustments are required when used concomitantly with these products.

Effect of Posaconazole on Other Drugs *In vitro* studies with human hepatic microsomes and clinical studies indicate that posaconazole is an inhibitor primarily of CYP3A4. A clinical study in healthy volunteers also indicates that posaconazole is a strong CYP3A4 inhibitor as evidenced by a >5-fold increase in midazolam AUC. Therefore, plasma concentrations of drugs predominantly metabolized by CYP3A4 may be increased by posaconazole. A summary of the drugs studied clinically, for which plasma concentrations were affected by posaconazole, is provided in **Table 4** (see **CONTRAINDICATIONS, WARNINGS,** and **PRECAUTIONS, Drug Interactions** section). [See table 4 at right and on next page]

Additional clinical studies demonstrated that no clinically significant effects on zidovudine, lamivudine, ritonavir, indinavir, or caffeine were observed when administered with posaconazole 200 mg QD; therefore, no dose adjustments are required for these coadministered drugs when coadministered with posaconazole 200 mg QD.

Posaconazole administration with glipizide does not require a dose adjustment in either drug; however, glucose concentrations decreased in some healthy volunteers administered the combination. Therefore, glucose concentrations should be monitored in accordance with the current standard of care for patients with diabetes when posaconazole is coadministered with glipizide.

MICROBIOLOGY

Mechanism of Action As a triazole antifungal agent, posaconazole blocks the synthesis of ergosterol, a key component of the fungal cell membrane, through the inhibition of the enzyme lanosterol 14α-demethylase and accumulation of methylated sterol precursors.

Activity In Vitro and In Vivo Posaconazole has shown *in vitro* activity against *Aspergillus fumigatus* and *Candida albicans*, including *Candida albicans* isolates from patients refractory to itraconazole or fluconazole or both drugs (see **CLINICAL STUDIES** and **INDICATIONS AND USAGE**).

In vitro susceptibility testing was performed according to the Clinical and Laboratory Standards Institute (CLSI) methods (M27-A2, M27-A, M38-A, M38-P). However, correlation between the results of susceptibility studies and clinical outcome has not been established. Posaconazole interpretive criteria/breakpoints have not been established for any fungi.

In immunocompetent and/or immunocompromised mice and rabbits with pulmonary or disseminated infection with *A. fumigatus*, posaconazole administered prophylactically was effective in prolonging survival and reducing mycological burden. Prophylactic posaconazole also prolonged survival

of immunocompetent mice challenged with *C. albicans* or *A. flavus* (see **CLINICAL STUDIES**).

Drug Resistance Clinical isolates of *Candida albicans* and *Candida glabrata* with decreases in posaconazole susceptibility were observed in oral swish samples taken during prophylaxis with posaconazole and fluconazole, suggesting a potential for development of resistance. These isolates also showed reduced susceptibility to other azoles, suggesting cross-resistance between azoles. The clinical significance of this finding is not known.

CLINICAL STUDIES

Prophylaxis of *Aspergillus* and *Candida* Infections Two randomized, controlled studies were conducted using

posaconazole as prophylaxis for the prevention of invasive fungal infections (IFIs) among patients at high risk due to severely compromised immune systems.

The first study (Study 1) was a randomized, double-blind trial that compared posaconazole oral suspension (200 mg 3 times a day) with fluconazole capsules (400 mg once daily) as prophylaxis against invasive fungal infections in allogeneic hematopoietic stem cell transplant (HSCT) recipients with graft-vs.-host disease (GVHD). Efficacy of prophylaxis was evaluated using a composite endpoint of proven/probable IFIs, death, or treatment with systemic antifungal therapy. (Patients may have met more than 1 of these criteria.) Study 1 assessed all patients while on study therapy plus 7 days and at 16 weeks postrandomization. The mean

TABLE 4: Summary of the Effect of Posaconazole on Coadministered Drugs in Healthy Volunteers and Patients

Coadministered Drug (Postulated Mechanism of Interaction)	Coadministered Drug Dose/ Schedule	Posaconazole Dose/Schedule	Effect on Bioavailability of Coadministered Drugs		Recommendations
			Change in Mean C_{max} (ratio estimate)*; 90% CI of the ratio estimate)	Change in Mean AUC (ratio estimate)*; 90% CI of the ratio estimate)	
Sirolimus (Inhibition of CYP3A4 by posaconazole)	2-mg single oral dose	400 mg (oral suspension) BID × 16 days	↑ 572% (6.72; 5.62-8.03)	↑788% (8.88; 7.26-10.9)	Coadministration of posaconazole with sirolimus is contraindicated (see **CONTRAINDICATIONS**).
Cyclosporine (Inhibition of CYP3A4 by posaconazole)	Stable maintenance dose in heart transplant recipients	200 mg (tablets) QD × 10 days	↑ Cyclosporine whole blood trough concentrations Cyclosporine dose reductions of up to 29% were required		At initiation of posaconazole treatment, reduce the cyclosporine dose to approximately three-fourths of the original dose. Frequent monitoring of cyclosporine whole blood trough concentrations should be performed during and at discontinuation of posaconazole treatment and the cyclosporine dose adjusted accordingly.
Tacrolimus (Inhibition of CYP3A4 by posaconazole)	0.05-mg/kg single oral dose	400 mg (oral suspension) BID × 7 days	↑ 121% (2.21; 2.01-2.42)	↑ 358% (4.58; 4.03-5.19)	At initiation of posaconazole treatment, reduce the tacrolimus dose to approximately one-third of the original dose. Frequent monitoring of tacrolimus whole blood trough concentrations should be performed during and at discontinuation of posaconazole treatment and the tacrolimus dose adjusted accordingly.
Rifabutin (Inhibition of CYP3A4 by posaconazole)	300 mg QD × 17 days	200 mg (tablets) QD × 10 days	↑ 31% (1.31; 1.10-1.57)	↑72% (1.72; 1.51-1.95)	Avoid concomitant use unless the benefit outweighs the risks. If the drugs are coadministered, frequent monitoring of rifabutin adverse effects (e.g., uveitis, leukopenia) should be performed.
Midazolam (Inhibition of CYP3A4 by posaconazole)	Single 30-min IV infusion of 0.05 mg/kg	200 mg (tablets) QD × 10 days	NA†	↑ 83% (1.83; 1.57-2.14)	Frequent monitoring of adverse effects of benzodiazepines metabolized by CYP3A4 should be performed and dose reduction of these benzodiazepines should be considered during coadministration with posaconazole.
	0.4-mg single IV dose‡	200 mg (oral suspension) BID × 7 days	↑ 30% (1.3; 1.13-1.48)	↑ 362% (4.62; 4.02-5.3)	
	2-mg single oral dose‡	200 mg (oral suspension) BID × 7 days	↑ 126% (2.26; 2.02-2.53)	↑ 362% (4.59; 4.12-5.11)	
	0.4-mg single IV dose‡	400 mg (oral suspension) BID × 7 days	↑ 62% (1.62; 1.41-1.86)	↑ 524% (6.24; 5.43-7.16)	
Phenytoin (Inhibition of CYP3A4 by posaconazole)	200 mg QD PO × 10 days	200 mg (tablets) QD × 10 days	↑ 16% (1.16; 0.85-1.57)	↑ 16% (1.16; 0.84-1.59)	Frequent monitoring of phenytoin concentrations should be performed while coadministered with posaconazole and dose reduction of phenytoin should be considered.

(Table continued on next page)

TABLE 4 (cont.): Summary of the Effect of Posaconazole on Coadministered Drugs in Healthy Volunteers and Patients

Coadministered Drug (Postulated Mechanism of Interaction)	Coadministered Drug Dose/Schedule	Posaconazole Dose/Schedule	Effect on Bioavailability of Coadministered Drugs		Recommendations
			Change in Mean C_{max} (ratio estimate[*]; 90% CI of the ratio estimate)	Change in Mean AUC (ratio estimate[*]; 90% CI of the ratio estimate)	
Ritonavir (Inhibition of CYP3A4 by posaconazole)	100 mg QD × 14 days	400 mg (oral suspension) BID × 7 days	↑ 49% (1.49; 1.04-2.15)	↑ 80% (1.8; 1.39-2.31)	Frequent monitoring of adverse effects and toxicity of ritonavir should be performed during coadministration with posaconazole.
Atazanavir (Inhibition of CYP3A4 by posaconazole)	300 mg QD × 14 days	400 mg (oral suspension) BID × 7 days	↑ 155% (2.55; 1.89-3.45)	↑ 268% (3.68; 2.89-4.70)	Frequent monitoring of adverse effects and toxicity of atazanavir should be performed during coadministration with posaconazole.
Atazanavir/ ritonavir boosted regimen (Inhibition of CYP3A4 by posaconazole)	300 mg/100 mg QD × 14 days	400 mg (oral suspension) BID × 7 days	↑ 53% (1.53; 1.13-2.07)	↑ 146% (2.46; 1.93-3.13)	

* Ratio Estimate is the ratio of coadministered drug plus posaconazole to coadministered drug alone for C_{max} or AUC.
† NA: Not applicable if administered as an IV.
‡ The mean terminal half-life of midazolam was increased from 3 hours to 8 to 10 hours during coadministration with posaconazole.

duration of therapy was comparable between the 2 treatment groups (80 days, posaconazole; 77 days, fluconazole). **Table 5** contains the results from Study 1.

TABLE 5: Results from Blinded Clinical Study 1 in Prophylaxis of IFI in All Randomized Patients with Hematopoietic Stem Cell Transplant (HSCT) and Graft-vs.-Host Disease (GVHD)

	Posaconazole n=301	Fluconazole n=299
On therapy plus 7 days		
Clinical Failure*	50 (17%)	55 (18%)
Failure due to:		
Proven/Probable IFI	7 (2%)	22 (7%)
(Aspergillus)	3 (1%)	17 (6%)
(Candida)	1 (<1%)	3 (1%)
(Other)	3 (1%)	2 (1%)
All Deaths	22 (7%)	24 (8%)
Proven/probable fungal infection prior to death	2 (<1%)	6 (2%)
SAF†	27 (9%)	25 (8%)
Through 16 weeks		
Clinical Failure*‡	99 (33%)	110 (37%)
Failure due to:		
Proven/Probable IFI	16 (5%)	27 (9%)
(Aspergillus)	7 (2%)	21 (7%)
(Candida)	4 (1%)	4 (1%)
(Other)	5 (2%)	2 (1%)
All Deaths	58 (19%)	59 (20%)
Proven/probable fungal infection prior to death	10 (3%)	16 (5%)
SAF†	26 (9%)	30 (10%)
Event-free lost to follow-up§	24 (8%)	30 (10%)

* Patients may have met more than 1 criterion defining failure.
† Use of systemic antifungal therapy (SAF) criterion is based on protocol definitions (empiric/IFI usage >4 consecutive days).
‡ 95% confidence interval (posaconazole-fluconazole) = (-11.5%, +3.7%).
§ Patients who are lost to follow-up (not observed for 112 days), and who did not meet another clinical failure endpoint. These patients were considered failures.

The second study (Study 2) was a randomized, open-label study that compared posaconazole oral suspension (200 mg 3 times a day) with fluconazole suspension (400 mg once daily) or itraconazole oral solution (200 mg twice a day) as prophylaxis against IFIs in neutropenic patients who were receiving cytotoxic chemotherapy for acute myelogenous leukemia or myelodysplastic syndromes. As in Study 1, efficacy of prophylaxis was evaluated using a composite endpoint of proven/probable IFIs, death, or treatment with systemic antifungal therapy. (Patients might have met more than 1 of these criteria.) Study 2 assessed patients while on treatment plus 7 days and 100 days postrandomization. The mean duration of therapy was comparable between the 2 treatment groups (29 days, posaconazole; 25 days, fluconazole or itraconazole). **Table 6** contains the results from Study 2.

TABLE 6: Results from Open-label Clinical Study 2 in Prophylaxis of IFI in All Randomized Patients with Hematologic Malignancy and Prolonged Neutropenia

	Posaconazole n=304	Fluconazole/ Itraconazole n=298
On therapy plus 7 days		
Clinical Failure*†	82 (27%)	126 (42%)
Failure due to:		
Proven/Probable IFI	7 (2%)	25 (8%)
(Aspergillus)	2 (1%)	20 (7%)
(Candida)	3 (1%)	2 (1%)
(Other)	2 (1%)	3 (1%)
All Deaths	17 (6%)	25 (8%)
Proven/probable fungal infection prior to death	1 (<1%)	2 (1%)
SAF‡	67 (22%)	98 (33%)
Through 100 days postrandomization		
Clinical Failure†	158 (52%)	191 (64%)
Failure due to:		
Proven/probable IFI	14 (5%)	33 (11%)
(Aspergillus)	2 (1%)	26 (9%)
(Candida)	10 (3%)	4 (1%)
(Other)	2 (1%)	3 (1%)
All Deaths	44 (14%)	64 (21%)
Proven/probable fungal infection prior to death	2 (1%)	16 (5%)
SAF‡	98 (32%)	125 (42%)
Event-free lost to follow-up§	34 (11%)	24 (8%)

* 95% confidence interval (posaconazole-fluconazole/ itraconazole) = (-22.9%, -7.8%).
† Patients may have met more than 1 criterion defining failure.
‡ Use of systemic antifungal therapy (SAF) criterion is based on protocol definitions (empiric/IFI usage >3 consecutive days).
§ Patients who are lost to follow-up (not observed for 100 days), and who did not meet another clinical failure endpoint. These patients were considered failures.

In summary, 2 clinical studies of prophylaxis were conducted. As seen in the accompanying tables (**Tables 5** and **6**), clinical failure represented a composite endpoint of breakthrough IFI, mortality, and use of systemic antifungal therapy. In Study 1 (**Table 5**), the clinical failure rate of posaconazole (33%) was similar to fluconazole (37%), (95% CI for the difference posaconazole-comparator -11.5% to 3.7%) while in Study 2 (**Table 6**) clinical failure was lower for patients treated with posaconazole (27%) when compared to patients treated with fluconazole or itraconazole (42%), (95% CI for the difference posaconazole-comparator -22.9% to -7.8%).

All-cause mortality was similar at 16 weeks for both treatment arms in Study 1 [POS 58/301 (19%) vs. FLU 59/299 (20%)]; all-cause mortality was lower at 100 days for posaconazole-treated patients in Study 2 [POS 44/304 (14%) vs. FLU/ITZ 64/298 (21%)]. Both studies demonstrated substantially fewer breakthrough infections caused by Aspergillus species in patients receiving posaconazole prophylaxis when compared to patients receiving fluconazole or itraconazole.

For information on a pharmacokinetic/pharmacodynamic analysis of patient data see **CLINICAL PHARMACOLOGY, Exposure Response Relationship** section.

Treatment of Oropharyngeal Candidiasis (OPC) Study 3 was a randomized, controlled, evaluator-blinded study in HIV-infected patients with oropharyngeal candidiasis. Patients were treated with posaconazole or fluconazole oral suspension (both posaconazole and fluconazole were given as follows: 100 mg twice a day for 1 day followed by 100 mg once a day for 13 days).

Clinical and mycological outcomes were assessed after 14 days of treatment and at 4 weeks after the end of treatment. Patients who received at least 1 dose of study medication and had a positive oral swish culture of Candida species at baseline were included in the analyses (**Table 7**). The majority of the subjects had C. albicans as the baseline pathogen. Clinical success at Day 14 (complete or partial resolution of all ulcers and/or plaques and symptoms) and clinical relapse rates (recurrence of signs or symptoms after initial cure or improvement) 4 weeks after the end of treatment were similar between the treatment arms (**Table 7**).

Mycologic eradication rates (absence of colony forming units in quantitative culture at the end of therapy, Day 14), as well as mycologic relapse rates (4 weeks after the end of treatment) were also similar between the treatment arms (see **Table 7**).

TABLE 7: Clinical Success, Mycological Eradication, and Relapse Rates in Oropharyngeal Candidiasis

	Posaconazole	Fluconazole
Clinical Success at End of Therapy (Day 14)	155/169 (91.7%)	148/160 (92.5%)
Clinical Relapse (4 Weeks after End of Therapy)	45/155 (29.0%)	52/148 (35.1%)
Mycological Eradication (absence of CFU) at End of Therapy (Day 14)	88/169 (52.1%)	80/160 (50.0%)
Mycological Relapse (4 Weeks after End of Treatment)	49/88 (55.6%)	51/80 (63.7%)

Mycologic response rates, using a criterion for success as a posttreatment quantitative culture with ≤20 colony-forming units (CFU/mL) were also similar between the 2 groups (posaconazole 68.0%, fluconazole 68.1%). The clinical significance of this finding is unknown.

Treatment of Oropharyngeal Candidiasis Refractory to Treatment with Fluconazole or Itraconazole Study 4 was a noncomparative study of posaconazole oral suspension in HIV-infected subjects with OPC that was refractory to treatment with fluconazole or itraconazole. An episode of OPC was considered refractory if there was failure to improve or worsening of OPC after a standard course of therapy with fluconazole ≥100 mg/day for at least 10 consecutive days or itraconazole 200 mg/day for at least 10 consecutive days and treatment with either fluconazole or itraconazole had not been discontinued for more than 14 days prior to treatment with posaconazole. Of the 199 subjects enrolled in this study, 89 subjects met these strict criteria for refractory infection.

Forty-five subjects with refractory OPC were treated with posaconazole 400 mg BID for 3 days, followed by 400 mg QD for 25 days with an option for further treatment during a 3-month maintenance period. Following a dosing amendment, a further 44 subjects were treated with posaconazole 400 mg BID for 28 days. The efficacy of posaconazole was assessed by the clinical success (cure or improvement) rate after 4 weeks of treatment. The clinical success rate was 74.2% (66/89). The clinical success rates for both the original and the amended dosing regimens were similar (73.3% and 75.0%, respectively).

For information on a pharmacokinetic/pharmacodynamic analysis of patient data see **CLINICAL PHARMACOLOGY, Exposure Response Relationship** section.

INDICATIONS AND USAGE

NOXAFIL® (posaconazole) Oral Suspension is indicated for prophylaxis of invasive *Aspergillus* and *Candida* infections in patients, 13 years of age and older, who are at high risk of developing these infections due to being severely immunocompromised, such as hematopoietic stem cell transplant (HSCT) recipients with graft-vs.-host disease (GVHD) or those with hematologic malignancies with prolonged neutropenia from chemotherapy (see **MICROBIOLOGY** and **CLINICAL STUDIES**).

NOXAFIL (posaconazole) is indicated for the treatment of oropharyngeal candidiasis, including oropharyngeal candidiasis refractory to itraconazole and/or fluconazole (see **MICROBIOLOGY** and **CLINICAL STUDIES**).

CONTRAINDICATIONS

Hypersensitivity to the active substance or to any of the excipients.

Coadministration of NOXAFIL® (posaconazole) with sirolimus is contraindicated (see **CLINICAL PHARMACOLOGY, Drug Interactions** section and **PRECAUTIONS, Drug Interactions** section).

Coadministration with ergot alkaloids (see **PRECAUTIONS, Drug Interactions** section).

Coadministration with the CYP3A4 substrates terfenadine, astemizole, cisapride, pimozide, halofantrine, or quinidine since this may result in increased plasma concentrations of these medicinal products, leading to QTc prolongation and rare occurrences of torsades de pointes (see **CLINICAL PHARMACOLOGY, Drug Interactions** section and **PRECAUTIONS, Drug Interactions** section).

WARNINGS

Hypersensitivity There is no information regarding cross-sensitivity between NOXAFIL® and other azole antifungal agents. Caution should be used when prescribing NOXAFIL to patients with hypersensitivity to other azoles.

Hepatic Toxicity In clinical trials, there were infrequent cases of hepatic reactions (e.g., mild to moderate elevations in ALT, AST, alkaline phosphatase, total bilirubin, and/or clinical hepatitis). The elevations in liver function tests were generally reversible on discontinuation of therapy, and in some instances these tests normalized without drug interruption and rarely required drug discontinuation. Rarely, more severe hepatic reactions including cholestasis or hepatic failure including fatalities were reported in patients with serious underlying medical conditions (e.g., hematologic malignancy) during treatment with posaconazole. These severe hepatic events were seen primarily in subjects receiving the 800 mg daily (400 mg BID or 200 mg QID) in another indication.

Monitoring of Hepatic Function Liver function tests should be evaluated at the start of and during the course of posaconazole therapy. Patients who develop abnormal liver function tests during posaconazole therapy should be monitored for the development of more severe hepatic injury. Patient management should include laboratory evaluation of hepatic function (particularly liver function tests and bilirubin). Discontinuation of posaconazole must be considered if clinical signs and symptoms consistent with liver disease develop that may be attributable to posaconazole.

Cyclosporine Drug Interaction Cases of elevated cyclosporine levels resulting in rare serious adverse events, including nephrotoxicity and leukoencephalopathy, and death were reported in clinical efficacy studies. Dose reduction and more frequent clinical monitoring of cyclosporine and tacrolimus should be performed when posaconazole therapy is initiated (see **PRECAUTIONS, Drug Interactions** section).

PRECAUTIONS

Arrhythmias and QT Prolongation Some azoles, including posaconazole, have been associated with prolongation of the QT interval on the electrocardiogram. Results from a multiple time-matched ECG analysis in healthy volunteers did not show any increase in the mean of the QTc interval. During clinical development there was 1 case of torsades de pointes in a patient taking posaconazole. This patient was seriously ill with multiple confounding risk factors including a history of cardiotoxic chemotherapy, hypokalemia, and concomitant medications that may have been contributory. Posaconazole should be administered with caution to patients with potentially proarrhythmic conditions and should not be administered with drugs that are known to prolong the QTc interval and are metabolized through CYP3A4 (see **CLINICAL PHARMACOLOGY, Electrocardiogram Evaluation** section, **CONTRAINDICATIONS**, and **PRECAUTIONS, Drug Interactions** section). Rigorous attempts to correct potassium, magnesium, and calcium should be made before starting posaconazole.

Information for Patients Patients should be advised to:
- Take each dose of NOXAFIL® Oral Suspension during or immediately (i.e., within 20 minutes) following a full meal or liquid nutritional supplement in order to enhance absorption.
- Inform their physician if they develop severe diarrhea or vomiting as these conditions may decrease the plasma concentrations of posaconazole.
- Inform their physician if they are taking other drugs or before they begin taking other drugs as certain drugs can decrease the plasma concentrations of posaconazole (see **CLINICAL PHARMACOLOGY, Drug Interactions** section).

Drug Interactions A summary of significant drug interactions with posaconazole that have been studied clinically are provided in **Tables 8** and **9**. Appropriate precautions for the coadministration of these drugs with posaconazole are provided (see **CLINICAL PHARMACOLOGY, Drug Interactions** section, **CONTRAINDICATIONS**, and **WARNINGS**).

TABLE 8: Summary of the Effect of Coadministered Drugs on Posaconazole

Coadministered Drug	Recommendations
Cimetidine	Avoid concomitant use unless the benefit outweighs the risks.
Rifabutin	Avoid concomitant use unless the benefit outweighs the risks.
Phenytoin	Avoid concomitant use unless the benefit outweighs the risks.
Efavirenz	Avoid concomitant use unless the benefit outweighs the risks.
Esomeprazole	Monitor closely for breakthrough fungal infections.
Metoclopramide	Monitor closely for breakthrough fungal infections.

Coadministration of these drugs listed in **Table 8** with posaconazole may result in lower plasma concentrations of posaconazole.

TABLE 9: Summary of the Effect of Posaconazole on Coadministered Drugs

Coadministered Drug	Recommendations
Sirolimus	Coadministration of posaconazole with sirolimus is contraindicated (see **CLINICAL PHARMACOLOGY, Drug Interactions** section and **CONTRAINDICATIONS**).
Cyclosporine	Increased cyclosporine concentrations resulted in cyclosporine dose reductions in heart transplant patients coadministered posaconazole. At initiation of posaconazole treatment, reduce the cyclosporine dose to approximately three-fourths of the original dose. Frequent monitoring of cyclosporine whole blood trough concentrations should be performed during and at discontinuation of posaconazole treatment and the cyclosporine dose adjusted accordingly.
Tacrolimus	Posaconazole has been shown to increase C_{max} and AUC of tacrolimus significantly. At initiation of posaconazole treatment, reduce the tacrolimus dose to approximately one-third of the original dose. Frequent monitoring of tacrolimus whole blood trough concentrations should be performed during and at discontinuation of posaconazole treatment and the tacrolimus dose adjusted accordingly.
Rifabutin	Concomitant use of posaconazole and rifabutin should be avoided unless the benefit to the patient outweighs the risk. However, if concomitant administration is required frequent monitoring of full blood counts and adverse events due to increased rifabutin levels (e.g., uveitis, leukopenia) is recommended.
Midazolam	Frequent monitoring of adverse effects of benzodiazepines metabolized by CYP3A4 should be performed and dose reduction of these benzodiazepines should be considered during coadministration with posaconazole.
Phenytoin	Frequent monitoring of phenytoin concentrations should be performed while coadministered with posaconazole and dose reduction of phenytoin should be considered.
Atazanavir	Frequent monitoring of adverse effects and toxicity of atazanavir should be performed during coadministration with posaconazole.
Ritonavir	Frequent monitoring of adverse effects and toxicity of ritonavir should be performed during coadministration with posaconazole.

Although not studied *in vitro* or *in vivo*, posaconazole may affect the plasma concentrations of the drugs or drug classes described in **Table 10**. Appropriate precautions for the coadministration of these drugs with posaconazole are provided (see **CONTRAINDICATIONS**).

TABLE 10: Drugs Not Studied In Vitro or In Vivo but Likely to Result in Significant Drug Interactions

Drug or Drug Class (CYP3A4 Substrates)	Recommendations
Terfenadine, Astemizole, Pimozide, Cisapride, Quinidine, Halofantrine	Increased plasma concentrations of these drugs can lead to QT prolongation with rare occurrences of torsade de pointes. **Coadministration with posaconazole is contraindicated** (see **CONTRAINDICATIONS**).
Ergot Alkaloids	Posaconazole may increase the plasma concentration of ergot alkaloids (ergotamine and dihydroergotamine) which may lead to ergotism. **Coadministration of posaconazole with ergot alkaloids is contraindicated** (see **CONTRAINDICATIONS**).
Vinca Alkaloids	Posaconazole may increase the plasma concentrations of vinca alkaloids (e.g., vincristine and vinblastine) which may lead to neurotoxicity. Therefore, it is recommended that the dose adjustment of the vinca alkaloid be considered.
HMG-CoA reductase inhibitors (statins) metabolized through CYP3A4	It is recommended that dose reduction of statins be considered during coadministration. Increased statin concentrations in plasma can be associated with rhabdomyolysis.
Calcium Channel Blockers metabolized through CYP3A4	Frequent monitoring for adverse events and toxicity related to calcium channel blockers is recommended during coadministration. Dose reduction of calcium channel blockers may be needed.
Digoxin	Increased plasma concentrations of digoxin have been reported in patients receiving digoxin and posaconazole. Therefore, monitoring of digoxin plasma concentrations is recommended during coadministration.

Carcinogenesis, Mutagenesis, Impairment of Fertility No drug-related neoplasms were recorded in rats or mice treated with posaconazole for 2 years at doses below the maximum tolerated dose. In a 2-year carcinogenicity study, rats were given posaconazole orally at doses up to 20 mg/kg (females), or 30 mg/kg (males). These doses are equivalent to 3.9 or 3.5 times the exposure achieved with a 400-mg BID regimen, respectively, based on steady-state AUC in healthy volunteers administered a high-fat meal (400-mg BID regimen). In the mouse study, mice were treated at oral doses up to 60 mg/kg/day or 4.8 times the exposure achieved with a 400-mg BID regimen.

Posaconazole was not genotoxic or clastogenic when evaluated in bacterial mutagenicity (Ames), a chromosome aberration study in human peripheral blood lymphocytes, a Chinese hamster ovary cell mutagenicity study, and a mouse bone marrow micronucleus study.

Posaconazole had no effect on fertility of male rats at a dose up to 180 mg/kg (1.7 times the 400-mg BID regimen based on steady-state plasma concentrations in healthy volunteers) or female rats at a dose up to 45 mg/kg (2.2 times the 400-mg BID regimen).

Pregnancy Pregnancy Category C. Posaconazole has been shown to cause skeletal malformations (cranial malformations and missing ribs) in rats when given in doses ≥27 mg/kg (≥1.4 times the 400-mg BID regimen based on steady-state plasma concentrations of drug in healthy volunteers). The no-effect dose for malformations in rats was 9 mg/kg, which is 0.7 times the exposure achieved with the 400-mg BID regimen. No malformations were seen in rabbits at doses up to 80 mg/kg. In the rabbit, the no-effect dose was 20 mg/kg, while high doses of 40 mg/kg and 80 mg/kg, 2.9 or 5.2 times the exposure achieved with the 400-mg BID regimen, caused an increase in resorptions. In rabbits dosed at 80 mg/kg, a reduction in body weight gain of females and a reduction in litter size was seen. There are no adequate and well-controlled studies in pregnant women. Posaconazole should be used in pregnancy only if the potential benefit justifies the potential risk to the fetus.

Nursing Mothers Posaconazole is excreted in milk of lactating rats. The excretion of posaconazole in human breast milk has not been investigated. NOXAFIL should not be used by nursing mothers unless the benefit to the mother clearly outweighs the potential risk to the infant.

Pediatric Use A total of 12 patients 13 to 17 years of age received 600 mg/day (200 mg 3 times a day) for prophylaxis of invasive fungal infections. The safety profile in these patients <18 years of age appears similar to the safety profile observed in adults. Based on pharmacokinetic data in 10 of these pediatric patients, the mean steady-state average posaconazole concentration (Cav) was similar between these patients and adults (≥18 years of age).

A total of 16 patients 8 to 17 years of age were treated with 800 mg/day (400 mg twice a day or 200 mg 4 times a day) in a study for another indication. Based on pharmacokinetic data in 12 of these pediatric patients, the mean steady-state average posaconazole concentration (Cav) was similar between these patients and adults (≥18 years of age) (see **CLINICAL PHARMACOLOGY, Pharmacokinetics in Special Populations, Pediatric** section).

Safety and effectiveness of posaconazole in pediatric patients below the age of 13 years have not been established.

TABLE 11: Study 1 and Study 2. Number (%) of Randomized Subjects Reporting Treatment-emergent Adverse Events: Frequency of at Least 10% in the Posaconazole or Fluconazole Treatment Groups (Pooled Prophylaxis Safety Analysis)

	Posaconazole (n=605)		Fluconazole (n=539)		Itraconazole (n=58)	
Subjects Reporting any Adverse Event	595	(98)	531	(99)	58	(100)
Body as a Whole – General Disorders						
Fever	274	(45)	254	(47)	32	(55)
Headache	171	(28)	141	(26)	23	(40)
Rigors	122	(20)	87	(16)	17	(29)
Fatigue	101	(17)	98	(18)	5	(9)
Edema Legs	93	(15)	67	(12)	11	(19)
Anorexia	92	(15)	94	(17)	16	(28)
Dizziness	64	(11)	56	(10)	5	(9)
Edema	54	(9)	68	(13)	8	(14)
Weakness	51	(8)	52	(10)	2	(3)
Cardiovascular Disorders, General						
Hypertension	106	(18)	88	(16)	3	(5)
Hypotension	83	(14)	79	(15)	10	(17)
Disorders of Blood and Lymphatic System						
Anemia	149	(25)	124	(23)	16	(28)
Neutropenia	141	(23)	122	(23)	23	(40)
Febrile Neutropenia	118	(20)	85	(16)	23	(40)
Disorders of the Reproductive System and Breast						
Vaginal Hemorrhage*	24	(10)	20	(9)	3	(12)
Gastrointestinal System Disorders						
Diarrhea	256	(42)	212	(39)	35	(60)
Nausea	232	(38)	198	(37)	30	(52)
Vomiting	174	(29)	173	(32)	24	(41)
Abdominal Pain	161	(27)	147	(27)	21	(36)
Constipation	126	(21)	94	(17)	10	(17)
Mucositis NOS	105	(17)	68	(13)	15	(26)
Dyspepsia	61	(10)	50	(9)	6	(10)
Heart Rate and Rhythm Disorders						
Tachycardia	72	(12)	75	(14)	3	(5)
Infection and Infestations						
Bacteremia	107	(18)	98	(18)	16	(28)
Herpes Simplex	88	(15)	61	(11)	10	(17)
Cytomegalovirus Infection	82	(14)	69	(13)	0	
Pharyngitis	71	(12)	60	(11)	12	(21)
Upper Respiratory Tract Infection	44	(7)	54	(10)	5	(9)
Liver and Biliary System Disorders						
Bilirubinemia	59	(10)	51	(9)	11	(19)
Metabolic and Nutritional Disorders						
Hypokalemia	181	(30)	142	(26)	30	(52)
Hypomagnesemia	110	(18)	84	(16)	11	(19)
Hyperglycemia	68	(11)	76	(14)	2	(3)
Hypocalcemia	56	(9)	55	(10)	5	(9)
Musculoskeletal System Disorders						
Musculoskeletal Pain	95	(16)	82	(15)	9	(16)
Arthralgia	69	(11)	67	(12)	5	(9)
Back Pain	63	(10)	66	(12)	4	(7)
Platelet, Bleeding and Clotting Disorders						
Thrombocytopenia	175	(29)	146	(27)	20	(34)
Petechiae	64	(11)	54	(10)	9	(16)
Psychiatric Disorders						
Insomnia	103	(17)	92	(17)	11	(19)
Anxiety	52	(9)	61	(11)	9	(16)
Respiratory System Disorders						
Coughing	146	(24)	130	(24)	14	(24)
Dyspnea	121	(20)	116	(22)	15	(26)
Epistaxis	82	(14)	73	(14)	12	(21)
Skin and Subcutaneous Tissue Disorders						
Rash	113	(19)	96	(18)	25	(43)
Pruritus	69	(11)	62	(12)	11	(19)

*Percentages of sex-specific adverse events are based on the number of males/females.
NOS = not otherwise specified.

IMPORTANT NOTICE: Updated drug information is sent bi-monthly via the PDR® Update Insert. For monthly email updates, register at PDR.net.

Geriatric Use Of the 605 patients randomized to posaconazole in the prophylaxis clinical trials, 63 (10%) were ≥65 years of age. In addition, 48 patients treated with ≥800 mg/day posaconazole in another indication were ≥65 years of age. No overall differences in safety were observed between the geriatric patients and younger patients; therefore, no dosage adjustment is recommended for geriatric patients (see **CLINICAL PHARMACOLOGY, Pharmacokinetics in Special Populations, *Geriatric* section).

ADVERSE REACTIONS

The safety of posaconazole therapy has been assessed in 1844 patients. This includes 605 patients in the prophylaxis studies, 796 in OPC/rOPC studies, and over 400 patients treated for other indications. Posaconazole therapy was given to 171 patients for ≥6 months, with 58 patients receiving posaconazole therapy for ≥12 months.

Prophylaxis of *Aspergillus* and *Candida* Table 11 presents treatment-emergent adverse events observed at an incidence >10% in posaconazole prophylaxis studies.

[See table 11 at top of previous page]

Tables 12 and **13** present treatment-related adverse events observed at an incidence ≥2% in the posaconazole prophylaxis studies.

TABLE 12: Study 1. Treatment-related Adverse Events, Occurring in Greater Than or Equal to 2% of Patients in Posaconazole or Fluconazole Treatment Group

Body System/Preferred Term	Posaconazole (n=301)	Fluconazole (n=299)
	n (%)	n (%)
Subjects Reporting Any Adverse Event	107 (36)	115 (38)
Body as a Whole – General Disorders		
Drug Level Altered	5 (2)	2 (1)
Dizziness	4 (1)	5 (2)
Fatigue	4 (1)	6 (2)
Anorexia	3 (1)	7 (2)
Headache	3 (1)	8 (3)
Weakness	3 (1)	5 (2)
Cardiovascular Disorders, General		
Hypertension	2 (1)	5 (2)
Central and Peripheral Nervous System Disorders		
Tremor	4 (1)	6 (2)
Disorders of the Eye		
Vision Blurred	3 (1)	5 (2)
Gastrointestinal System Disorders		
Nausea	22 (7)	28 (9)
Vomiting	13 (4)	15 (5)
Diarrhea	8 (3)	12 (4)
Abdominal Pain	4 (1)	7 (2)
Dyspepsia	3 (1)	6 (2)
Constipation	1 (<1)	5 (2)
Liver and Biliary System Disorders		
SGPT Increased	9 (3)	4 (1)
GGT Increased	9 (3)	7 (2)
Bilirubinemia	8 (3)	5 (2)
Hepatic Enzymes Increased	8 (3)	7 (2)
SGOT Increased	8 (3)	3 (1)
Metabolic and Nutritional Disorders		
Phosphatase Alkaline Increased	5 (2)	5 (2)
Renal and Urinary System Disorders		
Blood Creatinine Increased	6 (2)	5 (2)
Special Senses, Other Disorders		
Taste Perversion	3 (1)	5 (2)

GGT = gamma-glutamyl transpeptidase; SGOT = serum glutamic oxaloacetic transaminase; SGPT = serum glutamic pyruvic transaminase.

TABLE 13: Study 2. Treatment-related Adverse Events, Occurring in Greater Than or Equal to 2% of Patients in Posaconazole or Fluconazole/Itraconazole Treatment Group

Body System/Preferred Term	Number (%) of Patients			
	Posaconazole (n=304)	Fluconazole/Itraconazole (n=298)	Fluconazole (n=240)	Itraconazole (n=58)
Subjects Reporting Any Adverse Event	102 (34)	101 (34)	71 (30)	30 (52)
Body as a Whole – General Disorders				
Headache	5 (2)	1 (<1)	0	1 (2)
Gastrointestinal System Disorders				
Nausea	22 (7)	25 (8)	17 (7)	8 (14)
Diarrhea	20 (7)	21 (7)	12 (5)	9 (16)
Vomiting	14 (5)	20 (7)	14 (6)	6 (10)
Abdominal Pain	9 (3)	9 (3)	8 (3)	1 (2)
Mucositis NOS	7 (2)	0	0	0
Dyspepsia	5 (2)	3 (1)	3 (1)	0
Constipation	3 (1)	7 (2)	7 (3)	0
Heart Rate and Rhythm Disorders				
QT/QTc Prolongation	12 (4)	9 (3)	5 (2)	4 (7)
Liver and Biliary System Disorders				
Bilirubinemia	7 (2)	8 (3)	5 (2)	3 (5)
Hepatic Enzymes Increased	7 (2)	3 (1)	3 (1)	0
SGPT Increased	7 (2)	5 (2)	4 (2)	1 (2)
SGOT Increased	6 (2)	5 (2)	4 (2)	1 (2)
GGT Increased	5 (2)	2 (1)	1 (<1)	1 (2)
Metabolic and Nutritional Disorders				
Hypokalemia	9 (3)	6 (2)	5 (2)	1 (2)
Skin and Subcutaneous Tissue Disorders				
Rash	9 (3)	11 (4)	10 (4)	1 (2)

GGT = gamma-glutamyl transpeptidase; NOS = not otherwise specified; SGOT = serum glutamic oxaloacetic transaminase; SGPT = serum glutamic pyruvic transaminase.

[See table 13 above]

The most common treatment-related serious adverse events (1% each) in the combined prophylaxis studies were bilirubinemia, increased hepatic enzymes, hepatocellular damage, nausea, and vomiting.

Overview of Adverse Events in HIV-infected Subjects with OPC In 2 randomized comparative studies in OPC, the safety of posaconazole at a dose of ≤400 mg QD in 557 HIV-infected patients was compared to the safety of fluconazole in 262 HIV-infected patients at a dose of 100 mg QD.

An additional 239 HIV-infected patients with refractory OPC received posaconazole in 2 noncomparative trials for refractory OPC (rOPC). Of these subjects, 149 received the 800-mg/day dose and the remainder received the ≤400-mg QD dose.

Table 14 presents Treatment-emergent Adverse Events of Clinical Significance in the comparative and noncomparative studies of OPC.

[See table 14 at top of next page]

Treatment-related, treatment-emergent events observed in patients with OPC at an incidence of ≥2% are shown in **Table 15**.

[See table 15 at top of page 2201]

Adverse events were reported more frequently in the pool of patients with refractory OPC. Among these highly immunocompromised patients with advanced HIV disease, serious adverse events (SAEs) were reported in 55% (132/239). The most commonly reported SAEs were fever (13%) and neutropenia (10%).

Treatment-related SAEs were reported for 14% (34/239) of these patients and included neutropenia (5%) and abdominal pain (2%). Posaconazole was discontinued in 2 patients who developed neutropenia that was considered serious and treatment-related. All other reported treatment-related SAEs occurred in ≤1% of subjects on posaconazole.

Uncommon and rare treatment-related serious or medically significant adverse events reported during clinical trials in prophylaxis, OPC/rOPC or other indications with posaconazole have included adrenal insufficiency and allergic and/or hypersensitivity reactions.

Rare cases of hemolytic uremic syndrome, thrombotic thrombocytopenic purpura, and pulmonary embolus have been reported primarily among patients who had been receiving concomitant cyclosporine or tacrolimus for management of transplant rejection or graft-vs.-host disease.

During clinical development there was a single case of torsade de pointes in a patient taking posaconazole. This report involved a seriously ill patient with multiple confounding, potentially contributory risk factors, such as a history of palpitations, recent cardiotoxic chemotherapy, hypokalemia, and hypomagnesemia.

Additionally, in another indication, 428 patients were treated with ≥800 mg/day with a similar AE profile.

Clinical Laboratory Values In healthy volunteers and patients, elevation of liver function test values did not appear to be associated with higher plasma concentrations of posaconazole. The majority of abnormal liver function test results were minor, transient, and did not lead to discontinuation of therapy.

For the prophylaxis studies, the number of patients with changes in liver function test results from Common Toxicity Criteria (CTC) Grade 0, 1, or 2 at baseline to Grade 3 or 4 during the study is presented in **Table 16**.

TABLE 16: Study 1 and Study 2. Changes in Liver Function Test Results from CTC Grade 0, 1, or 2 at Baseline to Grade 3 or 4

Laboratory Parameter	Number (%) of Patients With Change*	
	Study 1	
	Posaconazole N=301	Fluconazole N=299
AST	11/266 (4)	13/266 (5)
ALT	47/271 (17)	39/272 (14)
Bilirubin	24/271 (9)	20/275 (7)
Alkaline Phosphatase	9/271 (3)	8/271 (3)
	Study 2	
	Posaconazole (n=304)	Fluconazole/Itraconazole (n=298)
AST	9/286 (3)	5/280 (2)
ALT	18/289 (6)	13/284 (5)

Bilirubin	20/290 (7)	25/285 (9)
Alkaline Phosphatase	4/281 (1)	1/276 (<1)

CTC = Common Toxicity Criteria; AST= Aspartate Aminotransferase; ALT= Alanine Aminotransferase.
*Change from Grade 0 to 2 at baseline to Grade 3 or 4 during the study. These data are presented in the form X/Y, where X represents the number of patients who met the criterion as indicated, and Y represents the number of patients who had a baseline observation and at least 1 post-baseline observation.

The number of patients treated for OPC with clinically significant liver function test (LFT) abnormalities at any time during the studies is provided in **Table 17** (LFT abnormalities were present in some of these patients prior to initiation of the study drug).
[See table 17 on next page]

OVERDOSAGE

During the clinical trials, some patients received posaconazole up to 1600 mg/day with no adverse events noted that were different from the lower doses. In addition, accidental overdose was noted in 1 patient who took 1200 mg BID for 3 days. No related adverse events were noted by the investigator.
Posaconazole is not removed by hemodialysis.

DOSAGE AND ADMINISTRATION

Indication	Dose and Duration of therapy
Prophylaxis of Invasive Fungal Infections	200 mg (5 mL) 3 times a day. The duration of therapy is based on recovery from neutropenia or immunosuppression.
Oropharyngeal Candidiasis	Loading dose of 100 mg (2.5 mL) twice a day on the first day, then 100 mg (2.5 mL) once a day for 13 days.
Oropharyngeal Candidiasis Refractory to Itraconazole and/or Fluconazole	400 mg (10 mL) twice a day. Duration of therapy should be based on the severity of the patient's underlying disease and clinical response.

Each dose of NOXAFIL® should be administered with a full meal or with a liquid nutritional supplement in patients who cannot eat a full meal (see **CLINICAL PHARMACOLOGY**).
Alternatively, NOXAFIL may be taken with an acidic carbonated beverage (e.g., ginger ale).
To enhance the oral absorption of posaconazole and optimize plasma concentrations:
• Each dose of NOXAFIL Oral Suspension should be administered during or immediately (i.e., within 20 minutes) following a full meal or liquid nutritional supplement. For patients who can not eat a full meal or tolerate an oral nutritional supplement, alternative antifungal therapy should be considered or patients should be monitored closely for breakthrough fungal infections.
• Patients who have severe diarrhea or vomiting should be monitored closely for breakthrough fungal infections.
• Coadministration of drugs that can decrease the plasma concentrations of posaconazole should generally be avoided unless the benefit outweighs the risk. If such drugs are necessary, patients should be monitored closely for breakthrough fungal infections (see **CLINICAL PHARMACOLOGY, Drug Interactions** section).
Shake NOXAFIL Oral Suspension well before use.
A measured dosing spoon is provided, marked for doses of 2.5 mL and 5 mL.

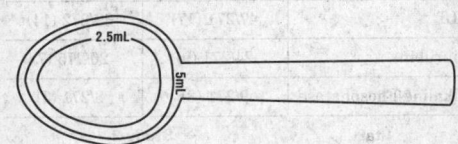

It is recommended that the spoon is rinsed with water after each administration and before storage.
Renal Insufficiency No dose adjustment is recommended for patients with renal dysfunction. However, the range of the posaconazole AUC estimates was highly variable (CV=96%) in subjects with severe renal insufficiency compared to that in the other renal impairment groups (CV<40%). Due to the variability in exposure, patients with severe renal impairment should be monitored closely for breakthrough IFIs (see **CLINICAL PHARMACOLOGY**).
Hepatic Insufficiency No dose adjustment of NOXAFIL is needed in patients with mild to severe hepatic insufficiency (Child-Pugh Class A, B, and C) (see **CLINICAL PHARMACOLOGY, Pharmacokinetics in Special Populations** section).

HOW SUPPLIED

NOXAFIL® (posaconazole) Oral Suspension is available in 4-ounce (123 mL) amber glass bottles with child-resistant closures (NDC 0085-1328-01) containing 105 mL of suspension (40 mg of posaconazole per mL).
Supplied with each bottle is a plastic dosing spoon calibrated for measuring 2.5-mL and 5-mL doses.
Store at 25°C (77°F); excursions permitted to 15°-30°C (59°-86°F) [see USP Controlled Room Temperature]. DO NOT FREEZE.
Schering-Plough
Kenilworth, NJ 07033 USA

TABLE 14: Treatment-emergent Adverse Events of Clinical Significance in OPC studies

	Number (%) of Subjects					
	Controlled OPC Pool				Refractory OPC Pool	
	Posaconazole n=557		Fluconazole n=262		Posaconazole n=239	
Subjects Reporting any Adverse Event*	356	(64)	175	(67)	221	(92)
Body as a Whole – General Disorders						
Fever	34	(6)	22	(8)	82	(34)
Headache	44	(8)	23	(9)	47	(20)
Anorexia	10	(2)	4	(2)	46	(19)
Fatigue	18	(3)	12	(5)	31	(13)
Asthenia	9	(2)	5	(2)	31	(13)
Rigors	2	(<1)	4	(2)	29	(12)
Pain	4	(1)	2	(1)	27	(11)
Disorders of Blood and Lymphatic System						
Neutropenia	21	(4)	8	(3)	39	(16)
Anemia	11	(2)	5	(2)	34	(14)
Neutropenia Aggravated	0		0		5	(2)
Gastrointestinal System Disorders						
Diarrhea	58	(10)	34	(13)	70	(29)
Nausea	48	(9)	30	(11)	70	(29)
Vomiting	37	(7)	18	(7)	67	(28)
Abdominal Pain	27	(5)	17	(6)	43	(18)
Infection and Infestations						
Candidiasis, Oral	3	(1)	1	(<1)	28	(12)
Herpes Simplex	16	(3)	8	(3)	26	(11)
Pneumonia	17	(3)	6	(2)	25	(10)
Liver and Biliary System Disorders						
Bilirubinemia	6	(1)	2	(1)	6	(3)
Hepatic Enzymes Increased	1	(<1)	1	(<1)	8	(3)
Hepatic Function Abnormal	8	(1)	4	(2)	0	
Hepatitis	3	(1)	0		5	(2)
Hepatomegaly	0		0		8	(3)
Jaundice	0		0		4	(2)
SGOT Increased	8	(1)	5	(2)	6	(3)
SGPT Increased	6	(1)	5	(2)	6	(3)
Metabolic and Nutritional Disorders						
Weight Decrease	4	(1)	2	(1)	33	(14)
Dehydration	4	(1)	7	(3)	27	(11)
Hypokalemia	6	(1)	3	(1)	15	(6)
Platelet, Bleeding, and Clotting Disorders						
Thrombocytopenia	4	(1)	1	(<1)	12	(5)
Psychiatric Disorders						
Insomnia	8	(1)	3	(1)	39	(16)
Renal & Urinary System Disorders						
Renal Failure Acute	0		0		7	(3)
Respiratory System Disorders						
Coughing	18	(3)	11	(4)	60	(25)
Dyspnea	8	(1)	8	(3)	28	(12)
Skin and Subcutaneous Tissue Disorders						
Rash	15	(3)	10	(4)	36	(15)
Sweating Increased	13	(2)	5	(2)	23	(10)

OPC=oropharyngeal candidiasis; SGOT=serum glutamic oxaloacetic transaminase (same as AST); SGPT=serum glutamic pyruvic transaminase (same as ALT).
*Number of subjects reporting treatment-emergent adverse events at least once during the study, without regard to relationship to treatment. Subjects may have reported more than 1 event.

PATIENT INFORMATION

NOXAFIL®
(posaconazole) ORAL SUSPENSION

Read the Patient Information that comes with NOXAFIL® Oral Suspension before you start taking it and each time you get a refill. There may be new information. This information does not replace talking with your doctor about your condition or treatment. Only your doctor can prescribe NOXAFIL and determine if it is right for you.

What is NOXAFIL®?

• NOXAFIL is a prescription medicine that is used to prevent invasive fungal infections (infections that can spread throughout the body) caused by *Aspergillus* or *Candida* in patients with weak immune systems because of medicines or diseases [such as stem cell transplantation with graft-vs.-host disease or chemotherapy for hematologic malignancy (blood cancers)].

- NOXAFIL is also used to treat fungal infections in the mouth or throat area (known as "thrush") caused by fungi called *Candida*. NOXAFIL can be used as initial treatment or as a treatment after itraconazole and/or fluconazole have failed.

NOXAFIL is for adults and children over 13 years of age.

What should I tell my doctor before taking NOXAFIL®?
Tell your doctor about all your health conditions, including if you:

- are taking certain drugs that suppress your immune system like cyclosporine (Neoral®), tacrolimus (Prograf®), or sirolimus (Rapamune®). Serious and rare fatal toxicity from cyclosporine has occurred when taken in combination with posaconazole and, therefore, reduction of the dose of drugs like cyclosporine, tacrolimus, or atazanavir and frequent monitoring of drug levels of these medicines is necessary when taking them in combination with posaconazole.
- have ever had an allergic reaction to other antifungal medicines such as ketoconazole, fluconazole, itraconazole, or voriconazole.
- are taking any other medicines, including prescription and nonprescription medicines, vitamins, and herbal supplements.
- have, or have had liver problems. Your doctor may do blood tests to make sure you should take NOXAFIL.
- have, or have had an abnormal heart rate or rhythm.
- are, or think you are pregnant. Do not use NOXAFIL during pregnancy unless specifically advised by your doctor. You should use effective birth control while you are taking NOXAFIL if you are a woman who could become pregnant.

Contact your doctor immediately if you become pregnant while being treated with NOXAFIL.
Do not breastfeed while being treated with NOXAFIL, unless specifically advised by your doctor.

Who should not take NOXAFIL®?
Do NOT take NOXAFIL if you are taking any of the medicines listed below.
If any of these medicines are taken together with NOXAFIL, serious or life-threatening side effects from these medicines, or a decrease in the effect of NOXAFIL can occur. Tell your doctor right away if you are taking any of these medicines:

- sirolimus
- ergot alkaloids (ergotamine, dihydroergotamine, methylsergide, methylergonovine, ergonovine, or bromocriptine)
- terfenadine
- astemizole
- cisapride
- pimozide
- halofantrine
- quinidine
- rifabutin
- phenytoin
- cimetidine

If you have questions or are uncertain about your medicines, talk with your doctor or pharmacist.
Do not take NOXAFIL if you are allergic to anything in it. There is a list of what is in NOXAFIL at the end of this leaflet.

Can I take other medicines with NOXAFIL®?
NOXAFIL and many medicines can interact with each other and some must not be taken together (see "**Who should not take NOXAFIL?**"). The dose of other medicines may need to be adjusted when taken with NOXAFIL [for example, **cyclosporine (Neoral®), tacrolimus (Prograf®), ritonavir, or atazanavir**] (see "**What should I tell my doctor before taking NOXAFIL?**").
Knowing the medicines that you are taking is important. **Tell your doctor** about all the medicines you take including prescription and nonprescription medicines, vitamins, and herbal supplements. Keep a list with you to show your doctor or pharmacist. Do not take any new medicine without talking to your doctor.

What are possible side effects of NOXAFIL®?
The most commonly reported side effects related to NOXAFIL use were nausea, diarrhea, vomiting, headache, stomach pain, bloating, liver problems, low blood potassium, and decrease in neutrophils (certain type of white blood cells that fight infection).
Rarely, NOXAFIL may cause serious or life-threatening side effects. It may also cause severe drug interactions as discussed above. Call your doctor right away if you have any of the symptoms listed below.
Changes in heart rate or rhythm. People who have certain heart conditions or who take certain other medicines have a higher chance for this problem.
Rarely, very serious liver problems were reported in patients with serious underlying medical conditions. Your doctor may test your liver function while you are taking NOXAFIL. Call your doctor if you have any of these symptoms, as these may be signs of liver problems: you have itching, your eyes or skin turn yellow, you feel more tired than usual or feel like you have the flu, or you have nausea or vomiting.
Rarely, an increase in blood clots may occur in patients with blood cancers or post-stem cell transplantation. These events may or may not be further increased in patients also on posaconazole and primarily occurred in patients also receiving cyclosporine or tacrolimus. If you notice swelling of one leg or shortness of breath, notify your doctor immediately.

These are not all the side effects associated with NOXAFIL. For more information, ask your doctor or pharmacist. If you experience any unusual effects while taking NOXAFIL, contact your doctor immediately.

How do I take NOXAFIL®?
- NOXAFIL comes in cherry-flavored liquid form. Shake NOXAFIL Oral Suspension well before use.
- Take NOXAFIL for as long as your doctor tells you. Take each dose of NOXAFIL during or immediately (i.e., within 20 minutes) following a full meal, or with a liquid nutritional supplement if you are unable to eat a full meal. Alternatively, NOXAFIL may be taken with an acidic carbonated beverage (e.g., ginger ale).

TABLE 15: Treatment-related Adverse Events (Any Grade) ≥2%

Adverse Event	Controlled OPC Pool Posaconazole n=557		Controlled OPC Pool Fluconazole n=262		Refractory OPC Pool Posaconazole n=239	
Subjects Reporting any Adverse Event*	150	(27)	70	(27)	135	(56)
Body As A Whole – General Disorders						
Headache	16	(3)	5	(2)	18	(8)
Anorexia	6	(1)	1	(<1)	7	(3)
Asthenia	4	(1)	2	(1)	6	(3)
Dizziness	9	(2)	5	(2)	8	(3)
Fatigue	8	(1)	5	(2)	7	(3)
Fever	10	(2)	1	(<1)	6	(3)
Central and Periph Nerv System						
Somnolence	4	(1)	5	(2)	3	(1)
Disorders of Blood and Lymphatic System						
Neutropenia	10	(2)	4	(2)	20	(8)
Anemia	2	(<1)	0		6	(3)
Gastrointestinal System Disorders						
Diarrhea	19	(3)	13	(5)	26	(11)
Nausea	27	(5)	18	(7)	20	(8)
Vomiting	20	(4)	4	(2)	16	(7)
Abdominal Pain	10	(2)	8	(3)	12	(5)
Flatulence	6	(1)	0		11	(5)
Mouth Dry	7	(1)	6	(2)	5	(2)
Liver and Biliary System Disorders						
Hepatic Enzymes Increased	1	(<1)	0		5	(2)
Hepatic Function Abnormal	3	(1)	4	(2)	0	
Metabolic and Nutritional Disorders						
Phosphatase Alkaline Increased	3	(1)	3	(1)	5	(2)
Musculoskeletal System Disorders						
Myalgia	1	(<1)	0		4	(2)
Platelet, Bleeding, and Clotting Disorders						
Thrombocytopenia	3	(1)	0		4	(2)
Psychiatric Disorders						
Insomnia	3	(1)	0		6	(3)
Skin and Subcutaneous Tissue Disorders						
Rash	8	(1)	4	(2)	10	(4)
Pruritus	6	(1)	2	(1)	5	(2)

OPC=oropharyngeal candidiasis; SGOT=serum glutamic oxaloacetic transaminase (same as AST); SGPT=serum glutamic pyruvic transaminase (same as ALT).
*Number of subjects reporting treatment-related adverse events at least once during the study, without regard to relationship to treatment. Subjects may have reported more than 1 event.

TABLE 17: Clinically Significant Laboratory Test Abnormalities Without Regard to Baseline Value

Laboratory Test	Controlled Posaconazole n=557	Controlled Fluconazole n=262	Refractory Posaconazole n=239
ALT > 3.0 × ULN	16/537(3)	13/254(5)	25/226(11)
AST > 3.0 × ULN	33/537(6)	26/254(10)	39/223(17)
Total Bilirubin > 1.5 × ULN	15/536(3)	5/254(2)	9/197(5)
Alkaline Phosphatase > 3.0 × ULN	17/535(3)	15/253(6)	24/190(13)

ALT= Alanine Aminotransferase; AST= Aspartate Aminotransferase.

- Follow your doctor's instructions on when and how much of NOXAFIL you should take.
If you miss a dose of NOXAFIL, take it as soon as you remember.
- If you take too much NOXAFIL, call your doctor or poison control center immediately.
- Tell your doctor right away if you develop severe diarrhea or vomiting.

A measured dosing spoon is provided, marked for doses of 2.5 mL and 5 mL.

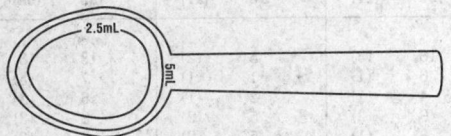

It is recommended that the spoon is rinsed with water after each administration and before storage.

How do I store NOXAFIL®?

- Store at 25°C (77°F); excursions permitted to 15°-30°C (59°-86°F) [see USP Controlled Room Temperature]. DO NOT FREEZE. Keep all containers tightly closed.
- **Keep NOXAFIL, as well as other medicines, out of the reach of children.**

General information about NOXAFIL®

Doctors can prescribe medicines for conditions that are not in this leaflet. Use NOXAFIL only as directed by your doctor. Do not give it to other people, even if they have the same symptoms as you. It may harm them.

This leaflet gives the most important information about NOXAFIL. For more information, talk to your doctor. You can ask your doctor or pharmacist for information about NOXAFIL that is written for health care professionals.

What is in NOXAFIL®?

Active ingredient: posaconazole

Inactive ingredients: polysorbate 80, simethicone, sodium benzoate, sodium citrate dihydrate, citric acid monohydrate, glycerin, xanthan gum, liquid glucose, titanium dioxide, artificial cherry flavor, and purified water.

Schering-Plough
Kenilworth, NJ 07033 USA
Rx only
© 2006, 2008, Schering Corporation. All rights reserved.
U.S. Patent Nos. 5,661,151; 5,703,079; and 6,958,337.
Rev. 2/09   **31157528T**
The trademarks depicted in this piece are owned by their respective companies.

Shown in Product Identification Guide, page 313

NUVARING®   ℞
(etonogestrel/ethinyl estradiol vaginal ring)
delivers 0.120 mg/0.015 mg per day

Women should be counseled that this product does not protect against HIV infection (AIDS) and other sexually transmitted diseases.
FOR VAGINAL USE ONLY

DESCRIPTION

NuvaRing® (etonogestrel/ethinyl estradiol vaginal ring) is a nonbiodegradable, flexible, transparent, colorless to almost colorless, combination contraceptive vaginal ring containing two active components, a progestin, etonogestrel (13-ethyl-17-hydroxy-11-methylene-18,19-dinor-17α-pregn-4-en-20-yn-3-one) and an estrogen, ethinyl estradiol (19-nor-17α-pregna-1,3,5(10)-trien-20-yne-3, 17-diol). When placed in the vagina, each ring releases on average 0.120 mg/day of etonogestrel and 0.015 mg/day of ethinyl estradiol over a three-week period of use. NuvaRing® is made of ethylene vinylacetate copolymers (28% and 9% vinylacetate) and magnesium stearate and contains 11.7 mg etonogestrel and 2.7 mg ethinyl estradiol. NuvaRing® is latex-free. NuvaRing® has an outer diameter of 54 mm and a cross-sectional diameter of 4 mm. The molecular weights for etonogestrel and ethinyl estradiol are 324.46 and 296.40, respectively.
The structural formulas are as follows:

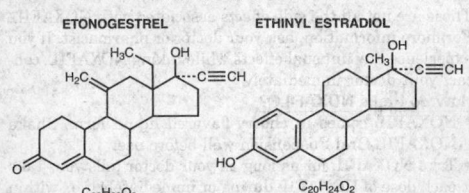

CLINICAL PHARMACOLOGY

Combination hormonal contraceptives act by suppression of gonadotropins. Although the primary effect of this action is inhibition of ovulation, other alterations include changes in the cervical mucus (which increase the difficulty of sperm entry into the uterus) and the endometrium (which reduce the likelihood of implantation).
Receptor binding studies, as well as studies in animals, have shown that etonogestrel, the biologically active metabolite of desogestrel, combines high progestational activity with low intrinsic androgenicity. The relevance of this latter finding in humans is unknown.

Pharmacokinetics

Absorption
Etonogestrel: Etonogestrel released by NuvaRing® is rapidly absorbed. The bioavailability of etonogestrel after vaginal administration is approximately 100%. The serum etonogestrel and ethinyl estradiol concentrations observed during three weeks of NuvaRing® use are summarized in Table I.
Ethinyl estradiol: Ethinyl estradiol released by NuvaRing® is rapidly absorbed. The bioavailability of ethinyl estradiol after vaginal administration is approximately 56%, which is comparable to that with oral administration of ethinyl estradiol. The serum ethinyl estradiol concentrations observed during three weeks of NuvaRing® use are summarized in Table I.

TABLE I: MEAN (SD) SERUM ETONOGESTREL AND ETHINYL ESTRADIOL CONCENTRATIONS (n=16).

	1 week	2 weeks	3 weeks
etonogestrel (pg/mL)	1578 (408)	1476 (362)	1374 (328)
ethinyl estradiol (pg/mL)	19.1 (4.5)	18.3 (4.3)	17.6 (4.3)

The pharmacokinetic profile of etonogestrel and ethinyl estradiol during use of NuvaRing® is shown in Figure 1.

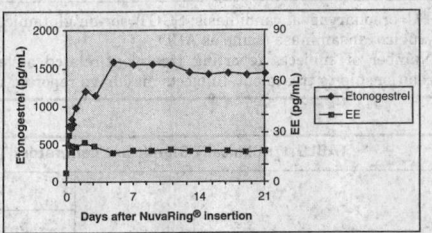

Figure 1. Mean serum concentration-time profile of etonogestrel and ethinyl estradiol during three weeks of NuvaRing® use.

The pharmacokinetic parameters of etonogestrel and ethinyl estradiol were determined during one cycle of NuvaRing® use in 16 healthy female subjects and are summarized in Table II.
[See table II above]

Distribution
Etonogestrel: Etonogestrel is approximately 32% bound to sex hormone-binding globulin (SHBG) and approximately 66% bound to albumin in blood.
Ethinyl estradiol: Ethinyl estradiol is highly but not specifically bound to serum albumin (98.5%) and induces an increase in the serum concentrations of SHBG.

Metabolism
In vitro data shows that both etonogestrel and ethinyl estradiol are metabolized in liver microsomes by the cytochrome P450 3A4 isoenzyme. Ethinyl estradiol is primarily metabolized by aromatic hydroxylation, but a wide variety of hydroxylated and methylated metabolites are formed. These are present as free metabolites and as sulfate and glucuronide conjugates. The hydroxylated ethinyl estradiol metabolites have weak estrogenic activity. The biological activity of etonogestrel metabolites is unknown.

Excretion
Etonogestrel and ethinyl estradiol are primarily eliminated in urine, bile and feces.

TABLE II: MEAN (SD) PHARMACOKINETIC PARAMETERS OF NuvaRing® (n=16).

Hormone	C_{max} pg/mL	T_{max} hr	$t_{1/2}$ hr	CL L/hr
etonogestrel	1716 (445)	200.3 (69.6)	29.3 (6.1)	3.4 (0.8)
ethinyl estradiol	34.7 (17.5)	59.3 (67.5)	44.7 (28.8)	34.8 (11.6)

C_{max} - maximum serum drug concentration
T_{max} - time at which maximum serum drug concentration occurs
$t_{1/2}$ - elimination half-life, calculated by $0.693/K_{elim}$
CL - apparent clearance

Special Populations

Race
No formal studies were conducted to evaluate the effect of race on the pharmacokinetics of NuvaRing®.
Hepatic Insufficiency
No formal studies were conducted to evaluate the effect of hepatic disease on the pharmacokinetics, safety, and efficacy of NuvaRing®. However, steroid hormones may be poorly metabolized in women with impaired liver function (see PRECAUTIONS).
Renal Insufficiency
No formal studies were conducted to evaluate the effect of renal disease on the pharmacokinetics, safety, and efficacy of NuvaRing®.
Drug-Drug Interactions
Interactions between contraceptive steroids and other drugs have been reported in the literature (see PRECAUTIONS). The drug interactions of NuvaRing® were evaluated in several studies.
A single-dose vaginal administration of an oil-based 1200 mg miconazole nitrate capsule increased the serum concentrations of etonogestrel and ethinyl estradiol by approximately 17% and 16%, respectively. Following multiple doses of 200 mg miconazole nitrate by vaginal suppository or vaginal cream, the mean serum concentrations of etonogestrel and ethinyl estradiol increased by up to 40%. A single-dose vaginal administration of 100 mg water-based nonoxynol-9 spermicide gel did not affect the serum concentrations of etonogestrel or ethinyl estradiol.
The serum concentrations of etonogestrel and ethinyl estradiol were not affected by concomitant administration of oral amoxicillin or doxycycline in standard dosages during 10 days of antibiotic treatment.
Tampon Use
The use of tampons had no effect on serum concentrations of etonogestrel and ethinyl estradiol during use of NuvaRing®.

INDICATIONS AND USAGE

NuvaRing® is indicated for the prevention of pregnancy in women who elect to use this product as a method of contraception. Like oral contraceptives, NuvaRing® is highly effective if used as recommended in this label.
In three large clinical trials of 13 cycles of NuvaRing® use, pregnancy rates were between one and two per 100 women-years of use. Table III lists the pregnancy rates for users of various contraceptive methods.
[See table III at top of next page]

CONTRAINDICATIONS

NuvaRing® should not be used in women who currently have the following conditions:
- Thrombophlebitis or thromboembolic disorders
- A past history of deep vein thrombophlebitis or thromboembolic disorders
- Cerebral vascular or coronary artery disease (current or history)
- Valvular heart disease with thrombogenic complications
- Severe hypertension
- Diabetes with vascular involvement
- Headaches with focal neurological symptoms
- Major surgery with prolonged immobilization
- Known or suspected carcinoma of the breast or personal history of breast cancer
- Carcinoma of the endometrium or other known or suspected estrogen-dependent neoplasia
- Undiagnosed abnormal genital bleeding
- Cholestatic jaundice of pregnancy or jaundice with prior hormonal contraceptive use
- Hepatic tumors (benign or malignant) or active liver disease
- Known or suspected pregnancy
- Heavy smoking (≥15 cigarettes per day) and over age 35
- Hypersensitivity to any of the components of NuvaRing®

WARNINGS

Cigarette smoking increases the risk of serious cardiovascular side effects from combination oral contraceptive use. This risk increases with age and with heavy

smoking (15 or more cigarettes per day) and is quite marked in women over 35 years of age. Women who use combination hormonal contraceptives, including NuvaRing®, should be strongly advised not to smoke.

NuvaRing® and other contraceptives that contain both an estrogen and a progestin are called combination hormonal contraceptives. There is no epidemiologic data available to determine whether safety and efficacy with the vaginal route of administration of combination hormonal contraceptives would be different than the oral route.

The use of oral contraceptives is associated with increased risks of several serious conditions including venous and arterial thrombotic and thromboembolic events (such as myocardial infarction, thromboembolism, and stroke), hepatic neoplasia, gallbladder disease, and hypertension, although the risk of serious morbidity or mortality is very small in healthy women without underlying risk factors. The risk of morbidity and mortality increases significantly in the presence of other underlying risk factors such as certain inherited thrombophilias, hypertension, hyperlipidemias, obesity, and diabetes.

The information contained in this package insert is principally based on studies carried out in women who used oral contraceptives with formulations of higher doses of estrogens and progestogens than those in common use today. The effect of long-term use of oral contraceptives with lower doses of both estrogens and progestogens remains to be determined.

Throughout this labeling, epidemiologic studies reported are of two types: retrospective or case control studies and prospective or cohort studies. Case control studies provide a measure of the relative risk of a disease, namely, a *ratio* of the incidence of a disease among oral contraceptive users to that among non-users. The relative risk does not provide information on the actual clinical occurrence of a disease. Cohort studies provide a measure of attributable risk, which is the *difference* in the incidence of disease between oral contraceptive users and non-users. The attributable risk does provide information about the actual occurrence of a disease in the population. For further information, the reader is referred to a text on epidemiologic methods.

1. THROMBOEMBOLIC DISORDERS AND OTHER VASCULAR PROBLEMS

a. Thromboembolism

An increased risk of thromboembolic and thrombotic disease associated with the use of oral contraceptives is well established. Case control studies have found the relative risk of users compared to non-users to be three for the first episode of superficial venous thrombosis, four to 11 for deep vein thrombosis or pulmonary embolism, and 1.5 to six for women with predisposing conditions for venous thromboembolic disease. Cohort studies have shown the relative risk to be somewhat lower, about three for new cases and about 4.5 for new cases requiring hospitalization. The risk of thromboembolic disease associated with oral contraceptives is not related to length of use and disappears after pill use is stopped.

Several epidemiology studies indicate that third generation oral contraceptives (those containing desogestrel (etonogestrel, the progestin in NuvaRing®, is the biologically active metabolite of desogestrel), are associated with a higher risk of venous thromboembolism than certain second generation oral contraceptives. In general, these studies indicate an approximate two-fold increased risk, which corresponds to an additional one to two cases of venous thromboembolism per 10,000 women-years of use. However, data from additional studies have not shown this two-fold increase in risk. It is unknown if NuvaRing® has a different risk of venous thromboembolism than second generation oral contraceptives.

A two- to four-fold increase in relative risk of post-operative thromboembolic complications has been reported with the use of oral contraceptives. The relative risk of venous thrombosis in women who have predisposing conditions is twice that of women without such medical conditions. If feasible, combination hormonal contraceptives, including NuvaRing®, should be discontinued at least four weeks prior to and for two weeks after elective surgery of a type associated with an increase in risk of thromboembolism and during and following prolonged immobilization. Since the immediate postpartum period is also associated with an increased risk of thromboembolism, combination hormonal contraceptives, such as NuvaRing®, should be started no earlier than four to six weeks after delivery in women who elect not to breast-feed.

The clinician should be alert to the earliest manifestations of thrombotic disorders (thrombophlebitis, pulmonary embolism, cerebrovascular disorders, and retinal thrombosis). Should any of these occur or be suspected, NuvaRing® should be discontinued immediately.

b. Myocardial infarction

An increased risk of myocardial infarction has been attributed to oral contraceptive use. This risk is primarily in

TABLE III: PERCENTAGE OF WOMEN EXPERIENCING AN UNINTENDED PREGNANCY DURING THE FIRST YEAR OF TYPICAL USE AND THE FIRST YEAR OF PERFECT USE OF CONTRACEPTION AND THE PERCENTAGE CONTINUING USE AT THE END OF THE FIRST YEAR: UNITED STATES.

Method (1)	% of Women Experiencing an Unintended Pregnancy within the First Year of Use		% of Women Continuing Use at One Year[3] (4)
	Typical Use[1] (2)	Perfect Use[2] (3)	
Chance[4]	85	85	
Spermicides[5]	26	6	40
Periodic abstinence	25		63
Calendar		9	
Ovulation Method		3	
Sympto-Thermal[6]		2	
Post-Ovulation		1	
Cap[7]			
Parous Women	40	26	42
Nulliparous Women	20	9	56
Sponge			
Parous Women	40	20	42
Nulliparous Women	20	9	56
Diaphragm[7]	20	6	56
Withdrawal	19	4	
Condom[8]			
Female (Reality)	21	5	56
Male	14	3	61
Pill	5		71
Progestin Only		0.5	
Combined		0.1	
IUD			
Progesterone T	2.0	1.5	81
Copper T 380A	0.8	0.6	78
LNg 20	0.1	0.1	81
Depo-Provera	0.3	0.3	70
Norplant and Norplant-2	0.05	0.05	88
Female sterilization	0.5	0.5	100
Male sterilization	0.15	0.10	100

Emergency Contraceptive Pills: Treatment initiated within 72 hours after unprotected intercourse reduces the risk of pregnancy by at least 75%.[9]

Lactation Amenorrhea Method: LAM is a highly effective, temporary method of contraception.[10]

Adapted from Hatcher et al., Contraceptive Technology, 17th Revised Edition. New York, NY: Irvington Publishers, 1998.

[1] Among *typical* couples who initiate use of a method (not necessarily for the first time), the percentage who experience an accidental pregnancy during the first year if they do not stop use for any other reason.

[2] Among couples who initiate use of a method (not necessarily for the first time) and who use it *perfectly* (both consistently and correctly), the percentage who experience an accidental pregnancy during the first year if they do not stop use for any other reason.

[3] Among couples attempting to avoid pregnancy, the percentage who continue to use a method for one year.

[4] The percents becoming pregnant in columns (2) and (3) are based on data from populations where contraception is not used and from women who cease using contraception in order to become pregnant. Among such populations, about 89% become pregnant within one year. This estimate was lowered slightly (to 85%) to represent the percent who would become pregnant within one year among women now relying on reversible methods of contraception if they abandoned contraception altogether.

[5] Foams, creams, gels, vaginal suppositories, and vaginal film.

[6] Cervical mucus (ovulation) method supplemented by calendar in the pre-ovulatory and basal body temperature in the post-ovulatory phases.

[7] With spermicidal cream or jelly.

[8] Without spermicides.

[9] The treatment schedule is one dose within 72 hours after unprotected intercourse, and a second dose 12 hours after the first dose. The FDA has declared the following brands of oral contraceptives to be safe and effective for emergency contraception: Ovral (one dose is two white pills), Alesse (one dose is five pink pills), Nordette or Levlen (one dose is four yellow pills).

[10] However, to maintain effective protection against pregnancy, another method of contraception must be used as soon as menstruation resumes, the frequency or duration of breast-feeds is reduced, bottle feeds are introduced, or the baby reaches six months of age.

TABLE IV: CIRCULATORY DISEASE MORTALITY RATES PER 100,000 WOMAN-YEARS BY AGE, SMOKING STATUS, AND COMBINATION ORAL CONTRACEPTIVE USE.

AGE	EVER-USERS NON-SMOKERS	EVER-USERS SMOKERS	CONTROLS NON-SMOKERS	CONTROLS SMOKERS
15–24	0.0	10.5	0.0	0.0
25–34	4.4	14.2	2.7	4.2
35–44	21.5	63.4	6.4	15.2
45+	52.4	206.7	11.4	27.9

(Adapted from P.M. Layde and V. Beral, Lancet, 1981;1:541–546.)

smokers or women with other underlying risk factors for coronary artery disease such as hypertension, hypercholesterolemia, morbid obesity, and diabetes. The relative risk of heart attack for current combination oral contraceptive users has been estimated to be two to six. The risk is very low in women under the age of 30.

Smoking in combination with oral contraceptive use has been shown to contribute substantially to the incidence of myocardial infarction in women in their mid-thirties or older with smoking accounting for the majority of excess cases. Mortality rates associated with circulatory disease have been shown to increase substantially in smokers, over the age of 35 and non-smokers over the age of 40 among women who use oral contraceptives (see Table IV).

[See table IV above]

Oral contraceptives may compound the effects of well-known risk factors, such as hypertension, diabetes, hyperlipidemias, age, and obesity. In particular, some progestogens are known to decrease HDL cholesterol and cause glucose intolerance, while estrogens may create a state of hyperinsulinism. Oral contraceptives have been shown to increase blood pressure among users (see WARNINGS).

TABLE V: ANNUAL NUMBER OF BIRTH-RELATED OR METHOD-RELATED DEATHS ASSOCIATED WITH CONTROL OF FERTILITY PER 100,000 NON-STERILE WOMEN, BY FERTILITY CONTROL METHOD ACCORDING TO AGE.

Method of control and outcome	15–19	20–24	25–29	30–34	35–39	40–44
No fertility control methods*	7.0	7.4	9.1	14.8	25.7	28.2
Oral contraceptives non-smoker**	0.3	0.5	0.9	1.9	13.8	31.6
Oral contraceptives smoker**	2.2	3.4	6.6	13.5	51.1	117.2
IUD**	0.8	0.8	1.0	1.0	1.4	1.4
Condom*	1.1	1.6	0.7	0.2	0.3	0.4
Diaphragm/spermicide*	1.9	1.2	1.2	1.3	2.2	2.8
Periodic abstinence*	2.5	1.6	1.6	1.7	2.9	3.6

* Deaths are birth related
** Deaths are method related

(Adapted from H.W. Ory, *Family Planning Perspectives* 1983;15:50–56.)

Similar effects on risk factors have been associated with an increased risk of heart disease. NuvaRing® must be used with caution in women with cardiovascular disease risk factors.

c. Cerebrovascular diseases

Oral contraceptives have been shown to increase both the relative and attributable risks of cerebrovascular events (thrombotic and hemorrhagic strokes), although, in general, the risk is greatest among older (>35 years), hypertensive women who also smoke. Hypertension was found to be a risk factor for both users and non-users, for both types of strokes, while smoking interacted to increase the risk for hemorrhagic strokes.

In a large study, the relative risk of thrombotic strokes has been shown to range from three for normotensive users to 14 for users with severe hypertension. The relative risk of hemorrhagic stroke is reported to be 1.2 for non-smokers who used oral contraceptives, 2.6 for smokers who did not use oral contraceptives, 7.6 for smokers who used oral contraceptives, 1.8 for normotensive users and 25.7 for users with severe hypertension. The attributable risk is also greater in older women. Oral contraceptives also increase the risk for stroke in women with other underlying risk factors such as certain inherited or acquired thrombophilias, hyperlipidemias, and obesity. Women with migraine (particularly migraine with aura) who take combination oral contraceptives may be at an increased risk of stroke.

d. Dose-related risk of vascular disease from oral contraceptives

A positive association has been observed between the amount of estrogen and progestogen in oral contraceptives and the risk of vascular disease. A decline in serum high-density lipoproteins (HDL) has been reported with many progestational agents. A decline in serum high-density lipoproteins has been associated with an increased incidence of ischemic heart disease. Because estrogens increase HDL cholesterol, the net effect of an oral contraceptive depends on a balance achieved between doses of estrogen and progestogen and the nature and absolute amount of progestogens used in the contraceptives. The activity and amount of both hormones should be considered in the choice of a hormonal contraceptive.

Minimizing exposure to estrogen and progestogen is in keeping with good principles of therapeutics. For any particular estrogen/progestogen combination, the dosage regimen prescribed should be one which contains the least amount of estrogen and progestogen that is compatible with a low failure rate and the needs of the individual patient. New acceptors of hormonal contraceptive agents should be started on a product containing the lowest hormone content that provides satisfactory results in the individual.

e. Persistence of risk of vascular disease

There are two studies that have shown persistence of risk of vascular disease for ever-users of oral contraceptives. In a study in the United States, the risk of developing myocardial infarction after discontinuing oral contraceptives persists for at least nine years for women 40-49 years old who had used oral contraceptives for five or more years, but this increased risk was not demonstrated in other age groups. In another study in Great Britain, the risk of developing cerebrovascular disease persisted for at least six years after discontinuation of oral contraceptives, although excess risk was very small. However, both studies were performed with oral contraceptive formulations containing 50 micrograms or more of estrogen.

It is unknown whether NuvaRing® is distinct from combination oral contraceptives with regard to the occurrence of venous or arterial thrombosis.

2. ESTIMATES OF MORTALITY FROM CONTRACEPTIVE USE

One study gathered data from a variety of sources that have estimated the mortality rate associated with different methods of contraception at different ages (Table V). These estimates include the combined risk of death associated with contraceptive methods plus the risk attributable to pregnancy in the event of method failure. Each method of contraception has its specific benefits and risks. The study concluded that with the exception of oral contraceptive users age 35 and older who smoke and age 40 and older who do not smoke, mortality associated with all methods of birth control is low and below that associated with childbirth.

The observation of a possible increase in risk of mortality with age for oral contraceptive users is based on data gathered in the 1970's, but not reported until 1983. However, current clinical practice involves the use of lower estrogen-dose formulations combined with careful restriction of hormonal contraceptive use to women who do not have the various risk factors listed in this labeling.

Because of these changes in practice and, also, because of some limited new data which suggest that the risk of cardiovascular disease with the use of oral contraceptives may now be less than previously observed, the Fertility and Maternal Health Drugs Advisory Committee was asked to review the topic in 1989. The Committee concluded that although cardiovascular disease risks may be increased with oral contraceptive use after age 40 in healthy nonsmoking women (even with the newer low-dose formulations), there are also greater potential health risks associated with pregnancy in older women and with the alternative surgical and medical procedures which may be necessary if such women do not have access to effective and acceptable means of contraception. Therefore, the Committee recommended that the benefits of low-dose hormonal oral contraceptive use by healthy non-smoking women over 40 may outweigh the possible risks. Older women, as all women who take hormonal contraceptives, should take the lowest possible dose formulation that is effective and meets the individual patient needs.

[See table V above]

3. CARCINOMA OF THE REPRODUCTIVE ORGANS AND BREASTS

Numerous epidemiologic studies have been performed on the incidence of breast, endometrial, ovarian, and cervical cancer in women using combination oral contraceptives. Although the risk of breast cancer may be slightly increased among current users of oral contraceptives (RR = 1.24), this excess risk decreases over time after oral contraceptive discontinuation and by 10 years after cessation the increased risk disappears. The risk does not increase with duration of use, and no relationships have been found with dose or type of steroid. The patterns of risk are also similar regardless of a woman's reproductive history or her family breast cancer history. The subgroup for whom risk has been found to be significantly elevated is women who first used oral contraceptives before age 20, but because breast cancer is so rare at these young ages, the number of cases attributable to this early oral contraceptive use is extremely small. Breast cancers diagnosed in current or previous oral contraceptive users tend to be less advanced clinically than in never-users. Women who currently have or have had breast cancer should not use hormonal contraceptives because breast cancer is a hormone-sensitive tumor.

Some studies suggest that combination oral contraceptive use has been associated with an increase in the risk of cervical intraepithelial neoplasia in some populations of women. However, there continues to be controversy about the extent to which such findings may be due to differences in sexual behavior and other factors.

In spite of many studies of the relationship between oral contraceptive use and breast and cervical cancers, a cause-and-effect relationship has not been established.

It is unknown whether NuvaRing® is distinct from oral contraceptives with regard to the above statements.

4. HEPATIC NEOPLASIA

Benign hepatic adenomas are associated with oral contraceptive use, although the incidence of benign tumors is rare in the United States. Indirect calculations have estimated the attributable risk to be in the range of 3.3 cases per 100,000 for users, a risk that increases after four or more years of use. Rupture of rare, benign, hepatic adenomas may cause death through intra-abdominal hemorrhage.

Studies from Britain have shown an increased risk of developing hepatocellular carcinoma in long term (>8 years) oral contraceptive users. However, these cancers are extremely rare in the US and the attributable risk (the excess incidence) of liver cancers in oral contraceptive users approaches less than one per million users. It is unknown whether NuvaRing® is distinct from oral contraceptives in this regard.

5. OCULAR LESIONS

There have been clinical case reports of retinal thrombosis associated with the use of oral contraceptives. NuvaRing® should be discontinued if there is unexplained partial or complete loss of vision, onset of proptosis or diplopia, papilledema, or retinal vascular lesions. Appropriate diagnostic and therapeutic measures should be undertaken immediately.

6. HORMONAL CONTRACEPTIVE USE BEFORE OR DURING EARLY PREGNANCY

Hormonal contraceptives should not be used during pregnancy.

Extensive epidemiologic studies have revealed no increased risk of birth defects in women who have used oral contraceptives prior to pregnancy. Studies also do not suggest a teratogenic effect, particularly in so far as cardiac anomalies and limb reduction defects are concerned, when oral contraceptives are taken inadvertently during early pregnancy.

Combination hormonal contraceptives, such as NuvaRing®, should not be used to induce withdrawal bleeding as a test for pregnancy. NuvaRing® should not be used during pregnancy to treat threatened or habitual abortion. It is recommended that for any woman who has not adhered to the prescribed regimen for use of NuvaRing® and has missed a menstrual period or who has missed two consecutive periods, pregnancy should be ruled out.

7. GALLBLADDER DISEASE

Combination hormonal contraceptives, such as NuvaRing®, may worsen existing gallbladder disease and may accelerate the development of this disease in previously asymptomatic women. Women with a history of combination hormonal contraceptive-related cholestasis are more likely to have the condition recur with subsequent combination hormonal contraceptive use.

8. CARBOHYDRATE AND LIPID METABOLIC EFFECTS

Hormonal contraceptives have been shown to cause a decrease in glucose tolerance in some users. However, in the non-diabetic woman, combination hormonal contraceptives appear to have no effect on fasting blood glucose. Prediabetic and diabetic women should be carefully observed while taking combination hormonal contraceptives, such as NuvaRing®. In a clinical study involving 37 NuvaRing®-treated subjects, glucose tolerance tests showed no clinically significant changes in serum glucose levels from baseline to cycle six.

A small proportion of women will have persistent hypertriglyceridemia while using oral contraceptives. Changes in serum triglycerides and lipoprotein levels have been reported in combination hormonal contraceptive users.

9. ELEVATED BLOOD PRESSURE

Women with severe hypertension should not be started on hormonal contraceptives. An increase in blood pressure has been reported in women taking oral contraceptives and this increase is more likely in older oral contraceptive users and with continued use. Data from the Royal College of General Practitioners and subsequent randomized trials have shown that the incidence of hypertension increases with increasing concentrations of progestogens.

Women with a history of hypertension or hypertension-related diseases, or renal disease should be encouraged to use another method of contraception. If these women elect to use NuvaRing®, they should be monitored closely and if significant elevation of blood pressure occurs, NuvaRing® should be discontinued. For most women, elevated blood pressure will return to normal after stopping hormonal contraceptives, and there is no difference in the occurrence of hypertension between former and never-users.

10. HEADACHE

The onset or exacerbation of migraine or development of headache with a new pattern which is recurrent, persistent, or severe requires discontinuation of NuvaRing® and evaluation of the cause.

11. BLEEDING IRREGULARITIES

Bleeding Patterns

Breakthrough bleeding and spotting are sometimes encountered in women using NuvaRing®. If abnormal bleeding while using NuvaRing® persists or is severe, appropriate investigation should be instituted to rule out the possibility of organic pathology or pregnancy, and appropriate treatment should be instituted when necessary. In the event of amenorrhea, pregnancy should be ruled out.

Bleeding patterns were evaluated in three large clinical studies. In the US-Canadian study (n=1177), the percentages of subjects with breakthrough bleeding/spotting ranged from 7.2 to 11.7% during cycles 1-13. In the two non-US studies, the percentages of subjects with breakthrough bleeding/spotting ranged from 2.6 to 6.4% (Study 1, n=1145 European and Israeli subjects) and from 2.0 to 8.7% (Study 2, n=512 European and South American subjects). In these three studies, the percentages of women who did not have withdrawal bleeding in a given cycle ranged from 0.3 to 3.8%.

Some women may encounter amenorrhea or oligomenorrhea after discontinuing use of NuvaRing®, especially when such a condition was pre-existent.

12. ECTOPIC PREGNANCY

Ectopic as well as intrauterine pregnancy may occur in contraceptive failures.

PRECAUTIONS

1. SEXUALLY TRANSMITTED DISEASES

Women should be counseled that this product does not protect against HIV infection (AIDS) and other sexually transmitted diseases.

2. PHYSICAL EXAMINATION AND FOLLOW-UP

It is routine medical practice for women using NuvaRing®, as for all women, to have an annual medical evaluation including physical examination and relevant laboratory tests. The physical examination should include special reference to blood pressure, breasts, abdomen, pelvic organs and vagina (including cervical cytology). In case of undiagnosed, persistent or recurrent abnormal vaginal bleeding, appropriate measures should be conducted to rule out malignancy. Women with a family history of breast cancer or who have breast nodules should be monitored with particular care.

3. LIPID DISORDERS

Women who are being treated for hyperlipidemias should be followed closely if they elect to use NuvaRing®. Some progestogens may elevate LDL levels and may render the control of hyperlipidemias more difficult.

In women with familial defects of lipoprotein metabolism receiving estrogen-containing preparations, there have been case reports of significant elevations of plasma triglycerides leading to pancreatitis.

4. LIVER FUNCTION

If jaundice develops in any woman using NuvaRing®, product use should be discontinued. The hormones in NuvaRing® may be poorly metabolized in women with impaired liver function.

5. FLUID RETENTION

Steroid hormones like those in NuvaRing®, may cause some degree of fluid retention. NuvaRing® should be prescribed with caution, and only with careful monitoring, in women with conditions which might be aggravated by fluid retention.

6. EMOTIONAL DISORDERS

Women becoming significantly depressed while taking hormonal contraceptives should stop the medication and use an alternate method of contraception in an attempt to determine whether the symptom is drug related. Women with a history of depression should be carefully observed and the drug discontinued if depression recurs to a serious degree.

7. TAMPON USE

On rare occasions, NuvaRing® may be expelled while removing a tampon (see EXPULSION). Pharmacokinetic data show that the use of tampons has no effect on the systemic absorption of the hormones released by NuvaRing®.

8. TOXIC SHOCK SYNDROME (TSS)

Cases of toxic shock syndrome have been associated with tampons and certain barrier contraceptives. Very rare cases of TSS have been reported by NuvaRing® users; in some cases the women were also using tampons. No causal relationship between the use of NuvaRing® and TSS has been established. If a patient exhibits signs or symptoms of TSS, the possibility of this diagnosis should not be excluded and appropriate medical evaluation and treatment initiated.

9. CONTACT LENSES

Contact lens wearers who develop visual changes or changes in lens tolerance should be assessed by an ophthalmologist.

10. DRUG INTERACTIONS

Changes in contraceptive effectiveness associated with co-administration of other drugs:

a. Anti-infective agents and anticonvulsants

Contraceptive effectiveness may be reduced when hormonal contraceptives are *co-administered* with some antifungals, anticonvulsants, and other drugs that increase metabolism of contraceptive steroids. This could result in unintended pregnancy or breakthrough bleeding. Examples include barbiturates, griseofulvin, rifampin, phenylbutazone, phenytoin, carbamazepine, felbamate, oxcarbazepine, topiramate, and modafinil. Women may need to use an additional contraceptive method when taking such medications.

b. Anti-HIV protease inhibitors

Several of the anti-HIV protease inhibitors have been studied with coadministration of oral combination hormonal contraceptives; significant changes (increases and decreases) in the plasma levels of the estrogen and progestin have been noted in some cases. The efficacy and safety of hormonal contraceptive products may be affected with coadministration of anti-HIV protease inhibitors. Healthcare providers should refer to the label of the individual anti-HIV protease inhibitors for further drug-drug interaction information.

c. Herbal products

Herbal products containing St. John's Wort (hypericum perforatum) may induce hepatic enzymes (cytochrome P450) and p-glycoprotein transporter and may reduce the effectiveness of contraceptive steroids. This may also result in breakthrough bleeding.

Increase in plasma hormone levels associated with co-administered drugs:

Co-administration of atorvastatin and certain oral contraceptives containing ethinyl estradiol increase AUC values for ethinyl estradiol by approximately 20%. Ascorbic acid and acetaminophen may increase plasma ethinyl estradiol levels, possibly by inhibition of conjugation. CYP 3A4 inhibitors such as itraconazole or ketoconazole may increase plasma hormone levels. Co-administration of vaginal miconazole nitrate and NuvaRing® increases the serum concentrations of etonogestrel and ethinyl estradiol by up to 40%.

Changes in plasma levels of co-administered drugs:

Combination hormonal contraceptives containing some synthetic estrogens (e.g., ethinyl estradiol) may inhibit the metabolism of other compounds. Increased plasma concentrations of cyclosporine, prednisolone, and theophylline have been reported with concomitant administration of oral contraceptives. In addition, oral contraceptives may induce the conjugation of other compounds. Decreased plasma concentrations of acetaminophen and increased clearance of temazepam, salicylic acid, morphine and clofibric acid have been noted when these drugs were administered with oral contraceptives.

11. INTERACTIONS WITH LABORATORY TESTS

Certain endocrine and liver function tests and blood components may be affected by combined hormonal contraceptives:

a. Increased prothrombin and factors VII, VIII, IX and X; decreased antithrombin 3, increased norepinephrine-induced platelet aggregability.
b. Increased thyroid-binding globulin (TBG) leading to increased circulating total thyroid hormone, as measured by protein-bound iodine (PBI), T4 by column or by radioimmunoassay. Free T3 resin uptake is decreased, reflecting the elevated TBG; free T4 concentration is unaltered.
c. Other binding proteins may be elevated in serum.
d. Sex hormone-binding globulins are increased and result in elevated levels of total circulating sex steroids; however, free or biologically active levels either decrease or remain unchanged.
e. Triglycerides may be increased and levels of various other lipids and lipoproteins may be affected.
f. Glucose tolerance may be decreased.
g. Serum folate levels may be depressed by oral contraceptive therapy. This may be of clinical significance if a woman becomes pregnant shortly after discontinuing NuvaRing®.

12. CARCINOGENESIS, MUTAGENESIS, IMPAIRMENT OF FERTILITY

In a 24-month carcinogenicity study in rats with subdermal implants releasing 10 and 20 µg etonogestrel per day, (approximately 0.3 and 0.6 times the systemic steady-state exposure of women using NuvaRing®), no drug-related carcinogenic potential was observed. Etonogestrel was not genotoxic in the *in vitro* Ames/Salmonella reverse mutation assay, the chromosomal aberration assay in Chinese hamster ovary cells or in the *in vivo* mouse micronucleus test. Fertility returned after withdrawal from treatment (see WARNINGS).

13. PREGNANCY

Pregnancy Category X (see CONTRAINDICATIONS and WARNINGS).

Teratology studies have been performed in rats and rabbits using the oral route of administration at doses up to 130 and 260 times, respectively, the human NuvaRing® dose (based on body surface area) and have revealed no evidence of harm to the fetus due to etonogestrel.

14. NURSING MOTHERS

The effects of NuvaRing® in nursing mothers have not been evaluated and are unknown. Small amounts of contraceptive steroids have been identified in the milk of nursing mothers and a few adverse effects on the child have been reported, including jaundice and breast enlargement. In addition, contraceptive steroids given in the postpartum period may interfere with lactation by decreasing the quantity and quality of breast milk. Long-term follow-up of children whose mothers used combination hormonal contraceptives while breast-feeding has shown no deleterious effects on infants. However, women who are breastfeeding should be advised not to use NuvaRing® but to use other forms of contraception until the child is weaned.

15. PEDIATRIC USE

Safety and efficacy of NuvaRing® have been established in women of reproductive age. Safety and efficacy are expected to be the same for postpubertal adolescents under the age of 16 and for users 16 years and older. Use of this product before menarche is not indicated.

16. GERIATRIC USE

This product has not been studied in women over 65 years of age and is not indicated in this population.

17. VAGINAL USE

NuvaRing® may not be suitable for women with conditions that make the vagina more susceptible to vaginal irritation or ulceration. Vaginal/cervical erosion or ulceration in women using NuvaRing® has been rarely reported. In some cases, the ring adhered to vaginal tissue, necessitating removal by a healthcare provider.

Some women are aware of the ring at random times during the 21 days of use or during intercourse. During intercourse some sexual partners may feel NuvaRing® in the vagina. However, clinical studies revealed that 90% of couples did not find this to be a problem.

NuvaRing® may interfere with the correct placement and position of a diaphragm. A diaphragm is therefore not recommended as a back-up method with NuvaRing® use.

18. URINARY BLADDER INSERTION

There have been rare reports of inadvertent insertions of NuvaRing® into the urinary bladder, which required cystoscopic removal. Healthcare providers should assess for ring insertion into the urinary bladder in NuvaRing® users who present with persistent urinary symptoms and are unable to locate the ring.

19. EXPULSION

NuvaRing® can be accidentally expelled, for example, while removing a tampon, during intercourse, or with straining during a bowel movement. NuvaRing® should be left in the vagina for a continuous period of three weeks. If the ring is accidentally expelled and is left outside of the vagina for **less than three hours** contraceptive efficacy is not reduced. NuvaRing® can be rinsed with cool to lukewarm (not hot) water and reinserted as soon as possible, but at the latest within three hours. If NuvaRing® is lost, a new vaginal ring should be inserted and the regimen should be continued without alteration.

If NuvaRing® is out of the vagina for more than three continuous hours:

During Weeks 1 and 2: If NuvaRing® has been out of the vagina for more than three continuous hours during the 1st or 2nd week of use, contraceptive efficacy may be reduced. The woman should reinsert the ring as soon as she remembers. A barrier method such as condoms or spermicides must be used until the ring has been used continuously for seven days.

During Week 3: If NuvaRing® has been out of the vagina for more than three continuous hours during the 3rd week of the three-week use period, the woman should discard that ring. One of the following two options should be chosen:

1. Insert a new ring immediately. Inserting a new ring will start the next three-week use period. The woman may not experience a withdrawal bleed from her previous cycle. However, breakthrough spotting or bleeding may occur.
2. Have a withdrawal bleeding and insert a new ring no later than seven days (7×24 hours) from the time the previous ring was removed or expelled. This option should only be chosen if the ring was used continuously for the preceding seven days.

A barrier method such as condoms or spermicides must be used until the new ring has been used continuously for seven days.

20. DISCONNECTED RING

There have been reported cases of NuvaRing® disconnecting at the weld joint. This is not expected to affect the contraceptive effectiveness of NuvaRing®. In the event of a disconnected ring, vaginal discomfort or expulsion (slipping out) is more likely to occur (see EXPULSION). If a woman discovers that her NuvaRing® has disconnected, she should discard the ring and replace it with a new ring.

INFORMATION FOR THE PATIENT

The woman should be instructed regarding the proper use of NuvaRing® (see PATIENT INFORMATION printed below).

ADVERSE REACTIONS

The most common adverse events reported by five to 14% of women using NuvaRing® in clinical trials (n=2501) were the following: vaginitis, headache, upper respiratory tract infection, vaginal secretion, sinusitis, weight gain, and nausea.

The most frequent system-organ class adverse events leading to discontinuation in one to 2.5% of women using NuvaRing® in the trials included the following: device-related events (foreign body sensation, coital problems, device expulsion), vaginal symptoms (discomfort/vaginitis/vaginal secretion), headache, emotional lability, and weight gain.

Listed below are adverse reactions that have been associated with the use of combination hormonal contraceptives. These are also likely to apply to combination vaginal hormonal contraceptives, such as NuvaRing®.

An increased risk of the following serious adverse reactions has been associated with the use of combination hormonal contraceptives (see CONTRAINDICATIONS and WARNINGS):

- Thrombophlebitis and venous thrombosis with or without embolism
- Arterial thromboembolism
- Pulmonary embolism
- Myocardial infarction
- Cerebral hemorrhage
- Cerebral thrombosis
- Hypertension
- Gallbladder disease
- Hepatic adenomas or benign liver tumors

There is evidence of an association between the following conditions and the use of combination hormonal contraceptives:

- Mesenteric thrombosis
- Retinal thrombosis

The following additional adverse reactions have been reported in users of combination hormonal contraceptives and are believed to be drug-related:

- Nausea
- Vomiting
- Gastrointestinal symptoms (such as abdominal pain, cramps and bloating)
- Breakthrough bleeding
- Spotting
- Change in menstrual flow
- Amenorrhea
- Temporary infertility after discontinuation of treatment
- Edema/fluid retention
- Melasma/chloasma which may persist
- Breast changes: tenderness, pain, enlargement, and secretion
- Decrease in serum folate levels
- Exacerbation of porphyria
- Aggravation of varicose veins
- Change in weight or appetite (increase or decrease)
- Change in cervical ectropion and secretion
- Possible diminution in lactation when given immediately postpartum
- Cholestatic jaundice
- Migraine headache
- Rash (allergic)
- Mood changes, including depression
- Vaginitis, including candidiasis
- Change in corneal curvature (steepening)
- Intolerance to contact lenses
- Exacerbation of systemic lupus erythematosus
- Exacerbation of chorea
- Anaphylactic/anaphylactoid reactions, including urticaria, angioedema, and severe reactions with respiratory and circulatory symptoms

The following additional adverse reactions have been reported in users of combination hormonal contraceptives and a causal association has been neither confirmed nor refuted:

- Pre-menstrual syndrome
- Cataracts
- Cystitis-like syndrome
- Headache
- Nervousness
- Dizziness
- Hirsutism
- Loss of scalp hair
- Erythema multiforme
- Dysmenorrhea
- Pancreatitis
- Erythema nodosum
- Hemorrhagic eruption
- Impaired renal function
- Hemolytic uremic syndrome
- Acne
- Changes in libido
- Colitis
- Budd-Chiari Syndrome
- Optic neuritis, which may lead partial or complete loss of vision

OVERDOSAGE

Overdosage of combination hormonal contraceptives may cause nausea, vomiting, vaginal bleeding, or other menstrual irregularities. Given the nature and design of NuvaRing® it is unlikely that overdosage will occur. If NuvaRing® is broken, it does not release a higher dose of hormones. Serious ill effects have not been reported following acute ingestion of large doses of oral contraceptives by young children. There are no antidotes and further treatment should be symptomatic.

DOSAGE AND ADMINISTRATION

To achieve maximum contraceptive effectiveness, NuvaRing® must be used as directed (see When to Start NuvaRing® below). One NuvaRing® is inserted in the vagina. **The ring is to remain in place continuously for three weeks.** It is removed for a one-week break, during which a withdrawal bleed usually occurs. A new ring is inserted one week after the last ring was removed.

The user can choose the insertion position that is most comfortable to her, for example, standing with one leg up, squatting, or lying down. The ring is to be compressed and inserted into the vagina. The exact position of NuvaRing® inside the vagina is not critical for its function. The vaginal ring must be inserted on the appropriate day and left in place for three consecutive weeks. This means that the ring is removed three weeks later on the same day of the week as it was inserted and at about the same time. NuvaRing® can be removed by hooking the index finger under the forward rim or by grasping the rim between the index and middle finger and pulling it out. The used ring should be placed in the sachet (foil pouch) and discarded in a waste receptacle out of the reach of children and pets (do not flush in toilet). After a one-week break, during which a withdrawal bleed usually occurs, a new ring is inserted on the same day of the week as it was inserted in the previous cycle. The withdrawal bleed usually starts on day 2-3 after removal of the ring and may not have finished before the next ring is inserted. In order to maintain contraceptive effectiveness, the new ring must be inserted one week after the previous one was removed even if menstrual bleeding has not finished.

When to Start NuvaRing®

IMPORTANT: The possibility of ovulation and conception prior to the first use of NuvaRing® should be considered.

<u>No hormonal contraceptive use in the preceding cycle</u>

Insert NuvaRing® on the first day of the woman's natural cycle (i.e., the first day of her menstrual bleeding). NuvaRing® may also be started on days 2-5 of the woman's cycle, but in this case a barrier method, such as male condoms or spermicide, is recommended for the first seven days of NuvaRing® use in the first cycle.

<u>Changing from a combined hormonal contraceptive</u>

The woman may switch from her previous combined hormonal contraceptive on any day, but at the latest on the day following the usual hormone-free interval, if she has been using her hormonal method consistently and correctly, or if it is reasonably certain that she is not pregnant.

<u>Changing from a progestagen-only method (minipill, implant, or injection) or from a progestagen-releasing intrauterine system (IUS)</u>

The woman may switch on any day from the minipill. She should switch from an implant or the IUS on the day of its removal and from an injectable on the day when the next injection would be due. In all of these cases, the woman should use an additional barrier method such as a male condom or spermicide, for the first seven days.

<u>Following complete first trimester abortion</u>

The woman may start using NuvaRing® within the first five days following a complete first trimester abortion and does not need to use an additional method of contraception. If use of NuvaRing® is not started within five days following a first trimester abortion, the woman should follow the instructions for "No hormonal contraceptive use in the preceding cycle." In the meantime she should be advised to use a non-hormonal contraceptive method.

<u>Following delivery or second trimester abortion</u>

The use of NuvaRing® for contraception may be initiated four weeks postpartum in women who elect not to breastfeed. Women who are breast-feeding should be advised not to use NuvaRing® but to use other forms of contraception until the child is weaned. NuvaRing® use may be initiated four weeks after a second trimester abortion. When NuvaRing® is used postpartum or postabortion, the increased risk of thromboembolic disease must be considered. (See CONTRAINDICATIONS and WARNINGS concerning thromboembolic disease. See PRECAUTIONS for "Nursing Mothers".) If a woman begins using NuvaRing® postpartum, she should be instructed to use an additional method of contraception, such as male condoms or spermicide, for the first seven days. If she has not yet had a period, the possibility of ovulation and conception occurring prior to initiation of NuvaRing® should be considered.

Deviations from the Recommended Regimen

To prevent loss of contraceptive efficacy, women should not deviate from the recommended regimen. NuvaRing® should be left in the vagina for a continuous period of three weeks.

<u>Inadvertent removal, expulsion, or prolonged ring-free interval</u>

If the ring is accidentally expelled and is left outside of the vagina for **less than three hours** contraceptive efficacy is not reduced. NuvaRing® can be rinsed with cool to lukewarm (not hot) water and **reinserted as soon as possible,** but at the latest within three hours. If NuvaRing® is lost, a new vaginal ring should be inserted and the regimen should be continued without alteration. If NuvaRing® is out of the vagina for more than three hours, the directions listed under PRECAUTIONS, EXPULSION should be followed.

If the ring-free interval has been extended beyond one week, the possibility of pregnancy should be considered, and an additional method of contraception, such as male condoms or spermicide, **MUST** be used until NuvaRing® has been used **continuously for seven days.**

<u>Prolonged Use of NuvaRing®</u>

If NuvaRing® has been left in place for up to one extra week (i.e., up to four weeks total), the woman will remain protected. NuvaRing® should be removed and the woman should insert a new ring after a one-week ring-free interval. The mean serum etonogestrel concentration during the fourth week of continuous use of NuvaRing® was 1272 ± 311 pg/mL compared to a mean concentration range of 1578 ± 408 to 1374 ± 328 pg/mL during weeks one to three. The mean serum ethinyl estradiol concentration during the fourth week of continuous use of NuvaRing® was 16.8 ± 4.6 pg/mL compared to a mean concentration range of 19.1 ± 4.5 to 17.6 ± 4.3 pg/mL during weeks one to three.

If NuvaRing® has been left in place for longer than four weeks, pregnancy should be ruled out, and an additional method of contraception, such as male condoms or spermicide, **MUST** be used until a new NuvaRing® has been used **continuously for seven days.**

In the event of a missed menstrual period

1. If the woman has not adhered to the prescribed regimen (NuvaRing® has been out of the vagina for more than three hours or the preceding ring-free interval was extended beyond one week) the possibility of pregnancy should be considered at the time of the first missed period and NuvaRing® use should be discontinued if pregnancy is confirmed.
2. If the woman has adhered to the prescribed regimen and misses two consecutive periods, pregnancy should be ruled out.
3. If the woman has retained one NuvaRing® for longer than four weeks, pregnancy should be ruled out.

HOW SUPPLIED

Each NuvaRing® (etonogestrel/ethinyl estradiol vaginal ring) is individually packaged in a reclosable aluminum laminate sachet consisting of three layers, from outside to inside: polyester, aluminum foil, and low-density polyethylene. The ring should be replaced in this reclosable sachet after use for convenient disposal.

Box of 3 sachets NDC 0052-0273-03
Box of 1 sachet NDC 0052-0273-01

Storage

Prior to dispensing to the user, store refrigerated 2–8°C (36–46°F). After dispensing to the user, NuvaRing® can be stored for up to four months at 25°C (77°F); excursions permitted to 15–30°C (59–86°F) [see USP Controlled Room Temperature]. Avoid storing NuvaRing® in direct sunlight or at temperatures above 30°C (86°F). For the Dispenser: When NuvaRing® is dispensed to the user, place an expiration date on the label. The date should not exceed either four months from the date of dispensing or the expiration date, whichever comes first.

℞ only

REFERENCES FURNISHED UPON REQUEST

Manufactured for Organon USA Inc.
Roseland, NJ 07068
by N.V. Organon, Oss, The Netherlands
 NUV-76928 6/08 00

NuvaRing®

(etonogestrel/ethinyl estradiol vaginal ring)
delivers 0.120 mg/0.015 mg per day

PATIENT INFORMATION

℞ only

Read this leaflet carefully before you use NuvaRing® so that you understand the benefits and risks of using this form of birth control. The leaflet gives you information about the possible serious side effects of NuvaRing®. This leaflet will also tell you how to use NuvaRing® properly so that it will give you the best possible protection against pregnancy. Read the information you get whenever you get a new prescription or refill, because there may be new information. This information does not take the place of talking with your healthcare provider.

<u>What is NuvaRing®?</u>

NuvaRing® (NEW-vah-ring) is a flexible combined contraceptive vaginal ring. It is used to prevent pregnancy. **It does not protect against HIV infection (AIDS) and other sexually** transmitted diseases (STD's) such as chlamydia, genital herpes, genital warts, gonorrhea, hepatitis B, and syphilis. NuvaRing® contains a combination of a progestin and estrogen, two kinds of female hormones. You insert the ring in your vagina and leave it there for three weeks. After the ring is inserted, it releases a continuous low dose of hormones into your body. You then remove it for a one-week ring-free period.

Contraceptives that contain both an estrogen and a progestin are called combination hormonal contraceptives. Most studies on combination contraceptives have used oral (taken by mouth) contraceptives. NuvaRing® may have the same risks that have been found for combination oral contraceptives. This leaflet will tell you about risks of taking combination oral contraceptives that may also apply to NuvaRing® users. In addition, it will tell you how to use NuvaRing® properly so that it will give you the best possible protection against pregnancy.

Who should not use NuvaRing®?

Cigarette smoking increases the risk of serious cardiovascular side effects when you use combination oral contraceptives. This risk increases even more if you are over age 35 and if you smoke 15 or more cigarettes a day. Women who use combination hormonal contraceptives, including NuvaRing®, are strongly advised not to smoke.

Do not use **NuvaRing®** if you have any of the following conditions:
- a history of heart attack or stroke
- a history of blood clots in your legs (thrombophlebitis), lungs (pulmonary embolism), or eyes
- a history of blood clots in the deep veins of your legs
- chest pain (angina pectoris)
- severe high blood pressure
- diabetes with complications of the kidneys, eyes, nerves, or blood vessels
- headaches with neurological symptoms
- known or suspected breast cancer or cancer of the lining of the uterus, cervix, or vagina (now or in the past)
- unexplained vaginal bleeding (until a diagnosis is reached by your healthcare provider)
- yellowing of the whites of the eyes or of the skin (jaundice) during pregnancy or during previous use of hormonal birth control of any kind (the pill, patch, vaginal ring, injection, or implant)
- liver tumor (benign or cancerous)
- heart valve or heart rhythm disorders that may be associated with formation of blood clots
- need for a long period of bed rest following major surgery
- known or suspected pregnancy
- active liver disease with abnormal liver function tests
- an allergy or hypersensitivity to any of the components of NuvaRing®

Tell your healthcare provider if you have ever had any of the conditions just listed. Your healthcare provider can suggest another method of birth control.

Talk with your healthcare provider about using NuvaRing® if you:
- smoke
- recently had a baby
- recently had a miscarriage or abortion
- are breast-feeding
- are taking other medications

In addition, talk to your healthcare provider about using NuvaRing® if you have any of the following conditions. Women with any of these conditions should be checked often by their doctor or healthcare provider if they choose to use NuvaRing®.
- a family history of breast cancer
- breast nodules, fibrocystic disease, an abnormal breast x-ray, or abnormal mammogram
- diabetes
- elevated cholesterol or triglycerides
- high blood pressure
- migraine or other headaches or epilepsy
- depression
- gallbladder, liver, heart, or kidney disease
- scanty or irregular menstrual periods
- plan to have major surgery (You may need to stop using NuvaRing® for a while to reduce your chance of getting blood clots.)
- any condition that makes the vagina get irritated easily
- prolapsed (dropped) uterus, dropped bladder (cystocele), or rectal prolapse (rectocele)
- severe constipation
- history of toxic shock syndrome

How should I use NuvaRing®?

For the best protection from pregnancy, use NuvaRing® exactly as directed. Insert one NuvaRing® in the vagina and **keep it in place for three weeks in a row.** Remove it for a one-week break and then insert a new ring. During the one-week break, you will usually have your menstrual period.

Your healthcare provider should examine you at least once a year to see if there are any signs of side effects of NuvaRing® use.

When should I start NuvaRing®?

Follow the instructions in one of the sections below to find out when to start using NuvaRing®:

If you **did not** use a hormonal contraceptive in the preceding cycle

Insert NuvaRing® on the first day of your cycle, (i.e., the first day of menstrual bleeding). NuvaRing® will work immediately; it is not necessary to use an additional contraceptive method. You may also start on days 2-5 of your cycle, but in this case make sure you also use an extra method of birth control (barrier method), such as male condoms or spermicide for the first seven days of NuvaRing® use in the first cycle.

If you are changing from a combined hormonal contraceptive pill or patch (containing both progestin and estrogen)

Switch from your previous combined hormonal contraceptive on any day, but at the latest on the day following the usual hormone-free interval by inserting NuvaRing®. If you have been using your hormonal contraceptive method consistently and correctly, no extra birth control method should be needed.

If you are changing from a progestagen-only method (minipill, implant or injection) or from a progestagen-releasing intrauterine system (IUS)

You may switch on any day from a minipill. You should switch from an implant or the IUS on the day of its removal and from an injectable on the day when the next injection would be due. In all of these cases, you should use an extra method of birth control, such as male condom or spermicide, for the first seven days of ring use.

Following first trimester abortion or miscarriage

If you start using NuvaRing® within five days after a complete first trimester abortion or miscarriage, you do not need to use an extra method of contraception.

If NuvaRing® is not started within five days after a first trimester abortion or miscarriage, begin NuvaRing® at the time of your next menstrual period. Counting the first day of your menstrual period as "Day 1", insert NuvaRing® on or before Day 5 of the cycle, even if you have not finished bleeding. During this first cycle, use an extra method of birth control, such as male condoms or spermicide, for the first seven days of ring use.

How do I insert NuvaRing®?

1. Each NuvaRing® comes in a reclosable foil pouch. After washing and drying your hands, remove NuvaRing® from its foil pouch. Keep the foil pouch for proper disposal of the ring after use. Choose the position that is most comfortable for you. For example, lying down, squatting, or standing with one leg up (Figures 1a, 1b, and 1c, respectively).

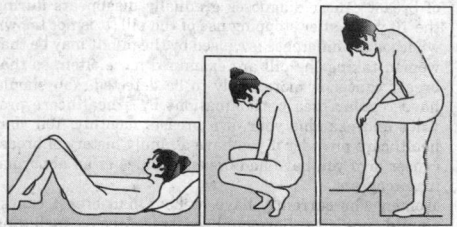

Figures 1a, 1b, and 1c. Positions for NuvaRing® insertion.

2. Hold NuvaRing® between your thumb and index finger (Figure 2a) and press the opposite sides of the ring together (Figure 2b).

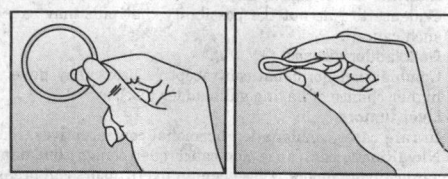

Figures 2a and 2b. Holding NuvaRing® and pressing the sides together.

3. Gently push the folded ring into your vagina (Figures 3a and 3b). The exact position of NuvaRing® in the vagina is not important for it to work (Figures 3c and 3d).
[See figures 3a, 3b, 3c and 3d at top of next column]

Although some women may be aware of NuvaRing® in the vagina, most women do not feel it once it is in place. If you feel discomfort, NuvaRing® is probably not inserted back far enough in the vagina. Use your finger to gently push the NuvaRing® farther into your vagina. **There is no danger of NuvaRing® being pushed too far up in the vagina or get-**

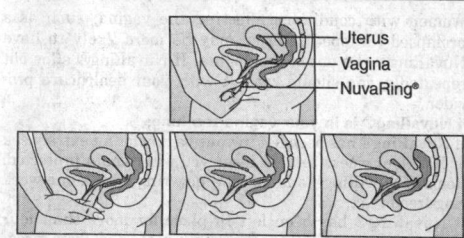

Figures 3a, 3b, 3c, and 3d. Inserting and positioning of NuvaRing®.

ting lost. NuvaRing® can be inserted only as far as the end of the vagina, where the cervix (the narrow, lower end of the uterus) will block NuvaRing® from going any farther.

4. Once inserted, keep NuvaRing® in place for three weeks in a row.

How do I remove NuvaRing®?

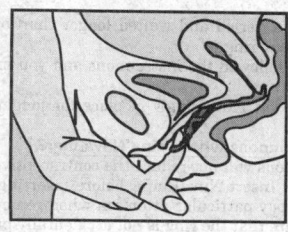

Figure 4. Removing NuvaRing®.

1. Remove the ring three weeks after insertion on the same day of the week as it was inserted, at about the same time of day.
   You can remove NuvaRing® by hooking the index finger under the forward rim or by holding the rim between the index and middle finger and pulling it out (Figure 4).
2. Place the used ring in the foil pouch and properly dispose of it in a waste receptacle out of the reach of children and pets. Do not throw it in the toilet.
   Your menstrual period will usually start two to three days after the ring is removed and may not have finished before the next ring is inserted. **To continue to have pregnancy protection, you must insert the new ring one week after the last one was removed, even if your menstrual period has not stopped.**

If you locate the ring in your vagina, but are unable to remove it, please contact your healthcare provider.

When do I insert a new ring?

After no more than a one-week ring-free break, insert a new ring on the same day of the week as it was removed in the last cycle. If the ring-free interval has been extended beyond one week, the possibility of pregnancy should be considered, and an extra method of birth control, such as male condoms or spermicide, **MUST** be used until NuvaRing® has been used **continuously for seven days.**

If NuvaRing® slips out:

NuvaRing® can accidentally slip out of the vagina while removing a tampon, during intercourse, or straining during a bowel movement. If NuvaRing® slips out of the vagina **and it has been out for less than three hours**, you should still be protected from pregnancy. NuvaRing® can be rinsed with cool to lukewarm (not hot) water and reinserted as soon as possible, and at the latest within three hours of removal or expulsion (slipping out).

If NuvaRing® is out of the vagina for more than three continuous hours:

During Weeks 1 and 2:   If the ring **has been out of the vagina for more than three continuous hours** during the 1st or 2nd week of use, contraceptive effectiveness may be reduced. Reinsert ring as soon as you remember and use an extra method of birth control, such as male condoms or spermicide, until the ring has been used continuously for seven days.

During Week 3:   If NuvaRing® slips **out of the vagina for more than three continuous hours** during the 3rd week of the three-week use period, throw the ring away and choose one of the following two options:
1. Insert a new ring immediately. Inserting a new ring will start the next three-week use period. You may not experience a period from your previous cycle. However, breakthrough spotting or bleeding may occur.
2. Have your period and insert a new ring no later than seven days (7×24 hours) from the time the previous ring was removed or expelled. This option should only be chosen if the ring was used continuously for the preceding seven days.

In addition, a barrier method such as condoms or spermicides must be used until the ring has been used continuously for seven days.

Women with conditions affecting the vagina, such as a prolapsed (dropped) uterus, may be more likely to have NuvaRing® slip out of the vagina. If NuvaRing® slips out repeatedly, you should consult with your healthcare provider.

If NuvaRing® is in your vagina too long:
If NuvaRing® has been left in your vagina for an extra week or less (four weeks total or less), you will remain protected. Remove NuvaRing® and insert a new ring after a one-week ring-free break.

If NuvaRing® has been left in place for more than four weeks, you may not be adequately protected from pregnancy and you must check to be sure you are not pregnant. You **MUST** use an extra method of birth control, such as male condoms or spermicide, until the new NuvaRing® has been in place for **seven days in a row.**

If you miss a menstrual period:
You must check to be sure that you are not pregnant if:
1. you miss a period and NuvaRing® was out of the vagina for more than three hours during the three weeks of ring use
2. you miss a period and waited longer than one week to insert a new ring
3. you have followed the instructions and you miss two periods in a row
4. you have left NuvaRing® in place for longer than four weeks

Can I use tampons when using NuvaRing®?
Use of tampons will not reduce the contraceptive efficacy of NuvaRing®. Insert NuvaRing® before inserting a tampon. You should pay particular attention when removing a tampon to be sure that the ring is not accidentally pulled out. If this should occur, simply rinse the ring in cool to lukewarm (not hot) water and immediately reinsert it.

Can I use vaginal medications?
Use of spermicides or vaginal yeast products will not reduce the contraceptive efficacy of NuvaRing®.

What should I do if my NuvaRing® disconnects?
There have been reported cases of NuvaRing® disconnecting at the weld joint causing the ring to change shape and straighten out. This is not expected to affect the contraceptive effectiveness of NuvaRing®. If NuvaRing® disconnects, expulsion (slipping out) is more likely to occur (see "If NuvaRing® slips out"). If you discover the ring has disconnected, you should discard the ring and replace it with a new ring.

Overdose
NuvaRing® is unlikely to cause an overdose because the ring holding the medicine releases a steady amount of contraceptive hormones. Do not use more than one ring at a time. Overdose of combination hormonal contraceptives may cause nausea, vomiting, or vaginal bleeding.

What should I avoid while using NuvaRing®?
Cigarette smoking increases the risk of serious cardiovascular side effects when you use combination oral contraceptives, including NuvaRing®. This risk increases even more if you are over age 35 and if you smoke 15 or more cigarettes a day. Women who use combination hormonal contraceptives, like NuvaRing®, are strongly advised not to smoke.

Do not breast-feed while using NuvaRing®. Some of the medicine may pass through the milk to the baby and could cause yellowing of the skin (jaundice) and breast enlargement in your baby. NuvaRing® could also decrease the amount and quality of your breast milk.

The hormones in NuvaRing® can interact with many other medicines and herbal supplements. Tell your healthcare provider about any medicines you are taking, including prescription medicines, over-the-counter medicines, herbal remedies, and vitamins.

The blood levels of the hormones released by NuvaRing® were increased when women used a vaginal medication (miconazole nitrate) for a yeast infection while NuvaRing® was in place. The pregnancy protection of NuvaRing® is not likely to be changed by use of these products. The blood levels of these hormones were not changed when women used vaginal, water-based spermicides (nonoxynol or N-9 products) along with NuvaRing®.

Certain drugs and herbal supplements may interact with combined hormonal contraceptives to make them less effective in preventing pregnancy or cause an increase in breakthrough bleeding. Such drugs include rifampin, drugs used for epilepsy such as barbiturates (for example, phenobarbital), carbamazepine, and phenytoin, primidone, topiramate, phenylbutazone, modafinil, and some drugs used for HIV such as ritonavir. Pregnancies and breakthrough bleeding have been reported by users of combined hormonal contraceptives who also used the herbal supplement St. John's Wort. You may need to use a non-hormonal method of contraception during any cycle in which you take drugs that can make oral contraceptives less effective. Be sure to tell your healthcare provider if you are taking or start taking any other medications, including non-prescription products or herbal products while using NuvaRing®.

While using NuvaRing®, you should not rely upon a diaphragm when you need a back-up method of birth control because NuvaRing® may interfere with the correct placement and position of a diaphragm.

If you are scheduled for any laboratory tests, tell your doctor or healthcare provider you are using NuvaRing®. Contraceptive hormones may change certain blood tests results.

What are the possible risks and side effects of NuvaRing®?
• **Blood clots**
The hormones in NuvaRing® may cause changes in your blood clotting system which may allow your blood to clot more easily. If blood clots form in your legs, they can travel to the lungs and cause a sudden blockage of a vessel carrying blood to the lungs. Rarely, clots occur in the blood vessels of the eye and may cause blindness, double vision, or other vision problems. The risk of getting blood clots may be greater with the type of progestin in NuvaRing® than with some other progestins in certain low-dose birth control pills. It is unknown if the risk of blood clots is different with NuvaRing® use than with the use of certain birth control pills.

If you take hormonal contraceptives and need elective surgery, need to stay in bed for a prolonged illness or have recently delivered a baby, you may be at risk of developing blood clots. You should consult your doctor or healthcare provider about stopping hormonal contraceptives three to four weeks before surgery and not taking hormonal contraceptives for two weeks after surgery or during bed rest. You should also not take hormonal contraceptives soon after delivery of a baby. It is advisable to wait for at least four weeks after delivery if you are not breast-feeding. If you are breast-feeding, you should wait until you have weaned your child before using the pill (see PRECAUTIONS, NURSING MOTHERS).

• **Strokes and heart attacks**
Hormonal contraceptives may increase your risk of strokes (blockage of blood flow to the brain) or heart attacks (blockage of blood flow to the heart). Any of these conditions can cause death or serious disability. Smoking greatly increases the risk of having strokes and heart attacks. Furthermore, smoking and the use of combination hormonal contraceptives, like NuvaRing®, greatly increases the chances of developing and dying of heart disease. If you use combination hormonal contraceptives, including NuvaRing®, you should not smoke.

• **High blood pressure and heart disease**
Combination hormonal contraceptives, including NuvaRing®, can worsen conditions like high blood pressure, diabetes, and problems with cholesterol and triglycerides.

• **Cancer of the reproductive organs and breast**
Breast cancer has been diagnosed slightly more often in women who use the pill than in women of the same age who do not use the pill. This small increase in the number of breast cancer diagnoses gradually disappears during the 10 years after stopping use of the pill. It is not known whether the difference is caused by the pill. It may be that women taking the pill are examined more often, so that breast cancer is more likely to be detected. You should have regular breast examinations by a healthcare provider and examine your own breasts monthly. Tell your healthcare provider if you have a family history of breast cancer or if you have had breast nodules or an abnormal mammogram.

Women who currently have or have had breast cancer should not use hormonal contraceptives, including NuvaRing®, because breast cancer is usually a hormone-sensitive tumor.

Some studies have found an increase in the incidence of cancer of the cervix in women who use oral contraceptives. However, this finding be related to factors other than the use of oral contraceptives. There is insufficient evidence to rule out the possibility that pills may cause such cancers.

• **Gallbladder disease**
Combination hormonal contraceptive users may have a higher chance of having gallbladder disease.

• **Liver tumors**
In rare cases, combination hormonal contraceptives, like NuvaRing®, can cause non-cancerous (benign) but dangerous liver tumors. These benign liver tumors can break and cause fatal internal bleeding. In addition, it is possible that women who use combination hormonal contraceptives, like NuvaRing®, have a higher chance of getting liver cancer. However, liver cancers are extremely rare.

• **Lipid metabolism and inflammation of the pancreas**
In women with inherited defects of lipid metabolism, there have been reports of significant elevations of plasma triglycerides during estrogen therapy. This has led to pancreatitis in some cases.

The common side effects reported by NuvaRing® users are:
• vaginal infections and irritation
• vaginal secretion
• headache

• weight gain
• nausea
In addition to the risks and side effects listed above, users of combination hormonal contraceptives have reported the following side effects:
• vomiting
• change in appetite
• abdominal cramps and bloating
• breast tenderness or enlargement
• irregular vaginal bleeding or spotting
• changes in menstrual cycle
• temporary infertility after treatment
• fluid retention (edema)
• spotty darkening of the skin, particularly on the face
• rash
• weight changes
• depression
• intolerance to contact lenses
• nervousness
• dizziness
• loss of scalp hair
Call your healthcare provider right away if you get any of the symptoms listed below. They may be signs of a serious problem:
• sharp chest pain, coughing blood, or sudden shortness of breath (possible clot in the lung)
• pain in the calf (back of lower leg; possible clot in the leg)
• crushing chest pain or heaviness in the chest (possible heart attack)
• sudden severe headache or vomiting, dizziness or fainting, problems with vision or speech, weakness, or numbness in an arm or leg (possible stroke)
• sudden partial or complete loss of vision (possible clot in the eye)
• yellowing of the skin or whites of the eyes (jaundice), especially with fever, tiredness, loss of appetite, dark colored urine, or light colored bowel movements (possible liver problems)
• severe pain, swelling, or tenderness in the abdomen (gallbladder or liver problems)
• sudden fever (usually 102°F or more), vomiting, diarrhea, dizziness, fainting, or a sunburn-like rash on the face or body (very rarely, toxic shock syndrome)
• breast lumps (possible breast cancer or benign breast disease)
• irregular vaginal bleeding or spotting that happens in more than one menstrual cycle or lasts for more than a few days
• urgent, frequent, burning and/or painful urination, and cannot locate the ring in the vagina (rarely, accidental placement of NuvaRing® into the urinary bladder)
• swelling (edema) of your fingers or ankles
• difficulty in sleeping, weakness, lack of energy, fatigue, or a change in mood (possible severe depression)
How effective is NuvaRing®?
If NuvaRing® is used according to the directions, your chance of getting pregnant is about 1 to 2% a year. This means that, for every 100 women who use NuvaRing® for a year, one or two will become pregnant. Your chance of getting pregnant increases if NuvaRing® is not used exactly according to the directions.

By comparison, the chances of getting pregnant in the first year of typical use (not always following directions exactly) of other methods of birth control are as follows:

No birth control method:	85%
Spermicides alone:	26%
Periodic abstinence methods (calendar, ovulation, thermometer):	25%
Withdrawal:	19%
Cervical Cap with spermicides:	20 to 40%
Vaginal sponge:	20 to 40%
Diaphragm with spermicides:	20%
Condom alone (male):	14%
Condom alone (female):	21%
Oral contraceptives:	5%
IUD:	less than 1 to 2%
Implants:	less than 1%
Injection:	less than 1%
Sterilization:	less than 1%

Other Information
• Store NuvaRing® at room temperature, 25°C (77°F). Temperatures can be from 59–86°F (15–30°C). Avoid direct sunlight or storing above 86°F (30°C).
• Medicines are sometimes prescribed for conditions that are not mentioned in patient information leaflets. Do not use NuvaRing® for a condition for which it was not prescribed. Do not give NuvaRing® to anyone else who may want to use it.
• Place the used ring in the reclosable foil pouch and properly dispose of it in a waste receptacle out of the reach of children and pets.
This leaflet summarizes the most important information about NuvaRing®. If you would like more information, talk with your healthcare provider. You can ask your pharmacist or healthcare provider for information about NuvaRing® that is written for health professionals.

1-877-NUVARING
Manufactured for Organon USA Inc.
Roseland, NJ 07068
by N.V. Organon, Oss, The Netherlands
© 2008 Organon USA Inc.   NUV-76926   6/08 00
Shown in Product Identification Guide, page 313

PEDVAXHIB® LIQUID ℞

[ped-vax-hib]

[Haemophilus b Conjugate Vaccine
(Meningococcal Protein Conjugate)]

DESCRIPTION

PedvaxHIB[1] [Haemophilus b Conjugate Vaccine (Meningococcal Protein Conjugate)] is a highly purified capsular polysaccharide (polyribosylribitol phosphate or PRP) of *Haemophilus influenzae* type b (Haemophilus b, Ross strain) that is covalently bound to an outer membrane protein complex (OMPC) of the B11 strain of *Neisseria meningitidis* serogroup B. The covalent bonding of the PRP to the OMPC which is necessary for enhanced immunogenicity of the PRP is confirmed by quantitative analysis of the conjugate's components following chemical treatment which yields a unique amino acid. The potency of PedvaxHIB is determined by assay of PRP.

Haemophilus influenzae type b and *Neisseria meningitidis* serogroup B are grown in complex fermentation media. The PRP is purified from the culture broth by purification procedures which include ethanol fractionation, enzyme digestion, phenol extraction and diafiltration. The OMPC from *Neisseria meningitidis* is purified by detergent extraction, ultracentrifugation, diafiltration and sterile filtration.

Liquid PedvaxHIB is ready to use and does not require a diluent. Each 0.5 mL dose of Liquid PedvaxHIB is a sterile product formulated to contain: 7.5 mcg of Haemophilus b PRP, 125 mcg of *Neisseria meningitidis* OMPC and 225 mcg of aluminum as amorphous aluminum hydroxyphosphate sulfate (previously referred to as aluminum hydroxide), in 0.9% sodium chloride, but does not contain lactose or thimerosal. Liquid PedvaxHIB is a slightly opaque white suspension.

This vaccine is for intramuscular administration and not for intravenous injection. (See DOSAGE AND ADMINISTRATION.)

---

[1] Registered trademark of MERCK & CO., Inc. COPYRIGHT © MERCK & CO., Inc., 1998 All rights reserved

CLINICAL PHARMACOLOGY

Prior to the introduction of Haemophilus b Conjugate Vaccines, *Haemophilus influenzae* type b (Hib) was the most frequent cause of bacterial meningitis and a leading cause of serious, systemic bacterial disease in young children worldwide.[1,2,3,4]

Hib disease occurred primarily in children under 5 years of age in the United States prior to the initiation of a vaccine program and was estimated to account for nearly 20,000 cases of invasive infections annually, approximately 12,000 of which were meningitis. The mortality rate from Hib meningitis is about 5%. In addition, up to 35% of survivors develop neurologic sequelae including seizures, deafness, and mental retardation.[5,6] Other invasive diseases caused by this bacterium include cellulitis, epiglottitis, sepsis, pneumonia, septic arthritis, osteomyelitis and pericarditis.

Prior to the introduction of the vaccine, it was estimated that 17% of all cases of Hib disease occurred in infants less than 6 months of age.[7] The peak incidence of Hib meningitis occurs between 6 to 11 months of age. Forty-seven percent of all cases occur by one year of age with the remaining 53% of cases occurring over the next four years.[2,20]

Among children under 5 years of age, the risk of invasive Hib disease is increased in certain populations including the following:

- Daycare attendees[8,9]
- Lower socio-economic groups[10]
- Blacks[11] (especially those who lack the Km(1) immunoglobulin allotype)[12]
- Caucasians who lack the G2m(n or 23) immunoglobulin allotype[13]
- Native Americans[14,15,16]
- Household contacts of cases[17]
- Individuals with asplenia, sickle cell disease, or antibody deficiency syndromes[18,19]

An important virulence factor of the Hib bacterium is its polysaccharide capsule (PRP). Antibody to PRP (anti-PRP) has been shown to correlate with protection against Hib disease.[3,21] While the anti-PRP level associated with protection using conjugated vaccines has not yet been determined, the level of anti-PRP associated with protection in studies using bacterial polysaccharide immune globulin or nonconjugated PRP vaccines ranged from >0.15 to >1.0 mcg/mL.[22-28]

Nonconjugated PRP vaccines are capable of stimulating B-lymphocytes to produce antibody without the help of T-lymphocytes (T-independent). The responses to many other antigens are augmented by helper T-lymphocytes (T-dependent). PedvaxHIB is a PRP-conjugate vaccine in which the PRP is covalently bound to the OMPC carrier[29] producing an antigen which is postulated to convert the T-independent antigen (PRP alone) into a T-dependent antigen resulting in both an enhanced antibody response and immunologic memory.

Clinical Evaluation of PedvaxHIB

PedvaxHIB, in a lyophilized formulation (lyophilized PedvaxHIB), was initially evaluated in 3,486 Native American (Navajo) infants, who completed the primary two-dose regimen in a randomized, double-blind, placebo-controlled study (The Protective Efficacy Study). At the time of the study, this population had a much higher incidence of Hib disease than the United States population as a whole and also had a lower antibody response to Haemophilus b Conjugate Vaccines, including PedvaxHIB.[14,15,16,30,33] Each infant in this study received two doses of either placebo or lyophilized PedvaxHIB with the first dose administered at a mean of 8 weeks of age and the second administered approximately two months later; DTP and OPV were administered concomitantly. Antibody levels were measured in a subset of each group (TABLE 1).

[See table 1 above]

Most subjects were initially followed until 15 to 18 months of age. During this time, 22 cases of invasive Hib disease occurred in the placebo group (8 cases after the first dose and 14 cases after the second dose) and only 1 case in the vaccine group (none after the first dose and 1 after the second dose). Following the primary two-dose regimen, the protective efficacy of lyophilized PedvaxHIB was calculated to be 93% with a 95% confidence interval of 57%-98% (p=0.001, two-tailed). In the two months between the first and second doses, the difference in number of cases of disease between placebo and vaccine recipients (8 vs. 0 cases, respectively) was statistically significant (p=0.008, two-tailed); however, a primary two-dose regimen is required for infants 2-14 months of age.

At termination of the study, placebo recipients were offered vaccine. All original participants were then followed two years and nine months from termination of the study. During this extended follow-up, invasive Hib disease occurred in an additional seven of the original placebo recipients prior to receiving vaccine and in one of the original vaccine recipients (who had received only one dose of vaccine). No cases of invasive Hib disease were observed in placebo recipients after they received at least one dose of vaccine. Efficacy for this follow-up period, estimated from person-days at risk, was 96.6% (95 C.I., 72.2-99.9%) in children under 18 months of age and 100% (95 C.I., 23.5-100%) in children over 18 months of age.[33]

Since protective efficacy with lyophilized PedvaxHIB was demonstrated in such a high risk population, it would be expected to be predictive of efficacy in other populations. The safety and immunogenicity of lyophilized PedvaxHIB were evaluated in infants and children in other clinical studies that were conducted in various locations throughout the United States. PedvaxHIB was highly immunogenic in all age groups studied.[31,32]

Lyophilized PedvaxHIB induced antibody levels greater than 1.0 mcg/mL in children who were poor responders to nonconjugated PRP vaccines. In a study involving such a subpopulation,[33,34] 34 children ranging in age from 27 to 61 months who developed invasive Hib disease despite previous vaccination with nonconjugated PRP vaccines were randomly assigned to 2 groups. One group (n=14) was vaccinated with lyophilized PedvaxHIB and the other group (n=20) with a nonconjugated PRP vaccine at a mean interval of approximately 12 months after recovery from disease. All 14 children vaccinated with lyophilized PedvaxHIB but only 6 of 20 children re-vaccinated with a nonconjugated PRP vaccine achieved an antibody level of >1.0 mcg/mL. The 14 children who had not responded to revaccination with the nonconjugated PRP vaccine were then vaccinated with a single dose of lyophilized PedvaxHIB; following this vaccination, all achieved antibody levels of >1.0 mcg/mL.

In addition, lyophilized PedvaxHIB has been studied in children at high risk of Hib disease because of genetically-related deficiencies [Blacks who were Km(1) allotype negative and Caucasians who were G2m(23) allotype negative] and are considered hyporesponsive to nonconjugated PRP vaccines on this basis.[35] The hyporesponsive children had anti-PRP responses comparable to those of allotype positive children of similar age range when vaccinated with lyophilized PedvaxHIB. All children achieved anti-PRP levels of >1.0 mcg/mL.

The safety and immunogenicity of Liquid PedvaxHIB were compared with those of lyophilized PedvaxHIB in a randomized clinical study involving 903 infants 2 to 6 months of age from the general U.S. population. DTP and OPV were administered concomitantly to most subjects. The antibody responses induced by each formulation of PedvaxHIB were similar. TABLE 2 shows antibody responses from this clinical study in subjects who received their first dose at 2 to 3 months of age.

[See table 2 above]

A booster dose of PedvaxHIB is required in infants who complete the primary two-dose regimen before 12 months of age. This booster dose will help maintain antibody levels

---

TABLE 1: Antibody Responses in Navajo Infants

Vaccine	No. of Subjects	Time	% Subjects with >0.15 mcg/mL	% Subjects with >1.0 mcg/mL	Anti-PRP GMT (mcg/mL)
Lyophilized PedvaxHIB*	416[†]	Pre-Vaccination	44	10	0.16
	416	Post-Dose 1	88	52	0.95
	416	Post-Dose 2	91	60	1.43
Placebo*	461[†]	Pre-Vaccination	44	9	0.16
	461	Post-Dose 1	21	2	0.09
	461	Post-Dose 2	14	1	0.08
Lyophilized PedvaxHIB	27[‡]	Prebooster	70	33	0.51
	27	Postbooster§	100	89	8.39

* Post-Vaccination values obtained approximately 1–3 months after each dose.
† The Protective Efficacy Study
‡ Immunogenicity Trial[34]
§ Booster given at 12 months of age; Post-Vaccination values obtained 1 month after administration of booster dose.

TABLE 2: Antibody Responses to Liquid and Lyophilized PedvaxHIB in Infants From the General U.S. Population

Formulation	Age (Months)	Time	No. of Subjects	% Subjects with anti-PRP >0.15 mcg/mL	% Subjects with anti-PRP >1.0 mcg/mL	Anti-PRP GMT (mcg/mL)
Liquid PedvaxHIB		Pre-Vaccination	487	32	7	0.12
	2-3	Post-Dose 1*	480	94	64	1.55
(7.5 mcg PRP)		Post-Dose 2†	393	97	80	3.22
	12-15	Prebooster	284	80	30	0.49
		Postbooster†	284	99	95	10.23
	24‡	Persistence	94	97	55	1.29
Lyophilized PedvaxHIB		Pre-Vaccination	171	37	6	0.13
	2-3	Post-Dose 1*	169	97	72	1.88
(15 mcg PRP)		Post-Dose 2†	133	99	81	2.69
	12-15	Prebooster	87	71	28	0.39
		Postbooster†	87	99	91	7.64
	24‡	Persistence	37	97	54	1.10

* Approximately two months Post-Vaccination
† Approximately one month Post-Vaccination
‡ Approximately

TABLE 3: Antibody Responses* After Two Doses of Lyophilized PedvaxHIB Among Infants Initially Vaccinated at 2–3 Months of Age By Racial/Ethnic Group

Racial/Ethnic Groups	No. of Subjects	LYOPHILIZED % Subjects With Anti-PRP >0.15 mcg/mL	>1.0 mcg/mL	Anti-PRP GMT (mcg/mL)
Native American[†]	54	96	70	2.47
Caucasian	201	99	82	3.52
Hispanic	76	99	88	3.54
Black	23	100	96	5.40

* One month after the second dose
† Apache and Navajo

TABLE 4: Antibody Responses* After Two Doses of Liquid PedvaxHIB Among Infants Initially Vaccinated at 2–3 Months of Age By Racial/Ethnic Group

Racial/Ethnic Groups	No. of Subjects	LIQUID % Subjects with Anti-PRP >0.15 mcg/mL	>1.0 mcg/mL	Anti-PRP GMT (mcg/mL)
Native American[†]	90	97	78	2.76
Caucasian	143	94	72	2.16
Hispanic	184	98	85	4.34
Black	18	100	94	7.58

* One month after the second dose
† Apache and Navajo

during the first two years of life when children are at highest risk for invasive Hib disease. (See TABLE 2 and DOSAGE AND ADMINISTRATION.)

In four United States studies, antibody responses to lyophilized PedvaxHIB were evaluated in several subpopulations of infants initially vaccinated between 2 to 3 months of age. (See TABLE 3.)

[See table 3 above]

In two United States studies, antibody responses to Liquid PedvaxHIB were evaluated in several subpopulations of infants initially vaccinated between 2 to 3 months of age. (See TABLE 4.)

[See table 4 above]

Antibodies to the OMPC of *N. meningitidis* have been demonstrated in vaccinee sera, but the clinical relevance of these antibodies has not been established.[33]

Interchangeability of Licensed Haemophilus b Conjugate Vaccines and PedvaxHIB

Published studies have examined the interchangeability of other licensed Haemophilus b Conjugate Vaccines and PedvaxHIB.[42,43,44,45,52] According to the American Academy of Pediatrics, excellent immune responses have been achieved when different vaccines have been interchanged in the primary series. If PedvaxHIB is given in a series with one of the other products licensed for infants, the recommended number of doses to complete the series is determined by the other product and not by PedvaxHIB. PedvaxHIB may be interchanged with other licensed Haemophilus b Conjugate Vaccines for the booster dose.[52]

Use with Other Vaccines

Results from clinical studies indicate that Liquid PedvaxHIB can be administered concomitantly with DTP, OPV, eIPV (enhanced inactivated poliovirus vaccine), VARIVAX[1] [Varicella Virus Vaccine Live (Oka/Merck)], M-M-R[1] II (Measles, Mumps, and Rubella Virus Vaccine Live) or RECOMBIVAX HB[1] [Hepatitis B Vaccine (Recombinant)].[33] No impairment of immune response to individual tested vaccine antigens was demonstrated.

The type, frequency and severity of adverse experiences observed in these studies with PedvaxHIB were similar to those seen when the other vaccines were given alone.

In addition, a PRP-OMPC-containing product, COMVAX[1] [Haemophilus b Conjugate (Meningococcal Protein Conjugate) and Hepatitis B (Recombinant) Vaccine], was given concomitantly with a booster dose of DTaP [diphtheria, tetanus, acellular pertussis] at approximately 15 months of age, using separate sites and syringes for injectable vaccines. No impairment of immune response to these individually tested vaccine antigens was demonstrated. COMVAX has also been administered concomitantly with the primary series of DTaP to a limited number of infants. PRP antibody responses are satisfactory for COMVAX, but immune responses are currently unavailable for DTaP (see Manufacturer's Product Circular for COMVAX). No serious vaccine-related adverse events were reported.[33]

INDICATIONS AND USAGE

Liquid PedvaxHIB is indicated for routine vaccination against invasive disease caused by *Haemophilus influenzae* type b in infants and children 2 to 71 months of age.

Liquid PedvaxHIB will not protect against disease caused by *Haemophilus influenzae* other than type b or against other microorganisms that cause invasive disease such as meningitis or sepsis. As with any vaccine, vaccination with Liquid PedvaxHIB may not result in a protective antibody response in all individuals given the vaccine.

BECAUSE OF THE POTENTIAL FOR IMMUNE TOLERANCE, Liquid PedvaxHIB IS NOT RECOMMENDED FOR USE IN INFANTS YOUNGER THAN 6 WEEKS OF AGE. (See PRECAUTIONS.)

Revaccination

Infants completing the primary two-dose regimen before 12 months of age should receive a booster dose (see DOSAGE AND ADMINISTRATION).

CONTRAINDICATIONS

Hypersensitivity to any component of the vaccine or the diluent. Persons who develop symptoms suggestive of hypersensitivity after an injection should not receive further injections of the vaccine.

PRECAUTIONS

General

As for any vaccine, adequate treatment provisions, including epinephrine, should be available for immediate use should an anaphylactoid reaction occur.

Special care should be taken to ensure that the injection does not enter a blood vessel.

It is important to use a separate sterile syringe and needle for each patient to prevent transmission of hepatitis B or other infectious agents from one person to another.

As with other vaccines, Liquid PedvaxHIB may not induce protective antibody levels immediately following vaccination.

As reported with Haemophilus b Polysaccharide Vaccine[36] and another Haemophilus b Conjugate Vaccine[37], cases of Hib disease may occur in the week after vaccination, prior to the onset of the protective effects of the vaccines.

There is insufficient evidence that Liquid PedvaxHIB given immediately after exposure to natural *Haemophilus influenzae* type b will prevent illness.

The decision to administer or delay vaccination because of current or recent febrile illness depends on the severity of symptoms and on the etiology of the disease. The Advisory Committee on Immunization Practices (ACIP) has recommended that vaccination should be delayed during the course of an acute febrile illness. All vaccines can be administered to persons with minor illnesses such as diarrhea, mild upper-respiratory infection with or without low-grade fever, or other low-grade febrile illness. Persons with moderate or severe febrile illness should be vaccinated as soon as they have recovered from the acute phase of the illness.[46]

If PedvaxHIB is used in persons with malignancies or those receiving immunosuppressive therapy or who are otherwise immunocompromised, the expected immune response may not be obtained.

Instructions to Healthcare Provider

The healthcare provider should determine the current health status and previous vaccination history of the vaccinee.

The healthcare provider should question the patient, parent, or guardian about reactions to a previous dose of PedvaxHIB or other Haemophilus b Conjugate Vaccines.

Information for Patients

The healthcare provider should provide the vaccine information required to be given with each vaccination to the patient, parent, or guardian.

The healthcare provider should inform the patient, parent, or guardian of the benefits and risks associated with vaccination. For risks associated with vaccination, see ADVERSE REACTIONS.

Patients, parents, and guardians should be instructed to report any serious adverse reactions to their healthcare provider who in turn should report such events to the U. S. Department of Health and Human Services through the Vaccine Adverse Event Reporting System (VAERS), 1-800-822-7967.[47]

Laboratory Test Interactions

Sensitive tests (e.g., Latex Agglutination Kits) may detect PRP derived from the vaccine in urine of some vaccinees for at least 30 days following vaccination with lyophilized PedvaxHIB;[38] in clinical studies with lyophilized PedvaxHIB, such children demonstrated normal immune response to the vaccine.

Carcinogenesis, Mutagenesis, Impairment of Fertility

Liquid PedvaxHIB has not been evaluated for carcinogenic or mutagenic potential, or potential to impair fertility.

Pregnancy

Pregnancy Category C

Animal reproduction studies have not been conducted with PedvaxHIB. Liquid PedvaxHIB is not recommended for use in individuals 6 years of age and older.

Pediatric Use

Safety and effectiveness in infants below the age of 2 months and in children 6 years of age and older have not been established. In addition, Liquid PedvaxHIB should not be used in infants younger than 6 weeks of age because this will lead to a reduced anti-PRP response and may lead to immune tolerance (impaired ability to respond to subsequent exposure to the PRP antigen).[49-51] Liquid PedvaxHIB is not recommended for use in individuals 6 years of age and older because they are generally not at risk of Hib disease.

Geriatric Use

This vaccine is NOT recommended for use in adult populations.

ADVERSE REACTIONS

Liquid PedvaxHIB

In a multicenter clinical study (n=903) comparing the effects of Liquid PedvaxHIB with those of lyophilized PedvaxHIB, 1,699 doses of Liquid PedvaxHIB were administered to 678 healthy infants 2 to 6 months of age from the general U.S. population. DTP and OPV were administered concomitantly to most subjects. Both formulations of PedvaxHIB were generally well tolerated and no serious vaccine-related adverse reactions were reported.

During a three-day period following primary vaccination with Liquid PedvaxHIB in these infants, the most frequently reported (>1%) adverse reactions, without regard to causality, excluding those shown in TABLE 5, in decreasing order of frequency, were: irritability, sleepiness, injection site pain/soreness, injection site erythema (≤2.5 cm diameter, see also TABLE 5), injection site swelling/induration (≤2.5 cm diameter, see also TABLE 5), unusual high-pitched crying, prolonged crying (>4 hr), diarrhea, vomiting, crying, pain, otitis media, rash, and upper respiratory infection.

Selected objective observations reported by parents over a 48-hour period in these infants following primary vaccination with Liquid PedvaxHIB are summarized in TABLE 5.

[See table 5 at top of next page]

Adverse reactions during a three-day period following administration of the booster dose were generally similar in type and frequency to those seen following primary vaccination.

Lyophilized PedvaxHIB

In The Protective Efficacy Study (see CLINICAL PHARMACOLOGY), 4,459 healthy Navajo infants 6 to 12 weeks of age received lyophilized PedvaxHIB or placebo. Most of these infants received DTP/OPV concomitantly. No differences were seen in the type and frequency of serious health problems expected in this Navajo population or in serious adverse experiences reported among those who received lyophilized PedvaxHIB and those who received placebo, and none was reported to be related to lyophilized PedvaxHIB. Only one serious reaction (tracheitis) was reported as possibly related to lyophilized PedvaxHIB and only one (diarrhea) as possibly related to placebo. Seizures occurred infrequently in both groups (9 occurred in vaccine recipients, 8 of whom also received DTP; 8 occurred in placebo recipients, 7 of whom also received DTP) and were not reported to be related to lyophilized PedvaxHIB.

In early clinical studies involving the administration of 8,086 doses of lyophilized PedvaxHIB alone to 5,027 healthy infants and children 2 months to 71 months of age, lyophilized PedvaxHIB was generally well tolerated. No serious adverse reactions were reported. In a subset of these infants, urticaria was reported in two children, and thrombocytopenia was seen in one child. A cause and effect relationship between these side effects and the vaccination has not been established.

Potential Adverse Reactions

The use of Haemophilus b Polysaccharide Vaccines and another Haemophilus b Conjugate Vaccine has been associated with the following additional adverse effects: early onset Hib disease and Guillain-Barré syndrome. A cause and effect relationship between these side effects and the vaccination was not established.(36,37,39,40,41,49)

Post-Marketing Adverse Reactions

The following additional adverse reactions have been reported with the use of the lyophilized and liquid formulations of PedvaxHIB:

Hemic and Lymphatic System
Lymphadenopathy
Hypersensitivity
Rarely, angioedema
Nervous System
Febrile seizures
Skin
Sterile injection site abscess

DOSAGE AND ADMINISTRATION

Liquid PedvaxHIB

FOR INTRAMUSCULAR ADMINISTRATION
DO NOT INJECT INTRAVENOUSLY

If there is an interruption or delay between doses in the primary series, there is no need to repeat the series, but dosing should be continued at the next clinic visit. (See CONTRAINDICATIONS and PRECAUTIONS.)

2 to 14 Months of Age

Infants 2 to 14 months of age should receive a 0.5 mL dose of vaccine ideally beginning at 2 months of age followed by a 0.5 mL dose 2 months later (or as soon as possible thereafter). When the primary two-dose regimen is completed before 12 months of age, a booster dose is required (see below and TABLE 6). Infants born prematurely, regardless of birth weight, should be vaccinated at the same chronological age and according to the same schedule and precautions as full-term infants and children.(46)

15 Months of Age and Older

Children 15 months of age and older previously unvaccinated against Hib disease should receive a single 0.5 mL dose of vaccine.

Booster Dose

In infants completing the primary two-dose regimen before 12 months of age, a booster dose (0.5 mL) should be administered at 12 to 15 months of age, but not earlier than 2 months after the second dose.

Vaccination regimens for Liquid PedvaxHIB by age group are outlined in TABLE 6.

TABLE 6: Vaccination Regimens for Liquid PedvaxHIB By Age Groups

Age (Months) at First Dose	Primary	Age (Months) at Booster Dose
2–10	2 doses, 2 mo. apart	12–15
11–14	2 doses, 2 mo. apart	—
15–71	1 dose	—

Interchangeability

PedvaxHIB may be interchanged with other licensed Haemophilus b Conjugate Vaccines for the primary and booster doses.(52) (See CLINICAL PHARMACOLOGY.)

Use with Other Vaccines

Results from clinical studies indicate that Liquid PedvaxHIB can be administered concomitantly with DTP, OPV, eIPV (enhanced inactivated poliovirus vaccine), VARIVAX [Varicella Virus Vaccine Live (Oka/Merck)], M-M-R II (Measles, Mumps, and Rubella Virus Vaccine Live) or RECOMBIVAX HB [Hepatitis B Vaccine (Recombinant)]. No impairment of immune response to these individually tested vaccine antigens was demonstrated.

The type, frequency and severity of adverse experiences observed in these studies with PedvaxHIB were similar to those seen with the other vaccines when given alone. (See CLINICAL PHARMACOLOGY.)

In addition, a PRP-OMPC-containing product, COMVAX [Haemophilus b Conjugate (Meningococcal Protein Conjugate) and Hepatitis B (Recombinant) Vaccine], was given concomitantly with a booster dose of DTaP [diphtheria, tetanus, acellular pertussis] at approximately 15 months of age, using separate sites and syringes for injectable vaccines. No impairment of immune response to these individually tested vaccine antigens was demonstrated. COMVAX has also been administered concomitantly with the primary series of DTaP to a limited number of infants. PRP antibody responses are satisfactory for COMVAX, but immune responses are currently unavailable for DTaP (see *Manufacturer's Product Circular for COMVAX*). No serious vaccine-related adverse events were reported.(33)

Parenteral drug products should be inspected visually for extraneous particulate matter and discoloration prior to administration whenever solution and container permit.

Liquid PedvaxHIB is a slightly opaque white suspension. (See DESCRIPTION.)

The vaccine should be used as supplied; no reconstitution is necessary.

Shake well before withdrawal and use. Thorough agitation is necessary to maintain suspension of the vaccine.

Inject 0.5 mL intramuscularly, preferably into the anterolateral thigh or the outer aspect of the upper arm. The buttocks should not be used for active vaccination of infants and children, because of the potential risk of injury to the sciatic nerve.

HOW SUPPLIED

Liquid PedvaxHIB is supplied as follows:
No. 4897—A box of 10 single-dose vials of liquid vaccine, **NDC** 0006-4897-00.

Storage

Store vaccine at 2-8°C (36-46°F).
DO NOT FREEZE.

TABLE 5: Fever or Local Reactions in Subjects First Vaccinated at 2 to 6 Months of Age with Liquid PedvaxHIB*

Reaction	No. of Subjects Evaluated	Post-Dose 1 (hr)			No. of Subjects Evaluated	Post-Dose 2 (hr)		
		6	24	48		6	24	48
		Percentage				Percentage		
Fever[†] >38.3°C (≥101°F) Rectal	222	18.1	4.4	0.5	206	14.1	9.4	2.8
Erythema >2.5 cm diameter	674	2.2	1.0	0.5	562	1.6	1.1	0.4
Swelling >2.5 cm diameter	674	2.5	1.9	0.9	562	0.9	0.9	1.3

* DTP and OPV were administered concomitantly to most subjects.
† Fever was also measured by another method or reported as normal for an additional 345 infants after dose 1 and for an additional 249 infants after dose 2; however, these data are not included in this table.

REFERENCES

1. Cochi, S. L., et al: Immunization of U.S. children with Haemophilus influenzae type b polysaccharide vaccine: A cost-effectiveness model of strategy assessment. JAMA 253: 521-529, 1985.
2. Schlech, W. F., III, et al: Bacterial meningitis in the United States, 1978 through 1981. The National Bacterial Meningitis Surveillance Study. JAMA 253: 1749-1754, 1985.
3. Peltola, H., et al: Prevention of Haemophilus influenzae type b bacteremic infections with the capsular polysaccharide vaccine. N Engl J Med 310: 1561-1566, 1984.
4. Cadoz, M., et al: Etude epidemiologique des cas de meningitis purulentes hospitalises a Dakar pendant la decemie 1970-1979. Bull WHO 59: 575-584, 1981.
5. Sell, S. H., et al: Long-term Sequelae of Haemophilus influenzae meningitis. Pediatr 49: 206-217, 1972.
6. Taylor, H. G., et al: Intellectual, neuropsychological, and achievement outcomes in children six to eight years after recovery from Haemophilus influenzae meningitis. Pediatr 74: 198-205, 1984.
7. Hay, J. W., et al: Cost-benefit analysis of two strategies for prevention of Haemophilus influenzae type b infection. Pediatr 80(3): 319-329, 1987.
8. Redmond, S. R., et al: Haemophilus influenzae type b disease: an epidemiologic study with special reference to daycare centers. JAMA 252: 2581-2584, 1984.
9. Istre, G. R., et al: Risk factors for primary invasive Haemophilus influenzae disease: increased risk from day-care attendance and school age household members. J Pediatr 106: 190-195, 1985.
10. Fraser, D.W., et al: Risk factors in bacterial meningitis: Charleston County, South Carolina. J Infect Dis 127: 271-277, 1973.
11. Tarr, P. I., et al: Demographic factors in the epidemiology of Haemophilus influenzae meningitis in young children. J Pediatr 92: 884-888, 1978.
12. Granoff, D. M., et al: Response to immunization with Haemophilus influenzae type b polysaccharide-pertussis vaccine and risk of Haemophilus meningitis in children with Km(1) immunoglobulin allotype. J Clin Invest 74: 1708-1714, 1984.
13. Ambrosino, D. M., et al: Correlation between G2m(n) immunoglobulin allotype and human antibody response and susceptibility to polysaccharide encapsulated bacteria. J Clin Invest 75: 1935-1942, 1985.
14. Coulehan, J. L., et al: Epidemiology of Haemophilus influenzae type b disease among Navajo Indians. Pub Health Rep 99: 404-409, 1984.
15. Losonsky, G. A., et al: Haemophilus influenzae disease in the White Mountain Apaches: molecular epidemiology of a high risk population. Pediatr Infect Dis J 3: 539-547, 1985.
16. Ward, J. I., et al: Haemophilus influenzae disease in Alaskan Eskimos: characteristics of a population with an unusual incidence of disease. Lancet 1: 1281-1285, 1981.
17. Ward, J. I., et al: Haemophilus influenzae meningitis: a national study of secondary spread in household contacts. N Engl J Med 301: 122-126, 1979.
18. Ward, J., et al: Haemophilus influenzae bacteremia in children with sickle cell disease. J Pediatr 88: 261-263, 1976.
19. Bartlett, A. V., et al: Unusual presentations of Haemophilus influenzae infections in immunocompromised patients. J Pediatr 102: 55-58, 1983.
20. Recommendations of the Immunization Practices Advisory Committee. Polysaccharide vaccine for prevention of Haemophilus influenzae type b disease. MMWR 34(15): 201-205, 1985.
21. Santosham, M., et al: Prevention of Haemophilus influenzae type b infections in high-risk infants treated with bacterial polysaccharide immune globulin. N Engl J Med 317: 923-929, 1987.
22. Siber, G. R., et al: Preparation of human hyperimmune globulin to Haemophilus influenzae b, Streptococcus pneumoniae, and Neisseria meningitidis. Infect Immun 45: 248-254, 1984.
23. Smith, D. H., et al: Responses of children immunized with the capsular polysaccharide of Haemophilus influenzae type b. Pediatr 52: 637-645, 1973.
24. Robbins, J. B., et al: Quantitative measurement of 'natural' and immunization-induced Haemophilus influenzae type b capsular polysaccharide antibodies. Pediatr Res 7: 103-110, 1973.
25. Kaythy, H., et al: The protective level of serum antibodies to the capsular polysaccharide of Haemophilus influenzae type b. J Infect Dis 147: 1100, 1983.
26. Peltola, H., et al: Haemophilus influenzae type b capsular polysaccharide vaccine in children: a double-blind field study of 100,000 vaccinees 3 months to 5 years of age in Finland. Pediatr 60: 730-737, 1977.
27. Ward, J. I., et al: Haemophilus influenzae type b vaccines: Lessons For the Future. Pediatr 81: 886-893, 1988.
28. Daum, R. S., et al: Haemophilus influenzae type b vaccines: Lessons From the Past. Pediatr 81: 893-897, 1988.
29. Marburg, S., et al: Bimolecular chemistry of macromolecules: Synthesis of bacterial polysaccharide conjugates with Neisseria meningitidis membrane protein. J Am Chem Soc 108: 5282-5287, 1986.
30. Letson, G. W., et al: Comparison of active and combined passive/active immunization of Navajo children against Haemophilus influenzae type b. Pediatr Infect Dis J 7(111): 747-752, 1988.
31. Einhorn, M. S., et al: Immunogenicity in infants of Haemophilus influenza type b polysaccharide in a conjugate vaccine with Neisseria meningitidis outer-membrane protein. Lancet 2: 299-302, 1986.
32. Ahonkhai, V.I., et al: Haemophilus influenzae type b Conjugate Vaccine (Meningococcal Protein Conjugate) (PedvaxHIB TM): Clinical Evaluation. Pediatr 85(4): 676-681, 1990.
33. Data on file at Merck Research Laboratories.
34. Granoff, D. M., et al: Immunogenicity of Haemophilus influenzae type b polysaccharide—outer membrane protein conjugate vaccine in patients who acquired Haemophilus disease despite previous vaccination with type b polysaccharide vaccine. J. Pediatr. 114(6): 925-933, June 1989.
35. Lenoir, A. A., et al: Response to Haemophilus influenzae type b (H. influenzae type b) polysaccharide N. meningitidis outer membrane protein (PS-OMP) conjugate vaccine in relation to Km(1) and G2m(23) allotypes.

Twenty-sixth Interscience Conference on Antimicrobial Agents and Chemotherapy (Abstract #216) 133, 1986.

36. Mortimer, E. A.: Efficacy of Haemophilus b polysaccharide vaccine: An enigma. JAMA 260: 1454, 1988.

37. Meekison, W., et al: Post-marketing surveillance of adverse effects following ProHIBiT vaccine. British Columbia Canada Diseases Weekly Report 15-28: 143-145, 1989.

38. Goepp, J. G., et al: Persistent urinary antigen excretion in infants vaccinated with Haemophilus influenzae type b capsular polysaccharide conjugated with outer membrane protein from Neisseria meningitidis. Pediatr Infect Dis J 11(1): 2-5, 1992.

39. Milstein, J. B., et al: Adverse reactions reported following receipt of Haemophilus influenzae type b vaccine: An analysis after one year of marketing. Pediatr 80: 270, 1987.

40. Black, S., et al: b-CAPSA 1 Haemophilus influenzae type b capsular polysaccharide vaccine safety. Pediatr 79: 321-325, 1987.

41. D'Cruz, O. F., et al: Acute inflammatory demyelinating polyradiculoneuropathy (Guillain-Barré syndrome) after immunization with Haemophilus influenzae type b Conjugate Vaccine. J Pediatr 115: 743-746, 1989.

42. Recommendations of the Immunization Practices Advisory Committee. Recommendations for use of Haemophilus b Conjugate Vaccines and a combined diphtheria, tetanus, pertussis, and Haemophilus b vaccine. MMWR 42(RR-13): 1-15, 1993.

43. Daum, R. S., et al: Interchangeability of Haemophilus influenzae type b vaccines for the primary series (mix and match): a preliminary analysis [Abstract 976]. Pediatr Res 33: 166A, 1993.

44. Greenberg, D. P., et al: Enhanced antibody responses in infants given different sequences of heterogeneous Haemophilus influenzae type b Conjugate Vaccines. J Pediatr 126: 206-211, 1995.

45. Anderson, E. L., et al: Interchangeability of Conjugated Haemophilus influenzae type b Vaccines in Infants. JAMA 273: 849-853, 1995.

46. Recommendations of the Immunization Practices Advisory Committee. General Recommendations on Immunization. MMWR 43(RR-1), 1994.

47. Vaccine Adverse Event Reporting System - United States. MMWR 39(41): 730-733, October 19, 1990.

48. Institute of Medicine Adverse Events Associated With Childhood Vaccines Evidence Bearing on Causality. National Academy Press, Washington, D.C., 260-261, 1994.

49. Keyserling, H.L., et al: Program and Abstracts of the 30th ICAAC, (Abstract #63), 1990.

50. Ward, J.I., et al: Program and Abstracts of the 32nd ICAAC, (Abstract #984), 1992.

51. Lieberman, J.M., et al: Infect Dis, (Abstract #1028), 1993.

52. American Academy of Pediatrics. Recommended Childhood Immunization Schedule - United States, January-December 1998. Pediatr 101(1): 154-157, 1998.

Manuf and Dist by:
MERCK & CO., INC., West Point, PA 19486, USA
Issued January 2001
Printed in USA
9018902

PEGINTRON®   ℞
[pĕg-ĭn-trŏn]
(Peginterferon alfa-2b)
Injection, Powder for Solution for Subcutaneous Use

HIGHLIGHTS OF PRESCRIBING INFORMATION
These highlights do not include all the information needed to use PegIntron safely and effectively. See full prescribing information for PegIntron.
PegIntron (Peginterferon alfa-2b) Injection, Powder for Solution for Subcutaneous Use
Initial U.S. Approval: 2001

WARNING: RISK OF SERIOUS DISORDERS AND RIBAVIRIN-ASSOCIATED EFFECTS
See full prescribing information for complete boxed warning.
- May cause or aggravate fatal or life-threatening neuropsychiatric, autoimmune, ischemic, and infectious disorders. Monitor closely and withdraw therapy

---

with persistently severe or worsening signs or symptoms of the above disorders. (5)
Use with Ribavirin
- Ribavirin may cause birth defects and fetal death; avoid pregnancy in female patients and female partners of male patients. (5.1)
- Ribavirin is a potential carcinogen. (5.1, 13.1)

──────INDICATIONS AND USAGE──────
PegIntron is an antiviral indicated for
- **Combination therapy with REBETOL (ribavirin):** Chronic Hepatitis C (CHC) in patients ≥3 years with compensated liver disease. (1.1) Patients with the following characteristics are less likely to benefit from re-treatment after failing a course of therapy: previous nonresponse, previous pegylated interferon treatment, significant bridging fibrosis or cirrhosis, and genotype 1 infection. (1.1)
- **Monotherapy:** CHC in patients (≥18 years) with compensated liver disease previously untreated with interferon alpha. (1.1)

──────DOSAGE AND ADMINISTRATION──────
- PegIntron is administered by subcutaneous injection. [See table below]
- Dose reduction is recommended in patients experiencing certain adverse reactions or renal dysfunction. (2.3, 2.5)

──────DOSAGE FORMS AND STRENGTHS──────
Single-use vial (with 1.25 mL diluent) and REDIPEN® (3):
- 50 mcg per 0.5 mL, 80 mcg per 0.5 mL, 120 mcg per 0.5 mL, 150 mcg per 0.5 mL.

──────CONTRAINDICATIONS──────
- Known hypersensitivity reactions, such as urticaria, angioedema, bronchoconstriction, anaphylaxis, Stevens-Johnson syndrome, and toxic epidermal necrolysis to interferon alpha or any other product component. (4)
- Autoimmune hepatitis. (4)
- Hepatic decompensation (Child-Pugh score >6 [class B and C]) in cirrhotic CHC patients before or during treatment. (4)
Additional contraindications for combination therapy with ribavirin:
- Pregnant women and men whose female partners are pregnant. (4, 8.1)
- Hemoglobinopathies (e.g., thalassemia major, sickle-cell anemia). (4)
- Creatinine clearance <50 mL/min. (4)

──────WARNINGS AND PRECAUTIONS──────
- Birth defects and fetal death with ribavirin: Patients must have a negative pregnancy test prior to therapy, use at least 2 forms of contraception, and undergo monthly pregnancy tests. (5.1)
Patients exhibiting the following conditions should be closely monitored and may require dose reduction or discontinuation of therapy:
- Hemolytic anemia with ribavirin. (5.1)
- Neuropsychiatric events. (5.2)
- History of significant or unstable cardiac disease. (5.3)
- Hypothyroidism, hyperthyroidism, hyperglycemia, diabetes mellitus that cannot be effectively treated by medication. (5.4)
- New or worsening ophthalmologic disorders. (5.5)
- Ischemic and hemorrhagic cerebrovascular events. (5.6)
- Severe decreases in neutrophil or platelet counts. (5.7)
- History of autoimmune disorders. (5.8)
- Pancreatitis and ulcerative or hemorrhagic/ischemic colitis and pancreatitis. (5.9, 5.10)

- Pulmonary infiltrates or pulmonary function impairment. (5.11)
- Child-Pugh score >6 (class B and C). (4, 5.12)
- Increased creatinine levels in patients with renal insufficiency. (5.13)
- Serious, acute hypersensitivity reactions and cutaneous eruptions. (5.14)
- Dental/periodontal disorders reported with combination therapy. (5.16)
- Hypertriglyceridemia may result in pancreatitis (e.g., triglycerides >1000 mg/dL). (5.17)
- Weight loss and growth inhibition reported with combination therapy in pediatric patients. (5.18)
- Peripheral neuropathy when used in combination with telbivudine. (5.19)

──────ADVERSE REACTIONS──────
Most common adverse reactions (>40%) in adult patients receiving either PegIntron or PegIntron/REBETOL are injection site inflammation/reaction, fatigue/asthenia, headache, rigors, fevers, nausea, myalgia and anxiety/emotional lability/irritability (6.1). Most common adverse reactions (>25%) in pediatric patients receiving PegIntron/REBETOL are pyrexia, headache, neutropenia, fatigue, anorexia, injection-site erythema, vomiting (6.1).
To report SUSPECTED ADVERSE REACTIONS, contact Schering Corporation at 1-800-526-4099 or FDA at 1-800-FDA-1088 or www.fda.gov/medwatch.

──────DRUG INTERACTIONS──────
- Drug metabolized by CYP450: Caution with drugs metabolized by CYP2C8/9 (e.g., warfarin, phenytoin) or CYP2D6 (e.g., flecainide). (7.1)
- Methadone: Monitor for increased narcotic effect. (7.2)
- Nucleoside analogues: Closely monitor for toxicities. Discontinue nucleoside reverse transcriptase inhibitors or reduce dose or discontinue interferon, ribavirin, or both with worsening toxicities. (7.3)
- Didanosine: Concurrent use with REBETOL is not recommended. (7.3)

──────USE IN SPECIFIC POPULATIONS──────
- Ribavirin Pregnancy Registry: 1-800-593-2214. (8.1)
- Pediatrics: safety and efficacy in pediatrics <3 years old have not been established (8.4)
- Geriatrics: neuropsychiatric, cardiac, pulmonary, GI, and systemic (flu-like) adverse reactions may be more severe (8.5)
- Organ transplant: safety and efficacy have not been studied (8.6)
- HIV or HBV coinfection: safety and efficacy have not been established (8.7)

See 17 for PATIENT COUNSELING INFORMATION and Medication Guide

Revised: 01/2010

FULL PRESCRIBING INFORMATION: CONTENTS*
WARNING: RISK OF SERIOUS DISORDERS AND RIBAVIRIN-ASSOCIATED EFFECTS

	PegIntron Dose (Adults)*	PegIntron Dose (Pediatric Patients)	REBETOL Dose* (Adults)	REBETOL Dose (Pediatric Patients)
PegIntron/REBETOL Combination Therapy (2.1)	1.5 mcg/kg/week	60 mcg/m²/week	800–1400 mg orally daily with food	15 mg/kg/day orally with food in 2 divided doses

*Refer to Tables 1–7 of the full Prescribing Information.

FULL PRESCRIBING INFORMATION

> **WARNING: RISK OF SERIOUS DISORDERS AND RIBAVIRIN-ASSOCIATED EFFECTS**
>
> Alpha interferons, including PegIntron, may cause or aggravate fatal or life-threatening neuropsychiatric, autoimmune, ischemic, and infectious disorders. Patients should be monitored closely with periodic clinical and laboratory evaluations. Patients with persistently severe or worsening signs or symptoms of these conditions should be withdrawn from therapy. In many, but not all cases, these disorders resolve after stopping PegIntron therapy *[see Warnings and Precautions (5) and Adverse Reactions (6.1)]*.
>
> **Use with Ribavirin**
>
> Ribavirin may cause birth defects and death of the unborn child. Extreme care must be taken to avoid pregnancy in female patients and in female partners of male patients. Ribavirin causes hemolytic anemia. The anemia associated with REBETOL therapy may result in a worsening of cardiac disease. Ribavirin is genotoxic and mutagenic and should be considered a potential carcinogen. *[See REBETOL package insert]*

1 INDICATIONS AND USAGE

1.1 Chronic Hepatitis C

Combination therapy:

PegIntron® in combination with REBETOL® (ribavirin) is indicated for the treatment of chronic hepatitis C in patients 3 years of age and older with compensated liver disease.

The following points should be considered when initiating therapy with PegIntron in combination with REBETOL:

- These indications are based on achieving undetectable HCV-RNA after treatment for 24 or 48 weeks and maintaining a Sustained Virologic Response (SVR) 24 weeks after the last dose.
- Patients with the following characteristics are less likely to benefit from retreatment after failing a course of therapy: previous nonresponse, previous pegylated interferon treatment, significant bridging fibrosis or cirrhosis, and genotype 1 infection *[see Clinical Studies (14)]*.
- No safety and efficacy data are available for treatment of longer than 1 year.

Monotherapy (for patients who are intolerant to ribavirin):

PegIntron (peginterferon alfa-2b) is indicated for use alone for the treatment of chronic hepatitis C in patients with compensated liver disease previously untreated with interferon alpha and who are at least 18 years of age.

The following point should be considered when initiating therapy with PegIntron alone:

- Combination therapy with REBETOL is preferred over PegIntron monotherapy unless there are contraindications to or significant intolerance of REBETOL.

Combination therapy provides substantially better response rates than monotherapy *[see Clinical Studies (14)]*.

2 DOSAGE AND ADMINISTRATION

2.1 PegIntron/REBETOL Combination Therapy

REBETOL® should be taken with food. REBETOL should not be used in patients with creatinine clearance <50 mL/min.

TABLE 1 Recommended PegIntron Combination Therapy Dosing (Adults)

Body weight kg (lbs)	PegIntron REDIPEN® or Vial Strength to Use	Amount of PegIntron (mcg) to Administer	Volume (mL)* of PegIntron to Administer	REBETOL Daily Dose	REBETOL Number of Capsules
<40 (<88)	50 mcg per 0.5 mL	50	0.5	800 mg/day	2 × 200 mg capsules A.M. / 2 × 200 mg capsules P.M.
40–50 (88–111)	80 mcg per 0.5 mL	64	0.4	800 mg/day	2 × 200 mg capsules A.M. / 2 × 200 mg capsules P.M.
51–60 (112–133)		80	0.5	800 mg/day	2 × 200 mg capsules A.M. / 2 × 200 mg capsules P.M.
61–65 (134–144)		96	0.4	800 mg/day	2 × 200 mg capsules A.M. / 2 × 200 mg capsules P.M.
66–75 (145–166)	120 mcg per 0.5 mL	96	0.4	1000 mg/day	2 × 200 mg capsules A.M. / 3 × 200 mg capsules P.M.
76–80 (167–177)		120	0.5	1000 mg/day	2 × 200 mg capsules A.M. / 3 × 200 mg capsules P.M.
81–85 (178–187)				1200 mg/day	3 × 200 mg capsules A.M. / 3 × 200 mg capsules P.M.
86–105 (188–231)	150 mcg per 0.5 mL	150	0.5	1200 mg/day	3 × 200 mg capsules A.M. / 3 × 200 mg capsules P.M.
>105 (>231)	†	†	†	1400 mg/day	3 × 200 mg capsules A.M. / 4 × 200 mg capsules P.M.

* When reconstituted as directed.
† For patients weighing >105 kg (>231 pounds), the PegIntron dose of 1.5 mcg/kg/week should be calculated based on the individual patient weight. Two vials of PegIntron may be necessary to provide the dose.

Adults

The recommended dose of PegIntron is 1.5 mcg/kg/week subcutaneously in combination with 800 to 1400 mg of REBETOL orally based on patient body weight. The volume of PegIntron to be injected depends on the strength of PegIntron and patient's body weight (*see Table 1*).

Duration of Treatment – Interferon Alpha-naïve Patients

The treatment duration for patients with genotype 1 is 48 weeks. Discontinuation of therapy should be considered in patients who do not achieve at least a 2 log$_{10}$ drop or loss of HCV-RNA at 12 weeks, or if HCV-RNA remains detectable after 24 weeks of therapy. Patients with genotype 2 and 3 should be treated for 24 weeks.

Duration of Treatment – Re-treatment with PegIntron/REBETOL of Prior Treatment Failures

The treatment duration for patients who previously failed therapy is 48 weeks, regardless of HCV genotype. Retreated patients who fail to achieve undetectable HCV-RNA at Week 12 of therapy, or whose HCV-RNA remains detectable after 24 weeks of therapy, are highly unlikely to achieve SVR and discontinuation of therapy should be considered *[see Clinical Studies (14.1)]*.

[See table 1 above]

Pediatric Patients

Dosing for pediatric patients is determined by body surface area for PegIntron and by body weight for REBETOL. The recommended dose of PegIntron is 60 mcg/m^2/week subcutaneously in combination with 15 mg/kg/day of REBETOL orally in 2 divided doses (*see Table 2*) for pediatric patients ages 3 to 17 years. Patients who reach their 18th birthday while receiving PegIntron/REBETOL, should remain on the pediatric dosing regimen. The treatment duration for patients with genotype 1 is 48 weeks. Patients with genotype 2 and 3 should be treated for 24 weeks.

TABLE 2 Recommended REBETOL* Dosing in Combination Therapy (Pediatrics)

Body weight kg (lbs)	REBETOL Daily Dose	REBETOL Number of Capsules
<47 (<103)	15 mg/kg/day	Use REBETOL Oral Solution†
47–59 (103–131)	800 mg/day	2 × 200 mg capsules A.M. / 2 × 200 mg capsules P.M.
60–73 (132–162)	1000 mg/day	2 × 200 mg capsules A.M. / 3 × 200 mg capsules P.M.
>73 (>162)	1200 mg/day	3 × 200 mg capsules A.M. / 3 × 200 mg capsules P.M.

* REBETOL to be used in combination with PegIntron 60 mcg/m^2 weekly.
† REBETOL Oral Solution may be used for any patient regardless of body weight.

2.2 PegIntron Monotherapy

The recommended dose of PegIntron regimen is 1 mcg/kg/week subcutaneously for 1 year administered on the same day of the week. Discontinuation of therapy should be considered in patients who do not achieve at least a 2 log$_{10}$ drop or loss of HCV-RNA at 12 weeks of therapy, or whose HCV-RNA levels remain detectable after 24 weeks of therapy. The volume of PegIntron to be injected depends on patient weight (*see Table 3*).

[See table 3 at top of next page]

2.3 Dose Reduction

If a serious adverse reaction develops during the course of treatment *[see Warnings and Precautions (5)]* discontinue or modify the dosage of PegIntron and REBETOL until the adverse event abates or decreases in severity. If persistent or recurrent serious adverse events develop despite adequate dosage adjustment, discontinue treatment. For guidelines for dose modifications and discontinuation based on depression or laboratory parameters, *see Tables 4 and 5*. Dose reduction of PegIntron in adult patients on PegIntron/REBETOL combination therapy is accomplished in a two-step process from the original starting dose of 1.5 mcg/kg/week, to 1 mcg/kg/week, then to 0.5 mcg/kg/week, if needed. Dose reduction in patients on PegIntron monotherapy is accomplished by reducing the original starting dose of 1 mcg/kg/week to 0.5 mcg/kg/week. Dose reduction of PegIntron in adults may be accomplished by utilizing a lower dose strength or administering a lesser volume as shown in *Table 6 or 7*.

In the adult combination therapy Study 2, dose reductions occurred in 42% of subjects receiving PegIntron 1.5 mcg/kg plus REBETOL 800 mg daily, including 57% of those subjects weighing 60 kg or less. In Study 4, 16% of subjects had a dose reduction of PegIntron to 1 mcg/kg in combination with REBETOL, with an additional 4% requiring the second dose reduction of PegIntron to 0.5 mcg/kg due to adverse events *[see Adverse Reactions (6.1)]*.

Dose reduction in pediatric patients is accomplished by modifying the recommended dose in a 2-step process from the original starting dose of 60 mcg/m^2/week, to 40 mcg/m^2/week, then to 20 mcg/m^2/week, if needed (*see Tables 4 and 5*). In the pediatric combination therapy trial, dose reduc-

tions occurred in 25% of subjects receiving PegIntron 60 mcg/m² weekly plus REBETOL 15 mg/kg daily.
[See table 4 at right]
[See table 5 at right]
[See table 6 at top of next page]
[See table 7 on next page]

2.4 Discontinuation of Dosing

Adults

It is recommended that HCV genotype 1 interferon-alfa-naïve patients receiving PegIntron, alone or in combination with ribavirin, be discontinued from therapy if there is not at least a 2 $\log_{10}$ drop or loss of HCV-RNA at 12 weeks of therapy, or whose HCV-RNA levels remain detectable after 24 weeks of therapy. Regardless of genotype, previously treated patients who have detectable HCV-RNA at Week 12 or 24, are highly unlikely to achieve SVR and discontinuation of therapy should be considered.

Pediatrics (3–17 years of age)

It is recommended that patients receiving PegIntron/REBETOL combination (excluding those with HCV Genotype 2 and 3) be discontinued from therapy at 12 weeks if their treatment Week 12 HCV-RNA dropped <2 $\log_{10}$ compared to pretreatment or at 24 weeks if they have detectable HCV-RNA at treatment Week 24.

2.5 Renal Function

In patients with moderate renal dysfunction (creatinine clearance 30–50 mL/min), the PegIntron dose should be reduced by 25%. Patients with severe renal dysfunction (creatinine clearance 10–29 mL/min), including those on hemodialysis, should have the PegIntron dose reduced by 50%. If renal function decreases during treatment, PegIntron therapy should be discontinued. When PegIntron is administered in combination with REBETOL, subjects with impaired renal function or those over the age of 50 should be more carefully monitored with respect to the development of anemia. PegIntron/REBETOL should not be used in patients with creatinine clearance <50 mL/min.

2.6 Preparation and Administration

PegIntron REDIPEN

PegIntron REDIPEN consists of a dual-chamber glass cartridge with sterile, lyophilized peginterferon alfa-2b in the active chamber and Sterile Water for Injection USP in the diluent chamber. The PegIntron in the glass cartridge should appear as a white to off-white tablet-shaped solid that is whole or in pieces, or powder.

To reconstitute the lyophilized peginterferon alfa-2b in the REDIPEN:

- Hold the REDIPEN upright (dose button down) and press the 2 halves of the pen together until there is an audible click.
- Gently invert the pen to mix the solution. **DO NOT SHAKE.** The reconstituted solution has a concentration of either 50 mcg per 0.5 mL, 80 mcg per 0.5 mL, 120 mcg per 0.5 mL, or 150 mcg per 0.5 mL for a single subcutaneous injection.
- Visually inspect the solution for particulate matter and discoloration prior to administration. The reconstituted solution should be clear and colorless. Do not use the solution if it is discolored or not clear, or if particulates are present.

Keeping the pen upright, attach the supplied needle and select the appropriate PegIntron dose by pulling back on the dosing button until the dark bands are visible and turning the button until the dark band is aligned with the correct dose. The prepared PegIntron solution is to be injected subcutaneously.

The PegIntron REDIPEN is a single-use pen and does not contain a preservative. The reconstituted solution should be used immediately and cannot be stored for more than 24 hours at 2°–8° C [see How Supplied/Storage and Handling (16)]. **DO NOT REUSE THE REDIPEN.** The sterility of any remaining product can no longer be guaranteed. **DISCARD THE UNUSED PORTION.** Pooling of unused portions of some medications has been linked to bacterial contamination and morbidity.

PegIntron Vials

Two BD® Safety-Lok® syringes are provided in the package; one syringe is for the reconstitution steps and one for the patient injection. There is a plastic safety sleeve to be pulled over the needle after use. The syringe locks with an audible click when the green stripe on the safety sleeve covers the red stripe on the needle. Instructions for the preparation and administration of PegIntron Powder for Injection are provided below.

- **Reconstitute the PegIntron lyophilized product with only 0.7 mL of the 1.25 mL of supplied diluent (Sterile Water for Injection USP). The diluent vial is for single use only. The remaining diluent should be discarded.** No other medications should be added to solutions containing

PegIntron, and PegIntron should not be reconstituted with other diluents.
- Swirl gently to hasten complete dissolution of the powder. The reconstituted solution should be clear and colorless.
- Visually inspect the solution for particulate matter and discoloration prior to administration. The solution should not be used if discolored or cloudy, or if particulates are present.

TABLE 3 Recommended PegIntron Monotherapy Dosing

Body weight kg (lbs)	PegIntron REDIPEN or Vial Strength to Use	Amount of PegIntron (mcg) to Administer	Volume (mL)* of PegIntron to Administer
≤45 (≤100)	50 mcg per 0.5 mL	40	0.4
46–56 (101–124)		50	0.5
57–72 (125–159)	80 mcg per 0.5 mL	64	0.4
73–88 (160–195)		80	0.5
89–106 (196–234)	120 mcg per 0.5 mL	96	0.4
107–136 (235–300)		120	0.5
137–160 (301–353)	150 mcg per 0.5 mL	150	0.5

*When reconstituted as directed.

TABLE 4 Guidelines for Modification or Discontinuation of PegIntron or PegIntron/REBETOL and for Scheduling Visits for Patients with Depression

Depression Severity*	Initial Management (4–8 Weeks)		Depression Status		
	Dose Modification	Visit Schedule	Remains Stable	Improves	Worsens
Mild	No change	Evaluate once weekly by visit or phone.	Continue weekly visit schedule.	Resume normal visit schedule.	See moderate or severe depression
Moderate	Adults: Adjust Dose† Pediatrics: Decrease dose to 40 mcg/m²/week, then to 20 mcg/m²/week, if needed	Evaluate once weekly (office visit at least every other week).	Consider psychiatric consultation. Continue reduced dosing.	If symptoms improve and are stable for 4 weeks, may resume normal visit schedule. Continue reduced dosing or return to normal dose.	See severe depression
Severe	Discontinue PegIntron/ REBETOL permanently.	Obtain immediate psychiatric consultation.	Psychiatric therapy as necessary		

* See DSM-IV for definitions.
† For patients on PegIntron/REBETOL combination therapy: 1st dose reduction of PegIntron is to 1 mcg/kg/week, 2nd dose reduction (if needed) of PegIntron is to 0.5 mcg/kg/week. For patients on PegIntron monotherapy: decrease PegIntron dose to 0.5 mcg/kg/week.

TABLE 5. Guidelines for Dose Modification and Discontinuation of PegIntron or PegIntron/REBETOL Based on Laboratory Parameters in Adults and Pediatrics

Laboratory Values		PegIntron		REBETOL	
		Adults	Pediatrics	Adults	Pediatrics
Hgb	< 10 g/dL	For patients with cardiac disease, reduce by 50%*	See footnote*	Adjust Dose†	1st reduction to 12 mg/kg/day 2nd reduction to 8 mg/kg/day
WBC Neutrophils Platelets	< 1.5 × 10⁹/L < 0.75 × 10⁹/L < 50 × 10⁹/L (Adults) < 70 × 10⁹/L (Pediatrics)	Adjust Dose‡	1st reduction to 40 mcg/m²/week 2nd reduction to 20 mcg/m²/week	No Dose Change	No Dose Change
Hgb WBC Neutrophils Platelets Creatinine	< 8.5 g/dL <1 × 10⁹/L < 0.5 × 10⁹/L < 25 × 10⁹/L (Adults) < 50 ×10⁹/L (Pediatrics) > 2 mg/dL (Pediatrics)	Permanently Discontinue	Permanently Discontinue	Permanently Discontinue	Permanently Discontinue

* For adult patients with a history of stable cardiac disease receiving PegIntron in combination with ribavirin, the PegIntron dose should be reduced by half and the ribavirin dose by 200 mg/day if a >2 g/dL decrease in hemoglobin is observed during any 4-week period. Both PegIntron and ribavirin should be permanently discontinued if patients have hemoglobin levels <12 g/dL after this ribavirin dose reduction. Pediatric patients who have pre-existing cardiac conditions and experience a hemoglobin decrease ≥2 g/dL during any 4-week period during treatment should have weekly evaluations and hematology testing.
† 1st dose reduction of REBETOL is by 200 mg/day, except in patients receiving the 1400 mg dose it is by 400 mg/day; 2nd dose reduction of REBETOL (if needed) is by an additional 200 mg/day.
‡ For patients on PegIntron/REBETOL combination therapy: 1st dose reduction of PegIntron is to 1 mcg/kg/week, 2nd dose reduction (if needed) of PegIntron is to 0.5 mcg/kg/week. For patients on PegIntron monotherapy: decrease PegIntron dose to 0.5 mcg/kg/week.

- The appropriate PegIntron dose should be withdrawn and injected subcutaneously. PegIntron vials are for single use only and do not contain a preservative.

The reconstituted solution should be used immediately and cannot be stored for more than 24 hours at 2°–8° C [see How Supplied/Storage and Handling (16)]. **DO NOT REUSE THE VIAL.** The sterility of any remaining product can no longer be guaranteed. **DISCARD THE UNUSED PORTION.** Pooling of unused portions of some medications has been linked to bacterial contamination and morbidity.

3 DOSAGE FORMS AND STRENGTHS

- Single-use vial: 1.25 mL diluent vial: 50 mcg per 0.5 mL, 80 mcg per 0.5 mL, 120 mcg per 0.5 mL, 150 mcg per 0.5 mL.
- Single-use REDIPEN: 50 mcg per 0.5 mL, 80 mcg per 0.5 mL, 120 mcg per 0.5 mL, 150 mcg per 0.5 mL.

4 CONTRAINDICATIONS

PegIntron is contraindicated in patients with:

- known hypersensitivity reactions, such as urticaria, angioedema, bronchoconstriction, anaphylaxis, Stevens-Johnson syndrome, and toxic epidermal necrolysis to interferon alpha or any other component of the product
- autoimmune hepatitis
- hepatic decompensation (Child-Pugh score >6 [class B and C]) in cirrhotic CHC patients before or during treatment

PegIntron/REBETOL combination therapy is additionally contraindicated in:

- women who are pregnant. REBETOL may cause fetal harm when administered to a pregnant woman. REBETOL is contraindicated in women who are or may become pregnant. If this drug is used during pregnancy, or if the patient becomes pregnant while taking this drug the patient should be apprised of the potential hazard to a fetus [see Use in Specific Populations (8.1)].
- men whose female partners are pregnant
- patients with hemoglobinopathies (e.g., thalassemia major, sickle-cell anemia)
- patients with creatinine clearance <50 mL/min

5 WARNINGS AND PRECAUTIONS

Patients should be monitored for the following serious conditions, some of which may become life threatening. Patients with persistently severe or worsening signs or symptoms should be withdrawn from therapy.

5.1 Use with Ribavirin

Pregnancy

REBETOL may cause birth defects and death of the unborn child. REBETOL therapy should not be started until a report of a negative pregnancy test has been obtained immediately prior to planned initiation of therapy. Patients should use at least 2 forms of contraception and have monthly pregnancy tests [see BOXED WARNING, Contraindications (4), Patient Counseling Information (17), and REBETOL package insert].

Anemia

Ribavirin caused hemolytic anemia in 10% of PegIntron/REBETOL-treated subjects within 1 to 4 weeks of initiation of therapy. Complete blood counts should be obtained pretreatment and at Week 2 and Week 4 of therapy or more frequently if clinically indicated. Anemia associated with REBETOL therapy may result in a worsening of cardiac disease. Decrease in dosage or discontinuation of REBETOL may be necessary [see Dosage and Administration (2.3) and REBETOL package insert].

5.2 Neuropsychiatric Events

Life-threatening or fatal neuropsychiatric events, including suicide, suicidal and homicidal ideation, depression, relapse of drug addiction/overdose, and aggressive behavior sometimes directed towards others have occurred in patients with and without a previous psychiatric disorder during PegIntron treatment and follow-up. Psychoses, hallucinations, bipolar disorders, and mania have been observed in patients treated with interferon alpha. PegIntron should be used with extreme caution in patients with a history of psychiatric disorders. Patients should be advised to report immediately any symptoms of depression or suicidal ideation to their prescribing physicians. Physicians should monitor all patients for evidence of depression and other psychiatric symptoms. If patients develop psychiatric problems, including clinical depression, it is recommended that the patients be carefully monitored during treatment and in the 6-month follow-up period. If psychiatric symptoms persist or worsen, or suicidal ideation or aggressive behavior towards others is identified, it is recommended that treatment with PegIntron be discontinued, and the patient followed, with psychiatric intervention as appropriate. In severe cases, PegIntron should be stopped immediately and psychiatric intervention instituted [see Dosage and Administration (2.3)]. Cases of encephalopathy have been observed in some patients, usually elderly, treated at higher doses of PegIntron.

TABLE 6 Reduced PegIntron Dose (0.5 mcg/kg) for (1 mcg/kg) Monotherapy in Adults

Body weight kg (lbs)	PegIntron REDIPEN/Vial Strength to Use	Amount of PegIntron (mcg) to Administer	Volume (mL)* of PegIntron to Administer
≤45 (≤100)	50 mcg per 0.5 mL†	20	0.2
46–56 (101–124)		25	0.25
57–72 (125–159)	50 mcg per 0.5 mL	30	0.3
73–88 (160–195)		40	0.4
89–106 (196–234)	50 mcg per 0.5 mL	50	0.5
107–136 (235–300)	80 mcg per 0.5 mL	64	0.4
≥137 (≥301)		80	0.5

* When reconstituted as directed.
† Must use vial. Minimum delivery for REDIPEN 0.3 mL.

TABLE 7 Two-Step Dose Reduction of PegIntron in Combination Therapy in Adults

First Dose Reduction to PegIntron 1 mcg/kg				Second Dose Reduction to PegIntron 0.5 mcg/kg			
Body weight kg (lbs)	PegIntron REDIPEN/Vial Strength to Use	Amount of PegIntron (mcg) to Administer	Volume (mL)* of PegIntron to Administer	Body weight kg (lbs)	PegIntron REDIPEN/Vial Strength to Use	Amount of PegIntron (mcg) to Administer	Volume (mL)* of PegIntron to Administer
<40 (<88)	50 mcg per 0.5 mL	35	0.35	<40 (<88)	50 mcg per 0.5 mL†	20	0.2
40–50 (88–111)		45	0.45	40–50 (88–111)		25	0.25
51–60 (112–133)		50	0.5	51–60 (112–133)		30	0.3
61–75 (134–166)	80 mcg per 0.5 mL	64	0.4	61–75 (134–166)	50 mcg per 0.5 mL	35	0.35
76–85 (167–187)		80	0.5	76–85 (167–187)		45	0.45
86–104 (188–230)	120 mcg per 0.5 mL	96	0.4	86–104 (188–230)		50	0.5
105–125 (231–275)		108	0.45	105–125 (231–275)	80 mcg per 0.5 mL	64	0.4
>125 (>275)	150 mcg per 0.5 mL	135	0.45	>125 (>275)		72	0.45

* When reconstituted as directed.
† Must use vial. Minimum delivery for REDIPEN 0.3 mL

5.3 Cardiovascular Events

Cardiovascular events, which include hypotension, arrhythmia, tachycardia, cardiomyopathy, angina pectoris, and myocardial infarction, have been observed in patients treated with PegIntron. PegIntron should be used cautiously in patients with cardiovascular disease. Patients with a history of myocardial infarction and arrhythmic disorder who require PegIntron therapy should be closely monitored [see Warnings and Precautions (5.15)]. Patients with a history of significant or unstable cardiac disease should not be treated with PegIntron/REBETOL combination therapy [see REBETOL package insert].

5.4 Endocrine Disorders

PegIntron causes or aggravates hypothyroidism and hyperthyroidism. Hyperglycemia has been observed in patients treated with PegIntron. Diabetes mellitus, including cases of new onset Type 1 diabetes, has been observed in patients treated with alpha interferons, including PegIntron. Patients with these conditions who cannot be effectively treated by medication should not begin PegIntron therapy. Patients who develop these conditions during treatment and cannot be controlled with medication should not continue PegIntron therapy.

5.5 Ophthalmologic Disorders

Decrease or loss of vision, retinopathy including macular edema, retinal artery or vein thrombosis, retinal hemorrhages and cotton wool spots, optic neuritis, papilledema, and serous retinal detachment may be induced or aggravated by treatment with peginterferon alfa-2b or other alpha interferons. All patients should receive an eye examination at baseline. Patients with preexisting ophthalmologic disorders (e.g., diabetic or hypertensive retinopathy) should receive periodic ophthalmologic exams during interferon alpha treatment. Any patient who develops ocular symptoms should receive a prompt and complete eye examination. Peginterferon alfa-2b treatment should be discontinued in patients who develop new or worsening ophthalmologic disorders.

5.6 Cerebrovascular Disorders

Ischemic and hemorrhagic cerebrovascular events have been observed in patients treated with interferon alfa-based therapies, including PegIntron. Events occurred in patients with few or no reported risk factors for stroke, including patients less than 45 years of age. Because these are spontaneous reports, estimates of frequency cannot be made, and a causal relationship between interferon alfa-based therapies and these events is difficult to establish.

5.7 Bone Marrow Toxicity

PegIntron suppresses bone marrow function, sometimes resulting in severe cytopenias. PegIntron should be discontinued in patients who develop severe decreases in neutrophil or platelet counts [see Dosage and Administration (2.3)]. Ribavirin may potentiate the neutropenia induced by interferon alpha. Very rarely alpha interferons may be associated with aplastic anemia.

5.8 Autoimmune Disorders

Development or exacerbation of autoimmune disorders (e.g., thyroiditis, thrombotic thrombocytopenic purpura, idiopathic thrombocytopenic purpura, rheumatoid arthritis, interstitial nephritis, systemic lupus erythematosus, and psoriasis) have been observed in patients receiving PegIntron. PegIntron should be used with caution in patients with autoimmune disorders.

5.9 Pancreatitis

Fatal and nonfatal pancreatitis have been observed in patients treated with alpha interferon. PegIntron therapy should be suspended in patients with signs and symptoms suggestive of pancreatitis and discontinued in patients diagnosed with pancreatitis.

TABLE 8 Adverse Reactions Occurring in > 5% of Subjects

Adverse Events	Percentage of Subjects Reporting Adverse Reactions*			
	Study 1		Study 2	
	PegIntron 1 mcg/kg (n=297)	INTRON A 3 MIU (n=303)	PegIntron 1.5 mcg/kg/REBETOL (n=511)	INTRON A/ REBETOL (n=505)
Application Site				
Injection Site Inflammation/Reaction	47	20	75	49
Autonomic Nervous System				
Dry Mouth	6	7	12	8
Increased Sweating	6	7	11	7
Flushing	6	3	4	3
Body as a Whole				
Fatigue/Asthenia	52	54	66	63
Headache	56	52	62	58
Rigors	23	19	48	41
Fever	22	12	46	33
Weight Loss	11	13	29	20
Right Upper Quadrant Pain	8	8	12	6
Chest Pain	6	4	8	7
Malaise	7	6	4	6
Central/Peripheral Nervous System				
Dizziness	12	10	21	17
Endocrine				
Hypothyroidism	5	3	5	4
Gastrointestinal				
Nausea	26	20	43	33
Anorexia	20	17	32	27
Diarrhea	18	16	22	17
Vomiting	7	6	14	12
Abdominal Pain	15	11	13	13
Dyspepsia	6	7	9	8
Constipation	1	3	5	5
Hematologic Disorders				
Neutropenia	6	2	26	14
Anemia	0	0	12	17
Leukopenia	<1	0	6	5
Thrombocytopenia	7	<1	5	2
Liver and Biliary System				
Hepatomegaly	6	5	4	4
Musculoskeletal				
Myalgia	54	53	56	50
Arthralgia	23	27	34	28
Musculoskeletal Pain	28	22	21	19

(Table continued on next page)

5.10   Colitis
Fatal and nonfatal ulcerative or hemorrhagic/ischemic colitis have been observed within 12 weeks of the start of alpha interferon treatment. Abdominal pain, bloody diarrhea, and fever are the typical manifestations. PegIntron treatment should be discontinued immediately in patients who develop these signs and symptoms. The colitis usually resolves within 1 to 3 weeks of discontinuation of alpha interferons.

5.11   Pulmonary Disorders
Dyspnea, pulmonary infiltrates, pneumonia, bronchiolitis obliterans, interstitial pneumonitis, pulmonary hypertension, and sarcoidosis, some resulting in respiratory failure or patient deaths, may be induced or aggravated by PegIntron or alpha interferon therapy. Recurrence of respiratory failure has been observed with interferon rechallenge. PegIntron combination treatment should be sus-

pended in patients who develop pulmonary infiltrates or pulmonary function impairment. Patients who resume interferon treatment should be closely monitored.

5.12   Hepatic Failure
Chronic hepatitis C (CHC) patients with cirrhosis may be at risk of hepatic decompensation and death when treated with alpha interferons, including PegIntron. Cirrhotic CHC patients coinfected with HIV receiving highly active antiretroviral therapy (HAART) and alpha interferons with or without ribavirin appear to be at increased risk for the development of hepatic decompensation compared to patients not receiving HAART. During treatment, patients' clinical status and hepatic function should be closely monitored, and PegIntron treatment should be immediately discontinued if decompensation (Child-Pugh score >6) is observed *[see Contraindications (4)]*.

5.13   Patients with Renal Insufficiency
Increases in serum creatinine levels have been observed in patients with renal insufficiency receiving interferon alpha products, including PegIntron. Patients with impaired renal function should be closely monitored for signs and symptoms of interferon toxicity, including increases in serum creatinine, and PegIntron dosing should be adjusted accordingly or discontinued *[see Clinical Pharmacology (12.3) and Dosage and Administration (2.3)]*. PegIntron monotherapy should be used with caution in patients with creatinine clearance <50 mL/min; the potential risks should be weighed against the potential benefits in these patients. Combination therapy with REBETOL must not be used in patients with creatinine clearance <50 mL/min *[see REBETOL Package Insert]*.

5.14   Hypersensitivity
Serious, acute hypersensitivity reactions (e.g., urticaria, angioedema, bronchoconstriction, anaphylaxis) and cutaneous eruptions (Stevens-Johnson syndrome, toxic epidermal necrolysis) have been rarely observed during alpha interferon therapy. If such a reaction develops during treatment with PegIntron, discontinue treatment and institute appropriate medical therapy immediately. Transient rashes do not necessitate interruption of treatment.

5.15   Laboratory Tests
PegIntron alone or in combination with ribavirin may cause severe decreases in neutrophil and platelet counts, and hematologic, endocrine (e.g., TSH), and hepatic abnormalities. Transient elevations in ALT (2- to 5-fold above baseline) were observed in 10% of subjects treated with PegIntron, and were not associated with deterioration of other liver functions. Triglyceride levels are frequently elevated in patients receiving alpha interferon therapy including PegIntron and should be periodically monitored.

Patients on PegIntron or PegIntron/REBETOL combination therapy should have hematology and blood chemistry testing before the start of treatment and then periodically thereafter. In the adult clinical trial CBC (including hemoglobin, neutrophil, and platelet counts) and chemistries (including AST, ALT, bilirubin, and uric acid) were measured during the treatment period at Weeks 2, 4, 8, and 12, and then at 6-week intervals or more frequently if abnormalities developed. In pediatric subjects, the same laboratory parameters were evaluated with additional assessment of hemoglobin at treatment Week 6. TSH levels were measured every 12 weeks during the treatment period. HCV-RNA should be measured periodically during treatment *[see Dosage and Administration (2)]*.

Patients who have pre-existing cardiac abnormalities should have electrocardiograms done before treatment with PegIntron/REBETOL.

5.16   Dental and Periodontal Disorders
Dental and periodontal disorders have been reported in patients receiving PegIntron/REBETOL combination therapy. In addition, dry mouth could have a damaging effect on teeth and mucous membranes of the mouth during long-term treatment with the combination of REBETOL and PegIntron. Patients should brush their teeth thoroughly twice daily and have regular dental examinations. If vomiting occurs, patients should be advised to rinse out their mouth thoroughly afterwards.

5.17   Triglycerides
Elevated triglyceride levels have been observed in patients treated with interferon alpha, including PegIntron therapy. Hypertriglyceridemia may result in pancreatitis *[see Warnings and Precautions (5.9)]*. Elevated triglyceride levels should be managed as clinically appropriate. Discontinuation of PegIntron therapy should be considered for patients with symptoms of potential pancreatitis, such as abdominal pain, nausea, or vomiting, and persistently elevated triglycerides (e.g., triglycerides >1000 mg/dL).

5.18   Impact on Growth-Pediatric Use
Data on the effects of PegIntron plus REBETOL on growth come from an open-label study in subjects 3 through 17 years of age, and weight and height changes are compared to US normative population data. In general, the weight and height gain of pediatric subjects treated with PegIntron plus REBETOL lags behind that predicted by normative

population data for the entire length of treatment. After about 6 months post-treatment (follow-up Week 24), subjects had weight gain rebounds and regained their weight to 53rd percentile, above the average of the normative population and similar to that predicted by their average baseline weight (57th percentile). After about 6 months post-treatment, height gain stabilized and subjects treated with PegIntron plus REBETOL had an average height percentile of 44th percentile, which was less than the average of the normative population and less than their average baseline height (51st percentile). Severely inhibited growth velocity (< 3rd percentile) was observed in 70% of the subjects while on treatment. Of the subjects experiencing severely inhibited growth, 20% had continued inhibited growth velocity (< 3rd percentile) after 6 months of follow-up.

Among the boys studied, the age groups of 3 to 11 years old and 12 to 17 years old had similar height percentile decreases of approximately 5 percentiles after 6 months post-treatment; weight gain continued to be similar to their average baseline percentile. Girls who were 3 to 11 years old and treated for 48 weeks had the largest average drop in height and weight percentiles (13 percentiles and 7 percentiles, respectively), whereas girls 12 to 17 years old continued along their average baseline height and weight percentiles after 6 months post-treatment.

5.19 Peripheral Neuropathy

Peripheral neuropathy has been reported when alpha interferons were given in combination with telbivudine. In one clinical trial, an increased risk and severity of peripheral neuropathy was observed with the combination use of telbivudine and pegylated interferon alfa-2a as compared to telbivudine alone. The safety and efficacy of telbivudine in combination with interferons for the treatment of chronic hepatitis B has not been demonstrated.

6 ADVERSE REACTIONS

Clinical trials with PegIntron alone or in combination with REBETOL have been conducted in over 6900 subjects from 3 to 75 years of age.

Serious adverse reactions have occurred in approximately 12% of subjects in clinical trials with PegIntron with or without REBETOL [see BOXED WARNING, Warnings and Precautions (5)]. The most common serious events occurring in subjects treated with PegIntron and REBETOL were depression and suicidal ideation [see Warnings and Precautions (5.2)], each occurring at a frequency of less than 1%. The most common fatal events occurring in subjects treated with PegIntron and REBETOL were cardiac arrest, suicidal ideation, and suicide attempt [see Warnings and Precautions (5.2, 5.5)], all occurring in less than 1% of subjects.

Greater than 96% of all subjects in clinical trials experienced one or more adverse events. The most commonly reported adverse reactions in adult subjects receiving either PegIntron or PegIntron/REBETOL were injection-site inflammation/reaction, fatigue/asthenia, headache, rigors, fevers, nausea, myalgia, and emotional lability/irritability. The most common adverse events in pediatric subjects, ages 3 and older, were pyrexia, headache, vomiting, neutropenia, fatigue, anorexia, injection-site erythema, and abdominal pain.

6.1 Clinical Trials Experience

Because clinical trials are conducted under widely varying conditions, adverse reaction rates observed in the clinical trials of a drug cannot be directly compared to rates in the clinical trials of another drug and may not reflect the rates observed in clinical practice.

Adults

Study 1 compared PegIntron monotherapy with INTRON® A monotherapy. Study 2 compared combination therapy of PegIntron/REBETOL with combination therapy with INTRON A/REBETOL. In these studies, nearly all study subjects in clinical trials experienced one or more adverse reactions. Study 3 compared a PegIntron/weight-based REBETOL combination to a PegIntron/flat dose REBETOL regimen. Study 4 compared 2 PegIntron (1.5 mcg/kg/week and 1 mcg/kg/week) doses in combination with REBETOL and a third treatment group receiving Pegasys® (180 mcg/week)/Copegus® (1000–1200 mg/day).

Adverse reactions that occurred in Studies 1 and 2 at >5% incidence are provided in Table 8 by treatment group. Due to potential differences in ascertainment procedures, adverse reaction rate comparisons across studies should not be made. Table 9 summarizes the treatment-related/treatment emergent adverse reactions in Study 4 that occurred at a ≥10% incidence.

[See table 8 on previous page and above]

[See table 9 at top of next page]

The adverse reaction profile in Study 3, which compared PegIntron/weight-based REBETOL combination to a PegIntron/flat-dose REBETOL regimen, revealed an increased rate of anemia with weight-based dosing (29% vs.

TABLE 8 (cont.) Adverse Reactions Occurring in > 5% of Subjects

| Adverse Events | Percentage of Subjects Reporting Adverse Reactions* | | | |
| | Study 1 | | Study 2 | |
	PegIntron 1 mcg/kg (n=297)	INTRON A 3 MIU (n=303)	PegIntron 1.5 mcg/kg/REBETOL (n=511)	INTRON A/ REBETOL (n=505)
Psychiatric				
Insomnia	23	23	40	41
Depression	29	25	31	34
Anxiety/Emotional Lability/Irritability	28	34	47	47
Concentration Impaired	10	8	17	21
Agitation	2	2	8	5
Nervousness	4	3	6	6
Reproductive, Female				
Menstrual Disorder	4	3	7	6
Resistance Mechanism				
Viral Infection	11	10	12	12
Fungal Infection	<1	3	6	1
Respiratory System				
Dyspnea	4	2	26	24
Coughing	8	5	23	16
Pharyngitis	10	7	12	13
Rhinitis	2	2	8	6
Sinusitis	7	7	6	5
Skin and Appendages				
Alopecia	22	22	36	32
Pruritus	12	8	29	28
Rash	6	7	24	23
Skin Dry	11	9	24	23
Special Senses, Other				
Taste Perversion	<1	2	9	4
Vision Disorders				
Vision Blurred	2	3	5	6
Conjunctivitis	4	2	4	5

*Subjects reporting one or more adverse reactions. A subject may have reported more than one adverse reaction within a body system/organ class category.

19% for weight-based vs. flat-dose regimens, respectively). However, the majority of cases of anemia were mild and responded to dose reductions.

The incidence of serious adverse reactions was comparable in all studies. In the PEG monotherapy trial (Study 1) the incidence of serious adverse reactions was similar (about 12%) in all treatment groups. In Study 2, the incidence of serious adverse reactions was 17% in the PegIntron/REBETOL groups compared to 14% in the INTRON A/REBETOL group. In Study 3, there was a similar incidence of serious adverse reactions reported for the weight-based REBETOL group (12%) and with the flat-dose REBETOL regimen.

In many but not all cases, adverse reactions resolved after dose reduction or discontinuation of therapy. Some subjects experienced ongoing or new serious adverse reactions during the 6-month follow-up period.

There have been 31 subject deaths which occurred during treatment or during follow-up in these clinical trials. In Study 1, there was 1 suicide in a subject receiving PegIntron monotherapy and 2 deaths among subjects receiving INTRON A monotherapy (1 murder/suicide and 1 sudden death). In Study 2, there was 1 suicide in a subject receiving PegIntron/REBETOL combination therapy, and 1 subject death in the INTRON A/REBETOL group (motor vehicle accident). In Study 3, there were 14 deaths, 2 of which were probable suicides, and 1 was an unexplained death in

a person with a relevant medical history of depression. In Study 4, there were 12 deaths, 6 of which occurred in subjects who received PegIntron/REBETOL combination therapy, 5 in the PegIntron 1.5 mcg/REBETOL arm (N=1019) and 1 in the PegIntron 1 mcg/REBETOL arm (N=1016), and 6 of which occurred in subjects receiving Pegasys/Copegus (N=1035). There were 3 suicides which occurred during the off-treatment follow-up period in subjects who received PegIntron (1.5 mcg/kg)/REBETOL combination therapy.

In Studies 1 and 2, 10% to 14% of subjects receiving PegIntron, alone or in combination with REBETOL, discontinued therapy compared with 6% treated with INTRON A alone and 13% treated with INTRON A in combination with REBETOL. Similarly in Study 3, 15% of subjects receiving PegIntron in combination with weight-based REBETOL and 14% of subjects receiving PegIntron and flat-dose REBETOL discontinued therapy due to an adverse reaction. The most common reasons for discontinuation of therapy were related to known interferon effects of psychiatric, systemic (e.g., fatigue, headache), or gastrointestinal adverse reactions. In Study 4, 13% of subjects in the PegIntron 1.5 mcg/REBETOL arm, 10% in the PegIntron 1 mcg/REBETOL arm, and 13% in the Pegasys 180 mcg/Copegus arm discontinued due to adverse events.

In Study 2, dose reductions due to adverse reactions occurred in 42% of subjects receiving PegIntron (1.5 mcg/kg)/REBETOL and in 34% of those receiving

TABLE 9 Summary of Treatment-related/Treatment-emergent Adverse Reactions (≥10% Incidence) By Descending Frequency

	Percentage of Patients Reporting Treatment-Related/ Treatment-emergent Adverse Reactions		
	Study 4		
Adverse Reactions	PegIntron 1.5 mcg/kg with REBETOL (n=1019)	PegIntron 1 mcg/kg with REBETOL (n=1016)	Pegasys 180 mcg with Copegus (n=1035)
Fatigue	67	68	64
Headache	50	47	41
Nausea	40	35	34
Chills	39	36	23
Insomnia	38	37	41
Anemia	35	30	34
Pyrexia	35	32	21
Injection Site Reactions	34	35	23
Anorexia	29	25	21
Rash	29	25	34
Myalgia	27	26	22
Neutropenia	26	19	31
Irritability	25	25	25
Depression	25	19	20
Alopecia	23	20	17
Dyspnea	21	20	22
Arthralgia	21	22	22
Pruritus	18	15	19
Influenza-like Illness	16	15	15
Dizziness	16	14	13
Diarrhea	15	16	14
Cough	15	16	17
Weight Decreased	13	10	10
Vomiting	12	10	9
Unspecified Pain	12	13	9
Dry Skin	11	11	12
Anxiety	11	11	10
Abdominal Pain	10	10	10
Leukopenia	9	7	10

INTRON A/REBETOL. The majority of subjects (57%) weighing 60 kg or less receiving PegIntron (1.5 mcg/kg)/REBETOL required dose reduction. Reduction of interferon was dose-related (PegIntron 1.5 mcg/kg > PegIntron 0.5 mcg/kg or INTRON A), 40%, 27%, 28%, respectively. Dose reduction for REBETOL was similar across all 3 groups, 33% to 35%. The most common reasons for dose modifications were neutropenia (18%) or anemia (9%). Other common reasons included depression, fatigue, nausea, and thrombocytopenia. In Study 3, dose modifications due to adverse reactions occurred more frequently with WBD compared to flat dosing (29% and 23%, respectively). In Study 4, 16% of subjects had a dose reduction of PegIntron to 1 mcg/kg in combination with REBETOL, with an additional 4% requiring the second dose reduction of PegIntron to 0.5 mcg/kg due to adverse events, compared to 15% of subjects in the Pegasys/Copegus arm, who required a dose reduction to 135 mcg/week with Pegasys, with an additional 7% in the Pegasys/Copegus arm requiring a second dose reduction to 90 mcg/week with Pegasys.

In the PegIntron/REBETOL combination trials the most common adverse reactions were psychiatric which occurred among 77% of subjects in Study 2 and 68% to 69% of subjects in Study 3. These psychiatric adverse reactions included most commonly depression, irritability, and insomnia, each reported by approximately 30% to 40% of subjects in all treatment groups. Suicidal behavior (ideation, attempts, and suicides) occurred in 2% of all subjects during treatment or during follow-up after treatment cessation [see Warnings and Precautions (5.2)]. In Study 4, psychiatric adverse reactions occurred in 58% of subjects in the PegIntron 1.5 mcg/REBETOL arm, 55% of subjects in the PegIntron 1 mcg/REBETOL arm, and 57% of subjects in the Pegasys 180 mcg/Copegus arm.

PegIntron induced fatigue or headache in approximately two-thirds of subjects, with fever or rigors in approximately half of the subjects. The severity of some of these systemic symptoms (e.g., fever and headache) tends to decrease as treatment continues. In Studies 1 and 2, application site inflammation and reaction (e.g., bruise, itchiness, and irritation) occurred at approximately twice the incidence with PegIntron therapies (in up to 75% of subjects) compared with INTRON A. However, injection-site pain was infrequent (2–3%) in all groups. In Study 3 there was a 23% to 24% incidence overall for injection-site reactions or inflammation.

In Study 2, many subjects continued to experience adverse reactions several months after discontinuation of therapy.

By the end of the 6-month follow-up period, the incidence of ongoing adverse reactions by body class in the PegIntron 1.5/REBETOL group was 33% (psychiatric), 20% (musculoskeletal), and 10% (for endocrine and for GI). In approximately 10% to 15% of subjects, weight loss, fatigue, and headache had not resolved.

Individual serious adverse reactions in Study 2 occurred at a frequency ≤1% and included suicide attempt, suicidal ideation, severe depression; psychosis, aggressive reaction, relapse of drug addiction/overdose; nerve palsy (facial, oculomotor); cardiomyopathy, myocardial infarction, angina, pericardial effusion, retinal ischemia, retinal artery or vein thrombosis, blindness, decreased visual acuity, optic neuritis, transient ischemic attack, supraventricular arrhythmias, loss of consciousness; neutropenia, infection (sepsis, pneumonia, abscess, cellulitis); emphysema, bronchiolitis obliterans, pleural effusion, gastroenteritis, pancreatitis, gout, hyperglycemia, hyperthyroidism and hypothyroidism, autoimmune thrombocytopenia with or without purpura, rheumatoid arthritis, interstitial nephritis, lupus-like syndrome, sarcoidosis, aggravated psoriasis; urticaria, injection-site necrosis, vasculitis, and phototoxicity.

Subjects receiving PegIntron/REBETOL as re-treatment after failing a previous interferon combination regimen reported adverse reactions similar to those previously associated with this regimen during clinical trials of treatment-naïve subjects.

Pediatric Subjects

In general, the adverse-reaction profile in the pediatric population was similar to that observed in adults. In the pediatric study, the most prevalent adverse reactions in all subjects were pyrexia (80%), headache (62%), neutropenia (33%), fatigue (30%), anorexia (29%), injection-site erythema (29%), and vomiting (27%). The majority of adverse reactions reported in the study were mild or moderate in severity. Severe adverse reactions were reported in 7% (8/107) of all subjects and included injection-site pain (1%), pain in extremity (1%), headache (1%), neutropenia (1%), and pyrexia (4%). Important adverse reactions that occurred in this subject population were nervousness (7%; 7/107), aggression (3%; 3/107), anger (2%; 2/107), and depression (1%; 1/107). Five subjects received levothyroxine treatment; 3 with clinical hypothyroidism and 2 with asymptomatic TSH elevations.

Dose modifications were required in 25% of subjects, most commonly for anemia, neutropenia, and weight loss. Two subjects (2%; 2/107) discontinued therapy as the result of an adverse reaction.

Adverse reactions that occurred with a ≥10% incidence in the pediatric trial subjects are provided in Table 10.

TABLE 10 Percentage of Pediatric Subjects With Treatment-emergent/Treatment-related Adverse Reactions (in at Least 10% of All Subjects)

System Organ Class Preferred Term	All Subjects n=107
Blood and Lymphatic System Disorders	
Neutropenia	33%
Anemia	11%
Leukopenia	10%
Gastrointestinal Disorders	
Abdominal Pain	21%
Abdominal Pain Upper	12%
Vomiting	27%
Nausea	18%
General Disorders and Administration Site Conditions	
Pyrexia	80%
Fatigue	30%
Injection-site Erythema	29%
Chills	21%
Asthenia	15%
Irritability	14%
Investigations	
Weight Decreased	19%

Metabolism and Nutrition Disorders

Anorexia	29%
Decreased Appetite	22%

Musculoskeletal and Connective Tissue Disorders

Arthralgia	17%
Myalgia	17%

Nervous System Disorders

Headache	62%
Dizziness	14%

Skin and Subcutaneous Tissue Disorders

Alopecia	17%

Laboratory Values
Adults
Changes in selected laboratory values during treatment with PegIntron alone or in combination with REBETOL treatment are described below. **Decreases in hemoglobin, neutrophils, and platelets may require dose reduction or permanent discontinuation from therapy** *[see Dosage and Administration (2.3) and Warnings and Precautions (5.1, 5.7)].*
Hemoglobin. Hemoglobin levels decreased to <11 g/dL in about 30% of subjects in Study 2. In Study 3, 47% of subjects receiving WBD REBETOL and 33% on flat-dose REBETOL had decreases in hemoglobin levels <11 g/dL. Reductions in hemoglobin to <9 g/dL occurred more frequently in subjects receiving WBD compared to flat dosing (4% and 2%, respectively). In Study 2, dose modification was required in 9% and 13% of subjects in the PegIntron/REBETOL and INTRON A/REBETOL groups. In Study 4, patients receiving PegIntron (1.5 mcg/kg)/REBETOL had decreases in hemoglobin levels to between 8.5 to <10 g/dL (28%) and to <8.5 g/dL (3%), whereas in patients receiving Pegasys 180 mcg/Copegus these decreases occurred in 26% and 4% of subjects, respectively. Hemoglobin levels become stable by treatment Weeks 4 to 6 on average. The typical pattern observed was a decrease in hemoglobin levels by treatment Week 4 followed by stabilization and a plateau, which was maintained to the end of treatment. In the PegIntron monotherapy trial, hemoglobin decreases were generally mild, and dose modifications were rarely necessary *[see Dosage and Administration (2.3)].*
Neutrophils. Decreases in neutrophil counts were observed in a majority of subjects treated with PegIntron alone (70%) or as combination therapy with REBETOL in Study 2 (85%) and INTRON A/REBETOL (60%). Severe potentially life-threatening neutropenia (<0.5 × 10⁹/L) occurred in 1% of subjects treated with PegIntron monotherapy, 2% of subjects treated with INTRON A/REBETOL, and in approximately 4% of subjects treated with PegIntron/REBETOL in Study 2. Two percent of subjects receiving PegIntron monotherapy and 18% of subjects receiving PegIntron/REBETOL in Study 2 required modification of interferon dosage. Few subjects (<1%) required permanent discontinuation of treatment. Neutrophil counts generally return to pretreatment levels 4 weeks after cessation of therapy *[see Dosage and Administration (2.3)].*
Platelets. Platelet counts decreased to <100,000/mm³ in approximately 20% of subjects treated with PegIntron alone or with REBETOL and in 6% of subjects treated with INTRON A/REBETOL. Severe decreases in platelet counts (<50,000/mm³) occur in <4% of subjects. Patients may require discontinuation or dose modification as a result of platelet decreases *[see Dosage and Administration (2.3)].* In Study 2, 1% or 3% of subjects required dose modification of INTRON A or PegIntron, respectively. Platelet counts generally returned to pretreatment levels 4 weeks after the cessation of therapy.
Triglycerides. Elevated triglyceride levels have been observed in patients treated with interferon alphas, including PegIntron *[see Warnings and Precautions (5.17)].*
Thyroid Function. Development of TSH abnormalities, with and without clinical manifestations, are associated with interferon therapies. In Study 2, clinically apparent thyroid disorders occur among subjects treated with either INTRON A or *PegIntron (with or without REBETOL)* at a similar incidence (5% for hypothyroidism and 3% for hyperthyroidism). Subjects developed new-onset TSH abnormalities while on treatment and during the follow-up period. At the end of the follow-up period, 7% of subjects still had abnormal TSH values *[see Warnings and Precautions (5.4)].*
Bilirubin and Uric Acid. In Study 2, 10% to 14% of subjects developed hyperbilirubinemia and 33% to 38% developed

hyperuricemia in association with hemolysis. Six subjects developed mild to moderate gout.
Pediatric Subjects
Decreases in hemoglobin, white blood cells, platelets, and neutrophils may require dose reduction or permanent discontinuation from therapy *[see Dosage and Administration (2.3)].* Changes in selected laboratory values during treatment of 107 pediatric subjects with PegIntron/REBETOL combination therapy are described in Table 11. Most of the changes in laboratory values in this study were mild or moderate.

TABLE 11: Selected Hematological Abnormalities During Treatment Phase with PegIntron Plus REBETOL in Previously Untreated Pediatric Subjects

Laboratory Parameter*	All Subjects (n=107)
Hemoglobin (g/dL)	
9.5–<11.0	30%
8.0–<9.5	2%
WBC (×10⁹/L)	
2.0–2.9	39%
1.5–<2.0	3%
Platelets (×10⁹/L)	
70–100	1%
50–<70	-
25–<50	1%
Neutrophils (×10⁹/L)	
1.0–1.5	35%
0.75–<1.0	26%
0.5–<0.75	13%
<0.5	3%
Total Bilirubin	
1.26–2.59 ×N†	7%
Evidence of Hepatic Failure	-

* The table summarizes the worst category observed within the period per subject per laboratory test. Only subjects with at least one treatment value for a given laboratory test are included.
† N=Upper limit of normal

6.2 Immunogenicity
As with all therapeutic proteins, there is potential for immunogenicity. Approximately 2% of subjects receiving PegIntron (32/1759) or INTRON A (11/728) with or without REBETOL developed low-titer (≤160) neutralizing antibodies to PegIntron or INTRON A. The clinical and pathological significance of the appearance of serum-neutralizing antibodies is unknown. The incidence of antibody formation is highly dependent on the sensitivity and specificity of the assay. Additionally, the observed incidence of antibody (including neutralizing antibody) positivity in an assay may be influenced by several factors, including assay methodology, sample handling, timing of sample collection, concomitant medications, and underlying disease. For these reasons, comparison of the incidence of antibodies to PegIntron with the incidence of antibodies to other products may be misleading.
6.3 Postmarketing Experience
The following adverse reactions have been identified during post-approval use of PegIntron therapy. Because these reactions are reported voluntarily from a population of uncertain size, it is not always possible to reliably estimate their frequency or establish a causal relationship to drug exposure.
Blood and Lymphatic System Disorders
pure red cell aplasia, thrombotic thrombocytopenic purpura
Cardiac Disorders
palpitations
Ear and Labyrinth Disorders
hearing loss, vertigo, hearing impairment
Eye Disorders
Vogt-Koyanagi-Harada syndrome, serous retinal detachment

Endocrine disorders
diabetic ketoacidosis, diabetes
Gastrointestinal Disorders
aphthous stomatitis
General Disorders and Administration Site Conditions
asthenic conditions (including asthenia, malaise, fatigue)
Immune System Disorders
cases of acute hypersensitivity reactions (including anaphylaxis, angioedema, urticaria); Stevens Johnson syndrome, toxic epidermal necrolysis, systemic lupus erythematosus, erythema multiforme
Infections and Infestations
bacterial infection including sepsis
Metabolism and Nutrition Disorders
dehydration, hypertriglyceridemia
Musculoskeletal and Connective Tissue Disorders
rhabdomylosis, myositis
Nervous System Disorders
seizures, memory loss, peripheral neuropathy, paraesthesia, migraine headache
Psychiatric Disorders
homicidal ideation
Respiratory, thoracic and mediastinal disorders
Pulmonary hypertension
Renal and Urinary Disorders
renal failure, renal insufficiency
Skin and Subcutaneous Tissue Disorders
psoriasis
Vascular Disorders
hypertension, hypotension

7 DRUG INTERACTIONS
7.1 Drugs Metabolized by Cytochrome P-450
When administering PegIntron with medications metabolized by CYP2C8/9 (e.g., warfarin and phenytoin) or CYP2D6 (e.g., flecainide), the therapeutic effect of these substrates may be decreased *[see Clinical Pharmacology (12.3)].*
7.2 Methadone
PegIntron may increase methadone concentrations *[see Clinical Pharmacology (12.3)].* The clinical significance of this finding is unknown; however, patients should be monitored for the signs and symptoms of increased narcotic effect.
7.3 Use with Ribavirin (Nucleoside Analogues)
Hepatic decompensation (some fatal) has occurred in cirrhotic HIV/HCV co-infected patients receiving combination antiretroviral therapy for HIV and interferon alpha and ribavirin. Adding treatment with alpha interferons alone or in combination with ribavirin may increase the risk in this patient subset. Patients receiving interferon with ribavirin and nucleoside reverse transcriptase inhibitors (NRTIs) should be closely monitored for treatment-associated toxicities, especially hepatic decompensation and anemia. Discontinuation of NRTIs should be considered as medically appropriate *[see Individual NRTI Product Information].* Dose reduction or discontinuation of interferon, ribavirin, or both should also be considered if worsening clinical toxicities are observed, including hepatic decompensation (e.g., Child-Pugh >6).
Stavudine, Lamivudine, and Zidovudine
In vitro studies have shown ribavirin can reduce the phosphorylation of pyrimidine nucleoside analogues such as stavudine, lamivudine, and zidovudine. In a study with another pegylated interferon alpha, no evidence of a pharmacokinetic or pharmacodynamic (e.g., loss of HIV/HCV virologic suppression) interaction was seen when ribavirin was co-administered with zidovudine, lamivudine, or stavudine in HIV/HCV co-infected subjects *[see Clinical Pharmacology (12.3)].*
HIV/HCV co-infected subjects who were administered zidovudine in combination with pegylated interferon alpha and ribavirin developed severe neutropenia (ANC <500) and severe anemia (hemoglobin <8 g/dL) more frequently than similar subjects not receiving zidovudine.
Didanosine
Co-administration of REBETOL Capsules or Oral Solution and didanosine is not recommended. Reports of fatal hepatic failure, as well as peripheral neuropathy, pancreatitis, and symptomatic hyperlactactemia/lactic acidosis have been reported in clinical trials *[see Clinical Pharmacology (12.3)].*

8 USE IN SPECIFIC POPULATIONS
8.1 Pregnancy
PegIntron Monotherapy
Pregnancy Category C: Nonpegylated interferon alfa-2b has been shown to have abortifacient effects in *Macaca mulatta* (rhesus monkeys) at 15 and 30 million IU/kg (estimated human equivalent of 5 and 10 million IU/kg, based on body surface area adjustment for a 60-kg adult). PegIntron should be assumed to also have abortifacient potential. There are no adequate and well-controlled studies in

pregnant women. PegIntron therapy is to be used during pregnancy only if the potential benefit justifies the potential risk to the fetus. Therefore, PegIntron is recommended for use in fertile women only when they are using effective contraception during the treatment period.

Use with Ribavirin
Pregnancy Category X: Significant teratogenic and/or embryocidal effects have been demonstrated in all animal species exposed to ribavirin. REBETOL therapy is contraindicated in women who are pregnant and in the male partners of women who are pregnant [see Contraindications (4) and the REBETOL Package Insert].

A Ribavirin Pregnancy Registry has been established to monitor maternal-fetal outcomes of pregnancies in female patients and female partners of male patients exposed to ribavirin during treatment and for 6 months following cessation of treatment. Physicians and patients are encouraged to report such cases by calling 1-800-593-2214.

8.3 Nursing Mothers
It is not known whether the components of PegIntron and/or REBETOL are excreted in human milk. Studies in mice have shown that mouse interferons are excreted in breast milk. Because of the potential for adverse reactions from the drug in nursing infants, a decision must be made whether to discontinue nursing or discontinue the PegIntron and REBETOL treatment, taking into account the importance of the therapy to the mother.

8.4 Pediatric Use
Safety and effectiveness in pediatric patients below the age of 3 years have not been established. Clinical trials in pediatric patients < 3 years of age are not considered feasible due to the small proportion of patients in this age group requiring treatment for CHC.

8.5 Geriatric Use
In general, younger patients tend to respond better than older patients to interferon-based therapies. Clinical studies of PegIntron alone or in combination with REBETOL did not include sufficient numbers of subjects aged 65 and over, however, to determine whether they respond differently than younger subjects. Treatment with alpha interferons, including PegIntron, is associated with neuropsychiatric, cardiac, pulmonary, GI, and systemic (flu-like) adverse effects. Because these adverse reactions may be more severe in the elderly, caution should be exercised in the use of PegIntron in this population. This drug is known to be substantially excreted by the kidney. Because elderly patients are more likely to have decreased renal function, the risk of toxic reactions to this drug may be greater in patients with impaired renal function [see Clinical Pharmacology (12.3)]. When using PegIntron/REBETOL therapy, refer also to the REBETOL Package Insert.

8.6 Organ Transplant Recipients
The safety and efficacy of PegIntron alone or in combination with REBETOL for the treatment of hepatitis C in liver or other organ transplant recipients have not been studied. In a small (n=16) single-center, uncontrolled case experience, renal failure in renal allograft recipients receiving interferon alpha and ribavirin combination therapy was more frequent than expected from the center's previous experience with renal allograft recipients not receiving combination therapy. The relationship of the renal failure to renal allograft rejection is not clear.

8.7 HIV or HBV Co-infection
The safety and efficacy of PegIntron/REBETOL for the treatment of patients with HCV co-infected with HIV or HBV have not been established.

10 OVERDOSAGE
There is limited experience with overdosage. In the clinical studies, a few subjects accidentally received a dose greater than that prescribed. There were no instances in which a participant in the monotherapy or combination therapy trials received more than 10.5 times the intended dose of PegIntron. The maximum dose received by any subject was 3.45 mcg/kg weekly over a period of approximately 12 weeks. The maximum known overdosage of REBETOL was an intentional ingestion of 10 g (fifty 200 mg capsules). There were no serious reactions attributed to these overdosages. In cases of overdosing, symptomatic treatment and close observation of the patient are recommended.

11 DESCRIPTION
PegIntron, peginterferon alfa-2b, Powder for Injection is a covalent conjugate of recombinant alfa-2b interferon with monomethoxy polyethylene glycol (PEG). The average molecular weight of the PEG portion of the molecule is 12,000 daltons. The average molecular weight of the PegIntron molecule is approximately 31,000 daltons. The specific activity of peginterferon alfa-2b is approximately 0.7×10^8 IU/mg protein.

Interferon alfa-2b is a water-soluble protein with a molecular weight of 19,271 daltons produced by recombinant DNA techniques. It is obtained from the bacterial fermentation of

a strain of *Escherichia coli* bearing a genetically engineered plasmid containing an interferon gene from human leukocytes.

PegIntron is supplied in both vials and the REDIPEN for subcutaneous use.
Vials
Each vial contains either 74 mcg, 118.4 mcg, 177.6 mcg, or 222 mcg of PegIntron as a white to off-white tablet-like solid that is whole/in pieces or as a loose powder, and 1.11 mg dibasic sodium phosphate anhydrous, 1.11 mg monobasic sodium phosphate dihydrate, 59.2 mg sucrose, and 0.074 mg polysorbate 80. Following reconstitution with 0.7 mL of the supplied Sterile Water for Injection USP, each vial contains PegIntron at strengths of either 50 mcg per 0.5 mL, 80 mcg per 0.5 mL, 120 mcg per 0.5 mL, or 150 mcg per 0.5 mL.
REDIPEN
REDIPEN is a dual-chamber glass cartridge containing lyophilized PegIntron as a white to off-white tablet or powder that is whole or in pieces in the sterile active chamber and a second chamber containing Sterile Water for Injection USP. Each PegIntron REDIPEN contains either 67.5 mcg, 108 mcg, 162 mcg, or 202.5 mcg of PegIntron, and 1.013 mg dibasic sodium phosphate anhydrous, 1.013 mg monobasic sodium phosphate dihydrate, 54 mg sucrose, and 0.0675 mg polysorbate 80. Each cartridge is reconstituted to allow for the administration of up to 0.5 mL of solution. Following reconstitution, each REDIPEN contains PegIntron at strengths of either 50 mcg per 0.5 mL, 80 mcg per 0.5 mL, 120 mcg per 0.5 mL, or 150 mcg per 0.5 mL for a single use. Because a small volume of reconstituted solution is lost during preparation of PegIntron, each REDIPEN contains an excess amount of PegIntron powder and diluent to ensure delivery of the labeled dose.

12 CLINICAL PHARMACOLOGY
12.1 Mechanism of Action
Pegylated recombinant human interferon alfa-2b is an inducer of the innate antiviral immune response [see Clinical Pharmacology (12.4)].
12.2 Pharmacodynamics
The pharmacodynamic effects of peginterferon alfa-2b include inhibition of viral replication in virus-infected cells, the suppression of cell cycle progression/cell proliferation, induction of apoptosis, anti-angiogenic activities, and numerous immunomodulating activities, such as enhancement of the phagocytic activity of macrophages, activation of NK cells, stimulation of cytotoxic T-lymphocytes, and the upregulation of the Th1 T-helper cell subset.

PegIntron raises concentrations of effector proteins such as serum neopterin and 2'5' oligoadenylate synthetase, raises body temperature, and causes reversible decreases in leukocyte and platelet counts. The correlation between the *in vitro* and *in vivo* pharmacologic and pharmacodynamic and clinical effects is unknown.
12.3 Pharmacokinetics
Following a single subcutaneous dose of PegIntron, the mean absorption half-life (t½ k_a) was 4.6 hours. Maximal serum concentrations (C_{max}) occur between 15 and 44 hours postdose, and are sustained for up to 48 to 72 hours. The C_{max} and AUC measurements of PegIntron increase in a dose-related manner. After multiple dosing, there is an increase in bioavailability of PegIntron. Week 48 mean trough concentrations (320 pg/mL; range 0, 2960) are approximately 3-fold higher than Week 4 mean trough concentrations (94 pg/mL; range 0, 416). The mean PegIntron elimination half-life is approximately 40 hours (range 22–60 hours) in patients with HCV infection. The apparent clearance of PegIntron is estimated to be approximately 22 mL/hr•kg. Renal elimination accounts for 30% of the clearance. Pegylation of interferon alfa-2b produces a product (PegIntron) whose clearance is lower than that of non-pegylated interferon alfa-2b. When compared to INTRON A, PegIntron (1 mcg/kg) has approximately a 7-fold lower mean apparent clearance and a 5-fold greater mean half-life, permitting a reduced dosing frequency. At effective therapeutic doses, PegIntron has approximately 10-fold greater C_{max} and 50-fold greater AUC than interferon alfa-2b.
Renal Dysfunction
Following multiple dosing of PegIntron (1 mcg/kg subcutaneously given every week for 4 weeks) the clearance of PegIntron is reduced by a mean of 17% in subjects with moderate renal impairment (creatinine clearance 30–49 mL/min) and by a mean of 44% in subjects with severe renal impairment (creatinine clearance 10–29 mL/min) compared to subjects with normal renal function. Clearance was similar in subjects with severe renal impairment not on dialysis and subjects who are receiving hemodialysis. The dose of PegIntron for monotherapy should be reduced in patients with moderate or severe renal impairment [see Dosage and Administration (2.3) and REBETOL Package Insert]. REBETOL should not be used in patients with creatinine clearance <50 mL/min [see REBETOL Package Insert, WARNINGS].

Gender
During the 48-week treatment period with PegIntron, no differences in the pharmacokinetic profiles were observed between male and female subjects with chronic hepatitis C infection.
Geriatric Patients
The pharmacokinetics of geriatric subjects (>65 years of age) treated with a single subcutaneous dose of 1 mcg/kg of PegIntron were similar in C_{max}, AUC, clearance, or elimination half-life as compared to younger subjects (28–44 years of age).
Pediatric Patients
Population pharmacokinetics for PegIntron and REBETOL (Capsules and Oral Solution) were evaluated in pediatric subjects with chronic hepatitis C between 3 and 17 years of age. In pediatric patients receiving PegIntron 60 mcg/m²/week subcutaneously, exposure may be approximately 50% higher than observed in adults receiving 1.5 mcg/kg/week subcutaneously. The pharmacokinetics of REBETOL (dose-normalized) in this trial were similar to those reported in a prior study of REBETOL in combination with INTRON A in pediatric subjects and in adult subjects.
Effect of Food on Absorption of Ribavirin
Both AUC_{tf} and C_{max} increased by 70% when REBETOL Capsules were administered with a high-fat meal (841 kcal, 53.8 g fat, 31.6 g protein, and 57.4 g carbohydrate) in a single-dose pharmacokinetic study [see Dosage and Administration (2.2)].
Drug Interactions
Drugs Metabolized by Cytochrome P-450
The pharmacokinetics of representative drugs metabolized by CYP1A2 (caffeine), CYP2C8/9 (tolbutamide), CYP2D6 (dextromethorphan), CYP3A4 (midazolam), and N-acetyltransferase (dapsone) were studied in 22 subjects with chronic hepatitis C who received PegIntron (1.5 mcg/kg) once weekly for 4 weeks. PegIntron treatment resulted in a 28% (mean) increase in a measure of CYP2C8/9 activity. PegIntron treatment also resulted in a 66% (mean) increase in a measure of CYP2D6 activity; however, the effect was variable as 13 subjects had an increase, 5 subjects had a decrease, and 4 subjects had no significant change [see Drug Interactions (7.1)].
No significant effect was observed on the pharmacokinetics of representative drugs metabolized by CYP1A2, CYP3A4, or N-acetyltransferase. The effects of PegIntron on CYP2C19 activity were not assessed.
Methadone
The pharmacokinetics of concomitant administration of methadone and PegIntron were evaluated in 18 PegIntron-naïve chronic hepatitis C subjects receiving 1.5 mcg/kg PegIntron subcutaneously weekly. All subjects were on stable methadone maintenance therapy receiving ≥40 mg/day prior to initiating PegIntron. Mean methadone AUC was approximately 16% higher after 4 weeks of PegIntron treatment as compared to baseline. In 2 subjects, methadone AUC was approximately double after 4 weeks of PegIntron treatment as compared to baseline [see Drug Interactions (7.2)].
Use with Ribavirin
Zidovudine, Lamivudine, and Stavudine
Ribavirin has been shown in vitro to inhibit phosphorylation of zidovudine, lamivudine, and stavudine. However, in a study with another pegylated interferon in combination with ribavirin, no pharmacokinetic (e.g., plasma concentrations or intracellular triphosphorylated active metabolite concentrations) or pharmacodynamic (e.g., loss of HIV/HCV virologic suppression) interaction was observed when ribavirin and lamivudine (n=18), stavudine (n=10), or zidovudine (n=6) were co-administered as part of a multi-drug regimen to HIV/HCV coinfected subjects [see Drug Interactions (7.3)].
Didanosine
Exposure to didanosine or its active metabolite (dideoxyadenosine 5'-triphosphate) is increased when didanosine is co-administered with ribavirin, which could cause or worsen clinical toxicities [see Drug Interactions (7.3)].
12.4 Microbiology
Mechanism of Action
The biological activity of PegIntron is derived from its interferon alfa-2b moiety. Peginterferon alfa-2b binds to and activates the human type 1 interferon receptor. Upon binding, the receptor subunits dimerize, and activate multiple intracellular signal transduction pathways. Signal transduction is initially mediated by the JAK/STAT activation, which may occur in a wide variety of cells. Interferon receptor activation also activates NFκB in many cell types. Given the diversity of cell types that respond to interferon alfa-2b, and the multiplicity of potential intracellular responses to interferon receptor activation, peginterferon alfa-2b is expected to have pleiotropic biological effects in the body.
The mechanism by which ribavirin contributes to its antiviral efficacy in the clinic is not fully understood. Ribavirin has direct antiviral activity in tissue culture against many RNA viruses. Ribavirin increases the mutation frequency in the genomes of several viruses and ribavirin triphosphate inhibits HCV polymerase in a biochemical reaction.

Antiviral Activity

The anti-HCV activity of interferon was demonstrated in cell culture using self-replicating HCV-RNA (HCV replicon cells) or HCV infection and resulted in an effective concentration (EC_{50}) value of 1 to 10 IU/mL.

The antiviral activity of ribavirin in the HCV-replicon is not well understood and has not been defined because of the cellular toxicity of ribavirin.

Resistance

HCV genotypes show wide variability in their response to pegylated recombinant human interferon/ribavirin therapy. Genetic changes associated with the variable response have not been identified.

Cross-resistance

There is no reported cross-resistance between pegylated/non-pegylated interferons and ribavirin.

13 NONCLINICAL TOXICOLOGY

13.1 Carcinogenesis, Mutagenesis, Impairment of Fertility

Carcinogenesis and Mutagenesis

PegIntron has not been tested for its carcinogenic potential. Neither PegIntron nor its components, interferon or methoxypolyethylene glycol, caused damage to DNA when tested in the standard battery of mutagenesis assays, in the presence and absence of metabolic activation.

Use with Ribavirin: Ribavirin is genotoxic and mutagenic and should be considered a potential carcinogen. See REBETOL package insert for additional warnings relevant to PegIntron therapy in combination with ribavirin.

Impairment of Fertility

PegIntron may impair human fertility. Irregular menstrual cycles were observed in female cynomolgus monkeys given subcutaneous injections of 4239 mcg/m^2 PegIntron alone every other day for 1 month (approximately 345 times the recommended weekly human dose based upon body surface area). These effects included transiently decreased serum levels of estradiol and progesterone, suggestive of anovulation. Normal menstrual cycles and serum hormone levels resumed in these animals 2 to 3 months following cessation of PegIntron treatment. Every other day dosing with 262 mcg/m^2 (approximately 21 times the weekly human dose) had no effects on cycle duration or reproductive hormone status. The effects of PegIntron on male fertility have not been studied.

14 CLINICAL STUDIES

14.1 Chronic Hepatitis C in Adults

PegIntron Monotherapy-Study 1

A randomized study compared treatment with PegIntron (0.5, 1, or 1.5 mcg/kg once weekly subcutaneously) to treatment with INTRON A (3 million units 3 times weekly subcutaneously) in 1219 adults with chronic hepatitis from HCV infection. The subjects were not previously treated with interferon alpha, had compensated liver disease, detectable HCV-RNA, elevated ALT, and liver histopathology consistent with chronic hepatitis. Subjects were treated for 48 weeks and were followed for 24 weeks post-treatment. Seventy percent of all subjects were infected with HCV genotype 1, and 74 percent of all subjects had high baseline levels of HCV-RNA (more than 2 million copies per mL of serum), 2 factors known to predict poor response to treatment.

Response to treatment was defined as undetectable HCV-RNA and normalization of ALT at 24 weeks post-treatment. The response rates to the 1 and 1.5 mcg/kg PegIntron doses were similar (approximately 24%) to each other and were both higher than the response rate to INTRON A (12%) *(see Table 12)*.

[See table 12 above]

Subjects with both viral genotype 1 and high serum levels of HCV-RNA at baseline were less likely to respond to treatment with PegIntron. Among subjects with the 2 unfavorable prognostic variables, 8% (12/157) responded to PegIntron treatment and 2% (4/169) responded to INTRON A. Doses of PegIntron higher than the recommended dose did not result in higher response rates in these subjects. Subjects receiving PegIntron with viral genotype 1 had a response rate of 14% (28/199) while subjects with other viral genotypes had a 45% (43/96) response rate. Ninety-six percent of the responders in the PegIntron groups and 100% of responders in the INTRON A group first cleared their viral RNA by Week 24 of treatment *[see Dosage and Administration (2)]*.

The treatment response rates were similar in men and women. Response rates were lower in African-American and Hispanic subjects and higher in Asians compared to Caucasians. Although African Americans had a higher proportion of poor prognostic factors compared to Caucasians, the number of non-Caucasians studied (9% of the total) was insufficient to allow meaningful conclusions about differences in response rates after adjusting for prognostic factors.

Liver biopsies were obtained before and after treatment in 60% of subjects. A modest reduction in inflammation compared to baseline that was similar in all 4 treatment groups was observed.

PegIntron/REBETOL Combination Therapy-Study 2

A randomized study compared treatment with 2 PegIntron/REBETOL regimens [PegIntron 1.5 mcg/kg subcutaneously once weekly/REBETOL 800 mg orally daily (in divided doses); PegIntron 1.5 mcg/kg subcutaneously once weekly for 4 weeks then 0.5 mcg/kg subcutaneously once weekly for 44 weeks/REBETOL 1000 or 1200 mg orally daily (in divided doses)] with INTRON A [3 MIU subcutaneously thrice weekly/REBETOL 1000 or 1200 mg orally daily (in divided doses)] in 1530 adults with chronic hepatitis C. Interferon-naïve subjects were treated for 48 weeks and followed for 24 weeks post-treatment. Eligible subjects had compensated liver disease, detectable HCV-RNA, elevated ALT, and liver histopathology consistent with chronic hepatitis.

Response to treatment was defined as undetectable HCV-RNA at 24 weeks post-treatment. The response rate to the PegIntron 1.5 mcg/kg plus ribavirin 800 mg dose was higher than the response rate to INTRON A/REBETOL *(see Table 13)*. The response rate to PegIntron 1.5→0.5 mcg/kg/REBETOL was essentially the same as the response to INTRON A/REBETOL (data not shown).

[See table 13 above]

Subjects with viral genotype 1, regardless of viral load, had a lower response rate to PegIntron (1.5 mcg/kg)/REBETOL (800 mg) compared to subjects with other viral genotypes. Subjects with both poor prognostic factors (genotype 1 and high viral load) had a response rate of 30% (78/256) compared to a response rate of 29% (71/247) with INTRON A/REBETOL.

Subjects with lower body weight tended to have higher adverse reaction rates *[see Adverse Reactions (6.1)]* and higher response rates than subjects with higher body weights. Differences in response rates between treatment arms did not substantially vary with body weight.

Treatment response rates with PegIntron/REBETOL were 49% in men and 56% in women. Response rates were lower in African American and Hispanic subjects and higher in Asians compared to Caucasians. Although African Americans had a higher proportion of poor prognostic factors compared to Caucasians, the number of non-Caucasians studied (11% of the total) was insufficient to allow meaningful conclusions about differences in response rates after adjusting for prognostic factors in this study.

Liver biopsies were obtained before and after treatment in 68% of subjects. Compared to baseline, approximately two-thirds of subjects in all treatment groups were observed to have a modest reduction in inflammation.

PegIntron/REBETOL Combination Therapy-Study 3

In a large United States community-based study (Study 3), 4913 subjects with chronic hepatitis C were randomized to receive PegIntron 1.5 mcg/kg subcutaneously once weekly in combination with a REBETOL dose of 800 to 1400 mg (weight-based dosing [WBD]) or 800 mg (flat) orally daily (in divided doses) for 24 or 48 weeks based on genotype. Response to treatment was defined as undetectable HCV-RNA (based on an assay with a lower limit of detection of 125 IU/mL) at 24 weeks post-treatment.

Treatment with PegIntron 1.5 mcg/kg and REBETOL 800 to 1400 mg resulted in a higher sustained virologic response compared to PegIntron in combination with a flat 800 mg daily dose of REBETOL. Subjects weighing >105 kg obtained the greatest benefit with WBD, although a modest benefit was also observed in subjects weighing >85 to 105 kg *(see Table 14)*. The benefit of WBD in subjects weighing >85 kg was observed with HCV genotypes 1 through 3. Insufficient data were available to reach conclusions regarding other genotypes. Use of WBD resulted in an increased incidence of anemia *[see Adverse Reactions (6.1)]*.

[See table 14 above]

A total of 1552 subjects weighing >65 kg in Study 3 had genotype 2 or 3 and were randomized to 24 or 48 weeks of therapy. No additional benefit was observed with the longer treatment duration.

PegIntron/REBETOL Combination Therapy-Study 4

A large randomized study compared the safety and efficacy of treatment for 48 weeks with two PegIntron/REBETOL regimens [PegIntron 1.5 mcg/kg and 1 mcg/kg subcutaneously once weekly both in combination with REBETOL 800 to 1400 mg PO daily (in two divided doses)] and Pegasys 180 mcg subcutaneously once weekly in combination with Copegus 1000 to 1200 mg PO daily (in two divided doses) in 3070 treatment-naïve adults with chronic hepatitis C genotype 1. In this study, lack of early virologic response by treatment Week 12 (subjects who do not achieve undetectable HCV-RNA or ≥2 log$_{10}$ reduction from baseline) was the

TABLE 12 Rates of Response to Treatment – Study 1

	A PegIntron 0.5 mcg/kg (N=315)	B PegIntron 1 mcg/kg (N=298)	C INTRON A 3 MIU three times weekly (N=307)	B - C (95% CI) Difference between PegIntron 1 mcg/kg and INTRON A
Treatment Response (Combined Virologic Response and ALT Normalization)	17%	24%	12%	11 (5, 18)
Virologic Response *	18%	25%	12%	12 (6, 19)
ALT Normalization	24%	29%	18%	11 (5, 18)

*Serum HCV is measured by a research-based quantitative polymerase chain reaction assay by a central laboratory.

TABLE 13 Rates of Response to Treatment – Study 2

	PegIntron 1.5 mcg/kg once weekly REBETOL 800 mg daily	INTRON A 3 MIU three times weekly REBETOL 1000/1200 mg daily
Overall response*†	52% (264/511)	46% (231/505)
Genotype 1	41% (141/348)	33% (112/343)
Genotype 2–6	75% (123/163)	73% (119/162)

* Serum HCV-RNA is measured with a research-based quantitative polymerase chain reaction assay by a central laboratory.
† Difference in overall treatment response (PegIntron/REBETOL vs. INTRON A/REBETOL) is 6% with 95% confidence interval of (0.18, 11.63) adjusted for viral genotype and presence of cirrhosis at baseline. Response to treatment was defined as undetectable HCV-RNA at 24 weeks posttreatment.

TABLE 14 SVR Rate by Treatment and Baseline Weight - Study 3

Treatment Group	Subject Baseline Weight			
	<65 kg (<143 lb)	65–85 kg (143–188 lb)	>85–105 kg (>188–231 lb)	>105 kg (>231 lb)
WBD*	50% (173/348)	45% (449/994)	42% (351/835)	47% (138/292)
Flat	51% (173/342)	44% (443/1011)	39% (318/819)	33% (91/272)

*$P=0.01$, primary efficacy comparison (based on data from subjects weighing 65 kg or higher at baseline and utilizing a logistic regression analysis that includes treatment [WBD or Flat], genotype and presence/absence of advanced fibrosis, in the model).

TABLE 16 SVR Rates by Baseline Characteristics of Prior Treatment Failures.

HCV Genotype/ Metavir Fibrosis Score	Overall SVR by Previous Response and Treatment			
	Nonresponder		Relapser	
	alfa interferon/ ribavirin % (number of patients)	peginterferon (2a and 2b combined)/ribavirin % (number of patients)	alfa interferon/ ribavirin % (number of patients)	peginterferon (2a and 2b combined)/ribavirin % (number of patients)
Overall	18 (158/903)	6 (30/476)	43 (130/300)	35 (113/344)
HCV 1	13 (98/761)	4 (19/431)	32 (67/208)	23 (56/243)
F2	18 (36/202)	6 (7/117)	42 (33/79)	32 (23/72)
F3	16 (38/233)	4 (4/112)	28 (16/58)	21 (14/67)
F4	7 (24/325)	4 (8/202)	26 (18/70)	18 (19/104)
HCV 2/3	49 (53/109)	36 (10/28)	67 (54/81)	57 (52/92)
F2	68 (23/34)	56 (5/9)	76 (19/25)	61 (11/18)
F3	39 (11/28)	38 (3/8)	67 (18/27)	62 (18/29)
F4	40 (19/47)	18 (2/11)	59 (17/29)	51 (23/45)
HCV 4	17 (5/29)	7 (1/15)	88 (7/8)	50 (4/8)

criteria for discontinuation of treatment. Sustained Virologic Response (SVR) to the treatment was defined as undetectable HCV-RNA (Roche COBAS TaqMan assay, a lower limit of quantitation of 27 IU/mL) at 24 weeks posttreatment [see Table 15].

TABLE 15 Response Rate by Treatment

Treatment Group	% (number) of Patients		
	PegIntron 1.5 mcg/kg/ REBETOL	PegIntron 1 mcg/kg/ REBETOL	Pegasys 180 mcg/ Copegus
SVR	40 (406/1019)	38 (386/1016)	41 (423/1035)

In all three treatment groups, overall SVR rates were similar. In subjects with poor prognostic factors, subjects randomized to PegIntron (1.5 mcg/kg)/REBETOL or Pegasys/Copegus achieved higher SVR rates compared to those randomized to the PegIntron 1 mcg/kg/REBETOL arm. In all arms, SVR rates were lower in subjects with poor prognostic factors compared to those without. For the PegIntron 1.5 mcg/kg plus REBETOL dose, SVR rates for those with and without, respectively, the following baseline factors were as follows: cirrhosis (10% vs. 42%), normal ALT levels (32% vs. 42%), baseline viral load >600,000 IU/mL (35% vs. 61%), >40 years old (38% vs. 50%), and African American subjects (23% vs. 44%). In subjects with undetectable HCV-RNA at treatment week 12 who received PegIntron (1.5 mcg/kg)/REBETOL, the SVR rate was 81% (328/407).

PegIntron/REBETOL Combination Therapy in Prior Treatment Failures-Study 5
In a noncomparative trial, 2293 patients with moderate to severe fibrosis who failed previous treatment with combination alpha interferon/ribavirin were retreated with PegIntron, 1.5 mcg/kg subcutaneously, once weekly, in combination with weight adjusted ribavirin. Eligible patients included prior nonresponders (patients who were HCV-RNA positive at the end of a minimum 12 weeks of treatment) and prior relapsers (patients who were HCV-RNA negative at the end of a minimum 12 weeks of treatment and subsequently relapsed after posttreatment follow-up). Patients who were negative at week 12 were treated for 48 weeks and followed for 24 weeks posttreatment. Response to treatment was defined as undetectable HCV-RNA at 24 weeks posttreatment (measured using a research-based test, limit of detection 125 IU/mL). The overall response rate was 22% (497/2293) (99% CI: 19.5, 23.9). Patients with the following characteristics were less likely to benefit from retreatment: previous nonresponse, previous pegylated interferon treatment, significant bridging fibrosis or cirrhosis, and genotype 1 infection.
The retreatment sustained virologic response rates by baseline characteristics are summarized in *Table 16*.
[See table 16 above]
Achievement of an undetectable HCV-RNA at treatment week 12 was a strong predictor of sustained virologic response (SVR). In this trial, 1470 (64%) subjects did not achieve an undetectable HCV-RNA at treatment week 12, and were offered enrollment into long-term treatment trials, due to an inadequate treatment response. Of the 823 (36%) subjects who were HCV-RNA undetectable at treatment week 12, those infected with genotype 1 had an SVR of 48% (245/507), with a range of responses by fibrosis scores (F4–F2) of 39–55%. Subjects infected with genotype 2/3 who were HCV-RNA undetectable at treatment week 12 had an overall SVR of 70% (196/281), with a range of responses by fibrosis scores (F4–F2) of 60–83%. For all genotypes, higher fibrosis scores were associated with a decreased likelihood of achieving SVR.

14.2 Chronic Hepatitis C in Pediatrics
PegIntron/REBETOL Combination Therapy-Pediatric Study
Previously untreated pediatric subjects 3 to 17 years of age with compensated chronic hepatitis C and detectable HCV-RNA were treated with REBETOL 15 mg/kg/day plus PegIntron 60 mcg/m^2 once weekly for 24 or 48 weeks based on HCV genotype and baseline viral load. All subjects were to be followed for 24 weeks post-treatment. A total of 107 subjects received treatment of whom 52% were female, 89% were Caucasian, and 67% were infected with HCV Genotype 1. Subjects infected with Genotype 1, 4 or Genotype 3 with HCV-RNA ≥ 600,000 IU/mL received 48 weeks of therapy while those infected with Genotype 2 or Genotype 3 with HCV-RNA < 600,000 IU/mL received 24 weeks of therapy. The study results are summarized in Table 17.

TABLE 17 Sustained Virologic Response Rates by Genotype and Treatment Duration – Pediatric Study

	All Subjects n=107	
	24 Weeks	48 Weeks
	Virologic Response n*† (%)	Virologic Response n*† (%)
Genotype		
All	26/27 (96.3)	44/80 (55.0)
1	-	38/72 (52.8)
2	14/15 (93.3)	-
3‡	12/12 (100)	2/3 (66.7)
4	-	4/5 (80.0)

* Response to treatment was defined as undetectable HCV-RNA at 24 weeks post-treatment.
† n = number of responders/number of subjects with given genotype, and assigned treatment duration.
‡ Subjects with genotype 3 low viral load (<600,000 IU/ mL) were to receive 24 weeks of treatment while those with genotype 3 and high viral load were to receive 48 weeks of treatment.

16 HOW SUPPLIED/STORAGE AND HANDLING
PegIntron REDIPEN

Each PegIntron REDIPEN Package Contains:

A box containing one 50 mcg per 0.5 mL PegIntron REDIPEN and 1 BD needle and 2 alcohol swabs.	(NDC 0085-1323-01)
A box containing one 80 mcg per 0.5 mL PegIntron REDIPEN and 1 BD needle and 2 alcohol swabs.	(NDC 0085-1316-01)
A box containing one 120 mcg per 0.5 mL PegIntron REDIPEN and 1 BD needle and 2 alcohol swabs.	(NDC 0085-1297-01)
A box containing one 150 mcg per 0.5 mL PegIntron REDIPEN and 1 BD needle and 2 alcohol swabs.	(NDC 0085-1370-01)

Each PegIntron REDIPEN PAK 4 Contains:

A box containing four 50 mcg per 0.5 mL PegIntron REDIPEN Units, each containing 1 BD needle and 2 alcohol swabs.	(NDC 0085-1323-02)
A box containing four 80 mcg per 0.5 mL PegIntron REDIPEN Units, each containing 1 BD needle and 2 alcohol swabs.	(NDC 0085-1316-02)
A box containing four 120 mcg per 0.5 mL PegIntron REDIPEN Units, each containing 1 BD needle and 2 alcohol swabs.	(NDC 0085-1297-02)
A box containing four 150 mcg per 0.5 mL PegIntron REDIPEN Units, each containing 1 BD needle and 2 alcohol swabs.	(NDC 0085-1370-02)

PegIntron Vials

Each PegIntron Package Contains:

A box containing one 50 mcg per 0.5 mL vial of PegIntron Powder for Injection and one 1.25 mL vial of Diluent (Sterile Water for Injection USP), 2 BD Safety-Lok syringes with a safety sleeve and 2 alcohol swabs.	(NDC 0085-1368-01)
A box containing one 80 mcg per 0.5 mL vial of PegIntron Powder for Injection and one 1.25 mL vial of Diluent (Sterile Water for Injection USP), 2 BD Safety-Lok syringes with a safety sleeve and 2 alcohol swabs.	(NDC 0085-1291-01)
A box containing one 120 mcg per 0.5 mL vial of PegIntron Powder for Injection and one 1.25 mL vial of Diluent (Sterile Water for Injection USP), 2 BD Safety-Lok syringes with a safety sleeve and 2 alcohol swabs.	(NDC 0085-1304-01)
A box containing one 150 mcg per 0.5 mL vial of PegIntron Powder for Injection and one 1.25 mL vial of Diluent (Sterile Water for Injection USP), 2 BD Safety-Lok syringes with a safety sleeve and 2 alcohol swabs.	(NDC 0085-1279-01)

Storage
PegIntron REDIPEN
PegIntron REDIPEN should be stored at 2°–8°C (36°–46°F). After reconstitution, the solution should be used immediately, but may be stored up to 24 hours at 2°–8°C (36°–46°F). The reconstituted solution contains no preservative, and is clear and colorless. **DO NOT FREEZE.**

PegIntron Vials

PegIntron should be stored at 25°C (77°F); excursions permitted to 15°–30°C (59°–86°F) [see USP Controlled Room Temperature]. After reconstitution with supplied Diluent the solution should be used immediately, but may be stored up to 24 hours at 2°–8°C (36°–46°F). The reconstituted solution contains no preservative, and is clear and colorless.
DO NOT FREEZE.
Disposal Instructions

Patients should be thoroughly instructed in the importance of proper disposal. After preparation and administration of PegIntron for Injection, patients should be advised to use a puncture-resistant container for the disposal of used syringes, needles, and the REDIPEN. The full container should be disposed of in accordance with state and local laws. Patients should also be cautioned against reusing or sharing needles, syringes, or the REDIPEN.

17 PATIENT COUNSELING INFORMATION

A patient should self-inject PegIntron only if it has been determined that it is appropriate, the patient agrees to medical follow-up as necessary, and training in proper injection technique has been given to him/her.
17.1 Medication Guide
Patients receiving PegIntron alone or in combination with REBETOL should be directed in its appropriate use, informed of the benefits and risks associated with treatment, and referred to the MEDICATION GUIDES for PegIntron and, if applicable, REBETOL (ribavirin).
17.2 Pregnancy
Patients must be informed that REBETOL may cause birth defects and death of the unborn child. Extreme care must be taken to avoid pregnancy in female patients and in female partners of male patients during treatment with combination PegIntron/REBETOL therapy and for 6 months post-therapy. Combination PegIntron/REBETOL therapy should not be initiated until a report of a negative pregnancy test has been obtained immediately prior to initiation of therapy. It is recommended that patients undergo monthly pregnancy tests during therapy and for 6 months post-therapy [see Contraindications (4), Use in Specific Populations (8.1), and REBETOL package insert].
17.3 HCV Transmission
Inform patients that there are no data regarding whether PegIntron therapy will prevent transmission of HCV infection to others. Also, it is not known if treatment with PegIntron will cure hepatitis C or prevent cirrhosis, liver failure, or liver cancer that may be the result of infection with the hepatitis C virus.
17.4 Laboratory Evaluations, Hydration, "Flu-like" Symptoms
Patients should be advised that laboratory evaluations are required before starting therapy and periodically thereafter [see Warnings and Precautions (5.15)]. It is advised that patients be well hydrated, especially during the initial stages of treatment. "Flu-like" symptoms associated with administration of PegIntron may be minimized by bedtime administration of PegIntron or by use of antipyretics.
Manufactured by Schering Corporation, a subsidiary of Schering-Plough Corporation, Kenilworth, NJ 07033 USA.
Schering-Plough
U.S. Patent Nos. 5,908,621; 5,951,974; 6,042,822; 6,177,074; 6,180,096; 6,250,469; 6,482,613; 6,524,570; and 6,610,830.
© 2001, 2009, Schering Corporation. All rights reserved.
BD and Safety-Lok are registered trademarks of Becton, Dickinson and Company.
Rev 1/2010
B-335388XXT
278535XXT
MEDICATION GUIDE
PegIntron®
(Peginterferon alfa-2b)
Including appendix with instructions for using PegIntron® Powder for Injection

Read this Medication Guide carefully before you start taking PegIntron (**Peg In-tron**) or PegIntron/REBETOL (**REB-eh-tole**) combination therapy. Read the Medication Guide each time you refill your prescription because there may be new information. The information in this Medication Guide does not take the place of talking with your health care provider (doctor, nurse, nurse practitioner, or physician's assistant).

If you are taking PegIntron/REBETOL combination therapy, also read the Medication Guide for REBETOL (ribavirin, USP) Capsules and Oral Solution.

What is the most important information I should know about PegIntron and PegIntron/REBETOL combination therapy?
PegIntron (peginterferon) is a treatment for some people who are infected with hepatitis C virus. However, PegIntron and PegIntron/REBETOL combination therapy can have serious side effects that may cause death in rare cases. Before you decide to start treatment, you should talk to your health care provider about the possible benefits and side effects of

PegIntron or PegIntron/REBETOL combination therapy. If you begin treatment you will need to see your health care provider regularly for medical examinations and lab tests to make sure your treatment is working and to check for side effects.

REBETOL may cause birth defects and/or death of an unborn child. If you are pregnant, you or your male partner must not take PegIntron/REBETOL combination therapy. You must not become pregnant while either you or your partner are being treated with the combination PegIntron/REBETOL therapy, or for 6 months after stopping therapy. Men and women should use birth control while taking the combination therapy and for 6 months afterwards. If you or your partner are being treated and you become pregnant either during treatment or within 6 months of stopping treatment, call your health care provider right away. There is a Ribavirin Pregnancy Registry that collects information about pregnancy outcomes in female patients and female partners of male patients exposed to ribavirin. You or your healthcare provider are encouraged to contact the Registry at 1-800-593-2214.
If you are taking PegIntron or PegIntron/REBETOL therapy you should call your health care provider immediately if you develop any of these symptoms:
New or worsening mental health problems such as thoughts about killing or hurting yourself or others, trouble breathing, chest pain, severe stomach or lower back pain, bloody diarrhea or bloody bowel movements, high fever, bruising, bleeding, or decreased vision.
The most serious possible side effects of PegIntron and PegIntron/REBETOL therapy include:
Problems with Pregnancy. Combination PegIntron/REBETOL therapy can cause death, serious birth defects, or other harm to your unborn child. If you are a woman of childbearing age you must not become pregnant during treatment, and for 6 months after you have stopped therapy. You must have a negative pregnancy test immediately before beginning treatment, during treatment and for 6 months after you have stopped therapy. Both male and female patients must use effective forms of birth control during treatment and for the 6 months after treatment is completed. Male patients should use a condom. If you are a female, you must use birth control even if you believe that you are not fertile or that your fertility is low. You should talk to your health care provider about birth control for you and your partner.
Mental health problems and suicide. PegIntron and PegIntron/REBETOL therapies may cause patients to develop mood or behavioral problems. These can include irritability (getting easily upset) and depression (feeling low, feeling bad about yourself, or feeling hopeless). Some patients may have aggressive behavior. Former drug addicts may fall back into drug addiction or overdose. Some patients think about hurting or killing themselves or other people and some have killed (suicide) or hurt themselves or others. You must tell your health care provider if you are being treated for a mental illness or had treatment in the past for any mental illness, including depression and suicidal behavior. You should tell your health care provider if you have ever been addicted to drugs or alcohol.
Heart problems. Some patients taking PegIntron or PegIntron/REBETOL therapy may develop problems with their heart, including low blood pressure, fast heart rate, and very rarely, heart attacks. Tell your health care provider if you have had any heart problems in the past.
Blood problems. PegIntron and PegIntron/REBETOL therapies commonly lower two types of blood cells (white blood cells and platelets). In some patients, these blood counts may fall to dangerously low levels. If your blood counts become very low, this could lead to infections or bleeding. REBETOL therapy causes a decrease in the number of red blood cells you have (anemia). This can be dangerous, especially for patients who already have heart or circulatory (cardiovascular) problems. Talk with your health care provider before taking combination PegIntron/REBETOL therapy if you have or have ever had any cardiovascular problems.
Body organ problems. Certain symptoms like severe stomach pain may mean that your internal organs are being damaged. PegIntron may cause lung problems including: trouble breathing, pneumonia, inflammation of lung tissue, and new or worse high blood pressure of the lungs (pulmonary hypertension), which can be severe and may in some cases lead to death. Cases of weakness, loss of coordination, and numbness due to stroke have been reported in patients taking PegIntron, including patients with few or no reported risk factors for stroke.
Eye problems. Changes in vision such as a decrease or loss of vision (blindness) may happen in some patients. You should have an eye exam before you take PegIntron. If you have eye problems or have had them in the past, you may need eye exams while you are taking PegIntron. Tell your healthcare provider or eye doctor right away if you have changes in your vision while taking PegIntron.

For other possible side effects, see "What are the possible side effects of PegIntron and PegIntron/REBETOL combination therapy?" in this Medication Guide.
What is PegIntron and PegIntron/REBETOL combination therapy?
The PegIntron product is a drug used to treat adults who have a lasting (chronic) infection with hepatitis C virus and who show signs that the virus is damaging the liver. PegIntron/REBETOL combination therapy consists of two medications also used to treat hepatitis C infection in adults and children 3 years of age and older. Patients with hepatitis C have the virus in their blood and in their liver. PegIntron reduces the amount of virus in the body and helps the body's immune system fight the virus. REBETOL (ribavirin) is a drug that helps to fight the viral infection but does not work when used by itself to treat chronic hepatitis C.
It is not known if PegIntron or PegIntron/REBETOL therapies can cure hepatitis C (permanently eliminate the virus) or if it can prevent liver failure or liver cancer that is caused by hepatitis C infection.
It is also not known if PegIntron or PegIntron/REBETOL combination therapy will prevent one infected person from infecting another person with hepatitis C.
Who should not take PegIntron or PegIntron/REBETOL therapy?
Do not take PegIntron or PegIntron/REBETOL therapy if you:
- are pregnant, planning to get pregnant during treatment or during the 6 months after treatment, or breast-feeding
- are a male patient with a female sexual partner who is pregnant or plans to become pregnant at any time while you are being treated with REBETOL or during the 6 months after your treatment has ended
- have hepatitis caused by your immune system attacking your liver (autoimmune hepatitis) or unstable liver disease
- had an allergic reaction to another alpha interferon or are allergic to any of the ingredients in PegIntron or REBETOL Capsules or Oral Solution. If you have any doubts, ask your health care provider
- Do not take PegIntron/REBETOL combination therapy if you have abnormal red blood cells such as is seen in sickle-cell anemia or thalassemia major
If you have any of the following conditions or serious medical problems, discuss them with your health care provider before taking PegIntron or PegIntron/REBETOL therapy:
- depression or anxiety
- sleep problems
- high blood pressure
- previous heart attack, or other heart problems
- liver problems (other than hepatitis C infection)
- any kind of autoimmune disease (where the body's immune system attacks the body's own cells), such as psoriasis, systemic lupus erythematosus, rheumatoid arthritis
- thyroid problems
- diabetes
- colitis (inflammation of the bowels)
- cancer
- hepatitis B infection
- HIV infection
- kidney problems
- bleeding problems
- alcoholism
- drug abuse or addiction
- body organ transplant and are taking medicine that keeps your body from rejecting your transplant (suppresses your immune system)
Tell your healthcare provider about all the medicines you take, including prescription and non-prescription medicines, vitamins, and herbal supplements. PegIntron and certain other medicines may affect each other and cause side effects.
Especially tell your doctor if you take the anti-hepatitis B medicine telbivudine (Tyzeka). See "What are the possible side effects of PegIntron?"
Know the medicines you take. Keep a list of them and show it to your healthcare provider and pharmacist when you get a new medicine.
How should I take PegIntron or PegIntron/REBETOL?
Your health care provider will decide whether you will take PegIntron therapy alone or the combination of PegIntron/REBETOL, as well as the correct dose (for adults the dose of PegIntron is based on weight). For children 3 years of age and older, your healthcare provider will recommend the dose of PegIntron based on body surface area. PegIntron and PegIntron/REBETOL are given for up to one year. Take your prescribed dose of PegIntron ONCE A WEEK, on the same day of each week and at approximately the same time. Take the medicine for the full course of prescribed therapy and do not take more than the prescribed dose. REBETOL should be taken with food. When you take REBETOL with food, more of the medicine (70% more on average) is taken up by your body. You should take REBETOL the same way

every day (twice a day with food) to keep the medicine in your body at a steady level. This will help your health care provider to decide how your treatment is working and how to change the dose of REBETOL you take if you have side effects from REBETOL. **Be sure to read the Medication Guide for REBETOL (ribavirin, USP) for complete instructions on how to take the REBETOL capsules and oral solution.**

You should be completely comfortable with how to prepare PegIntron; how to set the dose you take, and how to inject yourself before you use PegIntron for the first time. PegIntron comes in two different forms, a powder in a single-use vial and a REDIPEN® single-use delivery system. See the attached appendix for detailed instructions for preparing and giving a dose of PegIntron.

If you miss a dose of the PegIntron product, take the missed dose as soon as possible during the same day or the next day, then continue on your regular dosing schedule. If several days go by after you miss a dose, check with your health care provider about what to do. Do not double the next dose or take more than one dose a week without talking to your health care provider. Call your health care provider right away if you take more than your prescribed PegIntron dose. Your health care provider may wish to examine you more closely, and take blood for testing.

If you miss a dose of REBETOL, take the missed dose as soon as possible during the same day. If an entire day has gone by, check with your health care provider about what to do. Do not double the next dose.

You must get regular blood tests to help your health care provider check how the treatment is working and to check for side effects.

Tell your health care provider if you are taking or planning to take other prescription or non-prescription medicines, including vitamin and mineral supplements and herbal medicines.

What should I avoid while taking PegIntron or PegIntron/REBETOL therapies?

• If you are pregnant do not start taking PegIntron/REBETOL combination therapy.

• Avoid becoming pregnant while taking PegIntron or PegIntron/REBETOL.

PegIntron and PegIntron/REBETOL may harm your unborn child (death or serious birth defects) or cause you to lose your baby (miscarry). **If you or your partner become pregnant during treatment or during the 6 months after treatment with PegIntron/REBETOL combination therapy, immediately report the pregnancy to your health care provider. You or your health care provider should call 1-800-593-2214.** By calling this number, information about you and/or your partner will be added to a pregnancy registry that will be used to help you and your health care provider make decisions about your treatment for hepatitis in the future. You, your partner and/or your health care provider will be asked to provide follow-up information on the outcome of the pregnancy.

• Do not breast-feed your baby while taking PegIntron.

What are the possible side effects of PegIntron and PegIntron/REBETOL combination therapy?

PegIntron may cause serious side effects including:

• See "What is the most important information I should know about PegIntron and PegIntron/REBETOL combination therapy?"

• **Other body organ problems.** A few patients have inflammation of the kidney.

• **New or worsening autoimmune disease.** Some patients taking PegIntron or PegIntron/REBETOL develop autoimmune diseases (a condition where the body's immune cells attack other cells or organs in the body), including rheumatoid arthritis, systemic lupus erythematosus, and psoriasis. In some patients who already have an autoimmune disease, the disease worsens on PegIntron and PegIntron/REBETOL combination therapy.

• **Growth problems in children.** Weight loss and slowed growth are common in children during treatment with PegIntron/REBETOL. Catch-up weight gain and some catch-up in growth happen after treatment stops, but some children may not reach the height that they were expected to have before treatment.

• **Nerve problems.** People who take PegIntron or other alpha interferon products with telbivudine (Tyzeka) can have nerve problems such as continuing numbness, tingling, or burning sensation in the arms or legs (peripheral neuropathy). Call your healthcare provider if you have any of these symptoms.

Common but less serious side effects include:

• **Flu-like symptoms.** Most patients who take PegIntron or PegIntron/REBETOL therapy have "flu-like" symptoms (headache, muscle aches, tiredness and fever). Some of these symptoms (fever, headache) usually lessen after the first few weeks of therapy. You can reduce some of these symptoms by injecting your PegIntron dose at bedtime.

Over-the-counter pain and fever reducers, such as acetaminophen or ibuprofen, can be used to prevent or reduce the fever and headache.

• **Extreme fatigue (tiredness).** Many patients become extremely tired while on PegIntron or PegIntron/REBETOL combination therapy.

• **Appetite problems.** Nausea, loss of appetite, and weight loss occur commonly.

• **Thyroid problems.** Some patients develop changes in the function of their thyroid. Symptoms of thyroid changes include the inability to concentrate, feeling cold or hot all the time, a change in your weight and changes to your skin.

• **Blood sugar problems.** Some patients develop problems with the way their body controls their blood sugar and may develop high blood sugar or diabetes.

• **Skin reactions.** Redness, swelling, and itching are common at the site of injection. If after several days these symptoms do not disappear contact your health care provider. You may get a rash during treatment. If this occurs, your health care provider may recommend medicine to treat the rash.

• **Hair thinning.** Hair thinning is common during PegIntron and PegIntron/REBETOL treatment. Hair loss stops and hair growth returns after therapy is stopped.

These are not all of the side effects of PegIntron or PegIntron/REBETOL combination therapy. Your health care provider or pharmacist can give you a more complete list.

Call your doctor for medical advice about side effects. You may report side effects to FDA at 1–800–FDA–1088.

General advice about prescription medicines:

Medicines are sometimes prescribed for purposes other than those listed in a Medication Guide. If you have any concerns about PegIntron, ask your health care provider. Your health care provider or pharmacist can give you information about PegIntron that was written for health care professionals. Do not use PegIntron for a condition for which it was not prescribed. Do not share this medication with other people.

If you are taking PegIntron/REBETOL combination therapy, also read the Medication Guide for REBETOL (ribavirin, USP) Capsules and Oral Solution.

This Medication Guide has been approved by the U.S. Food and Drug Administration.

Revised August 2009

How do I prepare and inject the PegIntron Dose?

Before you inject PegIntron, the powder must be mixed with **0.7 mL of the supplied DILUENT for PegIntron, Sterile Water for Injection (diluent).** This product can also be administered by a parent or care-taker as instructed by your healthcare provider. You should carefully follow the directions given to you by your health care provider.

The vial of mixed PegIntron should be used immediately. DO NOT prepare more than one vial at a time. If you don't use the vial of the prepared solution right away, it must be stored in a refrigerator and used within 24 hours.

Storing PegIntron

PegIntron Powder should be stored at room temperature (25°C, 77°F); avoid exposure to heat. After mixing, the PegIntron solution should be used immediately but may be stored in the refrigerator up to 24 hours. The solution contains no preservatives. DO NOT FREEZE.

Preparing the PegIntron solution:

1. Find a clean, well-lit, non-slip flat working surface and assemble all of the supplies you will need for an injection. All of the supplies you will need for an injection are in the PegIntron Powder for Injection package. The package contains:
    ■ a vial of PegIntron powder
    ■ a 1.25 mL vial of DILUENT
    ■ 2 disposable syringes, and
    ■ alcohol swabs

2. Check the date printed on the PegIntron carton to make sure that the expiration date has not passed. Remove one vial and look at the contents. The PegIntron in the vial should appear as a white to off-white tablet-like solid that is whole/in pieces or as a loose powder.

    If you have already mixed the PegIntron solution and it has been stored properly in the refrigerator, take it out of the refrigerator and allow the solution to come to room temperature.

3. Wash your hands thoroughly with soap and water, rinse and towel dry. It is important to keep your work area, your hands, and injection site clean to minimize the risk of infection.

    The disposable syringes have needles that are already attached and cannot be removed. Each syringe has a clear plastic safety sleeve that is pulled over the needle for disposal after use. The safety sleeve should remain tight against the flange while using the syringe and moved over the needle only when ready for disposal.

Figure A.
The syringes and needles are for single use only.

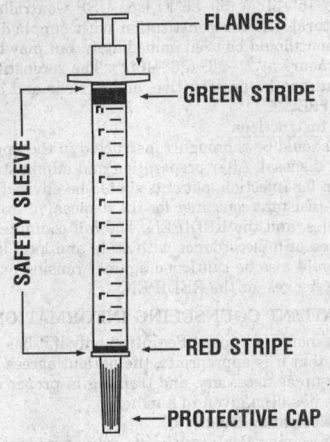

Figure A

4. Remove the protective wrapper from ONE of the syringes provided and use for the following steps 5–7. Make sure that the syringe safety sleeve is sitting against the flange (see **Figure A**).

5. Remove the protective plastic cap from the tops of both the supplied DILUENT and the PegIntron vials. Clean the rubber stopper on the top of both vials with an alcohol swab.

6. Carefully remove the protective cap straight off of the needle to avoid damaging the needle point. Fill the syringe with air by pulling the plunger to 0.7 mL (**Figure B**). Hold the DILUENT vial upright. Do not touch the cleaned top of the vial with your hands (**Figure C**). Insert the needle through the center of the rubber stopper of the DILUENT vial, and inject the air from the syringe into the vial (**Figure D**). Turn the vial upside down and make sure the tip of the needle is in the liquid. **Withdraw only 0.7 mL of DILUENT** by pulling the plunger back to the 0.7 mL mark on the side of the syringe (**Figure E**). Remove the needle from the vial (**Figure F**). Discard the remaining DILUENT.

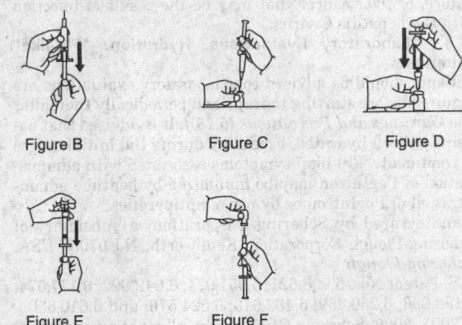

Figure B   Figure C   Figure D

Figure E   Figure F

7. Insert the needle through the center of the rubber stopper of the PegIntron vial, and place the needle tip against the glass wall of the vial (**Figure G**). SLOWLY inject the 0.7 mL DILUENT so that the stream of DILUENT runs down the side of the vial. To prevent bubbles from forming, DO NOT AIM THE STREAM of diluent directly on the tablet-like SOLID or POWDER in the bottom of the vial. Remove the needle from the vial.

    Firmly grasp the safety sleeve and pull it over the exposed needle until you hear a click. The green stripe on the safety sleeve will completely cover the red stripe on the needle. (See **Figure O** in the section: "Injecting the PegIntron dose.") Discard the syringe and needle in the puncture-proof container.

8. GENTLY swirl the vial in a gentle circular motion (**Figure H**), until the PegIntron is completely dissolved. **DO NOT SHAKE** the vial. If any powder remains undissolved in the vial, gently turn the vial upside down until all of the powder is dissolved. It is not unusual for the solution to appear cloudy or bubbly for a few minutes. If air bubbles do form, wait until the solution has settled and all bubbles have risen to the top before withdrawing your dose from the vial.

[See figure H at top of next page]

9. After the solution has settled and is completely dissolved it should be clear, colorless and without particles, but there may be a ring of foam or bubbles on the surface, this is normal. Do not use it if you see particles or the color is not correct.

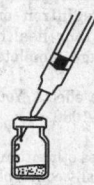

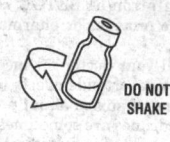

DO NOT SHAKE

Figure G   Figure H

10. After the PegIntron powder is dissolved but before you withdraw your dose, clean the rubber stopper again with an alcohol swab.

11. Unwrap the second syringe provided. You will use it to give yourself the injection. Carefully remove the protective cap from the needle and fill the syringe with air by pulling the plunger to the number on the side of the syringe (mL) that corresponds to your prescribed dose (**Figure J**). Hold the PegIntron vial upright. DO NOT touch the cleaned top of the vial with your hands (**Figure K**). Insert the needle into the vial containing the PegIntron solution and inject the air into the center of the vial (**Figure L**).

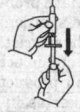 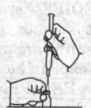 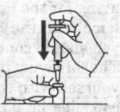

Figure J   Figure K   Figure L

12. Turn the PegIntron vial upside down. Be sure the tip of the needle is in the PegIntron solution. While holding the vial and syringe with one hand slowly pull the plunger back to withdraw the exact amount of PegIntron into the syringe your health care provider told you to use (**Figure M**).

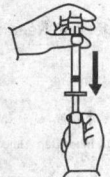

Figure M

13. Remove the needle from the vial (**Figure N**) and check for air bubbles in the syringe. If you see any bubbles, hold the syringe with the needle pointing up and gently tap the syringe until the bubbles rise. Then push the plunger in slowly until the bubbles disappear.

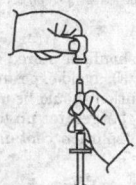

Figure N

Injecting the PegIntron Dose
Selecting the Site for Injection.
The best sites for giving yourself an injection are those areas with a layer of fat between the skin and muscle, like your thigh, the outer surface of your upper arm, and abdomen. Do not inject yourself in the area near your navel or waistline. If you are very thin, you should only use the thigh or outer surface of the arm for injection.
You should use a different site each time you inject PegIntron to avoid soreness at any one site. Do not inject PegIntron solution into an area where the skin is irritated, red, bruised, infected or has scars, stretch marks or lumps.

14. Clean the skin where the injection is to be given with an alcohol swab, and wait for the area to dry. Remove the protective cap from the needle. Make sure the safety sleeve of the syringe is pushed firmly against the syringe flange so that the needle is fully exposed (see **Figure A**).

15. *With one hand, pinch a 2-inch fold of loose skin. With your other hand, pick up the syringe and hold it like a pencil. Position the bevel of the needle facing up and insert the needle approximately ¼ inch into the pinched skin at approximately a 45 to 90 degree angle with a quick dart-like thrust. After the needle is in, remove the hand that you used to pinch your skin and use it to hold the syringe barrel. Pull the plunger of the sy-*ringe back very slightly. If blood comes into the syringe, the needle has entered a blood vessel. **Do not inject.** Withdraw the needle and discard the syringe as outlined in step 17. Repeat the above steps with a new vial to prepare a new syringe and inject the medicine at a new site. If no blood is present in the syringe, inject the medicine by gently pressing the plunger all the way down the syringe barrel.

16. Hold an alcohol swab near the needle and pull the needle straight out of the skin. Press the alcohol swab over the injection site for several seconds. Do not massage the injection site. If there is bleeding, cover it with a bandage.

17. After injecting your dose, firmly grasp the safety sleeve and pull it over the exposed needle until you hear a click, and the green stripe on the safety sleeve covers the red stripe on the needle (**Figure O**). Discard the syringe and needle in the Sharp's container supplied to you.

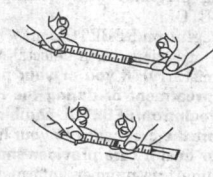

Figure O

18. After 2 hours, check the injection site for redness, swelling, or tenderness. If you have a skin reaction and it doesn't clear up in a few days, contact your health care provider or nurse.

How do I dispose of the used syringes and needles?
Discard used safety lock syringes and needles in a Sharp's container or other puncture-proof container like a coffee can. DO NOT USE glass or clear plastic containers. Your health care provider or nurse will tell you how to dispose of a full container. Always keep the container out of reach of children.
Manufactured by Schering Corporation, a subsidiary of Schering-Plough Corporation, Kenilworth, NJ 07033 USA.
© 2001, 2008, Schering Corporation. All rights reserved.
Rev 8/09
278535XXT
276624XXT

MEDICATION GUIDE
PegIntron® REDIPEN® Single-dose Delivery System (Peginterferon alfa-2b)
Including appendix with instructions for using PegIntron® REDIPEN® Single-dose Delivery System
Read this Medication Guide carefully before you start taking PegIntron® (**Peg In-tron**) or PegIntron/REBETOL® (**REB-eh-tole**) combination therapy. Read the Medication Guide each time you refill your prescription because there may be new information. The information in this Medication Guide does not take the place of talking with your health care provider (doctor, nurse, nurse practitioner, or physician's assistant).
If you are taking PegIntron/REBETOL combination therapy, also read the Medication Guide for REBETOL (ribavirin USP) Capsules and Oral Solution.
What is the most important information I should know about PegIntron and PegIntron/REBETOL combination therapy?
PegIntron (peginterferon) is a treatment for some people who are infected with hepatitis C virus. However, PegIntron and PegIntron/REBETOL combination therapy can have serious side effects that may cause death in rare cases. Before you decide to start treatment, you should talk to your health care provider about the possible benefits and side effects of PegIntron or PegIntron/REBETOL combination therapy. If you begin treatment you will need to see your health care provider regularly for medical examinations and lab tests to make sure your treatment is working and to check for side effects.

REBETOL may cause birth defects and/or death of an unborn child. If you are pregnant, you or your male partner must not take PegIntron/REBETOL combination therapy. You must not become pregnant while either you or your partner are being treated with the combination PegIntron/REBETOL therapy, or for 6 months after stopping therapy. Men and women should use birth control while taking the combination therapy and for 6 months afterwards. If you or your partner are being treated and you become pregnant, either during treatment or within 6 months of stopping treatment, call your health care provider right away. There is a Ribavirin Pregnancy Registry that collects information about pregnancy outcomes of female patients and female partners of male patients exposed to ribavirin. You or your healthcare provider are encouraged to contact the Registry at 1-800-593-2214.

If you are taking PegIntron or PegIntron/REBETOL therapy you should call your health care provider immediately if you develop any of these symptoms:
New or worsening mental health problems such as thoughts about killing or hurting yourself or others, trouble breathing, chest pain, severe stomach or lower back pain, bloody diarrhea or bloody bowel movements, high fever, bruising, bleeding, or decreased vision.
The most serious possible side effects of PegIntron and PegIntron/REBETOL therapy include:
Problems with Pregnancy. Combination PegIntron/REBETOL therapy can cause death, serious birth defects, or other harm to your unborn child. If you are a woman of childbearing age, you must not become pregnant during treatment and for 6 months after you have stopped therapy. You must have a negative pregnancy test immediately before beginning treatment, during treatment, and for 6 months after you have stopped therapy. Both male and female patients must use effective forms of birth control during treatment and for the 6 months after treatment is completed. Male patients should use a condom. If you are a female, you must use birth control even if you believe that you are not fertile or that your fertility is low. You should talk to your health care provider about birth control for you and your partner.
Mental health problems and suicide. PegIntron and PegIntron/REBETOL therapies may cause patients to develop mood or behavioral problems. These can include irritability (getting easily upset) and depression (feeling low, feeling bad about yourself, or feeling hopeless). Some patients may have aggressive behavior. Former drug addicts may fall back into drug addiction or overdose. Some patients think about hurting or killing themselves or other people and some have killed (suicide) or hurt themselves or others. You must tell your health care provider if you are being treated for a mental illness or had treatment in the past for any mental illness, including depression and suicidal behavior. You should tell your health care provider if you have ever been addicted to drugs or alcohol.
Heart problems. Some patients taking PegIntron or PegIntron/REBETOL therapy may develop problems with their heart, including low blood pressure, fast heart rate, and very rarely, heart attacks. Tell your health care provider if you have had any heart problems in the past.
Blood problems. PegIntron and PegIntron/REBETOL therapies commonly lower two types of blood cells (white blood cells and platelets). In some patients, these blood counts may fall to dangerously low levels. If your blood counts become very low, this could lead to infections or bleeding. REBETOL therapy causes a decrease in the number of red blood cells you have (anemia). This can be dangerous, especially for patients who already have heart or circulatory (cardiovascular) problems. Talk with your health care provider before taking combination PegIntron/REBETOL therapy if you have or have ever had any cardiovascular problems.
Body organ problems. Certain symptoms like severe stomach pain may mean that your internal organs are being damaged. PegIntron may cause lung problems including: trouble breathing, pneumonia, inflammation of lung tissue, and new or worse high blood pressure of the lungs (pulmonary hypertension), which can be severe and may in some cases lead to death. Cases of weakness, loss of coordination, and numbness due to stroke have been reported in patients taking PegIntron, including patients with few or no reported risk factors for stroke.
Eye problems. Changes in vision such as a decrease or loss of vision (blindness) may happen in some patients. You should have an eye exam before you take PegIntron. If you have eye problems or have had them in the past, you may need eye exams while you are taking PegIntron. Tell your healthcare provider or eye doctor right away if you have changes in your vision while taking PegIntron.
For other possible side effects, see "What are the possible side effects of PegIntron and PegIntron/REBETOL combination therapy?" in this Medication Guide.
What is PegIntron and PegIntron/REBETOL combination therapy?
The PegIntron product is a drug used to treat adults who have a lasting (chronic) infection with hepatitis C virus and who show signs that the virus is damaging the liver. PegIntron/REBETOL combination therapy consists of two medications also used to treat hepatitis C infection in adults and children 3 years of age and older. Patients with hepatitis C have the virus in their blood and in their liver. PegIntron reduces the amount of virus in the body and helps the body's immune system fight the virus. REBETOL (ribavirin) is a drug that helps to fight the viral infection, but does not work when used by itself to treat chronic hepatitis C.
It is not known if PegIntron or PegIntron/REBETOL therapies can cure hepatitis C (permanently eliminate the virus), or if it can prevent liver failure or liver cancer that is caused by hepatitis C infection.

It is also not known if PegIntron or PegIntron/REBETOL combination therapy will prevent one infected person from infecting another person with hepatitis C.

Who should not take PegIntron or PegIntron/REBETOL therapy?

Do not take PegIntron or PegIntron/REBETOL therapy if you:
- are pregnant, planning to get pregnant during treatment or during the 6 months after treatment, or breastfeeding.
- are a male patient with a female sexual partner who is pregnant, or plans to become pregnant at any time while you are being treated with REBETOL, or during the 6 months after your treatment has ended.
- have hepatitis caused by your immune system attacking your liver (autoimmune hepatitis) or unstable liver disease
- had an allergic reaction to another alpha interferon or are allergic to any of the ingredients in PegIntron or REBETOL Capsules or Oral Solution. If you have any doubts, ask your health care provider.
- Do not take PegIntron/REBETOL combination therapy if you have abnormal red blood cells such as is seen in sickle-cell anemia or thalassemia major.

If you have any of the following conditions or serious medical problems, discuss them with your health care provider before taking PegIntron or PegIntron/REBETOL therapy:
- depression or anxiety
- sleep problems
- high blood pressure
- previous heart attack, or other heart problems
- liver problems (other than hepatitis C infection)
- any kind of autoimmune disease (where the body's immune system attacks the body's own cells), such as psoriasis, systemic lupus erythematosus, rheumatoid arthritis
- thyroid problems
- diabetes
- colitis (inflammation of the bowels)
- cancer
- hepatitis B infection
- HIV infection
- kidney problems
- bleeding problems
- alcoholism
- drug abuse or addiction
- body organ transplant and are taking medicine that keeps your body from rejecting your transplant (suppresses your immune system)

Tell your healthcare provider about all the medicines you take, including prescription and non-prescription medicines, vitamins, and herbal supplements. PegIntron and certain other medicines may affect each other and cause side effects.

Especially tell your doctor if you take the anti-hepatitis B medicine telbivudine (Tyzeka). See "What are the possible side effects of PegIntron?"

Know the medicines you take. Keep a list of them and show it to your healthcare provider and pharmacist when you get a new medicine.

How should I take PegIntron or PegIntron/REBETOL?

Your health care provider will decide whether you will take PegIntron therapy alone or the combination of PegIntron/REBETOL, as well as the correct dose (for adults the dose of PegIntron is based on weight). For children 3 years of age and older, your healthcare provider will recommend the dose of PegIntron based on body surface area. PegIntron and PegIntron/REBETOL are given for up to 1 year. Take your prescribed dose of PegIntron ONCE A WEEK, on the same day of each week and at approximately the same time. Take the medicine for the full course of prescribed therapy and do not take more than the prescribed dose. REBETOL should be taken with food. When you take REBETOL with food, more of the medicine (70% more on average) is taken up by your body. You should take REBETOL the same way every day (twice a day with food) to keep the medicine in your body at a steady level. This will help your health care provider to decide how your treatment is working and how to change the dose of REBETOL you take if you have side effects from REBETOL. **Be sure to read the Medication Guide for REBETOL (ribavirin USP) for complete instructions on how to take the REBETOL capsules and oral solution.**

You should be completely comfortable with how to prepare PegIntron, how to set the dose you take, and how to inject yourself before you use PegIntron for the first time. PegIntron comes in two different forms, a powder in a single-use vial and a REDIPEN® single-use delivery system. See the attached appendix for detailed instructions for preparing and giving a dose of PegIntron.

If you miss a dose of the PegIntron product, take the missed dose as soon as possible during the same day or the next day, then continue on your regular dosing schedule. If several days go by after you miss a dose, check with your health care provider about what to do. Do not double the next dose or take more than one dose a week without talking to your health care provider. Call your health care provider right away if you take more than your prescribed PegIntron dose. Your health care provider may wish to examine you more closely, and take blood for testing.

If you miss a dose of REBETOL, take the missed dose as soon as possible during the same day. If an entire day has gone by, check with your health care provider about what to do. Do not double the next dose.

You must get regular blood tests to help your health care provider check how the treatment is working and to check for side effects.

Tell your health care provider if you are taking or planning to take other prescription or non-prescription medicines, including vitamin and mineral supplements and herbal medicines.

What should I avoid while taking PegIntron or PegIntron/REBETOL therapies?
- If you are pregnant do not start taking PegIntron/REBETOL combination therapy.
- Avoid becoming pregnant while taking PegIntron or PegIntron/REBETOL.

PegIntron and PegIntron/REBETOL may harm your unborn child (death or serious birth defects) or cause you to lose your baby (miscarry). **If you or your partner become pregnant during treatment or during the 6 months after treatment with PegIntron/REBETOL combination therapy, immediately report the pregnancy to your health care provider. You or your health care provider should call 1-800-593-2214.** By calling this number, information about you and/or your partner will be added to a pregnancy registry that will be used to help you and your health care provider make decisions about your treatment for hepatitis in the future. You, your partner, and/or your health care provider will be asked to provide follow-up information on the outcome of the pregnancy.
- Do not breastfeed your baby while taking PegIntron.

What are the possible side effects of PegIntron and PegIntron/REBETOL combination therapy?

PegIntron may cause serious side effects including:

See "What is the most important information I should know about PegIntron and PegIntron/REBETOL combination therapy?"

Other body organ problems. A few patients have inflammation of the kidney.

New or worsening autoimmune disease. Some patients taking PegIntron or PegIntron/REBETOL develop autoimmune diseases (a condition where the body's immune cells attack other cells or organs in the body), including rheumatoid arthritis, systemic lupus erythematosus, and psoriasis. In some patients who already have an autoimmune disease, the disease worsens on PegIntron and PegIntron/REBETOL combination therapy.

Growth problems in children. Weight loss and slowed growth are common in children during treatment with PegIntron/REBETOL. Catch-up weight gain and some catch-up in growth happen after treatment stops, but some children may not reach the height that they were expected to have before treatment.

Nerve problems. People who take PegIntron or other alpha interferon products with telbivudine (Tyzeka) can have nerve problems such as continuing numbness, tingling, or burning sensation in the arms or legs (peripheral neuropathy). Call your healthcare provider if you have any of these symptoms.

Common but less serious side effects include:

Flu-like symptoms. Most patients who take PegIntron or PegIntron/REBETOL therapy have "flu-like" symptoms (headache, muscle aches, tiredness, and fever). Some of these symptoms (fever, headache) usually lessen after the first few weeks of therapy. You can reduce some of these symptoms by injecting your PegIntron dose at bedtime. Over-the-counter pain and fever reducers, such as acetaminophen or ibuprofen, can be used to prevent or reduce the fever and headache.

Extreme fatigue (tiredness). Many patients become extremely tired while on PegIntron or PegIntron/REBETOL combination therapy.

Appetite problems. Nausea, loss of appetite, and weight loss occur commonly.

Thyroid problems. Some patients develop changes in the function of their thyroid. Symptoms of thyroid changes include the inability to concentrate, feeling cold or hot all the time, a change in your weight, and changes to your skin.

Blood sugar problems. Some patients develop problems with the way their body controls their blood sugar, and may develop high blood sugar or diabetes.

Skin reactions. Redness, swelling, and itching are common at the site of injection. If after several days these symptoms do not disappear contact your health care provider. You may get a rash during therapy. If this occurs, your health care provider may recommend medicine to treat the rash.

Hair thinning. Hair thinning is common during PegIntron and PegIntron/REBETOL treatment. Hair loss stops and hair growth returns after therapy is stopped.

These are not all of the side effects of PegIntron or PegIntron/REBETOL combination therapy. Your health care provider or pharmacist can give you a more complete list.

Call your doctor for medical advice about side effects. You may report side effects to FDA at 1–800–FDA–1088.

General advice about prescription medicines:

Medicines are sometimes prescribed for purposes other than those listed in a Medication Guide. If you have any concerns about PegIntron, ask your health care provider. Your health care provider or pharmacist can give you information about PegIntron that was written for health care professionals. Do not use PegIntron for a condition for which it was not prescribed. Do not share this medication with other people.

If you are taking PegIntron/REBETOL combination therapy, also read the Medication Guide for REBETOL (ribavirin USP) Capsules and Oral Solution.

This Medication Guide has been approved by the U.S. Food and Drug Administration.

Revised: August 2009

How do I prepare and inject the PegIntron REDIPEN dose?

The PegIntron REDIPEN system is for a single use, by one person only, ONCE A WEEK. The REDIPEN must not be shared. Use only the injection needle provided in the packaging for the PegIntron REDIPEN system. If you have problems with the REDIPEN system or the PegIntron solution, you should contact your health care provider or pharmacist. The following instructions explain how to prepare and inject yourself with the PegIntron REDIPEN system. This product can also be administered by a parent or caretaker as instructed by your healthcare provider. Please read the instructions carefully and follow them step by step. Your health care provider will instruct you on how to self-inject with the PegIntron REDIPEN. Do not attempt to inject yourself unless you are sure you understand the procedure and requirements for self-injection.

How to Use the PegIntron® REDIPEN® Single-dose Delivery System.

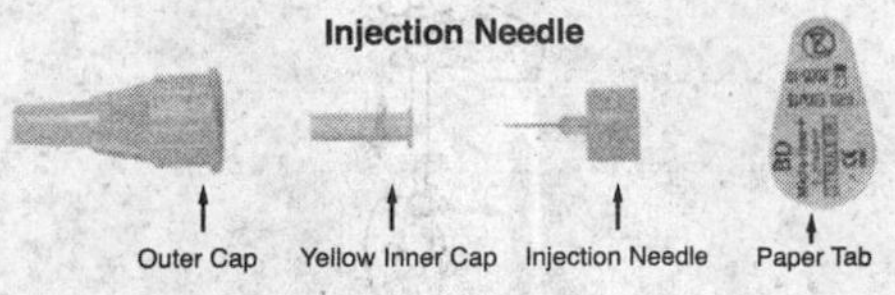
Injection Needle
Outer Cap
Yellow Inner Cap
Injection Needle
Paper Tab

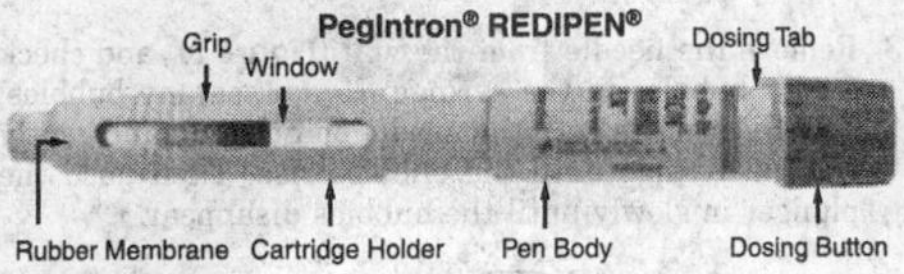
PegIntron® REDIPEN®
Grip
Window
Dosing Tab
Rubber Membrane
Cartridge Holder
Pen Body
Dosing Button

Storing PegIntron

PegIntron REDIPEN should be stored in the refrigerator at 2°C to 8°C (36°F to 46°F); avoid exposure to heat. After mixing, the PegIntron solution should be used immediately but may be stored in the refrigerator up to 24 hours at 2°C to 8°C (36°F–46°F). The solution contains no preservatives. DO NOT FREEZE.

Preparation

1. Find a clean, well-lit, non-slip flat working surface and assemble all of the supplies you will need for an injection. All of the supplies you will need are in the PegIntron REDIPEN package. The package contains:
   - a PegIntron REDIPEN single-dose delivery system
   - one disposable needle
   - two alcohol swabs, and
   - dosing tray (the dosing tray is the bottom half of the REDIPEN package).
2. Take the PegIntron REDIPEN out of the refrigerator and allow the medicine to come to room temperature. Before removing the REDIPEN from the carton, check the expiration date printed on the PegIntron REDIPEN carton to make sure that the expiration date has not passed. Do not use if the expiration date has passed.
3. After taking the PegIntron REDIPEN out of the carton, look in the window of the REDIPEN and make sure the PegIntron in the cartridge holder window is a white to off white tablet that is whole, or in pieces, or powdered.
4. Wash your hands thoroughly with soap and water, rinse, and towel dry. It is important to keep your work area, your hands, and the injection site clean to minimize the risk of infection.

1. **Mix the Drug**

   Key points:

   Before you mix the PegIntron, make sure it is at room temperature. It is important that you keep the PegIntron REDIPEN UPRIGHT (dosing button down) as shown in Figure 1.

a. Hold the PegIntron REDIPEN **UPRIGHT (Figure 1a)** in the dosing tray on a hard, flat, non-slip surface with the dosing button **down.** You may want to hold the REDIPEN using the grip.

b. To mix the powder and the liquid, keep the REDIPEN upright in the dosing tray and press the top half of the REDIPEN downward toward the hard, flat, non-slip surface <u>until you hear the click</u> (Figure 1b). Once you've heard the click, you will notice in the window that both dark stoppers are now touching. The dosing button should be flush with the pen body.

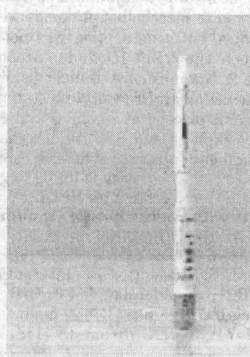

Figure 1a

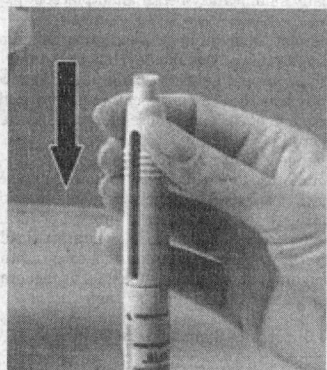

Figure 1b

c. Wait several seconds for the powder to completely dissolve.

d. Gently turn the PegIntron REDIPEN upside down twice (Figure 2). To avoid excessive foaming, DO NOT SHAKE.

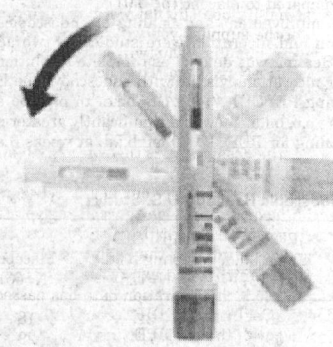

Figure 2

e. Keep the PegIntron REDIPEN **UPRIGHT,** with the dosing button down. Then, look through the REDIPEN window to see that the mixed PegIntron solution is completely dissolved. The solution should be clear and colorless <u>before use</u>. Before attaching the needle, it is normal to see some small bubbles in the REDIPEN window, near the top of the solution. Do not use the solution if it is discolored, or not clear, or if particulates are present.

f. Place the PegIntron REDIPEN back into the dosing tray provided in the packaging (Figure 3). The dosing button will be on the bottom.

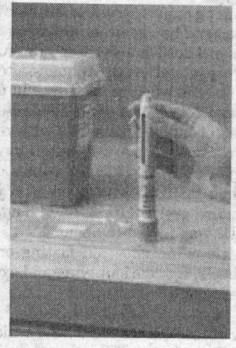

Figure 3

2. Attach the Needle

a. Wipe the rubber membrane of the PegIntron REDIPEN with one alcohol swab.

b. Remove the protective paper tab from the injection needle, but do NOT remove either the outer cap or the yellow inner cap from the injection needle. Keeping the PegIntron REDIPEN UPRIGHT in the dosing tray, FIRMLY push the injection needle straight into the REDIPEN rubber membrane, and screw it firmly in place, in a clockwise direction (Figure 4). Remember to leave the needle caps in place when you attach the needle to the REDIPEN. Pushing the needle through the rubber membrane "primes" the needle and allows the extra liquid and air in the pen to be removed.

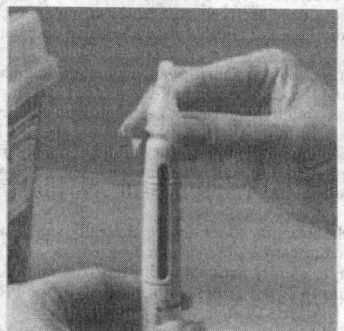

Figure 4

NOTE: Some fluid will trickle out. This is **normal.** The dark stoppers move up and you will no longer see the fluid in the window once the needle is successfully primed.

3. Dialing the Dose

a. **Remove the PegIntron REDIPEN from the dosing tray (Figure 5a).** Holding the PegIntron REDIPEN firmly, pull the dosing button out as far as it will go. You will see a dark band.
Do not push the dosing button in until you are ready to self-inject the PegIntron dose.

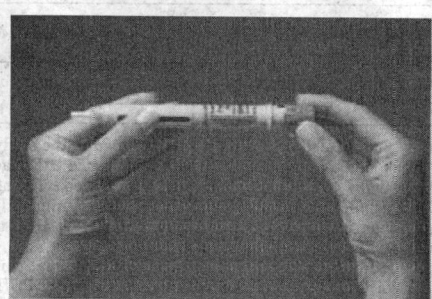

Figure 5a

b. Turn the dosing button until your prescribed dose is lined up with the dosing tab (**Figure 5b**). The dosing button will turn freely. If you have trouble dialing your dose, check to make sure the dosing button has been pulled out **as far** as it will go (**Figure 5c**).

[See figures 5b and 5c at top of next column]

c. Carefully lay the PegIntron REDIPEN down on a hard, flat, non-slip surface. Do NOT remove either of

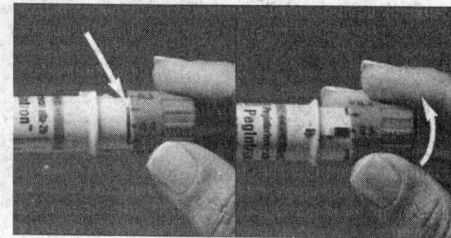

Figure 5b   Figure 5c

the needle caps and do NOT push the dosing button in until you are ready to self-inject the PegIntron dose.

4. Injecting the PegIntron Dose
Choosing an Injection Site
The best sites for giving yourself an injection are those areas with a layer of fat between the skin and muscle, like your thigh, the outer surface of your upper arm, and abdomen. Do not inject yourself in the area near your navel or waistline. If you are very thin, you should only use the thigh or outer surface of the arm for injection.

You should use a different site each time you inject PegIntron to avoid soreness at any one site. Do not inject PegIntron into an area where the skin is irritated, red, bruised, infected, or has scars, stretch marks, or lumps.

a. Clean the skin where the injection is to be given with the second alcohol swab provided, and wait for the area to dry.

b. Remove the **outer** cap from the needle (**Figure 6a**). There may be some liquid around the yellow inner needle cap (**Figure 6b**). This is normal.

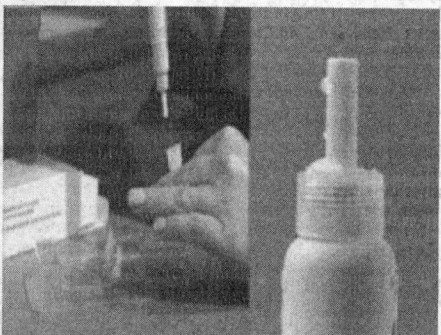

Figure 6a   Figure 6b

c. Once the injection site is dry, remove the **yellow** inner needle cap (**Figure 6c**). You are now ready to inject.

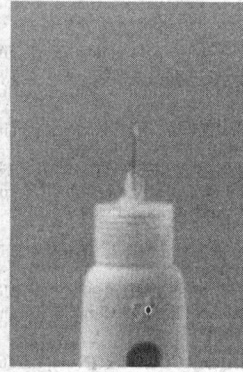

Figure 6c

d. **Hold the PegIntron REDIPEN with your fingers wrapped around the pen body barrel and your thumb on the dosing button (Figure 7).**
• With your other hand, pinch the skin in the area you have cleaned for injection.
• Insert the needle into the pinched skin at an angle of 45° to 90°.
• Press the dosing button down slowly and firmly until you can't push it any further.
• Keep your thumb pressed down on the dosing button for an additional 5 seconds to ensure that you get the complete dose.

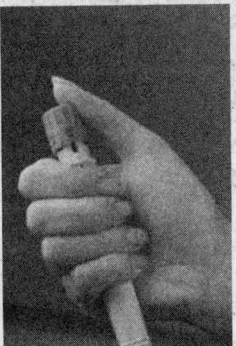

Figure 7

- Remove the needle from your skin.

e. **Gently press the injection site with a small bandage or sterile gauze if necessary for a few seconds but** do not massage the injection site. If there is bleeding, cover with an adhesive bandage. **DO NOT RECAP THE NEEDLE and DO NOT REUSE the REDIPEN.**

How do I dispose of the REDIPEN?
Discard the REDIPEN and needle and any solution remaining in the REDIPEN in a Sharp's container or other puncture-resistant container like a metal coffee can. DO NOT use glass or clear plastic containers. Ask your health care provider how to dispose of a full container. Always keep the container out of reach of children.

After 2 hours, check the injection site for redness, swelling, or tenderness. If you have a skin reaction and it doesn't clear up in a few days, contact your health care provider.
Manufactured by Schering Corporation, a subsidiary of Schering-Plough Corporation, Kenilworth, NJ 07033 USA.
© 2003, 2008, Schering Corporation. All rights reserved.
Rev 8/09
276624XXT
Shown in Product Identification Guide, page 313

PEPCID® ℞
[pep' sid]
(famotidine)
Tablets

DESCRIPTION
The active ingredient in PEPCID[1] (famotidine) is a histamine H_2-receptor antagonist. Famotidine is N'-(aminosulfonyl)-3-[[[2-[(diaminomethylene)amino]-4-thiazolyl]methyl]thio]propanimidamide. The empirical formula of famotidine is $C_8H_{15}N_7O_2S_3$ and its molecular weight is 337.43. Its structural formula is:

Famotidine is a white to pale yellow crystalline compound that is freely soluble in glacial acetic acid, slightly soluble in methanol, very slightly soluble in water, and practically insoluble in ethanol.

Each tablet for oral administration contains either 20 mg or 40 mg of famotidine and the following inactive ingredients: hydroxypropyl cellulose, hypromellose, iron oxides, magnesium stearate, microcrystalline cellulose, corn starch, talc, titanium dioxide, and carnauba wax.

[1] Registered trademark of Merck Sharp & Dohme Corp., a subsidiary of **Merck & Co., Inc.**
Copyright © 1986, 1988, 1991, 1995, 1996 Merck Sharp & Dohme Corp., a subsidiary of **Merck & Co., Inc.**
All rights reserved

CLINICAL PHARMACOLOGY IN ADULTS
GI Effects
PEPCID is a competitive inhibitor of histamine H_2-receptors. The primary clinically important pharmacologic activity of PEPCID is inhibition of gastric secretion. Both the acid concentration and volume of gastric secretion are suppressed by PEPCID, while changes in pepsin secretion are proportional to volume output.
In normal volunteers and hypersecretors, PEPCID inhibited basal and nocturnal gastric secretion, as well as secretion stimulated by food and pentagastrin. After oral administration, the onset of the antisecretory effect occurred within one hour; the maximum effect was dose-dependent, occurring within one to three hours. Duration of inhibition of secretion by doses of 20 and 40 mg was 10 to 12 hours.

Single evening oral doses of 20 and 40 mg inhibited basal and nocturnal acid secretion in all subjects; mean nocturnal gastric acid secretion was inhibited by 86% and 94%, respectively, for a period of at least 10 hours. The same doses given in the morning suppressed food-stimulated acid secretion in all subjects. The mean suppression was 76% and 84%, respectively, 3 to 5 hours after administration, and 25% and 30%, respectively, 8 to 10 hours after administration. In some subjects who received the 20-mg dose, however, the antisecretory effect was dissipated within 6-8 hours. There was no cumulative effect with repeated doses. The nocturnal intragastric pH was raised by evening doses of 20 and 40 mg of PEPCID to mean values of 5.0 and 6.4, respectively. When PEPCID was given after breakfast, the basal daytime interdigestive pH at 3 and 8 hours after 20 or 40 mg of PEPCID was raised to about 5.
PEPCID had little or no effect on fasting or postprandial serum gastrin levels. Gastric emptying and exocrine pancreatic function were not affected by PEPCID.
Other Effects
Systemic effects of PEPCID in the CNS, cardiovascular, respiratory or endocrine systems were not noted in clinical pharmacology studies. Also, no antiandrogenic effects were noted. (See ADVERSE REACTIONS.) Serum hormone levels, including prolactin, cortisol, thyroxine (T_4), and testosterone, were not altered after treatment with PEPCID.
Pharmacokinetics
PEPCID is incompletely absorbed. The bioavailability of oral doses is 40-45%. Bioavailability may be slightly increased by food, or slightly decreased by antacids; however, these effects are of no clinical consequence. PEPCID undergoes minimal first-pass metabolism. After oral doses, peak plasma levels occur in 1-3 hours. Plasma levels after multiple doses are similar to those after single doses. Fifteen to 20% of PEPCID in plasma is protein bound. PEPCID has an elimination half-life of 2.5-3.5 hours. PEPCID is eliminated by renal (65-70%) and metabolic (30-35%) routes. Renal clearance is 250-450 mL/min, indicating some tubular excretion. Twenty-five to 30% of an oral dose and 65-70% of an intravenous dose are recovered in the urine as unchanged compound. The only metabolite identified in man is the S-oxide.
There is a close relationship between creatinine clearance values and the elimination half-life of PEPCID. In patients with severe renal insufficiency, i.e., creatinine clearance less than 10 mL/min, the elimination half-life of PEPCID may exceed 20 hours and adjustment of dose or dosing intervals in moderate and severe renal insufficiency may be necessary (see PRECAUTIONS, DOSAGE AND ADMINISTRATION).
In elderly patients, there are no clinically significant age-related changes in the pharmacokinetics of PEPCID. However, in elderly patients with decreased renal function, the clearance of the drug may be decreased (see PRECAUTIONS, Geriatric Use).
Clinical Studies
Duodenal Ulcer
In a U.S. multicenter, double-blind study in outpatients with endoscopically confirmed duodenal ulcer, orally administered PEPCID was compared to placebo. As shown in Table 1, 70% of patients treated with PEPCID 40 mg h.s. were healed by week 4.

Table 1: Outpatients with Endoscopically Confirmed Healed Duodenal Ulcers

	PEPCID 40 mg h.s. (N = 89)	PEPCID 20 mg b.i.d. (N = 84)	Placebo h.s. (N = 97)
Week 2	*32%	*38%	17%
Week 4	*70%	*67%	31%

*Statistically significantly different than placebo (p<0.001)

Patients not healed by week 4 were continued in the study. By week 8, 83% of patients treated with PEPCID had healed versus 45% of patients treated with placebo. The incidence of ulcer healing with PEPCID was significantly higher than with placebo at each time point based on proportion of endoscopically confirmed healed ulcers.
In this study, time to relief of daytime and nocturnal pain was significantly shorter for patients receiving PEPCID than for patients receiving placebo; patients receiving PEPCID also took less antacid than the patients receiving placebo.
Long-Term Maintenance
Treatment of Duodenal Ulcers
PEPCID, 20 mg p.o. h.s., was compared to placebo h.s. as maintenance therapy in two double-blind, multicenter studies of patients with endoscopically confirmed healed duodenal ulcers. In the U.S. study the observed ulcer incidence within 12 months in patients treated with placebo was 2.4

times greater than in the patients treated with PEPCID. The 89 patients treated with PEPCID had a cumulative observed ulcer incidence of 23.4% compared to an observed ulcer incidence of 56.6% in the 89 patients receiving placebo (p<0.01). These results were confirmed in an international study where the cumulative observed ulcer incidence within 12 months in the 307 patients treated with PEPCID was 35.7%, compared to an incidence of 75.5% in the 325 patients treated with placebo (p<0.01).
Gastric Ulcer
In both a U.S. and an international multicenter, double-blind study in patients with endoscopically confirmed active benign gastric ulcer, orally administered PEPCID, 40 mg h.s., was compared to placebo h.s. Antacids were permitted during the studies, but consumption was not significantly different between the PEPCID and placebo groups. As shown in Table 2, the incidence of ulcer healing (dropouts counted as unhealed) with PEPCID was statistically significantly better than placebo at weeks 6 and 8 in the U.S. study, and at weeks 4, 6 and 8 in the international study, based on the number of ulcers that healed, confirmed by endoscopy.

Table 2: Patients with Endoscopically Confirmed Healed Gastric Ulcers

	U.S. Study		International Study	
	PEPCID 40 mg h.s. (N=74)	Placebo h.s. (N=75)	PEPCID 40 mg h.s. (N=149)	Placebo h.s. (N=145)
Week 4	45%	39%	*47%	31%
Week 6	*66%	44%	*65%	46%
Week 8	†78%	64%	*80%	54%

* Statistically significantly better than placebo (p≤0.01)
† Statistically significantly better than placebo (p≤0.05)

Time to complete relief of daytime and nighttime pain was statistically significantly shorter for patients receiving PEPCID than for patients receiving placebo; however, in neither study was there a statistically significant difference in the proportion of patients whose pain was relieved by the end of the study (week 8).
Gastroesophageal Reflux Disease (GERD)
Orally administered PEPCID was compared to placebo in a U.S. study that enrolled patients with symptoms of GERD and without endoscopic evidence of erosion or ulceration of the esophagus. PEPCID 20 mg b.i.d. was statistically significantly superior to 40 mg h.s. and to placebo in providing a successful symptomatic outcome, defined as moderate or excellent improvement of symptoms (Table 3).

Table 3: % Successful Symptomatic Outcome

	PEPCID 20 mg b.i.d. (N=154)	PEPCID 40 mg h.s. (N=149)	Placebo (N=73)
Week 6	82*	69	62

*p≤0.01 vs Placebo

By two weeks of treatment, symptomatic success was observed in a greater percentage of patients taking PEPCID 20 mg b.i.d. compared to placebo (p≤0.01).
Symptomatic improvement and healing of endoscopically verified erosion and ulceration were studied in two additional trials. Healing was defined as complete resolution of all erosions or ulcerations visible with endoscopy. The U.S. study comparing PEPCID 40 mg p.o. b.i.d. to placebo and PEPCID 20 mg p.o. b.i.d. showed a significantly greater percentage of healing for PEPCID 40 mg b.i.d. at weeks 6 and 12 (Table 4).

Table 4: % Endoscopic Healing - U.S. Study

	PEPCID 40 mg b.i.d. (N=127)	PEPCID 20 mg b.i.d. (N=125)	Placebo (N=66)
Week 6	48*,†	32	18
Week 12	69*,‡	54*	29

* p≤0.01 vs Placebo
† p≤0.01 vs PEPCID 20 mg b.i.d.
‡ p≤0.05 vs PEPCID 20 mg b.i.d.

As compared to placebo, patients who received PEPCID had faster relief of daytime and nighttime heartburn and a greater percentage of patients experienced complete relief of nighttime heartburn. These differences were statistically significant.
In the international study, when PEPCID 40 mg p.o. b.i.d. was compared to ranitidine 150 mg p.o. b.i.d., a statistically

significantly greater percentage of healing was observed with PEPCID 40 mg b.i.d. at week 12 (Table 5). There was, however, no significant difference among treatments in symptom relief.

Table 5: % Endoscopic Healing - International Study

	PEPCID 40 mg b.i.d. (N=175)	PEPCID 20 mg b.i.d. (N=93)	Ranitidine 150 mg b.i.d. (N=172)
Week 6	48	52	42
Week 12	71*	68	60

*p≤0.05 vs Ranitidine 150 mg b.i.d.

Pathological Hypersecretory Conditions (e.g., Zollinger-Ellison Syndrome, Multiple Endocrine Adenomas)
In studies of patients with pathological hypersecretory conditions such as Zollinger-Ellison Syndrome with or without multiple endocrine adenomas, PEPCID significantly inhibited gastric acid secretion and controlled associated symptoms. Orally administered doses from 20 to 160 mg q 6 h maintained basal acid secretion below 10 mEq/hr; initial doses were titrated to the individual patient need and subsequent adjustments were necessary with time in some patients. PEPCID was well tolerated at these high dose levels for prolonged periods (greater than 12 months) in eight patients, and there were no cases reported of gynecomastia, increased prolactin levels, or impotence which were considered to be due to the drug.

CLINICAL PHARMACOLOGY IN PEDIATRIC PATIENTS
Pharmacokinetics
Table 6 presents pharmacokinetic data from clinical trials and a published study in pediatric patients (<1 year of age; N=27) given famotidine I.V. 0.5 mg/kg and from published studies of small numbers of pediatric patients (1-15 years of age) given famotidine intravenously. Areas under the curve (AUCs) are normalized to a dose of 0.5 mg/kg I.V. for pediatric patients 1-15 years of age and compared with an extrapolated 40 mg intravenous dose in adults (extrapolation based on results obtained with a 20 mg I.V. adult dose).
[See table 6 above]
Plasma clearance is reduced and elimination half-life is prolonged in pediatric patients 0-3 months of age compared to older pediatric patients. The pharmacokinetic parameters for pediatric patients, ages >3 months-15 years, are comparable to those obtained for adults.
Bioavailability studies of 8 pediatric patients (11-15 years of age) showed a mean oral bioavailability of 0.5 compared to adult values of 0.42 to 0.49. Oral doses of 0.5 mg/kg achieved AUCs of 645 ± 249 ng-hr/mL and 580 ± 60 ng-hr/mL in pediatric patients <1 year of age (N=5) and in pediatric patients 11-15 years of age, respectively, compared to 482 ± 181 ng-hr/mL in adults treated with 40 mg orally.
Pharmacodynamics
Pharmacodynamics of famotidine were evaluated in 5 pediatric patients 2-13 years of age using the sigmoid E_{max} model. These data suggest that the relationship between serum concentration of famotidine and gastric acid suppression is similar to that observed in one study of adults (Table 7).

Table 7: Pharmacodynamics of famotidine using the sigmoid E_{max} model

	EC_{50} (ng/mL)*
Pediatric Patients Data from one study	26 ± 13
a) healthy adult subjects	26.5 ± 10.3
b) adult patients with upper GI bleeding	18.7 ± 10.8

*Serum concentration of famotidine associated with 50% maximum gastric acid reduction. Values are presented as means ± SD.

Five published studies (Table 8) examined the effect of famotidine on gastric pH and duration of acid suppression in pediatric patients. While each study had a different design, acid suppression data over time are summarized as follows:
[See table 8 above]
The duration of effect of famotidine I.V. 0.5 mg/kg on gastric pH and acid suppression was shown in one study to be longer in pediatric patients <1 month of age than in older pediatric patients. This longer duration of gastric acid suppression is consistent with the decreased clearance in pediatric patients <3 months of age (see Table 6).

Table 6: Pharmacokinetic Parameters* of Intravenous Famotidine

Age (N=number of patients)	Area Under the Curve (AUC) (ng-hr/mL)	Total Clearance (Cl) (L/hr/kg)	Volume of Distribution (V_d) (L/kg)	Elimination Half-life ($T_{1/2}$) (hours)
0-1 month† (N=10)	NA	0.13 ± 0.06	1.4 ± 0.4	10.5 ± 5.4
0-3 months‡ (N=6)	2688 ± 847	0.21 ± 0.06	1.8 ± 0.3	8.1 ± 3.5
>3-12 months‡ (N=11)	1160 ± 474	0.49 ± 0.17	2.3 ± 0.7	4.5 ± 1.1
1-11 yrs (N=20)	1089 ± 834	0.54 ± 0.34	2.07 ± 1.49	3.38 ± 2.60
11-15 yrs (N=6)	1140 ± 320	0.48 ± 0.14	1.5 ± 0.4	2.3 ± 0.4
Adult (N=16)	1726§	0.39 ± 0.14	1.3 ± 0.2	2.83 ± 0.99

* Values are presented as means ± SD unless indicated otherwise.
† Single center study.
‡ Multicenter study.
§ Mean value only.

Table 8

Dosage	Route	Effect*	Number of Patients (age range)
0.5 mg/kg, single dose	I.V.	gastric pH >4 for 19.5 hours (17.3, 21.8)†	11 (5-19 days)
0.3 mg/kg, single dose	I.V.	gastric pH >3.5 for 8.7 ± 4.7‡ hours	6 (2-7 years)
0.4-0.8 mg/kg	I.V.	gastric pH >4 for 6-9 hours	18 (2-69 months)
0.5 mg/kg, single dose	I.V.	a >2 pH unit increase above baseline in gastric pH for >8 hours	9 (2-13 years)
0.5 mg/kg b.i.d.	I.V.	gastric pH >5 for 13.5 ± 1.8‡ hours	4 (6-15 years)
0.5 mg/kg b.i.d.	oral	gastric pH >5 for 5.0 ± 1.1‡ hours	4 (11-15 years)

* Values reported in published literature.
† Mean (95% confidence interval).
‡ Means ± SD.

INDICATIONS AND USAGE
PEPCID is indicated in:
1. *Short-term treatment of active duodenal ulcer.* Most adult patients heal within 4 weeks; there is rarely reason to use PEPCID at full dosage for longer than 6 to 8 weeks. Studies have not assessed the safety of famotidine in uncomplicated active duodenal ulcer for periods of more than eight weeks.
2. *Maintenance therapy for duodenal ulcer patients at reduced dosage after healing of an active ulcer.* Controlled studies in adults have not extended beyond one year.
3. *Short-term treatment of active benign gastric ulcer.* Most adult patients heal within 6 weeks. Studies have not assessed the safety or efficacy of famotidine in uncomplicated active benign gastric ulcer for periods of more than 8 weeks.
4. *Short-term treatment of gastroesophageal reflux disease (GERD).* PEPCID is indicated for short-term treatment of patients with symptoms of GERD (see CLINICAL PHARMACOLOGY IN ADULTS, *Clinical Studies*).
   PEPCID is also indicated for the short-term treatment of esophagitis due to GERD including erosive or ulcerative disease diagnosed by endoscopy (see CLINICAL PHARMACOLOGY IN ADULTS, *Clinical Studies*).
5. *Treatment of pathological hypersecretory conditions (e.g., Zollinger-Ellison Syndrome, multiple endocrine adenomas)* (see CLINICAL PHARMACOLOGY IN ADULTS, *Clinical Studies*).

CONTRAINDICATIONS
Hypersensitivity to any component of these products. Cross sensitivity in this class of compounds has been observed. Therefore, PEPCID should not be administered to patients with a history of hypersensitivity to other H_2-receptor antagonists.

PRECAUTIONS
General
Symptomatic response to therapy with PEPCID does not preclude the presence of gastric malignancy.
Patients with Moderate or Severe Renal Insufficiency
Since CNS adverse effects have been reported in patients with moderate and severe renal insufficiency, longer intervals between doses or lower doses may need to be used in patients with moderate (creatinine clearance <50 mL/min) or severe (creatinine clearance <10 mL/min) renal insufficiency to adjust for the longer elimination half-life of famotidine (see CLINICAL PHARMACOLOGY IN ADULTS and DOSAGE AND ADMINISTRATION).
Drug Interactions
No drug interactions have been identified. Studies with famotidine in man, in animal models, and *in vitro* have shown no significant interference with the disposition of compounds metabolized by the hepatic microsomal enzymes, e.g., cytochrome P450 system. Compounds tested in man include warfarin, theophylline, phenytoin, diazepam,

aminopyrine and antipyrine. Indocyanine green as an index of hepatic drug extraction has been tested and no significant effects have been found.
Carcinogenesis, Mutagenesis, Impairment of Fertility
In a 106-week study in rats and a 92-week study in mice given oral doses of up to 2000 mg/kg/day (approximately 2500 times the recommended human dose for active duodenal ulcer), there was no evidence of carcinogenic potential for PEPCID.
Famotidine was negative in the microbial mutagen test (Ames test) using *Salmonella typhimurium* and *Escherichia coli* with or without rat liver enzyme activation at concentrations up to 10,000 mcg/plate. In *in vivo* studies in mice, with a micronucleus test and a chromosomal aberration test, no evidence of a mutagenic effect was observed.
In studies with rats given oral doses of up to 2000 mg/kg/day or intravenous doses of up to 200 mg/kg/day, fertility and reproductive performance were not affected.
Pregnancy
Pregnancy Category B
Reproductive studies have been performed in rats and rabbits at oral doses of up to 2000 and 500 mg/kg/day, respectively, and in both species at I.V. doses of up to 200 mg/kg/day, and have revealed no significant evidence of impaired fertility or harm to the fetus due to PEPCID. While no direct fetotoxic effects have been observed, sporadic abortions occurring only in mothers displaying marked decreased food intake were seen in some rabbits at oral doses of 200 mg/kg/day (250 times the usual human dose) or higher. There are, however, no adequate or well-controlled studies in pregnant women. Because animal reproductive studies are not always predictive of human response, this drug should be used during pregnancy only if clearly needed.
Nursing Mothers
Studies performed in lactating rats have shown that famotidine is secreted into breast milk. Transient growth depression was observed in young rats suckling from mothers treated with maternotoxic doses of at least 600 times the usual human dose. Famotidine is detectable in human milk. Because of the potential for serious adverse reactions in nursing infants from PEPCID, a decision should be made whether to discontinue nursing or discontinue the drug, taking into account the importance of the drug to the mother.
Pediatric Patients <1 year of age
Use of PEPCID in pediatric patients <1 year of age is supported by evidence from adequate and well-controlled studies of PEPCID in adults, and by the following studies in pediatric patients <1 year of age.
Two pharmacokinetic studies in pediatric patients <1 year of age (N=48) demonstrated that clearance of famotidine in patients >3 months to 1 year of age is similar to that seen in older pediatric patients (1-15 years of age) and adults. In contrast, pediatric patients 0-3 months of age had famotidine clearance values that were 2- to 4-fold less than

those in older pediatric patients and adults. These studies also show that the mean bioavailability in pediatric patients <1 year of age after oral dosing is similar to older pediatric patients and adults. Pharmacodynamic data in pediatric patients 0-3 months of age suggest that the duration of acid suppression is longer compared with older pediatric patients, consistent with the longer famotidine half-life in pediatric patients 0-3 months of age. (See CLINICAL PHARMACOLOGY IN PEDIATRIC PATIENTS, *Pharmacokinetics* and *Pharmacodynamics*.)

In a double-blind, randomized, treatment-withdrawal study, 35 pediatric patients <1 year of age who were diagnosed as having gastroesophageal reflux disease were treated for up to 4 weeks with famotidine oral suspension (0.5 mg/kg/dose or 1 mg/kg/dose). Although an intravenous famotidine formulation was available, no patients were treated with intravenous famotidine in this study. Also, caregivers were instructed to provide conservative treatment including thickened feedings. Enrolled patients were diagnosed primarily by history of vomiting (spitting up) and irritability (fussiness). The famotidine dosing regimen was once daily for patients <3 months of age and twice daily for patients ≥3 months of age. After 4 weeks of treatment, patients were randomly withdrawn from the treatment and followed an additional 4 weeks for adverse events and symptomatology. Patients were evaluated for vomiting (spitting up), irritability (fussiness) and global assessments of improvement. The study patients ranged in age at entry from 1.3 to 10.5 months (mean 5.6 ± 2.9 months), 57% were female, 91% were white and 6% were black. Most patients (27/35) continued into the treatment-withdrawal phase of the study. Two patients discontinued famotidine due to adverse events. Most patients improved during the initial treatment phase of the study. Results of the treatment-withdrawal phase were difficult to interpret because of small numbers of patients. Of the 35 patients enrolled in the study, agitation was observed in 5 patients on famotidine that resolved when the medication was discontinued; agitation was not observed in patients on placebo (see ADVERSE REACTIONS, *Pediatric Patients*).

These studies suggest that a starting dose of 0.5 mg/kg/dose of famotidine oral suspension may be of benefit for the treatment of GERD for up to 4 weeks once daily in patients <3 months of age and twice daily in patients 3 months to <1 year of age; the safety and benefit of famotidine treatment beyond 4 weeks have not been established. Famotidine should be considered for the treatment of GERD only if conservative measures (e.g., thickened feedings) are used concurrently and if the potential benefit outweighs the risk.

Pediatric Patients 1-16 years of age
Use of PEPCID in pediatric patients 1-16 years of age is supported by evidence from adequate and well-controlled studies of PEPCID in adults, and by the following studies in pediatric patients: In published studies in small numbers of pediatric patients 1-15 years of age, clearance of famotidine was similar to that seen in adults. In pediatric patients 11-15 years of age, oral doses of 0.5 mg/kg were associated with a mean area under the curve (AUC) similar to that seen in adults treated orally with 40 mg. Similarly, in pediatric patients 1-15 years of age, intravenous doses of 0.5 mg/kg were associated with a mean AUC similar to that seen in adults treated intravenously with 40 mg. Limited published studies also suggest that the relationship between serum concentration and acid suppression is similar in pediatric patients 1-15 years of age as compared with adults. These studies suggest a starting dose for pediatric patients 1-16 years of age as follows:
Peptic ulcer — 0.5 mg/kg/day p.o. at bedtime or divided b.i.d. up to 40 mg/day.
Gastroesophageal Reflux Disease with or without esophagitis including erosions and ulcerations—1.0 mg/kg/day p.o. divided b.i.d. up to 40 mg b.i.d.
While published uncontrolled studies suggest effectiveness of famotidine in the treatment of gastroesophageal reflux disease and peptic ulcer, data in pediatric patients are insufficient to establish percent response with dose and duration of therapy. Therefore, treatment duration (initially based on adult duration recommendations) and dose should be individualized based on clinical response and/or pH determination (gastric or esophageal) and endoscopy. Published uncontrolled clinical studies in pediatric patients have employed doses up to 1 mg/kg/day for peptic ulcer and 2 mg/kg/day for GERD with or without esophagitis including erosions and ulcerations.
Geriatric Use
Of the 4,966 subjects in clinical studies who were treated with famotidine, 488 subjects (9.8%) were 65 and older, and 88 subjects (1.7%) were greater than 75 years of age. No overall differences in safety or effectiveness were observed between these subjects and younger subjects. However, greater sensitivity of some older individuals cannot be ruled out.

No dosage adjustment is required based on age (see CLINICAL PHARMACOLOGY IN ADULTS, *Pharmacokinetics*).

This drug is known to be substantially excreted by the kidney, and the risk of toxic reactions to this drug may be greater in patients with impaired renal function. Because elderly patients are more likely to have decreased renal function, care should be taken in dose selection, and it may be useful to monitor renal function. Dosage adjustment in the case of moderate or severe renal impairment is necessary (see PRECAUTIONS, *Patients with Moderate or Severe Renal Insufficiency* and DOSAGE AND ADMINISTRATION, *Dosage Adjustment for Patients with Moderate or Severe Renal Insufficiency*).

ADVERSE REACTIONS

The adverse reactions listed below have been reported during domestic and international clinical trials in approximately 2500 patients. In those controlled clinical trials in which PEPCID Tablets were compared to placebo, the incidence of adverse experiences in the group which received PEPCID Tablets, 40 mg at bedtime, was similar to that in the placebo group.

The following adverse reactions have been reported to occur in more than 1% of patients on therapy with PEPCID in controlled clinical trials, and may be causally related to the drug: headache (4.7%), dizziness (1.3%), constipation (1.2%) and diarrhea (1.7%).

The following other adverse reactions have been reported infrequently in clinical trials or since the drug was marketed. The relationship to therapy with PEPCID has been unclear in many cases. Within each category the adverse reactions are listed in order of decreasing severity:
Body as a Whole: fever, asthenia, fatigue
Cardiovascular: arrhythmia, AV block, palpitation
Gastrointestinal: cholestatic jaundice, hepatitis, liver enzyme abnormalities, vomiting, nausea, abdominal discomfort, anorexia, dry mouth
Hematologic: rare cases of agranulocytosis, pancytopenia, leukopenia, thrombocytopenia
Hypersensitivity: anaphylaxis, angioedema, orbital or facial edema, urticaria, rash, conjunctival injection
Musculoskeletal: musculoskeletal pain including muscle cramps, arthralgia
Nervous System/Psychiatric: grand mal seizure; psychic disturbances, which were reversible in cases for which follow-up was obtained, including hallucinations, confusion, agitation, depression, anxiety, decreased libido; paresthesia; insomnia; somnolence. Convulsions, in patients with impaired renal function, have been reported very rarely.
Respiratory: bronchospasm, interstitial pneumonia
Skin: toxic epidermal necrolysis/Stevens-Johnson syndrome (very rare), alopecia, acne, pruritus, dry skin, flushing
Special Senses: tinnitus, taste disorder
Other: rare cases of impotence and rare cases of gynecomastia have been reported; however, in controlled clinical trials, the incidences were not greater than those seen with placebo.

The adverse reactions reported for PEPCID Tablets may also occur with PEPCID for Oral Suspension.
Pediatric Patients
In a clinical study in 35 pediatric patients <1 year of age with GERD symptoms [e.g., vomiting (spitting up), irritability (fussing)], agitation was observed in 5 patients on famotidine that resolved when the medication was discontinued.

OVERDOSAGE

The adverse reactions in overdose cases are similar to the adverse reactions encountered in normal clinical experience (see **ADVERSE REACTIONS**). Oral doses of up to 640 mg/day have been given to adult patients with pathological hypersecretory conditions with no serious adverse effects. In the event of overdosage, treatment should be symptomatic and supportive. Unabsorbed material should be removed from the gastrointestinal tract, the patient should be monitored, and supportive therapy should be employed.
The oral LD_{50} of famotidine in male and female rats and mice was greater than 3000 mg/kg and the minimum lethal acute oral dose in dogs exceeded 2000 mg/kg. Famotidine did not produce overt effects at high oral doses in mice, rats, cats and dogs, but induced significant anorexia and growth depression in rabbits starting with 200 mg/kg/day orally. The intravenous LD_{50} of famotidine for mice and rats ranged from 254-563 mg/kg and the minimum lethal single I.V. dose in dogs was approximately 300 mg/kg. Signs of acute intoxication in I.V. treated dogs were emesis, restlessness, pallor of mucous membranes or redness of mouth and ears, hypotension, tachycardia and collapse.

DOSAGE AND ADMINISTRATION
Duodenal Ulcer
Acute Therapy: The recommended adult oral dosage for active duodenal ulcer is 40 mg once a day at bedtime. Most patients heal within 4 weeks; there is rarely reason to use PEPCID at full dosage for longer than 6 to 8 weeks. A regimen of 20 mg b.i.d. is also effective.
Maintenance Therapy: The recommended adult oral dose is 20 mg once a day at bedtime.

Benign Gastric Ulcer
Acute Therapy: The recommended adult oral dosage for active benign gastric ulcer is 40 mg once a day at bedtime.
Gastroesophageal Reflux Disease (GERD)
The recommended oral dosage for treatment of adult patients with symptoms of GERD is 20 mg b.i.d. for up to 6 weeks. The recommended oral dosage for the treatment of adult patients with esophagitis including erosions and ulcerations and accompanying symptoms due to GERD is 20 or 40 mg b.i.d. for up to 12 weeks (see CLINICAL PHARMACOLOGY IN ADULTS, *Clinical Studies*).
Dosage for Pediatric Patients <1 year of age Gastroesophageal Reflux Disease (GERD)
See PRECAUTIONS, *Pediatric Patients <1 year of age.*
The studies described in PRECAUTIONS, *Pediatric Patients <1 year of age* suggest the following starting doses in pediatric patients <1 year of age: *Gastroesophageal Reflux Disease (GERD)* - 0.5 mg/kg/dose of famotidine oral suspension for the treatment of GERD for up to 8 weeks once daily in patients <3 months of age and 0.5 mg/kg/dose twice daily in patients 3 months to <1 year of age. Patients should also be receiving conservative measures (e.g., thickened feedings). The use of intravenous famotidine in pediatric patients <1 year of age with GERD has not been adequately studied.
Dosage for Pediatric Patients 1-16 years of age
See PRECAUTIONS, *Pediatric Patients 1-16 years of age.*
The studies described in PRECAUTIONS, *Pediatric Patients 1-16 years of age* suggest the following starting doses in pediatric patients 1-16 years of age:
Peptic ulcer — 0.5 mg/kg/day p.o. at bedtime or divided b.i.d. up to 40 mg/day.
Gastroesophageal Reflux Disease with or without esophagitis including erosions and ulcerations — 1.0 mg/kg/day p.o. divided b.i.d. up to 40 mg b.i.d.
While published uncontrolled studies suggest effectiveness of famotidine in the treatment of gastroesophageal reflux disease and peptic ulcer, data in pediatric patients are insufficient to establish percent response with dose and duration of therapy. Therefore, treatment duration (initially based on adult duration recommendations) and dose should be individualized based on clinical response and/or pH determination (gastric or esophageal) and endoscopy. Published uncontrolled clinical studies in pediatric patients 1-16 years of age have employed doses up to 1 mg/kg/day for peptic ulcer and 2 mg/kg/day for GERD with or without esophagitis including erosions and ulcerations.
Pathological Hypersecretory Conditions (e.g., Zollinger-Ellison Syndrome, Multiple Endocrine Adenomas)
The dosage of PEPCID in patients with pathological hypersecretory conditions varies with the individual patient. The recommended adult oral starting dose for pathological hypersecretory conditions is 20 mg q 6 h. In some patients, a higher starting dose may be required. Doses should be adjusted to individual patient needs and should continue as long as clinically indicated. Doses up to 160 mg q 6 h have been administered to some adult patients with severe Zollinger-Ellison Syndrome.
Concomitant Use of Antacids
Antacids may be given concomitantly if needed.
Dosage Adjustment for Patients with Moderate or Severe Renal Insufficiency
In adult patients with moderate (creatinine clearance <50 mL/min) or severe (creatinine clearance <10 mL/min) renal insufficiency, the elimination half-life of PEPCID is increased. For patients with severe renal insufficiency, it may exceed 20 hours, reaching approximately 24 hours in anuric patients. Since CNS adverse effects have been reported in patients with moderate and severe renal insufficiency, to avoid excess accumulation of the drug in patients with moderate or severe renal insufficiency, the dose of PEPCID may be reduced to half the dose or the dosing interval may be prolonged to 36-48 hours as indicated by the patient's clinical response.
Based on the comparison of pharmacokinetic parameters for PEPCID in adults and pediatric patients, dosage adjustment in pediatric patients with moderate or severe renal insufficiency should be considered.

HOW SUPPLIED
No. 9786—PEPCID Tablets, 20 mg, are beige colored, rounded square shaped, film-coated tablets coded MSD 963 on one side and plain on the other. They are supplied as follows:
NDC 0006-0963-31 unit of use bottles of 30
NDC 0006-0963-58 unit of use bottles of 100.
No. 9788—PEPCID Tablets, 40 mg, are tan, rounded square shaped, film-coated tablets coded MSD 964 on one side and plain on the other. They are supplied as follows:
NDC 0006-0964-31 unit of use bottles of 30
NDC 0006-0964-58 unit of use bottles of 100.
Storage
Preserve in well-closed, light-resistant containers. Store at controlled room temperature.
PEPCID (famotidine) Tablets 20 mg and Tablets 40 mg are manufactured for:
Merck Sharp & Dohme Corp., a subsidiary of
MERCK & CO., INC., Whitehouse Station, NJ 08889, USA

By:
MERCK SHARP & DOHME Pty., Ltd.
South Granville, NSW, Australia 2142.
Issued February 2010
Printed in USA
9883041

Shown in Product Identification Guide, page 313

PNEUMOVAX® 23
(PNEUMOCOCCAL VACCINE POLYVALENT) ℞

DESCRIPTION

PNEUMOVAX[1] 23 (Pneumococcal Vaccine Polyvalent) is a sterile, liquid vaccine for intramuscular or subcutaneous injection. It consists of a mixture of highly purified capsular polysaccharides from the 23 most prevalent or invasive pneumococcal types of *Streptococcus pneumoniae,* including the six serotypes that most frequently cause invasive drug-resistant pneumococcal infections among children and adults in the United States.{1} (See Table 1.) The 23-valent vaccine accounts for at least 90% of pneumococcal blood isolates and at least 85% of all pneumococcal isolates from sites which are generally sterile as determined by ongoing surveillance of U.S. data.{2}

PNEUMOVAX 23 is manufactured according to methods developed by the Merck Research Laboratories. Each 0.5 mL dose of vaccine contains 25 µg of each polysaccharide type in isotonic saline solution containing 0.25% phenol as a preservative.

[See table 1 above]

Table 1: 23 Pneumococcal Capsular Types Included in PNEUMOVAX 23

Nomenclature	Pneumococcal Types
Danish	1 2 3 4 5 6B* 7F 8 9N 9V* 10A 11A 12F 14* 15B 17F 18C 19F* 19A* 20 22F 23F* 33F

*These serotypes most frequently cause drug-resistant pneumococcal infections{1}

[1] Registered trademark of MERCK & CO., Inc.
COPYRIGHT © 1986, 2007 MERCK & CO., Inc.
All rights reserved

CLINICAL PHARMACOLOGY

Pneumococcal infection is a leading cause of death throughout the world{3} and a major cause of pneumonia, bacteremia, meningitis, and otitis media.

Strains of drug-resistant *S. pneumoniae* have become increasingly common in the United States and in other parts of the world. In some areas as many as 35% of pneumococcal isolates have been reported to be resistant to penicillin. Many penicillin-resistant pneumococci are also resistant to other antimicrobial drugs (e.g., erythromycin, trimethoprim-sulfamethoxazole and extended-spectrum cephalosporins), therefore emphasizing the importance of vaccine prophylaxis against pneumococcal disease.

Epidemiology

Pneumococcal infection causes approximately 40,000 deaths annually in the United States.{1}

At least 500,000 cases of pneumococcal pneumonia are estimated to occur annually in the United States; *S. pneumoniae* accounts for approximately 25-35% of cases of community-acquired bacterial pneumonia in persons who require hospitalization.{1}

Pneumococcal disease accounts for an estimated 50,000 cases of pneumococcal bacteremia annually in the United States. Some studies suggest the overall annual incidence of bacteremia to be approximately 15 to 30 cases/100,000 population with 50 to 83 cases/100,000 for persons 65 years of age and older and 160 cases/100,000 for children less than two years of age.

The incidence of pneumococcal bacteremia is as high as 1% (940 cases/100,000 population) among persons with acquired immunodeficiency syndrome (AIDS).

In the United States, the risk of acquiring bacteremia is lower among whites than among persons in some other racial/ethnic groups (i.e., blacks, Alaskan Natives, and American Indians).

Despite appropriate antimicrobial therapy and intensive medical care, the overall case-fatality rate for pneumococcal bacteremia is 15-20% among adults{4}, and among elderly patients this rate is approximately 30-40%. An overall case-fatality rate of 36% was documented for adult inner-city residents who were hospitalized for pneumococcal bacteremia.{1}

In the United States, pneumococcal disease accounts for an estimated 3,000 cases of meningitis annually. The estimated overall annual incidence of pneumococcal meningitis is approximately 1 to 2 cases per 100,000 population. The incidence of pneumococcal meningitis is highest among children six to 24 months and persons aged ≥ 65 years; rates for blacks are twice as high as those for whites or Hispanics.

Recurrent pneumococcal meningitis may occur in patients who have chronic cerebrospinal fluid leakage resulting from congenital lesions, skull fractures, or neurosurgical procedures.{1}

Invasive pneumococcal disease (e.g., bacteremia or meningitis) and pneumonia cause high morbidity and mortality in spite of effective antimicrobial control by antibiotics.{4} These effects of pneumococcal disease appear due to irreversible physiologic damage caused by the bacteria during the first 5 days following onset of illness,{5,6} and occur regardless of antimicrobial therapy.{5,7} Vaccination offers an effective means of further reducing the mortality and morbidity of this disease.

Risk Factors

In addition to the very young and persons 65 years of age or older, patients with certain chronic conditions are at increased risk of developing pneumococcal infection and severe pneumococcal illness.

Patients with chronic cardiovascular diseases (e.g., congestive heart failure or cardiomyopathy), chronic pulmonary diseases (e.g., chronic obstructive pulmonary disease or emphysema), or chronic liver diseases (e.g., cirrhosis), diabetes mellitus, alcoholism or asthma (when it occurs with chronic bronchitis, emphysema, or long-term use of systemic corticosteroids) have an increased risk of pneumococcal disease. In adults, this population is generally immunocompetent.{1}

Patients at high risk are those who have a decreased responsiveness to polysaccharide antigen or an increased rate of decline in serum antibody concentrations as a result of: immunosuppressive conditions (congenital immunodeficiency, human immunodeficiency virus [HIV] infection, leukemia, lymphoma, multiple myeloma, Hodgkin's disease, or generalized malignancy); organ or bone marrow transplantation; therapy with alkylating agents, antimetabolites, or systemic corticosteroids; chronic renal failure or nephrotic syndrome.{1,8}

Patients at the highest risk of pneumococcal infection are those with functional or anatomic asplenia (e.g., sickle cell disease{9} or splenectomy), because this condition leads to reduced clearance of encapsulated bacteria from the bloodstream. Children who have sickle cell disease or have had a splenectomy are at increased risk for fulminant pneumococcal sepsis associated with high mortality.{1}

Immunogenicity

It has been established that the purified pneumococcal capsular polysaccharides induce antibody production and that such antibody is effective in preventing pneumococcal disease.{6,10} Clinical studies have demonstrated the immunogenicity of each of the 23 capsular types when tested in polyvalent vaccines.

Studies with 12-, 14-, and 23-valent pneumococcal vaccines in children two years of age and older and in adults of all ages showed immunogenic responses.{10,11-14} Protective capsular type-specific antibody levels generally develop by the third week following vaccination.{13}

Bacterial capsular polysaccharides induce antibodies primarily by T-cell-independent mechanisms. Therefore, antibody response to most pneumococcal capsular types is generally poor or inconsistent in children aged < 2 years whose immune systems are immature.{1}

Efficacy

The protective efficacy of pneumococcal vaccines containing 6 or 12 capsular polysaccharides was investigated in two controlled studies of young, healthy gold miners in South Africa, in whom there was a high attack rate for pneumococcal pneumonia and bacteremia.{13} Capsular type-specific attack rates for pneumococcal pneumonia were observed for the period from 2 weeks through about 1 year after vaccination. Protective efficacy was 76% and 92%, respectively, in the two studies for the capsular types represented.

In similar studies carried out by Dr. R. Austrian and associates,{15} using similar pneumococcal vaccines prepared for the National Institute of Allergy and Infectious Diseases, the reduction in pneumonia caused by the capsular types contained in the vaccines was 79%. Reduction in type-specific pneumococcal bacteremia was 82%.

A prospective study in France found pneumococcal vaccine to be 77% effective in reducing the incidence of pneumonia among nursing home residents.{16}

In the United States, two postlicensure randomized controlled trials, in the elderly or patients with chronic medical conditions who received a multivalent polysaccharide vaccine, did not support the efficacy of the vaccine for nonbacteremic pneumonia.{17,18} However, these studies may have lacked sufficient statistical power to detect a difference in the incidence of laboratory-confirmed, nonbacteremic pneumococcal pneumonia between the vaccinated and nonvaccinated study groups.{1,19}

A meta-analysis of nine randomized controlled trials of pneumococcal vaccine concluded that pneumococcal vaccine is efficacious in reducing the frequency of nonbacteremic pneumococcal pneumonia among adults in low-risk groups but not in high-risk groups.{20} These studies may have been limited because of the lack of specific and sensitive diagnostic tests for nonbacteremic pneumococcal pneumonia. The pneumococcal polysaccharide vaccine is not effective for the prevention of common upper respiratory disease in children.{1}

More recently, multiple case-control studies have shown pneumococcal vaccine is effective in the prevention of serious pneumococcal disease, with point estimates of efficacy ranging from 56% to 81% in immunocompetent persons.{1,21-26}

Only one case-control study did not document effectiveness against bacteremic disease possibly due to study limitations, including small sample size and incomplete ascertainment of vaccination status in patients.{27} In addition, case-patients and persons who served as controls may not have been comparable regarding the severity of their underlying medical conditions, potentially creating a biased underestimate of vaccine effectiveness.{1,19}

A serotype prevalence study, based on the Centers for Disease Control pneumococcal surveillance system, demonstrated 57% overall protective effectiveness against invasive infections caused by serotypes included in the vaccine in persons ≥ 6 years of age, 65-84% effectiveness among specific patient groups (e.g., persons with diabetes mellitus, coronary vascular disease, congestive heart failure, chronic pulmonary disease, and anatomic asplenia) and 75% effectiveness in immunocompetent persons aged ≥ 65 years of age. Vaccine effectiveness could not be confirmed for certain groups of immunocompromised patients; however, the study could not recruit sufficient numbers of unvaccinated patients from each disease group.

In an earlier study, vaccinated children and young adults aged 2 to 25 years who had sickle cell disease, congenital asplenia, or undergone a splenectomy experienced significantly less bacteremic pneumococcal disease than patients who were not vaccinated.{1,28}

Duration of Immunity

Following pneumococcal vaccination, serotype-specific antibody levels decline after 5-10 years.{1} A more rapid decline in antibody levels may occur in some groups (e.g., children).{1} Limited published data suggest that antibody levels may decline in the elderly > 60 years of age.{29,30}

The Advisory Committee on Immunization Practices (ACIP) states that these findings indicate that revaccination may be needed to provide continued protection.{1} (See INDICATIONS AND USAGE, *Revaccination.*)

The results from one epidemiologic study suggest that vaccination may provide protection for at least nine years after receipt of the initial dose.{22} Decreasing estimates of effectiveness with increasing interval since vaccination, particularly among the very elderly (persons aged ≥ 85 years) have been reported.{23}

INDICATIONS AND USAGE

PNEUMOVAX 23 is indicated for vaccination against pneumococcal disease caused by those pneumococcal types included in the vaccine. Effectiveness of the vaccine in the prevention of pneumococcal pneumonia and pneumococcal bacteremia has been demonstrated in controlled trials in South Africa, France and in case-control studies.

PNEUMOVAX 23 will not prevent disease caused by capsular types of pneumococcus other than those contained in the vaccine.

Vaccination with PNEUMOVAX 23 is recommended for selected individuals as follows:

— routine vaccination for persons 50 years of age or older[2]
— persons aged ≥ 2 years with certain chronic conditions or in special environments or social settings.{1,31}

The ACIP has vaccine specific recommendations for the prevention of pneumococcal disease. Available from: http://www.cdc.gov/mmwr/PDF/rr/rr4608.pdf{1} and http://www.cdc.gov/vaccines/recs/provisional/downloads/pneumo-Oct-2008-508.pdf{31}

[2] NOTE: The ACIP recommends routine vaccination for immunocompetent persons 65 years of age and older.

Timing of Vaccination

Pneumococcal vaccine should be given at least two weeks before elective splenectomy, if possible.

For planning cancer chemotherapy or other immunosuppressive therapy (e.g., for patients with Hodgkin's disease or those who undergo organ or bone marrow transplantation), pneumococcal vaccination should be administered at least two weeks prior to the initiation of immunosuppressive therapy. Vaccination during chemotherapy or radiation therapy should be avoided. Based on literature reports, pneumococcal vaccine may be given as early as several months following completion of chemotherapy or radiation therapy for neoplastic disease.{32,33} In Hodgkin's disease, immune response to vaccination may be impaired for two years or longer after intensive chemotherapy (with or without radiation). During the two years following the completion of chemotherapy or other immunosuppressive therapy, antibody responses improve in some patients as the interval between the end of treatment and pneumococcal vaccination increases.{32}

Persons with asymptomatic or symptomatic HIV infection should be vaccinated as soon as possible after their diagnosis is confirmed.

Use With Other Vaccines

The ACIP states that pneumococcal vaccine may be administered at the same time as influenza vaccine (by separate injection in the other arm) without an increase in side effects or decreased antibody response to either vaccine.{1} In contrast to pneumococcal vaccine, influenza vaccine is recommended annually, for appropriate populations.{34}

Revaccination

The ACIP has recommendations for revaccination against pneumococcal disease in persons at high risk who were previously vaccinated with PNEUMOVAX 23 or the pneumococcal conjugate vaccine.{1,31,35}

If PNEUMOVAX 23 is used for revaccination, a single 0.5 mL dose is administered subcutaneously or intramuscularly.

CONTRAINDICATIONS

Hypersensitivity to any component of the vaccine. Epinephrine injection (1:1000) must be immediately available should an acute anaphylactoid reaction occur due to any component of the vaccine.

WARNINGS

For planning cancer chemotherapy or other immunosuppressive therapy (e.g., for patients with Hodgkin's disease or those who undergo organ or bone marrow transplantation), the timing of the vaccination is critical. (See INDICATIONS AND USAGE, *Timing of Vaccination*.)

If the vaccine is used in persons receiving immunosuppressive therapy, the expected serum antibody response may not be obtained and potential impairment of future immune responses to pneumococcal antigens may occur.{36} (See INDICATIONS AND USAGE, *Timing of Vaccination*.)

Intradermal administration may cause severe local reactions.

PRECAUTIONS

General

Caution and appropriate care should be exercised in administering PNEUMOVAX 23 to individuals with severely compromised cardiovascular and/or pulmonary function in whom a systemic reaction would pose a significant risk.

Any febrile respiratory illness or other active infection is reason for delaying use of PNEUMOVAX 23, except when, in the opinion of the physician, withholding the agent entails even greater risk.

In patients who require penicillin (or other antibiotic) prophylaxis against pneumococcal infection, such prophylaxis should not be discontinued after vaccination with PNEUMOVAX 23.

PNEUMOVAX 23 may not be effective in preventing pneumococcal meningitis in patients who have chronic cerebrospinal fluid (CSF) leakage resulting from congenital lesions, skull fractures, or neurosurgical procedures.

Routine revaccination of immunocompetent persons previously vaccinated with a 23-valent vaccine is not recommended. However, revaccination once is recommended for persons aged ≥ 2 years who are at highest risk for serious pneumococcal infections and those likely to have a rapid decline in pneumococcal antibody levels. (See INDICATIONS AND USAGE, *Revaccination*.)

Instructions to Health Care Provider

The health care provider should determine the current health status and previous vaccination history of the vaccinee. (See INDICATIONS AND USAGE, *Revaccination*.)

The health care provider should question the patient, parent or guardian about reactions to a previous dose of PNEUMOVAX 23 or other pneumococcal vaccine.

Information for Patients

The health care provider should inform the patient, parent or guardian of the benefits and risks associated with vaccination. For risks associated with vaccination, see WARNINGS, PRECAUTIONS, and ADVERSE REACTIONS. Patients, parents, or guardians should be told that vaccination with PNEUMOVAX 23 may not offer 100% protection from pneumococcal infection.

Patients, parents and guardians should be instructed to report any serious adverse reactions to their health care provider who in turn should report such events to the vaccine

manufacturer or the U.S. Department of Health and Human Services through the Vaccine Adverse Event Reporting System (VAERS), 1-800-822-7967.{37}

Pregnancy

Pregnancy Category C:

Animal reproduction studies have not been conducted with PNEUMOVAX 23. It is also not known whether PNEUMOVAX 23 can cause fetal harm when administered to a pregnant woman or can affect reproduction capacity. PNEUMOVAX 23 should be given to a pregnant woman only if clearly needed.

Nursing Mothers

It is not known whether this drug is excreted in human milk. Because many drugs are excreted in human milk, caution should be exercised when PNEUMOVAX 23 is administered to a nursing woman.

Pediatric Use

PNEUMOVAX 23 is not indicated in children less than 2 years of age. Safety and effectiveness in children below the age of 2 years have not been established. Children in this age group respond poorly to the capsular types contained in this polysaccharide vaccine. (See CLINICAL PHARMACOLOGY, *Immunogenicity*.)

Geriatric Use

Persons 65 years of age or older were enrolled in several clinical studies of PNEUMOVAX 23 that were conducted pre- and post-licensure. In the largest of these studies, the safety of PNEUMOVAX 23 in adults 65 years of age and older was compared to the safety of PNEUMOVAX 23 in adults 50 to 64 years of age. Of 1007 subjects enrolled in this study, 433 subjects were 65 to 74 years of age, and 195 subjects were 75 years of age or older. No overall difference in safety was observed between these subjects and younger subjects. However, since elderly individuals may not tolerate medical interventions as well as younger individuals, a higher frequency and/or a greater severity of reactions in some older individuals cannot be ruled out.

ADVERSE REACTIONS

The most common adverse experiences reported with PNEUMOVAX 23 in clinical trials were:

Local reaction at injection site including soreness, erythema, warmth, swelling and induration

Fever ≤102°F

Other adverse experiences reported in clinical trials and/or in post-marketing experience with PNEUMOVAX 23 include:

General disorders and administration site conditions

Cellulitis

Asthenia

Malaise

Fever (> 102°F)

Chills

Pain

Decreased limb mobility

Peripheral edema in the injected extremity

Digestive System

Nausea

Vomiting

Hematologic/Lymphatic

Lymphadenitis

Lymphadenopathy

Thrombocytopenia in patients with stabilized idiopathic thrombocytopenic purpura{38}

Hemolytic anemia in patients who have had other hematologic disorders

Leukocytosis

Hypersensitivity reactions including

Anaphylactoid reactions

Serum Sickness

Angioneurotic edema

Musculoskeletal System

Arthralgia

Arthritis

Myalgia

Nervous System

Headache

Paresthesia

Radiculoneuropathy

Guillain-Barré syndrome

Febrile convulsion

Skin

Rash

Urticaria

Investigations

Increased serum C-reactive protein

In post-marketing experience, injection site cellulitis-like reactions were reported rarely; between 1989 and 2002, when approximately 43 million doses were distributed, the annual reporting rate was <2/100,000 doses. These cellulitis-like reactions occurred with initial and repeat vaccination at a median onset time of 2 days after vaccine administration.

Systemic signs and symptoms including fever, leukocytosis and an increase in the laboratory value for serum C-reactive protein may be associated with local reactions.

In a clinical trial, an increased rate of local reactions has been observed with revaccination at 3-5 years following primary vaccination.

For subjects aged ≥65 years, it was reported that the overall injection-site adverse experiences rate was higher following revaccination (79.3%) than following primary vaccination (52.9%). For subjects aged 50-64 years, the reported overall injection-site adverse experiences rate for re-vaccinees and primary vaccinees were similar (79.6% and 72.8% respectively).

In both age groups, re-vaccinees reported a higher rate of a composite endpoint (any of the following: moderate pain, severe pain, and/or large induration at the injection site) than primary vaccinees. Among subjects ≥65 years of age, the composite endpoint was reported by 30.6% and 10.4% of revaccination and primary vaccination subjects, respectively, while among subjects 50-64 years of age, the endpoint was reported by 35.5% and 18.9% respectively. The injection site reactions occurred within the 3 day monitoring period and typically resolved by day 5.

The rate of overall systemic adverse experiences was similar among both primary vaccinees and re-vaccinees within each age group. The rate of vaccine-related systemic adverse experiences was higher following revaccination (33.1%) than following primary vaccination (21.7%) in subjects ≥65 years of age, and was similar following revaccination (37.5%) and primary vaccination (35.5%) in subjects 50-64 years of age. The most common systemic adverse experiences reported after PNEUMOVAX 23 were as follows: asthenia/fatigue, myalgia and headache.

Regardless of age, the observed increase in post vaccination use of analgesics (≤13% in the re-vaccinees and ≤4% in the primary vaccinees) returned to baseline by day 5.

DOSAGE AND ADMINISTRATION

Do not inject intravenously or intradermally.

Parenteral drug products should be inspected visually for particulate matter and discoloration prior to administration, whenever solution and container permit. PNEUMOVAX 23 is a clear, colorless solution. The vaccine is used directly as supplied. No dilution or reconstitution is necessary. Phenol 0.25% has been added as a preservative. It is important to use a separate sterile syringe and needle for each individual patient to prevent transmission of infectious agents from one person to another.

Withdraw 0.5 mL from the vial using a sterile needle and syringe free of preservatives, antiseptics, and detergents.

Administer a single 0.5 mL dose of PNEUMOVAX 23 subcutaneously or intramuscularly (preferably in the deltoid muscle or lateral mid-thigh), with appropriate precautions to avoid intravascular administration.

Store unopened and opened vials at 2-8°C (36-46°F). All vaccine must be discarded after the expiration date.

Use With Other Vaccines

The ACIP states that pneumococcal vaccine may be administered at the same time as influenza vaccine (by separate injection in the other arm) without an increase in side effects or decreased antibody response to either vaccine.{1} In contrast to pneumococcal vaccine, influenza vaccine is recommended annually, for appropriate populations.{35}

HOW SUPPLIED

No. 4739—PNEUMOVAX 23 is supplied as one 5-dose vial of liquid vaccine, color coded with a purple cap and stripe on the vial labels and cartons, **NDC** 0006-4739-00.

No. 4943—PNEUMOVAX 23 is supplied as a single-dose vial of liquid vaccine, in a box of 10 single-dose vials, color coded with a purple cap and stripe on the vial labels and cartons, **NDC** 0006-4943-00.

REFERENCES

1. Centers for Disease Control and Prevention. Prevention of Pneumococcal Disease. Recommendations of the Advisory Committee on Immunization Practices (ACIP). MMWR 1997; 46 (No. RR-8): 1-25. Available from: http://www.cdc.gov/mmwr/PDF/rr/rr4608.pdf
2. Robbins, J.B.; Lee, C.J.; Schiffman, G.; Austrian, R.; Henrichsen, J.; Mäkelä, P.H.; Broome, C.V.; Facklam, R.R.; Tiesjema, R.H.; Rastogi, S.C.: Considerations for formulating the second-generation pneumococcal capsular polysaccharide vaccine with emphasis on the cross-reactive types within groups, J. Infect. Dis. *148*: 1136-1159, 1983.
3. WHO: Vital statistics and causes of death, World Health Statistics Annual, 1, 1976.
4. Austrian, R.; Gold, J.: Pneumococcal bacteremia with especial reference to bacteremic pneumococcal pneumonia, Ann. Intern. Med. *60*: 759-776, 1964.
5. Austrian, R.: Random gleanings from a life with the pneumococcus, J. Infect. Dis. *131*: 474-484, 1975.
6. Austrian, R.: Vaccines of pneumococcal capsular polysaccharides and the prevention of pneumococcal

pneumonia in, "The role of immunological factors in infectious, allergic and autoimmune processes", R.F. Beers, Jr. and E.G. Bassett (eds.), New York, Raven Press: 79-89, 1976.
7. Mufson, M.A.; Kruss, D.M.; Wasil, R.E.; Metzger, W.I.: Capsular types and outcome of bacteremic pneumococcal disease in the antibiotic era, Arch. Intern. Med. *134:* 505-510, 1974.
8. Mufson, M.A.: Pneumococcal infections, J.A.M.A. *246*(17): 1942-1948, 1981.
9. Barrett-Connor, E.: Bacterial infection and sickle cell anemia: an analysis of 250 infections in 166 patients and a review of the literature, Medicine. *50:* 97-112, 1971.
10. Unpublished data; files of Merck Research Laboratories.
11. Borgono, J.M.; McLean, A.A.; Vella, P.P.; Woodhour, A.F.; Canepa, I.; Davidson, W.L.; Hilleman, M.R.: Vaccination and revaccination with polyvalent pneumococcal polysaccharide vaccines in adults and infants (40010), Proc. Soc. Exper. Biol. & Med. *157:* 148-154, 1978.
12. Hilleman, M.R.; McLean, A.A.; Vella, P.P.; Weibel, R.E.; Woodhour, A.F.: Polyvalent pneumococcal polysaccharide vaccines, Bull. WHO. *56:* 371-375, 1978.
13. Smit, P.; Oberholzer, D.; Hayden-Smith, S.; Koornhof, H.J.; Hilleman, M.R.: Protective efficacy of pneumococcal polysaccharide vaccines, J.A.M.A. *238:* 2613-2616, 1977.
14. Weibel, R.E.; Vella, P.P.; McLean, A.A.; Woodhour, A.F.; Hilleman, M.R.: Studies in human subjects of polyvalent pneumococcal vaccines (39894), Proc. Soc. Exper. Biol. & Med. *156:* 144-150, 1977.
15. Austrian, R.; Douglas, R.M.; Schiffman, G.; Coetzee, A.M.; Koornhof, H.J.; Hayden-Smith, S.; Reid, R.D.W.: Prevention of pneumococcal pneumonia by vaccination, Trans. Assoc. Am. Physicians. *89:* 184-194, 1976.
16. Gaillat, J.; Zmirou, D.; Mallaret, M.R.: Essai clinique du vaccin antipneuomococcique chez des personnes agees vivant en institution, Rev. Epidemiol. Sante Publique. *33:* 437-44, 1985.
17. Simberkoff, M.S.; Cross, A.P.; Al-Ibrahim, M.: Efficacy of pneumococcal vaccine in high risk patients: results of a Veterans Administration cooperative study, N. Engl. J. Med. *315:* 1318-27, 1986.
18. Broome, C.V.: Efficacy of pneumococcal polysaccharide vaccines, Rev. Infect. Dis. *3*(suppl): S82-S96, 1981.
19. Spika, J.S.; Fedson, D.S.; Facklam, R.R.: Pneumococcal vaccination-controversies and opportunities, Infect. Dis. Clin. North Am. *4:* 11-27, 1990.
20. Fine, M.J.; Smith, M.A.; Carson, C.A.; Meffe, F.; Sankey, S.S.; Weissfeld, L.A.; Detsky, A.S.; Kapoor, W.N.: Efficacy of pneumococcal vaccination in adults: a meta-analysis of randomized controlled trials, Arch. Intern. Med. *154:* 2666-77, 1994.
21. Fedson, D.S.; Shapiro, E.D.; LaForce, F.M.; Mufson, M.A.; Musher, D.M.; Spika, J.S.; Breiman, R.F.: Pneumococcal vaccine after 15 years of use: another view, Arch. Intern. Med. *154:* 2531-35, 1994.
22. Butler, J.C.; Breiman, R.F.; Campbell, J.F.; Lipman, H.B.; Broome, C.V.; Facklam, R.R.: Pneumococcal polysaccharide vaccine efficacy. An evaluation of current recommendations, J.A.M.A. *270:* 1826-31, 1993.
23. Shapiro, E.D.; Berg, A.T.; Austrian, R.; Schroeder, D.; Parcells, V.; Margolis, A.; Adair, R.K.; Clemens, J.D.: The protective efficacy of polyvalent pneumococcal polysaccharide vaccine, N. Engl. J. Med. *325:* 1453-60, 1991.
24. Farr, B.M.; Johnston, B.L.; Cobb, D.K.; Fisch, M.J.; Germanson, T.P.; Adal, K.A.; Anglim, A.M.: Preventing pneumococcal bacteremia in patients at risk. Results of a matched case-control study, Arch. Intern. Med. *155:* 2336-2340, 1995.
25. Shapiro, E.D.; Clemens, J.D.: A controlled evaluation of the protective efficacy of pneumococcal vaccine for patients at high risk of serious pneumococcal infections, Ann. Intern. Med. *101:* 325-30, 1984.
26. Sims, R.V.; Steinmann, W.C.; McConville, J.H.; King, L.R.; Zwick, W.C.; Schwartz, J.S.: The clinical effectiveness of pneumococcal vaccine in the elderly, Ann. Intern. Med. *108:* 653-7, 1988.
27. Forrester, H.L.; Jahnigen, D.W.; LaForce, F.M.: Inefficacy of pneumococcal vaccine in a high-risk population, Am. J. Med. *83:* 425-30, 1987.
28. Ammann, A.J.; Addiego, J.; Wara, D.W.; Lubin, B.; Smith, W.B.; Mentzer, W.C.: Polyvalent pneumococcal-polysaccharide immunization of patients with sickle-cell anemia and patients with splenectomy, N. Engl. J. Med. *297:* 897-900, 1977.
29. Musher, D.M.; Groover, J.E.; Rowland, J.M.; Watson, D.A.; Struewing, J.B.; Baughn, R.E.; Mufson, M.A.: Antibody to capsular polysaccharides of *Streptococcus pneumoniae:* prevalence, persistence, and response to revaccination, Clin. Infect. Dis. *17:* 66-73, 1993.
30. Konradsen, H.B.: Quantity and avidity of pneumococcal antibodies before and up to five years after pneumococcal vaccination of elderly persons, Clin. Infect. Dis. *21:* 616-20, 1995.
31. Centers for Disease Control and Prevention. ACIP Provisional Recommendations for Use of Pneumococcal Vaccines. [Internet]. 2008 October 22 [cited 2009 June 5]. Available from: http://www.cdc.gov/vaccines/recs/provisional/downloads/pneumo-oct-2008-508.pdf
32. Siber, G.R.; Weitzman, S.A.; Aisenberg, A.C.: Antibody response of patients with Hodgkin's disease to protein and polysaccharide antigens, Rev. Infect. Dis. (Suppl): S144-S159, March-April 1981.
33. Shildt, R.A.; Boyd, J.F.; McCracken, G.S.; Schiffman, G.; Giolma, J.P.: Antibody response to pneumococcal vaccine in patients with solid tumors and lymphomas, Med. Ped. Oncol. *11:* 305-309, 1983.
34. Carlson, A.J.; Davidson, W.L.; McLean, A.A.; Vella, P.P.; Weibel, R.E.; Woodhour, A.F.; Hilleman, M.R.: Pneumococcal vaccine dose, revaccination, and coadministration with influenza vaccine (40596), Proc. Soc. Exper. Biol. & Med. *161:* 558-563, 1979.
35. Centers for Disease Control and Prevention. Preventing Pneumococcal Disease Among Infants and Young Children, MMWR 2000; 49 (No. RR-9): Pages 25-27. Available from: http://www.cdc.gov/mmwr/PDF/rr/rr4909.pdf
36. Siber, G.R.; Gorham, C.; Martin, P.; Corkery, J.C.; Schiffman, G.: Antibody response to pretreatment immunization and post-treatment boosting with bacterial polysaccharide vaccines in patients with Hodgkin's disease, Ann. Intern. Med. *104:* 467-475, 1986.
37. Vaccine Adverse Event Reporting System - United States, Morbidity and Mortality Weekly Report. *39*(41): 730-33, October 19, 1990.
38. Kelton, J.G.: Vaccination-associated relapse of immune thrombocytopenia, J.A.M.A. *245*(4): 369-371, 1981.

Manuf. and Dist. by:
MERCK & CO., INC., Whitehouse Station, NJ 08889, USA
Issued March 2010
Printed in USA
9850934

PRIMAXIN® I.M. ℞

(imipenem and cilastatin for injectable suspension)

To reduce the development of drug-resistant bacteria and maintain the effectiveness of PRIMAXIN I.M.† and other antibacterial drugs, PRIMAXIN I.M. should be used only to treat or prevent infections that are proven or strongly suspected to be caused by bacteria.

For Intramuscular Injection Only

† Registered trademark of Merck Sharp & Dohme Corp., a subsidiary of **Merck & Co., Inc.**

DESCRIPTION

PRIMAXIN I.M. (Imipenem and Cilastatin for Injectable Suspension) is a formulation of imipenem (a thienamycin antibiotic) and cilastatin sodium (the inhibitor of the renal dipeptidase, dehydropeptidase I). PRIMAXIN I.M. is a potent broad spectrum antibacterial agent for intramuscular administration.

Imipenem (N-formimidoylthienamycin monohydrate) is a crystalline derivative of thienamycin, which is produced by *Streptomyces cattleya.* Its chemical name is [5*R*-[5α, 6α (*R**)]]-6-(1-hydroxyethyl) -3-[[2-[(iminomethyl) amino] ethyl]thio]-7-oxo-1-azabicyclo [3.2.0] hept-2-ene-2-carboxylic acid monohydrate. It is an off-white, nonhygroscopic crystalline compound with a molecular weight of 317.37. It is sparingly soluble in water, and slightly soluble in methanol. Its empirical formula is $C_{12}H_{17}N_3O_4S \bullet H_2O$, and its structural formula is:

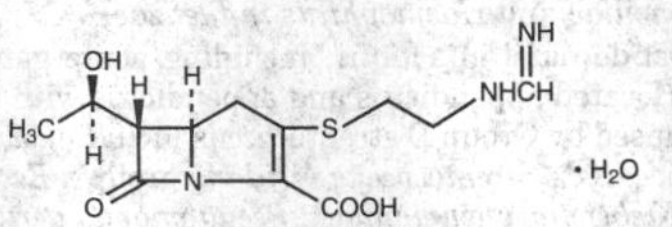

Cilastatin sodium is the sodium salt of a derivatized heptenoic acid. Its chemical name is [*R*-[*R**, *S**-(*Z*)]]-7-[(2-carboxyethyl)thio]2-[[2,2-dimethylcyclopropyl)carbonyl]amino]-2-heptenoic acid, monosodium salt. It is an off-white to yellowish-white, hygroscopic, amorphous compound with a molecular weight of 380.43. It is very soluble in water and in methanol. Its empirical formula is $C_{16}H_{25}N_2O_5SNa$, and its structural formula is:

[See chemical structure at top of next column]

PRIMAXIN I.M. 500 contains 32 mg of sodium (1.4 mEq) and PRIMAXIN I.M. 750 contains 48 mg of sodium (2.1 mEq). Prepared PRIMAXIN I.M. suspensions are white to light tan in color. Variations of color within this range do not affect the potency of the product.

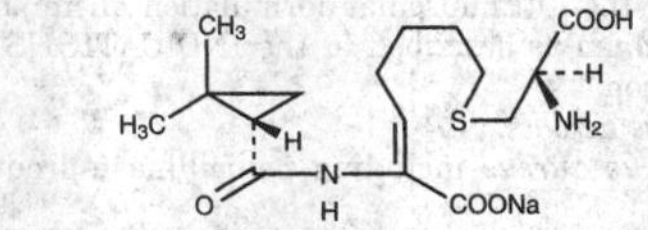

CLINICAL PHARMACOLOGY

Following intramuscular administrations of 500 or 750 mg doses of imipenem-cilastatin sodium in a 1:1 ratio with 1% lidocaine, peak plasma levels of imipenem antimicrobial activity occur within 2 hours and average 10 and 12 µg/mL, respectively. For cilastatin, peak plasma levels average 24 and 33 µg/mL, respectively, and occur within 1 hour. When compared to intravenous administration of imipenem-cilastatin sodium, imipenem is approximately 75% bioavailable following intramuscular administration while cilastatin is approximately 95% bioavailable. The absorption of imipenem from the IM injection site continues for 6 to 8 hours while that for cilastatin is essentially complete within 4 hours. This prolonged absorption of imipenem following the administration of the intramuscular formulation of imipenem-cilastatin sodium results in an effective plasma half-life of imipenem of approximately 2 to 3 hours and plasma levels of the antibiotic which remain above 2 µg/mL for at least 6 or 8 hours, following a 500 mg or 750 mg dose, respectively. This plasma profile for imipenem permits IM administration of the intramuscular formulation of imipenem-cilastatin sodium every 12 hours with no accumulation of cilastatin and only slight accumulation of imipenem.

A comparison of plasma levels of imipenem after a single dose of 500 mg or 750 mg of imipenem-cilastatin sodium (intravenous formulation) administered intravenously or of imipenem-cilastatin sodium (intramuscular formulation) diluted with 1% lidocaine and administered intramuscularly is as follows:

PLASMA CONCENTRATIONS OF IMIPENEM (µg/mL)

	500 MG		750 MG	
TIME	I.V.	I.M.	I.V.	I.M.
25 min	45.1	6.0	57.0	6.7
1 hr	21.6	9.4	28.1	10.0
2 hr	10.0	9.9	12.0	11.4
4 hr	2.6	5.6	3.4	7.3
6 hr	0.6	2.5	1.1	3.8
12 hr	ND**	0.5	ND**	0.8

** ND: Not Detectable (<0.3 µg/mL)

Imipenem urine levels remain above 10 µg/mL for the 12-hour dosing interval following the administration of 500 mg or 750 mg doses of the intramuscular formulation of imipenem-cilastatin sodium. Total urinary excretion of imipenem averages 50% while that for cilastatin averages 75% following either dose of the intramuscular formulation of imipenem-cilastatin sodium.

Imipenem, when administered alone, is metabolized in the kidneys by dehydropeptidase I resulting in relatively low levels in urine. Cilastatin sodium, an inhibitor of this enzyme, effectively prevents renal metabolism of imipenem so that when imipenem and cilastatin sodium are given concomitantly, increased levels of imipenem are achieved in the urine. The binding of imipenem to human serum proteins is approximately 20% and that of cilastatin is approximately 40%.

In a clinical study in which a 500-mg dose of the intramuscular formulation of imipenem-cilastatin sodium was administered to healthy subjects, the average peak level of imipenem in interstitial fluid (skin blister fluid) was approximately 5.0 µg/mL within 3.5 hours after administration.

Imipenem-cilastatin sodium is hemodialyzable. However, usefulness of this procedure in the overdosage setting is questionable. (See **OVERDOSAGE.**)

Microbiology

The bactericidal activity of imipenem results from the inhibition of cell wall synthesis. Its greatest affinity is for penicillin-binding proteins (PBPs) 1A, 1B, 2, 4, 5 and 6 of *Escherichia coli*, and 1A, 1B, 2, 4 and 5 of *Pseudomonas aeruginosa.* The lethal effect is related to binding to PBP 2 and PBP 1B.

Imipenem has a high degree of stability in the presence of beta-lactamases, including penicillinases and cephalosporinases produced by gram-negative and gram-positive bacteria. It is a potent inhibitor of beta-lactamases from certain gram-negative bacteria which are inherently resistant to many beta-lactam antibiotics, e.g., *Pseudomonas aeruginosa, Serratia* spp. and *Enterobacter* spp.

Imipenem has *in vitro* activity against a wide range of gram-positive and gram-negative organisms. Imipenem has been shown to be active against most strains of the following microorganisms both *in vitro* and in clinical infections treated with the intramuscular formulation of imipenem-cilastatin sodium as described in the INDICATIONS AND USAGE section.

Gram-positive aerobes:
Staphylococcus aureus including penicillinase-producing strains
(NOTE: Methicillin-resistant staphylococci should be reported as resistant to imipenem.)
Group D streptococcus including *Enterococcus faecalis* (formerly *S. faecalis*)
(NOTE: Imipenem is inactive *in vitro* against *Enterococcus faecium* [formerly *S. faecium*].)
Streptococcus pneumoniae
Streptococcus pyogenes (Group A streptococci)
Streptococcus viridans group
Gram-negative aerobes:
Acinetobacter spp., including *A. calcoaceticus*
Citrobacter spp.
Enterobacter cloacae
Escherichia coli
Haemophilus influenzae
Klebsiella pneumoniae
Pseudomonas aeruginosa
(NOTE: Imipenem is inactive *in vitro* against *Xanthomonas (Pseudomonas) maltophilia* and *P. cepacia*.)
Gram-positive anaerobes:
Peptostreptococcus spp.
Gram-negative anaerobes:
Bacteroides spp., including
Bacteroides distasonis
Bacteroides intermedius
(formerly *B. melaninogenicus intermedius*)
Bacteroides fragilis
Bacteroides thetaiotaomicron
Fusobacterium spp.
Imipenem exhibits *in vitro* minimal inhibitory concentrations (MICs) of 4 µg/mL or less against most (≥90%) strains of the following microorganisms; however, the safety and effectiveness of imipenem in treating clinical infections due to these microorganisms have not been established in adequate and well-controlled clinical trials.

Gram-positive aerobes:
Bacillus spp.
Listeria monocytogenes
Nocardia spp.
Group C streptococci
Group G streptococci
Gram-negative aerobes:
Aeromonas hydrophila
Alcaligenes spp.
Capnocytophaga spp.
Enterobacter agglomerans
Haemophilus ducreyi
Klebsiella oxytoca
Neisseria gonorrhoeae including penicillinase-producing strains
Pasteurella spp.
Proteus mirabilis
Providencia stuartii
Gram-positive anaerobes:
Clostridium perfringens
Gram-negative anaerobes:
Prevotella bivia
Prevotella disiens
Prevotella melaninogenica
Veillonella spp.
In vitro tests show imipenem to act synergistically with aminoglycoside antibiotics against some isolates of *Pseudomonas aeruginosa.*

Susceptibility Tests:
Dilution techniques:
Use a standardized dilution method[1] (broth, agar, microdilution) or equivalent with imipenem powder. The MIC values obtained should be interpreted according to the following criteria:

MIC (µg/mL)	Interpretation
≤4	Susceptible
8	Moderately Susceptible
≥16	Resistant

A report of "susceptible" indicates that the pathogen is likely to be inhibited by generally achievable blood levels. A report of "moderately susceptible" suggests that the organism would be susceptible if high dosage is used or if the infection is confined to tissues and fluids in which high antibiotic levels are attained. A report of "resistant" indicates that achievable concentrations are unlikely to be inhibitory and other therapy should be selected.

Standardized susceptibility test procedures require the use of laboratory control organisms. Standard imipenem powder should provide the following MIC values:

Organism	MIC (µg/mL)
E. coli ATCC 25922	0.06-0.25
S. aureus ATCC 29213	0.015-0.06
E. faecalis ATCC 29212	0.5-2.0
P. aeruginosa ATCC 27853	1.0-4.0

Diffusion techniques:
Quantitative methods that require measurement of zone diameters give the most precise estimate of antibiotic susceptibility. One such standard procedure[2], which has been recommended for use with disks to test susceptibility of organisms to imipenem, uses the 10-µg imipenem disk. Interpretation involves the correlation of the diameters obtained in the disk test with the minimum inhibitory concentration (MIC) for imipenem.
Reports from the laboratory giving results of the standard single-disk susceptibility test with a 10-µg imipenem disk should be interpreted according to the following criteria:

Zone Diameter (mm)	Interpretation
≥16	Susceptible
14-15	Moderately Susceptible
≤13	Resistant

Standardized procedures require the use of laboratory control organisms. The 10-µg imipenem disk should give the following zone diameters:

Organism	Zone Diameter (mm)
E. coli ATCC 25922	26-32
P. aeruginosa ATCC 27853	20-28

For anaerobic bacteria, the MIC of imipenem can be determined by agar or broth dilution (including microdilution) techniques[3].
The MIC values obtained should be interpreted according to the following criteria:

MIC (µg/mL)	Interpretation
≤4	Susceptible
8	Moderately Susceptible
≥16	Resistant

·

INDICATIONS AND USAGE

PRIMAXIN I.M. is indicated for the treatment of serious infections (listed below) of mild to moderate severity for which intramuscular therapy is appropriate. **PRIMAXIN I.M. is not intended for the therapy of severe or life-threatening infections, including bacterial sepsis or endocarditis, or in instances of major physiological impairments such as shock.**
PRIMAXIN I.M. is indicated for the treatment of infections caused by susceptible strains of the designated microorganisms in the conditions listed below:
1. **Lower respiratory tract infections**, including pneumonia and bronchitis as an exacerbation of COPD (chronic obstructive pulmonary disease), caused by *Streptococcus pneumoniae* and *Haemophilus influenzae.*
2. **Intra-abdominal infections**, including acute gangrenous or perforated appendicitis and appendicitis with peritonitis, caused by Group D streptococcus including *Enterococcus faecalis**; *Streptococcus viridans group*; *Escherichia coli*; *Klebsiella pneumoniae**; *Pseudomonas aeruginosa**; *Bacteroides* species including *B. fragilis, B. distasonis**, *B. intermedius** and *B. thetaiotaomicron**; *Fusobacterium* species and *Peptostreptococcu** species.
3. **Skin and skin structure infections**, including abscesses, cellulitis, infected skin ulcers and wound infections caused by *Staphylococcus aureus* including penicillinase-producing strains; *Streptococcus pyogenes**; Group D streptococcus including *Enterococcus faecalis*; *Acinetobacter* species* including *A. calcoaceticus**; *Citrobacter* species*; *Escherichia coli*; *Enterobacter cloacae*; *Klebsiella pneumoniae**; *Pseudomonas aeruginosa**; and *Bacteroides* species* including *B. fragilis*.
4. **Gynecologic infections**, including postpartum endomyometritis, caused by Group D streptococcus including

*Enterococcus faecalis**; *Escherichia coli*; *Klebsiella pneumoniae**; *Bacteroides intermedius**; and *Peptostreptococcus* species*.
As with other beta-lactam antibiotics, some strains of *Pseudomonas aeruginosa* may develop resistance fairly rapidly during treatment with PRIMAXIN I.M. During therapy of *Pseudomonas aeruginosa* infections, periodic susceptibility testing should be done when clinically appropriate.
To reduce the development of drug-resistant bacteria and maintain the effectiveness of PRIMAXIN I.M. and other antibacterial drugs, PRIMAXIN I.M. should be used only to treat or prevent infections that are proven or strongly suspected to be caused by susceptible bacteria. When culture and susceptibility information are available, they should be considered in selecting or modifying antibacterial therapy. In the absence of such data, local epidemiology and susceptibility patterns may contribute to the empiric selection of therapy.

* Efficacy for this organism in this organ system was studied in fewer than 10 infections.

CONTRAINDICATIONS

PRIMAXIN I.M. is contraindicated in patients who have shown hypersensitivity to any component of this product. Due to the use of lidocaine hydrochloride diluent, this product is contraindicated in patients with a known hypersensitivity to local anesthetics of the amide type and in patients with severe shock or heart block. (Refer to the package circular for lidocaine hydrochloride.)

WARNINGS

SERIOUS AND OCCASIONALLY FATAL HYPERSENSITIVITY (anaphylactic) REACTIONS HAVE BEEN REPORTED IN PATIENTS RECEIVING THERAPY WITH BETA-LACTAMS. THESE REACTIONS ARE MORE LIKELY TO OCCUR IN INDIVIDUALS WITH A HISTORY OF SENSITIVITY TO MULTIPLE ALLERGENS. THERE HAVE BEEN REPORTS OF INDIVIDUALS WITH A HISTORY OF PENICILLIN HYPERSENSITIVITY WHO HAVE EXPERIENCED SEVERE REACTIONS WHEN TREATED WITH ANOTHER BETA-LACTAM. BEFORE INITIATING THERAPY WITH PRIMAXIN® I.M., CAREFUL INQUIRY SHOULD BE MADE CONCERNING PREVIOUS HYPERSENSITIVITY REACTIONS TO PENICILLINS, CEPHALOSPORINS, OTHER BETA-LACTAMS, AND OTHER ALLERGENS. IF AN ALLERGIC REACTION OCCURS, PRIMAXIN® SHOULD BE DISCONTINUED. **SERIOUS ANAPHYLACTIC REACTIONS REQUIRE IMMEDIATE EMERGENCY TREATMENT WITH EPINEPHRINE. OXYGEN, INTRAVENOUS STEROIDS, AND AIRWAY MANAGEMENT, INCLUDING INTUBATION, MAY ALSO BE ADMINISTERED AS INDICATED.**

Seizure Potential
Seizures and other CNS adverse experiences, such as myoclonic activity, have been reported during treatment with PRIMAXIN I.M. (See **PRECAUTIONS** and **ADVERSE REACTIONS**.)
Case reports in the literature have shown that co-administration of carbapenems, including imipenem, to patients receiving valproic acid or divalproex sodium results in a reduction in valproic acid concentrations. The valproic acid concentrations may drop below the therapeutic range as a result of this interaction, therefore increasing the risk of breakthrough seizures. Increasing the dose of valproic acid or divalproex sodium may not be sufficient to overcome this interaction. The concomitant use of imipenem and valproic acid/divalproex sodium is generally not recommended. Anti-bacterials other than carbapenems should be considered to treat infections in patients whose seizures are well controlled on valproic acid or divalproex sodium. If administration of PRIMAXIN I.M. is necessary, supplemental anti-convulsant therapy should be considered (see **PRECAUTIONS**, Drug Interactions).
Clostridium difficile associated diarrhea (CDAD) has been reported with use of nearly all antibacterial agents, including PRIMAXIN I.M., and may range in severity from mild diarrhea to fatal colitis. Treatment with antibacterial agents alters the normal flora of the colon leading to overgrowth of *C. difficile.*
C. difficile produces toxins A and B which contribute to the development of CDAD.
Hypertoxin producing strains of *C. difficile* cause increased morbidity and mortality, as these infections can be refractory to antimicrobial therapy and may require colectomy. CDAD must be considered in all patients who present with diarrhea following antibiotic use. Careful medical history is necessary since CDAD has been reported to occur over two months after the administration of antibacterial agents.
If CDAD is suspected or confirmed, ongoing antibiotic use not directed against *C. difficile* may need to be discontinued. Appropriate fluid and electrolyte management, protein supplementation, antibiotic treatment of *C. difficile*, and surgical evaluation should be instituted as clinically indicated.

Lidocaine HCl—Refer to the package circular for lidocaine HCl.

PRECAUTIONS

General

CNS adverse experiences such as myoclonic activity or seizures have been reported with PRIMAXIN I.M. These experiences have occurred most commonly in patients with CNS disorders (e.g., brain lesions or history of seizures) who also have compromised renal function. However, there were reports in which there was no recognized or documented underlying CNS disorder. Anticonvulsant therapy should be continued in patients with a known seizure disorder.

As with other antibiotics, prolonged use of PRIMAXIN I.M. may result in overgrowth of nonsusceptible organisms. Repeated evaluation of the patient's condition is essential. If superinfection occurs during therapy, appropriate measures should be taken.

Prescribing PRIMAXIN I.M. in the absence of a proven or strongly suspected bacterial infection or a prophylactic indication is unlikely to provide benefit to the patient and increases the risk of the development of drug-resistant bacteria.

Caution should be taken to avoid inadvertent injection into a blood vessel. (See **DOSAGE AND ADMINISTRATION**.) For additional precautions, refer to the package circular for lidocaine HCl.

Information for Patients

Patients should be counseled to inform their physician if they are taking valproic acid or divalproex sodium. Valproic acid concentrations in the blood may drop below the therapeutic range upon co-administration with PRIMAXIN I.M. If treatment with PRIMAXIN I.M. is necessary and continued, alternative or supplemental anti-convulsant medication to prevent and/or treat seizures may be needed.

Patients should be counseled that antibacterial drugs including PRIMAXIN I.M. should only be used to treat bacterial infections. They do not treat viral infections (e.g., the common cold). When PRIMAXIN I.M. is prescribed to treat a bacterial infection, patients should be told that although it is common to feel better early in the course of therapy, the medication should be taken exactly as directed. Skipping doses or not completing the full course of therapy may (1) decrease the effectiveness of the immediate treatment and (2) increase the likelihood that bacteria will develop resistance and will not be treatable by PRIMAXIN I.M. or other antibacterial drugs in the future.

Diarrhea is a common problem caused by antibiotics, which usually ends when the antibiotic is discontinued. Sometimes after starting treatment with antibiotics, patients can develop watery and bloody stools (with or without stomach cramps and fever) even as late as two or more months after having taken the last dose of the antibiotic. If this occurs, patients should contact their physician as soon as possible.

Drug Interactions

Since concomitant administration of PRIMAXIN (Imipenem-Cilastatin Sodium) and probenecid results in only minimal increases in plasma levels of imipenem and plasma half-life, it is not recommended that probenecid be given with PRIMAXIN I.M.

PRIMAXIN I.M. should not be mixed with or physically added to other antibiotics. However, PRIMAXIN I.M. may be administered concomitantly with other antibiotics, such as aminoglycosides.

Case reports in the literature have shown that co-administration of carbapenems, including imipenem, to patients receiving valproic acid or divalproex sodium results in a reduction in valproic acid concentrations. The valproic acid concentrations may drop below the therapeutic range as a result of this interaction, therefore increasing the risk of breakthrough seizures. Although the mechanism of this interaction is unknown, data from in vitro and animal studies suggest that carbapenems may inhibit the hydrolysis of valproic acid's glucuronide metabolite (VPA-g) back to valproic acid, thus decreasing the serum concentrations of valproic acid (see **WARNINGS**, Seizure Potential).

Carcinogenesis, Mutagenesis, Impairment of Fertility

Long term studies in animals have not been performed to evaluate carcinogenic potential of imipenem-cilastatin. Genetic toxicity studies were performed in a variety of bacterial and mammalian tests in vivo and in vitro. The tests used were: V79 mammalian cell mutagenesis assay (imipenem-cilastatin sodium alone and imipenem alone), Ames test (cilastatin sodium alone and imipenem alone), unscheduled DNA synthesis assay (imipenem-cilastatin sodium) and in vivo mouse cytogenetics test (imipenem-cilastatin sodium). None of these tests showed any evidence of genetic alterations.

Reproductive tests in male and female rats were performed with imipenem-cilastatin sodium at intravenous doses up to 80 mg/kg/day and at a subcutaneous dose of 320 mg/kg/day, 2.1 times*** the maximum recommended daily human dose of the intramuscular formulation (on a mg/m² body surface area basis). Slight decreases in live fetal body weight were restricted to the highest dosage level. No other adverse effects were observed on fertility, reproductive performance, fetal viability, growth, or postnatal development of pups.

***Based on patient body surface area of 1.6 m² (weight of 60 kg).

Pregnancy: Teratogenic Effects

Pregnancy Category C: Teratology studies with cilastatin sodium at doses of 30, 100, and 300 mg/kg/day administered intravenously to rabbits and 40, 200, and 1000 mg/kg/day administered subcutaneously to rats, up to approximately 3.9 and 6.5 times*** the maximum recommended daily human dose (on a mg/m² body surface area basis) of the intramuscular formulation of PRIMAXIN (25 mg/kg/day) in the two species, respectively, showed no evidence of adverse effects on the fetus. No evidence of teratogenicity was observed in rabbits given imipenem at intravenous doses of 15, 30, or 60 mg/kg/day and rats given imipenem at intravenous doses of 225, 450, or 900 mg/kg/day, up to approximately 0.8 and 5.8 times*** the maximum recommended daily human dose (on a mg/m² body surface area basis) in the two species, respectively.

Teratology studies with imipenem-cilastatin sodium at intravenous doses of 20 and 80 and a subcutaneous dose of 320 mg/kg/day, approximately equal to (mice) and up to 2.1 times*** (rats) the maximum recommended daily intramuscular human dose (on a mg/m² body surface area basis) in pregnant rodents during the period of major organogenesis, revealed no evidence of teratogenicity.

Imipenem-cilastatin sodium, when administered to pregnant rabbits subcutaneously at dosages above the usual human dose of the intramuscular formulation (1000-1500 mg/day), caused body weight loss, diarrhea, and maternal deaths. When comparable doses of imipenem-cilastatin sodium were given to non-pregnant rabbits, body weight loss, diarrhea, and deaths were also observed. This intolerance is not unlike that seen with other beta-lactam antibiotics in this species and is probably due to alteration of gut flora.

A teratology study in pregnant cynomolgus monkeys given imipenem-cilastatin sodium at doses of 40 mg/kg/day (bolus intravenous injection) or 160 mg/kg/day (subcutaneous injection) resulted in maternal toxicity including emesis, inappetence, body weight loss, diarrhea, abortion and death in some cases. In contrast, no significant toxicity was observed when non-pregnant cynomolgus monkeys were given doses of imipenem-cilastatin sodium up to 180 mg/kg/day (subcutaneous injection). When doses of imipenem-cilastatin sodium (approximately 100 mg/kg/day or approximately 1.3 times*** the maximum recommended daily human dose of the intramuscular formulation) were administered to pregnant cynomolgus monkeys at an intravenous infusion rate which mimics human clinical use, there was minimal maternal intolerance (occasional emesis), no maternal deaths, no evidence of teratogenicity, but an increase in embryonic loss relative to the control groups.

No adverse effects on the fetus or on lactation were observed when imipenem-cilastatin sodium was administered subcutaneously to rats late in gestation at dosages up to 320 mg/kg/day, 2.1 times the maximum recommended daily human dose (on a mg/m² body surface area basis).

There are, however, no adequate and well-controlled studies in pregnant women. PRIMAXIN I.M. should be used during pregnancy only if the potential benefit justifies the potential risk to the mother and fetus.

Nursing Mothers

It is not known whether imipenem-cilastatin sodium or lidocaine HCl (diluent) is excreted in human milk. Because many drugs are excreted in human milk, caution should be exercised when PRIMAXIN I.M. is administered to a nursing woman.

Pediatric Use

Safety and effectiveness in pediatric patients below the age of 12 years have not been established.

Geriatric Use

Clinical studies of PRIMAXIN I.M. did not include sufficient numbers of subjects aged 65 and over to determine whether they respond differently from younger subjects; however, clinical studies of PRIMAXIN I.V. in a sufficient number of subjects aged 65 and over have not revealed overall differences in safety or effectiveness between these subjects and younger subjects (refer to the package circular for PRIMAXIN I.V.). Other reported clinical experience has not identified differences in responses between the elderly and younger patients. In general, dose selection for an elderly patient should be cautious, usually starting at the low end of the dosing range, reflecting the greater frequency of decreased hepatic, renal, or cardiac function, and of concomitant disease or other drug therapy.

This drug is known to be substantially excreted by the kidney, and the risk of toxic reactions to this drug may be greater in patients with impaired renal function. Because elderly patients are more likely to have decreased renal function, care should be taken in dose selection, and it may be useful to monitor renal function. Dosage adjustment in the case of renal impairment is necessary (see **DOSAGE AND ADMINISTRATION**, ADULTS WITH IMPAIRED RENAL FUNCTION).

ADVERSE REACTIONS

PRIMAXIN I.M.

In 686 patients in multiple dose clinical trials of PRIMAXIN I.M., the following adverse reactions were reported:

Local Adverse Reactions

The most frequent adverse local clinical reaction that was reported as possibly, probably, or definitely related to therapy with PRIMAXIN I.M. was pain at the injection site (1.2%).

Systemic Adverse Reactions

The most frequently reported systemic adverse clinical reactions that were reported as possibly, probably, or definitely related to PRIMAXIN I.M. were nausea (0.6%), diarrhea (0.6%), vomiting (0.3%) and rash (0.4%).

Adverse Laboratory Changes

Adverse laboratory changes without regard to drug relationship that were reported during clinical trials were:

Hemic: decreased hemoglobin and hematocrit, eosinophilia, increased and decreased WBC, increased and decreased platelets, decreased erythrocytes, and increased prothrombin time.

Hepatic: increased AST, ALT, alkaline phosphatase, and bilirubin.

Renal: increased BUN and creatinine.

Urinalysis: presence of red blood cells, white blood cells, casts, and bacteria in the urine.

Potential ADVERSE EFFECTS:

In addition, a variety of adverse effects, not observed in clinical trials with PRIMAXIN I.M., have been reported with intravenous administration of PRIMAXIN I.V. (Imipenem and Cilastatin for Injection). Those listed below are to serve as alerting information to physicians.

Systemic Adverse Reactions

The most frequently reported systemic adverse clinical reactions that were reported as possibly, probably, or definitely related to PRIMAXIN I.V. (Imipenem and Cilastatin for Injection) were fever, hypotension, seizures (see **PRECAUTIONS**), dizziness, pruritus, urticaria, and somnolence.

Additional adverse systemic clinical reactions reported possibly, probably, or definitely drug related or reported since the drug was marketed are listed within each body system in order of decreasing severity: *Gastrointestinal:* pseudomembranous colitis (the onset of pseudomembranous colitis symptoms may occur during or after antibiotic treatment, see **WARNINGS**), hemorrhagic colitis, hepatitis (including fulminant hepatitis), hepatic failure, jaundice, gastroenteritis, abdominal pain, glossitis, tongue papillar hypertrophy, staining of the teeth and/or tongue, heartburn, pharyngeal pain, increased salivation; *Hematologic:* pancytopenia, bone marrow depression, thrombocytopenia, neutropenia, leukopenia, hemolytic anemia; *CNS:* encephalopathy, tremor, confusion, myoclonus, seizures, paresthesia, vertigo, headache, psychic disturbances including hallucinations; *Special Senses:* hearing loss, tinnitus, taste perversion; *Respiratory:* chest discomfort, dyspnea, hyperventilation, thoracic spine pain; *Cardiovascular:* palpitations, tachycardia; *Renal:* acute renal failure, oliguria/anuria, polyuria, urine discoloration; *Skin:* toxic epidermal necrolysis, Stevens-Johnson syndrome, erythema multiforme, angioneurotic edema, flushing, cyanosis, hyperhidrosis, skin texture changes, candidiasis, pruritus vulvae; *Body as a whole:* polyarthralgia, asthenia/weakness, drug fever.

Adverse Laboratory Changes

Adverse laboratory changes without regard to drug relationship that were reported during clinical trials or reported since the drug was marketed were:

Hepatic: increased LDH; *Hemic:* positive Coombs test, decreased neutrophils, agranulocytosis, increased monocytes, abnormal prothrombin time, increased lymphocytes, increased basophils; *Electrolytes:* decreased serum sodium, increased potassium, increased chloride; *Urinalysis:* presence of urine protein, urine bilirubin, and urine urobilinogen.

Lidocaine HCl—Refer to the package circular for lidocaine HCl.

OVERDOSAGE

The acute intravenous toxicity of imipenem-cilastatin sodium in a ratio of 1:1 was studied in mice at doses of 751 to 1359 mg/kg. Following drug administration, ataxia was rapidly produced and clonic convulsions were noted in about 45 minutes. Deaths occurred within 4-56 minutes at all doses.

The acute intravenous toxicity of imipenem-cilastatin sodium was produced within 5-10 minutes in rats at doses of 771 to 1583 mg/kg. In all dosage groups, females had decreased activity, bradypnea and ptosis with clonic convulsions preceding death; in males, ptosis was seen at all dose levels while tremors and clonic convulsions were seen at all but the lowest dose (771 mg/kg). In another rat study, female rats showed ataxia, bradypnea and decreased activity

DOSAGE GUIDELINES

Type[††]/Location of Infection	Severity	Dosage Regimen
Lower respiratory tract Skin and skin structure Gynecologic	Mild/Moderate	500 or 750 mg q 12 h depending on the severity of infection
Intra-abdominal	Mild/Moderate	750 mg q 12 h

[††] See INDICATIONS AND USAGE section.

in all but the lowest dose (550 mg/kg); deaths were preceded by clonic convulsions. Male rats showed tremors at all doses and clonic convulsions and ptosis were seen at the two highest doses (1130 and 1734 mg/kg). Deaths occurred between 6 and 88 minutes with doses of 771 to 1734 mg/kg.

In the case of overdosage, discontinue PRIMAXIN I.M., treat symptomatically, and institute supportive measures as required. Imipenem-cilastatin sodium is hemodialyzable. However, usefulness of this procedure in the overdosage setting is questionable.

DOSAGE AND ADMINISTRATION

PRIMAXIN I.M. is for intramuscular use only.

The dosage recommendations for PRIMAXIN I.M. represent the quantity of imipenem to be administered. An equivalent amount of cilastatin is also present.

Patients with lower respiratory tract infections, skin and skin structure infections, and gynecologic infections of mild to moderate severity may be treated with 500 mg or 750 mg administered every 12 hours depending on the severity of the infection.

Intra-abdominal infection may be treated with 750 mg every 12 hours.

[See table above]

Total daily IM dosages greater than 1500 mg per day are not recommended.

The dosage for any particular patient should be based on the location of and severity of the infection, the susceptibility of the infecting pathogen(s), and renal function.

The duration of therapy depends upon the type and severity of the infection. Generally, PRIMAXIN I.M. should be continued for at least two days after the signs and symptoms of infection have resolved. Safety and efficacy of treatment beyond fourteen days have not been established.

PRIMAXIN I.M. should be administered by deep intramuscular injection into a large muscle mass (such as the gluteal muscles or lateral part of the thigh) with a 21 gauge 2″ needle. Aspiration is necessary to avoid inadvertent injection into a blood vessel.

ADULTS WITH IMPAIRED RENAL FUNCTION

The safety and efficacy of PRIMAXIN I.M. have not been studied in patients with creatinine clearance of less than 20 mL/min/1.73 m². Serum creatinine alone may not be a sufficiently accurate measure of renal function. Creatinine clearance (T_{cc}) may be estimated from the following equation:

$$T_{cc} \text{ (Males)} = \frac{\text{(wt. in kg)}(140 - \text{age})}{(72)(\text{creatinine in mg/dL})}$$

$$T_{cc} \text{ (Females)} = 0.85 \times \text{above value}$$

PREPARATION FOR ADMINISTRATION

PRIMAXIN I.M. should be prepared for use with 1.0% lidocaine HCl solution[†††] (without epinephrine). PRIMAXIN I.M. 500 should be prepared with 2 mL and PRIMAXIN I.M. 750 with 3 mL of lidocaine HCl. Agitate to form a suspension, then withdraw and inject the entire contents of vial intramuscularly. The suspension of PRIMAXIN I.M. in lidocaine HCl should be used within one hour after preparation.

Note: The IM formulation is not for IV use.

[†††] Refer to the package circular for lidocaine HCl for detailed information concerning CONTRAINDICATIONS, WARNINGS, PRECAUTIONS, and ADVERSE REACTIONS.

COMPATIBILITY AND STABILITY

Before Reconstitution

The dry powder should be stored at a temperature below 25°C (77°F).

Suspensions for IM Administration

Suspensions of PRIMAXIN I.M. are white to light tan in color. Variations of color within this range do not affect the potency of the product.

The suspension of PRIMAXIN I.M. in lidocaine HCl should be used within one hour after preparation.

PRIMAXIN I.M. should not be mixed with or physically added to other antibiotics. However, PRIMAXIN I.M. may be administered concomitantly but at separate sites with other antibiotics, such as aminoglycosides.

HOW SUPPLIED

PRIMAXIN I.M. is supplied as a sterile powder mixture in vials for IM administration as follows:

No. 3582—500 mg imipenem equivalent and 500 mg cilastatin equivalent

NDC 0006-3582-75 in trays of 10 vials.

No. 3583—750 mg imipenem equivalent and 750 mg cilastatin equivalent

NDC 0006-3583-76 in trays of 10 vials.

REFERENCES

1. National Committee for Clinical Laboratory Standards, Methods for Dilution Antimicrobial Susceptibility Tests for Bacteria that Grow Aerobically—Fourth Edition. Approved Standard NCCLS Document M7-A4, Vol. 17, No. 2 NCCLS, Villanova, PA, 1997.
2. National Committee for Clinical Laboratory Standards, Performance Standards for Antimicrobial Disk Susceptibility Tests—Sixth Edition. Approved Standard NCCLS Document M2-A6, Vol. 17, No. 1 NCCLS, Villanova, PA, 1997.
3. National Committee for Clinical Laboratory Standards, Method for Antimicrobial Susceptibility Testing of Anaerobic Bacteria—Third Edition. Approved Standard NCCLS Document M11-A3, Vol. 13, No. 26 NCCLS, Villanova, PA, 1993.

Merck Sharp & Dohme Corp., a subsidiary of
MERCK & CO., INC., Whitehouse Station, NJ 08889, USA
Issued February 2010
9882821

PRIMAXIN® I.V.   ℞
(IMIPENEM AND CILASTATIN FOR INJECTION)

To reduce the development of drug-resistant bacteria and maintain the effectiveness of PRIMAXIN I.V.[†] and other antibacterial drugs, PRIMAXIN I.V. should be used only to treat or prevent infections that are proven or strongly suspected to be caused by bacteria.

For Intravenous Injection Only

[†] Registered trademark of Merck Sharp & Dohme Corp., a subsidiary of **Merck & Co., Inc.**
Copyright © 1987, 1994, 1998 Merck Sharp & Dohme Corp., a subsidiary of **Merck & Co., Inc.**
All rights reserved

DESCRIPTION

PRIMAXIN I.V. (Imipenem and Cilastatin for Injection) is a sterile formulation of imipenem (a thienamycin antibiotic) and cilastatin sodium (the inhibitor of the renal dipeptidase, dehydropeptidase I), with sodium bicarbonate added as a buffer. PRIMAXIN I.V. is a potent broad spectrum antibacterial agent for intravenous administration.

Imipenem (N-formimidoylthienamycin monohydrate) is a crystalline derivative of thienamycin, which is produced by *Streptomyces cattleya*. Its chemical name is (5R,6S)-3-[[2-(formimidoylamino)ethyl]thio]-6-[(R)-1-hydroxyethyl]-7-oxo-1-azabicyclo[3.2.0]hept-2-ene-2-carboxylic acid monohydrate. It is an off-white, nonhygroscopic crystalline compound with a molecular weight of 317.37. It is sparingly soluble in water and slightly soluble in methanol. Its empirical formula is $C_{12}H_{17}N_3O_4S \cdot H_2O$, and its structural formula is:

Cilastatin sodium is the sodium salt of a derivatized heptenoic acid. Its chemical name is sodium (Z)-7-[[(R)-2-amino-2-carboxyethyl]thio]-2-[(S)-2,2-dimethylcyclopropanecarboxamido]-2-heptenoate. It is an off-white to yellowish-white, hygroscopic, amorphous compound with a molecular weight of 380.43. It is very soluble in water and in methanol. Its empirical formula is $C_{16}H_{25}N_2O_5SNa$, and its structural formula is:

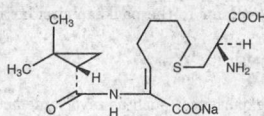

PRIMAXIN I.V. is buffered to provide solutions in the pH range of 6.5 to 8.5. There is no significant change in pH when solutions are prepared and used as directed. (See **COMPATIBILITY AND STABILITY**.) PRIMAXIN I.V. 250 contains 18.8 mg of sodium (0.8 mEq) and PRIMAXIN I.V. 500 contains 37.5 mg of sodium (1.6 mEq). Solutions of PRIMAXIN I.V. range from colorless to yellow. Variations of color within this range do not affect the potency of the product.

CLINICAL PHARMACOLOGY

Adults

Intravenous Administration

Intravenous infusion of PRIMAXIN I.V. over 20 minutes results in peak plasma levels of imipenem antimicrobial activity that range from 14 to 24 μg/mL for the 250 mg dose, from 21 to 58 μg/mL for the 500 mg dose, and from 41 to 83 μg/mL for the 1000 mg dose. At these doses, plasma levels of imipenem antimicrobial activity decline to below 1 μg/mL or less in 4 to 6 hours. Peak plasma levels of cilastatin following a 20-minute intravenous infusion of PRIMAXIN I.V. range from 15 to 25 μg/mL for the 250 mg dose, from 31 to 49 μg/mL for the 500 mg dose, and from 56 to 88 μg/mL for the 1000 mg dose.

The plasma half-life of each component is approximately 1 hour. The binding of imipenem to human serum proteins is approximately 20% and that of cilastatin is approximately 40%. Approximately 70% of the administered imipenem is recovered in the urine within 10 hours after which no further urinary excretion is detectable. Urine concentrations of imipenem in excess of 10 μg/mL can be maintained for up to 8 hours with PRIMAXIN I.V. at the 500-mg dose. Approximately 70% of the cilastatin sodium dose is recovered in the urine within 10 hours of administration of PRIMAXIN I.V. No accumulation of imipenem/cilastatin in plasma or urine is observed with regimens administered as frequently as every 6 hours in patients with normal renal function.

In healthy elderly volunteers (65 to 75 years of age with normal renal function for their age), the pharmacokinetics of a single dose of imipenem 500 mg and cilastatin 500 mg administered intravenously over 20 minutes are consistent with those expected in subjects with slight renal impairment for which no dosage alteration is considered necessary. The mean plasma half-lives of imipenem and cilastatin are 91 ± 7.0 minutes and 69 ± 15 minutes, respectively. Multiple dosing has no effect on the pharmacokinetics of either imipenem or cilastatin, and no accumulation of imipenem/cilastatin is observed.

Imipenem, when administered alone, is metabolized in the kidneys by dehydropeptidase I resulting in relatively low levels in urine. Cilastatin sodium, an inhibitor of this enzyme, effectively prevents renal metabolism of imipenem so that when imipenem and cilastatin sodium are given concomitantly, fully adequate antibacterial levels of imipenem are achieved in the urine.

After a 1 gram dose of PRIMAXIN I.V., the following average levels of imipenem were measured (usually at 1 hour post dose except where indicated) in the tissues and fluids listed:

[See table at top of next page]

Imipenem-cilastatin sodium is hemodialyzable. However, usefulness of this procedure in the overdosage setting is questionable. (See **OVERDOSAGE**.)

Microbiology

The bactericidal activity of imipenem results from the inhibition of cell wall synthesis. Its greatest affinity is for penicillin binding proteins (PBPs) 1A, 1B, 2, 4, 5 and 6 of *Escherichia coli*, and 1A, 1B, 2, 4 and 5 of *Pseudomonas aeruginosa*. The lethal effect is related to binding to PBP 2 and PBP 1B.

Imipenem has a high degree of stability in the presence of beta-lactamases, both penicillinases and cephalosporinases produced by gram-negative and gram-positive bacteria. It is a potent inhibitor of beta-lactamases from certain gram-negative bacteria which are inherently resistant to most beta-lactam antibiotics, e.g., *Pseudomonas aeruginosa, Serratia* spp., and *Enterobacter* spp.

Imipenem has *in vitro* activity against a wide range of gram-positive and gram-negative organisms. Imipenem has been shown to be active against most strains of the following microorganisms, both *in vitro* and in clinical infections treated with the intravenous formulation of imipenem-cilastatin sodium as described in the **INDICATIONS AND USAGE** section.

Gram-positive aerobes:

Enterococcus faecalis (formerly S. faecalis)
(NOTE: Imipenem is inactive *in vitro* against *Enterococcus faecium* [formerly S. faecium].)

Staphylococcus aureus including penicillinase-producing strains

Staphylococcus epidermidis including penicillinase-producing strains

(NOTE: Methicillin-resistant staphylococci should be reported as resistant to imipenem.)

Streptococcus agalactiae (Group B streptococci)
Streptococcus pneumoniae
Streptococcus pyogenes
Gram-negative aerobes:
Acinetobacter spp.
Citrobacter spp.
Enterobacter spp.
Escherichia coli
Gardnerella vaginalis
Haemophilus influenzae
Haemophilus parainfluenzae
Klebsiella spp.
Morganella morganii
Proteus vulgaris
Providencia rettgeri
Pseudomonas aeruginosa
(NOTE: Imipenem is inactive *in vitro* against *Xanthomonas (Pseudomonas) maltophilia* and some strains of *P. cepacia*.)
Serratia spp., including *S. marcescens*
Gram-positive anaerobes:
Bifidobacterium spp.
Clostridium spp.
Eubacterium spp.
Peptococcus spp.
Peptostreptococcus spp.
Propionibacterium spp.
Gram-negative anaerobes:
Bacteroides spp., including *B. fragilis*
Fusobacterium spp.
The following *in vitro* data are available, **but their clinical significance is unknown**.
Imipenem exhibits *in vitro* minimum inhibitory concentrations (MICs) of 4 µg/mL or less against most (≥90%) strains of the following microorganisms; however, the safety and effectiveness of imipenem in treating clinical infections due to these microorganisms have not been established in adequate and well-controlled clinical trials.
Gram-positive aerobes:
Bacillus spp.
Listeria monocytogenes
Nocardia spp.
Staphylococcus saprophyticus
Group C streptococci
Group G streptococci
Viridans group streptococci
Gram-negative aerobes:
Aeromonas hydrophila
Alcaligenes spp.
Capnocytophaga spp.
Haemophilus ducreyi
Neisseria gonorrhoeae including penicillinase-producing strains
Pasteurella spp.
Providencia stuartii
Gram-negative anaerobes:
*Prevotella bivia**
Prevotella disiens
Prevotella melaninogenica
Veillonella spp.
In vitro tests show imipenem to act synergistically with aminoglycoside antibiotics against some isolates of *Pseudomonas aeruginosa*.
Susceptibility Tests:
Measurement of MIC or minimum bactericidal concentration (MBC) and achieved antimicrobial compound concentrations may be appropriate to guide therapy in some infections. (See **CLINICAL PHARMACOLOGY** section for further information on drug concentrations achieved in infected body sites and other pharmacokinetic properties of this antimicrobial drug product.)
Dilution Techniques:
Quantitative methods that are used to determine MICs provide reproducible estimates of the susceptibility of bacteria to antimicrobial compounds. One such procedure uses a standardized dilution method[1] (broth, agar, or microdilution) or equivalent with imipenem powder.
The MIC values obtained should be interpreted according to the following criteria:

MIC (µg/mL)	Interpretation
≤4	Susceptible (S)
8	Intermediate (I)
≥16	Resistant (R)

A report of "Susceptible" indicates that the pathogen is likely to be inhibited by usually achievable concentrations of the antimicrobial compound in blood. A report of "Intermediate" indicates that the result should be considered equivocal, and, if the microorganism is not fully susceptible to alternative, clinically feasible drugs, the test should be repeated. This category implies possible clinical applicability in body sites where the drug is physiologically concentrated or in situations where high dosage of drug can be used. This category also provides a buffer zone that prevents small uncontrolled technical factors from causing major discrepancies in interpretation. A report of "Resistant" indicates that usually achievable concentrations of the antimicrobial compound in the blood are unlikely to be inhibitory and that other therapy should be selected.
Standardized susceptibility test procedures require the use of laboratory control microorganisms. Standard imipenem powder should provide the following MIC values:

Microorganism	MIC (µg/mL)
E. coli ATCC 25922	0.06–0.25
S. aureus ATCC 29213	0.015–0.06
E. faecalis ATCC 29212	0.5–2.0
P. aeruginosa ATCC 27853	1.0–4.0

Diffusion Techniques:
Quantitative methods that require measurement of zone diameters provide reproducible estimates of the susceptibility of bacteria to antimicrobial compounds. One such standardized procedure[2] that has been recommended for use with disks to test the susceptibility of microorganisms to imipenem uses the 10-µg imipenem disk. Interpretation involves correlation of the diameter obtained in the disk test with the MIC for imipenem.
Reports from the laboratory providing results of the standard single-disk susceptibility test with a 10-µg imipenem disk should be interpreted according to the following criteria:

Zone Diameter (mm)	Interpretation
≥16	Susceptible (S)
14–15	Intermediate (I)
≤13	Resistant (R)

Interpretation should be as stated above for results using dilution techniques.
Standardized susceptibility test procedures require the use of laboratory control microorganisms. The 10-µg imipenem disk should provide the following diameters in these laboratory test quality control strains:

Microorganism	Zone Diameter (mm)
E. coli ATCC 25922	26–32
P. aeruginosa ATCC 27853	20–28

Anaerobic Techniques:
For anaerobic bacteria, the susceptibility to imipenem can be determined by the reference agar dilution method or by alternate standardized test methods.[3]
The MIC values obtained should be interpreted according to the following criteria:

MIC (µg/mL)	Interpretation
≤4	Susceptible (S)
8	Intermediate (I)
≥16	Resistant (R)

Tissue or Fluid	N	Imipenem Level µg/mL or µg/g	Range
Vitreous Humor	3	3.4 (3.5 hours post dose)	2.88–3.6
Aqueous Humor	5	2.99 (2 hours post dose)	2.4–3.9
Lung Tissue	8	5.6 (median)	3.5–15.5
Sputum	1	2.1	—
Pleural	1	22.0	—
Peritoneal	12	23.9 S.D.±5.3 (2 hours post dose)	—
Bile	2	5.3 (2.25 hours post dose)	4.6–6.0
CSF (uninflamed)	5	1.0 (4 hours post dose)	0.26–2.0
CSF (inflamed)	7	2.6 (2 hours post dose)	0.5–5.5
Fallopian Tubes	1	13.6	—
Endometrium	1	11.1	—
Myometrium	1	5.0	—
Bone	10	2.6	0.4–5.4
Interstitial Fluid		16.4	10.0–22.6
Skin	12	4.4	NA
Fascia	12	4.4	NA

As with other susceptibility techniques, the use of laboratory control microorganisms is required. Standard imipenem powder should provide the following MIC values: Reference Agar Dilution Testing:

Microorganism	MIC (µg/mL)
B. fragilis ATCC 25285	0.03–0.12
B. thetaiotaomicron ATCC 29741	0.06–0.25
E. lentum ATCC 43055	0.25–1.0

Broth Microdilution Testing:

Microorganism	MIC (µg/mL)
B. thetaiotaomicron ATCC 29741	0.06–0.25
E. lentum ATCC 43055	0.12–0.5

INDICATIONS AND USAGE

PRIMAXIN I.V. is indicated for the treatment of serious infections caused by susceptible strains of the designated microorganisms in the conditions listed below:

1. **Lower respiratory tract infections**. *Staphylococcus aureus* (penicillinase-producing strains), *Acinetobacter* species, *Enterobacter* species, *Escherichia coli*, *Haemophilus influenzae*, *Haemophilus parainfluenzae**, *Klebsiella* species, *Serratia marcescens*

2. **Urinary tract infections** (complicated and uncomplicated). *Enterococcus faecalis*, *Staphylococcus aureus* (penicillinase-producing strains)*, *Enterobacter* species, *Escherichia coli*, *Klebsiella* species, *Morganella morganii**, *Proteus vulgaris**, *Providencia rettgeri**, *Pseudomonas aeruginosa*

3. **Intra-abdominal infections**. *Enterococcus faecalis*, *Staphylococcus aureus* (penicillinase-producing strains)*, *Staphylococcus epidermidis*, *Citrobacter* species, *Enterobacter* species, *Escherichia coli*, *Klebsiella* species, *Morganella morganii**, *Proteus* species, *Pseudomonas aeruginosa*, *Bifidobacterium* species, *Clostridium* species, *Eubacterium* species, *Peptococcus* species, *Peptostreptococcus* species, *Propionibacterium* species*, *Bacteroides* species including *B. fragilis*, *Fusobacterium* species

4. **Gynecologic infections**. *Enterococcus faecalis*, *Staphylococcus aureus* (penicillinase-producing strains)*, *Staphylococcus epidermidis*, *Streptococcus agalactiae* (Group B streptococci), *Enterobacter* species*, *Escherichia coli*, *Gardnerella vaginalis*, *Klebsiella* species*, *Proteus* species, *Bifidobacterium* species*, *Peptococcus* species*, *Peptostreptococcus* species, *Propionibacterium* species*, *Bacteroides* species including *B. fragilis**

5. **Bacterial septicemia**. *Enterococcus faecalis*, *Staphylococcus aureus* (penicillinase-producing strains), *Enterobacter* species, *Escherichia coli*, *Klebsiella* species, *Pseudomonas aeruginosa*, *Serratia* species*, *Bacteroides* species including *B. fragilis**

6. **Bone and joint infections**. *Enterococcus faecalis*, *Staphylococcus aureus* (penicillinase-producing strains), *Staphylococcus epidermidis*, *Enterobacter* species, *Pseudomonas aeruginosa*

7. **Skin and skin structure infections**. *Enterococcus faecalis*, *Staphylococcus aureus* (penicillinase-producing strains), *Staphylococcus epidermidis*, *Acinetobacter* species, *Citrobacter* species, *Enterobacter* species, *Escherichia coli*, *Klebsiella* species, *Morganella morganii*, *Proteus vulgaris*, *Providencia rettgeri**, *Pseudomonas aeruginosa*,

Serratia species, *Peptococcus* species, *Peptostreptococcus* species, *Bacteroides* species including *B. fragilis, Fusobacterium* species*

8. **Endocarditis.** *Staphylococcus aureus* (penicillinase-producing strains)

9. **Polymicrobic infections.** PRIMAXIN I.V. is indicated for polymicrobic infections including those in which *S. pneumoniae* (pneumonia, septicemia), *S. pyogenes* (skin and skin structure), or nonpenicillinase-producing *S. aureus* is one of the causative organisms. However, monobacterial infections due to these organisms are usually treated with narrower spectrum antibiotics, such as penicillin G. PRIMAXIN I.V. is not indicated in patients with meningitis because safety and efficacy have not been established.

For Pediatric Use information, see **PRECAUTIONS,** *Pediatric Use*, and **DOSAGE AND ADMINISTRATION** sections.

Because of its broad spectrum of bactericidal activity against gram-positive and gram-negative aerobic and anaerobic bacteria, PRIMAXIN I.V. is useful for the treatment of mixed infections and as presumptive therapy prior to the identification of the causative organisms.

Although clinical improvement has been observed in patients with cystic fibrosis, chronic pulmonary disease, and lower respiratory tract infections caused by *Pseudomonas aeruginosa*, bacterial eradication may not necessarily be achieved.

As with other beta-lactam antibiotics, some strains of *Pseudomonas aeruginosa* may develop resistance fairly rapidly during treatment with PRIMAXIN I.V. During therapy of *Pseudomonas aeruginosa* infections, periodic susceptibility testing should be done when clinically appropriate.

Infections resistant to other antibiotics, for example, cephalosporins, penicillin, and aminoglycosides, have been shown to respond to treatment with PRIMAXIN I.V.

To reduce the development of drug-resistant bacteria and maintain the effectiveness of PRIMAXIN I.V. and other antibacterial drugs, PRIMAXIN I.V. should be used only to treat or prevent infections that are proven or strongly suspected to be caused by susceptible bacteria. When culture and susceptibility information are available, they should be considered in selecting or modifying antibacterial therapy. In the absence of such data, local epidemiology and susceptibility patterns may contribute to the empiric selection of therapy.

---

* Efficacy for this organism in this organ system was studied in fewer than 10 infections.

CONTRAINDICATIONS

PRIMAXIN I.V. is contraindicated in patients who have shown hypersensitivity to any component of this product.

WARNINGS

SERIOUS AND OCCASIONALLY FATAL HYPERSENSITIVITY (ANAPHYLACTIC) REACTIONS HAVE BEEN REPORTED IN PATIENTS RECEIVING THERAPY WITH BETA-LACTAMS. THESE REACTIONS ARE MORE APT TO OCCUR IN PERSONS WITH A HISTORY OF SENSITIVITY TO MULTIPLE ALLERGENS.

THERE HAVE BEEN REPORTS OF PATIENTS WITH A HISTORY OF PENICILLIN HYPERSENSITIVITY WHO HAVE EXPERIENCED SEVERE HYPERSENSITIVITY REACTIONS WHEN TREATED WITH ANOTHER BETA-LACTAM. BEFORE INITIATING THERAPY WITH PRIMAXIN I.V., CAREFUL INQUIRY SHOULD BE MADE CONCERNING PREVIOUS HYPERSENSITIVITY REACTIONS TO PENICILLINS, CEPHALOSPORINS, OTHER BETA-LACTAMS, AND OTHER ALLERGENS. IF AN ALLERGIC REACTION OCCURS, PRIMAXIN SHOULD BE DISCONTINUED.

SERIOUS ANAPHYLACTIC REACTIONS REQUIRE IMMEDIATE EMERGENCY TREATMENT WITH EPINEPHRINE. OXYGEN, INTRAVENOUS STEROIDS, AND AIRWAY MANAGEMENT, INCLUDING INTUBATION, MAY ALSO BE ADMINISTERED AS INDICATED.

Seizure Potential

Seizures and other CNS adverse experiences, such as confusional states and myoclonic activity, have been reported during treatment with PRIMAXIN I.V. (See **PRECAUTIONS and ADVERSE REACTIONS.**)

Case reports in the literature have shown that co-administration of carbapenems, including imipenem, to patients receiving valproic acid or divalproex sodium results in a reduction in valproic acid concentrations. The valproic acid concentrations may drop below the therapeutic range as a result of this interaction, therefore increasing the risk of breakthrough seizures. Increasing the dose of valproic acid or divalproex sodium may not be sufficient to overcome this interaction. The concomitant use of imipenem and valproic acid/divalproex sodium is generally not recommended. Anti-bacterials other than carbapenems should be considered to treat infections in patients whose seizures are well controlled on valproic acid or divalproex sodium. If admin-

istration of PRIMAXIN I.V. is necessary, supplemental anticonvulsant therapy should be considered (see **PRECAUTIONS,** *Drug Interactions*).

Clostridium difficile associated diarrhea (CDAD) has been reported with use of nearly all antibacterial agents, including PRIMAXIN I.V., and may range in severity from mild diarrhea to fatal colitis. Treatment with antibacterial agents alters the normal flora of the colon leading to overgrowth of *C. difficile*.

C. difficile produces toxins A and B which contribute to the development of CDAD.

Hypertoxin producing strains of *C. difficile* cause increased morbidity and mortality, as these infections can be refractory to antimicrobial therapy and may require colectomy. CDAD must be considered in all patients who present with diarrhea following antibiotic use. Careful medical history is necessary since CDAD has been reported to occur over two months after the administration of antibacterial agents.

If CDAD is suspected or confirmed, ongoing antibiotic use not directed against *C. difficile* may need to be discontinued. Appropriate fluid and electrolyte management, protein supplementation, antibiotic treatment of *C. difficile*, and surgical evaluation should be instituted as clinically indicated.

PRECAUTIONS

General

CNS adverse experiences such as confusional states, myoclonic activity, and seizures have been reported during treatment with PRIMAXIN I.V., especially when recommended dosages were exceeded. These experiences have occurred most commonly in patients with CNS disorders (e.g., brain lesions or history of seizures) and/or compromised renal function. However, there have been reports of CNS adverse experiences in patients who had no recognized or documented underlying CNS disorder or compromised renal function.

When recommended doses were exceeded, adult patients with creatinine clearances of ≤20 mL/min/1.73 m², whether or not undergoing hemodialysis, had a higher risk of seizure activity than those without impairment of renal function. Therefore, close adherence to the dosing guidelines for these patients is recommended. (See **DOSAGE AND ADMINISTRATION.**)

Patients with creatinine clearances of ≤5 mL/min/1.73 m² should not receive PRIMAXIN I.V. unless hemodialysis is instituted within 48 hours.

For patients on hemodialysis, PRIMAXIN I.V. is recommended only when the benefit outweighs the potential risk of seizures.

Close adherence to the recommended dosage and dosage schedules is urged, especially in patients with known factors that predispose to convulsive activity. Anticonvulsant therapy should be continued in patients with known seizure disorders. If focal tremors, myoclonus, or seizures occur, patients should be evaluated neurologically, placed on anticonvulsant therapy if not already instituted, and the dosage of PRIMAXIN I.V. re-examined to determine whether it should be decreased or the antibiotic discontinued.

As with other antibiotics, prolonged use of PRIMAXIN I.V. may result in overgrowth of nonsusceptible organisms. Repeated evaluation of the patient's condition is essential. If superinfection occurs during therapy, appropriate measures should be taken.

Prescribing PRIMAXIN I.V. in the absence of a proven or strongly suspected bacterial infection or a prophylactic indication is unlikely to provide benefit to the patient and increases the risk of the development of drug-resistant bacteria.

Information for Patients

Patients should be counseled to inform their physician if they are taking valproic acid or divalproex sodium. Valproic acid concentrations in the blood may drop below the therapeutic range upon co-administration with PRIMAXIN I.V. If treatment with PRIMAXIN I.V. is necessary and continued, alternative or supplemental anti-convulsant medication to prevent and/or treat seizures may be needed.

Patients should be counseled that antibacterial drugs including PRIMAXIN I.V. should only be used to treat bacterial infections. They do not treat viral infections (e.g., the common cold). When PRIMAXIN I.V. is prescribed to treat a bacterial infection, patients should be told that although it is common to feel better early in the course of therapy, the medication should be taken exactly as directed. Skipping doses or not completing the full course of therapy may (1) decrease the effectiveness of the immediate treatment and (2) increase the likelihood that bacteria will develop resistance and will not be treatable by PRIMAXIN I.V. or other antibacterial drugs in the future.

Diarrhea is a common problem caused by antibiotics, which usually ends when the antibiotic is discontinued. Sometimes after starting treatment with antibiotics, patients can develop watery and bloody stools (with or without stomach cramps and fever) even as late as two or more months after

having taken the last dose of the antibiotic. If this occurs, patients should contact their physician as soon as possible.

Laboratory Tests

While PRIMAXIN I.V. possesses the characteristic low toxicity of the beta-lactam group of antibiotics, periodic assessment of organ system functions, including renal, hepatic, and hematopoietic, is advisable during prolonged therapy.

Drug Interactions

Generalized seizures have been reported in patients who received ganciclovir and PRIMAXIN. These drugs should not be used concomitantly unless the potential benefits outweigh the risks.

Since concomitant administration of PRIMAXIN and probenecid results in only minimal increases in plasma levels of imipenem and plasma half-life, it is not recommended that probenecid be given with PRIMAXIN.

PRIMAXIN should not be mixed with or physically added to other antibiotics. However, PRIMAXIN may be administered concomitantly with other antibiotics, such as aminoglycosides.

Case reports in the literature have shown that co-administration of carbapenems, including imipenem, to patients receiving valproic acid or divalproex sodium results in a reduction in valproic acid concentrations. The valproic acid concentrations may drop below the therapeutic range as a result of this interaction, therefore increasing the risk of breakthrough seizures. Although the mechanism of this interaction is unknown, data from *in vitro* and animal studies suggest that carbapenems may inhibit the hydrolysis of valproic acid's glucuronide metabolite (VPA-g) back to valproic acid, thus decreasing the serum concentrations of valproic acid (see **WARNINGS,** *Seizure Potential*).

Carcinogenesis, Mutagenesis, Impairment of Fertility

Long term studies in animals have not been performed to evaluate carcinogenic potential of imipenem-cilastatin. Genetic toxicity studies were performed in a variety of bacterial and mammalian tests *in vivo* and *in vitro*. The tests used were: V79 mammalian cell mutagenesis assay (imipenem-cilastatin sodium alone and imipenem alone), Ames test (cilastatin sodium alone and imipenem alone), unscheduled DNA synthesis assay (imipenem-cilastatin sodium) and *in vivo* mouse cytogenetics test (imipenem-cilastatin sodium). None of these tests showed any evidence of genetic alterations.

Reproductive tests in male and female rats were performed with imipenem-cilastatin sodium at intravenous doses up to 80 mg/kg/day and at a subcutaneous dose of 320 mg/kg/day, approximately equal to the highest recommended human dose of the intravenous formulation (on a mg/m² body surface area basis). Slight decreases in live fetal body weight were restricted to the highest dosage level. No other adverse effects were observed on fertility, reproductive performance, fetal viability, growth or postnatal development of pups.

Pregnancy: Teratogenic Effects

Pregnancy Category C: Teratology studies with cilastatin sodium at doses of 30, 100, and 300 mg/kg/day administered intravenously to rabbits and 40, 200, and 1000 mg/kg/day administered subcutaneously to rats, up to approximately 1.9 and 3.2 times[††] the maximum recommended daily human dose (on a mg/m² body surface area basis) of the intravenous formulation of imipenem-cilastatin sodium (50 mg/kg/day) in the two species, respectively, showed no evidence of adverse effect on the fetus. No evidence of teratogenicity was observed in rabbits given imipenem at intravenous doses of 15, 30 or 60 mg/kg/day and rats given imipenem at intravenous doses of 225, 450, or 900 mg/kg/day, up to approximately 0.4 and 2.9 times[††] the maximum recommended daily human dose (on a mg/m² body surface area basis) in the two species, respectively.

Teratology studies with imipenem-cilastatin sodium at intravenous doses of 20 and 80, and a subcutaneous dose of 320 mg/kg/day, up to 0.5 times[††] (mice) to approximately equal to (rats) the highest recommended daily intravenous human dose (on a mg/m² body surface area basis) in pregnant rodents during the period of major organogenesis, revealed no evidence of teratogenicity.

Imipenem-cilastatin sodium, when administered subcutaneously to pregnant rabbits at dosages equivalent to the usual human dose of the intravenous formulation and higher (1000-4000 mg/day), caused body weight loss, diarrhea, and maternal deaths. When comparable doses of imipenem-cilastatin sodium were given to non-pregnant rabbits, body weight loss, diarrhea, and deaths were also observed. This intolerance is not unlike that seen with other beta-lactam antibiotics in this species and is probably due to alteration of gut flora.

A teratology study in pregnant cynomolgus monkeys given imipenem-cilastatin sodium at doses of 40 mg/kg/day (bolus intravenous injection) or 160 mg/kg/day (subcutaneous injection) resulted in maternal toxicity including emesis, inappetence, body weight loss, diarrhea, abortion, and death in some cases. In contrast, no significant toxicity was observed when non-pregnant cynomolgus monkeys were given doses of imipenem-cilastatin sodium up to 180 mg/kg/day

Patients (≥3 Months of Age) With Normal Pretherapy but Abnormal During Therapy Laboratory Values

Laboratory Parameter	Abnormality			No. of Patients With Abnormalities/No. of Patients With Lab Done (%)
Hemoglobin	Age	<5 mos.:	<10 gm %	19/129 (14.7)
		6 mos.–12 yrs.:	<11.5 gm %	
Hematocrit	Age	<5 mos.:	<30 vol %	23/129 (17.8)
		6 mos.–12 yrs.:	<34.5 vol %	
Neutrophils	≤1000/mm^3 (absolute)			4/123 (3.3)
Eosinophils	≥7%			15/117 (12.8)
Platelet Count	≥500 ths/mm^3			16/119 (13.4)
Urine Protein	≥1			8/97 (8.2)
Serum Creatinine	>1.2 mg/dL			0/105 (0)
BUN	>22 mg/dL			0/108 (0)
AST (SGOT)	>36 IU/L			14/78 (17.9)
ALT (SGPT)	>30 IU/L			10/93 (10.8)

(subcutaneous injection). When doses of imipenem-cilastatin sodium (approximately 100 mg/kg/day or approximately 0.6 times[††] the maximum recommended daily human dose of the intravenous formulation) were administered to pregnant cynomolgus monkeys at an intravenous infusion rate which mimics human clinical use, there was minimal maternal intolerance (occasional emesis), no maternal deaths, no evidence of teratogenicity, but an increase in embryonic loss relative to control groups.

No adverse effects on the fetus or on lactation were observed when imipenem-cilastatin sodium was administered subcutaneously to rats late in gestation at dosages up to 320 mg/kg/day, approximately equal to the highest recommended human dose (on a mg/m^2 body surface area basis).

There are, however, no adequate and well-controlled studies in pregnant women. PRIMAXIN I.V. should be used during pregnancy only if the potential benefit justifies the potential risk to the mother and fetus.

[††] Based on patient body surface area of 1.6 m^2 (weight of 60 kg).

Nursing Mothers

It is not known whether imipenem-cilastatin sodium is excreted in human milk. Because many drugs are excreted in human milk, caution should be exercised when PRIMAXIN I.V. is administered to a nursing woman.

Pediatric Use

Use of PRIMAXIN I.V. in pediatric patients, neonates to 16 years of age, is supported by evidence from adequate and well-controlled studies of PRIMAXIN I.V. in adults and by the following clinical studies and published literature in pediatric patients: Based on published studies of 178** pediatric patients ≥3 months of age (with non-CNS infections), the recommended dose of PRIMAXIN I.V. is 15-25 mg/kg/dose administered every six hours. Doses of 25 mg/kg/dose in patients 3 months to <3 years of age, and 15 mg/kg/dose in patients 3-12 years of age were associated with mean trough plasma concentrations of imipenem of 1.1±0.4 μg/mL and 0.6±0.2 μg/mL following multiple 60-minute infusions, respectively; trough urinary concentrations of imipenem were in excess of 10 μg/mL for both doses. These doses have provided adequate plasma and urine concentrations for the treatment of non-CNS infections. Based on studies in adults, the maximum daily dose for treatment of infections with fully susceptible organisms is 2.0 g per day, and of infections with moderately susceptible organisms (primarily some strains of *P. aeruginosa*) is 4.0 g/day. (See Table 1, **DOSAGE AND ADMINISTRATION**.) Higher doses (up to 90 mg/kg/day in older children) have been used in patients with cystic fibrosis. (See **DOSAGE AND ADMINISTRATION**.)

Based on studies of 135*** pediatric patients ≤3 months of age (weighing ≥1,500 gms), the following dosage schedule is recommended for non-CNS infections:

<1 wk of age: 25 mg/kg every 12 hrs
1-4 wks of age: 25 mg/kg every 8 hrs
4 wks-3 mos. of age: 25 mg/kg every 6 hrs.

In a published dose-ranging study of smaller premature infants (670-1,890 gms) in the first week of life, a dose of 20 mg/kg q12h by 15-30 minutes infusion was associated with mean peak and trough plasma imipenem concentrations of 43 μg/mL and 1.7 μg/mL after multiple doses, respectively. However, moderate accumulation of cilastatin in neonates may occur following multiple doses of PRIMAXIN I.V. The safety of this accumulation is unknown.

PRIMAXIN I.V. is not recommended in pediatric patients with CNS infections because of the risk of seizures.

PRIMAXIN I.V. is not recommended in pediatric patients <30 kg with impaired renal function, as no data are available.

** Two patients were less than 3 months of age.
*** One patient was greater than 3 months of age.

Geriatric Use

Of the approximately 3600 subjects ≥18 years of age in clinical studies of PRIMAXIN I.V., including postmarketing studies, approximately 2800 received PRIMAXIN I.V. Of the subjects who received PRIMAXIN I.V., data are available on approximately 800 subjects who were 65 and over, including approximately 300 subjects who were 75 and over. No overall differences in safety or effectiveness were observed between these subjects and younger subjects. Other reported clinical experience has not identified differences in responses between the elderly and younger patients, but greater sensitivity of some older individuals cannot be ruled out.

This drug is known to be substantially excreted by the kidney, and the risk of toxic reactions to this drug may be greater in patients with impaired renal function. Because elderly patients are more likely to have decreased renal function, care should be taken in dose selection, and it may be useful to monitor renal function.

No dosage adjustment is required based on age (see **CLINICAL PHARMACOLOGY**, *Adults*). Dosage adjustment in the case of renal impairment is necessary (see **DOSAGE AND ADMINISTRATION**, *Reduced Intravenous Schedule for Adults with Impaired Renal Function and/or Body Weight <70 kg*):

ADVERSE REACTIONS

Adults

PRIMAXIN I.V. is generally well tolerated. Many of the 1,723 patients treated in clinical trials were severely ill and had multiple background diseases and physiological impairments, making it difficult to determine causal relationship of adverse experiences to therapy with PRIMAXIN I.V.

Local Adverse Reactions

Adverse local clinical reactions that were reported as possibly, probably, or definitely related to therapy with PRIMAXIN I.V. were:

Phlebitis/thrombophlebitis—3.1%
Pain at the injection site—0.7%
Erythema at the injection site—0.4%
Vein induration—0.2%
Infused vein infection—0.1%

Systemic Adverse Reactions

The most frequently reported systemic adverse clinical reactions that were reported as possibly, probably, or definitely related to PRIMAXIN I.V. were nausea (2.0%), diarrhea (1.8%), vomiting (1.5%), rash (0.9%), fever (0.5%), hypotension (0.4%), seizures (0.4%) (see **PRECAUTIONS**), dizziness (0.3%), pruritus (0.3%), urticaria (0.2%), somnolence (0.2%).

Additional adverse systemic clinical reactions reported as possibly, probably, or definitely drug related occurring in less than 0.2% of the patients or reported since the drug was marketed are listed within each body system in order of decreasing severity: *Gastrointestinal*—pseudomembranous colitis (the onset of pseudomembranous colitis symptoms may occur during or after antibacterial treatment, see **WARNINGS**), hemorrhagic colitis, hepatitis (including fulminant hepatitis), hepatic failure, jaundice, gastroenteritis, abdominal pain, glossitis, tongue papillar hypertrophy, staining of the teeth and/or tongue, heartburn, pharyngeal pain, increased salivation; *Hematologic*—pancytopenia, bone marrow depression, thrombocytopenia, neutropenia, leukopenia, hemolytic anemia; *CNS*—encephalopathy, tremor, confusion, myoclonus, paresthesia, vertigo, headache, psychic disturbances including hallucinations; *Special Senses*—hearing loss, tinnitus, taste perversion; *Respiratory*—chest discomfort, dyspnea, hyperventilation, thoracic spine pain; *Cardiovascular*—palpitations, tachycardia; *Skin*—Stevens-Johnson syndrome, toxic epidermal necrolysis, erythema multiforme, angioneurotic edema, flushing, cyanosis, hyperhidrosis, skin texture changes, candidiasis, pruritus vulvae; *Body as a whole*—polyarthralgia, asthenia/weakness, drug fever; *Renal*—acute renal failure, oliguria/anuria, polyuria, urine discoloration. The role of PRIMAXIN I.V. in changes in renal function is difficult to assess, since factors predisposing to pre-renal azotemia or to impaired renal function usually have been present.

Adverse Laboratory Changes

Adverse laboratory changes without regard to drug relationship that were reported during clinical trials or reported since the drug was marketed were:

Hepatic: Increased ALT (SGPT), AST (SGOT), alkaline phosphatase, bilirubin, and LDH

Hemic: Increased eosinophils, positive Coombs test, increased WBC, increased platelets, decreased hemoglobin and hematocrit, agranulocytosis, increased monocytes, abnormal prothrombin time, increased lymphocytes, increased basophils

Electrolytes: Decreased serum sodium, increased potassium, increased chloride

Renal: Increased BUN, creatinine

Urinalysis: Presence of urine protein, urine red blood cells, urine white blood cells, urine casts, urine bilirubin, and urine urobilinogen.

Pediatric Patients

In studies of 178 pediatric patients ≥3 months of age, the following adverse events were noted:

The Most Common Clinical Adverse Experiences Without Regard to Drug Relationship (Patient Incidence >1%)

Adverse Experience	No. of Patients (%)
Digestive System	
Diarrhea	7* (3.9)
Gastroenteritis	2 (1.1)
Vomiting	2* (1.1)
Skin	
Rash	4 (2.2)
Irritation, I.V. site	2 (1.1)
Urogenital System	
Urine discoloration	2 (1.1)
Cardiovascular System	
Phlebitis	4 (2.2)

* One patient had both vomiting and diarrhea and is counted in each category.

In studies of 135 patients (newborn to 3 months of age), the following adverse events were noted:

The Most Common Clinical Adverse Experiences Without Regard to Drug Relationship (Patient Incidence >1%)

Adverse Experience	No. of Patients (%)
Digestive System	
Diarrhea	4 (3.0%)
Oral Candidiasis	2 (1.5%)
Skin	
Rash	2 (1.5%)
Urogenital System	
Oliguria/anuria	3 (2.2%)
Cardiovascular System	
Tachycardia	2 (1.5%)
Nervous System	
Convulsions	8 (5.9%)

[See table above]

Patients (<3 Months of Age) With Normal Pretherapy but Abnormal During Therapy Laboratory Values

Laboratory Parameter	No. of Patients With Abnormalities* (%)
Eosinophil Count↑	11 (9.0%)
Hematocrit↓	3 (2.0%)
Hematocrit↑	1 (1.0%)
Platelet Count↑	5 (4.0%)
Platelet Count↓	2 (2.0%)
Serum Creatinine↑	5 (5.0%)
Bilirubin↑	3 (3.0%)
Bilirubin↓	1 (1.0%)
AST (SGOT)↑	5 (6.0%)
ALT (SGPT)↑	3 (3.0%)
Serum Alkaline Phosphate↑	2 (3.0%)

*The denominator used for percentages was the number of patients for whom the test was performed during or post-treatment and, therefore, varies by test.

Examination of published literature and spontaneous adverse event reports suggested a similar spectrum of adverse events in adult and pediatric patients.

TABLE I: INTRAVENOUS DOSAGE SCHEDULE FOR ADULTS WITH NORMAL RENAL FUNCTION AND BODY WEIGHT ≥70 kg

Type or Severity of Infection	A Fully susceptible organisms including gram-positive and gram-negative aerobes and anaerobes	B Moderately susceptible organisms, primarily some strains of *P. aeruginosa*
Mild	250 mg q6h (TOTAL DAILY DOSE = 1.0g)	500 mg q6h (TOTAL DAILY DOSE = 2.0g)
Moderate	500 mg q8h (TOTAL DAILY DOSE = 1.5g) or 500 mg q6h TOTAL DAILY DOSE = 2.0g)	500 mg q6h (TOTAL DAILY DOSE = 2.0g) or 1 g q8h (TOTAL DAILY DOSE = 3.0g)
Severe, life threatening only	500 mg q6h (TOTAL DAILY DOSE = 2.0g)	1 g q8h (TOTAL DAILY DOSE = 3.0g) or 1 g q6h (TOTAL DAILY DOSE = 4.0g)
Uncomplicated urinary tract infection	250 mg q6h (TOTAL DAILY DOSE = 1.0g)	250 mg q6h (TOTAL DAILY DOSE = 1.0g)
Complicated urinary tract infection	500 mg q6h (TOTAL DAILY DOSE = 2.0g)	500 mg q6h (TOTAL DAILY DOSE = 2.0g)

TABLE II: REDUCED INTRAVENOUS DOSAGE OF PRIMAXIN I.V. IN ADULT PATIENTS WITH IMPAIRED RENAL FUNCTION AND/OR BODY WEIGHT <70 kg

And Body Weight (kg) is:	1.0 g/day and creatinine clearance (mL/min/1.73m²) is:				1.5 g/day and creatinine clearance (mL/min/1.73m²) is:				2.0 g/day and creatinine clearance (mL/min/1.73m²) is:			
	≥71	41-70	21-40	6-20	≥71	41-70	21-40	6-20	≥71	41-70	21-40	6-20
	then the reduced dosage regimen (mg) is:				then the reduced dosage regimen (mg) is:				then the reduced dosage regimen (mg) is:			
≥70	250 q6h	250 q8h	250 q12h	250 q12h	500 q8h	250 q6h	250 q8h	250 q12h	500 q6h	500 q8h	250 q6h	250 q12h
60	250 q8h	125 q6h	250 q12h	125 q12h	250 q6h	250 q8h	250 q8h	250 q12h	500 q8h	250 q6h	250 q8h	250 q12h
50	125 q6h	125 q6h	125 q8h	125 q12h	250 q6h	250 q8h	250 q8h	250 q12h	250 q6h	250 q8h	250 q8h	250 q12h
40	125 q6h	125 q8h	125 q12h	125 q12h	250 q6h	125 q8h	125 q12h	125 q12h	250 q6h	250 q8h	250 q12h	250 q12h
30	125 q8h	125 q8h	125 q12h	125 q12h	125 q6h	125 q8h	125 q8h	125 q12h	250 q8h	125 q6h	125 q8h	125 q12h

TABLE III: REDUCED INTRAVENOUS DOSAGE OF PRIMAXIN I.V. IN ADULT PATIENTS WITH IMPAIRED RENAL FUNCTION AND/OR BODY WEIGHT <70 kg

And Body Weight (kg) is:	3.0 g/day and creatinine clearance (mL/min/1.73m²) is:				4.0 g/day and creatinine clearance (mL/min/1.73m²) is:			
	≥71	41-70	21-40	6-20	≥71	41-70	21-40	6-20
	then the reduced dosage regimen (mg) is:				then the reduced dosage regimen (mg) is:			
≥70	1000 q8h	500 q6h	500 q8h	500 q12h	1000 q6h	750 q8h	500 q6h	500 q12h
60	750 q8h	500 q8h	500 q8h	500 q12h	1000 q8h	750 q8h	500 q8h	500 q12h
50	500 q6h	500 q8h	250 q6h	250 q12h	750 q8h	500 q6h	500 q8h	500 q12h
40	500 q8h	250 q6h	250 q8h	250 q12h	500 q6h	500 q8h	250 q6h	250 q12h
30	250 q6h	250 q8h	250 q8h	250 q12h	500 q8h	250 q6h	250 q8h	250 q12h

OVERDOSAGE

The acute intravenous toxicity of imipenem-cilastatin sodium in a ratio of 1:1 was studied in mice at doses of 751 to 1359 mg/kg. Following drug administration, ataxia was rapidly produced and clonic convulsions were noted in about 45 minutes. Deaths occurred within 4-56 minutes at all doses. The acute intravenous toxicity of imipenem-cilastatin sodium was produced within 5-10 minutes in rats at doses of 771 to 1583 mg/kg. In all dosage groups, females had decreased activity, bradypnea, and ptosis with clonic convulsions preceding death; in males, ptosis was seen at all dose levels while tremors and clonic convulsions were seen at all but the lowest dose (771 mg/kg). In another rat study, female rats showed ataxia, bradypnea, and decreased activity in all but the lowest dose (550 mg/kg); deaths were preceded by clonic convulsions. Male rats showed tremors at all doses

and clonic convulsions and ptosis were seen at the two highest doses (1130 and 1734 mg/kg). Deaths occurred between 6 and 88 minutes with doses of 771 to 1734 mg/kg.

In the case of overdosage, discontinue PRIMAXIN I.V., treat symptomatically, and institute supportive measures as required. Imipenem-cilastatin sodium is hemodialyzable. However, usefulness of this procedure in the overdosage setting is questionable.

DOSAGE AND ADMINISTRATION

Adults

The dosage recommendations for PRIMAXIN I.V. represent the quantity of imipenem to be administered. An equivalent amount of cilastatin is also present in the solution. Each 125 mg, 250 mg, or 500 mg dose should be given by intravenous administration over 20 to 30 minutes. Each 750 mg or

1000 mg dose should be infused over 40 to 60 minutes. In patients who develop nausea during the infusion, the rate of infusion may be slowed.

The total daily dosage for PRIMAXIN I.V. should be based on the type or severity of infection and given in equally divided doses based on consideration of degree of susceptibility of the pathogen(s), renal function, and body weight. Adult patients with impaired renal function, as judged by creatinine clearance ≤70 mL/min/1.73 m², require adjustment of dosage as described in the succeeding section of these guidelines.

Intravenous Dosage Schedule for Adults with Normal Renal Function and Body Weight ≥70 kg

Doses cited in Table I are based on a patient with normal renal function and a body weight of 70 kg. These doses should be used for a patient with a creatinine clearance of ≥71 mL/min/1.73 m² and a body weight of ≥70 kg. A reduction in dose must be made for a patient with a creatinine clearance of ≤70 mL/min/1.73 m² and/or a body weight less than 70 kg. (See Tables II and III.)

Dosage regimens in column A of Table I are recommended for infections caused by fully susceptible organisms which represent the majority of pathogenic species. Dosage regimens in column B of Table I are recommended for infections caused by organisms with moderate susceptibility to imipenem, primarily some strains of *P. aeruginosa*.

[See table I at left]

Due to the high antimicrobial activity of PRIMAXIN I.V., it is recommended that the maximum total daily dosage not exceed 50 mg/kg/day or 4.0 g/day, whichever is lower. There is no evidence that higher doses provide greater efficacy. However, patients over twelve years of age with cystic fibrosis and normal renal function have been treated with PRIMAXIN I.V. at doses up to 90 mg/kg/day in divided doses, not exceeding 4.0 g/day.

Reduced Intravenous Schedule for Adults with Impaired Renal Function and/or Body Weight <70 kg

Patients with creatinine clearance of ≤70 mL/min/1.73 m² and/or body weight less than 70 kg require dosage reduction of PRIMAXIN I.V. as indicated in the tables below. Creatinine clearance may be calculated from serum creatinine concentration by the following equation:

$$T_{cc} \text{ (Males)} = \frac{(\text{wt. in kg}) (140 - \text{age})}{(72) (\text{creatinine in mg/dL})}$$

$$T_{cc} \text{ (Females)} = 0.85 \times \text{above value}$$

To determine the dose for adults with impaired renal function and/or reduced body weight:

1. Choose a total daily dose from Table I based on infection characteristics.
2. a) If the total daily dose is 1.0 g, 1.5 g, or 2.0 g, use the appropriate subsection of Table II and continue with step 3.

   b) If the total daily dose is 3.0 g or 4.0 g, use the appropriate subsection of Table III and continue with step 3.
3. From Table II or III:

   a) Select the body weight on the far left which is closest to the patient's body weight (kg).

   b) Select the patient's creatinine clearance category.

   c) Where the row and column intersect is the reduced dosage regimen.

[See table II at left]

[See table III at left]

Patients with creatinine clearances of 6 to 20 mL/min/1.73 m² should be treated with PRIMAXIN I.V. 125 mg or 250 mg every 12 hours for most pathogens. There may be an increased risk of seizures when doses of 500 mg every 12 hours are administered to these patients.

Patients with creatinine clearance ≤5 mL/min/1.73 m² should not receive PRIMAXIN I.V. unless hemodialysis is instituted within 48 hours. There is inadequate information to recommend usage of PRIMAXIN I.V. for patients undergoing peritoneal dialysis.

Hemodialysis

When treating patients with creatinine clearances of ≤5 mL/min/1.73 m² who are undergoing hemodialysis, use the dosage recommendations for patients with creatinine clearances of 6-20 mL/min/1.73 m². (See *Reduced Intravenous Dosage Schedule for Adults with Impaired Renal Function and/or Body Weight <70 kg*.) Both imipenem and cilastatin are cleared from the circulation during hemodialysis. The patient should receive PRIMAXIN I.V. after hemodialysis and at 12 hour intervals timed from the end of that hemodialysis session. Dialysis patients, especially those with background CNS disease, should be carefully monitored; for patients on hemodialysis, PRIMAXIN I.V. is recommended only when the benefit outweighs the potential risk of seizures. (See **PRECAUTIONS**.)

Pediatric Patients

See **PRECAUTIONS**, *Pediatric Patients*.

For pediatric patients ≥3 months of age, the recommended dose for non-CNS infections is 15-25 mg/kg/dose administered every six hours. Based on studies in adults, the maximum daily dose for treatment of infections with fully susceptible organisms is 2.0 g per day, and of infections with moderately susceptible organisms (primarily some strains of *P. aeruginosa*) is 4.0 g/day. Higher doses (up to 90 mg/kg/day in older children) have been used in patients with cystic fibrosis.

For pediatric patients ≤3 months of age (weighing ≥1,500 gms), the following dosage schedule is recommended for non-CNS infections:

<1 wk of age: 25 mg/kg every 12 hrs
1-4 wks of age: 25 mg/kg every 8 hrs
4 wks-3 mos. of age: 25 mg/kg every 6 hrs.

Doses less than or equal to 500 mg should be given by intravenous infusion over 15 to 30 minutes. Doses greater than 500 mg should be given by intravenous infusion over 40 to 60 minutes.

PRIMAXIN I.V. is not recommended in pediatric patients with CNS infections because of the risk of seizures.

PRIMAXIN I.V. is not recommended in pediatric patients <30 kg with impaired renal function, as no data are available.

PREPARATION OF SOLUTION

Vials

Contents of the vials must be suspended and transferred to 100 mL of an appropriate infusion solution.

A suggested procedure is to add approximately 10 mL from the appropriate infusion solution (see list of diluents under **COMPATIBILITY AND STABILITY**) to the vial. Shake well and transfer the resulting suspension to the infusion solution container.

Benzyl alcohol as a preservative has been associated with toxicity in neonates. While toxicity has not been demonstrated in pediatric patients greater than three months of age, small pediatric patients in this age range may also be at risk for benzyl alcohol toxicity. Therefore, diluents containing benzyl alcohol should not be used when PRIMAXIN I.V. is constituted for administration to pediatric patients in this age range.

CAUTION: THE SUSPENSION IS NOT FOR DIRECT INFUSION.

Repeat with an additional 10 mL of infusion solution to ensure complete transfer of vial contents to the infusion solution. **The resulting mixture should be agitated until clear.**

ADD-Vantage®††† Vials

See separate INSTRUCTIONS FOR USE OF 'PRIMAXIN I.V.' IN ADD-Vantage® VIALS. PRIMAXIN I.V. in ADD-Vantage® vials should be reconstituted with ADD-Vantage® diluent containers containing 100 mL of either 0.9% Sodium Chloride Injection or 100 mL 5% Dextrose Injection.

††† Registered trademark of Abbott Laboratories, Inc.

COMPATIBILITY AND STABILITY

Before Reconstitution:

The dry powder should be stored at a temperature below 25°C (77°F).

Reconstituted Solutions:

Solutions of PRIMAXIN I.V. range from colorless to yellow. Variations of color within this range do not affect the potency of the product

Vials

PRIMAXIN I.V., as supplied in single use vials and reconstituted with the following diluents (see **PREPARATION OF SOLUTION**), maintains satisfactory potency for 4 hours at room temperature or for 24 hours under refrigeration (5°C). Solutions of PRIMAXIN I.V. should not be frozen.

0.9% Sodium Chloride Injection
5% or 10% Dextrose Injection
5% Dextrose and 0.9% Sodium Chloride Injection
5% Dextrose Injection with 0.225% or 0.45% saline solution
5% Dextrose Injection with 0.15% potassium chloride solution
Mannitol 5% and 10%

ADD-Vantage® vials

PRIMAXIN I.V., as supplied in single dose ADD–Vantage® vials and reconstituted with the following diluents (see **PREPARATION OF SOLUTION**), maintains satisfactory potency for 4 hours at room temperature.

0.9% Sodium Chloride Injection
5% Dextrose Injection

PRIMAXIN I.V. should not be mixed with or physically added to other antibiotics. However, PRIMAXIN I.V. may be administered concomitantly with other antibiotics, such as aminoglycosides.

HOW SUPPLIED

PRIMAXIN I.V. is supplied as a sterile powder mixture in single dose containers including vials and ADD-Vantage® vials containing imipenem (anhydrous equivalent) and cilastatin sodium as follows:

No. 3514—250 mg imipenem equivalent and 250 mg cilastatin equivalent and 10 mg sodium bicarbonate as a buffer
NDC 0006-3514-58 in trays of 25 vials.

No. 3516—500 mg imipenem equivalent and 500 mg cilastatin equivalent and 20 mg sodium bicarbonate as a buffer
NDC 0006-3516-59 in trays of 25 vials.

No. 3551—250 mg imipenem equivalent and 250 mg cilastatin equivalent and 10 mg sodium bicarbonate as a buffer
NDC 0006-3551-58 in trays of 25 ADD-Vantage® vials.

No. 3552—500 mg imipenem equivalent and 500 mg cilastatin equivalent and 20 mg sodium bicarbonate as a buffer
NDC 0006-3552-59 in trays of 25 ADD-Vantage® vials.

REFERENCES

1. National Committee for Clinical Laboratory Standards, Methods for Dilution Antimicrobial Susceptibility Tests for Bacteria that Grow Aerobically-Fourth Edition. Approved Standard NCCLS Document M7-A4, Vol. 17, No. 2 NCCLS, Villanova, PA, 1997.
2. National Committee for Clinical Laboratory Standards, Performance Standards for Antimicrobial Disk Susceptibility Tests-Sixth Edition. Approved Standard NCCLS Document M2-A6, Vol. 17, No. 1 NCCLS, Villanova, PA, 1997.
3. National Committee for Clinical Laboratory Standards, Method for Antimicrobial Susceptibility Testing of Anaerobic Bacteria-Third Edition. Approved Standard NCCLS Document M11-A3, Vol. 13, No. 26 NCCLS, Villanova, PA, 1993.

Merck Sharp & Dohme Corp., a subsidiary of
MERCK & CO., INC., Whitehouse Station, NJ 08889, USA
Issued February 2010
9813936

PRINIVIL® TABLETS ℞

[pri-ni-vil]
(lisinopril)

USE IN PREGNANCY

When used in pregnancy during the second and third trimesters, ACE inhibitors can cause injury and even death to the developing fetus. When pregnancy is detected, PRINIVIL should be discontinued as soon as possible. See WARNINGS, Fetal/Neonatal Morbidity and Mortality.

DESCRIPTION

PRINIVIL[1] (Lisinopril), a synthetic peptide derivative, is an oral long-acting angiotensin converting enzyme inhibitor. Lisinopril is chemically described as (*S*)-1-[*N*^{2}-(1-carboxy-3-phenylpropyl)-L-lysyl]-L-proline dihydrate. Its empirical formula is $C_{21}H_{31}N_3O_5 \cdot 2H_2O$ and its structural formula is:

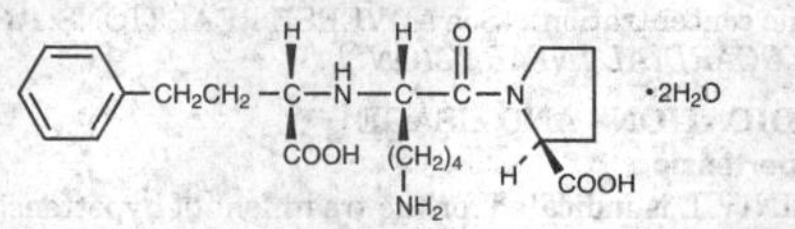

Lisinopril is a white to off-white, crystalline powder, with a molecular weight of 441.52. It is soluble in water and sparingly soluble in methanol and practically insoluble in ethanol.

PRINIVIL is supplied as 5 mg, 10 mg, and 20 mg tablets for oral administration. In addition to the active ingredient lisinopril, each tablet contains the following inactive ingredients: calcium phosphate, mannitol, magnesium stearate, and starch. The 10 mg and 20 mg tablets also contain iron oxide.

[1] Registered trademark of Merck Sharp & Dohme Corp., a subsidiary of **Merck & Co., Inc.**

Copyright © 1988, 1989, 1992, 1993, 1995, 2005, 2006 Merck Sharp & Dohme Corp., a subsidiary of **Merck & Co., Inc.**
All rights reserved

CLINICAL PHARMACOLOGY

Mechanism of Action

Lisinopril inhibits angiotensin converting enzyme (ACE) in human subjects and animals. ACE is a peptidyl dipeptidase that catalyzes the conversion of angiotensin I to the vasoconstrictor substance, angiotensin II. Angiotensin II also stimulates aldosterone secretion by the adrenal cortex. The beneficial effects of lisinopril in hypertension and heart failure appear to result primarily from suppression of the renin-angiotensin-aldosterone system. Inhibition of ACE results in decreased plasma angiotensin II which leads to decreased vasopressor activity and to decreased aldosterone secretion. The latter decrease may result in a small increase of serum potassium. In hypertensive patients with normal renal function treated with PRINIVIL alone for up to 24 weeks, the mean increase in serum potassium was approximately 0.1 mEq/L; however, approximately 15 percent of patients had increases greater than 0.5 mEq/L and approximately six percent had a decrease greater than 0.5 mEq/L. In the same study, patients treated with PRINIVIL and hydrochlorothiazide for up to 24 weeks had a mean decrease in serum potassium of 0.1 mEq/L; approximately 4 percent of patients had increases greater than 0.5 mEq/L and approximately 12 percent had a decrease greater than 0.5 mEq/L. (See PRECAUTIONS.) Removal of angiotensin II negative feedback on renin secretion leads to increased plasma renin activity.

ACE is identical to kininase, an enzyme that degrades bradykinin. Whether increased levels of bradykinin, a potent vasodepressor peptide, play a role in the therapeutic effects of PRINIVIL remains to be elucidated.

While the mechanism through which PRINIVIL lowers blood pressure is believed to be primarily suppression of the renin-angiotensin-aldosterone system, PRINIVIL is antihypertensive even in patients with low-renin hypertension. Although PRINIVIL was antihypertensive in all races studied, Black hypertensive patients (usually a low-renin hypertensive population) had a smaller average response to monotherapy than non-Black patients.

Concomitant administration of PRINIVIL and hydrochlorothiazide further reduced blood pressure in Black and non-Black patients and any racial difference in blood pressure response was no longer evident.

Pharmacokinetics and Metabolism

Adult Patients: Following oral administration of PRINIVIL, peak serum concentrations of lisinopril occur within about 7 hours, although there was a trend to a small delay in time taken to reach peak serum concentrations in acute myocardial infarction patients. Declining serum concentrations exhibit a prolonged terminal phase which does not contribute to drug accumulation. This terminal phase probably represents saturable binding to ACE and is not proportional to dose. Lisinopril does not appear to be bound to other serum proteins.

Lisinopril does not undergo metabolism and is excreted unchanged entirely in the urine. Based on urinary recovery, the mean extent of absorption of lisinopril is approximately 25 percent, with large inter-subject variability (6-60 percent) at all doses tested (5-80 mg). Lisinopril absorption is not influenced by the presence of food in the gastrointestinal tract. The absolute bioavailability of lisinopril is reduced to about 16 percent in patients with stable NYHA Class II-IV congestive heart failure, and the volume of distribution appears to be slightly smaller than that in normal subjects.

The oral bioavailability of lisinopril in patients with acute myocardial infarction is similar to that in healthy volunteers.

Upon multiple dosing, lisinopril exhibits an effective half-life of accumulation of 12 hours.

Impaired renal function decreases elimination of lisinopril, which is excreted principally through the kidneys, but this decrease becomes clinically important only when the glomerular filtration rate is below 30 mL/min. Above this glomerular filtration rate, the elimination half-life is little changed. With greater impairment, however, peak and trough lisinopril levels increase, time to peak concentration increases and time to attain steady state is prolonged. Older patients, on average, have (approximately doubled) higher blood levels and area under the plasma concentration time curve (AUC) than younger patients. (See DOSAGE AND ADMINISTRATION.) Lisinopril can be removed by hemodialysis.

Studies in rats indicate that lisinopril crosses the blood-brain barrier poorly. Multiple doses of lisinopril in rats do not result in accumulation in any tissues. Milk of lactating rats contains radioactivity following administration of ^{14}C lisinopril. By whole body autoradiography, radioactivity was found in the placenta following administration of labeled drug to pregnant rats, but none was found in the fetuses.

Pediatric Patients: The pharmacokinetics of lisinopril were studied in 29 pediatric hypertensive patients between 6 years and 16 years with glomerular filtration rate >30 mL/min/1.73 m^2. After doses of 0.1 to 0.2 mg/kg, steady state peak plasma concentrations of lisinopril occurred within 6 hours and the extent of absorption based on urinary recovery was about 28%. These values are similar to those obtained previously in adults. The typical value of lisinopril oral clearance (systemic clearance/absolute bioavailability) in a child weighing 30 kg is 10 L/h, which increases in proportion to renal function.

Pharmacodynamics and Clinical Effects

Hypertension:

Adult Patients: Administration of PRINIVIL to patients with hypertension results in a reduction of supine and standing blood pressure to about the same extent with no compensatory tachycardia. Symptomatic postural hypotension is usually not observed although it can occur and should be anticipated in volume and/or salt-depleted patients. (See WARNINGS.) When given together with thiazide-type diuretics, the blood pressure lowering effects of the two drugs are approximately additive.

In most patients studied, onset of antihypertensive activity was seen at one hour after oral administration of an individual dose of PRINIVIL, with peak reduction of blood pressure achieved by six hours. Although an antihypertensive effect was observed 24 hours after dosing with recommended single daily doses, the effect was more consistent and the mean effect was considerably larger in some studies with doses of 20 mg or more than with lower doses. However, at all doses studied, the mean antihypertensive effect was substantially smaller 24 hours after dosing than it was six hours after dosing.

In some patients achievement of optimal blood pressure reduction may require two to four weeks of therapy.

The antihypertensive effects of PRINIVIL are maintained during long-term therapy. Abrupt withdrawal of PRINIVIL has not been associated with a rapid increase in blood pressure or a significant increase in blood pressure compared to pretreatment levels.

Two dose-response studies utilizing a once daily regimen were conducted in 438 mild to moderate hypertensive patients not on a diuretic. Blood pressure was measured 24 hours after dosing. An antihypertensive effect of PRINIVIL was seen with 5 mg in some patients. However, in both studies blood pressure reduction occurred sooner and was greater in patients treated with 10, 20, or 80 mg of PRINIVIL. In controlled clinical studies, PRINIVIL 20-80 mg has been compared in patients with mild to moderate hypertension to hydrochlorothiazide 12.5-50 mg and with atenolol 50-500 mg; and in patients with moderate to severe hypertension to metoprolol 100-200 mg. It was superior to hydrochlorothiazide in effects on systolic and diastolic blood pressure in a population that was ¾ Caucasian. PRINIVIL was approximately equivalent to atenolol and metoprolol in effects on diastolic blood pressure and had somewhat greater effects on systolic blood pressure.

PRINIVIL had similar effectiveness and adverse effects in younger and older (>65 years) patients. It was less effective in Blacks than in Caucasians.

In hemodynamic studies in patients with essential hypertension, blood pressure reduction was accompanied by a reduction in peripheral arterial resistance with little or no change in cardiac output and in heart rate. In a study in nine hypertensive patients, following administration of PRINIVIL, there was an increase in mean renal blood flow that was not significant. Data from several small studies are inconsistent with respect to the effect of PRINIVIL on glomerular filtration rate in hypertensive patients with normal renal function, but suggest that changes, if any, are not large.

In patients with renovascular hypertension PRINIVIL has been shown to be well tolerated and effective in controlling blood pressure (see PRECAUTIONS).

Pediatric Patients: In a clinical study involving 115 hypertensive pediatric patients 6 to 16 years of age, patients who weighed <50 kg received either 0.625, 2.5, or 20 mg of lisinopril daily and patients who weighed ≥ 50 kg received either 1.25, 5, or 40 mg of lisinopril daily. At the end of 2 weeks, lisinopril administered once daily lowered trough blood pressure in a dose-dependent manner with consistent antihypertensive efficacy demonstrated at doses >1.25 mg (0.02 mg/kg). This effect was confirmed in a withdrawal phase, where the diastolic pressure rose by about 9 mmHg more in patients randomized to placebo than it did in patients who were randomized to remain on the middle and high doses of lisinopril. The dose-dependent antihypertensive effect of lisinopril was consistent across several demographic subgroups: age, Tanner stage, gender, race. In this study, lisinopril was generally well-tolerated.

In the above pediatric studies, lisinopril was given either as tablets or in a suspension for those children and infants who were unable to swallow tablets or who required a lower dose than is available in tablet form (see DOSAGE AND ADMINISTRATION, **Preparation of Suspension**).

Heart Failure:
During baseline-controlled clinical trials, in patients receiving digitalis and diuretics, single doses of PRINIVIL resulted in decreases in pulmonary capillary wedge pressure, systemic vascular resistance and blood pressure accompanied by an increase in cardiac output and no change in heart rate.

In two placebo-controlled, 12-week clinical studies using doses of PRINIVIL up to 20 mg, PRINIVIL as adjunctive therapy to digitalis and diuretics improved the following signs and symptoms due to congestive heart failure: edema, rales, paroxysmal nocturnal dyspnea and jugular venous distention. In one of the studies beneficial response was also noted for: orthopnea, presence of third heart sound and the number of patients classified as NYHA Class III and IV. Exercise tolerance was also improved in this study. The effect of lisinopril on mortality in patients with heart failure has not been evaluated.

The once daily dosing for the treatment of congestive heart failure was the only dosage regimen used during clinical trial development and was determined by the measurement of hemodynamic responses.

Acute Myocardial Infarction:
The Gruppo Italiano per lo Studio della Sopravvivenza nell'Infarto Miocardico (GISSI-3) study was a multicenter, controlled, randomized, unblinded clinical trial conducted in 19,394 patients with acute myocardial infarction admitted to a coronary care unit. It was designed to examine the effects of short-term (6 week) treatment with lisinopril, nitrates, their combination, or no therapy on short-term (6 week) mortality and on long-term death and markedly impaired cardiac function. Patients presenting within 24 hours of the onset of symptoms who were hemodynamically stable were randomized, in a 2 × 2 factorial design, to six weeks of either

1. PRINIVIL alone (n = 4841),
2. nitrates alone (n = 4869),
3. PRINIVIL plus nitrates (n = 4841), or
4. open control (n = 4843).

All patients received routine therapies, including thrombolytics (72%), aspirin (84%), and a beta-blocker (31%), as appropriate, normally utilized in acute myocardial infarction (MI) patients.

The protocol excluded patients with hypotension (systolic blood pressure ≤100 mmHg), severe heart failure, cardiogenic shock and renal dysfunction (serum creatinine >2 mg/dL and/or proteinuria >500 mg/24 h). Doses of PRINIVIL were adjusted as necessary according to protocol. (See DOSAGE AND ADMINISTRATION.)

Study treatment was withdrawn at six weeks except where clinical conditions indicated continuation of treatment.

The primary outcomes of the trial were the overall mortality at six weeks and a combined endpoint at six months after the myocardial infarction, consisting of the number of patients who died, had late (day 4) clinical congestive heart failure, or had extensive left ventricular damage defined as ejection fraction ≤35%, or an akinetic-dyskinetic [A-D] score ≥45%. Patients receiving PRINIVIL (n = 9646) alone or with nitrates, had an 11 percent lower risk of death (2p [two-tailed] = 0.04) compared to patients receiving no PRINIVIL (n = 9672) (6.4 percent versus 7.2 percent, respectively) at six weeks. Although patients randomized to receive PRINIVIL for up to six weeks also fared numerically better on the combined end-point at 6 months, the open nature of the assessment of heart failure, substantial loss to follow-up echocardiography, and substantial excess use of lisinopril between 6 weeks and 6 months in the group randomized to 6 weeks of lisinopril, preclude any conclusion about this endpoint.

Patients with acute myocardial infarction, treated with PRINIVIL had a higher (9.0 percent versus 3.7 percent, respectively) incidence of persistent hypotension (systolic blood pressure <90 mmHg for more than 1 hour) and renal dysfunction (2.4 percent versus 1.1 percent) in-hospital and at six weeks (increasing creatinine concentration to over 3 mg/dL or a doubling or more of the baseline serum creatinine concentration). (See ADVERSE REACTIONS, *ACUTE MYOCARDIAL INFARCTION*.)

INDICATIONS AND USAGE
Hypertension
PRINIVIL is indicated for the treatment of hypertension. It may be used alone as initial therapy or concomitantly with other classes of antihypertensive agents.

Heart Failure
PRINIVIL is indicated as adjunctive therapy in the management of heart failure in patients who are not responding adequately to diuretics and digitalis.

Acute Myocardial Infarction
PRINIVIL is indicated for the treatment of hemodynamically stable patients within 24 hours of acute myocardial infarction, to improve survival. Patients should receive, as appropriate, the standard recommended treatments such as thrombolytics, aspirin and beta-blockers.

In using PRINIVIL, consideration should be given to the fact that another angiotensin converting enzyme inhibitor, captopril, has caused agranulocytosis, particularly in patients with renal impairment or collagen vascular disease, and that available data are insufficient to show that PRINIVIL does not have a similar risk. (See WARNINGS.)

In considering use of PRINIVIL, it should be noted that in controlled clinical trials ACE inhibitors have an effect on blood pressure that is less in Black patients than in non-Blacks. In addition, it should be noted that Black patients receiving ACE inhibitors have been reported to have a higher incidence of angioedema compared to non-Blacks (see WARNINGS, **Anaphylactoid and Possibly Related Reactions, Head and Neck Angioedema**).

CONTRAINDICATIONS
PRINIVIL is contraindicated in patients who are hypersensitive to this product and in patients with a history of angioedema related to previous treatment with an angiotensin converting enzyme inhibitor and in patients with hereditary or idiopathic angioedema.

WARNINGS
Anaphylactoid and Possibly Related Reactions
Presumably because angiotensin converting enzyme inhibitors affect the metabolism of eicosanoids and polypeptides, including endogenous bradykinin, patients receiving ACE inhibitors (including PRINIVIL) may be subject to a variety of adverse reactions, some of them serious.

Head and Neck Angioedema: Angioedema of the face, extremities, lips, tongue, glottis and/or larynx has been reported in patients treated with angiotensin converting enzyme inhibitors, including PRINIVIL. This may occur at any time during treatment. ACE inhibitors have been associated with a higher rate of angioedema in Black than in non-Black patients. In such cases PRINIVIL should be promptly discontinued and appropriate therapy and monitoring should be provided until complete and sustained resolution of signs and symptoms has occurred. Even in those instances where swelling of only the tongue is involved, without respiratory distress, patients may require prolonged observation since treatment with antihistamines and corticosteroids may not be sufficient. Very rarely, fatalities have been reported due to angioedema associated with laryngeal edema or tongue edema. Patients with involvement of the tongue, glottis or larynx are likely to experience airway obstruction, especially those with a history of airway surgery. **Where there is involvement of the tongue, glottis or larynx, likely to cause airway obstruction, appropriate therapy, e.g., subcutaneous epinephrine solution 1:1000 (0.3 mL to 0.5 mL) and/or measures necessary to ensure a patent airway, should be promptly provided.** (See ADVERSE REACTIONS.)

Patients with a history of angioedema unrelated to ACE inhibitor therapy may be at increased risk of angioedema while receiving an ACE inhibitor (see also INDICATIONS AND USAGE and CONTRAINDICATIONS.)

Intestinal Angioedema: Intestinal angioedema has been reported in patients treated with ACE inhibitors. These patients presented with abdominal pain (with or without nausea or vomiting); in some cases there was no prior history of facial angioedema and C-1 esterase levels were normal. The angioedema was diagnosed by procedures including abdominal CT scan or ultrasound, or at surgery, and symptoms resolved after stopping the ACE inhibitor. Intestinal angioedema should be included in the differential diagnosis of patients on ACE inhibitors presenting with abdominal pain.

Anaphylactoid reactions during desensitization: Two patients undergoing desensitizing treatment with hymenoptera venom while receiving ACE inhibitors sustained life-threatening anaphylactoid reactions. In the same patients, these reactions were avoided when ACE inhibitors were temporarily withheld, but they reappeared upon inadvertent rechallenge.

Anaphylactoid reactions during membrane exposure: Sudden and potentially life-threatening anaphylactoid reactions have been reported in some patients dialyzed with high-flux membranes (e.g., AN69®) and treated concomitantly with an ACE inhibitor. In such patients, dialysis must be stopped immediately, and aggressive therapy for anaphylactoid reactions be initiated. Symptoms have not been relieved by antihistamines in these situations. In these patients, consideration should be given to using a different type of dialysis membrane or a different class of antihypertensive agent. Anaphylactoid reactions have also been reported in patients undergoing low-density lipoprotein apheresis with dextran sulfate absorption.

Hypotension
Excessive hypotension is rare in patients with uncomplicated hypertension treated with PRINIVIL alone.

Patients with heart failure given PRINIVIL commonly have some reduction in blood pressure with peak blood pressure reduction occurring 6 to 8 hours post dose, but discontinuation of therapy because of continuing symptomatic hypotension usually is not necessary when dosing instructions are followed; caution should be observed when initiating therapy. (See DOSAGE AND ADMINISTRATION.)

Patients at risk of excessive hypotension, sometimes associated with oliguria and/or progressive azotemia, and rarely with acute renal failure and/or death, include those with the following conditions or characteristics: heart failure with systolic blood pressure below 100 mmHg, hyponatremia, high-dose diuretic therapy, recent intensive diuresis or increase in diuretic dose, renal dialysis, or severe volume and/or salt depletion of any etiology. It may be advisable to eliminate the diuretic (except in patients with heart failure), reduce the diuretic dose or increase salt intake cautiously before initiating therapy with PRINIVIL in patients at risk for excessive hypotension who are able to tolerate such adjustments. (See PRECAUTIONS, **Drug Interactions**, and ADVERSE REACTIONS.)

Patients with acute myocardial infarction in the GISSI-3 study had a higher (9.0 percent versus 3.7 percent) incidence of persistent hypotension (systolic blood pressure <90 mmHg for more than 1 hour) when treated with PRINIVIL. Treatment with PRINIVIL must not be initiated in acute myocardial infarction patients at risk of further serious hemodynamic deterioration after treatment with a vasodilator (e.g., systolic blood pressure of 100 mmHg or lower) or cardiogenic shock.

In patients at risk of excessive hypotension, therapy should be started under very close medical supervision and such patients should be followed closely for the first two weeks of treatment and whenever the dose of PRINIVIL and/or diuretic is increased. Similar considerations may apply to patients with ischemic heart or cerebrovascular disease, or in patients with acute myocardial infarction, in whom an excessive fall in blood pressure could result in a myocardial infarction or cerebrovascular accident.

If excessive hypotension occurs, the patient should be placed in the supine position and, if necessary, receive an intravenous infusion of normal saline. A transient hypotensive response is not a contraindication to further doses of PRINIVIL which usually can be given without difficulty once the blood pressure has stabilized. If symptomatic hypotension develops, a dose reduction or discontinuation of PRINIVIL or concomitant diuretic may be necessary.

Leukopenia/Neutropenia/Agranulocytosis
Another angiotensin converting enzyme inhibitor, captopril, has been shown to cause agranulocytosis and bone marrow depression, rarely in uncomplicated patients but more frequently in patients with renal impairment especially if they also have a collagen vascular disease. Available data from clinical trials of PRINIVIL are insufficient to show that PRINIVIL does not cause agranulocytosis at similar rates. Marketing experience has revealed rare cases of leukopenia/neutropenia and bone marrow depression in which a causal relationship to lisinopril cannot be excluded. Periodic monitoring of white blood cell counts in patients with collagen vascular disease and renal disease should be considered.

Hepatic Failure
Rarely, ACE inhibitors have been associated with a syndrome that starts with cholestatic jaundice or hepatitis and progresses to fulminant hepatic necrosis, and (sometimes) death. The mechanism of this syndrome is not understood. Patients receiving ACE inhibitors who develop jaundice or marked elevations of hepatic enzymes should discontinue the ACE inhibitor and receive appropriate medical follow-up.

Fetal/Neonatal Morbidity and Mortality
ACE inhibitors can cause fetal and neonatal morbidity and death when administered to pregnant women. Several dozen cases have been reported in the world literature. When pregnancy is detected, ACE inhibitors should be discontinued as soon as possible.

In a published retrospective epidemiological study, infants whose mothers had taken an ACE inhibitor drug during the first trimester of pregnancy appeared to have an increased risk of major congenital malformations compared with infants whose mothers had not undergone first trimester exposure to ACE inhibitor drugs. The number of cases of birth defects is small and the findings of this study have not yet been repeated.

The use of ACE inhibitors during the second and third trimesters of pregnancy has been associated with fetal and neonatal injury, including hypotension, neonatal skull hypoplasia, anuria, reversible or irreversible renal failure, and death. Oligohydramnios has also been reported, presumably resulting from decreased fetal renal function; oligohydramnios in this setting has been associated with fetal limb contractures, craniofacial deformation, and hypoplastic lung development. Prematurity, intrauterine growth retardation, and patent ductus arteriosus have also been reported, although it is not clear whether these occurrences were due to the ACE-inhibitor exposure.

These adverse effects do not appear to have resulted from intrauterine ACE-inhibitor exposure that has been limited to the first trimester. Mothers whose embryos and fetuses are exposed to ACE inhibitors only during the first trimester should be so informed. Nonetheless, when patients become pregnant, physicians should make every effort to discontinue the use of PRINIVIL as soon as possible.

Rarely (probably less often than once in every thousand pregnancies), no alternative to ACE inhibitors will be found. In these rare cases, the mothers should be apprised of the potential hazards to their fetuses, and serial ultrasound examinations should be performed to assess the intraamniotic environment.

If oligohydramnios is observed, PRINIVIL should be discontinued unless it is considered lifesaving for the mother. Contraction stress testing (CST), a non-stress test (NST), or biophysical profiling (BPP) may be appropriate, depending upon the week of pregnancy. Patients and physicians should be aware, however, that oligohydramnios may not appear until after the fetus has sustained irreversible injury.

Infants with histories of *in utero* exposure to ACE inhibitors should be closely observed for hypotension, oliguria, and hyperkalemia. If oliguria occurs, attention should be directed toward support of blood pressure and renal perfusion. Ex-

change transfusion or dialysis may be required as means of reversing hypotension and/or substituting for disordered renal function. Lisinopril, which crosses the placenta, has been removed from neonatal circulation by peritoneal dialysis with some clinical benefit, and theoretically may be removed by exchange transfusion, although there is no experience with the latter procedure.

No teratogenic effects of lisinopril were seen in studies of pregnant mice, rats and rabbits. On a body surface area basis, the doses used were 55 times, 33 times, and 0.15 times, respectively, the maximum recommended human daily dose (MRHDD).

PRECAUTIONS
General
Aortic Stenosis/Hypertrophic Cardiomyopathy: As with all vasodilators, lisinopril should be given with caution to patients with obstruction in the outflow tract of the left ventricle.

Impaired Renal Function: As a consequence of inhibiting the renin-angiotensin-aldosterone system, changes in renal function may be anticipated in susceptible individuals. In patients with severe congestive heart failure whose renal function may depend on the activity of the renin-angiotensin-aldosterone system, treatment with angiotensin converting enzyme inhibitors, including PRINIVIL, may be associated with oliguria and/or progressive azotemia and rarely with acute renal failure and/or death.

In hypertensive patients with unilateral or bilateral renal artery stenosis, increases in blood urea nitrogen and serum creatinine may occur. Experience with another angiotensin converting enzyme inhibitor suggests that these increases are usually reversible upon discontinuation of PRINIVIL and/or diuretic therapy. In such patients renal function should be monitored during the first few weeks of therapy. Some patients with hypertension or heart failure with no apparent pre-existing renal vascular disease have developed increases in blood urea nitrogen and serum creatinine, usually minor and transient, especially when PRINIVIL has been given concomitantly with a diuretic. This is more likely to occur in patients with pre-existing renal impairment. Dosage reduction and/or discontinuation of the diuretic and/or PRINIVIL may be required.

Patients with acute myocardial infarction in the GISSI-3 study, treated with PRINIVIL, had a higher (2.4 percent versus 1.1 percent) incidence of renal dysfunction in-hospital and at six weeks (increasing creatinine concentration to over 3 mg/dL or a doubling or more of the baseline serum creatinine concentration). In acute myocardial infarction, treatment with PRINIVIL should be initiated with caution in patients with evidence of renal dysfunction, defined as serum creatinine concentration exceeding 2 mg/dL. If renal dysfunction develops during treatment with PRINIVIL (serum creatinine concentration exceeding 3 mg/dL or a doubling from the pre-treatment value) then the physician should consider withdrawal of PRINIVIL.

Evaluation of patients with hypertension, heart failure, or myocardial infarction should always include assessment of renal function. (See DOSAGE AND ADMINISTRATION.)

Hyperkalemia: In clinical trials hyperkalemia (serum potassium greater than 5.7 mEq/L) occurred in approximately 2.2 percent of hypertensive patients and 4.8 percent of patients with heart failure. In most cases these were isolated values which resolved despite continued therapy. Hyperkalemia was a cause of discontinuation of therapy in approximately 0.1 percent of hypertensive patients, 0.6 percent of patients with heart failure and 0.1 percent of patients with myocardial infarction. Risk factors for the development of hyperkalemia include renal insufficiency, diabetes mellitus, and the concomitant use of potassium-sparing diuretics, potassium supplements and/or potassium-containing salt substitutes. Hyperkalemia can cause serious, sometimes fatal, arrhythmias. PRINIVIL should be used cautiously, if at all, with these agents and with frequent monitoring of serum potassium. (See **Drug Interactions**.)

Cough: Presumably due to the inhibition of the degradation of endogenous bradykinin, persistent nonproductive cough has been reported with all ACE inhibitors, always resolving after discontinuation of therapy. ACE inhibitor-induced cough should be considered in the differential diagnosis of cough.

Surgery/Anesthesia: In patients undergoing major surgery or during anesthesia with agents that produce hypotension, PRINIVIL may block angiotensin II formation secondary to compensatory renin release. If hypotension occurs and is considered to be due to this mechanism, it can be corrected by volume expansion.

Information for Patients
Angioedema: Angioedema, including laryngeal edema, may occur at any time during treatment with angiotensin converting enzyme inhibitors, including lisinopril. Patients should be so advised and told to report immediately any signs or symptoms suggesting angioedema (swelling of face, extremities, eyes, lips, tongue, difficulty in swallowing or

breathing) and to take no more drug until they have consulted with the prescribing physician.

Symptomatic Hypotension: Patients should be cautioned to report lightheadedness especially during the first few days of therapy. If actual syncope occurs, the patients should be told to discontinue the drug until they have consulted with the prescribing physician.

All patients should be cautioned that excessive perspiration and dehydration may lead to an excessive fall in blood pressure because of reduction in fluid volume. Other causes of volume depletion such as vomiting or diarrhea may also lead to a fall in blood pressure; patients should be advised to consult with their physician.

Hyperkalemia: Patients should be told not to use salt substitutes containing potassium without consulting their physician.

Hypoglycemia: Diabetic patients treated with oral antidiabetic agents or insulin starting an ACE inhibitor should be told to closely monitor for hypoglycemia, especially during the first month of combined use. (See **Drug Interactions**.)

Leukopenia/Neutropenia: Patients should be told to report promptly any indication of infection (e.g., sore throat, fever) which may be a sign of leukopenia/neutropenia.

Pregnancy: Female patients of childbearing age should be told about the consequences of exposure to ACE inhibitors during pregnancy. These patients should be asked to report pregnancies to their physicians as soon as possible.

NOTE: As with many other drugs, certain advice to patients being treated with PRINIVIL is warranted. This information is intended to aid in the safe and effective use of this medication. It is not a disclosure of all possible adverse or intended effects.

Drug Interactions
Hypotension - Patients on Diuretic Therapy: Patients on diuretics, and especially those in whom diuretic therapy was recently instituted, may occasionally experience an excessive reduction of blood pressure after initiation of therapy with PRINIVIL. The possibility of hypotensive effects with PRINIVIL can be minimized by either discontinuing the diuretic or increasing the salt intake prior to initiation of treatment with PRINIVIL. If it is necessary to continue the diuretic, initiate therapy with PRINIVIL at a dose of 5 mg daily, and provide close medical supervision after the initial dose until blood pressure has stabilized. (See WARNINGS and DOSAGE AND ADMINISTRATION.) When a diuretic is added to the therapy of a patient receiving PRINIVIL, an additional antihypertensive effect is usually observed. Studies with ACE inhibitors in combination with diuretics indicate that the dose of the ACE inhibitor can be reduced when it is given with a diuretic. (See DOSAGE AND ADMINISTRATION.)

Antidiabetics: Epidemiological studies have suggested that concomitant administration of ACE inhibitors and antidiabetic medicines (insulins, oral hypoglycemic agents) may cause an increased blood-glucose-lowering effect with risk of hypoglycemia. This phenomenon appeared to be more likely to occur during the first weeks of combined treatment and in patients with renal impairment. In diabetic patients treated with oral antidiabetic agents or insulin, glycemic control should be closely monitored for hypoglycemia, especially during the first month of treatment with an ACE inhibitor.

Non-steroidal Anti-inflammatory Agents Including Selective Cyclooxygenase-2 (COX-2) Inhibitors: Reports suggest that NSAIDs including selective COX-2 inhibitors may diminish the antihypertensive effect of ACE inhibitors, including lisinopril. This interaction should be given consideration in patients taking NSAIDs or selective COX-2 inhibitors concomitantly with ACE inhibitors.

In a study in 36 patients with mild to moderate hypertension where the antihypertensive effects of PRINIVIL alone were compared to PRINIVIL given concomitantly with indomethacin, the use of indomethacin was associated with a reduced antihypertensive effect, although the difference between the two regimens was not significant.

In some patients with compromised renal function (e.g., elderly patients or patients who are volume-depleted including those on diuretic therapy) who are being treated with non-steroidal anti-inflammatory drugs, including selective COX-2 inhibitors, the co-administration of angiotensin II receptor antagonists or ACE inhibitors may result in a further deterioration of renal function, including possible acute renal failure. These effects are usually reversible.

These interactions should be considered in patients taking NSAIDS including selective COX-2 inhibitors concomitantly with diuretics and angiotensin II antagonists or ACE inhibitors. Therefore, monitor effects on blood pressure and renal function when administering the combination, especially in the elderly.

Other Agents: PRINIVIL has been used concomitantly with nitrates and/or digoxin without evidence of clinically significant adverse interactions. This included post myocardial infarction patients who were receiving intravenous or transdermal nitroglycerin. No clinically important pharmacokinetic interactions occurred when PRINIVIL was used concomitantly with propranolol or hydrochlorothiazide. The presence of food in the stomach does not alter the bioavailability of PRINIVIL.

Agents Increasing Serum Potassium: PRINIVIL attenuates potassium loss caused by thiazide-type diuretics. Use of PRINIVIL with potassium-sparing diuretics (e.g., spironolactone, eplerenone, triamterene, or amiloride), potassium supplements, or potassium-containing salt substitutes may lead to significant increases in serum potassium. Therefore, if concomitant use of these agents is indicated because of demonstrated hypokalemia, they should be used with caution and with frequent monitoring of serum potassium. Potassium-sparing agents should generally not be used in patients with heart failure who are receiving PRINIVIL.

Lithium: Lithium toxicity has been reported in patients receiving lithium concomitantly with drugs which cause elimination of sodium, including ACE inhibitors. Lithium toxicity was usually reversible upon discontinuation of lithium and the ACE inhibitor. It is recommended that serum lithium levels be monitored frequently if PRINIVIL is administered concomitantly with lithium.

Gold: Nitritoid reactions (symptoms include facial flushing, nausea, vomiting and hypotension) have been reported rarely in patients on therapy with injectable gold (sodium aurothiomalate) and concomitant ACE inhibitor therapy including PRINIVIL.

Carcinogenesis, Mutagenesis, Impairment of Fertility
There was no evidence of a tumorigenic effect when lisinopril was administered orally for 105 weeks to male and female rats at doses up to 90 mg/kg/day or for 92 weeks to male and female mice at doses up to 135 mg/kg/day. These doses are 10 times and 7 times, respectively, the maximum recommended human daily dose (MRHDD) when compared on a body surface area basis.

Lisinopril was not mutagenic in the Ames microbial mutagen test with or without metabolic activation. It was also negative in a forward mutation assay using Chinese hamster lung cells. Lisinopril did not produce single strand DNA breaks in an *in vitro* alkaline elution rat hepatocyte assay. In addition, lisinopril did not produce increases in chromosomal aberrations in an *in vitro* test in Chinese hamster ovary cells or in an *in vivo* study in mouse bone marrow.

There were no adverse effects on reproductive performance in male and female rats treated with up to 300 mg/kg/day of lisinopril (33 times the MRHDD when compared on a body surface area basis).

Pregnancy
Pregnancy Categories C (first trimester) **and D** (second and third trimesters). See WARNINGS, **Fetal/Neonatal Morbidity and Mortality**.

Nursing Mothers
Milk of lactating rats contains radioactivity following administration of ^{14}C lisinopril. It is not known whether this drug is secreted in human milk. Because many drugs are secreted in human milk, and because of the potential for serious adverse reactions in nursing infants from ACE inhibitors, a decision should be made whether to discontinue nursing or discontinue PRINIVIL, taking into account the importance of the drug to the mother.

Pediatric Use
Antihypertensive effects of PRINIVIL have been established in hypertensive pediatric patients aged 6 to 16 years. There are no data on the effect of PRINIVIL on blood pressure in pediatric patients under the age of 6 or in pediatric patients with glomerular filtration rate <30 mL/min/1.73 m² (see CLINICAL PHARMACOLOGY, **Pharmacokinetics and Metabolism and Pharmacodynamics and Clinical Effects**, and DOSAGE AND ADMINISTRATION).

Geriatric Use
Clinical studies of PRINIVIL in patients with hypertension and congestive heart failure did not include sufficient numbers of subjects aged 65 and over to determine whether they respond differently from younger subjects. Other clinical experience in this population has not identified differences in responses between the elderly and younger patients. In general, dose selection for an elderly patient should be cautious, usually starting at the low end of the dosing range, reflecting the greater frequency of decreased hepatic, renal, or cardiac function, and of concomitant disease or other drug therapy.

In a clinical study of PRINIVIL in patients with myocardial infarctions 4413 (47 percent) were 65 and over, while 1656 (18 percent) were 75 and over. No overall differences in safety or efficacy were observed between elderly and younger patients.

Other reported clinical experience has not identified differences in responses between the elderly and younger patients, but greater sensitivity of some older individuals cannot be ruled out.

Pharmacokinetic studies indicate that maximum blood levels and area under plasma concentration time curve (AUC) are doubled in elderly patients.

This drug is known to be substantially excreted by the kidney, and the risk of toxic reactions to this drug may be greater in patients with impaired renal function. Because elderly patients are more likely to have decreased renal function, care should be taken in dose selection. Evaluation of patients with hypertension, congestive heart failure, or myocardial infarction should always include assessment of renal function. (See DOSAGE AND ADMINISTRATION.)

ADVERSE REACTIONS
PRINIVIL has been found to be generally well tolerated in controlled clinical trials involving 1969 patients with hypertension or heart failure. For the most part, adverse experiences were mild and transient.

HYPERTENSION
In clinical trials in patients with hypertension treated with PRINIVIL, discontinuation of therapy due to clinical adverse experiences occurred in 5.7 percent of patients. The overall frequency of adverse experiences could not be related to total daily dosage within the recommended therapeutic dosage range.

For adverse experiences occurring in greater than one percent of patients with hypertension treated with PRINIVIL or PRINIVIL plus hydrochlorothiazide in controlled clinical trials and more frequently with PRINIVIL and/or PRINIVIL plus hydrochlorothiazide than placebo, comparative incidence data are listed in the table below:
[See table at left]
Chest pain and back pain were also seen but were more common on placebo than PRINIVIL.

HEART FAILURE
In patients with heart failure treated with PRINIVIL for up to four years, discontinuation of therapy due to clinical adverse experiences occurred in 11.0 percent of patients. In controlled studies in patients with heart failure, therapy was discontinued in 8.1 percent of patients treated with PRINIVIL for up to 12 weeks, compared to 7.7 percent of patients treated with placebo for 12 weeks.

The following table lists those adverse experiences which occurred in greater than one percent of patients with heart failure treated with PRINIVIL or placebo for up to 12 weeks in controlled clinical trials and more frequently on PRINIVIL than placebo.

Controlled Trials

	PRINIVIL (n=407) Incidence (discontinuation)	Placebo (n=155) Incidence (discontinuation)
	12 weeks	12 weeks
Body As A Whole		
Chest Pain	3.4 (0.2)	1.3 (0.0)
Abdominal Pain	2.2 (0.7)	1.9 (0.0)
Cardiovascular		
Hypotension	4.4 (1.7)	0.6 (0.6)
Digestive		
Diarrhea	3.7 (0.5)	1.9 (0.0)
Nervous/Psychiatric		
Dizziness	11.8 (1.2)	4.5 (1.3)
Headache	4.4 (0.2)	3.9 (0.0)
Respiratory		
Upper Respiratory Infection	1.5 (0.0)	1.3 (0.0)
Skin		
Rash	1.7 (0.5)	0.6 (0.6)

Also observed at >1% with PRINIVIL but more frequent or as frequent on placebo than PRINIVIL in controlled trials were asthenia, angina pectoris, nausea, dyspnea, cough and pruritus.

Worsening of heart failure, anorexia, increased salivation, muscle cramps, back pain, myalgia, depression, chest sound abnormalities and pulmonary edema were also seen in controlled clinical trials, but were more common on placebo than PRINIVIL.

ACUTE MYOCARDIAL INFARCTION
In the GISSI-3 trial, in patients treated with PRINIVIL for six weeks following acute myocardial infarction, discontinuation of therapy occurred in 17.6 percent of patients.

Patients treated with PRINIVIL had a significantly higher incidence of hypotension and renal dysfunction compared with patients not taking PRINIVIL.

In the GISSI-3 trial, hypotension (9.7 percent), renal dysfunction (2.0 percent), cough (0.5 percent), post-infarction angina (0.3 percent), skin rash and generalized edema (0.01 percent), and angioedema (0.01 percent) resulted in

Percent of Patients in Controlled Studies

	PRINIVIL (n = 1349) Incidence (discontinuation)	PRINIVIL/ Hydrochlorothiazide (n = 629) Incidence (discontinuation)	Placebo (n = 207) Incidence (discontinuation)
Body As A Whole			
Fatigue	2.5 (0.3)	4.0 (0.5)	1.0 (0.0)
Asthenia	1.3 (0.5)	2.1 (0.2)	1.0 (0.0)
Orthostatic Effects	1.2 (0.0)	3.5 (0.2)	1.0 (0.0)
Cardiovascular			
Hypotension	1.2 (0.5)	1.6 (0.5)	0.5 (0.5)
Digestive			
Diarrhea	2.7 (0.2)	2.7 (0.3)	2.4 (0.0)
Nausea	2.0 (0.4)	2.5 (0.2)	2.4 (0.0)
Vomiting	1.1 (0.2)	1.4 (0.1)	0.5 (0.0)
Dyspepsia	0.9 (0.0)	1.9 (0.0)	0.0 (0.0)
Musculoskeletal			
Muscle Cramps	0.5 (0.0)	2.9 (0.8)	0.5 (0.0)
Nervous/Psychiatric			
Headache	5.7 (0.2)	4.5 (0.5)	1.9 (0.0)
Dizziness	5.4 (0.4)	9.2 (1.0)	1.9 (0.0)
Paresthesia	0.8 (0.1)	2.1 (0.2)	0.0 (0.0)
Decreased Libido	0.4 (0.1)	1.3 (0.1)	0.0 (0.0)
Vertigo	0.2 (0.1)	1.1 (0.2)	0.0 (0.0)
Respiratory			
Cough	3.5 (0.7)	4.6 (0.8)	1.0 (0.0)
Upper Respiratory Infection	2.1 (0.1)	2.7 (0.1)	0.0 (0.0)
Common Cold	1.1 (0.1)	1.3 (0.1)	0.0 (0.0)
Nasal Congestion	0.4 (0.1)	1.3 (0.1)	0.0 (0.0)
Influenza	0.3 (0.1)	1.1 (0.1)	0.0 (0.0)
Skin			
Rash	1.3 (0.4)	1.6 (0.2)	0.5 (0.5)
Urogenital			
Impotence	1.0 (0.4)	1.6 (0.5)	0.0 (0.0)

withdrawal of treatment. In elderly patients treated with PRINIVIL, discontinuation due to renal dysfunction was 4.2 percent.

Other clinical adverse experiences occurring in 0.3 to 1.0 percent of patients with hypertension or heart failure treated with PRINIVIL in controlled trials and rarer, serious, possibly drug-related events reported in uncontrolled studies or marketing experience are listed below, and within each category, are in order of decreasing severity:

Body as a Whole: Anaphylactoid reactions (see WARNINGS, **Anaphylactoid and Possibly Related Reactions**), syncope, orthostatic effects, chest discomfort, pain, pelvic pain, flank pain, edema, facial edema, virus infection, fever, chills, malaise.

Cardiovascular: Cardiac arrest; myocardial infarction or cerebrovascular accident, possibly secondary to excessive hypotension in high-risk patients (see WARNINGS, **Hypotension**); pulmonary embolism and infarction, arrhythmias (including ventricular tachycardia, atrial tachycardia, atrial fibrillation, bradycardia and premature ventricular contractions), palpitations, transient ischemic attacks, paroxysmal nocturnal dyspnea, orthostatic hypotension, decreased blood pressure, peripheral edema, vasculitis.

Digestive: Pancreatitis, hepatitis (hepatocellular or cholestatic jaundice) (see WARNINGS, **Hepatic Failure**), vomiting, gastritis, dyspepsia, heartburn, gastrointestinal cramps, constipation, flatulence, dry mouth.

Hematologic: Rare cases of bone marrow depression, hemolytic anemia, leukopenia/neutropenia, and thrombocytopenia.

Endocrine: Diabetes mellitus, syndrome of inappropriate antidiuretic hormone secretion (SIADH).

Metabolic: Weight loss, dehydration, fluid overload, gout, weight gain. Cases of hypoglycemia in diabetic patients on oral antidiabetic agents or insulin have been reported (see PRECAUTIONS, **Drug Interactions**).

Musculoskeletal: Arthritis, arthralgia, neck pain, hip pain, low back pain, joint pain, leg pain, knee pain, shoulder pain, arm pain, lumbago.

Nervous System/Psychiatric: Stroke, ataxia, memory impairment, tremor, peripheral neuropathy (e.g., dysesthesia), spasm, paresthesia, confusion, insomnia, somnolence, hypersomnia, irritability, and nervousness.

Respiratory System: Malignant lung neoplasms, hemoptysis, pulmonary infiltrates, eosinophilic pneumonitis, bronchospasm, asthma, pleural effusion, pneumonia, bronchitis, wheezing, orthopnea, painful respiration, epistaxis, laryngitis, sinusitis, pharyngeal pain, pharyngitis, rhinitis, rhinorrhea.

Skin: Urticaria, alopecia, herpes zoster, photosensitivity, skin lesions, skin infections, pemphigus, erythema, flushing, diaphoresis. Other severe skin reactions (including toxic epidermal necrolysis, Stevens-Johnson syndrome and cutaneous pseudolymphoma) have been reported rarely; causal relationship has not been established.

Special Senses: Visual loss, diplopia, blurred vision, tinnitus, photophobia, taste disturbances.

Urogenital System: Acute renal failure, oliguria, anuria, uremia, progressive azotemia, renal dysfunction (see PRECAUTIONS and DOSAGE AND ADMINISTRATION), pyelonephritis, dysuria, urinary tract infection, breast pain.

Miscellaneous: A symptom complex has been reported which may include a positive ANA, an elevated erythrocyte sedimentation rate, arthralgia/arthritis, myalgia, fever, vasculitis, eosinophilia and leukocytosis. Rash, photosensitivity or other dermatological manifestations may occur alone or in combination with these symptoms.

Angioedema: Angioedema has been reported in patients receiving PRINIVIL (0.1%) with an incidence higher in Black than in non-Black patients. Angioedema associated with laryngeal edema may be fatal. If angioedema of the face, extremities, lips, tongue, glottis and/or larynx occurs, treatment with PRINIVIL should be discontinued and appropriate therapy instituted immediately. In rare cases, intestinal angioedema has been reported with angiotensin converting enzyme inhibitors including lisinopril. (See WARNINGS.)

Hypotension: In hypertensive patients, hypotension occurred in 1.2 percent and syncope occurred in 0.1 percent of patients. Hypotension or syncope was a cause for discontinuation of therapy in 0.5 percent of hypertensive patients. In patients with heart failure, hypotension occurred in 5.3 percent and syncope occurred in 1.8 percent of patients. These adverse experiences were causes for discontinuation of therapy in 1.8 percent of these patients. In patients treated with PRINIVIL for six weeks after acute myocardial infarction, hypotension (systolic blood pressure ≤100 mmHg) resulted in discontinuation of therapy in 9.7 percent of the patients. (See WARNINGS.)

Fetal/Neonatal Morbidity and Mortality: See WARNINGS, **Fetal/Neonatal Morbidity and Mortality**.

Cough: See PRECAUTIONS, **Cough**.

Pediatric Patients: No relevant differences between the adverse experience profile for pediatric patients and that previously reported for adult patients were identified.

Clinical Laboratory Test Findings

Serum Electrolytes: Hyperkalemia (see PRECAUTIONS), hyponatremia.

Creatinine, Blood Urea Nitrogen: Minor increases in blood urea nitrogen and serum creatinine, reversible upon discontinuation of therapy, were observed in about 2.0 percent of patients with essential hypertension treated with PRINIVIL alone. Increases were more common in patients receiving concomitant diuretics and in patients with renal artery stenosis. (See PRECAUTIONS.) Reversible minor increases in blood urea nitrogen and serum creatinine were observed in approximately 11.6 percent of patients with heart failure on concomitant diuretic therapy. Frequently, these abnormalities resolved when the dosage of the diuretic was decreased.

Hemoglobin and Hematocrit: Small decreases in hemoglobin and hematocrit (mean decreases of approximately 0.4 g percent and 1.3 vol percent, respectively) occurred frequently in patients treated with PRINIVIL but were rarely of clinical importance in patients without some other cause of anemia. In clinical trials, less than 0.1 percent of patients discontinued therapy due to anemia. Hemolytic anemia has been reported; a causal relationship to lisinopril cannot be excluded.

Liver Function Tests: Rarely, elevations of liver enzymes and/or serum bilirubin have occurred (see WARNINGS, **Hepatic Failure**).

In hypertensive patients, 2.0 percent discontinued therapy due to laboratory adverse experiences, principally elevations in blood urea nitrogen (0.6 percent), serum creatinine (0.5 percent) and serum potassium (0.4 percent). In the heart failure trials, 3.4 percent of patients discontinued therapy due to laboratory adverse experiences, 1.8 percent due to elevations in blood urea nitrogen and/or creatinine and 0.6 percent due to elevations in serum potassium. In the myocardial infarction trial, 2.0 percent of patients receiving PRINIVIL discontinued therapy due to renal dysfunction (increasing creatinine concentration to over 3 mg/dL or a doubling or more of the baseline serum creatinine concentration); less than 1.0 percent of patients discontinued therapy due to other laboratory adverse experiences: 0.1 percent with hyperkalemia and less than 0.1 percent with hepatic enzyme alterations.

OVERDOSAGE

Following a single oral dose of 20 g/kg, no lethality occurred in rats and death occurred in one of 20 mice receiving the same dose. The most likely manifestation of overdosage would be hypotension, for which the usual treatment would be intravenous infusion of normal saline solution.

Lisinopril can be removed by hemodialysis. (See WARNINGS, **Anaphylactoid reactions during membrane exposure**.)

DOSAGE AND ADMINISTRATION

Hypertension

Initial Therapy: In patients with uncomplicated essential hypertension not on diuretic therapy, the recommended initial dose is 10 mg once a day. Dosage should be adjusted according to blood pressure response. The usual dosage range is 20 to 40 mg per day administered in a single daily dose. The antihypertensive effect may diminish toward the end of the dosing interval regardless of the administered dose, but most commonly with a dose of 10 mg daily. This can be evaluated by measuring blood pressure just prior to dosing to determine whether satisfactory control is being maintained for 24 hours. If it is not, an increase in dose should be considered. Doses up to 80 mg have been used but do not appear to give a greater effect. If blood pressure is not controlled with PRINIVIL alone, a low dose of a diuretic may be added. Hydrochlorothiazide 12.5 mg has been shown to provide an additive effect. After the addition of a diuretic, it may be possible to reduce the dose of PRINIVIL.

Diuretic Treated Patients: In hypertensive patients who are currently being treated with a diuretic, symptomatic hypotension may occur occasionally following the initial dose of PRINIVIL. The diuretic should be discontinued, if possible, for two to three days before beginning therapy with PRINIVIL to reduce the likelihood of hypotension. (See WARNINGS.) The dosage of PRINIVIL should be adjusted according to blood pressure response. If the patient's blood pressure is not controlled with PRINIVIL alone, diuretic therapy may be resumed as described above.

If the diuretic cannot be discontinued, an initial dose of 5 mg should be used under medical supervision for at least two hours and until blood pressure has stabilized for at least an additional hour. (See WARNINGS and PRECAUTIONS, **Drug Interactions**.)

Concomitant administration of PRINIVIL with potassium supplements, potassium salt substitutes, or potassium-sparing diuretics may lead to increases of serum potassium (see PRECAUTIONS).

Dosage Adjustment in Renal Impairment: The usual dose of PRINIVIL (10 mg) is recommended for patients with a creatinine clearance >30 mL/min (serum creatinine of up to approximately 3 mg/dL). For patients with creatinine clearance ≥10 mL/min ≤30 mL/min (serum creatinine ≥3 mg/dL), the first dose is 5 mg once daily. For patients with creatinine clearance <10 mL/min (usually on hemodialysis) the recommended initial dose is 2.5 mg. The dosage may be titrated upward until blood pressure is controlled or to a maximum of 40 mg daily.

Renal Status	Creatinine-Clearance mL/min	Initial Dose mg/day
Normal Renal Function to Mild Impairment	>30 mL/min	10 mg
Moderate to Severe Impairment	≥10 ≤30 mL/min	5 mg
Dialysis Patients*	<10 mL/min	2.5 mg[†]

* See WARNINGS, **Anaphylactoid reactions during membrane exposure**

† *Dosage or dosing interval should be adjusted depending on the blood pressure response.*

Heart Failure

PRINIVIL is indicated as adjunctive therapy with diuretics and (usually) digitalis. The recommended starting dose is 5 mg once a day.

When initiating treatment with lisinopril in patients with heart failure, the initial dose should be administered under medical observation, especially in those patients with low blood pressure (systolic blood pressure below 100 mmHg). The mean peak blood pressure lowering occurs six to eight hours after dosing. Observation should continue until blood pressure is stable. The concomitant diuretic dose should be reduced, if possible, to help minimize hypovolemia which may contribute to hypotension. (See WARNINGS and PRECAUTIONS, **Drug Interactions**.) The appearance of hypotension after the initial dose of PRINIVIL does not preclude subsequent careful dose titration with the drug, following effective management of the hypotension.

The usual effective dosage range is 5 to 20 mg per day administered as a single daily dose.

Dosage Adjustment in Patients with Heart Failure and Renal Impairment or Hyponatremia: In patients with heart failure who have hyponatremia (serum sodium <130 mEq/L) or moderate to severe renal impairment (creatinine clearance ≤30 mL/min or serum creatinine >3 mg/dL), therapy with PRINIVIL should be initiated at a dose of 2.5 mg once a day under close medical supervision. (See WARNINGS and PRECAUTIONS, **Drug Interactions**.)

Acute Myocardial Infarction

In hemodynamically stable patients within 24 hours of the onset of symptoms of acute myocardial infarction, the first dose of PRINIVIL is 5 mg given orally, followed by 5 mg after 24 hours, 10 mg after 48 hours and then 10 mg of PRINIVIL once daily. Dosing should continue for six weeks. Patients should receive, as appropriate, the standard recommended treatments such as thrombolytics, aspirin and beta-blockers. Patients with a low systolic blood pressure (≤120 mmHg) when treatment is started or during the first 3 days after the infarct should be given a lower 2.5 mg oral dose of PRINIVIL (see WARNINGS). If hypotension occurs (systolic blood pressure ≤100 mmHg) a daily maintenance dose of 5 mg may be given with temporary reductions to 2.5 mg if needed. If prolonged hypotension occurs (systolic blood pressure <90 mmHg for more than 1 hour) PRINIVIL should be withdrawn. For patients who develop symptoms of heart failure, see DOSAGE AND ADMINISTRATION, **Heart Failure**.

Dosage Adjustment in Patients with Myocardial Infarction with Renal Impairment: In acute myocardial infarction, treatment with PRINIVIL should be initiated with caution in patients with evidence of renal dysfunction, defined as serum creatinine concentration exceeding 2 mg/dL. No evaluation of dosage adjustment in myocardial infarction patients with severe renal impairment has been performed.

Use in Elderly

In general, blood pressure response and adverse experiences were similar in younger and older patients given similar doses of PRINIVIL. Pharmacokinetic studies, however, indicate that maximum blood levels and area under the plasma concentration time curve (AUC) are doubled in older patients, so that dosage adjustments should be made with particular caution.

Pediatric Hypertensive Patients ≥6 years of age

The usual recommended starting dose is 0.07 mg/kg once daily (up to 5 mg total). Dosage should be adjusted according to blood pressure response. Doses above 0.61 mg/kg (or in excess of 40 mg) have not been studied in pediatric patients. (See CLINICAL PHARMACOLOGY, **Pharmacokinetics and Metabolism and Pharmacodynamics and Clinical Effects.**)

PRINIVIL is not recommended in pediatric patients <6 years or in pediatric patients with glomerular filtration rate <30 mL/min/1.73 m^2 (see CLINICAL PHARMACOLOGY, **Pharmacokinetics and Metabolism, Pharmacodynamics and Clinical Effects** and PRECAUTIONS).

Preparation of Suspension (for 200 mL of a 1.0 mg/mL suspension)

Add 10 mL of Purified Water USP to a polyethylene terephthalate (PET) bottle containing ten 20-mg tablets of PRINIVIL and shake for at least one minute. Add 30 mL of Bicitra®[2] diluent and 160 mL of Ora-Sweet SF™[3] to the concentrate in the PET bottle and gently shake for several seconds to disperse the ingredients. The suspension should be stored at or below 25°C (77°F) and can be stored for up to four weeks. Shake the suspension before each use.

[2] Registered trademark of Alza Corporation
[3] Trademark of Paddock Laboratories, Inc.

HOW SUPPLIED

No. 8110—Tablets PRINIVIL, 5 mg, are white, oval shaped compressed tablets with code MSD 19 on one side and scored on the other side. They are supplied as follows:
NDC 0006-0019-54 unit of use bottles of 90.

No. 8111—Tablets PRINIVIL, 10 mg, are light yellow, oval shaped compressed tablets with code MSD 106 on one side and scored on the other side. They are supplied as follows:
NDC 0006-0106-54 unit of use bottles of 90.

No. 8112—Tablets PRINIVIL, 20 mg, are peach, oval shaped compressed tablets with code MSD 207 on one side and scored on the other side. They are supplied as follows:
NDC 0006-0207-54 unit of use bottles of 90.

Storage

Store at controlled room temperature, 15-30°C (59-86°F), and protect from moisture.

Dispense in a tight container, if product package is subdivided.

Manuf. for: Merck Sharp & Dohme Corp., a subsidiary of **MERCK & CO., INC.**, Whitehouse Station, NJ 08889, USA
by:
MERCK SHARP & DOHME LTD.
Cramlington, Northumberland, UK NE23 3JU
Issued February 2010
9763204

Shown in Product Identification Guide, page 313

PRINZIDE® TABLETS ℞

[prin-zide]
(lisinopril-hydrochlorothiazide)

> **USE IN PREGNANCY**
> **When used in pregnancy during the second and third trimesters, ACE inhibitors can cause injury and even death to the developing fetus.** When pregnancy is detected, PRINZIDE should be discontinued as soon as possible. See WARNINGS, **Pregnancy, Lisinopril, Fetal/Neonatal Morbidity and Mortality.**

DESCRIPTION

PRINZIDE[1] (Lisinopril-Hydrochlorothiazide) combines an angiotensin converting enzyme inhibitor, lisinopril, and a diuretic, hydrochlorothiazide.

Lisinopril, a synthetic peptide derivative, is an oral long-acting angiotensin converting enzyme inhibitor. It is chemically described as (*S*)-1-[N^2-(1-carboxy-3-phenylpropyl)-L-lysyl]-L-proline dihydrate. Its empirical formula is $C_{21}H_{31}N_3O_5 \cdot 2H_2O$ and its structural formula is:

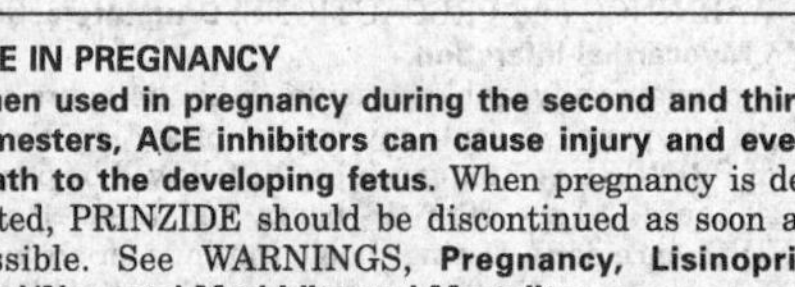

Lisinopril is a white to off-white, crystalline powder, with a molecular weight of 441.52. It is soluble in water, sparingly soluble in methanol, and practically insoluble in ethanol.

Hydrochlorothiazide is 6-chloro-3,4-dihydro-2*H*-1,2,4-benzothiadiazine-7-sulfonamide 1,1-dioxide. Its empirical formula is $C_7H_8ClN_3O_4S_2$ and its structural formula is:

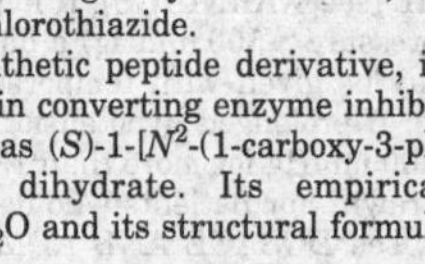

Hydrochlorothiazide is a white, or practically white, crystalline powder with a molecular weight of 297.73, which is slightly soluble in water, but freely soluble in sodium hydroxide solution.

PRINZIDE is available for oral use in three tablet combinations of lisinopril with hydrochlorothiazide: PRINZIDE 10-12.5, containing 10 mg lisinopril and 12.5 mg hydrochlorothiazide, PRINZIDE 20-12.5, containing 20 mg lisinopril and 12.5 mg hydrochlorothiazide and PRINZIDE 20-25, containing 20 mg lisinopril and 25 mg hydrochlorothiazide.

Inactive ingredients are calcium phosphate, magnesium stearate, mannitol, and starch. PRINZIDE 10-12.5 also contains FD&C Blue #2 aluminum lake. PRINZIDE 20-12.5 and PRINZIDE 20-25 also contain iron oxide.

[1] Registered trademark of Merck Sharp & Dohme Corp., a subsidiary of **Merck & Co., Inc.**
Copyright © 1989, 1992, 2005, 2006 Merck Sharp & Dohme Corp., a subsidiary of **Merck & Co., Inc.**
All rights reserved

CLINICAL PHARMACOLOGY

Lisinopril-Hydrochlorothiazide

As a result of its diuretic effects, hydrochlorothiazide increases plasma renin activity, increases aldosterone secretion, and decreases serum potassium. Administration of lisinopril blocks the renin-angiotensin-aldosterone axis and tends to reverse the potassium loss associated with the diuretic.

In clinical studies, the extent of blood pressure reduction seen with the combination of lisinopril and hydrochlorothiazide was approximately additive. The PRINZIDE 10-12.5 combination worked equally well in Black and Caucasian patients. The PRINZIDE 20-12.5 and PRINZIDE 20-25 combinations appeared somewhat less effective in Black patients, but relatively few Black patients were studied. In most patients, the antihypertensive effect of PRINZIDE was sustained for at least 24 hours.

In a randomized, controlled comparison, the mean antihypertensive effects of PRINZIDE 20-12.5 and PRINZIDE 20-25 were similar, suggesting that many patients who respond adequately to the latter combination may be controlled with PRINZIDE 20-12.5. (See DOSAGE AND ADMINISTRATION.)

Concomitant administration of lisinopril and hydrochlorothiazide has little or no effect on the bioavailability of either drug. The combination tablet is bioequivalent to concomitant administration of the separate entities.

Lisinopril

Mechanism of Action

Lisinopril inhibits angiotensin-converting enzyme (ACE) in human subjects and animals. ACE is a peptidyl dipeptidase that catalyzes the conversion of angiotensin I to the vasoconstrictor substance, angiotensin II. Angiotensin II also stimulates aldosterone secretion by the adrenal cortex. Inhibition of ACE results in decreased plasma angiotensin II which leads to decreased vasopressor activity and to decreased aldosterone secretion. The latter decrease may result in a small increase of serum potassium. Removal of angiotensin II negative feedback on renin secretion leads to increased plasma renin activity. In hypertensive patients with normal renal function treated with lisinopril alone for up to 24 weeks, the mean increase in serum potassium was less than 0.1 mEq/L; however, approximately 15 percent of patients had increases greater than 0.5 mEq/L and approximately six percent had a decrease greater than 0.5 mEq/L. In the same study, patients treated with lisinopril plus a thiazide diuretic showed essentially no change in serum potassium. (See PRECAUTIONS.)

ACE is identical to kininase, an enzyme that degrades bradykinin. Whether increased levels of bradykinin, a potent vasodepressor peptide, play a role in the therapeutic effects of lisinopril remains to be elucidated.

While the mechanism through which lisinopril lowers blood pressure is believed to be primarily suppression of the renin-angiotensin-aldosterone system, lisinopril is antihypertensive even in patients with low-renin hypertension. Although lisinopril was antihypertensive in all races studied, Black hypertensive patients (usually a low-renin hypertensive population) had a smaller average response to lisinopril monotherapy than non-Black patients.

Pharmacokinetics and Metabolism

Following oral administration of lisinopril, peak serum concentrations occur within about 7 hours. Declining serum concentrations exhibit a prolonged terminal phase which does not contribute to drug accumulation. This terminal phase probably represents saturable binding to ACE and is not proportional to dose. Lisinopril does not appear to be bound to other serum proteins.

Lisinopril does not undergo metabolism and is excreted unchanged entirely in the urine. Based on urinary recovery, the mean extent of absorption of lisinopril is approximately 25 percent, with large intersubject variability (6-60 percent) at all doses tested (5-80 mg). Lisinopril absorption is not influenced by the presence of food in the gastrointestinal tract.

Upon multiple dosing, lisinopril exhibits an effective half-life of accumulation of 12 hours.

Impaired renal function decreases elimination of lisinopril, which is excreted principally through the kidneys, but this decrease becomes clinically important only when the glomerular filtration rate is below 30 mL/min. Above this glomerular filtration rate, the elimination half-life is little changed. With greater impairment, however, peak and trough lisinopril levels increase, time to peak concentration increases and time to attain steady state is prolonged. Older patients, on average, have (approximately doubled) higher blood levels and area under the plasma concentration time curve (AUC) than younger patients. (See DOSAGE AND ADMINISTRATION.) Lisinopril can be removed by hemodialysis.

Studies in rats indicate that lisinopril crosses the blood-brain barrier poorly. Multiple doses of lisinopril in rats do not result in accumulation in any tissues. However, milk of lactating rats contains radioactivity following administration of ^{14}C lisinopril. By whole body autoradiography, radioactivity was found in the placenta following administration of labeled drug to pregnant rats, but none was found in the fetuses.

Pharmacodynamics

Administration of lisinopril to patients with hypertension results in a reduction of supine and standing blood pressure to about the same extent with no compensatory tachycardia. Symptomatic postural hypotension is usually not observed although it can occur and should be anticipated in volume and/or salt-depleted patients. (See WARNINGS.)

In most patients studied, onset of antihypertensive activity was seen at one hour after oral administration of an individual dose of lisinopril, with peak reduction of blood pressure achieved by six hours.

In some patients achievement of optimal blood pressure reduction may require two to four weeks of therapy.

At recommended single daily doses, antihypertensive effects have been maintained for at least 24 hours after dosing, although the effect at 24 hours was substantially smaller than the effect six hours after dosing.

The antihypertensive effects of lisinopril have continued during long-term therapy. Abrupt withdrawal of lisinopril has not been associated with a rapid increase in blood pressure; nor with a significant overshoot of pretreatment blood pressure.

In hemodynamic studies in patients with essential hypertension, blood pressure reduction was accompanied by a reduction in peripheral arterial resistance with little or no change in cardiac output and in heart rate. In a study in nine hypertensive patients, following administration of lisinopril, there was an increase in mean renal blood flow that was not significant. Data from several small studies are inconsistent with respect to the effect of lisinopril on glomerular filtration rate in hypertensive patients with normal renal function, but suggest that changes, if any, are not large.

In patients with renovascular hypertension lisinopril has been shown to be well tolerated and effective in controlling blood pressure (see PRECAUTIONS).

Hydrochlorothiazide

The mechanism of the antihypertensive effect of thiazides is unknown. Thiazides do not usually affect normal blood pressure.

Hydrochlorothiazide is a diuretic and antihypertensive. It affects the distal renal tubular mechanism of electrolyte reabsorption. Hydrochlorothiazide increases excretion of sodium and chloride in approximately equivalent amounts. Natriuresis may be accompanied by some loss of potassium and bicarbonate.

After oral use diuresis begins within two hours, peaks in about four hours and lasts about 6 to 12 hours.

Hydrochlorothiazide is not metabolized but is eliminated rapidly by the kidney. When plasma levels have been followed for at least 24 hours, the plasma half-life has been observed to vary between 5.6 and 14.8 hours. At least 61 percent of the oral dose is eliminated unchanged within 24 hours. Hydrochlorothiazide crosses the placental but not the blood-brain barrier.

INDICATIONS AND USAGE

PRINZIDE is indicated for the treatment of hypertension.

These fixed-dose combinations are not indicated for initial therapy (see DOSAGE AND ADMINISTRATION).

In using PRINZIDE, consideration should be given to the fact that an angiotensin converting enzyme inhibitor, captopril, has caused agranulocytosis, particularly in patients with renal impairment or collagen vascular disease, and that available data are insufficient to show that lisinopril does not have a similar risk. (See WARNINGS.)

In considering use of PRINZIDE, it should be noted that Black patients receiving ACE inhibitors have been reported to have a higher incidence of angioedema compared to non-Blacks. (See WARNINGS, **Head and Neck Angioedema.**)

CONTRAINDICATIONS

PRINZIDE is contraindicated in patients who are hypersensitive to any component of this product and in patients with a history of angioedema related to previous treatment with an angiotensin converting enzyme inhibitor and in patients with hereditary or idiopathic angioedema. Because of the hydrochlorothiazide component, this product is contraindicated in patients with anuria or hypersensitivity to other sulfonamide-derived drugs.

WARNINGS

General

Lisinopril

Anaphylactoid and Possibly Related Reactions:
Presumably because angiotensin-converting enzyme inhibitors affect the metabolism of eicosanoids and polypeptides, including endogenous bradykinin, patients receiving ACE inhibitors (including PRINZIDE) may be subject to a variety of adverse reactions, some of them serious.

Head and Neck Angioedema: Angioedema of the face, extremities, lips, tongue, glottis and/or larynx has been reported rarely in patients treated with angiotensin converting enzyme inhibitors, including lisinopril. This may occur at any time during treatment. ACE inhibitors have been associated with a higher rate of angioedema in Black than in non-Black patients. In such cases PRINZIDE should be promptly discontinued and appropriate therapy and monitoring should be provided until complete and sustained resolution of signs and symptoms has occurred. Even in those instances where swelling of only the tongue is involved, without respiratory distress, patients may require prolonged observation since treatment with antihistamines and corticosteroids may not be sufficient. Very rarely, fatalities have been reported due to angioedema associated with laryngeal edema or tongue edema. Patients with involvement of the tongue, glottis or larynx are likely to experience airway obstruction, especially those with a history of airway surgery. **Where there is involvement of the tongue, glottis or larynx, likely to cause airway obstruction, subcutaneous epinephrine solution 1:1000 (0.3 mL to 0.5 mL) and/or measures necessary to ensure a patent airway, should be promptly provided.** (See ADVERSE REACTIONS.)

Patients with a history of angioedema unrelated to ACE-inhibitor therapy may be at increased risk of angioedema while receiving an ACE inhibitor (see also INDICATIONS AND USAGE and CONTRAINDICATIONS).

Intestinal Angioedema: Intestinal angioedema has been reported in patients treated with ACE inhibitors. These patients presented with abdominal pain (with or without nausea or vomiting); in some cases there was no prior history of facial angioedema and C-1 esterase levels were normal. The angioedema was diagnosed by procedures including abdominal CT scan or ultrasound, or at surgery, and symptoms resolved after stopping the ACE inhibitor. Intestinal angioedema should be included in the differential diagnosis of patients on ACE inhibitors presenting with abdominal pain.

Anaphylactoid reactions during desensitization: Two patients undergoing desensitizing treatment with hymenoptera venom while receiving ACE inhibitors sustained life-threatening anaphylactoid reactions. In the same patients, these reactions were avoided when ACE inhibitors were temporarily withheld, but they reappeared upon inadvertent rechallenge.

Anaphylactoid reactions during membrane exposure:
Anaphylactoid reactions have been reported in patients dialyzed with high-flux membranes and treated concomitantly with an ACE inhibitor. Anaphylactoid reactions have also been reported in patients undergoing low-density lipoprotein apheresis with dextran sulfate absorption.

Hypotension and Related Effects

Excessive hypotension was rarely seen in uncomplicated hypertensive patients but is a possible consequence of lisinopril use in salt/volume-depleted persons, such as those treated vigorously with diuretics or patients on dialysis. (See PRECAUTIONS, **Drug Interactions** and ADVERSE REACTIONS.)

Syncope has been reported in 0.8 percent of patients receiving PRINZIDE. In patients with hypertension receiving lisinopril alone, the incidence of syncope was 0.1 percent. The overall incidence of syncope may be reduced by proper titration of the individual components. (See PRECAUTIONS, **Drug Interactions**, ADVERSE REACTIONS and DOSAGE AND ADMINISTRATION.)

In patients with severe congestive heart failure, with or without associated renal insufficiency, excessive hypotension has been observed and may be associated with oliguria and/or progressive azotemia, and rarely with acute renal failure and/or death. Because of the potential fall in blood pressure in these patients, therapy should be started under very close medical supervision. Such patients should be followed closely for the first two weeks of treatment and whenever the dose of lisinopril and/or diuretic is increased. Similar considerations apply to patients with ischemic heart or cerebrovascular disease in whom an excessive fall in blood pressure could result in a myocardial infarction or cerebrovascular accident.

If hypotension occurs, the patient should be placed in supine position and, if necessary, receive an intravenous infusion of normal saline. A transient hypotensive response is not a contraindication to further doses which usually can be given without difficulty once the blood pressure has increased after volume expansion.

Neutropenia/Agranulocytosis

Another angiotensin converting enzyme inhibitor, captopril, has been shown to cause agranulocytosis and bone marrow depression, rarely in uncomplicated patients but more frequently in patients with renal impairment, especially if they also have a collagen vascular disease. Available data from clinical trials of lisinopril are insufficient to show that lisinopril does not cause agranulocytosis at similar rates. Marketing experience has revealed rare cases of neutropenia and bone marrow depression in which a causal relationship to lisinopril cannot be excluded. Periodic monitoring of white blood cell counts in patients with collagen vascular disease and renal disease should be considered.

Hepatic Failure

Rarely, ACE inhibitors have been associated with a syndrome that starts with cholestatic jaundice or hepatitis and progresses to fulminant hepatic necrosis, and (sometimes) death. The mechanism of this syndrome is not understood. Patients receiving ACE inhibitors who develop jaundice or marked elevations of hepatic enzymes should discontinue the ACE inhibitor and receive appropriate medical follow-up.

Hydrochlorothiazide

Thiazides should be used with caution in severe renal disease. In patients with renal disease, thiazides may precipitate azotemia. Cumulative effects of the drug may develop in patients with impaired renal function.

Thiazides should be used with caution in patients with impaired hepatic function or progressive liver disease, since minor alterations of fluid and electrolyte balance may precipitate hepatic coma.

Sensitivity reactions may occur in patients with or without a history of allergy or bronchial asthma.

The possibility of exacerbation or activation of systemic lupus erythematosus has been reported.

Lithium generally should not be given with thiazides (see PRECAUTIONS, **Drug Interactions, Lisinopril** and **Hydrochlorothiazide**).

Pregnancy

Lisinopril-Hydrochlorothiazide

Teratogenicity studies were conducted in mice and rats with up to 90 mg/kg/day of lisinopril in combination with 10 mg/kg/day of hydrochlorothiazide. This dose of lisinopril is 5 times (in mice) and 10 times (in rats) the maximum recommended human daily dose (MRHDD) when compared on a body surface area basis (mg/m^2); the dose of hydrochlorothiazide is 0.9 times (in mice) and 1.8 times (in rats) the MRHDD. Maternal or fetotoxic effects were not seen in mice with the combination. In rats decreased maternal weight gain and decreased fetal weight occurred down to 3/10 mg/kg/day (the lowest dose tested). Associated with the decreased fetal weight was a delay in fetal ossification. The decreased fetal weight and delay in fetal ossification were not seen in saline-supplemented animals given 90/10 mg/kg/day.

When used in pregnancy during the second and third trimesters, ACE inhibitors can cause injury and even death to the developing fetus. When pregnancy is detected, PRINZIDE should be discontinued as soon as possible. (See **Lisinopril, Fetal/Neonatal Morbidity and Mortality,** below.)

Lisinopril

Fetal/Neonatal Morbidity and Mortality: ACE inhibitors can cause fetal and neonatal morbidity and death when administered to pregnant women. Several dozen cases have been reported in the world literature. When pregnancy is detected, ACE inhibitors should be discontinued as soon as possible.

In a published retrospective epidemiological study, infants whose mothers had taken an ACE inhibitor drug during the first trimester of pregnancy appeared to have an increased risk of major congenital malformations compared with infants whose mothers had not undergone first trimester exposure to ACE inhibitor drugs. The number of cases of birth defects is small and the findings of this study have not yet been repeated.

The use of ACE inhibitors during the second and third trimesters of pregnancy has been associated with fetal and neonatal injury, including hypotension, neonatal skull hypoplasia, anuria, reversible or irreversible renal failure, and death. Oligohydramnios has also been reported, presumably resulting from decreased fetal renal function; oligohydramnios in this setting has been associated with fetal limb contractures, craniofacial deformation, and hypoplastic lung development. Prematurity, intrauterine growth retardation, and patent ductus arteriosus have also been reported, although it is not clear whether these occurrences were due to the ACE-inhibitor exposure.

These adverse effects do not appear to have resulted from intrauterine ACE-inhibitor exposure that has been limited to the first trimester. Mothers whose embryos and fetuses are exposed to ACE inhibitors only during the first trimester should be so informed. Nonetheless, when patients become pregnant, physicians should make every effort to discontinue the use of PRINZIDE as soon as possible.

Rarely (probably less often than once in every thousand pregnancies), no alternative to ACE inhibitors will be found. In these rare cases, the mothers should be apprised of the potential hazards to their fetuses, and serial ultrasound examinations should be performed to assess the intraamniotic environment.

If oligohydramnios is observed, PRINZIDE should be discontinued unless it is considered lifesaving for the mother. Contraction stress testing (CST), a non-stress test (NST), or biophysical profiling (BPP) may be appropriate, depending upon the week of pregnancy. Patients and physicians should be aware, however, that oligohydramnios may not appear until after the fetus has sustained irreversible injury.

Infants with histories of *in utero* exposure to ACE inhibitors should be closely observed for hypotension, oliguria, and hyperkalemia. If oliguria occurs, attention should be directed toward support of blood pressure and renal perfusion. Exchange transfusion or dialysis may be required as means of reversing hypotension and/or substituting for disordered renal function. Lisinopril, which crosses the placenta, has been removed from neonatal circulation by peritoneal dialysis with some clinical benefit, and theoretically may be removed by exchange transfusion, although there is no experience with the latter procedure.

No teratogenic effects of lisinopril were seen in studies of pregnant mice, rats, and rabbits. On a body surface area basis, the doses used were up 55 times, 33 times, and 0.15 times, respectively, the MRHDD.

Hydrochlorothiazide

Studies in which hydrochlorothiazide was orally administered to pregnant mice and rats during their respective periods of major organogenesis at doses up to 3000 and 1000 mg/kg/day, respectively, provided no evidence of harm to the fetus. These doses are more than 150 times the MRHDD on a body surface area basis. Thiazides cross the placental barrier and appear in cord blood. There is a risk of fetal or neonatal jaundice, thrombocytopenia and possibly other adverse reactions that have occurred in adults.

PRECAUTIONS

General

Lisinopril

Aortic Stenosis/Hypertrophic Cardiomyopathy: As with all vasodilators, lisinopril should be given with caution to patients with obstruction in the outflow tract of the left ventricle.

Impaired Renal Function: As a consequence of inhibiting the renin-angiotensin-aldosterone system, changes in renal function may be anticipated in susceptible individuals. In patients with severe congestive heart failure whose renal function may depend on the activity of the renin-angiotensin-aldosterone system, treatment with angiotensin converting enzyme inhibitors, including lisinopril, may be associated with oliguria and/or progressive azotemia and rarely with acute renal failure and/or death.

In hypertensive patients with unilateral or bilateral renal artery stenosis, increases in blood urea nitrogen and serum creatinine may occur. Experience with another angiotensin converting enzyme inhibitor suggests that these increases are usually reversible upon discontinuation of lisinopril and/or diuretic therapy. In such patients renal function should be monitored during the first few weeks of therapy.

Some hypertensive patients with no apparent pre-existing renal vascular disease have developed increases in blood urea and serum creatinine, usually minor and transient, especially when lisinopril has been given concomitantly with a diuretic. This is more likely to occur in patients with pre-existing renal impairment. Dosage reduction of lisinopril and/or discontinuation of the diuretic may be required.

Evaluation of the hypertensive patient should always include assessment of renal function. (See DOSAGE AND ADMINISTRATION.)

Hyperkalemia: In clinical trials hyperkalemia (serum potassium greater than 5.7 mEq/L) occurred in approximately 1.4 percent of hypertensive patients treated with lisinopril plus hydrochlorothiazide. In most cases these were isolated values which resolved despite continued therapy. Hyperkalemia was not a cause of discontinuation of therapy. Risk factors for the development of hyperkalemia include renal insufficiency, diabetes mellitus, and the concomitant use of potassium-sparing diuretics, potassium supplements and/or potassium-containing salt substitutes. Hyperkalemia can cause serious, sometimes fatal, arrhythmias. PRINZIDE should be used cautiously, if at all, with these agents and with frequent monitoring of serum potassium. (See **Drug Interactions.**)

Cough: Presumably due to the inhibition of the degradation of endogenous bradykinin, persistent nonproductive cough has been reported with all ACE inhibitors, always resolving after discontinuation of therapy. ACE inhibitor-induced cough should be considered in the differential diagnosis of cough.

Surgery/Anesthesia: In patients undergoing major surgery or during anesthesia with agents that produce hypotension, lisinopril may block angiotensin II formation secondary to compensatory renin release. If hypotension occurs and is considered to be due to this mechanism, it can be corrected by volume expansion.

Hydrochlorothiazide Periodic determination of serum electrolytes to detect possible electrolyte imbalance should be performed at appropriate intervals.

All patients receiving thiazide therapy should be observed for clinical signs of fluid or electrolyte imbalance: namely, hyponatremia, hypochloremic alkalosis, and hypokalemia. Serum and urine electrolyte determinations are particularly important when the patient is vomiting excessively or receiving parenteral fluids. Warning signs or symptoms of fluid and electrolyte imbalance, irrespective of cause, include dryness of mouth, thirst, weakness, lethargy, drowsiness, restlessness, confusion, seizures, muscle pains or cramps, muscular fatigue, hypotension, oliguria, tachycardia, and gastrointestinal disturbances such as nausea and vomiting.

Hypokalemia may develop, especially with brisk diuresis, when severe cirrhosis is present, or after prolonged therapy. Interference with adequate oral electrolyte intake will also contribute to hypokalemia. Hypokalemia may cause cardiac arrhythmia and may also sensitize or exaggerate the response of the heart to the toxic effects of digitalis (e.g., increased ventricular irritability). Because lisinopril reduces the production of aldosterone, concomitant therapy with lisinopril attenuates the diuretic-induced potassium loss (see **Drug Interactions, Agents Increasing Serum Potassium**).

Although any chloride deficit is generally mild and usually does not require specific treatment, except under extraordinary circumstances (as in liver disease or renal disease), chloride replacement may be required in the treatment of metabolic alkalosis.

Dilutional hyponatremia may occur in edematous patients in hot weather; appropriate therapy is water restriction, rather than administration of salt except in rare instances when the hyponatremia is life-threatening. In actual salt depletion, appropriate replacement is the therapy of choice.

Hyperuricemia may occur or frank gout may be precipitated in certain patients receiving thiazide therapy.

In diabetic patients dosage adjustments of insulin or oral hypoglycemic agents may be required. Hyperglycemia may occur with thiazide diuretics. Thus latent diabetes mellitus may become manifest during thiazide therapy.

The antihypertensive effects of the drug may be enhanced in the postsympathectomy patient.

If progressive renal impairment becomes evident consider withholding or discontinuing diuretic therapy.

Thiazides have been shown to increase the urinary excretion of magnesium; this may result in hypomagnesemia.

Thiazides may decrease urinary calcium excretion. Thiazides may cause intermittent and slight elevation of serum calcium in the absence of known disorders of calcium metabolism. Marked hypercalcemia may be evidence of hidden hyperparathyroidism. Thiazides should be discontinued before carrying out tests for parathyroid function.

Increases in cholesterol and triglyceride levels may be associated with thiazide diuretic therapy.

Information for Patients

Angioedema:

Angioedema, including laryngeal edema, may occur at any time during treatment with angiotensin converting enzyme inhibitors, including lisinopril. Patients should be so advised and told to report immediately any signs or symptoms suggesting angioedema (swelling of face, extremities, eyes, lips, tongue, difficulty in swallowing or breathing) and to take no more drug until they have consulted with the prescribing physician.

Symptomatic Hypotension: Patients should be cautioned to report lightheadedness especially during the first few days of therapy. If actual syncope occurs, the patients should be told to discontinue the drug until they have consulted with the prescribing physician.

All patients should be cautioned that excessive perspiration and dehydration may lead to an excessive fall in blood pressure because of reduction in fluid volume. Other causes of volume depletion such as vomiting or diarrhea may also lead to a fall in blood pressure; patients should be advised to consult with their physician.

Hyperkalemia: Patients should be told not to use salt substitutes containing potassium without consulting their physician.

Neutropenia: Patients should be told to report promptly any indication of infection (e.g., sore throat, fever) which may be a sign of neutropenia.

Pregnancy: Female patients of childbearing age should be told about the consequences of exposure to ACE inhibitors during pregnancy. These patients should be asked to report pregnancies to their physicians as soon as possible.

NOTE: As with many other drugs, certain advice to patients being treated with PRINZIDE is warranted. This information is intended to aid in the safe and effective use of this medication. It is not a disclosure of all possible adverse or intended effects.

Drug Interactions

Lisinopril

Hypotension — Patients on Diuretic Therapy: Patients on diuretics, and especially those in whom diuretic therapy was recently instituted, may occasionally experience an excessive reduction of blood pressure after initiation of therapy with lisinopril. The possibility of hypotensive effects with lisinopril can be minimized by either discontinuing the diuretic or increasing the salt intake prior to initiation of treatment with lisinopril. If it is necessary to continue the diuretic, initiate therapy with lisinopril at a dose of 5 mg daily, and provide close medical supervision after the initial dose for at least two hours and until blood pressure has stabilized for at least an additional hour. (See WARNINGS and DOSAGE AND ADMINISTRATION.) When a diuretic is added to the therapy of a patient receiving lisinopril, an additional antihypertensive effect is usually observed. (See DOSAGE AND ADMINISTRATION.)

Non-steroidal Anti-inflammatory Agents Including Selective Cyclooxygenase-2 (COX-2) Inhibitors: Reports suggest that NSAIDs including selective COX-2 inhibitors may diminish the antihypertensive effect of ACE inhibitors, including lisinopril. This interaction should be given consideration in patients taking NSAIDs or selective COX-2 inhibitors concomitantly with ACE inhibitors.

In some patients with compromised renal function (e.g., elderly patients or patients who are volume-depleted, including those on diuretic therapy) who are being treated with non-steroidal anti-inflammatory drugs, including selective COX-2 inhibitors, the co-administration of angiotensin II receptor antagonists or ACE inhibitors, may result in a further deterioration of renal function, including possible acute renal failure. These effects are usually reversible.

These interactions should be considered in patients taking NSAIDS including selective COX-2 inhibitors concomitantly with diuretics and angiotensin II antagonists or ACE inhibitors. Therefore, monitor effects on blood pressure and renal function when administering the combination, especially in the elderly.

Other Agents: Lisinopril has been used concomitantly with nitrates

and/or digoxin without evidence of clinically significant adverse interactions. No meaningful clinically important pharmacokinetic interactions occurred when lisinopril was used concomitantly with propranolol, digoxin, or hydrochlorothiazide. The presence of food in the stomach does not alter the bioavailability of lisinopril.

Agents Increasing Serum Potassium: Lisinopril attenuates potassium loss caused by thiazide-type diuretics. Use of lisinopril with potassium-sparing diuretics (e.g., spironolactone, eplerenone, triamterene, or amiloride), potassium supplements, or potassium-containing salt substitutes may lead to significant increases in serum potassium. Therefore, if concomitant use of these agents is indicated, because of demonstrated hypokalemia, they should be used with caution and with frequent monitoring of serum potassium.

Lithium: Lithium toxicity has been reported in patients receiving lithium concomitantly with drugs which cause elimination of sodium, including ACE inhibitors. Lithium toxicity was usually reversible upon discontinuation of lithium and the ACE inhibitor. It is recommended that serum lithium levels be monitored frequently if lisinopril is administered concomitantly with lithium.

Gold: Nitritoid reactions (symptoms include facial flushing, nausea, vomiting and hypotension) have been reported rarely in patients on therapy with injectable gold (sodium aurothiomalate) and concomitant ACE inhibitor therapy including PRINZIDE.

Hydrochlorothiazide

When administered concurrently the following drugs may interact with thiazide diuretics.

Alcohol, barbiturates, or narcotics—potentiation of orthostatic hypotension may occur.

Antidiabetic drugs (oral agents and insulin)—dosage adjustment of the antidiabetic drug may be required.

Other antihypertensive drugs—additive effect or potentiation.

Cholestyramine and colestipol resins—Absorption of hydrochlorothiazide is impaired in the presence of anionic exchange resins. Single doses of either cholestyramine or colestipol resins bind the hydrochlorothiazide and reduce its absorption from the gastrointestinal tract by up to 85 and 43 percent, respectively.

Corticosteroids, ACTH—intensified electrolyte depletion, particularly hypokalemia.

Pressor amines (e.g., norepinephrine)—possible decreased response to pressor amines but not sufficient to preclude their use.

Skeletal muscle relaxants, nondepolarizing (e.g., tubocurarine)—possible increased responsiveness to the muscle relaxant.

Lithium—should not generally be given with diuretics. Diuretic agents reduce the renal clearance of lithium and add a high risk of lithium toxicity. Refer to the package insert for lithium preparations before use of such preparations with PRINZIDE.

Non-steroidal Anti-inflammatory Drugs—In some patients, the administration of a non-steroidal anti-inflammatory agent can reduce the diuretic, natriuretic, and antihypertensive effects of loop, potassium-sparing and thiazide diuretics. Therefore, when PRINZIDE and non-steroidal anti-inflammatory agents are used concomitantly, the patient should be observed closely to determine if the desired effect of PRINZIDE is obtained.

Carcinogenesis, Mutagenesis, Impairment of Fertility

Lisinopril-Hydrochlorothiazide

Lisinopril in combination with hydrochlorothiazide was not mutagenic in a microbial mutagen test using *Salmonella typhimurium* (Ames test) or *Escherichia coli* with or without metabolic activation or in a forward mutation assay using Chinese hamster lung cells. Lisinopril-hydrochlorothiazide did not produce DNA single strand breaks in an *in vitro* alkaline elution rat hepatocyte assay. In addition, it did not produce increases in chromosomal aberrations in an *in vitro* test in Chinese hamster ovary cells or in an *in vivo* study in mouse bone marrow.

Lisinopril

There was no evidence of a tumorigenic effect when lisinopril was administered orally for 105 weeks to male and female rats at doses up to 90 mg/kg/day or for 92 weeks to male and female mice at doses up to 135 mg/kg/day. These doses are 10 times and 7 times, respectively, the maximum recommended human daily dose (MRHDD) when compared on a body surface area basis.

Lisinopril was not mutagenic in the Ames microbial mutagen test with or without metabolic activation. It was also negative in a forward mutation assay using Chinese hamster lung cells. Lisinopril did not produce single strand DNA breaks in an *in vitro* alkaline elution rat hepatocyte assay. In addition, lisinopril did not produce increases in chromosomal aberrations in an *in vitro* test in Chinese hamster ovary cells or in an *in vivo* study in mouse bone marrow.

There were no adverse effects on reproductive performance in male and female rats treated with up to 300 mg/kg/day of lisinopril (33 times the MRHDD when compared on a body surface area basis).

Hydrochlorothiazide

Two-year feeding studies in mice and rats conducted under the auspices of the National Toxicology Program (NTP) uncovered no evidence of a carcinogenic potential of hydrochlorothiazide in female mice at doses of up to approximately 600 mg/kg/day (53 times the MRHDD when compared on a body surface area basis) or in male and female rats at doses of up to approximately 100 mg/kg/day (18 times the MRHDD when compared on a body surface area basis). The NTP, however, found equivocal evidence for hepatocarcinogenicity in male mice.

Hydrochlorothiazide was not genotoxic *in vitro* in the Ames mutagenicity assay of *Salmonella typhimurium* strains TA 98, TA 100, TA 1535, TA 1537, and TA 1538 and in the Chinese Hamster Ovary (CHO) test for chromosomal aberrations, or *in vivo* in assays using mouse germinal cell chromosomes, Chinese hamster bone marrow chromosomes, and the *Drosophila* sex-linked recessive lethal trait gene. Positive test results were obtained only in the *in vitro* CHO Sister Chromatid Exchange (clastogenicity) and in the Mouse Lymphoma Cell (mutagenicity) assays, using concentrations of hydrochlorothiazide from 43 to 1300 µg/mL, and in the *Aspergillus nidulans* non-disjunction assay at an unspecified concentration.

Hydrochlorothiazide had no adverse effects on the fertility of mice and rats of either sex in studies wherein these species were exposed, via their diet, to doses of up to 100 and 4 mg/kg, respectively, prior to conception and throughout gestation. In mice and rats these doses are 9 times and 0.7 times, respectively, the MRHDD when compared on a body surface area basis.

Pregnancy

Pregnancy Categories C (first trimester) **and D** (second and third trimesters). See WARNINGS, **Pregnancy, Lisinopril, Fetal/Neonatal Morbidity and Mortality.**

Nursing Mothers

It is not known whether lisinopril is secreted in human milk. However, milk of lactating rats contains radioactivity following administration of ^{14}C lisinopril. In another study, lisinopril was present in rat milk at levels similar to plasma levels in the dams. Thiazides do appear in human milk. Because of the potential for serious reactions in nursing infants from ACE inhibitors and hydrochlorothiazide, a decision should be made whether to discontinue nursing or to discontinue PRINZIDE, taking into account the importance of the drug to the mother.

Pediatric Use

Safety and effectiveness in pediatric patients have not been established.

Geriatric Use

Clinical studies of PRINZIDE did not include sufficient numbers of subjects aged 65 and over to determine whether they respond differently from younger subjects. Other reported clinical experience has not identified differences in responses between the elderly and younger patients. In general, dose selection for an elderly patient should be cautious, usually starting at the low end of the dosing range, reflecting the greater frequency of decreased hepatic, renal, or cardiac function, and of concomitant disease or other drug therapy. In a multiple-dose pharmacokinetic study in elderly versus young hypertensive patients using the lisinopril/hydrochlorothiazide combination, area under the plasma concentration time curve (AUC) increased approximately 120% for lisinopril and approximately 80% for hydrochlorothiazide in older patients.

This drug is known to be substantially excreted by the kidney, and the risk of toxic reactions to this drug may be greater in patients with impaired renal function. Because elderly patients are more likely to have decreased renal function, care should be taken in dose selection. Evaluation of the hypertensive patient should always include assessment of renal function. (See DOSAGE AND ADMINISTRATION.)

ADVERSE REACTIONS

PRINZIDE has been evaluated for safety in 930 patients, including 100 patients treated for 50 weeks or more.

In clinical trials with PRINZIDE no adverse experiences peculiar to this combination drug have been observed. Adverse experiences that have occurred have been limited to those that have been previously reported with lisinopril or hydrochlorothiazide.

The most frequent clinical adverse experiences in controlled trials (including open label extensions) with any combination of lisinopril and hydrochlorothiazide were: dizziness (7.5 percent), headache (5.2 percent), cough (3.9 percent), fatigue (3.7 percent) and orthostatic effects (3.2 percent), all of which were more common than in placebo-treated patients. Generally, adverse experiences were mild and transient in nature; but see WARNINGS regarding angioedema and excessive hypotension or syncope. Discontinuation of therapy due to adverse effects was required in 4.4 percent of patients, principally because of dizziness, cough, fatigue and muscle cramps.

Adverse experiences occurring in greater than one percent of patients treated with lisinopril plus hydrochlorothiazide in controlled clinical trials are shown below.

Percent of Patients in Controlled Studies

	Lisinopril-Hydrochlorothiazide (n=930) Incidence (discontinuation)	Placebo (n=207) Incidence
Dizziness	7.5 (0.8)	1.9
Headache	5.2 (0.3)	1.9
Cough	3.9 (0.6)	1.0
Fatigue	3.7 (0.4)	1.0
Orthostatic Effects	3.2 (0.1)	1.0
Diarrhea	2.5 (0.2)	2.4
Nausea	2.2 (0.1)	2.4
Upper Respiratory Infection	2.2 (0.0)	0.0
Muscle Cramps	2.0 (0.4)	0.5
Asthenia	1.8 (0.2)	1.0
Paresthesia	1.5 (0.1)	0.0
Hypotension	1.4 (0.3)	0.5
Vomiting	1.4 (0.1)	0.5
Dyspepsia	1.3 (0.0)	0.0
Rash	1.2 (0.1)	0.5
Impotence	1.2 (0.3)	0.0

Clinical adverse experiences occurring in 0.3 to 1.0 percent of patients in controlled trials included: **Body as a Whole:** Chest pain, abdominal pain, syncope, chest discomfort, fever, trauma, virus infection. **Cardiovascular:** Palpitation, orthostatic hypotension. **Digestive:** Gastrointestinal cramps, dry mouth, constipation, heartburn. **Musculoskeletal:** Back pain, shoulder pain, knee pain, back strain, myalgia, foot pain. **Nervous/Psychiatric:** Decreased libido, vertigo, depression, somnolence. **Respiratory:** Common cold, nasal congestion, influenza, bronchitis, pharyngeal pain, dyspnea, pulmonary congestion, chronic sinusitis, allergic rhinitis, pharyngeal discomfort. **Skin:** Flushing, pruritus, skin inflammation, diaphoresis. **Special Senses:** Blurred vision, tinnitus, otalgia. **Urogenital:** Urinary tract infection.

Angioedema: Angioedema has been reported in patients receiving PRINZIDE, with an incidence higher in Black than in non-Black patients. Angioedema associated with laryngeal edema may be fatal. If angioedema of the face, extremities, lips, tongue, glottis and/or larynx occurs, treatment with PRINZIDE should be discontinued and appropriate therapy instituted immediately. In rare cases, intestinal angioedema has been reported with angiotensin converting enzyme inhibitors including lisinopril. (See WARNINGS.)

Hypotension: In clinical trials, adverse effects relating to hypotension occurred as follows: hypotension (1.4), orthostatic hypotension (0.5), other orthostatic effects (3.2). In addition syncope occurred in 0.8 percent of patients. (See WARNINGS.)

Cough: See PRECAUTIONS, Cough.

Clinical Laboratory Test Findings

Serum Electrolytes: See PRECAUTIONS.

Creatinine, Blood Urea Nitrogen: Minor reversible increases in blood urea nitrogen and serum creatinine were observed in patients with essential hypertension treated with PRINZIDE. More marked increases have also been reported and were more likely to occur in patients with renal artery stenosis. (See PRECAUTIONS.)

Serum Uric Acid, Glucose, Magnesium, Cholesterol, Triglycerides and Calcium: See PRECAUTIONS.

Hemoglobin and Hematocrit: Small decreases in hemoglobin and hematocrit (mean decreases of approximately 0.5 g percent and 1.5 vol percent, respectively) occurred frequently in hypertensive patients treated with PRINZIDE but were rarely of clinical importance unless another cause of anemia coexisted. In clinical trials, 0.4 percent of patients discontinued therapy due to anemia.

Liver Function Tests: Rarely, elevations of liver enzymes and/or serum bilirubin have occurred (see WARNINGS, Hepatic Failure).

Other adverse reactions that have been reported with the individual components are listed below:

Lisinopril — In clinical trials adverse reactions which occurred with lisinopril were also seen with PRINZIDE. In addition, and since lisinopril has been marketed, the following adverse reactions have been reported with lisinopril and should be considered potential adverse reactions for PRINZIDE: **Body as a Whole:** Anaphylactoid reactions (see WARNINGS, **Anaphylactoid and Possibly Related Reactions**), malaise, edema, facial edema, pain, pelvic pain, flank pain, chills; **Cardiovascular:** Cardiac arrest, myocardial infarction or cerebrovascular accident, possibly secondary to excessive hypotension in high-risk patients (see WARNINGS, **Hypotension**), pulmonary embolism and infarction, worsening of heart failure, arrhythmias (including tachycardia, ventricular tachycardia, atrial tachycardia, atrial fibrillation, bradycardia, and premature ventricular contractions), angina pectoris, transient ischemic attacks, paroxysmal nocturnal dyspnea, decreased blood pressure, peripheral edema, vasculitis; **Digestive:** Pancreatitis, hepatitis (hepatocellular or cholestatic jaundice) (see WARNINGS, **Hepatic Failure**), gastritis, anorexia, flatulence, increased salivation; **Endocrine:** Diabetes mellitus, syndrome of inappropriate antidiuretic hormone secretion (SIADH); **Hematologic:** Rare cases of neutropenia, thrombocytopenia, and bone marrow depression have been reported. Hemolytic anemia has been reported; a causal relationship to lisinopril cannot be excluded; **Metabolic:** Gout, weight loss, dehydration, fluid overload, weight gain; **Musculoskeletal:** Arthritis, arthralgia, neck pain, hip pain, joint pain, leg pain, arm pain, lumbago; **Nervous System/Psychiatric:** Ataxia, memory impairment, tremor, insomnia, stroke, nervousness, confusion, peripheral neuropathy (e.g., paresthesia, dysesthesia), spasm, hypersomnia, irritability; **Respiratory:** Malignant lung neoplasms, hemoptysis, pulmonary edema, pulmonary infiltrates, eosinophilic pneumonitis, bronchospasm, asthma, pleural effusion, pneumonia, wheezing, orthopnea, painful respiration, epistaxis, laryngitis, sinusitis, pharyngitis, rhinitis, rhinorrhea, chest sound abnormalities; **Skin:** Urticaria, alopecia, herpes zoster, photosensitivity, skin lesions, skin infections, pemphigus, erythema. Other severe skin reactions (including toxic epidermal necrolysis, Stevens-Johnson syndrome and cutaneous pseudolymphoma) have been reported rarely; causal relationship has not been established; **Special Senses:** Visual loss, diplopia, photophobia, taste disturbances; **Urogenital:** Acute renal failure, oliguria, anuria, uremia, progressive azotemia, renal dysfunction (see PRECAUTIONS and DOSAGE AND ADMINISTRATION), pyelonephritis, dysuria, breast pain.

Miscellaneous: A symptom complex has been reported which may include a positive ANA, an elevated erythrocyte sedimentation rate, arthralgia/arthritis, myalgia, fever, vasculitis, leukocytosis, eosinophilia, photosensitivity, rash, and other dermatological manifestations.

Fetal/Neonatal Morbidity and Mortality: See WARNINGS, **Pregnancy, Lisinopril, Fetal/Neonatal Morbidity and Mortality.**

Hydrochlorothiazide — Body as a Whole: Weakness; *Digestive:* Anorexia, gastric irritation, cramping, jaundice (intrahepatic cholestatic jaundice), pancreatitis, sialadenitis, constipation; **Hematologic:** Leukopenia, agranulocytosis, thrombocytopenia, aplastic anemia, hemolytic anemia; **Musculoskeletal:** Muscle spasm; **Nervous System/Psychiatric:** Restlessness; **Renal:** Renal failure, renal dysfunction, interstitial nephritis (see WARNINGS); **Skin:** Erythema multiforme including Stevens-Johnson syndrome, exfoliative dermatitis including toxic epidermal necrolysis, alopecia; **Special Senses:** Xanthopsia; **Hypersensitivity:** Purpura, photosensitivity, urticaria, necrotizing angiitis (vasculitis and cutaneous vasculitis), respiratory distress including pneumonitis and pulmonary edema, anaphylactic reactions.

OVERDOSAGE

No specific information is available on the treatment of overdosage with PRINZIDE. Treatment is symptomatic and supportive. Therapy with PRINZIDE should be discontinued and the patient observed closely. Suggested measures include induction of emesis and/or gastric lavage, and correction of dehydration, electrolyte imbalance and hypotension by established procedures.

Lisinopril

Following a single oral dose of 20 mg/kg, no lethality occurred in rats and death occurred in one of 20 mice receiving the same dose. The most likely manifestation of overdosage would be hypotension, for which the usual treatment would be intravenous infusion of normal saline solution.

Lisinopril can be removed by hemodialysis. (See WARNINGS, **Anaphylactoid reactions during membrane exposure.**)

Hydrochlorothiazide

Oral administration of a single oral dose of 10 mg/kg to mice and rats was not lethal. The most common signs and symptoms observed are those caused by electrolyte depletion (hypokalemia, hypochloremia, hyponatremia) and dehydration resulting from excessive diuresis. If digitalis has also been administered, hypokalemia may accentuate cardiac arrhythmias.

DOSAGE AND ADMINISTRATION

Lisinopril is an effective treatment of hypertension in once-daily doses of 10-80 mg, while hydrochlorothiazide is effective in doses of 12.5-50 mg. In clinical trials of lisinopril/hydrochlorothiazide combination therapy using lisinopril doses of 10-80 mg and hydrochlorothiazide doses of 6.25-50 mg, the antihypertensive response rates generally increased with increasing dose of either component.

The side effects (see WARNINGS) of lisinopril are generally rare and apparently independent of dose; those of hydrochlorothiazide are a mixture of dose-dependent phenomena (primarily hypokalemia) and dose-independent phenomena (e.g., pancreatitis), the former much more common than the latter. Therapy with any combination of lisinopril and hydrochlorothiazide will be associated with both sets of dose-independent side effects, but addition of lisinopril in clinical trials blunted the hypokalemia normally seen with diuretics.

To minimize dose-independent side effects, it is usually appropriate to begin combination therapy only after a patient has failed to achieve the desired effect with monotherapy.

Dose Titration Guided by Clinical Effect

A patient whose blood pressure is not adequately controlled with either lisinopril or hydrochlorothiazide monotherapy may be switched to PRINZIDE 10/12.5 or PRINZIDE 20/12.5. Further increases of either or both components could depend on clinical response. The hydrochlorothiazide dose should generally not be increased until 2-3 weeks have elapsed. Patients whose blood pressures are adequately controlled with 25 mg of daily hydrochlorothiazide, but who experience significant potassium loss with this regimen, may achieve similar or greater blood pressure control with less potassium loss if they are switched to PRINZIDE 10/12.5. Dosage higher than lisinopril 80 mg and hydrochlorothiazide 50 mg should not be used.

Replacement Therapy

The combination may be substituted for the titrated individual components.

Use in Renal Impairment

The usual regimens of therapy with PRINZIDE need not be adjusted as long as the patient's creatinine clearance is >30 mL/min/1.73 m^2 (serum creatinine approximately ≤3 mg/dL or 265 μmol/L). In patients with more severe renal impairment, loop diuretics are preferred to thiazides, so PRINZIDE is not recommended (see WARNINGS, **Anaphylactoid reactions during membrane exposure**).

HOW SUPPLIED

No. 8439—Tablets PRINZIDE 10-12.5 are blue hexagon-shaped tablets with code 145 on one side and plain on the other side. Each tablet contains 10 mg of lisinopril and 12.5 mg of hydrochlorothiazide. They are supplied as follows:

NDC 0006-0145-58 unit of use bottles of 100.

No. 8247—Tablets PRINZIDE 20-12.5, are yellow, hexagon-shaped tablets with code MSD/140 on one side and scored on the other side. Each tablet contains 20 mg of lisinopril and 12.5 mg of hydrochlorothiazide. They are supplied as follows:

NDC 0006-0140-58 unit of use bottles of 100.

No. 3595—Tablets PRINZIDE 20-25, are peach, round, fluted-edge tablets, coded MSD 142 on one side and PRINZIDE on the other. Each tablet contains 20 mg of lisinopril and 25 mg of hydrochlorothiazide. They are supplied as follows:

NDC 0006-0142-58 unit of use bottles of 100.

Storage

Store at controlled room temperature, 15-30°C (59-86°F). Protect from excessive light and humidity.

Dispense in a well-closed container, if product package is subdivided.

Tablets PRINZIDE (lisinopril-hydrochlorothiazide) 10-12.5 mg and 20-12.5 mg are manufactured for:

Merck Sharp & Dohme Corp., a subsidiary of

MERCK & CO., INC., Whitehouse Station, NJ 08889, USA by:

MERCK SHARP & DOHME LTD.

Cramlington, Northumberland, UK NE23 3JU

Tablets PRINZIDE (lisinopril-hydrochlorothiazide) 20-25 mg are manufactured for:

Merck Sharp & Dohme Corp., a subsidiary of

MERCK & CO., INC., Whitehouse Station, NJ 08889, USA by:

MERCK FROSST CANADA LTD.

Kirkland, Quebec, Canada H9H 3L1

Issued February 2010

9763304

Shown in Product Identification Guide, page 313

PROPECIA®   ℞
[*Pro-pee-sha*]
(finasteride)
Tablets, 1 mg

DESCRIPTION

PROPECIA[1] (finasteride), a synthetic 4-azasteroid compound, is a specific inhibitor of steroid Type II 5α-reductase, an intracellular enzyme that converts the androgen testosterone into 5α-dihydrotestosterone (DHT).

Finasteride is 4-azaandrost-1-ene-17-carboxamide,N-(1,1-dimethylethyl)-3-oxo-,(5α,17β)-. The empirical formula of finasteride is $C_{23}H_{36}N_2O_2$ and its molecular weight is 372.55. Its structural formula is:

Finasteride is a white crystalline powder with a melting point near 250°C. It is freely soluble in chloroform and in lower alcohol solvents but is practically insoluble in water. PROPECIA tablets for oral administration are film-coated tablets that contain 1 mg of finasteride and the following inactive ingredients: lactose monohydrate, microcrystalline cellulose, pregelatinized starch, sodium starch glycolate, hydroxypropyl methylcellulose, hydroxypropyl cellulose LF, titanium dioxide, magnesium stearate, talc, docusate sodium, yellow ferric oxide, and red ferric oxide.

---

[1] Registered trademark of Merck Sharp & Dohme Corp., a subsidiary of **Merck & Co., Inc.**

Copyright © 1997 Merck Sharp & Dohme Corp., a subsidiary of **Merck & Co., Inc.**

All rights reserved

CLINICAL PHARMACOLOGY

Finasteride is a competitive and specific inhibitor of Type II 5α-reductase, an intracellular enzyme that converts the androgen testosterone into DHT. Two distinct isozymes are found in mice, rats, monkeys, and humans: Type I and II. Each of these isozymes are differentially expressed in tissues and developmental stages. In humans, Type I 5α-reductase is predominant in the sebaceous glands of most regions of skin, including scalp, and liver. Type I 5α-reductase is responsible for approximately one-third of circulating DHT. The Type II 5α-reductase isozyme is primarily found in

prostate, seminal vesicles, epididymides, and hair follicles as well as liver, and is responsible for two-thirds of circulating DHT.

In humans, the mechanism of action of finasteride is based on its preferential inhibition of the Type II isozyme. Using native tissues (scalp and prostate), *in vitro* binding studies examining the potential of finasteride to inhibit either isozyme revealed a 100-fold selectivity for the human Type II 5α-reductase over Type I isozyme (IC_{50}=500 and 4.2 nM for Type I and II, respectively). For both isozymes, the inhibition by finasteride is accompanied by reduction of the inhibitor to dihydrofinasteride and adduct formation with NADP+. The turnover for the enzyme complex is slow ($t_{1/2}$ approximately 30 days for the Type II enzyme complex and 14 days for the Type I complex).

Finasteride has no affinity for the androgen receptor and has no androgenic, antiandrogenic, estrogenic, antiestrogenic, or progestational effects. Inhibition of Type II 5α-reductase blocks the peripheral conversion of testosterone to DHT, resulting in significant decreases in serum and tissue DHT concentrations. Finasteride produces a rapid reduction in serum DHT concentration, reaching 65% suppression within 24 hours of oral dosing with a 1-mg tablet. Mean circulating levels of testosterone and estradiol were increased by approximately 15% as compared to baseline, but these remained within the physiologic range.

In men with male pattern hair loss (androgenetic alopecia), the balding scalp contains miniaturized hair follicles and increased amounts of DHT compared with hairy scalp. Administration of finasteride decreases scalp and serum DHT concentrations in these men. The relative contributions of these reductions to the treatment effect of finasteride have not been defined. By this mechanism, finasteride appears to interrupt a key factor in the development of androgenetic alopecia in those patients genetically predisposed.

A 48-week, placebo-controlled study designed to assess by phototrichogram the effect of PROPECIA on total and actively growing (anagen) scalp hairs in vertex baldness enrolled 212 men with androgenetic alopecia. At baseline and 48 weeks, total and anagen hair counts were obtained in a 1-cm² target area of the scalp. Men treated with PROPECIA showed increases from baseline in total and anagen hair counts of 7 hairs and 18 hairs, respectively, whereas men treated with placebo had decreases of 10 hairs and 9 hairs, respectively. These changes in hair counts resulted in a between-group difference of 17 hairs in total hair count (p<0.001) and 27 hairs in anagen hair count (p<0.001), and an improvement in the proportion of anagen hairs from 62% at baseline to 68% for men treated with PROPECIA.

Pharmacokinetics

Absorption

In a study in 15 healthy young male subjects, the mean bioavailability of finasteride 1-mg tablets was 65% (range 26-170%), based on the ratio of area under the curve (AUC) relative to an intravenous (IV) reference dose. At steady state following dosing with 1 mg/day (n=12), maximum finasteride plasma concentration averaged 9.2 ng/mL (range, 4.9-13.7 ng/mL) and was reached 1 to 2 hours postdose; $AUC_{(0-24 hr)}$ was 53 ng•hr/mL (range, 20-154 ng•hr/mL). Bioavailability of finasteride was not affected by food.

Distribution

Mean steady-state volume of distribution was 76 liters (range, 44-96 liters; n=15). Approximately 90% of circulating finasteride is bound to plasma proteins. There is a slow accumulation phase for finasteride after multiple dosing. Finasteride has been found to cross the blood-brain barrier. Semen levels have been measured in 35 men taking finasteride 1 mg/day for 6 weeks. In 60% (21 of 35) of the samples, finasteride levels were undetectable (<0.2 ng/mL). The mean finasteride level was 0.26 ng/mL and the highest level measured was 1.52 ng/mL. Using the highest semen level measured and assuming 100% absorption from a 5-mL ejaculate per day, human exposure through vaginal absorption would be up to 7.6 ng per day, which is 750 times lower than the exposure from the no-effect dose for developmental abnormalities in Rhesus monkeys and 650-fold less than the dose of finasteride (5 µg) that had no effect on circulating DHT levels in men (see PRECAUTIONS, Pregnancy).

Metabolism

Finasteride is extensively metabolized in the liver, primarily via the cytochrome P450 3A4 enzyme subfamily. Two metabolites, the t-butyl side chain monohydroxylated and monocarboxylic acid metabolites, have been identified that possess no more than 20% of the 5α-reductase inhibitory activity of finasteride.

Excretion

Following intravenous infusion in healthy young subjects (n=15), mean plasma clearance of finasteride was 165 mL/min (range, 70-279 mL/min). Mean terminal half-life in plasma was 4.5 hours (range, 3.3-13.4 hours; n=12). Following an oral dose of ¹⁴C-finasteride in man (n=6), a mean of 39% (range, 32-46%) of the dose was excreted in the urine in the form of metabolites; 57% (range, 51-64%) was excreted in the feces.

Mean terminal half-life is approximately 5-6 hours in men 18-60 years of age and 8 hours in men more than 70 years of age.

Special Populations

Pediatric:

Finasteride pharmacokinetics have not been investigated in patients <18 years of age.

Gender:

PROPECIA is not indicated for use in women.

Geriatric:

No dosage adjustment is necessary in the elderly. Although the elimination rate of finasteride is decreased in the elderly, these findings are of no clinical significance. See also Pharmacokinetics, Excretion, and PRECAUTIONS, Geriatric Use sections.

Race:

The effect of race on finasteride pharmacokinetics has not been studied.

Renal Insufficiency:

No dosage adjustment is necessary in patients with renal insufficiency. In patients with chronic renal impairment, with creatinine clearances ranging from 9.0 to 55 mL/min, AUC, maximum plasma concentration, half-life, and protein binding after a single dose of ¹⁴C-finasteride were similar to those obtained in healthy volunteers. Urinary excretion of metabolites was decreased in patients with renal impairment. This decrease was associated with an increase in fecal excretion of metabolites. Plasma concentrations of metabolites were significantly higher in patients with renal impairment (based on a 60% increase in total radioactivity AUC). However, finasteride has been well tolerated in men with normal renal function receiving up to 80 mg/day for 12 weeks where exposure of these patients to metabolites would presumably be much greater.

Hepatic Insufficiency:

The effect of hepatic insufficiency on finasteride pharmacokinetics has not been studied. Caution should be used in the administration of PROPECIA in patients with liver function abnormalities, as finasteride is metabolized extensively in the liver.

Drug Interactions

(also see PRECAUTIONS, Drug Interactions)

No drug interactions of clinical importance have been identified. Finasteride does not appear to affect the cytochrome P450-linked drug-metabolizing enzyme system. Compounds that have been tested in man include antipyrine, digoxin, propranolol, theophylline, and warfarin and no clinically meaningful interactions were found.

Mean (SD) Pharmacokinetic Parameters in Healthy Men (ages 18-26)

	Mean (± SD) n=15
Bioavailability	65% (26-170%)*
Clearance (mL/min)	165 (55)
Volume of Distribution (L)	76 (14)

* Range

Mean (SD) Noncompartmental Pharmacokinetic Parameters After Multiple Doses of 1 mg/day in Healthy Men (ages 19-42)

	Mean (± SD) (n=12)
AUC (ng•hr/mL)	53 (33.8)
Peak Concentration (ng/mL)	9.2 (2.6)
Time to Peak (hours)	1.3 (0.5)
Half-Life (hours)*	4.5 (1.6)

* First-dose values; all other parameters are last-dose values

Clinical Studies

Studies in Men

The efficacy of PROPECIA was demonstrated in men (88% Caucasian) with mild to moderate androgenetic alopecia (male pattern hair loss) between 18 and 41 years of age. In order to prevent seborrheic dermatitis which might confound the assessment of hair growth in these studies, all men, whether treated with finasteride or placebo, were instructed to use a specified, medicated, tar-based shampoo (Neutrogena T/Gel² Shampoo) during the first 2 years of the studies.

There were three double-blind, randomized, placebo-controlled studies of 12-month duration. The two primary endpoints were hair count and patient self-assessment; the two secondary endpoints were investigator assessment and ratings of photographs. In addition, information was collected regarding sexual function (based on a self-administered questionnaire) and non-scalp body hair growth. The three studies were conducted in 1879 men with mild to moderate, but not complete, hair loss. Two of the studies enrolled men with predominantly mild to moderate vertex hair loss (n=1553). The third enrolled men having mild to moderate hair loss in the anterior mid-scalp area with or without vertex balding (n=326).

[2] Registered trademark of Johnson & Johnson
Studies in Men with Vertex Baldness
Of the men who completed the first 12 months of the two vertex baldness trials, 1215 elected to continue in double-blind, placebo-controlled, 12-month extension studies. There were 547 men receiving PROPECIA for both the initial study and first extension periods (up to 2 years of treatment) and 60 men receiving placebo for the same periods. The extension studies were continued for 3 additional years, with 323 men on PROPECIA and 23 on placebo entering the fifth year of the study.
In order to evaluate the effect of discontinuation of therapy, there were 65 men who received PROPECIA for the initial 12 months followed by placebo in the first 12-month extension period. Some of these men continued in additional extension studies and were switched back to treatment with PROPECIA, with 32 men entering the fifth year of the study. Lastly, there were 543 men who received placebo for the initial 12 months followed by PROPECIA in the first 12-month extension period. Some of these men continued in additional extension studies receiving PROPECIA, with 290 men entering the fifth year of the study (see Figure below). Hair counts were assessed by photographic enlargements of a representative area of active hair loss. In these two studies in men with vertex baldness, significant increases in hair count were demonstrated at 6 and 12 months in men treated with PROPECIA, while significant hair loss from baseline was demonstrated in those treated with placebo. At 12 months there was a 107-hair difference between groups (p<0.001, PROPECIA [n=679] vs placebo [n=672]) within a 1-inch diameter circle (5.1 cm^2). Hair count was maintained in those men taking PROPECIA for up to 2 years, resulting in a 138-hair difference between treatment groups (p<0.001, PROPECIA [n=433] vs placebo [n=47]) within the same area. In men treated with PROPECIA, the maximum improvement in hair count compared to baseline was achieved during the first 2 years. Although the initial improvement was followed by a slow decline, hair count was maintained above baseline throughout the 5 years of the studies. Furthermore, because the decline in the placebo group was more rapid, the difference between treatment groups also continued to increase throughout the studies, resulting in a 277-hair difference (p<0.001, PROPECIA [n=219] vs placebo [n=15]) at 5 years (see Figure below).
Patients who switched from placebo to PROPECIA (n=425) had a decrease in hair count at the end of the initial 12-month placebo period, followed by an increase in hair count after 1 year of treatment with PROPECIA. This increase in hair count was less (56 hairs above original baseline) than the increase (91 hairs above original baseline) observed after 1 year of treatment in men initially randomized to PROPECIA. Although the increase in hair count, relative to when therapy was initiated, was comparable between these two groups, a higher absolute hair count was achieved in patients who were started on treatment with PROPECIA in the initial study. This advantage was maintained through the remaining 3 years of the studies. A change of treatment from PROPECIA to placebo (n=48) at the end of the initial 12 months resulted in reversal of the increase in hair count 12 months later, at 24 months (see Figure below).
At 12 months, 58% of men in the placebo group had further hair loss (defined as any decrease in hair count from baseline), compared with 14% of men treated with PROPECIA. In men treated for up to 2 years, 72% of men in the placebo group demonstrated hair loss, compared with 17% of men treated with PROPECIA. At 5 years, 100% of men in the placebo group demonstrated hair loss, compared with 35% of men treated with PROPECIA.
[See figure above]
Patient self-assessment was obtained at each clinic visit from a self-administered questionnaire, which included questions on their perception of hair growth, hair loss, and appearance. This self-assessment demonstrated an increase in amount of hair, a decrease in hair loss, and improvement in appearance in men treated with PROPECIA. Overall improvement compared with placebo was seen as early as 3 months (p<0.05), with improvement maintained over 5 years.
Investigator assessment was based on a 7-point scale evaluating increases or decreases in scalp hair at each patient

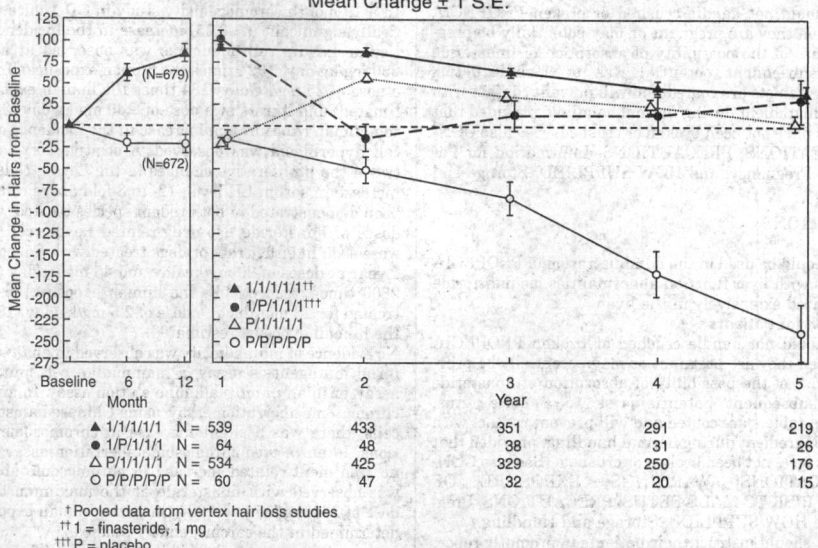

Effect on Hair Count[†]
Number of Hairs in a 1-Inch Diameter Circle
Mean Change ± 1 S.E.

	Baseline	6	12	1	2	3	4	5
		Month				Year		
▲ 1/1/1/1/1 N =	539			433	351		291	219
● 1/P/1/1/1 N =	64			48	38		31	26
△ P/1/1/1/1 N =	534			425	329		250	176
○ P/P/P/P/P N =	60			47	32		20	15

Legend:
▲ 1/1/1/1/1[††]
● 1/P/1/1/1[†††]
△ P/1/1/1/1
○ P/P/P/P/P

[†] Pooled data from vertex hair loss studies
[††] 1 = finasteride, 1 mg
[†††] P = placebo

visit. This assessment showed significantly greater increases in hair growth in men treated with PROPECIA compared with placebo as early as 3 months (p<0.001). At 12 months, the investigators rated 65% of men treated with PROPECIA as having increased hair growth compared with 37% in the placebo group. At 2 years, the investigators rated 80% of men treated with PROPECIA as having increased hair growth compared with 47% of men treated with placebo. At 5 years, the investigators rated 77% of men treated with PROPECIA as having increased hair growth, compared with 15% of men treated with placebo.
An independent panel rated standardized photographs of the head in a blinded fashion based on increases or decreases in scalp hair using the same 7-point scale as the investigator assessment. At 12 months, 48% of men treated with PROPECIA had an increase as compared with 7% of men treated with placebo. At 2 years, an increase in hair growth was demonstrated in 66% of men treated with PROPECIA, compared with 7% of men treated with placebo. At 5 years, 48% of men treated with PROPECIA demonstrated an increase in hair growth, 42% were rated as having no change (no further visible progression of hair loss from baseline) and 10% were rated as having lost hair when compared to baseline. In comparison, 6% of men treated with placebo demonstrated an increase in hair growth, 19% were rated as having no change and 75% were rated as having lost hair when compared to baseline.
Other Results in Vertex Baldness Studies
A sexual function questionnaire was self-administered by patients participating in the two vertex baldness trials to detect more subtle changes in sexual function. At Month 12, statistically significant differences in favor of placebo were found in 3 of 4 domains (sexual interest, erections, and perception of sexual problems). However, no significant difference was seen in the question on overall satisfaction with sex life.
In one of the two vertex baldness studies, patients were questioned on non-scalp body hair growth. PROPECIA did not appear to affect non-scalp body hair.
Study in Men with Hair Loss in the Anterior Mid-Scalp Area
A study of 12-month duration, designed to assess the efficacy of PROPECIA in men with hair loss in the anterior mid-scalp area, also demonstrated significant increases in hair count compared with placebo. Increases in hair count were accompanied by improvements in patient self-assessment, investigator assessment, and ratings based on standardized photographs. Hair counts were obtained in the anterior mid-scalp area, and did not include the area of bitemporal recession or the anterior hairline.
Summary of Clinical Studies in Men
Clinical studies were conducted in men aged 18 to 41 with mild to moderate degrees of androgenetic alopecia. All men treated with PROPECIA or placebo received a tar-based shampoo (Neutrogena T/Gel®[2] Shampoo) during the first 2 years of the studies. Clinical improvement was seen as early as 3 months in the patients treated with PROPECIA and led to a net increase in scalp hair count and hair regrowth. In clinical studies for up to 5 years, treatment with PROPECIA slowed the further progression of hair loss observed in the placebo group. In general, the difference between treatment groups continued to increase throughout the 5 years of the studies.
Ethnic Analysis of Clinical Data from Men
In a combined analysis of the two studies on vertex baldness, mean hair count changes from baseline were 91 vs -19 hairs (PROPECIA vs placebo) among Caucasians (n=1185), 49 vs -27 hairs among Blacks (n=84), 53 vs -38 hairs among Asians (n=17), 67 vs 5 hairs among Hispanics (n=45) and 67 vs -15 hairs among other ethnic groups (n=20). Patient self-assessment showed improvement across racial groups with PROPECIA treatment, except for satisfaction of the frontal hairline and vertex in Black men, who were satisfied overall.
Study in Women
In a study involving 137 postmenopausal women with androgenetic alopecia who were treated with PROPECIA (n=67) or placebo (n=70) for 12 months, effectiveness could not be demonstrated. There was no improvement in hair counts, patient self-assessment, investigator assessment, or ratings of standardized photographs in the women treated with PROPECIA when compared with the placebo group (see INDICATIONS AND USAGE).

INDICATIONS AND USAGE

PROPECIA is indicated for the treatment of male pattern hair loss (androgenetic alopecia) in **MEN ONLY**. Safety and efficacy were demonstrated in men between 18 to 41 years of age with mild to moderate hair loss of the vertex and anterior mid-scalp area (see CLINICAL PHARMACOLOGY, Clinical Studies).
Efficacy in bitemporal recession has not been established.
PROPECIA is not indicated in women (see CLINICAL PHARMACOLOGY, Clinical Studies and CONTRAINDICATIONS).
PROPECIA is not indicated in children (see PRECAUTIONS, Pediatric Use).

CONTRAINDICATIONS

PROPECIA is contraindicated in the following:
Pregnancy. Finasteride use is contraindicated in women when they are or may potentially be pregnant. Because of the ability of Type II 5α-reductase inhibitors to inhibit the conversion of testosterone to DHT, finasteride may cause abnormalities of the external genitalia of a male fetus of a pregnant woman who receives finasteride. If this drug is used during pregnancy, or if pregnancy occurs while taking this drug, the pregnant woman should be apprised of the potential hazard to the male fetus. (See also WARNINGS, EXPOSURE OF WOMEN - RISK TO MALE FETUS; and PRECAUTIONS, Information for Patients and Pregnancy.) In female rats, low doses of finasteride administered during pregnancy have produced abnormalities of the external genitalia in male offspring.
Hypersensitivity to any component of this medication.

WARNINGS

PROPECIA is not indicated for use in pediatric patients (see INDICATIONS AND USAGE; and PRECAUTIONS, Pediatric Use) or women (see also WARNINGS, EXPOSURE OF

WOMEN - RISK TO MALE FETUS; PRECAUTIONS, Information for Patients and Pregnancy; and HOW SUPPLIED, Storage and Handling).

EXPOSURE OF WOMEN - RISK TO MALE FETUS

Women should not handle crushed or broken PROPECIA tablets when they are pregnant or may potentially be pregnant because of the possibility of absorption of finasteride and the subsequent potential risk to a male fetus. PROPECIA tablets are coated and will prevent contact with the active ingredient during normal handling, provided that the tablets have not been broken or crushed. (See also CONTRAINDICATIONS; PRECAUTIONS, Information for Patients and Pregnancy; and HOW SUPPLIED, Storage and Handling.)

PRECAUTIONS

General

Caution should be used in the administration of PROPECIA in patients with liver function abnormalities, as finasteride is metabolized extensively in the liver.

Information for Patients

Women should not handle crushed or broken PROPECIA tablets when they are pregnant or may potentially be pregnant because of the possibility of absorption of finasteride and the subsequent potential risk to a male fetus. PROPECIA tablets are coated and will prevent contact with the active ingredient during normal handling, provided that the tablets have not been broken or crushed. (See also CONTRAINDICATIONS; WARNINGS, EXPOSURE OF WOMEN - RISK TO MALE FETUS; PRECAUTIONS, Pregnancy; and HOW SUPPLIED, Storage and Handling.)

Physicians should instruct their patients to promptly report any changes in their breasts such as lumps, pain or nipple discharge. Breast changes including breast enlargement, tenderness and neoplasm have been reported (see ADVERSE REACTIONS).

See also PATIENT PACKAGE INSERT.

Physicians should instruct their patients to read the patient package insert before starting therapy with PROPECIA and to read it again each time the prescription is renewed so that they are aware of current information for patients regarding PROPECIA.

Drug/Laboratory Test Interactions

Finasteride had no effect on circulating levels of cortisol, thyroid-stimulating hormone, or thyroxine, nor did it affect the plasma lipid profile (e.g., total cholesterol, low-density lipoproteins, high-density lipoproteins and triglycerides) or bone mineral density. In studies with finasteride, no clinically meaningful changes in luteinizing hormone (LH), follicle-stimulating hormone (FSH) or prolactin were detected. In healthy volunteers, treatment with finasteride did not alter the response of LH and FSH to gonadotropin-releasing hormone indicating that the hypothalamic-pituitary-testicular axis was not affected.

In clinical studies with PROPECIA (finasteride, 1 mg) in men 18-41 years of age, the mean value of serum prostate-specific antigen (PSA) decreased from 0.7 ng/mL at baseline to 0.5 ng/mL at Month 12. Further, in clinical studies with PROSCAR (finasteride, 5 mg) when used in older men who have benign prostatic hyperplasia (BPH), PSA levels are decreased by approximately 50%. Other studies with PROSCAR showed it may also cause decreases in serum PSA in the presence of prostate cancer. These findings should be taken into account for proper interpretation of serum PSA when evaluating men treated with finasteride. Any confirmed increases in PSA levels from nadir while on PROPECIA may signal the presence of prostate cancer and should be carefully evaluated, even if those values are still within the normal range for men not taking a 5α-reductase inhibitor. Non-compliance to therapy with PROPECIA may also affect PSA test results.

Drug Interactions

No drug interactions of clinical importance have been identified. Finasteride does not appear to affect the cytochrome P450-linked drug-metabolizing enzyme system. Compounds that have been tested in man include antipyrine, digoxin, propranolol, theophylline, and warfarin and no clinically meaningful interactions were found.

Other concomitant therapy:

Although specific interaction studies were not performed, finasteride doses of 1 mg or more were concomitantly used in clinical studies with acetaminophen, acetylsalicylic acid, α-blockers, analgesics, angiotensin-converting enzyme (ACE) inhibitors, anticonvulsants, benzodiazepines, beta blockers, calcium-channel blockers, cardiac nitrates, diuretics, H_2 antagonists, HMG-CoA reductase inhibitors, prostaglandin synthetase inhibitors (also referred to as NSAIDs), and quinolone anti-infectives without evidence of clinically significant adverse interactions.

Carcinogenesis, Mutagenesis, Impairment of Fertility

No evidence of a tumorigenic effect was observed in a 24-month study in Sprague-Dawley rats receiving doses of finasteride up to 160 mg/kg/day in males and 320 mg/kg/day in females. These doses produced respective systemic exposure in rats of 888 and 2192 times those observed in man receiving the recommended human dose of 1 mg/day. All exposure calculations were based on calculated $AUC_{(0-24\ hr)}$ for animals and mean $AUC_{(0-24\ hr)}$ for man (0.05 µg•hr/mL).

In a 19-month carcinogenicity study in CD-1 mice, a statistically significant (p≤0.05) increase in the incidence of testicular Leydig cell adenomas was observed at a dose of 250 mg/kg/day (1824 times the human exposure). In mice at a dose of 25 mg/kg/day (184 times the human exposure, estimated) and in rats at a dose of ≥40 mg/kg/day (312 times the human exposure) an increase in the incidence of Leydig cell hyperplasia was observed. A positive correlation between the proliferative changes in the Leydig cells and an increase in serum LH levels (2- to 3-fold above control) has been demonstrated in both rodent species treated with high doses of finasteride. No drug-related Leydig cell changes were seen in either rats or dogs treated with finasteride for 1 year at doses of 20 mg/kg/day and 45 mg/kg/day (240 and 2800 times, respectively, the human exposure) or in mice treated for 19 months at a dose of 2.5 mg/kg/day (18.4 times the human exposure, estimated).

No evidence of mutagenicity was observed in an *in vitro* bacterial mutagenesis assay, a mammalian cell mutagenesis assay, or in an *in vitro* alkaline elution assay. In an *in vitro* chromosome aberration assay, using Chinese hamster ovary cells, there was a slight increase in chromosome aberrations. In an *in vivo* chromosome aberration assay in mice, no treatment-related increase in chromosome aberration was observed with finasteride at the maximum tolerated dose of 250 mg/kg/day (1824 times the human exposure) as determined in the carcinogenicity studies.

In sexually mature male rabbits treated with finasteride at 80 mg/kg/day (4344 times the human exposure) for up to 12 weeks, no effect on fertility, sperm count, or ejaculate volume was seen. In sexually mature male rats treated with 80 mg/kg/day of finasteride (488 times the human exposure), there were no significant effects on fertility after 6 or 12 weeks of treatment; however, when treatment was continued for up to 24 or 30 weeks, there was an apparent decrease in fertility, fecundity, and an associated significant decrease in the weights of the seminal vesicles and prostate. All these effects were reversible within 6 weeks of discontinuation of treatment. No drug-related effect on testes or on mating performance has been seen in rats or rabbits. This decrease in fertility in finasteride-treated rats is secondary to its effect on accessory sex organs (prostate and seminal vesicles) resulting in failure to form a seminal plug. The seminal plug is essential for normal fertility in rats but is not relevant in man.

Pregnancy

Teratogenic Effects:

Pregnancy Category X

See CONTRAINDICATIONS.

PROPECIA is not indicated for use in women.

Administration of finasteride to pregnant rats on gestational days 6-20 at doses ranging from 100 µg/kg/day to 100 mg/kg/day (1-684 times the human exposure, estimated) resulted in dose-dependent development of hypospadias in 3.6 to 100% of male offspring. Pregnant rats produced male offspring with decreased prostatic and seminal vesicular weights, delayed preputial separation, and transient nipple development when given finasteride at ≥30 µg/kg/day (0.2 times the human exposure, estimated) and decreased anogenital distance when given finasteride at ≥3 µg/kg/day (0.02 times the human exposure, estimated). The critical period during which these effects can be induced in male rats has been defined to be days 16-17 of gestation. The changes described above are expected pharmacological effects of drugs belonging to the class of Type II 5α-reductase inhibitors and are similar to those reported in male infants with a genetic deficiency of Type II 5α-reductase. No abnormalities were observed in female offspring exposed to any dose of finasteride *in utero*.

No developmental abnormalities have been observed in first filial generation (F_1) male or female offspring resulting from mating finasteride-treated male rats (80 mg/kg/day; 488 times the human exposure) with untreated females. Administration of finasteride at 3 mg/kg/day (20 times the human exposure, estimated) during the late gestation and lactation period resulted in slightly decreased fertility in F_1 male offspring. No effects were seen in female offspring.

No evidence of malformations has been observed in rabbit fetuses exposed to finasteride *in utero* from days 6-18 of gestation at doses up to 100 mg/kg/day (1908 times the recommended human dose of 1 mg/day, based on body surface area comparison). However, effects on male genitalia would not be expected since the rabbits were not exposed during the critical period of genital system development.

The *in utero* effects of finasteride exposure during the period of embryonic and fetal development were evaluated in the rhesus monkey (gestation days 20-100), a species more predictive of human development than rats or rabbits. Intravenous administration of finasteride to pregnant monkeys at doses up to 800 ng/day (at least 250 times the highest estimated exposure of pregnant women to finasteride from semen of men taking 1 mg/day, based on body surface area comparison) resulted in no abnormalities in male fetuses. In confirmation of the relevance of the rhesus model for human fetal development, oral administration of a 2 mg/kg/day dose of finasteride to pregnant monkeys resulted in external genital abnormalities in male fetuses. No other abnormalities were observed in male fetuses and no finasteride-related abnormalities were observed in female fetuses at any dose.

Nursing Mothers

PROPECIA is not indicated for use in women.

It is not known whether finasteride is excreted in human milk.

Pediatric Use

PROPECIA is not indicated for use in pediatric patients. Safety and effectiveness in pediatric patients have not been established.

Geriatric Use

Clinical efficacy studies with PROPECIA did not include subjects aged 65 and over. Based on the pharmacokinetics of finasteride 5 mg, no dosage adjustment is necessary in the elderly for PROPECIA (see CLINICAL PHARMACOLOGY, Pharmacokinetics). However the efficacy of PROPECIA in the elderly has not been established.

ADVERSE REACTIONS

Clinical Studies for PROPECIA (finasteride 1 mg) in the Treatment of Male Pattern Hair Loss

In three controlled clinical trials for PROPECIA of 12-month duration, 1.4% of patients taking PROPECIA (n=945) were discontinued due to adverse experiences that were considered to be possibly, probably or definitely drug-related (1.6% for placebo; n=934).

Clinical adverse experiences that were reported as possibly, probably or definitely drug-related in ≥1% of patients treated with PROPECIA or placebo are presented in Table 1.

TABLE 1. Drug-Related Adverse Experiences for PROPECIA (finasteride 1 mg) in Year 1 (%) MALE PATTERN HAIR LOSS

	PROPECIA N=945	Placebo N=934
Decreased Libido	1.8	1.3
Erectile Dysfunction	1.3	0.7
Ejaculation Disorder *(Decreased Volume of Ejaculate)*	1.2 *(0.8)*	0.7 *(0.4)*
Discontinuation due to drug-related sexual adverse experiences	1.2	0.9

Integrated analysis of clinical adverse experiences showed that during treatment with PROPECIA, 36 (3.8%) of 945 men had reported one or more of these adverse experiences as compared to 20 (2.1%) of 934 men treated with placebo (p=0.04). Resolution occurred in men who discontinued therapy with PROPECIA due to these side effects and in most of those who continued therapy. The incidence of each of the above adverse experiences decreased to ≤0.3% by the fifth year of treatment with PROPECIA.

In a study of finasteride 1 mg daily in healthy men, a median decrease in ejaculate volume of 0.3 mL (-11%) compared with 0.2 mL (−8%) for placebo was observed after 48 weeks of treatment. Two other studies showed that finasteride at 5 times the dosage of PROPECIA (5 mg daily) produced significant median decreases of approximately 0.5 mL (-25%) compared to placebo in ejaculate volume, but this was reversible after discontinuation of treatment.

In the clinical studies with PROPECIA, the incidences for breast tenderness and enlargement, hypersensitivity reactions, and testicular pain in finasteride-treated patients were not different from those in patients treated with placebo.

Postmarketing Experience for PROPECIA (finasteride 1 mg)

Breast tenderness and enlargement; depression; hypersensitivity reactions including rash, pruritus, urticaria, and swelling of the lips and face; and testicular pain. See Controlled Clinical Trials and Long-Term Open Extension Studies for PROSCAR (finasteride 5 mg) in the Treatment of Benign Prostatic Hyperplasia.

Controlled Clinical Trials and Long-Term Open Extension Studies for PROSCAR[1] (finasteride 5 mg) in the Treatment of Benign Prostatic Hyperplasia

In the PROSCAR Long-Term Efficacy and Safety Study (PLESS), a 4-year controlled clinical study, 3040 patients between the ages of 45 and 78 with symptomatic BPH and an enlarged prostate were evaluated for safety over a period of 4 years (1524 on PROSCAR 5 mg/day and 1516 on placebo). 3.7% (57 patients) treated with PROSCAR 5 mg and 2.1% (32 patients) treated with placebo discontinued therapy as a result of adverse reactions related to sexual function, which are the most frequently reported adverse reactions.

Table 2 presents the only clinical adverse reactions considered possibly, probably or definitely drug related for which the incidence on PROSCAR was ≥1% and greater than placebo over the 4 years of the study. In years 2-4 of the study, there was no significant difference between treatment groups in the incidences of impotence, decreased libido and ejaculation disorder.

[See table 2 at right]

The adverse experience profiles in the 1-year, placebo-controlled, Phase III BPH studies and the 5-year open extensions with PROSCAR 5 mg and PLESS were similar.

There is no evidence of increased adverse experiences with increased duration of treatment with PROSCAR 5 mg. New reports of drug-related sexual adverse experiences decreased with duration of therapy.

The relationship between long-term use of finasteride and male breast neoplasia is currently unknown. During a 4- to 6-year placebo- and comparator-controlled study that enrolled 3047 men, there were 4 cases of breast cancer in men treated with PROSCAR but no cases in men not treated with PROSCAR. In another 4-year, placebo-controlled study that enrolled 3040 men, there were 2 cases of breast cancer in placebo-treated men, but no cases were reported in men treated with PROSCAR.

In a 7-year placebo-controlled trial that enrolled 18,882 healthy men, 9060 had prostate needle biopsy data available for analysis. In the PROSCAR group, 280 (6.4%) men had prostate cancer with Gleason scores of 7-10 detected on needle biopsy vs. 237 (5.1%) men in the placebo group. Of the total cases of prostate cancer diagnosed in this study, approximately 98% were classified as intracapsular (stage T1 or T2). The clinical significance of these findings is unknown. This information from the literature (Thompson IM, Goodman PJ, Tangen CM, et al. The influence of finasteride on the development of prostate cancer. *N Engl J Med* 2003;349:213-22) is provided for consideration by physicians when PROSCAR is used as indicated. PROSCAR is not approved to reduce the risk of developing prostate cancer.

OVERDOSAGE

In clinical studies, single doses of finasteride up to 400 mg and multiple doses of finasteride up to 80 mg/day for three months did not result in adverse reactions. Until further experience is obtained, no specific treatment for an overdose with finasteride can be recommended.

Significant lethality was observed in male and female mice at single oral doses of 1500 mg/m² (500 mg/kg) and in female and male rats at single oral doses of 2360 mg/m² (400 mg/kg) and 5900 mg/m² (1000 mg/kg), respectively.

DOSAGE AND ADMINISTRATION

The recommended dosage is 1 mg orally once a day.
PROPECIA may be administered with or without meals.
In general, daily use for three months or more is necessary before benefit is observed. Continued use is recommended to sustain benefit, which should be re-evaluated periodically. Withdrawal of treatment leads to reversal of effect within 12 months.

HOW SUPPLIED

No. 6642—PROPECIA tablets, 1 mg, are tan, octagonal, film-coated convex tablets with "stylized P" logo on one side and PROPECIA on the other. They are supplied as follows:
NDC 0006-0071-31 unit of use bottles of 30 (with desiccant).
NDC 0006-0071-54 PROPAK®[3] - unit of use bottles of 90 (with desiccant).

Storage and Handling

Store at room temperature, 15-30°C (59-86°F). Keep container closed and protect from moisture.
Women should not handle crushed or broken PROPECIA tablets when they are pregnant or may potentially be pregnant because of the possibility of absorption of finasteride and the subsequent potential risk to a male fetus. PROPECIA tablets are coated and will prevent contact with the active ingredient during normal handling, provided that the tablets are not broken or crushed. (See WARNINGS, EXPOSURE OF WOMEN - RISK TO MALE FETUS; and PRECAUTIONS, Information for Patients and Pregnancy.)
Dist. by: Merck Sharp & Dohme Corp., a subsidiary of **MERCK & CO., INC.**, Whitehouse Station, NJ 08889, USA
Issued July 2010
9636006
US Patent Nos.: 5,547,957; 5,571,817

---

[3] Registered trademark of Merck Sharp & Dohme Corp., a subsidiary of **Merck & Co., Inc.**

TABLE 2. Drug-Related Adverse Experiences for PROSCAR (finasteride 5 mg) BENIGN PROSTATIC HYPERPLASIA

	Year 1 (%)		Years 2, 3 and 4* (%)	
	Finasteride, 5 mg	Placebo	Finasteride, 5 mg	Placebo
Impotence	8.1	3.7	5.1	5.1
Decreased Libido	6.4	3.4	2.6	2.6
Decreased Volume of Ejaculate	3.7	0.8	1.5	0.5
Ejaculation Disorder	0.8	0.1	0.2	0.1
Breast Enlargement	0.5	0.1	1.8	1.1
Breast Tenderness	0.4	0.1	0.7	0.3
Rash	0.5	0.2	0.5	0.1

N = 1524 and 1516, finasteride vs placebo, respectively
* Combined Years 2-4

PATIENT PACKAGE INSERT

PROPECIA®
(finasteride) Tablets, 1 mg
Patient Information about
PROPECIA® (Pro-pee-sha)
Generic name: finasteride
(fin-AS-tur-eyed)
PROPECIA[1] is for use by MEN ONLY.
Please read this leaflet before you start taking PROPECIA. Also, read the information included with PROPECIA each time you renew your prescription, just in case anything has changed. Remember, this leaflet does not take the place of careful discussions with your doctor. You and your doctor should discuss PROPECIA when you start taking your medication and at regular checkups.

What is PROPECIA used for?
PROPECIA is used for the treatment of male pattern hair loss on the vertex and the anterior mid-scalp area.
PROPECIA is for use by **MEN ONLY** and should **NOT** be used by women or children.

What is male pattern hair loss?
Male pattern hair loss is a common condition in which men experience thinning of the hair on the scalp. Often, this results in a receding hairline and/or balding on the top of the head. These changes typically begin gradually in men in their 20s.
Doctors believe male pattern hair loss is due to heredity and is dependent on hormonal effects. Doctors refer to this type of hair loss as androgenetic alopecia.

Results of clinical studies:
For 12 months, doctors studied over 1800 men aged 18 to 41 with mild to moderate amounts of ongoing hair loss. Of these men, approximately 1200 with hair loss at the top of the head participated in additional extension studies, resulting in a total study time of up to five years. In general, men who took PROPECIA maintained or increased the number of visible scalp hairs and noticed improvement in their hair in the first year. Improvement, compared to the start of the study, was maintained through the remaining years of treatment. Hair counts in men who did not take PROPECIA continued to decrease.
In one study, patients were questioned on the growth of body hair. PROPECIA did not appear to affect hair in places other than the scalp.

Will PROPECIA work for me?
For most men, PROPECIA increases the number of scalp hairs in the first year of treatment, helping to fill in thin or balding areas of the scalp. In addition, men taking PROPECIA may note a slowing of hair loss. Although results will vary, generally you will not be able to grow back all of the hair you have lost. There is not sufficient evidence that PROPECIA works in the treatment of receding hairline in the temporal area on both sides of the head.
Male pattern hair loss occurs gradually over time. On average, healthy hair grows only about half an inch each month. Therefore, it will take time to see any effect.
You may need to take PROPECIA daily for three months or more before you see a benefit from taking PROPECIA. PROPECIA can only work over the long term if you continue taking it. If the drug has not worked for you in twelve months, further treatment is unlikely to be of benefit. If you stop taking PROPECIA, you will likely lose the hair you have gained within 12 months of stopping treatment. You should discuss this with your doctor.
PROPECIA is not effective in the treatment of hair loss due to androgenetic alopecia in postmenopausal women. PROPECIA should not be taken by women.

How should I take PROPECIA?
Follow your doctor's instructions.
• Take one tablet by mouth each day.
• You may take PROPECIA with or without food.
• If you forget to take PROPECIA, do not take an extra tablet. Just take the next tablet as usual.
PROPECIA will not work faster or better if you take it more than once a day.

Who should NOT take PROPECIA?
• PROPECIA is for the treatment of male pattern hair loss in **MEN ONLY** and should not be taken by women (see **A warning about PROPECIA and pregnancy**).
• PROPECIA should not be taken by children.
• Anyone allergic to any of the ingredients.
A warning about PROPECIA and pregnancy.
• **Women who are or may potentially be pregnant:**
   • **must not use PROPECIA**
   • **should not handle crushed or broken tablets of PROPECIA.**
If a woman who is pregnant with a male baby absorbs the active ingredient in PROPECIA, either by swallowing or through the skin, it may cause abnormalities of a male baby's sex organs. If a woman who is pregnant comes into contact with the active ingredient in PROPECIA, a doctor should be consulted. PROPECIA tablets are coated and will prevent contact with the active ingredient during normal handling, provided that the tablets are not broken or crushed.

What are the possible side effects of PROPECIA?
Like all prescription products, PROPECIA may cause side effects. In clinical studies, side effects from PROPECIA were uncommon and did not affect most men. A small number of men experienced certain sexual side effects. These men reported one or more of the following: less desire for sex; difficulty in achieving an erection; and, a decrease in the amount of semen. Each of these side effects occurred in less than 2% of men. These side effects went away in men who stopped taking PROPECIA. They also disappeared in most men who continued taking PROPECIA.
In general use, the following have been reported: allergic reactions including rash, itching, hives and swelling of the lips and face; problems with ejaculation; breast tenderness and enlargement; depression; and testicular pain. You should promptly report to your doctor any changes in your breasts such as lumps, pain or nipple discharge. Tell your doctor promptly about these or any other unusual side effects.
• **PROPECIA can affect a blood test called PSA (Prostate-Specific Antigen) for the screening of prostate cancer. If you have a PSA test done, you should tell your doctor(s) that you are taking PROPECIA. Because PROPECIA decreases PSA levels, changes in PSA levels will need to be carefully evaluated by your doctor(s). Any increase in follow-up PSA levels from their lowest point should be carefully evaluated even if the test results are still within the normal range for men not taking PROPECIA. You should also tell your doctor if you have not been taking PROPECIA as prescribed because this may affect the PSA test results. For more information, talk to your doctor.**

Storage and handling.
Keep PROPECIA in the original container and keep the container closed. Store it in a dry place at room temperature.
PROPECIA tablets are coated and will prevent contact with the active ingredient during normal handling, provided that the tablets are not broken or crushed.

Do not give your PROPECIA tablets to anyone else. It has been prescribed only for you. Keep PROPECIA and all medications out of the reach of children.

THIS LEAFLET PROVIDES A SUMMARY OF INFORMATION ABOUT PROPECIA. IF AFTER READING THIS LEAFLET YOU HAVE ANY QUESTIONS OR ARE NOT SURE ABOUT ANYTHING, TALK TO YOUR DOCTOR, PHARMACIST, OR HEALTH CARE PROVIDER.
1-888-637-2522, Monday through Friday, 8:30 A.M. TO 7:00 P.M. (ET).
www.propecia.com
Dist. by: Merck Sharp & Dohme Corp., a subsidiary of
MERCK & CO., INC., Whitehouse Station, NJ 08889, USA
Issued July 2010
9636006
US Patent Nos.: 5,547,957; 5,571,817
Revised: 07/2010
Distributed by: Merck Sharp & Dohme Corp.
Shown in Product Identification Guide, page 313

ProQuad   ℞
[prō-kwăd]
Measles, Mumps, Rubella and Varicella Virus Vaccine Live
Lyophilized preparation for subcutaneous injection

HIGHLIGHTS OF PRESCRIBING INFORMATION
These highlights do not include all the information needed to use ProQuad safely and effectively. See full prescribing information for ProQuad.
ProQuad
Measles, Mumps, Rubella and Varicella Virus Vaccine Live
Lyophilized preparation for subcutaneous injection
Initial U.S. Approval: 2005

RECENT MAJOR CHANGES
Indications and Usage (1)	10/2009
Contraindications (4.2)	10/2009
Warnings and Precautions (5.1)	10/2009

INDICATIONS AND USAGE
ProQuad is a vaccine indicated for active immunization for the prevention of measles, mumps, rubella, and varicella in children 12 months through 12 years of age. (1)

DOSAGE AND ADMINISTRATION
A 0.5-mL dose for subcutaneous injection only. (2.1)
• The first dose is usually administered at 12 to 15 months of age. (2.1)
• A second dose, if needed, is usually administered at 4 to 6 years of age. (2.1)

DOSAGE FORMS AND STRENGTHS
Suspension for injection (0.5-mL dose) supplied as a lyophilized vaccine to be reconstituted using only accompanying sterile diluent. (2.2, 3)

CONTRAINDICATIONS
• History of anaphylactic reaction to neomycin or hypersensitivity to gelatin or any other component of the vaccine. (4.1)
• Primary or acquired immunodeficiency states. (4.2)
• Family history of congenital or hereditary immunodeficiency. (4.2)
• Immunosuppressive therapy. (4.2, 7.3)
• Active untreated tuberculosis or febrile illness (>101.3°F or >38.5°C). (4.3)
• Pregnancy. (4.4, 8.1, 17.1)

WARNINGS AND PRECAUTIONS
• Administration of ProQuad (dose 1) to children 12 to 23 months old who have not been previously vaccinated against measles, mumps, rubella, or varicella, nor had a history of the wild-type infections, is associated with higher rates of fever and febrile seizures at 5 to 12 days after vaccination when compared to children vaccinated with M-M-R II and VARIVAX administered separately. (5.1, 6.1, 6.3)
• Use caution when administering ProQuad to children with a history of cerebral injury or seizures or any other condition in which stress due to fever should be avoided. (5.2)
• Use caution when administering ProQuad to children with anaphylaxis or immediate hypersensitivity to eggs (5.3) or contact hypersensitivity to neomycin. (5.4)
• Use caution when administering ProQuad to children with thrombocytopenia. (5.5)
• Avoid close contact with high-risk individuals susceptible to varicella since transmission of varicella vaccine virus may occur between vaccinees and susceptible contacts. (5.8)
• Avoid pregnancy for 3 months following vaccination with measles, mumps, rubella, and/or varicella vaccines. (8.1, 17.1)
• Defer vaccination for at least 3 months following blood or plasma transfusions, or administration of immune globulins (IG). (5.9, 7.1)
• Avoid using salicylates for 6 weeks after vaccination with ProQuad. (6.1, 7.2, 17.1)

ADVERSE REACTIONS
• The most frequent vaccine-related adverse events reported in ≥5% of subjects vaccinated with ProQuad were:
  • injection-site reactions (pain/tenderness/soreness, erythema, and swelling)
  • fever
  • irritability. (6.1)
• Systemic vaccine-related adverse events that were reported at a significantly greater rate in recipients of ProQuad than in recipients of the component vaccines administered concomitantly were:
  • fever
  • measles-like rash. (6.1)
To report SUSPECTED ADVERSE REACTIONS, contact Merck & Co., Inc. at 1-877-888-4231 or VAERS at 1-800-822-7967 or www.vaers.hhs.gov.

DRUG INTERACTIONS
• Tuberculin testing should be administered anytime before, simultaneously with, or at least 4 to 6 weeks after ProQuad. (7.4)
• ProQuad may be administered concomitantly with *Haemophilus influenzae* type b conjugate vaccine and/or hepatitis B vaccine at separate injection sites. (7.5)
• ProQuad may be administered concomitantly with pneumococcal 7-valent conjugate vaccine and/or hepatitis A vaccine (inactivated) at separate injection sites. (7.5)

USE IN SPECIFIC POPULATIONS
Pregnancy: Do not administer ProQuad to females who are pregnant; the possible effects of the vaccine on fetal development are unknown at this time. (8.1)
To report vaccine exposure during pregnancy call 1-800-986-8999.

See 17 for PATIENT COUNSELING INFORMATION
Revised: 09/2010

FULL PRESCRIBING INFORMATION: CONTENTS*

FULL PRESCRIBING INFORMATION

1 INDICATIONS AND USAGE
ProQuad[1] is a vaccine indicated for active immunization for the prevention of measles, mumps, rubella, and varicella in children 12 months through 12 years of age.

[1] Registered trademark of Merck & Co., Inc.

2 DOSAGE AND ADMINISTRATION
2.1 Recommended Dose and Schedule
FOR SUBCUTANEOUS ADMINISTRATION ONLY
Each 0.5-mL dose of ProQuad is administered subcutaneously.
The first dose is usually administered at 12 to 15 months of age but may be given anytime through 12 years of age.
If a second dose of measles, mumps, rubella, and varicella vaccine is needed, ProQuad may be used. This dose is usually administered at 4 to 6 years of age. At least 1 month should elapse between a dose of a measles-containing vaccine such as M-M-R II (measles, mumps, and rubella virus vaccine live) and a dose of ProQuad. At least 3 months should elapse between a dose of varicella-containing vaccine and ProQuad.
2.2 Preparation for Administration
CAUTION: Preservatives, antiseptics, detergents, and other anti-viral substances may inactivate the vaccine. Use only sterile syringes that are free of preservatives, antiseptics, detergents, and other anti-viral substances for reconstitution and injection of ProQuad. Withdraw the entire volume of the supplied diluent into a syringe. Use only the diluent supplied with the vaccine since it is free of preservatives or other anti-viral substances.
Inject the entire content of the syringe into the vial containing the powder. Gently agitate to dissolve completely.
Parenteral drug products should be inspected visually for particulate matter and discoloration prior to administration. Visually inspect the vaccine before and after reconstitution prior to administration. Before reconstitution, the lyophilized vaccine is a white to pale yellow compact crystalline plug. ProQuad, when reconstituted, is a clear pale yellow to light pink liquid.
Withdraw the entire amount of the reconstituted vaccine from the vial into the same syringe and inject the entire volume.
TO MINIMIZE LOSS OF POTENCY, THE VACCINE SHOULD BE ADMINISTERED IMMEDIATELY AFTER RECONSTITUTION. IF NOT USED IMMEDIATELY, THE RECONSTITUTED VACCINE MAY BE STORED AT ROOM TEMPERATURE, PROTECTED FROM LIGHT, FOR UP TO 30 MINUTES. DISCARD RECONSTITUTED VACCINE IF IT IS NOT USED WITHIN 30 MINUTES.
2.3 Method of Administration
Inject the vaccine subcutaneously into the outer aspect of the deltoid region of the upper arm or into the higher anterolateral area of the thigh.
Use With Other Vaccines
Use different injection sites to administer each vaccine if other vaccines are administered concomitantly. [See Drug Interactions (7.5).]

3 DOSAGE FORMS AND STRENGTHS
ProQuad is a suspension for injection supplied as a 0.5-mL single dose vial of lyophilized vaccine to be reconstituted using the sterile diluent supplied [see How Supplied/Storage and Handling (16)].

4 CONTRAINDICATIONS
4.1 Hypersensitivity
Do not administer ProQuad to individuals with a history of anaphylactic reactions to neomycin. If vaccination with ProQuad is medically necessary for such individuals, they are advised to consult an allergist or immunologist and should receive ProQuad only in settings where anaphylactic reactions can be appropriately managed.
Do not administer ProQuad to individuals with a history of hypersensitivity to gelatin or any other component of the vaccine or following previous vaccination with ProQuad, VARIVAX (varicella virus vaccine live), or any measles-, mumps-, or rubella-containing vaccine [see Description (11) and Warnings and Precautions (5) for exceptions].
4.2 Immunosuppression
Do not administer ProQuad to individuals with blood dyscrasias, leukemia, lymphomas of any type, or other malignant neoplasms affecting the bone marrow or lymphatic system; or to individuals on immunosuppressive therapy (including high-dose systemic corticosteroids) [see Drug Interactions (7.3)]. Vaccination with a live, attenuated vaccine, such as varicella, can result in a more extensive vaccine-associated rash or disseminated disease in individuals on immunosuppressive drugs. ProQuad may be used by individuals who are receiving topical corticosteroids or low-dose corticosteroids, as are commonly used for asthma prophylaxis or in patients who are receiving corticosteroids as replacement therapy, e.g., for Addison's disease.

Do not administer ProQuad to individuals with primary and acquired immunodeficiency states, including AIDS or other clinical manifestations of infection with human immunodeficiency viruses; cellular immune deficiencies; and hypogammaglobulinemic and dysgammaglobulinemic states. Measles inclusion body encephalitis, pneumonitis, and death as a direct consequence of disseminated measles vaccine virus infection have been reported in severely immunocompromised individuals inadvertently vaccinated with measles-containing vaccine. In addition, disseminated varicella vaccine virus infection has been reported in children with underlying immunodeficiency disorders who were inadvertently vaccinated with a varicella-containing vaccine.{1}

Do not administer ProQuad to individuals with a family history of congenital or hereditary immunodeficiency, unless the immune competence of the potential vaccine recipient is demonstrated.

4.3 Concurrent Illness

Do not administer ProQuad to individuals with active untreated tuberculosis or to individuals with an active febrile illness with fever >101.3°F (>38.5°C).

4.4 Pregnancy

Do not administer ProQuad to individuals who are pregnant; the possible effects of the vaccine on fetal development are unknown at this time *[see Use in Specific Populations (8.1)]*.

5 WARNINGS AND PRECAUTIONS

5.1 Fever and Febrile Seizures

Administration of ProQuad (dose 1) to children 12 to 23 months old who have not been previously vaccinated against measles, mumps, rubella, or varicella, nor had a history of the wild-type infections, is associated with higher rates of fever and febrile seizures at 5 to 12 days after vaccination when compared to children vaccinated with dose 1 of both M-M-R II and VARIVAX administered separately *[see Adverse Reactions (6.3)]*.

5.2 History of Cerebral Injury or Seizures

Exercise caution when administering ProQuad to persons with a history of cerebral injury, individual or family history of convulsions, or any other condition in which stress due to fever should be avoided. Healthcare providers should be alert to the temperature elevations that may occur following vaccination.

5.3 Hypersensitivity to Eggs

Live measles vaccine and live mumps vaccine are produced in chick embryo cell culture. Persons with a history of anaphylactic or other immediate hypersensitivity reactions (*e.g.*, hives, swelling of the mouth and throat, difficulty breathing, hypotension, or shock) subsequent to egg ingestion may be at an enhanced risk of immediate-type hypersensitivity reactions after receiving vaccines containing traces of chick embryo antigen. Carefully evaluate the potential risk-to-benefit ratio before considering vaccination in such cases. Such individuals may be vaccinated with extreme caution; adequate treatment should be readily available should a reaction occur *[see Contraindications (4.1)]*.{2}

Children with egg allergy are at low risk for anaphylactic reactions to measles-containing vaccines (including M-M-R II), and skin testing of children allergic to eggs is not predictive of reactions to M-M-R II vaccine. Persons with allergies to chickens or feathers are not at increased risk of reaction to the vaccine.{2}

5.4 Contact Hypersensitivity to Neomycin

Most often, neomycin allergy manifests as a contact dermatitis, which is not a contraindication to receiving measles-, mumps-, rubella-, or varicella-containing vaccine.

5.5 Thrombocytopenia

Carefully evaluate the potential risk-to-benefit ratio before considering vaccination with ProQuad in children with thrombocytopenia or in those who experienced thrombocytopenia after vaccination with a previous dose of measles, mumps, rubella, and/or varicella vaccine. No clinical data are available regarding the development or worsening of thrombocytopenia in individuals vaccinated with ProQuad. Cases of thrombocytopenia have been reported after primary vaccination with measles vaccine, measles, mumps, and rubella vaccine, after varicella vaccination, and following re-vaccination with measles vaccine or M-M-R II *[see Adverse Reactions (6.2)]*.

5.6 Use for Post-Exposure Prophylaxis

The safety and efficacy of ProQuad for use after exposure to measles, mumps, rubella, or varicella have not been established.

5.7 Use in HIV-Infected Children

The safety and efficacy of ProQuad for use in children known to be infected with human immunodeficiency viruses have not been established.

5.8 Risk of Vaccine Virus Transmission

Post-licensing experience with VARIVAX suggests that transmission of varicella vaccine virus may occur between healthy vaccine recipients (who develop or do not develop a varicella-like rash) and contacts susceptible to varicella, as well as high-risk individuals susceptible to varicella.

High-risk individuals susceptible to varicella include:

- Immunocompromised individuals;
- Pregnant women without documented positive history of varicella (chickenpox) or laboratory evidence of prior infection;
- Newborn infants of mothers without documented positive history of varicella or laboratory evidence of prior infection and all newborn infants born at <28 weeks gestation regardless of maternal varicella immunity.

Vaccine recipients should attempt to avoid, to the extent possible, close association with high-risk individuals susceptible to varicella for up to 6 weeks following vaccination. In circumstances where contact with high-risk individuals susceptible to varicella is unavoidable, the potential risk of transmission of the varicella vaccine virus should be weighed against the risk of acquiring and transmitting wild-type varicella virus.

Excretion of small amounts of the live, attenuated rubella virus from the nose or throat has occurred in the majority of susceptible individuals 7 to 28 days after vaccination. There is no confirmed evidence to indicate that such virus is transmitted to susceptible persons who are in contact with the vaccinated individuals. Consequently, transmission through close personal contact, while accepted as a theoretical possibility, is not regarded as a significant risk. However, transmission of the rubella vaccine virus to infants via breast milk has been documented *[see Use in Specific Populations (8.3)]*.

There are no reports of transmission of the more attenuated Enders' Edmonston strain of measles virus or the Jeryl Lynn™ strain of mumps virus from vaccine recipients to susceptible contacts.

5.9 Immune Globulins and Transfusions

Immune globulins (IG) administered concomitantly with ProQuad contain antibodies that may interfere with vaccine virus replication and decrease the expected immune response. Vaccination should be deferred for at least 3 months following blood or plasma transfusions, or administration of IG.

The appropriate suggested interval between transfusion or IG administration and vaccination will vary with the type of transfusion or indication for, and dose of, IG (*e.g.*, 5 months for Varicella Zoster Immune Globulin [VZIG]).{2} Following administration of ProQuad, any IG including VZIG should not be given for 1 month thereafter unless its use outweighs the benefits of vaccination.{2} *[See Drug Interactions (7.1).]*

5.10 Risk of Transmission of Creutzfeldt-Jakob Disease and other Adventitious Agents

This product contains albumin, a derivative of human blood. Based on effective donor screening and product manufacturing processes, it carries an extremely remote risk for transmission of viral diseases. Although there is a theoretical risk for transmission of Creutzfeldt-Jakob disease (CJD), no cases of transmission of CJD or viral disease have ever been identified that were associated with the use of albumin. The cells, virus pools, bovine serum, and human albumin used in manufacturing are all evaluated and tested to provide assurance that the final product is free of potential adventitious agents *[see Description (11)]*.

6 ADVERSE REACTIONS

6.1 Clinical Trials Experience

Because clinical trials are conducted under widely varying conditions, adverse reaction rates observed in the clinical trials of a vaccine cannot be directly compared to rates in the clinical trials of another vaccine and may not reflect the rates observed in clinical practice. Vaccine-related adverse reactions reported during clinical trials were assessed by the study investigators to be possibly, probably, or definitely vaccine-related and are summarized below.

Children 12 Through 23 Months of Age Who Received a Single Dose of ProQuad

ProQuad was administered to 4497 children 12 through 23 months of age involved in 4 randomized clinical trials without concomitant administration with other vaccines. The safety of ProQuad was compared with the safety of M-M-R II and VARIVAX given concomitantly (N=2038) at separate injection sites. The safety profile for ProQuad was similar to the component vaccines. Children in these studies were monitored for up to 42 days postvaccination using vaccination report card-aided surveillance. Safety follow-up was obtained for 98% of children in each group. Few subjects (<0.1%) who received ProQuad discontinued the study due to an adverse reaction. The race distribution of the study subjects across these studies following a first dose of ProQuad was as follows: 65.2% White; 13.1% African-American; 11.1% Hispanic; 5.8% Asian/Pacific; 4.5% other; and 0.2% American Indian. The racial distribution of the control group was similar to that of the group who received ProQuad. The gender distribution across the studies following a first dose of ProQuad was 52.5% male and 47.5% female. The gender distribution of the control group was similar to that of the group who received ProQuad. Vaccine-related injection-site and systemic adverse reactions observed among recipients of ProQuad or M-M-R II and VARIVAX at a rate of at least 1% are shown in Table 1. Systemic vaccine-related adverse reactions that were reported at a significantly greater rate in individuals who received a first dose of ProQuad than in individuals who received first doses of M-M-R II and VARIVAX concomitantly at separate injection sites were fever (≥102°F [≥38.9°C] oral equivalent or abnormal) (21.5% versus 14.9%, respectively, risk difference 6.6%, 95% CI: 4.6, 8.5), and measles-like rash (3.0% versus 2.1%, respectively, risk difference 1.0%, 95% CI: 0.1, 1.8). Both fever and measles-like rash usually occurred within 5 to 12 days following the vaccination, were of short duration, and resolved with no long-term sequelae. Pain/tenderness/soreness at the injection site was reported at a statistically lower rate in individuals who received ProQuad than in individuals who received M-M-R II and VARIVAX concomitantly at separate injection sites (22.0% versus 26.8%, respectively, risk difference -4.8%, 95% CI: -7.1, -2.5). The only vaccine-related injection-site adverse reaction that was more frequent among recipients of ProQuad than recipients of M-M-R II and VARIVAX was rash at the injection site (2.4% versus 1.6%, respectively, risk difference 0.9%, 95% CI: 0.1, 1.5).

Table 1: Vaccine-Related Injection-Site and Systemic Adverse Reactions Reported in ≥1% of Children Who Received ProQuad Dose 1 or M-M-R II and VARIVAX at 12 to 23 Months of Age (0 to 42 Days Postvaccination)

Adverse Reactions	ProQuad (N=4497) (n=4424) %	M-M-R II and VARIVAX (N=2038) (n=1997) %
*Injection Site**		
Pain/tenderness/soreness†	22.0	26.7
Erythema†	14.4	15.8
Swelling†	8.4	9.8
Ecchymosis	1.5	2.3
Rash	2.3	1.5
Systemic		
Fever†,‡	21.5	14.9
Irritability	6.7	6.7
Measles-like rash†	3.0	2.1
Varicella-like rash†	2.1	2.2
Rash (not otherwise specified)	1.6	1.4
Upper respiratory infection	1.3	1.1
Viral exanthema	1.2	1.1
Diarrhea	1.2	1.3

* Injection-site adverse reactions for M-M-R II and VARIVAX are based on occurrence with either of the vaccines administered.
† Designates a solicited adverse reaction. Injection-site adverse reactions were solicited only from Days 0 to 4 postvaccination.
‡ Temperature reported as elevated (≥102°F, oral equivalent) or abnormal.
N = number of subjects vaccinated.
n = number of subjects with safety follow-up.

Rubella-like rashes were observed in <1% of subjects following a first dose of ProQuad.

In these clinical trials, two cases of herpes zoster were reported among 2108 healthy subjects 12 through 23 months of age who were vaccinated with their first dose of ProQuad and followed for 1 year. Both cases were unremarkable and no sequelae were reported.

Children 15 to 31 Months of Age Who Received a Second Dose of ProQuad

In 5 clinical trials, 2780 healthy children were vaccinated with ProQuad (dose 1) at 12 to 23 months of age and then administered a second dose approximately 3 to 9 months later. The race distribution of the study subjects across these studies following a second dose of ProQuad was as follows: 64.4% White; 14.1% African-American; 12.0% Hispanic; 5.9% other; 3.5% Asian/Pacific; and 0.1% American Indian. The gender distribution across the studies following a second dose of ProQuad was 51.5% male and 48.5% female. Children in these open-label studies were monitored for at least 28 days postvaccination using vaccination report card-aided surveillance. Safety follow-up was obtained for approximately 97% of children overall. Vaccine-related injection-site and systemic adverse reactions observed after Dose 1 and 2 of ProQuad at a rate of at least 1% are shown in Table 2. In these trials, the overall rates of systemic adverse reactions after ProQuad (dose 2) were comparable to, or lower than, those seen with the first dose. In the subset of children who received both ProQuad dose 1 and dose 2 in these trials (N=2408) with follow-up for fever, fever ≥102.2°F (≥38.9°C) was observed significantly less frequently days 1 to 28 after the second dose (10.8%) than after the first dose (19.1%) (risk difference 8.3%, 95% CI: 6.4, 10.3). Fevers ≥102.2°F (≥38.9°C) days 5 to 12 after vaccinations were also reported significantly less frequently after dose 2 (3.9%) than after dose 1 (13.6%) (risk difference 9.7%, 95% CI: 8.1, 11.3). In the subset of children who received both doses and for whom injection-site reactions were reported (N=2679), injection-site erythema was noted significantly more frequently after ProQuad (dose 2) as compared to ProQuad (dose 1) (12.6% and 10.8%, respectively, risk difference -1.8, 95% CI: -3.3, -0.3); however, pain and tenderness at the injection site was significantly lower after dose 2 (16.1%) as compared with after dose 1 (21.9%) (risk difference, 5.8%, 95% CI: 4.1, 7.6). Two children had febrile seizures after ProQuad (dose 2); both febrile seizures were thought to be related to a concurrent viral illness [see Adverse Reactions (6.3) and Clinical Studies (14)]. These studies were not designed or statistically powered to detect a difference in rates of febrile seizure between recipients of ProQuad as compared to M-M-R II and VARIVAX. The risk of febrile seizure has not been evaluated in a clinical study comparing the incidence rate after ProQuad (dose 2) with the incidence rate after concomitant M-M-R II (dose 2) and VARIVAX (dose 2). [See Adverse Reactions (6.1), Children 4 to 6 Years of Age Who Received ProQuad After Primary Vaccination with M-M-R II and VARIVAX.]

Table 2: Vaccine-Related Injection-Site and Systemic Adverse Reactions Reported in ≥1% of Children Who Received ProQuad Dose 1 at 12 to 23 Months of Age and Dose 2 at 15 to 31 Months of Age (1 to 28 Days Postvaccination)

Adverse Reactions	ProQuad Dose 1 (N=3112) (n=3019) %	ProQuad Dose 2 (N=2780) (n=2695) %
Injection Site		
Pain/tenderness/soreness*	21.4	15.9
Erythema*	10.7	12.4
Swelling*	8.0	8.5
Injection-site bruising	1.1	0.0
Systemic		
Fever*,†	20.4	8.3
Irritability	6.0	2.4
Measles-like/Rubella-like rash	4.3	0.9
Varicella-like/Vesicular rash	1.5	0.1
Diarrhea	1.3	0.6
Upper respiratory infection	1.3	1.4
Rash (not otherwise specified)	1.2	0.6
Rhinorrhea	1.1	1.0

* Designates a solicited adverse reaction. Injection-site adverse reactions were solicited only from Days 1 to 5 postvaccination.
† Temperature reported as elevated or abnormal.
N = number of subjects vaccinated.
n = number of subjects with safety follow-up

Children 4 to 6 Years of Age Who Received ProQuad After Primary Vaccination with M-M-R II and VARIVAX
In a double-blind clinical trial, 799 healthy 4- to 6-year-old children who received M-M-R II and VARIVAX at least 1 month prior to study entry were randomized to receive ProQuad and placebo (N=399), M-M-R II and placebo concomitantly (N=205) at separate injection sites, or M-M-R II and VARIVAX (N=195) concomitantly at separate injection sites [see Clinical Studies (14)]. Children in these studies were monitored for up to 42 days postvaccination using vaccination report card-aided surveillance. Safety follow-up was obtained for >98% of children in each group. The race distribution of the study subjects following a dose of ProQuad was as follows: 78.4% White; 12.3% African-American; 3.8% Hispanic; 3.5% other; and 2.0% Asian/Pacific. The gender distribution following a dose of ProQuad was 52.1% male and 47.9% female. Injection-site and systemic adverse reactions observed after Dose 1 and 2 of ProQuad at a rate of at least 1% are shown in Table 3. [See Clinical Studies (14).]
[See table 3 above]

Safety in Trials that Evaluated Concomitant Use with Other Vaccines
ProQuad Administered with Diphtheria and Tetanus Toxoids and Acellular Pertussis Vaccine Adsorbed (DTaP) and Haemophilus influenzae type b Conjugate (Meningococcal Protein Conjugate) and Hepatitis B (Recombinant) Vaccine
In an open-label clinical trial, 1434 children were randomized to receive ProQuad given with diphtheria and tetanus toxoids and acellular pertussis vaccine adsorbed (DTaP) and Haemophilus influenzae type b conjugate (meningococcal protein conjugate) and hepatitis B (recombinant) vaccine concomitantly (N=949) or non-concomitantly with ProQuad given first and the other vaccines 6 weeks later (N=485). No clinically significant differences in adverse events were reported between treatment groups [see Clinical Studies (14)]. The race distribution of the study subjects who received ProQuad was as follows: 70.7% White; 10.9% Asian/Pacific; 10.7% African-American; 4.5% Hispanic; 3.0% other; and 0.2% American Indian. The gender distribution of the study subjects who received ProQuad was 53.6% male and 46.4% female.
ProQuad Administered with Pneumococcal 7-valent Conjugate Vaccine and/or Hepatitis A Vaccine, Inactivated
In an open-label clinical trial, 1027 healthy children 12 to 23 months of age were randomized to receive ProQuad (dose 1) and pneumococcal 7-valent conjugate vaccine (dose 4) concomitantly (N=510) or non-concomitantly at different clinic visits (N=517). The race distribution of the study subjects was as follows: 65.2% White; 15.1% African-American; 10.0% Hispanic; 6.6% other; and 3.0% Asian/Pacific. The gender distribution of the study subjects was 54.5% male and 45.5% female. Injection-site and systemic adverse reactions observed among recipients of ProQuad administered concomitantly or non-concomitantly with pneumococcal 7-valent conjugate vaccine at a rate of at least 1% are shown in Table 4. No clinically significant differences in adverse reactions were reported between the concomitant and non-concomitant treatment groups [see Clinical Studies (14)].

Table 4: Vaccine-Related Injection-Site and Systemic Adverse Reactions Reported in ≥1% of Children Who Received ProQuad (dose 1) Concomitantly or Non-Concomitantly with PCV7* (dose 4) at the First Visit (1 to 28 Days Postvaccination)

Adverse Reactions	ProQuad + PCV7 (N=510) (n=498) %	PCV7 (N=258) (n=250) %	ProQuad (N=259) (n=255) %
Injection-Site - ProQuad			
Pain†	24.9	N/A	24.7
Erythema†	12.4	N/A	11.0
Swelling†	10.8	N/A	7.5
Bruising	2.0	N/A	1.6
Injection-Site - PCV7			
Pain†	30.5	29.6	N/A
Erythema†	21.1	24.4	N/A
Swelling†	17.9	20.0	N/A
Bruising	1.6	1.2	N/A
Systemic			
Fever†,‡	15.5	10.0	15.3
Measles-like rash	4.4	0.8	5.1
Irritability	3.8	3.6	3.5
Upper respiratory infection	1.6	0.8	1.2
Varicella-like/vesicular rash	1.6	0.0	1.2
Diarrhea	0.8	1.2	1.2
Vomiting	0.6	0.8	1.2
Rash	0.4	0.0	1.2
Somnolence	0.0	0.0	1.2

* PCV7 = Pneumococcal 7-valent conjugate vaccine, dose 4.
† Designates a solicited adverse reaction. Injection-site adverse reactions were solicited only from Days 1 to 5 postvaccination.
‡ Temperature reported as elevated (≥102°F, oral equivalent) or abnormal.
N/A = Not applicable.
N = number of subjects vaccinated.
n = number of subjects with safety follow-up.

In an open-label clinical trial, 699 healthy children 12 to 23 months of age were randomized to receive 2 doses of VAQTA (hepatitis A vaccine, inactivated) (N=352) or 2 doses of VAQTA concomitantly with 2 doses of ProQuad (N=347) at least 6 months apart. An additional 1101 subjects received 2 doses of VAQTA alone at least 6 months apart (non-randomized), resulting in 1453 subjects receiving 2 doses of VAQTA alone (1101 non-randomized and 352 randomized) and 347 subjects receiving 2 doses of VAQTA concomitantly with ProQuad (all randomized). The race distribution of the study subjects following a dose of ProQuad was as follows: 47.3% White; 42.7% Hispanic; 5.5% other; 2.9% African-American; and 1.7% Asian/Pacific. The gender distribution of the study subjects following a dose of ProQuad was 49.3% male and 50.7% female. Vaccine-related injection-site adverse reactions (days 1 to 5 postvaccination) and systemic adverse events (days 1 to 14 post VAQTA and days 1 to 28 post ProQuad vaccination) observed among recipients of VAQTA and ProQuad administered concomitantly with VAQTA at a rate of at least 1% are shown in Tables 5 and 6, respectively. In addition, among the randomized cohort, in the 14 days after each vaccination, the rates of fever (including all vaccine- and non-vaccine-related reports) were significantly higher in subjects who received ProQuad with VAQTA concomitantly after dose 1 (22.0%) as compared to subjects given dose 1 of VAQTA without ProQuad (10.8%). However, rates of fever were not significantly higher in subjects who received ProQuad with VAQTA concomitantly after dose 2 (12.5%) as compared to subjects given dose 2 of VAQTA without ProQuad (9.4%). In post-hoc analyses, these rates were significantly different for dose 1 (RR 2.03 [95% CI: 1.42, 2.94]), but not dose 2 (RR 1.32 [95% CI: 0.82, 2.13]). Rates of injection-site adverse reactions and other systemic

Table 3: Vaccine-Related Injection-Site and Systemic Adverse Reactions Reported in ≥1% of Children Previously Vaccinated with M-M-R II and VARIVAX Who Received ProQuad + Placebo, M-M-R II + Placebo, or M-M-R II + VARIVAX at 4 to 6 Years of Age (1 to 43 Days Postvaccination)

Adverse Reactions	ProQuad + Placebo (N=399) (n=397) %	M-M-R II + Placebo (N=205) (n=205) %	M-M-R II + VARIVAX (N=195) (n=193) %
Systemic			
Fever*,†	2.5	2.0	4.1
Cough	1.3	0.5	0.5
Irritability	1.0	0.5	1.0
Headache	0.8	1.5	1.6
Rhinorrhea	0.5	1.0	1.0
Nasopharyngitis	0.3	1.0	1.0
Vomiting	0.3	1.0	0.5
Upper respiratory infection	0.0	0.0	1.0

	ProQuad %	Placebo %	M-M-R II %	Placebo %	M-M-R II %	VARIVAX %
Injection-Site						
Pain*	41.1	34.5	36.6	34.1	35.2	36.8
Erythema*	24.4	13.4	15.6	14.1	14.5	15.5
Swelling*	15.6	8.1	10.2	8.8	7.8	10.9
Bruising	3.5	3.8	2.4	3.4	1.6	2.1
Rash	1.5	1.3	0.0	0.0	0.5	0.0
Pruritus	1.0	0.3	0.0	0.0	0.0	1.0
Nodule	0.0	0.0	0.0	0.0	0.0	1.0

* Designates a solicited adverse reaction. Injection-site adverse reactions were solicited only from Days 1 to 5 postvaccination.
† Temperature reported as elevated (≥102°F, oral equivalent) or abnormal.
N = number of subjects vaccinated.
n = number of subjects with safety follow-up.

adverse events were lower following a second dose than following the first dose of both vaccines given concomitantly.
[See table 5 at right]
[See table 6 at right]
In an open-label clinical trial, 653 children 12 to 23 months of age were randomized to receive a first dose of ProQuad with VAQTA and pneumococcal 7-valent conjugate vaccine concomitantly (N=330) or a first dose of ProQuad and pneumococcal 7-valent conjugate vaccine concomitantly and then vaccinated with VAQTA 6 weeks later (N=323). Approximately 6 months later, subjects received either the second doses of ProQuad and VAQTA concomitantly or the second doses of ProQuad and VAQTA separately. The race distribution of the study subjects was as follows: 60.3% White; 21.6% African-American; 9.5% Hispanic; 7.2% other, 1.1% Asian/Pacific; and 0.3% American Indian. The gender distribution of the study subjects was 50.7% male and 49.3% female. Vaccine-related injection-site and systemic adverse reactions observed among recipients of concomitant ProQuad, VAQTA, and pneumococcal 7-valent conjugate vaccine and ProQuad and pneumococcal 7-valent conjugate vaccine at a rate of at least 1% are shown in Tables 7 and 8. In the 28 days after vaccination with the first dose of ProQuad, the rates of fever (including all vaccine- and non-vaccine-related reports) were comparable in subjects who received the 3 vaccines together (38.6%) as compared with subjects given ProQuad and pneumococcal 7-valent conjugate vaccine (42.7%). The rates of fever in the 28 days following the second dose of ProQuad were also comparable in subjects who received ProQuad and VAQTA together (17.4%) as compared with subjects given ProQuad separately from VAQTA (17.0%). In a post-hoc analysis, these differences were not statistically significant after ProQuad (dose 1) (RR 0.90 [95% CI: 0.75, 1.09]) nor after dose 2 (RR 1.02 [95% CI: 0.70, 1.51]). No clinically significant differences in adverse reactions were reported among treatment groups [see Clinical Studies (14)].
[See table 7 at top of next page]
[See table 8 on next page]
Reye's syndrome following wild-type varicella infection has occurred in children and adolescents, the majority of whom had received salicylates. In all clinical studies of ProQuad or VARIVAX, the recommendation was made to avoid the use of salicylates for 6 weeks after vaccination. There were no reports of Reye's syndrome in recipients of ProQuad or VARIVAX during these studies [see Drug Interactions (7.2) and Patient Counseling Information (17.1)].

6.2   Post-Marketing Experience
The following adverse events have been identified during post-approval use of either the components of ProQuad or ProQuad. Because the reactions are in some cases described in the literature or reported voluntarily from a population of uncertain size, it is not always possible to reliably estimate their frequency or establish a causal relationship.

Post-Marketing Reports
Adverse events reported with post-marketing use of ProQuad and/or in clinical studies and/or post-marketing use of M-M-R II, the component vaccines, and VARIVAX without regard to causality or frequency are summarized below.

Infections and infestations
Atypical measles, candidiasis, cellulitis, herpes zoster, infection, influenza, measles, orchitis, parotitis, respiratory infection, skin infection, varicella.

Blood and the lymphatic system disorders
Aplastic anemia, lymphadenitis, regional lymphadenopathy, thrombocytopenia.

Immune system disorders
Anaphylactoid reaction, anaphylaxis and related phenomena such as angioneurotic edema, facial edema, and peripheral edema, anaphylaxis in individuals with or without an allergic history.

Psychiatric disorders
Agitation, apathy, nervousness.

Nervous system disorders
Afebrile convulsions or seizures, aseptic meningitis (see below), ataxia, Bell's palsy, cerebrovascular accident, convulsion, dizziness, dream abnormality, encephalitis (see below), encephalopathy (see below), febrile seizure, Guillain-Barré syndrome, headache, hypersomnia, measles inclusion body encephalitis [see Contraindications (4.2)], ocular palsies, paraesthesia, polyneuritis, polyneuropathy, subacute sclerosing panencephalitis (see below), syncope, transverse myelitis, tremor.

Eye disorders
Edema of the eyelid, irritation, optic neuritis, retinitis, retrobulbar neuritis.

Ear and labyrinth disorders
Ear pain, nerve deafness.

Vascular disorders
Extravasation.

Table 5: Vaccine-Related Injection-Site Adverse Reactions Reported in ≥1% of Children Who Received VAQTA or ProQuad Concomitantly with VAQTA 1 to 5 Days After Vaccination with VAQTA or VAQTA and ProQuad

Adverse Reactions	Dose 1		Dose 2	
	VAQTA (N=1453) (n=1412) %	ProQuad + VAQTA (N=347) (n=328) %	VAQTA (N=1301) (n=1254) %	ProQuad + VAQTA (N=292) (n=264) %
Injection-Site VAQTA				
Pain/tenderness*	29.2	27.1	30.1	25.0
Erythema*	13.5	12.5	14.3	11.7
Swelling*	7.1	9.1	9.0	8.0
Injection-site bruising	1.9	2.4	1.0	0.8
Injection-Site ProQuad				
Pain/tenderness*	N/A	30.5	N/A	26.2
Erythema*	N/A	13.4	N/A	12.9
Swelling*	N/A	6.7	N/A	6.5
Injection-site bruising	N/A	1.5	N/A	0.4

* Designates a solicited adverse reaction. Injection-site adverse reactions were solicited only from Days 1 to 5 postvaccination.
N/A = Not applicable.
N = number of subjects vaccinated.
n = number of subjects with safety follow-up.

Table 6: Vaccine-Related Systemic Adverse Reactions Reported in ≥1% of Children Who Received VAQTA* or ProQuad Concomitantly with VAQTA 1 to 14 Days After VAQTA or Vaccination with ProQuad and VAQTA and 1 to 28 Days After Vaccination with ProQuad and VAQTA

Adverse Reactions	Dose 1			Dose 2		
	Days 1 to 14		Days 1 to 28	Days 1 to 14		Days 1 to 28
	VAQTA[†] (N=1453) (n=1412) %	ProQuad + VAQTA[†] (N=347) (n=328) %	ProQuad + VAQTA (N=347) (n=328) %	VAQTA (N=1301) (n=1254) %	ProQuad + VAQTA[†] (N=292) (n=264) %	ProQuad + VAQTA[†] (N=291) (n=263) %
Fever[‡,§]	5.7	14.9	15.2	4.1	8.0	8.4
Irritability	5.8	7.0	7.3	3.5	5.3	5.3
Measles-like rash	0.0	3.4	3.4	0.0	1.1	1.1
Rhinorrhea	0.6	2.7	3.0	0.6	1.1	2.7
Diarrhea	1.5	1.8	2.4	1.7	0.4	0.8
Cough	0.6	2.1	2.1	0.2	0.8	1.5
Vomiting	1.1	0.3	0.9	0.6	0.8	1.1

* Systemic adverse events for subjects given VAQTA alone were collected for 14 days postvaccination.
† Safety follow-up for systemic adverse reactions was 14 days for VAQTA and 28 days for ProQuad + VAQTA.
‡ Designates a solicited adverse reaction.
§ Temperature reported as elevated or abnormal.
N = number of subjects vaccinated.
n = number of subjects with safety follow-up.

Respiratory, thoracic and mediastinal disorders
Bronchial spasm, bronchitis, epistaxis, pneumonitis [see Contraindications (4.3)], pneumonia, pulmonary congestion, rhinitis, sinusitis, sneezing, sore throat, wheezing.

Gastrointestinal disorders
Abdominal pain, flatulence, hematochezia, mouth ulcer.

Skin and subcutaneous tissue disorders
Erythema multiforme, Henoch-Schönlein purpura, herpes simplex, impetigo, panniculitis, pruritus, purpura, skin induration, Stevens-Johnson syndrome, sunburn.

Musculoskeletal, connective tissue and bone disorders
Arthritis and/or arthralgia (usually transient and rarely chronic, see below), musculoskeletal pain, myalgia, pain of the hip, leg, or neck, swelling.

Reproductive system and breast disorders
Epididymitis.

General disorders and administration site conditions
Injection-site complaints (burning and/or stinging of short duration, eczema, edema/swelling, hive-like rash, discoloration, hematoma, induration, lump, vesicles, wheal and flare), inflammation, lip abnormality, papillitis, roughness/dryness, stiffness, trauma, varicella-like rash, venipuncture site hemorrhage, warm sensation, warm to touch.
Deaths have been reported following vaccination with measles, mumps, and rubella vaccines; however, a causal relationship has not been established in healthy individuals. Death as a direct consequence of disseminated measles vaccine virus infection has been reported in severely immunocompromised individuals in whom a measles-containing vaccine is contraindicated and who were inadvertently vaccinated. However, there were no deaths or permanent sequelae reported in a published post-marketing surveillance study in Finland involving 1.5 million children and adults who were vaccinated with M-M-R II during 1982 to 1993.[3]

Encephalitis and encephalopathy have been reported approximately once for every 3 million doses of the combination of measles, mumps, and rubella vaccine contained in M-M-R II. In no case has it been shown conclusively that reactions were actually caused by the vaccine; however, the data suggest the possibility that some of these cases may have been caused by measles vaccines. The risk of such serious neurological disorders following live measles virus vaccine administration remains far less than that for encephalitis and encephalopathy with wild-type measles (1 per 2000 reported cases).
Recipients of rubella vaccine may develop chronic joint symptoms. Arthralgia and/or arthritis, and polyneuritis after wild-type rubella virus infection vary in frequency and severity with age and gender, being greatest in adult females and least in pre-pubertal children. Following vaccination in children, reactions in joints are uncommon (0 to 3%) and of brief duration. In women, incidence rates for arthritis and arthralgia are higher than those seen in children (12 to 26%), and the reactions tend to be more marked and of longer duration (e.g., months or years). In adolescent girls, the reactions appear to be intermediate in incidence between those seen in children and adult women.
Chronic arthritis has been associated with wild-type rubella infection and has been related to persistent virus and/or viral antigen isolated from body tissues. Chronic joint symptoms have been reported following administration of rubella-containing vaccine. There have been reports of subacute sclerosing panencephalitis (SSPE) in children who did not have a history of infection with wild-type measles but did receive measles vaccine. Some of these cases may have resulted from unrecognized measles in the first year of life or possibly from the measles vaccination. Based on estimated measles vaccine distribution in the United States (US), the association of SSPE cases to measles vaccination

Table 7: Vaccine-Related Injection-Site Adverse Reactions Reported in ≥1% of Children Who Received ProQuad + VAQTA + PCV7* Concomitantly or VAQTA Alone Followed by ProQuad + PCV7 Concomitantly (1 to 5 Days After a Dose of ProQuad)

Adverse Reactions	Dose 1		Dose 2	
	VAQTA + ProQuad + PCV7 (N=330) (n=311) %	VAQTA Alone Followed by ProQuad + PCV7 (N=323) (n=302) %	VAQTA + ProQuad (N=273) (n=265) %	VAQTA Alone Followed by ProQuad (N=240) (n=230) %
Injection-Site - ProQuad				
Pain/tenderness[†]	21.2	24.2	18.1	17.0
Erythema[†]	13.5	11.9	10.6	13.0
Swelling[†]	7.4	10.9	8.3	11.7
Bruising	1.9	1.3	0.8	0.4
Injection-Site - VAQTA				
Pain/tenderness[†]	20.6	15.3	17.5	20.3
Erythema[†]	9.6	11.7	9.1	12.7
Swelling[†]	6.8	9.5	6.1	7.6
Bruising	1.3	1.1	1.1	1.6
Rash	1.0	0.0	0.4	0.4
Injection-Site - PCV7				
Pain/tenderness[†]	25.4	27.6	N/A	N/A
Erythema[†]	16.4	16.6	N/A	N/A
Swelling[†]	13.2	14.3	N/A	N/A
Bruising	0.6	1.7	N/A	N/A

* PCV7 = Pneumococcal 7-valent conjugate vaccine.
† Designates a solicited adverse reaction. Injection-site adverse reactions were solicited only from Days 1 to 5 postvaccination at each vaccine injection site.
N/A = Not applicable.
N = number of subjects vaccinated.
n = number of subjects with safety follow-up.

Table 8: Vaccine-Related Systemic Adverse Reactions Reported in ≥1% of Children Who Received ProQuad + VAQTA + PCV7* Concomitantly, or VAQTA Alone Followed By ProQuad + PCV7 Concomitantly (1 to 28 Days After a Dose of ProQuad)

Adverse Reactions	Dose 1		Dose 2	
	VAQTA + ProQuad + PCV7 (N=330) (n=311) %	VAQTA Alone Followed by ProQuad + PCV7 (N=323) (n=302) %	VAQTA + ProQuad (N=273) (n=265) %	VAQTA Alone Followed by ProQuad (N=240) (n=230) %
Fever[†,‡]	26.4	27.2	9.1	9.6
Irritability	4.8	6.3	1.9	1.3
Measles-like rash[†]	2.3	4.0	0.0	0.0
Varicella-like rash[†]	1.3	1.7	0.0	0.0
Rash (not otherwise specified)	1.3	1.3	0.0	0.9
Diarrhea	1.0	1.3	0.4	1.3
Upper respiratory infection	1.0	1.3	1.1	0.9
Viral infection	0.0	0.7	0.0	0.0
Rhinorrhea	0.0	0.7	1.1	0.0

* PCV7 = Pneumococcal 7-valent conjugate vaccine.
† Designates a solicited adverse reaction.
‡ Temperature reported as elevated or abnormal.
N = number of subjects vaccinated.
n = number of subjects with safety follow-up.

Table 9: Confirmed Febrile Seizures Days 5 to 12 and 0 to 30 After Vaccination with ProQuad (dose 1) Compared to Concomitant Vaccination with M-M-R II and VARIVAX (dose 1) in Children 12 to 60 Months of Age

Time Period	ProQuad cohort (N=31,298)		MMR+V cohort (N=31,298)		Relative risk (95% CI)
	n	Incidence per 1,000	n	Incidence per 1,000	
5 to 12 Days	22	0.70	10	0.32	2.20 (1.04, 4.65)
0 to 30 Days	44	1.41	40	1.28	1.10 (0.72, 1.69)

is about one case per million vaccine doses distributed. The association with wild-type measles virus infection is 6 to 22 cases of SSPE per million cases of measles. The results of a retrospective case-controlled study suggest that the overall effect of measles vaccine has been to protect against SSPE by preventing measles with its inherent higher risk of SSPE.

Cases of aseptic meningitis have been reported to VAERS following measles, mumps, and rubella vaccination. Although a causal relationship between other strains of mumps vaccine and aseptic meningitis has been shown, there is no evidence to link Jeryl Lynn™ mumps vaccine to aseptic meningitis.

Cases of thrombocytopenia have been reported after use of measles vaccine, measles, mumps, and rubella vaccine, and after varicella vaccination. Post-marketing experience with live measles, mumps, and rubella vaccine indicates that individuals with current thrombocytopenia may develop more severe thrombocytopenia following vaccination. In addition, individuals who experienced thrombocytopenia following the first dose of a live measles, mumps, and rubella vaccine may develop thrombocytopenia with repeat doses. Serologic testing for antibody to measles, mumps, or rubella should be considered in order to determine if additional doses of vaccine are needed *[see Warnings and Precautions (5.5)]*.

The reported rate of zoster in recipients of VARIVAX appears not to exceed that previously determined in a population-based study of healthy children who had experienced wild-type varicella.{4} In clinical trials, 8 cases of herpes zoster were reported in 9454 vaccinated individuals 12 months to 12 years of age during 42,556 person-years of follow-up. This resulted in a calculated incidence of at least 18.8 cases per 100,000 person-years. All 8 cases reported after VARIVAX were mild and no sequelae were reported. The long-term effect of VARIVAX on the incidence of herpes zoster is unknown at present.

6.3 Post-Marketing Observational Safety Surveillance Study
Safety was evaluated in an observational study that included 69,237 children vaccinated with ProQuad 12 months to 12 years old. A historical comparison group included 69,237 age-, gender-, and date-of-vaccination (day and month) matched subjects who were given M-M-R II and VARIVAX concomitantly. The primary objective was to assess the incidence of febrile seizures occurring within various time intervals after vaccination in 12- to 60-month-old children who had neither been vaccinated against measles, mumps, rubella, or varicella, nor had a history of the wild-type infections (N=31,298 vaccinated with ProQuad, including 31,043 who were 12 to 23 months old). The incidence of febrile seizures was also assessed in a historical control group of children who had received their first vaccination with M-M-R II and VARIVAX concomitantly (N=31,298, including 31,019 who were 12 to 23 months old). The secondary objective was to assess the general safety of ProQuad in the 30-day period after vaccination in children 12 months to 12 years old.

In pre-licensure clinical studies, an increase in fever was observed 5 to 12 days after vaccination with ProQuad (dose 1) compared to M-M-R II and VARIVAX (dose 1) given concomitantly. In the post-marketing observational surveillance study, results from the primary safety analysis revealed an approximate two-fold increase in the risk of febrile seizures in the same 5 to 12 day timeframe after vaccination with ProQuad (dose 1). The incidence of febrile seizures 5 to 12 days after ProQuad (dose 1) (0.70 per 1000 children) was higher than that in children receiving M-M-R II and VARIVAX concomitantly (0.32 per 1000 children) [relative risk (RR) 2.20, 95% confidence interval (CI): 1.04, 4.65]. The incidence of febrile seizures 0 to 30 days after ProQuad (dose 1) (1.41 per 1000 children) was similar to that observed in children receiving M-M-R II and VARIVAX concomitantly [RR 1.10 (95% CI: 0.72, 1.69)]. See Table 9. General safety analyses revealed that the risks of fever (RR=1.89; 95% CI: 1.67, 2.15) and skin eruption (RR=1.68; 95% CI: 1.07, 2.64) were significantly higher after ProQuad (dose 1) compared with those who received concomitant first doses of M-M-R II and VARIVAX, respectively. All medical events that resulted in hospitalization or emergency room visits were compared between the group given ProQuad and the historical comparison group, and no other safety concerns were identified in this study.
[See table 9 at left]
In this observational post-marketing study, no case of febrile seizure was observed during the 5 to 12 day postvaccination time period among 26,455 children who received ProQuad as a second dose of M-M-R II and VARIVAX. In addition, detailed general safety data were available from more than 25,000 children who received ProQuad as a second dose of M-M-R II and VARIVAX, most of them (95%) between 4 and 6 years of age, and an analysis of these data by an independent, external safety monitoring committee did not identify any specific safety concern.

7 DRUG INTERACTIONS
7.1 Immune Globulins and Transfusions
Immune globulins (IG) administered concomitantly with ProQuad contain antibodies that may interfere with vaccine virus replication and decrease the expected immune response. Vaccination should be deferred for at least 3 months following blood or plasma transfusions, or administration of IG.
The appropriate suggested interval between transfusion or IG administration and vaccination will vary with the type of transfusion or indication for, and dose of, IG (*e.g.*, 5 months for Varicella Zoster Immune Globulin [VZIG]).{2} Following administration of ProQuad, any IG including VZIG should not be given for 1 month thereafter unless its use outweighs the benefits of vaccination.{2} *[See Warnings and Precautions (5.9).]*

7.2 Salicylates
Reye's syndrome has been reported following the use of salicylates during wild-type varicella infection. Vaccine recipients should avoid use of salicylates for 6 weeks after vaccination with ProQuad. *[See Adverse Reactions (6.1) and Patient Counseling Information (17.1).]*

7.3 Corticosteroids and Immunosuppressive Drugs

ProQuad may be used in individuals who are receiving topical corticosteroids or low-dose corticosteroids for asthma prophylaxis or replacement therapy, *e.g.,* for Addison's disease. ProQuad should not be given to individuals receiving immunosuppressive doses of corticosteroids or other immunosuppressive drugs. Vaccination with a live, attenuated vaccine, such as varicella or measles, can result in a more extensive vaccine-associated rash or disseminated disease in individuals on immunosuppressive drugs *[see Contraindications (4.2)].*

7.4 Drug/Laboratory Test Interactions

Live, attenuated measles, mumps, and rubella virus vaccines given individually may result in a temporary depression of tuberculin skin sensitivity. Therefore, if a tuberculin test is to be done, it should be administered either any time before, simultaneously with, or at least 4 to 6 weeks after ProQuad.

7.5 Use With Other Vaccines

At least 1 month should elapse between a dose of a measles-containing vaccine such as M-M-R II and a dose of ProQuad, and at least 3 months should elapse between administration of 2 doses of ProQuad or varicella-containing vaccines.

ProQuad may be administered concomitantly with *Haemophilus influenzae* type b conjugate (meningococcal protein conjugate) and hepatitis B (recombinant). Additionally, ProQuad may be administered concomitantly with pneumococcal 7-valent conjugate vaccine, and/or hepatitis A (inactivated) vaccines. *[See Clinical Studies (14.)]*

There are no data regarding the administration of ProQuad with inactivated poliovirus vaccine or with other live virus vaccines.

There are insufficient data to support concomitant vaccination with diphtheria and tetanus toxoids and acellular pertussis vaccine adsorbed. *[See Clinical Studies (14.)]*

Children under treatment for tuberculosis have not experienced exacerbation of the disease when vaccinated with live measles virus vaccine; no studies have been reported to date of the effect of measles virus vaccines on children with untreated tuberculosis.

8 USE IN SPECIFIC POPULATIONS

8.1 Pregnancy

Pregnancy Category C: Animal reproduction studies have not been conducted with ProQuad.

Do not administer ProQuad to pregnant females. It is also not known whether ProQuad can cause fetal harm when administered to a pregnant woman or can affect reproduction capacity. If vaccination of post-pubertal females is undertaken, pregnancy should be avoided for 3 months following vaccination. *[See Contraindications (4.4).]*

In counseling women who are inadvertently vaccinated when pregnant or who become pregnant within 3 months of vaccination, the healthcare provider should be aware of the following: (1) Reports have indicated that contracting wild-type measles during pregnancy enhances fetal risk. Increased rates of spontaneous abortion, stillbirth, congenital defects, and prematurity have been observed subsequent to wild-type measles during pregnancy. There are no adequate studies of the attenuated (vaccine) strain of measles virus in pregnancy. However, it would be prudent to assume that the vaccine strain of virus is also capable of inducing adverse fetal effects; (2) Mumps infection during the first trimester of pregnancy may increase the rate of spontaneous abortion. Although mumps vaccine virus has been shown to infect the placenta and fetus, there is no evidence that it causes congenital malformations in humans;[5] (3) In a 10-year survey involving over 700 pregnant women who received rubella vaccine within 3 months before or after conception (of whom 189 received the Wistar RA 27/3 strain), none of the newborns had abnormalities compatible with congenital rubella syndrome;[6] and (4) Wild-type varicella can sometimes cause congenital varicella infection.

Merck & Co., Inc. maintains a Pregnancy Registry to monitor fetal outcomes of pregnant women exposed to varicella-containing vaccine (Oka/Merck). In the first 9 years of the Pregnancy Registry for varicella vaccine (Oka/Merck), of 129 seronegative women and 423 women of unknown serostatus who received varicella vaccine during pregnancy or within 3 months before pregnancy, none had newborns with abnormalities compatible with congenital varicella syndrome.

Patients and health care providers are encouraged to report any exposure to varicella-containing vaccine (Oka/Merck) during pregnancy by calling 1-800-986-8999.

8.3 Nursing Mothers

Do not administer ProQuad to nursing women. It is not known whether ProQuad is excreted in human milk. Because many drugs are excreted in human milk, caution should be exercised when ProQuad is administered to a nursing woman. The secretion of measles and mumps viruses in human milk has not been studied; however, studies have shown that lactating postpartum women vaccinated with live rubella vaccine may secrete the virus in breast

milk and transmit it to breast-fed infants. Limited evidence in the literature suggests that virus, viral DNA, or viral antigen could not be detected in the breast milk of women who were vaccinated postpartum with the vaccine strain of varicella virus.[7,8] *[See Warnings and Precautions (5.8).]*

8.4 Pediatric Use

Do not administer ProQuad to infants younger than 12 months of age or to children 13 years and older. Safety and effectiveness of ProQuad in infants younger than 12 months of age and in children 13 years and older have not been studied. ProQuad is not approved for use in persons in these age groups. *[See Adverse Reactions (6) and Clinical Studies (14.)]*

8.5 Geriatric Use

ProQuad is not indicated for use in the geriatric population (≥age 65).

11 DESCRIPTION

ProQuad (Measles, Mumps, Rubella and Varicella Virus Vaccine Live) is a combined, attenuated, live virus vaccine containing measles, mumps, rubella, and varicella viruses. ProQuad is a sterile lyophilized preparation of (1) the components of M-M-R II (Measles, Mumps, and Rubella Virus Vaccine Live): Measles Virus Vaccine Live, a more attenuated line of measles virus, derived from Enders' attenuated Edmonston strain and propagated in chick embryo cell culture; Mumps Virus Vaccine Live, the Jeryl Lynn™ (B level) strain of mumps virus propagated in chick embryo cell culture; Rubella Virus Vaccine Live, the Wistar RA 27/3 strain of live attenuated rubella virus propagated in WI-38 human diploid lung fibroblasts; and (2) Varicella Virus Vaccine Live (Oka/Merck), the Oka/Merck strain of varicella-zoster virus propagated in MRC-5 cells. The cells, virus pools, bovine serum, and human albumin used in manufacturing are all tested to provide assurance that the final product is free of potential adventitious agents.

ProQuad, when reconstituted as directed, is a sterile suspension for subcutaneous administration. Each 0.5-mL dose contains not less than 3.00 log$_{10}$ TCID$_{50}$ of measles virus; 4.30 log$_{10}$ TCID$_{50}$ of mumps virus; 3.00 log$_{10}$ TCID$_{50}$ of rubella virus; and a minimum of 3.99 log$_{10}$ PFU of Oka/Merck varicella virus.

Each 0.5-mL dose of the vaccine contains no more than 21 mg of sucrose, 11 mg of hydrolyzed gelatin, 2.4 mg of sodium chloride, 1.8 mg of sorbitol, 0.40 mg of monosodium L-glutamate, 0.34 mg of sodium phosphate dibasic, 0.31 mg of human albumin, 0.17 mg of sodium bicarbonate, 72 mcg of potassium phosphate monobasic, 60 mcg of potassium chloride; 36 mcg of potassium phosphate dibasic; residual components of MRC-5 cells including DNA and protein; <16 mcg of neomycin, bovine calf serum (0.5 mcg), and other buffer and media ingredients. The product contains no preservative.

12 CLINICAL PHARMACOLOGY

12.1 Mechanism of Action

ProQuad has been shown to induce measles-, mumps-, rubella-, and varicella-specific immunity, which is thought to be the mechanism by which it protects against these four childhood diseases.

The efficacy of ProQuad was established through the use of immunological correlates for protection against measles, mumps, rubella, and varicella. Results from efficacy studies or field effectiveness studies that were previously conducted for the component vaccines were used to define levels of serum antibodies that correlated with protection against measles, mumps, and rubella. Also, in previous studies with varicella vaccine, antibody responses against varicella virus ≥5 gpELISA units/mL in a glycoprotein enzyme-linked immunosorbent assay (gpELISA) (not commercially available) similarly correlated with long-term protection. In these efficacy studies, the clinical endpoint for measles and mumps was a clinical diagnosis of either disease confirmed by a 4-fold or greater rise in serum antibody titers between either postvaccination or acute and convalescent titers; for rubella, a 4-fold or greater rise in antibody titers with or without clinical symptoms of rubella; and for varicella, varicella-like rash that occurred >42 days postvaccination and for which varicella was not excluded by either viral cultures of the lesion or serological tests. Specific laboratory evidence of varicella either by serology or culture was not required to confirm the diagnosis of varicella. Clinical studies with a single dose of ProQuad have shown that vaccination elicited rates of antibody responses against measles, mumps, and rubella that were similar to those observed after vaccination with a single dose of M-M-R II *[see Clinical*

Table 10: Summary of Combined Immunogenicity Results 6 Weeks Following the Administration of a Single Dose of ProQuad (Varicella Virus Potency ≥3.97 log$_{10}$ PFU) or M-M-R II and VARIVAX (Per-Protocol Population)

Group	Antigen	n	Observed Response Rate (95% CI)	Observed GMT (95% CI)
ProQuad (N=5446*)	Varicella	4381	91.2% (90.3%, 92.0%)	15.5 (15.0, 15.9)
	Measles	4733	97.4% (96.9%, 97.9%)	3124.9 (3038.9, 3213.3)
	Mumps (OD cutoff)[†]	973	98.8% (97.9%, 99.4%)	105.3 (98.0, 113.1)
	Mumps (wild-type ELISA)[†]	3735	95.8% (95.1%, 96.4%)	93.1 (90.2, 96.0)
	Rubella	4773	98.5% (98.1%, 98.8%)	91.8 (89.6, 94.1)
M-M-R II + VARIVAX (N=2038*)	Varicella	1417	94.1% (92.8%, 95.3%)	16.6 (15.9, 17.4)
	Measles	1516	98.2% (97.4%, 98.8%)	2239.6 (2138.3, 2345.6)
	Mumps (OD cutoff)[†]	50	99.4% (98.3%, 99.9%)	87.5 (79.7, 96.0)
	Mumps (wild-type ELISA)[†]	1017	98.0% (97.0%, 98.8%)	90.8 (86.2, 95.7)
	Rubella	1528	98.5% (97.7%, 99.0%)	102.2 (97.8, 106.7)

* Includes ProQuad + Placebo followed by ProQuad (Visit 1) (Protocol 009), ProQuad Middle and High Doses (Visit 1) (Protocol 011), ProQuad (Lot 1, Lot 2, Lot 3) (Protocol 012), both the Concomitant and Non-concomitant groups (Protocol 013).
† The mumps antibody response was assessed by a vaccine-strain ELISA in Protocols 009 and 011 and by a wild-type ELISA in Protocols 012 and 013. In the former assay, the serostatus was based on the OD cutoff of the assay. In the latter assay, 10 mumps ELISA units was used as the serostatus cutoff.
n = Number of per-protocol subjects with evaluable serology.
CI = Confidence interval.
GMT = Geometric mean titer.
ELISA = Enzyme-linked immunosorbent assay.
PFU = Plaque-forming units.
OD = Optical density.

Table 11: Summary of Immune Response to a First and Second Dose of ProQuad in Subjects < 3 Years of Age Who Received ProQuad with a Varicella Virus Dose ≥3.97 Log_{10} PFU*

		Dose 1 N=1097			Dose 2 N=1097		
Antigen	Serostatus Cutoff/ Response Criteria	n	Observed Response Rate (95% CI)	Observed GMT (95% CI)	n	Observed Response Rate (95% CI)	Observed GMT (95% CI)
Measles	≥120 mIU/mL†	915	98.1% (97.0%, 98.9%)	2956.8 (2786.3, 3137.7)	915	99.5% (98.7%, 99.8%)	5958.0 (5518.9, 6432.1)
	≥255 mIU/mL	943	97.8% (96.6%, 98.6%)	2966.0 (2793.4, 3149.2)	943	99.4% (98.6%, 99.8%)	5919.3 (5486.2, 6386.6)
Mumps	≥OD Cutoff (ELISA antibody units)	920	98.7% (97.7%, 99.3%)	106.7 (99.1, 114.8)	920	99.9% (99.4%, 100%)	253.1 (237.9, 269.2)
Rubella	≥10 IU/mL	937	97.7% (96.5%, 98.5%)	91.1 (85.9, 96.6)	937	98.3% (97.2%, 99.0%)	158.8 (149.1, 169.2)
Varicella	<1.25 to ≥5 gpELISA units	864	86.6% (84.1%, 88.8%)	11.6 (10.9, 12.3)	864	99.4% (98.7%, 99.8%)	477.5 (437.8, 520.7)
	≥OD Cutoff (gpELISA units)	695	87.2% (84.5%, 89.6%)	11.6 (10.9, 12.4)	695	99.4% (98.5%, 99.8%)	478.7 (434.8, 527.1)

* Includes the following treatment groups: ProQuad + Placebo followed by ProQuad (Visit 1) (Protocol 009) and ProQuad (Middle and High Dose) (Protocol 011).
† Samples from Protocols 009 and 011 were assayed in the legacy format Measles ELISA, which reported antibody titers in Measles ELISA units. To convert titers from ELISA units to mIU/mL, titers for these 2 protocols were divided by 0.1025. The lowest measurable titer postvaccination is 207.5 mIU/mL. The response rate for measles in the legacy format is the percent of subjects with a negative baseline measles antibody titer, as defined by the optical density (OD) cutoff, with a postvaccination measles antibody titer ≥207.5 mIU/mL. Samples from Protocols 009 and 011 were assayed in the legacy format Rubella ELISA, which reported antibody titers in Rubella ELISA units. To convert titers from ELISA units to IU/mL, titers for these 2 protocols were divided by 1.28.
ProQuad (Middle Dose) = ProQuad containing a varicella virus dose of 3.97 log_{10} PFU.
ProQuad (High Dose) = ProQuad containing a varicella virus dose of 4.25 log_{10} PFU.
ELISA = Enzyme-linked immunosorbent assay.
gpELISA = Glycoprotein enzyme-linked immunosorbent assay.
N = Number vaccinated at baseline.
n = Number of subjects who were per-protocol Postdose 1 and Postdose 2 and satisfied the given prevaccination serostatus cutoff.
CI = Confidence interval.
GMT = Geometric mean titer.
PFU = Plaque-forming units.

Studies (14)] and seroresponse rates for varicella virus were similar to those observed after vaccination with a single dose of VARIVAX *[see Clinical Studies (14)]*. The duration of protection from measles, mumps, rubella, and varicella infections after vaccination with ProQuad is unknown.

12.4 Persistence of Antibody Responses After Vaccination

The persistence of antibody at 1 year after vaccination was evaluated in a subset of 2107 children enrolled in the clinical trials. Antibody was detected in 98.9% (1722/1741) for measles, 96.7% (1676/1733) for mumps, 99.6% (1796/1804) for rubella, and 97.5% (1512/1550) for varicella (≥5 gpELISA units/mL) of vaccinees following a single dose of ProQuad.

Experience with M-M-R II demonstrates that antibodies to measles, mumps, and rubella viruses are still detectable in most individuals 11 to 13 years after primary vaccination.(9) Varicella antibodies were present for up to ten years postvaccination in most of the individuals tested who received 1 dose of VARIVAX.

13 NONCLINICAL TOXICOLOGY

13.1 Carcinogenesis, Mutagenesis, Impairment of Fertility

ProQuad has not been evaluated for its carcinogenic, mutagenic, or teratogenic potential, or its potential to impair fertility.

14 CLINICAL STUDIES

Formal studies to evaluate the clinical efficacy of ProQuad have not been performed.

Efficacy of the measles, mumps, rubella, and varicella components of ProQuad was previously established in a series of clinical studies with the monovalent vaccines. A high degree of protection from infection was demonstrated in these studies.(10-17)

Immunogenicity in Children 12 Months to 6 Years of Age

Prior to licensure, immunogenicity was studied in 5845 healthy children 12 months to 6 years of age with a negative clinical history of measles, mumps, rubella, and varicella who participated in 5 randomized clinical trials. The immunogenicity of ProQuad was similar to that of its individual component vaccines (M-M-R II and VARIVAX), which are currently used in routine vaccination.

The presence of detectable antibody was assessed by an appropriately sensitive enzyme-linked immunosorbent assay (ELISA) for measles, mumps (wild-type and vaccine-type strains), and rubella, and by gpELISA for varicella. For evaluation of vaccine response rates, a positive result in the measles ELISA corresponded to measles antibody concentrations of ≥255 mIU/mL when compared to the WHO II (66/202) Reference Immunoglobulin for Measles.

Children were positive for mumps antibody if the antibody level was ≥10 ELISA units/mL. A positive result in the rubella ELISA corresponded to concentrations of ≥10 IU rubella antibody/mL when compared to the WHO International Reference Serum for Rubella; children with varicella antibody levels ≥5 gpELISA units/mL were considered to be seropositive since a response rate based on ≥5 gpELISA units/mL has been shown to be highly correlated with long-term protection.

Immunogenicity in Children 12 to 23 Months of Age After a Single Dose

In 4 randomized clinical trials, 5446 healthy children 12 to 23 months of age were administered ProQuad, and 2038 children were vaccinated with M-M-R II and VARIVAX given concomitantly at separate injection sites. Subjects enrolled in each of these trials had a negative clinical history, no known recent exposure, and no vaccination history for varicella, measles, mumps, and rubella. Children were excluded from study participation if they had an immune impairment or had a history of allergy to components of the vaccine(s). Except for in 1 trial *[see ProQuad Administered with Diphtheria and Tetanus Toxoids and Acellular Pertussis Vaccine Adsorbed (DTaP) and Haemophilus influenzae type b Conjugate (Meningococcal Protein Conjugate) and Hepatitis B (Recombinant) Vaccine below]*, no concomitant vaccines were permitted during study participation. The race distribution of the study subjects across these studies following a first dose of ProQuad was as follows: 66.3% White; 12.7% African-American; 9.9% Hispanic; 6.7% Asian/Pacific; 4.2% other; and 0.2% American Indian. The gender distribution of the study subjects across these studies following a first dose of ProQuad was 52.6% male and 47.4% female. A summary of combined immunogenicity results 6 weeks following administration of a single dose of ProQuad or M-M-R II and VARIVAX is shown in Table 10. These results were similar to the immune response rates induced by concomitant administration of single doses of M-M-R II and VARIVAX at separate injection sites (lower bound of the 95% CI for the risk difference in measles, mumps, and rubella seroconversion rates were >-5.0 percentage points and the lower bound of the 95% CI for the risk difference in varicella seroprotection rates was either >-15 percentage points [one study] or >-10.0 percentage points [three studies]).

[See table 10 at top of previous page]

Immunogenicity in Children 15 to 31 Months of Age After a Second Dose of ProQuad

In 2 of the 4 randomized clinical trials described above, a subgroup (N=1035) of the 5446 children administered a single dose of ProQuad were administered a second dose of ProQuad approximately 3 to 9 months after the first dose. Children were excluded from receiving a second dose of ProQuad if they were recently exposed to or developed varicella, measles, mumps, and/or rubella prior to receipt of the second dose. No concomitant vaccines were administered to these children. The race distribution across these studies following a second dose of ProQuad was as follows: 67.3% White; 14.3% African-American; 8.3% Hispanic; 5.4% Asian/Pacific; 4.4% other; 0.2% American Indian; and 0.10% mixed. The gender distribution of the study subjects across these studies following a second dose of ProQuad was 50.4% male and 49.6% female. A summary of immune responses following a second dose of ProQuad is presented in Table 11. Results from this study showed that 2 doses of ProQuad administered at least 3 months apart elicited a positive antibody response to all four antigens in greater than 98% of subjects. The geometric mean titers (GMTs) following the second dose of ProQuad increased approximately 2-fold each for measles, mumps, and rubella, and approximately 41-fold for varicella.

[See table 11 at left]

Immunogenicity in Children 4 to 6 Years of Age Who Received a First Dose of ProQuad After Primary Vaccination With M-M-R II and VARIVAX

In a clinical trial, 799 healthy 4- to 6-year-old children who had received M-M-R II and VARIVAX at least 1 month prior to study entry were randomized to receive ProQuad and placebo (N=399), M-M-R II and placebo concomitantly at separate injection sites (N=205), or M-M-R II and VARIVAX concomitantly at separate injection sites (N=195). Children were eligible if they were previously administered primary doses of M-M-R II and VARIVAX, either concomitantly or non-concomitantly, at 12 months of age or older. Children were excluded if they were recently exposed to measles, mumps, rubella, and/or varicella, had an immune impairment, or had a history of allergy to components of the vaccine(s). No concomitant vaccines were permitted during study participation. *[See Adverse Reactions (6.1) for ethnicity and gender information.]*

A summary of antibody responses to measles, mumps, rubella, and varicella at 6 weeks postvaccination in subjects who had previously received M-M-R II and VARIVAX is shown in Table 12. Results from this study showed that a first dose of ProQuad after primary vaccination with M-M-R II and VARIVAX elicited a positive antibody response to all four antigens in greater than 98% of subjects. Postvaccination GMTs for recipients of ProQuad were similar to those following a second dose of M-M-R II and VARIVAX administered concomitantly at separate injection sites (the lower bound of the 95% CI around the fold difference in measles, mumps, rubella, and varicella GMTs excluded 0.5). Additionally, GMTs for measles, mumps, and rubella were similar to those following a second dose of M-M-R II given concomitantly with placebo (the lower bound of the 95% CI around the fold difference for the comparison of measles, mumps, and rubella GMTs excluded 0.5).

[See table 12 at top of next page]

Immunogenicity Following Concomitant Use with Other Vaccines

ProQuad with Pneumococcal 7-valent Conjugate Vaccine and/or VAQTA

In a clinical trial, 1027 healthy children 12 to 15 months of age were randomized to receive ProQuad and pneumococcal 7-valent conjugate vaccine concomitantly (N=510) at separate injection sites or ProQuad and pneumococcal 7-valent conjugate vaccine non-concomitantly (N=517) at separate clinic visits. *[See Adverse Reactions (6.1) for ethnicity and gender information.]* The statistical analysis of non-inferiority in antibody response rates to measles, mumps, rubella, and varicella at 6 weeks postvaccination for subjects are shown in Table 13. In the per-protocol population, seroconversion rates were not inferior in children given ProQuad and pneumococcal 7-valent conjugate vaccine concomitantly when compared to seroconversion rates seen in children given these vaccines non-concomitantly for measles, mumps, and rubella. In children with baseline varicella antibody titers <1.25 gpELISA units/mL, the varicella seroprotection rates were not inferior when rates after concomitant and non-concomitant vaccination were compared 6 weeks postvaccination. Statistical analysis of non-inferiority in GMTs to *S. pneumoniae* serotypes at 6 weeks postvaccination are shown in Table 14. Geometric mean antibody titers (GMTs) for *S. pneumoniae* types 4, 6B, 9V,

14, 18C, 19F, and 23F were not inferior when antibody titers in the concomitant and non-concomitant groups were compared 6 weeks postvaccination.
[See table 13 below]
[See table 14 at top of next page]
In a clinical trial, 653 healthy children 12 to 15 months of age were randomized to receive VAQTA, ProQuad, and pneumococcal 7-valent conjugate vaccine concomitantly (N=330) or ProQuad and pneumococcal 7-valent conjugate vaccine concomitantly followed by VAQTA 6 weeks later (N=323). *[See Adverse Reactions (6.1) for ethnicity and gender information.]* Statistical analysis of non-inferiority of the response rate for varicella antibody at 6 weeks postvaccination among subjects who received VAQTA concomitantly or non-concomitantly with ProQuad and pneumococcal 7-valent conjugate vaccine is shown in Table 15. For the varicella component of ProQuad, in subjects with baseline antibody titers <1.25 gpELISA units/mL, the proportion with a titer ≥5 gpELISA units/mL 6 weeks after their first dose of ProQuad was non-inferior when ProQuad was administered with VAQTA and pneumococcal 7-valent conjugate vaccine as compared to the proportion with a titer ≥5 gpELISA units/mL when ProQuad was administered with pneumococcal 7-valent conjugate vaccine alone. Statistical analysis of non-inferiority of the seropositivity rate for hepatitis A antibody at 4 weeks postdose 2 of VAQTA among subjects who received VAQTA concomitantly or non-concomitantly with ProQuad and pneumococcal 7-valent conjugate vaccine is shown in Table 16. The seropositivity rate to hepatitis A 4 weeks after a second dose of VAQTA given concomitantly with ProQuad and pneumococcal 7-valent conjugate vaccine (defined as the percent of subjects with a titer ≥10 mIU/mL) was non-inferior to the seropositivity rate observed when VAQTA was administered separately from ProQuad and pneumococcal 7-valent conjugate vaccine. Statistical analysis of non-inferiority in GMT to *S. pneumoniae* serotypes at 6 weeks postvaccination among subjects who received VAQTA concomitantly or non-concomitantly with ProQuad and pneumococcal 7-valent conjugate vaccine is shown in Table 17. Additionally, the GMTs for *S. pneumoniae* types 4, 6B, 9V, 14, 18C, 19F, and 23F 6 weeks after vaccination with pneumococcal 7-valent conjugate vaccine administered concomitantly with ProQuad and VAQTA were non-inferior as compared to GMTs observed in the group given pneumococcal 7-valent conjugate vaccine with ProQuad alone. An earlier clinical study involving 617 healthy children provided data that indicated that the seroresponse rates 6 weeks post vaccination for measles, mumps, and rubella in those given M-M-R II and VAQTA concomitantly (N=309) were non-inferior as compared to historical controls.
[See table 15 on next page]
[See table 16 on next page]
[See table 17 at top of page 2263]
ProQuad Administered with Diphtheria and Tetanus Toxoids and Acellular Pertussis Vaccine Adsorbed (DTaP) and Haemophilus influenzae type b Conjugate (Meningococcal Protein Conjugate) and Hepatitis B (Recombinant) Vaccine
In a clinical trial, 1913 healthy children 12 to 15 months of age were randomized to receive ProQuad plus diphtheria and tetanus toxoids and acellular pertussis vaccine adsorbed (DTaP) and *Haemophilus influenzae* type b conjugate (meningococcal protein conjugate) and hepatitis B (recombinant) vaccine concomitantly at separate injection sites (N=949), ProQuad at the initial visit followed by DTaP and *Haemophilus* b conjugate and hepatitis B (recombinant) vaccine given concomitantly 6 weeks later (N=485), or M-M-R II and VARIVAX given concomitantly at separate injection sites (N=479) at the first visit. *[See Adverse Reactions (6.1) for ethnicity and gender information.]* Seroconversion rates and antibody titers for measles, mumps, rubella, varicella, anti-PRP, and hepatitis B were comparable between the 2 groups given ProQuad at approximately 6 weeks postvaccination indicating that ProQuad and *Haemophilus* b conjugate (meningococcal protein conjugate) and hepatitis B (recombinant) vaccine may be administered concomitantly at separate injection sites (see Table 18 below). Response rates for measles, mumps, rubella, varicella, *Haemophilus influenzae* type b, and hepatitis B were not inferior in children given ProQuad plus *Haemophilus influenzae* type b conjugate (meningococcal protein conjugate) and hepatitis B (recombinant) vaccines concomitantly when compared to ProQuad at the initial visit and *Haemophilus influenzae* type b conjugate (meningococcal protein conjugate) and hepatitis B (recombinant) vaccines given concomitantly 6 weeks later. There are insufficient data to support concomitant vaccination with diphtheria and tetanus toxoids and acellular pertussis vaccine adsorbed (data not shown).
[See table 18 on page 2263]

15 REFERENCES

1. Levy O, et al. Disseminated varicella infection due to the vaccine strain of varicella-zoster virus, in a patient with a novel deficiency in natural killer T cells. *J Infect Dis.* 188(7):948-53, 2003.

Table 12: Summary of Antibody Responses to Measles, Mumps, Rubella, and Varicella at 6 Weeks Postvaccination in Subjects 4 to 6 Years of Age Who Had Previously Received M-M-R II and VARIVAX (Per-Protocol Population)

Group Number (Description)	n	GMT (95% CI)	Seropositivity Rate (95% CI)	% ≥4-Fold Rise in Titer (95% CI)	Geometric Mean Fold Rise (95% CI)
Measles*					
Group 1 (N=399) (ProQuad + placebo)	367	1985.9 (1817.6, 2169.9)	100% (99.0%, 100%)	4.9% (2.9%, 7.6%)	1.21 (1.13, 1.30)
Group 2 (N=205) (M-M-R II + placebo)	185	2046.9 (1815.2, 2308.2)	100% (98.0%, 100%)	4.3% (1.9%, 8.3%)	1.28 (1.17, 1.40)
Group 3 (N=195) (M-M-R II + VARIVAX)	171	2084.3 (1852.3, 2345.5)	99.4% (96.8%, 100%)	4.7% (2.0%, 9.0%)	1.31 (1.17, 1.46)
Mumps†					
Group 1 (N=399) (ProQuad + placebo)	367	206.0 (188.2, 225.4)	99.5% (98.0%, 99.9%)	27.2% (22.8%, 32.1%)	2.43 (2.19, 2.69)
Group 2 (N=205) (M-M-R II + placebo)	185	308.5 (269.6, 352.9)	100% (98.0%, 100%)	41.1% (33.9%, 48.5%)	3.69 (3.14, 4.32)
Group 3 (N=195) (M-M-R II + VARIVAX)	171	295.9 (262.5, 333.5)	100% (97.9%, 100%)	41.5% (34.0%, 49.3%)	3.36 (2.84, 3.97)
Rubella‡					
Group 1 (N=399) (ProQuad + placebo)	367	217.3 (200.1, 236.0)	100% (99.0%, 100%)	32.7% (27.9%, 37.8%)	3.00 (2.72, 3.31)
Group 2 (N=205) (M-M-R II + placebo)	185	174.0 (157.3, 192.6)	100% (98.0%, 100%)	31.9% (25.2%, 39.1%)	2.81 (2.41, 3.27)
Group 3 (N=195) (M-M-R II + VARIVAX)	171	154.1 (138.9, 170.9)	99.4% (96.8%, 100%)	26.9% (20.4%, 34.2%)	2.47 (2.17, 2.81)
Varicella§					
Group 1 (N=399) (ProQuad + placebo)	367	322.2 (278.9, 372.2)	98.9% (97.2%, 99.7%)	80.7 (76.2%, 84.6%)	12.43 (10.63, 14.53)
Group 2 (N=205) (M-M-R II + placebo)	185	N/A	N/A	N/A	N/A
Group 3 (N=195) (M-M-R II + VARIVAX)	171	209.3 (171.2, 255.9)	99.4% (96.8%, 100%)	71.9% (64.6%, 78.5%)	8.50 (6.69, 10.81)

* Measles GMTs are reported in mIU/mL; seropositivity corresponds to ≥120 mIU/mL.
† Mumps GMTs are reported in mumps Ab units/mL; seropositivity corresponds to ≥10 Ab units/mL.
‡ Rubella titers obtained by the legacy format were converted to their corresponding titers in the modified format. Rubella serostatus was determined after the conversion to IU/mL: seropositivity corresponds to ≥10 IU/mL.
§ Varicella GMTs are reported in gpELISA units/mL; seropositivity rate is reported by % of subjects with postvaccination antibody titers ≥5 gpELISA units/mL. Percentages are calculated as the number of subjects who met the criterion divided by the number of subjects contributing to the per-protocol analysis.
gpELISA = Glycoprotein enzyme-linked immunosorbent assay; ELISA = Enzyme-linked immunosorbent assay; CI = Confidence interval; GMT = Geometric mean titer; N/A = Not applicable; N = Number of subjects vaccinated; n = number of subjects in the per-protocol analysis.

Table 13: Statistical Analysis of Non-Inferiority in Antibody Response Rates to Measles, Mumps, Rubella, and Varicella at 6 Weeks Postvaccination for Subjects Initially Seronegative to Measles, Mumps, or Rubella, or With Varicella Antibody Titer <1.25 gpELISA units at Baseline in the ProQuad + PCV7* Treatment Group and the ProQuad followed by PCV7 Control Group (Per-Protocol Analysis)

Assay Parameter	ProQuad + PCV7 (N=510)		ProQuad followed by PCV7 (N=259)		Difference (percentage points)†, ‡ (95% CI)
	n	Estimated Response†	n	Estimated Response†	
Measles % ≥255 mIU/mL	406	97.3%	204	99.5%	-2.2 (-4.6, 0.2)
Mumps % ≥10 Ab units/mL	403	96.6%	208	98.6%	-1.9 (-4.5, 1.0)
Rubella % ≥10 IU/mL	377	98.7%	195	97.9%	0.9 (-1.3, 4.1)
Varicella % ≥5 gpELISA units/mL	379	92.5%	192	87.9%	4.5 (-0.4, 10.4)

* PCV7 = Pneumococcal 7-valent conjugate vaccine.
† Estimated responses and their differences were based on statistical analysis models adjusting for study center.
‡ ProQuad + PCV7 - ProQuad followed by PCV7.
Seronegative defined as baseline measles antibody titer <255 mIU/mL for measles, baseline mumps antibody titer <10 ELISA Ab units/mL for mumps, and baseline rubella antibody titer <10 IU/mL for rubella.
The conclusion of non-inferiority is based on the lower bound of the 2-sided 95% CI on the risk difference being greater than -10 percentage points (*i.e.* excluding a decrease equal to or more than the prespecified criterion of 10.0 percentage points). This indicates that the difference is statistically significantly less than the prespecified clinically relevant decrease of 10.0 percentage points at the 1-sided alpha = 0.025 level.
N = Number of subjects vaccinated in each treatment group.
n = Number of subjects with measles antibody titer <255 mIU/mL, mumps antibody titer <10 ELISA Ab units/mL, rubella antibody titer <10 IU/mL, or varicella antibody titer <1.25 gpELISA units/mL at baseline and with postvaccination serology contributing to the per-protocol analysis.
Ab = antibody; ELISA = Enzyme-linked immunosorbent assay; gpELISA = Glycoprotein enzyme-linked immunosorbent assay; CI = Confidence interval.

2. Committee on Infectious Diseases, American Academy of Pediatrics. In: Pickering LK, Baker CJ, Overturf GD, et al., eds. Red Book: 2003 Report of the Committee on Infectious Diseases. 26th ed. Elk Grove Village, IL: American Academy of Pediatrics. 419-29, 2003.
3. Peltola H, et al. The elimination of indigenous measles, mumps, and rubella from Finland by a 12-year, two-dose vaccination program. *N Engl J Med.* 331(21):1397-1402, 1994.
4. Guess HA, et al. Population-based studies of varicella complications. *Pediatrics.* 78(4 Pt 2):723-727, 1986.
5. Recommendations of the Immunization Practices Advisory Committee (ACIP), Mumps Prevention. *MMWR.* 38(22):388-392, 397-400, 1989.
6. Rubella vaccination during pregnancy—United States, 1971-1986. *MMWR Morb Mortal Wkly Rep.* 36(28):457-61, 1987.
7. Bohlke K, Galil K, Jackson LA, et al. Postpartum varicella vaccination: Is the vaccine virus excreted in breast milk? *Obstetrics and Gynecology.* 102(5):970-977, 2003.
8. Dolbear GL, Moffat J, Falkner C and Wojtowycz M. A Pilot Study: Is attenuated varicella virus present in breast milk after postpartum immunization? *Obstetrics and Gynecology.* 101(4 Suppl.):47S-47S, 2003.
9. Weibel RE, et al. Clinical and laboratory studies of combined live measles, mumps, and rubella vaccines using the RA 27/3 rubella virus. *Proc Soc Exp Biol Med.* 165(2):323-326, 1980.
10. Hilleman MR, Stokes J, Jr., Buynak EB, Weibel R, Halenda R, Goldner H. Studies of live attenuated measles virus vaccine in man: II. appraisal of efficacy. *Am J Public Health.* 52(2):44-56, 1962.
11. Krugman S, Giles JP, Jacobs AM. Studies on an attenuated measles-virus vaccine: VI. clinical, antigenic and prophylactic effects of vaccine in institutionalized children. *N Engl J Med.* 263(4):174-7, 1960.
12. Hilleman MR, Weibel RE, Buynak EB, Stokes J, Jr., Whitman JE, Jr. Live, attenuated mumps-virus vaccine. 4. Protective efficacy as measured in a field evaluation. *N Engl J Med.* 276(5):252-8, 1967.
13. Sugg WC, Finger JA, Levine RH, Pagano JS. Field evaluation of live virus mumps vaccine. *J Pediatr.* 72(4): 461-6, 1968.
14. The Benevento and Compobasso Pediatricians Network for the Control of Vaccine-Preventable Diseases, D'Argenio P, Citarella A, Selvaggi MTM. Field evaluation of the clinical effectiveness of vaccines against pertussis, measles, rubella and mumps. *Vaccine.* 16(8):818-22, 1998.
15. Furukawa T, Miyata T, Kondo K, Kuno K, Isomura S, Takekoshi T. Rubella vaccination during an epidemic. *JAMA.* 213(6):987-90, 1970.
16. Vazquez M, et al. The effectiveness of the varicella vaccine in clinical practice. *N Engl J Med.* 344(13):955-960, 2001.
17. Kuter B, et al. Ten year follow-up of healthy children who received one or two injections of varicella vaccine. *Pediatr Infect Dis J.* 23(2):132-137, 2004.

16   HOW SUPPLIED/STORAGE AND HANDLING

No. 4999—ProQuad is supplied as follows:
(1) a package of 10 single-dose vials of lyophilized vaccine, NDC 0006-4999-00 (package A)
(2) a separate package of 10 vials of sterile water diluent (package B).

Storage

To maintain potency, ProQuad must be stored frozen between -58°F and +5°F (-50°C to -15°C). Use of dry ice may subject ProQuad to temperatures colder than -58°F (-50°C).

Before reconstitution, store the lyophilized vaccine continuously in a reliably maintained freezer (*e.g.*, chest, frost-free) for up to 18 months.

ProQuad may be stored at refrigerator temperature (36° to 46°F, 2° to 8°C) for up to 72 hours prior to reconstitution. Discard any ProQuad vaccine stored at 36° to 46°F which is not used within 72 hours of removal from 5°F (-15°C) storage.

Protect the vaccine from light at all times since such exposure may inactivate the vaccine viruses.

IF NOT USED IMMEDIATELY, THE RECONSTITUTED VACCINE MAY BE STORED AT ROOM TEMPERATURE, PROTECTED FROM LIGHT, FOR UP TO 30 MINUTES.

DISCARD RECONSTITUTED VACCINE IF IT IS NOT USED WITHIN 30 MINUTES.

DO NOT FREEZE RECONSTITUTED VACCINE.

Diluent should be stored separately at room temperature (68° to 77°F, 20° to 25°C), or in a refrigerator (36° to 46°F, 2° to 8°C).

For information regarding stability under conditions other than those recommended, call 1-800-MERCK-90.

17   PATIENT COUNSELING INFORMATION

17.1   Instructions

Provide the required vaccine information to the patient, parent, or guardian.

Table 14: Statistical Analysis of Non-Inferiority in GMTs to S. pneumoniae Serotypes at 6 Weeks Postvaccination in the ProQuad + PCV7* Treatment Group and the PCV7 Followed by ProQuad Control Group (Per-Protocol Analysis)

Serotype	Parameter	Group 1 ProQuad + PCV7 (N=510)		Group 2 PCV7 followed by ProQuad (N=258)		Fold-Difference[†*] (95% CI)
		n	Estimated Response[‡]	n	Estimated Response[‡]	
4	GMT	410	1.5	193	1.3	1.2 (1.0, 1.4)
6B	GMT	410	8.9	192	8.4	1.1 (0.9, 1.2)
9V	GMT	409	2.9	193	2.5	1.2 (1.0, 1.3)
14	GMT	408	6.5	193	5.7	1.1 (1.0, 1.3)
18C	GMT	408	2.3	193	2.0	1.2 (1.0, 1.3)
19F	GMT	408	3.5	192	3.1	1.1 (1.0, 1.3)
23F	GMT	413	4.1	197	3.7	1.1 (1.0, 1.3)

* PCV7 = Pneumococcal 7-valent conjugate vaccine.
† ProQuad + PCV7 / PCV7 followed by ProQuad.
‡ Estimated responses and their fold-difference were based on statistical analysis models adjusting for study center and prevaccination titer.
The conclusion of non-inferiority is based on the lower bound of the 2-sided 95% CI on the fold-difference being greater than 0.5, (*i.e.* excluding a decrease of 2-fold or more). This indicates that the fold-difference is statistically significantly less than the pre-specified clinically relevant 2-fold difference at the 1-sided alpha = 0.025 level.
N = Number of subjects vaccinated in each treatment group; n = Number of subjects contributing to the per-protocol analysis for the given serotype; GMT = geometric mean titer; CI = Confidence interval.

Table 15: Statistical Analysis of Non-Inferiority of the Response Rate for Varicella Antibody at 6 Weeks Postvaccination Among Subjects Who Received VAQTA Concomitantly or Non-Concomitantly With ProQuad and PCV7* (Per-Protocol Analysis Set)

Parameter	Group 1: Concomitant VAQTA with ProQuad + PCV7 (N=330)		Group 2: Non-concomitant VAQTA separate from ProQuad + PCV7 (N=323)		Difference[†] (percentage points): Group 1 – Group 2 (95% CI)
	n	Estimated Response[†]	n	Estimated Response[†]	
% ≥5 gpELISA units/mL[‡]	225[§]	93.2%	232[§]	98.3%	-5.1 (-9.3, -1.4)

*PCV7 = Pneumococcal 7-valent conjugate vaccine
N = Number of subjects enrolled/randomized; n = Number of subjects contributing to the per protocol analysis for varicella; CI = Confidence interval.
† Estimated responses and their differences were based on a statistical analysis model adjusting for combined study center.
‡ 6 weeks following Dose 1.
§ Initial Serostatus <1.25 gpELISA units/mL.
The conclusion of similarity (non-inferiority) was based on the lower bound of the 2-sided 95% CI on the risk difference excluding a decrease of 10 percentage points or more (lower bound >-10.0). This indicated that the risk difference was statistically significantly greater than the pre-specified clinically relevant difference of -10 percentage points at the 1-sided alpha = 0.025 level.

Table 16: Statistical Analysis of Non-Inferiority of the Seropositivity Rate (SPR) for Hepatitis A Antibody at 4 Weeks Postdose 2 of VAQTA Among Subjects Who Received VAQTA Concomitantly or Non-Concomitantly With ProQuad and PCV7* (Per-Protocol Analysis Set)

Parameter	Group 1: Concomitant VAQTA with ProQuad + PCV7 (N=330)		Group 2: Non-concomitant VAQTA separate from ProQuad + PCV7 (N=323)		Difference[†] (percentage points): Group 1 – Group 2 (95% CI)
	n	Estimated Response[†]	n	Estimated Response[†]	
% ≥10 mIU/mL[‡]	182[§]	100.0%	159[§]	99.3%	0.7 (-1.4, 3.8)

* PCV7 = Pneumococcal 7-valent conjugate vaccine
CI = Confidence interval; N = Number of subjects enrolled/randomized; n = Number of subjects contributing to the per-protocol analysis for hepatitis A.
† Estimated responses and their differences were based on a statistical analysis model adjusting for combined study center.
‡ 4 weeks following receipt of 2 doses of VAQTA.
§ Regardless of initial serostatus.
The conclusion of non-inferiority was based on the lower bound of the 2-sided 95% CI on the risk difference being greater than -10 percentage points (*i.e.* excluding a decrease of 10 percentage points or more) (lower bound >-10.0). This indicated that the risk difference was statistically significantly greater than the pre-specified clinically relevant difference of -10 percentage points at the 1-sided alpha = 0.025 level.

Inform the patient, parent, or guardian of the benefits and risks associated with vaccination.

Inform the patient, parent, or guardian that the vaccine recipient should avoid use of salicylates for 6 weeks after vaccination with ProQuad [see Adverse Reactions (6.1) and Drug Interactions (7.2)].

Instruct post-pubertal females to avoid pregnancy for 3 months following vaccination [see Indications and Usage (1) and Use In Specific Populations (8.1)].

Inform patients, parents, or guardians that vaccination with ProQuad may not offer 100% protection from measles, mumps, rubella, and varicella infection.

Table 17: Statistical Analysis of Non-Inferiority in Geometric Mean Titers (GMT) to S. pneumoniae Serotypes at 6 Weeks Postvaccination Among Subjects Who Received VAQTA Concomitantly or Non-Concomitantly With ProQuad and PCV7* (Per-Protocol Analysis Set)

Serotype	Group 1: Concomitant VAQTA with ProQuad + PCV7 (N=330)		Group 2: Non-concomitant VAQTA separate from ProQuad + PCV7 (N=323)		Fold-Difference[†] (95% CI)
	n	Estimated Response[†]	n	Estimated Response[†]	
4	246	1.9	247	1.7	1.1 (0.9, 1.3)
6B	246	9.9	246	9.9	1.0 (0.8, 1.2)
9V	247	3.7	247	4.2	0.9 (0.8, 1.0)
14	248	7.8	247	7.6	1.0 (0.9, 1.2)
18C	247	2.9	247	2.7	1.1 (0.9, 1.3)
19F	248	4.0	248	3.8	1.1 (0.9, 1.2)
23F	247	5.1	247	4.4	1.1 (1.0, 1.3)

* PCV7 = Pneumococcal 7-valent conjugate vaccine.
CI = Confidence interval; GMT = Geometric mean titer; N = Number of subjects enrolled/randomized; n = Number of subjects contributing to the per-protocol analysis for *S. pneumoniae* serotypes.
[†] Estimated responses and their fold-difference were based on statistical analysis models adjusting for combined study center and prevaccination titer.
The conclusion of non-inferiority was based on the lower bound of the 2-sided 95% CI on the fold-difference being greater than 0.5 (*i.e.* excluding a decrease of 2-fold or more). This indicates that the fold-difference was statistically significantly less than the prespecified clinically relevant 2-fold difference at the 1-sided alpha = 0.025 level.

Table 18: Summary of the Comparison of the Immunogenicity Endpoints for Measles, Mumps, Rubella, Varicella, Haemophilus influenzae type b, and Hepatitis B Responses Following Vaccination with ProQuad, Haemophilus influenzae type b Conjugate (Meningococcal Protein Conjugate), and Hepatitis B (Recombinant) Vaccine and DTaP Administered Concomitantly Versus Non-Concomitant Vaccination with ProQuad Followed by These Vaccines

Vaccine Antigen	Parameter	Concomitant Group N=949 Response	Non-Concomitant Group N=485 Response	Risk Difference (95% CI)	Criterion for Non-inferiority
Measles	% ≥120 mIU/mL	97.8%	98.7%	-0.9 (-2.3, 0.6)	LB >-5.0
Mumps	% ≥10 ELISA Ab units/mL	95.4%	95.1%	0.3 (-1.7, 2.6)	LB >-5.0
Rubella	% ≥10 IU/mL	98.6%	99.3%	-0.7 (-1.8, 0.5)	LB >-5.0
Varicella	% ≥5 gpELISA units/mL	89.6%	90.8%	-1.2 (-4.1, 2.0)	LB >-10.0
HiB-PRP	% ≥1.0 mcg/mL	94.6%	96.5%	-1.9 (-4.1, 0.8)	LB >-10.0
HepB	% ≥10 mIU/mL	95.9%	98.8%	-2.8 (-4.8, -0.8)	LB >10.0

HiB-PRP = *Haemophilus influenzae* type b, polyribosyl phosphate; HepB = hepatitis B; LB = lower bound, limit for non-inferiority comparison.

Instruct patients, parents, or guardians to report any adverse reactions to their health care provider. The U.S. Department of Health and Human Services has established a Vaccine Adverse Event Reporting System (VAERS) to accept all reports of suspected adverse events after the administration of any vaccine, including but not limited to the reporting of events required by the National Childhood Vaccine Injury Act of 1986. For information or a copy of the vaccine reporting form, call the VAERS toll-free number at 1-800-822-7967, or report online at http://www.vaers.hhs.gov.
Dist. by:
MERCK & CO., INC., Whitehouse Station, NJ 08889, USA
Issued September 2010
Printed in USA
9950903

PROSCAR®
(finasteride)
Tablets

℞

DESCRIPTION
PROSCAR[1] (finasteride), a synthetic 4-azasteroid compound, is a specific inhibitor of steroid Type II 5α-reductase, an intracellular enzyme that converts the androgen testosterone into 5α-dihydrotestosterone (DHT).

Finasteride is 4-azaandrost-1-ene-17-carboxamide, *N*-(1,1-dimethylethyl)-3-oxo-,(5α,17β)-. The empirical formula of finasteride is $C_{23}H_{36}N_2O_2$ and its molecular weight is 372.55. Its structural formula is:

Finasteride is a white crystalline powder with a melting point near 250°C. It is freely soluble in chloroform and in lower alcohol solvents, but is practically insoluble in water. PROSCAR (finasteride) tablets for oral administration are film-coated tablets that contain 5 mg of finasteride and the following inactive ingredients: hydrous lactose, microcrystalline cellulose, pregelatinized starch, sodium starch glycolate, hydroxypropyl cellulose LF, hydroxypropyl methylcellulose, titanium dioxide, magnesium stearate, talc, docusate sodium, FD&C Blue 2 aluminum lake and yellow iron oxide.

[1] Registered trademark of Merck Sharp & Dohme Corp., a subsidiary of **Merck & Co., Inc.**
Copyright © Merck Sharp & Dohme Corp., a subsidiary of **Merck & Co., Inc.,** 1992, 1995, 1998
All rights reserved

CLINICAL PHARMACOLOGY
The development and enlargement of the prostate gland is dependent on the potent androgen, 5α-dihydrotestosterone (DHT). Type II 5α-reductase metabolizes testosterone to DHT in the prostate gland, liver and skin. DHT induces androgenic effects by binding to androgen receptors in the cell nuclei of these organs.
Finasteride is a competitive and specific inhibitor of Type II 5α-reductase with which it slowly forms a stable enzyme complex. Turnover from this complex is extremely slow ($t_{1/2}$~ 30 days). This has been demonstrated both *in vivo* and *in vitro*. Finasteride has no affinity for the androgen receptor. In man, the 5α-reduced steroid metabolites in blood and urine are decreased after administration of finasteride.
In man, a single 5-mg oral dose of PROSCAR produces a rapid reduction in serum DHT concentration, with the maximum effect observed 8 hours after the first dose. The suppression of DHT is maintained throughout the 24-hour dosing interval and with continued treatment. Daily dosing of PROSCAR at 5 mg/day for up to 4 years has been shown to reduce the serum DHT concentration by approximately 70%. The median circulating level of testosterone increased by approximately 10-20% but remained within the physiologic range.
Adult males with genetically inherited Type II 5α-reductase deficiency also have decreased levels of DHT. Except for the associated urogenital defects present at birth, no other clinical abnormalities related to Type II 5α-reductase deficiency have been observed in these individuals. These individuals have a small prostate gland throughout life and do not develop BPH.
In patients with BPH treated with finasteride (1-100 mg/day) for 7-10 days prior to prostatectomy, an approximate 80% lower DHT content was measured in prostatic tissue removed at surgery, compared to placebo; testosterone tissue concentration was increased up to 10 times over pretreatment levels, relative to placebo. Intraprostatic content of prostate-specific antigen (PSA) was also decreased.
In healthy male volunteers treated with PROSCAR for 14 days, discontinuation of therapy resulted in a return of DHT levels to pretreatment levels in approximately 2 weeks. In patients treated for three months, prostate volume, which declined by approximately 20%, returned to close to baseline value after approximately three months of discontinuation of therapy.
Pharmacokinetics
Absorption
In a study of 15 healthy young subjects, the mean bioavailability of finasteride 5-mg tablets was 63% (range 34-108%), based on the ratio of area under the curve (AUC) relative to an intravenous (IV) reference dose. Maximum finasteride plasma concentration averaged 37 ng/mL (range, 27-49 ng/mL) and was reached 1-2 hours postdose. Bioavailability of finasteride was not affected by food.
Distribution
Mean steady-state volume of distribution was 76 liters (range, 44-96 liters). Approximately 90% of circulating finasteride is bound to plasma proteins. There is a slow accumulation phase for finasteride after multiple dosing. After dosing with 5 mg/day of finasteride for 17 days, plasma concentrations of finasteride were 47 and 54% higher than after the first dose in men 45-60 years old (n=12) and ≥70 years old (n=12), respectively. Mean trough concentrations after 17 days of dosing were 6.2 ng/mL (range, 2.4-9.8 ng/mL) and 8.1 ng/mL (range, 1.8-19.7 ng/mL), respectively, in the two age groups. Although steady state was not reached in this study, mean trough plasma concentration in another study in patients with BPH (mean age, 65 years) receiving 5 mg/day was 9.4 ng/mL (range, 7.1-13.3 ng/mL; n=22) after over a year of dosing.
Finasteride has been shown to cross the blood brain barrier but does not appear to distribute preferentially to the CSF. In 2 studies of healthy subjects (n=69) receiving PROSCAR 5 mg/day for 6-24 weeks, finasteride concentrations in semen ranged from undetectable (<0.1 ng/mL) to 10.54 ng/mL. In an earlier study using a less sensitive assay, finasteride concentrations in the semen of 16 subjects receiving PROSCAR 5 mg/day ranged from undetectable (<1.0 ng/mL) to 21 ng/mL. Thus, based on a 5-mL ejaculate volume, the amount of finasteride in semen was estimated to be 50- to 100-fold less than the dose of finasteride (5 μg) that had no effect on circulating DHT levels in men (see also PRECAUTIONS, Pregnancy).
Metabolism
Finasteride is extensively metabolized in the liver, primarily via the cytochrome P450 3A4 enzyme subfamily. Two

Mean (SD) Noncompartmental Pharmacokinetic Parameters After Multiple Doses of 5 mg/day in Older Men

	Mean (± SD)	
	45-60 years old (n=12)	≥70 years old (n=12)
AUC (ng•hr/mL)	389 (98)	463 (186)
Peak Concentration (ng/mL)	46.2 (8.7)	48.4 (14.7)
Time to Peak (hours)	1.8 (0.7)	1.8 (0.6)
Half-Life (hours)*	6.0 (1.5)	8.2 (2.5)

* First-dose values; all other parameters are last-dose values

Table 1: All Treatment Failures in PLESS

Event	Patients (%) *		Relative Risk[†]	95% CI	P Value[†]
	Placebo N=1503	Finasteride N=1513			
All Treatment Failures	37.1	26.2	0.68	(0.57 to 0.79)	<0.001
Surgical Interventions for BPH	10.1	4.6	0.45	(0.32 to 0.63)	<0.001
Acute Urinary Retention Requiring Catheterization	6.6	2.8	0.43	(0.28 to 0.66)	<0.001
Two consecutive symptoms scores ≥20	9.2	6.7			
Bladder Stone	0.4	0.5			
Incontinence	2.1	1.7			
Renal Failure	0.5	0.6			
UTI	5.7	4.9			
Discontinuation due to worsening of BPH, lack of improvement, or to receive other medical treatment	21.8	13.3			

* patients with multiple events may be counted more than once for each type of event
† Hazard ratio based on log rank test

metabolites, the t-butyl side chain monohydroxylated and monocarboxylic acid metabolites, have been identified that possess no more than 20% of the 5α-reductase inhibitory activity of finasteride.

Excretion
In healthy young subjects (n=15), mean plasma clearance of finasteride was 165 mL/min (range, 70-279 mL/min) and mean elimination half-life in plasma was 6 hours (range, 3-16 hours). Following an oral dose of ^{14}C-finasteride in man (n=6), a mean of 39% (range, 32-46%) of the dose was excreted in the urine in the form of metabolites; 57% (range, 51-64%) was excreted in the feces.
The mean terminal half-life of finasteride in subjects ≥70 years of age was approximately 8 hours (range, 6-15 hours; n=12), compared with 6 hours (range, 4-12 hours; n=12) in subjects 45-60 years of age. As a result, mean $AUC_{(0-24 hr)}$ after 17 days of dosing was 15% higher in subjects ≥70 years of age than in subjects 45-60 years of age (p=0.02).
Special Populations
Pediatric: Finasteride pharmacokinetics have not been investigated in patients <18 years of age.
Gender: Finasteride pharmacokinetics in women are not available.
Geriatric: No dosage adjustment is necessary in the elderly. Although the elimination rate of finasteride is decreased in the elderly, these findings are of no clinical significance. See also Pharmacokinetics, Excretion, PRECAUTIONS, Geriatric Use and DOSAGE AND ADMINISTRATION.
Race: The effect of race on finasteride pharmacokinetics has not been studied.
Renal Insufficiency: No dosage adjustment is necessary in patients with renal insufficiency. In patients with chronic renal impairment, with creatinine clearances ranging from 9.0 to 55 mL/min, AUC, maximum plasma concentration, half-life, and protein binding after a single dose of ^{14}C-finasteride were similar to values obtained in healthy volunteers. Urinary excretion of metabolites was decreased in patients with renal impairment. This decrease was associated with an increase in fecal excretion of metabolites. Plasma concentrations of metabolites were significantly higher in patients with renal impairment (based on a 60% increase in total radioactivity AUC). However, finasteride has been well tolerated in BPH patients with normal renal function receiving up to 80 mg/day for 12 weeks, where exposure of these patients to metabolites would presumably be much greater.

Hepatic Insufficiency: The effect of hepatic insufficiency on finasteride pharmacokinetics has not been studied. Caution should be used in the administration of PROSCAR in those patients with liver function abnormalities, as finasteride is metabolized extensively in the liver.
Drug Interactions (also see PRECAUTIONS, Drug Interactions)
No drug interactions of clinical importance have been identified. Finasteride does not appear to affect the cytochrome P450-linked drug metabolism enzyme system. Compounds that have been tested in man have included antipyrine, digoxin, propranolol, theophylline, and warfarin, and no clinically meaningful interactions were found.

Mean (SD) Pharmacokinetic Parameters in Healthy Young Subjects (n=15)

	Mean (± SD)
Bioavailability	63% (34-108%)*
Clearance (mL/min)	165 (55)
Volume of Distribution (L)	76 (14)
Half-Life (hours)	6.2 (2.1)

* Range

[See first table above]
Clinical Studies
PROSCAR 5 mg/day was initially evaluated in patients with symptoms of BPH and enlarged prostates by digital rectal examination in two 1-year, placebo-controlled, randomized, double-blind studies and their 5-year open extensions.
PROSCAR was further evaluated in the PROSCAR Long-Term Efficacy and Safety Study (PLESS), a double-blind, randomized, placebo-controlled, 4-year, multicenter study. 3040 patients between the ages of 45 and 78, with moderate to severe symptoms of BPH and an enlarged prostate upon digital rectal examination, were randomized into the study (1524 to finasteride, 1516 to placebo) and 3016 patients were evaluable for efficacy. 1883 patients completed the 4-year study (1000 in the finasteride group, 883 in the placebo group).
Effect on Symptom Score
Symptoms were quantified using a score similar to the American Urological Association Symptom Score, which

evaluated both obstructive symptoms (impairment of size and force of stream, sensation of incomplete bladder emptying, delayed or interrupted urination) and irritative symptoms (nocturia, daytime frequency, need to strain or push the flow of urine) by rating on a 0 to 5 scale for six symptoms and a 0 to 4 scale for one symptom, for a total possible score of 34.
Patients in PLESS had moderate to severe symptoms at baseline (mean of approximately 15 points on a 0-34 point scale). Patients randomized to PROSCAR who remained on therapy for 4 years had a mean (± 1 SD) decrease in symptom score of 3.3 (± 5.8) points compared with 1.3 (± 5.6) points in the placebo group. (See Figure 1.) A statistically significant improvement in symptom score was evident at 1 year in patients treated with PROSCAR vs placebo (−2.3 vs −1.6), and this improvement continued through Year 4.

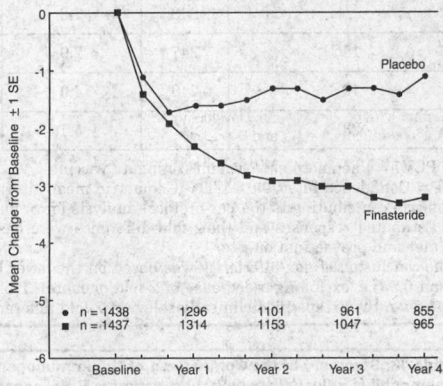

Figure 1: Symptom Score in PLESS

Results seen in earlier studies were comparable to those seen in PLESS. Although an early improvement in urinary symptoms was seen in some patients, a therapeutic trial of at least 6 months was generally necessary to assess whether a beneficial response in symptom relief had been achieved. The improvement in BPH symptoms was seen during the first year and maintained throughout an additional 5 years of open extension studies.
Effect on Acute Urinary Retention and the Need for Surgery
In PLESS, efficacy was also assessed by evaluating treatment failures. Treatment failure was prospectively defined as BPH-related urological events or clinical deterioration, lack of improvement and/or the need for alternative therapy. BPH-related urological events were defined as urological surgical intervention and acute urinary retention requiring catheterization. Complete event information was available for 92% of the patients. The following table (Table 1) summarizes the results.
[See table 1 above]
Compared with placebo, PROSCAR was associated with a significantly lower risk for acute urinary retention or the need for BPH-related surgery [13.2% for placebo vs 6.6% for PROSCAR; 51% reduction in risk, 95% CI: (34 to 63%)]. Compared with placebo, PROSCAR was associated with a significantly lower risk for surgery [10.1% for placebo vs 4.6% for PROSCAR; 55% reduction in risk, 95% CI: (37 to 68%)] and with a significantly lower risk of acute urinary retention [6.6% for placebo vs 2.8% for PROSCAR; 57% reduction in risk, 95% CI: (34 to 72%)]; see Figures 2 and 3.

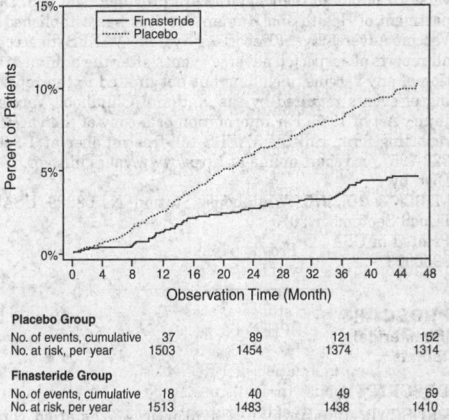

Placebo Group				
No. of events, cumulative	37	89	121	152
No. at risk, per year	1503	1454	1374	1314

Finasteride Group				
No. of events, cumulative	18	40	49	69
No. at risk, per year	1513	1483	1438	1410

Figure 2: Percent of Patients Having Surgery for BPH, Including TURP

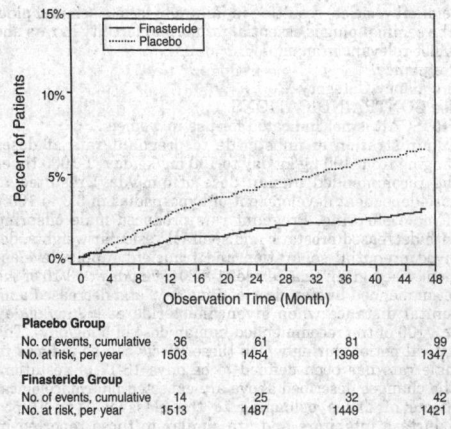

Placebo Group
No. of events, cumulative   36   61   81   99
No. at risk, per year   1503 1454 1398 1347

Finasteride Group
No. of events, cumulative   14   25   32   42
No. at risk, per year   1513 1487 1449 1421

Figure 3: Percent of Patients Developing Acute Urinary Retention (Spontaneous and Precipitated)

Effect on Maximum Urinary Flow Rate
In the patients in PLESS who remained on therapy for the duration of the study and had evaluable urinary flow data, PROSCAR increased maximum urinary flow rate by 1.9 mL/sec compared with 0.2 mL/sec in the placebo group. There was a clear difference between treatment groups in maximum urinary flow rate in favor of PROSCAR by month 4 (1.0 vs 0.3 mL/sec) which was maintained throughout the study. In the earlier 1-year studies, increase in maximum urinary flow rate was comparable to PLESS and was maintained through the first year and throughout an additional 5 years of open extension studies.

Effect on Prostate Volume
In PLESS, prostate volume was assessed yearly by magnetic resonance imaging (MRI) in a subset of patients. In patients treated with PROSCAR who remained on therapy, prostate volume was reduced compared with both baseline and placebo throughout the 4-year study. PROSCAR decreased prostate volume by 17.9% (from 55.9 cc at baseline to 45.8 cc at 4 years) compared with an increase of 14.1% (from 51.3 cc to 58.5 cc) in the placebo group (p<0.001). (See Figure 4.)

Results seen in earlier studies were comparable to those seen in PLESS. Mean prostate volume at baseline ranged between 40-50 cc. The reduction in prostate volume was seen during the first year and maintained throughout an additional five years of open extension studies.

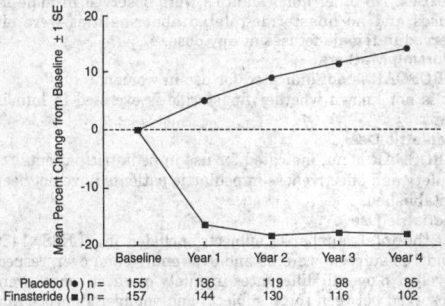

Placebo (●) n =   155   136   119   98   85
Finasteride (■) n = 157   144   130   116   102

Figure 4: Prostate Volume in PLESS

Prostate Volume as a Predictor of Therapeutic Response
A meta-analysis combining 1-year data from seven double-blind, placebo-controlled studies of similar design, including 4491 patients with symptomatic BPH, demonstrated that, in patients treated with PROSCAR, the magnitude of symptom response and degree of improvement in maximum urinary flow rate were greater in patients with an enlarged prostate at baseline.

Medical Therapy of Prostatic Symptoms
The Medical Therapy of Prostatic Symptoms (MTOPS) Trial was a double-blind, randomized, placebo-controlled, multi-center, 4- to 6-year study (average 5 years) in 3047 men with symptomatic BPH, who were randomized to receive PROSCAR 5 mg/day (n=768), doxazosin 4 or 8 mg/day (n=756), the combination of PROSCAR 5 mg/day and doxazosin 4 or 8 mg/day (n=786), or placebo (n=737). All participants underwent weekly titration of doxazosin (or its placebo) from 1 to 2 to 4 to 8 mg/day. Only those who tolerated the 4 or 8 mg dose level were kept on doxazosin (or its placebo) in the study. The participant's final tolerated dose (ei-

ther 4 mg or 8 mg) was administered beginning at end-Week 4. The final doxazosin dose was administered once per day, at bedtime.

The mean patient age at randomization was 62.6 years (±7.3 years). Patients were Caucasian (82%), African American (9%), Hispanic (7%), Asian (1%) or Native American (<1%). The mean duration of BPH symptoms was 4.7 years (±4.6 years). Patients had moderate to severe BPH symptoms at baseline with a mean AUA symptom score of approximately 17 out of 35 points. Mean maximum urinary flow rate was 10.5 mL/sec (±2.6 mL/sec). The mean prostate volume as measured by transrectal ultrasound was 36.3 mL (±20.1 mL). Prostate volume was ≤20 mL in 16% of patients, ≥50 mL in 18% of patients and between 21 and 49 mL in 66% of patients.

The primary endpoint was a composite measure of the first occurrence of any of the following five outcomes: a ≥4 point confirmed increase from baseline in symptom score, acute urinary retention, BPH-related renal insufficiency (creatinine rise), recurrent urinary tract infections or urosepsis, or incontinence. Compared to placebo, treatment with PROSCAR, doxazosin, or combination therapy resulted in a reduction in the risk of experiencing one of these five outcome events by 34% (p=0.002), 39% (p<0.001), and 67% (p<0.001), respectively. Combination therapy resulted in a significant reduction in the risk of the primary endpoint compared to treatment with PROSCAR alone (49%; p≤0.001) or doxazosin alone (46%; p≤0.001). (See Table 2.) [See table 2 above]

The majority of the events (274 out of 351; 78%) was a confirmed ≥4 point increase in symptom score, referred to as symptom score progression. The risk of symptom score progression was reduced by 30% (p=0.016), 46% (p<0.001), and 64% (p<0.001) in patients treated with PROSCAR, doxazosin, or the combination, respectively, compared to patients treated with placebo (see Figure 5). Combination therapy significantly reduced the risk of symptom score progression compared to the effect of PROSCAR alone (p<0.001) and compared to doxazosin alone (p=0.037). [See figure 5 at top of next column]

Treatment with PROSCAR, doxazosin or the combination of PROSCAR with doxazosin, reduced the mean symptom score from baseline at year 4. Table 3 provides the mean change from baseline for AUA symptom score by treatment group for patients who remained on therapy for four years. [See table 3 above]

The results of MTOPS are consistent with the findings of the 4-year, placebo-controlled study PLESS (see CLINICAL PHARMACOLOGY, Clinical Studies) in that treatment with PROSCAR reduces the risk of acute urinary retention and the need for BPH-related surgery. In MTOPS, the risk of developing acute urinary retention was reduced by 67% in patients treated with PROSCAR compared to patients treated with placebo (0.8% for PROSCAR and 2.4% for placebo). Also, the risk of requiring BPH-related invasive ther-

Table 2: Count and Percent Incidence of Primary Outcome Events by Treatment Group in MTOPS

Event	Placebo N=737 N (%)	Doxazosin N=756 N (%)	Finasteride N=768 N (%)	Combination N=786 N (%)	Total N=3047 N (%)
AUA 4-point rise	100 (13.6)	59 (7.8)	74 (9.6)	41 (5.2)	274 (9.0)
Acute urinary retention	18 (2.4)	13 (1.7)	6 (0.8)	4 (0.5)	41 (1.3)
Incontinence	8 (1.1)	11 (1.5)	9 (1.2)	3 (0.4)	31 (1.0)
Recurrent UTI/urosepsis	2 (0.3)	2 (0.3)	0 (0.0)	1 (0.1)	5 (0.2)
Creatinine rise	0 (0.0)	0 (0.0)	0 (0.0)	0 (0.0)	0 (0.0)
Total events	128 (17.4)	85 (11.2)	89 (11.6)	49 (6.2)	351 (11.5)

Table 3: Change From Baseline in AUA Symptom Score by Treatment Group at Year 4 in MTOPS

	Placebo N=534	Doxazosin N=582	Finasteride N=565	Combination N=598
Baseline Mean (SD)	16.8 (6.0)	17.0 (5.9)	17.1 (6.0)	16.8 (5.8)
Mean Change AUA Symptom Score (SD)	-4.9 (5.8)	-6.6 (6.1)	-5.6 (5.9)	-7.4 (6.3)
Comparison to Placebo (95% CI)		-1.8 (-2.5, -1.1)	-0.7 (-1.4, 0.0)	-2.5 (-3.2, -1.8)
Comparison to Doxazosin alone (95% CI)				-0.7 (-1.4, 0.0)
Comparison to Finasteride alone (95% CI)				-1.8 (-2.5, -1.1)

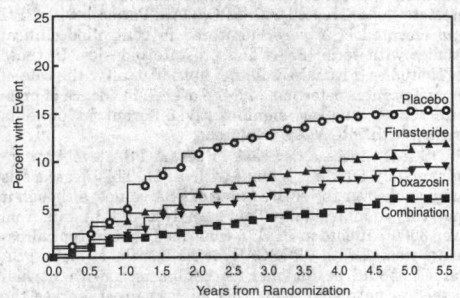

Figure 5: Cumulative Incidence of a 4-Point Rise in AUA Symptom Score by Treatment Group

apy was reduced by 64% in patients treated with PROSCAR compared to patients treated with placebo (2.0% for PROSCAR and 5.4% for placebo).

Summary of Clinical Studies
The data from these studies, showing improvement in BPH-related symptoms, reduction in treatment failure (BPH-related urological events), increased maximum urinary flow rates, and decreasing prostate volume, suggest that PROSCAR arrests the disease process of BPH in men with an enlarged prostate.

INDICATIONS AND USAGE

PROSCAR is indicated for the treatment of symptomatic benign prostatic hyperplasia (BPH) in men with an enlarged prostate to:
- Improve symptoms
- Reduce the risk of acute urinary retention
- Reduce the risk of the need for surgery including transurethral resection of the prostate (TURP) and prostatectomy.

PROSCAR administered in combination with the alpha-blocker doxazosin is indicated to reduce the risk of symptomatic progression of BPH (a confirmed ≥4 point increase in AUA symptom score).

CONTRAINDICATIONS

PROSCAR is contraindicated in the following:
Hypersensitivity to any component of this medication.
Pregnancy. Finasteride use is contraindicated in women when they are or may potentially be pregnant. Because of the ability of Type II 5α-reductase inhibitors to inhibit the conversion of testosterone to DHT, finasteride may cause abnormalities of the external genitalia of a male fetus of a pregnant woman who receives finasteride. If this drug is used during pregnancy, or if pregnancy occurs while taking this drug, the pregnant woman should be apprised of the potential hazard to the male fetus. (See also WARNINGS,

EXPOSURE OF WOMEN — RISK TO MALE FETUS and PRECAUTIONS, Information for Patients and Pregnancy.) In female rats, low doses of finasteride administered during pregnancy have produced abnormalities of the external genitalia in male offspring.

WARNINGS

PROSCAR is not indicated for use in pediatric patients (see PRECAUTIONS, Pediatric Use) or women (see also WARNINGS, EXPOSURE OF WOMEN — RISK TO MALE FETUS; PRECAUTIONS, Information for Patients and Pregnancy; and HOW SUPPLIED).

EXPOSURE OF WOMEN — RISK TO MALE FETUS

Women should not handle crushed or broken PROSCAR tablets when they are pregnant or may potentially be pregnant because of the possibility of absorption of finasteride and the subsequent potential risk to a male fetus. PROSCAR tablets are coated and will prevent contact with the active ingredient during normal handling, provided that the tablets have not been broken or crushed. (See CONTRAINDICATIONS; PRECAUTIONS, Information for Patients and Pregnancy; and HOW SUPPLIED.)

PRECAUTIONS

General

Prior to initiating therapy with PROSCAR, appropriate evaluation should be performed to identify other conditions such as infection, prostate cancer, stricture disease, hypotonic bladder or other neurogenic disorders that might mimic BPH.

Patients with large residual urinary volume and/or severely diminished urinary flow should be carefully monitored for obstructive uropathy. These patients may not be candidates for finasteride therapy.

Caution should be used in the administration of PROSCAR in those patients with liver function abnormalities, as finasteride is metabolized extensively in the liver.

Effects on PSA and Prostate Cancer Detection

No clinical benefit has been demonstrated in patients with prostate cancer treated with PROSCAR. Patients with BPH and elevated PSA were monitored in controlled clinical studies with serial PSAs and prostate biopsies. In these BPH studies, PROSCAR did not appear to alter the rate of prostate cancer detection, and the overall incidence of prostate cancer was not significantly different in patients treated with PROSCAR or placebo.

PROSCAR causes a decrease in serum PSA levels by approximately 50% in patients with BPH. This decrease is predictable over the entire range of PSA values, although it may vary in individual patients. Analysis of PSA data from over 3000 patients in PLESS confirmed that in typical patients treated with PROSCAR for six months or more, PSA values should be doubled for comparison with normal ranges in untreated men. This adjustment preserves the sensitivity and specificity of the PSA assay and maintains its ability to detect prostate cancer. PROSCAR may also cause decreases in serum PSA in the presence of prostate cancer.

Any confirmed increases in PSA levels from nadir while on PROSCAR may signal the presence of prostate cancer and should be carefully evaluated, even if those values are still within the normal range for men not taking a 5α-reductase inhibitor. Non-compliance with PROSCAR therapy may also affect PSA test results.

Percent free PSA (free to total PSA ratio) is not significantly decreased by PROSCAR. The ratio of free to total PSA remains constant even under the influence of PROSCAR. If clinicians elect to use percent free PSA as an aid in the detection of prostate cancer in men undergoing finasteride therapy, no adjustment to its value appears necessary.

Information for Patients

Women should not handle crushed or broken PROSCAR tablets when they are pregnant or may potentially be pregnant because of the possibility of absorption of finasteride and the subsequent potential risk to the male fetus (see CONTRAINDICATIONS; WARNINGS, EXPOSURE OF WOMEN — RISK TO MALE FETUS; PRECAUTIONS, Pregnancy and HOW SUPPLIED).

Physicians should inform patients that the volume of ejaculate may be decreased in some patients during treatment with PROSCAR. This decrease does not appear to interfere with normal sexual function. However, impotence and decreased libido may occur in patients treated with PROSCAR (see ADVERSE REACTIONS).

Physicians should instruct their patients to promptly report any changes in their breasts such as lumps, pain or nipple discharge. Breast changes including breast enlargement, tenderness and neoplasm have been reported (see ADVERSE REACTIONS).

Physicians should instruct their patients to read the patient package insert before starting therapy with PROSCAR and to reread it each time the prescription is renewed so that they are aware of current information for patients regarding PROSCAR.

Drug/Laboratory Test Interactions

In patients with BPH, PROSCAR has no effect on circulating levels of cortisol, estradiol, prolactin, thyroid-stimulating hormone, or thyroxine. No clinically meaningful effect was observed on the plasma lipid profile (i.e., total cholesterol, low density lipoproteins, high density lipoproteins and triglycerides) or bone mineral density. Increases of about 10% were observed in luteinizing hormone (LH) and follicle-stimulating hormone (FSH) in patients receiving PROSCAR, but levels remained within the normal range. In healthy volunteers, treatment with PROSCAR did not alter the response of LH and FSH to gonadotropin-releasing hormone indicating that the hypothalamic-pituitary-testicular axis was not affected.

Treatment with PROSCAR for 24 weeks to evaluate semen parameters in healthy male volunteers revealed no clinically meaningful effects on sperm concentration, mobility, morphology, or pH. A 0.6 mL (22.1%) median decrease in ejaculate volume with a concomitant reduction in total sperm per ejaculate was observed. These parameters remained within the normal range and were reversible upon discontinuation of therapy with an average time to return to baseline of 84 weeks.

Drug Interactions

No drug interactions of clinical importance have been identified. Finasteride does not appear to affect the cytochrome P450-linked drug metabolizing enzyme system. Compounds that have been tested in man have included antipyrine, digoxin, propranolol, theophylline, and warfarin and no clinically meaningful interactions were found.

Other Concomitant Therapy: Although specific interaction studies were not performed, PROSCAR was concomitantly used in clinical studies with acetaminophen, acetylsalicylic acid, α-blockers, angiotensin-converting enzyme (ACE) inhibitors, analgesics, anti-convulsants, beta-adrenergic blocking agents, diuretics, calcium channel blockers, cardiac nitrates, HMG-CoA reductase inhibitors, nonsteroidal anti-inflammatory drugs (NSAIDs), benzodiazepines, H_2 antagonists and quinolone anti-infectives without evidence of clinically significant adverse interactions.

Carcinogenesis, Mutagenesis, Impairment of Fertility

No evidence of a tumorigenic effect was observed in a 24-month study in Sprague-Dawley rats receiving doses of finasteride up to 160 mg/kg/day in males and 320 mg/kg/day in females. These doses produced respective systemic exposure in rats of 111 and 274 times those observed in man receiving the recommended human dose of 5 mg/day. All exposure calculations were based on calculated $AUC_{(0\text{-}24\ hr)}$ for animals and mean $AUC_{(0\text{-}24\ hr)}$ for man (0.4 μg•hr/mL).

In a 19-month carcinogenicity study in CD-1 mice, a statistically significant ($p \leq 0.05$) increase in the incidence of testicular Leydig cell adenomas was observed at a dose of 250 mg/kg/day (228 times the human exposure). In mice at a dose of 25 mg/kg/day (23 times the human exposure, estimated) and in rats at a dose of ≥40 mg/kg/day (39 times the human exposure) an increase in the incidence of Leydig cell hyperplasia was observed. A positive correlation between the proliferative changes in the Leydig cells and an increase in serum LH levels (2- to 3-fold above control) has been demonstrated in both rodent species treated with high doses of finasteride. No drug-related Leydig cell changes were seen in either rats or dogs treated with finasteride for 1 year at doses of 20 mg/kg/day and 45 mg/kg/day (30 and 350 times, respectively, the human exposure) or in mice treated for 19 months at a dose of 2.5 mg/kg/day (2.3 times the human exposure, estimated).

No evidence of mutagenicity was observed in an *in vitro* bacterial mutagenesis assay, a mammalian cell mutagenesis assay, or in an *in vitro* alkaline elution assay. In an *in vitro* chromosome aberration assay, using Chinese hamster ovary cells, there was a slight increase in chromosome aberrations. These concentrations correspond to 4000-5000 times the peak plasma levels in man given a total dose of 5 mg. In an *in vivo* chromosome aberration assay in mice, no treatment-related increase in chromosome aberration was observed with finasteride at the maximum tolerated dose of 250 mg/kg/day (228 times the human exposure) as determined in the carcinogenicity studies.

In sexually mature male rabbits treated with finasteride at 80 mg/kg/day (543 times the human exposure) for up to 12 weeks, no effect on fertility, sperm count, or ejaculate volume was seen. In sexually mature male rats treated with 80 mg/kg/day of finasteride (61 times the human exposure), there were no significant effects on fertility after 6 or 12 weeks of treatment; however, when treatment was continued for up to 24 or 30 weeks, there was an apparent decrease in fertility, fecundity and an associated significant decrease in the weights of the seminal vesicles and prostate. All these effects were reversible within 6 weeks of discontinuation of treatment. No drug-related effect on testes or on mating performance has been seen in rats or rabbits. This decrease in fertility in finasteride-treated rats is secondary to its effect on accessory sex organs (prostate and seminal vesicles) resulting in failure to form a seminal plug. The seminal plug is essential for normal fertility in rats and is not relevant in man.

Pregnancy

Pregnancy Category X

See CONTRAINDICATIONS.

PROSCAR is not indicated for use in women.

Administration of finasteride to pregnant rats at doses ranging from 100 μg/kg/day to 100 mg/kg/day (1-1000 times the recommended human dose of 5 mg/day) resulted in dose-dependent development of hypospadias in 3.6 to 100% of male offspring. Pregnant rats produced male offspring with decreased prostatic and seminal vesicular weights, delayed preputial separation and transient nipple development when given finasteride at ≥30 μg/kg/day (≥3/10 of the recommended human dose of 5 mg/day) and decreased anogenital distance when given finasteride at ≥3 μg/kg/day (≥3/100 of the recommended human dose of 5 mg/day). The critical period during which these effects can be induced in male rats has been defined to be days 16-17 of gestation. The changes described above are expected pharmacological effects of drugs belonging to the class of Type II 5α-reductase inhibitors and are similar to those reported in male infants with a genetic deficiency of Type II 5α-reductase. No abnormalities were observed in female offspring exposed to any dose of finasteride *in utero*.

No developmental abnormalities have been observed in first filial generation (F_1) male or female offspring resulting from mating finasteride-treated male rats (80 mg/kg/day; 61 times the human exposure) with untreated females. Administration of finasteride at 3 mg/kg/day (30 times the recommended human dose of 5 mg/day) during the late gestation and lactation period resulted in slightly decreased fertility in F_1 male offspring. No effects were seen in female offspring. No evidence of malformations has been observed in rabbit fetuses exposed to finasteride *in utero* from days 6-18 of gestation at doses up to 100 mg/kg/day (1000 times the recommended human dose of 5 mg/day). However, effects on male genitalia would not be expected since the rabbits were not exposed during the critical period of genital system development.

The *in utero* effects of finasteride exposure during the period of embryonic and fetal development were evaluated in the rhesus monkey (gestation days 20-100), a species more predictive of human development than rats or rabbits. Intravenous administration of finasteride to pregnant monkeys at doses as high as 800 ng/day (at least 60 to 120 times the highest estimated exposure of pregnant women to finasteride from semen of men taking 5 mg/day) resulted in no abnormalities in male fetuses. In confirmation of the relevance of the rhesus model for human fetal development, oral administration of a dose of finasteride (2 mg/kg/day; 20 times the recommended human dose of 5 mg/day or approximately 1-2 million times the highest estimated exposure to finasteride from semen of men taking 5 mg/day) to pregnant monkeys resulted in external genital abnormalities in male fetuses. No other abnormalities were observed in male fetuses and no finasteride-related abnormalities were observed in female fetuses at any dose.

Nursing Mothers

PROSCAR is not indicated for use in women.

It is not known whether finasteride is excreted in human milk.

Pediatric Use

PROSCAR is not indicated for use in pediatric patients.

Safety and effectiveness in pediatric patients have not been established.

Geriatric Use

Of the total number of subjects included in PLESS, 1480 and 105 subjects were 65 and over and 75 and over, respectively. No overall differences in safety or effectiveness were observed between these subjects and younger subjects, and other reported clinical experience has not identified differences in responses between the elderly and younger patients. No dosage adjustment is necessary in the elderly (see CLINICAL PHARMACOLOGY, Pharmacokinetics and Clinical Studies).

ADVERSE REACTIONS

PROSCAR is generally well tolerated; adverse reactions usually have been mild and transient.

4-Year Placebo-Controlled Study

In PLESS, 1524 patients treated with PROSCAR and 1516 patients treated with placebo were evaluated for safety over a period of 4 years. The most frequently reported adverse reactions were related to sexual function. 3.7% (57 patients) treated with PROSCAR and 2.1% (32 patients) treated with placebo discontinued therapy as a result of adverse reactions related to sexual function, which are the most frequently reported adverse reactions.

Table 4 presents the only clinical adverse reactions considered possibly, probably or definitely drug related by the investigator, for which the incidence on PROSCAR was ≥1% and greater than placebo over the 4 years of the study. In years 2-4 of the study, there was no significant difference between treatment groups in the incidences of impotence, decreased libido and ejaculation disorder.

[See table 4 at right]

Phase III Studies and 5-Year Open Extensions

The adverse experience profile in the 1-year, placebo-controlled, Phase III studies, the 5-year open extensions, and PLESS were similar.

Medical Therapy of Prostatic Symptoms (MTOPS) Study

The incidence rates of drug-related adverse experiences reported by ≥2% of patients in any treatment group in the MTOPS Study are listed in Table 5.

The individual adverse effects which occurred more frequently in the combination group compared to either drug alone were: asthenia, postural hypotension, peripheral edema, dizziness, decreased libido, rhinitis, abnormal ejaculation, impotence and abnormal sexual function (see Table 5). Of these, the incidence of abnormal ejaculation in patients receiving combination therapy was comparable to the sum of the incidences of this adverse experience reported for the two monotherapies.

Combination therapy with finasteride and doxazosin was associated with no new clinical adverse experience.

Four patients in MTOPS reported the adverse experience breast cancer. Three of these patients were on finasteride only and one was on combination therapy. (See ADVERSE REACTIONS, Long-Term Data.)

The MTOPS Study was not specifically designed to make statistical comparisons between groups for reported adverse experiences. In addition, direct comparisons of safety data between the MTOPS study and previous studies of the single agents may not be appropriate based upon differences in patient population, dosage or dose regimen, and other procedural and study design elements.

[See table 5 at right]

Long-Term Data

There is no evidence of increased adverse experiences with increased duration of treatment with PROSCAR. New reports of drug-related sexual adverse experiences decreased with duration of therapy.

During the 4- to 6-year placebo- and comparator-controlled MTOPS study that enrolled 3047 men, there were 4 cases of breast cancer in men treated with finasteride but no cases in men not treated with finasteride. During the 4-year, placebo-controlled PLESS study that enrolled 3040 men, there were 2 cases of breast cancer in placebo-treated men, but no cases were reported in men treated with finasteride. The relationship between long-term use of finasteride and male breast neoplasia is currently unknown.

In a 7-year placebo-controlled trial that enrolled 18,882 healthy men, 9060 had prostate needle biopsy data available for analysis. In the PROSCAR group, 280 (6.4%) men had prostate cancer with Gleason scores of 7-10 detected on needle biopsy vs. 237 (5.1%) men in the placebo group. Of the total cases of prostate cancer diagnosed in this study, approximately 98% were classified as intracapsular (stage T1 or T2). The clinical significance of these findings is unknown. This information from the literature (Thompson IM, Goodman PJ, Tangen CM, et al. The influence of finasteride on the development of prostate cancer. *N Engl J Med* 2003;349:213-22) is provided for consideration by physicians when PROSCAR is used as indicated (see INDICATIONS AND USAGE). PROSCAR is not approved to reduce the risk of developing prostate cancer.

Post-Marketing Experience

The following additional adverse effects have been reported in post-marketing experience:

- hypersensitivity reactions, including pruritus, urticaria, and swelling of the lips and face
- testicular pain.

OVERDOSAGE

Patients have received single doses of PROSCAR up to 400 mg and multiple doses of PROSCAR up to 80 mg/day for three months without adverse effects. Until further experience is obtained, no specific treatment for an overdose with PROSCAR can be recommended.

Significant lethality was observed in male and female mice at single oral doses of 1500 mg/m^2 (500 mg/kg) and in female and male rats at single oral doses of 2360 mg/m^2 (400 mg/kg) and 5900 mg/m^2 (1000 mg/kg), respectively.

DOSAGE AND ADMINISTRATION

The recommended dose is 5 mg orally once a day.

PROSCAR can be administered alone or in combination with the alpha-blocker doxazosin (see CLINICAL PHARMACOLOGY, Clinical Studies).

PROSCAR may be administered with or without meals.

No dosage adjustment is necessary for patients with renal impairment or for the elderly (see CLINICAL PHARMACOLOGY, Pharmacokinetics).

HOW SUPPLIED

No. 3094—PROSCAR tablets 5 mg are blue, modified apple-shaped, film-coated tablets, with the code MSD 72 on one side and PROSCAR on the other. They are supplied as follows:

NDC 0006-0072-31 unit of use bottles of 30
NDC 0006-0072-58 unit of use bottles of 100

TABLE 4: Drug-Related Adverse Experiences

	Year 1 (%)		Years 2, 3 and 4* (%)	
	Finasteride	Placebo	Finasteride	Placebo
Impotence	8.1	3.7	5.1	5.1
Decreased Libido	6.4	3.4	2.6	2.6
Decreased Volume of Ejaculate	3.7	0.8	1.5	0.5
Ejaculation Disorder	0.8	0.1	0.2	0.1
Breast Enlargement	0.5	0.1	1.8	1.1
Breast Tenderness	0.4	0.1	0.7	0.3
Rash	0.5	0.2	0.5	0.1

N = 1524 and 1516, finasteride vs placebo, respectively

* Combined Years 2-4

Table 5: Incidence ≥2% in One or More Treatment Groups: Drug-Related Clinical Adverse Experiences in MTOPS

Adverse Experience	Placebo (N=737) (%)	Doxazosin 4 mg or 8 mg* (N=756) (%)	Finasteride (N= 768) (%)	Combination (N=786) (%)
Body as a whole				
Asthenia	7.1	15.7	5.3	16.8
Headache	2.3	4.1	2.0	2.3
Cardiovascular				
Hypotension	0.7	3.4	1.2	1.5
Postural Hypotension	8.0	16.7	9.1	17.8
Metabolic and Nutritional				
Peripheral Edema	0.9	2.6	1.3	3.3
Nervous				
Dizziness	8.1	17.7	7.4	23.2
Libido Decreased	5.7	7.0	10.0	11.6
Somnolence	1.5	3.7	1.7	3.1
Respiratory				
Dyspnea	0.7	2.1	0.7	1.9
Rhinitis	0.5	1.3	1.0	2.4
Urogenital				
Abnormal Ejaculation	2.3	4.5	7.2	14.1
Gynecomastia	0.7	1.1	2.2	1.5
Impotence	12.2	14.4	18.5	22.6
Sexual Function Abnormal	0.9	2.0	2.5	3.1

* Doxazosin dose was achieved by weekly titration (1 to 2 to 4 to 8 mg). The final tolerated dose (4 mg or 8 mg) was administered at end-Week 4. Only those patients tolerating at least 4 mg were kept on doxazosin. The majority of patients received the 8-mg dose over the duration of the study.

Storage and Handling

Store at room temperatures below 30°C (86°F). Protect from light and keep container tightly closed.

Women should not handle crushed or broken PROSCAR tablets when they are pregnant or may potentially be pregnant because of the possibility of absorption of finasteride and the subsequent potential risk to a male fetus (see WARNINGS, EXPOSURE OF WOMEN — RISK TO MALE FETUS, and PRECAUTIONS, Information for Patients and Pregnancy).

Dist. by: Merck Sharp & Dohme Corp., a subsidiary of **MERCK & CO., INC.,** Whitehouse Station, NJ 08889, USA
Issued March 2010
Printed in USA
9631304

PATIENT PACKAGE INSERT

PROSCAR® (Finasteride) Tablets
Patient Information about
PROSCAR® (Prahs-car)
Generic name: finasteride
(fin-AS-tur-eyed)
PROSCAR[1] is for use by men only.
Please read this leaflet before you start taking PROSCAR. Also, read it each time you renew your prescription, just in case anything has changed. Remember, this leaflet does not take the place of careful discussions with your doctor. You and your doctor should discuss PROSCAR when you start taking your medication and at regular checkups.

[1] Registered trademark of Merck Sharp & Dohme Corp., a subsidiary of **Merck & Co., Inc.**

Copyright © Merck Sharp & Dohme Corp., a subsidiary of **Merck & Co., Inc.,** 1992, 1995, 1998
All rights reserved

What is PROSCAR?

PROSCAR is a medication used to treat symptoms of benign prostatic hyperplasia (BPH) in men with an enlarged prostate. PROSCAR may also be used to reduce the risk of a sudden inability to pass urine and the need for surgery related to BPH in men with an enlarged prostate.

PROSCAR may be prescribed along with another medicine, an alpha-blocker called doxazosin, to help you better manage your BPH symptoms.

Who should NOT take PROSCAR?

PROSCAR is for use by MEN only.

Do Not Take PROSCAR if you are:

• a woman who is pregnant or may potentially be pregnant. PROSCAR may harm your unborn baby. Do not touch or handle crushed or broken PROSCAR tablets (see **"A warning about PROSCAR and pregnancy"**).

• allergic to finasteride or any of the ingredients in PROSCAR. See the end of this leaflet for a complete list of ingredients in PROSCAR.

A warning about PROSCAR and pregnancy.

Women who are or may potentially be pregnant must not use PROSCAR. They should also not handle crushed or broken tablets of PROSCAR. PROSCAR tablets are coated and will prevent contact with the active ingredient during normal handling, provided that the tablets are not broken or crushed.

If a woman who is pregnant with a male baby absorbs the active ingredient in PROSCAR after oral use or through the skin, it may cause the male baby to be born with abnormalities of the sex organs. If a woman who is pregnant comes into contact with the active ingredient in PROSCAR, a doctor should be consulted.

How should I take PROSCAR?

Follow your doctor's instruction.

• Take one tablet by mouth each day. To avoid forgetting to take PROSCAR, you can take it at the same time every day.
• If you forget to take PROSCAR, do not take an extra tablet. Just take the next tablet as usual.
• You may take PROSCAR with or without food.
• Do not share PROSCAR with anyone else; it was prescribed only for you.

What are the possible side effects of PROSCAR?

The most common side effects of PROSCAR include:

• trouble getting or keeping an erection (impotence)
• decrease in sex drive
• decreased volume of ejaculate
• ejaculation disorders
• enlarged or painful breast. You should promptly report to your doctor any changes in your breasts such as lumps, pain or nipple discharge.

Allergic reactions: Call your doctor if you get any signs of an allergic reaction while taking PROSCAR, including rash, itching, hives, and swelling of the lips and face.

Testicular pain: Rarely, some men may have testicular pain while taking PROSCAR.

You should discuss side effects with your doctor before taking PROSCAR and anytime you think you are having a side effect. These are not all the possible side effects with PROSCAR. For more information, ask your doctor or pharmacist.

Call your doctor for medical advice about side effects. You may report side effects to FDA at: 1-800-FDA-1088.

What you need to know while taking PROSCAR

• **You should see your doctor regularly while taking PROSCAR.** Follow your doctor's advice about when to have these checkups.
• **Checking for prostate cancer.** Your doctor has prescribed PROSCAR for BPH and not for treatment of prostate cancer—but a man can have BPH and prostate cancer at the same time. Checking for prostate cancer should continue while you take PROSCAR.
• **About Prostate-Specific Antigen (PSA).** Your doctor may have done a blood test called PSA for the screening of prostate cancer. Because PROSCAR decreases PSA levels, you should tell your doctor(s) that you are taking PROSCAR. Changes in PSA levels will need to be carefully evaluated by your doctor(s). Any increase in follow-up PSA levels from their lowest point should be carefully evaluated, even if the test results are still within the normal range. You should also tell your doctor if you have not been taking PROSCAR as prescribed because this may affect the PSA test results. For more information, talk to your doctor.

How should I store PROSCAR?

• Store PROSCAR tablets in a dry place at room temperature.
• Keep PROSCAR in the original container and keep the container closed.

PROSCAR tablets are coated and will prevent contact with the active ingredient during normal handling, provided that the tablets are not broken or crushed.

Keep PROSCAR and all medications out of the reach of children.

Do not give your PROSCAR tablets to anyone else. It has been prescribed only for you.

For more information call 1-800-633-4477.

What are the ingredients in PROSCAR?

Active ingredients: finasteride

Inactive ingredients: hydrous lactose, microcrystalline cellulose, pregelatinized starch, sodium starch glycolate, hydroxypropyl cellulose LF, hydroxypropyl methylcellulose, titanium dioxide, magnesium stearate, talc, docusate sodium, FD&C Blue 2 aluminum lake and yellow iron oxide.

What is BPH?

BPH is an enlargement of the prostate gland. The prostate is located below the bladder. As the prostate enlarges, it may slowly restrict the flow of urine. This can lead to symptoms such as:

• a weak or interrupted urinary stream
• a feeling that you cannot empty your bladder completely
• a feeling of delay or hesitation when you start to urinate
• a need to urinate often, especially at night
• a feeling that you must urinate right away.

In some men, BPH can lead to serious problems, including urinary tract infections, a sudden inability to pass urine (acute urinary retention), as well as the need for surgery.

What PROSCAR does

PROSCAR lowers levels of a hormone called DHT (dihydrotestosterone), which is a cause of prostate growth. Lowering DHT leads to shrinkage of the enlarged prostate gland in most men. This can lead to gradual improvement in urine flow and symptoms over the next several months. PROSCAR will help reduce the risk of developing a sudden inability to pass urine and the need for surgery related to an enlarged prostate. However, since each case of BPH is different, you should know that:

• Even though the prostate shrinks, you may NOT notice an improvement in urine flow or symptoms.
• You may need to take PROSCAR for six (6) months or more to see whether it improves your symptoms.
• Therapy with PROSCAR may reduce your risk for a sudden inability to pass urine and the need for surgery for an enlarged prostate.

Dist. by: Merck Sharp & Dohme Corp., a subsidiary of
MERCK & CO., INC., Whitehouse Station, NJ 08889, USA
Issued March 2010
9631304
Revised: 03/2010

Distributed by: Merck Sharp & Dohme Corp.
Shown in Product Identification Guide, page 313

PROVENTIL® HFA ℞

[*prō-vĕn-tĭl H-F-A*]
(albuterol sulfate)
Inhalation Aerosol

FOR ORAL INHALATION ONLY
Prescribing Information

DESCRIPTION

The active component of PROVENTIL® HFA (albuterol sulfate) Inhalation Aerosol is albuterol sulfate, USP racemic α^1[(*tert*-Butylamino)methyl]-4-hydroxy-*m*-xylene-α,α'-diol sulfate (2:1)(salt), a relatively selective beta$_2$-adrenergic bronchodilator having the following chemical structure:

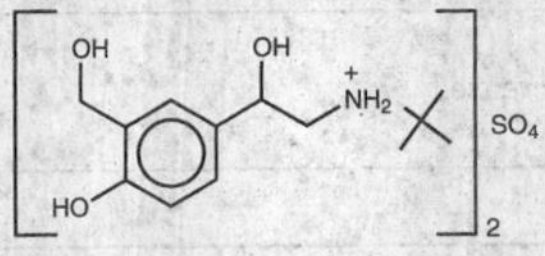

Albuterol sulfate is the official generic name in the United States. The World Health Organization recommended name for the drug is salbutamol sulfate. The molecular weight of albuterol sulfate is 576.7, and the empirical formula is (C13H21 NO3)2•H2SO4. Albuterol sulfate is a white to off-white crystalline solid. It is soluble in water and slightly soluble in ethanol. PROVENTIL HFA Inhalation Aerosol is a pressurized metered-dose aerosol unit for oral inhalation. It contains a microcrystalline suspension of albuterol sulfate in propellant HFA-134a (1,1,1,2-tetrafluoroethane), ethanol, and oleic acid.

Each actuation delivers 120 mcg albuterol sulfate, USP from the valve and 108 mcg albuterol sulfate, USP from the mouthpiece (equivalent to 90 mcg of albuterol base from the mouthpiece). Each canister provides 200 inhalations. It is recommended to prime the inhaler before using for the first time and in cases where the inhaler has not been used for more than 2 weeks by releasing four "test sprays" into the air, away from the face.

This product does not contain chlorofluorocarbons (CFCs) as the propellant.

CLINICAL PHARMACOLOGY

Mechanism of Action *In vitro* studies and *in vivo* pharmacologic studies have demonstrated that albuterol has a preferential effect on beta$_2$-adrenergic receptors compared with isoproterenol. While it is recognized that beta$_2$-adrenergic receptors are the predominant receptors on bronchial smooth muscle, data indicate that there is a population of beta$_2$-receptors in the human heart existing in a concentration between 10% and 50% of cardiac beta-adrenergic receptors. The precise function of these receptors has not been established. (See **WARNINGS, Cardiovascular Effects** section.)

Activation of beta$_2$-adrenergic receptors on airway smooth muscle leads to the activation of adenylcyclase and to an increase in the intra-cellular concentration of cyclic-3′,5′-adenosine monophosphate (cyclic AMP). This increase of cyclic AMP leads to the activation of protein kinase A, which inhabits the phosphorylation of myosin and lowers intracellular ionic calcium concentrations, resulting in relaxation. Albuterol relaxes the smooth muscles of all airways, from the trachea to the terminal bronchioles. Albuterol acts as a functional antagonist to relax the airway irrespective of the spasmogen involved, thus protecting against all bronchoconstrictor challenges. Increased cyclic AMP concentrations are also associated with the inhibition of release of mediators from mast cells in the airway.

Albuterol has been shown in most clinical trials to have more effect on the respiratory tract, in the form of bronchial smooth muscle relaxation, than isoproterenol at comparable doses while producing fewer cardiovascular effects. Controlled clinical studies and other clinical experience have shown that inhaled albuterol, like other beta-adrenergic agonist drugs, can produce a significant cardiovascular effect in some patients, as measured by pulse rate, blood pressure, symptoms, and/or electrocardiographic changes.

Preclinical Intravenous studies in rats with albuterol sulfate have demonstrated that albuterol crosses the blood-brain barrier and reaches brain concentrations amounting to approximately 5% of the plasma concentrations. In structures outside the blood-brain barrier (pineal and pituitary glands), albuterol concentrations were found to be 100 times those in the whole brain.

Studies in laboratory animals (minipigs, rodents, and dogs) have demonstrated the occurrence of cardiac arrhythmias and sudden death (with histologic evidence of myocardial necrosis) when beta$_2$-agonist and methylxanthines were administered concurrently. The clinical significance of these findings is unknown.

Propellant HFA-134a is devoid of pharmacological activity except at very high doses in animals (380-1300 times the maximum human exposure based on comparisons of AUC values), primarily producing ataxia, tremors, dyspnea, or salivation. These are similar to effects produced by the structurally related chlorofluorocarbons (CFCs), which have been used extensively in metered dose inhalers.

In animals and humans, propellant HFA-134a was found to be rapidly absorbed and rapidly eliminated, with an elimination half-life of 3 to 27 minutes in animals and 5 to 7 minutes in humans. Time to maximum plasma concentration (Tmax) and mean residence time are both extremely short, leading to a transient appearance of HFA-134a in the blood with no evidence of accumulation.

Pharmacokinetics In a single-dose bioavailability study which enrolled six healthy, male volunteers, transient low albuterol levels (close to the lower limit of quantitation) were observed after administration of two puffs from both PROVENTIL® HFA Inhalation Aerosol and a CFC 11/12 propelled albuterol inhaler. No formal pharmacokinetic analyses were possible for either treatment, but systemic albuterol levels appeared similar.

Clinical Trials In a 12-week, randomized, double-blind, double-dummy, active- and placebo-controlled trial, 565 patients with asthma were evaluated for the bronchodilator efficacy of PROVENTIL HFA Inhalation Aerosol (193 patients) in comparison to a CFC 11/12 propelled albuterol inhaler (186 patients) and an HFA-134a placebo inhaler (186 patients).

Serial FEV1 measurements (shown below as percent change from test-day baseline) demonstrated that two inhalations of PROVENTIL HFA Inhalation Aerosol produced significantly greater improvement in pulmonary function than placebo and produced outcomes which were clinically comparable to a CFC 11/12 propelled albuterol inhaler.

The mean time to onset of a 15% increase in FEV1 was 6 minutes and the mean time to peak effect was 50 to 55 minutes. The mean duration of effect as measured by a 15% increase in FEV1 was 3 hours. In some patients, duration of effect was as long as 6 hours.

In another clinical study in adults, two inhalations of PROVENTIL HFA Inhalation Aerosol taken 30 minutes before exercise prevented exercise-induced bronchospasm as demonstrated by the maintenance of FEV1 within 80% of baseline values in the majority of patients.

In a 4-week, randomized, open-label trial, 63 children, 4 to 11 years of age, with asthma were evaluated for the bronchodilator efficacy of PROVENTIL HFA Inhalation Aerosol (33 pediatric patients) in comparison to a CFC 11/12 propelled albuterol inhaler (30 pediatric patients).

[See figure at top of next page]

Serial FEV1 measurements as percent change from test-day baseline demonstrated that two inhalations of PROVENTIL HFA Inhalation Aerosol produced outcomes which were clinically comparable to a CFC 11/12 propelled albuterol inhaler.

The mean time to onset of a 12% increase in FEV1 for PROVENTIL HFA Inhalation Aerosol was 7 minutes and the mean time to peak effect was approximately 50 minutes. The mean duration of effect as measured by a 12% increase in FEV1 was 2.3 hours. In some pediatric patients, duration of effect was as long as 6 hours.

FEV_1 as Percent Change from Predose in a Large 12-Week Clinical Trial

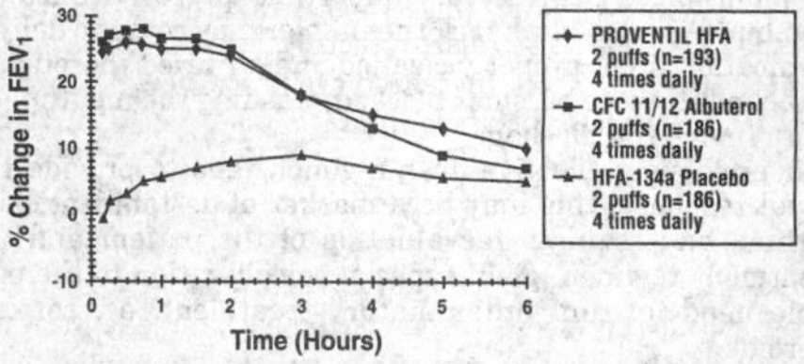
% Change in FEV_1
30
20
10
0
-10
0
1
2
3
4
5
6
Time (Hours)
PROVENTIL HFA 2 puffs (n=193) 4 times daily
CFC 11/12 Albuterol 2 puffs (n=186) 4 times daily
HFA-134a Placebo 2 puffs (n=186) 4 times daily

In another clinical study in pediatric patients, two inhalations of PROVENTIL HFA Inhalation Aerosol taken 30 minutes before exercise provided comparable protection against exercise-induced bronchospasm as a CFC 11/12 propelled albuterol inhaler.

INDICATIONS AND USAGE

PROVENTIL® HFA Inhalation Aerosol is indicated in adults and children 4 years of age and older for the treatment or prevention of bronchospasm with reversible obstructive airway disease and for the prevention of exercise-induced bronchospasm.

CONTRAINDICATIONS

PROVENTIL® HFA Inhalation Aerosol is contraindicated in patients with a history of hypersensitivity to albuterol or any other PROVENTIL HFA components.

WARNINGS

1. **Paradoxical Bronchospasm:** Inhaled albuterol sulfate can produce paradoxical bronchospasm that may be life threatening. If paradoxical bronchospasm occur, PROVENTIL® HFA Inhalation Aerosol should be discontinued immediately and alternative therapy instituted. It should be recognized that paradoxical bronchospasm, when associated with inhaled formulations, frequently occurs with the first use of a new canister.
2. **Deterioration of Asthma:** Asthma may deteriorate acutely over a period of hours or chronically over several days or longer. If the patient needs more doses of PROVENTIL HFA Inhalation Aerosol than usual, this may be a marker of destabilization of asthma and requires re-evaluation of the patient and treatment regimen, giving special consideration to the possible need for anti-inflammatory treatment, eg, corticosteroids.
3. **Use of Anti-inflammatory Agents:** The use of beta-adrenergic-agonist bronchodilators alone may not be adequate to control asthma in many patients. Early consideration should be given to adding anti-inflammatory agents, eg, corticosteroids, to the therapeutic regimen.
4. **Cardiovascular Effects:** PROVENTIL HFA Inhalation Aerosol, like other beta-adrenergic agonist, can produce clinically significant cardiovascular effects in some patients as measured by pulse rate, blood pressure, and/or symptoms. Although such effects are uncommon after administration of PROVENTIL HFA Inhalation Aerosol at recommended doses, if they occur, the drug may need to be discontinued. In addition, beta-agonists have been reported to produce ECG changes, such as flattening of the T wave, prolongation of the QTc interval, and ST segment depression. The clinical significance of these findings is unknown. Therefore, PROVENTIL HFA Inhalation Aerosol, like all sympathomimetic amines, should be used with caution in patients with cardiovascular disorders, especially coronary insufficiency, cardiac arrhythmias, and hypertension.
5. **Do Not Exceed Recommended Dose:** Fatalities have been reported in association with excessive use of inhaled sympathomimetic drugs in patients with asthma. The exact cause of death is unknown, but cardiac arrest following an unexpected development of a severe acute asthmatic crisis and subsequent hypoxia is suspected.
6. **Immediate Hypersensitivity Reactions:** Immediate hypersensitivity reactions may occur after administration of albuterol sulfate, as demonstrated by rare cases of urticaria, angioedema, rash, bronchospasm, anaphylaxis, and oropharyngeal edema.

PRECAUTIONS

General Albuterol sulfate, as with all sympathomimetic amines, should be used with caution in patients with cardiovascular disorders, especially coronary insufficiency, cardiac arrhythmias, and hypertension; in patients with convulsive disorders, hyperthyroidism, or diabetes mellitus; and in patients who are unusually responsive to sympathomimetic amines. Clinically significant changes in systolic and diastolic blood pressure have been seen in individual patients and could be expected to occur in some patients after use of any beta-adrenergic bronchodilator.

Large doses of intravenous albuterol have been reported to aggravate preexisting diabetes mellitus and ketoacidosis. As with other beta-agonists, albuterol may produce significant hypokalemia in some patients, possibly through intracellular shunting, which has the potential to produce adverse cardiovascular effects. The decrease is usually transient, not requiring supplementation.

Information for Patients See illustrated Patient's Instructions for Use. SHAKE WELL BEFORE USING. Patients should be given the following information:

It is recommended to prime the inhaler before using for the first time and in cases where the inhaler has not been used for more than 2 weeks by releasing four "test sprays" into the air, away from the face.

KEEPING THE PLASTIC MOUTHPIECE CLEAN IS VERY IMPORTANT TO PREVENT MEDICATION BUILD-UP AND BLOCKAGE. THE MOUTHPIECE SHOULD BE WASHED, SHAKEN TO REMOVE EXCESS WATER, AND AIR DRIED THOROUGHLY AT LEASE ONCE A WEEK. INHALER MAY CEASE TO DELIVER MEDICATION IF NOT PROPERLY CLEANED.

The mouthpiece should be cleaned (with the canister removed) by running warm water through the top and bottom for 30 seconds at least once a week. The mouthpiece must be shaken to remove excess water, then air dried thoroughly (such as overnight). Blockage from medication build-up or improper medication delivery may result from failure to thoroughly air dry the mouthpiece.

If the mouthpiece should become blocked (little or no medication coming out of the mouthpiece), the blockage may be removed by washing as described above.

If it is necessary to use the inhaler before it is completely dry, shake off excess water, replace canister, test spray twice away from face, and take the prescribed dose. After such use, the mouthpiece should be rewashed and allowed to air dry thoroughly.

The action of PROVENTIL® HFA Inhalation Aerosol should last up to 4 to 6 hours. PROVENTIL HFA Inhalation Aerosol should not be used more frequently than recommended. Do not increase the dose or frequency of doses of PROVENTIL HFA Inhalation Aerosol without consulting your physician. If you find that treatment with PROVENTIL HFA Inhalation Aerosol becomes less effective for symptomatic relief, your symptoms become worse, and/or you need to use the product more frequently than usual, medical attention should be sought immediately. While you are taking PROVENTIL HFA Inhalation Aerosol, other inhaled drugs and asthma medications should be taken only as directed by your physician.

Common adverse effects of treatment with inhaled albuterol include palpitations, chest pain, rapid heart rate, tremor, or nervousness. If you are pregnant or nursing, contact your physician about use of PROVENTIL HFA Inhalation Aerosol. Effective and safe use of PROVENTIL HFA Inhalation Aerosol includes an understanding of the way that it should be administered. Use PROVENTIL HFA Inhalation Aerosol only with the actuator supplied with the product. Discard the canister after 200 sprays have been used.

In general, the technique for administering PROVENTIL HFA Inhalation Aerosol to children is similar to that for adults. Children should use PROVENTIL HFA Inhalation Aerosol under adult supervision, as instructed by the patient's physician. (See Patient's Instructions for Use).

Drug Interactions

1. **Beta-Blockers:** Beta-adrenergic-receptor blocking agents not only block the pulmonary effect of beta-agonists, such as PROVENTIL HFA Inhalation Aerosol, but may produce severe bronchospasm in asthmatic patients. Therefore, patients with asthma should not normally be treated with beta-blockers. However, under certain circumstances, eg, as prophylaxis after myocardial infarction, there may be no acceptable alternatives to the use of beta-adrenergic blocking agents in patients with asthma. In this setting, cardioselective beta blockers should be considered, although they should be administered with caution.
2. **Diuretics:** The ECG changes and/or hypokalemia which may result from the administration of nonpotassium-sparing diuretics (such as loop or thiazide diuretics) can be acutely worsened by beta-agonists, especially when the recommended dose of the beta-agonist is exceeded. Although the clinical significance of these effects is not known, caution is advised in the coadministration of beta agonists with nonpotassium-sparing diuretics.
3. **Albuterol-Digoxin:** Mean decreases of 16% and 22% in serum digoxin levels were demonstrated after single-dose intravenous and oral administration of albuterol, respectively, to normal volunteers who had received digoxin for 10 days. The clinical significance of these findings for patients with obstructive airway disease who are receiving albuterol and digoxin on a chronic basis is unclear; nevertheless, it would be prudent to carefully evaluate the serum digoxin levels in patients who are currently receiving digoxin and albuterol.
4. **Monoamine Oxidase Inhibitors or Tricyclic Antidepressants:** PROVENTIL HFA Inhalation Aerosol should be administered with extreme caution to patients being treated with monoamine oxidase inhibitors or tricyclic antidepressants, or within 2 weeks of discontinuation of such agents, because the action of albuterol on the cardiovascular system may be potentiated.

Carcinogenesis, Mutagenesis, and Impairment of Fertility

In a 2-year study in SPRAGUE-DAWLEY® rats, albuterol sulfate caused a dose-related increase in the incidence of benign leiomyomas of the mesovarium at the above dietary doses of 2 mg/kg (approximately 15 times the maximum recommended daily inhalation dose for adults on a mg/m_2 basis and approximately 6 times the maximum recommended daily inhalation dose for children on a mg/m_2 basis). In another study this effect was blocked by the coadministration of propranolol, a nonselective beta-adrenergic antagonist. In an 18-month study in CD-1 mice, albuterol sulfate showed no evidence of tumorigenicity at dietary doses of up to 500 mg/kg (approximately 1700 times the maximum recommended daily inhalation dose for adults on a mg/m_2 basis and approximately 800 times the maximum recommended daily inhalation dose for children on a mg/m_2 basis). In a 22-month study in Golden Hamsters, albuterol sulfate showed no evidence of tumorigenicity at dietary doses of up to 50 mg/kg (approximately 225 times the maximum recommended daily inhalation dose for adults on a mg/m_2 basis and approximately 110 times the maximum recommended daily inhalation dose for children on a mg/m_2 basis).

Albuterol sulfate was not mutagenic in the Ames test or a mutation test in yeast. Albuterol sulfate was not clastogenic in a human peripheral lymphocyte assay or in an AH1 strain mouse micronucleus assay.

Reproduction studies in rats demonstrated no evidence of impaired fertility at oral doses up to 50 mg/kg (approximately 340 times the maximum recommended daily inhalation dose for adults on a mg/m_2 basis).

Pregnancy: ***Teratogenic Effects:*** **Pregnancy Category C**

Albuterol sulfate has been shown to be teratogenic in mice. A study in CD-1 mice given albuterol sulfate subcutaneously showed cleft palate formation in 5 of 111 (4.5%) fetuses at 0.25 mg/kg (less than the maximum recommended daily inhalation dose for adults on a mg/m_2 basis) and in 10 of 108 (9.3%) fetuses at 2.5 mg/kg (approximately 8 times the maximum recommended daily inhalation dose for adults on a mg/m_2 basis). The drug did not induce cleft palate formation at a dose of 0.025 mg/kg (less than the maximum recommended daily inhalation dose for adults on a mg/m_2 basis). Cleft palate also occurred in 22 of 72 (30.5%) fetuses from females treated subcutaneously with 2.5 mg/kg of isoproterenol (positive control).

A reproduction study in Stride Dutch rabbits revealed cranioschisis in 7 of 19 (37%) fetuses when albuterol sulfate was administered orally at 50 mg/kg dose (approximately 680 times the maximum recommended daily inhalation dose for adults on a mg/m_2 basis).

In an inhalation reproduction study in SPRAGUE-DAWLEY rats, the albuterol sulfate/HFA-134a formulation did not exhibit any teratogenic effects at 10.5 mg/kg (approximately 70 times the maximum recommended daily inhalation dose for adults on a mg/m_2 basis).

A study in which pregnant rats were dosed with radiolabeled albuterol sulfate demonstrated that drug-related material is transferred from the maternal circulation to the fetus.

There are no adequate and well-controlled studies of PROVENTIL HFA Inhalation Aerosol or albuterol sulfate in pregnant women. PROVENTIL HFA Inhalation Aerosol should be used during pregnancy only if the potential benefit justifies the potential risk to the fetus.

During worldwide marketing experience, various congenital anomalies, including cleft palate and limb defects, have been reported in the offspring of patients being treated with albuterol. Some of the mothers were taking multiple medications during their pregnancies. Because no consistent pattern of defects can be discerned, a relationship between albuterol use and congenital anomalies has not been established.

Use in Labor and Delivery

Because of the potential for beta-agonist interference with uterine contractility, use of PROVENTIL HFA Inhalation Aerosol for relief of bronchospesm during labor should be restricted to those patients in whom the benefits clearly outweigh the risk.

Tocolysis: Albuterol has not been approved for the management of preterm labor. The benefit:risk ratio when albuterol is administered for tocolysis has not been established. Serious adverse reactions, including pulmonary edema, have been reported during the following treatment of premature labor with $beta_2$-agonists, including albuterol.

Nursing Mothers

Plasma levels of albuterol sulfate and HFA-134a after inhaled therapeutic doses are very low in humans, but it is not known whether the components of PROVENTIL HFA Inhalation Aerosol are excreated in human milk.

Because of the potential for tumorigenicity shown for albuterol in animal studies and lack of experience with the

Adverse Experience Incidences (% of patients) in a Large 12-week Clinical Trial*

Body System/ Adverse Event (Preferred Term)		PROVENTIL® HFA Inhalation Aerosol (N=193)	CFC 11/12 Propelled Albuterol Inhaler (N=186)	HFA-134a Placebo Inhaler (N=186)
Application Site Disorders	Inhalation Site Sensation	6	9	2
	Inhalation Taste Sensation	4	3	3
Body as a Whole	Allergic Reaction/Symptoms	6	4	<1
	Back Pain	4	2	3
	Fever	6	2	5
Central and Peripheral Nervous System	Tremor	7	8	2
Gastrointestinal System	Nausea	10	9	5
	Vomiting	7	2	3
Heart Rate and Rhythm Disorder	Tachycardia	7	2	<1
Psychiatric Disorders	Nervousness	7	9	3
Respiratory System Disorders	Respiratory Disorder (unspecified)	6	4	5
	Rhinitis	16	22	14
	Upper Resp Tract Infection	21	20	18
Urinary System Disorder	Urinary Tract Infection	3	4	2

*This table includes all adverse events (whether considered by the investigator drug related or unrelated to drug) which occurred at an incidence rate of at least 3.0% in the PROVENTIL HFA Inhalation Aerosol group and more frequently in the PROVENTIL HFA Inhalation Aerosol group than in the HFA-134a placebo inhaler group.

use of PROVENTIL HFA Inhalation Aerosol by nursing mothers, a decision should be made whether to discontinue nursing or to discontinue the drug, taking into account the importance of the drug to the mother. Caution should be exercised when albuterol sulfate is administered to a nursing woman.

Pediatrics
The safety and effectiveness of PROVENTIL HFA Inhalation Aerosol in pediatric patients below the age of 4 years have not been established.

Geriatrics
PROVENTIL HFA Inhalation Aerosol has not been studied in a geriatric population. As with other beta$_2$-agonists, special caution should be observed when using PROVENTIL HFA Inhalation Aerosol in elderly patients who have concomitant cardiovascular disease that could be adversely affected by this class of drug.

ADVERSE REACTIONS
Adverse reaction information concerning PROVENTIL® HFA Inhalation Aerosol is derived from a 12-week, double-blind, double-dummy study which compared PROVENTIL HFA Inhalation Aerosol, a CFC 11/12 propelled albuterol inhaler, and an HFA-134a placebo inhaler in 565 asthmatic patients. The following table lists the incidence of all adverse events (whether considered by the investigator drug related or unrelated to drug) from this study which occurred at a rate of 3% or greater in the PROVENTIL HFA Inhalation Aerosol treatment group and more frequently in the PROVENTIL HFA Inhalation Aerosol treatment group than in the placebo group. Overall, the incidence and nature of the adverse reactions reported for PROVENTIL HFA Inhalation Aerosol and a CFC 11/12 propelled albuterol inhaler were comparable.
[See table above]
Adverse events reported by less than 3% of the patients receiving PROVENTIL HFA Inhalation Aerosol, and by a greater proportion of PROVENTIL HFA Inhalation Aerosol patients than placebo patients, which have the potential to be related to PROVENTIL HFA Inhalation Aerosol include: dysphonia, increased sweating, dry mouth, chest pain, edema, rigors, ataxia, leg cramps, hyperkinesia, eructation, flatulence, tinnitus, diabetes mellitus, anxiety, depression, somnolence, rash. Palpitation and dizziness have also been observed with PROVENTIL HFA Inhalation Aerosol.
Adverse events reported in a 4-week pediatric clinical trail comparing PROVENTIL HFA Inhalation Aerosol and a CFC 11/12 propelled albuterol inhaler occurred at a low incidence rate and were similar to those seen in the adult trials.
In small, cumulative dose studies, tremor, nervousness, and headache appeared to be dose related.
Rare cases of urticaria, angioedema, rash, bronchospasm, and oropharyngeal edema have been reported after the use of inhaled albuterol. In addition, albuterol, like other sympathomimetic agents, can cause adverse reactions such as hypertension, angina, vertigo, central nervous system stimulation, insomnia, headache, and drying or irritation of the oropharynx.

OVERDOSE
The expected symptoms with overdosage are those of excessive beta-adrenergic stimulation and/or occurrence or exaggeration of any of the symptoms listed under **ADVERSE REACTIONS**, eg, seizures, angina, hypertension or hypotension, tachycardia with rates up to 200 beats per minute, arrhythmias, nervousness, headache, tremor, dry mouth, palpitation, nausea, dizziness, fatigue, malaise, and insomnia.
Hypokalemia may also occur. As with all sympathomimetic medications, cardiac arrest and even death may be associated with abuse of PROVENTIL® HFA Inhalation Aerosol. Treatment consists of discontinuation of PROVENTIL HFA Inhalation Aerosol together with appropriate symptomatic therapy. The judicious use of a cardioselective beta-receptor blocker may be considered, bearing in mind that such medication can produce bronchospasm. There is insufficient evidence to determine if dialysis is beneficial for overdosage of PROVENTIL HFA Inhalation Aerosol.
The oral median lethal dose of albuterol sulfate in mice is greater than 2000 mg/kg (approximately 6800 times the maximum recommended daily inhalation dose for adults on a mg/m$_2$ basis and approximately 3200 times the maximum recommended daily inhalation dose for children on a mg/m$_2$ basis). In mature rats, the subcutaneous median lethal dose of albuterol sulfate is approximately 450 mg/kg (approximately 3000 times the maximum recommended daily inhalation dose for adults on a mg/m$_2$ basis and approximately 1400 times the maximum recommended daily inhalation dose for children on a mg/m$_2$ basis). In young rats, the subcutaneous median lethal dose is approximately 2000 mg/kg (approximately 14,000 times the maximum recommended daily inhalation dose for adults on a mg/m$_2$ basis and approximately 6400 times the maximum recommended daily inhalation dose for children on a mg/m$_2$ basis). The inhalation median lethal dose has not been determined in animals.

DOSAGE AND ADMINISTRATION
For treatment of acute episodes of bronchospasm or prevention of asthmatic symptoms, the usual dosage for adults and children 4 years of age and older is two inhalations repeated every 4 to 6 hours. More frequent administration or a larger number of inhalations is not recommended. In some patients, one inhalation every 4 hours may be sufficient. Each actuation of PROVENTIL® HFA Inhalation Aerosol delivers 108 mcg of albuterol sulfate (equivalent to 90 mcg of albuterol base) from the mouthpiece. It is recommended to prime the inhaler before using for the first time and in cases where the inhaler has not been used for more than 2 weeks by releasing four "test sprays" into the air, away from the face.
Exercise Induced Bronchospasm Prevention: The usual dosage for adults and children 4 years of age and older is two inhalations 15 to 30 minutes before exercise.
To maintain proper use of this product, it is important that the mouthpiece be washed and dried thoroughly at least once a week. The inhaler may cease to deliver medication if

not properly cleaned and dried thoroughly (see **PRECAUTIONS, Information for Patients** section). Keeping the plastic mouthpiece clean is very important to prevent medication build-up and blockage. The inhaler may cease to deliver medication if not properly cleaned and air dried thoroughly. If the mouthpiece becomes blocked, washing the mouthpiece will remove the blockage.
If a previously effective dose regimen fails to provide the usual response, this may be a marker of destabilization of asthma and requires reevaluation of the patient and the treatment regimen, giving special consideration to the possible need for anti-inflammatory treatment, eg, corticosteroids.

HOW SUPPLIED
PROVENTIL® HFA (albuterol sulfate) Inhalation Aerosol is supplied as a pressurized aluminum canister with a yellow plastic actuator and orange dust cap each in boxes of one. Each actuation delivers 120 mcg of albuterol sulfate from the valve and 108 mcg of albuterol sulfate from the mouthpiece (equivalent to 90 mcg of albuterol base). Canisters with a labeled net weight of 6.7 g contain 200 inhalations (NDC 0085-1132-01).
Rx only. Store between 15°-25°C (59°-77°F). For best results, canister should be at room temperature before use. SHAKE WELL BEFORE USING.
The yellow actuator supplied with PROVENTIL HFA Inhalation Aerosol should not be used with any other product canister, and actuator from other products should not be used with a PROVENTIL HFA Inhalation Aerosol canister. The correct amount of medication in each canister cannot be assured after 200 actuations, even though the canister is not completely empty. The canister should be discarded when the labeled number of actuations have been used.
• **WARNING: Avoid spraying in eyes. Contents under pressure. Do not puncture or incinerate. Exposure to temperatures above 120°F may cause bursting. Keep out of reach of children.**
PROVENTIL® HFA Inhalation Aerosol does not contain chlorofluorocarbons (CFCs) as the propellant.
Developed and Manufactured by
3M Health Care Limited
Loughborough UK
or
3M Drug Delivery Systems
Northridge, CA 91324
for
Schering Corporation,
a subsidiary of
Schering-Plough Corporation,
Kenilworth, NJ 07033 USA
Schering-Plough
© 1996, 1998, Schering Corporation.
All rights reserved.
The trademarks depicted in this piece are owned by their respective companies.
673700
Rev. 02/09
Attention Health Care Professional
Detach Patient's Instructions for Use from package insert and dispense with the product.

PROVENTIL® HFA
(albuterol sulfate)
Inhalation Aerosol
FOR ORAL INHALATION ONLY
Patient's Instructions for Use

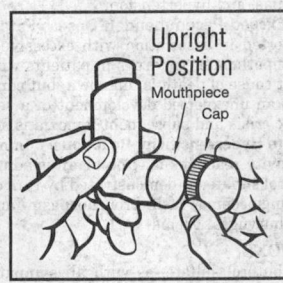

Figure 1

[See figure 2 at top of next page]
Before using your PROVENTIL® HFA (albuterol Sulfate) Inhalation Aerosol, read complete instructions carefully. Children should use PROVENTIL HFA Inhalation Aerosol under adult supervision, as instructed by the patient's doctor
Please note that ⊘ indicates that this inhalation aerosol does not contain chlorofluorocarbons (CFCs) as the propellant.
1. SHAKE THE INHALER WELL immediately before each use. **Then remove the cap from the mouthpiece (see

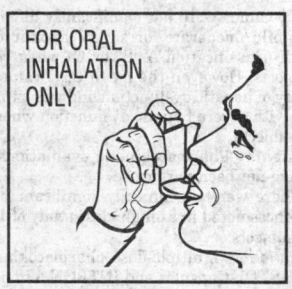

Figure 2

Figure 1). **Check mouthpiece for foreign objects prior to use.** Make sure the canister is fully inserted into the actuator.

2. As with all aerosol medications, it is recommended to prime the inhaler before using for the first time and in cases where the inhaler has not been used for more than 2 weeks. Prime by releasing four "test sprays" into the air, away from your face.

3. BREATH OUT FULLY THROUGH THE MOUTH, expelling as much air from your lungs as possible. Place the mouthpiece fully into the mouth holding the inhaler in its upright position (see Figure 2) and closing the lips around it.

4. WHILE BREATHING IN DEEPLY AND SLOWLY THROUGH THE MOUTH, FULLY DEPRESS THE TOP OF THE METAL CANISTER with your index finger (see Figure 2).

5. HOLD YOUR BREATH AS LONG AS POSSIBLE, up to 10 seconds. Before breathing out, remove the inhaler from your mouth and release your finger from the canister.

6. If your physician has prescribed additional puffs, wait 1 minute, shake the inhaler again, and repeat steps 3 through 5. Replace the cap after use.

7. KEEPING THE PLACTIC MOUTHPIECE CLEAN IS EXTREMELY IMPORTANT TO PREVENT MEDICATION BUILD-UP AND BLOCKAGE. THE MOUTHPIECE SHOULD BE WASHED, SHAKEN TO REMOVE EXCESS WATER, AND AIR DRIED THOROUGHLY AT LEAST ONCE A WEEK. INHALER MAY STOP SPRAYING IF NOT PROPERLY CLEANED.
- **Routine cleaning instructions:**
- Step 1. To clean, remove the canister and mouthpiece cap. Wash the mouthpiece through the top and bottom with warm running water for 30 seconds at lease once a week (see Figure A). **Never immerse the metal canister in water.**

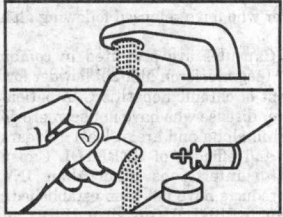

Figure A

- Wash mouthpiece under warm running water.

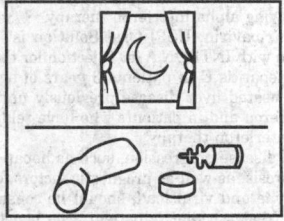

Figure B

- Allow mouthpiece to dry, such as overnight.
[See figure C at top of next column]
- When blocked, little or no medicine comes out.
- Step 2. To dry, shake off excess water and let the mouthpiece air dry thoroughly, such as overnight (see Figure B). When the mouthpiece is dry, replace the canister and the mouthpiece cap. Blockage from medication buildup is more likely to occur if the mouthpiece is not allowed to air dry thoroughly.
- **IF YOUR INHALER HAS BECOME BLOCKED** (little or no medication coming out of the mouthpiece, see Fig-

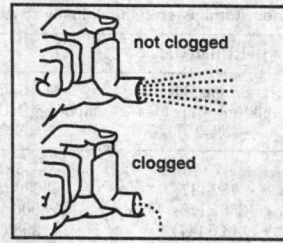

not clogged

clogged

Figure C

ure C), wash the mouthpiece as described in Step 1 and air dry thoroughly as described in Step 2.
- **IF YOU NEED TO USE YOUR INHALER BEFORE IT IS COMPLETELY DRY, SHAKE OFF EXCESS WATER,** replace the canister, and test spray twice into the air, away from your face, to remove most of the water remaining in the mouthpiece. Then take your dose as prescribed. **After such use, rewash and air dry thoroughly as described in Step 1 and 2.**

8. The correct amount of medication in each inhalation cannot be assured after 200 actuations, even though the canister is not completely empty. The canister should be discarded when the labeled number of actuations have been used. Before you reach the specific number of actuations, you should consult your physician to determine whether a refill is needed. Just as you should not take extra doses without consulting your physician, you also should not stop using PROVENTIL HFA Inhalation Aerosol without consulting your physician.

You may notice a slightly different taste or spray force than you are used to with PROVENTIL HFA Inhalation Aerosol, compared to other albuterol inhalation aerosol products.

DOSAGE:
Use only as directed by your physician.

WARNINGS:
The action of PROVENTIL® HFA Inhalation Aerosol should last up to 4 to 6 hours. PROVENTIL HFA Inhalation Aerosol should not be used more frequently than recommended. Do not increase the number of puffs or frequency of doses of PROVENTIL HFA Inhalation Aerosol without consulting your physician. If you find that treatment with PROVENTIL HFA Inhalation Aerosol becomes less effective for symptomatic relief, your symptoms become worse, and/or you need to use the product more frequently than usual, medical attention should be sought immediately. While you are taking PROVENTIL HFA Inhalation Aerosol, other inhaled drugs should be taken only as directed by your physician. If you are pregnant or nursing, contact your physician about the use of PROVENTIL HFA Inhalation Aerosol.

Common adverse effects of treatment with PROVENTIL HFA Inhalation Aerosol include palpitations, chest pain, rapid heart rate, tremor, or nervousness. Effective and safe use of PROVENTIL HFA Inhalation Aerosol includes an understanding of the way that it should be administered. Use PROVENTIL HFA Inhalation Aerosol only with the yellow actuator supplied with the product. The PROVENTIL HFA Inhalation Aerosol actuator should not be used with other aerosol medications.

For best results, use at room temperature. Avoid exposing product to extreme heat and cold.

Shake well before use.

Contents Under Pressure.

Do not puncture. Do not store near hear or open flame. Exposure to temperatures above 120°F may cause bursting. Never throw container into fire or incinerator. Store between 15°-25°C (59°-77°F). Avoid spraying in eyes. Keep out of reach of children.

Further Information: Your PROVENTIL® HFA (albuterol sulfate) Inhalation Aerosol does not contain chlorofluorocarbons (CFCs) as the propellant. Instead, the inhaler contains a hydrofluoroalkane (HFA-134a) as the propellant.

Developed and Manufactured by
3M Health Care Limited
Loughborough UK
or
3M Drug Delivery Systems
Northridge, CA 91324
For Schering Corporation
a subsidiary of
Schering-Plough Corporation,
Kenilworth, NJ 07033 USA
Schering-Plough
Rev. 02/09
673800
© 1996, 1999, Schering Corporation
All rights reserved.

U.S. Patent No. 5,225,183; 5,439,670; 5,605,674; 5,695,743; 5,766,573; and 6,352,684.
Shown in Product Identification Guide, page 313

REBETOL®   ℞
[rē' bə-tōl]
(ribavirin, USP)
Capsules and Oral Solution
PRODUCT INFORMATION

- **REBETOL® monotherapy is not effective for the treatment of chronic hepatitis C virus infection and should not be used alone for this indication** (see **WARNINGS**).
- **The primary toxicity of ribavirin is hemolytic anemia. The anemia associated with REBETOL therapy may result in worsening of cardiac disease that has led to fatal and nonfatal myocardial infarctions. Patients with a history of significant or unstable cardiac disease should not be treated with REBETOL** (see **WARNINGS, ADVERSE REACTIONS,** and **DOSAGE AND ADMINISTRATION**).
- **Significant teratogenic and/or embryocidal effects have been demonstrated in all animal species exposed to ribavirin. In addition, ribavirin has a multiple-dose half-life of 12 days, and so it may persist in nonplasma compartments for as long as 6 months. Therefore, REBETOL therapy is contraindicated in women who are pregnant and in the male partners of women who are pregnant. Extreme care must be taken to avoid pregnancy during therapy and for 6 months after completion of treatment in both female patients and in female partners of male patients who are taking REBETOL therapy. At least two reliable forms of effective contraception must be utilized during treatment and during the 6-month posttreatment follow-up period** (see **CONTRAINDICATIONS, WARNINGS,** and **PRECAUTIONS, Information for Patients** and **Pregnancy Category X** sections).

DESCRIPTION
REBETOL® REBETOL is Schering Corporation's brand name for ribavirin, a nucleoside analog. The chemical name of ribavirin is 1-β-D-ribofuranosyl-1*H*-1,2,4-triazole-3-carboxamide and has the following structural formula:

HO, OH, OH, NH₂ (structural formula)

Ribavirin is a white, crystalline powder. It is freely soluble in water and slightly soluble in anhydrous alcohol. The empirical formula is $C_8H_{12}N_4O_5$ and the molecular weight is 244.21.

REBETOL Capsules consist of a white powder in a white, opaque, gelatin capsule. Each capsule contains 200 mg ribavirin and the inactive ingredients microcrystalline cellulose, lactose monohydrate, croscarmellose sodium, and magnesium stearate. The capsule shell consists of gelatin, sodium lauryl sulfate, silicon dioxide, and titanium dioxide. The capsule is printed with edible blue pharmaceutical ink which is made of shellac, anhydrous ethyl alcohol, isopropyl alcohol, n-butyl alcohol, propylene glycol, ammonium hydroxide, and FD&C Blue #2 aluminum lake.

REBETOL Oral Solution is a clear, colorless to pale or light yellow bubble gum-flavored liquid. Each milliliter of the solution contains 40 mg of ribavirin and the inactive ingredients sucrose, glycerin, sorbitol, propylene glycol, sodium citrate, citric acid, sodium benzoate, natural and artificial flavor for bubble gum #15864, and water.

Mechanism of Action The mechanism of inhibition of hepatitis C virus (HCV) RNA by combination therapy with ribavirin and interferon products has not been established.

CLINICAL PHARMACOLOGY
Pharmacokinetics *Ribavirin* Single- and multiple-dose pharmacokinetic properties in adults are summarized in **TABLE 1.** Ribavirin was rapidly and extensively absorbed following oral administration. However, due to first-pass metabolism, the absolute bioavailability averaged 64% (44%). There was a linear relationship between dose and AUC_{tf} (AUC from time zero to last measurable concentration) following single doses of 200-1200 mg ribavirin. The relationship between dose and C_{max} was curvilinear, tending to asymptote above single doses of 400-600 mg.

Upon multiple oral dosing, based on AUC_{12hr}, a sixfold accumulation of ribavirin was observed in plasma. Following

TABLE 1. Mean (% CV) Pharmacokinetic Parameters for REBETOL When Administered Individually to Adults

Parameter	REBETOL		
	Single Dose 600-mg Oral Solution (N=14)	Single Dose 600-mg Capsules (N=12)	Multiple Dose 600-mg BID Capsules (N=12)
T_{max} (hr)	1.00 (34)	1.7 (46)***	3 (60)
C_{max} *	872 (42)	782 (37)	3680 (85)
AUC_{tf} **	14098 (38)	13400 (48)	228000 (25)
$T_{1/2}$ (hr)		43.6 (47)	298 (30)
Apparent Volume of Distribution (L)		2825 (9)†	
Apparent Clearance (L/hr)		38.2 (40)	
Absolute Bioavailability		64% (44)††	

* ng/mL
** ng•hr/mL
*** N = 11
† data obtained from a single-dose pharmacokinetic study using ^{14}C labeled ribavirin; N = 5
†† N = 6

TABLE 3. Virologic and Histologic Responses: Previously Untreated Patients*

	US Study				International Study		
	24 weeks of treatment		48 weeks of treatment		24 weeks of treatment	48 weeks of treatment	
	INTRON A plus REBETOL (N=228)	INTRON A plus Placebo (N=231)	INTRON A plus REBETOL (N=228)	INTRON A plus Placebo (N=225)	INTRON A plus REBETOL (N=265)	INTRON A plus REBETOL (N=268)	INTRON A plus Placebo (N=266)
Virologic Response							
-Responder[1]	65 (29)	13 (6)	85 (37)	27 (12)	86 (32)	113 (42)	46 (17)
-Nonresponder	147 (64)	194 (84)	110 (48)	168 (75)	158 (60)	120 (45)	196 (74)
-Missing Data	16 (7)	24 (10)	33 (14)	30 (13)	21 (8)	35 (13)	24 (9)
Histologic Response							
-Improvement[2]	102 (45)	77 (33)	96 (42)	65 (29)	103 (39)	102 (38)	69 (26)
-No improvement	77 (34)	99 (43)	61 (27)	93 (41)	85 (32)	58 (22)	111 (41)
-Missing Data	49 (21)	55 (24)	71 (31)	67 (30)	77 (29)	108 (40)	86 (32)

* Number (%) of patients.
1. Defined as HCV RNA below limit of detection using a research-based RT-PCR assay at end of treatment and during follow-up period.
2. Defined as posttreatment (end of follow-up) minus pretreatment liver biopsy Knodell HAI score (I+II+III) improvement of ≥2 points.

mean AUC_{tf} values were not significantly different in subjects with mild, moderate, or severe hepatic dysfunction (Child-Pugh Classification A, B, or C) when compared to control subjects. However, the mean C_{max} values increased with severity of hepatic dysfunction and was twofold greater in subjects with severe hepatic dysfunction when compared to control subjects.

Elderly Patients Pharmacokinetic evaluations in elderly subjects have not been performed.

Gender There were no clinically significant pharmacokinetic differences noted in a single-dose study of 18 male and 18 female subjects.

Pediatric Patients Multiple-dose pharmacokinetic properties for REBETOL Capsules and INTRON A in pediatric patients with chronic hepatitis C between 5 and 16 years of age are summarized in **TABLE 2**. The pharmacokinetics of REBETOL and INTRON A (dose-normalized) are similar in adults and pediatric patients.

Complete pharmacokinetic characteristics of REBETOL Oral Solution have not been determined in pediatric patients. Ribavirin C_{min} values were similar following administration of REBETOL Oral Solution or REBETOL Capsules during 48 weeks of therapy in pediatric patients (3 to 16 years of age).

TABLE 2. Mean (% CV) Multiple-Dose Pharmacokinetic Parameters for INTRON A and REBETOL Capsules When Administered to Pediatric Patients With Chronic Hepatitis C

Parameter	REBETOL 15 mg/kg/day as 2 divided doses (n=17)	INTRON A 3 MIU/m² TIW (n=54)
T_{max} (hr)	1.9 (83)	5.9 (36)
C_{max} (ng/mL)	3275 (25)	51 (48)
AUC*	29774 (26)	622 (48)
Apparent clearance L/hr/kg	0.27 (27)	ND

* AUC_{12} (ng•hr/mL) for REBETOL; AUC_{0-24} (IU•hr/mL) for INTRON A
ND=not done

In this section of the label, numbers in parenthesis indicate % coefficient of variation.

INDICATIONS AND USAGE

Adult Use REBETOL® (ribavirin, USP) Capsules and Oral Solution are indicated in combination with INTRON® A (interferon alfa-2b, recombinant) for the treatment of chronic hepatitis C in patients 18 years of age and older with compensated liver disease previously untreated with alpha interferon and in patients 18 years of age and older who have relapsed following alpha interferon therapy.

REBETOL Capsules are indicated in combination with PegIntron™ (peginterferon alfa-2b) Powder for Injection for the treatment of chronic hepatitis C in patients with compensated liver disease who have not been previously treated with interferon alpha and are at least 18 years of age.

The safety and efficacy of REBETOL Capsules or Oral Solution with interferons other than INTRON A or PegIntron products have not been established.

Pediatric Use REBETOL (ribavirin, USP) Capsules are indicated in combination with INTRON A for Injection for the treatment of chronic hepatitis C in patients 5 years of age and older with compensated liver disease previously untreated with alpha interferon and in patients who have relapsed following alpha interferon therapy.

REBETOL (ribavirin, USP) Oral Solution is indicated in combination with INTRON A for Injection for the treatment of chronic hepatitis C in patients 3 years of age and older with compensated liver disease previously untreated with alpha interferon and in patients who have relapsed following alpha interferon therapy.

Evidence of disease progression, such as hepatic inflammation and fibrosis, as well as prognostic factors for response, HCV genotype and viral load, should be considered when deciding to treat a pediatric patient. The benefits of treatment should be weighed against the safety findings observed (see **PRECAUTIONS, Pediatric Use** section) for pediatric subjects in the clinical trials.

Description of Clinical Studies REBETOL/INTRON A Combination Therapy **Adult Patients** *Previously Untreated Patients* Adults with compensated chronic hepatitis C and detectable HCV RNA (assessed by a central laboratory using a research-based RT-PCR assay) who were previously untreated with alpha interferon therapy were enrolled into two multicenter, double-blind trials (US and International) and randomized to receive REBETOL Capsules 1200 mg/day (1000 mg/day for patients weighing ≤75 kg) plus INTRON A for Injection 3 MIU TIW or INTRON A for

oral dosing with 600 mg BID, steady-state was reached by approximately 4 weeks, with mean steady-state plasma concentrations of 2200 (37%) ng/mL. Upon discontinuation of dosing, the mean half-life was 298 (30%) hours, which probably reflects slow elimination from nonplasma compartments.

Effect of Food on Absorption of Ribavirin Both AUC_{tf} and C_{max} increased by 70% when REBETOL® Capsules were administered with a high-fat meal (841 kcal, 53.8 g fat, 31.6 g protein, and 57.4 g carbohydrate) in a single-dose pharmacokinetic study. There are insufficient data to address the clinical relevance of these results. Clinical efficacy studies with REBETOL/INTRON® A were conducted without instructions with respect to food consumption. During clinical studies with REBETOL/PegIntron™, all subjects were instructed to take REBETOL Capsules with food (see **DOSAGE AND ADMINISTRATION**).

Effect of Antacid on Absorption of Ribavirin Coadministration of REBETOL Capsules with an antacid containing magnesium, aluminum, and simethicone (Mylanta®) resulted in a 14% decrease in mean ribavirin AUC_{tf}. The clinical relevance of results from this single-dose study is unknown.

[See table above]

Ribavirin transport into nonplasma compartments has been most extensively studied in red blood cells, and has been identified to be primarily via an e_s-type equilibrative nucleoside transporter. This type of transporter is present on virtually all cell types and may account for the extensive volume of distribution. Ribavirin does not bind to plasma proteins.

Ribavirin has two pathways of metabolism: (i) a reversible phosphorylation pathway in nucleated cells; and (ii) a degradative pathway involving deribosylation and amide hydrolysis to yield a triazole carboxylic acid metabolite. Ribavirin and its triazole carboxamide and triazole carboxylic acid metabolites are excreted renally. After oral administration of 600 mg of ^{14}C-ribavirin, approximately 61% and

12% of the radioactivity was eliminated in the urine and feces, respectively, in 336 hours. Unchanged ribavirin accounted for 17% of the administered dose.

Results of *in vitro* studies using both human and rat liver microsome preparations indicated little or no cytochrome P450 enzyme-mediated metabolism of ribavirin, with minimal potential for P450 enzyme-based drug interactions.

No pharmacokinetic interactions were noted between INTRON A for Injection and REBETOL Capsules in a multiple-dose pharmacokinetic study.

Drug Interactions Ribavirin has been shown *in vitro* to inhibit phosphorylation of zidovudine and stavudine, which could lead to decreased antiretroviral activity. Exposure to didanosine or its active metabolite (dideoxyadenosine 5'-triphosphate) is increased when didanosine is coadministered with ribavirin, which could cause or worsen clinical toxicities (see **PRECAUTIONS, Drug Interactions** section).

Special Populations *Renal Dysfunction* The pharmacokinetics of ribavirin were assessed after administration of a single oral dose (400 mg) of ribavirin to non HCV-infected subjects with varying degrees of renal dysfunction. The mean AUC_{tf} value was threefold greater in subjects with creatinine clearance values between 10 to 30 mL/min when compared to control subjects (creatinine clearance >90 mL/min). In subjects with creatinine clearance values between 30 to 60 mL/min, AUC_{tf} was twofold greater when compared to control subjects. The increased AUC_{tf} appears to be due to reduction of renal and nonrenal clearance in these patients. Phase III efficacy trials included subjects with creatinine clearance values >50 mL/min. The multiple-dose pharmacokinetics of ribavirin cannot be accurately predicted in patients with renal dysfunction. Ribavirin is not effectively removed by hemodialysis. Patients with creatinine clearance <50 mL/min should not be treated with REBETOL (see **WARNINGS**).

Hepatic Dysfunction The effect of hepatic dysfunction was assessed after a single oral dose of ribavirin (600 mg). The

Injection plus placebo for 24 or 48 weeks followed by 24 weeks of off-therapy follow-up. The International study did not contain a 24-week INTRON A plus placebo treatment arm. The US study enrolled 912 patients who, at baseline, were 67% male, 89% Caucasian with a mean Knodell HAI score (I+II+III) of 7.5, and 72% genotype 1. The International study, conducted in Europe, Israel, Canada, and Australia, enrolled 799 patients (65% male, 95% Caucasian, mean Knodell score 6.8, and 58% genotype 1).

Study results are summarized in **TABLE 3**.

[See table 3 on previous page]

Of patients who had not achieved HCV RNA below the limit of detection of the research-based assay by Week 24 of REBETOL/INTRON A treatment, less than 5% responded to an additional 24 weeks of combination treatment.

Among patients with HCV Genotype 1 treated with REBETOL/INTRON A therapy who achieved HCV RNA below the detection limit of the research-based assay by 24 weeks, those randomized to 48 weeks of treatment had higher virologic responses compared to those in the 24-week treatment group. There was no observed increase in response rates for patients with HCV nongenotype 1 randomized to REBETOL/INTRON A therapy for 48 weeks compared to 24 weeks.

Relapse Patients Patients with compensated chronic hepatitis C and detectable HCV RNA (assessed by a central laboratory using a research-based RT-PCR assay) who had relapsed following one or two courses of interferon therapy (defined as abnormal serum ALT levels) were enrolled into two multicenter, double-blind trials (US and International) and randomized to receive REBETOL 1200 mg/day (1000 mg/day for patients weighing ≤75 kg) plus INTRON A 3 MIU TIW or INTRON A plus placebo for 24 weeks followed by 24 weeks of off-therapy follow-up. The US study enrolled 153 patients who, at baseline, were 67% male, 92% Caucasian with a mean Knodell HAI score (I+II+III) of 6.8, and 58% genotype 1. The International study, conducted in Europe, Israel, Canada, and Australia, enrolled 192 patients (64% male, 95% Caucasian, mean Knodell score 6.6, and 56% genotype 1).

Study results are summarized in **TABLE 4**.

[See table 4 above]

Virologic and histologic responses were similar among male and female patients in both the previously untreated and relapse studies.

Pediatric Patients Pediatric patients 3 to 16 years of age with compensated chronic hepatitis C and detectable HCV RNA (assessed by a central laboratory using a research-based RT-PCR assay) were treated with REBETOL 15 mg/kg per day plus INTRON A 3 MIU/m^2 TIW for 48 weeks followed by 24 weeks of off-therapy follow-up. A total of 118 patients received treatment who were 57% male, 80% Caucasian, and 78% genotype 1. Patients <5 years of age received REBETOL Oral Solution and those ≥5 years of age received either REBETOL Oral Solution or Capsules.

Study results are summarized in **TABLE 5**.

TABLE 5. Virologic Response: Previously Untreated Pediatric Patients*

	INTRON A 3 MIU/m^2 TIW Plus REBETOL 15 mg/kg/day
Overall Response[1] (n=118)	54 (46)
Genotype 1 (n=92)	33 (36)
Genotype non-1 (n=26)	21 (81)

* Number (%) of patients.
1. Defined as HCV RNA below limit of detection using a research-based RT-PCR assay at end of treatment and during follow-up period.

Patients with viral genotype 1, regardless of viral load, had a lower response rate to INTRON A/REBETOL combination therapy compared to patients with genotype non-1, 36% versus 81%. Patients with both poor prognostic factors (genotype 1 and high viral load) had a response rate of 26% (13/50).

REBETOL/PegIntron Combination Therapy A randomized study compared treatment with two PegIntron/REBETOL regimens [PegIntron 1.5 mcg/kg SC once weekly (QW)/REBETOL 800 mg PO daily (in divided doses); PegIntron 1.5 mcg/kg SC QW for 4 weeks then 0.5 mcg/kg SC QW for 44 weeks/REBETOL 1000/1200 mg PO daily (in divided doses)] with INTRON A [3 MIU SC thrice weekly (TIW)/REBETOL 1000/1200 mg PO daily (in divided doses)] in 1530 adults with chronic hepatitis C. Interferon-naïve patients were treated for 48 weeks and followed for 24 weeks posttreatment. Eligible patients had compensated liver dis-

TABLE 4. Virologic and Histologic Responses: Relapse Patients*

	US Study		International Study	
	INTRON A plus REBETOL (N=77)	INTRON A plus Placebo (N=76)	INTRON A plus REBETOL (N=96)	INTRON A plus Placebo (N=96)
Virologic Response				
-Responder[1]	33 (43)	3 (4)	46 (48)	5 (5)
-Nonresponder	36 (47)	66 (87)	45 (47)	91 (95)
-Missing Data	8 (10)	7 (9)	5 (5)	0 (0)
Histologic Response				
-Improvement[2]	38 (49)	27 (36)	49 (51)	30 (31)
-No improvement	23 (30)	37 (49)	29 (30)	44 (46)
-Missing Data	16 (21)	12 (16)	18 (19)	22 (23)

* Number (%) of patients.
1. Defined as HCV RNA below limit of detection using a research-based RT-PCR assay at end of treatment and during follow-up period.
2. Defined as posttreatment (end of follow-up) minus pretreatment liver biopsy Knodell HAI score (I+II+III) improvement of ≥2 points.

ease, detectable HCV RNA, elevated ALT, and liver histopathology consistent with chronic hepatitis.

Response to treatment was defined as undetectable HCV RNA at 24 weeks posttreatment (see **TABLE 6**).

TABLE 6. Rates of Response to Combination Treatment

	PegIntron 1.5 mcg/kg QW REBETOL 800 mg QD	INTRON A 3 MIU TIW REBETOL 1000/1200 mg QD
Overall Response[1,2]	52% (264/511)	46% (231/505)
Genotype 1	41% (141/348)	33% (112/343)
Genotype 2-6	75% (123/163)	73% (119/162)

1. Serum HCV RNA was measured with a research-based quantitative polymerase chain reaction assay by a central laboratory.
2. Difference in overall treatment response (PegIntron/REBETOL vs. INTRON A/REBETOL) is 6% with 95% confidence interval of (0.18, 11.63) adjusted for viral genotype and presence of cirrhosis at baseline.

The response rate to PegIntron 1.5→0.5 mcg/kg/REBETOL was essentially the same as the response to INTRON A/REBETOL (data not shown).

Patients with viral genotype 1, regardless of viral load, had a lower response rate to PegIntron (1.5 mcg/kg)/REBETOL combination therapy compared to patients with other viral genotypes. Patients with both poor prognostic factors (genotype 1 and high viral load) had a response rate of 30% (78/256) compared to a response rate of 29% (71/247) with INTRON A/REBETOL combination therapy.

Patients with lower body weight tended to have higher adverse event rates (see **ADVERSE REACTIONS**) and higher response rates than patients with higher body weights. Differences in response rates between treatment arms did not substantially vary with body weight.

Treatment response rates with PegIntron/REBETOL combination therapy were 49% in men and 56% in women. Response rates were lower in African American and Hispanic patients and higher in Asians compared to Caucasians. Although African Americans had a higher proportion of poor prognostic factors compared to Caucasians, the number of non-Caucasians studied (11% of the total) was insufficient to allow meaningful conclusions about differences in response rates after adjusting for prognostic factors.

Liver biopsies were obtained before and after treatment in 68% of patients. Compared to baseline approximately 2/3 of patients in all treatment groups were observed to have a modest reduction in inflammation.

CONTRAINDICATIONS

Pregnancy REBETOL® Capsules and Oral Solution may cause birth defects and/or death of the exposed fetus. REBETOL therapy is contraindicated for use in women who are pregnant or in men whose female partners are pregnant (see **WARNINGS and PRECAUTIONS**, **Information for Patients** and **Pregnancy Category X** sections).

REBETOL Capsules and Oral Solution are contraindicated in patients with a history of hypersensitivity to ribavirin or any component of the capsule.

Patients with autoimmune hepatitis must not be treated with combination REBETOL/INTRON® A therapy because using these medicines can make the hepatitis worse.

Patients with hemoglobinopathies (eg, thalassemia major, sickle-cell anemia) should not be treated with REBETOL Capsules or Oral Solution.

WARNINGS

Based on results of clinical trials ribavirin monotherapy is not effective for the treatment of chronic hepatitis C virus infection; therefore, REBETOL® Capsules or Oral Solution must not be used alone. The safety and efficacy of REBETOL Capsules and Oral Solution have only been established when used together with INTRON® A as a combination therapy or with PegIntron™ Injection.

There are significant adverse events caused by REBETOL/INTRON A or PegIntron therapy, including severe depression and suicidal ideation, hemolytic anemia, suppression of bone marrow function, autoimmune and infectious disorders, pulmonary dysfunction, pancreatitis, and diabetes. Suicidal ideation or attempts occurred more frequently among pediatric patients, primarily adolescents, compared to adult patients (2.4% versus 1%) during treatment and off-therapy follow-up. The INTRON A and PegIntron package inserts should be reviewed in their entirety prior to initiation of combination treatment for additional safety information.

Pregnancy: REBETOL Capsules and Oral Solution may cause birth defects and/or death of the exposed fetus. Extreme care must be taken to avoid pregnancy in female patients and in female partners of male patients. REBETOL has demonstrated significant teratogenic and/or embryocidal effects in all animal species in which adequate studies have been conducted. These effects occurred at doses as low as one twentieth of the recommended human dose of ribavirin. REBETOL THERAPY SHOULD NOT BE STARTED UNTIL A REPORT OF A NEGATIVE PREGNANCY TEST HAS BEEN OBTAINED IMMEDIATELY PRIOR TO PLANNED INITIATION OF THERAPY. Patients should be instructed to use at least two forms of effective contraception during treatment and during the 6-month period after treatment has been stopped based on multiple-dose half-life of ribavirin of 12 days. Pregnancy testing should occur monthly during REBETOL therapy and for 6 months after therapy has stopped (see **CONTRAINDICATIONS** and **PRECAUTIONS**, **Information for Patients** and **Pregnancy Category X** sections).

Anemia: The primary toxicity of ribavirin is hemolytic anemia, which was observed in approximately 10% of REBETOL/INTRON A-treated patients in clinical trials (see **ADVERSE REACTIONS**, Laboratory Values, *REBETOL/INTRON A Combination Therapy, Hemoglobin* section). The anemia associated with REBETOL capsules occurs within 1 - 2 weeks of initiation of therapy. BECAUSE THE INITIAL DROP IN HEMOGLOBIN MAY BE SIGNIFICANT, IT IS ADVISED THAT HEMOGLOBIN OR HEMATOCRIT BE OBTAINED PRETREATMENT AND AT WEEK 2 AND WEEK 4 OF THERAPY, OR MORE FREQUENTLY IF CLINICALLY INDICATED. Patients should then be followed as clinically appropriate.

Fatal and nonfatal myocardial infarctions have been reported in patients with anemia caused by REBETOL. Patients should be assessed for underlying cardiac disease before initiation of ribavirin therapy. Patients with pre-existing cardiac disease should have electrocardiograms administered before treatment, and should be appropriately monitored during therapy. If there is any deterioration of cardiovascular status, therapy should be suspended or discontinued (see DOSAGE AND ADMINISTRATION, Guidelines for Dose Modifications section). Because cardiac disease may be worsened by drug-induced anemia, patients with a history of significant or unstable cardiac disease should not use REBETOL (see ADVERSE REACTIONS).

REBETOL and INTRON A or PegIntron therapy should be suspended in patients with signs and symptoms of pancreatitis and discontinued in patients with confirmed pancreatitis.

REBETOL should not be used in patients with creatinine clearance <50 mL/min (see CLINICAL PHARMACOLOGY, Special Populations section).

Pulmonary Pulmonary symptoms, including dyspnea, pulmonary infiltrates, pneumonitis and pneumonia, have been reported during therapy with REBETOL/INTRON A; occasional cases of fatal pneumonia have occurred. In addition, sarcoidosis or the exacerbation of sarcoidosis has been reported. If there is evidence of pulmonary infiltrates or pulmonary function impairment, the patient should be closely monitored, and if appropriate, combination REBETOL/INTRON A treatment should be discontinued.

Dental and Periodontal Disorders Dental and periodontal disorders have been reported in patients receiving ribavirin and interferon or peginterferon combination therapy. In addition, dry mouth could have a damaging effect on teeth and mucous membranes of the mouth during long-term treatment with the combination of REBETOL and interferon alfa-2b or pegylated interferon alfa-2b. Patients should brush their teeth thoroughly twice daily and have regular dental examinations. In addition, some patients may experience vomiting. If this reaction occurs, they should be advised to rinse out their mouth thoroughly afterwards.

PRECAUTIONS

The safety and efficacy of REBETOL®/INTRON® A and PegIntron™ therapy for the treatment of HIV infection, adenovirus, RSV, parainfluenza, or influenza infections have not been established. REBETOL Capsules should not be used for these indications. Ribavirin for inhalation has a separate package insert, which should be consulted if ribavirin inhalation therapy is being considered.

The safety and efficacy of REBETOL/INTRON A therapy has not been established in liver or other organ transplant patients, patients with decompensated liver disease due to hepatitis C infection, patients who are nonresponders to interferon therapy, or patients coinfected with HBV or HIV.

Information for Patients Patients must be informed that REBETOL Capsules and Oral Solution may cause birth defects and/or death of the exposed fetus. REBETOL must not be used by women who are pregnant or by men whose female partners are pregnant. Extreme care must be taken to avoid pregnancy in female patients and in female partners of male patients taking REBETOL. REBETOL should not be initiated until a report of a negative pregnancy test has been obtained immediately prior to initiation of therapy. Patients must perform a pregnancy test monthly during therapy and for 6 months posttherapy. Women of childbearing potential must be counseled about use of effective contraception (two reliable forms) prior to initiating therapy. Patients (male and female) must be advised of the teratogenic/embryocidal risks and must be instructed to practice effective contraception during REBETOL and for 6 months posttherapy. Patients (male and female) should be advised to notify the physician immediately in the event of a pregnancy (see CONTRAINDICATIONS and WARNINGS).

If pregnancy does occur during treatment or during 6 months posttherapy, the patient must be advised of the teratogenic risk of REBETOL therapy to the fetus. Patients, or partners of patients, should immediately report any pregnancy that occurs during treatment or within 6 months after treatment cessation to their physician. Physicians should report such cases by calling 1-800-593-2214.

Patients receiving REBETOL Capsules should be informed of the benefits and risks associated with treatment, directed in its appropriate use, and referred to the patient MEDICATION GUIDE. Patients should be informed that the effect of treatment of hepatitis C infection on transmission is not known, and that appropriate precautions to prevent transmission of the hepatitis C virus should be taken.

The most common adverse experience occurring with REBETOL Capsules is anemia, which may be severe (see ADVERSE REACTIONS). Patients should be advised that laboratory evaluations are required prior to starting therapy and periodically thereafter (see PRECAUTIONS, Laboratory Tests section). It is advised that patients be well hydrated, especially during the initial stages of treatment.

Laboratory Tests The following laboratory tests are recommended for all patients treated with REBETOL Capsules, prior to beginning treatment and then periodically thereafter.

- Standard hematologic tests - including hemoglobin (pretreatment, Week 2 and Week 4 of therapy, and as clinically appropriate [see WARNINGS]), complete and differential white blood cell counts, and platelet count.
- Blood chemistries - liver function tests and TSH.
- Pregnancy - including monthly monitoring for women of childbearing potential.
- ECG (see WARNINGS).

Carcinogenesis and Mutagenesis Ribavirin did not cause an increase in any tumor type when administered for 6 months in the transgenic p53 deficient mouse model at doses up to 300 mg/kg (estimated human equivalent of 25 mg/kg based on body surface area adjustment for a 60 kg adult; approximately 1.9 times the maximum recommended human daily dose). Ribavirin was noncarcinogenic when administered for 2 years to rats at doses up to 40 mg/kg (estimated human equivalent of 5.71 mg/kg based on body surface area adjustment for a 60 kg adult). However, this dose was less than the maximum tolerated dose, and therefore the study was not adequate to fully characterize the carcinogenic potential of ribavirin.

Ribavirin demonstrated increased incidences of mutation and cell transformation in multiple genotoxicity assays. Ribavirin was active in the Balb/3T3 *In Vitro* Cell Transformation Assay. Mutagenic activity was observed in the mouse lymphoma assay, and at doses of 20-200 mg/kg (estimated human equivalent of 1.67-16.7 mg/kg, based on body surface area adjustment for a 60 kg adult; 0.1-1 × the maximum recommended human 24-hour dose of ribavirin) in a

TABLE 7. Selected Treatment-Emergent Adverse Events: Previously Untreated and Relapse Adult Patients and Previously Untreated Pediatric Patients

Patients Reporting Adverse Events*	US Previously Untreated Study				US Relapse Study		Pediatric Patients
	24 weeks of treatment		48 weeks of treatment		24 weeks of treatment		48 weeks of treatment
	INTRON A plus REBETOL (N=228)	INTRON A plus Placebo (N=231)	INTRON A plus REBETOL (N=228)	INTRON A plus Placebo (N=225)	INTRON A plus REBETOL (N=77)	INTRON A plus Placebo (N=76)	INTRON A plus REBETOL (N=118)
Application Site Disorders							
Injection Site Inflammation	13	10	12	14	6	8	14
Injection Site Reaction	7	9	8	9	5	3	19
Body as a Whole – General Disorders							
Headache	63	63	66	67	66	68	69
Fatigue	68	62	70	72	60	53	58
Rigors	40	32	42	39	43	37	25
Fever	37	35	41	40	32	36	61
Influenza-Like Symptoms	14	18	18	20	13	13	31
Asthenia	9	4	9	9	10	4	5
Chest Pain	5	4	9	8	6	7	5
Central & Peripheral Nervous System Disorders							
Dizziness	17	15	23	19	26	21	20
Gastrointestinal System Disorders							
Nausea	38	35	46	33	47	33	33
Anorexia	27	16	25	19	21	14	51
Dyspepsia	14	6	16	9	16	9	<1
Vomiting	11	10	9	13	12	8	42
Musculoskeletal System Disorders							
Myalgia	61	57	64	63	61	58	32
Arthralgia	30	27	33	36	29	29	15
Musculoskeletal Pain	20	26	28	32	22	28	21
Psychiatric Disorders							
Insomnia	39	27	39	30	26	25	14
Irritability	23	19	32	27	25	20	10
Depression	32	25	36	37	23	14	13
Emotional Lability	7	6	11	8	12	8	16
Concentration Impaired	11	14	14	14	10	12	5
Nervousness	4	2	4	4	5	4	3
Respiratory System Disorders							
Dyspnea	19	9	18	10	17	12	5
Sinusitis	9	7	10	14	12	7	<1
Skin and Appendages Disorders							
Alopecia	28	27	32	28	27	26	23
Rash	20	9	28	8	21	5	17
Pruritus	21	9	19	8	13	4	12
Special Senses, Other Disorders							
Taste Perversion	7	4	8	4	6	5	<1

*Patients reporting one or more adverse events. A patient may have reported more than one adverse event within a body system/organ class category.

mouse micronucleus assay. A dominant lethal assay in rats was negative, indicating that if mutations occurred in rats they were not transmitted through male gametes.

Impairment of Fertility Ribavirin demonstrated significant embryocidal and/or teratogenic effects at doses well below the recommended human dose in all animal species in which adequate studies have been conducted.

Fertile women and partners of fertile women should not receive REBETOL unless the patient and his/her partner are using effective contraception (two reliable forms). Based on a multiple-dose half-life (t1/2) of ribavirin of 12 days, effective contraception must be utilized for 6 months posttherapy (eg, 15 half-lives of clearance for ribavirin).

REBETOL should be used with caution in fertile men. In studies in mice to evaluate the time course and reversibility of ribavirin-induced testicular degeneration at doses of 15 to 150 mg/kg/day (estimated human equivalent of 1.25-12.5 mg/kg/day, based on body surface area adjustment for a 60 kg adult; 0.1-0.8 × the maximum human 24-hour dose of ribavirin) administered for 3 or 6 months, abnormalities in sperm occurred. Upon cessation of treatment, essentially total recovery from ribavirin-induced testicular toxicity was apparent within 1 or 2 spermatogenesis cycles.

Animal Toxicology Long-term studies in the mouse and rat (18-24 months; doses of 20-75 and 10-40 mg/kg/day, respectively (estimated human equivalent doses of 1.67-6.25 and 1.43-5.71 mg/kg/day, respectively, based on body surface area adjustment for a 60 kg adult; approximately 0.1-0.4 × the maximum human 24-hour dose of ribavirin)) have demonstrated a relationship between chronic ribavirin exposure and increased incidences of vascular lesions (microscopic hemorrhages) in mice. In rats, retinal degeneration occurred in controls, but the incidence was increased in ribavirin-treated rats.

In a study in which rat pups were dosed postnatally with ribavirin at doses of 10, 25, and 50 mg/kg/day, drug-related deaths occurred at 50 mg/kg (at rat pup plasma concentrations below human plasma concentrations at the human therapeutic dose) between study Days 13 and 48. Rat pups dosed from postnatal Day 7 through 63 demonstrated a minor, dose-related decrease in overall growth at all doses, which was subsequently manifested as slight decreases in body weight, crown-rump length, and bone length. These effects showed evidence of reversibility, and no histopathological effects on bone were observed. No ribavirin effects were observed regarding neurobehavioral or reproductive development.

Pregnancy Category X (see **CONTRAINDICATIONS**) Ribavirin produced significant embryocidal and/or teratogenic effects in all animal species in which adequate studies have been conducted. Malformations of the skull, palate, eye, jaw, limbs, skeleton, and gastrointestinal tract were noted. The incidence and severity of teratogenic effects increased with escalation of the drug dose. Survival of fetuses and offspring was reduced. In conventional embryotoxicity/teratogenicity studies in rats and rabbits, observed no-effect dose levels were well below those for proposed clinical use (0.3 mg/kg/day for both the rat and rabbit; approximately 0.06 × the recommended human 24-hour dose of ribavirin). No maternal toxicity or effects on offspring were observed in a peri/postnatal toxicity study in rats dosed orally at up to 1 mg/kg/day (estimated human equivalent dose of 0.17 mg/kg based on body surface area adjustment for a 60 kg adult; approximately 0.01 × the maximum recommended human 24-hour dose of ribavirin).

Treatment and Posttreatment Potential Risk to the Fetus Ribavirin is known to accumulate in intracellular components from where it is cleared very slowly. It is not known whether ribavirin contained in sperm will exert a potential teratogenic effect upon fertilization of the ova. In a study in rats, it was concluded that dominant lethality was not induced by ribavirin at doses up to 200 mg/kg for 5 days (estimated human equivalent doses of 7.14-28.6 mg/kg, based on body surface area adjustment for a 60 kg adult; up to 1.7 × the maximum recommended human dose of ribavirin). However, because of the potential human teratogenic effects of ribavirin, male patients should be advised to take every precaution to avoid risk of pregnancy for their female partners.

Women of childbearing potential should not receive REBETOL unless they are using effective contraception (two reliable forms) during the therapy period. In addition, effective contraception should be utilized for 6 months posttherapy based on a multiple-dose half-life (t1/2) of ribavirin of 12 days.

Male patients and their female partners must practice effective contraception (two reliable forms) during treatment with REBETOL and for the 6-month posttherapy period (eg, 15 half-lives for ribavirin clearance from the body).

Ribavirin Pregnancy Registry A Ribavirin Pregnancy Registry has been established to monitor maternal-fetal outcomes of pregnancies in female patients and female partners of male patients exposed to ribavirin during treatment and for 6 months following cessation of treatment. Physi-

cians and patients are encouraged to report such cases by calling 1-800-593-2214.

Nursing Mothers It is not known whether the REBETOL product is excreted in human milk. Because of the potential for serious adverse reactions from the drug in nursing infants, a decision should be made whether to discontinue nursing or to delay or discontinue REBETOL.

Geriatric Use Clinical studies of REBETOL/INTRON A or PegIntron therapy did not include sufficient numbers of subjects aged 65 and over to determine if they respond differently from younger subjects.

REBETOL is known to be substantially excreted by the kidney, and the risk of toxic reactions to this drug may be greater in patients with impaired renal function. Because elderly patients often have decreased renal function, care should be taken in dose selection. Renal function should be monitored and dosage adjustments should be made accordingly. REBETOL should not be used in patients with creatinine clearance <50 mL/min (see **WARNINGS**).

In general, REBETOL Capsules should be administered to elderly patients cautiously, starting at the lower end of the dosing range, reflecting the greater frequency of decreased hepatic and/or cardiac function, and of concomitant disease or other drug therapy. In clinical trials, elderly subjects had a higher frequency of anemia (67%) than did younger patients (28%) (see **WARNINGS**).

Pediatric Use: Suicidal ideation or attempts occurred more frequently among pediatric patients, primarily adolescents, compared to adult patients (2.4% versus 1%) during treatment and off-therapy follow-up (see WARNINGS). As in adult patients, pediatric patients experienced other psychiatric adverse events (eg, depression, emotional lability, somnolence), anemia, and neutropenia (see **WARNINGS**). During a 48-week course of therapy there was a decrease in the rate of linear growth (mean percentile assignment decrease of 9%) and a decrease in the rate of weight gain (mean percentile assignment decrease of 13%). A general reversal of these trends was noted during the 24-week posttreatment period.

Drug Interactions *Didanosine* Coadministration of REBETOL Capsules or Oral Solution and didanosine is not recommended. Reports of fatal hepatic failure, as well as peripheral neuropathy, pancreatitis, and symptomatic hyperlactactemia/lactic acidosis have been reported in clinical trials (see **CLINICAL PHARMACOLOGY, Pharmacokinetics,** *Drug Interactions* section).

Stavudine and Zidovudine Ribavirin may antagonize the *in vitro* antiviral activity of stavudine and zidovudine against HIV. Therefore, concomitant use of ribavirin with either of these drugs should be used with caution (see **CLINICAL PHARMACOLOGY, Pharmacokinetics,** *Drug Interactions* section).

ADVERSE REACTIONS

The primary toxicity of ribavirin is hemolytic anemia. Reductions in hemoglobin levels occurred within the first 1-2 weeks of oral therapy (see WARNINGS).Cardiac and pulmonary events associated with anemia occurred in approximately 10% of patients (see WARNINGS).

REBETOL®/INTRON® A Combination Therapy In clinical trials, 19% and 6% of previously untreated and relapse patients, respectively, discontinued therapy due to adverse events in the combination arms compared to 13% and 3% in the interferon arms. Selected treatment-emergent adverse events that occurred in the US studies with ≥5% incidence are provided in **TABLE 7** by treatment group. In general, the selected treatment-emergent adverse events were reported with lower incidence in the international studies as compared to the US studies with the exception of asthenia, influenza-like symptoms, nervousness, and pruritus.

Pediatric Patients In clinical trials of 118 pediatric patients 3 to 16 years of age, 6% discontinued therapy due to adverse events. Dose modifications were required in 30% of patients, most commonly for anemia and neutropenia. In general, the adverse-event profile in the pediatric population was similar to that observed in adults. Injection site disorders, fever, anorexia, vomiting, and emotional lability occurred more frequently in pediatric patients compared to adult patients. Conversely, pediatric patients experienced less fatigue, dyspepsia, arthralgia, insomnia, irritability, impaired concentration, dyspnea, and pruritus compared to adult patients. Selected treatment-emergent adverse events that occurred with ≥5% incidence among all pediatric patients who received the recommended dose of REBETOL/INTRON A combination therapy are provided in **TABLE 7**.

[See table 7 at top of previous page]

In addition, the following spontaneous adverse events have been reported during the marketing surveillance of REBETOL/INTRON A therapy: hearing disorder and vertigo.

REBETOL/PegIntron™ Combination Therapy Overall, in clinical trials, 14% of patients receiving REBETOL in combination with PegIntron discontinued therapy compared with 13% treated with REBETOL in combination with

INTRON A. The most common reasons for discontinuation of therapy were related to psychiatric, systemic (eg, fatigue, headache), or gastrointestinal adverse events. Adverse events that occurred in clinical trial at >5% incidence are provided in **TABLE 8** by treatment group. Safety and effectiveness of REBETOL in combination with PegIntron have not been established in pediatric patients.

TABLE 8. Adverse Events Occurring in >5% of Patients

Percentage of Patients Reporting Adverse Events*

Adverse Events	PegIntron 1.5 mcg/kg/ REBETOL (N=511)	INTRON A/ REBETOL (N=505)
Application Site		
Injection Site Inflammation	25	18
Injection Site Reaction	58	36
Autonomic Nervous System		
Mouth Dry	12	8
Sweating Increased	11	7
Flushing	4	3
Body as a Whole		
Fatigue/Asthenia	66	63
Headache	62	58
Rigors	48	41
Fever	46	33
Weight Decrease	29	20
RUQ Pain	12	6
Chest Pain	8	7
Malaise	4	6
Central/Peripheral Nervous System		
Dizziness	21	17
Endocrine		
Hypothyroidism	5	4
Gastrointestinal		
Nausea	43	33
Anorexia	32	27
Diarrhea	22	17
Vomiting	14	12
Abdominal Pain	13	13
Dyspepsia	9	8
Constipation	5	5
Hematologic Disorders		
Neutropenia	26	14
Anemia	12	17
Leukopenia	6	5
Thrombocytopenia	5	2
Liver and Biliary System		
Hepatomegaly	4	4
Musculoskeletal		
Myalgia	56	50
Arthralgia	34	28
Musculoskeletal Pain	21	19
Psychiatric		
Insomnia	40	41
Depression	31	34
Anxiety/Emotional Lability/Irritability	47	47
Concentration Impaired	17	21
Agitation	8	5
Nervousness	6	6
Reproductive, Female		
Menstrual Disorder	7	6
Resistance Mechanism		
Infection Viral	12	12
Infection Fungal	6	1
Respiratory System		
Dyspnea	26	24
Coughing	23	16
Pharyngitis	12	13
Rhinitis	8	6
Sinusitis	6	5

Skin and Appendages		
Alopecia	36	32
Pruritus	29	28
Rash	24	23
Skin Dry	24	23
Special Senses, Other		
Taste Perversion	9	4
Vision Disorders		
Vision blurred	5	6
Conjunctivitis	4	5

*Patients reporting one or more adverse events. A patient may have reported more than one adverse event within a body system/organ class category.

Laboratory Values *REBETOL/INTRON A Combination Therapy* Changes in selected hematologic values (hemoglobin, white blood cells, neutrophils, and platelets) during therapy are described below (see **TABLE 9**).

Hemoglobin Hemoglobin decreases among patients receiving REBETOL therapy began at Week 1, with stabilization by Week 4. In previously untreated patients treated for 48 weeks the mean maximum decrease from baseline was 3.1 g/dL in the US study and 2.9 g/dL in the International study. In relapse patients the mean maximum decrease from baseline was 2.8 g/dL in the US study and 2.6 g/dL in the International study. Hemoglobin values returned to pretreatment levels within 4-8 weeks of cessation of therapy in most patients.

Bilirubin and Uric Acid Increases in both bilirubin and uric acid, associated with hemolysis, were noted in clinical trials. Most were moderate biochemical changes and were reversed within 4 weeks after treatment discontinuation. This observation occurs most frequently in patients with a previous diagnosis of Gilbert's syndrome. This has not been associated with hepatic dysfunction or clinical morbidity. [See table 9 above]

REBETOL/PegIntron Combination Therapy Changes in selected hematologic values (hemoglobin, white blood cells, neutrophils, and platelets) during therapy are described below (see **TABLE 10**).

Hemoglobin REBETOL induced a decrease in hemoglobin levels in approximately two thirds of patients. Hemoglobin levels decreased to <11 g/dL in about 30% of patients. Severe anemia (<8 g/dL) occurred in <1% of patients. Dose modification was required in 9% and 13% of patients in the PegIntron/REBETOL and INTRON A/REBETOL groups.

Bilirubin and Uric Acid In the REBETOL/PegIntron combination trial 10-14% of patients developed hyperbilirubinemia and 33-38% developed hyperuricemia in association with hemolysis. Six patients developed mild to moderate gout.

TABLE 10. Selected Hematologic Values During Treatment With REBETOL Plus PegIntron

	Number (%) of Subjects	
	PegIntron plus REBETOL (N=511)	INTRON A plus REBETOL (N=505)
Hemoglobin (g/dL)		
9.5 - 10.9	26	27
8.0 - 9.4	3	3
6.5 - 7.9	0.2	0.2
<6.5	0	0
Leukocytes (×10⁹/L)		
2.0 - 2.9	46	41
1.5 - 1.9	24	8
1.0 - 1.4	5	1
<1.0	0	0
Neutrophils (×10⁹/L)		
1.0 - 1.49	33	37
0.75 - 0.99	25	13
0.5 - 0.74	18	7
<0.5	4	2
Platelets (×10⁹/L)		
70 - 99	15	5
50 - 69	3	0.8
30 - 49	0.2	0.2
<30	0	0
Total Bilirubin (mg/dL)		
1.5 - 3.0	10	13
3.1 - 6.0	0.6	0.2

TABLE 9. Selected Hematologic Values During Treatment with REBETOL Plus INTRON A: Previously Untreated and Relapse Adult Patients and Previously Untreated Pediatric Patients

Percentage of Patients

	US Previously Untreated Study				US Relapse Study		Pediatric Patients
	24 weeks of treatment		48 weeks of treatment		24 weeks of treatment		48 weeks of treatment
	INTRON A plus REBETOL (N=228)	INTRON A plus Placebo (N=231)	INTRON A plus REBETOL (N=228)	INTRON A plus Placebo (N=225)	INTRON A plus REBETOL (N=77)	INTRON A plus Placebo (N=76)	INTRON A plus REBETOL (N=118)
Hemoglobin (g/dL)							
9.5 - 10.9	24	1	32	1	21	3	24
8.0 - 9.4	5	0	4	0	4	0	3
6.5 - 7.9	0	0	0	0.4	0	0	0
<6.5	0	0	0	0	0	0	0
Leukocytes (×10⁹/L)							
2.0 - 2.9	40	20	38	23	45	26	35
1.5 - 1.9	4	1	9	2	5	3	8
1.0 - 1.4	0.9	0	2	0	0	0	0
<1.0	0	0	0	0	0	0	0
Neutrophils (×10⁹/L)							
1.0 - 1.49	30	32	31	44	42	34	37
0.75 - 0.99	14	15	14	11	16	18	15
0.5 - 0.74	9	9	14	7	8	4	16
<0.5	11	8	11	5	5	8	3
Platelets (×10⁹/L)							
70 - 99	9	11	11	14	6	12	0.8
50 - 69	2	3	2	3	0	5	2
30 - 49	0	0.4	0	0.4	0	0	0
<30	0.9	0	1	0.9	0	0	0
Total Bilirubin (mg/dL)							
1.5 - 3.0	27	13	32	13	21	7	2
3.1 - 6.0	0.9	0.4	2	0	3	0	0
6.1 - 12.0	0	0	0.4	0	0	0	0
>12.0	0	0	0	0	0	0	0

6.1 - 12.0	0	0.2
>12.0	0	0
ALT (SGPT)		
2 × Baseline	0.6	0.2
2.1 - 5 × Baseline	3	1
5.1 - 10 × Baseline	0	0
>10 × Baseline	0	0

Postmarketing Experiences The following adverse reactions have been identified during postapproval use of REBETOL in combination with INTRON A or PegIntron therapy: hearing disorder, vertigo, aplastic anemia, pure red cell aplasia. Because these reactions are reported voluntarily from a population of uncertain size, it is not always possible to reliably estimate their frequency or establish a causal relationship to drug exposure.

OVERDOSAGE

There is limited experience with overdosage. Acute ingestion of up to 20 grams of REBETOL® Capsules, INTRON® A ingestion of up to 120 million units, and subcutaneous doses of INTRON A up to 10 times the recommended doses have been reported. Primary effects that have been observed are increased incidence and severity of the adverse events related to the therapeutic use of INTRON A and REBETOL. However, hepatic enzyme abnormalities, renal failure, hemorrhage, and myocardial infarction have been reported with administration of single subcutaneous doses of INTRON A that exceed dosing recommendations. There is no specific antidote for INTRON A or REBETOL overdose, and hemodialysis and peritoneal dialysis are not effective for treatment of overdose of either agent.

DOSAGE AND ADMINISTRATION
(see **CLINICAL PHARMACOLOGY, Special Populations** section and **WARNINGS**)
REBETOL®/INTRON® A Combination Therapy *Adults* The recommended dose of REBETOL Capsules depends on the patient's body weight. The recommended dose of REBETOL is provided in **TABLE 11**.
The recommended duration of treatment for patients previously untreated with interferon is 24 to 48 weeks. The duration of treatment should be individualized to the patient depending on baseline disease characteristics, response to therapy, and tolerability of the regimen (see **INDICA-**

TIONS AND USAGE, **Description of Clinical Studies** section and **ADVERSE REACTIONS**). After 24 weeks of treatment virologic response should be assessed. Treatment discontinuation should be considered in any patient who has not achieved an HCV RNA below the limit of detection of the assay by 24 weeks. There are no safety and efficacy data on treatment for longer than 48 weeks in the previously untreated patient population.
In patients who relapse following non-pegylated interferon monotherapy, the recommended duration of treatment is 24 weeks. There are no safety and efficacy data on treatment for longer than 24 weeks in the relapse patient population.

TABLE 11. Recommended Dosing

Body weight	REBETOL Capsules
≤ 75 kg	2 × 200-mg capsules AM, 3 × 200-mg capsules PM daily p.o.
> 75 kg	3 × 200-mg capsules AM, 3 × 200-mg capsules PM daily p.o.

Pediatrics The recommended dose of REBETOL is 15 mg/kg per day orally (divided dose AM and PM). For children weighing ≤25 kg or who cannot swallow capsules, REBETOL Oral Solution is supplied in a concentration of 40 mg/mL. For children weighing >25 kg, either the Oral Solution or 200-mg capsule may be administered. Refer to **TABLE 12** for dosing recommendations for the 200-mg capsule to achieve the recommended dose.
The recommended duration of treatment is 48 weeks for pediatric patients with genotype 1. After 24 weeks of treatment virologic response should be assessed. Treatment discontinuation should be considered in any patient who has not achieved an HCV RNA below the limit of detection of the assay by this time. The recommended duration of treatment for pediatric patients with genotype 2/3 is 24 weeks. There are no safety and efficacy data on treatment for longer than 48 weeks in pediatrics.
[See table 12 at top of next page]
REBETOL may be administered without regard to food, but should be administered in a consistent manner with respect to food intake (see **CLINICAL PHARMACOLOGY**).

Under no circumstances should REBETOL Capsules be opened, crushed, or broken (see **CONTRAINDICATIONS** and **WARNINGS**).

REBETOL/PegIntron™ Combination Therapy The recommended dose of REBETOL Capsules is 800 mg/day in 2 divided doses: two capsules (400 mg) in the morning with food and two capsules (400 mg) in the evening with food.

Dose Modifications (**TABLE 13**) If severe adverse reactions or laboratory abnormalities develop during combination REBETOL/INTRON A therapy the dose should be modified, or discontinued if appropriate, until the adverse reactions abate. If intolerance persists after dose adjustment, REBETOL/INTRON A therapy should be discontinued.

REBETOL should not be used in patients with creatinine clearance <50 mL/min. Subjects with impaired renal function and/or those over the age of 50 should be carefully monitored with respect to development of anemia (see **CLINICAL PHARMACOLOGY, Special Populations** section and **WARNINGS**).

REBETOL should be administered with caution to patients with pre-existing cardiac disease. Patients should be assessed before commencement of therapy and should be appropriately monitored during therapy. If there is any deterioration of cardiovascular status, therapy should be stopped (see **WARNINGS**).

For patients with a history of stable cardiovascular disease, a permanent dose reduction is required if the hemoglobin decreases by ≥2 g/dL during any 4-week period. In addition, for these cardiac history patients, if the hemoglobin remains <12 g/dL after 4 weeks on a reduced dose, the patient should discontinue combination REBETOL/INTRON A therapy.

It is recommended that a patient whose hemoglobin level falls below 10 g/dL have his/her REBETOL dose reduced to 600 mg daily (1 × 200-mg capsule AM, 2 × 200-mg capsules PM) for adults and 7.5 mg/kg per day (divided dose AM and PM) for pediatric patients. A patient whose hemoglobin level falls below 8.5 g/dL should be permanently discontinued from REBETOL therapy (see **WARNINGS**).

[See table 13 above]

TABLE 12. Pediatric Dosing

Body weight	REBETOL Capsules	INTRON A for Injection
25-36 kg	1 × 200-mg capsule AM, 1 × 200-mg capsule PM daily p.o.	3 million IU/m^2 3 times weekly s.c.
37-49 kg	1 × 200-mg capsule AM, 2 × 200-mg capsules PM daily p.o.	3 million IU/m^2 3 times weekly s.c.
50-61 kg	2 × 200-mg capsules AM, 2 × 200-mg capsules PM daily p.o.	3 million IU/m^2 3 times weekly s.c.
>61 kg	Refer to adult dosing table	Refer to adult dosing table

TABLE 13. Guidelines for Dose Modifications and Discontinuation for Anemia

Hemoglobin	Dose Reduction REBETOL — 600 mg daily adults 7.5 mg/kg daily for pediatrics	Permanent Discontinuation of REBETOL Treatment
No Cardiac History	**<10 g/dL**	**<8.5 g/dL**
Cardiac History Patients	**≥ 2 g/dL decrease during any 4-week period during treatment**	**<12 g/dL after 4 weeks of dose reduction**

HOW SUPPLIED

REBETOL® 200-mg Capsules are white, opaque capsules with REBETOL, 200 mg, and the Schering Corporation logo imprinted on the capsule shell; the capsules are packaged in a bottle containing 42 capsules (NDC 0085-1327-04), 56 capsules (NDC 0085-1351-05), 70 capsules (NDC 0085-1385-07), and 84 capsules (NDC 0085-1194-03).

REBETOL Oral Solution 40 mg/mL is a clear, colorless to pale or light yellow bubble gum-flavored liquid and it is packaged in 4-oz amber glass bottles (100 mL/bottle) with child-resistant closures (NDC 0085-1318-01).

Storage Conditions: The bottle of REBETOL Capsules should be stored at 25°C (77°F); excursions permitted to 15°-30°C (59°-86°F) [see USP Controlled Room Temperature].

REBETOL Oral Solution should be stored between 2°-8°C (36°-46°F) or at 25°C (77°F); excursions permitted to 15°-30°C (59°-86°F) [see USP Controlled Room Temperature].

Schering Corporation
Kenilworth, NJ 07033 USA

U.S. Patent Nos. 5,767,097; 5,914,128; 6,051,252; 6,063,772; 6,172,046; 6,177,074; 6,335,032; 6,337,090; 6,461,605; 6,472,373; and 6,524,570.

Copyright © 2003, Schering Corporation. All rights reserved.

Trademarks depicted herein are the property of their respective owners.

Rev. 1/08
27002455T

MEDICATION GUIDE

REBETOL®

(ribavirin, USP) Capsules and Oral Solution

Read this medication guide carefully before you or your child begin taking REBETOL® [REB-eh-tol] Capsules or Oral Solution, and each time you refill your prescription in case new information has been included. This summary does not tell you everything about REBETOL Capsules or Oral Solution. Your health care provider is the best source of information about this medicine. After reading this medication guide, talk with your health care provider if you have any questions about REBETOL.

What is the most important information I should know about therapy with REBETOL® Capsules or Oral Solution?

• **REBETOL Capsules and Oral Solution may cause birth defects or death of an unborn child. Therefore, if you are pregnant or your sexual partner is pregnant, do not take REBETOL.** If you could become pregnant, you must not become pregnant during therapy and for 6 months after you have stopped therapy. During this time you must use 2 forms of birth control, and you must have pregnancy tests that show that you are not pregnant.

Female sexual partners of male patients being treated with REBETOL must not become pregnant during treatment and for 6 months after treatment has stopped. Therefore, you must use 2 forms of birth control during this time.

If you or a female sexual partner becomes pregnant, you should tell your health care provider. There is a Ribavirin Pregnancy Registry that collects information about pregnancy outcomes in female patients and female partners of male patients exposed to ribavirin. You or your health care provider are encouraged to contact the Registry at 1-800-593-2214. Be assured that any information you tell the Registry will be kept confidential (see **"What should I avoid while taking REBETOL Capsules or Oral Solution?"**).

• After each use of REBETOL Oral Solution, wash the measuring cup or spoon to avoid swallowing of the medicine by someone other than the person to whom it was prescribed.

• **REBETOL Capsules and Oral Solution can cause a dangerous drop in your red blood cell count.** REBETOL Capsules and Oral Solution can cause anemia, which is a decrease in the number of red blood cells. This can be dangerous, especially if you have heart or breathing problems. Tell your health care provider before taking REBETOL if you have ever had any of these problems. Your health care provider should check your red blood cell count before you start therapy and often during the first 4 weeks of therapy. Your red blood cell count may be checked more often if you have any heart or breathing problems.

• **Do not take REBETOL Capsules or Oral Solution alone to treat hepatitis C infection.** REBETOL Capsules should be used in combination with interferon alfa-2b (INTRON® A) or in combination with peginterferon alfa-2b (PegIntron®) for treating chronic hepatitis C infection in adults. In children, safety and effectiveness of REBETOL Capsules or Oral Solution have only been shown when used in combination with interferon alfa-2b (INTRON A). Your health care provider or pharmacist should give you a copy of the INTRON A or PegIntron Medication Guide. They have additional important information about combination therapy not covered in this guide.

What is REBETOL® (ribavirin)?

"REBETOL" is a form of the antiviral drug ribavirin. It is used in combination with interferon alfa-2b to treat some patients with chronic hepatitis C infection. It is not known how REBETOL and interferon alfa-2b work together to fight hepatitis C infection (see the **INTRON® A** or **PegIntron® Medication Guide**).

It is not known if treatment with REBETOL and interferon alfa-2b will cure hepatitis C virus infections or prevent cirrhosis, liver failure, or liver cancer that can be caused by hepatitis C virus infections. It is not known if treatment with REBETOL and interferon alfa-2b will prevent an infected person from infecting another person with the hepatitis C virus.

Who should not take REBETOL® Capsules or Oral Solution?

Do not use these medicines if:

• You are a female and you are pregnant or plan to become pregnant at any time during your treatment with REBETOL or during the 6 months after your treatment has ended.

• You are a male patient with a female sexual partner who is pregnant or plans to become pregnant at any time while you are being treated with REBETOL or during the 6 months after your treatment has ended (see **"What is the most important information I should know about therapy with REBETOL Capsules or Oral Solution?"** and **"What should I avoid while taking REBETOL Capsules or Oral Solution?"**).

• You are breastfeeding. REBETOL may pass through your milk and harm your baby. Talk with your provider about whether you should stop breast-feeding.

• You are allergic to any of the ingredients in REBETOL Capsules or Oral Solution. See the ingredients listed at the end of this Medication Guide.

Tell your health care provider before starting treatment with REBETOL Capsules or Oral Solution in combination with PegIntron®/INTRON® A if you have any of the following medical conditions:

• **mental health problems, such as depression or anxiety.** REBETOL/PegIntron/INTRON A therapy may make them worse. Tell your health care provider if you are being treated or had treatment in the past for any mental problems, including depression, suicidal behavior, or a feeling of loss of contact with reality, such as hearing voices or seeing things that are not there (psychosis). Tell your health care provider if you take any medicines for these problems.

• **high blood pressure, heart problems, or have had a heart attack.** REBETOL Capsules and Oral Solution may worsen heart problems. Patients who have had certain heart problems should not take REBETOL Capsules or Oral Solution.

• **blood disorders,** including anemia (low red blood cell count), thalassemia (Mediterranean anemia), and sickle-cell anemia. REBETOL Capsules and Oral Solution can reduce the number of red blood cells you have. This may make you feel dizzy or weak and could worsen any heart problems you might have.

• **kidney problems.** If your kidneys do not work properly, you may experience worse side effects from REBETOL therapy and require a lower dose.

• **liver problems** (other than hepatitis C infection).

• **organ transplant,** and are taking medicine that keeps your body from rejecting your transplant (suppresses your immune system).

• **thyroid disease.** REBETOL/PegIntron/INTRON A therapy may make your thyroid disease worse or harder to treat. REBETOL/PegIntron/INTRON A therapy may be stopped if you develop thyroid problems that cannot be controlled by medicine.

• **lung problems.** REBETOL/PegIntron/INTRON A therapy can cause breathing problems or worsen breathing problems you already have.

• **alcoholism or drug abuse or addiction.**

• **cancer.**

• **infection with hepatitis B virus and/or human immunodeficiency virus** (the virus that causes AIDS).

• **diabetes.** REBETOL/PegIntron/INTRON A therapy may make your diabetes worse or harder to treat.

• **past interferon treatment for hepatitis C virus infection that did not work for you.**

For more information see the INTRON A or PegIntron Medication Guides.

How should I take REBETOL® Capsules or Oral Solution?

Your health care provider has determined the correct dose of REBETOL Capsules or Oral Solution based on your weight. Your health care provider may lower your dose of REBETOL if you have side effects.

• It is important to follow your dosing schedule and your health care provider's instructions on how to take your medicines.

• Under no circumstances should REBETOL Capsules be opened, crushed, or broken.

• You should take REBETOL with food. Taking REBETOL with food helps your body take up more of the medicine. Taking REBETOL at the same time of day every day will help keep the amount of medicine in your body at a steady level. This can help your health care provider decide how your treatment is working and how to change the number of REBETOL Capsules you take if you have side effects.

• Take the medicine for as long as prescribed and do not take more than the recommended dose.

• If you miss a dose of REBETOL Capsules or Oral Solution, take the missed dose as soon as possible during the same day. If an entire day has gone by, check with your health care provider about what to do. Do not double the next dose.

• Tell your health care provider if you are taking or planning to take other prescription or nonprescription medicines, including vitamin and mineral supplements, and herbal medicines.

• Tell your provider before taking REBETOL Capsules or Oral Solution if you have ever had any heart or breathing problems. Your provider should check your red blood cell count before starting therapy and often during the first 4 weeks of therapy. Your red blood cell count may be checked more frequently if you have had heart or breathing problems.

• Females taking REBETOL Capsules or Oral Solution or female sexual partners of male patients taking REBETOL Capsules or Oral Solution must have a pregnancy test before treatment begins, every month during treatment, and for 6 months after treatment ends to make sure there is no pregnancy.

What should I avoid while taking REBETOL® Capsules or Oral Solution?

Avoid the following during REBETOL Capsule or Oral Solution treatment:

• **Pregnancy.** If you or your sexual partner gets pregnant during treatment with REBETOL Capsules or Oral Solution or in the 6 months after treatment ends, tell your health care provider right away (see "**What is the most important information I should know about therapy with REBETOL Capsules or Oral Solution?**").

Talk with your health care provider about how to avoid pregnancy. If you or your sexual partner gets pregnant while on REBETOL or during the 6 months after your treatment ends, you must report the pregnancy to your health care provider right away. Your health care provider should call 1-800-593-2214. Your health care provider will be asked to give follow-up information about the pregnancy. Any information about your pregnancy that is reported will be confidential.

• **Breastfeeding.** The medicine may pass through your milk and harm the baby.

• **Drinking alcohol,** including beer, wine, and liquor. This may make your liver disease worse.

• **Taking other medicines.** Take only medicines prescribed or approved by your health care provider. These include prescription and nonprescription medicines and herbal supplements.

What are the most common side effects of REBETOL® Capsules and Oral Solution?

The most serious possible side effects of REBETOL Capsules and Oral Solution are:

• **Harm to unborn children.** REBETOL Capsules and Oral Solution may cause birth defects or death of an unborn child. (For more details, see "**What is the most important information I should know about REBETOL Capsules or Oral Solution?**")

• **Anemia.** Anemia is a reduction in the number of red blood cells you have which can be dangerous, especially if you have heart or breathing problems. Tell your health care provider right away if you feel tired, have chest pain, or shortness of breath. These may be signs of low red blood cell counts.

Tell your provider right away if you have any of the following symptoms. They may be signs of a serious side effect:

• trouble breathing
• hives or swelling
• chest pain
• severe stomach or low back pain
• bloody diarrhea or bloody stools (bowel movements). These may appear black and tarry.
• bruising
• other bleeding

The most common side effects of REBETOL Capsules and Oral Solution are:

• feeling tired
• nausea and appetite loss
• rash and itching
• cough

This summary does not include all possible side effects of REBETOL therapy. Talk to your health care provider if you do not feel well while taking REBETOL. Your health care provider can give you more information about managing your side effects.

Call your doctor for medical advice about side effects. You may report side effects to FDA at 1-800-FDA-1088.

What should I know about hepatitis C infection?

Hepatitis C infection is a disease caused by a virus that infects the liver. This liver infection becomes a continuing (chronic) condition in most patients. Patients with chronic hepatitis C infection may develop cirrhosis, liver cancer, and liver failure. The virus is spread from one person to another by contact with the infected person's blood. You should talk to your health care provider about ways to prevent you from infecting others.

How do I store my REBETOL® Capsules?

Store REBETOL Capsules at room temperature 77°F (25°C).

How do I store my REBETOL® Oral Solution?

Store REBETOL Oral Solution at room temperature 77°F (25°C) or in the refrigerator 36°-46°F (2°-8°C).

General advice about prescription medicines

Do not use REBETOL® Capsules or Oral Solution for conditions for which they were not prescribed. If you have any concern about REBETOL Capsules or Oral Solution, ask your health care provider. Your health care provider or pharmacist can give you information about REBETOL Capsules or Oral Solution that was written for health care professionals. Do not give this medicine to other people, even if they have the same condition you have.

Ingredients:

REBETOL® Capsules contain ribavirin and the inactive ingredients micro-crystalline cellulose, lactose monohydrate, croscarmellose sodium, and magnesium stearate. The capsule shell consists of gelatin and titanium dioxide. The capsule is printed with edible blue pharmaceutical ink which is made of shellac, anhydrous ethyl alcohol, isopropyl alcohol, n-butyl alcohol, propylene glycol, ammonium hydroxide, and FD&C Blue #2 aluminum lake.

REBETOL Oral Solution contains ribavirin and the inactive ingredients sodium citrate, citric acid, sodium benzoate, glycerin, sucrose, sorbitol, propylene glycol, and water.

This Medication Guide has been approved by the U.S. Food and Drug Administration.

Revised: April 2009

Manufactured by Schering Corporation, a subsidiary of Schering-Plough Corporation, Kenilworth, NJ 07033 USA. © 2001, 2002, 2003, Schering Corporation. All rights reserved.

Rev. 4/09   27002560T

Shown in Product Identification Guide, page 313

RECOMBIVAX HB®   ℞

[re-com-biv-ax]

hepatitis b vaccine (recombinant)

DESCRIPTION

RECOMBIVAX HB[1] Hepatitis B Vaccine (Recombinant) is a non-infectious subunit viral vaccine derived from hepatitis B surface antigen (HBsAg) produced in yeast cells. A portion of the hepatitis B virus gene, coding for HBsAg, is cloned into yeast, and the vaccine for hepatitis B is produced from cultures of this recombinant yeast strain according to methods developed in the Merck Research Laboratories.

The antigen is harvested and purified from fermentation cultures of a recombinant strain of the yeast *Saccharomyces cerevisiae* containing the gene for the *adw* subtype of HBsAg. The fermentation process involves growth of *Saccharomyces cerevisiae* on a complex fermentation medium which consists of an extract of yeast, soy peptone, dextrose, amino acids and mineral salts. The HBsAg protein is released from the yeast cells by cell disruption and purified by a series of physical and chemical methods. The purified protein is treated in phosphate buffer with formaldehyde and then coprecipitated with alum (potassium aluminum sulfate) to form bulk vaccine adjuvanted with amorphous aluminum hydroxyphosphate sulfate. The vaccine contains no detectable yeast DNA but may contain not more than 1% yeast protein. The vaccine produced by the Merck method has been shown to be comparable to the plasma-derived vaccine in terms of animal potency (mouse, monkey, and chimpanzee) and protective efficacy (chimpanzee and human).

The vaccine against hepatitis B, prepared from recombinant yeast cultures, is free of association with human blood or blood products.

Each lot of hepatitis B vaccine is tested for sterility.

RECOMBIVAX HB is a sterile suspension for intramuscular injection. However, for persons at risk of hemorrhage following intramuscular injection, the vaccine may be administered subcutaneously. (See DOSAGE AND ADMINISTRATION).

RECOMBIVAX HB Hepatitis B Vaccine (Recombinant) is supplied in three formulations. (See HOW SUPPLIED.)

Pediatric/Adolescent Formulation (Without Preservative), 10 mcg/mL: each 0.5 mL dose contains 5 mcg of hepatitis B surface antigen.

Adult Formulation (Without Preservative), 10 mcg/mL: each 1 mL dose contains 10 mcg of hepatitis B surface antigen.

Dialysis Formulation (Without Preservative), 40 mcg/mL: each 1 mL dose contains 40 mcg of hepatitis B surface antigen.

All formulations contain approximately 0.5 mg of aluminum (provided as amorphous aluminum hydroxyphosphate sulfate, previously referred to as aluminum hydroxide) per mL of vaccine. In each formulation, hepatitis B surface antigen is adsorbed onto approximately 0.5 mg of aluminum (provided as amorphous aluminum hydroxyphosphate sulfate) per mL of vaccine. The vaccine is of the *adw* subtype. RECOMBIVAX HB is indicated for vaccination of persons at risk of infection from hepatitis B virus including all known subtypes. RECOMBIVAX HB Dialysis Formulation is indicated for vaccination of adult predialysis and dialysis patients against infection caused by all known subtypes of hepatitis B virus.

[1] Registered trademark of MERCK & CO., Inc.
   COPYRIGHT © 1998 MERCK & CO., Inc.
   All rights reserved

CLINICAL PHARMACOLOGY

Hepatitis B virus is one of several hepatitis viruses that cause a systemic infection, with a major pathology in the liver. These include hepatitis A virus, hepatitis D virus, and hepatitis C and E viruses, previously referred to as non-A, non-B hepatitis viruses.

Hepatitis B virus is an important cause of viral hepatitis. There is no specific treatment for this disease. The incubation period for hepatitis B is relatively long; six weeks to six months may elapse between exposure and the onset of clinical symptoms. The prognosis following infection with hepatitis B virus is variable and dependent on at least three factors: (1) Age — Infants and younger children usually experience milder initial disease than older persons;[1] (2) Dose of virus — The higher the dose, the more likely acute icteric hepatitis B will result;[1] and, (3) Severity of associated underlying disease — Underlying malignancy or pre-existing hepatic disease predisposes to increased morbidity and mortality.[1]

Persistence of viral infection (the chronic hepatitis B virus carrier state) occurs in 5-10% of persons following acute hepatitis B, and occurs more frequently after initial anicteric hepatitis B than after initial icteric disease. Consequently, carriers of hepatitis B surface antigen (HBsAg) frequently give no history of having had recognized acute hepatitis. The Centers for Disease Control and Prevention (CDC) estimates that there are more than 300 million chronic carriers worldwide and 1.25 million chronic carriers of hepatitis B virus in the USA.[29,30] Chronic carriers represent the largest human reservoir of hepatitis B virus.

Serious complications and sequelae of hepatitis B virus infection include massive hepatic necrosis, cirrhosis of the liver and chronic active hepatitis. More than one million people worldwide die each year of hepatitis B-associated acute and chronic liver disease.[33] In the United States, hepatitis B-virus-related acute and chronic liver disease causes approximately 4-5000 deaths annually.[29,30]

Reduced Risk of Hepatocellular Carcinoma

Hepatocellular carcinoma is another serious complication of hepatitis B virus infection. Studies have demonstrated the link between chronic hepatitis B infection and hepatocellular carcinoma; 80% of primary liver cancers are caused by hepatitis B virus infection. The CDC has recognized hepatitis B vaccine as the first anti-cancer vaccine because it can prevent primary liver cancer.[34]

There is also evidence that several diseases other than hepatitis have been associated with hepatitis B virus infection through an immunologic mechanism involving antigen-antibody complexes. Such diseases include a syndrome with rash, urticaria, and arthralgia resembling serum sickness; periarteritis nodosa; membranous glomerulonephritis; and infantile papular acrodermatitis.[3,4]

Although the vehicles for transmission of the virus are often blood and blood products, viral antigen has also been found in tears, saliva, breast milk, urine, semen and vaginal secretions. Hepatitis B virus is capable of surviving at least a month[29] on environmental surfaces exposed to body fluids containing hepatitis B virus. Infection may occur when hepatitis B virus, transmitted by infected body fluids, is implanted via mucous surfaces or percutaneously introduced through accidental or deliberate breaks in the skin. Transmission of hepatitis B virus infection is often associated with close interpersonal contact with an infected individual and with crowded living conditions. In such circumstances, transmission by inoculation via routes other than overt percutaneous ones may be quite common.[1] Perinatal transmission of hepatitis B infection from infected mother to child, at or shortly after birth, can occur if the mother is a hepatitis B surface antigen (HBsAg) carrier or if the mother has an acute hepatitis B infection in the third trimester. Infection in infancy by the hepatitis B virus usually leads to the chronic carrier state. Without prophylaxis, infants born to women whose sera are positive for both the hepatitis B surface antigen and the e antigen have an 85-90% likelihood of being infected and becoming a chronic carrier.[5,6] Well-controlled studies have shown that administration of three 0.5 mL doses of Hepatitis B Immune Globulin (Human) - HBIG starting at birth is 75% effective in preventing establishment of the chronic carrier state in these infants during the first year of life.[6] However, the protective effect of HBIG is transient.

Hepatitis B is endemic throughout the world and is a serious medical problem in population groups at increased risk. Because vaccination limited to high-risk individuals has failed to substantially lower the overall incidence of hepatitis B infection, both the Advisory Committee on Immunization Practices (ACIP) and the Committee on Infectious Diseases of the American Academy of Pediatrics (AAP) have also endorsed universal infant immunization as part of a comprehensive strategy for the control of hepatitis B infection.[7,8] In addition, the ACIP also recommends hepatitis B vaccination for all infants and children born after November 21, 1991 and catch-up vaccination of children at high risk of infection (children <11 years of age in households of Pacific Islander ethnicity or of first generation immigrants/refugees from countries with an intermediate or high endemicity of infection).[30] These advisory groups further recommend broad-based vaccination of adolescents. The ACIP recommends that all individuals not previously vaccinated with hepatitis B vaccine be vaccinated at 11-12 years of age with the age-appropriate dose of vaccine and that the vaccination schedule take into account the feasibility of delivering three doses of vaccine to this age group. In addition, older unvaccinated adolescents with identified risk factors for hepatitis B virus infection should also be vaccinated.[30] Similarly, the AAP recommends that universal immunization of all adolescents should be implemented when resources permit with emphasis on those individuals in high-risk settings.[8] A National Institutes of Health Consensus Development Conference Panel on the management of hepatitis C recommends the immunization of all hepatitis C virus (HCV) positive individuals with hepatitis B vaccine.[35] (Refer to INDICATIONS AND USAGE.)

Numerous epidemiological studies have shown that persons who develop anti-HBs following active infection with the hepatitis B virus are protected against the disease on re-exposure to the virus.[9]

Clinical studies have shown that RECOMBIVAX HB when injected into the deltoid muscle induced protective levels of antibody in 96% of 1213 healthy adults who received the recommended 3-dose regimen. Antibody responses varied with age; a protective level of antibody was induced in 98% of 787 young adults 20-29 years of age, 94% of 249 adults 30-39 years of age and in 89% of 177 adults ≥40 years of age.[10] Studies with hepatitis B vaccine derived from plasma have shown that a lower response rate (81%) to vaccine may be obtained if the vaccine is administered as a buttock injection.[11] Seroconversion rates and geometric mean antibody titers were measured 1 to 2 months after the third dose. Multiple clinical studies have defined a protective antibody (anti-HBs) level as 1) 10 or more sample ratio units (SRU) as determined by radioimmunoassay or 2) a positive result as determined by enzyme immunoassay. [2] Note: 10 SRU is comparable to 10 mIU/mL of antibody.[12,13,14,15]

RECOMBIVAX HB was shown to be highly immunogenic in clinical studies involving infants, children, and adolescents. Three 5 mcg doses of vaccine induced a protective level of antibody in 100% of 92 infants, 99% of 129 children, and in 99% of 112 adolescents[10] (see DOSAGE AND ADMINISTRATION).

The protective efficacy of three 5 mcg doses of RECOMBIVAX HB has been demonstrated in neonates born of mothers positive for both HBsAg and HBeAg (a core-associated antigenic complex which correlates with high infectivity). In a clinical study of infants who received one dose of HBIG at birth followed by the recommended three-dose regimen of RECOMBIVAX HB, chronic infection had not occurred in 96% of 130 infants after nine months of follow-up.[16] The estimated efficacy in prevention of chronic hepatitis B infection was 95% as compared to the infection rate in untreated historical controls.[17] Significantly fewer neonates became chronically infected when given one dose of HBIG at birth followed by the recommended three-dose regimen of RECOMBIVAX HB when compared to historical controls who received only a single dose of HBIG.[6] Testing for HBsAg and anti-HBs is recommended at 12-15 months of age. If HBsAg is not detectable, and anti-HBs is present, the child has been protected.

As demonstrated in the above study, HBIG, when administered simultaneously with RECOMBIVAX HB at separate body sites, did not interfere with the induction of protective antibodies against hepatitis B virus elicited by the vaccine.

For adolescents (11 through 15 years of age), the immunogenicity of a two-dose regimen (10 mcg at 0 and 4-6 months) was compared with that of the standard three-dose regimen (5 mcg at 0, 1, and 6 months) in an open, randomized, multicenter study. The proportion of adolescents receiving the two-dose regimen who developed a protective level of antibody one month after the last dose (99% of 255 subjects) appears similar to that among adolescents who received the three-dose regimen (98% of 121 subjects). After adolescents (11 through 15 years of age) received the first 10-mcg dose of the two-dose regimen, the proportion who developed a protective level of antibody was approximately 72%.[10]

In one published study, the seroprotection rates in individuals with chronic HCV infection given the standard regimen of RECOMBIVAX HB was approximately 70%.[36] In a second published study of intravenous drug users given an accelerated schedule of RECOMBIVAX HB, infection with HCV did not affect the response to RECOMBIVAX HB.[37]

As with other hepatitis B vaccines, the duration of the protective effect of RECOMBIVAX HB in healthy vaccinees is unknown at present, and the need for booster doses is not yet defined. However, long-term follow-up (5 to 9 years) of approximately 3000 high-risk vaccinees (infants of carrier mothers, male homosexuals, Alaskan Natives) who developed an anti-HBs titer of ≥10 mIU/mL when given a similar plasma-derived vaccine at intervals of 0, 1, and 6 months showed that no subjects developed clinically apparent hepatitis B infection and that 5 subjects developed antigenemia, even though up to half of the subjects failed to maintain a titer at this level.[18-21] Persistence of vaccine-induced immunologic memory among healthy vaccinees who responded to a primary course of plasma-derived or recombinant hepatitis B vaccine has been demonstrated by an anamnestic antibody response to a booster dose of RECOMBIVAX HB given 5-12 years later.[22]

Predialysis and Dialysis Patients

Predialysis and dialysis adult patients respond less well to hepatitis B vaccines than do healthy individuals; however, vaccination of adult patients early in the course of their renal disease produces higher seroconversion rates than vaccination after dialysis has been initiated.[30] In addition, the responses to these vaccines may be lower if the vaccine is administered as a buttock injection. When 40 mcg of Hepatitis B Vaccine (Recombinant), was administered in the deltoid muscle, 89% of 28 participants developed anti-HBs with 86% achieving levels ≥10 mIU/mL. However, when the same dosage of this vaccine was administered inappropriately either in the buttock or a combination of buttock and deltoid, 62% of 47 participants developed anti-HBs with 55% achieving levels of ≥10 mIU/mL.[10]

A booster dose or revaccination with RECOMBIVAX HB Dialysis Formulation may be considered in predialysis/dialysis patients if the anti-HBs level is less than 10 mIU/mL.[23]

Reports in the literature describe a more virulent form of hepatitis B associated with superinfections or coinfections by delta virus, an incomplete RNA virus. Delta virus can only infect and cause illness in persons infected with hepatitis B virus since the delta agent requires a coat of HBsAg in order to become infectious. Therefore, persons immune to hepatitis B virus infection should also be immune to delta virus infection.[2]

Interchangeability of Plasma-Derived and Recombinant Hepatitis B Vaccines

Although there have been no clinical studies in which a three-dose vaccine series was initiated with HEPTAVAX-B* (Hepatitis B Vaccine) and completed with RECOMBIVAX HB, or vice versa, extensive *in vitro* and *in vivo* studies have demonstrated that these two vaccines are immunologically comparable.[22,24-28]

INDICATIONS AND USAGE

RECOMBIVAX HB is indicated for vaccination against infection caused by all known subtypes of hepatitis B virus. **RECOMBIVAX HB Dialysis Formulation** is indicated for vaccination of adult predialysis and dialysis patients against infection caused by all known subtypes of hepatitis B virus.

Vaccination with RECOMBIVAX HB is recommended for:

1. Infants including those born to HBsAg positive mothers (high-risk infants).
2. Children born after November 21, 1991.[30]
3. Adolescents (see CLINICAL PHARMACOLOGY).
4. Other persons of all ages in areas of high prevalence or those who are or may be at increased risk of infection with hepatitis B virus, such as:[30]

- *Health Care Personnel*
  Dentists and oral surgeons.
  Physicians and surgeons.
  Nurses.
  Paramedical personnel and custodial staff who may be exposed to the virus via blood or other patient specimens.
  Dental hygienists and dental nurses.
  Laboratory personnel handling blood, blood products, and other patient specimens.
  Dental, medical and nursing students.
- *Selected Patients and Patient Contacts*
  Staff in hemodialysis units and hematology/oncology units.
  Hemodialysis patients and patients with early renal failure before they require hemodialysis.
  Patients requiring frequent and/or large volume blood transfusions or clotting factor concentrates (e.g., persons with hemophilia, thalassemia).
  Individuals with hepatitis C virus infection.[35]
  Clients (residents) and staff of institutions for the mentally handicapped.
  Classroom contacts of deinstitutionalized mentally handicapped persons who have persistent hepatitis B surface antigenemia and who show aggressive behavior.
  Household and other intimate contacts of persons with persistent hepatitis B surface antigenemia.
- *Sub-populations with a known high incidence of the disease, such as:*
  Alaskan Natives.
  Pacific Islanders.
  Refugees from areas where hepatitis B virus infection is endemic.
  Adoptees from countries where hepatitis B virus infection is endemic.
- *International Travelers*
- *Military Personnel identified as being at increased risk*
- *Morticians and Embalmers*
- *Blood bank and plasma fractionation workers*
- *Persons at Increased Risk of the Disease Due to Their Sexual Practices, such as:*
  Persons who have heterosexual activity with multiple partners.
  Persons who repeatedly contract sexually transmitted diseases.
  Homosexual and bisexual adolescent and adult men.
  Female prostitutes.
- *Prisoners*
- *Injection drug users*

Neither dosage strength will prevent hepatitis caused by other agents, such as hepatitis A virus, hepatitis C virus, hepatitis E virus or other viruses known to infect the liver.

Revaccination

See CLINICAL PHARMACOLOGY.

Use with Other Vaccines

Results from clinical studies indicate that RECOMBIVAX HB can be administered concomitantly with DTP (Diphtheria, Tetanus and whole cell Pertussis), OPV (oral Poliomyelitis vaccine), M-M-R* II (Measles, Mumps, and Rubella Virus Vaccine Live), Liquid PedvaxHIB* [Haemophilus b Conjugate Vaccine (Meningococcal Protein Conjugate)] or a booster dose of DTaP [Diphtheria, Tetanus, acellular Pertussis], using separate sites and syringes for injectable vaccines. No impairment of immune response to individually tested vaccine antigens was demonstrated.

The type, frequency and severity of adverse experiences observed in these studies with RECOMBIVAX HB were similar to those seen when the other vaccines were given alone.

In addition, an HBsAg-containing product, COMVAX* [Haemophilus b Conjugate (Meningococcal Protein Conjugate) and Hepatitis B (Recombinant) Vaccine], was given concomitantly with eIPV (enhanced inactivated Poliovirus vaccine) or VARIVAX* [Varicella Virus Vaccine Live (Oka/Merck)], using separate sites and syringes for injectable vaccines. No impairment of immune response to these individually tested vaccine antigens was demonstrated. No serious vaccine-related adverse events were reported.

COMVAX has also been administered concomitantly with the primary series of DTaP to a limited number of infants. No serious vaccine-related adverse events were reported.[10]

Separate sites and syringes should be used for simultaneous administration of injectable vaccines.

CONTRAINDICATIONS

Hypersensitivity to yeast or any component of the vaccine.

WARNINGS

Patients who develop symptoms suggestive of hypersensitivity after an injection should not receive further injections of the vaccine (see CONTRAINDICATIONS).

Because of the long incubation period for hepatitis B, it is possible for unrecognized infection to be present at the time the vaccine is given. The vaccine may not prevent hepatitis B in such patients.

PRECAUTIONS

General

As with any percutaneous vaccine, epinephrine (1:1000) should be available for immediate use should an anaphylactoid reaction occur.

Any serious active infection including febrile illness is reason for delaying use of the vaccine except when in the opinion of the physician, withholding the vaccine entails a greater risk.

Caution and appropriate care should be exercised in administering the vaccine to individuals with severely compromised cardiopulmonary status or to others in whom a febrile or systemic reaction could pose a significant risk.

Instructions to Healthcare Provider

The healthcare provider should determine the current health status and previous vaccination history of the vaccinee.

The healthcare provider should question the patient, parent or guardian about reactions to a previous dose of RECOMBIVAX HB or other hepatitis B vaccines.

The healthcare provider must record in the patient's permanent record: the manufacturer, lot number, date of administration, and the name and address of the person administering the vaccine.

Injection of a blood vessel should be avoided.

Information for Vaccine Recipients and Parents / Guardians

The healthcare provider should provide the vaccine information required to be given with each vaccination to the patient, parent or guardian.

The healthcare provider should inform the patient, parent or guardian of the benefits and risks associated with vaccination, as well as the importance of completing the immunization series. For risks associated with vaccination, see WARNINGS, PRECAUTIONS, and ADVERSE REACTIONS.

Patients, parents and guardians should be instructed to report any serious adverse reactions to their healthcare provider, who in turn should report such events to the U.S. Department of Health and Human Services through the Vaccine Adverse Event Reporting System (VAERS), 1-800-822-7967.[31] The healthcare provider should inform the parent or guardian of the National Vaccine Injury Compensation Program (NVICP), 1-800-338-2382.

Drug Interactions

There are no known drug interactions. (See INDICATIONS AND USAGE, *Use with Other Vaccines*.)

Carcinogenesis, Mutagenesis, Impairment of Fertility

RECOMBIVAX HB has not been evaluated for its carcinogenic or mutagenic potential, or its potential to impair fertility.

Pregnancy

Pregnancy Category C: Animal reproduction studies have not been conducted with the vaccine. It is also not known whether the vaccine can cause fetal harm when administered to a pregnant woman or can affect reproduction capacity. The vaccine should be given to a pregnant woman only if clearly needed.

Nursing Mothers

It is not known whether the vaccine is excreted in human milk. Because many drugs are excreted in human milk, caution should be exercised when the vaccine is administered to a nursing woman.

Pediatric Use

RECOMBIVAX HB has been shown to be usually well-tolerated and highly immunogenic in infants and children of all ages. Newborns also respond well; maternally transferred antibodies do not interfere with the active immune response to the vaccine. See DOSAGE AND ADMINISTRATION for recommended pediatric dosage and for recommended dosage for infants born to HBsAg positive mothers. The safety and effectiveness of RECOMBIVAX HB Dialysis Formulation in children have not been established.

Geriatric Use

Clinical studies of RECOMBIVAX HB did not include sufficient numbers of subjects aged 65 and over to determine whether they respond differently from younger subjects. Other reports from the clinical literature indicate that hepatitis B vaccines are less immunogenic in adults aged 65 years or older than in younger individuals.[32] No overall differences in safety were observed between these subjects and younger subjects.

ADVERSE REACTIONS

RECOMBIVAX HB and RECOMBIVAX HB Dialysis Formulation are generally well-tolerated. No adverse experiences were reported during clinical trials which could be related to changes in the titers of antibodies to yeast. As with any vaccine, there is the possibility that broad use of the vaccine could reveal adverse reactions not observed in clinical trials.

In three clinical studies, 434 doses of RECOMBIVAX HB, 5 mcg, were administered to 147 healthy infants and children (up to 10 years of age) who were monitored for 5 days after each dose. Injection site reactions and systemic complaints were reported following 0.2% and 10.4% of the injections, respectively. The most frequently reported systemic adverse reactions (>1% injections), in decreasing order of frequency, were irritability, fever (≥101°F oral equivalent), diarrhea, fatigue/weakness, diminished appetite, and rhinitis.[10]

In a study that compared the three-dose regimen (5 mcg) with the two-dose regimen (10 mcg) of RECOMBIVAX HB in adolescents, the overall frequency of adverse reactions was generally similar.

In a group of studies, 3258 doses of RECOMBIVAX HB, 10 mcg, were administered to 1252 healthy adults who were monitored for 5 days after each dose. Injection site reactions and systemic complaints were reported following 17% and 15% of the injections, respectively. The following adverse reactions were reported:

Incidence Equal To or Greater Than 1% of Injections

LOCAL REACTION (INJECTION SITE)

Injection site reactions consisting principally of soreness, and including pain, tenderness, pruritus, erythema, ecchymosis, swelling, warmth, and nodule formation.

BODY AS A WHOLE

The most frequent systemic complaints include fatigue/weakness; headache; fever (≥100°F); and malaise.

DIGESTIVE SYSTEM

Nausea; and diarrhea

RESPIRATORY SYSTEM

Pharyngitis; and upper respiratory infection

Incidence Less Than 1% of Injections

BODY AS A WHOLE

Sweating; achiness; sensation of warmth; lightheadedness; chills; and flushing

DIGESTIVE SYSTEM

Vomiting; abdominal pains/cramps; dyspepsia; and diminished appetite

RESPIRATORY SYSTEM

Rhinitis; influenza; and cough

NERVOUS SYSTEM

Vertigo/dizziness; and paresthesia

INTEGUMENTARY SYSTEM

Pruritus; rash (non-specified); angioedema; and urticaria

MUSCULOSKELETAL SYSTEM

Arthralgia including monoarticular; myalgia; back pain; neck pain; shoulder pain; and neck stiffness

HEMIC / LYMPHATIC SYSTEM

Lymphadenopathy

PSYCHIATRIC / BEHAVIORAL

Insomnia/disturbed sleep

SPECIAL SENSES

Earache

UROGENITAL SYSTEM

Dysuria

CARDIOVASCULAR SYSTEM

Hypotension

Marketed Experience

The following additional adverse reactions have been reported with use of the marketed vaccine. In many instances, the relationship to the vaccine was unclear.

Hypersensitivity

Anaphylaxis and symptoms of immediate hypersensitivity reactions including rash, pruritus, urticaria, edema, angioedema, dyspnea, chest discomfort, bronchial spasm, palpitation, or symptoms consistent with a hypotensive episode have been reported within the first few hours after vaccination. An apparent hypersensitivity syndrome (serum-sickness-like) of delayed onset has been reported days to weeks after vaccination, including: arthralgia/arthritis (usually transient), fever, and dermatologic reactions such as urticaria, erythema multiforme, ecchymoses and erythema nodosum (see WARNINGS and PRECAUTIONS).

Digestive System

Elevation of liver enzymes; constipation

Nervous System

Guillain-Barré Syndrome; multiple sclerosis; exacerbation of multiple sclerosis; myelitis including transverse myelitis; seizure; febrile seizure; peripheral neuropathy including Bell's Palsy; radiculopathy; herpes zoster; migraine; muscle weakness; hypesthesia; encephalitis

Integumentary System

Stevens-Johnson Syndrome; alopecia; petechiae; eczema

Musculoskeletal System

Arthritis

Pain in extremity

Hematologic

Increased erythrocyte sedimentation rate; thrombocytopenia

Immune System

Systemic lupus erythematosus (SLE); lupus-like syndrome; vasculitis; polyarteritis nodosa

Psychiatric / Behavioral

Irritability; agitation; somnolence

Special Senses

Optic neuritis; tinnitus; conjunctivitis; visual disturbances

Cardiovascular System

Syncope; tachycardia.

The following adverse reaction has been reported with another Hepatitis B Vaccine (Recombinant) but not with RECOMBIVAX HB: keratitis.

Patients, parents and guardians should be instructed to report any serious adverse reactions to their healthcare provider, who in turn should report such events to the U.S. Department of Health and Human Services through the Vaccine Adverse Event Reporting System (VAERS), 1-800-822-7967.[31]

DOSAGE AND ADMINISTRATION

Do not inject intravenously or intradermally.

RECOMBIVAX HB Hepatitis B Vaccine (Recombinant) DIALYSIS FORMULATION [(40 mcg/mL) (WITHOUT PRESERVATIVE)] IS INTENDED ONLY FOR ADULT PREDIALYSIS / DIALYSIS PATIENTS.

RECOMBIVAX HB Hepatitis B Vaccine (Recombinant) PEDIATRIC / ADOLESCENT (WITHOUT PRESERVATIVE) and ADULT FORMULATIONS (WITHOUT PRESERVATIVE) ARE NOT INTENDED FOR USE IN PREDIALYSIS / DIALYSIS PATIENTS.

Three-Dose Regimen

The vaccination regimen for each population consists of 3 doses of vaccine given according to the following schedule:

First dose: at elected date

Second dose: 1 month later

Third dose: 6 months after the first dose

For infants born of mothers who are HBsAg positive or mothers of unknown HBsAg status, treatment recommendations are described in the subsection titled: *Guidelines for Treatment of Infants Born of HBsAg Positive Mothers or Mothers of Unknown HBsAg Status.*

Two-Dose Regimen – Adolescents (11 through 15 years of age)

An alternate two-dose regimen is available for routine vaccination of adolescents (11 through 15 years of age). The regimen consists of two doses of vaccine (10 mcg) given according to the following schedule:

First injection: at elected date

Second injection: 4-6 months later

Table 1 summarizes the dose and formulation of RECOMBIVAX HB for specific populations, regardless of the risk of infection with hepatitis B virus.

[See table 1 at left]

RECOMBIVAX HB is for intramuscular injection. The *deltoid muscle* is the preferred site for intramuscular injection in adults. Data suggest that injections given in the buttocks frequently are given into fatty tissue instead of into muscle. Such injections have resulted in a lower seroconversion rate than was expected. The *anterolateral thigh* is the recommended site for intramuscular injection in infants and young children.

Table 1

Group	Dose/Regimen	Formulation	Color Code
Infants, Children, and Adolescents 0-19 years of age	5 mcg (0.5 mL) 3 × 5 mcg	Pediatric/Adolescent	Yellow
Adolescents* 11 through 15 years of age	10 mcg[†] (1.0 mL) 2 × 10 mcg	Adult	Green
Adults ≥20 years of age	10 mcg[†] (1.0 mL) 3 × 10 mcg	Adult	Green
Predialysis and Dialysis Patients[‡]	40 mcg (1.0 mL) 3 × 40 mcg	Dialysis	Blue

* Adolescents (11 through 15 years of age) may receive either regimen: the 3 × 5 mcg (Pediatric/Adolescent Formulation) or the 2 × 10 mcg (Adult Formulation).

† If the suggested formulation is not available, the appropriate dosage can be achieved from another formulation provided that the total volume of vaccine administered does not exceed 1 mL. However, the Dialysis Formulation may be used only for adult predialysis/dialysis patients.

‡ See also recommendations for revaccination of predialysis and dialysis patients in DOSAGE AND ADMINISTRATION, Revaccination.

For persons at risk of hemorrhage following intramuscular injection, RECOMBIVAX HB may be administered subcutaneously. However, when other aluminum-adsorbed vaccines have been administered subcutaneously, an increased incidence of local reactions including subcutaneous nodules has been observed. Therefore, subcutaneous administration should be used only in persons (e.g., hemophiliacs) who are at risk of hemorrhage following intramuscular injections.

The vaccine should be used as supplied; no dilution or reconstitution is necessary. The full recommended dose of the vaccine should be used.

For All Formulations: Since none of the formulations contain a preservative, once the single-dose vial has been penetrated, the withdrawn vaccine should be used promptly, and the vial must be discarded.

Shake well before use. Thorough agitation at the time of administration is necessary to maintain suspension of the vaccine.

Parenteral drug products should be inspected visually for particulate matter and discoloration prior to administration. After thorough agitation, the vaccine is a slightly opaque, white suspension.

Withdraw the recommended dose from the vial using a sterile needle and syringe free of preservatives, antiseptics, and detergents.

It is important to use a separate sterile syringe and needle for each individual patient to prevent transmission of hepatitis and other infectious agents from one person to another. Needles should be disposed of properly and should not be recapped.

Injection must be accomplished with a needle long enough to ensure intramuscular deposition of the vaccine.

Guidelines for Treatment of Infants Born of HBsAg Positive Mothers or Mothers of Unknown HBsAg Status

Each infant should receive three 5 mcg doses of RECOMBIVAX HB irrespective of the mother's HBsAg status (see Table 1). The ACIP recommends that if the mother is determined to be HBsAg positive within 7 days of delivery, the infant also should be given a dose of HBIG (0.5 mL) immediately. The first dose of RECOMBIVAX HB may be given at the same time as HBIG, but it should be administered in the opposite anterolateral thigh.[7]

Revaccination

The duration of the protective effect of RECOMBIVAX HB in healthy vaccinees is unknown at present and the need for booster doses is not yet defined (see CLINICAL PHARMACOLOGY).

A booster dose or revaccination with RECOMBIVAX HB Dialysis Formulation (blue color code) may be considered in predialysis/dialysis patients if the anti-HBs level is less than 10 mIU/mL 1 to 2 months after the third dose.[23] The ACIP recommends that the need for booster doses of vaccine should be assessed by annual antibody testing and a booster dose given when antibody levels decline to <10 mIU/mL.[30]

Known or Presumed Exposure to HBsAg

There are no prospective studies directly testing the efficacy of a combination of HBIG and RECOMBIVAX HB in preventing clinical hepatitis B following percutaneous, ocular or mucous membrane exposure to hepatitis B virus. However, since most persons with such exposures (e.g., healthcare workers) are candidates for RECOMBIVAX HB and since combined HBIG plus vaccine is more efficacious than HBIG alone in perinatal exposures, the following guidelines are recommended for persons who have been exposed to hepatitis B virus such as through (1) percutaneous (needlestick), ocular, mucous membrane exposure to blood known or presumed to contain HBsAg, (2) human bites by known or presumed HBsAg carriers, that penetrate the skin, or (3) following intimate sexual contact with known or presumed HBsAg carriers.

HBIG (0.06 mL/kg) should be given intramuscularly as soon as possible after exposure and within 24 hours if possible. RECOMBIVAX HB (see dosage recommendation) should be given intramuscularly at a separate site within 7 days of exposure and second and third doses given one and six months, respectively, after the first dose.

Prefilled Syringe

Shake well before use. Attach the needle by twisting in a clockwise direction until the needle fits securely on the syringe. Administer the entire dose as per standard protocol.

HOW SUPPLIED

PEDIATRIC/ADOLESCENT FORMULATION (PRESERVATIVE FREE)

Vials

No. 4980—RECOMBIVAX HB for use in infants, children, and adolescents is supplied as 5 mcg/0.5 mL of HBsAg in a 0.5 mL single-dose vial, color coded with a yellow cap and stripe on the vial labels and cartons and an orange banner on the vial labels and cartons stating "Preservative Free", **NDC** 0006-4980-00.

No. 4981—RECOMBIVAX HB for use in infants, children, and adolescents is supplied as 5 mcg/0.5 mL of HBsAg in a 0.5 mL single-dose vial, in a box of 10 single-dose vials, color coded with a yellow cap and stripe on the vial labels and cartons and an orange banner on the vial labels and cartons stating "Preservative Free", **NDC** 0006-4981-00.

Syringes

No. 4093—RECOMBIVAX HB for use in infants, children and adolescents is supplied as 5 mcg/0.5 mL of HBsAg in a carton of 6 prefilled single-dose Luer Lock syringes with tip caps, color coded with a yellow plunger rod and stripe on the peel-off syringe labels and cartons and an orange banner on the cartons stating "Preservative Free", **NDC** 0006-4093-09.

ADULT FORMULATION (PRESERVATIVE FREE)

Vials

No. 4995—RECOMBIVAX HB for use in adults and adolescents (11 through 15 years of age) is supplied as 10 mcg/mL of HBsAg in a 1 mL single-dose vial, color coded with a green cap and stripe on the vial labels and cartons and an orange banner on the vial labels and cartons stating "Preservative Free", **NDC** 0006-4995-00.

No. 4995—RECOMBIVAX HB for use in adults and adolescents (11 through 15 years of age) is supplied as 10 mcg/mL of HBsAg in a 1 mL single-dose vial, in a box of 10 single-dose vials, color coded with a green cap and stripe on the vial labels and cartons and an orange banner on the vial labels and cartons stating "Preservative Free", **NDC** 0006-4995-41.

Syringes

No. 4094—RECOMBIVAX HB for use in adults and adolescents (11 through 15 years of age) is supplied as 10 mcg/1.0 mL HBsAg in a carton of 6 single-dose prefilled Luer Lock syringes with tip caps, color coded with a green plunger rod and stripe on the peel-off syringe labels and cartons and an orange banner on the carton stating "Preservative Free", **NDC** 0006-4094-09.

DIALYSIS FORMULATION (PRESERVATIVE FREE)

Vials

No. 4992—RECOMBIVAX 4992—RECOMBIVAX HB Dialysis Formulation is supplied as 40 mcg/mL of HBsAg in a 1 mL single-dose vial, color coded with a blue cap and stripe on the vial labels and cartons and an orange banner on the vial labels and cartons stating "Preservative Free", **NDC** 0006-4992-00.

Storage

Store vials and syringes at 2-8°C (36-46°F). Storage above or below the recommended temperature may reduce potency.

Do not freeze since freezing destroys potency.

REFERENCES

1. Robinson, W.S.: Hepatitis B Virus and the Delta Virus, in "Principles and Practice of Infectious Diseases," G.L. Mandell; R.G. Douglas; J.E. Bennett (eds), vol. 2, New York, John Wiley & Sons, 1002-1029, 1985.
2. Recommendation of the Immunization Practices Advisory Committee (ACIP): Protection Against Viral Hepatitis, MMWR *39*(RR-2): 5-22, Feb. 9, 1990.
3. Balistreri, W.F.: Viral Hepatitis, Unique Aspects of Infection During Childhood, Consultant *24*(4): 131-153 passim, April 1984.
4. Robinson, W.S.: Hepatitis B Virus and Hepatitis Delta Virus, in "Principles and Practice of Infectious Diseases," G.L. Mandell, R.G. Douglas, and J.E. Bennett (eds), Churchill Livingstone, 1204-1231, 1990.
5. Stevens, C.E.; Toy, P.T.; Tong, M.J.; Taylor, P.E.; Vyas, G.N.; Nair, P.V.; Gudavalli, M.; Krugman, S.: Perinatal Hepatitis B Virus Transmission in the United States, JAMA *253*(12): 1740-1745, 1985.
6. Beasley, R.P.; Hwang, L.; Stevens, C.E.; Lin, C.; Hsieh, F.; Wang, K.; Sun, T.; Szmuness, W.: Efficacy of Hepatitis B Immune Globulin for Prevention of Perinatal Transmission of the Hepatitis B Virus Carrier State: Final Report of a Randomized Double-Blind, Placebo-Controlled Trial, Hepatology *3:* 135-141, 1983.
7. Recommendations of the Immunization Practices Advisory Committee (ACIP): Hepatitis B Virus: A Comprehensive Strategy for Eliminating Transmission in the United States Through Universal Childhood Vaccination, MMWR *40*(RR-13): 1-25, November 22, 1991.
8. Universal Hepatitis B Immunization, Committee on Infectious Diseases, Pediatrics *89*(4): 795-800, 1992.
9. Melnick, J.L.: Historical Aspects of Hepatitis B Vaccine, in "Hepatitis B Vaccine INSERM Symposium No. 18," P. Maupas and P. Guesry (eds), Elsevier/North-Holland Biomedical Press, 23-31, 1981.
10. Data on file at Merck Research Laboratories.
11. Centers for Disease Control: Suboptimal Response to Hepatitis B Vaccine Given by Injection into the Buttock. MMWR *34*(8): 105-113, March 1, 1985.
12. Hadler, S.C., et al.: Long-term Immunogenicity and Efficacy of Hepatitis B Vaccine in Homosexual Men, NEJM *315:* 209-214, 1986.
13. Szmuness, W.; Stevens, C.E.; Horley, H.J., et al.: Hepatitis B Vaccine. Demonstration of Efficacy in a Controlled Clinical Trial in a High-risk Population in the United States. NEJM *303:* 833-841, 1980.
14. Francis, D.P.; Hadler, S.C.; Thompson, S.E., et al.: The Prevention of Hepatitis B with Vaccine. Report of the Centers for Disease Control Multi-center Efficacy Trial among Homosexual Men. Ann. Int. Med. *97:* 362-366, 1982.
15. Szmuness, W.; Stevens, C.E.; Horley, H.J., et al.: Hepatitis B Vaccine in Medical Staff of Hemodialysis Units. Efficacy and Subtype Cross-protection, NEJM *307:* 1481-1486, 1982.
16. Stevens, C.E.; Taylor, P.E.; Tong, M.J., et al.: Prevention of Perinatal Hepatitis B Virus Infection with Hepatitis B Immune Globulin and Hepatitis B Vaccine, in Zuckerman, A.J. (ed.), "Viral Hepatitis and Liver Diseases", Alan R. Liss, 982-983, 1988.
17. Stevens, C.E.; Taylor, P.E.; Tong, M.J., et al.: Yeast-Recombinant Hepatitis B Vaccine, Efficacy with Hepatitis B Immune Globulin in Prevention of Perinatal Hepatitis B Virus Transmission, JAMA *257*(19): 2612-2616, 1987.
18. Wainwright, R.B.; McMahon, B.J.; Bulkow, L.R., et al.: Duration of Immunogenicity and Efficacy of Hepatitis B Vaccine in a Yupik Eskimo Population, Preliminary Results of an 8-Year Study, in "Viral Hepatitis and Liver Disease," F.B. Hollinger, S.M. Lemon, and H. Margolis (eds), Williams & Wilkins, 762-766, 1990.
19. Hadler, S.C.; Coleman, P.J.; O'Malley, P., et al.: Evaluation of Long-Term Protection by Hepatitis B Vaccine for Seven to Nine Years in Homosexual Men, in "Viral Hepatitis and Liver Disease," F.B. Hollinger, S.M. Lemon, and H. Margolis (eds), Williams & Wilkins, 766-768, 1990.
20. Tong, M.J.; Stevens, C.E.; Taylor, P.E., et al.: Prevention of Hepatitis B Infection in Infants Born to HBeAg Positive HBsAg Carrier Mothers in the United States, in "An Update, 1989, Progress in Hepatitis B Immunization," P. Coursaget and M.J. Tong (eds), Colloque INSERM/John Libbey Eurotext Ltd., Vol. 194, 339-345, 1990.
21. Hwang, L-Y.; Lee, C-Y.; and Beasley, R.P.: Five-Year Follow-up of HBV Vaccination with Plasma-derived Vaccine in Neonates: Evaluation of Immunogenicity and Efficacy Against Perinatal Transmission, in "Viral Hepatitis and Liver Disease," F.B. Hollinger, S.M. Lemon, and H. Margolis (eds), Williams & Wilkins, 759-761, 1990.
22. West, D.J.; Calandra, G.B.: Vaccine Induced Immunologic Memory for Hepatitis B Surface Antigen; Implications for Policy on Booster Vaccination, Vaccine, *14*(11): 1019-1027, 1996.
23. Recommendations of the Immunization Practices Advisory Committee (ACIP): Update on Hepatitis B Prevention, MMWR *36*(23): 353-366, June 19, 1987.
24. Emini, E.A.; Ellis, R.W.; Miller, W.J.; McAleer, W.J.; Scolnick, E.M. and Gerety, R.J.: Production and Immunological Analysis of Recombinant Hepatitis B Vaccine, J. Infection, *13*(Sup. A): 3-9, 1986.
25. Brown, S.E.; Stanley, C.; Howard, C.R.; Zuckerman, A.J.; Steward, M.W.: Antibody Responses to Recombinant and Plasma-derived Hepatitis B Vaccines, Brit. Med. J., *292:* 159-161, 1986.
26. Yamamoto, S.; Kuroki, T.; Kurai, K.; Iino, S.: Comparison of Results for Phase I Studies with Recombinant and Plasma-derived Hepatitis B Vaccines, and Controlled Study Comparing Intramuscular and Subcutaneous Injections of Recombinant Hepatitis B Vaccine, J. Infection, *13*(Sup. A): 53-60, 1986.
27. Jilg, W.; Schmidt, M.; Zoulek, G.; Lorbeer, B.; Wilske, B.; Deinhardt, F.: Clinical Evaluation of a Recombinant Hepatitis B Vaccine, Lancet, 1174-1175, Nov. 24, 1984.
28. Schalm, S.W.; Heytink, R.A.; Kruining, H.; Bakker-Bendik, M.: Immunogenicity of Recombinant Yeast Hepatitis-B Vaccine, Neth. J. Med. *29:* 28, 1986.
29. Centers for Disease Control: Epidemiology and Prevention of Vaccine-preventative Diseases, W. Atkinson, L. Furphy, J. Gantt, M. Mayfield, G. Phyne (eds), chapter 9.
30. Recommendations of the Advisory Committee on Immunization Practices (ACIP): Hepatitis B Virus Infection: A Comprehensive Strategy to Eliminate Transmission in the United States, 1996 update, MMWR (draft January 13, 1996).
31. Vaccine Adverse Event Reporting System - United States. MMWR *39*(41): 730-733, October 19, 1990.
32. Zajac, B.A.; West, D.J.; McAleer, W.J.; Scolnick, E.M.: Overview of Clinical Studies with Hepatitis B Vaccine Made by Recombinant DNA, J. Infection, *13*(Sup. A): 39-45, July 1986.
33. WHO Bulletin, Expanded Programme on Immunization, Hepatitis B Vaccine – Making Global Progress. October, 1996.
34. Centers for Disease Control and Prevention, Federal Register, February 23, 1999, *64*(35): 9044-9045.
35. National Institutes of Health, National Institutes of Health Consensus Development Conference Panel

Statement: Management of Hepatitis C, Hepatology, *26*(Suppl. 1): 2S-10S, 1997.

36. Wiedmann, M.; Liebert, U.G.; Oesen, U.; Porst, H.; Wiese, M.; Schroeder, S.; Halm, U.; Mossner, J.; Berr, F.: Decreased Immunogenicity of Recombinant Hepatitis B Vaccine in Chronic Hepatitis C, Hepatology, *31:* 230-234, 2000.
37. Minniti, F.; Baldo, V.; Trivello, R.; Bricolo, R.; Di Furia, L.; Renzulli, G.; Chiaramonte, M.: Response to HBV vaccine in Relation to anti-HCV and anti-HBc Positivity: a Study in Intravenous Drug Addicts, Vaccine, *17:* 3083-3085, 1999.

Manuf. and Dist. by:
MERCK & CO., INC., Whitehouse Station, NJ 08889, USA
Issued March 2010
Printed in USA
9987433

REMERON® ℞

[rem-er-on]
(mirtazapine)
Tablets

Suicidality and Antidepressant Drugs

Antidepressants increased the risk compared to placebo of suicidal thinking and behavior (suicidality) in children, adolescents, and young adults in short-term studies of major depressive disorder (MDD) and other psychiatric disorders. Anyone considering the use of REMERON® (mirtazapine) Tablets or any other antidepressant in a child, adolescent, or young adult must balance this risk with the clinical need. Short-term studies did not show an increase in the risk of suicidality with antidepressants compared to placebo in adults beyond age 24; there was a reduction in risk with antidepressants compared to placebo in adults aged 65 and older. Depression and certain other psychiatric disorders are themselves associated with increases in the risk of suicide. Patients of all ages who are started on antidepressant therapy should be monitored appropriately and observed closely for clinical worsening, suicidality, or unusual changes in behavior. Families and caregivers should be advised of the need for close observation and communication with the prescriber. REMERON is not approved for use in pediatric patients. (See WARNINGS: Clinical Worsening and Suicide Risk, PRECAUTIONS: Information for Patients, and PRECAUTIONS: Pediatric Use)

DESCRIPTION

REMERON® (mirtazapine) Tablets are an orally administered drug. Mirtazapine has a tetracyclic chemical structure and belongs to the piperazino-azepine group of compounds. It is designated 1,2,3,4,10,14b-hexahydro-2-methylpyrazino [2,1-a] pyrido [2,3-c] benzazepine and has the empirical formula of $C_{17}H_{19}N_3$. Its molecular weight is 265.36. The structural formula is the following and it is the racemic mixture:

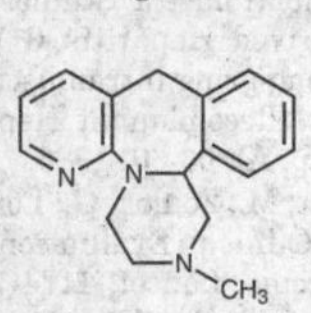

Mirtazapine is a white to creamy white crystalline powder which is slightly soluble in water.

REMERON is supplied for oral administration as scored film-coated tablets containing 15 or 30 mg of mirtazapine, and unscored film-coated tablets containing 45 mg of mirtazapine. Each tablet also contains corn starch, hydroxypropyl cellulose, magnesium stearate, colloidal silicon dioxide, lactose, and other inactive ingredients.

CLINICAL PHARMACOLOGY

Pharmacodynamics

The mechanism of action of REMERON® (mirtazapine) Tablets, as with other drugs effective in the treatment of major depressive disorder, is unknown.

Evidence gathered in preclinical studies suggests that mirtazapine enhances central noradrenergic and serotonergic activity. These studies have shown that mirtazapine acts as an antagonist at central presynaptic α_2 adrenergic inhibitory autoreceptors and heteroreceptors, an action that is postulated to result in an increase in central noradrenergic and serotonergic activity.

Mirtazapine is a potent antagonist of 5-HT_2 and 5-HT_3 receptors. Mirtazapine has no significant affinity for the 5-HT_{1A} and 5-HT_{1B} receptors.

Mirtazapine is a potent antagonist of histamine (H_1) receptors, a property that may explain its prominent sedative effects.

Mirtazapine is a moderate peripheral α_1 adrenergic antagonist, a property that may explain the occasional orthostatic hypotension reported in association with its use.

Mirtazapine is a moderate antagonist at muscarinic receptors, a property that may explain the relatively low incidence of anticholinergic side effects associated with its use.

Pharmacokinetics

REMERON (mirtazapine) Tablets are rapidly and completely absorbed following oral administration and have a half-life of about 20 to 40 hours. Peak plasma concentrations are reached within about 2 hours following an oral dose. The presence of food in the stomach has a minimal effect on both the rate and extent of absorption and does not require a dosage adjustment.

Mirtazapine is extensively metabolized after oral administration. Major pathways of biotransformation are demethylation and hydroxylation followed by glucuronide conjugation. *In vitro* data from human liver microsomes indicate that cytochrome 2D6 and 1A2 are involved in the formation of the 8-hydroxy metabolite of mirtazapine, whereas cytochrome 3A is considered to be responsible for the formation of the N-desmethyl and N-oxide metabolite. Mirtazapine has an absolute bioavailability of about 50%. It is eliminated predominantly via urine (75%) with 15% in feces. Several unconjugated metabolites possess pharmacological activity but are present in the plasma at very low levels. The (–) enantiomer has an elimination half-life that is approximately twice as long as the (+) enantiomer and therefore achieves plasma levels that are about 3 times as high as that of the (+) enantiomer.

Plasma levels are linearly related to dose over a dose range of 15 to 80 mg. The mean elimination half-life of mirtazapine after oral administration ranges from approximately 20 to 40 hours across age and gender subgroups, with females of all ages exhibiting significantly longer elimination half-lives than males (mean half-life of 37 hours for females vs 26 hours for males). Steady state plasma levels of mirtazapine are attained within 5 days, with about 50% accumulation (accumulation ratio = 1.5).

Mirtazapine is approximately 85% bound to plasma proteins over a concentration range of 0.01 to 10 mcg/mL.

Special Populations

Geriatric

Following oral administration of REMERON (mirtazapine) Tablets 20 mg/day for 7 days to subjects of varying ages (range, 25–74), oral clearance of mirtazapine was reduced in the elderly compared to the younger subjects. The differences were most striking in males, with a 40% lower clearance in elderly males compared to younger males, while the clearance in elderly females was only 10% lower compared to younger females. Caution is indicated in administering REMERON to elderly patients (see PRECAUTIONS and DOSAGE AND ADMINISTRATION).

Pediatrics

Safety and effectiveness of mirtazapine in the pediatric population have not been established (see PRECAUTIONS).

Gender

The mean elimination half-life of mirtazapine after oral administration ranges from approximately 20 to 40 hours across age and gender subgroups, with females of all ages exhibiting significantly longer elimination half-lives than males (mean half-life of 37 hours for females vs. 26 hours for males) (see Pharmacokinetics).

Race

There have been no clinical studies to evaluate the effect of race on the pharmacokinetics of REMERON.

Renal Insufficiency

The disposition of mirtazapine was studied in patients with varying degrees of renal function. Elimination of mirtazapine is correlated with creatinine clearance. Total body clearance of mirtazapine was reduced approximately 30% in patients with moderate (Clcr = 11–39 mL/min/1.73 m^2) and approximately 50% in patients with severe (Clcr = <10 mL/min/1.73 m^2) renal impairment when compared to normal subjects. Caution is indicated in administering REMERON to patients with compromised renal function (see PRECAUTIONS and DOSAGE AND ADMINISTRATION).

Hepatic Insufficiency

Following a single 15-mg oral dose of REMERON, the oral clearance of mirtazapine was decreased by approximately 30% in hepatically impaired patients compared to subjects with normal hepatic function. Caution is indicated in administering REMERON to patients with compromised hepatic function (see PRECAUTIONS and DOSAGE AND ADMINISTRATION).

Clinical Trials Showing Effectiveness

The efficacy of REMERON (mirtazapine) Tablets as a treatment for major depressive disorder was established in 4 placebo-controlled, 6-week trials in adult outpatients meeting DSM-III criteria for major depressive disorder. Patients were titrated with mirtazapine from a dose range of 5 mg up to 35 mg/day. Overall, these studies demonstrated mirtazapine to be superior to placebo on at least 3 of the following 4 measures: 21-Item Hamilton Depression Rating Scale (HDRS) total score; HDRS Depressed Mood Item; CGI Severity score; and Montgomery and Asberg Depression Rating Scale (MADRS). Superiority of mirtazapine over placebo was also found for certain factors of the HDRS, including anxiety/somatization factor and sleep disturbance factor. The mean mirtazapine dose for patients who completed these 4 studies ranged from 21 to 32 mg/day. A fifth study of similar design utilized a higher dose (up to 50 mg) per day and also showed effectiveness.

Examination of age and gender subsets of the population did not reveal any differential responsiveness on the basis of these subgroupings.

In a longer-term study, patients meeting (DSM-IV) criteria for major depressive disorder who had responded during an initial 8 to 12 weeks of acute treatment on REMERON were randomized to continuation of REMERON or placebo for up to 40 weeks of observation for relapse. Response during the open phase was defined as having achieved a HAM-D 17 total score of ≤8 and a CGI-Improvement score of 1 or 2 at 2 consecutive visits beginning with week 6 of the 8 to 12 weeks in the open-label phase of the study. Relapse during the double-blind phase was determined by the individual investigators. Patients receiving continued REMERON treatment experienced significantly lower relapse rates over the subsequent 40 weeks compared to those receiving placebo. This pattern was demonstrated in both male and female patients.

INDICATIONS AND USAGE

REMERON® (mirtazapine) Tablets are indicated for the treatment of major depressive disorder.

The efficacy of REMERON in the treatment of major depressive disorder was established in 6-week controlled trials of outpatients whose diagnoses corresponded most closely to the Diagnostic and Statistical Manual of Mental Disorders – 3rd edition (DSM-III) category of major depressive disorder (see CLINICAL PHARMACOLOGY).

A major depressive episode (DSM-IV) implies a prominent and relatively persistent (nearly every day for at least 2 weeks) depressed or dysphoric mood that usually interferes with daily functioning, and includes at least 5 of the following 9 symptoms: depressed mood, loss of interest in usual activities, significant change in weight and/or appetite, insomnia or hypersomnia, psychomotor agitation or retardation, increased fatigue, feelings of guilt or worthlessness, slowed thinking or impaired concentration, a suicide attempt, or suicidal ideation.

The effectiveness of REMERON in hospitalized depressed patients has not been adequately studied.

The efficacy of REMERON in maintaining a response in patients with major depressive disorder for up to 40 weeks following 8 to 12 weeks of initial open-label treatment was demonstrated in a placebo-controlled trial. Nevertheless, the physician who elects to use REMERON for extended periods should periodically re-evaluate the long-term usefulness of the drug for the individual patient (see CLINICAL PHARMACOLOGY).

CONTRAINDICATIONS

Hypersensitivity

REMERON® (mirtazapine) Tablets are contraindicated in patients with a known hypersensitivity to mirtazapine or to any of the excipients.

Monoamine Oxidase Inhibitors

The concomitant use of REMERON Tablets and a monoamine oxidase (MAO) inhibitor is contraindicated. REMERON should not be used within 14 days of initiating or discontinuing therapy with a monoamine oxidase inhibitor (MAOI) (see WARNINGS, PRECAUTIONS: Drug Interactions, and DOSAGE AND ADMINISTRATION).

WARNINGS

Clinical Worsening and Suicide Risk

Patients with major depressive disorder (MDD), both adult and pediatric, may experience worsening of their depression and/or the emergence of suicidal ideation and behavior (suicidality) or unusual changes in behavior, whether or not they are taking antidepressant medications, and this risk may persist until significant remission occurs. Suicide is a known risk of depression and certain other psychiatric disorders, and these disorders themselves are the strongest predictors of suicide. There has been a long-standing concern, however, that antidepressants may have a role in inducing worsening of depression and the emergence of suicidality in certain patients during the early phases of treatment. Pooled analyses of short-term placebo-controlled trials of antidepressant drugs (SSRIs and others) showed that these drugs increase the risk of suicidal thinking and behavior (suicidality) in children, adolescents, and young adults (ages 18–24) with major depressive disorder (MDD) and other psychiatric disorders. Short-term studies did not show an increase in the risk of suicidality with antidepressants compared to placebo in adults beyond age 24; there was a reduction in risk with antidepressants compared to placebo in adults aged 65 and older.

The pooled analyses of placebo-controlled trials in children and adolescents with MDD, obsessive compulsive disorder (OCD), or other psychiatric disorders included a total of 24 short-term trials of 9 antidepressant drugs in over 4400 patients. The pooled analyses of placebo-controlled trials in adults with MDD or other psychiatric disorders included a total of 295 short-term trials (median duration of 2 months) of 11 antidepressant drugs in over 77,000 patients. There was considerable variation in risk of suicidality among drugs, but a tendency toward an increase in the younger patients for almost all drugs studied. There were differences in absolute risk of suicidality across different indications, with the highest incidence in MDD. The risk differences (drug vs. placebo), however, were relatively stable within age strata and across indications. These risk differences (drug-placebo difference in the number of cases of suicidality per 1000 patients treated) are provided in Table 1.

Table 1

Age Range	Drug-Placebo Difference in Number of Cases of Suicidality per 1000 Patients Treated
	Increases Compared to Placebo
<18	14 additional cases
18–24	5 additional cases
	Decreases Compared to Placebo
25–64	1 fewer case
≥65	6 fewer cases

No suicides occurred in any of the pediatric trials. There were suicides in the adult trials, but the number was not sufficient to reach any conclusion about drug effect on suicide.

It is unknown whether the suicidality risk extends to longer-term use, i.e., beyond several months. However, there is substantial evidence from placebo-controlled maintenance trials in adults with depression that the use of antidepressants can delay the recurrence of depression.

All patients being treated with antidepressants for any indication should be monitored appropriately and observed closely for clinical worsening, suicidality, and unusual changes in behavior, especially during the initial few months of a course of drug therapy, or at times of dose changes, either increases or decreases.

The following symptoms, anxiety, agitation, panic attacks, insomnia, irritability, hostility, aggressiveness, impulsivity, akathisia (psychomotor restlessness), hypomania, and mania, have been reported in adult and pediatric patients being treated with antidepressants for major depressive disorder as well as for other indications, both psychiatric and nonpsychiatric. Although a causal link between the emergence of such symptoms and either the worsening of depression and/or the emergence of suicidal impulses has not been established, there is concern that such symptoms may represent precursors to emerging suicidality.

Consideration should be given to changing the therapeutic regimen, including possibly discontinuing the medication, in patients whose depression is persistently worse, or who are experiencing emergent suicidality or symptoms that might be precursors to worsening depression or suicidality, especially if these symptoms are severe, abrupt in onset, or were not part of the patient's presenting symptoms.

Families and caregivers of patients being treated with antidepressants for major depressive disorder or other indications, both psychiatric and nonpsychiatric, should be alerted about the need to monitor patients for the emergence of agitation, irritability, unusual changes in behavior, and the other symptoms described above, as well as the emergence of suicidality, and to report such symptoms immediately to health care providers. Such monitoring should include daily observation by families and caregivers. Prescriptions for REMERON® (mirtazapine) Tablets should be written for the smallest quantity of tablets consistent with good patient management, in order to reduce the risk of overdose.

Screening Patients for Bipolar Disorder

A major depressive episode may be the initial presentation of bipolar disorder. It is generally believed (though not established in controlled trials) that treating such an episode with an antidepressant alone may increase the likelihood of precipitation of a mixed/manic episode in patients at risk for bipolar disorder. Whether any of the symptoms described above represent such a conversion is unknown. However, prior to initiating treatment with an antidepressant, patients with depressive symptoms should be adequately screened to determine if they are at risk for bipolar disorder; such screening should include a detailed psychiatric history, including a family history of suicide, bipolar disorder, and depression. It should be noted that REMERON (mirtazapine) Tablets are not approved for use in treating bipolar depression.

Agranulocytosis

In premarketing clinical trials, 2 (1 with Sjögren's Syndrome) out of 2796 patients treated with REMERON (mirtazapine) Tablets developed agranulocytosis [absolute neutrophil count (ANC) <500/mm^3 with associated signs and symptoms, e.g., fever, infection, etc.] and a third patient developed severe neutropenia (ANC <500/mm^3 without any associated symptoms). For these 3 patients, onset of severe neutropenia was detected on days 61, 9, and 14 of treatment, respectively. All 3 patients recovered after REMERON was stopped. These 3 cases yield a crude incidence of severe neutropenia (with or without associated infection) of approximately 1.1 per thousand patients exposed, with a very wide 95% confidence interval, i.e., 2.2 cases per 10,000 to 3.1 cases per 1000. If a patient develops a sore throat, fever, stomatitis, or other signs of infection, along with a low WBC count, treatment with REMERON should be discontinued and the patient should be closely monitored.

MAO Inhibitors

In patients receiving other drugs for major depressive disorder in combination with a monoamine oxidase inhibitor (MAOI) and in patients who have recently discontinued a drug for major depressive disorder and then are started on an MAOI, there have been reports of serious and sometimes fatal reactions, including nausea, vomiting, flushing, dizziness, tremor, myoclonus, rigidity, diaphoresis, hyperthermia, autonomic instability with rapid fluctuations of vital signs, seizures, and mental status changes ranging from agitation to coma. Although there are no human data pertinent to such an interaction with REMERON (mirtazapine) Tablets, it is recommended that REMERON not be used in combination with an MAOI, or within 14 days of initiating or discontinuing therapy with an MAOI.

Serotonin Syndrome

On rare occasions serotonin syndrome has occurred in association with treatment of REMERON Tablets, particularly when given in combination with other serotonergic drugs. As serotonin syndrome may result in potentially life-threatening conditions, treatment with REMERON should be discontinued if patients develop a combination of symptoms possibly including hyperthermia, rigidity, myoclonus, autonomic instability with possible rapid fluctuations of vital signs, mental status changes including confusion, irritability, extreme agitation progressing to delirium and coma, and supportive symptomatic treatment should be initiated. Due to the risk of serotonin syndrome, REMERON should not be used in combination with MAO inhibitors or serotonin-precursors (such as L-tryptophan and oxitriptan) and should be used with caution in patients receiving other serotonergic drugs (e.g., triptans, lithium, tramadol, St. John's wort, and most tricyclic antidepressants) (see CONTRAINDICATIONS and PRECAUTIONS: Drug Interactions).

PRECAUTIONS

General

Discontinuation Symptoms

There have been reports of adverse reactions upon the discontinuation of REMERON® (mirtazapine) Tablets (particularly when abrupt), including but not limited to the following: dizziness, abnormal dreams, sensory disturbances (including paresthesia and electric shock sensations), agitation, anxiety, fatigue, confusion, headache, tremor, nausea, vomiting, and sweating, or other symptoms which may be of clinical significance. The majority of the reported cases are mild and self-limiting. Even though these have been reported as adverse reactions, it should be realized that these symptoms may be related to underlying disease.

Patients currently taking REMERON should NOT discontinue treatment abruptly, due to risk of discontinuation symptoms. At the time that a medical decision is made to discontinue treatment with REMERON, a gradual reduction in the dose, rather than an abrupt cessation, is recommended.

Akathisia/Psychomotor Restlessness

The use of antidepressants has been associated with the development of akathisia, characterized by a subjectively unpleasant or distressing restlessness and need to move, often accompanied by an inability to sit or stand still. This is most likely to occur within the first few weeks of treatment. In patients who develop these symptoms, increasing the dose may be detrimental.

Hyponatremia

Hyponatremia has been reported very rarely with the use of mirtazapine. Caution should be exercised in patients at risk, such as elderly patients or patients concomitantly treated with medications known to cause hyponatremia.

Somnolence

In US controlled studies, somnolence was reported in 54% of patients treated with REMERON (mirtazapine) Tablets, compared to 18% for placebo and 60% for amitriptyline. In these studies, somnolence resulted in discontinuation for 10.4% of REMERON-treated patients, compared to 2.2% for placebo. It is unclear whether or not tolerance develops to the somnolent effects of REMERON. Because of the potentially significant effects of REMERON on impairment of performance, patients should be cautioned about engaging in activities requiring alertness until they have been able to assess the drug's effect on their own psychomotor performance (see Information for Patients).

Dizziness

In US controlled studies, dizziness was reported in 7% of patients treated with REMERON, compared to 3% for placebo and 14% for amitriptyline. It is unclear whether or not tolerance develops to the dizziness observed in association with the use of REMERON.

Increased Appetite/Weight Gain

In US controlled studies, appetite increase was reported in 17% of patients treated with REMERON, compared to 2% for placebo and 6% for amitriptyline. In these same trials, weight gain of ≥7% of body weight was reported in 7.5% of patients treated with mirtazapine, compared to 0% for placebo and 5.9% for amitriptyline. In a pool of premarketing US studies, including many patients for long-term, open-label treatment, 8% of patients receiving REMERON discontinued for weight gain. In an 8-week-long pediatric clinical trial of doses between 15 to 45 mg/day, 49% of REMERON-treated patients had a weight gain of at least 7%, compared to 5.7% of placebo-treated patients (see PRECAUTIONS: Pediatric Use).

Cholesterol/Triglycerides

In US controlled studies, nonfasting cholesterol increases to ≥20% above the upper limits of normal were observed in 15% of patients treated with REMERON, compared to 7% for placebo and 8% for amitriptyline. In these same studies, nonfasting triglyceride increases to ≥ 500 mg/dL were observed in 6% of patients treated with mirtazapine, compared to 3% for placebo and 3% for amitriptyline.

Transaminase Elevations

Clinically significant ALT (SGPT) elevations (≥3 times the upper limit of the normal range) were observed in 2.0% (8/424) of patients exposed to REMERON in a pool of short-term US controlled trials, compared to 0.3% (1/328) of placebo patients and 2.0% (3/181) of amitriptyline patients. Most of these patients with ALT increases did not develop signs or symptoms associated with compromised liver function. While some patients were discontinued for the ALT increases, in other cases, the enzyme levels returned to normal despite continued REMERON treatment. REMERON should be used with caution in patients with impaired hepatic function (see CLINICAL PHARMACOLOGY and DOSAGE AND ADMINISTRATION).

Activation of Mania/Hypomania

Mania/hypomania occurred in approximately 0.2% (3/1299 patients) of REMERON-treated patients in US studies. Although the incidence of mania/hypomania was very low during treatment with mirtazapine, it should be used carefully in patients with a history of mania/hypomania.

Seizure

In premarketing clinical trials, only 1 seizure was reported among the 2796 US and non-US patients treated with REMERON. However, no controlled studies have been carried out in patients with a history of seizures. Therefore, care should be exercised when mirtazapine is used in these patients.

Use in Patients with Concomitant Illness

Clinical experience with REMERON in patients with concomitant systemic illness is limited. Accordingly, care is advisable in prescribing mirtazapine for patients with diseases or conditions that affect metabolism or hemodynamic responses.

REMERON has not been systematically evaluated or used to any appreciable extent in patients with a recent history of myocardial infarction or other significant heart disease. REMERON was associated with significant orthostatic hypotension in early clinical pharmacology trials with normal volunteers. Orthostatic hypotension was infrequently observed in clinical trials with depressed patients. REMERON should be used with caution in patients with known cardiovascular or cerebrovascular disease that could be exacerbated by hypotension (history of myocardial infarction, angina, or ischemic stroke) and conditions that would predispose patients to hypotension (dehydration, hypovolemia, and treatment with antihypertensive medication).

Mirtazapine clearance is decreased in patients with moderate [glomerular filtration rate (GFR) = 11–39 mL/min/1.73 m^2] and severe [GFR <10 mL/min/1.73 m^2] renal impairment, and also in patients with hepatic impairment.

Caution is indicated in administering REMERON to such patients (see CLINICAL PHARMACOLOGY and DOSAGE AND ADMINISTRATION).

Information for Patients
Prescribers or other health professionals should inform patients, their families, and their caregivers about the benefits and risks associated with treatment with REMERON (mirtazapine) Tablets and should counsel them in its appropriate use. A patient Medication Guide about "Antidepressant Medicines, Depression and other Serious Mental Illnesses, and Suicidal Thoughts or Actions" is available for REMERON. The prescriber or health professional should instruct patients, their families, and their caregivers to read the Medication Guide and should assist them in understanding its contents. Patients should be given the opportunity to discuss the contents of the Medication Guide and to obtain answers to any questions they may have. The complete text of the Medication Guide is reprinted at the end of this document.

Patients should be advised of the following issues and asked to alert their prescriber if these occur while taking REMERON.

Clinical Worsening and Suicide Risk
Patients, their families, and their caregivers should be encouraged to be alert to the emergence of anxiety, agitation, panic attacks, insomnia, irritability, hostility, aggressiveness, impulsivity, akathisia (psychomotor restlessness), hypomania, mania, other unusual changes in behavior, worsening of depression, and suicidal ideation, especially early during antidepressant treatment and when the dose is adjusted up or down. Families and caregivers of patients should be advised to look for the emergence of such symptoms on a day-to-day basis, since changes may be abrupt. Such symptoms should be reported to the patient's prescriber or health professional, especially if they are severe, abrupt in onset, or were not part of the patient's presenting symptoms. Symptoms such as these may be associated with an increased risk for suicidal thinking and behavior and indicate a need for very close monitoring and possibly changes in the medication.

Agranulocytosis
Patients who are to receive REMERON should be warned about the risk of developing agranulocytosis. Patients should be advised to contact their physician if they experience any indication of infection such as fever, chills, sore throat, mucous membrane ulceration, or other possible signs of infection. Particular attention should be paid to any flu-like complaints or other symptoms that might suggest infection.

Interference with Cognitive and Motor Performance
REMERON may impair judgment, thinking, and particularly, motor skills, because of its prominent sedative effect. The drowsiness associated with mirtazapine use may impair a patient's ability to drive, use machines, or perform tasks that require alertness. Thus, patients should be cautioned about engaging in hazardous activities until they are reasonably certain that REMERON therapy does not adversely affect their ability to engage in such activities.

Completing Course of Therapy
While patients may notice improvement with REMERON therapy in 1 to 4 weeks, they should be advised to continue therapy as directed.

Concomitant Medication
Patients should be advised to inform their physician if they are taking, or intend to take, any prescription or over-the-counter drugs, since there is a potential for REMERON to interact with other drugs.

Alcohol
The impairment of cognitive and motor skills produced by REMERON has been shown to be additive with those produced by alcohol. Accordingly, patients should be advised to avoid alcohol while taking mirtazapine.

Pregnancy
Patients should be advised to notify their physician if they become pregnant or intend to become pregnant during REMERON therapy.

Nursing
Patients should be advised to notify their physician if they are breast-feeding an infant.

Laboratory Tests
There are no routine laboratory tests recommended.

Drug Interactions
As with other drugs, the potential for interaction by a variety of mechanisms (e.g., pharmacodynamic, pharmacokinetic inhibition or enhancement, etc.) is a possibility (see CLINICAL PHARMACOLOGY).

Monoamine Oxidase Inhibitors
(See CONTRAINDICATIONS, WARNINGS, and DOSAGE AND ADMINISTRATION.)

Serotonergic drugs
Based on the mechanism of action of mirtazapine and the potential for serotonin syndrome, caution is advised when REMERON Tablets are coadministered with other drugs or agents that may affect the serotonergic neurotransmitter systems, such as tryptophan, triptans, linezolid, serotonin reuptake inhibitors, venlafaxine, lithium, tramadol, or St. John's wort (see CONTRAINDICATIONS and WARNINGS).

Drugs Affecting Hepatic Metabolism
The metabolism and pharmacokinetics of REMERON (mirtazapine) Tablets may be affected by the induction or inhibition of drug-metabolizing enzymes.

Drugs that are Metabolized by and/or Inhibit Cytochrome P450 Enzymes
CYP Enzyme Inducers (these studies used both drugs at steady state)
Phenytoin
In healthy male patients (n=18), phenytoin (200 mg daily) increased mirtazapine (30 mg daily) clearance about 2-fold, resulting in a decrease in average plasma mirtazapine concentrations of 45%. Mirtazapine did not significantly affect the pharmacokinetics of phenytoin.

Carbamazepine
In healthy male patients (n=24), carbamazepine (400 mg b.i.d.) increased mirtazapine (15 mg b.i.d.) clearance about 2-fold, resulting in a decrease in average plasma mirtazapine concentrations of 60%.

When phenytoin, carbamazepine, or another inducer of hepatic metabolism (such as rifampicin) is added to mirtazapine therapy, the mirtazapine dose may have to be increased. If treatment with such a medicinal product is discontinued, it may be necessary to reduce the mirtazapine dose.

CYP Enzyme Inhibitors
Cimetidine
In healthy male patients (n=12), when cimetidine, a weak inhibitor of CYP1A2, CYP2D6, and CYP3A4, given at 800 mg b.i.d. at steady state was coadministered with mirtazapine (30 mg daily) at steady state, the Area Under the Curve (AUC) of mirtazapine increased more than 50%. Mirtazapine did not cause relevant changes in the pharmacokinetics of cimetidine. The mirtazapine dose may have to be decreased when concomitant treatment with cimetidine is started, or increased when cimetidine treatment is discontinued.

Ketoconazole
In healthy, male, Caucasian patients (n=24), coadministration of the potent CYP3A4 inhibitor ketoconazole (200 mg b.i.d. for 6.5 days) increased the peak plasma levels and the AUC of a single 30-mg dose of mirtazapine by approximately 40% and 50%, respectively.

Caution should be exercised when coadministering mirtazapine with potent CYP3A4 inhibitors, HIV protease inhibitors, azole antifungals, erythromycin, or nefazodone.

Paroxetine
In an *in vivo* interaction study in healthy, CYP2D6 extensive metabolizer patients (n=24), mirtazapine (30 mg/day), at steady state, did not cause relevant changes in the pharmacokinetics of steady state paroxetine (40 mg/day), a CYP2D6 inhibitor.

Other Drug-Drug Interactions
Amitriptyline
Amitriptyline: In healthy, CYP2D6 extensive metabolizer patients (n=32), amitriptyline (75 mg daily), at steady state, did not cause relevant changes to the pharmacokinetics of steady state mirtazapine (30 mg daily); mirtazapine also did not cause relevant changes to the pharmacokinetics of amitriptyline.

Warfarin
In healthy male subjects (n=16), mirtazapine (30 mg daily), at steady state, caused a small (0.2) but statistically significant increase in the International Normalized Ratio (INR) in subjects treated with warfarin. As at a higher dose of mirtazapine, a more pronounced effect can not be excluded. It is advisable to monitor the INR in case of concomitant treatment of warfarin with mirtazapine.

Lithium
No relevant clinical effects or significant changes in pharmacokinetics have been observed in healthy male subjects on concurrent treatment with subtherapeutic levels of lithium (600 mg/day for 10 days) at steady state and a single 30 mg dose of mirtazapine. The effects of higher doses of lithium on the pharmacokinetics of mirtazapine are unknown.

Risperidone
In an *in vivo*, nonrandomized, interaction study, subjects (n=6) in need of treatment with an antipsychotic and antidepressant drug, showed that mirtazapine (30 mg daily) at steady state did not influence the pharmacokinetics of risperidone (up to 3 mg b.i.d.).

Alcohol
Concomitant administration of alcohol (equivalent to 60 g) had a minimal effect on plasma levels of mirtazapine (15 mg) in 6 healthy male subjects. However, the impairment of cognitive and motor skills produced by REMERON were shown to be additive with those produced by alcohol. Accordingly, patients should be advised to avoid alcohol while taking REMERON.

Diazepam
Concomitant administration of diazepam (15 mg) had a minimal effect on plasma levels of mirtazapine (15 mg) in 12 healthy subjects. However, the impairment of motor skills produced by REMERON has been shown to be additive with those caused by diazepam. Accordingly, patients should be advised to avoid diazepam and other similar drugs while taking REMERON.

Carcinogenesis, Mutagenesis, Impairment of Fertility
Carcinogenesis
Carcinogenicity studies were conducted with mirtazapine given in the diet at doses of 2, 20, and 200 mg/kg/day to mice and 2, 20, and 60 mg/kg/day to rats. The highest doses used are approximately 20 and 12 times the maximum recommended human dose (MRHD) of 45 mg/day on an mg/m² basis in mice and rats, respectively. There was an increased incidence of hepatocellular adenoma and carcinoma in male mice at the high dose. In rats, there was an increase in hepatocellular adenoma in females at the mid and high doses and in hepatocellular tumors and thyroid follicular adenoma/cystadenoma and carcinoma in males at the high dose. The data suggest that the above effects could possibly be mediated by non-genotoxic mechanisms, the relevance of which to humans is not known.

The doses used in the mouse study may not have been high enough to fully characterize the carcinogenic potential of REMERON (mirtazapine) Tablets.

Mutagenesis
Mirtazapine was not mutagenic or clastogenic and did not induce general DNA damage as determined in several genotoxicity tests: Ames test, *in vitro* gene mutation assay in Chinese hamster V 79 cells, *in vitro* sister chromatid exchange assay in cultured rabbit lymphocytes, *in vivo* bone marrow micronucleus test in rats, and unscheduled DNA synthesis assay in HeLa cells.

Impairment of Fertility
In a fertility study in rats, mirtazapine was given at doses up to 100 mg/kg [20 times the maximum recommended human dose (MRHD) on an mg/m² basis]. Mating and conception were not affected by the drug, but estrous cycling was disrupted at doses that were 3 or more times the MRHD, and pre-implantation losses occurred at 20 times the MRHD.

Pregnancy
Teratogenic Effects – Pregnancy Category C
Reproduction studies in pregnant rats and rabbits at doses up to 100 mg/kg and 40 mg/kg, respectively [20 and 17 times the maximum recommended human dose (MRHD) on an mg/m² basis, respectively], have revealed no evidence of teratogenic effects. However, in rats, there was an increase in postimplantation losses in dams treated with mirtazapine. There was an increase in pup deaths during the first 3 days of lactation and a decrease in pup birth weights. The cause of these deaths is not known. The effects occurred at doses that were 20 times the MRHD, but not at 3 times the MRHD, on an mg/m² basis. There are no adequate and well-controlled studies in pregnant women. Because animal reproduction studies are not always predictive of human response, this drug should be used during pregnancy only if clearly needed.

Nursing Mothers
It is not known whether mirtazapine is excreted in human milk. Because many drugs are excreted in human milk, caution should be exercised when REMERON (mirtazapine) Tablets are administered to nursing women.

Pediatric Use
Safety and effectiveness in the pediatric population have not been established (see BOX WARNING and WARNINGS: Clinical Worsening and Suicide Risk). Two placebo-controlled trials in 258 pediatric patients with MDD have been conducted with REMERON (mirtazapine) Tablets, and the data were not sufficient to support a claim for use in pediatric patients. Anyone considering the use of REMERON in a child or adolescent must balance the potential risks with the clinical need.

In an 8-week-long pediatric clinical trial of doses between 15 to 45 mg/day, 49% of REMERON-treated patients had a weight gain of at least 7%, compared to 5.7% of placebo-treated patients. The mean increase in weight was 4 kg (2 kg SD) for REMERON-treated patients versus 1 kg (2 kg SD) for placebo-treated patients (see PRECAUTIONS: Increased Appetite/Weight Gain).

Geriatric Use
Approximately 190 elderly individuals (≥65 years of age) participated in clinical studies with REMERON (mirtazapine) Tablets. This drug is known to be substantially excreted by the kidney (75%), and the risk of decreased clearance of this drug is greater in patients with impaired renal function. Because elderly patients are more likely to have decreased renal function, care should be taken in dose selection. Sedating drugs may cause confusion and over-sedation in the elderly. No unusual adverse age-related phenomena were identified in this group. Pharmacokinetic studies revealed a decreased clearance in the

elderly. Caution is indicated in administering REMERON to elderly patients (see CLINICAL PHARMACOLOGY and DOSAGE AND ADMINISTRATION).

ADVERSE REACTIONS
Associated with Discontinuation of Treatment
Approximately 16% of the 453 patients who received REMERON® (mirtazapine) Tablets in US 6-week controlled clinical trials discontinued treatment due to an adverse experience, compared to 7% of the 361 placebo-treated patients in those studies. The most common events (≥1%) associated with discontinuation and considered to be drug related (i.e., those events associated with dropout at a rate at least twice that of placebo) included:

Common Adverse Events Associated with Discontinuation of Treatment in 6-Week US REMERON Trials

Adverse Event	Percentage of Patients Discontinuing with Adverse Event	
	REMERON (n=453)	Placebo (n=361)
Somnolence	10.4%	2.2%
Nausea	1.5%	0%

Commonly Observed Adverse Events in US Controlled Clinical Trials
The most commonly observed adverse events associated with the use of REMERON (mirtazapine) Tablets (incidence of 5% or greater) and not observed at an equivalent incidence among placebo-treated patients (REMERON incidence at least twice that for placebo) were:

Common Treatment-Emergent Adverse Events Associated with the Use of REMERON in 6-Week US Trials

Adverse Event	Percentage of Patients Reporting Adverse Event	
	REMERON (n=453)	Placebo (n=361)
Somnolence	54%	18%
Increased Appetite	17%	2%
Weight Gain	12%	2%
Dizziness	7%	3%

Adverse Events Occurring at an Incidence of 1% or More Among REMERON-Treated Patients
The table that follows enumerates adverse events that occurred at an incidence of 1% or more, and were more frequent than in the placebo group, among REMERON (mirtazapine) Tablets-treated patients who participated in short-term US placebo-controlled trials in which patients were dosed in a range of 5 to 60 mg/day. This table shows the percentage of patients in each group who had at least 1 episode of an event at some time during their treatment. Reported adverse events were classified using a standard COSTART-based dictionary terminology.

The prescriber should be aware that these figures cannot be used to predict the incidence of side effects in the course of usual medical practice where patient characteristics and other factors differ from those which prevailed in the clinical trials. Similarly, the cited frequencies cannot be compared with figures obtained from other investigations involving different treatments, uses, and investigators. The cited figures, however, do provide the prescribing physician with some basis for estimating the relative contribution of drug and nondrug factors to the side-effect incidence rate in the population studied.

INCIDENCE OF ADVERSE CLINICAL EXPERIENCES* (≥1%) IN SHORT-TERM US CONTROLLED STUDIES

Body System Adverse Clinical Experience	REMERON (n=453)	Placebo (n=361)
Body as a Whole		
Asthenia	8%	5%
Flu Syndrome	5%	3%
Back Pain	2%	1%

Digestive System

Dry Mouth	25%	15%
Increased Appetite	17%	2%
Constipation	13%	7%

Metabolic and Nutritional Disorders

Weight Gain	12%	2%
Peripheral Edema	2%	1%
Edema	1%	0%

Musculoskeletal System

Myalgia	2%	1%

Nervous System

Somnolence	54%	18%
Dizziness	7%	3%
Abnormal Dreams	4%	1%
Thinking Abnormal	3%	1%
Tremor	2%	1%
Confusion	2%	0%

Respiratory System

Dyspnea	1%	0%

Urogenital System

Urinary Frequency	2%	1%

*Events reported by at least 1% of patients treated with REMERON are included, except the following events which had an incidence on placebo greater than or equal to REMERON: headache, infection, pain, chest pain, palpitation, tachycardia, postural hypotension, nausea, dyspepsia, diarrhea, flatulence, insomnia, nervousness, libido decreased, hypertonia, pharyngitis, rhinitis, sweating, amblyopia, tinnitus, taste perversion.

ECG Changes
The electrocardiograms for 338 patients who received REMERON (mirtazapine) Tablets and 261 patients who received placebo in 6-week, placebo-controlled trials were analyzed. Prolongation in QTc ≥500 msec was not observed among mirtazapine-treated patients; mean change in QTc was +1.6 msec for mirtazapine and –3.1 msec for placebo. Mirtazapine was associated with a mean increase in heart rate of 3.4 bpm, compared to 0.8 bpm for placebo. The clinical significance of these changes is unknown.

Other Adverse Events Observed During the Premarketing Evaluation of REMERON
During its premarketing assessment, multiple doses of REMERON (mirtazapine) Tablets were administered to 2796 patients in clinical studies. The conditions and duration of exposure to mirtazapine varied greatly, and included (in overlapping categories) open and double-blind studies, uncontrolled and controlled studies, inpatient and outpatient studies, fixed-dose and titration studies. Untoward events associated with this exposure were recorded by clinical investigators using terminology of their own choosing. Consequently, it is not possible to provide a meaningful estimate of the proportion of individuals experiencing adverse events without first grouping similar types of untoward events into a smaller number of standardized event categories.

In the tabulations that follow, reported adverse events were classified using a standard COSTART-based dictionary terminology. The frequencies presented, therefore, represent the proportion of the 2796 patients exposed to multiple doses of REMERON who experienced an event of the type cited on at least 1 occasion while receiving REMERON. All reported events are included except those already listed in the previous table, those adverse experiences subsumed under COSTART terms that are either overly general or excessively specific so as to be uninformative, and those events for which a drug cause was very remote.

It is important to emphasize that, although the events reported occurred during treatment with REMERON, they were not necessarily caused by it.

Events are further categorized by body system and listed in order of decreasing frequency according to the following definitions: frequent adverse events are those occurring on 1

or more occasions in at least 1/100 patients; infrequent adverse events are those occurring in 1/100 to 1/1000 patients; rare events are those occurring in fewer than 1/1000 patients. Only those events not already listed in the previous table appear in this listing. Events of major clinical importance are also described in the WARNINGS and PRECAUTIONS sections.

Body as a Whole: *frequent:* malaise, abdominal pain, abdominal syndrome acute; *infrequent:* chills, fever, face edema, ulcer, photosensitivity reaction, neck rigidity, neck pain, abdomen enlarged; *rare:* cellulitis, chest pain substernal.

Cardiovascular System: *frequent:* hypertension, vasodilatation; *infrequent:* angina pectoris, myocardial infarction, bradycardia, ventricular extrasystoles, syncope, migraine, hypotension; *rare:* atrial arrhythmia, bigeminy, vascular headache, pulmonary embolus, cerebral ischemia, cardiomegaly, phlebitis, left heart failure.

Digestive System: *frequent:* vomiting, anorexia; *infrequent:* eructation, glossitis, cholecystitis, nausea and vomiting, gum hemorrhage, stomatitis, colitis, liver function tests abnormal; *rare:* tongue discoloration, ulcerative stomatitis, salivary gland enlargement, increased salivation, intestinal obstruction, pancreatitis, aphthous stomatitis, cirrhosis of liver, gastritis, gastroenteritis, oral moniliasis, tongue edema.

Endocrine System: *rare:* goiter, hypothyroidism.

Hemic and Lymphatic System: *rare:* lymphadenopathy, leukopenia, petechia, anemia, thrombocytopenia, lymphocytosis, pancytopenia.

Metabolic and Nutritional Disorders: *frequent:* thirst; *infrequent:* dehydration, weight loss; *rare:* gout, SGOT increased, healing abnormal, acid phosphatase increased, SGPT increased, diabetes mellitus, hyponatremia.

Musculoskeletal System: *frequent:* myasthenia, arthralgia; *infrequent:* arthritis, tenosynovitis; *rare:* pathologic fracture, osteoporosis fracture, bone pain, myositis, tendon rupture, arthrosis, bursitis.

Nervous System: *frequent:* hypesthesia, apathy, depression, hypokinesia, vertigo, twitching, agitation, anxiety, amnesia, hyperkinesia, paresthesia; *infrequent:* ataxia, delirium, delusions, depersonalization, dyskinesia, extrapyramidal syndrome, libido increased, coordination abnormal, dysarthria, hallucinations, manic reaction, neurosis, dystonia, hostility, reflexes increased, emotional lability, euphoria, paranoid reaction; *rare:* aphasia, nystagmus, akathisia (psychomotor restlessness), stupor, dementia, diplopia, drug dependence, paralysis, grand mal convulsion, hypotonia, myoclonus, psychotic depression, withdrawal syndrome, serotonin syndrome.

Respiratory System: *frequent:* cough increased, sinusitis; *infrequent:* epistaxis, bronchitis, asthma, pneumonia; *rare:* asphyxia, laryngitis, pneumothorax, hiccup.

Skin and Appendages: *frequent:* pruritus, rash; *infrequent:* acne, exfoliative dermatitis, dry skin, herpes simplex, alopecia; *rare:* urticaria, herpes zoster, skin hypertrophy, seborrhea, skin ulcer.

Special Senses: *infrequent:* eye pain, abnormality of accommodation, conjunctivitis, deafness, keratoconjunctivitis, lacrimation disorder, glaucoma, hyperacusis, ear pain; *rare:* blepharitis, partial transitory deafness, otitis media, taste loss, parosmia.

Urogenital System: *frequent:* urinary tract infection; *infrequent:* kidney calculus, cystitis, dysuria, urinary incontinence, urinary retention, vaginitis, hematuria, breast pain, amenorrhea, dysmenorrhea, leukorrhea, impotence; *rare:* polyuria, urethritis, metrorrhagia, menorrhagia, abnormal ejaculation, breast engorgement, breast enlargement, urinary urgency.

Other Adverse Events Observed During Postmarketing Evaluation of REMERON
Adverse events reported since market introduction, which were temporally (but not necessarily causally) related to mirtazapine therapy, include 4 cases of the ventricular arrhythmia torsades de pointes. In 3 of the 4 cases, however, concomitant drugs were implicated. All patients recovered. Cases of severe skin reactions, including Stevens-Johnson Syndrome, bullous dermatitis, erythema multiforme and toxic epidermal necrolysis have also been reported.

DRUG ABUSE AND DEPENDENCE
Controlled Substance Class
REMERON® (mirtazapine) Tablets are not a controlled substance.

Physical and Psychologic Dependence
REMERON (mirtazapine) Tablets have not been systematically studied in animals or humans for its potential for abuse, tolerance, or physical dependence. While the clinical trials did not reveal any tendency for any drug-seeking behavior, these observations were not systematic and it is not possible to predict on the basis of this limited experience the extent to which a CNS-active drug will be misused, diverted and/or abused once marketed. Consequently, patients should be evaluated carefully for history of drug abuse, and

such patients should be observed closely for signs of REMERON misuse or abuse (e.g., development of tolerance, incrementations of dose, drug-seeking behavior).

OVERDOSAGE

Human Experience
There is very limited experience with REMERON® (mirtazapine) Tablets overdose. In premarketing clinical studies, there were 8 reports of REMERON overdose alone or in combination with other pharmacological agents. The only drug overdose death reported while taking REMERON was in combination with amitriptyline and chlorprothixene in a non-US clinical study. Based on plasma levels, the REMERON dose taken was 30 to 45 mg, while plasma levels of amitriptyline and chlorprothixene were found to be at toxic levels. All other premarketing overdose cases resulted in full recovery. Signs and symptoms reported in association with overdose included disorientation, drowsiness, impaired memory, and tachycardia. There were no reports of ECG abnormalities, coma, or convulsions following overdose with REMERON alone.

Overdose Management
Treatment should consist of those general measures employed in the management of overdose with any drug effective in the treatment of major depressive disorder. Ensure an adequate airway, oxygenation, and ventilation. Monitor cardiac rhythm and vital signs. General supportive and symptomatic measures are also recommended. Induction of emesis is not recommended. Gastric lavage with a large-bore orogastric tube with appropriate airway protection, if needed, may be indicated if performed soon after ingestion, or in symptomatic patients.

Activated charcoal should be administered. There is no experience with the use of forced diuresis, dialysis, hemoperfusion, or exchange transfusion in the treatment of mirtazapine overdosage. No specific antidotes for mirtazapine are known.

In managing overdosage, consider the possibility of multiple-drug involvement. The physician should consider contacting a poison control center for additional information on the treatment of any overdose. Telephone numbers for certified poison control centers are listed in the *Physicians' Desk Reference* (PDR).

DOSAGE AND ADMINISTRATION

Initial Treatment
The recommended starting dose for REMERON® (mirtazapine) Tablets is 15 mg/day, administered in a single dose, preferably in the evening prior to sleep. In the controlled clinical trials establishing the efficacy of REMERON in the treatment of major depressive disorder, the effective dose range was generally 15 to 45 mg/day. While the relationship between dose and satisfactory response in the treatment of major depressive disorder for REMERON has not been adequately explored, patients not responding to the initial 15-mg dose may benefit from dose increases up to a maximum of 45 mg/day. REMERON has an elimination half-life of approximately 20 to 40 hours; therefore, dose changes should not be made at intervals of less than 1 to 2 weeks in order to allow sufficient time for evaluation of the therapeutic response to a given dose.

Elderly and Patients with Renal or Hepatic Impairment
The clearance of mirtazapine is reduced in elderly patients and in patients with moderate to severe renal or hepatic impairment. Consequently, the prescriber should be aware that plasma mirtazapine levels may be increased in these patient groups, compared to levels observed in younger adults without renal or hepatic impairment (see PRECAUTIONS and CLINICAL PHARMACOLOGY).

Maintenance/Extended Treatment
It is generally agreed that acute episodes of depression require several months or longer of sustained pharmacological therapy beyond response to the acute episode. Systematic evaluation of REMERON (mirtazapine) Tablets has demonstrated that its efficacy in major depressive disorder is maintained for periods of up to 40 weeks following 8 to 12 weeks of initial treatment at a dose of 15 to 45 mg/day (see CLINICAL PHARMACOLOGY). Based on these limited data, it is unknown whether or not the dose of REMERON needed for maintenance treatment is identical to the dose needed to achieve an initial response. Patients should be periodically reassessed to determine the need for maintenance treatment and the appropriate dose for such treatment.

Switching Patients To or From a Monoamine Oxidase Inhibitor
Concomitant use of REMERON (mirtazapine) Tablets with MAOIs is contraindicated. At least 14 days should elapse between discontinuation of an MAOI and initiation of therapy with REMERON (mirtazapine) Tablets. In addition, at least 14 days should be allowed after stopping REMERON before starting an MAOI.

Discontinuation of Remeron Treatment
Symptoms associated with the discontinuation or dose reduction of REMERON Tablets have been reported. Patients should be monitored for these and other symptoms when discontinuing treatment or during dosage reduction. A gradual reduction in the dose over several weeks, rather than abrupt cessation, is recommended whenever possible. If intolerable symptoms occur following a decrease in the dose or upon discontinuation of treatment, dose titration should be managed on the basis of the patient's clinical response (see PRECAUTIONS and ADVERSE REACTIONS).

HOW SUPPLIED
REMERON® (mirtazapine) Tablets are supplied as:
15 mg Tablets—oval, scored, yellow, coated, with "Organon" debossed on 1 side and "$^T_3Z^n$" on the other side.
Bottles of 30   NDC 0052-0105-30
30 mg Tablets—oval, scored, red-brown, coated, with "Organon" debossed on 1 side and "$^T_5Z^n$" on the other side.
Bottles of 30   NDC 0052-0107-30
45 mg Tablets—oval, white, coated, with "Organon" debossed on 1 side and "$^T_7Z^n$" on the other side.
Bottles of 30   NDC 0052-0109-30

Storage
Store at 25°C (77°F); excursions permitted to 15°–30°C (59°–86°F) [see USP Controlled Room Temperature]. Protect from light and moisture.

Rx only
Manufactured by N.V. Organon, Oss, The Netherlands. Distributed by Schering Corporation, a subsidiary of Schering-Plough Corporation, Kenilworth, NJ 07033 USA. © 1996, 2007, Schering Corporation. All rights reserved. Rev. 5/10

MEDICATION GUIDE
Antidepressant Medicines, Depression and other Serious Mental Illnesses, and Suicidal Thoughts or Actions
Read the Medication Guide that comes with you or your family member's antidepressant medicine. This Medication Guide is only about the risk of suicidal thoughts and actions with antidepressant medicines. Talk to your, or your family member's, healthcare provider about:
- all risks and benefits of treatment with antidepressant medicines
- all treatment choices for depression or other serious mental illness

What is the most important information I should know about antidepressant medicines, depression and other serious mental illnesses, and suicidal thoughts or actions?
1. **Antidepressant medicines may increase suicidal thoughts or actions in some children, teenagers, and young adults within the first few months of treatment.**
2. **Depression and other serious mental illnesses are the most important causes of suicidal thoughts and actions. Some people may have a particularly high risk of having suicidal thoughts or actions.** These include people who have (or have a family history of) bipolar illness (also called manic-depressive illness) or suicidal thoughts or actions.
3. **How can I watch for and try to prevent suicidal thoughts and actions in myself or a family member?**
   - Pay close attention to any changes, especially sudden changes, in mood, behaviors, thoughts, or feelings. This is very important when an antidepressant medicine is started or when the dose is changed.
   - Call the healthcare provider right away to report new or sudden changes in mood, behavior, thoughts, or feelings.
   - Keep all follow-up visits with the healthcare provider as scheduled. Call the healthcare provider between visits as needed, especially if you have concerns about symptoms.

Call a healthcare provider right away if you or your family member has any of the following symptoms, especially if they are new, worse, or worry you:
- thoughts about suicide or dying
- attempts to commit suicide
- new or worse depression
- new or worse anxiety
- feeling very agitated or restless
- panic attacks
- trouble sleeping (insomnia)
- new or worse irritability
- acting aggressive, being angry, or violent
- acting on dangerous impulses
- an extreme increase in activity and talking (mania)
- other unusual changes in behavior or mood

Call your doctor for medical advice about side effects. You may report side effects to FDA at 1-800-FDA-1088.

What else do I need to know about antidepressant medicines?
- **Never stop an antidepressant medicine without first talking to a healthcare provider.** Stopping an antidepressant medicine suddenly can cause other symptoms.
- **Antidepressants are medicines used to treat depression and other illnesses.** It is important to discuss all the risks of treating depression and also the risks of not treating it.

Patients and their families or other caregivers should discuss all treatment choices with the healthcare provider, not just the use of antidepressants.
- **Antidepressant medicines have other side effects.** Talk to the healthcare provider about the side effects of the medicine prescribed for you or your family member.
- **Antidepressant medicines can interact with other medicines.** Know all of the medicines that you or your family member takes. Keep a list of all medicines to show the healthcare provider. Do not start new medicines without first checking with your healthcare provider.
- **Not all antidepressant medicines prescribed for children are FDA approved for use in children.** Talk to your child's healthcare provider for more information.

This Medication Guide has been approved by the U.S. Food and Drug Administration for all antidepressants.

Shown in Product Identification Guide, page 314

REMERONSolTab®   ℞
[rem-er-on]
(mirtazapine)
Orally Disintegrating Tablets
ONCE-A-DAY

Suicidality and Antidepressant Drugs
Antidepressants increased the risk compared to placebo of suicidal thinking and behavior (suicidality) in children, adolescents, and young adults in short-term studies of major depressive disorder (MDD) and other psychiatric disorders. Anyone considering the use of REMERONSolTab® (mirtazapine) Orally Disintegrating Tablets or any other antidepressant in a child, adolescent, or young adult must balance this risk with the clinical need. Short-term studies did not show an increase in the risk of suicidality with antidepressants compared to placebo in adults beyond age 24; there was a reduction in risk with antidepressants compared to placebo in adults aged 65 and older. Depression and certain other psychiatric disorders are themselves associated with increases in the risk of suicide. Patients of all ages who are started on antidepressant therapy should be monitored appropriately and observed closely for clinical worsening, suicidality, or unusual changes in behavior. Families and caregivers should be advised of the need for close observation and communication with the prescriber. REMERONSolTab is not approved for use in pediatric patients. (See WARNINGS: Clinical Worsening and Suicide Risk, PRECAUTIONS: Information for Patients, and PRECAUTIONS: Pediatric Use)

DESCRIPTION
REMERONSolTab® (mirtazapine) Orally Disintegrating Tablets are an orally administered drug. Mirtazapine has a tetracyclic chemical structure and belongs to the piperazino-azepine group of compounds. It is designated 1,2,3,4,10,14b-hexahydro-2-methylpyrazino [2,1-a] pyrido [2,3-c] benzazepine and has the empirical formula of $C_{17}H_{19}N_3$. Its molecular weight is 265.36. The structural formula is the following and it is the racemic mixture:

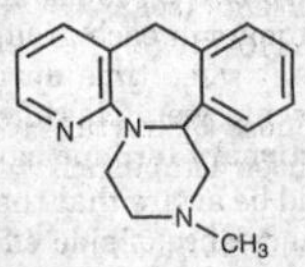

Mirtazapine is a white to creamy white crystalline powder which is slightly soluble in water. REMERONSolTab is available for oral administration as an orally disintegrating tablet containing 15, 30, or 45 mg of mirtazapine. It disintegrates in the mouth within seconds after placement on the tongue, allowing its contents to be subsequently swallowed with or without water. REMERONSolTab also contains the following inactive ingredients: aspartame, citric acid, crospovidone, hypromellose, magnesium stearate, mannitol, microcrystalline cellulose, natural and artificial orange flavor, polymethacrylate, povidone, sodium bicarbonate, starch, and sucrose.

CLINICAL PHARMACOLOGY
Pharmacodynamics
The mechanism of action of REMERONSolTab® (mirtazapine) Orally Disintegrating Tablets, as with other drugs effective in the treatment of major depressive disorder, is unknown.
Evidence gathered in preclinical studies suggests that mirtazapine enhances central noradrenergic and serotonergic activity. These studies have shown that mirtazapine acts as an antagonist at central presynaptic α_2 adrenergic

inhibitory autoreceptors and heteroreceptors, an action that is postulated to result in an increase in central noradrenergic and serotonergic activity.
Mirtazapine is a potent antagonist of 5-HT_2 and 5-HT_3 receptors. Mirtazapine has no significant affinity for the 5-HT_{1A} and 5-HT_{1B} receptors.
Mirtazapine is a potent antagonist of histamine (H_1) receptors, a property that may explain its prominent sedative effects.
Mirtazapine is a moderate peripheral α_1 adrenergic antagonist, a property that may explain the occasional orthostatic hypotension reported in association with its use.
Mirtazapine is a moderate antagonist at muscarinic receptors, a property that may explain the relatively low incidence of anticholinergic side effects associated with its use.

Pharmacokinetics

REMERONSolTab (mirtazapine) Orally Disintegrating Tablets are rapidly and completely absorbed following oral administration and have a half-life of about 20 to 40 hours. Peak plasma concentrations are reached within about 2 hours following an oral dose. The presence of food in the stomach has a minimal effect on both the rate and extent of absorption and does not require a dosage adjustment. REMERONSolTab Orally Disintegrating Tablets are bioequivalent to REMERON® (mirtazapine) Tablets.
Mirtazapine is extensively metabolized after oral administration. Major pathways of biotransformation are demethylation and hydroxylation followed by glucuronide conjugation. *In vitro* data from human liver microsomes indicate that cytochrome 2D6 and 1A2 are involved in the formation of the 8-hydroxy metabolite of mirtazapine, whereas cytochrome 3A is considered to be responsible for the formation of the N-desmethyl and N-oxide metabolite. Mirtazapine has an absolute bioavailability of about 50%. It is eliminated predominantly via urine (75%) with 15% in feces. Several unconjugated metabolites possess pharmacological activity but are present in the plasma at very low levels. The (−) enantiomer has an elimination half-life that is approximately twice as long as the (+) enantiomer and therefore achieves plasma levels that are about 3 times as high as that of the (+) enantiomer.
Plasma levels are linearly related to dose over a dose range of 15 to 80 mg. The mean elimination half-life of mirtazapine after oral administration ranges from approximately 20 to 40 hours across age and gender subgroups, with females of all ages exhibiting significantly longer elimination half-lives than males (mean half-life of 37 hours for females vs 26 hours for males). Steady state plasma levels of mirtazapine are attained within 5 days, with about 50% accumulation (accumulation ratio = 1.5).
Mirtazapine is approximately 85% bound to plasma proteins over a concentration range of 0.01 to 10 mcg/mL.

Special Populations

Geriatric

Following oral administration of REMERON (mirtazapine) Tablets 20 mg/day for 7 days to subjects of varying ages (range, 25–74), oral clearance of mirtazapine was reduced in the elderly compared to the younger subjects. The differences were most striking in males, with a 40% lower clearance in elderly males compared to younger males, while the clearance in elderly females was only 10% lower compared to younger females. Caution is indicated in administering REMERONSolTab (mirtazapine) Orally Disintegrating Tablets to elderly patients (see PRECAUTIONS and DOSAGE AND ADMINISTRATION).

Pediatrics

Safety and effectiveness of mirtazapine in the pediatric population have not been established (see PRECAUTIONS).

Gender

The mean elimination half-life of mirtazapine after oral administration ranges from approximately 20 to 40 hours across age and gender subgroups, with females of all ages exhibiting significantly longer elimination half-lives than males (mean half-life of 37 hours for females vs. 26 hours for males) (see Pharmacokinetics).

Race

There have been no clinical studies to evaluate the effect of race on the pharmacokinetics of REMERONSolTab.

Renal Insufficiency

The disposition of mirtazapine was studied in patients with varying degrees of renal function. Elimination of mirtazapine is correlated with creatinine clearance. Total body clearance of mirtazapine was reduced approximately 30% in patients with moderate (Clcr = 11–39 mL/min/1.73 m^2) and approximately 50% in patients with severe (Clcr = <10 mL/min/1.73 m^2) renal impairment when compared to normal subjects. Caution is indicated in administering REMERONSolTab to patients with compromised renal function (see PRECAUTIONS and DOSAGE AND ADMINISTRATION).

Hepatic Insufficiency

Following a single 15-mg oral dose of REMERON, the oral clearance of mirtazapine was decreased by approximately 30% in hepatically impaired patients compared to subjects with normal hepatic function. Caution is indicated in administering REMERONSolTab to patients with compromised hepatic function (see PRECAUTIONS and DOSAGE AND ADMINISTRATION).

Clinical Trials Showing Effectiveness

The efficacy of REMERON (mirtazapine) Tablets as a treatment for major depressive disorder was established in 4 placebo-controlled, 6-week trials in adult outpatients meeting DSM-III criteria for major depressive disorder. Patients were titrated with mirtazapine from a dose range of 5 mg up to 35 mg/day. Overall, these studies demonstrated mirtazapine to be superior to placebo on at least 3 of the following 4 measures: 21-Item Hamilton Depression Rating Scale (HDRS) total score; HDRS Depressed Mood Item; CGI Severity score; and Montgomery and Asberg Depression Rating Scale (MADRS). Superiority of mirtazapine over placebo was also found for certain factors of the HDRS, including anxiety/somatization factor and sleep disturbance factor. The mean mirtazapine dose for patients who completed these 4 studies ranged from 21 to 32 mg/day. A fifth study of similar design utilized a higher dose (up to 50 mg) per day and also showed effectiveness.
Examination of age and gender subsets of the population did not reveal any differential responsiveness on the basis of these subgroupings.
In a longer-term study, patients meeting (DSM-IV) criteria for major depressive disorder who had responded during an initial 8 to 12 weeks of acute treatment on REMERON were randomized to continuation of REMERON or placebo for up to 40 weeks of observation for relapse. Response during the open phase was defined as having achieved a HAM-D 17 total score of ≤8 and a CGI-Improvement score of 1 or 2 at 2 consecutive visits beginning with week 6 of the 8 to 12 weeks in the open-label phase of the study. Relapse during the double-blind phase was determined by the individual investigators. Patients receiving continued REMERON treatment experienced significantly lower relapse rates over the subsequent 40 weeks compared to those receiving placebo. This pattern was demonstrated in both male and female patients.

INDICATIONS AND USAGE

REMERONSolTab® (mirtazapine) Orally Disintegrating Tablets are indicated for the treatment of major depressive disorder.
The efficacy of REMERON® (mirtazapine) Tablets in the treatment of major depressive disorder was established in 6-week controlled trials of outpatients whose diagnoses corresponded most closely to the Diagnostic and Statistical Manual of Mental Disorders – 3rd edition (DSM-III) category of major depressive disorder (see CLINICAL PHARMACOLOGY).
A major depressive episode (DSM-IV) implies a prominent and relatively persistent (nearly every day for at least 2 weeks) depressed or dysphoric mood that usually interferes with daily functioning, and includes at least 5 of the following 9 symptoms: depressed mood, loss of interest in usual activities, significant change in weight and/or appetite, insomnia or hypersomnia, psychomotor agitation or retardation, increased fatigue, feelings of guilt or worthlessness, slowed thinking or impaired concentration, a suicide attempt, or suicidal ideation.
The effectiveness of REMERONSolTab in hospitalized depressed patients has not been adequately studied.
The efficacy of REMERON in maintaining a response in patients with major depressive disorder for up to 40 weeks following 8 to 12 weeks of initial open-label treatment was demonstrated in a placebo-controlled trial. Nevertheless, the physician who elects to use REMERON for extended periods should periodically re-evaluate the long-term usefulness of the drug for the individual patient (see CLINICAL PHARMACOLOGY).

CONTRAINDICATIONS

Hypersensitivity

REMERONSolTab® (mirtazapine) Orally Disintegrating Tablets are contraindicated in patients with a known hypersensitivity to mirtazapine or to any of the excipients.

Monoamine Oxidase Inhibitors

The concomitant use of REMERONSolTab Orally Disintegrating Tablets and a monoamine oxidase (MAO) inhibitor is contraindicated. REMERON® should not be used within 14 days of initiating or discontinuing therapy with a monoamine oxidase inhibitor (MAOI) (see WARNINGS, PRECAUTIONS: Drug Interactions, and DOSAGE AND ADMINISTRATION).

WARNINGS

Clinical Worsening and Suicide Risk

Patients with major depressive disorder (MDD), both adult and pediatric, may experience worsening of their depression and/or the emergence of suicidal ideation and behavior (suicidality) or unusual changes in behavior, whether or not they are taking antidepressant medications, and this risk may persist until significant remission occurs. Suicide is a known risk of depression and certain other psychiatric disorders, and these disorders themselves are the strongest predictors of suicide. There has been a long-standing concern, however, that antidepressants may have a role in inducing worsening of depression and the emergence of suicidality in certain patients during the early phases of treatment. Pooled analyses of short-term placebo-controlled trials of antidepressant drugs (SSRIs and others) showed that these drugs increase the risk of suicidal thinking and behavior (suicidality) in children, adolescents, and young adults (ages 18–24) with major depressive disorder (MDD) and other psychiatric disorders. Short-term studies did not show an increase in the risk of suicidality with antidepressants compared to placebo in adults beyond age 24; there was a reduction in risk with antidepressants compared to placebo in adults aged 65 and older.
The pooled analyses of placebo-controlled trials in children and adolescents with MDD, obsessive compulsive disorder (OCD), or other psychiatric disorders included a total of 24 short-term trials of 9 antidepressant drugs in over 4400 patients. The pooled analyses of placebo-controlled trials in adults with MDD or other psychiatric disorders included a total of 295 short-term trials (median duration of 2 months) of 11 antidepressant drugs in over 77,000 patients. There was considerable variation in risk of suicidality among drugs, but a tendency toward an increase in the younger patients for almost all drugs studied. There were differences in absolute risk of suicidality across different indications, with the highest incidence in MDD. The risk differences (drug vs. placebo), however, were relatively stable within age strata and across indications. These risk differences (drug-placebo difference in the number of cases of suicidality per 1000 patients treated) are provided in Table 1.

Table 1

Age Range	Drug-Placebo Difference in Number of Cases of Suicidality per 1000 Patients Treated
Increases Compared to Placebo	
<18	14 additional cases
18–24	5 additional cases
Decreases Compared to Placebo	
25–64	1 fewer case
≥65	6 fewer cases

No suicides occurred in any of the pediatric trials. There were suicides in the adult trials, but the number was not sufficient to reach any conclusion about drug effect on suicide.
It is unknown whether the suicidality risk extends to longer-term use, i.e., beyond several months. However, there is substantial evidence from placebo-controlled maintenance trials in adults with depression that the use of antidepressants can delay the recurrence of depression.
All patients being treated with antidepressants for any indication should be monitored appropriately and observed closely for clinical worsening, suicidality, and unusual changes in behavior, especially during the initial few months of a course of drug therapy, or at times of dose changes, either increases or decreases.
The following symptoms, anxiety, agitation, panic attacks, insomnia, irritability, hostility, aggressiveness, impulsivity, akathisia (psychomotor restlessness), hypomania, and mania, have been reported in adult and pediatric patients being treated with antidepressants for major depressive disorder as well as for other indications, both psychiatric and nonpsychiatric. Although a causal link between the emergence of such symptoms and either the worsening of depression and/or the emergence of suicidal impulses has not been established, there is concern that such symptoms may represent precursors to emerging suicidality.
Consideration should be given to changing the therapeutic regimen, including possibly discontinuing the medication, in patients whose depression is persistently worse, or who are experiencing emergent suicidality or symptoms that might be precursors to worsening depression or suicidality, especially if these symptoms are severe, abrupt in onset, or were not part of the patient's presenting symptoms.
Families and caregivers of patients being treated with antidepressants for major depressive disorder or other indications, both psychiatric and nonpsychiatric, should be alerted about the need to monitor patients for the emergence of agitation, irritability, unusual changes in behavior, and the other symptoms described above, as well as the emergence of suicidality, and to report such symptoms immediately to health care providers. Such monitoring should include daily observation by families and

caregivers. Prescriptions for REMERONSolTab® (mirtazapine) Orally Disintegrating Tablets should be written for the smallest quantity of tablets consistent with good patient management, in order to reduce the risk of overdose.

Screening Patients for Bipolar Disorder

A major depressive episode may be the initial presentation of bipolar disorder. It is generally believed (though not established in controlled trials) that treating such an episode with an antidepressant alone may increase the likelihood of precipitation of a mixed/manic episode in patients at risk for bipolar disorder. Whether any of the symptoms described above represent such a conversion is unknown. However, prior to initiating treatment with an antidepressant, patients with depressive symptoms should be adequately screened to determine if they are at risk for bipolar disorder; such screening should include a detailed psychiatric history, including a family history of suicide, bipolar disorder, and depression. It should be noted that REMERONSolTab (mirtazapine) Orally Disintegrating Tablets are not approved for use in treating bipolar depression.

Agranulocytosis

In premarketing clinical trials, 2 (1 with Sjögren's Syndrome) out of 2796 patients treated with REMERON® (mirtazapine) Tablets developed agranulocytosis [absolute neutrophil count (ANC) <500/mm³ with associated signs and symptoms, e.g., fever, infection, etc.] and a third patient developed severe neutropenia (ANC <500/mm³ without any associated symptoms). For these 3 patients, onset of severe neutropenia was detected on days 61, 9, and 14 of treatment, respectively. All 3 patients recovered after REMERON was stopped. These 3 cases yield a crude incidence of severe neutropenia (with or without associated infection) of approximately 1.1 per thousand patients exposed, with a very wide 95% confidence interval, i.e., 2.2 cases per 10,000 to 3.1 cases per 1000. If a patient develops a sore throat, fever, stomatitis, or other signs of infection, along with a low WBC count, treatment with REMERONSolTab (mirtazapine) Orally Disintegrating Tablets should be discontinued and the patient should be closely monitored.

MAO Inhibitors

In patients receiving other drugs for major depressive disorder in combination with a monoamine oxidase inhibitor (MAOI) and in patients who have recently discontinued a drug for major depressive disorder and then are started on an MAOI, there have been reports of serious and sometimes fatal reactions, including nausea, vomiting, flushing, dizziness, tremor, myoclonus, rigidity, diaphoresis, hyperthermia, autonomic instability with rapid fluctuations of vital signs, seizures, and mental status changes ranging from agitation to coma. Although there are no human data pertinent to such an interaction with REMERONSolTab (mirtazapine) Orally Disintegrating Tablets, it is recommended that REMERONSolTab not be used in combination with an MAOI, or within 14 days of initiating or discontinuing therapy with an MAOI.

Serotonin Syndrome

On rare occasions, serotonin syndrome has occurred in association with treatment of REMERONSolTab Orally Disintegrating Tablets, particularly when given in combination with other serotonergic drugs. As serotonin syndrome may result in potentially life-threatening conditions, treatment with REMERON should be discontinued if patients develop a combination of symptoms possibly including hyperthermia, rigidity, myoclonus, autonomic instability with possible rapid fluctuations of vital signs, mental status changes including confusion, irritability, extreme agitation progressing to delirium and coma, and supportive symptomatic treatment should be initiated. Due to the risk of serotonin syndrome, REMERON should not be used in combination with MAO inhibitors or serotonin-precursors (such as L-tryptophan and oxitriptan) and should be used with caution in patients receiving other serotonergic drugs (e.g., triptans, lithium, tramadol, St. John's wort, and most tricyclic antidepressants) (see CONTRAINDICATIONS and PRECAUTIONS: Drug Interactions).

PRECAUTIONS

General

Discontinuation Symptoms

There have been reports of adverse reactions upon the discontinuation of REMERON®/REMERONSolTab® (mirtazapine) Orally Disintegrating Tablets (particularly when abrupt), including but not limited to the following: dizziness, abnormal dreams, sensory disturbances (including paresthesia and electric shock sensations), agitation, anxiety, fatigue, confusion, headache, tremor, nausea, vomiting, and sweating, or other symptoms which may be of clinical significance. The majority of the reported cases are mild and self-limiting. Even though these have been reported as adverse reactions, it should be realized that these symptoms may be related to underlying disease.

Patients currently taking REMERON should NOT discontinue treatment abruptly, due to risk of discontinuation symptoms. At the time that a medical decision is made to discontinue treatment with REMERON, a gradual reduction in the dose, rather than an abrupt cessation, is recommended.

Akathisia/Psychomotor Restlessness

The use of antidepressants has been associated with the development of akathisia, characterized by a subjectively unpleasant or distressing restlessness and need to move, often accompanied by an inability to sit or stand still. This is most likely to occur within the first few weeks of treatment. In patients who develop these symptoms, increasing the dose may be detrimental.

Hyponatremia

Hyponatremia has been reported very rarely with the use of mirtazapine. Caution should be exercised in patients at risk, such as elderly patients or patients concomitantly treated with medications known to cause hyponatremia.

Somnolence

In US controlled studies, somnolence was reported in 54% of patients treated with REMERON® (mirtazapine) Tablets, compared to 18% for placebo and 60% for amitriptyline. In these studies, somnolence resulted in discontinuation for 10.4% of REMERON-treated patients, compared to 2.2% for placebo. It is unclear whether or not tolerance develops to the somnolent effects of REMERON. Because of the potentially significant effects of REMERON on impairment of performance, patients should be cautioned about engaging in activities requiring alertness until they have been able to assess the drug's effect on their own psychomotor performance (see Information for Patients).

Dizziness

In US controlled studies, dizziness was reported in 7% of patients treated with REMERON, compared to 3% for placebo and 14% for amitriptyline. It is unclear whether or not tolerance develops to the dizziness observed in association with the use of REMERON.

Increased Appetite/Weight Gain

In US controlled studies, appetite increase was reported in 17% of patients treated with REMERON, compared to 2% for placebo and 6% for amitriptyline. In these same trials, weight gain of ≥ 7% of body weight was reported in 7.5% of patients treated with mirtazapine, compared to 0% for placebo and 5.9% for amitriptyline. In a pool of premarketing US studies, including many patients for long-term, open-label treatment, 8% of patients receiving REMERON discontinued for weight gain. In an 8-week-long pediatric clinical trial of doses between 15 to 45 mg/day, 49% of REMERON-treated patients had a weight gain of at least 7%, compared to 5.7% of placebo-treated patients (see PRECAUTIONS: Pediatric Use).

Cholesterol/Triglycerides

In US controlled studies, nonfasting cholesterol increases to ≥20% above the upper limits of normal were observed in 15% of patients treated with REMERON, compared to 7% for placebo and 8% for amitriptyline. In these same studies, nonfasting triglyceride increases to ≥ 500 mg/dL were observed in 6% of patients treated with mirtazapine, compared to 3% for placebo and 3% for amitriptyline.

Transaminase Elevations

Clinically significant ALT (SGPT) elevations (≥3 times the upper limit of the normal range) were observed in 2.0% (8/424) of patients exposed to REMERON in a pool of short-term US controlled trials, compared to 0.3% (1/328) of placebo patients and 2.0% (3/181) of amitriptyline patients. Most of these patients with ALT increases did not develop signs or symptoms associated with compromised liver function. While some patients were discontinued for the ALT increases, in other cases, the enzyme levels returned to normal despite continued REMERON treatment. REMERONSolTab® (mirtazapine) Orally Disintegrating Tablets should be used with caution in patients with impaired hepatic function (see CLINICAL PHARMACOLOGY and DOSAGE AND ADMINISTRATION).

Activation of Mania/Hypomania

Mania/hypomania occurred in approximately 0.2% (3/1299 patients) of REMERON-treated patients in US studies. Although the incidence of mania/hypomania was very low during treatment with mirtazapine, it should be used carefully in patients with a history of mania/hypomania.

Seizure

In premarketing clinical trials, only 1 seizure was reported among the 2796 US and non-US patients treated with REMERON. However, no controlled studies have been carried out in patients with a history of seizures. Therefore, care should be exercised when mirtazapine is used in these patients.

Use in Patients with Concomitant Illness

Clinical experience with REMERONSolTab in patients with concomitant systemic illness is limited. Accordingly, care is advisable in prescribing mirtazapine for patients with diseases or conditions that affect metabolism or hemodynamic responses.

REMERONSolTab has not been systematically evaluated or used to any appreciable extent in patients with a recent history of myocardial infarction or other significant heart disease. REMERON was associated with significant orthostatic hypotension in early clinical pharmacology trials with normal volunteers. Orthostatic hypotension was infrequently observed in clinical trials with depressed patients. REMERONSolTab should be used with caution in patients with known cardiovascular or cerebrovascular disease that could be exacerbated by hypotension (history of myocardial infarction, angina, or ischemic stroke) and conditions that would predispose patients to hypotension (dehydration, hypovolemia, and treatment with antihypertensive medication).

Mirtazapine clearance is decreased in patients with moderate [glomerular filtration rate (GFR) = 11–39 mL/min/1.73 m²] and severe [GFR <10 mL/min/1.73 m²] renal impairment, and also in patients with hepatic impairment. Caution is indicated in administering REMERONSolTab to such patients (see CLINICAL PHARMACOLOGY and DOSAGE AND ADMINISTRATION).

Information for Patients

Prescribers or other health professionals should inform patients, their families, and their caregivers about the benefits and risks associated with treatment with REMERONSolTab (mirtazapine) Orally Disintegrating Tablets and should counsel them in its appropriate use. A patient Medication Guide about "Antidepressant Medicines, Depression and other Serious Mental Illnesses, and Suicidal Thoughts or Actions" is available for REMERONSolTab. The prescriber or health professional should instruct patients, their families, and their caregivers to read the Medication Guide and should assist them in understanding its contents. Patients should be given the opportunity to discuss the contents of the Medication Guide and to obtain answers to any questions they may have. The complete text of the Medication Guide is reprinted at the end of this document.

Patients should be advised of the following issues and asked to alert their prescriber if these occur while taking REMERONSolTab.

Clinical Worsening and Suicide Risk

Patients, their families, and their caregivers should be encouraged to be alert to the emergence of anxiety, agitation, panic attacks, insomnia, irritability, hostility, aggressiveness, impulsivity, akathisia (psychomotor restlessness), hypomania, mania, other unusual changes in behavior, worsening of depression, and suicidal ideation, especially early during antidepressant treatment and when the dose is adjusted up or down. Families and caregivers of patients should be advised to look for the emergence of such symptoms on a day-to-day basis, since changes may be abrupt. Such symptoms should be reported to the patient's prescriber or health professional, especially if they are severe, abrupt in onset, or were not part of the patient's presenting symptoms. Symptoms such as these may be associated with an increased risk for suicidal thinking and behavior and indicate a need for very close monitoring and possibly changes in the medication.

Agranulocytosis

Patients who are to receive REMERONSolTab should be warned about the risk of developing agranulocytosis. Patients should be advised to contact their physician if they experience any indication of infection such as fever, chills, sore throat, mucous membrane ulceration, or other possible signs of infection. Particular attention should be paid to any flu-like complaints or other symptoms that might suggest infection.

Interference with Cognitive and Motor Performance

REMERONSolTab may impair judgment, thinking, and particularly, motor skills, because of its prominent sedative effect. The drowsiness associated with mirtazapine use may impair a patient's ability to drive, use machines, or perform tasks that require alertness. Thus, patients should be cautioned about engaging in hazardous activities until they are reasonably certain that REMERONSolTab therapy does not adversely affect their ability to engage in such activities.

Completing Course of Therapy

While patients may notice improvement with REMERONSolTab therapy in 1 to 4 weeks, they should be advised to continue therapy as directed.

Concomitant Medication

Patients should be advised to inform their physician if they are taking, or intend to take, any prescription or over-the-counter drugs, since there is a potential for REMERONSolTab to interact with other drugs.

Alcohol

The impairment of cognitive and motor skills produced by REMERON has been shown to be additive with those produced by alcohol. Accordingly, patients should be advised to avoid alcohol while taking any dosage form of mirtazapine.

Phenylalanine

Phenylketonuric patients should be informed that REMERONSolTab contains phenylalanine 2.6 mg per 15-mg tablet, 5.2 mg per 30-mg tablet, and 7.8 mg per 45-mg tablet.

Pregnancy
Patients should be advised to notify their physician if they become pregnant or intend to become pregnant during REMERONSolTab therapy.

Nursing
Patients should be advised to notify their physician if they are breast-feeding an infant.

Laboratory Tests
There are no routine laboratory tests recommended.

Drug Interactions
As with other drugs, the potential for interaction by a variety of mechanisms (e.g., pharmacodynamic, pharmacokinetic inhibition or enhancement, etc.) is a possibility (see CLINICAL PHARMACOLOGY).

Monoamine Oxidase Inhibitors
(See CONTRAINDICATIONS, WARNINGS, and DOSAGE AND ADMINISTRATION.)

Serotonergic drugs
Based on the mechanism of action of mirtazapine and the potential for serotonin syndrome, caution is advised when REMERONSolTab Orally Disintegrating Tablets are coadministered with other drugs or agents that may affect the serotonergic neurotransmitter systems, such as tryptophan, triptans, linezolid, serotonin reuptake inhibitors, venlafaxine, lithium, tramadol, or St. John's wort (see CONTRAINDICATIONS and WARNINGS).

Drugs Affecting Hepatic Metabolism
The metabolism and pharmacokinetics of REMERONSolTab (mirtazapine) Orally Disintegrating Tablets may be affected by the induction or inhibition of drug-metabolizing enzymes.

Drugs that are Metabolized by and/or Inhibit Cytochrome P450 Enzymes
CYP Enzyme Inducers (these studies used both drugs at steady state)

Phenytoin
In healthy male patients (n=18), phenytoin (200 mg daily) increased mirtazapine (30 mg daily) clearance about 2-fold, resulting in a decrease in average plasma mirtazapine concentrations of 45%. Mirtazapine did not significantly affect the pharmacokinetics of phenytoin.

Carbamazepine
In healthy male patients (n=24), carbamazepine (400 mg b.i.d.) increased mirtazapine (15 mg b.i.d.) clearance about 2-fold, resulting in a decrease in average plasma mirtazapine concentrations of 60%.

When phenytoin, carbamazepine, or another inducer of hepatic metabolism (such as rifampicin) is added to mirtazapine therapy, the mirtazapine dose may have to be increased. If treatment with such a medicinal product is discontinued, it may be necessary to reduce the mirtazapine dose.

CYP Enzyme Inhibitors

Cimetidine
In healthy male patients (n=12), when cimetidine, a weak inhibitor of CYP1A2, CYP2D6, and CYP3A4, given at 800 mg b.i.d. at steady state was coadministered with mirtazapine (30 mg daily) at steady state, the Area Under the Curve (AUC) of mirtazapine increased more than 50%. Mirtazapine did not cause relevant changes in the pharmacokinetics of cimetidine. The mirtazapine dose may have to be decreased when concomitant treatment with cimetidine is started, or increased when cimetidine treatment is discontinued.

Ketoconazole
In healthy, male, Caucasian patients (n=24), coadministration of the potent CYP3A4 inhibitor ketoconazole (200 mg b.i.d. for 6.5 days) increased the peak plasma levels and the AUC of a single 30-mg dose of mirtazapine by approximately 40% and 50%, respectively.

Caution should be exercised when coadministering mirtazapine with potent CYP3A4 inhibitors, HIV protease inhibitors, azole antifungals, erythromycin, or nefazodone.

Paroxetine
In an *in vivo* interaction study in healthy, CYP2D6 extensive metabolizer patients (n=24), mirtazapine (30 mg/day), at steady state, did not cause relevant changes in the pharmacokinetics of steady state paroxetine (40 mg/day), a CYP2D6 inhibitor.

Other Drug-Drug Interactions
Amitriptyline
In healthy, CYP2D6 extensive metabolizer patients (n=32), amitriptyline (75 mg daily), at steady state, did not cause relevant changes to the pharmacokinetics of steady state mirtazapine (30 mg daily); mirtazapine also did not cause relevant changes to the pharmacokinetics of amitriptyline.

Warfarin
In healthy male subjects (n=16), mirtazapine (30 mg daily), at steady state, caused a small (0.2) but statistically significant increase in the International Normalized Ratio (INR) in subjects treated with warfarin. As at a higher dose of mirtazapine, a more pronounced effect can not be excluded. It is advisable to monitor the INR in case of concomitant treatment of warfarin with mirtazapine.

Lithium
No relevant clinical effects or significant changes in pharmacokinetics have been observed in healthy male subjects on concurrent treatment with subtherapeutic levels of lithium (600 mg/day for 10 days) at steady state and a single 30 mg dose of mirtazapine. The effects of higher doses of lithium on the pharmacokinetics of mirtazapine are unknown.

Risperidone
In an *in vivo*, nonrandomized, interaction study, subjects (n=6) in need of treatment with an antipsychotic and antidepressant drug, showed that mirtazapine (30 mg daily) at steady state did not influence the pharmacokinetics of risperidone (up to 3 mg b.i.d.).

Alcohol
Concomitant administration of alcohol (equivalent to 60 g) had a minimal effect on plasma levels of mirtazapine (15 mg) in 6 healthy male subjects. However, the impairment of cognitive and motor skills produced by REMERON were shown to be additive with those produced by alcohol. Accordingly, patients should be advised to avoid alcohol while taking REMERONSolTab.

Diazepam
Concomitant administration of diazepam (15 mg) had a minimal effect on plasma levels of mirtazapine (15 mg) in 12 healthy subjects. However, the impairment of motor skills produced by REMERON has been shown to be additive with those caused by diazepam. Accordingly, patients should be advised to avoid diazepam and other similar drugs while taking REMERONSolTab.

Carcinogenesis, Mutagenesis, Impairment of Fertility
Carcinogenesis
Carcinogenicity studies were conducted with mirtazapine given in the diet at doses of 2, 20, and 200 mg/kg/day to mice and 2, 20, and 60 mg/kg/day to rats. The highest doses used are approximately 20 and 12 times the maximum recommended human dose (MRHD) of 45 mg/day on an mg/m^2 basis in mice and rats, respectively. There was an increased incidence of hepatocellular adenoma and carcinoma in male mice at the high dose. In rats, there was an increase in hepatocellular adenoma in females at the mid and high doses and in hepatocellular tumors and thyroid follicular adenoma/cystadenoma and carcinoma in males at the high dose. The data suggest that the above effects could possibly be mediated by non-genotoxic mechanisms, the relevance of which to humans is not known.

The doses used in the mouse study may not have been high enough to fully characterize the carcinogenic potential of REMERON (mirtazapine) Tablets.

Mutagenesis
Mirtazapine was not mutagenic or clastogenic and did not induce general DNA damage as determined in several genotoxicity tests: Ames test, *in vitro* gene mutation assay in Chinese hamster V 79 cells, *in vitro* sister chromatid exchange assay in cultured rabbit lymphocytes, *in vivo* bone marrow micronucleus test in rats, and unscheduled DNA synthesis assay in HeLa cells.

Impairment of Fertility
In a fertility study in rats, mirtazapine was given at doses up to 100 mg/kg [20 times the maximum recommended human dose (MRHD) on an mg/m^2 basis]. Mating and conception were not affected by the drug, but estrous cycling was disrupted at doses that were 3 or more times the MRHD, and pre-implantation losses occurred at 20 times the MRHD.

Pregnancy
Teratogenic Effects – Pregnancy Category C
Reproduction studies in pregnant rats and rabbits at doses up to 100 mg/kg and 40 mg/kg, respectively [20 and 17 times the maximum recommended human dose (MRHD) on an mg/m^2 basis, respectively], have revealed no evidence of teratogenic effects. However, in rats, there was an increase in postimplantation losses in dams treated with mirtazapine. There was an increase in pup deaths during the first 3 days of lactation and a decrease in pup birth weights. The cause of these deaths is not known. The effects occurred at doses that were 20 times the MRHD, but not at 3 times the MRHD, on an mg/m^2 basis. There are no adequate and well-controlled studies in pregnant women. Because animal reproduction studies are not always predictive of human response, this drug should be used during pregnancy only if clearly needed.

Nursing Mothers
It is not known whether mirtazapine is excreted in human milk. Because many drugs are excreted in human milk, caution should be exercised when REMERONSolTab (mirtazapine) Orally Disintegrating Tablets are administered to nursing women.

Pediatric Use
Safety and effectiveness in the pediatric population have not been established (see BOX WARNING and WARNINGS: Clinical Worsening and Suicide Risk). Two placebo-controlled trials in 258 pediatric patients with MDD have been conducted with REMERON (mirtazapine) Tablets, and the data were not sufficient to support a claim for use in pediatric patients. Anyone considering the use of REMERONSolTab (mirtazapine) Orally Disintegrating Tablets in a child or adolescent must balance the potential risks with the clinical need.

In an 8-week-long pediatric clinical trial of doses between 15 to 45 mg/day, 49% of REMERON-treated patients had a weight gain of at least 7%, compared to 5.7% of placebo-treated patients. The mean increase in weight was 4 kg (2 kg SD) for REMERON-treated patients versus 1 kg (2 kg SD) for placebo-treated patients (see PRECAUTIONS: Increased Appetite/Weight Gain).

Geriatric Use
Approximately 190 elderly individuals (≥65 years of age) participated in clinical studies with REMERON (mirtazapine) Tablets. This drug is known to be substantially excreted by the kidney (75%), and the risk of decreased clearance of this drug is greater in patients with impaired renal function. Because elderly patients are more likely to have decreased renal function, care should be taken in dose selection. Sedating drugs may cause confusion and over-sedation in the elderly. No unusual adverse age-related phenomena were identified in this group. Pharmacokinetic studies revealed a decreased clearance in the elderly. Caution is indicated in administering REMERONSolTab (mirtazapine) Orally Disintegrating Tablets to elderly patients (see CLINICAL PHARMACOLOGY and DOSAGE AND ADMINISTRATION).

ADVERSE REACTIONS
Associated with Discontinuation of Treatment
Approximately 16% of the 453 patients who received REMERON® (mirtazapine) Tablets in US 6-week controlled clinical trials discontinued treatment due to an adverse experience, compared to 7% of the 361 placebo-treated patients in those studies. The most common events (≥1%) associated with discontinuation and considered to be drug related (i.e., those events associated with dropout at a rate at least twice that of placebo) included:

Common Adverse Events Associated with Discontinuation of Treatment in 6-Week US REMERON Trials

Adverse Event	Percentage of Patients Discontinuing with Adverse Event	
	REMERON (n=453)	Placebo (n=361)
Somnolence	10.4%	2.2%
Nausea	1.5%	0%

Commonly Observed Adverse Events in US Controlled Clinical Trials
The most commonly observed adverse events associated with the use of REMERON (mirtazapine) Tablets (incidence of 5% or greater) and not observed at an equivalent incidence among placebo-treated patients (REMERON incidence at least twice that for placebo) were:

Common Treatment-Emergent Adverse Events Associated with the Use of REMERON in 6-Week US Trials

Adverse Event	Percentage of Patients Reporting Adverse Event	
	REMERON (n=453)	Placebo (n=361)
Somnolence	54%	18%
Increased Appetite	17%	2%
Weight Gain	12%	2%
Dizziness	7%	3%

Adverse Events Occurring at an Incidence of 1% or More Among REMERON-Treated Patients
The table that follows enumerates adverse events that occurred at an incidence of 1% or more, and were more frequent than in the placebo group, among REMERON (mirtazapine) Tablets-treated patients who participated in short-term US placebo-controlled trials in which patients were dosed in a range of 5 to 60 mg/day. This table shows the percentage of patients in each group who had at least 1 episode of an event at some time during their treatment. Reported adverse events were classified using a standard COSTART-based dictionary terminology.

The prescriber should be aware that these figures cannot be used to predict the incidence of side effects in the course of usual medical practice where patient characteristics and other factors differ from those which prevailed in the clinical trials. Similarly, the cited frequencies cannot be compared with figures obtained from other investigations involving different treatments, uses, and investigators. The cited figures, however, do provide the prescribing physician with some basis for estimating the relative contribution of drug and nondrug factors to the side-effect incidence rate in the population studied.

INCIDENCE OF ADVERSE CLINICAL EXPERIENCES* (≥1%) IN SHORT-TERM US CONTROLLED STUDIES

Body System / Adverse Clinical Experience	REMERON (n=453)	Placebo (n=361)
Body as a Whole		
Asthenia	8%	5%
Flu Syndrome	5%	3%
Back Pain	2%	1%
Digestive System		
Dry Mouth	25%	15%
Increased Appetite	17%	2%
Constipation	13%	7%
Metabolic and Nutritional Disorders		
Weight Gain	12%	2%
Peripheral Edema	2%	1%
Edema	1%	0%
Musculoskeletal System		
Myalgia	2%	1%
Nervous System		
Somnolence	54%	18%
Dizziness	7%	3%
Abnormal Dreams	4%	1%
Thinking Abnormal	3%	1%
Tremor	2%	1%
Confusion	2%	0%
Respiratory System		
Dyspnea	1%	0%
Urogenital System		
Urinary Frequency	2%	1%

*Events reported by at least 1% of patients treated with REMERON are included, except the following events which had an incidence on placebo greater than or equal to REMERON: headache, infection, pain, chest pain, palpitation, tachycardia, postural hypotension, nausea, dyspepsia, diarrhea, flatulence, insomnia, nervousness, libido decreased, hypertonia, pharyngitis, rhinitis, sweating, amblyopia, tinnitus, taste perversion.

ECG Changes

The electrocardiograms for 338 patients who received REMERON (mirtazapine) Tablets and 261 patients who received placebo in 6-week, placebo-controlled trials were analyzed. Prolongation in QTc ≥500 msec was not observed among mirtazapine-treated patients; mean change in QTc was +1.6 msec for mirtazapine and −3.1 msec for placebo. Mirtazapine was associated with a mean increase in heart rate of 3.4 bpm, compared to 0.8 bpm for placebo. The clinical significance of these changes is unknown.

Other Adverse Events Observed During the Premarketing Evaluation of REMERON

During its premarketing assessment, multiple doses of REMERON (mirtazapine) Tablets were administered to 2796 patients in clinical studies. The conditions and duration of exposure to mirtazapine varied greatly, and included (in overlapping categories) open and double-blind studies, uncontrolled and controlled studies, inpatient and outpatient studies, fixed-dose and titration studies. Untoward events associated with this exposure were recorded by clinical investigators using terminology of their own choosing. Consequently, it is not possible to provide a meaningful estimate of the proportion of individuals experiencing adverse events without first grouping similar types of untoward events into a smaller number of standardized event categories.

In the tabulations that follow, reported adverse events were classified using a standard COSTART-based dictionary terminology. The frequencies presented, therefore, represent the proportion of the 2796 patients exposed to multiple doses of REMERON who experienced an event of the type cited on at least 1 occasion while receiving REMERON. All reported events are included except those already listed in the previous table, those adverse experiences subsumed under COSTART terms that are either overly general or excessively specific so as to be uninformative, and those events for which a drug cause was very remote. It is important to emphasize that, although the events reported occurred during treatment with REMERON, they were not necessarily caused by it.

Events are further categorized by body system and listed in order of decreasing frequency according to the following definitions: frequent adverse events are those occurring on 1 or more occasions in at least 1/100 patients; infrequent adverse events are those occurring in 1/100 to 1/1000 patients; rare events are those occurring in fewer than 1/1000 patients. Only those events not already listed in the previous table appear in this listing. Events of major clinical importance are also described in the WARNINGS and PRECAUTIONS sections.

Body as a Whole: *frequent:* malaise, abdominal pain, abdominal syndrome acute; *infrequent:* chills, fever, face edema, ulcer, photosensitivity reaction, neck rigidity, neck pain, abdomen enlarged; *rare:* cellulitis, chest pain substernal.

Cardiovascular System: *frequent:* hypertension, vasodilatation; *infrequent:* angina pectoris, myocardial infarction, bradycardia, ventricular extrasystoles, syncope, migraine, hypotension; *rare:* atrial arrhythmia, bigeminy, vascular headache, pulmonary embolus, cerebral ischemia, cardiomegaly, phlebitis, left heart failure.

Digestive System: *frequent:* vomiting, anorexia; *infrequent:* eructation, glossitis, cholecystitis, nausea and vomiting, gum hemorrhage, stomatitis, colitis, liver function tests abnormal; *rare:* tongue discoloration, ulcerative stomatitis, salivary gland enlargement, increased salivation, intestinal obstruction, pancreatitis, aphthous stomatitis, cirrhosis of liver, gastritis, gastroenteritis, oral moniliasis, tongue edema.

Endocrine System: *rare:* goiter, hypothyroidism.

Hemic and Lymphatic System: *rare:* lymphadenopathy, leukopenia, petechia, anemia, thrombocytopenia, lymphocytosis, pancytopenia.

Metabolic and Nutritional Disorders: *frequent:* thirst; *infrequent:* dehydration, weight loss; *rare:* gout, SGOT increased, healing abnormal, acid phosphatase increased, SGPT increased, diabetes mellitus, hyponatremia.

Musculoskeletal System: *frequent:* myasthenia, arthralgia; *infrequent:* arthritis, tenosynovitis; *rare:* pathologic fracture, osteoporosis fracture, bone pain, myositis, tendon rupture, arthrosis, bursitis.

Nervous System: *frequent:* hypesthesia, apathy, depression, hypokinesia, vertigo, twitching, agitation, anxiety, amnesia, hyperkinesia, paresthesia; *infrequent:* ataxia, delirium, delusions, depersonalization, dyskinesia, extrapyramidal syndrome, libido increased, coordination abnormal, dysarthria, hallucinations, manic reaction, neurosis, dystonia, hostility, reflexes increased, emotional lability, euphoria, paranoid reaction; *rare:* aphasia, nystagmus, akathisia (psychomotor restlessness), stupor, dementia, diplopia, drug dependence, paralysis, grand mal convulsion, hypotonia, myoclonus, psychotic depression, withdrawal syndrome, serotonin syndrome.

Respiratory System: *frequent:* cough increased, sinusitis; *infrequent:* epistaxis, bronchitis, asthma, pneumonia; *rare:* asphyxia, laryngitis, pneumothorax, hiccup.

Skin and Appendages: *frequent:* pruritus, rash; *infrequent:* acne, exfoliative dermatitis, dry skin, herpes simplex, alopecia; *rare:* urticaria, herpes zoster, skin hypertrophy, seborrhea, skin ulcer.

Special Senses: *infrequent:* eye pain, abnormality of accommodation, conjunctivitis, deafness, keratoconjunctivitis, lacrimation disorder, glaucoma, hyperacusis, ear pain; *rare:* blepharitis, partial transitory deafness, otitis media, taste loss, parosmia.

Urogenital System: *frequent:* urinary tract infection; *infrequent:* kidney calculus, cystitis, dysuria, urinary incontinence, urinary retention, vaginitis, hematuria, breast pain, amenorrhea, dysmenorrhea, leukorrhea, impotence; *rare:* polyuria, urethritis, metrorrhagia, menorrhagia, abnormal ejaculation, breast engorgement, breast enlargement, urinary urgency.

Other Adverse Events Observed During Postmarketing Evaluation of REMERON

Adverse events reported since market introduction, which were temporally (but not necessarily causally) related to mirtazapine therapy, include 4 cases of the ventricular arrhythmia torsades de pointes. In 3 of the 4 cases, however, concomitant drugs were implicated. All patients recovered. Cases of severe skin reactions, including Stevens-Johnson Syndrome, bullous dermatitis, erythema multiforme and toxic epidermal necrolysis have also been reported.

DRUG ABUSE AND DEPENDENCE

Controlled Substance Class

REMERONSolTab® (mirtazapine) Orally Disintegrating Tablets are not a controlled substance.

Physical and Psychologic Dependence

REMERONSolTab (mirtazapine) Orally Disintegrating Tablets have not been systematically studied in animals or humans for its potential for abuse, tolerance, or physical dependence. While the clinical trials did not reveal any tendency for any drug-seeking behavior, these observations were not systematic and it is not possible to predict on the basis of this limited experience the extent to which a CNS-active drug will be misused, diverted and/or abused once marketed. Consequently, patients should be evaluated carefully for history of drug abuse, and such patients should be observed closely for signs of REMERONSolTab misuse or abuse (e.g., development of tolerance, incrementations of dose, drug-seeking behavior).

OVERDOSAGE

Human Experience

There is very limited experience with REMERONSolTab® (mirtazapine) Orally Disintegrating Tablets overdose. In premarketing clinical studies, there were 8 reports of REMERON® overdose alone or in combination with other pharmacological agents. The only drug overdose death reported while taking REMERON was in combination with amitriptyline and chlorprothixene in a non-US clinical study. Based on plasma levels, the REMERON dose taken was 30 to 45 mg, while plasma levels of amitriptyline and chlorprothixene were found to be at toxic levels. All other premarketing overdose cases resulted in full recovery. Signs and symptoms reported in association with overdose included disorientation, drowsiness, impaired memory, and tachycardia. There were no reports of ECG abnormalities, coma, or convulsions following overdose with REMERON alone.

Overdose Management

Treatment should consist of those general measures employed in the management of overdose with any drug effective in the treatment of major depressive disorder. Ensure an adequate airway, oxygenation, and ventilation. Monitor cardiac rhythm and vital signs. General supportive and symptomatic measures are also recommended. Induction of emesis is not recommended. Gastric lavage with a large-bore orogastric tube with appropriate airway protection, if needed, may be indicated if performed soon after ingestion, or in symptomatic patients. Because of the rapid disintegration of REMERONSolTab (mirtazapine) Orally Disintegrating Tablets, pill fragments may not appear in gastric contents obtained with lavage. Activated charcoal should be administered. There is no experience with the use of forced diuresis, dialysis, hemoperfusion, or exchange transfusion in the treatment of mirtazapine overdosage. No specific antidotes for mirtazapine are known.

In managing overdosage, consider the possibility of multiple-drug involvement. The physician should consider contacting a poison control center for additional information on the treatment of any overdose. Telephone numbers for certified poison control centers are listed in the *Physicians' Desk Reference* (PDR).

DOSAGE AND ADMINISTRATION

Initial Treatment

The recommended starting dose for REMERONSolTab® (mirtazapine) Orally Disintegrating Tablets is 15 mg/day, administered in a single dose, preferably in the evening prior to sleep. In the controlled clinical trials establishing the efficacy of REMERON® in the treatment of major depressive disorder, the effective dose range was generally 15 to 45 mg/day. While the relationship between dose and satisfactory response in the treatment of major depressive disorder for REMERON has not been adequately explored, patients not responding to the initial 15-mg dose may benefit from dose increases up to a maximum of 45 mg/day. REMERON has an elimination half-life of approximately 20 to 40 hours; therefore, dose changes should not be made at intervals of less than 1 to 2 weeks in order to allow sufficient time for evaluation of the therapeutic response to a given dose.

Administration of REMERONSolTab (mirtazapine) Orally Disintegrating Tablets

Patients should be instructed to open tablet blister pack with dry hands and place the tablet on the tongue. The tablet should be used immediately after removal from its blister; once removed, it cannot be stored. REMERONSolTab (mirtazapine) Orally Disintegrating Tablets will disintegrate rapidly on the tongue and can be swallowed with saliva. No water is needed for taking the tablet. Patients should not attempt to split the tablet.

Elderly and Patients with Renal or Hepatic Impairment

The clearance of mirtazapine is reduced in elderly patients and in patients with moderate to severe renal or hepatic impairment. Consequently, the prescriber should be aware that plasma mirtazapine levels may be increased in these patient groups, compared to levels observed in younger adults without renal or hepatic impairment (see PRECAUTIONS and CLINICAL PHARMACOLOGY).

Maintenance/Extended Treatment

It is generally agreed that acute episodes of depression require several months or longer of sustained pharmacological therapy beyond response to the acute episode. Systematic evaluation of REMERON (mirtazapine) Tablets has demonstrated that its efficacy in major depressive disorder is maintained for periods of up to 40 weeks following 8 to 12 weeks of initial treatment at a dose of 15 to 45 mg/day (see CLINICAL PHARMACOLOGY). Based on these limited data, it is unknown whether or not the dose of REMERON needed for maintenance treatment is identical to the dose needed to achieve an initial response. Patients should be periodically reassessed to determine the need for maintenance treatment and the appropriate dose for such treatment.

Switching Patients To or From a Monoamine Oxidase Inhibitor

Concomitant use of REMERONSolTab Orally Disintegrating Tablets with MAOIs is contraindicated. At least 14 days should elapse between discontinuation of an MAOI and initiation of therapy with REMERONSolTab Orally Disintegrating Tablets. In addition, at least 14 days should be allowed after stopping REMERONSolTab before starting an MAOI.

Discontinuation of Remeron Treatment

Symptoms associated with the discontinuation or dose reduction of REMERONSolTab Orally Disintegrating Tablets have been reported. Patients should be monitored for these and other symptoms when discontinuing treatment or during dosage reduction. A gradual reduction in the dose over several weeks, rather than abrupt cessation, is recommended whenever possible. If intolerable symptoms occur following a decrease in the dose or upon discontinuation of treatment, dose titration should be managed on the basis of the patient's clinical response (see PRECAUTIONS and ADVERSE REACTIONS).

HOW SUPPLIED

REMERONSolTab® (mirtazapine) Orally Disintegrating Tablets are supplied as:

15 mg Tablets—round, white, with "ᵀ₁ᶻ" debossed on 1 side.

Box of 30	5 × 6 Unit Dose Blisters	NDC 0052-0106-30
Long Term Care Carton		
Box of 30	5 × 6 Unit Dose Blisters	NDC 0052-0106-93

30 mg Tablets—round, white, with "ᵀ₂ᶻ" debossed on 1 side.

Box of 30	5 × 6 Unit Dose Blisters	NDC 0052-0108-30
Long Term Care Carton		
Box of 30	5 × 6 Unit Dose Blisters	NDC 0052-0108-93

45 mg Tablets—round, white, with "ᵀ₄ᶻ" debossed on 1 side.

Box of 30	5 × 6 Unit Dose Blisters	NDC 0052-0110-30

Storage

Store at 25°C (77°F); excursions permitted to 15°–30°C (59°–86°F) [see USP Controlled Room Temperature]. Protect from light and moisture. Use immediately upon opening individual tablet blister.

Rx only

Manufactured by CIMA Labs Inc., Eden Prairie, MN 55344 USA.

Distributed by Schering Corporation, a subsidiary of Schering-Plough Corporation, Kenilworth, NJ 07033 USA. © 2001, 2007, 20XX Schering Corporation. All rights reserved.

Rev. 5/10

MEDICATION GUIDE

Antidepressant Medicines, Depression and other Serious Mental Illnesses, and Suicidal Thoughts or Actions

Read the Medication Guide that comes with you or your family member's antidepressant medicine. This Medication Guide is only about the risk of suicidal thoughts and actions with antidepressant medicines. **Talk to your, or your family member's, healthcare provider about:**

• all risks and benefits of treatment with antidepressant medicines

• all treatment choices for depression or other serious mental illness

What is the most important information I should know about antidepressant medicines, depression and other serious mental illnesses, and suicidal thoughts or actions?

1. Antidepressant medicines may increase suicidal thoughts or actions in some children, teenagers, and young adults within the first few months of treatment.

2. Depression and other serious mental illnesses are the most important causes of suicidal thoughts and actions. Some people may have a particularly high risk of having suicidal thoughts or actions. These include people who have (or have a family history of) bipolar illness (also called manic-depressive illness) or suicidal thoughts or actions.

3. How can I watch for and try to prevent suicidal thoughts and actions in myself or a family member?
   • Pay close attention to any changes, especially sudden changes, in mood, behaviors, thoughts, or feelings. This is very important when an antidepressant medicine is started or when the dose is changed.
   • Call the healthcare provider right away to report new or sudden changes in mood, behavior, thoughts, or feelings.
   • Keep all follow-up visits with the healthcare provider as scheduled. Call the healthcare provider between visits as needed, especially if you have concerns about symptoms.

Call a healthcare provider right away if you or your family member has any of the following symptoms, especially if they are new, worse, or worry you:

• thoughts about suicide or dying
• attempts to commit suicide
• new or worse depression
• new or worse anxiety
• feeling very agitated or restless
• panic attacks
• trouble sleeping (insomnia)
• new or worse irritability
• acting aggressive, being angry, or violent
• acting on dangerous impulses
• an extreme increase in activity and talking (mania)
• other unusual changes in behavior or mood

Call your doctor for medical advice about side effects. You may report side effects to FDA at 1-800-FDA-1088.

What else do I need to know about antidepressant medicines?

• **Never stop an antidepressant medicine without first talking to a healthcare provider.** Stopping an antidepressant medicine suddenly can cause other symptoms.
• **Antidepressants are medicines used to treat depression and other illnesses.** It is important to discuss all the risks of treating depression and also the risks of not treating it. Patients and their families or other caregivers should discuss all treatment choices with the healthcare provider, not just the use of antidepressants.
• **Antidepressant medicines have other side effects.** Talk to the healthcare provider about the side effects of the medicine prescribed for you or your family member.
• **Antidepressant medicines can interact with other medicines.** Know all of the medicines that you or your family member takes. Keep a list of all medicines to show the healthcare provider. Do not start new medicines without first checking with your healthcare provider.
• **Not all antidepressant medicines prescribed for children are FDA approved for use in children.** Talk to your child's healthcare provider for more information.

This Medication Guide has been approved by the U.S. Food and Drug Administration for all antidepressants.

Shown in Product Identification Guide, page 314

RotaTeq® ℞

[*Row-ta-tech*]
(Rotavirus Vaccine, Live, Oral, Pentavalent)
Oral Solution

HIGHLIGHTS OF PRESCRIBING INFORMATION

These highlights do not include all the information needed to use RotaTeq safely and effectively. See full prescribing information for RotaTeq.

RotaTeq (Rotavirus Vaccine, Live, Oral, Pentavalent) Oral Solution
Initial U.S. Approval: 2006

——RECENT MAJOR CHANGES——

Contraindications (4)	12/2009
Warnings and Precautions (5)	
Immunocompromised Populations (5.1)	09/2010
Shedding and Transmission (5.4)	09/2010

——INDICATIONS AND USAGE——

RotaTeq® is indicated for the prevention of rotavirus gastroenteritis caused by the G1, G2, G3 and G4 serotypes contained in the vaccine. (1)

RotaTeq is approved for use in infants 6 weeks to 32 weeks of age.

——DOSAGE AND ADMINISTRATION——

• FOR ORAL USE ONLY. NOT FOR INJECTION. (2)
• The vaccination series consists of three ready-to-use liquid doses of RotaTeq administered orally starting at 6 to 12 weeks of age, with the subsequent doses administered at 4- to 10-week intervals. The third dose should not be given after 32 weeks of age. (2)

——DOSAGE FORMS AND STRENGTHS——

2 mL solution for oral administration of 5 live human-bovine reassortant rotaviruses which contains a minimum of $2.0–2.8 \times 10^6$ infectious units (IU) per reassortant dose, depending on the serotype, and not greater than 116×10^6 IU per aggregate dose. (3)

——CONTRAINDICATIONS——

• A demonstrated history of hypersensitivity to the vaccine or any component of the vaccine. (4)
• History of Severe Combined Immunodeficiency Disease (SCID). (4) (6.2)

——WARNINGS AND PRECAUTIONS——

• No safety or efficacy data are available from clinical trials regarding the administration of RotaTeq to infants who are potentially immunocompromised (e.g., HIV/AIDS). (5.1)
• No safety or efficacy data are available for the administration of RotaTeq to infants with a history of gastrointestinal disorders (e.g., active acute gastrointestinal illness, chronic diarrhea, failure to thrive, history of congenital abdominal disorders, abdominal surgery and intussusception). (5.2)
• Vaccine virus transmission from vaccine recipient to non-vaccinated contacts has been reported. Caution is advised when considering whether to administer RotaTeq to individuals with immunodeficient contacts. (5.4)

——ADVERSE REACTIONS——

Most common adverse events included diarrhea, vomiting, irritability, otitis media, nasopharyngitis, and bronchospasm. (6.1)

To report SUSPECTED ADVERSE REACTIONS, contact Merck & Co., Inc. at 1-877-888-4231 or VAERS at 1-800-822-7967 or www.vaers.hhs.gov².

——USE IN SPECIFIC POPULATIONS——

Pediatric Use: Safety and efficacy have not been established in infants less than 6 weeks of age or greater than 32 weeks of age. Data are available from clinical studies to support the use of RotaTeq in:
• Pre-term infants according to their age in weeks since birth
• Infants with controlled gastroesophageal reflux disease. (8.4)

See 17 for PATIENT COUNSELING INFORMATION and FDA-approved patient labeling.

Revised: 09/2010

15 REFERENCES
16 HOW SUPPLIED/STORAGE AND HANDLING
  16.1 Storage and Handling
17 PATIENT COUNSELING INFORMATION
  17.1 Information for Parents/Guardians
  17.2 FDA-Approved Patient Labeling
*Sections or subsections omitted from the full prescribing information are not listed.

FULL PRESCRIBING INFORMATION

1 INDICATIONS AND USAGE

RotaTeq[1] is indicated for the prevention of rotavirus gastroenteritis in infants and children caused by the serotypes G1, G2, G3, and G4 when administered as a 3-dose series to infants between the ages of 6 to 32 weeks. The first dose of RotaTeq should be administered between 6 and 12 weeks of age [see Dosage and Administration (2)].

___
[1] Registered trademark MERCK & CO., Inc., Whitehouse Station, New Jersey 08889 USA
COPYRIGHT © 2006, 2007 MERCK & CO., Inc.
All rights reserved

2 DOSAGE AND ADMINISTRATION

FOR ORAL USE ONLY. NOT FOR INJECTION.
The vaccination series consists of three ready-to-use liquid doses of RotaTeq administered orally starting at 6 to 12 weeks of age, with the subsequent doses administered at 4- to 10-week intervals. The third dose should not be given after 32 weeks of age [see Clinical Studies (14)].
There are no restrictions on the infant's consumption of food or liquid, including breast milk, either before or after vaccination with RotaTeq.
Do not mix the RotaTeq vaccine with any other vaccines or solutions. Do not reconstitute or dilute [see Dosage and Administration (2.2)].
For storage instructions [see How Supplied/Storage and Handling (16.1)].
Each dose is supplied in a container consisting of a squeezable plastic dosing tube with a twist-off cap, allowing for direct oral administration. The dosing tube is contained in a pouch [see Dosage and Administration (2.2)].

2.1 Use with Other Vaccines

In clinical trials, RotaTeq was administered concomitantly with other licensed pediatric vaccines [see Adverse Reactions (6.1), Drug Interactions (7.1), and Clinical Studies (14)].

2.2 Instructions for Use

To administer the vaccine:

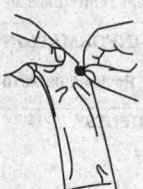

Tear open the pouch and remove the dosing tube.

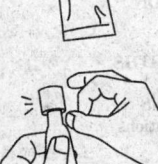

Clear the fluid from the dispensing tip by holding tube vertically and tapping cap.
Open the dosing tube in 2 easy motions:

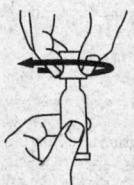

1. Puncture the dispensing tip by screwing cap *clockwise* until it becomes tight.

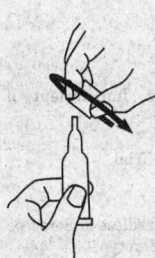

2. Remove cap by turning it *counterclockwise*.

Administer dose by gently squeezing liquid into infant's mouth toward the inner cheek until dosing tube is empty. (A residual drop may remain in the tip of the tube.)
If for any reason an incomplete dose is administered (e.g., infant spits or regurgitates the vaccine), a replacement dose is not recommended, since such dosing was not studied in the clinical trials. The infant should continue to receive any remaining doses in the recommended series.
Discard the empty tube and cap in approved biological waste containers according to local regulations.

3 DOSAGE FORMS AND STRENGTHS

RotaTeq, 2 mL for oral use, is a ready-to-use solution of live reassortant rotaviruses, containing G1, G2, G3, G4 and P1A[8] which contains a minimum of $2.0–2.8 \times 10^6$ infectious units (IU) per individual reassortant dose, depending on the serotype, and not greater than 116×10^6 IU per aggregate dose.
Each dose is supplied in a container consisting of a squeezable plastic dosing tube with a twist-off cap, allowing for direct oral administration. The dosing tube is contained in a pouch.

4 CONTRAINDICATIONS

A demonstrated history of hypersensitivity to any component of the vaccine.
Infants who develop symptoms suggestive of hypersensitivity after receiving a dose of RotaTeq should not receive further doses of RotaTeq.
Infants with Severe Combined Immunodeficiency Disease (SCID) should not receive RotaTeq. Post-marketing reports of gastroenteritis, including severe diarrhea and prolonged shedding of vaccine virus, have been reported in infants who were administered RotaTeq and later identified as having SCID [see Adverse Reactions (6.2)].

5 WARNINGS AND PRECAUTIONS

5.1 Immunocompromised Populations

No safety or efficacy data are available from clinical trials regarding the administration of RotaTeq to infants who are potentially immunocompromised including:
- Infants with blood dyscrasias, leukemia, lymphomas of any type, or other malignant neoplasms affecting the bone marrow or lymphatic system.
- Infants on immunosuppressive therapy (including high-dose systemic corticosteroids). RotaTeq may be administered to infants who are being treated with topical corticosteroids or inhaled steroids.
- Infants with primary and acquired immunodeficiency states, including HIV/AIDS or other clinical manifestations of infection with human immunodeficiency viruses; cellular immune deficiencies; and hypogammaglobulinemic and dysgammaglobulinemic states. There are insufficient data from the clinical trials to support administration of RotaTeq to infants with indeterminate HIV status who are born to mothers with HIV/AIDS.
- Infants who have received a blood transfusion or blood products, including immunoglobulins within 42 days.

Vaccine virus transmission from vaccine recipient to non-vaccinated contacts has been reported [see Warnings and Precautions (5.4)].

5.2 Gastrointestinal Illness

No safety or efficacy data are available for administration of RotaTeq to infants with a history of gastrointestinal disorders including infants with active acute gastrointestinal illness, infants with chronic diarrhea and failure to thrive, and infants with a history of congenital abdominal disorders, abdominal surgery, and intussusception. Caution is advised when considering administration of RotaTeq to these infants.

5.3 Intussusception

Following administration of a previously licensed live rhesus rotavirus-based vaccine, an increased risk of intussusception was observed.[1] In the Rotavirus Efficacy and Safety Trial [REST] (n=69,625), the data did not show an increased risk of intussusception for RotaTeq when compared to placebo. In post-marketing experience, cases of intussusception have been reported in temporal association with RotaTeq. [See Adverse Reactions (6.1 and 6.2).]

5.4 Shedding and Transmission

Shedding of vaccine virus was evaluated among a subset of subjects in REST 4 to 6 days after each dose and among all subjects who submitted a stool antigen rotavirus positive sample at any time. RotaTeq was shed in the stools of 32 of 360 [8.9%, 95% CI (6.2%, 12.3%)] vaccine recipients tested after dose 1; 0 of 249 [0.0%, 95% CI (0.0%, 1.5%)] vaccine recipients tested after dose 2; and in 1 of 385 [0.3%, 95% CI (<0.1%, 1.4%)] vaccine recipients after dose 3. In phase 3 studies, shedding was observed as early as 1 day and as late as 15 days after a dose. Transmission of vaccine virus was not evaluated in phase 3 studies.
Transmission of vaccine virus strains from vaccinees to non-vaccinated contacts has been observed post-marketing.

The potential risk of transmission of vaccine virus should be weighed against the risk of acquiring and transmitting natural rotavirus.
Caution is advised when considering whether to administer RotaTeq to individuals with immunodeficient close contacts such as:
- Individuals with malignancies or who are otherwise immunocompromised;
- Individuals with primary immunodeficiency; or
- Individuals receiving immunosuppressive therapy.

5.5 Febrile Illness

Febrile illness may be reason for delaying use of RotaTeq except when, in the opinion of the physician, withholding the vaccine entails a greater risk. Low-grade fever (<100.5°F [38.1°C]) itself and mild upper respiratory infection do not preclude vaccination with RotaTeq.

5.6 Incomplete Regimen

The clinical studies were not designed to assess the level of protection provided by only one or two doses of RotaTeq.

5.7 Limitations of Vaccine Effectiveness

RotaTeq may not protect all vaccine recipients against rotavirus.

5.8 Post-Exposure Prophylaxis

No clinical data are available for RotaTeq when administered after exposure to rotavirus.

6 ADVERSE REACTIONS

6.1 Clinical Studies Experience

71,725 infants were evaluated in 3 placebo-controlled clinical trials including 36,165 infants in the group that received RotaTeq and 35,560 infants in the group that received placebo. Parents/guardians were contacted on days 7, 14, and 42 after each dose regarding intussusception and any other serious adverse events. The racial distribution was as follows: White (69% in both groups); Hispanic-American (14% in both groups); Black (8% in both groups); Multiracial (5% in both groups); Asian (2% in both groups); Native American (RotaTeq 2%, placebo 1%); and Other (<1% in both groups). The gender distribution was 51% male and 49% female in both vaccination groups.
Because clinical trials are conducted under conditions that may not be typical of those observed in clinical practice, the adverse reaction rates presented below may not be reflective of those observed in clinical practice.

Serious Adverse Events

Serious adverse events occurred in 2.4% of recipients of RotaTeq when compared to 2.6% of placebo recipients within the 42-day period of a dose in the phase 3 clinical studies of RotaTeq. The most frequently reported serious adverse events for RotaTeq compared to placebo were:

bronchiolitis	(0.6% RotaTeq vs. 0.7% Placebo),
gastroenteritis	(0.2% RotaTeq vs. 0.3% Placebo),
pneumonia	(0.2% RotaTeq vs. 0.2% Placebo),
fever	(0.1% RotaTeq vs. 0.1% Placebo), and
urinary tract infection	(0.1% RotaTeq vs. 0.1% Placebo).

Deaths

Across the clinical studies, 52 deaths were reported. There were 25 deaths in the RotaTeq recipients compared to 27 deaths in the placebo recipients. The most commonly reported cause of death was sudden infant death syndrome, which was observed in 8 recipients of RotaTeq and 9 placebo recipients.

Intussusception

In REST, 34,837 vaccine recipients and 34,788 placebo recipients were monitored by active surveillance to identify potential cases of intussusception at 7, 14, and 42 days after each dose, and every 6 weeks thereafter for 1 year after the first dose.
For the primary safety outcome, cases of intussusception occurring within 42 days of any dose, there were 6 cases among RotaTeq recipients and 5 cases among placebo recipients (see Table 1). The data did not suggest an increased risk of intussusception relative to placebo.

Table 1
Confirmed cases of intussusception in recipients of RotaTeq as compared with placebo recipients during REST

	RotaTeq (n=34,837)	Placebo (n=34,788)
Confirmed intussusception cases within 42 days of any dose	6	5
Relative risk (95% CI) *	1.6 (0.4, 6.4)	
Confirmed intussusception cases within 365 days of dose 1	13	15
Relative risk (95% CI)	0.9 (0.4, 1.9)	

*Relative risk and 95% confidence interval based upon group sequential design stopping criteria employed in REST.

Among vaccine recipients, there were no confirmed cases of intussusception within the 42-day period after the first dose, which was the period of highest risk for the rhesus rotavirus-based product (see Table 2).
[See table 2 at right]
All of the children who developed intussusception recovered without sequelae with the exception of a 9-month-old male who developed intussusception 98 days after dose 3 and died of post-operative sepsis. There was a single case of intussusception among 2,470 recipients of RotaTeq in a 7-month-old male in the phase 1 and 2 studies (716 placebo recipients).

Hematochezia
Hematochezia reported as an adverse experience occurred in 0.6% (39/6,130) of vaccine and 0.6% (34/5,560) of placebo recipients within 42 days of any dose. Hematochezia reported as a serious adverse experience occurred in <0.1% (4/36,150) of vaccine and <0.1% (7/35,536) of placebo recipients within 42 days of any dose.

Seizures
All seizures reported in the phase 3 trials of RotaTeq (by vaccination group and interval after dose) are shown in Table 3.

Table 3
Seizures reported by day range in relation to any dose in the phase 3 trials of RotaTeq

Day range	1-7	1-14	1-42
RotaTeq	10	15	33
Placebo	5	8	24

Seizures reported as serious adverse experiences occurred in <0.1% (27/36,150) of vaccine and <0.1% (18/35,536) of placebo recipients (not significant). Ten febrile seizures were reported as serious adverse experiences, 5 were observed in vaccine recipients and 5 in placebo recipients.

Kawasaki Disease
In the phase 3 clinical trials, infants were followed for up to 42 days of vaccine dose. Kawasaki disease was reported in 5 of 36,150 vaccine recipients and in 1 of 35,536 placebo recipients with unadjusted relative risk 4.9 (95% CI 0.6, 239.1).

Most Common Adverse Events
Solicited Adverse Events
Detailed safety information was collected from 11,711 infants (6,138 recipients of RotaTeq) which included a subset of subjects in REST and all subjects from Studies 007 and 009 (Detailed Safety Cohort). A Vaccination Report Card was used by parents/guardians to record the child's temperature and any episodes of diarrhea and vomiting on a daily basis during the first week following each vaccination. Table 4 summarizes the frequencies of these adverse events and irritability.
[See table 4 above]

Other Adverse Events
Parents/guardians of the 11,711 infants were also asked to report the presence of other events on the Vaccination Report Card for 42 days after each dose.
Fever was observed at similar rates in vaccine (N=6,138) and placebo (N=5,573) recipients (42.6% vs. 42.8%). Adverse events that occurred at a statistically higher incidence (i.e., 2-sided p-value <0.05) within the 42 days of any dose among recipients of RotaTeq as compared with placebo recipients are shown in Table 5.

Table 5
Adverse events that occurred at a statistically higher incidence within 42 days of any dose among recipients of RotaTeq as compared with placebo recipients

Adverse event	RotaTeq N=6,138 n (%)	Placebo N=5,573 n (%)
Diarrhea	1,479 (24.1%)	1,186 (21.3%)
Vomiting	929 (15.2%)	758 (13.6%)
Otitis media	887 (14.5%)	724 (13.0%)
Nasopharyngitis	422 (6.9%)	325 (5.8%)
Bronchospasm	66 (1.1%)	40 (0.7%)

Safety in Pre-Term Infants
RotaTeq or placebo was administered to 2,070 pre-term infants (25 to 36 weeks gestational age, median 34 weeks) according to their age in weeks since birth in REST. All pre-term infants were followed for serious adverse experiences; a subset of 308 infants was monitored for all adverse experiences. There were 4 deaths throughout the study, 2 among vaccine recipients (1 SIDS and 1 motor vehicle accident) and 2 among placebo recipients (1 SIDS and 1 unknown

Table 2
Intussusception cases by day range in relation to dose in REST

Day Range	Dose 1 RotaTeq	Dose 1 Placebo	Dose 2 RotaTeq	Dose 2 Placebo	Dose 3 RotaTeq	Dose 3 Placebo	Any Dose RotaTeq	Any Dose Placebo
1-7	0	0	1	0	0	0	1	0
1-14	0	0	1	0	0	1	1	1
1-21	0	0	3	0	0	1	3	1
1-42	0	1	4	1	2	3	6	5

Table 4
Solicited adverse experiences within the first week after doses 1, 2, and 3 (Detailed Safety Cohort)

Adverse experience	Dose 1 RotaTeq	Dose 1 Placebo	Dose 2 RotaTeq	Dose 2 Placebo	Dose 3 RotaTeq	Dose 3 Placebo
Elevated temperature*	n=5,616 17.1%	n=5,077 16.2%	n=5,215 20.0%	n=4,725 19.4%	n=4,865 18.2%	n=4,382 17.6%
	n=6,130	n=5,560	n=5,703	n=5,173	n=5,496	n=4,989
Vomiting	6.7%	5.4%	5.0%	4.4%	3.6%	3.2%
Diarrhea	10.4%	9.1%	8.6%	6.4%	6.1%	5.4%
Irritability	7.1%	7.1%	6.0%	6.5%	4.3%	4.5%

* Temperature ≥100.5°F [38.1°C] rectal equivalent obtained by adding 1 degree F to otic and oral temperatures and 2 degrees F to axillary temperatures

Table 6
Solicited adverse experiences within the first week of doses 1, 2, and 3 among pre-term infants

Adverse event	Dose 1 RotaTeq	Dose 1 Placebo	Dose 2 RotaTeq	Dose 2 Placebo	Dose 3 RotaTeq	Dose 3 Placebo
Elevated temperature*	N=127 18.1%	N=133 17.3%	N=124 25.0%	N=121 28.1%	N=115 14.8%	N=108 20.4%
	N=154	N=154	N=137	N=137	N=135	N=129
Vomiting	5.8%	7.8%	2.9%	2.2%	4.4%	4.7%
Diarrhea	6.5%	5.8%	7.3%	7.3%	3.7%	3.9%
Irritability	3.9%	5.2%	2.9%	4.4%	8.1%	5.4%

* Temperature ≥100.5°F [38.1°C] rectal equivalent obtained by adding 1 degree F to otic and oral temperatures and 2 degrees F to axillary temperatures

cause). No cases of intussusception were reported. Serious adverse experiences occurred in 5.5% of vaccine and 5.8% of placebo recipients. The most common serious adverse experience was bronchiolitis, which occurred in 1.4% of vaccine and 2.0% of placebo recipients. Parents/guardians were asked to record the child's temperature and any episodes of vomiting and diarrhea daily for the first week following vaccination. The frequencies of these adverse experiences and irritability within the week after dose 1 are summarized in Table 6.
[See table 6 above]

6.2   Post-Marketing Experience
The following adverse events have been identified during post-approval use of RotaTeq from reports to the Vaccine Adverse Event Reporting System (VAERS).
Reporting of adverse events following immunization to VAERS is voluntary, and the number of doses of vaccine administered is not known; therefore, it is not always possible to reliably estimate the adverse event frequency or establish a causal relationship to vaccine exposure using VAERS data.
In post-marketing experience, the following adverse events have been reported following the use of RotaTeq:
Gastrointestinal disorders:
Intussusception (including death)
Hematochezia
Gastroenteritis with vaccine viral shedding in infants with Severe Combined Immunodeficiency Disease (SCID)
Skin and subcutaneous tissue disorders:
Urticaria
Infections and infestations:
Kawasaki disease
Transmission of vaccine virus strains from vaccine recipient to non-vaccinated contacts.
Reporting Adverse Events
Parents or guardians should be instructed to report any adverse reactions to their health care provider.
Health care providers should report all adverse events to the U.S. Department of Health and Human Services' Vaccine Adverse Events Reporting System (VAERS). VAERS accepts all reports of suspected adverse events after the administration of any vaccine, including but not limited to the reporting of events required by the National Childhood Vaccine Injury Act of 1986. For information or a copy of the vaccine reporting form, call the VAERS toll-free number at 1-800-822-7967 or report on line to **www.vaers.hhs.gov**.[2]

7   DRUG INTERACTIONS
Immunosuppressive therapies including irradiation, antimetabolites, alkylating agents, cytotoxic drugs and corticosteroids (used in greater than physiologic doses), may reduce the immune response to vaccines.

7.1   Concomitant Vaccine Administration
In clinical trials, RotaTeq was administered concomitantly with diphtheria and tetanus toxoids and acellular pertussis (DTaP), inactivated poliovirus vaccine (IPV), H. influenzae type b conjugate (Hib), hepatitis B vaccine, and pneumococcal conjugate vaccine *[see Clinical Studies (14)]*. The safety data available are in the ADVERSE REACTIONS section *[see Adverse Reactions (6.1)]*. There was no evidence for reduced antibody responses to the vaccines that were concomitantly administered with RotaTeq.

8   USE IN SPECIFIC POPULATIONS
8.1   Pregnancy
Pregnancy Category C: Animal reproduction studies have not been conducted with RotaTeq. It is also not known whether RotaTeq can cause fetal harm when administered to a pregnant woman or can affect reproduction capacity. RotaTeq is not indicated in women of child-bearing age and should not be administered to pregnant females.

8.4   Pediatric Use
Safety and efficacy have not been established in infants less than 6 weeks of age or greater than 32 weeks of age.
Data are available from clinical studies to support the use of RotaTeq in pre-term infants according to their age in weeks since birth *[see Adverse Reactions (6.1)]*.
Data are available from clinical studies to support the use of RotaTeq in infants with controlled gastroesophageal reflux disease.

11   DESCRIPTION
RotaTeq is a live, oral pentavalent vaccine that contains 5 live reassortant rotaviruses. The rotavirus parent strains of the reassortants were isolated from human and bovine

Table 7

Name of Reassortant	Human Rotavirus Parent Strains and Outer Surface Protein Compositions	Bovine Rotavirus Parent Strain and Outer Surface Protein Composition	Reassortant Outer Surface Protein Composition (Human Rotavirus Component in Bold)	Minimum Dose Levels (10^6 infectious units)
G1	WI79 – G1P1A[8]		**G1**P7[5]	2.2
G2	SC2 – G2P2[6]		**G2**P7[5]	2.8
G3	WI78 – G3P1A[8]	WC3 - G6, P7[5]	**G3**P7[5]	2.2
G4	BrB – G4P2[6]		**G4**P7[5]	2.0
P1A[8]	WI79 – G1P1A[8]		G6**P1A[8]**	2.3

Table 8
Efficacy of RotaTeq against any grade of severity of and severe* G1-4 rotavirus gastroenteritis through the first rotavirus season postvaccination in REST

	Per Protocol		Intent-to-Treat†	
	RotaTeq	Placebo	RotaTeq	Placebo
Subjects vaccinated	2,834	2,839	2,834	2,839
	Gastroenteritis cases			
Any grade of severity	82	315	150	371
Severe*	1	51	2	55
	Efficacy estimate % and (95% confidence interval)			
Any grade of severity	74.0 (66.8, 79.9)		60.0 (51.5, 67.1)	
Severe*	98.0 (88.3, 100.0)		96.4 (86.2, 99.6)	

* Severe gastroenteritis defined by a clinical scoring system based on the intensity and duration of symptoms of fever, vomiting, diarrhea, and behavioral changes
† ITT analysis includes all subjects in the efficacy cohort who received at least one dose of vaccine.

Table 9
Efficacy of RotaTeq in reducing G1-4 rotavirus-related hospitalizations in REST

	Per Protocol		Intent-to-Treat*	
	RotaTeq	Placebo	RotaTeq	Placebo
Subjects vaccinated	34,035	34,003	34,035	34,003
Number of hospitalizations	6	144	10	187
Efficacy estimate % and (95% confidence interval)	95.8 (90.5, 98.2)		94.7 (89.3, 97.3)	

*ITT analysis includes all subjects who received at least one dose of vaccine.

hosts. Four reassortant rotaviruses express one of the outer capsid proteins (G1, G2, G3, or G4) from the human rotavirus parent strain and the attachment protein (serotype P7) from the bovine rotavirus parent strain. The fifth reassortant virus expresses the attachment protein, P1A (genotype P[8]), herein referred to as serotype P1A[8], from the human rotavirus parent strain and the outer capsid protein of serotype G6 from the bovine rotavirus parent strain (see Table 7).
[See table 7 above]
The reassortants are propagated in Vero cells using standard cell culture techniques in the absence of antifungal agents.
The reassortants are suspended in a buffered stabilizer solution. Each vaccine dose contains sucrose, sodium citrate, sodium phosphate monobasic monohydrate, sodium hydroxide, polysorbate 80, cell culture media, and trace amounts of fetal bovine serum. RotaTeq contains no preservatives.
In the manufacturing process for RotaTeq, a porcine-derived material is used. DNA from porcine circoviruses (PCV) 1 and 2 has been detected in RotaTeq. PCV-1 and PCV-2 are not known to cause disease in humans.
RotaTeq is a pale yellow clear liquid that may have a pink tint.
The plastic dosing tube and cap do not contain latex.

12   CLINICAL PHARMACOLOGY
Rotavirus is a leading cause of severe acute gastroenteritis in infants and young children, with over 95% of these children infected by the time they are 5 years old.[3] The most severe cases occur among infants and young children between 6 months and 24 months of age.[4]
12.1   Mechanism of Action
The exact immunologic mechanism by which RotaTeq protects against rotavirus gastroenteritis is unknown *[see Clinical Studies (14.6)]*. RotaTeq is a live viral vaccine that replicates in the small intestine and induces immunity.

13   NONCLINICAL TOXICOLOGY
13.1   Carcinogenesis, Mutagenesis, Impairment of Fertility
RotaTeq has not been evaluated for its carcinogenic or mutagenic potential or its potential to impair fertility.

14   CLINICAL STUDIES
Overall, 72,324 infants were randomized in 3 placebo-controlled, phase 3 studies conducted in 11 countries on 3 continents. The data demonstrating the efficacy of RotaTeq in preventing rotavirus gastroenteritis come from 6,983 of these infants from the US (including Navajo and White Mountain Apache Nations) and Finland who were enrolled in 2 of these studies: REST and Study 007. The third trial, Study 009, provided clinical evidence supporting the consistency of manufacture and contributed data to the overall safety evaluation.
The racial distribution of the efficacy subset was as follows: White (RotaTeq 68%, placebo 69%); Hispanic-American (RotaTeq 10%, placebo 9%); Black (2% in both groups); Multiracial (RotaTeq 4%, placebo 5%); Asian (<1% in both groups); Native American (RotaTeq 15%, placebo 14%); and Other (<1% in both groups). The gender distribution was 52% male and 48% female in both vaccination groups.
The efficacy evaluations in these studies included: 1) Prevention of any grade of severity of rotavirus gastroenteritis; 2) Prevention of severe rotavirus gastroenteritis, as defined by a clinical scoring system; and 3) Reduction in hospitalizations due to rotavirus gastroenteritis.
The vaccine was given as a three-dose series to healthy infants with the first dose administered between 6 and 12 weeks of age and followed by two additional doses administered at 4- to 10-week intervals. The age of infants receiving the third dose was 32 weeks of age or less. Oral polio vaccine administration was not permitted; however, other childhood vaccines could be concomitantly administered. Breast-feeding was permitted in all studies.

The case definition for rotavirus gastroenteritis used to determine vaccine efficacy required that a subject meet both of the following clinical and laboratory criteria: (1) greater than or equal to 3 watery or looser-than-normal stools within a 24-hour period and/or forceful vomiting; and (2) rotavirus antigen detection by enzyme immunoassay (EIA) in a stool specimen taken within 14 days of onset of symptoms. The severity of rotavirus acute gastroenteritis was determined by a clinical scoring system that took into account the intensity and duration of symptoms of fever, vomiting, diarrhea, and behavioral changes.
The primary efficacy analyses included cases of rotavirus gastroenteritis caused by serotypes G1, G2, G3, and G4 that occurred at least 14 days after the third dose through the first rotavirus season post vaccination.
Analyses were also done to evaluate the efficacy of RotaTeq against rotavirus gastroenteritis caused by serotypes G1, G2, G3, and G4 at any time following the first dose through the first rotavirus season postvaccination among infants who received at least one vaccination (Intent-to-treat, ITT).
14.1   Rotavirus Efficacy and Safety Trial
Primary efficacy against any grade of severity of rotavirus gastroenteritis caused by naturally occurring serotypes G1, G2, G3, or G4 through the first rotavirus season after vaccination was 74.0% (95% CI: 66.8, 79.9) and the ITT efficacy was 60.0% (95% CI: 51.5, 67.1). Primary efficacy against severe rotavirus gastroenteritis caused by naturally occurring serotypes G1, G2, G3, or G4 through the first rotavirus season after vaccination was 98.0% (95% CI: 88.3, 100.0), and ITT efficacy was 96.4% (95% CI: 86.2, 99.6). See Table 8.
[See table 8 at left]
The efficacy of RotaTeq against severe disease was also demonstrated by a reduction in hospitalizations for rotavirus gastroenteritis among all subjects enrolled in REST. RotaTeq reduced hospitalizations for rotavirus gastroenteritis caused by serotypes G1, G2, G3, and G4 through the first two years after the third dose by 95.8% (95% CI: 90.5, 98.2). The ITT efficacy in reducing hospitalizations was 94.7% (95% CI: 89.3, 97.3) as shown in Table 9.
[See table 9 at left]
14.2   Study 007
Primary efficacy against any grade of severity of rotavirus gastroenteritis caused by naturally occurring serotypes G1, G2, G3, or G4 through the first rotavirus season after vaccination was 72.5% (95% CI: 50.6, 85.6) and the ITT efficacy was 58.4% (95% CI: 33.8, 74.5). Primary efficacy against severe rotavirus gastroenteritis caused by naturally occurring serotypes G1, G2, G3, or G4 through the first rotavirus season after vaccination was 100% (95% CI: 13.0, 100.0) and ITT efficacy against severe rotavirus disease was 100% (95% CI: 30.2, 100.0) as shown in Table 10.
[See table 10 at top of next page]
14.3   Multiple Rotavirus Seasons
The efficacy of RotaTeq through a second rotavirus season was evaluated in a single study (REST). Efficacy against any grade of severity of rotavirus gastroenteritis caused by rotavirus serotypes G1, G2, G3, and G4 through the two rotavirus seasons after vaccination was 71.3% (95% CI: 64.7, 76.9). The efficacy of RotaTeq in preventing cases occurring only during the second rotavirus season postvaccination was 62.6% (95% CI: 44.3, 75.4). The efficacy of RotaTeq beyond the second season postvaccination was not evaluated.
14.4   Rotavirus Gastroenteritis Regardless of Serotype
The rotavirus serotypes identified in the efficacy subset of REST and Study 007 were G1P1A[8]; G2P1[4]; G3P1A[8]; G4P1A[8]; and G9P1A[8].
In REST, the efficacy of RotaTeq against any grade of severity of naturally occurring rotavirus gastroenteritis regardless of serotype was 71.8% (95% CI: 64.5, 77.8) and efficacy against severe rotavirus disease was 98.0% (95% CI: 88.3, 99.9). The ITT efficacy starting at dose 1 was 50.9% (95% CI: 41.6, 58.9) for any grade of severity of rotavirus disease and was 96.4% (95% CI: 86.3, 99.6) for severe rotavirus disease.
In Study 007, the primary efficacy of RotaTeq against any grade of severity of rotavirus gastroenteritis regardless of serotype was 72.7% (95% CI: 51.9, 85.4) and efficacy against severe rotavirus disease was 100% (95% CI: 12.7, 100). The ITT efficacy starting at dose 1 was 48.0% (95% CI: 21.6, 66.1) for any grade of severity of rotavirus disease and was 100% (95% CI: 30.4, 100.0) for severe rotavirus disease.
14.5   Rotavirus Gastroenteritis by Serotype
The efficacy against any grade of severity of rotavirus gastroenteritis by serotype in the REST efficacy cohort is shown in Table 11.
[See table 11 on next page]
In a separate post hoc analysis of health care utilization data from 68,038 infants (RotaTeq 34,035 and placebo 34,003) in REST, using a case definition that included culture confirmation, hospitalization and emergency departments visits due to G9P1A[8] rotavirus gastroenteritis were reduced (RotaTeq 0 cases: placebo 14 cases) by 100% (95% CI: 69.6%, 100.0%).

14.6 Immunogenicity

A relationship between antibody responses to RotaTeq and protection against rotavirus gastroenteritis has not been established. In phase 3 studies, 92.9% to 100% of 439 recipients of RotaTeq achieved a 3-fold or more rise in serum anti-rotavirus IgA after a three-dose regimen when compared to 12.3%-20.0% of 397 placebo recipients.

15 REFERENCES

1. Murphy TV, Gargiullo PM, Massoudi MS et al. Intussusception among infants given an oral rotavirus vaccine. N Engl J Med 2001;344:564-572.
2. Centers for Disease Control and Prevention. General recommendations on immunization: recommendations of the Advisory Committee on Immunization Practices (ACIP) and the American Academy of Family Physicians (AAFP). MMWR 2002;51(RR-2):1-35.
3. Parashar UD et al. Global illness and deaths caused by rotavirus disease in children. Emerg Infect Dis 2003;9(5):565-572.
4. Parashar UD, Holman RC, Clarke MJ, Bresee JS, Glass RI. Hospitalizations associated with rotavirus diarrhea in the United States, 1993 through 1995: surveillance based on the new ICD-9-CM rotavirus-specific diagnostic code. J Infect Dis 1998;177:13-7.

16 HOW SUPPLIED/STORAGE AND HANDLING

No. 4047—RotaTeq, 2 mL, a solution for oral use, is a pale yellow clear liquid that may have a pink tint. It is supplied as follows:

NDC 0006-4047-41 package of 10 individually pouched single-dose tubes.

The plastic dosing tube and cap do not contain latex.

16.1 Storage and Handling

Store and transport refrigerated at 2-8°C (36-46°F). RotaTeq should be administered as soon as possible after being removed from refrigeration. For information regarding stability under conditions other than those recommended, call 1-800-MERCK-90.

Protect from light.

RotaTeq should be discarded in approved biological waste containers according to local regulations.

The product must be used before the expiration date.

17 PATIENT COUNSELING INFORMATION

[See FDA-Approved Patient Labeling (17.2).]

17.1 Information for Parents/Guardians

Parents or guardians should be given a copy of the required vaccine information and be given the "Patient Information" appended to this insert. Parents and/or guardians should be encouraged to read the patient information that describes the benefits and risks associated with the vaccine and ask any questions they may have during the visit. See PRECAUTIONS and Patient Information.

Manuf. and Dist. by:
MERCK & CO., INC., Whitehouse Station, NJ 08889, USA
Issued September 2010
Printed in USA
9714310

17.2 FDA-Approved Patient Labeling

Patient Information

RotaTeq®* (pronounced "RŌ-tuh-tek")
rotavirus vaccine, live, oral, pentavalent

Read this information carefully before your child receives each dose of RotaTeq in case any information about the vaccine changes. Your child will need 3 doses of the vaccine over the course of a few months. This leaflet is a summary of certain information about RotaTeq and does not take the place of talking with your child's doctor, who can give you more complete information written for health care professionals.

* Registered trademark of MERCK & Co., Inc., Whitehouse Station, NJ, 08889 USA
COPYRIGHT © 2008, 2009 MERCK & Co., Inc.
All rights reserved

What is RotaTeq?

RotaTeq is an oral vaccine used to help prevent rotavirus infection in children. Rotavirus infection can cause fever, vomiting, and diarrhea that can be severe and can lead to loss of body fluids (dehydration), hospitalization and even death in some children. RotaTeq may not fully protect all children that get the vaccine, and if your child already has the virus it will not help them.

Who should not receive RotaTeq?

Your child should not get RotaTeq if:
• He or she had an allergic reaction after getting a dose of this vaccine.
• He or she is allergic to any of the ingredients of the vaccine. A list of ingredients can be found at the end of this leaflet.
• He or she has Severe Combined Immunodeficiency Disease (SCID).

Table 10
Efficacy of RotaTeq against any grade of severity of and severe* G1-4 rotavirus gastroenteritis through the first rotavirus season postvaccination in Study 007

| | Per Protocol | | Intent-to-Treat[†] | |
	RotaTeq	Placebo	RotaTeq	Placebo
Subjects vaccinated	650	660	650	660
Gastroenteritis cases				
Any grade of severity	15	54	27	64
Severe*	0	6	0	7

Efficacy estimate % and (95% confidence interval)

	Per Protocol	Intent-to-Treat
Any grade of severity	72. (50.6, 85.6)	58.4 (33.8, 74.5)
Severe*	100.0 (13.0, 100.0)	100.0 (30.2, 100.0)

* Severe gastroenteritis defined by a clinical scoring system based on the intensity and duration of symptoms of fever, vomiting, diarrhea, and behavioral change
[†] ITT analysis includes all subjects in the efficacy cohort who received at least one dose of vaccine.

Table 11
Serotype-specific efficacy of RotaTeq against any grade of severity of rotavirus gastroenteritis among infants in the REST efficacy cohort through the first rotavirus season postvaccination (Per Protocol)

| | Number of cases | | |
Serotype identified by PCR	RotaTeq (N=2,834)	Placebo (N=2,839)	% Efficacy (95% Confidence Interval)
Serotypes present in RotaTeq			
G1P1A[8]	72	286	74.9 (67.3, 80.9)
G2P1[4]	6	17	63.4 (2.6, 88.2)
G3P1A[8]	1	6	NS
G4P1A[8]	3	6	NS
Serotypes not present in RotaTeq			
G9P1A[8]	1	3	NS
Unidentified*	11	15	NS

N=number vaccinated
NS=not significant

* Includes rotavirus antigen-positive samples in which the specific serotype could not be identified by PCR

What should I tell the doctor before my child gets RotaTeq?
Tell your doctor if your child:
• Has illness with fever. A mild fever or cold by itself is not reason to delay taking the vaccine.
• Has diarrhea or has been vomiting.
• Has not been gaining weight or is not growing as expected.
• Has a blood disorder.
• Has any type of cancer.
• Has a weak immune system because of a disease (this includes HIV/AIDS).
• Gets treatment or takes medicines that may weaken the immune system (such as high doses of steroids) or has received a blood transfusion or blood products within the past 42 days.
• Was born with gastrointestinal problems, or has had a blockage or abdominal surgery.
• Has regular close contact with a member of family or household who has a weak immune system such as someone with cancer or someone taking medicines that weaken their immune system.

What are the possible side effects of RotaTeq?
The most common side effects reported after taking RotaTeq were diarrhea, vomiting, fever, runny nose and sore throat, wheezing or coughing, and ear infection.

Other reported side effects include: hives; Kawasaki disease (a serious condition that can affect the heart; symptoms may include fever, rash, red eyes, red mouth, swollen glands, swollen hands and feet and, if not treated, death can occur).

Call your doctor right away if your child has any side effects that concern you or seem to get worse.

These are NOT all the possible side effects of RotaTeq. You can ask your doctor for a more complete list.

You, as a parent or guardian, may also report any adverse reactions to your child's doctor or directly to the Vaccine Adverse Event Reporting System (VAERS). The VAERS toll-free number is 1-800-822-7967 or report online to www.vaers.hhs.gov.

What other important information should I know?
Call your child's doctor or go to the emergency department right away if, following any dose of RotaTeq, your child has vomiting, diarrhea, severe stomach pain, blood in their stool or change in their bowel movements. These symptoms may be signs of a serious and life-threatening problem, called intussusception, that happens when a part of the intestine gets blocked or twisted. Intussusception can happen even when no vaccine has been given and the cause is usually unknown.

Since FDA approval, reports of infants with intussusception have been received by Vaccine Adverse Event Reporting System (VAERS). Intussusception occurred days and sometimes weeks after vaccination. Some infants needed hospitalization, surgery on their intestines, or a special enema to treat this problem. Death due to intussusception has occurred.

Contact your doctor or go to the emergency department right away if your child has any symptoms of intussusception, even if it has been several weeks since the last vaccine dose.

Since FDA approval, the spread of vaccine virus to non-vaccinated contacts has been reported. Tell your doctor if you have someone in your household who has a weak immune system, cancer or is taking medications that can weaken the immune system so that your doctor can provide further advice. Hand washing is recommended after diaper changes to help prevent the spread of vaccine virus.

Can RotaTeq be given with other vaccines?
Your child may get RotaTeq at the same time as other childhood vaccines.

How is RotaTeq given?
The vaccine is given by mouth. Your child will receive 3 doses of the vaccine. The first dose is given when your child is 6 to 12 weeks of age, the second dose is given 4 to 10 weeks later and the third dose is given 4 to 10 weeks after the second dose. The last (third) dose should be given to your child by 32 weeks of age.

Your doctor will gently squeeze the vaccine into your child's mouth (see Figure 1). Your infant may spit out some or all of it. If this happens, the dose does not need to be given again during that visit.

Figure 1:

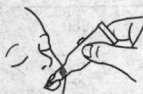

What do I do if my child misses a dose of RotaTeq?
All 3 doses of the vaccine should be given to your child by 32 weeks of age. Your doctor will tell you when your child should come for the follow-up doses. It is important to keep those appointments. If you forget or are not able to go back at the planned time, ask your doctor for advice.

What else should I know about RotaTeq?
This leaflet gives a summary of certain information about the vaccine. If you have any questions or concerns about RotaTeq, talk to your doctor.

What are the ingredients in RotaTeq?
5 live rotavirus strains (G1, G2, G3, G4, and P1).
Sucrose, sodium citrate, sodium phosphate monobasic monohydrate, sodium hydroxide, polysorbate 80 and also fetal bovine serum.
Parts of porcine circovirus (a virus that infects pigs) types 1 and 2 have been found in RotaTeq. Porcine circovirus type 1 (PCV-1) and porcine circovirus type 2 (PCV-2) are not known to cause disease in humans.
Rx only
Issued September 2010
Manuf. and Dist. by:
MERCK & CO., INC., Whitehouse Station, NJ 08889, USA

SAPHRIS®   ℞
[sa-ph-ris]
(asenapine)
sublingual tablets

HIGHLIGHTS OF PRESCRIBING INFORMATION
These highlights do not include all the information needed to use SAPHRIS® (asenapine) safely and effectively. See full prescribing information for SAPHRIS.
SAPHRIS (asenapine) sublingual tablets
Initial U.S. Approval: 2009

> **WARNING: INCREASED MORTALITY IN ELDERLY PATIENTS WITH DEMENTIA-RELATED PSYCHOSIS**
> *See full prescribing information for complete boxed warning.*
> Elderly patients with dementia-related psychosis treated with antipsychotic drugs are at an increased risk of death. SAPHRIS is not approved for the treatment of patients with dementia-related psychosis. (5.1)

————INDICATIONS AND USAGE————
SAPHRIS is an atypical antipsychotic indicated for:
• Acute treatment of schizophrenia in adults (1.1)
• Acute treatment of manic or mixed episodes associated with bipolar I disorder in adults (1.2)
————DOSAGE AND ADMINISTRATION————
Schizophrenia: The recommended starting and target dose of SAPHRIS is 5 mg sublingually twice daily. (2.1)
Bipolar Disorder: The recommended starting dose of SAPHRIS is 10 mg sublingually twice daily. The dose can be decreased to 5 mg twice daily if there are adverse effects. (2.2)
Administration: Do not swallow tablet. SAPHRIS sublingual tablets should be placed under the tongue and left to dissolve completely. The tablet will dissolve in saliva within seconds. Eating and drinking should be avoided for 10 minutes after administration. (2.3, 17.1)
————DOSAGE FORMS AND STRENGTHS————
Sublingual tablets: 5 mg and 10 mg (3)
Sublingual tablets, black cherry flavor: 5 mg and 10 mg (3)
————CONTRAINDICATIONS————
None (4)
————WARNINGS AND PRECAUTIONS————
• *Cerebrovascular Adverse Events:* An increased incidence of cerebrovascular adverse events (e.g., stroke, transient ischemic attack) has been seen in elderly patients with dementia-related psychoses treated with atypical antipsychotic drugs. (5.2)
• *Neuroleptic Malignant Syndrome:* Manage with immediate discontinuation and close monitoring. (5.3)
• *Tardive Dyskinesia:* Discontinue if clinically appropriate. (5.4)
• *Hyperglycemia and Diabetes Mellitus:* Monitor glucose regularly in patients with, and at risk for, diabetes. (5.5)

• *Orthostatic Hypotension and Syncope:* Dizziness, tachycardia or bradycardia, and syncope may occur, especially early in treatment. Use with caution in patients with known cardiovascular or cerebrovascular disease, and in antipsychotic-naïve patients. (5.7)
• *Leukopenia, Neutropenia, and Agranulocytosis* have been reported with antipsychotics. Patients with a pre-existing low white blood cell count (WBC) or a history of leukopenia/neutropenia should have their complete blood count (CBC) monitored frequently during the first few months of therapy and SAPHRIS should be discontinued at the first sign of a decline in WBC in the absence of other causative factors. (5.8)
• *QT Prolongation:* Increases in QT interval; avoid use with drugs that also increase the QT interval and in patients with risk factors for prolonged QT interval. (5.9)
• *Seizures:* Use cautiously in patients with a history of seizures or with conditions that lower the seizure threshold. (5.11)
• *Potential for Cognitive and Motor Impairment:* Use caution when operating machinery. (5.12)
• *Suicide:* The possibility of a suicide attempt is inherent in schizophrenia and bipolar disorder. Closely supervise high-risk patients. (5.14)
————ADVERSE REACTIONS————
Commonly observed adverse reactions (incidence ≥5% and at least twice that for placebo) were (6.2):
• Patients with Schizophrenia: akathisia, oral hypoesthesia, and somnolence.
• Patients with Bipolar Disorder: somnolence, dizziness, extrapyramidal symptoms other than akathisia, and weight increased.
To report SUSPECTED ADVERSE REACTIONS, contact Schering-Plough at 1-800-526-4099 or FDA at 1-800-FDA-1088 or www.fda.gov/medwatch.
————DRUG INTERACTIONS————
• *Fluvoxamine (strong CYP1A2 inhibitor) and Paroxetine (CYP2D6 substrate and inhibitor):* cautiously approach coadministration with SAPHRIS. (7.1, 7.2)
————USE IN SPECIFIC POPULATIONS————
• *Pregnancy:* Use SAPHRIS during pregnancy only if the potential benefit justifies the potential risk. (8.1)
• *Nursing Mothers:* Breast feeding is not recommended. (8.3)
• *Pediatric Use:* Safety and effectiveness have not been established. (8.4)
• *Renal Impairment:* No dose adjustment needed. (8.6)
• *Hepatic Impairment:* SAPHRIS is not recommended in patients with severe hepatic impairment (Child-Pugh C). (2.4, 8.7, 12.3)
See 17 for PATIENT COUNSELING INFORMATION
                                                    Revised: 06/2010

FULL PRESCRIBING INFORMATION: CONTENTS*
WARNING: INCREASED MORTALITY IN ELDERLY PATIENTS WITH DEMENTIA-RELATED PSYCHOSIS
* Sections or subsections omitted from the full prescribing information are not listed

---

FULL PRESCRIBING INFORMATION

> **WARNING: INCREASED MORTALITY IN ELDERLY PATIENTS WITH DEMENTIA-RELATED PSYCHOSIS**
> Elderly patients with dementia-related psychosis treated with antipsychotic drugs are at an increased risk of death. Analyses of 17 placebo-controlled trials (modal duration of 10 weeks), largely in patients taking atypical antipsychotic drugs, revealed a risk of death in the drug-treated patients of between 1.6 and 1.7 times that seen in placebo-treated patients. Over the course of a typical 10-week controlled trial, the rate of death in drug-treated patients was about 4.5%, compared to a rate of about 2.6% in the placebo group. Although the causes of death were varied, most of the deaths appeared to be either cardiovascular (e.g., heart failure, sudden death) or infectious (e.g., pneumonia) in nature. Observational studies suggest that, similar to atypical antipsychotic drugs, treatment with conventional antipsychotic drugs may increase mortality. The extent to which the findings of increased mortality in observational studies may be attributed to the antipsychotic drug as opposed to some characteristic(s) of the patients is not clear. SAPHRIS® (asenapine) is not approved for the treatment of patients with dementia-related psychosis *[see Warnings and Precautions (5.1)]*.

1   INDICATIONS AND USAGE
1.1   Schizophrenia
SAPHRIS is indicated for the acute treatment of schizophrenia in adults *[see Clinical Studies (14.1)]*. The physician who elects to use SAPHRIS for extended periods in schizophrenia should periodically re-evaluate the long-term risks and benefits of the drug for the individual patient *[see Dosage and Administration (2.1)]*.
1.2   Bipolar Disorder
SAPHRIS is indicated for the acute treatment of manic or mixed episodes associated with bipolar I disorder with or without psychotic features in adults *[see Clinical Studies (14.2)]*. If SAPHRIS is used for extended periods in bipolar disorder, the physician should periodically re-evaluate the long-term risks and benefits of the drug for the individual patient *[see Dosage and Administration (2.2)]*.

2   DOSAGE AND ADMINISTRATION
2.1   Schizophrenia
Usual Dose for Acute Treatment in Adults: The recommended starting and target dose of SAPHRIS is 5 mg given twice daily. In controlled trials, there was no suggestion of added benefit with the higher dose, but there was a clear increase in certain adverse reactions. The safety of doses above 10 mg twice daily has not been evaluated in clinical studies.
Maintenance Treatment: While there is no body of evidence available to answer the question of how long the

schizophrenic patient should remain on SAPHRIS, it is generally recommended that responding patients be continued beyond the acute response.

2.2 Bipolar Disorder

Usual Dose for Acute Treatment in Adults: The recommended starting dose of SAPHRIS, and the dose maintained by 90% of the patients studied, is 10 mg twice daily. The dose can be decreased to 5 mg twice daily if there are adverse effects.

In controlled trials, the starting dose for SAPHRIS was 10 mg twice daily. On the second and subsequent days of the trials, the dose could be lowered to 5 mg twice daily, based on tolerability, but less than 10% of patients had their dose reduced. The safety of doses above 10 mg twice daily has not been evaluated in clinical trials.

Maintenance Treatment: While there is no body of evidence available to answer the question of how long the bipolar patient should remain on SAPHRIS, it is generally recommended that responding patients be continued beyond the acute response.

2.3 Administration Instructions

SAPHRIS is a sublingual tablet. To ensure optimal absorption, patients should be instructed to place the tablet under the tongue and allow it to dissolve completely. The tablet will dissolve in saliva within seconds. SAPHRIS sublingual tablets should not be crushed, chewed, or swallowed *[see Clinical Pharmacology (12.3)]*. Patients should be instructed to not eat or drink for 10 minutes after administration *[see Clinical Pharmacology (12.3) and Patient Counseling Information (17.1)]*.

2.4 Dosage in Special Populations

In a study of subjects with hepatic impairment who were treated with a single dose of SAPHRIS 5 mg, there were increases in asenapine exposures (compared to subjects with normal hepatic function), that correlated with the degree of hepatic impairment. While the results indicated that no dosage adjustments are required in patients with mild (Child-Pugh A) or moderate (Child-Pugh B) hepatic impairment, there was a 7-fold increase (on average) in asenapine concentrations in subjects with severe hepatic impairment (Child-Pugh C) compared to the concentrations of those in subjects with normal hepatic function. Therefore, SAPHRIS is not recommended in patients with severe hepatic impairment *[see Use in Special Populations (8.7)]*. Dosage adjustments are not routinely required on the basis of age, gender, race, or renal impairment status *[see Use in Specific Populations (8.4, 8.5, 8.6) and Clinical Pharmacology (12.3)]*.

2.5 Switching from Other Antipsychotics

There are no systematically collected data to specifically address switching patients with schizophrenia or bipolar mania from other antipsychotics to SAPHRIS or concerning concomitant administration with other antipsychotics. While immediate discontinuation of the previous antipsychotic treatment may be acceptable for some patients with schizophrenia, more gradual discontinuation may be most appropriate for others. In all cases, the period of overlapping antipsychotic administration should be minimized.

3 DOSAGE FORMS AND STRENGTHS

- SAPHRIS 5-mg tablets are round, white- to off-white sublingual tablets, with "5" on one side.
- SAPHRIS 10-mg tablets are round, white- to off-white sublingual tablets, with "10" on one side.
- SAPHRIS 5-mg tablets, black cherry flavor, are round, white- to off-white sublingual tablets, with "5" on one side within a circle.
- SAPHRIS 10-mg tablets, black cherry flavor, are round, white- to off-white sublingual tablets, with "10" on one side within a circle.

4 CONTRAINDICATIONS

None

5 WARNINGS AND PRECAUTIONS

5.1 Increased Mortality in Elderly Patients with Dementia-Related Psychosis

Elderly patients with dementia-related psychosis treated with antipsychotic drugs are at an increased risk of death. SAPHRIS is not approved for the treatment of patients with dementia-related psychosis *[see Boxed Warning]*.

5.2 Cerebrovascular Adverse Events, Including Stroke, In Elderly Patients with Dementia-Related Psychosis

In placebo-controlled trials with risperidone, aripiprazole, and olanzapine in elderly subjects with dementia, there was a higher incidence of cerebrovascular adverse reactions (cerebrovascular accidents and transient ischemic attacks) including fatalities compared to placebo-treated subjects. SAPHRIS is not approved for the treatment of patients with dementia-related psychosis *[see also Boxed Warning and Warnings and Precautions (5.1)]*.

5.3 Neuroleptic Malignant Syndrome

A potentially fatal symptom complex sometimes referred to as Neuroleptic Malignant Syndrome (NMS) has been reported in association with administration of antipsychotic drugs, including SAPHRIS. Clinical manifestations of NMS are hyperpyrexia, muscle rigidity, altered mental status, and evidence of autonomic instability (irregular pulse or blood pressure, tachycardia, diaphoresis, and cardiac dysrhythmia). Additional signs may include elevated creatine phosphokinase, myoglobinuria (rhabdomyolysis), and acute renal failure.

The diagnostic evaluation of patients with this syndrome is complicated. It is important to exclude cases where the clinical presentation includes both serious medical illness (e.g. pneumonia, systemic infection) and untreated or inadequately treated extrapyramidal signs and symptoms (EPS). Other important considerations in the differential diagnosis include central anticholinergic toxicity, heat stroke, drug fever, and primary central nervous system pathology.

The management of NMS should include: 1) immediate discontinuation of antipsychotic drugs and other drugs not essential to concurrent therapy; 2) intensive symptomatic treatment and medical monitoring; and 3) treatment of any concomitant serious medical problems for which specific treatments are available. There is no general agreement about specific pharmacological treatment regimens for NMS.

If a patient requires antipsychotic drug treatment after recovery from NMS, the potential reintroduction of drug therapy should be carefully considered. The patient should be carefully monitored, since recurrences of NMS have been reported.

5.4 Tardive Dyskinesia

A syndrome of potentially irreversible, involuntary, dyskinetic movements can develop in patients treated with antipsychotic drugs. Although the prevalence of the syndrome appears to be highest among the elderly, especially elderly women, it is impossible to rely upon prevalence estimates to predict, at the inception of antipsychotic treatment, which patients are likely to develop the syndrome. Whether antipsychotic drug products differ in their potential to cause Tardive Dyskinesia (TD) is unknown.

The risk of developing TD and the likelihood that it will become irreversible are believed to increase as the duration of treatment and the total cumulative dose of antipsychotic drugs administered to the patient increase. However, the syndrome can develop, although much less commonly, after relatively brief treatment periods at low doses.

There is no known treatment for established cases of TD, although the syndrome may remit, partially or completely, if antipsychotic treatment is withdrawn. Antipsychotic treatment, itself, however, may suppress (or partially suppress) the signs and symptoms of the syndrome and thereby may possibly mask the underlying process. The effect that symptomatic suppression has upon the long-term course of the syndrome is unknown.

Given these considerations, SAPHRIS should be prescribed in a manner that is most likely to minimize the occurrence of TD. Chronic antipsychotic treatment should generally be reserved for patients who suffer from a chronic illness that (1) is known to respond to antipsychotic drugs, and (2) for whom alternative, equally effective, but potentially less harmful treatments are not available or appropriate. In patients who do require chronic treatment, the smallest dose and the shortest duration of treatment producing a satisfactory clinical response should be sought. The need for continued treatment should be reassessed periodically.

If signs and symptoms of TD appear in a patient on SAPHRIS, drug discontinuation should be considered. However, some patients may require treatment with SAPHRIS despite the presence of the syndrome.

5.5 Hyperglycemia and Diabetes Mellitus

Hyperglycemia, in some cases extreme and associated with ketoacidosis or hyperosmolar coma or death, has been reported in patients treated with atypical antipsychotics. In clinical trials of SAPHRIS, the occurrence of any adverse reaction related to glucose metabolism was less than 1% in both the SAPHRIS and placebo treatment groups. Assessment of the relationship between atypical antipsychotic use and glucose abnormalities is complicated by the possibility of an increased background risk of diabetes mellitus in patients with schizophrenia and the increasing incidence of diabetes mellitus in the general population. Given these confounders, the relationship between atypical antipsychotic use and hyperglycemia-related adverse reactions is not completely understood. However, epidemiological studies, which did not include SAPHRIS, suggest an increased risk of treatment-emergent hyperglycemia-related adverse reactions in patients treated with the atypical antipsychotics included in these studies.

Patients with an established diagnosis of diabetes mellitus who are started on atypical antipsychotics should be monitored regularly for worsening of glucose control. Patients with risk factors for diabetes mellitus (e.g., obesity, family history of diabetes) who are starting treatment with atypical antipsychotics should undergo fasting blood glucose testing at the beginning of treatment and periodically during treatment. Any patient treated with atypical antipsychotics should be monitored for symptoms of hyperglycemia including polydipsia, polyuria, polyphagia, and weakness. Patients who develop symptoms of hyperglycemia during treatment with atypical antipsychotics should undergo fasting blood glucose testing. In some cases, hyperglycemia has resolved when the atypical antipsychotic was discontinued; however, some patients required continuation of anti-diabetic treatment despite discontinuation of the antipsychotic drug.

5.6 Weight Gain

In short-term schizophrenia and bipolar mania trials, there were differences in mean weight gain between SAPHRIS-treated and placebo-treated patients. In short-term, placebo-controlled schizophrenia trials, the mean weight gain was 1.1 kg for SAPHRIS-treated patients compared to 0.1 kg for placebo-treated patients. The proportion of patients with a ≥7% increase in body weight (at Endpoint) was 4.9% for SAPHRIS-treated patients versus 2% for placebo-treated patients. In short-term, placebo-controlled bipolar mania trials, the mean weight gain for SAPHRIS-treated patients was 1.3 kg compared to 0.2 kg for placebo-treated patients. The proportion of patients with a ≥7% increase in body weight (at Endpoint) was 5.8% for SAPHRIS-treated patients versus 0.5% for placebo-treated patients.

In a 52-week, double-blind, comparator-controlled trial of patients with schizophrenia or schizoaffective disorder, the mean weight gain from baseline was 0.9 kg. The proportion of patients with a ≥7% increase in body weight (at Endpoint) was 14.7%. Table 1 provides the mean weight change from baseline and the proportion of patients with a weight gain of ≥7% categorized by Body Mass Index (BMI) at baseline:

[See table 1 above]

TABLE 1: Weight Change Results Categorized by BMI at Baseline: Comparator-Controlled 52-Week Study in Schizophrenia

	BMI < 23 SAPHRIS N=295	BMI 23-≤ 27 SAPHRIS N=290	BMI > 27 SAPHRIS N=302
Mean change from Baseline (kg)	1.7	1	0
% with ≥ 7% increase in body weight	22%	13%	9%

5.7 Orthostatic Hypotension, Syncope, and Other Hemodynamic Effects

SAPHRIS may induce orthostatic hypotension and syncope in some patients, especially early in treatment, because of its α1-adrenergic antagonist activity. In short-term schizophrenia trials, syncope was reported in 0.2% (1/572) of patients treated with therapeutic doses (5 mg or 10 mg twice daily) of SAPHRIS, compared to 0.3% (1/378) of patients treated with placebo. In short-term bipolar mania trials, syncope was reported in 0.3% (1/379) of patients treated with therapeutic doses (5 mg or 10 mg twice daily) of SAPHRIS, compared to 0% (0/203) of patients treated with placebo. During clinical trials with SAPHRIS, including long-term trials without comparison to placebo, syncope was reported in 0.6% (11/1953) of patients treated with SAPHRIS.

Four normal volunteers in clinical pharmacology studies treated with either intravenous, oral, or sublingual SAPHRIS experienced hypotension, bradycardia, and sinus pauses. These spontaneously resolved in 3 cases, but the fourth subject received external cardiac massage. The risk of this sequence of hypotension, bradycardia, and sinus pause might be greater in nonpsychiatric patients compared to psychiatric patients who are possibly more adapted to certain effects of psychotropic drugs.

Patients should be instructed about nonpharmacologic interventions that help to reduce the occurrence of orthostatic hypotension (e.g., sitting on the edge of the bed for several minutes before attempting to stand in the morning and slowly rising from a seated position). SAPHRIS should be used with caution in (1) patients with known cardiovascular disease (history of myocardial infarction or ischemic heart disease, heart failure or conduction abnormalities), cerebrovascular disease, or conditions which would predispose patients to hypotension (dehydration, hypovolemia, and treatment with antihypertensive medications); and (2) in the elderly. SAPHRIS should be used cautiously when treating patients who receive treatment with other drugs that can induce hypotension, bradycardia, respiratory or central nervous system depression *[see Drug Interactions (7)]*. Monitoring of orthostatic vital signs should be considered in all such patients, and a dose reduction should be considered if hypotension occurs.

5.8 Leukopenia, Neutropenia, and Agranulocytosis

In clinical trial and postmarketing experience, events of leukopenia/neutropenia have been reported temporally related to antipsychotic agents, including SAPHRIS. Agranulocytosis (including fatal cases) has been reported with other agents in the class.

Possible risk factors for leukopenia/neutropenia include pre-existing low white blood cell count (WBC) and history of drug induced leukopenia/neutropenia. Patients with a pre-existing low WBC or a history of drug induced leukopenia/neutropenia should have their complete blood count (CBC) monitored frequently during the first few months of therapy and SAPHRIS should be discontinued at the first sign of decline in WBC in the absence of other causative factors. Patients with neutropenia should be carefully monitored for fever or other symptoms or signs of infection and treated promptly if such symptoms or signs occur. Patients with severe neutropenia (absolute neutrophil count <1000/mm^3) should discontinue SAPHRIS and have their WBC followed until recovery.

5.9 QT Prolongation

The effects of SAPHRIS on the QT/QTc interval were evaluated in a dedicated QT study. This trial involved SAPHRIS doses of 5 mg, 10 mg, 15 mg, and 20 mg twice daily, and placebo, and was conducted in 151 clinically stable patients with schizophrenia, with electrocardiographic assessments throughout the dosing interval at baseline and steady state. At these doses, SAPHRIS was associated with increases in QTc interval ranging from 2 to 5 msec compared to placebo. No patients treated with SAPHRIS experienced QTc increases ≥60 msec from baseline measurements, nor did any patient experience a QTc of ≥500 msec.

Electrocardiogram (ECG) measurements were taken at various time points during the SAPHRIS clinical trial program (5 mg or 10 mg twice daily doses). Post-baseline QT prolongations exceeding 500 msec were reported at comparable rates for SAPHRIS and placebo in these short-term trials. There were no reports of Torsade de Pointes or any other adverse reactions associated with delayed ventricular repolarization.

The use of SAPHRIS should be avoided in combination with other drugs known to prolong QTc including Class 1A antiarrhythmics (e.g., quinidine, procainamide) or Class 3 antiarrhythmics (e.g., amiodarone, sotalol), antipsychotic medications (e.g., ziprasidone, chlorpromazine, thioridazine), and antibiotics (e.g., gatifloxacin, moxifloxacin). SAPHRIS should also be avoided in patients with a history of cardiac arrhythmias and in other circumstances that may increase the risk of the occurrence of torsade de pointes and/or sudden death in association with the use of drugs that prolong the QTc interval, including bradycardia; hypokalemia or hypomagnesemia; and presence of congenital prolongation of the QT interval.

5.10 Hyperprolactinemia

Like other drugs that antagonize dopamine D_2 receptors, SAPHRIS can elevate prolactin levels, and the elevation can persist during chronic administration. Hyperprolactinemia may suppress hypothalamic GnRH, resulting in reduced pituitary gonadotropin secretion. This, in turn, may inhibit reproductive function by impairing gonadal steroidogenesis in both female and male patients. Galactorrhea, amenorrhea, gynecomastia, and impotence have been reported in patients receiving prolactin-elevating compounds. Long-standing hyperprolactinemia when associated with hypogonadism may lead to decreased bone density in both female and male subjects. In SAPHRIS clinical trials, the incidences of adverse events related to abnormal prolactin levels were 0.4% versus 0% for placebo *[see Adverse Reactions (6.2)]*.

Tissue culture experiments indicate that approximately one-third of human breast cancers are prolactin-dependent *in vitro*, a factor of potential importance if the prescription of these drugs is considered in a patient with previously-detected breast cancer. Neither clinical studies nor epidemiologic studies conducted to date have shown an association between chronic administration of this class of drugs and tumorigenesis in humans, but the available evidence is too limited to be conclusive.

5.11 Seizures

Seizures were reported in 0% and 0.3% (0/572, 1/379) of patients treated with doses of 5 mg and 10 mg twice daily of SAPHRIS, respectively, compared to 0% (0/503, 0/203) of patients treated with placebo in short-term schizophrenia and bipolar mania trials, respectively. During clinical trials with SAPHRIS, including long-term trials without comparison to placebo, seizures were reported in 0.3% (5/1953) of patients treated with SAPHRIS. As with other antipsychotic drugs, SAPHRIS should be used with caution in patients with a

history of seizures or with conditions that potentially lower the seizure threshold, e.g., Alzheimer's dementia. Conditions that lower the seizure threshold may be more prevalent in patients 65 years or older.

5.12 Potential for Cognitive and Motor Impairment

Somnolence was reported in patients treated with SAPHRIS. It was usually transient with the highest incidence reported during the first week of treatment. In short-term, fixed-dose, placebo-controlled schizophrenia trials, somnolence was reported in 15% (41/274) of patients on SAPHRIS 5 mg twice daily and 13% (26/208) of patients on SAPHRIS 10 mg twice daily compared to 7% (26/378) of placebo patients. In short-term, placebo-controlled bipolar mania trials of therapeutic doses (5-10 mg twice daily), somnolence was reported in 24% (90/379) of patients on SAPHRIS compared to 6% (13/203) of placebo patients. During clinical trials with SAPHRIS, including long-term trials without comparison to placebo, somnolence was reported in 18% (358/1953) of patients treated with SAPHRIS. Somnolence (including sedation) led to discontinuation in 0.6% (12/1953) of patients in short-term, placebo-controlled trials.

Patients should be cautioned about performing activities requiring mental alertness, such as operating hazardous machinery or operating a motor vehicle, until they are reasonably certain that SAPHRIS therapy does not affect them adversely.

5.13 Body Temperature Regulation

Disruption of the body's ability to reduce core body temperature has been attributed to antipsychotic agents. In the short-term placebo-controlled trials for both schizophrenia and acute bipolar disorder, the incidence of adverse reactions suggestive of body temperature increases was low

(≤1%) and comparable to placebo. During clinical trials with SAPHRIS, including long-term trials without comparison to placebo, the incidence of adverse reactions suggestive of body temperature increases (pyrexia and feeling hot) was ≤1%. Appropriate care is advised when prescribing SAPHRIS for patients who will be experiencing conditions that may contribute to an elevation in core body temperature, e.g., exercising strenuously, exposure to extreme heat, receiving concomitant medication with anticholinergic activity, or being subject to dehydration.

5.14 Suicide

The possibility of a suicide attempt is inherent in psychotic illnesses and bipolar disorder, and close supervision of high-risk patients should accompany drug therapy. Prescriptions for SAPHRIS should be written for the smallest quantity of tablets consistent with good patient management in order to reduce the risk of overdose.

5.15 Dysphagia

Esophageal dysmotility and aspiration have been associated with antipsychotic drug use. Dysphagia was reported in 0.2% and 0% (1/572, 0/379) of patients treated with therapeutic doses (5-10 mg twice daily) of SAPHRIS as compared to 0% (0/378, 0/203) of patients treated with placebo in short-term schizophrenia and bipolar mania trials, respectively. During clinical trials with SAPHRIS, including long-term trials without comparison to placebo, dysphagia was reported in 0.1% (2/1953) of patients treated with SAPHRIS.

Aspiration pneumonia is a common cause of morbidity and mortality in elderly patients, in particular those with advanced Alzheimer's dementia. SAPHRIS is not indicated for the treatment of dementia-related psychosis, and should not be used in patients at risk for aspiration pneumonia *[see also Warnings and Precautions (5.1)]*.

TABLE 2: Adverse Reactions Reported in 2% or More of Subjects in one of the SAPHRIS Dose Groups and Which Occurred at Greater Incidence Than in the Placebo group in 6-Week Schizophrenia Trials

System Organ Class/ Preferred Term	Placebo N=378	SAPHRIS 5 mg twice daily N=274	SAPHRIS 10 mg twice daily N=208	All SAPHRIS* 5 or 10 mg twice daily N=572
Gastrointestinal disorders				
Constipation	6%	7%	4%	5%
Dry mouth	1%	3%	1%	2%
Oral hypoesthesia	1%	6%	7%	5%
Salivary hypersecretion	0%	<1%	4%	2%
Stomach discomfort	1%	<1%	3%	2%
Vomiting	5%	4%	7%	5%
General disorders				
Fatigue	3%	4%	3%	3%
Irritability	<1%	2%	1%	2%
Investigations				
Weight increased	<1%	2%	2%	3%
Metabolism disorders				
Increased appetite	<1%	3%	0%	2%
Nervous system disorders				
Akathisia[†]	3%	4%	11%	6%
Dizziness	4%	7%	3%	5%
Extrapyramidal symptoms (excluding akathisia)[‡]	7%	9%	12%	10%
Somnolence[§]	7%	15%	13%	13%
Psychiatric disorders				
Insomnia	13%	16%	15%	15%
Vascular disorders				
Hypertension	2%	2%	3%	2%

*Also includes the Flexible-dose trial (N=90).
†Akathisia includes: akathisia and hyperkinesia.
‡Extrapyramidal symptoms included dystonia, oculogyration, dyskinesia, tardive dyskinesia, muscle rigidity, parkinsonism, tremor, and extrapyramidal disorder (excluding akathisia).
§Somnolence includes the following events: somnolence, sedation, and hypersomnia.

5.16 Use in Patients with Concomitant Illness

Clinical experience with SAPHRIS in patients with certain concomitant systemic illnesses is limited [see Clinical Pharmacology (12.3)].

SAPHRIS has not been evaluated in patients with a recent history of myocardial infarction or unstable heart disease. Patients with these diagnoses were excluded from premarketing clinical trials. Because of the risk of orthostatic hypotension with SAPHRIS, caution should be observed in cardiac patients [see Warnings and Precautions (5.6)].

6 ADVERSE REACTIONS

6.1 Overall Adverse Reactions Profile

The following adverse reactions are discussed in more detail in other sections of the labeling:

- Use in Elderly Patients with Dementia-Related Psychosis [see Boxed Warning and Warnings and Precautions (5.1 and 5.2)]
- Neuroleptic Malignant Syndrome [see Warnings and Precautions (5.3)]
- Tardive Dyskinesia [see Warnings and Precautions (5.4)]
- Hyperglycemia and Diabetes Mellitus [see Warnings and Precautions (5.5)]
- Weight Gain [see Warnings and Precautions (5.6)]
- Orthostatic Hypotension, Syncope, and other Hemodynamic Effects [see Warnings and Precautions (5.7)]
- Leukopenia, Neutropenia, and Agranulocytosis [see Warnings and Precautions (5.8)]
- QT Interval Prolongation [see Warnings and Precautions (5.9)]
- Hyperprolactinemia [see Warnings and Precautions (5.10)]
- Seizures [see Warnings and Precautions (5.11)]
- Potential for Cognitive and Motor Impairment [see Warnings and Precautions (5.12)]
- Body Temperature Regulation [see Warnings and Precautions (5.13)]
- Suicide [see Warnings and Precautions (5.14)]
- Dysphagia [see Warnings and Precautions (5.15)]
- Use in Patients with Concomitant Illness [see Warnings and Precautions (5.16)]

The most common adverse reactions (≥5% and at least twice the rate on placebo) in schizophrenia were akathisia, oral hypoesthesia, and somnolence.

The most common adverse reactions (≥5% and at least twice the rate on placebo) in bipolar disorder were somnolence, dizziness, extrapyramidal symptoms other than akathisia, and weight increased.

The information below is derived from a clinical trial database for SAPHRIS consisting of over 3350 patients and/or normal subjects exposed to one or more sublingual doses of SAPHRIS. Of these subjects, 1953 (1480 in schizophrenia and 473 in acute bipolar mania) were patients who participated in multiple-dose effectiveness trials of therapeutic doses (5 or 10 mg twice daily, with a total experience of approximately 611 patient-years). A total of 486 SAPHRIS-treated patients were treated for at least 24 weeks and 293 SAPHRIS-treated patients had at least 52 weeks of exposure.

The stated frequencies of adverse reactions represent the proportion of individuals who experienced a treatment-emergent adverse event of the type listed. A reaction was considered treatment emergent if it occurred for the first time or worsened while receiving therapy following baseline evaluation.

The figures in the tables and tabulations cannot be used to predict the incidence of side effects in the course of usual medical practice where patient characteristics and other factors differ from those that prevailed in the clinical trials. Similarly, the cited frequencies cannot be compared with figures obtained from other clinical investigations involving different treatment, uses, and investigators. The cited figures, however, do provide the prescriber with some basis for estimating the relative contribution of drug and nondrug factors to the adverse reaction incidence in the population studied.

6.2 Clinical Studies Experience

Adult Patients with Schizophrenia: The following findings are based on the short-term placebo-controlled premarketing trials for schizophrenia (a pool of three 6-week fixed-dose trials and one 6-week flexible-dose trial) in which sublingual SAPHRIS was administered in doses ranging from 5 to 10 mg twice daily.

Adverse Reactions Associated with Discontinuation of Treatment: A total of 9% of SAPHRIS-treated subjects and 10% of placebo subjects discontinued due to adverse reactions. There were no drug-related adverse reactions associated with discontinuation in subjects treated with SAPHRIS at the rate of at least 1% and at least twice the placebo rate.

Adverse Reactions Occurring at an Incidence of 2% or More in SAPHRIS-Treated Schizophrenic Patients: Adverse reactions associated with the use of SAPHRIS (incidence of 2% or greater, rounded to the nearest percent, and

SAPHRIS incidence greater than placebo) that occurred during acute therapy (up to 6-weeks in patients with schizophrenia) are shown in Table 2.

[See table 2 at top of previous page]

Dose-Related Adverse Reactions: Of all the adverse reactions listed in Table 2, the only apparent dose-related adverse reaction was akathisia.

Adult Patients with Bipolar Mania: The following findings are based on the short-term placebo-controlled trials for bipolar mania (a pool of two 3-week flexible-dose trials) in which sublingual SAPHRIS was administered in doses of 5 mg or 10 mg twice daily.

Adverse Reactions Associated with Discontinuation of Treatment: Approximately 10% (38/379) of SAPHRIS-treated patients in short-term, placebo-controlled trials discontinued treatment due to an adverse reaction, compared with about 6% (12/203) on placebo. The most common adverse reactions associated with discontinuation in subjects treated with SAPHRIS (rates at least 1% and at least twice the placebo rate) were anxiety (1.1%) and oral hypoesthesia (1.1%) compared to placebo (0%).

Adverse Reactions Occurring at an Incidence of 2% or More Among SAPHRIS-Treated Bipolar Patients: Adverse reactions associated with the use of SAPHRIS (incidence of 2% or greater, rounded to the nearest percent, and SAPHRIS incidence greater than placebo) that occurred during acute therapy (up to 3-weeks in patients with bipolar mania) are shown in Table 3.

TABLE 3: Adverse Reactions Reported in 2% or More of Subjects in one of the SAPHRIS Dose Groups and Which Occurred at Greater Incidence Than in the Placebo Group in 3-Week Bipolar Mania Trials

System Organ Class/ Preferred Term	Placebo (N=203)	SAPHRIS 5 or 10 mg twice daily* (N=379)
Gastrointestinal disorders		
Dry mouth	1%	3%
Dyspepsia	2%	4%
Oral hypoesthesia	<1%	4%
Toothache	2%	3%
General disorders		
Fatigue	2%	4%
Investigations		
Weight increased	<1%	5%
Metabolism disorders		
Increased appetite	1%	4%
Musculoskeletal and connective tissue disorders		
Arthralgia	1%	3%
Pain in extremity	<1%	2%
Nervous system disorders		
Akathisia	2%	4%
Dizziness	3%	11%
Dysgeusia	<1%	3%
Headache	11%	12%
Other extrapyramidal symptoms (excluding akathisia)†	2%	7%
Somnolence‡	6%	24%
Psychiatric disorders		
Anxiety	2%	4%
Depression	1%	2%
Insomnia	5%	6%

*SAPHRIS 5 to 10 mg twice daily with flexible dosing.

†Extrapyramidal symptoms included: dystonia, blepharospasm, torticollis, dyskinesia, tardive dyskinesia, muscle rigidity, parkinsonism, gait disturbance, masked facies, and tremor (excluding akathisia).

‡Somnolence includes the following events: somnolence, sedation, and hypersomnia.

Dystonia: Antipsychotic Class Effect: Symptoms of dystonia, prolonged abnormal contractions of muscle groups, may occur in susceptible individuals during the first few days of treatment. Dystonic symptoms include: spasm of the neck muscles, sometimes progressing to tightness of the throat, swallowing difficulty, difficulty breathing, and/or protrusion of the tongue. While these symptoms can occur at low doses, they occur more frequently and with greater severity with high potency and at higher doses of first generation antipsychotic drugs. An elevated risk of acute dystonia is observed in males and younger age groups.

Extrapyramidal Symptoms: In the short-term, placebo-controlled schizophrenia and bipolar mania trials, data was objectively collected on the Simpson Angus Rating Scale for extrapyramidal symptoms (EPS), the Barnes Akathisia Scale (for akathisia) and the Assessments of Involuntary Movement Scales (for dyskinesias). The mean change from baseline for the all-SAPHRIS 5 mg or 10 mg twice daily treated group was comparable to placebo in each of the rating scale scores.

In the short-term, placebo-controlled schizophrenia trials, the incidence of reported EPS-related events, excluding events related to akathisia, for SAPHRIS-treated patients was 10% versus 7% for placebo; and the incidence of akathisia-related events for SAPHRIS-treated patients was 6% versus 3% for placebo. In short-term placebo-controlled bipolar mania trials, the incidence of EPS-related events, excluding events related to akathisia, for SAPHRIS-treated patients was 7% versus 2% for placebo; and the incidence of akathisia-related events for SAPHRIS-treated patients was 4% versus 2% for placebo.

Laboratory Test Abnormalities: *Glucose:* The effects on fasting serum glucose levels in the short-term schizophrenia and bipolar mania trials revealed no clinically relevant mean changes [see also Warnings and Precautions (5.5)]. In the short-term placebo-controlled schizophrenia trials, the mean increase in fasting glucose levels for SAPHRIS-treated patients was 3.2 mg/dL compared to a decrease of 1.6 mg/dL for placebo-treated patients. The proportion of patients with fasting glucose elevations ≥126 mg/dL (at Endpoint), was 7.4% for SAPHRIS-treated patients versus 6% for placebo-treated patients. In the short-term, placebo-controlled bipolar mania trials, the mean decreases in fasting glucose levels for both SAPHRIS-treated and placebo-treated patients were 0.6 mg/dL. The proportion of patients with fasting glucose elevations ≥126 mg/dL (at Endpoint), was 4.9% for SAPHRIS-treated patients versus 2.2% for placebo-treated patients.

In a 52-week, double-blind, comparator-controlled trial of patients with schizophrenia and schizoaffective disorder, the mean increase from baseline of fasting glucose was 2.4 mg/dL.

Lipids: The effects on total cholesterol and fasting triglycerides in the short-term schizophrenia and bipolar mania trials revealed no clinically relevant mean changes. In short-term, placebo-controlled schizophrenia trials, the mean increase in total cholesterol levels for SAPHRIS-treated patients was 0.4 mg/dL compared to a decrease of 3.6 mg/dL for placebo-treated patients. The proportion of patients with total cholesterol elevations ≥240 mg/dL (at Endpoint) was 8.3% for SAPHRIS-treated patients versus 7% for placebo-treated patients. In short-term, placebo-controlled bipolar mania trials, the mean increase in total cholesterol levels for SAPHRIS-treated patients was 1.1 mg/dL compared to a decrease of 1.5 mg/dL in placebo-treated patients. The proportion of patients with total cholesterol elevations ≥240 mg/dL (at Endpoint) was 8.7% for SAPHRIS-treated patients versus 8.6% for placebo-treated patients. In short-term, placebo-controlled schizophrenia trials, the mean increase in triglyceride levels for SAPHRIS-treated patients was 3.8 mg/dL compared to a decrease of 13.5 mg/dL for placebo-treated patients. The proportion of patients with elevations in triglycerides ≥200 mg/dL (at Endpoint) was 13.2% for SAPHRIS-treated patients versus 10.5% for placebo-treated patients. In short-term, placebo-controlled bipolar mania trials, the mean decrease in triglyceride levels for SAPHRIS-treated patients was 3.5 mg/dL versus 17.9 mg/dL for placebo-treated subjects. The proportion of patients with elevations in triglycerides ≥200 mg/dL (at Endpoint) was 15.2% for SAPHRIS-treated patients versus 11.4% for placebo-treated patients. In a 52-week, double-blind, comparator-controlled trial of patients with schizophrenia and schizoaffective disorder, the mean decrease from baseline of total cholesterol was 6 mg/dL and the mean decrease from baseline of fasting triglycerides was 9.8 mg/dL.

Transaminases: Transient elevations in serum transaminases (primarily ALT) in the short-term schizophrenia and bipolar mania trials were more common in treated patients but mean changes were not clinically relevant. In short-term, placebo-controlled schizophrenia trials, the mean increase in transaminase levels for SAPHRIS-treated patients was 1.6 units/L compared to a decrease of 0.4 units/L for placebo-treated patients. The proportion of patients with transaminase elevations ≥3 times ULN (at Endpoint) was 0.9% for SAPHRIS-treated patients versus 1.3% for placebo-treated patients. In short-term, placebo-controlled bipolar mania trials, the mean increase in transaminase levels for SAPHRIS-treated patients was 8.9 units/L compared to a decrease of 4.9 units/L in placebo-treated patients. The proportion of patients with transaminase elevations ≥3 times upper limit of normal (ULN) (at Endpoint) was 2.5% for SAPHRIS-treated patients versus 0.6% for placebo-treated patients. No cases of more severe liver injury were seen.

In a 52-week, double-blind, comparator-controlled trial of patients with schizophrenia and schizoaffective disorder, the mean increase from baseline of ALT was 1.7 units/L.

Prolactin: The effects on prolactin levels in the short-term schizophrenia and bipolar mania trials revealed no clinically relevant changes in mean change in baseline. In short-term, placebo-controlled schizophrenia trials, the mean decreases in prolactin levels were 6.5 ng/mL for SAPHRIS-treated patients compared to 10.7 ng/mL for placebo-treated patients. The proportion of patients with prolactin elevations ≥4 times ULN (at Endpoint) were 2.6% for SAPHRIS-treated patients versus 0.6% for placebo-treated patients. In short-term, placebo-controlled bipolar mania trials, the mean increase in prolactin levels was 4.9 ng/mL for SAPHRIS-treated patients compared to a decrease of 0.2 ng/mL for placebo-treated patients. The proportion of patients with prolactin elevations ≥4 times ULN (at Endpoint) were 2.3% for SAPHRIS-treated patients versus 0.7% for placebo-treated patients.

In a long-term (52-week), double-blind, comparator-controlled trial of patients with schizophrenia and schizoaffective disorder, the mean decrease in prolactin from baseline for SAPHRIS-treated patients was 26.9 ng/mL.

Other Adverse Reactions Observed During the Premarketing Evaluation of SAPHRIS: Following is a list of MedDRA terms that reflect adverse reactions reported by patients treated with sublingual SAPHRIS at multiple doses of ≥5 mg twice daily during any phase of a trial within the database of adult patients. The reactions listed are those that could be of clinical importance, as well as reactions that are plausibly drug-related on pharmacologic or other grounds. Reactions already listed in other parts of *Adverse Reactions (6)*, or those considered in *Warnings and Precautions (5)* or *Overdosage (10)* are not included. Although the reactions reported occurred during treatment with SAPHRIS, they were not necessarily caused by it. Reactions are further categorized by MedDRA system organ class and listed in order of decreasing frequency according to the following definitions: those occurring in at least 1/100 patients (only those not already listed in the tabulated results from placebo-controlled trials appear in this listing); those occurring in 1/100 to 1/1000 patients; and those occurring in fewer than 1/1000 patients.

Blood and lymphatic disorders: *<1/1000 patients:* thrombocytopenia; *≥1/1000 patients and <1/100 patients:* anemia

Cardiac disorders: *≥1/1000 patients and <1/100 patients:* tachycardia, temporary bundle branch block

Eye disorders: *≥1/1000 patients and <1/100 patients:* accommodation disorder

Gastrointestinal disorders: *≥1/1000 patients and <1/100 patients:* oral paraesthesia, glossodynia, swollen tongue

General disorders: *<1/1000 patients:* idiosyncratic drug reaction

Investigations: *≥1/1000 patients and <1/100 patients:* hyponatremia

Nervous system disorders: *≥1/1000 patients and <1/100 patients:* dysarthria

7 DRUG INTERACTIONS

The risks of using SAPHRIS in combination with other drugs have not been extensively evaluated. Given the primary CNS effects of SAPHRIS, caution should be used when it is taken in combination with other centrally-acting drugs or alcohol.

Because of its α1-adrenergic antagonism with potential for inducing hypotension, SAPHRIS may enhance the effects of certain antihypertensive agents.

7.1 Potential for Other Drugs to Affect SAPHRIS

Asenapine is cleared primarily through direct glucuronidation by UGT1A4 and oxidative metabolism by cytochrome P450 isoenzymes (predominantly CYP1A2). The potential effects of inhibitors of several of these enzyme pathways on asenapine clearance were studied.

[See table 4 below]

7.2 Potential for SAPHRIS to Affect Other Drugs

Coadministration with CYP2D6 Substrates: *In vitro* studies indicate that asenapine weakly inhibits CYP2D6. Following coadministration of dextromethorphan and SAPHRIS in healthy subjects, the ratio of dextrorphan/dextromethorphan (DX/DM) as a marker of CYP2D6 activity was measured. Indicative of CYP2D6 inhibition, treatment with SAPHRIS 5 mg twice daily decreased the DX/DM ratio to 0.43. In the same study, treatment with paroxetine 20 mg daily decreased the DX/DM ratio to 0.032. In a separate study, coadministration of a single 75-mg dose of imipramine with a single 5-mg dose of SAPHRIS did not affect the plasma concentrations of the metabolite desipramine (a CYP2D6 substrate). Thus, *in vivo*, SAPHRIS appears to be at most a weak inhibitor of CYP2D6. Coadministration of a single 20-mg dose of paroxetine (a CYP2D6 substrate and inhibitor) during treatment with 5 mg SAPHRIS twice daily in 15 healthy male subjects resulted in an almost 2-fold increase in paroxetine exposure. Asenapine may enhance the inhibitory effects of paroxetine on its own metabolism.

SAPHRIS should be coadministered cautiously with drugs that are both substrates and inhibitors for CYP2D6.

8 USE IN SPECIFIC POPULATIONS

8.1 Pregnancy

Pregnancy Category C: There are no adequate and well-controlled studies of SAPHRIS in pregnant women. In animal studies, asenapine increased post-implantation loss and decreased pup weight and survival at doses similar to or less than recommended clinical doses. In these studies there was no increase in the incidence of structural abnormalities caused by asenapine. SAPHRIS should be used during pregnancy only if the potential benefit justifies the potential risk to the fetus.

Asenapine was not teratogenic in reproduction studies in rats and rabbits at intravenous doses up to 1.5 mg/kg in rats and 0.44 mg/kg in rabbits. These doses are 0.7 and 0.4 times, respectively, the maximum recommended human dose (MRHD) of 10 mg twice daily given sublingually on a mg/m^2 basis. Plasma levels of asenapine were measured in the rabbit study, and the area under the curve (AUC) at the highest dose tested was 2 times that in humans receiving the MRHD.

In a study in which rats were treated from day 6 of gestation through day 21 postpartum with intravenous doses of asenapine of 0.3, 0.9, and 1.5 mg/kg/day (0.15, 0.4, and 0.7 times the MRHD of 10 mg twice daily given sublingually on a mg/m^2 basis), increases in post-implantation loss and early pup deaths were seen at all doses, and decreases in subsequent pup survival and weight gain were seen at the two higher doses. A cross-fostering study indicated that the decreases in pup survival were largely due to prenatal drug effects. Increases in post-implantation loss and decreases in pup weight and survival were also seen when pregnant rats were dosed orally with asenapine.

8.2 Labor and Delivery

The effect of SAPHRIS on labor and delivery in humans is unknown.

8.3 Nursing Mothers

Asenapine is excreted in milk of rats during lactation. It is not known whether asenapine or its metabolites are excreted in human milk. Because many drugs are excreted in human milk, caution should be exercised when SAPHRIS is administered to a nursing woman. It is recommended that women receiving SAPHRIS should not breast feed.

8.4 Pediatric Use

Safety and effectiveness in pediatric patients have not been established.

8.5 Geriatric Use

Clinical studies of SAPHRIS in the treatment of schizophrenia and bipolar mania did not include sufficient numbers of patients aged 65 and over to determine whether or not they respond differently than younger patients. Of the approximately 2250 patients in premarketing clinical studies of SAPHRIS, 1.1% (25) were 65 years of age or over. Multiple factors that might increase the pharmacodynamic response to SAPHRIS, causing poorer tolerance or orthostasis, could be present in elderly patients, and these patients should be monitored carefully.

Elderly patients with dementia-related psychosis treated with SAPHRIS are at an increased risk of death compared to placebo. SAPHRIS is not approved for the treatment of patients with dementia-related psychosis *[see Boxed Warning]*.

8.6 Renal Impairment

The exposure of asenapine following a single dose of 5 mg was similar among subjects with varying degrees of renal impairment and subjects with normal renal function *[see Clinical Pharmacology (12.3)]*.

8.7 Hepatic Impairment

In subjects with severe hepatic impairment who were treated with a single dose of SAPHRIS 5 mg, asenapine exposures (on average), were 7-fold higher than the exposures observed in subjects with normal hepatic function. Thus, SAPHRIS is not recommended in patients with severe hepatic impairment (Child-Pugh C) *[see Dosage and Administration (2.4) and Clinical Pharmacology (12.3)]*.

9 DRUG ABUSE AND DEPENDENCE

9.1 Controlled Substance

SAPHRIS is not a controlled substance.

9.2 Abuse

SAPHRIS has not been systematically studied in animals or humans for its abuse potential or its ability to induce tolerance or physical dependence. Thus, it is not possible to predict the extent to which a CNS-active drug will be misused, diverted and/or abused once it is marketed. Patients should be evaluated carefully for a history of drug abuse, and such patients should be observed carefully for signs that they are misusing or abusing SAPHRIS (e.g., drug-seeking behavior, increases in dose).

10 OVERDOSAGE

Human Experience: In premarketing clinical studies involving more than 3350 patients and/or healthy subjects, accidental or intentional acute overdosage of SAPHRIS was identified in 3 patients. Among these few reported cases of overdose, the highest estimated ingestion of SAPHRIS was 400 mg. Reported adverse reactions at the highest dosage included agitation and confusion.

Management of Overdosage: There is no specific antidote to SAPHRIS. The possibility of multiple drug involvement should be considered. An electrocardiogram should be obtained and management of overdose should concentrate on

TABLE 4: Summary of Effect of Coadministered Drugs on Exposure to Asenapine in Healthy Volunteers

Coadministered drug (Postulated effect on CYP450/UGT)	Dose schedules		Effect on asenapine pharmacokinetics		Recommendation
	Coadministered drug	Asenapine	C_{max}	$AUC_{0-\infty}$	
Fluvoxamine (CYP1A2 inhibitor)	25 mg twice daily for 8 days	5 mg Single Dose	+13%	+29%	Coadminister with caution*
Paroxetine (CYP2D6 inhibitor)	20 mg once daily for 9 days	5 mg Single Dose	−13%	−9%	No SAPHRIS dose adjustment required *[see Drug Interactions (7.2)]*
Imipramine (CYP1A2/2C19/3A4 inhibitor)	75 mg Single Dose	5 mg Single Dose	+17%	+10%	No SAPHRIS dose adjustment required
Cimetidine (CYP3A4/2D6/1A2 inhibitor)	800 mg twice daily for 8 days	5 mg Single Dose	−13%	+1%	No SAPHRIS dose adjustment required
Carbamazepine (CYP3A4 inducer)	400 mg twice daily for 15 days	5 mg Single Dose	−16%	−16%	No SAPHRIS dose adjustment required
Valproate (UGT1A4 inhibitor)	500 mg twice daily for 9 days	5 mg Single Dose	2%	−1%	No SAPHRIS dose adjustment required

*The full therapeutic dose of fluvoxamine would be expected to cause a greater increase in asenapine plasma concentrations. AUC: Area under the curve.

supportive therapy, maintaining an adequate airway, oxygenation and ventilation, and management of symptoms. Hypotension and circulatory collapse should be treated with appropriate measures, such as intravenous fluids and/or sympathomimetic agents (epinephrine and dopamine should not be used, since beta stimulation may worsen hypotension in the setting of SAPHRIS-induced alpha blockade). In case of severe extrapyramidal symptoms, anticholinergic medication should be administered. Close medical supervision and monitoring should continue until the patient recovers.

11 DESCRIPTION

SAPHRIS is a psychotropic agent that is available for sublingual administration. Asenapine belongs to the class dibenzo-oxepino pyrroles. The chemical designation is (3a*RS*,12b*RS*)-5-Chloro-2-methyl-2,3,3a,12b-tetrahydro-1*H*dibenzo[2,3:6,7]oxepino[4,5-c]pyrrole (2*Z*)-2-butenedioate (1:1). Its molecular formula is $C_{17}H_{16}ClNO \bullet C_4H_4O_4$ and its molecular weight is 401.84 (free base: 285.8). The chemical structure is:

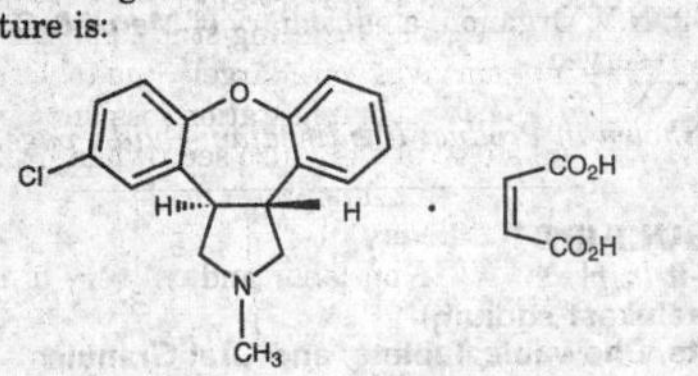

Asenapine is a white- to off-white powder.
SAPHRIS is supplied for sublingual administration in tablets containing 5-mg or 10-mg asenapine; inactive ingredients include gelatin and mannitol.
SAPHRIS, black cherry flavor, is supplied for sublingual administration in tablets containing 5-mg or 10-mg asenapine; inactive ingredients include gelatin, mannitol, sucralose, and black cherry flavor.

12 CLINICAL PHARMACOLOGY

12.1 Mechanism of Action

The mechanism of action of asenapine, as with other drugs having efficacy in schizophrenia and bipolar disorder, is unknown. It has been suggested that the efficacy of asenapine in schizophrenia is mediated through a combination of antagonist activity at D_2 and $5\text{-}HT_{2A}$ receptors.

12.2 Pharmacodynamics

Asenapine exhibits high affinity for serotonin $5\text{-}HT_{1A}$, $5\text{-}HT_{1B}$, $5\text{-}HT_{2A}$, $5\text{-}HT_{2B}$, $5\text{-}HT_{2C}$, $5\text{-}HT_5$, $5\text{-}HT_6$, and $5\text{-}HT_7$ receptors (Ki values of 2.5, 4.0, 0.06, 0.16, 0.03, 1.6, 0.25, and 0.13 nM), dopamine D_2, D_3, D_4, and D_1 receptors (Ki values of 1.3, 0.42, 1.1, and 1.4 nM), α_1 and α_2-adrenergic receptors (Ki values of 1.2 and 1.2 nM), and histamine H_1 receptors (Ki value 1.0 nM), and moderate affinity for H_2 receptors (Ki value of 6.2 nM). In *in vitro* assays asenapine acts as an antagonist at these receptors. Asenapine has no appreciable affinity for muscarinic cholinergic receptors (e.g., Ki value of 8128 nM for M_1).

12.3 Pharmacokinetics

Following a single 5-mg dose of SAPHRIS, the mean C_{max} was approximately 4 ng/mL and was observed at a mean t_{max} of 1 hr. Elimination of asenapine is primarily through direct glucuronidation by UGT1A4 and oxidative metabolism by cytochrome P450 isoenzymes (predominantly CYP1A2). Following an initial more rapid distribution phase, the mean terminal half-life is approximately 24 hrs. With multiple-dose twice-daily dosing, steady-state is attained within 3 days. Overall, steady-state asenapine pharmacokinetics are similar to single-dose pharmacokinetics.

Absorption: Following sublingual administration, asenapine is rapidly absorbed with peak plasma concentrations occurring within 0.5 to 1.5 hours. The absolute bioavailability of sublingual asenapine at 5 mg is 35%. Increasing the dose from 5 to 10 mg twice daily (a two-fold increase) results in less than linear (1.7 times) increases in both the extent of exposure and maximum concentration. The absolute bioavailability of asenapine when swallowed is low (<2% with an oral tablet formulation).

The intake of water several (2 or 5) minutes after asenapine administration resulted in decreased asenapine exposure. Therefore, eating and drinking should be avoided for 10 minutes after administration *[see Dosage and Administration (2.3)]*.

Distribution: Asenapine is rapidly distributed and has a large volume of distribution (approximately 20 - 25 L/kg), indicating extensive extravascular distribution. Asenapine is highly bound (95%) to plasma proteins, including albumin and α1-acid glycoprotein.

Metabolism and Elimination: Direct glucuronidation by UGT1A4 and oxidative metabolism by cytochrome P450 isoenzymes (predominantly CYP1A2) are the primary metabolic pathways for asenapine.

Asenapine is a high clearance drug with a clearance after intravenous administration of 52 L/h. In this circumstance, hepatic clearance is influenced primarily by changes in liver blood flow rather than by changes in the intrinsic clearance, i.e., the metabolizing enzymatic activity. Following an initial more rapid distribution phase, the terminal half life of asenapine is approximately 24 hours. Steady-state concentrations of asenapine are reached within 3 days of twice daily dosing.

After administration of a single dose of [^{14}C]-labeled asenapine, about 90% of the dose was recovered; approximately 50% was recovered in urine, and 40% recovered in feces. About 50% of the circulating species in plasma have been identified. The predominant species was asenapine N^+-glucuronide; others included N-desmethylasenapine, N-desmethylasenapine N-carbamoyl glucuronide, and unchanged asenapine in smaller amounts. SAPHRIS activity is primarily due to the parent drug.

In vitro studies indicate that asenapine is a substrate for UGT1A4, CYP1A2 and to a lesser extent CYP3A4 and CYP2D6. Asenapine is a weak inhibitor of CYP2D6. Asenapine does not cause induction of CYP1A2 or CYP3A4 activities in cultured human hepatocytes. Coadministration of asenapine with known inhibitors, inducers or substrates of these metabolic pathways has been studied in a number of drug-drug interaction studies *[see Drug Interactions (7)]*.

Smoking: A population pharmacokinetic analysis indicated that smoking, which induces CYP1A2, had no effect on the clearance of asenapine in smokers. In a crossover study in which 24 healthy male subjects (who were smokers) were administered a single 5-mg sublingual dose, concomitant smoking had no effect on the pharmacokinetics of asenapine.

Food: A crossover study in 26 healthy male subjects was performed to evaluate the effect of food on the pharmacokinetics of a single 5-mg dose of asenapine. Consumption of food immediately prior to sublingual administration decreased asenapine exposure by 20%; consumption of food 4 hours after sublingual administration decreased asenapine exposure by about 10%. These effects are probably due to increased hepatic blood flow.

In clinical trials establishing the efficacy and safety of SAPHRIS, patients were instructed to avoid eating for 10 minutes following sublingual dosing. There were no other restrictions with regard to the timing of meals in these trials *[see Dosage and Administration (2.3) and Patient Counseling Information (17.1)]*.

Water: In clinical trials establishing the efficacy and safety of SAPHRIS, patients were instructed to avoid drinking for 10 minutes following sublingual dosing. The effect of water administration following 10 mg sublingual SAPHRIS dosing was studied at different time points of 2, 5, 10, and 30 minutes in 15 healthy male subjects. The exposure of asenapine following administration of water 10 minutes after sublingual dosing was equivalent to that when water was administered 30 minutes after dosing. Reduced exposure to asenapine was observed following water administration at 2 minutes (19% decrease) and 5 minutes (10% decrease) *[see Dosage and Administration (2.3) and Patient Counseling Information (17.1)]*.

Special Populations:

Hepatic Impairment: The effect of decreased hepatic function on the pharmacokinetics of asenapine, administered as a single 5-mg sublingual dose, was studied in 30 subjects (8 each in those with normal hepatic function and Child-Pugh A and B groups, and 6 in the Child Pugh C group). In subjects with mild or moderate hepatic impairment (Child-Pugh A or B), asenapine exposure was 12% higher than that in subjects with normal hepatic function, indicating that dosage adjustment is not required for these subjects. In subjects with severe hepatic impairment, asenapine exposures were on average 7 times higher than the exposures of those in subjects with normal hepatic function. Thus, SAPHRIS is not recommended in patients with severe hepatic impairment (Child-Pugh C) *[see Dosage in Specific Populations (2.4) and Use in Specific Populations (8.7) and Warnings and Precautions (5.14)]*.

Renal Impairment: The effect of decreased renal function on the pharmacokinetics of asenapine was studied in subjects with mildly (creatinine clearance (CrCl) 51 to 80 mL/min; N=8), moderately (CrCl 30 to 50 mL/min; N=8), and severely (CrCl less than 30 mL/min but not on dialysis; N=8) impaired renal function and compared to normal subjects (CrCl greater than 80 mL/min; N=8). The exposure of asenapine following a single dose of 5 mg was similar among subjects with varying degrees of renal impairment and subjects with normal renal function. Dosage adjustment based upon degree of renal impairment is not required. The effect of renal function on the excretion of other metabolites and the effect of dialysis on the pharmacokinetics of asenapine has not been studied *[see Use in Specific Populations (8.6)]*.

Geriatric Patients: In elderly patients with psychosis (65-85 years of age), asenapine concentrations were on average 30 to 40% higher compared to younger adults. When the range of exposures in the elderly was examined, the highest exposure for asenapine was up to 2-fold higher than the highest exposure in younger subjects. In a population pharmacokinetic analysis, a decrease in clearance with increasing age was observed, implying a 30% higher exposure in elderly as compared to adult patients *[see Use in Specific Populations (8.5)]*.

Gender: The potential difference in asenapine pharmacokinetics between males and females was not studied in a dedicated trial. In a population pharmacokinetic analysis, no significant differences between genders were observed.

Race: In a population pharmacokinetic analysis, no effect of race on asenapine concentrations was observed. In a dedicated study, the pharmacokinetics of SAPHRIS were similar in Caucasian and Japanese subjects.

13 NONCLINICAL TOXICOLOGY

13.1 Carcinogenesis, Mutagenesis, Impairment of Fertility

Carcinogenesis: In a lifetime carcinogenicity study in CD-1 mice asenapine was administered subcutaneously at doses up to those resulting in plasma levels (AUC) estimated to be 5 times those in humans receiving the MRHD of 10 mg twice daily. The incidence of malignant lymphomas was increased in female mice, with a no-effect dose resulting in plasma levels estimated to be 1.5 times those in humans receiving the MRHD. The mouse strain used has a high and variable incidence of malignant lymphomas, and the significance of these results to humans is unknown. There were no increases in other tumor types in female mice. In male mice, there were no increases in any tumor type.

In a lifetime carcinogenicity study in Sprague-Dawley rats, asenapine did not cause any increases in tumors when administered subcutaneously at doses up to those resulting in plasma levels (AUC) estimated to be 5 times those in humans receiving the MRHD.

Mutagenesis: No evidence for genotoxic potential of asenapine was found in the *in vitro* bacterial reverse mutation assay, the *in vitro* forward gene mutation assay in mouse lymphoma cells, the *in vitro* chromosomal aberration assays in human lymphocytes, the *in vitro* sister chromatid exchange assay in rabbit lymphocytes, or the *in vivo* micronucleus assay in rats.

Impairment of Fertility: Asenapine did not impair fertility in rats when tested at doses up to 11 mg/kg twice daily given orally. This dose is 10 times the maximum recommended human dose of 10 mg twice daily given sublingually on a mg/m^2 basis.

14 CLINICAL STUDIES

14.1 Schizophrenia

The efficacy of SAPHRIS in the treatment of schizophrenia in adults was evaluated in three fixed-dose, short-term (6 week), randomized, double-blind, placebo-controlled, and active-controlled (haloperidol, risperidone, and olanzapine) trials of adult patients who met DSM-IV criteria for schizophrenia and were having an acute exacerbation of their schizophrenic illness. In two of the three trials SAPHRIS demonstrated superior efficacy to placebo. In a third trial, SAPHRIS could not be distinguished from placebo; however, an active control in that trial was superior to placebo.

In the two positive trials for SAPHRIS, the primary efficacy rating scale was the Positive and Negative Syndrome Scale (PANSS), which assesses the symptoms of schizophrenia. The primary endpoint was change from baseline to endpoint on the PANSS total score. The results of the SAPHRIS trials in schizophrenia follow:

In trial 1, a 6-week trial (n=174), comparing SAPHRIS (5 mg twice daily) to placebo, SAPHRIS 5 mg twice daily was statistically superior to placebo on the PANSS total score.

In trial 2, a 6-week trial (n=448), comparing two fixed doses of SAPHRIS (5 mg and 10 mg twice daily) to placebo, SAPHRIS 5 mg twice daily was statistically superior to placebo on the PANSS total score. SAPHRIS 10 mg twice daily showed no added benefit compared to 5 mg twice daily and was not significantly different from placebo.

An examination of population subgroups did not reveal any clear evidence of differential responsiveness on the basis of age, gender or race.

14.2 Bipolar Disorder

The efficacy of SAPHRIS in the treatment of acute mania was established in two similarly designed 3-week, randomized, double-blind, placebo-controlled, and active-controlled (olanzapine) trials of adult patients who met DSM-IV criteria for Bipolar I Disorder with an acute manic or mixed episode with or without psychotic features.

The primary rating instrument used for assessing manic symptoms in these trials was the Young Mania Rating Scale (YMRS). Patients were also assessed on the Clinical Global Impression–Bipolar (CGI-BP) scale. In both trials, all patients randomized to SAPHRIS were initially administered 10 mg twice daily, and the dose could be adjusted within the dose range of 5 to 10 mg twice daily from Day 2 onward based on efficacy and tolerability. Ninety percent of patients remained on the 10 mg twice daily dose. SAPHRIS was

5-mg Tablets
Round, white- to off-white sublingual tablets, with "5" on one side.

Child-resistant packaging		
Box of 60	6 blisters with 10 tablets	NDC 0052-0118-06
Hospital Unit Dose		
Box of 100	10 blisters with 10 tablets	NDC 0052-0118-90

10-mg Tablets
Round, white- to off-white sublingual tablets, with "10" on one side.

Child-resistant packaging		
Box of 60	6 blisters with 10 tablets	NDC 0052-0119-06
Hospital Unit Dose		
Box of 100	10 blisters with 10 tablets	NDC 0052-0119-90

5-mg Tablets, black cherry flavor
Round, white- to off-white sublingual tablets, with "5" on one side within a circle.

Child-resistant packaging		
Box of 60	6 blisters with 10 tablets	NDC 0052-2139-03
Hospital Unit Dose		
Box of 100	10 blisters with 10 tablets	NDC 0052-2139-04

10-mg Tablets, black cherry flavor
Round, white- to off-white sublingual tablets, with "10" on one side within a circle.

Child-resistant packaging		
Box of 60	6 blisters with 10 tablets	NDC 0052-2142-03
Hospital Unit Dose		
Box of 100	10 blisters with 10 tablets	NDC 0052-2142-04

statistically superior to placebo on the YMRS total score and the CGI-BP Severity of Illness score (mania) in both studies.

An examination of subgroups did not reveal any clear evidence of differential responsiveness on the basis of age, gender or race.

16 HOW SUPPLIED/STORAGE AND HANDLING

SAPHRIS (asenapine) sublingual tablets are supplied as:
[See table above]
Storage
Store at 15°-30°C (59°-86°F) [*see* USP Controlled Room Temperature].

17 PATIENT COUNSELING INFORMATION

17.1 Tablet Administration

IMPORTANT:
- **Do not remove tablet until ready to administer.**
- **Use dry hands when handling tablet.**

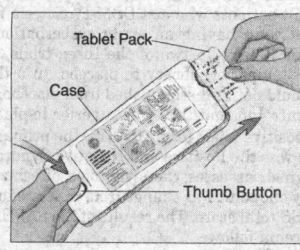

Tablet Pack
Case
Thumb Button

Step 1. Firmly press and hold thumb button, then pull out tablet pack.
Do not push tablet through tablet pack.
Do not cut or tear tablet pack.

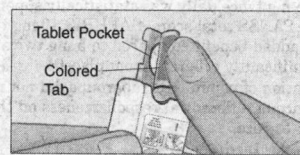

Tablet Pocket
Colored Tab

Step 2. Peel back colored tab.

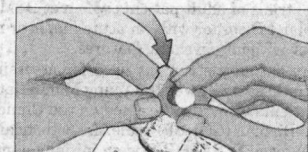

Step 3. Gently remove tablet.
Do not crush tablet.
[See figure Step 3 above]

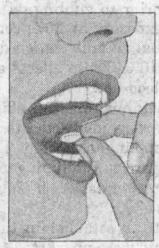

Step 4. Place tablet **under** tongue and allow it to dissolve completely.

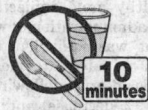

10 minutes

Do not chew or swallow tablet.
Do not eat or drink for 10 minutes.

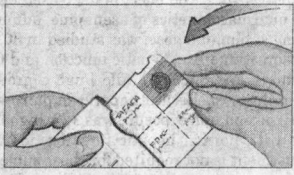

Step 5. Slide tablet pack into case until it clicks.
[*see Drug Interactions (7) and Clinical Pharmacology (12.3)*].

17.2 Interference with Cognitive and Motor Performance

Patients should be cautioned about performing activities requiring mental alertness, such as operating hazardous machinery or operating a motor vehicle, until they are reasonably certain that SAPHRIS therapy does not affect them adversely [*see Warnings and Precautions (5.12)*].

17.3 Neuroleptic Malignant Syndrome

Patients and caregivers should be counseled that a potentially fatal symptom complex sometimes referred to as Neuroleptic Malignant Syndrome (NMS) has been reported in association with administration of antipsychotic drugs. Signs and symptoms of NMS include hyperpyrexia, muscle rigidity, altered mental status, and evidence of autonomic instability (irregular pulse or blood pressure, tachycardia, diaphoresis, and cardiac dysrhythmia) [*see Warnings and Precautions (5.3)*].

17.4 Orthostatic Hypotension

Patients should be advised of the risk of orthostatic hypotension (symptoms include feeling dizzy or lightheaded upon standing) especially early in treatment, and also at times of re-initiating treatment or increases in dose [*see Warnings and Precautions (5.7)*].

17.5 Pregnancy and Nursing

Patients should be advised to notify their physician if they become pregnant or intend to become pregnant during therapy with SAPHRIS. Patients should be advised not to breast feed if they are taking SAPHRIS [*see Use in Special Populations (8.1, 8.3)*].

17.6 Concomitant Medication and Alcohol

Patients should be advised to inform their physicians if they are taking, or plan to take, any prescription or over-the-counter medications since there is a potential for interactions. Patients should be advised to avoid alcohol while taking SAPHRIS [*see Drug Interactions (7)*].

17.7 Heat Exposure and Dehydration

Patients should be advised regarding appropriate care in avoiding overheating and dehydration [*see Warnings and Precautions (5.13)*].

Manufactured by Catalent UK Swindon Zydis Ltd., Blagrove, Swindon, Wiltshire, SN5 8RU, UK.
Distributed by Schering Corporation, a subsidiary of **Merck & Co., Inc.**, Whitehouse Station, NJ 08889 USA.
U.S. Patent No. 5,763,476.
XX/XXXX

Shown in Product Identification Guide, page 314

SINGULAIR®   ℞

[*sing-u-lair*]
(montelukast sodium)
Tablets, Chewable Tablets, and Oral Granules

HIGHLIGHTS OF PRESCRIBING INFORMATION
These highlights do not include all the information needed to use SINGULAIR safely and effectively. See full prescribing information for SINGULAIR.
SINGULAIR® (montelukast sodium) tablets, chewable tablets, and oral granules
Initial U.S. Approval: 1998

——————RECENT MAJOR CHANGES——————

Warnings and Precautions,
  Neuropsychiatric Events (5.4)   04/2010

——————INDICATIONS AND USAGE——————

SINGULAIR® is a leukotriene receptor antagonist indicated for:
- Prophylaxis and chronic treatment of asthma in patients 12 months of age and older (1.1).
- Acute prevention of exercise-induced bronchoconstriction (EIB) in patients 15 years of age and older (1.2).
- Relief of symptoms of allergic rhinitis (AR): seasonal allergic rhinitis (SAR) in patients 2 years of age and older, and perennial allergic rhinitis (PAR) in patients 6 months of age and older (1.3).

——————DOSAGE AND ADMINISTRATION——————

Administration (by indications):
- Asthma (2.1): Once daily in the evening for patients 12 months and older.
- Acute prevention of EIB (2.2): 10 mg tablet at least 2 hours before exercise for patients 15 years of age and older.
- Seasonal allergic rhinitis (2.3): Once daily for patients 2 years and older.
- Perennial allergic rhinitis (2.3): Once daily for patients 6 months and older.

Dosage (by age):
- 15 years and older: one 10-mg tablet.
- 6 to 14 years: one 5-mg chewable tablet.
- 2 to 5 years: one 4-mg chewable tablet or one packet of 4-mg oral granules.
- 6 to 23 months: one packet of 4-mg oral granules.

Patients with both asthma and allergic rhinitis should take only one dose daily in the evening (2.4). For oral granules: Must administer within 15 minutes after opening the packet (with or without mixing with food) (2.5).

——————DOSAGE FORMS AND STRENGTHS——————

- SINGULAIR 10-mg Film-Coated Tablets
- SINGULAIR 5-mg and 4-mg Chewable Tablets
- SINGULAIR 4-mg Oral Granules

——————CONTRAINDICATIONS——————

- Hypersensitivity to any component of this product (4).

——————WARNINGS AND PRECAUTIONS——————

- Do not prescribe SINGULAIR to treat an acute asthma attack.
- Advise patients to have appropriate rescue medication available (5.1).
- Inhaled corticosteroid may be reduced gradually. Do not abruptly substitute SINGULAIR for inhaled or oral corticosteroids (5.2).
- Patients with known aspirin sensitivity should continue to avoid aspirin or non-steroidal anti-inflammatory agents while taking SINGULAIR (5.3).
- Neuropsychiatric events have been reported with SINGULAIR. Instruct patients to be alert for neuropsychiatric events. Evaluate the risks and benefits of continuing treatment with SINGULAIR if such events occur (5.4 and 6.2).
- Systemic eosinophilia, sometimes presenting with clinical features of vasculitis consistent with Churg-Strauss

syndrome, has been reported. These events usually, but not always, have been associated with the reduction of oral corticosteroid therapy (5.5 and 6.2).

• Inform patients with phenylketonuria that the 4-mg and 5-mg chewable tablets contain phenylalanine (5.6).

ADVERSE REACTIONS

Most common adverse reactions (incidence ≥5% and greater than placebo listed in descending order of frequency): upper respiratory infection, fever, headache, pharyngitis, cough, abdominal pain, diarrhea, otitis media, influenza, rhinorrhea, sinusitis, otitis (6.1).

To report SUSPECTED ADVERSE REACTIONS, contact Merck Sharp & Dohme Corp., a subsidiary of Merck & Co., Inc., at 1-877-888-4231 or FDA at 1-800-FDA-1088 or www.fda.gov/medwatch.

See 17 for PATIENT COUNSELING INFORMATION and FDA-approved patient labeling.

Revised: 07/2010

FULL PRESCRIBING INFORMATION

1 INDICATIONS AND USAGE

1.1 Asthma

SINGULAIR[1] is indicated for the prophylaxis and chronic treatment of asthma in adults and pediatric patients 12 months of age and older.

---

[1] Registered trademark of Merck Sharp & Dohme Corp., a subsidiary of **Merck & Co., Inc.**
Copyright © 1998-2010 Merck Sharp & Dohme Corp., a subsidiary of **Merck & Co., Inc.**
All rights reserved

1.2 Exercise-Induced Bronchoconstriction

SINGULAIR is indicated for prevention of exercise-induced bronchoconstriction (EIB) in patients 15 years of age and older.

1.3 Allergic Rhinitis

SINGULAIR is indicated for the relief of symptoms of seasonal allergic rhinitis in patients 2 years of age and older and perennial allergic rhinitis in patients 6 months of age and older.

---

2 DOSAGE AND ADMINISTRATION

2.1 Asthma

SINGULAIR should be taken once daily in the evening. The following doses are recommended:

For adults and adolescents 15 years of age and older: one 10-mg tablet.

For pediatric patients 6 to 14 years of age: one 5-mg chewable tablet.

For pediatric patients 2 to 5 years of age: one 4-mg chewable tablet or one packet of 4-mg oral granules.

For pediatric patients 12 to 23 months of age: one packet of 4-mg oral granules.

Safety and effectiveness in pediatric patients less than 12 months of age with asthma have not been established.

There have been no clinical trials in patients with asthma to evaluate the relative efficacy of morning versus evening dosing. The pharmacokinetics of montelukast are similar whether dosed in the morning or evening. Efficacy has been demonstrated for asthma when montelukast was administered in the evening without regard to time of food ingestion.

2.2 Exercise-Induced Bronchoconstriction (EIB) in Patients 15 Years of Age and Older

For prevention of EIB, a single 10 mg dose of SINGULAIR should be taken at least 2 hours before exercise. An additional dose of SINGULAIR should not be taken within 24 hours of a previous dose. Patients already taking SINGULAIR daily for another indication (including chronic asthma) should not take an additional dose to prevent EIB. All patients should have available for rescue a short-acting β-agonist. Safety and effectiveness in patients younger than 15 years of age have not been established. Daily administration of SINGULAIR for the chronic treatment of asthma has not been established to prevent acute episodes of EIB.

2.3 Allergic Rhinitis

For allergic rhinitis, SINGULAIR should be taken once daily. Efficacy was demonstrated for seasonal allergic rhinitis when montelukast was administered in the morning or the evening without regard to time of food ingestion. The time of administration may be individualized to suit patient needs.

The following doses for the treatment of symptoms of seasonal allergic rhinitis are recommended:

For adults and adolescents 15 years of age and older: one 10-mg tablet.

For pediatric patients 6 to 14 years of age: one 5-mg chewable tablet.

For pediatric patients 2 to 5 years of age: one 4-mg chewable tablet or one packet of 4-mg oral granules.

Safety and effectiveness in pediatric patients younger than 2 years of age with seasonal allergic rhinitis have not been established.

The following doses for the treatment of symptoms of perennial allergic rhinitis are recommended:

For adults and adolescents 15 years of age and older: one 10-mg tablet.

For pediatric patients 6 to 14 years of age: one 5-mg chewable tablet.

For pediatric patients 2 to 5 years of age: one 4-mg chewable tablet or one packet of 4-mg oral granules.

For pediatric patients 6 to 23 months of age: one packet of 4-mg oral granules.

Safety and effectiveness in pediatric patients younger than 6 months of age with perennial allergic rhinitis have not been established.

2.4 Asthma and Allergic Rhinitis

Patients with both asthma and allergic rhinitis should take only one SINGULAIR dose daily in the evening.

2.5 Instructions for Administration of Oral Granules

SINGULAIR 4-mg oral granules can be administered either directly in the mouth, dissolved in 1 teaspoonful (5 mL) of cold or room temperature baby formula or breast milk, or mixed with a spoonful of cold or room temperature soft foods; based on stability studies, only applesauce, carrots, rice, or ice cream should be used. The packet should not be opened until ready to use. After opening the packet, the full dose (with or without mixing with baby formula, breast milk, or food) must be administered within 15 minutes. If mixed with baby formula, breast milk, or food, SINGULAIR oral granules must not be stored for future use. Discard any unused portion. SINGULAIR oral granules are not intended to be dissolved in any liquid other than baby formula or breast milk for administration. However, liquids may be taken subsequent to administration. SINGULAIR oral granules can be administered without regard to the time of meals.

---

3 DOSAGE FORMS AND STRENGTHS

• SINGULAIR 10-mg Film-Coated Tablets are beige, rounded square-shaped tablets, with code MRK 117 on one side and SINGULAIR on the other.

• SINGULAIR 5-mg Chewable Tablets are pink, round, bi-convex-shaped tablets, with code MRK 275 on one side and SINGULAIR on the other.

• SINGULAIR 4-mg Chewable Tablets are pink, oval, bi-convex-shaped tablets, with code MRK 711 on one side and SINGULAIR on the other.

• SINGULAIR 4-mg Oral Granules are white granules with 500 mg net weight, packed in a child-resistant foil packet.

---

4 CONTRAINDICATIONS

Hypersensitivity to any component of this product.

---

5 WARNINGS AND PRECAUTIONS

5.1 Acute Asthma

SINGULAIR is not indicated for use in the reversal of bronchospasm in acute asthma attacks, including status asthmaticus. Patients should be advised to have appropriate rescue medication available. Therapy with SINGULAIR can be continued during acute exacerbations of asthma. Patients who have exacerbations of asthma after exercise should have available for rescue a short-acting inhaled β-agonist.

5.2 Concomitant Corticosteroid Use

While the dose of inhaled corticosteroid may be reduced gradually under medical supervision, SINGULAIR should not be abruptly substituted for inhaled or oral corticosteroids.

5.3 Aspirin Sensitivity

Patients with known aspirin sensitivity should continue avoidance of aspirin or non-steroidal anti-inflammatory agents while taking SINGULAIR. Although SINGULAIR is effective in improving airway function in asthmatics with documented aspirin sensitivity, it has not been shown to truncate bronchoconstrictor response to aspirin and other non-steroidal anti-inflammatory drugs in aspirin-sensitive asthmatic patients *[see Clinical Studies (14.1)]*.

5.4 Neuropsychiatric Events

Neuropsychiatric events have been reported in adult, adolescent, and pediatric patients taking SINGULAIR. Postmarketing reports with SINGULAIR use include agitation, aggressive behavior or hostility, anxiousness, depression, disorientation, dream abnormalities, hallucinations, insomnia, irritability, restlessness, somnambulism, suicidal thinking and behavior (including suicide), and tremor. The clinical details of some post-marketing reports involving SINGULAIR appear consistent with a drug-induced effect. Patients and prescribers should be alert for neuropsychiatric events. Patients should be instructed to notify their prescriber if these changes occur. Prescribers should carefully evaluate the risks and benefits of continuing treatment with SINGULAIR if such events occur *[see Adverse Reactions (6.2)]*.

5.5 Eosinophilic Conditions

Patients with asthma on therapy with SINGULAIR may present with systemic eosinophilia, sometimes presenting with clinical features of vasculitis consistent with Churg-Strauss syndrome, a condition which is often treated with systemic corticosteroid therapy. These events usually, but not always, have been associated with the reduction of oral corticosteroid therapy. Physicians should be alert to eosinophilia, vasculitic rash, worsening pulmonary symptoms, cardiac complications, and/or neuropathy presenting in their patients. A causal association between SINGULAIR and these underlying conditions has not been established *[see Adverse Reactions (6.2)]*.

5.6 Phenylketonuria

Phenylketonuric patients should be informed that the 4-mg and 5-mg chewable tablets contain phenylalanine (a component of aspartame), 0.674 and 0.842 mg per 4-mg and 5-mg chewable tablet, respectively.

---

6 ADVERSE REACTIONS

6.1 Clinical Trials Experience

Because clinical trials are conducted under widely varying conditions, adverse reaction rates observed in the clinical trials of a drug cannot be directly compared to rates in the clinical trials of another drug and may not reflect the rates observed in clinical practice. In the following description of clinical trials experience, adverse reactions are listed regardless of causality assessment.

The most common adverse reactions (incidence ≥5% and greater than placebo; listed in descending order of frequency) in controlled clinical trials were: upper respiratory infection, fever, headache, pharyngitis, cough, abdominal pain, diarrhea, otitis media, influenza, rhinorrhea, sinusitis, otitis.

Adults and Adolescents 15 Years of Age and Older with Asthma

SINGULAIR has been evaluated for safety in approximately 2950 adult and adolescent patients 15 years of age and older in clinical trials. In placebo-controlled clinical trials, the following adverse experiences reported with SINGULAIR occurred in greater than or equal to 1% of patients and at an incidence greater than that in patients treated with placebo:

TABLE 1: Adverse Experiences Occurring in ≥1% of Patients with an Incidence Greater than that in Patients Treated with Placebo

	SINGULAIR 10 mg/day (%) (n=1955)	Placebo (%) (n=1180)
Body As A Whole		
Pain, abdominal	2.9	2.5
Asthenia/fatigue	1.8	1.2
Fever	1.5	0.9
Trauma	1.0	0.8
Digestive System Disorders		
Dyspepsia	2.1	1.1
Pain, dental	1.7	1.0
Gastroenteritis, infectious	1.5	0.5
Nervous System / Psychiatric		
Headache	18.4	18.1
Dizziness	1.9	1.4
Respiratory System Disorders		
Influenza	4.2	3.9
Cough	2.7	2.4
Congestion, nasal	1.6	1.3
Skin / Skin Appendages Disorder		
Rash	1.6	1.2
*Laboratory Adverse Experiences**		
ALT increased	2.1	2.0
AST increased	1.6	1.2
Pyuria	1.0	0.9

* Number of patients tested (SINGULAIR and placebo, respectively): ALT and AST, 1,935, 1,170; pyuria, 1,924, 1,159.

The frequency of less common adverse events was comparable between SINGULAIR and placebo.

The safety profile of SINGULAIR, when administered as a single dose for prevention of EIB in adult and adolescent patients 15 years of age and older, was consistent with the safety profile previously described for SINGULAIR.

Cumulatively, 569 patients were treated with SINGULAIR for at least 6 months, 480 for one year, and 49 for two years in clinical trials. With prolonged treatment, the adverse experience profile did not significantly change.

Pediatric Patients 6 to 14 Years of Age with Asthma
SINGULAIR has been evaluated for safety in 476 pediatric patients 6 to 14 years of age. Cumulatively, 289 pediatric patients were treated with SINGULAIR for at least 6 months, and 241 for one year or longer in clinical trials. The safety profile of SINGULAIR in the 8-week, double-blind, pediatric efficacy trial was generally similar to the adult safety profile. In pediatric patients 6 to 14 years of age receiving SINGULAIR, the following events occurred with a frequency ≥2% and more frequently than in pediatric patients who received placebo: pharyngitis, influenza, fever, sinusitis, nausea, diarrhea, dyspepsia, otitis, viral infection, and laryngitis. The frequency of less common adverse events was comparable between SINGULAIR and placebo. With prolonged treatment, the adverse experience profile did not significantly change.

In studies evaluating growth rate, the safety profile in these pediatric patients was consistent with the safety profile previously described for SINGULAIR. In a 56-week, double-blind study evaluating growth rate in pediatric patients 6 to 8 years of age receiving SINGULAIR, the following events not previously observed with the use of SINGULAIR in this age group occurred with a frequency ≥2% and more frequently than in pediatric patients who received placebo: headache, rhinitis (infective), varicella, gastroenteritis, atopic dermatitis, acute bronchitis, tooth infection, skin infection, and myopia.

Pediatric Patients 2 to 5 Years of Age with Asthma
SINGULAIR has been evaluated for safety in 573 pediatric patients 2 to 5 years of age in single- and multiple-dose studies. Cumulatively, 426 pediatric patients 2 to 5 years of age were treated with SINGULAIR for at least 3 months, 230 for 6 months or longer, and 63 patients for one year or longer in clinical trials. In pediatric patients 2 to 5 years of age receiving SINGULAIR, the following events occurred with a frequency ≥2% and more frequently than in pediatric patients who received placebo: fever, cough, abdominal pain, diarrhea, headache, rhinorrhea, sinusitis, otitis, influenza, rash, ear pain, gastroenteritis, eczema, urticaria, varicella, pneumonia, dermatitis, and conjunctivitis.

Pediatric Patients 6 to 23 Months of Age with Asthma
Safety and effectiveness in pediatric patients younger than 12 months of age with asthma have not been established. SINGULAIR has been evaluated for safety in 175 pediatric patients 6 to 23 months of age. The safety profile of SINGULAIR in a 6-week, double-blind, placebo-controlled clinical study was generally similar to the safety profile in adults and pediatric patients 2 to 14 years of age. In pediatric patients 6 to 23 months of age receiving SINGULAIR, the following events occurred with a frequency ≥2% and more frequently than in pediatric patients who received placebo: upper respiratory infection, wheezing; otitis media; pharyngitis, tonsillitis, cough; and rhinitis. The frequency of less common adverse events was comparable between SINGULAIR and placebo.

Adults and Adolescents 15 Years of Age and Older with Seasonal Allergic Rhinitis
SINGULAIR has been evaluated for safety in 2199 adult and adolescent patients 15 years of age and older in clinical trials. SINGULAIR administered once daily in the morning or in the evening had a safety profile similar to that of placebo. In placebo-controlled clinical trials, the following event was reported with SINGULAIR with a frequency ≥1% and at an incidence greater than placebo: upper respiratory infection, 1.9% of patients receiving SINGULAIR vs. 1.5% of patients receiving placebo. In a 4-week, placebo-controlled clinical study, the safety profile was consistent with that observed in 2-week studies. The incidence of somnolence was similar to that of placebo in all studies.

Pediatric Patients 2 to 14 Years of Age with Seasonal Allergic Rhinitis
SINGULAIR has been evaluated in 280 pediatric patients 2 to 14 years of age in a 2-week, multicenter, double-blind, placebo-controlled, parallel-group safety study. SINGULAIR administered once daily in the evening had a safety profile similar to that of placebo. In this study, the following events occurred with a frequency ≥2% and at an incidence greater than placebo: headache, otitis media, pharyngitis, and upper respiratory infection.

Adults and Adolescents 15 Years of Age and Older with Perennial Allergic Rhinitis
SINGULAIR has been evaluated for safety in 3357 adult and adolescent patients 15 years of age and older with perennial allergic rhinitis of whom 1632 received SINGULAIR in two, 6-week, clinical studies. SINGULAIR administered once daily had a safety profile consistent with that observed in patients with seasonal allergic rhinitis and similar to that of placebo. In these two studies, the following events were reported with SINGULAIR with a frequency ≥1% and at an incidence greater than placebo: sinusitis, upper respiratory infection, sinus headache, cough, epistaxis, and increased ALT. The incidence of somnolence was similar to that of placebo.

Pediatric Patients 6 Months to 14 Years of Age with Perennial Allergic Rhinitis
The safety in patients 2 to 14 years of age with perennial allergic rhinitis is supported by the safety in patients 2 to 14 years of age with seasonal allergic rhinitis. The safety in patients 6 to 23 months of age is supported by data from pharmacokinetic and safety and efficacy studies in asthma in this pediatric population and from adult pharmacokinetic studies.

6.2 Post-Marketing Experience
The following adverse reactions have been identified during post-approval use of SINGULAIR. Because these reactions are reported voluntarily from a population of uncertain size, it is not always possible to reliably estimate their frequency or establish a causal relationship to drug exposure.
Blood and lymphatic system disorders: increased bleeding tendency.
Immune system disorders: hypersensitivity reactions including anaphylaxis, hepatic eosinophilic infiltration.
Psychiatric disorders: agitation including aggressive behavior or hostility, anxiousness, depression, disorientation, dream abnormalities, hallucinations, insomnia, irritability, restlessness, somnambulism, suicidal thinking and behavior (including suicide), tremor *[see Warnings and Precautions (5.4)].*
Nervous system disorders: drowsiness, paraesthesia/ hypoesthesia, seizures.
Cardiac disorders: palpitations.
Respiratory, thoracic and mediastinal disorders: epistaxis.
Gastrointestinal disorders: diarrhea, dyspepsia, nausea, pancreatitis, vomiting.
Hepatobiliary disorders: Cases of cholestatic hepatitis, hepatocellular liver-injury, and mixed-pattern liver injury have been reported in patients treated with SINGULAIR. Most of these occurred in combination with other confounding factors, such as use of other medications, or when SINGULAIR was administered to patients who had underlying potential for liver disease such as alcohol use or other forms of hepatitis.
Skin and subcutaneous tissue disorders: angioedema, bruising, erythema nodosum, pruritus, urticaria.
Musculoskeletal and connective tissue disorders: arthralgia, myalgia including muscle cramps.
General disorders and administration site conditions: edema.
Patients with asthma on therapy with SINGULAIR may present with systemic eosinophilia, sometimes presenting with clinical features of vasculitis consistent with Churg-Strauss syndrome, a condition which is often treated with systemic corticosteroid therapy. These events usually, but not always, have been associated with the reduction of oral corticosteroid therapy. Physicians should be alert to eosinophilia, vasculitic rash, worsening pulmonary symptoms, cardiac complications, and/or neuropathy presenting in their patients *[see Warnings and Precautions (5.5)].*

7 DRUG INTERACTIONS
No dose adjustment is needed when SINGULAIR is co-administered with theophylline, prednisone, prednisolone, oral contraceptives, terfenadine, digoxin, warfarin, thyroid hormones, sedative hypnotics, non-steroidal anti-inflammatory agents, benzodiazepines, decongestants, and Cytochrome P450 (CYP) enzyme inducers *[see Clinical Pharmacology (12.3)].*

8 USE IN SPECIFIC POPULATIONS
8.1 Pregnancy
Pregnancy Category B: There are no adequate and well-controlled studies in pregnant women. Because animal reproduction studies are not always predictive of human response, SINGULAIR should be used during pregnancy only if clearly needed.
Teratogenic Effect: No teratogenicity was observed in rats and rabbits at doses approximately 100 and 110 times, respectively, the maximum recommended daily oral dose in adults based on AUCs *[see Nonclinical Toxicology (13.2)].* During worldwide marketing experience, congenital limb defects have been rarely reported in the offspring of women being treated with SINGULAIR during pregnancy. Most of these women were also taking other asthma medications during their pregnancy. A causal relationship between these events and SINGULAIR has not been established.
Merck Sharp & Dohme Corp., a subsidiary of Merck & Co., Inc., maintains a registry to monitor the pregnancy outcomes of women exposed to SINGULAIR while pregnant. Patients and healthcare providers are encouraged to report any prenatal exposure to SINGULAIR by calling the Pregnancy Registry at 1-800-986-8999.
8.3 Nursing Mothers
Studies in rats have shown that montelukast is excreted in milk. It is not known if montelukast is excreted in human milk. Because many drugs are excreted in human milk, caution should be exercised when SINGULAIR is given to a nursing mother.
8.4 Pediatric Use
Safety and efficacy of SINGULAIR have been established in adequate and well-controlled studies in pediatric patients with asthma 6 to 14 years of age. Safety and efficacy profiles in this age group are similar to those seen in adults *[see Adverse Reactions (6.1), Clinical Pharmacology, Special Populations (12.3), and Clinical Studies (14.1)].*
The efficacy of SINGULAIR for the treatment of seasonal allergic rhinitis in pediatric patients 2 to 14 years of age and for the treatment of perennial allergic rhinitis in pediatric patients 6 months to 14 years of age is supported by extrapolation from the demonstrated efficacy in patients 15 years of age and older with allergic rhinitis as well as the assumption that the disease course, pathophysiology and the drug's effect are substantially similar among these populations.
The safety of SINGULAIR 4-mg chewable tablets in pediatric patients 2 to 5 years of age with asthma has been demonstrated by adequate and well-controlled data *[see Adverse Reactions (6.1)].* Efficacy of SINGULAIR in this age group is extrapolated from the demonstrated efficacy in patients 6 years of age and older with asthma and is based on similar pharmacokinetic data, as well as the assumption that the disease course, pathophysiology and the drug's effect are substantially similar among these populations. Efficacy in this age group is supported by exploratory efficacy assessments from a large, well-controlled safety study conducted in patients 2 to 5 years of age.
The safety of SINGULAIR 4-mg oral granules in pediatric patients 12 to 23 months of age with asthma has been demonstrated in an analysis of 172 pediatric patients, 124 of whom were treated with SINGULAIR, in a 6-week, double-blind, placebo-controlled study *[see Adverse Reactions (6.1)].* Efficacy of SINGULAIR in this age group is extrapolated from the demonstrated efficacy in patients 6 years of age and older with asthma based on similar mean systemic exposure (AUC), and that the disease course, pathophysiology and the drug's effect are substantially similar among these populations, supported by efficacy data from a safety trial in which efficacy was an exploratory assessment.
The safety of SINGULAIR 4-mg and 5-mg chewable tablets in pediatric patients aged 2 to 14 years with allergic rhinitis is supported by data from studies conducted in pediatric patients aged 2 to 14 years with asthma. A safety study in pediatric patients 2 to 14 years of age with seasonal allergic rhinitis demonstrated a similar safety profile *[see Adverse Reactions (6.1)].* The safety of SINGULAIR 4-mg oral granules in pediatric patients as young as 6 months of age with perennial allergic rhinitis is supported by extrapolation from safety data obtained from studies conducted in

pediatric patients 6 months to 23 months of age with asthma and from pharmacokinetic data comparing systemic exposures in patients 6 months to 23 months of age to systemic exposures in adults.

The safety and effectiveness in pediatric patients below the age of 12 months with asthma and 6 months with perennial allergic rhinitis have not been established. The safety and effectiveness in pediatric patients below the age of 15 years with exercise-induced bronchoconstriction have not been established.

Growth Rate in Pediatric Patients

A 56-week, multi-center, double-blind, randomized, active- and placebo-controlled parallel group study was conducted to assess the effect of SINGULAIR on growth rate in 360 patients with mild asthma, aged 6 to 8 years. Treatment groups included SINGULAIR 5 mg once daily, placebo, and beclomethasone dipropionate administered as 168 mcg twice daily with a spacer device. For each subject, a growth rate was defined as the slope of a linear regression line fit to the height measurements over 56 weeks. The primary comparison was the difference in growth rates between SINGULAIR and placebo groups. Growth rates, expressed as least-squares (LS) mean (95% CI) in cm/year, for the SINGULAIR, placebo, and beclomethasone treatment groups were 5.67 (5.46, 5.88), 5.64 (5.42, 5.86), and 4.86 (4.64, 5.08), respectively. The differences in growth rates, expressed as least-squares (LS) mean (95% CI) in cm/year, for SINGULAIR minus placebo, beclomethasone minus placebo, and SINGULAIR minus beclomethasone treatment groups were 0.03 (-0.26, 0.31), -0.78 (-1.06, -0.49); and 0.81 (0.53, 1.09), respectively. Growth rate (expressed as mean change in height over time) for each treatment group is shown in FIGURE 1.

FIGURE 1: Change in Height (cm) from Randomization Visit by Scheduled Week (Treatment Group Mean ± Standard Error* of the Mean)

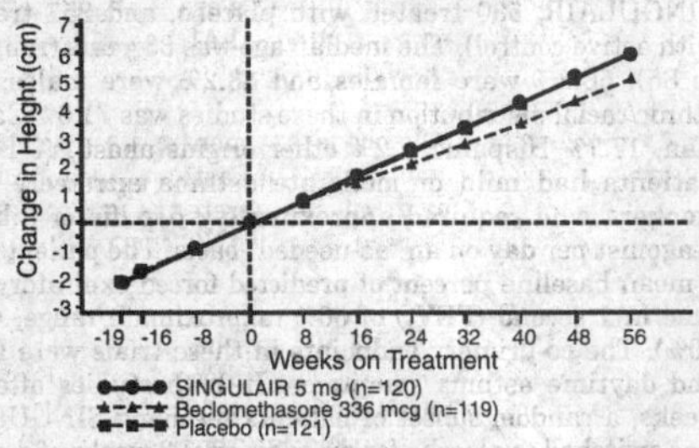

*The standard errors of the treatment group means in change in height are too small to be visible on the plot

8.5 Geriatric Use

Of the total number of subjects in clinical studies of montelukast, 3.5% were 65 years of age and over, and 0.4% were 75 years of age and over. No overall differences in safety or effectiveness were observed between these subjects and younger subjects, and other reported clinical experience has not identified differences in responses between the elderly and younger patients, but greater sensitivity of some older individuals cannot be ruled out. The pharmacokinetic profile and the oral bioavailability of a single 10-mg oral dose of montelukast are similar in elderly and younger adults. The plasma half-life of montelukast is slightly longer in the elderly. No dosage adjustment in the elderly is required.

8.6 Hepatic Insufficiency

No dosage adjustment is required in patients with mild-to-moderate hepatic insufficiency *[see Clinical Pharmacology (12.3)]*.

8.7 Renal Insufficiency

No dosage adjustment is recommended in patients with renal insufficiency *[see Clinical Pharmacology (12.3)]*.

10 OVERDOSAGE

No mortality occurred following single oral doses of montelukast up to 5000 mg/kg in mice (estimated exposure was approximately 335 and 210 times the AUC for adults and children, respectively, at the maximum recommended daily oral dose) and rats (estimated exposure was approximately 230 and 145 times the AUC for adults and children, respectively, at the maximum recommended daily oral dose).

No specific information is available on the treatment of overdosage with SINGULAIR. In chronic asthma studies, montelukast has been administered at doses up to 200 mg/day to adult patients for 22 weeks and, in short-term studies, up to 900 mg/day to patients for approximately a week without clinically important adverse experiences. In the event of overdose, it is reasonable to employ the usual supportive measures; e.g., remove unabsorbed material from the gastrointestinal tract, employ clinical monitoring, and institute supportive therapy, if required.

There have been reports of acute overdosage in post-marketing experience and clinical studies with SINGULAIR. These include reports in adults and children with a dose as high as 1000 mg. The clinical and laboratory findings observed were consistent with the safety profile in adults and pediatric patients. There were no adverse experiences in the majority of overdosage reports. The most frequently occurring adverse experiences were consistent with the safety profile of SINGULAIR and included abdominal pain, somnolence, thirst, headache, vomiting and psychomotor hyperactivity.

It is not known whether montelukast is removed by peritoneal dialysis or hemodialysis.

11 DESCRIPTION

Montelukast sodium, the active ingredient in SINGULAIR, is a selective and orally active leukotriene receptor antagonist that inhibits the cysteinyl leukotriene $CysLT_1$ receptor.

Montelukast sodium is described chemically as [*R*-(*E*)]-1-[[[1-[3-[2-(7-chloro-2-quinolinyl)ethenyl]phenyl]-3-[2-(1-hydroxy-1-methylethyl)phenyl]propyl]thio]methyl]cyclopropaneacetic acid, monosodium salt.

The empirical formula is $C_{35}H_{35}ClNNaO_3S$, and its molecular weight is 608.18. The structural formula is:

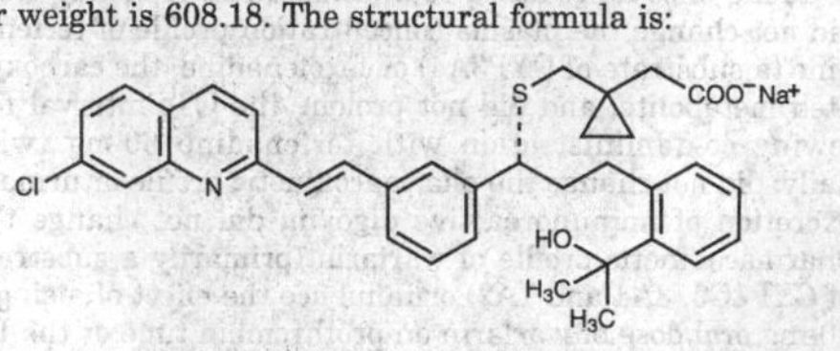

Montelukast sodium is a hygroscopic, optically active, white to off-white powder. Montelukast sodium is freely soluble in ethanol, methanol, and water and practically insoluble in acetonitrile.

Each 10-mg film-coated SINGULAIR tablet contains 10.4 mg montelukast sodium, which is equivalent to 10 mg of montelukast, and the following inactive ingredients: microcrystalline cellulose, lactose monohydrate, croscarmellose sodium, hydroxypropyl cellulose, and magnesium stearate. The film coating consists of: hydroxypropyl methylcellulose, hydroxypropyl cellulose, titanium dioxide, red ferric oxide, yellow ferric oxide, and carnauba wax.

Each 4-mg and 5-mg chewable SINGULAIR tablet contains 4.2 and 5.2 mg montelukast sodium, respectively, which are equivalent to 4 and 5 mg of montelukast, respectively. Both chewable tablets contain the following inactive ingredients: mannitol, microcrystalline cellulose, hydroxypropyl cellulose, red ferric oxide, croscarmellose sodium, cherry flavor, aspartame, and magnesium stearate.

Each packet of SINGULAIR 4-mg oral granules contains 4.2 mg montelukast sodium, which is equivalent to 4 mg of montelukast. The oral granule formulation contains the following inactive ingredients: mannitol, hydroxypropyl cellulose, and magnesium stearate.

12 CLINICAL PHARMACOLOGY

12.1 Mechanism of Action

The cysteinyl leukotrienes (LTC_4, LTD_4, LTE_4) are products of arachidonic acid metabolism and are released from various cells, including mast cells and eosinophils. These eicosanoids bind to cysteinyl leukotriene (CysLT) receptors. The CysLT type-1 ($CysLT_1$) receptor is found in the human airway (including airway smooth muscle cells and airway macrophages) and on other pro-inflammatory cells (including eosinophils and certain myeloid stem cells). CysLTs have been correlated with the pathophysiology of asthma and allergic rhinitis. In asthma, leukotriene-mediated effects include airway edema, smooth muscle contraction, and altered cellular activity associated with the inflammatory process. In allergic rhinitis, CysLTs are released from the nasal mucosa after allergen exposure during both early- and late-phase reactions and are associated with symptoms of allergic rhinitis.

Montelukast is an orally active compound that binds with high affinity and selectivity to the $CysLT_1$ receptor (in preference to other pharmacologically important airway receptors, such as the prostanoid, cholinergic, or β-adrenergic receptor). Montelukast inhibits physiologic actions of LTD_4 at the $CysLT_1$ receptor without any agonist activity.

12.2 Pharmacodynamics

Montelukast causes inhibition of airway cysteinyl leukotriene receptors as demonstrated by the ability to inhibit bronchoconstriction due to inhaled LTD_4 in asthmatics. Doses as low as 5 mg cause substantial blockage of LTD_4-induced bronchoconstriction. In a placebo-controlled, crossover study (n=12), SINGULAIR inhibited early- and late-phase bronchoconstriction due to antigen challenge by 75% and 57%, respectively.

The effect of SINGULAIR on eosinophils in the peripheral blood was examined in clinical trials. In patients with asthma aged 2 years and older who received SINGULAIR, a decrease in mean peripheral blood eosinophil counts ranging from 9% to 15% was noted, compared with placebo, over the double-blind treatment periods. In patients with seasonal allergic rhinitis aged 15 years and older who received SINGULAIR, a mean increase of 0.2% in peripheral blood eosinophil counts was noted, compared with a mean increase of 12.5% in placebo-treated patients, over the double-blind treatment periods; this reflects a mean difference of 12.3% in favor of SINGULAIR. The relationship between these observations and the clinical benefits of montelukast noted in the clinical trials is not known *[see Clinical Studies (14)]*.

12.3 Pharmacokinetics

Absorption

Montelukast is rapidly absorbed following oral administration. After administration of the 10-mg film-coated tablet to fasted adults, the mean peak montelukast plasma concentration (C_{max}) is achieved in 3 to 4 hours (T_{max}). The mean oral bioavailability is 64%. The oral bioavailability and C_{max} are not influenced by a standard meal in the morning.

For the 5-mg chewable tablet, the mean C_{max} is achieved in 2 to 2.5 hours after administration to adults in the fasted state. The mean oral bioavailability is 73% in the fasted state versus 63% when administered with a standard meal in the morning.

For the 4-mg chewable tablet, the mean C_{max} is achieved 2 hours after administration in pediatric patients 2 to 5 years of age in the fasted state.

The 4-mg oral granule formulation is bioequivalent to the 4-mg chewable tablet when administered to adults in the fasted state. The co-administration of the oral granule formulation with applesauce did not have a clinically significant effect on the pharmacokinetics of montelukast. A high fat meal in the morning did not affect the AUC of montelukast oral granules; however, the meal decreased C_{max} by 35% and prolonged T_{max} from 2.3 ± 1.0 hours to 6.4 ± 2.9 hours.

The safety and efficacy of SINGULAIR in patients with asthma were demonstrated in clinical trials in which the 10-mg film-coated tablet and 5-mg chewable tablet formulations were administered in the evening without regard to the time of food ingestion. The safety of SINGULAIR in patients with asthma was also demonstrated in clinical trials in which the 4-mg chewable tablet and 4-mg oral granule formulations were administered in the evening without regard to the time of food ingestion. The safety and efficacy of SINGULAIR in patients with seasonal allergic rhinitis were demonstrated in clinical trials in which the 10-mg film-coated tablet was administered in the morning or evening without regard to the time of food ingestion.

The comparative pharmacokinetics of montelukast when administered as two 5-mg chewable tablets versus one 10-mg film-coated tablet have not been evaluated.

Distribution

Montelukast is more than 99% bound to plasma proteins. The steady state volume of distribution of montelukast averages 8 to 11 liters. Studies in rats with radiolabeled montelukast indicate minimal distribution across the blood-brain barrier. In addition, concentrations of radiolabeled material at 24 hours postdose were minimal in all other tissues.

Metabolism

Montelukast is extensively metabolized. In studies with therapeutic doses, plasma concentrations of metabolites of montelukast are undetectable at steady state in adults and pediatric patients.

In vitro studies using human liver microsomes indicate that CYP3A4 and 2C9 are involved in the metabolism of montelukast. Clinical studies investigating the effect of known inhibitors of CYP3A4 (e.g., ketoconazole, erythromycin) or 2C9 (e.g., fluconazole) on montelukast pharmacokinetics have not been conducted. Based on further *in vitro* results in human liver microsomes, therapeutic plasma concentrations of montelukast do not inhibit CYP3A4, 2C9, 1A2, 2A6, 2C19, or 2D6 *[see Drug Interactions (7) and Clinical Pharmacology, Drug-Drug Interactions (12.3)]*. *In vitro* studies have shown that montelukast is a potent inhibitor of CYP2C8; however, data from a clinical drug-drug interaction study involving montelukast and rosiglitazone (a probe substrate representative of drugs primarily metabolized by CYP2C8) demonstrated that montelukast does not inhibit CYP2C8 *in vivo*, and therefore is not anticipated to alter the metabolism of drugs metabolized by this enzyme *[see Drug Interactions (7) and Clinical Pharmacology, Drug-Drug Interactions (12.3)]*.

Elimination

The plasma clearance of montelukast averages 45 mL/min in healthy adults. Following an oral dose of radiolabeled montelukast, 86% of the radioactivity was recovered in 5-day fecal collections and <0.2% was recovered in urine. Coupled with estimates of montelukast oral bioavailability, this indicates that montelukast and its metabolites are excreted almost exclusively via the bile.

In several studies, the mean plasma half-life of montelukast ranged from 2.7 to 5.5 hours in healthy young adults. The pharmacokinetics of montelukast are nearly linear for oral doses up to 50 mg. During once-daily dosing with 10-mg montelukast, there is little accumulation of the parent drug in plasma (14%).

Special Populations

Hepatic Insufficiency: Patients with mild-to-moderate hepatic insufficiency and clinical evidence of cirrhosis had evidence of decreased metabolism of montelukast resulting in 41% (90% CI=7%, 85%) higher mean montelukast AUC following a single 10-mg dose. The elimination of montelukast was slightly prolonged compared with that in healthy subjects (mean half-life, 7.4 hours). No dosage adjustment is required in patients with mild-to-moderate hepatic insufficiency. The pharmacokinetics of SINGULAIR in patients with more severe hepatic impairment or with hepatitis have not been evaluated.

Renal Insufficiency: Since montelukast and its metabolites are not excreted in the urine, the pharmacokinetics of montelukast were not evaluated in patients with renal insufficiency. No dosage adjustment is recommended in these patients.

Gender: The pharmacokinetics of montelukast are similar in males and females.

Race: Pharmacokinetic differences due to race have not been studied.

Adolescents and Pediatric Patients: Pharmacokinetic studies evaluated the systemic exposure of the 4-mg oral granule formulation in pediatric patients 6 to 23 months of age, the 4-mg chewable tablets in pediatric patients 2 to 5 years of age, the 5-mg chewable tablets in pediatric patients 6 to 14 years of age, and the 10-mg film-coated tablets in young adults and adolescents ≥15 years of age.

The plasma concentration profile of montelukast following administration of the 10-mg film-coated tablet is similar in adolescents ≥15 years of age and young adults. The 10-mg film-coated tablet is recommended for use in patients ≥15 years of age.

The mean systemic exposure of the 4-mg chewable tablet in pediatric patients 2 to 5 years of age and the 5-mg chewable tablets in pediatric patients 6 to 14 years of age is similar to the mean systemic exposure of the 10-mg film-coated tablet in adults. The 5-mg chewable tablet should be used in pediatric patients 6 to 14 years of age and the 4-mg chewable tablet should be used in pediatric patients 2 to 5 years of age.

In children 6 to 11 months of age, the systemic exposure to montelukast and the variability of plasma montelukast concentrations were higher than those observed in adults. Based on population analyses, the mean AUC (4296 ng•hr/mL [range 1200 to 7153]) was 60% higher and the mean C_{max} (667 ng/mL [range 201 to 1058]) was 89% higher than those observed in adults (mean AUC 2689 ng•hr/mL [range 1521 to 4595]) and mean C_{max} (353 ng/mL [range 180 to 548]). The systemic exposure in children 12 to 23 months of age was less variable, but was still higher than that observed in adults. The mean AUC (3574 ng•hr/mL [range 2229 to 5408]) was 33% higher and the mean C_{max} (562 ng/mL [range 296 to 814]) was 60% higher than those observed in adults. Safety and tolerability of montelukast in a single-dose pharmacokinetic study in 26 children 6 to 23 months of age were similar to that of patients two years and above *[see Adverse Reactions (6.1)]*. The 4-mg oral granule formulation should be used for pediatric patients 12 to 23 months of age for the treatment of asthma, or for pediatric patients 6 to 23 months of age for the treatment of perennial allergic rhinitis. Since the 4-mg oral granule formulation is bioequivalent to the 4-mg chewable tablet, it can also be used as an alternative formulation to the 4-mg chewable tablet in pediatric patients 2 to 5 years of age.

Drug-Drug Interactions

Theophylline, Prednisone, and Prednisolone: SINGULAIR has been administered with other therapies routinely used in the prophylaxis and chronic treatment of asthma with no apparent increase in adverse reactions. In drug-interaction studies, the recommended clinical dose of montelukast did not have clinically important effects on the pharmacokinetics of the following drugs: theophylline, prednisone, and prednisolone.

Montelukast at a dose of 10 mg once daily dosed to pharmacokinetic steady state, did not cause clinically significant changes in the kinetics of a single intravenous dose of theophylline [predominantly a cytochrome P450 (CYP) 1A2 substrate]. Montelukast at doses of ≥100 mg daily dosed to pharmacokinetic steady state, did not cause any clinically significant change in plasma profiles of prednisone or prednisolone following administration of either oral prednisone or intravenous prednisolone.

Oral Contraceptives, Terfenadine, Digoxin, and Warfarin: In drug interaction studies, the recommended clinical dose of montelukast did not have clinically important effects on the pharmacokinetics of the following drugs: oral contraceptives (norethindrone 1 mg/ethinyl estradiol 35 mcg), terfenadine, digoxin, and warfarin. Montelukast at doses of ≥100 mg daily dosed to pharmacokinetic steady state did not significantly alter the plasma concentrations of either component of an oral contraceptive containing norethindrone 1 mg/ethinyl estradiol 35 mcg. Montelukast at a dose of 10 mg once daily dosed to pharmacokinetic steady state did not change the plasma concentration profile of terfenadine (a substrate of CYP3A4) or fexofenadine, the carboxylated metabolite, and did not prolong the QTc interval following co-administration with terfenadine 60 mg twice daily; did not change the pharmacokinetic profile or urinary excretion of immunoreactive digoxin; did not change the pharmacokinetic profile of warfarin (primarily a substrate of CYP2C9, 3A4 and 1A2) or influence the effect of a single 30-mg oral dose of warfarin on prothrombin time or the International Normalized Ratio (INR).

Thyroid Hormones, Sedative Hypnotics, Non-Steroidal Anti-Inflammatory Agents, Benzodiazepines, and Decongestants: Although additional specific interaction studies were not performed, SINGULAIR was used concomitantly with a wide range of commonly prescribed drugs in clinical studies without evidence of clinical adverse interactions. These medications included thyroid hormones, sedative hypnotics, non-steroidal anti-inflammatory agents, benzodiazepines, and decongestants.

Cytochrome P450 (CYP) Enzyme Inducers: Phenobarbital, which induces hepatic metabolism, decreased the area under the plasma concentration curve (AUC) of montelukast approximately 40% following a single 10-mg dose of montelukast. No dosage adjustment for SINGULAIR is recommended. It is reasonable to employ appropriate clinical monitoring when potent CYP enzyme inducers, such as phenobarbital or rifampin, are co-administered with SINGULAIR.

Montelukast is a potent inhibitor of CYP2C8 *in vitro*. However, data from a clinical drug-drug interaction study involving montelukast and rosiglitazone (a probe substrate representative of drugs primarily metabolized by CYP2C8) in 12 healthy individuals demonstrated that the pharmacokinetics of rosiglitazone are not altered when the drugs are coadministered, indicating that montelukast does not inhibit CYP2C8 *in vivo*. Therefore, montelukast is not anticipated to alter the metabolism of drugs metabolized by this enzyme (e.g., paclitaxel, rosiglitazone, and repaglinide).

13 NONCLINICAL TOXICOLOGY

13.1 Carcinogenesis, Mutagenesis, Impairment of Fertility

No evidence of tumorigenicity was seen in carcinogenicity studies of either 2 years in Sprague-Dawley rats or 92 weeks in mice at oral gavage doses up to 200 mg/kg/day or 100 mg/kg/day, respectively. The estimated exposure in rats was approximately 120 and 75 times the AUC for adults and children, respectively, at the maximum recommended daily oral dose. The estimated exposure in mice was approximately 45 and 25 times the AUC for adults and children, respectively, at the maximum recommended daily oral dose.

Montelukast demonstrated no evidence of mutagenic or clastogenic activity in the following assays: the microbial mutagenesis assay, the V-79 mammalian cell mutagenesis assay, the alkaline elution assay in rat hepatocytes, the chromosomal aberration assay in Chinese hamster ovary cells, and in the *in vivo* mouse bone marrow chromosomal aberration assay.

In fertility studies in female rats, montelukast produced reductions in fertility and fecundity indices at an oral dose of 200 mg/kg (estimated exposure was approximately 70 times the AUC for adults at the maximum recommended daily oral dose). No effects on female fertility or fecundity were observed at an oral dose of 100 mg/kg (estimated exposure was approximately 20 times the AUC for adults at the maximum recommended daily oral dose). Montelukast had no effects on fertility in male rats at oral doses up to 800 mg/kg (estimated exposure was approximately 160 times the AUC for adults at the maximum recommended daily oral dose).

13.2 Animal Toxicology and/or Pharmacology

Reproductive Toxicology Studies

No teratogenicity was observed at oral doses up to 400 mg/kg/day and 300 mg/kg/day in rats and rabbits, respectively. These doses were approximately 100 and 110 times the maximum recommended daily oral dose in adults, respectively, based on AUCs. Montelukast crosses the placenta following oral dosing in rats and rabbits *[see Pregnancy (8.1)]*.

14 CLINICAL STUDIES

14.1 Asthma

Adults and Adolescents 15 Years of Age and Older with Asthma

Clinical trials in adults and adolescents 15 years of age and older demonstrated there is no additional clinical benefit to montelukast doses above 10 mg once daily.

The efficacy of SINGULAIR for the chronic treatment of asthma in adults and adolescents 15 years of age and older was demonstrated in two (U.S. and Multinational) similarly designed, randomized, 12-week, double-blind, placebo-controlled trials in 1576 patients (795 treated with SINGULAIR, 530 treated with placebo, and 251 treated with active control). The median age was 33 years (range 15 to 85); 56.8% were females and 43.2% were males. The ethnic/racial distribution in these studies was 71.6% Caucasian, 17.7% Hispanic, 7.2% other origins and 3.5% Black. Patients had mild or moderate asthma and were non-smokers who required approximately 5 puffs of inhaled β-agonist per day on an "as-needed" basis. The patients had a mean baseline percent of predicted forced expiratory volume in 1 second (FEV_1) of 66% (approximate range, 40 to 90%). The co-primary endpoints in these trials were FEV_1 and daytime asthma symptoms. In both studies after 12 weeks, a random subset of patients receiving SINGULAIR was switched to placebo for an additional 3 weeks of double-blind treatment to evaluate for possible rebound effects.

The results of the U.S. trial on the primary endpoint, morning FEV_1, expressed as mean percent change from baseline averaged over the 12-week treatment period, are shown in FIGURE 2. Compared with placebo, treatment with one SINGULAIR 10-mg tablet daily in the evening resulted in a statistically significant increase in FEV_1 percent change from baseline (13.0%-change in the group treated with SINGULAIR vs. 4.2%-change in the placebo group, p<0.001); the change from baseline in FEV_1 for SINGULAIR was 0.32 liters compared with 0.10 liters for placebo, corresponding to a between-group difference of 0.22 liters (p<0.001, 95% CI 0.17 liters, 0.27 liters). The results of the Multinational trial on FEV_1 were similar.

FIGURE 2: FEV_1 Mean Percent Change from Baseline (U.S. Trial: SINGULAIR N=406; Placebo N=270) (ANOVA Model)

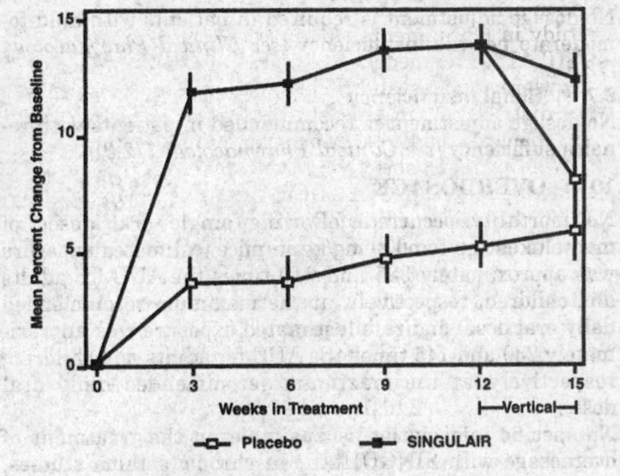

The effect of SINGULAIR on other primary and secondary endpoints, represented by the Multinational study is shown in TABLE 2. Results on these endpoints were similar in the US study.

[See table 2 at left]

Both studies evaluated the effect of SINGULAIR on secondary outcomes, including asthma attack (utilization of

TABLE 2: Effect of SINGULAIR on Primary and Secondary Endpoints in a Multinational Placebo-controlled Trial (ANOVA Model)

	SINGULAIR			Placebo		
Endpoint	N	Baseline	Mean Change from Baseline	N	Baseline	Mean Change from Baseline
Daytime Asthma Symptoms (0 to 6 scale)	372	2.35	-0.49*	245	2.40	-0.26
β-agonist (puffs per day)	371	5.35	-1.65*	241	5.78	-0.42
AM PEFR (L/min)	372	339.57	25.03*	244	335.24	1.83
PM PEFR (L/min)	372	355.23	20.13*	244	354.02	-0.49
Nocturnal Awakenings (#/week)	285	5.46	-2.03*	195	5.57	-0.78

* p<0.001, compared with placebo

health-care resources such as an unscheduled visit to a doctor's office, emergency room, or hospital; or treatment with oral, intravenous, or intramuscular corticosteroid), and use of oral corticosteroids for asthma rescue. In the Multinational study, significantly fewer patients (15.6% of patients) on SINGULAIR experienced asthma attacks compared with patients on placebo (27.3%, p < 0.001). In the US study, 7.8% of patients on SINGULAIR and 10.3% of patients on placebo experienced asthma attacks, but the difference between the two treatment groups was not significant (p = 0.334). In the Multinational study, significantly fewer patients (14.8% of patients) on SINGULAIR were prescribed oral corticosteroids for asthma rescue compared with patients on placebo (25.7%, p < 0.001). In the US study, 6.9% of patients on SINGULAIR and 9.9% of patients on placebo were prescribed oral corticosteroids for asthma rescue, but the difference between the two treatment groups was not significant (p = 0.196).

Onset of Action and Maintenance of Effects

In each placebo-controlled trial in adults, the treatment effect of SINGULAIR, measured by daily diary card parameters, including symptom scores, "as-needed" β-agonist use, and PEFR measurements, was achieved after the first dose and was maintained throughout the dosing interval (24 hours). No significant change in treatment effect was observed during continuous once-daily evening administration in non-placebo-controlled extension trials for up to one year. Withdrawal of SINGULAIR in asthmatic patients after 12 weeks of continuous use did not cause rebound worsening of asthma.

Pediatric Patients 6 to 14 Years of Age with Asthma

The efficacy of SINGULAIR in pediatric patients 6 to 14 years of age was demonstrated in one 8-week, double-blind, placebo-controlled trial in 336 patients (201 treated with SINGULAIR and 135 treated with placebo) using an inhaled β-agonist on an "as-needed" basis. The patients had a mean baseline percent predicted FEV_1 of 72% (approximate range, 45 to 90%) and a mean daily inhaled β-agonist requirement of 3.4 puffs of albuterol. Approximately 36% of the patients were on inhaled corticosteroids. The median age was 11 years (range 6 to 15); 35.4% were females and 64.6% were males. The ethnic/racial distribution in this study was 80.1% Caucasian, 12.8% Black, 4.5% Hispanic, and 2.7% other origins.

Compared with placebo, treatment with one 5-mg SINGULAIR chewable tablet daily resulted in a significant improvement in mean morning FEV_1 percent change from baseline (8.7% in the group treated with SINGULAIR vs. 4.2% change from baseline in the placebo group, p<0.001). There was a significant decrease in the mean percentage change in daily "as-needed" inhaled β-agonist use (11.7% decrease from baseline in the group treated with SINGULAIR vs. 8.2% increase from baseline in the placebo group, p<0.05). This effect represents a mean decrease from baseline of 0.56 and 0.23 puffs per day for the montelukast and placebo groups, respectively. Subgroup analyses indicated that younger pediatric patients aged 6 to 11 had efficacy results comparable to those of the older pediatric patients aged 12 to 14.

Similar to the adult studies, no significant change in the treatment effect was observed during continuous once-daily administration in one open-label extension trial without a concurrent placebo group for up to 6 months.

Pediatric Patients 2 to 5 Years of Age with Asthma

The efficacy of SINGULAIR for the chronic treatment of asthma in pediatric patients 2 to 5 years of age was explored in a 12-week, placebo-controlled safety and tolerability study in 689 patients, 461 of whom were treated with SINGULAIR. The median age was 4 years (range 2 to 6); 41.5% were females and 58.5% were males. The ethnic/racial distribution in this study was 56.5% Caucasian, 20.9% Hispanic, 14.4% other origins, and 8.3% Black.

While the primary objective was to determine the safety and tolerability of SINGULAIR in this age group, the study included exploratory efficacy evaluations, including daytime and overnight asthma symptom scores, β-agonist use, oral corticosteroid rescue, and the physician's global evaluation. The findings of these exploratory efficacy evaluations, along with pharmacokinetics and extrapolation of efficacy data from older patients, support the overall conclusion that SINGULAIR is efficacious in the maintenance treatment of asthma in patients 2 to 5 years of age.

Effects in Patients on Concomitant Inhaled Corticosteroids

Separate trials in adults evaluated the ability of SINGULAIR to add to the clinical effect of inhaled corticosteroids and to allow inhaled corticosteroid tapering when used concomitantly.

One randomized, placebo-controlled, parallel-group trial (n=226) enrolled adults with stable asthma with a mean FEV_1 of approximately 84% of predicted who were previously maintained on various inhaled corticosteroids (delivered by metered-dose aerosol or dry powder inhalers). The median age was 41.5 years (range 16 to 70); 52.2% were females and 47.8% were males. The ethnic/racial distribution in this study was 92.0% Caucasian, 3.5% Black, 2.2% Hispanic, and 2.2% Asian. The types of inhaled corticosteroids and their mean baseline requirements included beclomethasone dipropionate (mean dose, 1203 mcg/day), triamcinolone acetonide (mean dose, 2004 mcg/day), flunisolide (mean dose, 1971 mcg/day), fluticasone propionate (mean dose, 1083 mcg/day), or budesonide (mean dose, 1192 mcg/day). Some of these inhaled corticosteroids were non-U.S.-approved formulations, and doses expressed may not be ex-actuator. The pre-study inhaled corticosteroid requirements were reduced by approximately 37% during a 5- to 7-week placebo run-in period designed to titrate patients toward their lowest effective inhaled corticosteroid dose. Treatment with SINGULAIR resulted in a further 47% reduction in mean inhaled corticosteroid dose compared with a mean reduction of 30% in the placebo group over the 12-week active treatment period (p≤0.05). It is not known whether the results of this study can be generalized to patients with asthma who require higher doses of inhaled corticosteroids or systemic corticosteroids.

In another randomized, placebo-controlled, parallel-group trial (n=642) in a similar population of adult patients previously maintained, but not adequately controlled, on inhaled corticosteroids (beclomethasone 336 mcg/day), the addition of SINGULAIR to beclomethasone resulted in statistically significant improvements in FEV_1 compared with those patients who were continued on beclomethasone alone or those patients who were withdrawn from beclomethasone and treated with montelukast or placebo alone over the last 10 weeks of the 16-week, blinded treatment period. Patients who were randomized to treatment arms containing beclomethasone had statistically significantly better asthma control than those patients randomized to SINGULAIR alone or placebo alone as indicated by FEV_1, daytime asthma symptoms, PEFR, nocturnal awakenings due to asthma, and "as-needed" β-agonist requirements.

In adult patients with asthma with documented aspirin sensitivity, nearly all of whom were receiving concomitant inhaled and/or oral corticosteroids, a 4-week, randomized, parallel-group trial (n=80) demonstrated that SINGULAIR, compared with placebo, resulted in significant improvement in parameters of asthma control. The magnitude of effect of SINGULAIR in aspirin-sensitive patients was similar to the effect observed in the general population of asthma patients studied. The effect of SINGULAIR on the bronchoconstrictor response to aspirin or other non-steroidal anti-inflammatory drugs in aspirin-sensitive asthmatic patients has not been evaluated *[see Warnings and Precautions (5.3)]*.

14.2 Exercise-Induced Bronchoconstriction (EIB)

Exercise-Induced Bronchoconstriction - Single-Dose Administration (Adults and Adolescents 15 years of age and older)

The efficacy of SINGULAIR, 10 mg, when given as a single dose 2 hours before exercise for the prevention of EIB was investigated in three (U.S. and Multinational), randomized, double-blind, placebo-controlled crossover studies that included a total of 160 adult and adolescent patients 15 years of age and older with EIB. Exercise challenge testing was conducted at 2 hours, 8.5 or 12 hours, and 24 hours following administration of a single dose of study drug (SINGULAIR 10 mg or placebo). The primary endpoint was the mean maximum percent fall in FEV_1 following the 2 hours post-dose exercise challenge in all three studies (Study A, Study B, and Study C). In Study A, a single dose of SINGULAIR 10 mg demonstrated a statistically significant protective benefit against EIB when taken 2 hours prior to exercise. Some patients were protected from EIB at 8.5 and 24 hours after administration; however, some patients were not. The results for the mean maximum percent fall at each timepoint in Study A are shown in TABLE 3 and are representative of the results from the other two studies.

[See table 3 above]

TABLE 3: Mean Maximum Percent Fall in FEV_1 Following Exercise Challenge in Study A (N=47) ANOVA Model

Time of exercise challenge following medication administration	Mean Maximum percent fall in FEV_1*		Treatment difference % for SINGULAIR versus Placebo (95%CI)*
	SINGULAIR	Placebo	
2 hours	13	22	-9 (-12, -5)
8.5 hours	12	17	-5 (-9, -2)
24 hours	10	14	-4 (-7, -1)

* Least squares-mean

Daily administration of SINGULAIR for the chronic treatment of asthma has not been established to prevent acute episodes of EIB. The efficacy of SINGULAIR for prevention of EIB in patients below 15 years of age has not been established.

In a 12-week, randomized, double-blind, parallel group study of 110 adult and adolescent asthmatics 15 years of age and older, with a mean baseline FEV_1 percent of predicted of 83% and with documented exercise-induced exacerbation of asthma, treatment with SINGULAIR, 10 mg, once daily in the evening, resulted in a statistically significant reduction in mean maximal percent fall in FEV_1 and mean time to recovery to within 5% of the pre-exercise FEV_1. Exercise challenge was conducted at the end of the dosing interval (i.e., 20 to 24 hours after the preceding dose). This effect was maintained throughout the 12-week treatment period indicating that tolerance did not occur. SINGULAIR did not, however, prevent clinically significant deterioration in maximal percent fall in FEV_1 after exercise (i.e., ≥20% decrease from pre-exercise baseline) in 52% of patients studied. In a separate crossover study in adults, a similar effect was observed after two once-daily 10-mg doses of SINGULAIR.

In pediatric patients 6 to 14 years of age, using the 5-mg chewable tablet, a 2-day crossover study demonstrated effects similar to those observed in adults when exercise challenge was conducted at the end of the dosing interval (i.e., 20 to 24 hours after the preceding dose).

14.3 Allergic Rhinitis (Seasonal and Perennial)

Seasonal Allergic Rhinitis

The efficacy of SINGULAIR tablets for the treatment of seasonal allergic rhinitis was investigated in 5 similarly designed, randomized, double-blind, parallel-group, placebo- and active-controlled (loratadine) trials conducted in North America. The 5 trials enrolled a total of 5029 patients, of whom 1799 were treated with SINGULAIR tablets. Patients were 15 to 82 years of age with a history of seasonal allergic rhinitis, a positive skin test to at least one relevant seasonal allergen, and active symptoms of seasonal allergic rhinitis at study entry.

The period of randomized treatment was 2 weeks in 4 trials and 4 weeks in one trial. The primary outcome variable was mean change from baseline in daytime nasal symptoms score (the average of individual scores of nasal congestion,

TABLE 4: Effects of SINGULAIR on Daytime Nasal Symptoms Score* in a Placebo- and Active-controlled Trial in Patients with Seasonal Allergic Rhinitis (ANCOVA Model)

Treatment Group (N)	Baseline Mean Score	Mean Change from Baseline	Difference Between Treatment and Placebo (95% CI) Least-Squares Mean
SINGULAIR 10 mg (344)	2.09	-0.39	-0.13† (-0.21, -0.06)
Placebo (351)	2.10	-0.26	N.A.
Active Control‡ (Loratadine 10 mg) (599)	2.06	-0.46	-0.24† (-0.31, -0.17)

* Average of individual scores of nasal congestion, rhinorrhea, nasal itching, sneezing as assessed by patients on a 0-3 categorical scale.
† Statistically different from placebo (p≤0.001).
‡ The study was not designed for statistical comparison between SINGULAIR and the active control (loratadine).

TABLE 5: Effects of SINGULAIR on Daytime Nasal Symptoms Score* in a Placebo-controlled Trial in Patients with Perennial Allergic Rhinitis (ANCOVA Model)

Treatment Group (N)	Baseline Mean Score	Mean Change from Baseline	Difference Between Treatment and Placebo (95% CI) Least-Squares Mean
SINGULAIR 10 mg (1000)	2.09	-0.42	-0.08[†] (-0.12, -0.04)
Placebo (980)	2.10	-0.35	N.A.

* Average of individual scores of nasal congestion, rhinorrhea, sneezing as assessed by patients on a 0-3 categorical scale.

† Statistically different from placebo (p≤0.001).

rhinorrhea, nasal itching, sneezing) as assessed by patients on a 0-3 categorical scale.

Four of the five trials showed a significant reduction in daytime nasal symptoms scores with SINGULAIR 10-mg tablets compared with placebo. The results of one trial are shown below. The median age in this trial was 35.0 years (range 15 to 81); 65.4% were females and 34.6% were males. The ethnic/racial distribution in this study was 83.1% Caucasian, 6.4% other origins, 5.8% Black, and 4.8% Hispanic. The mean changes from baseline in daytime nasal symptoms score in the treatment groups that received SINGULAIR tablets, loratadine, and placebo are shown in TABLE 4. The remaining three trials that demonstrated efficacy showed similar results.

[See table 4 on previous page]

Perennial Allergic Rhinitis

The efficacy of SINGULAIR tablets for the treatment of perennial allergic rhinitis was investigated in 2 randomized, double-blind, placebo-controlled studies conducted in North America and Europe. The two studies enrolled a total of 3357 patients, of whom 1632 received SINGULAIR 10-mg tablets. Patients 15 to 82 years of age with perennial allergic rhinitis as confirmed by history and a positive skin test to at least one relevant perennial allergen (dust mites, animal dander, and/or mold spores), who had active symptoms at the time of study entry, were enrolled.

In the study in which efficacy was demonstrated, the median age was 35 years (range 15 to 81); 64.1% were females and 35.9% were males. The ethnic/racial distribution in this study was 83.2% Caucasian, 8.1% Black, 5.4% Hispanic, 2.3% Asian, and 1.0% other origins. SINGULAIR 10-mg tablets once daily was shown to significantly reduce symptoms of perennial allergic rhinitis over a 6-week treatment period (TABLE 5); in this study the primary outcome variable was mean change from baseline in daytime nasal symptoms score (the average of individual scores of nasal congestion, rhinorrhea, and sneezing).

[See table 5 above]

The other 6-week study evaluated SINGULAIR 10 mg (n=626), placebo (n=609), and an active-control (cetirizine 10 mg; n=120). The primary analysis compared the mean change from baseline in daytime nasal symptoms score for SINGULAIR vs. placebo over the first 4 weeks of treatment; the study was not designed for statistical comparison between SINGULAIR and the active-control. The primary outcome variable included nasal itching in addition to nasal congestion, rhinorrhea, and sneezing. The estimated difference between SINGULAIR and placebo was -0.04 with a 95% CI of (-0.09, 0.01). The estimated difference between the active-control and placebo was -0.10 with a 95% CI of (-0.19, -0.01).

16   HOW SUPPLIED/STORAGE AND HANDLING

No. 3841—SINGULAIR Oral Granules, 4 mg, are white granules with 500 mg net weight, packed in a child-resistant foil packet. They are supplied as follows:

NDC 0006-3841-30 unit of use carton with 30 packets.
No. 3796—SINGULAIR Tablets, 4 mg, are pink, oval, biconvex-shaped chewable tablets, with code MRK 711 on one side and SINGULAIR on the other. They are supplied as follows:

NDC 0006-0711-31 unit of use high-density polyethylene (HDPE) bottles of 30 with a polypropylene child-resistant cap, an aluminum foil induction seal, and silica gel desiccant

NDC 0006-0711-54 unit of use high-density polyethylene (HDPE) bottles of 90 with a polypropylene child-resistant cap, an aluminum foil induction seal, and silica gel desiccant

NDC 0006-0711-28 unit dose paper and aluminum foil-backed aluminum foil peelable blister packs of 100.
No. 3760—SINGULAIR Tablets, 5 mg, are pink, round, biconvex-shaped chewable tablets, with code MRK 275 on one side and SINGULAIR on the other. They are supplied as follows:

NDC 0006-0275-31 unit of use high-density polyethylene (HDPE) bottles of 30 with a polypropylene child-resistant cap, an aluminum foil induction seal, and silica gel desiccant

NDC 0006-0275-54 unit of use high-density polyethylene (HDPE) bottles of 90 with a polypropylene child-resistant cap, an aluminum foil induction seal, and silica gel desiccant

NDC 0006-0275-28 unit dose paper and aluminum foil-backed aluminum foil peelable blister packs of 100

NDC 0006-0275-82 bulk packaging high-density polyethylene (HDPE) bottles of 1000 with a non-child-resistant white plastic closure with a wax paper/pulp liner, an aluminum foil induction seal, and silica gel desiccant.
No. 3761—SINGULAIR Tablets, 10 mg, are beige, rounded square-shaped, film-coated tablets, with code MRK 117 on one side and SINGULAIR on the other. They are supplied as follows:

NDC 0006-0117-31 unit of use high-density polyethylene (HDPE) bottles of 30 with a polypropylene child-resistant cap, an aluminum foil induction seal, and silica gel desiccant

NDC 0006-0117-54 unit of use high-density polyethylene (HDPE) bottles of 90 with a polypropylene child-resistant cap, an aluminum foil induction seal, and silica gel desiccant

NDC 0006-0117-28 unit dose paper and aluminum foil-backed aluminum foil peelable blister pack of 100

NDC 0006-0117-80 bulk packaging high-density polyethylene (HDPE) bottles of 8000 with a non-child-resistant white plastic closure with a wax paper/pulp liner, an aluminum foil induction seal, and silica gel desiccant.

Storage

Store SINGULAIR 4-mg oral granules, 4-mg chewable tablets, 5-mg chewable tablets and 10-mg film-coated tablets at 25°C (77°F), excursions permitted to 15-30°C (59-86°F) [see USP Controlled Room Temperature]. Protect from moisture and light. Store in original package.

Storage for Bulk Bottles

Store bottles of 1000 SINGULAIR 5-mg chewable tablets and 8000 SINGULAIR 10-mg film-coated tablets at 25°C (77°F), excursions permitted to 15-30°C (59-86°F) [see USP Controlled Room Temperature]. Protect from moisture and light. Store in original container. When product container is subdivided, repackage into a well-closed, light-resistant container.

US Patent No.: 5,565,473

Dist. by: Merck Sharp & Dohme Corp., a subsidiary of **MERCK & CO., INC.,** Whitehouse Station, NJ 08889, USA
Issued July 2010
9989619

17   PATIENT COUNSELING INFORMATION

[See FDA-Approved Patient Labeling (17.2).]

17.1   Information for Patients

- Patients should be advised to take SINGULAIR daily as prescribed, even when they are asymptomatic, as well as during periods of worsening asthma, and to contact their physicians if their asthma is not well controlled.

- Patients should be advised that oral SINGULAIR is not for the treatment of acute asthma attacks. They should have appropriate short-acting inhaled β-agonist medication available to treat asthma exacerbations. Patients who have exacerbations of asthma after exercise should be instructed to have available for rescue a short-acting inhaled β-agonist. Daily administration of SINGULAIR for the chronic treatment of asthma has not been established to prevent acute episodes of EIB.

- Patients should be advised that, while using SINGULAIR, medical attention should be sought if short-acting inhaled bronchodilators are needed more often than usual, or if more than the maximum number of inhalations of short-acting bronchodilator treatment prescribed for a 24-hour period are needed.

- Patients receiving SINGULAIR should be instructed not to decrease the dose or stop taking any other anti-asthma medications unless instructed by a physician.

- Patients should be instructed to notify their physician if neuropsychiatric events occur while using SINGULAIR.

- Patients with known aspirin sensitivity should be advised to continue avoidance of aspirin or non-steroidal anti-inflammatory agents while taking SINGULAIR.

17.2   FDA-Approved Patient Labeling

See the full patient prescribing information for SINGULAIR.

Patient Information
SINGULAIR® (SING-u-lair)
(montelukast sodium)
Tablets
SINGULAIR®
(montelukast sodium)
Chewable Tablets
SINGULAIR®
(montelukast sodium)
Oral Granules

Read the Patient Information Leaflet that comes with SINGULAIR before you start taking it and each time you get a refill. There may be new information. This leaflet does not take the place of talking with your healthcare provider about your medical condition or your treatment.

What is SINGULAIR?

- SINGULAIR is a prescription medicine that blocks substances in the body called leukotrienes. This may help to improve symptoms of asthma and allergic rhinitis. SINGULAIR does not contain a steroid.

SINGULAIR is used to:

1. Prevent asthma attacks and for the long-term treatment of asthma in adults and children ages 12 months and older.
   Do not take SINGULAIR if you need relief right away for a sudden asthma attack. If you get an asthma attack, you should follow the instructions your healthcare provider gave you for treating asthma attacks.
2. Prevent exercise-induced asthma in people 15 years of age and older.
3. Help control the symptoms of allergic rhinitis (sneezing, stuffy nose, runny nose, itching of the nose). SINGULAIR is used to treat:
   - outdoor allergies that happen part of the year (seasonal allergic rhinitis) in adults and children ages 2 years and older, **and**
   - indoor allergies that happen all year (perennial allergic rhinitis) in adults and children ages 6 months and older.

Who should not take SINGULAIR?

Do not take SINGULAIR if you are allergic to any of its ingredients.

See the end of this leaflet for a complete list of the ingredients in SINGULAIR.

What should I tell my healthcare provider before taking SINGULAIR?

Before taking SINGULAIR, tell your healthcare provider if you:

- are allergic to aspirin
- have phenylketonuria. SINGULAIR chewable tablets contain aspartame, a source of phenylalanine
- have any other medical conditions
- are pregnant or plan to become pregnant. If you are pregnant or plan to become pregnant, SINGULAIR may not be right for you. If you become pregnant while taking SINGULAIR, talk to your healthcare provider about reporting your pregnancy to the Pregnancy Registry for SINGULAIR, or you can enroll in this registry by calling 1-800-986-8999.
- are breast-feeding or plan to breast-feed. It is not known if SINGULAIR passes into your breast milk. Talk to your healthcare provider about the best way to feed your baby while taking SINGULAIR.

Tell your healthcare provider about all the medicines you take, including prescription and non-prescription medicines, vitamins, and herbal supplements. Some medicines may affect how SINGULAIR works, or SINGULAIR may affect how your other medicines work.

How should I take SINGULAIR?

For anyone who takes SINGULAIR:

- Take SINGULAIR exactly as prescribed by your healthcare provider. Your healthcare provider will tell you how much SINGULAIR to take, and **when to take it.**
- Do not stop taking SINGULAIR or change when you take it without talking with your healthcare provider.
- You can take SINGULAIR with food or without food. See the information below in the section "How should I give SINGULAIR oral granules to my child?" for information about what foods and liquids can be taken with SINGULAIR oral granules.
- **If you or your child misses a dose of SINGULAIR, just take the next dose at your regular time. Do not take 2 doses at the same time.**
- If you take too much SINGULAIR, call your doctor.

For adults and children 12 months of age and older with asthma:

- Take SINGULAIR 1 time each day, in the evening. Continue to take SINGULAIR every day for as long as your healthcare provider prescribes it, even if you have no asthma symptoms.

- Tell your healthcare provider right away if your asthma symptoms get worse, or if you need to use your rescue inhaler medicine more often for asthma attacks.
- **Do not take SINGULAIR if you need relief right away from a sudden asthma attack.** If you get an asthma attack, you should follow the instructions your healthcare provider gave you for treating asthma attacks.
- Always have your rescue inhaler medicine with you for asthma attacks.
- Do not stop taking or lower the dose of your other asthma medicines unless your healthcare provider tells you to.

For patients 15 years of age and older for the prevention of exercise-induced asthma:
- Take SINGULAIR at least 2 hours before exercise.
- Always have your rescue inhaler medicine with you for asthma attacks.
- If you take SINGULAIR every day for chronic asthma or allergic rhinitis, **do not** take another dose to prevent exercise-induced asthma. Talk to your healthcare provider about your treatment for exercise-induced asthma.
- **Do not take 2 doses of SINGULAIR within 24 hours (1 day).**

For adults and children 2 years of age and older with seasonal allergic rhinitis, or for adults and children 6 months of age and older with perennial allergic rhinitis:
- Take SINGULAIR 1 time each day, at about the same time each day.

How should I give SINGULAIR oral granules to my child?
Give SINGULAIR oral granules to your child exactly as instructed by your healthcare provider.
Do not open the packet until ready to use.
SINGULAIR 4-mg oral granules can be given:
- right in the mouth; or
- dissolved in 1 teaspoonful (5 mL) of cold or room temperature baby formula or breast milk; or
- mixed with 1 spoonful of one of the following soft foods at cold or room temperature: applesauce, mashed carrots, rice, or ice cream.

Give the child all of the mixture right away, within 15 minutes.
Do not store any leftover SINGULAIR mixture (oral granules mixed with food, baby formula, or breast milk) for use at a later time. Throw away any unused portion.
Do not mix SINGULAIR oral granules with any liquid drink other than baby formula or breast milk. Your child may drink other liquids after swallowing the mixture.

What is the dose of SINGULAIR?
The dose of SINGULAIR prescribed for your or your child's condition is based on age:
- 6 to 23 months: one packet of 4-mg oral granules.
- 2 to 5 years: one 4-mg chewable tablet or one packet of 4-mg oral granules.
- 6 to 14 years: one 5-mg chewable tablet.
- 15 years and older: one 10-mg tablet.

What should I avoid while taking SINGULAIR?
If you have asthma and aspirin makes your asthma symptoms worse, continue to avoid taking aspirin or other medicines called non-steroidal anti-inflammatory drugs (NSAIDs) while taking SINGULAIR.

What are the possible side effects of SINGULAIR?
SINGULAIR may cause serious side effects.
- **Behavior and mood-related changes.** Tell your healthcare provider right away if you or your child have any of these symptoms while taking SINGULAIR:

• agitation including aggressive behavior or hostility	• irritability
	• restlessness
• bad or vivid dreams	• sleep walking
• depression	• suicidal thoughts and actions (including suicide)
• disorientation (confusion)	
• feeling anxious	• tremor
• hallucinations (seeing or hearing things that are not really there)	• trouble sleeping

- **Increase in certain white blood cells (eosinophils) and possible inflamed blood vessels throughout the body (systemic vasculitis).** Rarely, this can happen in people with asthma who take SINGULAIR. This usually, but not always, happens in people who also take a steroid medicine by mouth that is being stopped or the dose is being lowered.

Tell your healthcare provider right away if you get one or more of these symptoms:
- a feeling of pins and needles or numbness of arms or legs
- a flu-like illness
- rash
- severe inflammation (pain and swelling) of the sinuses (sinusitis)

The most common side effects with SINGULAIR include:
- upper respiratory infection
- fever

- headache
- sore throat
- cough
- stomach pain
- diarrhea
- earache or ear infection
- flu
- runny nose
- sinus infection

Other side effects with SINGULAIR include:
- increased bleeding tendency
- allergic reactions [including swelling of the face, lips, tongue, and/or throat (which may cause trouble breathing or swallowing), hives and itching]
- dizziness, drowsiness, pins and needles/numbness, seizures (convulsions or fits)
- palpitations
- nose bleed, stuffy nose
- diarrhea, heartburn, indigestion, inflammation of the pancreas, nausea, stomach or intestinal upset, vomiting
- hepatitis
- bruising, rash
- joint pain, muscle aches and muscle cramps
- tiredness, swelling

Tell your healthcare provider if you have any side effect that bothers you or that does not go away.
These are not all the possible side effects of SINGULAIR. For more information ask your healthcare provider or pharmacist.
Call your healthcare provider for medical advice about side effects. You may report side effects to FDA at 1-800-FDA-1088.

How should I store SINGULAIR?
- Store SINGULAIR at 59°F to 86°F (15°C to 30°C).
- Keep SINGULAIR in the container it comes in.
- Keep SINGULAIR in a dry place and away from light.

General Information about the safe and effective use of SINGULAIR
Medicines are sometimes prescribed for purposes other than those mentioned in Patient Information Leaflets. Do not use SINGULAIR for a condition for which it was not prescribed. Do not give SINGULAIR to other people even if they have the same symptoms you have. It may harm them. **Keep SINGULAIR and all medicines out of the reach of children.**
This leaflet summarizes information about SINGULAIR. If you would like more information, talk to your healthcare provider. You can ask your pharmacist or healthcare provider for information about SINGULAIR that is written for health professionals. For more information, go to www.singulair.com or call the Merck National Service Center at 1-800-NSC-Merck (1-800-672-6372).

What are the ingredients in SINGULAIR?
Active ingredient: montelukast sodium
Inactive ingredients:
- **4-mg oral granules:** mannitol, hydroxypropyl cellulose, and magnesium stearate.
- **4-mg and 5-mg chewable tablets:** mannitol, microcrystalline cellulose, hydroxypropyl cellulose, red ferric oxide, croscarmellose sodium, cherry flavor, aspartame, and magnesium stearate.
  People with Phenylketonuria: SINGULAIR 4-mg chewable tablets contain 0.674 mg of phenylalanine, and SINGULAIR 5-mg chewable tablets contain 0.842 mg of phenylalanine.
- **10-mg tablet:** microcrystalline cellulose, lactose monohydrate, croscarmellose sodium, hydroxypropyl cellulose, and magnesium stearate. The film coating contains: hydroxypropyl methylcellulose, hydroxypropyl cellulose, titanium dioxide, red ferric oxide, yellow ferric oxide, and carnauba wax.

SINGULAIR is a registered trademark of Merck Sharp & Dohme Corp., a subsidiary of **Merck & Co., Inc.**
Copyright © 1998-2010 Merck Sharp & Dohme Corp., a subsidiary of **Merck & Co., Inc.**
All rights reserved
Dist. by: Merck Sharp & Dohme Corp., a subsidiary of **MERCK & CO., INC.,** Whitehouse Station, NJ 08889, USA
Issued July 2010
US Patent No.: 5,565,473
9989619
Shown in Product Identification Guide, page 314

STROMECTOL® ℞
[stro-mec-tol]
(ivermectin)
Tablets

DESCRIPTION
STROMECTOL[1] (Ivermectin) is a semisynthetic, anthelmintic agent for oral administration. Ivermectin is derived from the avermectins, a class of highly active broad-spectrum, anti-parasitic agents isolated from the fermentation products of *Streptomyces avermitilis*. Ivermectin is a

mixture containing at least 90% 5-O-demethyl-22, 23-dihydroavermectin A_{1a} and less than 10% 5-O-demethyl-25-de(1-methylpropyl)-22,23-dihydro-25-(1-methylethyl)avermectin A_{1a}, generally referred to as 22, 23-dihydroavermectin B_{1a} and B_{1b}, or H_2B_{1a} and H_2B_{1b}, respectively. The respective empirical formulas are $C_{48}H_{74}O_{14}$ and $C_{47}H_{72}O_{14}$, with molecular weights of 875.10 and 861.07, respectively. The structural formulas are:

Component B_{1a}, R = C_2H_5 Component B_{1b}, R = CH_3

Ivermectin is a white to yellowish-white, nonhygroscopic, crystalline powder with a melting point of about 155°C. It is insoluble in water but is freely soluble in methanol and soluble in 95% ethanol.
STROMECTOL is available in 3-mg tablets containing the following inactive ingredients: microcrystalline cellulose, pregelatinized starch, magnesium stearate, butylated hydroxyanisole, and citric acid powder (anhydrous).

[1] Registered trademark of Merck Sharp & Dohme Corp., a subsidiary of **Merck & Co., Inc.**
Copyright © 1996, 2007 Merck Sharp & Dohme Corp., a subsidiary of **Merck & Co., Inc.**
All rights reserved

CLINICAL PHARMACOLOGY
Pharmacokinetics
Following oral administration of ivermectin, plasma concentrations are approximately proportional to the dose. In two studies, after single 12-mg doses of STROMECTOL in fasting healthy volunteers (representing a mean dose of 165 mcg/kg), the mean peak plasma concentrations of the major component (H_2B_{1a}) were 46.6 (±21.9) (range: 16.4-101.1) and 30.6 (±15.6) (range: 13.9-68.4) ng/mL, respectively, at approximately 4 hours after dosing. Ivermectin is metabolized in the liver, and ivermectin and/or its metabolites are excreted almost exclusively in the feces over an estimated 12 days, with less than 1% of the administered dose excreted in the urine. The plasma half-life of ivermectin in man is approximately 18 hours following oral administration.
The safety and pharmacokinetic properties of ivermectin were further assessed in a multiple-dose clinical pharmacokinetic study involving healthy volunteers. Subjects received oral doses of 30 to 120 mg (333 to 2000 mcg/kg) ivermectin in a fasted state or 30 mg (333 to 600 mcg/kg) ivermectin following a standard high-fat (48.6 g of fat) meal. Administration of 30 mg ivermectin following a high-fat meal resulted in an approximate 2.5-fold increase in bioavailability relative to administration of 30 mg ivermectin in the fasted state.
In vitro studies using human liver microsomes and recombinant CYP450 enzymes have shown that ivermectin is primarily metabolized by CYP3A4. Depending on the *in vitro* method used, CYP2D6 and CYP2E1 were also shown to be involved in the metabolism of ivermectin but to a significantly lower extent compared to CYP3A4. The findings of *in vitro* studies using human liver microsomes suggest that clinically relevant concentrations of ivermectin do not significantly inhibit the metabolizing activities of CYP3A4, CYP2D6, CYP2C9, CYP1A2, and CYP2E1.
Microbiology
Ivermectin is a member of the avermectin class of broad-spectrum antiparasitic agents which have a unique mode of action. Compounds of the class bind selectively and with high affinity to glutamate-gated chloride ion channels which occur in invertebrate nerve and muscle cells. This leads to an increase in the permeability of the cell membrane to chloride ions with hyperpolarization of the nerve or muscle cell, resulting in paralysis and death of the parasite. Compounds of this class may also interact with other ligand-gated chloride channels, such as those gated by the neurotransmitter gamma-aminobutyric acid (GABA).
The selective activity of compounds of this class is attributable to the facts that some mammals do not have glutamate-gated chloride channels and that the avermec-

tins have a low affinity for mammalian ligand-gated chloride channels. In addition, ivermectin does not readily cross the blood-brain barrier in humans.

Ivermectin is active against various life-cycle stages of many but not all nematodes. It is active against the tissue microfilariae of *Onchocerca volvulus* but not against the adult form. Its activity against *Strongyloides stercoralis* is limited to the intestinal stages.

Clinical Studies
Strongyloidiasis

Two controlled clinical studies using albendazole as the comparative agent were carried out in international sites where albendazole is approved for the treatment of strongyloidiasis of the gastrointestinal tract, and three controlled studies were carried out in the U.S. and internationally using thiabendazole as the comparative agent. Efficacy, as measured by cure rate, was defined as the absence of larvae in at least two follow-up stool examinations 3 to 4 weeks post-therapy. Based on this criterion, efficacy was significantly greater for STROMECTOL (a single dose of 170 to 200 mcg/kg) than for albendazole (200 mg b.i.d. for 3 days). STROMECTOL administered as a single dose of 200 mcg/kg for 1 day was as efficacious as thiabendazole administered at 25 mg/kg b.i.d. for 3 days.

Summary of Cure Rates for Ivermectin Versus Comparative Agents in the Treatment of Strongyloidiasis

	Cure Rate* (%)	
	Ivermectin[†]	Comparative Agent
Albendazole[‡] Comparative		
International Study	24/26 (92)	12/22 (55)
WHO Study	126/152 (83)	67/149 (45)
Thiabendazole[§] Comparative		
International Study	9/14 (64)	13/15 (87)
US Studies	14/14 (100)	16/17 (94)

* Number and % of evaluable patients
† 170-200 mcg/kg
‡ 200 mg b.i.d. for 3 days
§ 25 mg/kg b.i.d. for 3 days

In one study conducted in France, a non-endemic area where there was no possibility of reinfection, several patients were observed to have recrudescence of *Strongyloides* larvae in their stool as long as 106 days following ivermectin therapy. Therefore, at least three stool examinations should be conducted over the three months following treatment to ensure eradication. If recrudescence of larvae is observed, retreatment with ivermectin is indicated. Concentration techniques (such as using a Baermann apparatus) should be employed when performing these stool examinations, as the number of *Strongyloides* larvae per gram of feces may be very low.

Onchocerciasis

The evaluation of STROMECTOL in the treatment of onchocerciasis is based on the results of clinical studies involving 1278 patients. In a double-blind, placebo-controlled study involving adult patients with moderate to severe onchocercal infection, patients who received a single dose of 150 mcg/kg STROMECTOL experienced an 83.2% and 99.5% decrease in skin microfilariae count (geometric mean) 3 days and 3 months after the dose, respectively. A marked reduction of >90% was maintained for up to 12 months after the single dose. As with other microfilaricidal drugs, there was an increase in the microfilariae count in the anterior chamber of the eye at day 3 after treatment in some patients. However, at 3 and 6 months after the dose, a significantly greater percentage of patients treated with STROMECTOL had decreases in microfilariae count in the anterior chamber than patients treated with placebo.

In a separate open study involving pediatric patients ages 6 to 13 (n=103; weight range: 17-41 kg), similar decreases in skin microfilariae counts were observed for up to 12 months after dosing.

INDICATIONS AND USAGE

STROMECTOL is indicated for the treatment of the following infections:

Strongyloidiasis of the intestinal tract. STROMECTOL is indicated for the treatment of intestinal (i.e., nondisseminated) strongyloidiasis due to the nematode parasite *Strongyloides stercoralis*.

This indication is based on clinical studies of both comparative and open-label designs, in which 64-100% of infected patients were cured following a single 200-mcg/kg dose of ivermectin. (See CLINICAL PHARMACOLOGY, Clinical Studies.)

Onchocerciasis. STROMECTOL is indicated for the treatment of onchocerciasis due to the nematode parasite *Onchocerca volvulus*.

This indication is based on randomized, double-blind, placebo-controlled and comparative studies conducted in 1427 patients in onchocerciasis-endemic areas of West Africa. The comparative studies used diethylcarbamazine citrate (DEC-C).

NOTE: STROMECTOL has no activity against adult *Onchocerca volvulus* parasites. The adult parasites reside in subcutaneous nodules which are infrequently palpable. Surgical excision of these nodules (nodulectomy) may be considered in the management of patients with onchocerciasis, since this procedure will eliminate the microfilariae-producing adult parasites.

CONTRAINDICATIONS

STROMECTOL is contraindicated in patients who are hypersensitive to any component of this product.

WARNINGS

Historical data have shown that microfilaricidal drugs, such as diethylcarbamazine citrate (DEC-C), might cause cutaneous and/or systemic reactions of varying severity (the Mazzotti reaction) and ophthalmological reactions in patients with onchocerciasis. These reactions are probably due to allergic and inflammatory responses to the death of microfilariae. Patients treated with STROMECTOL for onchocerciasis may experience these reactions in addition to clinical adverse reactions possibly, probably, or definitely related to the drug itself. (See ADVERSE REACTIONS, Onchocerciasis.)

The treatment of severe Mazzotti reactions has not been subjected to controlled clinical trials. Oral hydration, recumbency, intravenous normal saline, and/or parenteral corticosteroids have been used to treat postural hypotension. Antihistamines and/or aspirin have been used for most mild to moderate cases.

PRECAUTIONS
General

After treatment with microfilaricidal drugs, patients with hyperreactive onchodermatitis (sowda) may be more likely than others to experience severe adverse reactions, especially edema and aggravation of onchodermatitis.

Rarely, patients with onchocerciasis who are also heavily infected with *Loa loa* may develop a serious or even fatal encephalopathy either spontaneously or following treatment with an effective microfilaricide. In these patients, the following adverse experiences have also been reported: pain (including neck and back pain), red eye, conjunctival hemorrhage, dyspnea, urinary and/or fecal incontinence, difficulty in standing/walking, mental status changes, confusion, lethargy, stupor, seizures, or coma. This syndrome has been seen very rarely following the use of ivermectin. In individuals who warrant treatment with ivermectin for any reason and have had significant exposure to *Loa loa*-endemic areas of West or Central Africa, pretreatment assessment for loiasis and careful post-treatment follow-up should be implemented.

Information for Patients

STROMECTOL should be taken on an empty stomach with water. (See CLINICAL PHARMACOLOGY, Pharmacokinetics.)

Strongyloidiasis: The patient should be reminded of the need for repeated stool examinations to document clearance of infection with *Strongyloides stercoralis*.

Onchocerciasis: The patient should be reminded that treatment with STROMECTOL does not kill the adult *Onchocerca* parasites, and therefore repeated follow-up and retreatment is usually required.

Drug Interactions

Post-marketing reports of increased INR (International Normalized Ratio) have been rarely reported when ivermectin was co-administered with warfarin.

Carcinogenesis, Mutagenesis, Impairment of Fertility

Long-term studies in animals have not been performed to evaluate the carcinogenic potential of ivermectin.

Ivermectin was not genotoxic *in vitro* in the Ames microbial mutagenicity assay of *Salmonella typhimurium* strains TA1535, TA1537, TA98, and TA100 with and without rat liver enzyme activation, the Mouse Lymphoma Cell Line L5178Y (cytotoxicity and mutagenicity) assays, or the unscheduled DNA synthesis assay in human fibroblasts.

Ivermectin had no adverse effects on the fertility in rats in studies at repeated doses of up to 3 times the maximum recommended human dose of 200 mcg/kg (on a mg/m^2/day basis).

Pregnancy, *Teratogenic Effects*
Pregnancy Category C

Ivermectin has been shown to be teratogenic in mice, rats, and rabbits when given in repeated doses of 0.2, 8.1, and 4.5 times the maximum recommended human dose, respectively (on a mg/m^2/day basis). Teratogenicity was characterized in the three species tested by cleft palate; clubbed forepaws were additionally observed in rabbits. These developmental effects were found only at or near doses that were maternotoxic to the pregnant female. Therefore, ivermectin does not appear to be selectively fetotoxic to the developing fetus. There are, however, no adequate and well-controlled studies in pregnant women. Ivermectin should not be used during pregnancy since safety in pregnancy has not been established.

Nursing Mothers

STROMECTOL is excreted in human milk in low concentrations. Treatment of mothers who intend to breast-feed should only be undertaken when the risk of delayed treatment to the mother outweighs the possible risk to the newborn.

Pediatric Use

Safety and effectiveness in pediatric patients weighing less than 15 kg have not been established.

Geriatric Use

Clinical studies of STROMECTOL did not include sufficient numbers of subjects aged 65 and over to determine whether they respond differently from younger subjects. Other reported clinical experience has not identified differences in responses between the elderly and younger patients. In general, treatment of an elderly patient should be cautious, reflecting the greater frequency of decreased hepatic, renal, or cardiac function, and of concomitant disease or other drug therapy.

Strongyloidiasis in Immunocompromised Hosts

In immunocompromised (including HIV-infected) patients being treated for intestinal strongyloidiasis, repeated courses of therapy may be required. Adequate and well-controlled clinical studies have not been conducted in such patients to determine the optimal dosing regimen. Several treatments, i.e., at 2-week intervals, may be required, and cure may not be achievable. Control of extra-intestinal strongyloidiasis in these patients is difficult, and suppressive therapy, i.e., once per month, may be helpful.

ADVERSE REACTIONS
Strongyloidiasis

In four clinical studies involving a total of 109 patients given either one or two doses of 170 to 200 mcg/kg of STROMECTOL, the following adverse reactions were reported as possibly, probably, or definitely related to STROMECTOL:

Body as a Whole: asthenia/fatigue (0.9%), abdominal pain (0.9%)

Gastrointestinal: anorexia (0.9%), constipation (0.9%), diarrhea (1.8%), nausea (1.8%), vomiting (0.9%)

Nervous System/Psychiatric: dizziness (2.8%), somnolence (0.9%), vertigo (0.9%), tremor (0.9%)

Skin: pruritus (2.8%), rash (0.9%), and urticaria (0.9%).

In comparative trials, patients treated with STROMECTOL experienced more abdominal distention and chest discomfort than patients treated with albendazole. However, STROMECTOL was better tolerated than thiabendazole in comparative studies involving 37 patients treated with thiabendazole.

The Mazzotti-type and ophthalmologic reactions associated with the treatment of onchocerciasis or the disease itself would not be expected to occur in strongyloidiasis patients treated with STROMECTOL. (See ADVERSE REACTIONS, Ochocerciasis.)

Laboratory Test Findings

In clinical trials involving 109 patients given either one or two doses of 170 to 200 mcg/kg STROMECTOL, the following laboratory abnormalities were seen regardless of drug relationship: elevation in ALT and/or AST (2%), decrease in leukocyte count (3%). Leukopenia and anemia were seen in one patient.

Onchocerciasis

In clinical trials involving 963 adult patients treated with 100 to 200 mcg/kg STROMECTOL, worsening of the following Mazzotti reactions during the first 4 days post-treatment were reported: arthralgia/synovitis (9.3%), axillary lymph node enlargement and tenderness (11.0% and 4.4%, respectively), cervical lymph node enlargement and tenderness (5.3% and 1.2%, respectively), inguinal lymph node enlargement and tenderness (12.6% and 13.9%, respectively), other lymph node enlargement and tenderness (3.0% and 1.9%, respectively), pruritus (27.5%), skin involvement including edema, papular and pustular or frank urticarial rash (22.7%), and fever (22.6%). (See WARNINGS.)

In clinical trials, ophthalmological conditions were examined in 963 adult patients before treatment, at day 3, and months 3 and 6 after treatment with 100 to 200 mcg/kg STROMECTOL. Changes observed were primarily deterioration from baseline 3 days post-treatment. Most changes either returned to baseline condition or improved over baseline severity at the month 3 and 6 visits. The percentages of patients with worsening of the following conditions at day 3, month 3 and 6, respectively, were: limbitis: 5.5%, 4.8%, and 3.5% and punctate opacity: 1.8%, 1.8%, and 1.4%. The corresponding percentages for patients treated with placebo were: limbitis: 6.2%, 9.9%, and 9.4% and punctate opacity: 2.0%, 6.4%, and 7.2%. (See WARNINGS.)

In clinical trials involving 963 adult patients who received 100 to 200 mcg/kg STROMECTOL, the following clinical adverse reactions were reported as possibly, probably, or definitely related to the drug in ≥1% of the patients: facial edema (1.2%), peripheral edema (3.2%), orthostatic hypotension (1.1%), and tachycardia (3.5%). Drug-related headache and myalgia occurred in <1% of patients (0.2% and

0.4%, respectively). However, these were the most common adverse experiences reported overall during these trials regardless of causality (22.3% and 19.7%, respectively).

A similar safety profile was observed in an open study in pediatric patients ages 6 to 13.

The following ophthalmological side effects do occur due to the disease itself but have also been reported after treatment with STROMECTOL: abnormal sensation in the eyes, eyelid edema, anterior uveitis, conjunctivitis, limbitis, keratitis, and chorioretinitis or choroiditis. These have rarely been severe or associated with loss of vision and have generally resolved without corticosteroid treatment.

Laboratory Test Findings

In controlled clinical trials, the following laboratory adverse experiences were reported as possibly, probably, or definitely related to the drug in ≥1% of the patients: eosinophilia (3%) and hemoglobin increase (1%).

Post-Marketing Experience

The following adverse reactions have been reported since the drug was registered overseas:

Onchocerciasis

Conjunctival hemorrhage

All Indications

Hypotension (mainly orthostatic hypotension), worsening of bronchial asthma, toxic epidermal necrolysis, Stevens-Johnson syndrome, seizures, hepatitis, elevation of liver enzymes, and elevation of bilirubin.

OVERDOSAGE

Significant lethality was observed in mice and rats after single oral doses of 25 to 50 mg/kg and 40 to 50 mg/kg, respectively. No significant lethality was observed in dogs after single oral doses of up to 10 mg/kg. At these doses, the treatment-related signs that were observed in these animals include ataxia, bradypnea, tremors, ptosis, decreased activity, emesis, and mydriasis.

In accidental intoxication with, or significant exposure to, unknown quantities of veterinary formulations of ivermectin in humans, either by ingestion, inhalation, injection, or exposure to body surfaces, the following adverse effects have been reported most frequently: rash, edema, headache, dizziness, asthenia, nausea, vomiting, and diarrhea. Other adverse effects that have been reported include: seizure, ataxia, dyspnea, abdominal pain, paresthesia, urticaria, and contact dermatitis.

In case of accidental poisoning, supportive therapy, if indicated, should include parenteral fluids and electrolytes, respiratory support (oxygen and mechanical ventilation if necessary) and pressor agents if clinically significant hypotension is present. Induction of emesis and/or gastric lavage as soon as possible, followed by purgatives and other routine anti-poison measures, may be indicated if needed to prevent absorption of ingested material.

DOSAGE AND ADMINISTRATION

Strongyloidiasis

The recommended dosage of STROMECTOL for the treatment of strongyloidiasis is a single oral dose designed to provide approximately 200 mcg of ivermectin per kg of body weight. See Table 1 for dosage guidelines. Patients should take tablets on an empty stomach with water. (See CLINICAL PHARMACOLOGY, Pharmacokinetics.) In general, additional doses are not necessary. However, follow-up stool examinations should be performed to verify eradication of infection. (See CLINICAL PHARMACOLOGY, Clinical Studies.)

Table 1: Dosage Guidelines for STROMECTOL for Strongyloidiasis

Body Weight (kg)	Single Oral Dose Number of 3-mg Tablets
15-24	1 tablet
25-35	2 tablets
36-50	3 tablets
51-65	4 tablets
66-79	5 tablets
≥80	200 mcg/kg

Onchocerciasis

The recommended dosage of STROMECTOL for the treatment of onchocerciasis is a single oral dose designed to provide approximately 150 mcg of ivermectin per kg of body weight. See Table 2 for dosage guidelines. Patients should take tablets on an empty stomach with water. (See CLINICAL PHARMACOLOGY, Pharmacokinetics.) In mass distribution campaigns in international treatment programs, the most commonly used dose interval is 12 months. For the treatment of individual patients, retreatment may be considered at intervals as short as 3 months.

Table 2: Dosage Guidelines for STROMECTOL for Onchocerciasis

Body Weight (kg)	Single Oral Dose Number of 3-mg Tablets
15-25	1 tablet
26-44	2 tablets
45-64	3 tablets
65-84	4 tablets
≥85	150 mcg/kg

HOW SUPPLIED

No. 8495—Tablets STROMECTOL 3 mg are white, round, flat, bevel-edged tablets coded MSD on one side and 32 on the other side. They are supplied as follows:

NDC 0006-0032-20 unit dose packages of 20.

Storage

Store at temperatures below 30°C (86°F).

Dist. by: Merck Sharp & Dohme Corp., a subsidiary of **MERCK & CO., INC.**, Whitehouse Station, NJ 08889, USA

Manufactured by:

Merck Sharp & Dohme BV

Waarderweg 39

2031 BN Haarlem

Netherlands

Issued May 2010

Printed in the Netherlands

9032319

87447/080610

8495

Shown in Product Identification Guide, page 314

TEMODAR® ℞

[tĕm-ō-dăr]

(temozolomide)

Capsules

TEMODAR®

(temozolomide)

for Injection administered via intravenous infusion

HIGHLIGHTS OF PRESCRIBING INFORMATION

These highlights do not include all the information needed to use TEMODAR safely and effectively. See full prescribing information for TEMODAR.

TEMODAR (temozolomide) Capsules

TEMODAR (temozolomide) for Injection administered via intravenous infusion

Initial U.S. Approval: 1999

————INDICATIONS AND USAGE————

TEMODAR is an alkylating drug indicated for the treatment of adult patients with:

- Newly diagnosed glioblastoma multiforme (GBM) concomitantly with radiotherapy and then as maintenance treatment. (1.1)
- Refractory anaplastic astrocytoma patients who have experienced disease progression on a drug regimen containing nitrosourea and procarbazine. (1.2)

————DOSAGE AND ADMINISTRATION————

- Newly Diagnosed GBM: 75 mg/m² for 42 days concomitant with focal radiotherapy followed by initial maintenance dose of 150 mg/m² once daily for Days 1–5 of a 28-day cycle of TEMODAR for 6 cycles. (2.1)
- Refractory Anaplastic Astrocytoma: Initial dose 150 mg/m² once daily for 5 consecutive days per 28-day treatment cycle. (2.1)
- The recommended dose for TEMODAR as an intravenous infusion over 90 minutes is the same as the dose for the oral capsule formulation. Bioequivalence has been established only when TEMODAR for Injection was given over 90 minutes. (2.1, 12.3)

————DOSAGE FORMS AND STRENGTHS————

- 5-mg, 20-mg, 100-mg, 140-mg, 180-mg, and 250-mg capsules. (3)
- 100-mg powder for injection. (3)

————CONTRAINDICATIONS————

- Known hypersensitivity to any TEMODAR component or to dacarbazine (DTIC). (4.1)

————WARNINGS AND PRECAUTIONS————

- Myelosuppression - monitor Absolute Neutrophil Count (ANC) and platelet count prior to dosing and throughout treatment. Geriatric patients and women have a higher risk of developing myelosuppression. (5.1)
- Cases of myelodysplastic syndrome and secondary malignancies, including myeloid leukemia, have been observed. (5.2)
- *Pneumocystis carinii* pneumonia (PCP) – prophylaxis required for all patients receiving concomitant TEMODAR and radiotherapy for the 42-day regimen for the treatment of newly diagnosed glioblastoma multiforme. (5.3)

- All patients, particularly those receiving steroids, should be observed closely for the development of lymphopenia and PCP. (5.4)
- Complete blood counts should be obtained throughout the treatment course as specified. (5.4)
- Fetal harm can occur when administered to a pregnant woman. Women should be advised to avoid becoming pregnant when receiving TEMODAR. (5.5)
- As bioequivalence has been established only when given over 90 minutes, infusion over a shorter or longer period of time may result in suboptimal dosing; the possibility of an increase in infusion related adverse reactions cannot be ruled out. (5.6)

————ADVERSE REACTIONS————

- The most common adverse reactions (≥10% incidence) are: alopecia, fatigue, nausea, vomiting, headache, constipation, anorexia, convulsions, rash, hemiparesis, diarrhea, asthenia, fever, dizziness, coordination abnormal, viral infection, amnesia, and insomnia. (6.1)
- The most common Grade 3 to 4 hematologic laboratory abnormalities (≥10% incidence) that have developed during treatment with temozolomide are: lymphopenia, thrombocytopenia, neutropenia, and leukopenia. (6.1)
- Allergic reactions have also been reported. (6)

To report **SUSPECTED ADVERSE REACTIONS**, contact Schering Corporation, a subsidiary of Merck & Co., Inc. at 1-800-526-4099 or FDA at 1-800-FDA-1088 or www.fda.gov/medwatch

————DRUG INTERACTIONS————

- Valproic acid: decreases oral clearance of temozolomide. (7.1)

————USE IN SPECIFIC POPULATIONS————

- Nursing mothers: Not recommended. (8.3)
- Pediatric use: No established use. (8.4)
- Hepatic/Renal Impairment: Caution should be exercised when TEMODAR is administered to patients with severe renal or hepatic impairment. (8.6, 8.7)

See 17 for **PATIENT COUNSELING INFORMATION** and FDA-approved patient labeling

Revised: 04/2010

FULL PRESCRIBING INFORMATION: CONTENTS*

1 INDICATIONS AND USAGE
   1.1 Newly Diagnosed Glioblastoma Multiforme
   1.2 Refractory Anaplastic Astrocytoma
2 DOSAGE AND ADMINISTRATION
   2.1 Recommended Dosing and Dose Modification Guidelines
   2.2 Preparation and Administration
3 DOSAGE FORMS AND STRENGTHS
4 CONTRAINDICATIONS
   4.1 Hypersensitivity
5 WARNINGS AND PRECAUTIONS
   5.1 Myelosuppression
   5.2 Myelodysplastic Syndrome
   5.3 *Pneumocystis carinii* Pneumonia
   5.4 Laboratory Tests
   5.5 Use in Pregnancy
   5.6 Infusion Time
6 ADVERSE REACTIONS
   6.1 Clinical Trials Experience
   6.2 Postmarketing Experience
7 DRUG INTERACTIONS
   7.1 Valproic Acid
8 USE IN SPECIFIC POPULATIONS
   8.1 Pregnancy
   8.3 Nursing Mothers
   8.4 Pediatric Use
   8.5 Geriatric Use
   8.6 Renal Impairment
   8.7 Hepatic Impairment
10 OVERDOSAGE
11 DESCRIPTION
12 CLINICAL PHARMACOLOGY
   12.1 Mechanism of Action
   12.3 Pharmacokinetics
13 NONCLINICAL TOXICOLOGY
   13.1 Carcinogenesis, Mutagenesis, Impairment of Fertility
   13.2 Animal Toxicology and/or Pharmacology
14 CLINICAL STUDIES
   14.1 Newly Diagnosed Glioblastoma Multiforme
   14.2 Refractory Anaplastic Astrocytoma
15 REFERENCES
16 HOW SUPPLIED/STORAGE AND HANDLING
   16.1 Safe Handling and Disposal
   16.2 How Supplied
   16.3 Storage
17 PATIENT COUNSELING INFORMATION
   17.1 Information for the Patient
   17.2 FDA-approved Patient Labeling

* Sections or subsections omitted from the full prescribing information are not listed

FULL PRESCRIBING INFORMATION

1 INDICATIONS AND USAGE

1.1 Newly Diagnosed Glioblastoma Multiforme

TEMODAR® (temozolomide) is indicated for the treatment of adult patients with newly diagnosed glioblastoma multiforme concomitantly with radiotherapy and then as maintenance treatment.

1.2 Refractory Anaplastic Astrocytoma

TEMODAR is indicated for the treatment of adult patients with refractory anaplastic astrocytoma, i.e., patients who have experienced disease progression on a drug regimen containing nitrosourea and procarbazine.

2 DOSAGE AND ADMINISTRATION

2.1 Recommended Dosing and Dose Modification Guidelines

The recommended dose for TEMODAR as an intravenous infusion over 90 minutes is the same as the dose for the oral capsule formulation. Bioequivalence has been established only when TEMODAR for Injection was given over 90 minutes [see Clinical Pharmacology (12.3)]. Dosage of TEMODAR must be adjusted according to nadir neutrophil and platelet counts in the previous cycle and the neutrophil and platelet counts at the time of initiating the next cycle. For TEMODAR dosage calculations based on body surface area (BSA) see **Table 5**. For suggested capsule combinations on a daily dose see **Table 6**.

Patients with Newly Diagnosed High Grade Glioma:
Concomitant Phase:
TEMODAR is administered at 75 mg/m² daily for 42 days concomitant with focal radiotherapy (60 Gy administered in 30 fractions) followed by maintenance TEMODAR for 6 cycles. Focal RT includes the tumor bed or resection site with a 2- to 3-cm margin. No dose reductions are recommended during the concomitant phase; however, dose interruptions or discontinuation may occur based on toxicity. The TEMODAR dose should be continued throughout the 42-day concomitant period up to 49 days if all of the following conditions are met: absolute neutrophil count ≥1.5 × 10⁹/L, platelet count ≥100 × 10⁹/L, common toxicity criteria (CTC) nonhematologic toxicity ≤Grade 1 (except for alopecia, nausea, and vomiting). During treatment a complete blood count should be obtained weekly. Temozolomide dosing should be interrupted or discontinued during concomitant phase according to the hematological and nonhematological toxicity criteria as noted in **Table 1**. PCP prophylaxis is required during the concomitant administration of TEMODAR and radiotherapy and should be continued in patients who develop lymphocytopenia until recovery from lymphocytopenia (CTC Grade ≤1).

TABLE 1: Temozolomide Dosing Interruption or Discontinuation During Concomitant Radiotherapy and Temozolomide

Toxicity	TMZ Interruption*	TMZ Discontinuation
Absolute Neutrophil Count	≥0.5 and <1.5 × 10⁹/L	<0.5 × 10⁹/L
Platelet Count	≥10 and <100 × 10⁹/L	<10 × 10⁹/L
CTC Nonhematological Toxicity (except for alopecia, nausea, vomiting)	CTC Grade 2	CTC Grade 3 or 4

TMZ = temozolomide; CTC = Common Toxicity Criteria.
*Treatment with concomitant TMZ could be continued when all of the following conditions were met: absolute neutrophil count ≥1.5 × 10⁹/L; platelet count ≥100 × 10⁹/L; CTC non-hematological toxicity ≤Grade 1 (except for alopecia, nausea, vomiting).

Maintenance Phase:
Cycle 1:
Four weeks after completing the TEMODAR+RT phase, TEMODAR is administered for an additional 6 cycles of maintenance treatment. Dosage in Cycle 1 (maintenance) is 150 mg/m² once daily for 5 days followed by 23 days without treatment.
Cycles 2–6:
At the start of Cycle 2, the dose can be escalated to 200 mg/m², if the CTC nonhematologic toxicity for Cycle 1 is Grade ≤2 (except for alopecia, nausea, and vomiting), absolute neutrophil count (ANC) is ≥1.5 × 10⁹/L, and the platelet count is ≥100 × 10⁹/L. The dose remains at 200 mg/m² per day for the first 5 days of each subsequent cycle except if toxicity occurs. If the dose was not escalated at Cycle 2, escalation should not be done in subsequent cycles.

Dose Reduction or Discontinuation During Maintenance:
Dose reductions during the maintenance phase should be applied according to **Tables 2** and **3**.
During treatment, a complete blood count should be obtained on Day 22 (21 days after the first dose of TEMODAR) or within 48 hours of that day, and weekly until the ANC is above 1.5 × 10⁹/L (1500/μL) and the platelet count exceeds 100 × 10⁹/L (100,000/μL). The next cycle of TEMODAR should not be started until the ANC and platelet count exceed these levels. Dose reductions during the next cycle should be based on the lowest blood counts and worst nonhematologic toxicity during the previous cycle. Dose reductions or discontinuations during the maintenance phase should be applied according to **Tables 2** and **3**.

TABLE 2: Temozolomide Dose Levels for Maintenance Treatment

Dose Level	Dose (mg/m²/day)	Remarks
–1	100	Reduction for prior toxicity
0	150	Dose during Cycle 1
1	200	Dose during Cycles 2–6 in absence of toxicity

TABLE 3: Temozolomide Dose Reduction or Discontinuation During Maintenance Treatment

Toxicity	Reduce TMZ by 1 Dose Level*	Discontinue TMZ
Absolute Neutrophil Count	<1.0 × 10⁹/L	See footnote †
Platelet Count	<50 × 10⁹/L	See footnote †
CTC Nonhematological Toxicity (except for alopecia, nausea, vomiting)	CTC Grade 3	CTC Grade 4†

TMZ = temozolomide; CTC = Common Toxicity Criteria.
*TMZ dose levels are listed in **Table 2**.
†TMZ is to be discontinued if dose reduction to <100 mg/m² is required or if the same Grade 3 non-hematological toxicity (except for alopecia, nausea, vomiting) recurs after dose reduction.

Patients with Refractory Anaplastic Astrocytoma:
For adults the initial dose is 150 mg/m² once daily for 5 consecutive days per 28-day treatment cycle. For adult patients, if both the nadir and day of dosing (Day 29, Day 1 of next cycle) ANC are ≥1.5 × 10⁹/L (1500/μL) and both the nadir and Day 29, Day 1 of next cycle platelet counts are ≥100 × 10⁹/L (100,000/μL), the TEMODAR dose may be increased to 200 mg/m²/day for 5 consecutive days per 28-day treatment cycle. During treatment, a complete blood count should be obtained on Day 22 (21 days after the first dose) or within 48 hours of that day, and weekly until the ANC is above 1.5 × 10⁹/L (1500/μL) and the platelet count exceeds 100 × 10⁹/L (100,000/μL). The next cycle of TEMODAR should not be started until the ANC and platelet count exceed these levels. If the ANC falls to <1.0 × 10⁹/L (1000/μL) or the platelet count is <50 × 10⁹/L (50,000/μL) during any cycle, the next cycle should be reduced by 50 mg/m², but not below 100 mg/m², the lowest recommended dose (see **Table 4**). TEMODAR therapy can be continued until disease progression. In the clinical trial, treatment could be continued for a maximum of 2 years, but the optimum duration of therapy is not known.
[See table at top of next column]

TABLE 5: Daily Dose Calculations by Body Surface Area (BSA)

Total BSA (m²)	75 mg/m² (mg daily)	150 mg/m² (mg daily)	200 mg/m² (mg daily)
1.0	75	150	200
1.1	82.5	165	220
1.2	90	180	240
1.3	97.5	195	260
1.4	105	210	280
1.5	112.5	225	300
1.6	120	240	320
1.7	127.5	255	340
1.8	135	270	360
1.9	142.5	285	380
2.0	150	300	400
2.1	157.5	315	420
2.2	165	330	440
2.3	172.5	345	460
2.4	180	360	480
2.5	187.5	375	500

TABLE 4: Dosing Modification Table

TABLE 6: Suggested Capsule Combinations Based on Daily Dose in Adults

Number of Daily Capsules by Strength (mg)

Total Daily Dose (mg)	250 mg	180 mg	140 mg	100 mg	20 mg	5 mg
75	0	0	0	0	3	3
82.5	0	0	0	0	4	0
90	0	0	0	0	4	2
97.5	0	0	0	1	0	0
105	0	0	0	1	0	1
112.5	0	0	0	1	0	2
120	0	0	0	1	1	0
127.5	0	0	0	1	1	1
135	0	0	0	1	1	3
142.5	0	0	1	0	0	0
150	0	0	1	0	0	2
157.5	0	0	1	0	1	0
165	0	0	1	0	1	1
172.5	0	0	1	0	1	2
180	0	1	0	0	0	0
187.5	0	1	0	0	0	1
195	0	1	0	0	1	0
200	0	1	0	0	1	0
210	0	0	0	2	0	2
220	0	0	0	2	1	0
225	0	0	0	2	1	1
240	0	0	1	1	0	0
255	1	0	0	0	0	1
260	0	0	1	0	0	0
270	1	0	0	0	1	0
280	0	0	2	0	0	0
285	0	0	2	0	0	1
300	0	0	0	3	0	0
315	0	0	0	3	0	3
320	0	1	1	0	0	0
330	0	1	1	0	1	0
340	0	1	0	0	1	0
345	0	1	0	0	1	1
360	0	2	0	0	0	0
375	0	2	0	0	0	1
380	0	1	0	0	1	0
400	0	0	0	4	0	0
420	0	0	3	0	0	0

440	0	0	3	0	1	0
460	0	2	0	1	0	0
480	0	1	0	3	0	0
500	2	0	0	0	0	0

2.2 Preparation and Administration

TEMODAR Capsules:

In clinical trials, TEMODAR was administered under both fasting and nonfasting conditions; however, absorption is affected by food [see Clinical Pharmacology (12)], and consistency of administration with respect to food is recommended. There are no dietary restrictions with TEMODAR. To reduce nausea and vomiting, TEMODAR should be taken on an empty stomach. Bedtime administration may be advised. Antiemetic therapy may be administered prior to and/or following administration of TEMODAR.

TEMODAR (temozolomide) Capsules should not be opened or chewed. They should be swallowed whole with a glass of water.

If capsules are accidentally opened or damaged, precautions should be taken to avoid inhalation or contact with the skin or mucous membranes [see How Supplied/Storage and Handling (16.1)].

TEMODAR for Injection:

Each vial of TEMODAR for Injection contains sterile and pyrogen-free temozolomide lyophilized powder. When reconstituted with 41 mL Sterile Water for Injection, the resulting solution will contain 2.5 mg/mL temozolomide. Bring the vial to room temperature prior to reconstitution with Sterile Water for Injection. The vials should be gently swirled and not shaken. Vials should be inspected, and any vial containing visible particulate matter should not be used. Do not further dilute the reconstituted solution. After reconstitution, store at room temperature (25°C [77°F]). Reconstituted product must be used within 14 hours, including infusion time.

Using aseptic technique, withdraw up to 40 mL from each vial to make up the total dose based on **Table 5** above and transfer into an empty 250 mL PVC infusion bag.[2] Compatibility studies with non-PVC bags have not been conducted. TEMODAR for Injection should be infused intravenously using a pump over a period of 90 minutes. TEMODAR for Injection should be administered only by intravenous infusion. Flush the lines before and after each TEMODAR infusion.

Because no data are available on the compatibility of TEMODAR for Injection with other intravenous substances or additives, other medications should not be infused simultaneously through the same intravenous line.

3 DOSAGE FORMS AND STRENGTHS

- TEMODAR (temozolomide) Capsules for oral administration
  - –5-mg capsules have opaque white bodies with green caps. The capsule body is imprinted with two stripes, the dosage strength, and the Schering-Plough logo. The cap is imprinted with "TEMODAR."
  - –20-mg capsules have opaque white bodies with yellow caps. The capsule body is imprinted with two stripes, the dosage strength, and the Schering-Plough logo. The cap is imprinted with "TEMODAR."
  - –100-mg capsules have opaque white bodies with pink caps. The capsule body is imprinted with two stripes, the dosage strength, and the Schering-Plough logo. The cap is imprinted with "TEMODAR."
  - –140-mg capsules have opaque white bodies with blue caps. The capsule body is imprinted with two stripes, the dosage strength, and the Schering-Plough logo. The cap is imprinted with "TEMODAR."
  - –180-mg capsules have opaque white bodies with orange caps. The capsule body is imprinted with two stripes, the dosage strength, and the Schering-Plough logo. The cap is imprinted with "TEMODAR."
  - –250-mg capsules have opaque white bodies with white caps. The capsule body is imprinted with two stripes, the dosage strength, and the Schering-Plough logo. The cap is imprinted with "TEMODAR."
- TEMODAR (temozolomide) is available as 100-mg/vial powder for injection. The lyophilized powder is white to light tan/light pink.

4 CONTRAINDICATIONS

4.1 Hypersensitivity

TEMODAR (temozolomide) is contraindicated in patients who have a history of hypersensitivity reaction (such as urticaria, allergic reaction including anaphylaxis, toxic epidermal necrolysis, and Stevens-Johnson syndrome) to any of its components. TEMODAR is also contraindicated in patients who have a history of hypersensitivity to DTIC, since both drugs are metabolized to 5-(3-methyltriazen-1-yl)-imidazole-4-carboxamide (MTIC).

TABLE 7: Number (%) of Patients with Adverse Reactions: All and Severe/Life Threatening (Incidence of 5% or Greater)

	Concomitant Phase RT Alone (n=285)		Concomitant Phase RT+TMZ (n=288)*		Maintenance Phase TMZ (n=224)	
	All	Grade ≥3	All	Grade ≥3	All	Grade ≥3
Subjects Reporting any Adverse Reaction	258 (91)	74 (26)	266 (92)	80 (28)	206 (92)	82 (37)
Body as a Whole - General Disorders						
Anorexia	25 (9)	1 (<1)	56 (19)	2 (1)	61 (27)	3 (1)
Dizziness	10 (4)	0	12 (4)	2 (1)	12 (5)	0
Fatigue	139 (49)	15 (5)	156 (54)	19 (7)	137 (61)	20 (9)
Headache	49 (17)	11 (4)	56 (19)	5 (2)	51 (23)	9 (4)
Weakness	9 (3)	3 (1)	10 (3)	5 (2)	16 (7)	4 (2)
Central and Peripheral Nervous System Disorders						
Confusion	12 (4)	6 (2)	11 (4)	4 (1)	12 (5)	4 (2)
Convulsions	20 (7)	9 (3)	17 (6)	10 (3)	25 (11)	7 (3)
Memory Impairment	12 (4)	1 (<1)	8 (3)	1 (<1)	16 (7)	2 (1)
Disorders of the Eye						
Vision Blurred	25 (9)	4 (1)	26 (9)	2 (1)	17 (8)	0
Disorders of the Immune System						
Allergic Reaction	7 (2)	1 (<1)	13 (5)	0	6 (3)	0
Gastrointestinal System Disorders						
Abdominal Pain	2 (1)	0	7 (2)	1 (<1)	11 (5)	1 (<1)
Constipation	18 (6)	0	53 (18)	3 (1)	49 (22)	0
Diarrhea	9 (3)	0	18 (6)	0	23 (10)	2 (1)
Nausea	45 (16)	1 (<1)	105 (36)	2 (1)	110 (49)	3 (1)
Stomatitis	14 (5)	1 (<1)	19 (7)	0	20 (9)	3 (1)
Vomiting	16 (6)	1 (<1)	57 (20)	1 (<1)	66 (29)	4 (2)
Injury and Poisoning						
Radiation Injury NOS	11 (4)	1 (<1)	20 (7)	0	5 (2)	0
Musculoskeletal System Disorders						
Arthralgia	2 (1)	0	7 (2)	1 (<1)	14 (6)	0
Platelet, Bleeding and Clotting Disorders						
Thrombocytopenia	3 (1)	0	11 (4)	8 (3)	19 (8)	8 (4)
Psychiatric Disorders						
Insomnia	9 (3)	1 (<1)	14 (5)	0	9 (4)	0
Respiratory System Disorders						
Coughing	3 (1)	0	15 (5)	2 (1)	19 (8)	1 (<1)
Dyspnea	9 (3)	4 (1)	11 (4)	5 (2)	12 (5)	1 (<1)
Skin and Subcutaneous Tissue Disorders						
Alopecia	179 (63)	0	199 (69)	0	124 (55)	0
Dry Skin	6 (2)	0	7 (2)	0	11 (5)	1 (<1)
Erythema	15 (5)	0	14 (5)	0	2 (1)	0
Pruritus	4 (1)	0	11 (4)	0	11 (5)	0
Rash	42 (15)	0	56 (19)	3 (1)	29 (13)	3 (1)
Special Senses Other, Disorders						
Taste Perversion	6 (2)	0	18 (6)	0	11 (5)	0

RT+TMZ=radiotherapy plus temozolomide; NOS=not otherwise specified.
Note: Grade 5 (fatal) adverse reactions are included in the Grade ≥3 column.
*One patient who was randomized to RT only arm received RT+temozolomide.

5 WARNINGS AND PRECAUTIONS

5.1 Myelosuppression

Patients treated with TEMODAR may experience myelosuppression, including prolonged pancytopenia, which may result in aplastic anemia, which in some cases has resulted in a fatal outcome. In some cases, exposure to concomitant medications associated with aplastic anemia, including carbamazepine, phenytoin, and sulfamethoxazole/trimethoprim, complicates assessment. Prior to dosing, patients must have an absolute neutrophil count (ANC) ≥1.5 × 10⁹/L and a platelet count ≥100 × 10⁹/L. A complete blood count should be obtained on Day 22 (21 days after the first dose) or within 48 hours of that day, and weekly until the ANC is above 1.5 × 10⁹/L and platelet count exceeds 100 × 10⁹/L. Geriatric patients and women have been shown in clinical trials to have a higher risk of developing myelosuppression.

5.2 Myelodysplastic Syndrome

Cases of myelodysplastic syndrome and secondary malignancies, including myeloid leukemia, have been observed.

5.3 *Pneumocystis carinii* Pneumonia

For treatment of newly diagnosed glioblastoma multiforme: Prophylaxis against *Pneumocystis carinii* pneumonia is required for all patients receiving concomitant TEMODAR and radiotherapy for the 42-day regimen.

There may be a higher occurrence of PCP when temozolomide is administered during a longer dosing regimen. However, all patients receiving temozolomide, particularly patients receiving steroids, should be observed closely for the development of PCP regardless of the regimen.

5.4 Laboratory Tests

For the concomitant treatment phase with RT, a complete blood count should be obtained prior to initiation of treatment and weekly during treatment.

For the 28-day treatment cycles, a complete blood count should be obtained prior to treatment on Day 1 and on Day 22 (21 days after the first dose) of each cycle. Blood counts should be performed weekly until recovery if the ANC falls below 1.5 × 10⁹/L and the platelet count falls below 100 × 10⁹/L [see Recommended Dosing and Dose Modification Guidelines (2.1)].

5.5 Use in Pregnancy

TEMODAR can cause fetal harm when administered to a pregnant woman. Administration of TEMODAR to rats and rabbits during organogenesis at 0.38 and 0.75 times the maximum recommended human dose (75 and 150 mg/m²), respectively, caused numerous fetal malformations of the external organs, soft tissues, and skeleton in both species [see Use in Specific Populations (8.1)].

5.6 Infusion Time

As bioequivalence has been established only when TEMODAR for Injection was given over 90 minutes, infusion over a shorter or longer period of time may result in suboptimal dosing. Additionally, the possibility of an increase in infusion-related adverse reactions cannot be ruled out.

6 ADVERSE REACTIONS

6.1 Clinical Trials Experience

Because clinical trials are conducted under widely varying conditions, adverse reaction rates observed in the clinical trials of a drug cannot be directly compared to rates in the clinical trials of another drug and may not reflect the rates observed in practice.

Newly Diagnosed Glioblastoma Multiforme:

During the concomitant phase (TEMODAR+radiotherapy), adverse reactions including thrombocytopenia, nausea, vomiting, anorexia, and constipation were more frequent in the TEMODAR+RT arm. The incidence of other adverse reactions was comparable in the two arms. The most common adverse reactions across the cumulative TEMODAR experience were alopecia, nausea, vomiting, anorexia, headache, and constipation (see **Table 7**). Forty-nine percent (49%) of patients treated with TEMODAR reported one or more severe or life-threatening reactions, most commonly fatigue

(13%), convulsions (6%), headache (5%), and thrombocytopenia (5%). Overall, the pattern of reactions during the maintenance phase was consistent with the known safety profile of TEMODAR.

[See table 7 at top of previous page]

Myelosuppression (neutropenia and thrombocytopenia), which is a known dose-limiting toxicity for most cytotoxic agents, including TEMODAR, was observed. When laboratory abnormalities and adverse reactions were combined, Grade 3 or Grade 4 neutrophil abnormalities including neutropenic reactions were observed in 8% of the patients, and Grade 3 or Grade 4 platelet abnormalities, including thrombocytopenic reactions, were observed in 14% of the patients treated with TEMODAR.

Refractory Anaplastic Astrocytoma:

Tables 8 and 9 show the incidence of adverse reactions in the 158 patients in the anaplastic astrocytoma study for whom data are available. In the absence of a control group, it is not clear in many cases whether these reactions should be attributed to temozolomide or the patients' underlying conditions, but nausea, vomiting, fatigue, and hematologic effects appear to be clearly drug-related. The most frequently occurring adverse reactions were nausea, vomiting, headache, and fatigue. The adverse reactions were usually NCI Common Toxicity Criteria (CTC) Grade 1 or 2 (mild to moderate in severity) and were self-limiting, with nausea and vomiting readily controlled with antiemetics. The incidence of severe nausea and vomiting (CTC Grade 3 or 4) was 10% and 6%, respectively. Myelosuppression (thrombocytopenia and neutropenia) was the dose-limiting adverse reaction. It usually occurred within the first few cycles of therapy and was not cumulative.

Myelosuppression occurred late in the treatment cycle and returned to normal, on average, within 14 days of nadir counts. The median nadirs occurred at 26 days for platelets (range: 21–40 days) and 28 days for neutrophils (range: 1–44 days). Only 14% (22/158) of patients had a neutrophil nadir and 20% (32/158) of patients had a platelet nadir, which may have delayed the start of the next cycle. Less than 10% of patients required hospitalization, blood transfusion, or discontinuation of therapy due to myelosuppression.

In clinical trial experience with 110 to 111 women and 169 to 174 men (depending on measurements), there were higher rates of Grade 4 neutropenia (ANC<500 cells/µL) and thrombocytopenia (<20,000 cells/µL) in women than in men in the first cycle of therapy (12% vs. 5% and 9% vs. 3%, respectively).

In the entire safety database for which hematologic data exist (N=932), 7% (4/61) and 9.5% (6/63) of patients over age 70 experienced Grade 4 neutropenia or thrombocytopenia in the first cycle, respectively. For patients less than or equal to age 70, 7% (62/871) and 5.5% (48/879) experienced Grade 4 neutropenia or thrombocytopenia in the first cycle, respectively. Pancytopenia, leukopenia, and anemia have also been reported.

TABLE 8: Adverse Reactions in the Anaplastic Astrocytoma Trial in Adults (≥5%)

	No. (%) of TEMODAR Patients (N=158)	
	All Reactions	Grade 3/4
Any Adverse Reaction	153 (97)	79 (50)
Body as a Whole		
Headache	65 (41)	10 (6)
Fatigue	54 (34)	7 (4)
Asthenia	20 (13)	9 (6)
Fever	21 (13)	3 (2)
Back pain	12 (8)	4 (3)
Cardiovascular		
Edema peripheral	17 (11)	1 (1)
Central and Peripheral Nervous System		
Convulsions	36 (23)	8 (5)
Hemiparesis	29 (18)	10 (6)
Dizziness	19 (12)	1 (1)
Coordination abnormal	17 (11)	2 (1)
Amnesia	16 (10)	6 (4)
Insomnia	16 (10)	0
Paresthesia	15 (9)	1 (1)
Somnolence	15 (9)	5 (3)
Paresis	13 (8)	4 (3)
Urinary incontinence	13 (8)	3 (2)
Ataxia	12 (8)	3 (2)
Dysphasia	11 (7)	1 (1)
Convulsions local	9 (6)	0

Gait abnormal	9 (6)	1 (1)
Confusion	8 (5)	0
Endocrine		
Adrenal hypercorticism	13 (8)	0
Gastrointestinal System		
Nausea	84 (53)	16 (10)
Vomiting	66 (42)	10 (6)
Constipation	52 (33)	1 (1)
Diarrhea	25 (16)	3 (2)
Abdominal pain	14 (9)	2 (1)
Anorexia	14 (9)	1 (1)
Metabolic		
Weight increase	8 (5)	0
Musculoskeletal System		
Myalgia	8 (5)	
Psychiatric Disorders		
Anxiety	11 (7)	1 (1)
Depression	10 (6)	0
Reproductive Disorders		
Breast pain, female	4 (6)	
Resistance Mechanism Disorders		
Infection viral	17 (11)	0
Respiratory System		
Upper respiratory tract infection	13 (8)	0
Pharyngitis	12 (8)	0
Sinusitis	10 (6)	0
Coughing	8 (5)	0
Skin and Appendages		
Rash	13 (8)	0
Pruritus	12 (8)	2 (1)
Urinary System		
Urinary tract infection	12 (8)	0
Micturition increased frequency	9 (6)	0
Vision		
Diplopia	8 (5)	0
Vision abnormal*	8 (5)	

*Blurred vision; visual deficit; vision changes; vision troubles

TABLE 9: Adverse Hematologic Effects (Grade 3 to 4) in the Anaplastic Astrocytoma Trial in Adults

	TEMODAR*
Hemoglobin	7/158 (4%)
Lymphopenia	83/152 (55%)
Neutrophils	20/142 (14%)
Platelets	29/156 (19%)
WBC	18/158 (11%)

*Change from Grade 0 to 2 at baseline to Grade 3 or 4 during treatment.

TEMODAR for injection delivers equivalent temozolomide dose and exposure to both temozolomide and 5-(3-methyltriazen-1-yl)-imidazole-4-carboxamide (MTIC) as the corresponding TEMODAR capsules. Adverse reactions probably related to treatment that were reported from the 2 studies with the intravenous formulation (n=35) that were not reported in studies using the TEMODAR capsules were: pain, irritation, pruritus, warmth, swelling, and erythema at infusion site as well as the following adverse reactions: petechiae and hematoma.

6.2 Postmarketing Experience

The following adverse reactions have been identified during postapproval use of TEMODAR. Because these reactions are reported voluntarily from a population of uncertain size, it is not always possible to reliably estimate their frequency or establish a causal relationship to the drug exposure.

TEMODAR Capsules: allergic reactions, including anaphylaxis, have been reported. Erythema multiforme has been reported, which resolved after discontinuation of TEMODAR, and, in some cases, recurred upon rechallenge. Cases of toxic epidermal necrolysis and Stevens-Johnson syndrome have been reported. Opportunistic infections including *Pneumocystis carinii* pneumonia (PCP) have also been reported. Cases of interstitial pneumonitis/

pneumonitis, alveolitis, and pulmonary fibrosis have been reported. Prolonged pancytopenia, which may result in aplastic anemia, has been reported, and in some cases has resulted in a fatal outcome.

7 DRUG INTERACTIONS

7.1 Valproic Acid

Administration of valproic acid decreases oral clearance of temozolomide by about 5%. The clinical implication of this effect is not known [see Clinical Pharmacology (12.3)].

8 USE IN SPECIFIC POPULATIONS

8.1 Pregnancy

Pregnancy Category D. See Warnings and Precautions section.

TEMODAR can cause fetal harm when administered to a pregnant woman. Five consecutive days of oral temozolomide administration of 0.38 and 0.75 times the highest recommended human dose (75 and 150 mg/m^2) in rats and rabbits, respectively, during the period of organogenesis caused numerous malformations of the external and internal soft tissues and skeleton in both species. Doses equivalent to 0.75 times the highest recommended human dose (150 mg/m^2) caused embryolethality in rats and rabbits as indicated by increased resorptions. There are no adequate and well-controlled studies in pregnant women. If this drug is used during pregnancy, or if the patient becomes pregnant while taking this drug, the patient should be apprised of the potential hazard to a fetus. Women of childbearing potential should be advised to avoid becoming pregnant during therapy with TEMODAR.

8.3 Nursing Mothers

It is not known whether this drug is excreted in human milk. Because many drugs are excreted in human milk and because of the potential for serious adverse reactions in nursing infants and tumorigenicity shown for temozolomide in animal studies, a decision should be made whether to discontinue nursing or to discontinue the drug, taking into account the importance of the drug to the mother from TEMODAR.

8.4 Pediatric Use

Safety and effectiveness in pediatric patients have not been established. TEMODAR Capsules have been studied in 2 open-label studies in pediatric patients (aged 3–18 years) at a dose of 160 to 200 mg/m^2 daily for 5 days every 28 days. In one trial, 29 patients with recurrent brain stem glioma and 34 patients with recurrent high grade astrocytoma were enrolled. All patients had recurrence following surgery and radiation therapy, while 31% also had disease progression following chemotherapy. In a second study conducted by the Children's Oncology Group (COG), 122 patients were enrolled, including patients with medulloblastoma/PNET (29), high grade astrocytoma (23), low grade astrocytoma (22), brain stem glioma (16), ependymoma (14), other CNS tumors (9), and non-CNS tumors (9). The TEMODAR toxicity profile in pediatric patients is similar to adults. Table 10 shows the adverse reactions in 122 children in the COG study.

TABLE 10: Adverse Reactions Reported in the Pediatric Cooperative Group Trial (≥10%)

Body System/Organ Class Adverse Reaction	No. (%) of TEMODAR Patients (N=122)*	
	All Reactions	Grade 3/4
Subjects Reporting an AE	107 (88)	69 (57)
Body as a Whole		
Central and Peripheral Nervous System		
Central cerebral CNS cortex	22 (18)	13 (11)
Gastrointestinal System		
Nausea	56 (46)	5 (4)
Vomiting	62 (51)	4 (3)
Platelet, Bleeding and Clotting		
Thrombocytopenia	71 (58)	31 (25)
Red Blood Cell Disorders		
Decreased Hemoglobin	62 (51)	7 (6)
White Cell and RES Disorders		
Decreased WBC	71 (58)	21 (17)
Lymphopenia	73 (60)	48 (39)
Neutropenia	62 (51)	24 (20)

*These various tumors included the following: PNET-medulloblastoma, glioblastoma, low grade astrocytoma, brain stem tumor, ependymoma, mixed glioma, oligodendroglioma, neuroblastoma, Ewing's sarcoma, pineoblastoma, alveolar soft part sarcoma, neurofibrosarcoma, optic glioma, and osteosarcoma.

8.5 Geriatric Use

Clinical studies of temozolomide did not include sufficient numbers of subjects aged 65 and over to determine whether they responded differently from younger subjects. Other reported clinical experience has not identified differences in responses between the elderly and younger patients. In general, dose selection for an elderly patient should be cautious, reflecting the greater frequency of decreased hepatic, renal, or cardiac function, and of concomitant disease or other drug therapy.

In the anaplastic astrocytoma study population, patients 70 years of age or older had a higher incidence of Grade 4 neutropenia and Grade 4 thrombocytopenia (2/8; 25%, P=0.31 and 2/10; 20%, P=0.09, respectively) in the first cycle of therapy than patients under 70 years of age *[see Warnings and Precautions (5) and Adverse Reactions (6)]*.

In newly diagnosed patients with glioblastoma multiforme, the adverse reaction profile was similar in younger patients (<65 years) vs. older (≥65 years).

8.6 Renal Impairment

Caution should be exercised when TEMODAR is administered to patients with severe renal impairment *[see Clinical Pharmacology (12.3)]*.

8.7 Hepatic Impairment

Caution should be exercised when TEMODAR is administered to patients with severe hepatic impairment *[see Clinical Pharmacology (12.3)]*.

10 OVERDOSAGE

Doses of 500, 750, 1000, and 1250 mg/m^2 (total dose per cycle over 5 days) have been evaluated clinically in patients. Dose-limiting toxicity was hematologic and was reported with any dose but is expected to be more severe at higher doses. An overdose of 2000 mg per day for 5 days was taken by one patient and the adverse reactions reported were pancytopenia, pyrexia, multi-organ failure, and death. There are reports of patients who have taken more than 5 days of treatment (up to 64 days), with adverse reactions reported including bone marrow suppression, which in some cases was severe and prolonged, and infections and resulted in death. In the event of an overdose, hematologic evaluation is needed. Supportive measures should be provided as necessary.

11 DESCRIPTION

TEMODAR contains temozolomide, an imidazotetrazine derivative. The chemical name of temozolomide is 3,4-dihydro-3-methyl-4-oxoimidazo[5,1-d]-as-tetrazine-8-carboxamide. The structural formula is:

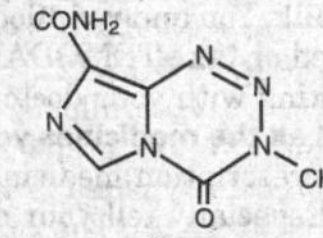

The material is a white to light tan/light pink powder with a molecular formula of $C_6H_6N_6O_2$ and a molecular weight of 194.15. The molecule is stable at acidic pH (<5) and labile at pH >7; hence TEMODAR can be administered orally and intravenously. The prodrug, temozolomide, is rapidly hydrolyzed to the active 5-(3-methyltriazen-1-yl) imidazole-4-carboxamide (MTIC) at neutral and alkaline pH values, with hydrolysis taking place even faster at alkaline pH.

TEMODAR Capsules:

Each capsule for oral use contains either 5 mg, 20 mg, 100 mg, 140 mg, 180 mg, or 250 mg of temozolomide.

The inactive ingredients for TEMODAR Capsules are as follows:

- *TEMODAR 5 mg*: lactose anhydrous (132.8 mg), colloidal silicon dioxide (0.2 mg), sodium starch glycolate (7.5 mg), tartaric acid (1.5 mg), and stearic acid (3 mg).
- *TEMODAR 20 mg*: lactose anhydrous (182.2 mg), colloidal silicon dioxide (0.2 mg), sodium starch glycolate (11 mg), tartaric acid (2.2 mg), and stearic acid (4.4 mg).
- *TEMODAR 100 mg*: lactose anhydrous (175.7 mg), colloidal silicon dioxide (0.3 mg), sodium starch glycolate (15 mg), tartaric acid (3 mg), and stearic acid (6 mg).
- *TEMODAR 140 mg*: lactose anhydrous (246 mg), colloidal silicon dioxide (0.4 mg), sodium starch glycolate (21 mg), tartaric acid (4.2 mg), and stearic acid (8.4 mg).
- *TEMODAR 180 mg*: lactose anhydrous (316.3 mg), colloidal silicon dioxide (0.5 mg), sodium starch glycolate (27 mg), tartaric acid (5.4 mg), and stearic acid (10.8 mg).
- *TEMODAR 250 mg*: lactose anhydrous (154.3 mg), colloidal silicon dioxide (0.7 mg), sodium starch glycolate (22.5 mg), tartaric acid (9 mg), and stearic acid (13.5 mg).

The body of the capsules are made of gelatin, and are opaque white. The cap is also made of gelatin, and the colors vary based on the dosage strength. The capsule body and cap are imprinted with pharmaceutical branding ink, which contains shellac, dehydrated alcohol, isopropyl alcohol, butyl alcohol, propylene glycol, purified water, strong ammonia solution, potassium hydroxide, and ferric oxide.

- *TEMODAR 5 mg:* The green cap contains gelatin, titanium dioxide, iron oxide yellow, sodium lauryl sulfate, and FD&C Blue #2.
- *TEMODAR 20 mg:* The yellow cap contains gelatin, sodium lauryl sulfate, and iron oxide yellow.
- *TEMODAR 100 mg:* The pink cap contains gelatin, titanium dioxide, sodium lauryl sulfate, and iron oxide red.
- *TEMODAR 140 mg:* The blue cap contains gelatin, sodium lauryl sulfate, and FD&C Blue #2.
- *TEMODAR 180 mg:* The orange cap contains gelatin, iron oxide red, iron oxide yellow, titanium dioxide, and sodium lauryl sulfate.
- *TEMODAR 250 mg:* The white cap contains gelatin, titanium dioxide, and sodium lauryl sulfate.

TEMODAR for Injection:

Each vial contains 100 mg of sterile and pyrogen-free temozolomide lyophilized powder for intravenous injection. The inactive ingredients are: mannitol (600 mg), L-threonine (160 mg), polysorbate 80 (120 mg), sodium citrate dihydrate (235 mg), and hydrochloric acid (160 mg).

12 CLINICAL PHARMACOLOGY

12.1 Mechanism of Action

Temozolomide is not directly active but undergoes rapid nonenzymatic conversion at physiologic pH to the reactive compound 5-(3-methyltriazen-1-yl)-imidazole-4-carboxamide (MTIC). The cytotoxicity of MTIC is thought to be primarily due to alkylation of DNA. Alkylation (methylation) occurs mainly at the O^6 and N^7 positions of guanine.

12.3 Pharmacokinetics

Absorption:

Temozolomide is rapidly and completely absorbed after oral administration with a peak plasma concentration (C_{max}) achieved in a median T_{max} of 1 hour. Food reduces the rate and extent of temozolomide absorption. Mean peak plasma concentration and AUC decreased by 32% and 9%, respectively, and median T_{max} increased by 2-fold (from 1–2.25 hours) when temozolomide was administered after a modified high-fat breakfast.

A pharmacokinetic study comparing oral and intravenous temozolomide in 19 patients with primary CNS malignancies showed that 150 mg/m^2 TEMODAR for injection administered over 90 minutes is bioequivalent to 150 mg/m^2 TEMODAR oral capsules with respect to both C_{max} and AUC of temozolomide and MTIC. Following a single 90-minute intravenous infusion of 150 mg/m^2, the geometric mean C_{max} values for temozolomide and MTIC were 7.3 mcg/mL and 276 ng/mL, respectively. Following a single oral dose of 150 mg/m^2, the geometric mean C_{max} values for temozolomide and MTIC were 7.5 mcg/mL and 282 ng/mL, respectively. Following a single 90-minute intravenous infusion of 150 mg/m^2, the geometric mean AUC values for temozolomide and MTIC were 24.6 mcg•hr/mL and 891 ng•hr/mL, respectively. Following a single oral dose of 150 mg/m^2, the geometric mean AUC values for temozolomide and MTIC were 23.4 mcg•hr/mL and 864 ng•hr/mL, respectively.

Distribution:

Temozolomide has a mean apparent volume of distribution of 0.4 L/kg (%CV=13%). It is weakly bound to human plasma proteins; the mean percent bound of drug-related total radioactivity is 15%.

Metabolism and Elimination:

Temozolomide is spontaneously hydrolyzed at physiologic pH to the active species, MTIC and to temozolomide acid metabolite. MTIC is further hydrolyzed to 5-amino-imidazole-4-carboxamide (AIC), which is known to be an intermediate in purine and nucleic acid biosynthesis, and to methylhydrazine, which is believed to be the active alkylating species. Cytochrome P450 enzymes play only a minor role in the metabolism of temozolomide and MTIC. Relative to the AUC of temozolomide, the exposure to MTIC and AIC is 2.4% and 23%, respectively.

Excretion:

About 38% of the administered temozolomide total radioactive dose is recovered over 7 days: 37.7% in urine and 0.8% in feces. The majority of the recovery of radioactivity in urine is unchanged temozolomide (5.6%), AIC (12%), temozolomide acid metabolite (2.3%), and unidentified polar metabolite(s) (17%). Overall clearance of temozolomide is about 5.5 L/hr/m^2. Temozolomide is rapidly eliminated, with a mean elimination half-life of 1.8 hours, and exhibits linear kinetics over the therapeutic dosing range of 75 to 250 mg/m^2/day.

Effect of Age:

A population pharmacokinetic analysis indicated that age (range: 19–78 years) has no influence on the pharmacokinetics of temozolomide.

Effect of Gender:

A population pharmacokinetic analysis indicated that women have an approximately 5% lower clearance (adjusted for body surface area) for temozolomide than men.

Effect of Race:

The effect of race on the pharmacokinetics of temozolomide has not been studied.

Tobacco Use:

A population pharmacokinetic analysis indicated that the oral clearance of temozolomide is similar in smokers and nonsmokers.

Effect of Renal Impairment:

A population pharmacokinetic analysis indicated that creatinine clearance over the range of 36 to 130 mL/min/m^2 has no effect on the clearance of temozolomide after oral administration. The pharmacokinetics of temozolomide have not been studied in patients with severely impaired renal function (CLcr <36 mL/min/m^2). Caution should be exercised when TEMODAR is administered to patients with severe renal impairment *[see Use in Special Populations (8.6)]*. TEMODAR has not been studied in patients on dialysis.

Effect of Hepatic Impairment:

A study showed that the pharmacokinetics of temozolomide in patients with mild-to-moderate hepatic impairment (Child-Pugh Class I–II) were similar to those observed in patients with normal hepatic function. Caution should be exercised when temozolomide is administered to patients with severe hepatic impairment *[see Use in Special Populations (8.7)]*.

Effect of Other Drugs on Temozolomide Pharmacokinetics:

In a multiple-dose study, administration of TEMODAR Capsules with ranitidine did not change the C_{max} or AUC values for temozolomide or MTIC.

A population analysis indicated that administration of valproic acid decreases the clearance of temozolomide by about 5% *[see Drug Interactions (7)]*.

A population analysis did not demonstrate any influence of coadministered dexamethasone, prochlorperazine, phenytoin, carbamazepine, ondansetron, H_2-receptor antagonists, or phenobarbital on the clearance of orally administered temozolomide.

13 NONCLINICAL TOXICOLOGY

13.1 Carcinogenesis, Mutagenesis, Impairment of Fertility

Temozolomide is carcinogenic in rats at doses less than the maximum recommended human dose. Temozolomide induced mammary carcinomas in both males and females at doses 0.13 to 0.63 times the maximum human dose (25–125 mg/m^2) when administered orally on 5 consecutive days every 28 days for 6 cycles. Temozolomide also induced fibrosarcomas of the heart, eye, seminal vesicles, salivary glands, abdominal cavity, uterus, and prostate, carcinomas of the seminal vesicles, schwannomas of the heart, optic nerve, and harderian gland, and adenomas of the skin, lung, pituitary, and thyroid at doses 0.5 times the maximum daily dose. Mammary tumors were also induced following 3 cycles of temozolomide at the maximum recommended daily dose.

Temozolomide is a mutagen and a clastogen. In a reverse bacterial mutagenesis assay (Ames assay), temozolomide increased revertant frequency in the absence and presence of metabolic activation. Temozolomide was clastogenic in human lymphocytes in the presence and absence of metabolic activation.

Temozolomide impairs male fertility. Temozolomide caused syncytial cells/immature sperm formation at 0.25 and 0.63 times the maximum recommended human dose (50 and 125 mg/m^2) in rats and dogs, respectively, and testicular atrophy in dogs at 0.63 times the maximum recommended human dose (125 mg/m^2).

13.2 Animal Toxicology and/or Pharmacology

Toxicology studies in rats and dogs identified a low incidence of hemorrhage, degeneration, and necrosis of the retina at temozolomide doses equal to or greater than 0.63 times the maximum recommended human dose (125 mg/m^2). These changes were most commonly seen at doses where mortality was observed.

14 CLINICAL STUDIES

14.1 Newly Diagnosed Glioblastoma Multiforme

Five hundred and seventy-three patients were randomized to receive either TEMODAR (TMZ)+Radiotherapy (RT) (n=287) or RT alone (n=286). Patients in the TEMODAR+RT arm received concomitant TEMODAR (75 mg/m^2) once daily, starting the first day of RT until the last day of RT, for 42 days (with a maximum of 49 days). This was followed by 6 cycles of TEMODAR alone (150 or 200 mg/m^2) on Days 1 to 5 of every 28-day cycle, starting 4 weeks after the end of RT. Patients in the control arm received RT only. In both arms, focal radiation therapy was delivered as 60 Gy/30 fractions. Focal RT includes the tumor bed or resection site with a 2- to 3-cm margin. *Pneumocystis carinii* pneumonia (PCP) prophylaxis was required during the TMZ + RT, regardless of lymphocyte count, and was to continue until recovery of lymphocyte count to less than or equal to Grade 1.

At the time of disease progression, TEMODAR was administered as salvage therapy in 161 patients of the 282 (57%) in the RT alone arm, and 62 patients of the 277 (22%) in the TEMODAR+RT arm.

The addition of concomitant and maintenance TEMODAR to radiotherapy in the treatment of patients with newly diagnosed GBM showed a statistically significant improvement in overall survival compared to radiotherapy alone (**Figure 1**). The hazard ratio (HR) for overall survival was 0.63 (95% CI for HR=0.52-0.75) with a log-rank $P<0.0001$ in favor of the TEMODAR arm. The median survival was increased by 2.5 months in the TEMODAR arm.

FIGURE 1: Kaplan-Meier Curves for Overall Survival (ITT Population)

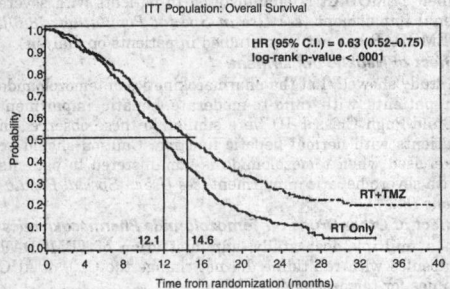

14.2 Refractory Anaplastic Astrocytoma

A single-arm, multicenter study was conducted in 162 patients who had anaplastic astrocytoma at first relapse and who had a baseline Karnofsky performance status of 70 or greater. Patients had previously received radiation therapy and may also have previously received a nitrosourea with or without other chemotherapy. Fifty-four patients had disease progression on prior therapy with both a nitrosourea and procarbazine, and their malignancy was considered refractory to chemotherapy (refractory anaplastic astrocytoma population). Median age of this subgroup of 54 patients was 42 years (19–76). Sixty-five percent were male. Seventy-two percent of patients had a KPS of >80. Sixty-three percent of patients had surgery other than a biopsy at the time of initial diagnosis. Of those patients undergoing resection, 73% underwent a subtotal resection and 27% underwent a gross total resection. Eighteen percent of patients had surgery at the time of first relapse. The median time from initial diagnosis to first relapse was 13.8 months (4.2–75.4).

TEMODAR Capsules were given for the first 5 consecutive days of a 28-day cycle at a starting dose of 150 mg/m²/day. If the nadir and day of dosing (Day 29, Day 1 of next cycle) absolute neutrophil count was ≥1.5 × 10⁹/L (1500/µL) and the nadir and Day 29, Day 1 of next cycle platelet count was ≥100 × 10⁹/L (100,000/µL), the TEMODAR dose was increased to 200 mg/m²/day for the first 5 consecutive days of a 28-day cycle.

In the refractory anaplastic astrocytoma population, the overall tumor response rate (CR + PR) was 22% (12/54 patients) and the complete response rate was 9% (5/54 patients). The median duration of all responses was 50 weeks (range: 16–114 weeks) and the median duration of complete responses was 64 weeks (range: 52–114 weeks). In this population, progression-free survival at 6 months was 45% (95% CI: 31%–58%) and progression-free survival at 12 months was 29% (95% CI: 16%–42%). Median progression-free survival was 4.4 months. Overall survival at 6 months was 74% (95% CI: 62%–86%) and 12-month overall survival was 65% (95% CI: 52%–78%). Median overall survival was 15.9 months.

15 REFERENCES

1. OSHA Technical Manual, TED 1-0.15A, Section VI: Chapter 2. Controlling Occupational Exposure to Hazardous Drugs. OSHA, 1999.
2. American Society of Health-System Pharmacists. ASHP guidelines on handling hazardous drugs. *Am J Health-Syst Pharm.* 2006; 63:1172–1193.
3. NIOSH Alert: Preventing occupational exposures to antineoplastic and other hazardous drugs in healthcare settings. 2004. U.S. Department of Health and Human Services, Public Health Service, Centers for Disease Control and Prevention, National Institute for Occupational Safety and Health, DHHS (NIOSH) Publication No. 2004-165.[3]
4. Polovich, M., White, J. M., & Kelleher, L.O. (eds.) 2005. Chemotherapy and biotherapy guidelines and recommendations for practice (2nd. ed.) Pittsburgh, PA: Oncology.

16 HOW SUPPLIED/STORAGE AND HANDLING

16.1 Safe Handling and Disposal

Care should be exercised in the handling and preparation of TEMODAR. Vials and capsules should not be opened. If vials or capsules are accidentally opened or damaged, rigorous precautions should be taken with the contents to avoid inhalation or contact with the skin or mucous membranes. The use of gloves and safety glasses is recommended to avoid exposure in case of breakage of the vial or capsules.

Procedures for proper handling and disposal of anticancer drugs should be considered[1-4]. Several guidelines on this subject have been published.

16.2 How Supplied

TEMODAR Capsules:
TEMODAR (temozolomide) Capsules are supplied in amber glass bottles with child-resistant polypropylene caps containing the following capsule strengths:

TEMODAR Capsules 5 mg: have opaque white bodies with green caps. The capsule body is imprinted with two stripes, the dosage strength, and the Schering-Plough logo. The cap is imprinted with "TEMODAR".
They are supplied as follows:
5-count - NDC 0085-3004-02
14-count - NDC 0085-3004-01

TEMODAR Capsules 20 mg: have opaque white bodies with yellow caps. The capsule body is imprinted with two stripes, the dosage strength, and the Schering-Plough logo. The cap is imprinted with "TEMODAR".
They are supplied as follows:
5-count - NDC 0085-1519-02
14-count - NDC 0085-1519-01

TEMODAR Capsules 100 mg: have opaque white bodies with pink caps. The capsule body is imprinted with two stripes, the dosage strength, and the Schering-Plough logo. The cap is imprinted with "TEMODAR".
They are supplied as follows:
5-count - NDC 0085-1366-02
14-count - NDC 0085-1366-01

TEMODAR Capsules 140 mg: have opaque white bodies with blue caps. The capsule body is imprinted with two stripes, the dosage strength, and the Schering-Plough logo. The cap is imprinted with "TEMODAR".
They are supplied as follows:
5-count - NDC 0085-1425-01
14-count - NDC 0085-1425-02

TEMODAR Capsules 180 mg: have opaque white bodies with orange caps. The capsule body is imprinted with two stripes, the dosage strength, and the Schering-Plough logo. The cap is imprinted with "TEMODAR".
They are supplied as follows:
5-count - NDC 0085-1430-01
14-count - NDC 0085-1430-02

TEMODAR Capsules 250 mg: have opaque white bodies with white caps. The capsule body is imprinted with two stripes, the dosage strength, and the Schering-Plough logo. The cap is imprinted with "TEMODAR".
They are supplied as follows:
5-count - NDC 0085-1417-01

TEMODAR for Injection:
TEMODAR (temozolomide) for Injection is supplied in single-use glass vials containing 100 mg temozolomide. The lyophilized powder is white to light tan/light pink.
TEMODAR for Injection 100 mg:
NDC 0085-1381-01

16.3 Storage

Store TEMODAR Capsules at 25°C (77°F); excursions permitted to 15°–30°C (59°–86°F)
[see USP Controlled Room Temperature].
Store TEMODAR for Injection refrigerated at 2°–8°C (36°–46°F). After reconstitution, store reconstituted product at room temperature (25°C [77°F]). Reconstituted product must be used within 14 hours, including infusion time.

17 PATIENT COUNSELING INFORMATION

17.1 Information for the Patient

Physicians should discuss the following with their patients:
- Nausea and vomiting are the most frequently occurring adverse reactions. Nausea and vomiting are usually either self-limiting or readily controlled with standard antiemetic therapy.
- Capsules should not be opened. If capsules are accidentally opened or damaged, rigorous precautions should be taken with the capsule contents to avoid inhalation or contact with the skin or mucous membranes.
- The medication should be kept away from children and pets.

17.2 FDA-approved Patient Labeling

TEMODAR Capsules
Manufactured by: Schering Corporation, a subsidiary of **MERCK & CO., INC.**, Whitehouse Station, NJ 08889, USA.
TEMODAR for Injection
Manufactured by: Baxter Oncology GmbH, Halle/Westfalen, Germany. Distributed by: Schering Corporation, a subsidiary of **MERCK & CO., INC.**, Whitehouse Station, NJ 08889, USA.

U.S. Patent Nos. 5,260,291 and 6,987,108.
Rev 4/10
318509XXT

Tear patient package insert at perforation and give to patient.
Patient Package Insert
TEMODAR® (tĕm-ō-dăr)
(temozolomide)
Capsules
TEMODAR® (tĕm-ō-dăr)
for Injection
What is the most important information I should know about TEMODAR?
- **TEMODAR may cause birth defects.** Male and female patients who take TEMODAR should use effective birth control. Female patients and female partners of male patients should avoid becoming pregnant while taking TEMODAR.
See the section "What are the possible side effects of TEMODAR?" for more information about side effects.
What is TEMODAR?
TEMODAR (temozolomide) is a prescription medicine used to treat adults with certain brain cancer tumors. TEMODAR blocks cell growth, especially cells that grow fast, such as cancer cells. TEMODAR may decrease the size of certain brain tumors in some patients.
It is not known if TEMODAR is safe and effective in children.
Who should not take TEMODAR?
Do not take TEMODAR if you:
- have had an allergic reaction to DTIC (dacarbazine), another cancer medicine.
- have had a red itchy rash, or a severe allergic reaction, such as trouble breathing, swelling of the face, throat, or tongue, or severe skin reaction to TEMODAR or any of the ingredients in TEMODAR. If you are not sure, ask your doctor. See the end of the leaflet for a list of ingredients in TEMODAR.
What should I tell my doctor before taking TEMODAR?
Tell your doctor about all your medical conditions, including if you:
- are allergic to DTIC (dacarbazine) or have had a severe allergic reaction to TEMODAR. See "Who should not take TEMODAR?"
- have kidney problems
- have liver problems
- are pregnant. See "What is the most important information I should know about TEMODAR?"
- are breast-feeding. It is not known whether TEMODAR passes into breast milk. You and your doctor should decide if you will breast-feed or take TEMODAR. You should not do both without talking with your doctor.
Tell your doctor about all the medicines you take, including prescription and non-prescription medicines, vitamins, and herbal supplements. Especially tell your doctor if you take a medicine that contains valproic acid (Stavzor®, Depakene®).
Know the medicines you take. Keep a list of them and show it to your doctor and pharmacist when you get a new medicine.
How should I take TEMODAR?
Temodar may be taken by mouth as a capsule at home, or you may receive TEMODAR by injection into a vein (intravenous). Your doctor will decide the best way for you to take TEMODAR.
There are two common dosing schedules for taking TEMODAR.
- Some people take TEMODAR for 42 days in a row (possibly 49 days depending on side effects) with radiation treatment. This is one cycle of treatment. After this, you may have "maintenance" treatment. Your doctor may prescribe 6 more cycles of TEMODAR. For each of these cycles, you take TEMODAR one time each day for 5 days in a row and then you stop taking it for the next 23 days. This is a 28-day maintenance treatment cycle.
- Another way to take TEMODAR is to take it one time each day for 5 days in a row only, and then you stop taking it for the next 23 days. This is one cycle of treatment (28 days). Your doctor will watch your progress on TEMODAR and decide how long you should take it. You might take TEMODAR until your tumor gets worse or for possibly up to 2 years.
- Your dose is based on your height and weight, and the number of treatment cycles will depend on how you respond to and tolerate this treatment.
- Your doctor may modify your schedule based on how you tolerate the treatment.
- If your doctor prescribes a treatment regimen that is different from the information in this leaflet, make sure you follow the specific instructions given to you by your doctor.
TEMODAR Capsules:
- Take TEMODAR Capsules exactly as prescribed.
- TEMODAR Capsules come in different strengths. Each strength has a different color cap. Your doctor may prescribe more than one strength of TEMODAR Capsules for you, so it is important that you understand how to take your medicine the right way. Be sure that you understand

exactly how many capsules you need to take on each day of your treatment, and what strengths to take. This may be different whenever you start a new cycle.

- Talk to your doctor before you take your dose if you are not sure how much to take. This will help to prevent taking too much TEMODAR and decrease your chances of getting serious side effects.
- Take each day's dose of TEMODAR Capsules at one time, with a full glass of water.
- **Swallow TEMODAR Capsules whole. Do not chew, open, or split the capsules.**
- If TEMODAR capsules are accidentally opened or damaged, be careful not to breathe in (inhale) the powder from the capsules or get the powder on your skin or mucous membranes (for example, in your nose or mouth). If contact with any of these areas happens, flush the area with water.
- If you vomit TEMODAR Capsules, do not take any more capsules. Wait and take your next planned dose.
- The medicine is used best by your body if you take it at the same time every day in relation to a meal.
- To lessen nausea, try to take TEMODAR on an empty stomach or at bedtime. Your doctor may prescribe medicine to prevent or treat nausea, or other medicines to lessen side effects with TEMODAR.
- See your doctor regularly to check your progress. Your doctor will check you for side effects that you might not notice.
- If you miss a dose of TEMODAR, talk with your doctor for instructions about when to take your next dose of TEMODAR.
- Call your doctor right away if you take more than the prescribed amount of TEMODAR. It is important that you do not take more than the amount of TEMODAR prescribed for you.

TEMODAR for Injection:
- You will receive TEMODAR as an infusion directly into your vein. Your treatment will take about 90 minutes.
- Your doctor may prescribe medicine to prevent or treat nausea, or other medicines to relieve side effects with TEMODAR.

What should I avoid while taking TEMODAR?
- Female patients and female partners of male patients should avoid becoming pregnant while taking TEMODAR. See "What is the most important information I should know about TEMODAR?"

What are the possible side effects of TEMODAR?
TEMODAR can cause serious side effects.
- See "What is the most important information I should know about TEMODAR?"
- **Decreased blood cells.** TEMODAR affects cells that grow rapidly, including bone marrow cells. This can cause you to have a decrease in blood cells. Your doctor can monitor your blood for these effects.
  - White blood cells are needed to fight infections. Neutrophils are a type of white blood cell that help prevent bacterial infections. Decreased neutrophils can lead to serious infections that can lead to death. Other white blood cells called lymphocytes may also be decreased.
  - Platelets are blood cells needed for normal blood clotting. Low platelet counts can lead to bleeding. Tell your doctor about any unusual bruising or bleeding.

Your doctor will check your blood regularly while you are taking TEMODAR to see if these side effects are happening. Your doctor may need to change the dose of TEMODAR or when you get it depending on your blood cell counts. People who are age 70 or older and women may be more likely to have their blood cells affected.
- *Pneumocystis carinii* **Pneumonia (PCP).** PCP is an infection that people can get when their immune system is weak. TEMODAR decreases white blood cells, which makes your immune system weaker and can increase your risk of getting PCP. **All patients** taking TEMODAR will be watched carefully by their doctor for this infection, especially patients who take steroids. Tell your doctor if you have any of the following signs and symptoms of PCP infection: shortness of breath and/or fever, chills, dry cough.
- **Secondary cancers.** Blood problems such as myelodysplastic syndrome and secondary cancers, such as a certain kind of leukemia, can happen in people who take TEMODAR. Your doctor will watch you for this.
- **Convulsions.** Convulsions may be severe or life-threatening in people who take TEMODAR.

Common side effects with TEMODAR include:
- nausea and vomiting. Your doctor can prescribe medicines that may help reduce these symptoms.
- headache
- feeling tired
- loss of appetite
- hair loss
- constipation
- bruising
- rash

- paralysis on one side of the body
- diarrhea
- weakness
- fever
- dizziness
- coordination problems
- viral infection
- sleep problems
- memory loss
- pain, irritation, itching, warmth, swelling or redness at the site of infusion
- bruising or small red or purple spots under the skin

Tell your doctor about any side effect that bothers you or that does not go away.
These are not all the possible side effects with TEMODAR. For more information, ask your doctor or pharmacist.
Call your doctor for medical advice about side effects. You may report side effects to FDA at 1-800-FDA-1088.

How should I store TEMODAR Capsules?
- Store TEMODAR Capsules at 77°F (controlled room temperature). Storage at 59° to 86°F (15° to 30°C) is permitted occasionally.
- **Keep TEMODAR Capsules out of the reach of children and pets.**

General information about TEMODAR.
Medicines are sometimes prescribed for purposes other than those listed in a Patient Package Insert. Do not use TEMODAR for a condition for which it was not prescribed. Do not give TEMODAR to other people, even if they have the same symptoms that you have. It may harm them.
This leaflet summarizes the most important information about TEMODAR. If you would like more information, talk with your doctor. You can ask your pharmacist or doctor for information about TEMODAR that is written for health professionals.
For more information, go to www.TEMODAR.com or call 1-800-526-4099.

How are TEMODAR Capsules supplied?
TEMODAR Capsules contain a white capsule body with a color cap and the colors vary based on the dosage strength. The capsules are available in six different strengths.

TEMODAR Capsule Strength	Color
5 mg	Green Cap
20 mg	Yellow Cap
100 mg	Pink Cap
140 mg	Blue Cap
180 mg	Orange Cap
250 mg	White Cap

What are the ingredients in TEMODAR?
TEMODAR Capsules:
Active ingredient: temozolomide.
Inactive ingredients: lactose anhydrous, colloidal silicon dioxide, sodium starch glycolate, tartaric acid, stearic acid. The body of the capsules are made of gelatin and are opaque white. The cap is also made of gelatin, and the colors vary based on the dosage strength. The capsule body and cap are imprinted with pharmaceutical branding ink, which contains shellac, dehydrated alcohol, isopropyl alcohol, butyl alcohol, propylene glycol, purified water, strong ammonia, potassium hydroxide, and ferric oxide.
TEMODAR 5 mg: The green cap contains gelatin, titanium dioxide, iron oxide yellow, sodium lauryl sulfate, and FD&C Blue #2.
TEMODAR 20 mg: The yellow cap contains gelatin, sodium lauryl sulfate, and iron oxide yellow.
TEMODAR 100 mg: The pink cap contains gelatin, titanium dioxide, sodium lauryl sulfate, and iron oxide red.
TEMODAR 140 mg: The blue cap contains gelatin, sodium lauryl sulfate, and FD&C Blue #2.
TEMODAR 180 mg: The orange cap contains gelatin, iron oxide red, iron oxide yellow, titanium dioxide, and sodium lauryl sulfate.
TEMODAR 250 mg: The white cap contains gelatin, titanium dioxide, and sodium lauryl sulfate.
TEMODAR for Injection:
Active ingredient: temozolomide.
Inactive ingredients: mannitol, L-threonine, polysorbate 80, sodium citrate dihydrate, and hydrochloric acid.
Issued: February 2009
TEMODAR Capsules
Manufactured by: Schering Corporation, a subsidiary of **MERCK & CO. INC.**, Whitehouse Station, NJ 08889, USA.
TEMODAR for Injection
Manufactured by: Baxter Oncology GmbH, Halle/Westfalen, Germany. Distributed by: Schering Corporation, a subsidiary of **MERCK & CO., INC.**, Whitehouse Station, NJ 08889, USA.

U.S. Patent Nos. 5,260,291 and 6,987,108.
Rev. 04/10
318511XXT
The trademarks depicted in this piece are owned by their respective companies.

PHARMACIST INFORMATION SHEET
What is TEMODAR? [See Full Prescribing Information, Indications and Usage (1)].
TEMODAR® (temozolomide) is an alkylating drug for the treatment of adult patients with newly diagnosed glioblastoma multiforme and refractory anaplastic astrocytoma.
How is TEMODAR dosed? [See Full Prescribing Information, Recommended Dosing and Dose Modification Guidelines (2.1)].
The daily dose of TEMODAR for a given patient is calculated by the physician, based on the patient's body surface area (BSA) [see Table 5 in the Full Prescribing Information, Recommended Dosing and Dose Modification Guidelines (2.1)]. The recommended dose for TEMODAR as an intravenous infusion over 90 minutes is the same as the dose for the oral capsule formulation. Bioequivalence has been established only when TEMODAR for Injection was given over 90 minutes. The dose for subsequent cycles may be adjusted according to nadir neutrophil and platelet counts in the previous cycle and at the time of initiating the next cycle.
Dosing for Patients with Refractory Anaplastic Astrocytoma [See Full Prescribing Information, Recommended Dosing and Dose Modification Guidelines, Patients with Refractory Anaplastic Astrocytoma (2.1)].
Dosage of TEMODAR must be adjusted according to nadir neutrophil and platelet counts in the previous cycle and neutrophil and platelet counts at the time of initiating the next cycle. The initial dose is 150 mg/m^2 orally once daily for 5 consecutive days per 28-day treatment cycle. If both the nadir and day of dosing (Day 29, Day 1 of next cycle) absolute neutrophil counts (ANC) are ≥1.5 × 10^9/L (1500/µL) and both the nadir and Day 29, Day 1 of next cycle platelet counts are ≥100 × 10^9/L (100,000/µL), the TEMODAR dose may be increased to 200 mg/m^2/day for 5 consecutive days per 28-day treatment cycle. During treatment, a complete blood count should be obtained on Day 22 (21 days after the first dose) or within 48 hours of that day, and weekly until the ANC is above 1.5 × 10^9/L (1500/µL) and the platelet count exceeds 100 × 10^9/L (100,000/µL). The next cycle of TEMODAR should not be started until the ANC and platelet count exceed these levels. If the ANC falls to <1.0 × 10^9/L (1000/µL) or the platelet count is <50 × 10^9/L (50,000/µL) during any cycle, the next cycle should be reduced by 50 mg/m^2, but not below 100 mg/m^2, the lowest recommended dose [see Table 4 in the Full Prescribing Information, Recommended Dosing and Dose Modification Guidelines (2.1)].
Patients should continue to receive TEMODAR until their physician determines that their disease has progressed, or until unacceptable side effects or toxicities occur. Physicians may alter the treatment regimen for a given patient.
Dosing for Patients with Newly Diagnosed Glioblastoma Multiforme [See Full Prescribing Information, Recommended Dosing and Dose Modification Guidelines, Patients with Newly Diagnosed High Grade Glioma (2.1)].
Concomitant Phase Treatment Schedule
TEMODAR is administered at 75 mg/m^2 daily for 42 days concomitant with focal radiotherapy (60 Gy administered in 30 fractions), followed by maintenance TEMODAR for 6 cycles. No dose reductions are recommended; however, dose interruptions may occur based on patient tolerance. The TEMODAR dose can be continued throughout the 42-day concomitant period up to 49 days if all of the following conditions are met: absolute neutrophil count ≥1.5 × 10^9/L, platelet count ≥100 ×10^9/L, common toxicity criteria (CTC) non-hematological toxicity ≤ Grade 1 (except for alopecia, nausea, and vomiting). During treatment a complete blood count should be obtained weekly. Temozolomide dosing should be interrupted or discontinued during concomitant phase according to the hematological and non-hematological toxicity criteria as noted in **Table 1** of the Full Prescribing Information under 2.1 Recommended Dosing and Dose Modification Guidelines. PCP prophylaxis is required during the concomitant administration of TEMODAR and radiotherapy and should be continued in patients who develop lymphocytopenia until recovery from lymphocytopenia (CTC Grade ≤1).
Maintenance Phase Treatment Schedule
Four weeks after completing the TEMODAR + RT phase, TEMODAR is administered for an additional 6 cycles of maintenance treatment. Dosage in Cycle 1 (maintenance) is 150 mg/m^2 once daily for 5 days followed by 23 days without treatment. At the start of Cycle 2, the dose can be escalated to 200 mg/m^2, if the CTC non-hematologic toxicity for Cycle 1 is Grade ≤2 (except for alopecia, nausea, and vomiting), absolute neutrophil count (ANC) is ≥1.5 × 10^9/L, and the platelet count is ≥100 × 10^9/L. If the dose was not escalated at Cycle 2, escalation should not be done in subse-

quent cycles. The dose remains at 200 mg/m² per day for the first 5 days of each subsequent cycle except if toxicity occurs.

During treatment a complete blood count should be obtained on Day 22 (21 days after the first dose) or within 48 hours of that day, and weekly until the ANC is above 1.5 × 10⁹/L (1500/μL) and the platelet count exceeds 100 × 10⁹/L (100,000/μL). The next cycle of TEMODAR should not be started until the ANC and platelet count exceed these levels. Dose reductions during the next cycle should be based on the lowest blood counts and worst non-hematologic toxicity during the previous cycle. Dose reductions or discontinuations during the maintenance phase should be applied according to **Tables 2** and **3** in the Full Prescribing Information under 2.1 Recommended Dosing and Dose Modification Guidelines.

How is TEMODAR for Injection prepared? *[See Full Prescribing Information, Preparation and Administration, TEMODAR for Injection (2.2)].*

Care should be exercised in the handling and preparation of TEMODAR. Vials should not be opened. If vials are accidentally opened or damaged, rigorous precautions should be taken with the contents to avoid inhalation or contact with the skin or mucous membranes. The use of gloves and safety glasses is recommended to avoid exposure in case of breakage of the vial. Procedures for proper handling and disposal of anticancer drugs should be considered[1–4]. Several guidelines on this subject have been published.

1. TEMODAR for Injection vials should be stored refrigerated at 2°–8°C (36°–46°F).
2. Bring the vial to room temperature prior to reconstitution with Sterile Water for Injection.
3. Using aseptic technique, reconstitute each vial with 41 mL Sterile Water for Injection. The resulting solution will contain 2.5 mg/mL temozolomide.
4. Vial should be gently swirled and not shaken. Inspect vials, and any vial containing visible particulate matter should not be used. Do not further dilute the reconstituted solution. Upon reconstitution, store at room temperature for up to 14 hours, including infusion time.
5. Using aseptic technique, withdraw up to 40 mL from each vial to make up the total dose and transfer into an empty 250 mL PVC infusion bag. Studies with non-PVC bags have not been conducted.
6. Attach the pump tubing to the bag, purge the tubing and then cap.

How is TEMODAR for Injection administered? *[See Full Prescribing Information, Preparation and Administration, TEMODAR for Injection (2.2)].*

TEMODAR for Injection is administered as an intravenous infusion over 90 minutes. Bioequivalence has been established only when TEMODAR for Injection was given over 90 minutes. TEMODAR for Injection should be administered only by intravenous infusion. Flush the lines before and after each TEMODAR infusion.

Because no data are available on the compatibility of TEMODAR for Injection with other intravenous substances or additives, other medications should not be infused simultaneously through the same intravenous line.

What should the patient avoid during treatment with TEMODAR? *[See Full Prescribing Information, Use in Specific Populations, Pregnancy (8.1) and Nursing Mothers (8.3)].*

There are no dietary restrictions for patients taking TEMODAR. TEMODAR may affect testicular function, so male patients should exercise adequate birth control measures. TEMODAR may cause birth defects. Female patients should avoid becoming pregnant while receiving this drug. It is not known whether TEMODAR is excreted into breast milk. Because many drugs are excreted in human milk, and because of the potential for serious adverse reactions in nursing infants and tumorigenicity shown for temozolomide in animal studies, a decision should be made whether to discontinue nursing or to discontinue the drug, taking into account the importance of the drug to the mother from TEMODAR.

What are the side effects of TEMODAR? *[See Full Prescribing Information, Adverse Reactions (6)].*

Nausea and vomiting are the most common side effects associated with TEMODAR. Noncumulative myelosuppression is the dose-limiting toxicity. Patients should be evaluated periodically by their physician to monitor blood counts.

Other commonly reported side effects reported by patients taking TEMODAR are fatigue, constipation, alopecia, anorexia, headache, and bruising, as well as pain, irritation, itching, warmth, swelling, and redness at the site of infusion.

How is TEMODAR supplied? *[See Full Prescribing Information, How Supplied/Storage and Handling (16)].*

TEMODAR for Injection is supplied in single-use glass vials containing 100 mg temozolomide. TEMODAR is also available as capsules in 5-mg, 20-mg, 100-mg, 140-mg, 180-mg, and 250-mg strengths.

1. OSHA Technical Manual, TED 1-0.15A, Section VI: Chapter 2. Controlling Occupational Exposure to Hazardous Drugs. OSHA, 1999.
2. American Society of Health-System Pharmacists. ASHP guidelines on handling hazardous drugs. *Am J Health-Syst Pharm.* 2006; 63:1172–1193.
3. NIOSH Alert: Preventing occupational exposures to antineoplastic and other hazardous drugs in healthcare settings. 2004. U.S. Department of Health and Human Services, Public Health Service, Centers for Disease Control and Prevention, National Institute for Occupational Safety and Health, DHHS (NIOSH) Publication No. 2004-165.[3]
4. Polovich, M., White, J. M., & Kelleher, L.O. (eds.) 2005. Chemotherapy and biotherapy guidelines and recommendations for practice (2nd. ed.) Pittsburgh, PA: Oncology.

TEMODAR for Injection

Manufactured by: Baxter Oncology GmbH, Halle/Westfalen, Germany. Distributed by: Schering Corporation, a subsidiary of **MERCK & CO., INC.**, Whitehouse Station, NJ 08889, USA.

PHARMACIST:

Tear at perforation and give to patient.

PHARMACIST INFORMATION SHEET

IMPORTANT DISPENSING INFORMATION

For every patient, TEMODAR must be dispensed in a separate vial or in its original glass bottle making sure each container lists the strength per capsule and that patients take the appropriate number of capsules from each bottle or vial.

Please see the dispensing instructions below for more information.

What is TEMODAR?

TEMODAR® (temozolomide) is an oral alkylating agent for the treatment of newly diagnosed glioblastoma multiforme and refractory anaplastic astrocytoma.

How is TEMODAR dosed?

The daily dose of TEMODAR Capsules for a given patient is calculated by the physician, based on the patient's body surface area (BSA). The resulting dose is then rounded off to the nearest 5 mg. An example of the dosing may be as follows: the initial daily dose of TEMODAR in milligrams is the BSA multiplied by mg/m²/day, (a patient with a BSA of 1.84 is 1.84 × 75 mg = 138, or 140 mg/day). The dose for subsequent cycles may be adjusted according to nadir neutrophil and platelet counts in the previous cycle and at the time of initiating the next cycle.

How might the dose of TEMODAR be modified for Refractory Anaplastic Astrocytoma?

Dosage of TEMODAR must be adjusted according to nadir neutrophil and platelet counts in the previous cycle and neutrophil and platelet counts at the time of initiating the next cycle. The initial dose is 150 mg/m² orally once daily for 5 consecutive days per 28-day treatment cycle. If both the nadir and day of dosing (Day 29, Day 1 of next cycle) absolute neutrophil counts (ANC) are ≥1.5 × 10⁹/L (1,500/μL) and both the nadir and Day 29, Day 1 of next cycle platelet counts are ≥100 × 10⁹/L (100,000/μL), the TEMODAR dose may be increased to 200 mg/m²/day for 5 consecutive days per 28-day treatment cycle. During treatment, a complete blood count should be obtained on Day 22 (21 days after the first dose) or within 48 hours of that day, and weekly until the ANC is above 1.5 × 10⁹/L (1,500/μL) and the platelet count exceeds 100 × 10⁹/L (100,000/μL). The next cycle of TEMODAR should not be started until the ANC and platelet count exceed these levels. If the ANC falls to <1.0 × 10⁹/L (1,000/μL) or the platelet count is <50 × 10⁹/L (50,000/μL) during any cycle, the next cycle should be reduced by 50 mg/m², but not below 100 mg/m², the lowest recommended dose (see **Table 1** below).

[See table at top of next column]

What is the TEMODAR Capsules treatment regimen?

TEMODAR is given for 5 consecutive days on a 28-day cycle. Patients should continue taking TEMODAR until their physician determines that their disease has progressed, up to 2 years, or until unacceptable side effects or toxicities occur. Physicians may alter the treatment regimen for a given patient.

Newly Diagnosed Concomitant Phase Treatment Schedule

TEMODAR is administered orally at 75 mg/m² daily for 42 days concomitant with focal radiotherapy (60Gy administered in 30 fractions), followed by maintenance TEMODAR for 6 cycles. No dose reductions are recommended, however, dose interruptions may occur based on patient tolerance. The TEMODAR dose can be continued throughout the 42 day concomitant period up to 49 days if all of the following

TABLE 1: Dosing Modification Table for Refractory Anaplastic Astrocytoma

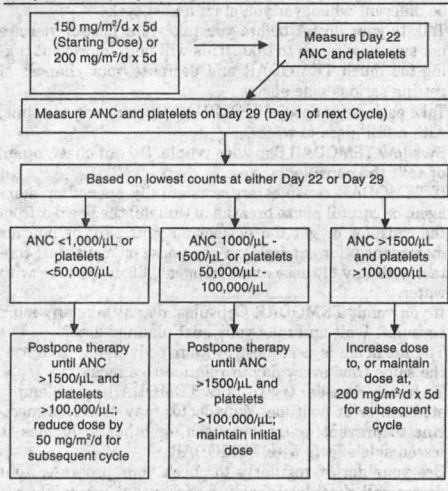

conditions are met: absolute neutrophil count ≥1.5 × 10⁹/L, platelet count ≥100 ×10⁹/L, common toxicity criteria (CTC) nonhematological toxicity ≤Grade 1 (except for alopecia, nausea and vomiting). During treatment a complete blood count should be obtained weekly. Temozolomide dosing should be interrupted or discontinued during concomitant phase according to the hematological and nonhematological toxicity criteria as noted in **Table 2**. PCP prophylaxis is required during the concomitant administration of TEMODAR and radiotherapy and should be continued in patients who develop lymphocytopenia until recovery from lymphocytopenia (CTC grade ≤1).

TABLE 2: Temozolomide Dosing Interruption or Discontinuation During Concomitant Radiotherapy and Temozolomide

Toxicity	TMZ Interruption*	TMZ Discontinuation
Absolute Neutrophil Count	≥0.5 and <1.5 × 10⁹/L	<0.5 × 10⁹/L
Platelet Count	≥10 and <100 × 10⁹/L	<10 × 10⁹/L
CTC Non-hematological Toxicity (except for alopecia, nausea, vomiting)	CTC Grade 2	CTC Grade 3 or 4

TMZ = temozolomide; CTC = Common Toxicity Criteria.
*Treatment with concomitant TMZ could be continued when all of the following conditions were met: absolute neutrophil count ≥1.5 × 10⁹/L; platelet count ≥100 × 10⁹/L; CTC non-hematological toxicity ≤Grade 1 (except for alopecia, nausea, vomiting).

Maintenance Phase Treatment Schedule

Four weeks after completing the TEMODAR + RT phase, TEMODAR is administered for an additional 6 cycles of maintenance treatment. Dosage in Cycle 1 (maintenance) is 150 mg/m² once daily for 5 days followed by 23 days without treatment. At the start of Cycle 2, the dose is escalated to 200 mg/m², if the CTC nonhematologic toxicity for Cycle 1 is Grade ≤2 (except for alopecia, nausea and vomiting), absolute neutrophil count (ANC) is ≥1.5 × 10⁹/L, and the platelet count is ≥100 × 10⁹/L. If the dose was not escalated at Cycle 2, escalation should not be done in subsequent cycles. The dose remains at 200 mg/m² per day for the first 5 days of each subsequent cycle except if toxicity occurs.

During treatment a complete blood count should be obtained on Day 22 (21 days after the first dose) or within 48 hours of that day, and weekly until the ANC is above 1.5 × 10⁹/L (1,500/μL) and the platelet count exceeds 100 × 10⁹/L (100,000/μL). The next cycle of TEMODAR should not be started until the ANC and platelet count exceed these levels. Dose reductions during the next cycle should be based on the lowest blood counts and worst non-hematologic toxicity during the previous cycle. Dose reductions or discontinuations during the maintenance phase should be applied according to Tables 3 and 4.

TABLE 3: Temozolomide Dose Levels for Maintenance Treatment

Dose Level	Dose (mg/m²/day)	Remarks
–1	100	Reduction for prior toxicity
0	150	Dose during Cycle 1
1	200	Dose during Cycles 2–6 in absence of toxicity

TABLE 4: Temozolomide Dose Reduction or Discontinuation During Maintenance Treatment

Toxicity	Reduce TMZ by 1 Dose Level*	Discontinue TMZ
Absolute Neutrophil Count	$<1.0 \times 10^9$/L	See footnote †
Platelet Count	$<50 \times 10^9$/L	See footnote †
CTC Non-hematological Toxicity (except for alopecia, nausea, vomiting)	CTC Grade 3	CTC Grade 4†

TMZ = temozolomide; CTC = Common Toxicity Criteria.
*TMZ dose levels are listed in Table 3.
†TMZ is to be discontinued if dose reduction to <100 mg/m² is required or if the same Grade 3 non-hematological toxicity (except for alopecia, nausea, vomiting) recurs after dose reduction.

How is TEMODAR taken?
Patients should take each day's dose with a full glass of water at the same time each day. Taking the medication on an empty stomach or at bedtime may help ease nausea. If patients are also taking antinausea or other medications to relieve the side effects associated with TEMODAR, they should be advised to take these medications 30 minutes before they take TEMODAR. Temozolomide causes the rapid appearance of malignant tumors in rats. Patients **SHOULD NOT** open or split the capsules. If capsules are accidentally opened or damaged, rigorous precautions should be taken with the capsule contents to avoid inhalation or contact with the skin or mucous membranes. The medication should be kept away from children and pets. The TEMODAR capsules should be swallowed whole and **NEVER CHEWED.**
What should the patient avoid during treatment with TEMODAR?
There are no dietary restrictions for patients taking TEMODAR. TEMODAR may affect testicular function, so male patients should exercise adequate birth control measures. TEMODAR may cause birth defects. Female patients should avoid becoming pregnant while receiving this drug. Women who are nursing prior to receiving TEMODAR should discontinue nursing. It is not known whether TEMODAR is excreted into breast milk.
What are the side effects of TEMODAR?
Nausea and vomiting are the most common side effects associated with TEMODAR. Noncumulative myelosuppression is the dose-limiting toxicity. Patients should be evaluated periodically by their physician to monitor blood counts. **Other commonly reported side effects reported by patients taking TEMODAR** are fatigue, constipation, alopecia, anorexia, and headache.
How is TEMODAR supplied?
TEMODAR Capsules are available in 5-mg, 20-mg, 100-mg, 140-mg, 180-mg, and 250-mg strengths. The capsules contain a white capsule body with a color cap, and the colors vary based on the dosage strength.

TEMODAR Capsule Strength	Color
5 mg	Green Cap
20 mg	Yellow Cap
100 mg	Pink Cap
140 mg	Blue Cap
180 mg	Orange Cap
250 mg	White Cap

The 5-mg, 20-mg, 100-mg, 140-mg, and 180-mg capsule strengths are available in 5-count and 14-count packages. The 250-mg capsule strength is available in a 5-count package.
How is TEMODAR dispensed?
Each strength of TEMODAR must be dispensed in a separate vial or in its original glass bottle (one strength per one container). Follow the instructions below:
Based on the dose prescribed, determine the number of each strength of TEMODAR capsules needed for the full 42- or 5-day cycle as prescribed by the physician. For example, in a 5-day cycle, 275 mg/day would be dispensed as five 250-mg capsules, five 20-mg capsules and five 5-mg capsules. Label each container with the appropriate number of capsules to be taken each day. Dispense to the patient, making sure each container lists the strength (mg) per capsule and that he or she understands to take the appropriate number of capsules of TEMODAR from each bottle or vial to equal the total daily dose prescribed by the physician.
How can TEMODAR be ordered?
TEMODAR can be ordered from your wholesaler. It is important to understand if TEMODAR is being used as part of a 42-day regimen or as part of a 5-day course. Remember to order enough TEMODAR for the appropriate cycle.
For example:
- a 5-day course of 360-mg/day would require the following to be ordered: two 5-count packages of 180-mg capsules.
- a 42-day course of 140-mg/day would require the following to be ordered: three 14-count packages of 140-mg capsules.

For examples of other dosing regimens, please refer to the full Prescribing Information (Table 10)

TEMODAR Product	NDC Number
5-mg capsules (5 count)	0085-3004-02
5-mg capsules (14 count)	0085-3004-01
20-mg capsules (5 count)	0085-1519-02
20-mg capsules (14 count)	0085-1519-01
100-mg capsules (5 count)	0085-1366-02
100-mg capsules (14 count)	0085-1366-01
140 mg capsules (5 count)	0085-1425-01
140 mg capsules (14 count)	0085-1425-02
180 mg capsules (5 count)	0085-1430-01
180 mg capsules (14 count)	0085-1430-02
250-mg capsules (5 count)	0085-1417-01

TEMODAR Capsules
Manufactured by: Schering Corporation, a subsidiary of **MERCK & CO., INC.**, Whitehouse Station, NJ 08889, USA.
Copyright© 2005 Schering Corporation, a subsidiary of **Merck & Co., Inc.** All rights reserved.
U.S. Patent No. 5,260,291. Rev. 4/10 332769XXT
Shown in Product Identification Guide, page 314

TICE® BCG ℞
[tīss BCG]
BCG LIVE
(FOR INTRAVESICAL USE)

WARNING
TICE® BCG contains live, attenuated mycobacteria. Because of the potential risk for transmission, it should be prepared, handled, and disposed of as a biohazard material (see PRECAUTIONS and DOSAGE AND ADMINISTRATION sections).
BCG infections have been reported in health care workers, primarily from exposures resulting from accidental needle sticks or skin lacerations during the preparation of BCG for administration. Nosocomial infections have been reported in patients receiving parenteral drugs that were prepared in areas in which BCG was reconstituted. BCG is capable of dissemination when administered by the intravesical route, and serious infections, including fatal infections, have been reported in patients receiving intravesical BCG (see WARNINGS, PRECAUTIONS, and ADVERSE REACTIONS sections).

DESCRIPTION
TICE® BCG for intravesical use, is an attenuated, live culture preparation of the Bacillus of Calmette and Guerin (BCG) strain of *Mycobacterium bovis*.[1] The TICE strain was developed at the University of Illinois from a strain originated at the Pasteur Institute.
The medium in which the BCG organism is grown for preparation of the freeze-dried cake is composed of the following ingredients: glycerin, asparagine, citric acid, potassium phosphate, magnesium sulfate, and iron ammonium citrate. The final preparation prior to freeze drying also contains lactose. The freeze-dried BCG preparation is delivered in glass vials, each containing 1 to 8×10^8 colony forming units (CFU) of TICE BCG which is equivalent to approximately 50 mg wet weight. Determination of *in vitro* potency is achieved through colony counts derived from a serial dilution assay. A single dose consists of 1 reconstituted vial (see **DOSAGE AND ADMINISTRATION**).
For intravesical use the entire vial is reconstituted with sterile saline. TICE BCG is viable upon reconstitution.
No preservatives have been added.

CLINICAL PHARMACOLOGY
TICE® BCG induces a granulomatous reaction at the local site of administration. Intravesical TICE BCG has been used as a therapy for, and prophylaxis against, recurrent tumors in patients with carcinoma *in situ* (CIS) of the urinary bladder, and to prevent recurrence of Stage TaT1 papillary tumors of the bladder at high risk of recurrence. The precise mechanism of action is unknown.

CLINICAL STUDIES
To evaluate the efficacy of intravesical administration of TICE® BCG in the treatment of carcinoma *in situ*, patients were identified who had been treated with TICE BCG under 6 different Investigational New Drug (IND) applications in which the most important shared aspect was the use of an induction plus maintenance schedule. Patients received TICE BCG (50 mg; 1 to 8×10^8 CFU) intravesically, once weekly for at least 6 weeks and once monthly thereafter for up to 12 months. A longer maintenance was given in some cases. The study population consisted of 153 patients, 132 males, 19 females, and 2 unidentified as to gender. Thirty patients lacking baseline documentation of CIS and 4 patients lost to follow-up were not evaluable for treatment response. Therefore, 119 patients were available for efficacy evaluation. The mean age was 69 years (range: 38-97 years). There were 2 categories of clinical response: (1) Complete Histological Response (CR), defined as complete resolution of carcinoma *in situ* documented by cystoscopy and cytology, with or without biopsy; and (2) Complete Clinical Response Without Cytology (CRNC), defined as an apparent complete disappearance of tumor upon cystoscopy. The results of a 1987 analysis of the evaluable patients are shown in **Table I.**
[See table I below]
A 1989 update of these data is presented in **Table II.** The median duration of follow-up was 47 months.
[See table II at top of next page]
There was no significant difference in response rates between patients with or without prior intravesical chemotherapy. The median duration of response, calculated from the Kaplan-Meier curve as median time to recurrence, is estimated at 4 years or greater. The incidence of cystectomy for 90 patients who achieved a complete response (CR or CRNC) was 11%. The median time to cystectomy in patients who achieved a complete response (CR or CRNC) exceeded 74 months.
The efficacy of intravesical TICE BCG in preventing the recurrence of a TaT1 bladder cancer after complete transurethral resection of all papillary tumors was evaluated in 2 open-label, randomized phase III clinical trials. Initial diagnosis of patients included in the studies was determined by cystoscopic biopsies. One was conducted by the Southwestern Oncology Group (SWOG) in patients at high risk of recurrence. High risk was defined as 2 occurrences of tumor within 56 weeks, any stage T1 tumor, or 3 or more tumors presenting simultaneously. The second study was conducted at the Nijmegen University Hospital; Nijmegen, The Netherlands. In this study patients were not selected for high risk of recurrence. In both studies treatment was initiated between 1 and 2 weeks after transurethral resection (TUR). In the SWOG trial (study 8795) patients were randomized to TICE BCG or mitomycin C (MMC). Both drugs were given intravesically weekly for 6 weeks, at 8 and 12 weeks, and then monthly for a total treatment duration of 1 year. Cystoscopy and urinary cytology were performed every 3 months for 2 years. Patients with progressive disease or residual or recurrent disease at or after the 6 month follow-up were removed from the study and were classified as treatment failures.
A total of 469 patients was entered into the study: 237 to the TICE BCG arm and 232 to the MMC arm. Twenty-two patients were subsequently found to be ineligible, and 66 patients had concurrent CIS, and were analyzed separately. Four patients were lost to follow-up, leaving 191 evaluable patients in the TICE BCG arm and 186 in the MMC arm. Of the patients, 84% were male and 16% were female. The average age of these patients was 65 years old.
The Kaplan-Meier estimates of 2-year disease-free survival are shown in **Table III.** The difference in disease-free survival time between the 2 groups was statistically significant by the log rank test (*P*=0.03). The 95% confidence interval of

TABLE I: The Response of Patients With CIS Bladder Cancer in 6 IND Studies

	Entered	Evaluable	CR	CRNC	Overall response
No. (%) of patients	153	119 (78%)	54 (46%)	36 (30%)	90 (76%)

TABLE II: Follow-up Response of Patients With CIS Bladder Cancer in 6 IND Studies
1989 Status of 90 Responders (CR or CRNC)

Response	1987/CR n=54	1987/CRNC n=36	1987 Response n=90	Percent
CR	30	15	45	50
CRNC	0	0	0	0
Unrelated deaths	6	6	12	13
Failure	18	15	33	37

TABLE IV: Results of Nijmegen Study

	TICE BCG Arm N=117	BCG-RIVM Arm N=134	MMC Arm N=136
Estimated disease-free survival at 2 years	53%	62%	64%
95% Confidence Interval (CI)	(44%, 64%)	(53%, 72%)	(55%, 74%)

the difference in 2-year disease-free survival was 12% ± 10%. No statistically significant differences between the groups were noted in time to tumor progression, tumor invasion, or overall survival.

TABLE III: Results of SWOG Study 8795

	TICE BCG Arm N=191	MMC Arm N=186
Estimated disease-free survival at 2 years	57%	45%
95% Confidence Interval (CI)	(50%, 65%)	(38%, 53%)

In the Nijmegen study, the efficacy of 3 treatments was compared: TICE substrain BCG, *Rijksinstituut voor Volksgezondheid en Milieuhygiene* substrain BCG (BCG-RIVM), and MMC.
TICE BCG and BCG-RIVM were given intravesically weekly for 6 weeks. In contrast to the SWOG study, maintenance BCG was not given. Mitomycin C was given intravesically weekly for 4 weeks and then monthly for a total duration of treatment of 6 months. Cystoscopy and urinary cytology were performed every 3 months until recurrence.
A total of 469 patients was enrolled and randomized. Thirty-two patients were not evaluable, 17 were ineligible, 15 were withdrawn before treatment, and 50 had concurrent CIS and were analyzed separately, leaving 387 evaluable patients: 117 in the TICE BCG arm, 134 in the BCG-RIVM arm, and 136 in the MMC arm. Twenty-eight patients (24%) in the TICE BCG arm, 32 patients (24%) in the BCG-RIVM arm, and 24 patients (18%) in the MMC arm had TaG1 tumors. The median duration of follow-up was 22 months (range: 3-54 months).
The Kaplan-Meier estimates of 2-year disease-free survival are shown in **Table IV**. The differences in disease-free survival among the 3 arms were not statistically significant by the log-rank test (P=0.08).
[See table IV above]
In both the SWOG 8795 study and the Nijmegen study, acute toxicity was more common, and usually more severe, with TICE BCG than with MMC (see **ADVERSE REACTIONS**).

INDICATIONS AND USAGE

TICE® BCG is indicated for the treatment and prophylaxis of carcinoma *in situ* (CIS) of the urinary bladder, and for the prophylaxis of primary or recurrent stage Ta and/or T1 papillary tumors following transurethral resection (TUR). TICE BCG is not recommended for stage TaG1 papillary tumors, unless they are judged to be at high risk of tumor recurrence.
TICE BCG is not indicated for papillary tumors of stages higher than T1.

CONTRAINDICATIONS

TICE® BCG should not be used in immunosuppressed patients or persons with congenital or acquired immune deficiencies, whether due to concurrent disease (e.g., AIDS, leukemia, lymphoma) cancer therapy (e.g., cytotoxic drugs, radiation), or immunosuppressive therapy (e.g., corticosteroids).
Treatment should be postponed until resolution of a concurrent febrile illness, urinary tract infection, or gross hematuria. Seven to 14 days should elapse before BCG is administered following biopsy, TUR, or traumatic catheterization.
TICE BCG should not be administered to persons with active tuberculosis. Active tuberculosis should be ruled out in individuals who are PPD positive before starting treatment with TICE BCG.

WARNINGS

BCG LIVE (TICE® BCG) is not a vaccine for the prevention of cancer. BCG Vaccine USP, not BCG LIVE (TICE BCG), should be used for the prevention of tuberculosis. For vaccination use, refer to BCG Vaccine USP prescribing information.
TICE BCG is an infectious agent. Physicians using this product should be familiar with the literature on the prevention and treatment of BCG-related complications, and should be prepared in such emergencies to contact an infectious disease specialist with experience in treating the infectious complications of intravesical BCG. The treatment of the infectious complications of BCG requires long-term, multiple-drug antibiotic therapy. Special culture media are required for mycobacteria, and physicians administering intravesical BCG or those caring for these patients should have these media readily available.
Instillation of TICE BCG with an actively bleeding mucosa may promote systemic BCG infection. Treatment should be postponed for at least 1 week following transurethral resection, biopsy, traumatic catheterization, or gross hematuria. Deaths have been reported as a result of systemic BCG infection and sepsis.[2,3] Patients should be monitored for the presence of symptoms and signs of toxicity after each intravesical treatment. Febrile episodes with flu-like symptoms lasting more than 72 hours, fever ≥103°F, systemic manifestations increasing in intensity with repeated instillations, or persistent abnormalities of liver function tests suggest systemic BCG infection and may require antituberculous therapy. Local symptoms (prostatitis, epididymitis, orchitis) lasting more than 2 to 3 days may also suggest active infection (see **WARNINGS, Management of Serious BCG Complications** section).
The use of TICE BCG may cause tuberculin sensitivity. Since this is a valuable aid in the diagnosis of tuberculosis, it is advisable to determine the tuberculin reactivity by PPD skin testing before treatment.
Intravesical instillations of BCG should be postponed during treatment with antibiotics, since antimicrobial therapy may interfere with the effectiveness of TICE BCG (see **PRECAUTIONS**). TICE BCG should not be used in individuals with concurrent infections.
Small bladder capacity has been associated with increased risk of severe local reactions and should be considered in deciding to use TICE BCG therapy.
Management of Serious BCG Complications.
Acute, localized irritative toxicities of TICE BCG may be accompanied by systemic manifestations, consistent with a "flu-like" syndrome. Systemic adverse effects of 1 to 2 days' duration such as malaise, fever, and chills often reflect hypersensitivity reactions. However, **symptoms such as fever of ≥38.5°C (101.3°F), or acute localized inflammation such as epididymitis, prostatitis, or orchitis persisting longer than 2 to 3 days suggest active infection, and evaluation for serious infectious complication should be considered.**
In patients who develop persistent fever or experience an acute febrile illness consistent with BCG infection, 2 or more antimycobacterial agents should be administered while diagnostic evaluation, including cultures, is conducted. **BCG treatment should be discontinued.** Negative cultures do not necessarily rule out infection. Physicians using this product should be familiar with the literature on prevention, diagnosis, and treatment of BCG-related complications and, when appropriate, should consult an infectious disease specialist or other physician with experience in the diagnosis and treatment of mycobacterial infections. TICE BCG is sensitive to the most commonly used antituberculous agents (isoniazid, rifampin, and ethambutol). **TICE BCG is not sensitive to pyrazinamide.**

PRECAUTIONS

General

TICE® BCG contains live mycobacteria and should be prepared and handled using aseptic technique (see **DOSAGE AND ADMINISTRATION, Preparation of Agent** section).
BCG infections have been reported in health care workers preparing BCG for administration. Needle stick injuries should be avoided during the handling and mixing of TICE BCG. Nosocomial infections have been reported in patients receiving parenteral drugs which were prepared in areas in which BCG was prepared.[4]
BCG is capable of dissemination when administered by intravesical route, and serious reactions, including fatal infections, have been reported in patients receiving intravesical BCG.[3] Care should be taken not to traumatize the urinary tract or to introduce contaminants into the urinary system. Seven to 14 days should elapse before TICE BCG is administered following TUR, biopsy, or traumatic catheterization. TICE BCG should be administered with caution to persons in groups at high risk for HIV infection.

Laboratory Tests

The use of TICE BCG may cause tuberculin sensitivity. It is advisable to determine the tuberculin reactivity of patients receiving TICE BCG by PPD skin testing before treatment is initiated.

Information for Patients

TICE BCG is retained in the bladder for 2 hours and then voided. Patients should void while seated in order to avoid splashing of urine. For the 6 hours after treatment, urine voided should be disinfected for 15 minutes with an equal volume of household bleach before flushing. Patients should be instructed to increase fluid intake in order to "flush" the bladder in the hours following BCG treatment. Patients may experience burning with the first void after treatment. Patients should be attentive to side effects, such as fever, chills, malaise, flu-like symptoms, or increased fatigue. If the patient experiences severe urinary side effects, such as burning or pain on urination, urgency, frequency of urination, blood in urine, or other symptoms such as joint pain, cough, or skin rash, the physician should be notified.

Drug Interaction

Drug combinations containing immunosuppressants and/or bone marrow depressants and/or radiation interfere with the development of the immune response and should not be used in combination with TICE BCG. Antimicrobial therapy for other infections may interfere with the effectiveness of TICE BCG. There are no data to suggest that the acute, local urinary tract toxicity common with BCG is due to mycobacterial infection, and **antituberculosis drugs (e.g., isoniazid) should not be used to prevent or treat the local, irritative toxicities of TICE BCG.**

Carcinogenesis, Mutagenesis, Impairment of Fertility

TICE BCG has not been evaluated for its carcinogenic, mutagenic potentials, or impairment of fertility.

Pregnancy

Teratogenic Effects – Pregnancy Category C
Animal reproduction studies have not been conducted with TICE BCG. It is also not known whether TICE BCG can cause fetal harm when administered to a pregnant woman or can affect reproductive capacity. TICE BCG should not be given to a pregnant woman except when clearly needed. Women should be advised not to become pregnant while on therapy.

Nursing Mothers

It is not known whether TICE BCG is excreted in human milk. Because many drugs are excreted in human milk and because of the potential for serious adverse reactions from TICE BCG in nursing infants, it is advisable to discontinue nursing or to discontinue the drug, taking into account the importance of the drug to the mother.

Pediatric Use

Safety and effectiveness of TICE BCG for the treatment of superficial bladder cancer in pediatric patients have not been established.

Geriatric Use

Of the total number of subjects in clinical studies of TICE BCG, the average age was 66 years old. No overall difference in safety or effectiveness was observed between older and younger subjects. Other reported clinical experience has not identified differences in response between elderly and younger patients, but greater sensitivity of some older individuals to BCG cannot be ruled out.

ADVERSE REACTIONS

Symptoms of bladder irritability, related to the inflammatory response induced, are reported in approximately 60% of patients receiving TICE® BCG. The symptoms typically begin 4 to 6 hours after instillation and last 24 to 72 hours. The irritative side effects are usually seen following the third instillation, and tend to increase in severity after each administration.
The irritative bladder adverse effects can usually be managed symptomatically with products such as pyridium, propantheline bromide, oxybutynin chloride, and acetaminophen. The mechanism of action of the irritative side effects has not been firmly established, but is most consistent with an immunological mechanism.[3] There is no evidence that dose reduction or antituberculous drug therapy can prevent or lessen the irritative toxicity of TICE BCG.

"Flu-like" symptoms (malaise, fever, and chills) which may accompany the localized, irritative toxicities often reflect hypersensitivity reactions which can be treated symptomatically. Antihistamines have also been used.[5]

Adverse reactions to TICE BCG tend to be progressive in frequency and severity with subsequent instillation. Delay or postponement of subsequent treatment may or may not reduce the severity of a reaction during subsequent instillation.

Although uncommon, serious infectious complications of intravesical BCG have been reported.[2,3,6] The most serious infectious complication of BCG is disseminated sepsis with associated mortality. In addition, *M. bovis* infections have been reported in lung, liver, bone, bone marrow, kidney, regional lymph nodes, and prostate in patients who have received intravesical BCG. Some male genitourinary tract infections (orchitis/epididymitis) have been resistant to multiple-drug antituberculous therapy and required orchiectomy.

If a patient develops persistent fever or experiences an acute febrile illness consistent with BCG infection, BCG treatment should be discontinued and the patient immediately evaluated and treated for systemic infection (see WARNINGS).

The local and systemic adverse reactions reported in a review of 674 patients with superficial bladder cancer, including 153 patients with carcinoma *in situ*, are summarized in **Table V.**

[See table V above]

The following adverse events were reported in ≤1% of patients: anemia, BCG sepsis, coagulopathy, contracted bladder, diarrhea, epididymitis/prostatitis, hepatic granuloma, hepatitis, leukopenia, neurologic (unclassified), orchitis, pneumonitis, pyuria, rash, thrombocytopenia, urethritis, and urinary obstruction.

In SWOG study 8795, toxicity evaluations were available on a total of 222 TICE BCG-treated patients and 220 MMC-treated patients. Direct bladder toxicity (cramps, dysuria, frequency, urgency, hematuria, hemorrhagic cystitis, or incontinence) was seen more often with TICE BCG with 356 events, compared to 234 events for MMC. Grade ≤2 toxicity was seen significantly more frequently following TICE BCG treatment (P=0.003). No life-threatening toxicity was seen in either arm. Systemic toxicity with TICE BCG was markedly increased compared to that of MMC, with 181 events for TICE BCG compared to 80 for MMC. The frequency of toxicity was increased in all grades, particularly for grades 2 and 3. The most common complaints were malaise, fatigue and lethargy, fever, and abdominal pain. Thirty-two TICE BCG patients were reported to have been treated with isoniazid. Five TICE BCG patients had liver enzyme elevation, including 2 with grade 3 elevations. Eighteen of the 222 (8.1%) TICE BCG patients failed to complete the prescribed protocol compared to 6.2% in the MMC group. **Table VI** summarizes the most common adverse reactions reported in this trial.[7]

[See table VI above]

OVERDOSAGE

Overdosage occurs if more than 1 vial of TICE® BCG is administered per instillation. If overdosage occurs, the patient should be closely monitored for signs of active local or systemic BCG infection. For acute local or systemic reactions suggesting active infection, an infectious disease specialist experienced in BCG complications should be consulted.

DOSAGE AND ADMINISTRATION

The dose for the intravesical treatment of carcinoma *in situ* and for the prophylaxis of recurrent papillary tumors consists of 1 vial of TICE® BCG suspended in 50 mL preservative-free saline.

Do not inject subcutaneously or intravenously.

Preparation of Agent

The preparation of the TICE BCG suspension should be done using aseptic technique. To avoid cross-contamination, parenteral drugs should not be prepared in areas where BCG has been prepared. A separate area for the preparation of the TICE BCG suspension is recommended. All equipment, supplies, and receptacles in contact with TICE BCG should be handled and disposed of as biohazardous. The pharmacist or individual responsible for mixing the agent should wear gloves and take precautions to avoid contact of BCG with broken skin. If preparation cannot be performed in a biocontainment hood, then a mask and gown should be worn to avoid inhalation of BCG organisms and inadvertent exposure to broken skin.

Option 1 (Using Syringe Method)

Draw 1 mL of sterile, preservative-free saline (0.9% Sodium Chloride Injection USP) at 4°-25°C into a small syringe (e.g., 3 mL) and add to 1 vial of TICE BCG to resuspend. Gently swirl the vial until a homogenous suspension is obtained. Avoid forceful agitation which may cause clumping of the mycobacteria. Dispense the cloudy TICE BCG suspension into the top end of a catheter-tip syringe which contains 49 mL of saline diluent, bringing the total volume to 50 mL. To mix, gently rotate the syringe.

Option 2 (Using Reconstitution Accessories)

Reconstitution Accessories may be provided with each TICE BCG product order. Please refer to the Reconstitution Accessories Instructions provided with the accessories for a full description of the product reconstitution procedures using these accessories.

The reconstituted TICE BCG should be kept refrigerated (2°-8°C), protected from exposure to direct sunlight, and used within 2 hours. Unused solution should be discarded after 2 hours.

Note: DO NOT filter the contents of the TICE BCG vial. Precautions should be taken to avoid exposing the TICE BCG to direct sunlight. Bacteriostatic solutions must be avoided. In addition, use only sterile, preservative-free saline, 0.9% Sodium Chloride Injection USP as diluent.

Treatment and Schedule

Allow 7 to 14 days to elapse after bladder biopsy before TICE BCG is administered. Patients should not drink fluids for 4 hours before treatment and should empty their bladder prior to TICE BCG administration. The reconstituted TICE BCG is instilled into the bladder by gravity flow via the catheter. **DO NOT** depress plunger and force the flow of the TICE BCG. The TICE BCG is retained in the bladder 2 hours and then voided. Patients unable to retain the suspension for 2 hours should be allowed to void sooner, if necessary.

While the BCG is retained in the bladder, the patient ideally should be repositioned from left side to right side and also should lie upon the back and the abdomen, changing these positions every 15 minutes to maximize bladder surface exposure to the agent.

A standard treatment schedule consists of 1 intravesical instillation per week for 6 weeks. This schedule may be repeated once if tumor remission has not been achieved and if the clinical circumstances warrant. Thereafter, intravesical TICE BCG administration should continue at approximately monthly intervals for at least 6 to 12 months. There are no data to support the interchangeability of BCG LIVE products.

HOW SUPPLIED

TICE® BCG is supplied in a box of 1 vial of TICE BCG. Each vial contains 1 to 8×10^8 CFU, which is equivalent to approximately 50 mg (wet weight), as lyophilized (freeze-dried) powder, NDC 0052-0602-02.

STORAGE

The intact vials of TICE® BCG should be stored refrigerated, at 2-8°C (36-46°F).

This agent contains live bacteria and should be protected from **direct** sunlight.

The product should not be used after the expiration date printed on the label.

Rx Only

TABLE V: Summary of Adverse Effects Seen in 674 Patients with Superficial Bladder Cancer, Including 153 With Carcinoma *in Situ*

Adverse event	N	Percent of patients Overall (Grade ≥3)	Adverse event	N	Percent of patients Overall (Grade ≥3)
Dysuria	401	60% (11%)	Arthritis/myalgia	18	3% (<1%)
Urinary frequency	272	40% (7%)	Headache/dizziness	16	2% (0)
Flu-like syndrome	224	33% (9%)	Urinary incontinence	16	2% (0)
Hematuria	175	26% (7%)	Anorexia/weight loss	15	2% (<1%)
Fever	134	20% (8%)	Urinary debris	15	2% (<1%)
Malaise/fatigue	50	7% (0)	Allergy	14	2% (<1%)
Cystitis	40	6% (2%)	Cardiac (unclassified)	13	2% (1%)
Urgency	39	6% (1%)	Genital inflammation/ abscess	12	2% (<1%)
Nocturia	30	5% (1%)	Respiratory (unclassified)	11	2% (<1%)
Cramps/pain	27	4% (1%)	Urinary tract infection	10	2% (1%)
Rigors	22	3% (1%)	Abdominal pain	10	2% (1%)
Nausea/vomiting	20	3% (<1%)			

TABLE VI: Most Common Adverse Reactions in SWOG Study 8795*

	Study Arm				
	TICE BCG (N=222)		MMC (N=220)		
Adverse event	All Grades	Grade ≥3	All Grades	Grade ≥3	
Dysuria	115 (52%)	6 (3%)	77 (35%)	5 (2%)	
Urgency/frequency	112 (50%)	5 (2%)	63 (29%)	7 (3%)	
Hematuria	85 (38%)	6 (3%)	56 (25%)	5 (2%)	
Flu-like symptoms	54 (24%)	1 (<1%)	29 (13%)	0	
Fever	37 (17%)	1 (<1%)	7 (3%)	0	
Pain (not specified)	37 (17%)	4 (2%)	22 (10%)	1 (<1%)	
Hemorrhagic cystitis	19 (9%)	3 (1%)	10 (5%)	0	
Chills	19 (9%)	0	2 (1%)	0	
Bladder cramps	18 (8%)	0	9 (4%)	0	
Nausea	16 (7%)	0	12 (5%)	0	
Incontinence	8 (4%)	0	3 (1%)	0	
Myalgia/arthralgia	7 (3%)	0	0	0	
Diaphoresis	7 (3%)	0	1 (<1%)	0	
Rash	6 (3%)	1 (<1%)	16 (7%)	2 (1%)	

*The adverse reaction profile of TICE BCG was similar in the Nijmegen study.[8]

REFERENCES

1. DeJager R, Guinan P, Lamm D, Khanna O, Brosman S, DeKernion J, et al. Long-Term Complete Remission in Bladder Carcinoma in Situ with Intravesical TICE Bacillus Calmette Guerin. *Urology* 1991;38:507-513.
2. Rawls WH, Lamm DL, Lowe BA, Crawford ED, Sarosdy MF, Montie JE, Grossman HB, Scardino PT. Fatal Sepsis Following Intravesical Bacillus Calmette-Guerin Administration For Bladder Cancer. *J Urol* 1990; 144: 1328-1330.
3. Lamm DL, van der Meijden APM, Morales A, Brosman SA, Catalona WJ, Herr HW, et al. Incidence and Treatment of Complications of Bacillus Calmette-Guerin Intravesical Therapy in Superficial Bladder Cancer. *J. Urol* 1992;147:596-600.
4. Stone MM, Vannier AM, Storch SK, Nitta AT, Zhang Y. Brief Report: Meningitis Due to Iatrogenic BCG Infection in Two Immunocompromised Children. *NEJM* 1995:333: 561-563.
5. Steg A, Leleu C, Debre B, Gibod-Boccon L, Sicard D. Systemic Bacillus Calmette-Guerin Infection in Patients Treated by Intravesical BCG Therapy for Superficial Bladder Cancer. *EORTC Genitourinary Group Monograph 6: BCG in Superficial Bladder Cancer.* Edited by F.M. J. Debruyne, L. Denis and A.P.M. van der Meijden. New York: Alan R. Liss Inc., pp. 325-334.
6. van der Meijden, APM. Practical Approaches to the Prevention and Treatment of Adverse Reactions to BCG. *Eur Urol* 1995;27(suppl 1):23-28.
7. Lamm DL, Blumenstein BA, Crawford ED, Crissman JD, Lowe BA, Smith JA, Sarosdy MF, Schellhammer PF, Sagalowsky AI, Messing EM, et al. Randomized Intergroup Comparison of Bacillus Calmette-Guerin Immunotherapy and Mitomycin C Chemotherapy Prophylaxis in Superficial Transitional Cell Carcinoma of the Bladder. *Urol Oncol* 1995;1:119-126.
8. Witjes JA, van der Meijden APM, Witjes WPJ, et al. A Randomized Prospective Study Comparing Intravesical Instillations of Mitomycin-C, BCG-Tice, and BCG-RIVM in pTa-pT1 Tumours and Primary Carcinoma *In Situ* of the Urinary Bladder. *Eur J Cancer* 1993;29A(12): 1672-1676.

Manufactured for:
Organon USA Inc.
Roseland, NJ 07068

Manufactured by:
Organon Teknika
Corporation LLC
Durham, NC 27712
U.S. License No. 1747
TICE® is a registered trademark owned by the University of Illinois and licensed to Organon Teknika Corporation LLC.
Rev. 6/09 33639309T
Shown in Product Identification Guide, page 314

TRUSOPT® ℞
(dorzolamide hydrochloride ophthalmic solution)
Sterile Ophthalmic Solution 2%

DESCRIPTION

TRUSOPT[1] (dorzolamide hydrochloride ophthalmic solution) is a carbonic anhydrase inhibitor formulated for topical ophthalmic use.
Dorzolamide hydrochloride is described chemically as: (4*S*-*trans*)-4-(ethylamino)-5,6-dihydro-6-methyl-4*H*-thieno[2,3-*b*]thiopyran-2-sulfonamide 7,7-dioxide monohydrochloride. Dorzolamide hydrochloride is optically active. The specific rotation is

$$\alpha^{25°}_{405} \text{ (C=1, water)} = \sim -17°.$$

Its empirical formula is $C_{10}H_{16}N_2O_4S_3$•HCl and its structural formula is:

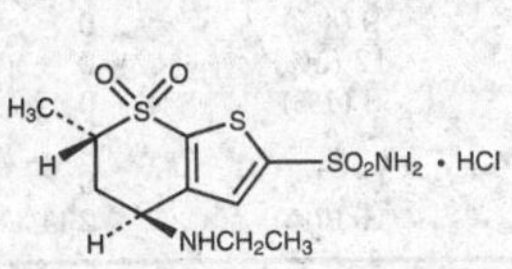

Dorzolamide hydrochloride has a molecular weight of 360.9 and a melting point of about 264°C. It is a white to off-white, crystalline powder, which is soluble in water and slightly soluble in methanol and ethanol.
TRUSOPT Sterile Ophthalmic Solution is supplied as a sterile, isotonic, buffered, slightly viscous, aqueous solution of dorzolamide hydrochloride. The pH of the solution is approximately 5.6, and the osmolarity is 260-330 mOsM. Each mL of TRUSOPT 2% contains 20 mg dorzolamide (22.3 mg of dorzolamide hydrochloride). Inactive ingredients are hydroxyethyl cellulose, mannitol, sodium citrate dihydrate, sodium hydroxide (to adjust pH) and water for injection. Benzalkonium chloride 0.0075% is added as a preservative.

[1] Registered trademark of Merck Sharp & Dohme Corp., a subsidiary of **Merck & Co., Inc.**
Copyright © 1994, 2003 Merck Sharp & Dohme Corp., a subsidiary of **Merck & Co., Inc.**
All rights reserved

CLINICAL PHARMACOLOGY

Mechanism of Action
Carbonic anhydrase (CA) is an enzyme found in many tissues of the body including the eye. It catalyzes the reversible reaction involving the hydration of carbon dioxide and the dehydration of carbonic acid. In humans, carbonic anhydrase exists as a number of isoenzymes, the most active being carbonic anhydrase II (CA-II), found primarily in red blood cells (RBCs), but also in other tissues. Inhibition of carbonic anhydrase in the ciliary processes of the eye decreases aqueous humor secretion, presumably by slowing the formation of bicarbonate ions with subsequent reduction in sodium and fluid transport. The result is a reduction in intraocular pressure (IOP).
TRUSOPT Ophthalmic Solution contains dorzolamide hydrochloride, an inhibitor of human carbonic anhydrase II. Following topical ocular administration, TRUSOPT reduces elevated intraocular pressure. Elevated intraocular pressure is a major risk factor in the pathogenesis of optic nerve damage and glaucomatous visual field loss.

Pharmacokinetics/Pharmacodynamics
When topically applied, dorzolamide reaches the systemic circulation. To assess the potential for systemic carbonic anhydrase inhibition following topical administration, drug and metabolite concentrations in RBCs and plasma and carbonic anhydrase inhibition in RBCs were measured. Dorzolamide accumulates in RBCs during chronic dosing as a result of binding to CA-II. The parent drug forms a single N-desethyl metabolite, which inhibits CA-II less potently than the parent drug but also inhibits CA-I. The metabolite also accumulates in RBCs where it binds primarily to CA-I. Plasma concentrations of dorzolamide and metabolite are generally below the assay limit of quantitation (15nM). Dorzolamide binds moderately to plasma proteins (approximately 33%). Dorzolamide is primarily excreted unchanged in the urine; the metabolite also is excreted in urine. After dosing is stopped, dorzolamide washes out of RBCs nonlinearly, resulting in a rapid decline of drug concentration initially, followed by a slower elimination phase with a half-life of about four months.
To simulate the systemic exposure after long-term topical ocular administration, dorzolamide was given orally to eight healthy subjects for up to 20 weeks. The oral dose of 2 mg b.i.d. closely approximates the amount of drug delivered by topical ocular administration of TRUSOPT 2% t.i.d. Steady state was reached within 8 weeks. The inhibition of CA-II and total carbonic anhydrase activities was below the degree of inhibition anticipated to be necessary for a pharmacological effect on renal function and respiration in healthy individuals.

Clinical Studies
The efficacy of TRUSOPT was demonstrated in clinical studies in the treatment of elevated intraocular pressure in patients with glaucoma or ocular hypertension (baseline IOP ≥ 23 mmHg). The IOP-lowering effect of TRUSOPT was approximately 3 to 5 mmHg throughout the day and this was consistent in clinical studies of up to one year duration.
The efficacy of TRUSOPT when dosed less frequently than three times a day (alone or in combination with other products) has not been established.
In a one year clinical study, the effect of TRUSOPT 2% t.i.d. on the corneal endothelium was compared to that of betaxolol ophthalmic solution b.i.d. and timolol maleate ophthalmic solution 0.5% b.i.d. There were no statistically significant differences between groups in corneal endothelial cell counts or in corneal thickness measurements. There was a mean loss of approximately 4% in the endothelial cell counts for each group over the one year period.

INDICATIONS AND USAGE

TRUSOPT Ophthalmic Solution is indicated in the treatment of elevated intraocular pressure in patients with ocular hypertension or open-angle glaucoma.

CONTRAINDICATIONS

TRUSOPT is contraindicated in patients who are hypersensitive to any component of this product.

WARNINGS

TRUSOPT is a sulfonamide and, although administered topically, is absorbed systemically. Therefore, the same types of adverse reactions that are attributable to sulfonamides may occur with topical administration with TRUSOPT. Fatalities have occurred, although rarely, due to severe reactions to sulfonamides including Stevens-Johnson syndrome, toxic epidermal necrolysis, fulminant hepatic necrosis, agranulocytosis, aplastic anemia, and other blood dyscrasias. Sensitization may recur when a sulfonamide is readministered irrespective of the route of administration. If signs of serious reactions or hypersensitivity occur, discontinue the use of this preparation.

PRECAUTIONS

General
The management of patients with acute angle-closure glaucoma requires therapeutic interventions in addition to ocular hypotensive agents. TRUSOPT has not been studied in patients with acute angle-closure glaucoma.
TRUSOPT has not been studied in patients with severe renal impairment (CrCl < 30 mL/min). Because TRUSOPT and its metabolite are excreted predominantly by the kidney, TRUSOPT is not recommended in such patients.
TRUSOPT has not been studied in patients with hepatic impairment and should therefore be used with caution in such patients.
In clinical studies, local ocular adverse effects, primarily conjunctivitis and lid reactions, were reported with chronic administration of TRUSOPT. Many of these reactions had the clinical appearance and course of an allergic-type reaction that resolved upon discontinuation of drug therapy. If such reactions are observed, TRUSOPT should be discontinued and the patient evaluated before considering restarting the drug. (See ADVERSE REACTIONS.)
There is a potential for an additive effect on the known systemic effects of carbonic anhydrase inhibition in patients receiving an oral carbonic anhydrase inhibitor and TRUSOPT. The concomitant administration of TRUSOPT and oral carbonic anhydrase inhibitors is not recommended.
There have been reports of bacterial keratitis associated with the use of multiple-dose containers of topical ophthalmic products. These containers had been inadvertently contaminated by patients who, in most cases, had a concurrent corneal disease or a disruption of the ocular epithelial surface.
Choroidal detachment has been reported with administration of aqueous suppressant therapy (e.g., dorzolamide) after filtration procedures.
There is an increased potential for developing corneal edema in patients with low endothelial cell counts. Precautions should be used when prescribing TRUSOPT to this group of patients.

Information for Patients
TRUSOPT is a sulfonamide and although administered topically is absorbed systemically. Therefore the same types of adverse reactions that are attributable to sulfonamides may occur with topical administration. Patients should be advised that if serious or unusual reactions including severe skin reactions or signs of hypersensitivity occur, they should discontinue the use of the product (see WARNINGS).
Patients should be advised that if they develop any ocular reactions, particularly conjunctivitis and lid reactions, they should discontinue use and seek their physician's advice.
Patients should be instructed to avoid allowing the tip of the dispensing container to contact the eye or surrounding structures.
Patients should also be instructed that ocular solutions, if handled improperly or if the tip of the dispensing container contacts the eye or surrounding structures, can become contaminated by common bacteria known to cause ocular infections. Serious damage to the eye and subsequent loss of vision may result from using contaminated solutions.
Patients also should be advised that if they have ocular surgery or develop an intercurrent ocular condition (e.g., trauma or infection), they should immediately seek their physician's advice concerning the continued use of the present multidose container.
If more than one topical ophthalmic drug is being used, the drugs should be administered at least ten minutes apart.
Patients should be advised that TRUSOPT contains benzalkonium chloride which may be absorbed by soft contact lenses. Contact lenses should be removed prior to administration of the solution. Lenses may be reinserted 15 minutes following TRUSOPT administration.

Drug Interactions
Although acid-base and electrolyte disturbances were not reported in the clinical trials with TRUSOPT, these disturbances have been reported with oral carbonic anhydrase inhibitors and have, in some instances, resulted in drug interactions (e.g., toxicity associated with high-dose salicylate therapy). Therefore, the potential for such drug interactions should be considered in patients receiving TRUSOPT.

Carcinogenesis, Mutagenesis, Impairment of Fertility
In a two-year study of dorzolamide hydrochloride administered orally to male and female Sprague-Dawley rats, urinary bladder papillomas were seen in male rats in the highest dosage group of 20 mg/kg/day (250 times the recommended human ophthalmic dose). Papillomas were not seen in rats given oral doses equivalent to approximately 12 times the recommended human ophthalmic dose. No treatment-related tumors were seen in a 21-month study in female and male mice given oral doses up to 75 mg/kg/day (~900 times the recommended human ophthalmic dose).
The increased incidence of urinary bladder papillomas seen in the high-dose male rats is a class-effect of carbonic anhydrase inhibitors in rats. Rats are particularly prone to developing papillomas in response to foreign bodies, compounds causing crystalluria, and diverse sodium salts.
No changes in bladder urothelium were seen in dogs given oral dorzolamide hydrochloride for one year at 2 mg/kg/day (25 times the recommended human ophthalmic dose) or monkeys dosed topically to the eye at 0.4 mg/kg/day (~5 times the recommended human ophthalmic dose) for one year.
The following tests for mutagenic potential were negative: (1) *in vivo* (mouse) cytogenetic assay; (2) *in vitro* chromosomal aberration assay; (3) alkaline elution assay; (4) V-79 assay; and (5) Ames test.
In reproduction studies of dorzolamide hydrochloride in rats, there were no adverse effects on the reproductive capacity of males or females at doses up to 188 or 94 times, respectively, the recommended human ophthalmic dose.

Pregnancy
Teratogenic Effects
Pregnancy Category C
Developmental toxicity studies with dorzolamide hydrochloride in rabbits at oral doses of ≥ 2.5 mg/kg/day (31 times the recommended human ophthalmic dose) revealed malformations of the vertebral bodies. These malformations occurred at doses that caused metabolic acidosis with decreased body weight gain in dams and decreased fetal weights. No treatment-related malformations were seen at 1.0 mg/kg/day (13 times the recommended human ophthalmic dose). There are no adequate and well-controlled studies in pregnant women. TRUSOPT should be used during pregnancy only if the potential benefit justifies the potential risk to the fetus.

Nursing Mothers

In a study of dorzolamide hydrochloride in lactating rats, decreases in body weight gain of 5 to 7% in offspring at an oral dose of 7.5 mg/kg/day (94 times the recommended human ophthalmic dose) were seen during lactation. A slight delay in postnatal development (incisor eruption, vaginal canalization and eye openings), secondary to lower fetal body weight, was noted.

It is not known whether this drug is excreted in human milk. Because many drugs are excreted in human milk and because of the potential for serious adverse reactions in nursing infants from TRUSOPT, a decision should be made whether to discontinue nursing or to discontinue the drug, taking into account the importance of the drug to the mother.

Pediatric Use

Safety and IOP-lowering effects of TRUSOPT have been demonstrated in pediatric patients in a 3-month, multicenter, double-masked, active-treatment-controlled trial.

Geriatric Use

No overall differences in safety or effectiveness have been observed between elderly and younger patients.

ADVERSE REACTIONS

Controlled clinical trials

The most frequent adverse events associated with TRUSOPT were ocular burning, stinging, or discomfort immediately following ocular administration (approximately one-third of patients). Approximately one-quarter of patients noted a bitter taste following administration. Superficial punctate keratitis occurred in 10-15% of patients and signs and symptoms of ocular allergic reaction in approximately 10%. Events occurring in approximately 1-5% of patients were conjunctivitis and lid reactions (see PRECAUTIONS, General), blurred vision, eye redness, tearing, dryness, and photophobia. Other ocular events and systemic events were reported infrequently, including headache, nausea, asthenia/fatigue; and, rarely, skin rashes, urolithiasis, and iridocyclitis.

In a 3-month, double-masked, active-treatment-controlled, multicenter study in pediatric patients, the adverse experience profile of TRUSOPT was comparable to that seen in adult patients.

Clinical practice

The following adverse events have occurred either at low incidence (<1%) during clinical trials or have been reported during the use of TRUSOPT in clinical practice where these events were reported voluntarily from a population of unknown size and frequency of occurrence cannot be determined precisely. They have been chosen for inclusion based on factors such as seriousness, frequency of reporting, possible causal connection to TRUSOPT, or a combination of these factors: signs and symptoms of systemic allergic reactions including angioedema, bronchospasm, pruritus, and urticaria; Stevens-Johnson syndrome and toxic epidermal necrolysis; dizziness, paresthesia; ocular pain, transient myopia, choroidal detachment following filtration surgery, eyelid crusting; dyspnea; contact dermatitis, epistaxis, dry mouth and throat irritation.

OVERDOSAGE

Electrolyte imbalance, development of an acidotic state, and possible central nervous system effects may occur. Serum electrolyte levels (particularly potassium) and blood pH levels should be monitored.

DOSAGE AND ADMINISTRATION

The dose is one drop of TRUSOPT Ophthalmic Solution in the affected eye(s) three times daily.

TRUSOPT may be used concomitantly with other topical ophthalmic drug products to lower intraocular pressure. If more than one topical ophthalmic drug is being used, the drugs should be administered at least ten minutes apart.

HOW SUPPLIED

TRUSOPT Ophthalmic Solution is a slightly opalescent, nearly colorless, slightly viscous solution.

No. 3519—TRUSOPT Ophthalmic Solution 2% is supplied in an OCUMETER® PLUS container, a white, translucent, HDPE plastic ophthalmic dispenser with a controlled drop tip and a white polystyrene cap with orange label as follows:
NDC 0006-3519-36, 10 mL, in an 18 mL capacity bottle.

Storage

Store TRUSOPT Ophthalmic Solution at 15-30°C (59-86°F). Protect from light.

Rx only

[2] Registered trademark of Merck Sharp & Dohme Corp., a subsidiary of **Merck & Co., Inc.**

Manuf. for: Merck Sharp & Dohme Corp., a subsidiary of **MERCK & CO., INC.**, Whitehouse Station, NJ 08889, USA
By: Laboratories Merck Sharp & Dohme-Chibret
  63963 Clermont-Ferrand Cedex 9, France
Issued December 2009
221A-12/09 514297Z
9368211

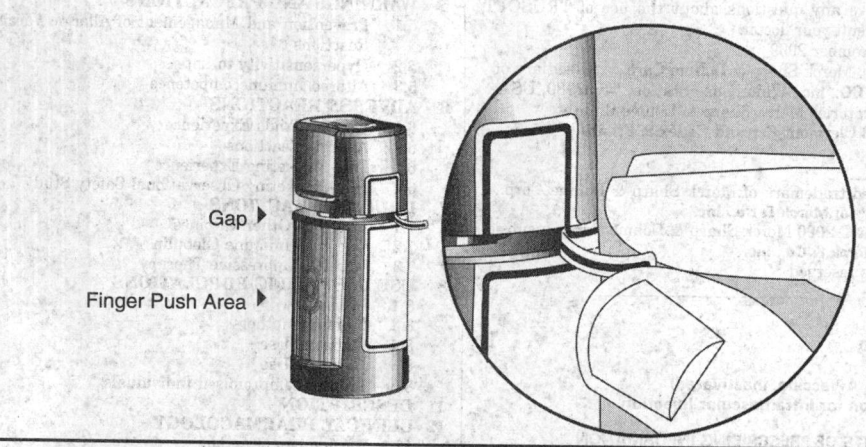

Gap ▶

Finger Push Area ▶

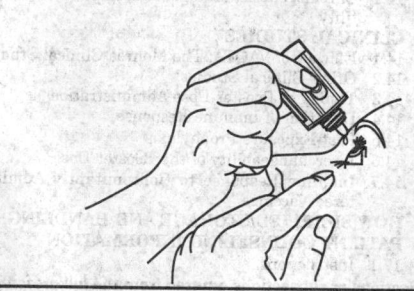

◀ Finger Push Area

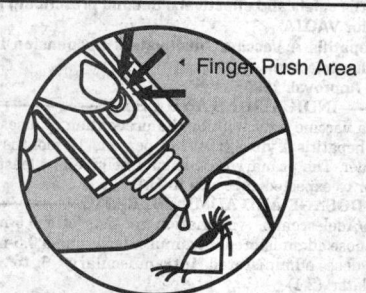

INSTRUCTIONS FOR USE

TRUSOPT®
(dorzolamide hydrochloride ophthalmic solution)
Sterile Ophthalmic Solution 2%
Please follow these instructions carefully when using TRUSOPT[3]. Use TRUSOPT as prescribed by your doctor.

1. If you use other topically applied ophthalmic medications, they should be administered at least 10 minutes before or after TRUSOPT.
2. Wash hands before each use.
3. Before using the medication for the first time, be sure the Safety Strip on the front of the bottle is unbroken. A gap between the bottle and the cap is normal for an unopened bottle.

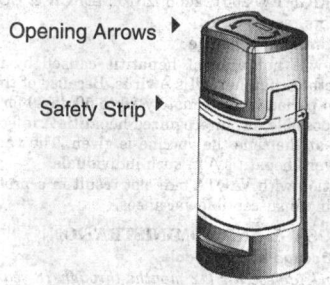

Opening Arrows ▶

Safety Strip ▶

4. Tear off the Safety Strip to break the seal.
[See first figure above]
5. To open the bottle, unscrew the cap by turning as indicated by the arrows on the top of the cap. Do not pull the cap directly up and away from the bottle. Pulling the cap directly up will prevent your dispenser from operating properly.

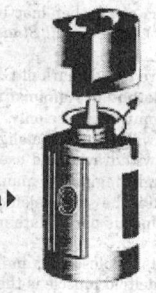

Finger Push Area ▶

6. Tilt your head back and pull your lower eyelid down slightly to form a pocket between your eyelid and your eye.

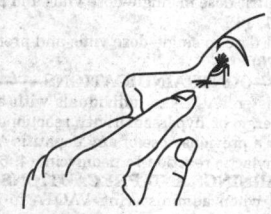

7. Invert the bottle, and press lightly with the thumb or index finger over the "Finger Push Area" (as shown) until a single drop is dispensed into the eye as directed by your doctor.
[See second figure above]
  DO NOT TOUCH YOUR EYE OR EYELID WITH THE DROPPER TIP.
  OPHTHALMIC MEDICATIONS, IF HANDLED IMPROPERLY, CAN BECOME CONTAMINATED BY COMMON BACTERIA KNOWN TO CAUSE EYE INFECTIONS. SERIOUS DAMAGE TO THE EYE AND SUBSEQUENT LOSS OF VISION MAY RESULT FROM USING CONTAMINATED OPHTHALMIC MEDICATIONS. IF YOU THINK YOUR MEDICATION MAY BE CONTAMINATED, OR IF YOU DEVELOP AN EYE INFECTION, CONTACT YOUR DOCTOR IMMEDIATELY CONCERNING CONTINUED USE OF THIS BOTTLE.
8. If drop dispensing is difficult after opening for the first time, replace the cap on the bottle and tighten (DO NOT OVERTIGHTEN) and then remove by turning the cap in the opposite direction as indicated by the arrows on the top of the cap.
9. Repeat steps 6 & 7 with the other eye if instructed to do so by your doctor.
10. Replace the cap by turning until it is firmly touching the bottle. The arrow on the left side of the cap must be aligned with the arrow on the left side of the bottle label for proper closure. Do not overtighten or you may damage the bottle and cap.
11. The dispenser tip is designed to provide a single drop; therefore, do NOT enlarge the hole of the dispenser tip.
12. After you have used all doses, there will be some TRUSOPT left in the bottle. You should not be concerned since an extra amount of TRUSOPT has been added and you will get the full amount of TRUSOPT that your doctor prescribed. Do not attempt to remove excess medicine from the bottle.

WARNING: Keep out of reach of children.

If you have any questions about the use of TRUSOPT, please consult your doctor.

Issued December 2009

Manuf. for: Merck Sharp & Dohme Corp., a subsidiary of **MERCK & CO., Inc.**, Whitehouse Station, NJ 08889, USA

By: Laboratories Merck Sharp & Dohme-Chibret
63963 Clermont-Ferrand Cedex 9, France
9368211

[3] Registered trademark of Merck Sharp & Dohme Corp., a subsidiary of **Merck & Co., Inc.**

Copyright © 2000 Merck Sharp & Dohme Corp., a subsidiary of **Merck & Co., Inc.**

All rights reserved

VAQTA®

[va-q-ta]

(Hepatitis A Vaccine, Inactivated)
Suspension for Intramuscular Injection

R

HIGHLIGHTS OF PRESCRIBING INFORMATION
These highlights do not include all the information needed to use VAQTA safely and effectively. See full prescribing information for VAQTA.

VAQTA (Hepatitis A Vaccine, Inactivated) Suspension for Intramuscular Injection
Initial U.S. Approval: 1996

————INDICATIONS AND USAGE————
VAQTA is a vaccine indicated for the prevention of disease caused by hepatitis A virus (HAV) in persons 12 months of age and older. The primary dose should be given at least 2 weeks prior to expected exposure to HAV. (1.1)

————DOSAGE AND ADMINISTRATION————
• Children/Adolescents: vaccination consists of a 0.5-mL primary dose administered intramuscularly, and a 0.5-mL booster dose administered intramuscularly 6 to 18 months later. (2.1)
• Adults: vaccination consists of a 1.0-mL primary dose administered intramuscularly, and a 1.0-mL booster dose administered intramuscularly 6 to 18 months later. (2.1)

————DOSAGE FORMS AND STRENGTHS————
Sterile suspension supplied in four presentations:
• 0.5-mL pediatric dose in single-dose vials and prefilled syringes. (3, 11, 16)
• 1.0-mL adult dose in single-dose vials and prefilled syringes. (3, 11, 16)

————CONTRAINDICATIONS————
Do not administer VAQTA to individuals with a history of immediate allergic or hypersensitivity reactions (e.g., anaphylaxis) after a previous dose of any hepatitis A vaccine or with an anaphylactic reaction to neomycin. (4, 6.2, 11)

————WARNINGS AND PRECAUTIONS————
• Use caution when administering VAQTA to individuals with latex allergies. (5.2)

————ADVERSE REACTIONS————
The most common local adverse reactions and systemic adverse events reported in different clinical trials across different age groups were:
• Children—12 through 23 months of age: injection-site pain/tenderness (6.8%-42.1%) and fever (12.3%-18.5%)
• Children/Adolescents—2 through 18 years of age: injection-site pain (18.7%) and headache (2.3%)
• Adults—19 years of age and older: injection-site pain, tenderness, or soreness (67.0%) and headache (16.1%) (6.1)

To report SUSPECTED ADVERSE REACTIONS, contact Merck & Co., Inc. at 1-877-888-4231 or VAERS at 1-800-822-7967 or www.vaers.hhs.gov.

————DRUG INTERACTIONS————
• VAQTA may be given concomitantly with measles, mumps, rubella, varicella, and pneumococcal 7-valent conjugate vaccines. (6.1, 7.1, 14.7)
• VAQTA may be given to adults concomitantly with typhoid Vi polysaccharide and yellow fever vaccines. (6.1, 7.1, 14.7)
• VAQTA may be administered concomitantly with immune globulin. (7.2, 14.5)

————USE IN SPECIFIC POPULATIONS————
• Safety and effectiveness of VAQTA have not been established in children less than 12 months of age, pregnant women, and nursing mothers. (8.1, 8.3, 8.4)

See 17 for PATIENT COUNSELING INFORMATION
Revised: 06/2010

FULL PRESCRIBING INFORMATION: CONTENTS*

FULL PRESCRIBING INFORMATION

1 INDICATIONS AND USAGE

1.1 Indications and Use

VAQTA[1] [Hepatitis A Vaccine, Inactivated] is indicated for the prevention of disease caused by hepatitis A virus (HAV) in persons 12 months of age and older. The primary dose should be given at least 2 weeks prior to expected exposure to HAV.

VAQTA may be administered along with immune globulin (IG) at a separate site with a separate syringe for post-exposure prophylaxis [see Clinical Studies (14.5)].

[1] Registered trademark of MERCK & CO., Inc.
COPYRIGHT © 2001, 2005, 2010 MERCK & CO., Inc.
All rights reserved

1.2 Limitations of Use

VAQTA will not prevent hepatitis caused by infectious agents other than hepatitis A virus. Because of the long incubation period (approximately 20 to 50 days) for hepatitis A, it is possible for unrecognized hepatitis A infection to be present at the time the vaccine is given. The vaccine may not prevent hepatitis A in such individuals.

Vaccination with VAQTA may not result in a protective response in all susceptible vaccinees.

2 DOSAGE AND ADMINISTRATION

2.1 Dosage and Schedule

Children/Adolescents (12 months through 18 years of age): Vaccination consists of a primary 0.5-mL dose administered intramuscularly, and a 0.5-mL booster dose administered intramuscularly 6 to 18 months later.

Adults (≥19 years of age): Vaccination consists of a primary 1.0-mL dose administered intramuscularly, and a 1.0-mL booster dose administered intramuscularly 6 to 18 months later.

Interchangeability of the Booster Dose: A booster dose of VAQTA may be given at 6 to 12 months following the primary dose of another inactivated hepatitis A vaccine (i.e., HAVRIX[2]) [see Clinical Studies (14.6)].

[2] Registered trademark of GlaxoSmithKline

2.2 Method of Administration

For intramuscular use only.
• Shake well to obtain a slightly opaque, white suspension before withdrawal and use.
• Thoroughly agitate to maintain suspension of the vaccine.
• Discard if the suspension does not appear homogenous or if extraneous particulate matter remains or discoloration is observed.

For adults, adolescents, and children older than 2 years of age, the deltoid muscle is the preferred site for intramuscular injection. For children 12 through 23 months of age, the anterolateral area of the thigh is the preferred site for intramuscular injection.

Single-Dose Vial Use
• Withdraw dose of vaccine from the single-dose vial using a sterile needle and syringe.

Prefilled Syringe Use
The following are instructions for using the prefilled single-dose syringes:
• Shake well before use.
• Attach the needle by twisting in a clockwise direction until the needle fits securely on the syringe.
• Administer the entire dose as per standard protocol as stated above under DOSAGE AND ADMINISTRATION.
• Dispose of the syringe and needle in approved sharps container.

3 DOSAGE FORMS AND STRENGTHS

Sterile suspension available in four presentations:
• 0.5-mL pediatric dose in single-dose vials and prefilled syringes
• 1.0-mL adult dose in single-dose vials and prefilled syringes

[See Description (11) for listing of vaccine components and How Supplied/Storage and Handling (16).]

4 CONTRAINDICATIONS

Do not administer VAQTA to individuals with a history of immediate allergic or hypersensitivity reactions (e.g., anaphylaxis) after a previous dose of any hepatitis A vaccine, or to individuals who have had an anaphylactic reaction to any component of VAQTA, including neomycin [see Description (11)].

5 WARNINGS AND PRECAUTIONS

5.1 Prevention and Management of Allergic Vaccine Reactions

Have appropriate medical treatment and supervision available to manage possible immediate-type hypersensitivity reactions, such as anaphylaxis, should an acute reaction occur.

5.2 Hypersensitivity to Latex

Use caution when vaccinating latex-sensitive individuals since the vial stopper and the syringe plunger stopper contain dry natural latex rubber that may cause allergic reactions.

5.3 Altered Immunocompetence

Immunocompromised persons, including individuals receiving immunosuppressive therapy, may have a diminished immune response to VAQTA and may not be protected against HAV infection after vaccination [see Drug Interactions (7.3) and Use in Specific Populations (8.6)].

6 ADVERSE REACTIONS

Because clinical trials are conducted under widely varying conditions, adverse reaction rates observed in the clinical trials of a vaccine cannot be directly compared to rates in the clinical trials of another vaccine and may not reflect the rates observed in practice.

The most common local adverse reactions and systemic adverse events reported in different clinical trials across different age groups were:
• Children—12 through 23 months of age: injection-site pain/tenderness (6.8%-42.1%) and fever (12.3%-18.5%)
• Children/Adolescents—2 through 18 years of age: injection-site pain (18.7%) and headache (2.3%)
• Adults—19 years of age and older: injection-site pain, tenderness, or soreness (67.0%) and headache (16.1%) (6.1)

6.1 Clinical Trials Experience

The safety of VAQTA has been evaluated in over 10,000 subjects 1 year to 85 years of age. Subjects were given one or two doses of the vaccine. The second (booster dose) was given 6 months or more after the first dose.

Children—12 through 23 Months of Age

In two open-label clinical trials involving 706 healthy children 12 through 23 months of age who received one or two 25U doses of VAQTA, subjects were monitored for local adverse reactions and fever for 5 days and systemic adverse events for 14 days after each vaccination by diary cards. In one trial, 89 children were enrolled and received VAQTA alone. In the other trial, children were randomized to receive the first dose of VAQTA with or without M-M-R® II[1] (Measles, Mumps, and Rubella Virus Vaccine, Live) and VARIVAX®[1] (Varicella Virus Vaccine Live) (N=617) and the second dose of VAQTA with or without Tripedia[3] (Diphtheria and Tetanus Toxoids and Acellular Pertussis Vaccine Adsorbed) (DTaP) and optionally either ORIMUNE[4] (Poliovirus vaccine live oral trivalent) (OPV) or IPOL[3] (Poliovirus Vaccine Inactivated) (IPV) (N=555). The race distribution of the study subjects who received at least one dose of VAQTA in these studies was as follows: 62.2% Caucasian; 15.3% Hispanic-American; 12.4% African-American; 6.1% Native

American; 3.0% other; 0.7% Oriental, 0.1% Asian; and 0.1% Indian. The distribution of subjects by gender was 53.2% male and 46.8% female. Listed below are the solicited local adverse reactions and systemic adverse events (with 95% Confidence Interval (CI)) (Table 1) and unsolicited local adverse reactions and systemic adverse events (Table 2) reported at ≥1.0% in children who received one or two doses of VAQTA alone and for subjects who received VAQTA concomitantly with other vaccines.

Table 1: Incidences of Solicited Local Adverse Reactions and Systemic Adverse Events in Healthy Infants 12 through 23 Months of Age Occurring at ≥1% After Any Dose

Adverse Event	VAQTA administered alone (N=241)	VAQTA + vaccines administered concomitantly* (N=706)
	Rate (n/total n) (95% CI)	
Injection-site†		
Pain/tenderness/ soreness	6.8% (16/236) (3.9%, 10.8%)	8.6% (59/683) (6.6%, 11.0%)
Swelling	4.2% (10/236) (2.1%, 7.7%)	5.1% (35/683) (3.6%, 7.1%)
Erythema	3.8% (9/236) (1.8%, 7.1%)	5.9% (40/683) (4.2%, 7.9%)
Warmth	2.5% (6/236) (0.9%, 5.5%)	3.2% (22/683) (2.0%, 4.8%)
Systemic‡		
Fever§		
≥100.4°F, Oral	12.3% (29/236) (8.4%, 17.2%)	14.6% (99/679) (12.0%, 17.5%)
≥102.0°F, Oral	3.4% (8/236) (1.5%, 6.6%)	4.9% (33/679) (3.4%, 6.8%)
Abnormal	1.7% (4/236) (0.5%, 4.3%)	0.9% (6/679) (0.3%, 1.9%)
Rash (measles-like, rubella-like, varicella-like)	0.0% (0/236) (0.0%, 1.5%)	1.8% (12/683) (0.9%, 3.1%)

N=Number of subjects enrolled/randomized.
n=Number of subjects in each category.

* VAQTA administered alone or concomitantly with M-M-R II and VARIVAX at Dose 1. VAQTA administered alone or concomitantly with DTaP and poliovirus vaccine optionally at Dose 2.
† Adverse Reactions at the injection site (VAQTA) Days 1-5 after vaccination
‡ Systemic Adverse Events reported Days 1-14 after vaccination, regardless of causality.
§ Monitored Days 1-5 after vaccination.

[See table 2 above]
Serious Adverse Events: Subjects in an open-label study were randomized to receive VAQTA (Dose 1) alone (N=308) or VAQTA concomitantly with M-M-R II and VARIVAX (N=309). Seven children experienced a total of 9 seizures between 9 days and 81 days following the administration of the vaccines. None of the events was considered to be related to VAQTA by the investigator. Other serious events that occurred during the study included bronchiolitis (N=1), dehydration (N=2), RLL (Right Lower Lobe) pneumonia and asthma (N=1), and asthma exacerbation (N=1), which occurred 9 days to 46 days following the administration of VAQTA and were also considered by the investigator to be unrelated to VAQTA.
In an open-label clinical trial of 1800 subjects, 699 healthy children 12 to 23 months of age were randomized to receive two doses of VAQTA (N=352) or two doses of VAQTA concomitantly with two doses of ProQuad[1] (Measles, Mumps, Rubella and Varicella Virus Vaccine Live) (N=347) at least 6 months apart. An additional 1101 subjects received two doses of VAQTA alone at least 6 months apart (non-randomized), resulting in 1453 subjects receiving two doses of VAQTA alone (1101 non-randomized and 352 randomized) and 347 subjects receiving two doses of VAQTA concomitantly with ProQuad (all randomized). The race distribution of the study subjects who received VAQTA with or without ProQuad was as follows: 66.4% Caucasian; 19.7% Hispanic-American; 6.7% African-American; 5.0% other; 2.1% Asian; and 0.1% Native American. The distribution of subjects by gender was 51.2% male and 48.8% female. Tables 3 and 4 present injection-site adverse reactions and fever ≥100.4°C (≥38.0°C) and ≥102.2°F (≥39.0°C) (Days 1 to 5 postvacci-

Table 2: Incidences of Unsolicited Local Adverse Reactions and Systemic Adverse Events in Healthy Infants 12 through 23 Months of Age Occurring at ≥1%

Body System Adverse Event	VAQTA administered alone (N=241)	VAQTA + vaccines administered concomitantly* (N=706)
	Rate (n/total n) (95% CI)	
Eye disorders†		
Conjunctivitis	0.4% (1/236) (0.0%, 2.3%)	1.3% (9/683) (0.6%, 2.5%)
Respiratory, thoracic and mediastinal disorders†		
Rhinorrhea	3.7% (9/236) (1.8%, 7.1%)	5.7% (39/683) (4.1%, 7.7%)
Cough	3.7% (9/236) (1.8%, 7.1%)	5.1% (35/683) (3.6%, 7.1%)
Asthma	1.2% (3/236) (0.3%, 3.7%)	0.7% (5/683) (0.2%, 1.7%)
Respiratory congestion	0.4% (1/236) (0.0%, 2.3%)	1.6% (11/683) (0.8%, 2.9%)
Nasal congestion	0.4% (1/236) (0.0%, 2.3%)	1.2% (8/683) (0.5%, 2.3%)
Laryngotracheobronchitis	0.4% (1/236) (0.0%, 2.3%)	1.2% (8/683) (0.5%, 2.3%)
Gastrointestinal disorders†		
Diarrhea	3.3% (8/236) (1.5%, 6.6%)	5.9% (40/683) (4.2%, 7.9%)
Vomiting	2.9% (7/236) (1.2%, 6.0%)	4.0% (27/683) (2.6%, 5.7%)
Skin and subcutaneous tissue disorders†		
Rash	1.7% (4/236) (0.5%, 4.3%)	4.5% (31/683) (3.1%, 6.4%)
Metabolism and nutrition disorders†		
Anorexia	1.7% (4/236) (0.5%, 4.3%)	1.2% (8/683) (0.5%, 2.3%)
Infections and infestations†		
Upper respiratory infection	10.0% (24/236) (6.6%, 14.8%)	10.1% (69/683) (8.0%, 12.6%)
Otitis Media	4.1% (10/236) (2.1%, 7.7%)	7.6% (52/683) (5.7%, 9.9%)
Otitis	0.8% (2/236) (0.1%, 3.0%)	1.8% (12/683) (0.9%, 3.1%)
Viral exanthema	0.4% (1/236) (0.0%, 2.3%)	1.0% (7/683) (0.4%, 2.1%)
General disorders and administration site conditions†		
Irritability	7.1% (17/236) (4.3%, 11.3%)	10.8% (74/683) (8.6%, 13.4%)
Injection-site ecchymosis‡	0.0% (0/236) (0.0%, 1.6%)	1.0% (7/683) (0.4%, 2.2%)
Psychiatric disorders†		
Insomnia	1.7% (4/236) (0.5%, 4.3%)	0.7% (5/683) (0.2%, 1.7%)
Crying	1.2% (3/236) (0.3%, 3.7%)	1.8% (12/683) (0.9%, 3.1%)

N=Number of subjects enrolled/randomized.
n=Number of subjects in each category.

* VAQTA administered alone or concomitantly with M-M-R II and VARIVAX at Dose 1. VAQTA administered alone or concomitantly with DTaP and poliovirus vaccine optionally at Dose 2.
† Systemic Adverse Events reported Days 1-14 after vaccination, regardless of causality.
‡ Adverse Reactions at the injection site (VAQTA) Days 1-5 after vaccination.

nation) and systemic adverse events, including fever or feverish >98.6°F (>37.0°C) (Days 1 to 14 postvaccination) observed among recipients of VAQTA alone or concomitantly with ProQuad at a rate of at least 1% following any dose of VAQTA. Among all subjects, fever (>98.6°F (>37.0°C) or feverish) was the most common systemic adverse event and injection-site pain/tenderness was the most common injection-site adverse reaction. Based on a post-hoc analysis, the rate of fever (>98.6°F (>37.0°C) or feverish) after any dose of VAQTA was increased in subjects who received VAQTA with ProQuad as compared to VAQTA alone in the 14 days after vaccination {risk difference (11.8% [95% CI: 6.8, 17.2]) and relative risk (1.72 [95% CI: 1.40, 2.12])}. The difference in rate of fever (>98.6°F (>37.0°C) or feverish)

was higher after Dose 1 (11.5%) as compared to Dose 2 (4.0%). The rates of fever ≥100.4°F (≥38.0°C) and ≥102.2°F (≥39.0°C) in the 5 days after any dose of VAQTA were similar in both treatment groups.
[See table 3 at top of next page]
[See table 4 on next page]
In an open-label clinical trial, 653 children 12 to 23 months of age were randomized to receive a first dose of VAQTA with ProQuad and Prevnar[4] (Pneumococcal 7-valent Conjugate Vaccine) concomitantly (N=330) or a first dose of ProQuad and pneumococcal 7-valent conjugate vaccine concomitantly and then vaccinated with VAQTA 6 weeks later (N=323). Approximately 6 months later, subjects received either the second doses of ProQuad and VAQTA

Table 3: Incidences of Unsolicited and Solicited Local Adverse Reactions at the Injection Site for VAQTA Occurring at ≥1% in Healthy Infants 12 through 23 Months of Age After Any Dose of VAQTA Alone or Concomitantly With ProQuad

Adverse Reaction	VAQTA administered alone (N=1453)	VAQTA + ProQuad (N=347)
	Rate (n/total n)	
Injection-site erythema*	21.2% (300/1415)	17.7% (59/334)
Injection-site pain/tenderness*	42.1% (596/1415)	35.9% (120/334)
Injection-site swelling*	12.6% (178/1415)	13.5% (45/334)
Injection-site bruising*,†	2.6% (37/1415)	3.0% (10/334)

N=Number of subjects enrolled/randomized.
n=Number of subjects in each category.

* Adverse Reactions at the injection site (VAQTA) Days 1-5 after vaccination
† Unsolicited Reaction.

Table 4: Incidences of Unsolicited and Solicited Systemic Adverse Events by Body System Occurring at ≥1% in Healthy Infants 12 through 23 Months of Age After Any Dose of VAQTA Alone or Concomitantly With ProQuad

Body System Adverse Event	VAQTA administered alone (N=1453)	VAQTA + ProQuad (N=347)
	Rate (n/total n)	
Eye disorders*		
Conjunctivitis	0.9% (13/1415)	1.5% (5/334)
Gastrointestinal disorders*		
Constipation	1.1% (15/1415)	0.3% (1/334)
Diarrhea	10.1% (143/1415)	6.9% (23/334)
Vomiting	6.4% (90/1415)	4.8% (16/334)
General disorders and administration site conditions*		
Irritability	11.2% (158/1415)	10.8% (36/334)
Fever ≥102.2°F (≥39.0°C) (Days 1-5 postvaccination)†	4.0% (56/1383)	4.1% (13/320)
Fever ≥100.4°F (≥38.0&°C) (Days 1-5 postvaccination)†	16.3% (226/1383)	15.9% (51/320)
Fever >98.6°F or feverish (>37.0°C) (Days 1-14 postvaccination)‡	16.3% (231/1415)	28.1% (94/334)
Infections and infestations*		
Ear infection	1.1% (15/1415)	0.0% (0/334)
Gastroenteritis	1.1% (16/1415)	0.6% (2/334)
Gastroenteritis viral	0.8% (11/1415)	1.8% (6/334)
Nasopharyngitis	4.7% (66/1415)	4.8% (16/334)
Otitis media	4.0% (56/1415)	3.3% (11/334)
Rhinitis	3.2% (45/1415)	0.3% (1/334)
Upper respiratory tract infection	6.6% (93/1415)	9.0% (30/334)
Viral infection	1.1% (16/1415)	0.9% (3/334)
Metabolism and nutrition disorders*		
Anorexia	1.1% (15/1415)	0.9% (3/334)
Respiratory, thoracic and mediastinal disorders*		
Cough	7.8% (111/1415)	6.0% (20/334)
Nasal congestion	2.6% (37/1415)	2.1% (7/334)
Rhinorrhea	7.6% (107/1415)	6.6% (22/334)
Skin and subcutaneous tissue disorders*		
Dermatitis diaper	1.7% (24/1415)	5.7% (19/334)
Rash	2.0% (29/1415)	5.7% (19/334)
Rash morbilliform	0.0% (0/1415)	4.8% (16/334)

N=Number of subjects enrolled/randomized.
n=Number of subjects in each category.

* Systemic Adverse Events reported Days 1-14 after vaccination, regardless of causality.
† T≥100.4°F and T≥102.2°F, recorded Days 1-5 after vaccination.
‡ Risk Difference (11.8% [95% CI: 6.8, 17.2]) and relative risk (1.72 [95% CI: 1.40, 2.12]) in post-hoc analysis.

concomitantly or the second doses of ProQuad and VAQTA separately. The race distribution of the study subjects who received VAQTA with or without ProQuad and pneumococcal 7-valent conjugate vaccine was as follows: 60.3% Caucasian; 21.6% African-American; 9.5% Hispanic-American; 7.2% other; 1.1% Asian; and 0.3% Native American. The distribution of subjects by gender was 50.7% male and 49.3% female.

Tables 5 and 6 present injection-site adverse reactions (Days 1 to 5 postvaccination with VAQTA) and systemic adverse events (Days 1 to 14 postvaccination with VAQTA) observed among recipients of VAQTA concomitantly with ProQuad and pneumococcal 7-valent conjugate vaccine and VAQTA administered separately from ProQuad and pneumococcal 7-valent conjugate vaccine at a rate of at least 1% following any dose of VAQTA. Among all subjects, fever (>98.6°F or feverish) was the most common systemic adverse event, and injection-site pain/tenderness was the most common injection-site adverse reaction.

In the 14 days after vaccination with any dose of VAQTA, the rate of fever (>98.6°F or feverish) was increased in subjects who received VAQTA with ProQuad and pneumococcal 7-valent conjugate vaccine as compared to VAQTA alone {risk difference (20.0% [95% CI: 13.0, 26.8]) and relative risk (2.10 [95% CI: 1.59, 2.79] in post-hoc analysis)}. A difference in rates of fever was noted after Dose 1 of VAQTA with ProQuad and pneumococcal 7-valent conjugate vaccine, but not after Dose 2 of VAQTA with ProQuad. The rates of fever ≥100.4°F and ≥102.2°F in the five days after vaccination were similar in both treatment groups (Table 6).

In the 28 days after vaccination, the administration of Dose 1 of VAQTA with Dose 1 of ProQuad and Dose 4 of pneumococcal 7-valent conjugate vaccine does not increase incidence rates of fever (>98.6°F or feverish) as compared to when ProQuad is administered with pneumococcal 7-valent conjugate vaccine alone {38.6% and 42.7%, respectively; relative risk (0.9 [95% CI: 0.75, 1.09])} in post-hoc analysis. Similarly, the administration of Dose 2 of VAQTA with Dose 2 of ProQuad does not increase incidence rates of fever (>98.6°F or feverish) as compared to when Dose 2 of ProQuad is administered alone {17.4% and 17.0%, respectively; relative risk (1.02 [95% CI: 0.70, 1.51])}.

[See table 5 on next page]
[See table 6 on next page]

Children/Adolescents—2 through 18 Years of Age
The Monroe Efficacy Study
The Monroe Efficacy Study was a double-blind, randomized, placebo-controlled study of the protective efficacy, safety, and immunogenicity of VAQTA in 1037 healthy children and adolescents, 2 through 16 years of age, who were initially seronegative for hepatitis A. Placebo control was alum diluent. These children were randomized to receive a primary dose of 25U of hepatitis A vaccine and a booster 6, 12, or 18 months later, or placebo (alum diluent). All of these children were Caucasian and there were 51.5% males and 48.5% females. In this blinded study, subjects were followed days 1 to 5 postvaccination for fever and local adverse reactions and days 1 to 14 for systemic adverse events. The most common adverse events/reactions were injection-site reactions, reported by 6.4% of subjects. Table 7 summarizes the local adverse reactions and systemic adverse events (≥1%) reported in this study. There were no significant differences in the rates of any adverse events or adverse reactions between vaccine and placebo recipients after Dose 1.
[See table 7 at top of page 2328]
Combined Clinical Trials
In eleven randomized clinical trials (including Monroe Efficacy Study participants) involving 2615 healthy children (≥2 years of age) and adolescents who received at least one dose of hepatitis A vaccine, subjects were followed for fever and local adverse reactions days 1 to 5 and for systemic adverse events 1 to 14 days postvaccination. These studies included administration of VAQTA in varying doses and regimens (N=404 received 25U/0.5 mL), the Monroe Efficacy Study (N=973), and comparison studies for process and formulation changes (N=1238). The race distribution of the study subjects who received at least one dose of VAQTA in these studies was as follows: 84.7% Caucasian; 10.6% American Indian; 2.3% African-American; 1.5% Hispanic-American; 0.6% other; 0.2% Oriental. The distribution of subjects by gender was 51.2% male and 48.8% female. The most common adverse events/reactions were injection-site reactions reported by 24.3% of subjects. Of all reported injection-site reactions, 99.4% were mild (i.e., easily tolerated with no medical intervention) or moderate (i.e., minimally interfered with usual activity possibly requiring little medical intervention). Listed below in Table 8 are the local adverse reactions and systemic adverse events reported by ≥1% of subjects, in decreasing order of frequency within each body system.
[See table 8 on page 2328]
Adults—19 Years of Age and Older
In an open-label clinical trial, 240 healthy adults 18 to 54 years of age were randomized to receive either VAQTA (50U/1.0 mL) with Typhim Vi[3] (Typhoid Vi polysaccharide vaccine) and YF-Vax[3] (yellow fever vaccine) concomitantly (N=80), typhoid Vi polysaccharide and yellow fever vaccines concomitantly (N=80), or VAQTA alone (N=80). Approximately 6 months later, subjects who received VAQTA were administered a second dose of VAQTA. The race distribution of the study subjects who received VAQTA with or without typhoid Vi polysaccharide and yellow fever vaccine was as follows: 78.3% Caucasian; 14.2% Oriental; 3.3% other; 2.1% African-American; 1.7% Indian; 0.4% Hispanic-American. The distribution of subjects by gender was 40.8% male and 59.2% female. Subjects were monitored for local adverse reactions and fever for 5 days and systemic adverse events for 14 days after each vaccination. In the 14 days after the first dose of VAQTA was given with or without typhoid Vi polysaccharide and yellow fever vaccines, the proportion of subjects with adverse events was similar between recipients of VAQTA concomitantly with typhoid Vi polysaccharide and yellow fever vaccines compared to recipients of typhoid Vi

polysaccharide and yellow fever vaccines, but higher compared to recipients of VAQTA alone. Listed below are the solicited local adverse reactions and systemic adverse events (Table 9) and unsolicited systemic adverse events (Table 10) reported at ≥5% in adults who received one or two doses of VAQTA alone and for subjects who received VAQTA concomitantly with typhoid Vi polysaccharide and yellow fever vaccines.

Table 5: Incidences of Unsolicited and Solicited Local Adverse Reactions Occurring at ≥1% at the Injection Site for VAQTA in Healthy Infants 12 through 23 Months of Age Receiving VAQTA Alone or Concomitantly With ProQuad and PCV7*

Adverse Reaction	VAQTA alone (N=323)	VAQTA with ProQuad + PCV7 (N=330)
	Rate (n/total n)	
Injection-site erythema[†]	17.8% (51/286)	13.3% (44/330)
Injection-site pain/tenderness[†]	25.5% (73/286)	25.8% (85/330)
Injection-site swelling[†,‡]	13.3% (38/286)	9.7% (32/330)
Injection-site bruising[†,‡]	2.4% (7/286)	1.8% (6/330)
Injection-site rash [†,‡]	0.3% (1/286)	1.2% (4/330)

N=Number of subjects enrolled/randomized.
n=Number of subjects in each category.

* PCV7 = Pneumococcal 7-valent conjugate.
† Adverse Reactions at the injection site (VAQTA) Days 1-5 after vaccination.
‡ Unsolicited Reaction.

Table 6: Incidences of Unsolicited and Solicited Systemic Adverse Events by Body System Occurring at ≥1% in Healthy Infants 12 through 23 Months of Age After Any Dose of VAQTA Alone or Concomitantly With ProQuad and PCV7*

Body System Adverse Event[†]	VAQTA alone (N=323)	VAQTA with ProQuad + PCV7 (N=330)
	Rate (n/total n)	
Eye disorders[‡]		
Conjunctivitis	1.4% (4/286)	0.9% (3/330)
Gastrointestinal disorders[‡]		
Diarrhea	2.8% (8/286)	4.8% (16/330)
Vomiting	2.1% (6/286)	3.0% (10/330)
General disorders and administration site conditions[‡]		
Irritability	5.9% (17/286)	7.3% (24/330)
Fever ≥102.2°F (≥39.0°C) (Days 1-5 postvaccination)[§]	3.9% (10/257)	5.5% (16/293)
Fever ≥100.4°F (≥38.0°C) (Days 1-5 postvaccination)[§]	16.7% (43/257)	18.1% (53/293)
Fever >98.6°F or feverish (Days 1-14 postvaccination)[¶]	18.5% (53/286)	38.2% (126/330)
Infections and infestations[‡]		
Croup infectious	1.4% (4/286)	0.9% (3/330)
Ear infection	0.3% (1/286)	1.8% (6/330)
Gastroenteritis	1.0% (3/286)	0.9% (3/330)
Gastroenteritis viral	1.0% (3/286)	0.6% (2/330)
Nasopharyngitis	2.4% (7/286)	3.6% (12/330)
Otitis media	5.9% (17/286)	7.6% (25/330)
Otitis media acute	1.0% (3/286)	0.6% (2/330)
Pharyngitis	1.0% (3/286)	0.9% (3/330)
Pharyngitis streptococcal	1.0% (3/286)	0.6% (2/330)
Rhinitis	2.4% (7/286)	2.1% (7/330)
Roseola	0.3% (1/286)	1.5% (5/330)
Upper respiratory tract infection	6.6% (19/286)	10.3% (34/330)
Viral infection	0.3% (1/286)	2.7% (9/330)
Respiratory, thoracic and mediastinal disorders[‡]		
Cough	3.1% (9/286)	4.5% (15/330)
Nasal congestion	1.0% (3/286)	2.1% (7/330)
Rhinorrhea	3.1% (9/286)	4.8% (16/330)
Skin and subcutaneous tissue disorders[‡]		
Dermatitis diaper	3.1% (9/286)	7.9% (26/330)
Rash	1.4% (4/286)	3.0% (10/330)
Rash morbilliform	0.3% (1/286)	2.4% (8/330)
Rash vesicular	0.7% (2/286)	1.2% (4/330)

N=Number of subjects enrolled/randomized.
n=Number of subjects in each category.

* PCV7 = Pneumococcal 7-valent conjugate.
† Following administration of VAQTA either with or without other vaccines.
‡ Systemic Adverse Events reported Days 1-14 after vaccination, regardless of causality.
§ T≥100.4°F and T≥102.2°F, recorded Days 1-5 after vaccination
¶ Risk difference (20.0% [95% CI: 13.0, 26.8]) and relative risk (2.10 [95% CI: 1.59, 2.79]) in post-hoc analysis.

Table 9: Incidences of Solicited Local Adverse Reactions and Systemic Adverse Events in Healthy Adults ≥19 Years of Age Occurring at ≥5% After Any Dose

Adverse Event	VAQTA administered alone (N=80)	VAQTA + ViCPS* and Yellow Fever vaccines administered concomitantly[†] (N=80)
	Rate (n/total n)	
Injection-site[‡]		
Pain/tenderness/soreness	78.8% (63/80)	70.3% (56/80)
Warmth	23.7% (19/80)	23.7% (19/80)
Swelling	16.2% (13/80)	8.8% (7/80)
Erythema	17.5% (14/80)	6.3% (5/80)
Systemic[§]		

N=Number of subjects enrolled/randomized.
n=Number of subjects in each category.

* ViCPS = Typhoid Vi polysaccharide vaccine.
† VAQTA administered concomitantly with typhoid Vi polysaccharide (ViCPS) and yellow fever vaccines.
‡ Adverse Reactions at the injection site (VAQTA) Days 1-5 after vaccination
§ There were no solicited systemic complaints ≥5%. Fever (≥101°F, Oral) was reported at 1.3% (1/80) in both groups.

Table 10: Incidences of Unsolicited Systemic Adverse Events in Adults ≥19 Years of Age Occurring at ≥5% After Any Dose

Body System Adverse Event	VAQTA administered alone (N=80)	VAQTA + ViCPS* and Yellow Fever vaccines administered concomitantly[†] (N=80)
	Rate (n/total n)	
General disorders and administration site reactions		
Asthenia/fatigue	7.5% (6/80)	11.3% (9/80)
Chills	1.3% (1/80)	7.5% (6/80)
Gastrointestinal disorders		
Nausea	7.5% (6/80)	12.5% (10/80)
Musculoskeletal and connective tissue disorders		
Myalgia	5.0% (4/80)	10.0% (8/80)
Arm pain	0.0% (0/80)	6.3% (5/80)
Nervous system disorders		
Headache	23.8% (19/80)	26.3% (21/80)
Infections and infestations		
Upper respiratory infection	7.5% (6/80)	3.8% (3/80)
Pharyngitis	2.5% (2/80)	6.3% (5/80)

N=Number of subjects enrolled/randomized.
n=Number of subjects in each category.

* ViCPS = Typhoid Vi polysaccharide vaccine.
† VAQTA administered concomitantly with typhoid Vi polysaccharide (ViCPS) and yellow fever vaccines.
†Systemic Adverse Events reported Days 1-15 after vaccination, regardless of causality.

Combined Clinical Trials

In four randomized clinical trials involving 1645 healthy adults 19 years of age and older who received one or more 50U doses of hepatitis A vaccine, subjects were followed for fever and local adverse reactions 1 to 5 days postvaccination and for systemic adverse events 1 to 14 days postvaccination. One single-blind study evaluated doses of VAQTA with varying amounts of viral antigen and/or alum content in healthy adults ≥170 pounds and ≥30 years of age (N=210 adults administered 50U/1.0 mL dose). One open-label study evaluated VAQTA given with immune globulin or

Table 7: Local Adverse Reactions and Systemic Adverse Events (≥1%) in Healthy Children and Adolescents from the Monroe Efficacy Study

Adverse Event	VAQTA (N=519)		Placebo (Alum Diluent)*,†,‡ (N=518)
	Dose 1* Rate (n/total n)	Booster Rate (n/total n)	Rate (n/total n)
Injection-site§			
Pain	6.4% (33/515)	3.4% (16/475)	6.3% (32/510)
Tenderness	4.9% (25/515)	1.7% (8/475)	6.1% (31/510)
Erythema	1.9% (10/515)	0.8% (4/475)	1.8% (9/510)
Swelling	1.7% (9/515)	1.5% (7/475)	1.6% (8/510)
Warmth	1.7% (9/515)	0.6% (3/475)	1.6% (8/510)
Systemic¶			
Abdominal pain	1.2% (6/519)	1.1% (5/475)	1.0% (5/518)
Pharyngitis	1.2% (6/519)	0% (0/475)	0.8% (4/518)
Headache	0.4% (2/519)	0.8% (4/475)	1.0% (5/518)

N=Number of subjects enrolled/randomized.
n=Number of subjects in each category.

* No statistically significant differences between the two groups.
† Second injection of placebo not administered because code for the trial was broken.
‡ Placebo (Alum diluent) = amorphous aluminum hydroxyphosphate sulfate.
§ Adverse Reactions at the injection site (VAQTA) Days 1-5 after vaccination with VAQTA
¶ Systemic adverse events reported Days 1-15 after vaccination, regardless of causality.

Table 8: Incidences of Local Adverse Reactions and Systemic Adverse Events ≥1% in Healthy Children and Adolescents 2 through 18 Years of Age

Body System Adverse Event	VAQTA Alone (N=2615)	Placebo (Alum Diluent)* (N=542)
	Rate (n/total n) 95% CI	
Respiratory, thoracic, and mediastinal disorders†		
Pharyngitis	1.5% (40/2609) (1.1%, 2.1%)	0.9% (5/542) (0.3%, 2.1%)
Upper respiratory infection	1.1% (29/2609) (0.8%, 1.6%)	0.0% (0/542) (0.0%, 0.7%)
Cough	1.0% (26/2609) (0.7%, 1.5%)	0.0% (0/542) (0.0%, 0.7%)
Gastrointestinal disorders†		
Abdominal pain	1.6% (42/2609) (1.2%, 2.2%)	0.9% (5/542) (0.3%, 2.1%)
Diarrhea	1.0% (26/2609) (0.7%, 1.5%)	0.0% (0/542) (0.0%, 0.7%)
Vomiting	1.0% (27/2609) (0.7%, 1.5%)	0.2% (1/542) (0.0%, 1.0%)
Nervous system disorders†		
Headache	2.3% (60/2609) (1.8%, 3.0%)	1.1% (6/542) (0.4%, 2.4%)
General disorders and administration site reactions†,‡		
Injection-site pain	18.7% (488/2608) (17.2%, 20.3%)	6.4% (34/534) (4.5%, 8.8%)
Injection-site tenderness	16.9% (441/2608) (15.5%, 18.4%)	6.6% (35/534) (4.6%, 9.0%)
Injection-site warmth	8.6% (223/2608) (7.5%, 9.7%)	1.7% (9/534) (0.8%, 3.2%)
Injection-site erythema	7.5% (195/2608) (6.5%, 8.6%)	1.7% (9/534) (0.8%, 3.2%)
Injection-site swelling	7.3% (190/2608) (6.3%, 8.4%)	1.7% (9/534) (0.8%, 3.2%)
Fever (≥102°F, oral)†	1.1% (28/2591) (0.7%, 1.6%)	0.9% (5/542) (0.3%, 2.1%)
Injection-site ecchymosis	1.3% (35/2608) (0.9%, 1.9%)	0.4% (2/534) (0.1%, 1.4%)

N=Number of subjects enrolled/randomized.
n=Number of subjects in each category.

* Placebo (Alum diluent) = amorphous aluminum hydroxyphosphate sulfate. Data represent adverse events following a single dose of placebo, since they were subsequently unblinded and received vaccine.
† Systemic Adverse Events reported Days 1 to 14 after vaccination, regardless of causality.
‡ Adverse Reactions at the injection site (VAQTA) and measured fevers Days 1 to 5 after vaccination

The race distribution of the study subjects who received at least one dose of VAQTA in these studies was as follows: 94.2% Caucasian; 2.2% Black; 1.5% Hispanic; 1.5% Oriental; 0.4% other; 0.2% American Indian. The distribution of subjects by gender was 47.6% male and 52.4% female. The most common adverse event/reaction was injection-site pain/soreness/tenderness reported by 67.0% of subjects. Of all reported injection-site reactions 99.8% were mild (i.e., easily tolerated with no medical intervention) or moderate (i.e., minimally interfered with usual activity possibly requiring little medical intervention). Listed below in Table 11 are the local adverse reactions and systemic adverse events reported by ≥1% of subjects, in decreasing order of frequency within each body system.

Table 11: Incidences of Local Adverse Reactions and Systemic Adverse Events ≥1% in Adults 19 Years of Age and Older

Body System Adverse Events	VAQTA (Any Dose) (N=1645) Rate (n/total n) (95% CI)
Nervous system disorders*	
Headache	16.1% (265/1641) (14.4%, 18.0%)
Gastrointestinal disorders*	
Abdominal pain	1.3% (22/1641) (0.8%, 2.0%)
Diarrhea	2.6% (43/1641) (1.9%, 3.5%)
Nausea	2.4% (40/1641) (1.8%, 3.3%)
Musculoskeletal and connective tissue disorders*	
Myalgia	1.9% (31/1641) (1.3%, 2.7%)
Arm pain	1.5% (25/1641) (1.0%, 2.2%)
Back pain	1.1% (18/1641) (0.7%, 1.7%)
Stiffness	1.0% (17/1641) (0.6%, 1.7%)
Infections and infestations*	
Pharyngitis	2.9% (47/1641) (2.1%, 3.8%)
Upper respiratory infection	2.7% (45/1641) (2.0%, 3.7%)
General disorders and administration site reactions†	
Injection-site pain/tenderness/soreness	67.0% (1099/1640) (64.6%, 69.3%)
Injection-site warmth	18.2% (298/1640) (16.3%, 20.1%)
Injection-site swelling	14.7% (242/1640) (13.1%, 16.6%)
Injection-site erythema	13.7% (224/1640) (12.0%, 15.4%)
Asthenia/fatigue	4.0% (67/1641)† (3.2%, 5.2%)
Injection-site ecchymosis	1.3% (22/1640) (0.8%, 2.0%)
Fever (≥101°F, oral)†	1.0% (17/1626) (0.6%, 1.7%)
Reproductive system and breast disorders*	
Menstruation disorders	1.0% (17/1641) (0.6%, 1.7%)

N=Number of subjects enrolled/randomized.
n=Number of subjects in each category.

* Systemic Adverse Events reported Days 1 to 14 after vaccination, regardless of causality.
† Adverse Reactions at the injection site (VAQTA) and measured fever Days 1 to 5 after vaccination.

alone (N=164 adults who received VAQTA alone). A third study was single-blind and evaluated 3 different lots of VAQTA (N=1112). The fourth study that was also single-blind evaluated doses of VAQTA with varying amounts of viral antigen in healthy adults ≥170 pounds and ≥30 years of age (N=159 adults administered the 50U/1.0 mL dose).

³ Registered trademark of Sanofi Pasteur, Inc.
⁴ Registered trademark of Wyeth Pharmaceuticals, Inc.

6.2 Allergic Reactions

Local and/or systemic allergic reactions that occurred in <1% of over 10,000 children/adolescents or adults in clinical trials regardless of causality included:

Local
Injection-site pruritus and/or rash.

Systemic
Bronchial constriction; asthma; wheezing; edema/swelling; rash; generalized erythema; urticaria; pruritus; eye irritation/itching; dermatitis [see Contraindications (4) and Warnings and Precautions (5.1)].

6.3 Post-Marketing Experience

The following additional adverse events have been reported with use of the marketed vaccine. Because these reactions are reported voluntarily from a population of uncertain size, it is not possible to reliably estimate their frequency or establish a causal relationship to a vaccine exposure.

Blood and lymphatic disorders: Thrombocytopenia.
Nervous system disorders: Guillain-Barré syndrome; cerebellar ataxia; encephalitis.

6.4 Post-Marketing Observational Safety Study

In a post-marketing, short-term safety surveillance study, conducted at a large health maintenance organization in the United States, a total of 42,110 individuals ≥2 years of age received 1 or 2 doses of VAQTA (13,735 children/adolescents and 28,375 adult subjects). Safety was passively monitored by electronic search of the automated medical records database for emergency room and outpatient visits, hospitalizations, and deaths. Medical charts were reviewed when indicated. There was no serious, vaccine-related adverse reaction identified among the 42,110 vaccine recipients in this study. Diarrhea/gastroenteritis, resulting in outpatient visits, was determined by the investigator to be the only vaccine-related nonserious adverse reaction in the study. There was no vaccine-related adverse reaction identified that had not been reported in earlier clinical trials with VAQTA.

7 DRUG INTERACTIONS

7.1 Use with Other Vaccines

Do not mix VAQTA with any other vaccine in the same syringe or vial. Use separate injection sites and syringes for each vaccine. Please refer to package inserts of coadministered vaccines.

VAQTA may be given concomitantly with measles, mumps, rubella, varicella, and pneumococcal 7-valent conjugate vaccines [see Adverse Reactions (6.1) and Clinical Studies (14.7)].

VAQTA may be given to adults concomitantly with typhoid Vi polysaccharide and yellow fever vaccines [see Adverse Reactions (6.1) and Clinical Studies (14.7)].

Data on concomitant use of VAQTA with other vaccines such as combination diphtheria toxoid, tetanus toxoid and acellular pertussis vaccine and poliovirus vaccine are insufficient to support coadministration with VAQTA [see Clinical Studies (14.7)].

7.2 Use with Immune Globulin

VAQTA may be administered concomitantly with Immune Globulin, human, using separate sites and syringes. The recommended vaccination regimen for VAQTA should be followed. Consult the manufacturer's product circular for the appropriate dosage of IG. A booster dose of VAQTA should be administered at the appropriate time as outlined in the recommended regimen for VAQTA [see Clinical Studies (14.5)].

7.3 Immunosuppressive Therapy

If VAQTA is administered to a person receiving immunosuppressive therapy, an adequate immunologic response may not be obtained.

8 USE IN SPECIFIC POPULATIONS

8.1 Pregnancy

Pregnancy Category C: Animal reproduction studies have not been conducted with VAQTA. It is also not known whether VAQTA can cause fetal harm when administered to a pregnant woman or can affect reproduction capacity. VAQTA should be given to a pregnant woman only if clearly needed.

8.3 Nursing Mothers

It is not known whether VAQTA is excreted in human milk. Because many drugs are excreted in human milk, caution should be exercised when VAQTA is administered to a woman who is breast-feeding.

8.4 Pediatric Use

The safety of VAQTA has been evaluated in 3159 children 12 through 23 months of age, and 2615 children/adolescents 2 through 18 years of age who received at least one 25U dose of VAQTA [see Adverse Reactions (6) and Dosage and Administration (2)].

Safety and effectiveness in infants below 12 months of age have not been established.

8.5 Geriatric Use

In a large post-marketing observational safety study in 42,110 individuals, 4769 were 65 years of age or older, of whom 1073 were 75 years of age or older. There were no adverse events judged by the investigator to be vaccine-related in the geriatric study population. In other clinical studies of VAQTA, conducted pre- and post-licensure, 68 subjects were vaccinated with VAQTA who were 65 years of age or older, 10 of whom were 75 years of age or older. No overall differences in safety and immunogenicity were observed between these subjects and younger subjects; however, greater sensitivity of some older individuals cannot be ruled out. Other reported clinical experience has not identified differences in responses between the elderly and younger subjects.

8.6 Immunocompromised Individuals

Immunocompromised persons may have a diminished immune response to VAQTA and may not be protected against HAV infection [see Drug Interactions (7.3)].

11 DESCRIPTION

VAQTA is an inactivated whole virus vaccine derived from hepatitis A virus grown in cell culture in human MRC-5 diploid fibroblasts. It contains inactivated virus of a strain which was originally derived by further serial passage of a proven attenuated strain. The virus is grown, harvested, purified by a combination of physical and high performance liquid chromatographic techniques developed at the Merck Research Laboratories, formalin inactivated, and then adsorbed onto amorphous aluminum hydroxyphosphate sulfate.

VAQTA is a sterile suspension for intramuscular injection. One milliliter of the vaccine contains approximately 50U of hepatitis A virus antigen, which is purified and formulated without a preservative. Within the limits of current assay variability, the 50U dose of VAQTA contains less than 0.1 mcg of non-viral protein, less than 4×10^{-6} mcg of DNA, less than 10^{-4} mcg of bovine albumin, and less than 0.8 mcg of formaldehyde. Other process chemical residuals are less than 10 parts per billion (ppb), including neomycin.

Each 0.5-mL pediatric dose contains 25U of hepatitis A virus antigen and adsorbed onto approximately 0.225 mg of aluminum provided as amorphous aluminum hydroxyphosphate sulfate, and 35 mcg of sodium borate as a pH stabilizer, in 0.9% sodium chloride.

Each 1.0-mL adult dose contains 50U of hepatitis A virus antigen and adsorbed onto approximately 0.45 mg of aluminum provided as amorphous aluminum hydroxyphosphate sulfate, and 70 mcg of sodium borate as a pH stabilizer, in 0.9% sodium chloride.

12 CLINICAL PHARMACOLOGY

12.1 Mechanism of Action

Hepatitis A Disease

Hepatitis A virus is one of several hepatitis viruses that cause a systemic infection with pathology in the liver. The incubation period ranges from approximately 20 to 50 days. The course of the disease following infection ranges from asymptomatic infection to fulminant hepatitis and death. Protection from hepatitis A disease has been shown to be related to the presence of antibody. However, the lowest titer needed to confer protection has not been determined.

13 NONCLINICAL TOXICOLOGY

13.1 Carcinogenesis, Mutagenesis, Impairment of Fertility

VAQTA has not been evaluated for its carcinogenic or mutagenic potential, or its potential to impair fertility.

14 CLINICAL STUDIES

14.1 Efficacy of VAQTA: The Monroe Clinical Study

The immunogenicity and protective efficacy of VAQTA were evaluated in a randomized, double-blind, placebo-controlled study involving 1037 susceptible healthy children and adolescents 2 through 16 years of age in a U.S. community with recurrent outbreaks of hepatitis A (The Monroe Efficacy Study). All of these children were Caucasian, and there were 51.5% male and 48.5% female. Each child received an intramuscular dose of VAQTA (25U) (N=519) or placebo (alum diluent) (N=518). Among those individuals who were initially seronegative (measured by a modification of the HAVAB[5] radioimmunoassay [RIA]), seroconversion was achieved in >99% of vaccine recipients within 4 weeks after vaccination. The onset of seroconversion following a single dose of VAQTA was shown to parallel the onset of protection against clinical hepatitis A disease.

Because of the long incubation period of the disease (approximately 20 to 50 days, or longer in children), clinical efficacy was based on confirmed cases[6] of hepatitis A occurring ≥50 days after vaccination in order to exclude any children incubating the infection before vaccination. In subjects who were initially seronegative, the protective efficacy of a single dose of VAQTA was observed to be 100% with 21 cases of clinically confirmed hepatitis A occurring in the placebo group and none in the vaccine group (p<0.001). The number of clinically confirmed cases of hepatitis A ≥30 days after vaccination were also compared. In this analysis, 28 cases of clinically confirmed hepatitis A occurred in the placebo group while none occurred in the vaccine group ≥30 days after vaccination. In addition, it was observed in this trial that no cases of clinically confirmed hepatitis A occurred in the vaccine group after day 16.[7] Following demonstration of protection with a single dose and termination of the study, a booster dose was administered to a subset of vaccinees 6, 12, or 18 months after the primary dose.

No cases of clinically confirmed hepatitis A disease ≥50 days after vaccination have occurred in those vaccinees from The Monroe Efficacy Study monitored for up to 9 years.

[5] Trademark of Abbott Laboratories
[6] The clinical case definition included all of the following occurring at the same time: 1) one or more typical clinical signs or symptoms of hepatitis A (e.g., jaundice, malaise, fever ≥38.3°C); 2) elevation of hepatitis A IgM antibody (HAVAB-M); 3) elevation of alanine transferase (ALT) ≥2 times the upper limit of normal.
[7] One vaccinee did not meet the pre-defined criteria for clinically confirmed hepatitis A but did have positive hepatitis A IgM and borderline liver enzyme (ALT) elevations on days 34, 50, and 58 after vaccination with mild clinical symptoms observed on days 49 and 50.

14.2 Other Clinical Studies

The efficacy of VAQTA in other age groups was based upon immunogenicity measured 4 to 6 weeks following vaccination. VAQTA was found to be immunogenic in all age groups.

Children—12 through 23 Months of Age

In one study children were randomized to receive the first dose of VAQTA with or without M-M-R II and VARIVAX (N=617) and the second dose of VAQTA with or without DTaP and optionally either oral or inactivated poliovirus vaccine (N=555). The race distribution of the study subjects who received at least one dose of VAQTA in this study was as follows: 56.7% Caucasian; 17.5% Hispanic-American; 14.3% African-American; 7.0% Native American; 3.4% other; 0.8% Oriental; 0.2% Asian; and 0.2% Indian. The distribution of subjects by gender was 53.6% male and 46.4% female. In the analysis population, there were 471 initially seronegative children 12 through 23 months of age, who received the first dose of VAQTA with (N=237) or without (N=234) M-M-R II and VARIVAX of whom 96% (95% CI: 93.7%, 97.5%) seroconverted (defined as having a titer ≥10 mIU/mL) post dose 1 with a GMT of 48 mIU/mL (95% CI: 44.7, 51.6). There were 343 children in the analysis population who received the second dose of VAQTA with (N=168) or without (N=175) DTaP and optional oral or inactivated poliovirus vaccine of whom 100% (95% CI: 99.3%, 100%) seroconverted post dose 2 with a GMT of 6920 mIU/mL (95% CI: 6136, 7801). Of children who received only VAQTA at both visits, 100% (n=97) seroconverted after the second dose of VAQTA. This rate was similar to the expected rate of 99% in 2- to 3-year-old children.

In a clinical trial involving 653 healthy children 12 to 15 months of age, 330 were randomized to receive VAQTA, ProQuad, and pneumococcal 7-valent conjugate vaccine concomitantly, and 323 were randomized to receive ProQuad and pneumococcal 7-valent conjugate vaccine concomitantly followed by VAQTA 6 weeks later. The race distribution of the study subjects was as follows: 60.3% Caucasian; 21.6% African-American; 9.5% Hispanic-American; 7.2% other; 1.1% Asian/Pacific; and 0.3% Native American. The distribution of subjects by gender was 50.7% male and 49.3% female. In the analysis population, the seropositivity rate for hepatitis A antibody (defined as the percent of subjects with a titer ≥10 mIU/mL) was 100% (n=182; 95% CI: 98.0%, 100%) post dose 2 with a GMT of 4977 mIU/mL (95% CI: 4068, 6089) when VAQTA was given with ProQuad and pneumococcal 7-valent conjugate vaccine and 99.4% (n=159, 95% CI: 96.5%, 100%) post dose 2 with a GMT of 6123 mIU/mL (95% CI: 4826, 7770) when VAQTA alone was given. These seropositivity rates were similar whether VAQTA was given with or without ProQuad and pneumococcal 7-valent conjugate vaccine.

Children/Adolescents—2 through 18 Years of Age

Immunogenicity data were combined from eleven randomized clinical studies in children and adolescents 2 through 18 years of age who received VAQTA (25U/0.5 mL). These included administration of VAQTA in varying doses and regimens (N=404 received 25U/0.5 mL), the Monroe Efficacy Study (N=973), and comparison studies for process and formulation changes (N=1238). The race distribution of the study subjects who received at least one dose of VAQTA in these studies was as follows: 84.8% Caucasian; 10.6% American Indian; 2.3% African-American; 1.5% Hispanic-American; 0.6% other; 0.2% Oriental. The distribution of subjects by gender was 51.2% male and 48.8% female. The proportions of subjects who seroconverted 4 weeks after the first and second doses administered 6 months apart were 97% (n=1230; 95% CI: 96%, 98%) and 100% (n=1057; 95% CI: 99.5%, 100%) of subjects with GMTs of 43 mIU/mL (95% CI: 40, 45) and 10,077 mIU/mL (95% CI: 9394, 10,810), respectively.

Adults—19 Years of Age and Older

Immunogenicity data were combined from five randomized clinical studies in adults 19 years of age and older who received VAQTA (50U/1.0 mL). One single-blind study evaluated doses of VAQTA with varying amounts of viral antigen and/or alum content in healthy adults ≥170 pounds and ≥30 years of age (N=208 adults administered 50U/1.0 mL dose). One open-label study evaluated VAQTA given with immune globulin or alone (N=164 adults who received VAQTA alone). A third study was single-blind and evaluated 3 different lots of VAQTA (N=1112). The fourth study was single-blind and evaluated doses of VAQTA with varying amounts of viral antigen in healthy adults ≥170 pounds and ≥30 years of age (N=159 adults administered the 50U/1.0 mL dose). The fifth study was an open-label study to evaluate various regimens for time of administration of the booster dose of VAQTA (6, 12, and 18 months post dose 1, N=354). The race distribution of the study subjects who received at least one dose of VAQTA in these studies was as follows: 93.2% Caucasian; 2.5% African-American; 2.1% Hispanic-American; 1.4% Oriental; 0.5% other; 0.3% American Indian. The distribution of subjects by gender was 44.8% male and 55.2% female. The proportion of subjects who seroconverted 4 weeks after the first and second doses administered 6 months apart was 95% (n=1411; 95% CI: 94%, 96%) and 99.9% (n=1244; 95% CI: 99.4%, 100%) with GMTs of 37 mIU/mL (95% CI: 35, 38) and 6013 mIU/mL (95% CI: 5592, 6467), respectively. Furthermore, at 2 weeks postvaccination, 69.2% (n=744; 95% CI: 65.7%, 72.5%) of adults seroconverted with a GMT of 16 mIU/mL after a single dose of VAQTA.

14.3 Timing of Booster Dose Administration

Children/Adolescents—2 through 18 Years of Age

In the Monroe Efficacy Study, children were administered a second dose of VAQTA (25U/0.5 mL) 6, 12, or 18 months following the initial dose. For subjects who received both doses of VAQTA, the GMTs and proportions of subjects who seroconverted 4 weeks after the booster dose administered 6, 12, and 18 months after the first dose are presented in Table 12.

[See table 12 above]

Adults—19 years of age and older

Among the 5 randomized clinical studies in adults 19 years of age and older described in Section 14.2, there were additional data in which a booster dose of VAQTA (50U/1.0 mL) was administered 12 or 18 months after the first dose. For subjects in these studies who received both doses of VAQTA, the proportions who seroconverted 4 weeks after the booster dose administered 6, 12, and 18 months after the first dose were 100% of 1201 subjects, 98% of 91 subjects, and 100% of 84 subjects, respectively. GMTs in mIU/mL one month after the subjects received the booster dose at 6, 12, or 18 months after the primary dose were 5987 mIU/mL (95% CI: 5561, 6445), 4896 mIU/mL (95% CI: 3589, 6679), and 6043 mIU/mL (95% CI: 4687, 7793), respectively.

14.4 Duration of Immune Response

In follow-up of subjects in The Monroe Efficacy Study, in children (≥2 years of age) and adolescents who received two doses (25U) of VAQTA, detectable levels of anti-HAV antibodies (≥10 mIU/mL) were present in 100% of subjects for at least 10 years postvaccination. In subjects who received VAQTA at 0 and 6 months, the GMT was 819 mIU/mL (n=175) at 2.5 to 3.5 years and 505 mIU/mL (n=174) at 5 to 6 years, and 574 mIU/mL (n=114) at 10 years postvaccination. In subjects who received VAQTA at 0 and 12 months, the GMT was 2224 mIU/mL (n=49) at 2.5 to 3.5 years, 1191 mIU/mL (n=47) at 5 to 6 years, and 1005 mIU/mL (n=36) at 10 years postvaccination. In subjects who received VAQTA at 0 and 18 months, the GMT was 2501 mIU/mL (n=53) at 2.5 to 3.5 years, 1614 mIU/mL (n=56) at 5 to 6 years, and 1507 mIU/mL (n=41) at 10 years postvaccination.

In adults that were administered VAQTA at 0 and 6 months, the hepatitis A antibody response to date has been shown to persist at least 6 years. Detectable levels of anti-HAV antibodies (≥10 mIU/mL) were present in 100% (378/378) of subjects with a GMT of 1734 mIU/mL at 1 year, 99.2% (252/254) of subjects with a GMT of 687 mIU/mL at 2 to 3 years, 99.1% (219/221) of subjects with a GMT of 605 mIU/mL at 4 years, and 99.4% (170/171) of subjects with a GMT of 684 mIU/mL at 6 years postvaccination.

The total duration of the protective effect of VAQTA in healthy vaccinees is unknown at present.

14.5 Post-Exposure Prophylaxis

The concurrent use of VAQTA (50U) and immune globulin (IG, 0.06 mL/kg) was evaluated in an open-label, randomized clinical study involving 294 healthy adults 18 to 39 years of age. Adults were randomized to receive 2 doses of VAQTA 24 weeks apart (N=129), the first dose of VAQTA concomitant with a dose of IG followed by the second dose of VAQTA alone 24 weeks later (N=135), or IG alone (N=30). The race distribution of the study subjects who received at least one dose of VAQTA or IG in this study was as follows: 92.3% Caucasian; 4.0% Hispanic-American; 3.0% African-American; 0.3% Native American; 0.3% Asian/Pacific. The distribution of subjects by gender was 28.7% male and 71.3% female. Table 13 provides seroconversion rates and

Table 12: Children/Adolescents from the Monroe Efficacy Study: Seroconversion Rates (%) and Geometric Mean Titers (GMT) for Cohorts of Initially Seronegative Vaccinees at the Time of the Booster (25U) and 4 Weeks Later

Months Following Initial 25U Dose	Cohort* (n=960) 0 and 6 Months	Cohort* (n=35) 0 and 12 Months	Cohort* (n=39) 0 and 18 Months
	Seroconversion Rate GMT (mIU/mL) (95% CI)		
6	97% 107 (98, 117)	—	—
7	100% 10433 (9681, 11243)	—	—
12	—	91% 48 (33, 71)	—
13	—	100% 12308 (9337, 16226)	—
18	—	—	90% 50 (28, 89)
19	—	—	100% 9591 (7613, 12082)

* Blood samples were taken at prebooster and postbooster time points.

Table 14: VAQTA versus HAVRIX: Seropositivity Rate, Booster Response Rate* and Geometric Mean Titer at 4 Weeks Postbooster

First Dose	Booster Dose	Seropositivity Rate	Booster Response Rate*	Geometric Mean Titer
HAVRIX 1440 EL.U.	VAQTA 50 U	99.7% (n=313)	86.1% (n=310)	3272 (n=313)
HAVRIX 1440 EL.U.	HAVRIX 1440 EL.U.	99.3% (n=151)	80.1% (n=151)	2423 (n=151)

* Booster Response Rate is defined as greater than or equal to a tenfold rise from prebooster to postbooster titer and postbooster titer ≥100 mIU/mL.

geometric mean titers (GMTs) at 4 and 24 weeks after the first dose in each treatment group and at one month after a booster dose of VAQTA (administered at 24 weeks).

Table 13: Seroconversion Rates (%) and Geometric Mean Titers (GMT) After Vaccination with VAQTA Plus IG, VAQTA Alone, and IG Alone

Weeks	VAQTA plus IG	VAQTA	IG
	Seroconversion Rate GMT (mIU/mL) (95% CI)		
4	100% 42 (39, 45) (n=129)	96% 38 (33, 42) (n=135)	87% 19 (15, 23) (n=30)
24	92% 83 (65, 105) (n=125)	97%* 137* (112, 169) (n=132)	0% Undetectable† (n=28)
28	100% 4872 (3716, 6388) (n=114)	100% 6498 (5111, 8261) (n=128)	N/A

N/A = Not Applicable.

* The seroconversion rate and the GMT in the group receiving VAQTA alone were significantly higher than in the group receiving VAQTA plus IG (p=0.05, p<0.001, respectively).
† Undetectable is defined as <10mIU/mL.

14.6 Interchangeability of the Booster Dose

A randomized, double-blind clinical study in 537 healthy adults, 18 to 83 years of age, evaluated the immune response to a booster dose of VAQTA and HAVRIX (Hepatitis A vaccine, inactivated) given at 6 or 12 months following an initial dose of HAVRIX. Subjects were randomized to receive VAQTA (50U) as a booster dose 6 months (N=232) or 12 months (N=124) following an initial dose of HAVRIX or HAVRIX (1440 EL. U) as a booster dose 6 months (N=118) or 12 months (N=63) following an initial dose of HAVRIX. The race distribution of the study subjects who received the booster dose of VAQTA or HAVRIX in this study was as follows: 87.2% Caucasian; 8.0% African-American; 1.9% Hispanic-American; 1.3% Oriental; 0.9% Asian; 0.4% Indian; 0.4% other. The distribution of subjects by gender was 44.9% male and 55.1% female. When VAQTA was given as a booster dose following HAVRIX, the vaccine produced an adequate immune response (see Table 14) *[see Dosage and Administration (2.1)]*.

[See table 14 above]

14.7 Immune Response to Concomitantly Administered Vaccines

Clinical Studies of VAQTA with M-M-R II, VARIVAX, and DTaP

Concomitant administration of routinely administered recommended childhood vaccines with VAQTA was assessed in a study of 617 children. In this study, the immune response to VAQTA (25U) was assessed in 471 children randomized to receive VAQTA with (N=237) or without M-M-R II and VARIVAX (N=234) at 12 months of age. The race distribution of the study subjects who received at least one dose of VAQTA in these studies was as follows: 56.7% Caucasian; 17.5% Hispanic-American; 14.3% African-American; 7.0% Native American; 3.4% other; 0.8% Oriental; 0.2% Asian; and 0.2% Indian. The distribution of subjects by gender was 53.6% male and 46.4% female. Rates of seroprotection to hepatitis A were similar between the two groups who received VAQTA with or without M-M-R II and VARIVAX. Measles, mumps, and rubella immune responses were 98.8% [95% CI: 96.4%, 99.7%], 99.6% [95% CI: 97.9%, 100%], and 100% [95% CI: 98.6%, 100%], respectively, which were similar to historical rates observed following vaccination with a first dose of M-M-R II in this age group. Data on the varicella immune response were insufficient to adequately assess its immunogenicity when VARIVAX was administered concomitantly with VAQTA. In this same study, immune responses were evaluated in 183 subjects who were administered VAQTA with (N=86) and without DTaP (N=97) at 18 months of age. Rates of seroprotection to hepatitis A were similar between the two groups who received VAQTA with or without DTaP. However, data are insufficient to assess the immune response of DTaP when administered with VAQTA.

Clinical Studies of VAQTA with ProQuad and Pneumococcal 7-valent Conjugate Vaccine

In a clinical trial involving 653 healthy children 12 to 15 months of age, 330 were randomized to receive VAQTA, ProQuad, and pneumococcal 7-valent conjugate vaccine concomitantly, and 323 were randomized to receive ProQuad and pneumococcal 7-valent conjugate vaccine concomitantly followed by VAQTA 6 weeks later. The race distribution of the study subjects was as follows: 60.3% Caucasian; 21.6% African-American; 9.5% Hispanic-American; 7.2% other; 1.1% Asian/Pacific; and 0.3% Native American. The distribution of subjects by gender was 50.7% male and 49.3% female. The GMTs for *S. pneumoniae* types 4, 6B, 9V, 14, 18C, 19F, and 23F 6 weeks after vaccination with pneumococcal 7-valent conjugate vaccine administered concomitantly with ProQuad and VAQTA were non-inferior as compared to GMTs observed in the group given pneumococcal 7-valent conjugate vaccine with ProQuad alone (the lower bounds of the 95% CI around the fold-difference for the 7 serotypes excluded 0.5). For the varicella component of ProQuad, in subjects with baseline antibody titers <1.25 gpELISA units/

mL, the proportion with a titer ≥5 gpELISA units/mL 6 weeks after their first dose of ProQuad was non-inferior (defined as -10 percentage point change) when ProQuad was administered with VAQTA and pneumococcal 7-valent conjugate vaccine as compared to the proportion with a titer ≥5 gpELISA units/mL when ProQuad was administered with pneumococcal 7-valent conjugate vaccine alone (difference in seroprotection rate -5.1% [95% CI: -9.3, -1.4%]). Hepatitis A responses were similar when compared between the two groups who received VAQTA with or without ProQuad and pneumococcal 7-valent conjugate vaccine. Seroconversion rates and antibody titers for varicella and *S. pneumoniae* types 4, 6B, 9V, 14, 18C, 19F, and 23F were similar between groups at 6 weeks postvaccination.

Clinical Studies of VAQTA with Typhoid Vi Polysaccharide Vaccine and Yellow Fever Vaccine, Live Attenuated

In an open-label clinical trial, 240 healthy adults 18 to 54 years of age were randomized to receive either VAQTA with typhoid Vi polysaccharide and yellow fever vaccines concomitantly (N=80), typhoid Vi polysaccharide and yellow fever vaccines concomitantly (N=80), or VAQTA alone (N=80). Approximately 6 months later, subjects who received VAQTA were administered a booster dose. The race distribution of the study subjects who received VAQTA with or without typhoid Vi polysaccharide and yellow fever vaccine was as follows: 78.3% Caucasian; 14.2% Oriental; 3.3% other; 2.1% African-American; 1.7% Indian; 0.4% Hispanic-American. The distribution of subjects by gender was 40.8% male and 59.2% female. The seropositivity rate for hepatitis A when VAQTA, typhoid Vi polysaccharide, and yellow fever vaccines were administered concomitantly was generally similar to when VAQTA was given alone. The antibody response rates for typhoid Vi polysaccharide and yellow fever were adequate when typhoid Vi polysaccharide and yellow fever vaccines were administered concomitantly with and without VAQTA. The GMTs for hepatitis A when VAQTA, typhoid Vi polysaccharide, and yellow fever vaccines were administered concomitantly were reduced when compared to VAQTA alone. Following receipt of the booster dose of VAQTA, the GMTs for hepatitis A in these two groups were observed to be comparable *[see Drug Interactions (7.1)]*.

Data are insufficient to assess the immune response to VAQTA and poliovirus vaccine following concomitant administration of the vaccines.

There are no data to assess concomitant use of Haemophilus influenzae type b conjugate vaccine with VAQTA *[see Drug Interactions (7.1)]*.

16 HOW SUPPLIED/STORAGE AND HANDLING

VAQTA is available in single-dose vials and prefilled Luer Lock syringes.

Pediatric/Adolescent Formulations

25U/0.5 mL in single-dose vials and prefilled Luer Lock syringes.

NDC 0006-4831-41–box of ten 0.5-mL single dose vials.

NDC 0006-4095-09–carton of six 0.5-mL prefilled single-dose Luer Lock syringes with tip caps.

Adult Formulations

50U/1.0 mL in single-dose vials and prefilled Luer Lock syringes.

NDC 0006-4841-00–1.0-mL single dose vial.

NDC 0006-4841-41–box of ten 1.0-mL single dose vials.

NDC 0006-4096-09–carton of six 1.0-mL prefilled single-dose Luer Lock syringes with tip caps.

Store vaccine at 2-8°C (36-46°F).

DO NOT FREEZE since freezing destroys potency.

17 PATIENT COUNSELING INFORMATION

17.1 Instructions

Information for Vaccine Recipients and Parents or Guardians

- Inform the patient, parent or guardian of the potential benefits and risks of the vaccine.
- Question the vaccine recipient, parent, or guardian about the occurrence of any symptoms and/or signs of an adverse reaction after a previous dose of hepatitis A vaccine.
- Inform the patient, parent, or guardian about the potential for adverse events that have been temporally associated with administration of VAQTA.
- Tell the patient, parent, or guardian accompanying the recipient, to report severe or unusual adverse events to the physician or clinic where the vaccine was administered.
- Prior to vaccination, give the patient, parent, or guardian the Vaccine Information Statements which are required by the National Childhood Vaccine Injury Act of 1986. These materials are available free of charge at the Centers for Disease Control and Prevention (CDC) website (www.cdc.gov/vaccines).
- Tell the patient, parent, or guardian that the United States Department of Health and Human Services has established a Vaccine Adverse Event Reporting System (VAERS) to accept all reports of suspected adverse events after the administration of any vaccine, including but not limited to the reporting of events required by the National Childhood Vaccine Injury Act of 1986. The VAERS toll-free number is 1-800-822-7967. Reporting forms may also be obtained at the VAERS website at (www.vaers.hhs.gov).

Manuf. and Dist. by:
MERCK & CO., INC., Whitehouse Station, NJ 08889, USA
Issued June 2010
Printed in USA
9987012

VARIVAX® ℞

[*var-i-vax*]

Varicella Virus Vaccine Live

DESCRIPTION

VARIVAX[1] [Varicella Virus Vaccine Live] is a preparation of the Oka/Merck strain of live, attenuated varicella virus. The virus was initially obtained from a child with natural varicella, then introduced into human embryonic lung cell cultures, adapted to and propagated in embryonic guinea pig cell cultures and finally propagated in human diploid cell cultures (WI-38). Further passage of the virus for varicella vaccine was performed at Merck Research Laboratories (MRL) in human diploid cell cultures (MRC-5) that were free of adventitious agents. This live, attenuated varicella vaccine is a lyophilized preparation containing sucrose, phosphate, glutamate, and processed gelatin as stabilizers.

VARIVAX, when reconstituted as directed, is a sterile preparation for subcutaneous administration. Each 0.5 mL dose contains the following: a minimum of 1350 PFU (plaque forming units) of Oka/Merck varicella virus when reconstituted and stored at room temperature for 30 minutes, approximately 25 mg of sucrose, 12.5 mg hydrolyzed gelatin, 3.2 mg sodium chloride, 0.5 mg monosodium L-glutamate, 0.45 mg of sodium phosphate dibasic, 0.08 mg of potassium phosphate monobasic, 0.08 mg of potassium chloride; residual components of MRC-5 cells including DNA and protein; and trace quantities of sodium phosphate monobasic, EDTA, neomycin, and fetal bovine serum. The product contains no preservative.

To maintain potency, the lyophilized vaccine must be kept frozen at an average temperature of –15°C (+5°F) or colder and must be used before the expiration date (see HOW SUPPLIED, Stability and Storage). Storage in any freezer (e.g., chest, frost-free) that reliably maintains an average temperature of –15°C (+5°F) or colder and has a separate sealed freezer door is acceptable.

[1] Registered trademark of MERCK & CO., Inc.

CLINICAL PHARMACOLOGY

Varicella is a highly communicable disease in children, adolescents, and adults caused by the varicella-zoster virus (VZV). The disease usually consists of 300 to 500 maculopapular and/or vesicular lesions accompanied by a fever (oral temperature ≥100°F) in up to 70% of individuals.(1,2) Approximately 3.5 million cases of varicella occurred annually from 1980-1994 in the United States with the peak incidence occurring in children five to nine years of age.(3) The incidence rate of chickenpox in the total population was 8.3-9.1% per year in children 1-9 years of age before licensure of VARIVAX.(4,6) The attack rate of natural varicella following household exposure among healthy susceptible children was shown to be 87% in unvaccinated populations.(2) Although it is generally a benign, self-limiting disease, varicella may be associated with serious complications (e.g., bacterial superinfection, pneumonia, encephalitis, Reye's Syndrome), and/or death.

Evaluation of Clinical Efficacy Afforded by VARIVAX

The following section presents clinical efficacy data on a 1-dose regimen and a 2-dose regimen in children, and a 2-dose regimen in adolescents and adults.

Clinical Data in Children

One-Dose Regimen in Children

In combined clinical trials(5) of VARIVAX at doses ranging from 1000-17,000 PFU, the majority of subjects who received VARIVAX and were exposed to wild-type virus were either completely protected from chickenpox or developed a milder form (for clinical description see below) of the disease. The protective efficacy of VARIVAX was evaluated in three different ways: 1) by comparing chickenpox rates in vaccinees versus historical controls, 2) by assessment of protection from disease following household exposure, and 3) by a placebo-controlled, double-blind clinical trial.

In early clinical trials,(5) a total of 4240 children 1 to 12 years of age received 1000-1625 PFU of attenuated virus per dose of VARIVAX and have been followed for up to nine years post single-dose vaccination. In this group there was considerable variation in chickenpox rates among studies and study sites, and much of the reported data was acquired by passive follow-up. It was observed that 0.3%-3.8% of vaccinees per year reported chickenpox (called breakthrough cases). This represents an approximate 83% (95% confidence interval [CI], 82%, 84%) decrease from the age-adjusted expected incidence rates in susceptible subjects over this same period.(19) In those who developed breakthrough chickenpox postvaccination, the majority experienced mild disease (median of the maximum number of lesions <50). In one study, a total of 47% (27/58) of breakthrough cases had <50 lesions compared with 8% (7/92) in unvaccinated individuals, and 7% (4/58) of breakthrough cases had >300 lesions compared with 50% (46/92) in unvaccinated individuals.(7)

Among a subset of vaccinees who were actively followed in these early trials for up to nine years postvaccination, 179 individuals had household exposure to chickenpox. There were no reports of breakthrough chickenpox in 84% (150/179) of exposed children, while 16% (29/179) reported a mild form of chickenpox (38% [11/29] of the cases with a maximum total number of <50 lesions; no individuals with >300 lesions). This represents an 81% reduction in the expected number of varicella cases utilizing the historical attack rate of 87% following household exposure to chickenpox in unvaccinated individuals in the calculation of efficacy.

In later clinical trials(5) with the current vaccine, a total of 1114 children 1 to 12 years of age received 2900-9000 PFU of attenuated virus per dose of VARIVAX and have been actively followed for up to 10 years post single-dose vaccination. It was observed that 0.2%-2.3% of vaccinees per year reported breakthrough chickenpox for up to 10 years post single-dose vaccination. This represents an estimated efficacy of 94% (95% CI, 93%, 96%), compared with the age-adjusted expected incidence rates in susceptible subjects over the same period.(4,6,19) In those who developed breakthrough chickenpox postvaccination, the majority experienced mild disease, with the median of the maximum total number of lesions <50. The severity of reported breakthrough chickenpox, as measured by number of lesions and maximum temperature, appeared not to increase with time since vaccination.

Among a subset of vaccinees who were actively followed in these later trials for up to 10 years postvaccination, 95 individuals were exposed to an unvaccinated individual with wild-type chickenpox in a household setting. There were no reports of breakthrough chickenpox in 92% (87/95) of exposed children, while 8% (8/95) reported a mild form of chickenpox (maximum total number of lesions <50; observed range, 10 to 34). This represents an estimated efficacy of 90% (95% CI, 82%, 96%) based on the historical attack rate of 87% following household exposure to chickenpox in unvaccinated individuals in the calculation of efficacy.

Although no placebo-controlled trial was carried out with VARIVAX using the current vaccine, a placebo-controlled trial was conducted using a formulation containing 17,000 PFU per dose.(4,8) In this trial, a single dose of VARIVAX protected 96-100% of children against chickenpox over a two-year period. The study enrolled healthy individuals 1 to 14 years of age (n=491 vaccine, n=465 placebo). In the first year, 8.5% of placebo recipients contracted chickenpox, while no vaccine recipient did, for a calculated protection rate of 100% during the first varicella season. In the second year, when only a subset of individuals agreed to remain in the blinded study (n=163 vaccine, n=161 placebo), 96% protective efficacy was calculated for the vaccine group as compared to placebo.

There are insufficient data to assess the rate of protection against the complications of chickenpox (e.g., encephalitis, hepatitis, pneumonia) in children.

Two-Dose Regimen in Children

In a clinical trial, a total of 2216 children 12 months to 12 years of age with a negative history of varicella were randomized to receive either 1 dose of VARIVAX (n=1114) or 2 doses of VARIVAX (n=1102) given 3 months apart. Subjects were actively followed for varicella, any varicella-like illness, or herpes zoster and any exposures to varicella or herpes zoster on an annual basis for 10 years after vaccination. Persistence of VZV antibody was measured annually for 9 years. Most cases of varicella reported in recipients of 1 dose or 2 doses of vaccine were mild.(26) The estimated vaccine efficacy for the 10-year observation period was 94% for 1 dose and 98% for 2 doses (p<0.001). This translates to a 3.4-fold lower risk of developing varicella >42 days postvaccination during the 10-year observation period in children who received 2 doses than in those who received 1 dose (2.2% vs. 7.5%, respectively).

Clinical Data in Adolescents and Adults

Two-Dose Regimen in Adolescents and Adults

In early clinical trials, a total of 796 adolescents and adults received 905-1230 PFU of attenuated virus per dose of

	VARIVAX 1-Dose Regimen (N = 1114)	VARIVAX 2-Dose Regimen (N = 1102)	
	6 Weeks Postvaccination	6 Weeks Postdose 1	6 Weeks Postdose 2
Seroconversion Rate	98.9% (882/892)	99.5% (847/851)	99.9% (768/769)
Percent with VZV Antibody Titer ≥5 gpELISA units/mL	84.9% (757/892)	87.3% (743/851)	99.5% (765/769)
Geometric mean titers (gpELISA units/mL)	12.0	12.8	141.5

VARIVAX and have been followed for up to six years following 2-dose vaccination. A total of 50 clinical varicella cases were reported >42 days following 2-dose vaccination. Based on passive follow-up, the annual chickenpox breakthrough event rate ranged from <0.1% to 1.9%. The median of the maximum total number of lesions ranged from 15 to 42 per year.

Although no placebo-controlled trial was carried out in adolescents and adults, the protective efficacy of VARIVAX was determined by evaluation of protection when vaccinees received 2 doses of VARIVAX 4 or 8 weeks apart and were subsequently exposed to chickenpox in a household setting.{5} Among the subset of vaccinees who were actively followed in these early trials for up to six years, 76 individuals had household exposure to chickenpox. There were no reports of breakthrough chickenpox in 83% (63/76) of exposed vaccinees, while 17% (13/76) reported a mild form of chickenpox. Among 13 vaccinated individuals who developed breakthrough chickenpox after a household exposure, 62% (8/13) of the cases reported maximum total number of lesions <50, while no individual reported >75 lesions. The attack rate of unvaccinated adults exposed to a single contact in a household has not been previously studied. Utilizing the previously reported historical attack rate of 87% for natural varicella following household exposure to chickenpox among unvaccinated children in the calculation of efficacy, this represents an approximate 80% reduction in the expected number of cases in the household setting.

In later clinical trials, a total of 220 adolescents and adults received 3315-9000 PFU of attenuated virus per dose of VARIVAX and have been actively followed for up to six years following 2-dose vaccination. A total of 3 clinical varicella cases were reported >42 days following 2-dose vaccination. Two cases reported <50 lesions and none reported >75. The annual chickenpox breakthrough event rate ranged from 0% to 1.2%. Among the subset of vaccinees who were actively followed in these later trials for up to five years, 16 individuals were exposed to an unvaccinated individual with wild-type chickenpox in a household setting. There were no reports of breakthrough chickenpox among the exposed vaccinees.

There are insufficient data to assess the rate of protection of VARIVAX against the serious complications of chickenpox in adults (e.g., encephalitis, hepatitis, pneumonitis) and during pregnancy (congenital varicella syndrome).

Immunogenicity of VARIVAX

The following section presents immunogenicity data on a 1-dose regimen and a 2-dose regimen in children, and a 2-dose regimen in adolescents and adults.

One-Dose Regimen in Children

Clinical trials with several formulations of the vaccine containing attenuated virus ranging from 1000 to 17,000 PFU per dose have demonstrated that VARIVAX induces detectable immune responses in a high proportion of individuals and is generally well tolerated in healthy individuals ranging from 12 months to 55 years of age.{4,5,9-15}

Seroconversion is defined by the acquisition of any detectable VZV antibodies, based on an optical density (OD) cutoff, corresponding approximately to a lower limit of 0.6 glycoprotein enzyme-linked immunosorbent assay (gpELISA) units/mL.

The gpELISA is a highly sensitive assay that is not commercially available. Seroconversion was observed in 97% of vaccinees at approximately 4-6 weeks postvaccination in 6889 susceptible children 12 months to 12 years of age. Rates of breakthrough disease were significantly lower among children with VZV antibody titers ≥5 gpELISA units/mL compared with children with titers <5 gpELISA units/mL. Titers ≥5 gpELISA units/mL were induced in approximately 76% of children vaccinated with a single dose of vaccine at 1000-17,000 PFU per dose.

VARIVAX also induces cell-mediated immune responses in vaccinees. The relative contributions of humoral immunity and cell-mediated immunity to protection from chickenpox are unknown.

Two-Dose Regimen in Children

In a multicenter study, healthy children 12 months to 12 years of age received either 1 dose of VARIVAX or 2 doses administered 3 months apart. The immunogenicity results are shown in the following table.

[See table above]

The results from this study and other studies in which a second dose of vaccine was administered 3 to 6 years after the initial dose demonstrate significant boosting of the VZV antibody response with a second dose. VZV antibody levels after 2 doses given 3 to 6 years apart are comparable to those obtained when the 2 doses are given 3 months apart.

Two-Dose Regimen in Adolescents and Adults

In a multicenter study involving susceptible adolescents and adults 13 years of age and older, 2 doses of VARIVAX administered 4 to 8 weeks apart induced a seroconversion rate of approximately 75% in 539 individuals 4 weeks after the first dose and of 99% in 479 individuals 4 weeks after the second dose. The average antibody response in vaccinees who received the second dose 8 weeks after the first dose was higher than that in vaccinees who received the second dose 4 weeks after the first dose. In another multicenter study involving adolescents and adults, 2 doses of VARIVAX administered 8 weeks apart induced a seroconversion rate of 94% in 142 individuals 6 weeks after the first dose and 99% in 122 individuals 6 weeks after the second dose.

Persistence of Immune Response

The following section presents immune persistence data on a 1-dose regimen and a 2-dose regimen in children, and a 2-dose regimen in adolescents and adults.

One-Dose Regimen in Children

In clinical studies involving healthy children who received 1 dose of vaccine, detectable VZV antibodies were present in 99.0% (3886/3926) at 1 year, 99.3% (1555/1566) at 2 years, 98.6% (1106/1122) at 3 years, and 99.4% (1168/1175) at 4 years, 99.2% (737/743) at 5 years, 100% (142/142) at 6 years, 97.4% (38/39) at 7 years, 100% (34/34) at 8 years, and 100% (16/16) at 10 years postvaccination.

Two-Dose Regimen in Children

In recipients of 1 dose of VARIVAX over 9 years of follow-up, the geometric mean titer (GMT) and the percent of subjects with VZV antibody titers ≥5 gpELISA units/mL generally increased. The GMTs and percent of subjects with VZV antibody titers ≥5 gpELISA units/mL in the 2-dose recipients were higher than those in the 1-dose recipients for the first year of follow-up and generally comparable thereafter. The cumulative rate of VZV antibody persistence with both regimens remained very high at year 9 (99.0% for the 1-dose group and 98.8% for the 2-dose group).

Two-Dose Regimen in Adolescents and Adults

In clinical studies involving healthy adolescents and adults who received 2 doses of vaccine, detectable VZV antibodies were present in 97.9% (568/580) at 1 year, 97.1% (34/35) at 2 years, 100% (144/144) at 3 years, 97.0% (98/101) at 4 years, 97.4% (76/78) at 5 years, and 100% (34/34) at 6 years postvaccination.

A boost in antibody levels has been observed in vaccinees following exposure to natural varicella which could account for the apparent long-term persistence of antibody levels after vaccination in these studies. The duration of protection from varicella obtained using VARIVAX in the absence of wild-type boosting is unknown. VARIVAX also induces cell-mediated immune responses in vaccinees. The relative contributions of humoral immunity and cell-mediated immunity to protection from chickenpox are unknown.

Transmission

In the placebo-controlled trial, transmission of vaccine virus was assessed in household settings (during the 8-week post-vaccination period) in 416 susceptible placebo recipients who were household contacts of 445 vaccine recipients. Of the 416 placebo recipients, three developed chickenpox and seroconverted, nine reported a varicella-like rash and did not seroconvert, and six had no rash but seroconverted. If vaccine virus transmission occurred, it did so at a very low rate and possibly without recognizable clinical disease in contacts. These cases may represent either natural varicella from community contacts or a low incidence of transmission of vaccine virus from vaccinated contacts (see PRECAUTIONS, Transmission).{4,16} Post-marketing experience suggests that transmission of vaccine virus may occur rarely between healthy vaccinees who develop a varicella-like rash and healthy susceptible contacts. Transmission of vaccine virus from vaccinees who do not develop a varicella-like rash has also been reported.

Herpes Zoster

Overall, 9454 healthy children (12 months to 12 years of age) and 1648 adolescents and adults (13 years of age and older) have been vaccinated with VARIVAX in clinical trials. Eight cases of herpes zoster have been reported in children during 42,556 person years of follow-up in clinical trials, resulting in a calculated incidence of at least 18.8 cases per 100,000 person years. The completeness of this reporting has not been determined. One case of herpes zoster has been reported in the adolescent and adult age group during 5410 person years of follow-up in clinical trials resulting in a calculated incidence of 18.5 cases per 100,000 person years.{5}

All nine cases were mild and without sequelae. Two cultures (one child and one adult) obtained from vesicles were positive for wild-type VZV as confirmed by restriction endonuclease analysis.{5,17} The long-term effect of VARIVAX on the incidence of herpes zoster, particularly in those vaccinees exposed to natural varicella, is unknown at present.

In children, the reported rate of herpes zoster in vaccine recipients appears not to exceed that previously determined in a population-based study of healthy children who had experienced natural varicella.{5,18,19} The incidence of herpes zoster in adults who have had natural varicella infection is higher than that in children.{20}

Reye's Syndrome

Reye's Syndrome has occurred in children and adolescents following natural varicella infection, the majority of whom had received salicylates.{21} In clinical studies in healthy children and adolescents in the United States, physicians advised varicella vaccine recipients not to use salicylates for six weeks after vaccination. There were no reports of Reye's Syndrome in varicella vaccine recipients during these studies.

Studies with Other Vaccines

In combined clinical studies involving 1080 children 12 to 36 months of age, 653 received VARIVAX and M-M-R[1] II (Measles, Mumps, and Rubella Virus Vaccine Live) concomitantly at separate sites and 427 received the vaccines six weeks apart. Seroconversion rates and antibody levels were comparable between the two groups at approximately six weeks post-vaccination to each of the virus vaccine components. No differences were noted in adverse reactions reported in those who received VARIVAX concomitantly with M-M-R II at separate sites and those who received VARIVAX and M-M-R II at different times (see PRECAUTIONS, Drug Interactions, Use with Other Vaccines).{5}

In a clinical study involving 318 children 12 months to 42 months of age, 160 received an investigational vaccine (a formulation combining measles, mumps, rubella, and varicella in one syringe) concomitantly with booster doses of DTaP (diphtheria, tetanus, acellular pertussis) and OPV (oral poliovirus vaccine) while 144 received M-M-R II concomitantly with booster doses of DTaP and OPV followed by VARIVAX 6 weeks later. At six weeks postvaccination, seroconversion rates for measles, mumps, rubella, and VZV and the percentage of vaccinees whose titers were boosted for diphtheria, tetanus, pertussis, and polio were comparable between the two groups, but anti-VZV levels were decreased when the investigational vaccine containing varicella was administered concomitantly with DTaP. No clinically significant differences were noted in adverse reactions between the two groups.{5}

In another clinical study involving 307 children 12 to 18 months of age, 150 received an investigational vaccine (a formulation combining measles, mumps, rubella, and varicella in one syringe) concomitantly with a booster dose of PedvaxHIB[1] [Haemophilus b Conjugate Vaccine (Meningococcal Protein Conjugate)] while 130 received M-M-R II concomitantly with a booster dose of PedvaxHIB followed by VARIVAX 6 weeks later. At six weeks postvaccination, seroconversion rates for measles, mumps, rubella, and VZV, and geometric mean titers for PedvaxHIB were comparable between the two groups, but anti-VZV levels were decreased when the investigational vaccine containing varicella was administered concomitantly with PedvaxHIB. No clinically significant differences in adverse reactions were seen between the two groups.{5}

In a clinical study involving 609 children 12 to 23 months of age, 305 received VARIVAX, M-M-R II, and TETRAMUNE[2] (*Haemophilus influenzae* type b, diphtheria, tetanus, and pertussis vaccines) concomitantly at separate sites, and 304 received M-M-R II and TETRAMUNE concomitantly at separate sites, followed by VARIVAX 6 weeks later. At six weeks postvaccination, seroconversion rates for measles, mumps, rubella and VZV were similar between the two groups. Postvaccination GMTs for all antigens were similar in both treatment groups except for VZV, which was lower when VARIVAX was administered concomitantly with M-M-R II and TETRAMUNE, but within the range of GMTs seen in previous clinical experience when VARIVAX was administered alone. At 1 year postvaccination, GMTs for measles, mumps, rubella, VZV and *Haemophilus influenzae* type b were similar between the two groups. All three vaccines were well tolerated regardless of whether they were administered concomitantly at separate sites or 6 weeks apart. There were no clinically important differences in reaction rates when the three vaccines were administered concomitantly versus 6 weeks apart.

In a clinical study involving 822 children 12 to 15 months of age, 410 received COMVAX[1] [Haemophilus b Conjugate (Meningococcal Protein Conjugate) and Hepatitis B (Recombinant) vaccine], M-M-R II, and VARIVAX concomitantly at separate sites, and 412 received COMVAX followed by M-M-R II and VARIVAX given concomitantly at separate sites, 6 weeks later. At six weeks postvaccination, the immune responses for the subjects who received the concomitant doses of COMVAX, M-M-R II, and VARIVAX were similar to those of the subjects who received COMVAX followed 6 weeks later by M-M-R II and VARIVAX with respect to all antigens administered. All three vaccines were generally well tolerated regardless of whether they were administered concomitantly at separate sites or 6 weeks apart. There were no clinically important differences in reaction rates when the three vaccines were administered concomitantly versus 6 weeks apart.

VARIVAX is recommended for subcutaneous administration. However, during clinical trials, some children received VARIVAX intramuscularly resulting in seroconversion rates similar to those in children who received the vaccine by the subcutaneous route.[22] Persistence of antibody and efficacy in those receiving intramuscular doses have not been defined.

[2] Registered trademark of Lederle Laboratories

INDICATIONS AND USAGE

VARIVAX is indicated for vaccination against varicella in individuals 12 months of age and older.

The duration of protection of VARIVAX is unknown; however, long-term efficacy studies have demonstrated continued protection up to 10 years after vaccination.[26] In addition, a boost in antibody levels has been observed in vaccinees following exposure to natural varicella as well as following a second dose of VARIVAX.[5]

In a highly vaccinated population, immunity for some individuals may wane due to lack of exposure to natural varicella as a result of shifting epidemiology. Postmarketing surveillance studies are ongoing to evaluate the need and timing for booster vaccination.

Vaccination with VARIVAX may not result in protection of all healthy, susceptible children, adolescents, and adults (see CLINICAL PHARMACOLOGY).

CONTRAINDICATIONS

A history of hypersensitivity to any component of the vaccine, including gelatin.

A history of anaphylactoid reaction to neomycin (each dose of reconstituted vaccine contains trace quantities of neomycin).

Individuals with blood dyscrasias, leukemia, lymphomas of any type, or other malignant neoplasms affecting the bone marrow or lymphatic systems.

Individuals receiving immunosuppressive therapy. Individuals who are on immunosuppressant drugs are more susceptible to infections than healthy individuals. Vaccination with live attenuated varicella vaccine can result in a more extensive vaccine-associated rash or disseminated disease in individuals on immunosuppressant doses of corticosteroids.

Individuals with primary and acquired immunodeficiency states, including those who are immunosuppressed in association with AIDS or other clinical manifestations of infection with human immunodeficiency virus,[23] cellular immune deficiencies; and hypogammaglobulinemic and dysgammaglobulinemic states.

A family history of congenital or hereditary immunodeficiency, unless the immune competence of the potential vaccine recipient is demonstrated.

Active untreated tuberculosis.

Any febrile respiratory illness or other active febrile infection.

Pregnancy; the possible effects of the vaccine on fetal development are unknown at this time. However, natural varicella is known to sometimes cause fetal harm. If vaccination of postpubertal females is undertaken, pregnancy should be avoided for three months following vaccination (See PRECAUTIONS, Pregnancy).

Table 1: Fever, Local Reactions, or Rashes (%) in Children 0 to 42 Days Postvaccination

Reaction	N	Post Dose 1	Peak Occurrence in Postvaccination Days
Fever ≥102°F (39°C) Oral	8827	14.7%	0-42
Injection-site complaints (pain/soreness, swelling and/or erythema, rash, pruritus, hematoma, induration, stiffness)	8916	19.3%	0-2
Varicella-like rash (injection site) Median number of lesions	8916	3.4% 2	8-19
Varicella-like rash (generalized) Median number of lesions	8916	3.8% 5	5-26

PRECAUTIONS
General

Adequate treatment provisions, including epinephrine injection (1:1000), should be available for immediate use should an anaphylactoid reaction occur.

The duration of protection from varicella infection after vaccination with VARIVAX is unknown.

It is not known whether VARIVAX given immediately after exposure to natural varicella virus will prevent illness.

Vaccination should be deferred for at least 5 months following blood or plasma transfusions, or administration of immune globulin or varicella zoster immune globulin (VZIG).[24]

Following administration of VARIVAX, any immune globulin, including VZIG, should not be given for 2 months thereafter unless its use outweighs the benefits of vaccination.[24]

Vaccine recipients should avoid use of salicylates for 6 weeks after vaccination with VARIVAX as Reye's Syndrome has been reported following the use of salicylates during natural varicella infection (see CLINICAL PHARMACOLOGY, Reye's Syndrome).

The safety and efficacy of VARIVAX have not been established in children and young adults who are known to be infected with human immunodeficiency viruses with and without evidence of immunosuppression (see also CONTRAINDICATIONS).

Care is to be taken by the health care provider for safe and effective use of VARIVAX.

The health care provider should question the patient, parent, or guardian about reactions to a previous dose of VARIVAX or a similar product.

The health care provider should obtain the previous immunization history of the vaccinee.

VARIVAX should not be injected into a blood vessel.

Vaccination should be deferred in patients with a family history of congenital or hereditary immunodeficiency until the patient's own immune system has been evaluated.

A separate sterile needle and syringe should be used for administration of each dose of VARIVAX to prevent transfer of infectious diseases.

Needles should be disposed of properly and should not be recapped.

Transmission

Post-marketing experience suggests that transmission of vaccine virus may occur rarely between healthy vaccinees who develop a varicella-like rash and healthy susceptible contacts. Transmission of vaccine virus from vaccinees who do not develop a varicella-like rash has also been reported. Therefore, vaccine recipients should attempt to avoid, whenever possible, close association with susceptible high-risk individuals for up to six weeks. In circumstances where contact with high-risk individuals is unavoidable, the potential risk of transmission of vaccine virus should be weighed against the risk of acquiring and transmitting natural varicella virus. Susceptible high-risk individuals include:

* immunocompromised individuals
* pregnant women without documented history of chickenpox or laboratory evidence of prior infection
* newborn infants of mothers without documented history of chickenpox or laboratory evidence of prior infection.

Information for Patients

The health care provider should inform the patient, parent, or guardian of the benefits and risks of VARIVAX.

Patients, parents, or guardians should be instructed to report any adverse reactions to their health care provider.

The U.S. Department of Health and Human Services has established a Vaccine Adverse Event Reporting System (VAERS) to accept all reports of suspected adverse events after the administration of any vaccine, including but not limited to the reporting of events required by the National Childhood Vaccine Injury Act of 1986.[25] The VAERS toll-free number for VAERS forms and information is 1-800-822-7967.

Pregnancy should be avoided for three months following vaccination.

Drug Interactions

See PRECAUTIONS, General, regarding the administration of immune globulins, salicylates, and transfusions.

Drug Interactions, Use with Other Vaccines

Results from clinical studies indicate that VARIVAX can be administered concomitantly with M-M-R II, COMVAX, or TETRAMUNE (see CLINICAL PHARMACOLOGY, Studies with Other Vaccines).

Limited data from an experimental product containing varicella vaccine suggest that VARIVAX can be administered concomitantly with DTaP (diphtheria, tetanus, acellular pertussis) and PedvaxHIB using separate sites and syringes (see CLINICAL PHARMACOLOGY, Studies with Other Vaccines).[5] However, there are no data relating to simultaneous administration of VARIVAX with DTP or OPV.

Carcinogenesis, Mutagenesis, Impairment of Fertility

VARIVAX has not been evaluated for its carcinogenic or mutagenic potential, or its potential to impair fertility.

Pregnancy

Pregnancy Category C:

Animal reproduction studies have not been conducted with VARIVAX. It is also not known whether VARIVAX can cause fetal harm when administered to a pregnant woman or can affect reproduction capacity. Therefore, VARIVAX should not be administered to pregnant females; furthermore, pregnancy should be avoided for three months following vaccination (see CONTRAINDICATIONS).

Merck & Co., Inc. maintains a Pregnancy Registry to monitor fetal outcomes of pregnant women exposed to VARIVAX. Patients and healthcare providers are encouraged to report any exposure to VARIVAX during pregnancy by calling (800) 986-8999.

Nursing Mothers

It is not known whether varicella vaccine virus is secreted in human milk. Therefore, because some viruses are secreted in human milk, caution should be exercised if VARIVAX is administered to a nursing woman.

Geriatric Use

Clinical studies of VARIVAX did not include sufficient numbers of seronegative subjects aged 65 and over to determine whether they respond differently from younger subjects. Other reported clinical experience has not identified differences in responses between the elderly and younger subjects.

Pediatric Use

No clinical data are available on safety or efficacy of VARIVAX in children less than one year of age and administration to infants under twelve months of age is not recommended.

ADVERSE REACTIONS

In clinical trials,[4,5,9-15] VARIVAX was administered to over 11,000 healthy children, adolescents, and adults. VARIVAX was generally well tolerated.

In a double-blind, placebo-controlled study among 914 healthy children and adolescents who were serologically confirmed to be susceptible to varicella, the only adverse reactions that occurred at a significantly (p<0.05) greater rate in vaccine recipients than in placebo recipients were pain and redness at the injection site.[4]

Children 1 to 12 Years of Age

One-Dose Regimen in Children

In clinical trials involving healthy children monitored for up to 42 days after a single dose of VARIVAX, the frequency of fever, injection-site complaints, or rashes were reported as follows:

[See table 1 above]

In addition, the most frequently (≥1%) reported adverse experiences, without regard to causality, are listed in decreasing order of frequency: upper respiratory illness, cough, irritability/nervousness, fatigue, disturbed sleep, diarrhea, loss of appetite, vomiting, otitis, diaper rash/contact rash, headache, teething, malaise, abdominal pain, other rash, nausea, eye complaints, chills, lymphadenopathy, myalgia,

Table 2: Fever, Local Reactions, or Rashes (%) in Adolescents and Adults 0 to 42 Days Postvaccination

Reaction	N	Post Dose 1	Peak Occurrence in Postvaccination Days	N	Post Dose 2	Peak Occurrence in Postvaccination Days
Fever ≥100°F (37.7°C) Oral	1584	10.2%	14-27	956	9.5%	0-42
Injection-site complaints (soreness, erythema, swelling, rash, pruritus, pyrexia, hematoma, induration, numbness)	1606	24.4%	0-2	955	32.5%	0-2
Varicella-like rash (injection site) Median number of lesions	1606	3% 2	6-20	955	1% 2	0-6
Varicella-like rash (generalized) Median number of lesions	1606	5.5% 5	7-21	955	0.9% 5.5	0-23

lower respiratory illness, allergic reactions (including allergic rash, hives), stiff neck, heat rash/prickly heat, arthralgia, eczema/dry skin/dermatitis, constipation, itching.

Pneumonitis has been reported rarely (<1%) in children vaccinated with VARIVAX; a causal relationship has not been established.

Febrile seizures have occurred rarely (<0.1%) in children vaccinated with VARIVAX; a causal relationship has not been established.

Two-Dose Regimen in Children
Nine hundred eighty-one (981) subjects in a clinical trial received 2 doses of VARIVAX 3 months apart and were actively followed for 42 days after each dose. The 2-dose regimen of varicella vaccine was generally well tolerated, with a safety profile generally comparable to that of the 1-dose regimen. The incidence of injection-site clinical complaints (primarily erythema and swelling) observed in the first 4 days following vaccination was slightly higher Postdose 2 (overall incidence 25.4%) than Postdose 1 (overall incidence 21.7%), whereas the incidence of systemic clinical complaints in the 42-day follow-up period was lower Postdose 2 (66.3%) than Postdose 1 (85.8%).

Adolescents and Adults 13 Years of Age and Older
In clinical trials involving healthy adolescents and adults, the majority of whom received two doses of VARIVAX and were monitored for up to 42 days after any dose, the frequency of fever, injection-site complaints, or rashes were reported as follows:
[See table 2 above]

In addition, the most frequently (≥1%) reported adverse experiences, without regard to causality, are listed in decreasing order of frequency: upper respiratory illness, headache, fatigue, cough, myalgia, disturbed sleep, nausea, malaise, diarrhea, stiff neck, irritability/nervousness, lymphadenopathy, chills, eye complaints, abdominal pain, loss of appetite, arthralgia, otitis, itching, vomiting, other rashes, constipation, lower respiratory illness, allergic reactions (including allergic rash, hives), contact rash, cold/canker sore.

As with any vaccine, there is the possibility that broad use of the vaccine could reveal adverse reactions not observed in clinical trials.

The following additional adverse reactions have been reported since the vaccine has been marketed:

Body as a Whole
Anaphylaxis (including anaphylactic shock) and related phenomena such as angioneurotic edema, facial edema, and peripheral edema.

Hemic and Lymphatic System
Aplastic anemia, thrombocytopenia (including idiopathic thrombocytopenic purpura (ITP)).

Nervous/Psychiatric
Encephalitis; cerebrovascular accident; transverse myelitis; Guillain-Barré syndrome; Bell's palsy; ataxia; non-febrile seizures; aseptic meningitis; dizziness; paresthesia.

Respiratory
Pharyngitis, pneumonia/pneumonitis.

Skin
Stevens-Johnson syndrome; erythema multiforme; Henoch-Schönlein purpura; secondary bacterial infections of skin and soft tissue, including impetigo and cellulitis; herpes zoster.

DOSAGE AND ADMINISTRATION
FOR SUBCUTANEOUS ADMINISTRATION
Do not inject intravascularly
Children
Children 12 months to 12 years of age should receive a 0.5-mL dose administered subcutaneously. If a second 0.5-mL dose is administered, it should be given a minimum of 3 months later.
Adolescents and Adults
Adolescents and adults 13 years of age and older should receive a 0.5-mL dose administered subcutaneously at elected date and a second 0.5-mL dose 4 to 8 weeks later.

VARIVAX is for subcutaneous administration. The outer aspect of the upper arm (deltoid) is the preferred site of injection.

VARIVAX **SHOULD BE STORED FROZEN** at an average temperature of –15°C (+5°F) or colder until it is reconstituted for injection (see HOW SUPPLIED, Storage). Any freezer (e.g., chest, frost-free) that reliably maintains an average temperature of –15°C and has a separate sealed freezer door is acceptable for storing VARIVAX. The diluent should be stored separately at room temperature or in the refrigerator. To reconstitute the vaccine, first withdraw 0.7 mL of diluent into a syringe. Inject all the diluent in the syringe into the vial of lyophilized vaccine and gently agitate to mix thoroughly. Withdraw the entire contents into a syringe and inject the total volume (about 0.5 mL) of reconstituted vaccine subcutaneously, preferably into the outer aspect of the upper arm (deltoid) or the anterolateral thigh. **IT IS RECOMMENDED THAT THE VACCINE BE ADMINISTERED IMMEDIATELY AFTER RECONSTITUTION, TO MINIMIZE LOSS OF POTENCY. DISCARD IF RECONSTITUTED VACCINE IS NOT USED WITHIN 30 MINUTES.**
CAUTION: A sterile syringe free of preservatives, antiseptics, and detergents should be used for each injection and/or reconstitution of VARIVAX because these substances may inactivate the vaccine virus.
It is important to use a separate sterile syringe and needle for each patient to prevent transmission of infectious agents from one individual to another.
To reconstitute the vaccine, use only the Merck sterile diluent supplied with VARIVAX, M-M-R II, or the component vaccines of M-M-R II, since it is free of preservatives or other anti-viral substances which might inactivate the vaccine virus.
Do not freeze reconstituted vaccine.
Do not give immune globulin, including Varicella Zoster Immune Globulin, concurrently with VARIVAX (see also PRECAUTIONS).
Parenteral drug products should be inspected visually for particulate matter and discoloration prior to administration, whenever solution and container permit. VARIVAX when reconstituted is a clear, colorless to pale yellow liquid.

HOW SUPPLIED
No. 4826/4309—VARIVAX is supplied as follows: (1) a single-dose vial of lyophilized vaccine, **NDC** 0006-4826-00 (package A); and (2) a box of 10 vials of diluent (package B). No. 4827/4309—VARIVAX is supplied as follows: (1) a box of 10 single-dose vials of lyophilized vaccine (package A), **NDC** 0006-4827-00; and (2) a box of 10 vials of diluent (package B).
Stability
VARIVAX retains a potency level of 1500 PFU or higher per dose for at least 24 months in a frost-free freezer with an average temperature of –15°C (+5°F) or colder.
VARIVAX has a minimum potency level of approximately 1350 PFU 30 minutes after reconstitution at room temperature (20-25°C, 68-77°F).
Prior to reconstitution, VARIVAX retains potency when stored for up to 72 continuous hours at refrigerator temperature (2-8°C, 36-46°F).
For information regarding stability under conditions other than those recommended, call 1-800-9-VARIVAX.
Storage
During shipment, to ensure that there is no loss of potency, the vaccine must be maintained at a temperature of –15°C (+5°F) or colder.
Before reconstitution, store the lyophilized vaccine in a freezer at an average temperature of –15°C (+5°F) or colder. Any freezer (e.g., chest, frost-free) that reliably maintains an average temperature of –15°C and has a separate sealed freezer door is acceptable for storing VARIVAX.
VARIVAX may be stored at refrigerator temperature (2-8°C, 36-46°F) for up to 72 continuous hours prior to reconstitution. Vaccine stored at 2-8°C which is not used within 72 hours of removal from –15°C storage should be discarded.

Before reconstitution, protect from light.
The diluent should be stored separately at room temperature (20-25°C, 68-77°F), or in the refrigerator.

REFERENCES
1. Balfour, H.H.; et al.: Acyclovir Treatment of Varicella in Otherwise Healthy Children, Pediatrics., *116*: 633-639, 1990.
2. Ross, A.H.: Modification of Chickenpox in Family Contacts by Administration of Gamma Globulin, N Engl J Med. *267*: 369-376, 1962.
3. Preblud, S.R.: Varicella: Complications and Costs, Pediatrics, *78*(4 Pt 2): 728-735, 1986.
4. Weibel, R.E.; et al.: Live Attenuated Varicella Virus Vaccine, N Engl J Med. *310*(22): 1409-1415, 1984.
5. Unpublished data; files of Merck Research Laboratories.
6. Wharton, M.; et al.: Health Impact of Varicella in the 1980's. Thirtieth Interscience Conference on Antimicrobial Agents and Chemotherapy, (Abstract #1138), 1990.
7. Bernstein, H.H.; et al.: Clinical Survey of Natural Varicella Compared with Breakthrough Varicella After Immunization with Live Attenuated Oka/Merck Varicella Vaccine. Pediatrics *92*: 833-837, 1993.
8. Kuter, B.J.; et al.: Oka/Merck Varicella Vaccine in Healthy Children: Final Report of a 2-Year Efficacy Study and 7-Year Follow-up Studies, Vaccine, *9*: 643-647, 1991.
9. Arbeter, A.M.; et al.: Varicella Vaccine Trials in Healthy Children, A Summary of Comparative and Follow-up Studies, AJDC *138*: 434-438, 1984.
10. Weibel, R.E.; et al.: Live Oka/Merck Varicella Vaccine in Healthy Children, JAMA *254*(17): 2435-2439, 1985.
11. Chartrand, D.M.; et al.: New Varicella Vaccine Production Lots in Healthy Children and Adolescents, Abstracts of the 1988 Inter-Science Conference Antimicrobial Agents and Chemotherapy: 237(Abstract #731).
12. Johnson, C.E.; et al.: Live Attenuated Vaccine in Healthy 12 to 24 month old Children, Pediatrics *81*: 512-518, 1988.
13. Gershon, A.A.; et al.: Immunization of Healthy Adults with Live Attenuated Varicella Vaccine, J Infect Dis, *158*(1): 132-137, 1988.
14. Gershon, A.A.; et al.: Live Attenuated Varicella Vaccine: Protection in Healthy Adults Compared with Leukemic Children, J Infect Dis, *161*: 661-666, 1990.
15. White, C.J.; et al.: Varicella Vaccine (VARIVAX) in Healthy Children and Adolescents: Results From Clinical Trials, 1987 to 1989, Pediatrics, *87*(5): 604-610, 1991.
16. Asano, Y.; et al.: Contact Infection from Live Varicella Vaccine Recipients, Lancet *1*(7966): 965, 1976.
17. Hammerschlag, M.R.; et al.: Herpes Zoster in an Adult Recipient of Live Attenuated Varicella Vaccine, J Infect Dis *160*(3): 535-537, 1989.
18. White, C.J.: Letters to the Editor, Pediatrics *318*: 354, 1992.
19. Guess, H.A.; et al.: Population-Based Studies of Varicella Complications, Pediatrics *78*(4 Pt 2): 723-727, 1986.
20. Ragozzino, M.; et al.: Population-Based Study of Herpes Zoster and Its Sequelae, Medicine *61*(5): 310-316, 1982.
21. Morbidity and Mortality Weekly Report *34*(1): 13-16, Jan. 11, 1985.
22. Dennehy, P.H.; et al.: Immunogenicity of Subcutaneous Versus Intramuscular Oka/Merck Varicella Vaccination in Healthy Children, Pediatrics *88*(3): 604-607, 1991.
23. Center for Disease Control: Immunization of Children Infected with Human T-Lymphotropic Virus Type III/Lymphadenopathy—Associated Virus, Ann Intern Med, *106*: 75-78, 1987.
24. Recommendations of the Advisory Committee on Immunization Practices (ACIP); General Recommendations on Immunization, MMWR *43*(No. RR-1): 15-18, Jan. 28, 1994.
25. Vaccine Adverse Event Reporting System—United States, MMWR *39*(41): 730-733, 1990.
26. Kuter, B.J.; et al.: Ten Year Follow-up of Healthy Children who Received One or Two Injections of Varicella Vaccine, Pediatr Infect Dis J, 23:132-37, 2004.

Dist. by:
MERCK & CO., INC., Whitehouse Station, NJ 08889, USA
Issued June 2010
Printed in USA
9904701

PATIENT PACKAGE INSERT
Patient Information about
VARIVAX® (pronounced "VAR ih vax")
Generic name: Varicella Virus Vaccine Live
This is a summary of information about VARIVAX[3]. You should read it before you or your child get the vaccine. If you have any questions about the vaccine after reading this leaflet, you should ask your health care provider. This is a summary only. It does not take the place of talking about VARIVAX with your doctor, nurse, or other health care provider. Only your health care provider can decide if VARIVAX is right for you or your child.

What is VARIVAX and how does it work?

VARIVAX is also known as Varicella Virus Vaccine Live. It is a live virus vaccine that is given as a shot. It is meant to help prevent chickenpox. Chickenpox is sometimes called varicella (pronounced VAR ih sell a).

VARIVAX contains a weakened form of chickenpox virus. VARIVAX works by helping the immune system protect you or your child from getting chickenpox.

VARIVAX may not protect everyone who gets it.

VARIVAX does not treat chickenpox once you or your child have it.

What do I need to know about chickenpox?

Chickenpox is an illness that occurs most often in children who are 5 to 9 years old. It can be passed to others. The illness can include headache, fever, and general discomfort. Then an itchy rash occurs, which can turn into blisters. The most common complication is that the blisters can get infected. Less common but very serious complications can occur. These include pneumonia, inflammation of the brain, Reye's syndrome (which affects the liver and the brain), and death. Severe disease and serious complications are more likely to occur in adolescents and adults.

Who should not get VARIVAX?

Do not take VARIVAX if you or your child:
* are allergic to any of its ingredients. (This includes gelatin or neomycin. See the ingredient list at the end of this leaflet.)
* have a weakened immune system, such as an immune deficiency, an inherited immune disorder, leukemia, lymphoma, or HIV/AIDS.
* take high doses of steroids by mouth or in a shot.
* have active tuberculosis that is not treated.
* have a fever.
* are pregnant or plan to get pregnant within the next three months.

What should I tell my health care provider before getting VARIVAX?

Tell your health care provider if you or your child:
* have or have had any medical problems.
* have received blood or plasma transfusions or human serum globulin within the last 5 months.
* take any medicines. (This includes non-prescription medicines and dietary supplements.)
* have any allergies. (This includes allergies to neomycin or gelatin.)
* had an allergic reaction to any other vaccine.
* are pregnant or plan to become pregnant within the next three months.
* are breast-feeding.

How is VARIVAX given?

VARIVAX is given as a shot to people who are 12 months old or older. If your child is 12 months to 12 years old and your doctor gives a second dose, the second dose must be given at least 3 months after the first shot.

A second dose should be given to those who first get the vaccine when they are 13 years old or older. This second dose should be given 4 to 8 weeks after the first dose.

Your doctor or health care provider will use the official recommendations to decide the number of shots needed and when to get them.

If a dose is missed, your health care provider will let you know when you should have it.

What should you or your child avoid when getting VARIVAX?

Do not take aspirin or aspirin-containing products for 6 weeks after getting VARIVAX.

It is rare, but possible, that once you have the vaccine, you could spread the chickenpox virus to others. Whenever possible, try to avoid contact with certain groups of people for up to six weeks after getting the vaccine. This is because the disease for these groups may be quite serious. These groups include:
* people who have a weakened immune system.
* pregnant women who have never had chickenpox.
* newborn babies whose mothers have never had chickenpox.

Tell your doctor or healthcare provider if you or your child expect to have contact with someone who falls into one of these groups.

What are the possible side effects of VARIVAX?

The most common side effects reported after taking VARIVAX are:
* Fever
* Pain, swelling, itching, or redness at the site of the shot
* Chickenpox-like rash on the body or at the site of the shot
* Irritability

Other less common side effects have also been reported.
* Tingling of the skin
* Shingles

Tell your healthcare provider if you have any of the following symptoms within a short time after getting VARIVAX because they may be signs of an allergic reaction:
* Shortness of breath or wheezing
* Rash or hives

Other side effects have been reported. Some of them were serious. These include bruising more easily than normal; red or purple, flat, pinhead spots under the skin; severe paleness; difficulty walking; severe skin disorders; and skin infection. Rarely, swelling of the brain, stroke, inflammation of the lungs (known as pneumonia or pneumonitis), and seizures with or without a fever have been reported. It is not known if these rare side effects are related to the vaccine. Your doctor has a more complete list of side effects for VARIVAX.

Tell your doctor or health care provider if you or your child have any new or unusual symptoms after getting VARIVAX. You may also report any adverse reactions to your doctor or your child's doctor or directly to the Vaccine Adverse Event Reporting System (VAERS). The VAERS toll-free number is 1-800-822-7967 or report online to www.vaers.hhs.gov.

What are the ingredients of VARIVAX?

Active Ingredient: a weakened form of chickenpox virus.
Inactive Ingredients: sucrose, hydrolyzed gelatin, sodium chloride, monosodium L-glutamate, sodium phosphate dibasic, potassium phosphate monobasic, potassium chloride, residual components of MRC-5 cells including DNA and protein, sodium phosphate monobasic, EDTA, neomycin, fetal bovine serum.

What else should I know about VARIVAX?

If you get VARIVAX while you are pregnant, please call 1-800-986-8999. Or, you can have your health care provider call.

This leaflet summarizes important information about VARIVAX.

If you would like more information, talk to your health care provider, visit the web site at www.merckvaccines.com, or call 1-800-Merck-90.

Rx Only
Issued June 2010
Dist. by:
MERCK & CO., INC., Whitehouse Station, NJ 08889, USA
9904701

³ Registered trademark of MERCK & CO., Inc.
COPYRIGHT © 2008 MERCK & CO., Inc.
All rights reserved

VYTORIN®
[vī-tŏr-in]
(ezetimibe/simvastatin)
Tablets   ℞

HIGHLIGHTS OF PRESCRIBING INFORMATION
These highlights do not include all the information needed to use VYTORIN safely and effectively. See full prescribing information for VYTORIN.
VYTORIN (ezetimibe/simvastatin) Tablets
Initial U.S. Approval: 2004

RECENT MAJOR CHANGES
Dosage and Administration
  Chinese Patients Taking Lipid-Modifying Doses (≥1 g/day Niacin) of Niacin-Containing Products (2.6)
      03/2010
  Coadministration with Other Drugs (2.7) 03/2010
Warnings and Precautions
  Myopathy/Rhabdomyolysis (5.1)   03/2010

INDICATIONS AND USAGE
VYTORIN®, which contains a cholesterol absorption inhibitor and an HMG-CoA reductase inhibitor (statin), is indicated as adjunctive therapy to diet to:
* reduce elevated total-C, LDL-C, Apo B, TG, and non-HDL-C, and to increase HDL-C in patients with primary (heterozygous familial and non-familial) hyperlipidemia or mixed hyperlipidemia. (1.1)
* reduce elevated total-C and LDL-C in patients with homozygous familial hypercholesterolemia (HoFH), as an adjunct to other lipid-lowering treatments. (1.2)
Limitations of Use (1.3)
* No incremental benefit of VYTORIN on cardiovascular morbidity and mortality over and above that demonstrated for simvastatin has been established. VYTORIN has not been studied in Fredrickson Type I, III, IV, and V dyslipidemias.

DOSAGE AND ADMINISTRATION
* Dosage range is 10/10 mg/day through 10/80 mg/day. (2.1)
* Recommended usual starting dose is 10/20 mg/day. (2.1)
* Dosing of VYTORIN should occur either ≥2 hours before or ≥4 hours after administration of a bile acid sequestrant. (2.7, 7.5)

DOSAGE FORMS AND STRENGTHS
* Tablets (ezetimibe mg/simvastatin mg): 10/10, 10/20, 10/40, 10/80 (3)

CONTRAINDICATIONS
* Hypersensitivity to any component of this medication (4, 6.2)
* Active liver disease or unexplained persistent elevations of hepatic transaminase levels (4, 5.2)

* Women who are pregnant or may become pregnant (4, 8.1)
* Nursing mothers (4, 8.3)

WARNINGS AND PRECAUTIONS
* Patients should be advised to report promptly any symptoms of myopathy. VYTORIN should be discontinued immediately if myopathy is diagnosed or suspected. (5.1)
* Skeletal muscle effects (e.g., myopathy and rhabdomyolysis): Risks increase with higher doses and concomitant use of certain CYP3A4 inhibitors, gemfibrozil, cyclosporine, danazol, amiodarone, verapamil, and diltiazem. Predisposing factors include advanced age (≥65), uncontrolled hypothyroidism, and renal impairment. (5.1, 8.5, 8.6)
* Liver enzyme abnormalities and monitoring: Persistent elevations in hepatic transaminase can occur. Monitor liver enzymes before and during treatment. Patients titrated to the 10/80-mg dose should receive additional liver function tests. (5.2)
* VYTORIN is not recommended in patients with moderate or severe hepatic impairment. (5.3, 12.3)

ADVERSE REACTIONS
* Common (incidence ≥2% and greater than placebo) adverse reactions in clinical trials: headache, increased ALT, myalgia, upper respiratory tract infection, and diarrhea. (6.1)
To report SUSPECTED ADVERSE REACTIONS, contact Merck/Schering-Plough Pharmaceuticals at 1-866-637-2501 or FDA at 1-800-FDA-1088 or www.fda.gov/medwatch.

DRUG INTERACTIONS
Drug Interactions Associated with Increased Risk of Myopathy/Rhabdomyolysis (2.7, 5.1, 7.1, 7.2, 7.3, 7.6, 7.8)

Interacting Agents	Prescribing Recommendations
Itraconazole, ketoconazole, erythromycin, clarithromycin, telithromycin, HIV protease inhibitors, nefazodone, fibrates	Avoid VYTORIN
Cyclosporine, danazol	Do not exceed 10/10 mg VYTORIN daily
Amiodarone, verapamil	Do not exceed 10/20 mg VYTORIN daily
Diltiazem	Do not exceed 10/40 mg VYTORIN daily
Grapefruit juice	Avoid large quantities of grapefruit juice (>1 quart daily)

* Cyclosporine: Combination increases exposure of ezetimibe and cyclosporine. Cyclosporine concentrations should be monitored. (7.6, 12.3)
* Coumarin anticoagulants: simvastatin prolongs INR. Achieve stable INR prior to starting VYTORIN. Monitor INR frequently until stable upon initiation or alteration of VYTORIN therapy. (7.9)
* Cholestyramine: Combination decreases exposure of ezetimibe. (2.7, 7.5)

USE IN SPECIFIC POPULATIONS
* Severe renal impairment: Caution should be exercised and the patient should be closely monitored. (2.4, 8.6)

See 17 for PATIENT COUNSELING INFORMATION and FDA-approved patient labeling

Revised: 05/2010

FULL PRESCRIBING INFORMATION: CONTENTS*

FULL PRESCRIBING INFORMATION

1 INDICATIONS AND USAGE

Therapy with lipid-altering agents should be only one component of multiple risk factor intervention in individuals at significantly increased risk for atherosclerotic vascular disease due to hypercholesterolemia. Drug therapy is indicated as an adjunct to diet when the response to a diet restricted in saturated fat and cholesterol and other nonpharmacologic measures alone has been inadequate.

1.1 Primary Hyperlipidemia

VYTORIN is indicated for the reduction of elevated total cholesterol (total-C), low-density lipoprotein cholesterol (LDL-C), apolipoprotein B (Apo B), triglycerides (TG), and non-high-density lipoprotein cholesterol (non-HDL-C), and to increase high-density lipoprotein cholesterol (HDL-C) in patients with primary (heterozygous familial and nonfamilial) hyperlipidemia or mixed hyperlipidemia.

1.2 Homozygous Familial Hypercholesterolemia (HoFH)

VYTORIN is indicated for the reduction of elevated total-C and LDL-C in patients with homozygous familial hypercholesterolemia, as an adjunct to other lipid-lowering treatments (e.g., LDL apheresis) or if such treatments are unavailable.

1.3 Limitations of Use

No incremental benefit of VYTORIN on cardiovascular morbidity and mortality over and above that demonstrated for simvastatin has been established. VYTORIN has not been studied in Fredrickson type I, III, IV, and V dyslipidemias.

2 DOSAGE AND ADMINISTRATION

2.1 Recommended Dosing

The dosage range is 10/10 mg/day through 10/80 mg/day. The recommended usual starting dose is 10/20 mg/day. VYTORIN should be taken as a single daily dose in the evening, with or without food. Initiation of therapy with 10/10 mg/day may be considered for patients requiring less aggressive LDL-C reductions. Patients who require a larger reduction in LDL-C (greater than 55%) may be started at 10/40 mg/day. After initiation or titration of VYTORIN, lipid levels may be analyzed after 2 or more weeks and dosage adjusted, if needed.

2.2 Patients with Homozygous Familial Hypercholesterolemia

The recommended dosage for patients with homozygous familial hypercholesterolemia is VYTORIN 10/40 mg/day or 10/80 mg/day in the evening. VYTORIN should be used as an adjunct to other lipid-lowering treatments (e.g., LDL apheresis) in these patients or if such treatments are unavailable.

2.3 Patients with Hepatic Impairment

No dosage adjustment is necessary in patients with mild hepatic impairment [see Warnings and Precautions (5.3)].

2.4 Patients with Renal Impairment

No dosage adjustment is necessary in patients with mild or moderate renal impairment. However, for patients with severe renal insufficiency, VYTORIN should not be started unless the patient has already tolerated treatment with simvastatin at a dose of 5 mg or higher. Caution should be exercised when VYTORIN is administered to these patients; and they should be closely monitored [see Warnings and Precautions (5.1); Clinical Pharmacology (12.3)].

2.5 Geriatric Patients

No dosage adjustment is necessary in geriatric patients [see Clinical Pharmacology (12.3)].

2.6 Chinese Patients Taking Lipid-Modifying Doses (≥1 g/day Niacin) of Niacin-Containing Products

Because of an increased risk for myopathy, caution should be used when treating Chinese patients with VYTORIN coadministered with lipid-modifying doses (≥1 g/day niacin) of niacin-containing products. Because the risk for myopathy is dose-related, Chinese patients should not receive VYTORIN 10/80 mg coadministered with lipid-modifying doses of niacin-containing products. The cause of the increased risk of myopathy is not known. It is also unknown if the risk for myopathy with coadministration of simvastatin with lipid-modifying doses of niacin-containing products observed in Chinese patients applies to other Asian patients. [See Warnings and Precautions (5.1).]

2.7 Coadministration with Other Drugs

[See Warnings and Precautions (5.1) and Drug Interactions (7).]

Bile Acid Sequestrants

Dosing of VYTORIN should occur either ≥2 hours before or ≥4 hours after administration of a bile acid sequestrant [see Drug Interactions (7.5)].

Cyclosporine or Danazol

Caution should be exercised when initiating VYTORIN in the setting of cyclosporine. In patients taking cyclosporine or danazol, VYTORIN should not be started unless the patient has already tolerated treatment with simvastatin at a dose of 5 mg or higher. The dose of VYTORIN should not exceed 10/10 mg/day [see Drug Interactions (7.6)].

Amiodarone or Verapamil

In patients taking amiodarone or verapamil concomitantly with VYTORIN, the dose should not exceed 10/20 mg/day [see Warnings and Precautions (5.1) and Drug Interactions (7.3)].

Diltiazem

The dose of VYTORIN should not exceed 10/40 mg/day [see Warnings and Precautions (5.1), Drug Interactions (7.3), and Clinical Pharmacology (12.3)].

Other Concomitant Lipid-Lowering Therapy

The safety and effectiveness of VYTORIN administered with fibrates have not been established. Therefore, the combination of VYTORIN and fibrates should be avoided [see Warnings and Precautions (5.1) and Drug Interactions (7.2 and 7.8)].

There is an increased risk of myopathy when simvastatin is used concomitantly with fibrates (especially gemfibrozil). Combination therapy with gemfibrozil should be avoided because of an increase in simvastatin exposure with concomitant use. [See Warnings and Precautions (5.1) and Drug Interactions (7.2 and 7.8).]

3 DOSAGE FORMS AND STRENGTHS

- VYTORIN® 10/10, (ezetimibe 10 mg/simvastatin 10 mg tablets) are white to off-white capsule-shaped tablets with code "311" on one side.
- VYTORIN® 10/20, (ezetimibe 10 mg/simvastatin 20 mg tablets) are white to off-white capsule-shaped tablets with code "312" on one side.
- VYTORIN® 10/40, (ezetimibe 10 mg/simvastatin 40 mg tablets) are white to off-white capsule-shaped tablets with code "313" on one side.
- VYTORIN® 10/80, (ezetimibe 10 mg/simvastatin 80 mg tablets) are white to off-white capsule-shaped tablets with code "315" on one side.

4 CONTRAINDICATIONS

Hypersensitivity to any component of this medication [see Adverse Reactions (6.2)].

Active liver disease or unexplained persistent elevations in hepatic transaminase levels [see Warnings and Precautions (5.2)].

Women who are pregnant or may become pregnant. Serum cholesterol and triglycerides increase during normal pregnancy, and cholesterol or cholesterol derivatives are essential for fetal development. Because HMG-CoA reductase inhibitors (statins), such as simvastatin, decrease cholesterol synthesis and possibly the synthesis of other biologically active substances derived from cholesterol, VYTORIN may cause fetal harm when administered to a pregnant woman. Atherosclerosis is a chronic process and the discontinuation of lipid-lowering drugs during pregnancy should have little impact on the outcome of long-term therapy of primary hypercholesterolemia. There are no adequate and well-controlled studies of VYTORIN use during pregnancy; however, in rare reports congenital anomalies were observed following intrauterine exposure to statins. In rat and rabbit animal reproduction studies, simvastatin revealed no evidence of teratogenicity. VYTORIN should be administered to women of childbearing age only when such patients are highly unlikely to conceive. If the patient becomes pregnant while taking this drug, VYTORIN should be discontinued immediately and the patient should be apprised of the potential hazard to the fetus [see Use in Specific Populations (8.1)].

Nursing mothers. It is not known whether simvastatin is excreted into human milk; however, a small amount of another drug in this class does pass into breast milk. Because statins have the potential for serious adverse reactions in nursing infants, women who require VYTORIN treatment should not breast-feed their infants [see Use in Specific Populations (8.3)].

5 WARNINGS AND PRECAUTIONS

5.1 Myopathy/Rhabdomyolysis

In clinical trials, there was no excess of myopathy or rhabdomyolysis associated with ezetimibe compared with the relevant control arm (placebo or statin alone). However, myopathy and rhabdomyolysis are known adverse reactions to statins and other lipid-lowering drugs. In clinical trials, the incidence of CK >10 × the upper limit of normal (ULN) was 0.2% for VYTORIN, 0.6% for placebo, 0.0% for ezetimibe, and 0.3% for all simvastatin doses.

Simvastatin, like other statins, occasionally causes myopathy manifested as muscle pain, tenderness or weakness with creatine kinase above 10 × ULN. Myopathy sometimes takes the form of rhabdomyolysis with or without acute renal failure secondary to myoglobinuria, and rare fatalities have occurred. The risk of myopathy is increased by high levels of statin activity in plasma. Predisposing factors for myopathy include advanced age (≥65 years), uncontrolled hypothyroidism, and renal impairment.

As with other statins, the risk of myopathy/rhabdomyolysis is dose related. In a clinical trial database in which 41,050 patients were treated with simvastatin with 24,747 (approximately 60%) treated for at least 4 years, the incidence of myopathy was approximately 0.02%, 0.08% and 0.53% at 20, 40 and 80 mg/day, respectively. In these trials, patients were carefully monitored and some interacting medicinal products were excluded.

In post-marketing experience with ezetimibe, cases of myopathy and rhabdomyolysis have been reported. Most patients who developed rhabdomyolysis were taking a statin prior to initiating ezetimibe. However, rhabdomyolysis has been reported very rarely with ezetimibe monotherapy and very rarely with the addition of ezetimibe to agents known to be associated with increased risk of rhabdomyolysis, such as fibrates.

All patients starting therapy with VYTORIN or whose dose of VYTORIN is being increased should be advised of the risk of myopathy and told to report promptly any unexplained muscle pain, tenderness or weakness. VYTORIN therapy should be discontinued immediately if myopathy is diagnosed or suspected. In most cases, muscle symptoms and CK increases resolved when simvastatin treatment was promptly discontinued. Periodic CK determinations may be considered in patients starting therapy with simvastatin or whose dose is being increased, but there is no assurance that such monitoring will prevent myopathy.

Many of the patients who have developed rhabdomyolysis on therapy with simvastatin have had complicated medical histories, including renal insufficiency usually as a consequence of long-standing diabetes mellitus. Such patients taking VYTORIN merit closer monitoring. Therapy with VYTORIN should be temporarily stopped a few days prior to elective major surgery and when any major medical or surgical condition supervenes.

Drug Interactions

The risk of myopathy and rhabdomyolysis is increased by high levels of statin activity in plasma. Simvastatin is metabolized by the cytochrome P450 isoform 3A4. Certain drugs that inhibit this metabolic pathway can raise the plasma levels of simvastatin and may increase the risk of myopathy. These include itraconazole, ketoconazole, and other antifungal azoles, the macrolide antibiotics erythromycin and clarithromycin, and the ketolide antibiotic telithromycin, HIV protease inhibitors, the antidepressant nefazodone, or large quantities of grapefruit juice (>1 quart daily). The use of VYTORIN concomitantly with these CYP3A4 inhibitors should be avoided. If treatment with itraconazole, ketoconazole, erythromycin, clarithromycin or telithromycin is unavoidable, therapy with VYTORIN should be suspended during the course of treatment. [See Drug Interactions (7).]

The benefits of the combined use of VYTORIN with the following drugs should be carefully weighed against the potential risks of combinations: gemfibrozil, other lipid-lowering drugs (other fibrates or ≥1 g/day of niacin), cyclosporine, danazol, amiodarone, verapamil, or diltiazem.

Caution should be used when prescribing other fibrates with VYTORIN, as these agents can cause myopathy when given alone.

Cases of myopathy/rhabdomyolysis have been observed with simvastatin coadministered with lipid-modifying doses (≥1 g/day niacin) of niacin-containing products. In an ongoing, double-blind, randomized cardiovascular outcomes trial, an independent safety monitoring committee identified that the incidence of myopathy is higher in Chinese compared with non-Chinese patients taking simvastatin 40 mg or ezetimibe/simvastatin 10/40 mg coadministered with lipid-modifying doses of a niacin-containing product. Because the risk for myopathy is dose-related, Chinese patients should not receive VYTORIN 10/80 mg coadministered with lipid-modifying doses of niacin-containing products. It is unknown if the risk for myopathy with coadministration of simvastatin with lipid-modifying doses of niacin-containing products observed in Chinese patients applies to other Asian patients.

Prescribing recommendations for interacting agents are summarized in Table 1 [see also Dosage and Administration (2.7), Drug Interactions (7), and Clinical Pharmacology (12.3)].

Table 1: Drug Interactions Associated with Increased Risk of Myopathy/Rhabdomyolysis

Interacting Agents	Prescribing Recommendations
Itraconazole Ketoconazole Erythromycin Clarithromycin Telithromycin HIV protease inhibitors Nefazodone Fibrates*	Avoid VYTORIN
Cyclosporine† Danazol†	Do not exceed 10/10 mg VYTORIN daily
Amiodarone‡ Verapamil‡	Do not exceed 10/20 mg VYTORIN daily
Diltiazem§	Do not exceed 10/40 mg VYTORIN daily
Grapefruit juice	Avoid large quantities of grapefruit juice (>1 quart daily)

* Combination therapy with fibrates should be avoided; however, although not recommended, if VYTORIN is used in combination with gemfibrozil, the dose should not exceed 10/10 mg daily.
† The benefits of the use of VYTORIN in patients receiving cyclosporine or danazol should be carefully weighed against the risks of these combinations.
‡ The combined use of VYTORIN at doses higher than 10/20 mg daily with amiodarone or verapamil should be avoided unless the clinical benefit is likely to outweigh the increased risk of myopathy.
§ The combined use of VYTORIN at doses higher than 10/40 mg daily with diltiazem should be avoided unless the clinical benefit is likely to outweigh the increased risk of myopathy.

5.2   Liver Enzymes

In three placebo-controlled, 12-week trials, the incidence of consecutive elevations (≥3 × ULN) in serum transaminases was 1.7% overall for patients treated with VYTORIN and appeared to be dose-related with an incidence of 2.6% for patients treated with VYTORIN 10/80. In controlled long-term (48-week) extensions, which included both newly-treated and previously-treated patients, the incidence of consecutive elevations (≥3 × ULN) in serum transaminases was 1.8% overall and 3.6% for patients treated with VYTORIN 10/80. These elevations in transaminases were generally asymptomatic, not associated with cholestasis, and returned to baseline after discontinuation of therapy or with continued treatment.

It is recommended that liver function tests be performed before the initiation of treatment with VYTORIN, and thereafter when clinically indicated. Patients titrated to the 10/80-mg dose should receive an additional test prior to titration, 3 months after titration to the 10/80-mg dose, and periodically thereafter (e.g., semiannually) for the first year of treatment. Patients who develop increased transaminase levels should be monitored with a second liver function eval-

uation to confirm the finding and be followed thereafter with frequent liver function tests until the abnormality(ies) return to normal. Should an increase in AST or ALT of 3 × ULN or greater persist, withdrawal of therapy with VYTORIN is recommended.

VYTORIN should be used with caution in patients who consume substantial quantities of alcohol and/or have a past history of liver disease. Active liver diseases or unexplained persistent transaminase elevations are contraindications to the use of VYTORIN.

5.3   Hepatic Impairment

Due to the unknown effects of the increased exposure to ezetimibe in patients with moderate or severe hepatic impairment, VYTORIN is not recommended in these patients. [See Clinical Pharmacology (12.3).]

6   ADVERSE REACTIONS

The following serious adverse reactions are discussed in greater detail in other sections of the label:
• Rhabdomyolysis and myopathy [see Warnings and Precautions (5.1)]
• Liver enzyme abnormalities [see Warnings and Precautions (5.2)]

6.1   Clinical Trials Experience

VYTORIN

Because clinical studies are conducted under widely varying conditions, adverse reaction rates observed in the clinical studies of a drug cannot be directly compared to rates in the clinical studies of another drug and may not reflect the rates observed in practice.

In the VYTORIN (ezetimibe/simvastatin) placebo-controlled clinical trials database of 1420 patients (age range 20-83 years, 52% women, 87% Caucasians, 3% Blacks, 5% Hispanics, 3% Asians) with a median treatment duration of 27 weeks, 5% of patients on VYTORIN and 2.2% of patients on placebo discontinued due to adverse reactions.

The most common adverse reactions in the group treated with VYTORIN that led to treatment discontinuation and occurred at a rate greater than placebo were:
• Increased ALT (0.9%)
• Myalgia (0.6%)
• Increased AST (0.4%)
• Back pain (0.4%)

The most commonly reported adverse reactions (incidence ≥2% and greater than placebo) in controlled clinical trials were: headache (5.8%), increased ALT (3.7%), myalgia (3.6%), upper respiratory tract infection (3.6%), and diarrhea (2.8%).

VYTORIN has been evaluated for safety in more than 10,189 patients in clinical trials.

Table 2 summarizes the frequency of clinical adverse reactions reported in ≥2% of patients treated with VYTORIN (n=1420) and at an incidence greater than placebo, regardless of causality assessment, from four placebo-controlled trials.

[See table 2 above]

Ezetimibe

Other adverse reactions reported with ezetimibe in placebo-controlled studies, regardless of causality assessment: Musculoskeletal system disorders: arthralgia; Infections and infestations: sinusitis; Body as a whole–general disorders: fatigue.

Simvastatin

Other adverse reactions reported with simvastatin in placebo-controlled clinical studies, regardless of causality assessment: Cardiac disorders: atrial fibrillation; Ear and labyrinth disorders: vertigo; Gastrointestinal disorders: abdominal pain, constipation, dyspepsia, flatulence, gastritis; Skin and subcutaneous tissue disorders: eczema, rash; Endocrine disorders: diabetes mellitus; Infections and infesta-

Table 2*: Clinical Adverse Reactions Occurring in ≥2% of Patients Treated with VYTORIN and at an Incidence Greater than Placebo, Regardless of Causality

Body System/Organ Class Adverse Reaction	Placebo (%) n=371	Ezetimibe 10 mg (%) n=302	Simvastatin† (%) n=1234	VYTORIN† (%) n=1420
Body as a whole–general disorders				
Headache	5.4	6.0	5.9	5.8
Gastrointestinal system disorders				
Diarrhea	2.2	5.0	3.7	2.8
Infections and infestations				
Influenza	0.8	1.0	1.9	2.3
Upper respiratory tract infection	2.7	5.0	5.0	3.6
Musculoskeletal and connective tissue disorders				
Myalgia	2.4	2.3	2.6	3.6
Pain in extremity	1.3	3.0	2.0	2.3

* Includes two placebo-controlled combination studies in which the active ingredients equivalent to VYTORIN were coadministered and two placebo-controlled studies in which VYTORIN was administered.
† All doses.

tions: bronchitis, sinusitis, urinary tract infections; Body as a whole–general disorders: asthenia, edema/swelling; Psychiatric disorders: insomnia.

Laboratory Tests

Marked persistent increases of hepatic serum transaminases have been noted [see Warnings and Precautions (5.2)]. Elevated alkaline phosphatase and γ-glutamyl transpeptidase have been reported. About 5% of patients taking simvastatin had elevations of CK levels of 3 or more times the normal value on one or more occasions. This was attributable to the noncardiac fraction of CK [see Warnings and Precautions (5.1)].

6.2   Post-Marketing Experience

Because the below reactions are reported voluntarily from a population of uncertain size, it is generally not possible to reliably estimate their frequency or establish a causal relationship to drug exposure.

The following adverse reactions have been reported in post-marketing experience for VYTORIN or ezetimibe or simvastatin: pruritus; alopecia; erythema multiforme; a variety of skin changes (e.g., nodules, discoloration, dryness of skin/mucous membranes, changes to hair/nails); dizziness; muscle cramps; myalgia; arthralgia; pancreatitis; memory impairment; paresthesia; peripheral neuropathy; vomiting; nausea; anemia; erectile dysfunction; interstitial lung disease; myopathy/rhabdomyolysis [see Warnings and Precautions (5.1)]; hepatitis/jaundice; hepatic failure; depression; cholelithiasis; cholecystitis; thrombocytopenia; elevations in liver transaminases; elevated creatine phosphokinase.

Hypersensitivity reactions, including anaphylaxis, angioedema, rash, and urticaria have been reported.

In addition, an apparent hypersensitivity syndrome has been reported rarely that has included one or more of the following features: anaphylaxis, angioedema, lupus erythematous-like syndrome, polymyalgia rheumatica, dermatomyositis, vasculitis, purpura, thrombocytopenia, leukopenia, hemolytic anemia, positive ANA, ESR increase, eosinophilia, arthritis, arthralgia, urticaria, asthenia, photosensitivity, fever, chills, flushing, malaise, dyspnea, toxic epidermal necrolysis, erythema multiforme, including Stevens-Johnson syndrome.

7   DRUG INTERACTIONS

[See Clinical Pharmacology (12.3).]
VYTORIN

7.1   CYP3A4 Interactions

The risk of myopathy is increased by reducing the elimination of the simvastatin component of VYTORIN. Hence when VYTORIN is used with an inhibitor of CYP3A4 (e.g., as listed below), elevated plasma levels of HMG-CoA reductase inhibitory activity can increase the risk of myopathy and rhabdomyolysis, particularly with higher doses of VYTORIN. [See Warnings and Precautions (5.1) and Clinical Pharmacology (12.3).]
Itraconazole, ketoconazole, and other antifungal azoles
Macrolide antibiotics erythromycin, clarithromycin, and the ketolide antibiotic telithromycin
HIV protease inhibitors
Antidepressant nefazodone
Grapefruit juice in large quantities (>1 quart daily)
Concomitant use of these drugs and any medication labeled as having a strong inhibitory effect on CYP3A4 should be avoided unless the benefits of combined therapy outweigh the increased risk. If treatment with itraconazole, ketoconazole, erythromycin, clarithromycin or telithromycin is unavoidable, therapy with VYTORIN should be suspended during the course of treatment.

7.2   Lipid-Lowering Drugs That Can Cause Myopathy When Given Alone

The risk of myopathy is increased by gemfibrozil and to a lesser extent by other fibrates [see Warnings and Precautions (5.1)].

Table 3: Mean Percent Difference at Week 6 Between the Pooled Ezetimibe Coadministered with Simvastatin Group and the Pooled Simvastatin Monotherapy Group in Adolescent Patients with Heterozygous Familial Hypercholesterolemia

	Total-C	LDL-C	Apo B	Non-HDL-C	TG*	HDL-C
Mean percent difference between treatment groups	-12%	-15%	-12%	-14%	-2%	+0.1%
95% Confidence Interval	(-15%, -9%)	(-18%, -12%)	(-15%, -9%)	(-17%, -11%)	(-9, +4)	(-3, +3)

* For triglycerides, median % change from baseline

7.3 Amiodarone, Verapamil, or Diltiazem
The risk of myopathy/rhabdomyolysis is increased by concomitant administration of amiodarone, verapamil, or diltiazem with higher doses of VYTORIN *[see Warnings and Precautions (5.1)]*.

7.4 Niacin
Cases of myopathy/rhabdomyolysis have been observed with simvastatin coadministered with lipid-modifying doses (≥1 g/day niacin) of niacin-containing products. In particular, caution should be used when treating Chinese patients with VYTORIN coadministered with lipid-modifying doses of niacin-containing products. Because the risk for myopathy is dose-related, Chinese patients should not receive VYTORIN 10/80 mg coadministered with lipid-modifying doses of niacin-containing products. *[See Warnings and Precautions (5.1).]*

7.5 Cholestyramine
Concomitant cholestyramine administration decreased the mean AUC of total ezetimibe approximately 55%. The incremental LDL-C reduction due to adding VYTORIN to cholestyramine may be reduced by this interaction.

7.6 Cyclosporine or Danazol
The risk of myopathy/rhabdomyolysis is increased by concomitant administration of cyclosporine or danazol particularly with higher doses of VYTORIN *[see Warnings and Precautions (5.1) and Clinical Pharmacology (12.3)]*.
Caution should be exercised when using VYTORIN and cyclosporine concomitantly due to increased exposure to both ezetimibe and cyclosporine *[see Dosage and Administration (2.7)]*. Cyclosporine concentrations should be monitored in patients receiving VYTORIN and cyclosporine *[see Clinical Pharmacology (12.3)]*.
The degree of increase in ezetimibe exposure may be greater in patients with severe renal impairment. In patients treated with cyclosporine, the potential effects of the increased exposure to ezetimibe from concomitant use should be carefully weighed against the benefits of alterations in lipid levels provided by ezetimibe. *[See Warnings and Precautions (5.1) and Clinical Pharmacology (12.3).]*

7.7 Digoxin
In one study, concomitant administration of digoxin with simvastatin resulted in a slight elevation in plasma digoxin concentrations. Patients taking digoxin should be monitored appropriately when VYTORIN is initiated.

7.8 Fibrates
The safety and effectiveness of VYTORIN administered with fibrates have not been established.
Fibrates may increase cholesterol excretion into the bile, leading to cholelithiasis. In a preclinical study in dogs, ezetimibe increased cholesterol in the gallbladder bile *[see Animal Toxicology and/or Pharmacology (13.2)]*. Coadministration of VYTORIN with fibrates is not recommended until use in patients is studied. *[See Warnings and Precautions (5.1).]*

7.9 Coumarin Anticoagulants
Simvastatin 20-40 mg/day modestly potentiated the effect of coumarin anticoagulants: the prothrombin time, reported as International Normalized Ratio (INR), increased from a baseline of 1.7 to 1.8 and from 2.6 to 3.4 in a normal volunteer study and in a hypercholesterolemic patient study, respectively. With other statins, clinically evident bleeding and/or increased prothrombin time has been reported in a few patients taking coumarin anticoagulants concomitantly. In such patients, prothrombin time should be determined before starting VYTORIN and frequently enough during early therapy to ensure that no significant alteration of prothrombin time occurs. Once a stable prothrombin time has been documented, prothrombin times can be monitored at the intervals usually recommended for patients on coumarin anticoagulants. If the dose of VYTORIN is changed or discontinued, the same procedure should be repeated. Simvastatin therapy has not been associated with bleeding or with changes in prothrombin time in patients not taking anticoagulants.
Concomitant administration of ezetimibe (10 mg once daily) had no significant effect on bioavailability of warfarin and prothrombin time in a study of twelve healthy adult males. There have been post-marketing reports of increased INR in patients who had ezetimibe added to warfarin. Most of these patients were also on other medications.
The effect of VYTORIN on the prothrombin time has not been studied.

8 USE IN SPECIFIC POPULATIONS

8.1 Pregnancy
Pregnancy Category X.
[See Contraindications (4).]
VYTORIN
VYTORIN is contraindicated in women who are or may become pregnant. Lipid-lowering drugs offer no benefit during pregnancy, because cholesterol and cholesterol derivatives are needed for normal fetal development. Atherosclerosis is a chronic process, and discontinuation of lipid-lowering drugs during pregnancy should have little impact on long-term outcomes of primary hypercholesterolemia therapy. There are no adequate and well-controlled studies of VYTORIN use during pregnancy; however, there are rare reports of congenital anomalies in infants exposed to statins *in utero*. Animal reproduction studies of simvastatin in rats and rabbits showed no evidence of teratogenicity. Serum cholesterol and triglycerides increase during normal pregnancy, and cholesterol or cholesterol derivatives are essential for fetal development. Because statins, such as simvastatin, decrease cholesterol synthesis and possibly the synthesis of other biologically active substances derived from cholesterol, VYTORIN may cause fetal harm when administered to a pregnant woman. If VYTORIN is used during pregnancy or if the patient becomes pregnant while taking this drug, the patient should be apprised of the potential hazard to the fetus.
Women of childbearing potential, who require VYTORIN treatment for a lipid disorder, should be advised to use effective contraception. For women trying to conceive, discontinuation of VYTORIN should be considered. If pregnancy occurs, VYTORIN should be immediately discontinued.
Ezetimibe
In oral (gavage) embryo-fetal development studies of ezetimibe conducted in rats and rabbits during organogenesis, there was no evidence of embryolethal effects at the doses tested (250, 500, 1000 mg/kg/day). In rats, increased incidences of common fetal skeletal findings (extra pair of thoracic ribs, unossified cervical vertebral centra, shortened ribs) were observed at 1000 mg/kg/day (~10 times the human exposure at 10 mg daily based on $AUC_{0\text{-}24hr}$ for total ezetimibe). In rabbits treated with ezetimibe, an increased incidence of extra thoracic ribs was observed at 1000 mg/kg/day (150 times the human exposure at 10 mg daily based on $AUC_{0\text{-}24hr}$ for total ezetimibe). Ezetimibe crossed the placenta when pregnant rats and rabbits were given multiple oral doses.
Multiple-dose studies of ezetimibe coadministered with statins in rats and rabbits during organogenesis result in higher ezetimibe and statin exposures. Reproductive findings occur at lower doses in coadministration therapy compared to monotherapy.
Simvastatin
Simvastatin was not teratogenic in rats or rabbits at doses (25, 10 mg/kg/day, respectively) that resulted in 3 times the human exposure based on mg/m^2 surface area. However, in studies with another structurally-related statin, skeletal malformations were observed in rats and mice.
There are rare reports of congenital anomalies following intrauterine exposure to statins. In a review[1] of approximately 100 prospectively followed pregnancies in women exposed to simvastatin or another structurally-related statin, the incidences of congenital anomalies, spontaneous abortions and fetal deaths/stillbirths did not exceed what would be expected in the general population. The number of cases is adequate only to exclude a 3- to 4-fold increase in congenital anomalies over the background incidence. In 89% of the prospectively followed pregnancies, drug treatment was initiated prior to pregnancy and was discontinued at some point in the first trimester when pregnancy was identified.

[1] Manson, J.M., Freyssinges, C., Ducrocq, M.B., Stephenson, W.P., Postmarketing Surveillance of Lovastatin and Simvastatin Exposure During Pregnancy, *Reproductive Toxicology*, 10(6):439-446, 1996.

8.3 Nursing Mothers
It is not known whether simvastatin is excreted in human milk. Because a small amount of another drug in this class is excreted in human milk and because of the potential for serious adverse reactions in nursing infants, women taking simvastatin should not nurse their infants. A decision should be made whether to discontinue nursing or discontinue drug, taking into account the importance of the drug to the mother *[see Contraindications (4)]*.
In rat studies, exposure to ezetimibe in nursing pups was up to half of that observed in maternal plasma. It is not known whether ezetimibe or simvastatin are excreted into human breast milk. Because a small amount of another drug in the same class as simvastatin is excreted in human milk and because of the potential for serious adverse reactions in nursing infants, women who are nursing should not take VYTORIN *[see Contraindications (4)]*.

8.4 Pediatric Use
The effects of ezetimibe coadministered with simvastatin (n=126) compared to simvastatin monotherapy (n=122) have been evaluated in adolescent boys and girls with heterozygous familial hypercholesterolemia (HeFH). In a multicenter, double-blind, controlled study followed by an open-label phase, 142 boys and 106 postmenarchal girls, 10 to 17 years of age (mean age 14.2 years, 43% females, 82% Caucasians, 4% Asian, 2% Blacks, 13% multi-racial) with HeFH were randomized to receive either ezetimibe coadministered with simvastatin or simvastatin monotherapy. Inclusion in the study required 1) a baseline LDL-C level between 160 and 400 mg/dL and 2) a medical history and clinical presentation consistent with HeFH. The mean baseline LDL-C value was 225 mg/dL (range: 161-351 mg/dL) in the ezetimibe coadministered with simvastatin group compared to 219 mg/dL (range: 149-336 mg/dL) in the simvastatin monotherapy group. The patients received coadministered ezetimibe and simvastatin (10 mg, 20 mg, or 40 mg) or simvastatin monotherapy (10 mg, 20 mg, or 40 mg) for 6 weeks, coadministered ezetimibe and 40 mg simvastatin or 40 mg simvastatin monotherapy for the next 27 weeks, and open-label coadministered ezetimibe and simvastatin (10 mg, 20 mg, or 40 mg) for 20 weeks thereafter.
The results of the study at Week 6 are summarized in Table 3. Results at Week 33 were consistent with those at Week 6.
[See table 3 above]
From the start of the trial to the end of Week 33, discontinuations due to an adverse reaction occurred in 7 (6%) patients in the ezetimibe coadministered with simvastatin group and in 2 (2%) patients in the simvastatin monotherapy group.
During the trial, hepatic transaminase elevations (two consecutive measurements for ALT and/or AST ≥3 × ULN) occurred in four (3%) individuals in the ezetimibe coadministered with simvastatin group and in two (2%) individuals in the simvastatin monotherapy group. Elevations of CPK (≥10 × ULN) occurred in two (2%) individuals in the ezetimibe coadministered with simvastatin group and in zero individuals in the simvastatin monotherapy group.
In this limited controlled study, there was no significant effect on growth or sexual maturation in the adolescent boys or girls, or on menstrual cycle length in girls.
Coadministration of ezetimibe with simvastatin at doses greater than 40 mg/day has not been studied in adolescents. Also, VYTORIN has not been studied in patients younger than 10 years of age or in pre-menarchal girls.
Ezetimibe
Based on total ezetimibe (ezetimibe + ezetimibe-glucuronide) there are no pharmacokinetic differences between adolescents and adults. Pharmacokinetic data in the pediatric population <10 years of age are not available.
Simvastatin
The pharmacokinetics of simvastatin has not been studied in the pediatric population.

8.5 Geriatric Use
Of the 10,189 patients who received VYTORIN in clinical studies, 3242 (32%) were 65 and older (this included 844 (8%) who were 75 and older). No overall differences in safety or effectiveness were observed between these subjects and younger subjects, and other reported clinical experience has not identified differences in responses between the elderly and younger patients but greater sensitivity of some older individuals cannot be ruled out. Since advanced age (≥65 years) is a predisposing factor for myopathy, VYTORIN should be prescribed with caution in the elderly. *[See Clinical Pharmacology (12.3).]*

8.6 Renal Impairment
Caution should be exercised when VYTORIN is administered to patients with severe renal impairment. *[See Dosage and Administration (2.4).]*

8.7 Hepatic Impairment
VYTORIN is contraindicated in patients with active liver disease or unexplained persistent elevations of hepatic transaminases. VYTORIN is not recommended in patients with moderate to severe hepatic impairment. *[See Contraindications (4) and Warnings and Precautions (5.2).]*

10 OVERDOSAGE

VYTORIN

No specific treatment of overdosage with VYTORIN can be recommended. In the event of an overdose, symptomatic and supportive measures should be employed.

Ezetimibe

In clinical studies, administration of ezetimibe, 50 mg/day to 15 healthy subjects for up to 14 days, or 40 mg/day to 18 patients with primary hyperlipidemia for up to 56 days, was generally well tolerated.

A few cases of overdosage have been reported; most have not been associated with adverse experiences. Reported adverse experiences have not been serious.

Simvastatin

Significant lethality was observed in mice after a single oral dose of 9 g/m^2. No evidence of lethality was observed in rats or dogs treated with doses of 30 and 100 g/m^2, respectively. No specific diagnostic signs were observed in rodents. At these doses the only signs seen in dogs were emesis and mucoid stools.

A few cases of overdosage with simvastatin have been reported; the maximum dose taken was 3.6 g. All patients recovered without sequelae.

The dialyzability of simvastatin and its metabolites in man is not known at present.

11 DESCRIPTION

VYTORIN contains ezetimibe, a selective inhibitor of intestinal cholesterol and related phytosterol absorption, and simvastatin, an HMG-CoA reductase inhibitor.

The chemical name of ezetimibe is 1-(4-fluorophenyl)-3(R)-[3-(4-fluorophenyl)-3(S)-hydroxypropyl]-4(S)-(4-hydroxyphenyl)-2-azetidinone. The empirical formula is $C_{24}H_{21}F_2NO_3$ and its molecular weight is 409.4.

Ezetimibe is a white, crystalline powder that is freely to very soluble in ethanol, methanol, and acetone and practically insoluble in water. Its structural formula is:

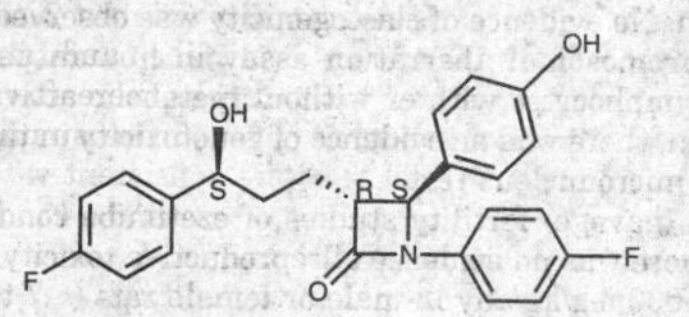

Simvastatin, an inactive lactone, is hydrolyzed to the corresponding β-hydroxyacid form, which is an inhibitor of HMG-CoA reductase. Simvastatin is butanoic acid, 2,2-dimethyl-,1,2,3,7,8,8a-hexahydro-3,7-dimethyl-8-[2-(tetrahydro-4-hydroxy-6-oxo-2*H*-pyran-2-yl)-ethyl]-1-naphthalenyl ester, [1*S*-[1α,3α,7β,8β(2*S**,4*S**),-8aβ]]. The empirical formula of simvastatin is $C_{25}H_{38}O_5$ and its molecular weight is 418.57.

Simvastatin is a white to off-white, nonhygroscopic, crystalline powder that is practically insoluble in water and freely soluble in chloroform, methanol and ethanol. Its structural formula is:

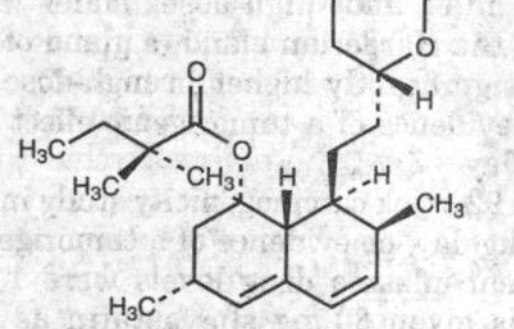

VYTORIN is available for oral use as tablets containing 10 mg of ezetimibe, and 10 mg of simvastatin (VYTORIN 10/10), 20 mg of simvastatin (VYTORIN 10/20), 40 mg of simvastatin (VYTORIN 10/40), or 80 mg of simvastatin (VYTORIN 10/80). Each tablet contains the following inactive ingredients: butylated hydroxyanisole NF, citric acid monohydrate USP, croscarmellose sodium NF, hypromellose USP, lactose monohydrate NF, magnesium stearate NF, microcrystalline cellulose NF, and propyl gallate NF.

12 CLINICAL PHARMACOLOGY

12.1 Mechanism of Action

VYTORIN

Plasma cholesterol is derived from intestinal absorption and endogenous synthesis. VYTORIN contains ezetimibe and simvastatin, two lipid-lowering compounds with complementary mechanisms of action. VYTORIN reduces elevated total-C, LDL-C, Apo B, TG, and non-HDL-C, and increases HDL-C through dual inhibition of cholesterol absorption and synthesis.

Ezetimibe

Ezetimibe reduces blood cholesterol by inhibiting the absorption of cholesterol by the small intestine. The molecular target of ezetimibe has been shown to be the sterol transporter, Niemann-Pick C1-Like 1 (NPC1L1), which is involved in the intestinal uptake of cholesterol and phytosterols. In a 2-week clinical study in 18 hypercholesterolemic patients, ezetimibe inhibited intestinal cholesterol absorption by 54%, compared with placebo. Ezetimibe had no clinically meaningful effect on the plasma concentrations of the fat-soluble vitamins A, D, and E and did not impair adrenocortical steroid hormone production.

Ezetimibe localizes at the brush border of the small intestine and inhibits the absorption of cholesterol, leading to a decrease in the delivery of intestinal cholesterol to the liver. This causes a reduction of hepatic cholesterol stores and an increase in clearance of cholesterol from the blood; this distinct mechanism is complementary to that of statins *[see Clinical Studies (14)]*.

Simvastatin

Simvastatin is a prodrug and is hydrolyzed to its active β-hydroxyacid form, simvastatin acid, after administration. Simvastatin is a specific inhibitor of 3-hydroxy-3-methylglutaryl-coenzyme A (HMG-CoA) reductase, the enzyme that catalyzes the conversion of HMG-CoA to mevalonate, an early and rate limiting step in the biosynthetic pathway for cholesterol. In addition, simvastatin reduces very-low-density lipoproteins (VLDL) and TG and increases HDL-C.

12.2 Pharmacodynamics

Clinical studies have demonstrated that elevated levels of total-C, LDL-C and Apo B, the major protein constituent of LDL, promote human atherosclerosis. In addition, decreased levels of HDL-C are associated with the development of atherosclerosis. Epidemiologic studies have established that cardiovascular morbidity and mortality vary directly with the level of total-C and LDL-C and inversely with the level of HDL-C. Like LDL, cholesterol-enriched triglyceride-rich lipoproteins, including VLDL, intermediate-density lipoproteins (IDL), and remnants, can also promote atherosclerosis. The independent effect of raising HDL-C or lowering TG on the risk of coronary and cardiovascular morbidity and mortality has not been determined.

12.3 Pharmacokinetics

The results of a bioequivalence study in healthy subjects demonstrated that the VYTORIN (ezetimibe/simvastatin) 10 mg/10 mg to 10 mg/80 mg combination tablets are bioequivalent to coadministration of corresponding doses of ezetimibe (ZETIA®) and simvastatin (ZOCOR®) as individual tablets.

Absorption

Ezetimibe

After oral administration, ezetimibe is absorbed and extensively conjugated to a pharmacologically active phenolic glucuronide (ezetimibe-glucuronide).

Simvastatin

The availability of the β-hydroxyacid to the systemic circulation following an oral dose of simvastatin was found to be less than 5% of the dose, consistent with extensive hepatic first-pass extraction.

Effect of Food on Oral Absorption

Ezetimibe

Concomitant food administration (high-fat or non-fat meals) had no effect on the extent of absorption of ezetimibe when administered as 10-mg tablets. The C_{max} value of ezetimibe was increased by 38% with consumption of high-fat meals.

Simvastatin

Relative to the fasting state, the plasma profiles of both active and total inhibitors of HMG-CoA reductase were not affected when simvastatin was administered immediately before an American Heart Association recommended low-fat meal.

Distribution

Ezetimibe

Ezetimibe and ezetimibe-glucuronide are highly bound (>90%) to human plasma proteins.

Simvastatin

Both simvastatin and its β-hydroxyacid metabolite are highly bound (approximately 95%) to human plasma proteins. When radiolabeled simvastatin was administered to rats, simvastatin-derived radioactivity crossed the blood-brain barrier.

Metabolism and Excretion

Ezetimibe

Ezetimibe is primarily metabolized in the small intestine and liver via glucuronide conjugation with subsequent biliary and renal excretion. Minimal oxidative metabolism has been observed in all species evaluated.

In humans, ezetimibe is rapidly metabolized to ezetimibe-glucuronide. Ezetimibe and ezetimibe-glucuronide are the major drug-derived compounds detected in plasma, constituting approximately 10 to 20% and 80 to 90% of the total drug in plasma, respectively. Both ezetimibe and ezetimibe-glucuronide are eliminated from plasma with a half-life of approximately 22 hours for both ezetimibe and ezetimibe-glucuronide. Plasma concentration-time profiles exhibit multiple peaks, suggesting enterohepatic recycling.

Following oral administration of ^{14}C-ezetimibe (20 mg) to human subjects, total ezetimibe (ezetimibe + ezetimibe-glucuronide) accounted for approximately 93% of the total radioactivity in plasma. After 48 hours, there were no detectable levels of radioactivity in the plasma.

Approximately 78% and 11% of the administered radioactivity were recovered in the feces and urine, respectively, over a 10-day collection period. Ezetimibe was the major component in feces and accounted for 69% of the administered dose, while ezetimibe-glucuronide was the major component in urine and accounted for 9% of the administered dose.

Simvastatin

Simvastatin is a lactone that is readily hydrolyzed *in vivo* to the corresponding β-hydroxyacid, a potent inhibitor of HMG-CoA reductase. Inhibition of HMG-CoA reductase is a basis for an assay in pharmacokinetic studies of the β-hydroxyacid metabolites (active inhibitors) and, following base hydrolysis, active plus latent inhibitors (total inhibitors) in plasma following administration of simvastatin. The major active metabolites of simvastatin present in human plasma are the β-hydroxyacid of simvastatin and its 6′-hydroxy, 6′-hydroxymethyl, and 6′-exomethylene derivatives.

Following an oral dose of ^{14}C-labeled simvastatin in man, 13% of the dose was excreted in urine and 60% in feces. Plasma concentrations of total radioactivity (simvastatin plus ^{14}C-metabolites) peaked at 4 hours and declined rapidly to about 10% of peak by 12 hours postdose.

Specific Populations

Geriatric Patients

Ezetimibe

In a multiple-dose study with ezetimibe given 10 mg once daily for 10 days, plasma concentrations for total ezetimibe were about 2-fold higher in older (≥65 years) healthy subjects compared to younger subjects.

Simvastatin

In a study including 16 elderly patients between 70 and 78 years of age who received simvastatin 40 mg/day, the mean plasma level of HMG-CoA reductase inhibitory activity was increased approximately 45% compared with 18 patients between 18-30 years of age.

Pediatric Patients: *[See Pediatric Use (8.4).]*

Gender

Ezetimibe

In a multiple-dose study with ezetimibe given 10 mg once daily for 10 days, plasma concentrations for total ezetimibe were slightly higher (<20%) in women than in men.

Race

Ezetimibe

Based on a meta-analysis of multiple-dose pharmacokinetic studies, there were no pharmacokinetic differences between Black and Caucasian subjects. Studies in Asian subjects indicated that the pharmacokinetics of ezetimibe was similar to those seen in Caucasian subjects.

Hepatic Impairment

Ezetimibe

After a single 10-mg dose of ezetimibe, the mean exposure (based on area under the curve [AUC]) to total ezetimibe was increased approximately 1.7-fold in patients with mild hepatic impairment (Child-Pugh score 5 to 6), compared to healthy subjects. The mean AUC values for total ezetimibe and ezetimibe increased approximately 3- to 4-fold and 5- to 6-fold, respectively, in patients with moderate (Child-Pugh score 7 to 9) or severe hepatic impairment (Child-Pugh score 10 to 15). In a 14-day, multiple-dose study (10 mg daily) in patients with moderate hepatic impairment, the mean AUC for total ezetimibe and ezetimibe increased approximately 4-fold compared to healthy subjects.

Renal Impairment

Ezetimibe

After a single 10-mg dose of ezetimibe in patients with severe renal disease (n=8; mean CrCl ≤30 mL/min/1.73 m^2), the mean AUC for total ezetimibe and ezetimibe increased approximately 1.5-fold, compared to healthy subjects (n=9).

Simvastatin

Pharmacokinetic studies with another statin having a similar principal route of elimination to that of simvastatin have suggested that for a given dose level higher systemic exposure may be achieved in patients with severe renal impairment (as measured by creatinine clearance).

Drug Interactions [See also Drug Interactions (7).]

No clinically significant pharmacokinetic interaction was seen when ezetimibe was coadministered with simvastatin. No specific pharmacokinetic drug interaction studies with VYTORIN have been conducted other than the following study with NIASPAN (Niacin extended-release tablets).

Niacin: The effect of VYTORIN (10/20 mg daily for 7 days) on the pharmacokinetics of NIASPAN extended-release tablets (1000 mg for 2 days and 2000 mg for 5 days following a low-fat breakfast) was studied in healthy subjects. The mean C_{max} and AUC of niacin increased 9% and 22%, respectively. The mean C_{max} and AUC of nicotinuric acid increased 10% and 19%, respectively (N=13). In the same study, the effect of NIASPAN on the pharmacokinetics of

Table 4: Effect of Coadministered Drugs on Total Ezetimibe

Coadministered Drug and Dosing Regimen	Total Ezetimibe* Change in AUC	Total Ezetimibe* Change in C_{max}
Cyclosporine-stable dose required (75-150 mg BID)[†,‡]	↑240%	↑290%
Fenofibrate, 200 mg QD, 14 days[‡]	↑48%	↑64%
Gemfibrozil, 600 mg BID, 7 days[‡]	↑64%	↑91%
Cholestyramine, 4 g BID, 14 days[‡]	↓55%	↓4%
Aluminum & magnesium hydroxide combination antacid, single dose[§]	↓4%	↓30%
Cimetidine, 400 mg BID, 7 days	↑6%	↑22%
Glipizide, 10 mg, single dose	↑4%	↓8%
Statins		
Lovastatin 20 mg QD, 7 days	↑9%	↑3%
Pravastatin 20 mg QD, 14 days	↑7%	↑23%
Atorvastatin 10 mg QD, 14 days	↓2%	↑12%
Rosuvastatin 10 mg QD, 14 days	↑13%	↑18%
Fluvastatin 20 mg QD, 14 days	↓19%	↑7%

* Based on 10 mg-dose of ezetimibe
† Post-renal transplant patients with mild impaired or normal renal function. In a different study, a renal transplant patient with severe renal insufficiency (creatinine clearance of 13.2 mL/min/1.73 m²) who was receiving multiple medications, including cyclosporine, demonstrated a 12-fold greater exposure to total ezetimibe compared to healthy subjects.
‡ See 7. Drug Interactions
§ Supralox®, 20 mL

Table 5: Effect of Ezetimibe Coadministration on Systemic Exposure to Other Drugs

Coadministered Drug and its Dosage Regimen	Ezetimibe Dosage Regimen	Change in AUC of Coadministered Drug	Change in C_{max} of Coadministered Drug
Warfarin, 25 mg single dose on Day 7	10 mg QD, 11 days	↓2% (R-warfarin) ↓4% (S-warfarin)	↑3% (R-warfarin) ↑1% (S-warfarin)
Digoxin, 0.5 mg single dose	10 mg QD, 8 days	↑2%	↓7%
Gemfibrozil, 600 mg BID, 7 days*	10 mg QD, 7 days	↓1%	↓11%
Ethinyl estradiol & Levonorgestrel QD, 21 days	10 mg QD, Days 8–14 of 21 day oral contraceptive cycle	Ethinyl estradiol 0% Levonorgestrel 0%	Ethinyl estradiol ↓9% Levonorgestrel ↓5%
Glipizide, 10 mg on Days 1 and 9	10 mg QD, Days 2-9	↓3%	↓5%
Fenofibrate, 200 mg QD, 14 days*	10 mg QD, 14 days	↑11%	↑7%
Cyclosporine, 100 mg single dose Day 7*	20 mg QD, 8 days	↑15%	↑10%
Statins			
Lovastatin 20 mg QD, 7 days	10 mg QD, 7 days	↑19%	↑3%
Pravastatin 20 mg QD, 14 days	10 mg QD, 14 days	↓20%	↓24%
Atorvastatin 10 mg QD, 14 days	10 mg QD, 14 days	↓4%	↑7%
Rosuvastatin 10 mg QD, 14 days	10 mg QD, 14 days	↑19%	↑17%
Fluvastatin 20 mg QD, 14 days	10 mg QD, 14 days	↓39%	↓27%

* See 7. Drug Interactions

VYTORIN was evaluated (N=15). While concomitant NIASPAN decreased the mean C_{max} of total ezetimibe (1%), and simvastatin (2%), it increased the mean C_{max} of simvastatin acid (18%). In addition, concomitant NIASPAN increased the mean AUC of total ezetimibe (26%), simvastatin (20%), and simvastatin acid (35%).
Cases of myopathy/rhabdomyolysis have been observed with simvastatin coadministered with lipid-modifying doses (≥1 g/day niacin) of niacin-containing products. [See Warnings and Precautions (5.1) and Drug Interactions (7.4).]
Cytochrome P450: Ezetimibe had no significant effect on a series of probe drugs (caffeine, dextromethorphan, tolbutamide, and IV midazolam) known to be metabolized by cytochrome P450 (1A2, 2D6, 2C8/9 and 3A4) in a "cocktail" study of twelve healthy adult males. This indicates that ezetimibe is neither an inhibitor nor an inducer of these cytochrome P450 isozymes, and it is unlikely that ezetimibe will affect the metabolism of drugs that are metabolized by these enzymes.
In a study of 12 healthy volunteers, simvastatin at the 80-mg dose had no effect on the metabolism of the probe cytochrome P450 isoform 3A4 (CYP3A4) substrates midazolam and erythromycin. This indicates that simvastatin is not an inhibitor of CYP3A4 and, therefore, is not expected to affect the plasma levels of other drugs metabolized by CYP3A4.
Although the mechanism is not fully understood, cyclosporine has been shown to increase the AUC of statins. The increase in AUC for simvastatin acid is presumably due, in part, to inhibition of CYP3A4.
Simvastatin is a substrate for CYP3A4. Inhibitors of CYP3A4 can raise the plasma levels of HMG-CoA reductase

inhibitory activity and increase the risk of myopathy. [See Warnings and Precautions (5.1); Drug Interactions (7.1).]
Ezetimibe
[See table 4 at left]
[See table 5 at left]
Simvastatin
[See table 6 at top of next page]

13 NONCLINICAL TOXICOLOGY
13.1 Carcinogenesis, Mutagenesis, Impairment of Fertility
VYTORIN
No animal carcinogenicity or fertility studies have been conducted with the combination of ezetimibe and simvastatin. The combination of ezetimibe with simvastatin did not show evidence of mutagenicity *in vitro* in a microbial mutagenicity (Ames) test with *Salmonella typhimurium* and *Escherichia coli* with or without metabolic activation. No evidence of clastogenicity was observed *in vitro* in a chromosomal aberration assay in human peripheral blood lymphocytes with ezetimibe and simvastatin with or without metabolic activation. There was no evidence of genotoxicity at doses up to 600 mg/kg with the combination of ezetimibe and simvastatin (1:1) in the *in vivo* mouse micronucleus test.
Ezetimibe
A 104-week dietary carcinogenicity study with ezetimibe was conducted in rats at doses up to 1500 mg/kg/day (males) and 500 mg/kg/day (females) (~20 times the human exposure at 10 mg daily based on AUC_{0-24hr} for total ezetimibe). A 104-week dietary carcinogenicity study with ezetimibe was also conducted in mice at doses up to 500 mg/kg/day (>150 times the human exposure at 10 mg daily based on AUC_{0-24hr} for total ezetimibe). There were no statistically significant increases in tumor incidences in drug-treated rats or mice.
No evidence of mutagenicity was observed *in vitro* in a microbial mutagenicity (Ames) test with *Salmonella typhimurium* and *Escherichia coli* with or without metabolic activation. No evidence of clastogenicity was observed *in vitro* in a chromosomal aberration assay in human peripheral blood lymphocytes with or without metabolic activation. In addition, there was no evidence of genotoxicity in the *in vivo* mouse micronucleus test.
In oral (gavage) fertility studies of ezetimibe conducted in rats, there was no evidence of reproductive toxicity at doses up to 1000 mg/kg/day in male or female rats (~7 times the human exposure at 10 mg daily based on AUC_{0-24hr} for total ezetimibe).
Simvastatin
In a 72-week carcinogenicity study, mice were administered daily doses of simvastatin of 25, 100, and 400 mg/kg body weight, which resulted in mean plasma drug levels approximately 1, 4, and 8 times higher than the mean human plasma drug level, respectively, (as total inhibitory activity based on AUC) after an 80-mg oral dose. Liver carcinomas were significantly increased in high-dose females and mid- and high-dose males with a maximum incidence of 90% in males. The incidence of adenomas of the liver was significantly increased in mid- and high-dose females. Drug treatment also significantly increased the incidence of lung adenomas in mid- and high-dose males and females. Adenomas of the Harderian gland (a gland of the eye of rodents) were significantly higher in high-dose mice than in controls. No evidence of a tumorigenic effect was observed at 25 mg/kg/day.
In a separate 92-week carcinogenicity study in mice at doses up to 25 mg/kg/day, no evidence of a tumorigenic effect was observed (mean plasma drug levels were 1 times higher than humans given 80 mg simvastatin as measured by AUC).
In a two-year study in rats at 25 mg/kg/day, there was a statistically significant increase in the incidence of thyroid follicular adenomas in female rats exposed to approximately 11 times higher levels of simvastatin than in humans given 80 mg simvastatin (as measured by AUC).
A second two-year rat carcinogenicity study with doses of 50 and 100 mg/kg/day produced hepatocellular adenomas and carcinomas (in female rats at both doses and in males at 100 mg/kg/day). Thyroid follicular cell adenomas were increased in males and females at both doses; thyroid follicular cell carcinomas were increased in females at 100 mg/kg/day. The increased incidence of thyroid neoplasms appears to be consistent with findings from other statins. These treatment levels represented plasma drug levels (AUC) of approximately 7 and 15 times (males) and 22 and 25 times (females) the mean human plasma drug exposure after an 80-mg daily dose.
No evidence of mutagenicity was observed in a microbial mutagenicity (Ames) test with or without rat or mouse liver metabolic activation. In addition, no evidence of damage to genetic material was noted in an *in vitro* alkaline elution assay using rat hepatocytes, a V-79 mammalian cell forward mutation study, an *in vitro* chromosome aberration study in CHO cells, or an *in vivo* chromosomal aberration assay in mouse bone marrow.

There was decreased fertility in male rats treated with simvastatin for 34 weeks at 25 mg/kg body weight (4 times the maximum human exposure level, based on AUC, in patients receiving 80 mg/day); however, this effect was not observed during a subsequent fertility study in which simvastatin was administered at this same dose level to male rats for 11 weeks (the entire cycle of spermatogenesis including epididymal maturation). No microscopic changes were observed in the testes of rats from either study. At 180 mg/kg/day, (which produces exposure levels 22 times higher than those in humans taking 80 mg/day based on surface area, mg/m²), seminiferous tubule degeneration (necrosis and loss of spermatogenic epithelium) was observed. In dogs, there was drug-related testicular atrophy, decreased spermatogenesis, spermatocytic degeneration and giant cell formation at 10 mg/kg/day (approximately 2 times the human exposure, based on AUC, at 80 mg/day). The clinical significance of these findings is unclear.

13.2 Animal Toxicology and/or Pharmacology

CNS Toxicity

Optic nerve degeneration was seen in clinically normal dogs treated with simvastatin for 14 weeks at 180 mg/kg/day, a dose that produced mean plasma drug levels about 12 times higher than the mean plasma drug level in humans taking 80 mg/day.

A chemically similar drug in this class also produced optic nerve degeneration (Wallerian degeneration of retinogeniculate fibers) in clinically normal dogs in a dose-dependent fashion starting at 60 mg/kg/day, a dose that produced mean plasma drug levels about 30 times higher than the mean plasma drug level in humans taking the highest recommended dose (as measured by total enzyme inhibitory activity). This same drug also produced vestibulocochlear Wallerian-like degeneration and retinal ganglion cell chromatolysis in dogs treated for 14 weeks at 180 mg/kg/day, a dose that resulted in a mean plasma drug level similar to that seen with the 60 mg/kg/day dose.

CNS vascular lesions, characterized by perivascular hemorrhage and edema, mononuclear cell infiltration of perivascular spaces, perivascular fibrin deposits and necrosis of small vessels, were seen in dogs treated with simvastatin at a dose of 360 mg/kg/day, a dose that produced mean plasma drug levels that were about 14 times higher than the mean plasma drug levels in humans taking 80 mg/day. Similar CNS vascular lesions have been observed with several other drugs of this class.

There were cataracts in female rats after two years of treatment with 50 and 100 mg/kg/day (22 and 25 times the human AUC at 80 mg/day, respectively) and in dogs after three months at 90 mg/kg/day (19 times) and at two years at 50 mg/kg/day (5 times).

Ezetimibe

The hypocholesterolemic effect of ezetimibe was evaluated in cholesterol-fed Rhesus monkeys, dogs, rats, and mouse models of human cholesterol metabolism. Ezetimibe was found to have an ED_{50} value of 0.5 µg/kg/day for inhibiting the rise in plasma cholesterol levels in monkeys. The ED_{50} values in dogs, rats, and mice were 7, 30, and 700 µg/kg/day, respectively. These results are consistent with ezetimibe being a potent cholesterol absorption inhibitor.

In a rat model, where the glucuronide metabolite of ezetimibe (ezetimibe-glucuronide) was administered intraduodenally, the metabolite was as potent as ezetimibe in inhibiting the absorption of cholesterol, suggesting that the glucuronide metabolite had activity similar to the parent drug.

In 1-month studies in dogs given ezetimibe (0.03 to 300 mg/kg/day), the concentration of cholesterol in gallbladder bile increased ~2- to 4-fold. However, a dose of 300 mg/kg/day administered to dogs for one year did not result in gallstone formation or any other adverse hepatobiliary effects. In a 14-day study in mice given ezetimibe (0.3 to 5 mg/kg/day) and fed a low-fat or cholesterol-rich diet, the concentration of cholesterol in gallbladder bile was either unaffected or reduced to normal levels, respectively.

A series of acute preclinical studies was performed to determine the selectivity of ezetimibe for inhibiting cholesterol absorption. Ezetimibe inhibited the absorption of ¹⁴C-cholesterol with no effect on the absorption of triglycerides, fatty acids, bile acids, progesterone, ethinyl estradiol, or the fat-soluble vitamins A and D.

In 4- to 12-week toxicity studies in mice, ezetimibe did not induce cytochrome P450 drug-metabolizing enzymes. In toxicity studies, a pharmacokinetic interaction of ezetimibe with statins (parents or their active hydroxy acid metabolites) was seen in rats, dogs, and rabbits.

14 CLINICAL STUDIES

14.1 Primary Hyperlipidemia

VYTORIN

VYTORIN reduces total-C, LDL-C, Apo B, TG, and non-HDL-C, and increases HDL-C in patients with hyperlipidemia. Maximal to near maximal response is generally achieved within 2 weeks and maintained during chronic therapy.

Table 6: Effect of Coadministered Drugs or Grapefruit Juice on Simvastatin Systemic Exposure

Coadministered Drug or Grapefruit Juice	Dosing of Coadministered Drug or Grapefruit Juice	Dosing of Simvastatin	Geometric Mean Ratio (Ratio* with/without coadministered drug) No Effect = 1.00		
				AUC	C_{max}
Avoid taking with VYTORIN [*see Warnings and Precautions (5.1)*]					
Telithromycin[†]	200 mg QD for 4 days	80 mg	simvastatin acid[‡] simvastatin	12 8.9	15 5.3
Nelfinavir[†]	1250 mg BID for 14 days	20 mg QD for 28 days	simvastatin acid[‡] simvastatin	6	6.2
Itraconazole[†]	200 mg QD for 4 days	80 mg	simvastatin acid[‡] simvastatin		13.1 13.1
Avoid >1 quart of grapefruit juice with VYTORIN [*see Warnings and Precautions (5.1)*]					
Grapefruit Juice[§] (high dose)	200 mL of double-strength TID[¶]	60 mg single dose	simvastatin acid simvastatin	7 16	
Grapefruit Juice[§] (low dose)	8 oz (about 237 mL) of single-strength[#]	20 mg single dose	simvastatin acid simvastatin	1.3 1.9	
Avoid taking with VYTORIN. If VYTORIN is used in combination with gemfibrozil, the dose should not exceed 10/10 mg daily, based on clinical and/or post-marketing simvastatin experience [*see Warnings and Precautions (5.1)*]					
Gemfibrozil	600 mg BID for 3 days	40 mg	simvastatin acid simvastatin	2.85 1.35	2.18 0.91
Avoid taking with >10/20 mg VYTORIN, based on clinical and/or post-marketing simvastatin experience [*see Warnings and Precautions (5.1)*]					
Verapamil SR	240 mg QD Days 1-7 then 240 mg BID on Days 8-10	80 mg on Day 10	simvastatin acid simvastatin	2.3 2.5	2.4 2.1
Avoid taking with >10/40 mg VYTORIN, based on clinical and/or post-marketing simvastatin experience [*see Warnings and Precautions (5.1)*]					
Diltiazem	120 mg BID for 10 days	80 mg on Day 10	simvastatin acid simvastatin	2.69 3.10	2.69 2.88
Diltiazem	120 mg BID for 14 days	20 mg on Day 14	simvastatin	4.6	3.6
No dosing adjustments required for the following:					
Fenofibrate	160 mg QD ×14 days	80 mg QD on Days 8-14	simvastatin acid simvastatin	0.64 0.89	0.89 0.83
Amlodipine	10 mg QD × 10 days	80 mg on Day 10	simvastatin acid simvastatin	1.58 1.77	1.56 1.47
Propranolol	80 mg single dose	80 mg single dose	total inhibitor active inhibitor	0.79 0.79	↓ from 33.6 to 21.1 ng•eq/mL ↓ from 7.0 to 4.7 ng•eq/mL

* Results based on a chemical assay except results with propranolol as indicated.
† Results could be representative of the following CYP3A4 inhibitors: ketoconazole, erythromycin, clarithromycin, HIV protease inhibitors, and nefazodone.
‡ Simvastatin acid refers to the β-hydroxyacid of simvastatin.
§ The effect of amounts of grapefruit juice between those used in these two studies on simvastatin pharmacokinetics has not been studied.
¶ Double-strength: one can of frozen concentrate diluted with one can of water. Grapefruit juice was administered TID for 2 days, and 200 mL together with single dose simvastatin and 30 and 90 minutes following single dose simvastatin on Day 3.
# Single-strength: one can of frozen concentrate diluted with 3 cans of water. Grapefruit juice was administered with breakfast for 3 days, and simvastatin was administered in the evening on Day 3.

VYTORIN is effective in men and women with hyperlipidemia. Experience in non-Caucasians is limited and does not permit a precise estimate of the magnitude of the effects of VYTORIN.

Five multicenter, double-blind studies conducted with either VYTORIN or coadministered ezetimibe and simvastatin equivalent to VYTORIN in patients with primary hyperlipidemia are reported: two were comparisons with simvastatin, two were comparisons with atorvastatin, and one was a comparison with rosuvastatin.

In a multicenter, double-blind, placebo-controlled, 12-week trial, 1528 hyperlipidemic patients were randomized to one of ten treatment groups: placebo, ezetimibe (10 mg), simvastatin (10 mg, 20 mg, 40 mg, or 80 mg), or VYTORIN (10/10, 10/20, 10/40, or 10/80).

When patients receiving VYTORIN were compared to those receiving all doses of simvastatin, VYTORIN significantly lowered total-C, LDL-C, Apo B, TG, and non-HDL-C. The effects of VYTORIN on HDL-C were similar to the effects seen with simvastatin. Further analysis showed VYTORIN

significantly increased HDL-C compared with placebo. (See Table 7.) The lipid response to VYTORIN was similar in patients with TG levels greater than or less than 200 mg/dL. [See table 7 at top of next page]

In a multicenter, double-blind, controlled, 23-week study, 710 patients with known CHD or CHD risk equivalents, as defined by the NCEP ATP III guidelines, and an LDL-C ≥130 mg/dL were randomized to one of four treatment groups: coadministered ezetimibe and simvastatin equivalent to VYTORIN (10/10, 10/20, and 10/40) or simvastatin 20 mg. Patients not reaching an LDL-C <100 mg/dL had their simvastatin dose titrated at 6-week intervals to a maximal dose of 80 mg.

At Week 5, the LDL-C reductions with VYTORIN 10/10, 10/20, or 10/40 were significantly larger than with simvastatin 20 mg (see Table 8).

[See table 8 on next page]

In a multicenter, double-blind, 6-week study, 1902 patients with primary hyperlipidemia, who had not met their NCEP

Table 7: Response to VYTORIN in Patients with Primary Hyperlipidemia (Mean* % Change from Untreated Baseline[†])

Treatment (Daily Dose)	N	Total-C	LDL-C	Apo B	HDL-C	TG*	Non-HDL-C
Pooled data (All VYTORIN doses)[‡]	609	-38	-53	-42	+7	-24	-49
Pooled data (All simvastatin doses)[‡]	622	-28	-39	-32	+7	-21	-36
Ezetimibe 10 mg	149	-13	-19	-15	+5	-11	-18
Placebo	148	-1	-2	0	0	-2	-2
VYTORIN by dose							
10/10	152	-31	-45	-35	+8	-23	-41
10/20	156	-36	-52	-41	+10	-24	-47
10/40	147	-39	-55	-44	+6	-23	-51
10/80	154	-43	-60	-49	+6	-31	-56
Simvastatin by dose							
10 mg	158	-23	-33	-26	+5	-17	-30
20 mg	150	-24	-34	-28	+7	-18	-32
40 mg	156	-29	-41	-33	+8	-21	-38
80 mg	158	-35	-49	-39	+7	-27	-45

* For triglycerides, median % change from baseline
† Baseline - on no lipid-lowering drug
‡ VYTORIN doses pooled (10/10-10/80) significantly reduced total-C, LDL-C, Apo B, TG, and non-HDL-C compared to simvastatin and significantly increased HDL-C compared to placebo.

Table 8: Response to VYTORIN after 5 Weeks in Patients with CHD or CHD Risk Equivalents and an LDL-C ≥130 mg/dL

	Simvastatin 20 mg	VYTORIN 10/10	VYTORIN 10/20	VYTORIN 10/40
N	253	251	109	97
Mean baseline LDL-C	174	165	167	171
Percent change LDL-C	-38	-47	-53	-59

Table 9: Response to VYTORIN and Atorvastatin in Patients with Primary Hyperlipidemia (Mean* % Change from Untreated Baseline[†])

Treatment (Daily Dose)	N	Total-C[‡]	LDL-C[‡]	Apo B[‡]	HDL-C	TG*	Non-HDL-C[‡]
VYTORIN by dose							
10/10	230	-34[§]	-47[§]	-37[§]	+8	-26	-43[§]
10/20	233	-37[§]	-51[§]	-40[§]	+7	-25	-46[§]
10/40	236	-41[§]	-57[§]	-46[§]	+9[§]	-27	-52[§]
10/80	224	-43[§]	-59[§]	-48[§]	+8[§]	-31	-54[§]
Atorvastatin by dose							
10 mg	235	-27	-36	-31	+7	-21	-34
20 mg	230	-32	-44	-37	+5	-25	-41
40 mg	232	-36	-48	-40	+4	-24	-45
80 mg	230	-40	-53	-44	+1	-32	-50

* For triglycerides, median % change from baseline
† Baseline - on no lipid-lowering drug
‡ VYTORIN doses pooled (10/10-10/80) provided significantly greater reductions in total-C, LDL-C, Apo B, and non-HDL-C compared to atorvastatin doses pooled (10-80)
§ p<0.05 for difference with atorvastatin at equal mg doses of the simvastatin component

ATP III target LDL-C goal, were randomized to one of eight treatment groups: VYTORIN (10/10, 10/20, 10/40, or 10/80) or atorvastatin (10 mg, 20 mg, 40 mg, or 80 mg).
Across the dosage range, when patients receiving VYTORIN were compared to those receiving milligram-equivalent statin doses of atorvastatin, VYTORIN lowered total-C, LDL-C, Apo B, and non-HDL-C significantly more than atorvastatin. Only the 10/40 mg and 10/80 mg VYTORIN doses increased HDL-C significantly more than the corresponding milligram-equivalent statin dose of atorvastatin. The effects of VYTORIN on TG were similar to the effects seen with atorvastatin. (See Table 9.)
[See table 9 above]

In a multicenter, double-blind, 24-week, forced-titration study, 788 patients with primary hyperlipidemia, who had not met their NCEP ATP III target LDL-C goal, were randomized to receive coadministered ezetimibe and simvastatin equivalent to VYTORIN (10/10 and 10/20) or atorvastatin 10 mg. For all three treatment groups, the dose of the statin was titrated at 6-week intervals to 80 mg. At each pre-specified dose comparison, VYTORIN lowered LDL-C to a greater degree than atorvastatin (see Table 10).
[See table 10 at top of next page]
In a multicenter, double-blind, 6-week study, 2959 patients with primary hyperlipidemia, who had not met their NCEP

ATP III target LDL-C goal, were randomized to one of six treatment groups: VYTORIN (10/20, 10/40, or 10/80) or rosuvastatin (10 mg, 20 mg, or 40 mg).
The effects of VYTORIN and rosuvastatin on total-C, LDL-C, Apo B, TG, non-HDL-C and HDL-C are shown in Table 11.
[See table 11 on next page]
In a multicenter, double-blind, 24-week trial, 214 patients with type 2 diabetes mellitus treated with thiazolidinediones (rosiglitazone or pioglitazone) for a minimum of 3 months and simvastatin 20 mg for a minimum of 6 weeks were randomized to receive either simvastatin 40 mg or the coadministered active ingredients equivalent to VYTORIN 10/20. The median LDL-C and HbA1c levels at baseline were 89 mg/dL and 7.1%, respectively.
VYTORIN 10/20 was significantly more effective than doubling the dose of simvastatin to 40 mg. The median percent changes from baseline for VYTORIN vs. simvastatin were: LDL-C -25% and -5%; total-C -16% and -5%; Apo B -19% and -5%; and non-HDL-C -23% and -5%. Results for HDL-C and TG between the two treatment groups were not significantly different.
Ezetimibe
In two multicenter, double-blind, placebo-controlled, 12-week studies in 1719 patients with primary hyperlipidemia, ezetimibe significantly lowered total-C (-13%), LDL-C (-19%), Apo B (-14%), and TG (-8%), and increased HDL-C (+3%) compared to placebo. Reduction in LDL-C was consistent across age, sex, and baseline LDL-C.
Simvastatin
In two large, placebo-controlled clinical trials, the Scandinavian Simvastatin Survival Study (N=4,444 patients) and the Heart Protection Study (N=20,536 patients), the effects of treatment with simvastatin were assessed in patients at high risk of coronary events because of existing coronary heart disease, diabetes, peripheral vessel disease, history of stroke or other cerebrovascular disease. Simvastatin was proven to reduce: the risk of total mortality by reducing CHD deaths; the risk of non-fatal myocardial infarction and stroke; and the need for coronary and non-coronary revascularization procedures.
No incremental benefit of VYTORIN on cardiovascular morbidity and mortality over and above that demonstrated for simvastatin has been established.
14.2 Homozygous Familial Hypercholesterolemia (HoFH)
A double-blind, randomized, 12-week study was performed in patients with a clinical and/or genotypic diagnosis of HoFH. Data were analyzed from a subgroup of patients (n=14) receiving simvastatin 40 mg at baseline. Increasing the dose of simvastatin from 40 to 80 mg (n=5) produced a reduction of LDL-C of 13% from baseline on simvastatin 40 mg. Coadministered ezetimibe and simvastatin equivalent to VYTORIN (10/40 and 10/80 pooled, n=9), produced a reduction of LDL-C of 23% from baseline on simvastatin 40 mg. In those patients coadministered ezetimibe and simvastatin equivalent to VYTORIN (10/80, n=5), a reduction of LDL-C of 29% from baseline on simvastatin 40 mg was produced.

16 HOW SUPPLIED/STORAGE AND HANDLING
No. 3873—Tablets VYTORIN 10/10 are white to off-white capsule-shaped tablets with code "311" on one side.
They are supplied as follows:
NDC 66582-311-31 bottles of 30
NDC 66582-311-54 bottles of 90
NDC 66582-311-82 bottles of 1000 (If repackaged in blisters, then opaque or light-resistant blisters should be used.)
NDC 66582-311-87 bottles of 10,000 (If repackaged in blisters, then opaque or light-resistant blisters should be used.)
NDC 66582-311-28 unit dose packages of 100.
No. 3874—Tablets VYTORIN 10/20 are white to off-white capsule-shaped tablets with code "312" on one side.
They are supplied as follows:
NDC 66582-312-31 bottles of 30
NDC 66582-312-54 bottles of 90
NDC 66582-312-82 bottles of 1000 (If repackaged in blisters, then opaque or light-resistant blisters should be used.)
NDC 66582-312-87 bottles of 10,000 (If repackaged in blisters, then opaque or light-resistant blisters should be used.)
NDC 66582-312-28 unit dose packages of 100.
No. 3875—Tablets VYTORIN 10/40 are white to off-white capsule-shaped tablets with code "313" on one side.
They are supplied as follows:
NDC 66582-313-31 bottles of 30
NDC 66582-313-54 bottles of 90
NDC 66582-313-74 bottles of 500 (If repackaged in blisters, then opaque or light-resistant blisters should be used.)
NDC 66582-313-86 bottles of 5000 (If repackaged in blisters, then opaque or light-resistant blisters should be used.)
NDC 66582-313-52 unit dose packages of 50.

Table 10: Response to VYTORIN and Atorvastatin in Patients with Primary Hyperlipidemia (Mean* % Change from Untreated Baseline[†])

Treatment	N	Total-C	LDL-C	Apo B	HDL-C	TG*	Non-HDL-C
Week 6							
Atorvastatin 10 mg[‡]	262	-28	-37	-32	+5	-23	-35
VYTORIN 10/10[§]	263	-34[¶]	-46[¶]	-38[¶]	+8[¶]	-26	-43[¶]
VYTORIN 10/20[#]	263	-36[¶]	-50[¶]	-41[¶]	+10[¶]	-25	-46[¶]
Week 12							
Atorvastatin 20 mg	246	-33	-44	-38	+7	-28	-42
VYTORIN 10/20	250	-37[¶]	-50[¶]	-41[¶]	+9	-28	-46[¶]
VYTORIN 10/40	252	-39[¶]	-54[¶]	-45[¶]	+12[¶]	-31	-50[¶]
Week 18							
Atorvastatin 40 mg	237	-37	-49	-42	+8	-31	-47
VYTORIN 10/40[Þ]	482	-40[¶]	-56[¶]	-45[¶]	+11[¶]	-32	-52[¶]
Week 24							
Atorvastatin 80 mg	228	-40	-53	-45	+6	-35	-50
VYTORIN 10/80[Þ]	459	-43[¶]	-59[¶]	-49[¶]	+12[¶]	-35	-55[¶]

* For triglycerides, median % change from baseline
† Baseline - on no lipid-lowering drug
‡ Atorvastatin: 10 mg start dose titrated to 20 mg, 40 mg, and 80 mg through Weeks 6, 12, 18, and 24
§ VYTORIN: 10/10 start dose titrated to 10/20, 10/40, and 10/80 through Weeks 6, 12, 18, and 24
¶ p≤0.05 for difference with atorvastatin in the specified week
# VYTORIN: 10/20 start dose titrated to 10/40, 10/40, and 10/80 through Weeks 6, 12, 18, and 24
Þ Data pooled for common doses of VYTORIN at Weeks 18 and 24.

Table 11: Response to VYTORIN and Rosuvastatin in Patients with Primary Hyperlipidemia (Mean* % Change from Untreated Baseline[†])

Treatment (Daily Dose)	N	Total-C[‡]	LDL-C[‡]	Apo B[‡]	HDL-C	TG*	Non-HDL-C[‡]
VYTORIN by dose							
10/20	476	-37[§]	-52[§]	-42[§]	+7	-23[§]	-47[§]
10/40	477	-39[¶]	-55[¶]	-44[¶]	+8	-27	-50[¶]
10/80	474	-44[#]	-61[#]	-50[#]	+8	-30[#]	-56[#]
Rosuvastatin by dose							
10 mg	475	-32	-46	-37	+7	-20	-42
20 mg	478	-37	-52	-43	+8	-26	-48
40 mg	475	-41	-57	-47	+8	-28	-52

* For triglycerides, median % change from baseline
† Baseline - on no lipid-lowering drug
‡ VYTORIN doses pooled (10/20-10/80) provided significantly greater reductions in total-C, LDL-C, Apo B, and non-HDL-C compared to rosuvastatin doses pooled (10-40 mg).
§ p<0.05 vs. rosuvastatin 10 mg
¶ p<0.05 vs. rosuvastatin 20 mg
# p<0.05 vs. rosuvastatin 40 mg

No. 3876—Tablets VYTORIN 10/80 are white to off-white capsule-shaped tablets with code "315" on one side.
They are supplied as follows:
NDC 66582-315-31 bottles of 30
NDC 66582-315-54 bottles of 90
NDC 66582-315-74 bottles of 500 (If repackaged in blisters, then opaque or light-resistant blisters should be used.)
NDC 66582-315-66 bottles of 2500 (If repackaged in blisters, then opaque or light-resistant blisters should be used.)
NDC 66582-315-52 unit dose packages of 50.
Storage
Store at 20-25°C (68-77°F). [See USP Controlled Room Temperature.] Keep container tightly closed.
Storage of 10,000, 5000, and 2500 count bottles
Store bottle of 10,000 VYTORIN 10/10 and 10/20, 5000 VYTORIN 10/40, and 2500 VYTORIN 10/80 capsule-shaped tablets at 20-25°C (68-77°F). [See USP Controlled Room Temperature.] Store in original container until time of use. When product container is subdivided, repackage into a tightly-closed, light-resistant container. Entire contents must be repackaged immediately upon opening.

17   PATIENT COUNSELING INFORMATION
[See FDA-Approved Patient Labeling (17.5).]
Patients should be advised to adhere to their National Cholesterol Education Program (NCEP)-recommended diet, a regular exercise program, and periodic testing of a fasting lipid panel.
Patients should be advised about substances they should not take concomitantly with VYTORIN [see Warnings and Precautions (5.1)]. Patients should also be advised to inform other physicians prescribing a new medication that they are taking VYTORIN.
17.1   Muscle Pain
All patients starting therapy with VYTORIN should be advised of the risk of myopathy and told to report promptly any unexplained muscle pain, tenderness or weakness. The risk of this occurring is increased when taking certain types of medication or consuming larger quantities of grapefruit juice. They should discuss all medication, both prescription and over the counter, with their healthcare professional.
17.2   Liver Enzymes
It is recommended that liver function tests be performed before the initiation of VYTORIN, and thereafter when clini-

cally indicated. Patients titrated to the 10/80-mg dose should receive an additional test prior to titration, 3 months after titration to the 10/80-mg dose, and periodically thereafter (e.g., semiannually) for the first year of treatment.
17.3   Pregnancy
Women of childbearing age should be advised to use an effective method of birth control to prevent pregnancy while using VYTORIN. Discuss future pregnancy plans with your patients, and discuss when to stop taking VYTORIN if they are trying to conceive. Patients should be advised that if they become pregnant they should stop taking VYTORIN and call their healthcare professional.
17.4   Breast-feeding
Women who are breast-feeding should be advised to not use VYTORIN. Patients who have a lipid disorder and are breast-feeding should be advised to discuss the options with their healthcare professional.
17.5   FDA-Approved Patient Labeling
Issued May 2010
9619517
Manufactured for:
MERCK/Schering-Plough Pharmaceuticals
North Wales, PA 19454, USA
By:
MSD Technology Singapore Pte. Ltd.
Singapore 637766
Or
Merck Sharp & Dohme (Italia) S.p.A.
Via Emilia, 21
27100–Pavia, Italy
Or
Merck Sharp & Dohme Ltd.
Cramlington, Northumberland, UK NE23 3JU
Or
Jointly manufactured by:
Merck Sharp & Dohme (Italia) S.p.A.
Via Emilia, 21
27100–Pavia, Italy
and
MSD Technology Singapore Pte. Ltd.
Singapore 637766
U.S. Patent Nos. 5,846,966 and RE37,721
VYTORIN® (ezetimibe/simvastatin) Tablets
Patient Information about VYTORIN (VI-tor-in)
Generic name: ezetimibe/simvastatin tablets
Read this information carefully before you start taking VYTORIN. Review this information each time you refill your prescription for VYTORIN as there may be new information. This information does not take the place of talking with your doctor about your medical condition or your treatment. If you have any questions about VYTORIN, ask your doctor. Only your doctor can determine if VYTORIN is right for you.
What is VYTORIN?
VYTORIN contains two cholesterol-lowering medications, ezetimibe and simvastatin, available as a tablet in four strengths:
• VYTORIN 10/10 (ezetimibe 10 mg/simvastatin 10 mg)
• VYTORIN 10/20 (ezetimibe 10 mg/simvastatin 20 mg)
• VYTORIN 10/40 (ezetimibe 10 mg/simvastatin 40 mg)
• VYTORIN 10/80 (ezetimibe 10 mg/simvastatin 80 mg)
VYTORIN is a medicine used to lower levels of total cholesterol, LDL (bad) cholesterol, and fatty substances called triglycerides in the blood. In addition, VYTORIN raises levels of HDL (good) cholesterol. VYTORIN is for patients who cannot control their cholesterol levels by diet and exercise alone. You should stay on a cholesterol-lowering diet while taking this medicine.
VYTORIN works to reduce your cholesterol in two ways. It reduces the cholesterol absorbed in your digestive tract, as well as the cholesterol your body makes by itself. VYTORIN does not help you lose weight. VYTORIN has not been shown to reduce heart attacks or strokes more than simvastatin alone.
For more information about cholesterol, see the section called "What should I know about high cholesterol?"
Who should not take VYTORIN?
Do not take VYTORIN:
• If you are allergic to ezetimibe or simvastatin, the active ingredients in VYTORIN, or to the inactive ingredients. For a list of inactive ingredients, see the "Inactive ingredients" section at the end of this information sheet.
• If you have active liver disease or repeated blood tests indicating possible liver problems.
• If you are pregnant, or think you may be pregnant, or planning to become pregnant or breast-feeding.
• If you are a woman of childbearing age, you should use an effective method of birth control to prevent pregnancy while using VYTORIN.
VYTORIN has not been studied in children under 10 years of age.

What should I tell my doctor before and while taking VYTORIN?

Tell your doctor right away if you experience unexplained muscle pain, tenderness, or weakness. This is because on rare occasions, muscle problems can be serious, including muscle breakdown resulting in kidney damage.

The risk of muscle breakdown is greater at higher doses of VYTORIN.

The risk of muscle breakdown is greater in patients with kidney problems.

Taking VYTORIN with certain substances can increase the risk of muscle problems. It is particularly important to tell your doctor if you are taking any of the following:

- cyclosporine
- danazol
- antifungal agents (such as itraconazole or ketoconazole)
- fibric acid derivatives (such as gemfibrozil, bezafibrate, or fenofibrate)
- the antibiotics erythromycin, clarithromycin, and telithromycin
- HIV protease inhibitors (such as indinavir, nelfinavir, ritonavir, and saquinavir)
- the antidepressant nefazodone
- amiodarone (a drug used to treat an irregular heartbeat)
- verapamil or diltiazem (a drug used to treat high blood pressure, chest pain associated with heart disease, or other heart conditions)
- large quantities of grapefruit juice (>1 quart daily)
- large doses (≥1 g/day) of niacin or nicotinic acid

Tell your doctor if you are taking niacin or a niacin-containing product, as this may increase your risk of muscle problems, especially if you are Chinese.

It is also important to tell your doctor if you are taking coumarin anticoagulants (drugs that prevent blood clots, such as warfarin).

Tell your doctor about any prescription and nonprescription medicines you are taking or plan to take, including natural or herbal remedies.

Tell your doctor about all your medical conditions including allergies.

Tell your doctor if you:

- drink substantial quantities of alcohol or ever had liver problems. VYTORIN may not be right for you.
- are pregnant or plan to become pregnant. Do not use VYTORIN if you are pregnant, trying to become pregnant or suspect that you are pregnant. If you become pregnant while taking VYTORIN, stop taking it and contact your doctor immediately.
- are breast-feeding. Do not use VYTORIN if you are breast-feeding.

Tell other doctors prescribing a new medication that you are taking VYTORIN.

How should I take VYTORIN?

Your doctor has prescribed your dose of VYTORIN. The available doses of VYTORIN are 10/10, 10/20, 10/40, and 10/80. The usual daily starting dose is VYTORIN 10/20.

- Take VYTORIN once a day, in the evening, with or without food.
- Try to take VYTORIN as prescribed. If you miss a dose, do not take an extra dose. Just resume your usual schedule.
- Continue to follow a cholesterol-lowering diet while taking VYTORIN. Ask your doctor if you need diet information.
- Keep taking VYTORIN unless your doctor tells you to stop. If you stop taking VYTORIN, your cholesterol may rise again.

What should I do in case of an overdose?

Contact your doctor immediately.

What are the possible side effects of VYTORIN?

See your doctor regularly to check your cholesterol level and to check for side effects. Your doctor may do blood tests to check your liver before you start taking VYTORIN and during treatment.

In clinical studies patients reported the following common side effects while taking VYTORIN: headache, muscle pain, and diarrhea (see What should I tell my doctor before and while taking VYTORIN?).

The following side effects have been reported in general use with VYTORIN or with ezetimibe or simvastatin tablets (tablets that contain the active ingredients of VYTORIN):

- allergic reactions including swelling of the face, lips, tongue, and/or throat that may cause difficulty in breathing or swallowing (which may require treatment right away), rash, hives; raised red rash, sometimes with target-shaped lesions; joint pain; muscle pain; alterations in some laboratory blood tests; liver problems (sometimes serious); inflammation of the pancreas; nausea; dizziness; tingling sensation; depression; gallstones; inflammation of the gallbladder; trouble sleeping; poor memory; erectile dysfunction; breathing problems including persistent cough and/or shortness of breath or fever.

Tell your doctor if you are having these or any other medical problems while on VYTORIN. This is not a complete list of side effects. For a complete list, ask your doctor or pharmacist.

What should I know about high cholesterol?

Cholesterol is a type of fat found in your blood. Cholesterol comes from two sources. It is produced by your body and it comes from the food you eat. Your total cholesterol is made up of both LDL and HDL cholesterol.

LDL cholesterol is called "bad" cholesterol because it can build up in the wall of your arteries and form plaque. Over time, plaque build-up can cause a narrowing of the arteries. This narrowing can slow or block blood flow to your heart, brain, and other organs. High LDL cholesterol is a major cause of heart disease and one of the causes for stroke.

HDL cholesterol is called "good" cholesterol because it keeps the bad cholesterol from building up in the arteries.

Triglycerides also are fats found in your body.

General Information about VYTORIN

Medicines are sometimes prescribed for conditions that are not mentioned in patient information leaflets. Do not use VYTORIN for a condition for which it was not prescribed. Do not give VYTORIN to other people, even if they have the same condition you have. It may harm them.

This summarizes the most important information about VYTORIN. If you would like more information, talk with your doctor. You can ask your pharmacist or doctor for information about VYTORIN that is written for health professionals. For additional information, visit the following web site: vytorin.com.

Inactive ingredients:

Butylated hydroxyanisole NF, citric acid monohydrate USP, croscarmellose sodium NF, hypromellose USP, lactose monohydrate NF, magnesium stearate NF, microcrystalline cellulose NF, and propyl gallate NF.

Issued May 2010

9619517

Manufactured for:

Merck/Schering-Plough Pharmaceuticals

North Wales, PA 19454, USA

By:

MSD Technology Singapore Pte. Ltd.

Singapore 637766

Or

Merck Sharp & Dohme (Italia) S.p.A.

Via Emilia, 21

27100–Pavia, Italy

Or

Merck Sharp & Dohme Ltd.

Cramlington, Northumberland, UK NE23 3JU

Or

Jointly manufactured by:

Merck Sharp & Dohme (Italia) S.p.A.

Via Emilia, 21

27100–Pavia, Italy

and

MSD Technology Singapore Pte. Ltd.

Singapore 637766

U.S. Patent Nos. 5,846,966 and RE37,721

Shown in Product Identification Guide, page 314

ZEMURON®
(rocuronium bromide)
Injection
PRODUCT INFORMATION

℞

HIGHLIGHTS OF PRESCRIBING INFORMATION

These highlights do not include all the information needed to use ZEMURON safely and effectively. See full prescribing information for ZEMURON.

ZEMURON (rocuronium bromide) injection solution for intravenous use

Initial U.S. Approval: 1994

———————RECENT MAJOR CHANGES———————

Dosage and Administration, Dosage in Specific Populations (2.5)	8/2008
Warnings and Precautions,	
Residual Paralysis (5.4)	8/2008
Long-term Use in an Intensive Care Unit (5.5)	8/2008
QT Interval Prolongation (5.8)	8/2008

———————INDICATIONS AND USAGE———————

ZEMURON is a nondepolarizing neuromuscular blocking agent indicated as an adjunct to general anesthesia to facilitate both rapid sequence and routine tracheal intubation, and to provide skeletal muscle relaxation during surgery or mechanical ventilation. (1)

———————DOSAGE AND ADMINISTRATION———————

To be administered only by experienced clinicians or adequately trained individuals supervised by an experienced clinician familiar with the use, actions, characteristics, and complications of neuromuscular blocking agents. (2)

- Individualize the dose for each patient. (2)
- Peripheral nerve stimulator recommended for determination of drug response and need for additional doses, and to evaluate recovery. (2)
- Tracheal intubation: Recommended initial dose is 0.6 mg/kg. (2.1)
- Rapid sequence intubation: 0.6 to 1.2 mg/kg. (2.2)
- Maintenance doses: Guided by response to prior dose, not administered until recovery is evident. (2.3)
- Continuous infusion: Initial rate of 10 to 12 mcg/kg/min. Start only after early evidence of spontaneous recovery from an intubating dose. (2.4)

———————DOSAGE FORMS AND STRENGTHS———————

- 5 mL multiple dose vials containing 50 mg rocuronium bromide injection (10 mg/mL). (3)
- 10 mL multiple dose vials containing 100 mg rocuronium bromide injection (10 mg/mL). (3)

———————CONTRAINDICATIONS———————

- Hypersensitivity (e.g., anaphylaxis) to rocuronium bromide or other neuromuscular blocking agents. (4)

———————WARNINGS AND PRECAUTIONS———————

- Appropriate Administration and Monitoring: Use only if facilities for intubation, mechanical ventilation, oxygen therapy, and an antagonist are immediately available. (5.1)
- Anaphylaxis: Severe anaphylaxis has been reported. Consider cross-reactivity among neuromuscular blocking agents. (5.2)
- Need for Adequate Anesthesia: Must be accompanied by adequate anesthesia or sedation. (5.3)
- Residual Paralysis: Consider using a reversal agent in cases where residual paralysis is more likely to occur. (5.4)

———————ADVERSE REACTIONS———————

Most common adverse reactions (2%) are transient hypotension and hypertension. (6.1)

To report SUSPECTED ADVERSE REACTIONS, contact Schering-Plough at 1-800-526-4099 or FDA at 1-800-FDA-1088 or www.fda.gov/medwatch.

———————DRUG INTERACTIONS———————

- Succinylcholine: Use before succinylcholine has not been studied. (7.11)
- Nondepolarizing muscle relaxants: Interactions have been observed. (7.7)
- Enhanced ZEMURON activity possible: Inhalation anesthetics (7.3), certain antibiotics (7.1), quinidine (7.10), magnesium (7.6), lithium (7.4), local anesthetics (7.5), procainamide (7.8).
- Reduced ZEMURON activity possible: Anticonvulsants. (7.2)

———————USE IN SPECIFIC POPULATIONS———————

- Labor and Delivery: Not recommended for rapid sequence induction in patients undergoing Cesarean section. (8.2)
- Pediatric Use: Onset time and duration will vary with dose, age, and anesthetic technique. Not recommended for rapid sequence intubation in pediatric patients. (8.4)

See 17 for PATIENT COUNSELING INFORMATION and FDA-approved labeling.

Revised: 8/2008

FULL PRESCRIBING INFORMATION: CONTENTS*

TABLE 1: Infusion Rates Using ZEMURON Injection (0.5 mg/mL)*

Patient Weight		Drug Delivery Rate (mcg/kg/min)									
(kg)	(lbs)	4	5	6	7	8	9	10	12	14	16
		Infusion Delivery Rate (mL/hr)									
10	22	4.8	6	7.2	8.4	9.6	10.8	12	14.4	16.8	19.2
15	33	7.2	9	10.8	12.6	14.4	16.2	18	21.6	25.2	28.8
20	44	9.6	12	14.4	16.8	19.2	21.6	24	28.8	33.6	38.4
25	55	12	15	18	21	24	27	30	36	42	48
35	77	16.8	21	25.2	29.4	33.6	37.8	42	50.4	58.8	67.2
50	110	24	30	36	42	48	54	60	72	84	96
60	132	28.8	36	43.2	50.4	57.6	64.8	72	86.4	100.8	115.2
70	154	33.6	42	50.4	58.8	67.2	75.6	84	100.8	117.6	134.4
80	176	38.4	48	57.6	67.2	76.8	86.4	96	115.2	134.4	153.6
90	198	43.2	54	64.8	75.6	86.4	97.2	108	129.6	151.2	172.8
100	220	48	60	72	84	96	108	120	144	168	192

*50 mg ZEMURON in 100 mL solution

TABLE 2: Infusion Rates Using ZEMURON Injection (1 mg/mL)*

Patient Weight		Drug Delivery Rate (mcg/kg/min)									
(kg)	(lbs)	4	5	6	7	8	9	10	12	14	16
		Infusion Delivery Rate (mL/hr)									
10	22	2.4	3	3.6	4.2	4.8	5.4	6	7.2	8.4	9.6
15	33	3.6	4.5	5.4	6.3	7.2	8.1	9	10.8	12.6	14.4
20	44	4.8	6	7.2	8.4	9.6	10.8	12	14.4	16.8	19.2
25	55	6	7.5	9	10.5	12	13.5	15	18	21	24
35	77	8.4	10.5	12.6	14.7	16.8	18.9	21	25.2	29.4	33.6
50	110	12	15	18	21	24	27	30	36	42	48
60	132	14.4	18	21.6	25.2	28.8	32.4	36	43.2	50.4	57.6
70	154	16.8	21	25.2	29.4	33.6	37.8	42	50.4	58.8	67.2
80	176	19.2	24	28.8	33.6	38.4	43.2	48	57.6	67.2	76.8
90	198	21.6	27	32.4	37.8	43.2	48.6	54	64.8	75.6	86.4
100	220	24	30	36	42	48	54	60	72	84	96

*100 mg ZEMURON in 100 mL solution

FULL PRESCRIBING INFORMATION

1 INDICATIONS AND USAGE

ZEMURON® (rocuronium bromide) Injection is indicated for inpatients and outpatients as an adjunct to general anesthesia to facilitate both rapid sequence and routine tracheal intubation, and to provide skeletal muscle relaxation during surgery or mechanical ventilation.

2 DOSAGE AND ADMINISTRATION

ZEMURON is for intravenous use only. **This drug should only be administered by experienced clinicians or trained individuals supervised by an experienced clinician familiar with the use, actions, characteristics and complications of neuromuscular blocking agents. Doses of ZEMURON injection should be individualized and a peripheral nerve stimulator should be used to monitor drug effect, need for additional doses, adequacy of spontaneous recovery or antagonism, and to decrease the complications of overdosage if additional doses are administered.**

The dosage information which follows is derived from studies based upon units of drug per unit of body weight. It is intended to serve as an initial guide to clinicians familiar with other neuromuscular blocking agents to acquire experience with ZEMURON.

In patients in whom potentiation of, or resistance to, neuromuscular block is anticipated, a dose adjustment should be considered [see Dosage and Administration (2.5), Warnings and Precautions (5.9, 5.12), Drug Interactions (7.2, 7.3, 7.4, 7.5, 7.6, 7.8, 7.10), and Use in Specific Populations (8.6)].

2.1 Dose for Tracheal Intubation

The recommended initial dose of ZEMURON, regardless of anesthetic technique, is 0.6 mg/kg. Neuromuscular block sufficient for intubation (80% block or greater) is attained in a median (range) time of 1 (0.4-6) minute(s) and most patients have intubation completed within 2 minutes. Maximum blockade is achieved in most patients in less than 3 minutes. This dose may be expected to provide 31 (15-85) minutes of clinical relaxation under opioid/nitrous oxide/oxygen anesthesia. Under halothane, isoflurane, and enflurane anesthesia, some extension of the period of clinical relaxation should be expected [see Drug Interactions (7.3)].

A lower dose of ZEMURON (0.45 mg/kg) may be used. Neuromuscular block sufficient for intubation (80% block or greater) is attained in a median (range) time of 1.3 (0.8-6.2) minute(s) and most patients have intubation completed within 2 minutes. Maximum blockade is achieved in most patients in less than 4 minutes. This dose may be expected to provide 22 (12-31) minutes of clinical relaxation under opioid/nitrous oxide/oxygen anesthesia. Patients receiving this low dose of 0.45 mg/kg who achieve less than 90% block (about 16% of these patients) may have a more rapid time to 25% recovery, 12 to 15 minutes.

A large bolus dose of 0.9 or 1.2 mg/kg can be administered under opioid/nitrous oxide/oxygen anesthesia without adverse effects to the cardiovascular system [see Clinical Pharmacology (12.2)].

2.2 Rapid Sequence Intubation

In appropriately premedicated and adequately anesthetized patients, ZEMURON 0.6 to 1.2 mg/kg will provide excellent or good intubating conditions in most patients in less than 2 minutes [see Clinical Studies (14.1)].

2.3 Maintenance Dosing

Maintenance doses of 0.1, 0.15, and 0.2 mg/kg ZEMURON, administered at 25% recovery of control T_1 (defined as 3 twitches of train-of-four), provide a median (range) of 12 (2-31), 17 (6-50) and 24 (7-69) minutes of clinical duration under opioid/nitrous oxide/oxygen anesthesia [see Clinical Pharmacology (12.2)]. In all cases, dosing should be guided based on the clinical duration following initial dose or prior maintenance dose and not administered until recovery of neuromuscular function is evident. A clinically insignificant cumulation of effect with repetitive maintenance dosing has been observed [see Clinical Pharmacology (12.2)].

2.4 Use by Continuous Infusion

Infusion at an initial rate of 10 to 12 mcg/kg/min of ZEMURON should be initiated only after early evidence of spontaneous recovery from an intubating dose. Due to rapid redistribution [see Clinical Pharmacology (12.3)] and the associated rapid spontaneous recovery, initiation of the infusion after substantial return of neuromuscular function (more than 10% of control T_1) may necessitate additional bolus doses to maintain adequate block for surgery.

Upon reaching the desired level of neuromuscular block, the infusion of ZEMURON must be individualized for each patient. The rate of administration should be adjusted according to the patient's twitch response as monitored with the use of a peripheral nerve stimulator. In clinical trials, infusion rates have ranged from 4 to 16 mcg/kg/min.

Inhalation anesthetics, particularly enflurane and isoflurane, may enhance the neuromuscular blocking action of nondepolarizing muscle relaxants. In the presence of steady-state concentrations of enflurane or isoflurane, it may be necessary to reduce the rate of infusion by 30% to 50%, at 45 to 60 minutes after the intubating dose.

Spontaneous recovery and reversal of neuromuscular blockade following discontinuation of ZEMURON infusion may be expected to proceed at rates comparable to that following comparable total doses administered by repetitive bolus injections [see Clinical Pharmacology (12.2)].

Infusion solutions of ZEMURON can be prepared by mixing ZEMURON with an appropriate infusion solution such as 5% glucose in water or lactated Ringers [see Dosage and Administration (2.6)]. These infusion solutions should be used within 24 hours of mixing. Unused portions of infusion solutions should be discarded.

Infusion rates of ZEMURON can be individualized for each patient using the following tables for three different concentrations of ZEMURON solution as guidelines:

[See table 1 above]
[See table 2 above]
[See table 3 at top of next page]

2.5 Dosage in Specific Populations

Pediatric Patients: The recommended initial intubation dose of ZEMURON is 0.6 mg/kg; however, a lower dose of 0.45 mg/kg may be used depending on anesthetic technique and the age of the patient.

For sevoflurane (induction) ZEMURON doses of 0.45 mg/kg and 0.6 mg/kg in general produce excellent to good intubat-

TABLE 3: Infusion Rates Using ZEMURON Injection (5 mg/mL)*

Patient Weight		Drug Delivery Rate (mcg/kg/min)									
(kg)	(lbs)	4	5	6	7	8	9	10	12	14	16
		Infusion Delivery Rate (mL/hr)									
10	22	0.5	0.6	0.7	0.8	1	1.1	1.2	1.4	1.7	1.9
15	33	0.7	0.9	1.1	1.3	1.4	1.6	1.8	2.2	2.5	2.9
20	44	1	1.2	1.4	1.7	1.9	2.2	2.4	2.9	3.4	3.8
25	55	1.2	1.5	1.8	2.1	2.4	2.7	3	3.6	4.2	4.8
35	77	1.7	2.1	2.5	2.9	3.4	3.8	4.2	5	5.9	6.7
50	110	2.4	3	3.6	4.2	4.8	5.4	6	7.2	8.4	9.6
60	132	2.9	3.6	4.3	5	5.8	6.5	7.2	8.6	10.1	11.5
70	154	3.4	4.2	5	5.9	6.7	7.6	8.4	10.1	11.8	13.4
80	176	3.8	4.8	5.8	6.7	7.7	8.6	9.6	11.5	13.4	15.4
90	198	4.3	5.4	6.5	7.6	8.6	9.7	10.8	13	15.1	17.3
100	220	4.8	6	7.2	8.4	9.6	10.8	12	14.4	16.8	19.2

*500 mg ZEMURON in 100 mL solution

ing conditions within 75 seconds. When halothane is used, a 0.6 mg/kg dose of ZEMURON resulted in excellent to good intubating conditions within 60 seconds.

The time to maximum block for an intubating dose was shortest in infants (28 days up to 3 months) and longest in neonates (birth to less than 28 days). The duration of clinical relaxation following an intubating dose is shortest in children (greater than 2 years up to 11 years) and longest in infants.

When sevoflurane is used for induction and isoflurane/nitrous oxide for maintenance of general anesthesia, maintenance dosing of ZEMURON can be administered as bolus doses of 0.15 mg/kg at reappearance of T_3 in all pediatric age groups. Maintenance dosing can also be administered at the reappearance of T_2 at a rate of 7-10 mcg/kg/min, with the lowest dose requirement for neonates (birth to less than 28 days) and the highest dose requirement for children (greater than 2 years up to 11 years).

When halothane is used for general anesthesia, patients ranging from 3 months old through adolescence can be administered ZEMURON maintenance doses of 0.075 to 0.125 mg/kg upon return of T_1 to 0.25% to provide clinical relaxation for 7 to 10 minutes. Alternatively, a continuous infusion of ZEMURON initiated at a rate of 12 mcg/kg/min upon return of T_1 to 10% (one twitch present in train-of-four) may also be used to maintain neuromuscular blockade in pediatric patients.

Additional information for administration to pediatric patients of all age groups is presented elsewhere in the label [see Clinical Pharmacology (12.2)].

The infusion of ZEMURON must be individualized for each patient. The rate of administration should be adjusted according to the patient's twitch response as monitored with the use of a peripheral nerve stimulator. Spontaneous recovery and reversal of neuromuscular blockade following discontinuation of ZEMURON infusion may be expected to proceed at rates comparable to that following similar total exposure to single bolus doses [see Clinical Pharmacology (12.2)].

ZEMURON is not recommended for rapid sequence intubation in pediatric patients.

Geriatric Patients: Geriatric patients (65 years or older) exhibited a slightly prolonged median (range) clinical duration of 46 (22-73), 62 (49-75), and 94 (64-138) minutes under opioid/nitrous oxide/oxygen anesthesia following doses of 0.6, 0.9, and 1.2 mg/kg, respectively. No differences in duration of neuromuscular blockade following maintenance doses of ZEMURON were observed between these subjects and younger subjects, and other reported clinical experience has not identified differences in response between elderly and younger patients, but greater sensitivity of some older individuals cannot be ruled out [see Clinical Pharmacology (12.2, 12.3)].

Patients with Renal or Hepatic Impairment: No differences from patients with normal hepatic and kidney function were observed for onset time at a dose of 0.6 mg/kg ZEMURON. When compared to patients with normal renal and hepatic function, the mean clinical duration is similar in patients with end-stage renal disease undergoing renal transplant, and is about 1.5 times longer in patients with hepatic disease. Patients with renal failure may have a greater varia-

tion in duration of effect [see Use in Specific Populations (8.6, 8.7) and Clinical Pharmacology (12.3)].

Obese Patients: In obese patients, the initial dose of ZEMURON 0.6 mg/kg should be based upon the patient's actual body weight [see Clinical Studies (14.1)].

An analysis across all US controlled clinical studies indicates that the pharmacodynamics of ZEMURON are not different between obese and non-obese patients when dosed based upon their actual body weight.

Patients with Reduced Plasma Cholinesterase Activity: Rocuronium metabolism does not depend on plasma cholinesterase so dosing adjustments are not needed in patients with reduced plasma cholinesterase activity.

Patients with Prolonged Circulation Time: Because higher doses of ZEMURON produce a longer duration of action, the initial dosage should usually not be increased in these patients to reduce onset time; instead, in these situations, when feasible, more time should be allowed for the drug to achieve onset of effect [see Warnings and Precautions (5.7)].

Patients with Drugs or Conditions Causing Potentiation of Neuromuscular Block: The neuromuscular blocking action of ZEMURON is potentiated by isoflurane and enflurane anesthesia. Potentiation is minimal when administration of the recommended dose of ZEMURON occurs prior to the administration of these potent inhalation agents. The median clinical duration of a dose of 0.57 to 0.85 mg/kg was 34, 38, and 42 minutes under opioid/nitrous oxide/oxygen, enflurane and isoflurane maintenance anesthesia, respectively. During 1 to 2 hours of infusion, the infusion rate of ZEMURON required to maintain about 95% block was decreased by as much as 40% under enflurane and isoflurane anesthesia [see Drug Interactions (7.3)].

2.6 Preparation for Administration of ZEMURON

Diluent Compatibility: ZEMURON is compatible in solution with:

0.9% NaCl solution   sterile water for injection
5% glucose in water   lactated Ringers
5% glucose in saline

ZEMURON is compatible in the above solutions at concentrations up to 5 mg/mL for 24 hours at room temperature in plastic bags, glass bottles, and plastic syringe pumps.

Drug Admixture Incompatibility: ZEMURON is physically incompatible when mixed with the following drugs:

amphotericin	hydrocortisone sodium succinate
amoxicillin	insulin
azathioprine	intralipid
cefazolin	ketorolac
cloxacillin	lorazepam
dexamethasone	methohexital
diazepam	methylprednisolone
erythromycin	thiopental
famotidine	trimethoprim
furosemide	vancomycin

If ZEMURON is administered via the same infusion line that is also used for other drugs, it is important that this infusion line is adequately flushed between administration of ZEMURON and drugs for which incompatibility with ZEMURON has been demonstrated or for which compatibility with ZEMURON has not been established.

Infusion solutions should be used within 24 hours of mixing. Unused portions of infusion solutions should be discarded.

ZEMURON should not be mixed with alkaline solutions [see Warnings and Precautions (5.10)].

Visual Inspection: Parenteral drug products should be inspected visually for particulate matter and clarity prior to administration whenever solution and container permit. Do not use solution if particulate matter is present.

3 DOSAGE FORMS AND STRENGTHS

ZEMURON (rocuronium bromide) injection is available as

- 5 mL multiple dose vials containing 50 mg rocuronium bromide injection (10 mg/mL)
- 10 mL multiple dose vials containing 100 mg rocuronium bromide injection (10 mg/mL)

4 CONTRAINDICATIONS

ZEMURON is contraindicated in patients known to have hypersensitivity (e.g., anaphylaxis) to rocuronium bromide or other neuromuscular blocking agents [see Warnings and Precautions (5.2)].

5 WARNINGS AND PRECAUTIONS

5.1 Appropriate Administration and Monitoring

ZEMURON should be administered in carefully adjusted dosages by or under the supervision of experienced clinicians who are familiar with the drug's actions and the possible complications of its use. The drug should not be administered unless facilities for intubation, mechanical ventilation, oxygen therapy, and an antagonist are immediately available. It is recommended that clinicians administering neuromuscular blocking agents such as ZEMURON employ a peripheral nerve stimulator to monitor drug effect, need for additional doses, adequacy of spontaneous recovery or antagonism, and to decrease the complications of overdosage if additional doses are administered.

5.2 Anaphylaxis

Severe anaphylactic reactions to neuromuscular blocking agents, including ZEMURON, have been reported. These reactions have, in some cases (including cases with ZEMURON), been life threatening. Due to the potential severity of these reactions, the necessary precautions, such as the immediate availability of appropriate emergency treatment, should be taken.

5.3 Need for Adequate Anesthesia

ZEMURON has no known effect on consciousness, pain threshold, or cerebration. Therefore, its administration must be accompanied by adequate anesthesia or sedation.

5.4 Residual Paralysis

In order to prevent complications resulting from residual paralysis, it is recommended to extubate only after the patient has recovered sufficiently from neuromuscular block. Other factors which could cause residual paralysis after extubation in the post-operative phase (such as drug interactions or patient condition) should also be considered. If not used as part of standard clinical practice the use of a reversal agent should be considered, especially in those cases where residual paralysis is more likely to occur.

5.5 Long-term Use in an Intensive Care Unit

ZEMURON has not been studied for long-term use in the intensive care unit (ICU). As with other nondepolarizing neuromuscular blocking drugs, apparent tolerance to ZEMURON may develop during chronic administration in the ICU. While the mechanism for development of this resistance is not known, receptor up-regulation may be a contributing factor. **It is strongly recommended that neuromuscular transmission be monitored continuously during administration and recovery with the help of a nerve stimulator. Additional doses of ZEMURON or any other neuromuscular blocking agent should not be given until there is a definite response (one twitch of the train-of-four) to nerve stimulation.** Prolonged paralysis and/or skeletal muscle weakness may be noted during initial attempts to wean from the ventilator patients who have chronically received neuromuscular blocking drugs in the ICU.

Myopathy after long-term administration of other nondepolarizing neuromuscular blocking agents in the ICU alone or in combination with corticosteroid therapy has been reported. Therefore, for patients receiving both neuromuscular blocking agents and corticosteroids, the period of use of the neuromuscular blocking agent should be limited as much as possible and only used in the setting where in the opinion of the prescribing physician, the specific advantages of the drug outweigh the risk.

5.6 Malignant Hyperthermia (MH)

ZEMURON has not been studied in MH-susceptible patients. Because ZEMURON is always used with other agents, and the occurrence of malignant hyperthermia during anesthesia is possible even in the absence of known triggering agents, clinicians should be familiar with early signs, confirmatory diagnosis and treatment of malignant hyperthermia prior to the start of any anesthetic.

In an animal study in MH-susceptible swine, the administration of ZEMURON Injection did not appear to trigger malignant hyperthermia.

5.7 Prolonged Circulation Time

Conditions associated with an increased circulatory delayed time, e.g., cardiovascular disease or advanced age, may be associated with a delay in onset time [see Dosage and Administration (2.5)].

5.8 QT Interval Prolongation
The overall analysis of ECG data in pediatric patients indicates that the concomitant use of ZEMURON with general anesthetic agents can prolong the QTc interval *[see Clinical Studies (14.3)]*.

5.9 Conditions/Drugs Causing Potentiation of, or Resistance to, Neuromuscular Block
Potentiation: Nondepolarizing neuromuscular blocking agents have been found to exhibit profound neuromuscular blocking effects in cachectic or debilitated patients, patients with neuromuscular diseases, and patients with carcinomatosis.
Certain inhalation anesthetics, particularly enflurane and isoflurane, antibiotics, magnesium salts, lithium, local anesthetics, procainamide, and quinidine have been shown to increase the duration of neuromuscular block and decrease infusion requirements of neuromuscular blocking agents *[see Drug Interactions (7.3)]*.
In these or other patients in whom potentiation of neuromuscular block or difficulty with reversal may be anticipated, a decrease from the recommended initial dose of ZEMURON should be considered *[see Dosage and Administration (2.5)]*.
Resistance: Resistance to nondepolarizing agents, consistent with up-regulation of skeletal muscle acetylcholine receptors, is associated with burns, disuse atrophy, denervation, and direct muscle trauma. Receptor up-regulation may also contribute to the resistance to nondepolarizing muscle relaxants which sometimes develops in patients with cerebral palsy, patients chronically receiving anticonvulsant agents such as carbamazepine or phenytoin or with chronic exposure to nondepolarizing agents. When ZEMURON is administered to these patients, shorter durations of neuromuscular block may occur and infusion rates may be higher due to the development of resistance to nondepolarizing muscle relaxants.
Potentiation or Resistance: Severe acid-base and/or electrolyte abnormalities may potentiate or cause resistance to the neuromuscular blocking action of ZEMURON. No data are available in such patients and no dosing recommendations can be made.
ZEMURON-induced neuromuscular blockade was modified by alkalosis and acidosis in experimental pigs. Both respiratory and metabolic acidosis prolonged the recovery time. The potency of ZEMURON was significantly enhanced in metabolic acidosis and alkalosis, but was reduced in respiratory alkalosis. In addition, experience with other drugs has suggested that acute (e.g., diarrhea) or chronic (e.g., adrenocortical insufficiency) electrolyte imbalance may alter neuromuscular blockade. Since electrolyte imbalance and acid-base imbalance are usually mixed, either enhancement or inhibition may occur.

5.10 Incompatibility with Alkaline Solutions
ZEMURON, which has an acid pH, should not be mixed with alkaline solutions (e.g., barbiturate solutions) in the same syringe or administered simultaneously during intravenous infusion through the same needle.

5.11 Increase in Pulmonary Vascular Resistance
ZEMURON may be associated with increased pulmonary vascular resistance, so caution is appropriate in patients with pulmonary hypertension or valvular heart disease *[see Clinical Studies (14.1)]*.

5.12 Use In Patients with Myasthenia
In patients with myasthenia gravis or myasthenic (Eaton-Lambert) syndrome, small doses of nondepolarizing neuromuscular blocking agents may have profound effects. In such patients, a peripheral nerve stimulator and use of a small test dose may be of value in monitoring the response to administration of muscle relaxants.

5.13 Extravasation
If extravasation occurs, it may be associated with signs or symptoms of local irritation. The injection or infusion should be terminated immediately and restarted in another vein.

6 ADVERSE REACTIONS

In clinical trials, the most common adverse reactions (2%) are transient hypotension and hypertension.
The following adverse reactions are described, or described in greater detail, in other sections:
- Anaphylaxis *[see Warnings and Precautions (5.2)]*
- Residual paralysis *[see Warnings and Precautions (5.4)]*
- Myopathy *[see Warnings and Precautions (5.5)]*
- Increased pulmonary vascular resistance *[see Warnings and Precautions (5.11)]*

6.1 Clinical Trials Experience
Because clinical trials are conducted under widely varying conditions, adverse reaction rates observed in the clinical trials of a drug cannot be directly compared to rates in the clinical trials of another drug and may not reflect the rates observed in practice.
Clinical studies in the US (n=1137) and Europe (n=1394) totaled 2531 patients. The patients exposed in the US clinical studies provide the basis for calculation of adverse reaction rates. The following adverse reactions were reported in patients administered ZEMURON (all events judged by investigators during the clinical trials to have a possible causal relationship):
Adverse reactions in greater than 1% of patients: None
Adverse reactions in less than 1% of patients (probably related or relationship unknown):
Cardiovascular: arrhythmia, abnormal electrocardiogram, tachycardia
Digestive: nausea, vomiting
Respiratory: asthma (bronchospasm, wheezing, or rhonchi), hiccup
Skin and Appendages: rash, injection site edema, pruritus
In the European studies, the most commonly reported reactions were transient hypotension (2%) and hypertension (2%); these are in greater frequency than the US studies (0.1% and 0.1%). Changes in heart rate and blood pressure were defined differently from in the US studies in which changes in cardiovascular parameters were not considered as adverse events unless judged by the investigator as unexpected, clinically significant, or thought to be histamine related.
In a clinical study in patients with clinically significant cardiovascular disease undergoing coronary artery bypass graft, hypertension and tachycardia were reported in some patients, but these occurrences were less frequent in patients receiving beta or calcium channel-blocking drugs. In some patients, ZEMURON was associated with transient increases (30% or greater) in pulmonary vascular resistance. In another clinical study of patients undergoing abdominal aortic surgery, transient increases (30% or greater) in pulmonary vascular resistance were observed in about 24% of patients receiving ZEMURON 0.6 or 0.9 mg/kg.
In pediatric patient studies worldwide (n=704), tachycardia occurred at an incidence of 5.3% (n=37) and it was judged by the investigator as related in 10 cases (1.4%).

6.2 Post-marketing Experience
In clinical practice, there have been reports of severe allergic reactions (anaphylactic and anaphylactoid reactions and shock) with ZEMURON, including some that have been life-threatening and fatal *[see Warnings and Precautions (5.2)]*. Because these reactions were reported voluntarily from a population of uncertain size, it is not possible to reliably estimate their frequency.

7 DRUG INTERACTIONS

7.1 Antibiotics
Drugs which may enhance the neuromuscular blocking action of nondepolarizing agents such as ZEMURON include certain antibiotics (e.g., aminoglycosides; vancomycin; tetracyclines; bacitracin; polymyxins; colistin; and sodium colistimethate). If these antibiotics are used in conjunction with ZEMURON, prolongation of neuromuscular block may occur.

7.2 Anticonvulsants
In 2 of 4 patients receiving chronic anticonvulsant therapy, apparent resistance to the effects of ZEMURON was observed in the form of diminished magnitude of neuromuscular block, or shortened clinical duration. As with other nondepolarizing neuromuscular blocking drugs, if ZEMURON is administered to patients chronically receiving anticonvulsant agents such as carbamazepine or phenytoin, shorter durations of neuromuscular block may occur and infusion rates may be higher due to the development of resistance to nondepolarizing muscle relaxants. While the mechanism for development of this resistance is not known, receptor up-regulation may be a contributing factor *[see Warnings and Precautions (5.9)]*.

7.3 Inhalation Anesthetics
Use of inhalation anesthetics has been shown to enhance the activity of other neuromuscular blocking agents (enflurane > isoflurane > halothane).
Isoflurane and enflurane may also prolong the duration of action of initial and maintenance doses of ZEMURON and decrease the average infusion requirement of ZEMURON by 40% compared to opioid/nitrous oxide/oxygen anesthesia. No definite interaction between ZEMURON and halothane has been demonstrated. In one study, use of enflurane in 10 patients resulted in a 20% increase in mean clinical duration of the initial intubating dose, and a 37% increase in the duration of subsequent maintenance doses, when compared in the same study to 10 patients under opioid/nitrous oxide/oxygen anesthesia. The clinical duration of initial doses of ZEMURON of 0.57 to 0.85 mg/kg under enflurane or isoflurane anesthesia, as used clinically, was increased by 11% and 23%, respectively. The duration of maintenance doses was affected to a greater extent, increasing by 30% to 50% under either enflurane or isoflurane anesthesia.
Potentiation by these agents is also observed with respect to the infusion rates of ZEMURON required to maintain approximately 95% neuromuscular block. Under isoflurane and enflurane anesthesia, the infusion rates are decreased by approximately 40% compared to opioid/nitrous oxide/oxygen anesthesia. The median spontaneous recovery time (from 25% to 75% of control T_1) is not affected by halothane, but is prolonged by enflurane (15% longer) and isoflurane (62% longer). Reversal-induced recovery of ZEMURON neuromuscular block is minimally affected by anesthetic technique *[see Dosage and Administration (2.5) and Warnings and Precautions (5.9)]*.

7.4 Lithium Carbonate
Lithium has been shown to increase the duration of neuromuscular block and decrease infusion requirements of neuromuscular blocking agents *[see Warnings and Precautions (5.9)]*.

7.5 Local Anesthetics
Local anesthetics have been shown to increase the duration of neuromuscular block and decrease infusion requirements of neuromuscular blocking agents *[see Warnings and Precautions (5.9)]*.

7.6 Magnesium
Magnesium salts administered for the management of toxemia of pregnancy may enhance neuromuscular blockade *[see Warnings and Precautions (5.9)]*.

7.7 Nondepolarizing Muscle Relaxants
There are no controlled studies documenting the use of ZEMURON before or after other nondepolarizing muscle relaxants. Interactions have been observed when other nondepolarizing muscle relaxants have been administered in succession.

7.8 Procainamide
Procainamide has been shown to increase the duration of neuromuscular block and decrease infusion requirements of neuromuscular blocking agents *[see Warnings and Precautions (5.9)]*.

7.9 Propofol
The use of propofol for induction and maintenance of anesthesia does not alter the clinical duration or recovery characteristics following recommended doses of ZEMURON.

7.10 Quinidine
Injection of quinidine during recovery from use of muscle relaxants is associated with recurrent paralysis. This possibility must also be considered for ZEMURON *[see Warnings and Precautions (5.9)]*.

7.11 Succinylcholine
The use of ZEMURON before succinylcholine, for the purpose of attenuating some of the side effects of succinylcholine, has not been studied.
If ZEMURON is administered following administration of succinylcholine, it should not be given until recovery from succinylcholine has been observed. The median duration of action of ZEMURON 0.6 mg/kg administered after a 1 mg/kg dose of succinylcholine when T_1 returned to 75% of control was 36 minutes (range 14-57, n=12) vs. 28 minutes (17-51, n=12) without succinylcholine.

8 USE IN SPECIFIC POPULATIONS

8.1 Pregnancy
Pregnancy Category C: Developmental toxicology studies have been performed with rocuronium bromide in pregnant, conscious, nonventilated rabbits and rats. Inhibition of neuromuscular function was the endpoint for high-dose selection. The maximum tolerated dose served as the high dose and was administered intravenously three times a day to rats (0.3 mg/kg, 15% to 30% of human intubation dose of 0.6 to 1.2 mg/kg based on the body surface unit of mg/m^2) from day 6 to 17 and to rabbits (0.02 mg/kg, 25% human dose) from day 6 to 18 of pregnancy. High-dose treatment caused acute symptoms of respiratory dysfunction due to the pharmacological activity of the drug. Teratogenicity was not observed in these animal species. The incidence of late embryonic death was increased at the high dose in rats, most likely due to oxygen deficiency. Therefore, this finding probably has no relevance for humans because immediate mechanical ventilation of the intubated patient will effectively prevent embryo-fetal hypoxia. However, there are no adequate and well-controlled studies in pregnant women. ZEMURON should be used during pregnancy only if the potential benefit justifies the potential risk to the fetus.

8.2 Labor and Delivery
The use of ZEMURON in Cesarean section has been studied in a limited number of patients *[see Clinical Studies (14.5)]*. ZEMURON is not recommended for rapid sequence induction in Cesarean section patients.

8.4 Pediatric Use
The use of ZEMURON has been studied in pediatric patients 3 months to 14 years of age under halothane anesthesia. Of the pediatric patients anesthetized with halothane who did not receive atropine for induction, about 80% experienced a transient increase (30% or greater) in heart rate after intubation. One of the 19 infants anesthetized with halothane and fentanyl who received atropine for induction experienced this magnitude of change *[see Dosage and Administration (2.5) and Clinical Studies (14.3)]*.
ZEMURON was also studied in pediatric patients up to 17 years of age, including neonates, under sevoflurane (induction) and isoflurane/nitrous oxide (maintenance) anesthesia. Onset time and clinical duration varied with dose, the

age of the patient, and anesthetic technique. The overall analysis of ECG data in pediatric patients indicates that the concomitant use of ZEMURON with general anesthetic agents can prolong the QTc interval. The data also suggest that ZEMURON may increase heart rate. However, it was not possible to conclusively identify an effect of ZEMURON independent of that of anesthesia and other factors. Additionally, when examining plasma levels of ZEMURON in correlation to QTc interval prolongation, no relationship was observed [see Dosage and Administration (2.5), Warnings and Precautions (5.8) and Clinical Studies (14.3)].

ZEMURON is not recommended for rapid sequence intubation in pediatric patients. Recommendations for use in pediatric patients are discussed in other sections [see Dosage and Administration (2.5) and Clinical Pharmacology (12.2)].

8.5   Geriatric Use
ZEMURON was administered to 140 geriatric patients (65 years or greater) in US clinical trials and 128 geriatric patients in European clinical trials. The observed pharmacokinetic profile for geriatric patients (n=20) was similar to that for other adult surgical patients [see Clinical Pharmacology (12.3)]. Onset time and duration of action were slightly longer for geriatric patients (n=43) in clinical trials. Clinical experiences and recommendations for use in geriatric patients are discussed in other sections [see Dosage and Administration (2.5), Clinical Pharmacology (12.2), and Clinical Studies (14.2)].

8.6   Patients with Hepatic Impairment
Since ZEMURON is primarily excreted by the liver, it should be used with caution in patients with clinically significant hepatic impairment. ZEMURON 0.6 mg/kg has been studied in a limited number of patients (n=9) with clinically significant hepatic impairment under steady-state isoflurane anesthesia. After ZEMURON 0.6 mg/kg, the median (range) clinical duration of 60 (35-166) minutes was moderately prolonged compared to 42 minutes in patients with normal hepatic function. The median recovery time of 53 minutes was also prolonged in patients with cirrhosis compared to 20 minutes in patients with normal hepatic function. Four of eight patients with cirrhosis, who received ZEMURON 0.6 mg/kg under opioid/nitrous oxide/oxygen anesthesia, did not achieve complete block. These findings are consistent with the increase in volume of distribution at steady state observed in patients with significant hepatic impairment [see Clinical Pharmacology (12.3)]. If used for rapid sequence induction in patients with ascites, an increased initial dosage may be necessary to assure complete block. Duration will be prolonged in these cases. The use of doses higher than 0.6 mg/kg has not been studied [see Dosage and Administration (2.5)].

8.7   Patients with Renal Impairment
Due to the limited role of the kidney in the excretion of ZEMURON, usual dosing guidelines should be followed. In patients with renal dysfunction, the duration of neuromuscular blockade was not prolonged; however, there was substantial individual variability (range, 22-90 minutes) [see Clinical Pharmacology (12.3)].

10   OVERDOSAGE
Overdosage with neuromuscular blocking agents may result in neuromuscular block beyond the time needed for surgery and anesthesia. The primary treatment is maintenance of a patent airway, controlled ventilation and adequate sedation until recovery of normal neuromuscular function is assured.

Once evidence of recovery from neuromuscular block is observed, further recovery may be facilitated by administration of an anticholinesterase agent in conjunction with an appropriate anticholinergic agent.

Patients should be evaluated for adequate clinical evidence of neuromuscular recovery, e.g., 5-second head lift, adequate phonation, ventilation, and upper airway patency. Ventilation must be supported while patients exhibit any signs of muscle weakness.

Reversal of Neuromuscular Blockade: Anticholinesterase agents should not be administered prior to the demonstration of some spontaneous recovery from neuromuscular blockade. The use of a nerve stimulator to document recovery is recommended.

Patients should be evaluated for adequate clinical evidence of neuromuscular recovery, e.g., 5-second head lift, adequate phonation, ventilation, and upper airway patency. Ventilation must be supported while patients exhibit any signs of muscle weakness.

Recovery may be delayed in the presence of debilitation, carcinomatosis, and concomitant use of certain drugs which enhance neuromuscular blockade or separately cause respiratory depression. Under such circumstances the management is the same as that of prolonged neuromuscular blockade.

11   DESCRIPTION
ZEMURON (rocuronium bromide) injection is a nondepolarizing neuromuscular blocking agent with a rapid to intermediate onset depending on dose and intermediate duration. Rocuronium bromide is chemically designated as 1-[17β-(acetyloxy)-3α-hydroxy-2β-(4-morpholinyl)-5α-androstan-16β-yl]-1-(2-propenyl)pyrrolidinium bromide. The structural formula is:

The chemical formula is $C_{32}H_{53}BrN_2O_4$ with a molecular weight of 609.70. The partition coefficient of rocuronium bromide in n-octanol/water is 0.5 at 20°C.

ZEMURON is supplied as a sterile, nonpyrogenic, isotonic solution that is clear, colorless to yellow/orange, for intravenous injection only. Each mL contains 10 mg rocuronium bromide and 2 mg sodium acetate. The aqueous solution is adjusted to isotonicity with sodium chloride and to a pH of 4 with acetic acid and/or sodium hydroxide.

12   CLINICAL PHARMACOLOGY
12.1   Mechanism of Action
ZEMURON is a nondepolarizing neuromuscular blocking agent with a rapid to intermediate onset depending on dose and intermediate duration. It acts by competing for cholinergic receptors at the motor end-plate. This action is antagonized by acetylcholinesterase inhibitors, such as neostigmine and edrophonium.

12.2   Pharmacodynamics
The ED_{95} (dose required to produce 95% suppression of the first [T_1] mechanomyographic [MMG] response of the adductor pollicis muscle [thumb] to indirect supramaximal train-of-four stimulation of the ulnar nerve) during opioid/nitrous oxide/oxygen anesthesia is approximately 0.3 mg/kg. Patient variability around the ED_{95} dose suggests that 50% of patients will exhibit T_1 depression of 91% to 97%. **Table 4** presents intubating conditions in patients with intubation initiated at 60 to 70 seconds.

TABLE 4: Percent of Excellent or Good Intubating Conditions and Median (Range) Time to Completion of Intubation in Patients with Intubation Initiated at 60 to 70 Seconds

ZEMURON Dose (mg/kg) Administered over 5 sec	Percent of Patients With Excellent or Good Intubating Conditions	Time to Completion of Intubation (min)
Adults* 18 to 64 yrs 0.45 (n=43) 0.6 (n=51)	86% 96%	1.6 (1.0-7.0) 1.6 (1.0-3.2)
Infants** 3 mo to 1 yr 0.6 (n=18)	100%	1.0 (1.0-1.5)
Pediatric** 1 to 12 yrs 0.6 (n=12)	100%	1.0 (0.5-2.3)

*Excludes patients undergoing Cesarean section
**Pediatric patients were under halothane anesthesia
Excellent intubating conditions=jaw relaxed, vocal cords apart and immobile, no diaphragmatic movement
Good intubating conditions=same as excellent but with some diaphragmatic movement

Table 5 presents the time to onset and clinical duration for the initial dose of ZEMURON (rocuronium bromide) injection under opioid/nitrous oxide/oxygen anesthesia in adults and geriatric patients, and under halothane anesthesia in pediatric patients.
[See table 5 below]
Table 6 presents the time to onset and clinical duration for the initial dose of ZEMURON (rocuronium bromide) Injection under sevoflurane (induction) and isoflurane/nitrous oxide (maintenance) anesthesia in pediatric patients.
[See table 6 at top of next page]
The time to 80% or greater block and clinical duration as a function of dose are presented in **Figures 1** and **2**.

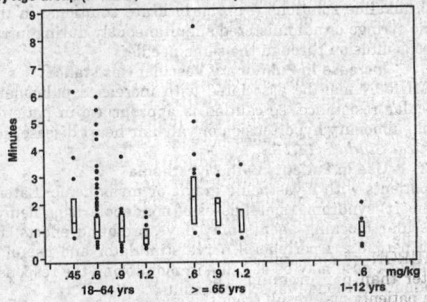

FIGURE 1: Time to 80% or Greater Block vs. Initial Dose of ZEMURON by Age Group (Median, 25th and 75th percentile, and individual values)

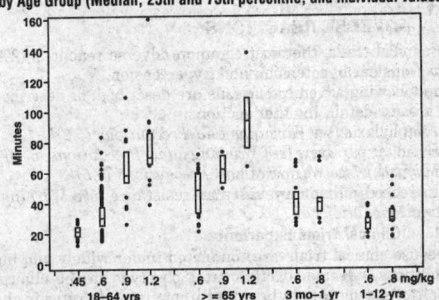

FIGURE 2: Duration of Clinical Effect vs. Initial Dose of ZEMURON by Age Group (Median, 25th and 75th percentile, and individual values)

The clinical durations for the first five maintenance doses, in patients receiving five or more maintenance doses are represented in **Figure 3** [see Dosage and Administration (2.3)].

TABLE 5: Median (Range) Time to Onset and Clinical Duration Following Initial (Intubating) Dose During Opioid/Nitrous Oxide/Oxygen Anesthesia (Adults) and Halothane Anesthesia (Pediatric Patients)

ZEMURON Dose (mg/kg) Administered over 5 sec	Time to ≥80% Block (min)	Time to Maximum Block (min)	Clinical Duration (min)
Adults 18 to 64 yrs			
0.45 (n=50)	1.3 (0.8-6.2)	3.0 (1.3-8.2)	22 (12-31)
0.6 (n=142)	1.0 (0.4-6.0)	1.8 (0.6-13.0)	31 (15-85)
0.9 (n=20)	1.1 (0.3-3.8)	1.4 (0.8-6.2)	58 (27-111)
1.2 (n=18)	0.7 (0.4-1.7)	1.0 (0.6-4.7)	67 (38-160)
Geriatric ≥65 yrs			
0.6 (n=31)	2.3 (1.0-8.3)	3.7 (1.3-11.3)	46 (22-73)
0.9 (n=5)	2.0 (1.0-3.0)	2.5 (1.2-5.0)	62 (49-75)
1.2 (n=7)	1.0 (0.8-3.5)	1.3 (1.2-4.7)	94 (64-138)
Infants 3 mo to 1 yr			
0.6 (n=17)	—	0.8 (0.3-3.0)	41 (24-68)
0.8 (n=9)	—	0.7 (0.5-0.8)	40 (27-70)
Pediatric 1 to 12 yrs			
0.6 (n=27)	0.8 (0.4-2.0)	1.0 (0.5-3.3)	26 (17-39)
0.8 (n=18)		0.5 (0.3-1.0)	30 (17-56)

n=the number of patients who had time to maximum block recorded
Clinical duration=time until return to 25% of control T_1. Patients receiving doses of 0.45 mg/kg who achieved less than 90% block (16% of these patients) had about 12 to 15 minutes to 25% recovery.

FIGURE 3: Duration of Clinical Effect vs. Number of ZEMURON Maintenance Doses, by Dose

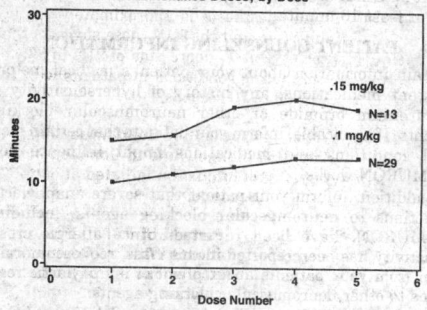

Once spontaneous recovery has reached 25% of control T_1, the neuromuscular block produced by ZEMURON is readily reversed with anticholinesterase agents, e.g., edrophonium or neostigmine.

The median spontaneous recovery from 25% to 75% T_1 was 13 minutes in adult patients. When neuromuscular block was reversed in 36 adults at a T_1 of 22% to 27%, recovery to a T_1 of 89 (50-132)% and T_4/T_1 of 69 (38-92)% was achieved within 5 minutes. Only five of 320 adults reversed received an additional dose of reversal agent. The median (range) dose of neostigmine was 0.04 (0.01-0.09) mg/kg and the median (range) dose of edrophonium was 0.5 (0.3-1.0) mg/kg. In geriatric patients (n=51) reversed with neostigmine, the median T_4/T_1 increased from 40% to 88% in 5 minutes. In clinical trials with halothane, pediatric patients (n=27) who received 0.5 mg/kg edrophonium had increases in the median T_4/T_1 from 37% at reversal to 93% after 2 minutes. Pediatric patients (n=58) who received 1 mg/kg edrophonium had increases in the median T_4/T_1 from 72% at reversal to 100% after 2 minutes. Infants (n=10) who were reversed with 0.03 mg/kg neostigmine recovered from 25% to 75% T_1 within 4 minutes.

There were no reports of less than satisfactory clinical recovery of neuromuscular function.

The neuromuscular blocking action of ZEMURON may be enhanced in the presence of potent inhalation anesthetics [see Drug Interactions (7.3)].

Hemodynamics: There were no dose-related effects on the incidence of changes from baseline (30% or greater) in mean arterial blood pressure (MAP) or heart rate associated with ZEMURON administration over the dose range of 0.12 to 1.2 mg/kg ($4 \times ED_{95}$) within 5 minutes after ZEMURON administration and prior to intubation. Increases or decreases in MAP were observed in 2% to 5% of geriatric and other adult patients, and in about 1% of pediatric patients. Heart rate changes (30% or greater) occurred in 0% to 2% of geriatric and other adult patients. Tachycardia (30% or greater) occurred in 12 of 127 pediatric patients. Most of the pediatric patients developing tachycardia were from a single study where the patients were anesthetized with halothane and who did not receive atropine for induction [see Clinical Studies (14.3)]. In US studies, laryngoscopy and tracheal intubation following ZEMURON administration were accompanied by transient tachycardia (30% or greater increases) in about one-third of adult patients under opioid/nitrous oxide/oxygen anesthesia. Animal studies have indicated that the ratio of vagal:neuromuscular block following ZEMURON administration is less than vecuronium but greater than pancuronium. The tachycardia observed in some patients may result from this vagal blocking activity.

Histamine Release: In studies of histamine release, clinically significant concentrations of plasma histamine occurred in 1 of 88 patients. Clinical signs of histamine release (flushing, rash, or bronchospasm) associated with the administration of ZEMURON were assessed in clinical trials and reported in 9 of 1137 (0.8%) patients.

12.3 Pharmacokinetics

Adult and Geriatric Patients: In an effort to maximize the information gathered in the *in vivo* pharmacokinetic studies, the data from the studies was used to develop population estimates of the parameters for the subpopulations represented (e.g., geriatric, pediatric, renal and hepatic impairment). These population-based estimates and a measure of the estimate variability are contained in the following section.

Following intravenous administration of ZEMURON, plasma levels of rocuronium follow a three-compartment open model. The rapid distribution half-life is 1 to 2 minutes and the slower distribution half-life is 14 to 18 minutes. Rocuronium is approximately 30% bound to human plasma proteins. In geriatric and other adult surgical patients undergoing either opioid/nitrous oxide/oxygen or inhalational anesthesia, the observed pharmacokinetic profile was essentially unchanged.

TABLE 6: Median (Range) Time to Onset and Clinical Duration Following Initial (Intubating) Dose During Sevoflurane (induction) and Isoflurane/Nitrous Oxide (maintenance) Anesthesia (Pediatric Patients)

ZEMURON Dose (mg/kg) Administered over 5 sec	Time to Maximum Block (min)	Time to Reappearance T_3 (min)
Neonates birth to <28 days		
0.45 (n=5)	1.1 (0.6-2.2)	40.3 (32.5-62.6)
0.6 (n=10)	1.0 (0.2-2.1)	49.7 (16.6-119.0)
1 (n=6)	0.6 (0.3-1.8)	114.4 (92.6-136.3)
Infants 28 days to ≤3 mo		
0.45 (n=9)	0.5 (0.4-1.3)	49.1 (13.5-79.9)
0.6 (n=11)	0.4 (0.2-0.8)	59.8 (32.3-87.8)
1 (n=5)	0.3 (0.2-0.7)	103.3 (90.8-155.4)
Toddlers >3 mo to ≤2 yrs		
0.45 (n=17)	0.8 (0.3-1.9)	39.2 (16.9-59.4)
0.6 (n=29)	0.6 (0.2-1.6)	44.2 (18.9-68.8)
1 (n=15)	0.5 (0.2-1.5)	72.0 (36.2-128.2)
Children >2 yrs to ≤11 yrs		
0.45 (n=14)	0.9 (0.4-1.9)	21.5 (17.5-38.0)
0.6 (n=37)	0.8 (0.3-1.7)	36.7 (20.1-65.9)
1 (n=16)	0.7 (0.4-1.2)	53.1 (31.2-89.9)
Adolescents >11 to ≤17 yrs		
0.45 (n=18)	1.0 (0.5-1.7)	37.5 (18.3-65.7)
0.6 (n=31)	0.9 (0.2-2.1)	41.4 (16.3-91.2)
1 (n=14)	0.7 (0.5-1.2)	67.1 (25.6-93.8)

n=the number of patients with the highest number of observations for time to maximum block or reappearance T_3.

TABLE 8: Mean (SD) Pharmacokinetic Parameters in Adults with Normal Renal and Hepatic Function (n=10, ages 23 to 65), Renal Transplant Patients (n=10, ages 21 to 45) and Hepatic Dysfunction Patients (n=9, ages 31 to 67) During Isoflurane Anesthesia

PK Parameters	Normal Renal and Hepatic Function	Renal Transplant Patients	Hepatic Dysfunction Patients
Clearance (L/kg/hr)	0.16 (0.05)*	0.13 (0.04)	0.13 (0.06)
Volume of Distribution at Steady State (L/kg)	0.26 (0.03)	0.34 (0.11)	0.53 (0.14)
$t_{1/2} \beta$ Elimination (hr)	2.4 (0.8)*	2.4 (1.1)	4.3 (2.6)

* Differences in the calculated $t_{1/2} \beta$ and Cl between this study and the study in young adults vs. geriatrics (≥65 years) is related to the different sample populations and anesthetic techniques.

TABLE 7: Mean (SD) Pharmacokinetic Parameters in Adults (n=22; ages 27 to 58 yrs) and Geriatric (n=20; 65 yrs or greater) During Opioid/Nitrous Oxide/Oxygen Anesthesia

PK Parameters	Adults (Ages 27 to 58 yrs)	Geriatrics (≥65 yrs)
Clearance (L/kg/hr)	0.25 (0.08)	0.21 (0.06)
Volume of Distribution at Steady State (L/kg)	0.25 (0.04)	0.22 (0.03)
$t_{1/2} \beta$ Elimination (hr)	1.4 (0.4)	1.5 (0.4)

In general, studies with normal adult subjects did not reveal any differences in the pharmacokinetics of rocuronium due to gender.

Studies of distribution, metabolism, and excretion in cats and dogs indicate that rocuronium is eliminated primarily by the liver. The rocuronium analog 17-desacetyl-rocuronium, a metabolite, has been rarely observed in the plasma or urine of humans administered single doses of 0.5 to 1 mg/kg with or without a subsequent infusion (for up to 12 hr) of rocuronium. In the cat, 17-desacetyl-rocuronium has approximately one-twentieth the neuromuscular blocking potency of rocuronium. The effects of renal failure and hepatic disease on the pharmacokinetics and pharmacodynamics of rocuronium in humans are consistent with these findings.

In general, patients undergoing cadaver kidney transplant have a small reduction in clearance which is offset pharmacokinetically by a corresponding increase in volume, such that the net effect is an unchanged plasma half-life. Patients with demonstrated liver cirrhosis have a marked increase in their volume of distribution resulting in a plasma half-life approximately twice that of patients with normal hepatic function. **Table 8** shows the pharmacokinetic parameters in subjects with either impaired renal or hepatic function.

[See table 8 above]
The net result of these findings is that subjects with renal failure have clinical durations that are similar to but somewhat more variable than the duration that one would expect in subjects with normal renal function. Hepatically impaired patients, due to the large increase in volume, may demonstrate clinical durations approaching 1.5 times that of subjects with normal hepatic function. In both populations the clinician should individualize the dose to the needs of the patient [see Dosage and Administration (2.5)].

Tissue redistribution accounts for most (about 80%) of the initial amount of rocuronium administered. As tissue compartments fill with continued dosing (4 to 8 hours), less drug is redistributed away from the site of action and, for an infusion-only dose, the rate to maintain neuromuscular blockade falls to about 20% of the initial infusion rate. The use of a loading dose and a smaller infusion rate reduces the need for adjustment of dose.

Pediatric Patients: Under halothane anesthesia, the clinical duration of effects of ZEMURON did not vary with age in patients 4 months to 8 years of age. The terminal half-life and other pharmacokinetic parameters of rocuronium in these pediatric patients are presented in **Table 9**.
[See table 9 at top of next page]
Pharmacokinetics of ZEMURON were evaluated using a population analysis of the pooled pharmacokinetic datasets from two trials under sevoflurane (induction) and isoflurane/nitrous oxide (maintenance) anesthesia. All pharmacokinetic parameters were found to be linearly proportional to body weight. In patients under the age of 18 years clearance (CL) and volume of distribution (Vss) increase with body-weight (kg) and age (years). As a result the terminal half-life of ZEMURON decreases with increasing age from 1.1 hour to 0.7-0.8 hour. Table 10 presents the pharmacokinetic parameters in the different age groups in the studies with sevoflurane (induction) and isoflurane/nitrous oxide (maintenance) anesthesia.
[See table 10 on next page]

13 NONCLINICAL TOXICOLOGY

13.1 Carcinogenesis, Mutagenesis, Impairment of Fertility

Studies in animals have not been performed with rocuronium bromide to evaluate carcinogenic potential or

TABLE 9: Mean (SD) Pharmacokinetic Parameters of Rocuronium in Pediatric Patients (ages 3 to less than 12 mos, n=6; 1 to less than 3 yrs, n=5; 3 to less than 8 yrs, n=7) During Halothane Anesthesia

PK Parameters	Patient Age Range		
	3 to <12 mos	1 to <3 yrs	3 to <8 yrs
Clearance (L/kg/hr)	0.35 (0.08)	0.32 (0.07)	0.44 (0.16)
Volume of Distribution at Steady State (L/kg)	0.30 (0.04)	0.26 (0.06)	0.21 (0.03)
$t_{1/2}$ β Elimination (hr)	1.3 (0.5)	1.1 (0.7)	0.8 (0.3)

TABLE 10: Mean (SD) Pharmacokinetic Parameters of Rocuronium in Pediatric Patients During Sevoflurane (induction) and Isoflurane/Nitrous Oxide (maintenance) Anesthesia

PK Parameters	Patient Age Range				
	Birth to <28 days	28 days to ≤3 mos	3 mos to ≤2 yrs	2 to ≤11 yrs	11 to ≤17 yrs
CL (L/kg/hr)	0.31 (0.07)	0.30 (0.08)	0.33 (0.10)	0.35 (0.09)	0.29 (0.14)
Volume of Distribution (L/kg)	0.42 (0.06)	0.31 (0.03)	0.23 (0.03)	0.18 (0.02)	0.18 (0.01)
$t_{1/2}$ β (hr)	1.1 (0.2)	0.9 (0.3)	0.8 (0.2)	0.7 (0.2)	0.8 (0.3)

impairment of fertility. Mutagenicity studies (Ames test, analysis of chromosomal aberrations in mammalian cells, and micronucleus test) conducted with rocuronium bromide did not suggest mutagenic potential.

14   CLINICAL STUDIES
In US clinical studies, a total of 1137 patients received ZEMURON, including 176 pediatric, 140 geriatric, 55 obstetric, and 766 other adults. Most patients (90%) were ASA physical status I or II, about 9% were ASA III, and 10 patients (undergoing coronary artery bypass grafting or valvular surgery) were ASA IV. In European clinical studies, a total of 1394 patients received ZEMURON, including 52 pediatric, 128 geriatric (65 years or greater) and 1214 other adults.

14.1   Adult Patients
Intubation using doses of ZEMURON 0.6 to 0.85 mg/kg was evaluated in 203 adults in 11 clinical studies. Excellent to good intubating conditions were generally achieved within 2 minutes and maximum block occurred within 3 minutes in most patients. Doses within this range provide clinical relaxation for a median (range) time of 33 (14-85) minutes under opioid/nitrous oxide/oxygen anesthesia. Larger doses (0.9 and 1.2 mg/kg) were evaluated in two studies with 19 and 16 patients under opioid/nitrous oxide/oxygen anesthesia and provided 58 (27-111) and 67 (38-160) minutes of clinical relaxation, respectively.

Cardiovascular Disease: In one clinical study, 10 patients with clinically significant cardiovascular disease undergoing coronary artery bypass graft received an initial dose of 0.6 mg/kg ZEMURON. Neuromuscular block was maintained during surgery with bolus maintenance doses of 0.3 mg/kg. Following induction, continuous 8 mcg/kg/min infusion of ZEMURON produced relaxation sufficient to support mechanical ventilation for 6 to 12 hours in the surgical intensive care unit (SICU) while the patients were recovering from surgery.

Rapid Sequence Intubation: Intubating conditions were assessed in 230 patients in six clinical studies where anesthesia was induced with either thiopental (3 to 6 mg/kg) or propofol (1.5 to 2.5 mg/kg) in combination with either fentanyl (2 to 5 mcg/kg) or alfentanil (1 mg). Most of the patients also received a premedication such as midazolam or temazepam. Most patients had intubation attempted within 60 to 90 seconds of administration of ZEMURON 0.6 mg/kg or succinylcholine 1 to 1.5 mg/kg. Excellent or good intubating conditions were achieved in 119/120 (99% [95% confidence interval 95%-99.9%]) patients receiving ZEMURON and in 108/110 (98% [94%-99.8%]) patients receiving succinylcholine. The duration of action of ZEMURON 0.6 mg/kg is longer than succinylcholine and at this dose is approximately equivalent to the duration of other intermediate-acting neuromuscular blocking drugs.

Obese Patients: ZEMURON was dosed according to actual body weight (ABW) in most clinical studies. The administration of ZEMURON in the 47 of 330 (14%) patients who were at least 30% or more above their ideal body weight (IBW) was not associated with clinically significant differences in the onset, duration, recovery, or reversal of ZEMURON-induced neuromuscular block.

In one clinical study in obese patients, ZEMURON 0.6 mg/kg was dosed according to ABW (n=12) or IBW (n=11). Obese patients dosed according to IBW had a longer time to maximum block, a shorter median (range) clinical duration of 25 (14-29) minutes, and did not achieve intubat-

ing conditions comparable to those dosed based on ABW. These results support the recommendation that obese patients be dosed based on actual body weight *[see Dosage and Administration (2.5)].*

Obstetric Patients: ZEMURON 0.6 mg/kg was administered with thiopental, 3 to 4 mg/kg (n=13) or 4 to 6 mg/kg (n=42), for rapid sequence induction of anesthesia for Cesarean section. No neonate had APGAR scores greater than 7 at 5 minutes. The umbilical venous plasma concentrations were 18% of maternal concentrations at delivery. Intubating conditions were poor or inadequate in 5 of 13 women receiving 3 to 4 mg/kg thiopental when intubation was attempted 60 seconds after drug injection. Therefore, ZEMURON is not recommended for rapid sequence induction in Cesarean section patients.

14.2   Geriatric Patients
ZEMURON was evaluated in 55 geriatric patients (ages 65 to 80 years) in six clinical studies. Doses of 0.6 mg/kg provided excellent to good intubating conditions in a median (range) time of 2.3 (1-8) minutes. Recovery times from 25% to 75% after these doses were not prolonged in geriatric patients compared to other adult patients *[see Dosage and Administration (2.5) and Use in Specific Populations (8.5)].*

14.3   Pediatric Patients
ZEMURON 0.45, 0.6 or 1 mg/kg was evaluated under sevoflurane (induction) and isoflurane/nitrous oxide (maintenance) anesthesia for intubation in 326 patients in two studies. In one of these studies maintenance bolus and infusion requirements were evaluated in 137 patients. In all age groups, doses of 0.6 mg/kg provided time to maximum block in about 1 minute. Across all age groups, median (range) time to reappearance of T_3 for doses of 0.6 mg/kg was shortest in the children [36.7 (20.1-65.9) minutes] and longest in infants [59.8 (32.3-87.8) minutes]. For pediatric patients older than 3 months, the time to recovery was shorter after stopping infusion maintenance when compared with bolus maintenance *[see Dosage and Administration (2.5) and Use in Specific Populations (8.4)].*

ZEMURON 0.6 or 0.8 mg/kg was evaluated for intubation in 75 pediatric patients (n=28; age 3 to 12 months, n=47; age 1 to 12 years) in three studies using halothane (1% to 5%) and nitrous oxide (60% to 70%) in oxygen. Doses of 0.6 mg/kg provided a median (range) time to maximum block of 1 (0.5-3.3) minute(s). This dose provided a median (range) time of clinical relaxation of 41 (24-68) minutes in 3-month to 1-year-old infants and 26 (17-39) minutes in 1-to 12-year-old pediatric patients *[see Dosage and Administration (2.5) and Use in Specific Populations (8.4)].*

16   HOW SUPPLIED/STORAGE AND HANDLING
ZEMURON (rocuronium bromide) injection is available in the following:
- ZEMURON 5 mL multiple dose vials containing 50 mg rocuronium bromide injection (10 mg/mL)
  Box of 10   NDC 0052-0450-15
- ZEMURON 10 mL multiple dose vials containing 100 mg rocuronium bromide injection (10 mg/mL)
  Box of 10   NDC 0052-0450-16

The packaging of this product contains **no** natural rubber (latex).

ZEMURON should be stored in a refrigerator, 2°-8°C (36°-46°F). DO NOT FREEZE. Upon removal from refrigeration to room temperature storage conditions (25°C/77°F), use ZEMURON within 60 days. Use opened vials of ZEMURON within 30 days.

Safety and Handling: There is no specific work exposure limit for ZEMURON. In case of eye contact, flush with water for at least 10 minutes.

17   PATIENT COUNSELING INFORMATION
Obtain information about your patient's medical history, current medications, any history of hypersensitivity to rocuronium bromide or other neuromuscular blocking agents. If applicable, inform your patients that certain medical conditions and medications might influence how ZEMURON works.

In addition, inform your patient that severe anaphylactic reactions to neuromuscular blocking agents, including ZEMURON, have been reported. Since allergic cross-reactivity has been reported in this class, request information from your patients about previous anaphylactic reactions to other neuromuscular blocking agents.

Manufactured by Baxter Pharmaceutical Solutions LLC
Bloomington, IN 47403
or Organon (Ireland) Ltd., Swords, Co. Dublin, Ireland
Distributed by Schering Corporation,
a subsidiary of Schering-Plough Corporation.
ZEM-76952 9/08

Shown in Product Identification Guide, page 314

ZETIA®   ℞
[zĕt′-ē-ă]
(ezetimibe)
Tablets

HIGHLIGHTS OF PRESCRIBING INFORMATION
These highlights do not include all the information needed to use ZETIA safely and effectively. See full prescribing information for ZETIA.

ZETIA (ezetimibe) Tablets
Initial U.S. Approval: 2002

————INDICATIONS AND USAGE————
ZETIA® is an inhibitor of intestinal cholesterol (and related phytosterol) absorption indicated as an adjunct to diet to:
- Reduce elevated total-C, LDL-C, and Apo B in patients with primary hyperlipidemia, alone or in combination with an HMG-CoA reductase inhibitor (statin) (1.1)
- Reduce elevated total-C, LDL-C, Apo B, and non-HDL-C in patients with mixed hyperlipidemia in combination with fenofibrate (1.1)
- Reduce elevated total-C and LDL-C in patients with homozygous familial hypercholesterolemia (HoFH), in combination with atorvastatin or simvastatin (1.2)
- Reduce elevated sitosterol and campesterol in patients with homozygous sitosterolemia (phytosterolemia) (1.3)

Limitations of Use (1.4)
- The effect of ZETIA on cardiovascular morbidity and mortality has not been determined.
- ZETIA has not been studied in Fredrickson Type I, III, IV, and V dyslipidemias.

————DOSAGE AND ADMINISTRATION————
- One 10-mg tablet once daily, with or without food (2.1)
- Dosing of ZETIA should occur either ≥2 hours before or ≥4 hours after administration of a bile acid sequestrant. (2.3, 7.4)

————DOSAGE FORMS AND STRENGTHS————
- Tablets: 10 mg (3)

————CONTRAINDICATIONS————
- Statin contraindications apply when ZETIA is used with a statin:
  ○ Active liver disease, which may include unexplained persistent elevations in hepatic transaminase levels (4, 5.2)
  ○ Women who are pregnant or may become pregnant (4, 8.1)
  ○ Nursing mothers (4, 8.3)
- Known hypersensitivity to product components (4, 6.2)

————WARNINGS AND PRECAUTIONS————
- ZETIA is not recommended in patients with moderate or severe hepatic impairment. (5.4, 8.6, 12.3)
- Liver enzyme abnormalities and monitoring: Persistent elevations in hepatic transaminase can occur when ZETIA is added to a statin. Therefore, when ZETIA is added to statin therapy, monitor hepatic transaminase levels before and during treatment according to the recommendations for the individual statin used. (5.2)
- Skeletal muscle effects (e.g., myopathy and rhabdomyolysis):
  ○ Cases of myopathy and rhabdomyolysis have been reported in patients treated with ZETIA co-administered with a statin and with ZETIA administered alone. Risk for skeletal muscle toxicity increases with higher doses of statin, advanced age (>65), hypothyroidism, renal impairment, and depending on the statin used, concomitant use of other drugs. (5.3, 6.2)

ADVERSE REACTIONS
- Common adverse reactions in clinical trials:
  - ZETIA co-administered with a statin (incidence ≥2% and greater than statin alone):
    - nasopharyngitis, myalgia, upper respiratory tract infection, arthralgia, and diarrhea (6)
  - ZETIA administered alone (incidence ≥2% and greater than placebo):
    - upper respiratory tract infection, diarrhea, arthralgia, sinusitis, and pain in extremity (6)

To report SUSPECTED ADVERSE REACTIONS, contact Merck/Schering-Plough Pharmaceuticals at 1-866-637-2501 or FDA at 1-800-FDA-1088 or www.fda.gov/medwatch.

DRUG INTERACTIONS
- Cyclosporine: Combination increases exposure of ZETIA and cyclosporine. Cyclosporine concentrations should be monitored in patients taking ZETIA concomitantly. (7.1, 12.3)
- Fenofibrate: Combination increases exposure of ZETIA. If cholelithiasis is suspected in a patient receiving ZETIA and fenofibrate, gallbladder studies are indicated and alternative lipid-lowering therapy should be considered. (6.1, 7.3)
- Fibrates: Co-administration of ZETIA with fibrates other than fenofibrate is not recommended until use in patients is adequately studied. (7.2)
- Cholestyramine: Combination decreases exposure of ZETIA. (2.3, 7.4, 12.3)

See 17 for PATIENT COUNSELING INFORMATION and FDA-approved patient labeling.

Revised: 07/2009

FULL PRESCRIBING INFORMATION

1 INDICATIONS AND USAGE
Therapy with lipid-altering agents should be only one component of multiple risk factor intervention in individuals at significantly increased risk for atherosclerotic vascular disease due to hypercholesterolemia. Drug therapy is indicated as an adjunct to diet when the response to a diet restricted in saturated fat and cholesterol and other nonpharmacologic measures alone has been inadequate.

1.1 Primary Hyperlipidemia
Monotherapy
ZETIA[1], administered alone, is indicated as adjunctive therapy to diet for the reduction of elevated total cholesterol (total-C), low-density lipoprotein cholesterol (LDL-C), and apolipoprotein B (Apo B) in patients with primary (heterozygous familial and non-familial) hyperlipidemia.

---

[1] COPYRIGHT © 2001, 2002, 2005, 2007, 2008 Merck/Schering-Plough Pharmaceuticals. All rights reserved.

Combination Therapy with HMG-CoA Reductase Inhibitors (Statins)
ZETIA, administered in combination with a 3-hydroxy-3-methylglutaryl-coenzyme A (HMG-CoA) reductase inhibitor (statin), is indicated as adjunctive therapy to diet for the reduction of elevated total-C, LDL-C, and Apo B in patients with primary (heterozygous familial and non-familial) hyperlipidemia.

Combination Therapy with Fenofibrate
ZETIA, administered in combination with fenofibrate, is indicated as adjunctive therapy to diet for the reduction of elevated total-C, LDL-C, Apo B, and non-high-density lipoprotein cholesterol (non-HDL-C) in adult patients with mixed hyperlipidemia.

1.2 Homozygous Familial Hypercholesterolemia (HoFH)
The combination of ZETIA and atorvastatin or simvastatin is indicated for the reduction of elevated total-C and LDL-C levels in patients with HoFH, as an adjunct to other lipid-lowering treatments (e.g., LDL apheresis) or if such treatments are unavailable.

1.3 Homozygous Sitosterolemia
ZETIA is indicated as adjunctive therapy to diet for the reduction of elevated sitosterol and campesterol levels in patients with homozygous familial sitosterolemia.

1.4 Limitations of Use
The effect of ZETIA on cardiovascular morbidity and mortality has not been determined.
ZETIA has not been studied in Fredrickson Type I, III, IV, and V dyslipidemias.

2 DOSAGE AND ADMINISTRATION
2.1 General Dosing Information
The recommended dose of ZETIA is 10 mg once daily. ZETIA can be administered with or without food.
2.2 Concomitant Lipid-Lowering Therapy
ZETIA may be administered with a statin (in patients with primary hyperlipidemia) or with fenofibrate (in patients with mixed hyperlipidemia) for incremental effect. For convenience, the daily dose of ZETIA may be taken at the same time as the statin or fenofibrate, according to the dosing recommendations for the respective medications.
2.3 Co-Administration with Bile Acid Sequestrants
Dosing of ZETIA should occur either ≥2 hours before or ≥4 hours after administration of a bile acid sequestrant *[see Drug Interactions (7.4)]*.
2.4 Patients with Hepatic Impairment
No dosage adjustment is necessary in patients with mild hepatic impairment *[see Warnings and Precautions (5.4)]*.
2.5 Patients with Renal Impairment
No dosage adjustment is necessary in patients with renal impairment *[see Clinical Pharmacology (12.3)]*.
2.6 Geriatric Patients
No dosage adjustment is necessary in geriatric patients *[see Clinical Pharmacology (12.3)]*.

3 DOSAGE FORMS AND STRENGTHS
10-mg tablets are white to off-white, capsule-shaped tablets debossed with "414" on one side.

4 CONTRAINDICATIONS
ZETIA is contraindicated in the following conditions:
- The combination of ZETIA with a statin is contraindicated in patients with active liver disease or unexplained persistent elevations in hepatic transaminase levels.
- Women who are pregnant or may become pregnant. Because statins decrease cholesterol synthesis and possibly the synthesis of other biologically active substances derived from cholesterol, ZETIA in combination with a statin may cause fetal harm when administered to pregnant women. Additionally, there is no apparent benefit to therapy during pregnancy, and safety in pregnant women has not been established. If the patient becomes pregnant while taking this drug, the patient should be apprised of the potential hazard to the fetus and the lack of known clinical benefit with continued use during pregnancy. *[see Use in Specific Populations (8.1).]*
- Nursing mothers. Because statins may pass into breast milk, and because statins have the potential to cause serious adverse reactions in nursing infants, women who require ZETIA treatment in combination with a statin should be advised not to nurse their infants *[see Use in Specific Populations (8.3)]*.
- Patients with a known hypersensitivity to any component of this product. Hypersensitivity reactions including anaphylaxis, angioedema, rash and urticaria have been reported with ZETIA *[see Adverse Reactions (6.2)]*.

5 WARNINGS AND PRECAUTIONS
5.1 Use with Statins or Fenofibrate
Concurrent administration of ZETIA with a specific statin or fenofibrate should be in accordance with the product labeling for that medication.
5.2 Liver Enzymes
In controlled clinical monotherapy studies, the incidence of consecutive elevations (≥3 × the upper limit of normal [ULN]) in hepatic transaminase levels was similar between ZETIA (0.5%) and placebo (0.3%).
In controlled clinical combination studies of ZETIA initiated concurrently with a statin, the incidence of consecutive elevations (≥3 × ULN) in hepatic transaminase levels was 1.3% for patients treated with ZETIA administered with statins and 0.4% for patients treated with statins alone. These elevations in transaminases were generally asymptomatic, not associated with cholestasis, and returned to baseline after discontinuation of therapy or with continued treatment. When ZETIA is co-administered with a statin, liver tests should be performed at initiation of therapy and according to the recommendations of the statin. Should an increase in ALT or AST ≥3 × ULN persist, consider withdrawal of ZETIA and/or the statin.
5.3 Myopathy/Rhabdomyolysis
In clinical trials, there was no excess of myopathy or rhabdomyolysis associated with ZETIA compared with the relevant control arm (placebo or statin alone). However, myopathy and rhabdomyolysis are known adverse reactions to statins and other lipid-lowering drugs. In clinical trials, the incidence of creatine phosphokinase (CPK) >10 × ULN was 0.2% for ZETIA vs 0.1% for placebo, and 0.1% for ZETIA co-administered with a statin vs 0.4% for statins alone. Risk for skeletal muscle toxicity increases with higher doses of statin, advanced age (>65), hypothyroidism, renal impairment, and depending on the statin used, concomitant use of other drugs.
In post-marketing experience with ZETIA, cases of myopathy and rhabdomyolysis have been reported. Most patients who developed rhabdomyolysis were taking a statin prior to initiating ZETIA. However, rhabdomyolysis has been reported with ZETIA monotherapy and with the addition of ZETIA to agents known to be associated with increased risk of rhabdomyolysis, such as fibrates. ZETIA and any statin or fibrate that the patient is taking concomitantly should be immediately discontinued if myopathy is diagnosed or suspected. The presence of muscle symptoms and a CPK level >10 × the ULN indicates myopathy.
5.4 Hepatic Impairment
Due to the unknown effects of the increased exposure to ezetimibe in patients with moderate to severe hepatic impairment, ZETIA is not recommended in these patients. *[See Clinical Pharmacology (12.3).]*

6 ADVERSE REACTIONS
The following serious adverse reactions are discussed in greater detail in other sections of the label:
- Liver enzyme abnormalities *[see Warnings and Precautions (5.2)]*
- Rhabdomyolysis and myopathy *[see Warnings and Precautions (5.3)]*

Monotherapy Studies: In the ZETIA controlled clinical trials database (placebo-controlled) of 2396 patients with a median treatment duration of 12 weeks (range 0 to 39 weeks), 3.3% of patients on ZETIA and 2.9% of patients on placebo discontinued due to adverse reactions. The most common adverse reactions in the group of patients treated with ZETIA that led to treatment discontinuation and occurred at a rate greater than placebo were:
- Arthralgia (0.3%)
- Dizziness (0.2%)
- Gamma-glutamyltransferase increased (0.2%)
The most commonly reported adverse reactions (incidence ≥2% and greater than placebo) in the ZETIA monotherapy controlled clinical trial database of 2396 patients were:

upper respiratory tract infection (4.3%), diarrhea (4.1%), arthralgia (3.0%), sinusitis (2.8%), and pain in extremity (2.7%).

Statin Co-administration Studies: In the ZETIA + statin controlled clinical trials database of 11,308 patients with a median treatment duration of 8 weeks (range 0 to 112 weeks), 4.0% of patients on ZETIA + statin and 3.3% of patients on statin alone discontinued due to adverse reactions. The most common adverse reactions in the group of patients treated with ZETIA + statin that led to treatment discontinuation and occurred at a rate greater than statin alone were:

- Alanine aminotransferase increased (0.6%)
- Myalgia (0.5%)
- Fatigue, aspartate aminotransferase increased, headache, and pain in extremity (each at 0.2%)

The most commonly reported adverse reactions (incidence ≥2% and greater than statin alone) in the ZETIA + statin controlled clinical trial database of 11,308 patients were: nasopharyngitis (3.7%), myalgia (3.2%), upper respiratory tract infection (2.9%), arthralgia (2.6%) and diarrhea (2.5%).

6.1 Clinical Trials Experience

Because clinical studies are conducted under widely varying conditions, adverse reaction rates observed in the clinical studies of a drug cannot be directly compared to rates in the clinical studies of another drug and may not reflect the rates observed in clinical practice.

Monotherapy

In 10 double-blind, placebo-controlled clinical trials, 2396 patients with primary hyperlipidemia (age range 9–86 years, 50% women, 90% Caucasians, 5% Blacks, 3% Hispanics, 2% Asians) and elevated LDL-C were treated with ZETIA 10 mg/day for a median treatment duration of 12 weeks (range 0 to 39 weeks).

Adverse reactions reported in ≥2% of patients treated with ZETIA and at an incidence greater than placebo in placebo-controlled studies of ZETIA, regardless of causality assessment, are shown in Table 1.

TABLE 1: Clinical Adverse Reactions Occurring in ≥2% of Patients Treated with ZETIA and at an Incidence Greater than Placebo, Regardless of Causality

Body System/Organ Class Adverse Reaction	ZETIA 10 mg (%) n = 2396	Placebo (%) n = 1159
Gastrointestinal disorders		
Diarrhea	4.1	3.7
General disorders and administration site conditions		
Fatigue	2.4	1.5
Infections and infestations		
Influenza	2.0	1.5
Sinusitis	2.8	2.2
Upper respiratory tract infection	4.3	2.5
Musculoskeletal and connective tissue disorders		
Arthralgia	3.0	2.2
Pain in extremity	2.7	2.5

The frequency of less common adverse reactions was comparable between ZETIA and placebo.

Combination with a Statin

In 28 double-blind, controlled (placebo- or active-controlled) clinical trials, 11,308 patients with primary hyperlipidemia (age range 10–93 years, 48% women, 85% Caucasians, 7% Blacks, 4% Hispanics, 3% Asians) and elevated LDL-C were treated with ZETIA 10 mg/day concurrently with or added to on-going statin therapy for a median treatment duration of 8 weeks (range 0 to 112 weeks).

The incidence of consecutive increased transaminases (≥3 × ULN) was higher in patients receiving ZETIA administered with statins (1.3%) than in patients treated with statins alone (0.4%). [See Warnings and Precautions (5.2).] Clinical adverse reactions reported in ≥2% of patients treated with ZETIA + statin and at an incidence greater than statin, regardless of causality assessment, are shown in Table 2.

TABLE 2: Clinical Adverse Reactions Occurring in ≥2% of Patients Treated with ZETIA Co-Administered with a Statin and at an Incidence Greater than Statin, Regardless of Causality

Body System/Organ Class Adverse Reaction	All Statins* (%) n = 9361	ZETIA + All Statins* (%) n = 11,308
Gastrointestinal disorders		
Diarrhea	2.2	2.5
General disorders and administration site conditions		
Fatigue	1.6	2.0
Infections and infestations		
Influenza	2.1	2.2
Nasopharyngitis	3.3	3.7
Upper respiratory tract infection	2.8	2.9
Musculoskeletal and connective tissue disorders		
Arthralgia	2.4	2.6
Back pain	2.3	2.4
Myalgia	2.7	3.2
Pain in extremity	1.9	2.1

* All Statins = all doses of all statins

Combination with Fenofibrate

This clinical study involving 625 patients with mixed dyslipidemia (age range 20–76 years, 44% women, 79% Caucasians, 0.1% Blacks, 11% Hispanics, 5% Asians) treated for up to 12 weeks and 576 patients treated for up to an additional 48 weeks evaluated co-administration of ZETIA and fenofibrate. This study was not designed to compare treatment groups for infrequent events. Incidence rates (95% CI) for clinically important elevations (≥3 × ULN, consecutive) in hepatic transaminase levels were 4.5% (1.9, 8.8) and 2.7% (1.2, 5.4) for fenofibrate monotherapy (n=188) and ZETIA co-administered with fenofibrate (n=183), respectively, adjusted for treatment exposure. Corresponding incidence rates for cholecystectomy were 0.6% (95% CI: 0.0%, 3.1%) and 1.7% (95% CI: 0.6%, 4.0%) for fenofibrate monotherapy and ZETIA co-administered with fenofibrate, respectively [see Drug Interactions (7.3)]. The numbers of patients exposed to co-administration therapy as well as fenofibrate and ezetimibe monotherapy were inadequate to assess gallbladder disease risk. There were no CPK elevations >10 × ULN in any of the treatment groups.

6.2 Post-Marketing Experience

Because the reactions below are reported voluntarily from a population of uncertain size, it is generally not possible to reliably estimate their frequency or establish a causal relationship to drug exposure.

The following additional adverse reactions have been identified during post-approval use of ZETIA:

Hypersensitivity reactions, including anaphylaxis, angioedema, rash, and urticaria; erythema multiforme; arthralgia; myalgia; elevated creatine phosphokinase; myopathy/rhabdomyolysis [see Warnings and Precautions (5.3)]; elevations in liver transaminases; hepatitis; abdominal pain; thrombocytopenia; pancreatitis; nausea; dizziness; paresthesia; depression; headache; cholelithiasis; cholecystitis.

7 DRUG INTERACTIONS

[See Clinical Pharmacology (12.3).]

7.1 Cyclosporine

Caution should be exercised when using ZETIA and cyclosporine concomitantly due to increased exposure to both ezetimibe and cyclosporine. Cyclosporine concentrations should be monitored in patients receiving ZETIA and cyclosporine.

The degree of increase in ezetimibe exposure may be greater in patients with severe renal insufficiency. In patients treated with cyclosporine, the potential effects of the increased exposure to ezetimibe from concomitant use should be carefully weighed against the benefits of alterations in lipid levels provided by ezetimibe.

7.2 Fibrates

The efficacy and safety of co-administration of ezetimibe with fibrates other than fenofibrate have not been studied. Fibrates may increase cholesterol excretion into the bile, leading to cholelithiasis. In a preclinical study in dogs, ezetimibe increased cholesterol in the gallbladder bile [see Nonclinical Toxicology (13.2)]. Co-administration of ZETIA with fibrates other than fenofibrate is not recommended until use in patients is adequately studied.

7.3 Fenofibrate

If cholelithiasis is suspected in a patient receiving ZETIA and fenofibrate, gallbladder studies are indicated and alternative lipid-lowering therapy should be considered [see Adverse Reactions (6.1) and the product labeling for fenofibrate].

7.4 Cholestyramine

Concomitant cholestyramine administration decreased the mean area under the curve (AUC) of total ezetimibe approximately 55%. The incremental LDL-C reduction due to adding ezetimibe to cholestyramine may be reduced by this interaction.

7.5 Coumarin Anticoagulants

If ezetimibe is added to warfarin, a coumarin anticoagulant, the International Normalized Ratio (INR) should be appropriately monitored.

8 USE IN SPECIFIC POPULATIONS

8.1 Pregnancy

Pregnancy Category C:

There are no adequate and well-controlled studies of ezetimibe in pregnant women. Ezetimibe should be used during pregnancy only if the potential benefit justifies the risk to the fetus.

In oral (gavage) embryo-fetal development studies of ezetimibe conducted in rats and rabbits during organogenesis, there was no evidence of embryolethal effects at the doses tested (250, 500, 1000 mg/kg/day). In rats, increased incidences of common fetal skeletal findings (extra pair of thoracic ribs, unossified cervical vertebral centra, shortened ribs) were observed at 1000 mg/kg/day (~10 × the human exposure at 10 mg daily based on AUC_{0-24hr} for total ezetimibe). In rabbits treated with ezetimibe, an increased incidence of extra thoracic ribs was observed at 1000 mg/kg/day (150 × the human exposure at 10 mg daily based on AUC_{0-24hr} for total ezetimibe). Ezetimibe crossed the placenta when pregnant rats and rabbits were given multiple oral doses.

Multiple-dose studies of ezetimibe given in combination with statins in rats and rabbits during organogenesis result in higher ezetimibe and statin exposures. Reproductive findings occur at lower doses in combination therapy compared to monotherapy.

All statins are contraindicated in pregnant and nursing women. When ZETIA is administered with a statin in a woman of childbearing potential, refer to the pregnancy category and product labeling for the statin. [See Contraindications (4).]

8.3 Nursing Mothers

It is not known whether ezetimibe is excreted into human breast milk. In rat studies, exposure to total ezetimibe in nursing pups was up to half of that observed in maternal plasma. Because many drugs are excreted in human milk, caution should be exercised when ZETIA is administered to a nursing woman. ZETIA should not be used in nursing mothers unless the potential benefit justifies the potential risk to the infant.

8.4 Pediatric Use

The effects of ZETIA co-administered with simvastatin (n=126) compared to simvastatin monotherapy (n=122) have been evaluated in adolescent boys and girls with heterozygous familial hypercholesterolemia (HeFH). In a multicenter, double-blind, controlled study followed by an open-label phase, 142 boys and 106 postmenarchal girls, 10 to 17 years of age (mean age 14.2 years, 43% females, 82% Caucasians, 4% Asian, 2% Blacks, 13% multi-racial) with HeFH were randomized to receive either ZETIA co-administered with simvastatin or simvastatin monotherapy. Inclusion in the study required 1) a baseline LDL-C level between 160 and 400 mg/dL and 2) a medical history and clinical presentation consistent with HeFH. The mean baseline LDL-C value was 225 mg/dL (range: 161–351 mg/dL) in the ZETIA co-administered with simvastatin group compared to 219 mg/dL (range: 149–336 mg/dL) in the simvastatin monotherapy group. The patients received co-administered ZETIA and simvastatin (10 mg, 20 mg, or 40 mg) or simvastatin monotherapy (10 mg, 20 mg, or 40 mg) for 6 weeks, co-administered ZETIA and 40 mg simvastatin or 40 mg simvastatin monotherapy for the next 27 weeks, and open-label co-administered ZETIA and simvastatin (10 mg, 20 mg, or 40 mg) for 20 weeks thereafter.

The results of the study at Week 6 are summarized in Table 3. Results at Week 33 were consistent with those at Week 6.

[See table 3 at left]

TABLE 3: Mean Percent Difference at Week 6 Between the Pooled ZETIA Co-Administered with Simvastatin Group and the Pooled Simvastatin Monotherapy Group in Adolescent Patients with Heterozygous Familial Hypercholesterolemia

	Total-C	LDL-C	Apo B	Non-HDL-C	TG*	HDL-C
Mean percent difference between treatment groups	-12%	-15%	-12%	-14%	-2%	+0.1%
95% Confidence Interval	(-15%, -9%)	(-18%, -12%)	(-15%, -9%)	(-17%, -11%)	(-9%, +4%)	(-3%, +3%)

*For triglycerides, median % change from baseline

From the start of the trial to the end of Week 33, discontinuations due to an adverse reaction occurred in 7 (6%) patients in the ZETIA co-administered with simvastatin group and in 2 (2%) patients in the simvastatin monotherapy group.

During the trial, hepatic transaminase elevations (two consecutive measurements for ALT and/or AST ≥3 × ULN) occurred in four (3%) individuals in the ZETIA co-administered with simvastatin group and in two (2%) individuals in the simvastatin monotherapy group. Elevations of CPK (≥10 × ULN) occurred in two (2%) individuals in the ZETIA co-administered with simvastatin group and in zero individuals in the simvastatin monotherapy group.

In this limited controlled study, there was no significant effect on growth or sexual maturation in the adolescent boys or girls, or on menstrual cycle length in girls.

Co-administration of ZETIA with simvastatin at doses greater than 40 mg/day has not been studied in adolescents. Also, ZETIA has not been studied in patients younger than 10 years of age or in pre-menarchal girls.

Based on total ezetimibe (ezetimibe + ezetimibe-glucuronide), there are no pharmacokinetic differences between adolescents and adults. Pharmacokinetic data in the pediatric population <10 years of age are not available.

8.5 Geriatric Use

Monotherapy Studies

Of the 2396 patients who received ZETIA in clinical studies, 669 (28%) were 65 and older, and 111 (5%) were 75 and older.

Statin Co-Administration Studies

Of the 11,308 patients who received ZETIA + statin in clinical studies, 3587 (32%) were 65 and older, and 924 (8%) were 75 and older.

No overall differences in safety and effectiveness were observed between these patients and younger patients, and other reported clinical experience has not identified differences in responses between the elderly and younger patients, but greater sensitivity of some older individuals cannot be ruled out *[see Clinical Pharmacology (12.3)]*.

8.6 Hepatic Impairment

ZETIA is not recommended in patients with moderate to severe hepatic impairment *[see Warnings and Precautions (5.4) and Clinical Pharmacology (12.3)]*.

ZETIA given concomitantly with a statin is contraindicated in patients with active liver disease or unexplained persistent elevations of hepatic transaminase levels *[see Contraindications (4); Warnings and Precautions (5.2) and Clinical Pharmacology (12.3)]*.

10 OVERDOSAGE

In clinical studies, administration of ezetimibe, 50 mg/day to 15 healthy subjects for up to 14 days, or 40 mg/day to 18 patients with primary hyperlipidemia for up to 56 days, was generally well tolerated.

A few cases of overdosage with ZETIA have been reported; most have not been associated with adverse experiences. Reported adverse experiences have not been serious. In the event of an overdose, symptomatic and supportive measures should be employed.

11 DESCRIPTION

ZETIA (ezetimibe) is in a class of lipid-lowering compounds that selectively inhibits the intestinal absorption of cholesterol and related phytosterols. The chemical name of ezetimibe is 1-(4-fluorophenyl)-3(R)-[3-(4-fluorophenyl)-3(S)-hydroxypropyl]-4(S)-(4-hydroxyphenyl)-2-azetidinone. The empirical formula is $C_{24}H_{21}F_2NO_3$. Its molecular weight is 409.4 and its structural formula is:

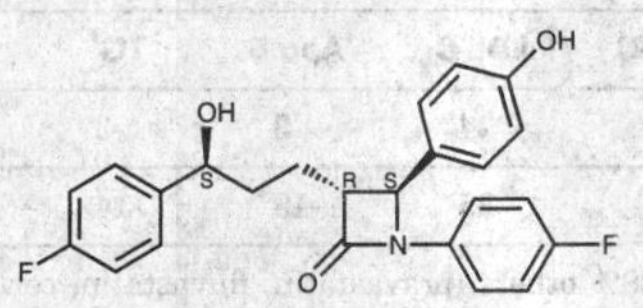

Ezetimibe is a white, crystalline powder that is freely to very soluble in ethanol, methanol, and acetone and practically insoluble in water. Ezetimibe has a melting point of about 163°C and is stable at ambient temperature. ZETIA is available as a tablet for oral administration containing 10 mg of ezetimibe and the following inactive ingredients: *croscarmellose sodium NF, lactose monohydrate NF*, magnesium stearate NF, microcrystalline cellulose NF, povidone USP, and sodium lauryl sulfate NF.

12 CLINICAL PHARMACOLOGY

12.1 Mechanism of Action

Ezetimibe reduces blood cholesterol by inhibiting the absorption of cholesterol by the small intestine. In a 2-week clinical study in 18 hypercholesterolemic patients, ZETIA inhibited intestinal cholesterol absorption by 54%, compared with placebo. ZETIA had no clinically meaningful effect on the plasma concentrations of the fat-soluble vitamins A, D, and E (in a study of 113 patients), and did not impair adrenocortical steroid hormone production (in a study of 118 patients).

The cholesterol content of the liver is derived predominantly from three sources. The liver can synthesize cholesterol, take up cholesterol from the blood from circulating lipoproteins, or take up cholesterol absorbed by the small intestine. Intestinal cholesterol is derived primarily from cholesterol secreted in the bile and from dietary cholesterol.

Ezetimibe has a mechanism of action that differs from those of other classes of cholesterol-reducing compounds (statins, bile acid sequestrants [resins], fibric acid derivatives, and plant stanols). The molecular target of ezetimibe has been shown to be the sterol transporter, Niemann-Pick C1-Like 1 (NPC1L1), which is involved in the intestinal uptake of cholesterol and phytosterols.

Ezetimibe does not inhibit cholesterol synthesis in the liver, or increase bile acid excretion. Instead, ezetimibe localizes at the brush border of the small intestine and inhibits the absorption of cholesterol, leading to a decrease in the delivery of intestinal cholesterol to the liver. This causes a reduction of hepatic cholesterol stores and an increase in clearance of cholesterol from the blood; this distinct mechanism is complementary to that of statins and of fenofibrate *[see Clinical Studies (14.1)]*.

12.2 Pharmacodynamics

Clinical studies have demonstrated that elevated levels of total-C, LDL-C and Apo B, the major protein constituent of LDL, promote human atherosclerosis. In addition, decreased levels of HDL-C are associated with the development of atherosclerosis. Epidemiologic studies have established that cardiovascular morbidity and mortality vary directly with the level of total-C and LDL-C and inversely with the level of HDL-C. Like LDL, cholesterol-enriched triglyceride-rich lipoproteins, including very-low-density lipoproteins (VLDL), intermediate-density lipoproteins (IDL), and remnants, can also promote atherosclerosis. The independent effect of raising HDL-C or lowering TG on the risk of coronary and cardiovascular morbidity and mortality has not been determined.

ZETIA reduces total-C, LDL-C, Apo B, and TG, and increases HDL-C in patients with hyperlipidemia. Administration of ZETIA with a statin is effective in improving serum total-C, LDL-C, Apo B, TG, and HDL-C beyond either treatment alone. Administration of ZETIA with fenofibrate is effective in improving serum total-C, LDL-C, Apo B, and non-HDL-C in patients with mixed hyperlipidemia as compared to either treatment alone. The effects of ezetimibe given either alone or in addition to a statin or fenofibrate on cardiovascular morbidity and mortality have not been established.

12.3 Pharmacokinetics

Absorption

After oral administration, ezetimibe is absorbed and extensively conjugated to a pharmacologically active phenolic glucuronide (ezetimibe-glucuronide). After a single 10-mg dose of ZETIA to fasted adults, mean ezetimibe peak plasma concentrations (C_{max}) of 3.4 to 5.5 ng/mL were attained within 4 to 12 hours (T_{max}). Ezetimibe-glucuronide mean C_{max} values of 45 to 71 ng/mL were achieved between 1 and 2 hours (T_{max}). There was no substantial deviation from dose proportionality between 5 and 20 mg. The absolute bioavailability of ezetimibe cannot be determined, as the compound is virtually insoluble in aqueous media suitable for injection.

Effect of Food on Oral Absorption

Concomitant food administration (high-fat or non-fat meals) had no effect on the extent of absorption of ezetimibe when administered as ZETIA 10-mg tablets. The C_{max} value of ezetimibe was increased by 38% with consumption of high-fat meals. ZETIA can be administered with or without food.

Distribution

Ezetimibe and ezetimibe-glucuronide are highly bound (>90%) to human plasma proteins.

Metabolism and Excretion

Ezetimibe is primarily metabolized in the small intestine and liver via glucuronide conjugation (a phase II reaction) with subsequent biliary and renal excretion. Minimal oxidative metabolism (a phase I reaction) has been observed in all species evaluated.

In humans, ezetimibe is rapidly metabolized to ezetimibe-glucuronide. Ezetimibe and ezetimibe-glucuronide are the major drug-derived compounds detected in plasma, constituting approximately 10 to 20% and 80 to 90% of the total drug in plasma, respectively. Both ezetimibe and ezetimibe-glucuronide are eliminated from plasma with a half-life of approximately 22 hours for both ezetimibe and ezetimibe-glucuronide. Plasma concentration-time profiles exhibit multiple peaks, suggesting enterohepatic recycling.

Following oral administration of ^{14}C-ezetimibe (20 mg) to human subjects, total ezetimibe (ezetimibe + ezetimibe-glucuronide) accounted for approximately 93% of the total radioactivity in plasma. After 48 hours, there were no detectable levels of radioactivity in the plasma.

Approximately 78% and 11% of the administered radioactivity were recovered in the feces and urine, respectively, over a 10-day collection period. Ezetimibe was the major component in feces and accounted for 69% of the administered dose, while ezetimibe-glucuronide was the major component in urine and accounted for 9% of the administered dose.

Specific Populations

Geriatric Patients: In a multiple-dose study with ezetimibe given 10 mg once daily for 10 days, plasma concentrations for total ezetimibe were about 2-fold higher in older (≥65 years) healthy subjects compared to younger subjects.

Pediatric Patients: *[See Use in Specific Populations (8.4).]*

Gender: In a multiple-dose study with ezetimibe given 10 mg once daily for 10 days, plasma concentrations for total ezetimibe were slightly higher (<20%) in women than in men.

Race: Based on a meta-analysis of multiple-dose pharmacokinetic studies, there were no pharmacokinetic differences between Black and Caucasian subjects. Studies in Asian subjects indicated that the pharmacokinetics of ezetimibe were similar to those seen in Caucasian subjects.

Hepatic Impairment: After a single 10-mg dose of ezetimibe, the mean AUC for total ezetimibe was increased approximately 1.7-fold in patients with mild hepatic impairment (Child-Pugh score 5 to 6), compared to healthy subjects. The mean AUC values for total ezetimibe and ezetimibe were increased approximately 3- to 4-fold and 5- to 6-fold, respectively, in patients with moderate (Child-Pugh score 7 to 9) or severe hepatic impairment (Child-Pugh score 10 to 15). In a 14-day, multiple-dose study (10 mg daily) in patients with moderate hepatic impairment, the mean AUC values for total ezetimibe and ezetimibe were increased approximately 4-fold on Day 1 and Day 14 compared to healthy subjects. Due to the unknown effects of the increased exposure to ezetimibe in patients with moderate or severe hepatic impairment, ZETIA is not recommended in these patients *[see Warnings and Precautions (5.4)]*.

Renal Impairment: After a single 10-mg dose of ezetimibe in patients with severe renal disease (n=8; mean CrCl ≤30 mL/min/1.73 m^2), the mean AUC values for total ezetimibe, ezetimibe-glucuronide, and ezetimibe were increased approximately 1.5-fold, compared to healthy subjects (n=9).

Drug Interactions [See also Drug Interactions (7)]

ZETIA had no significant effect on a series of probe drugs (caffeine, dextromethorphan, tolbutamide, and IV midazolam) known to be metabolized by cytochrome P450 (1A2, 2D6, 2C8/9 and 3A4) in a "cocktail" study of twelve healthy adult males. This indicates that ezetimibe is neither an inhibitor nor an inducer of these cytochrome P450 isozymes, and it is unlikely that ezetimibe will affect the metabolism of drugs that are metabolized by these enzymes.

TABLE 4: Effect of Co-Administered Drugs on Total Ezetimibe

Co-Administered Drug and Dosing Regimen	Total Ezetimibe* Change in AUC	Change in C_{max}
Cyclosporine-stable dose required (75–150 mg BID)[†,‡]	↑240%	↑290%
Fenofibrate, 200 mg QD, 14 days[†]	↑48%	↑64%
Gemfibrozil, 600 mg BID, 7 days[†]	↑64%	↑91%
Cholestyramine, 4 g BID, 14 days[†]	↓55%	↓4%
Aluminum & magnesium hydroxide combination antacid, single dose[§]	↓4%	↓30%
Cimetidine, 400 mg BID, 7 days	↑6%	↑22%
Glipizide, 10 mg, single dose	↑4%	↓8%
Statins		
Lovastatin 20 mg QD, 7 days	↑9%	↑3%
Pravastatin 20 mg QD, 14 days	↑7%	↑23%
Atorvastatin 10 mg QD, 14 days	↓2%	↑12%

Rosuvastatin 10 mg QD, 14 days	↑13%	↑18%
Fluvastatin 20 mg QD, 14 days	↓19%	↑7%

* Based on 10 mg dose of ezetimibe
† See Drug Interactions (7)
‡ Post-renal transplant patients with mild impaired or normal renal function. In a different study, a renal transplant patient with severe renal insufficiency (creatinine clearance of 13.2 mL/min/1.73 m²) who was receiving multiple medications, including cyclosporine, demonstrated a 12-fold greater exposure to total ezetimibe compared to healthy subjects.
§ Supralox®, 20 mL

[See table 5 at right]

13 NONCLINICAL TOXICOLOGY
13.1 Carcinogenesis, Mutagenesis, Impairment of Fertility
A 104-week dietary carcinogenicity study with ezetimibe was conducted in rats at doses up to 1500 mg/kg/day (males) and 500 mg/kg/day (females) (~20 × the human exposure at 10 mg daily based on AUC_{0-24hr} for total ezetimibe). A 104-week dietary carcinogenicity study with ezetimibe was also conducted in mice at doses up to 500 mg/kg/day (>150 × the human exposure at 10 mg daily based on AUC_{0-24hr} for total ezetimibe). There were no statistically significant increases in tumor incidences in drug-treated rats or mice.

No evidence of mutagenicity was observed *in vitro* in a microbial mutagenicity (Ames) test with *Salmonella typhimurium* and *Escherichia coli* with or without metabolic activation. No evidence of clastogenicity was observed *in vitro* in a chromosomal aberration assay in human peripheral blood lymphocytes with or without metabolic activation. In addition, there was no evidence of genotoxicity in the *in vivo* mouse micronucleus test.

In oral (gavage) fertility studies of ezetimibe conducted in rats, there was no evidence of reproductive toxicity at doses up to 1000 mg/kg/day in male or female rats (~7 × the human exposure at 10 mg daily based on AUC_{0-24hr} for total ezetimibe).

13.2 Animal Toxicology and/or Pharmacology
The hypocholesterolemic effect of ezetimibe was evaluated in cholesterol-fed Rhesus monkeys, dogs, rats, and mouse models of human cholesterol metabolism. Ezetimibe was found to have an ED_{50} value of 0.5 µg/kg/day for inhibiting the rise in plasma cholesterol levels in monkeys. The ED_{50} values in dogs, rats, and mice were 7, 30, and 700 µg/kg/day, respectively. These results are consistent with ZETIA being a potent cholesterol absorption inhibitor.

In a rat model, where the glucuronide metabolite of ezetimibe (SCH 60663) was administered intraduodenally, the metabolite was as potent as the parent compound (SCH 58235) in inhibiting the absorption of cholesterol, suggesting that the glucuronide metabolite had activity similar to the parent drug.

In 1-month studies in dogs given ezetimibe (0.03 to 300 mg/kg/day), the concentration of cholesterol in gallbladder bile increased ~2- to 4-fold. However, a dose of 300 mg/kg/day administered to dogs for one year did not result in gallstone formation or any other adverse hepatobiliary effects. In a 14-day study in mice given ezetimibe (0.3 to 5 mg/kg/day) and fed a low-fat or cholesterol-rich diet, the concentration of cholesterol in gallbladder bile was either unaffected or reduced to normal levels, respectively.

A series of acute preclinical studies was performed to determine the selectivity of ZETIA for inhibiting cholesterol absorption. Ezetimibe inhibited the absorption of ¹⁴C-cholesterol with no effect on the absorption of triglycerides, fatty acids, bile acids, progesterone, ethinyl estradiol, or the fat-soluble vitamins A and D.

In 4- to 12-week toxicity studies in mice, ezetimibe did not induce cytochrome P450 drug metabolizing enzymes. In toxicity studies, a pharmacokinetic interaction of ezetimibe with statins (parents or their active hydroxy acid metabolites) was seen in rats, dogs, and rabbits.

14 CLINICAL STUDIES
14.1 Primary Hyperlipidemia
ZETIA reduces total-C, LDL-C, Apo B, and TG, and increases HDL-C in patients with hyperlipidemia. Maximal to near maximal response is generally achieved within 2 weeks and maintained during chronic therapy.

Monotherapy
In two multicenter, double-blind, placebo-controlled, 12-week studies in 1719 patients with primary hyperlipidemia, ZETIA significantly lowered total-C, LDL-C, Apo B, and TG, and increased HDL-C compared to placebo (see **Table 6**). Reduction in LDL-C was consistent across age, sex, and baseline LDL-C.
[See table 6 above]

Combination with Statins
ZETIA Added to On-going Statin Therapy
In a multicenter, double-blind, placebo-controlled, 8-week study, 769 patients with primary hyperlipidemia, known coronary heart disease or multiple cardiovascular risk factors who were already receiving statin monotherapy, but who had not met their NCEP ATP II target LDL-C goal were randomized to receive either ZETIA or placebo in addition to their on-going statin.
ZETIA, added to on-going statin therapy, significantly lowered total-C, LDL-C, Apo B, and TG, and increased HDL-C

compared with a statin administered alone (see **Table 7**). LDL-C reductions induced by ZETIA were generally consistent across all statins.
[See table 7 above]
ZETIA Initiated Concurrently with a Statin
In four multicenter, double-blind, placebo-controlled, 12-week trials, in 2382 hyperlipidemic patients, ZETIA or placebo was administered alone or with various doses of atorvastatin, simvastatin, pravastatin, or lovastatin.
When all patients receiving ZETIA with a statin were compared to all those receiving the corresponding statin alone,

TABLE 5: Effect of Ezetimibe Co-Administration on Systemic Exposure to Other Drugs

Co-Administered Drug and its Dosage Regimen	Ezetimibe Dosage Regimen	Change in AUC of Co-Administered Drug	Change in C_{max} of Co-Administered Drug
Warfarin, 25 mg single dose on day 7	10 mg QD, 11 days	↓2% (R-warfarin) ↓4% (S-warfarin)	↑3% (R-warfarin) ↑1% (S-warfarin)
Digoxin, 0.5 mg single dose	10 mg QD, 8 days	↑2%	↓7%
Gemfibrozil, 600 mg BID, 7 days*	10 mg QD, 7 days	↓1%	↓11%
Ethinyl estradiol & Levonorgestrel, QD, 21 days	10 mg QD, days 8–14 of 21d oral contraceptive cycle	Ethinyl estradiol 0% Levonorgestrel 0%	Ethinyl estradiol ↓9% Levonorgestrel ↓5%
Glipizide, 10 mg on days 1 and 9	10 mg QD, days 2–9	↓3%	↓5%
Fenofibrate, 200 mg QD, 14 days*	10 mg QD, 14 days	↑11%	↑7%
Cyclosporine, 100 mg single dose day 7*	20 mg QD, 8 days	↑15%	↑10%
Statins			
Lovastatin 20 mg QD, 7 days	10 mg QD, 7 days	↑19%	↑3%
Pravastatin 20 mg QD, 14 days	10 mg QD, 14 days	↓20%	↓24%
Atorvastatin 10 mg QD, 14 days	10 mg QD, 14 days	↓4%	↑7%
Rosuvastatin 10 mg QD, 14 days	10 mg QD, 14 days	↑19%	↑17%
Fluvastatin 20 mg QD, 14 days	10 mg QD, 14 days	↓39%	↓27%

*See Drug Interactions (7)

TABLE 6: Response to ZETIA in Patients with Primary Hyperlipidemia (Mean* % Change from Untreated Baseline[†])

Treatment Group		N	Total-C	LDL-C	Apo B	TG*	HDL-C
Study 1[‡]	Placebo	205	+1	+1	-1	-1	-1
	Ezetimibe	622	-12	-18	-15	-7	+1
Study 2[‡]	Placebo	226	+1	+1	-1	+2	-2
	Ezetimibe	666	-12	-18	-16	-9	+1
Pooled Data[‡] (Studies 1 & 2)	Placebo	431	0	+1	-2	0	-2
	Ezetimibe	1288	-13	-18	-16	-8	+1

* For triglycerides, median % change from baseline
† Baseline - on no lipid-lowering drug
‡ ZETIA significantly reduced total-C, LDL-C, Apo B, and TG, and increased HDL-C compared to placebo.

TABLE 7: Response to Addition of ZETIA to On-Going Statin Therapy* in Patients with Hyperlipidemia (Mean[†] % Change from Treated Baseline[‡])

Treatment (Daily Dose)	N	Total-C	LDL-C	Apo B	TG[†]	HDL-C
On-going Statin + Placebo[§]	390	-2	-4	-3	-3	+1
On-going Statin + ZETIA[§]	379	-17	-25	-19	-14	+3

* Patients receiving each statin: 40% atorvastatin, 31% simvastatin, 29% others (pravastatin, fluvastatin, cerivastatin, lovastatin)
† For triglycerides, median % change from baseline
‡ Baseline - on a statin alone
§ ZETIA + statin significantly reduced total-C, LDL-C, Apo B, and TG, and increased HDL-C compared to statin alone.

TABLE 8: Response to ZETIA and Atorvastatin Initiated Concurrently in Patients with Primary Hyperlipidemia (Mean* % Change from Untreated Baseline†)

Treatment (Daily Dose)	N	Total-C	LDL-C	Apo B	TG*	HDL-C
Placebo	60	+4	+4	+3	-6	+4
ZETIA	65	-14	-20	-15	-5	+4
Atorvastatin 10 mg	60	-26	-37	-28	-21	+6
ZETIA + Atorvastatin 10 mg	65	-38	-53	-43	-31	+9
Atorvastatin 20 mg	60	-30	-42	-34	-23	+4
ZETIA + Atorvastatin 20 mg	62	-39	-54	-44	-30	+9
Atorvastatin 40 mg	66	-32	-45	-37	-24	+4
ZETIA + Atorvastatin 40 mg	65	-42	-56	-45	-34	+5
Atorvastatin 80 mg	62	-40	-54	-46	-31	+3
ZETIA + Atorvastatin 80 mg	63	-46	-61	-50	-40	+7
Pooled data (All Atorvastatin Doses)‡	248	-32	-44	-36	-24	+4
Pooled data (All ZETIA + Atorvastatin Doses)‡	255	-41	-56	-45	-33	+7

* For triglycerides, median % change from baseline
† Baseline - on no lipid-lowering drug
‡ ZETIA + all doses of atorvastatin pooled (10–80 mg) significantly reduced total-C, LDL-C, Apo B, and TG, and increased HDL-C compared to all doses of atorvastatin pooled (10–80 mg).

TABLE 9: Response to ZETIA and Simvastatin Initiated Concurrently in Patients with Primary Hyperlipidemia (Mean* % Change from Untreated Baseline†)

Treatment (Daily Dose)	N	Total-C	LDL-C	Apo B	TG*	HDL-C
Placebo	70	-1	-1	0	+2	+1
ZETIA	61	-13	-19	-14	-11	+5
Simvastatin 10 mg	70	-18	-27	-21	-14	+8
ZETIA + Simvastatin 10 mg	67	-32	-46	-35	-26	+9
Simvastatin 20 mg	61	-26	-36	-29	-18	+6
ZETIA + Simvastatin 20 mg	69	-33	-46	-36	-25	+9
Simvastatin 40 mg	65	-27	-38	-32	-24	+6
ZETIA + Simvastatin 40 mg	73	-40	-56	-45	-32	+11
Simvastatin 80 mg	67	-32	-45	-37	-23	+8
ZETIA + Simvastatin 80 mg	65	-41	-58	-47	-31	+8
Pooled data (All Simvastatin Doses)‡	263	-26	-36	-30	-20	+7
Pooled data (All ZETIA + Simvastatin Doses)‡	274	-37	-51	-41	-29	+9

* For triglycerides, median % change from baseline
† Baseline - on no lipid-lowering drug
‡ ZETIA + all doses of simvastatin pooled (10–80 mg) significantly reduced total-C, LDL-C, Apo B, and TG, and increased HDL-C compared to all doses of simvastatin pooled (10–80 mg).

ZETIA significantly lowered total-C, LDL-C, Apo B, and TG, and, with the exception of pravastatin, increased HDL-C compared to the statin administered alone. LDL-C reductions induced by ZETIA were generally consistent across all statins. (See footnote‡, **Tables 8 to 11**.)
[See table 8 above]
[See table 9 above]
[See table 10 at top of next page]
[See table 11 on next page]
Combination with Fenofibrate
In a multicenter, double-blind, placebo-controlled, clinical study in patients with mixed hyperlipidemia, 625 patients were treated for up to 12 weeks and 576 for up to an additional 48 weeks. Patients were randomized to receive placebo, ZETIA alone, 160 mg fenofibrate alone, or ZETIA plus 160 mg fenofibrate in the 12-week study. After completing the 12-week study, eligible patients were assigned to ZETIA co-administered with fenofibrate or fenofibrate monotherapy for an additional 48 weeks.
ZETIA co-administered with fenofibrate significantly lowered total-C, LDL-C, Apo B, and non-HDL-C compared to fenofibrate administered alone. The percent decrease in TG and percent increase in HDL-C for ZETIA co-administered with fenofibrate were comparable to those for fenofibrate administered alone (see **Table 12**).

[See table 12 on next page]
The changes in lipid endpoints after an additional 48 weeks of treatment with ZETIA co-administered with fenofibrate or with fenofibrate alone were consistent with the 12-week data displayed above.

14.2   Homozygous Familial Hypercholesterolemia (HoFH)
A study was conducted to assess the efficacy of ZETIA in the treatment of HoFH. This double-blind, randomized, 12-week study enrolled 50 patients with a clinical and/or genotypic diagnosis of HoFH, with or without concomitant LDL apheresis, already receiving atorvastatin or simvastatin (40 mg). Patients were randomized to one of three treatment groups, atorvastatin or simvastatin (80 mg), ZETIA administered with atorvastatin or simvastatin (40 mg), or ZETIA administered with atorvastatin or simvastatin (80 mg). Due to decreased bioavailability of ezetimibe in patients concomitantly receiving cholestyramine *[see Drug Interactions (7.1)]*, ezetimibe was dosed at least 4 hours before or after administration of resins. Mean baseline LDL-C was 341 mg/dL in those patients randomized to atorvastatin 80 mg or simvastatin 80 mg alone and 316 mg/dL in the group randomized to ZETIA plus atorvastatin 40 or 80 mg or simvastatin 40 or 80 mg. ZETIA, administered with atorvastatin or simvastatin (40 and 80 mg statin groups,

pooled), significantly reduced LDL-C (21%) compared with increasing the dose of simvastatin or atorvastatin monotherapy from 40 to 80 mg (7%). In those treated with ZETIA plus 80 mg atorvastatin or with ZETIA plus 80 mg simvastatin, LDL-C was reduced by 27%.

14.3   Homozygous Sitosterolemia (Phytosterolemia)
A study was conducted to assess the efficacy of ZETIA in the treatment of homozygous sitosterolemia. In this multi-center, double-blind, placebo-controlled, 8-week trial, 37 patients with homozygous sitosterolemia with elevated plasma sitosterol levels (>5 mg/dL) on their current therapeutic regimen (diet, bile-acid-binding resins, statins, ileal bypass surgery and/or LDL apheresis), were randomized to receive ZETIA (n=30) or placebo (n=7). Due to decreased bioavailability of ezetimibe in patients concomitantly receiving cholestyramine *[see Drug Interactions (7.1)]*, ezetimibe was dosed at least 2 hours before or 4 hours after resins were administered. Excluding the one subject receiving LDL apheresis, ZETIA significantly lowered plasma sitosterol and campesterol, by 21% and 24% from baseline, respectively. In contrast, patients who received placebo had increases in sitosterol and campesterol of 4% and 3% from baseline, respectively. For patients treated with ZETIA, mean plasma levels of plant sterols were reduced progressively over the course of the study. The effects of reducing plasma sitosterol and campesterol on reducing the risks of cardiovascular morbidity and mortality have not been established.
Reductions in sitosterol and campesterol were consistent between patients taking ZETIA concomitantly with bile acid sequestrants (n=8) and patients not on concomitant bile acid sequestrant therapy (n=21).

Limitations of Use
The effect of ZETIA on cardiovascular morbidity and mortality has not been determined.

16   HOW SUPPLIED/STORAGE AND HANDLING
No. 3861—Tablets ZETIA, 10 mg, are white to off-white, capsule-shaped tablets debossed with "414" on one side. They are supplied as follows:
NDC 66582-414-31 bottles of 30
NDC 66582-414-54 bottles of 90
NDC 66582-414-74 bottles of 500
NDC 66582-414-76 bottles of 5000
NDC 66582-414-28 unit dose packages of 100.
Storage
Store at 25°C (77°F); excursions permitted to 15–30°C (59–86°F). [See USP Controlled Room Temperature.] Protect from moisture.

17   PATIENT COUNSELING INFORMATION
[See FDA-approved Patient Labeling (17.5).]
Patients should be advised to adhere to their National Cholesterol Education Program (NCEP)-recommended diet, a regular exercise program, and periodic testing of a fasting lipid panel.

17.1   Muscle Pain
All patients starting therapy with ezetimibe should be advised of the risk of myopathy and told to report promptly any unexplained muscle pain, tenderness or weakness. The risk of this occurring is increased when taking certain types of medication. Patients should discuss all medication, both prescription and over-the-counter, with their physician.

17.2   Liver Enzymes
Liver tests should be performed when ZETIA is added to statin therapy and according to statin recommendations.

17.3   Pregnancy
Women of childbearing age should be advised to use an effective method of birth control to prevent pregnancy while using ZETIA added to statin therapy. Discuss future pregnancy plans with your patients, and discuss when to stop combination ZETIA and statin therapy if they are trying to conceive. Patients should be advised that if they become pregnant they should stop taking combination ZETIA and statin therapy and call their healthcare professional.

17.4   Breastfeeding
Women who are breastfeeding should be advised to not use ZETIA added to statin therapy. Patients who have a lipid disorder and are breastfeeding should be advised to discuss the options with their healthcare professionals.

17.5   FDA-approved Patient Labeling
32147054T
REV 21
Issued July 2009
U.S. Patent Nos. 5,846,966; 7,030,106 and RE37,721.
Manufactured for:
Merck/Schering-Plough Pharmaceuticals
North Wales, PA 19454, USA
By:
Schering Corporation
Kenilworth, NJ 07033, USA
or
Merck & Co., Inc.
Whitehouse Station, NJ 08889, USA

TABLE 10: Response to ZETIA and Pravastatin Initiated Concurrently in Patients with Primary Hyperlipidemia
(Mean* % Change from Untreated Baseline†)

Treatment (Daily Dose)	N	Total-C	LDL-C	Apo B	TG*	HDL-C
Placebo	65	0	-1	-2	-1	+2
ZETIA	64	-13	-20	-15	-5	+4
Pravastatin 10 mg	66	-15	-21	-16	-14	+6
ZETIA + Pravastatin 10 mg	71	-24	-34	-27	-23	+8
Pravastatin 20 mg	69	-15	-23	-18	-8	+8
ZETIA + Pravastatin 20 mg	66	-27	-40	-31	-21	+8
Pravastatin 40 mg	70	-22	-31	-26	-19	+6
ZETIA + Pravastatin 40 mg	67	-30	-42	-32	-21	+8
Pooled data (All Pravastatin Doses)‡	205	-17	-25	-20	-14	+7
Pooled data (All ZETIA + Pravastatin Doses)‡	204	-27	-39	-30	-21	+8

* For triglycerides, median % change from baseline
† Baseline - on no lipid-lowering drug
‡ ZETIA + all doses of pravastatin pooled (10–40 mg) significantly reduced total-C, LDL-C, Apo B, and TG compared to all doses of pravastatin pooled (10–40 mg).

TABLE 11: Response to ZETIA and Lovastatin Initiated Concurrently in Patients with Primary Hyperlipidemia
(Mean* % Change from Untreated Baseline†)

Treatment (Daily Dose)	N	Total-C	LDL-C	Apo B	TG*	HDL-C
Placebo	64	+1	0	+1	+6	0
ZETIA	72	-13	-19	-14	-5	+3
Lovastatin 10 mg	73	-15	-20	-17	-11	+5
ZETIA + Lovastatin 10 mg	65	-24	-34	-27	-19	+8
Lovastatin 20 mg	74	-19	-26	-21	-12	+3
ZETIA + Lovastatin 20 mg	62	-29	-41	-34	-27	+9
Lovastatin 40 mg	73	-21	-30	-25	-15	+5
ZETIA + Lovastatin 40 mg	65	-33	-46	-38	-27	+9
Pooled data (All Lovastatin Doses)‡	220	-18	-25	-21	-12	+4
Pooled data (All ZETIA + Lovastatin Doses)‡	192	-29	-40	-33	-25	+9

* For triglycerides, median % change from baseline
† Baseline - on no lipid-lowering drug
‡ ZETIA + all doses of lovastatin pooled (10–40 mg) significantly reduced total-C, LDL-C, Apo B, and TG, and increased HDL-C compared to all doses of lovastatin pooled (10–40 mg).

TABLE 12: Response to ZETIA and Fenofibrate Initiated Concurrently in Patients with Mixed Hyperlipidemia
(Mean* % Change from Untreated Baseline† at 12 weeks)

Treatment (Daily Dose)	N	Total-C	LDL-C	Apo B	TG*	HDL-C	Non-HDL-C
Placebo	63	0	0	-1	-9	+3	0
ZETIA	185	-12	-13	-11	-11	+4	-15
Fenofibrate 160 mg	188	-11	-6	-15	-43	+19	-16
ZETIA + Fenofibrate 160 mg	183	-22	-20	-26	-44	+19	-30

* For triglycerides, median % change from baseline
† Baseline - on no lipid-lowering drug

ZETIA® (ezetimibe) Tablets
Patient Information about ZETIA (zĕt´-ē-ă)
Generic name: ezetimibe (ĕ-zĕt´-ē-mīb)
Read this information carefully before you start taking ZETIA and each time you get more ZETIA. There may be new information. This information does not take the place of talking with your doctor about your medical condition or your treatment. If you have any questions about ZETIA, ask your doctor. Only your doctor can determine if ZETIA is right for you.
What is ZETIA?
ZETIA is a medicine used to lower levels of total cholesterol and LDL (bad) cholesterol in the blood. ZETIA is for patients who cannot control their cholesterol levels by diet and exercise alone. It can be used by itself or with other medicines to treat high cholesterol. You should stay on a cholesterol-lowering diet while taking this medicine.
ZETIA works to reduce the amount of cholesterol your body absorbs. ZETIA does not help you lose weight. ZETIA has not been shown to prevent heart disease or heart attacks. For more information about cholesterol, see the "What should I know about high cholesterol?"section that follows.
Who should not take ZETIA?
• Do not take ZETIA if you are allergic to ezetimibe, the active ingredient in ZETIA, or to the inactive ingredients. For a list of inactive ingredients, see the "Inactive ingredients"section that follows.

• If you have active liver disease, do not take ZETIA while taking cholesterol-lowering medicines called statins.
• If you are pregnant or breast-feeding, do not take ZETIA while taking a statin.
• If you are a woman of childbearing age, you should use an effective method of birth control to prevent pregnancy while using ZETIA added to statin therapy.
ZETIA has not been studied in children under age 10.
What should I tell my doctor before and while taking ZETIA?
Tell your doctor about any prescription and non-prescription medicines you are taking or plan to take, including natural or herbal remedies.
Tell your doctor about all your medical conditions including allergies.
Tell your doctor if you:
• ever had liver problems. ZETIA may not be right for you.
• are pregnant or plan to become pregnant. Your doctor will discuss with you whether ZETIA is right for you.
• are breast-feeding. We do not know if ZETIA can pass to your baby through your milk. Your doctor will discuss with you whether ZETIA is right for you.
• experience unexplained muscle pain, tenderness, or weakness.
How should I take ZETIA?
• Take ZETIA once a day, with or without food. It may be easier to remember to take your dose if you do it at the same time every day, such as with breakfast, dinner, or at bedtime. If you also take another medicine to reduce your cholesterol, ask your doctor if you can take them at the same time.
• If you forget to take ZETIA, take it as soon as you remember. However, do not take more than one dose of ZETIA a day.
• Continue to follow a cholesterol-lowering diet while taking ZETIA. Ask your doctor if you need diet information.
• Keep taking ZETIA unless your doctor tells you to stop. It is important that you keep taking ZETIA even if you do not feel sick.
See your doctor regularly to check your cholesterol level and to check for side effects. Your doctor may do blood tests to check your liver before you start taking ZETIA with a statin and during treatment.
What are the possible side effects of ZETIA?
In clinical studies patients reported few side effects while taking ZETIA. These included diarrhea, joint pains, and feeling tired.
Patients have experienced severe muscle problems while taking ZETIA, usually when ZETIA was added to a statin drug. If you experience unexplained muscle pain, tenderness, or weakness while taking ZETIA, contact your doctor immediately. You need to do this promptly, because on rare occasions, these muscle problems can be serious, with muscle breakdown resulting in kidney damage.
Additionally, the following side effects have been reported in general use: allergic reactions (which may require treatment right away) including swelling of the face, lips, tongue, and/or throat that may cause difficulty in breathing or swallowing, rash, and hives; raised red rash, sometimes with target-shaped lesions; joint pain; muscle aches; alterations in some laboratory blood tests; liver problems; stomach pain; inflammation of the pancreas; nausea; dizziness; tingling sensation; depression; headache; gallstones; inflammation of the gallbladder.
Tell your doctor if you are having these or any other medical problems while on ZETIA. For a complete list of side effects, ask your doctor or pharmacist.
What should I know about high cholesterol?
Cholesterol is a type of fat found in your blood. Your total cholesterol is made up of LDL and HDL cholesterol.
LDL cholesterol is called "bad" cholesterol because it can build up in the wall of your arteries and form plaque. Over time, plaque build-up can cause a narrowing of the arteries. This narrowing can slow or block blood flow to your heart, brain, and other organs. High LDL cholesterol is a major cause of heart disease and one of the causes for stroke.
HDL cholesterol is called "good" cholesterol because it keeps the bad cholesterol from building up in the arteries.
Triglycerides also are fats found in your blood.
General information about ZETIA
Medicines are sometimes prescribed for conditions that are not mentioned in patient information leaflets. Do not use ZETIA for a condition for which it was not prescribed. Do not give ZETIA to other people, even if they have the same condition you have. It may harm them.
This summarizes the most important information about ZETIA. If you would like more information, talk with your doctor. You can ask your pharmacist or doctor for information about ZETIA that is written for health professionals.
Inactive ingredients:
Croscarmellose sodium, lactose monohydrate, magnesium stearate, microcrystalline cellulose, povidone, and sodium lauryl sulfate.

29480885T
REV 21
Issued July 2009
U.S. Patent Nos. 5,846,966; 7,030,106 and RE37,721.
Manufactured for:
Merck/Schering-Plough Pharmaceuticals
North Wales, PA 19454, USA
By:
Schering Corporation
Kenilworth, NJ 07033, USA
or
Merck & Co., Inc.
Whitehouse Station, NJ 08889, USA
COPYRIGHT © 2001, 2002, 2007, 2008, 2009, Merck/
Schering-Plough Pharmaceuticals. All rights reserved.
Shown in Product Identification Guide, page 314

ZOCOR® ℞
[zō′kōr]
(simvastatin)
Tablets

HIGHLIGHTS OF PRESCRIBING INFORMATION
These highlights do not include all the information needed to use ZOCOR safely and effectively. See full prescribing information for ZOCOR.
ZOCOR (simvastatin) Tablets
Initial U.S. Approval: 1991

——————RECENT MAJOR CHANGES——————

Dosage and Administration
Chinese Patients Taking Lipid-Modifying Doses
(≥1 g/day Niacin) of Niacin-Containing
Products (2.5) — 03/2010
Coadministration with Other Drugs (2.6) — 03/2010
Warnings and Precautions
Myopathy/Rhabdomyolysis (5.1) — 03/2010

——————INDICATIONS AND USAGE——————

ZOCOR® is an HMG-CoA reductase inhibitor (statin) indicated as an adjunctive therapy to diet to:
• Reduce the risk of total mortality by reducing CHD deaths and reduce the risk of non-fatal myocardial infarction, stroke, and the need for revascularization procedures in patients at high risk of coronary events. (1.1)
• Reduce elevated total-C, LDL-C, Apo B, TG and increase HDL-C in patients with primary hyperlipidemia (heterozygous familial and nonfamilial) and mixed dyslipidemia. (1.2)
• Reduce elevated TG in patients with hypertriglyceridemia and reduce TG and VLDL-C in patients with primary dysbetalipoproteinemia. (1.2)
• Reduce total-C and LDL-C in adult patients with homozygous familial hypercholesterolemia. (1.2)
• Reduce elevated total-C, LDL-C, and Apo B in boys and postmenarchal girls, 10 to 17 years of age with heterozygous familial hypercholesterolemia after failing an adequate trial of diet therapy. (1.2, 1.3)

Limitations of Use
ZOCOR has not been studied in Fredrickson Types I and V dyslipidemias. (1.4)

——————DOSAGE AND ADMINISTRATION——————

• Dose range is 5-80 mg/day. (2.1)
• Recommended usual starting dose is 20-40 mg once a day in the evening. (2.1)
• Recommended starting dose for patients at high risk of CHD is 40 mg/day. (2.1)
• Adolescents (10-17 years of age) with HeFH: starting dose is 10 mg/day; maximum recommended dose is 40 mg/day. (2.3)

——————DOSAGE FORMS AND STRENGTHS——————

Tablets: 5 mg; 10 mg; 20 mg; 40 mg; 80 mg (3)

——————CONTRAINDICATIONS——————

• Hypersensitivity to any component of this medication. (4, 6.2)
• Active liver disease, which may include unexplained persistent elevations in hepatic transaminase levels. (4, 5.2)
• Women who are pregnant or may become pregnant. (4, 8.1)
• Nursing mothers. (4, 8.3)

——————WARNINGS AND PRECAUTIONS——————

• Skeletal muscle effects (e.g., myopathy and rhabdomyolysis): Risks increase with higher doses and concomitant use of certain CYP3A4 inhibitors, gemfibrozil, cyclosporine, danazol, amiodarone, verapamil and diltiazem. Predisposing factors include advanced age (≥65), uncontrolled hypothyroidism, and renal impairment. (5.1, 8.5, 8.6)
• Patients should be advised to report promptly any symptoms of myopathy. Simvastatin therapy should be discontinued immediately if myopathy is diagnosed or suspected. See Drug Interaction table. (5.1)
• Liver enzyme abnormalities and monitoring: Persistent elevations in hepatic transaminase can occur. Monitor liver enzymes before and during treatment. Patients titrated to the 80-mg dose should receive more frequent liver function tests than patients on lower doses. (5.2)

——————ADVERSE REACTIONS——————

Most common adverse reactions (incidence ≥5.0%) are: upper respiratory infection, headache, abdominal pain, constipation, and nausea. (6.1)

To report SUSPECTED ADVERSE REACTIONS, contact Merck Sharp & Dohme Corp., a subsidiary of Merck & Co., Inc., at 1-877-888-4231 or FDA at 1-800-FDA-1088 or www.fda.gov/medwatch.

——————DRUG INTERACTIONS——————

Drug Interactions Associated with Increased Risk of Myopathy/Rhabdomyolysis (2.6, 5.1, 7.1, 7.2, 7.3, 7.4)

Interacting Agents	Prescribing Recommendations
Itraconazole, ketoconazole, erythromycin, clarithromycin, telithromycin, HIV protease inhibitors, nefazodone	Avoid simvastatin
Gemfibrozil, cyclosporine, danazol	Do not exceed 10 mg simvastatin daily
Amiodarone, verapamil	Do not exceed 20 mg simvastatin daily
Diltiazem	Do not exceed 40 mg simvastatin daily
Grapefruit juice	Avoid large quantities of grapefruit juice (>1 quart daily)

• Coumarin anticoagulants: Concomitant use with ZOCOR prolongs INR. Achieve stable INR prior to starting ZOCOR. Monitor INR frequently until stable upon initiation or alteration of ZOCOR therapy. (7.7)

——————USE IN SPECIFIC POPULATIONS——————

• Severe renal impairment: patients should be started at 5 mg/day and be closely monitored. (2.4, 8.6)

See 17 for PATIENT COUNSELING INFORMATION
Revised: 05/2010

——————————————————————————————

FULL PRESCRIBING INFORMATION: CONTENTS*

——————————————————————————————

FULL PRESCRIBING INFORMATION

1 INDICATIONS AND USAGE

Therapy with lipid-altering agents should be only one component of multiple risk factor intervention in individuals at significantly increased risk for atherosclerotic vascular disease due to hypercholesterolemia. Drug therapy is indicated as an adjunct to diet when the response to a diet restricted in saturated fat and cholesterol and other nonpharmacologic measures alone has been inadequate. In patients with coronary heart disease (CHD) or at high risk of CHD, ZOCOR[1] can be started simultaneously with diet.

[1] Registered trademark of Merck Sharp & Dohme Corp., a subsidiary of Merck & Co., Inc.
Copyright © 1999-2008 Merck Sharp & Dohme Corp., a subsidiary of Merck & Co., Inc.
All rights reserved

1.1 Reductions in Risk of CHD Mortality and Cardiovascular Events

In patients at high risk of coronary events because of existing coronary heart disease, diabetes, peripheral vessel disease, history of stroke or other cerebrovascular disease, ZOCOR is indicated to:
• Reduce the risk of total mortality by reducing CHD deaths.
• Reduce the risk of non-fatal myocardial infarction and stroke.
• Reduce the need for coronary and non-coronary revascularization procedures.

1.2 Hyperlipidemia

ZOCOR is indicated to:
• Reduce elevated total cholesterol (total-C), low-density lipoprotein cholesterol (LDL-C), apolipoprotein B (Apo B), and triglycerides (TG), and to increase high-density lipoprotein cholesterol (HDL-C) in patients with primary hyperlipidemia (Fredrickson type IIa, heterozygous familial and nonfamilial) or mixed dyslipidemia (Fredrickson type IIb).
• Reduce elevated TG in patients with hypertriglyceridemia (Fredrickson type IV hyperlipidemia).
• Reduce elevated TG and VLDL-C in patients with primary dysbetalipoproteinemia (Fredrickson type III hyperlipidemia).
• Reduce total-C and LDL-C in patients with homozygous familial hypercholesterolemia as an adjunct to other lipid-lowering treatments (e.g., LDL apheresis) or if such treatments are unavailable.

1.3 Adolescent Patients with Heterozygous Familial Hypercholesterolemia (HeFH)

ZOCOR is indicated as an adjunct to diet to reduce total-C, LDL-C, and Apo B levels in adolescent boys and girls who are at least one year post-menarche, 10-17 years of age, with HeFH, if after an adequate trial of diet therapy the following findings are present:
1. LDL cholesterol remains ≥190 mg/dL; or
2. LDL cholesterol remains ≥160 mg/dL and
• There is a positive family history of premature cardiovascular disease (CVD) or
• Two or more other CVD risk factors are present in the adolescent patient.
The minimum goal of treatment in pediatric and adolescent patients is to achieve a mean LDL-C <130 mg/dL. The optimal age at which to initiate lipid-lowering therapy to decrease the risk of symptomatic adulthood CAD has not been determined.

1.4 Limitations of Use

ZOCOR has not been studied in conditions where the major abnormality is elevation of chylomicrons (i.e., hyperlipidemia Fredrickson types I and V).

2 DOSAGE AND ADMINISTRATION

2.1 Recommended Dosing

The dosage range is 5-80 mg/day. In patients with CHD or at high risk of CHD, ZOCOR can be started simultaneously with diet. The recommended usual starting dose is 20 to 40 mg once a day in the evening. For patients at high risk for a CHD event due to existing CHD, diabetes, peripheral vessel disease, history of stroke or other cerebrovascular disease, the recommended starting dose is 40 mg/day. Lipid determinations should be performed after 4 weeks of therapy and periodically thereafter.

2.2 Patients with Homozygous Familial Hypercholesterolemia

The recommended dosage is 40 mg/day in the evening or 80 mg/day in 3 divided doses of 20 mg, 20 mg, and an evening dose of 40 mg. ZOCOR should be used as an adjunct to other lipid-lowering treatments (e.g., LDL apheresis) in these patients or if such treatments are unavailable.

2.3 Adolescents (10-17 years of age) with Heterozygous Familial Hypercholesterolemia

The recommended usual starting dose is 10 mg once a day in the evening. The recommended dosing range is 10-40 mg/day; the maximum recommended dose is 40 mg/day. Doses should be individualized according to the recommended goal of therapy [see NCEP Pediatric Panel Guidelines[2] and Clinical Studies (14.2)]. Adjustments should be made at intervals of 4 weeks or more.

[2] National Cholesterol Education Program (NCEP): Highlights of the Report of the Expert Panel on Blood Cholesterol Levels in Children and Adolescents. *Pediatrics.* 89(3):495-501. 1992.

2.4 Patients with Renal Impairment

Because ZOCOR does not undergo significant renal excretion, modification of dosage should not be necessary in patients with mild to moderate renal impairment. However, caution should be exercised when ZOCOR is administered to patients with severe renal impairment; such patients should be started at 5 mg/day and be closely monitored [see Warnings and Precautions (5.1) and Clinical Pharmacology (12.3)].

2.5 Chinese Patients Taking Lipid-Modifying Doses (≥1 g/day Niacin) of Niacin-Containing Products

Because of an increased risk for myopathy, caution should be used when treating Chinese patients with simvastatin coadministered with lipid-modifying doses (≥1 g/day niacin) of niacin-containing products. Because the risk for myopathy is dose-related, Chinese patients should not receive simvastatin 80 mg coadministered with lipid-modifying doses of niacin-containing products. The cause of the increased risk of myopathy is not known. It is also unknown if the risk for myopathy with coadministration of simvastatin with lipid-modifying doses of niacin-containing products observed in Chinese patients applies to other Asian patients. [See Warnings and Precautions (5.1).]

2.6 Coadministration with Other Drugs

Concomitant Lipid-Lowering Therapy
- ZOCOR may be used concomitantly with bile acid sequestrants.
- Combination therapy with gemfibrozil increases simvastatin exposure. Therefore, if ZOCOR is used in combination with gemfibrozil, the dose of ZOCOR should not exceed 10 mg/day [see Warnings and Precautions (5.1), Drug Interactions (7.2), and Clinical Pharmacology (12.3)].

Patients taking Cyclosporine or Danazol
- ZOCOR therapy should begin with 5 mg/day and should not exceed 10 mg/day [see Warnings and Precautions (5.1) and Drug Interactions (7.3)].

Patients taking Amiodarone or Verapamil
- The dose of ZOCOR should not exceed 20 mg/day [see Warnings and Precautions (5.1), Drug Interactions (7.4), and Clinical Pharmacology (12.3)].

Patients taking Diltiazem
- The dose of ZOCOR should not exceed 40 mg/day [see Warnings and Precautions (5.1), Drug Interactions (7.4), and Clinical Pharmacology (12.3)].

3 DOSAGE FORMS AND STRENGTHS

- Tablets ZOCOR 5 mg are buff, oval, film-coated tablets, coded MSD 726 on one side and ZOCOR 5 on the other.
- Tablets ZOCOR 10 mg are peach, oval, film-coated tablets, coded MSD 735 on one side and plain on the other.
- Tablets ZOCOR 20 mg are tan, oval, film-coated tablets, coded MSD 740 on one side and plain on the other.
- Tablets ZOCOR 40 mg are brick red, oval, film-coated tablets, coded MSD 749 on one side and plain on the other.
- Tablets ZOCOR 80 mg are brick red, capsule-shaped, film-coated tablets, coded 543 on one side and 80 on the other.

4 CONTRAINDICATIONS

ZOCOR is contraindicated in the following conditions:
- Hypersensitivity to any component of this medication [see Adverse Reactions (6.2)].
- Active liver disease, which may include unexplained persistent elevations in hepatic transaminase levels [see Warnings and Precautions (5.2)].
- Women who are pregnant or may become pregnant. Serum cholesterol and triglycerides increase during normal pregnancy, and cholesterol or cholesterol derivatives

are essential for fetal development. Because HMG-CoA reductase inhibitors (statins) decrease cholesterol synthesis and possibly the synthesis of other biologically active substances derived from cholesterol, ZOCOR may cause fetal harm when administered to a pregnant woman. Atherosclerosis is a chronic process and the discontinuation of lipid-lowering drugs during pregnancy should have little impact on the outcome of long-term therapy of primary hypercholesterolemia. There are no adequate and well-controlled studies of use with ZOCOR during pregnancy; however, in rare reports congenital anomalies were observed following intrauterine exposure to statins. In rat and rabbit animal reproduction studies, simvastatin revealed no evidence of teratogenicity. **ZOCOR should be administered to women of childbearing age only when such patients are highly unlikely to conceive.** If the patient becomes pregnant while taking this drug, ZOCOR should be discontinued immediately and the patient should be apprised of the potential hazard to the fetus [see Use in Specific Populations (8.1)].
- Nursing mothers. It is not known whether simvastatin is excreted into human milk; however, a small amount of another drug in this class does pass into breast milk. Because statins have the potential for serious adverse reactions in nursing infants, women who require treatment with ZOCOR should not breastfeed their infants [see Use in Specific Populations (8.3)].

5 WARNINGS AND PRECAUTIONS

5.1 Myopathy/Rhabdomyolysis

Simvastatin, like other statins, occasionally causes myopathy manifested as muscle pain, tenderness or weakness with creatine kinase (CK) above ten times the upper limit of normal (ULN). Myopathy sometimes takes the form of rhabdomyolysis with or without acute renal failure secondary to myoglobinuria, and rare fatalities have occurred. The risk of myopathy is increased by high levels of statin activity in plasma. Predisposing factors for myopathy include advanced age (≥65 years), uncontrolled hypothyroidism, and renal impairment.

As with other statins, the risk of myopathy/rhabdomyolysis is dose related. In a clinical trial database in which 41,050 patients were treated with ZOCOR with 24,747 (approximately 60%) treated for at least 4 years, the incidence of myopathy was approximately 0.02%, 0.08% and 0.53% at 20, 40 and 80 mg/day, respectively. In these trials, patients were carefully monitored and some interacting medicinal products were excluded.

All patients starting therapy with simvastatin, or whose dose of simvastatin is being increased, should be advised of the risk of myopathy and told to report promptly any unexplained muscle pain, tenderness or weakness. Simvastatin therapy should be discontinued immediately if myopathy is diagnosed or suspected. In most cases, muscle symptoms and CK increases resolved when treatment was promptly discontinued. Periodic CK determinations may be considered in patients starting therapy with simvastatin or whose dose is being increased, but there is no assurance that such monitoring will prevent myopathy.

Many of the patients who have developed rhabdomyolysis on therapy with simvastatin have had complicated medical histories, including renal insufficiency usually as a consequence of long-standing diabetes mellitus. Such patients merit closer monitoring. Therapy with simvastatin should be temporarily stopped a few days prior to elective major surgery and when any major medical or surgical condition supervenes.

Drug Interactions
The risk of myopathy and rhabdomyolysis is increased by high levels of statin activity in plasma. Simvastatin is metabolized by the cytochrome P450 isoform 3A4. Certain drugs which inhibit this metabolic pathway can raise the plasma levels of simvastatin and may increase the risk of myopathy. These include itraconazole, ketoconazole, and other antifungal azoles, the macrolide antibiotics erythromycin and clarithromycin, and the ketolide antibiotic telithromycin, HIV protease inhibitors, the antidepressant nefazodone, or large quantities of grapefruit juice (>1 quart daily). The use of ZOCOR concomitantly with these CYP3A4 inhibitors should be avoided. If treatment with itraconazole, ketoconazole, erythromycin, clarithromycin or telithromycin is unavoidable, therapy with ZOCOR should be suspended during the course of treatment. [See Drug Interactions (7).]

The benefits of the combined use of simvastatin with the following drugs should be carefully weighed against the potential risks of combinations: gemfibrozil, other lipid-lowering drugs (other fibrates or ≥1 g/day of niacin), cyclosporine, danazol, amiodarone, verapamil or diltiazem. Caution should be used when prescribing other fibrates with simvastatin, as these agents can cause myopathy when given alone.

Cases of myopathy/rhabdomyolysis have been observed with simvastatin coadministered with lipid-modifying doses

(≥1 g/day niacin) of niacin-containing products. In an ongoing, double-blind, randomized cardiovascular outcomes trial, an independent safety monitoring committee identified that the incidence of myopathy is higher in Chinese compared with non-Chinese patients taking simvastatin 40 mg coadministered with lipid-modifying doses of a niacin-containing product. Because the risk for myopathy is dose-related, Chinese patients should not receive simvastatin 80 mg coadministered with lipid-modifying doses of niacin-containing products. It is unknown if the risk for myopathy with coadministration of simvastatin with lipid-modifying doses of niacin-containing products observed in Chinese patients applies to other Asian patients. Prescribing recommendations for interacting agents are summarized in Table 1 [see also Dosage and Administration (2.6), Drug Interactions (7), Clinical Pharmacology (12.3)].

TABLE 1: Drug Interactions Associated with Increased Risk of Myopathy/Rhabdomyolysis

Interacting Agents	Prescribing Recommendations
Itraconazole Ketoconazole Erythromycin Clarithromycin Telithromycin HIV protease inhibitors Nefazodone	Avoid simvastatin
Gemfibrozil* Cyclosporine[†] Danazol[†]	Do not exceed 10 mg simvastatin daily
Amiodarone[‡] Verapamil[‡]	Do not exceed 20 mg simvastatin daily
Diltiazem[§]	Do not exceed 40 mg simvastatin daily
Grapefruit juice	Avoid large quantities of grapefruit juice (>1 quart daily)

* The combined use of simvastatin with gemfibrozil should be avoided, unless the benefits are likely to outweigh the increased risks of this drug combination.
† The benefits of the use of simvastatin in patients receiving cyclosporine or danazol should be carefully weighed against the risks of these combinations.
‡ The combined use of simvastatin at doses higher than 20 mg daily with amiodarone or verapamil should be avoided unless the clinical benefit is likely to outweigh the increased risk of myopathy.
§ The combined use of simvastatin in patients receiving diltiazem should not exceed 40 mg daily unless the clinical benefit is likely to outweigh the increased risk of myopathy.

5.2 Liver Dysfunction

Persistent increases (to more than 3× the ULN) in serum transaminases have occurred in approximately 1% of patients who received simvastatin in clinical studies. When drug treatment was interrupted or discontinued in these patients, the transaminase levels usually fell slowly to pretreatment levels. The increases were not associated with jaundice or other clinical signs or symptoms. There was no evidence of hypersensitivity.

In the Scandinavian Simvastatin Survival Study (4S) [see Clinical Studies (14.1)], the number of patients with more than one transaminase elevation to >3× ULN, over the course of the study, was not significantly different between the simvastatin and placebo groups (14 [0.7%] vs. 12 [0.6%]). Elevated transaminases resulted in the discontinuation of 8 patients from therapy in the simvastatin group (n=2,221) and 5 in the placebo group (n=2,223). Of the 1,986 simvastatin treated patients in 4S with normal liver function tests (LFTs) at baseline, 8 (0.4%) developed consecutive LFT elevations to >3× ULN and/or were discontinued due to transaminase elevations during the 5.4 years (median follow-up) of the study. Among these 8 patients, 5 initially developed these abnormalities within the first year. All of the patients in this study received a starting dose of 20 mg of simvastatin; 37% were titrated to 40 mg.

In 2 controlled clinical studies in 1,105 patients, the 12-month incidence of persistent hepatic transaminase elevation without regard to drug relationship was 0.9% and 2.1% at the 40- and 80-mg dose, respectively. No patients developed persistent liver function abnormalities following the initial 6 months of treatment at a given dose.

It is recommended that liver function tests be performed before the initiation of treatment, and thereafter when clinically indicated. Patients titrated to the 80-mg dose should

receive an additional test prior to titration, 3 months after titration to the 80-mg dose, and periodically thereafter (e.g., semiannually) for the first year of treatment. Patients who develop increased transaminase levels should be monitored with a second liver function evaluation to confirm the finding and be followed thereafter with frequent liver function tests until the abnormality(ies) return to normal. Should an increase in AST or ALT of 3× ULN or greater persist, withdrawal of therapy with ZOCOR is recommended.

The drug should be used with caution in patients who consume substantial quantities of alcohol and/or have a past history of liver disease. Active liver diseases or unexplained transaminase elevations are contraindications to the use of simvastatin.

As with other lipid-lowering agents, moderate (less than 3× ULN) elevations of serum transaminases have been reported following therapy with simvastatin. These changes appeared soon after initiation of therapy with simvastatin, were often transient, were not accompanied by any symptoms and did not require interruption of treatment.

6 ADVERSE REACTIONS

6.1 Clinical Trials Experience

Because clinical studies are conducted under widely varying conditions, adverse reaction rates observed in the clinical studies of a drug cannot be directly compared to rates in the clinical studies of another drug and may not reflect the rates observed in practice.

In the pre-marketing controlled clinical studies and their open extensions (2,423 patients with median duration of follow-up of approximately 18 months), 1.4% of patients were discontinued due to adverse reactions. The most common adverse reactions that led to treatment discontinuation were: gastrointestinal disorders (0.5%), myalgia (0.1%), and arthralgia (0.1%). The most commonly reported adverse reactions (incidence ≥5%) in simvastatin controlled clinical trials were: upper respiratory infections (9.0%), headache (7.4%), abdominal pain (7.3%), constipation (6.6%), and nausea (5.4%).

Scandinavian Simvastatin Survival Study

In 4S involving 4,444 (age range 35-71 years, 19% women, 100% Caucasians) treated with 20-40 mg/day of ZOCOR (n=2,221) or placebo (n=2,223) over a median of 5.4 years, adverse reactions reported in ≥2% of patients and at a rate greater than placebo are shown in Table 2.

TABLE 2: Adverse Reactions Reported Regardless of Causality by ≥2% of Patients Treated with ZOCOR and Greater than Placebo in 4S

	ZOCOR (N = 2,221) %	Placebo (N = 2,223) %
Body as a Whole		
Edema/swelling	2.7	2.3
Abdominal pain	5.9	5.8
Cardiovascular System Disorders		
Atrial fibrillation	5.7	5.1
Digestive System Disorders		
Constipation	2.2	1.6
Gastritis	4.9	3.9
Endocrine Disorders		
Diabetes mellitus	4.2	3.6
Musculoskeletal Disorders		
Myalgia	3.7	3.2
Nervous System / Psychiatric Disorders		
Headache	2.5	2.1
Imsomnia	4.0	3.8
Vertigo	4.5	4.2
Respiratory System Disorders		
Bronchitis	6.6	6.3
Sinusitis	2.3	1.8
Skin / Skin Appendage Disorders		
Eczema	4.5	3.0
Urogenital System Disorders		
Infection, urinary tract	3.2	3.1

Heart Protection Study

In the Heart Protection Study (HPS), involving 20,536 patients (age range 40-80 years, 25% women, 97% Caucasians, 3% other races) treated with ZOCOR 40 mg/day (n=10,269) or placebo (n=10,267) over a mean of 5 years, only serious adverse reactions and discontinuations due to any adverse reactions were recorded. Discontinuation rates due to adverse reactions were 4.8% in patients treated with ZOCOR compared with 5.1% in patients treated with placebo. The incidence of myopathy/rhabdomyolysis was <0.1% in patients treated with ZOCOR.

Other Clinical Studies

Other adverse reactions reported in clinical trials were: diarrhea, rash, dyspepsia, flatulence, and asthenia.

Laboratory Tests

Marked persistent increases of hepatic transaminases have been noted *[see Warnings and Precautions (5.2)]*. Elevated alkaline phosphatase and γ-glutamyl transpeptidase have also been reported. About 5% of patients had elevations of CK levels of 3 or more times the normal value on one or more occasions. This was attributable to the noncardiac fraction of CK. *[See Warnings and Precautions (5.1).]*

Adolescent Patients (ages 10-17 years)

In a 48-week, controlled study in adolescent boys and girls who were at least 1 year post-menarche, 10-17 years of age (43.4% female, 97.7% Caucasians, 1.7% Hispanics, 0.6% Multiracial) with heterozygous familial hypercholesterolemia (n=175), treated with placebo or ZOCOR (10-40 mg daily), the most common adverse reactions observed in both groups were upper respiratory infection, headache, abdominal pain, and nausea *[see Use in Specific Populations (8.4) and Clinical Studies (14.2)]*.

6.2 Post-Marketing Experience

Because the below reactions are reported voluntarily from a population of uncertain size, it is generally not possible to reliably estimate their frequency or establish a causal relationship to drug exposure. The following additional adverse reactions have been identified during postapproval use of simvastatin: pruritus, alopecia, a variety of skin changes (e.g., nodules, discoloration, dryness of skin/mucous membranes, changes to hair/nails), dizziness, muscle cramps, myalgia, pancreatitis, memory impairment, paresthesia, peripheral neuropathy, vomiting, anemia, erectile dysfunction, interstitial lung disease, rhabdomyolysis, hepatitis/jaundice, hepatic failure, and depression.

An apparent hypersensitivity syndrome has been reported rarely which has included some of the following features: anaphylaxis, angioedema, lupus erythematous-like syndrome, polymyalgia rheumatica, dermatomyositis, vasculitis, purpura, thrombocytopenia, leukopenia, hemolytic anemia, positive ANA, ESR increase, eosinophilia, arthritis, arthralgia, urticaria, asthenia, photosensitivity, fever, chills, flushing, malaise, dyspnea, toxic epidermal necrolysis, erythema multiforme, including Stevens-Johnson syndrome.

7 DRUG INTERACTIONS

7.1 CYP3A4 Interactions

Simvastatin, like several other inhibitors of HMG-CoA reductase, is a substrate of CYP3A4. Simvastatin is metabolized by CYP3A4 but has no CYP3A4 inhibitory activity; therefore it is not expected to affect the plasma concentrations of other drugs metabolized by CYP3A4.

The risk of myopathy is increased by reducing the elimination of simvastatin. Hence when simvastatin is used with an inhibitor of CYP3A4 (e.g., as listed below), elevated plasma levels of HMG-CoA reductase inhibitory activity can increase the risk of myopathy and rhabdomyolysis, particularly with higher doses of simvastatin. *[See Warnings and Precautions (5.1) and Clinical Pharmacology (12.3).]*

Itraconazole, ketoconazole, and other antifungal azoles
Macrolide antibiotics erythromycin, clarithromycin, and the ketolide antibiotic telithromycin
HIV protease inhibitors
Antidepressant nefazodone
Grapefruit juice in large quantities (>1 quart daily)

Concomitant use of these drugs and any medication labeled as having a strong inhibitory effect on CYP3A4 should be avoided unless the benefits of combined therapy outweigh the increased risk. If treatment with itraconazole, ketoconazole, erythromycin, clarithromycin or telithromycin is unavoidable, therapy with ZOCOR should be suspended during the course of treatment.

7.2 Lipid-Lowering Drugs That Can Cause Myopathy When Given Alone

The risk of myopathy is increased by gemfibrozil *[see Dosage and Administration (2.6)]* and to a lesser extent by other fibrates *[see Warnings and Precautions (5.1)]*.

7.3 Cyclosporine or Danazol

The risk of myopathy/rhabdomyolysis is increased by concomitant administration of cyclosporine or danazol particularly with higher doses of simvastatin *[see Warnings and Precautions (5.1) and Clinical Pharmacology (12.3)]*.

7.4 Amiodarone, Verapamil, or Diltiazem

The risk of myopathy/rhabdomyolysis is increased by concomitant administration of amiodarone, verapamil, or diltiazem with higher doses of simvastatin *[see Warnings and Precautions (5.1)]*.

7.5 Niacin

Cases of myopathy/rhabdomyolysis have been observed with simvastatin coadministered with lipid-modifying doses (≥1 g/day niacin) of niacin-containing products. In particular, caution should be used when treating Chinese patients with simvastatin coadministered with lipid-modifying doses of niacin-containing products. Because the risk for myopathy is dose-related, Chinese patients should not receive simvastatin 80 mg coadministered with lipid-modifying doses of niacin-containing products. *[See Warnings and Precautions (5.1) and Clinical Pharmacology (12.3).]*

7.6 Digoxin

In one study, concomitant administration of digoxin with simvastatin resulted in a slight elevation in digoxin concentrations in plasma. Patients taking digoxin should be monitored appropriately when simvastatin is initiated *[see Clinical Pharmacology (12.3)]*.

7.7 Coumarin Anticoagulants

In two clinical studies, one in normal volunteers and the other in hypercholesterolemic patients, simvastatin 20-40 mg/day modestly potentiated the effect of coumarin anticoagulants: the prothrombin time, reported as International Normalized Ratio (INR), increased from a baseline of 1.7 to 1.8 and from 2.6 to 3.4 in the volunteer and patient studies, respectively. With other statins, clinically evident bleeding and/or increased prothrombin time has been reported in a few patients taking coumarin anticoagulants concomitantly. In such patients, prothrombin time should be determined before starting simvastatin and frequently enough during early therapy to ensure that no significant alteration of prothrombin time occurs. Once a stable prothrombin time has been documented, prothrombin times can be monitored at the intervals usually recommended for patients on coumarin anticoagulants. If the dose of simvastatin is changed or discontinued, the same procedure should be repeated. Simvastatin therapy has not been associated with bleeding or with changes in prothrombin time in patients not taking anticoagulants.

8 USE IN SPECIFIC POPULATIONS

8.1 Pregnancy

Pregnancy Category X

[See Contraindications (4).]

ZOCOR is contraindicated in women who are or may become pregnant. Lipid lowering drugs offer no benefit during pregnancy, because cholesterol and cholesterol derivatives are needed for normal fetal development. Atherosclerosis is a chronic process, and discontinuation of lipid-lowering drugs during pregnancy should have little impact on long-term outcomes of primary hypercholesterolemia therapy. There are no adequate and well-controlled studies of use with ZOCOR during pregnancy; however, there are rare reports of congenital anomalies in infants exposed to statins *in utero*. Animal reproduction studies of simvastatin in rats and rabbits showed no evidence of teratogenicity. Serum cholesterol and triglycerides increase during normal pregnancy, and cholesterol or cholesterol derivatives are essential for fetal development. Because statins decrease cholesterol synthesis and possibly the synthesis of other biologically active substances derived from cholesterol, ZOCOR may cause fetal harm when administered to a pregnant woman. If ZOCOR is used during pregnancy or if the patient becomes pregnant while taking this drug, the patient should be apprised of the potential hazard to the fetus.

There are rare reports of congenital anomalies following intrauterine exposure to statins. In a review[3] of approximately 100 prospectively followed pregnancies in women exposed to simvastatin or another structurally related statin, the incidences of congenital anomalies, spontaneous abortions, and fetal deaths/stillbirths did not exceed those expected in the general population. However, the study was only able to exclude a 3- to 4-fold increased risk of congenital anomalies over the background rate. In 89% of these cases, drug treatment was initiated prior to pregnancy and was discontinued during the first trimester when pregnancy was identified.

Simvastatin was not teratogenic in rats or rabbits at doses (25, 10 mg/kg/day, respectively) that resulted in 3 times the human exposure based on mg/m^2 surface area. However, in studies with another structurally-related statin, skeletal malformations were observed in rats and mice.

Women of childbearing potential, who require treatment with ZOCOR for a lipid disorder, should be advised to use effective contraception. For women trying to conceive, discontinuation of ZOCOR should be considered. If pregnancy occurs, ZOCOR should be immediately discontinued.

[3] Manson, J.M., Freyssinges, C., Ducrocq, M.B., Stephenson, W.P., Postmarketing Surveillance of Lovastatin and Simvastatin Exposure During Pregnancy, *Reproductive Toxicology*, 10(6):439-446, 1996.

8.3 Nursing Mothers

It is not known whether simvastatin is excreted in human milk. Because a small amount of another drug in this class is excreted in human milk and because of the potential for serious adverse reactions in nursing infants, women taking simvastatin should not nurse their infants. A decision should be made whether to discontinue nursing or discontinue drug, taking into account the importance of the drug to the mother *[see Contraindications (4)]*.

8.4 Pediatric Use

Safety and effectiveness of simvastatin in patients 10-17 years of age with heterozygous familial hypercholesterolemia have been evaluated in a controlled clinical trial in adolescent boys and in girls who were at least 1 year postmenarche. Patients treated with simvastatin had an adverse reaction profile similar to that of patients treated with placebo. **Doses greater than 40 mg have not been studied in this population.** In this limited controlled study, there was no significant effect on growth or sexual maturation in the adolescent boys or girls, or on menstrual cycle length in girls. *[See Dosage and Administration (2.3), Adverse Reactions (6.1), Clinical Studies (14.2).]* Adolescent females should be counseled on appropriate contraceptive methods while on simvastatin therapy *[see Contraindications (4) and Use in Specific Populations (8.1)]*. Simvastatin has not been studied in patients younger than 10 years of age, nor in pre-menarchal girls.

8.5 Geriatric Use

Of the 2,423 patients who received ZOCOR in Phase III clinical studies and the 10,269 patients in the Heart Protection Study who received ZOCOR, 363 (15%) and 5,366 (52%), respectively were ≥65 years old. In HPS, 615 (6%) were ≥75 years old. No overall differences in safety or effectiveness were observed between these subjects and younger subjects, and other reported clinical experience has not identified differences in responses between the elderly and younger patients, but greater sensitivity of some older individuals cannot be ruled out. Since advanced age (≥65 years) is a predisposing factor for myopathy, ZOCOR should be prescribed with caution in the elderly. *[See Clinical Pharmacology (12.3).]*

A pharmacokinetic study with simvastatin showed the mean plasma level of statin activity to be approximately 45% higher in elderly patients between 70-78 years of age compared with patients between 18-30 years of age. In 4S, 1,021 (23%) of 4,444 patients were 65 or older. Lipid-lowering efficacy was at least as great in elderly patients compared with younger patients, and ZOCOR significantly reduced total mortality and CHD mortality in elderly patients with a history of CHD. In HPS, 52% of patients were elderly (4,891 patients 65-69 years and 5,806 patients 70 years or older). The relative risk reductions of CHD death, non-fatal MI, coronary and non-coronary revascularization procedures, and stroke were similar in older and younger patients *[see Clinical Studies (14.1)]*. In HPS, among 32,145 patients entering the active run-in period, there were 2 cases of myopathy/rhabdomyolysis; these patients were aged 67 and 73. Of the 7 cases of myopathy/rhabdomyolysis among 10,269 patients allocated to simvastatin, 4 were aged 65 or more (at baseline), of whom one was over 75. There were no overall differences in safety between older and younger patients in either 4S or HPS.

8.6 Renal Impairment

Caution should be exercised when ZOCOR is administered to patients with severe renal impairment. *[See Dosage and Administration (2.4).]*

8.7 Hepatic Impairment

ZOCOR is contraindicated in patients with active liver disease which may include unexplained persistent elevations in hepatic transaminase levels *[see Contraindications (4) and Warnings and Precautions (5.2)]*.

10 OVERDOSAGE

Significant lethality was observed in mice after a single oral dose of 9 g/m². No evidence of lethality was observed in rats or dogs treated with doses of 30 and 100 g/m², respectively. No specific diagnostic signs were observed in rodents. At these doses the only signs seen in dogs were emesis and mucoid stools.

A few cases of overdosage with ZOCOR have been reported; the maximum dose taken was 3.6 g. All patients recovered without sequelae. Supportive measures should be taken in the event of an overdose. The dialyzability of simvastatin and its metabolites in man is not known at present.

11 DESCRIPTION

ZOCOR (simvastatin) is a lipid-lowering agent that is derived synthetically from a fermentation product of *Aspergillus terreus*. After oral ingestion, simvastatin, which is an inactive lactone, is hydrolyzed to the corresponding β-hydroxyacid form. This is an inhibitor of 3-hydroxy-3-methylglutaryl-coenzyme A (HMG-CoA) reductase. This enzyme catalyzes the conversion of HMG-CoA to mevalonate, which is an early and rate-limiting step in the biosynthesis of cholesterol.

Simvastatin is butanoic acid, 2,2-dimethyl-,1,2,3,7,8,8a-hexahydro-3,7-dimethyl-8-[2-(tetrahydro-4-hydroxy-6-oxo-2*H*-pyran-2-yl)-ethyl]-1-naphthalenyl ester, [1*S*-[1α,3α,7β,8β(2*S**,4*S**),-8aβ]]. The empirical formula of simvastatin is $C_{25}H_{38}O_5$ and its molecular weight is 418.57. Its structural formula is:

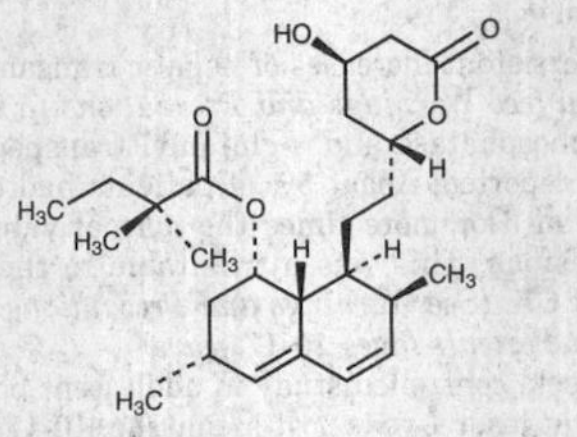

Simvastatin is a white to off-white, nonhygroscopic, crystalline powder that is practically insoluble in water, and freely soluble in chloroform, methanol and ethanol.

Tablets ZOCOR for oral administration contain either 5 mg, 10 mg, 20 mg, 40 mg or 80 mg of simvastatin and the following inactive ingredients: ascorbic acid, citric acid, hydroxypropyl cellulose, hypromellose, iron oxides, lactose, magnesium stearate, microcrystalline cellulose, starch, talc, and titanium dioxide. Butylated hydroxyanisole is added as a preservative.

12 CLINICAL PHARMACOLOGY

12.1 Mechanism of Action

Simvastatin is a prodrug and is hydrolyzed to its active β-hydroxyacid form, simvastatin acid, after administration. Simvastatin is a specific inhibitor of 3-hydroxy-3-methylglutaryl-coenzyme A (HMG-CoA) reductase, the enzyme that catalyzes the conversion of HMG-CoA to mevalonate, an early and rate limiting step in the biosynthetic pathway for cholesterol. In addition, simvastatin reduces VLDL and TG and increases HDL-C.

12.2 Pharmacodynamics

Epidemiological studies have demonstrated that elevated levels of total-C, LDL-C, as well as decreased levels of HDL-C are associated with the development of atherosclerosis and increased cardiovascular risk. Lowering LDL-C decreases this risk. However, the independent effect of raising HDL-C or lowering TG on the risk of coronary and cardiovascular morbidity and mortality has not been determined.

12.3 Pharmacokinetics

Simvastatin is a lactone that is readily hydrolyzed *in vivo* to the corresponding β-hydroxyacid, a potent inhibitor of HMG-CoA reductase. Inhibition of HMG-CoA reductase is the basis for an assay in pharmacokinetic studies of the β-hydroxyacid metabolites (active inhibitors) and, following base hydrolysis, active plus latent inhibitors (total inhibitors) in plasma following administration of simvastatin.

Following an oral dose of ^{14}C-labeled simvastatin in man, 13% of the dose was excreted in urine and 60% in feces. Plasma concentrations of total radioactivity (simvastatin plus ^{14}C-metabolites) peaked at 4 hours and declined rapidly to about 10% of peak by 12 hours postdose. Since simvastatin undergoes extensive first-pass extraction in the liver, the availability of the drug to the general circulation is low (<5%).

Both simvastatin and its β-hydroxyacid metabolite are highly bound (approximately 95%) to human plasma proteins. Rat studies indicate that when radiolabeled simvastatin was administered, simvastatin-derived radioactivity crossed the blood-brain barrier.

The major active metabolites of simvastatin present in human plasma are the β-hydroxyacid of simvastatin and its 6′-hydroxy, 6′-hydroxymethyl, and 6′-exomethylene derivatives. Peak plasma concentrations of both active and total inhibitors were attained within 1.3 to 2.4 hours postdose. While the recommended therapeutic dose range is 5 to 80 mg/day, there was no substantial deviation from linearity of AUC of inhibitors in the general circulation with an increase in dose to as high as 120 mg. Relative to the fasting state, the plasma profile of inhibitors was not affected when simvastatin was administered immediately before an American Heart Association recommended low-fat meal.

In a study including 16 elderly patients between 70 and 78 years of age who received ZOCOR 40 mg/day, the mean plasma level of HMG-CoA reductase inhibitory activity was increased approximately 45% compared with 18 patients between 18-30 years of age. Clinical study experience in the elderly (n=1522), suggests that there were no overall differences in safety between elderly and younger patients *[see Use in Specific Populations (8.5)]*.

Kinetic studies with another statin, having a similar principal route of elimination, have suggested that for a given dose level higher systemic exposure may be achieved in patients with severe renal insufficiency (as measured by creatinine clearance).

Although the mechanism is not fully understood, cyclosporine has been shown to increase the AUC of statins. The increase in AUC for simvastatin acid is presumably due, in part, to inhibition of CYP3A4.

The risk of myopathy is increased by high levels of HMG-CoA reductase inhibitory activity in plasma. Inhibitors of CYP3A4 can raise the plasma levels of HMG-CoA reductase inhibitory activity and increase the risk of myopathy *[see Warnings and Precautions (5.1) and Drug Interactions (7.1)]*.

[See table 3 at top of next page]

In a study of 12 healthy volunteers, simvastatin at the 80-mg dose had no effect on the metabolism of the probe cytochrome P450 isoform 3A4 (CYP3A4) substrates midazolam and erythromycin. This indicates that simvastatin is not an inhibitor of CYP3A4, and, therefore, is not expected to affect the plasma levels of other drugs metabolized by CYP3A4.

Coadministration of simvastatin (40 mg QD for 10 days) resulted in an increase in the maximum mean levels of cardioactive digoxin (given as a single 0.4 mg dose on day 10) by approximately 0.3 ng/mL.

13 NONCLINICAL TOXICOLOGY

13.1 Carcinogenesis, Mutagenesis, Impairment of Fertility

In a 72-week carcinogenicity study, mice were administered daily doses of simvastatin of 25, 100, and 400 mg/kg body weight, which resulted in mean plasma drug levels approximately 1, 4, and 8 times higher than the mean human plasma drug level, respectively (as total inhibitory activity based on AUC) after an 80-mg oral dose. Liver carcinomas were significantly increased in high-dose females and mid- and high-dose males with a maximum incidence of 90% in males. The incidence of adenomas of the liver was significantly increased in mid- and high-dose females. Drug treatment also significantly increased the incidence of lung adenomas in mid- and high-dose males and females. Adenomas of the Harderian gland (a gland of the eye of rodents) were significantly higher in high-dose mice than in controls. No evidence of a tumorigenic effect was observed at 25 mg/kg/day.

In a separate 92-week carcinogenicity study in mice at doses up to 25 mg/kg/day, no evidence of a tumorigenic effect was observed (mean plasma drug levels were 1 times higher than humans given 80 mg simvastatin as measured by AUC).

In a two-year study in rats at 25 mg/kg/day, there was a statistically significant increase in the incidence of thyroid follicular adenomas in female rats exposed to approximately 11 times higher levels of simvastatin than in humans given 80 mg simvastatin (as measured by AUC).

A second two-year rat carcinogenicity study with doses of 50 and 100 mg/kg/day produced hepatocellular adenomas and carcinomas (in female rats at both doses and in males at 100 mg/kg/day). Thyroid follicular cell adenomas were increased in males and females at both doses; thyroid follicular cell carcinomas were increased in females at 100 mg/kg/day. The increased incidence of thyroid neoplasms appears to be consistent with findings from other statins. These treatment levels represented plasma drug levels (AUC) of approximately 7 and 15 times (males) and 22 and 25 times (females) the mean human plasma drug exposure after an 80 milligram daily dose.

No evidence of mutagenicity was observed in a microbial mutagenicity (Ames) test with or without rat or mouse liver metabolic activation. In addition, no evidence of damage to genetic material was noted in an *in vitro* alkaline elution assay using rat hepatocytes, a V-79 mammalian cell forward mutation study, an *in vitro* chromosome aberration study in CHO cells, or an *in vivo* chromosomal aberration assay in mouse bone marrow.

There was decreased fertility in male rats treated with simvastatin for 34 weeks at 25 mg/kg body weight (4 times the maximum human exposure level, based on AUC, in patients receiving 80 mg/day); however, this effect was not observed during a subsequent fertility study in which simvastatin was administered at this same dose level to male rats for 11 weeks (the entire cycle of spermatogenesis including epididymal maturation). No microscopic changes were observed in the testes of rats from either study. At 180 mg/kg/day, (which produces exposure levels 22 times higher than those in humans taking 80 mg/day based on surface area, mg/m²), seminiferous tubule degeneration (necrosis and loss of spermatogenic epithelium) was observed. In dogs, there was drug-related testicular atrophy, decreased spermatogenesis, spermatocytic degeneration and giant cell formation at 10 mg/kg/day, (approximately 2 times the human exposure, based on AUC, at 80 mg/day). The clinical significance of these findings is unclear.

13.2 Animal Toxicology and/or Pharmacology

CNS Toxicity

Optic nerve degeneration was seen in clinically normal dogs treated with simvastatin for 14 weeks at 180 mg/kg/day, a dose that produced mean plasma drug levels about 12 times higher than the mean plasma drug level in humans taking 80 mg/day.

A chemically similar drug in this class also produced optic nerve degeneration (Wallerian degeneration of retinogeniculate fibers) in clinically normal dogs in a dose-dependent fashion starting at 60 mg/kg/day, a dose that produced mean plasma drug levels about 30 times higher than the mean plasma drug level in humans taking the highest recommended dose (as measured by total enzyme inhibitory activity). This same drug also produced vestibulocochlear Wallerian-like degeneration and retinal ganglion cell chromatolysis in dogs treated for 14 weeks at 180 mg/kg/day, a dose that resulted in a mean plasma drug level similar to that seen with the 60 mg/kg/day dose.

CNS vascular lesions, characterized by perivascular hemorrhage and edema, mononuclear cell infiltration of perivascular spaces, perivascular fibrin deposits and necrosis of small vessels were seen in dogs treated with simvastatin at a dose of 360 mg/kg/day, a dose that produced mean plasma drug levels that were about 14 times higher than the mean plasma drug levels in humans taking 80 mg/day. Similar CNS vascular lesions have been observed with several other drugs of this class.

There were cataracts in female rats after two years of treatment with 50 and 100 mg/kg/day (22 and 25 times the human AUC at 80 mg/day, respectively) and in dogs after three months at 90 mg/kg/day (19 times) and at two years at 50 mg/kg/day (5 times).

14   CLINICAL STUDIES

14.1   Clinical Studies in Adults

Reductions in Risk of CHD Mortality and Cardiovascular Events

In 4S, the effect of therapy with ZOCOR on total mortality was assessed in 4,444 patients with CHD and baseline total cholesterol 212-309 mg/dL (5.5-8.0 mmol/L). In this multicenter, randomized, double-blind, placebo-controlled study, patients were treated with standard care, including diet, and either ZOCOR 20-40 mg/day (n=2,221) or placebo (n=2,223) for a median duration of 5.4 years. Over the course of the study, treatment with ZOCOR led to mean reductions in total-C, LDL-C and TG of 25%, 35%, and 10%, respectively, and a mean increase in HDL-C of 8%. ZOCOR significantly reduced the risk of mortality by 30% (p=0.0003, 182 deaths in the ZOCOR group vs 256 deaths in the placebo group). The risk of CHD mortality was significantly reduced by 42% (p=0.00001, 111 vs 189 deaths). There was no statistically significant difference between groups in non-cardiovascular mortality. ZOCOR significantly decreased the risk of having major coronary events (CHD mortality plus hospital-verified and silent non-fatal myocardial infarction [MI]) by 34% (p<0.00001, 431 vs 622 patients with one or more events). The risk of having a hospital-verified non-fatal MI was reduced by 37%. ZOCOR significantly reduced the risk for undergoing myocardial revascularization procedures (coronary artery bypass grafting or percutaneous transluminal coronary angioplasty) by 37% (p<0.00001, 252 vs 383 patients). ZOCOR significantly reduced the risk of fatal plus non-fatal cerebrovascular events (combined stroke and transient ischemic attacks) by 28% (p=0.033, 75 vs 102 patients). ZOCOR reduced the risk of major coronary events to a similar extent across the range of baseline total and LDL cholesterol levels. Because there were only 53 female deaths, the effect of ZOCOR on mortality in women could not be adequately assessed. However, ZOCOR significantly lessened the risk of having major coronary events by 34% (60 vs 91 women with one or more event). The randomization was stratified by angina alone (21% of each treatment group) or a previous MI. Because there were only 57 deaths among the patients with angina alone at baseline, the effect of ZOCOR on mortality in this subgroup could not be adequately assessed. However, trends in reduced coronary mortality, major coronary events and revascularization procedures were consistent between this group and the total study cohort. Additionally, ZOCOR resulted in similar decreases in relative risk for total mortality, CHD mortality, and major coronary events in elderly patients (≥65 years), compared with younger patients.

The Heart Protection Study (HPS) was a large, multicenter, placebo-controlled, double-blind study with a mean duration of 5 years conducted in 20,536 patients (10,269 on ZOCOR 40 mg and 10,267 on placebo). Patients were allocated to treatment using a covariate adaptive method[4] which took into account the distribution of 10 important baseline characteristics of patients already enrolled and minimized the imbalance of those characteristics across the groups. Patients had a mean age of 64 years (range 40-80 years), were 97% Caucasian and were at high risk of developing a major coronary event because of existing CHD (65%), diabetes (Type 2, 26%; Type 1, 3%), history of stroke or other cerebrovascular disease (16%), peripheral vessel disease (33%), or hypertension in males ≥65 years (6%). At baseline, 3,421 patients (17%) had LDL-C levels below 100 mg/dL, of whom 953 (5%) had LDL-C levels below 80 mg/dL; 7,068 patients (34%) had levels between 100 and 130 mg/dL; and 10,047 patients (49%) had levels greater than 130 mg/dL.

TABLE 3: Effect of Coadministered Drugs or Grapefruit Juice on Simvastatin Systemic Exposure

Coadministered Drug or Grapefruit Juice	Dosing of Coadministered Drug or Grapefruit Juice	Dosing of Simvastatin	Geometric Mean Ratio (Ratio* with/without coadministered drug) No Effect = 1.00		
				AUC	C_{max}
Avoid taking with simvastatin *[see Warnings and Precautions (5.1)]*					
Telithromycin[†]	200 mg QD for 4 days	80 mg	simvastatin acid[‡]	12	15
			simvastatin	8.9	5.3
Nelfinavir[†]	1250 mg BID for 14 days	20 mg QD for 28 days	simvastatin acid[‡] simvastatin	6	6.2
Itraconazole[†]	200 mg QD for 4 days	80 mg	simvastatin acid[‡] simvastatin	13.1	13.1
Avoid >1 quart of grapefruit juice with simvastatin *[see Warnings and Precautions (5.1)]*					
Grapefruit Juice[§] (high dose)	200 mL of double-strength TID[¶]	60 mg single dose	simvastatin acid	7	
			simvastatin	16	
Grapefruit Juice[§] (low dose)	8 oz (about 237mL) of single-strength[#]	20 mg single dose	simvastatin acid	1.3	
			simvastatin	1.9	
Avoid taking with >10 mg simvastatin, based on clinical and/or post-marketing experience *[see Warnings and Precautions (5.1)]*					
Gemfibrozil	600 mg BID for 3 days	40 mg	simvastatin acid	2.85	2.18
			simvastatin	1.35	0.91
Avoid taking with >20 mg simvastatin, based on clinical and/or post-marketing experience *[see Warnings and Precautions (5.1)]*					
Verapamil SR	240 mg QD Days 1-7 then 240 mg BID on Days 8-10	80 mg on Day 10	simvastatin acid	2.3	2.4
			simvastatin	2.5	2.1
Avoid taking with >40 mg simvastatin, based on clinical and/or post-marketing experience *[see Warnings and Precautions (5.1)]*					
Diltiazem	120 mg BID for 10 days	80 mg on Day 10	simvastatin acid	2.69	2.69
			simvastatin	3.10	2.88
Diltiazem	120 mg BID for 14 days	20 mg on Day 14	simvastatin	4.6	3.6
No dosing adjustments required for the following:					
Fenofibrate	160 mg QD × 14 days	80 mg QD on Days 8-14	simvastatin acid	0.64	0.89
			simvastatin	0.89	0.83
Niacin extended-release[Þ]	2 g single dose	20 mg single dose	simvastatin acid	1.6	1.84
			simvastatin	1.4	1.08
Amlodipine	10 mg QD × 10 days	80 mg on Day 10	simvastatin acid	1.58	1.56
			simvastatin	1.77	1.47
Propranolol	80 mg single dose	80 mg single dose	total inhibitor	0.79	↓ from 33.6 to 21.1 ng·eq/mL
			active inhibitor	0.79	↓ from 7.0 to 4.7 ng·eq/mL

* Results based on a chemical assay except results with propranolol as indicated.
† Results could be representative of the following CYP3A4 inhibitors: ketoconazole, erythromycin, clarithromycin, HIV protease inhibitors, and nefazodone.
‡ Simvastatin acid refers to the β-hydroxyacid of simvastatin.
§ The effect of amounts of grapefruit juice between those used in these two studies on simvastatin pharmacokinetics has not been studied.
¶ Double-strength: one can of frozen concentrate diluted with one can of water. Grapefruit juice was administered TID for 2 days, and 200 mL together with single dose simvastatin and 30 and 90 minutes following single dose simvastatin on Day 3.
# Single-strength: one can of frozen concentrate diluted with 3 cans of water. Grapefruit juice was administered with breakfast for 3 days, and simvastatin was administered in the evening on Day 3.
Þ Because Chinese patients have an increased risk for myopathy with simvastatin coadministered with lipid-modifying doses (≥ 1 gram/day niacin) of niacin-containing products, and the risk is dose-related, Chinese patients should not receive simvastatin 80 mg coadministered with lipid-modifying doses of niacin-containing products *[see Warnings and Precautions (5.1) and Drug Interactions (7.5)]*.

The HPS results showed that ZOCOR 40 mg/day significantly reduced: total and CHD mortality; non-fatal MI, stroke, and revascularization procedures (coronary and non-coronary) (see Table 4).

[See table 4 at top of next page]

Two composite endpoints were defined in order to have sufficient events to assess relative risk reductions across a range of baseline characteristics (see Figure 1). A composite of major coronary events (MCE) was comprised of CHD mortality and non-fatal MI (analyzed by time-to-first event; 898 patients treated with ZOCOR had events and 1,212 patients on placebo had events). A composite of major vascular events (MVE) was comprised of MCE, stroke and revascularization procedures including coronary, peripheral and other non-coronary procedures (analyzed by time-to-first event; 2,033 patients treated with ZOCOR had events and 2,585 patients on placebo had events). Significant relative risk reductions were observed for both composite endpoints (27% for MCE and 24% for MVE, p<0.0001). Treatment with ZOCOR produced significant relative risk reductions for all

TABLE 4: Summary of Heart Protection Study Results

Endpoint	ZOCOR (N=10,269) n (%)*	Placebo (N=10,267) n (%)*	Risk Reduction (%) (95% CI)	p-Value
Primary				
Mortality	1,328 (12.9)	1,507 (14.7)	13 (6-19)	p=0.0003
CHD mortality	587 (5.7)	707 (6.9)	18 (8-26)	p=0.0005
Secondary				
Non-fatal MI	357 (3.5)	574 (5.6)	38 (30-46)	p<0.0001
Stroke	444 (4.3)	585 (5.7)	25 (15-34)	p<0.0001
Tertiary				
Coronary revascularization	513 (5)	725 (7.1)	30 (22-38)	p<0.0001
Peripheral and other non-coronary revascularization	450 (4.4)	532 (5.2)	16 (5-26)	p=0.006

* n = number of patients with indicated event

Figure 1: The Effects of Treatment with ZOCOR on Major Vascular Events and Major Coronary Events in HPS

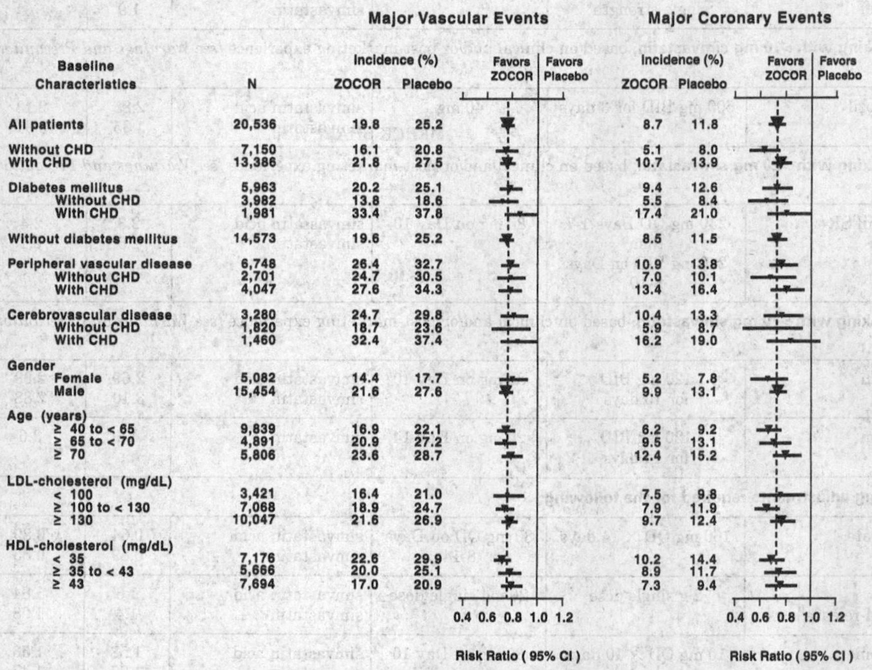

Baseline Characteristics	N	Major Vascular Events Incidence (%) ZOCOR	Placebo	Major Coronary Events Incidence (%) ZOCOR	Placebo
All patients	20,536	19.8	25.2	8.7	11.8
Without CHD	7,150	16.1	20.8	5.1	8.0
With CHD	13,386	21.8	27.5	10.7	13.9
Diabetes mellitus	5,963	20.2	25.1	9.4	12.6
Without CHD	3,982	13.8	18.6	5.5	8.4
With CHD	1,981	33.4	37.8	17.4	21.0
Without diabetes mellitus	14,573	19.6	25.2	8.5	11.5
Peripheral vascular disease	6,748	26.4	32.7	10.9	13.8
Without CHD	2,701	24.7	30.5	7.0	10.1
With CHD	4,047	27.6	34.3	13.4	16.4
Cerebrovascular disease	3,280	24.7	29.8	10.4	13.3
Without CHD	1,820	18.7	23.6	5.9	8.7
With CHD	1,460	32.4	37.4	16.2	19.0
Gender					
Female	5,082	14.4	17.7	5.2	7.8
Male	15,454	21.6	27.6	9.9	13.1
Age (years)					
≥ 40 to < 65	9,839	16.9	22.1	6.2	9.2
≥ 65 to < 70	4,891	20.9	27.2	9.5	13.1
≥ 70	5,806	23.6	28.7	12.4	15.2
LDL-cholesterol (mg/dL)					
< 100	3,421	16.4	21.0	7.5	9.8
≥ 100 to < 130	7,068	18.9	24.7	7.9	11.9
≥ 130	10,047	21.6	26.9	9.7	12.4
HDL-cholesterol (mg/dL)					
< 35	7,176	22.6	29.9	10.2	14.4
≥ 35 to < 43	5,666	20.0	25.1	8.9	11.7
≥ 43	7,694	17.0	20.9	7.3	9.4

Risk Ratio (95% CI)   Risk Ratio (95% CI)

N = number of patients in each subgroup. The inverted triangles are point estimates of the relative risk, with their 95% confidence intervals represented as a line. The area of a triangle is proportional to the number of patients with MVE or MCE in the subgroup relative to the number with MVE or MCE, respectively, in the entire study population. The vertical solid line represents a relative risk of one. The vertical dashed line represents the point estimate of relative risk in the entire study population.

components of the composite endpoints. The risk reductions produced by ZOCOR in both MCE and MVE were evident and consistent regardless of cardiovascular disease related medical history at study entry (i.e., CHD alone; or peripheral vascular disease, cerebrovascular disease, diabetes or treated hypertension, with or without CHD), gender, age, creatinine levels up to the entry limit of 2.3 mg/dL, baseline levels of LDL-C, HDL-C, apolipoprotein B and A-1, baseline concomitant cardiovascular medications (i.e., aspirin, beta blockers, or calcium channel blockers), smoking status, alcohol intake, or obesity. Diabetics showed risk reductions for MCE and MVE due to ZOCOR treatment regardless of baseline HbA1c levels or obesity with the greatest effects seen for diabetics without CHD.
[See figure 1 above]

Angiographic Studies
In the Multicenter Anti-Atheroma Study, the effect of simvastatin on atherosclerosis was assessed by quantitative coronary angiography in hypercholesterolemic patients with CHD. In this randomized, double-blind, controlled study, patients were treated with simvastatin 20 mg/day or placebo. Angiograms were evaluated at baseline, two and four years. The co-primary study endpoints were mean change per-patient in minimum and mean lumen diameters, indicating focal and diffuse disease, respectively. ZOCOR significantly slowed the progression of lesions as measured in the Year 4 angiogram by both parameters, as

well as by change in percent diameter stenosis. In addition, simvastatin significantly decreased the proportion of patients with new lesions and with new total occlusions.
Modifications of Lipid Profiles
Primary Hyperlipidemia (Fredrickson type IIa and IIb)
ZOCOR has been shown to be effective in reducing total-C and LDL-C in heterozygous familial and non-familial forms of hyperlipidemia and in mixed hyperlipidemia. Maximal to near maximal response is generally achieved within 4-6 weeks and maintained during chronic therapy. ZOCOR consistently and significantly decreased total-C, LDL-C, total-C/HDL-C ratio, and LDL-C/HDL-C ratio; ZOCOR also decreased TG and increased HDL-C (see Table 5).
[See table 5 on next page]
Hypertriglyceridemia (Frederickson type IV)
The results of a subgroup analysis in 74 patients with type IV hyperlipidemia from a 130-patient, double-blind, placebo-controlled, 3-period crossover study are presented in Table 6.
[See table 6 on next page]
Dysbetalipoproteinemia (Fredrickson type III)
The results of a subgroup analysis in 7 patients with type III hyperlipidemia (dysbetalipoproteinemia) (apo E2/2) (VLDL-C/TG>0.25) from a 130-patient, double-blind, placebo-controlled, 3-period crossover study are presented in Table 7.
[See table 7 on next page]

Homozygous Familial Hypercholesterolemia
In a controlled clinical study, 12 patients 15-39 years of age with homozygous familial hypercholesterolemia received simvastatin 40 mg/day in a single dose or in 3 divided doses, or 80 mg/day in 3 divided doses. In 11 patients with reductions in LDL-C, the mean LDL-C changes for the 40- and 80-mg doses were 14% (range 8% to 23%, median 12%) and 30% (range 14% to 46%, median 29%), respectively. One patient had an increase of 15% in LDL-C. Another patient with absent LDL-C receptor function had an LDL-C reduction of 41% with the 80-mg dose.
Endocrine Function
In clinical studies, simvastatin did not impair adrenal reserve or significantly reduce basal plasma cortisol concentration. Small reductions from baseline in basal plasma testosterone in men were observed in clinical studies with simvastatin, an effect also observed with other statins and the bile acid sequestrant cholestyramine. There was no effect on plasma gonadotropin levels. In a placebo-controlled, 12-week study there was no significant effect of simvastatin 80 mg on the plasma testosterone response to human chorionic gonadotropin. In another 24-week study, simvastatin 20-40 mg had no detectable effect on spermatogenesis. In 4S, in which 4,444 patients were randomized to simvastatin 20-40 mg/day or placebo for a median duration of 5.4 years, the incidence of male sexual adverse events in the two treatment groups was not significantly different. Because of these factors, the small changes in plasma testosterone are unlikely to be clinically significant. The effects, if any, on the pituitary-gonadal axis in pre-menopausal women are unknown.

[4] D.R. Taves, Minimization: a new method of assigning patients to treatment and control groups. Clin. Pharmacol. Ther. 15 (1974), pp. 443-453

14.2   Clinical Studies in Adolescents
In a double-blind, placebo-controlled study, 175 patients (99 adolescent boys and 76 post-menarchal girls) 10-17 years of age (mean age 14.1 years) with heterozygous familial hypercholesterolemia (HeFH) were randomized to simvastatin (n=106) or placebo (n=67) for 24 weeks (base study). Inclusion in the study required a baseline LDL-C level between 160 and 400 mg/dL and at least one parent with an LDL-C level >189 mg/dL. The dosage of simvastatin (once daily in the evening) was 10 mg for the first 8 weeks, 20 mg for the second 8 weeks, and 40 mg thereafter. In a 24-week extension, 144 patients elected to continue therapy with simvastatin 40 mg or placebo.
ZOCOR significantly decreased plasma levels of total-C, LDL-C, and Apo B (see Table 8). Results from the extension at 48 weeks were comparable to those observed in the base study.
[See table 8 on next page]
After 24 weeks of treatment, the mean achieved LDL-C value was 124.9 mg/dL (range: 64.0-289.0 mg/dL) in the ZOCOR 40 mg group compared to 207.8 mg/dL (range: 128.0-334.0 mg/dL) in the placebo group.
The safety and efficacy of doses above 40 mg daily have not been studied in children with HeFH. The long-term efficacy of simvastatin therapy in childhood to reduce morbidity and mortality in adulthood has not been established.

16   HOW SUPPLIED/STORAGE AND HANDLING
No. 8360—Tablets ZOCOR 5 mg are buff, oval, film-coated tablets, coded MSD 726 on one side and ZOCOR 5 on the other. They are supplied as follows:
NDC 0006-0726-31 unit of use bottles of 30
NDC 0006-0726-54 unit of use bottles of 90.
No. 8146—Tablets ZOCOR 10 mg are peach, oval, film-coated tablets, coded MSD 735 on one side and plain on the other. They are supplied as follows:
NDC 0006-0735-31 unit of use bottles of 30
NDC 0006-0735-54 unit of use bottles of 90
NDC 0006-0735-82 bottles of 1000.
No. 8147—Tablets ZOCOR 20 mg are tan, oval, film-coated tablets, coded MSD 740 on one side and plain on the other. They are supplied as follows:
NDC 0006-0740-31 unit of use bottles of 30
NDC 0006-0740-54 unit of use bottles of 90
NDC 0006-0740-82 bottles of 1000.
No. 8148—Tablets ZOCOR 40 mg are brick red, oval, film-coated tablets, coded MSD 749 on one side and plain on the other. They are supplied as follows:
NDC 0006-0749-31 unit of use bottles of 30
NDC 0006-0749-54 unit of use bottles of 90
NDC 0006-0749-82 bottles of 1000.
No. 6577—Tablets ZOCOR 80 mg are brick red, capsule-shaped, film-coated tablets, coded 543 on one side and 80 on the other. They are supplied as follows:
NDC 0006-0543-31 unit of use bottles of 30
NDC 0006-0543-54 unit of use bottles of 90
NDC 0006-0543-28 unit dose packages of 100
NDC 0006-0543-82 bottles of 1000.
Storage
Store between 5-30°C (41-86°F).
Storage of 1,000 count bottles
Dispense in a tightly-closed container.

17 PATIENT COUNSELING INFORMATION

Patients should be advised to adhere to their National Cholesterol Education Program (NCEP)-recommended diet, a regular exercise program, and periodic testing of a fasting lipid panel.

Patients should be advised about substances they should not take concomitantly with simvastatin *[see Warnings and Precautions (5.1)]*. Patients should also be advised to inform other healthcare professionals prescribing a new medication that they are taking ZOCOR.

TABLE 5: Mean Response in Patients with Primary Hyperlipidemia and Combined (mixed) Hyperlipidemia (Mean Percent Change from Baseline After 6 to 24 Weeks)

TREATMENT	N	TOTAL-C	LDL-C	HDL-C	TG*
Lower Dose Comparative Study[†] (Mean % Change at Week 6)					
ZOCOR 5 mg q.p.m.	109	-19	-26	10	-12
ZOCOR 10 mg q.p.m.	110	-23	-30	12	-15
Scandinavian Simvastatin Survival Study[‡] (Mean % Change at Week 6)					
Placebo	2223	-1	-1	0	-2
ZOCOR 20 mg q.p.m.	2221	-28	-38	8	-19
Upper Dose Comparative Study[§] (Mean % Change Averaged at Weeks 18 and 24)					
ZOCOR 40 mg q.p.m.	433	-31	-41	9	-18
ZOCOR 80 mg q.p.m.[¶]	664	-36	-47	8	-24
Multi-Center Combined Hyperlipidemia Study[#] (Mean % Change at Week 6)					
Placebo	125	1	2	3	-4
ZOCOR 40 mg q.p.m.	123	-25	-29	13	-28
ZOCOR 80 mg q.p.m.	124	-31	-36	16	-33

* median percent change
† mean baseline LDL-C 244 mg/dL and median baseline TG 168 mg/dL
‡ mean baseline LDL-C 188 mg/dL and median baseline TG 128 mg/dL
§ mean baseline LDL-C 226 mg/dL and median baseline TG 156 mg/dL
¶ 21% and 36% median reduction in TG in patients with TG ≤ 200 mg/dL and TG > 200 mg/dL, respectively. Patients with TG > 350 mg/dL were excluded
# mean baseline LDL-C 156 mg/dL and median baseline TG 391 mg/dL.

TABLE 6: Six-week, Lipid-lowering Effects of Simvastatin in Type IV Hyperlipidemia Median Percent Change (25th and 75th percentile) from Baseline*

TREATMENT	N	Total-C	LDL-C	HDL-C	TG	VLDL-C	Non-HDL-C
Placebo	74	+2 (-7, +7)	+1 (-8, +14)	+3 (-3, +10)	-9 (-25, +13)	-7 (-25, +11)	+1 (-9, +8)
ZOCOR 40 mg/day	74	-25 (-34, -19)	-28 (-40, -17)	+11 (+5, +23)	-29 (-43, -16)	-37 (-54, -23)	-32 (-42, -23)
ZOCOR 80 mg/day	74	-32 (-38, -24)	-37 (-46, -26)	+15 (+5, +23)	-34 (-45, -18)	-41 (-57, -28)	-38 (-49, -32)

* The median baseline values (mg/dL) for the patients in this study were: total-C = 254, LDL-C = 135, HDL-C = 36, TG = 404, VLDL-C = 83, and non-HDL-C = 215.

TABLE 7: Six-week, Lipid-lowering Effects of Simvastatin in Type III Hyperlipidemia Median Percent Change (min, max) from Baseline*

TREATMENT	N	Total-C	LDL-C + IDL	HDL-C	TG	VLDL-C + IDL	Non-HDL-C
Placebo	7	-8 (-24, +34)	-8 (-27, +23)	-2 (-21, +16)	+4 (-22, +90)	-4 (-28, +78)	-8 (-26, -39)
ZOCOR 40 mg/day	7	-50 (-66, -39)	-50 (-60, -31)	+7 (-8, +23)	-41 (-74, -16)	-58 (-90, -37)	-57 (-72, -44)
ZOCOR 80 mg/day	7	-52 (-55, -41)	-51 (-57, -28)	+7 (-5, +29)	-38 (-58, +2)	-60 (-72, -39)	-59 (-61, -46)

* The median baseline values (mg/dL) were: total-C = 324, LDL-C = 121, HDL-C = 31, TG = 411, VLD-C = 170, and non-HDL-C = 291.

TABLE 8: Lipid-Lowering Effects of Simvastatin in Adolescent Patients with Heterozygous Familial Hypercholesterolemia (Mean Percent Change from Baseline)

Dosage	Duration	N		Total-C	LDL-C	HDL-C	TG*	Apo B
Placebo	24 Weeks	67	% Change from Baseline	1.6	1.1	3.6	-3.2	-0.5
			(95% CI)	(-2.2, 5.3)	(-3.4, 5.5)	(-0.7, 8.0)	(-11.8, 5.4)	(-4.7, 3.6)
			Mean baseline, mg/dL	278.6	211.9	46.9	90.0	186.3
			(SD)	(51.8)	(49.0)	(11.9)	(50.7)	(38.1)
ZOCOR	24 Weeks	106	% Change from Baseline	-26.5	-36.8	8.3	-7.9	-32.4
			(95% CI)	(-29.6, -23.3)	(-40.5, -33.0)	(4.6, 11.9)	(-15.8, 0.0)	(-35.9, -29.0)
			Mean baseline, mg/dL	270.2	203.8	47.7	78.3	179.9
			(SD)	(44.0)	(41.5)	(9.0)	(46.0)	(33.8)

* median percent change

17.1 Muscle Pain
All patients starting therapy with ZOCOR should be advised of the risk of myopathy and told to report promptly any unexplained muscle pain, tenderness or weakness. The risk of this occurring is increased when taking certain types of medication or consuming larger quantities of grapefruit juice. They should discuss all medication, both prescription and over the counter, with their healthcare professional.

17.2 Liver Enzymes
It is recommended that liver function tests be performed before the initiation of ZOCOR, and thereafter when clinically indicated. Patients titrated to the 80-mg dose should receive an additional test prior to titration, 3 months after titration to the 80-mg dose, and periodically thereafter (e.g., semiannually) for the first year of treatment.

17.3 Pregnancy
Women of childbearing age should be advised to use an effective method of birth control to prevent pregnancy while using ZOCOR. Discuss future pregnancy plans with your patients, and discuss when to stop taking ZOCOR if they are trying to conceive. Patients should be advised that if they become pregnant they should stop taking ZOCOR and call their healthcare professional.

17.4 Breastfeeding
Women who are breastfeeding should not use ZOCOR. Patients who have a lipid disorder and are breastfeeding should be advised to discuss the options with their healthcare professional.

Manuf. for: Merck Sharp & Dohme Corp., a subsidiary of **MERCK & CO., INC.**, Whitehouse Station, NJ 08889, USA
By:
MERCK SHARP & DOHME LTD.
Cramlington, Northumberland, UK NE23 3JU
Issued May 2010
9992855
Shown in Product Identification Guide, page 314

ZOLINZA®   Rx
[zō-linz'-a]
(vorinostat)
Capsules

HIGHLIGHTS OF PRESCRIBING INFORMATION
These highlights do not include all the information needed to use ZOLINZA safely and effectively. See full prescribing information for ZOLINZA.
ZOLINZA® (vorinostat) Capsules
Initial U.S. Approval: 2006
————————RECENT MAJOR CHANGES————————
Warnings and Precautions
  QTc Prolongation (5.5) 09/2009
  Monitoring: Laboratory Tests (5.5) 09/2009
————————INDICATIONS AND USAGE————————
ZOLINZA is a histone deacetylase (HDAC) inhibitor indicated for:
• Treatment of cutaneous manifestations in patients with cutaneous T-cell lymphoma (CTCL) who have progressive, persistent or recurrent disease on or following two systemic therapies. (1)
————————DOSAGE AND ADMINISTRATION————————
• 400 mg orally once daily with food. (2.1)
• If patient is intolerant to therapy, the dose may be reduced to 300 mg orally once daily with food. If necessary, the dose may be further reduced to 300 mg once daily with food for 5 consecutive days each week. (2.2, 5)
————————DOSAGE FORMS AND STRENGTHS————————
• Capsules: 100 mg (3)
————————CONTRAINDICATIONS————————
• None (4)
————————WARNINGS AND PRECAUTIONS————————
• Pulmonary embolism and deep vein thrombosis have been reported. Monitor patient for pertinent signs and symptoms. (5.1)
• Dose-related thrombocytopenia and anemia have occurred and may require dose modification or discontinuation. (2.2, 5.2, 6)
• Gastrointestinal disturbances (e.g., nausea, vomiting and diarrhea) have been reported. Patients may require antiemetics, antidiarrheals and fluid and electrolyte replacement (to prevent dehydration). (5.3, 6, 17.1)
• Hyperglycemia has been observed. Adjustment of diet and/or therapy for increased glucose may be necessary. (5.4, 5.5)
• Monitor electrolytes at baseline and periodically during treatment. (5.5)
• Monitor blood cell counts and chemistry tests, including electrolytes, glucose and serum creatinine, every 2 weeks during the first 2 months of therapy and monthly thereafter. (5.5)
• Severe thrombocytopenia and gastrointestinal bleeding have been reported with concomitant use of ZOLINZA and other HDAC inhibitors (e.g., valproic acid). Monitor platelet count. (5.6, 7.2)

- Fetal harm can occur when administered to a pregnant woman. Women should be apprised of the potential harm to the fetus. (5.7)

---ADVERSE REACTIONS---

- The most common adverse reactions (incidence ≥20%) are diarrhea, fatigue, nausea, thrombocytopenia, anorexia and dysgeusia. (6)

To report SUSPECTED ADVERSE REACTIONS, contact Merck Sharp & Dohme Corp., a subsidiary of Merck & Co., Inc., at 1-877-888-4231 or FDA at 1-800-FDA-1088 or www.fda.gov/medwatch.

---DRUG INTERACTIONS---

- Coumarin-derivative anticoagulants: Prolongation of prothrombin time and International Normalized Ratio have been observed with concomitant use. Monitor carefully. (7.1)

See 17 for PATIENT COUNSELING INFORMATION and FDA-approved patient labeling

Revised: 02/2010

FULL PRESCRIBING INFORMATION: CONTENTS*

FULL PRESCRIBING INFORMATION

1 INDICATIONS AND USAGE

ZOLINZA[1] is indicated for the treatment of cutaneous manifestations in patients with cutaneous T-cell lymphoma who have progressive, persistent or recurrent disease on or following two systemic therapies.

2 DOSAGE AND ADMINISTRATION

2.1 Dosing Information

The recommended dose is 400 mg orally once daily with food.

Treatment may be continued as long as there is no evidence of progressive disease or unacceptable toxicity.

ZOLINZA capsules should not be opened or crushed [see How Supplied/Storage and Handling (16)].

2.2 Dose Modifications

If a patient is intolerant to therapy, the dose may be reduced to 300 mg orally once daily with food. The dose may be further reduced to 300 mg once daily with food for 5 consecutive days each week, as necessary.

2.3 Dosing in Special Populations

No information is available in patients with renal or hepatic impairment [see Pharmacokinetics (12.3)].

3 DOSAGE FORMS AND STRENGTHS

100 mg white, opaque, hard gelatin capsules with "568" over "100 mg" printed within radial bar in black ink on the capsule body.

4 CONTRAINDICATIONS

None

5 WARNINGS AND PRECAUTIONS

5.1 Thromboembolism

As pulmonary embolism and deep vein thrombosis have been reported as adverse reactions, physicians should be alert to the signs and symptoms of these events, particularly in patients with a prior history of thromboembolic events [see Adverse Reactions (6)].

5.2 Hematologic

Treatment with ZOLINZA can cause dose-related thrombocytopenia and anemia. If platelet counts and/or hemoglobin are reduced during treatment with ZOLINZA, the dose should be modified or therapy discontinued. [See Dosage and Administration (2.2), Warnings and Precautions (5.6) and Adverse Reactions (6).]

5.3 Gastrointestinal

Gastrointestinal disturbances, including nausea, vomiting and diarrhea, have been reported [see Adverse Reactions (6)] and may require the use of antiemetic and antidiarrheal medications. Fluid and electrolytes should be replaced to prevent dehydration [see Adverse Reactions (6.1)]. Pre-existing nausea, vomiting, and diarrhea should be adequately controlled before beginning therapy with ZOLINZA.

5.4 Hyperglycemia

Hyperglycemia has been observed in patients receiving ZOLINZA [see Adverse Reactions (6.1)]. Serum glucose should be monitored, especially in diabetic or potentially diabetic patients. Adjustment of diet and/or therapy for increased glucose may be necessary.

5.5 Monitoring: Laboratory Tests

Careful monitoring of blood cell counts and chemistry tests, including electrolytes, glucose and serum creatinine, should be performed every 2 weeks during the first 2 months of therapy and monthly thereafter. Electrolyte monitoring should include potassium, magnesium and calcium. Hypokalemia or hypomagnesemia should be corrected prior to administration of ZOLINZA, and consideration should be given to monitoring potassium and magnesium in symptomatic patients (e.g., patients with nausea, vomiting, diarrhea, fluid imbalance or cardiac symptoms).

5.6 Other Histone Deacetylase (HDAC) Inhibitors

Severe thrombocytopenia and gastrointestinal bleeding have been reported with concomitant use of ZOLINZA and other HDAC inhibitors (e.g., valproic acid). Monitor platelet count every 2 weeks during the first 2 months. [See Drug Interactions (7.2)].

5.7 Pregnancy

Pregnancy Category D

ZOLINZA can cause fetal harm when administered to a pregnant woman. There are no adequate and well-controlled studies of ZOLINZA in pregnant women. Results of animal studies indicate that vorinostat crosses the placenta and is found in fetal tissue at levels up to 50% of maternal concentrations. Doses up to 50 and 150 mg/kg/day were tested in rats and rabbits, respectively (~0.5 times the human exposure based on $AUC_{0-24\ hours}$). Treatment-related developmental effects including decreased mean live fetal weights, incomplete ossifications of the skull, thoracic vertebra, sternebra, and skeletal variations (cervical ribs, supernumerary ribs, vertebral count and sacral arch variations) in rats at the highest dose of vorinostat tested. Reductions in mean live fetal weight and an elevated incidence of incomplete ossification of the metacarpals were seen in rabbits dosed at 150 mg/kg/day. The no observed effect levels (NOELs) for these findings were 15 and 50 mg/kg/day (<0.1 times the human exposure based on AUC) in rats and rabbits, respectively. A dose-related increase in the incidence of malformations of the gall bladder was noted in all drug treatment groups in rabbits versus the concurrent control. If this drug is used during pregnancy, or if the patient becomes pregnant while taking this drug, the patient should be apprised of the potential hazard to the fetus.

6 ADVERSE REACTIONS

The most common drug-related adverse reactions can be classified into 4 symptom complexes: gastrointestinal symptoms (diarrhea, nausea, anorexia, weight decrease, vomiting, constipation), constitutional symptoms (fatigue, chills), hematological abnormalities (thrombocytopenia, anemia), and taste disorders (dysgeusia, dry mouth). The most common serious drug-related adverse reactions were pulmonary embolism and anemia.

6.1 Clinical Trials Experience

The safety of ZOLINZA was evaluated in 107 CTCL patients in two single arm clinical studies in which 86 patients received 400 mg once daily.

The data described below reflect exposure to ZOLINZA 400 mg once daily in the 86 patients for a median number of 97.5 days on therapy (range 2 to 480+ days). Seventeen (19.8%) patients were exposed beyond 24 weeks and 8 (9.3%) patients were exposed beyond 1 year. The population of CTCL patients studied was 37 to 83 years of age, 47.7% female, 52.3% male, and 81.4% white, 16.3% black, and 1.2% Asian or multi-racial.

Because clinical trials are conducted under widely varying conditions, adverse reaction rates observed in the clinical trials of a drug cannot be directly compared to rates in the clinical trials of another drug and may not reflect the rates observed in practice.

Common Adverse Reactions

Table 1 summarizes the frequency of CTCL patients with specific adverse events, regardless of causality, using the National Cancer Institute-Common Terminology Criteria for Adverse Events (NCI-CTCAE, version 3.0).

Table 1: Clinical or Laboratory Adverse Events Occurring in CTCL Patients (Incidence ≥10% of patients)

| Adverse Events | ZOLINZA 400 mg once daily (N=86) | | | |
| | All Grades | | Grades 3-5* | |
	n	%	n	%
Fatigue	45	52.3	3	3.5
Diarrhea	45	52.3	0	0.0
Nausea	35	40.7	3	3.5
Dysgeusia	24	27.9	0	0.0
Thrombocytopenia	22	25.6	5	5.8
Anorexia	21	24.4	2	2.3
Weight Decreased	18	20.9	1	1.2
Muscle Spasms	17	19.8	2	2.3
Alopecia	16	18.6	0	0.0
Dry Mouth	14	16.3	0	0.0
Blood Creatinine Increased	14	16.3	0	0.0
Chills	14	16.3	1	1.2
Vomiting	13	15.1	1	1.2
Constipation	13	15.1	0	0.0
Dizziness	13	15.1	1	1.2
Anemia	12	14.0	2	2.3
Decreased Appetite	12	14.0	1	1.2
Peripheral Edema	11	12.8	0	0.0
Headache	10	11.6	0	0.0
Pruritus	10	11.6	1	1.2
Cough	9	10.5	0	0.0
Upper Respiratory Infection	9	10.5	0	0.0
Pyrexia	9	10.5	1	1.2

* No Grade 5 events were reported.

The frequencies of more severe thrombocytopenia, anemia [see Warnings and Precautions (5.2)] and fatigue were increased at doses higher than 400 mg once daily of ZOLINZA.

Serious Adverse Reactions

The most common serious adverse events, regardless of causality, in the 86 CTCL patients in two clinical studies were pulmonary embolism reported in 4.7% (4/86) of patients, squamous cell carcinoma reported in 3.5% (3/86) of patients and anemia reported in 2.3% (2/86) of patients. There were single events of cholecystitis, death (of unknown cause), deep vein thrombosis, enterococcal infection, exfoliative dermatitis, gastrointestinal hemorrhage, infection, lobar pneumonia, myocardial infarction, ischemic stroke, pelviureteric obstruction, sepsis, spinal cord injury, streptococcal bacteremia, syncope, T-cell lymphoma, thrombocytopenia and ureteral obstruction.

Discontinuations

Of the CTCL patients who received the 400-mg once daily dose, 9.3% (8/86) of patients discontinued ZOLINZA due to adverse events. These adverse events, regardless of causality, included anemia, angioneurotic edema, asthenia, chest pain, exfoliative dermatitis, death, deep vein thrombosis, ischemic stroke, lethargy, pulmonary embolism, and spinal cord injury.

Dose Modifications

Of the CTCL patients who received the 400-mg once daily dose, 10.5% (9/86) of patients required a dose modification of ZOLINZA due to adverse events. These adverse events included increased serum creatinine, decreased appetite, hypokalemia, leukopenia, nausea, neutropenia, thrombocytopenia and vomiting. The median time to the first adverse event resulting in dose reduction was 42 days (range 17 to 263 days).

Laboratory Abnormalities

Laboratory abnormalities were reported in all of the 86 CTCL patients who received the 400-mg once-daily dose. Increased serum glucose was reported as a laboratory abnormality in 69% (59/86) of CTCL patients who received the 400-mg once daily dose; only 4 of these abnormalities were severe (Grade 3). Increased serum glucose was reported as an adverse event in 8.1% (7/86) of CTCL patients who received the 400-mg once daily dose. [See Warnings and Precautions (5.4).]

Transient increases in serum creatinine were detected in 46.5% (40/86) of CTCL patients who received the 400-mg once daily dose. Of these laboratory abnormalities, 34 were NCI CTCAE Grade 1, 5 were Grade 2, and 1 was Grade 3. Proteinuria was detected as a laboratory abnormality (51.4%) in 38 of 74 patients tested. The clinical significance of this finding is unknown.

Dehydration

Based on reports of dehydration as a serious drug-related adverse event in clinical trials, patients were instructed to drink at least 2 L/day of fluids for adequate hydration. *[See Warnings and Precautions (5.3, 5.5).]*

Adverse Reactions in Non-CTCL Patients

The frequencies of individual adverse events were substantially higher in the non-CTCL population. Drug-related serious adverse events reported in the non-CTCL population which were not observed in the CTCL population included single events of blurred vision, asthenia, hyponatremia, tumor hemorrhage, Guillain-Barré syndrome, renal failure, urinary retention, cough, hemoptysis, hypertension, and vasculitis.

7 DRUG INTERACTIONS

7.1 Coumarin-Derivative Anticoagulants

Prolongation of prothrombin time (PT) and International Normalized Ratio (INR) were observed in patients receiving ZOLINZA concomitantly with coumarin-derivative anticoagulants. Physicians should carefully monitor PT and INR in patients concurrently administered ZOLINZA and coumarin derivatives.

7.2 Other HDAC Inhibitors

Severe thrombocytopenia and gastrointestinal bleeding have been reported with concomitant use of ZOLINZA and other HDAC inhibitors (e.g., valproic acid). Monitor platelet count every 2 weeks for the first 2 months. *[See Warnings and Precautions (5.6).]*

8 USE IN SPECIFIC POPULATIONS

8.1 Pregnancy

Pregnancy Category D [See Warnings and Precautions (5.7)]

8.3 Nursing Mothers

It is not known whether this drug is excreted in human milk. Because many drugs are excreted in human milk and because of the potential for serious adverse reactions in nursing infants from ZOLINZA, a decision should be made whether to discontinue nursing or discontinue the drug, taking into account the importance of the drug to the mother.

8.4 Pediatric Use

The safety and effectiveness of ZOLINZA in pediatric patients have not been established.

8.5 Geriatric Use

Of the total number of patients with CTCL in trials (N=107), 46 percent were 65 years of age and over, while 15 percent were 75 years of age and over. No overall differences in safety or effectiveness were observed between these subjects and younger subjects, and other reported clinical experience has not identified differences in responses between the elderly and younger patients, but greater sensitivity of some older individuals cannot be ruled out.

8.6 Use in Patients with Hepatic Impairment

Vorinostat was not evaluated in patients with hepatic impairment. As vorinostat is predominantly eliminated through metabolism, patients with hepatic impairment should be treated with caution. *[See Clinical Pharmacology (12.3).]*

8.7 Use in Patients with Renal Impairment

Vorinostat was not evaluated in patients with renal impairment. However, renal excretion does not play a role in the elimination of vorinostat. Patients with pre-existing renal impairment should be treated with caution. *[See Clinical Pharmacology (12.3).]*

10 OVERDOSAGE

No specific information is available on the treatment of overdosage of ZOLINZA.

In the event of overdose, it is reasonable to employ the usual supportive measures, e.g., remove unabsorbed material from the gastrointestinal tract, employ clinical monitoring, and institute supportive therapy, if required. It is not known if vorinostat is dialyzable.

11 DESCRIPTION

ZOLINZA contains vorinostat, which is described chemically as *N*-hydroxy-*N'*-phenyloctanediamide.

The empirical formula is $C_{14}H_{20}N_2O_3$. The molecular weight *is 264.32 and the structural formula is:*

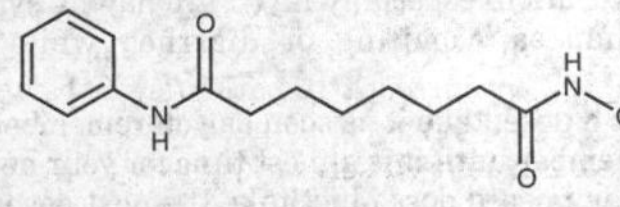

Vorinostat is a white to light orange powder. It is very slightly soluble in water, slightly soluble in ethanol, isopropanol and acetone, freely soluble in dimethyl sulfoxide and insoluble in methylene chloride. It has no chiral centers and is non-hygroscopic. The differential scanning calorimetry ranged from 161.7 (endotherm) to 163.9°C. The pH of saturated water solutions of vorinostat drug substance was 6.6. The pKa of vorinostat was determined to be 9.2.

Each 100 mg ZOLINZA capsule for oral administration contains 100 mg vorinostat and the following inactive ingredients: microcrystalline cellulose, sodium croscarmellose and magnesium stearate. The capsule shell excipients are titanium dioxide, gelatin and sodium lauryl sulfate.

12 CLINICAL PHARMACOLOGY

12.1 Mechanism of Action

Vorinostat inhibits the enzymatic activity of histone deacetylases HDAC1, HDAC2 and HDAC3 (Class I) and HDAC6 (Class II) at nanomolar concentrations (IC_{50}<86 nM). These enzymes catalyze the removal of acetyl groups from the lysine residues of proteins, including histones and transcription factors. In some cancer cells, there is an overexpression of HDACs, or an aberrant recruitment of HDACs to oncogenic transcription factors causing hypoacetylation of core nucleosomal histones. Hypoacetylation of histones is associated with a condensed chromatin structure and repression of gene transcription. Inhibition of HDAC activity allows for the accumulation of acetyl groups on the histone lysine residues resulting in an open chromatin structure and transcriptional activation. *In vitro*, vorinostat causes the accumulation of acetylated histones and induces cell cycle arrest and/or apoptosis of some transformed cells. The mechanism of the antineoplastic effect of vorinostat has not been fully characterized.

12.2 Pharmacodynamics

Cardiac Electrophysiology

A randomized, partially-blind, placebo-controlled, 2-period crossover study was performed to assess the effects of a single 800-mg dose of vorinostat on the QTc interval in 24 patients with advanced cancer. This study was conducted to assess the impact of vorinostat on ventricular repolarization. The upper bound of the 90% confidence interval of the placebo-adjusted mean QTc interval change-from-baseline was less than 10 msec at every time point through 24 hours. Based on these study results, administration of a single supratherapeutic 800-mg dose of vorinostat does not appear to prolong the QTc interval in patients with advanced cancer; however the study did not include a positive control to demonstrate assay sensitivity. In the fasted state, oral administration of a single 800-mg dose of vorinostat resulted in a mean AUC and C_{max} and median T_{max} of 8.6±5.7 μM•hr and 1.7±0.67 μM and 2.1 (0.5-6) hours, respectively.

In clinical studies in patients with CTCL, three of 86 CTCL patients exposed to 400 mg once daily had Grade 1 (>450-470 msec) or 2 (>470-500 msec or increase of >60 msec above baseline) clinical adverse events of QTc prolongation. In a retrospective analysis of three Phase 1 and two Phase 2 studies, 116 patients had a baseline and at least one follow-up ECG. Four patients had Grade 2 (>470-500 msec or increase of >60 msec above baseline) and 1 patient had Grade 3 (>500 msec) QTc prolongation. In 49 non-CTCL patients from 3 clinical trials who had complete evaluation of QT interval, 2 had QTc measurements of >500 msec and 1 had a QTc prolongation of >60 msec.

12.3 Pharmacokinetics

Absorption

The pharmacokinetics of vorinostat were evaluated in 23 patients with relapsed or refractory advanced cancer. After oral administration of a single 400-mg dose of vorinostat with a high-fat meal, the mean ± standard deviation area under the curve (AUC) and peak serum concentration (C_{max}) and the median (range) time to maximum concentration (T_{max}) were 5.5±1.8 μM•hr, 1.2±0.62 μM and 4 (2-10) hours, respectively.

In the fasted state, oral administration of a single 400-mg dose of vorinostat resulted in a mean AUC and C_{max} and median T_{max} of 4.2±1.9 μM•hr and 1.2±0.35 μM and 1.5 (0.5-10) hours, respectively. Therefore, oral administration of vorinostat with a high-fat meal resulted in an increase (33%) in the extent of absorption and a modest decrease in the rate of absorption (T_{max} delayed 2.5 hours) compared to the fasted state. However, these small effects are not expected to be clinically meaningful. In clinical trials of patients with CTCL, vorinostat was taken with food.

At steady state in the fed-state, oral administration of multiple 400-mg doses of vorinostat resulted in a mean AUC and C_{max} and a median T_{max} of 6.0±2.0 μM•hr, 1.2±0.53 μM and 4 (0.5-14) hours, respectively.

Distribution

Vorinostat is approximately 71% bound to human plasma proteins over the range of concentrations of 0.5 to 50 μg/mL.

Metabolism

The major pathways of vorinostat metabolism involve glucuronidation and hydrolysis followed by β-oxidation. Human serum levels of two metabolites, *O*-glucuronide of vorinostat and 4-anilino-4-oxobutanoic acid were measured. Both metabolites are pharmacologically inactive. Compared to vorinostat, the mean steady state serum exposures in humans of the *O*-glucuronide of vorinostat and 4-anilino-4-oxobutanoic acid were 4-fold and 13-fold higher, respectively.

In vitro studies using human liver microsomes indicate negligible biotransformation by cytochromes P450 (CYP).

Excretion

Vorinostat is eliminated predominantly through metabolism with less than 1% of the dose recovered as unchanged drug in urine, indicating that renal excretion does not play a role in the elimination of vorinostat. The mean urinary recovery of two pharmacologically inactive metabolites at steady state was 16±5.8% of vorinostat dose as the *O*–glucuronide of vorinostat, and 36±8.6% of vorinostat dose as 4-anilino-4-oxobutanoic acid. Total urinary recovery of vorinostat and these two metabolites averaged 52±13.3% of vorinostat dose. The mean terminal half-life ($t_{1/2}$) was ~2.0 hours for both vorinostat and the *O*-glucuronide metabolite, while that of the 4-anilino-4-oxobutanoic acid metabolite was 11 hours.

Special Populations

Based upon an exploratory analysis of limited data, gender, race and age do not appear to have meaningful effects on the pharmacokinetics of vorinostat.

Pediatric

Vorinostat was not evaluated in patients <18 years of age.

Hepatic Insufficiency

Vorinostat was not evaluated in patients with hepatic impairment. *[See Use in Specific Populations (8.6).]*

Renal Insufficiency

Vorinostat was not evaluated in patients with renal impairment. However, renal excretion does not play a role in the elimination of vorinostat. *[See Use in Specific Populations (8.7).]*

Pharmacokinetic effects of vorinostat with other agents

Vorinostat is not an inhibitor of CYP drug metabolizing enzymes in human liver microsomes at steady state C_{max} of the 400 mg dose (C_{max} of 1.2 μM vs IC_{50} of >75 μM). Gene expression studies in human hepatocytes detected some potential for suppression of CYP2C9 and CYP3A4 activities by vorinostat at concentrations higher (≥10 μM) than pharmacologically relevant. Thus, vorinostat is not expected to affect the pharmacokinetics of other agents. As vorinostat is not eliminated via the CYP pathways, it is anticipated that vorinostat will not be subject to drug-drug interactions when co-administered with drugs that are known CYP inhibitors or inducers. However, no formal clinical studies have been conducted to evaluate drug interactions with vorinostat.

In vitro studies indicate that vorinostat is not a substrate of human P-glycoprotein (P-gp). In addition, vorinostat has no inhibitory effect on human P-gp-mediated transport of vinblastine (a marker P-gp substrate) at concentrations of up to 100 μM. Thus, vorinostat is not likely to inhibit P-gp at the pharmacologically relevant serum concentration of 2 μM (C_{max}) in humans.

13 NONCLINICAL TOXICOLOGY

13.1 Carcinogenesis, Mutagenesis, Impairment of Fertility

Carcinogenicity studies have not been performed with vorinostat.

Vorinostat was mutagenic *in vitro* in the bacterial reverse mutation assays (Ames test), caused chromosomal aberrations *in vitro* in Chinese hamster ovary (CHO) cells and increased the incidence of micro-nucleated erythrocytes when administered to mice (Mouse Micronucleus Assay).

Effects on the female reproductive system were identified in the oral fertility study when females were dosed for 14 days prior to mating through gestational day 7. Doses of 15, 50 and 150 mg/kg/day to rats resulted in approximate exposures of 0.15, 0.36 and 0.70 times the expected clinical exposure based on AUC. Dose dependent increases in corpora lutea were noted at ≥15 mg/kg/day, which resulted in increased peri-implantation losses were noted at ≥50 mg/kg/day. At 150 mg/kg/day, there were increases in the incidences of dead fetuses and in resorptions.

No effects on reproductive performance were observed in male rats dosed (20, 50, 150 mg/kg/day; approximate exposures of 0.15, 0.36 and 0.70 times the expected clinical exposure based on AUC), for 70 days prior to mating with untreated females. *[See Warnings and Precautions (5.7).]*

14 CLINICAL STUDIES

Cutaneous T-cell Lymphoma

In two open-label clinical studies, patients with refractory CTCL have been evaluated to determine their response rate to oral ZOLINZA. One study was a single-arm clinical study and the other assessed several dosing regimens. In both studies, patients were treated until disease progression or intolerable toxicity.

Study 1

In an open-label, single–arm, multicenter non-randomized study, 74 patients with advanced CTCL were treated with

ZOLINZA at a dose of 400 mg once daily. The primary endpoint was response rate to oral ZOLINZA in the treatment of skin disease in patients with advanced CTCL (Stage IIB and higher) who had progressive, persistent, or recurrent disease on or following two systemic therapies. Enrolled patients should have received, been intolerant to or not a candidate for bexarotene. Extent of skin disease was quantitatively assessed by investigators using a modified Severity Weighted Assessment Tool (SWAT). The investigator measured the percentage total body surface area (%TBSA) involvement separately for patches, plaques, and tumors within 12 body regions using the patient's palm as a "ruler". The total %TBSA for each lesion type was multiplied by a severity weighting factor (1=patch, 2=plaque and 4=tumor) and summed to derive the SWAT score. Efficacy was measured as either a Complete Clinical Response (CCR) defined as no evidence of disease, or Partial Response (PR) defined as a ≥50% decrease in SWAT skin assessment score compared to baseline. Both CCR and PR had to be maintained for at least 4 weeks.

Secondary efficacy endpoints included response duration, time to progression, and time to objective response.

The population had been exposed to a median of three prior therapies (range 1 to 12).

Table 2 summarizes the demographic and disease characteristics of the Study 1 population.

Table 2: Baseline Patient Characteristics (All Patients As Treated)

Characteristics	Vorinostat (N=74)
Age (year)	
Mean (SD)	61.2 (11.3)
Median (Range)	60.0 (39.0, 83.0)
Gender, n (%)	
Male	38 (51.4%)
Female	36 (48.6%)
CTCL stage, n (%)	
IB	11 (14.9%)
IIA	2 (2.7%)
IIB	19 (25.7%)
III	22 (29.7%)
IVA	16 (21.6%)
IVB	4 (5.4%)
Racial Origin, n (%)	
Asian	1 (1.4%)
Black	11 (14.9%)
Other	1 (1.4%)
White	61 (82.4%)
Time from Initial CTCL Diagnosis (year)	
Median (Range)	2.6 (0.0, 27.3)
Clinical Characteristics	
Number of prior systemic treatments, median (range)	3.0 (1.0, 12.0)

The overall objective response rate was 29.7% (22/74, 95% CI [19.7 to 41.5%]) in all patients treated with ZOLINZA. In patients with Stage IIB and higher CTCL, the overall objective response rate was 29.5% (18/61). One patient with Stage IIB CTCL achieved a CCR. Median times to response were 55 and 56 days (range 28 to 171 days), respectively in the overall population and in patients with Stage IIB and higher CTCL. However, in rare cases it took up to 6 months for patients to achieve an objective response to ZOLINZA. The median response duration was not reached since the majority of responses continued at the time of analysis, but was estimated to exceed 6 months for both the overall population and in patients with Stage IIB and higher CTCL. When end of response was defined as a 50% increase in SWAT score from the nadir, the estimated median response duration was 168 days and the median time to tumor progression was 202 days.

Using a 25% increase in SWAT score from the nadir as criterion for tumor progression, the estimated median time-to-progression was 148 days for the overall population and 169 days in the 61 patients with Stage IIB and higher CTCL. Response to any previous systemic therapy does not appear to be predictive of response to ZOLINZA.

Study 2

In an open-label, non-randomized study, ZOLINZA was evaluated to determine the response rate for patients with CTCL who were refractory or intolerant to at least one treatment. In this study, 33 patients were assigned to one of 3 cohorts: Cohort 1, 400 mg once daily; Cohort 2, 300 mg twice daily 3 days/week; or Cohort 3, 300 mg twice daily for 14 days followed by a 7-day rest (induction). In Cohort 3, if at least a partial response was not observed then patients were dosed with a maintenance regimen of 200 mg twice daily. The primary efficacy endpoint, objective response, was measured by the 7-point Physician's Global Assessment (PGA) scale. The investigator assessed improvement or worsening in overall disease compared to baseline based on overall clinical impression. Index and non-index cutaneous lesions as well as cutaneous tumors, lymph nodes and all other disease manifestations were also assessed and included in the overall clinical impression. CCR required 100% clearing of all findings, and PR required at least 50% improvement in disease findings.

The median age was 67.0 years (range 26.0 to 82.0). Fifty-five percent of patients were male, and 45% of patients were female. Fifteen percent of patients had Stage IA, IB, or IIA CTCL and 85% of patients had Stage IIB, III, IVA, or IVB CTCL. The median number of prior systemic therapies was 4 (range 0.0 to 11.0).

In all patients treated, the objective response was 24.2% (8/33) in the overall population, 25% (7/28) in patients with Stage IIB or higher disease and 36.4% (4/11) in patients with Sezary syndrome. The overall response rates were 30.8%, 9.1% and 33.3% in Cohort 1, Cohort 2 and Cohort 3, respectively. The 300 mg twice daily regimen had higher toxicity with no additional clinical benefit over the 400 mg once daily regimen. No CCR was observed.

Among the 8 patients who responded to study treatment, the median time to response was 83.5 days (range 25 to 153 days). The median response duration was 106 days (range 66 to 136 days). Median time to progression was 211.5 days (range 94 to 255 days).

15 REFERENCES

1. NIOSH Alert: Preventing occupational exposures to antineoplastic and other hazardous drugs in healthcare settings. 2004. U.S. Department of Health and Human Services, Public Health Service, Centers for Disease Control and Prevention, National Institute for Occupational Safety and Health, DHHS (NIOSH) Publication No. 2004-165.
2. OSHA Technical Manual, TED 1-0.15A, Section VI: Chapter 2. Controlling Occupational Exposure to Hazardous Drugs. OSHA, 1999. http://www.osha.gov/dts/osta/otm/otm_vi/otm_vi_2.html
3. NIH [2002]. 1999 recommendations for the safe handling of cytotoxic drugs. U.S. Department of Health and Human Services, Public Health Service, National Institutes of Health, NIH Publication No. 92-2621.
4. American Society of Health-System Pharmacists. (2006) ASHP Guidelines on Handling Hazardous Drugs.
5. Polovich, M., White, J. M., & Kelleher, L.O. (eds.) 2005. Chemotherapy and biotherapy guidelines and recommendations for practice (2nd. ed.) Pittsburgh, PA: Oncology Nursing Society.

16 HOW SUPPLIED/STORAGE AND HANDLING

ZOLINZA capsules, 100 mg, are white, opaque hard gelatin capsules with "568" over "100 mg" printed within the radial bar in black ink on the capsule body. They are supplied as follows:

NDC 0006-0568-40.

Each bottle contains 120 capsules.

Storage and Handling

Store at 20-25°C (68-77°F), excursions permitted between 15-30°C (59-86°F). [See USP Controlled Room Temperature.]

Procedures for proper handling and disposal of anticancer drugs should be considered. Several guidelines on this subject have been published.(1-5) There is no general agreement that all of the procedures recommended in the guidelines are necessary or appropriate.

ZOLINZA (vorinostat) capsules should not be opened or crushed. Direct contact of the powder in ZOLINZA capsules with the skin or mucous membranes should be avoided. If such contact occurs, wash thoroughly as outlined in the references. Personnel should avoid exposure to crushed and/or broken capsules *[see Nonclinical Toxicology (13.1)]*.

Manufactured for:

Merck Sharp & Dohme Corp., a subsidiary of Merck & Co., Inc.

Whitehouse Station, NJ 08889, USA

Manufactured by:

Patheon, Inc.

Mississauga, Ontario, Canada L5N 7K9

Printed in USA

9762603

U.S. Patent Nos. RE 38,506 E, 6,087,367

¹Registered trademark of Merck Sharp & Dohme Corp., a subsidiary of **Merck & Co., Inc.**

17 PATIENT COUNSELING INFORMATION

[See FDA-Approved Patient Labeling (17.2)]

17.1 Instructions

Patients should be instructed to drink at least 2 L/day of fluid to prevent dehydration and should promptly report excessive vomiting or diarrhea to their physician. Patients should be instructed about the signs of deep vein thrombosis and should consult their physician should any evidence of deep vein thrombosis develop. Patients receiving ZOLINZA should seek immediate medical attention if unusual bleeding occurs. ZOLINZA capsules should not be opened or crushed.

Patients should be instructed to read the patient insert carefully.

17.2 FDA-Approved Patient Labeling

Patient Information

ZOLINZA® (zo LINZ ah)

(vorinostat)

Capsules

Read the patient information that comes with ZOLINZA² before you start taking it and each time you get a refill. There may be new information. This leaflet is a summary of the information for patients. Your doctor or pharmacist can give you additional information. This leaflet does not take the place of talking with your doctor about your medical condition or your treatment.

What is ZOLINZA?

ZOLINZA is a prescription medicine used to treat a type of cancer called cutaneous T-cell lymphoma (CTCL) in patients when the CTCL gets worse, does not go away, or comes back after treatment with other medicines.

ZOLINZA has not been studied in children under the age of 18.

What should I tell my doctor before taking ZOLINZA?

Tell your doctor about all of your medical conditions, including if you:

• Have any allergies

• Have had a blood clot in your lung (pulmonary embolus)

• Have had a blood clot in a vein (a blood vessel) anywhere in your body (deep vein thrombosis)

• Have nausea, vomiting, or diarrhea

• Have high blood sugar or diabetes

• Are pregnant or plan to become pregnant. ZOLINZA may harm your unborn baby. ZOLINZA has not been studied in pregnant women. If you use ZOLINZA during pregnancy, tell your doctor immediately.

• Are breast-feeding or plan to breast-feed. It is not known if ZOLINZA will pass into your breast milk. Talk to your doctor about the best way to feed your baby while you are taking ZOLINZA.

Tell your doctor about all of the medicines you take, including prescription and non-prescription medicines, vitamins and herbal supplements. Some medicines may affect how ZOLINZA works, or ZOLINZA may affect how your other medicines work. **Especially tell your doctor if you take:**

• **Valproic acid:** a medicine used to treat seizures. Your doctor will decide if you should continue to take valproic acid and may want to test your blood more frequently.

• **COUMADIN®:** (warfarin) or any other blood thinner. Ask your doctor if you are not sure if you are taking a blood thinner. Your doctor may want to test your blood more frequently.

Know the medicines you take. Keep a list of your medicines and show it to your doctor and pharmacist when you get a new medicine.

How should I take ZOLINZA?

• Take ZOLINZA exactly as your doctor tells you to.

• Your doctor will tell you how many ZOLINZA capsules to take and when to take them.

• Swallow each capsule whole. Do not chew or break open the capsule. If you can't swallow ZOLINZA capsules whole, tell your doctor. You may need a different medicine.

• Take ZOLINZA with food.

• If ZOLINZA capsules are accidentally opened or crushed, do not touch the capsules or the powder contents of the capsules. If the powder from an open or crushed capsule gets on your skin or in your eyes, wash the contacted area well with plenty of plain water. Call your doctor.

• **Drink at least eight 8-ounce glasses of liquids every day while taking ZOLINZA.** Drinking enough fluids may help to decrease the chances of losing too much fluid from your body (dehydration) especially if you are having symptoms such as nausea, vomiting or diarrhea while taking ZOLINZA.

• If you miss a dose, take it as soon as you remember. If you do not remember until it is almost time for your next dose, just skip the missed dose. Just take the next dose at your regular time. Do not take two doses of ZOLINZA at the same time.

- If you take too much ZOLINZA, call your doctor, local emergency room, or poison control center right away.
- Your doctor will check your blood cell counts, blood sugar, blood electrolytes, and other chemistries every two weeks for the first two months of your treatment with ZOLINZA and then monthly. Your doctor may decide to do other tests to check your health as needed.
- If you have high blood sugar (hyperglycemia) or diabetes, continue to monitor your blood sugar as your doctor tells you to. Your doctor may need to change your diet or medicine to help control your blood sugar while you take ZOLINZA. Be sure to tell your doctor if you are unable to eat or drink normally due to nausea, vomiting or diarrhea.

What are the possible side effects of ZOLINZA?
ZOLINZA may cause **serious side effects**. Tell your doctor right away if you have any of the following symptoms:
- **Blood clots in the legs (deep vein thrombosis)**
  - sudden swelling in a leg
  - pain or tenderness in the leg. The pain may only be felt when standing or walking.
  - increased warmth in the area where the swelling is.
  - skin redness or change in skin color
- **Blood clots that travel to the lungs (pulmonary embolus)**
  - sudden sharp chest pain
  - shortness of breath
  - cough with bloody secretions
  - sweating
  - rapid pulse
  - fainting
  - feeling anxious
- **Dehydration** (loss of too much fluid from the body). This can happen if you are having nausea, vomiting or diarrhea and can not drink fluids well.
- **Changes in blood tests:** Your doctor will periodically do blood tests to check your blood counts and electrolytes.
  - **Low red blood cells.** Low red blood cells may make you feel tired and get tired easily. You may look pale, and feel short of breath.
  - **Low platelets.** Low platelets can cause unusual bleeding or bruising under the skin. Talk to your doctor right away if this happens.
- **High blood sugar** (blood glucose). If you have high blood sugar or diabetes, monitor your blood sugar frequently as directed by your doctor. Tell your doctor right away if your blood sugar is higher than normal.

In addition, the most common side effects with ZOLINZA include:
- **Stomach and intestinal problems,** including diarrhea, nausea, vomiting, loss of appetite, constipation and weight loss
- **Tiredness**
- **Dizziness**
- **Headache**
- **Changes in the way things taste and dry mouth**
- **Muscle aches**
- **Hair loss**
- **Chills**
- **Fever**
- **Upper respiratory infection**
- **Cough**
- **Increase in blood creatinine**
- **Swelling in the foot, ankle and leg**
- **Itching**

Tell your doctor if you have any side effect that bothers you or that does not go away.

These are not all the possible side effects of ZOLINZA. For more information, ask your doctor or pharmacist.

General information about ZOLINZA
Medicines are sometimes prescribed for conditions that are not mentioned in patient information leaflets. Do not use ZOLINZA for a condition for which it was not prescribed. Do not give ZOLINZA to other people, even if they have the same symptoms you have. It may harm them.

Keep ZOLINZA and all medicines out of the reach of children.

This leaflet summarizes the most important information about ZOLINZA. If you would like to know more information, talk to your doctor. You can ask your doctor or pharmacist for information about ZOLINZA that is written for health professionals.

What are the ingredients in ZOLINZA?
Active ingredient: vorinostat
Inactive ingredients: microcrystalline cellulose, sodium croscarmellose and magnesium stearate. The inactive ingredients in the capsule shell are titanium dioxide, gelatin, and sodium lauryl sulfate.

How should I store ZOLINZA?
Store ZOLINZA at room temperature, 68°F to 77°F (20°C to 25°C).

Issued: February 2010
Merck Sharp & Dohme Corp., a subsidiary of Merck & Co., Inc.
Whitehouse Station, NJ 08889, USA

9762603
[2]Registered trademark of Merck Sharp & Dohme Corp., a subsidiary of **Merck & Co., Inc.**
Copyright © 2006, 2009 Merck Sharp & Dohme Corp., a subsidiary of **Merck & Co., Inc.**
All rights reserved
Revised: 02/2010
Distributed by: Merck Sharp & Dohme Corp.
Shown in Product Identification Guide, page 314

ZOSTAVAX®   ℞
[ZOS tah vax]
(Zoster Vaccine Live)

HIGHLIGHTS OF PRESCRIBING INFORMATION
These highlights do not include all the information needed to use ZOSTAVAX[1] safely and effectively. See full prescribing information for ZOSTAVAX.
ZOSTAVAX®
Zoster Vaccine Live
Suspension for subcutaneous injection
Initial U.S. Approval: 2006

———————**INDICATIONS AND USAGE**———————
ZOSTAVAX is a live attenuated virus vaccine indicated for prevention of herpes zoster (shingles) in individuals 60 years of age and older (1).
ZOSTAVAX is not indicated for the treatment of zoster or postherpetic neuralgia (PHN) (1).

————**DOSAGE AND ADMINISTRATION**————
Single 0.65 mL subcutaneous injection (2.1)

————**DOSAGE FORMS AND STRENGTHS**————
Single dose vials with not less than 19,400 plaque-forming units [PFU] per 0.65 mL dose when reconstituted to a suspension (2.1, 3, 16).

———————**CONTRAINDICATIONS**———————
- History of anaphylactic/anaphylactoid reaction to gelatin, neomycin, or any other component of the vaccine (4.1).
- History of primary or acquired immunodeficiency states (4.2).
- On immunosuppressive therapy (4.2).
- ZOSTAVAX is not indicated in women of child-bearing age and should not be administered to pregnant females (4.3, 8.1, 17.1).

————**WARNINGS AND PRECAUTIONS**————
- ZOSTAVAX is not indicated for prevention of primary varicella infection (Chickenpox) (5.2, 8.4).
- Transmission of vaccine virus may occur rarely between vaccinees and susceptible contacts (5.1).
- Defer vaccination in patients with active untreated tuberculosis (5.5).

———————**ADVERSE REACTIONS**———————
The rate of serious adverse events (SAEs) from Days 0 to 42 postvaccination may be increased in recipients of ZOSTAVAX compared to recipients of placebo (Table 1, 6.1.1).
The most frequent vaccine-related adverse events, reported in ≥1% of subjects vaccinated with ZOSTAVAX, were headache and injection site reactions (6.1.1).
ZOSTAVAX and PNEUMOVAX®[2] 23 should not be given concurrently because concomitant use resulted in reduced immunogenicity of ZOSTAVAX (7.1, 14).
To report vaccine exposure during pregnancy call 1-800-986-8999.
To report SUSPECTED ADVERSE REACTIONS, contact Merck & Co., Inc. at 1-877-888-4231 or VAERS at 1-800-822-7967 and www.fda.gov/vaers.
See 17 for PATIENT COUNSELING INFORMATION and FDA-Approved Patient Labeling.
Revised: 12/2009

---

[1] Registered trademark of Merck & Co., Inc.
Copyright © 2006 Merck & Co., Inc. Whitehouse Station, NJ, USA
All rights reserved
[2] Registered trademark of Merck & Co., Inc.

FULL PRESCRIBING INFORMATION: CONTENTS*
1 INDICATIONS AND USAGE
2 DOSAGE AND ADMINISTRATION
2.1 Recommended Dose and Schedule
2.2 Preparation for Administration
3 DOSAGE FORMS AND STRENGTHS
4 CONTRAINDICATIONS
4.1 Hypersensitivity
4.2 Immunosuppression
4.3 Pregnancy
5 WARNINGS AND PRECAUTIONS
5.1 Transmission of Vaccine Virus
5.2 Primary Varicella Disease
5.3 Preventing and Managing Allergic Vaccine Reactions
5.4 Limitations of Vaccine Effectiveness
5.5 Concurrent Illness

6 ADVERSE REACTIONS
6.1 Clinical Trials Experience
6.2 Post-Marketing Experience
7 DRUG INTERACTIONS
7.1 Concomitant Administration with Other Vaccines
8 USE IN SPECIFIC POPULATIONS
8.1 Pregnancy
8.3 Nursing Mothers
8.4 Pediatric Use
8.5 Geriatric Use
11 DESCRIPTION
12 CLINICAL PHARMACOLOGY
12.1 Mechanism of Action
13 NONCLINICAL TOXICOLOGY
13.1 Carcinogenesis, Mutagenesis, Impairment of Fertility
14 CLINICAL STUDIES
15 REFERENCES
16 HOW SUPPLIED/STORAGE AND HANDLING
17 PATIENT COUNSELING INFORMATION
17.1 Instructions
17.2 FDA-Approved Patient Labeling

*SECTIONS OR SUBSECTIONS OMITTED FROM THE FULL PRESCRIBING INFORMATION ARE NOT LISTED.

FULL PRESCRIBING INFORMATION

1 INDICATIONS AND USAGE
ZOSTAVAX is a live attenuated virus vaccine indicated for prevention of herpes zoster (shingles) in individuals 60 years of age and older.
ZOSTAVAX is not indicated for the treatment of zoster or postherpetic neuralgia (PHN).

2 DOSAGE AND ADMINISTRATION
2.1 Recommended Dose and Schedule
ZOSTAVAX should be administered as a single 0.65 mL dose subcutaneously in the deltoid region of the upper arm.
Do not inject intravascularly or intramuscularly. Use only sterile syringes free of preservatives, antiseptics, and detergents for each injection and/or reconstitution of ZOSTAVAX. Preservatives, antiseptics and detergents may inactivate the vaccine virus.
2.2 Preparation for Administration
ZOSTAVAX is stored frozen and should be reconstituted immediately upon removal from the freezer. The diluent should be stored separately at room temperature or in the refrigerator.
Use separate sterile needles for reconstitution and administration of ZOSTAVAX.
To reconstitute the vaccine: Use only the diluent supplied. Withdraw the entire contents of the diluent into a syringe. To avoid excessive foaming, slowly inject all of the diluent in the syringe into the vial of lyophilized vaccine and gently agitate to mix thoroughly.
ZOSTAVAX when reconstituted is a semi-hazy to translucent, off-white to pale yellow liquid.
Withdraw the entire contents of reconstituted vaccine into a syringe and inject the total volume subcutaneously.
THE VACCINE SHOULD BE ADMINISTERED IMMEDIATELY AFTER RECONSTITUTION, TO MINIMIZE LOSS OF POTENCY.
DISCARD RECONSTITUTED VACCINE IF IT IS NOT USED WITHIN 30 MINUTES.
DO NOT FREEZE RECONSTITUTED VACCINE.
Needles should be disposed of properly and should not be recapped.

3 DOSAGE FORMS AND STRENGTHS
ZOSTAVAX is a lyophilized preparation of live, attenuated varicella-zoster virus (Oka/Merck) to be reconstituted with sterile diluent to give a single dose suspension with a minimum of 19,400 PFU (plaque forming units) when stored at room temperature for up to 30 minutes.

4 CONTRAINDICATIONS
4.1 Hypersensitivity
Do not administer ZOSTAVAX to individuals with a history of anaphylactic/anaphylactoid reaction to gelatin, neomycin or any other component of the vaccine. Neomycin allergy manifested as contact dermatitis is not a contraindication to receiving this vaccine.[1]
4.2 Immunosuppression
Do not administer ZOSTAVAX to individuals with a history of primary or acquired immunodeficiency states including leukemia; lymphomas of any type, or other malignant neoplasms affecting the bone marrow or lymphatic system; or AIDS or other clinical manifestations of infection with human immunodeficiency viruses. ZOSTAVAX is a live attenuated varicella-zoster vaccine and administration may result in disseminated disease in individuals who are immunosuppressed. Do not administer ZOSTAVAX to individuals on immunosuppressive therapy.

Table 1
Number of Subjects with ≥1 Serious Adverse Events
(0-42 Days Postvaccination) in the Shingles Prevention Study

Cohort	ZOSTAVAX n/N %	Placebo n/N %	Relative Risk (95% CI)
Overall Study Cohort (all ages)	255/18671 1.4%	254/18717 1.4%	1.01 (0.85, 1.20)
60-69 years old	113/10100 1.1%	101/10095 1.0%	1.12 (0.86, 1.46)
70-79 years old	115/7351 1.6%	132/7333 1.8%	0.87 (0.68, 1.11)
≥80 years old	27/1220 2.2%	21/1289 1.6%	1.36 (0.78, 2.37)
AE Monitoring Substudy Cohort (all ages)	64/3326 1.9%	41/3249 1.3%	1.53 (1.04, 2.25)
60-69 years old	22/1726 1.3%	18/1709 1.1%	1.21 (0.66, 2.23)
70-79 years old	31/1383 2.2%	19/1367 1.4%	1.61 (0.92, 2.82)
≥80 years old	11/217 5.1%	4/173 2.3%	2.19 (0.75, 6.45)

N=number of subjects in cohort with safety follow-up
n=number of subjects reporting an SAE 0-42 Days postvaccination

Table 2
Injection-Site and Systemic Adverse Experiences
Reported by Vaccine Report Card in ≥1% of Adults Who
Received ZOSTAVAX or Placebo (0-42 Days
Postvaccination) in the AE Monitoring Substudy of the
Shingles Prevention Study

Adverse Experience	ZOSTAVAX (N = 3345) %	Placebo (N = 3271) %
Injection Site		
Erythema[†]	33.7	6.4
Pain/tenderness[†]	33.4	8.3
Swelling[†]	24.9	4.3
Hematoma	1.4	1.4
Pruritus	6.6	1.0
Warmth	1.5	0.3
Systemic		
Headache	1.4	0.8

[†] Designates a solicited adverse experience. Injection-site adverse experiences were solicited only from Days 0-4 postvaccination.

The numbers of subjects with elevated temperature (≥38.3°C [≥101.0°F]) within 42 days postvaccination were similar in the ZOSTAVAX and the placebo vaccination groups [27 (0.8%) vs. 27 (0.9%), respectively].

The following adverse experiences in the AE Monitoring Substudy of the SPS (Days 0 to 42 postvaccination) were reported at an incidence ≥1% and greater in subjects who received ZOSTAVAX than in subjects who received placebo, respectively: respiratory infection (65 [1.9%] vs. 55 [1.7%]), fever (59 [1.8%] vs. 53 [1.6%]), flu syndrome (57 [1.7%] vs. 52 [1.6%]), diarrhea (51 [1.5%] vs. 41 [1.3%]), rhinitis (46 [1.4%] vs. 36 [1.1%]), skin disorder (35 [1.1%] vs. 31 [1.0%]), respiratory disorder (35 [1.1%] vs. 27 [0.8%]), asthenia (32 [1.0%] vs. 14 [0.4%]).

6.1.2 VZV Rashes Following Vaccination
Within the 42-day post vaccination reporting period in the SPS, non-injection-site zoster-like rashes were reported by 53 subjects (17 for ZOSTAVAX and 36 for placebo). Of 41 specimens that were adequate for Polymerase Chain Reaction (PCR) testing, wild-type VZV was detected in 25 (5 for ZOSTAVAX, 20 for placebo) of these specimens. The Oka/Merck strain of VZV was not detected from any of these specimens.

Of reported varicella-like rashes (n=59), 10 had specimens that were available and adequate for PCR testing. VZV was not detected in any of these specimens.

In clinical trials in support of the initial licensure of the frozen formulation of ZOSTAVAX, the reported rates of noninjection-site zoster-like and varicella-like rashes within 42 days postvaccination were also low in both zoster vaccine and placebo recipients. Of 17 reported varicella-like rashes and noninjection-site, zoster-like rashes, 10 specimens were available and adequate for PCR testing. The Oka/Merck strain was identified by PCR analysis from the lesion specimens of two subjects who reported varicella-like rashes (onset on Day 8 and 17).

6.2 Post-Marketing Experience
The following additional adverse reactions have been identified during post-marketing use of ZOSTAVAX. Because these reactions are reported voluntarily from a population of uncertain size, it is generally not possible to reliably estimate their frequency or establish a causal relationship to the vaccine.

Skin and subcutaneous tissue disorders: rash
Musculoskeletal and connective tissue disorders: arthralgia; myalgia
General disorders and administration site conditions: injection-site rash; injection-site urticaria; pyrexia; transient injection-site lymphadenopathy
Hypersensitivity: hypersensitivity reactions including anaphylactic reactions
Reporting Adverse Events
The U.S. Department of Health and Human Services has established a Vaccine Adverse Event Reporting System (VAERS) to accept all reports of suspected adverse events after the administration of any vaccine. For information or a copy of the vaccine reporting form, call the VAERS toll-free number at 1-800-822-7967 or report online to www.vaers.hhs.gov.[2]

7 DRUG INTERACTIONS
Concurrent administration of ZOSTAVAX and antiviral medications known to be effective against VZV has not been evaluated.

7.1 Concomitant Administration with Other Vaccines
ZOSTAVAX and PNEUMOVAX® 23 should not be given concurrently because concomitant use resulted in reduced immunogenicity of ZOSTAVAX [see Clinical Studies (14)].

4.3 Pregnancy
ZOSTAVAX is not indicated in women of child-bearing age and should not be administered to pregnant females [see Pregnancy (8.1)].

5 WARNINGS AND PRECAUTIONS
5.1 Transmission of Vaccine Virus
Transmission of vaccine virus may occur rarely between vaccinees and susceptible contacts.

5.2 Primary Varicella Disease
ZOSTAVAX is not indicated for prevention of primary varicella infection (Chickenpox).

5.3 Preventing and Managing Allergic Vaccine Reactions
As with any vaccine, adequate treatment provisions, including epinephrine injection (1:1000), should be available for immediate use should an anaphylactic/anaphylactoid reaction occur.

5.4 Limitations of Vaccine Effectiveness
The duration of protection beyond 4 years after vaccination with ZOSTAVAX is unknown. The need for revaccination has not been defined.
Vaccination with ZOSTAVAX may not result in protection of all vaccine recipients.

5.5 Concurrent Illness
Vaccination should be deferred in patients with active untreated tuberculosis. Deferral should be considered in acute illness, for example, in the presence of fever.

6 ADVERSE REACTIONS
6.1 Clinical Trials Experience
Because clinical trials are conducted under widely varying conditions, adverse event rates observed in the clinical trials of a vaccine cannot be directly compared to rates in the clinical trials of another vaccine and may not reflect the rates observed in practice.

6.1.1 Shingles Prevention Study
In clinical trials, ZOSTAVAX has been evaluated for safety in approximately 21,000 adults. In the largest of these trials, the Shingles Prevention Study (SPS), subjects received a single dose of either ZOSTAVAX (n=19,270) or placebo (n=19,276). The racial distribution across both vaccination groups was similar: White (95%); Black (2.0%); Hispanic (1.0%) and Other (1.0%) in both vaccination groups. The gender distribution was 59% male and 41% female in both vaccination groups. The age distribution of subjects enrolled, 59-99 years, was similar in both vaccination groups.

The Adverse Event Monitoring Substudy of the SPS, designed to provide detailed data on the safety profile of the zoster vaccine (n=3,345 received ZOSTAVAX and n=3,271 received placebo) used vaccination report cards (VRC) to record adverse events occurring from Days 0 to 42 postvaccination (97% of subjects completed VRC in both vaccination groups). In addition, monthly surveillance for hospitalization was conducted through the end of the study, 2 to 5 years postvaccination.

The remainder of subjects in the SPS (n=15,925 received ZOSTAVAX and n=16,005 received placebo) were actively followed for safety outcomes through Day 42 postvaccination and passively followed for safety after Day 42.

Serious Adverse Events Occurring 0-42 Days Postvaccination
In the overall SPS study population, serious adverse events occurred at a similar rate (1.4%) in subjects vaccinated with ZOSTAVAX or placebo.
In the AE Monitoring Substudy, the rate of SAEs was increased in the group of subjects who received ZOSTAVAX as compared to the group of subjects who received placebo (Table 1).
[See table 1 above]
Among reported serious adverse events in the SPS (Days 0 to 42 postvaccination), serious cardiovascular events occurred more frequently in subjects who received ZOSTAVAX (20 [0.6%]) than in subjects who received placebo (12 [0.4%]) in the AE Monitoring Substudy. The frequencies of serious cardiovascular events were similar in subjects who received ZOSTAVAX (81 [0.4%]) and in subjects who received placebo (72 [0.4%]) in the entire study cohort (Days 0 to 42 postvaccination).
Serious Adverse Events Occurring Over the Entire Course of the Study
Rates of hospitalization were similar among subjects who received ZOSTAVAX and subjects who received placebo in the AE Monitoring Substudy, throughout the entire study. Fifty-one individuals (1.5%) receiving ZOSTAVAX were reported to have congestive heart failure (CHF) or pulmonary edema compared to 39 individuals (1.2%) receiving placebo in the AE Monitoring Substudy; 58 individuals (0.3%) receiving ZOSTAVAX were reported to have congestive heart failure (CHF) or pulmonary edema compared to 45 (0.2%) individuals receiving placebo in the overall study.
In the SPS, all subjects were monitored for vaccine-related SAEs. Investigator-determined, vaccine-related adverse experiences were reported for 2 subjects vaccinated with ZOSTAVAX (asthma exacerbation and polymyalgia rheumatica) and 3 subjects who received placebo (Goodpasture's syndrome, anaphylactic reaction, and polymyalgia rheumatica).
Deaths
The incidence of death was similar in the groups receiving ZOSTAVAX or placebo during the Days 0-42 postvaccination period; 14 deaths occurred in the group of subjects who received ZOSTAVAX and 16 deaths occurred in the group of subjects who received placebo. The most common reported cause of death was cardiovascular disease (10 in the group of subjects who received ZOSTAVAX, 8 in the group of subjects who received placebo). The overall incidence of death occurring at any time during the study was similar between vaccination groups: 793 deaths (4.1%) occurred in subjects who received ZOSTAVAX and 795 deaths (4.1%) in subjects who received placebo.
Most Common Adverse Reactions
Adverse Events Reported in the AE Monitoring Substudy of the SPS
Injection-site and systemic adverse events reported at an incidence ≥1% are shown in Table 2. Most of these adverse events were reported as mild in intensity. The overall incidence of vaccine-related injection-site adverse reactions was significantly greater for subjects vaccinated with ZOSTAVAX versus subjects who received placebo (48% for ZOSTAVAX and 17% for placebo).

For concomitant administration of ZOSTAVAX with trivalent inactivated influenza vaccine, [see Clinical Studies (14)].

8 USE IN SPECIFIC POPULATIONS

8.1 Pregnancy
Pregnancy Category C: Animal reproduction studies have not been conducted with ZOSTAVAX. It is also not known whether ZOSTAVAX can cause fetal harm when administered to a pregnant woman or can affect reproduction capacity. However, naturally occurring VZV infection is known to sometimes cause fetal harm. ZOSTAVAX is not indicated in women of child-bearing age and should not be administered to pregnant females.

Vaccinees and health care providers are encouraged to report any exposure to ZOSTAVAX during pregnancy by calling (800) 986-8999.

8.3 Nursing Mothers
ZOSTAVAX is not indicated in women who are nursing. It is not known whether VZV is secreted in human milk. Therefore, because some viruses are secreted in human milk, caution should be exercised if ZOSTAVAX is administered to a nursing woman.

8.4 Pediatric Use
ZOSTAVAX is not indicated for prevention of primary varicella infection (Chickenpox) and should not be used in children and adolescents.

8.5 Geriatric Use
The median age of subjects enrolled in the largest (N=38,546) clinical study of ZOSTAVAX was 69 years (range 59-99 years). Of the 19,270 subjects who received ZOSTAVAX, 10,378 were 60-69 years of age, 7,629 were 70-79 years of age, and 1,263 were 80 years of age or older.

11 DESCRIPTION
ZOSTAVAX is a lyophilized preparation of the Oka/Merck strain of live, attenuated varicella-zoster virus (VZV). ZOSTAVAX, when reconstituted as directed, is a sterile suspension for subcutaneous administration. Each 0.65-mL dose contains a minimum of 19,400 PFU (plaque-forming units) of Oka/Merck strain of VZV when reconstituted and stored at room temperature for up to 30 minutes.

Each dose contains 31.16 mg of sucrose, 15.58 mg of hydrolyzed porcine gelatin, 3.99 mg of sodium chloride, 0.62 mg of monosodium L-glutamate, 0.57 mg of sodium phosphate dibasic, 0.10 mg of potassium phosphate monobasic, 0.10 mg of potassium chloride; residual components of MRC-5 cells including DNA and protein; and trace quantities of neomycin and bovine calf serum. The product contains no preservatives.

12 CLINICAL PHARMACOLOGY
12.1 Mechanism of Action
The risk of developing zoster appears to be related to a decline in VZV-specific immunity. ZOSTAVAX was shown to boost VZV-specific immunity, which is thought to be the mechanism by which it protects against zoster and its complications. [See Clinical Studies (14).]

Herpes zoster (HZ), commonly known as shingles or zoster, is a manifestation of the reactivation of varicella zoster virus (VZV), which, as a primary infection, produces chickenpox (varicella). Following initial infection, the virus remains latent in the dorsal root or cranial sensory ganglia until it reactivates, producing zoster. Zoster is characterized by a unilateral, painful, vesicular cutaneous eruption with a dermatomal distribution.

Pain associated with zoster may occur during the prodrome, the acute eruptive phase, and the postherpetic phase of the infection. Pain occurring in the postherpetic phase of infection is commonly referred to as postherpetic neuralgia (PHN).

Serious complications, such as PHN, scarring, bacterial superinfection, allodynia, cranial and motor neuron palsies, pneumonia, encephalitis, visual impairment, hearing loss, and death can occur as the result of zoster.

13 NONCLINICAL TOXICOLOGY
13.1 Carcinogenesis, Mutagenesis, Impairment of Fertility
ZOSTAVAX has not been evaluated for its carcinogenic or mutagenic potential, or its potential to impair fertility.

14 CLINICAL STUDIES
Efficacy of ZOSTAVAX was evaluated in the Shingles Prevention Study (SPS), a placebo-controlled, double-blind clinical trial in which 38,546 subjects 60 years of age or older were randomized to receive a single dose of either ZOSTAVAX (n=19,270) or placebo (n=19,276). Subjects were followed for the development of zoster for a median of 3.1 years (range 31 days to 4.90 years). The study excluded people who were immunocompromised or using corticosteroids on a regular basis, anyone with a previous history of HZ, and those with conditions that might interfere with study evaluations, including people with cognitive impairment, severe hearing loss, those who were non-ambulatory and those whose survival was not considered to be at least 5 years. Randomization was stratified by age, 60-69 and ≥70 years of age. Suspected zoster cases were confirmed by Polymerase Chain Reaction (PCR) [93%], viral culture [1%], or in the absence of viral detection, as determined by the Clinical Evaluation Committee [6%]. Individuals in both vaccination groups who developed zoster were given famciclovir, and, as necessary, pain medications. The primary efficacy analysis included all subjects randomized in the study who were followed for at least 30 days postvaccination and did not develop an evaluable case of HZ within the first 30 days postvaccination (Modified Intent-To-Treat [MITT] analysis). ZOSTAVAX significantly reduced the risk of developing zoster when compared with placebo (Table 3). Vaccine efficacy for the prevention of HZ was highest for those subjects 60-69 years of age and declined with increasing age.

[See table 3 above]

Forty-five subjects were excluded from the MITT analysis (16 in the group of subjects who received ZOSTAVAX and 29 in the group of subjects who received placebo), including 24 subjects with evaluable HZ cases that occurred in the first 30 days postvaccination (6 evaluable HZ cases in the group of subjects who received ZOSTAVAX and 18 evaluable HZ cases in the group of subjects who received placebo).

Suspected HZ cases were followed prospectively for the development of HZ-related complications. Table 4 compares the rates of PHN defined as HZ-associated pain (rated as 3 or greater on a 10-point scale by the study subject and occurring or persisting at least 90 days) following the onset of rash in evaluable cases of HZ.

[See table 4 below]

The median duration of clinically significant pain (defined as ≥3 on a 0-10 point scale) among HZ cases in the group of subjects who received ZOSTAVAX as compared to the group of subjects who received placebo was 20 days vs. 22 days based on the confirmed HZ cases.

Overall, the benefit of ZOSTAVAX in the prevention of PHN can be primarily attributed to the effect of the vaccine on the prevention of herpes zoster. Vaccination with ZOSTAVAX in the SPS reduced the incidence of PHN in individuals 70 years of age and older who developed zoster postvaccination. Other prespecified zoster-related complications were reported less frequently in subjects who received ZOSTAVAX compared to subjects who received placebo. Among HZ cases, zoster-related complications were reported at similar rates in both vaccination groups (Table 5).

[See table 5 at top of next page]

Table 3
Efficacy of ZOSTAVAX on HZ Incidence Compared with Placebo in the Shingles Prevention Study*

Age group** (yrs.)	ZOSTAVAX			Placebo			Vaccine Efficacy (95% CI)
	# subjects	# HZ cases	Incidence rate of HZ per 1000 person-yrs.	# subjects	# HZ cases	Incidence rate of HZ per 1000 person-yrs.	
Overall	19254	315	5.4	19247	642	11.1	51% (44%, 58%)
60-69	10370	122	3.9	10356	334	10.8	64% (56%, 71%)
70-79	7621	156	6.7	7559	261	11.4	41% (28%, 52%)
≥80	1263	37	9.9	1332	47	12.2	18% (-29%, 48%)

* The analysis was performed on the Modified Intent-To-Treat (MITT) population that included all subjects randomized in the study who were followed for at least 30 days postvaccination and did not develop an evaluable case of HZ within the first 30 days postvaccination.

** Age strata at randomization were 60-69 and ≥70 years of age.

Table 4
Postherpetic Neuralgia (PHN)* in the Shingles Prevention Study*

Age group (yrs.)†	ZOSTAVAX					Placebo					Vaccine efficacy against PHN in subjects who develop HZ postvaccination (95% CI)
	# subjects	# HZ cases	# PHN cases	Incidence rate of PHN per 1,000 person-yrs.	% HZ cases with PHN	# subjects	# HZ cases	# PHN cases	Incidence rate of PHN per 1,000 person-yrs.	% HZ cases with PHN	
Overall	19254	315	27	0.5	8.6%	19247	642	80	1.4	12.5%	39%†† (7%, 59%)
60-69	10370	122	8	0.3	6.6%	10356	334	23	0.7	6.9%	5% (-107%, 56%)
70-79	7621	156	12	0.5	7.7%	7559	261	45	2.0	17.2%	55% (18%, 76%)
≥80	1263	37	7	1.9	18.9%	1332	47	12	3.1	25.5%	26% (-69%, 68%)

* PHN was defined as HZ-associated pain rated as ≥3 (on a 0-10 scale), persisting or appearing more than 90 days after onset of HZ rash using Zoster Brief Pain Inventory (ZBPI)[3].

**The table is based on the Modified Intent-To-Treat (MITT) population that included all subjects randomized in the study who were followed for at least 30 days postvaccination and did not develop an evaluable case of HZ within the first 30 days postvaccination.

† Age strata at randomization were 60-69 and ≥70 years of age.

†† Age-adjusted estimate based on the age strata (60-69 and ≥70 years of age) at randomization.

Table 5
Specific complications* of zoster among HZ cases in the Shingles Prevention Study

Complication	ZOSTAVAX (N = 19,270)		Placebo (N = 19,276)	
	(n = 321)	% Among Zoster Cases	(n = 659)	% Among Zoster Cases
Allodynia	135	42.1	310	47.0
Bacterial Superinfection	3	0.9	7	1.1
Dissemination	5	1.6	11	1.7
Impaired Vision	2	0.6	9	1.4
Ophthalmic Zoster	35	10.9	69	10.5
Peripheral Nerve Palsies (motor)	5	1.6	12	1.8
Ptosis	2	0.6	9	1.4
Scarring	24	7.5	57	8.6
Sensory Loss	7	2.2	12	1.8

N=number of subjects randomized
n=number of zoster cases, including those cases occurring within 30 days postvaccination, with these data available
*Complications reported at a frequency of ≥1% in at least one vaccination group among subjects with zoster.

Visceral complications reported by fewer than 1% of subjects with zoster included 3 cases of pneumonitis and 1 case of hepatitis in the placebo group, and 1 case of meningoencephalitis in the vaccine group.

Immune responses to vaccination were evaluated in a subset of subjects enrolled in the Shingles Prevention Study (N=1395). VZV antibody levels (Geometric Mean Titers, GMT), as measured by glycoprotein enzyme-linked immunosorbent assay (gpELISA) 6 weeks postvaccination, were increased 1.7-fold (95% CI: [1.6 to 1.8]) in the group of subjects who received ZOSTAVAX compared to subjects who received placebo; the specific antibody level that correlates with protection from zoster has not been established.

In a double-blind, controlled substudy, 374 adults in the US, 60 years of age and older (median age = 66 years), were randomized to receive trivalent inactivated influenza vaccine (TIV) and ZOSTAVAX concurrently (N=188), or TIV alone followed 4 weeks later by ZOSTAVAX alone (N=186). The antibody responses to both vaccines at 4 weeks postvaccination were similar in both groups.

In a double-blind, controlled clinical trial, 473 adults, 60 years of age or older, were randomized to receive ZOSTAVAX and PNEUMOVAX® 23 concomitantly (N=237), or PNEUMOVAX® 23 alone followed 4 weeks later by ZOSTAVAX alone (N=236). At four weeks postvaccination, the VZV antibody levels following concomitant use were significantly lower than the VZV antibody levels following non-concomitant administration (GMTs of 338 vs. 484 gpELISA units/mL, respectively; GMT ratio = 0.70 (95% CI: [0.61, 0.80]).

15 REFERENCES

1. Reitschel RL, Bernier R. Neomycin sensitivity and the MMR vaccine. JAMA 1981;245(6):571.
2. Atkinson WL, Pickering LK, Schwartz B, Weniger BG, Iskander JK, Watson JC. General recommendations on immunization: Recommendations of the Advisory Committee on Immunization Practices (ACIP) and the American Academy of Family Physicians (AAFP). MMWR 2002;51(RR02):1-36.
3. Coplan PM, Schmader K, Nikas A, Chan ISF, Choo P, Levin MJ, et al. Development of a measure of the burden of pain due to herpes zoster and postherpetic neuralgia for prevention trials: Adaptation of the brief pain inventory. J Pain 2004;5(6):344-56.

16 HOW SUPPLIED/STORAGE AND HANDLING

No. 4963-00 — ZOSTAVAX is supplied as follows: (1) a package of 1 single-dose vial of lyophilized vaccine, **NDC** 0006-4963-00 (package A); and (2) a separate package of 10 vials of diluent (package B).

No. 4963-41 — ZOSTAVAX is supplied as follows: (1) a package of 10 single-dose vials of lyophilized vaccine, **NDC** 0006-4963-41 (package A); and (2) a separate package of 10 vials of diluent (package B).

Handling and Storage
During shipment, to ensure that there is no loss of potency, the vaccine must be maintained at a temperature of −15°C (+5°F) or colder.

ZOSTAVAX SHOULD BE STORED FROZEN at an average temperature of −15°C (+5°F) or colder until it is reconstituted for injection. Any freezer, including frost-free, that has a separate sealed freezer door and reliably maintains an average temperature of −15°C or colder is acceptable for storing ZOSTAVAX.

ZOSTAVAX may be stored and/or transported at refrigerator temperature (2 to 8°C, 36 to 46°F) for up to 72 continuous hours prior to reconstitution. Vaccine stored at 2 to 8°C (36 to 46°F) that is not used within 72 hours of removal from -15°C (+5°F) storage should be discarded.

For information regarding stability under conditions other than those recommended, call 1-800-MERCK-90.

Before reconstitution, protect from light.

The diluent should be stored separately at room temperature (20 to 25°C, 68 to 77°F), or in the refrigerator (2 to 8°C, 36 to 46°F).

17 PATIENT COUNSELING INFORMATION

[See FDA-Approved Patient Labeling (17.2).]

17.1 Instructions

The health care provider should question the vaccine recipient about reactions to previous vaccines. The health care provider should also inform the vaccine recipient of the benefits and risks of ZOSTAVAX. Patients should be provided with a copy of the Patient Information about ZOSTAVAX at the end of this insert, and be given an opportunity to discuss any questions or concerns.

Vaccinees should also be informed of the potential risk of transmitting the vaccine virus to varicella-susceptible individuals, including pregnant women who have not had chickenpox.

Patients should be instructed to report any adverse reactions to their health care provider.

Dist. by:
MERCK & CO., INC., Whitehouse Station, NJ 08889, USA
Issued December 2009
Printed in USA
9815611

17.2 FDA-Approved Patient Labeling

**Patient Information about
ZOSTAVAX®
(pronounced "ZOS tah vax")
Generic name: Zoster Vaccine Live**

You should read this summary of information about ZOSTAVAX[1] before you are vaccinated. If you have any questions about ZOSTAVAX after reading this leaflet, you should ask your health care provider. This information does not take the place of talking about ZOSTAVAX with your doctor, nurse, or other health care provider. Only your health care provider can decide if ZOSTAVAX is right for you.

What is ZOSTAVAX and how does it work?

ZOSTAVAX is a vaccine that is used for adults 60 years of age or older to prevent shingles (also known as zoster).

ZOSTAVAX contains a weakened chickenpox virus (varicella-zoster virus).

ZOSTAVAX works by helping your immune system protect you from getting shingles. If you do get shingles even though you have been vaccinated, ZOSTAVAX may help prevent the nerve pain that can follow shingles in some people. ZOSTAVAX may not protect everyone who gets the vaccine. ZOSTAVAX cannot be used to treat shingles once you have it.

What do I need to know about shingles and the virus that causes it?

Shingles is caused by the same virus that causes chickenpox. Once you have had chickenpox, the virus can stay in your nervous system for many years. For reasons that are not fully understood, the virus may become active again and give you shingles. Age and problems with the immune system may increase your chances of getting shingles.

Shingles is a rash that is usually on one side of the body. The rash begins as a cluster of small red spots that often blister. The rash can be painful. Shingles rashes usually last up to 30 days and, for most people, the pain associated with the rash lessens as it heals.

Who should not get ZOSTAVAX?

You should not get ZOSTAVAX if you:
• are allergic to any of its ingredients.
• are allergic to gelatin or neomycin.
• have a weakened immune system (for example, an immune deficiency, leukemia, lymphoma, or HIV/AIDS).
• take high doses of steroids by injection or by mouth.
• are pregnant or plan to get pregnant.
You should not get ZOSTAVAX to prevent chickenpox.
Children should not get ZOSTAVAX.

How is ZOSTAVAX given?

ZOSTAVAX is given as a single dose by injection under the skin.

What should I tell my health care provider before I get ZOSTAVAX?

You should tell your health care provider if you:
• have or have had any medical problems.
• take any medicines, including non-prescription medicines, and dietary supplements.
• have any allergies, including allergies to neomycin or gelatin.
• had an allergic reaction to another vaccine.
• are pregnant or plan to become pregnant.
• are breast-feeding.

Tell your health care provider if you expect to be in close contact (including household contact) with newborn infants, someone who may be pregnant and has not had chickenpox or been vaccinated against chickenpox, or someone who has problems with their immune system. Your health care provider can tell you what situations you may need to avoid.

Can I receive ZOSTAVAX with other vaccines?

Talk to your health care provider if you plan to get ZOSTAVAX at the same time as the flu vaccine. ZOSTAVAX should not be given at the same time as the PNEUMOVAX®[2] 23 vaccine. For more information about these vaccines, talk to your health care provider.

What are the possible side effects of ZOSTAVAX?

The most common side effects that people in the clinical studies reported after receiving the vaccine include:
• redness, pain, itching, swelling, warmth, or bruising where the shot was given.
• headache.

The following additional side effects have been reported in general use with ZOSTAVAX:
• allergic reactions, which may be serious and may include difficulty in breathing or swallowing. If you have an allergic reaction, call your doctor right away.
• fever
• hives at the injection site
• joint pain
• muscle pain
• rash
• Rash at the injection site
• Swollen glands near the injection site (that may last a few days to a few weeks)

Tell your healthcare provider if you have any new or unusual symptoms after you receive ZOSTAVAX. For a complete list of side effects, ask your health care provider.

What are the ingredients of ZOSTAVAX?

Active Ingredient: a weakened form of the varicella-zoster virus.

Inactive Ingredients: sucrose, hydrolyzed porcine gelatin, sodium chloride, monosodium L-glutamate, sodium phosphate dibasic, potassium phosphate monobasic, potassium chloride.

What else should I know about ZOSTAVAX?

Vaccinees and their health care providers are encouraged to call (800) 986-8999 to report any exposure to ZOSTAVAX during pregnancy.

This leaflet summarizes important information about ZOSTAVAX.

If you would like more information, talk to your health care provider or visit the website at www.ZOSTAVAX.com or call 1-800-622-4477.

[1] Registered trademark of Merck & Co., Inc.
Copyright © 2006 Merck & Co., Inc. Whitehouse Station, NJ, USA
All rights reserved

Rx Only
Issued December 2009
9815611
Dist. by:
MERCK & CO., INC., Whitehouse Station, NJ 08889, USA

Merck/Schering Plough Pharmaceuticals Inc.

for product information, please see Merck

Merz Pharmaceuticals

Division of Merz, Inc.
4215 TUDOR LANE (27410)
P.O. BOX 18806
GREENSBORO, NC 27419

Direct Inquiries to:
Medical/Regulatory Affairs
(336) 856-2003
FAX: (336) 217-2439
For Medical Information Contact:
(336) 856-2003
FAX: (336) 217-2439
To report
suspected
Adverse Events,
contact Merz
Pharmaceuticals, LLC
at 888-493-6646 •
or the FDA at
1-800-FDA-1088

NAFTIN®

(naftifine hydrochloride) 1% Cream
Rx Only

℞

DESCRIPTION

Naftin® Cream, 1% contains the synthetic, broad-spectrum, antifungal agent naftifine hydrochloride.
Naftin® Cream, 1% is for topical use only.
Chemical Name:
(E)-N-Cinnamyl-N-methyl-1-naphthalenemethylamine hydrochloride.
Naftifine hydrochloride has an empirical formula of $C_{21}H_{21}N \cdot HCl$ and a molecular weight of 323.86.

naftifine hydrochloride

Active Ingredient: Naftifine hydrochloride 1%
Inactive Ingredients: benzyl alcohol, cetyl alcohol, cetyl esters wax, isopropyl myristate, polysorbate 60, purified water, sodium hydroxide, sorbitan monostearate, and stearyl alcohol. Hydrochloric acid may be added to adjust pH.

CLINICAL PHARMACOLOGY

Naftifine hydrochloride is a synthetic allylamine derivative. The following *in vitro* data are available, but their clinical significance is unknown. Naftifine hydrochloride has been shown to exhibit fungicidal activity *in vitro* against a broad spectrum of organisms, including *Trichophyton rubrum, Trichophyton mentagrophytes, Trichophyton tonsurans, Epidermophyton floccosum, Microsporum canis, Microsporum audouini,* and *Microsporum gypseum;* and fungistatic activity against *Candida* species, including *Candida albicans*. Naftin® Cream, 1% has only been shown to be clinically effective against the disease entities listed in the INDICATIONS AND USAGE section.
Although the exact mechanism of action against fungi is not known, naftifine hydrochloride appears to interfere with sterol biosynthesis by inhibiting the enzyme squalene 2, 3-epoxidase. This inhibition of enzyme activity results in decreased amounts of sterols, especially ergosterol, and a corresponding accumulation of squalene in the cells.
Pharmacokinetics: *In vitro* and *in vivo* bioavailability studies have demonstrated that naftifine penetrates the stratum corneum in sufficient concentration to inhibit the growth of dermatophytes.
Following a single topical application of 1% naftifine cream to the skin of healthy subjects, systemic absorption of naftifine was approximately 6% of the applied dose. Naftifine and/or its metabolites are excreted via the urine and feces with a half-life of approximately two to three days.

INDICATIONS AND USAGE

Naftin® Cream, 1% is indicated for the topical treatment of tinea pedis, tinea cruris and tinea corporis caused by the organisms *Trichophyton rubrum, Trichophyton mentagrophytes,* and *Epidermophyton floccosum.*

CONTRAINDICATIONS

Naftin® Cream, 1% is contraindicated in individuals who have shown hypersensitivity to any of its components.

WARNINGS

Naftin® Cream, 1% is for topical use only and not for ophthalmic use.

PRECAUTIONS

General: Naftin® Cream, 1% is for external use only. If irritation or sensitivity develops with the use of Naftin® Cream, 1%, treatment should be discontinued and appropriate therapy instituted. Diagnosis of the disease should be confirmed either by direct microscopic examination of a mounting of infected tissue in a solution of potassium hydroxide or by culture on an appropriate medium.
Information for patients: The patient should be told to:
1. Avoid the use of occlusive dressings or wrappings unless otherwise directed by the physician.
2. Keep Naftin® Cream, 1% away from the eyes, nose, mouth and other mucous membranes.
Carcinogenesis, mutagenesis, impairment of fertility: Long-term animal studies to evaluate the carcinogenic potential of Naftin® Cream, 1% have not been performed. *In vitro* and animal studies have not demonstrated any mutagenic effect or effect on fertility.
Pregnancy: Teratogenic Effects: Pregnancy Category B: Reproduction studies have been performed in rats and rabbits (via oral administration) at doses 150 times or more the topical human dose and have revealed no evidence of impaired fertility or harm to the fetus due to naftifine. There are, however, no adequate and well-controlled studies in pregnant women. Because animal reproduction studies are not always predictive of human response, this drug should be used during pregnancy only if clearly needed.
Nursing mothers: It is not known whether this drug is excreted in human milk. Because many drugs are excreted in human milk, caution should be exercised when Naftin® Cream, 1% is administered to a nursing woman.
Pediatric use: Safety and effectiveness in pediatric patients have not been established.

ADVERSE REACTIONS

During clinical trials with Naftin® Cream, 1%, the incidence of adverse reactions was as follows: burning/stinging (6%), dryness (3%), erythema (2%), itching (2%), local irritation (2%).

DOSAGE AND ADMINISTRATION

A sufficient quantity of Naftin® Cream, 1% should be gently massaged into the affected and surrounding skin areas once a day. The hands should be washed after application.
If no clinical improvement is seen after four weeks of treatment with Naftin® Cream, 1%, the patient should be re-evaluated.

HOW SUPPLIED

Naftin® (naftifine hydrochloride) 1% Cream is supplied in the following sizes:

    30g – NDC 0259-4126-30 (tube)
    60g – NDC 0259-4126-60 (tube)
    90g – NDC 0259-4126-90 (tube)

    30g – NDC 0259-4126-03 (pump)
    90g – NDC 0259-4126-09 (pump)

Tubes: Store below 30°C (86°F).
Pumps: Store at controlled room temperature: 25°C (77°F); excursions permitted between 15°–30°C (59°–86°F)
Manufactured for: **Merz Pharmaceuticals, Greensboro, NC 27410**

©2009 Merz Pharmaceuticals
Rev 2/09 Printed in U.S.A.

NAFTIN®

(naftifine hydrochloride) 1% Gel
Rx Only

℞

DESCRIPTION

Naftin® Gel, 1% contains the synthetic, broad-spectrum, antifungal agent naftifine hydrochloride.
Naftin® Gel, 1% is for topical use only.
Chemical Name:
(E)-N-Cinnamyl-N-methyl-1-naphthalenemethylamine hydrochloride.
Naftifine hydrochloride has an empirical formula of $C_{21}H_{21}N \cdot HCl$ and a molecular weight of 323.86.

naftifine hydrochloride

Contains:
Active Ingredient: Naftifine hydrochloride 1%
Inactive Ingredients: polysorbate 80, carbomer 934P, diisopropanolamine, edetate disodium, alcohol (52%v/v) and purified water.

CLINICAL PHARMACOLOGY

Naftifine hydrochloride is a synthetic allylamine derivative. The following *in vitro* data are available, but their clinical significance is unknown. Naftifine hydrochloride has been shown to exhibit fungicidal activity *in vitro* against a broad spectrum of organisms, including *Trichophyton rubrum, Trichophyton mentagrophytes, Trichophyton tonsurans, Epidermophyton floccosum, Microsporum canis, Microsporum audouini,* and *Microsporum gypseum;* and fungistatic activity against *Candida* species, including *Candida albicans*. Naftin® Gel, 1% has only been shown to be clinically effective against the disease entities listed in the INDICATIONS AND USAGE section.
Although the exact mechanism of action against fungi is not known, naftifine hydrochloride appears to interfere with sterol biosynthesis by inhibiting the enzyme squalene 2, 3-epoxidase. This inhibition of enzyme activity results in decreased amounts of sterols, especially ergosterol, and a corresponding accumulation of squalene in the cells.
Pharmacokinetics: *In vitro* and *in vivo* bioavailability studies have demonstrated that naftifine penetrates the stratum corneum in sufficient concentration to inhibit the growth of dermatophytes.
Following single topical applications of ^{3}H-labeled naftifine gel 1% to the skin of healthy subjects, up to 4.2% of the applied dose was absorbed. Naftifine and/or its metabolites are excreted via the urine and feces with a half-life of approximately two to three days.

INDICATIONS AND USAGE

Naftin® Gel, 1% is indicated for the topical treatment of tinea pedis, tinea cruris and tinea corporis caused by the organisms *Trichophyton rubrum, Trichophyton mentagrophytes, Trichophyton tonsurans** and *Epidermophyton floccosum.**
*Efficacy for this organism in this organ system was studied in fewer than 10 infections.

CONTRAINDICATIONS

Naftin® Gel, 1% is contraindicated in individuals who have shown hypersensitivity to any of its components.

WARNINGS

Naftin® Gel, 1% is for topical use only and not for ophthalmic use.

PRECAUTIONS

General: Naftin® Gel, 1% is for external use only. If irritation or sensitivity develops with the use of Naftin® Gel, 1%, treatment should be discontinued and appropriate therapy instituted. Diagnosis of the disease should be confirmed either by direct microscopic examination of a mounting of infected tissue in a solution of potassium hydroxide or by culture on an appropriate medium.
Information for patients: The patient should be told to:
1. Avoid the use of occlusive dressings or wrappings unless otherwise directed by the physician.
2. Keep Naftin® Gel, 1% away from the eyes, nose, mouth and other mucous membranes.
Carcinogenesis, mutagenesis, impairment of fertility: Long-term studies to evaluate the carcinogenic potential of Naftin® Gel, 1% have not been performed. *In vitro* and animal studies have not demonstrated any mutagenic effect or effect on fertility.
Pregnancy: Teratogenic Effects: Pregnancy Category B: Reproduction studies have been performed in rats and rabbits (via oral administration) at doses 150 times or more than the topical human dose and have revealed no evidence of impaired fertility or harm to the fetus due to naftifine. There are, however, no adequate and well-controlled studies in pregnant women. Because animal reproduction studies are not always predictive of human response, this drug should be used during pregnancy only if clearly needed.
Nursing mothers: It is not known whether this drug is excreted in human milk. Because many drugs are excreted in human milk, caution should be exercised when Naftin® Gel, 1% is administered to a nursing woman.
Pediatric use: Safety and effectiveness in pediatric patients have not been established.

ADVERSE REACTIONS

During clinical trials with Naftin® Gel, 1%, the incidence of adverse reactions was as follows: burning/stinging (5.0%), itching (1.0%), erythema (0.5%), rash (0.5%), skin tenderness (0.5%).

DOSAGE AND ADMINISTRATION

A sufficient quantity of Naftin® Gel, 1% should be gently massaged into the affected and surrounding skin areas twice a day in the morning and evening. The hands should be washed after application.

If no clinical improvement is seen after four weeks of treatment with Naftin® Gel, 1%, the patient should be re-evaluated.

HOW SUPPLIED

Naftin® (naftifine hydrochloride) 1% Gel is supplied in collapsible tubes in the following sizes:

    40g – NDC 0259-4770-40
    60g – NDC 0259-4770-60
    90g – NDC 0259-4770-90

Note: Store at room temperature.
Manufactured for: **Merz Pharmaceuticals, Greensboro, NC 27410**

©2009 Merz Pharmaceuticals
Rev 2/09 Printed in U.S.A.

Millennium Pharmaceuticals, Inc.

**40 LANDSDOWNE STREET
CAMBRIDGE, MA 02139**

Direct Inquiries to:
Medical Information:
Call 1-866-VELCADE

VELCADE®   ℞
[věl-kād]
(bortezomib)
for Injection

HIGHLIGHTS OF PRESCRIBING INFORMATION
These highlights do not include all the information needed to use VELCADE safely and effectively. See full prescribing information for VELCADE.
VELCADE® (bortezomib) for Injection
Initial U.S. Approval: 2003

──────RECENT MAJOR CHANGES──────
Dosage and Administration (2.5)	12/2009
Warnings and Precautions,	
Hepatic Impairment (5.11)	12/2009
Patients with Hepatic Impairment (8.7)	12/2009
Clinical Studies, Multiple Myeloma (14.1)	12/2009

──────INDICATIONS AND USAGE──────
VELCADE is a proteasome inhibitor indicated for:
• treatment of patients with multiple myeloma (1.1)
• treatment of patients with mantle cell lymphoma who have received at least 1 prior therapy (1.2)

──────DOSAGE AND ADMINISTRATION──────
The recommended dose of VELCADE is 1.3 mg/m² administered as a 3 to 5 second bolus intravenous injection. (2.1, 2.3)
Dose adjustment may be used to manage adverse events that occur during treatment (2.2, 2.4)

──────DOSAGE FORMS AND STRENGTHS──────
• 1 single use vial contains 3.5 mg of bortezomib. Dose must be individualized to prevent overdose. (3)

──────CONTRAINDICATIONS──────
• VELCADE is contraindicated in patients with hypersensitivity to bortezomib, boron, or mannitol. (4)

──────WARNINGS AND PRECAUTIONS──────
• Women should avoid becoming pregnant while being treated with VELCADE. Pregnant women should be apprised of the potential harm to the fetus. (5.1, 8.1)

• Peripheral neuropathy, including severe cases, may occur - manage with dose modification or discontinuation. (2.2, 2.4) Patients with preexisting severe neuropathy should be treated with VELCADE only after careful risk-benefit assessment. (2.2, 2.4, 5.2)
• Hypotension can occur. Caution should be used when treating patients receiving antihypertensives, those with a history of syncope, and those who are dehydrated. (5.3)
• Patients with risk factors for, or existing heart disease, should be closely monitored. (5.4)
• Acute diffuse infiltrative pulmonary disease has been reported. (5.5)
• Nausea, diarrhea, constipation, and vomiting have occurred and may require use of antiemetic and antidiarrheal medications or fluid replacement. (5.7)
• Thrombocytopenia or neutropenia can occur; complete blood counts should be regularly monitored throughout treatment. (5.8)
• Tumor Lysis Syndrome (5.9), Reversible Posterior Leukoencephalopathy Syndrome (5.6), and acute hepatic failure (5.10) have been reported.

──────ADVERSE REACTIONS──────
Most commonly reported adverse reactions (incidence ≥30%) in clinical studies include asthenic conditions, diarrhea, nausea, constipation, peripheral neuropathy, vomiting, pyrexia, thrombocytopenia, psychiatric disorders, anorexia and decreased appetite, neutropenia, neuralgia, leukopenia and anemia. Other adverse reactions, including serious adverse reactions, have been reported. (6.1)
To report SUSPECTED ADVERSE REACTIONS, contact Millennium Pharmaceuticals at 1-866 VELCADE or FDA at 1-800-FDA-1088 or *www.fda.gov/medwatch*.

──────USE IN SPECIFIC POPULATIONS──────
• Women should be advised against breast feeding or becoming pregnant while being treated with VELCADE. (5.1, 8.1, 8.3)
• Patients with diabetes may require close monitoring of blood glucose and adjustment of anti-diabetic medication. (8.8)
• Hepatic Impairment: In patients with moderate or severe hepatic impairment, use a lower starting dose (2.5, 5.11, 8.7, 12.3)

See 17 for PATIENT COUNSELING INFORMATION.
Revised: [12/2009]

FULL PRESCRIBING INFORMATION: CONTENTS*

FULL PRESCRIBING INFORMATION

1   INDICATIONS AND USAGE
1.1   Multiple Myeloma
VELCADE® (bortezomib) for Injection is indicated for the treatment of patients with multiple myeloma.
1.2   Mantle Cell Lymphoma
VELCADE (bortezomib) for Injection is indicated for the treatment of patients with mantle cell lymphoma who have received at least 1 prior therapy.

2   DOSAGE AND ADMINISTRATION
2.1   Dosage in Previously Untreated Multiple Myeloma
VELCADE (bortezomib) is administered as a 3-5 second bolus IV injection in combination with oral melphalan and oral prednisone for nine 6-week treatment cycles as shown in Table 1. In Cycles 1-4, VELCADE is administered twice weekly (days 1, 4, 8, 11, 22, 25, 29 and 32). In Cycles 5-9, VELCADE is administered once weekly (days 1, 8, 22 and 29). At least 72 hours should elapse between consecutive doses of VELCADE.
[See table 1 below]
2.2   Dose Modification Guidelines for Combination Therapy with VELCADE, Melphalan and Prednisone
Prior to initiating any cycle of therapy with VELCADE in combination with melphalan and prednisone:
• Platelet count should be ≥ 70 × 10⁹/L and the ANC should be ≥ 1.0 × 10⁹/L
• Non-hematological toxicities should have resolved to Grade 1 or baseline
[See table 2 at top of next page]
2.3   Dosage in Relapsed Multiple Myeloma and Mantle Cell Lymphoma
VELCADE (1.3 mg/m²/dose) is administered as a 3 to 5 second bolus intravenous injection twice weekly for 2 weeks (Days 1, 4, 8, and 11) followed by a 10-day rest period (Days 12-21). For extended therapy of more than 8 cycles, VELCADE may be administered on the standard schedule or on a maintenance schedule of once weekly for 4 weeks (Days 1, 8, 15, and 22) followed by a 13-day rest period (Days 23 to 35) *[see Clinical Studies section (14) for a description of dose administration during the trials]*. At least 72 hours should elapse between consecutive doses of VELCADE.
2.4   Dose Modification Guidelines for Relapsed Multiple Myeloma and Mantle Cell Lymphoma
VELCADE therapy should be withheld at the onset of any Grade 3 non-hematological or Grade 4 hematological toxicities excluding neuropathy as discussed below [*see Warnings and Precautions* (5)]. Once the symptoms of the toxicity have resolved, VELCADE therapy may be reinitiated at a 25% reduced dose (1.3 mg/m²/dose reduced to 1 mg/m²/dose; 1 mg/m²/dose reduced to 0.7 mg/m²/dose).

Table 1-Dosage Regimen for Patients with Previously Untreated Multiple Myeloma

Twice Weekly VELCADE (Cycles 1-4)

Week		1				2	3	4		5	6
VELCADE (1.3 mg/m²)	Day 1	—	—	Day 4	Day 8	Day 11	rest period	Day 22	Day 25	Day 29	Day 32	rest period
Melphalan (9 mg/m²) Prednisone (60 mg/m²)	Day 1	Day 2	Day 3	Day 4	—	—	rest period	—	—	—	—	rest period

Once Weekly VELCADE (Cycles 5-9 when used in combination with Melphalan and Prednisone)

Week		1				2	3	4	5	6
VELCADE (1.3 mg/m²)	Day 1	—	—		Day 8	rest period	Day 22	Day 29	rest period
Melphalan (9 mg/m²) Prednisone (60 mg/m²)	Day 1	Day 2	Day 3	Day 4	—	rest period	—	—	rest period

For the management of patients who experience VELCADE related neuropathic pain and/or peripheral neuropathy see Table 3. Patients with preexisting severe neuropathy should be treated with VELCADE only after careful risk-benefit assessment.

[See table 3 at right]

2.5 Dosage in Patients with Hepatic Impairment

Patients with mild hepatic impairment do not require a starting dose adjustment and should be treated per the recommended VELCADE dose. Patients with moderate or severe hepatic impairment should be started on VELCADE at a reduced dose of 0.7 mg/m^2 per injection during the first cycle, and a subsequent dose escalation to 1.0 mg/m^2 or further dose reduction to 0.5 mg/m^2 may be considered based on patient tolerance (see Table 4). *[see Warnings and Precautions (5.11), Use in Specific Populations (8.7) and Clinical Pharmacology (12.3)]*

[See table 4 below]

2.6 Administration Precautions

The drug quantity contained in one vial (3.5 mg) may exceed the usual dose required. Caution should be used in calculating the dose to prevent overdose.

VELCADE is an antineoplastic. Procedures for proper handling and disposal should be considered. *[see How Supplied/Storage and Handling (16)]*

In clinical trials, local skin irritation was reported in 5% of patients, but extravasation of VELCADE was not associated with tissue damage.

2.7 Reconstitution/Preparation for Intravenous Administration

Proper aseptic technique should be used. Reconstitute with 3.5 mL of 0.9% Sodium Chloride resulting in a final concentration of 1 mg/mL of bortezomib. The reconstituted product should be a clear and colorless solution.

Parenteral drug products should be inspected visually for particulate matter and discoloration prior to administration whenever solution and container permit. If any discoloration or particulate matter is observed, the reconstituted product should not be used.

Stability: Unopened vials of VELCADE are stable until the date indicated on the package when stored in the original package protected from light.

VELCADE contains no antimicrobial preservative. Reconstituted VELCADE should be administered within 8 hours of preparation. When reconstituted as directed, VELCADE may be stored at 25°C (77°F). The reconstituted material may be stored in the original vial and/or the syringe prior to administration. The product may be stored for up to 8 hours in a syringe; however total storage time for the reconstituted material must not exceed 8 hours when exposed to normal indoor lighting.

3 DOSAGE FORMS AND STRENGTHS

Each single use vial of VELCADE contains 3.5 mg of bortezomib as a sterile lyophilized powder.

4 CONTRAINDICATIONS

VELCADE is contraindicated in patients with hypersensitivity to bortezomib, boron, or mannitol.

5 WARNINGS AND PRECAUTIONS

VELCADE should be administered under the supervision of a physician experienced in the use of antineoplastic therapy. Complete blood counts (CBC) should be monitored frequently during treatment with VELCADE.

5.1 Use in Pregnancy

Pregnancy Category D

Women of childbearing potential should avoid becoming pregnant while being treated with VELCADE. Bortezomib administered to rabbits during organogenesis at a dose approximately 0.5 times the clinical dose of 1.3 mg/m^2 based on body surface area caused post-implantation loss and a decreased number of live fetuses. *[see Use in Specific Populations (8.1)]*

5.2 Peripheral Neuropathy

VELCADE treatment causes a peripheral neuropathy that is predominantly sensory. However, cases of severe sensory and motor peripheral neuropathy have been reported. Patients with pre-existing symptoms (numbness, pain or a burning feeling in the feet or hands) and/or signs of peripheral neuropathy may experience worsening peripheral neuropathy (including ≥Grade 3) during treatment with VELCADE. Patients should be monitored for symptoms of neuropathy, such as a burning sensation, hyperesthesia, hypoesthesia, paresthesia, discomfort, neuropathic pain or weakness. Patients experiencing new or worsening peripheral neuropathy may require change in the dose and schedule of VELCADE *[see Dosage and Administration (2.2, 2.4)]*. Following dose adjustments, improvement in or resolution of peripheral neuropathy was reported in 51% of patients with ≥Grade 2 peripheral neuropathy in the relapsed multiple myeloma study. Improvement in or resolution of peripheral neuropathy was reported in 73% of patients who discontinued due to Grade 2 neuropathy or who had ≥Grade 3 peripheral neuropathy in the phase 2 multiple

myeloma studies *[see Adverse Reactions (6)]*. The long-term outcome of peripheral neuropathy has not been studied in mantle cell lymphoma.

5.3 Hypotension

The incidence of hypotension (postural, orthostatic, and hypotension NOS) was 13%. These events are observed throughout therapy. Caution should be used when treating patients with a history of syncope, patients receiving medications known to be associated with hypotension, and patients who are dehydrated. Management of orthostatic/postural hypotension may include adjustment of antihypertensive medications, hydration, and administration of mineralocorticoids and/or sympathomimetics. *[see Adverse Reactions (6)]*

5.4 Cardiac Disorders

Acute development or exacerbation of congestive heart failure and new onset of decreased left ventricular ejection fraction have been reported, including reports in patients with no risk factors for decreased left ventricular ejection fraction. Patients with risk factors for, or existing heart disease should be closely monitored. In the relapsed multiple myeloma study, the incidence of any treatment-emergent cardiac disorder was 15% and 13% in the VELCADE and dexamethasone groups, respectively. The incidence of heart failure events (acute pulmonary edema, cardiac failure, congestive cardiac failure, cardiogenic shock, pulmonary edema) was similar in the VELCADE and dexamethasone

groups, 5% and 4%, respectively. There have been isolated cases of QT-interval prolongation in clinical studies; causality has not been established.

5.5 Pulmonary Disorders

There have been reports of acute diffuse infiltrative pulmonary disease of unknown etiology such as pneumonitis, interstitial pneumonia, lung infiltration and Acute Respiratory Distress Syndrome (ARDS) in patients receiving VELCADE. Some of these events have been fatal.

In a clinical trial, the first two patients given high-dose cytarabine (2g/m^2 per day) by continuous infusion with daunorubicin and VELCADE for relapsed acute myelogenous leukemia died of ARDS early in the course of therapy. There have been reports of pulmonary hypertension associated with VELCADE administration in the absence of left heart failure or significant pulmonary disease.

In the event of new or worsening cardiopulmonary symptoms, a prompt comprehensive diagnostic evaluation should be conducted.

5.6 Reversible Posterior Leukoencephalopathy Syndrome (RPLS)

There have been reports of RPLS in patients receiving VELCADE. RPLS is a rare, reversible, neurological disorder which can present with seizure, hypertension, headache, lethargy, confusion, blindness, and other visual and neurological disturbances. Brain imaging, preferably MRI (Magnetic Resonance Imaging), is used to confirm the diagnosis.

Table 2-Dose Modifications During Cycles of Combination VELCADE, Melphalan and Prednisone Therapy

Toxicity	Dose modification or delay
Hematological toxicity during a cycle: If prolonged Grade 4 neutropenia or thrombocytopenia, or thrombocytopenia with bleeding is observed in the previous cycle	Consider reduction of the melphalan dose by 25% in the next cycle
If platelet count ≤30 × 10^9/L or ANC ≤0.75 × 10^9/L on a VELCADE dosing day (other than day 1)	VELCADE dose should be withheld
If several VELCADE doses in consecutive cycles are withheld due to toxicity	VELCADE dose should be reduced by 1 dose level (from 1.3 mg/m^2 to 1 mg/m^2, or from 1 mg/m^2 to 0.7 mg/m^2)
Grade ≥ 3 non-hematological toxicities	VELCADE therapy should be withheld until symptoms of the toxicity have resolved to Grade 1 or baseline. Then, VELCADE may be reinitiated with one dose level reduction (from 1.3 mg/m^2 to 1 mg/m^2, or from 1 mg/m^2 to 0.7 mg/m^2). For VELCADE-related neuropathic pain and/or peripheral neuropathy, hold or modify VELCADE as outlined in Table 3.

For information concerning melphalan and prednisone, see manufacturer's prescribing information.

Table 3: Recommended Dose Modification for VELCADE related Neuropathic Pain and/or Peripheral Sensory or Motor Neuropathy

Severity of Peripheral Neuropathy Signs and Symptoms	Modification of Dose and Regimen
Grade 1 (paresthesias, weakness and/or loss of reflexes) without pain or loss of function	No action
Grade 1 with pain or Grade 2 (interfering with function but not with activities of daily living)	Reduce VELCADE to 1 mg/m^2
Grade 2 with pain or Grade 3 (interfering with activities of daily living)	Withhold VELCADE therapy until toxicity resolves. When toxicity resolves reinitiate with a reduced dose of VELCADE at 0.7 mg/m^2 and change treatment schedule to once per week.
Grade 4 (sensory neuropathy which is disabling or motor neuropathy that is life threatening or leads to paralysis)	Discontinue VELCADE

Grading based on NCI Common Toxicity Criteria CTCAE v3.0

Table 4: Recommended Starting Dose Modification for VELCADE in Patients with Hepatic Impairment

	Bilirubin Level	SGOT (AST) Levels	Modification of Starting Dose
Mild	≤ 1.0× ULN	> ULN	None
	> 1.0×–1.5× ULN	Any	None
Moderate	> 1.5×–3× ULN	Any	Reduce VELCADE to 0.7 mg/m^2 in the first cycle. Consider dose escalation to 1.0 mg/m^2 or further dose reduction to 0.5 mg/m^2 in subsequent cycles based on patient tolerability.
Severe	> 3× ULN	Any	

Abbreviations: SGOT = serum glutamic oxaloacetic transaminase; AST = aspartate aminotransferase; ULN = upper limit of the normal range.

Table 5: Severity of Thrombocytopenia Related to Pretreatment Platelet Count in the Relapsed Multiple Myeloma Study

Pretreatment Platelet Count*	Number of Patients (N=331)**	Number (%) of Patients with Platelet Count <10,000/µL	Number (%) of Patients with Platelet Count 10,000-25,000/µL
≥75,000/µL	309	8 (3%)	36 (12%)
≥50,000/µL-<75,000/µL	14	2 (14%)	11 (79%)
≥10,000/µL-<50,000/µL	7	1 (14%)	5 (71%)

* A baseline platelet count of 50,000/µL was required for study eligibility
** Data were missing at baseline for 1 patient

Table 6-Most Commonly Reported Adverse Events (≥ 10% in VELCADE, Melphalan and Prednisone arm) with Grades 3 and ≥4 Intensity in the Previously Untreated Multiple Myeloma Study

MedDRA System Organ Class Preferred Term	VELCADE, Melphalan and Prednisone (N=340) Total n (%)	Toxicity Grade, n (%) 3	≥4	Melphalan and Prednisone (N=337) Total n (%)	Toxicity Grade, n (%) 3	≥4
Blood and Lymphatic System Disorders						
Thrombocytopenia	178 (52)	68 (20)	59 (17)	159 (47)	55 (16)	47 (14)
Neutropenia	165 (49)	102 (30)	35 (10)	155 (46)	79 (23)	49 (15)
Anemia	147 (43)	53 (16)	9 (3)	187 (55)	66 (20)	26 (8)
Leukopenia	113 (33)	67 (20)	10 (3)	100 (30)	55 (16)	13 (4)
Lymphopenia	83 (24)	49 (14)	18 (5)	58 (17)	30 (9)	7 (2)
Gastrointestinal Disorders						
Nausea	164 (48)	14 (4)	0	94 (28)	1 (<1)	0
Diarrhea	157 (46)	23 (7)	2 (1)	58 (17)	2 (1)	0
Constipation	125 (37)	2 (1)	0	54 (16)	0	0
Vomiting	112 (33)	14 (4)	0	55 (16)	2 (1)	0
Abdominal Pain	49 (14)	7 (2)	0	22 (7)	1 (<1)	0
Abdominal Pain Upper	40 (12)	1 (<1)	0	29 (9)	0	0
Dyspepsia	39 (11)	0	0	23 (7)	0	0
Nervous System Disorders						
Peripheral Neuropathy	159 (47)	43 (13)	2 (1)	18 (5)	0	0
Neuralgia	121 (36)	28 (8)	2 (1)	5 (1)	1 (<1)	0
Dizziness	56 (16)	7 (2)	0	37 (11)	1 (<1)	0
Headache	49 (14)	2 (1)	0	35 (10)	4 (1)	0
Paresthesia	45 (13)	6 (2)	0	15 (4)	0	0
General Disorders and Administration Site Conditions						
Pyrexia	99 (29)	8 (2)	2 (1)	64 (19)	6 (2)	2 (1)
Fatigue	98 (29)	23 (7)	2 (1)	86 (26)	7 (2)	0
Asthenia	73 (21)	20 (6)	1 (<1)	60 (18)	9 (3)	0
Edema Peripheral	68 (20)	2 (1)	0	34 (10)	0	0
Infections and Infestations						
Pneumonia	56 (16)	16 (5)	13 (4)	36 (11)	13 (4)	9 (3)
Herpes Zoster	45 (13)	11 (3)	0	14 (4)	6 (2)	0
Bronchitis	44 (13)	4 (1)	0	27 (8)	4 (1)	0
Nasopharyngitis	39 (11)	1 (<1)	0	27 (8)	0	0
Musculoskeletal and Connective Tissue Disorders						
Back Pain	58 (17)	9 (3)	1 (<1)	62 (18)	11 (3)	1 (<1)
Pain In Extremity	47 (14)	8 (2)	0	32 (9)	3 (1)	1 (<1)
Bone Pain	37 (11)	7 (2)	1 (<1)	35 (10)	7 (2)	0
Arthralgia	36 (11)	4 (1)	0	50 (15)	2 (1)	1 (<1)
Metabolism and Nutrition Disorders						
Anorexia	77 (23)	9 (3)	1 (<1)	34 (10)	4 (1)	0
Hypokalemia	44 (13)	19 (6)	3 (1)	25 (7)	8 (2)	2 (1)
Skin and Subcutaneous Tissue Disorders						
Rash	66 (19)	2 (1)	0	24 (7)	1 (<1)	0
Pruritus	35 (10)	3 (1)	0	18 (5)	0	0
Respiratory, Thoracic and Mediastinal Disorders						
Cough	71 (21)	0	0	45 (13)	2 (1)	0
Dyspnea	50 (15)	11 (3)	2 (1)	44 (13)	5 (1)	4 (1)
Psychiatric Disorders						
Insomnia	69 (20)	1 (<1)	0	43 (13)	0	0
Vascular Disorders						
Hypertension	45 (13)	8 (2)	1 (<1)	25 (7)	2 (1)	0
Hypotension	41 (12)	4 (1)	3 (1)	10 (3)	2 (1)	2 (1)

In patients developing RPLS, discontinue VELCADE. The safety of reinitiating VELCADE therapy in patients previously experiencing RPLS is not known.

5.7 Gastrointestinal Adverse Events
VELCADE treatment can cause nausea, diarrhea, constipation, and vomiting [see *Adverse Reactions (6)*] sometimes requiring use of antiemetic and antidiarrheal medications. Ileus can occur. Fluid and electrolyte replacement should be administered to prevent dehydration.

5.8 Thrombocytopenia/Neutropenia
VELCADE is associated with thrombocytopenia and neutropenia that follow a cyclical pattern with nadirs occurring following the last dose of each cycle and typically recovering prior to initiation of the subsequent cycle. The cyclical pattern of platelet and neutrophil decreases and recovery remained consistent over the 8 cycles of twice weekly dosing, and there was no evidence of cumulative thrombocytopenia or neutropenia. The mean platelet count nadir measured was approximately 40% of baseline. The severity of thrombocytopenia related to pretreatment platelet count is shown in **Table 5**. In the relapsed multiple myeloma study, the incidence of significant bleeding events (≥Grade 3) was similar on both the VELCADE (4%) and dexamethasone (5%) arms. Platelet count should be monitored prior to each dose of VELCADE. Patients experiencing thrombocytopenia may require change in the dose and schedule of VELCADE [see *Table 2 and Dosage and Administration (2.4)*]. There have been reports of gastrointestinal and intracerebral hemorrhage in association with VELCADE. Transfusions may be considered. The incidence of febrile neutropenia was <1%.
[See table 5 at left]

5.9 Tumor Lysis Syndrome
Because VELCADE is a cytotoxic agent and can rapidly kill malignant cells, the complications of tumor lysis syndrome may occur. Patients at risk of tumor lysis syndrome are those with high tumor burden prior to treatment. These patients should be monitored closely and appropriate precautions taken.

5.10 Hepatic Events
Cases of acute liver failure have been reported in patients receiving multiple concomitant medications and with serious underlying medical conditions. Other reported hepatic events include increases in liver enzymes, hyperbilirubinemia, and hepatitis. Such changes may be reversible upon discontinuation of VELCADE. There is limited re-challenge information in these patients.

5.11 Patients with Hepatic Impairment:
Bortezomib is metabolized by liver enzymes. Bortezomib exposure is increased in patients with moderate or severe hepatic impairment; these patients should be treated with VELCADE at reduced starting doses and closely monitored for toxicities. [see *Dosage and Administration (2.5), Use In Specific Populations (8.7) and Clinical Pharmacology (12.3)*]

6 ADVERSE REACTIONS
The following adverse reactions are also discussed in other sections of the labeling:
- Peripheral Neuropathy [see *Warnings and Precautions (5.2); Dosage and Administration (Table 3)*]
- Hypotension [see *Warnings and Precautions (5.3)*]
- Cardiac Disorders [see *Warnings and Precautions (5.4)*]
- Pulmonary Disorders [see *Warnings and Precautions (5.5)*]
- Reversible Posterior Leukoencephalopathy Syndrome (RPLS) [see *Warnings and Precautions (5.6)*]
- Gastrointestinal Adverse Events [see *Warnings and Precautions (5.7)*]
- Thrombocytopenia/Neutropenia [see *Warnings and Precautions (5.8)*]
- Tumor Lysis Syndrome [see *Warnings and Precautions (5.9)*]
- Hepatic Events [see *Warnings and Precautions (5.10)*]

6.1 Clinical Trials Safety Experience
Because clinical trials are conducted under widely varying conditions, adverse reaction rates observed in the clinical trials of a drug cannot be directly compared to rates in the clinical trials of another drug and may not reflect the rates observed in practice.

Summary of Clinical Trial in Patients with Previously Untreated Multiple Myeloma:
Table 6 describes safety data from 340 patients with previously untreated multiple myeloma who received VELCADE (1.3 mg/m²) in combination with melphalan (9 mg/m²) and prednisone (60 mg/m²) in a prospective randomized study. The safety profile of VELCADE in combination with melphalan/prednisone is consistent with the known safety profiles of both VELCADE and melphalan/prednisone.
[See table 6 at left]

Relapsed Multiple Myeloma Randomized Study
The safety data described below and in Table 7 reflect exposure to either VELCADE (n=331) or dexamethasone (n=332) in a study of patients with multiple myeloma. VELCADE was administered intravenously at doses of 1.3 mg/m² twice weekly for 2 out of 3 weeks (21 day cycle). After eight 21-day cycles patients continued therapy for three 35-day cycles on a weekly schedule. Duration of treatment was up to 11 cycles (9 months) with a median duration of 6 cycles (4.1 months). For inclusion in the trial, patients must have had measurable disease and 1 to 3 prior therapies. There was no upper age limit for entry. Creatinine clearance could be as low as 20 mL/min and bilirubin levels as high as 1.5 times the upper limit of normal. The overall frequency of adverse events was similar in men and women, and in patients <65 and ≥65 years of age. Most patients were Caucasian. [see *Clinical Studies (14.1)*]
Among the 331 VELCADE treated patients, the most commonly reported events overall were asthenic conditions (61%), diarrhea and nausea (each 57%), constipation (42%), peripheral neuropathy NEC (36%), vomiting, pyrexia, thrombocytopenia, and psychiatric disorders (each 35%), anorexia and appetite decreased (34%), paresthesia and dysesthesia (27%), anemia and headache (each 26%), and cough (21%). The most commonly reported adverse events reported among the 332 patients in the dexamethasone group were psychiatric disorders (49%), asthenic conditions (45%), insomnia (27%), anemia (22%), and diarrhea and lower respiratory/lung infections (each 21%). Fourteen

percent (14%) of patients in the VELCADE treated arm experienced a Grade 4 adverse event; the most common toxicities were thrombocytopenia (4%), 10/34 neutropenia (2%) and hypercalcemia (2%). Sixteen percent (16%) of dexamethasone treated patients experienced a Grade 4 adverse event; the most common toxicity was hyperglycemia (2%).

Serious Adverse Events (SAEs) and Events Leading to Treatment Discontinuation in the Relapsed Multiple Myeloma Study

Serious adverse events are defined as any event, regardless of causality, that results in death, is life-threatening, requires hospitalization or prolongs a current hospitalization, results in a significant disability, or is deemed to be an important medical event. A total of 144 (44%) patients from the VELCADE treatment arm experienced an SAE during the study, as did 144 (43%) dexamethasone-treated patients. The most commonly reported SAEs in the VELCADE treatment arm were pyrexia (6%), diarrhea (5%), dyspnea and pneumonia (4%), and vomiting (3%). In the dexamethasone treatment group, the most commonly reported SAEs were pneumonia (7%), pyrexia (4%), and hyperglycemia (3%).

A total of 145 patients, including 84 (25%) of 331 patients in the VELCADE treatment group and 61 (18%) of 332 patients in the dexamethasone treatment group were discontinued from treatment due to adverse events assessed as drug-related by the investigators. Among the 331 VELCADE treated patients, the most commonly reported drug-related event leading to discontinuation was peripheral neuropathy (8%). Among the 332 patients in the dexamethasone group, the most commonly reported drug-related events leading to treatment discontinuation were psychotic disorder and hyperglycemia (2% each).

Four deaths were considered to be VELCADE related in this relapsed multiple myeloma study: 1 case each of cardiogenic shock, respiratory insufficiency, congestive heart failure and cardiac arrest. Four deaths were considered dexamethasone-related: 2 cases of sepsis, 1 case of bacterial meningitis, and 1 case of sudden death at home.

Most Commonly Reported Adverse Events in the Relapsed Multiple Myeloma Study

The most common adverse events from the relapsed multiple myeloma study are shown in **Table 7**. All adverse events with incidence ≥10% in the VELCADE arm are included.

[See table 7 above]

Table 7: Most Commonly Reported Adverse Events (≥10% in VELCADE arm), with Grades 3 and 4 Intensity in the Relapsed Multiple Myeloma Study (N=663)

	Treatment Group					
	VELCADE (n=331) [n (%)]			Dexamethasone (n=332) [n (%)]		
	All Events	Grade 3 Events	Grade 4 Events	All Events	Grade 3 Events	Grade 4 Events
Adverse Event	331 (100)	203 (61)	45 (14)	327 (98)	146 (44)	52 (16)
Asthenic conditions	201 (61)	39 (12)	1 (<1)	148 (45)	20 (6)	0
Diarrhea	190 (57)	24 (7)	0	69 (21)	6 (2)	0
Nausea	190 (57)	8 (2)	0	46 (14)	0	0
Constipation	140 (42)	7 (2)	0	49 (15)	4 (1)	0
Peripheral neuropathy	120 (36)	24 (7)	2 (<1)	29 (9)	1 (<1)	1 (<1)
Vomiting	117 (35)	11 (3)	0	20 (6)	4 (1)	0
Pyrexia	116 (35)	6 (2)	0	54 (16)	4 (1)	1 (<1)
Thrombocytopenia	115 (35)	85 (26)	12 (4)	36 (11)	18 (5)	4 (1)
Psychiatric disorders	117 (35)	9 (3)	2 (<1)	163 (49)	26 (8)	3 (<1)
Anorexia and appetite decreased	112 (34)	9 (3)	0	31 (9)	1 (<1)	0
Paresthesia and dysesthesia	91 (27)	6 (2)	0	38 (11)	1 (<1)	0
Anemia	87 (26)	31 (9)	2 (<1)	74 (22)	32 (10)	3 (<1)
Headache	85 (26)	3 (<1)	0	43 (13)	2 (<1)	0
Cough	70 (21)	2 (<1)	0	35 (11)	1 (<1)	0
Dyspnea	65 (20)	16 (5)	1 (<1)	58 (17)	9 (3)	2 (<1)
Neutropenia	62 (19)	40 (12)	8 (2)	5 (2)	4 (1)	0
Rash	61 (18)	4 (1)	0	20 (6)	0	0
Insomnia	60 (18)	1 (<1)	0	90 (27)	5 (2)	0
Abdominal pain	53 (16)	6 (2)	0	12 (4)	1 (<1)	0
Bone pain	52 (16)	12 (4)	0	50 (15)	9 (3)	0
Lower respiratory/lung infections	48 (15)	12 (4)	2 (<1)	69 (21)	24 (7)	1 (<1)
Pain in limb	50 (15)	5 (2)	0	24 (7)	2 (<1)	0
Back pain	46 (14)	10 (3)	0	33 (10)	4 (1)	0
Arthralgia	45 (14)	3 (<1)	0	35 (11)	5 (2)	0
Dizziness (excl. vertigo)	45 (14)	3 (<1)	0	34 (10)	0	0
Nasopharyngitis	45 (14)	1 (<1)	0	22 (7)	0	0
Herpes zoster	42 (13)	6 (2)	0	15 (5)	4 (1)	1 (<1)
Muscle cramps	41 (12)	0	0	50 (15)	3 (<1)	0
Myalgia	39 (12)	1 (<1)	0	18 (5)	1 (<1)	0
Rigors	37 (11)	0	0	8 (2)	0	0
Edema lower limb	35 (11)	0	0	43 (13)	1 (<1)	0

Safety Experience from the Phase 2 Open-Label Extension Study in Relapsed Multiple Myeloma

In the phase 2 extension study of 63 patients, no new cumulative or new long-term toxicities were observed with prolonged VELCADE treatment. These patients were treated for a total of 5.3 to 23 months, including time on VELCADE in the prior VELCADE study. **[*see Clinical Studies (14)*]**

Integrated Summary of Safety (Relapsed Multiple Myeloma and Mantle Cell Lymphoma)

Safety data from phase 2 and 3 studies of single agent VELCADE 1.3 mg/m^2/dose twice weekly for 2 weeks followed by a 10-day rest period in 1163 patients with previously treated multiple myeloma (N=1008) and previously treated mantle cell lymphoma (N=155) were integrated and tabulated. In these studies, the safety profile of VELCADE was similar in patients with multiple myeloma and mantle cell lymphoma. **[*see Clinical Studies (14)*]**

In the integrated analysis, the most commonly reported adverse events were asthenic conditions (including fatigue, malaise, and weakness) (64%), nausea (55%), diarrhea (52%), constipation (41%), peripheral neuropathy NEC (including peripheral sensory neuropathy and peripheral neuropathy aggravated) (39%), thrombocytopenia and appetite decreased (including anorexia) (each 36%), pyrexia (34%), vomiting (33%), and anemia (29%). Twenty percent (20%) of patients experienced at least 1 episode of ≥Grade 4 toxicity, most commonly thrombocytopenia (5%) and neutropenia (3%).

Serious Adverse Events (SAEs) and Events Leading to Treatment Discontinuation in the Integrated Summary of Safety

A total of 50% of patients experienced SAEs during the studies. The most commonly reported SAEs included pneumonia (7%), pyrexia (6%), diarrhea (5%), vomiting (4%), and nausea, dehydration, dyspnea and thrombocytopenia (each 3%).

Adverse events thought by the investigator to be drug-related and leading to discontinuation occurred in 22% of patients. The reasons for discontinuation included peripheral neuropathy (8%), asthenic conditions (3%) and thrombocytopenia and diarrhea (each 2%).

In total, 2% of the patients died and the cause of death was considered by the investigator to be possibly related to study drug: including reports of cardiac arrest, congestive heart failure, respiratory failure, renal failure, pneumonia and sepsis.

Most Commonly Reported Adverse Events in the Integrated Summary of Safety

The most common adverse events are shown in Table 8. All adverse events occurring at ≥10% are included. In the absence of a randomized comparator arm, it is often not possible to distinguish between adverse events that are drug-caused and those that reflect the patient's underlying disease. Please see the discussion of specific adverse reactions that follows.

[See table 8 at top of next page]

Description of Selected Adverse Events from the Phase 2 and 3 Relapsed Multiple Myeloma and Phase 2 Mantle Cell Lymphoma Studies

Gastrointestinal Events

A total of 87% of patients experienced at least one GI disorder. The most common GI disorders included nausea, diarrhea, constipation, vomiting, and appetite decreased. Other GI disorders included dyspepsia and dysgeusia. Grade 3 GI events occurred in 18% of patients; Grade 4 events were 1%. GI events were considered serious in 11% of patients. Five percent (5%) of patients discontinued due to a GI event. Nausea was reported more often in patients with multiple myeloma (57%) compared to patients with mantle cell lymphoma (44%). **[*see Warnings and Precautions (5.7)*]**

Thrombocytopenia

Across the studies, VELCADE associated thrombocytopenia was characterized by a decrease in platelet count during the dosing period (days 1 to 11) and a return toward baseline during the 10-day rest period during each treatment cycle. Overall, thrombocytopenia was reported in 36% of patients. Thrombocytopenia was Grade 3 in 24%, ≥Grade 4 in 5%, and serious in 3% of patients, and the event resulted in VELCADE discontinuation in 2% of patients **[*see Warnings and Precautions (5.8)*]**. Thrombocytopenia was reported more often in patients with multiple myeloma (38%) compared to patients with mantle cell lymphoma (21%). The incidence of ≥Grade 3 thrombocytopenia also was higher in patients with multiple myeloma (32%) compared to patients with mantle cell lymphoma (11%). **[*see Warnings and Precautions (5.8)*]**

Peripheral Neuropathy

Overall, peripheral neuropathy NEC occurred in 39% of patients. Peripheral neuropathy was Grade 3 for 11% of patients and Grade 4 for <1% of patients. Eight percent (8%) of patients discontinued VELCADE due to peripheral neuropathy. The incidence of peripheral neuropathy was higher among patients with mantle cell lymphoma (55%) compared to patients with multiple myeloma (37%).

In the relapsed multiple myeloma study, among the 87 patients who experienced ≥ Grade 2 peripheral neuropathy, 51% had improved or resolved with a median of 3.5 months from first onset.

Among the patients with peripheral neuropathy in the phase 2 multiple myeloma studies that was Grade 2 and led to discontinuation or was ≥Grade 3, 73% (24 of 33) reported improvement or resolution following VELCADE dose adjustment, with a median time to improvement of one Grade or more from the last dose of VELCADE of 33 days. **[*see Warnings and Precautions (5.2)*]**

Hypotension

The incidence of hypotension (postural hypotension, orthostatic hypotension and hypotension NOS) was 13% in patients treated with VELCADE. Hypotension was Grade 1 or 2 in the majority of patients and Grade 3 in 3% and ≥Grade 4 in <1%. Three percent (3%) of patients had hypotension reported as an SAE, and 1% discontinued due to hypotension. The incidence of hypotension was similar in patients with multiple myeloma (12%) and those with mantle cell lymphoma (15%). In addition, 2% of patients experienced hypotension and had a syncopal event. Doses of antihypertensive medications may need to be adjusted in patients receiving VELCADE. **[*see Warnings and Precautions (5.3)*]**

Neutropenia

Neutrophil counts decreased during the VELCADE dosing period (days 1 to 11) and returned toward baseline during the 10-day rest period during each treatment cycle. Overall, neutropenia occurred in 17% of patients and was Grade 3 in 9% of patients and ≥Grade 4 in 3%. Neutropenia was reported as a serious event in <1% of patients and <1% of patients discontinued due to neutropenia. The incidence of neutropenia was higher in patients with multiple myeloma (18%) compared to patients with mantle cell lymphoma (6%). The incidence of ≥Grade 3 neutropenia also was higher in patients with multiple myeloma (14%) compared to patients with mantle cell lymphoma (4%). **[*see Warnings and Precautions (5.8)*]**

Asthenic conditions (Fatigue, Malaise, Weakness)

Asthenic conditions were reported in 64% of patients. Asthenia was Grade 3 for 16% and ≥Grade 4 in <1% of patients. Four percent (4%) of patients discontinued treatment due to asthenia. Asthenic conditions were reported in 62% of patients with multiple myeloma and 72% of patients with mantle cell lymphoma.

Pyrexia

Pyrexia (>38°C) was reported as an adverse event for 34% of patients. The event was Grade 3 in 3% and ≥Grade 4 in

Table 8: Most Commonly Reported (≥10% Overall) Adverse Events in Integrated Analyses of Relapsed Multiple Myeloma and Mantle Cell Lymphoma Studies using the 1.3 mg/m² Dose (N=1163)

Adverse Events	All Patients (N=1163)		Multiple Myeloma (N=1008)		Mantle Cell Lymphoma (N=155)	
	All Events	≥Grade 3	All Events	≥Grade 3	All Events	≥Grade 3
Asthenic conditions	740 (64)	189 (16)	628 (62)	160 (16)	112 (72)	29 (19)
Nausea	640 (55)	43 (4)	572 (57)	39 (4)	68 (44)	4 (3)
Diarrhea	604 (52)	96 (8)	531 (53)	85 (8)	73 (47)	11 (7)
Constipation	481 (41)	26 (2)	404 (40)	22 (2)	77 (50)	4 (3)
Peripheral neuropathy	457 (39)	134 (12)	372 (37)	114 (11)	85 (55)	20 (13)
Thrombocytopenia	421 (36)	337 (29)	388 (38)	320 (32)	33 (21)	17 (11)
Appetite decreased	417 (36)	30 (3)	357 (35)	25 (2)	60 (39)	5 (3)
Pyrexia	401 (34)	36 (3)	371 (37)	34 (3)	30 (19)	2 (1)
Vomiting	385 (33)	57 (5)	343 (34)	53 (5)	42 (27)	4 (3)
Anemia	333 (29)	124 (11)	306 (30)	120 (12)	27 (17)	4 (3)
Edema	262 (23)	10 (<1)	218 (22)	6 (<1)	44 (28)	4 (3)
Paresthesia and dysesthesia	254 (22)	16 (1)	240 (24)	14 (1)	14 (9)	2 (1)
Headache	253 (22)	17 (1)	227 (23)	17 (2)	26 (17)	0
Dyspnea	244 (21)	59 (5)	209 (21)	52 (5)	35 (23)	7 (5)
Cough	232 (20)	5 (<1)	202 (20)	5 (<1)	30 (19)	0
Insomnia	232 (20)	7 (<1)	199 (20)	6 (<1)	33 (21)	1 (<1)
Rash	213 (18)	10 (<1)	170 (17)	6 (<1)	43 (28)	4 (3)
Arthralgia	199 (17)	27 (2)	179 (18)	25 (2)	20 (13)	2 (1)
Neutropenia	195 (17)	143 (12)	185 (18)	137 (14)	10 (6)	6 (4)
Dizziness (excluding vertigo)	195 (17)	18 (2)	159 (16)	13 (1)	36 (23)	5 (3)
Pain in limb	179 (15)	36 (3)	172 (17)	36 (4)	7 (5)	0
Abdominal pain	170 (15)	30 (3)	146 (14)	22 (2)	24 (15)	8 (5)
Bone pain	166 (14)	37 (3)	163 (16)	37 (4)	3 (2)	0
Back pain	151 (13)	39 (3)	150 (15)	39 (4)	1 (<1)	0
Hypotension	147 (13)	37 (3)	124 (12)	32 (3)	23 (15)	5 (3)
Herpes zoster	145 (12)	22 (2)	131 (13)	21 (2)	14 (9)	1 (<1)
Nasopharyngitis	139 (12)	2 (<1)	126 (13)	2 (<1)	13 (8)	0
Upper respiratory tract infection	138 (12)	2 (<1)	114 (11)	1 (<1)	24 (15)	1 (<1)
Myalgia	136 (12)	9 (<1)	121 (12)	9 (<1)	15 (10)	0
Pneumonia	134 (12)	72 (6)	120 (12)	65 (6)	14 (9)	7 (5)
Muscle cramps	125 (11)	1 (<1)	118 (12)	1 (<1)	7 (5)	0
Dehydration	120 (10)	40 (3)	109 (11)	33 (3)	11 (7)	7 (5)
Anxiety	118 (10)	6 (<1)	111 (11)	6 (<1)	7 (5)	0

<1%. Pyrexia was reported as a serious adverse event in 6% of patients and led to VELCADE discontinuation in <1% of patients. The incidence of pyrexia was higher among patients with multiple myeloma (37%) compared to patients with mantle cell lymphoma (19%). The incidence of ≥Grade 3 pyrexia was 3% in patients with multiple myeloma and 1% in patients with mantle cell lymphoma.

Herpes Virus Infection
Physicians should consider using antiviral prophylaxis in subjects being treated with VELCADE. In the randomized studies in previously untreated and relapsed multiple myeloma, herpes zoster reactivation was more common in subjects treated with VELCADE (13%) than in the control groups (4-5%). Herpes simplex was seen in 2-8% in subjects treated with VELCADE and 1-5% in the control groups. In the previously untreated multiple myeloma study, herpes zoster virus reactivation in the VELCADE, melphalan and prednisone arm was less common in subjects receiving prophylactic antiviral therapy (3%) than in subjects who did not receive prophylactic antiviral therapy (17%). In the postmarketing experience, rare cases of herpes meningoencephalitis and ophthalmic herpes have been reported.

Additional Adverse Events from Clinical Studies
The following clinically important SAEs that are not described above have been reported in clinical trials in patients treated with VELCADE administered as monotherapy or in combination with other chemotherapeutics. These studies were conducted in patients with hematological malignancies and in solid tumors.

Blood and lymphatic system disorders: Disseminated intravascular coagulation, lymphopenia, leukopenia
Cardiac disorders: Angina pectoris, atrial fibrillation aggravated, atrial flutter, bradycardia, sinus arrest, cardiac amyloidosis, complete atrioventricular block, myocardial ischemia, myocardial infarction, pericarditis, pericardial effusion, Torsades de pointes, ventricular tachycardia
Ear and labyrinth disorders: Hearing impaired, vertigo
Eye disorders: Diplopia and blurred vision, conjunctival infection, irritation
Gastrointestinal disorders: Ascites, dysphagia, fecal impaction, gastroenteritis, gastritis hemorrhagic, hematemesis, hemorrhagic duodenitis, ileus paralytic, large intestinal obstruction, paralytic intestinal obstruction, peritonitis, small intestinal obstruction, large intestinal perforation, stomatitis, melena, pancreatitis acute, oral mucosal petechiae, gastroesophageal reflux

General disorders and administration site conditions: Injection site erythema, neuralgia, injection site pain, irritation, phlebitis
Hepatobiliary disorders: Cholestasis, hepatic hemorrhage, hyperbilirubinemia, portal vein thrombosis, hepatitis, liver failure
Immune system disorders: Anaphylactic reaction, drug hypersensitivity, immune complex mediated hypersensitivity, angioedema, laryngeal edema
Infections and infestations: Aspergillosis, bacteremia, urinary tract infection, herpes viral infection, listeriosis, septic shock, toxoplasmosis, oral candidiasis, sinusitis, catheter related infection
Injury, poisoning and procedural complications: Catheter related complication, skeletal fracture, subdural hematoma
Metabolism and nutrition disorders: Hypocalcemia, hyperuricemia, hypokalemia, hyperkalemia, hyponatremia, hypernatremia
Nervous system disorders: Ataxia, coma, dysarthria, dysautonomia, encephalopathy, cranial palsy, grand mal convulsion, hemorrhagic stroke, motor dysfunction, spinal cord compression, paralysis, postherpetic neuralgia, transient ischemic attack, reversible posterior leukoencephalopathy syndrome
Psychiatric disorders: Agitation, confusion, mental status change, psychotic disorder, suicidal ideation
Renal and urinary disorders: Calculus renal, bilateral hydronephrosis, bladder spasm, hematuria, hemorrhagic cystitis, urinary incontinence, urinary retention, renal failure (acute and chronic), glomerular nephritis proliferative
Respiratory, thoracic and mediastinal disorders: Acute respiratory distress syndrome, aspiration pneumonia, atelectasis, chronic obstructive airways disease exacerbated, dysphagia, dyspnea, dyspnea exertional, epistaxis, hemoptysis, hypoxia, lung infiltration, pleural effusion, pneumonitis, respiratory distress, pulmonary hypertension
Skin and subcutaneous tissue disorders: Urticaria, face edema, rash (which may be pruritic), leukocytoclastic vasculitis
Vascular disorders: Cerebrovascular accident, cerebral hemorrhage, deep venous thrombosis, peripheral embolism, pulmonary embolism, pulmonary hypertension
6.2 Postmarketing Experience
The following adverse drug reactions have been identified from the worldwide post-marketing experience with VELCADE. Because these reactions are reported volun-

tarily from a population of uncertain size, it is not always possible to reliably estimate their frequency or establish a causal relationship to drug exposure: atrioventricular block complete, cardiac tamponade, ischemic colitis, encephalopathy, dysautonomia, deafness bilateral, disseminated intravascular coagulation, hepatitis, acute pancreatitis, acute diffuse infiltrative pulmonary disease, toxic epidermal necrolysis, herpes meningoencephalitis and ophthalmic herpes.

7   DRUG INTERACTIONS
7.1   Ketoconazole: Co-administration of ketoconazole, a potent CYP3A inhibitor, increased the exposure of bortezomib. *[see Pharmacokinetics (12.3)]* Therefore, patients should be closely monitored when given bortezomib in combination with potent CYP3A4 inhibitors (e.g. ketoconazole, ritonavir). *[see Pharmacokinetics (12.3)]*
7.2   Melphalan-Prednisone: Co-administration of melphalan-prednisone increased the exposure of bortezomib. However, this increase is unlikely to be clinically relevant. *[see Pharmacokinetics (12.3)]*
7.3   Omeprazole: Co-administration of omeprazole, a potent inhibitor of CYP2C19, had no effect on the exposure of bortezomib. *[see Pharmacokinetics (12.3)]*
7.4   Cytochrome P450: Patients who are concomitantly receiving VELCADE and drugs that are inhibitors or inducers of cytochrome P450 3A4 should be closely monitored for either toxicities or reduced efficacy. *[see Pharmacokinetics (12.3)]*

8   USE IN SPECIFIC POPULATIONS
8.1   Pregnancy
Pregnancy Category D *[see Warnings and Precautions (5.1)]*
Bortezomib was not teratogenic in nonclinical developmental toxicity studies in rats and rabbits at the highest dose tested (0.075 mg/kg; 0.5 mg/m² in the rat and 0.05 mg/kg; 0.6 mg/m² in the rabbit) when administered during organogenesis. These dosages are approximately half the clinical dose of 1.3 mg/m² based on body surface area.
Pregnant rabbits given bortezomib during organogenesis at a dose of 0.05mg/kg (0.6 mg/m²) experienced significant post-implantation loss and decreased number of live fetuses. Live fetuses from these litters also showed significant decreases in fetal weight. The dose is approximately 0.5 times the clinical dose of 1.3 mg/m² based on body surface area.
There are no adequate and well-controlled studies in pregnant women. If VELCADE is used during pregnancy, or if the patient becomes pregnant while receiving this drug, the patient should be apprised of the potential hazard to the fetus.
8.3   Nursing Mothers
It is not known whether bortezomib is excreted in human milk. Because many drugs are excreted in human milk and because of the potential for serious adverse reactions in nursing infants from VELCADE, a decision should be made whether to discontinue nursing or to discontinue the drug, taking into account the importance of the drug to the mother.
8.4   Pediatric Use
The safety and effectiveness of VELCADE in children have not been established.
8.5   Geriatric Use
Of the 669 patients enrolled in the relapsed multiple myeloma study, 245 (37%) were 65 years of age or older: 125 (38%) on the VELCADE arm and 120 (36%) on the dexamethasone arm. Median time to progression and median duration of response for patients ≥65 were longer on VELCADE compared to dexamethasone [5.5 mo versus 4.3 mo, and 8.0 mo versus 4.9 mo, respectively]. On the VELCADE arm, 40% (n=46) of evaluable patients aged ≥65 experienced response (CR+PR) versus 18% (n=21) on the dexamethasone arm. The incidence of Grade 3 and 4 events was 64%, 78% and 75% for VELCADE patients ≤50, 51-64 and ≥65 years old, respectively. *[see Adverse Reactions (6.1); Clinical Studies (14)]*
No overall differences in safety or effectiveness were observed between patients ≥ age 65 and younger patients receiving VELCADE; but greater sensitivity of some older individuals cannot be ruled out.
8.6   Patients with Renal Impairment
The pharmacokinetics of VELCADE are not influenced by the degree of renal impairment. Therefore, dosing adjustments of VELCADE are not necessary for patients with renal insufficiency. Since dialysis may reduce VELCADE concentrations, the drug should be administered after the dialysis procedure. For information concerning dosing of melphalan in patients with renal impairment see manufacturer's prescribing information. *[see Clinical Pharmacology (12.3)]*
8.7   Patients with Hepatic Impairment
The exposure of bortezomib is increased in patients with moderate and severe hepatic impairment. Starting dose

should be reduced in those patients. ***[see Dosage and Administration (2.5), Warnings and Precautions (5.11), and Pharmacokinetics (12.3)]***

8.8 Patients with Diabetes

During clinical trials, hypoglycemia and hyperglycemia were reported in diabetic patients receiving oral hypoglycemics. Patients on oral antidiabetic agents receiving VELCADE treatment may require close monitoring of their blood glucose levels and adjustment of the dose of their antidiabetic medication.

10 OVERDOSAGE

There is no known specific antidote for VELCADE overdosage ***[see Warnings and Precautions (5.3) and Dosage and Administration (2.5)]***. In humans, fatal outcomes following the administration of more than twice the recommended therapeutic dose have been reported, which were associated with the acute onset of symptomatic hypotension and thrombocytopenia. In the event of an overdosage, the patient's vital signs should be monitored and appropriate supportive care given.

Studies in monkeys and dogs showed that IV bortezomib doses as low as 2 times the recommended clinical dose on a mg/m^2 basis were associated with increases in heart rate, decreases in contractility, hypotension, and death. In dog studies, a slight increase in the corrected QT interval was observed at doses resulting in death. In monkeys, doses of 3.0 mg/m^2 and greater (approximately twice the recommended clinical dose) resulted in hypotension starting at 1 hour post-administration, with progression to death in 12 to 14 hours following drug administration.

11 DESCRIPTION

VELCADE® (bortezomib) for Injection is an antineoplastic agent available for intravenous injection (IV) use only. Each single use vial contains 3.5 mg of bortezomib as a sterile lyophilized powder. Inactive ingredient: 35 mg mannitol, USP.

Bortezomib is a modified dipeptidyl boronic acid. The product is provided as a mannitol boronic ester which, in reconstituted form, consists of the mannitol ester in equilibrium with its hydrolysis product, the monomeric boronic acid. The drug substance exists in its cyclic anhydride form as a trimeric boroxine.

The chemical name for bortezomib, the monomeric boronic acid, is [(1R)-3-methyl-1-[[(2S)-1-oxo-3-phenyl-2-[(pyrazinylcarbonyl) amino]propyl]amino]butyl] boronic acid.

Bortezomib has the following chemical structure:

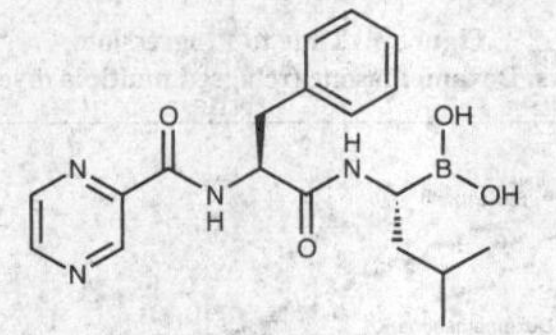

The molecular weight is 384.24. The molecular formula is $C_{19}H_{25}BN_4O_4$. The solubility of bortezomib, as the monomeric boronic acid, in water is 3.3 to 3.8 mg/mL in a pH range of 2 to 6.5.

12 CLINICAL PHARMACOLOGY

12.1 Mechanism of Action

Bortezomib is a reversible inhibitor of the chymotrypsin-like activity of the 26S proteasome in mammalian cells. The 26S proteasome is a large protein complex that degrades ubiquitinated proteins. The ubiquitin-proteasome pathway plays an essential role in regulating the intracellular concentration of specific proteins, thereby maintaining homeostasis within cells. Inhibition of the 26S proteasome prevents this targeted proteolysis, which can affect multiple signaling cascades within the cell. This disruption of normal homeostatic mechanisms can lead to cell death. Experiments have demonstrated that bortezomib is cytotoxic to a variety of cancer cell types *in vitro*. Bortezomib causes a delay in tumor growth *in vivo* in nonclinical tumor models, including multiple myeloma.

12.2 Pharmacodynamics

Following twice weekly administration of 1 mg/m^2 and 1.3 mg/m^2 bortezomib doses (n=12 per each dose level), the maximum inhibition of 20S proteasome activity (relative to baseline) in whole blood was observed 5 minutes after drug administration. Comparable maximum inhibition of 20S proteasome activity was observed between 1 and 1.3 mg/m^2 doses. Maximal inhibition ranged from 70% to 84% and from 73% to 83% for the 1 mg/m^2 and 1.3 mg/m^2 dose regimens, respectively.

12.3 Pharmacokinetics

Following intravenous administration of 1 mg/m^2 and 1.3 mg/m^2 doses to 24 patients with multiple myeloma (n=12, per each dose level), the mean maximum plasma concentrations of bortezomib (C_{max}) after the first dose (Day 1) were 57 and 112 ng/mL, respectively. In subsequent doses, when administered twice weekly, the mean maximum observed plasma concentrations ranged from 67 to 106 ng/mL for the 1 mg/m^2 dose and 89 to 120 ng/mL for the 1.3 mg/m^2 dose. The mean elimination half-life of bortezomib upon multiple dosing ranged from 40 to 193 hours after the 1 mg/m^2 dose and 76 to 108 hours after the 1.3mg/m^2 dose. The mean total body clearances was 102 and 112 L/h following the first dose for doses of 1 mg/m^2 and 1.3 mg/m^2, respectively, and ranged from 15 to 32 L/h following subsequent doses for doses of 1 and 1.3 mg/m^2, respectively.

Distribution: The mean distribution volume of bortezomib ranged from approximately 498 to 1884 L/m^2 following single- or repeat-dose administration of 1 mg/m^2 or 1.3mg/m^2 to patients with multiple myeloma. This suggests bortezomib distributes widely to peripheral tissues. The binding of bortezomib to human plasma proteins averaged 83% over the concentration range of 100 to 1000 ng/mL.

Metabolism: *In vitro* studies with human liver microsomes and human cDNA-expressed cytochrome P450 isozymes indicate that bortezomib is primarily oxidatively metabolized via cytochrome P450 enzymes 3A4, 2C19, and 1A2. Bortezomib metabolism by CYP 2D6 and 2C9 enzymes is minor. The major metabolic pathway is deboronation to form 2 deboronated metabolites that subsequently undergo hydroxylation to several metabolites. Deboronated bortezomib metabolites are inactive as 26S proteasome inhibitors. Pooled plasma data from 8 patients at 10 min and 30 min after dosing indicate that the plasma levels of metabolites are low compared to the parent drug.

Elimination: The pathways of elimination of bortezomib have not been characterized in humans.

Age: Analyses of data after the first dose of Cycle 1 (Day 1) in 39 multiple myeloma patients who had received intravenous doses of 1 mg/m^2 and 1.3 mg/m^2 showed that both dose-normalized AUC and C_{max} tend to be less in younger patients. Patients < 65 years of age (n=26) had about 25% lower mean dose-normalized AUC and C_{max} than those ≥ 65 years of age (n=13).

Gender: Mean dose-normalized AUC and C_{max} values were comparable between male (n=22) and female (n=17) patients after the first dose of Cycle 1 for the 1 and 1.3 mg/m^2 doses.

Race: The effect of race on exposure to bortezomib could not be assessed as most of the patients were Caucasian.

Hepatic Impairment: The effect of hepatic impairment (see **Table 4** for definition of hepatic impairment) on the pharmacokinetics of bortezomib was assessed in 51 cancer patients at bortezomib doses ranging from 0.5 to 1.3 mg/m^2. When compared to patients with normal hepatic function, mild hepatic impairment did not alter dose-normalized bortezomib AUC. However, the dose-normalized mean AUC values were increased by approximately 60% in patients with moderate or severe hepatic impairment. A lower starting dose is recommended in patients with moderate or severe hepatic impairment, and those patients should be monitored closely. ***[see Dosage and Administration (2.5), Warning and Precautions (5.11) and Use in Specific Populations (8.7)]***

Renal Impairment: A pharmacokinetic study was conducted in patients with various degrees of renal impairment who were classified according to their creatinine clearance values (CrCl) into the following groups: Normal (CrCl ≥60 mL/min/1.73 m^2, N=12), Mild (CrCl=40-59 mL/min/1.73 m^2, N=10), Moderate (CrCl=20-39 mL/min/1.73 m^2, N=9), and Severe (CrCl < 20 mL/min/1.73 m^2, N=3). A group of dialysis patients who were dosed after dialysis was also included in the study (N=8). Patients were administered intravenous doses of 0.7 to 1.3 mg/m^2 of bortezomib twice weekly. Exposure of bortezomib (dose-normalized AUC and C_{max}) was comparable among all the groups. ***[see Use in Specific Populations (8.6)]***

Pediatric: There are no pharmacokinetic data in pediatric patients.

Effect of Ketoconazole: Co-administration of ketoconazole, a potent CYP3A inhibitor, showed a 35% increase in mean bortezomib AUC, based on data from 12 patients. ***[see Drug Interactions (7.1)]***

Effect of Melphalan-Prednisone: Co-administration of melphalan-prednisone on VELCADE showed a 17% increase in mean bortezomib AUC based on data from 21 patients. This increase is unlikely to be clinically relevant. ***[see Drug Interactions (7.2)]***

Effect of Omeprazole: Co-administration of omeprazole, a potent inhibitor of CYP2C19, had no significant effect on the pharmacokinetics of bortezomib, based on data from 17 patients. ***[see Drug Interactions (7.3)]***

Cytochrome P450: Bortezomib is a poor inhibitor of human liver microsome cytochrome P450 1A2, 2C9, 2D6, and 3A4, with IC_{50} values of >30µM (>11.5µg/mL). Bortezomib may inhibit 2C19 activity (IC_{50} = 18 µM, 6.9 µg/mL) and increase exposure to drugs that are substrates for this enzyme. Bortezomib did not induce the activities of cytochrome P450 3A4 and 1A2 in primary cultured human hepatocytes. ***[see Drug Interactions (7.4)]***

13 NONCLINICAL TOXICOLOGY

13.1 Carcinogenesis, Mutagenesis, Impairment of Fertility

Carcinogenicity studies have not been conducted with bortezomib.

Bortezomib showed clastogenic activity (structural chromosomal aberrations) in the in vitro chromosomal aberration assay using Chinese hamster ovary cells. Bortezomib was not genotoxic when tested in the in vitro mutagenicity assay (Ames test) and in vivo micronucleus assay in mice.

Fertility studies with bortezomib were not performed but evaluation of reproductive tissues has been performed in the general toxicity studies. In the 6-month rat toxicity study, degenerative effects in the ovary were observed at doses ≥0.3 mg/m^2 (one-fourth of the recommended clinical dose), and degenerative changes in the testes occurred at 1.2 mg/m^2. VELCADE could have a potential effect on either male or female fertility.

13.2 Animal Toxicology

Cardiovascular Toxicity: Studies in monkeys showed that administration of dosages approximately twice the recommended clinical dose resulted in heart rate elevations, followed by profound progressive hypotension, bradycardia, and death 12 to 14 hours post dose. Doses ≥1.2 mg/m^2 induced dose-proportional changes in cardiac parameters. Bortezomib has been shown to distribute to most tissues in the body, including the myocardium. In a repeated dosing toxicity study in the monkey, myocardial hemorrhage, inflammation, and necrosis were also observed.

Chronic Administration: In animal studies at a dose and schedule similar to that recommended for patients (twice weekly dosing for 2 weeks followed by 1-week rest), toxicities observed included severe anemia and thrombocytopenia, and gastrointestinal, neurological and lymphoid system toxicities. Neurotoxic effects of bortezomib in animal studies included axonal swelling and degeneration in peripheral nerves, dorsal spinal roots, and tracts of the spinal cord. Additionally, multifocal hemorrhage and necrosis in the brain, eye, and heart were observed.

14 CLINICAL STUDIES

14.1 Multiple Myeloma

Randomized, Open-Label Clinical Study in Patients with Previously Untreated Multiple Myeloma:

A prospective, international, randomized (1:1), open-label clinical study of 682 patients was conducted to determine whether VELCADE (1.3 mg/m^2) in combination with melphalan (9 mg/m^2) and prednisone (60 mg/m^2) resulted in improvement in time to progression (TTP) when compared to melphalan (9 mg/m^2) and prednisone (60 mg/m^2) in patients with previously untreated multiple myeloma. Treatment was administered for a maximum of 9 cycles (approximately 54 weeks) and was discontinued early for disease progression or unacceptable toxicity. Antiviral prophylaxis was recommended for patients on the VELCADE study arm.

The median age of the patients in the study was 71 years (48;91), 50% were male, 88% were Caucasian and the median Karnofsky performance status score for the patients was 80 (60;100). Patients had IgG/IgA/Light chain myeloma in 63%/25%/8% instances, a median hemoglobin of 105 g/L (64;165), and a median platelet count of 221,500 /microliter (33,000;587,000).

Efficacy results for the trial are presented in Table 9. At a pre-specified interim analysis (with median follow-up of 16.3 months), the combination of VELCADE, Melphalan and Prednisone therapy resulted in significantly superior results for time to progression, progression free survival, overall survival and response rate. Further enrollment was halted, and patients receiving Melphalan and Prednisone were offered VELCADE in addition. A later, pre-specified analysis of overall survival (with median follow-up of 36.7 months) continued to show a statistically significant survival benefit for the VELCADE, Melphalan and Prednisone treatment arm despite subsequent therapies including VELCADE based regimens.

Table 9: Summary of Efficacy Analyses in the Previously Untreated Multiple Myeloma Study

Efficacy Endpoint	VELCADE, Melphalan and Prednisone n=344	Melphalan and Prednisone n=338
Time to Progression		
Events n (%)	101 (29)	152 (45)
Median[a] (months)	20.7	15.0
(95% CI)	(17.6, 24.7)	(14.1, 17.9)
Hazard ratio[b]	0.54	
(95% CI)	(0.42, 0.70)	

p-value[c]   0.000002

Progression-free Survival

Events n (%)	135 (39)	190 (56)
Median[a] (months)	18.3	14.0
(95% CI)	(16.6, 21.7)	(11.1, 15.0)
Hazard ratio[b]		0.61
(95% CI)		(0.49, 0.76)
p-value[c]		0.00001

Response Rate

CR[d] n (%)	102 (30)	12 (4)
PR[d] n (%)	136 (40)	103 (30)
nCR n (%)	5 (1)	0
CR + PR[d] n (%)	238 (69)	115 (34)
p-value[e]		<10^{-10}

Overall Survival

Events (deaths) n (%)	109 (32)	148 (44)
Median[a] (months)	Not Reached	43.1
(95% CI)	(46.2, NR)	(34.8, NR)
Hazard ratio[b]		0.65
(95% CI)		(0.51, 0.84)
p-value[c]		0.00084

Note: All results are based on the analysis performed at a median follow-up duration of 16.3 months except for the overall survival analysis that was performed at a median follow-up duration of 36.7 months.
[a] Kaplan-Meier estimate
[b] Hazard ratio estimate is based on a Cox proportional-hazard model adjusted for stratification factors: beta2-microglobulin, albumin, and region. A hazard ratio less than 1 indicates an advantage for VELCADE, Melphalan and Prednisone
[c] p-value based on the stratified log-rank test adjusted for stratification factors: beta2-microglobulin, albumin, and region
[d] EBMT criteria
[e] p-value for Response Rate (CR + PR) from the Cochran-Mantel-Haenszel chi-square test adjusted for the stratification factors

TTP was statistically significantly longer on the VELCADE, Melphalan and Prednisone arm (see **Figure 1**). (median follow up 16.3 months)

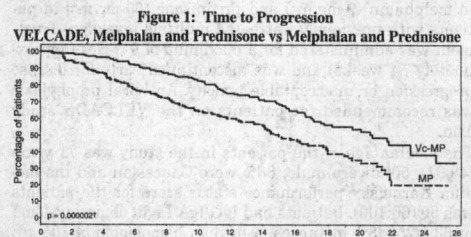

Figure 1: Time to Progression
VELCADE, Melphalan and Prednisone vs Melphalan and Prednisone

Overall survival was statistically significantly longer on the VELCADE, Melphalan and Prednisone arm (see **Figure 2**). (median follow up 36.7 months)

Figure 2: Overall Survival
VELCADE, Melphalan and Prednisone vs Melphalan and Prednisone

Randomized, Clinical Study in Relapsed Multiple Myeloma

A prospective phase 3, international, randomized (1:1), stratified, open-label clinical study enrolling 669 patients was designed to determine whether VELCADE resulted in improvement in time to progression (TTP) compared to high-dose dexamethasone in patients with progressive multiple myeloma following 1 to 3 prior therapies. Patients considered to be refractory to prior high-dose dexamethasone were excluded as were those with baseline grade ≥2 peripheral neuropathy or platelet counts <50,000/μL. A total of 627 patients were evaluable for response.

Table 10: Summary of Baseline Patient and Disease Characteristics in the Relapsed Multiple Myeloma Study

Patient Characteristics	VELCADE N=333	Dexamethasone N=336
Median age in years (range)	62.0 (33, 84)	61.0 (27, 86)
Gender: Male/female	56%/44%	60%/40%
Race: Caucasian/black/other	90%/6%/4%	88%/7%/5%
Karnofsky performance status score ≤70	13%	17%
Hemoglobin <100 g/L	32%	28%
Platelet count <75 × 10^9/L	6%	4%
Disease Characteristics		
Type of myeloma (%): IgG/IgA/Light chain	60%/23%/12%	59%/24%/13%
Median β_2-microglobulin (mg/L)	3.7	3.6
Median albumin (g/L)	39.0	39.0
Creatinine clearance ≤30 mL/min [n (%)]	17 (5%)	11 (3%)
Median Duration of Multiple Myeloma Since Diagnosis (Years)	3.5	3.1
Number of Prior Therapeutic Lines of Treatment		
Median	2	2
1 prior line	40%	35%
>1 prior line	60%	65%
Previous Therapy		
Any prior steroids, e.g., dexamethasone, VAD	98%	99%
Any prior anthracyclines, e.g., VAD, mitoxantrone	77%	76%
Any prior alkylating agents, e.g., MP, VBMCP	91%	92%
Any prior thalidomide therapy	48%	50%
Vinca alkaloids	74%	72%
Prior stem cell transplant/other high-dose therapy	67%	68%
Prior experimental or other types of therapy	3%	2%

Stratification factors were based on the number of lines of prior therapy the patient had previously received (1 previous line versus more than 1 line of therapy), time of progression relative to prior treatment (progression during or within 6 months of stopping their most recent therapy versus relapse >6 months after receiving their most recent therapy), and screening β_2-microglobulin levels (≤2.5 mg/L versus >2.5 mg/L).

Baseline patient and disease characteristics are summarized in **Table 10**.
[See table 10 above]

Patients in the VELCADE treatment group were to receive eight 3-week treatment cycles followed by three 5-week treatment cycles of VELCADE. Patients achieving a CR were treated for 4 cycles beyond first evidence of CR. Within each 3-week treatment cycle, VELCADE 1.3 mg/m^2/dose alone was administered by IV bolus twice weekly for 2 weeks on Days 1, 4, 8, and 11 followed by a 10-day rest period (Days 12 to 21). Within each 5-week treatment cycle, VELCADE 1.3 mg/m^2/dose alone was administered by IV bolus once weekly for 4 weeks on Days 1, 8, 15, and 22 followed by a 13-day rest period (Days 23 to 35). [*see Dosage and Administration (2.1)*]

Patients in the dexamethasone treatment group were to receive four 5-week treatment cycles followed by five 4-week treatment cycles. Within each 5-week treatment cycle, dexamethasone 40 mg/day PO was administered once daily on Days 1 to 4, 9 to 12, and 17 to 20 followed by a 15-day rest period (Days 21-35). Within each 4-week treatment cycle, dexamethasone 40 mg/day PO was administered once daily on Days 1 to 4 followed by a 24-day rest period (Days 5 to 28). Patients with documented progressive disease on dexamethasone were offered VELCADE at a standard dose and schedule on a companion study. Following a preplanned interim analysis of time to progression, the dexamethasone arm was halted and all patients randomized to dexamethasone were offered VELCADE, regardless of disease status. In the VELCADE arm, 34% of patients received at least one VELCADE dose in all 8 of the 3-week cycles of therapy, and 13% received at least one dose in all 11 cycles. The average number of VELCADE doses during the study was 22, with a range of 1 to 44. In the dexamethasone arm, 40% of patients received at least one dose in all 4 of the 5-week treatment cycles of therapy, and 6% received at least one dose in all 9 cycles.

The time to event analyses and response rates from the relapsed multiple myeloma study are presented in **Table 11**. Response and progression were assessed using the European Group for Blood and Marrow Transplantation (EBMT) criteria.[1] Complete response (CR) required <5% plasma cells in the marrow, 100% reduction in M-protein, and a negative immunofixation test (IF-). Partial response (PR) requires ≥50% reduction in serum myeloma protein and ≥90% reduction of urine myeloma protein on at least 2 occasions for a minimum of at least 6 weeks along with stable bone disease and normal calcium. Near complete response (nCR) was defined as meeting all the criteria for complete response including 100% reduction in M-protein by protein electrophoresis, however M-protein was still detectable by immunofixation (IF+).

[See table 11 at top of next page]

TTP was statistically significantly longer on the VELCADE arm (see Figure 3).

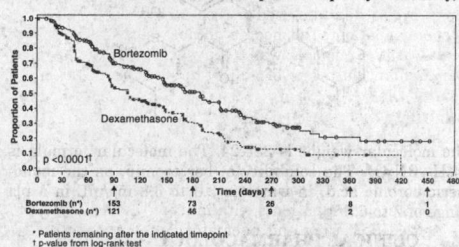

Figure 3: Time to Progression
Bortezomib vs. Dexamethasone (relapsed multiple myeloma study)

As shown in **Figure 4** VELCADE had a significant survival advantage relative to dexamethasone (p<0.05). The median follow-up was 8.3 months.

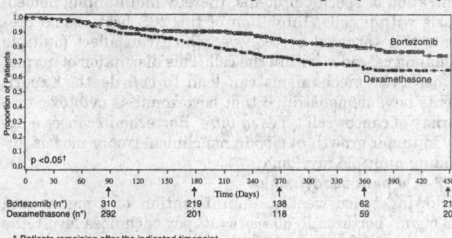

Figure 4: Overall Survival
Bortezomib vs. Dexamethasone (relapsed multiple myeloma study)

For the 121 patients achieving a response (CR or PR) on the VELCADE arm, the median duration was 8.0 months (95% CI: 6.9, 11.5 months) compared to 5.6 months (95% CI: 4.8, 9.2 months) for the 56 responders on the dexamethasone arm. The response rate was significantly higher on the VELCADE arm regardless of β_2-microglobulin levels at baseline.

A Randomized Phase 2 Dose-Response Study in Relapsed Multiple Myeloma

An open-label, multicenter study randomized 54 patients with multiple myeloma who had progressed or relapsed on or after front-line therapy to receive VELCADE 1 mg/m^2 or

1.3 mg/m² IV bolus twice weekly for 2 weeks on Days 1, 4, 8, and 11 followed by a 10-day rest period (Days 12 to 21). The median duration of time between diagnosis of multiple myeloma and first dose of VELCADE on this trial was 2.0 years, and patients had received a median of 1 prior line of treatment (median of 3 prior therapies). A single complete response was seen at each dose. The overall response rates (CR + PR) were 30% (8/27) at 1 mg/m² and 38% (10/26) at 1.3 mg/m².

A Phase 2 Open-Label Extension Study in Relapsed Multiple Myeloma

Patients from the two phase 2 studies who in the investigators' opinion would experience additional clinical benefit continued to receive VELCADE beyond 8 cycles on an extension study. Sixty-three (63) patients from the phase 2 multiple myeloma studies were enrolled and received a median of 7 additional cycles of VELCADE therapy for a total median of 14 cycles (range 7 to 32). The overall median dosing intensity was the same in both the parent protocol and extension study. Sixty-seven percent (67%) of patients initiated the extension study at the same or higher dose intensity at which they completed the parent protocol, and 89% of patients maintained the standard 3-week dosing schedule during the extension study. No new cumulative or new long-term toxicities were observed with prolonged VELCADE treatment. [see Adverse Reactions (6.1)]

14.2   Mantle Cell Lymphoma

A Phase 2 Single-arm Clinical Study in Relapsed Mantle Cell Lymphoma After Prior Therapy

The safety and efficacy of VELCADE in relapsed or refractory mantle cell lymphoma were evaluated in an open-label, single-arm, multicenter study of 155 patients with progressive disease who had received at least 1 prior therapy. The median age of the patients was 65 years (42, 89), 81% were male, and 92% were Caucasian. Of the total, 75% had one or more extra-nodal sites of disease, and 77% were stage 4. In 91% of the patients, prior therapy included all of the following: an anthracycline or mitoxantrone, cyclophosphamide, and rituximab. A total of thirty seven percent (37%) of patients were refractory to their last prior therapy. An IV bolus injection of VELCADE 1.3 mg/m²/dose was administered twice weekly for 2 weeks on Days 1, 4, 8, and 11 followed by a 10-day rest period (Days 12 to 21) for a maximum of 17 treatment cycles. Patients achieving a CR or CRu were treated for 4 cycles beyond first evidence of CR or CRu. The study employed dose modifications for toxicity. [see Dosage and Administration (2.4)]

Responses to VELCADE are shown in Table 12. Response rates to VELCADE were determined according to the International Workshop Response Criteria (IWRC)[2] based on independent radiologic review of CT scans. The median number of cycles administered across all patients was 4; in responding patients the median number of cycles was 8. The median time to response was 40 days (range 31 to 204 days). The median duration of follow-up was more than 13 months.

[See table 12 at right]

15   REFERENCES

1. Bladé J, Samson D, Reece D, Apperley J, Bjorkstrand B, Gahrton G et al. Criteria for evaluating disease response and progression in patients with multiple myeloma treated by high-dose therapy and haematopoietic stem cell transplantation. Myeloma Subcommittee of the EBMT. European Group for Blood and Marrow Transplant. British Journal of Haematology 1998;102(5):1115-1123.

2. Cheson BD, Horning SJ, Coiffier B, Shipp MA, Fisher RI, Connors JM et al. Report of an international workshop to standardize response criteria for non-Hodgkin's lymphomas. NCI Sponsored International Working Group. Journal of Clinical Oncology 1999; 17 (4):1244.

3. Preventing Occupational Exposures to Antineoplastic and Other Hazardous Drugs in Health Care Settings. NIOSH Alert 2004-165.

4. OSHA Technical Manual, TED 1-0.15A, Section VI: Chapter 2. Controlling Occupational Exposure to Hazardous Drugs. OSHA, 1999.http://www.osha.gov/dts/osta/otm/otm_vi/otm_vi_2.html.

5. American Society of Health-System Pharmacists. ASHP guidelines on handling hazardous drugs. Am J Health-Syst Pharm. 2006;63:1172-1193.

6. Polovich, M., White, J. M., & Kelleher, L.O. (eds.) 2005. Chemotherapy and biotherapy guidelines and recommendations for practice (2nd. ed.) Pittsburgh, PA: Oncology Nursing Society.

16   HOW SUPPLIED/STORAGE AND HANDLING

VELCADE® (bortezomib) for Injection is supplied as individually cartoned 10 mL vials containing 3.5 mg of bortezomib as a white to off-white cake or powder.
NDC 63020-049-01
3.5 mg single use vial
Unopened vials may be stored at controlled room temperature 25°C (77°F); excursions permitted from 15 to 30°C (59 to 86°F) [see USP Controlled Room Temperature]. Retain in original package to protect from light.

Table 11: Summary of Efficacy Analyses in the Relapsed Multiple Myeloma Study

Efficacy Endpoint	All Patients		1 Prior Line of Therapy		> 1 Prior Line of Therapy	
	VELCADE	Dex	VELCADE	Dex	VELCADE	Dex
	n=333	n=336	n=132	n=119	n=200	n=217
Time to Progression						
Events n (%)	147 (44)	196 (58)	55 (42)	64 (54)	92 (46)	132 (61)
Median[a] (95% CI)	6.2 mo (4.9, 6.9)	3.5 mo (2.9, 4.2)	7.0 mo (6.2, 8.8)	5.6 mo (3.4, 6.3)	4.9 mo (4.2, 6.3)	2.9 mo (2.8, 3.5)
Hazard ratio[b] (95% CI)	0.55 (0.44, 0.69)		0.55 (0.38, 0.81)		0.54 (0.41, 0.72)	
p-value[c]	<0.0001		0.0019		<0.0001	
Overall Survival						
Events (deaths) n (%)	51 (15)	84 (25)	12 (9)	24 (20)	39 (20)	60 (28)
Hazard ratio[b] (95% CI)	0.57 (0.40, 0.81)		0.39 (0.19, 0.81)		0.65 (0.43, 0.97)	
p-value[c,d]	<0.05		<0.05		<0.05	
Response Rate Population[e] n = 627	n=315	n=312	n=128	n=110	n=187	n=202
CR[f] n (%)	20 (6)	2 (<1)	8 (6)	2 (2)	12 (6)	0 (0)
PR[f] n(%)	101 (32)	54 (17)	49 (38)	27 (25)	52 (28)	27 (13)
nCR[f,g] n(%)	21 (7)	3(<1)	8 (6)	2 (2)	13 (7)	1 (<1)
CR + PR[f] n (%)	121 (38)	56 (18)	57 (45)	29 (26)	64 (34)	27 (13)
p-value[h]	<0.0001		0.0035		<0.0001	

[a] Kaplan-Meier estimate
[b] Hazard ratio is based on Cox proportional-hazard model with the treatment as single independent variable. A hazard ratio less than 1 indicates an advantage for VELCADE
[c] p-value based on the stratified log-rank test including randomization stratification factors
[d] Precise p-value cannot be rendered
[e] Response population includes patients who had measurable disease at baseline and received at least 1 dose of study drug
[f] EBMT criteria[1]; nCR meets all EBMT criteria for CR but has positive IF. Under EBMT criteria nCR is in the PR category
[g] In 2 patients, the IF was unknown
[h] p-value for Response Rate (CR + PR) from the Cochran-Mantel-Haenszel chi-square test adjusted for the stratification factors

Table 12: Response Outcomes in a Phase 2 Mantle Cell Lymphoma Study

Response Analyses (N = 155)	N (%)	95% CI
Overall Response Rate (IWRC) (CR + CRu + PR)	48 (31)	(24, 39)
Complete Response (CR + CRu)	12 (8)	(4, 13)
CR	10 (6)	(3, 12)
CRu	2 (1)	(0, 5)
Partial Response (PR)	36 (23)	(17, 31)
Duration of Response	**Median**	**95% CI**
CR + CRu + PR (N = 48)	9.3 months	(5.4, 13.8)
CR + CRu (N = 12)	15.4 months	(13.4, 15.4)
PR (N=36)	6.1 months	(4.2, 9.3)

Consider handling and disposal of VELCADE according to guidelines issued for cytotoxic drugs, including the use of gloves and other protective clothing to prevent skin contact[3-6].

Caution: Rx only
U.S. Patents: 5,780,454; 6,083,903; 6,297,217 B1; 6,617,317 B1; 6,713, 446 B2; 6,958,319 B2

Distributed and Marketed by:
Millennium Pharmaceuticals, Inc.
40 Landsdowne Street
Cambridge, MA 02139
MILLENNIUM
VELCADE, and MILLENNIUM are registered trademarks of Millennium Pharmaceuticals, Inc.
©2009 Millennium Pharmaceuticals, Inc. All rights reserved. Printed in USA.
Issued December 2009
Rev 10

17   PATIENT COUNSELING INFORMATION

Physicians are advised to discuss the following with patients prior to treatment with VELCADE:

Ability to Drive or Operate Machinery or Impairment of Mental Ability: VELCADE may cause fatigue, dizziness, syncope, orthostatic/postural hypotension. Patients should be advised not to drive or operate machinery if they experience any of these symptoms.

Dehydration/Hypotension: Since patients receiving VELCADE therapy may experience vomiting and/or diarrhea, patients should be advised regarding appropriate measures to avoid dehydration. Patients should be instructed to seek medical advice if they experience symptoms of dizziness, light headedness or fainting spells.

Pregnancy/Nursing: Patients should be advised to use effective contraceptive measures to prevent pregnancy during treatment with VELCADE. If a patient becomes pregnant during treatment she should be instructed to inform her physician immediately. Patients should also be advised not to take VELCADE treatment while pregnant or breastfeeding. If a patient wishes to restart breastfeeding after treatment, she should be advised to discuss the appropriate timing with her physician.

Concomitant Medications: Patients should be advised to speak with their physician about any other medication they are currently taking.

Diabetic Patients: Patients should be advised to check their blood sugar frequently if using an oral antidiabetic medication and notify their physician of any changes in blood sugar level.

Peripheral Neuropathy: Patients should be advised to contact their physician if they experience new or worsening symptoms of peripheral neuropathy such as tingling, numbness, pain, a burning feeling in the feet or hands, or weakness in the arms or legs.

Other: Patients should be instructed to contact their physician if they develop a rash, experience shortness of breath, cough, or swelling of the feet, ankles, or legs, convulsion, persistent headache, reduced eyesight, an increase in blood pressure or blurred vision.

Millennium Pharmaceuticals, Inc.
40 Landsdowne Street
Cambridge, MA 02139
MILLENNIUM
VELCADE, and MILLENNIUM are registered trademarks of Millennium Pharmaceuticals, Inc.
©2009 Millennium Pharmaceuticals, Inc. All rights reserved. Printed in USA.
Issued December 2009   Rev10
Shown in Product Identification Guide, page 314

Mission Pharmacal Company
**10999 IH 10 WEST, SUITE 1000
SAN ANTONIO, TX 78230-1355**

Direct All Inquiries to:
PO Box 786099
San Antonio, TX 78278–6099
TOLL FREE: (800) 292-7364
Customer Service (M–W 7A–5:30P Central Time
               Th 7:30A–5P Central Time)
(210) 696-8400; FAX: (210) 696-6010

CITRANATAL ASSURE®   ℞
Rx Prenatal Vitamin Tablet and 300 mg DHA capsule

DESCRIPTION
CitraNatal Assure® is a prescription prenatal/postnatal multivitamin/mineral tablet with FERR-EASE™, a patented dual-iron delivery comprising both a quick release and slow release iron, and a capsule of an essential fatty acid. The prenatal vitamin is a white, coated, oval multivitamin/mineral tablet. The tablet is debossed "0893" on one side and is blank on the other. The essential fatty acid DHA capsule is clear and contains an amber to light/dark orange semi-solid mixture.

Each prenatal tablet contains:
Vitamin C (Ascorbic acid)	120 mg
Calcium (Calcium citrate)	125 mg
Iron (Carbonyl iron, ferrous gluconate)	35 mg
Vitamin D₃ (Cholecalciferol)	400 IU
Vitamin E (dl-alpha tocopheryl acetate)	30 IU
Thiamin (Vitamin B₁)	3 mg
Riboflavin (Vitamin B₂)	3.4 mg
Niacinamide (Vitamin B₃)	20 mg
Vitamin B₆ (Pyridoxine HCl)	25 mg
Folic Acid	1 mg
Iodine (Potassium iodide)	150 mcg
Zinc (Zinc oxide)	25 mg
Copper (Cupric oxide)	2 mg
Docusate Sodium	50 mg

Each DHA gelatin capsule contains:
Docosahexaenoic Acid (DHA)	300 mg
Eicosapentaenoic Acid (EPA)	Not more than 0.750 mg

DHA is contained in the oil derived from microalgae.
Other ingredients in DHA gelatin capsule: Gelatin, Glycerin USP, Water.

INDICATIONS
CitraNatal Assure® is a multivitamin/mineral prescription drug indicated for use in improving the nutritional status of women prior to conception, throughout pregnancy, and in the postnatal period for both lactating and nonlactating mothers.

CONTRAINDICATIONS
This product is contraindicated in patients with a known hypersensitivity to any of the ingredients.

> **WARNING:** Accidental overdose of **iron-containing** products is a leading cause of fatal poisoning in children under 6. KEEP THIS PRODUCT OUT OF THE REACH OF CHILDREN. In case of accidental overdose, call a doctor or poison control center immediately.

WARNING
Ingestion of more than 3 grams of omega-3 fatty acids per day has been shown to have potential antithrombotic effects, including an increased bleeding time and INR. Administration of omega-3 fatty acids should be avoided in patients on anticoagulants and in those known to have an inherited or acquired bleeding diathesis.

WARNING
Folic acid alone is improper therapy in the treatment of pernicious anemia and other megaloblastic anemias where vitamin B₁₂ is deficient.

PRECAUTIONS
Folic acid in doses above 0.1 mg daily may obscure pernicious anemia in that hematologic remission can occur while neurological manifestations progress.

ADVERSE REACTIONS
Allergic sensitization has been reported following both oral and parenteral administration of folic acid.
CAUTION: Exercise caution to ensure that the prescribed dosage of DHA does not exceed 1 gram (1000 mg) per day.

DOSAGE AND ADMINISTRATION
One tablet and one capsule daily or as directed by a physician.
Store at controlled room temperature.
NOTICE: Contact with moisture can discolor or erode the tablet.

HOW SUPPLIED
Six child-resistant blister packs of 5 tablets and 5 capsules each - NDC 0178-0893-30
To report a serious adverse event or obtain product information, call (210) 696-8400.
Rev 1009

CITRANATAL B-CALM®   ℞
Rx Prenatal Vitamin with two 25 mg each Vitamin B₆ tablets

A prescription prenatal supplement with 1 mg folic acid and a high level of vitamin B₆ which may act as an antiemetic.

DESCRIPTION
CitraNatal B-Calm® is a prescription prenatal multivitamin/mineral tablet with a high level of B₆, along with two vitamin B₆ tablets. The prenatal tablet is white, coated, modified oval, and is debossed with "0866" on one side and is blank on the other. The B₆ 25 mg tablets are white to off-white, uncoated, round, and are debossed with "B" on one side and "6" on the other.

Each prenatal tablet contains:
Vitamin C (Ascorbic acid)	120 mg
Calcium (Calcium citrate)	125 mg
Iron (Carbonyl iron)	20 mg
Vitamin D₃ (Cholecalciferol)	400 IU
Vitamin B₆ (Pyridoxine HCl)	25 mg
Folic Acid	1 mg

Each vitamin B₆ tablet contains:
Vitamin B₆ (Pyridoxine HCl)	25 mg

INDICATIONS
CitraNatal B-Calm® is a multivitamin/mineral prescription drug indicated for use in improving the nutritional status of women prior to conception, throughout pregnancy, and in the postnatal period for both lactating and nonlactating mothers. CitraNatal B-Calm® may be used in conjunction with a physician prescribed regimen to help minimize pregnancy related nausea and vomiting.

CONTRAINDICATIONS
This product is contraindicated in patients with a known hypersensitivity to any of the ingredients.

> **WARNING:** Accidental overdose of **iron-containing** products is a leading cause of fatal poisoning in children under 6. KEEP THIS AND ALL DRUGS OUT OF THE REACH OF CHILDREN. In case of accidental overdose, call a doctor or poison control center immediately.

WARNING
Folic acid alone is improper therapy in the treatment of pernicious anemia and other megaloblastic anemias where vitamin B₁₂ is deficient.

PRECAUTION
Folic acid in doses above 0.1 mg daily may obscure pernicious anemia, in that hematologic remission can occur while neurological manifestations remain progressive.

ADVERSE REACTIONS
Allergic sensitization has been reported following both oral and parenteral administration of folic acid.

DOSAGE AND ADMINISTRATION
One tablet every eight hours, beginning with "Tablet 1", or as directed by a physician.
Store at controlled room temperature.
NOTICE: Contact with moisture can discolor or erode tablets.

HOW SUPPLIED
Six child-resistant blister packs of 5 multivitamin/multimineral tablets and 10 vitamin B₆ tablets each - NDC 0178-0866-30.
To report a serious adverse event or obtain product information, call (210) 696-8400.
Rev. 1009

CITRANATAL® 90 DHA   ℞
Rx Prenatal Vitamin Tablet and 300 mg DHA Capsule

DESCRIPTION
CitraNatal® 90 DHA is a prescription prenatal/postnatal multivitamin/mineral tablet with FERR-EASE™, a patented dual-iron delivery comprising both a quick release and slow release iron, and a capsule of an essential fatty acid. The prenatal vitamin is a scored, white, oval multivitamin/mineral tablet. The tablet is debossed "CN 90" on one side and "08" bisect "29" on the other. The essential fatty acid DHA capsule is clear and contains an amber to light/dark orange semi-solid mixture.

Each prenatal tablet contains:
Vitamin C (Ascorbic acid)	120 mg
Calcium (Calcium citrate)	160 mg
Iron (Carbonyl iron, ferrous gluconate)	90 mg
Vitamin D₃ (Cholecalciferol)	400 IU
Vitamin E (dl-alpha tocopheryl acetate)	30 IU
Thiamin (Vitamin B₁)	3 mg
Riboflavin (Vitamin B₂)	3.4 mg
Niacinamide (Vitamin B₃)	20 mg
Vitamin B₆ (Pyridoxine HCl)	20 mg
Folic Acid	1 mg
Iodine (Potassium iodide)	150 mcg
Zinc (Zinc oxide)	25 mg
Copper (Cupric oxide)	2 mg
Docusate Sodium	50 mg

Each DHA gelatin capsule contains:
Docosahexaenoic Acid (DHA)	300 mg
Eicosapentaenoic Acid (EPA)	Not more than 0.750 mg

DHA is contained in the oil derived from microalgae.
Other ingredients in DHA gelatin capsule: Gelatin, Glycerin USP, Water.

INDICATIONS
CitraNatal® 90 DHA is a multivitamin/mineral prescription drug indicated for use in improving the nutritional status of women prior to conception, throughout pregnancy, and in the postnatal period for both lactating and nonlactating mothers.

CONTRAINDICATIONS
This product is contraindicated in patients with a known hypersensitivity to any of the ingredients.

> **WARNING**
> Accidental overdose of **iron-containing** products is a leading cause of fatal poisoning in children under 6. KEEP THIS PRODUCT OUT OF THE REACH OF CHILDREN. In case of accidental overdose, call a doctor or poison control center immediately.

WARNING
Ingestion of more than 3 grams of omega-3 fatty acids per day has been shown to have potential antithrombotic effects, including an increased bleeding time and INR. Administration of omega-3 fatty acids should be avoided in patients on anticoagulants and in those known to have an inherited or acquired bleeding diathesis.

WARNING
Folic acid alone is improper therapy in the treatment of pernicious anemia and other megaloblastic anemias where vitamin B₁₂ is deficient.

PRECAUTIONS
Folic acid in doses above 0.1 mg daily may obscure pernicious anemia in that hematologic remission can occur while neurological manifestations progress.

ADVERSE REACTIONS
Allergic sensitization has been reported following both oral and parenteral administration of folic acid.

CAUTION

Exercise caution to ensure that the prescribed dosage of DHA does not exceed 1 gram (1000 mg) per day.

DOSAGE AND ADMINISTRATION

One tablet and one capsule daily or as directed by a physician.

Store at controlled room temperature.

NOTICE

Contact with moisture can discolor or erode the tablet.

HOW SUPPLIED

Six child-resistant blister packs of 5 tablets and 5 capsules each - **NDC 0178-0829-30**

Rev 0110

CITRANATAL HARMONY®   Rx

Rx Prenatal Vitamin Gel Cap

DESCRIPTION

CitraNatal Harmony®; is a prescription prenatal/postnatal multivitamin/mineral soft gelatin capsule. The prenatal vitamin is a purple, opaque soft gelatin capsule containing a greenish-gray liquid to semi-solid fill. The capsule is printed "0812" in white ink.

Each prenatal capsule contains:

Calcium (Calcium citrate) .... 100 mg
Iron (Carbonyl iron) .... 27 mg
Vitamin D₃ (Cholecalciferol) .... 400 IU
Vitamin E (dl-alpha tocopheryl acetate) ...... 30 IU
Vitamin B₆ (Pyridoxine HCl) .... 25 mg
Folic Acid .... 1 mg
Docusate Sodium .... 50 mg
Docosahexaenoic Acid (DHA) .... 250 mg
DHA is contained in the oil derived from microalgae.

INDICATIONS

CitraNatal Harmony® is a multivitamin/mineral prescription drug indicated for use in improving the nutritional status of women prior to conception, throughout pregnancy, and in the postnatal period for both lactating and nonlactating mothers.

CONTRAINDICATIONS

This product is contraindicated in patients with a known hypersensitivity to any of the ingredients.

> **WARNING**
> Accidental overdose of **iron-containing** products is a leading cause of fatal poisoning in children under 6. KEEP THIS PRODUCT OUT OF THE REACH OF CHILDREN. In case of accidental overdose, call a doctor or poison control center immediately.

WARNING

Ingestion of more than 3 grams of omega-3 fatty acids per day has been shown to have potential antithrombotic effects, including an increased bleeding time and INR. Administration of omega-3 fatty acids should be avoided in patients on anticoagulants and in those known to have an inherited or acquired bleeding diathesis.

WARNING

Folic acid alone is improper therapy in the treatment of pernicious anemia and other megaloblastic anemias where vitamin B₁₂ is deficient.

PRECAUTIONS

Folic acid in doses above 0.1 mg daily may obscure pernicious anemia in that hematologic remission can occur while neurological manifestations progress.

ADVERSE REACTIONS

Allergic sensitization has been reported following both oral and parenteral administration of folic acid.

CAUTION: Exercise caution to ensure that the prescribed dosage of DHA does not exceed 1 gram (1000 mg) per day.

DOSAGE AND ADMINISTRATION

One capsule daily or as directed by a physician.

Store at controlled room temperature.

NOTICE: Contact with moisture can discolor or erode the capsule.

HOW SUPPLIED

Bottles of 30 capsules each—**NDC 0178-0812-30.**

To report a serious adverse event or obtain product information, call (210) 696-8400.

Rev 1009

FERRALET® 90   Rx

Carbonyl Iron/ferrous gluconate tablet

DESCRIPTION

Each green film-coated tablet for oral administration contains:

Iron (Carbonyl iron, ferrous gluconate) .... 90 mg
Folic Acid .... 1 mg
Vitamin B₁₂ (Cyanocobalamin) .... 12 mcg
Vitamin C (Ascorbic acid) .... 120 mg
Docusate sodium .... 50 mg

Inactive Ingredients: Povidone, croscarmellose sodium, acrylic resin, color added, magnesium stearate, FD&C Yellow No. 5, magnesium silicate, FD&C Blue No. 1, polyethylene glycol, vitamin A palmitate, ethyl vanillin.

CLINICAL PHARMACOLOGY

Oral iron is absorbed most efficiently when administered between meals. Iron is critical for normal hemoglobin synthesis to maintain oxygen transport energy production and proper function of cells. Adequate amounts of iron are necessary for effective erythropoiesis. Iron also serves as a cofactor of several essential enzymes, including cytochromes, which are involved in electron transport.

Folic acid is required for nucleoprotein synthesis and the maintenance of normal erythropoiesis. Folic acid is the precursor of tetrahydrofolic acid, which is involved as a cofactor for transformylation reactions in the biosynthesis of purines and thymidylates of nucleic acids. Deficiency of folic acid may account for the defective deoxyribonucleic acid (DNA) synthesis that leads to megaloblast formation and megaloblastic macrocytic anemias. Vitamin B₁₂ is essential to growth, cell reproduction, hematopoiesis, nucleic acid, and myelin synthesis. Deficiency may result in megaloblastic anemia or pernicious anemia.

INDICATIONS AND USAGE

Ferralet® 90 is indicated for the treatment of all anemias that are responsive to oral iron therapy. These include: hypochromic anemia associated with pregnancy, chronic and/or acute blood loss, metabolic disease, post-surgical convalescence, and dietary needs.

CONTRAINDICATIONS

Hypersensitivity to any of the ingredients. Hemolytic anemia, hemochromatosis, and hemosiderosis are contraindications to iron therapy.

WARNING

Folic acid alone is improper therapy in the treatment of pernicious anemia and other megaloblastic anemias where vitamin B₁₂ is deficient.

> **WARNING:** Accidental overdose of iron-containing products is a leading cause of fatal poisoning in children under 6. KEEP THIS PRODUCT OUT OF REACH OF CHILDREN. In case of accidental overdose, call a doctor or poison control center immediately.

PRECAUTIONS

General: Take 2 hours after meals. Do not exceed recommended dose. Discontinue use if symptoms of intolerance appear. The type of anemia and underlying cause or causes should be determined before starting therapy with Ferralet® 90 tablets. Ensure Hgb, Hct, reticulocyte count are determined before starting therapy and periodically thereafter during prolonged treatment. Periodically review therapy to determine if it needs to be continued without change or if a dose change is indicated. This product contains FD&C Yellow No. 5 (tartrazine) which may cause allergic-type reactions (including bronchial asthma) in certain susceptible persons. Although the overall incidence of FD&C Yellow No. 5 (tartrazine) sensitivity in the general population is low, it is frequently seen in patients who also have aspirin hypersensitivity.

Folic Acid: Folic acid in doses above 0.1 mg daily may obscure pernicious anemia in that hematologic remission can occur while neurological manifestations remain progressive. Pernicious anemia should be excluded before using these products since folic acid may mask the symptoms of pernicious anemia.

Pediatric Use: Safety and effectiveness in pediatric patients have not been established.

Geriatric Use: Dosing for elderly patients should be cautious. Due to the greater frequency of decreased hepatic, renal, or cardiac function, and of concomitant disease or other drug therapy, dosing should start at the lower end of the dosing range.

ADVERSE REACTIONS

Adverse reactions with iron therapy may include GI irritation, constipation, diarrhea, nausea, vomiting, and dark stools. Adverse reactions with iron therapy are usually transient. Allergic sensitization has been reported following both oral and parenteral administration of folic acid.

DRUG INTERACTIONS: Prescriber should be aware of a number of iron/drug interactions, including antacids, tetracyclines, or fluoroquinolones.

OVERDOSAGE

Symptoms: abdominal pain, metabolic acidosis, anuria, CNS damage, coma, convulsions, death, dehydration, diffuse vascular congestion, hepatic cirrhosis, hypotension, hypothermia, lethargy, nausea, vomiting, diarrhea, tarry stools, melena, hematemesis, tachycardia, hyperglycemia, drowsiness, pallor, cyanosis, lassitude, seizures, and shock.

DOSAGE AND ADMINISTRATION

One tablet daily or as directed by a physician.

NOTICE: Contact with moisture can discolor or erode the tablet. Do not chew tablet.

HOW SUPPLIED

Ferralet® 90 (NDC 0178-0089-90) is a green, modified rectangle shaped, film-coated tablet, debossed with "F6" on one side and blank on the other, and packaged in bottles of 90. Store at 25°C (77°F). Excursions permitted to 15°-30°C (59°-86°F). (See USP Controlled Room Temperature.)

To report a serious adverse event or obtain product information, call (210) 696-8400.

Rev 1209

TINDAMAX®   Rx

[tin-da-max]
(tinidazole)

HIGHLIGHTS OF PRESCRIBING INFORMATION

These highlights do not include all the information needed to use Tindamax® safely and effectively. See full prescribing information for Tindamax®.

Tindamax® (tinidazole) tablets for oral use

Initial U.S. Approval: 2004

To reduce the development of drug-resistant bacteria and maintain the effectiveness of Tindamax and other antibacterial drugs, Tindamax should be used only to treat or prevent infections that are proven or strongly suspected to be caused by bacteria.

> **WARNING: POTENTIAL RISK FOR CARCINOGENICITY**
> *See full prescribing information for complete boxed warning.*
> Carcinogenicity has been seen in mice and rats treated chronically with metronidazole, another nitroimidazole agent (13.1). Although such data have not been reported for tinidazole, the two drugs are structurally related and have similar biologic effects. Use should be limited to approved indications only.

──────RECENT MAJOR CHANGES──────

Indications and Usage, Bacterial Vaginosis (1.4)   5/2007
Dosage and Administration, Bacterial Vaginosis (2.6) 5/2007

──────INDICATIONS AND USAGE──────

Tindamax is a nitroimidazole antimicrobial indicated for:
• Trichomoniasis (1.1)
• Giardiasis: in patients age 3 and older (1.2)
• Amebiasis: in patients age 3 and older (1.3)
• Bacterial Vaginosis: in non-pregnant, adult women (1.4, 8.1)

──────DOSAGE AND ADMINISTRATION──────

• Trichomoniasis: a single 2 g oral dose taken with food. Treat sexual partners with the same dose and at the same time (2.3)
• Giardiasis: Adults: a single 2 g dose taken with food. Pediatric patients older than three years of age: a single dose of 50 mg/kg (up to 2 g) with food (2.4)
• Amebiasis, *Intestinal:* Adults: 2 g per day for 3 days with food. Pediatric patients older than three years of age: 50 mg/kg/day (up to 2 g per day) for 3 days with food (2.5). *Amebic liver abscess:* Adults: 2 g per day for 3-5 days with food. Pediatric patients older than three years of age: 50 mg/kg/day (up to 2 g per day) for 3-5 days with food (2.5)
• Bacterial vaginosis: Non-pregnant, adult women: 2 g once daily for 2 days taken with food, or 1 g once daily for 5 days taken with food (2.6)

──────DOSAGE FORMS AND STRENGTHS──────

Tablets: 250 mg and 500 mg (3)

──────CONTRAINDICATIONS──────

• Prior history of hypersensitivity to tinidazole or other nitroimidazole derivatives (4, 6.1, 6.2)
• First trimester of pregnancy (4, 8.1)
• Nursing mothers, unless breast-feeding is interrupted during tinidazole therapy and for 3 days following the last dose (4, 8.3)

WARNINGS AND PRECAUTIONS

- Seizures and neuropathy have been reported. Discontinue Tindamax if abnormal neurologic signs develop (5.1)
- Vaginal candidiasis may develop with Tindamax and require treatment with an antifungal agent (5.2)
- Use Tindamax with caution in patients with blood dyscrasias. Tindamax may produce transient leukopenia and neutropenia (5.3, 7.3)

ADVERSE REACTIONS

Most common adverse reactions for a single 2 g dose of tinidazole (incidence >1%) are metallic/bitter taste, nausea, weakness/fatigue/malaise, dyspepsia/ cramps/epigastric discomfort, vomiting, anorexia, headache, dizziness and constipation (6.1)

To report SUSPECTED ADVERSE REACTIONS, contact Mission Pharmacal Company at 1-800-298-1087 or FDA at 1-800-FDA-1088 or www.fda.gov/medwatch

DRUG INTERACTIONS

The following drug interactions were reported for metronidazole, a chemically-related nitroimidazole and may therefore occur with tinidazole:

- Warfarin and other oral coumarin anticoagulants: Anticoagulant dosage may need adjustment during and up to 8 days after tinidazole therapy (7.1)
- Alcohol-containing beverages/preparations: Avoid during and up to 3 days after tinidazole therapy (7.1)
- Lithium: Monitor serum lithium concentrations (7.1)
- Cyclosporine, tacrolimus: Monitor for toxicities of these immunosuppressive drugs (7.1)
- Fluorouracil: Monitor for fluorouracil-associated toxicities (7.1)
- Phenytoin, fosphenytoin: Adjustment of anticonvulsant and/or tinidazole dose(s) may be needed (7.1, 7.2)
- CYP3A4 inducers/inhibitors: Monitor for decreased tinidazole effect or increased adverse reactions (7.2)

USE IN SPECIFIC POPULATIONS

- Pediatric Use: Data on tinidazole use in children is limited to treatment of giardiasis and amebiasis in patients age 3 and older (8.4)
- Hemodialysis patients: If tinidazole is administered the same day and prior to hemodialysis, administer an additional ½ dose after end of hemodialysis (8.6, 12.3)

See 17 for PATIENT COUNSELING INFORMATION
Revised: 8/2007

FULL PRESCRIBING INFORMATION: CONTENTS*
WARNING: POTENTIAL RISK FOR CARCINOGENICITY

FULL PRESCRIBING INFORMATION

WARNING: POTENTIAL RISK FOR CARCINOGENICITY

Carcinogenicity has been seen in mice and rats treated chronically with metronidazole, another nitroimidazole agent (13.1). Although such data have not been reported for tinidazole, the two drugs are structurally related and have similar biologic effects. **Its use should be reserved for the conditions described in INDICATIONS AND USAGE (1).**

---

1 INDICATIONS AND USAGE

1.1 Trichomoniasis

Tinidazole is indicated for the treatment of trichomoniasis caused by *Trichomonas vaginalis*. The organism should be identified by appropriate diagnostic procedures. Because trichomoniasis is a sexually transmitted disease with potentially serious sequelae, partners of infected patients should be treated simultaneously in order to prevent re-infection *[see Clinical Studies (14.1)]*.

1.2 Giardiasis

Tinidazole is indicated for the treatment of giardiasis caused by *Giardia duodenalis* (also termed *G. lamblia*) in both adults and pediatric patients older than three years of age *[see Clinical Studies (14.2)]*.

1.3 Amebiasis

Tinidazole is indicated for the treatment of intestinal amebiasis and amebic liver abscess caused by *Entamoeba histolytica* in both adults and pediatric patients older than three years of age. It is not indicated in the treatment of asymptomatic cyst passage *[see Clinical Studies (14.3, 14.4)]*.

1.4 Bacterial Vaginosis

Tinidazole is indicated for the treatment of bacterial vaginosis (formerly referred to as *Haemophilus* vaginitis, *Gardnerella* vaginitis, nonspecific vaginitis, or anaerobic vaginosis) in non-pregnant women *[see Use in Specific Populations (8.1) and Clinical Studies (14.5)]*.

Other pathogens commonly associated with vulvovaginitis such as *Trichomonas vaginalis*, *Chlamydia trachomatis*, *Neisseria gonorrhoeae*, *Candida albicans* and *Herpes simplex* virus should be ruled out.

To reduce the development of drug-resistant bacteria and maintain the effectiveness of Tindamax and other antibacterial drugs, Tindamax should be used only to treat or prevent infections that are proven or strongly suspected to be caused by susceptible bacteria. When culture and susceptibility information are available, they should be considered in selecting or modifying antibacterial therapy. In the absence of such data, local epidemiology and susceptibility patterns may contribute to the empiric selection of therapy.

2 DOSAGE AND ADMINISTRATION

2.1 Dosing Instructions

It is advisable to take tinidazole with food to minimize the incidence of epigastric discomfort and other gastrointestinal side-effects. Food does not affect the oral bioavailability of tinidazole *[see Clinical Pharmacology (12.3)]*.

Alcoholic beverages should be avoided when taking tinidazole and for 3 days afterwards *[see Drug Interactions (7.1)]*.

2.2 Compounding of the Oral Suspension

For those unable to swallow tablets, tinidazole tablets may be crushed in artificial cherry syrup to be taken with food.

Procedure for Extemporaneous Pharmacy Compounding of the Oral Suspension: Pulverize four 500 mg oral tablets with a mortar and pestle. Add approximately 10 mL of cherry syrup to the powder and mix until smooth. Transfer the suspension to a graduated amber container. Use several small rinses of cherry syrup to transfer any remaining drug in the mortar to the final suspension for a final volume of 30 mL. The suspension of crushed tablets in artificial cherry syrup is stable for 7 days at room temperature. When this suspension is used, it should be shaken well before each administration.

2.3 Trichomoniasis

The recommended dose in both females and males is a single 2 g oral dose taken with food. Since trichomoniasis is a sexually transmitted disease, sexual partners should be treated with the same dose and at the same time.

2.4 Giardiasis

The recommended dose in adults is a single 2 g dose taken with food. In pediatric patients older than three years of age, the recommended dose is a single dose of 50 mg/kg (up to 2 g) with food.

2.5 Amebiasis

Intestinal: The recommended dose in adults is a 2 g dose per day for 3 days taken with food. In pediatric patients older than three years of age, the recommended dose is 50 mg/kg/day (up to 2 g per day) for 3 days with food.

Amebic Liver Abscess: The recommended dose in adults is a 2 g dose per day for 3-5 days taken with food. In pediatric patients older than three years of age, the recommended dose is 50 mg/kg/day (up to 2 g per day) for 3-5 days with food. There are limited pediatric data on durations of therapy exceeding 3 days, although a small number of children were treated for 5 days without additional reported adverse reactions. Children should be closely monitored when treatment durations exceed 3 days.

2.6 Bacterial Vaginosis

The recommended dose in non-pregnant females is a 2 g oral dose once daily for 2 days taken with food or a 1 g oral dose once daily for 5 days taken with food. The use of tinidazole in pregnant patients has not been studied for bacterial vaginosis.

3 DOSAGE FORMS AND STRENGTHS

- 250 mg tablets are pink, round, scored tablets, with TM debossed on one side and 250 on the other
- 500 mg tablets are pink, oval, scored tablets, with TM debossed on one side and 500 on the other

4 CONTRAINDICATIONS

The use of tinidazole is contraindicated:
- In patients with a previous history of hypersensitivity to tinidazole or other nitroimidazole derivatives. Reported reactions have ranged in severity from urticaria to Stevens-Johnson syndrome *[see Adverse Reactions (6.1, 6.2)]*.
- During first trimester of pregnancy *[see Use in Specific Populations (8.1)]*.
- In nursing mothers: Interruption of breast-feeding is recommended during tinidazole therapy and for 3 days following the last dose *[see Use in Specific Populations (8.3)]*.

5 WARNINGS AND PRECAUTIONS

5.1 Neurological Adverse Reactions

Convulsive seizures and peripheral neuropathy, the latter characterized mainly by numbness or paresthesia of an extremity, have been reported in patients treated with tinidazole. The appearance of abnormal neurologic signs demands the prompt discontinuation of tinidazole therapy.

5.2 Vaginal Candidiasis

The use of tinidazole may result in *Candida* vaginitis. In a clinical study of 235 women who received tinidazole for bacterial vaginosis, a vaginal fungal infection developed in 11 (4.7%) of all study subjects *[see Clinical Studies (14.5)]*.

5.3 Blood Dyscrasia

Tinidazole should be used with caution in patients with evidence of or history of blood dyscrasia *[see Drug Interactions (7.3)]*.

5.4 Drug Resistance

Prescribing Tindamax in the absence of a proven or strongly suspected bacterial infection or a prophylactic indication is unlikely to provide benefit to the patient and increases the risk of the development of drug-resistant bacteria.

6 ADVERSE REACTIONS

6.1 Clinical Studies Experience

Because clinical trials are conducted under widely varying conditions, adverse reaction rates observed in the clinical trials of a drug cannot be directly compared to rates in the clinical trials of another drug and may not reflect the rates observed in practice.

Among 3669 patients treated with a single 2 g dose of tinidazole, in both controlled and uncontrolled trichomoniasis and giardiasis clinical studies, adverse reactions were reported by 11.0% of patients. For multi-day dosing in controlled and uncontrolled amebiasis studies, adverse reactions were reported by 13.8% of 1765 patients. Common (≥ 1% incidence) adverse reactions reported by body system are as follows. (Note: Data described in Table 1 below are pooled from studies with variable designs and safety evaluations.)

Other adverse reactions reported with tinidazole include:
Central Nervous System: Two serious adverse reactions reported include convulsions and transient peripheral neuropathy including numbness and paresthesia *[see Warnings and Precautions (5.1)]*. Other CNS reports include vertigo, ataxia, giddiness, insomnia, drowsiness.
Gastrointestinal: tongue discoloration, stomatitis, diarrhea
Hypersensitivity: urticaria, pruritus, rash, flushing, sweating, dryness of mouth, fever, burning sensation, thirst, salivation, angioedema
Renal: darkened urine
Cardiovascular: palpitations
Hematopoietic: transient neutropenia, transient leukopenia

Other: *Candida* overgrowth, increased vaginal discharge, oral candidiasis, hepatic abnormalities including raised transaminase level, arthralgias, myalgias, and arthritis. [See table 1 at right]

Rare reported adverse reactions include bronchospasm, dyspnea, coma, confusion, depression, furry tongue, pharyngitis and reversible thrombocytopenia.

Adverse Reactions in Pediatric Patients: In pooled pediatric studies, adverse reactions reported in pediatric patients taking tinidazole were similar in nature and frequency to adult findings including nausea, vomiting, diarrhea, taste change, anorexia, and abdominal pain.

Bacterial vaginosis: The most common adverse reactions in treated patients (incidence >2%), which were not identified in the trichomoniasis, giardiasis and amebiasis studies, are gastrointestinal: decreased appetite, and flatulence; renal: urinary tract infection, painful urination, and urine abnormality; and other reactions including pelvic pain, vulvo-vaginal discomfort, vaginal odor, menorrhagia, and upper respiratory tract infection *[See Clinical Studies (14.5)]*.

6.2 Postmarketing Experience

The following adverse reactions have been identified and reported during post-approval use of Tindamax. Because the reports of these reactions are voluntary and the population is of uncertain size, it is not always possible to reliably estimate the frequency of the reaction or establish a causal relationship to drug exposure.

Severe acute hypersensitivity reactions have been reported on initial or subsequent exposure to tinidazole. Hypersensitivity reactions may include urticaria, pruritis, angioedema, Stevens-Johnson syndrome and erythema multiforme.

7 DRUG INTERACTIONS

Although not specifically identified in studies with tinidazole, the following drug interactions were reported for metronidazole, a chemically-related nitroimidazole. Therefore, these drug interactions may occur with tinidazole.

7.1 Potential Effects of Tinidazole on Other Drugs

Warfarin and Other Oral Coumarin Anticoagulants: As with metronidazole, tinidazole may enhance the effect of warfarin and other coumarin anticoagulants, resulting in a prolongation of prothrombin time. The dosage of oral anticoagulants may need to be adjusted during tinidazole co-administration and up to 8 days after discontinuation.

Alcohols, Disulfiram: Alcoholic beverages and preparations containing ethanol or propylene glycol should be avoided during tinidazole therapy and for 3 days afterward because abdominal cramps, nausea, vomiting, headaches, and flushing may occur. Psychotic reactions have been reported in alcoholic patients using metronidazole and disulfiram concurrently. Though no similar reactions have been reported with tinidazole, tinidazole should not be given to patients who have taken disulfiram within the last two weeks.

Lithium: Metronidazole has been reported to elevate serum lithium levels. It is not known if tinidazole shares this property with metronidazole, but consideration should be given to measuring serum lithium and creatinine levels after several days of simultaneous lithium and tinidazole treatment to detect potential lithium intoxication.

Phenytoin, Fosphenytoin: Concomitant administration of oral metronidazole and intravenous phenytoin was reported to result in prolongation of the half-life and reduction in the clearance of phenytoin. Metronidazole did not significantly affect the pharmacokinetics of orally-administered phenytoin.

Cyclosporine, Tacrolimus: There are several case reports suggesting that metronidazole has the potential to increase the levels of cyclosporine and tacrolimus. During tinidazole co-administration with either of these drugs, the patient should be monitored for signs of calcineurin-inhibitor associated toxicities.

Fluorouracil: Metronidazole was shown to decrease the clearance of fluorouracil, resulting in an increase in side-effects without an increase in therapeutic benefits. If the concomitant use of tinidazole and fluorouracil cannot be avoided, the patient should be monitored for fluorouracil-associated toxicities.

7.2 Potential Effects of Other Drugs on Tinidazole

CYP3A4 Inducers and Inhibitors: Simultaneous administration of tinidazole with drugs that induce liver microsomal enzymes, i.e., CYP3A4 inducers such as *phenobarbital, rifampin, phenytoin,* and *fosphenytoin* (a pro-drug of phenytoin), may accelerate the elimination of tinidazole, decreasing the plasma level of tinidazole. Simultaneous administration of drugs that inhibit the activity of liver microsomal enzymes, i.e., CYP3A4 inhibitors such as *cimetidine* and *ketoconazole,* may prolong the half-life and decrease the plasma clearance of tinidazole, increasing the plasma concentrations of tinidazole.

Cholestyramine: Cholestyramine was shown to decrease the oral bioavailability of metronidazole by 21%. Thus, it is

Table 1. Adverse Reactions Summary of Published Reports

		2 g single dose	Multi-day dose
GI:	Metallic/bitter taste	3.7%	6.3%
	Nausea	3.2%	4.5%
	Anorexia	1.5%	2.5%
	Dyspepsia/cramps/epigastric discomfort	1.8%	1.4%
	Vomiting	1.5%	0.9%
	Constipation	0.4%	1.4%
CNS:	Weakness/fatigue/malaise	2.1%	1.1%
	Dizziness	1.1%	0.5%
Other:	Headache	1.3%	0.7%
Total patients with adverse reactions		11.0% (403/3669)	13.8% (244/1765)

advisable to separate dosing of cholestyramine and tinidazole to minimize any potential effect on the oral bioavailability of tinidazole.

Oxytetracycline: Oxytetracycline was reported to antagonize the therapeutic effect of metronidazole.

7.3 Laboratory Test Interactions

Tinidazole, like metronidazole, may interfere with certain types of determinations of serum chemistry values, such as aspartate aminotransferase (AST, SGOT), alanine aminotransferase (ALT, SGPT), lactate dehydrogenase (LDH), triglycerides, and hexokinase glucose. Values of zero may be observed. All of the assays in which interference has been reported involve enzymatic coupling of the assay to oxidation-reduction of nicotinamide adenine dinucleotide ($NAD^+ \leftrightarrow NADH$). Potential interference is due to the similarity of absorbance peaks of NADH and tinidazole.

Tinidazole, like metronidazole, may produce transient leukopenia and neutropenia; however, no persistent hematological abnormalities attributable to tinidazole have been observed in clinical studies. Total and differential leukocyte counts are recommended if re-treatment is necessary.

8 USE IN SPECIFIC POPULATIONS

8.1 Pregnancy

Teratogenic effects: Pregnancy Category C

The use of tinidazole in pregnant patients has not been studied. Since tinidazole crosses the placental barrier and enters fetal circulation it should not be administered to pregnant patients in the first trimester.

Embryo-fetal developmental toxicity studies in pregnant mice indicated no embryo-fetal toxicity or malformations at the highest dose level of 2,500 mg/kg (approximately 6.3-fold the highest human therapeutic dose based upon body surface area conversions). In a study with pregnant rats a slightly higher incidence of fetal mortality was observed at a maternal dose of 500 mg/kg (2.5-fold the highest human therapeutic dose based upon body surface area conversions). No biologically relevant neonatal developmental effects were observed in rat neonates following maternal doses as high as 600 mg/kg (3-fold the highest human therapeutic dose based upon body surface area conversions). Although there is some evidence of mutagenic potential and animal reproduction studies are not always predictive of human response, the use of tinidazole after the first trimester of pregnancy requires that the potential benefits of the drug be weighed against the possible risks to both the mother and the fetus.

8.3 Nursing Mothers

Tinidazole is excreted in breast milk in concentrations similar to those seen in serum. Tinidazole can be detected in breast milk for up to 72 hours following administration. Interruption of breast-feeding is recommended during tinidazole therapy and for 3 days following the last dose.

8.4 Pediatric Use

Other than for use in the treatment of giardiasis and amebiasis in pediatric patients older than three years of age, safety and effectiveness of tinidazole in pediatric patients have not been established.

Pediatric Administration: For those unable to swallow tablets, tinidazole tablets may be crushed in artificial cherry syrup, to be taken with food *[see Dosage and Administration (2.2)]*.

8.5 Geriatric Use

Clinical studies of tinidazole did not include sufficient numbers of subjects aged 65 and over to determine whether they respond differently from younger subjects. In general, dose selection for an elderly patient should be cautious, reflecting the greater frequency of decreased hepatic, renal, or cardiac function, and of concomitant disease or other drug therapy.

8.6 Renal Impairment

Because the pharmacokinetics of tinidazole in patients with severe renal impairment (CrCL < 22 mL/min) are not significantly different from those in healthy subjects, no dose adjustments are necessary in these patients.

Patients undergoing hemodialysis: If tinidazole is administered on the same day as and prior to hemodialysis, it is recommended that an additional dose of tinidazole equivalent to one-half of the recommended dose be administered after the end of the hemodialysis *[see Clinical Pharmacology (12.3)]*.

8.7 Hepatic Impairment

There are no data on tinidazole pharmacokinetics in patients with impaired hepatic function. Reduced elimination of metronidazole, a chemically-related nitroimidazole, has been reported in this population. Usual recommended doses of tinidazole should be administered cautiously in patients with hepatic dysfunction *[see Clinical Pharmacology (12.3)]*.

10 OVERDOSAGE

There are no reported overdoses with tinidazole in humans.

Treatment of Overdosage: There is no specific antidote for the treatment of overdosage with tinidazole; therefore, treatment should be symptomatic and supportive. Gastric lavage may be helpful. Hemodialysis can be considered because approximately 43% of the amount present in the body is eliminated during a 6-hour hemodialysis session.

11 DESCRIPTION

Tinidazole is a synthetic antiprotozoal and antibacterial agent. It is 1-(2-ethylsulfonylethyl)-2-methyl-5-nitroimidazole, a second-generation 2-methyl-5-nitroimidazole, which has the following chemical structure:

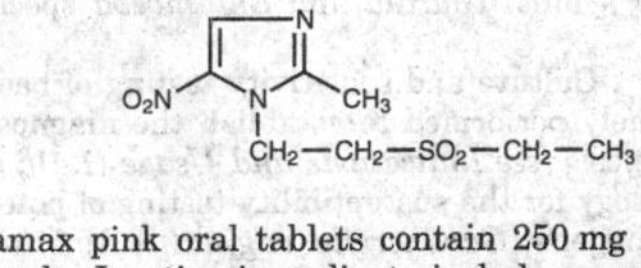

Tindamax pink oral tablets contain 250 mg or 500 mg of tinidazole. Inactive ingredients include croscarmellose sodium, FD&C Red 40 lake, FD&C Yellow 6 lake, hypromellose, magnesium stearate, microcrystalline cellulose, polydextrose, polyethylene glycol, pregelatinized corn starch, titanium dioxide, and triacetin.

12 CLINICAL PHARMACOLOGY

12.1 Mechanism of Action

Tinidazole is an antiprotozoal, antibacterial agent. *[See Clinical Pharmacology (12.4)]*.

12.3 Pharmacokinetics

Absorption: After oral administration, tinidazole is rapidly and completely absorbed. A bioavailability study of Tindamax tablets was conducted in adult healthy volunteers. All subjects received a single oral dose of 2 g (four 500 mg tablets) of Tindamax following an overnight fast. Oral administration of four 500 mg tablets of Tindamax under fasted conditions produced a mean peak plasma concentration (C_{max}) of 47.7 (±7.5) μg/mL with a mean time to peak concentration (T_{max}) of 1.6 (±0.7) hours, and a mean area under the plasma concentration-time curve (AUC, 0-∞) of 901.6 (± 126.5) μg.hr/mL at 72 hours. The elimination half-life ($T_{1/2}$) was 13.2 (±1.4) hours. Mean plasma levels decreased to 14.3 μg/mL at 24 hours, 3.8 μg/mL at 48 hours and 0.8 μg/mL at 72 hours following administration. Steady-state conditions are reached in 2½-3 days of multi-day dosing.

Administration of Tindamax tablets with food resulted in a delay in T_{max} of approximately 2 hours and a decline in C_{max}

of approximately 10%, compared to fasted conditions. However, administration of Tindamax with food did not affect AUC or $T_{1/2}$ in this study.

In healthy volunteers, administration of crushed Tindamax tablets in artificial cherry syrup, [prepared as described in *Dosage and Administration (2.2)*] after an overnight fast had no effect on any pharmacokinetic parameter as compared to tablets swallowed whole under fasted conditions.

Distribution: Tinidazole is distributed into virtually all tissues and body fluids and also crosses the blood-brain barrier. The apparent volume of distribution is about 50 liters. Plasma protein binding of tinidazole is 12%. Tinidazole crosses the placental barrier and is secreted in breast milk.

Metabolism: Tinidazole is significantly metabolized in humans prior to excretion. Tinidazole is partly metabolized by oxidation, hydroxylation, and conjugation. Tinidazole is the major drug-related constituent in plasma after human treatment, along with a small amount of the 2-hydroxymethyl metabolite.

Tinidazole is biotransformed mainly by CYP3A4. In an *in vitro* metabolic drug interaction study, tinidazole concentrations of up to 75 µg/mL did not inhibit the enzyme activities of CYP1A2, CYP2B6, CYP2C9, CYP2D6, CYP2E1, and CYP3A4.

The potential of tinidazole to induce the metabolism of other drugs has not been evaluated.

Elimination: The plasma half-life of tinidazole is approximately 12-14 hours. Tinidazole is excreted by the liver and the kidneys. Tinidazole is excreted in the urine mainly as unchanged drug (approximately 20-25% of the administered dose). Approximately 12% of the drug is excreted in the feces.

Patients with impaired renal function: The pharmacokinetics of tinidazole in patients with severe renal impairment (CrCL < 22 mL/min) are not significantly different from the pharmacokinetics seen in healthy subjects. However, during hemodialysis, clearance of tinidazole is significantly increased; the half-life is reduced from 12.0 hours to 4.9 hours. Approximately 43% of the amount present in the body is eliminated during a 6-hour hemodialysis session *[see Use in Specific Populations (8.6)]*. The pharmacokinetics of tinidazole in patients undergoing routine continuous peritoneal dialysis have not been investigated.

Patients with impaired hepatic function: There are no data on tinidazole pharmacokinetics in patients with impaired hepatic function. Reduction of metabolic elimination of metronidazole, a chemically-related nitroimidazole, in patients with hepatic dysfunction has been reported in several studies *[see Use in Specific Populations (8.7)]*.

12.4 Microbiology

Mechanism of Action: Tinidazole is an antiprotozoal, antibacterial agent. The nitro-group of tinidazole is reduced by cell extracts of *Trichomonas*. The free nitro-radical generated as a result of this reduction may be responsible for the antiprotozoal activity. Chemically reduced tinidazole was shown to release nitrites and cause damage to purified bacterial DNA *in vitro*. Additionally, the drug caused DNA base changes in bacterial cells and DNA strand breakage in mammalian cells. The mechanism by which tinidazole exhibits activity against *Giardia* and *Entamoeba* species is not known.

Antibacterial: Culture and sensitivity testing of bacteria are not routinely performed to establish the diagnosis of bacterial vaginosis *[see Indications and Usage (1.4)]*; standard methodology for the susceptibility testing of potential bacterial pathogens, *Gardnerella vaginalis, Mobiluncus spp.* or *Mycoplasma hominis*, has not been defined. The following *in vitro* data are available, but their clinical significance is unknown. Tinidazole is active *in vitro* against most strains of the following organisms that have been reported to be associated with bacterial vaginosis:

- *Bacteroides spp.*
- *Gardnerella vaginalis*
- *Prevotella spp.*

Tinidazole does not appear to have activity against most strains of vaginal lactobacilli.

Antiprotozoal: Tinidazole demonstrates activity both *in vitro* and in clinical infections against the following protozoa: *Trichomonas vaginalis; Giardia duodenalis* (also termed *G. lamblia*); and *Entamoeba histolytica*.

For protozoal parasites, standardized susceptibility tests do not exist for use in clinical microbiology laboratories.

Drug Resistance: The development of resistance to tinidazole by *G. duodenalis, E. histolytica*, or bacteria associated with bacterial vaginosis has not been examined.

Cross-resistance: Approximately 38% of *T. vaginalis* isolates exhibiting reduced susceptibility to metronidazole also show reduced susceptibility to tinidazole *in vitro*. The clinical significance of such an effect is not known.

13 NONCLINICAL TOXICOLOGY

13.1 Carcinogenesis, Mutagenesis, Impairment of Fertility

Metronidazole, a chemically-related nitroimidazole, has been reported to be carcinogenic in mice and rats but not hamsters. In several studies metronidazole showed evidence of pulmonary, hepatic, and lymphatic tumorigenesis in mice and mammary and hepatic tumors in female rats. Tinidazole carcinogenicity studies in rats, mice or hamsters have not been reported.

Tinidazole was mutagenic in the TA 100, *S. typhimurium* tester strain both with and without the metabolic activation system and was negative for mutagenicity in the TA 98 strain. Mutagenicity results were mixed (positive and negative) in the TA 1535, 1537, and 1538 strains. Tinidazole was also mutagenic in a tester strain of *Klebsiella pneumonia*. Tinidazole was negative for mutagenicity in a mammalian cell culture system utilizing Chinese hamster lung V79 cells (HGPRT test system) and negative for genotoxicity in the Chinese hamster ovary (CHO) sister chromatid exchange assay. Tinidazole was positive for *in vivo* genotoxicity in the mouse micronucleus assay.

In a 60-day fertility study, tinidazole reduced fertility and produced testicular histopathology in male rats at a 600 mg/kg/day dose level (approximately 3-fold the highest human therapeutic dose based upon body surface area conversions). Spermatogenic effects resulted from 300 and 600 mg/kg/day dose levels. The no observed adverse reaction level for testicular and spermatogenic effects was 100 mg/kg/day (approximately 0.5-fold the highest human therapeutic dose based upon body surface area conversions). This effect is characteristic of agents in the 5-nitroimidazole class.

13.2 Animal Toxicology and/or Pharmacology

In acute studies with mice and rats, the LD_{50} for mice was generally > 3,600 mg/kg for oral administration and was > 2,300 mg/kg for intraperitoneal administration. In rats, the LD_{50} was > 2,000 mg/kg for both oral and intraperitoneal administration.

A repeated-dose toxicology study has been performed in beagle dogs using oral dosing of tinidazole at 100 mg/kg/day, 300 mg/kg/day, and 1000 mg/kg/day for 28-days. On Day 18 of the study, the highest dose was lowered to 600 mg/kg/day due to severe clinical symptoms. The two compound-related effects observed in the dogs treated with tinidazole were increased atrophy of the thymus in both sexes at the middle and high doses, and atrophy of the prostate at all doses in the males. A no-adverse-effect level (NOAEL) of 100 mg/kg/day for females was determined. There was no NOAEL identified for males because of minimal atrophy of the prostate at 100 mg/kg/day (approximately 0.9-fold the highest human dose based upon plasma AUC comparisons).

14 CLINICAL STUDIES

14.1 Trichomoniasis

Tinidazole (2 g single oral dose) use in trichomoniasis has been well documented in 34 published reports from the world literature involving over 2,800 patients treated with tinidazole. In four published, blinded, randomized, comparative studies of the 2 g tinidazole single oral dose where efficacy was assessed by culture at time points post-treatment ranging from one week to one month, reported cure rates ranged from 92% (37/40) to 100% (65/65) (n=172 total subjects). In four published, blinded, randomized, comparative studies where efficacy was assessed by wet mount between 7-14 days post-treatment, reported cure rates ranged from 80% (8/10) to 100% (16/16) (n=116 total subjects). In these studies, tinidazole was superior to placebo and comparable to other anti-trichomonal drugs. The single oral 2 g tinidazole dose was also assessed in four open-label trials in men (one comparative to metronidazole and 3 single-arm studies). Parasitological evaluation of the urine was performed both pre- and post-treatment and reported cure rates ranged from 83% (25/30) to 100% (80/80) (n=142 total subjects).

14.2 Giardiasis

Tinidazole (2 g single dose) use in giardiasis has been documented in 19 published reports from the world literature involving over 1,600 patients (adults and pediatric patients). In eight controlled studies involving a total of 619 subjects of whom 299 were given the 2 g × 1 day (50 mg/kg × 1 day in pediatric patients) oral dose of tinidazole, reported cure rates ranged from 80% (40/50) to 100% (15/15). In three of these trials where the comparator was 2 to 3 days of various doses of metronidazole, reported cure rates for metronidazole were 76% (19/25) to 93% (14/15). Data comparing a single 2 g dose of tinidazole to usually recommended 5-7 days of metronidazole are limited.

14.3 Intestinal Amebiasis

Tinidazole use in intestinal amebiasis has been documented in 26 published reports from the world literature involving over 1,400 patients. Most reports utilized tinidazole 2 g/day × 3 days. In four published, randomized, controlled studies (1 investigator single- blind, 3 open-label) of the 2 g/day × 3 days oral dose of tinidazole, reported cure rates after 3 days of therapy among a total of 220 subjects ranged from 86% (25/29) to 93% (25/27).

14.4 Amebic Liver Abscess

Tinidazole use in amebic liver abscess has been documented in 18 published reports from the world literature involving over 470 patients. Most reports utilized tinidazole 2 g/day × 2-5 days. In seven published, randomized, controlled studies (1 double-blind, 1 single-blind, 5 open-label) of the 2 g/day × 2-5 days oral dose of tinidazole accompanied by aspiration of the liver abscess when clinically necessary, reported cure rates among 133 subjects ranged from 81% (17/21) to 100% (16/16). Four of these studies utilized at least 3 days of tinidazole.

14.5 Bacterial Vaginosis

A randomized, double-blind, placebo-controlled clinical trial in 235 non-pregnant women was conducted to evaluate the efficacy of tinidazole for the treatment of bacterial vaginosis. A clinical diagnosis of bacterial vaginosis was based on Amsel's criteria and defined by the presence of an abnormal homogeneous vaginal discharge that (a) has a pH of greater than 4.5, (b) emits a "fishy" amine odor when mixed with a 10% KOH solution, and (c) contains ≥20% clue cells on microscopic examination. Clinical cure required a return to normal vaginal discharge and resolution of all Amsel's criteria. A microbiologic diagnosis of bacterial vaginosis was based on Gram stain of the vaginal smear demonstrating (a) markedly reduced or absent *Lactobacillus* morphology, (b) predominance of *Gardnerella* morphotype, and (c) absent or few white blood cells, with quantification of these bacterial morphotypes to determine the Nugent score, where a score ≥4 was required for study inclusion and a score of 0-3 considered a microbiologic cure. Therapeutic cure was a composite endpoint, consisting of both a clinical cure and microbiologic cure. In patients with all four Amsel's criteria and with a baseline Nugent score ≥4, tinidazole oral tablets given as either 2 g once daily for 2 days or 1 g once daily for 5 days demonstrated superior efficacy over placebo tablets as measured by therapeutic cure, clinical cure, and a microbiologic cure.

[See table 2 at left]

The therapeutic cure rates reported in this clinical study conducted with Tindamax were based on resolution of 4 out

Table 2. Efficacy of Tindamax in the Treatment of Bacterial Vaginosis in a Randomized, Double-Blind, Double-Dummy, Placebo-Controlled Trial: Modified Intent-to-Treat Population[1] (n=227)

Outcome	Tindamax 1 g × 5 days (n=76)	Tindamax 2 g × 2 days (n=73)	Placebo (n=78)
	% Cure	% Cure	% Cure
Therapeutic Cure	36.8	27.4	5.1
Difference[2]	31.7	22.3	
97.5% CI[3]	(16.8, 46.6)	(8.0, 36.6)	
Clinical Cure	51.3	35.6	11.5
Difference[2]	39.8	24.1	
97.5% CI[3]	(23.3, 56.3)	(7.8, 40.3)	
Nugent Score Cure	38.2	27.4	5.1
Difference[2]	33.1	22.3	
97.5% CI[3]	(18.1, 48.0)	(8.0, 36.6)	

[1] Modified Intent-to-Treat defined as all patients randomized with a baseline Nugent score of at least 4

[2] Difference in cure rates (Tindamax-placebo)

[3] CI: confidence interval

p-values for both Tindamax regimens vs. placebo for therapeutic, clinical and Nugent score cure rates for both 2 and 5 days <0.001

of 4 Amsel's criteria and a Nugent score of <4. The cure rates for previous clinical studies with other products approved for bacterial vaginosis were based on resolution of either 2 or 3 out of 4 Amsel's criteria. At the time of approval for other products for bacterial vaginosis, there was no requirement for a Nugent score on Gram stain, resulting in higher reported rates of cure for bacterial vaginosis for those products than for those reported here for tinidazole.

16   HOW SUPPLIED/STORAGE AND HANDLING

Tindamax 250 mg tablets are pink, round, scored tablets, with TM debossed on one side and 250 on the other, supplied in bottles with child-resistant caps as:

NDC 0178-8250-40   Bottle of 40

Tindamax 500 mg tablets are pink, oval, scored tablets, with TM debossed on one side and 500 on the other, supplied in bottles with child-resistant caps as:

NDC 0178-8500-60   Bottle of 60
NDC 0178-8500-20   Bottle of 20

Professional Samples:
NDC 0178-8500-02   Bottle of 2

Storage: Store at controlled room temperature 20-25° C (68-77° F); excursions permitted to 15-30° C (59-86° F) [see USP]. Protect contents from light.

17   PATIENT COUNSELING INFORMATION
17.1   Administration of Drug

Patients should be told to take Tindamax with food to minimize the incidence of epigastric discomfort and other gastrointestinal side-effects. Food does not affect the oral bioavailability of tinidazole.

17.2   Alcohol Avoidance

Patients should be told to avoid alcoholic beverages and preparations containing ethanol or propylene glycol during Tindamax therapy and for 3 days afterward because abdominal cramps, nausea, vomiting, headaches, and flushing may occur.

17.3   Drug Resistance

Patients should be counseled that antibacterial drugs including Tindamax should only be used to treat bacterial infections. They do not treat viral infections (e.g., the common cold). When Tindamax is prescribed to treat a bacterial infection, patients should be told that although it is common to feel better early in the course of therapy, the medication should be taken exactly as directed. Skipping doses or not completing the full course of therapy may (1) decrease the effectiveness of the immediate treatment and (2) increase the likelihood that bacteria will develop resistance and will not be treatable by Tindamax or other antibacterial drugs in the future.

Rev 0907

UROCIT®-K   ℞

[yu 'ro-cĭt kay]
(Potassium Citrate)
Extended-release tablets for oral use

HIGHLIGHTS OF PRESCRIBING INFORMATION

These highlights do not include all the information needed to use Urocit®-K safely and effectively. See full prescribing information for Urocit®-K.

Urocit®-K (Potassium Citrate) Extended-release tablets for oral use
Initial U.S. Approval: 1985

————RECENT MAJOR CHANGES————

Dosage and Administration, Urocit®-K 15 mEq (2.2, 2.3)	12/2009
Dosage Forms and Strengths, Urocit®-K 15 mEq (3)	12/2009
Description, Urocit®-K 15 mEq (11)	12/2009
Clinical Studies (14)	12/2009
How Supplied/Storage and Handling, Urocit®-K 15 mEq (16)	12/2009

————INDICATIONS AND USAGE————

Urocit®-K is a citrate salt of potassium indicated for the management of:
- Renal tubular acidosis (RTA) with calcium stones (1.1)
- Hypocitraturic calcium oxalate nephrolithiasis of any etiology (1.2)
- Uric acid lithiasis with or without calcium stones (1.3)

————DOSAGE AND ADMINISTRATION————

Objective: To restore normal urinary citrate (greater than 320 mg/day and as close to the normal mean of 640 mg/day as possible), and to increase urinary pH to a level of 6.0 to 7.0.
- Severe hypocitraturia (urinary citrate < 150 mg/day): therapy should be initiated at 60 mEq per day; a dose of 30 mEq two times per day or 20 mEq three times per day with meals or within 30 minutes after meals or bedtime snack (2.2)
- Mild to moderate hypocitraturia (urinary citrate >150 mg/day): therapy should be initiated at 30 mEq per day; a dose of 15 mEq two times per day or 10 mEq three times per day with meals or within 30 minutes after meals or bedtime snack (2.3)

————DOSAGE FORMS AND STRENGTHS————

Tablets: 5 mEq, 10 mEq and 15 mEq (3)

————CONTRAINDICATIONS————

- Patients with hyperkalemia (or who have conditions predisposing them to hyperkalemia). Such conditions include chronic renal failure, uncontrolled diabetes mellitus, acute dehydration, strenuous physical exercise in unconditioned individuals, adrenal insufficiency, extensive tissue breakdown (4)
- Patients for whom there is cause for arrest or delay in tablet passage through the gastrointestinal tract such as those suffering from delayed gastric emptying, esophageal compression, intestinal obstruction or stricture (4)
- Patients with peptic ulcer disease (4)
- Patients with active urinary tract infection (4)
- Patients with renal insufficiency (glomerular filtration rate of less than 0.7 ml/kg/min) (4)

————WARNINGS AND PRECAUTIONS————

- Hyperkalemia: In patients with impaired mechanisms for excreting potassium, Urocit®-K administration can produce hyperkalemia and cardiac arrest. Potentially fatal hyperkalemia can develop rapidly and be asymptomatic. The use of Urocit®-K in patients with chronic renal failure, or any other condition which impairs potassium excretion such as severe myocardial damage or heart failure, should be avoided (5.1)
- Gastrointestinal lesions: if there is severe vomiting, abdominal pain or gastrointestinal bleeding, Urocit®-K should be discontinued immediately and the possibility of bowel perforation or obstruction investigated (5.2)

————ADVERSE REACTIONS————

Some patients may develop minor gastrointestinal complaints such as abdominal discomfort, vomiting, diarrhea, loose bowel movements or nausea. These may be alleviated by taking the dose with meals or snacks or by reducing the dosage (6.1)

To report SUSPECTED ADVERSE REACTIONS, contact Mission Pharmacal Company at 1-800-298-1087 or FDA at 1-800-FDA-1088 or www.fda.gov/medwatch

————DRUG INTERACTIONS————

The following drug interactions may occur with potassium citrate:
- Potassium-sparing diuretics: concomitant administration should be avoided since the simultaneous administration of these agents can produce severe hyperkalemia (7.1)
- Drugs that slow gastrointestinal transit time: These agents (such as anticholinergics) can be expected to increase the gastrointestinal irritation produced by potassium salts (7.2)

————USE IN SPECIFIC POPULATIONS————

- Pregnant women: Pregnancy Category C; animal reproduction studies have not been conducted. It is not known whether Urocit®-K can cause fetal harm when administered to a pregnant woman or can affect reproduction capacity. Urocit®-K should be given to a pregnant woman only if clearly needed (8.1)
- Nursing mothers: The normal potassium ion content of human milk is about 13 mEq/L. It is not known if Urocit®-K has an effect on this content. Urocit®-K should be given to a woman who is breast feeding only if clearly needed (8.3)
- Pediatric Use: Safety and effectiveness in children have not been established (8.4)

See 17 for PATIENT COUNSELING INFORMATION
Revised: 04/2010

————FULL PRESCRIBING INFORMATION: CONTENTS*————

FULL PRESCRIBING INFORMATION

1   INDICATIONS AND USAGE
1.1   Renal tubular acidosis (RTA) with calcium stones

Potassium citrate is indicated for the management of renal tubular acidosis *[see Clinical Studies (14.1)]*.

1.2   Hypocitraturic calcium oxalate nephrolithiasis of any etiology

Potassium citrate is indicated for the management of Hypocitraturic calcium oxalate nephrolithiasis *[see Clinical Studies (14.2)]*.

1.3   Uric acid lithiasis with or without calcium stones

Potassium citrate is indicated for the management of Uric acid lithiasis with or without calcium stones *[see Clinical Studies (14.3)]*.

2   DOSAGE AND ADMINISTRATION
2.1   Dosing Instructions

Treatment with extended release potassium citrate should be added to a regimen that limits salt intake (avoidance of foods with high salt content and of added salt at the table) and encourages high fluid intake (urine volume should be at least two liters per day). The objective of treatment with Urocit®-K is to provide Urocit®-K in sufficient dosage to restore normal urinary citrate (greater than 320 mg/day and as close to the normal mean of 640 mg/day as possible), and to increase urinary pH to a level of 6.0 or 7.0.

Monitor serum electrolytes (sodium, potassium, chloride and carbon dioxide), serum creatinine and complete blood counts every four months and more frequently in patients with cardiac disease, renal disease or acidosis. Perform electrocardiograms periodically. Treatment should be discontinued if there is hyperkalemia, a significant rise in serum creatinine or a significant fall in blood hemocrit or hemoglobin.

2.2   Severe Hypocitraturia

In patients with severe hypocitraturia (urinary citrate < 150 mg/day), therapy should be initiated at a dosage of 60 mEq/day (30 mEq two times/day or 20 mEq three times/day with meals or within 30 minutes after meals or bedtime snack). Twenty-four hour urinary citrate and/or urinary pH measurements should be used to determine the adequacy of the initial dosage and to evaluate the effectiveness of any dosage change. In addition, urinary citrate and/or pH should be measured every four months. Doses of Urocit®-K greater than 100 mEq/day have not been studied and should be avoided.

2.3   Mild to Moderate Hypocitraturia

In patients with mild to moderate hypocitraturia (urinary citrate > 150 mg/day) therapy should be initiated at 30 mEq/day (15 mEq two times/day or 10 mEq three times/day within 30 minutes after meals or bedtime snack). Twenty-four hour urinary citrate and/or urinary pH measurements should be used to determine the adequacy of the initial dosage and to evaluate the effectiveness of any dosage change. Doses of Urocit®-K greater than 100 mEq/day have not been studied and should be avoided.

3   DOSAGE FORMS AND STRENGTHS

- 5 mEq tablets are uncoated, tan to yellowish in color, modified ball shaped, with MPC 600 debossed on one side and blank on the other
- 10 mEq tablets are uncoated, tan to yellowish in color, elliptical shaped, with 610 debossed on one side and MISSION on the other
- 15 mEq tablets are uncoated, tan to yellowish in color, modified rectangle shaped, with M15 debossed on one side and blank on the other

4   CONTRAINDICATIONS

Urocit®-K is contraindicated:
- In patients with hyperkalemia (or who have conditions pre-disposing them to hyperkalemia), as a further rise in serum potassium concentration may produce cardiac arrest. Such conditions include: chronic renal failure, uncontrolled diabetes mellitus, acute dehydration, strenuous physical exercise in unconditioned individuals, adrenal insufficiency, extensive tissue breakdown or the administration of a potassium-sparing agent (such as triamterene, spironolactone or amiloride).
- In patients in whom there is cause for arrest or delay in tablet passage through the gastrointestinal tract, such as

those suffering from delayed gastric emptying, esophageal compression, intestinal obstruction or stricture, or those taking anticholinergic medication.
- In patients with peptic ulcer disease because of its ulcerogenic potential.
- In patients with active urinary tract infection (with either urea-splitting or other organisms, in association with either calcium or struvite stones). The ability of Urocit®-K to increase urinary citrate may be attenuated by bacterial enzymatic degradation of citrate. Moreover, the rise in urinary pH resulting from Urocit®-K therapy might promote further bacterial growth.
- In patients with renal insufficiency (glomerular filtration rate of less than 0.7 ml/kg/min), because of the danger of soft tissue calcification and increased risk for the development of hyperkalemia.

5 WARNINGS AND PRECAUTIONS

5.1 Hyperkalemia

In patients with impaired mechanisms for excreting potassium, Urocit®-K administration can produce hyperkalemia and cardiac arrest. Potentially fatal hyperkalemia can develop rapidly and be asymptomatic. The use of Urocit®-K in patients with chronic renal failure, or any other condition which impairs potassium excretion such as severe myocardial damage or heart failure, should be avoided. Closely monitor for signs of hyperkalemia with periodic blood tests and ECGs.

5.2 Gastrointestinal Lesions

Because of reports of upper gastrointestinal mucosal lesions following administration of potassium chloride (wax-matrix), an endoscopic examination of the upper gastrointestinal mucosa was performed in 30 normal volunteers after they had taken glycopyrrolate 2 mg p.o. t.i.d., Urocit®-K 95 mEq/day, wax-matrix potassium chloride 96 mEq/day or wax-matrix placebo, in thrice daily schedule in the fasting state for one week. Urocit®-K and the wax-matrix formulation of potassium chloride were indistinguishable but both were significantly more irritating than the wax-matrix placebo. In a subsequent, similar study, lesions were less severe when glycopyrrolate was omitted.

Solid dosage forms of potassium chlorides have produced stenotic and/or ulcerative lesions of the small bowel and deaths. These lesions are caused by a high local concentration of potassium ions in the region of the dissolving tablets, which injured the bowel. In addition, perhaps because wax-matrix preparations are not enteric-coated and release some of their potassium content in the stomach, there have been reports of upper gastrointestinal bleeding associated with these products. The frequency of gastrointestinal lesions with wax-matrix potassium chloride products is estimated at one per 100,000 patient-years. Experience with Urocit®-K is limited, but a similar frequency of gastrointestinal lesions should be anticipated.

If there is severe vomiting, abdominal pain or gastrointestinal bleeding, Urocit®-K should be discontinued immediately and the possibility of bowel perforation or obstruction investigated.

6 ADVERSE REACTIONS

6.1 Postmarketing Experience

Some patients may develop minor gastrointestinal complaints during Urocit®-K therapy, such as abdominal discomfort, vomiting, diarrhea, loose bowel movements or nausea. These symptoms are due to the irritation of the gastrointestinal tract, and may be alleviated by taking the dose with meals or snacks, or by reducing the dosage. Patients may find intact matrices in their feces.

7 DRUG INTERACTIONS

7.1 Potential Effects of Potassium citrate on Other Drugs

Potassium-sparing Diuretics: Concomitant administration of Urocit®-K and a potassium-sparing diuretic (such as triamterene, spironolactone or amiloride) should be avoided since the simultaneous administration of these agents can produce severe hyperkalemia.

7.2 Potential Effects of Other Drugs on Potassium citrate

Drugs that slow gastrointestinal transit time: These agents (such as anticholinergics) can be expected to increase the gastrointestinal irritation produced by potassium salts.

8 USE IN SPECIFIC POPULATIONS

8.1 Pregnancy

Pregnancy Category C

Animal reproduction studies have not been conducted. It is also not known whether Urocit®-K can cause fetal harm when administered to a pregnant woman or can affect reproduction capacity. Urocit®-K should be given to a pregnant woman only if clearly needed.

8.3 Nursing Mothers

The normal potassium ion content of human milk is about 13 mEq/L. It is not known if Urocit®-K has an effect on this content. Urocit®-K should be given to a woman who is breast feeding only if clearly needed.

Table 1. Effect of Urocit®-K In Patients With Calcium Oxalate Nephrolithiasis.

	Stones Formed Per Year			
Group	**Baseline**	**On Treatment**	**Remission***	**Any Decrease**
I (n=19)	12 ± 30	0.9 ± 1.3	58%	95%
II (n=37)	1.2 ± 2	0.4 ± 1.5	89%	97%
III (n=15)	4.2 ± 7	0.7 ± 2	67%	100%
IV (n=18)	3.4 ± 8	0.5 ± 2	94%	100%
Total (n=89)	4.3 ±15	0.6 ± 2	80%	98%

*Remission defined as "the percentage of patients remaining free of newly formed stones during treatment".

8.4 Pediatric Use

Safety and effectiveness in children have not been established.

10 OVERDOSAGE

Treatment of Overdosage: The administration of potassium salts to persons without predisposing conditions for hyperkalemia rarely causes serious hyperkalemia at recommended dosages. It is important to recognize that hyperkalemia is usually asymptomatic and may be manifested only by an increased serum potassium concentration and characteristic electrocardiographic changes (peaking of T-wave, loss of P-wave, depression of S-T segment and prolongation of the QT interval). Late manifestations include muscle paralysis and cardiovascular collapse from cardiac arrest.

Treatment measures for hyperkalemia include the following:

1. Patients should be closely monitored for arrhythmias and electrolyte changes.
2. Elimination of medications containing potassium and of agents with potassium-sparing properties such as potassium-sparing diuretics, ARBs, ACE inhibitors, NSAIDs, certain nutritional supplements and many others.
3. Elimination of foods containing high levels of potassium such as almonds, apricots, bananas, beans (lima, pinto, white), cantaloupe, carrot juice (canned), figs, grapefruit juice, halibut, milk, oat bran, potato (with skin), salmon, spinach, tuna and many others.
4. Intravenous calcium gluconate if the patient is at no risk or low risk of developing digitalis toxicity.
5. Intravenous administration of 300-500 mL/hr of 10% dextrose solution containing 10-20 units of crystalline insulin per 1,000 mL.
6. Correction of acidosis, if present, with intravenous sodium bicarbonate.
7. Hemodialysis or peritoneal dialysis.
8. Exchange resins may be used. However, this measure alone is not sufficient for the acute treatment of hyperkalemia.

Lowering potassium levels too rapidly in patients taking digitalis can produce digitalis toxicity.

11 DESCRIPTION

Urocit®-K is a citrate salt of potassium. Its empirical formula is $K_3C_6H_5O_7 \bullet H_2O$, and it has the following chemical structure:

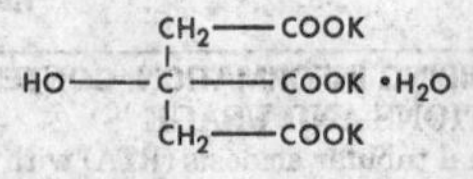

Urocit®-K yellowish to tan, oral wax-matrix tablets, contain 5 mEq (540 mg) potassium citrate, 10 mEq (1080 mg) potassium citrate and 15 mEq (1620 mg) potassium citrate each. Inactive ingredients include carnauba wax and magnesium stearate.

12 CLINICAL PHARMACOLOGY

12.1 Mechanism of Action

When Urocit®-K is given orally, the metabolism of absorbed citrate produces an alkaline load. The induced alkaline load in turn increases urinary pH and raises urinary citrate by augmenting citrate clearance without measurably altering ultrafilterable serum citrate. Thus, Urocit®-K therapy appears to increase urinary citrate principally by modifying the renal handling of citrate, rather than by increasing the filtered load of citrate. The increased filtered load of citrate may play some role, however, as in small comparisons of oral citrate and oral bicarbonate, citrate had a greater effect on urinary citrate.

In addition to raising urinary pH and citrate, Urocit®-K increases urinary potassium by approximately the amount contained in the medication. In some patients, Urocit®-K causes a transient reduction in urinary calcium.

The changes induced by Urocit®-K produce urine that is less conducive to the crystallization of stone-forming salts (calcium oxalate, calcium phosphate and uric acid). Increased citrate in the urine, by complexing with calcium, decreases calcium ion activity and thus the saturation of calcium oxalate. Citrate also inhibits the spontaneous nucleation of calcium oxalate and calcium phosphate (brushite).

The increase in urinary pH also decreases calcium ion activity by increasing calcium complexation to dissociated anions. The rise in urinary pH also increases the ionization of uric acid to the more soluble urate ion.

Urocit®-K therapy does not alter the urinary saturation of calcium phosphate, since the effect of increased citrate complexation of calcium is opposed by the rise in pH-dependent dissociation of phosphate. Calcium phosphate stones are more stable in alkaline urine.

In the setting of normal renal function, the rise in urinary citrate following a single dose begins by the first hour and lasts for 12 hours. With multiple doses the rise in citrate excretion reaches its peak by the third day and averts the normally wide circadian fluctuation in urinary citrate, thus maintaining urinary citrate at a higher, more constant level throughout the day. When the treatment is withdrawn, urinary citrate begins to decline toward the pre-treatment level on the first day.

The rise in citrate excretion is directly dependent on the Urocit®-K dosage. Following long-term treatment, Urocit®-K at a dosage of 60 mEq/day raises urinary citrate by approximately 400 mg/day and increases urinary pH by approximately 0.7 units.

In patients with severe renal tubular acidosis or chronic diarrheal syndrome where urinary citrate may be very low (<100 mg/day), Urocit®-K may be relatively ineffective in raising urinary citrate. A higher dose of Urocit®-K may therefore be required to produce a satisfactory citraturic response. In patients with renal tubular acidosis in whom urinary pH may be high, Urocit®-K produces a relatively small rise in urinary pH.

14 CLINICAL STUDIES

The pivotal Urocit®-K trials were non-randomized and non-placebo controlled where dietary management may have changed coincidentally with pharmacological treatment. Therefore, the results as presented in the following sections may overstate the effectiveness of the product.

14.1 Renal tubular acidosis (RTA) with calcium stones

The effect of oral potassium citrate therapy in a non-randomized, non-placebo controlled clinical study of five men and four women with calcium oxalate/calcium phosphate nephrolithiasis and documented incomplete distal renal tubular acidosis was examined. The main inclusion criterion was a history of stone passage or surgical removal of stones during the 3 years prior to initiation of potassium citrate therapy. All patients began alkali treatment with 60-80 mEq potassium citrate daily in 3 or 4 divided doses. Throughout treatment, patients were instructed to stay on a sodium restricted diet (100 mEq/day) and to reduce oxalate intake (limited intake of nuts, dark roughage, chocolate and tea). A moderate calcium restriction (400-800 mg/day) was imposed on patients with hypercalciuria.

X-rays of the urinary tract, available in all patients, were reviewed to determine presence of pre-existing stones, appearance of new stones, or change in the number of stones. Potassium citrate therapy was associated with inhibition of new stone formation in patients with distal tubular acidosis. Three of the nine patients continued to pass stones during the on-treatment phase. While it is likely that these patients passed pre-existing stones during therapy, the most conservative assumption is that the passed stones were newly formed. Using this assumption, the stone-passage remission rate was 67%. All patients had a reduced stone formation rate. Over the first 2 years of treatment, the on-treatment stone formation rate was reduced from 13±27 to 1±2 per year.

14.2 Hypocitraturic calcium oxalate nephrolithiasis of any etiology

Eighty-nine patients with hypocitraturic calcium nephrolithiasis or uric acid lithiasis with or without calcium nephrolithiasis participated in this non-randomized, non-placebo controlled clinical study. Four groups of patients were treated with potassium citrate: Group 1 was comprised of 19 patients, 10 with renal tubular acidosis and 9 with chronic diarrheal syndrome, Group 2 was comprised of 37 patients, 5 with uric acid stones alone, 6 with uric acid lithiasis and calcium stones, 3 with type 1 absorptive hypercalciuria, 9 with type 2 absorptive hypercalciuria and 14 with hypocitraturia. Group 3 was comprised of 15 patients with history of relapse on other therapy and Group 4 was comprised of 18 patients, 9 with type 1 absorptive hypercalciuria and calcium stones, 1 with type 2 absorptive hypercalciuria and calcium stones, 2 with hyperuricosuric calcium oxalate nephrolithiasis, 4 with uric acid lithiasis accompanied by calcium stones and 2 with hypocitraturia and hyperuricemia accompanied by calcium stones. The dose of potassium citrate ranged from 30 to 100 mEq per day, and usually was 20 mEq administered orally 3 times daily. Patients were followed in an outpatient setting every 4 months during treatment and were studied over a period from 1 to 4.33 years. A three-year retrospective pre-study history for stone passage or removal was obtained and corroborated by medical records. Concomitant therapy (with thiazide or allopurinol) was allowed if patients had hypercalciuria, hyperuricosuria or hyperuricemia. Group 2 was treated with potassium citrate alone.

In all groups, treatment that included potassium citrate was associated with a sustained increase in urinary citrate excretion from subnormal values to normal values (400 to 700 mg/day), and a sustained increase in urinary pH from 5.6-6.0 to approximately 6.5. The stone formation rate was reduced in all groups as shown in **Table 1**.

[See table 1 at top of previous page]

14.3 Uric acid lithiasis with or without calcium stones

A long-term non-randomized, non-placebo controlled clinical trial with eighteen adult patients with uric acid lithiasis participated in the study. Six patients formed only uric acid stones, and the remaining 12 patients formed mixed stones containing both uric acid and calcium salts or formed both uric acid stones (without calcium salts) and calcium stones (without uric acid) on separate occasions.

Eleven of the 18 patients received potassium citrate alone. Six of the 7 other patients also received allopurinol for hyperuricemia with gouty arthritis, symptomatic hyperuricemia, or hyperuricosuria. One patient also received hydrochlorothiazide because of unclassified hypercalciuria. The main inclusion criterion was a history of stone passage or surgical removal of stones during the 3 years prior to initiation of potassium citrate therapy. All patients received potassium citrate at a dosage of 30-80 mEq/day in three-to-four divided doses and were followed every four months for up to 5 years.

While on potassium citrate treatment, urinary pH rose significantly from a low value of 5.3 ± 0.3 to within normal limits (6.2 to 6.5). Urinary citrate which was low before treatment rose to the high normal range and only one stone was formed in the entire group of 18 patients.

15 REFERENCES

1. Pak, C. (1987). Citrate and Renal Calculi. *Mineral and Electrolyte Metabolism* 13, 257-266.
2. Pak, C. (1985). Long-Term Treatment of Calcium Nephrolithiasis with Potassium Citrate. *The Journal of Urology* 134, 11-19.
3. Preminger, G.M., K. Sakhaee, C. Skurla and C.Y.C. Pak. (1985). Prevention of Recurrent Calcium Stone Formation with Potassium Citrate Therapy in Patients with Distal Renal Tubular Acidosis. *The Journal of Urology* 134, 20-23.
4. Pak, C.Y.C., K. Sakhaee and C. Fuller. (1986). Successful Management of Uric Acid Nephrolithiasis with Potassium Citrate. *Kidney International* 30, 422-428.
5. Hollander-Rodriguez, J et al. (2006). Hyperkalemia, *American Family Physician*, Vol. 73/No. 2.
6. Greenberg, A et al. (1998). Hyperkalemia: treatment options. *Semen Nephrol.* Jan; 18 (1): 46-57.

16 HOW SUPPLIED/STORAGE AND HANDLING

Urocit®-K 5 mEq tablets are uncoated, tan to yellowish in color, modified ball shaped, with MPC 600 debossed on one side and blank on the other, supplied in bottles as:
NDC 0178-0600-01   Bottle of 100
Urocit®-K 10 mEq tablets are uncoated, tan to yellowish in color, elliptical shaped, with 610 debossed on one side and MISSION on the other, supplied in bottles as:
NDC 0178-0610-01   Bottle of 100
Urocit®-K 15 mEq tablets are uncoated, tan to yellowish in color, modified rectangle shaped, with M15 debossed on one side and blank on the other, supplied in bottles as:
NDC 0178-0615-01   Bottle of 100
Storage: Store in a tight container.

17 PATIENT COUNSELING INFORMATION

17.1 Administration of Drug

Tell patients to take each dose without crushing, chewing or sucking the tablet.

Tell patients to take this medicine only as directed. This is especially important if the patient is also taking both diuretics and digitalis preparations.

Tell patients to check with the doctor if there is trouble swallowing tablets or if the tablet seems to stick in the throat.

Tell patients to check with the doctor at once if tarry stools or other evidence of gastrointestinal bleeding is noticed.

Tell patients that their doctor will perform regular blood tests and electrocardiograms to ensure safety.

Rev 0410

Monarch Pharmaceuticals
Please see King Pharmaceuticals, Inc.

Mylan Pharmaceuticals Inc.
**781 CHESTNUT RIDGE ROAD
P.O. BOX 4310
MORGANTOWN, WV 26504-4310**

Direct Inquiries to:
304.599.2595
For Medical Information Contact:
Clinical Research Department
877.446.3679
877.4INFO.RX
Sales and Ordering:
Sales Department
800.RX.MYLAN

Product List - Mylan

The following list of Mylan products is provided to facilitate identification. It includes the color(s) and identification codes for all tablets and capsules.

PRODUCT GENERIC NAME Description Color(s)	IDENTIFICATION CODE (Front/Back*)
ACEBUTOLOL HYDROCHLORIDE Capsules, USP, 200 mg ℞ *Med. Orange & Med. Orange*	MYLAN 1200
ACEBUTOLOL HYDROCHLORIDE Capsules, USP, 400 mg ℞ *Med. Orange & Med. Orange*	MYLAN 1400
ACTICIN® (permethrin) Cream 5%, ℞ *White to Off-white (vanishing)*	N/A
ACYCLOVIR Capsules, USP, 200 mg ℞ *Lavender Opaque & Lavender Opaque*	MYLAN 2200
ACYCLOVIR Tablets, USP, 400 mg ℞ *White*	M253/Blank
ACYCLOVIR Tablets, USP, 800 mg ℞ *White*	MYLAN/302
ALBUTEROL Tablets, USP, 2 mg ℞ *White*	M255/Blank
ALBUTEROL Tablets, USP, 4 mg ℞ *White*	M572/Blank
ALBUTEROL SULFATE Extended-release Tablets, 4 mg ℞ *White*	M/22
ALBUTEROL SULFATE Extended-release Tablets, 8 mg ℞ *Blue*	M/24
ALBUTEROL SULFATE Inhalation Solution, 0.63 mg/3 mL ℞	N/A
ALBUTEROL SULFATE Inhalation Solution, 1.25 mg/3 mL ℞	N/A
ALBUTEROL SULFATE Inhalation Solution, 0.083% ℞	N/A
ALENDRONATE SODIUM Tablets, USP, 5 mg ℞ *White*	M/A6
ALENDRONATE SODIUM Tablets, USP, 10 mg ℞ *White*	M/A7
ALENDRONATE SODIUM Tablets, USP, 35 mg ℞ *White*	M A11/Blank
ALENDRONATE SODIUM Tablets, USP, 70 mg ℞ *White*	M A12/Blank
ALLOPURINOL Tablets, USP, 100 mg ℞ *White*	M31/Blank
ALLOPURINOL Tablets, USP, 300 mg ℞ *White*	M71/Blank
ALPRAZOLAM Extended-release Tablets, 0.5 mg ℂ/℞ *White*	M/A21
ALPRAZOLAM Extended-release Tablets, 1 mg ℂ/℞ *Light Orange*	M/A22
ALPRAZOLAM Extended-release Tablets, 2 mg ℂ/℞ *Light Lavender*	M/A23
ALPRAZOLAM Extended-release Tablets, 3 mg ℂ/℞ *Light Pink*	M/A24
ALPRAZOLAM Tablets, USP, 0.25 mg ℂ/℞ *White*	MYLAN A/Scored
ALPRAZOLAM Tablets, USP, 0.5 mg ℂ/℞ *Peach*	MYLAN A3/Scored
ALPRAZOLAM Tablets, USP, 1 mg ℂ/℞ *Blue*	MYLAN A1/Scored
ALPRAZOLAM Tablets, USP, 2 mg ℂ/℞ *White*	MYLAN A4/Scored
AMILORIDE HYDROCHLORIDE and HYDROCHLOROTHIAZIDE Tablets, USP, 5 mg/50 mg ℞ *Lt. Orange*	M577/Blank
AMITRIPTYLINE HYDROCHLORIDE Tablets, USP, 10 mg ℞ *White*	M77/Blank
AMITRIPTYLINE HYDROCHLORIDE Tablets, USP, 25 mg ℞ *Lt. Green*	M51/Blank
AMITRIPTYLINE HYDROCHLORIDE Tablets, USP, 50 mg ℞ *Brown*	M36/Blank
AMITRIPTYLINE HYDROCHLORIDE Tablets, USP, 75 mg ℞ *Blue*	M37/Blank
AMITRIPTYLINE HYDROCHLORIDE Tablets, USP, 100 mg ℞ *Orange*	M38/Blank
AMITRIPTYLINE HYDROCHLORIDE Tablets, USP, 150 mg ℞ *Flesh*	M39/Blank
AMLODIPINE BESYLATE Tablets, 2.5 mg ℞ *Blue*	M/A8
AMLODIPINE BESYLATE Tablets, 5 mg ℞ *Blue*	M/A9
AMLODIPINE BESYLATE Tablets, 10 mg ℞ *Blue*	M/A10
AMNESTEEM® (isotretinoin) Capsules, USP, 10 mg ℞ *Reddish Brown*	I10
AMNESTEEM® (isotretinoin) Capsules, USP, 20 mg ℞ *Reddish Brown & Cream*	I20
AMNESTEEM® (isotretinoin) Capsules, USP, 40 mg ℞ *Orange-brown*	I40
ANAGRELIDE HYDROCHLORIDE Capsules, 0.5 mg ℞ *Light Gray & Coral*	MYLAN 6868
ANAGRELIDE HYDROCHLORIDE Capsules, 1 mg ℞ *Light Gray & Aqua Blue*	MYLAN 6869
ANASTROZOLE Tablets, 1 mg ℞ *White*	M/34
ATENOLOL Tablets, USP, 25 mg ℞ *White*	M/A2
ATENOLOL Tablets, USP, 50 mg ℞ *White*	M/231
ATENOLOL Tablets, USP, 100 mg ℞ *White*	M/757

Drug	Code
ATENOLOL and CHLORTHALIDONE Tablets, USP, 50 mg/25 mg ℞ *White*	M63/Blank
ATENOLOL and CHLORTHALIDONE Tablets, USP, 100 mg/25 mg ℞ *White*	M64/Blank
AVITA® (tretinoin) Cream 0.025%, ℞	N/A
AVITA® (tretinoin) Gel 0.025%, ℞	N/A
AZATHIOPRINE Tablets, USP, 50 mg ℞ *Yellow*	A Score Z/Blank
AZITHROMYCIN Tablets, USP, 250 mg ℞ *Blue*	M 533/Blank
AZITHROMYCIN Tablets, USP, 500 mg ℞ *Blue*	M 534/Blank
AZITHROMYCIN Tablets, USP, 600 mg ℞ *Blue*	M 535/Blank
BACLOFEN Tablets, USP, 10 mg ℞ *Light Yellow*	MX/23
BACLOFEN Tablets, USP, 20 mg ℞ *Light Yellow*	MX/24
BALSALAZIDE DISODIUM Capsules, 750 mg ℞ *Orange & Orange*	MYLAN 6750
BENAZEPRIL HYDROCHLORIDE Tablets, USP, 5 mg ℞ *White*	M/441
BENAZEPRIL HYDROCHLORIDE Tablets, USP, 10 mg ℞ *White*	M/443
BENAZEPRIL HYDROCHLORIDE Tablets, USP, 20 mg ℞ *White*	M444/Blank
BENAZEPRIL HYDROCHLORIDE Tablets, USP, 40 mg ℞ *White*	M447/Blank
BENAZEPRIL HYDROCHLORIDE and HYDROCHLOROTHIAZIDE Tablets, 5 mg/6.25 mg ℞ *Beige*	M725/Scored
BENAZEPRIL HYDROCHLORIDE and HYDROCHLOROTHIAZIDE Tablets, 10 mg/12.5 mg ℞ *Beige*	M735/Blank
BENAZEPRIL HYDROCHLORIDE and HYDROCHLOROTHIAZIDE Tablets, 20 mg/12.5 mg ℞ *Beige*	M745/Blank
BENAZEPRIL HYDROCHLORIDE and HYDROCHLOROTHIAZIDE Tablets, 20 mg/25 mg ℞ *Beige*	M775/Blank
BICALUTAMIDE Tablets, USP, 50 mg ℞ *White*	M/C17
BISOPROLOL FUMARATE Tablets, USP, 5 mg ℞ *Purple*	M/523
BISOPROLOL FUMARATE Tablets, USP, 10 mg ℞ *White*	M/524
BISOPROLOL FUMARATE and HYDROCHLOROTHIAZIDE Tablets, USP, 2.5 mg/6.25 mg ℞ *Orange*	M/501
BISOPROLOL FUMARATE and HYDROCHLOROTHIAZIDE Tablets, USP, 5 mg/6.25 mg ℞ *Blue*	M/503
BISOPROLOL FUMARATE and HYDROCHLOROTHIAZIDE Tablets, USP, 10 mg/6.25 mg ℞ *White*	M/505
BROMOCRIPTINE MESYLATE Capsules, USP, 5 mg ℞ *Light Brown / Ivory*	MYLAN 7096
BROMOCRIPTINE MESYLATE Tablets, USP, 2.5 mg ℞ *White to Off-White*	M42/Scored
BUMETANIDE Tablets, USP, 0.5 mg ℞ *Green*	E128/Blank
BUMETANIDE Tablets, USP, 1 mg ℞ *Yellow*	E129/Blank
BUMETANIDE Tablets, USP, 2 mg ℞ *Beige to Lt. Brown*	E130/Blank
BUPROPION HYDROCHLORIDE Tablets, USP, 75 mg ℞ *Peach*	M/433
BUPROPION HYDROCHLORIDE Tablets, USP, 100 mg ℞ *Lt. Blue*	M/435
BUPROPION HYDROCHLORIDE Extended-release Tablets, USP (SR), 100 mg ℞ *Lt. Green*	MU11/Blank
BUPROPION HYDROCHLORIDE Extended-release Tablets, USP (SR), 150 mg ℞ *Lt. Green*	MU12/Blank
BUPROPION HYDROCHLORIDE Extended-release Tablets, USP (SR), 200 mg ℞ *Lt. Green*	MU13/Blank
BUSPIRONE HYDROCHLORIDE Tablets, USP, 5 mg ℞ *White*	MB1/Blank
BUSPIRONE HYDROCHLORIDE Tablets, USP, 10 mg ℞ *White*	MB2/Blank
BUSPIRONE HYDROCHLORIDE Tablets, USP, 15 mg ℞ *White*	MB3/555 (Trisect)
BUSPIRONE HYDROCHLORIDE Tablets, USP, 30 mg ℞ *White*	MB4/10 10 10 (Trisect)
BUTORPHANOL TARTRATE Nasal Solution, 10 mg/mL ℅/℞	—
CAPTOPRIL Tablets, USP, 12.5 mg ℞ *White*	MC1/Scored
CAPTOPRIL Tablets, USP, 25 mg ℞ *White*	MC2/(Quadrisect)
CAPTOPRIL Tablets, USP, 50 mg ℞ *White*	MC3/Blank
CAPTOPRIL Tablets, USP, 100 mg ℞ *White*	MC4/Blank
CAPTOPRIL and HYDROCHLOROTHIAZIDE Tablets, USP, 25 mg/15 mg ℞ *White*	M81/Scored
CAPTOPRIL and HYDROCHLOROTHIAZIDE Tablets, USP, 25 mg/25 mg ℞ *Peach*	M83/Scored
CAPTOPRIL and HYDROCHLOROTHIAZIDE Tablets, USP, 50 mg/15 mg ℞ *White*	M84/Scored
CAPTOPRIL and HYDROCHLOROTHIAZIDE Tablets, USP, 50 mg/25 mg ℞ *Peach*	M86/Scored
CARBIDOPA and LEVODOPA Tablets, USP, 10 mg/100 mg ℞ *Blue*	M score CL1/Blank
CARBIDOPA and LEVODOPA Tablets, USP, 25 mg/100 mg ℞ *Yellow*	M score CL2/Blank
CARBIDOPA and LEVODOPA Tablets, USP, 25 mg/250 mg ℞ *Blue*	M score CL3/Blank
CARBIDOPA and LEVODOPA Extended-release Tablets, 25 mg/100 mg ℞ *Purple*	MYLAN/88
CARBIDOPA and LEVODOPA Extended-release Tablets, 50 mg/200 mg ℞ *Purple*	MYLAN/94
CARBIDOPA and LEVODOPA ORALLY DISINTEGRATING Tablets, 10 mg/100 mg ℞ *Green*	M (score) C51/Blank
CARBIDOPA and LEVODOPA ORALLY DISINTEGRATING Tablets, 25 mg/100 mg ℞ *Blue*	M (score) C52/Blank
CARBIDOPA and LEVODOPA ORALLY DISINTEGRATING Tablets, 25 mg/250 mg ℞ *Green*	M (score) C53/Blank
CARVEDILOL Tablets, 3.125 mg ℞ *Blue*	M/C31
CARVEDILOL Tablets, 6.25 mg ℞ *White*	M/C32
CARVEDILOL Tablets, 12.5 mg ℞ *White*	M/C33
CARVEDILOL Tablets, 25 mg ℞ *White*	M/C34
CETIRIZINE HYDROCHLORIDE Tablets (OTC), 5 mg ℞ *White*	M/C35
CETIRIZINE HYDROCHLORIDE Tablets (OTC), 10 mg ℞ *White*	M/C37
CHLORDIAZEPOXIDE and AMITRIPTYLINE HYDROCHLORIDE Tablets, USP, 5 mg/12.5 mg ℅/℞ *Green*	MYLAN/211
CHLORDIAZEPOXIDE and AMITRIPTYLINE HYDROCHLORIDE Tablets, USP, 10 mg/25 mg ℅/℞ *White*	MYLAN/277
CHLOROTHIAZIDE Tablets, USP, 250 mg ℞ *White*	M50/Blank
CHLOROTHIAZIDE Tablets, USP, 500 mg ℞ *White*	MYLAN 162/Blank
CHLORPROPAMIDE Tablets, USP, 100 mg ℞ *Green*	MYLAN 197/100
CHLORPROPAMIDE Tablets, USP, 250 mg ℞ *Green*	MYLAN 210/250
CHLORTHALIDONE Tablets, USP, 25 mg ℞ *Lt. Yellow*	M35/Blank
CHLORTHALIDONE Tablets, USP, 50 mg ℞ *Lt. Green*	M75/Blank
CILOSTAZOL Tablets, USP, 50 mg ℞ *White to Off-White*	MC41/Blank
CILOSTAZOL Tablets, USP, 100 mg ℞ *White to Off-White*	MC42/Blank
CIMETIDINE Tablets, USP, 200 mg ℞ *Green*	M/53
CIMETIDINE Tablets, USP, 300 mg ℞ *Green*	M/317
CIMETIDINE Tablets, USP, 400 mg ℞ *Green*	M/372
CIMETIDINE Tablets, USP, 800 mg ℞ *Green*	M541/Blank
CIPROFLOXACIN Extended-release Tablets, 500 mg ℞ *Orange*	M 1743/Blank
CIPROFLOXACIN Extended-release Tablets, 1000 mg ℞ *Orange*	M 1745/Blank
CIPROFLOXACIN Tablets, 500 mg ℞ *White*	CF500
CITALOPRAM Tablets, USP, 10 mg ℞ *Beige*	MX31/Blank
CITALOPRAM Tablets, USP, 20 mg ℞ *Pink*	MX32/Blank
CITALOPRAM Tablets, USP, 40 mg ℞ *White*	MX33/Blank
CLARITHROMYCIN Tablets, USP, 250 mg ℞ *White to Off-white*	G/C250
CLARITHROMYCIN Tablets, USP, 500 mg ℞ *White to Off-white*	G/C500
CLINDAMYCIN PHOSPHATE and BENZOYL PEROXIDE Gel, 1%/5% ℞	N/A
CLOMIPRAMINE HYDROCHLORIDE Capsules, USP, 25 mg ℞ *Medium Orange & Flesh*	MYLAN 3025
CLOMIPRAMINE HYDROCHLORIDE Capsules, USP, 50 mg ℞ *Yellow & Flesh*	MYLAN 3050
CLOMIPRAMINE HYDROCHLORIDE Capsules, USP, 75 mg ℞ *Swedish Orange & Flesh*	MYLAN 3075
CLONAZEPAM Tablets, USP, 0.5 mg ℅/℞ *Yellow*	M/C13
CLONAZEPAM Tablets, USP, 1 mg ℅/℞ *Lt. Green*	M/C14

IMPORTANT NOTICE: Updated drug information is sent bi-monthly via the PDR® Update Insert. For *monthly* email updates, register at PDR.net.

CLONAZEPAM — M/C15
Tablets, USP, 2 mg ℭ/Ṙ
White

CLONIDINE HYDROCHLORIDE — MYLAN 152/Blank
Tablets, USP, 0.1 mg Ṙ
White

CLONIDINE HYDROCHLORIDE — MYLAN 186/Blank
Tablets, USP, 0.2 mg Ṙ
White

CLONIDINE HYDROCHLORIDE — MYLAN 199/Blank
Tablets, USP, 0.3 mg Ṙ
White

CLONIDINE TRANSDERMAL — N/A
SYSTEM, USP, 0.1 mg/day Ṙ

CLONIDINE TRANSDERMAL — N/A
SYSTEM, USP, 0.2 mg/day Ṙ

CLONIDINE TRANSDERMAL — N/A
SYSTEM, USP, 0.3 mg/day Ṙ

CLORAZEPATE DIPOTASSIUM — M30/Blank
Tablets, USP, 3.75 mg ℭ/Ṙ
Blue

CLORAZEPATE DIPOTASSIUM — M40/Blank
Tablets, USP, 7.5 mg ℭ/Ṙ
Peach

CLORAZEPATE DIPOTASSIUM — M70/Blank
Tablets, USP, 15 mg ℭ/Ṙ
White

CLORPRES® — M1/Blank
(clonidine hydrochloride and chlorthalidone)
Tablets, USP, 0.1 mg/15 mg Ṙ
Yellow

CLORPRES® — M27/Blank
(clonidine hydrochloride and chlorthalidone)
Tablets, USP, 0.2 mg/15 mg Ṙ
Yellow

CLORPRES® — M72/Blank
(clonidine hydrochloride and chlorthalidone)
Tablets, USP, 0.3 mg/15 mg Ṙ
Yellow

CLOZAPINE — M/C7
Tablets, USP, 25 mg Ṙ
Peach

CLOZAPINE — M/C72
Tablets, USP, 50 mg Ṙ
Green

CLOZAPINE — M/C11
Tablets, USP, 100 mg Ṙ
Green

CLOZAPINE — M/C73
Tablets, USP, 200 mg Ṙ
Green

CYCLOBENZAPRINE HYDROCHLORIDE — M/771
Tablets, USP, 5 mg Ṙ
Blue

CYCLOBENZAPRINE HYDROCHLORIDE — M/751
Tablets, USP, 10 mg Ṙ
Butterscotch-Yellow

DIAZEPAM — MYLAN 271/Scored
Tablets, USP, 2 mg ℭ/Ṙ
White

DIAZEPAM — MYLAN 345/Scored
Tablets, USP, 5 mg ℭ/Ṙ
Orange

DIAZEPAM — MYLAN 477/Scored
Tablets, USP, 10 mg ℭ/Ṙ
Green

DICLOFENAC POTASSIUM — M/D5
Tablets, USP, 50 mg Ṙ
White

DICLOFENAC SODIUM — G-DS-50/Blank
Delayed-release Tablets, USP, 50 mg Ṙ
Light Brown

DICLOFENAC SODIUM — G-DS-75/Blank
Delayed-release Tablets, USP, 75 mg Ṙ
Light Pink

DICLOFENAC SODIUM — M355/Blank
Extended-release Tablets, USP, 100 mg Ṙ
Yellow

DICYCLOMINE HYDROCHLORIDE — MYLAN 1610
Capsules, USP, 10 mg Ṙ
Lt. Turquoise Blue and Lt. Turquoise Blue

DICYCLOMINE HYDROCHLORIDE — MD6/Blank
Tablets, USP, 20 mg Ṙ
Blue

DIDANOSINE — M159
Delayed-release Capsules, 125 mg Ṙ
White Opaque & White Opaque

DIDANOSINE — M160
Delayed-release Capsules, 200 mg Ṙ
Yellow Opaque & White Opaque

DIDANOSINE — M161
Delayed-release Capsules, 250 mg Ṙ
Yellow Opaque & Yellow Opaque

DIDANOSINE — M162
Delayed-release Capsules, 400 mg Ṙ
White Opaque & Yellow Opaque

DILTIAZEM HYDROCHLORIDE — MYLAN 5220
Extended-release Capsules, USP (once-a-day),
120 mg Ṙ
Lt. Pink & Flesh

DILTIAZEM HYDROCHLORIDE — MYLAN 5280
Extended-release Capsules, USP (once-a-day),
180 mg Ṙ
Lavender & Flesh

DILTIAZEM HYDROCHLORIDE — MYLAN 5340
Extended-release Capsules, USP (once-a-day),
240 mg Ṙ
Lt. Blue & Flesh

DILTIAZEM HYDROCHLORIDE — MYLAN 6060
Extended-release Capsules, USP (twice-a-day),
60 mg Ṙ
Coral & White

DILTIAZEM HYDROCHLORIDE — MYLAN 6090
Extended-release Capsules, USP (twice-a-day),
90 mg Ṙ
Coral & Ivory

DILTIAZEM HYDROCHLORIDE — MYLAN 6120
Extended-release Capsules, USP (twice-a-day),
120 mg Ṙ
Coral & Coral

DILTIAZEM HYDROCHLORIDE — M23/Blank
Tablets, USP, 30 mg Ṙ
White

DILTIAZEM HYDROCHLORIDE — M45/Scored
Tablets, USP, 60 mg Ṙ
White

DILTIAZEM HYDROCHLORIDE — M135/Scored
Tablets, USP, 90 mg Ṙ
White

DILTIAZEM HYDROCHLORIDE — M525/Scored
Tablets, USP, 120 mg Ṙ
White

DIPHENOXYLATE HYDROCHLORIDE — M15/Blank
and ATROPINE SULFATE
Tablets, USP, 2.5 mg/0.025 mg ℭ/Ṙ
White

DIVALPROEX SODIUM — M over 943/Blank
Delayed-release Tablets, USP, 125 mg Ṙ
Blue

DIVALPROEX SODIUM — M over 944/Blank
Delayed-release Tablets, USP, 250 mg Ṙ
Blue

DIVALPROEX SODIUM — M945/Blank
Delayed-release Tablets, USP, 500 mg Ṙ
Blue

DIVALPROEX SODIUM — M over 177/Blank
Extended-release Tablets, 250 mg Ṙ
White

DIVALPROEX SODIUM — M473/Blank
Extended-release Tablets, 500 mg Ṙ
White

DOXAZOSIN — MD9/Scored
Tablets, USP, 1 mg Ṙ
White to Off-white

DOXAZOSIN — MD10/Scored
Tablets, USP, 2 mg Ṙ
Pink

DOXAZOSIN — MD11/Scored
Tablets, USP, 4 mg Ṙ
Blue

DOXAZOSIN — MD12/Scored
Tablets, USP, 8 mg Ṙ
Purple

DOXEPIN HYDROCHLORIDE — MYLAN 1049
Capsules, USP, 10 mg Ṙ
Buff & Buff

DOXEPIN HYDROCHLORIDE — MYLAN 3125
Capsules, USP, 25 mg Ṙ
Ivory & White

DOXEPIN HYDROCHLORIDE — MYLAN 4250
Capsules, USP, 50 mg Ṙ
Ivory & Ivory

DOXEPIN HYDROCHLORIDE — MYLAN 5375
Capsules, USP, 75 mg Ṙ
Brite Lite Green & Brite Lite Green

DOXEPIN HYDROCHLORIDE — MYLAN 6410
Capsules, USP, 100 mg Ṙ
Brite Lite Green & White

DOXYCYCLINE — M/D21
Tablets, 50 mg Ṙ
Light Yellow

DOXYCYCLINE — M/D22
Tablets, 75 mg Ṙ
Orange

DOXYCYCLINE — M/D23
Tablets, 100 mg Ṙ
Light Yellow

DOXYCYCLINE — M/D (score) 24
Tablets, 150 mg Ṙ
Orange

ENALAPRIL MALEATE — ME15/Scored
Tablets, USP, 2.5 mg Ṙ
White

ENALAPRIL MALEATE — ME16/Scored
Tablets, USP, 5 mg Ṙ
White

ENALAPRIL MALEATE — ME17/Scored
Tablets, USP, 10 mg Ṙ
Lt. Blue

ENALAPRIL MALEATE — ME18/Scored
Tablets, USP, 20 mg Ṙ
Med. Blue

ENALAPRIL MALEATE — M/712
and HYDROCHLOROTHIAZIDE
Tablets, USP, 5 mg /12.5 mg Ṙ
White

ENALAPRIL MALEATE — M/723
and HYDROCHLOROTHIAZIDE
Tablets, USP, 10 mg/25 mg Ṙ
White

ESTRADIOL — M/E3
Tablets, USP, 0.5 mg Ṙ
White to Off-White

ESTRADIOL — M/E4
Tablets, USP, 1 mg Ṙ
Pink

ESTRADIOL — M/E5
Tablets, USP, 2 mg Ṙ
Pale Blue

ESTRADIOL TRANSDERMAL — Estradiol
SYSTEM Continuous Delivery — 0.025 mg/day
Patches, 0.025 mg/day Ṙ — (once weekly)
Peach

ESTRADIOL TRANSDERMAL — Estradiol
SYSTEM Continuous Delivery — 0.0375 mg/day
Patches, 0.0375 mg/day Ṙ — (once weekly)
Peach

ESTRADIOL TRANSDERMAL — Estradiol
SYSTEM Continuous Delivery — 0.05 mg/day
Patches, 0.05 mg/day Ṙ — (once weekly)
Peach

ESTRADIOL TRANSDERMAL — Estradiol
SYSTEM Continuous Delivery — 0.06 mg/day
Patches, 0.06 mg/day Ṙ — (once weekly)
Peach

ESTRADIOL TRANSDERMAL — Estradiol
SYSTEM Continuous Delivery — 0.075 mg/day
Patches, 0.075 mg/day Ṙ — (once weekly)
Peach

ESTRADIOL TRANSDERMAL — Estradiol
SYSTEM Continuous Delivery — 0.1 mg/day
Patches, 0.1 mg/day Ṙ — (once weekly)
Peach

ESTROPIPATE — ME7/Blank
Tablets, USP, 0.75 mg Ṙ
Yellow

ESTROPIPATE — ME8/Blank
Tablets, USP, 1.5 mg Ṙ
Peach

ETIDRONATE DISODIUM — ED 200/G
Tablets, USP, 200 mg Ṙ
White

ETIDRONATE DISODIUM — ED 400/G
Tablets, USP, 400 mg Ṙ
White

ETOPOSIDE — E50
Capsules, USP, 50 mg Ṙ
Dark Pink

FAMOTIDINE — MF1/Blank
Tablets, USP, 20 mg Ṙ
Yellow

FAMOTIDINE — MF2/Blank
Tablets, USP, 40 mg Ṙ
Green

FELODIPINE — M/F11
Extended-release Tablets, USP, 2.5 mg Ṙ
White

FELODIPINE — M/F12
Extended-release Tablets, USP, 5 mg Ṙ
Yellow

FELODIPINE — M/F13
Extended-release Tablets, USP, 10 mg Ṙ
Blue

FENOFIBRATE — KLX/170
Tablets, 54 mg Ṙ
Yellow

FENOFIBRATE — KLX/171
Tablets, 160 mg Ṙ
White

FENOPROFEN CALCIUM	M471/Scored
Tablets, USP, 600 mg ℞	
Orange	
FENTANYL TRANSDERMAL	
SYSTEM	Fentanyl
Patches, 12 mcg/hr ⓒⅡ/℞	12 mcg/hr
Translucent	
FENTANYL TRANSDERMAL	
SYSTEM	Fentanyl
Patches, 25 mcg/hr ⓒⅡ/℞	25 mcg/hr
Translucent	
FENTANYL TRANSDERMAL	
SYSTEM	Fentanyl
Patches, 50 mcg/hr ⓒⅡ/℞	50 mcg/hr
Translucent	
FENTANYL TRANSDERMAL	
SYSTEM	Fentanyl
Patches, 75 mcg/hr ⓒⅡ/℞	75 mcg/hr
Translucent	
FENTANYL TRANSDERMAL	
SYSTEM	Fentanyl
Patches, 100 mcg/hr ⓒⅡ/℞	100 mcg/hr
Translucent	
FEXOFENADINE HYDROCHLORIDE	M/752
Tablets, USP, 30 mg ℞	
Blue	
FEXOFENADINE HYDROCHLORIDE	M over 753/Blank
Tablets, USP, 60 mg ℞	
Blue	
FEXOFENADINE HYDROCHLORIDE	M 755/Blank
Tablets, USP, 180 mg ℞	
Blue	
FINASTERIDE	M/151
Tablets, USP, 5 mg ℞	
White	
FLUCONAZOLE	M/F3
Tablets, 50 mg ℞	
Yellow	
FLUCONAZOLE	M over F4/Blank
Tablets, 100 mg ℞	
Yellow	
FLUCONAZOLE	M over F5/Blank
Tablets, 150 mg ℞	
Yellow	
FLUCONAZOLE	M over F6/Blank
Tablets, 200 mg ℞	
Yellow	
FLUOXETINE	MYLAN 4210
Capsules, USP, 10 mg ℞	
White & Flesh	
FLUOXETINE	MYLAN 4220
Capsules, USP, 20 mg ℞	
Lt. Turquoise Blue & Flesh	
FLUOXETINE	MYLAN 4350
Capsules, USP, 40 mg ℞	
Lt. Blue & White	
FLUOXETINE	MYLAN over 5410
Capsules, USP, 10 mg ℞	
Blue Green & Blue Green	
FLUOXETINE	MYLAN over 5420
Capsules, USP, 20 mg ℞	
Red & Red	
FLUPHENAZINE HYDROCHLORIDE	M/4
Tablets, USP, 1 mg ℞	
White	
FLUPHENAZINE HYDROCHLORIDE	M/9
Tablets, USP, 2.5 mg ℞	
Yellow	
FLUPHENAZINE HYDROCHLORIDE	M/74
Tablets, USP, 5 mg ℞	
Green	
FLUPHENAZINE HYDROCHLORIDE	M/97
Tablets, USP, 10 mg ℞	
Orange	
FLURAZEPAM HYDROCHLORIDE	MYLAN 4415
Capsules, USP, 15 mg ⓒⅣ/℞	
White & Powder Blue	
FLURAZEPAM HYDROCHLORIDE	MYLAN 4430
Capsules, USP, 30 mg ⓒⅣ/℞	
Powder Blue & Powder Blue	
FLURBIPROFEN	M76/Blank
Tablets, USP, 50 mg ℞	
Beige	
FLURBIPROFEN	M93/Blank
Tablets, USP, 100 mg ℞	
Beige	
FLUVOXAMINE MALEATE	M407/Blank
Tablets, USP, 25 mg ℞	
Orange	
FLUVOXAMINE MALEATE	M412/Scored
Tablets, USP, 50 mg ℞	
Orange	
FLUVOXAMINE MALEATE	M414/Scored
Tablets, USP, 100 mg ℞	
Orange	

FUROSEMIDE	M2/Blank
Tablets, USP, 20 mg ℞	
White	
FUROSEMIDE	MYLAN 216/40
Tablets, USP, 40 mg ℞	
White	
FUROSEMIDE	MYLAN 232/80
Tablets, USP, 80 mg ℞	
White	
GALANTAMINE	M/G21
Tablets, USP, 4 mg ℞	
Blue	
GALANTAMINE	M/G22
Tablets, USP, 8 mg ℞	
Blue	
GALANTAMINE	M/G23
Tablets, USP, 12 mg ℞	
Blue	
GLIMEPIRIDE	MYLAN/G11
Tablets, USP, 1 mg ℞	
White	
GLIMEPIRIDE	MYLAN/G12
Tablets, USP, 2 mg ℞	
Light Yellow	
GLIMEPIRIDE	MYLAN/G13
Tablets, USP, 4 mg ℞	
Peach	
GLIPIZIDE	MYLAN G1/Blank
Tablets, USP, 5 mg ℞	
White	
GLIPIZIDE	MYLAN G2/Blank
Tablets, USP, 10 mg ℞	
White	
GLIPIZIDE and METFORMIN	M/G31
HYDROCHLORIDE	
Tablets, USP, 2.5 mg/250 mg ℞	
White	
GLIPIZIDE and METFORMIN	M/G32
HYDROCHLORIDE	
Tablets, USP, 2.5 mg/500 mg ℞	
White	
GLIPIZIDE and METFORMIN	M/G33
HYDROCHLORIDE	
Tablets, USP, 5 mg/500 mg ℞	
Peach	
GLYBURIDE	M113/Blank
Tablets, USP (micronized), 1.5 mg ℞	
White	
GLYBURIDE	M125/Blank
Tablets, USP (micronized), 3 mg ℞	
Lt. Yellow	
GLYBURIDE	M142/Blank
Tablets, USP (micronized), 6 mg ℞	
Green	
GRANISETRON HYDROCHLORIDE	M/G3
Tablets, 1 mg ℞	
White	
GUANFACINE	M/G4
Tablets, USP, 1 mg ℞	
White	
GUANFACINE	M/G5
Tablets, USP, 2 mg ℞	
Blue	
HALOPERIDOL	MYLAN 351/Scored
Tablets, USP, 0.5 mg ℞	
Orange	
HALOPERIDOL	MYLAN 257/Scored
Tablets, USP, 1 mg ℞	
Orange	
HALOPERIDOL	MYLAN 214/Scored
Tablets, USP, 2 mg ℞	
Orange	
HALOPERIDOL	MYLAN 327/Scored
Tablets, USP, 5 mg ℞	
Orange	
HALOPERIDOL	MYLAN 334/Scored
Tablets, USP, 10 mg ℞	
Light Green	
HALOPERIDOL	MYLAN 335/Scored
Tablets, USP, 20 mg ℞	
Light Blue	
HYDROCHLOROTHIAZIDE	MYLAN 810
Capsules, 12.5 mg ℞	
White	
HYDROCHLOROTHIAZIDE	M/H (score) 1
Tablets, USP, 25 mg ℞	
White to Off-White	
HYDROCHLOROTHIAZIDE	M/H (score) 2
Tablets, USP, 50 mg ℞	
White to Off-White	
HYDROXYCHLOROQUINE SULFATE	M/373
Tablets, USP, 200 mg ℞	
White	

HYDROXYZINE HYDROCHLORIDE	M/H10
Tablets, USP, 10 mg ℞	
Light Blue	
HYDROXYZINE HYDROCHLORIDE	M/H25
Tablets, USP, 25 mg ℞	
Blue	
HYDROXYZINE HYDROCHLORIDE	M/H50
Tablets, USP, 50 mg ℞	
Blue	
INDAPAMIDE	M/69
Tablets, USP, 1.25 mg ℞	
Pink	
INDAPAMIDE	M/80
Tablets, USP, 2.5 mg ℞	
White	
INDOMETHACIN	MYLAN 143
Capsules, USP, 25 mg ℞	
Lt. Green & Lt. Green	
INDOMETHACIN	MYLAN 147
Capsules, USP, 50 mg ℞	
Lt. Green & Lt. Green	
IPRATROPIUM BROMIDE and	3-mL sterile solution
ALBUTEROL SULFATE Inhalation Solution,	
0.5 mg/3.0 mg ℞	
IPRATROPIUM BROMIDE	N/A
Inhalation Solution, 0.02% ℞	
KETOCONAZOLE	M261/Blank
Tablets, USP, 200 mg ℞	
White to Off-white	
KETOPROFEN	MYLAN 8200
Extended-release Capsules, 200 mg ℞	
Blue Green & Iron Gray	
KETOPROFEN	MYLAN 4070
Capsules, 50 mg ℞	
Lt. Celery & Lt. Celery	
KETOPROFEN	MYLAN 5750
Capsules, 75 mg ℞	
Lt. Aqua & Lt. Aqua	
KETOROLAC TROMETHAMINE	M134
Tablets, USP, 10 mg ℞	
White	
LAMOTRIGINE	M/L (score) 51
Tablets, 25 mg ℞	
White to Off-white	
LAMOTRIGINE	M (score) L52/Blank
Tablets, 100 mg ℞	
White to Off-white	
LAMOTRIGINE	M (score) L53/Blank
Tablets, 150 mg ℞	
White to Off-white	
LAMOTRIGINE	M (score) L54/Blank
Tablets, 200 mg ℞	
Green	
LAMOTRIGINE	G/LY over 5
Tablets, (Chewable, Dispersible) 5 mg ℞	
White to Off-white	
LAMOTRIGINE	G/LY over 25
Tablets, (Chewable, Dispersible) 25 mg ℞	
White to Off-white	
LANSOPRAZOLE	MYLAN over 8015
Delayed-release Capsules, USP, 15 mg ℞	
Green Opaque & Green Opaque	
LANSOPRAZOLE	MYLAN over 8030
Delayed-release Capsules, USP, 30 mg ℞	
Pink Opaque & Pink Opaque	
LEVALBUTEROL	N/A
Inhalation Solution, USP, Concentrate, 1.25 mg ℞	
LEVETIRACETAM	M (score) 613/Blank
Tablets, 250 mg ℞	
White	
LEVETIRACETAM	M (score) 615/Blank
Tablets, 500 mg ℞	
White	
LEVETIRACETAM	M (score) 617/Blank
Tablets, 750 mg ℞	
White	
LEVETIRACETAM	M (score) 619/Blank
Tablets, 1000 mg ℞	
White	
LEVOTHYROXINE SODIUM	M/L (score) 4
Tablets, USP, 25 mcg ℞	
Orange	
LEVOTHYROXINE SODIUM	M/L (score) 5
Tablets, USP, 50 mcg ℞	
White	
LEVOTHYROXINE SODIUM	M/L (score) 6
Tablets, USP, 75 mcg ℞	
Violet	
LEVOTHYROXINE SODIUM	M/L (score) 7
Tablets, USP, 88 mcg ℞	
Olive	
LEVOTHYROXINE SODIUM	M/L (score) 8
Tablets, USP, 100 mcg ℞	
Yellow	
LEVOTHYROXINE SODIUM	M/L (score) 9
Tablets, USP, 112 mcg ℞	
Rose	

IMPORTANT NOTICE: Updated drug information is sent bi-monthly via the PDR® Update Insert. For *monthly* email updates, register at PDR.net.

LEVOTHYROXINE SODIUM — M/L (score) 10
Tablets, USP, 125 mcg ℞
Gray

LEVOTHYROXINE SODIUM — M/L (score) 15
Tablets, USP, 137 mcg ℞
Turquoise

LEVOTHYROXINE SODIUM — M/L (score) 11
Tablets, USP, 150 mcg ℞
Blue

LEVOTHYROXINE SODIUM — M/L (score) 12
Tablets, USP, 175 mcg ℞
Lilac

LEVOTHYROXINE SODIUM — M/L (score) 13
Tablets, USP, 200 mcg ℞
Pink

LEVOTHYROXINE SODIUM — M/L (score) 14
Tablets, USP, 300 mcg ℞
Green

LIOTHYRONINE SODIUM — ML/11
Tablets, USP, 5 mcg ℞
White to Off-white

LIOTHYRONINE SODIUM — M (score) L/12
Tablets, USP, 25 mcg ℞
White to Off-white

LIOTHYRONINE SODIUM — M (score) L/13
Tablets, USP, 50 mcg ℞
White to Off-white

LISINOPRIL — LH1/M
and HYDROCHLOROTHIAZIDE
Tablets, USP, 10 mg/12.5 mg ℞
White

LISINOPRIL — LH2/M
and HYDROCHLOROTHIAZIDE
Tablets, USP, 20 mg/12.5 mg ℞
Yellow

LISINOPRIL — LH3/M
and HYDROCHLOROTHIAZIDE
Tablets, USP, 20 mg/25 mg ℞
Green

LISINOPRIL — L22/M
Tablets, USP, 2.5 mg ℞
Blue

LISINOPRIL — ML23/M
Tablets, USP, 5 mg ℞
Peach

LISINOPRIL — L24/M
Tablets, USP, 10 mg ℞
White

LISINOPRIL — L25/M
Tablets, USP, 20 mg ℞
Yellow

LISINOPRIL — L27/M
Tablets, USP, 30 mg ℞
Blue

LISINOPRIL — L26/M
Tablets, USP, 40 mg ℞
Green

LOPERAMIDE HYDROCHLORIDE — MYLAN 2100
Capsules, USP, 2 mg ℞
Lt. Brown & Lt. Brown

LORAZEPAM — M/321
Tablets, USP, 0.5 mg Ⓒ/℞
White to Off-White

LORAZEPAM — MYLAN 457/Blank
Tablets, USP, 1 mg Ⓒ/℞
White to Off-White

LORAZEPAM — MYLAN 777/Blank
Tablets, USP, 2 mg Ⓒ/℞
White to Off-White

LOSARTAN POTASSIUM & — M/LH5
HYDROCHLOROTHIAZIDE
Tablets, 100 mg/12.5 mg ℞
Orange

LOVASTATIN — ML19/Blank
Tablets, USP, 10 mg ℞
White to Off-White

LOVASTATIN — ML20/Blank
Tablets, USP, 20 mg ℞
Yellow

LOVASTATIN — ML21/Blank
Tablets, USP, 40 mg ℞
Pink

LOXAPINE — MYLAN 7005
Capsules, USP, 5 mg ℞
Olive & Olive

LOXAPINE — MYLAN 7010
Capsules, USP, 10 mg ℞
Olive & Yellow

LOXAPINE — MYLAN 7025
Capsules, USP, 25 mg ℞
Olive & Lt. Green

LOXAPINE — MYLAN 7050
Capsules, USP, 50 mg ℞
Olive & Lt. Blue

MAPROTILINE HYDROCHLORIDE — M/60
Tablets, USP, 25 mg ℞
White

MAPROTILINE HYDROCHLORIDE — M/87
Tablets, USP, 50 mg ℞
Lt. Blue

MAPROTILINE HYDROCHLORIDE — M/92
Tablets, USP, 75 mg ℞
White

MAXZIDE® — MAXZIDE/B(score)M8
(triamterene & hydrochlorothiazide)
Tablets, 75 mg/50 mg ℞
Lt. Yellow

MAXZIDE®-25 mg Tablets — MAXZIDE/B(score)M9
(triamterene & hydrochlorothiazide)
Tablets, 37.5 mg/25 mg ℞
Lt. Green

MECLOFENAMATE SODIUM — MYLAN 2150
Capsules, USP, 50 mg ℞
Coral & Coral

MECLOFENAMATE SODIUM — MYLAN 3000
Capsules, USP, 100 mg ℞
Coral & White

MELOXICAM — M66/Blank
Tablets, USP, 7.5 mg ℞
Yellow

MELOXICAM — M89/Blank
Tablets, USP, 15 mg ℞
Yellow

MENTAX® — N/A
(butenafine hydrochloride)
Cream, 1% ℞
Lt. Yellow

MERCAPTOPURINE — M547/Blank
Tablets, USP, 50 mg ℞
Off-White to Light Yellow

METFORMIN HYDROCHLORIDE — M352/Blank
Extended-release Tablets, USP, 500 mg ℞
Tan

METFORMIN HYDROCHLORIDE — M350/Blank
Extended-release Tablets, USP, 750 mg ℞
Tan

METFORMIN HYDROCHLORIDE — M/234
Tablets, USP, 500 mg ℞
White

METFORMIN HYDROCHLORIDE — M/240
Tablets, USP, 850 mg ℞
White

METFORMIN HYDROCHLORIDE — M244/Scored
Tablets, USP, 1000 mg ℞
White

METFORMIN HYDROCHLORIDE — MF over 1/G
Tablets, USP, *Blackberry-scented*, 500 mg ℞
White to Off-White

METFORMIN HYDROCHLORIDE — MF over 2/G
Tablets, USP, *Blackberry-scented*, 850 mg ℞
White to Off-White

METFORMIN HYDROCHLORIDE — MF over 3/G score G
Tablets, USP, *Blackberry-scented*, 1000 mg ℞
White to Off-White

METHAMPHETAMINE HYDROCHLORIDE — 115/Blank
Tablets, USP, Ⓒ, 5 mg ℞
White

METHOTREXATE — M14/Blank
Tablets, USP, 2.5 mg ℞
Orange

METHYCLOTHIAZIDE — M29/Blank
Tablets, USP, 5 mg ℞
Blue

METHYLDOPA — MYLAN/611
Tablets, USP, 250 mg ℞
Beige

METHYLDOPA — MYLAN/421
Tablets, USP, 500 mg ℞
Beige

METHYLDOPA — MYLAN/507
and HYDROCHLOROTHIAZIDE
Tablets, USP, 250 mg/15 mg ℞
Green

METHYLDOPA — MYLAN/711
and HYDROCHLOROTHIAZIDE
Tablets, USP, 250 mg/25 mg ℞
Green

METOLAZONE — M/172
Tablets, USP, 2.5 mg ℞
Peach

METOLAZONE — M/173
Tablets, USP, 5 mg ℞
Orange

METOLAZONE — M/174
Tablets, USP, 10 mg ℞
Lt. Green

METOPROLOL TARTRATE — M424/Blank
and HYDROCHLOROTHIAZIDE
Tablets, USP, 50 mg/25 mg ℞
Peach

METOPROLOL TARTRATE — M434/Blank
and HYDROCHLOROTHIAZIDE
Tablets, USP, 100 mg/25 mg ℞
Peach

METOPROLOL TARTRATE — M445/Blank
and HYDROCHLOROTHIAZIDE
Tablets, USP, 100 mg/50 mg ℞
Peach

METOPROLOL TARTRATE — M18/Scored
Tablets, USP, 25 mg ℞
White

METOPROLOL TARTRATE — M32/Scored
Tablets, USP, 50 mg ℞
Pink

METOPROLOL TARTRATE — M47/Scored
Tablets, USP, 100 mg ℞
Lt. Blue

MIDODRINE HYDROCHLORIDE — MH1/M
Tablets, 2.5 mg ℞
White to Off-white

MIDODRINE HYDROCHLORIDE — MH2/M
Tablets, 5 mg ℞
White to Off-white

MIDODRINE HYDROCHLORIDE — MH3/M
Tablets, 10 mg ℞
White to Off-white

MIRTAZAPINE — M515/Scored
Tablets, USP, 15 mg ℞
Beige

MIRTAZAPINE — M530/Scored
Tablets, USP, 30 mg ℞
Beige

MIRTAZAPINE — M545/Blank
Tablets, USP, 45 mg ℞
Beige

MYCOPHENOLATE MOFETIL — MYLAN over 2250
Capsules, 250 mg ℞
Caramel & Lavender

MYCOPHENOLATE MOFETIL — MYLAN/472
Tablets, 500 mg ℞
Light Pink

NADOLOL and — M score 96/Blank
BENDROFLUMETHIAZIDE
Tablets, USP, 40 mg/5g ℞
Yellow

NADOLOL and — M score 99/Blank
BENDROFLUMETHIAZIDE
Tablets, USP, 80 mg/5g ℞
Yellow

NADOLOL — M28/Blank
Tablets, USP, 20 mg ℞
Yellow

NADOLOL — M171/Blank
Tablets, USP, 40 mg ℞
Yellow

NADOLOL — M132/Blank
Tablets, USP, 80 mg ℞
Yellow

NAPROXEN — MYLAN/377
Tablets, USP, 250 mg ℞
White

NAPROXEN — MYLAN/555
Tablets, USP, 375 mg ℞
White

NAPROXEN — MYLAN/451
Tablets, USP, 500 mg ℞
White

NICARDIPINE HYDROCHLORIDE — MYLAN 1020
Capsules, 20 mg ℞
Med. Blue Green & Ivory

NICARDIPINE HYDROCHLORIDE — MYLAN 1430
Capsules, 30 mg ℞
Bluish Green & Rich Yellow

NIFEDIPINE — M over 030/Blank
Extended-release Tablets, USP, 30 mg ℞
Light Pink

NIFEDIPINE — M over 060/Blank
Extended-release Tablets, USP, 60 mg ℞
Light Pink

NIFEDIPINE — M over 090/Blank
Extended-release Tablets, USP, 90 mg ℞
Light Pink

NISOLDIPINE — M/N over 22
Extended-release Tablets, 20 mg ℞
Beige

NISOLDIPINE — M/N over 23
Extended-release Tablets, 30 mg ℞
Orange

NISOLDIPINE — M/N over 24
Extended-release Tablets, 40 mg ℞
Yellow

Drug	Code
NITROFURANTOIN Monohydrate/Macrocrystals Capsules, USP, 100 mg Rx *Lt. gray & Lt. brown*	MYLAN 3422
NITROFURANTOIN (Macrocrystals) Capsules, USP, 50 mg Rx *Lt. Brown & Lt. Brown*	MYLAN 1650
NITROFURANTOIN (Macrocrystals) Capsules, USP, 100 mg Rx *Gray & Gray*	MYLAN 1700
NITROGLYCERIN TRANSDERMAL SYSTEM Patches, 0.1 mg/hr Rx *Translucent*	Nitroglycerin 0.1 mg/hr
NITROGLYCERIN TRANSDERMAL SYSTEM Patches, 0.2 mg/hr Rx *Translucent*	Nitroglycerin 0.2 mg/hr
NITROGLYCERIN TRANSDERMAL SYSTEM Patches, 0.4 mg/hr Rx *Translucent*	Nitroglycerin 0.4 mg/hr
NITROGLYCERIN TRANSDERMAL SYSTEM Patches, 0.6 mg/hr Rx *Translucent*	Nitroglycerin 0.6 mg/hr
NIZATIDINE Capsules, USP, 150 mg Rx *Lavender & Lt. Lavender*	MYLAN 5150
NIZATIDINE Capsules, USP, 300 mg Rx *Lavender & Lavender*	MYLAN 5300
OMEPRAZOLE Delayed-release Capsules, USP, 10 mg Rx *Dark Green & Dark Green*	MYLAN 5211
OMEPRAZOLE Delayed-release Capsules, USP, 20 mg Rx *Dark Green & Blue-Green*	MYLAN 6150
OMEPRAZOLE Delayed-release Capsules, USP, 40 mg Rx *Dark Green & Light Blue*	MYLAN over 5222
ONDANSETRON HYDROCHLORIDE Tablets, 4 mg Rx *White*	M/315
ONDANSETRON HYDROCHLORIDE Tablets, 8 mg Rx *Orange*	M/344
ONDANSETRON ORALLY DISINTEGRATING Tablets, USP, 4 mg Rx *White to Off-White*	M/732
ONDANSETRON ORALLY DISINTEGRATING Tablets, USP, 8 mg Rx *White to Off-White*	M/734
OXYBUTYNIN CHLORIDE Extended-release Tablets, USP, 5 mg Rx *Light Green*	M O5/Blank
OXYBUTYNIN CHLORIDE Extended-release Tablets, USP, 10 mg Rx *Peach*	M O10/Blank
OXYBUTYNIN CHLORIDE Extended-release Tablets, USP, 15 mg Rx *Gray*	M O17/Blank
OXYCODONE and ACETAMINOPHEN Tablets, USP, 2.5 mg/325 mg CII/Rx *White*	103/Blank
OXYCODONE and ACETAMINOPHEN Tablets, USP, 5 mg/325 mg CII/Rx *White*	104 (score) Blank/Blank
OXYCODONE and ACETAMINOPHEN Tablets, USP, 7.5 mg/325 mg CII/Rx *White*	105/Blank
OXYCODONE and ACETAMINOPHEN Tablets, USP, 10 mg/325 mg CII/Rx *White*	106/Blank
OXYCODONE and ACETAMINOPHEN Tablets, USP, 7.5 mg/500 mg CII/Rx *White*	107/Blank
OXYCODONE and ACETAMINOPHEN Tablets, USP, 10 mg/650 mg CII/Rx *White*	108/Blank
PAROXETINE HYDROCHLORIDE Extended-release Tablets, 12.5 mg Rx *White*	M P3/Blank
PAROXETINE HYDROCHLORIDE Extended-release Tablets, 25 mg Rx *Lavender*	M P4/Blank
PAROXETINE HYDROCHLORIDE Controlled-release Tablets, 37.5 mg Rx *Blue*	PL PCR/375
PAROXETINE Tablets, USP, 10 mg Rx *Blue*	M/N score 1
PAROXETINE Tablets, USP, 20 mg Rx *Blue*	M/N score 2
PAROXETINE Tablets, USP, 30 mg Rx *Blue*	M over N3/Blank
PAROXETINE Tablets, USP, 40 mg Rx *Blue*	M over N4/Blank
PEG-3350, SODIUM CHLORIDE, SODIUM BICARBONATE & POTASSIUM CHLORIDE for Oral Solution with Flavor Packs Rx	N/A
PENTOXIFYLLINE Extended-release Tablets, USP, 400 mg Rx *Lavender*	MYLAN/357
PERPHENAZINE and AMITRIPTYLINE HYDROCHLORIDE Tablets, USP, 2 mg/10 mg Rx *White*	MYLAN/330
PERPHENAZINE and AMITRIPTYLINE HYDROCHLORIDE Tablets, USP, 2 mg/25 mg Rx *Purple*	MYLAN/442
PERPHENAZINE and AMITRIPTYLINE HYDROCHLORIDE Tablets, USP, 4 mg/10 mg Rx *Blue*	MYLAN/727
PERPHENAZINE and AMITRIPTYLINE HYDROCHLORIDE Tablets, USP, 4 mg/25 mg Rx *Orange*	MYLAN/574
PERPHENAZINE and AMITRIPTYLINE HYDROCHLORIDE Tablets, USP, 4 mg/50 mg Rx *Purple*	MYLAN/73
PHENYTEK® (extended phenytoin sodium) Capsules, 200 mg Rx *Dark Blue & Blue*	BERTEK/670
PHENYTEK® (extended phenytoin sodium) Capsules, 300 mg Rx *Blue & Blue*	BERTEK/750
EXTENDED PHENYTOIN SODIUM Capsules, USP, 100 mg Rx *Lt. Lavender & White*	MYLAN 1560
PINDOLOL Tablets, USP, 5 mg Rx *White*	M52/Blank
PINDOLOL Tablets, USP, 10 mg Rx *White*	M127/Blank
POLYETHYLENE GLYCOL 3350 and ELECTROLYTES for Oral Solution, USP Rx	N/A
PRAVASTATIN SODIUM Tablets, USP, 10 mg Rx *Light Pink*	P 14/Blank
PRAVASTATIN SODIUM Tablets, USP, 20 mg Rx *Light Yellow*	P 15/Blank
PRAVASTATIN SODIUM Tablets, USP, 40 mg Rx *Light Blue*	P 16/Blank
PRAVASTATIN SODIUM Tablets, USP, 80 mg Rx *Peach*	P 18/Blank
PRAZOSIN HYDROCHLORIDE Capsules, USP, 1 mg Rx *Dark Green & Lt. Brown*	MYLAN 1101
PRAZOSIN HYDROCHLORIDE Capsules, USP, 2 mg Rx *Brown & Lt. Brown*	MYLAN 2302
PRAZOSIN HYDROCHLORIDE Capsules, USP, 5 mg Rx *Lt. Blue & Lt. Brown*	MYLAN 3205
PROBENECID Tablets, USP, 500 mg Rx *Yellow*	MYLAN 156/500
PROCHLORPERAZINE MALEATE Tablets, USP, 5 mg Rx *Maroon*	M/P1
PROCHLORPERAZINE MALEATE Tablets, USP, 10 mg Rx *Maroon*	M/P2
PROPOXYPHENE HYDROCHLORIDE Capsules, USP, 65 mg CIV/Rx *Rose & Rose*	MYLAN 7065
PROPOXYPHENE HYDROCHLORIDE and ACETAMINOPHEN Tablets, USP, 65 mg/650 mg CIV/Rx *Orange*	MYLAN/130
PROPOXYPHENE NAPSYLATE and ACETAMINOPHEN Tablets, USP, 100 mg/650 mg CIV/Rx *Pink*	MYLAN/155
PROPRANOLOL HYDROCHLORIDE Extended-release Capsules, USP, 60 mg Rx *Blue Violet & Pink*	MYLAN/6160
PROPRANOLOL HYDROCHLORIDE Extended-release Capsules, USP, 80 mg Rx *Orange & Pink*	MYLAN/6180
PROPRANOLOL HYDROCHLORIDE Extended-release Capsules, USP, 120 mg Rx *Blue Violet & Blue Violet*	MYLAN/6220
PROPRANOLOL HYDROCHLORIDE Extended-release Capsules, USP, 160 mg Rx *Pink & Pink*	MYLAN/6260
PROPRANOLOL HYDROCHLORIDE Tablets, USP, 10 mg Rx *Orange*	MYLAN 182/10
PROPRANOLOL HYDROCHLORIDE Tablets, USP, 20 mg Rx *Blue*	MYLAN 183/20
PROPRANOLOL HYDROCHLORIDE Tablets, USP, 40 mg Rx *Green*	MYLAN 184/40
PROPRANOLOL HYDROCHLORIDE Tablets, USP, 80 mg Rx *Yellow*	MYLAN 185/80
PROPRANOLOL HYDROCHLORIDE and HYDROCHLOROTHIAZIDE Tablets, USP, 40 mg/25 mg Rx *White*	MYLAN 731/Scored
PROPRANOLOL HYDROCHLORIDE and HYDROCHLOROTHIAZIDE Tablets, USP, 80 mg/25 mg Rx *White*	MYLAN 347/Scored
QUINAPRIL HYDROCHLORIDE and HYDROCHLOROTHIAZIDE Tablets, 10 mg/12.5 mg Rx *Pink*	M (score) 542/Blank
QUINAPRIL HYDROCHLORIDE and HYDROCHLOROTHIAZIDE Tablets, 20 mg/12.5 mg Rx *Yellow*	M (score) 543/Blank
QUINAPRIL HYDROCHLORIDE and HYDROCHLOROTHIAZIDE Tablets, 20 mg/25 mg Rx *Pink*	M (score) 544/Blank
QUINAPRIL Tablets, USP, 5 mg Rx *Orange*	M/1 Score 7
QUINAPRIL Tablets, USP, 10 mg Rx *Orange*	M/226
QUINAPRIL Tablets, USP, 20 mg Rx *Orange*	M/254
QUINAPRIL Tablets, USP, 40 mg Rx *Orange*	M/272
RISPERIDONE Tablets, USP, 0.25 mg Rx *White*	M/R
RISPERIDONE Tablets, USP, 0.5 mg Rx *Beige*	M/R5
RISPERIDONE Tablets, USP, 1 mg Rx *White*	M/R11
RISPERIDONE Tablets, USP, 2 mg Rx *Beige*	M/R12
RISPERIDONE Tablets, USP, 3 mg Rx *White*	M/R13
RISPERIDONE Tablets, USP, 4 mg Rx *Beige*	M/R14
ROPINIROLE HYDROCHLORIDE Tablets, 0.25 mg Rx *White*	M/N over 25
ROPINIROLE HYDROCHLORIDE Tablets, 0.5 mg Rx *Yellow*	M/N over 5
ROPINIROLE HYDROCHLORIDE Tablets, 1 mg Rx *Green*	M/N over 10
ROPINIROLE HYDROCHLORIDE Tablets, 2 mg Rx *Orange*	M/N over 20
ROPINIROLE HYDROCHLORIDE Tablets, 3 mg Rx *Lavender*	M/N over 30
ROPINIROLE HYDROCHLORIDE Tablets, 4 mg Rx *Grayish Beige*	M/N over 40

ROPINIROLE HYDROCHLORIDE	M/N over 50
Tablets, 5 mg ℞	
Blue	
SELEGILINE HYDROCHLORIDE	SE over 5/G
Tablets, USP, 5 mg ℞	
White	
SERTRALINE HYDROCHLORIDE	M (score) S1/Blank
Tablets, 25 mg ℞	
Light Green	
SERTRALINE HYDROCHLORIDE	M (score) S2/Blank
Tablets, 50 mg ℞	
Light Green	
SERTRALINE HYDROCHLORIDE	M (score) S3/Blank
Tablets, 100 mg ℞	
Light Green	
SODIUM CHLORIDE	N/A
Inhalation Solution, USP, 3.0%/15 mL ℞	
SODIUM CHLORIDE	N/A
Inhalation Solution, USP, 10.0%/15 mL ℞	
SODIUM CHLORIDE	N/A
Inhalation Solution, USP, 0.9%/3 mL ℞	
SODIUM CHLORIDE	N/A
Inhalation Solution, USP, 0.9%/5 mL ℞	
SODIUM CHLORIDE	N/A
Inhalation Solution, USP, 0.9%/15 mL ℞	
SOTALOL HYDROCHLORIDE	M305/Blank
Tablets, USP, 80 mg ℞	
Lt. Orange	
SOTALOL HYDROCHLORIDE	M310/Blank
Tablets, USP, 120 mg ℞	
Lt. Orange	
SOTALOL HYDROCHLORIDE	M314/Blank
Tablets, USP, 160 mg ℞	
Lt. Orange	
SOTALOL HYDROCHLORIDE	M (score) S23/Blank
Tablets, USP (AF), 80 mg ℞	
Lt. Orange	
SOTALOL HYDROCHLORIDE	M (score) S24/Blank
Tablets, USP (AF), 120 mg ℞	
Lt. Orange	
SOTALOL HYDROCHLORIDE	M (score) S25/Blank
Tablets, USP (AF), 160 mg ℞	
Lt. Orange	
SPIRONOLACTONE	M146/Blank
Tablets, USP, 25 mg ℞	
White	
SPIRONOLACTONE	M243/Scored
Tablets, USP, 50 mg ℞	
White	
SPIRONOLACTONE	M437/Scored
Tablets, USP, 100 mg ℞	
White	
SPIRONOLACTONE and	M41/Blank
HYDROCHLOROTHIAZIDE	
Tablets, USP, 25 mg/25 mg ℞	
Ivory	
STAVUDINE	M 154
Capsules, USP, 15 mg ℞	
Off-white & Pink	
STAVUDINE	M 155
Capsules, USP, 20 mg ℞	
Pink & Pink	
STAVUDINE	M 137
Capsules, USP, 30 mg ℞	
Off-white & Light Orange	
STAVUDINE	M 138
Capsules, USP, 40 mg ℞	
Light Orange & Light Orange	
SULINDAC	MYLAN/427
Tablets, USP, 150 mg ℞	
Yellow-Orange	
SULINDAC	MYLAN 531/Blank
Tablets, USP, 200 mg ℞	
Yellow-Orange	
SUMATRIPTAN SUCCINATE	M/S4
Tablets, 25 mg ℞	
White	
SUMATRIPTAN SUCCINATE	M over S7/Blank
Tablets, 50 mg ℞	
White	
SUMATRIPTAN SUCCINATE	M over S12/Blank
Tablets, 100 mg ℞	
White	
TAMOXIFEN CITRATE	M/144
Tablets, USP, 10 mg ℞	
White	
TAMOXIFEN CITRATE	M/274
Tablets, USP, 20 mg ℞	
White to Off-White	
TAMSULOSIN HYDROCHLORIDE	MYLAN over 2500
Capsules, USP, 0.4 mg ℞	
Blue Opaque & Blue Opaque	
TEMAZEPAM	MYLAN over 3110
Capsules, USP, 7.5 mg ℞	
Peach Opaque & Ivory Opaque	

TEMAZEPAM	MYLAN 4010
Capsules, USP, 15 mg Ⓒ/℞	
Peach & Peach	
TEMAZEPAM	MYLAN 3120
Capsules, USP, 22.5 mg ℞	
Yellow and Peach	
TEMAZEPAM	MYLAN 5050
Capsules, USP, 30 mg Ⓒ/℞	
Yellow & Yellow	
TERAZOSIN HYDROCHLORIDE	MYLAN 2260
Capsules, 1 mg ℞	
Rich Yellow & Lt. Lavender	
TERAZOSIN HYDROCHLORIDE	MYLAN 2264
Capsules, 2 mg ℞	
Black & Lt. Lavender	
TERAZOSIN HYDROCHLORIDE	MYLAN 2268
Capsules, 5 mg ℞	
Iron Gray & Lt. Lavender	
TERAZOSIN HYDROCHLORIDE	MYLAN 1570
Capsules, 10 mg ℞	
Lt. Lavender & Lt. Lavender	
TERBINAFINE HYDROCHLORIDE	M 571/Blank
Tablets, 250 mg ℞	
White to Off-White	
THIORIDAZINE HYDROCHLORIDE	M54/10
Tablets, USP, 10 mg ℞	
Orange	
THIORIDAZINE HYDROCHLORIDE	M58/25
Tablets, USP, 25 mg ℞	
Orange	
THIORIDAZINE HYDROCHLORIDE	M59/50
Tablets, USP, 50 mg ℞	
Orange	
THIORIDAZINE HYDROCHLORIDE	M61/100
Tablets, USP, 100 mg ℞	
Orange	
THIOTHIXENE	MYLAN 1001
Capsules, USP, 1 mg ℞	
Caramel & Powder Blue	
THIOTHIXENE	MYLAN 2002
Capsules, USP, 2 mg ℞	
Caramel & Yellow	
THIOTHIXENE	MYLAN 3005
Capsules, USP, 5 mg ℞	
Caramel & White	
THIOTHIXENE	MYLAN 5010
Capsules, USP, 10 mg ℞	
Caramel & Peach	
TIMOLOL MALEATE	M55/Blank
Tablets, USP, 5 mg ℞	
Green	
TIMOLOL MALEATE	M221/Blank
Tablets, USP, 10 mg ℞	
Green	
TIMOLOL MALEATE	M715/Blank
Tablets, USP, 20 mg ℞	
Green	
TIZANIDINE	M 722/Scored
Tablets, USP, 2 mg ℞	
White to Off-White	
TIZANIDINE	M 724/Quadrisect Scored
Tablets, USP, 4 mg ℞	
White to Off-White	
TOLAZAMIDE	MYLAN 217/250
Tablets, USP, 250 mg ℞	
White to Off-white	
TOLAZAMIDE	MYLAN 551/Blank
Tablets, USP, 500 mg ℞	
White to Off-white	
TOLBUTAMIDE	M13/Blank
Tablets, USP, 500 mg ℞	
White to Off-white	
TOLMETIN SODIUM	MYLAN 5200
Capsules, USP, 400 mg ℞	
Lt. Blue & Lt. Blue	
TOLMETIN SODIUM	M313/Blank
Tablets, USP, 600 mg ℞	
Beige	
TOPIRAMATE	Mylan over 2035
Capsules (Sprinkle), 15 mg ℞	
Natural & Flesh Opaque	
TOPIRAMATE	Mylan over 2036
Capsules (Sprinkle), 25 mg ℞	
Natural & Flesh Opaque	
TOPIRAMATE	M over T11/Blank
Tablets, 25 mg ℞	
White	
TOPIRAMATE	M over T12/Blank
Tablets, 50 mg ℞	
White	
TOPIRAMATE	M over T13/Blank
Tablets, 100 mg ℞	
White	

TOPIRAMATE	M T15/Blank
Tablets, 200 mg ℞	
White	
TRAMADOL HYDROCHLORIDE	M/T7
Tablets, 50 mg ℞	
White	
TRAMADOL HYDROCHLORIDE	M/P/T
and ACETAMINOPHEN	
Tablets, 37.5 mg/325 mg ℞	
Yellow	
TRANDOLAPRIL	M/T (score) 41
Tablets, 1 mg ℞	
White to Off-white	
TRANDOLAPRIL	M/T42
Tablets, 2 mg ℞	
White to Off-white	
TRANDOLAPRIL	M/T43
Tablets, 4 mg ℞	
Beige	
TRAZODONE HYDROCHLORIDE	MX score 71/Blank
Tablets, USP, 50 mg ℞	
Light Yellow	
TRAZODONE HYDROCHLORIDE	MX score 72/Blank
Tablets, USP, 100 mg ℞	
Light Yellow	
TRAZODONE HYDROCHLORIDE	MX 73/Bisect and Partial Trisects
Tablets, USP, 150 mg ℞	
Light Yellow	
TRAZODONE HYDROCHLORIDE	MX 74/Bisect and Partial Trisects
Tablets, USP, 300 mg ℞	
Light Yellow	
TRIAMTERENE and	MYLAN 2537
HYDROCHLOROTHIAZIDE	
Capsules, USP, 37.5 mg/25 mg ℞	
Olive & Rich Yellow	
TRIAMTERENE and	MYLAN/TH1
HYDROCHLOROTHIAZIDE	
Tablets, USP, 37.5 mg/25 mg ℞	
Green	
TRIAMTERENE and	MYLAN/TH2
HYDROCHLOROTHIAZIDE	
Tablets, USP, 75 mg/50 mg ℞	
Yellow	
TRIFLUOPERAZINE HYDROCHLORIDE	M/T3
Tablets, USP, 1 mg ℞	
White	
TRIFLUOPERAZINE HYDROCHLORIDE	M/T4
Tablets, USP, 2 mg ℞	
White	
TRIFLUOPERAZINE HYDROCHLORIDE	M/T5
Tablets, USP, 5 mg ℞	
Lavender	
TRIFLUOPERAZINE HYDROCHLORIDE	M/T6
Tablets, USP, 10 mg ℞	
Lavender	
URSODIOL	MYLAN over 1930
Capsules, USP, 300 mg ℞	
Peach Opaque & White Opaque	
VALACYCLOVIR HYDROCHLORIDE	M122/Blank
Tablets, 500 mg ℞	
White	
VALACYCLOVIR HYDROCHLORIDE	M123/Blank
Tablets, 1 gram ℞	
White	
VENLAFAXINE HYDROCHLORIDE	V score 1/M
Tablets, 25 mg ℞	
Yellow	
VENLAFAXINE HYDROCHLORIDE	V score 2/M
Tablets, 37.5 mg ℞	
Yellow	
VENLAFAXINE HYDROCHLORIDE	V score 3/M
Tablets, 50 mg ℞	
Yellow	
VENLAFAXINE HYDROCHLORIDE	M score V4/Blank
Tablets, 75 mg ℞	
Yellow	
VENLAFAXINE HYDROCHLORIDE	M score V5/Blank
Tablets, 100 mg ℞	
Yellow	
VERAPAMIL HYDROCHLORIDE	MYLAN 6320
Extended-release Capsules, 120 mg ℞	
Bluish Green & White	
VERAPAMIL HYDROCHLORIDE	MYLAN 6380
Extended-release Capsules, 180 mg ℞	
Bluish Green & Lt. Green	
VERAPAMIL HYDROCHLORIDE	MYLAN 6440
Extended-release Capsules, 240 mg ℞	
Bluish Green & Bluish Green	
VERAPAMIL HYDROCHLORIDE	Mylan/6201
Extended-release Capsules (PM)	
(Controlled-Onset), 100 mg ℞	
Red & White	
VERAPAMIL HYDROCHLORIDE	Mylan/6202
Extended-release Capsules (PM)	
(Controlled-Onset), 200 mg ℞	
Red & Light Orange	

VERAPAMIL HYDROCHLORIDE Mylan/6203
Extended-release Capsules (PM)
(Controlled-Onset), 300 mg ℞
Red & Red
VERAPAMIL HYDROCHLORIDE MYLAN/244
Extended-release Tablets, USP, 120 mg ℞
Blue
VERAPAMIL HYDROCHLORIDE M312/Blank
Extended-release Tablets, USP, 180 mg ℞
Blue
VERAPAMIL HYDROCHLORIDE M411/Blank
Extended-release Tablets, USP, 240 mg ℞
Blue
VERAPAMIL HYDROCHLORIDE MYLAN 512/Blank
Tablets, USP, 80 mg ℞
White
VERAPAMIL HYDROCHLORIDE MYLAN 772/Blank
Tablets, USP, 120 mg ℞
White
ZALEPLON G/ZA5
Capsules, 5 mg CIV/℞
Peach & Peach
ZALEPLON G/ZA10
Capsules, 10 mg CIV/℞
White & White
ZIDOVUDINE M 106/Blank
Tablets, USP, 300 mg ℞
White to Off-white
ZOLPIDEM TARTRATE MZ1/Blank
Tablets, 5 mg CIV/℞
Lavender
ZOLPIDEM TARTRATE MZ2/Blank
Tablets, 10 mg CIV/℞
Lavender
ZONISAMIDE MYLAN/6725
Capsules, 25 mg ℞
Violet & Lavender
ZONISAMIDE MYLAN/6726
Capsules, 50 mg ℞
Violet & White
ZONISAMIDE MYLAN/6727
Capsules, 100 mg ℞
Violet & Light Blue

*Front/Back Side for Tablets or Both Cap and Body for Capsules.

CAPTOPRIL TABLETS, USP ℞
12.5 mg, 25 mg, 50 mg and 100 mg

> **USE IN PREGNANCY**
> **When used in pregnancy during the second and third trimesters, ACE inhibitors can cause injury and even death to the developing fetus.** When pregnancy is detected, captopril should be discontinued as soon as possible. **See WARNINGS: Fetal/Neonatal Morbidity and Mortality.**

DESCRIPTION

Captopril is a specific competitive inhibitor of angiotensin I-converting enzyme (ACE), the enzyme responsible for the conversion of angiotensin I to angiotensin II.
Captopril is designated chemically as 1-[(2S)-3-mercapto-2-methylpropionyl]-L-proline (MW 217.29).
Captopril is a white to off-white crystalline powder that may have a slight sulfurous odor; it is soluble in water (approx. 160 mg/mL), methanol, and ethanol and sparingly soluble in chloroform and ethyl acetate.
The structural formula is:

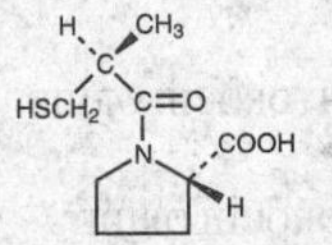

$C_9H_{15}NO_3S$

Each tablet for oral administration contains 12.5 mg, 25 mg, 50 mg or 100 mg of captopril and the following inactive ingredients: anhydrous lactose, colloidal silicon dioxide, crospovidone, microcrystalline cellulose and stearic acid.

CLINICAL PHARMACOLOGY

Mechanism of Action: The mechanism of action of captopril has not yet been fully elucidated. Its beneficial effects in hypertension and heart failure appear to result primarily from suppression of the renin-angiotensin-aldosterone system. However, there is no consistent correlation between renin levels and response to the drug. Renin, an enzyme synthesized by the kidneys, is released into the circulation where it acts on a plasma globulin substrate to produce angiotensin I, a relatively inactive decapeptide. Angiotensin I is then converted by angiotensin converting enzyme (ACE) to angiotensin II, a potent endogenous vasoconstrictor substance. Angiotensin II also stimulates aldosterone secretion from the adrenal cortex, thereby contributing to sodium and fluid retention.
Captopril prevents the conversion of angiotensin I to angiotensin II by inhibition of ACE, a peptidyldipeptide carboxy hydrolase. This inhibition has been demonstrated in both healthy human subjects and in animals by showing that the elevation of blood pressure caused by exogenously administered angiotensin I was attenuated or abolished by captopril. In animal studies, captopril did not alter the pressor responses to a number of other agents, including angiotensin II and norepinephrine, indicating specificity of action.
ACE is identical to "bradykininase", and captopril may also interfere with the degradation of the vasodepressor peptide, bradykinin. Increased concentrations of bradykinin or prostaglandin E_2 may also have a role in the therapeutic effect of captopril.
Inhibition of ACE results in decreased plasma angiotensin II and increased plasma renin activity (PRA), the latter resulting from loss of negative feedback on renin release caused by reduction in angiotensin II. The reduction of angiotensin II leads to decreased aldosterone secretion, and, as a result, small increases in serum potassium may occur along with sodium and fluid loss.
The antihypertensive effects persist for a longer period of time than does demonstrable inhibition of circulating ACE. It is not known whether the ACE present in vascular endothelium is inhibited longer than the ACE in circulating blood.

Pharmacokinetics: After oral administration of therapeutic doses of captopril, rapid absorption occurs with peak blood levels at about one hour. The presence of food in the gastrointestinal tract reduces absorption by about 30 to 40 percent; captopril therefore should be given one hour before meals. Based on carbon-14 labeling, average minimal absorption is approximately 75 percent. In a 24-hour period, over 95 percent of the absorbed dose is eliminated in the urine; 40 to 50 percent is unchanged drug; most of the remainder is the disulfide dimer of captopril and captopril-cysteine disulfide.
Approximately 25 to 30 percent of the circulating drug is bound to plasma proteins. The apparent elimination half-life for total radioactivity in blood is probably less than 3 hours. An accurate determination of half-life of unchanged captopril is not, at present, possible, but it is probably less than 2 hours. In patients with renal impairment, however, retention of captopril occurs (see DOSAGE AND ADMINISTRATION).

Pharmacodynamics: Administration of captopril results in a reduction of peripheral arterial resistance in hypertensive patients with either no change, or an increase, in cardiac output. There is an increase in renal blood flow following administration of captopril and glomerular filtration rate is usually unchanged.
Reductions of blood pressure are usually maximal 60 to 90 minutes after oral administration of an individual dose of captopril. The duration of effect is dose related. The reduction in blood pressure may be progressive, so to achieve maximal therapeutic effects, several weeks of therapy may be required. The blood pressure lowering effects of captopril and thiazide-type diuretics are additive. In contrast, captopril and beta-blockers have a less than additive effect. Blood pressure is lowered to about the same extent in both standing and supine positions. Orthostatic effects and tachycardia are infrequent but may occur in volume-depleted patients. Abrupt withdrawal of captopril has not been associated with a rapid increase in blood pressure.
In patients with heart failure, significantly decreased peripheral (systemic vascular) resistance and blood pressure (afterload), reduced pulmonary capillary wedge pressure (preload) and pulmonary vascular resistance, increased cardiac output, and increased exercise tolerance time (ETT) have been demonstrated. These hemodynamic and clinical effects occur after the first dose and appear to persist for the duration of therapy. Placebo controlled studies of 12 weeks duration in patients who did not respond adequately to diuretics and digitalis show no tolerance to beneficial effects on ETT; open studies, with exposure up to 18 months in some cases, also indicate that ETT benefit is maintained. Clinical improvement has been observed in some patients where acute hemodynamic effects were minimal.
The Survival and Ventricular Enlargement (SAVE) study was a multicenter, randomized, double-blind, placebo-controlled trial conducted in 2,231 patients (age 21 to 79 years) who survived the acute phase of a myocardial infarction and did not have active ischemia. Patients had left ventricular dysfunction (LVD), defined as a resting left ventricular ejection fraction ≤ 40%, but at the time of randomization were not sufficiently symptomatic to require ACE inhibitor therapy for heart failure. About half of the patients had had symptoms of heart failure in the past. Patients were given a test dose of 6.25 mg oral captopril and were within 3 to 16 days post-infarction to receive either captopril or placebo in addition to conventional therapy. Captopril was initiated at 6.25 mg or 12.5 mg tid and after two weeks titrated to a target maintenance dose of 50 mg tid. About 80% of patients were receiving the target dose at the end of the study. Patients were followed for a minimum of two years and for up to five years, with an average follow-up of 3.5 years.
Baseline blood pressure was 113/70 mm Hg and 112/70 mm Hg for the placebo and captopril groups, respectively. Blood pressure increased slightly in both treatment groups during the study and was somewhat lower in the captopril group (119/74 vs. 125/77 mm Hg at 1 yr).
Therapy with captopril improved long-term survival and clinical outcomes compared to placebo. The risk reduction for all cause mortality was 19% (P = 0.02) and for cardiovascular death was 21% (P = 0.014). Captopril treated subjects had 22% (P = 0.034) fewer first hospitalizations for heart failure. Compared to placebo, 22% fewer patients receiving captopril developed symptoms of overt heart failure. There was no significant difference between groups in total hospitalizations for all cause (2056 placebo; 2036 captopril).
In a multicenter study, a marketed brand of captopril tablets, USP were well tolerated in the presence of other therapies such as aspirin, beta blockers, nitrates, vasodilators, calcium antagonists and diuretics.
Studies in rats and cats indicate that captopril does not cross the blood-brain barrier to any significant extent.

INDICATIONS AND USAGE

Hypertension: Captopril tablets, USP are indicated for the treatment of hypertension.
In using captopril, consideration should be given to the risk of neutropenia/agranulocytosis (see WARNINGS).
Captopril may be used as initial therapy for patients with normal renal function, in whom the risk is relatively low. In patients with impaired renal function, particularly those with collagen vascular disease, captopril should be reserved for hypertensives who have either developed unacceptable side effects on other drugs, or have failed to respond satisfactorily to drug combinations.
Captopril is effective alone and in combination with other antihypertensive agents, especially thiazide-type diuretics. The blood pressure lowering effects of captopril and thiazides are approximately additive.

Heart Failure: Captopril tablets, USP are indicated in the treatment of congestive heart failure usually in combination with diuretics and digitalis. The beneficial effect of captopril in heart failure does not require the presence of digitalis, however, most controlled clinical trial experience with captopril has been in patients receiving digitalis, as well as diuretic treatment.

Left Ventricular Dysfunction After Myocardial Infarction: Captopril tablets, USP are indicated to improve survival following myocardial infarction in clinically stable patients with left ventricular dysfunction manifested as an ejection fraction ≤ 40% and to reduce the incidence of overt heart failure and subsequent hospitalizations for congestive heart failure in these patients.
In considering use of captopril tablets, USP it should be noted that in controlled trials ACE inhibitors have an effect on blood pressure that is less in black patients than in non-blacks. In addition, ACE inhibitors (for which adequate data are available) cause a higher rate of angioedema in black than in non-black patients (see WARNINGS: Head and Neck Angioedema and Intestinal Angioedema).

CONTRAINDICATIONS

Captopril tablets, USP are contraindicated in patients who are hypersensitive to this product or any other angiotensin-converting enzyme inhibitor (e.g., a patient who has experienced angioedema during therapy with any other ACE inhibitor).

WARNINGS

Anaphylactoid and Possibly Related Reactions: Presumably because angiotensin-converting enzyme inhibitors affect the metabolism of eicosanoids and polypeptides, including endogenous bradykinin, patients receiving ACE inhibitors (including captopril) may be subject to a variety of adverse reactions, some of them serious.

Head and Neck Angioedema: Angioedema involving the extremities, face, lips, mucous membranes, tongue, glottis or larynx has been seen in patients treated with ACE inhibitors, including captopril. If angioedema involves the tongue, glottis or larynx, airway obstruction may occur and be fatal. Emergency therapy, including but not necessarily limited to, subcutaneous administration of a 1:1000 solution of epinephrine should be promptly instituted.
Swelling confined to the face, mucous membranes of the mouth, lips and extremities has usually resolved with

discontinuation of captopril; some cases required medical therapy. (See PRECAUTIONS: Information for Patients and ADVERSE REACTIONS.)

Intestinal Angioedema: Intestinal angioedema has been reported in patients treated with ACE inhibitors. These patients presented with abdominal pain (with or without nausea or vomiting); in some cases there was no prior history of facial angioedema and C-1 esterase levels were normal. The angioedema was diagnosed by procedures including abdominal CT scan or ultrasound, or at surgery, and symptoms resolved after stopping the ACE inhibitor. Intestinal angioedema should be included in the differential diagnosis of patients on ACE inhibitors presenting with abdominal pain.

Anaphylactoid Reactions During Desensitization: Two patients undergoing desensitizing treatment with hymenoptera venom while receiving ACE inhibitors sustained life-threatening anaphylactoid reactions. In the same patients, these reactions were avoided when ACE inhibitors were temporarily withheld, but they reappeared upon inadvertent rechallenge.

Anaphylactoid Reactions During Membrane Exposure: Anaphylactoid reactions have been reported in patients dialyzed with high-flux membranes and treated concomitantly with an ACE inhibitor. Anaphylactoid reactions have also been reported in patients undergoing low-density lipoprotein apheresis with dextran sulfate absorption.

Neutropenia/Agranulocytosis: Neutropenia (< 1000/mm^3) with myeloid hypoplasia has resulted from use of captopril. About half of the neutropenic patients developed systemic or oral cavity infections or other features of the syndrome of agranulocytosis.

The risk of neutropenia is dependent on the clinical status of the patient:

In clinical trials in patients with hypertension who have normal renal function (serum creatinine less than 1.6 mg/dL and no collagen vascular disease), neutropenia has been seen in one patient out of over 8,600 exposed.

In patients with some degree of renal failure (serum creatinine at least 1.6 mg/dL) but no collagen vascular disease, the risk of neutropenia in clinical trials was about 1 per 500, a frequency over 15 times that for uncomplicated hypertension. Daily doses of captopril were relatively high in these patients, particularly in view of their diminished renal function. In foreign marketing experience in patients with renal failure, use of allopurinol concomitantly with captopril has been associated with neutropenia but this association has not appeared in U.S. reports. In patients with collagen vascular diseases (e.g., systemic lupus erythematosus, scleroderma) and impaired renal function, neutropenia occurred in 3.7 percent of patients in clinical trials.

While none of the over 750 patients in formal clinical trials of heart failure developed neutropenia, it has occurred during the subsequent clinical experience. About half of the reported cases had serum creatinine ≥ 1.6 mg/dL and more than 75 percent were in patients also receiving procainamide. In heart failure, it appears that the same risk factors for neutropenia are present.

The neutropenia has usually been detected within three months after captopril was started. Bone marrow examinations in patients with neutropenia consistently showed myeloid hypoplasia, frequently accompanied by erythroid hypoplasia and decreased numbers of megakaryocytes (e.g., hypoplastic bone marrow and pancytopenia); anemia and thrombocytopenia were sometimes seen.

In general, neutrophils returned to normal in about two weeks after captopril was discontinued, and serious infections were limited to clinically complex patients. About 13 percent of the cases of neutropenia have ended fatally, but almost all fatalities were in patients with serious illness, having collagen vascular disease, renal failure, heart failure or immunosuppressant therapy, or a combination of these complicating factors.

Evaluation of the hypertensive or heart failure patient should always include assessment of renal function.

If captopril is used in patients with impaired renal function, white blood cell and differential counts should be evaluated prior to starting treatment and at approximately two-week intervals for about three months, then periodically.

In patients with collagen vascular disease or who are exposed to other drugs known to affect the white cells or immune response, particularly when there is impaired renal function, captopril should be used only after an assessment of benefit and risk, and then with caution.

All patients treated with captopril should be told to report *any signs of infection (e.g., sore throat, fever). If infection is suspected, white cell counts should be performed without delay.*

Since discontinuation of captopril and other drugs has generally led to prompt return of the white count to normal, upon confirmation of neutropenia (neutrophil count < 1000/mm^3) the physician should withdraw captopril and closely follow the patient's course.

Proteinuria: Total urinary proteins greater than 1 g per day were seen in about 0.7 percent of patients receiving captopril. About 90 percent of affected patients had evidence of prior renal disease or received relatively high doses of captopril (in excess of 150 mg/day), or both. The nephrotic syndrome occurred in about one-fifth of proteinuric patients. In most cases, proteinuria subsided or cleared within six months whether or not captopril was continued. Parameters of renal function, such as BUN and creatinine, were seldom altered in the patients with proteinuria.

Hypotension: Excessive hypotension was rarely seen in hypertensive patients but is a possible consequence of captopril use in salt/volume depleted persons (such as those treated vigorously with diuretics), patients with heart failure or those patients undergoing renal dialysis. (See PRECAUTIONS: Drug Interactions.)

In heart failure, where the blood pressure was either normal or low, transient decreases in mean blood pressure greater than 20 percent were recorded in about half of the patients. This transient hypotension is more likely to occur after any of the first several doses and is usually well tolerated, producing either no symptoms or brief mild lightheadedness, although in rare instances it has been associated with arrhythmia or conduction defects. Hypotension was the reason for discontinuation of drug in 3.6 percent of patients with heart failure.

BECAUSE OF THE POTENTIAL FALL IN BLOOD PRESSURE IN THESE PATIENTS, THERAPY SHOULD BE STARTED UNDER VERY CLOSE MEDICAL SUPERVISION. A starting dose of 6.25 or 12.5 mg tid may minimize the hypotensive effect. Patients should be followed closely for the first two weeks of treatment and whenever the dose of captopril and/or diuretic is increased. In patients with heart failure, reducing the dose of diuretic, if feasible, may minimize the fall in blood pressure.

Hypotension is not *per se* a reason to discontinue captopril. Some decrease of systemic blood pressure is a common and desirable observation upon initiation of captopril treatment in heart failure. The magnitude of the decrease is greatest early in the course of treatment; this effect stabilizes within a week or two, and generally returns to pretreatment levels, without a decrease in therapeutic efficacy, within two months.

Fetal/Neonatal Morbidity and Mortality: ACE inhibitors can cause fetal and neonatal morbidity and death when administered to pregnant women. Several dozen cases have been reported in the world literature. When pregnancy is detected, ACE inhibitors should be discontinued as soon as possible.

The use of ACE inhibitors during the second and third trimesters of pregnancy has been associated with fetal and neonatal injury, including hypotension, neonatal skull hypoplasia, anuria, reversible or irreversible renal failure, and death. Oligohydramnios has also been reported, presumably resulting from decreased fetal renal function; oligohydramnios in this setting has been associated with fetal limb contractures, craniofacial deformation, and hypoplastic lung development. Prematurity, intrauterine growth retardation, and patent ductus arteriosus have also been reported, although it is not clear whether these occurrences were due to the ACE-inhibitor exposure.

These adverse effects do not appear to have resulted from intrauterine ACE-inhibitor exposure that has been limited to the first trimester. Mothers whose embryos and fetuses are exposed to ACE inhibitors only during the first trimester should be so informed. Nonetheless, when patients become pregnant, physicians should make every effort to discontinue the use of captopril as soon as possible.

Rarely (probably less often than once in every thousand pregnancies), no alternative to ACE inhibitors will be found. In these rare cases, the mothers should be apprised of the potential hazards to their fetuses, and serial ultrasound examinations should be performed to assess the intraamniotic environment.

If oligohydramnios is observed, captopril should be discontinued unless it is considered life-saving for the mother. Contraction stress testing (CST), a non-stress test (NST), or biophysical profiling (BPP) may be appropriate, depending upon the week of pregnancy. Patients and physicians should be aware, however, that oligohydramnios may not appear until after the fetus has sustained irreversible injury.

Infants with histories of *in utero* exposure to ACE inhibitors should be closely observed for hypotension, oliguria, and hyperkalemia. If oliguria occurs, attention should be directed toward support of blood pressure and renal perfusion. Exchange transfusion or dialysis may be required as a means of reversing hypotension and/or substituting for disordered renal function. While captopril may be removed from the adult circulation by hemodialysis, there is inadequate data concerning the effectiveness of hemodialysis for removing it from the circulation of neonates or children. Peritoneal dialysis is not effective for removing captopril; there is no information concerning exchange transfusion for removing captopril from the general circulation.

When captopril was given to rabbits at doses about 0.8 to 70 times (on a mg/kg basis) the maximum recommended human dose, low incidences of craniofacial malformations were seen. No teratogenic effects of captopril were seen in studies of pregnant rats and hamsters. On a mg/kg basis, the doses used were up to 150 times (in hamsters) and 625 times (in rats) the maximum recommended human dose.

Hepatic Failure: Rarely, ACE inhibitors have been associated with a syndrome that starts with cholestatic jaundice and progresses to fulminant hepatic necrosis and (sometimes) death. The mechanism of this syndrome is not understood. Patients receiving ACE inhibitors who develop jaundice or marked elevations of hepatic enzymes should discontinue the ACE inhibitor and receive appropriate medical follow-up.

PRECAUTIONS

General: *Impaired Renal Function: Hypertension:* Some patients with renal disease, particularly those with severe renal artery stenosis have developed increases in BUN and serum creatinine after reduction of blood pressure with captopril. Captopril dosage reduction and/or discontinuation of diuretic may be required. For some of these patients, it may not be possible to normalize blood pressure and maintain adequate renal perfusion.

Heart Failure: About 20 percent of patients develop stable elevations of BUN and serum creatinine greater than 20 percent above normal or baseline upon long-term treatment with captopril. Less than 5 percent of patients, generally those with severe preexisting renal disease, required discontinuation of treatment due to progressively increasing creatinine; subsequent improvement probably depends upon the severity of the underlying renal disease. See CLINICAL PHARMACOLOGY, DOSAGE AND ADMINISTRATION, ADVERSE REACTIONS: Altered Laboratory Findings.

Hyperkalemia: Elevations in serum potassium have been observed in some patients treated with ACE inhibitors, including captopril. When treated with ACE inhibitors, patients at risk for the development of hyperkalemia include those with: renal insufficiency; diabetes mellitus; and those using concomitant potassium-sparing diuretics, potassium supplements or potassium-containing salt substitutes; or other drugs associated with increases in serum potassium. (See PRECAUTIONS: Information for Patients and Drug Interactions; ADVERSE REACTION: Altered Laboratory Findings.)

Cough: Presumably due to the inhibition of the degradation of endogenous bradykinin, persistent nonproductive cough has been reported with all ACE inhibitors, always resolving after discontinuation of therapy. ACE inhibitor-induced cough should be considered in the differential diagnosis of cough.

Valvular Stenosis: There is concern, on theoretical grounds, that patients with aortic stenosis might be at particular risk of decreased coronary perfusion when treated with vasodilators because they do not develop as much afterload reduction as others.

Surgery/Anesthesia: In patients undergoing major surgery or during anesthesia with agents that produce hypotension, captopril will block angiotensin II formation secondary to compensatory renin release. If hypotension occurs and is considered to be due to this mechanism, it can be corrected by volume expansion.

Hemodialysis: Recent clinical observations have shown an association of hypersensitivity-like (anaphylactoid) reactions during hemodialysis with high-flux dialysis membranes (e.g., AN69) in patients receiving ACE inhibitors. In these patients, consideration should be given to using a different type of dialysis membrane or a different class of medication. (See WARNINGS: Anaphylactoid Reactions During Membrane Exposure.)

Information For Patients: Patients should be advised to immediately report to their physician any signs or symptoms suggesting angioedema (e.g., swelling of face, eyes, lips, tongue, larynx and extremities; difficulty in swallowing or breathing; hoarseness) and to discontinue therapy. (See WARNINGS: Head and Neck Angioedema and Intestinal Angioedema.)

Patients should be told to report promptly any indication of infection (e.g., sore throat, fever), which may be a sign of neutropenia, or of progressive edema which might be related to proteinuria and nephrotic syndrome.

All patients should be cautioned that excessive perspiration and dehydration may lead to an excessive fall in blood pressure because of reduction in fluid volume. Other causes of volume depletion such as vomiting or diarrhea may also lead to a fall in blood pressure; patients should be advised to consult with the physician.

Patients should be advised not to use potassium-sparing diuretics, potassium supplements or potassium-containing salt substitutes without consulting their physician. (See PRECAUTIONS: General and Drug Interactions; ADVERSE REACTIONS.)

Patients should be warned against interruption or discontinuation of medication unless instructed by the physician. Heart failure patients on captopril therapy should be cautioned against rapid increases in physical activity.

Patients should be informed that captopril should be taken one hour before meals (see DOSAGE AND ADMINISTRATION).

Pregnancy: Female patients of childbearing age should be told about the consequences of second- and third-trimester exposure to ACE inhibitors, and they should also be told that these consequences do not appear to have resulted from intrauterine ACE-inhibitor exposure that has been limited to the first trimester. These patients should be asked to report pregnancies to their physicians as soon as possible.

Drug Interactions: *Hypotension–Patients on Diuretic Therapy:* Patients on diuretics and especially those in whom diuretic therapy was recently instituted, as well as those on severe dietary salt restriction or dialysis, may occasionally experience a precipitous reduction of blood pressure usually within the first hour after receiving the initial dose of captopril.

The possibility of hypotensive effects with captopril can be minimized by either discontinuing the diuretic or increasing the salt intake approximately one week prior to initiation of treatment with captopril or initiating therapy with small doses (6.25 or 12.5 mg). Alternatively, provide medical supervision for at least one hour after the initial dose. If hypotension occurs, the patient should be placed in a supine position and, if necessary, receive an intravenous infusion of normal saline. This transient hypotensive response is not a contraindication to further doses which can be given without difficulty once the blood pressure has increased after volume expansion.

Agents Having Vasodilator Activity: Data on the effect of concomitant use of other vasodilators in patients receiving captopril for heart failure are not available; therefore, nitroglycerin or other nitrates (as used for management of angina) or other drugs having vasodilator activity should, if possible, be discontinued before starting captopril. If resumed during captopril therapy, such agents should be administered cautiously, and perhaps at lower dosage.

Agents Causing Renin Release: Captopril's effect will be augmented by antihypertensive agents that cause renin release. For example, diuretics (e.g., thiazides) may activate the renin-angiotensin-aldosterone system.

Agents Affecting Sympathetic Activity: The sympathetic nervous system may be especially important in supporting blood pressure in patients receiving captopril alone or with diuretics. Therefore, agents affecting sympathetic activity (e.g., ganglionic blocking agents or adrenergic neuron blocking agents) should be used with caution. Beta-adrenergic blocking drugs add some further antihypertensive effect to captopril, but the overall response is less than additive.

Agents Increasing Serum Potassium: Since captopril decreases aldosterone production, elevation of serum potassium may occur. Potassium-sparing diuretics such as spironolactone, triamterene, or amiloride, or potassium supplements should be given only for documented hypokalemia, and then with caution, since they may lead to a significant increase of serum potassium. Salt substitutes containing potassium should also be used with caution.

Inhibitors of Endogenous Prostaglandin Synthesis: It has been reported that indomethacin may reduce the antihypertensive effect of captopril, especially in cases of low renin hypertension. Other nonsteroidal anti-inflammatory agents (e.g., aspirin) may also have this effect.

Lithium: Increased serum lithium levels and symptoms of lithium toxicity have been reported in patients receiving concomitant lithium and ACE inhibitor therapy. These drugs should be coadministered with caution and frequent monitoring of serum lithium levels is recommended. If a diuretic is also used, it may increase the risk of lithium toxicity.

Cardiac Glycosides: In a study of young healthy male subjects no evidence of a direct pharmacokinetic captopril-digoxin interaction could be found.

Loop Diuretics: Furosemide administered concurrently with captopril does not alter the pharmacokinetics of captopril in renally impaired hypertensive patients.

Allopurinol: In a study of healthy male volunteers no significant pharmacokinetic interaction occurred when captopril and allopurinol were administered concomitantly for 6 days.

Drug/Laboratory Test Interactions: Captopril may cause a false-positive urine test for acetone.

Carcinogenesis, Mutagenesis and Impairment of Fertility: Two-year studies with doses of 50 to 1350 mg/kg/day in mice and rats failed to show any evidence of carcinogenic potential. The high dose in these studies is 150 times the maximum recommended human dose of 450 mg, assuming a 50 kg subject. On a body-surface area basis, the high doses for mice and rats are 13 and 26 times the maximum recommended human dose, respectively.

Studies in rats have revealed no impairment of fertility.

Animal Toxicology: Chronic oral toxicity studies were conducted in rats (2 years), dogs (47 weeks; 1 year), mice (2 years), and monkeys (1 year). Significant drug-related toxicity included effects on hematopoiesis, renal toxicity, erosion/ulceration of the stomach, and variation of retinal blood vessels.

Reductions in hemoglobin and/or hematocrit values were seen in mice, rats, and monkeys at doses 50 to 150 times the maximum recommended human dose (MRHD) of 450 mg, assuming a 50 kg subject. On a body-surface-area basis, these doses are 5 to 25 times maximum recommended human dose (MRHD). Anemia, leukopenia, thrombocytopenia, and bone marrow suppression occurred in dogs at doses 8 to 30 times MRHD on a body-weight basis (4 to 15 times MRHD on a surface-area basis). The reductions in hemoglobin and hematocrit values in rats and mice were only significant at 1 year and returned to normal with continued dosing by the end of the study. Marked anemia was seen at all dose levels (8 to 30 times MRHD) in dogs, whereas moderate to marked leukopenia was noted only at 15 and 30 times MRHD and thrombocytopenia at 30 times MRHD. The anemia could be reversed upon discontinuation of dosing. Bone marrow suppression occurred to a varying degree, being associated only with dogs that died or were sacrificed in a moribund condition in the 1 year study. However, in the 47-week study at a dose 30 times MRHD, bone marrow suppression was found to be reversible upon continued drug administration.

Captopril caused hyperplasia of the juxtaglomerular apparatus of the kidneys in mice and rats at doses 7 to 200 times MRHD on a body-weight basis (0.6 to 35 times MRHD on a surface-area basis); in monkeys at 20 to 60 times MRHD on a body-weight basis (7 to 20 times MRHD on a surface-area basis); and in dogs at 30 times MRHD on a body-weight basis (15 times MRHD on a surface-area basis).

Gastric erosions/ulcerations were increased in incidence in male rats at 20 to 200 times MRHD on a body-weight basis (3.5 and 35 times MRHD on a surface-area basis); in dogs at 30 times MRHD on a body-weight basis (15 times MRHD on a surface-area basis); and in monkeys at 65 times MRHD on a body-weight basis (20 times MRHD on a surface-area basis). Rabbits developed gastric and intestinal ulcers when given oral doses approximately 30 times MRHD on a body-weight basis (10 times MRHD on a surface-area basis) for only 5 to 7 days.

In the two-year rat study, irreversible and progressive variations in the caliber of retinal vessels (focal sacculations and constrictions) occurred at all dose levels (7 to 200 times MRHD) on a body-weight basis; 1 to 35 times MRHD on a surface-area basis in a dose-related fashion. The effect was first observed in the 88th week of dosing, with a progressively increased incidence thereafter, even after cessation of dosing.

Pregnancy Categories C (first trimester) and D (second and third trimesters): See WARNINGS: Fetal/Neonatal Morbidity and Mortality.

Nursing Mothers: Concentrations of captopril in human milk are approximately one percent of those in maternal blood. Because of the potential for serious adverse reactions in nursing infants from captopril, a decision should be made whether to discontinue nursing or to discontinue the drug, taking into account the importance of captopril to the mother. (See PRECAUTIONS: Pediatric Use.)

Pediatric Use: Safety and effectiveness in pediatric patients have not been established. There is limited experience reported in the literature with the use of captopril in the pediatric population; dosage, on a weight basis, was generally reported to be comparable to or less than that used in adults.

Infants, especially newborns, may be more susceptible to the adverse hemodynamic effects of captopril. Excessive, prolonged and unpredictable decreases in blood pressure and associated complications, including oliguria and seizures, have been reported.

Captopril should be used in pediatric patients only if other measures for controlling blood pressure have not been effective.

ADVERSE REACTIONS

Reported incidences are based on clinical trials involving approximately 7000 patients.

Renal: About one of 100 patients developed proteinuria (see WARNINGS).

Each of the following has been reported in approximately 1 to 2 of 1000 patients and are of uncertain relationship to drug use: renal insufficiency, renal failure, nephrotic syndrome, polyuria, oliguria, and urinary frequency.

Hematologic: Neutropenia/agranulocytosis has occurred (see WARNINGS). Cases of anemia, thrombocytopenia, and pancytopenia have been reported.

Dermatologic: Rash, often with pruritus, and sometimes with fever, arthralgia, and eosinophilia, occurred in about 4 to 7 (depending on renal status and dose) of 100 patients, usually during the first four weeks of therapy. It is usually maculopapular, and rarely urticarial. The rash is usually mild and disappears within a few days of dosage reduction, short-term treatment with an antihistaminic agent, and/or discontinuing therapy; remission may occur even if captopril is continued. Pruritus, without rash, occurs in about 2 of 100 patients. Between 7 and 10 percent of patients with skin rash have shown an eosinophilia and/or positive ANA titers. A reversible associated pemphigoid-like lesion, and photosensitivity, have also been reported.

Flushing or pallor has been reported in 2 to 5 of 1000 patients.

Cardiovascular: Hypotension may occur; see WARNINGS and PRECAUTIONS (Drug Interactions) for discussion of hypotension with captopril therapy.

Tachycardia, chest pain, and palpitations have each been observed in approximately 1 of 100 patients.

Angina pectoris, myocardial infarction, Raynaud's syndrome, and congestive heart failure have each occurred in 2 to 3 of 1000 patients.

Dysgeusia: Approximately 2 to 4 (depending on renal status and dose) of 100 patients developed a diminution or loss of taste perception. Taste impairment is reversible and usually self-limited (2 to 3 months) even with continued drug administration. Weight loss may be associated with the loss of taste.

Angioedema: Angioedema involving the extremities, face, lips, mucous membranes, tongue, glottis or larynx has been reported in approximately one in 1000 patients. Angioedema involving the upper airways has caused fatal airway obstruction. (See WARNINGS: Head and Neck Angioedema, Intestinal Angioedema and PRECAUTIONS: Information for Patients.)

Cough: Cough has been reported in 0.5 to 2% of patients treated with captopril in clinical trials (see : PRECAUTIONS: General *Cough*).

The following have been reported in about 0.5 to 2 percent of patients but did not appear at increased frequency compared to placebo or other treatments used in controlled trials: gastric irritation, abdominal pain, nausea, vomiting, diarrhea, anorexia, constipation, aphthous ulcers, peptic ulcer, dizziness, headache, malaise, fatigue, insomnia, dry mouth, dyspnea, alopecia, paresthesias.

Other clinical adverse effects reported since the drug was marketed are listed below by body system. In this setting, an incidence or causal relationship cannot be accurately determined.

Body as a Whole: Anaphylactoid reactions (see WARNINGS: Anaphylactoid and Possible Related Reactions and PRECAUTIONS: Hemodialysis.)

General: Asthenia, gynecomastia.

Cardiovascular: Cardiac arrest, cerebrovascular accident/insufficiency, rhythm disturbances, orthostatic hypotension, syncope.

Dermatologic: Bullous pemphigus, erythema multi-forme (including Stevens-Johnson syndrome), exfoliative dermatitis.

Gastrointestinal: Pancreatitis, glossitis, dyspepsia.

Hematologic: Anemia, including aplastic and hemolytic.

Hepatobiliary: Jaundice, hepatitis, including rare cases of necrosis, cholestasis.

Metabolic: Symptomatic hyponatremia.

Musculoskeletal: Myalgia, myasthenia.

Nervous/Psychiatric: Ataxia, confusion, depression, nervousness, somnolence.

Respiratory: Bronchospasm, eosinophilic pneumonitis, rhinitis.

Special Senses: Blurred vision.

Urogenital: Impotence.

As with other ACE inhibitors, a syndrome has been reported which may include: fever, myalgia, arthralgia, interstitial nephritis, vasculitis, rash or other dermatologic manifestations, eosinophilia and an elevated ESR.

Fetal/Neonatal Morbidity and Mortality: See WARNINGS: Fetal/Neonatal Morbidity and Mortality.

Altered Laboratory Findings: *Serum Electrolytes: Hyperkalemia:* small increases in serum potassium, especially in patients with renal impairment (see PRECAUTIONS).

Hyponatremia: particularly in patients receiving a low sodium diet or concomitant diuretics.

BUN/Serum Creatinine: Transient elevations of BUN or serum creatinine especially in volume or salt depleted patients or those with renovascular hypertension may occur. Rapid reduction of longstanding or markedly elevated blood pressure can result in decreases in the glomerular filtration rate and, in turn, lead to increases in BUN or serum creatinine.

Hematologic: A positive ANA has been reported.

Liver Function Tests: Elevations of liver transaminases, alkaline phosphatase, and serum bilirubin have occurred.

OVERDOSAGE

Correction of hypotension would be of primary concern. Volume expansion with an intravenous infusion of normal saline is the treatment of choice for restoration of blood pressure.

While captopril may be removed from the adult circulation by hemodialysis, there is inadequate data concerning the effectiveness of hemodialysis for removing it from the circulation of neonates or children. Peritoneal dialysis is not effective for removing captopril; there is no information concerning exchange transfusion for removing captopril from the general circulation.

DOSAGE AND ADMINISTRATION

Captopril should be taken one hour before meals. Dosage must be individualized.

Hypertension: Initiation of therapy requires consideration of recent antihypertensive drug treatment, the extent of blood pressure elevation, salt restriction, and other clinical circumstances. If possible, discontinue the patient's previous antihypertensive drug regimen for one week before starting captopril.

The initial dose of captopril is 25 mg bid or tid. If satisfactory reduction of blood pressure has not been achieved after one or two weeks, the dose may be increased to 50 mg bid or tid. Concomitant sodium restriction may be beneficial when captopril is used alone.

The dose of captopril in hypertension usually does not exceed 50 mg tid. Therefore, if the blood pressure has not been satisfactorily controlled after one to two weeks at this dose, (and the patient is not already receiving a diuretic), a modest dose of a thiazide-type diuretic (e.g., hydrochlorothiazide, 25 mg daily), should be added. The diuretic dose may be increased at one- to two-week intervals until its highest usual antihypertensive dose is reached.

If captopril is being started in a patient already receiving a diuretic, captopril therapy should be initiated under close medical supervision (see WARNINGS and PRECAUTIONS [Drug Interactions] regarding hypotension), with dosage and titration of captopril as noted above.

If further blood pressure reduction is required, the dose of captopril may be increased to 100 mg bid or tid and then, if necessary, to 150 mg bid or tid (while continuing the diuretic). The usual dose range is 25 to 150 mg bid or tid. A maximum daily dose of 450 mg captopril should not be exceeded.

For patients with severe hypertension (e.g., accelerated or malignant hypertension), when temporary discontinuation of current antihypertensive therapy is not practical or desirable, or when prompt titration to more normotensive blood pressure levels is indicated, diuretic should be continued but other current antihypertensive medication stopped and captopril dosage promptly initiated at 25 mg bid or tid, under close medical supervision.

When necessitated by the patient's clinical condition, the daily dose of captopril may be increased every 24 hours or less under continuous medical supervision until a satisfactory blood pressure response is obtained or the maximum dose of captopril is reached. In this regimen, addition of a more potent diuretic, e.g., furosemide, may also be indicated.

Beta-blockers may also be used in conjunction with captopril therapy (see PRECAUTIONS: Drug Interactions), but the effects of the two drugs are less than additive.

Heart Failure: Initiation of therapy requires consideration of recent diuretic therapy and the possibility of severe salt/volume depletion. In patients with either normal or low blood pressure, who have been vigorously treated with diuretics and who may be hyponatremic and/or hypovolemic, a starting dose of 6.25 or 12.5 mg tid may minimize the magnitude or duration of the hypotensive effect (see WARNINGS: Hypotension); for these patients, titration to the usual daily dosage can then occur within the next several days.

For most patients the usual initial daily dosage is 25 mg tid. After a dose of 50 mg tid is reached, further increases in dosage should be delayed, where possible, for at least two weeks to determine if a satisfactory response occurs. Most patients studied have had a satisfactory clinical improvement at 50 or 100 mg tid. A maximum daily dose of 450 mg of captopril should not be exceeded.

Captopril should generally be used in conjunction with a diuretic and digitalis. Captopril therapy must be initiated under very close medical supervision.

Left Ventricular Dysfunction After Myocardial Infarction: The recommended dose for long-term use in patients following a myocardial infarction is a target maintenance dose of 50 mg tid.

Therapy may be initiated as early as three days following a myocardial infarction. After a single dose of 6.25 mg, captopril therapy should be initiated at 12.5 mg tid. Captopril should then be increased to 25 mg tid during the next several days and to a target dose of 50 mg tid over the next several weeks as tolerated (see CLINICAL PHARMACOLOGY).

Captopril may be used in patients treated with other post-myocardial infarction therapies, e.g., thrombolytics, aspirin, beta-blockers.

Dosage Adjustment in Renal Impairment: Because captopril is excreted primarily by the kidneys, excretion rates are reduced in patients with impaired renal function. These patients will take longer to reach steady-state captopril levels and will reach higher steady-state levels for a given daily dose than patients with normal renal function. Therefore, these patients may respond to smaller or less frequent doses.

Accordingly, for patients with significant renal impairment, initial daily dosage of captopril should be reduced, and smaller increments utilized for titration, which should be quite slow (one- to two-week intervals). After the desired therapeutic effect has been achieved, the dose should be slowly back-titrated to determine the minimal effective dose. When concomitant diuretic therapy is required, a loop diuretic (e.g., furosemide), rather than a thiazide diuretic, is preferred in patients with severe renal impairment. (See WARNINGS: Anaphylactoid Reactions During Membrane Exposure and PRECAUTIONS: Hemodialysis.)

HOW SUPPLIED

Captopril tablets, USP are available containing 12.5 mg, 25 mg, 50 mg or 100 mg of captopril.

The 12.5 mg tablets are white, partially scored (both sides), oval tablets marked with **M** to the left of the score and **C1** to the right of the score on one side. They are available as follows:

NDC 0378-3007-01
bottles of 100 tablets
NDC 0378-3007-10
bottles of 1000 tablets

The 25 mg tablets are white, quadrisect scored, round tablets marked with **M** over **C2** on the non-scored side. They are available as follows:

NDC 0378-3012-01
bottles of 100 tablets
NDC 0378-3012-10
bottles of 1000 tablets

The 50 mg tablets are white, scored, round tablets marked with **M** over **C3** on the scored side. They are available as follows:

NDC 0378-3017-01
bottles of 100 tablets
NDC 0378-3017-10
bottles of 1000 tablets

The 100 mg tablets are white, scored, round tablets marked with **M** over **C4** on the scored side. They are available as follows:

NDC 0378-3022-01
bottles of 100 tablets

Captopril tablets, USP may exhibit a slight sulfurous odor. Bottles contain a desiccant-charcoal canister.

Store at 20° to 25°C (68° to 77°F). [See USP for Controlled Room Temperature.]

Protect from moisture.

Dispense in a tight, light-resistant container as defined in the USP using a child-resistant closure.

MYLAN®
Mylan Pharmaceuticals Inc.
Morgantown, WV 26505

REVISED JUNE 2004
CAPT:R9

CLINDAMYCIN PHOSPHATE AND BENZOYL PEROXIDE GEL, 1%*/5% ℞

[clin-da-my-cin]

Topical Gel: clindamycin (1%)
***as clindamycin phosphate, benzoyl peroxide (5%)**
For Dermatological Use Only - Not for Ophthalmic Use
Mix Before Dispensing
℞ only

DESCRIPTION

Clindamycin Phosphate and Benzoyl Peroxide Gel, 1%/5% contains clindamycin phosphate, (7(S)-chloro-7-deoxylincomycin-2-phosphate). Clindamycin phosphate is a water soluble ester of the semi-synthetic antibiotic produced by a 7(S)-chloro-substitution of the 7(R)-hydroxyl group of the parent antibiotic lincomycin.

Chemically, clindamycin phosphate is ($C_{18}H_{34}ClN_2O_8PS$). The structural formula for clindamycin is represented below:

[See chemical structure at top of next column]

Clindamycin phosphate has a molecular weight of 504.97 and its chemical name is Methyl 7-chloro-6,7,8-trideoxy-6-(1-methyl-trans-4-propyl-L-2-pyrrolidinecarboxamido)-1-thio-L-threo-alpha-D-galacto-octopyranoside 2-(dihydrogen phosphate).

Clindamycin Phosphate and Benzoyl Peroxide Gel, 1%/5% also contains benzoyl peroxide, for topical use.

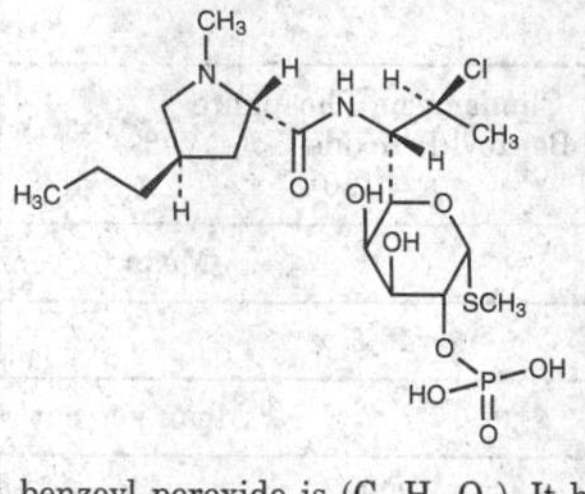

Chemically, benzoyl peroxide is ($C_{14}H_{10}O_4$). It has the following structural formula:

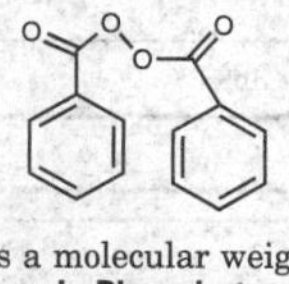

Benzoyl peroxide has a molecular weight of 242.23.

Each gram of **Clindamycin Phosphate and Benzoyl Peroxide Gel, 1%/5%** contains, as dispensed, 10 mg (1%) clindamycin as phosphate and 50 mg (5%) benzoyl peroxide in a base of carbomer, propylene glycol, potassium hydroxide, and purified water.

CLINICAL PHARMACOLOGY

An *in vitro* percutaneous penetration study comparing **Clindamycin Phosphate and Benzoyl Peroxide Gel, 1%/5%** and topical 1% clindamycin gel alone, demonstrated there was no statistical difference in penetration between the two drugs. Mean systemic bioavailability of topical clindamycin in **Clindamycin Phosphate and Benzoyl Peroxide Gel, 1%/5%** is suggested to be less than 1%.

Benzoyl peroxide has been shown to be absorbed by the skin where it is converted to benzoic acid. Less than 2% of the dose enters systemic circulation as benzoic acid. It is suggested that the lipophilic nature of benzoyl peroxide acts to concentrate the compound into the lipid-rich sebaceous follicle.

Microbiology:

The clindamycin and benzoyl peroxide components individually have been shown to have *in vitro* activity against *Propionibacterium acnes* an organism which has been associated with acne vulgaris; however, the clinical significance of this activity against *P. acnes* was not examined in clinical trials with this product.

CLINICAL STUDIES

In two adequate and well controlled clinical studies of 758 patients, 214 used Clindamycin Phosphate and Benzoyl Peroxide Gel, 1%/5%, 210 used benzoyl peroxide, 168 used clindamycin, and 166 used vehicle. Clindamycin Phosphate and Benzoyl Peroxide Gel, 1%/5% applied twice daily for 10 weeks was significantly more effective than vehicle in the treatment of moderate to moderately severe facial acne vulgaris. Patients were evaluated and acne lesions counted at each clinical visit; weeks 2, 4, 6, 8 and 10. The primary efficacy measures were the lesion counts and the investigator's global assessment evaluated at week 10. Patients were instructed to wash the face with a mild soap, using only the hands. Fifteen minutes after the face was thoroughly dry, application was made to the entire face. Non-medicated make-up could be applied at one hour after the Clindamycin Phosphate and Benzoyl Peroxide Gel, 1%/5% application. If a moisturizer was required, the patients were provided a moisturizer to be used as needed. Patients were instructed to avoid sun exposure. Percent reductions in lesion counts after treatment for 10 weeks in these two studies are shown below:

[See first table at top of next page]
[See second table on next page]

The Clindamycin Phosphate and Benzoyl Peroxide Gel, 1%/5% group showed greater overall improvement than the benzoyl peroxide, clindamycin and vehicle groups as rated by the investigator.

INDICATIONS AND USAGE

Clindamycin Phosphate and Benzoyl Peroxide Gel, 1%/5% is indicated for the topical treatment of acne vulgaris.

CONTRAINDICATIONS

Clindamycin Phosphate and Benzoyl Peroxide Gel, 1%/5% is contraindicated in those individuals who have shown hypersensitivity to any of its components or to lincomycin. It is also contraindicated in those having a history of regional enteritis, ulcerative colitis, or antibiotic-associated colitis.

WARNINGS

ORALLY AND PARENTERALLY ADMINISTERED CLINDAMYCIN HAS BEEN ASSOCIATED WITH SEVERE COLITIS WHICH MAY RESULT IN PATIENT DEATH. USE OF THE TOPICAL FORMULATION OF CLINDAMYCIN RESULTS IN ABSORPTION OF THE ANTIBIOTIC FROM THE SKIN SURFACE. DIARRHEA, BLOODY DIARRHEA, AND COLITIS (INCLUDING PSEUDOMEMBRANOUS COLITIS) HAVE BEEN REPORTED WITH THE USE OF TOPICAL AND SYSTEMIC

Study 1

Clindamycin Phosphate and Benzoyl Peroxide Gel, 1%/5% n = 120	Benzoyl peroxide n = 120	Clindamycin n = 120	Vehicle n = 120
Mean percent reduction in inflammatory lesion counts			
46%	32%	16%	+3%
Mean percent reduction in non-inflammatory lesion counts			
22%	22%	9%	+1%
Mean percent reduction in total lesion counts			
36%	28%	15%	0.2%

Study 2

Clindamycin Phosphate and Benzoyl Peroxide Gel, 1%/5% n = 95	Benzoyl peroxide n = 95	Clindamycin n = 49	Vehicle n = 48
Mean percent reduction in inflammatory lesion counts			
63%	53%	45%	42%
Mean percent reduction in non-inflammatory lesion counts			
54%	50%	39%	36%
Mean percent reduction in total lesion counts			
58%	52%	42%	39%

CLINDAMYCIN. STUDIES INDICATE A TOXIN(S) PRODUCED BY CLOSTRIDIA IS ONE PRIMARY CAUSE OF ANTIBIOTIC-ASSOCIATED COLITIS. THE COLITIS IS USUALLY CHARACTERIZED BY SEVERE PERSISTENT DIARRHEA AND SEVERE ABDOMINAL CRAMPS AND MAY BE ASSOCIATED WITH THE PASSAGE OF BLOOD AND MUCUS. ENDOSCOPIC EXAMINATION MAY REVEAL PSEUDOMEMBRANOUS COLITIS. STOOL CULTURE FOR *Clostridium Difficile* AND STOOL ASSAY FOR *C. difficile* TOXIN MAY BE HELPFUL DIAGNOSTICALLY. WHEN SIGNIFICANT DIARRHEA OCCURS, THE DRUG SHOULD BE DISCONTINUED. LARGE BOWEL ENDOSCOPY SHOULD BE CONSIDERED TO ESTABLISH A DEFINITIVE DIAGNOSIS IN CASES OF SEVERE DIARRHEA. ANTIPERISTALTIC AGENTS SUCH AS OPIATES AND DIPHENOXYLATE WITH ATROPINE MAY PROLONG AND/OR WORSEN THE CONDITION. DIARRHEA, COLITIS, AND PSEUDOMEMBRANOUS COLITIS HAVE BEEN OBSERVED TO BEGIN UP TO SEVERAL WEEKS FOLLOWING CESSATION OF ORAL AND PARENTERAL THERAPY WITH CLINDAMYCIN.

Mild cases of pseudomembranous colitis usually respond to drug discontinuation alone. In moderate to severe cases, consideration should be given to management with fluids and electrolytes, protein supplementation and treatment with an antibacterial drug clinically effective against *C. difficile* colitis.

PRECAUTIONS

General:
For dermatological use only; not for ophthalmic use. Concomitant topical acne therapy should be used with caution because a possible cumulative irritancy effect may occur, especially with the use of peeling, desquamating, or abrasive agents.

The use of antibiotic agents may be associated with the overgrowth of non-susceptible organisms including fungi. If this occurs, discontinue use of this medication and take appropriate measures.

Avoid contact with eyes and mucous membranes.

Clindamycin and erythromycin containing products should not be used in combination. *In vitro* studies have shown antagonism between these two anti-microbials. The clinical significance of this *in vitro* antagonism is not known.

Information for Patients:
Patients using **Clindamycin Phosphate and Benzoyl Peroxide Gel, 1%/5%** should receive the following information and instructions:
1. **Clindamycin Phosphate and Benzoyl Peroxide Gel, 1%/5%** is to be used as directed by the physician. It is for external use only. Avoid contact with eyes, and inside the nose, mouth, and all mucous membranes, as this product may be irritating.
2. This medication should not be used for any disorder other than that for which it was prescribed.
3. Patients should not use any other topical acne preparation unless otherwise directed by physician.

4. Patients should minimize or avoid exposure to natural or artificial sunlight (tanning beds or UVA/B treatment) while using Clindamycin Phospate and Benzoyl Peroxide Gel, 1%/5%. To minimize exposure to sunlight, a wide-brimmed hat or other protective clothing should be worn, and a sunscreen with SPF 15 rating or higher should be used.
5. Patients who develop allergic symptoms such as severe swelling or shortness of breath should discontinue **Clindamycin Phosphate and Benzoly Peroxide Gel, 1%/5%** and contact their physician immediately. In addition, patients should report any signs of local adverse reactions to their physician.
6. **Clindamycin Phosphate and Benzoyl Peroxide Gel, 1%/5%** may bleach hair or colored fabric.
7. **Clindamycin Phosphate and Benzoyl Peroxide Gel, 1%/5%** can be stored at room temperature up to 25°C (77°F) for 3 months. Do not freeze. Discard any unused product after 3 months.
8. Before applying **Clindamycin Phosphate and Benzoyl Peroxide Gel, 1%/5%** to affected areas wash the skin gently, then rinse with warm water and pat dry.

Carcinogenesis, Mutagenesis, Impairment of Fertility:
Benzoyl peroxide has been shown to be a tumor promoter and progression agent in a number of animal studies. The clinical significance of this is unknown. Benzoyl peroxide in acetone at doses of 5 and 10 mg administered twice per week induced skin tumors in transgenic Tg.AC mice in a study using 20 weeks of topical treatment.

In a 52 week dermal photocarcinogenicity study in hairless mice, the median time to onset of skin tumor formation was decreased and the number of tumors per mouse increased following chronic concurrent topical administration of Clindamycin Phosphate and Benzoyl Peroxide Gel, 1%/5% with exposure to ultraviolet radiation (40 weeks of treatment followed by 12 weeks of observation).

Genotoxicity studies were not conducted with Clindamycin Phosphate and Benzoyl Peroxide Gel, 1%/5%. Clindamycin phosphate was not genotoxic in *Salmonella typhimurium* or in a rat micronucleus test. Clindamycin phosphate sulfoxide, an oxidative degradation product of clindamycin phosphate and benzoyl peroxide, was not clastogenic in a mouse micronucleus test. Benzoyl peroxide has been found to cause DNA strand breaks in a variety of mammalian cell types, to be mutagenic in *S. typhimurium* tests by some but not all investigators, and to cause sister chromatid exchanges in Chinese hamster ovary cells. Studies have not been performed with **Clindamycin Phosphate and Benzoyl Peroxide Gel, 1%/5%** or benzoyl peroxide to evaluate the effect on fertility. Fertility studies in rats treated orally with up to 300 mg/kg/day of clindamycin (approximately 120 times the amount of clindamycin in the highest recommended adult human dose of 2.5 grams Clindamycin Phosphate and Benzoyl Peroxide Gel, 1%/5%, based on mg/m^2) revealed no effects on fertility or mating ability.

Pregnancy: Teratogenic Effects: Pregnancy Category C:
Animal reproductive/developmental toxicity studies have not been conducted with Clindamycin Phosphate and Benzoyl Peroxide Gel, 1%/5% or benzoyl peroxide. Developmental toxicity studies performed in rats and mice using oral doses of clindamycin up to 600 mg/kg/day (240 and 120 times amount of clindamycin in the highest recommended adult human dose based on mg/m^2, respectively) or subcutaneous doses of clindamycin up to 250 mg/kg/day (100 and 50 times the amount of clindamycin in the highest recommended adult human dose based on mg/m^2, respectively) revealed no evidence of teratogenicity.

There are no well-controlled trials in pregnant women treated with **Clindamycin Phosphate and Benzoyl Peroxide Gel, 1%/5%**. It also is not known whether **Clindamycin Phosphate and Benzoyl Peroxide Gel, 1%/5%** can cause fetal harm when administered to a pregnant woman.

Nursing Women:
It is not known whether **Clindamycin Phosphate and Benzoyl Peroxide Gel, 1%/5%** is excreted in human milk after topical application. However, orally and parenterally administered clindamycin has been reported to appear in breast milk. Because of the potential for serious adverse reactions in nursing infants, a decision should be made whether to discontinue nursing or to discontinue the drug, taking into account the importance of the drug to the mother.

Pediatric Use:
Safety and effectiveness of this product in pediatric patients below the age of 12 have not been established.

ADVERSE REACTIONS

During clinical trials, the most frequently reported adverse event in the Clindamycin Phosphate and Benzoyl Peroxide Gel, 1%/5% treatment group was dry skin (12%). The Table below lists local adverse events reported by at least 1% of patients in the Clindamycin Phosphate and Benzoyl Peroxide Gel, 1%/5% and vehicle groups.

Local Adverse Events - all causalities in >/= 1% of patients

	Clindamycin Phosphate and Benzoyl Peroxide Gel, 1%/5% n = 420	Vehicle n = 168
Application Site Reaction	13 (3%)	1 (< 1%)
Dry Skin	50 (12%)	10 (6%)
Pruritis	8 (2%)	1 (< 1%)
Peeling	9 (2%)	
Erythema	6 (1%)	1 (< 1%)
Sunburn	5 (1%)	

The actual incidence of dry skin might have been greater were it not for the use of a moisturizer in these studies. Anaphylaxis, as well as allergic reactions leading to hospitalization, have been reported during post-marketing use of clindamycin/benzoyl peroxide products. Because these reactions are reported voluntarily from a population of uncertain size, it is not always possible to reliably estimate their frequency or establish a causal relationship to drug exposure.

DOSAGE AND ADMINISTRATION

Clindamycin Phosphate and Benzoyl Peroxide Gel, 1%/5% should be applied twice daily, morning and evening, or as directed by a physician, to affected areas after the skin is gently washed, rinsed with warm water and patted dry.

HOW SUPPLIED AND COMPOUNDING INSTRUCTIONS

Size (Net Weight)	NDC #	Benzoyl Peroxide Gel	Clindamycin Phosphate Solution (in plastic bottle)
50 grams	0378-8688-54	40 grams	10 grams

Prior to dispensing, add the solution in the bottle to the gel and stir until homogenous in appearance (1 to 1½ minutes). **Clindamycin Phosphate and Benzoyl Peroxide Gel, 1%/5%** can be stored at room temperature up to 25°C (77°F) for 3 months. Place a 3 month expiration date on the labeling immediately following mixing.

Store at room temperature up to 25°C (77°F) [See USP]. Do not freeze. Keep tightly closed. Keep out of the reach of children.
US Patents 5,733,886; 6,117,843
Distributed by:
Mylan Pharmaceuticals Inc.
Morgantown, WV 26505
Manufactured by:
Contract Pharmaceuticals Ltd.
Buffalo, NY 14213

090068
REVISED JUNE 2009
DW-M-CLBZPX:R3

CLONIDINE TRANSDERMAL SYSTEM, USP ℞

[*Clon-i-dine*]
℞ **only**

Programmed delivery *in vivo* of 0.1 mg, 0.2 mg, or 0.3 mg clonidine per day, for one week.
Prescribing Information

DESCRIPTION

CLONIDINE TRANSDERMAL SYSTEM is a transdermal system providing continuous systemic delivery of clonidine for 7 days at an approximately constant rate. Clonidine is a centrally acting alpha-agonist hypotensive agent. It is an imidazoline derivative with the chemical name 2, 6-dichloro-N-2-imidazolidinylidenebenzenamine and has the following chemical structure:

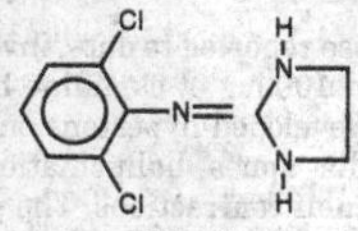

(Clonidine)

USP Drug Release Test Pending.

System Structure and Components: CLONIDINE TRANSDERMAL SYSTEM is a multi-layered film, 0.25 mm thick, containing clonidine as the active agent. The system areas are 3.33 cm^2 (0.1 mg/day), 6.67 cm^2 (0.2 mg/day), and 10.0 cm^2 (0.3 mg/day) and the amount of drug released is directly proportional to the area (see DESCRIPTION: Release Rate Concept). The composition per unit area is the same for all three doses.

Proceeding from the visible surface towards the surface attached to the skin, there are three consecutive layers: (1) a backing layer of pigmented polyethylene and polyester film, (2) a solid matrix reservoir of clonidine, mineral oil, polyisobutylene, and colloidal silicon dioxide, (3) an adhesive formulation of clonidine, mineral oil, polyisobutylene, and colloidal silicon dioxide. Prior to use, a protective slit release liner of polyester that covers the adhesive formulation layer is removed.

CLONIDINE TRANSDERMAL SYSTEMS are packaged with additional pieces of protective film above and below the system within each pouch. These pieces of protective film are removed and discarded at the time of use.

Cross Section of the System:

(Diagram Not to Scale)

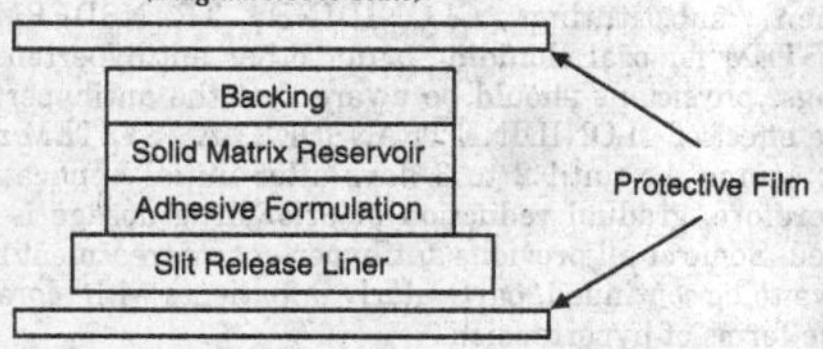

Release Rate Concept: CLONIDINE TRANSDERMAL SYSTEM is programmed to release clonidine at an approximately constant rate for 7 days. The energy for drug release is derived from the concentration gradient existing between the patch and the much lower concentration prevailing in the skin. Clonidine flows in the direction of the lower concentration at a constant rate.

Following system application to intact skin, clonidine in the adhesive formulation layer saturates the skin site below the system. Clonidine from the patch then begins to flow into the systemic circulation via the capillaries beneath the skin. Therapeutic plasma clonidine levels are achieved 2 to 3 days after initial application of CLONIDINE TRANSDERMAL SYSTEM.

The 3.33 cm^2, 6.67 cm^2, and 10.0 cm^2 systems deliver 0.1 mg, 0.2 mg, and 0.3 mg of clonidine per day, respectively. To ensure constant release of drug for 7 days, the total drug content of the system is higher than the total amount of drug delivered. Application of a new system to a fresh skin site at weekly intervals continuously maintains therapeutic plasma concentrations of clonidine. If the CLONIDINE TRANSDERMAL SYSTEM is removed and not replaced with a new system, therapeutic plasma clonidine levels will persist for about 8 hours and then decline slowly over several days. Over this time period, blood pressure returns gradually to pretreatment levels.

CLINICAL PHARMACOLOGY

Clonidine stimulates alpha-adrenoreceptors in the brain stem. This action results in reduced sympathetic outflow from the central nervous system and in decreases in peripheral resistance, renal vascular resistance, heart rate, and blood pressure. Renal blood flow and glomerular filtration rate remain essentially unchanged. Normal postural reflexes are intact; therefore, orthostatic symptoms are mild and infrequent.

Acute studies with clonidine hydrochloride in humans have demonstrated a moderate reduction (15% to 20%) of cardiac output in the supine position with no change in the peripheral resistance; at a 45° tilt there is a smaller reduction in cardiac output and a decrease of peripheral resistance.

During long-term therapy, cardiac output tends to return to control values, while peripheral resistance remains decreased. Slowing of the pulse rate has been observed in most patients given clonidine, but the drug does not alter normal hemodynamic responses to exercise.

Tolerance to the antihypertensive effect may develop in some patients, necessitating a reevaluation of therapy.

Other studies in patients have provided evidence of a reduction in plasma renin activity and in the excretion of aldosterone and catecholamines. The exact relationship of these pharmacologic actions to the antihypertensive effect of clonidine has not been fully elucidated.

Clonidine acutely stimulates the release of growth hormone in children as well as adults but does not produce a chronic elevation of growth hormone with long-term use.

Pharmacokinetics: The plasma half-life of clonidine is 12.7 ± 7 hours. Following oral administration, about 40% to 60% of the absorbed dose is recovered in the urine as unchanged drug within 24 hours. The remainder of the absorbed dose is metabolized in the liver.

INDICATIONS AND USAGE

CLONIDINE TRANSDERMAL SYSTEM, USP is indicated in the treatment of hypertension. It may be employed alone or concomitantly with other antihypertensive agents.

CONTRAINDICATIONS

CLONIDINE TRANSDERMAL SYSTEM should not be used in patients with known hypersensitivity to clonidine or to any other component of the therapeutic system.

WARNINGS

Withdrawal: Patients should be instructed not to discontinue therapy without consulting their physician. Sudden cessation of clonidine treatment has, in some cases, resulted in symptoms such as nervousness, agitation, headache, and confusion accompanied or followed by a rapid rise in blood pressure and elevated catecholamine concentrations in the plasma. The likelihood of such reactions to discontinuation of clonidine therapy appears to be greater after administration of higher doses or continuation of concomitant beta-blocker treatment and special caution is therefore advised in these situations. Rare instances of hypertensive encephalopathy, cerebrovascular accidents and death have been reported after clonidine withdrawal. When discontinuing therapy with CLONIDINE TRANSDERMAL SYSTEM, the physician should reduce the dose gradually over 2 to 4 days to avoid withdrawal symptomatology.

An excessive rise in blood pressure following discontinuation of CLONIDINE TRANSDERMAL SYSTEM therapy can be reversed by administration of oral clonidine hydrochloride or by intravenous phentolamine. If therapy is to be discontinued in patients receiving a beta-blocker and clonidine concurrently, the beta-blocker should be withdrawn several days before the gradual discontinuation of CLONIDINE TRANSDERMAL SYSTEM.

PRECAUTIONS

General: In patients who have developed localized contact sensitization to CLONIDINE TRANSDERMAL SYSTEM continuation of CLONIDINE TRANSDERMAL SYSTEM or substitution of oral clonidine hydrochloride therapy may be associated with development of a generalized skin rash.

In patients who develop an allergic reaction to CLONIDINE TRANSDERMAL SYSTEM, substitution of oral clonidine hydrochloride may also elicit an allergic reaction (including generalized rash, urticaria, or angioedema).

CLONIDINE TRANSDERMAL SYSTEM should be used with caution in patients with severe coronary insufficiency, conduction disturbances, recent myocardial infarction, cerebrovascular disease, or chronic renal failure.

In rare instances, loss of blood pressure control has been reported in patients using CLONIDINE TRANSDERMAL SYSTEM according to the instructions for use.

Perioperative Use: CLONIDINE TRANSDERMAL SYSTEM therapy should not be interrupted during the surgical period. Blood pressure should be carefully monitored during surgery and additional measures to control blood pressure should be available if required. Physicians considering starting CLONIDINE TRANSDERMAL SYSTEM therapy during the perioperative period must be aware that therapeutic plasma clonidine levels are not achieved until 2 to 3 days after initial application of CLONIDINE TRANSDERMAL SYSTEM (see DOSAGE AND ADMINISTRATION).

Defibrillation or Cardioversion: The transdermal clonidine systems should be removed before attempting defibrillation or cardioversion because of the potential for altered electrical conductivity which may increase the risk of arcing, a phenomenon associated with the use of defibrillators.

Information for Patients: Patients should be cautioned against interruption of CLONIDINE TRANSDERMAL SYSTEM therapy without their physician's advice.

Patients who engage in potentially hazardous activities, such as operating machinery or driving, should be advised of a possible sedative effect of clonidine. They should also be informed that this sedative effect may be increased by concomitant use of alcohol, barbiturates, or other sedating drugs.

Patients who wear contact lenses should be cautioned that treatment with CLONIDINE TRANSDERMAL SYSTEM may cause dryness of eyes.

Patients should be instructed to consult their physicians promptly about the possible need to remove the patch if they observe moderate to severe localized erythema and/or vesicle formation at the site of application or generalized skin rash.

If a patient experiences isolated, mild localized skin irritation before completing 7 days of use, the system may be removed and replaced with a new system applied to a fresh skin site.

If the system should begin to loosen from the skin after application, the patient should be instructed to place the adhesive cover directly over the system to ensure adhesion during its 7-day use.

Used CLONIDINE TRANSDERMAL SYSTEM PATCHES contain a substantial amount of their initial drug content which may be harmful to infants and children if accidentally applied or ingested. THEREFORE, PATIENTS SHOULD BE CAUTIONED TO KEEP BOTH USED AND UNUSED CLONIDINE TRANSDERMAL SYSTEM PATCHES OUT OF THE REACH OF CHILDREN. After use, CLONIDINE TRANSDERMAL SYSTEM should be folded in half with the adhesive sides together and discarded away from children's reach.

Instructions for use, storage and disposal of the system are provided at the end of this monograph. These instructions are also included in each box of CLONIDINE TRANSDERMAL SYSTEM.

Drug Interactions: Clonidine may potentiate the CNS-depressive effects of alcohol, barbiturates or other sedating drugs. If a patient receiving clonidine is also taking tricyclic antidepressants, the hypotensive effect of clonidine may be reduced, necessitating an increase in the clonidine dose.

Due to a potential for additive effects such as bradycardia and AV block, caution is warranted in patients receiving clonidine concomitantly with agents known to affect sinus node function or AV nodal conduction e.g., digitalis, calcium channel blockers and beta-blockers.

Amitriptyline in combination with clonidine enhances the manifestation of corneal lesions in rats (see PRECAUTIONS: Toxicology).

Toxicology: In several studies with oral clonidine hydrochloride, a dose-dependent increase in the incidence and severity of spontaneous retinal degeneration was seen in albino rats treated for 6 months or longer. Tissue distribution studies in dogs and monkeys showed a concentration of clonidine in the choroid.

In view of the retinal degeneration seen in rats, eye examinations were performed during clinical trials in 908 patients before, and periodically after, the start of clonidine therapy. In 353 of these 908 patients, the eye examinations were carried out over periods of 24 months or longer. Except for some dryness of the eyes, no drug-related abnormal ophthalmological findings were recorded and, according to specialized tests such as electroretinography and macular dazzle, retinal function was unchanged.

In combination with amitriptyline, clonidine hydrochloride administration led to the development of corneal lesions in rats within 5 days.

Carcinogenesis, Mutagenesis, Impairment of Fertility: Chronic dietary administration of clonidine was not carcinogenic to rats (132 weeks) or mice (78 weeks) dosed, respectively, at up to 46 to 70 times the maximum recommended daily human dose as mg/kg (9 or 6 times the MRDHD on a mg/m^2 basis). There was no evidence of genotoxicity in the Ames test for mutagenicity or mouse micronucleus test for clastogenicity.

Fertility of male and female rats was unaffected by clonidine doses as high as 150 mcg/kg (approximately 3 times the MRDHD). In a separate experiment, fertility of female rats appeared to be affected at dose levels of 500 to 2000 mcg/kg (10 to 40 times the oral MRDHD on a mg/kg basis; 2 to 8 times the MRDHD on a mg/m^2 basis).

Pregnancy: ***Teratogenic Effects.*** *Pregnancy Category C:* Reproduction studies performed in rabbits at doses up to approximately 3 times the oral maximum recommended daily human dose (MRDHD) of clonidine hydrochloride produced no evidence of a teratogenic or embryotoxic potential in rabbits. In rats, however, doses as low as 1/3 the oral MRDHD (1/15 the MRDHD on a mg/m^2 basis) of clonidine were associated with increased resorptions in a study in which dams were treated continuously from 2 months prior to mating. Increased resorptions were not associated with treatment at the same or at higher dose levels (up to 3 times the oral MRDHD) when the dams were treated on gestation days 6 to 15. Increases in resorption were observed at much higher dose levels (40 times the oral MRDHD on a mg/kg basis; 4 to 8 times the MRDHD on a mg/m^2 basis) in mice and rats treated on gestation days 1 to 14 (lowest dose employed in the study was 500 mcg/kg).

No adequate well controlled studies have been conducted in pregnant women. Because animal reproduction studies are not always predictive of human response, this drug should be used during pregnancy only if clearly needed.

Nursing Mothers: As clonidine is excreted in human milk, caution should be exercised when CLONIDINE TRANSDERMAL SYSTEM is administered to a nursing woman.

Pediatric Use: Safety and effectiveness in pediatric patients have not been established in adequate and well controlled trials (see WARNINGS: Withdrawal).

ADVERSE REACTIONS

Clinical trial experience with CLONIDINE TRANSDERMAL SYSTEM: Most systemic adverse effects during CLONIDINE TRANSDERMAL SYSTEM therapy have been mild and have tended to diminish with continued therapy. In a 3-month multiclinic trial of CLONIDINE TRANSDERMAL SYSTEM in 101 hypertensive patients, the systemic adverse reactions were, dry mouth (25 patients) and drowsiness (12), fatigue (6), headache (5), lethargy and sedation (3 each), insomnia, dizziness, impotence/sexual dysfunction, dry throat (2 each) and constipation, nausea, change in taste and nervousness (1 each).

In the above mentioned 3-month controlled clinical trial, as well as other uncontrolled clinical trials, the most frequent adverse reactions were dermatological and are described below.

In the 3-month trial, 51 of the 101 patients had localized skin reactions such as erythema (26 patients) and/or pruritus, particularly after using an adhesive cover throughout the 7-day dosage interval. Allergic contact sensitization to CLONIDINE TRANSDERMAL SYSTEM was observed in 5 patients. Other skin reactions were localized vesiculation (7 patients), hyperpigmentation (5), edema (3), excoriation (3), burning (3), papules (1), throbbing (1), blanching (1), and a generalized macular rash (1).

In additional clinical experience, contact dermatitis resulting in treatment discontinuation was observed in 128 of 673 patients (about 19 in 100) after a mean duration of treatment of 37 weeks. The incidence of contact dermatitis was about 34 in 100 among white women, about 18 in 100 in white men, about 14 in 100 in black women, and approximately 8 in 100 in black men. Analysis of skin reaction data showed that the risk of having to discontinue CLONIDINE TRANSDERMAL SYSTEM treatment because of contact dermatitis was greatest between treatment weeks 6 and 26, although sensitivity may develop either earlier or later in treatment.

In a large-scale clinical acceptability and safety study by 451 physicians in a total of 3,539 patients, other allergic reactions were recorded for which a causal relationship to CLONIDINE TRANSDERMAL SYSTEM was not established: maculopapular rash (10 cases); urticaria (2 cases); and angioedema of the face (2 cases), which also affected the tongue in one of the patients.

Marketing Experience with CLONIDINE TRANSDERMAL SYSTEM: The following adverse reactions have been identified during post-approval use of CLONIDINE TRANSDERMAL SYSTEM. Because these reactions are reported voluntarily from a population of uncertain size, it is not always possible to estimate reliably their frequency or establish a causal relationship to drug exposure. Decisions to include these reactions in labeling are typically based on one or more of the following factors: (1) seriousness of the reaction, (2) frequency of reporting, or (3) strength of causal connection to CLONIDINE TRANSDERMAL SYSTEM.

Body as a Whole: Fever; malaise; weakness; pallor; and withdrawal syndrome.

Cardiovascular: Congestive heart failure; cerebrovascular accident; electrocardiographic abnormalities (i.e., bradycardia, sick sinus syndrome disturbances and arrhythmias); chest pain; orthostatic symptoms; syncope; increases in blood pressure; sinus bradycardia and atrioventricular (AV) block with and without the use of concomitant digitalis; Raynaud's phenomenon; tachycardia; bradycardia; and palpitations.

Central and Peripheral Nervous System/Psychiatric: Delirium; mental depression; hallucinations (including visual and auditory); localized numbness; vivid dreams or nightmares; restlessness; anxiety; agitation; irritability; other behavioral changes; and drowsiness.

Dermatological: Angioneurotic edema; localized or generalized rash; hives; urticaria; contact dermatitis; pruritus; alopecia; and localized hypo or hyper pigmentation.

Gastrointestinal: Anorexia and vomiting.

Genitourinary: Difficult micturition; loss of libido; and decreased sexual activity.

Metabolic: Gynecomastia or breast enlargement and weight gain.

Musculoskeletal: Muscle or joint pain; and leg cramps.

Ophthalmological: Blurred vision; burning of the eyes and dryness of the eyes.

Adverse Events Associated with Oral Clonidine Therapy: Most adverse effects are mild and tend to diminish with continued therapy. The most frequent (which appear to be dose-related) are dry mouth, occurring in about 40 of 100 patients; drowsiness, about 33 in 100; dizziness, about 16 in 100; constipation and sedation, each about 10 in 100. The following less frequent adverse experiences have also been reported in patients receiving clonidine hydrochloride, USP tablets, but in many cases patients were receiving concomitant medication and a causal relationship has not been established.

Body as a Whole: Fatigue, fever, headache, pallor, weakness, and withdrawal syndrome. Also reported were a weakly positive Coombs' test and increased sensitivity to alcohol.

Cardiovascular: Bradycardia, congestive heart failure, electrocardiographic abnormalities (i.e., sinus node arrest, junctional bradycardia, high degree AV block and arrhythmias), orthostatic symptoms, palpitations, Raynaud's phenomenon, syncope, and tachycardia. Cases of sinus bradycardia and AV block have been reported, both with and without the use of concomitant digitalis.

Central Nervous System: Agitation, anxiety, delirium, delusional perception, hallucinations (including visual and auditory), insomnia, mental depression, nervousness, other behavioral changes, paresthesia, restlessness, sleep disorder, and vivid dreams or nightmares.

Dermatological: Alopecia, angioneurotic edema, hives, pruritus, rash, and urticaria.

Gastrointestinal: Abdominal pain, anorexia, constipation, hepatitis, malaise, mild transient abnormalities in liver function tests, nausea, parotitis, pseudoobstruction (including colonic pseudo-obstruction), salivary gland pain, and vomiting.

Genitourinary: Decreased sexual activity, difficulty in micturition, erectile dysfunction, loss of libido, nocturia, and urinary retention.

Hematologic: Thrombocytopenia.

Metabolic: Gynecomastia, transient elevation of blood glucose or serum creatine phosphokinase, and weight gain.

Musculoskeletal: Leg cramps and muscle or joint pain.

Oro-otolaryngeal: Dryness of the nasal mucosa.

Ophthalmological: Accommodation disorder, blurred vision, burning of the eyes, decreased lacrimation, and dryness of the eyes.

OVERDOSAGE

Hypertension may develop early and may be followed by hypotension, bradycardia, respiratory depression, hypothermia, drowsiness, decreased or absent reflexes, weakness, irritability and miosis. The frequency of CNS depression may be higher in children than adults. Large overdoses may result in reversible cardiac conduction defects or dysrhythmias, apnea, coma and seizures. Signs and symptoms of overdose generally occur within 30 minutes to 2 hours after exposure. As little as 0.1 mg of clonidine has produced signs of toxicity in children.

If symptoms of poisoning occur following dermal exposure, remove all CLONIDINE TRANSDERMAL SYSTEMS. After their removal, the plasma clonidine levels will persist for about 8 hours, then decline slowly over a period of several days. Rare cases of CLONIDINE TRANSDERMAL SYSTEM poisoning due to accidental or deliberate mouthing or ingestion of the patch have been reported, many of them involving children.

There is no specific antidote for clonidine overdosage. Ipecac syrup-induced vomiting and gastric lavage would not be expected to remove significant amounts of clonidine following dermal exposure. If the patch is ingested, whole bowel irrigation may be considered and the administration of activated charcoal and/or cathartic may be beneficial. Supportive care may include atropine sulfate for bradycardia, intravenous fluids and/or vasopressor agents for hypotension and vasodilators for hypertension. Naloxone may be a useful adjunct for the management of clonidine-induced respiratory depression, hypotension and/or coma; blood pressure should be monitored since the administration of naloxone has occasionally resulted in paradoxical hypertension. Tolazoline administration has yielded inconsistent results and is not recommended as first-line therapy. Dialysis is not likely to significantly enhance the elimination of clonidine.

The largest overdose reported to date, involved a 28-year old male who ingested 100 mg of clonidine hydrochloride powder. This patient developed hypertension followed by hypotension, bradycardia, apnea, hallucinations, semicoma, and premature ventricular contractions. The patient fully recovered after intensive treatment. Plasma clonidine levels were 60 ng/mL after 1 hour, 190 ng/mL after 1.5 hours, 370 ng/mL after 2 hours, and 120 ng/mL after 5.5 and 6.5 hours. In mice and rats, the oral LD_{50} of clonidine is 206 and 465 mg/kg, respectively.

DOSAGE AND ADMINISTRATION

Apply CLONIDINE TRANSDERMAL SYSTEM once every 7 days to a hairless area of intact skin on the upper outer arm or chest. Each new application of CLONIDINE TRANSDERMAL SYSTEM should be on a different skin site from the previous location. If the system loosens during 7-day wearing, the ADHESIVE COVER should be applied directly over the system to ensure good adhesion. There have been rare reports of the need for PATCH changes prior to 7 days to maintain blood pressure control.

To initiate therapy, CLONIDINE TRANSDERMAL SYSTEM dosage should be titrated according to individual therapeutic requirements, starting with CLONIDINE TRANSDERMAL SYSTEM 0.1 mg/day. If after one or two weeks the desired reduction in blood pressure is not achieved, increase the dosage by adding another CLONIDINE TRANSDERMAL SYSTEM, 0.1 mg/day or changing to a larger system. An increase in dosage above two CLONIDINE TRANSDERMAL SYSTEM 0.3 mg/day is usually not associated with additional efficacy.

When substituting CLONIDINE TRANSDERMAL SYSTEM for oral clonidine or for other antihypertensive drugs, physicians should be aware that the antihypertensive effect of CLONIDINE TRANSDERMAL SYSTEM may not commence until 2 to 3 days after initial application. Therefore, gradual reduction of prior drug dosage is advised. Some or all previous antihypertensive treatment may have to be continued, particularly in patients with more severe forms of hypertension.

Renal Impairment: Dosage must be adjusted according to the degree of impairment, and patients should be carefully monitored. Since only a minimal amount of clonidine is removed during routine hemodialysis, there is no need to give supplemental clonidine following dialysis.

HOW SUPPLIED

CLONIDINE TRANSDERMAL SYSTEM, USP, 0.1 mg/day, CLONIDINE TRANSDERMAL SYSTEM, USP, 0.2 mg/day and CLONIDINE TRANSDERMAL SYSTEM, USP, 0.3 mg/day are supplied as 4 pouched systems and 4 ADHESIVE COVERS per carton. See chart below.

[See table below]

	Programmed Delivery Clonidine *in vivo* Per Day Over 1 Week	Clonidine Content	Size
Clonidine Transdermal System, USP NDC 0378-0871-99	0.1 mg	2.52 mg	3.33 cm^2
Clonidine Transdermal System, USP NDC 0378-0872-99	0.2 mg	5.04 mg	6.67 cm^2
Clonidine Transdermal System, USP NDC 0378-0873-99	0.3 mg	7.56 mg	10.0 cm^2

STORAGE AND HANDLING: Store at 20° to 25°C (68° to 77°F). [See USP for Controlled Room Temperature.]

Address medical inquiries to: 1-877-446-3679 (1-877-4-INFO-RX)

MYLAN®

Mylan Pharmaceuticals Inc.
Morgantown, WV 26505

REVISED NOVEMBER 2009
CTS:R9

PATIENT INSTRUCTIONS

Clonidine Transdermal System, USP
(Read the following instructions carefully before using this medication. If you have any questions, please consult with your doctor.)

General Information

CLONIDINE TRANSDERMAL SYSTEM is a peach colored, rectangular PATCH with rounded corners, containing an active blood-pressure-lowering medication. It is designed to deliver the drug into the body through the skin smoothly and consistently for one full week. Normal exposure to water, as in showering, bathing, and swimming, should not affect the PATCH.

The optional ivory ADHESIVE COVER should be applied directly over the PATCH, should the PATCH begin to separate from the skin. The ADHESIVE COVER ensures that the PATCH sticks to the skin. The CLONIDINE TRANSDERMAL SYSTEM PATCH must be replaced with a new one on a fresh skin site if the one in use significantly loosens or falls off.

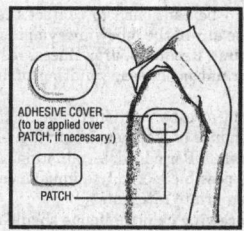

Figure 1

How to Apply the CLONIDINE TRANSDERMAL SYSTEM PATCH

1) Apply the peach colored, rectangular PATCH with rounded corners, once a week, preferably at a convenient time on the same day of the week (i.e., prior to bedtime on Tuesday of week one; prior to bedtime on Tuesday of week two, etc.).

Each box of CLONIDINE TRANSDERMAL SYSTEM contains two types of pouches:

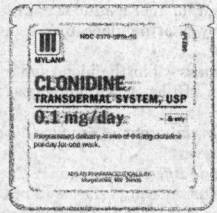

Contains PATCH with medication | Contains COVER for use if the PATCH becomes loose

Figure 2

2) Select a hairless area such as on the upper, outer arm or upper chest. The area chosen should be free of cuts, abrasions, irritation, scars or calluses and should not be shaved before applying the CLONIDINE TRANSDERMAL SYSTEM PATCH. Do not place the CLONIDINE TRANSDERMAL SYSTEM PATCH on skin folds or under tight undergarments, since premature loosening may occur.
3) Wash hands with soap and water and thoroughly dry them.
4) Clean the area chosen with soap and water. Rinse and wipe dry with a clean, dry tissue.
5) Select the pouch labeled CLONIDINE TRANSDERMAL SYSTEM, USP and open it as illustrated in Figure 3. Remove the contents of the pouch and discard the additional pieces of clear protective film above and below the PATCH.

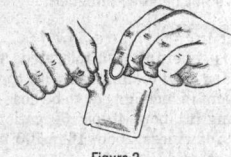

Figure 3

6) Remove the clear plastic protective backing from the peach colored, rectangular PATCH by gently peeling off one half of the backing at a time as shown in Figure 4. Avoid touching the sticky side of the CLONIDINE TRANSDERMAL SYSTEM PATCH.

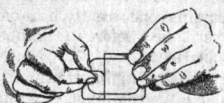

Figure 4

7) Place the CLONIDINE TRANSDERMAL SYSTEM PATCH on the prepared skin site (sticky side down) by applying firm pressure over the PATCH to ensure good contact with the skin, especially around the edges (Figure 5). Discard the clear plastic protective backing and wash your hands with soap and water to remove any drug from your hands.

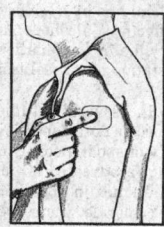

Figure 5

8) After one week, remove the old PATCH and discard it (refer to **Instructions for Disposal**). After choosing a different skin site, repeat instructions 2 through 7 for the application of your next CLONIDINE TRANSDERMAL SYSTEM PATCH.

What to do if your CLONIDINE TRANSDERMAL SYSTEM PATCH becomes loose while wearing:

How to Apply the ADHESIVE COVER

NOTE: The ivory ADHESIVE COVER **does not contain any drug** and should not be used alone. The COVER should be applied directly over the CLONIDINE TRANSDERMAL SYSTEM PATCH **only** if the PATCH begins to separate from the skin, thereby ensuring that it sticks to the skin for 7 full days.

1) Wash hands with soap and water and thoroughly dry them.
2) Using a clean, dry tissue, make sure that the area around the rectangular, peach CLONIDINE TRANSDERMAL SYSTEM PATCH is clean and dry. Press gently on the CLONIDINE TRANSDERMAL SYSTEM PATCH to ensure that the edges are in good contact with the skin.
3) Take the ivory ADHESIVE COVER (Figure 6) from the plain white pouch and remove the paper liner backing from the COVER.

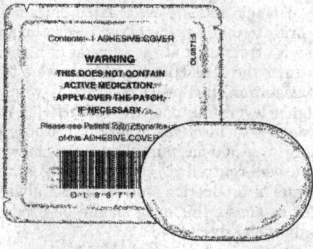

Figure 6

4) Carefully center the ivory ADHESIVE COVER over the rectangular, peach CLONIDINE TRANSDERMAL SYSTEM PATCH and apply firm pressure, especially around the edges in contact with the skin.

Instructions for Disposal

KEEP OUT OF REACH OF CHILDREN

During or even after use, a PATCH contains active medication which may be harmful to infants and children if accidentally applied or ingested. After use, fold in half with the sticky sides together. Dispose of carefully out of reach of children.

Call your doctor for medical advice about side effects. You may report side effects to FDA at 1-800-FDA-1088.

MYLAN®
Mylan Pharmaceuticals Inc.
Morgantown, WV 26505

REVISED MARCH 2009
PL:CTS:R7

CLORPRES® TABLETS ℞
[klŏr prĕs]
(Clonidine Hydrochloride and Chlorthalidone Tablets, USP)
0.1 mg/15 mg, 0.2 mg/15 mg and 0.3 mg/15 mg
℞ only

DESCRIPTION

CLORPRES® is a combination of clonidine hydrochloride (a centrally acting antihypertensive agent) and chlorthalidone (a diuretic). CLORPRES® is available as tablets for oral administration in three dosage strengths: 0.1 mg/15 mg, 0.2 mg/15 mg and 0.3 mg/15 mg of clonidine hydrochloride/chlorthalidone, respectively.

The inactive ingredients are ammonium chloride, colloidal silicon dioxide, croscarmellose sodium (Type A), magnesium stearate, microcrystalline cellulose, sodium lauryl sulfate, D&C yellow #10.

Clonidine Hydrochloride: Clonidine hydrochloride, USP is an imidazoline derivative and exists as a mesomeric compound. The chemical name is 2-[(2,6-dichlorophenyl)imino]imidazoline monohydrochloride. The following are the structural formula, molecular formula and molecular weight:

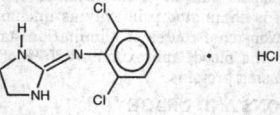

$C_9H_9Cl_2N_3 \cdot HCl$
M.W. 266.56

Clonidine hydrochloride is an odorless, bitter, white crystalline substance soluble in water and alcohol.

Chlorthalidone: Chlorthalidone, USP is a monosulfamyl diuretic that differs chemically from thiazide diuretics in that a double ring system is incorporated in its structure. It is 2-chloro-5-(1-hydroxy-3-oxo-1-isoindolinyl) benzenesulfonamide with the following structural formula, molecular formula and molecular weight:

$C_{14}H_{11}Cl N_2O_4S$
M.W. 338.76

Chlorthalidone is practically insoluble in water, in ether and in chloroform; soluble in methanol; slightly soluble in alcohol.

CLINICAL PHARMACOLOGY

CLORPRES®: CLORPRES® produces a more pronounced antihypertensive response than occurs after either clonidine hydrochloride or chlorthalidone alone in equivalent doses.

Clonidine Hydrochloride: Clonidine hydrochloride acts relatively rapidly. The patient's blood pressure declines within 30 to 60 minutes after an oral dose, the maximum decrease occurring within 2 to 4 hours. The plasma level of clonidine hydrochloride peaks in approximately 3 to 5 hours and the plasma half-life ranges from 12 to 16 hours. The half-life increases up to 41 hours in patients with severe impairment of renal function. Following oral administration about 40 to 60% of the absorbed dose is recovered in the urine as unchanged drug in 24 hours. About 50% of the absorbed dose is metabolized in the liver.

Clonidine stimulates alpha-adrenoreceptors in the brain stem, resulting in reduced sympathetic outflow from the central nervous system and a decrease in peripheral resistance, renal vascular resistance, heart rate, and blood pressure. Renal blood flow and glomerular filtration rate remain essentially unchanged. Normal postural reflexes are intact and therefore orthostatic symptoms are mild and infrequent.

Acute studies with clonidine hydrochloride in humans have demonstrated a moderate reduction (15 to 20%) of cardiac output in the supine position with no change in the peripheral resistance; at a 45° tilt there is a smaller reduction in cardiac output and a decrease of peripheral resistance. During long-term therapy, cardiac output tends to return to control values, while peripheral resistance remains decreased. Slowing of the pulse rate has been observed in most patients given clonidine but the drug does not alter normal hemodynamic response to exercise.

Other studies in patients have provided evidence of a reduction in plasma renin activity and in the excretion of aldosterone and catecholamines, but the exact relationship of these pharmacologic actions to the antihypertensive effect has not been fully elucidated.

Clonidine acutely stimulates growth hormone release in both children and adults, but does not produce a chronic elevation of growth hormone with long-term use.

Tolerance may develop in some patients, necessitating a reevaluation of therapy.

Chlorthalidone: Chlorthalidone is a long-acting oral diuretic with antihypertensive activity. Its diuretic action commences a mean of 2.6 hours after dosing and continues for up to 72 hours. The drug produces diuresis with increased excretion of sodium and chloride. The diuretic effects of chlorthalidone and the benzothiadiazine (thiazide) diuretics appear to arise from similar mechanisms and the maximal effect of chlorthalidone and the thiazides appears to be similar. The site of action appears to be the distal convoluted tubule of the nephron. The diuretic effects of chlorthalidone lead to decreased extracellular fluid volume, plasma volume, cardiac output, total exchangeable sodium, glomerular filtration rate, and renal plasma flow. Although the mechanism of action of chlorthalidone and related drugs is not wholly clear, sodium and water depletion appear to provide a basis for its antihypertensive effect. Like the thiazide diuretics, chlorthalidone produces dose-related reductions in serum potassium levels, elevations in serum uric acid and blood glucose, and it can lead to decreased sodium and chloride levels.

The mean plasma half-life of chlorthalidone is about 40 to 60 hours. It is eliminated primarily as unchanged drug in the urine. Non-renal routes of elimination have yet to be clarified. In the blood, approximately 75% of the drug is bound to plasma proteins.

INDICATIONS AND USAGE

CLORPRES® (clonidine hydrochloride USP/chlorthalidone USP) is indicated in the treatment of hypertension. **This fixed combination drug is not indicated for initial therapy of hypertension. Hypertension requires therapy titrated to the individual patient. If the fixed combination represents the dosage so determined, its use may be more convenient in patient management. The treatment of hypertension is not static, but must be reevaluated as conditions in each patient warrant.**

CONTRAINDICATIONS

Anuria: CLORPRES® is contraindicated in patients with known hypersensitivity to chlorthalidone or other sulfonamide-derived drugs.

WARNINGS

Chlorthalidone should be used with caution in severe renal disease. In patients with renal disease, chlorthalidone or related drugs may precipitate azotemia. Cumulative effects of the drug may develop in patients with impaired renal function. Chlorthalidone should be used with caution in patients with impaired hepatic function or progressive liver disease, because minor alterations of fluid and electrolyte balance may precipitate hepatic coma.

Sensitivity reactions may occur in patients with a history of allergy or bronchial asthma.

The possibility of exacerbation or activation of systemic lupus erythematosus has been reported with thiazide diuretics which are structurally related to chlorthalidone. However, systemic lupus erythematosus has not been reported following chlorthalidone administration.

PRECAUTIONS

Clonidine Hydrochloride: *General:* In patients who have developed localized contact sensitization to transdermal clonidine, substitution of oral clonidine hydrochloride therapy may be associated with the development of a generalized skin rash.

In patients who develop an allergic reaction from transdermal clonidine that extends beyond the local patch site (such as generalized skin rash, urticaria, or angioedema), oral clonidine hydrochloride substitution may elicit a similar reaction.

As with all antihypertensive therapy, clonidine hydrochloride should be used with caution in patients with severe coronary insufficiency, recent myocardial infarction, cerebrovascular disease or chronic renal failure.

Withdrawal: Patients should be instructed not to discontinue therapy without consulting their physician. Sudden cessation of clonidine treatment has resulted in subjective symptoms such as nervousness, agitation and headache, accompanied or followed by a rapid rise in blood pressure and elevated catecholamine concentrations in the plasma, but such occurrences have usually been associated with previous administration of high oral doses (exceeding 1.2 mg/day) and/or with continuation of concomitant beta-blocker therapy. Rare instances of hypertensive encephalopathy and death have been reported. When discontinuing therapy with clonidine hydrochloride, the physician should reduce the dose gradually over 2 to 4 days to avoid withdrawal symptomatology.

An excessive rise in blood pressure following clonidine hydrochloride discontinuance can be reversed by administration of oral clonidine or by intravenous phentolamine. If therapy is to be discontinued in patients receiving beta-blockers and clonidine concurrently, beta-blockers should be discontinued several days before the gradual withdrawal of clonidine hydrochloride.

Perioperative Use: Administration of clonidine hydrochloride should be continued to within four hours of surgery and resumed as soon as possible thereafter. The blood pressure should be carefully monitored and appropriate measures instituted to control it as necessary.

Information for Patients: Patients who engage in potentially hazardous activities, such as operating machinery or driving, should be advised of a potential sedative effect of clonidine. Patients should be cautioned against interruption of clonidine hydrochloride therapy without a physician's advice.

Drug Interactions: If a patient receiving clonidine hydrochloride is also taking tricyclic antidepressants, the effect of clonidine may be reduced, thus necessitating an increase in dosage. Clonidine hydrochloride may enhance the CNS-depressive effects of alcohol, barbiturates or other sedatives. Amitriptyline in combination with clonidine enhances the manifestation of corneal lesions in rats (see Ocular Toxicity).

Ocular Toxicity: In several studies, oral clonidine hydrochloride produced a dose-dependent increase in the incidence and severity of spontaneously occurring retinal degeneration in albino rats treated for six months or longer. Tissue distribution studies in dogs and monkeys revealed that clonidine hydrochloride was concentrated in the choroid of the eye. In view of the retinal degeneration observed in rats, eye examinations were performed in 908 patients prior to the start of clonidine hydrochloride therapy, who were then examined periodically thereafter. In 353 of these 908 patients, examinations were performed for periods of 24 months or longer. Except for some dryness of the eyes, no drug-related abnormal ophthalmologic findings were recorded and clonidine hydrochloride did not alter retinal function as shown by specialized tests such as the electroretinogram and macular dazzle.

In rats, clonidine hydrochloride in combination with amitriptyline produced corneal lesions within 5 days.

Carcinogenesis, Mutagenesis, Impairment of Fertility: In a 132-week (fixed concentration) dietary administration study in rats, clonidine hydrochloride administered at 32 to 46 times the maximum recommended daily human oral dose was unassociated with evidence of carcinogenic potential.

Fertility of male or female rats was unaffected by clonidine hydrochloride doses as high as 150 mcg/kg or about 3 times the maximum recommended daily human oral dose (MRDHD). Fertility of female rats did, however, appear to be affected (in another experiment) at dose levels of 500 to 2000 mcg/kg or 10 to 40 times the MRDHD.

Usage in Pregnancy: *Teratogenic Effect, Pregnancy Category C:* Reproduction studies performed in rabbits at doses up to approximately 3 times the maximum recommended daily human dose (MRDHD) of clonidine hydrochloride have revealed no evidence of teratogenic or embryotoxic potential. In rats however, doses as low as 1/3 the MRDHD were associated with increased resorptions in a study in which dams were treated continuously from 2 months prior to mating. Increased resorptions were not associated with treatment at the same or at higher dose levels (up to 3 times the MRDHD) when dams were treated days 6 to 15 of gestation. Increased resorptions were observed at much higher levels (40 times the MRDHD) in rats and mice treated days 1 to 14 of gestation (lowest dose employed in that study was 500 mcg/kg). There are, however, no adequate and well-controlled studies in pregnant women. Because animal reproduction studies are not always predictive of human response, this drug should be used during pregnancy only if clearly needed.

Nursing Mothers: As clonidine hydrochloride is excreted in human milk, caution should be exercised when it is administered to a nursing woman.

Pediatric Use: Safety and effectiveness in the pediatric population have not been established.

Chlorthalidone: *General:* Hypokalemia and other electrolyte abnormalities, including hyponatremia and hypochloremic alkalosis, are common in patients receiving chlorthalidone. These abnormalities are dose-related but may occur even at the lowest marketed doses of chlorthalidone. Serum electrolytes should be determined before initiating therapy and at periodic intervals during therapy. Serum and urine electrolyte determinations are particularly important when the patient is vomiting excessively or receiving parenteral fluids. All patients taking chlorthalidone should be observed for clinical signs of electrolyte imbalance, including dryness of mouth, thirst, weakness, lethargy, drowsiness, restlessness, muscle pains or cramps, muscular fatigue, hypotension, oliguria, tachycardia, palpitations and gastrointestinal disturbances, such as nausea and vomiting. Digitalis therapy may exaggerate metabolic effects of hypokalemia especially with reference to myocardial activity.

Any chloride deficit is generally mild and usually does not require specific treatment except under extraordinary circumstances (as in liver disease or renal disease). Dilutional hyponatremia may occur in edematous patients in hot weather: appropriate therapy is water restriction, rather than administration of salt, except in rare instances when the hyponatremia is life-threatening. In cases of actual salt depletion, appropriate replacement is the therapy of choice.

Uric Acid: Hyperuricemia may occur or frank gout may be precipitated in certain patients receiving chlorthalidone.

Other: Increases in serum glucose may occur and latent diabetes mellitus may become manifest during chlorthalidone therapy (see PRECAUTIONS: Chlorthalidone: Drug Interactions). Chlorthalidone and related drugs may decrease serum PBI levels without signs of thyroid disturbance.

Information for Patients: Patients should inform their doctor if they have: 1) had an allergic reaction to chlorthalidone or other diuretics or have asthma 2) kidney disease 3) liver disease 4) gout 5) systemic lupus erythematosus, or 6) been taking other drugs such as cortisone, digitalis, lithium carbonate, or drugs for diabetes.

Patients should be cautioned to contact their physician if they experience any of the following symptoms of potassium loss: excess thirst, tiredness, drowsiness, restlessness, muscle pains or cramps, nausea, vomiting or increased heart rate or pulse.

Patients should also be cautioned that taking alcohol can increase the chance of dizziness occurring.

Laboratory Tests: Periodic determination of serum electrolytes to detect possible electrolyte imbalance should be performed at appropriate intervals.

All patients receiving chlorthalidone should be observed for clinical signs of fluid or electrolyte imbalance: namely, hyponatremia, hypochloremic alkalosis and hypokalemia. Serum and urine electrolyte determinations are particularly important when the patient is vomiting excessively or receiving parenteral fluids.

Drug Interactions: Chlorthalidone may add to or potentiate the action of other antihypertensive drugs. Insulin requirements in diabetic patients may be increased, decreased or unchanged. Higher dosage of oral hypoglycemic agents may be required. Chlorthalidone and related drugs may increase the responsiveness to tubocurarine. Chlorthalidone and related drugs may decrease arterial responsiveness to norepinephrine. This diminution is not sufficient to preclude effectiveness of the pressor agent for therapeutic use. Lithium renal clearance is reduced by chlorthalidone, increasing the risk of lithium toxicity.

Drug/Laboratory Test Interactions: Chlorthalidone and related drugs may decrease serum PBI levels without signs of thyroid disturbance.

Carcinogenesis, Mutagenesis, Impairment of Fertility: No information is available.

Usage in Pregnancy: *Teratogenic Effects:* *Pregnancy Category B:* Reproduction studies have been performed in the rat and the rabbit at doses up to 420 times the human dose and have revealed no evidence of harm to the fetus due to chlorthalidone. There are, however, no adequate and well-controlled studies in pregnant women. Because animal reproduction studies are not always predictive of human response, this drug should be used during pregnancy only if clearly needed.

Non-Teratogenic Effects: Thiazides cross the placental barrier and appear in cord blood. The use of chlorthalidone and related drugs in pregnant women requires that the anticipated benefits of the drug be weighed against possible hazards to the fetus. These hazards include fetal or neonatal jaundice, thrombocytopenia, and possibly other adverse reactions that have occurred in the adult.

Nursing Mothers: Thiazides are excreted in human milk. Because of the potential for serious adverse reactions in nursing infants from chlorthalidone, a decision should be made whether to discontinue nursing or to discontinue the drug, taking into account the importance of the drug to the mother.

Pediatric Use: Safety and effectiveness in the pediatric population have not been established.

ADVERSE REACTIONS

CLORPRES® is generally well tolerated. Most adverse effects are mild and tend to diminish with continued therapy. The most frequent (which appear to be dose-related) are dry mouth, occurring in about 40 of 100 patients; drowsiness, about 33 in 100; dizziness, about 16 in 100; constipation and sedation, each about 10 in 100.

In addition to the reactions listed above, certain less frequent adverse experiences, which are shown below, have also been reported in patients receiving the component drugs of CLORPRES® but in many cases patients were receiving concomitant medication and a causal relationship has not been established:

Clonidine Hydrochloride: *Gastrointestinal:* Nausea and vomiting, about 5 in 100 patients; anorexia and malaise, each about 1 in 100; mild transient abnormalities in liver function tests, about 1 in 100; rare reports of hepatitis; parotitis, rarely.
Metabolic: Weight gain, about 1 in 100 patients; gynecomastia, about 1 in 1000, transient elevation of blood glucose or serum creatine phosphokinase, rarely.
Central Nervous System: Nervousness and agitation, about 3 in 100 patients; mental depression, about 1 in 100; headache, about 1 in 100; insomnia, about 5 in 1000. Vivid dreams or nightmares, other behavioral changes, restlessness, anxiety, visual and auditory hallucinations and delirium have been reported.
Cardiovascular: Orthostatic symptoms, about 3 in 100 patients; palpitations and tachycardia, and bradycardia, each about 5 in 1000. Raynaud's phenomenon, congestive heart failure, and electrocardiographic abnormalities, i.e., conduction disturbances and arrhythmias, have been reported rarely. Rare cases of sinus bradycardia and atrioventricular block have been reported, both with and without the use of concomitant digitalis.
Dermatological: Rash, about 1 in 100 patients; pruritus, about 7 in 1000; hives, angioneurotic edema and urticaria, about 5 in 1000, alopecia, about 2 in 1000.
Genitourinary: Decreased sexual activity, impotence and loss of libido, about 3 in 100 patients; nocturia, about 1 in 100; difficulty in micturition, about 2 in 1000; urinary retention, about 1 in 1000.
Other: Weakness, about 10 in 100 patients; fatigue, about 4 in 100; discontinuation syndrome, about 1 in 100; muscle or joint pain, about 6 in 1000 and cramps of the lower limbs, about 3 in 1000. Dryness, burning of the eyes, blurred vision, dryness of the nasal mucosa, pallor, weakly positive Coombs' test, increased sensitivity to alcohol and fever have been reported.
Chlorthalidone: *Gastrointestinal:* Anorexia, gastric irritation, nausea, vomiting, cramping, diarrhea, constipation, jaundice (intrahepatic cholestatic jaundice), pancreatitis.
Central Nervous System: Dizziness, vertigo, paresthesias, headache, xanthopsia.
Hematologic: Leukopenia, agranulocytosis, thrombocytopenia, aplastic anemia.
Dermatologic-Hypersensitivity: Purpura, photosensitivity, rash, urticaria, necrotizing angiitis (vasculitis) (cutaneous vasculitis), Lyell's syndrome (toxic epidermal necrolysis).
Cardiovascular: Orthostatic hypotension may occur and may be aggravated by alcohol, barbiturates or narcotics.
Other Adverse Reactions: Hyperglycemia, glycosuria, hyperuricemia, muscle spasm, weakness, restlessness, impotence.
Whenever adverse reactions are moderate or severe, chlorthalidone dosage should be reduced or therapy withdrawn.

OVERDOSAGE
Clonidine Hydrochloride: The signs and symptoms of clonidine hydrochloride overdosage include hypotension, bradycardia, lethargy, irritability, weakness, somnolence, diminished or absent reflexes, miosis, vomiting and hypoventilation. With large overdoses, reversible cardiac conduction defects or arrhythmias, apnea, seizures and transient hypertension have been reported. The oral LD_{50} of clonidine in rats was 465 mg/kg, and in mice 206 mg/kg.
The general treatment of clonidine hydrochloride overdosage may include intravenous fluids as indicated. Bradycardia can be treated with intravenous atropine sulfate and hypotension with dopamine infusion in addition to intravenous fluids. Hypertension, associated with overdosage, has been treated with intravenous furosemide or diazoxide or alpha-blocking agents such as phentolamine. Tolazoline, an alpha-blocker, in intravenous doses of 10 mg at 30-minute intervals, may reverse clonidine's effects if other efforts fail. Routine hemodialysis is of limited benefit, since a maximum of 5% of circulating clonidine is removed.
In a patient who ingested 100 mg clonidine hydrochloride, plasma clonidine levels were 60 ng/mL (one hour), 190 ng/mL (1.5 hours), 370 ng/mL (two hours) and 120 ng/mL (5.5 and 6.5 hours). This patient developed hypertension followed by hypotension, bradycardia, apnea, hallucinations, semicoma, and premature ventricular contractions. The patient fully recovered after intensive treatment.
Chlorthalidone: Symptoms of acute overdosage include nausea, weakness, dizziness and disturbances of electrolyte balance. The oral LD_{50} of the drug in the mouse and the rat is more than 25,000 mg/kg body weight. The minimum lethal dose (MLD) in humans has not been established. There is no specific antidote but gastric lavage is recommended, followed by supportive treatment. Where necessary, this may include intravenous dextrose-saline with potassium, administered with caution.

DOSAGE AND ADMINISTRATION
The dosage must be determined by individual titration. (See INDICATIONS AND USAGE.)

Chlorthalidone is usually initiated at a dose of 25 mg once daily and may be increased to 50 mg if the response is insufficient after a suitable trial.
Clonidine hydrochloride is usually initiated at a dose of 0.1 mg twice daily. Elderly patients may benefit from a lower initial dose. Further increments of 0.1 mg/day may be made if necessary until the desired response is achieved. The therapeutic doses most commonly employed have ranged from 0.2 to 0.6 mg per day in divided doses.
One CLORPRES® (clonidine hydrochloride/chlorthalidone) Tablet administered once or twice daily can be used to administer a minimum of 0.1 mg clonidine hydrochloride and 15 mg chlorthalidone to a maximum of 0.6 mg clonidine hydrochloride and 30 mg chlorthalidone.

HOW SUPPLIED
CLORPRES® TABLETS (Clonidine Hydrochloride and Chlorthalidone Tablets, USP) are available containing:
0.1 mg clonidine hydrochloride, USP and 15 mg chlorthalidone, USP
or
0.2 mg clonidine hydrochloride, USP and 15 mg chlorthalidone, USP
or
0.3 mg clonidine hydrochloride, USP and 15 mg chlorthalidone, USP
The 0.1 mg/15 mg product is a yellow, round, scored tablet debossed with **M** above the score and **1** below the score on one side of the tablet and blank on the other side. They are available as follows:
NDC 0378-0001-01
bottles of 100 tablets
The 0.2 mg/15 mg product is a yellow, round, scored tablet debossed with **M** above the score and **27** below the score on one side of the tablet and blank on the other side. They are available as follows:
NDC 0378-0027-01
bottles of 100 tablets
The 0.3 mg/15 mg product is a yellow, round, scored tablet debossed with **M** above the score and **72** below the score on one side of the tablet and blank on the other side. They are available as follows:
NDC 0378-0072-01
bottles of 100 tablets
Dispense in tight, light-resistant container as defined in the USP using a child-resistant closure.
Keep this and all medication out of the reach of children.
Store at 20° to 25°C (68° to 77°F). [See USP for Controlled Room Temperature.]
Avoid excessive humidity.
Mylan Pharmaceuticals Inc.
Morgantown, WV 26505

REVISED APRIL 2009
BKCLCH:R5

FENTANYL TRANSDERMAL SYSTEM ℂ ℞
[fen-tan-yl]
℞ only
Full PrescribingInformation
FOR USE IN OPIOID-TOLERANT PATIENTS ONLY

Fentanyl transdermal system contains a high concentration of a potent Schedule II opioid agonist, fentanyl. Schedule II opioid substances which include fentanyl, hydromorphone, methadone, morphine, oxycodone, and oxymorphone have the highest potential for abuse and associated risk of fatal overdose due to respiratory depression. Fentanyl can be abused and is subject to criminal diversion. The high content of fentanyl in the patches (fentanyl transdermal system) may be a particular target for abuse and diversion.
Fentanyl transdermal system is indicated for management of persistent, moderate to severe chronic pain that:

• requires continuous, around-the-clock opioid administration for an extended period of time, and
• cannot be managed by other means such as non-steroidal analgesics, opioid combination products, or immediate-release opioids

Fentanyl transdermal system should ONLY be used in patients who are already receiving opioid therapy, who have demonstrated opioid tolerance, and who require a total daily dose at least equivalent to fentanyl transdermal system 25 mcg/hr. Patients who are considered opioid-tolerant are those who have been taking, for a week or longer, at least 60 mg of morphine daily, or at least 30 mg of oral oxycodone daily, or at least 8 mg of oral hydromorphone daily or an equianalgesic dose of another opioid.
Because serious or life-threatening hypoventilation could occur, fentanyl transdermal system is contraindicated:

• in patients who are not opioid-tolerant
• in the management of acute pain or in patients who require opioid analgesia for a short period of time
• in the management of postoperative pain, including use after out-patient or day surgeries (e.g., tonsillectomies)
• in the management of mild pain
• in the management of intermittent pain [e.g., use on an as needed basis (prn)]
(See CONTRAINDICATIONS for further information.)
Since the peak fentanyl concentrations generally occur between 20 and 72 hours of treatment; prescribers should be aware that serious or life-threatening hypoventilation may occur, even in opioid-tolerant patients, during the initial application period.
The concomitant use of fentanyl transdermal system with all cytochrome P450 3A4 inhibitors (such as ritonavir, ketoconazole, itraconazole, troleandomycin, clarithromycin, nelfinavir, nefazodone, amiodarone, amprenavir, aprepitant, diltiazem, erythromycin, fluconazole, fosamprenavir, grapefruit juice, and verapamil) may result in an increase in fentanyl plasma concentrations, which could increase or prolong adverse drug effects and may cause potentially fatal respiratory depression. Patients receiving fentanyl transdermal system and any CYP3A4 inhibitor should be carefully monitored for an extended period of time and dosage adjustments should be made if warranted (see CLINICAL PHARMACOLOGY: Drug Interactions, WARNINGS, PRECAUTIONS and DOSAGE AND ADMINISTRATION for further information).
The safety of fentanyl transdermal system has not been established in children under 2 years of age. Fentanyl transdermal system should be administered to children only if they are opioid-tolerant and 2 years of age or older (see PRECAUTIONS: Pediatric Use).
Fentanyl transdermal system is ONLY for use in patients who are already tolerant to opioid therapy of comparable potency. Use in non-opioid-tolerant patients may lead to fatal respiratory depression. Overestimating the fentanyl transdermal system dose when converting patients from another opioid medication can result in fatal overdose with the first dose (see DOSAGE AND ADMINISTRATION: Initial Fentanyl Transdermal System Dose Selection). Due to the mean half-life of approximately 20 to 27 hours, patients who are thought to have had a serious adverse event, including overdose, will require monitoring and treatment for at least 24 hours.
Fentanyl transdermal system can be abused in a manner similar to other opioid agonists, legal or illicit. This risk should be considered when administering, prescribing, or dispensing fentanyl transdermal system in situations where the healthcare professional is concerned about increased risk of misuse, abuse or diversion.
Persons at increased risk for opioid abuse include those with a personal or family history of substance abuse (including drug or alcohol abuse or addiction) or mental illness (e.g., major depression). Patients should be assessed for their clinical risks for opioid abuse or addiction prior to being prescribed opioids. All patients receiving opioids should be routinely monitored for signs of misuse, abuse and addiction. Patients at increased risk of opioid abuse may still be appropriately treated with modified-release opioid formulations; however, these patients will require intensive monitoring for signs of misuse, abuse, or addiction.
Fentanyl transdermal system patches are intended for transdermal use (on intact skin) only. Do not use a fentanyl transdermal system if the pouch seal is broken or the patch is cut, damaged, or changed in any way.
Avoid exposing the fentanyl transdermal system application site and surrounding area to direct external heat sources, such as heating pads or electric blankets, heat or tanning lamps, saunas, hot tubs, and heated water beds, while wearing the system. Avoid taking hot baths or sunbathing. There is a potential for temperature-dependent increases in fentanyl released from the system resulting in possible overdose and death. Patients wearing fentanyl transdermal systems who develop fever or increased core body temperature due to strenuous exertion should be monitored for opioid side effects and the fentanyl transdermal system dose should be adjusted if necessary.

DESCRIPTION
Fentanyl transdermal system is a transdermal system providing continuous systemic delivery of fentanyl, a potent opioid analgesic, for 72 hours. The chemical name is N-Phenyl-N-(1-(2-phenylethyl)-4-piperidinyl) propanamide.

The structural formula is:

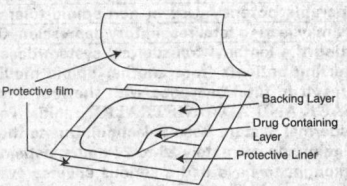

The molecular weight of fentanyl base is 336.5, and the molecular formula is $C_{22}H_{28}N_2O$. The n-octanol:water partition coefficient is 860:1. The pKa is 8.4.

System Components and Structure: The amount of fentanyl released from each system per hour is proportional to the surface area (25 mcg/hr per 6.25 cm^2). The composition per unit area of all system sizes is identical.

Dose* (mcg/hr)	Size (cm^2)	Fentanyl Content (mg)
12**	3.13	1.28
25	6.25	2.55
50	12.5	5.10
75	18.75	7.65
100	25	10.20

* Nominal delivery rate per hour
** Nominal delivery rate is 12.5 mcg/hr

Fentanyl transdermal system is a translucent rectangular patch with rounded corners comprising a protective liner and two functional layers. Proceeding from the outer surface toward the surface adhering to skin, these layers are: 1) a backing layer of polyolefin film; and 2) a drug-in-adhesive layer. Before use, a protective liner covering the adhesive layer is removed and discarded.
Fentanyl transdermal systems are packaged with additional pieces of protective film above and below the system within each pouch. These are also discarded at the time of use.

The active component of the system is fentanyl. The remaining components are pharmacologically inactive.

CLINICAL PHARMACOLOGY

Pharmacology: Fentanyl is an opioid analgesic. Fentanyl interacts predominately with the opioid mu-receptor. These mu-binding sites are discretely distributed in the human brain, spinal cord, and other tissues. In clinical settings, fentanyl exerts its principal pharmacologic effects on the central nervous system.
In addition to analgesia, alterations in mood, euphoria, dysphoria, and drowsiness commonly occur. Fentanyl depresses the respiratory centers, depresses the cough reflex, and constricts the pupils. Analgesic blood concentrations of fentanyl may cause nausea and vomiting directly by stimulating the chemoreceptor trigger zone, but nausea and vomiting are significantly more common in ambulatory than in recumbent patients, as is postural syncope.
Opioids increase the tone and decrease the propulsive contractions of the smooth muscle of the gastrointestinal tract. The resultant prolongation in gastrointestinal transit time may be responsible for the constipating effect of fentanyl. Because opioids may increase biliary tract pressure, some patients with biliary colic may experience worsening rather than relief of pain.
While opioids generally increase the tone of urinary tract smooth muscle, the net effect tends to be variable, in some cases producing urinary urgency, in others, difficulty in urination. At therapeutic dosages, fentanyl usually does not exert major effects on the cardiovascular system. However, some patients may exhibit orthostatic hypotension and fainting.
Histamine assays and skin wheal testing in clinical studies indicate that clinically significant histamine release rarely occurs with fentanyl administration. Clinical assays show no clinically significant histamine release in dosages up to 50 mcg/kg.
Pharmacokinetics (see graph and tables): Fentanyl transdermal system is a drug-in-adhesive matrix designed formulation. Fentanyl is released from the matrix at a nearly constant amount per unit time. The concentration gradient existing between the matrix and the lower concentration in the skin drives drug release. Fentanyl moves in the direction of the lower concentration at a rate deter-

mined by the matrix and the diffusion of fentanyl through the skin layers. While the actual rate of fentanyl delivery to the skin varies over the 72 hour application period, each system is labeled with a nominal flux which represents the average amount of drug delivered to the systemic circulation per hour across average skin.
While there is variation in dose delivered among patients, the nominal flux of the systems (12.5, 25, 50, 75, and 100 mcg of fentanyl per hour) is sufficiently accurate as to allow individual titration of dosage for a given patient.
Following fentanyl transdermal system application, the skin under the system absorbs fentanyl, and a depot of fentanyl concentrates in the upper skin layers. Fentanyl then becomes available to the systemic circulation. Serum fentanyl concentrations increase gradually following initial fentanyl transdermal system application, generally leveling off between 12 and 24 hours and remaining relatively constant, with some fluctuation, for the remainder of the 72 hour application period. Peak serum concentrations of fentanyl generally occurred between 20 and 72 hours after initial application (see Table A). Serum fentanyl concentrations achieved are proportional to the fentanyl transdermal system delivery rate. With continuous use, serum fentanyl concentrations continue to rise for the first two system applications. By the end of the second 72 hour application, a steady-state serum concentration is reached and is maintained during subsequent applications of a patch of the same size. Patients reach and maintain a steady-state serum concentration that is determined by individual variation in skin permeability and body clearance of fentanyl.
The kinetics of fentanyl in normal subjects following application of a 25 mcg/hr fentanyl transdermal system were bioequivalent with or without either a Bioclusive® or Askina®Derm overlay (polyurethane film dressing).
After system removal, serum fentanyl concentrations decline gradually, falling about 50% in approximately 20 to 27 hours. Continued absorption of fentanyl from the skin accounts for a slower disappearance of the drug from the serum than is seen after an IV infusion, where the apparent half-life is approximately 7 (range 3 to 12) hours.

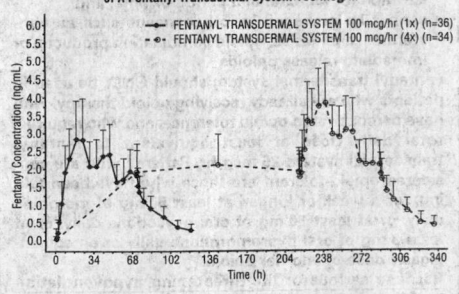

Serum Fentanyl Concentrations Following Single and Multiple Applications of A Fentanyl Transdermal System 100 mcg/hr

— FENTANYL TRANSDERMAL SYSTEM 100 mcg/hr (1x) (n=36)
-- FENTANYL TRANSDERMAL SYSTEM 100 mcg/hr (4x) (n=34)

[See table A above]

NOTE: After system removal there is continued systemic absorption from residual fentanyl in the skin so that serum concentrations fall 50%, on average, in approximately 20 to 27 hours.
[See table B above]
NOTE: Information on volume of distribution and half-life not available for renally impaired patients.
Fentanyl plasma protein binding capacity decreases with increasing ionization of the drug. Alterations in pH may affect its distribution between plasma and the central nervous system. Fentanyl accumulates in the skeletal muscle and fat and is released slowly into the blood. The average volume of distribution for fentanyl is 6 L/kg (range 3 to 8; N = 8).
Fentanyl is metabolized primarily via human cytochrome P450 3A4 isoenzyme system. In humans, the drug appears to be metabolized primarily by oxidative N-dealkylation to norfentanyl and other inactive metabolites that do not contribute materially to the observed activity of the drug. Within 72 hours of IV fentanyl administration, approximately 75% of the dose is excreted in urine, mostly as metabolites with less than 10% representing unchanged drug. Approximately 9% of the dose is recovered in the feces, primarily as metabolites. Mean values for unbound fractions of fentanyl in plasma are estimated to be between 13% and 21%.
Skin does not appear to metabolize fentanyl delivered transdermally. This was determined in a human keratinocyte cell assay and in clinical studies in which 92% of the dose delivered from the system was accounted for as unchanged fentanyl that appeared in the systemic circulation.
Special Populations: *Hepatic or Renal Disease:* Insufficient information exists to make recommendations regarding the use of fentanyl transdermal system in patients with impaired renal or hepatic function. Fentanyl is metabolized primarily via human cytochrome P450 3A4 isoenzyme system and mostly eliminated in urine. If the drug is used in these patients, it should be used with caution because of the hepatic metabolism and renal excretion of fentanyl.
Pediatric Use: In 1.5 to 5 year old, non-opioid-tolerant pediatric patients, the fentanyl plasma concentrations were approximately twice as high as that of adult patients. In older pediatric patients, the pharmacokinetic parameters were similar to that of adults. However, these findings have been taken into consideration in determining the dosing recommendations for opioid-tolerant pediatric patients (2 years of age and older). For pediatric dosing information, refer to DOSAGE AND ADMINISTRATION section.
Geriatric Use: Data from intravenous studies with fentanyl suggest that the elderly patients may have reduced clearance and a prolonged half-life. Moreover elderly patients may be more sensitive to the active substance than younger patients. A study conducted with fentanyl transdermal system in elderly patients demonstrated that fentanyl pharmacokinetics did not differ significantly from young adult subjects, although peak serum concentrations tended to be lower and mean half-life values were prolonged to approximately 34 hours.
Respiratory depression is the chief hazard in elderly or debilitated patients, usually following large initial doses in non-tolerant patients or when opioids are given in conjunction with other agents that depress respiration.

TABLE A
FENTANYL PHARMACOKINETIC PARAMETERS FOLLOWING FIRST 72 HOUR APPLICATION OF A FENTANYL TRANSDERMAL SYSTEM

	Mean (SD) Time to Maximal Concentration T_{max} (hr)	Mean (SD) Maximal Concentration C_{max} (ng/mL)
Fentanyl Transdermal System 12 mcg/hr	28.8 (13.7)	0.38 (0.13)*
Fentanyl Transdermal System 25 mcg/hr	31.7 (16.5)	0.85 (0.26)
Fentanyl Transdermal System 50 mcg/hr	32.8 (15.6)	1.72 (0.53)
Fentanyl Transdermal System 75 mcg/hr	35.8 (14.1)	2.32 (0.86)
Fentanyl Transdermal System 100 mcg/hr	29.9 (13.3)	3.36 (1.28)

* C_{max} values dose normalized from 4×12.5 mcg/hr

TABLE B
RANGE OF PHARMACOKINETIC PARAMETERS OF INTRAVENOUS FENTANYL IN PATIENTS

	Clearance (L/hr) Range [70 kg]	Volume of Distribution V_{ss} (L/kg) Range	Half-Life $t_{1/2}$ (hr) Range
Surgical Patients	27 to 75	3 to 8	3 to 12
Hepatically Impaired Patients	3 to 80+	0.8 to 8+	4 to 12+
Renally Impaired Patients	30 to 78	—	—

+Estimated

Fentanyl transdermal system should be used with caution in elderly, cachectic or debilitated patients as they may have altered pharmacokinetics due to poor fat stores, muscle wasting, or altered clearance (see DOSAGE AND ADMINISTRATION).

Drug Interactions: The interaction between ritonavir, a CYP3A4 inhibitor, and fentanyl was investigated in 11 healthy volunteers in a randomized crossover study. Subjects received oral ritonavir or placebo for 3 days. The ritonavir dose was 200 mg tid on Day 1 and 300 mg tid on Day 2 followed by one morning dose of 300 mg on Day 3. On Day 2, fentanyl was given as a single IV dose at 5 mcg/kg 2 hours after the afternoon dose of oral ritonavir or placebo. Naloxone was administered to counteract the side effects of fentanyl. The results suggested that ritonavir might decrease the clearance of fentanyl by 67%, resulting in a 174% (range 52% to 420%) increase in fentanyl $AUC_{0-\infty}$. Coadministration of ritonavir in patients receiving fentanyl transdermal system has not been studied; however, an increase in fentanyl AUC is expected (see BOX WARNING, WARNINGS, PRECAUTIONS, and DOSAGE AND ADMINISTRATION).

Fentanyl is metabolized mainly via the human cytochrome P450 3A4 isoenzyme system (CYP3A4), therefore, potential interactions may occur when fentanyl transdermal system is given concurrently with agents that affect CYP3A4 activity. Coadminstration with agents that induce CYP3A4 activity may reduce the efficacy of fentanyl transdermal system. The concomitant use of transdermal fentanyl with all CYP3A4 inhibitors (such as ritonavir, ketoconazole, itraconazole, troleandomycin, clarithromycin, nelfinavir, nefazadone, amiodarone, amprenavir, aprepitant, diltiazem, erythromycin, fluconazole, fosamprenavir, grapefruit juice, and verapamil) may result in an increase in fentanyl plasma concentrations, which could increase or prolong adverse drug effects and may cause potentially fatal respiratory depression. Patients receiving fentanyl transdermal system and any CYP3A4 inhibitor should be carefully monitored for an extended period of time and dosage adjustments should be made if warranted (see BOX WARNING, WARNINGS, PRECAUTIONS, and DOSAGE AND ADMINISTRATION for further information).

Pharmacodynamics: *Ventilatory Effects:* Because of the risk for serious or life-threatening hypoventilation, fentanyl transdermal system is CONTRAINDICATED in the treatment of postoperative and acute pain and in patients who are not opioid-tolerant. In clinical trials of 357 patients with acute pain treated with fentanyl transdermal system, 13 patients experienced hypoventilation. Hypoventilation was manifested by respiratory rates of less than 8 breaths/minute or a pCO_2 greater than 55 mm Hg. In these studies, the incidence of hypoventilation was higher in non-tolerant women (10) than in men (3) and in patients weighing less than 63 kg (9 of 13). Although patients with impaired respiration were not common in the trials, they had higher rates of hypoventilation. In addition, post-marketing reports have been received that describe opioid-naive post-operative patients who have experienced clinically significant hypoventilation and death with fentanyl transdermal system.

While most adult and pediatric patients using fentanyl transdermal system chronically develop tolerance to fentanyl-induced hypoventilation, episodes of slowed respirations may occur at any time during therapy.

Hypoventilation can occur throughout the therapeutic range of fentanyl serum concentrations, especially for patients who have an underlying pulmonary condition or who receive usual doses of opioids or other CNS drugs associated with hypoventilation in addition to fentanyl transdermal system. The use of fentanyl transdermal system is contraindicated in patients who are not tolerant to opioid therapy. The use of fentanyl transdermal system should be monitored by clinical evaluation, especially within the initial 24 to 72 hours when serum concentrations from the initial patch will peak, and following increases in dosage. Fentanyl transdermal system should be administered to children only if they are opioid-tolerant and 2 years of age or older.

See BOX WARNING, CONTRAINDICATIONS, WARNINGS, PRECAUTIONS, ADVERSE REACTIONS, and OVERDOSAGE for additional information on hypoventilation.

Cardiovascular Effects: Fentanyl may infrequently produce bradycardia. The incidence of bradycardia in clinical trials with fentanyl transdermal system was less than 1%.

CNS Effects: Central nervous system effects increase with increasing serum fentanyl concentrations.

INDICATIONS AND USAGE

Fentanyl transdermal system is indicated for management of persistent, moderate to severe chronic pain that:
- requires continuous, around-the-clock opioid administration for an extended period of time, and
- cannot be managed by other means such as non-steroidal analgesics, opioid combination products, or immediate-release opioids

Fentanyl transdermal system should ONLY be used in patients who are already receiving opioid therapy, who have demonstrated opioid tolerance, and who require a total daily dose at least equivalent to fentanyl transdermal system 25 mcg/hr (see DOSAGE AND ADMINISTRATION). Patients who are considered opioid-tolerant are those who have been taking, for a week or longer, at least 60 mg of morphine daily, or at least 30 mg of oral oxycodone daily, or at least 8 mg of oral hydromorphone daily, or an equianalgesic dose of another opioid.

Because serious or life-threatening hypoventilation could result, fentanyl transdermal system is contraindicated for use on an as needed basis (i.e., prn), for the management of postoperative or acute pain, or in patients who are not opioid-tolerant or who require opioid analgesia for a short period of time (see BOX WARNING and CONTRAINDICATIONS).

An evaluation of the appropriateness and adequacy of treating with immediate-release opioids is advisable prior to initiating therapy with any modified-release opioid. Prescribers should individualize treatment in every case, initiating therapy at the appropriate point along a progression from non-opioid analgesics, such as non-steroidal anti-inflammatory drugs and acetaminophen, to opioids, in a plan of pain management such as outlined by the World Health Organization, the Agency for Health Research and Quality, the Federation of State Medical Boards Model Policy, or the American Pain Society.

Patients should be assessed for their clinical risks for opioid abuse or addiction prior to being prescribed opioids. Patients receiving opioids should be routinely monitored for signs of misuse, abuse, and addiction. Persons at increased risk for opioid abuse include those with a personal or family history of substance abuse (including drug or alcohol abuse or addiction) or mental illness (e.g., major depression). Patients at increased risk may still be appropriately treated with modified-release opioid formulations; however these patients will require intensive monitoring for signs of misuse, abuse, or addiction.

CONTRAINDICATIONS

Because serious or life-threatening hypoventilation could occur, fentanyl transdermal system is contraindicated:
- **in patients who are not opioid-tolerant**
- **in the management of acute pain or in patients who require opioid analgesia for a short period of time**
- **in the management of postoperative pain, including use after out-patient or day surgeries (e.g., tonsillectomies)**
- **in the management of mild pain**
- **in the management of intermittent pain [e.g., use on an as needed basis (prn)]**
- **in situations of significant respiratory depression, especially in unmonitored settings where there is a lack of resuscitative equipment**
- **in patients who have acute or severe bronchial asthma**

Fentanyl transdermal system is contraindicated in patients who have or are suspected of having paralytic ileus.

Fentanyl transdermal system is contraindicated in patients with known hypersensitivity to fentanyl or any components of this product.

WARNINGS

Fentanyl transdermal systems are intended for transdermal use (on intact skin) only. Do not use a fentanyl transdermal system if the pouch seal is broken or the patch is cut, damaged, or changed in any way.

The safety of fentanyl transdermal system has not been established in children under 2 years of age. Fentanyl transdermal system should be administered to children only if they are opioid-tolerant and 2 years of age or older (see PRECAUTIONS: Pediatric Use).

Fentanyl transdermal system is ONLY for use in patients who are already tolerant to opioid therapy of comparable potency. Use in non-opioid-tolerant patients may lead to fatal respiratory depression. Overestimating the fentanyl transdermal system dose when converting patients from another opioid medication can result in fatal overdose with the first dose. The mean half-life is approximately 20 to 27 hours. Therefore, patients who have experienced serious adverse events, including overdose, will require monitoring for at least 24 hours after fentanyl transdermal system removal since serum fentanyl concentrations decline gradually and reach an approximate 50% reduction in serum concentrations 20 to 27 hours after system removal.

Fentanyl transdermal system should be prescribed only by persons knowledgeable in the continuous administration of potent opioids, in the management of patients receiving potent opioids for treatment of pain, and in the detection and management of hypoventilation including the use of opioid antagonists.

All patients and their caregivers should be advised to avoid exposing the fentanyl transdermal system application site and surrounding area to direct external heat sources, such as heating pads or electric blankets, heat or tanning lamps, saunas, hot tubs, and heated water beds, etc., while wearing the system. Patients should be advised against taking hot baths or sunbathing. There is a potential for temperature-dependent increases in fentanyl released from the system resulting in possible overdose and death. A clinical pharmacology trial conducted in healthy adult subjects has shown that the application of heat over the fentanyl transdermal system increased mean fentanyl AUC values by 120% and mean C_{max} values by 61%.

Based on a pharmacokinetic model, serum fentanyl concentrations could theoretically increase by approximately one-third for patients with a body temperature of 40°C (104°F) due to temperature-dependent increases in fentanyl released from the system and increased skin permeability. **Patients wearing fentanyl transdermal systems who develop fever or increased core body temperature due to strenuous exertion should be monitored for opioid side effects and the fentanyl transdermal system dose should be adjusted if necessary.**

Death and other serious medical problems have occurred when people were accidentally exposed to fentanyl transdermal system. Examples of accidental exposure include transfer of a fentanyl transdermal system from an adult's body to a child while hugging, accidental sitting on a patch and possible accidental exposure of a caregiver's skin to the medication in the patch while the caregiver was applying or removing the patch.

Placing fentanyl transdermal system in the mouth, chewing it, swallowing it, or using it in ways other than indicated may cause choking or overdose that could result in death.

Misuse, Abuse and Diversion of Opioids

Fentanyl is an opioid agonist of the morphine-type. Such drugs are sought by drug abusers and people with addiction disorders and are subject to criminal diversion.

Fentanyl can be abused in a manner similar to other opioids, legal or illicit. This should be considered when prescribing or dispensing fentanyl transdermal system in situations where the physician or pharmacist is concerned about an increased risk of misuse, abuse or diversion.

Fentanyl transdermal system has been reported as being abused by other methods and routes of administration. These practices will result in uncontrolled delivery of the opioid and pose a significant risk to the abuser that could result in overdose and death (see WARNINGS and DRUG ABUSE AND ADDICTION).

Concerns about abuse, addiction and diversion should not prevent the proper management of pain. However, all patients treated with opioids require careful monitoring for signs of abuse and addiction, since use of opioid analgesic products carries the risk of addiction even under appropriate medical use.

Healthcare professionals should contact their state professional licensing board or state controlled substances authority for information on how to prevent and detect abuse or diversion of this product.

Hypoventilation (Respiratory Depression): Serious or life-threatening hypoventilation may occur at any time during the use of fentanyl transdermal system especially during the initial 24 to 72 hours following initiation of therapy and following increases in dose.

Because significant amounts of fentanyl continue to be absorbed from the skin for 20 to 27 hours or more after the patch is removed, hypoventilation may persist beyond the removal of fentanyl transdermal system. Consequently, patients with hypoventilation should be carefully observed for degree of sedation and their respiratory rate monitored until respiration has stabilized.

The use of concomitant CNS active drugs requires special patient care and observation.

Respiratory depression is the chief hazard of opioid agonists, including fentanyl the active ingredient in fentanyl transdermal system. Respiratory depression is more likely to occur in elderly or debilitated patients, usually following large initial doses in non-tolerant patients, or when opioids are given in conjunction with other drugs that depress respiration.

Respiratory depression from opioids is manifested by a reduced urge to breathe and a decreased rate of respiration, often associated with the "sighing" pattern of breathing (deep breaths separated by abnormally long pauses). Carbon dioxide retention from opioid-induced respiratory depression can exacerbate the sedating effects of opioids. This makes overdoses involving drugs with sedative properties and opioids especially dangerous.

Fentanyl transdermal system should be used with extreme caution in patients with significant chronic obstructive pulmonary disease or cor pulmonale, and in patients having a substantially decreased respiratory reserve, hypoxia, hypercapnia, or preexisting respiratory depression. In such patients, even usual therapeutic doses of fentanyl transdermal system may decrease respiratory drive to the point of apnea. In these patients, alternative non-opioid analgesics should be considered, and opioids should be employed only under careful medical supervision at the lowest effective dose.

Chronic Pulmonary Disease: Because potent opioids can cause serious or life-threatening hypoventilation, fentanyl transdermal system should be administered with caution to patients with preexisting medical conditions predisposing them to hypoventilation. In such patients, normal analgesic doses of opioids may further decrease respiratory drive to the point of respiratory failure.

Head Injuries and Increased Intracranial Pressure: Fentanyl transdermal system should not be used in patients who may be particularly susceptible to the intracranial effects of CO_2 retention such as those with evidence of increased intracranial pressure, impaired consciousness, or coma. Opioids may obscure the clinical course of patients with head injury. Fentanyl transdermal system should be used with caution in patients with brain tumors.

Interactions with other CNS Depressants: The concomitant use of fentanyl transdermal system with other central nervous system depressants, including but not limited to other opioids, sedatives, hypnotics, tranquilizers (e.g., benzodiazepines), general anesthetics, phenothiazines, skeletal muscle relaxants, and alcohol, may cause respiratory depression, hypotension, and profound sedation or potentially result in coma. When such combined therapy is contemplated, the dose of one or both agents should be significantly reduced.

Interactions with Alcohol and Drugs of Abuse: Fentanyl may be expected to have additive CNS depressant effects when used in conjunction with alcohol, other opioids, or illicit drugs that cause central nervous system depression.

Interactions with CYP3A4 Inhibitors: The concomitant use of transdermal fentanyl with all CYP3A4 inhibitors (such as ritonavir, ketoconazole, itraconazole, troleandomycin, clarithromycin, nelfinavir, nefazadone, amiodarone, amprenavir, aprepitant, diltiazem, erythromycin, fluconazole, fosamprenavir, grapefruit juice, and verapamil) may result in an increase in fentanyl plasma concentrations, which could increase or prolong adverse drug effects and may cause potentially fatal respiratory depression. Patients receiving fentanyl transdermal system and any CYP3A4 inhibitor should be carefully monitored for an extended period of time, and dosage adjustments should be made if warranted (see BOX WARNING, CLINICAL PHARMACOLOGY: Drug Interactions, PRECAUTIONS, and DOSAGE AND ADMINISTRATION for further information).

PRECAUTIONS

General: Fentanyl transdermal system should not be used to initiate opioid therapy in patients who are not opioid-tolerant. Children converting to fentanyl transdermal system should be opioid-tolerant and 2 years of age or older (see BOX WARNING).

Patients, family members and caregivers should be instructed to keep patches (new and used) out of the reach of children and others for whom fentanyl transdermal system was not prescribed. A considerable amount of active fentanyl remains in fentanyl transdermal system even after use as directed. Accidental or deliberate application or ingestion by a child or adolescent will cause respiratory depression that could result in death.

Cardiac Disease: Fentanyl may produce bradycardia. Fentanyl should be administered with caution to patients with bradyarrhythmias.

Hepatic or Renal Disease: Insufficient information exists to make recommendations regarding the use of fentanyl transdermal system in patients with impaired renal or hepatic function. If the drug is used in these patients, it should be used with caution because of the hepatic metabolism and renal excretion of fentanyl.

Use in Pancreatic/Biliary Tract Disease: Fentanyl transdermal system may cause spasm of the sphincter of Oddi and should be used with caution in patients with biliary tract disease, including acute pancreatitis. Opioids like fentanyl transdermal system may cause increases in the serum amylase concentration.

Tolerance: Tolerance is a state of adaptation in which exposure to a drug induces changes that result in a diminution of one or more of the drug's effects over time. Tolerance may occur to both the desired and undesired effects of drugs, and may develop at different rates for different effects.

Physical Dependence: Physical dependence is a state of adaptation that is manifested by an opioid specific withdrawal syndrome that can be produced by abrupt cessation, rapid dose reduction, decreasing blood concentration of the drug, and/or administration of an antagonist. The opioid abstinence or withdrawal syndrome is characterized by some or all of the following: restlessness, lacrimation, rhinorrhea, yawning, perspiration, chills, piloerection, myalgia, mydriasis, irritability, anxiety, backache, joint pain, weakness, abdominal cramps, insomnia, nausea, anorexia, vomiting, diarrhea, or increased blood pressure, respiratory rate, or heart rate. In general, opioids should not be abruptly discontinued (see DOSAGE AND ADMINISTRATION: Discontinuation of Fentanyl Transdermal System).

Ambulatory Patients: Strong opioid analgesics impair the mental or physical abilities required for the performance of potentially dangerous tasks, such as driving a car or operating machinery. Patients who have been given fentanyl transdermal system should not drive or operate dangerous machinery unless they are tolerant to the effects of the drug.

Information for Patients: Patients and their caregivers should be provided with a Medication Guide each time fentanyl transdermal system is dispensed because new information may be available.

Patients receiving fentanyl transdermal system should be given the following instructions by the physician:

1. Patients should be advised that fentanyl transdermal systems contain fentanyl, an opioid pain medicine similar to morphine, hydromorphone, methadone, oxycodone, and oxymorphone.
2. Patients should be advised that each fentanyl transdermal system may be worn continuously for 72 hours, and that each patch should be applied to a different skin site after removal of the previous transdermal patch.
3. Patients should be advised that fentanyl transdermal system should be applied to intact, nonirritated, and nonirradiated skin on a flat surface such as the chest, back, flank, or upper arm. Additionally, patients should be advised of the following:
   - In young children or persons with cognitive impairment, the patch should be put on the upper back to lower the chances that the patch will be removed and placed in the mouth.
   - Hair at the application site should be clipped (not shaved) prior to patch application.
   - If the site of fentanyl transdermal system application must be cleansed prior to application of the patch, do so with clear water.
   - Do not use soaps, oils, lotions, alcohol, or any other agents that might irritate the skin or alter its characteristics.
   - Allow the skin to dry completely prior to patch application.
4. Patients should be advised that fentanyl transdermal system should be applied immediately upon removal from the sealed pouch and after removal of the protective liner. Additionally the patient should be advised of the following:
   - The fentanyl transdermal system should not be used if the pouch seal is broken or if the patch is cut, damaged, or changed in any way.
   - The transdermal patch should be pressed firmly in place with the palm of the hand for 30 seconds, making sure the contact is complete, especially around the edges.
   - The patch should not be folded so that only part of the patch is exposed.
5. Patients should be advised that the dose of fentanyl transdermal system or the number of patches applied to the skin should NEVER be adjusted without the prescribing healthcare professional's instruction.
6. Patients should be advised that while wearing the patch, they should avoid exposing the fentanyl transdermal system application site and surrounding area to direct external heat sources, such as:
   - heating pads,
   - electric blankets,
   - sunbathing,
   - heat or tanning lamps,
   - saunas,
   - hot tubs or hot baths, and
   - heated water beds, etc.
7. Patients should also be advised of a potential for temperature-dependent increases in fentanyl release from the patch that could result in an overdose of fentanyl; therefore, patients who develop a high fever or increased body temperature due to strenuous exertion while wearing the patch should contact their physician.
8. Patients should be advised that if they experience problems with adhesion of the fentanyl transdermal system, they may tape the edges of the patch with first aid tape. If problems with adhesion persist, patients may overlay the patch with a transparent adhesive film dressing (e.g., Bioclusive® or Askina®Derm).
9. Patients should be advised that if the patch falls off before 72 hours a new patch may be applied to a different skin site.
10. Patients should be advised to fold (so that the adhesive side adheres to itself) and immediately flush down the toilet used fentanyl transdermal systems after removal from the skin.
11. Patients should be advised that fentanyl transdermal system may impair mental and/or physical ability required for the performance of potentially hazardous tasks (e.g., driving, operating machinery).
12. Patients should be advised to refrain from any potentially dangerous activity when starting on fentanyl transdermal system or when their dose is being adjusted, until it is established that they have not been adversely affected.
13. Patients should be advised that fentanyl transdermal system should not be combined with alcohol or other CNS depressants (e.g., sleep medications, tranquilizers) because dangerous additive effects may occur, resulting in serious injury or death.
14. Patients should be advised to consult their physician or pharmacist if other medications are being or will be used with fentanyl transdermal system.
15. Patients should be advised of the potential for severe constipation.
16. Patients should be advised that if they have been receiving treatment with fentanyl transdermal system and cessation of therapy is indicated, it may be appropriate to taper the fentanyl transdermal system dose, rather than abruptly discontinue it, due to the risk of precipitating withdrawal symptoms.
17. Patients should be advised that fentanyl transdermal system contains fentanyl, a drug with high potential for abuse.
18. Patients, family members and caregivers should be advised to protect fentanyl transdermal system from theft or misuse in the work or home environment.
19. Patients should be instructed to keep fentanyl transdermal system in a secure place out of the reach of children due to the high risk of **fatal respiratory depression**.
20. Patients should be advised that fentanyl transdermal system should never be given to anyone other than the individual for whom it was prescribed because of the risk of death or other serious medical problems to that person for whom it was not intended.
21. Patients should be informed that, if the patch dislodges and accidentally sticks to the skin of another person, they should immediately take the patch off, wash the exposed area with water and seek medical attention for the accidentally exposed individual.
22. When fentanyl transdermal system is no longer needed, the unused patches should be removed from their pouches, folded so that the adhesive side of the patch adheres to itself, and flushed down the toilet.
23. Women of childbearing potential who become, or are planning to become pregnant, should be advised to consult a physician prior to initiating or continuing therapy with fentanyl transdermal system.
24. Patients should be informed that accidental exposure or misuse may lead to death or other serious medical problems.

Drug Interactions: ***Agents Affecting Cytochrome P450 3A4 Isoenzyme System:*** Fentanyl is metabolized mainly via the human cytochrome P450 3A4 isoenzyme system (CYP3A4), therefore potential interactions may occur when fentanyl transdermal system is given concurrently with agents that affect CYP3A4 activity. Coadministration with agents that induce CYP3A4 activity may reduce the efficacy of fentanyl transdermal system. The concomitant use of transdermal fentanyl with all CYP3A4 inhibitors (such as ritonavir, ketoconazole, itraconazole, troleandomycin, clarithromycin, nelfanivir, nefazadone, amiodarone, amprenavir, aprepitant, diltiazem, erythromycin, fluconazole, fosamprenavir, grapefruit juice, and verapamil) may result in an increase in fentanyl plasma concentrations, which could increase or prolong adverse drug effects and may cause fatal respiratory depression. Patients receiving fentanyl transdermal system and any CYP3A4 inhibitor should be carefully monitored for an extended period of time, and dosage adjustments should be made if warranted (see BOX WARNING, CLINICAL PHARMACOLOGY: Drug Interactions, WARNINGS, and DOSAGE AND ADMINISTRATION for further information).

Central Nervous System Depressants: The concomitant use of fentanyl transdermal system with other central nervous system depressants, including but not limited to other opioids, sedatives, hypnotics, tranquilizers (e.g., benzodiazepines), general anesthetics, phenothiazines, skeletal muscle relaxants, and alcohol, may cause respiratory depression, hypotension, and profound sedation, or potentially result in coma or death. When such combined therapy is contemplated, the dose of one or both agents should be significantly reduced.

MAO Inhibitors: Fentanyl transdermal system is not recommended for use in patients who have received MAOI within 14 days because severe and unpredictable potentiation by MAO inhibitors has been reported with opioid analgesics.

Carcinogenesis, Mutagenesis, and Impairment of Fertility: In a 2-year carcinogenicity study conducted in rats, fentanyl was not associated with an increased incidence of tumors at subcutaneous doses up to 33 mcg/kg/day in males or 100 mcg/kg/day in females (0.16 and 0.39 times the human daily exposure obtained via the 100 mcg/hr patch based on $AUC_{0\text{-}24h}$ comparison). There was no evidence of mutagenicity in the Ames Salmonella mutagenicity assay, the primary rat hepatocyte unscheduled DNA synthesis assay, the BALB/c 3T3 transformation test, and the human lymphocyte and CHO chromosomal aberration *in vitro* assays.

The potential effects of fentanyl on male and female fertility were examined in the rat model via two separate experiments. In the male fertility study, male rats were treated with fentanyl (0, 0.025, 0.1 or 0.4 mg/kg/day) via continuous intravenous infusion for 28 days prior to mating; female rats were not treated. In the female fertility study, female rats were treated with fentanyl (0, 0.025, 0.1 or 0.4 mg/kg/day) via continuous intravenous infusion for 14 days prior to mating until day 16 of pregnancy; male rats were not treated. Analysis of fertility parameters in both studies indicated that an intravenous dose of fentanyl up to 0.4 mg/kg/day to either the male or the female alone produced no effects on fertility (this dose is approximately 1.6 times the daily human dose administered by a 100 mcg/hr patch on a mg/m² basis). In a separate study, a single daily bolus dose of fentanyl was shown to impair fertility in rats when given in intravenous doses of 0.3 times the human dose for a period of 12 days.

Pregnancy: ***Teratogenic Effects:*** *Pregnancy Category C:* No epidemiological studies of congenital anomalies in infants born to women treated with fentanyl during pregnancy have been reported.

The potential effects of fentanyl on embryo-fetal development were studied in the rat, mouse, and rabbit models. Published literature reports that administration of fentanyl (0, 10, 100, or 500 mcg/kg/day) to pregnant female Sprague-Dawley rats from day 7 to 21 via implanted microosmotic minipumps did not produce any evidence of teratogenicity (the high dose is approximately 2 times the daily human dose administered by a 100 mcg/hr patch on a mg/m² basis). In contrast, the intravenous administration of fentanyl (0, 0.01, or 0.03 mg/kg) to bred female rats from gestation day 6 to 18 suggested evidence of embryotoxicity and a slight increase in mean delivery time in the 0.03 mg/kg/day group. There was no clear evidence of teratogenicity noted.

Pregnant female New Zealand White rabbits were treated with fentanyl (0, 0.025, 0.1, 0.4 mg/kg) via intravenous infusion from day 6 to day 18 of pregnancy. Fentanyl produced a slight decrease in the body weight of the live fetuses at the high dose, which may be attributed to maternal toxicity. Under the conditions of the assay, there was no evidence for fentanyl-induced adverse effects on embryo-fetal development at doses up to 0.4 mg/kg (approximately 3 times the daily human dose administered by a 100 mcg/hr patch on a mg/m² basis).

There are no adequate and well controlled studies in pregnant women. Fentanyl transdermal system should be used during pregnancy only if the potential benefit justifies the potential risk to the fetus.

Nonteratogenic Effects: Chronic maternal treatment with fentanyl during pregnancy has been associated with transient respiratory depression, behavioral changes, or seizures characteristic of neonatal abstinence syndrome in newborn infants. Symptoms of neonatal respiratory or neurological depression were no more frequent than expected in most studies of infants born to women treated acutely during labor with intravenous or epidural fentanyl. Transient neonatal muscular rigidity has been observed in infants whose mothers were treated with intravenous fentanyl.

The potential effects of fentanyl on prenatal and postnatal development were examined in the rat model. Female Wistar rats were treated with 0, 0.025, 0.1, or 0.4 mg/kg/day fentanyl via intravenous infusion from day 6 of pregnancy through 3 weeks of lactation. Fentanyl treatment (0.4 mg/kg/day) significantly decreased body weight in male and female pups and also decreased survival in pups at day 4. Both the mid-dose and high-dose of fentanyl animals demonstrated alterations in some physical landmarks of development (delayed incisor eruption and eye opening) and transient behavioral development (decreased locomotor activity at day 28 which recovered by day 50). The mid-dose and the high-dose are 0.4 and 1.6 times the daily human dose administered by a 100 mcg/hr patch on a mg/m² basis.

Labor and Delivery: Fentanyl readily passes across the placenta to the fetus; therefore, fentanyl transdermal system is not recommended for analgesia during labor and delivery.

Nursing Mothers: Fentanyl is excreted in human milk; therefore, fentanyl transdermal system is not recommended for use in nursing women because of the possibility of effects in their infants.

Pediatric Use: The safety of fentanyl transdermal system was evaluated in three open-label trials in 291 pediatric patients with chronic pain, 2 years of age through 18 years of age. Starting doses of 25 mcg/hr and higher were used by 181 patients who had been on prior daily opioid doses of at least 45 mg/day of oral morphine or an equianalgesic dose of another opioid. Initiation of fentanyl transdermal system therapy in pediatric patients taking less than 60 mg/day of oral morphine or an equianalgesic dose of another opioid has not been evaluated in controlled clinical trials. Approximately 90% of the total daily opioid requirement (fentanyl transdermal system plus rescue medication) was provided by fentanyl transdermal system.

Fentanyl transdermal system was not studied in children under 2 years of age.

Fentanyl transdermal system should be administered to children only if they are opioid-tolerant and 2 years of age or older (see DOSAGE AND ADMINISTRATION and BOX WARNING).

To guard against accidental ingestion by children, use caution when choosing the application site for fentanyl transdermal system (see DOSAGE AND ADMINISTRATION) and monitor adhesion of the system closely.

Geriatric Use: Data from intravenous studies with fentanyl suggest that the elderly patients may have reduced clearance and a prolonged half-life. Moreover elderly patients may be more sensitive to the active substance than younger patients. A study conducted with fentanyl transdermal system in elderly patients demonstrated that fentanyl pharmacokinetics did not differ significantly from young adult subjects, although peak serum concentrations tended to be lower and mean half-life values were prolonged to approximately 34 hours.

Respiratory depression is the chief hazard in elderly or debilitated patients, usually following large initial doses in non-tolerant patients, or when opioids are given in conjunction with other agents that depress respiration.

Fentanyl transdermal system should be used with caution in elderly, cachectic, or debilitated patients as they may have altered pharmacokinetics due to poor fat stores, muscle wasting or altered clearance (see DOSAGE AND ADMINISTRATION).

ADVERSE REACTIONS

In post-marketing experience, deaths from hypoventilation due to use of fentanyl transdermal system have been reported (see BOX WARNING and CONTRAINDICATIONS).

Premarketing Clinical Trial Experience: Although fentanyl transdermal system use in postoperative or acute pain and in patients who are not opioid-tolerant is CONTRAINDICATED, the safety of fentanyl transdermal system was originally evaluated in 357 postoperative adult patients for 1 to 3 days and 153 cancer patients for a total of 510 patients. The duration of fentanyl transdermal system use varied in cancer patients; 56% of patients used fentanyl transdermal system for over 30 days, 28% continued treatment for more than 4 months, and 10% used fentanyl transdermal system for more than 1 year.

Hypoventilation was the most serious adverse reaction observed in 13 (4%) postoperative patients and in 3 (2%) of the cancer patients. Hypotension and hypertension were observed in 11 (3%) and 4 (1%) of the opioid-naive patients.

Various adverse events were reported; a causal relationship to fentanyl transdermal system was not always determined. The frequencies presented here reflect the actual frequency of each adverse effect in patients who received fentanyl transdermal system. There has been no attempt to correct for a placebo effect, concomitant use of other opioids, or to subtract the frequencies reported by placebo-treated patients in controlled trials.

Adverse reactions reported in 153 cancer patients at a frequency of 1% or greater are presented in Table 1; similar reactions were seen in the 357 postoperative patients.

In the pediatric population, the safety of fentanyl transdermal system has been evaluated in 291 patients with chronic pain 2 to 18 years of age. The duration of fentanyl transdermal system use varied; 20% of pediatric patients were treated for ≤ 15 days; 46% for 16 to 30 days; 16% for 31 to 60 days; and 17% for at least 61 days. Twenty-five patients were treated with fentanyl transdermal system for at least 4 months and 9 patients for more than 9 months.

There was no apparent pediatric-specific risk associated with fentanyl transdermal system use in children as young as 2 years old when used as directed. The most common adverse events were fever (35%), vomiting (33%), and nausea (24%).

Adverse events reported in pediatric patients at a rate of ≥ 1% are presented in Table 1.

[See table 1 above]

TABLE 1: ADVERSE EVENTS (at rate of ≥ 1%)
Adults (N = 380) and Pediatric (N = 291) Clinical Trial Experience

Body System	Adults	Pediatrics
Body as a Whole	Abdominal pain*, headache*, fatigue*, back pain, fever, influenza-like symptoms*, accidental injury, rigors	Pain*, headache*, fever, syncope, abdominal pain, allergic reaction, flushing
Cardiovascular	Arrhythmia, chest pain	Hypertension, tachycardia
Digestive	Nausea**, vomiting**, constipation**, dry mouth**, anorexia*, diarrhea*, dyspepsia*, flatulence	Nausea**, vomiting**, constipation*, dry mouth, diarrhea
Nervous	Somnolence**, insomnia, confusion**, asthenia**, dizziness*, nervousness*, hallucinations*, anxiety*, depression*, euphoria*, tremor, abnormal coordination, speech disorder, abnormal thinking, abnormal gait, abnormal dreams, agitation, paresthesia, amnesia, syncope, paranoid reaction	Somnolence*, nervousness*, insomnia*, asthenia*, hallucinations, anxiety, depression, convulsions, dizziness, tremor, speech disorder, agitation, stupor, confusion, paranoid reaction
Respiratory	Dyspnea*, hypoventilation*, apnea*, hemoptysis, pharyngitis*, hiccups, bronchitis, rhinitis, sinusitis, upper respiratory tract infection*	Dyspnea, respiratory depression, rhinitis, coughing
Skin and Appendages	Sweating**, pruritus*, rash, application site reaction – erythema, papules, itching, edema	Pruritus*, application site reaction*, sweating increased, rash, rash erythematous, skin reaction localized
Urogenital	Urinary retention*, micturition disorder	Urinary retention

* Reactions occurring in 3% to 10% of fentanyl transdermal system patients
** Reactions occurring in 10% or more of fentanyl transdermal system patients

The following adverse effects have been reported in less than 1% of the 510 adult postoperative and cancer patients studied:

Cardiovascular: bradycardia
Digestive: abdominal distention
Nervous: aphasia, hypertonia, vertigo, stupor, hypotonia, depersonalization, hostility
Respiratory: stertorous breathing, asthma, respiratory disorder
Skin and Appendages, General: exfoliative dermatitis, pustules
Special Senses: amblyopia
Urogenital: bladder pain, oliguria, urinary frequency

Post-Marketing Experience: Adults: The following adverse reactions have been reported in association with the use of fentanyl transdermal system and not reported in the premarketing adverse reactions section above:

Body as a Whole: edema
Cardiovascular: tachycardia
Metabolic and Nutritional: weight loss
Special Senses: blurred vision
Urogenital: decreased libido, anorgasmia, ejaculatory difficulty

DRUG ABUSE AND ADDICTION

Fentanyl transdermal system contains a high concentration of fentanyl, a potent Schedule II opioid agonist. Schedule II opioid substances, which include hydromorphone, methadone, morphine, oxycodone, and oxymorphone, have the highest potential for abuse and risk of fatal overdose due to respiratory depression. Fentanyl, like morphine and other opioids used in analgesia, can be abused and is subject to criminal diversion.

The high content of fentanyl in the patches (fentanyl transdermal system) may be a particular target for abuse and diversion.

Addiction is a primary, chronic, neurobiologic disease, with genetic, psychosocial, and environmental factors influencing its development and manifestations. It is characterized by behaviors that include one or more of the following: impaired control over drug use, compulsive use, continued use despite harm, and craving. Drug addiction is a treatable disease, utilizing a multidisciplinary approach, but relapse is common.

"Drug seeking" behavior is very common in addicts and drug abusers. Drug-seeking tactics include emergency calls or visits near the end of office hours, refusal to undergo appropriate examination, testing or referral, repeated "loss" of prescriptions, tampering with prescriptions and reluctance to provide prior medical records or contact information for other treating physician(s). "Doctor shopping" to obtain additional prescriptions is common among drug abusers and people suffering from untreated addiction.

Abuse and addiction are separate and distinct from physical dependence and tolerance. Physicians should be aware that addiction may be accompanied by concurrent tolerance and symptoms of physical dependence. In addition, abuse of opioids can occur in the absence of true addiction and is characterized by misuse for nonmedical purposes, often in combination with other psychoactive substances. Since fentanyl transdermal system may be diverted for nonmedical use, careful record keeping of prescribing information, including quantity, frequency, and renewal requests is strongly advised.

Proper assessment of the patient, proper prescribing practices, periodic re-evaluation of therapy, and proper dispensing and storage are appropriate measures that help to limit abuse of opioid drugs.

Fentanyl transdermal systems are intended for transdermal use (to be applied on the skin) only. Do not use a fentanyl transdermal system if the pouch seal is broken or the patch is cut, damaged, or changed in any way.

OVERDOSAGE

Clinical Presentation: The manifestations of fentanyl overdosage are an extension of its pharmacologic actions with the most serious significant effect being hypoventilation.

Treatment: For the management of hypoventilation, immediate countermeasures include removing the fentanyl transdermal system and physically or verbally stimulating the patient. These actions can be followed by administration of a specific narcotic antagonist such as naloxone. The duration of hypoventilation following an overdose may be longer than the effects of the narcotic antagonist's action (the half-life of naloxone ranges from 30 to 81 minutes). The interval between IV antagonist doses should be carefully chosen because of the possibility of renarcotization after system removal; repeated administration of naloxone may be necessary. Reversal of the narcotic effect may result in acute onset of pain and the release of catecholamines.

Always ensure a patent airway is established and maintained, administer oxygen and assist or control respiration as indicated and use an oropharyngeal airway or endotracheal tube if necessary. Adequate body temperature and fluid intake should be maintained.

If severe or persistent hypotension occurs, the possibility of hypovolemia should be considered and managed with appropriate parenteral fluid therapy.

DOSAGE AND ADMINISTRATION

Special Precautions: Fentanyl transdermal system contains a high concentration of a potent Schedule II opioid agonist, fentanyl. Schedule II opioid substances which include fentanyl, hydromorphone, methadone, morphine, oxycodone, and oxymorphone have the highest potential for abuse and associated risk of fatal overdose due to respiratory depression. Fentanyl can be abused and is subject to criminal diversion. The high content of fentanyl in the patches (fentanyl transdermal system) may be a particular target for abuse and diversion.

Fentanyl transdermal systems are intended for transdermal use (on intact skin) only. The fentanyl transdermal system should not be used if the pouch seal is broken, or the patch is cut, damaged, or changed in any way.

Each fentanyl transdermal system may be worn continuously for 72 hours. The next patch should be applied to a different skin site after removal of the previous transdermal system.

If problems with adhesion of the fentanyl transdermal system patch occur, the edges of the patch may be taped with first aid tape. If problems with adhesion persist, the patch may be overlayed with a transparent adhesive film dressing (e.g., Bioclusive® or Askina®Derm).

If the patch falls off before 72 hours, dispose of it by folding in half and flushing down the toilet. A new patch may be applied to a different skin site.

Fentanyl transdermal system is ONLY for use in patients who are already tolerant to opioid therapy of comparable potency. Use in non-opioid-tolerant patients may lead to fatal respiratory depression. Overestimating the fentanyl

transdermal system dose when converting patients from another opioid medication can result in fatal overdose with the first dose. Due to the mean half-life of approximately 20 to 27 hours, patients who are thought to have had a serious adverse event, including overdose, will require monitoring and treatment for at least 24 hours.

The concomitant use of fentanyl transdermal system with all cytochrome P450 3A4 inhibitors (such as ritonavir, ketoconazole, itraconazole, troleandomycin, clarithromycin, nelfinavir, nefazodone, amiodarone, amprenavir, aprepitant, diltiazem, erythromycin, fluconazole, fosamprenavir, grapefruit juice, and verapamil) may result in an increase in fentanyl plasma concentrations, which could increase or prolong adverse drug effects and may cause potentially fatal respiratory depression. Patients receiving fentanyl transdermal system and any CYP3A4 inhibitor should be carefully monitored for an extended period of time and dosage adjustments should be made if warranted (see BOX WARNING, CLINICAL PHARMACOLOGY: Drug Interactions, WARNINGS, and PRECAUTIONS for further information).

Pediatric patients converting to fentanyl transdermal system with a 25 mcg/hr patch should be opioid-tolerant and receiving at least 60 mg of oral morphine or the equivalent per day. The dose conversion schedule described in Table C, and method of titration described below are recommended in opioid-tolerant pediatric patients over 2 years of age with chronic pain (see PRECAUTIONS: Pediatric Use). Respiratory depression is the chief hazard in elderly or debilitated patients, usually following large initial doses in non-tolerant patients, or when opioids are given in conjunction with other agents that depress respiration.

Fentanyl transdermal system should be used with caution in elderly, cachectic, or debilitated patients as they may have altered pharmacokinetics due to poor fat stores, muscle wasting, or altered clearance (see CLINICAL PHARMACOLOGY: Special Populations: *Geriatric Use*).

General Principles: Fentanyl transdermal system is indicated for management of **persistent**, moderate to severe chronic pain that:

- requires continuous, around-the-clock opioid administration for an extended period of time
- cannot be managed by other means such as non-steroidal analgesics, opioid combination products, or immediate-release opioids

Fentanyl transdermal system should ONLY be used in patients who are already receiving opioid therapy, who have demonstrated opioid tolerance, and who require a total daily dose at least equivalent to fentanyl transdermal system 25 mcg/hr. Patients who are considered opioid-tolerant are those who have been taking, for a week or longer, at least 60 mg of morphine daily, or at least 30 mg of oral oxycodone daily, or at least 8 mg oral hydromorphone daily, or an equianalgesic dose of another opioid.

Because serious or life-threatening hypoventilation could occur, fentanyl transdermal system is contraindicated:

- in patients who are not opioid-tolerant
- in the management of acute pain or in patients who require opioid analgesia for a short period of time
- in the management of postoperative pain, including use after out patient or day surgeries (e.g., tonsillectomies)
- in the management of mild pain
- in the management of intermittent pain [e.g., use on an as needed basis (prn)]

(See CONTRAINDICATIONS for further information.)

Safety of fentanyl transdermal system has not been established in children under 2 years of age. Fentanyl transdermal system should be administered to children only if they are opioid-tolerant and 2 years of age or older (see PRECAUTIONS: Pediatric Use).

Prescribers should individualize treatment using a progressive plan of pain management such as outlined by the World Health Organization, the Agency for Health Research and Quality, the Federation of State Medical Boards Model Policy, or the American Pain Society.

With all opioids, the safety of patients using the products is dependent on healthcare practitioners prescribing them in strict conformity with their approved labeling with respect to patient selection, dosing, and proper conditions for use. As with all opioids, dosage should be individualized. The most important factor to be considered in determining the appropriate dose is the extent of preexisting opioid-tolerance (see BOX WARNING and CONTRAINDICATIONS). Initial doses should be reduced in elderly or debilitated patients (see PRECAUTIONS).

Fentanyl transdermal system should be applied to intact, nonirritated, and nonirradiated skin on a flat surface such as the chest, back, flank or upper arm. In young children and persons with cognitive impairment, adhesion should be monitored and the upper back is the preferred location to minimize the potential of inappropriate patch removal. Hair at the application site should be clipped (not shaved) prior to system application. If the site of fentanyl transdermal system application must be cleansed prior to application of

the patch, do so with clear water. Do not use soaps, oils, lotions, alcohol, or any other agents that might irritate the skin or alter its characteristics. Allow the skin to dry completely prior to patch application.

Fentanyl transdermal system should be applied immediately upon removal from the sealed package. Do not use if the pouch seal is broken. Do not alter the patch (e.g., cut) in any way prior to application and do not use cut or damaged patches.

The transdermal system should be pressed firmly in place with the palm of the hand for 30 seconds, making sure the contact is complete, especially around the edges.

Fentanyl transdermal system should be kept out of the reach of children. Used patches should be folded so that the adhesive side of the patch adheres to itself, then the patch should be flushed down the toilet immediately upon removal. Patients should dispose of any patches remaining from a prescription as soon as they are no longer needed. Unused patches should be removed from their pouches, folded so that the adhesive side of the patch adheres to itself, and flushed down the toilet.

Dose Selection: Doses must be individualized based upon the status of each patient and should be assessed at regular intervals after fentanyl transdermal system application. Reduced doses of fentanyl transdermal system are suggested for the elderly and other groups discussed in PRECAUTIONS.

Fentanyl transdermal system is ONLY for use in patients who are already tolerant to opioid therapy of comparable potency. Use in non-opioid-tolerant patients may lead to fatal respiratory depression.

In selecting an initial fentanyl transdermal system dose, attention should be given to 1) the daily dose, potency, and characteristics of the opioid the patient has been taking previously (e.g., whether it is a pure agonist or mixed agonist-antagonist), 2) the reliability of the relative potency estimates used to calculate the fentanyl transdermal system dose needed (potency estimates may vary with the route of administration), 3) the degree of opioid tolerance, and 4) the general condition and medical status of the patient. Each patient should be maintained at the lowest dose providing acceptable pain control.

Initial Fentanyl Transdermal System Dose Selection: Overestimating the fentanyl transdermal system dose when converting patients from another opioid medication can result in fatal overdose with the first dose. Due to the mean half-life of approximately 20 to 27 hours, patients who are thought to have had a serious adverse event, including overdose, will require monitoring and treatment for at least 24 hours.

There has been no systematic evaluation of fentanyl transdermal system as an initial opioid analgesic in the management of chronic pain, since most patients in the clinical trials were converted to fentanyl transdermal system from other narcotics. The efficacy of fentanyl transdermal system 12 mcg/hr as an initiating dose has not been determined. In addition, patients who are not opioid-tolerant have experienced hypoventilation and death during use of fentanyl transdermal system. Therefore, fentanyl transdermal system should be used only in patients who are opioid-tolerant.

To convert adult and pediatric patients from oral or parenteral opioids to fentanyl transdermal system, use Table C. Alternatively, for adult and pediatric patients taking opioids or doses not listed in Table C, use the following methodology:

1. Calculate the previous 24 hour analgesic requirement.
2. Convert this amount to the equianalgesic oral morphine dose using Table D.
3. Table E displays the range of 24 hour oral morphine doses that are recommended for conversion to each fentanyl transdermal system dose. Use this table to find the calculated 24 hour morphine dose and the corresponding fentanyl transdermal system dose. Initiate fentanyl transdermal system treatment using the recommended dose and titrate patients upwards (no more frequently than every 3 days after the initial dose or than every 6 days thereafter) until analgesic efficacy is attained. The recommended starting dose when converting from other opioids to fentanyl transdermal system is likely too low for 50% of patients. This starting dose is recommended to minimize the potential for overdosing patients with the first dose. For delivery rates in excess of 100 mcg/hr, multiple systems may be used.

[See table C at top of next page]

Alternatively, for adult and pediatric patients taking opioids or doses not listed in Table C, use the conversion methodology outlined above with Table D.

[1] Table C should not be used to convert from fentanyl transdermal system to other therapies because this conversion to fentanyl transdermal system is conservative. Use of Table C for conversion to other analgesic therapies can overestimate the dose of the new agent. Overdosage

of the new analgesic agent is possible (see DOSAGE AND ADMINISTRATION: Discontinuation of Fentanyl Transdermal System).

TABLE D[1,a]
EQUIANALGESIC POTENCY CONVERSION

Name	Equianalgesic Dose (mg)	
	IM[b,c]	PO
Morphine	10	60 (30)[d]
Hydromorphone (Dilaudid®)	1.5	7.5
Methadone (Dolophine®)	10	20
Oxycodone	15	30
Levorphanol (Levo-Dromoran®)	2	4
Oxymorphone (Numorphan®)	1	10 (PR)
Meperidine (Demerol®)	75	—
Codeine	130	200

[1] Table D should not be used to convert from fentanyl transdermal system to other therapies because this conversion to fentanyl transdermal system is conservative. Use of Table D for conversion to other analgesic therapies can overestimate the dose of the new agent. Overdosage of the new analgesic agent is possible (see DOSAGE AND ADMINISTRATION: Discontinuation of Fentanyl Transdermal System).

[a] All IM and PO doses in this chart are considered equivalent to 10 mg of IM morphine in analgesic effect. IM denotes intramuscular, PO oral, and PR rectal.

[b] Based on single-dose studies in which an intramuscular dose of each drug listed was compared with morphine to establish the relative potency. Oral doses are those recommended when changing from parenteral to an oral route. Reference: Foley, K.M. (1985) The treatment of cancer pain. NEJM 313(2):84-95.

[c] Although controlled studies are not available, in clinical practice it is customary to consider the doses of opioid given IM, IV, or subcutaneously to be equivalent. There may be some differences in pharmacokinetic parameters such as C_{max} and T_{max}.

[d] The conversion ratio of 10 mg parenteral morphine = 30 mg oral morphine is based on clinical experience in patients with chronic pain. The conversion ratio of 10 mg parenteral morphine = 60 mg oral morphine is based on a potency study in acute pain. Reference: Ashburn and Lipman (1993) Management of pain in the cancer patient. Anesth Analg 76:402-416.

TABLE E[1]
RECOMMENDED INITIAL FENTANYL TRANSDERMAL SYSTEM DOSE BASED UPON DAILY ORAL MORPHINE DOSE

Oral 24 hour Morphine (mg/day)	Fentanyl Transdermal System Dose (mcg/hr)
60 to 134	25
135 to 224	50
225 to 314	75
315 to 404	100
405 to 494	125
495 to 584	150
585 to 674	175
675 to 764	200
765 to 854	225
855 to 944	250
945 to 1034	275
1035 to 1124	300

NOTE: In clinical trials, these ranges of daily oral morphine doses were used as a basis for conversion to fentanyl transdermal system.

[1] Table E should not be used to convert from fentanyl transdermal system to other therapies because this conversion to fentanyl transdermal system is conservative. Use of Table E for conversion to other analgesic therapies can overestimate the dose of the new agent. Overdosage of the new analgesic agent is possible (see DOSAGE AND ADMINISTRATION: Discontinuation of Fentanyl Transdermal System).

The majority of patients are adequately maintained with fentanyl transdermal system administered every 72 hours. Some patients may not achieve adequate analgesia using this dosing interval and may require systems to be applied every 48 hours rather than every 72 hours. An increase in the fentanyl transdermal system dose should be evaluated before changing dosing intervals in order to maintain patients on a 72-hour regimen. Dosing intervals less than every 72 hours were not studied in children and adolescents and are not recommended.

TABLE C[1]
DOSE CONVERSION GUIDELINES

Current Analgesic	Daily Dosage (mg/d)			
Oral morphine	60 to 134	135 to 224	225 to 314	315 to 404
IM/IV morphine	10 to 22	23 to 37	38 to 52	53 to 67
Oral oxycodone	30 to 67	67.5 to 112	112.5 to 157	157.5 to 202
IM/IV oxycodone	15 to 33	33.1 to 56	56.1 to 78	78.1 to 101
Oral codeine	150 to 447	448 to 747	748 to 1047	1048 to 1347
Oral hydromorphone	8 to 17	17.1 to 28	28.1 to 39	39.1 to 51
IV hydromorphone	1.5 to 3.4	3.5 to 5.6	5.7 to 7.9	8 to 10
IM meperidine	75 to 165	166 to 278	279 to 390	391 to 503
Oral methadone	20 to 44	45 to 74	75 to 104	105 to 134
IM methadone	10 to 22	23 to 37	38 to 52	53 to 67
	⇓	⇓	⇓	⇓
Recommended Fentanyl Transdermal System Dose	25 mcg/hr	50 mcg/hr	75 mcg/hr	100 mcg/hr

Fentanyl Transdermal System Dose (mcg/hr)	System Size (cm²)	Fentanyl Content (mg)	NDC Number
Fentanyl Transdermal System – 12	3.13	1.28	0378-9119-98
Fentanyl Transdermal System – 25	6.25	2.55	0378-9121-98
Fentanyl Transdermal System – 50	12.5	5.10	0378-9122-98
Fentanyl Transdermal System – 75	18.75	7.65	0378-9123-98
Fentanyl Transdermal System – 100	25	10.20	0378-9124-98

Because of the increase in serum fentanyl concentration over the first 24 hours following initial system application, the initial evaluation of the maximum analgesic effect of fentanyl transdermal system cannot be made before 24 hours of wearing. The initial fentanyl transdermal system dose may be increased after 3 days (see DOSAGE AND ADMINISTRATION: Dose Titration).

During the initial application of fentanyl transdermal system, patients should use short acting analgesics as needed until analgesic efficacy with fentanyl transdermal system is attained. Thereafter, some patients still may require periodic supplemental doses of other short acting analgesics for "breakthrough" pain.

Dose Titration: The recommended initial fentanyl transdermal system dose based upon the daily oral morphine dose is conservative, and 50% of patients are likely to require a dose increase after initial application of fentanyl transdermal system. The initial fentanyl transdermal system dose may be increased after 3 days based on the daily dose of supplemental opioid analgesics required by the patient in the second or third day of the initial application. Physicians are advised that it may take up to 6 days after increasing the dose of fentanyl transdermal system for the patient to reach equilibrium on the new dose (see graph in CLINICAL PHARMACOLOGY). Therefore, patients should wear a higher dose through two applications before any further increase in dosage is made on the basis of the average daily use of a supplemental analgesic.

Appropriate dosage increments should be based on the daily dose of supplementary opioids, using the ratio of 45 mg/24 hours of oral morphine to a 12.5 mcg/hr increase in fentanyl transdermal system dose. Fentanyl transdermal system 12 mcg/hr delivers 12.5 mcg/hr of fentanyl.

Discontinuation of Fentanyl Transdermal System: To convert patients to another opioid, remove fentanyl transdermal system and titrate the dose of the new analgesic based upon the patient's report of pain until adequate analgesia has been attained. Upon system removal, 17 hours or more are required for a 50% decrease in serum fentanyl concentrations. Opioid withdrawal symptoms (such as nausea, vomiting, diarrhea, anxiety, and shivering) are possible in some patients after conversion or dose adjustment. For patients requiring discontinuation of opioids, a gradual downward titration is recommended since it is not known at what dose level the opioid may be discontinued without producing the signs and symptoms of abrupt withdrawal.

Tables C, D, and E should not be used to convert from fentanyl transdermal system to other therapies. Because the conversion to fentanyl transdermal system is conservative, use of Tables C, D, and E for conversion to other analgesic therapies can overestimate the dose of the new agent. Overdosage of the new analgesic agent is possible.

HOW SUPPLIED

Fentanyl transdermal system is supplied in cartons containing 5 individually packaged systems. See chart for information regarding individual systems.

[See second table above]

Safety and Handling: Fentanyl transdermal systems are supplied in sealed pouches which pose little risk of exposure to healthcare workers. Do not use a fentanyl transdermal system if the pouch seal is broken or the patch is cut, damaged, or changed in any way.

KEEP FENTANYL TRANSDERMAL SYSTEM OUT OF THE REACH OF CHILDREN AND PETS.
Store in original unopened pouch. Store at 20° to 25°C (68° to 77°F). [See USP Controlled Room Temperature.] Apply immediately after removal from individually sealed pouch. Do not use if the pouch seal is broken. **For transdermal use only.**

A schedule CII narcotic. DEA order form required.

BIOCLUSIVE® is a registered trademark of Systagenix Wound Management, Inc.
Askina®Derm is a registered trademark of BBraun Melsungen AG
DILAUDID® is a registered trademark of Purdue Pharmaceutical Products L.P.
DOLOPHINE® is a registered trademark of Roxane Laboratories, Inc.
LEVO-DROMORAN® is a registered trademark of Valeant Pharmaceuticals
NUMORPHAN® is a registered trademark of Endo Pharmaceuticals, Inc.
DEMEROL® is a registered trademark of Sanofi-Synthelabo Inc. of Sanofi-Aventis U.S.
Mylan Pharmaceuticals Inc.
Morgantown, WV 26505

REVISED DECEMBER 2009
FTS:R17

MEDICATION GUIDE
Fentanyl Transdermal System
℞ only

IMPORTANT:
- Keep fentanyl transdermal system in a safe place away from children and pets. Accidental use by a child or pet is a medical emergency and may result in death. If a child or pet accidentally uses fentanyl transdermal system, get emergency help right away.
- Make sure you read the separate "Instructions for Applying a Fentanyl Transdermal System." Always use a fentanyl transdermal system the right way. Fentanyl transdermal system can cause serious breathing problems and death, especially if it is used the wrong way.
- Fentanyl transdermal system is a federally controlled substance (C-II) because it can be abused. Keep fentanyl transdermal system in a safe place to prevent theft. Selling or giving away fentanyl transdermal system may harm others, and is against the law.
- Tell your doctor if you (or a family member) have ever abused or been dependent on alcohol, prescription medicines or street drugs.

Read the Medication Guide that comes with fentanyl transdermal system before you start using it and each time you get a new prescription. There may be new information. This Medication Guide does not take the place of talking to your healthcare provider about your medical condition or your treatment. Make sure you read and understand all the instructions for using fentanyl transdermal system. Do not use fentanyl transdermal system unless you understand everything. Talk to your healthcare provider if you have questions.

What is the most important information I should know about fentanyl transdermal system?

Fentanyl transdermal system is a skin patch that contains fentanyl. **Fentanyl is a very strong opioid narcotic pain medicine that can cause serious and life-threatening breathing problems.** Serious and life-threatening breathing problems can happen because of an overdose or if the dose you are using is too high for you. Call your doctor right away or get emergency medical help if you:

- have trouble breathing, or have slow or shallow breathing
- have a slow heartbeat
- have severe sleepiness
- have cold, clammy skin
- feel faint, dizzy, confused, or cannot think, walk, or talk normally
- have a seizure
- have hallucinations

Fentanyl transdermal system is only for adults and children over the age of two with persistent, moderate to severe chronic pain and who:

- are already using another strong opioid narcotic pain medicine around-the-clock, and have been using the medicine regularly for a week or longer. This is called being opioid-tolerant.
- have pain that cannot be controlled with other medicines

Do not use fentanyl transdermal system:

- **if you are not already using another opioid narcotic medicine and are not opioid-tolerant**
- if you need opioid pain medicines for only a short time
- for pain from surgery, medical or dental procedures
- if your pain can be taken care of by occasional use of other pain medicines
- in children who are less than 2 years of age
- if you have asthma symptoms or have severe asthma

A fentanyl transdermal system must be used only on the skin of the person for whom it was prescribed. If the patch comes off and accidentally sticks to the skin of another person, take the patch off of that person right away, wash the area with water, and get medical care for them right away.

Fentanyl transdermal system is not safe for everyone. Tell your doctor about all of your medical conditions.

Tell your doctor if you are planning to become pregnant, are pregnant, or breast-feeding. Fentanyl transdermal system may cause serious harm to a baby.

Tell your doctor about all the medicines you take. Some medicines may cause serious or life-threatening side effects when used with fentanyl transdermal system. Your doctor will tell you if it is safe to take other medicines while you are using fentanyl transdermal system.

Know the medicines you take. Keep a list of your medicines to show to your doctor and pharmacist.

How should I use fentanyl transdermal system?

Read the separate "Instructions for Applying a Fentanyl Transdermal System".

- **You must always use** fentanyl transdermal systems the right way:
  - **Do not** use a fentanyl transdermal system if the pouch seal is broken or the patch is cut, damaged, or changed in any way.
  - **Do not** use heat sources such as heating pads, electric blankets, heat lamps, tanning lamps, saunas, hot tubs, or heated waterbeds while wearing a fentanyl transdermal system.
  - **Do not** take hot baths or sunbathe while wearing a fentanyl transdermal system.
- **If you have problems with the fentanyl transdermal system not sticking:**
  1. Apply first aid tape only to the edges of the patch.
  2. If problems with the patch not sticking persist, cover the patch with Bioclusive® or Askina®Derm. These are special see-through adhesive dressings. **Never cover a fentanyl transdermal system with any other bandage or tape.**
- **If your fentanyl transdermal system falls off before 3 days or 72 hours,** fold the sticky side together and flush down a toilet. Put a new one on at a different skin site.
- **Do not change your dose unless your doctor tells you to.** Your doctor may change your dose after seeing how the medicine affects you. Do not use fentanyl transdermal system more often than prescribed. Call your doctor if your pain is not well controlled while using fentanyl transdermal system.
- **Do not stop using fentanyl transdermal system suddenly.** Stopping fentanyl transdermal system suddenly can make you sick with withdrawal symptoms (for example, nausea, vomiting, diarrhea, anxiety, and shivering). Your body can develop a physical dependence on fentanyl transdermal system. If your doctor decides you no longer need fentanyl transdermal system, ask how to slowly reduce this medicine so you don't have withdrawal symptoms. Do not stop taking fentanyl transdermal system without talking to your doctor.
- **Do not wear more than one fentanyl transdermal system at a time,** unless your doctor tells you to do so.

- **Call your doctor right away if**
  - **You get a fever higher than 102°F**
  - **Your body temperature increases from exercise**
  A fever or increase in body temperature may cause too much of the medicine in fentanyl transdermal system to pass into your body.
- **If you use more fentanyl transdermal system than your doctor has prescribed, get emergency medical help right away.**
- **Do not drink any alcohol while using fentanyl transdermal system.** Alcohol can increase your chances of having serious side effects.
- **Do not drive, operate heavy machinery, or do other possibly dangerous activities until you know how fentanyl transdermal system affects you.** Fentanyl transdermal system can make you sleepy. Ask your doctor to tell you when it is okay to do these activities.
- When you remove your fentanyl transdermal system, fold the sticky sides of the used fentanyl transdermal system together and flush it down the toilet. **Do not put used fentanyl transdermal systems in a trash can.**

What are the possible side effects of fentanyl transdermal system?

Serious side effects include:

- **Life-threatening breathing problems.** See "What is the most important information I should know about fentanyl transdermal system?"
- **Low blood pressure.** This can make you feel dizzy if you get up too fast from sitting or lying down.

The common side effects with fentanyl transdermal system are nausea, vomiting, constipation, dry mouth, sleepiness, confusion, weakness, sweating, and pain and redness where the patch was applied.

Constipation is a very common side effect of all opioid medicines. Talk to your doctor about the use of laxatives and stool softeners to prevent or treat constipation while taking fentanyl transdermal system.

Talk to your doctor about any side effect that concerns you. These are not all the possible side effects of fentanyl transdermal system. For a complete list, ask your doctor or pharmacist.

Call your doctor for medical advice about side effects. You may report side effects to FDA at 1-800-FDA-1088.

How should I store fentanyl transdermal system?

- Store fentanyl transdermal system in original unopened pouch at 20° to 25°C (68° to 77°F). [See USP Controlled Room Temperature.]
- Keep fentanyl transdermal system in its protective pouch until you are ready to use it.
- **Keep fentanyl transdermal system in a safe place out of the reach of children and pets.**
- Dispose of fentanyl transdermal systems you no longer need. Open the unused packages, fold the sticky sides of the patches together, and flush them down the toilet.

General information about the safe and effective use of fentanyl transdermal system

- Do not use fentanyl transdermal system for a condition for which it was not prescribed.
- **Do not give fentanyl transdermal system to other people, even if they have the same symptoms you have. Fentanyl transdermal system can harm other people and even cause death. Sharing fentanyl transdermal system is against the law.**
- This Medication Guide summarizes the most important information about fentanyl transdermal system. If you would like more information, talk with your doctor. You can ask your doctor or pharmacist for information about fentanyl transdermal system that is written for doctors.

For questions about fentanyl transdermal system, call Mylan Pharmaceuticals Inc. Product Information at 1-877-446-3679. If this is a medical emergency, please call 911.

What are the ingredients of fentanyl transdermal system?

Active Ingredient: fentanyl

Inactive ingredients: Dimethicone NF and silicone adhesive and polyolefin film backing.

This Medication Guide has been approved by the United States Food and Drug Administration.

BIOCLUSIVE® is a registered trademark of Systagenix Wound Management, Inc.

Askina®Derm is a registered trademark of BBraun Melsungen AG

Mylan Pharmaceuticals Inc.
Morgantown, WV 26505

REVISED DECEMBER 2009
MG:FTS:R3

Fentanyl Transdermal System CII
Instructions for Applying a Fentanyl Transdermal System
℞ only
[See figure at top of next column]
Before Applying Fentanyl Transdermal System

- **Each fentanyl transdermal system is sealed in its own protective pouch. Do not remove fentanyl transdermal system from the pouch until you are ready to use it.**
- **Do not use a fentanyl transdermal system if the pouch seal is broken or the patch is cut, damaged or changed in any way.**

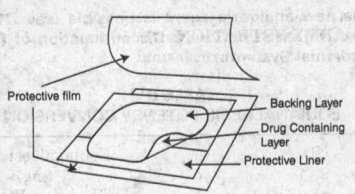

Protective film — Backing Layer — Drug Containing Layer — Protective Liner

- **Fentanyl transdermal systems are available in 5 different doses and patch sizes. Make sure you have the right dose patch or patches that have been prescribed for you.**

Applying a Fentanyl Transdermal System

1. Skin Areas Where the Fentanyl Transdermal System May Be Applied:

For adults:

- Put the patch on the chest, back, flank (sides of the waist), or upper arm in a place where there is no hair (see Figures 1-4).

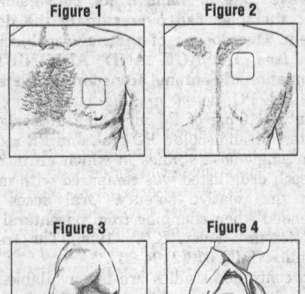

Figure 1   Figure 2

Figure 3   Figure 4

For children (and adults with mental impairment):

- Put the patch on the upper back (see Figure 2). This will lower the chances that the child will remove the patch and put it in their mouth.

For adults and children

- Do not put a fentanyl transdermal system on skin that is very oily, burned, broken out, cut, irritated, or damaged in any way.
- Avoid sensitive areas or those that move around a lot. If there is hair, **do not shave (shaving irritates the skin)**. Instead, clip hair as close to the skin as possible (see Figure 5).
- **Talk to your doctor if you have questions about skin application sites.**

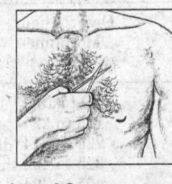

Figure 5

2. Prepare to Apply a Fentanyl Transdermal System:

- Choose the time of day that is best for you to apply fentanyl transdermal system. Change it at about the same time of day (3 days or 72 hours after you apply the patch) or as directed by your doctor.
- Do not wear more than one fentanyl transdermal system at a time unless your doctor tells you to do so. Before putting on a new fentanyl transdermal system, remove the patch you have been wearing.
- Clean the skin area with clear water **only**. Pat skin **completely dry.** Do not use anything on the skin such as soaps, lotions, oils, or alcohol before the patch is applied.

3. Open the Pouch: Tear at notch and remove the fentanyl transdermal system. Each fentanyl transdermal system is packaged with additional pieces of protective film above and below the patch and is sealed in its own protective pouch. Do not remove fentanyl transdermal system from the pouch until you are ready to use it (see Figure 6). The additional pieces of protective film are discarded at time of use (see Figure 7).

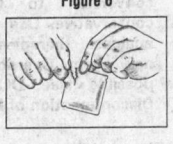

Figure 6

Figure 7

4. Peel: Peel off both parts of the protective liner from the patch. Each fentanyl transdermal system has a clear plastic liner that can be peeled off in two pieces. This covers the sticky side of the patch. Carefully peel this liner off. Throw the clear plastic liner away. **Touch the sticky side of a fentanyl transdermal system as little as possible** (see Figure 8).

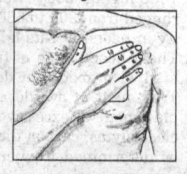

Figure 8

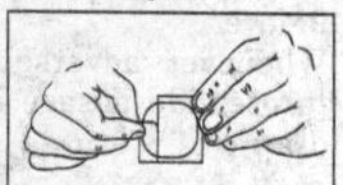

5. Press: Press the patch onto the chosen skin site **with the palm of your hand and hold there for at least 30 seconds** (see Figure 9). Make sure it sticks well, especially at the edges.

Figure 9

- Fentanyl transdermal system may not stick to all patients. You need to check the patches often to make sure that they are sticking well to the skin.
- If the patch falls off right away after applying, throw it away and put a new one on at a different skin site (see Disposing a Fentanyl Transdermal System).
- If you have a problem with the patch not sticking
  ◦ Apply first aid tape only to the edges of the patch.
  ◦ If you continue to have problems with the patch sticking, you may cover the patch with Bioclusive® or Askina®Derm. These are special see-through adhesive dressings. **Never cover a fentanyl transdermal system with any other bandage or tape.** Remove the backing from the Bioclusive® or Askina®Derm dressing and place it carefully over the fentanyl transdermal system, smoothing it over the patch and your skin.
- **If your patch falls off later, but before 3 days (72 hours) of use, discard it properly (see Disposing a Fentanyl Transdermal System) and put a new one on at a different skin site. Be sure to let your doctor know that this has happened, and do not replace the new patch until 3 days (72 hours) after you put it on (or as directed by your doctor).**
6. Wash your hands when you have finished applying a fentanyl transdermal system.
7. Remove a fentanyl transdermal system after wearing it for 3 days (72 hours) (see "Disposing a Fentanyl Transdermal System"). Choose a **different** place on the skin to apply a new fentanyl transdermal system and repeat Steps 2 through 6.

Do not apply the new patch to the same place as the last one.

Water and Fentanyl Transdermal System

- You can bathe, swim or shower while you are wearing a fentanyl transdermal system. If the patch falls off before 3 days (72 hours) after application, discard it properly (see Disposing a Fentanyl Transdermal System) and put a new one on at a different skin site. Be sure to let your doctor know that this has happened, and do not replace the new patch until 3 days (72 hours) after you put it on (or as directed by your doctor).

Disposing a Fentanyl Transdermal System

- Fold the used fentanyl transdermal system in half so that the sticky side sticks to itself (Figure 10). Flush the used fentanyl transdermal system down the toilet right away (Figure 11).

Figure 10

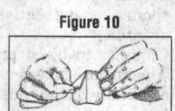

A used fentanyl transdermal system CAN be VERY dangerous for or even lead to death in babies, children, pets, and adults who have not been prescribed fentanyl transdermal system.

Figure 11

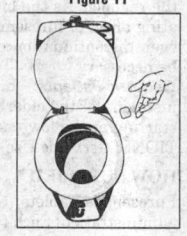

- Throw away any fentanyl transdermal systems that are left over from your prescription as soon as they are no longer needed. Remove the leftover patches from their protective pouch and remove the protective liner. **Fold the patches in half with the sticky sides together, and flush the patches down the toilet.** Do not flush the pouch or the protective liner down the toilet. These items can be thrown away in a trash can.

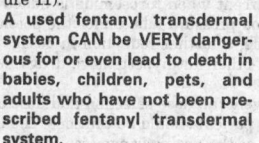

BIOCLUSIVE® is a registered trademark of Systagenix Wound Management, Inc.
Askina®Derm is a registered trademark of BBraun Melsungen AG
Mylan Pharmaceuticals Inc.
Morgantown, WV 26505

REVISED DECEMBER 2009
MG:FTS:R3

FUROSEMIDE TABLETS, USP ℞
20 mg, 40 mg and 80 mg
℞ only

> **WARNING**
> **Furosemide is a potent diuretic which, if given in excessive amounts, can lead to a profound diuresis with water and electrolyte depletion. Therefore, careful medical supervision is required and dose and dose schedule must be adjusted to the individual patient's needs. (See DOSAGE AND ADMINISTRATION.)**

DESCRIPTION

Furosemide is a diuretic which is an anthranilic acid derivative. Chemically, it is 4-chloro-N-furfuryl-5-sulfamoylanthranilic acid. Furosemide, USP is a white to slightly yellow odorless, crystalline powder. It is practically insoluble in water, sparingly soluble in alcohol, freely soluble in dilute alkali solutions and insoluble in dilute acids. The structural formula is as follows:

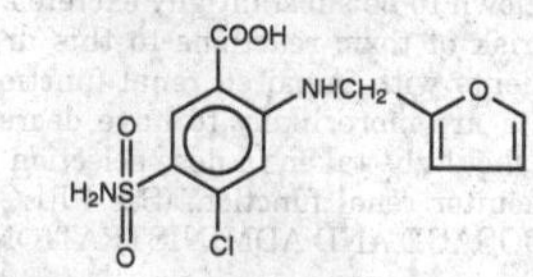

$C_{12}H_{11}ClN_2O_5S$
M.W. 330.75

Each tablet for oral administration contains 20 mg, 40 mg or 80 mg of furosemide, USP and the following inactive ingredients: colloidal silicon dioxide, lactose monohydrate, microcrystalline cellulose, pregelatinized starch and stearic acid.
Furosemide Tablets, USP 20 mg, 40 mg and 80 mg meet *USP DISSOLUTION TEST 1.*

CLINICAL PHARMACOLOGY

Investigations into the mode of action of furosemide have utilized micropuncture studies in rats, stop flow experiments in dogs and various clearance studies in both humans and experimental animals. It has been demonstrated that furosemide inhibits primarily the absorption of sodium and chloride not only in the proximal and distal tubules but also in the loop of Henle. The high degree of efficacy is largely due to the unique site of action. The action on the distal tubule is independent of any inhibitory effect on carbonic anhydrase and aldosterone.
Recent evidence suggests that furosemide glucuronide is the only or at least the major biotransformation product of furosemide in man. Furosemide is extensively bound to plasma proteins, mainly to albumin. Plasma concentrations ranging from 1 to 400 mcg/mL are 91% to 99% bound in healthy individuals. The unbound fraction averages 2.3% to 4.1% at therapeutic concentrations.
The onset of diuresis following oral administration is within one hour. The peak effect occurs within the first or second hour. The duration of diuretic effect is 6 to 8 hours.
In fasted normal men, the mean bioavailability of furosemide from furosemide tablets and furosemide oral solution is 64% to 60%, respectively, of that from an intravenous injection of the drug. Although furosemide is more rapidly absorbed from the oral solution (50 minutes) than from the tablet (87 minutes), peak plasma levels and area under the plasma concentration-time curves do not differ significantly. Peak plasma concentrations increase with increasing dose but times-to-peak do not differ among doses. The terminal half-life of furosemide is approximately 2 hours.
Significantly more furosemide is excreted in urine following the IV injection than after the tablet or oral solution. There are no significant differences between the two oral formulations in the amount of unchanged drug excreted in urine.

Geriatric Population: Furosemide binding to albumin may be reduced in elderly patients. Furosemide is predominantly excreted unchanged in the urine. The renal clearance of furosemide after intravenous administration in older healthy male subjects (60 to 70 years of age) is statistically significantly smaller than in younger healthy male subjects (20 to 35 years of age). The initial diuretic effect of

furosemide in older subjects is decreased relative to younger subjects. (See PRECAUTIONS: Geriatric Use.)

INDICATIONS AND USAGE

Edema: Furosemide is indicated in adults and pediatric patients for the treatment of edema associated with congestive heart failure, cirrhosis of the liver, and renal disease, including the nephrotic syndrome. Furosemide is particularly useful when an agent with greater diuretic potential is desired.
Hypertension: Oral furosemide may be used in adults for the treatment of hypertension alone or in combination with other antihypertensive agents. Hypertensive patients who cannot be adequately controlled with thiazides will probably also not be adequately controlled with furosemide alone.

CONTRAINDICATIONS

Furosemide is contraindicated in patients with anuria and in patients with a history of hypersensitivity to furosemide.

WARNINGS

In patients with hepatic cirrhosis and ascites, furosemide therapy is best initiated in the hospital. In hepatic coma and in states of electrolyte depletion, therapy should not be instituted until the basic condition is improved. Sudden alteration of fluid and electrolyte balance in patients with cirrhosis may precipitate hepatic coma; therefore, strict observation is necessary during the period of diuresis. Supplemental potassium chloride and, if required, an aldosterone antagonist are helpful in preventing hypokalemia and metabolic alkalosis.
If increasing azotemia and oliguria occur during treatment of severe progressive renal disease, furosemide should be discontinued.
Cases of tinnitus and reversible or irreversible hearing impairment have been reported. Usually, reports indicate that furosemide ototoxicity is associated with rapid injection, severe renal impairment, doses exceeding several times the usual recommended dose, or concomitant therapy with aminoglycoside antibiotics, ethacrynic acid, or other ototoxic drugs. If the physician elects to use high dose parenteral therapy, controlled intravenous infusion is advisable (for adults, an infusion rate not exceeding 4 mg furosemide per minute has been used).

PRECAUTIONS

General: Excessive diuresis may cause dehydration and blood volume reduction with circulatory collapse and possibly vascular thrombosis and embolism, particularly in elderly patients. As with any effective diuretic, electrolyte depletion may occur during furosemide therapy, especially in patients receiving higher doses and a restricted salt intake.
Hypokalemia may develop with furosemide, especially with brisk diuresis, inadequate oral electrolyte intake, when cirrhosis is present, or during concomitant use of corticosteroids or ACTH. Digitalis therapy may exaggerate metabolic effects of hypokalemia, especially myocardial effects.
All patients receiving furosemide therapy should be observed for these signs or symptoms of fluid or electrolyte imbalance (hyponatremia, hypochloremic alkalosis, hypokalemia, hypomagnesemia or hypocalcemia): dryness of mouth, thirst, weakness, lethargy, drowsiness, restlessness, muscle pains or cramps, muscular fatigue, hypotension, oliguria, tachycardia, arrhythmia, or gastrointestinal disturbances such as nausea and vomiting. Increases in blood glucose and alterations in glucose tolerance tests (with abnormalities of the fasting and 2-hour postprandial sugar) have been observed, and rarely, precipitation of diabetes mellitus has been reported.
Asymptomatic hyperuricemia can occur and gout may rarely be precipitated.
Patients allergic to sulfonamides may also be allergic to furosemide. The possibility exists of exacerbation or activation of systemic lupus erythematosus.
As with many other drugs, patients should be observed regularly for the possible occurrence of blood dyscrasias, liver or kidney damage or other idiosyncratic reactions.
Information for Patients: Patients receiving furosemide should be advised that they may experience symptoms from excessive fluid and/or electrolyte losses. The postural hypotension that sometimes occurs can usually be managed by getting up slowly. Potassium supplements and/or dietary measures may be needed to control or avoid hypokalemia.
Patients with diabetes mellitus should be told that furosemide may increase blood glucose levels and thereby affect urine glucose tests. The skin of some patients may be more sensitive to the effects of sunlight while taking furosemide.
Hypertensive patients should avoid medications that may increase blood pressure, including over-the-counter products for appetite suppression and cold symptoms.
Laboratory Tests: Serum electrolytes, (particularly potassium), CO_2, creatinine and BUN should be determined frequently during the first few months of furosemide therapy and periodically thereafter. Serum and urine electrolyte determinations are particularly important when the patient is

vomiting profusely or receiving parenteral fluids. Abnormalities should be corrected or the drug temporarily withdrawn. Other medications may also influence serum electrolytes.

Reversible elevations of BUN may occur and are associated with dehydration which should be avoided, particularly in patients with renal insufficiency.

Urine and blood glucose should be checked periodically in diabetics receiving furosemide, even in those suspected of latent diabetes.

Furosemide may lower serum levels of calcium (rarely cases of tetany have been reported) and magnesium. Accordingly, serum levels of these electrolytes should be determined periodically.

Drug Interactions: Furosemide may increase the ototoxic potential of aminoglycoside antibiotics, especially in the presence of impaired renal function. Except in life threatening situations, avoid this combination.

Furosemide should not be used concomitantly with ethacrynic acid because of the possibility of ototoxicity. Patients receiving high doses of salicylates concomitantly with furosemide, as in rheumatic disease, may experience salicylate toxicity at lower doses because of competitive renal excretory sites.

Furosemide has a tendency to antagonize the skeletal muscle relaxing effect of tubocurarine and may potentiate the action of succinylcholine.

Lithium generally should not be given with diuretics because they reduce lithium's renal clearance and add a high risk of lithium toxicity.

Furosemide may add to or potentiate the therapeutic effect of other antihypertensive drugs. Potentiation occurs with ganglionic or peripheral adrenergic blocking drugs.

Furosemide may decrease arterial responsiveness to norepinephrine. However, norepinephrine may still be used effectively.

Simultaneous administration of sucralfate and furosemide tablets may reduce the natriuretic and antihypertensive effects of furosemide. Patients receiving both drugs should be observed closely to determine if the desired diuretic and/or antihypertensive effect of furosemide is achieved. The intake of furosemide and sucralfate should be separated by at least 2 hours.

One study in six subjects demonstrated that the combination of furosemide and acetylsalicylic acid temporarily reduced creatinine clearance in patients with chronic renal insufficiency. There are case reports of patients who developed increased BUN, serum creatinine and serum potassium levels, and weight gain when furosemide was used in conjunction with NSAIDs.

Literature reports indicate that coadministration of indomethacin may reduce the natriuretic and antihypertensive effects of furosemide in some patients by inhibiting prostaglandin synthesis. Indomethacin may also affect plasma renin levels, aldosterone excretion, and renin profile evaluation. Patients receiving both indomethacin and furosemide should be observed closely to determine if the desired diuretic and/or antihypertensive effect of furosemide is achieved.

Carcinogenesis, Mutagenesis, Impairment of Fertility: Furosemide was tested for carcinogenicity by oral administration in one strain of mice and one strain of rats. A small but significantly increased incidence of mammary gland carcinomas occurred in female mice at a dose 17.5 times the maximum human dose of 600 mg. There were marginal increases in uncommon tumors in male rats at a dose of 15 mg/kg (slightly greater than the maximum human dose) but not at 30 mg/kg.

Furosemide was devoid of mutagenic activity in various strains of *Salmonella typhimurium* when tested in the presence or absence of an *in vitro* metabolic activation system, and questionably positive for gene mutation in mouse lymphoma cells in the presence of rat liver S9 at the highest dose tested. Furosemide did not induce sister chromatid exchange in human cells *in vitro*, but other studies on chromosomal aberrations in human cells *in vitro* gave conflicting results. In Chinese hamster cells it induced chromosomal damage but was questionably positive for sister chromatid exchange. Studies on the induction by furosemide of chromosomal aberrations in mice were inconclusive. The urine of rats treated with this drug did not induce gene conversion in *Saccharomyces cerevisiae*.

Furosemide produced no impairment of fertility in male or female rats at 100 mg/kg/day (the maximum effective diuretic dose in the rat and 8 times the maximal human dose of 600 mg/day).

Pregnancy: *Teratogenic Effects. Pregnancy Category C:* Furosemide has been shown to cause unexplained maternal deaths and abortions in rabbits at 2, 4 and 8 times the maximal recommended human dose. There are no adequate and well controlled studies in pregnant women. Furosemide should be used during pregnancy only if the potential benefit justifies the potential risk to the fetus.

The effects of furosemide on embryonic and fetal development and on pregnant dams were studied in mice, rats and rabbits.

Furosemide caused unexplained maternal deaths and abortions in the rabbit at the lowest dose of 25 mg/kg (two times the maximal recommended human dose of 600 mg/day). In another study, a dose of 50 mg/kg (four times the maximal recommended human dose of 600 mg/day) also caused maternal deaths and abortions when administered to rabbits between Days 12 and 17 of gestation. In a third study, none of the pregnant rabbits survived a dose of 100 mg/kg. Data from the above studies indicate fetal lethality that can precede maternal deaths.

The results of the mouse study and one of the three rabbit studies also showed an increased incidence and severity of hydronephrosis (distention of the renal pelvis and, in some cases, of the ureters) in fetuses derived from the treated dams as compared with the incidence in fetuses from the control group.

Nursing Mothers: Because it appears in breast milk, caution should be exercised when furosemide is administered to a nursing mother.

Geriatric Use: Controlled clinical studies of furosemide did not include sufficient numbers of subjects aged 65 and over to determine whether they respond differently from younger subjects. Other reported clinical experience has not identified differences in responses between the elderly and younger patients. In general, dose selection for the elderly patient should be cautious, usually starting at the low end of the dosing range, reflecting the greater frequency of decreased hepatic, renal or cardiac function and of concomitant disease or other drug therapy.

This drug is known to be substantially excreted by the kidney, and the risk of toxic reactions to this drug may be greater in patients with impaired renal function. Because elderly patients are more likely to have decreased renal function, care should be taken in dose selection and it may be useful to monitor renal function. (See PRECAUTIONS: General and DOSAGE AND ADMINISTRATION.)

ADVERSE REACTIONS

Adverse reactions are categorized below by organ system and listed by decreasing severity.

Gastrointestinal System Reactions
1. hepatic encephalopathy in patients with hepatocellular insufficiency
2. pancreatitis
3. jaundice (intrahepatic cholestatic jaundice)
4. anorexia
5. oral and gastric irritation
6. cramping
7. diarrhea
8. constipation
9. nausea
10. vomiting

Systemic Hypersensitivity Reactions
1. systemic vasculitis
2. interstitial nephritis
3. necrotizing angiitis

Central Nervous System Reactions
1. tinnitus and hearing loss
2. paresthesias
3. vertigo
4. dizziness
5. headache
6. blurred vision
7. xanthopsia

Hematologic Reactions
1. aplastic anemia (rare)
2. thrombocytopenia
3. agranulocytosis (rare)
4. hemolytic anemia
5. leukopenia
6. anemia

Dermatologic-Hypersensitivity Reactions
1. exfoliative dermatitis
2. bullous pemphigoid
3. erythema multiforme
4. purpura
5. photosensitivity
6. urticaria
7. rash
8. pruritus

Cardiovascular Reaction
Orthostatic hypotension may occur and be aggravated by alcohol, barbiturates or narcotics.

Other Reactions
1. hyperglycemia
2. glycosuria
3. hyperuricemia
4. muscle spasm
5. weakness
6. restlessness
7. urinary bladder spasm
8. thrombophlebitis
9. fever

Whenever adverse reactions are moderate or severe, furosemide dosage should be reduced or therapy withdrawn.

OVERDOSAGE

The principal signs and symptoms of overdosage with furosemide are dehydration, blood volume reduction, hypotension, electrolyte imbalance, hypokalemia and hypochloremic alkalosis, and are extensions of its diuretic action.

The acute toxicity of furosemide has been determined in mice, rats and dogs. In all three, the oral LD_{50} exceeded 1000 mg/kg body weight, while the intravenous LD_{50} ranged from 300 to 680 mg/kg. The acute intragastric toxicity in neonatal rats is 7 to 10 times that of adult rats.

The concentration of furosemide in biological fluids associated with toxicity or death is not known.

Treatment of overdosage is supportive and consists of replacement of excessive fluid and electrolyte losses. Serum electrolytes, carbon dioxide level and blood pressure should be determined frequently. Adequate drainage must be assured in patients with urinary bladder outlet obstruction (such as prostatic hypertrophy).

Hemodialysis does not accelerate furosemide elimination.

DOSAGE AND ADMINISTRATION

Edema: Therapy should be individualized according to patient response to gain maximal therapeutic response and to determine the minimal dose needed to maintain that response.

Adults: The usual initial dose of furosemide is 20 mg to 80 mg given as a single dose. Ordinarily a prompt diuresis ensues. If needed, the same dose can be administered 6 to 8 hours later or the dose may be increased. The dose may be raised by 20 mg or 40 mg and given not sooner than 6 to 8 hours after the previous dose until the desired diuretic effect has been obtained. The individually determined single dose should then be given once or twice daily (e.g., at 8 am and 2 pm). The dose of furosemide may be carefully titrated up to 600 mg/day in patients with clinically severe edematous states.

Edema may be most efficiently and safely mobilized by giving furosemide on 2 to 4 consecutive days each week.

When doses exceeding 80 mg/day are given for prolonged periods, careful clinical observation and laboratory monitoring are particularly advisable. (See PRECAUTIONS: Laboratory Tests.)

Geriatric Patients: In general, dose selection for the elderly patient should be cautious, usually starting at the low end of the dosing range (see PRECAUTIONS: Geriatric Use).

Pediatric Patients: The usual initial dose of oral furosemide in pediatric patients is 2 mg/kg body weight, given as a single dose. If the diuretic response is not satisfactory after the initial dose, dosage may be increased by 1 or 2 mg/kg no sooner than 6 to 8 hours after the previous dose. Doses greater than 6 mg/kg body weight are not recommended. For maintenance therapy in pediatric patients, the dose should be adjusted to the minimum effective level.

Hypertension: Therapy should be individualized according to the patient's response to gain maximal therapeutic response and to determine the minimal dose needed to maintain the therapeutic response.

Adults: The usual initial dose of furosemide for hypertension is 80 mg, usually divided into 40 mg twice a day. Dosage should then be adjusted according to response. If response is not satisfactory, add other antihypertensive agents.

Changes in blood pressure must be carefully monitored when furosemide is used with other antihypertensive drugs, especially during initial therapy. To prevent excessive drop in blood pressure, the dosage of other agents should be reduced by at least 50 percent when furosemide is added to the regimen. As the blood pressure falls under the potentiating effect of furosemide, a further reduction in dosage or even discontinuation of other antihypertensive drugs may be necessary.

Geriatric Patients: In general, dose selection and dose adjustment for the elderly patient should be cautious, usually starting at the low end of the dosing range (see PRECAUTIONS: Geriatric Use).

HOW SUPPLIED

Furosemide Tablets, USP are available as tablets for oral administration. Each tablet for oral administration contains 20 mg, 40 mg or 80 mg of furosemide, USP.

The 20 mg tablets are white, round, unscored tablets debossed with **M2**. They are available as follows:

NDC 0378-0208-93
bottles of 30 tablets
NDC 0378-0208-01
bottles of 100 tablets
NDC 0378-0208-10
bottles of 1000 tablets

The 40 mg tablets are white, round, scored tablets debossed with **MYLAN** over **216** on one side of the tablet and **40** on the other side. They are available as follows:
NDC 0378-0216-93
bottles of 30 tablets
NDC 0378-0216-01
bottles of 100 tablets
NDC 0378-0216-10
bottles of 1000 tablets
The 80 mg tablets are white, round, scored tablets debossed with **MYLAN** over **232** on one side of the tablet and **80** on the other side. They are available as follows:
NDC 0378-0232-93
bottles of 30 tablets
NDC 0378-0232-01
bottles of 100 tablets
NDC 0378-0232-05
bottles of 500 tablets
Store at 20° to 25°C (68° to 77°F). [See USP for Controlled Room Temperature.]
Protect from light.
Dispense in a tight, light-resistant container as defined in the USP using a child-resistant closure. Exposure to light may cause slight discoloration. Discolored tablets should not be dispensed.
Mylan Pharmaceuticals Inc.
Morgantown, WV 26505

REVISED JULY 2008
FUR:R26

INDAPAMIDE TABLETS, USP ℞

1.25 mg and 2.5 mg
℞ only

DESCRIPTION

Indapamide is an oral antihypertensive/diuretic. Its molecule contains both a polar sulfamoyl chlorobenzamide moiety and a lipid-soluble methylindoline moiety. It differs chemically from the thiazides in that it does not possess the thiazide ring system and contains only one sulfonamide group. The chemical name of indapamide is 4-Chloro-N-(2-methyl-1-indolinyl)-3-Sulfamoylbenzamide, and its molecular weight is 365.84. The compound is a weak acid, pK_a=8.8, and is soluble in aqueous solutions of strong bases. It is a white to yellow-white crystalline (tetragonal) powder.

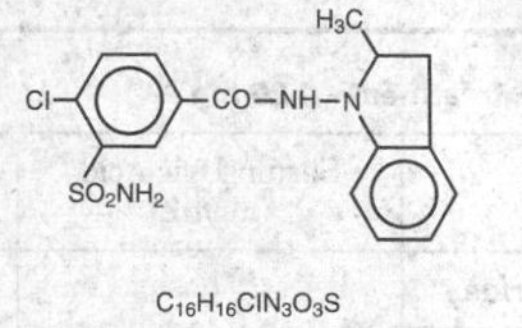

$C_{16}H_{16}ClN_3O_3S$

Each tablet, for oral administration, contains 1.25 mg or 2.5 mg of indapamide, USP and the following inactive ingredients: anhydrous lactose, colloidal silicon dioxide, hypromellose, magnesium stearate, microcrystalline cellulose, polydextrose, polyethylene glycol, pregelatinized starch, sodium lauryl sulfate, and titanium dioxide. Additionally, the 1.25 mg product contains glyceryl triacetate and D&C Red No. 30 Aluminum Lake and the 2.5 mg product contains triacetin.

CLINICAL PHARMACOLOGY

Indapamide is the first of a new class of antihypertensive/diuretics, the indolines. The oral administration of 2.5 mg (two 1.25 mg tablets) of indapamide to male subjects produced peak concentrations of approximately 115 ng/mL of the drug in the blood within 2 hours. The oral administration of 5 mg (two 2.5 mg tablets) of indapamide to healthy male subjects produced peak concentrations of approximately 260 ng/mL of the drug in the blood within 2 hours. A minimum of 70% of a single oral dose is eliminated by the kidneys and an additional 23% by the gastrointestinal tract, probably including the biliary route. The half-life of indapamide in whole blood is approximately 14 hours.
Indapamide is preferentially and reversibly taken up by the erythrocytes in the peripheral blood. The whole blood/plasma ratio is approximately 6:1 at the time of peak concentration and decreases to 3.5:1 at 8 hours. From 71% to 79% of the indapamide in plasma is reversibly bound to plasma proteins.
Indapamide is an extensively metabolized drug, with only *about 7% of the total* dose administered, recovered in the urine as unchanged drug during the first 48 hours after administration. The urinary elimination of ^{14}C-labeled indapamide and metabolites is biphasic with a terminal half-life of excretion of total radioactivity of 26 hours.
In a parallel design double-blind, placebo controlled trial in hypertension, daily doses of indapamide between 1.25 mg and 10 mg produced dose related antihypertensive effects. Doses of 5 mg and 10 mg were not distinguishable from each other although each was differentiated from placebo and 1.25 mg indapamide. At daily doses of 1.25 mg, 5 mg and 10 mg, a mean decrease of serum potassium of 0.28, 0.61 and 0.76 mEq/L, respectively, was observed and uric acid increased by about 0.69 mg/100 mL.
In other parallel design, dose-ranging clinical trials in hypertension and edema, daily doses of indapamide between 0.5 mg and 5 mg produced dose related effects. Generally, doses of 2.5 mg and 5 mg were not distinguishable from each other although each was differentiated from placebo and from 0.5 mg or 1 mg indapamide. At daily doses of 2.5 mg and 5 mg a mean decrease of serum potassium of 0.5 and 0.6 mEq/Liter, respectively, was observed and uric acid increased by about 1 mg/100 mL.
At these doses, the effects of indapamide on blood pressure and edema are approximately equal to those obtained with conventional doses of other antihypertensive/diuretics.
In hypertensive patients, daily doses of 1.25 mg, 2.5 mg and 5 mg of indapamide have no appreciable cardiac inotropic or chronotropic effect. The drug decreases peripheral resistance, with little or no effect on cardiac output, rate or rhythm. Chronic administration of indapamide to hypertensive patients has little or no effect on glomerular filtration rate or renal plasma flow.
Indapamide had an antihypertensive effect in patients with varying degrees of renal impairment, although in general, diuretic effects declined as renal function decreased.
In a small number of controlled studies, indapamide taken with other antihypertensive drugs such as hydralazine, propranolol, guanethidine and methyldopa, appeared to have the additive effect typical of thiazide-type diuretics.

INDICATIONS AND USAGE

Indapamide tablets are indicated for the treatment of hypertension, alone or in combination with other antihypertensive drugs.
Indapamide tablets are also indicated for the treatment of salt and fluid retention associated with congestive heart failure.
Usage in Pregnancy: The routine use of diuretics in an otherwise healthy woman is inappropriate and exposes mother and fetus to unnecessary hazard (see PRECAUTIONS below).
Diuretics do not prevent development of toxemia of pregnancy, and there is no satisfactory evidence that they are useful in the treatment of developed toxemia.
Edema during pregnancy may arise from pathological causes or from the physiologic and mechanical consequences of pregnancy. Indapamide is indicated in pregnancy when edema is due to pathologic causes, just as it is in the absence of pregnancy (however, see PRECAUTIONS below). Dependent edema in pregnancy, resulting from restriction of venous return by the expanded uterus, is properly treated through elevation of the lower extremities and use of support hose; use of diuretics to lower intravascular volume in this case is illogical and unnecessary. There is hypervolemia during normal pregnancy which is not harmful to either the fetus or the mother (in the absence of cardiovascular disease), but which is associated with edema, including generalized edema in the majority of pregnant women. If this edema produces discomfort, increased recumbency will often provide relief. In rare instances, this edema may cause extreme discomfort which is not relieved by rest. In these cases, a short course of diuretics may provide relief and may be appropriate.

CONTRAINDICATIONS

Anuria. Known hypersensitivity to indapamide or to other sulfonamide-derived drugs.

WARNINGS

Severe cases of hyponatremia, accompanied by hypokalemia have been reported with recommended doses of indapamide. This occurred primarily in elderly females. (See PRECAUTIONS: Geriatric Use.) This appears to be dose related. Also, a large case-controlled pharmacoepidemiology study indicates that there is an increased risk of hyponatremia with indapamide 2.5 mg and 5 mg doses. Hyponatremia considered possibly clinically significant (< 125 mEq/L) has not been observed in clinical trials with the 1.25 mg dosage (see PRECAUTIONS). Thus, patients should be started at the 1.25 mg dose and maintained at the lowest possible dose. (See DOSAGE AND ADMINISTRATION.)
Hypokalemia occurs commonly with diuretics (see ADVERSE REACTIONS: Hypokalemia), and electrolyte monitoring is essential, particularly in patients who would be at increased risk from hypokalemia, such as those with cardiac arrhythmias or who are receiving concomitant cardiac glycosides.
In general, diuretics should not be given concomitantly with lithium because they reduce its renal clearance and add a high risk of lithium toxicity. Read prescribing information for lithium preparations before use of such concomitant therapy.

PRECAUTIONS

General: ***Hypokalemia, Hyponatremia, and Other Fluid and Electrolyte Imbalances:*** Periodic determinations of serum electrolytes should be performed at appropriate intervals. In addition, patients should be observed for clinical signs of fluid or electrolyte imbalance, such as hyponatremia, hypochloremic alkalosis, or hypokalemia. Warning signs include dry mouth, thirst, weakness, fatigue, lethargy, drowsiness, restlessness, muscle pains or cramps, hypotension, oliguria, tachycardia, and gastrointestinal disturbance. Electrolyte determinations are particularly important in patients who are vomiting excessively or receiving parenteral fluids, in patients subject to electrolyte imbalance (including those with heart failure, kidney disease, and cirrhosis), and in patients on a salt-restricted diet.
The risk of hypokalemia secondary to diuresis and natriuresis is increased when larger doses are used, when the diuresis is brisk, when severe cirrhosis is present and during concomitant use of corticosteroids or ACTH. Interference with adequate oral intake of electrolytes will also contribute to hypokalemia. Hypokalemia can sensitize or exaggerate the response of the heart to the toxic effects of digitalis, such as increased ventricular irritability.
Dilutional hyponatremia may occur in edematous patients; the appropriate treatment is restriction of water rather than administration of salt, except in rare instances when the hyponatremia is life threatening. However, in actual salt depletion, appropriate replacement is the treatment of choice. Any chloride deficit that may occur during treatment is generally mild and usually does not require specific treatment except in extraordinary circumstances as in liver or renal disease. Thiazide-like diuretics have been shown to increase the urinary excretion of magnesium; this may result in hypomagnesemia.
Hyperuricemia and Gout: Serum concentrations of uric acid increased by an average of 0.69 mg/100 mL in patients treated with indapamide 1.25 mg, and by an average of 1 mg/100 mL in patients treated with indapamide 2.5 mg and 5 mg, and frank gout may be precipitated in certain patients receiving indapamide (see ADVERSE REACTIONS below). Serum concentrations of uric acid should, therefore, be monitored periodically during treatment.
Renal Impairment: Indapamide, like the thiazides, should be used with caution in patients with severe renal disease, as reduced plasma volume may exacerbate or precipitate azotemia. If progressive renal impairment is observed in a patient receiving indapamide, withholding or discontinuing diuretic therapy should be considered. Renal function tests should be performed periodically during treatment with indapamide.
Impaired Hepatic Function: Indapamide, like the thiazides, should be used with caution in patients with impaired hepatic function or progressive liver disease, since minor alterations of fluid and electrolyte balance may precipitate hepatic coma.
Glucose Tolerance: Latent diabetes may become manifest and insulin requirements in diabetic patients may be altered during thiazide administration. A mean increase in glucose of 6.47 mg/dL was observed in patients treated with indapamide 1.25 mg, which was not considered clinically significant in these trials. Serum concentrations of glucose should be monitored routinely during treatment with indapamide.
Calcium Excretion: Calcium excretion is decreased by diuretics pharmacologically related to indapamide. After 6 to 8 weeks of indapamide 1.25 mg treatment and in long-term studies of hypertensive patients with higher doses of indapamide, however, serum concentrations of calcium increased only slightly with indapamide. Prolonged treatment with drugs pharmacologically related to indapamide may in rare instances be associated with hypercalcemia and hypophosphatemia secondary to physiologic changes in the parathyroid gland; however, the common complications of hyperparathyroidism, such as renal lithiasis, bone resorption, and peptic ulcer, have not been seen. Treatment should be discontinued before tests for parathyroid function are performed. Like the thiazides, indapamide may decrease serum PBI levels without signs of thyroid disturbance.
Interaction with Systemic Lupus Erythematosus: Thiazides have exacerbated or activated systemic lupus erythematosus and this possibility should be considered with indapamide as well.
Drug Interactions:
Other Antihypertensives: Indapamide may add to or potentiate the action of other antihypertensive drugs. In limited controlled trials that compared the effect of indapamide combined with other antihypertensive drugs with the effect of the other drugs administered alone, there was no notable change in the nature or frequency of adverse reactions associated with the combined therapy.
Lithium: See WARNINGS.
Post-Sympathectomy Patient: The antihypertensive effect of the drug may be enhanced in the post-sympathectomized patient.

Norepinephrine: Indapamide, like the thiazides, may decrease arterial responsiveness to norepinephrine, but this diminution is not sufficient to preclude effectiveness of the pressor agent for therapeutic use.

Carcinogenesis, Mutagenesis, Impairment of Fertility: Both mouse and rat lifetime carcinogenicity studies were conducted. There was no significant difference in the incidence of tumors between the indapamide-treated animals and the control groups.

Pregnancy: *Teratogenic Effects. Pregnancy Category B:* Reproduction studies have been performed in rats, mice and rabbits at doses up to 6,250 times the therapeutic human dose and have revealed no evidence of impaired fertility or harm to the fetus due to indapamide. Postnatal development in rats and mice was unaffected by pretreatment of parent animals during gestation. There are, however, no adequate and well controlled studies in pregnant women. Moreover, diuretics are known to cross the placental barrier and appear in cord blood. Because animal reproduction studies are not always predictive of human response, this drug should be used during pregnancy only if clearly needed. There may be hazards associated with this use such as fetal or neonatal jaundice, thrombocytopenia, and possibly other adverse reactions that have occurred in the adult.

Nursing Mothers: It is not known whether this drug is excreted in human milk. Because most drugs are excreted in human milk, if use of this drug is deemed essential, the patient should stop nursing.

Pediatric Use: Safety and effectiveness of indapamide in pediatric patients have not been established.

Geriatric Use: Clinical studies of indapamide did not include sufficient numbers of subjects aged 65 and over to determine whether they respond differently from younger subjects. Other reported clinical experience has not identified differences in responses between the elderly and younger patients. In general, dose selection for an elderly patient should be cautious, usually starting at the low end of the dosing range, reflecting the greater frequency of decreased hepatic, renal, or cardiac function, and of concomitant disease or other drug therapy.

Severe cases of hyponatremia, accompanied by hypokalemia have been reported with recommended doses of indapamide in elderly females (see WARNINGS).

ADVERSE REACTIONS

Most adverse effects have been mild and transient.

The clinical adverse reactions listed in Table 1 represent data from Phase II/III placebo-controlled studies (306 patients given indapamide 1.25 mg). The clinical adverse reactions listed in Table 2 represent data from Phase II placebo-controlled studies and long-term controlled clinical trials (426 patients given indapamide 2.5 mg or 5 mg). The reactions are arranged into two groups: 1) a cumulative incidence equal to or greater than 5%; 2) a cumulative incidence less than 5%. Reactions are counted regardless of relation to drug.

TABLE 1: Adverse Reactions from Studies of 1.25 mg

Incidence ≥ 5%	Incidence < 5%*
BODY AS A WHOLE	
Headache	Asthenia
Infection	Flu Syndrome
Pain	Abdominal Pain
Back Pain	Chest Pain
GASTROINTESTINAL SYSTEM	
	Constipation
	Diarrhea
	Dyspepsia
	Nausea
METABOLIC SYSTEM	
	Peripheral Edema
CENTRAL NERVOUS SYSTEM	
Dizziness	Nervousness
	Hypertonia
RESPIRATORY SYSTEM	
Rhinitis	Cough
	Pharyngitis
	Sinusitis
SPECIAL SENSES	
	Conjunctivitis

*OTHER
All other clinical adverse reactions occurred at an incidence of < 1%.

Approximately 4% of patients given indapamide 1.25 mg compared to 5% of the patients given placebo discontinued treatment in the trials of up to 8 weeks because of adverse reactions.

In controlled clinical trials of 6 to 8 weeks in duration, 20% of patients receiving indapamide 1.25 mg, 61% of patients receiving indapamide 5 mg, and 80% of patients receiving indapamide 10 mg had at least one potassium value below 3.4 mEq/L. In the indapamide 1.25 mg group, about 40% of

TABLE 2: Adverse Reactions from Studies of 2.5 mg and 5 mg

Incidence ≥ 5%	Incidence < 5%
CENTRAL NERVOUS SYSTEM/NEUROMUSCULAR	
Headache	Lightheadedness
Dizziness	Drowsiness
Fatigue, weakness, loss of energy, lethargy, tiredness, or malaise	Vertigo
Muscle cramps or spasm, or numbness of the extremities	Insomnia
Nervousness, tension, anxiety, irritability, or agitation	Depression
	Blurred vision
GASTROINTESTINAL SYSTEM	
	Constipation
	Nausea
	Vomiting
	Diarrhea
	Gastric irritation
	Abdominal pain or cramps
	Anorexia
CARDIOVASCULAR SYSTEM	
	Orthostatic hypotension
	Premature ventricular contractions
	Irregular heart beat
	Palpitations
GENITOURINARY SYSTEM	
	Frequency of urination
	Nocturia
	Polyuria
DERMATOLOGIC/HYPERSENSITIVITY	
	Rash
	Hives
	Pruritus
	Vasculitis
OTHER	
	Impotence or reduced libido
	Rhinorrhea
	Flushing
	Hyperuricemia
	Hyperglycemia
	Hyponatremia
	Hypochloremia
	Increase in serum urea nitrogen (BUN) or creatinine
	Glycosuria
	Weight loss
	Dry mouth
	Tingling of extremities

Mean Changes From Baseline After 8 Weeks Of Treatment - 1.25 mg

	Serum Electrolytes (mEq/L)			Serum Uric Acid (mg/dL)	BUN (mg/dL)
	Potassium	Sodium	Chloride		
Indapamide 1.25 mg (n = 255 to 257)	-0.28	-0.63	-2.60	0.69	1.46
Placebo (n = 263 to 266)	0.00	-0.11	-0.21	0.06	0.06

Mean Changes From Baseline After 40 Weeks Of Treatment - 2.5 mg and 5 mg

	Serum Electrolytes (mEq/L)			Serum Uric Acid (mg/dL)	BUN (mg/dL)
	Potassium	Sodium	Chloride		
Indapamide 2.5 mg (n = 76)	-0.4	-0.6	-3.6	0.7	-0.1
Indapamide 5 mg (n = 81)	-0.6	-0.7	-5.1	1.1	1.4

those patients who reported hypokalemia as a laboratory adverse event returned to normal serum potassium values without intervention. Hypokalemia with concomitant clinical signs or symptoms occurred in 2% of patients receiving indapamide 1.25 mg.
[See table 2 above]
Because most of these data are from long-term studies (up to 40 weeks of treatment), it is probable that many of the adverse experiences reported are due to causes other than the drug. Approximately 10% of patients given indapamide discontinued treatment in long-term trials because of reactions either related or unrelated to the drug.
Hypokalemia with concomitant clinical signs or symptoms occurred in 3% of patients receiving indapamide 2.5 mg q.d. and 7% of patients receiving indapamide 5 mg q.d. In long-term controlled clinical trials comparing the hypokalemic

effects of daily doses of indapamide and hydrochlorothiazide, however, 47% of patients receiving indapamide 2.5 mg, 72% of patients receiving indapamide 5 mg, and 44% of patients receiving hydrochlorothiazide 50 mg had at least one potassium value (out of a total of 11 taken during the study) below 3.5 mEq/L. In the indapamide 2.5 mg group, over 50% of those patients returned to normal serum potassium values without intervention.
In clinical trials of 6 to 8 weeks, the mean changes in selected values were as shown in the tables below.
[See second table above]
No patients receiving indapamide 1.25 mg experienced hyponatremia considered possibly clinically significant (< 125 mEq/L).
Indapamide had no adverse effects on lipids.
[See third table above]

The following reactions have been reported with clinical usage of indapamide: jaundice (intrahepatic cholestatic jaundice), hepatitis, pancreatitis and abnormal liver function tests. These reactions were reversible with discontinuance of the drug.

Also reported are erythema multiforme, Stevens-Johnson Syndrome, bullous eruptions, purpura, photosensitivity, fever, pneumonitis, anaphylactic reactions, agranulocytosis, leukopenia, thrombocytopenia and aplastic anemia. Other adverse reactions reported with antihypertensive/diuretics are necrotizing angiitis, respiratory distress, sialadenitis, xanthopsia.

OVERDOSAGE

Symptoms of overdosage include nausea, vomiting, weakness, gastrointestinal disorders and disturbances of electrolyte balance. In severe instances, hypotension and depressed respiration may be observed. If this occurs, support of respiration and cardiac circulation should be instituted. There is no specific antidote. An evacuation of the stomach is recommended by emesis and gastric lavage after which the electrolyte and fluid balance should be evaluated carefully.

DOSAGE AND ADMINISTRATION

Hypertension: The adult starting indapamide dose for hypertension is 1.25 mg as a single daily dose taken in the morning. If the response to 1.25 mg is not satisfactory after 4 weeks, the daily dose may be increased to 2.5 mg taken once daily. If the response to 2.5 mg is not satisfactory after 4 weeks, the daily dose may be increased to 5 mg taken once daily, but adding another antihypertensive should be considered.

Edema of Congestive Heart Failure: The adult starting indapamide dose for edema of congestive heart failure is 2.5 mg as a single daily dose taken in the morning. If the response to 2.5 mg is not satisfactory after one week, the daily dose may be increased to 5 mg taken once daily.

If the antihypertensive response to indapamide is insufficient, indapamide may be combined with other antihypertensive drugs, with careful monitoring of blood pressure. It is recommended that the usual dose of other agents be reduced by 50% during initial combination therapy. As the blood pressure response becomes evident, further dosage adjustments may be necessary.

In general, doses of 5 mg and larger have not appeared to provide additional effects on blood pressure or heart failure, but are associated with a greater degree of hypokalemia. There is minimal clinical trial experience in patients with doses greater than 5 mg once a day.

HOW SUPPLIED

Indapamide Tablets, USP are available containing 1.25 mg or 2.5 mg of indapamide, USP.

The 1.25 mg tablets are pink film-coated, unscored, round tablets debossed with **M** on one side of the tablet and **69** on the other side. They are available as follows:

NDC 0378-0069-01
bottles of 100 tablets
NDC 0378-0069-05
bottles of 500 tablets

The 2.5 mg tablets are white film-coated, unscored, round tablets debossed with **M** on one side of the tablet and **80** on the other side. They are available as follows:

NDC 0378-0080-77
bottles of 90 tablets
NDC 0378-0080-01
bottles of 100 tablets
NDC 0378-0080-10
bottles of 1000 tablets

Store at 20° to 25°C (68° to 77°F). [See USP Controlled Room Temperature.]
Avoid excessive heat.

Dispense in a tight, light-resistant container as defined in the USP using a child-resistant closure.

Mylan Pharmaceuticals Inc.
Morgantown, WV 26505

REVISED JANUARY 2010
INDAP:R6

MENTAX®

[mĕn-tax]
(butenafine HCl)
Cream, 1%
Rx Only

DESCRIPTION

Mentax® Cream, 1%, contains the synthetic antifungal agent, butenafine hydrochloride. Butenafine is a member of the class of antifungal compounds known as benzylamines which are structurally related to the allylamines.

Butenafine HCl is designated chemically as N-4-tert-butylbenzyl-N-methyl-1-naphthalenemethylamine hydrochloride. The compound has the molecular formula

$C_{23}H_{27}N \cdot HCl$, a molecular weight of 353.93, and the following structural formula:

Butenafine HCl is a white, odorless, crystalline powder. It is freely soluble in methanol, ethanol, and chloroform, and slightly soluble in water. Each gram of Mentax® Cream, 1%, contains 10 mg of butenafine HCl in a white cream base of purified water USP, propylene glycol dicaprylate, glycerin USP, cetyl alcohol NF, glyceryl monostearate SE, white petrolatum USP, stearic acid NF, polyoxyethylene (23) cetyl ether, benzyl alcohol NF, diethanolamine NF, and sodium benzoate NF.

CLINICAL PHARMACOLOGY
Pharmacokinetics

In one study conducted in healthy subjects for 14 days, 6 grams of Mentax® Cream, 1%, was applied once daily to the dorsal skin (3,000 cm²) of 7 subjects, and 20 grams of the cream was applied once daily to the arms, trunk and groin areas (10,000 cm²) of another 12 subjects. After 14 days of topical applications, the 6-gram dose group yielded a mean peak plasma butenafine HCl concentration, Cmax of 1.4 ± 0.8 ng/mL, occurring at a mean time to the peak plasma concentration, Tmax, of 15 ± 8 hours, and a mean area under the plasma concentration-time curve, $AUC_{0-24 \text{ hrs}}$ of 23.9 ± 11.3 ng-hr/mL. For the 20-gram dose group, the mean Cmax was 5.0 ± 2.0 ng/mL, occurring at a mean Tmax of 6 ± 6 hours, and the mean $AUC_{0-24 \text{ hrs}}$ was 87.8 ± 45.3 ng-hr/mL. A biphasic decline of plasma butenafine HCl concentrations was observed with the half-lives estimated to be 35 hours and > 150 hours, respectively. At 72 hours after the last dose application, the mean plasma concentrations decreased to 0.3 ± 0.2 ng/mL for the 6-gram dose group and 1.1 ± 0.9 ng/mL for the 20-gram dose group. Low levels of butenafine HCl remained in the plasma 7 days after the last dose application (mean: 0.1 ± 0.2 ng/mL for the 6-gram dose group, and 0.7 ± 0.5 ng/mL for the 20-gram dose group). The total amount (or % dose) of butenafine HCl absorbed through the skin into the systemic circulation has not been quantitated. It was determined that the primary metabolite in urine was formed through hydroxylation at the terminal *t*-butyl side-chain.

In 11 patients with tinea pedis, butenafine HCl cream, 1%, was applied by the patients to cover the affected and immediately surrounding skin area once daily for 4 weeks, and a single blood sample was collected between 10 and 20 hours following single dosing at 1, 2 and 4 weeks after treatment. The plasma butenafine HCl concentration ranged from undetectable to 0.3 ng/mL.

In 24 patients with tinea cruris, butenafine HCl cream, 1%, was applied by the patients to cover the affected and immediately surrounding skin area once daily for 2 weeks (mean average daily dose: 1.3 ± 0.2 g). A single blood sample was collected between 0.5 and 65 hours after the last dose, and the plasma butenafine HCl concentration ranged from undetectable to 2.52 ng/mL (mean ± SD: 0.91 ± 0.15 ng/mL). Four weeks after cessation of treatment, the plasma butenafine HCl concentration ranged from undetectable to 0.28 ng/mL.

Microbiology

Butenafine HCl is a benzylamine derivative with a mode of action similar to that of the allylamine class of antifungal drugs. Butenafine HCl is hypothesized to act by inhibiting the epoxidation of squalene, thus blocking the biosynthesis of ergosterol, an essential component of fungal cell membranes. The benzylamine derivatives, like the allylamines, act at an earlier step in the ergosterol biosynthesis pathway than the azole class of antifungal drugs. Depending on the concentration of the drug and the fungal species tested, butenafine HCl may be fungicidal or fungistatic *in vitro*. However, the clinical significance of these *in vitro* data are unknown.

Butenafine HCl has been shown to be active against most strains of the following microorganisms, both *in vitro* and in clinical infections as described in the INDICATIONS AND USAGE section:

Epidermophyton floccosum   *Trichophyton rubrum*
Malassezia furfur   *Trichophyton tonsurans*
Trichophyton mentagrophytes

CLINICAL STUDIES
Tinea (pityriasis) versicolor

In the following data presentations, patients with tinea (pityriasis) versicolor were studied. The term **"Negative Mycology"** is defined as absence of hyphae in a KOH preparation of skin scrapings, i.e., no fungal forms seen or the presence of yeast cells (blastospores) only. The term **"Effective Treatment"** is defined as Negative Mycology plus total signs and symptoms score (on a scale from zero to three) for erythema, scaling, and pruritus equal to or less than 1 at Week 8. The term **"Complete Cure"** refers to patients who had Negative Mycology plus sign/symptoms score of zero for erythema, scaling, and pruritus.

Two separate studies compared Mentax® Cream to vehicle applied once daily for 2 weeks in the treatment of tinea (pityriasis) versicolor. Patients were treated for 2 weeks and were evaluated at the following weeks post-treatment: 2 (Week 4) and 6 (Week 8). All subjects with a positive baseline KOH and who were dispensed medications were included in the "intent-to-treat" analysis shown in the table below. Statistical significance (Mentax® vs. vehicle) was achieved for Effective Treatment, but not Complete Cure at 6 weeks post-treatment in Study 31. Marginal statistical significance (p = 0.051) (Mentax® vs. vehicle) was achieved for Effective Treatment, but not Complete Cure at 6 weeks post-treatment in Study 32. Data from these two controlled studies are presented in the table below.
[See table above]

Tinea (pityriasis) versicolor is a superficial, chronically recurring infection of the glabrous skin caused by *Malassezia furfur* (formerly *Pityrosporum orbiculare*). The commensal organism is part of the normal skin flora. In susceptible individuals, the condition may give rise to hyperpigmented or hypopigmented patches on the trunk which may extend to the neck, arms, and upper thighs.

Treatment of the infection may not immediately result in restoration of pigment of the affected sites. Normalization of pigment following successful therapy is variable and may take months, depending upon individual skin type and incidental sun exposure. The rate of recurrence of infection is variable.

INDICATIONS AND USAGE

Mentax® (butenafine HCl) Cream, 1% is indicated for the topical treatment of the dermatologic infection, tinea (pityriasis) versicolor due to *M. furfur* (formerly *P. orbiculare*).

Patient Response Category	Week @	Study 31		Study 32	
		Butenafine	Vehicle	Butenafine	Vehicle
Complete Cure*	2	41/87 (47%)	11/40 (28%)	29/85 (34%)	12/41 (29%)
	4	43/86 (50%)	15/42 (36%)	36/83 (43%)	13/41 (32%)
	8	44/87 (51%)	15/42 (36%)	30/86 (35%)	10/43 (23%)
Effective Treatment**	2	56/87 (64%)	16/40 (40%)	46/85 (54%)	16/41 (39%)
	4	50/86 (58%)	19/42 (45%)	45/83 (54%)	16/41 (39%)
	8	48/87 (55%)	15/42 (36%)	37/86 (43%)	11/43 (26%)
Negative Mycology***	2	57/87 (66%)	20/40 (50%)	57/85 (67%)	21/41 (51%)
	4	51/86 (59%)	20/42 (48%)	52/83 (63%)	18/41 (44%)
	8	48/87 (55%)	15/42 (36%)	43/86 (50%)	12/43 (28%)

Proportion (%) of responders in pivotal clinical trials (all randomized patients)

@Week 2 (end of treatment), Week 4 (2 weeks post-treatment), and Week 8 (6 weeks post-treatment)
*Negative Mycology plus absence of erythema, scaling, and pruritus
**Negative Mycology plus no or minimal involvement of erythema, scaling or pruritus
***Absence of hyphae in a KOH preparation of skin scrapings, i.e., no fungal forms seen or the presence of yeast cells (blastospores) only.

Butenafine HCl cream was not studied in immunocompromised patients. (See DOSAGE AND ADMINISTRATION.)

CONTRAINDICATIONS

Mentax® (butenafine HCl) Cream, 1%, is contraindicated in individuals who have known or suspected sensitivity to Mentax® Cream, 1%, or any of its components.

WARNINGS

Mentax® (butenafine HCl) Cream, 1%, is not for ophthalmic, oral, or intravaginal use.

PRECAUTIONS

General

Mentax® Cream, 1%, is for external use only. If irritation or sensitivity develops with the use of Mentax® Cream, 1%, treatment should be discontinued and appropriate therapy instituted. Diagnosis of the disease should be confirmed either by culture on an appropriate medium, [except *M. furfur* (formerly *P. orbiculare*)] or by direct microscopic examination of infected superficial epidermal tissue in a solution of potassium hydroxide.

Patients who are known to be sensitive to allylamine antifungals should use Mentax® (butenafine HCl) Cream, 1%, with caution since cross-reactivity may occur.

Use Mentax® Cream, 1%, as directed by the physician, and avoid contact with the eyes, nose, mouth, and other mucous membranes.

Information for Patients

The patient should be instructed to:

1. Use Mentax® Cream, 1%, as directed by the physician. The hands should be washed after applying the medication to the affected area(s). Avoid contact with the eyes, nose, mouth, and other mucous membranes. Mentax® Cream, 1%, is for external use only.
2. Dry the affected area(s) thoroughly before application, if you wish to apply Mentax® Cream, 1%, after bathing.
3. Use the medication for the full treatment time recommended by the physician, even though symptoms may have improved.
   Notify the physician if there is no improvement after the end of the prescribed treatment period, or sooner, if the condition worsens (see below).
4. Inform the physician if the area of application shows signs of increased irritation, redness, itching, burning, blistering, swelling, or oozing.
5. Avoid the use of occlusive dressings unless otherwise directed by the physician.
6. Do not use this medication for any disorder other than that for which it was prescribed.

Drug Interactions

Potential drug interactions between Mentax® (butenafine HCl) Cream, 1%, and other drugs have not been systematically evaluated.

Carcinogenesis, Mutagenesis, Impairment of Fertility

Long-term studies to evaluate the carcinogenic potential of Mentax® Cream, 1%, have not been conducted. Two *in vitro* assays (bacterial reverse mutation test and chromosome aberration test in Chinese hamster lymphocytes) and one *in vivo* study (rat micronucleus bioassay) revealed no mutagenic or clastogenic potential for butenafine.

In subcutaneous fertility studies conducted in rats at dose levels up to 25 mg/kg/day (0.5 times the maximum recommended dose in humans for tinea versicolor based on body surface area comparisons), butenafine did not produce any adverse effects on male or female fertility.

Pregnancy

Teratogenic Effects: Pregnancy Category C

Subcutaneous doses of butenafine (dose levels up to 25 mg/kg/day administered during organogenesis) (equivalent to 0.5 times the maximum recommended dose in humans for tinea versicolor based on body surface area comparisons) were not teratogenic in rats. In an oral embryofetal development study in rabbits (dose levels up to 400 mg butenafine HCl/kg/day administered during organogenesis) (equivalent to 16 times the maximum recommended dose in humans for tinea versicolor based on body surface area comparisons), no treatment-related external, visceral, skeletal malformations or variations were observed.

In an oral peri- and post-natal developmental study in rats (dose levels up to 125 mg butenafine HCl/kg/day) (equivalent to 2.5 times the maximum recommended dose in humans for tinea versicolor based on body surface area comparisons), no treatment-related effects on postnatal survival, development of the F1 generation or their subsequent maturation and fertility were observed.

There are, however, no adequate and well-controlled studies that have been conducted with topically applied butenafine in pregnant women. Because animal reproduction studies are not always predictive of human response, this drug should be used during pregnancy only if clearly needed.

Nursing Mothers

It is not known if butenafine HCl is excreted in human milk. Because many drugs are excreted in human milk, caution should be exercised in prescribing Mentax® Cream, 1%, to a nursing woman.

Pediatric Use

Safety and efficacy in pediatric patients below the age of 12 years have not been studied since tinea versicolor is uncommon in patients below the age of 12 years.

ADVERSE REACTIONS

In controlled clinical trials, 9 (approximately 1%) of 815 patients treated with Mentax® Cream, 1%, reported adverse events related to the skin. These included burning/stinging, itching and worsening of the condition. No patient treated with Mentax® Cream, 1%, discontinued treatment due to an adverse event. In the vehicle-treated patients, 2 of 718 patients discontinued because of treatment site adverse events, one of which was severe burning/stinging and itching at the site of application.

In uncontrolled clinical trials, the most frequently reported adverse events in patients treated with Mentax® Cream, 1%, were: contact dermatitis, erythema, irritation, and itching, each occurring in less than 2% of patients.

In provocative testing in over 200 subjects, there was no evidence of allergic-contact sensitization for either cream or vehicle base for Mentax® Cream, 1%.

OVERDOSAGE

Overdosage of butenafine HCl in humans has not been reported to date.

DOSAGE AND ADMINISTRATION

Patients with tinea (pityriasis) versicolor should apply Mentax® Cream, 1%, once daily for two weeks. Sufficient Mentax® Cream should be applied to cover affected areas and immediately surrounding skin of patients with tinea versicolor. If a patient shows no clinical improvement after the treatment period, the diagnosis and therapy should be reviewed.

HOW SUPPLIED

Mentax® (butenafine HCl) Cream, 1%, is supplied in tubes in the following sizes:
15-gram tube (NDC 0378-6151-46)
30-gram tube (NDC 0378-6151-49)
STORE BETWEEN 5° and 30°C (41° and 86°F).
Mylan Pharmaceuticals Inc.
Morgantown, WV 26505

REVISED FEBRUARY 2009

Patent #: 5,021,458 029.6

NADOLOL TABLETS, USP ℞

20 mg, 40 mg and 80 mg
℞ only

DESCRIPTION

Nadolol is a synthetic nonselective beta-adrenergic receptor blocking agent designated chemically as 1-(*tert*-butylamino)-3-[(5,6,7,8-tetrahydro-*cis*-6,7-dihydroxy-1-naphthyl)oxy]-2-propanol. Its structural formula is:

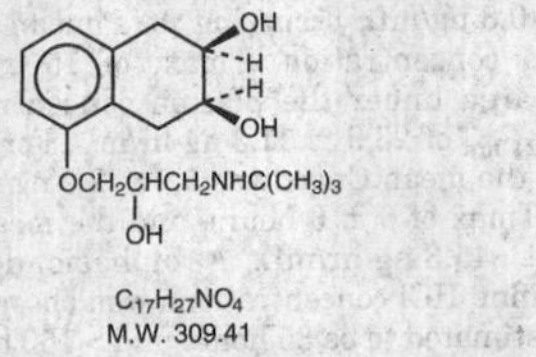

$C_{17}H_{27}NO_4$
M.W. 309.41

Nadolol is a white crystalline powder. It is freely soluble in ethanol, soluble in hydrochloric acid, slightly soluble in water and in chloroform, and very slightly soluble in sodium hydroxide.

Each tablet for oral administration contains 20 mg, 40 mg or 80 mg of nadolol, USP and the following inactive ingredients: croscarmellose sodium, lactose (anhydrous), magnesium stearate, microcrystalline cellulose, sodium lauryl sulfate, and D&C Yellow No. 10 aluminum lake.

CLINICAL PHARMACOLOGY

Nadolol is a nonselective beta-adrenergic receptor blocking agent. Clinical pharmacology studies have demonstrated beta-blocking activity by showing (1) reduction in heart rate and cardiac output at rest and on exercise, (2) reduction of systolic and diastolic blood pressure at rest and on exercise, (3) inhibition of isoproterenol-induced tachycardia, and (4) reduction of reflex orthostatic tachycardia.

Nadolol specifically competes with beta-adrenergic receptor agonists for available beta receptor sites; it inhibits both the $beta_1$ receptors located chiefly in cardiac muscle and the $beta_2$ receptors located chiefly in the bronchial and vascular musculature, inhibiting the chronotropic, inotropic, and vasodilator responses to beta-adrenergic stimulation proportionately. Nadolol has no intrinsic sympathomimetic activity and, unlike some other beta-adrenergic blocking agents, nadolol has little direct myocardial depressant activity and does not have an anesthetic-like membrane stabilizing action. Animal and human studies show that nadolol slows the sinus rate and depresses AV conduction. In dogs, only minimal amounts of nadolol were detected in the brain relative to amounts in blood and other organs and tissues. Nadolol has low lipophilicity as determined by octanol/water partition coefficient, a characteristic of certain beta-blocking agents that has been correlated with the limited extent to which these agents cross the blood-brain barrier, their low concentration in the brain, and low incidence of CNS-related side effects.

In controlled clinical studies, nadolol at doses of 40 to 320 mg/day has been shown to decrease both standing and supine blood pressure, the effect persisting for approximately 24 hours after dosing.

The mechanism of the antihypertensive effects of beta-adrenergic receptor blocking agents has not been established; however, factors that may be involved include (1) competitive antagonism of catecholamines at peripheral (non-CNS) adrenergic neuron sites (especially cardiac) leading to decreased cardiac output, (2) a central effect leading to reduced tonic-sympathetic nerve outflow to the periphery, and (3) suppression of renin secretion by blockade of the beta-adrenergic receptors responsible for renin release from the kidneys.

While cardiac output and arterial pressure are reduced by nadolol therapy, renal hemodynamics are stable, with preservation of renal blood flow and glomerular filtration rate.

By blocking catecholamine-induced increases in heart rate, velocity and extent of myocardial contraction, and blood pressure, nadolol generally reduces the oxygen requirements of the heart at any given level of effort, making it useful for many patients in the long-term management of angina pectoris. On the other hand, nadolol can increase oxygen requirements by increasing left ventricular fiber length and end diastolic pressure, particularly in patients with heart failure.

Although beta-adrenergic receptor blockade is useful in treatment of angina and hypertension, there are also situations in which sympathetic stimulation is vital. For example, in patients with severely damaged hearts, adequate ventricular function may depend on sympathetic drive. Beta-adrenergic blockade may worsen AV block by preventing the necessary facilitating effects of sympathetic activity on conduction. $Beta_2$-adrenergic blockade results in passive bronchial constriction by interfering with endogenous adrenergic bronchodilator activity in patients subject to bronchospasm and may also interfere with exogenous bronchodilators in such patients.

Absorption of nadolol after oral dosing is variable, averaging about 30%. Peak serum concentrations of nadolol usually occur in 3 to 4 hours after oral administration and the presence of food in the gastrointestinal tract does not affect the rate or extent of nadolol absorption. Approximately 30% of the nadolol present in serum is reversibly bound to plasma protein.

Unlike many other beta-adrenergic blocking agents, nadolol is not metabolized by the liver and is excreted unchanged, principally by the kidneys.

The half-life of therapeutic doses of nadolol is about 20 to 24 hours, permitting once daily dosage. Because nadolol is excreted predominantly in the urine, its half-life increases in renal failure (see PRECAUTIONS and DOSAGE AND ADMINISTRATION). Steady-state serum concentrations of nadolol are attained in 6 to 9 days with once daily dosage in persons with normal renal function. Because of variable absorption and different individual responsiveness, the proper dosage must be determined by titration.

Exacerbation of angina and, in some cases, myocardial infarction and ventricular dysrhythmias have been reported after abrupt discontinuation of therapy with beta-adrenergic blocking agents in patients with coronary artery disease. Abrupt withdrawal of these agents in patients without coronary artery disease has resulted in transient symptoms, including tremulousness, sweating, palpitation, headache, and malaise. Several mechanisms have been proposed to explain these phenomena, among them increased sensitivity to catecholamines because of increased numbers of beta receptors.

INDICATIONS AND USAGE

Angina Pectoris: Nadolol tablets are indicated for the long-term management of patients with angina pectoris.

Hypertension: Nadolol tablets are indicated in the management of hypertension; it may be used alone or in combination with other antihypertensive agents, especially thiazide-type diuretics.

CONTRAINDICATIONS

Nadolol tablets are contraindicated in bronchial asthma, sinus bradycardia and greater than first-degree conduction block, cardiogenic shock, and overt cardiac failure (see WARNINGS).

WARNINGS

Cardiac Failure: Sympathetic stimulation may be a vital component supporting circulatory function in patients with congestive heart failure, and its inhibition by beta-blockade may precipitate more severe failure. Although beta-blockers should be avoided in overt congestive heart failure, if necessary, they can be used with caution in patients with a history of failure who are well compensated, usually with digitalis and diuretics. Beta-adrenergic blocking agents do not abolish the inotropic action of digitalis on heart muscle. IN PATIENTS WITHOUT A HISTORY OF HEART FAILURE, continued use of beta-blockers can, in some cases, lead to cardiac failure. Therefore, at the first sign or symptom of heart failure, the patient should be digitalized and/or treated with diuretics, and the response observed closely, or nadolol should be discontinued (gradually, if possible).

Exacerbation of Ischemic Heart Disease Following Abrupt Withdrawal: Hypersensitivity to catecholamines has been observed in patients withdrawn from beta-blocker therapy; exacerbation of angina and, in some cases, myocardial infarction have occurred after *abrupt* discontinuation of such therapy. When discontinuing chronically administered nadolol, particularly in patients with ischemic heart disease, the dosage should be gradually reduced over a period of 1 to 2 weeks and the patient should be carefully monitored. If angina markedly worsens or acute coronary insufficiency develops, nadolol administration should be reinstituted promptly, at least temporarily, and other measures appropriate for the management of unstable angina should be taken. Patients should be warned against interruption or discontinuation of therapy without the physician's advice. Because coronary artery disease is common and may be unrecognized, it may be prudent not to discontinue nadolol therapy abruptly even in patients treated only for hypertension.

Nonallergic Bronchospasm (e.g., chronic bronchitis, emphysema): PATIENTS WITH BRONCHOSPASTIC DISEASES SHOULD IN GENERAL NOT RECEIVE BETA-BLOCKERS. Nadolol should be administered with caution since it may block bronchodilation produced by endogenous or exogenous catecholamine stimulation of beta$_2$ receptors.

Major Surgery: Because beta-blockade impairs the ability of the heart to respond to reflex stimuli and may increase the risks of general anesthesia and surgical procedures, resulting in protracted hypotension or low cardiac output, it has generally been suggested that such therapy should be withdrawn several days prior to surgery. Recognition of the increased sensitivity to catecholamines of patients recently withdrawn from beta-blocker therapy, however, has made this recommendation controversial. If possible, beta-blockers should be withdrawn well before surgery takes place. In the event of emergency surgery, the anesthesiologist should be informed that the patient is on beta-blocker therapy. The effects of nadolol can be reversed by administration of beta-receptor agonists such as isoproterenol, dopamine, dobutamine, or levarterenol. Difficulty in restarting and maintaining the heart beat has also been reported with beta-adrenergic receptor blocking agents.

Diabetes and Hypoglycemia: Beta-adrenergic blockade may prevent the appearance of premonitory signs and symptoms (e.g., tachycardia and blood pressure changes) of acute hypoglycemia. This is especially important with labile diabetics. Beta-blockade also reduces the release of insulin in response to hyperglycemia; therefore, it may be necessary to adjust the dose of antidiabetic drugs.

Thyrotoxicosis: Beta-adrenergic blockade may mask certain clinical signs (e.g., tachycardia) of hyperthyroidism. Patients suspected of developing thyrotoxicosis should be managed carefully to avoid abrupt withdrawal of beta-adrenergic blockade which might precipitate a thyroid storm.

PRECAUTIONS

Impaired Renal Function: Nadolol should be used with caution in patients with impaired renal function. (See DOSAGE AND ADMINISTRATION.)

Information for Patients: Patients, especially those with evidence of coronary artery insufficiency, should be warned against interruption or discontinuation of nadolol therapy without the physician's advice. Although cardiac failure rarely occurs in properly selected patients, patients being treated with beta-adrenergic blocking agents should be advised to consult the physician at the first sign or symptom of impending failure. The patient should also be advised of a proper course in the event of an inadvertently missed dose.

Drug Interactions: When administered concurrently, the following drugs may interact with beta-adrenergic receptor blocking agents:

Anesthetics, general: Exaggeration of the hypotension induced by general anesthetics (see WARNINGS, Major Surgery).

Antidiabetic drugs (oral agents and insulin): Hypoglycemia or hyperglycemia; adjust dosage of antidiabetic drug accordingly (see WARNINGS, Diabetes and Hypoglycemia).

Catecholamine-depleting drugs (e.g.,reserpine): Additive effect; monitor closely for evidence of hypotension and/or excessive bradycardia (e.g., vertigo, syncope, postural hypotension).

Response to Treatment for Anaphylactic Reaction: While taking beta-blockers, patients with a history of severe anaphylactic reaction to a variety of allergens may be more reactive to repeated challenge, either accidental, diagnostic, or therapeutic. Such patients may be unresponsive to the usual doses of epinephrine used to treat allergic reaction.

Carcinogenesis, Mutagenesis, Impairment of Fertility: In chronic oral toxicologic studies (1 to 2 years) in mice, rats, and dogs, nadolol did not produce any significant toxic effects. In 2 year oral carcinogenic studies in rats and mice, nadolol did not produce any neoplastic, preneoplastic, or nonneoplastic pathologic lesions. In fertility and general reproductive performance studies in rats, nadolol caused no adverse effects.

Pregnancy Category C: In animal reproduction studies with nadolol, evidence of embryotoxicity and fetotoxicity was found in rabbits, but not in rats or hamsters, at doses five to ten times greater (on a mg/kg basis) than the maximum indicated human dose. No teratogenic potential was observed in any of these species.

There are no adequate and well controlled studies in pregnant women. Nadolol should be used during pregnancy only if the potential benefit justifies the potential risk to the fetus. Neonates whose mothers are receiving nadolol at parturition have exhibited bradycardia, hypoglycemia, and associated symptoms.

Nursing Mothers: Nadolol is excreted in human milk. Because of the potential for adverse effects in nursing infants, a decision should be made whether to discontinue nursing or to discontinue therapy taking into account the importance of nadolol to the mother.

Pediatric Use: Safety and effectiveness in pediatric patients have not been established.

ADVERSE REACTIONS

Most adverse effects have been mild and transient and have rarely required withdrawal of therapy.

Cardiovascular: Bradycardia with heart rates of less than 60 beats per minute occurs commonly, and heart rates below 40 beats per minute and/or symptomatic bradycardia were seen in about 2 of 100 patients. Symptoms of peripheral vascular insufficiency, usually of the Raynaud type, have occurred in approximately 2 of 100 patients. Cardiac failure, hypotension, and rhythm/conduction disturbances have each occurred in about 1 of 100 patients. Single instances of first-degree and third-degree heart block have been reported; intensification of AV block is a known effect of beta-blockers (see also CONTRAINDICATIONS, WARNINGS, and PRECAUTIONS).

Central Nervous System: Dizziness or fatigue has been reported in approximately 2 of 100 patients; paresthesias, sedation, and change in behavior have each been reported in approximately 6 of 1,000 patients.

Respiratory: Bronchospasm has been reported in approximately 1 of 1,000 patients (see CONTRAINDICATIONS and WARNINGS).

Gastrointestinal: Nausea, diarrhea, abdominal discomfort, constipation, vomiting, indigestion, anorexia, bloating, and flatulence have been reported in 1 to 5 of 1,000 patients.

Miscellaneous: Each of the following has been reported in 1 to 5 of 1,000 patients: rash; pruritus; headache; dry mouth, eyes, or skin; impotence or decreased libido; facial swelling; weight gain; slurred speech; cough; nasal stuffiness; sweating; tinnitus; blurred vision. Reversible alopecia has been reported infrequently.

The following adverse reactions have been reported in patients taking nadolol and/or other beta-adrenergic blocking agents, but no causal relationship to nadolol has been established.

Central Nervous System: Reversible mental depression progressing to catatonia; visual disturbances; hallucinations; an acute reversible syndrome characterized by disorientation for time and place, short-term memory loss, emotional lability with slightly clouded sensorium, and decreased performance on neuropsychometrics.

Gastrointestinal: Mesenteric arterial thrombosis; ischemic colitis; elevated liver enzymes.

Hematologic: Agranulocytosis; thrombocytopenic or nonthrombocytopenic purpura.

Allergic: Fever combined with aching and sore throat; laryngospasm; respiratory distress.

Miscellaneous: Pemphigoid rash; hypertensive reaction in patients with pheochromocytoma; sleep disturbances; Peyronie's disease.

The oculomucocutaneous syndrome associated with the beta-blocker practolol has not been reported with nadolol.

OVERDOSAGE

Nadolol can be removed from the general circulation by hemodialysis.

In addition to gastric lavage, the following measures should be employed, as appropriate. In determining the duration of corrective therapy, note must be taken of the long duration of the effect of nadolol.

Excessive Bradycardia: Administer atropine (0.25 to 1.0 mg). If there is no response to vagal blockade, administer isoproterenol cautiously.

Cardiac Failure: Administer a digitalis glycoside and diuretic. It has been reported that glucagon may also be useful in this situation.

Hypotension: Administer vasopressors, e.g., epinephrine or levarterenol. (There is evidence that epinephrine may be the drug of choice.)

Bronchospasm: Administer a beta$_2$-stimulating agent and/or a theophylline derivative.

DOSAGE AND ADMINISTRATION

DOSAGE MUST BE INDIVIDUALIZED. NADOLOL MAY BE ADMINISTERED WITHOUT REGARD TO MEALS.

Angina Pectoris: The usual initial dose is 40 mg nadolol once daily. Dosage may be gradually increased in 40 to 80 mg increments at 3 to 7 day intervals until optimum clinical response is obtained or there is pronounced slowing of the heart rate. The usual maintenance dose is 40 or 80 mg administered once daily. Doses up to 160 or 240 mg administered once daily may be needed.

The usefulness and safety in angina pectoris of dosages exceeding 240 mg per day have not been established. If treatment is to be discontinued, reduce the dosage gradually over a period of 1 to 2 weeks (see WARNINGS).

Hypertension: The usual initial dose is 40 mg nadolol once daily, whether it is used alone or in addition to diuretic therapy. Dosage may be gradually increased in 40 to 80 mg increments until optimum blood pressure reduction is achieved. The usual maintenance dose is 40 or 80 mg administered once daily. Doses up to 240 or 320 mg administered once daily may be needed.

Dosage Adjustment in Renal Failure: Absorbed nadolol is excreted principally by the kidneys and, although nonrenal elimination does occur, dosage adjustments are necessary in patients with renal impairment. The following dose intervals are recommended:

Creatinine Clearance (mL/min/1.73^2)	Dosage Interval (hours)
>50	24
31 to 50	24 to 36
10 to 30	24 to 48
< 10	40 to 60

HOW SUPPLIED

Nadolol Tablets, USP are available containing 20 mg, 40 mg or 80 mg of nadolol, USP.

The 20 mg tablets are yellow, round, scored tablets debossed with **M** above the score and **28** below the score on one side of the tablet and blank on the other side. They are available as follows:

NDC 0378-0028-01
bottles of 100 tablets

The 40 mg tablets are yellow, round, scored tablets debossed with **M** above the score and **171** below the score on one side of the tablet and blank on the other side. They are available as follows:

NDC 0378-1171-01
bottles of 100 tablets
NDC 0378-1171-10
bottles of 1000 tablets

The 80 mg tablets are yellow, round, scored tablets debossed with **M** above the score and **132** below the score on one side of the tablet and blank on the other side. They are available as follows:

NDC 0378-1132-01
bottles of 100 tablets
NDC 0378-1132-10
bottles of 1000 tablets

Store at 20° to 25°C (68° to 77°F). [See USP for Controlled Room Temperature.]

Protect from light.

Dispense in a tight, light-resistant container as defined in the USP using a child-resistant closure.

MYLAN®

Mylan Pharmaceuticals Inc.
Morgantown, WV 26505

REVISED OCTOBER 2006
NAD:R9

PAROXETINE HYDROCHLORIDE ℞

[PA-rox-eh-tine HY-dro-chlo-ride]

Controlled-Release Tablets

37.5 mg

PRESCRIBING INFORMATION

Suicidality and Antidepressant Drugs

Antidepressants increased the risk compared to placebo of suicidal thinking and behavior (suicidality) in children, adolescents, and young adults in short-term studies of major depressive disorder (MDD) and other psychiatric disorders. Anyone considering the use of Paroxetine Hydrochloride Controlled-Release Tablets or any other antidepressant in a child, adolescent, or young adult must balance this risk with the clinical need. Short-term studies did not show an increase in the risk of suicidality with antidepressants compared to placebo in adults beyond age 24; there was a reduction in risk with antidepressants compared to placebo in adults aged 65 and older. Depression and certain other psychiatric disorders are themselves associated with increases in the risk of suicide. Patients of all ages who are started on antidepressant therapy should be monitored appropriately and observed closely for clinical worsening, suicidality, or unusual changes in behavior. Families and caregivers should be advised of the need for close observation and communication with the prescriber. Paroxetine Hydrochloride Controlled-Release Tablets are not approved for use in pediatric patients. (See WARNINGS: Clinical Worsening and Suicide Risk, PRECAUTIONS: Information for Patients, and PRECAUTIONS: Pediatric Use.)

DESCRIPTION

Paroxetine hydrochloride is an orally administered psychotropic drug with a chemical structure unrelated to other selective serotonin reuptake inhibitors or to tricyclic, tetracyclic, or other available antidepressant or antipanic agents. It is the hydrochloride salt of a phenylpiperidine compound identified chemically as (-)-*trans*-4*R*-(4'-fluorophenyl)-3*S*-[(3',4'-methylenedioxyphenoxy) methyl] piperidine hydrochloride hemihydrate and has the empirical formula of $C_{19}H_{20}FNO_3 \bullet HCl \bullet 1/2H_2O$. The molecular weight is 374.8 (329.4 as free base). The structural formula of paroxetine hydrochloride is:

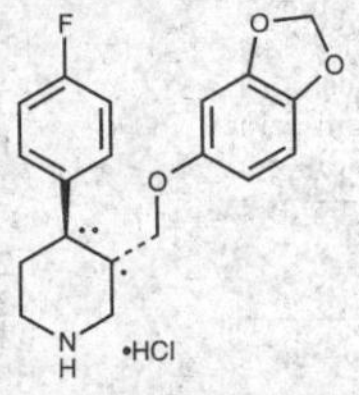

Paroxetine hydrochloride is an odorless, off-white powder, having a melting point range of 120° to 138°C and a solubility of 5.4 mg/mL in water.

Each enteric, film-coated, controlled-release, blue tablet contains paroxetine hydrochloride equivalent to 37.5 mg of paroxetine. One layer of the tablet consists of a degradable barrier layer and the other contains the active material in a hydrophilic matrix.

Inactive ingredients consist of hypromellose, polyvinylpyrrolidone, lactose monohydrate, magnesium stearate, silicon dioxide, glyceryl behenate, methacrylic acid copolymer type C, polysorbate 80, talc, triethyl citrate, titanium dioxide, polyethylene glycols, yellow ferric oxide, and FD&C Blue No. 2 aluminum lake.

CLINICAL PHARMACOLOGY

Pharmacodynamics: The efficacy of paroxetine in the treatment of major depressive disorder, panic disorder, social anxiety disorder, and premenstrual dysphoric disorder (PMDD) is presumed to be linked to potentiation of serotonergic activity in the central nervous system resulting from inhibition of neuronal reuptake of serotonin (5-hydroxy-tryptamine, 5-HT). Studies at clinically relevant doses in humans have demonstrated that paroxetine blocks the uptake of serotonin into human platelets. In vitro studies in animals also suggest that paroxetine is a potent and highly selective inhibitor of neuronal serotonin reuptake and has only very weak effects on norepinephrine and dopamine neuronal reuptake. In vitro radioligand binding studies indicate that paroxetine has little affinity for muscarinic, alpha$_1$-, alpha$_2$-, beta-adrenergic-, dopamine (D_2)-, 5-HT$_1$-, 5-HT$_2$-, and histamine (H_1)-receptors; antagonism of muscarinic, histaminergic, and alpha$_1$-adrenergic receptors has been associated with various anticholinergic, sedative, and cardiovascular effects for other psychotropic drugs. Because the relative potencies of paroxetine's major metabolites are at most 1/50 of the parent compound, they are essentially inactive.

Pharmacokinetics: Paroxetine hydrochloride is completely absorbed after oral dosing of a solution of the hydrochloride salt. The elimination half-life is approximately 15 to 20 hours after a single dose of Paroxetine Hydrochloride Controlled-Release Tablets. Paroxetine is extensively metabolized and the metabolites are considered to be inactive. Nonlinearity in pharmacokinetics is observed with increasing doses. Paroxetine metabolism is mediated in part by CYP2D6, and the metabolites are primarily excreted in the urine and to some extent in the feces. Pharmacokinetic behavior of paroxetine has not been evaluated in subjects who are deficient in CYP2D6 (poor metabolizers).

Absorption and Distribution: Paroxetine Hydrochloride Controlled-Release Tablets contain a degradable polymeric matrix (GEOMATRIX™) designed to control the dissolution rate of paroxetine over a period of approximately 4 to 5 hours. In addition to controlling the rate of drug release in vivo, an enteric coat delays the start of drug release until Paroxetine Hydrochloride Controlled-Release Tablets have left the stomach.

Paroxetine hydrochloride is completely absorbed after oral dosing of a solution of the hydrochloride salt. In a study in which normal male and female subjects (n = 23) received single oral doses of Paroxetine Hydrochloride Controlled-Release Tablets at 4 dosage strengths (12.5 mg, 25 mg, 37.5 mg, and 50 mg), paroxetine C_{max} and AUC_{0-inf} increased disproportionately with dose (as seen also with immediate-release formulations). Mean C_{max} and AUC_{0-inf} values at these doses were 2.0, 5.5, 9.0, and 12.5 ng/mL, and 121, 261, 338, and 540 ng•hr./mL, respectively. T_{max} was observed typically between 6 and 10 hours post-dose, reflecting a reduction in absorption rate compared with immediate-release formulations. The bioavailability of 25 mg Paroxetine Hydrochloride Controlled-Release Tablets is not affected by food.

Paroxetine distributes throughout the body, including the CNS, with only 1% remaining in the plasma.

Approximately 95% and 93% of paroxetine is bound to plasma protein at 100 ng/mL and 400 ng/mL, respectively. Under clinical conditions, paroxetine concentrations would normally be less than 400 ng/mL. Paroxetine does not alter the in vitro protein binding of phenytoin or warfarin.

Metabolism and Excretion: The mean elimination half-life of paroxetine was 15 to 20 hours throughout a range of single doses of Paroxetine Hydrochloride Controlled-Release Tablets (12.5 mg, 25 mg, 37.5 mg, and 50 mg). During repeated administration of Paroxetine Hydrochloride Controlled-Release Tablets (25 mg once daily), steady state was reached within 2 weeks (i.e., comparable to immediate-release formulations). In a repeat-dose study in which normal male and female subjects (n = 23) received Paroxetine Hydrochloride Controlled-Release Tablets (25 mg daily), mean steady state C_{max}, C_{min}, and AUC_{0-24} values were 30 ng/mL, 20 ng/mL, and 550 ng•hr./mL, respectively.

Based on studies using immediate-release formulations, steady-state drug exposure based on AUC_{0-24} was several-fold greater than would have been predicted from single-dose data. The excess accumulation is a consequence of the fact that 1 of the enzymes that metabolizes paroxetine is readily saturable.

In steady-state dose proportionality studies involving elderly and nonelderly patients, at doses of the immediate-release formulation of 20 mg to 40 mg daily for the elderly and 20 mg to 50 mg daily for the nonelderly, some nonlinearity was observed in both populations, again reflecting a saturable metabolic pathway. In comparison to C_{min} values after 20 mg daily, values after 40 mg daily were only about 2 to 3 times greater than doubled.

Paroxetine is extensively metabolized after oral administration. The principal metabolites are polar and conjugated products of oxidation and methylation, which are readily cleared. Conjugates with glucuronic acid and sulfate predominate, and major metabolites have been isolated and identified. Data indicate that the metabolites have no more than 1/50 the potency of the parent compound at inhibiting serotonin uptake. The metabolism of paroxetine is accomplished in part by CYP2D6. Saturation of this enzyme at clinical doses appears to account for the nonlinearity of paroxetine kinetics with increasing dose and increasing duration of treatment. The role of this enzyme in paroxetine metabolism also suggests potential drug-drug interactions (see PRECAUTIONS).

Approximately 64% of a 30-mg oral solution dose of paroxetine was excreted in the urine with 2% as the parent compound and 62% as metabolites over a 10-day post-dosing period. About 36% was excreted in the feces (probably via the bile), mostly as metabolites and less than 1% as the parent compound over the 10-day post-dosing period.

Other Clinical Pharmacology Information: *Specific Populations: Renal and Liver Disease:* Increased plasma concentrations of paroxetine occur in subjects with renal and hepatic impairment. The mean plasma concentrations in patients with creatinine clearance below 30 mL/min. were approximately 4 times greater than seen in normal volunteers. Patients with creatinine clearance of 30 to 60 mL/min. and patients with hepatic functional impairment had about a 2-fold increase in plasma concentrations (AUC, C_{max}).

The initial dosage should therefore be reduced in patients with severe renal or hepatic impairment, and upward titration, if necessary, should be at increased intervals (see DOSAGE AND ADMINISTRATION).

Elderly Patients: In a multiple-dose study in the elderly at daily doses of 20, 30, and 40 mg of the immediate-release formulation, C_{min} concentrations were about 70% to 80% greater than the respective C_{min} concentrations in nonelderly subjects. Therefore the initial dosage in the elderly should be reduced (see DOSAGE AND ADMINISTRATION).

Drug-Drug Interactions: In vitro drug interaction studies reveal that paroxetine inhibits CYP2D6. Clinical drug interaction studies have been performed with substrates of CYP2D6 and show that paroxetine can inhibit the metabolism of drugs metabolized by CYP2D6 including desipramine, risperidone, and atomoxetine (see PRECAUTIONS—Drug Interactions).

Clinical Trials

Major Depressive Disorder: The efficacy of Paroxetine Hydrochloride Controlled-Release Tablets as a treatment for major depressive disorder has been established in two 12-week, flexible-dose, placebo-controlled studies of patients with DSM-IV Major Depressive Disorder. One study included patients in the age range 18 to 65 years, and a second study included elderly patients, ranging in age from 60 to 88. In both studies, Paroxetine Hydrochloride Controlled-Release Tablets were shown to be significantly more effective than placebo in treating major depressive disorder as measured by the following: Hamilton Depression Rating Scale (HDRS), the Hamilton depressed mood item, and the Clinical Global Impression (CGI)–Severity of Illness score.

A study of outpatients with major depressive disorder who had responded to immediate-release paroxetine tablets (HDRS total score <8) during an initial 8-week open-treatment phase and were then randomized to continuation on immediate-release paroxetine tablets or placebo for 1 year demonstrated a significantly lower relapse rate for patients taking immediate-release paroxetine tablets (15%) compared to those on placebo (39%). Effectiveness was similar for male and female patients.

Panic Disorder: The effectiveness of Paroxetine Hydrochloride Controlled-Release Tablets in the treatment of panic disorder was evaluated in three 10-week, multicenter, flexible-dose studies (Studies 1, 2, and 3) comparing Paroxetine Hydrochloride Controlled-Release Tablets (12.5 to 75 mg daily) to placebo in adult outpatients who had panic disorder (DSM-IV), with or without agoraphobia. These trials were assessed on the basis of their outcomes on 3 variables: (1) the proportions of patients free of full panic attacks at endpoint; (2) change from baseline to endpoint in the median number of full panic attacks; and (3) change from baseline to endpoint in the median Clinical Global Impression Severity score. For Studies 1 and 2, Paroxetine Hydrochloride Controlled-Release Tablets were consistently superior to placebo on 2 of these 3 variables. Study 3 failed to consistently demonstrate a significant difference between Paroxetine Hydrochloride Controlled-Release Tablets and placebo on any of these variables.

For all 3 studies, the mean dose of Paroxetine Hydrochloride Controlled-Release Tablets for completers at endpoint was approximately 50 mg/day. Subgroup analyses did not indicate that there were any differences in treatment outcomes as a function of age or gender.

Long-term maintenance effects of the immediate-release formulation of paroxetine in panic disorder were demonstrated in an extension study. Patients who were responders during a 10-week double-blind phase with immediate-release paroxetine and during a 3-month double-blind extension phase were randomized to either immediate-release paroxetine or placebo in a 3-month double-blind relapse prevention phase. Patients randomized to paroxetine were significantly less likely to relapse than comparably treated patients who were randomized to placebo.

Social Anxiety Disorder: The efficacy of Paroxetine Hydrochloride Controlled-Release Tablets as a treatment for social anxiety disorder has been established, in part, on the basis of extrapolation from the established effectiveness of the immediate-release formulation of paroxetine. In addition, the effectiveness of Paroxetine Hydrochloride Controlled-Release Tablets in the treatment of social anxiety disorder was demonstrated in a 12-week, multicenter, double-blind, flexible-dose, placebo-controlled study of adult outpatients with a primary diagnosis of social anxiety disorder (DSM-IV). In the study, the effectiveness of Paroxetine Hydrochloride Controlled-Release Tablets (12.5 to 37.5 mg daily) compared to placebo was evaluated on the basis of (1) change from baseline in the Liebowitz Social Anxiety Scale (LSAS) total score and (2) the proportion of responders who scored 1 or 2 (very much improved or much improved) on the Clinical Global Impression (CGI) Global Improvement score.

Paroxetine Hydrochloride Controlled-Release Tablets demonstrated statistically significant superiority over placebo on both the LSAS total score and the CGI Improvement responder criterion. For patients who completed the trial, 64% of patients treated with Paroxetine Hydrochloride Controlled-Release Tablets compared to 34.7% of patients treated with placebo were CGI Improvement responders.

Subgroup analyses did not indicate that there were any differences in treatment outcomes as a function of gender. Subgroup analyses of studies utilizing the immediate-release formulation of paroxetine generally did not indicate differences in treatment outcomes as a function of age, race, or gender.

Premenstrual Dysphoric Disorder: The effectiveness of Paroxetine Hydrochloride Controlled-Release Tablets for the treatment of PMDD utilizing a continuous dosing regimen has been established in 2 placebo-controlled trials. Patients in these trials met DSM-IV criteria for PMDD. In a pool of 1,030 patients, treated with daily doses of Paroxetine Hydrochloride Controlled-Release Tablets 12.5 or 25 mg/day, or placebo the mean duration of the PMDD symptoms was approximately 11 ± 7 years. Patients on systemic hormonal contraceptives were excluded from these trials. Therefore, the efficacy of Paroxetine Hydrochloride Controlled-Release Tablets in combination with systemic (including oral) hormonal contraceptives for the continuous daily treatment of PMDD is unknown. In both positive studies, patients (N = 672) were treated with 12.5 mg/day or 25 mg/day of Paroxetine Hydrochloride Controlled-Release Tablets or placebo continuously throughout the menstrual cycle for a period of 3 menstrual cycles. The VAS-Total score is a patient-rated instrument that mirrors the diagnostic criteria of PMDD as identified in the DSM-IV, and includes assessments for mood, physical symptoms, and other symptoms. 12.5 mg/day and 25 mg/day of Paroxetine Hydrochloride Controlled-Release Tablets were significantly more effective than placebo as measured by change from baseline to the endpoint on the luteal phase VAS-Total score.

In a third study employing intermittent dosing, patients (N = 366) were treated for the 2 weeks prior to the onset of menses (luteal phase dosing, also known as intermittent dosing) with 12.5 mg/day or 25 mg/day of Paroxetine Hydrochloride Controlled-Release Tablets or placebo for a period of 3 months. 12.5 mg/day and 25 mg/day of Paroxetine Hydrochloride Controlled-Release Tablets, as luteal phase dosing, was significantly more effective than placebo as measured by change from baseline luteal phase VAS total score.

There is insufficient information to determine the effect of race or age on outcome in these studies.

INDICATIONS AND USAGE
Major Depressive Disorder: Paroxetine Hydrochloride Controlled-Release Tablets are indicated for the treatment of major depressive disorder.

The efficacy of Paroxetine Hydrochloride Controlled-Release Tablets in the treatment of a major depressive episode was established in two 12-week controlled trials of outpatients whose diagnoses corresponded to the DSM-IV category of major depressive disorder (see CLINICAL PHARMACOLOGY—Clinical Trials).

A major depressive episode (DSM-IV) implies a prominent and relatively persistent (nearly every day for at least 2 weeks) depressed mood or loss of interest or pleasure in nearly all activities, representing a change from previous functioning, and includes the presence of at least 5 of the following 9 symptoms during the same 2-week period: Depressed mood, markedly diminished interest or pleasure in usual activities, significant change in weight and/or appetite, insomnia or hypersomnia, psychomotor agitation or retardation, increased fatigue, feelings of guilt or worthlessness, slowed thinking or impaired concentration, a suicide attempt, or suicidal ideation.

The antidepressant action of paroxetine in hospitalized depressed patients has not been adequately studied.

Paroxetine Hydrochloride Controlled-Release Tablets have not been systematically evaluated beyond 12 weeks in controlled clinical trials; however, the effectiveness of immediate-release paroxetine hydrochloride in maintaining a response in major depressive disorder for up to 1 year has been demonstrated in a placebo-controlled trial (see CLINICAL PHARMACOLOGY—Clinical Trials). The physician who elects to use Paroxetine Hydrochloride Controlled-Release Tablets for extended periods should periodically re-evaluate the long-term usefulness of the drug for the individual patient.

Panic Disorder: Paroxetine Hydrochloride Controlled-Release Tablets are indicated for the treatment of panic disorder, with or without agoraphobia, as defined in DSM-IV. Panic disorder is characterized by the occurrence of unexpected panic attacks and associated concern about having additional attacks, worry about the implications or consequences of the attacks, and/or a significant change in behavior related to the attacks.

The efficacy of Paroxetine Hydrochloride Controlled-Release Tablets was established in two 10-week trials in panic disorder patients whose diagnoses corresponded to the DSM-IV category of panic disorder (see CLINICAL PHARMACOLOGY—Clinical Trials).

Panic disorder (DSM-IV) is characterized by recurrent unexpected panic attacks, i.e., a discrete period of intense fear or discomfort in which 4 (or more) of the following symptoms develop abruptly and reach a peak within 10 minutes: (1) palpitations, pounding heart, or accelerated heart rate; (2) sweating; (3) trembling or shaking; (4) sensations of shortness of breath or smothering; (5) feeling of choking; (6) chest pain or discomfort; (7) nausea or abdominal distress; (8) feeling dizzy, unsteady, lightheaded, or faint; (9) derealization (feelings of unreality) or depersonalization (being detached from oneself); (10) fear of losing control; (11) fear of dying; (12) paresthesias (numbness or tingling sensations); (13) chills or hot flushes.

Long-term maintenance of efficacy with the immediate-release formulation of paroxetine was demonstrated in a 3-month relapse prevention trial. In this trial, patients with panic disorder assigned to immediate-release paroxetine demonstrated a lower relapse rate compared to patients on placebo (see CLINICAL PHARMACOLOGY—Clinical Trials). Nevertheless, the physician who prescribes Paroxetine Hydrochloride Controlled-Release Tablets for extended periods should periodically re-evaluate the long-term usefulness of the drug for the individual patient.

Social Anxiety Disorder: Paroxetine Hydrochloride Controlled-Release Tablets are indicated for the treatment of social anxiety disorder, also known as social phobia, as defined in DSM-IV (300.23). Social anxiety disorder is characterized by a marked and persistent fear of 1 or more social or performance situations in which the person is exposed to unfamiliar people or to possible scrutiny by others. Exposure to the feared situation almost invariably provokes anxiety, which may approach the intensity of a panic attack. The feared situations are avoided or endured with intense anxiety or distress. The avoidance, anxious anticipation, or distress in the feared situation(s) interferes significantly with the person's normal routine, occupational or academic functioning, or social activities or relationships, or there is marked distress about having the phobias. Lesser degrees of performance anxiety or shyness generally do not require psychopharmacological treatment.

The efficacy of Paroxetine Hydrochloride Controlled-Release Tablets as a treatment for social anxiety disorder has been established, in part, on the basis of extrapolation from the established effectiveness of the immediate-release formulation of paroxetine. In addition, the efficacy of Paroxetine Hydrochloride Controlled-Release Tablets was established in a 12-week trial, in adult outpatients with social anxiety disorder (DSM-IV). Paroxetine Hydrochloride Controlled-Release Tablets have not been studied in children or adolescents with social phobia (see CLINICAL PHARMACOLOGY—Clinical Trials).

The effectiveness of Paroxetine Hydrochloride Controlled-Release Tablets in long-term treatment of social anxiety disorder, i.e., for more than 12 weeks, has not been systematically evaluated in adequate and well-controlled trials. Therefore, the physician who elects to prescribe Paroxetine Hydrochloride Controlled-Release Tablets for extended periods should periodically re-evaluate the long-term usefulness of the drug for the individual patient (see DOSAGE AND ADMINISTRATION).

Premenstrual Dysphoric Disorder: Paroxetine Hydrochloride Controlled-Release Tablets are indicated for the treatment of PMDD.

The efficacy of Paroxetine Hydrochloride Controlled-Release Tablets in the treatment of PMDD has been established in 3 placebo-controlled trials (see CLINICAL PHARMACOLOGY—Clinical Trials).

The essential features of PMDD, according to DSM-IV, include markedly depressed mood, anxiety or tension, affective lability, and persistent anger or irritability. Other features include decreased interest in usual activities, difficulty concentrating, lack of energy, change in appetite or sleep, and feeling out of control. Physical symptoms associated with PMDD include breast tenderness, headache, joint and muscle pain, bloating, and weight gain. These symptoms occur regularly during the luteal phase and remit within a few days following the onset of menses; the disturbance markedly interferes with work or school or with usual social activities and relationships with others. In making the diagnosis, care should be taken to rule out other cyclical mood disorders that may be exacerbated by treatment with an antidepressant.

The effectiveness of Paroxetine Hydrochloride Controlled-Release Tablets in long-term use, that is, for more than 3 menstrual cycles, has not been systematically evaluated in controlled trials. Therefore, the physician who elects to use Paroxetine Hydrochloride Controlled-Release Tablets for extended periods should periodically re-evaluate the long-term usefulness of the drug for the individual patient.

CONTRAINDICATIONS
Concomitant use in patients taking either monoamine oxidase inhibitors (MAOIs), including linezolid, an antibiotic which is a reversible non-selective MAOI, or thioridazine is contraindicated (see WARNINGS and PRECAUTIONS).

Concomitant use in patients taking pimozide is contraindicated (see PRECAUTIONS).

Paroxetine Hydrochloride Controlled-Release Tablets are contraindicated in patients with a hypersensitivity to paroxetine or to any of the inactive ingredients in Paroxetine Hydrochloride Controlled-Release Tablets.

WARNINGS
Clinical Worsening and Suicide Risk: Patients with major depressive disorder (MDD), both adult and pediatric, may experience worsening of their depression and/or the emergence of suicidal ideation and behavior (suicidality) or unusual changes in behavior, whether or not they are taking antidepressant medications, and this risk may persist until significant remission occurs. Suicide is a known risk of depression and certain other psychiatric disorders, and these disorders themselves are the strongest predictors of suicide. There has been a long-standing concern, however, that antidepressants may have a role in inducing worsening of depression and the emergence of suicidality in certain patients during the early phases of treatment. Pooled analyses of short-term placebo-controlled trials of antidepressant drugs (SSRIs and others) showed that these drugs increase the risk of suicidal thinking and behavior (suicidality) in children, adolescents, and young adults (ages 18-24) with major depressive disorder (MDD) and other psychiatric disorders. Short-term studies did not show an increase in the risk of suicidality with antidepressants compared to placebo in adults beyond age 24; there was a reduction with antidepressants compared to placebo in adults aged 65 and older. The pooled analyses of placebo-controlled trials in children and adolescents with MDD, obsessive compulsive disorder (OCD), or other psychiatric disorders included a total of 24 short-term trials of 9 antidepressant drugs in over 4,400 patients. The pooled analyses of placebo-controlled trials in adults with MDD or other psychiatric disorders included a total of 295 short-term trials (median duration of 2 months) of 11 antidepressant drugs in over 77,000 patients. There was considerable variation in risk of suicidality among drugs, but a tendency toward an increase in the younger patients for almost all drugs studied. There were differences in absolute risk of suicidality across the different indications, with the highest incidence in MDD. The risk differences (drug vs placebo), however, were relatively stable within age strata and across indications. These risk differences (drug-placebo difference in the number of cases of suicidality per 1,000 patients treated) are provided in Table 1.

Table 1

Age Range	Drug-Placebo Difference in Number of Cases of Suicidality per 1,000 Patients Treated
	Increases Compared to Placebo
<18	14 additional cases
18-24	5 additional cases
	Decreases Compared to Placebo
25-64	1 fewer case
≥65	6 fewer cases

No suicides occurred in any of the pediatric trials. There were suicides in the adult trials, but the number was not sufficient to reach any conclusion about drug effect on suicide.

It is unknown whether the suicidality risk extends to longer-term use, i.e., beyond several months. However, there is substantial evidence from placebo-controlled maintenance trials in adults with depression that the use of antidepressants can delay the recurrence of depression.

All patients being treated with antidepressants for any indication should be monitored appropriately and observed closely for clinical worsening, suicidality, and unusual changes in behavior, especially during the initial few months of a course of drug therapy, or at times of dose changes, either increases or decreases.

The following symptoms, anxiety, agitation, panic attacks, insomnia, irritability, hostility, aggressiveness, impulsivity, akathisia (psychomotor restlessness), hypomania, and mania, have been reported in adult and pediatric patients being treated with antidepressants for major depressive disorder as well as for other indications, both psychiatric and nonpsychiatric. Although a causal link between the emergence of such symptoms and either the worsening of depression and/or the emergence of suicidal impulses has not been established, there is concern that such symptoms may represent precursors to emerging suicidality.

Consideration should be given to changing the therapeutic regimen, including possibly discontinuing the medication, in patients whose depression is persistently worse, or who are experiencing emergent suicidality or symptoms that might be precursors to worsening depression or suicidality, especially if these symptoms are severe, abrupt in onset, or were not part of the patient's presenting symptoms.

If the decision has been made to discontinue treatment, medication should be tapered, as rapidly as is feasible, but with recognition that abrupt discontinuation can be associated with certain symptoms (see PRECAUTIONS and DOSAGE AND ADMINISTRATION—Discontinuation of Treatment With Paroxetine Hydrochloride Controlled-Release Tablets, for a description of the risks of discontinuation of Paroxetine Hydrochloride Controlled-Release Tablets).

Families and caregivers of patients being treated with antidepressants for major depressive disorder or other indications, both psychiatric and nonpsychiatric, should be alerted about the need to monitor patients for the emergence of agitation, irritability, unusual changes in behavior, and the other symptoms described above, as well as the emergence of suicidality, and to report such symptoms immediately to healthcare providers. Such monitoring should include daily observation by families and caregivers. Prescriptions for Paroxetine Hydrochloride Controlled-Release Tablets should be written for the smallest quantity of tablets consistent with good patient management, in order to reduce the risk of overdose.

Screening Patients for Bipolar Disorder: A major depressive episode may be the initial presentation of bipolar disorder. It is generally believed (though not established in controlled trials) that treating such an episode with an antidepressant alone may increase the likelihood of precipitation of a mixed/manic episode in patients at risk for bipolar disorder. Whether any of the symptoms described above represent such a conversion is unknown. However, prior to initiating treatment with an antidepressant, patients with depressive symptoms should be adequately screened to determine if they are at risk for bipolar disorder; such screening should include a detailed psychiatric history, including a family history of suicide, bipolar disorder, and depression. It should be noted that Paroxetine Hydrochloride Controlled-Release Tablets are not approved for use in treating bipolar depression.

Potential for Interaction With Monoamine Oxidase Inhibitors: In patients receiving another serotonin reuptake inhibitor drug in combination with an MAOI, there have been reports of serious, sometimes fatal, reactions including hyperthermia, rigidity, myoclonus, autonomic instability with possible rapid fluctuations of vital signs, and mental status changes that include extreme agitation progressing to delirium and coma. These reactions have also been reported in patients who have recently discontinued that drug and have been started on an MAOI. Some cases presented with features resembling neuroleptic malignant syndrome. While there are no human data showing such an interaction with paroxetine hydrochloride, limited animal data on the effects of combined use of paroxetine and MAOIs suggest that these drugs may act synergistically to elevate blood pressure and evoke behavioral excitation. Therefore, it is recommended that Paroxetine Hydrochloride Controlled-Release Tablets not be used in combination with an MAOI (including linezolid, an antibiotic which is a reversible non-selective MAOI), or within 14 days of discontinuing treatment with an MAOI (see CONTRAINDICATIONS). At least 2 weeks should be allowed after stopping Paroxetine Hydrochloride Controlled-Release Tablets before starting an MAOI.

Serotonin Syndrome or Neuroleptic Malignant Syndrome (NMS)-like Reactions: The development of a potentially life-threatening serotonin syndrome or Neuroleptic Malignant Syndrome (NMS)-like reactions have been reported with SNRIs and SSRIs alone, including treatment with Paroxetine Hydrochloride Controlled-Release Tablets, but particularly with concomitant use of serotonergic drugs (including triptans) with drugs which impair metabolism of serotonin (including MAOIs), or with antipsychotics or other dopamine antagonists. Serotonin syndrome symptoms may include mental status changes (e.g., agitation, hallucinations, coma), autonomic instability (e.g., tachycardia, labile blood pressure, hyperthermia), neuromuscular aberrations (e.g., hyperreflexia, incoordination) and/or gastrointestinal symptoms (e.g., nausea, vomiting, diarrhea). Serotonin syndrome, in its most severe form can resemble neuroleptic malignant syndrome, which includes hyperthermia, muscle rigidity, autonomic instability with possible rapid fluctuation of vital signs, and mental status changes. Patients should be monitored for the emergence of serotonin syndrome or NMS-like signs and symptoms. The concomitant use of Paroxetine Hydrochloride Controlled-Release Tablets with MAOIs intended to treat depression is contraindicated.

If concomitant treatment of Paroxetine Hydrochloride Controlled-Release Tablets with a 5-hydroxytryptamine receptor agonist (triptan) is clinically warranted, careful observation of the patient is advised, particularly during treatment initiation and dose increases.

The concomitant use of Paroxetine Hydrochloride Controlled-Release Tablets with serotonin precursors (such as tryptophan) is not recommended.

Treatment with Paroxetine Hydrochloride Controlled-Release Tablets and any concomitant serotonergic or antidopaminergic agents, including antipsychotics, should be discontinued immediately if the above events occur and supportive symptomatic treatment should be initiated.

Potential Interaction With Thioridazine: Thioridazine administration alone produces prolongation of the QTc interval, which is associated with serious ventricular arrhythmias, such as torsade de pointes–type arrhythmias, and sudden death. This effect appears to be dose related.

An in vivo study suggests that drugs which inhibit CYP2D6, such as paroxetine, will elevate plasma levels of thioridazine. Therefore, it is recommended that paroxetine not be used in combination with thioridazine (see CONTRAINDICATIONS and PRECAUTIONS).

Usage in Pregnancy: *Teratogenic Effects:* Epidemiological studies have shown that infants exposed to paroxetine in the first trimester of pregnancy have an increased risk of congenital malformations, particularly cardiovascular malformations. The findings from these studies are summarized below:

- A study based on Swedish national registry data demonstrated that infants exposed to paroxetine during pregnancy (n = 815) had an increased risk of cardiovascular malformations (2% risk in paroxetine-exposed infants) compared to the entire registry population (1% risk), for an odds ratio (OR) of 1.8 (95% confidence interval 1.1 to 2.8). No increase in the risk of overall congenital malformations was seen in the paroxetine-exposed infants. The cardiac malformations in the paroxetine-exposed infants were primarily ventricular septal defects (VSDs) and atrial septal defects (ASDs). Septal defects range in severity from those that resolve spontaneously to those which require surgery.

- A separate retrospective cohort study from the United States (United Healthcare data) evaluated 5,956 infants of mothers dispensed antidepressants during the first trimester (n = 815 for paroxetine). This study showed a trend towards an increased risk for cardiovascular malformations for paroxetine (risk of 1.5%) compared to other antidepressants (risk of 1%), for an OR of 1.5 (95% confidence interval 0.8 to 2.9). Of the 12 paroxetine- exposed infants with cardiovascular malformations, 9 had VSDs. This study also suggested an increased risk of overall major congenital malformations including cardiovascular defects for paroxetine (4% risk) compared to other (2% risk) antidepressants (OR 1.8; 95% confidence interval 1.2 to 2.8).

- Two large case-control studies using separate databases, each with >9,000 birth defect cases and >4,000 controls, found that maternal use of paroxetine during the first trimester of pregnancy was associated with a 2- to 3-fold increased risk of right ventricular outflow tract obstructions. In one study the OR was 2.5 (95% confidence interval, 1.0 to 6.0, 7 exposed infants) and in the other study the OR was 3.3 (95% confidence interval, 1.3 to 8.8, 6 exposed infants).

Other studies have found varying results as to whether there was an increased risk of overall, cardiovascular, or specific congenital malformations. A meta-analysis of epidemiological data over a 16-year period (1992 to 2008) on first trimester paroxetine use in pregnancy and congenital malformations included the above-noted studies in addition to others (n = 17 studies that included overall malformations and n = 14 studies that included cardiovascular malformations; n = 20 distinct studies). While subject to limitations, this meta-analysis suggested an increased occurrence of cardiovascular malformations (prevalence odds ratio [POR] 1.5; 95% confidence interval 1.2 to 1.9) and overall malformations (POR 1.2; 95% confidence interval 1.1 to 1.4) with paroxetine use during the first trimester. It was not possible in this meta-analysis to determine the extent to which the observed prevalence of cardiovascular malformations might have contributed to that of overall malformations, nor was it possible to determine whether any specific types of cardiovascular malformations might have contributed to the observed prevalence of all cardiovascular malformations.

If a patient becomes pregnant while taking paroxetine, she should be advised of the potential harm to the fetus. Unless the benefits of paroxetine to the mother justify continuing treatment, consideration should be given to either discontinuing paroxetine therapy or switching to another antidepressant (see PRECAUTIONS—Discontinuation of Treatment With Paroxetine HCl Controlled-Release Tablets). For women who intend to become pregnant or are in their first trimester of pregnancy, paroxetine should only be initiated after consideration of the other available treatment options.

Animal Findings: Reproduction studies were performed at doses up to 50 mg/kg/day in rats and 6 mg/kg/day in rabbits administered during organogenesis. These doses are approximately 8 (rat) and 2 (rabbit) times the maximum recommended human dose (MRHD) on an mg/m² basis. These studies have revealed no evidence of teratogenic effects. However, in rats, there was an increase in pup deaths during the first 4 days of lactation when dosing occurred during the last trimester of gestation and continued throughout lactation. This effect occurred at a dose of 1 mg/kg/day or approximately one-sixth of the MRHD on an mg/m² basis. The no-effect dose for rat pup mortality was not determined. The cause of these deaths is not known.

Nonteratogenic Effects: Neonates exposed to Paroxetine Hydrochloride Controlled-Release Tablets and other SSRIs or serotonin and norepinephrine reuptake inhibitors (SNRIs), late in the third trimester have developed complications requiring prolonged hospitalization, respiratory support, and tube feeding. Such complications can arise immediately upon delivery. Reported clinical findings have included respiratory distress, cyanosis, apnea, seizures, temperature instability, feeding difficulty, vomiting, hypoglycemia, hypotonia, hypertonia, hyperreflexia, tremor, jitteriness, irritability, and constant crying. These features are consistent with either a direct toxic effect of SSRIs and SNRIs or, possibly, a drug discontinuation syndrome. It should be noted that, in some cases, the clinical picture is consistent with serotonin syndrome (see WARNINGS—Potential for Interaction With Monoamine Oxidase Inhibitors).

Infants exposed to SSRIs in late pregnancy may have an increased risk for persistent pulmonary hypertension of the newborn (PPHN). PPHN occurs in 1–2 per 1,000 live births in the general population and is associated with substantial neonatal morbidity and mortality. In a retrospective case-control study of 377 women whose infants were born with PPHN and 836 women whose infants were born healthy, the risk for developing PPHN was approximately six-fold higher for infants exposed to SSRIs after the 20th week of gestation compared to infants who had not been exposed to antidepressants during pregnancy. There is currently no corroborative evidence regarding the risk for PPHN following exposure to SSRIs in pregnancy; this is the first study that has investigated the potential risk. The study did not include enough cases with exposure to individual SSRIs to determine if all SSRIs posed similar levels of PPHN risk.

There have also been postmarketing reports of premature births in pregnant women exposed to paroxetine or other SSRIs.

When treating a pregnant woman with paroxetine during the third trimester, the physician should carefully consider both the potential risks and benefits of treatment (see DOSAGE AND ADMINISTRATION). Physicians should note that in a prospective longitudinal study of 201 women with a history of major depression who were euthymic at the beginning of pregnancy, women who discontinued antidepressant medication during pregnancy were more likely to experience a relapse of major depression than women who continued antidepressant medication.

PRECAUTIONS

General: *Activation of Mania/Hypomania:* During premarketing testing of immediate-release paroxetine hydrochloride, hypomania or mania occurred in approximately 1.0% of paroxetine-treated unipolar patients compared to 1.1% of active-control and 0.3% of placebo-treated unipolar patients. In a subset of patients classified as bipolar, the rate of manic episodes was 2.2% for immediate-release paroxetine and 11.6% for the combined active-control groups. Among 1,627 patients with major depressive disorder, panic disorder, social anxiety disorder, or PMDD treated with Paroxetine Hydrochloride Controlled-Release Tablets in controlled clinical studies, there were no reports of mania or hypomania. As with all drugs effective in the treatment of major depressive disorder, Paroxetine Hydrochloride Controlled-Release Tablets should be used cautiously in patients with a history of mania.

Seizures: During premarketing testing of immediate-release paroxetine hydrochloride, seizures occurred in 0.1% of paroxetine-treated patients, a rate similar to that associated with other drugs effective in the treatment of major depressive disorder. Among 1,627 patients who received Paroxetine Hydrochloride Controlled-Release Tablets in controlled clinical trials in major depressive disorder, panic disorder, social anxiety disorder, or PMDD, 1 patient (0.1%) experienced a seizure. Paroxetine Hydrochloride Controlled-Release Tablets should be used cautiously in patients with a history of seizures. It should be discontinued in any patient who develops seizures.

Discontinuation of Treatment With Paroxetine Hydrochloride Controlled-Release Tablets: Adverse events while discontinuing therapy with Paroxetine Hydrochloride Controlled-Release Tablets were not systematically evaluated in most clinical trials; however, in recent placebo-controlled clinical trials utilizing daily doses of Paroxetine Hydrochloride Controlled-Release Tablets up to 37.5 mg/day, spontaneously reported adverse events while discontinuing therapy with Paroxetine Hydrochloride Controlled-Release Tablets were evaluated. Patients receiving 37.5 mg/day underwent an incremental decrease in the daily dose by 12.5 mg/day to a dose of 25 mg/day for 1 week before treatment was stopped. For patients receiving 25 mg/day or 12.5 mg/day, treatment was stopped without an incremental decrease in dose. With this regimen in those studies, the following adverse events were reported for Paroxetine Hydrochloride Controlled-Release Tablets, at an incidence of 2% or greater for Paroxetine Hydrochloride Controlled-Release Tablets and were at least twice that reported for placebo: Dizziness, nausea, nervousness, and additional symptoms described by the investigator as associated with tapering or discontinuing Paroxetine Hydrochloride Controlled-Release Tablets (e.g., emotional lability, headache, agitation, electric shock sensations, fatigue, and sleep disturbances). These events were reported as serious in 0.3% of patients who discontinued therapy with Paroxetine Hydrochloride Controlled-Release Tablets. During marketing of Paroxetine Hydrochloride Controlled-Release Tablets and other SSRIs and SNRIs, there have been spontaneous reports of adverse events occurring upon discontinuation of these drugs, (particularly when abrupt), including the following: Dysphoric mood, irritability, agitation, dizziness, sensory disturbances (e.g., paresthesias such as electric shock sensations and tinnitus), anxiety, confusion, headache, lethargy, emotional lability, insomnia, and hypomania. While these events are generally self-limiting, there have been reports of serious discontinuation symptoms.

Patients should be monitored for these symptoms when discontinuing treatment with Paroxetine Hydrochloride Controlled-Release Tablets. A gradual reduction in the dose rather than abrupt cessation is recommended whenever possible. If intolerable symptoms occur following a decrease in the dose or upon discontinuation of treatment, then resuming the previously prescribed dose may be considered. Subsequently, the physician may continue decreasing the dose but at a more gradual rate (see DOSAGE AND ADMINISTRATION).

See also PRECAUTIONS—Pediatric Use, for adverse events reported upon discontinuation of treatment with paroxetine in pediatric patients.

Akathisia: The use of paroxetine or other SSRIs has been associated with the development of akathisia, which is characterized by an inner sense of restlessness and psychomotor agitation such as an inability to sit or stand still usually associated with subjective distress. This is most likely to occur within the first few weeks of treatment.

Hyponatremia: Hyponatremia may occur as a result of treatment with SSRIs and SNRIs, including Paroxetine Hydrochloride Controlled-Release Tablets. In many cases, this hyponatremia appears to be the result of the syndrome of inappropriate antidiuretic hormone secretion (SIADH). Cases with serum sodium lower than 110 mmol/L have been reported. Elderly patients may be at greater risk of developing hyponatremia with SSRIs and SNRIs. Also, patients taking diuretics or who are otherwise volume depleted may be at greater risk (see Geriatric Use). Discontinuation of Paroxetine Hydrochloride Controlled-Release Tablets should be considered in patients with symptomatic hyponatremia and appropriate medical intervention should be instituted.

Signs and symptoms of hyponatremia include headache, difficulty concentrating, memory impairment, confusion, weakness, and unsteadiness, which may lead to falls. Signs and symptoms associated with more severe and/or acute cases have included hallucination, syncope, seizure, coma, respiratory arrest, and death.

Abnormal Bleeding: SSRIs and SNRIs, including paroxetine, may increase the risk of bleeding events. Concomitant use of aspirin, nonsteroidal anti-inflammatory drugs, warfarin, and other anticoagulants may add to this risk. Case reports and epidemiological studies (case-control and cohort design) have demonstrated an association between use of drugs that interfere with serotonin reuptake and the occurrence of gastrointestinal bleeding. Bleeding events related to SSRIs and SNRIs use have ranged from ecchymoses, hematomas, epistaxis, and petechiae to life-threatening hemorrhages. Patients should be cautioned about the risk of bleeding associated with the concomitant use of paroxetine and NSAIDs, aspirin, or other drugs that affect coagulation.

Use in Patients With Concomitant Illness: Clinical experience with immediate-release paroxetine hydrochloride in patients with certain concomitant systemic illness is limited. Caution is advisable in using Paroxetine Hydrochloride Controlled-Release Tablets in patients with diseases or conditions that could affect metabolism or hemodynamic responses.

As with other SSRIs, mydriasis has been infrequently reported in premarketing studies with paroxetine hydrochloride. A few cases of acute angle closure glaucoma associated with therapy with immediate-release paroxetine have been reported in the literature. As mydriasis can cause acute angle closure in patients with narrow angle glaucoma, caution should be used when Paroxetine Hydrochloride Controlled-Release Tablets are prescribed for patients with narrow angle glaucoma.

Paroxetine Hydrochloride Controlled-Release Tablets and the immediate-release formulation of paroxetine hydrochloride have not been evaluated or used to any appreciable extent in patients with a recent history of myocardial infarction or unstable heart disease. Patients with these diagnoses were excluded from clinical studies during premarket testing. Evaluation of electrocardiograms of 682 patients who received immediate-release paroxetine hydrochloride in double-blind, placebo-controlled trials, however, did not indicate that paroxetine is associated with the development of significant ECG abnormalities. Similarly, paroxetine hydrochloride does not cause any clinically important changes in heart rate or blood pressure.

Increased plasma concentrations of paroxetine occur in patients with severe renal impairment (creatinine clearance <30 mL/min.) or severe hepatic impairment. A lower starting dose should be used in such patients (see DOSAGE AND ADMINISTRATION).

Information for Patients: Paroxetine Hydrochloride Controlled-Release Tablets should not be chewed or crushed, and should be swallowed whole.

Patients should be cautioned about the risk of serotonin syndrome with the concomitant use of Paroxetine Hydrochloride Controlled-Release Tablets and triptans, tramadol, or other serotonergic agents.

Prescribers or other health professionals should inform patients, their families, and their caregivers about the benefits and risks associated with treatment with Paroxetine Hydrochloride Controlled-Release Tablets and should counsel them in its appropriate use. A patient Medication Guide about–Antidepressant Medicines, Depression and Other Serious Mental Illnesses, and Suicidal Thoughts or Actions is available for Paroxetine Hydrochloride Controlled-Release Tablets. The prescriber or health professional should instruct patients, their families, and their caregivers to read the Medication Guide and should assist them in understanding its contents. Patients should be given the opportunity to discuss the contents of the Medication Guide and to obtain answers to any questions they may have. The complete text of the Medication Guide is reprinted at the end of this document.

Patients should be advised of the following issues and asked to alert their prescriber if these occur while taking Paroxetine Hydrochloride Controlled-Release Tablets.

Clinical Worsening and Suicide Risk: Patients, their families, and their caregivers should be encouraged to be alert to the emergence of anxiety, agitation, panic attacks, insomnia, irritability, hostility, aggressiveness, impulsivity, akathisia (psychomotor restlessness), hypomania, mania, other unusual changes in behavior, worsening of depression, and suicidal ideation, especially early during antidepressant treatment and when the dose is adjusted up or down. Families and caregivers of patients should be advised to look for the emergence of such symptoms on a day-to-day basis, since changes may be abrupt. Such symptoms should be reported to the patient's prescriber or health professional, especially if they are severe, abrupt in onset, or were not part of the patient's presenting symptoms. Symptoms such as these may be associated with an increased risk for suicidal thinking and behavior and indicate a need for very close monitoring and possibly changes in the medication.

Drugs That Interfere With Hemostasis (e.g., NSAIDs, Aspirin, and Warfarin): Patients should be cautioned about the concomitant use of paroxetine and NSAIDs, aspirin, warfarin, or other drugs that affect coagulation since combined use of psychotropic drugs that interfere with serotonin reuptake and these agents has been associated with an increased risk of bleeding.

Interference With Cognitive and Motor Performance: Any psychoactive drug may impair judgment, thinking, or motor skills. Although in controlled studies immediate-release paroxetine hydrochloride has not been shown to impair psychomotor performance, patients should be cautioned about operating hazardous machinery, including automobiles, until they are reasonably certain that therapy with Paroxetine Hydrochloride Controlled-Release Tablets does not affect their ability to engage in such activities.

Completing Course of Therapy: While patients may notice improvement with use of Paroxetine Hydrochloride Controlled-Release Tablets in 1 to 4 weeks, they should be advised to continue therapy as directed.

Concomitant Medications: Patients should be advised to inform their physician if they are taking, or plan to take, any prescription or over-the-counter drugs, since there is a potential for interactions.

Alcohol: Although immediate-release paroxetine hydrochloride has not been shown to increase the impairment of mental and motor skills caused by alcohol, patients should be advised to avoid alcohol while taking Paroxetine Hydrochloride Controlled-Release Tablets.

Pregnancy: Patients should be advised to notify their physician if they become pregnant or intend to become pregnant during therapy (see WARNINGS—Usage in Pregnancy: Teratogenic Effects and Nonteratogenic Effects).

Nursing: Patients should be advised to notify their physician if they are breastfeeding an infant (see PRECAUTIONS—Nursing Mothers).

Laboratory Tests: There are no specific laboratory tests recommended.

Drug Interactions: *Tryptophan:* As with other serotonin reuptake inhibitors, an interaction between paroxetine and tryptophan may occur when they are coadministered. Adverse experiences, consisting primarily of headache, nausea, sweating, and dizziness, have been reported when tryptophan was administered to patients taking immediate-release paroxetine. Consequently, concomitant use of Paroxetine Hydrochloride Controlled-Release Tablets with tryptophan is not recommended (see WARNINGS—Serotonin Syndrome).

Monoamine Oxidase Inhibitors: See CONTRAINDICATIONS and WARNINGS.

Pimozide: In a controlled study of healthy volunteers, after immediate-release paroxetine hydrochloride was titrated to 60 mg daily, co-administration of a single dose of 2 mg pimozide was associated with mean increases in pimozide AUC of 151% and C_{max} of 62%, compared to pimozide administered alone. The increase in pimozide AUC and C_{max} is due to the CYP2D6 inhibitory properties of paroxetine. Due to the narrow therapeutic index of pimozide and its known ability to prolong the QT interval, concomitant use of pimozide and Paroxetine Hydrochloride Controlled-Release Tablets is contraindicated (see CONTRAINDICATIONS).

Serotonergic Drugs: Based on the mechanism of action of SNRIs and SSRIs, including paroxetine hydrochloride, and the potential for serotonin syndrome, caution is advised when Paroxetine Hydrochloride Controlled-Release Tablets are coadministered with other drugs that may affect the serotonergic neurotransmitter systems, such as triptans, linezolid (an antibiotic which is a reversible non-selective MAOI), lithium, tramadol, or St. John's Wort (see WARNINGS—Serotonin Syndrome). The concomitant use of Paroxetine Hydrochloride Controlled-Release Tablets with MAOIs (including linezolid) is contraindicated (see CONTRAINDICATIONS). The concomitant use of Paroxetine Hydrochloride Controlled-Release Tablets with other SSRIs, SNRIs or tryptophan is not recommended (see PRECAUTIONS—Drug Interactions, *Tryptophan*).

Thioridazine: See CONTRAINDICATIONS and WARNINGS.

Warfarin: Preliminary data suggest that there may be a pharmacodynamic interaction (that causes an increased bleeding diathesis in the face of unaltered prothrombin time) between paroxetine and warfarin. Since there is little clinical experience, the concomitant administration of Paroxetine Hydrochloride Controlled-Release Tablets and warfarin should be undertaken with caution (see Drugs That Interfere With Hemostasis).

Triptans: There have been rare postmarketing reports of serotonin syndrome with the use of an SSRI and a triptan. If concomitant use of Paroxetine Hydrochloride Controlled-Release Tablets with a triptan is clinically warranted, careful observation of the patient is advised, particularly during treatment initiation and dose increases (see WARNINGS—Serotonin Syndrome).

Drugs Affecting Hepatic Metabolism: The metabolism and pharmacokinetics of paroxetine may be affected by the induction or inhibition of drug-metabolizing enzymes.

Cimetidine: Cimetidine inhibits many cytochrome P_{450} (oxidative) enzymes. In a study where immediate-release paroxetine (30 mg once daily) was dosed orally for 4 weeks, steady-state plasma concentrations of paroxetine were increased by approximately 50% during coadministration with oral cimetidine (300 mg three times daily) for the final week. Therefore, when these drugs are administered concurrently, dosage adjustment of Paroxetine Hydrochloride Controlled-Release Tablets after the starting dose should be guided by clinical effect. The effect of paroxetine on cimetidine's pharmacokinetics was not studied.

Phenobarbital: Phenobarbital induces many cytochrome P_{450} (oxidative) enzymes. When a single oral 30-mg dose of immediate-release paroxetine was administered at phenobarbital steady state (100 mg once daily for 14 days), paroxetine AUC and $T_{1/2}$ were reduced (by an average of 25% and 38%, respectively) compared to paroxetine administered alone. The effect of paroxetine on phenobarbital pharmacokinetics was not studied. Since paroxetine exhibits nonlinear pharmacokinetics, the results of this study may not address the case where the 2 drugs are both being chronically dosed. No initial dosage adjustment with

Paroxetine Hydrochloride Controlled-Release Tablets is considered necessary when coadministered with phenobarbital; any subsequent adjustment should be guided by clinical effect.

Phenytoin: When a single oral 30-mg dose of immediate-release paroxetine was administered at phenytoin steady state (300 mg once daily for 14 days), paroxetine AUC and $T_{1/2}$ were reduced (by an average of 50% and 35%, respectively) compared to immediate-release paroxetine administered alone. In a separate study, when a single oral 300-mg dose of phenytoin was administered at paroxetine steady state (30 mg once daily for 14 days), phenytoin AUC was slightly reduced (12% on average) compared to phenytoin administered alone. Since both drugs exhibit nonlinear pharmacokinetics, the above studies may not address the case where the 2 drugs are both being chronically dosed. No initial dosage adjustments are considered necessary when Paroxetine Hydrochloride Controlled-Release Tablets are coadministered with phenytoin; any subsequent adjustments should be guided by clinical effect (see ADVERSE REACTIONS—Postmarketing Reports).

Drugs Metabolized by CYP2D6: Many drugs, including most drugs effective in the treatment of major depressive disorder (paroxetine, other SSRIs, and many tricyclics), are metabolized by the cytochrome P_{450} isozyme CYP2D6. Like other agents that are metabolized by CYP2D6, paroxetine may significantly inhibit the activity of this isozyme. In most patients (>90%), this CYP2D6 isozyme is saturated early during paroxetine dosing. In 1 study, daily dosing of immediate-release paroxetine (20 mg once daily) under steady-state conditions increased single-dose desipramine (100 mg) C_{max}, AUC, and $T_{1/2}$ by an average of approximately 2-, 5-, and 3-fold, respectively. Concomitant use of paroxetine with risperidone, a CYP2D6 substrate has also been evaluated. In 1 study, daily dosing of paroxetine 20 mg in patients stabilized on risperidone (4 to 8 mg/day) increased mean plasma concentrations of risperidone approximately 4-fold, decreased 9-hydroxyrisperidone concentrations approximately 10%, and increased concentrations of the active moiety (the sum of risperidone plus 9-hydroxyrisperidone) approximately 1.4-fold. The effect of paroxetine on the pharmacokinetics of atomoxetine has been evaluated when both drugs were at steady state. In healthy volunteers who were extensive metabolizers of CYP2D6, paroxetine 20 mg daily was given in combination with 20 mg atomoxetine every 12 hours. This resulted in increases in steady state atomoxetine AUC values that were 6- to 8-fold greater and in atomoxetine C_{max} values that were 3- to 4-fold greater than when atomoxetine was given alone. Dosage adjustment of atomoxetine may be necessary and it is recommended that atomoxetine be initiated at a reduced dose when given with paroxetine.

Concomitant use of Paroxetine Hydrochloride Controlled-Release Tablets with other drugs metabolized by cytochrome CYP2D6 has not been formally studied but may require lower doses than usually prescribed for either Paroxetine Hydrochloride Controlled-Release Tablets or the other drug.

Therefore, coadministration of Paroxetine Hydrochloride Controlled-Release Tablets with other drugs that are metabolized by this isozyme, including certain drugs effective in the treatment of major depressive disorder (e.g., nortriptyline, amitriptyline, imipramine, desipramine, and fluoxetine), phenothiazines, risperidone, tamoxifen, and Type 1C antiarrhythmics (e.g., propafenone, flecainide, and encainide), or that inhibit this enzyme (e.g., quinidine), should be approached with caution.

However, due to the risk of serious ventricular arrhythmias and sudden death potentially associated with elevated plasma levels of thioridazine, paroxetine and thioridazine should not be coadministered (see CONTRAINDICATIONS and WARNINGS).

Tamoxifen is a pro-drug requiring metabolic activation by CYP2D6. Inhibition of CYP2D6 by paroxetine may lead to reduced plasma concentrations of an active metabolite and hence reduced efficacy of tamoxifen.

At steady state, when the CYP2D6 pathway is essentially saturated, paroxetine clearance is governed by alternative P_{450} isozymes that, unlike CYP2D6, show no evidence of saturation (see PRECAUTIONS—Tricyclic Antidepressants).

Drugs Metabolized by Cytochrome CYP3A4: An in vivo interaction study involving the coadministration under steady-state conditions of paroxetine and terfenadine, a substrate for CYP3A4, revealed no effect of paroxetine on terfenadine pharmacokinetics. In addition, in vitro studies have shown ketoconazole, a potent inhibitor of CYP3A4 activity, to be at least 100 times more potent than paroxetine as an inhibitor of the metabolism of several substrates for this enzyme, including terfenadine, astemizole, cisapride, triazolam, and cyclosporine. Based on the assumption that the relationship between paroxetine's in vitro K_i and its lack of effect on terfenadine's in vivo clearance predicts its effect on other CYP3A4 substrates, paroxetine's extent of inhibition of CYP3A4 activity is not likely to be of clinical significance.

Tricyclic Antidepressants (TCAs): Caution is indicated in the coadministration of TCAs with Paroxetine Hydrochloride Controlled-Release Tablets, because paroxetine may inhibit TCA metabolism. Plasma TCA concentrations may need to be monitored, and the dose of TCA may need to be reduced, if a TCA is coadministered with Paroxetine Hydrochloride Controlled-Release Tablets (see PRECAUTIONS—Drugs Metabolized by Cytochrome CYP2D6).

Drugs Highly Bound to Plasma Protein: Because paroxetine is highly bound to plasma protein, administration of Paroxetine Hydrochloride Controlled-Release Tablets to a patient taking another drug that is highly protein bound may cause increased free concentrations of the other drug, potentially resulting in adverse events. Conversely, adverse effects could result from displacement of paroxetine by other highly bound drugs.

Drugs That Interfere With Hemostasis (e.g., NSAIDs, Aspirin, and Warfarin): Serotonin release by platelets plays an important role in hemostasis. Epidemiological studies of the case-control and cohort design that have demonstrated an association between use of psychotropic drugs that interfere with serotonin reuptake and the occurrence of upper gastrointestinal bleeding have also shown that concurrent use of an NSAID or aspirin may potentiate this risk of bleeding. Altered anticoagulant effects, including increased bleeding, have been reported when SSRIs or SNRIs are coadministered with warfarin. Patients receiving warfarin therapy should be carefully monitored when paroxetine is initiated or discontinued.

Alcohol: Although paroxetine does not increase the impairment of mental and motor skills caused by alcohol, patients should be advised to avoid alcohol while taking Paroxetine Hydrochloride Controlled-Release Tablets.

Lithium: A multiple-dose study with immediate-release paroxetine hydrochloride has shown that there is no pharmacokinetic interaction between paroxetine and lithium carbonate. However, due to the potential for serotonin syndrome, caution is advised when immediate-release paroxetine hydrochloride is coadministered with lithium.

Digoxin: The steady-state pharmacokinetics of paroxetine was not altered when administered with digoxin at steady state. Mean digoxin AUC at steady state decreased by 15% in the presence of paroxetine. Since there is little clinical experience, the concurrent administration of Paroxetine Hydrochloride Controlled-Release Tablets and digoxin should be undertaken with caution.

Diazepam: Under steady-state conditions, diazepam does not appear to affect paroxetine kinetics. The effects of paroxetine on diazepam were not evaluated.

Procyclidine: Daily oral dosing of immediate-release paroxetine (30 mg once daily) increased steady-state AUC_{0-24}, C_{max}, and C_{min} values of procyclidine (5 mg oral once daily) by 35%, 37%, and 67%, respectively, compared to procyclidine alone at steady state. If anticholinergic effects are seen, the dose of procyclidine should be reduced.

Beta-Blockers: In a study where propranolol (80 mg twice daily) was dosed orally for 18 days, the established steady-state plasma concentrations of propranolol were unaltered during coadministration with immediate-release paroxetine (30 mg once daily) for the final 10 days. The effects of propranolol on paroxetine have not been evaluated (see ADVERSE REACTIONS—Postmarketing Reports).

Theophylline: Reports of elevated theophylline levels associated with immediate-release paroxetine treatment have been reported. While this interaction has not been formally studied, it is recommended that theophylline levels be monitored when these drugs are concurrently administered.

Fosamprenavir/Ritonavir: Co-administration of fosamprenavir/ritonavir with paroxetine significantly decreased plasma levels of paroxetine. Any dose adjustment should be guided by clinical effect (tolerability and efficacy).

Electroconvulsive Therapy (ECT): There are no clinical studies of the combined use of ECT and Paroxetine Hydrochloride Controlled-Release Tablets.

Carcinogenesis, Mutagenesis, Impairment of Fertility: Carcinogenesis: Two-year carcinogenicity studies were conducted in rodents given paroxetine in the diet at 1, 5, and 25 mg/kg/day (mice) and 1, 5, and 20 mg/kg/day (rats). These doses are up to approximately 2 (mouse) and 3 (rat) times the MRHD on a mg/m² basis. There was a significantly greater number of male rats in the high-dose group with reticulum cell sarcomas (1/100, 0/50, 0/50, and 4/50 for control, low-, middle-, and high-dose groups, respectively) and a significantly increased linear trend across dose groups for the occurrence of lymphoreticular tumors in male rats. Female rats were not affected. Although there was a dose-related increase in the number of tumors in mice, there was no drug-related increase in the number of mice with tumors. The relevance of these findings to humans is unknown.

Mutagenesis: Paroxetine produced no genotoxic effects in a battery of 5 in vitro and 2 in vivo assays that included the following: Bacterial mutation assay, mouse lymphoma mutation assay, unscheduled DNA synthesis assay, and tests for cytogenetic aberrations in vivo in mouse bone marrow and in vitro in human lymphocytes and in a dominant lethal test in rats.

Impairment of Fertility: A reduced pregnancy rate was found in reproduction studies in rats at a dose of paroxetine of 15 mg/kg/day, which is approximately twice the MRHD on a mg/m² basis. Irreversible lesions occurred in the reproductive tract of male rats after dosing in toxicity studies for 2 to 52 weeks. These lesions consisted of vacuolation of epididymal tubular epithelium at 50 mg/kg/day and atrophic changes in the seminiferous tubules of the testes with arrested spermatogenesis at 25 mg/kg/day (approximately 8 and 4 times the MRHD on a mg/m² basis).

Pregnancy: Pregnancy Category D. See WARNINGS—Usage in Pregnancy: *Teratogenic Effects* and *Nonteratogenic Effects.*

Labor and Delivery: The effect of paroxetine on labor and delivery in humans is unknown.

Nursing Mothers: Like many other drugs, paroxetine is secreted in human milk, and caution should be exercised when Paroxetine Hydrochloride Controlled-Release Tablets are administered to a nursing woman.

Pediatric Use: Safety and effectiveness in the pediatric population have not been established (see BOX WARNING and WARNINGS—Clinical Worsening and Suicide Risk). Three placebo-controlled trials in 752 pediatric patients with MDD have been conducted with immediate-release paroxetine, and the data were not sufficient to support a claim for use in pediatric patients. Anyone considering the use of Paroxetine Hydrochloride Controlled-Release Tablets in a child or adolescent must balance the potential risks with the clinical need.

In placebo-controlled clinical trials conducted with pediatric patients, the following adverse events were reported in at least 2% of pediatric patients treated with immediate-release paroxetine hydrochloride and occurred at a rate at least twice that for pediatric patients receiving placebo: emotional lability (including self-harm, suicidal thoughts, attempted suicide, crying, and mood fluctuations), hostility, decreased appetite, tremor, sweating, hyperkinesia, and agitation.

Events reported upon discontinuation of treatment with immediate-release paroxetine hydrochloride in the pediatric clinical trials that included a taper phase regimen, which occurred in at least 2% of patients who received immediate-release paroxetine hydrochloride and which occurred at a rate at least twice that of placebo, were: emotional lability (including suicidal ideation, suicide attempt, mood changes, and tearfulness), nervousness, dizziness, nausea, and abdominal pain (see Discontinuation of Treatment With Paroxetine Hydrochloride Controlled-Release Tablets).

Geriatric Use: SSRIs and SNRIs, including Paroxetine Hydrochloride Controlled-Release Tablets, have been associated with cases of clinically significant hyponatremia in elderly patients, who may be at greater risk for this adverse event (see PRECAUTIONS, Hyponatremia).

In worldwide premarketing clinical trials with immediate-release paroxetine hydrochloride, 17% of paroxetine-treated patients (approximately 700) were 65 years or older. Pharmacokinetic studies revealed a decreased clearance in the elderly, and a lower starting dose is recommended; there were, however, no overall differences in the adverse event profile between elderly and younger patients, and effectiveness was similar in younger and older patients (see CLINICAL PHARMACOLOGY and DOSAGE AND ADMINISTRATION).

In a controlled study focusing specifically on elderly patients with major depressive disorder, Paroxetine Hydrochloride Controlled-Release Tablets were demonstrated to be safe and effective in the treatment of elderly patients (>60 years) with major depressive disorder. (See CLINICAL PHARMACOLOGY—Clinical Trials and ADVERSE REACTIONS—Table 2.)

ADVERSE REACTIONS

The information included under the "Adverse Findings Observed in Short-Term, Placebo-Controlled Trials With Paroxetine Hydrochloride Controlled-Release Tablets" subsection of ADVERSE REACTIONS is based on data from 11 placebo-controlled clinical trials. Three of these studies were conducted in patients with major depressive disorder, 3 studies were done in patients with panic disorder, 1 study was conducted in patients with social anxiety disorder, and 4 studies were done in female patients with PMDD. Two of the studies in major depressive disorder, which enrolled patients in the age range 18 to 65 years, are pooled. Information from a third study of major depressive disorder, which focused on elderly patients (60 to 88 years), is presented separately as is the information from the panic disorder studies and the information from the PMDD studies.

Information on additional adverse events associated with Paroxetine Hydrochloride Controlled-Release Tablets and the immediate-release formulation of paroxetine hydrochloride is included in a separate subsection (see Other Events).

Adverse Findings Observed in Short-Term, Placebo-Controlled Trials With Paroxetine Hydrochloride Controlled-Release Tablets:

Adverse Events Associated With Discontinuation of Treatment: *Major Depressive Disorder:* Ten percent (21/212) of patients treated with Paroxetine Hydrochloride Controlled-Release Tablets discontinued treatment due to an adverse event in a pool of 2 studies of patients with major depressive disorder. The most common events (≥1%) associated with discontinuation and considered to be drug related (i.e., those events associated with dropout at a rate approximately twice or greater for Paroxetine Hydrochloride Controlled-Release Tablets compared to placebo) included the following:

	Paroxetine Hydrochloride Controlled-Release Tablets (n = 212)	Placebo (n = 211)
Nausea	3.7%	0.5%
Asthenia	1.9%	0.5%
Dizziness	1.4%	0.0%
Somnolence	1.4%	0.0%

In a placebo-controlled study of elderly patients with major depressive disorder, 13% (13/104) of patients treated with Paroxetine Hydrochloride Controlled-Release Tablets discontinued due to an adverse event. Events meeting the above criteria included the following:

	Paroxetine Hydrochloride Controlled-Release Tablets (n = 104)	Placebo (n = 109)
Nausea	2.9%	0.0%
Headache	1.9%	0.9%
Depression	1.9%	0.0%
LFT's abnormal	1.9%	0.0%

Panic Disorder: Eleven percent (50/444) of patients treated with Paroxetine Hydrochloride Controlled-Release Tablets in panic disorder studies discontinued treatment due to an adverse event. Events meeting the above criteria included the following:

	Paroxetine Hydrochloride Controlled-Release Tablets (n = 444)	Placebo (n = 445)
Nausea	2.9%	0.4%
Insomnia	1.8%	0.0%
Headache	1.4%	0.2%
Asthenia	1.1%	0.0%

Social Anxiety Disorder: Three percent (5/186) of patients treated with Paroxetine Hydrochloride Controlled-Release Tablets in the social anxiety disorder study discontinued treatment due to an adverse event. Events meeting the above criteria included the following:

	Paroxetine Hydrochloride Controlled-Release Tablets (n = 186)	Placebo (n = 184)
Nausea	2.2%	0.5%
Headache	1.6%	0.5%
Diarrhea	1.1%	0.5%

Premenstrual Dysphoric Disorder: Spontaneously reported adverse events were monitored in studies of both continuous and intermittent dosing of Paroxetine Hydrochloride Controlled-Release Tablets in the treatment of PMDD. Generally, there were few differences in the adverse event profiles of the 2 dosing regimens. Thirteen percent (88/681) of patients treated with Paroxetine Hydrochloride Controlled-Release Tablets in PMDD studies of continuous dosing discontinued treatment due to an adverse event. The most common events (≥1%) associated with discontinuation in either group treated with Paroxetine Hydrochloride Controlled-Release Tablets with an incidence rate that is at least twice that of placebo in PMDD trials that employed a continuous dosing regimen are shown in the following table. This table also shows those events that were dose dependent (indicated with an asterisk) as defined as events

	Paroxetine Hydrochloride Controlled-Release Tablets 25 mg (n = 348)	Paroxetine Hydrochloride Controlled-Release Tablets 12.5 mg (n = 333)	Placebo (n = 349)
TOTAL	15%	9.9%	6.3%
Nausea*	6.0%	2.4%	0.9%
Asthenia	4.9%	3.0%	1.4%
Somnolence*	4.3%	1.8%	0.3%
Insomnia	2.3%	1.5%	0.0%
Concentration Impaired*	2.0%	0.6%	0.3%
Dry mouth*	2.0%	0.6%	0.3%
Dizziness*	1.7%	0.6%	0.6%
Decreased Appetite*	1.4%	0.6%	0.0%
Sweating*	1.4%	0.0%	0.3%
Tremor*	1.4%	0.3%	0.0%
Yawn*	1.1%	0.0%	0.0%
Diarrhea	0.9%	1.2%	0.0%

*Events considered to be dose dependent are defined as events having an incidence rate with 25 mg of Paroxetine Hydrochloride Controlled-Release Tablets that was at least twice that with 12.5 mg of Paroxetine Hydrochloride Controlled-Release Tablets (as well as the placebo group).

having an incidence rate with 25 mg of Paroxetine Hydrochloride Controlled-Release Tablets that was at least twice that with 12.5 mg of Paroxetine Hydrochloride Controlled-Release Tablets (as well as the placebo group). [See table above]

Commonly Observed Adverse Events: *Major Depressive Disorder:* The most commonly observed adverse events associated with the use of Paroxetine Hydrochloride Controlled-Release Tablets in a pool of 2 trials (incidence of 5.0% or greater and incidence for Paroxetine Hydrochloride Controlled-Release Tablets at least twice that for placebo, derived from Table 2) were: Abnormal ejaculation, abnormal vision, constipation, decreased libido, diarrhea, dizziness, female genital disorders, nausea, somnolence, sweating, trauma, tremor, and yawning.

Using the same criteria, the adverse events associated with the use of Paroxetine Hydrochloride Controlled-Release Tablets in a study of elderly patients with major depressive disorder were: Abnormal ejaculation, constipation, decreased appetite, dry mouth, impotence, infection, libido decreased, sweating, and tremor.

Panic Disorder: In the pool of panic disorder studies, the adverse events meeting these criteria were: Abnormal ejaculation, somnolence, impotence, libido decreased, tremor, sweating, and female genital disorders (generally anorgasmia or difficulty achieving orgasm).

Social Anxiety Disorder: In the social anxiety disorder study, the adverse events meeting these criteria were: Nausea, asthenia, abnormal ejaculation, sweating, somnolence, impotence, insomnia, and libido decreased.

Premenstrual Dysphoric Disorder: The most commonly observed adverse events associated with the use of Paroxetine Hydrochloride Controlled-Release Tablets either during continuous dosing or luteal phase dosing (incidence of 5% or greater and incidence for Paroxetine Hydrochloride Controlled-Release Tablets at least twice that for placebo, derived from Table 6) were: Nausea, asthenia, libido decreased, somnolence, insomnia, female genital disorders, sweating, dizziness, diarrhea, and constipation.

In the luteal phase dosing PMDD trial, which employed dosing of 12.5 mg/day or 25 mg/day of Paroxetine Hydrochloride Controlled-Release Tablets limited to the 2 weeks prior to the onset of menses over 3 consecutive menstrual cycles, adverse events were evaluated during the first 14 days of each off-drug phase. When the 3 off-drug phases were combined, the following adverse events were reported at an incidence of 2% or greater for Paroxetine Hydrochloride Controlled-Release Tablets and were at least twice the rate of that reported for placebo: Infection (5.3% versus 2.5%), depression (2.8% versus 0.8%), insomnia (2.4% versus 0.8%), sinusitis (2.4% versus 0%), and asthenia (2.0% versus 0.8%).

Incidence in Controlled Clinical Trials: Table 2 enumerates adverse events that occurred at an incidence of 1% or more among patients treated with Paroxetine Hydrochloride Controlled-Release Tablets, aged 18 to 65, who participated in 2 short-term (12-week) placebo-controlled trials in major depressive disorder in which patients were dosed in a range of 25 mg to 62.5 mg/day. Table 3 enumerates adverse events reported at an incidence of 5% or greater among elderly patients (ages 60 to 88) treated with Paroxetine Hydrochloride Controlled-Release Tablets who participated in a short-term (12-week) placebo-controlled trial in major depressive disorder in which patients were dosed in a range of 12.5 mg to 50 mg/day. Table 4 enumerates adverse events reported at an incidence of 1% or greater among patients (19 to 72 years) treated with Paroxetine Hydrochloride Controlled-Release Tablets who participated in short-term (10-week) placebo-controlled trials in panic disorder in which patients were dosed in a range of 12.5 mg to 75 mg/day. Table 5 enumerates adverse events reported at an incidence of 1% or greater among adult patients treated with Paroxetine

Hydrochloride Controlled-Release Tablets who participated in a short-term (12-week), double-blind, placebo-controlled trial in social anxiety disorder in which patients were dosed in a range of 12.5 to 37.5 mg/day. Table 6 enumerates adverse events that occurred at an incidence of 1% or more among patients treated with Paroxetine Hydrochloride Controlled-Release Tablets who participated in three, 12-week, placebo-controlled trials in PMDD in which patients were dosed at 12.5 mg/day or 25 mg/day and in one 12-week placebo-controlled trial in which patients were dosed for 2 weeks prior to the onset of menses (luteal phase dosing) at 12.5 mg/day or 25 mg/day. Reported adverse events were classified using a standard COSTART-based Dictionary terminology.

The prescriber should be aware that these figures cannot be used to predict the incidence of side effects in the course of usual medical practice where patient characteristics and other factors differ from those that prevailed in the clinical trials. Similarly, the cited frequencies cannot be compared with figures obtained from other clinical investigations involving different treatments, uses, and investigators. The cited figures, however, do provide the prescribing physician with some basis for estimating the relative contribution of drug and nondrug factors to the side effect incidence rate in the population studied.

Table 2. Treatment-Emergent Adverse Events Occurring in ≥1% of Patients Treated With Paroxetine Hydrochloride Controlled-Release Tablets in a Pool of 2 Studies in Major Depressive Disorder[1,2]

Body System/ Adverse Event	% Reporting Event Paroxetine Hydrochloride Controlled-Release Tablets (n = 212)	Placebo (n = 211)
Body as a Whole		
Headache	27%	20%
Asthenia	14%	9%
Infection[3]	8%	5%
Abdominal Pain	7%	4%
Back Pain	5%	3%
Trauma[4]	5%	1%
Pain[5]	3%	1%
Allergic Reaction[6]	2%	1%
Cardiovascular System		
Tachycardia	1%	0%
Vasodilatation[7]	2%	0%
Digestive System		
Nausea	22%	10%
Diarrhea	18%	7%
Dry Mouth	15%	8%
Constipation	10%	4%
Flatulence	6%	4%
Decreased Appetite	4%	2%
Vomiting	2%	1%
Nervous System		
Somnolence	22%	8%
Insomnia	17%	9%
Dizziness	14%	4%
Libido Decreased	7%	3%
Tremor	7%	1%
Hypertonia	3%	1%
Paresthesia	3%	1%
Agitation	2%	1%

	1%	0%
Confusion	1%	0%
Respiratory System		
Yawn	5%	0%
Rhinitis	4%	1%
Cough Increased	2%	1%
Bronchitis	1%	0%
Skin and Appendages		
Sweating	6%	2%
Photosensitivity	2%	0%
Special Senses		
Abnormal Vision[8]	5%	1%
Taste Perversion	2%	0%
Urogenital System		
Abnormal Ejaculation[9,10]	26%	1%
Female Genital Disorder[9,11]	10%	<1%
Impotence[9]	5%	3%
Urinary Tract Infection	3%	1%
Menstrual Disorder[9]	2%	<1%
Vaginitis[9]	2%	0%

1. Adverse events for which the Paroxetine Hydrochloride Controlled-Release Tablets reporting incidence was less than or equal to the placebo incidence are not included. These events are: Abnormal dreams, anxiety, arthralgia, depersonalization, dysmenorrhea, dyspepsia, hyperkinesia, increased appetite, myalgia, nervousness, pharyngitis, purpura, rash, respiratory disorder, sinusitis, urinary frequency, and weight gain.
2. <1% means greater than zero and less than 1%.
3. Mostly flu.
4. A wide variety of injuries with no obvious pattern.
5. Pain in a variety of locations with no obvious pattern.
6. Most frequently seasonal allergic symptoms.
7. Usually flushing.
8. Mostly blurred vision.
9. Based on the number of males or females.
10. Mostly anorgasmia or delayed ejaculation.
11. Mostly anorgasmia or delayed orgasm.

Table 3. Treatment-Emergent Adverse Events Occurring in ≥5% of Patients Treated With Paroxetine Hydrochloride Controlled-Release Tablets in a Study of Elderly Patients With Major Depressive Disorder[1,2]

	% Reporting Event	
Body System/ Adverse Event	Paroxetine Hydrochloride Controlled-Release Tablets (n = 104)	Placebo (n = 109)
Body as a Whole		
Headache	17%	13%
Asthenia	15%	14%
Trauma	8%	5%
Infection	6%	2%
Digestive System		
Dry Mouth	18%	7%
Diarrhea	15%	9%
Constipation	13%	5%
Dyspepsia	13%	10%
Decreased Appetite	12%	5%
Flatulence	8%	7%
Nervous System		
Somnolence	21%	12%
Insomnia	10%	8%
Dizziness	9%	5%
Libido Decreased	8%	<1%
Tremor	7%	0%
Skin and Appendages		
Sweating	10%	<1%
Urogenital System		
Abnormal Ejaculation[3,4]	17%	3%
Impotence[3]	9%	3%

1. Adverse events for which the Paroxetine Hydrochloride Controlled-Release Tablets reporting incidence was less than or equal to the placebo incidence are not included. These events are nausea and respiratory disorder.
2. <1% means greater than zero and less than 1%.
3. Based on the number of males.
4. Mostly anorgasmia or delayed ejaculation.

Table 4. Treatment-Emergent Adverse Events Occurring in ≥1% of Patients Treated With Paroxetine Hydrochloride Controlled-Release Tablets in a Pool of 3 Panic Disorder Studies[1,2]

	% Reporting Event	
Body System/ Adverse Event	Paroxetine Hydrochloride Controlled-Release Tablets (n = 444)	Placebo (n = 445)
Body as a Whole		
Asthenia	15%	10%
Abdominal Pain	6%	4%
Trauma[3]	5%	4%
Cardiovascular System		
Vasodilation[4]	3%	2%
Digestive System		
Nausea	23%	17%
Dry Mouth	13%	9%
Diarrhea	12%	9%
Constipation	9%	6%
Decreased Appetite	8%	6%
Metabolic/Nutritional Disorders		
Weight Loss	1%	0%
Musculoskeletal System		
Myalgia	5%	3%
Nervous System		
Insomnia	20%	11%
Somnolence	20%	9%
Libido Decreased	9%	4%
Nervousness	8%	7%
Tremor	8%	2%
Anxiety	5%	4%
Agitation	3%	2%
Hypertonia[5]	2%	<1%
Myoclonus	2%	<1%
Respiratory System		
Sinusitis	8%	5%
Yawn	3%	0%
Skin and Appendages		
Sweating	7%	2%
Special Senses		
Abnormal Vision[6]	3%	<1%
Urogenital System		
Abnormal Ejaculation[7,8]	27%	3%
Impotence[7]	10%	1%
Female Genital Disorders[9,10]	7%	1%
Urinary Frequency	2%	<1%
Urination Impaired	2%	<1%
Vaginitis[9]	1%	<1%

1. Adverse events for which the reporting rate for Paroxetine Hydrochloride Controlled-Release Tablets was less than or equal to the placebo rate are not included. These events are: Abnormal dreams, allergic reaction, back pain, bronchitis, chest pain, concentration impaired, confusion, cough increased, depression, dizziness, dysmenorrhea, dyspepsia, fever, flatulence, headache, increased appetite, infection, menstrual disorder, migraine, pain, paresthesia, pharyngitis, respiratory disorder, rhinitis, tachycardia, taste perversion, thinking abnormal, urinary tract infection, and vomiting.
2. <1% means greater than zero and less than 1%.
3. Various physical injuries.
4. Mostly flushing.
5. Mostly muscle tightness or stiffness.
6. Mostly blurred vision.
7. Based on the number of male patients.
8. Mostly anorgasmia or delayed ejaculation.
9. Based on the number of female patients.
10. Mostly anorgasmia or difficulty achieving orgasm.

Table 5. Treatment-Emergent Adverse Effects Occurring in ≥1% of Patients Treated With Paroxetine Hydrochloride Controlled-Release Tablets in a Social Anxiety Disorder Study[1,2]

	% Reporting Event	
Body System/ Adverse Event	Paroxetine Hydrochloride Controlled-Release Tablets (n = 186)	Placebo (n = 184)
Body as a Whole		
Headache	23%	17%
Asthenia	18%	7%
Abdominal Pain	5%	4%
Back Pain	4%	1%
Trauma[3]	3%	<1%
Allergic Reaction[4]	2%	<1%
Chest Pain	1%	<1%
Cardiovascular System		
Hypertension	2%	0%
Migraine	2%	1%
Tachycardia	2%	1%
Digestive System		
Nausea	22%	6%
Diarrhea	9%	8%
Constipation	5%	2%
Dry Mouth	3%	2%
Dyspepsia	2%	<1%
Decreased Appetite	1%	<1%
Tooth Disorder	1%	0%
Metabolic/Nutritional Disorders		
Weight Gain	3%	1%
Weight Loss	1%	0%
Nervous System		
Insomnia	9%	4%
Somnolence	9%	4%
Libido Decreased	8%	1%
Dizziness	7%	4%
Tremor	4%	2%
Anxiety	2%	1%
Concentration Impaired	2%	0%
Depression	2%	1%
Myoclonus	1%	<1%
Paresthesia	1%	<1%
Respiratory System		
Yawn	2%	0%
Skin and Appendages		
Sweating	14%	3%
Eczema	1%	0%
Special Senses		
Abnormal Vision[5]	2%	0%
Abnormality of Accommodation	2%	0%
Urogenital System		
Abnormal Ejaculation[6,7]	15%	1%
Impotence[6]	9%	0%
Female Genital Disorders[8,9]	3%	0%

1. Adverse events for which the reporting rate for Paroxetine Hydrochloride Controlled-Release Tablets was less than or equal to the placebo rate are not included. These events are: Dysmenorrhea, flatulence, gastroenteritis, hypertonia, infection, pain, pharyngitis, rash, respiratory disorder, rhinitis, and vomiting.
2. <1% means greater than zero and less than 1%.
3. Various physical injuries.
4. Most frequently seasonal allergic symptoms.
5. Mostly blurred vision.
6. Based on the number of male patients.
7. Mostly anorgasmia or delayed ejaculation.
8. Based on the number of female patients.
9. Mostly anorgasmia or difficulty achieving orgasm.

[See table 6 at top of next page]

Dose Dependency of Adverse Events: The following table shows results in PMDD trials of common adverse events, defined as events with an incidence of ≥1% with 25 mg of Paroxetine Hydrochloride Controlled-Release Tablets that was at least twice that with 12.5 mg of Paroxetine Hydrochloride Controlled-Release Tablets and with placebo.

[See table at top of next page]

A comparison of adverse event rates in a fixed-dose study comparing immediate-release paroxetine with placebo in the treatment of major depressive disorder revealed a clear dose dependency for some of the more common adverse events associated with the use of immediate-release paroxetine.

Male and Female Sexual Dysfunction With SSRIs: Although changes in sexual desire, sexual performance, and sexual satisfaction often occur as manifestations of a psychiatric disorder, they may also be a consequence of pharmacologic treatment. In particular, some evidence suggests that SSRIs can cause such untoward sexual experiences.

Reliable estimates of the incidence and severity of untoward experiences involving sexual desire, performance, and satisfaction are difficult to obtain; however, in part because patients and physicians may be reluctant to discuss them. Accordingly, estimates of the incidence of untoward sexual experience and performance cited in product labeling, are likely to underestimate their actual incidence.

The percentage of patients reporting symptoms of sexual dysfunction in the pool of 2 placebo-controlled trials in non-elderly patients with major depressive disorder, in the pool of 3 placebo-controlled trials in patients with panic disorder, in the placebo-controlled trial in patients with social anxiety disorder, and in the intermittent dosing and the pool of 3 placebo-controlled continuous dosing trials in female patients with PMDD are as follows:

[See table at bottom of next page]

There are no adequate, controlled studies examining sexual dysfunction with paroxetine treatment.

Paroxetine treatment has been associated with several cases of priapism. In those cases with a known outcome, patients recovered without sequelae.

While it is difficult to know the precise risk of sexual dysfunction associated with the use of SSRIs, physicians should routinely inquire about such possible side effects.

Weight and Vital Sign Changes: Significant weight loss may be an undesirable result of treatment with paroxetine for some patients but, on average, patients in controlled trials with Paroxetine Hydrochloride Controlled-Release Tablets or the immediate-release formulation of paroxetine hydrochloride, had minimal weight loss (about 1 pound). No significant changes in vital signs (systolic and diastolic blood pressure, pulse, and temperature) were observed in patients treated with Paroxetine Hydrochloride Controlled-Release Tablets, or immediate-release paroxetine hydrochloride, in controlled clinical trials.

ECG Changes: In an analysis of ECGs obtained in 682 patients treated with immediate-release paroxetine and 415 patients treated with placebo in controlled clinical trials, no clinically significant changes were seen in the ECGs of either group.

Liver Function Tests: In a pool of 2 placebo-controlled clinical trials, patients treated with Paroxetine Hydrochloride Controlled-Release Tablets or placebo exhibited abnormal values on liver function tests at comparable rates. In particular, the controlled-release paroxetine-versus-placebo comparisons for alkaline phosphatase, SGOT, SGPT, and bilirubin revealed no differences in the percentage of patients with marked abnormalities.

In a study of elderly patients with major depressive disorder, 3 of 104 patients treated with Paroxetine Hydrochloride Controlled-Release Tablets and none of 109 placebo patients experienced liver transaminase elevations of potential clinical concern.

Two of the patients treated with Paroxetine Hydrochloride Controlled-Release Tablets dropped out of the study due to abnormal liver function tests; the third patient experienced normalization of transaminase levels with continued treatment. Also, in the pool of 3 studies of patients with panic disorder, 4 of 444 patients treated with Paroxetine Hydrochloride Controlled-Release Tablets and none of 445 placebo patients experienced liver transaminase elevations of potential clinical concern. Elevations in all 4 patients decreased substantially after discontinuation of Paroxetine Hydrochloride Controlled-Release Tablets. The clinical significance of these findings is unknown.

In placebo-controlled clinical trials with the immediate-release formulation of paroxetine, patients exhibited abnormal values on liver function tests at no greater rate than that seen in placebo-treated patients.

Hallucinations: In pooled clinical trials of immediate-release paroxetine hydrochloride, hallucinations were observed in 22 of 9,089 patients receiving drug and in 4 of 3,187 patients receiving placebo.

Other Events Observed During the Clinical Development of Paroxetine: The following adverse events were reported during the clinical development of Paroxetine Hydrochloride Controlled-Release Tablets and/or the clinical development of the immediate-release formulation of paroxetine.

Table 6. Treatment-Emergent Adverse Events Occurring in ≥1% of Patients Treated With Paroxetine Hydrochloride Controlled-Release Tablets in a Pool of 3 Premenstrual Dysphoric Disorder Studies with Continuous Dosing or in 1 Premenstrual Dysphoric Disorder Study with Luteal Phase Dosing[1,2,3]

Body System/Adverse Event	% Reporting Event			
	Continuous Dosing		Luteal Phase Dosing	
	Paroxetine Hydrochloride Controlled-Release Tablets (n = 681)	Placebo (n = 349)	Paroxetine Hydrochloride Controlled-Release Tablets (n = 246)	Placebo (n = 120)
Body as a Whole				
Asthenia	17%	6%	15%	4%
Headache	15%	12%	-	-
Infection	6%	4%	-	-
Abdominal pain	-	-	3%	0%
Cardiovascular System				
Migraine	1%	<1%	-	-
Digestive System				
Nausea	17%	7%	18%	2%
Diarrhea	6%	2%	6%	0%
Constipation	5%	1%	2%	<1%
Dry Mouth	4%	2%	2%	<1%
Increased Appetite	3%	<1%	-	-
Decreased Appetite	2%	<1%	2%	0%
Dyspepsia	2%	1%	2%	2%
Gingivitis	-	-	1%	0%
Metabolic and Nutritional Disorders				
Generalized Edema	-	-	1%	<1%
Weight Gain	-	-	1%	<1%
Musculoskeletal System				
Arthralgia	2%	1%	-	-
Nervous System				
Libido Decreased	12%	5%	9%	6%
Somnolence	9%	2%	3%	<1%
Insomnia	8%	2%	7%	3%
Dizziness	7%	3%	6%	3%
Tremor	4%	<1%	5%	0%
Concentration Impaired	3%	<1%	1%	0%
Nervousness	2%	<1%	3%	2%
Anxiety	2%	1%	-	-
Lack of Emotion	2%	<1%	-	-
Depression	-	-	2%	<1%
Vertigo	-	-	2%	<1%
Abnormal Dreams	1%	<1%	-	-
Amnesia	-	-	1%	0%
Respiratory System				
Sinusitis	-	-	4%	2%
Yawn	2%	<1%	-	-
Bronchitis	-	-	2%	0%
Cough Increased	1%	<1%	-	-
Skin and Appendages				
Sweating	7%	<1%	6%	<1%
Special Senses				
Abnormal Vision	-	-	1%	0%
Urogenital System				
Female Genital Disorders[4]	8%	1%	2%	0%
Menorrhagia	1%	<1%	-	-
Vaginal Moniliasis	1%	<1%	-	-
Menstrual Disorder	-	-	1%	0%

1. Adverse events for which the reporting rate of Paroxetine Hydrochloride Controlled-Release Tablets was less than or equal to the placebo rate are not included. These events for continuous dosing are: Abdominal pain, back pain, pain, trauma, weight gain, myalgia, pharyngitis, respiratory disorder, rhinitis, sinusitis, pruritis, dysmenorrhea, menstrual disorder, urinary tract infection, and vomiting. The events for luteal phase dosing are: Allergic reaction, back pain, headache, infection, pain, trauma, myalgia, anxiety, pharyngitis, respiratory disorder, cystitis, and dysmenorrhea.
2. <1% means greater than zero and less than 1%.
3. The luteal phase and continuous dosing PMDD trials were not designed for making direct comparisons between the 2 dosing regimens. Therefore, a comparison between the 2 dosing regimens of the PMDD trials of incidence rates shown in Table 5 should be avoided.
4. Mostly anorgasmia or difficulty achieving orgasm.

Adverse events for which frequencies are provided below occurred in clinical trials with the controlled-release formulation of paroxetine. During its premarketing assessment in major depressive disorder, panic disorder, social anxiety disorder, and PMDD, multiple doses of Paroxetine Hydrochloride Controlled-Release Tablets were administered to 1,627 patients in phase 3 double-blind, controlled, outpatient studies. Untoward events associated with this exposure were recorded by clinical investigators using terminology of their own choosing. Consequently, it is not possible to provide a meaningful estimate of the proportion of individuals experiencing adverse events without first grouping similar types of untoward events into a smaller number of standardized event categories.

In the tabulations that follow, reported adverse events were classified using a COSTART-based dictionary. The frequencies presented, therefore, represent the proportion of the 1,627 patients exposed to Paroxetine Hydrochloride Controlled-Release Tablets who experienced an event of the type cited on at least 1 occasion while receiving Paroxetine

Hydrochloride Controlled-Release Tablets. All reported events are included except those already listed in Tables 2 through 6 and those events where a drug cause was remote. If the COSTART term for an event was so general as to be uninformative, it was deleted or, when possible, replaced with a more informative term. It is important to emphasize that although the events reported occurred during treatment with paroxetine, they were not necessarily caused by it.

Events are further categorized by body system and listed in order of decreasing frequency according to the following definitions: Frequent adverse events are those occurring on 1 or more occasions in at least 1/100 patients (only those not already listed in the tabulated results from placebo-controlled trials appear in this listing); infrequent adverse events are those occurring in 1/100 to 1/1,000 patients; rare events are those occurring in fewer than 1/1,000 patients. Adverse events for which frequencies are not provided occurred during the premarketing assessment of immediate-release paroxetine in phase 2 and 3 studies of major depressive disorder, obsessive compulsive disorder, panic disorder, social anxiety disorder, generalized anxiety disorder, and posttraumatic stress disorder. The conditions and duration of exposure to immediate-release paroxetine varied greatly and included (in overlapping categories) open and double-blind studies, uncontrolled and controlled studies, inpatient and outpatient studies, and fixed-dose and titration studies. Only those events not previously listed for controlled-release paroxetine are included. The extent to which these events may be associated with Paroxetine Hydrochloride Controlled-Release Tablets is unknown.

Events are listed alphabetically within the respective body system. Events of major clinical importance are also described in the PRECAUTIONS section.

Body as a Whole: Infrequent were chills, face edema, fever, flu syndrome, malaise; rare were abscess, anaphylactoid reaction, anticholinergic syndrome, hypothermia; also observed were adrenergic syndrome, neck rigidity, sepsis.

Cardiovascular System: Infrequent were angina pectoris, bradycardia, hematoma, hypertension, hypotension, palpitation, postural hypotension, supraventricular tachycardia, syncope; rare were bundle branch block; also observed were arrhythmia nodal, atrial fibrillation, cerebrovascular accident, congestive heart failure, low cardiac output, myocardial infarct, myocardial ischemia, pallor, phlebitis, pulmonary embolus, supraventricular extrasystoles, thrombophlebitis, thrombosis, vascular headache, ventricular extrasystoles.

Digestive System: Infrequent were bruxism, dysphagia, eructation, gastritis, gastroenteritis, gastroesophageal reflux, gingivitis, hemorrhoids, liver function test abnormal, melena, pancreatitis, rectal hemorrhage, toothache, ulcerative stomatitis; rare were colitis, glossitis, gum hyperplasia, hepatosplenomegaly, increased salivation, intestinal obstruction, peptic ulcer, stomach ulcer, throat tightness; also observed were aphthous stomatitis, bloody diarrhea, bulimia, cardiospasm, cholelithiasis, duodenitis, enteritis, esophagitis, fecal impactions, fecal incontinence, gum hemorrhage, hematemesis, hepatitis, ileitis, ileus, jaundice, mouth ulceration, salivary gland enlargement, sialadenitis, stomatitis, tongue discoloration, tongue edema.

Endocrine System: Infrequent were ovarian cyst, testes pain; rare were diabetes mellitus, hyperthyroidism; also observed were goiter, hypothyroidism, thyroiditis.

Hemic and Lymphatic System: Infrequent were anemia, eosinophilia, hypochromic anemia, leukocytosis, leukopenia, lymphadenopathy, purpura; rare were thrombocytopenia; also observed were anisocytosis, basophilia, bleeding time increased, lymphedema, lymphocytosis, lymphopenia, microcytic anemia, monocytosis, normocytic anemia, thrombocythemia.

Metabolic and Nutritional Disorders: Infrequent were generalized edema, hyperglycemia, hypokalemia, peripheral edema, SGOT increased, SGPT increased, thirst; rare were bilirubinemia, dehydration, hyperkalemia, obesity; also observed were alkaline phosphatase increased, BUN increased, creatinine phosphokinase increased, gamma globulins increased, gout, hypercalcemia, hypercholesteremia, hyperphosphatemia, hypocalcemia, hypoglycemia, hyponatremia, ketosis, lactic dehydrogenase increased, non-protein nitrogen (NPN) increased.

Musculoskeletal System: Infrequent were arthritis, bursitis, tendonitis; rare were myasthenia, myopathy, myositis; also observed were generalized spasm, osteoporosis, tenosynovitis, tetany.

Nervous System: Frequent were depression; infrequent were amnesia, convulsion, depersonalization, dystonia, emotional lability, hallucinations, hyperkinesia, hypesthesia, hypokinesia, incoordination, libido increased, neuralgia, neuropathy, nystagmus, paralysis, vertigo; rare were ataxia, coma, diplopia, dyskinesia, hostility, paranoid reaction, torticollis, withdrawal syndrome; also observed were abnormal gait, akathisia, akinesia, aphasia, choreoathetosis, circumoral paresthesia, delirium, delusions, dysarthria, euphoria, extrapyramidal syndrome, fasciculations, grand mal convulsion, hyperalgesia, irritability, manic reaction, manic-depressive reaction, meningitis, myelitis, peripheral neuritis, psychosis, psychotic depression, reflexes decreased, reflexes increased, stupor, trismus.

Respiratory System: Frequent were pharyngitis; infrequent were asthma, dyspnea, epistaxis, laryngitis, pneumonia; rare were stridor; also observed were dysphonia, emphysema, hemoptysis, hiccups, hyperventilation, lung fibrosis, pulmonary edema, respiratory flu, sputum increased.

Skin and Appendages: Frequent were rash; infrequent were acne, alopecia, dry skin, eczema, pruritus, urticaria; rare were exfoliative dermatitis, furunculosis, pustular rash, seborrhea; also observed were angioedema, ecchymosis, erythema multiforme, erythema nodosum, hirsutism, maculopapular rash, skin discoloration, skin hypertrophy, skin ulcer, sweating decreased, vesiculobullous rash.

Special Senses: Infrequent were conjunctivitis, earache, keratoconjunctivitis, mydriasis, photophobia, retinal hemorrhage, tinnitus; rare were blepharitis, visual field defect; also observed were amblyopia, anisocoria, blurred vision, cataract, conjunctival edema, corneal ulcer, deafness, exophthalmos, glaucoma, hyperacusis, night blindness, parosmia, ptosis, taste loss.

Urogenital System: Frequent were dysmenorrhea*; infrequent were albuminuria, amenorrhea*, breast pain*, cystitis, dysuria, prostatitis*, urinary retention; rare were breast enlargement*, breast neoplasm*, female lactation, hematuria, kidney calculus, metrorrhagia*, nephritis, nocturia, pregnancy and puerperal disorders*, salpingitis, urinary incontinence, uterine fibroids enlarged*; also observed were breast atrophy, ejaculatory disturbance, endometrial disorder, epididymitis, fibrocystic breast, leukorrhea, mastitis, oliguria, polyuria, pyuria, urethritis, urinary casts, urinary urgency, urolith, uterine spasm, vaginal hemorrhage.

* Based on the number of men and women as appropriate.

Postmarketing Reports: Voluntary reports of adverse events in patients taking immediate-release paroxetine hydrochloride that have been received since market introduction and not listed above that may have no causal relationship with the drug include acute pancreatitis, elevated liver function tests (the most severe cases were deaths due to liver necrosis, and grossly elevated transaminases associated with severe liver dysfunction), Guillain-Barré syndrome, toxic epidermal necrolysis, priapism, syndrome of inappropriate ADH secretion, symptoms suggestive of prolactinemia and galactorrhea; extrapyramidal symptoms which have included akathisia, bradykinesia, cogwheel rigidity, dystonia, hypertonia, oculogyric crisis which has been associated with concomitant use of pimozide; tremor and trismus; status epilepticus, acute renal failure, pulmonary hypertension, allergic alveolitis, anaphylaxis, eclampsia, laryngismus, optic neuritis, porphyria, ventricular fibrillation, ventricular tachycardia (including torsade de pointes), thrombocytopenia, hemolytic anemia, events related to impaired hematopoiesis (including aplastic anemia, pancytopenia, bone marrow aplasia, and agranulocytosis), and vasculitic syndromes (such as Henoch-Schönlein purpura). There has been a case report of an elevated phenytoin level after 4 weeks of immediate-release paroxetine and phenytoin coadministration. There has been a case report of severe hypotension when immediate-release paroxetine was added to chronic metoprolol treatment.

DRUG ABUSE AND DEPENDENCE

Controlled Substance Class: Paroxetine Hydrochloride Controlled-Release Tablets are not a controlled substance. **Physical and Psychologic Dependence:** Paroxetine Hydrochloride Controlled-Release Tablets have not been systematically studied in animals or humans for its potential for abuse, tolerance or physical dependence. While the clinical trials did not reveal any tendency for any drug-seeking behavior, these observations were not systematic and it is not possible to predict on the basis of this limited experience the extent to which a CNS-active drug will be misused, diverted, and/or abused once marketed. Consequently, patients should be evaluated carefully for history of drug abuse, and such patients should be observed closely for signs of misuse or abuse of Paroxetine Hydrochloride Controlled-Release Tablets (e.g., development of tolerance, incrementations of dose, drug-seeking behavior).

OVERDOSAGE

Human Experience: Since the introduction of immediate-release paroxetine hydrochloride in the United States, 342

Incidence of Common Adverse Events in Placebo, 12.5 mg and 25 mg of Paroxetine Hydrochloride Controlled-Release Tablets in a Pool of 3 Fixed-Dose PMDD Trials

Common Adverse Event	Paroxetine Hydrochloride Controlled-Release Tablets 25 mg (n = 348)	Paroxetine Hydrochloride Controlled-Release Tablets 12.5 mg (n = 333)	Placebo (n = 349)
Sweating	8.9%	4.2%	0.9%
Tremor	6.0%	1.5%	0.3%
Concentration Impaired	4.3%	1.5%	0.6%
Yawn	3.2%	0.9%	0.3%
Paresthesia	1.4%	0.3%	0.3%
Hyperkinesia	1.1%	0.3%	0.0%
Vaginitis	1.1%	0.3%	0.3%

	Major Depressive Disorder		Panic Disorder		Social Anxiety Disorder		PMDD Continuous Dosing		PMDD Luteal Phase Dosing	
	Controlled-Release Paroxetine	Placebo	Controlled-Release Paroxetine	Placebo	Controlled-Release Paroxetine	Placebo	Controlled-Release Paroxetine	Placebo	Controlled-Release Paroxetine	Placebo
n (males)	78	78	162	194	88	97	n/a	n/a	n/a	n/a
Decreased Libido	10%	5%	9%	6%	13%	1%	n/a	n/a	n/a	n/a
Ejaculatory Disturbance	26%	1%	27%	3%	15%	1%	n/a	n/a	n/a	n/a
Impotence	5%	3%	10%	1%	9%	0%	n/a	n/a	n/a	n/a
n (females)	134	133	282	251	98	87	681	349	246	120
Decreased Libido	4%	2%	8%	2%	4%	1%	12%	5%	9%	6%
Orgasmic Disturbance	10%	<1%	7%	1%	3%	0%	8%	1%	2%	0%

spontaneous cases of deliberate or accidental overdosage during paroxetine treatment have been reported worldwide (circa 1999). These include overdoses with paroxetine alone and in combination with other substances. Of these, 48 cases were fatal and of the fatalities, 17 appeared to involve paroxetine alone. Eight fatal cases that documented the amount of paroxetine ingested were generally confounded by the ingestion of other drugs or alcohol or the presence of significant comorbid conditions. Of 145 non-fatal cases with known outcome, most recovered without sequelae. The largest known ingestion involved 2,000 mg of paroxetine (33 times the maximum recommended daily dose) in a patient who recovered.

Commonly reported adverse events associated with paroxetine overdosage include somnolence, coma, nausea, tremor, tachycardia, confusion, vomiting, and dizziness. Other notable signs and symptoms observed with overdoses involving paroxetine (alone or with other substances) include mydriasis, convulsions (including status epilepticus), ventricular dysrhythmias (including torsade de pointes), hypertension, aggressive reactions, syncope, hypotension, stupor, bradycardia, dystonia, rhabdomyolysis, symptoms of hepatic dysfunction (including hepatic failure, hepatic necrosis, jaundice, hepatitis, and hepatic steatosis), serotonin syndrome, manic reactions, myoclonus, acute renal failure, and urinary retention.

Overdosage Management: Treatment should consist of those general measures employed in the management of overdosage with any drugs effective in the treatment of major depressive disorder.

Ensure an adequate airway, oxygenation, and ventilation. Monitor cardiac rhythm and vital signs. General supportive and symptomatic measures are also recommended. Induction of emesis is not recommended. Gastric lavage with a large-bore orogastric tube with appropriate airway protection, if needed, may be indicated if performed soon after ingestion, or in symptomatic patients.

Activated charcoal should be administered. Due to the large volume of distribution of this drug, forced diuresis, dialysis, hemoperfusion, and exchange transfusion are unlikely to be of benefit. No specific antidotes for paroxetine are known.

A specific caution involves patients taking or recently having taken paroxetine who might ingest excessive quantities of a tricyclic antidepressant. In such a case, accumulation of the parent tricyclic and an active metabolite may increase the possibility of clinically significant sequelae and extend the time needed for close medical observation (see PRECAUTIONS—*Drugs Metabolized by Cytochrome CYP2D6*). In managing overdosage, consider the possibility of multiple-drug involvement. The physician should consider contacting a poison control center for additional information on the treatment of any overdose. Telephone numbers for certified poison control centers are listed in the *Physicians' Desk Reference* (PDR).

DOSAGE AND ADMINISTRATION

Major Depressive Disorder: *Usual Initial Dosage:* Paroxetine Hydrochloride Controlled-Release Tablets should be administered as a single daily dose, usually in the morning, with or without food. The recommended initial dose is 25 mg/day. Patients were dosed in a range of 25 mg to 62.5 mg/day in the clinical trials demonstrating the effectiveness of Paroxetine Hydrochloride Controlled-Release Tablets in the treatment of major depressive disorder. As with all drugs effective in the treatment of major depressive disorder, the full effect may be delayed. Some patients not responding to a 25-mg dose may benefit from dose increases, in 12.5-mg/day increments, up to a maximum of 62.5 mg/day. Dose changes should occur at intervals of at least 1 week.

Patients should be cautioned that Paroxetine Hydrochloride Controlled-Release Tablets should not be chewed or crushed, and should be swallowed whole.

Maintenance Therapy: There is no body of evidence available to answer the question of how long the patient should be treated with Paroxetine Hydrochloride Controlled-Release Tablets. It is generally agreed that acute episodes of major depressive disorder require several months or longer of sustained pharmacologic therapy. Whether the dose of an antidepressant needed to induce remission is identical to the dose needed to maintain and/or sustain euthymia is unknown.

Systematic evaluation of the efficacy of immediate-release paroxetine hydrochloride has shown that efficacy is maintained for periods of up to 1 year with doses that averaged about 30 mg, which corresponds to a 37.5-mg dose of *Paroxetine Hydrochloride Controlled-Release Tablets*, based on relative bioavailability considerations (see CLINICAL PHARMACOLOGY—Pharmacokinetics).

Panic Disorder: *Usual Initial Dosage:* Paroxetine Hydrochloride Controlled-Release Tablets should be administered as a single daily dose, usually in the morning. Patients should be started on 12.5 mg/day. Dose changes should occur in 12.5-mg/day increments and at intervals of

at least 1 week. Patients were dosed in a range of 12.5 to 75 mg/day in the clinical trials demonstrating the effectiveness of Paroxetine Hydrochloride Controlled-Release Tablets. The maximum dosage should not exceed 75 mg/day. Patients should be cautioned that Paroxetine Hydrochloride Controlled-Release Tablets should not be chewed or crushed, and should be swallowed whole.

Maintenance Therapy: Long-term maintenance of efficacy with the immediate-release formulation of paroxetine was demonstrated in a 3-month relapse prevention trial. In this trial, patients with panic disorder assigned to immediate-release paroxetine demonstrated a lower relapse rate compared to patients on placebo. Panic disorder is a chronic condition, and it is reasonable to consider continuation for a responding patient. Dosage adjustments should be made to maintain the patient on the lowest effective dosage, and patients should be periodically reassessed to determine the need for continued treatment.

Social Anxiety Disorder: *Usual Initial Dosage:* Paroxetine Hydrochloride Controlled-Release Tablets should be administered as a single daily dose, usually in the morning, with or without food. The recommended initial dose is 12.5 mg/day. Patients were dosed in a range of 12.5 mg to 37.5 mg/day in the clinical trial demonstrating the effectiveness of Paroxetine Hydrochloride Controlled-Release Tablets in the treatment of social anxiety disorder. If the dose is increased, this should occur at intervals of at least 1 week, in increments of 12.5 mg/day, up to a maximum of 37.5 mg/day.

Patients should be cautioned that Paroxetine Hydrochloride Controlled-Release Tablets should not be chewed or crushed, and should be swallowed whole.

Maintenance Therapy: There is no body of evidence available to answer the question of how long the patient should be treated with Paroxetine Hydrochloride Controlled-Release Tablets. Although the efficacy of Paroxetine Hydrochloride Controlled-Release Tablets beyond 12 weeks of dosing has not been demonstrated in controlled clinical trials, social anxiety disorder is recognized as a chronic condition, and it is reasonable to consider continuation of treatment for a responding patient. Dosage adjustments should be made to maintain the patient on the lowest effective dosage, and patients should be periodically reassessed to determine the need for continued treatment.

Premenstrual Dysphoric Disorder: *Usual Initial Dosage:* Paroxetine Hydrochloride Controlled-Release Tablets should be administered as a single daily dose, usually in the morning, with or without food. Paroxetine Hydrochloride Controlled-Release Tablets may be administered either daily throughout the menstrual cycle or limited to the luteal phase of the menstrual cycle, depending on physician assessment. The recommended initial dose is 12.5 mg/day. In clinical trials, both 12.5 mg/day and 25 mg/day were shown to be effective. Dose changes should occur at intervals of at least 1 week.

Patients should be cautioned that Paroxetine Hydrochloride Controlled-Release Tablets should not be chewed or crushed, and should be swallowed whole.

Maintenance/Continuation Therapy: The effectiveness of Paroxetine Hydrochloride Controlled-Release Tablets for a period exceeding 3 menstrual cycles has not been systematically evaluated in controlled trials. However, women commonly report that symptoms worsen with age until relieved by the onset of menopause. Therefore, it is reasonable to consider continuation of a responding patient. Patients should be periodically reassessed to determine the need for continued treatment.

Special Populations: *Treatment of Pregnant Women During the Third Trimester:* Neonates exposed to Paroxetine Hydrochloride Controlled-Release Tablets and other SSRIs or SNRIs, late in the third trimester have developed complications requiring prolonged hospitalization, respiratory support, and tube feeding (see WARNINGS). When treating pregnant women with paroxetine during the third trimester, the physician should carefully consider the potential risks and benefits of treatment. The physician may consider tapering paroxetine in the third trimester.

Dosage for Elderly or Debilitated Patients, and Patients With Severe Renal or Hepatic Impairment: The recommended initial dose of Paroxetine Hydrochloride Controlled-Release Tablets is 12.5 mg/day for elderly patients, debilitated patients, and/or patients with severe renal or hepatic impairment. Increases may be made if indicated. Dosage should not exceed 50 mg/day.

Switching Patients to or From a Monoamine Oxidase Inhibitor: At least 14 days should elapse between discontinuation of an MAOI and initiation of therapy with Paroxetine Hydrochloride Controlled-Release Tablets. Similarly, at least 14 days should be allowed after stopping Paroxetine Hydrochloride Controlled-Release Tablets before starting an MAOI.

Discontinuation of Treatment With Paroxetine Hydrochloride Controlled-Release Tablets: Symptoms associated with discontinuation of immediate-release

paroxetine hydrochloride or Paroxetine Hydrochloride Controlled-Release Tablets have been reported (see PRECAUTIONS). Patients should be monitored for these symptoms when discontinuing treatment, regardless of the indication for which Paroxetine Hydrochloride Controlled-Release Tablets is being prescribed. A gradual reduction in the dose rather than abrupt cessation is recommended whenever possible. If intolerable symptoms occur following a decrease in the dose or upon discontinuation of treatment, then resuming the previously prescribed dose may be considered. Subsequently, the physician may continue decreasing the dose but at a more gradual rate.

HOW SUPPLIED

Enteric film-coated, controlled-release, round, blue tablets containing paroxetine hydrochloride equivalent to 37.5 mg of paroxetine, engraved with – "PL PCR" on one side and "37.5" on the other.

NDC 0378-2006-93 Bottles of 30

Store at or below 25C (77F) [see USP].

GEOMATRIX is a trademark of Jago Pharma, Muttenz, Switzerland.

MEDICATION GUIDE

Antidepressant Medicines, Depression and Other Serious Mental Illnesses, and Suicidal Thoughts or Actions Paroxetine Hydrochloride (PA-rox-eh-tine HY-dro-chlo-ride) Controlled-Release Tablets

Read the Medication Guide that comes with your or your family member's antidepressant medicine. This Medication Guide is only about the risk of suicidal thoughts and actions with antidepressant medicines. **Talk to your, or your family member's, healthcare provider about:**

- All risks and benefits of treatment with antidepressant medicines
- All treatment choices for depression or other serious mental illness

What is the most important information I should know about antidepressant medicines, depression and other serious mental illnesses, and suicidal thoughts or action?

1. **Antidepressant medicines may increase suicidal thoughts or actions in some children, teenagers, and young adults within the first few months of treatment.**
2. **Depression and other serious mental illnesses are the most important causes of suicidal thoughts and actions. Some people may have a particularly high risk of having suicidal thoughts or actions. These include people who have (or have a family history of) bipolar illness (also called manic-depressive illness) or suicidal thoughts or actions.**
3. **How can I watch for and try to prevent suicidal thoughts and actions in myself or a family member?**
   - Pay close attention to any changes, especially sudden changes, in mood, behaviors, thoughts, or feelings. This is very important when an antidepressant medicine is started or when the dose is changed.
   - Call the healthcare provider right away to report new or sudden changes in mood, behavior, thoughts, or feelings.
   - Keep all follow-up visits with the healthcare provider as scheduled. Call the healthcare provider between visits as needed, especially if you have concerns about symptoms.

Call a healthcare provider right away if you or your family member has any of the following symptoms, especially if they are new, worse, or worry you:

- Thoughts about suicide or dying
- Attempts to commit suicide
- New or worse depression
- New or worse anxiety
- Feeling very agitated or restless
- Panic attacks
- Trouble sleeping (insomnia)
- New or worse irritability
- Acting aggressive, being angry, or violent
- Acting on dangerous impulses
- An extreme increase in activity and talking (mania)
- Other unusual changes in behavior or mood

What else do I need to know about antidepressant medicines?

- **Never stop an antidepressant medicine without first talking to a healthcare provider.** Stopping an antidepressant medicine suddenly can cause other symptoms.
- **Antidepressants are medicines used to treat depression and other illnesses.** It is important to discuss all the risks of treating depression and also the risks of not treating it. Patients and their families or other caregivers should discuss all treatment choices with the healthcare provider, not just the use of antidepressants.
- **Antidepressant medicines have other side effects.** Call your doctor for medical advice about side effects. You may report side effects to FDA at 1-800-FDA-1088.
- **Antidepressant medicines can interact with other medicines.** Know all of the medicines that you or your family

member takes. Keep a list of all medicines to show the healthcare provider. Do not start new medicines without first checking with your healthcare provider.

- Not all antidepressant medicines prescribed for children are FDA approved for use in children. Talk to your child's healthcare provider for more information.

This Medication Guide has been approved by the U.S. Food and Drug Administration for all antidepressants.

January 2008 PCT:1MG

Manufactured by **Penn Labs Inc.** (a GlaxoSmithKline company), Cidra, PR 00739

Distributed by **Mylan Pharmaceuticals Inc.,**

GSK:PRXTER:R3

Morgantown, WV 26505 September, 2009

August 2009 PCT:4PI A073959

PAROXETINE HYDROCHLORIDE EXTENDED-RELEASE TABLETS ℞

[*PA-ro-xe-teen*]

12.5 mg and 25 mg*

(*containsparoxetine hydrochloride equivalent to 12.5 mg and 25 mg of paroxetine, respectively)

℞ only

Suicidality and Antidepressant Drugs

Antidepressants increased the risk compared to placebo of suicidal thinking and behavior (suicidality) in children, adolescents and young adults in short-term studies of major depressive disorder (MDD) and other psychiatric disorders. Anyone considering the use of paroxetine or any other antidepressant in a child, adolescent or young adult must balance this risk with the clinical need. Short-term studies did not show an increase in the risk of suicidality with antidepressants compared to placebo in adults beyond age 24; there was a reduction in risk with antidepressants compared to placebo in adults aged 65 and older. Depression and certain other psychiatric disorders are themselves associated with increases in the risk of suicide. Patients of all ages who are started on antidepressant therapy should be monitored appropriately and observed closely for clinical worsening, suicidality or unusual changes in behavior. Families and caregivers should be advised of the need for close observation and communication with the prescriber. Paroxetine is not approved for use in pediatric patients. (See WARNINGS: Clinical Worsening and Suicide Risk, PRECAUTIONS: Information for Patients and PRECAUTIONS: Pediatric Use.)

DESCRIPTION

Paroxetine hydrochloride extended-release tablets are an orally administered psychotropic drug with a chemical structure unrelated to other selective serotonin reuptake inhibitors or to tricyclic, tetracyclic or other available antidepressant or antipanic agents. It is the hydrochloride salt of a phenylpiperidine compound identified chemically as (3S-trans)-3-[(1,3-benzodioxol-5-yloxy)methyl)]4-(4-fluorophenyl)-piperidine hydrochloride hemihydrate and has the molecular formula of $C_{19}H_{20}FNO_3 \bullet HCl \bullet ½ H_2O$. The molecular weight is 374.8 (329.4 as free base). The structural formula of paroxetine hydrochloride is:

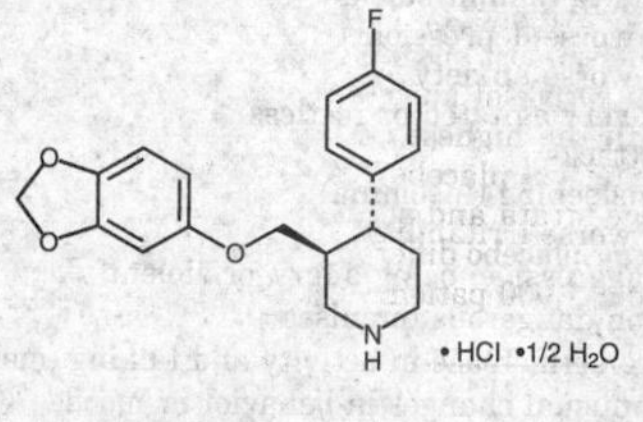

Paroxetine hydrochloride (hemihydrate), USP is an odorless, white to almost white crystalline powder, having a melting point range of 120° to 138°C and a solubility of 5.4 mg/mL in water.

Each enteric film-coated, extended-release tablet contains paroxetine hydrochloride hemihydrate equivalent to 12.5 mg or 25 mg paroxetine. Inactive ingredients consist of colloidal silicon dioxide, hydroxypropyl cellulose, hypromellose, lactose monohydrate, magnesium stearate, methacrylic acid copolymer type C, microcrystalline cellulose, polydextrose, polyethylene glycol, polysorbate 80, sodium hydroxide, talc, titanium dioxide, triacetin and triethyl citrate. In addition, the 25 mg product contains the following coloring agents: D&C Red No. 30 Aluminum Lake, FD&C Blue No. 2 Aluminum Lake, FD&C Yellow No. 6 Aluminum Lake.

In addition, paroxetine hydrochloride extended-release tablets may also contain imprinting ink consisting of either black pigment and natural resin or black iron oxide and propylene glycol.

Paroxetine hydrochloride complies with *USP Chromatographic Purity Test 1*.

CLINICAL PHARMACOLOGY

Pharmacodynamics: The efficacy of paroxetine in the treatment of major depressive disorder, panic disorder, social anxiety disorder and premenstrual dysphoric disorder (PMDD) is presumed to be linked to potentiation of serotonergic activity in the central nervous system resulting from inhibition of neuronal reuptake of serotonin (5-hydroxytryptamine, 5-HT). Studies at clinically relevant doses in humans have demonstrated that paroxetine blocks the uptake of serotonin into human platelets. *In vitro* studies in animals also suggest that paroxetine is a potent and highly selective inhibitor of neuronal serotonin reuptake and has only very weak effects on norepinephrine and dopamine neuronal reuptake. *In vitro* radioligand binding studies indicate that paroxetine has little affinity for muscarinic, alpha$_1$-, alpha$_2$-, beta-adrenergic-, dopamine (D_2)-, 5-HT_1-, 5-HT_2- and histamine (H_1)-receptors; antagonism of muscarinic, histaminergic and alpha$_1$-adrenergic receptors has been associated with various anticholinergic, sedative and cardiovascular effects for other psychotropic drugs.

Because the relative potencies of paroxetine's major metabolites are at most 1/50 of the parent compound, they are essentially inactive.

Pharmacokinetics: Paroxetine hydrochloride is completely absorbed after oral dosing of a solution of the hydrochloride salt. The elimination half-life is approximately 15 to 20 hours after a single dose of paroxetine hydrochloride extended-release tablets. Paroxetine is extensively metabolized and the metabolites are considered to be inactive. Nonlinearity in pharmacokinetics is observed with increasing doses. Paroxetine metabolism is mediated in part by CYP2D6 and the metabolites are primarily excreted in the urine and to some extent in the feces. Pharmacokinetic behavior of paroxetine has not been evaluated in subjects who are deficient in CYP2D6 (poor metabolizers).

Absorption and Distribution: Paroxetine hydrochloride is completely absorbed after oral dosing of a solution of the hydrochloride salt. In a study in which normal male and female subjects (n = 23) received single oral doses of paroxetine hydrochloride extended-release tablets at 4 dosage strengths (12.5 mg, 25 mg, 37.5 mg and 50 mg), paroxetine C_{max} and AUC_{0-inf} increased disproportionately with dose (as seen also with immediate-release formulations). Mean C_{max} and AUC_{0-inf} values at these doses were 2, 5.5, 9 and 12.5 ng/mL and 121, 261, 338 and 540 ng•hr/mL, respectively. T_{max} was observed typically between 6 and 10 hours post-dose, reflecting a reduction in absorption rate compared with immediate-release formulations. The bioavailability of 25 mg paroxetine hydrochloride extended-release tablets is not affected by food.

Paroxetine distributes throughout the body, including the CNS, with only 1% remaining in the plasma.

Approximately 95% and 93% of paroxetine is bound to plasma protein at 100 ng/mL and 400 ng/mL, respectively. Under clinical conditions, paroxetine concentrations would normally be less than 400 ng/mL. Paroxetine does not alter the *in vitro* protein binding of phenytoin or warfarin.

Metabolism and Excretion: The mean elimination half-life of paroxetine was 15 to 20 hours throughout a range of single doses of paroxetine hydrochloride extended-release tablets (12.5 mg, 25 mg, 37.5 mg and 50 mg). During repeated administration of paroxetine hydrochloride extended-release tablets (25 mg once daily), steady-state was reached within 2 weeks (i.e., comparable to immediate-release formulations). In a repeat dose study in which normal male and female subjects (n = 23) received paroxetine hydrochloride extended-release tablets (25 mg daily), mean steady-state C_{max}, C_{min} and AUC_{0-24} values were 30 ng/mL, 20 ng/mL and 550 ng•hr/mL, respectively.

Based on studies using immediate-release formulations, steady-state drug exposure based on AUC_{0-24} was several-fold greater than would have been predicted from single-dose data. The excess accumulation is a consequence of the fact that one of the enzymes that metabolizes paroxetine is readily saturable.

In steady-state dose proportionality studies involving elderly and nonelderly patients, at doses of the immediate-release formulation of 20 mg to 40 mg daily for the elderly and 20 mg to 50 mg daily for the nonelderly, some nonlinearity was observed in both populations, again reflecting a saturable metabolic pathway. In comparison to C_{min} values after 20 mg daily, values after 40 mg daily were only about 2 to 3 times greater than doubled.

Paroxetine is extensively metabolized after oral administration. The principal metabolites are polar and conjugated products of oxidation and methylation, which are readily cleared. Conjugates with glucuronic acid and sulfate predominate and major metabolites have been isolated and identified. Data indicate that the metabolites have no more than 1/50 the potency of the parent compound at inhibiting serotonin uptake. The metabolism of paroxetine is accomplished in part by CYP2D6. Saturation of this enzyme at clinical doses appears to account for the nonlinearity of paroxetine kinetics with increasing dose and increasing duration of treatment. The role of this enzyme in paroxetine metabolism also suggests potential drug-drug interactions (see PRECAUTIONS).

Approximately 64% of a 30 mg oral solution dose of paroxetine was excreted in the urine with 2% as the parent compound and 62% as metabolites over a 10 day post-dosing period. About 36% was excreted in the feces (probably via the bile), mostly as metabolites and less than 1% as the parent compound over the 10 day post-dosing period.

Other Clinical Pharmacology Information: ***Specific Populations:*** *Renal and Liver Disease:* Increased plasma concentrations of paroxetine occur in subjects with renal and hepatic impairment. The mean plasma concentrations in patients with creatinine clearance below 30 mL/min was approximately 4 times greater than seen in normal volunteers. Patients with creatinine clearance of 30 to 60 mL/min and patients with hepatic functional impairment had about a 2-fold increase in plasma concentrations (AUC, C_{max}).

The initial dosage should therefore be reduced in patients with severe renal or hepatic impairment and upward titration, if necessary, should be at increased intervals (see DOSAGE AND ADMINISTRATION).

Elderly Patients: In a multiple-dose study in the elderly at daily doses of 20 mg, 30 mg and 40 mg of the immediate-release formulation, C_{min} concentrations were about 70% to 80% greater than the respective C_{min} concentrations in nonelderly subjects. Therefore the initial dosage in the elderly should be reduced (see DOSAGE AND ADMINISTRATION).

Drug-Drug Interactions: *In vitro* drug interaction studies reveal that paroxetine inhibits CYP2D6. Clinical drug interaction studies have been performed with substrates of CYP2D6 and show that paroxetine can inhibit the metabolism of drugs metabolized by CYP2D6 including desipramine, risperidone and atomoxetine (see PRECAUTIONS: Drug Interactions).

Clinical Trials: ***Major Depressive Disorder:*** The efficacy of paroxetine hydrochloride extended-release tablets as a treatment for major depressive disorder has been established in two 12 week, flexible dose, placebo-controlled studies of patients with DSM-IV Major Depressive Disorder. One study included patients in the age range 18 to 65 years and a second study included elderly patients, ranging in age from 60 to 88. In both studies, paroxetine hydrochloride extended-release tablets were shown to be significantly more effective than placebo in treating major depressive disorder as measured by the following: Hamilton Depression Rating Scale (HDRS), the Hamilton depressed mood item and the Clinical Global Impression (CGI)–Severity of Illness score.

A study of outpatients with major depressive disorder who had responded to immediate-release paroxetine tablets (HDRS total score < 8) during an initial 8 week open treatment phase and were then randomized to continuation on immediate-release paroxetine tablets or placebo for one year demonstrated a significantly lower relapse rate for patients taking immediate-release paroxetine tablets (15%) compared to those on placebo (39%). Effectiveness was similar for male and female patients.

Panic Disorder: The effectiveness of paroxetine hydrochloride extended-release tablets in the treatment of panic disorder was evaluated in three 10 week, multicenter, flexible dose studies (Studies 1, 2 and 3) comparing paroxetine extended-release tablets (12.5 mg to 75 mg daily) to placebo in adult outpatients who had panic disorder (DSM-IV), with or without agoraphobia. These trials were assessed on the basis of their outcomes on three variables: (1) the proportions of patients free of full panic attacks at endpoint; (2) change from baseline to endpoint in the median number of full panic attacks; and (3) change from baseline to endpoint in the median Clinical Global Impression Severity score. For Studies 1 and 2, paroxetine hydrochloride extended-release tablets were consistently superior to placebo on 2 of these 3 variables. Study 3 failed to consistently demonstrate a significant difference between paroxetine hydrochloride extended-release tablets and placebo on any of these variables.

For all three studies, the mean dose of paroxetine hydrochloride extended-release tablets for completers at endpoint was approximately 50 mg/day. Subgroup analyses did not indicate that there were any differences in treatment outcomes as a function of age or gender.

Long-term maintenance effects of the immediate-release formulation of paroxetine in panic disorder were demonstrated in an extension study. Patients who were responders during a 10 week double-blind phase with immediate-release paroxetine and during a 3 month double-blind extension phase were randomized to either immediate-release paroxetine or placebo in a 3 month double-blind relapse prevention phase. Patients randomized to paroxetine were significantly less likely to relapse than comparably treated patients who were randomized to placebo.

Social Anxiety Disorder: The efficacy of paroxetine hydrochloride extended-release tablets as a treatment for social anxiety disorder has been established, in part, on the basis of extrapolation from the established effectiveness of the immediate-release formulation of paroxetine. In addition, the effectiveness of paroxetine hydrochloride extended-release tablets in the treatment of social anxiety disorder was demonstrated in a 12 week, multicenter, double-blind, flexible dose, placebo-controlled study of adult outpatients with a primary diagnosis of social anxiety disorder (DSM-IV). In the study, the effectiveness of paroxetine hydrochloride extended-release tablets (12.5 mg to 37.5 mg daily) compared to placebo was evaluated on the basis of (1) change from baseline in the Liebowitz Social Anxiety Scale (LSAS) total score and (2) the proportion of responders who scored 1 or 2 (very much improved or much improved) on the Clinical Global Impression (CGI) Global Improvement score.

Paroxetine hydrochloride extended-release tablets demonstrated statistically significant superiority over placebo on both the LSAS total score and the CGI Improvement responder criterion. For patients who completed the trial, 64% of patients treated with paroxetine hydrochloride extended-release tablets compared to 34.7% of patients treated with placebo were CGI Improvement responders.

Subgroup analyses did not indicate that there were any differences in treatment outcomes as a function of gender. Subgroup analyses of studies utilizing the immediate-release formulation of paroxetine generally did not indicate differences in treatment outcomes as a function of age, race or gender.

Premenstrual Dysphoric Disorder: The effectiveness of paroxetine hydrochloride extended-release tablets for the treatment of PMDD utilizing a continuous dosing regimen has been established in two placebo-controlled trials. Patients in these trials met DSM-IV criteria for PMDD. In a pool of 1,030 patients, treated with daily doses of paroxetine hydrochloride extended-release tablets 12.5 or 25 mg/day or placebo the mean duration of the PMDD symptoms was approximately 11 ± 7 years. Patients on systemic hormonal contraceptives were excluded from these trials. Therefore, the efficacy of paroxetine hydrochloride extended-release tablets in combination with systemic (including oral) hormonal contraceptives for the continuous daily treatment of PMDD is unknown. In both positive studies, patients (n = 672) were treated with 12.5 mg/day or 25 mg/day of paroxetine hydrochloride extended-release tablets or placebo continuously throughout the menstrual cycle for a period of 3 menstrual cycles. The VAS-Total score is a patient-rated instrument that mirrors the diagnostic criteria of PMDD as identified in the DSM-IV and includes assessments for mood, physical symptoms and other symptoms. 12.5 mg/day and 25 mg/day of paroxetine hydrochloride extended-release tablets were significantly more effective than placebo as measured by change from baseline to the endpoint on the luteal phase VAS-Total score.

In a third study employing intermittent dosing, patients (n = 366) were treated for the 2 weeks prior to the onset of menses (luteal phase dosing, also known as intermittent dosing) with 12.5 mg/day or 25 mg/day of paroxetine hydrochloride extended-release tablets or placebo for a period of 3 months. 12.5 mg/day and 25 mg/day of paroxetine hydrochloride extended-release tablets, as luteal phase dosing, was significantly more effective than placebo as measured by change from baseline luteal phase VAS total score. There is insufficient information to determine the effect of race or age on outcome in these studies.

INDICATIONS AND USAGE

Major Depressive Disorder: Paroxetine hydrochloride extended-release tablets are indicated for the treatment of major depressive disorder.

The efficacy of paroxetine hydrochloride extended-release tablets in the treatment of a major depressive episode was established in two 12 week controlled trials of outpatients whose diagnoses corresponded to the DSM-IV category of major depressive disorder (see CLINICAL PHARMACOLOGY: Clinical Trials).

A major depressive episode (DSM-IV) implies a prominent and relatively persistent (nearly every day for at least 2 weeks) depressed mood or loss of interest or pleasure in nearly all activities, representing a change from previous *functioning* and includes the presence of at least 5 of the following 9 symptoms during the same 2 week period: Depressed mood, markedly diminished interest or pleasure in usual activities, significant change in weight and/or appetite, insomnia or hypersomnia, psychomotor agitation or retardation, increased fatigue, feelings of guilt or worthlessness, slowed thinking or impaired concentration, a suicide attempt or suicidal ideation.

The antidepressant action of paroxetine in hospitalized depressed patients has not been adequately studied.

Paroxetine hydrochloride extended-release tablets have not been systematically evaluated beyond 12 weeks in controlled clinical trials; however, the effectiveness of immediate-release paroxetine hydrochloride in maintaining a response in major depressive disorder for up to one year has been demonstrated in a placebo-controlled trial (see CLINICAL PHARMACOLOGY: Clinical Trials). The physician who elects to use paroxetine hydrochloride extended-release tablets for extended periods should periodically reevaluate the long-term usefulness of the drug for the individual patient.

Panic Disorder: Paroxetine hydrochloride extended-release tablets are indicated for the treatment of panic disorder, with or without agoraphobia, as defined in DSM-IV. Panic disorder is characterized by the occurrence of unexpected panic attacks and associated concern about having additional attacks, worry about the implications or consequences of the attacks, and/or a significant change in behavior related to the attacks.

The efficacy of paroxetine hydrochloride extended-release tablets was established in two 10 week trials in panic disorder patients whose diagnoses corresponded to the DSM-IV category of panic disorder (see CLINICAL PHARMACOLOGY: Clinical Trials).

Panic disorder (DSM-IV) is characterized by recurrent unexpected panic attacks, i.e., a discrete period of intense fear or discomfort in which four (or more) of the following symptoms develop abruptly and reach a peak within 10 minutes: (1) palpitations, pounding heart or accelerated heart rate; (2) sweating; (3) trembling or shaking; (4) sensations of shortness of breath or smothering; (5) feeling of choking; (6) chest pain or discomfort; (7) nausea or abdominal distress; (8) feeling dizzy, unsteady, lightheaded or faint; (9) derealization (feelings of unreality) or depersonalization (being detached from oneself); (10) fear of losing control; (11) fear of dying; (12) paresthesias (numbness or tingling sensations); (13) chills or hot flushes.

Long-term maintenance of efficacy with the immediate-release formulation of paroxetine was demonstrated in a 3 month relapse prevention trial. In this trial, patients with panic disorder assigned to immediate-release paroxetine demonstrated a lower relapse rate compared to patients on placebo (see CLINICAL PHARMACOLOGY: Clinical Trials). Nevertheless, the physician who prescribes paroxetine hydrochloride extended-release tablets for extended periods should periodically reevaluate the long-term usefulness of the drug for the individual patient.

Social Anxiety Disorder: Paroxetine hydrochloride extended-release tablets are indicated for the treatment of social anxiety disorder, also known as social phobia, as defined in DSM-IV (300.23). Social anxiety disorder is characterized by a marked and persistent fear of one or more social or performance situations in which the person is exposed to unfamiliar people or to possible scrutiny by others. Exposure to the feared situation almost invariably provokes anxiety, which may approach the intensity of a panic attack. The feared situations are avoided or endured with intense anxiety or distress. The avoidance, anxious anticipation or distress in the feared situation(s) interferes significantly with the person's normal routine, occupational or academic functioning or social activities or relationships or there is marked distress about having the phobias. Lesser degrees of performance anxiety or shyness generally do not require psychopharmacological treatment.

The efficacy of paroxetine hydrochloride extended-release tablets as a treatment for social anxiety disorder has been established, in part, on the basis of extrapolation from the established effectiveness of the immediate-release formulation of paroxetine. In addition, the efficacy of paroxetine hydrochloride extended-release tablets was established in a 12 week trial, in adult outpatients with social anxiety disorder (DSM-IV). Paroxetine hydrochloride extended-release tablets have not been studied in children or adolescents with social phobia (see CLINICAL PHARMACOLOGY: Clinical Trials).

The effectiveness of paroxetine hydrochloride extended-release tablets in long-term treatment of social anxiety disorder, i.e., for more than 12 weeks, has not been systematically evaluated in adequate and well controlled trials. Therefore, the physician who elects to prescribe paroxetine hydrochloride extended-release tablets for extended periods should periodically reevaluate the long-term usefulness of the drug for the individual patient (see DOSAGE AND ADMINISTRATION).

Premenstrual Dysphoric Disorder: Paroxetine hydrochloride extended-release tablets are indicated for the treatment of PMDD.

The efficacy of paroxetine hydrochloride extended-release tablets in the treatment of PMDD has been established in 3 placebo-controlled trials (see CLINICAL PHARMACOLOGY: Clinical Trials).

The essential features of PMDD, according to DSM-IV, include markedly depressed mood, anxiety or tension, affective lability and persistent anger or irritability. Other features include decreased interest in usual activities, difficulty concentrating, lack of energy, change in appetite or sleep and feeling out of control. Physical symptoms associated with PMDD include breast tenderness, headache, joint and muscle pain, bloating and weight gain. These symptoms occur regularly during the luteal phase and remit within a few days following the onset of menses; the disturbance markedly interferes with work or school or with usual social activities and relationships with others. In making the diagnosis, care should be taken to rule out other cyclical mood disorders that may be exacerbated by treatment with an antidepressant.

The effectiveness of paroxetine hydrochloride extended-release tablets in long-term use, that is, for more than three menstrual cycles, has not been systematically evaluated in controlled trials. Therefore, the physician who elects to use paroxetine hydrochloride extended-release tablets for extended periods should periodically reevaluate the long-term usefulness of the drug for the individual patient.

CONTRAINDICATIONS

Concomitant use in patients taking either monoamine oxidase inhibitors (MAOIs), including linezolid, an antibiotic which is a reversible nonselective MAOI or thioridazine is contraindicated (see WARNINGS and PRECAUTIONS).

Concomitant use in patients taking pimozide is contraindicated (see PRECAUTIONS).

Paroxetine hydrochloride extended-release tablets are contraindicated in patients with a hypersensitivity to paroxetine or to any of the inactive ingredients in paroxetine hydrochloride extended-release tablets.

WARNINGS

Clinical Worsening and Suicide Risk: Patients with major depressive disorder (MDD), both adult and pediatric, may experience worsening of their depression and/or the emergence of suicidal ideation and behavior (suicidality) or unusual changes in behavior, whether or not they are taking antidepressant medications, and this risk may persist until significant remission occurs. Suicide is a known risk of depression and certain other psychiatric disorders and these disorders themselves are the strongest predictors of suicide. There has been a longstanding concern, however, that antidepressants may have a role in inducing worsening of depression and the emergence of suicidality in certain patients during the early phases of treatment. Pooled analyses of short-term placebo-controlled trials of antidepressant drugs (SSRIs and others) showed that these drugs increase the risk of suicidal thinking and behavior (suicidality) in children, adolescents and young adults (ages 18 to 24) with major depressive disorder (MDD) and other psychiatric disorders. Short-term studies did not show an increase in the risk of suicidality with antidepressants compared to placebo in adults beyond age 24; there was a reduction with antidepressants compared to placebo in adults aged 65 and older. The pooled analyses of placebo-controlled trials in children and adolescents with MDD, obsessive compulsive disorder (OCD) or other psychiatric disorders included a total of 24 short-term trials of nine antidepressant drugs in over 4,400 patients. The pooled analyses of placebo-controlled trials in adults with MDD or other psychiatric disorders included a total of 295 short-term trials (median duration of 2 months) of 11 antidepressant drugs in over 77,000 patients. There was considerable variation in risk of suicidality among drugs, but a tendency toward an increase in the younger patients for almost all drugs studied. There were differences in absolute risk of suicidality across the different indications, with the highest incidence in MDD. The risk differences (drug vs. placebo), however, were relatively stable within age strata and across indications. These risk differences (drug-placebo difference in the number of cases of suicidality per 1,000 patients treated) are provided in Table 1.

Table 1	
Age Range	Drug-Placebo Difference in Number of Cases of Suicidality Per 1,000 Patients Treated
Increases Compared to Placebo	
< 18	14 additional cases
18 to 24	5 additional cases
Decreases Compared to Placebo	
25 to 64	1 fewer case
≥ 65	6 fewer cases

No suicides occurred in any of the pediatric trials. There were suicides in the adult trials, but the number was not sufficient to reach any conclusion about drug effect on suicide.

It is unknown whether the suicidality risk extends to longer-term use, i.e., beyond several months. However, there is substantial evidence from placebo-controlled maintenance trials in adults with depression that the use of antidepressants can delay the recurrence of depression.

All patients being treated with antidepressants for any indication should be monitored appropriately and observed closely for clinical worsening, suicidality and unusual changes in behavior, especially during the initial few months of a course of drug therapy or at times of dose changes, either increases or decreases.

The following symptoms, anxiety, agitation, panic attacks, insomnia, irritability, hostility, aggressiveness, impulsivity, akathisia (psychomotor restlessness), hypomania and mania, have been reported in adult and pediatric patients being treated with antidepressants for major depressive disorder as well as for other indications, both psychiatric and nonpsychiatric. Although a causal link between the emergence of such symptoms and either the worsening of depression and/or the emergence of suicidal impulses has not been established, there is concern that such symptoms may represent precursors to emerging suicidality.

Consideration should be given to changing the therapeutic regimen, including possibly discontinuing the medication, in patients whose depression is persistently worse or who are experiencing emergent suicidality or symptoms that might be precursors to worsening depression or suicidality, especially if these symptoms are severe, abrupt in onset or were not part of the patient's presenting symptoms.

If the decision has been made to discontinue treatment, medication should be tapered, as rapidly as is feasible, but with recognition that abrupt discontinuation can be associated with certain symptoms (see PRECAUTIONS and DOSAGE AND ADMINISTRATION: Discontinuation of Treatment with Paroxetine Hydrochloride Extended-Release Tablets, for a description of the risks of discontinuation of paroxetine).

Families and caregivers of patients being treated with antidepressants for major depressive disorder or other indications, both psychiatric and nonpsychiatric, should be alerted about the need to monitor patients for the emergence of agitation, irritability, unusual changes in behavior and the other symptoms described above, as well as the emergence of suicidality and to report such symptoms immediately to healthcare providers. Such monitoring should include daily observation by families and caregivers. Prescriptions for paroxetine should be written for the smallest quantity of tablets consistent with good patient management, in order to reduce the risk of overdose.

Screening Patients for Bipolar Disorder: A major depressive episode may be the initial presentation of bipolar disorder. It is generally believed (though not established in controlled trials) that treating such an episode with an antidepressant alone may increase the likelihood of precipitation of a mixed/manic episode in patients at risk for bipolar disorder. Whether any of the symptoms described above represent such a conversion is unknown. However, prior to initiating treatment with an antidepressant, patients with depressive symptoms should be adequately screened to determine if they are at risk for bipolar disorder; such screening should include a detailed psychiatric history, including a family history of suicide, bipolar disorder and depression. It should be noted that paroxetine is not approved for use in treating bipolar depression.

Potential for Interaction With Monoamine Oxidase Inhibitors: In patients receiving another serotonin reuptake inhibitor drug in combination with an MAOI, there have been reports of serious, sometimes fatal, reactions including hyperthermia, rigidity, myoclonus, autonomic instability with possible rapid fluctuations of vital signs and mental status changes that include extreme agitation progressing to delirium and coma. These reactions have also been reported in patients who have recently discontinued that drug and have been started on an MAOI. Some cases presented with features resembling neuroleptic malignant syndrome. While there are no human data showing such an interaction with paroxetine hydrochloride, limited animal data on the effects of combined use of paroxetine and MAOIs suggest that these drugs may act synergistically to elevate blood pressure and evoke behavioral excitation. Therefore, it is recommended that paroxetine hydrochloride extended-release tablets not be used in combination with an MAOI (including linezolid, an antibiotic which is a reversible non-selective MAOI) or within 14 days of discontinuing treatment with an MAOI (see CONTRAINDICATIONS). At least 2 weeks should be allowed after stopping paroxetine hydrochloride extended-release tablets before starting an MAOI.**

Serotonin Syndrome or Neuroleptic Malignant Syndrome (NMS)-Like Reactions: The development of a potentially life threatening serotonin syndrome or Neuroleptic Malignant Syndrome (NMS)-like reactions have been reported with SNRIs and SSRIs alone, including paroxetine hydrochloride extended-release tablets treatment, but particularly with concomitant use of serotonergic drugs (including triptans) with drugs which impair metabolism of serotonin (including MAOIs) or with antipsychotics or other dopamine antagonists. Serotonin syndrome symptoms may include mental status changes (e.g., agitation, hallucinations, coma), autonomic instability (e.g., tachycardia, labile blood pressure, hyperthermia), neuromuscular aberrations (e.g., hyperreflexia, incoordination) and/or gastrointestinal symptoms (e.g., nausea, vomiting, diarrhea). Serotonin syndrome, in its most severe form can resemble neuroleptic malignant syndrome, which includes hyperthermia, muscle rigidity, autonomic instability with possible rapid fluctuation of vital signs and mental status changes. Patients should be monitored for the emergence of serotonin syndrome or NMS-like signs and symptoms. The concomitant use of paroxetine hydrochloride extended-release tablets with MAOIs intended to treat depression is contraindicated.**

If concomitant treatment of paroxetine hydrochloride extended-release tablets with a 5-hydroxytryptamine receptor agonist (triptan) is clinically warranted, careful observation of the patient is advised, particularly during treatment initiation and dose increases.

The concomitant use of paroxetine hydrochloride extended-release tablets with serotonin precursors (such as tryptophan) is not recommended.

Treatment with paroxetine hydrochloride extended-release tablets and any concomitant serotonergic or antidopaminergic agents, including antipsychotics, should be discontinued immediately if the above events occur and supportive symptomatic treatment should be initiated.

Potential Interaction with Thioridazine: Thioridazine administration alone produces prolongation of the QTc interval, which is associated with serious ventricular arrhythmias, such as Torsade de pointes type arrhythmias and sudden death. This effect appears to be dose related.

An *in vivo* study suggests that drugs which inhibit CYP2D6, such as paroxetine, will elevate plasma levels of thioridazine. Therefore, it is recommended that paroxetine not be used in combination with thioridazine (see CONTRAINDICATIONS and PRECAUTIONS).

Usage in Pregnancy: *Teratogenic Effects:* Epidemiological studies have shown that infants exposed to paroxetine in the first trimester of pregnancy have an increased risk of congenital malformations, particularly cardiovascular malformations. The findings from these studies are summarized below:

- A study based on Swedish national registry data demonstrated that infants exposed to paroxetine during pregnancy (n = 815) had an increased risk of cardiovascular malformations (2% risk in paroxetine-exposed infants) compared to the entire registry population (1% risk), for an odds ratio (OR) of 1.8 (95% confidence interval 1.1 to 2.8). No increase in the risk of overall congenital malformations was seen in the paroxetine-exposed infants. The cardiac malformations in the paroxetine-exposed infants were primarily ventricular septal defects (VSDs) and atrial septal defects (ASDs). Septal defects range in severity from those that resolve spontaneously to those which require surgery.
- A separate retrospective cohort study from the United States (United Healthcare data) evaluated 5,956 infants of mothers dispensed antidepressants during the first trimester (n = 815 for paroxetine). This study showed a trend towards an increased risk for cardiovascular malformations for paroxetine (risk of 1.5%) compared to other antidepressants (risk of 1%), for an OR of 1.5 (95% confidence interval 0.8 to 2.9). Of the 12 paroxetine-exposed infants with cardiovascular malformations, nine had VSDs. This study also suggested an increased risk of overall major congenital malformations including cardiovascular defects for paroxetine (4% risk) compared to other (2% risk) antidepressants (OR 1.8; 95% confidence interval 1.2 to 2.8).
- Two large case control studies using separate databases, each with > 9,000 birth defect cases and > 4,000 controls, found that maternal use of paroxetine during the first trimester of pregnancy was associated with a 2- to 3-fold increased risk of right ventricular outflow tract obstructions. In one study the OR was 2.5 (95% confidence interval, 1 to 6, seven exposed infants) and in the other study the OR was 3.3 (95% confidence interval, 1.3 to 8.8, six exposed infants).

Other studies have found varying results as to whether there was an increased risk of overall, cardiovascular or specific congenital malformations. A meta-analysis of epidemiological data over a 16-year period (1992 to 2008) on first trimester paroxetine use in pregnancy and congenital malformations included the above-noted studies in addition to others (n = 17 studies that included overall malformations and n = 14 studies that included cardiovascular malformations; n = 20 distinct studies). While subject to limitations, this meta-analysis suggested an increased occurrence of cardiovascular malformations (prevalence odds ratio [POR] 1.5; 95% confidence interval 1.2 to 1.9) and overall malformations (POR 1.2; 95% confidence interval 1.1 to 1.4) with paroxetine use during the first trimester. It was not possible in this meta-analysis to determine the extent to which the observed prevalence of cardiovascular malformations might have contributed to that of overall malformations, nor was it possible to determine whether any specific types of cardiovascular malformations might have contributed to the observed prevalence of all cardiovascular malformations.

If a patient becomes pregnant while taking paroxetine, she should be advised of the potential harm to the fetus. Unless the benefits of paroxetine to the mother justify continuing treatment, consideration should be given to either discontinuing paroxetine therapy or switching to another antidepressant (see PRECAUTIONS: General: Discontinuation of Treatment with Paroxetine Hydrochloride Extended-release Tablets). For women who intend to become pregnant or are in their first trimester of pregnancy, paroxetine should only be initiated after consideration of the other available treatment options.

Animal Findings: Reproduction studies were performed at doses up to 50 mg/kg/day in rats and 6 mg/kg/day in rabbits administered during organogenesis. These doses are approximately 8 (rat) and 2 (rabbit) times the maximum recommended human dose (MRHD) on a mg/m² basis. These studies have revealed no evidence of teratogenic effects. However, in rats, there was an increase in pup deaths during the first 4 days of lactation when dosing occurred during the last trimester of gestation and continued throughout lactation. This effect occurred at a dose of 1 mg/kg/day or approximately one-sixth of the MRHD on a mg/m² basis. The no effect dose for rat pup mortality was not determined. The cause of these deaths is not known.

Nonteratogenic Effects: Neonates exposed to paroxetine hydrochloride extended-release tablets and other SSRIs or serotonin and norepinephrine reuptake inhibitors (SNRIs), late in the third trimester have developed complications requiring prolonged hospitalization, respiratory support, and tube feeding. Such complications can arise immediately upon delivery. Reported clinical findings have included respiratory distress, cyanosis, apnea, seizures, temperature instability, feeding difficulty, vomiting, hypoglycemia, hypotonia, hypertonia, hyperreflexia, tremor, jitteriness, irritability and constant crying. These features are consistent with either a direct toxic effect of SSRIs and SNRIs or, possibly, a drug discontinuation syndrome. It should be noted that, in some cases, the clinical picture is consistent with serotonin syndrome (see WARNINGS: Potential for Interaction with Monoamine Oxidase Inhibitors).

Infants exposed to SSRIs in late pregnancy may have an increased risk for persistent pulmonary hypertension of the newborn (PPHN). PPHN occurs in 1 to 2 per 1,000 live births in the general population and is associated with substantial neonatal morbidity and mortality. In a retrospective case control study of 377 women whose infants were born with PPHN and 836 women whose infants were born healthy, the risk for developing PPHN was approximately 6-fold higher for infants exposed to SSRIs after the 20th week of gestation compared to infants who had not been exposed to antidepressants during pregnancy. There is currently no corroborative evidence regarding the risk for PPHN following exposure to SSRIs in pregnancy; this is the first study that has investigated the potential risk. The study did not include enough cases with exposure to individual SSRIs to determine if all SSRIs posed similar levels of PPHN risk.

There have also been post-marketing reports of premature births in pregnant women exposed to paroxetine or other SSRIs.

When treating a pregnant woman with paroxetine during the third trimester, the physician should carefully consider both the potential risks and benefits of treatment (see DOSAGE AND ADMINISTRATION). Physicians should note that in a prospective longitudinal study of 201 women with a history of major depression who were euthymic at the beginning of pregnancy, women who discontinued antidepressant medication during pregnancy were more likely to experience a relapse of major depression than women who continued antidepressant medication.

PRECAUTIONS

General: *Activation of Mania/Hypomania:* During premarketing testing of immediate-release paroxetine hydrochloride, hypomania or mania occurred in approximately 1% of paroxetine-treated unipolar patients compared to 1.1% of active control and 0.3% of placebo-treated unipolar patients. In a subset of patients classified as bipolar, the rate of manic episodes was 2.2% for immediate-release paroxetine and 11.6% for the combined active control groups. Among 1,627 patients with major depressive disorder, panic disorder, social anxiety disorder or PMDD treated with paroxetine hydrochloride extended-release tablets in controlled clinical studies, there were no reports of mania or hypomania. As with all drugs effective in the treatment of major depressive disorder, paroxetine hydrochloride extended-release tablets should be used cautiously in patients with a history of mania.

Seizures: During premarketing testing of immediate-release paroxetine hydrochloride, seizures occurred in 0.1% of paroxetine-treated patients, a rate similar to that associated with other drugs effective in the treatment of major depressive disorder. Among 1,627 patients who received paroxetine hydrochloride extended-release tablets in controlled clinical trials in major depressive disorder, panic disorder, social anxiety disorder or PMDD, one patient (0.1%) experienced a seizure. Paroxetine hydrochloride extended-release tablets should be used cautiously in patients with a history of seizures. It should be discontinued in any patient who develops seizures.

Discontinuation of Treatment with Paroxetine Hydrochloride Extended-Release Tablets: Adverse events while discontinuing therapy with paroxetine hydrochloride extended-release tablets were not systematically evaluated in most clinical trials; however, in recent placebo-controlled clinical trials utilizing daily doses of paroxetine hydrochloride extended-release tablets up to 37.5 mg/day, spontaneously reported adverse events while discontinuing therapy with paroxetine hydrochloride extended-release tablets were evaluated. Patients receiving 37.5 mg/day underwent an incremental decrease in the daily dose by 12.5 mg/day to a dose of 25 mg/day for one week before treatment was stopped. For patients receiving 25 mg/day or 12.5 mg/day, treatment was stopped without an incremental decrease in dose. With this regimen in those studies, the following adverse events were reported for paroxetine hydrochloride extended-release tablets, at an incidence of 2% or greater for paroxetine hydrochloride extended-release tablets and were at least twice that reported for placebo: Dizziness, nausea, nervousness and additional symptoms described by the investigator as associated with tapering or discontinuing paroxetine hydrochloride extended-release tablets (e.g., emotional lability, headache, agitation, electric shock sensations, fatigue and sleep disturbances). These events were reported as serious in 0.3% of patients who discontinued therapy with paroxetine hydrochloride extended-release tablets.

During marketing of paroxetine hydrochloride extended-release tablets and other SSRIs and SNRIs, there have been spontaneous reports of adverse events occurring upon discontinuation of these drugs (particularly when abrupt), including the following: Dysphoric mood, irritability, agitation, dizziness, sensory disturbances (e.g., paresthesias such as electric shock sensations and tinnitus), anxiety, confusion, headache, lethargy, emotional lability, insomnia and hypomania. While these events are generally self limiting, there have been reports of serious discontinuation symptoms.

Patients should be monitored for these symptoms when discontinuing treatment with paroxetine hydrochloride extended-release tablets. A gradual reduction in the dose rather than abrupt cessation is recommended whenever possible. If intolerable symptoms occur following a decrease in the dose or upon discontinuation of treatment, then resuming the previously prescribed dose may be considered. Subsequently, the physician may continue decreasing the dose but at a more gradual rate (see DOSAGE AND ADMINISTRATION).

See also PRECAUTIONS: Pediatric Use, for adverse events reported upon discontinuation of treatment with paroxetine in pediatric patients.

Akathisia: The use of paroxetine or other SSRIs has been associated with the development of akathisia, which is characterized by an inner sense of restlessness and psychomotor agitation such as an inability to sit or stand still usually associated with subjective distress. This is most likely to occur within the first few weeks of treatment.

Hyponatremia: Hyponatremia may occur as a result of treatment with SSRIs and SNRIs, including paroxetine hydrochloride extended-release tablets. In many cases, this hyponatremia appears to be the result of the syndrome of inappropriate antidiuretic hormone secretion (SIADH). Cases with serum sodium lower than 110 mmol/L have been reported. Elderly patients may be at greater risk of developing hyponatremia with SSRIs and SNRIs. Also, patients taking diuretics or who are otherwise volume depleted may be at greater risk (see Geriatric Use). Discontinuation of paroxetine hydrochloride extended-release tablets should be considered in patients with symptomatic hyponatremia and appropriate medical intervention should be instituted. Signs and symptoms of hyponatremia include headache, difficulty concentrating, memory impairment, confusion, weakness and unsteadiness, which may lead to falls. Signs and symptoms associated with more severe and/or acute cases have included hallucination, syncope, seizure, coma, respiratory arrest and death.

Abnormal Bleeding: SSRIs and SNRIs, including paroxetine, may increase the risk of bleeding events. Concomitant use of aspirin, nonsteroidal anti-inflammatory drugs, warfarin and other anticoagulants may add to this risk. Case reports and epidemiological studies (case control and cohort design) have demonstrated an association between use of drugs that interfere with serotonin reuptake and the occurrence of gastrointestinal bleeding. Bleeding events related to SSRIs and SNRIs use have ranged from ecchymoses, hematomas, epistaxis and petechiae to life threatening hemorrhages. Patients should be cautioned about the risk of bleeding associated with the concomitant use of paroxetine and NSAIDs, aspirin or other drugs that affect coagulation.

Use in Patients with Concomitant Illness: Clinical experience with immediate-release paroxetine hydrochloride in patients with certain concomitant systemic illness is limited. Caution is advisable in using paroxetine hydrochloride extended-release tablets in patients with diseases or conditions that could affect metabolism or hemodynamic responses.

As with other SSRIs, mydriasis has been infrequently reported in premarketing studies with paroxetine hydrochloride. A few cases of acute angle closure glaucoma associated with therapy with immediate-release paroxetine have been reported in the literature. As mydriasis can cause acute angle closure in patients with narrow angle glaucoma, caution should be used when paroxetine hydrochloride extended-release tablets are prescribed for patients with narrow angle glaucoma.

Paroxetine hydrochloride extended-release tablets or the immediate-release formulation has not been evaluated or used to any appreciable extent in patients with a recent history of myocardial infarction or unstable heart disease. Patients with these diagnoses were excluded from clinical studies during premarket testing. Evaluation of electrocardiograms of 682 patients who received immediate-release paroxetine hydrochloride in double-blind, placebo-controlled trials, however, did not indicate that paroxetine is associated with the development of significant ECG abnormalities. Similarly, paroxetine hydrochloride does not cause any clinically important changes in heart rate or blood pressure. Increased plasma concentrations of paroxetine occur in patients with severe renal impairment (creatinine clearance < 30 mL/min.) or severe hepatic impairment. A lower starting dose should be used in such patients (see DOSAGE AND ADMINISTRATION).

Information for Patients: Paroxetine hydrochloride extended-release tablets should not be chewed or crushed and should be swallowed whole.

Patients should be cautioned about the risk of serotonin syndrome with the concomitant use of paroxetine and triptans, tramadol or other serotonergic agents.

Prescribers or other health professionals should inform patients, their families and their caregivers about the benefits and risks associated with treatment with paroxetine and should counsel them in its appropriate use. A patient Medication Guide about "Antidepressant Medicines, Depression and other Serious Mental Illness and Suicidal Thoughts or Actions" is available for paroxetine. The prescriber or health professional should instruct patients, their families and their caregivers to read the Medication Guide and should assist them in understanding its contents. Patients should be given the opportunity to discuss the contents of the Medication Guide and to obtain answers to any questions they may have. The complete text of the Medication Guide is reprinted at the end of this document.

Patients should be advised of the following issues and asked to alert their prescriber if these occur while taking paroxetine.

Clinical Worsening and Suicide Risk: Patients, their families and their caregivers should be encouraged to be alert to the emergence of anxiety, agitation, panic attacks, insomnia, irritability, hostility, aggressiveness, impulsivity, akathisia (psychomotor restlessness), hypomania, mania, other unusual changes in behavior, worsening of depression and suicidal ideation, especially early during antidepressant treatment and when the dose is adjusted up or down. Families and caregivers of patients should be advised to look for the emergence of such symptoms on a day to day basis, since changes may be abrupt. Such symptoms should be reported to the patient's prescriber or health professional, especially if they are severe, abrupt in onset or were not part of the patient's presenting symptoms. Symptoms such as these may be associated with an increased risk for suicidal thinking and behavior and indicate a need for very close monitoring and possibly changes in the medication.

Drugs That Interfere with Hemostasis (e.g., NSAIDs, Aspirin and Warfarin): Patients should be cautioned about the concomitant use of paroxetine and NSAIDs, aspirin, warfarin or other drugs that affect coagulation since the combined use of psychotropic drugs that interfere with serotonin reuptake and these agents has been associated with an increased risk of bleeding.

Interference with Cognitive and Motor Performance: Any psychoactive drug may impair judgment, thinking or motor skills. Although in controlled studies immediate-release paroxetine hydrochloride has not been shown to impair psychomotor performance, patients should be cautioned about operating hazardous machinery, including automobiles, until they are reasonably certain that therapy with paroxetine hydrochloride extended-release tablets does not affect their ability to engage in such activities.

Completing Course of Therapy: While patients may notice improvement with use of paroxetine hydrochloride extended-release tablets in 1 to 4 weeks, they should be advised to continue therapy as directed.

Concomitant Medications: Patients should be advised to inform their physician if they are taking or plan to take, any prescription or over-the-counter drugs, since there is a potential for interactions.

Alcohol: Although immediate-release paroxetine hydrochloride has not been shown to increase the impairment of mental and motor skills caused by alcohol, patients should be advised to avoid alcohol while taking paroxetine hydrochloride extended-release tablets.

Pregnancy: Patients should be advised to notify their physician if they become pregnant or intend to become pregnant during therapy (see WARNINGS: Usage in Pregnancy: *Teratogenic* and *Nonteratogenic Effects*).

Nursing: Patients should be advised to notify their physician if they are breast-feeding an infant (see PRECAUTIONS: Nursing Mothers).

Laboratory Tests: There are no specific laboratory tests recommended.

Drug Interactions: *Tryptophan:* As with other serotonin reuptake inhibitors, an interaction between paroxetine and tryptophan may occur when they are coadministered. Adverse experiences, consisting primarily of headache, nausea, sweating and dizziness, have been reported when tryptophan was administered to patients taking immediate-release paroxetine. Consequently, concomitant use of paroxetine hydrochloride extended-release tablets with tryptophan is not recommended (see WARNINGS: Potential for Interaction with Monoamine Oxidase Inhibitors: *Serotonin Syndrome*).

Monoamine Oxidase Inhibitors: See CONTRAINDICATIONS and WARNINGS.

Pimozide: In a controlled study of healthy volunteers, after immediate-release paroxetine hydrochloride was titrated to 60 mg daily, coadministration of a single-dose of 2 mg pimozide was associated with mean increases in pimozide AUC of 151% and C_{max} of 62%, compared to pimozide administered alone. The increase in pimozide AUC and C_{max} is due to the CYP2D6 inhibitory properties of paroxetine. Due to the narrow therapeutic index of pimozide and its known ability to prolong the QT interval, concomitant use of pimozide and paroxetine hydrochloride extended-release tablets are contraindicated (see CONTRAINDICATIONS).

Serotonergic Drugs: Based on the mechanism of action of SNRIs and SSRIs, including paroxetine hydrochloride and the potential for serotonin syndrome, caution is advised when paroxetine hydrochloride extended-release tablets are coadministered with other drugs that may affect the serotonergic neurotransmitter systems, such as triptans, linezolid (an antibiotic which is a reversible nonselective MAOI), lithium, tramadol or St. John's Wort (see WARNINGS: Potential for Interaction with Monoamine Oxidase Inhibitors: *Serotonin Syndrome*). The concomitant use of paroxetine extended-release tablets with MAOIs (including linezolid) is contraindicated (see CONTRAINDICATIONS). The concomitant use of paroxetine extended-release tablets with other SSRI's, SNRIs or tryptophan is not recommended (see PRECAUTIONS: Drug Interactions: *Tryptophan*).

Thioridazine: See CONTRAINDICATIONS and WARNINGS.

Warfarin: Preliminary data suggest that there may be a pharmacodynamic interaction (that causes an increased bleeding diathesis in the face of unaltered prothrombin time) between paroxetine and warfarin. Since there is little clinical experience, the concomitant administration of paroxetine hydrochloride extended-release tablets and warfarin should be undertaken with caution (see PRECAUTIONS: Information for Patients: *Drugs That Interfere with Hemostasis*).

Triptans: There have been rare post-marketing reports of serotonin syndrome with the use of an SSRI and a triptan. If concomitant use of paroxetine hydrochloride extended-release tablets with a triptan is clinically warranted, careful observation of the patient is advised, particularly during treatment initiation and dose increases (see WARNINGS:

Potential for Interaction with Monoamine Oxidase Inhibitors: *Serotonin Syndrome*).

Drugs Affecting Hepatic Metabolism: The metabolism and pharmacokinetics of paroxetine may be affected by the induction or inhibition of drug-metabolizing enzymes.

Cimetidine: Cimetidine inhibits many cytochrome P450 (oxidative) enzymes. In a study where immediate-release paroxetine (30 mg once daily) was dosed orally for 4 weeks, steady-state plasma concentrations of paroxetine were increased by approximately 50% during coadministration with oral cimetidine (300 mg three times daily) for the final week. Therefore, when these drugs are administered concurrently, dosage adjustment of paroxetine hydrochloride extended-release tablets after the starting dose should be guided by clinical effect. The effect of paroxetine on cimetidine's pharmacokinetics was not studied.

Phenobarbital: Phenobarbital induces many cytochrome P$_{450}$ (oxidative) enzymes. When a single oral 30 mg dose of immediate-release paroxetine was administered at phenobarbital steady-state (100 mg once daily for 14 days), paroxetine AUC and T$_{1/2}$ were reduced (by an average of 25% and 38%, respectively) compared to paroxetine administered alone. The effect of paroxetine on phenobarbital pharmacokinetics was not studied. Since paroxetine exhibits nonlinear pharmacokinetics, the results of this study may not address the case where the two drugs are both being chronically dosed. No initial dosage adjustment with paroxetine hydrochloride extended-release tablets is considered necessary when coadministered with phenobarbital; any subsequent adjustment should be guided by clinical effect.

Phenytoin: When a single oral 30 mg dose of immediate-release paroxetine was administered at phenytoin steady-state (300 mg once daily for 14 days), paroxetine AUC and T$_{1/2}$ were reduced (by an average of 50% and 35%, respectively) compared to immediate-release paroxetine administered alone. In a separate study, when a single oral 300 mg dose of phenytoin was administered at paroxetine steady-state (30 mg once daily for 14 days), phenytoin AUC was slightly reduced (12% on average) compared to phenytoin administered alone. Since both drugs exhibit nonlinear pharmacokinetics, the above studies may not address the case where the two drugs are both being chronically dosed. No initial dosage adjustments are considered necessary when paroxetine hydrochloride extended-release tablets are coadministered with phenytoin; any subsequent adjustments should be guided by clinical effect (see ADVERSE REACTIONS: Post-marketing Reports).

Drugs Metabolized by CYP2D6: Many drugs, including most drugs effective in the treatment of major depressive disorder (paroxetine, other SSRIs and many tricyclics), are metabolized by the cytochrome P$_{450}$ isozyme CYP2D6. Like other agents that are metabolized by CYP2D6, paroxetine may significantly inhibit the activity of this isozyme. In most patients (> 90%), this CYP2D6 isozyme is saturated early during paroxetine dosing. In one study, daily dosing of immediate-release paroxetine (20 mg once daily) under steady-state conditions increased single dose desipramine (100 mg) C$_{max}$, AUC and T$_{1/2}$ by an average of approximately 2-, 5- and 3-fold, respectively. Concomitant use of paroxetine with risperidone, a CYP2D6 substrate has also been evaluated. In one study, daily dosing of paroxetine 20 mg in patients stabilized on risperidone (4 to 8 mg/day) increased mean plasma concentrations of risperidone approximately 4-fold, decreased 9-hydroxyrisperidone concentrations approximately 10% and increased concentrations of the active moiety (the sum of risperidone plus 9-hydroxyrisperidone) approximately 1.4-fold. The effect of paroxetine on the pharmacokinetics of atomoxetine has been evaluated when both drugs were at steady-state. In healthy volunteers who were extensive metabolizers of CYP2D6, paroxetine 20 mg daily was given in combination with 20 mg atomoxetine every 12 hours. This resulted in increases in steady-state atomoxetine AUC values that were 6- to 8-fold greater and in atomoxetine C$_{max}$ values that were 3- to 4-fold greater than when atomoxetine was given alone. Dosage adjustment of atomoxetine may be necessary and it is recommended that atomoxetine be initiated at a reduced dose when given with paroxetine.

Concomitant use of paroxetine hydrochloride extended-release tablets with other drugs metabolized by cytochrome CYP2D6 has not been formally studied but may require lower doses than usually prescribed for either paroxetine hydrochloride extended-release tablets or the other drug.

Therefore, coadministration of paroxetine hydrochloride extended-release tablets with other drugs that are metabolized by this isozyme, including certain drugs effective in the treatment of major depressive disorder (e.g., nortriptyline, amitriptyline, imipramine, desipramine and fluoxetine), phenothiazines, risperidone, tamoxifen and Type 1C antiarrhythmics (e.g., propafenone, flecainide and encainide) or that inhibit this enzyme (e.g., quinidine), should be approached with caution.

However, due to the risk of serious ventricular arrhythmias and sudden death potentially associated with elevated plasma levels of thioridazine, paroxetine and thioridazine should not be coadministered (see CONTRAINDICATIONS and WARNINGS).

Tamoxifen is a prodrug requiring metabolic activation by CYP2D6. Inhibition of CYP2D6 by paroxetine may lead to reduced plasma concentrations of an active metabolite and hence reduced efficacy of tamoxifen.

At steady-state, when the CYP2D6 pathway is essentially saturated, paroxetine clearance is governed by alternative P$_{450}$ isozymes that, unlike CYP2D6, show no evidence of saturation (see PRECAUTIONS: Drug Interactions: *Tricyclic Antidepressants*).

Drugs Metabolized by Cytochrome CYP3A4: An *in vivo* interaction study involving the coadministration under steady-state conditions of paroxetine and terfenadine, a substrate for CYP3A4, revealed no effect of paroxetine on terfenadine pharmacokinetics. In addition, *in vitro* studies have shown ketoconazole, a potent inhibitor of CYP3A4 activity, to be at least 100 times more potent than paroxetine as an inhibitor of the metabolism of several substrates for this enzyme, including terfenadine, astemizole, cisapride, triazolam and cyclosporine. Based on the assumption that the relationship between paroxetine's *in vitro* K$_i$ and its lack of effect on terfenadine's *in vivo* clearance predicts its effect on other CYP3A4 substrates, paroxetine's extent of inhibition of CYP3A4 activity is not likely to be of clinical significance.

Tricyclic Antidepressants (TCAs): Caution is indicated in the coadministration of TCAs with paroxetine hydrochloride extended-release tablets, because paroxetine may inhibit TCA metabolism. Plasma TCA concentrations may need to be monitored and the dose of TCA may need to be reduced, if a TCA is coadministered with paroxetine hydrochloride extended-release tablets (see PRECAUTIONS: Drug Interactions: *Drugs Metabolized by Cytochrome CYP2D6*).

Drugs Highly Bound to Plasma Protein: Because paroxetine is highly bound to plasma protein, administration of paroxetine hydrochloride extended-release tablets to a patient taking another drug that is highly protein bound may cause increased free concentrations of the other drug, potentially resulting in adverse events. Conversely, adverse effects could result from displacement of paroxetine by other highly bound drugs.

Drugs That Interfere with Hemostasis (e.g., NSAIDs, Aspirin and Warfarin): Serotonin release by platelets plays an important role in hemostasis. Epidemiological studies of the case control and cohort design that have demonstrated an association between use of psychotropic drugs that interfere with serotonin reuptake and the occurrence of upper gastrointestinal bleeding have also shown that concurrent use of an NSAID or aspirin may potentiate this risk of bleeding. Altered anticoagulant effects, including increased bleeding, have been reported when SSRIs or SNRIs are coadministered with warfarin. Patients receiving warfarin therapy should be carefully monitored when paroxetine is initiated or discontinued.

Alcohol: Although paroxetine does not increase the impairment of mental and motor skills caused by alcohol, patients should be advised to avoid alcohol while taking paroxetine hydrochloride extended-release tablets.

Lithium: A multiple-dose study with immediate-release paroxetine hydrochloride has shown that there is no pharmacokinetic interaction between paroxetine and lithium carbonate. However, due to the potential for serotonin syndrome, caution is advised when immediate-release paroxetine hydrochloride is coadministered with lithium.

Digoxin: The steady-state pharmacokinetics of paroxetine was not altered when administered with digoxin at steady-state. Mean digoxin AUC at steady-state decreased by 15% in the presence of paroxetine. Since there is little clinical experience, the concurrent administration of paroxetine hydrochloride extended-release tablets and digoxin should be undertaken with caution.

Diazepam: Under steady-state conditions, diazepam does not appear to affect paroxetine kinetics. The effects of paroxetine on diazepam were not evaluated.

Procyclidine: Daily oral dosing of immediate-release paroxetine (30 mg once daily) increased steady-state AUC$_{0-24}$, C$_{max}$, and C$_{min}$ values of procyclidine (5 mg oral once daily) by 35%, 37% and 67%, respectively, compared to procyclidine alone at steady-state. If anticholinergic effects are seen, the dose of procyclidine should be reduced.

Beta-Blockers: In a study where propranolol (80 mg twice daily) was dosed orally for 18 days, the established steady-state plasma concentrations of propranolol were unaltered during coadministration with immediate-release paroxetine (30 mg once daily) for the final 10 days. The effects of propranolol on paroxetine have not been evaluated (see ADVERSE REACTIONS: Post-marketing Reports).

Theophylline: Reports of elevated theophylline levels associated with immediate-release paroxetine treatment have been reported. While this interaction has not been formally studied, it is recommended that theophylline levels be monitored when these drugs are concurrently administered.

Fosamprenavir/Ritonavir: Coadministration of fosamprenavir/ritonavir with paroxetine significantly decreased plasma levels of paroxetine. Any dose adjustment should be guided by clinical effect (tolerability and efficacy).

Electroconvulsive Therapy (ECT): There are no clinical studies of the combined use of ECT and paroxetine hydrochloride extended-release tablets.

Carcinogenesis, Mutagenesis, Impairment of Fertility:
Carcinogenesis: Two year carcinogenicity studies were conducted in rodents given paroxetine in the diet at 1, 5 and 25 mg/kg/day (mice) and 1, 5 and 20 mg/kg/day (rats). These doses are up to approximately 2 (mouse) and 3 (rat) times the (MRHD) on a mg/m^2 basis. There was a significantly greater number of male rats in the high-dose group with reticulum cell sarcomas (1/100, 0/50, 0/50 and 4/50 for control, low-, middle-, and high-dose groups, respectively) and a significantly increased linear trend across dose groups for the occurrence of lymphoreticular tumors in male rats. Female rats were not affected. Although there was a dose related increase in the number of tumors in mice, there was no drug-related increase in the number of mice with tumors. The relevance of these findings to humans is unknown.

Mutagenesis: Paroxetine produced no genotoxic effects in a battery of five *in vitro* and two *in vivo* assays that included the following: Bacterial mutation assay, mouse lymphoma mutation assay, unscheduled DNA synthesis assay and tests for cytogenetic aberrations *in vivo* in mouse bone marrow and *in vitro* in human lymphocytes and in a dominant lethal test in rats.

Impairment of Fertility: A reduced pregnancy rate was found in reproduction studies in rats at a dose of paroxetine of 15 mg/kg/day, which is approximately twice the MRHD on a mg/m^2 basis. Irreversible lesions occurred in the reproductive tract of male rats after dosing in toxicity studies for 2 to 52 weeks. These lesions consisted of vacuolation of epididymal tubular epithelium at 50 mg/kg/day and atrophic changes in the seminiferous tubules of the testes with arrested spermatogenesis at 25 mg/kg/day (approximately 8 and 4 times the MRHD on a mg/m^2 basis).

Pregnancy: ***Pregnancy Category D:*** See WARNINGS: Usage in Pregnancy: *Teratogenic and Nonteratogenic Effects:*.

Labor and Delivery: The effect of paroxetine on labor and delivery in humans is unknown.

Nursing Mothers: Like many other drugs, paroxetine is secreted in human milk and caution should be exercised when paroxetine hydrochloride extended-release tablets are administered to a nursing woman.

Pediatric Use: Safety and effectiveness in the pediatric population have not been established (see BOX WARNING and WARNINGS: Clinical Worsening and Suicide Risk). Three placebo-controlled trials in 752 pediatric patients with MDD have been conducted with paroxetine hydrochloride and the data were not sufficient to support a claim for use in pediatric patients. Anyone considering the use of paroxetine hydrochloride extended-release tablets in a child or adolescent must balance the potential risks with the clinical need.

In placebo-controlled clinical trials conducted with pediatric patients, the following adverse events were reported in at least 2% of pediatric patients treated with immediate-release paroxetine hydrochloride and occurred at a rate at least twice that for pediatric patients receiving placebo: emotional lability (including self harm, suicidal thoughts, attempted suicide, crying and mood fluctuations), hostility, decreased appetite, tremor, sweating, hyperkinesia and agitation.

Events reported upon discontinuation of treatment with immediate-release paroxetine hydrochloride in the pediatric clinical trials that included a taper phase regimen, which occurred in at least 2% of patients who received immediate-release paroxetine hydrochloride and which occurred at a rate at least twice that of placebo, were: emotional lability (including suicidal ideation, suicide attempt, mood changes and tearfulness), nervousness, dizziness, nausea and abdominal pain (see DOSAGE AND ADMINISTRATION: Discontinuation of Treatment with Paroxetine Hydrochloride Extended-Release Tablets).

Geriatric Use: SSRIs and SNRIs, including paroxetine, have been associated with cases of clinically significant hyponatremia in elderly patients, who may be at greater risk for this adverse event (see PRECAUTIONS: Hyponatremia).

In worldwide premarketing clinical trials with immediate-release paroxetine hydrochloride, 17% of paroxetine-treated patients (approximately 700) were 65 years or older. Pharmacokinetic studies revealed a decreased clearance in the elderly and a lower starting dose is recommended; there were, however, no overall differences in the adverse event profile between elderly and younger patients and effectiveness was similar in younger and older patients (see CLINICAL PHARMACOLOGY and DOSAGE AND ADMINISTRATION).

In a controlled study focusing specifically on elderly patients with major depressive disorder, paroxetine hydrochloride extended-release tablets were demonstrated to be safe and effective in the treatment of elderly patients (> 60 years) with major depressive disorder. (See CLINICAL PHARMACOLOGY: Clinical Trials and ADVERSE REACTIONS: Table 3.)

ADVERSE REACTIONS

The information included under the "Adverse Findings Observed in Short-Term, Placebo-Controlled Trials with Paroxetine Hydrochloride Extended-Release Tablets" subsection of ADVERSE REACTIONS is based on data from eleven placebo-controlled clinical trials. Three of these studies were conducted in patients with major depressive disorder, three studies were done in patients with panic disorder, one study was conducted in patients with social anxiety disorder and four studies were done in female patients with PMDD. Two of the studies in major depressive disorder, which enrolled patients in the age range 18 to 65 years, are pooled. Information from a third study of major depressive disorder, which focused on elderly patients (60 to 88 years), is presented separately as is the information from the panic disorder studies and the information from the PMDD studies. Information on additional adverse events associated with paroxetine hydrochloride extended-release tablets and the immediate-release formulation of paroxetine hydrochloride is included in a separate subsection (see Other Events Observed During the Clinical Development of Paroxetine).

Adverse Findings Observed in Short-Term, Placebo-Controlled Trials With Paroxetine Hydrochloride Extended-Release Tablets: *Adverse Events Associated With Discontinuation of Treatment:* *Major Depressive Disorder:* Ten percent (21/212) of patients treated with paroxetine hydrochloride extended-release tablets discontinued treatment due to an adverse event in a pool of two studies of patients with major depressive disorder. The most common events (≥ 1%) associated with discontinuation and considered to be drug-related (i.e., those events associated with dropout at a rate approximately twice or greater for paroxetine hydrochloride extended-release tablets compared to placebo) included the following:

	Paroxetine Hydrochloride Extended-Release Tablets (n = 212)	Placebo (n = 211)
Nausea	3.7%	0.5%
Asthenia	1.9%	0.5%
Dizziness	1.4%	0%
Somnolence	1.4%	0%

In a placebo-controlled study of elderly patients with major depressive disorder, 13% (13/104) of patients treated with paroxetine hydrochloride extended-release tablets discontinued due to an adverse event. Events meeting the above criteria included the following:

	Paroxetine Hydrochloride Extended-Release Tablets (n = 104)	Placebo (n = 109)
Nausea	2.9%	0%
Headache	1.9%	0.9%
Depression	1.9%	0%
LFT's abnormal	1.9%	0%

Panic Disorder: Eleven percent (50/444) of patients treated with paroxetine hydrochloride extended-release tablets in panic disorder studies discontinued treatment due to an adverse event. Events meeting the above criteria included the following:

	Paroxetine Hydrochloride Extended-Release Tablets (n = 444)	Placebo (n = 445)
Nausea	2.9%	0.4%
Insomnia	1.8%	0%
Headache	1.4%	0.2%
Asthenia	1.1%	0%

Social Anxiety Disorder: Three percent (5/186) of patients treated with paroxetine hydrochloride extended-release tablets in the social anxiety disorder study discontinued treatment due to an adverse event. Events meeting the above criteria included the following:

	Paroxetine Hydrochloride Extended-Release Tablets 25 mg (n = 348)	Paroxetine Hydrochloride Extended-Release Tablets 12.5 mg (n = 333)	Placebo (n = 349)
TOTAL	15%	9.9%	6.3%
Nausea*	6%	2.4%	0.9%
Asthenia	4.9%	3%	1.4%
Somnolence*	4.3%	1.8%	0.3%
Insomnia	2.3%	1.5%	0%
Concentration Impaired*	2%	0.6%	0.3%
Dry mouth*	2%	0.6%	0.3%
Dizziness*	1.7%	0.6%	0.6%
Decreased Appetite*	1.4%	0.6%	0%
Sweating*	1.4%	0%	0.3%
Tremor*	1.4%	0.3%	0%
Yawn*	1.1%	0%	0%
Diarrhea	0.9%	1.2%	0%

*Events considered to be dose dependent are defined as events having an incidence rate with 25 mg of paroxetine hydrochloride extended-release tablets that was at least twice that with 12.5 mg of paroxetine hydrochloride extended-release tablets (as well as the placebo group).

	Paroxetine Hydrochloride Extended-Release Tablets (n = 186)	Placebo (n = 184)
Nausea	2.2%	0.5%
Headache	1.6%	0.5%
Diarrhea	1.1%	0.5%

Premenstrual Dysphoric Disorder: Spontaneously reported adverse events were monitored in studies of both continuous and intermittent dosing of paroxetine hydrochloride extended-release tablets in the treatment of PMDD. Generally, there were few differences in the adverse event profiles of the two dosing regimens. Thirteen percent (88/681) of patients treated with paroxetine hydrochloride extended-release tablets in PMDD studies of continuous dosing discontinued treatment due to an adverse event.

The most common events (≥ 1%) associated with discontinuation in either group treated with paroxetine hydrochloride extended-release tablets with an incidence rate that is at least twice that of placebo in PMDD trials that employed a continuous dosing regimen are shown in the following table. This table also shows those events that were dose dependent (indicated with an asterisk) as defined as events having an incidence rate with 25 mg of paroxetine hydrochloride extended-release tablets that was at least twice that with 12.5 mg of paroxetine hydrochloride extended-release tablets (as well as the placebo group). [See table above]

Commonly Observed Adverse Events: *Major Depressive Disorder:* The most commonly observed adverse events associated with the use of paroxetine hydrochloride extended-release tablets in a pool of two trials (incidence of 5% or greater and incidence for paroxetine hydrochloride extended-release tablets at least twice that for placebo, derived from Table 2) were: Abnormal ejaculation, abnormal vision, constipation, decreased libido, diarrhea, dizziness, female genital disorders, nausea, somnolence, sweating, trauma, tremor and yawning.

Using the same criteria, the adverse events associated with the use of paroxetine hydrochloride extended-release tablets in a study of elderly patients with major depressive disorder were: Abnormal ejaculation, constipation, decreased appetite, dry mouth, impotence, infection, libido decreased, sweating and tremor.

Panic Disorder: In the pool of panic disorder studies, the adverse events meeting these criteria were: Abnormal ejaculation, somnolence, impotence, libido decreased, tremor, sweating and female genital disorders (generally anorgasmia or difficulty achieving orgasm).

Social Anxiety Disorder: In the social anxiety disorder study, the adverse events meeting these criteria were: Nausea, asthenia, abnormal ejaculation, sweating, somnolence, impotence, insomnia and libido decreased.

Premenstrual Dysphoric Disorder: The most commonly observed adverse events associated with the use of paroxetine hydrochloride extended-release tablets either during continuous dosing or luteal phase dosing (incidence of 5% or greater and incidence for paroxetine hydrochloride extended-release tablets at least twice that for placebo, derived from Table 6) were: Nausea, asthenia, libido decreased, somnolence, insomnia, female genital disorders, sweating, dizziness, diarrhea and constipation.

In the luteal phase dosing PMDD trial, which employed dosing of 12.5 mg/day or 25 mg/day of paroxetine hydrochloride extended-release tablets limited to the 2 weeks prior to the onset of menses over 3 consecutive menstrual cycles, adverse events were evaluated during the first 14 days of each off-drug phase. When the three off-drug phases were combined, the following adverse events were reported at an incidence of 2% or greater for paroxetine hydrochloride extended-release tablets and were at least twice the rate of that reported for placebo: Infection (5.3% versus 2.5%), depression (2.8% versus 0.8%), insomnia (2.4% versus 0.8%), sinusitis (2.4% versus 0%) and asthenia (2% versus 0.8%).

Incidence in Controlled Clinical Trials: Table 2 enumerates adverse events that occurred at an incidence of 1% or more among patients treated with paroxetine hydrochloride extended-release tablets, aged 18 to 65, who participated in two short-term (12 week) placebo-controlled trials in major depressive disorder in which patients were dosed in a range of 25 mg to 62.5 mg/day. Table 3 enumerates adverse events reported at an incidence of 5% or greater among elderly patients (ages 60 to 88) treated with paroxetine hydrochloride extended-release tablets who participated in a short-term (12 week) placebo-controlled trial in major depressive disorder in which patients were dosed in a range of 12.5 mg to 50 mg/day. Table 4 enumerates adverse events reported at an incidence of 1% or greater among patients (19 to 72 years) treated with paroxetine hydrochloride extended-release tablets who participated in short-term (10 week) placebo-controlled trials in panic disorder in which patients were dosed in a range of 12.5 mg to 75 mg/day. Table 5 enumerates adverse events reported at an incidence of 1% or greater among adult patients treated with paroxetine hydrochloride extended-release tablets who participated in a short-term (12 week), double-blind, placebo-controlled trial in social anxiety disorder in which patients were dosed in a range of 12.5 to 37.5 mg/day. Table 6 enumerates adverse events that occurred at an incidence of 1% or more among patients treated with paroxetine hydrochloride extended-release tablets who participated in three, 12-week, placebo-controlled trials in PMDD in which patients were dosed at 12.5 mg/day or 25 mg/day and in one 12-week placebo-controlled trial in which patients were dosed for 2 weeks prior to the onset of menses (luteal phase dosing) at 12.5 mg/day or 25 mg/day. Reported adverse events were classified using a standard COSTART-based Dictionary terminology.

The prescriber should be aware that these figures cannot be used to predict the incidence of side effects in the course of usual medical practice where patient characteristics and other factors differ from those that prevailed in the clinical trials. Similarly, the cited frequencies cannot be compared with figures obtained from other clinical investigations involving different treatments, uses and investigators. The cited figures, however, do provide the prescribing physician with some basis for estimating the relative contribution of drug and nondrug factors to the side effect incidence rate in the population studied.

Table 2. Treatment Emergent Adverse Events Occurring in ≥ 1% of Patients Treated with Paroxetine Hydrochloride Extended-Release Tablets in a Pool of Two Studies in Major Depressive Disorder[1,2]

Body System/ Adverse Event	% Reporting Event	
	Paroxetine Hydrochloride Extended-Release Tablets (n = 212)	Placebo (n = 211)
Body as a Whole		
Headache	27%	20%
Asthenia	14%	9%
Infection[3]	8%	5%
Abdominal Pain	7%	4%
Back Pain	5%	3%
Trauma[4]	5%	1%
Pain[5]	3%	1%
Allergic Reaction[6]	2%	1%
Cardiovascular System		
Tachycardia	1%	0%
Vasodilatation[7]	2%	0%
Digestive System		
Nausea	22%	10%
Diarrhea	18%	7%
Dry Mouth	15%	8%
Constipation	10%	4%
Flatulence	6%	4%
Decreased Appetite	4%	2%
Vomiting	2%	1%
Nervous System		
Somnolence	22%	8%
Insomnia	17%	9%
Dizziness	14%	4%
Libido Decreased	7%	3%
Tremor	7%	1%
Hypertonia	3%	1%
Paresthesia	3%	1%
Agitation	2%	1%
Confusion	1%	0%
Respiratory System		
Yawn	5%	0%
Rhinitis	4%	1%
Cough Increased	2%	1%
Bronchitis	1%	0%
Skin and Appendages		
Sweating	6%	2%
Photosensitivity	2%	0%
Special Senses		
Abnormal Vision[8]	5%	1%
Taste Perversion	2%	0%
Urogenital System		
Abnormal Ejaculation[9,10]	26%	1%
Female Genital Disorder[9,11]	10%	< 1%
Impotence[9]	5%	3%
Urinary Tract Infection	3%	1%
Menstrual Disorder[9]	2%	< 1%
Vaginitis[9]	2%	0%

[1] Adverse events for which the paroxetine hydrochloride extended-release tablets reporting incidence was less than or equal to the placebo incidence are not included. These events are: Abnormal dreams, anxiety, arthralgia, depersonalization, dysmenorrhea, dyspepsia, hyperkinesia, increased appetite, myalgia, nervousness, pharyngitis, purpura, rash, respiratory disorder, sinusitis, urinary frequency, and weight gain.
[2] < 1% means greater than zero and less than 1%.
[3] Mostly flu.
[4] A wide variety of injuries with no obvious pattern.
[5] Pain in a variety of locations with no obvious pattern.
[6] Most frequently seasonal allergic symptoms.
[7] Usually flushing.
[8] Mostly blurred vision.
[9] Based on the number of males or females.
[10] Mostly anorgasmia or delayed ejaculation.
[11] Mostly anorgasmia or delayed orgasm.

Table 3. Treatment Emergent Adverse Events Occurring in ≥ 5% of Patients Treated with Paroxetine Hydrochloride Extended-Release Tablets in a Study of Elderly Patients with Major Depressive Disorder[1,2]

Body System/ Adverse Event	% Reporting Event	
	Paroxetine Hydrochloride Extended-Release Tablets (n = 104)	Placebo (n = 109)
Body as a Whole		
Headache	17%	13%
Asthenia	15%	14%
Trauma	8%	5%
Infection	6%	2%
Digestive System		
Dry Mouth	18%	7%
Diarrhea	15%	9%
Constipation	13%	5%
Dyspepsia	13%	10%
Decreased Appetite	12%	5%
Flatulence	8%	7%
Nervous System		
Somnolence	21%	12%
Insomnia	10%	8%
Dizziness	9%	5%
Libido Decreased	8%	< 1%
Tremor	7%	0%
Skin and Appendages		
Sweating	10%	< 1%
Urogenital System		
Abnormal Ejaculation[3,4]	17%	3%
Impotence[3]	9%	3%

[1] Adverse events for which the paroxetine hydrochloride extended-release tablets reporting incidence was less than or equal to the placebo incidence are not included. These events are nausea and respiratory disorder.
[2] < 1% means greater than zero and less than 1%.
[3] Based on the number of males.
[4] Mostly anorgasmia or delayed ejaculation.

Table 4. Treatment Emergent Adverse Events Occurring in ≥ 1% of Patients Treated with Paroxetine Hydrochloride Extended-Release Tablets in a Pool of Three Panic Disorder Studies[1,2]

Body System/ Adverse Event	% Reporting Event	
	Paroxetine Hydrochloride Extended-Release Tablets (n = 444)	Placebo (n = 445)
Body as a Whole		
Asthenia	15%	10%
Abdominal Pain	6%	4%
Trauma[3]	5%	4%
Cardiovascular System		
Vasodilation[4]	3%	2%
Digestive System		
Nausea	23%	17%
Dry Mouth	13%	9%
Diarrhea	12%	9%
Constipation	9%	6%
Decreased Appetite	8%	6%
Metabolic/Nutritional Disorders		
Weight Loss	1%	0%
Musculoskeletal System		
Myalgia	5%	3%
Nervous System		
Insomnia	20%	11%
Somnolence	20%	9%
Libido Decreased	9%	4%
Nervousness	8%	7%
Tremor	8%	2%

Anxiety	5%	4%
Agitation	3%	2%
Hypertonia[5]	2%	< 1%
Myoclonus	2%	< 1%
Respiratory System		
Sinusitis	8%	5%
Yawn	3%	0%
Skin and Appendages		
Sweating	7%	2%
Special Senses		
Abnormal Vision[6]	3%	< 1%
Urogenital System		
Abnormal Ejaculation[7,8]	27%	3%
Impotence[7]	10%	1%
Female Genital Disorders[9,10]	7%	1%
Urinary Frequency	2%	< 1%
Urination Impaired	2%	< 1%
Vaginitis[9]	1%	< 1%

[1] Adverse events for which the reporting rate for paroxetine hydrochloride extended-release tablets was less than or equal to the placebo rate are not included. These events are: Abnormal dreams, allergic reaction, back pain, bronchitis, chest pain, concentration impaired, confusion, cough increased, depression, dizziness, dysmenorrhea, dyspepsia, fever, flatulence, headache, increased appetite, infection, menstrual disorder, migraine, pain, paresthesia, pharyngitis, respiratory disorder, rhinitis, tachycardia, taste perversion, thinking abnormal, urinary tract infection, and vomiting.
[2] < 1% means greater than zero and less than 1%.
[3] Various physical injuries.
[4] Mostly flushing.
[5] Mostly muscle tightness or stiffness.
[6] Mostly blurred vision.
[7] Based on the number of male patients.
[8] Mostly anorgasmia or delayed ejaculation.
[9] Based on the number of female patients.
[10] Mostly anorgasmia or difficulty achieving orgasm.

Table 5. Treatment Emergent Adverse Effects Occurring in ≥ 1% of Patients Treated with Paroxetine Hydrochloride Extended-Release Tablets in a Social Anxiety Disorder Study[1,2]

Body System/ Adverse Event	% Reporting Event	
	Paroxetine Hydrochloride Extended-Release Tablets (n = 186)	Placebo (n = 184)
Body as a Whole		
Headache	23%	17%
Asthenia	18%	7%
Abdominal Pain	5%	4%
Back Pain	4%	1%
Trauma[3]	3%	< 1%
Allergic Reaction[4]	2%	< 1%
Chest Pain	1%	< 1%
Cardiovascular System		
Hypertension	2%	0%
Migraine	2%	1%
Tachycardia	2%	1%
Digestive System		
Nausea	22%	6%
Diarrhea	9%	8%
Constipation	5%	2%
Dry Mouth	3%	2%
Dyspepsia	2%	< 1%
Decreased Appetite	1%	< 1%
Tooth Disorder	1%	0%
Metabolic/ Nutritional Disorders		
Weight Gain	3%	1%
Weight Loss	1%	0%
Nervous System		
Insomnia	9%	4%
Somnolence	9%	4%

Libido Decreased	8%	1%
Dizziness	7%	4%
Tremor	4%	2%
Anxiety	2%	1%
Concentration Impaired	2%	0%
Depression	2%	1%
Myoclonus	1%	< 1%
Paresthesia	1%	< 1%
Respiratory System		
Yawn	2%	0%
Skin and Appendages		
Sweating	14%	3%
Eczema	1%	0%
Special Senses		
Abnormal Vision[5]	2%	0%
Abnormality of Accommodation	2%	0%
Urogenital System		
Abnormal Ejaculation[6,7]	15%	1%
Impotence[6]	9%	0%
Female Genital Disorders[8,9]	3%	0%

[1] Adverse events for which the reporting rate for paroxetine hydrochloride extended-release tablets was less than or equal to the placebo rate are not included. These events are: Dysmenorrhea, flatulence, gastroenteritis, hypertonia, infection, pain, pharyngitis, rash, respiratory disorder, rhinitis, and vomiting.

[2] < 1% means greater than zero and less than 1%.

[3] Various physical injuries.

[4] Most frequently seasonal allergic symptoms.

[5] Mostly blurred vision.

[6] Based on the number of male patients.

[7] Mostly anorgasmia or delayed ejaculation.

[8] Based on the number of female patients.

[9] Mostly anorgasmia or difficulty achieving orgasm.

[See table 6 above]

Dose Dependency of Adverse Events: The following table shows results in PMDD trials of common adverse events, defined as events with an incidence of ≥ 1% with 25 mg of paroxetine hydrochloride extended release tablets that was at least twice that with 12.5 mg of paroxetine hydrochloride extended release tablets and with placebo.

[See table at top of next page]

A comparison of adverse event rates in a fixed dose study comparing immediate-release paroxetine with placebo in the treatment of major depressive disorder revealed a clear dose dependency for some of the more common adverse events associated with the use of immediate-release paroxetine.

Male and Female Sexual Dysfunction with SSRIs: Although changes in sexual desire, sexual performance and sexual satisfaction often occur as manifestations of a psychiatric disorder, they may also be a consequence of pharmacologic treatment. In particular, some evidence suggests that SSRIs can cause such untoward sexual experiences.

Reliable estimates of the incidence and severity of untoward experiences involving sexual desire, performance and satisfaction are difficult to obtain; however, in part because patients and physicians may be reluctant to discuss them. Accordingly, estimates of the incidence of untoward sexual experience and performance cited in product labeling, are likely to underestimate their actual values.

The percentage of patients reporting symptoms of sexual dysfunction in the pool of two placebo-controlled trials in nonelderly patients with major depressive disorder, in the pool of three placebo-controlled trials in patients with panic disorder, in the placebo-controlled trial in patients with social anxiety disorder and in the intermittent dosing and the pool of three placebo-controlled continuous dosing trials in female patients with PMDD are as follows:

[See table at bottom of next page]

There are no adequate, controlled studies examining sexual dysfunction with paroxetine treatment.

Paroxetine treatment has been associated with several cases of priapism. In those cases with a known outcome, patients recovered without sequelae.

While it is difficult to know the precise risk of sexual dysfunction associated with the use of SSRIs, physicians should routinely inquire about such possible side effects.

Weight and Vital Sign Changes: Significant weight loss may be an undesirable result of treatment with paroxetine for some patients but, on average, patients in controlled trials with paroxetine hydrochloride extended-release tablets or the immediate-release formulation, had minimal weight loss (about 1 pound). No significant changes in vital signs (systolic and diastolic blood pressure, pulse and temperature) were observed in patients treated with paroxetine hydrochloride extended-release tablets or immediate-release paroxetine hydrochloride, in controlled clinical trials.

Table 6. Treatment-Emergent Adverse Events Occurring in ≥ 1% of Patients Treated With Paroxetine Hydrochloride Extended-Release Tablets in a Pool of Three Premenstrual Dysphoric Disorder Studies with Continuous Dosing or in One Premenstrual Dysphoric Disorder Study with Luteal Phase Dosing[1,2,3]

	% Reporting Event			
	Continuous Dosing		Luteal Phase Dosing	
Body System/Adverse Event	Paroxetine Hydrochloride Extended-Release Tablets (n = 681)	Placebo (n = 349)	Paroxetine Hydrochloride Extended-Release Tablets (n = 246)	Placebo (n = 120)
Body as a Whole				
Asthenia	17%	6%	15%	4%
Headache	15%	12%	-	-
Infection	6%	4%	-	-
Abdominal pain	-	-	3%	0%
Cardiovascular System				
Migraine	1%	< 1%	-	-
Digestive System				
Nausea	17%	7%	18%	2%
Diarrhea	6%	2%	6%	0%
Constipation	5%	1%	2%	< 1%
Dry Mouth	4%	2%	2%	< 1%
Increased Appetite	3%	< 1%	-	-
Decreased Appetite	2%	< 1%	2%	0%
Dyspepsia	2%	1%	2%	2%
Gingivitis	-	-	1%	0%
Metabolic and Nutritional Disorders				
Generalized Edema	-	-	1%	< 1%
Weight Gain	-	-	1%	< 1%
Musculoskeletal System				
Arthralgia	2%	1%	-	-
Nervous System				
Libido Decreased	12%	5%	9%	6%
Somnolence	9%	2%	3%	< 1%
Insomnia	8%	2%	7%	3%
Dizziness	7%	3%	6%	3%
Tremor	4%	< 1%	5%	0%
Concentration Impaired	3%	< 1%	1%	0%
Nervousness	2%	< 1%	3%	2%
Anxiety	2%	1%	-	-
Lack of Emotion	2%	< 1%	-	-
Depression	-	-	2%	< 1%
Vertigo	-	-	2%	< 1%
Abnormal Dreams	< 1%	< 1%	-	-
Amnesia	-	-	1%	0%
Respiratory System				
Sinusitis	-	-	4%	2%
Yawn	2%	< 1%	-	-
Bronchitis	-	-	2%	0%
Cough Increased	1%	< 1%	-	-
Skin and Appendages				
Sweating	7%	< 1%	6%	< 1%
Special Senses				
Abnormal Vision	-	-	1%	0%
Urogenital System				
Female Genital Disorders[4]	8%	1%	2%	0%
Menorrhagia	1%	1%	-	-
Vaginal Moniliasis	1%	1%	-	-
Menstrual Disorder	-	-	1%	0%

[1] Adverse events for which the reporting rate of paroxetine hydrochloride extended-release tablets was less than or equal to the placebo rate are not included. These events for continuous dosing are: Abdominal pain, back pain, pain, trauma, weight gain, myalgia, pharyngitis, respiratory disorder, rhinitis, sinusitis, pruritis, dysmenorrhea, menstrual disorder, urinary tract infection and vomiting. The events for luteal phase dosing are: Allergic reaction, back pain, headache, infection, pain, trauma, myalgia, anxiety, pharyngitis, respiratory disorder, cystitis and dysmenorrhea.

[2] < 1% means greater than zero and less than 1%.

[3] The luteal phase and continuous dosing PMDD trials were not designed for making direct comparisons between the two dosing regimens. Therefore, a comparison between the two dosing regimens of the PMDD trials of incidence rates shown in Table 5 should be avoided.

[4] Mostly anorgasmia or difficulty achieving orgasm.

ECG Changes: In an analysis of ECGs obtained in 682 patients treated with immediate-release paroxetine and 415 patients treated with placebo in controlled clinical trials, no clinically significant changes were seen in the ECGs of either group.

Liver Function Tests: In a pool of two placebo-controlled clinical trials, patients treated with paroxetine hydrochloride extended-release tablets or placebo exhibited

Incidence of Common Adverse Events in Placebo, 12.5 mg and 25 mg of Paroxetine Hydrochloride Extended-release Tablets in a Pool of Three Fixed-Dose PMDD Trials

Common Adverse Event	Paroxetine Hydrochloride Extended-Release Tablets 25 mg (n = 348)	Paroxetine Hydrochloride Extended-Release Tablets 12.5 mg (n = 333)	Placebo (n = 349)
Sweating	8.9%	4.2%	0.9%
Tremor	6%	1.5%	0.3%
Concentration Impaired	4.3%	1.5%	0.6%
Yawn	3.2%	0.9%	0.3%
Paresthesia	1.4%	0.3%	0.3%
Hyperkinesia	1.1%	0.3%	0%
Vaginitis	1.1%	0.3%	0.3%

abnormal values on liver function tests at comparable rates. In particular, the extended-release paroxetine versus placebo comparisons for alkaline phosphatase, SGOT, SGPT and bilirubin revealed no differences in the percentage of patients with marked abnormalities.

In a study of elderly patients with major depressive disorder, 3 of 104 patients treated with paroxetine hydrochloride extended-release tablets and none of 109 placebo patients experienced liver transaminase elevations of potential clinical concern.

Two of the patients treated with paroxetine hydrochloride extended-release tablets dropped out of the study due to abnormal liver function tests; the third patient experienced normalization of transaminase levels with continued treatment. Also, in the pool of three studies of patients with panic disorder, 4 of 444 patients treated with paroxetine hydrochloride extended-release tablets and none of 445 placebo patients experienced liver transaminase elevations of potential clinical concern. Elevations in all four patients decreased substantially after discontinuation of paroxetine hydrochloride extended-release tablets. The clinical significance of these findings is unknown.

In placebo-controlled clinical trials with the immediate-release formulation of paroxetine, patients exhibited abnormal values on liver function tests at no greater rate than that seen in placebo-treated patients.

Hallucinations: In pooled clinical trials of immediate-release paroxetine hydrochloride, hallucinations were observed in 22 of 9,089 patients receiving drug and in 4 of 3,187 patients receiving placebo.

Other Events Observed During the Clinical Development of Paroxetine: The following adverse events were reported during the clinical development of paroxetine hydrochloride extended-release tablet and/or the clinical development of the immediate-release formulation of paroxetine.

Adverse events for which frequencies are provided below occurred in clinical trials with the extended-release formulation of paroxetine. During its premarketing assessment in major depressive disorder, panic disorder, social anxiety disorder and PMDD, multiple doses of paroxetine hydrochloride extended-release tablets were administered to 1,627 patients in phase three double-blind, controlled, outpatient studies. Untoward events associated with this exposure were recorded by clinical investigators using terminology of their own choosing. Consequently, it is not possible to provide a meaningful estimate of the proportion of individuals experiencing adverse events without first grouping similar types of untoward events into a smaller number of standardized event categories.

In the tabulations that follow, reported adverse events were classified using a COSTART based dictionary. The frequencies presented, therefore, represent the proportion of the 1,627 patients exposed to paroxetine hydrochloride extended-release tablets who experienced an event of the type cited on at least one occasion while receiving paroxetine hydrochloride extended-release tablets. All reported events are included except those already listed in Tables 2 through 6 and those events where a drug cause was remote. If the COSTART term for an event was so general as to be uninformative, it was deleted or, when possible, replaced with a more informative term. It is important to emphasize that although the events reported occurred during treatment with paroxetine, they were not necessarily caused by it.

Events are further categorized by body system and listed in order of decreasing frequency according to the following definitions: Frequent adverse events are those occurring on one or more occasions in at least 1/100 patients (only those not already listed in the tabulated results from placebo-controlled trials appear in this listing); infrequent adverse events are those occurring in 1/100 to 1/1,000 patients; rare events are those occurring in fewer than 1/1,000 patients.

Adverse events for which frequencies are not provided occurred during the premarketing assessment of immediate-release paroxetine in phase two and three studies of major depressive disorder, obsessive compulsive disorder, panic disorder, social anxiety disorder, generalized anxiety disorder and posttraumatic stress disorder. The conditions and duration of exposure to immediate-release paroxetine varied greatly and included (in overlapping categories) open and double-blind studies, uncontrolled and controlled studies, inpatient and outpatient studies and fixed dose and titration studies. Only those events not previously listed for extended-release paroxetine are included. The extent to which these events may be associated with paroxetine hydrochloride extended-release tablets is unknown.

Events are listed alphabetically within the respective body system. Events of major clinical importance are also described in the PRECAUTIONS section.

Body as a Whole: Infrequent were chills, face edema, fever, flu syndrome, malaise; rare were abscess, anaphylactoid reaction, anticholinergic syndrome, hypothermia; also observed were adrenergic syndrome, neck rigidity, sepsis.

Cardiovascular System: Infrequent were angina pectoris, bradycardia, hematoma, hypertension, hypotension, palpitation, postural hypotension, supraventricular tachycardia, syncope; rare were bundle branch block; also observed were arrhythmia nodal, atrial fibrillation, cerebrovascular accident, congestive heart failure, low cardiac output, myocardial infarct, myocardial ischemia, pallor, phlebitis, pulmonary embolus, supraventricular extrasystoles, thrombophlebitis, thrombosis, vascular headache, ventricular extrasystoles.

Digestive System: Infrequent were bruxism, dysphagia, eructation, gastritis, gastroenteritis, gastroesophageal reflux, gingivitis, hemorrhoids, liver function test abnormal, melena, pancreatitis, rectal hemorrhage, toothache, ulcer-ative stomatitis; rare were colitis, glossitis, gum hyperplasia, hepatosplenomegaly, increased salivation, intestinal obstruction, peptic ulcer, stomach ulcer, throat tightness; also observed were aphthous stomatitis, bloody diarrhea, bulimia, cardiospasm, cholelithiasis, duodenitis, enteritis, esophagitis, fecal impactions, fecal incontinence, gum hemorrhage, hematemesis, hepatitis, ileitis, ileus, jaundice, mouth ulceration, salivary gland enlargement, sialadenitis, stomatitis, tongue discoloration, tongue edema.

Endocrine System: Infrequent were ovarian cyst, testes pain; rare were diabetes mellitus, hyperthyroidism; also observed were goiter, hypothyroidism, thyroiditis.

Hemic and Lymphatic System: Infrequent were anemia, eosinophilia, hypochromic anemia, leukocytosis, leukopenia, lymphadenopathy, purpura; rare were thrombocytopenia; also observed were anisocytosis, basophilia, bleeding time increased, lymphedema, lymphocytosis, lymphopenia, microcytic anemia, monocytosis, normocytic anemia, thrombocythemia.

Metabolic and Nutritional Disorders: Infrequent were generalized edema, hyperglycemia, hypokalemia, peripheral edema, SGOT increased, SGPT increased, thirst; rare were bilirubinemia, dehydration, hyperkalemia, obesity; also observed were alkaline phosphatase increased, BUN increased, creatinine phosphokinase increased, gamma globulins increased, gout, hypercalcemia, hypercholesteremia, hyperphosphatemia, hypocalcemia, hypoglycemia, hyponatremia, ketosis, lactic dehydrogenase increased, nonprotein nitrogen (NPN) increased.

Musculoskeletal System: Infrequent were arthritis, bursitis, tendonitis; rare were myasthenia, myopathy, myositis; also observed were generalized spasm, osteoporosis, tenosynovitis, tetany.

Nervous System: Frequent were depression; infrequent were amnesia, convulsion, depersonalization, dystonia, emotional lability, hallucinations, hyperkinesia, hypesthesia, hypokinesia, incoordination, libido increased, neuralgia, neuropathy, nystagmus, paralysis, vertigo; rare were ataxia, coma, diplopia, dyskinesia, hostility, paranoid reaction, torticollis, withdrawal syndrome; also observed were abnormal gait, akathisia, akinesia, aphasia, choreoathetosis, circumoral paresthesia, delirium, delusions, dysarthria, euphoria, extrapyramidal syndrome, fasciculations, grand mal convulsion, hyperalgesia, irritability, manic reaction, manic-depressive reaction, meningitis, myelitis, peripheral neuritis, psychosis, psychotic depression, reflexes decreased, reflexes increased, stupor, trismus.

Respiratory System: Frequent were pharyngitis; infrequent were asthma, dyspnea, epistaxis, laryngitis, pneumonia; rare were stridor; also observed were dysphonia, emphysema, hemoptysis, hiccups, hyperventilation, lung fibrosis, pulmonary edema, respiratory flu, sputum increased.

Skin and Appendages: Frequent were rash; infrequent were acne, alopecia, dry skin, eczema, pruritus, urticaria; rare were exfoliative dermatitis, furunculosis, pustular rash, seborrhea; also observed were angioedema, ecchymosis, erythema multiforme, erythema nodosum, hirsutism, maculopapular rash, skin discoloration, skin hypertrophy, skin ulcer, sweating decreased, vesiculobullous rash.

Special Senses: Infrequent were conjunctivitis, earache, keratoconjunctivitis, mydriasis, photophobia, retinal hemorrhage, tinnitus; rare were blepharitis, visual field defect; also observed were amblyopia, anisocoria, blurred vision, cataract, conjunctival edema, corneal ulcer, deafness, exophthalmos, glaucoma, hyperacusis, night blindness, parosmia, ptosis, taste loss.

Urogenital System: Frequent were dysmenorrhea*; infrequent were albuminuria, amenorrhea*, breast pain*, cystitis, dysuria, prostatitis*, urinary retention; rare were breast enlargement*, breast neoplasm*, female lactation, hematuria, kidney calculus, metrorrhagia*, nephritis, noc-

	Major Depressive Disorder		Panic Disorder		Social Anxiety Disorder		PMDD Continuous Dosing		PMDD Luteal Phase Dosing	
	Paroxetine HCl Extended-Release Tablets	Placebo	Paroxetine HCl Extended-Release Tablets	Placebo	Paroxetine HCl Extended-Release Tablets	Placebo	Paroxetine HCl Extended-Release Tablets	Placebo	Paroxetine HCl Extended-Release Tablets	Placebo
n (males)	78	78	162	194	88	97	n/a	n/a	n/a	n/a
Decreased Libido	10%	5%	9%	6%	13%	1%	n/a	n/a	n/a	n/a
Ejaculatory Disturbance	26%	1%	27%	3%	15%	1%	n/a	n/a	n/a	n/a
Impotence	5%	3%	10%	1%	9%	0%	n/a	n/a	n/a	n/a
n (females)	134	133	282	251	98	87	681	349	246	120
Decreased Libido	4%	2%	8%	2%	4%	1%	12%	5%	9%	6%
Orgasmic Disturbance	10%	< 1%	7%	1%	3%	0%	8%	1%	2%	0%

turia, pregnancy and puerperal disorders*, salpingitis, urinary incontinence, uterine fibroids enlarged*; also observed were breast atrophy, ejaculatory disturbance, endometrial disorder, epididymitis, fibrocystic breast, leukorrhea, mastitis, oliguria, polyuria, pyuria, urethritis, urinary casts, urinary urgency, urolith, uterine spasm, vaginal hemorrhage.
*Based on the number of men and women as appropriate.

Post-Marketing Reports: Voluntary reports of adverse events in patients taking immediate-release paroxetine hydrochloride that have been received since market introduction and not listed above that may have no causal relationship with the drug include acute pancreatitis, elevated liver function tests (the most severe cases were deaths due to liver necrosis and grossly elevated transaminases associated with severe liver dysfunction), Guillain-Barré syndrome, toxic epidermal necrolysis, priapism, syndrome of inappropriate ADH secretion, symptoms suggestive of prolactinemia and galactorrhea; extrapyramidal symptoms which have included akathisia, bradykinesia, cogwheel rigidity, dystonia, hypertonia, oculogyric crisis which has been associated with concomitant use of pimozide; tremor and trismus; status epilepticus, acute renal failure, pulmonary hypertension, allergic alveolitis, anaphylaxis, eclampsia, laryngismus, optic neuritis, porphyria, ventricular fibrillation, ventricular tachycardia (including Torsade de pointes), thrombocytopenia, hemolytic anemia, events related to impaired hematopoiesis (including aplastic anemia, pancytopenia, bone marrow aplasia and agranulocytosis) and vasculitic syndromes (such as Henoch-Schönlein purpura). There has been a case report of an elevated phenytoin level after 4 weeks of immediate-release paroxetine and phenytoin coadministration. There has been a case report of severe hypotension when immediate-release paroxetine was added to chronic metoprolol treatment.

DRUG ABUSE AND DEPENDENCE

Controlled Substance Class: Paroxetine hydrochloride is not a controlled substance.

Physical and Psychologic Dependence: Paroxetine hydrochloride extended-release tablets have not been systematically studied in animals or humans for its potential for abuse, tolerance or physical dependence. While the clinical trials did not reveal any tendency for any drug seeking behavior, these observations were not systematic and it is not possible to predict on the basis of this limited experience the extent to which a CNS active drug will be misused, diverted and/or abused once marketed. Consequently, patients should be evaluated carefully for history of drug abuse and such patients should be observed closely for signs of misuse or abuse of paroxetine hydrochloride extended-release tablets (e.g., development of tolerance, incrementations of dose, drug seeking behavior).

OVERDOSAGE

Human Experience: Since the introduction of immediate-release paroxetine hydrochloride in the United States, 342 spontaneous cases of deliberate or accidental overdosage during paroxetine treatment have been reported worldwide (circa 1999). These include overdoses with paroxetine alone and in combination with other substances. Of these, 48 cases were fatal and of the fatalities, 17 appeared to involve paroxetine alone. Eight fatal cases that documented the amount of paroxetine ingested were generally confounded by the ingestion of other drugs or alcohol or the presence of significant comorbid conditions. Of 145 nonfatal cases with known outcome, most recovered without sequelae. The largest known ingestion involved 2000 mg of paroxetine (33 times the maximum recommended daily dose) in a patient who recovered.

Commonly reported adverse events associated with paroxetine overdosage include somnolence, coma, nausea, tremor, tachycardia, confusion, vomiting and dizziness. Other notable signs and symptoms observed with overdoses involving paroxetine (alone or with other substances) include mydriasis, convulsions (including status epilepticus), ventricular dysrhythmias (including Torsade de pointes), hypertension, aggressive reactions, syncope, hypotension, stupor, bradycardia, dystonia, rhabdomyolysis, symptoms of hepatic dysfunction (including hepatic failure, hepatic necrosis, jaundice, hepatitis and hepatic steatosis), serotonin syndrome, manic reactions, myoclonus, acute renal failure and urinary retention.

Overdosage Management: Treatment should consist of those general measures employed in the management of overdosage with any drugs effective in the treatment of major depressive disorder.

Ensure an adequate airway, oxygenation and ventilation. *Monitor cardiac rhythm* and vital signs. General supportive and symptomatic measures are also recommended. Induction of emesis is not recommended. Gastric lavage with a large-bore orogastric tube with appropriate airway protection, if needed, may be indicated if performed soon after ingestion or in symptomatic patients.

Activated charcoal should be administered. Due to the large volume of distribution of this drug, forced diuresis, dialysis, hemoperfusion and exchange transfusion are unlikely to be of benefit. No specific antidotes for paroxetine are known.

A specific caution involves patients taking or recently having taken paroxetine who might ingest excessive quantities of a tricyclic antidepressant. In such a case, accumulation of the parent tricyclic and an active metabolite may increase the possibility of clinically significant sequelae and extend the time needed for close medical observation (see PRECAUTIONS: Drug Interactions: *Drugs Metabolized by Cytochrome CPY2D6*).

In managing overdosage, consider the possibility of multiple drug involvement. The physician should consider contacting a poison control center for additional information on the treatment of any overdose. Telephone numbers for certified poison control centers are listed in the *Physicians' Desk Reference* (PDR).

DOSAGE AND ADMINISTRATION

Major Depressive Disorder: ***Usual Initial Dosage:*** Paroxetine hydrochloride extended-release tablets should be administered as a single daily dose, usually in the morning, with or without food. The recommended initial dose is 25 mg/day. Patients were dosed in a range of 25 mg to 62.5 mg/day in the clinical trials demonstrating the effectiveness of paroxetine hydrochloride extended-release tablets in the treatment of major depressive disorder. As with all drugs effective in the treatment of major depressive disorder, the full effect may be delayed. Some patients not responding to a 25 mg dose may benefit from dose increases, in 12.5 mg/day increments, up to a maximum of 62.5 mg/day. Dose changes should occur at intervals of at least one week.

Patients should be cautioned that paroxetine hydrochloride extended-release tablets should not be chewed or crushed and should be swallowed whole.

Maintenance Therapy: There is no body of evidence available to answer the question of how long the patient treated with paroxetine hydrochloride extended-release tablets should remain on it. It is generally agreed that acute episodes of major depressive disorder require several months or longer of sustained pharmacologic therapy. Whether the dose of an antidepressant needed to induce remission is identical to the dose needed to maintain and/or sustain euthymia is unknown.

Systematic evaluation of the efficacy of immediate-release paroxetine hydrochloride has shown that efficacy is maintained for periods of up to one year with doses that averaged about 30 mg, which corresponds to a 37.5 mg dose of paroxetine hydrochloride extended-release tablets, based on relative bioavailability considerations (see CLINICAL PHARMACOLOGY: Pharmacokinetics).

Panic Disorder: ***Usual Initial Dosage:*** Paroxetine hydrochloride extended-release tablets should be administered as a single daily dose, usually in the morning. Patients should be started on 12.5 mg/day. Dose changes should occur in 12.5 mg/day increments and at intervals of at least one week. Patients were dosed in a range of 12.5 to 75 mg/day in the clinical trials demonstrating the effectiveness of paroxetine hydrochloride extended-release tablets. The maximum dosage should not exceed 75 mg/day.

Patients should be cautioned that paroxetine hydrochloride extended-release tablets should not be chewed or crushed and should be swallowed whole.

Maintenance Therapy: Long-term maintenance of efficacy with the immediate-release formulation of paroxetine was demonstrated in a 3 month relapse prevention trial. In this trial, patients with panic disorder assigned to immediate-release paroxetine demonstrated a lower relapse rate compared to patients on placebo. Panic disorder is a chronic condition and it is reasonable to consider continuation for a responding patient. Dosage adjustments should be made to maintain the patient on the lowest effective dosage and patients should be periodically reassessed to determine the need for continued treatment.

Social Anxiety Disorder: ***Usual Initial Dosage:*** Paroxetine hydrochloride extended-release tablets should be administered as a single daily dose, usually in the morning, with or without food. The recommended initial dose is 12.5 mg/day. Patients were dosed in a range of 12.5 mg to 37.5 mg/day in the clinical trial demonstrating the effectiveness of paroxetine hydrochloride extended-release tablets in the treatment of social anxiety disorder. If the dose is increased, this should occur at intervals of at least one week, in increments of 12.5 mg/day, up to a maximum of 37.5 mg/day.

Patients should be cautioned that paroxetine hydrochloride extended-release tablets should not be chewed or crushed and should be swallowed whole.

Maintenance Therapy: There is no body of evidence available to answer the question of how long the patient treated with paroxetine hydrochloride extended-release tablets should remain on it. Although the efficacy of paroxetine hydrochloride extended-release tablets beyond 12 weeks of dosing has not been demonstrated in controlled clinical trials, social anxiety disorder is recognized as a chronic condition and it is reasonable to consider continuation of treatment for a responding patient. Dosage adjustments should be made to maintain the patient on the lowest effective dosage and patients should be periodically reassessed to determine the need for continued treatment.

Premenstrual Dysphoric Disorder: ***Usual Initial Dosage:*** Paroxetine hydrochloride extended-release tablets should be administered as a single daily dose, usually in the morning, with or without food. Paroxetine hydrochloride extended-release tablets may be administered either daily throughout the menstrual cycle or limited to the luteal phase of the menstrual cycle, depending on physician assessment. The recommended initial dose is 12.5 mg/day. In clinical trials, both 12.5 mg/day and 25 mg/day were shown to be effective. Dose changes should occur at intervals of at least one week.

Patients should be cautioned that paroxetine hydrochloride extended-release tablets should not be chewed or crushed and should be swallowed whole.

Maintenance/Continuation Therapy: The effectiveness of Paroxetine hydrochloride extended-release tablets for a period exceeding three menstrual cycles has not been systematically evaluated in controlled trials. However, women commonly report that symptoms worsen with age until relieved by the onset of menopause. Therefore, it is reasonable to consider continuation of a responding patient. Patients should be periodically reassessed to determine the need for continued treatment.

Special Populations: ***Treatment of Pregnant Women During the Third Trimester:*** Neonates exposed to paroxetine hydrochloride extended-release tablets and other SSRIs or SNRIs, late in the third trimester have developed complications requiring prolonged hospitalization, respiratory support and tube feeding (see WARNINGS). When treating pregnant women with paroxetine during the third trimester, the physician should carefully consider the potential risks and benefits of treatment. The physician may consider tapering paroxetine in the third trimester.

Dosage for Elderly or Debilitated Patients and Patients with Severe Renal or Hepatic Impairment: The recommended initial dose of paroxetine hydrochloride extended-release tablets is 12.5 mg/day for elderly patients, debilitated patients and/or patients with severe renal or hepatic impairment. Increases may be made if indicated. Dosage should not exceed 50 mg/day.

Switching Patients to or From a Monoamine Oxidase Inhibitor: At least 14 days should elapse between discontinuation of an MAOI and initiation of therapy with paroxetine hydrochloride extended-release tablets. Similarly, at least 14 days should be allowed after stopping paroxetine hydrochloride extended-release tablets before starting an MAOI.

Discontinuation of Treatment with Paroxetine Hydrochloride Extended-Release Tablets: Symptoms associated with discontinuation of immediate-release paroxetine hydrochloride or paroxetine hydrochloride extended-release tablets have been reported (see PRECAUTIONS). Patients should be monitored for these symptoms when discontinuing treatment, regardless of the indication for which paroxetine hydrochloride extended-release tablets are being prescribed. A gradual reduction in the dose rather than abrupt cessation is recommended whenever possible. If intolerable symptoms occur following a decrease in the dose or upon discontinuation of treatment, then resuming the previously prescribed dose may be considered. Subsequently, the physician may continue decreasing the dose but at a more gradual rate.

HOW SUPPLIED

Paroxetine Hydrochloride Extended-release Tablets are available as 12.5 mg and 25 mg tablets.

The 12.5 mg tablet is a white film-coated, round, unscored tablet with **M** over **P3** imprinted in black ink on one side of the tablet and blank on the other side. They are available as follows:

NDC 0378-2003-93
bottles of 30 tablets
NDC 0378-2003-01
bottles of 100 tablets
NDC 0378-2003-05
bottles of 500 tablets

The 25 mg tablet is a lavender film-coated, round, unscored tablet with **M** over **P4** imprinted in black ink on one side of the tablet and blank on the other side. They are available as follows:

NDC 0378-2004-93
bottles of 30 tablets
NDC 0378-2004-01
bottles of 100 tablets
NDC 0378-2004-05
bottles of 500 tablets

Store at 20° to 25 °C (68° to 77°F). [See USP Controlled Room Temperature.]
Dispense in a tight, light-resistant container as defined in the USP using a child-resistant closure.
PHARMACIST: Dispense a Medication Guide with each prescription.
MYLAN®
Mylan Pharmaceuticals Inc.
Morgantown, WV 26505
REVISED JULY 2010
PRXT:R8mc

MEDICATION GUIDE

Antidepressant Medicines, Depression and other Serious Mental Illnesses, and Suicidal Thoughts or Actions

Read the Medication Guide that comes with your or your family member's antidepressant medicine. This Medication Guide is only about the risk of suicidal thoughts and actions with antidepressant medicines. **Talk to your, or your family member's, healthcare provider about:**

- all risks and benefits of treatment with antidepressant medicines
- all treatment choices for depression or other serious mental illness

What is the most important information I should know about antidepressant medicines, depression and other serious mental illnesses, and suicidal thoughts or actions?

1. **Antidepressant medicines may increase suicidal thoughts or actions in some children, teenagers, and young adults within the first few months of treatment.**
2. **Depression and other serious mental illnesses are the most important causes of suicidal thoughts and actions. Some people may have a particularly high risk of having suicidal thoughts or actions.** These include people who have (or have a family history of) bipolar illness (also called manic-depressive illness) or suicidal thoughts or actions.
3. **How can I watch for and try to prevent suicidal thoughts and actions in myself or a family member?**
   - Pay close attention to any changes, especially sudden changes, in mood, behaviors, thoughts, or feelings. This is very important when an antidepressant medicine is started or when the dose is changed.
   - Call the healthcare provider right away to report new or sudden changes in mood, behavior, thoughts, or feelings.
   - Keep all follow-up visits with the healthcare provider as scheduled. Call the healthcare provider between visits as needed, especially if you have concerns about symptoms.

Call a healthcare provider right away if you or your family member has any of the following symptoms, especially if they are new, worse, or worry you:

- thoughts about suicide or dying
- attempts to commit suicide
- new or worse depression
- new or worse anxiety
- feeling very agitated or restless
- panic attacks
- trouble sleeping (insomnia)
- new or worse irritability
- acting aggressive, being angry, or violent
- acting on dangerous impulses
- an extreme increase in activity and talking (mania)
- other unusual changes in behavior or mood

What else do I need to know about antidepressant medicines?

- **Never stop an antidepressant medicine without first talking to a healthcare provider.** Stopping an antidepressant medicine suddenly can cause other symptoms.
- **Antidepressants are medicines used to treat depression and other illnesses.** It is important to discuss all the risks of treating depression and also the risks of not treating it. Patients and their families or other caregivers should discuss all treatment choices with the healthcare provider, not just the use of antidepressants.
- **Antidepressant medicines have other side effects.** Talk to the healthcare provider about the side effects of the medicine prescribed for you or your family member.
- **Antidepressant medicines can interact with other medicines.** Know all of the medicines that you or your family member takes. Keep a list of all medicines to show the healthcare provider. Do not start new medicines without first checking with your healthcare provider.
- **Not all antidepressant medicines prescribed for children are FDA approved for use in children.** Talk to your child's healthcare provider for more information.

Call your doctor for medical advice about side effects. You may report side effects to FDA at 1-800-FDA-1088.
This Medication Guide has been approved by the U.S. Food and Drug Administration for all antidepressants.
Revised 1/2008

PHENYTEK® CAPSULES ℞

[fen EE tek]
(extended phenytoin sodium capsules, USP)
200 mg and 300 mg
℞ only

DESCRIPTION

PHENYTEK® (phenytoin sodium) is an antiepileptic drug. Phenytoin sodium is related to the barbiturates in chemical structure, but has a five-membered ring. The chemical name is 5,5-Diphenylhydantoin sodium salt, having a molecular weight of 274.25 and having the following structural formula and molecular formula:

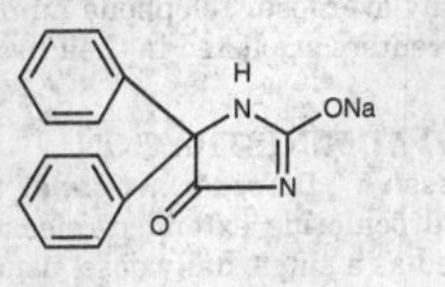

$C_{15}H_{11}N_2NaO_2$

Each PHENYTEK® CAPSULE (extended phenytoin sodium capsule, USP) for oral administration contains 200 mg or 300 mg of phenytoin sodium, USP. Each capsule also contains the following inactive ingredients: colloidal silicon dioxide, hydroxyethyl cellulose, magnesium oxide, magnesium stearate, microcrystalline cellulose, povidone and sodium lauryl sulfate. In addition, each of the empty gelatin capsules contains the following: FD&C Blue No. 1, gelatin, sodium lauryl sulfate and titanium dioxide.
The imprinting ink contains the following: black iron oxide, D&C Yellow No. 10 Aluminum Lake, FD&C Blue No. 1 Aluminum Lake, FD&C Blue No. 2 Aluminum Lake, FD&C Red No. 40 Aluminum Lake, propylene glycol and shellac glaze.
Product *in vivo* performance is characterized by a slow and extended rate of absorption with peak blood concentrations expected in 4 to 12 hours as contrasted to prompt phenytoin sodium capsules, USP with a rapid rate of absorption with peak blood concentration expected in 1½ to 3 hours.
PHENYTEK® CAPSULES, 200 mg and 300 mg meet *USP Dissolution Test 3.*

CLINICAL PHARMACOLOGY

Phenytoin is an antiepileptic drug which can be used in the treatment of epilepsy. The primary site of action appears to be the *motor cortex* where spread of *seizure* activity is inhibited. Possibly by promoting sodium efflux from neurons, phenytoin tends to stabilize the threshold against hyperexcitability caused by excessive stimulation or environmental changes capable of reducing membrane sodium gradient. This includes the reduction of posttetanic potentiation at synapses. Loss of posttetanic potentiation prevents cortical seizure foci from detonating adjacent cortical areas. Phenytoin reduces the maximal activity of brain stem centers responsible for the tonic phase of tonic-clonic (grand mal) seizures.
The plasma half-life in man after oral administration of phenytoin averages 22 hours, with a range of 7 to 42 hours. Steady-state therapeutic levels are achieved at least 7 to 10 days (5 to 7 half-lives) after initiation of therapy with recommended doses of 300 mg/day.
When serum level determinations are necessary, they should be obtained at least 5 to 7 half-lives after treatment initiation, dosage change, or addition or subtraction of another drug to the regimen so that equilibrium or steady-state will have been achieved. Trough levels provide information about clinically effective serum level range and confirm patient compliance and are obtained just prior to the patient's next scheduled dose. Peak levels indicate an individual's threshold for emergence of dose related side effects and are obtained at the time of expected peak concentration. For extended phenytoin sodium capsules peak serum levels occur 4 to 12 hours after administration.
Optimum control without clinical signs of toxicity occurs more often with serum levels between 10 and 20 mcg/mL, although some mild cases of tonic-clonic (grand mal) epilepsy may be controlled with lower serum levels of phenytoin.
In most patients maintained at a steady dosage, stable phenytoin serum levels are achieved. There may be wide interpatient variability in phenytoin serum levels with equivalent dosages. Patients with unusually low levels may be noncompliant or hypermetabolizers of phenytoin. Unusually high levels result from liver disease, congenital enzyme deficiency, or drug interactions which result in metabolic interference. The patient with large variations in phenytoin plasma levels, despite standard doses, presents a difficult clinical problem. Serum level determinations in such patients may be particularly helpful. As phenytoin is highly protein bound, free phenytoin levels may be altered in patients whose protein binding characteristics differ from normal.
Most of the drug is excreted in the bile as inactive metabolites which are then reabsorbed from the intestinal tract and excreted in the urine. Urinary excretion of phenytoin and its metabolites occurs partly with glomerular filtration but more importantly by tubular secretion. Because phenytoin is hydroxylated in the liver by an enzyme system which is saturable at high plasma levels, small incremental doses may increase the half-life and produce very substantial increases in serum levels, when these are in the upper range. The steady-state level may be disproportionately increased, with resultant intoxication, from an increase in dosage of 10% or more.

INDICATIONS AND USAGE

PHENYTEK® CAPSULES (extended phenytoin sodium capsules, USP) are indicated for the control of generalized tonic-clonic (grand mal) and complex partial (psychomotor, temporal lobe) seizures and prevention and treatment of seizures occurring during or following neurosurgery.
Phenytoin serum level determinations may be necessary for optimal dosage adjustments (see DOSAGE AND ADMINISTRATION and CLINICAL PHARMACOLOGY).

CONTRAINDICATIONS

PHENYTEK® CAPSULES (extended phenytoin sodium capsules) are contraindicated in those patients who are hypersensitive to phenytoin or other hydantoins.

WARNINGS

Abrupt withdrawal of phenytoin in epileptic patients may precipitate status epilepticus. When, in the judgment of the clinician, the need for dosage reduction, discontinuation, or substitution of alternative antiepileptic medication arises, this should be done gradually. However, in the event of an allergic or hypersensitivity reaction, rapid substitution of alternative therapy may be necessary. In this case, alternative therapy should be an antiepileptic drug not belonging to the hydantoin chemical class.
Suicidal Behavior and Ideation: Antiepileptic drugs (AEDs), including phenytoin sodium, may increase the risk of suicidal thoughts or behavior in patients taking these drugs for any indication. Patients treated with any AED for any indication should be monitored for the emergence or worsening of depression, suicidal thoughts or behavior, and/or any unusual changes in mood or behavior.
Pooled analyses of 199 placebo-controlled clinical trials (mono- and adjunctive therapy) of 11 different AEDs showed that patients randomized to one of the AEDs had approximately twice the risk (adjusted Relative Risk 1.8, 95% CI:1.2, 2.7) of suicidal thinking or behavior compared to patients randomized to placebo. In these trials, which had a median treatment duration of 12 weeks, the estimated incidence rate of suicidal behavior or ideation among 27,863 AED-treated patients was 0.43%, compared to 0.24% among 16,029 placebo-treated patients, representing an increase of approximately one case of suicidal thinking or behavior for every 530 patients treated. There were four suicides in drug-treated patients in the trials and none in placebo-treated patients, but the number is too small to allow any conclusion about drug effect on suicide.
The increased risk of suicidal thoughts or behavior with AEDs was observed as early as one week after starting drug treatment with AEDs and persisted for the duration of treatment assessed. Because most trials included in the analysis did not extend beyond 24 weeks, the risk of suicidal thoughts or behavior beyond 24 weeks could not be assessed.
The risk of suicidal thoughts or behavior was generally consistent among drugs in the data analyzed. The finding of increased risk with AEDs of varying mechanisms of action and across a range of indications suggests that the risk applies to all AEDs used for any indication. The risk did not vary substantially by age (5 to 100 years) in the clinical trials analyzed.
Table 1 shows absolute and relative risk by indication for all evaluated AEDs.

Table 1 Risk by Indication for Antiepileptic Drugs in the Pooled Analysis

Indication	Placebo Patients with Events per 1,000 Patients	Drug Patients with Events per 1,000 Patients	Relative Risk: Incidence of Events in Drug Patients/ Incidence in Placebo Patients	Risk Difference: Additional Drug Patients with Events per 1,000 Patients
Epilepsy	1	3.4	3.5	2.4
Psychiatric	5.7	8.5	1.5	2.9
Other	1	1.8	1.9	0.9
Total	2.4	4.3	1.8	1.9

The relative risk for suicidal thoughts or behavior was higher in clinical trials for epilepsy than in clinical trials for psychiatric or other conditions, but the absolute risk differences were similar for the epilepsy and psychiatric indications.

Anyone considering prescribing phenytoin sodium or any other AED must balance this risk with the risk of untreated illness. Epilepsy and many other illnesses for which AEDs are prescribed are themselves associated with morbidity and mortality and an increased risk of suicidal thoughts and behavior. Should suicidal thoughts and behavior emerge during treatment, the prescriber needs to consider whether the emergence of these symptoms in any given patient may be related to the illness being treated.

Patients, their caregivers, and families should be informed that AEDs increase the risk of suicidal thoughts and behavior and should be advised of the need to be alert for the emergence or worsening of the signs and symptoms of depression, any unusual changes in mood or behavior, or the emergence of suicidal thoughts, behavior, or thoughts about self-harm. Behaviors of concern should be reported immediately to healthcare providers.

There have been a number of reports suggesting a relationship between phenytoin and the development of lymphadenopathy (local or generalized) including benign lymph node hyperplasia, pseudolymphoma, lymphoma, and Hodgkin's Disease. Although a cause and effect relationship has not been established, the occurrence of lymphadenopathy indicates the need to differentiate such a condition from other types of lymph node pathology. Lymph node involvement may occur with or without symptoms and signs resembling serum sickness, e.g., fever, rash, and liver involvement.

In all cases of lymphadenopathy, follow-up observation for an extended period is indicated and every effort should be made to achieve seizure control using alternative antiepileptic drugs.

Acute alcoholic intake may increase phenytoin serum levels while chronic alcohol use may decrease serum levels.

In view of isolated reports associating phenytoin with exacerbation of porphyria, caution should be exercised in using this medication in patients suffering from this disease.

Usage in Pregnancy: *Clinical:*

A. *Risks to Mother:* An increase in seizure frequency may occur during pregnancy because of altered phenytoin pharmacokinetics. Periodic measurement of plasma phenytoin concentrations may be valuable in the management of pregnant women as a guide to appropriate adjustment of dosage (see PRECAUTIONS: Laboratory Tests). However, postpartum restoration of the original dosage will probably be indicated.

B. *Risks to the Fetus:* If this drug is used during pregnancy, or if the patient becomes pregnant while taking the drug, the patient should be apprised of the potential harm to the fetus.

Prenatal exposure to phenytoin may increase the risks for congenital malformations and other adverse developmental outcomes. Increased frequencies of major malformations (such as orofacial clefts and cardiac defects), minor anomalies (dysmorphic facial features, nail and digit hypoplasia), growth abnormalities (including microcephaly), and mental deficiency have been reported among children born to epileptic women who took phenytoin alone or in combination with other antiepileptic drugs during pregnancy. There have also been several reported cases of malignancies, including neuroblastoma, in children whose mothers received phenytoin during pregnancy. The overall incidence of malformations for children of epileptic women treated with antiepileptic drugs (phenytoin and/or others) during pregnancy is about 10%, or 2-to 3-fold that in the general population. However, the relative contributions of antiepileptic drugs and other factors associated with epilepsy to this increased risk are uncertain and in most cases it has not been possible to attribute specific developmental abnormalities to particular antiepileptic drugs.

Patients should consult with their physicians to weigh the risks and benefits of phenytoin during pregnancy.

C. *Postpartum Period:* A potentially life threatening bleeding disorder related to decreased levels of vitamin K-dependent clotting factors may occur in newborns exposed to phenytoin *in utero*. This drug-induced condition can be prevented with vitamin K administration to the mother before delivery and to the neonate after birth.

Preclinical: Increased resorption and malformation rates have been reported following administration of phenytoin doses of 75 mg/kg or higher (approximately 120% of the maximum human loading dose or higher on a mg/m^2 basis) to pregnant rabbits.

PRECAUTIONS

General: The liver is the chief site of biotransformation of phenytoin; patients with impaired liver function, elderly pa-

tients, or those who are gravely ill may show early signs of toxicity.

A small percentage of individuals who have been treated with phenytoin have been shown to metabolize the drug slowly. Slow metabolism may be due to limited enzyme availability and lack of induction; it appears to be genetically determined.

Phenytoin should be discontinued if a skin rash appears (see WARNINGS section regarding drug discontinuation). If the rash is exfoliative, purpuric, or bullous, or if lupus erythematosus, Stevens-Johnson Syndrome, or toxic epidermal necrolysis is suspected, use of this drug should not be resumed and alternative therapy should be considered. (See ADVERSE REACTIONS.) If the rash is of a milder type (measles-like or scarlatiniform), therapy may be resumed after the rash has completely disappeared. If the rash recurs upon reinstitution of therapy, further phenytoin medication is contraindicated.

Phenytoin and other hydantoins are contraindicated in patients who have experienced phenytoin hypersensitivity (see CONTRAINDICATIONS). Additionally, caution should be exercised if using structurally similar compounds (e.g., barbiturates, succinamides, oxazolidinediones and other related compounds) in these same patients.

Hyperglycemia, resulting from the drug's inhibitory effects on insulin release, has been reported. Phenytoin may also raise the serum glucose level in diabetic patients.

Osteomalacia has been associated with phenytoin therapy and is considered to be due to phenytoin's interference with Vitamin D metabolism.

Phenytoin is not indicated for seizures due to hypoglycemic or other metabolic causes. Appropriate diagnostic procedures should be performed as indicated.

Phenytoin is not effective for absence (petit mal) seizures. If tonic-clonic (grand mal) and absence (petit mal) seizures are present, combined drug therapy is needed.

Serum levels of phenytoin sustained above the optimal range may produce confusional states referred to as "delirium," "psychosis," or "encephalopathy," or rarely irreversible cerebellar dysfunction. Accordingly, at the first sign of acute toxicity, plasma levels are recommended. Dose reduction of phenytoin therapy is indicated if plasma levels are excessive; if symptoms persist, termination is recommended. (See WARNINGS.)

Information for Patients: Patients taking phenytoin should be advised of the importance of adhering strictly to the prescribed dosage regimen, and of informing the physician of any clinical condition in which it is not possible to take the drug orally as prescribed, e.g., surgery, etc.

Patients should also be cautioned on the use of other drugs or alcoholic beverages without first seeking the physician's advice.

Patients should be instructed to call their physician if skin rash develops.

The importance of good dental hygiene should be stressed in order to minimize the development of gingival hyperplasia and its complications.

Patients should be informed of the availability of a Medication Guide, and they should be instructed to read the Medication Guide prior to taking phenytoin sodium. Patients should be instructed to take phenytoin sodium only as prescribed.

Suicidal Thinking and Behavior: Patients, their caregivers, and families should be counseled that AEDs, including phenytoin sodium, may increase the risk of suicidal thoughts and behavior and should be advised of the need to be alert for the emergence or worsening of symptoms of depression, any unusual changes in mood or behavior, or the emergence of suicidal thoughts, behavior, or thoughts about self-harm. Behaviors of concern should be reported immediately to healthcare providers.

Patients should be encouraged to enroll in the North American Antiepileptic Drug (NAAED) Pregnancy Registry if they become pregnant. This Registry is collecting information about the safety of antiepileptic drugs during pregnancy. To enroll, patients can call the toll free number 1-888-233-2334 (see PRECAUTIONS: Pregnancy).

Laboratory Tests: Phenytoin serum level determinations may be necessary to achieve optimal dosage adjustments.

Drug Interactions: There are many drugs which may increase or decrease phenytoin levels or which phenytoin may affect. Serum level determinations for phenytoin are especially helpful when possible drug interactions are suspected. The most commonly occurring drug interactions are listed below.

1. Drugs which may increase phenytoin serum levels include: acute alcohol intake, amiodarone, chloramphenicol, chlordiazepoxide, cimetidine, diazepam, dicumarol, disulfiram, estrogens, ethosuximide, fluoxetine, H$_2$-antagonists, halothane, isoniazid, methylphenidate, phe-

nothiazines, phenylbutazone, salicylates, succinamides, sulfonamides, ticlopidine, tolbutamide, trazodone.

2. Drugs which may decrease phenytoin levels include: carbamazepine, chronic alcohol abuse, reserpine, and sucralfate. Moban® brand of molindone hydrochloride contains calcium ions which interfere with the absorption of phenytoin. Ingestion times of phenytoin and antacid preparations containing calcium should be staggered in patients with low serum phenytoin levels to prevent absorption problems.

3. Drugs which may either increase or decrease phenytoin serum levels include: phenobarbital, sodium valproate, and valproic acid. Similarly, the effect of phenytoin on phenobarbital, valproic acid and sodium valproate serum levels is unpredictable.

4. Although not a true drug interaction, tricyclic antidepressants may precipitate seizures in susceptible patients and phenytoin dosage may need to be adjusted.

5. Drugs whose efficacy is impaired by phenytoin include: corticosteroids, coumarin anticoagulants, digitoxin, doxycycline, estrogens, furosemide, oral contraceptives, paroxetine, quinidine, rifampin, theophylline, vitamin D.

Drug Enteral Feeding/Nutritional Preparations Interaction: Literature reports suggest that patients who have received enteral feeding preparations and/or related nutritional supplements have lower than expected phenytoin plasma levels. It is therefore suggested that phenytoin not be administered concomitantly with an enteral feeding preparation. More frequent serum phenytoin level monitoring may be necessary in these patients.

Drug/Laboratory Test Interactions: Phenytoin may decrease serum concentrations of T$_4$. It may also produce lower than normal values for dexamethasone or metyrapone tests. Phenytoin may cause increased serum levels of glucose, alkaline phosphatase, and gamma glutamyl transpeptidase (GGT).

Care should be taken when using immunoanalytical methods to measure plasma phenytoin concentrations.

Carcinogenesis: See WARNINGS section for information on carcinogenesis.

Pregnancy: Pregnancy Category D: See WARNINGS.

To provide information regarding the effects of *in utero* exposure to phenytoin sodium, physicians are advised to recommend that pregnant patients taking phenytoin sodium enroll in the North American Antiepileptic Drug (NAAED) Pregnancy Registry. This can be done by calling the toll free number 1-888-233-2334, and must be done by patients themselves. Information on the registry can also be found at the website http://www.aedpregnancyregistry.org/.

Nursing Mothers: Infant breast feeding is not recommended for women taking this drug because phenytoin appears to be secreted in low concentrations in human milk.

Pediatric Use: See DOSAGE AND ADMINISTRATION.

ADVERSE REACTIONS

Central Nervous System: The most common manifestations encountered with phenytoin therapy are referable to this system and are usually dose-related. These include nystagmus, ataxia, slurred speech, decreased coordination, and mental confusion. Dizziness, insomnia, transient nervousness, motor twitchings, and headaches have also been observed. There have also been rare reports of phenytoin induced dyskinesias, including chorea, dystonia, tremor and asterixis, similar to those induced by phenothiazine and other neuroleptic drugs.

A predominantly sensory peripheral polyneuropathy has been observed in patients receiving long-term phenytoin therapy.

Gastrointestinal System: Nausea, vomiting, constipation, toxic hepatitis and liver damage.

Integumentary System: Dermatological manifestations sometimes accompanied by fever have included scarlatiniform or morbilliform rashes. A morbilliform rash (measles-like) is the most common; other types of dermatitis are seen more rarely. Other more serious forms which may be fatal have included bullous, exfoliative or purpuric dermatitis, lupus erythematosus, Stevens-Johnson Syndrome, and toxic epidermal necrolysis (see PRECAUTIONS).

Hemopoietic System: Hemopoietic complications, some fatal, have occasionally been reported in association with administration of phenytoin. These have included thrombocytopenia, leukopenia, granulocytopenia, agranulocytosis, and pancytopenia with or without bone marrow suppression. While macrocytosis and megaloblastic anemia have occurred, these conditions usually respond to folic acid therapy. Lymphadenopathy including benign lymph node hyperplasia, pseudolymphoma, lymphoma, and Hodgkin's Disease have been reported (see WARNINGS).

Connective Tissue System: Coarsening of the facial features, enlargement of the lips, gingival hyperplasia, hypertrichosis, and Peyronie's Disease.

Immunologic: Hypersensitivity syndrome (which may include, but is not limited to, symptoms such as arthralgias, eosinophilia, fever, liver dysfunction, lymphadenopathy or rash), systemic lupus erythematosus, periarteritis nodosa and immunoglobulin abnormalities.

OVERDOSAGE

The lethal dose in pediatric patients is not known. The lethal dose in adults is estimated to be 2 to 5 grams. The initial symptoms are nystagmus, ataxia, and dysarthria. Other signs are tremor, hyperreflexia, lethargy, slurred speech, nausea, vomiting. The patient may become comatose and hypotensive. Death is due to respiratory and circulatory depression.

There are marked variations among individuals with respect to phenytoin plasma levels where toxicity may occur. Nystagmus, on lateral gaze, usually appears at 20 mcg/mL, ataxia at 30 mcg/mL, dysarthria and lethargy appear when the plasma concentration is over 40 mcg/mL, but as high a concentration as 50 mcg/mL has been reported without evidence of toxicity. As much as 25 times the therapeutic dose has been taken to result in a serum concentration over 100 mcg/mL with complete recovery.

Treatment: Treatment is nonspecific since there is no known antidote.

The adequacy of the respiratory and circulatory systems should be carefully observed and appropriate supportive measures employed. Hemodialysis can be considered since phenytoin is not completely bound to plasma proteins. Total exchange transfusion has been used in the treatment of severe intoxication in pediatric patients.

In acute overdosage, the possibility of other CNS depressants, including alcohol, should be borne in mind.

DOSAGE AND ADMINISTRATION

Serum concentrations should be monitored in changing from extended phenytoin sodium capsules, USP, to prompt phenytoin sodium capsules, USP, and from the sodium salt to the free acid form.

PHENYTEK® CAPSULES (extended phenytoin sodium capsules, USP) are formulated with the sodium salt of phenytoin. Because there is approximately an 8% increase in drug content with the free acid form over that of the sodium salt, dosage adjustments and serum level monitoring may be necessary when switching from a product formulated with the free acid to a product formulated with the sodium salt and vice versa.

General: Dosage should be individualized to provide maximum benefit. In some cases, serum blood level determinations may be necessary for optimal dosage adjustments — the clinically effective serum level is usually 10 to 20 mcg/mL. With recommended dosage, a period of 7 to 10 days may be required to achieve steadystate blood levels with phenytoin and changes in dosage (increase or decrease) should not be carried out at intervals shorter than 7 to 10 days.

Adult Dosage: ***Divided Daily Dosage:*** Patients who have received no previous treatment may be started on one 100 mg extended phenytoin sodium capsule three times daily and the dosage then adjusted to suit individual requirements. For most adults, the satisfactory maintenance dosage will be one 100 mg capsule three to four times a day. An increase up to one 200 mg PHENYTEK® three times a day may be made, if necessary.

Once-A-Day Dosage: In adults, if seizure control is established with divided doses of three 100 mg extended phenytoin sodium capsules daily, once-a-day dosage with 300 mg PHENYTEK® may be considered. Studies comparing divided doses of 300 mg with a single daily dose of this quantity indicated absorption, peak plasma levels, biologic half-life, difference between peak and minimum values, and urinary recovery were equivalent. Once-a-day dosage offers a convenience to the individual patient or to nursing personnel for institutionalized patients and is intended to be used only for patients requiring this amount of drug daily. A major problem in motivating noncompliant patients may also be lessened when the patient can take this drug once a day. However, patients should be cautioned not to miss a dose, inadvertently.

Only extended phenytoin sodium capsules are recommended for once-a-day dosing. Inherent differences in dissolution characteristics and resultant absorption rates of phenytoin due to different manufacturing procedures and/or dosage forms preclude such recommendation for other phenytoin products. When a change in the dosage form or brand is prescribed, careful monitoring of phenytoin serum levels should be carried out.

Loading Dose: Some authorities have advocated use of an oral loading dose of phenytoin in adults who require rapid steady-state serum levels and where intravenous administration is not desirable. This dosing regimen should be reserved for patients in a clinic or hospital setting where phenytoin serum levels can be closely monitored. Patients with a history of renal or liver disease should not receive the oral loading regimen.

Initially, one gram of phenytoin capsules is divided into three doses (400 mg, 300 mg, 300 mg) and administered at 2 hour intervals. Normal maintenance dosage is then instituted 24 hours after the loading dose, with frequent serum level determinations.

Pediatric Dosage: Initially, 5 mg/kg/day in two or three equally divided doses, with subsequent dosage individualized to a maximum of 300 mg daily. A recommended daily maintenance dosage is usually 4 to 8 mg/kg. Children over 6 years old and adolescents may require the minimum adult dose (300 mg/day).

HOW SUPPLIED

PHENYTEK® CAPSULES (extended phenytoin sodium capsules, USP) are available containing 200 mg or 300 mg of phenytoin sodium, USP.

The 200 mg capsule has a dark blue opaque cap and a blue opaque body. The hard-shell gelatin capsule is filled with two white to off-white round tablets. The capsule is rectified radial printed with **BERTEK** over **670** in black ink on both the cap and the body. They are available as follows:

NDC 0378-2670-93
bottles of 30 capsules
NDC 0378-2670-01
bottles of 100 capsules

The 300 mg capsule has a blue opaque cap and a blue opaque body. The hard-shell gelatin capsule is filled with three white to off-white round tablets. The capsule is rectified radial printed with **BERTEK** over **750** in black ink on both the cap and the body. They are available as follows:

NDC 0378-3750-93
bottles of 30 capsules
NDC 0378-3750-01
bottles of 100 capsules

Store at 20° to 25°C (68° to 77°F). [See USP Controlled Room Temperature.]

Protect from light and moisture.

Dispense in a tight, light-resistant container as defined in the USP using a child-resistant closure.

U.S. Patent No. 6,274,168
Mylan Pharmaceuticals Inc.
Morgantown, WV 26505

REVISED NOVEMBER 2009
BKPHTK:R10

SELEGILINE HYDROCHLORIDE TABLETS USP ℞

5 mg
℞ only

DESCRIPTION

Selegiline hydrochloride is a levorotatory acetylenic derivative of phenethylamine. It is commonly referred to in the clinical and pharmacological literature as l-deprenyl.

The chemical name is: (R)-(-)-N,2-dimethylpropynyl-phenethylamine hydrochloride. It is a white to near white crystalline powder, freely soluble in water, chloroform, and methanol, and has a molecular weight of 223.75. The structural formula is as follows:

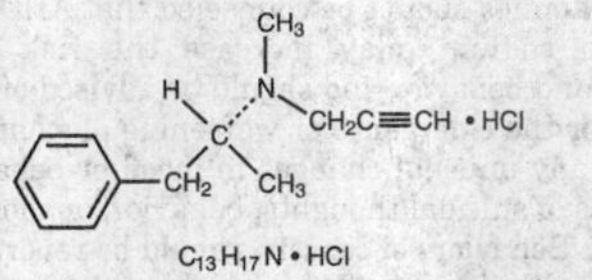

$C_{13}H_{17}N \cdot HCl$

Each tablet, for oral administration, contains 5 mg selegiline hydrochloride, USP. In addition, each tablet contains the following inactive ingredients: citric acid, lactose monohydrate, maize starch, magnesium stearate, povidone and talc.

CLINICAL PHARMACOLOGY

The mechanisms accounting for selegiline's beneficial adjunctive action in the treatment of Parkinson's disease are not fully understood. Inhibition of monoamine oxidase, type B, activity is generally considered to be of primary importance; in addition, there is evidence that selegiline may act through other mechanisms to increase dopaminergic activity.

Selegiline is best known as an irreversible inhibitor of monoamine oxidase (MAO), an intracellular enzyme associated with the outer membrane of mitochondria. Selegiline inhibits MAO by acting as a 'suicide' substrate for the enzyme; that is, it is converted by MAO to an active moiety which combines irreversibly with the active site and/or the enzyme's essential FAD cofactor. Because selegiline has greater affinity for type B rather than for type A active sites, it can serve as a selective inhibitor of MAO type B if it is administered at the recommended dose.

MAOs are widely distributed throughout the body; their concentration is especially high in liver, kidney, stomach, intestinal wall, and brain. MAOs are currently subclassified into two types, A and B, which differ in their substrate specificity and tissue distribution. In humans, intestinal MAO is predominantly type A, while most of that in brain is type B. In CNS neurons, MAO plays an important role in the catabolism of catecholamines (dopamine, norepinephrine and epinephrine) and serotonin. MAOs are also important in the catabolism of various exogenous amines found in a variety of foods and drugs. MAO in the GI tract and liver (primarily type A), for example, is thought to provide vital protection from exogenous amines (e.g., tyramine) that have the capacity, if absorbed intact, to cause a 'hypertensive crisis', the so-called 'cheese reaction.' (If large amounts of certain exogenous amines gain access to the systemic circulation - e.g., from fermented cheese, red wine, herring, over-the-counter cough/cold medications, etc. - they are taken up by adrenergic neurons and displace norepinephrine from storage sites within membrane bound vesicles. Subsequent release of the displaced norepinephrine causes the rise in systemic blood pressure, etc.)

In theory, since MAO-A of the gut is not inhibited, patients treated with selegiline at a dose of 10 mg a day should be able to take medications containing pharmacologically active amines and consume tyramine-containing foods without risk of uncontrolled hypertension. Although rare, a few reports of hypertensive reactions have occurred in patients receiving selegiline at the recommended dose, with tyramine-containing foods. In addition, one case of hypertensive crisis has been reported in a patient taking the recommended dose of selegiline and a sympathomimetic medication, ephedrine. The pathophysiology of the 'cheese reaction' is complicated and, in addition to its ability to inhibit MAO-B selectively, selegiline's relative freedom from this reaction has been attributed to an ability to prevent tyramine and other indirect acting sympathomimetics from displacing norepinephrine from adrenergic neurons. However, until the pathophysiology of the cheese reaction is more completely understood, it seems prudent to assume that selegiline can ordinarily only be used safely without dietary restrictions at doses where it presumably selectively inhibits MAO-B (e.g., 10 mg/day).

In short, attention to the dose dependent nature of selegiline's selectivity is critical if it is to be used without elaborate restrictions being placed on diet and concomitant drug use although, as noted above, a few cases of hypertensive reactions have been reported at the recommended dose (see WARNINGS and PRECAUTIONS).

It is important to be aware that selegiline may have pharmacological effects unrelated to MAO-B inhibition. As noted above, there is some evidence that it may increase dopaminergic activity by other mechanisms, including interfering with dopamine re-uptake at the synapse. Effects resulting from selegiline administration may also be mediated through its metabolites. Two of its three principal metabolites, amphetamine and methamphetamine, have pharmacological actions of their own; they interfere with neuronal uptake and enhance release of several neurotransmitters (e.g., norepinephrine, dopamine, serotonin). However, the extent to which these metabolites contribute to the effects of selegiline are unknown.

Rationale for the Use of a Selective Monoamine Oxidase Type B Inhibitor in Parkinson's Disease: Many of the prominent symptoms of Parkinson's disease are due to a deficiency of striatal dopamine that is the consequence of a progressive degeneration and loss of a population of dopaminergic neurons which originate in the substantia nigra of the midbrain and project to the basal ganglia or striatum. Early in the course of Parkinson's Disease, the deficit in the capacity of these neurons to synthesize dopamine can be overcome by administration of exogenous levodopa, usually given in combination with a peripheral decarboxylase inhibitor (carbidopa).

With the passage of time, due to the progression of the disease and/or the effect of sustained treatment, the efficacy and quality of the therapeutic response to levodopa diminishes. Thus, after several years of levodopa treatment, the response, for a given dose of levodopa, is shorter, has less predictable onset and offset (i.e., there is 'wearing off'), and is often accompanied by side effects (e.g., dyskinesia, akinesias, on-off phenomena, freezing, etc.).

This deteriorating response is currently interpreted as a manifestation of the inability of the ever decreasing population of intact nigrostriatal neurons to synthesize and release adequate amounts of dopamine.

MAO-B inhibition may be useful in this setting because, by blocking the catabolism of dopamine, it would increase the net amount of dopamine available (i.e., it would increase the pool of dopamine). Whether or not this mechanism or an alternative one actually accounts for the observed beneficial effects of adjunctive selegiline is unknown.

Selegiline's benefit in Parkinson's disease has only been documented as an adjunct to levodopa/carbidopa. Whether or not it might be effective as a sole treatment is unknown, but past attempts to treat Parkinson's disease with non-selective MAOI monotherapy are reported to have been unsuccessful. It is important to note that attempts to treat Parkinsonian patients with combinations of levodopa and currently marketed non-selective MAO inhibitors were abandoned because of multiple side effects including hypertension, increase in involuntary movement, and toxic delirium.

Pharmacokinetic Information (Absorption, Distribution, Metabolism and Elimination—ADME): The absolute bioavailability of selegiline following oral dosing is not known; however, selegiline undergoes extensive metabolism (presumably attributable to presystemic clearance in gut and liver). The major plasma metabolites are N-desmethylselegiline, L-amphetamine and L-methamphetamine. Only N-desmethylselegiline has MAO-B inhibiting activity. The peak plasma levels of these metabolites following a single oral dose of 10 mg are from 4 to almost 20 times greater than that of the maximum plasma concentration of selegiline [1 ng/mL]. The maximum concentrations of amphetamine and methamphetamine, however, are far below those ordinarily expected to produce clinically important effects.

Single oral dose studies do not predict multiple dose kinetics, however, at steady-state the peak plasma level of selegiline is 4-fold that obtained following a single dose. Metabolite concentrations increase to a lesser extent, averaging 2-fold that seen after a single dose.

The bioavailability of selegiline is increased 3- to 4-fold when it is taken with food.

The extent of systemic exposure to selegiline at a given dose varies considerably among individuals. Estimates of systemic clearance of selegiline are not available. Following a single oral dose, the mean elimination half-life of selegiline is 2 hours. Under steady-state conditions the elimination half-life increases to 10 hours.

Because selegiline's inhibition of MAO-B is irreversible, it is impossible to predict the extent of MAO-B inhibition from steady-state plasma levels. For the same reason, it is not possible to predict the rate of recovery of MAO-B activity as a function of plasma levels. The recovery of MAO-B activity is a function of de novo protein synthesis; however, information about the rate of de novo protein synthesis is not yet available. Although platelet MAO-B activity returns to the normal range within 5 to 7 days of selegiline discontinuation, the linkage between platelet and brain MAO-B inhibition is not fully understood nor is the relationship of MAO-B inhibition to the clinical effect established (see CLINICAL PHARMACOLOGY).

Special Populations:

Renal Impairment: No pharmacokinetic information is available on selegiline or its metabolites in renally impaired subjects.

Hepatic Impairment: No pharmacokinetic information is available on selegiline or its metabolites in hepatically impaired subjects.

Age: Although a general conclusion about the effects of age on the pharmacokinetics of selegiline is not warranted because of the size of the sample evaluated (12 subjects greater than 60 years of age, 12 subjects between the ages of 18 to 30), systemic exposure was about twice as great in older as compared to a younger population given a single oral dose of 10 mg.

Gender: No information is available on the effects of gender on the pharmacokinetics of selegiline.

INDICATIONS AND USAGE

Selegiline hydrochloride tablets are indicated as an adjunct in the management of Parkinsonian patients being treated with *levodopa/carbidopa* who exhibit deterioration in the quality of their response to this therapy. There is no evidence from controlled studies that selegiline hydrochloride tablets have any beneficial effect in the absence of concurrent levodopa therapy.

Evidence supporting this claim was obtained in randomized controlled clinical investigations that compared the effects of added selegiline hydrochloride tablets or placebo

in patients receiving levodopa/carbidopa. Selegiline hydrochloride tablets were significantly superior to placebo on all three principal outcome measures employed: change from baseline in daily levodopa/carbidopa dose, the amount of 'off' time, and patient self-rating of treatment success. Beneficial effects were also observed on other measures of treatment success (e.g., measures of reduced end of dose akinesia, decreased tremor and sialorrhea, improved speech and dressing ability and improved overall disability as assessed by walking and comparison to previous state).

CONTRAINDICATIONS

Selegiline hydrochloride tablets are contraindicated in patients with a known hypersensitivity to this drug.

Selegiline hydrochloride is contraindicated for use with meperidine (DEMEROL† and other trade names). This contraindication is often extended to other opioids (see PRECAUTIONS: Drug Interactions).

WARNINGS

Selegiline should not be used at daily doses exceeding those recommended (10 mg/day) because of the risks associated with non-selective inhibition of MAO (see CLINICAL PHARMACOLOGY).

The selectivity of selegiline for MAO-B may not be absolute even at the recommended daily dose of 10 mg a day. Rare cases of hypertensive reactions associated with ingestion of tyramine-containing foods have been reported in patients taking the recommended daily dose of selegiline. The selectivity is further diminished with increasing daily doses. The precise dose at which selegiline becomes a non-selective inhibitor of all MAO is unknown, but may be in the range of 30 mg to 40 mg a day.

Severe CNS toxicity associated with hyperpyrexia and death have been reported with the combination of tricyclic antidepressants and nonselective MAOIs [phenelzine (NARDIL†), tranylcypromine (PARNATE†)]. A similar reaction has been reported for a patient on amitriptyline and selegiline. Another patient receiving protriptyline and selegiline developed tremors, agitation and restlessness followed by unresponsiveness and death 2 weeks after selegiline was added. Related adverse events including hypertension, syncope, asystole, diaphoresis, seizures, changes in behavioral and mental status, and muscular rigidity have also been reported in some patients receiving selegiline and various tricyclic antidepressants.

Serious, sometimes fatal, reactions with signs and symptoms that may include hyperthermia, rigidity, myoclonus, autonomic instability with rapid fluctuations of the vital signs, and mental status changes that include extreme agitation progressing to delirium and coma have been reported with patients receiving a combination of fluoxetine hydrochloride (PROZAC†) and non-selective MAOIs. Similar signs have been reported in some patients on the combination of selegiline (10 mg a day) and selective serotonin re-uptake inhibitors including fluoxetine, sertraline and paroxetine.

Since the mechanisms of these reactions are not fully understood, it seems prudent, in general, to avoid this combination of selegiline and tricyclic antidepressants as well as selegiline and selective serotonin re-uptake inhibitors. At least 14 days should elapse between discontinuation of selegiline and initiation of treatment with a tricyclic antidepressant or selective serotonin re-uptake inhibitors. Because of the long half-lives of fluoxetine and its active metabolite, at least 5 weeks (perhaps longer, especially if fluoxetine has been prescribed chronically and/or at higher doses) should elapse between discontinuation of fluoxetine and initiation of treatment with selegiline.

PRECAUTIONS

General: Some patients given selegiline may experience an exacerbation of levodopa associated side effects, presumably due to the increased amounts of dopamine reaction with super sensitive, post-synaptic receptors. These effects may often be mitigated by reducing the dose of levodopa/carbidopa by approximately 10% to 30%.

The decision to prescribe selegiline should take into consideration that the MAO system of enzymes is complex and incompletely understood and there is only a limited amount of carefully documented clinical experience with selegiline. Consequently, the full spectrum of possible responses to selegiline may not have been observed in premarketing evaluation of the drug. It is advisable, therefore, to observe patients closely for atypical responses.

Melanoma: Epidemiological studies have shown that patients with Parkinson's disease have a higher risk (2- to approximately 6-fold higher) of developing melanoma than the general population. Whether the increased risk observed was due to Parkinson's disease or other factors, such as drugs used to treat Parkinson's disease, is unclear.

For the reasons stated above, patients and providers are advised to monitor for melanomas frequently and on a regular basis when using selegiline for any indication. Ideally, periodic skin examinations should be performed by appropriately qualified individuals (e.g., dermatologists).

Information for Patients: Patients should be advised of the possible need to reduce levodopa dosage after the initiation of selegiline hydrochloride therapy.

Patients (or their families if the patient is incompetent) should be advised not to exceed the daily recommended dose of 10 mg. The risk of using higher daily doses of selegiline should be explained, and a brief description of the 'cheese reaction' provided. Rare hypertensive reactions with selegiline at recommended doses associated with dietary influences have been reported.

Consequently, it may be useful to inform patients (or their families) about the signs and symptoms associated with MAOI induced hypertensive reactions. In particular, patients should be urged to report, immediately, any severe headache or other atypical or unusual symptoms not previously experienced.

There have been reports of patients experiencing intense urges to gamble, increased sexual urges, and other intense urges and the inability to control these urges while taking one or more of the medications that increase central dopaminergic tone, that are generally used for the treatment of Parkinson's disease, including selegiline. Although it is not proven that the medications caused these events, these urges were reported to have stopped in some cases when the dose was reduced or the medication was stopped. Prescribers should ask patients about the development of new or increased gambling urges, sexual urges or other urges while being treated with selegiline. Patients should inform their physician if they experience new or increased gambling urges, increased sexual urges or other intense urges while taking selegiline. Physicians should consider dose reduction or stopping the medication if a patient develops such urges while taking selegiline.

Laboratory Tests: No specific laboratory tests are deemed essential for the management of patients on selegiline hydrochloride. Periodic routine evaluation of all patients, however, is appropriate.

Drug Interactions: The occurrence of stupor, muscular rigidity, severe agitation and elevated temperature has been reported in some patients receiving the combination of selegiline and meperidine. Symptoms usually resolve over days when the combination is discontinued. This is typical of the interaction of meperidine and MAOIs. Other serious reactions (including severe agitation, hallucinations and death) have been reported in patients receiving this combination (see CONTRAINDICATIONS). Severe toxicity has also been reported in patients receiving the combination of tricyclic antidepressants and selegiline and selective serotonin re-uptake inhibitors and selegiline (see WARNINGS for details). One case of hypertensive crisis has been reported in a patient taking the recommended doses of selegiline and a sympathomimetic medication (ephedrine).

Carcinogenesis, Mutagenesis and Impairment of Fertility: Assessment of the carcinogenic potential of selegiline in mice and rats is ongoing for all dosage forms. Selegiline did not induce mutations or chromosomal damage when tested in the bacterial mutation assay in *Salmonella typhimurium* and in an *in vivo* chromosomal aberration assay. While these studies provide some reassurance that selegiline is not mutagenic or clastogenic, they are not definitive because of methodological limitations. No definitive *in vitro* chromosomal aberration or *in vitro* mammalian gene mutation assays have been performed.

The effect of selegiline on fertility has not been adequately assessed.

Pregnancy: *Pregnancy Category C:* No teratogenic effects were observed in a study of embryo-fetal development in Sprague-Dawley rats at oral doses of 4, 12 and 36 mg/kg or 4, 12 and 35 times the human therapeutic dose on a mg/m² basis. No teratogenic effects were observed in a study of embryo-fetal development in New Zealand White rabbits at oral doses of 5, 25 and 50 mg/kg or 10, 48 and 95 times the human therapeutic dose on a mg/m² basis; however, in this study, the number of litters produced at the two higher doses was less than recommended for assessing teratogenic potential. In the rat study, there was a decrease in fetal body weight at the highest dose tested. In the rabbit study, increases in total resorptions and % post-implantation loss, and a decrease in the number of live fetuses per dam occurred at the highest dose tested. In a peri- and postnatal development study in Sprague-Dawley rats (oral doses of 4, 16 and 64 mg/kg or 4, 15 and 62 times the human therapeutic dose on a mg/m² basis), an increase in the number of stillbirths and decreases in the number of pups per dam, pup survival and pup body weight (at birth and throughout the lactation period) were observed at the two highest doses. At the highest dose tested, no pups born alive survived to Day 4 postpartum. Postnatal development at the highest dose tested in dams could not be evaluated because of the lack of surviving pups. The reproductive performance of the untreated offspring was not assessed.

There are no adequate and well controlled studies in pregnant women. Selegiline should be used during pregnancy only if the potential benefit justifies the potential risk to the fetus.

Nursing Mothers: It is not known whether selegiline hydrochloride is excreted in human milk. Because many drugs are excreted in human milk, consideration should be given to discontinuing the use of all but absolutely essential drug treatments in nursing women.

Pediatric Use: The effects of selegiline hydrochloride in children have not been evaluated.

ADVERSE REACTIONS

Introduction: The number of patients who received selegiline in prospectively monitored premarketing studies is limited. While other sources of information about the use of selegiline are available (e.g., literature reports, foreign post-marketing reports, etc.) they do not provide the kind of information necessary to estimate the incidence of adverse events. Thus, overall incidence figures for adverse reactions associated with the use of selegiline cannot be provided. Many of the adverse reactions seen have also been reported as symptoms of dopamine excess.

Moreover, the importance and severity of various reactions reported often cannot be ascertained. One index of relative importance, however, is whether or not a reaction caused treatment discontinuation. In prospective premarketing studies, the following events led, in decreasing order of frequency, to discontinuation of treatment with selegiline: nausea, hallucinations, confusion, depression, loss of balance, insomnia, orthostatic hypotension, increased akinetic involuntary movements, agitation, arrhythmia, bradykinesia, chorea, delusions, hypertension, new or increased angina pectoris and syncope. Events reported only once as a cause of discontinuation are ankle edema, anxiety, burning lips/mouth, constipation, drowsiness/lethargy, dystonia, excess perspiration, increased freezing, gastrointestinal bleeding, hair loss, increased tremor, nervousness, weakness and weight loss.

Experience with selegiline hydrochloride obtained in parallel, placebo controlled, randomized studies provides only a limited basis for estimates of adverse reaction rates. The following reactions that occurred with greater frequency among the 49 patients assigned to selegiline as compared to the 50 patients assigned to placebo in the only parallel, placebo-controlled trial performed in patients with Parkinson's disease are shown in the following Table. None of these adverse reactions led to a discontinuation of treatment.

INCIDENCE OF TREATMENT-EMERGENT ADVERSE EXPERIENCES IN THE PLACEBO-CONTROLLED CLINICAL TRIAL

Adverse Event	Number of Patients Reporting Events	
	selegiline hydrochloride N = 49	placebo N = 50
Nausea	10	3
Dizziness/Light-headed/ Fainting	7	1
Abdominal Pain	4	2
Confusion	3	0
Hallucinations	3	1
Dry mouth	3	1
Vivid Dreams	2	0
Dyskinesias	2	5
Headache	2	1

The following events were reported once in either or both groups:

Ache, generalized	1	0
Anxiety/Tension	1	1
Anemia	0	1
Diarrhea	1	0
Hair Loss	0	1
Insomnia	1	1
Lethargy	1	0
Leg pain	1	0
Low back pain	1	0
Malaise	0	1
Palpitations	1	0
Urinary Retention	1	0
Weight Loss	1	0

In all prospectively monitored clinical investigations, enrolling approximately 920 patients, the following adverse events, classified by body system, were reported.

Central Nervous System: *Motor/Coordination/Extrapyramidal:* increased tremor, chorea, loss of balance, restlessness, blepharospasm, increased bradykinesia, facial grimace, falling down, heavy leg, muscle twitch*, myoclonic jerks*, stiff neck, tardive dyskinesia, dystonic symptoms, dyskinesia, involuntary movements, freezing, festination, increased apraxia, muscle cramps.

Mental Status/Behavioral/Psychiatric: hallucinations, dizziness, confusion, anxiety, depression, drowsiness, behavior/mood change, dreams/nightmares, tiredness, delusions, disorientation, lightheadedness, impaired memory*, increased energy*, transient high*, hollow feeling, lethargy/malaise, apathy, overstimulation, vertigo, personality change, sleep disturbance, restlessness, weakness, transient irritability.

Pain/Altered Sensation: headache, back pain, leg pain, tinnitus, migraine, supraorbital pain, throat burning, generalized ache, chills, numbness of toes/fingers, taste disturbance.

Autonomic Nervous System: dry mouth, blurred vision, sexual dysfunction.

Cardiovascular: orthostatic hypotension, hypertension, arrhythmia, palpitations, new or increased angina pectoris, hypotension, tachycardia, peripheral edema, sinus bradycardia, syncope.

Gastrointestinal: nausea/vomiting, constipation, weight loss, anorexia, poor appetite, dysphagia, diarrhea, heartburn, rectal bleeding, bruxism*, gastrointestinal bleeding (exacerbation of preexisting ulcer disease).

Genitourinary/Gynecologic/Endocrine: slow urination, transient anorgasmia*, nocturia, prostatic hypertrophy, urinary hesitancy, urinary retention, decreased penile sensation*, urinary frequency.

Skin and Appendages: increased sweating, diaphoresis, facial hair, hair loss, hematoma, rash, photosensitivity.

Miscellaneous: asthma, diplopia, shortness of breath, speech affected.

Post-Marketing Reports: The following experiences were described in spontaneous post-marketing reports. These reports do not provide sufficient information to establish a clear causal relationship with the use of selegiline hydrochloride.

CNS: Seizure in dialyzed chronic renal failure patient on concomitant medications.

* indicates events reported only at doses greater than 10 mg/day.

OVERDOSAGE

Selegiline: No specific information is available about clinically significant overdoses with selegiline hydrochloride. However, experience gained during selegiline's development reveals that some individuals exposed to doses of 600 mg of d,l-selegiline suffered severe hypotension and psychomotor agitation.

Since the selective inhibition of MAO-B by selegiline hydrochloride is achieved only at doses in the range recommended for the treatment of Parkinson's disease (e.g., 10 mg/day), overdoses are likely to cause significant inhibition of both MAO-A and MAO-B. Consequently, the signs and symptoms of overdose may resemble those observed with marketed non-selective MAO inhibitors [e.g., tranylcypromine (PARNATE†), isocarboxazide (MARPLAN†) and phenelzine (NARDIL†)].

Overdose with Non-Selective MAO Inhibition: NOTE: This section is provided for reference; it does not describe events that have actually been observed with selegiline in overdose.

Characteristically, signs and symptoms of non-selective MAOI overdose may not appear immediately. Delays of up to 12 hours between ingestion of drug and the appearance of signs may occur. Importantly, the peak intensity of the syndrome may not be reached for upwards of a day following the overdose. Death has been reported following overdosage. Therefore, immediate hospitalization, with continuous patient observation and monitoring for a period of at least 2 days following the ingestion of such drugs in overdose, is strongly recommended.

The clinical picture of MAOI overdose varies considerably; its severity may be a function of the amount of drug consumed. The central nervous and cardiovascular systems are prominently involved.

Signs and symptoms of overdosage may include, alone or in combination, any of the following: drowsiness, dizziness, faintness, irritability, hyperactivity, agitation, severe headache, hallucinations, trismus, opisthotonos, convulsions, and coma; rapid and irregular pulse, hypertension, hypotension and vascular collapse; precordial pain, respiratory depression and failure, hyperpyrexia, diaphoresis, and cool, clammy skin.

Treatment Suggestions for Overdose: NOTE: Because there is no recorded experience with selegiline overdose, the following suggestions are offered based upon the as-

sumption that selegiline overdose may be modeled by non-selective MAOI poisoning. In any case, up-to-date information about the treatment of overdose can often be obtained from a certified Regional Poison Control Center. Telephone numbers of certified Poison Control Centers are listed in the Physicians' Desk Reference (PDR).

Treatment of overdose with non-selective MAOIs is symptomatic and supportive. Induction of emesis or gastric lavage with instillation of charcoal slurry may be helpful in early poisoning, provided the airway has been protected against aspiration. Signs and symptoms of central nervous system stimulation, including convulsions, should be treated with diazepam, given slowly intravenously. Phenothiazine derivatives and central nervous system stimulants should be avoided. Hypotension and vascular collapse should be treated with intravenous fluids and, if necessary, blood pressure titration with an intravenous infusion of a dilute pressor agent. It should be noted that adrenergic agents may produce a markedly increased pressor response.

Respiration should be supported by appropriate measures, including management of the airway, use of supplemental oxygen and mechanical ventilatory assistance, as required. Body temperature should be monitored closely. Intensive management of hyperpyrexia may be required. Maintenance of fluid and electrolyte balance is essential.

DOSAGE AND ADMINISTRATION

Selegiline hydrochloride tablets are intended for administration to Parkinsonian patients receiving levodopa/carbidopa therapy who demonstrate a deteriorating response to this treatment. The recommended regimen for the administration of selegiline hydrochloride tablets are 10 mg per day administered as divided doses of 5 mg each taken at breakfast and lunch. There is no evidence that additional benefit will be obtained from the administration of higher doses. Moreover, higher doses should ordinarily be avoided because of the increased risk of side effects.

After 2 to 3 days of selegiline hydrochloride tablet treatment, an attempt may be made to reduce the dose of levodopa/carbidopa. A reduction of 10% to 30% was achieved with the typical participant in the domestic placebo-controlled trials who was assigned to selegiline hydrochloride tablet treatment. Further reductions of levodopa/carbidopa may be possible during continued selegiline hydrochloride tablet therapy.

HOW SUPPLIED

Selegiline Hydrochloride Tablets, USP are available containing 5 mg of selegiline hydrochloride, USP. Each white round, unscored tablet is debossed with **G** on one side and **SE** over **5** on the other side. They are available as follows:
NDC 0378-9290-91
bottles of 60 tablets
NDC 0378-9290-10
bottles of 1000 tablets
Store at 20° to 25°C (68° to 77°F). [See USP Controlled Room Temperature.]
Dispense in a tight, light-resistant container as defined in the USP using a child-resistant closure.
† The brand names mentioned are registered trademarks of their respective manufacturers.
Manufactured in Australia by:
ALPHAPHARM PTY. LTD.
15 Garnet Street,
Carole Park. Qld. 4300
Australia
Manufactured for:
Mylan Pharmaceuticals Inc.
Morgantown, WV 26505 U.S.A.

REVISED NOVEMBER 2009
ALP:SELG:R1

THIORIDAZINE HYDROCHLORIDE TABLETS, USP

℞

10 mg, 25 mg, 50 mg and 100 mg
℞ only

WARNING
Thioridazine has been shown to prolong the QTc interval in a dose related manner, and drugs with this potential, including thioridazine, have been associated with Torsades de pointes type arrhythmias and sudden death. Due to its potential for significant, possibly life threatening, proarrhythmic effects, thioridazine should be reserved for use in the treatment of schizophrenic patients who fail to show an acceptable response to adequate courses of treatment with other antipsychotic drugs, either because of insufficient effectiveness or the inability to achieve an effective dose due to intolerable adverse effects from those drugs (see WARNINGS, CONTRAINDICATIONS, and INDICATIONS).

Increased Mortality in Elderly Patients with Dementia-Related Psychosis: Elderly patients with dementia-related psychosis treated with antipsychotic drugs are at an increased risk of death. Analyses of seventeen placebo-controlled trials (modal duration of 10 weeks), largely in patients taking atypical antipsychotic drugs, revealed a risk of death in drug-treated patients of between 1.6 to 1.7 times the risk of death in placebo-treated patients. Over the course of a typical 10-week controlled trial, the rate of death in drug-treated patients was about 4.5%, compared to a rate of about 2.6% in the placebo group. Although the causes of death were varied, most of the deaths appeared to be either cardiovascular (e.g., heart failure, sudden death) or infectious (e.g., pneumonia) in nature. Observational studies suggest that, similar to atypical antipsychotic drugs, treatment with conventional antipsychotic drugs may increase mortality. The extent to which the findings of increased mortality in observational studies may be attributed to the antipsychotic drug as opposed to some characteristic(s) of the patients is not clear. Thioridazine hydrochloride is not approved for the treatment of patients with dementia-related psychosis (see WARNINGS).

DESCRIPTION

Thioridazine hydrochloride is 2-methylmercapto-10-[2-(N-methyl-2-piperidyl) ethyl] phenothiazine. Its structural formula, molecular weight and molecular formula are:

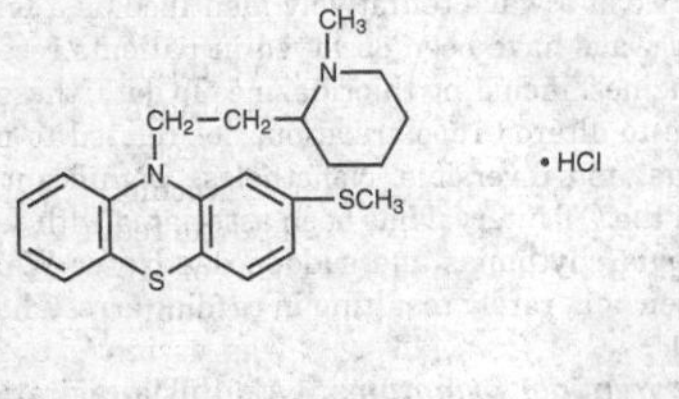

$C_{21}H_{26}N_2S_2 \cdot HCl$ M.Wt.: 407.05

Thioridazine hydrochloride, USP is available as tablets for oral administration containing 10 mg, 25 mg, 50 mg or 100 mg.

Each tablet for oral administration contains the following inactive ingredients: colloidal silicon dioxide, croscarmellose sodium, FD&C Yellow No. 6 Aluminum Lake, hydroxypropyl cellulose, hypromellose, magnesium stearate, microcrystalline cellulose, polyethylene glycol, sodium lauryl sulfate and titanium dioxide.

CLINICAL PHARMACOLOGY

The basic pharmacological activity of thioridazine is similar to that of other phenothiazines, but is associated with minimal extrapyramidal stimulation.

However, thioridazine has been shown to prolong the QTc interval in a dose dependent fashion. This effect may increase the risk of serious, potentially fatal, ventricular arrhythmias, such as Torsades de pointes type arrhythmias. Due to this risk, thioridazine is indicated only for schizophrenic patients who have not been responsive to or cannot tolerate other antipsychotic agents (see WARNINGS and CONTRAINDICATIONS). However, the prescriber should be aware that thioridazine has not been systematically evaluated in controlled trials in treatment refractory schizophrenic patients and its efficacy in such patients is unknown.

INDICATIONS AND USAGE

Thioridazine is indicated for the management of schizophrenic patients who fail to respond adequately to treatment with other antipsychotic drugs. Due to the risk of significant, potentially life threatening, proarrhythmic effects with thioridazine treatment, thioridazine should be used only in patients who have failed to respond adequately to treatment with appropriate courses of other antipsychotic drugs, either because of insufficient effectiveness or the inability to achieve an effective dose due to intolerable adverse effects from those drugs. Consequently, before initiating treatment with thioridazine, it is strongly recommended that a patient be given at least two trials, each with a different antipsychotic drug product, at an adequate dose, and for an adequate duration (see WARNINGS and CONTRAINDICATIONS).

However, the prescriber should be aware that thioridazine has not been systematically evaluated in controlled trials in treatment refractory schizophrenic patients and its efficacy in such patients is unknown.

CONTRAINDICATIONS

Thioridazine use should be avoided in combination with other drugs that are known to prolong the QTc interval and in patients with congenital long QT syndrome or a history of cardiac arrhythmias.

Reduced cytochrome P450 2D6 isozyme activity drugs that inhibit this isozyme (e.g., fluoxetine and paroxetine) and certain other drugs (e.g., fluvoxamine, propranolol, and pindolol) appear to appreciably inhibit the metabolism of thioridazine. The resulting elevated levels of thioridazine would be expected to augment the prolongation of the QTc interval associated with thioridazine and may increase the risk of serious, potentially fatal, cardiac arrhythmias, such as Torsades de pointes type arrhythmias. Such an increased risk may result also from the additive effect of coadministering thioridazine with other agents that prolong the QTc interval. Therefore, thioridazine is contraindicated with these drugs as well as in patients, comprising about 7% of the normal population, who are known to have a genetic defect leading to reduced levels of activity of P450 2D6 (see WARNINGS and PRECAUTIONS).

In common with other phenothiazines, thioridazine is contraindicated in severe central nervous system depression or comatose states from any cause including drug induced central nervous system depression (see WARNINGS). It should also be noted that hypertensive or hypotensive heart disease of extreme degree is a contraindication of phenothiazine administration.

WARNINGS

Increased Mortality in Elderly Patients with Dementia-Related Psychosis: Elderly patients with dementia-related psychosis treated with antipsychotic drugs are at an increased risk of death. Thioridazine hydrochloride is not approved for the treatment of patients with dementia-related psychosis (see BOXED WARNING).

Potential for Proarrhythmic Effects: DUE TO THE POTENTIAL FOR SIGNIFICANT, POSSIBLY LIFE THREATENING, PROARRHYTHMIC EFFECTS WITH THIORIDAZINE TREATMENT, THIORIDAZINE SHOULD BE RESERVED FOR USE IN THE TREATMENT OF SCHIZOPHRENIC PATIENTS WHO FAIL TO SHOW AN ACCEPTABLE RESPONSE TO ADEQUATE COURSES OF TREATMENT WITH OTHER ANTIPSYCHOTIC DRUGS, EITHER BECAUSE OF INSUFFICIENT EFFECTIVENESS OR THE INABILITY TO ACHIEVE AN EFFECTIVE DOSE DUE TO INTOLERABLE ADVERSE EFFECTS FROM THOSE DRUGS. CONSEQUENTLY, BEFORE INITIATING TREATMENT WITH THIORIDAZINE, IT IS STRONGLY RECOMMENDED THAT A PATIENT BE GIVEN AT LEAST TWO TRIALS, EACH WITH A DIFFERENT ANTIPSYCHOTIC DRUG PRODUCT, AT AN ADEQUATE DOSE, AND FOR AN ADEQUATE DURATION. THIORIDAZINE HAS NOT BEEN SYSTEMATICALLY EVALUATED IN CONTROLLED TRIALS IN THE TREATMENT OF REFRACTORY SCHIZOPHRENIC PATIENTS AND ITS EFFICACY IN SUCH PATIENTS IS UNKNOWN.

A crossover study in nine healthy males comparing single doses of thioridazine 10 mg and 50 mg with placebo demonstrated a dose related prolongation of the QTc interval. The mean maximum increase in QTc interval following the 50 mg dose was about 23 msec; greater prolongation may be observed in the clinical treatment of unscreened patients.

Prolongation of the QTc interval has been associated with the ability to cause Torsades de pointes type arrhythmias, a potentially fatal polymorphic ventricular tachycardia, and sudden death. There are several published case reports of Torsades de pointes and sudden death associated with thioridazine treatment. A causal relationship between these events and thioridazine therapy has not been established but, given the ability of thioridazine to prolong the QTc interval, such a relationship is possible.

Certain circumstances may increase the risk of Torsades de pointes and/or sudden death in association with the use of drugs that prolong the QTc interval, including 1) bradycardia, 2) hypokalemia, 3) concomitant use of other drugs that prolong the QTc interval, 4) presence of congenital prolongation of the QT interval, and 5) for thioridazine in particular, its use in patients with reduced activity of P450 2D6 or its coadministration with drugs that may inhibit P450 2D6 or by some other mechanism interfere with the clearance of thioridazine (see CONTRAINDICATIONS and PRECAUTIONS).

It is recommended that patients being considered for thioridazine treatment have a baseline ECG performed and serum potassium levels measured. Serum potassium should be normalized before initiating treatment and patients with a QTc interval greater than 450 msec should not receive thioridazine treatment. It may also be useful to periodically monitor ECG's and serum potassium during thioridazine treatment, especially during a period of dose adjustment. Thioridazine should be discontinued in patients who are found to have a QTc interval over 500 msec.

Patients taking thioridazine who experience symptoms that may be associated with the occurrence of Torsades de pointes (e.g., dizziness, palpitations, or syncope) may warrant further cardiac evaluation; in particular, Holter monitoring should be considered.

Tardive Dyskinesia: Tardive dyskinesia, a syndrome consisting of potentially irreversible, involuntary, dyskinetic movements may develop in patients treated with antipsychotic drugs. Although the prevalence of the syndrome appears to be highest among the elderly, especially elderly women, it is impossible to rely upon prevalence estimates to predict, at the inception of antipsychotic treatment, which patients are likely to develop the syndrome. Whether antipsychotic drug products differ in their potential to cause tardive dyskinesia is unknown.

Both the risk of developing the syndrome and the likelihood that it will become irreversible are believed to increase as the duration of treatment and the total cumulative dose of antipsychotic drugs administered to the patient increase. However, the syndrome can develop, although much less commonly, after relatively brief treatment periods at low doses.

There is no known treatment for established cases of tardive dyskinesia, although the syndrome may remit, partially or completely, if antipsychotic treatment is withdrawn. Antipsychotic treatment itself, however, may suppress (or partially suppress) the signs and symptoms of the syndrome and thereby may possibly mask the underlying disease process. The effect that symptomatic suppression has upon the long-term course of the syndrome is unknown.

Given these considerations, antipsychotics should be prescribed in a manner that is most likely to minimize the occurrence of tardive dyskinesia. Chronic antipsychotic treatment should generally be reserved for patients who suffer from a chronic illness that, 1) is known to respond to antipsychotic drugs, and, 2) for whom alternative, equally effective, but potentially less harmful treatments are *not* available or appropriate. In patients who do require chronic treatment, the smallest dose and the shortest duration of treatment producing a satisfactory clinical response should be sought. The need for continued treatment should be reassessed periodically.

If signs and symptoms of tardive dyskinesia appear in a patient on antipsychotics, drug discontinuation should be considered. However, some patients may require treatment despite the presence of the syndrome.

(For further information about the description of tardive dyskinesia and its clinical detection, please refer to the sections on Information for Patients and ADVERSE REACTIONS.)

It has been suggested in regard to phenothiazines in general, that people who have demonstrated a hypersensitivity reaction (e.g., blood dyscrasias, jaundice) to one may be more prone to demonstrate a reaction to others. Attention should be paid to the fact that phenothiazines are capable of potentiating central nervous system depressants (e.g., anesthetics, opiates, alcohol, etc.) as well as atropine and phosphorus insecticides. Physicians should carefully consider benefit versus risk when treating less severe disorders.

Reproductive studies in animals and clinical experience to date have failed to show a teratogenic effect with thioridazine. However, in view of the desirability of keeping the administration of all drugs to a minimum during pregnancy, thioridazine should be given only when the benefits derived from treatment exceed the possible risks to mother and fetus.

Neuroleptic Malignant Syndrome (NMS): A potentially fatal symptom complex sometimes referred to as Neuroleptic Malignant Syndrome (NMS) has been reported in association with antipsychotic drugs. Clinical manifestations of NMS are hyperpyrexia, muscle rigidity, altered mental status, and evidence of autonomic instability (irregular pulse or blood pressure, tachycardia, diaphoresis, and cardiac dysrhythmias).

The diagnostic evaluation of patients with this syndrome is complicated. In arriving at a diagnosis, it is important to identify cases where the clinical presentation includes both serious medical illness (e.g., pneumonia, systemic infection, etc.) and untreated or inadequately treated extrapyramidal signs and symptoms (EPS). Other important considerations in the differential diagnosis include central anticholinergic toxicity, heat stroke, drug fever, and primary central nervous system (CNS) pathology.

The management of NMS should include, 1) immediate discontinuation of antipsychotic drugs and other drugs not essential to concurrent therapy, 2) intensive symptomatic treatment and medical monitoring, and 3) treatment of any concomitant serious medical problems for which specific treatments are available. There is no general agreement about specific pharmacological treatment regimens for uncomplicated NMS.

If a patient requires antipsychotic drug treatment after recovery from NMS, the potential reintroduction of drug therapy should be carefully considered. The patient should be carefully monitored, since recurrences of NMS have been reported.

Central Nervous System Depressants: As in the case of other phenothiazines, thioridazine is capable of potentiating central nervous system depressants (e.g., alcohol, anesthetics, barbiturates, narcotics, opiates, other psychoactive drugs, etc.) as well as atropine and phosphorus insecticides. Severe respiratory depression and respiratory arrest have been reported when a patient was given a phenothiazine and a concomitant high dose of a barbiturate.

PRECAUTIONS

Leukopenia and/or agranulocytosis and convulsive seizures have been reported but are infrequent. In schizophrenic patients with epilepsy, anticonvulsant medication should be maintained during treatment with thioridazine. Pigmentary retinopathy, which has been observed primarily in patients taking larger than recommended doses, is characterized by diminution of visual acuity, brownish coloring of vision, and impairment of night vision; examination of the fundus discloses deposits of pigment. The possibility of this complication may be reduced by remaining within the recommended limits of dosage.

Where patients are participating in activities requiring complete mental alertness (e.g., driving) it is advisable to administer the phenothiazines cautiously and to increase the dosage gradually. Female patients appear to have a greater tendency to orthostatic hypotension than male patients. The administration of epinephrine should be avoided in the treatment of drug-induced hypotension in view of the fact that phenothiazines may induce a reversed epinephrine effect on occasion. Should a vasoconstrictor be required, the most suitable are levarterenol and phenylephrine.

Antipsychotic drugs elevate prolactin levels; the elevation persists during chronic administration. Tissue culture experiments indicate that approximately one-third of human breast cancers are prolactin dependent *in vitro*, a factor of potential importance if the prescription of these drugs is contemplated in a patient with a previously detected breast cancer. Although disturbances such as galactorrhea, amenorrhea, gynecomastia, and impotence have been reported, the clinical significance of elevated serum prolactin levels is unknown for most patients. An increase in mammary neoplasms has been found in rodents after chronic administration of neuroleptic drugs. Neither clinical studies nor epidemiologic studies conducted to date, however, have shown an association between chronic administration of these drugs and mammary tumorigenesis; the available evidence is considered too limited to be conclusive at this time.

Drug Interactions: Reduced cytochrome P450 2D6 isozyme activity, drugs which inhibit this isozyme (e.g., fluoxetine and paroxetine), and certain other drugs (e.g., fluvoxamine, propranolol, and pindolol) appear to appreciably inhibit the metabolism of thioridazine. The resulting elevated levels of thioridazine would be expected to augment the prolongation of the QTc interval associated with thioridazine and may increase the risk of serious, potentially fatal, cardiac arrhythmias, such as Torsades de pointes type arrhythmias. Such an increased risk may result also from the additive effect of coadministering thioridazine with other agents that prolong the QTc interval. Therefore, thioridazine is contraindicated with these drugs as well as in patients, comprising about 7% of the normal population, who are known to have a genetic defect leading to reduced levels of activity of P450 2D6 (see WARNINGS and CONTRAINDICATIONS).

Drugs That Inhibit Cytochrome P450 2D6: In a study of 19 healthy male subjects, which included 6 slow and 13 rapid hydroxylators of debrisoquin, a single 25 mg oral dose of thioridazine produced a 2.4-fold higher C_{max} and a 4.5-fold higher AUC for thioridazine in the slow hydroxylators compared to rapid hydroxylators. The rate of debrisoquin hydroxylation is felt to depend on the level of cytochrome P450 2D6 isozyme activity. Thus, this study suggests that drugs that inhibit P450 2D6 or the presence of reduced activity levels of this isozyme will produce elevated plasma levels of thioridazine. Therefore, the coadministration of drugs that inhibit P450 2D6 with thioridazine and the use of thioridazine in patients known to have reduced activity of P450 2D6 are contraindicated.

Drugs That Reduce the Clearance of Thioridazine Through Other Mechanisms: *Fluvoxamine:* The effect of fluvoxamine (25 mg b.i.d. for one week) on thioridazine steady-state concentration was evaluated in ten male inpatients with schizophrenia. Concentrations of thioridazine and its two active metabolites, mesoridazine and sulforidazine, increased 3-fold following coadministration of fluvoxamine. Fluvoxamine and thioridazine should not be coadministered.

Propranolol: Concurrent administration of propranolol (100 mg to 800 mg daily) has been reported to produce increases in plasma levels of thioridazine (approximately 50% to 400%) and its metabolites (approximately 80% to 300%). Propranolol and thioridazine should not be coadministered.

Pindolol: Concurrent administration of pindolol and thioridazine have resulted in moderate, dose related increases in the serum levels of thioridazine and two of its metabolites, as well as higher than expected serum pindolol levels. Pindolol and thioridazine should not be coadministered.

Drugs That Prolong the QTc Interval: There are no studies of the coadministration of thioridazine and other drugs that prolong the QTc interval. However, it is expected that such coadministration would produce additive prolongation of the QTc interval and, thus, such use is contraindicated.

Information for Patients: Patients should be informed that thioridazine has been associated with potentially fatal heart rhythm disturbances. The risk of such events may be increased when certain drugs are given together with thioridazine. Therefore, patients should inform the prescriber that they are receiving thioridazine treatment before taking any new medication.

Given the likelihood that some patients exposed chronically to antipsychotics will develop tardive dyskinesia, it is advised that all patients in whom chronic use is contemplated be given, if possible, full information about this risk. The decision to inform patients and/or their guardians must obviously take into account the clinical circumstances and the competency of the patient to understand the information provided.

Pediatric Use: See DOSAGE AND ADMINISTRATION: Pediatric Patients.

Leukopenia, Neutropenia and Agranulocytosis: In clinical trial and post-marketing experience, events of leukopenia/neutropenia and agranulocytosis have been reported temporally related to antipsychotic agents.

Possible risk factors for leukopenia/neutropenia include preexisting low white blood cell count (WBC) and history of drug induced leukopenia/neutropenia. Patients with a pre-existing low WBC or a history of drug induced leukopenia/neutropenia should have their complete blood count (CBC) monitored frequently during the first few months of therapy and should discontinue Thioridazine Hydrochloride Tablets, USP at the first sign of a decline in WBC in the absence of other causative factors.

Patients with neutropenia should be carefully monitored for fever or other symptoms or signs of infection and treated promptly if such symptoms occur. Patients with severe neutropenia (absolute neutrophil count < 1000/mm³) should discontinue Thioridazine Hydrochloride Tablets, USP and have their WBC followed until recovery.

ADVERSE REACTIONS

In the recommended dosage ranges with thioridazine hydrochloride most side effects are mild and transient.

Central Nervous System: Drowsiness may be encountered on occasion, especially where large doses are given early in treatment. Generally, this effect tends to subside with continued therapy or a reduction in dosage. Pseudoparkinsonism and other extrapyramidal symptoms may occur but are infrequent. Nocturnal confusion, hyperactivity, lethargy, psychotic reactions, restlessness, and headache have been reported but are extremely rare.

Autonomic Nervous System: Dryness of mouth, blurred vision, constipation, nausea, vomiting, diarrhea, nasal stuffiness, and pallor have been seen.

Endocrine System: Galactorrhea, breast engorgement, amenorrhea, inhibition of ejaculation, and peripheral edema have been described.

Skin: Dermatitis and skin eruptions of the urticarial type have been observed infrequently. Photosensitivity is extremely rare.

Cardiovascular System: Thioridazine produces a dose related prolongation of the QTc interval, which is associated with the ability to cause Torsades de pointes type arrhythmias, a potentially fatal polymorphic ventricular tachycardia, and sudden death (see WARNINGS). Both Torsades de pointes type arrhythmias and sudden death have been reported in association with thioridazine. A causal relationship between these events and thioridazine therapy has not been established but, given the ability of thioridazine to prolong the QTc interval, such a relationship is possible. Other ECG changes have been reported (see Phenothiazine Derivatives: *Cardiovascular Effects*).

Other: Rare cases described as parotid swelling have been reported following administration of thioridazine.

Post Introduction Reports: These are voluntary reports of adverse events temporally associated with thioridazine that were received since marketing, and there may be no causal relationship between thioridazine use and these events: priapism.

Phenothiazine Derivatives: It should be noted that efficacy, indications, and untoward effects have varied with the different phenothiazines. It has been reported that old age lowers the tolerance for phenothiazines. The most common neurological side effects in these patients are parkinsonism and akathisia. There appears to be an increased risk of agranulocytosis and leukopenia in the geriatric population. The physician should be aware that the following have occurred with one or more phenothiazines and should be considered whenever one of these drugs is used:

Autonomic Reactions: Miosis, obstipation, anorexia, paralytic ileus.

Cutaneous Reactions: Erythema, exfoliative dermatitis, contact dermatitis.

Blood Dyscrasias: Agranulocytosis, leukopenia, eosinophilia, thrombocytopenia, anemia, aplastic anemia, pancytopenia.

Allergic Reactions: Fever, laryngeal edema, angioneurotic edema, asthma.

Hepatotoxicity: Jaundice, biliary stasis.

Cardiovascular Effects: Changes in the terminal portion of the electrocardiogram to include prolongation of the QT interval, depression and inversion of the T wave, and the appearance of a wave tentatively identified as a bifid T wave or a U wave have been observed in patients receiving phenothiazines, including thioridazine. To date, these appear to be due to altered repolarization, not related to myocardial damage, and reversible. Nonetheless, significant prolongation of the QT interval has been associated with serious ventricular arrhythmias and sudden death (see WARNINGS). Hypotension, rarely resulting in cardiac arrest, has been reported.

Extrapyramidal Symptoms: Akathisia, agitation, motor restlessness, dystonic reactions, trismus, torticollis, opisthotonus, oculogyric crises, tremor, muscular rigidity, akinesia.

Tardive Dyskinesia: Chronic use of antipsychotics may be associated with the development of tardive dyskinesia. The salient features of this syndrome are described in the WARNINGS section and subsequently.

The syndrome is characterized by involuntary choreoathetoid movements which variously involve the tongue, face, mouth, lips, or jaw (e.g., protrusion of the tongue, puffing of cheeks, puckering of the mouth, chewing movements), trunk, and extremities. The severity of the syndrome and the degree of impairment produced vary widely.

The syndrome may become clinically recognizable either during treatment, upon dosage reduction, or upon withdrawal of treatment. Movements may decrease in intensity and may disappear altogether if further treatment with antipsychotics is withheld. It is generally believed that reversibility is more likely after short rather than long-term antipsychotic exposure. Consequently, early detection of tardive dyskinesia is important. To increase the likelihood of detecting the syndrome at the earliest possible time, the dosage of antipsychotic drug should be reduced periodically (if clinically possible) and the patient observed for signs of the disorder. This maneuver is critical, for antipsychotic drugs may mask the signs of the syndrome.

Neuroleptic Malignant Syndrome (NMS): Chronic use of antipsychotics may be associated with the development of Neuroleptic Malignant Syndrome. The salient features of this syndrome are described in the WARNINGS section and subsequently. Clinical manifestations of NMS are hyperpyrexia, muscle rigidity, altered mental status, and evidence of autonomic instability (irregular pulse or blood pressure, tachycardia, diaphoresis, and cardiac dysrhythmias).

Endocrine Disturbances: Menstrual irregularities, altered libido, gynecomastia, lactation, weight gain, edema. False positive pregnancy tests have been reported.

Urinary Disturbances: Retention, incontinence.

Others: Hyperpyrexia. Behavioral effects suggestive of a paradoxical reaction have been reported. These include excitement, bizarre dreams, aggravation of psychoses, and toxic confusional states. More recently, a peculiar skin-eye syndrome has been recognized as a side effect following long-term treatment with phenothiazines. This reaction is marked by progressive pigmentation of areas of the skin or conjunctiva and/or accompanied by discoloration of the exposed sclera and cornea. Opacities of the anterior lens and cornea described as irregular or stellate in shape have also been reported. Systemic lupus erythematosus-like syndrome.

OVERDOSAGE

Many of the symptoms observed are extensions of the side effects described under ADVERSE REACTIONS. Thioridazine can be toxic in overdose, with cardiac toxicity being of particular concern. Frequent ECG and vital sign monitoring of overdosed patients is recommended. Observation for several days may be required because of the risk of delayed effects.

Signs and Symptoms: Effects and clinical complications of acute overdose involving phenothiazines may include:

Cardiovascular: Cardiac arrhythmias, hypotension, shock, ECG changes, increased QT and PR intervals, non-specific ST and T wave changes, bradycardia, sinus tachycardia, atrioventricular block, ventricular tachycardia, ventricular fibrillation, Torsade de pointes, myocardial depression.

Central Nervous System: Sedation, extrapyramidal effects, confusion, agitation, hypothermia, hyperthermia, restlessness, seizures, areflexia, coma.

Autonomic Nervous System: Mydriasis, miosis, dry skin, dry mouth, nasal congestion, urinary retention, blurred vision.

Respiratory: Respiratory depression, apnea, pulmonary edema.

Gastrointestinal: Hypomotility, constipation, ileus.

Renal: Oliguria, uremia.

Toxic dose and blood concentration ranges for the phenothiazines have not been firmly established. It has been suggested that the toxic blood concentration range for thioridazine begins at 1 mg/dL, and 2 to 8 mg/dL is the lethal concentration range.

Treatment: An airway must be established and maintained. Adequate oxygenation and ventilation must be ensured.

Cardiovascular monitoring should commence immediately and should include continuous electrocardiographic monitoring to detect possible arrhythmias. Treatment may include one or more of the following therapeutic interventions: correction of electrolyte abnormalities and acid-base balance, lidocaine, phenytoin, isoproterenol, ventricular pacing, and defibrillation. Disopyramide, procainamide, and quinidine may produce additive QT-prolonging effects when administered to patients with acute overdosage of thioridazine and should be avoided (see WARNINGS and CONTRAINDICATIONS). Caution must be exercised when administering lidocaine, as it may increase the risk of developing seizures.

Treatment of hypotension may require intravenous fluids and vasopressors. Phenylephrine, levarterenol, or metaraminol are the appropriate pressor agents for use in the management of refractory hypotension. The potent α adrenergic blocking properties of the phenothiazines makes the use of vasopressors with mixed α and β adrenergic agonist properties inappropriate, including epinephrine and dopamine. Paradoxical vasodilation may result. In addition, it is reasonable to expect that the α adrenergic-blocking properties of bretylium might be additive to those of thioridazine, resulting in problematic hypotension.

In managing overdosage, the physician should always consider the possibility of multiple drug involvement. Gastric lavage and repeated doses of activated charcoal should be considered. Induction of emesis is less preferable to gastric lavage because of the risk of dystonia and the potential for aspiration of vomitus. Emesis should not be induced in patients expected to deteriorate rapidly, or those with impaired consciousness.

Acute extrapyramidal symptoms may be treated with diphenhydramine hydrochloride or benztropine mesylate.

Avoid the use of barbiturates when treating seizures, as they may potentiate phenothiazine-induced respiratory depression.

Forced diuresis, hemoperfusion, hemodialysis and manipulation of urine pH are of unlikely benefit in the treatment of phenothiazine overdose due to their large volume of distribution and extensive plasma protein binding.

Up-to-date information about the treatment of overdose can often be obtained from a certified Regional Poison Control Center. Telephone numbers of certified Regional Poison Control Centers are listed in the Physicians' Desk Reference®**.

DOSAGE AND ADMINISTRATION

Since thioridazine is associated with a dose related prolongation of the QTc interval, which is a potentially life threatening event, its use should be reserved for schizophrenic patients who fail to respond adequately to treatment with *other antipsychotic drugs.* Dosage must be individualized and the smallest effective dosage should be determined for each patient (see INDICATIONS and WARNINGS).

Adults: The usual starting dose for adult schizophrenic patients is 50 mg to 100 mg three times a day, with a gradual increment to a maximum of 800 mg daily if necessary. Once effective control of symptoms has been achieved, the dosage may be reduced gradually to determine the minimum maintenance dose. The total daily dosage ranges from 200 mg to 800 mg, divided into two to four doses.

Pediatric Patients: For pediatric patients with schizophrenia who are unresponsive to other agents, the recommended initial dose is 0.5 mg/kg/day given in divided doses. Dosage may be increased gradually until optimum therapeutic effect is obtained or the maximum dose of 3 mg/kg/day has been reached.

HOW SUPPLIED

Thioridazine Hydrochloride Tablets, USP are available containing 10 mg, 25 mg, 50 mg or 100 mg of thioridazine hydrochloride, USP.

The 10 mg tablets are orange film-coated, round, unscored tablets debossed with **M** over **54** on one side and **10** on the other side. They are available as follows:
NDC 0378-0612-01
bottles of 100 tablets
NDC 0378-0612-10
bottles of 1000 tablets

The 25 mg tablets are orange film-coated, round, unscored tablets debossed with **M** over **58** on one side and **25** on the other side. They are available as follows:
NDC 0378-0614-01
bottles of 100 tablets
NDC 0378-0614-10
bottles of 1000 tablets

The 50 mg tablets are orange film-coated, round, unscored tablets debossed with **M** over **59** on one side and **50** on the other side. They are available as follows:
NDC 0378-0616-01
bottles of 100 tablets
NDC 0378-0616-10
bottles of 1000 tablets

The 100 mg tablets are orange film-coated, round, unscored tablets debossed with **M** over **61** on one side and **100** on the other side. They are available as follows:
NDC 0378-0618-01
bottles of 100 tablets
NDC 0378-0618-10
bottles of 1000 tablets

Store at 20° to 25°C (68° to 77°F). [See USP Controlled Room Temperature.] Protect from light.

Dispense in a tight, light-resistant container as defined in the USP using a child-resistant closure.

**Trademark of Physicians' Desk Reference, Inc.

Mylan Pharmaceuticals Inc.
Morgantown, WV 26505

REVISED APRIL 2009
THIO:R14

THIOTHIXENE CAPSULES, USP ℞

[*thī-ō-thiks-ēn*]

1 mg, 2 mg, 5 mg and 10mg

℞ Only

> **WARNING**
>
> **Increased Mortality in Elderly Patients with Dementia-Related Psychosis:** Elderly patients with dementia-related psychosis treated with antipsychotic drugs are at an increased risk of death. Analyses of seventeen placebo-controlled trials (modal duration of 10 weeks), largely in patients taking atypical antipsychotic drugs, revealed a risk of death in drug-treated patients of between 1.6 to 1.7 times the risk of death in placebo-treated patients. Over the course of a typical 10-week controlled trial, the rate of death in drug-treated patients was about 4.5%, compared to a rate of about 2.6% in the placebo group. Although the causes of death were varied, most of the deaths appeared to be either cardiovascular (e.g., heart failure, sudden death) or infectious (e.g., pneumonia) in nature. Observational studies suggest that, similar to atypical antipsychotic drugs, treatment with conventional antipsychotic drugs may increase mortality. The extent to which the findings of increased mortality in observational studies may be attributed to the antipsychotic drug as opposed to some characteristic(s) of the patients is not clear. Thiothixene is not approved for the treatment of patients with dementia-related psychosis (see WARNINGS).

DESCRIPTION

Thiothixene is a thioxanthene derivative. Specifically, it is the *cis* isomer of *N,N*-dimethyl-9-[3-(4-methyl-1-piperazinyl)propylidene]thioxanthene-2-sulfonamide. It may be represented by the following structural formula:

[See chemical structure at top of next column]

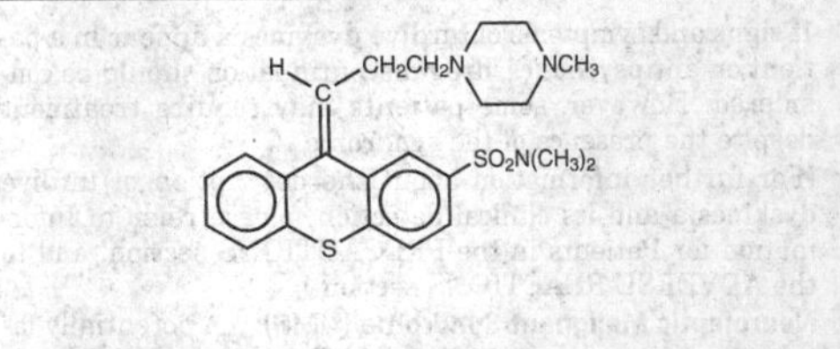

The thioxanthenes differ from the phenothiazines by the replacement of nitrogen in the central ring with a carbon-linked side chain fixed in space in a rigid structural configuration. An N,N-dimethyl sulfonamide functional group is bonded to the thioxanthene nucleus.

Each capsule contains 1 mg, 2 mg, 5 mg or 10 mg of thiothixene, USP and the following inactive ingredients: colloidal silicon dioxide, croscarmellose sodium, magnesium stearate, microcrystalline cellulose, powdered cellulose, pregelatinized starch and sodium lauryl sulfate. Each of the empty gelatin capsules contains FD&C Blue No. 1, FD&C Red No. 40, FD&C Yellow No. 6, gelatin and titanium dioxide. In addition, the 1 mg empty gelatin capsules contain D&C Red No. 28 and the 2 mg empty gelatin capsules contain D&C Yellow No. 10.

The imprinting ink contains the following: black iron oxide, D&C Yellow No. 10 Aluminum Lake, FD&C Blue No. 1 Aluminum Lake, FD&C Blue No. 2 Aluminum Lake, FD&C Red No. 40 Aluminum Lake, propylene glycol and shellac glaze.

CLINICAL PHARMACOLOGY

Thiothixene is an antipsychotic of the thioxanthene series. Thiothixene possesses certain chemical and pharmacological similarities to the piperazine phenothiazines and differences from the aliphatic group of phenothiazines.

INDICATIONS AND USAGE

Thiothixene capsules are effective in the management of schizophrenia. Thiothixene capsules have not been evaluated in the management of behavioral complications in patients with mental retardation.

CONTRAINDICATIONS

Thiothixene capsules are contraindicated in patients with circulatory collapse, comatose states, central nervous system depression due to any cause, and blood dyscrasias. Thiothixene is contraindicated in individuals who have shown hypersensitivity to the drug. It is not known whether there is a cross sensitivity between the thioxanthenes and the phenothiazine derivatives, but this possibility should be considered.

WARNINGS

Increased Mortality in Elderly Patients with Dementia-Related Psychosis: Elderly patients with dementia-related psychosis treated with antipsychotic drugs are at an increased risk of death. Thiothixene is not approved for the treatment of patients with dementia-related psychosis (see BOXED WARNING).

Tardive Dyskinesia: Tardive dyskinesia, a syndrome consisting of potentially irreversible, involuntary, dyskinetic movements may develop in patients treated with antipsychotic drugs, including thiothixene[1]. Although the prevalence of the syndrome appears to be highest among the elderly, especially elderly women, it is impossible to rely upon prevalence estimates to predict, at the inception of antipsychotic treatment, which patients are likely to develop the syndrome. Whether antipsychotic drug products differ in their potential to cause tardive dyskinesia is unknown.

Both the risk of developing the syndrome and the likelihood that it will become irreversible are believed to increase as the duration of treatment and the total cumulative dose of antipsychotic drugs administered to the patient increase. However, the syndrome can develop, although much less commonly, after relatively brief treatment periods at low doses.

There is no known treatment for established cases of tardive dyskinesia, although the syndrome may remit, partially or completely, if antipsychotic treatment is withdrawn. Antipsychotic treatment, itself, however, may suppress (or partially suppress) the signs and symptoms of the syndrome and thereby may possibly mask the underlying disease process. The effect that symptomatic suppression has upon the long-term course of the syndrome is unknown.

Given these considerations, antipsychotics should be prescribed in a manner that is most likely to minimize the occurrence of tardive dyskinesia. Chronic antipsychotic treatment should generally be reserved for patients who suffer from a chronic illness that, 1) is known to respond to antipsychotic drugs, and 2) for whom alternative, equally effective, but potentially less harmful treatments are not available or appropriate. In patients who do require chronic treatment, the smallest dose and the shortest duration of treatment producing a satisfactory clinical response should be sought. The need for continued treatment should be reassessed periodically.

If signs and symptoms of tardive dyskinesia appear in a patient on antipsychotics, drug discontinuation should be considered. However, some patients may require treatment despite the presence of the syndrome.

(For further information about the description of tardive dyskinesia and its clinical detection, please refer to Information for Patients in the PRECAUTIONS section, and to the ADVERSE REACTIONS section.)

Neuroleptic Malignant Syndrome (NMS): A potentially fatal symptom complex sometimes referred to as Neuroleptic Malignant Syndrome (NMS) has been reported in association with antipsychotic drugs, including thiothixene[2]. Clinical manifestations of NMS are hyperpyrexia, muscle rigidity, altered mental status and evidence of autonomic instability (irregular pulse or blood pressure, tachycardia, diaphoresis, and cardiac dysrhythmias).

The diagnostic evaluation of patients with this syndrome is complicated. In arriving at a diagnosis, it is important to identify cases where the clinical presentation includes both serious medical illness (e.g., pneumonia, systemic infection, etc.) and untreated or inadequately treated extrapyramidal signs and symptoms (EPS). Other important considerations in the differential diagnosis include central anticholinergic toxicity, heat stroke, drug fever and primary central nervous system (CNS) pathology.

The management of NMS should include 1) immediate discontinuation of antipsychotic drugs and other drugs not essential to concurrent therapy, 2) intensive symptomatic treatment and medical monitoring, and 3) treatment of any concomitant serious medical problems for which specific treatments are available. There is no general agreement about specific pharmacological treatment regimens for uncomplicated NMS.

If a patient requires antipsychotic drug treatment after recovery from NMS, the potential reintroduction of drug therapy should be carefully considered. The patient should be carefully monitored, since recurrences of NMS have been reported.

Usage in Pregnancy: Safe use of thiothixene during pregnancy has not been established. Therefore, this drug should be given to pregnant patients only when, in the judgment of the physician, the expected benefits from the treatment exceed the possible risks to mother and fetus. Animal reproduction studies and clinical experience to date have not demonstrated any teratogenic effects.

In the animal reproduction studies with thiothixene, there was some decrease in conception rate and litter size, and an increase in resorption rate in rats and rabbits. Similar findings have been reported with other psychotropic agents. After repeated oral administration of thiothixene to rats (5 to 15 mg/kg/day), rabbits (3 to 50 mg/kg/day), and monkeys (1 to 3 mg/kg/day) before and during gestation, no teratogenic effects were seen.

Usage in Children: The use of thiothixene in children under 12 years of age is not recommended because safe conditions for its use have not been established.

As is true with many CNS drugs, thiothixene may impair the mental and/or physical abilities required for the performance of potentially hazardous tasks such as driving a car or operating machinery, especially during the first few days of therapy. Therefore, the patient should be cautioned accordingly.

As in the case of other CNS-acting drugs, patients receiving thiothixene should be cautioned about the possible additive effects (which may include hypotension) with CNS depressants and with alcohol.

PRECAUTIONS

An antiemetic effect was observed in animal studies with thiothixene; since this effect may also occur in man, it is possible that thiothixene may mask signs of overdosage of toxic drugs and may obscure conditions such as intestinal obstruction and brain tumor.

In consideration of the known capability of thiothixene and certain other psychotropic drugs to precipitate convulsions, extreme caution should be used in patients with a history of convulsive disorders or those in a state of alcohol withdrawal, since it may lower the convulsive threshold. Although thiothixene potentiates the actions of the barbiturates, the dosage of the anticonvulsant therapy should not be reduced when thiothixene is administered concurrently. Though exhibiting rather weak anticholinergic properties, thiothixene should be used with caution in patients who might be exposed to extreme heat or who are receiving atropine or related drugs.

Use with caution in patients with cardiovascular disease.

Caution as well as careful adjustment of the dosages is indicated when thiothixene is used in conjunction with other CNS depressants.

Also, careful observation should be made for pigmentary retinopathy and lenticular pigmentation (fine lenticular pigmentation has been noted in a small number of patients treated with thiothixene for prolonged periods). Blood dyscrasias (agranulocytosis, pancytopenia, thrombocytopenic purpura), and liver damage (jaundice, biliary stasis), have been reported with related drugs.

Antipsychotic drugs, including thiothixene[3], elevate prolactin levels; the elevation persists during chronic administration. Tissue culture experiments indicate that approximately one-third of human breast cancers are prolactin dependent *in vitro*, a factor of potential importance if the prescription of these drugs is contemplated in a patient with a previously detected breast cancer. Although disturbances such as galactorrhea, amenorrhea, gynecomastia, and impotence have been reported, the clinical significance of elevated serum prolactin levels is unknown for most patients. An increase in mammary neoplasms has been found in rodents after chronic administration of antipsychotic drugs. Neither clinical studies nor epidemiologic studies conducted to date, however, have shown an association between chronic administration of these drugs and mammary tumorigenesis; the available evidence is considered too limited to be conclusive at this time.

Leukopenia, Neutropenia and Agranulocytosis: _Class Effect:_ In clinical trial and/or post-marketing experience, events of leukopenia/neutropenia and agranulocytosis have been reported temporally related to antipsychotic agents.

Possible risk factors for leukopenia/neutropenia include preexisting low white blood cell count (WBC) and history of drug induced leukopenia/neutropenia. Patients with a history of a clinically significant low WBC or drug induced leukopenia/neutropenia should have their complete blood count (CBC) monitored frequently during the first few months of therapy and discontinuation of thiothixene should be considered at the first sign of a clinically significant decline in WBC in the absence of other causative factors.

Patients with clinically significant neutropenia should be carefully monitored for fever or other symptoms or signs of infection and treated promptly if such symptoms or signs occur. Patients with severe neutropenia (absolute neutrophil count < 1000/mm[3]) should discontinue thiothixene and have their WBC followed until recovery.

Information for Patients: Given the likelihood that some patients exposed chronically to antipsychotics will develop tardive dyskinesia, it is advised that all patients in whom chronic use is contemplated be given, if possible, full information about this risk. The decision to inform patients and/or their guardians must obviously take into account the clinical circumstances and the competency of the patient to understand the information provided.

Drug Interactions: Hepatic microsomal enzyme inducing agents, such as carbamazepine, were found to significantly increase the clearance of thiothixene. Patients receiving these drugs should be observed for signs of reduced thiothixene effectiveness[4,5].

Due to a possible additive effect with hypotensive agents, patients receiving these drugs should be observed closely for signs of excessive hypotension when thiothixene is added to their drug regimen[6].

ADVERSE REACTIONS

NOTE: Not all of the following adverse reactions have been reported with thiothixene. However, since thiothixene has certain chemical and pharmacologic similarities to the phenothiazines, all of the known side effects and toxicity associated with phenothiazine therapy should be borne in mind when thiothixene is used.

Cardiovascular Effects: Tachycardia, hypotension, lightheadedness, and syncope. In the event hypotension occurs, epinephrine should not be used as a pressor agent since a paradoxical further lowering of blood pressure may result. Nonspecific EKG changes have been observed in some patients receiving thiothixene. These changes are usually reversible and frequently disappear on continued thiothixene therapy. The incidence of these changes is lower than that observed with some phenothiazines. The clinical significance of these changes is not known.

CNS Effects: Drowsiness, usually mild, may occur although it usually subsides with continuation of thiothixene therapy. The incidence of sedation appears similar to that of the piperazine group of phenothiazines but less than that of certain aliphatic phenothiazines. Restlessness, agitation and insomnia have been noted with thiothixene. Seizures and paradoxical exacerbation of psychotic symptoms have occurred with thiothixene infrequently.

Hyperreflexia has been reported in infants delivered from mothers having received structurally related drugs.

In addition, phenothiazine derivatives have been associated with cerebral edema and cerebrospinal fluid abnormalities.

Extrapyramidal Symptoms: Extrapyramidal symptoms, such as pseudoparkinsonism, akathisia and dystonia have been reported (see Adverse Reactions: Dystonia: Class Effect). Management of these extrapyramidal symptoms depends upon the type and severity. Rapid relief of acute symptoms may require the use of an injectable antiparkinson agent. More slowly emerging symptoms may be managed by reducing the dosage of thiothixene and/or administering an oral antiparkinson agent.

Dystonia: _Class Effect:_ Symptoms of dystonia, prolonged abnormal contractions of muscle groups, may occur in susceptible individuals during the first few days of treatment. Dystonic symptoms include: spasm of the neck muscles, sometimes progressing to tightness of the throat, swallowing difficulty, difficulty breathing, and/or protrusion of the tongue. While these symptoms can occur at low doses, they occur more frequently and with greater severity with high potency and at higher doses of first generation antipsychotic drugs. An elevated risk of acute dystonia is observed in males and younger age groups.

Persistent Tardive Dyskinesia: As with all antipsychotic agents, tardive dyskinesia may appear in some patients on long-term therapy with thiothixene, or may occur after drug therapy has been discontinued. The syndrome is characterized by rhythmical involuntary movements of the tongue, face, mouth or jaw (e.g., protrusion of tongue, puffing of cheeks, puckering of mouth, chewing movements). Sometimes these may be accompanied by involuntary movements of extremities.

Since early detection of tardive dyskinesia is important, patients should be monitored on an ongoing basis. It has been reported that fine vermicular movement of the tongue may be an early sign of the syndrome. If this or any other presentation of the syndrome is observed, the clinician should consider possible discontinuation of antipsychotic medication. (See WARNINGS.)

Hepatic Effects: Elevations of serum transaminase and alkaline phosphatase, usually transient, have been infrequently observed in some patients. No clinically confirmed cases of jaundice attributable to thiothixene have been reported.

Hematologic Effects: As is true with certain other psychotropic drugs, leukopenia and leukocytosis, which are usually transient, can occur occasionally with thiothixene. Other antipsychotic drugs have been associated with agranulocytosis, eosinophilia, hemolytic anemia, thrombocytopenia and pancytopenia.

Allergic Reactions: Rash, pruritus, urticaria, photosensitivity and rare cases of anaphylaxis have been reported with thiothixene. Undue exposure to sunlight should be avoided. Although not experienced with thiothixene, exfoliative dermatitis and contact dermatitis (in nursing personnel) have been reported with certain phenothiazines.

Endocrine/Reproductive: Hyperprolactinemia[3], lactation, menstrual irregularities, moderate breast enlargement and amenorrhea have occurred in a small percentage of females receiving thiothixene. If persistent, this may necessitate a reduction in dosage or the discontinuation of therapy. Phenothiazines have been associated with false positive pregnancy tests, gynecomastia, hypoglycemia, hyperglycemia and glycosuria.

Autonomic Effects: Dry mouth, blurred vision, nasal congestion, constipation, increased sweating, increased salivation and impotence have occurred infrequently with thiothixene therapy. Phenothiazines have been associated with miosis, mydriasis, and adynamic ileus.

Other Adverse Reactions: Hyperpyrexia, anorexia, nausea, vomiting, diarrhea, increase in appetite and weight, weakness or fatigue, polydipsia, and peripheral edema.

Although not reported with thiothixene, evidence indicates there is a relationship between phenothiazine therapy and the occurrence of a systemic lupus erythematosus-like syndrome.

Neuroleptic Malignant Syndrome (NMS): Please refer to the text regarding NMS in the WARNINGS section.

NOTE: Sudden deaths have occasionally been reported in patients who have received certain phenothiazine derivatives. In some cases the cause of death was apparently cardiac arrest or asphyxia due to failure of the cough reflex. In others, the cause could not be determined nor could it be established that death was due to phenothiazine administration.

OVERDOSAGE

Manifestations include muscular twitching, drowsiness and dizziness. Symptoms of gross overdosage may include CNS depression, rigidity, weakness, torticollis, tremor, salivation, dysphagia, hypotension, disturbances of gait, or coma.

Treatment: Essentially symptomatic and supportive. Early gastric lavage is helpful. Keep patient under careful observation and maintain an open airway, since involvement of the extrapyramidal system may produce dysphagia and respiratory difficulty in severe overdosage. If hypotension occurs, the standard measures for managing circulatory shock should be used (I.V. fluids and/or vasoconstrictors).

If a vasoconstrictor is needed, norepinephrine and phenylephrine are the most suitable drugs. Other pressor agents, including epinephrine, are not recommended, since phenothiazine derivatives may reverse the usual pressor action of these agents and cause further lowering of blood pressure.

If CNS depression is marked, symptomatic treatment is indicated. Extrapyramidal symptoms may be treated with antiparkinson drugs.

There are no data on the use of peritoneal or hemodialysis, but they are known to be of little value in phenothiazine intoxication.

DOSAGE AND ADMINISTRATION

Dosage of thiothixene capsules should be individually adjusted depending on the chronicity and severity of the symptoms of schizophrenia. In general, small doses should be used initially and gradually increased to the optimal effective level, based on patient response.

Some patients have been successfully maintained on once a day thiothixene capsule therapy.

The use of thiothixene capsules in children under 12 years of age is not recommended because safe conditions for its use have not been established.

In milder conditions, an initial dose of 2 mg three times daily is recommended. If indicated, a subsequent increase to 15 mg/day total daily dose is often effective.

In more severe conditions, an initial dose of 5 mg twice daily is recommended.

The usual optimal dose is 20 mg to 30 mg daily. If indicated, an increase to 60 mg/day total daily dose is often effective. Exceeding a total daily dose of 60 mg rarely increases the beneficial response.

HOW SUPPLIED

Thiothixene Capsules, USP are available containing 1 mg, 2 mg, 5 mg or 10 mg of thiothixene, USP.

The 1 mg capsule is a hard-shell gelatin capsule with a caramel opaque cap and a powder blue opaque body filled with white to off-white powder. The capsule is axially imprinted with **MYLAN** over **1001** in black ink on both the cap and body. They are available as follows:

NDC 0378-1001-01
bottles of 100 capsules

The 2 mg capsule is a hard-shell gelatin capsule with a caramel opaque cap and a yellow opaque body filled with white to off-white powder. The capsule is axially imprinted with **MYLAN** over **2002** in black ink on both the cap and body. They are available as follows:

NDC 0378-2002-01
bottles of 100 capsules
NDC 0378-2002-10
bottles of 1000 capsules

The 5 mg capsule is a hard-shell gelatin capsule with a caramel opaque cap and a white opaque body filled with white to off-white powder. The capsule is axially imprinted with **MYLAN** over **3005** in black ink on both the cap and body. They are available as follows:

NDC 0378-3005-01
bottles of 100 capsules
NDC 0378-3005-10
bottles of 1000 capsules

The 10 mg capsule is a hard-shell gelatin capsule with a caramel opaque cap and a peach opaque body filled with white to off-white powder. The capsule is axially imprinted with **MYLAN** over **5010** in black ink on both the cap and body. They are available as follows:

NDC 0378-5010-01
bottles of 100 capsules
NDC 0378-5010-10
bottles of 1000 capsules

Store at 20° to 25°C (68° to 77°F). [See USP Controlled Room Temperature.]

Protect from light.

Dispense in a tight, light-resistant container as defined in the USP using a child-resistant closure.

REFERENCES

1. Worldwide Labeling Safety Report: Dyskinesia and Dyskinesia Tardive and Thiothixene, (16Apr02).
2. Worldwide Labeling Safety Report: Neuroleptic Malignant Syndrome and Thiothixene, (16Apr02).
3. Worldwide Labeling Safety Report: Hyperprolactinemia and Thiothixene, (16Apr02).
4. Ereshefsky L, Saklad SR, Watanabe MD, et al. Thiothixene Pharmacokinetic Interactions: A Study of Hepatic Enzyme Inducers, Clearance Inhibitors, and Demographic Variables. *Journal of Clinical Psychopharmacology*, 11(5):296–301, (1991).
5. Worldwide Labeling Safety Report: Drug Interaction and Thiothixene, (09May02).
6. McEvoy GK, Miller JL, Snow EK, et al. AHFS Drug Information. American Society of Health-System Pharmacists, Inc., p. 2334-2336, (2002).
7. Worldwide Labeling Safety Report: Menstrual Disorder and Thiothixene, (16Apr02).

Mylan Pharmaceuticals Inc.
Morgantown, WV 26505

REVISED JANUARY 2010
THTX:R19

Novartis Consumer Health, Inc.
200 KIMBALL DRIVE
PARSIPPANY, NJ 07054-0622

Direct Inquiries to:
Novartis Consumer Relationship Center
Call: 800-452-0051
Fax: 973-503-8400
or write to 200 Kimball Drive
Parsippany, NJ 07054-0622

DENAVIR® ℞
brand of
penciclovir cream, 1%
For Dermatologic Use Only
Rx only
Prescribing Information

DESCRIPTION

Denavir contains penciclovir, an antiviral agent active against herpes viruses. *Denavir* is available for topical administration as a 1% white cream. Each gram of *Denavir* contains 10 mg of penciclovir and the following inactive ingredients: cetomacrogol 1000 BP, cetostearyl alcohol, mineral oil, propylene glycol, purified water and white petrolatum.

Chemically, penciclovir is known as 9-[4-hydroxy-3-(hydroxymethyl) butyl]guanine. Its molecular formula is $C_{10}H_{15}N_5O_3$; its molecular weight is 253.26. It is a synthetic acyclic guanine derivative and has the following structure:

Penciclovir is a white to pale yellow solid. At 20°C it has a solubility of 0.2 mg/mL in methanol, 1.3 mg/mL in propylene glycol, and 1.7 mg/mL in water. In aqueous buffer (pH 2) the solubility is 10.0 mg/mL. Penciclovir is not hygroscopic. Its partition coefficient in n-octanol/water at pH 7.5 is 0.024 (logP = -1.62).

CLINICAL PHARMACOLOGY
Microbiology

Mechanism of Antiviral Activity: The antiviral compound penciclovir has *in vitro* inhibitory activity against herpes simplex virus types 1 (HSV-1) and 1 (HSV-2). In cells infected with HSV-1 or HSV-2, viral thymidine kinase phosphorylates penciclovir to a monophosphate form which, in turn, is converted to penciclovir triphosphate by cellular kinases. *In vitro* studies demonstrate that penciclovir triphosphate inhibits HSV polymerase competitively with deoxyguanosine triphosphate. Consequently, herpes viral DNA synthesis and, therefore, replication are selectively inhibited.

Antiviral Activity *In Vitro* and *In Vivo*: In cell culture studies, penciclovir has antiviral activity against HSV-1 and HSV-2. Sensitivity test results, expressed as the concentration of the drug required to inhibit growth of the virus by 50% (IC_{50}) or 99% (IC_{99}) in cell culture, vary depending upon a number of factors, including the assay protocols. See Table 1.
[See table 1 below]

Drug Resistance: Penciclovir-resistant mutants of HSV can result from qualitative changes in viral thymidine kinase or DNA polymerase. The most commonly encountered acyclovir-resistant mutants that are deficient in viral thymidine kinase are also resistant to penciclovir.

Pharmacokinetics

Measurable penciclovir concentrations were not detected in plasma or urine of healthy male volunteers (n=12) following single or repeat application of the 1% cream at a dose of 180 mg penciclovir daily (approximately 67 times the estimated usual clinical dose).

Pediatric Patients: The systemic absorption of penciclovir following topical administration has not been evaluated in patients <18 years of age.

CLINICAL TRIALS

Denavir was studied in two double-blind, placebo (vehicle)-controlled trials for the treatment of recurrent herpes labialis in which otherwise healthy adults were randomized to either *Denavir* or placebo. Therapy was to be initiated by the subjects within 1 hour of noticing signs or symptoms and continued for 4 days, with application of study medication every 2 hours while awake. In both studies, the mean duration of lesions was approximately one-half-day shorter in the subjects treated with *Denavir* (N=1,516) as compared to subjects treated with placebo (N=1,541) (approximately 4.5 days versus 5 days, respectively). The mean duration of lesion pain was also approximately one-half-day shorter in the *Denavir* group compared to the placebo group.

INDICATIONS AND USAGE

Denavir (penciclovir cream) is indicated for the treatment of recurrent herpes labialis (cold sores) in adults and children 12 years of age and older.

CONTRAINDICATIONS

Denavir is contraindicated in patients with known hypersensitivity to the product or any of its components.

PRECAUTIONS
General

Denavir should only be used on herpes labialis on the lips and face. Because no data are available, application to human mucous membranes is not recommended. Particular care should be taken to avoid application in or near the eyes since it may cause irritation. Lesions that do not improve or that worsen on therapy should be evaluated for secondary bacterial infection. The effect of *Denavir* has not been established in immunocompromised patients.

Information for Patients

Denavir is a prescription topical cream for the treatment of cold sores (recurrent herpes labialis) that occur on the face and lips. It is not a cure for cold sores and not all patients respond to it. Do not use if you are allergic to *Denavir* (penciclovir) or any of the ingredients in *Denavir* cream. Before you use *Denavir*, tell your doctor if you are pregnant, planning to become pregnant, or are breast-feeding.

Directions: Wash your hands. Your face should be clean and dry. Apply a layer of *Denavir* cream to cover only the cold sore area or the area of tingling (or other symptoms) before the cold sore appears. Rub in the cream until it disappears. Apply the cream every 2 hours during waking hours for 4 days. Even though *Denavir* works at the blister stage, treatment should be started at the earliest sign of a cold sore (i.e. tingling, redness, itching, or bump). Wash your hands with soap and water after using *Denavir* cream. Store *Denavir* cream at controlled room temperature, 20°-25°C (68°-77°F). Keep out of reach of children.

Possible side effects: *Denavir* cream was well tolerated in clinical studies in patients with cold sores. The most frequently reported side effect was headache. Common skin-related side effects of *Denavir* cream are application site reactions, local anesthesia, taste perversion, and rash.

Carcinogenesis, Mutagenesis, Impairment of Fertility

In clinical trials, systemic drug exposure following the topical administration of penciclovir cream was negligible, as the penciclovir content of all plasma and urine samples was below the limit of assay detection (0.1 mcg/mL and

Table 1				
Method of Assay	**Virus Type**	**Cell Type**	**IC50 (mcg/mL)**	**IC99 (mcg/mL)**
Plaque Reduction	HSV-1 (c.i.)	MRC-5	0.2-0.6	
	HSV-1 (c.i.)	WISH	0.04-0.5	
	HSV-2 (c.i.)	MRC-5	0.9-2.1	
	HSV-2 (c.i.)	WISH	0.1-0.8	
Virus Yield Reduction	HSV-1 (c.i.)	MRC-5		0.4-0.5
	HSV-2 (c.i.)	MRC-5		0.6-0.7
DNA Synthesis Inhibition	HSV-1 (SC16)	MRC-5	0.04	
	HSV-2 (MS)	MRC-5	0.05	

(c.i.) = clinical isolates. The latent state of any herpes virus is not known to respond to any antiviral therapy.

10 mcg/mL, respectively). However, for the purpose of interspecies dose comparisons presented in the following sections, an assumption of 100% absorption of penciclovir from the topically applied product has been used. Based on use of the maximal recommended topical dose of penciclovir of 0.05 mg/kg/day and an assumption of 100% absorption, the maximum theoretical plasma $AUC_{0-24\ hrs}$ for penciclovir is approximately 0.129 mcg.hr/mL.

Carcinogenesis: Two-year carcinogenicity studies were conducted with famciclovir (the oral prodrug of penciclovir) in rats and mice. An increase in the incidence of mammary adenocarcinoma (a common tumor in female rats of the strain used) was seen in female rats receiving 600 mg/kg/day (approximately 395× the maximum theoretical human exposure to penciclovir following application of the topical product, based on area under the plasma concentration curve comparisons [24 hr. AUC]). No increases in tumor incidence were seen among male rats treated as doses up to 240 mg/kg/day (approximately 190× the maximum theoretical human AUC for penciclovir), or in male and female mice at doses up to 600 mg/kg/day (approximately 100× the maximum theoretical human AUC for penciclovir).

Mutagenesis: When tested *in vitro*, penciclovir did not cause an increase in gene mutation in the Ames assay using multiple strains of *S. typhimurium* or *E. coli* (at up to 20,000 mcg/plate), nor did it cause an increase in unscheduled DNA repair in mammalian HeLa S3 cells (at up to 5,000 mcg/mL). However, an increase in clastogenic responses was seen with penciclovir in the L5178Y mouse lymphoma cell assay (at doses ≥1000 mcg/mL) and, in human lymphocytes incubated *in vitro* at doses ≥250 mcg/mL. When tested *in vivo*, penciclovir caused an increase in micronuclei in mouse bone marrow following the intravenous administration of doses ≥500 mg/kg (≥810× the maximum human dose, based on body surface area conversion).

Impairment of Fertility: Testicular toxicity was observed in multiple animal species (rats and dogs) following repeated intravenous administration of penciclovir (160 mg/kg/day and 100 mg/kg/day, respectively, approximately 1155 and 3255× the maximum theoretical human AUC). Testicular changes seen in both species included atrophy of the seminiferous tubules and reductions in epididymal sperm counts and/or an increased incidence of sperm with abnormal morphology or reduced motility. Adverse testicular effects were related to an increasing dose or duration of exposure to penciclovir. No adverse testicular or reproductive effects (fertility and reproductive function) were observed in rats after 10 to 13 weeks dosing at 80 mg/kg/day, or testicular effects in dogs after 13 weeks dosing at 30 mg/kg/day (575 and 845× the maximum theoretical human AUC, respectively). Intravenously administered penciclovir had no effect on fertility or reproductive performance in female rats at doses of up to 80 mg/kg/day (260× the maximum human dose [BSA]).

There was no evidence of any clinically significant effects on sperm count, motility or morphology in 2 placebo-controlled clinical trials of Famvir® (famciclovir [the oral prodrug of penciclovir], 250 mg b.i.d.; n=66) in immunocompetent men with recurrent genital herpes, when dosing and follow-up were maintained for 18 and 8 weeks, respectively (approximately 2 and 1 spermatogenic cycles in the human).

Pregnancy

Teratogenic Effects-Pregnancy Category B. No adverse effects on the course and outcome of pregnancy or on fetal development were noted in rats and rabbits following the intravenous administration of penciclovir at doses of 80 and 60 mg/kg/day, respectively (estimated human equivalent doses of 13 and 18 mg/kg/day for the rat and rabbit, respectively, based on body surface area conversion; the body surface area doses being 260 and 355× the maximum recommended dose following topical application of the penciclovir cream). There are, however, no adequate and well-controlled studies in pregnant women. Because animal reproduction studies are not always predictive of human response, penciclovir should be used during pregnancy only if clearly needed.

Nursing Mothers

There is no information on whether penciclovir is excreted in human milk after topical administration. However, following oral administration of famciclovir (the oral prodrug of penciclovir) to lactating rats, penciclovir was excreted in breast milk at concentrations higher than those seen in the plasma. Therefore, a decision should be made whether to discontinue the drug, taking into account the importance of the drug to the mother. There are no data on the safety of penciclovir in newborns.

Pediatric Use

An open-label, uncontrolled trial with penciclovir cream 1% was conducted in 102 patients, ages 12-17 years, with recurrent herpes labialis. The frequency of adverse events was generally similar to the frequency previously reported for adult patients. Safety and effectiveness in pediatric patients less than 12 years of age have not been established.

Geriatric Use

In 74 patients ≥65 years of age, the adverse events profile was comparable to that observed in younger patients.

ADVERSE REACTIONS

In two double-blind, placebo-controlled trials, 1516 patients were treated with *Denavir* (penciclovir cream) and 1541 with placebo. The most frequently reported adverse event was headache, which occurred in 5.3% of the patients treated with *Denavir* and 5.8% of the placebo-treated patients. The rates of reported local adverse reactions are shown in Table 2 below. One or more local adverse reactions were reported by 2.7% of the patients treated with *Denavir* and 3.9% of placebo-treated patients.

Table 2—Local Adverse Reactions Reported in Phase III Trials

	Penciclovir n=1516 %	Placebo n=1541 %
Application site reaction	1.3	1.8
Hypesthesia/Local anesthesia	0.9	1.4
Taste perversion	0.2	0.3
Pruritus	0.0	0.3
Pain	0.0	0.1
Rash (erythematous)	0.1	0.1
Allergic reaction	0.0	0.1

Two studies, enrolling 108 healthy subjects, were conducted to evaluate the dermal tolerance of 5% penciclovir cream (a 5-fold higher concentration than the commercial formulation) compared to vehicle using repeated occluded patch testing methodology. The 5% penciclovir cream induced mild erythema in approximately one-half of the subjects exposed, an irritancy profile similar to the vehicle control in terms of severity and proportion of subjects with a response. No evidence of sensitization was observed.

Post-Marketing Experience

The following events have been identified from worldwide post-marketing use of *Denavir* in treatment of recurrent herpes labialis (cold sores) in adults. These events have been chosen for inclusion due to a combination of their seriousness, frequency of reporting, or potential causal connections to *Denavir* cream.

General: Headache, oral/pharyngeal edema, parosmia.

Skin: Application site reactions, aggravated condition, decreased therapeutic response, erythematous rash, local edema, pain, paresthesia, pruritus, skin discoloration and urticaria.

OVERDOSAGE

Since penciclovir is poorly absorbed following oral administration, adverse reactions related to penciclovir ingestion are unlikely. There is no information on overdose.

DOSAGE AND ADMINISTRATION

Denavir should be applied every 2 hours during waking hours for a period of 4 days. Treatment should be started as early as possible (i.e., during the prodrome or when lesions appear).

HOW SUPPLIED

Denavir is supplied in a 1.5 gram tube containing 10 mg of penciclovir per gram.
NDC 0067-6024-15
Store at controlled room temperature, 20°–25°C (68°–77°F) [see USP].
QUESTIONS? call **1-800-452-0051**
October 2003
Manufactured by Novartis Pharma GmbH,
Wehr, Germany for
Novartis Consumer Health, Inc.
Parsippany, NJ 07054-0622
©2010 Novartis

TRANSDERM SCŌP® ℞
scopolamine 1.5 mg
Transdermal Therapeutic System

Programmed to deliver *in-vivo* approximately 1.0 mg of scopolamine over 3 days

DESCRIPTION

The Transderm Scōp (transdermal scopolamine) system is a circular flat patch designed for continuous release of scopolamine following application to an area of intact skin on the head, behind the ear. Each system contains 1.5 mg of scopolamine base. Scopolamine is α-(hydroxymethyl) benzeneacetic acid 9-methyl-3-oxa-9-azatricyclo [3.3.1.0^{2,4}] non-7-yl ester. The empirical formula is $C_{17}H_{21}NO_4$ and its structural formula is

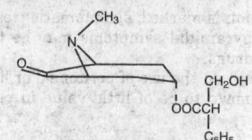

Scopolamine is a viscous liquid that has a molecular weight of 303.35 and a pKa of 7.55-7.81. The Transderm Scōp system is a film 0.2 mm thick and 2.5 cm², with four layers. Proceeding from the visible surface towards the surface attached to the skin, these layers are: (1) a backing layer of tan-colored, aluminized, polyester film; (2) a drug reservoir of scopolamine, light mineral oil, and polyisobutylene; (3) a microporous polypropylene membrane that controls the rate of delivery of scopolamine from the system to the skin surface; and (4) an adhesive formulation of mineral oil, polyisobutylene, and scopolamine. A protective peel strip of siliconized polyester, which covers the adhesive layer, is removed before the system is used. The inactive components, light mineral oil (12.4 mg) and polyisobutylene (11.4 mg), are not released from the system.

Cross section of the system:

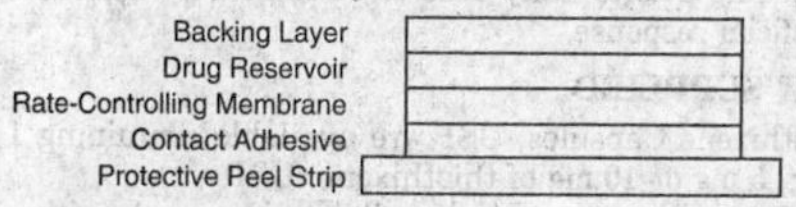

Backing Layer
Drug Reservoir
Rate-Controlling Membrane
Contact Adhesive
Protective Peel Strip

CLINICAL PHARMACOLOGY

Pharmacology
The sole active agent of Transderm Scōp is scopolamine, a belladonna alkaloid with well-known pharmacological properties. It is an anticholinergic agent which acts: i) as a competitive inhibitor at postganglionic muscarinic receptor sites of the parasympathetic nervous system, and ii) on smooth muscles that respond to acetylcholine but lack cholinergic innervation. It has been suggested that scopolamine acts in the central nervous system (CNS) by blocking cholinergic transmission from the vestibular nuclei to higher centers in the CNS and from the reticular formation to the vomiting center[1,2]. Scopolamine can inhibit the secretion of saliva and sweat, decrease gastrointestinal secretions and motility, cause drowsiness, dilate the pupils, increase heart rate, and depress motor function[2].

Pharmacokinetics
Scopolamine's activity is due to the parent drug. The pharmacokinetics of scopolamine delivered via the system are due to the characteristics of both the drug and dosage form. The system is programmed to deliver *in-vivo* approximately 1.0 mg of scopolamine at an approximately constant rate to the systemic circulation over 3 days. Upon application to the post-auricular skin, an initial priming dose of scopolamine is released from the adhesive layer to saturate skin binding sites. The subsequent delivery of scopolamine to the blood is determined by the rate-controlling membrane and is designed to produce stable plasma levels in a therapeutic range. Following removal of the used system, there is some degree of continued systemic absorption of scopolamine bound in the skin layers.

Absorption: Scopolamine is well-absorbed percutaneously. Following application to the skin behind the ear, circulating plasma levels are detected within 4 hours with peak levels being obtained, on average, within 24 hours. The average plasma concentration produced is 87 pg/mL for free scopolamine and 354 pg/mL for total scopolamine (free + conjugates).

Distribution: The distribution of scopolamine is not well characterized. It crosses the placenta and the blood brain barrier and may be reversibly bound to plasma proteins.

Metabolism: Although not well characterized, scopolamine is extensively metabolized and conjugated with less than 5% of the total dose appearing unchanged in the urine.

Elimination: The exact elimination pattern of scopolamine has not been determined. Following patch removal, plasma levels decline in a log linear fashion with an observed half-life of 9.5 hours. Less than 10% of the total dose is excreted in the urine as parent and metabolites over 108 hours.

Clinical Results: In 195 adult subjects of different racial origins who participated in clinical efficacy studies at sea or in a controlled motion environment, there was a 75% reduction in the incidence of motion-induced nausea and vomiting[3].

In two pivotal clinical efficacy studies in 391 adult female patients undergoing cesarean section or gynecological surgery with anesthesia and opiate analgesia, 66% of those treated with Transderm Scōp (compared to only 46% of those receiving placebo) reported no retching/vomiting within the 24-hour period following administration of anesthesia/opiate analgesia. When the need for additional antiemetic medication was assessed during the same period, there was no need for medication in 76% of patients treated with Transderm Scōp as compared to 59% of placebo-treated patients[4,5]

INDICATIONS AND USAGE

Transderm Scōp is indicated in adults for prevention of nausea and vomiting associated with motion sickness and recovery from anesthesia and surgery. The patch should be applied only to skin in the postauricular area.

CONTRAINDICATIONS

Transderm Scōp is contraindicated in persons who are hypersensitive to the drug scopolamine or to other belladonna alkaloids, or to any ingredient or component in the formulation or delivery system, or in patients with angle-closure (narrow angle) glaucoma.

WARNINGS

Glaucoma therapy in patients with chronic open-angle (wide-angle) glaucoma should be monitored and may need to be adjusted during Transderm Scōp use, as the mydriatic effect of scopolamine may cause an increase in intraocular pressure.

Transderm Scōp should not be used in children and should be used with caution in the elderly. See PRECAUTIONS.

Since drowsiness, disorientation, and confusion may occur with the use of scopolamine, patients should be warned of the possibility and cautioned against engaging in activities that require mental alertness, such as driving a motor vehicle or operating dangerous machinery.

Rarely, idiosyncratic reactions may occur with ordinary therapeutic doses of scopolamine. The most serious of these that have been reported are: acute toxic psychosis, including confusion, agitation, rambling speech, hallucinations, paranoid behaviors, and delusions.

PRECAUTIONS
General

Scopolamine should be used with caution in patients with pyloric obstruction or urinary bladder neck obstruction. Caution should be exercised when administering an antiemetic or antimuscarinic drug to patients suspected of having intestinal obstruction.

Transderm Scōp should be used with caution in the elderly or in individuals with impaired liver or kidney functions because of the increased likelihood of CNS effects.

Caution should be exercised in patients with a history of seizures or psychosis, since scopolamine can potentially aggravate both disorders.

Skin burns have been reported at the patch site in several patients wearing an aluminized transdermal systems during a Magnetic Resonance Imaging scan (MRI). Because Transderm Scōp contains aluminum, it is recommended to remove the system before undergoing an MRI.

Information for Patients

Since scopolamine can cause temporary dilation of the pupils and blurred vision if it comes in contact with the eyes, patients should be strongly advised to wash their hands thoroughly with soap and water immediately after handling the patch. In addition, it is important that used patches be disposed of properly to avoid contact with children or pets. Patients should be advised to remove the patch immediately and promptly contact a physician in the unlikely event that they experience symptoms of acute narrow-angle glaucoma (pain and reddening of the eyes, accompanied by dilated pupils). Patients should also be instructed to remove the patch if they develop any difficulties in urinating.

Patients who expect to participate in underwater sports should be cautioned regarding the potentially disorienting effects of scopolamine. A patient brochure is available.

Drug Interactions

The absorption of oral medications may be decreased during the concurrent use of scopolamine because of decreased gastric motility and delayed gastric emptying.

Scopolamine should be used with care in patients taking other drugs that are capable of causing CNS effects such as sedatives, tranquilizers, or alcohol. Special attention should be paid to potential interactions with drugs having anticholinergic properties; e.g., other belladonna alkaloids, antihistamines (including meclizine), tricyclic antidepressants, and muscle relaxants.

Laboratory Test Interactions

Scopolamine will interfere with the gastric secretion test.

Carcinogenesis, Mutagenesis, Impairment of Fertility

No long-term studies in animals have been completed to evaluate the carcinogenic potential of scopolamine. The mutagenic potential of scopolamine has not been evaluated. Fertility studies were performed in female rats and revealed no evidence of impaired fertility or harm to the fetus due to scopolamine hydrobromide administered by daily subcutaneous injection. Maternal body weights were reduced in the highest-dose group (plasma level approximately 500 times the level achieved in humans using a transdermal system).

Pregnancy Category C

Teratogenic studies were performed in pregnant rats and rabbits with scopolamine hydrobromide administered by daily intravenous injection. No adverse effects were recorded in rats.

Scopolamine hydrobromide has been shown to have a marginal embryotoxic effect in rabbits when administered by daily intravenous injection at doses producing plasma levels approximately 100 times the level achieved in humans using a transdermal system. During a clinical study among women undergoing cesarean section treated with Transderm Scōp in conjunction with epidural anesthesia and opiate analgesia, no evidence of CNS depression was found in the newborns. There are no other adequate and well-controlled studies in pregnant women.

Other than in the adjunctive use for delivery by cesarean section, Transderm Scōp should be used in pregnancy only if the potential benefit justifies the potential risk to the fetus.

Nursing Mothers

Because scopolamine is excreted in human milk, caution should be exercised when Transderm Scōp is administered to a nursing woman.

Labor and Delivery

Scopolamine administered parenterally at higher doses than the dose delivered by Transderm Scōp does not increase the duration of labor, nor does it affect uterine contractions. Scopolamine does cross the placenta.

Pediatric Use

The safety and effectiveness of Transderm Scōp in children has not been established. Children are particularly susceptible to the side effects of belladonna alkaloids. Transderm Scōp should not be used in children because it is not known whether this system will release an amount of scopolamine that could produce serious adverse effects in children.

ADVERSE DRUG EXPERIENCES

The adverse reactions for Transderm Scōp are provided separately for patients with motion sickness and with postoperative nausea and vomiting.

Motion Sickness: In motion sickness clinical studies of Transderm Scōp, the most frequent adverse reaction was dryness of the mouth. This occurred in about two thirds of patients on drug. A less frequent adverse drug reaction was drowsiness, which occurred in less than one sixth of patients on drug. Transient impairment of eye accommodation, including blurred vision and dilation of the pupils, was also observed.

Post-operative Nausea and Vomiting: In a total of five clinical studies in which Transderm Scōp was administered perioperatively to a total of 461 patients and safety was assessed, dry mouth was the most frequently reported adverse drug experience, which occurred in approximately 29% of patients on drug. Dizziness was reported by approximately 12% of patients on drug[6].

Postmarketing and Other Experience: In addition to the adverse experiences reported during clinical testing of Transderm Scōp, the following are spontaneously reported adverse events from postmarketing experience. Because the reports cite events reported spontaneously from worldwide postmarketing experience, frequency of events and the role of Transderm Scōp in their causation cannot be reliably determined: acute angle-closure (narrow-angle) glaucoma; confusion; difficulty urinating; dry, itchy, or conjunctival injection of eyes; restlessness; hallucinations; memory disturbances; rashes and erythema; and transient changes in heart rate.

Drug Withdrawal/Post-Removal Symptoms: Symptoms such as dizziness, nausea, vomiting, and headache occur following abrupt discontinuation of antimuscarinics. Similar symptoms, including disturbances of equilibrium, have been reported in some patients following discontinuation of use of the Transderm Scōp system. These symptoms usually do not appear until 24 hours or more after the patch has been removed. Some symptoms may be related to adaptation from a motion environment to a motion-free environment. More serious symptoms including muscle weakness, bradycardia and hypotension may occur following discontinuation of Transderm Scōp.

OVERDOSAGE

Because strategies for the management of drug overdose continually evolve, it is strongly recommended that a poison control center be contacted to obtain up-to-date information regarding the management of Transderm Scōp patch overdose. The prescriber should be mindful that antidotes used routinely in the past may no longer be considered optimal treatment. For example, physostigmine, used more or less routinely in the past, is seldom recommended for the routine management of anticholinergic syndromes.

Until up-to-date authoritative advice is obtained, routine supportive measures should be directed to maintaining adequate respiratory and cardiac function.

The signs and symptoms of anticholinergic toxicity include: lethargy, somnolence, coma, confusion, agitation, hallucinations, convulsion, visual disturbance, dry flushed skin, dry mouth, decreased bowel sounds, urinary retention, tachycardia, hypertension, and supraventricular arrhythmias.

Most cases of toxicity involving the use of the product will resolve with simple removal of the patch. Serious symptomatic cases of overdosage involving multiple patch applications and/or ingestion may be managed by initially ensuring the patient has an adequate airway, and supporting respiration and circulation. This should be rapidly followed by removal of all patches from the skin and the mouth. If there is evidence of patch ingestion, gastric lavage, endoscopic removal of swallowed patches, or administration of activated charcoal should be considered, as indicated by the clinical situation. In any case where there is serious overdosage or signs of evolving acute toxicity, continuous monitoring of vital signs and ECG, establishment of intravenous access, and administration of oxygen are all recommended.

The symptoms of overdose/toxicity due to scopolamine should be carefully distinguished from the occasionally observed syndrome of withdrawal (see Drug Withdrawal/Post Removal Symptoms). Although mental confusion and dizziness may be observed with both acute toxicity and withdrawal, other characteristic findings differ: tachyarrhythmias, dry skin, and decreased bowel sounds suggest anticholinergic toxicity, while bradycardia, headache, nausea and abdominal cramps, and sweating suggest postremoval withdrawal. Obtaining a careful history is crucial to making the correct diagnosis.

DOSAGE AND ADMINISTRATION

Initiation of Therapy: To prevent the nausea and vomiting associated with motion sickness, one Transderm Scōp patch (programmed to deliver approximately 1.0 mg of scopolamine over 3 days) should be applied to the hairless area behind one ear at least 4 hours before the antiemetic effect is required. To prevent post operative nausea and vomiting, the patch should be applied the evening before scheduled surgery. To minimize exposure of the newborn baby to the drug, apply the patch one hour prior to cesarean section. Only one patch should be worn at any time. Do not cut the patch.

Handling: After the patch is applied on dry skin behind the ear, the hands should be washed thoroughly with soap and water and dried. Upon removal, the patch should be discarded. To prevent any traces of scopolamine from coming into direct contact with the eyes, the hands and the application site should be washed thoroughly with soap and water and dried. (A patient brochure is available).

Continuation of Therapy: Should the patch become displaced, it should be discarded, and a fresh one placed on the hairless area behind the other ear. For motion sickness, if therapy is required for longer than 3 days, the first patch should be removed and a fresh one placed on the hairless area behind the other ear. For perioperative use, the patch should be kept in place for 24 hours following surgery at which time it should be removed and discarded.

HOW SUPPLIED

The Transderm Scōp system is a tan-colored circular patch, 2.5 cm², on a clear, oversized, hexagonal peel strip, which is removed prior to use.

Each Transderm Scōp system contains 1.5 mg of scopolamine and is programmed to deliver *in-vivo* approximately 1.0 mg of scopolamine over 3 days. Transderm Scōp is available in packages of four patches. Each patch is foil wrapped. Patient instructions are included.

1 Package (4 patches)   NDC 0067-4345-04
The system should be stored at controlled room temperature between 20°C–25°C (68°F–77°F).

Rx ONLY

REFERENCES

1. McEvoy, G.K. (ed.); AHSF Drug Information; American Society of Hospital Pharmacists, Bethesda, MD, pp. 608–611 (1990).
2. Gilman, A.G. et al (ed.); The Pharmacological Basis of Therapeutics (8th Ed.); Pergamon Press, New York, NY, pp. 150–165 (1990).
3. Pharmacokinetic Clinical data on file.
4. Kotelko, D.M. et al; "Transdermal scopolamine decreases nausea and vomiting following cesarean section in patients receiving epidural morphine", Anesthesiology 71(5): 675–678 (1989).
5. Bailey, P.L. et al; "Transdermal scopolamine reduces nausea and vomiting after outpatient laparoscopy", Anesthesiology 72(6): 977–980 (1990).
6. Clinical safety data on file.

Mfd by: ALZA Corporation
Mountain View, CA 94043

Distributed by:
Novartis Consumer Health, Inc.
Parsippany, NJ 07054-0622
©2010

42013C   Printed in U.S.A.   (Rev. 2/06)
Shown in Product Identification Guide, page 314

Novartis Pharmaceuticals Corporation
ONE HEALTH PLAZA
EAST HANOVER, NJ 07936
(for branded products)

For Information Contact (branded products):
Customer Response Department
(888) NOW-NOVA [888-669-6682]
www.novartis.com

AFINITOR® ℞
[a-fin-it-or]
(everolimus)
Tablets for Oral Administration

The following prescribing information is based on labeling in effect July 2010.

HIGHLIGHTS OF PRESCRIBING INFORMATION
These highlights do not include all the information needed to use AFINITOR safely and effectively. See full prescribing information for AFINITOR.

AFINITOR (everolimus) tablets for oral administration
Initial U.S. Approval: 2009

——RECENT MAJOR CHANGES——
- Dosage and Administration (2.2)   6/2010
- Warnings and Precautions: Infections (5.2)   6/2010

——INDICATIONS AND USAGE——
AFINITOR is a kinase inhibitor indicated for the treatment of patients with advanced renal cell carcinoma after failure of treatment with sunitinib or sorafenib. (1)

——DOSAGE AND ADMINISTRATION——
- 10 mg once daily with or without food. (2.1)
- Treatment interruption and/or dose reduction to 5 mg once daily may be needed to manage adverse drug reactions. (2.2)
- For patients with Child-Pugh class B hepatic impairment, reduce dose to 5 mg once daily. (2.2)
- If moderate inhibitors of CYP3A4 or P-glycoprotein (PgP) are required, reduce the dose of AFINITOR to 2.5 mg once daily; if tolerated, consider increasing to 5 mg once daily. (2.2)
- If strong inducers of CYP3A4 are required, increase AFINITOR dose in 5 mg increments to a maximum of 20 mg once daily. (2.2)

——DOSAGE FORMS AND STRENGTHS——
2.5 mg, 5 mg and 10 mg tablets with no score. (3)

——CONTRAINDICATIONS——
Hypersensitivity to everolimus, to other rapamycin derivatives, or to any of the excipients. (4)

——WARNINGS AND PRECAUTIONS——
- Non-infectious pneumonitis: Monitor for clinical symptoms or radiological changes; fatal cases have occurred. Manage by dose reduction or discontinuation until symptoms resolve, and consider use of corticosteroids. (5.1)
- Infections: Increased risk of infections, some fatal. Monitor for signs and symptoms, and treat promptly. (5.2)
- Oral ulceration: Mouth ulcers, stomatitis, and oral mucositis are common. Management includes mouthwashes (without alcohol or peroxide) and topical treatments. (5.3)
- Laboratory test alterations: Elevations of serum creatinine, blood glucose, and lipids may occur. Decreases in hemoglobin, neutrophils, and platelets may also occur. Monitor renal function, blood glucose, lipids, and hematologic parameters prior to treatment and periodically thereafter. (5.4)
- Vaccinations: Avoid live vaccines and close contact with those who have received live vaccines. (5.7)
- Use in pregnancy: Fetal harm can occur when administered to a pregnant woman. Apprise women of potential harm to the fetus. (5.8, 8.1)

——ADVERSE REACTIONS——
Most common adverse reactions (incidence ≥30%) are stomatitis, infections, asthenia, fatigue, cough, and diarrhea. (6.1)

To report SUSPECTED ADVERSE REACTIONS, contact Novartis Pharmaceuticals Corporation at 1-888-669-6682 or FDA at 1-800-FDA-1088 or www.fda.gov/medwatch

——DRUG INTERACTIONS——
- Strong CYP3A4 or PgP inhibitors: Avoid concomitant use. (2.2, 5.5, 7.1)
- Moderate CYP3A4 or PgP inhibitors: If combination is required, use caution and reduce dose of AFINITOR. (2.2, 5.5, 7.1)
- Strong CYP3A4 inducers: Avoid concomitant use. If combination cannot be avoided, increase dose of AFINITOR. (2.2, 5.5, 7.2)

——USE IN SPECIFIC POPULATIONS——
- Nursing mothers: Discontinue drug or nursing, taking into consideration the importance of drug to the mother. (8.3)
- Hepatic impairment: AFINITOR should not be used in patients with Child-Pugh class C hepatic impairment. For patients with Child-Pugh class B hepatic impairment, reduce dose to 5 mg daily. (2.2, 5.6, 8.7)

See 17 for PATIENT COUNSELING INFORMATION and FDA-approved patient labeling

Revised: 06/2010

FULL PRESCRIBING INFORMATION: CONTENTS*
1 INDICATIONS AND USAGE
2 DOSAGE AND ADMINISTRATION
   2.1 Recommended Dose
   2.2 Dose Modifications
3 DOSAGE FORMS AND STRENGTHS
4 CONTRAINDICATIONS
5 WARNINGS AND PRECAUTIONS
   5.1 Non-infectious Pneumonitis
   5.2 Infections
   5.3 Oral Ulceration
   5.4 Laboratory Tests and Monitoring
   5.5 Drug-drug Interactions
   5.6 Hepatic Impairment
   5.7 Vaccinations
   5.8 Use in Pregnancy
6 ADVERSE REACTIONS
   6.1 Clinical Studies Experience
7 DRUG INTERACTIONS
   7.1 Agents that may Increase Everolimus Blood Concentrations
   7.2 Agents that may Decrease Everolimus Blood Concentrations
   7.3 Agents whose Plasma Concentrations may be Altered by Everolimus
8 USE IN SPECIFIC POPULATIONS
   8.1 Pregnancy
   8.3 Nursing Mothers
   8.4 Pediatric Use
   8.5 Geriatric Use
   8.6 Renal Impairment
   8.7 Hepatic Impairment
10 OVERDOSAGE
11 DESCRIPTION
12 CLINICAL PHARMACOLOGY
   12.1 Mechanism of Action
   12.2 Pharmacodynamics
   12.3 Pharmacokinetics
13 NONCLINICAL TOXICOLOGY
   13.1 Carcinogenesis, Mutagenesis, Impairment of Fertility
14 CLINICAL STUDIES
15 REFERENCES
16 HOW SUPPLIED/STORAGE AND HANDLING
17 PATIENT COUNSELING INFORMATION
   17.1 Non-infectious Pneumonitis
   17.2 Infections
   17.3 Oral Ulceration
   17.4 Laboratory Tests and Monitoring
   17.5 Drug-drug Interactions
   17.6 Hepatic Impairment
   17.7 Vaccinations
   17.8 Pregnancy
   17.9 Dosing Instructions

*Sections or subsections omitted from the full prescribing information are not listed

FULL PRESCRIBING INFORMATION

1 INDICATIONS AND USAGE
AFINITOR® is indicated for the treatment of patients with advanced renal cell carcinoma after failure of treatment with sunitinib or sorafenib.

2 DOSAGE AND ADMINISTRATION
2.1 Recommended Dose
The recommended dose of AFINITOR for treatment of advanced renal cell carcinoma is 10 mg, to be taken once daily at the same time every day, either with or without food [see Clinical Pharmacology (12.3)]. AFINITOR tablets should be swallowed whole with a glass of water. The tablets should not be chewed or crushed.
Continue treatment as long as clinical benefit is observed or until unacceptable toxicity occurs.
2.2 Dose Modifications
Management of severe and/or intolerable adverse reactions may require temporary dose reduction and/or interruption of AFINITOR therapy. If dose reduction is required, the suggested dose is 5 mg daily [see Warnings and Precautions (5.1)].
Hepatic Impairment: For patients with moderate hepatic impairment (Child-Pugh class B), reduce the dose to 5 mg daily. AFINITOR has not been evaluated in patients with

severe hepatic impairment (Child-Pugh class C) and should not be used in this patient population [see Warnings and Precautions (5.6) and Use in Specific Populations (8.7)].
CYP3A4 or PgP inhibitors: Use caution when administered in combination with moderate CYP3A4 inhibitors (e.g., amprenavir, fosamprenavir, aprepitant, erythromycin, fluconazole, verapamil, diltiazem) or moderate P-glycoprotein (PgP) inhibitors. If patients require co-administration of a moderate CYP3A4 or PgP inhibitor, reduce the AFINITOR dose to 2.5 mg daily. The reduced dose of AFINITOR is predicted to adjust the area under the curve (AUC) to the range observed without inhibitors. An AFINITOR dose increase from 2.5 mg to 5 mg may be considered based on patient tolerance. If the moderate inhibitor is discontinued, a washout period of approximately 2 to 3 days should be allowed before the AFINITOR dose is increased. If the moderate inhibitor is discontinued, the AFINITOR dose should be returned to the dose used prior to initiation of the moderate CYP3A4 or PgP inhibitor.
Avoid the use of strong inhibitors of CYP3A4 (e.g., ketoconazole, itraconazole, clarithromycin, atazanavir, nefazodone, saquinavir, telithromycin, ritonavir, indinavir, nelfinavir, voriconazole) or PgP. Grapefruit, grapefruit juice, starfruit, Seville oranges and other foods that are known to affect cytochrome P450 and PgP activity should also be avoided during treatment [see Warnings and Precautions (5.5) and Drug Interactions (7.1)].
Strong CYP3A4 Inducers: Avoid the use of concomitant strong CYP3A4 inducers (e.g., dexamethasone, phenytoin, carbamazepine, rifampin, rifabutin, rifapentine, phenobarbital). If patients require co-administration of a strong CYP3A4 inducer, consider increasing the AFINITOR dose from 10 mg daily up to 20 mg daily (based on pharmacokinetic data), using 5 mg increments. This dose of AFINITOR is predicted to adjust the AUC to the range observed without inducers. However, there are no clinical data with this dose adjustment in patients receiving strong CYP3A4 inducers. If the strong inducer is discontinued, the AFINITOR dose should be returned to the dose used prior to initiation of the strong CYP3A4 inducer [see Warnings and Precautions (5.5) and Drug Interactions (7.2)].

3 DOSAGE FORMS AND STRENGTHS
2.5 mg tablet
White to slightly yellow, elongated tablets with a bevelled edge and no score, engraved with "LCL" on one side and "NVR" on the other.
5 mg tablet
White to slightly yellow, elongated tablets with a bevelled edge and no score, engraved with "5" on one side and "NVR" on the other.
10 mg tablet
White to slightly yellow, elongated tablets with a bevelled edge and no score, engraved with "UHE" on one side and "NVR" on the other.

4 CONTRAINDICATIONS
Hypersensitivity to the active substance, to other rapamycin derivatives, or to any of the excipients. Hypersensitivity reactions manifested by symptoms including, but not limited to, anaphylaxis, dyspnea, flushing, chest pain, or angioedema (e.g., swelling of the airways or tongue, with or without respiratory impairment) have been observed with everolimus and other rapamycin derivatives.

5 WARNINGS AND PRECAUTIONS
5.1 Non-infectious Pneumonitis
Non-infectious pneumonitis is a class effect of rapamycin derivatives, including AFINITOR. In the randomized study, non-infectious pneumonitis was reported in 14% of patients treated with AFINITOR. The incidence of Common Toxicity Criteria (CTC) grade 3 and 4 non-infectious pneumonitis was 4% and 0%, respectively [see Adverse Reactions (6.1)]. Fatal outcomes have been observed.
Consider a diagnosis of non-infectious pneumonitis in patients presenting with non-specific respiratory signs and symptoms such as hypoxia, pleural effusion, cough, or dyspnea, and in whom infectious, neoplastic, and other causes have been excluded by means of appropriate investigations. Advise patients to report promptly any new or worsening respiratory symptoms.
Patients who develop radiological changes suggestive of non-infectious pneumonitis and have few or no symptoms may continue AFINITOR therapy without dose alteration. If symptoms are moderate, consider interrupting therapy until symptoms improve. The use of corticosteroids may be indicated. AFINITOR may be reintroduced at 5 mg daily.
For cases where symptoms of non-infectious pneumonitis are severe, discontinue AFINITOR therapy and the use of corticosteroids may be indicated until clinical symptoms resolve. Therapy with AFINITOR may be re-initiated at a reduced dose of 5 mg daily depending on the individual clinical circumstances.

5.2 Infections

AFINITOR has immunosuppressive properties and may predispose patients to bacterial, fungal, viral, or protozoan infections, including infections with opportunistic pathogens [see Adverse Reactions (6.1)]. Localized and systemic infections, including pneumonia, other bacterial infections, invasive fungal infections, such as aspergillosis or candidiasis, and viral infections including reactivation of hepatitis B virus have occurred in patients taking AFINITOR. Some of these infections have been severe (e.g., leading to respiratory or hepatic failure) or fatal. Physicians and patients should be aware of the increased risk of infection with AFINITOR. Complete treatment of pre-existing invasive fungal infections prior to starting treatment with AFINITOR. While taking AFINITOR be vigilant for signs and symptoms of infection; if a diagnosis of an infection is made, institute appropriate treatment promptly and consider interruption or discontinuation of AFINITOR. If a diagnosis of invasive systemic fungal infection is made, discontinue AFINITOR and treat with appropriate antifungal therapy.

5.3 Oral Ulceration

Mouth ulcers, stomatitis, and oral mucositis have occurred in patients treated with AFINITOR. In the randomized study, approximately 44% of AFINITOR-treated patients developed mouth ulcers, stomatitis, or oral mucositis, which were mostly CTC grade 1 and 2 [see Adverse Reactions (6.1)]. In such cases, topical treatments are recommended, but alcohol- or peroxide-containing mouthwashes should be avoided as they may exacerbate the condition. Antifungal agents should not be used unless fungal infection has been diagnosed [see Drug Interactions (7.1)].

5.4 Laboratory Tests and Monitoring

Renal Function

Elevations of serum creatinine, usually mild, have been reported in clinical trials [see Adverse Reactions (6.1)]. Monitoring of renal function, including measurement of blood urea nitrogen (BUN) or serum creatinine, is recommended prior to the start of AFINITOR therapy and periodically thereafter.

Blood Glucose and Lipids

Hyperglycemia, hyperlipidemia, and hypertriglyceridemia have been reported in clinical trials [see Adverse Reactions (6.1)]. Monitoring of fasting serum glucose and lipid profile is recommended prior to the start of AFINITOR therapy and periodically thereafter. When possible, optimal glucose and lipid control should be achieved before starting a patient on AFINITOR.

Hematological Parameters

Decreased hemoglobin, lymphocytes, neutrophils, and platelets have been reported in clinical trials [see Adverse Reactions (6.1)]. Monitoring of complete blood count is recommended prior to the start of AFINITOR therapy and periodically thereafter.

5.5 Drug-drug Interactions

Due to significant increases in exposure of everolimus, co-administration with strong inhibitors of CYP3A4 (e.g., ketoconazole, itraconazole, clarithromycin, atazanavir, nefazodone, saquinavir, telithromycin, ritonavir, indinavir, nelfinavir, voriconazole) or P-glycoprotein (PgP) should be avoided. Grapefruit, grapefruit juice and other foods that are known to affect cytochrome P450 and PgP activity should also be avoided during treatment [see Dosage and Administration (2.2) and Drug Interactions (7.1)].

A reduction of the AFINITOR dose is recommended when co-administered with a moderate CYP3A4 inhibitor (e.g., amprenavir, fosamprenavir, aprepitant, erythromycin, fluconazole, verapamil, diltiazem) or PgP inhibitor [see Dosage and Administration (2.2) and Drug Interactions (7.1)].

An increase in the AFINITOR dose is recommended when co-administered with a strong CYP3A4 inducer (e.g., St. John's Wort (Hypericum perforatum), dexamethasone, prednisone, prednisolone, phenytoin, carbamazepine, rifampin, rifabutin, rifapentine, phenobarbital) [see Dosage and Administration (2.2) and Drug Interactions (7.2)].

5.6 Hepatic Impairment

The safety and pharmacokinetics of AFINITOR were evaluated in a study in eight patients with moderate hepatic impairment (Child-Pugh class B) and eight subjects with normal hepatic function. Exposure was increased in patients with moderate hepatic impairment, therefore a dose reduction is recommended.

AFINITOR has not been studied in patients with severe hepatic impairment (Child-Pugh class C) and should not be used in this population [see Dosage and Administration (2.2) and Use in Specific Populations (8.7)].

5.7 Vaccinations

The use of live vaccines and close contact with those who have received live vaccines should be avoided during treatment with AFINITOR. Examples of live vaccines are: intranasal influenza, measles, mumps, rubella, oral polio, BCG, yellow fever, varicella, and TY21a typhoid vaccines.

Table 1
Adverse Reactions Reported in at least 10% of Patients and at a Higher Rate in the AFINITOR Arm than in the Placebo Arm

	AFINITOR 10 mg/day N=274			Placebo N=137		
	All grades %	Grade 3 %	Grade 4 %	All grades %	Grade 3 %	Grade 4 %
Any Adverse Reaction	97	52	13	93	23	5
Gastrointestinal Disorders						
Stomatitis[a]	44	4	<1	8	0	0
Diarrhea	30	1	0	7	0	0
Nausea	26	1	0	19	0	0
Vomiting	20	2	0	12	0	0
Infections and Infestations[b]	37	7	3	18	1	0
General Disorders and Administration Site Conditions						
Asthenia	33	3	<1	23	4	0
Fatigue	31	5	0	27	3	<1
Edema peripheral	25	<1	0	8	<1	0
Pyrexia	20	<1	0	8	0	0
Mucosal inflammation	19	1	0	1	0	0
Respiratory, Thoracic and Mediastinal Disorders						
Cough	30	<1	0	16	0	0
Dyspnea	24	6	1	15	3	0
Epistaxis	18	0	0	0	0	0
Pneumonitis[c]	14	4	0	0	0	0
Skin and Subcutaneous Tissue Disorders						
Rash	29	1	0	7	0	0
Pruritus	14	<1	0	7	0	0
Dry skin	13	<1	0	5	0	0
Metabolism and Nutrition Disorders						
Anorexia	25	1	0	14	<1	0
Nervous System Disorders						
Headache	19	<1	<1	9	<1	0
Dysgeusia	10	0	0	2	0	0
Musculoskeletal and Connective Tissue Disorders						
Pain in extremity	10	1	0	7	0	0
Median Duration of Treatment (d)	141			60		

CTCAE Version 3.0
[a] Stomatitis (including aphthous stomatitis), and mouth and tongue ulceration.
[b] Includes all preferred terms within the 'infections and infestations' system organ class, the most common being nasopharyngitis (6%), pneumonia (6%), urinary tract infection (5%), bronchitis (4%), and sinusitis (3%), and also including aspergillosis (<1%), candidiasis (<1%), and sepsis (<1%).
[c] Includes pneumonitis, interstitial lung disease, lung infiltration, pulmonary alveolar hemorrhage, pulmonary toxicity, and alveolitis.

5.8 Use in Pregnancy

Pregnancy Category D

There are no adequate and well-controlled studies of AFINITOR in pregnant women. However, based on mechanism of action, AFINITOR may cause fetal harm when administered to a pregnant woman. Everolimus caused embryo-fetal toxicities in animals at maternal exposures that were lower than human exposures at the recommended dose of 10 mg daily. If this drug is used during pregnancy or if the patient becomes pregnant while taking the drug, the patient should be apprised of the potential hazard to the fetus. Women of childbearing potential should be advised to use an effective method of contraception while using AFINITOR and for up to 8 weeks after ending treatment [see Use in Specific Populations (8.1)].

6 ADVERSE REACTIONS

The following serious adverse reactions are discussed in greater detail in another section of the label:
• Non-infectious pneumonitis [see Warnings and Precautions (5.1)].
• Infections [see Warnings and Precautions (5.2)].

6.1 Clinical Studies Experience

Because clinical trials are conducted under widely varying conditions, the adverse reaction rates observed cannot be directly compared to rates in other trials and may not reflect the rates observed in clinical practice.

The data described below reflect exposure to AFINITOR (n=274) and placebo (n=137) in a randomized, controlled trial in patients with metastatic renal cell carcinoma who received prior treatment with sunitinib and/or sorafenib. The median age of patients was 61 years (range 27-85), 88% were Caucasian, and 78% were male. The median duration of blinded study treatment was 141 days (range 19-451) for patients receiving AFINITOR and 60 days (range 21-295) for those receiving placebo.

The most common adverse reactions (incidence ≥30%) were stomatitis, infections, asthenia, fatigue, cough, and diarrhea. The most common grade 3/4 adverse reactions (incidence ≥3%) were infections, dyspnea, fatigue, stomatitis, dehydration, pneumonitis, abdominal pain, and asthenia. The most common laboratory abnormalities (incidence ≥50%) were anemia, hypercholesterolemia, hypertriglyceridemia, hyperglycemia, lymphopenia, and increased creatinine. The most common grade 3/4 laboratory abnormalities (incidence ≥3%) were lymphopenia, hyperglycemia, anemia, hypophosphatemia, and hypercholesterolemia. Deaths due to acute respiratory failure (0.7%), infection (0.7%) and acute renal failure (0.4%) were observed on the AFINITOR arm but none on the placebo arm. The rates of treatment-emergent adverse events (irrespective of causality) resulting in permanent discontinuation were 14% and 3% for the AFINITOR and placebo treatment groups, respectively. The most common adverse reactions (irrespective of causality) leading to treatment discontinuation were pneumonitis and dyspnea. Infections, stomatitis, and pneumonitis were the most common reasons for treatment delay or dose reduction. The most common medical interventions required during AFINITOR treatment were for infections, anemia, and stomatitis.

Table 1 compares the incidence of treatment-emergent adverse reactions reported with an incidence of ≥10% for patients receiving AFINITOR 10 mg daily versus placebo. Within each MedDRA system organ class, the adverse reactions are presented in order of decreasing frequency. [See table above]

Other notable adverse reactions occurring more frequently with AFINITOR than with placebo, but with an incidence of <10% include:

Gastrointestinal disorders: Abdominal pain (9%), dry mouth (8%), hemorrhoids (5%), dysphagia (4%)

General disorders and administration site conditions: Weight decreased (9%), chest pain (5%), chills (4%), impaired wound healing (<1%)

Respiratory, thoracic and mediastinal disorders: Pleural effusion (7%), pharyngolaryngeal pain (4%), rhinorrhea (3%)

Skin and subcutaneous tissue disorders: Hand-foot syndrome (reported as palmar-plantar erythrodysesthesia syndrome) (5%), nail disorder (5%), erythema (4%), onychoclasis (4%), skin lesion (4%), acneiform dermatitis (3%)

Metabolism and nutrition disorders: Exacerbation of pre-existing diabetes mellitus (2%), new onset of diabetes mellitus (<1%)

Psychiatric disorders: Insomnia (9%)

Nervous system disorders: Dizziness (7%), paresthesia (5%)

Table 2
Key Laboratory Abnormalities Reported at a Higher Rate in the AFINITOR Arm than the Placebo Arm

Laboratory Parameter	AFINITOR 10 mg/day N=274			Placebo N=137		
	All grades %	Grade 3 %	Grade 4 %	All grades %	Grade 3 %	Grade 4 %
Hematology[a]						
Hemoglobin decreased	92	12	1	79	5	<1
Lymphocytes decreased	51	16	2	28	5	0
Platelets decreased	23	1	0	2	0	<1
Neutrophils decreased	14	0	<1	4	0	0
Clinical Chemistry						
Cholesterol increased	77	4	0	35	0	0
Triglycerides increased	73	<1	0	34	0	0
Glucose increased	57	15	<1	25	1	0
Creatinine increased	50	1	0	34	0	0
Phosphate decreased	37	6	0	8	0	0
Aspartate transaminase (AST) increased	25	<1	<1	7	0	0
Alanine transaminase (ALT) increased	21	1	0	4	0	0
Bilirubin increased	3	<1	<1	2	0	0

CTCAE Version 3.0
[a] Includes reports of anemia, leukopenia, lymphopenia, neutropenia, pancytopenia, thrombocytopenia.

Eye disorders: Eyelid edema (4%), conjunctivitis (2%)
Vascular disorders: Hypertension (4%)
Renal and urinary disorders: Renal failure (3%)
Cardiac disorders: Tachycardia (3%), congestive cardiac failure (1%)
Musculoskeletal and connective tissue disorders: Jaw pain (3%)
Hematologic disorders: Hemorrhage (3%)
Key treatment-emergent laboratory abnormalities are presented in Table 2.
[See table above]
Information from further clinical trials
In clinical trials, everolimus has been associated with serious cases of hepatitis B reactivation, including fatal outcomes.

7 DRUG INTERACTIONS
Everolimus is a substrate of CYP3A4, and also a substrate and moderate inhibitor of the multidrug efflux pump PgP. *In vitro*, everolimus is a competitive inhibitor of CYP3A4 and a mixed inhibitor of CYP2D6.
7.1 Agents that may Increase Everolimus Blood Concentrations
CYP3A4 Inhibitors and PgP Inhibitors: In healthy subjects, compared to AFINITOR treatment alone there were significant increases in everolimus exposure when AFINITOR was coadministered with:
- ketoconazole (a strong CYP3A4 inhibitor and a PgP inhibitor) - C_{max} and AUC increased by 3.9- and 15.0-fold, respectively.
- erythromycin (a moderate CYP3A4 inhibitor and a PgP inhibitor) - C_{max} and AUC increased by 2.0- and 4.4-fold, respectively.
- verapamil (a moderate CYP3A4 inhibitor and a PgP inhibitor) - C_{max} and AUC increased by 2.3- and 3.5-fold, respectively.
Concomitant strong inhibitors of CYP3A4 and PgP should not be used *[see Warnings and Precautions (5.5)]*.
Use caution when AFINITOR is used in combination with moderate CYP3A4 or PgP inhibitors. If alternative treatment cannot be administered reduce the AFINITOR dose. *[See Dosage and Administration (2.2)]*.
7.2 Agents that may Decrease Everolimus Blood Concentrations
CYP3A4 Inducers: In healthy subjects, co-administration of AFINITOR with rifampin, a strong inducer of CYP3A4, decreased everolimus AUC and C_{max} by 64% and 58% respectively, compared to everolimus treatment alone. Consider a dose increase of AFINITOR when co-administered with strong inducers of CYP3A4 (e.g., dexamethasone, phenytoin, carbamazepine, rifampin, rifabutin, phenobarbital) or PgP if alternative treatment cannot be administered. St. John's Wort may decrease everolimus exposure unpredictably and should be avoided *[see Dosage and Administration (2.2)]*.
7.3 Agents whose Plasma Concentrations may be Altered by Everolimus
Studies in healthy subjects indicate that there are no clinically significant pharmacokinetic interactions between AFINITOR and the HMG-CoA reductase inhibitors atorvastatin (a CYP3A4 substrate) and pravastatin (a non-CYP3A4 substrate) and population pharmacokinetic analyses also detected no influence of simvastatin (a CYP3A4 substrate) on the clearance of AFINITOR.

8 USE IN SPECIFIC POPULATIONS
8.1 Pregnancy
Pregnancy Category D *[see Warnings and Precautions (5.8)]*
There are no adequate and well-controlled studies of AFINITOR in pregnant women. However, based on mechanism of action, AFINITOR may cause fetal harm when administered to a pregnant woman. Everolimus caused embryo-fetal toxicities in animals at maternal exposures that were lower than human exposures at the recommended dose of 10 mg daily. If this drug is used during pregnancy or if the patient becomes pregnant while taking the drug, the patient should be apprised of the potential hazard to the fetus. Women of childbearing potential should be advised to use an effective method of contraception while receiving AFINITOR and for up to 8 weeks after ending treatment.
In animal reproductive studies, oral administration of everolimus to female rats before mating and through organogenesis induced embryo-fetal toxicities, including increased resorption, pre-implantation and post-implantation loss, decreased numbers of live fetuses, malformation (e.g., sternal cleft) and retarded skeletal development. These effects occurred in the absence of maternal toxicities. Embryo-fetal toxicities occurred at approximately 4% the exposure (AUC_{0-24h}) in patients receiving the recommended dose of 10 mg daily. In rabbits, embryotoxicity evident as an increase in resorptions occurred at an oral dose approximately 1.6 times the recommended human dose on a body surface area basis. The effect in rabbits occurred in the presence of maternal toxicities.
In a pre- and post-natal development study in rats, animals were dosed from implantation through lactation. At approximately 10% of the recommended human dose based on body surface area, there were no adverse effects on delivery and lactation and there were no signs of maternal toxicity. However, there was reduced body weight (up to 9% reduction from the control) and slight reduction in survival in offspring (~5% died or missing). There were no drug-related effects on the developmental parameters (morphological development, motor activity, learning, or fertility assessment) in the offspring.
Doses that resulted in embryo-fetal toxicities in rats and rabbits were ≥0.1 mg/kg (0.6 mg/m²) and 0.8 mg/kg (9.6 mg/m²), respectively. The dose in the pre- and post-natal development study in rats that caused reduction in body weights and survival of offspring was 0.1 mg/kg (0.6 mg/m²).
8.3 Nursing Mothers
It is not known whether everolimus is excreted in human milk. Everolimus and/or its metabolites passed into the milk of lactating rats at a concentration 3.5 times higher than in maternal serum. Because many drugs are excreted in human milk and because of the potential for serious adverse reactions in nursing infants from everolimus, a decision should be made whether to discontinue nursing or to discontinue the drug, taking into account the importance of the drug to the mother.
8.4 Pediatric Use
The safety and effectiveness in pediatric patients have not been established.
8.5 Geriatric Use
In the randomized study, 41% of AFINITOR-treated patients were ≥65 years in age, while 7% percent were 75 and over. No overall differences in safety or effectiveness were observed between these subjects and younger subjects, and other reported clinical experience has not identified differ-

ences in responses between the elderly and younger patients, but greater sensitivity of some older individuals cannot be ruled out *[see Clinical Pharmacology (12.3)]*.
No dosage adjustment is required in elderly patients *[see Clinical Pharmacology (12.3)]*.
8.6 Renal Impairment
No clinical studies were conducted with AFINITOR in patients with decreased renal function. Renal impairment is not expected to influence drug exposure and no dosage adjustment of everolimus is recommended in patients with renal impairment *[see Clinical Pharmacology (12.3)]*.
8.7 Hepatic Impairment
For patients with moderate hepatic impairment (Child-Pugh class B), the dose should be reduced to 5 mg daily *[see Dosage and Administration (2.2), Warnings and Precautions (5.6) and Clinical Pharmacology (12.3)]*.
The impact of severe hepatic impairment (Child-Pugh class C) has not been assessed and use in this patient population is not recommended *[see Warnings and Precautions (5.6)]*.

10 OVERDOSAGE
In animal studies, everolimus showed a low acute toxic potential. No lethality or severe toxicity were observed in either mice or rats given single oral doses of 2000 mg/kg (limit test).
Reported experience with overdose in humans is very limited. Single doses of up to 70 mg have been administered. The acute toxicity profile observed with the 70 mg dose was consistent with that for the 10 mg dose.

11 DESCRIPTION
AFINITOR (everolimus), an inhibitor of mTOR, is an antineoplastic agent.
The chemical name of everolimus is (1R,9S,12S, 15R,16E,18R,19R,21R,23S,24E,26E,28E,30S,32S,35R)-1,18-dihydroxy-12-[(1R)-2-[(1S,3R,4R)-4-(2-hydroxyethoxy)-3-methoxycyclohexyl]-1-methylethyl]-19,30-dimethoxy-15,17,21,23,29,35-hexamethyl-11,36-dioxa-4-aza-tricyclo[30.3.1.0⁴,⁹]hexatriaconta-16,24,26,28-tetraene-2,3,10,14,20-pentaone.
The molecular formula is $C_{53}H_{83}NO_{14}$ and the molecular weight is 958.2. The structural formula is

AFINITOR is supplied as tablets for oral administration containing 2.5 mg, 5 mg and 10 mg of everolimus together with butylated hydroxytoluene, magnesium stearate, lactose monohydrate, hypromellose, crospovidone and lactose anhydrous as inactive ingredients.

12 CLINICAL PHARMACOLOGY
12.1 Mechanism of Action
Everolimus is an inhibitor of mTOR (mammalian target of rapamycin), a serine-threonine kinase, downstream of the PI3K/AKT pathway. The mTOR pathway is dysregulated in several human cancers. Everolimus binds to an intracellular protein, FKBP-12, resulting in an inhibitory complex formation and inhibition of mTOR kinase activity. Everolimus reduced the activity of S6 ribosomal protein kinase (S6K1) and eukaryotic elongation factor 4E-binding protein (4E-BP), downstream effectors of mTOR, involved in protein synthesis. In addition, everolimus inhibited the expression of hypoxia-inducible factor (e.g., HIF-1) and reduced the expression of vascular endothelial growth factor (VEGF). Inhibition of mTOR by everolimus has been shown to reduce cell proliferation, angiogenesis, and glucose uptake in *in vitro* and/or *in vivo* studies.
12.2 Pharmacodynamics
QT/QTc Prolongation Potential
In a randomized, placebo-controlled, crossover study, 59 healthy subjects were administered a single oral dose of AFINITOR (20 mg and 50 mg) and placebo. There is no indication of a QT/QTc prolonging effect of AFINITOR in single doses up to 50 mg.
Exposure Response Relationships
Markers of protein synthesis show that inhibition of mTOR is complete after a 10 mg daily dose.
12.3 Pharmacokinetics
Absorption
In patients with advanced solid tumors, peak everolimus concentrations are reached 1 to 2 hours after administra-

tion of oral doses ranging from 5 mg to 70 mg. Following single doses, C_{max} is dose-proportional between 5 mg and 10 mg. At doses of 20 mg and higher, the increase in C_{max} is less than dose-proportional, however AUC shows dose-proportionality over the 5 mg to 70 mg dose range. Steady-state was achieved within two weeks following once-daily dosing.

Food effect: In healthy subjects, high fat meals reduced systemic exposure to AFINITOR 10 mg tablet (as measured by AUC) by 22% and the peak plasma concentration C_{max} by 54%. Light fat meals reduced AUC by 32% and C_{max} by 42%. Food, however, had no apparent effect on the post absorption phase concentration-time profile.

Distribution

The blood-to-plasma ratio of everolimus, which is concentration-dependent over the range of 5 to 5000 ng/mL, is 17% to 73%. The amount of everolimus confined to the plasma is approximately 20% at blood concentrations observed in cancer patients given AFINITOR 10 mg/day. Plasma protein binding is approximately 74% both in healthy subjects and in patients with moderate hepatic impairment.

Metabolism

Everolimus is a substrate of CYP3A4 and PgP. Following oral administration, everolimus is the main circulating component in human blood. Six main metabolites of everolimus have been detected in human blood, including three mono-hydroxylated metabolites, two hydrolytic ring-opened products, and a phosphatidylcholine conjugate of everolimus. These metabolites were also identified in animal species used in toxicity studies, and showed approximately 100-times less activity than everolimus itself.

In vitro, everolimus competitively inhibited the metabolism of CYP3A4 and was a mixed inhibitor of the CYP2D6 substrate dextromethorphan. The mean steady-state C_{max} following an oral dose of 10 mg daily is more than 12-fold below the Ki-values of the *in vitro* inhibition. Therefore, an effect of everolimus on the metabolism of CYP3A4 and CYP2D6 substrates is unlikely.

Excretion

No specific excretion studies have been undertaken in cancer patients. Following the administration of a 3 mg single dose of radiolabelled everolimus in patients who were receiving cyclosporine, 80% of the radioactivity was recovered from the feces, while 5% was excreted in the urine. The parent substance was not detected in urine or feces. The mean elimination half-life of everolimus is approximately 30 hours.

Patients with Renal Impairment

Approximately 5% of total radioactivity was excreted in the urine following a 3 mg dose of [^{14}C]-labeled everolimus. In a population pharmacokinetic analysis which included 170 patients with advanced cancer, no significant influence of creatinine clearance (25-178 mL/min) was detected on oral clearance (CL/F) of everolimus *[see Use in Specific Populations (8.6)]*.

Patients with Hepatic Impairment

The average AUC of everolimus in eight subjects with moderate hepatic impairment (Child-Pugh class B) was twice that found in eight subjects with normal hepatic function. AUC was positively correlated with serum bilirubin concentration and with prolongation of prothrombin time and negatively correlated with serum albumin concentration. A dose reduction for patients with Child-Pugh class B hepatic impairment is recommended. AFINITOR should not be used in patients with severe (Child-Pugh class C) hepatic impairment as the impact of severe hepatic impairment on everolimus exposure has not been assessed *[see Dosage and Administration (2.2), Warnings and Precautions (5.6) and Use in Specific Populations (8.7)]*.

Effects of Age and Gender

In a population pharmacokinetic evaluation in cancer patients, no relationship was apparent between oral clearance and patient age or gender.

Ethnicity

Based on a cross-study comparison, Japanese patients (n = 6) had on average exposures that were higher than non-Japanese patients receiving the same dose.

Based on analysis of population pharmacokinetics, oral clearance (CL/F) is on average 20% higher in Black patients than in Caucasians.

The significance of these differences on the safety and efficacy of everolimus in Japanese or Black patients has not been established.

13 NONCLINICAL TOXICOLOGY

13.1 Carcinogenesis, Mutagenesis, Impairment of Fertility

Administration of everolimus for up to 2 years did not indicate oncogenic potential in mice and rats up to the highest doses tested (0.9 mg/kg) corresponding respectively to 4.3 and 0.2 times the estimated clinical exposure (AUC_{0-24h}) at the recommended human dose of 10 mg daily.

Table 3
Efficacy Results by Central Radiologic Review

	AFINITOR N=277	Placebo N=139	Hazard Ratio (95% CI)	p-value[a]
Median Progression-free Survival (95% CI)	4.9 months (4.0 to 5.5)	1.9 months (1.8 to 1.9)	0.33 (0.25 to 0.43)	<0.0001
Objective Response Rate	2%	0%	n/a[b]	n/a[b]

[a]Log-rank test stratified by prognostic score.
[b]Not applicable.

Everolimus was not genotoxic in a battery of *in vitro* assays (Ames mutation test in *Salmonella*, mutation test in L5178Y mouse lymphoma cells, and chromosome aberration assay in V79 Chinese hamster cells). Everolimus was not genotoxic in an *in vivo* mouse bone marrow micronucleus test at doses up to 500 mg/kg/day (1500 mg/m²/day, approximately 255-fold the recommended human dose, based on the body surface area), administered as two doses, 24 hours apart.

Based on non-clinical findings, male fertility may be compromised by treatment with AFINITOR. In a 13-week male fertility study in rats, testicular morphology was affected at 0.5 mg/kg and above, and sperm motility, sperm count, and plasma testosterone levels were diminished at 5 mg/kg, which resulted in infertility at 5 mg/kg. Effects on male fertility occurred at the AUC_{0-24h} values below that of therapeutic exposure (approximately 10%-81% of the AUC_{0-24h} in patients receiving the recommended dose of 10 mg daily). After a 10-13 week non-treatment period, the fertility index increased from zero (infertility) to 60% (12/20 mated females were pregnant).

Oral doses of everolimus in female rats at ≥0.1 mg/kg (approximately 4% the AUC_{0-24h} in patients receiving the recommended dose of 10 mg daily) resulted in increases in pre-implantation loss, suggesting that the drug may reduce female fertility. Everolimus crossed the placenta and was toxic to the conceptus *[see Use in Specific Populations (8.1)]*.

14 CLINICAL STUDIES

An international, multicenter, randomized, double-blind trial comparing AFINITOR 10 mg daily and placebo, both in conjunction with best supportive care, was conducted in patients with metastatic renal cell carcinoma whose disease had progressed despite prior treatment with sunitinib, sorafenib, or both sequentially. Prior therapy with bevacizumab, interleukin 2, or interferon-α was also permitted. Randomization was stratified according to prognostic score[1] and prior anticancer therapy.

Progression-free survival (PFS), documented using RECIST (Response Evaluation Criteria in Solid Tumors) was assessed via a blinded, independent, central radiologic review. After documented radiological progression, patients could be unblinded by the investigator: those randomized to placebo were then able to receive open-label AFINITOR 10 mg daily.

In total, 416 patients were randomized 2:1 to receive AFINITOR (n=277) or placebo (n=139). Demographics were well balanced between the two arms (median age 61 years; 77% male, 88% Caucasian, 74% received prior sunitinib or sorafenib, and 26% received both sequentially).

AFINITOR was superior to placebo for progression-free survival *(see Table 3 and Figure 1)*. The treatment effect was similar across prognostic scores and prior sorafenib and/or sunitinib. The overall survival (OS) results were not mature and 32% of patients had died by the time of cut-off.

[See table above]

Figure 1
Kaplan-Meier Progression-free Survival Curves

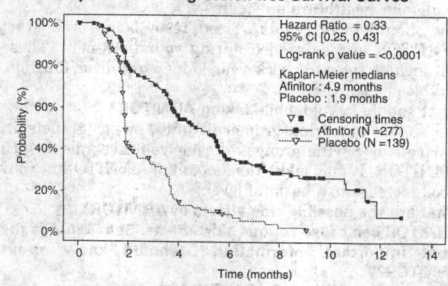

15 REFERENCES

1. Motzer RJ, Bacik J, Schwartz LH, et al. Prognostic factors for survival in previously treated patients with metastatic renal cell cancer. J Clin Oncol (2004) 22:454-63.
2. NIOSH Alert: Preventing occupational exposures to antineoplastic and other hazardous drugs in healthcare settings. 2004. U.S. Department of Health and Human Services, Public Health Service, Centers for Disease Control and Prevention, National Institute for Occupational Safety and Health, DHHS (NIOSH) Publication No. 2004-165.
3. OSHA Technical Manual, TED 1-0.15A, Section VI: Chapter 2. Controlling Occupational Exposure to Hazardous Drugs. OSHA, 1999. http://www.osha.gov/dts/osta/otm/otm_vi/otm_vi_2.html
4. American Society of Health-System Pharmacists. ASHP guidelines on handling hazardous drugs. Am J Health-Syst Pharm. (2006) 63:1172-1193.
5. Polovich, M., White, J.M., & Kelleher, L.O. (eds.) 2005. Chemotherapy and biotherapy guidelines and recommendations for practice (2nd. ed.) Pittsburgh, PA: Oncology Nursing Society.

16 HOW SUPPLIED/STORAGE AND HANDLING

2.5 mg tablets

White to slightly yellow, elongated tablets with a bevelled edge and no score, engraved with "LCL" on one side and "NVR" on the other; available in:

Blisters of 28 tablets .... NDC 0078-0594-51
Each carton contains 4 blister cards of 7 tablets each

5 mg tablets

White to slightly yellow, elongated tablets with a bevelled edge and no score, engraved with "5" on one side and "NVR" on the other; available in:

Blisters of 28 tablets .... NDC 0078-0566-51
Each carton contains 4 blister cards of 7 tablets each

10 mg tablets

White to slightly yellow, elongated tablets with a bevelled edge and no score, engraved with "UHE" on one side and "NVR" on the other; available in:

Blisters of 28 tablets .... NDC 0078-0567-51
Each carton contains 4 blister cards of 7 tablets each

Store AFINITOR (everolimus) tablets at 25° C (77°F); excursions permitted between 15°-30°C (59°-86°F). [See USP Controlled Room Temperature.] Store in the original container, protect from light and moisture. Keep this and all drugs out of the reach of children.

Procedures for proper handling and disposal of anticancer drugs should be considered. Several guidelines on this subject have been published.[2-5]

AFINITOR tablets should not be crushed. Do not take tablets which are crushed or broken.

17 PATIENT COUNSELING INFORMATION

17.1 Non-infectious Pneumonitis

Warn patients of the possibility of developing non-infectious pneumonitis. In clinical studies, some non-infectious pneumonitis cases have been severe and occasionally fatal. Advise patients to report promptly any new or worsening respiratory symptoms *[see Warnings and Precautions (5.1)]*.

17.2 Infections

Inform patients that they are more susceptible to infections while being treated with AFINITOR and that cases of hepatitis B reactivation have been associated with AFINITOR treatment. In clinical studies, some of these infections have been severe (e.g., leading to respiratory or hepatic failure) and occasionally fatal. Patients should be aware of the signs and symptoms of infection and should report any such signs or symptoms promptly to their physician *[see Warnings and Precautions (5.2)]*.

17.3 Oral Ulceration

Inform patients of the possibility of developing mouth ulcers, stomatitis and oral mucositis. In such cases, mouthwashes and/or topical treatments are recommended, but these should not contain alcohol or peroxide. *[See Warnings and Precautions (5.3)]*

17.4 Laboratory Tests and Monitoring

Inform patients of the need to monitor blood chemistry and hematology prior to the start of AFINITOR therapy and periodically thereafter *[see Warnings and Precautions (5.4)]*.

17.5 Drug-drug Interactions

Avoid concurrent treatment with **strong** CYP3A4 and PgP inhibitors. Use caution if AFINITOR must be co-administered with **moderate** CYP3A4 and PgP inhibitors; reduce the dose and carefully monitor the patient for undesirable effects. Avoid concurrent treatment with strong CYP3A4 and PgP inducers. If AFINITOR must be co-administered with strong CYP3A4 inducers, consider a dose increase and carefully monitor the patient for clinical response. Advise patients to inform their healthcare providers of all concomitant medications, including over-the-counter medications and dietary supplements *[see Dosage and Administration (2.2), Warnings and Precautions (5.5) and Drug-drug Interactions (7.1 and 7.2)].*

17.6 Hepatic Impairment

Advise patients that AFINITOR is not recommended in patients with severe hepatic impairment (Child-Pugh class C). Prescribe a reduced dose of 5 mg AFINITOR per day for patients with moderate hepatic impairment (Child-Pugh class B) *[see Dosage and Administration (2), Warnings and Precautions (5.6) and Clinical Pharmacology (12)].*

17.7 Vaccinations

Advise patients to avoid the use of live vaccines and close contact with those who have received live vaccines *[see Warnings and Precautions (5.7)].*

17.8 Pregnancy

Advise female patients of childbearing potential that AFINITOR may cause fetal harm and that an effective method of contraception should be used during therapy with AFINITOR and for 8 weeks after ending treatment.

17.9 Dosing Instructions

Inform patients to take AFINITOR once daily at the same time every day, either with or without food. The tablets should not be crushed or chewed. AFINITOR should be swallowed whole with a full glass of water.

Instruct patients that if they miss a dose of AFINITOR, they may still take it up to 6 hours after the time they would normally take it. If more than 6 hours have elapsed, they should be instructed to skip the dose for that day. The next day, they should take AFINITOR at the usual time. Warn patients to not take 2 doses to make up for the one that they missed.

PATIENT INFORMATION

AFINITOR® (a-fin-it-or)
(everolimus)
Tablets

Read this patient information leaflet that comes with AFINITOR before you start taking it and each time you get a refill. There may be new information. This information does not take the place of talking to your healthcare provider about your medical condition or treatment.

What is the most important information I should know about AFINITOR?

AFINITOR can cause serious side effects, including:

1. **You may develop lung or breathing problems.** In some people lung or breathing problems may be severe, and can even lead to death. You may need to stop taking AFINITOR for a while or use a lower dose.

   Tell your healthcare provider right away if you have any of these symptoms:
   - new or worsening cough
   - shortness of breath
   - difficulty breathing or wheezing

2. **You may be more likely to develop an infection**, such as pneumonia, or a bacterial, fungal or viral infection. Viral infections may include active hepatitis B in people who have had hepatitis B in the past (reactivation). In some people these infections may be severe, and can even lead to death. You may need to be treated as soon as possible. Tell your healthcare provider right away if you have a temperature of 100.5° F or above, chills, or do not feel well.

   Symptoms of hepatitis B or infection may include the following:
   - Fever
   - Skin rash
   - Joint pain and inflammation
   - Tiredness
   - Loss of appetite
   - Nausea
   - Pale stool or dark urine
   - Yellowing of the skin
   - Pain in your upper right side

What is AFINITOR?

AFINITOR is a prescription medicine used to treat people with advanced kidney cancer (renal cell carcinoma or RCC) when certain other treatments have not worked.

AFINITOR may slow the growth and spread of kidney cancer.

It is not known if AFINITOR is safe and effective in children.

Who should not take AFINITOR?

Do not take AFINITOR if you are allergic to AFINITOR or to any of its ingredients. See the end of this leaflet for a complete list of ingredients in AFINITOR. Talk to your healthcare provider before taking this medicine if you are allergic to:
- sirolimus (Rapamune®)
- temsirolimus (Torisel®)

Ask your healthcare provider if you do not know.

What should I tell my healthcare provider before taking AFINITOR?

Before taking AFINITOR, tell your healthcare provider about all of your medical conditions including if you:
- Have or have had liver problems
- Have diabetes or high blood sugar
- Have high blood cholesterol levels
- Have any infections
- Previously had hepatitis B
- Are scheduled to receive any vaccinations. You should not receive a live vaccine or be around people who have recently received a live vaccine during your treatment with AFINITOR. If you are not sure about the type of immunization or vaccine, ask your healthcare provider.
- Other medical conditions
- Are pregnant, or could become pregnant. It is not known if AFINITOR will harm your unborn baby. You should use effective birth control while using AFINITOR and for 8 weeks after stopping treatment.
- Are breast-feeding or plan to breast-feed. It is not known if AFINITOR passes into your breast milk. You and your healthcare provider should decide if you will take AFINITOR or breast-feed. You should not do both.

Tell your healthcare provider about all of the medicines you take, including prescription and non-prescription medicines, vitamins, and herbal supplements. AFINITOR may affect the way other medicines work, and other medicines can affect how AFINITOR works. Using AFINITOR with other medicines can cause serious side effects.

Know the medicines you take. Keep a list of them and show it to your healthcare provider and pharmacist when you get a new medicine. Especially tell your healthcare provider if you take:
- St. John's Wort (Hypericum perforatum)
- Medicine for:
  - Fungal infections
  - Bacterial infections
  - Tuberculosis
  - Seizures
  - HIV-AIDS
  - Heart conditions or high blood pressure
- Medicines that suppress your immune system

Ask your healthcare provider or pharmacist if you are not sure if your medicine is one of those taken for the conditions listed above. If you are taking any medicines for the conditions listed above, your healthcare provider might need to prescribe a different medicine. You should also tell your healthcare provider before you start taking any new medicine.

How should I take AFINITOR?
- Your healthcare provider will prescribe the dose of AFINITOR that is right for you.
- Take AFINITOR exactly as your healthcare provider tells you. Your healthcare provider may change your dose of AFINITOR if needed.
- Swallow AFINITOR tablets whole with a glass of water. Do not crush or chew the tablets. If you cannot swallow AFINITOR tablets whole, tell your healthcare provider.
- Take AFINITOR one time every day, at about the same time every day.
- You can take AFINITOR with or without food.
- Do not take any tablet that is broken or crushed.
- You may use scissors to open the blister to avoid spillage.
- If you take too much AFINITOR contact your healthcare provider or go to the nearest hospital emergency department right away. Take the pack of AFINITOR with you.
- If you miss a dose of AFINITOR, you may still take it up to 6 hours after the time you normally take it. If it is more than 6 hours after you normally take your AFINITOR, skip the dose for that day. The next day, take AFINITOR at your usual time. Do not take 2 doses to make up for the one that you missed. If you are not sure about what to do, call your healthcare provider.

You should have regular blood tests before you start AFINITOR and as needed during your treatment. These will include tests to check your kidney and liver function, and blood sugar levels.

What should I avoid while taking AFINITOR?

You should not drink grapefruit juice, or eat grapefruit, starfruit or Seville oranges during your treatment with AFINITOR. It may make the amount of AFINITOR in your blood increase to a harmful level.

What are the possible side effects of AFINITOR?

AFINITOR can cause serious side effects. See "What is the most important information I should know about AFINITOR?"

Common side effects of AFINITOR include:
- **mouth ulcers.** AFINITOR can cause mouth ulcers and sores. Tell your healthcare provider if you have pain, discomfort, or open sores in your mouth. Your healthcare provider may tell you to use a special mouthwash or mouth gel that does not contain alcohol or peroxide.
- **feeling weak or tired**
- **cough, shortness of breath**
- diarrhea
- rash, dry skin, and itching
- nausea and vomiting
- fever
- loss of appetite
- swelling of arms, hands, feet, ankles, face or other parts of the body
- abnormal taste
- inflammation of lining of the digestive system
- headache
- nose bleeds
- pain in arms and legs

Tell your healthcare provider if you have any side effect that bothers you or does not go away.

These are not all the possible side effects of AFINITOR. For more information, ask your healthcare provider or pharmacist.

Call your doctor for medical advice about side effects. You may report side effects to FDA at 1-800-FDA-1088.

How do I store AFINITOR?
- Keep AFINITOR at room temperature, between 59° to 86°F (15° to 30°C).
- Keep AFINITOR in the package it comes in.
- Open the blister package just before taking AFINITOR.
- Keep the blister package and tablets dry.
- Keep AFINITOR out of light.
- Throw away AFINITOR that is out of date or no longer needed.

Keep AFINITOR and all medicines out of the reach of children.

General information about AFINITOR

Medicines are sometimes prescribed for conditions that are not mentioned in a patient information leaflet. Do not use AFINITOR for a condition for which it was not prescribed. Do not give AFINITOR to other people, even if they have the same problem you have. It may harm them.

This leaflet summarizes the most important information about AFINITOR. If you would like more information, talk with your healthcare provider. You can ask your healthcare provider or pharmacist for information written for healthcare professionals.

For more information call 1-888-423-4648 or go to www.AFINITOR.com.

What are the ingredients in AFINITOR?

Active ingredient: everolimus.

Inactive ingredients: butylated hydroxytoluene, magnesium stearate, lactose monohydrate, hypromellose, crospovidone, lactose anhydrous.

The brands listed are the trademarks or register marks of their respective owners and are not trademarks or register marks of Novartis.

T2010-56/T2010-57

Manufactured by:
Novartis Pharma Stein AG
Stein, Switzerland
Distributed by:
Novartis Pharmaceuticals Corporation
East Hanover, New Jersey 07936
©Novartis

Shown in Product Identification Guide, page 314

COARTEM®   ℞

[co-AR-tem]
(artemether/lumefantrine)
Tablets

The following prescribing information is based on official labeling in effect July 2010.

HIGHLIGHTS OF PRESCRIBING INFORMATION
These highlights do not include all the information needed to use Coartem Tablets safely and effectively. See full prescribing information for Coartem Tablets.
Coartem (artemether/lumefantrine) Tablets
Initial U.S. Approval: 2009

————————RECENT MAJOR CHANGES————————
Dosage and Administration (2.4)   02/2010

————————INDICATIONS AND USAGE————————
- Coartem (artemether and lumefantrine) Tablets are indicated for treatment of acute, uncomplicated malaria infections due to *Plasmodium falciparum* in patients of 5 kg bodyweight and above. (1)
- Coartem Tablets have been shown to be effective in geographical regions where resistance to chloroquine has been reported. (1)
- Coartem Tablets should not be used to treat severe malaria or to prevent malaria. (1)

————————DOSAGE AND ADMINISTRATION————————
- Coartem Tablets should be taken with food. (2.1, 5.2)
- Tablets may be crushed and mixed with one to two teaspoons of water immediately prior to administration to patients, including children. (2.1)
- Coartem Tablets should be administered over 3-days for a total of 6 doses: an initial dose, second dose after 8 hours and then twice daily (morning and evening) for the following two days. (2.2, 2.3)

- The adult dosage for patients with bodyweight of 35 kg and above is 4 tablets per dose for a total of 6 doses. (2.2)
- The number of tablets per dose for children is determined by bodyweight, as shown in the chart below. (2.3)

Tablets per dose by bodyweight; total of 6 doses over 3 days

5 to <15 kg	1 tablet
15 to <25 kg	2 tablets
25 to <35 kg	3 tablets
35 kg and over	4 tablets

—DOSAGE FORMS AND STRENGTHS—
Tablets are scored and contain 20 mg artemether and 120 mg lumefantrine. (3)

—CONTRAINDICATIONS—
- Patients hypersensitive to artemether, lumefantrine, or to any of the excipients. (4.1)

—WARNINGS AND PRECAUTIONS—
- Avoid use in patients with known QT prolongation, those with hypokalemia or hypomagnesemia, and those taking other drugs that prolong the QT interval. (5.1, 12.5)
- Halofantrine and Coartem Tablets should not be administered within one month of each other due to potential additive effects on the QT interval. (5.1, 5.2, 12.3)
- Antimalarials should not be given concomitantly, unless there is no other treatment option, due to limited safety data. (5.2)
- QT prolonging drugs, including quinine and quinidine, should be used cautiously following Coartem Tablets. (5.1, 5.2, 7.6, 12.3)
- Substrates, inhibitors, or inducers of CYP3A4, including antiretroviral medications, should be used cautiously with Coartem Tablets, due to a potential loss of efficacy of the concomitant drug or additive QT prolongation. (5.3, 7.1, 7.3)

—ADVERSE REACTIONS—
The most common adverse reactions in adults (>30%) are headache, anorexia, dizziness, asthenia, arthralgia and myalgia. The most common adverse reactions in children (>12%) are pyrexia, cough, vomiting, anorexia and headache. (6.2)

To report SUSPECTED ADVERSE REACTIONS, contact Novartis Pharmaceuticals Corporation at 1-888-669-6682 or FDA at 1-800-FDA-1088 or www.fda.gov/medwatch

—DRUG INTERACTIONS—
- CYP3A4 Inhibitors: Use cautiously due to potential for QT prolongation. (5.3, 7.1)
- Mefloquine: If used immediately before treatment, monitor for decreased efficacy of Coartem Tablets and encourage food consumption. (2.1, 7.2)
- Hormonal Contraceptives: Effectiveness may be reduced; use an additional method of birth control. (5.3, 7.3)
- Anti-Retrovirals: Use cautiously due to potential for QT prolongation, loss of anti-viral efficacy, or loss of antimalarial efficacy of Coartem Tablets. (5.3, 7.3)
- CYP2D6 Substrates: Monitor for adverse reactions and potential QT prolongation. (5.1, 5.4, 7.4)

—USE IN SPECIFIC POPULATIONS—
- Pregnancy: Based on animal data, may increase fetal loss. (8.1)
- Nursing Mothers: Use caution when administering to a nursing woman. (8.3)
- Pediatric Use: Studied in children 2 months of age and older with a bodyweight of 5 kg and greater. (8.4)
- Geriatric Use: Not studied in geriatric patients. (8.5)

See 17 for PATIENT COUNSELING INFORMATION and FDA-approved patient labeling

Revised: 02/2010

FULL PRESCRIBING INFORMATION: CONTENTS*

FULL PRESCRIBING INFORMATION

1 INDICATIONS AND USAGE
Coartem (artemether/lumefantrine) Tablets are indicated for treatment of acute, uncomplicated malaria infections due to *Plasmodium falciparum* in patients of 5 kg bodyweight and above. Coartem Tablets have been shown to be effective in geographical regions where resistance to chloroquine has been reported [*see Clinical Studies (14.1)*].

Limitations of Use:
- Coartem Tablets are not approved for patients with severe or complicated *P. falciparum* malaria.
- Coartem Tablets are not approved for the prevention of malaria.

2 DOSAGE AND ADMINISTRATION
2.1 Administration Instructions
Coartem Tablets should be taken with food. Patients with acute malaria are frequently averse to food. Patients should be encouraged to resume normal eating as soon as food can be tolerated since this improves absorption of artemether and lumefantrine.

For patients who are unable to swallow the tablets such as infants and children, Coartem Tablets may be crushed and mixed with a small amount of water (one to two teaspoons) in a clean container for administration immediately prior to use. The container can be rinsed with more water and the contents swallowed by the patient. The crushed tablet preparation should be followed whenever possible by food/drink (e.g., milk, formula, pudding, broth, and porridge).

In the event of vomiting within 1 to 2 hours of administration, a repeat dose should be taken. If the repeat dose is vomited, the patient should be given an alternative antimalarial for treatment.

2.2 Dosage in Adult Patients (>16 years of age)
A 3-day treatment schedule with a total of 6 doses is recommended for adult patients with a bodyweight of 35 kg and above:

Four tablets as a single initial dose, 4 tablets again after 8 hours and then 4 tablets twice daily (morning and evening) for the following two days (total course of 24 tablets).

For patients weighing less than 35 kg, *see* Dosage in Pediatric Patients (2.3).

2.3 Dosage in Pediatric Patients
A 3-day treatment schedule with a total of 6 doses is recommended as below:

5 kg to less than 15 kg bodyweight: One tablet as an initial dose, 1 tablet again after 8 hours and then 1 tablet twice daily (morning and evening) for the following two days (total course of 6 tablets).

15 kg to less than 25 kg bodyweight: Two tablets as an initial dose, 2 tablets again after 8 hours and then 2 tablets twice daily (morning and evening) for the following two days (total course of 12 tablets).

25 kg to less than 35 kg bodyweight: Three tablets as an initial dose, 3 tablets again after 8 hours and then 3 tablets twice daily (morning and evening) for the following two days (total course of 18 tablets).

35 kg bodyweight and above: Four tablets as a single initial dose, 4 tablets again after 8 hours and then 4 tablets twice daily (morning and evening) for the following two days (total course of 24 tablets).

2.4 Dosage in Patients with Hepatic or Renal Impairment
No specific pharmacokinetic studies have been carried out in patients with hepatic or renal impairment. Most patients with acute malaria present with some degree of related hepatic and/or renal impairment. In clinical studies, the adverse event profile did not differ in patients with mild or moderate hepatic impairment compared to patients with normal hepatic function. No specific dose adjustments are needed for patients with mild or moderate hepatic impairment.

In clinical studies, the adverse event profile did not differ in patients with mild or moderate renal impairment compared to patients with normal renal function. There were few patients with severe renal impairment in clinical studies. There is no significant renal excretion of lumefantrine, artemether and dihydroartemisinin (DHA) in healthy volunteers and while clinical experience in this population is limited, no dose adjustment is recommended.

Caution should be exercised when administering Coartem Tablets in patients with severe hepatic or renal impairment [*see Warnings and Precautions (5.6)*].

3 DOSAGE FORMS AND STRENGTHS
Coartem Tablets contain 20 mg of artemether and 120 mg of lumefantrine. Coartem Tablets are supplied as yellow, round, flat tablets with beveled edges and scored on one side. Tablets are imprinted with N/C on one side and CG on the other side.

4 CONTRAINDICATIONS
4.1 Hypersensitivity
- Patients hypersensitive to artemether, lumefantrine, or to any of the excipients of Coartem Tablets [*see Adverse Reactions (6.3)*].

5 WARNINGS AND PRECAUTIONS
5.1 Prolongation of the QT Interval
Some antimalarials (e.g., halofantrine, quinine, quinidine) including Coartem Tablets have been associated with prolongation of the QT interval on the electrocardiogram. Coartem Tablets should be avoided in patients:
- with congenital prolongation of the QT interval (e.g., long QT syndrome) or any other clinical condition known to prolong the QTc interval such as patients with a history of symptomatic cardiac arrhythmias, with clinically relevant bradycardia or with severe cardiac disease.
- with a family history of congenital prolongation of the QT interval or sudden death.
- with known disturbances of electrolyte balance, e.g., hypokalemia or hypomagnesemia.
- receiving other medications that prolong the QT interval, such as class IA (quinidine, procainamide, disopyramide), or class III (amiodarone, sotalol) antiarrhythmic agents; antipsychotics (pimozide, ziprasidone); antidepressants; certain antibiotics (macrolide antibiotics, fluoroquinolone antibiotics, imidazole, and triazole antifungal agents); certain non-sedating antihistaminics (terfenadine, astemizole), or cisapride [*see Clinical Pharmacology (12.5)*].
- receiving medications that are metabolized by the cytochrome enzyme CYP2D6 which also have cardiac effects (e.g., flecainide, imipramine, amitriptyline, clomipramine) [*see Warnings and Precautions (5.4), Drug Interactions (7.4) and Clinical Pharmacology (12.3)*].

5.2 Use of QT Prolonging Drugs and Other Antimalarials
Halofantrine and Coartem Tablets should not be administered within one month of each other due to the long elimination half-life of lumefantrine (3-6 days) and potential additive effects on the QT interval [*see Warnings and Precautions (5.1), and Clinical Pharmacology (12.3)*].

Antimalarials should not be given concomitantly with Coartem Tablets, unless there is no other treatment option, due to limited safety data.

Drugs that prolong the QT interval, including antimalarials such as quinine and quinidine, should be used cautiously following Coartem Tablets, due to the long elimination half-life of lumefantrine (3-6 days) and the potential for additive effects on the QT interval [*see Warnings and Precautions (5.1), Drug Interactions (7.5), and Clinical Pharmacology (12.3)*].

If mefloquine is administered immediately prior to Coartem Tablets there may be a decreased exposure to lumefantrine, possibly due to a mefloquine-induced decrease in bile production. Therefore, patients should be monitored for

Table 1: Adverse Reactions Occurring in 3% or More of Adult Patients Treated in Clinical Trials with the 6-dose Regimen of Coartem Tablets

System Organ Class	Preferred Term	Adults* N=647 (%)
Nervous system disorders	Headache	360 (56)
	Dizziness	253 (39)
Metabolism and nutrition disorders	Anorexia	260 (40)
General disorders and administration site conditions	Asthenia	243 (38)
	Pyrexia	159 (25)
	Chills	147 (23)
	Fatigue	111 (17)
	Malaise	20 (3)
Musculoskeletal and connective tissue disorders	Arthralgia	219 (34)
	Myalgia	206 (32)
Gastrointestinal disorders	Nausea	169 (26)
	Vomiting	113 (17)
	Abdominal pain	112 (17)
	Diarrhea	46 (7)
Psychiatric disorders	Sleep disorder	144 (22)
	Insomnia	32 (5)
Cardiac disorders	Palpitations	115 (18)
Hepatobiliary disorders	Hepatomegaly	59 (9)
Blood and lymphatic system disorders	Splenomegaly	57 (9)
	Anemia	23 (4)
Respiratory, thoracic and mediastinal disorders	Cough	37 (6)
Skin and subcutaneous tissue disorders	Pruritus	24 (4)
	Rash	21 (3)
Ear and labyrinth disorders	Vertigo	21 (3)
Infections and infestations	Malaria	18 (3)
	Nasopharyngitis	17 (3)

*Adult patients defined as >16 years of age

Table 2: Adverse Reactions Occurring in 3% or More of Pediatric Patients Treated in Clinical Trials with the 6-dose Regimen of Coartem Tablets

System Organ Class	Preferred Term	Children* N=1,332 (%)
General disorders and administration site conditions	Pyrexia	381 (29)
	Chills	72 (5)
	Asthenia	63 (5)
	Fatigue	46 (3)
Respiratory, thoracic and mediastinal disorders	Cough	302 (23)
Gastrointestinal disorders	Vomiting	242 (18)
	Abdominal pain	112 (8)
	Diarrhea	100 (8)
	Nausea	61 (5)
Infections and infestations	Plasmodium falciparum infection	224 (17)
	Rhinitis	51 (4)
Metabolism and nutrition disorders	Anorexia	175 (13)
Nervous system disorders	Headache	168 (13)
	Dizziness	56 (4)
Blood and lymphatic system disorders	Splenomegaly	124 (9)
	Anemia	115 (9)
Hepatobiliary disorders	Hepatomegaly	75 (6)
Investigations	Aspartate aminotransferase increased	51 (4)
Musculoskeletal and connective tissue disorders	Arthralgia	39 (3)
	Myalgia	39 (3)
Skin and subcutaneous tissue disorders	Rash	38 (3)

*Children defined as patients ≤16 years of age

decreased efficacy and food consumption should be encouraged while taking Coartem Tablets [see *Dosage and Administration (2.1)*, *Drug Interactions (7.2)*, and *Clinical Pharmacology (12.3)*].

5.3   Drug Interactions with CYP3A4
When Coartem Tablets are co-administered with substrates of CYP3A4 it may result in decreased concentrations of the substrate and potential loss of substrate efficacy. When

Coartem Tablets are co-administered with an inhibitor of CYP3A4, including grapefruit juice it may result in increased concentrations of artemether and/or lumefantrine and potentiate QT prolongation. When Coartem Tablets are co-administered with inducers of CYP3A4 it may result in decreased concentrations of artemether and/or lumefantrine and loss of anti-malarial efficacy [see *Drug Interactions (7.1)*].

Drugs that have a mixed effect on CYP3A4, especially Anti-Retroviral drugs, and those that have an effect on the QT interval should be used with caution in patients taking Coartem Tablets [see *Drug Interactions (7.3)*].
Coartem Tablets may reduce the effectiveness of hormonal contraceptives. Therefore, patients using oral, transdermal patch, or other systemic hormonal contraceptives should be advised to use an additional non-hormonal method of birth control [see *Drug Interactions (7.3)*].

5.4   Drug Interactions with CYP2D6
Administration of Coartem Tablets with drugs that are metabolized by CYP2D6 may significantly increase plasma concentrations of the co-administered drug and increase the risk of adverse effects. Many of the drugs metabolized by CYP2D6 can prolong the QT interval and should not be administered with Coartem Tablets due to the potential additive effect on the QT interval (e.g., flecainide, imipramine, amitriptyline, clomipramine) [see *Warnings and Precautions (5.1)*, *Drug Interactions (7.4)* and *Clinical Pharmacology (12.3)*].

5.5   Recrudescence
Food enhances absorption of artemether and lumefantrine following administration of Coartem Tablets. Patients who remain averse to food during treatment should be closely monitored as the risk of recrudescence may be greater [see *Dosage and Administration (2.1)*].
In the event of recrudescent *P. falciparum* infection after treatment with Coartem Tablets, patients should be treated with a different antimalarial drug.

5.6   Hepatic and Renal Impairment
Coartem Tablets have not been studied for efficacy and safety in patients with severe hepatic and/or renal impairment [see *Dosage and Administration (2.4)*].

5.7   *Plasmodium vivax* Infection
Coartem Tablets have been shown in limited data (43 patients) to be effective in treating the erythrocytic stage of *P. vivax* infection. However, relapsing malaria caused by *P. vivax* requires additional treatment with other antimalarial agents to achieve radical cure i.e., eradicate any hypnozoites forms that may remain dormant in the liver.

6   ADVERSE REACTIONS
6.1   Serious Adverse Reactions
The following serious and otherwise important adverse reactions are discussed in greater detail in other sections of labeling:
• Hypersensitivity Reactions [see *Contraindications (4.1)* and *Postmarketing Experience (6.3)*].

6.2   Clinical Studies Experience
Because clinical trials are conducted under widely varying conditions, adverse reaction rates observed in the clinical trials of a drug cannot be directly compared to rates in the clinical trials of another drug and may not reflect the rate observed in practice.
The data described below reflect exposure to a 6-dose regimen of Coartem Tablets in 1,979 patients including 647 adults (older than 16 years) and 1,332 children (16 years and younger). For the 6-dose regimen, Coartem Tablets was studied in active-controlled (366 patients) and non-controlled, open-label trials (1,613 patients). The 6-dose Coartem Tablets population was patients with malaria between ages 2 months and 71 years: 67% (1,332) were 16 years and younger and 33% (647) were older than 16 years. Males represented 73% and 53% of the adult and pediatric populations, respectively. The majority of adult patients were enrolled in studies in Thailand, while the majority of pediatric patients were enrolled in Africa.
Tables 1 and 2 show the most frequently reported adverse reactions (≥3%) in adults and children respectively who received the 6-dose regimen of Coartem Tablets. Adverse reactions collected in clinical trials included signs and symptoms at baseline but only treatment emergent adverse events, defined as events that appeared or worsened after the start of treatment, are presented below. In adults, the most frequently reported adverse reactions were headache, anorexia, dizziness, and asthenia. In children, the adverse reactions were pyrexia, cough, vomiting, anorexia, and headache. Most adverse reactions were mild, did not lead to discontinuation of study medication, and resolved.
In limited comparative studies, the adverse reaction profile of Coartem Tablets appeared similar to that of another antimalarial regimen.
Discontinuation of Coartem Tablets due to adverse drug reactions occurred in 1.1% of patients treated with the 6-dose regimen overall: 0.2% (1/647) in adults and 1.6% (21/1,332) in children.
[See table 1 above]
[See table 2 at left]
Clinically significant adverse reactions reported in adults and/or children treated with the 6-dose regimen of Coartem Tablets which occurred in clinical studies at <3% regardless of causality are listed below:
Blood and lymphatic system disorders: eosinophilia
Ear and labyrinth disorders: tinnitus

Eye disorders: conjunctivitis
Gastrointestinal disorders: constipation, dyspepsia, dysphagia, peptic ulcer
General disorders: gait disturbance
Infections and infestations: abscess, acrodermatitis, bronchitis, ear infection, gastroenteritis, helminthic infection, hookworm infection, impetigo, influenza, lower respiratory tract infection, malaria, nasopharyngitis, oral herpes, pneumonia, respiratory tract infection, subcutaneous abscess, upper respiratory tract infection, urinary tract infection
Investigations: alanine aminotransferase increased, aspartate aminotransferase increased hematocrit decreased, lymphocyte morphology abnormal, platelet count decreased, platelet count increased, white blood cell count decreased, white blood cell count increased
Metabolism and nutrition disorders: hypokalemia
Musculoskeletal and connective tissue disorders: back pain
Nervous system disorders: ataxia, clonus, fine motor delay, hyperreflexia, hypoaesthesia, nystagmus, tremor
Psychiatric disorders: agitation, mood swings
Renal and urinary disorders: hematuria, proteinuria
Respiratory, thoracic and mediastinal disorders: asthma, pharyngo-laryngeal pain
Skin and subcutaneous tissue disorders: urticaria

6.3 Postmarketing Experience

The following adverse reactions have been identified during post-approval use of Coartem Tablets. Because these events are reported voluntarily from a population of uncertain size, it is not always possible to reliably estimate their frequency or establish a causal relationship to drug exposure.

- Hypersensitivity including urticaria and angioedema. Serious skin reactions (bullous eruption) have been rarely reported.

7 DRUG INTERACTIONS

7.1 Ketoconazole

Concurrent oral administration of ketoconazole, a potent CYP3A4 inhibitor, with a single dose of Coartem Tablets resulted in a moderate increase in exposure to artemether, dihydroartemisinin (DHA, metabolite of artemether), and lumefantrine in a study of 15 healthy subjects. No dose adjustment of Coartem Tablets is necessary when administered with ketoconazole or other potent CYP3A4 inhibitors. However, due to the potential for increased concentrations of lumefantrine which could lead to QT prolongation, Coartem Tablets should be used cautiously with drugs that inhibit CYP3A4 [*see Warnings and Precautions (5.1, 5.3)*].

7.2 Prior Use of Mefloquine

Administration of three doses of mefloquine followed 12 hours later by a 6-dose regimen of Coartem Tablets in 14 healthy volunteers demonstrated no effect of mefloquine on plasma concentrations of artemether or the artemether/DHA ratio. However, exposure to lumefantrine was reduced, possibly due to lower absorption secondary to a mefloquine-induced decrease in bile production. Patients should be monitored for decreased efficacy and food consumption should be encouraged with administration of Coartem Tablets [*see Warnings and Precautions (5.2)* and *Clinical Pharmacology (12.3)*].

7.3 CYP3A4 Metabolism: Hormonal Contraceptives and Anti-Retroviral Drugs

Artemether induces CYP3A4 and both artemether and lumefantrine are metabolized primarily by CYP3A4.
Coartem Tablets may reduce the effectiveness of hormonal contraceptives. Therefore, patients using oral, transdermal patch, or other systemic hormonal contraceptives should be advised to use an additional non-hormonal method of birth control [*see Warnings and Precautions (5.3)* and *Clinical Pharmacology (12.3)*].
Anti-Retroviral drugs (ARTs), such as protease inhibitors and non-nucleoside reverse transcriptase inhibitors, are known to have variable patterns of inhibition, induction or competition for CYP3A4. No formal drug-drug interaction studies between Coartem Tablets and ARTs have been performed. However, Coartem Tablets should be used cautiously in patients on ARTs as the result may be an increase in lumefantrine concentrations causing QT prolongation or a decrease in concentrations of the ART resulting in loss of efficacy, or a decrease in artemether and/or lumefantrine concentrations resulting in loss of antimalarial efficacy of Coartem Tablets [*see Warnings and Precautions (5.3)* and *Clinical Pharmacology (12.3)*].

7.4 CYP2D6 Substrates

Lumefantrine inhibits CYP2D6 *in vitro*. Administration of Coartem Tablets with drugs that are metabolized by CYP2D6 may significantly increase plasma concentrations of the co-administered drug and increase the risk of adverse effects. Many of the drugs metabolized by CYP2D6 can *prolong the QT interval and should not be administered with* Coartem Tablets due to the potential additive effect on the QT interval (e.g., flecainide, imipramine, amitriptyline, clomipramine) [*see Warnings and Precautions (5.1, 5.4)* and *Clinical Pharmacology (12.3)*].

7.5 Sequential Use of Quinine

A single dose of intravenous quinine (10 mg/kg bodyweight) concurrent with the final dose of a 6-dose regimen of Coartem Tablets demonstrated no effect of intravenous quinine on the systemic exposure of DHA or lumefantrine. Quinine exposure was also not altered. Exposure to artemether was decreased. This decrease in artemether exposure is not thought to be clinically significant. However, quinine and other drugs that prolong the QT interval should be used cautiously following treatment with Coartem Tablets due to the long elimination half life of lumefantrine and the potential for additive QT effects. [*see Warnings and Precautions (5.2)* and *Clinical Pharmacology (12.3)*].

8 USE IN SPECIFIC POPULATIONS

8.1 Pregnancy

Pregnancy Category C
Safety data from an observational pregnancy study of approximately 500 pregnant women who were exposed to Coartem Tablets (including a third of patients who were exposed in the first trimester), and published data of over 1,000 pregnant patients who were exposed to artemisinin derivatives, did not show an increase in adverse pregnancy outcomes or teratogenic effects over background rate.
The efficacy of Coartem Tablets in the treatment of acute, uncomplicated malaria in pregnant women has not been established.
Coartem Tablets should be used during pregnancy only if the potential benefit justifies the potential risk to the fetus. Pregnant rats dosed during the period of organogenesis at or higher than a dose of about half the highest clinical dose of 1120 mg artemether-lumefantrine per day (based on body surface area comparisons), showed increases in fetal loss, early resorptions and post implantation loss. No adverse effects were observed in animals dosed at about one-third the highest clinical dose. Similarly, dosing in pregnant rabbits at about three times the clinical dose (based on body surface area comparisons) resulted in abortions, preimplantation loss, post implantation loss and decreases in the number of live fetuses. No adverse reproductive effects were detected in rabbits at two times the clinical dose. Embryo-fetal loss is a significant reproductive toxicity. Other artemisinins are known to be embryotoxic in animals. However, because metabolic profiles in animals and humans are dissimilar, artemether exposures in animals may not be predictive of human exposures [*see Nonclinical Toxicology (13.2)*]. These data cannot rule out an increased risk for early pregnancy loss or fetal defects in humans.

8.3 Nursing Mothers

It is not known whether artemether or lumefantrine is excreted in human milk. Because many drugs are excreted in human milk, caution should be exercised when Coartem Tablets are administered to a nursing woman. Animal data suggest both artemether and lumefantrine are excreted into breast milk. The benefits of breastfeeding to mother and infant should be weighed against potential risk from infant exposure to artemether and lumefantrine through breast milk.

8.4 Pediatric Use

The safety and effectiveness of Coartem Tablets have been established for the treatment of acute, uncomplicated malaria in studies involving pediatric patients weighing 5 kg or more [*see Clinical Studies (14.1)*]. The safety and efficacy have not been established in pediatric patients who weigh less than 5 kg. Children from non-endemic countries were not included in clinical trials.

8.5 Geriatric Use

Clinical studies of Coartem Tablets did not include sufficient numbers of subjects aged 65 years and over to determine they respond differently from younger subjects. In general, the greater frequency of decreased hepatic, renal, or cardiac function, and of concomitant disease or other drug therapy in elderly patients should be considered when prescribing Coartem Tablets.

8.6 Hepatic and Renal Impairment

No specific pharmacokinetic studies have been performed in patients with either hepatic or renal impairment. Coartem Tablets have not been studied for efficacy and safety in patients with severe hepatic and/or renal impairment. Based on the pharmacokinetic data in 16 healthy subjects showing no or insignificant renal excretion of lumefantrine, artemether and DHA, no dose adjustment for the use of Coartem in patients with renal impairment is advised. No dosage adjustment is necessary in patients with mild to moderate hepatic impairment. [*see Dosage and Administration (2.4)* and *Warnings and Precautions (5.6)*].

10 OVERDOSAGE

There is no information on overdoses of Coartem Tablets higher than the doses recommended for treatment.
In cases of suspected overdosage, symptomatic and supportive therapy, which would include ECG and blood electrolyte monitoring, should be given as appropriate.

11 DESCRIPTION

Coartem Tablets contain a fixed combination of two antimalarial active ingredients, artemether, an artemisinin derivative, and lumefantrine. Both components are blood schizontocides. The chemical name of artemether is (3R,5aS,6R,8aS,9R,10S,12R,12aR)-decahydro-10-methoxy-3,6,9-trimethyl-3,12-epoxy-12H-pyrano[4,3-j]-1,2-benzodioxepine. Artemether is a white, crystalline powder that is freely soluble in acetone, soluble in methanol and ethanol, and practically insoluble in water. It has the empirical formula $C_{16}H_{26}O_5$ with a molecular weight of 298.4, and the following structural formula:

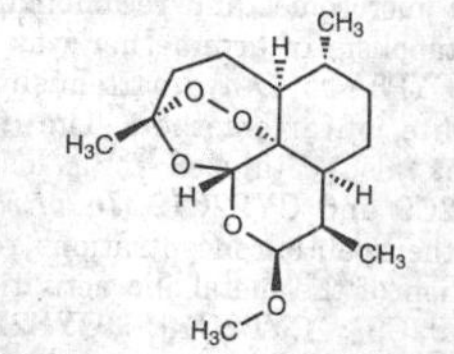

The chemical name of lumefantrine is (±)-2-dibutylamino-1-[2,7-dichloro-9-(4-chlorobenzylidene)-9H-fluorene-4-yl]-ethanol. Lumefantrine is a yellow, crystalline powder that is freely soluble in N,N-dimethylformamide, chloroform, and ethyl acetate; soluble in dichloromethane; slightly soluble in ethanol and methanol; and insoluble in water. It has the empirical formula $C_{30}H_{32}Cl_3NO$ with a molecular weight of 528.9, and the following structural formula:

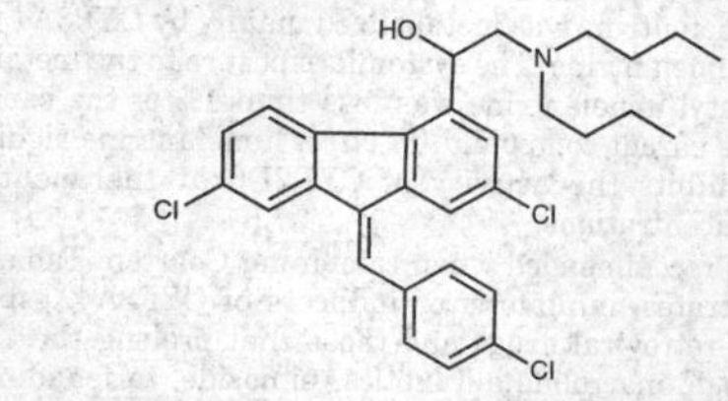

Coartem Tablets are for oral administration. Each Coartem Tablet contains 20 mg of artemether and 120 mg lumefantrine. The inactive ingredients are colloidal silicon dioxide, croscarmellose sodium, hypromellose, magnesium stearate, microcrystalline cellulose, and polysorbate 80.

12 CLINICAL PHARMACOLOGY

12.1 Mechanism of Action

Coartem Tablets, a fixed dose combination of artemether and lumefantrine in the ratio of 1:6, is an antimalarial agent [*see Clinical Pharmacology (12.4)*].

12.3 Pharmacokinetics

Absorption

Following administration of Coartem Tablets to healthy volunteers and patients with malaria, artemether is absorbed with peak plasma concentrations reached about 2 hours after dosing. Absorption of lumefantrine, a highly lipophilic compound, starts after a lag-time of up to 2 hours, with peak plasma concentrations about 6 to 8 hours after administration. The single dose (4 tablets) pharmacokinetic parameters for artemether, dihydroartemisinin (DHA), an active antimalarial metabolite of artemether, and lumefantrine in adult Caucasian healthy volunteers are given in Table 3. Multiple dose data after the 6-dose regimen of Coartem Tablets in adult malaria patients are given in Table 4.

Table 3: Single Dose Pharmacokinetic Parameters[a] for Artemether, Dihydroartemisinin (DHA), and Lumefantrine under Fed Conditions

	Study 2102 (n=50)	Study 2104 (n=48)
Artemether		
C_{max} (ng/mL)	60.0 ± 32.5	83.8 ± 59.7
t_{max} (h)	1.50	2.00
AUC_{last} (ng•h/mL)	146 ± 72.2	259 ± 150
$t_{1/2}$ (h)	1.6 ± 0.7	2.2 ± 1.9
DHA		
C_{max} (ng/mL)	104 ± 35.3	90.4 ± 48.9
t_{max} (h)	1.76	2.00
AUC_{last} (ng•h/mL)	284 ± 83.8	285 ± 98.0
$t_{1/2}$ (h)	1.6 ± 0.6	2.2 ± 1.5
Lumefantrine		
C_{max} (µg/mL)	7.38 ± 3.19	9.80 ± 4.20
t_{max} (h)	6.01	8.00
AUC_{last} (µg•h/mL)	158 ± 70.1	243 ± 117
$t_{1/2}$ (h)	101 ± 35.6	119 ± 51.0

[a] Mean ± SD C_{max}, AUC_{last}, $t_{1/2}$ and Median t_{max}

Food enhances the absorption of both artemether and lumefantrine. In healthy volunteers, the relative bioavailability of artemether was increased between two- to three-fold, and that of lumefantrine sixteen-fold when Coartem Tablets were taken after a high-fat meal compared under fasted conditions. . Patients should be encouraged to take Coartem Tablets with a meal as soon as food can be tolerated [*see Dosage and Administration (2.1)*].

Distribution

Artemether and lumefantrine are both highly bound to human serum proteins *in vitro* (95.4% and 99.7%, respectively). Dihydroartemisinin is also bound to human serum proteins (47% to 76%). Protein binding to human plasma proteins is linear.

Biotransformation

In human liver microsomes and recombinant CYP450 enzymes, the metabolism of artemether was catalyzed predominantly by CYP3A4/5. Dihydroartemisinin (DHA) is an active metabolite of artemether. The metabolism of artemether was also catalyzed to a lesser extent by CYP2B6, CYP2C9 and CYP2C19. *In vitro* studies with artemether at therapeutic concentrations revealed no significant inhibition of the metabolic activities of CYP1A2, CYP2A6, CYP2C9, CYP2C19, CYP2D6, CYP2E1, CYP3A4/5, and CYP4A9/11.

During repeated administration of Coartem Tablets, systemic exposure of artemether decreased significantly, while concentrations of DHA increased, although not to a statistically significant degree. The artemether/DHA AUC ratio is 1.2 after a single dose and 0.3 after 6 doses given over 3 days. This suggests that there was induction of CYP3A4/5 responsible for the metabolism of artemether.

In human liver microsomes and in recombinant CYP450 enzymes, lumefantrine was metabolized mainly by CYP3A4 to desbutyl-lumefantrine. The systemic exposure to the metabolite desbutyl-lumefantrine was less than 1% of the exposure to the parent compound. *In vitro*, lumefantrine significantly inhibits the activity of CYP2D6 at therapeutic plasma concentrations.

Caution is recommended when combining Coartem Tablets with substrates, inhibitors, or inducers of CYP3A4, especially anti-retroviral drugs and those that prolong the QT interval (e.g., macrolide antibiotics, pimozide, terfenadine, astemizole, cisapride) [*see Warnings and Precautions (5.1, 5.3)*].

Co-administration of Coartem Tablets with CYP2D6 substrates may result in increased plasma concentrations of the CYP2D6 substrate and increase the risk of adverse reactions. In addition, many of the drugs metabolized by CYP2D6 can prolong the QT interval and should not be administered with Coartem Tablets due to the potential additive effect on the QT interval (e.g., flecainide, imipramine, amitriptyline, clomipramine) [*see Warnings and Precautions (5.1, 5.4)*].

Elimination

Artemether and DHA are cleared from plasma with an elimination half-life of about 2 hours. Lumefantrine is eliminated more slowly, with a terminal half-life of 3-6 days in healthy volunteers and in patients with *falciparum* malaria. Demographic characteristics such as sex and weight appear to have no clinically relevant effects on the pharmacokinetics of artemether and lumefantrine.

In 16 healthy volunteers, neither lumefantrine nor artemether was found in the urine after administration of Coartem, and urinary excretion of DHA amounted to less than 0.01% of the artemether dose.

Hepatic and Renal Impairment

No specific pharmacokinetic studies have been performed in patients with either hepatic or renal impairment. There is no significant renal excretion of lumefantrine, artemether and DHA in healthy volunteers and while clinical experience in this population is limited, no dose adjustment in renal impairment is recommended [*see Dosage and Administration (2.4)*].

Pediatric Patients

The PK of artemether, DHA, and lumefantrine were obtained in two pediatric studies by sparse sampling using a population based approach. PK estimates derived from a composite plasma concentration profile for artemether, DHA, and lumefantrine are provided in Table 4.

Systemic exposure to artemether, DHA, and lumefantrine, when dosed on a mg/kg body weight basis in pediatric patients (≥5 to <35 kg body weight), is comparable to that of the recommended dosing regimen in adult patients. [See table 4 below]

Geriatric Patients

No specific pharmacokinetic studies have been performed in patients older than 65 years of age.

Drug Interactions

Ketoconazole (potent CYP3A4 inhibitor)

Concurrent oral administration of ketoconazole (400 mg on Day 1 followed by 200 mg on days 2, 3, 4 and 5) with Coartem Tablets (single dose of 4 tablets of 20 mg artemether/120 mg lumefantrine per tablet) with a meal led to an increase in exposure, in terms of area under the curve (AUC), of artemether (2.3-fold), DHA (1.5-fold), and lumefantrine (1.6-fold) in 13 healthy subjects. The pharmacokinetics of ketoconazole were not evaluated. Based on this study, dose adjustment of Coartem Tablets is considered unnecessary when administered with ketoconazole or other CYP3A4 inhibitors. However, due to the potential for increased concentrations of lumefantrine which could lead to QT prolongation, Coartem Tablets should be used cautiously with other drugs that inhibit CYP3A4 (e.g., anti-retroviral drugs, macrolide antibiotics, antidepressants, imidazole antifungal agents) [*see Warnings and Precautions (5.1, 5.3)*].

Antimalarials

The oral administration of mefloquine in 14 healthy volunteers administered as three doses of 500 mg, 250 mg and 250 mg, followed 12 hours later by Coartem Tablets (6 doses of 4 tablets of 20 mg artemether/120 mg lumefantrine per tablet), had no effect on plasma concentrations of artemether or the artemether/DHA ratio. In the same study, there was a 30% reduction in C_{max} and 40% reduction in AUC of lumefantrine, possibly due to lower absorption secondary to a mefloquine-induced decrease in bile production.

Intravenous administration of a single dose of quinine (10 mg/kg bodyweight) concurrent with the last dose of a 6-dose regimen of Coartem Tablets had no effect on systemic exposure of DHA, lumefantrine or quinine in 14 healthy volunteers. Mean AUC of artemether were 46% lower when administered with quinine compared to Coartem Tablets alone. This decrease in artemether exposure is not thought to be clinically significant. However, quinine should be used cautiously in patients following treatment with Coartem Tablets due to the long elimination half-life of lumefantrine and the potential for additive effects on the QT interval [*see Warnings and Precautions (5.2)*].

Anti-Retroviral Drugs

No formal drug-drug interaction studies between Coartem Tablets and Anti-Retroviral drugs (ARTs), such as protease inhibitors, non-nucleoside reverse transcriptase inhibitors, have been performed. Due to variable patterns of inhibition, induction or competition for CYP3A4 with anti-retroviral drugs, Coartem Tablets should be used cautiously in patients on ARTs as the result may be an increase in lumefantrine concentrations causing QT prolongation, a decrease in concentrations of the ART resulting in loss of efficacy, or a decrease in artemether and/or lumefantrine concentrations resulting in loss of antimalarial efficacy of Coartem Tablets [*see Warnings and Precautions (5.3)*].

Hormonal Contraceptives

No formal drug-drug interaction studies between Coartem Tablets and hormonal contraceptives have been performed. However, artemether may induce CYP3A4/5, reducing the effectiveness of hormonal contraceptives [*see Warnings and Precautions (5.3)*].

12.4   Microbiology

Mechanism of Action

Coartem Tablets, a fixed ratio of 1:6 parts of artemether and lumefantrine, respectively, is an antimalarial agent.

Artemether is rapidly metabolized into an active metabolite dihydroartemisinin (DHA). The anti-malarial activity of artemether and DHA has been attributed to endoperoxide moiety. The exact mechanism by which lumefantrine exerts its anti-malarial effect is not well defined. Available data suggest lumefantrine inhibits the formation of β-hematin by forming a complex with hemin. Both artemether and lumefantrine were shown to inhibit nucleic acid and protein synthesis.

Activity In Vitro and In Vivo

Artemether and lumefantrine are active against the erythrocytic stages of *Plasmodium falciparum*.

Drug Resistance

Strains of *P. falciparum* with a moderate decrease in susceptibility to artemether or lumefantrine alone can be selected *in vitro* or *in vivo*, but not maintained in the case of artemether. The clinical relevance of such an effect is not known.

12.5   Effects on the Electrocardiogram

In a healthy adult volunteer parallel group study including a placebo and moxifloxacin control group (n=42 per group), the administration of the 6-dose regimen of Coartem Tablets was associated with prolongation of QTcF (Fridericia). Following administration of a 6-dose regimen of Coartem Tablets consisting of 4 tablets per dose (total of 4 tablets of 80 mg artemether/480 mg lumefantrine) taken with food, the maximum mean change from baseline and placebo adjusted QTcF was 7.5 msec (1-sided 95% Upper CI: 11 msec). There was a concentration-dependent increase in QTcF for lumefantrine.

In clinical trials conducted in children, no patient had QTcF >500 msec. Over 5% of patients had an increase in QTcF of over 60 msec.

In clinical trials conducted in adults, QTcF prolongation of >500 msec was reported in 3 (0.3%) of patients. Over 6% of adults had a QTcF increase of over 60 msec from baseline.

13   NONCLINICAL TOXICOLOGY

13.1   Carcinogenesis, Mutagenesis, Impairment of Fertility

Carcinogenesis

Carcinogenicity studies were not conducted.

Mutagenesis

No evidence of mutagenicity was detected. The artemether:lumefantrine combination was evaluated using the *Salmonella* and *Escherichia*/mammalian-microsome mutagenicity test, the gene mutation test with Chinese hamster cells V79, the cytogenetic test on Chinese hamster cells *in vitro*, and the rat micronucleus test, *in vivo*.

Impairment of Fertility

Pregnancy rates were reduced by about one half in female rats dosed for 2 to 4 weeks with the artemether-lumefantrine combination at 1000 mg/kg (about 9 times the clinical dose based on body surface area comparisons). Male rats dosed for 70 days showed increases in abnormal sperm (87% abnormal) and increased testes weights at 30 mg/kg doses (about one third the clinical dose). Higher doses (about 9 times the clinical dose) resulted in decreased sperm motility and 100% abnormal sperm cells.

13.2   Animal Toxicology and/or Pharmacology

Reproductive Toxicity

Pregnant rats dosed during the period of organogenesis, at or higher than 60 mg/kg/day with the artemether-lumefantrine combination (a dose about half the highest clinical dose based on body surface area comparisons), showed increases in the number of dead fetuses, early resorptions and post implantation losses. No adverse effects were observed in animals dosed at 40 mg/kg (about one third the clinical dose). Similarly, dosing in pregnant rabbits at 175 mg/kg/day (about three times the highest clinical dose based on body surface area comparisons) resulted in abortions, preimplantation losses, post implantation losses, and decreases in the number of live fetuses. No adverse reproductive effects were detected in rabbits at 105 mg/kg/day, about two times the clinical dose based on body surface area comparisons.

Other artemisinins are known to be embryotoxic in animals. Reproductive toxicity studies with artemisinin derivatives (e.g, artesunate) demonstrated increased post-implantation loss and teratogenicity (a low incidence of cardiovascular and skeletal malformations) in rats and rabbits. Similar findings were not seen in animal reproductive studies using artemether.

Neurotoxicity

Studies in dogs and rats have shown that intramuscular injections of artemether resulted in brain lesions. Changes observed mainly in brainstem nuclei included chromatolysis, eosinophilic cytoplasmic granulation, spheroids, apoptosis, and dark neurons. Lesions were observed in rats dosed with artemether at 25 mg/kg for 7 or 14 days and dogs dosed at 20 mg/kg for 8 days or longer, but lesions were not observed after shorter courses of drug or after oral dosing. The estimated artemether 24 h AUC after 7 days of dosing at the no observed effect level (10 mg/kg/day given intramuscularly)

Table 4: Summary of Pharmacokinetic Parameters for Lumefantrine, Artemether and DHA in Pediatric and Adult Patients with Malaria Following Administration of a 6-dose Regimen of Coartem Tablets

Drug	Adults[1]	Pediatric patients (body weight, kg)[2]		
		5-<15	15-<25	25-<35
Lumefantrine				
Mean C_{max}, range (μg/mL)	5.60-9.0	4.71-12.6		Not Available
Mean AUC_{last}, range (μg•h/mL)	410-561	372-699		Not Available
Artemether				
Mean C_{max} ± SD (ng/mL)	186 ± 125	223 ± 309	198 ± 179	174 ± 145
Dihydroartemisinin				
Mean C_{max} ± SD (ng/mL)	101 ± 58	54.7 ± 58.9	79.8 ± 80.5	65.3 ± 23.6

[1] There are a total of 181 adults for lumefantrine pharmacokinetic parameters and a total of 25 adults for artemether and dihydroarthemisin pharmacokinetic parameters.

[2] There are 477 children for the lumefantrine pharmacokinetic parameters; for artemether and dihydroartemisinin pharmacokinetic parameters there are 55, 29, and 8 children for the 5 to <15, 15 to <25 and the 25 to <35 kg groups, respectively.

is approximately 7-fold greater than the estimated artemether 24 h AUC in humans on day 1 of the standard 3-day oral treatment regimen; oral exposure in humans decreases on subsequent days, thus the exposure margin increases. Dogs dosed orally with 143 mg/kg artemether showed a statistically measureable effect on the hearing threshold at 20 dB. This dose is equivalent to about 29 times the highest artemether clinical dose (160 mg/day) based on body surface area comparisons. Most nervous system disorder adverse events in the studies of the 6-dose regimen were mild in intensity and resolved by the end of the study [see Adverse Reactions (6.2)].

14 CLINICAL STUDIES

14.1 Treatment of Acute, Uncomplicated *P. falciparum* Malaria

The efficacy of Coartem Tablets was evaluated for the treatment of acute, uncomplicated malaria caused by *P. falciparum* in HIV negative patients in 8 clinical studies. Uncomplicated malaria was defined as symptomatic *P. falciparum* malaria without signs and symptoms of severe malaria or evidence of vital organ dysfunction. Baseline parasite density ranged from 500/µL-200,000/µL (0.01% to 4% parasitemia) in the majority of patients. Studies were conducted in partially immune and non-immune adults and children (≥5kg body weight) with uncomplicated malaria in China, Thailand, sub-Saharan Africa, Europe, and South America. Patients who had clinical features of severe malaria, severe cardiac, renal, or hepatic impairment were excluded.

The studies include two 4-dose studies assessing the efficacy of the components of the regimen, a study comparing a 4-dose versus a 6-dose regimen, and 5 additional 6-dose regimen studies.

Coartem Tablets were administered at 0, 8, 24, and 48 hours in the 4-dose regimen, and at 0, 8, 24, 36, 48, and 60 hours in the 6-dose regimen. Efficacy endpoints consisted of:

- 28 day cure rate, defined as clearance of asexual parasites (the erythrocytic stage) within 7 days without recrudescence by day 28
- parasite clearance time (PCT), defined as time from first dose until first total and continued disappearance of asexual parasite which continues for a further 48 hours
- fever clearance time (FCT), defined as time from first dose until the first time body temperature fell below 37.5°C and remained below 37.5°C for at least a further 48 hours (only for patients with temperature >37.5°C at baseline)

The modified intent to treat (mITT) population includes all patients with malaria diagnosis confirmation who received at least one dose of study drug. Evaluable patients generally are all patients who had a day 7 and a day 28 parasitological assessment or experienced treatment failure by day 28.

Studies 1 and 2: The two studies which assessed the efficacy of Coartem Tablets (4 doses of 4 tablets of 20 mg artemether/120 mg lumefantrine) compared to each component alone were randomized, double-blind, comparative, single center, conducted in China. The efficacy results (Table 5) support that the combination of artemether and lumefantrine in Coartem Tablets had a significantly higher 28-day cure rate compared to artemether and had a significantly faster parasite clearance time (PCT) and fever clearance time (FCT) compared to lumefantrine.
[See table 5 above]

Results of 4-dose studies conducted in areas with high resistance such as Thailand during 1995-96 showed lower efficacy results than the above studies. Therefore, Study 3 was conducted.

Study 3: Study 3 was a randomized, double-blind, two-center study conducted in Thailand in adults and children (aged ≥2 years), which compared the 4-dose regimen (administered over 48 hours) of Coartem Tablets to a 6-dose regimen (administered over 60 hours). Twenty-eight day cure rate in mITT subjects was 81% (96/118) for the Coartem Tablets 6-dose arm as compared to 71% (85/120) in the 4-dose arm.

Studies 4, 5, 6, 7, and 8: In these studies, Coartem Tablets were administered as the 6-dose regimen.

In study 4, a total of 150 adults and children aged ≥2 years received Coartem Tablets. In study 5, a total 164 adults and children ≥12 years received Coartem Tablets. Both studies were conducted in Thailand.

Study 6 was a study of 165 non-immune adults residing in regions non-endemic for malaria (Europe and Colombia) who contracted acute uncomplicated *falciparum* malaria when traveling in endemic regions.

Study 7 was conducted in Africa in 310 infants and children aged 2 months to 9 years, weighing 5 kg to 25 kg, with an axillary temperature ≥37.5°C.

Study 8 was conducted in Africa in 452 infants and children, aged 3 months to 12 years, weighing 5 kg to <35 kg, with fever (≥37.5°C axillary or ≥38°C rectally) or history of fever in the preceding 24 hours.

Table 5: Clinical Efficacy of Coartem Tablets versus Components (mITT Population)[1]

Study No. Region/patient ages	28-day cure rate[2] n/N (%) patients	Median FCT[3] [25th, 75th percentile]	Median PCT [25th, 75th percentile]
Study 1 China, ages 13-57 years			
Coartem Tablets	50/51 (98.0)	24 hours [9, 48]	30 hours [24, 36]
Artemether[4]	24/52 (46.2)	21 hours [12, 30]	30 hours [24, 33]
Lumefantrine[5]	47/52 (90.4)	60 hours [36, 78]	54 hours [45, 66]
Study 2 China, ages 12-65 years			
Coartem Tablets	50/52 (96.2)	21 hours [6, 33]	30 hours [24, 36]
Lumefantrine[6]	45/51 (88.2)	36 hours [12, 60]	48 hours [42, 60]

[1] In mITT analysis, patients whose status was uncertain were classified as treatment failures.
[2] Efficacy cure rate based on blood smear microscopy.
[3] For patients who had a body temperature >37.5°C at baseline only
[4] 95% CI (Coartem Tablets – artemether) on 28-day cure rate: 37.8%, 66.0%
[5] P-value comparing Coartem Tablets to lumefantrine on parasite clearance time (PCT) and fever clearance time (FCT): <0.001
[6] P-value comparing Coartem Tablets to lumefantrine on parasite clearance time (PCT): <0.001 and on fever clearance time (FCT): <0.05

Table 6: Clinical Efficacy of 6-dose Regimen of Coartem Tablets

Study No. Region/ages	28-day cure rate[1] n/N (%) patients		Median FCT[2] [25th, 75th percentile]	Median PCT [25th, 75th percentile]
	mITT[3]	Evaluable		
Study 3 Thailand, ages 3-62 years	96/118 (81.4)	93/96 (96.9)	35 hours [20, 46]	44 hours [22, 47]
Early failure[4]	0	0		
Late failure[5]	4 (3.4)	3 (3.1)		
Lost to follow up	18 (15.3)			
Other[6]	0			
Study 4 Thailand, ages 2-63 years	130/149 (87.2)	130/134 (97.0)	22 hours [19, 44]	NA
Early failure[4]	0	0		
Late failure[5]	4 (2.7)	4 (3.0)		
Lost to follow up	13 (8.7)			
Other[6]	2 (1.3)			
Study 5 Thailand, ages 12-71 years	148/164 (90.2)	148/155 (95.5)	29 hours [8, 51]	29 hours [18, 40]
Early failure[4]	0	0		
Late failure[5]	7 (4.3)	7 (4.5)		
Lost to follow up	9 (5.5)			
Other[6]	0			
Study 6 Europe/Columbia, ages 16-66 years	120/162 (74.1)	119/124 (96.0)	37 hours [18, 44]	42 hours [34, 63]
Early failure[4]	6 (3.7)	1 (0.8)		
Late failure[5]	3 (1.9)	3 (2.4)		
Lost to follow up	17 (10.5)			
Other[6]	16 (9.9)	1 (0.8)		
Study 7 Africa, ages 2 months-9 years	268/310 (86.5)	267/300 (89.0)	8 hours [8, 24]	24 hours [24, 36]
Early failure[4]	2 (0.6)	0		
Late failure[5]	34 (11.0)	33 (11.0)		
Lost to follow up	2 (0.6)			
Other[6]	4 (1.3)			
Study 8 Africa, ages 3 months-12 years	374/452 (82.7)	370/419 (88.3)	8 hours [8, 23]	35 hours [24, 36]
Early failure[4]	13 (2.9)	0		
Late failure[5]	49 (10.8)	49 (11.7)		
Lost to follow up	6 (1.3)			
Other[6]	10 (2.2)			

[1] Efficacy cure rate based on blood smear microscopy
[2] For patients who had a body temperature >37.5°C at baseline only
[3] In mITT analysis, patients whose status was uncertain were classified as treatment failures.
[4] Early failures were usually defined as patients withdrawn for unsatisfactory therapeutic effect within the first 7 days or because they received another antimalarial medication within the first 7 days
[5] Late failures were defined as patients achieving parasite clearance within 7 days but having parasite reappearance including recrudescence or new infection during the 28 day follow-up period
[6] Other includes withdrawn due to protocol violation or non-compliance, received additional medication after day 7, withdrew consent, missing day 7 or 28 assessment

Results of 28-day cure rate, median parasite clearance time (PCT), and fever clearance time (FCT) for Studies 3 to 8 are reported in Table 6.
[See table 6 above]

In all studies, patients' signs and symptoms of malaria resolved when parasites were cleared.

In studies conducted in areas with high transmission rates, such as Africa, reappearance of *P. falciparum* parasites may be due to recrudescence or a new infection.

The efficacy by body weight category for studies 7 and 8 is summarized in Table 7.
[See table 7 at top of next page]

The efficacy of Coartem Tablets for the treatment *P. falciparum* infections mixed with *P. vivax* was assessed in a small number of patients. Coartem Tablets are only active against the erythrocytic phase of *P. vivax* malaria. Of the 43 patients with mixed infections at baseline, all cleared their parasitemia within 48 hours. However, parasite relapse

Table 7: Clinical Efficacy by Weight for Pediatric Studies
Coartem Tablets 6-dose Regimen

Study No. Age category	mITT population[1]		Evaluable population
	Median PCT [25th,75th percentile]	28-day cure rate[2] n/N (%) patients	28-day cure rate[2] n/N (%) patients
Study 7			
5-<10 kg	24 [24, 36]	133/154 (86.4)	133/149 (89.3)
10-<15 kg	35 [24, 36]	94/110 (85.5)	94/107 (87.9)
15-25 kg	24 [24, 36]	41/46 (89.1)	40/44 (90.9)
Study 8[3]			
5-<10 kg	36 [24, 36]	61/83 (73.5)	61/69 (88.4)
10-<15 kg	35 [24, 36]	160/190 (84.2)	157/179 (87.7)
15-<25 kg	35 [24, 36]	123/145 (84.8)	123/140 (87.9)
25-<35 kg	26 [24, 36]	30/34 (88.2)	29/31 (93.5)

[1] In mITT analysis, patients whose status was uncertain were classified as treatment failures.
[2] Efficacy cure rate based on blood smear microscopy
[3] Coartem Tablets administered as crushed tablets

occurred commonly (14/43; 33%). Relapsing malaria caused by *P. vivax* requires additional treatment with other anti-malarial agents to achieve radical cure i.e., eradicate any hypnozoite forms that may remain dormant in the liver.

16   HOW SUPPLIED/STORAGE AND HANDLING

Coartem (artemether/lumefantrine) Tablets
20 mg/120 mg Tablets-yellow, round flat tablets with beveled edges and scored on one side. Tablets are imprinted with N/C on one side and CG on the other.
Bottle of 24   NDC 0078-0568-45
Store at 25°C (77°F); excursions permitted to 15-30°C (59-86°F) [*see USP Controlled Room Temperature*].
Dispense in tight container (USP).

17   PATIENT COUNSELING INFORMATION

See FDA-Approved Patient Labeling.
17.1   Information for Safe Use
- Instruct patients to take Coartem Tablets with food. Patients who do not have an adequate intake of food are at risk for recrudescence of malaria.
- Patients hypersensitive to artemether, lumefantrine, or to any of the excipients should not receive Coartem Tablets.
- Instruct patients to inform their physician of any personal or family history of QT prolongation or proarrhythmic conditions such as hypokalemia, bradycardia, or recent myocardial ischemia.
- Instruct patients to inform their physician if they are taking any other medications that prolong the QT interval, such as class IA (quinidine, procainamide, disopyramide), or class III (amiodarone, sotalol) antiarrhythmic agents; antipsychotics (pimozide, ziprasidone); antidepressants; certain antibiotics (macrolide antibiotics, fluoroquinolone antibiotics, imidazole, and triazole antifungal agents); certain non-sedating antihistamines (terfenadine, astemizole), or cisapride.
- Instruct patients to notify their physicians if they have any symptoms of prolongation of the QT interval, including prolonged heart palpitations or a loss of consciousness.
- Instruct patients to avoid medications that are metabolized by the cytochrome enzyme CYP2D6 while receiving Coartem Tablets since these drugs also have cardiac effects (e.g., flecainide, imipramine, amitriptyline, clomipramine).
- Inform patients that based on animal data, Coartem Tablets administered during pregnancy may result in fetal loss. Fetal defects have been reported when artemisinins are administered to animals.
- Halofantrine and Coartem Tablets should not be administered within one month of each other due to potential additive effects on the QT interval.
- Antimalarials should not be given concomitantly with Coartem Tablets, unless there is no other treatment option, due to limited safety data.
- QT prolonging drugs, including quinine and quinidine, should be used cautiously following Coartem Tablets due to the long elimination half-life of lumefantrine and the potential for additive effects on the QT interval.
- Closely monitor food intake in patients who received mefloquine immediately prior to treatment with Coartem Tablets.
- Use Coartem Tablets cautiously in patients receiving other drugs that are substrates, inhibitors or inducers of CYP3A4, including grapefruit juice, especially those that prolong the QT interval or are anti-retroviral drugs.
- Coartem Tablets may reduce the effectiveness of hormonal contraceptives. Therefore, patients using oral, transdermal patch, or other systemic hormonal contraceptives should be advised to use an additional non-hormonal method of birth control.
- Inform patients that Coartem Tablets can cause hypersensitivity reactions. Instruct patients to discontinue the drug at the first sign of a skin rash, hives or other skin reactions, a rapid heartbeat, difficulty in swallowing or breathing, any swelling suggesting angioedema (e.g., swelling of the lips, tongue, face, tightness of the throat, hoarseness), or other symptoms of an allergic reaction.

FDA-APPROVED PATIENT LABELING
Patient Information
Coartem®
(co-AR-tem)
(artemether and lumefantrine)
Tablets
Read this patient information before you start taking Coartem. There may be new information. This information does not take the place of talking to your healthcare provider about your medical condition or your treatment.
What is Coartem?
Coartem is a prescription medicine used to treat uncomplicated malaria in adults and children who weigh at least 11 pounds (5 kg).
Who should not take Coartem?
Do not take Coartem if you are allergic to any of the ingredients. See the end of this leaflet for a complete list of ingredients in Coartem.
What should I tell my healthcare provider before taking Coartem?
Before you take Coartem, tell your healthcare provider about all your medical conditions including if you have:
- heart disease or a family history of heart problems or heart disease
- liver or kidney problems
- recently taken other medicines used to treat malaria
- if you are pregnant or are planning to become pregnant. Coartem may increase your risk for loss of pregnancy. Fetal defects have been reported when artemisinins are administered to animals. Talk to your healthcare provider before taking Coartem.
- if you are breast-feeding. It is not known if Coartem passes into your breast milk. You and your doctor will decide the best way to feed your baby if you take Coartem.
Tell your doctor about all the medicines you take, including prescription and non-prescription medicines, vitamins, and herbal supplements. Coartem and other medicines may affect each other causing side effects. Coartem may affect the way other medicines work and other medicines may affect how Coartem works.
Especially tell your doctor if you take:
- any other medicines to treat or prevent malaria
- medicines for your heart
- antipsychotic medicines
- antidepressants
- antibiotics
- antihistamines
- Cisapride (Propulsid®)
- medicines to treat HIV-infection
- hormonal methods of birth control (for example, birth control pills or patch)
Ask your healthcare provider if you are not sure if your medicine is one that is listed above. Know the medicines you take. Keep a list of your medicines with you to show your healthcare providers when you get a new medicine.
How should I take Coartem?
- Take Coartem exactly as prescribed.
- If you weigh 77 pounds (35 kg) or more, one dose of Coartem is 4 tablets.
- If you weigh less than 77 pounds (35 kg), your healthcare provider will tell you how many tablets to take for each dose.
- A full course of treatment is 6 doses of Coartem taken over 3 days:
Day 1:   take 1 dose; 8 hours later take 1 dose
Day 2:   take 1 dose in the morning, 1 dose in the evening
Day 3:   take 1 dose in the morning, 1 dose in the evening

Take Coartem for 3 days even if you are feeling better.
- Every dose of Coartem should be taken with food, such as milk, infant formula pudding, porridge, or broth. It is important for you to eat as soon as you can so that your malaria will go away and not get worse.
- Do not drink grapefruit juice while you take Coartem. Drinking grapefruit juice during treatment with Coartem can cause you to have too much medicine in your blood.
- Coartem may be crushed and mixed with one to two teaspoons of water in a clean container.
- If you vomit within 1 hour of taking Coartem you should take another dose of Coartem. If you vomit the second dose, tell your healthcare provider. A different medicine may need to be prescribed for you.
Tell your healthcare provider right away if:
- your malaria does not get better
- you vomited any of your doses of Coartem
- you are not able to eat
- you get flu-like symptoms (chills, fever, muscle pains, or headaches) again after you have finished your treatment with Coartem.
- you have any change in the way your heart beats or a loss of consciousness (fainting).
What are the possible side effects of Coartem?
Coartem can cause serious side effects including:
- **A heart problem called QT prolongation** that can cause an abnormal heartbeat can happen in people who take Coartem. The chance of this happening is higher in people with a family history of prolonged QT interval, low potassium (hypokalemia), and in people who take medicines to control heartbeats.
- **Allergic reactions.** Symptoms of an allergic reaction include: rash, hives, fast heartbeat, trouble swallowing or breathing, swelling of lips, tongue, face, tightness of the throat, or trouble speaking. If you have a serious allergic reaction, stop taking Coartem and get emergency medical help right away.
The most common side effects in adults are:
- headache
- feeling dizzy
- feeling weak
- loss of appetite
- muscle and joint pain or stiffness
- feeling tired
- chills
- fever
The most common side effects in children are:
- fever
- cough
- vomiting
- headache
- loss of appetite
These are not all the possible side effects of Coartem. For more information, ask your doctor or pharmacist. Call your doctor for medical advice about side effects. You may report side effects to FDA at 1-800-FDA-1088.
How should I store Coartem?
Store Coartem between 59°F to 86°F (15°C to 30°C).
Keep Coartem and all medicines out of the reach of children.
General information about the safe and effective use of Coartem.
Medicines are sometimes prescribed for purposes other than those listed in patient information leaflets. Do not use Coartem for a condition for which it was not prescribed. Do not give Coartem to other people, even if they have the same symptoms that you have. It may harm them.
This patient information leaflet summarizes the most important information about Coartem. If you would like more information about Coartem talk with your healthcare provider. You can ask your healthcare provider or pharmacist for information about Coartem that is written for health professionals. For more information call 1-888-294-6287.
What are the ingredients in Coartem?
Active ingredients include: artemether, lumefantrine
Inactive ingredients include: colloidal silicon dioxide, croscarmellose sodium, hypromellose, magnesium stearate, microcrystalline cellulose, polysorbate 80
Distributed by:
Novartis Pharmaceuticals Corporation
East Hanover, New Jersey 07936
February 2010   T2010-30/T2010-31
© Novartis

COMTAN®   ℞
[cŏm-tăn]
(entacapone)
Tablets
Rx only
Prescribing Information

The following prescribing information is based on official labeling in effect July 2009.

DESCRIPTION
Comtan® (entacapone) is available as tablets containing 200-mg entacapone.

Entacapone is an inhibitor of catechol-O-methyltransferase (COMT), used in the treatment of Parkinson's Disease as an adjunct to levodopa/carbidopa therapy. It is a nitrocatechol-structured compound with a relative molecular mass of 305.29. The chemical name of entacapone is (E)-2-cyano-3-(3,4-dihydroxy-5-nitrophenyl)-N,N-diethyl-2-propenamide. Its empirical formula is $C_{14}H_{15}N_3O_5$ and its structural formula is:

The inactive ingredients of the Comtan tablet are microcrystalline cellulose, mannitol, croscarmellose sodium, hydrogenated vegetable oil, hydroxypropyl methylcellulose, polysorbate 80, glycerol 85%, sucrose, magnesium stearate, yellow iron oxide, red oxide, and titanium dioxide.

CLINICAL PHARMACOLOGY

Mechanism of Action

Entacapone is a selective and reversible inhibitor of catechol-O-methyltransferase (COMT).

In mammals, COMT is distributed throughout various organs with the highest activities in the liver and kidney. COMT also occurs in the heart, lung, smooth and skeletal muscles, intestinal tract, reproductive organs, various glands, adipose tissue, skin, blood cells, and neuronal tissues, especially in glial cells. COMT catalyzes the transfer of the methyl group of S-adenosyl-L-methionine to the phenolic group of substrates that contain a catechol structure. Physiological substrates of COMT include dopa, catecholamines (dopamine, norepinephrine, and epinephrine) and their hydroxylated metabolites. The function of COMT is the elimination of biologically active catechols and some other hydroxylated metabolites. In the presence of a decarboxylase inhibitor, COMT becomes the major metabolizing enzyme for levodopa, catalyzing the metabolism to 3-methoxy-4-hydroxy-L-phenylalanine (3-OMD) in the brain and periphery.

The mechanism of action of entacapone is believed to be through its ability to inhibit COMT and alter the plasma pharmacokinetics of levodopa. When entacapone is given in conjunction with levodopa and an aromatic amino acid decarboxylase inhibitor, such as carbidopa, plasma levels of levodopa are greater and more sustained than after administration of levodopa and an aromatic amino acid decarboxylase inhibitor alone. It is believed that at a given frequency of levodopa administration, these more sustained plasma levels of levodopa result in more constant dopaminergic stimulation in the brain, leading to greater effects on the signs and symptoms of Parkinson's Disease. The higher levodopa levels also lead to increased levodopa adverse effects, sometimes requiring a decrease in the dose of levodopa.

In animals, while entacapone enters the CNS to a minimal extent, it has been shown to inhibit central COMT activity. In humans, entacapone inhibits the COMT enzyme in peripheral tissues. The effects of entacapone on central COMT activity in humans have not been studied.

Pharmacodynamics

COMT Activity in Erythrocytes: Studies in healthy volunteers have shown that entacapone reversibly inhibits human erythrocyte catechol-O-methyltransferase (COMT) activity after oral administration. There was a linear correlation between entacapone dose and erythrocyte COMT inhibition, the maximum inhibition being 82% following an 800-mg single dose. With a 200-mg single dose of entacapone, maximum inhibition of erythrocyte COMT activity is on average 65% with a return to baseline level within 8 hours.

Effect on the Pharmacokinetics of Levodopa and its Metabolites

When 200 mg entacapone is administered together with levodopa/carbidopa, it increases the area under the curve (AUC) of levodopa by approximately 35% and the elimination half-life of levodopa is prolonged from 1.3 h-2.4 h. In general, the average peak levodopa plasma concentration and the time of its occurrence (T_{max} of 1 hour) are unaffected. The onset of effect occurs after the first administration and is maintained during long-term treatment. Studies in Parkinson's Disease patients suggest that the maximal effect occurs with 200-mg entacapone. Plasma levels of 3-OMD are markedly and dose-dependently decreased by entacapone when given with levodopa/carbidopa.

Pharmacokinetics of Entacapone

Entacapone pharmacokinetics are linear over the dose range of 5 mg-800 mg, and are independent of levodopa/carbidopa coadministration. The elimination of entacapone

is biphasic, with an elimination half-life of 0.4 h-0.7 h based on the β-phase and 2.4 h based on the γ-phase. The γ-phase accounts for approximately 10% of the total AUC. The total body clearance after i.v. administration is 850 mL/min. After a single 200-mg dose of Comtan (entacapone), the C_{max} is approximately 1.2 μg/mL.

Absorption: Entacapone is rapidly absorbed, with a T_{max} of approximately 1 hour. The absolute bioavailability following oral administration is 35%. Food does not affect the pharmacokinetics of entacapone.

Distribution: The volume of distribution of entacapone at steady state after i.v. injection is small (20 L). Entacapone does not distribute widely into tissues due to its high plasma protein binding. Based on *in vitro* studies, the plasma protein binding of entacapone is 98% over the concentration range of 0.4-50 μg/mL. Entacapone binds mainly to serum albumin.

Metabolism and Elimination: Entacapone is almost completely metabolized prior to excretion, with only a very small amount (0.2% of dose) found unchanged in urine. The main metabolic pathway is isomerization to the *cis*-isomer, followed by direct glucuronidation of the parent and *cis*-isomer; the glucuronide conjugate is inactive. After oral administration of a ^{14}C-labeled dose of entacapone, 10% of labeled parent and metabolite is excreted in urine and 90% in feces.

Special Populations: Entacapone pharmacokinetics are independent of age. No formal gender studies have been conducted. Racial representation in clinical trials was largely limited to Caucasians (there were only 4 blacks in one US trial and no Asians in any of the clinical trials); no conclusions can therefore be reached about the effect of Comtan on groups other than Caucasian.

Hepatic Impairment: A single 200-mg dose of entacapone, without levodopa/dopa decarboxylase inhibitor coadministration, showed approximately twofold higher AUC and

C_{max} values in patients with a history of alcoholism and hepatic impairment (n=10) compared to normal subjects (n=10). All patients had biopsy-proven liver cirrhosis caused by alcohol. According to Child-Pugh grading 7 patients with liver disease had mild hepatic impairment and 3 patients had moderate hepatic impairment. As only about 10% of the entacapone dose is excreted in urine as parent compound and conjugated glucuronide, biliary excretion appears to be the major route of excretion of this drug. Consequently, entacapone should be administered with care to patients with biliary obstruction.

Renal Impairment: The pharmacokinetics of entacapone have been investigated after a single 200-mg entacapone dose, without levodopa/dopa decarboxylase inhibitor coadministration, in a specific renal impairment study. There were three groups: normal subjects (n=7; creatinine clearance >1.12 mL/sec/1.73 m²), moderate impairment (n=10; creatinine clearance ranging from 0.60-0.89 mL/sec/ 1.73 m²), and severe impairment (n=7; creatinine clearance ranging from 0.20-0.44 mL/sec/1.73 m²). No important effects of renal function on the pharmacokinetics of entacapone were found.

Drug Interactions: See PRECAUTIONS, Drug Interactions.

Clinical Studies

The effectiveness of Comtan (entacapone) as an adjunct to levodopa in the treatment of Parkinson's Disease was established in three 24-week multicenter, randomized, double-blind placebo-controlled trials in patients with Parkinson's Disease. In two of these trials, the patients' disease was "fluctuating," i.e., was characterized by documented periods of "On" (periods of relatively good functioning) and "Off" (periods of relatively poor functioning), despite optimum levodopa therapy. There was also a withdrawal period following 6 months of treatment. In the third trial patients were not required to have been experiencing fluctuations.

Table 1. Nordic Study

Primary Measure from Home Diary (from an 18-hour Diary Day)

	Baseline	Change from Baseline at Month 6*	p-value vs. placebo
Hours of Awake Time "On"			
Placebo	9.2	+0.1	–
Comtan	9.3	+1.5	<0.001
Duration of "On" time after first AM dose (hrs)			
Placebo	2.2	0.0	–
Comtan	2.1	+0.2	<0.05

Secondary Measures from Home Diary (from an 18-hour Diary Day)

	Baseline	Change from Baseline at Month 6*	p-value vs. placebo
Hours of Awake Time "Off"			
Placebo	5.3	0.0	–
Comtan	5.5	-1.3	<0.001
Proportion of Awake Time "On" * (%)**			
Placebo	63.8	+0.6	–
Comtan	62.7	+9.3	<0.001
Levodopa Total Daily Dose (mg)			
Placebo	705	+14	–
Comtan	701	-87	<0.001
Frequency of Levodopa Daily Intakes			
Placebo	6.1	+0.1	–
Comtan	6.2	-0.4	<0.001

Other Secondary Measures

	Baseline	Change from Baseline at Month 6	p-value vs. placebo
Investigator's Global (overall) % Improved**			
Placebo	–	28	–
Comtan	–	56	<0.01
Patient's Global (overall) % Improved**			
Placebo	–	22	–
Comtan	–	39	N.S.‡
UPDRS Total			
Placebo	37.4	-1.1	–
Comtan	38.5	-4.8	<0.01
UPDRS Motor			
Placebo	24.6	-0.7	–
Comtan	25.5	-3.3	<0.05
UPDRS ADL			
Placebo	11.0	-0.4	–
Comtan	11.2	-1.8	<0.05

* Mean; the month 6 values represent the average of weeks 8, 16, and 24, by protocol-defined outcome measure.

** At least one category change at endpoint.

*** Not an endpoint for this study but primary endpoint in the North American Study.

‡ Not significant.

Table 2. North American Study

Primary Measure from Home Diary (for a 24-hour Diary Day)

	Baseline	Change from Baseline at Month 6*	p-value vs. placebo
Percent of Awake Time "On"			
Placebo	60.8	+2.0	–
Comtan	60.0	+6.7	<0.05

Secondary Measures from Home Diary (for a 24-hour Diary Day)

Hours of Awake Time "Off"			
Placebo	6.6	-0.3	–
Comtan	6.8	-1.2	<0.01
Hours of Awake Time "On"			
Placebo	10.3	+0.4	–
Comtan	10.2	+1.0	N.S.‡
Levodopa Total Daily Dose (mg)			
Placebo	758	+19	–
Comtan	804	-93	<0.001
Frequency of Levodopa Daily Intakes			
Placebo	6.0	+0.2	–
Comtan	6.2	0.0	N.S.‡

Other Secondary Measures

	Baseline	Change from Baseline at Month 6	p-value vs. placebo
Investigator's Global (overall) % Improved **			
Placebo	–	21	–
Comtan	–	34	<0.05
Patient's Global (overall) % Improved**			
Placebo	–	20	–
Comtan	–	31	<0.05
UPDRS Total*			
Placebo	35.6	+2.8	–
Comtan	35.1	-0.6	<0.05
UPDRS Motor*			
Placebo	22.6	+1.2	–
Comtan	22.0	-0.9	<0.05
UPDRS ADL*			
Placebo	11.7	+1.1	–
Comtan	11.9	0.0	<0.05

* Mean; the month 6 values represent the average of weeks 8, 16, and 24, by protocol-defined outcome measure.
** At least one category change at endpoint.
*** Score change at endpoint similarly to the Nordic Study.
‡ Not significant.

Prior to the controlled part of the trials, patients were stabilized on levodopa for 2-4 weeks. Comtan has not been systematically evaluated in patients who do not experience fluctuations.

In the first two studies to be described, patients were randomized to receive placebo or entacapone 200 mg administered concomitantly with each dose of levodopa/carbidopa (up to 10 times daily, but averaging 4-6 doses per day). The formal double-blind portion of both trials was 6 months long. Patients recorded the time spent in the "On" and "Off" states in home diaries periodically throughout the duration of the trial. In one study, conducted in the Nordic countries, the primary outcome measure was the total mean time spent in the "On" state during an 18-hour diary recorded day (6 AM to midnight). In the other study, the primary outcome measure was the proportion of awake time spent over 24 hours in the "On" state.

In addition to the primary outcome measure, the amount of time spent in the "Off" state was evaluated, and patients were also evaluated by subparts of the Unified Parkinson's Disease Rating Scale (UPDRS), a frequently used multi-item rating scale intended to assess mentation (Part I), activities of daily living (Part II), motor function (Part III), complications of therapy (Part IV), and disease staging (Part V & VI); an investigator's and patient's global assessment of clinical condition, a 7-point subjective scale designed to assess global functioning in Parkinson's Disease; and the change in daily levodopa/carbidopa dose.

In one of the studies, 171 patients were randomized in 16 centers in Finland, Norway, Sweden, and Denmark (Nordic study), all of whom received concomitant levodopa plus dopa-decarboxylase inhibitor (either levodopa/carbidopa or levodopa/benserazide). In the second trial, 205 patients were randomized in 17 centers in North America (US and Canada); all patients received concomitant levodopa/carbidopa.

The following tables display the results of these two trials:
[See table 1 at top of previous page]
[See table 2 above]

Effects on "On" time did not differ by age, sex, weight, disease severity at baseline, levodopa dose and concurrent treatment with dopamine agonists or selegiline.

Withdrawal of entacapone: In the North American study, abrupt withdrawal of entacapone, without alteration of the dose of levodopa/carbidopa, resulted in a significant worsening of fluctuations, compared to placebo. In some cases, symptoms were slightly worse than at baseline, but returned to approximately baseline severity within two weeks following levodopa dose increase on average by 80 mg. In the Nordic study, similarly, a significant worsening of parkinsonian symptoms was observed after entacapone withdrawal, as assessed two weeks after drug withdrawal. At this phase, the symptoms were approximately at baseline severity following levodopa dose increase by about 50 mg.

In the third placebo controlled trial, a total of 301 patients were randomized in 32 centers in Germany and Austria. In this trial, as in the other two trials, entacapone 200 mg was administered with each dose of levodopa/dopa decarboxylase inhibitor (up to 10 times daily) and UPDRS Parts II and III and total daily "On" time were the primary measures of effectiveness. The following results were seen for the primary measures, as well as for some secondary measures:
[See table 3 at top of next page]

INDICATIONS

Comtan (entacapone) is indicated as an adjunct to levodopa/carbidopa to treat patients with idiopathic Parkinson's Disease who experience the signs and symptoms of end-of-dose "wearing-off" (*see CLINICAL PHARMACOLOGY, Clinical Studies*).

Comtan's effectiveness has not been systematically evaluated in patients with idiopathic Parkinson's Disease who do not experience end-of-dose "wearing-off".

CONTRAINDICATIONS

Comtan (entacapone) tablets are contraindicated in patients who have demonstrated hypersensitivity to the drug or its ingredients.

WARNINGS

Monoamine oxidase (MAO) and COMT are the two major enzyme systems involved in the metabolism of catecholamines. It is theoretically possible, therefore, that the combination of Comtan (entacapone) and a non-selective MAO inhibitor (e.g., phenelzine and tranylcypromine) would result in inhibition of the majority of the pathways responsible for normal catecholamine metabolism. For this reason, patients should ordinarily not be treated concomitantly with Comtan and a non-selective MAO inhibitor.

Entacapone can be taken concomitantly with a selective MAO-B inhibitor (e.g., selegiline).

Drugs Metabolized by Catechol-*O*-methyltransferase (COMT)

When a single 400-mg dose of entacapone was given together with intravenous isoprenaline (isoproterenol) and epinephrine without coadministered levodopa/dopa decarboxylase inhibitor, the overall mean maximal changes in heart rate during infusion were about 50% and 80% higher than with placebo, for isoprenaline and epinephrine, respectively.

Therefore, drugs known to be metabolized by COMT, such as isoproterenol, epinephrine, norepinephrine, dopamine, dobutamine, alpha-methyldopa, apomorphine, isoetherine, and bitolterol should be administered with caution in patients receiving entacapone regardless of the route of administration (including inhalation), as their interaction may result in increased heart rates, possibly arrhythmias, and excessive changes in blood pressure.

Ventricular tachycardia was noted in one 32-year-old healthy male volunteer in an interaction study after epinephrine infusion and oral entacapone administration. Treatment with propranolol was required. A causal relationship to entacapone administration appears probable but cannot be attributed with certainty.

PRECAUTIONS

Hypotension/Syncope

Dopaminergic therapy in Parkinson's Disease patients has been associated with orthostatic hypotension. Entacapone enhances levodopa bioavailability and, therefore, might be expected to increase the occurrence of orthostatic hypotension. In Comtan (entacapone) clinical trials, however, no differences from placebo were seen for measured orthostasis or symptoms of orthostasis. Orthostatic hypotension was documented at least once in 2.7% and 3.0% of the patients treated with 200 mg Comtan and placebo, respectively. A total of 4.3% and 4.0% of the patients treated with 200 mg Comtan and placebo, respectively, reported orthostatic symptoms at some time during their treatment and also had at least one episode of orthostatic hypotension documented (however, the episode of orthostatic symptoms itself was not accompanied by vital sign measurements). Neither baseline treatment with dopamine agonists or selegiline, nor the presence of orthostasis at baseline, increased the risk of orthostatic hypotension in patients treated with Comtan compared to patients on placebo.

In the large controlled trials, approximately 1.2% and 0.8% of 200 mg entacapone and placebo patients, respectively, reported at least one episode of syncope. Reports of syncope were generally more frequent in patients in both treatment groups who had an episode of documented hypotension (although the episodes of syncope, obtained by history, were themselves not documented with vital sign measurement).

Diarrhea

In clinical trials, diarrhea developed in 60 of 603 (10.0%) and 16 of 400 (4.0%) of patients treated with 200 mg Comtan and placebo, respectively. In patients treated with Comtan, diarrhea was generally mild to moderate in severity (8.6%) but was regarded as severe in 1.3%. Diarrhea resulted in withdrawal in 10 of 603 (1.7%) patients, 7 (1.2%) with mild and moderate diarrhea and 3 (0.5%) with severe diarrhea. Diarrhea generally resolved after discontinuation of Comtan. Two patients with diarrhea were hospitalized. Typically, diarrhea presents within 4-12 weeks after entacapone is started, but it may appear as early as the first week and as late as many months after the initiation of treatment.

Hallucinations

Dopaminergic therapy in Parkinson's Disease patients has been associated with hallucinations. In clinical trials, hallucinations developed in approximately 4.0% of patients treated with 200 mg Comtan or placebo. Hallucinations led to drug discontinuation and premature withdrawal from clinical trials in 0.8% and 0% of patients treated with 200 mg Comtan and placebo, respectively. Hallucinations led to hospitalization in 1.0% and 0.3% of patients in the 200 mg Comtan and placebo groups, respectively.

Dyskinesia

Comtan may potentiate the dopaminergic side effects of levodopa and may cause and/or exacerbate preexisting dyskinesia. Although decreasing the dose of levodopa may ameliorate this side effect, many patients in controlled trials continued to experience frequent dyskinesias despite a reduction in their dose of levodopa. The rates of withdrawal for dyskinesia were 1.5% and 0.8% for 200 mg Comtan and placebo, respectively.

Other Events Reported with Dopaminergic Therapy
The events listed below are rare events known to be associated with the use of drugs that increase dopaminergic activity, although they are most often associated with the use of direct dopamine agonists.

Rhabdomyolysis: Cases of severe rhabdomyolysis have been reported with Comtan use. The complicated nature of these cases makes it impossible to determine what role, if any, Comtan played in their pathogenesis. Severe prolonged motor activity including dyskinesia may account for rhabdomyolysis. One case, however, included fever and alteration of consciousness. It is therefore possible that the rhabdomyolysis may be a result of the syndrome described in Hyperpyrexia and Confusion *(see PRECAUTIONS, Other Events Reported with Dopaminergic Therapy).*

Hyperpyrexia and Confusion: Cases of a symptom complex resembling the neuroleptic malignant syndrome characterized by elevated temperature, muscular rigidity, altered consciousness, and elevated CPK have been reported in association with the rapid dose reduction or withdrawal of other dopaminergic drugs. Several cases with similar signs and symptoms have been reported in association with Comtan therapy, although no information about dose manipulation is available. The complicated nature of these cases makes it difficult to determine what role, if any, Comtan may have played in their pathogenesis. No cases have been reported following the abrupt withdrawal or dose reduction of entacapone treatment during clinical studies. Prescribers should exercise caution when discontinuing entacapone treatment. When considered necessary, withdrawal should proceed slowly. If a decision is made to discontinue treatment with Comtan, recommendations include monitoring the patient closely and adjusting other dopaminergic treatments as needed. This syndrome should be considered in the differential diagnosis for any patient who develops a high fever or severe rigidity. Tapering Comtan has not been systematically evaluated.

Fibrotic Complications: Cases of retroperitoneal fibrosis, pulmonary infiltrates, pleural effusion, and pleural thickening have been reported in some patients treated with ergot derived dopaminergic agents. These complications may resolve when the drug is discontinued, but complete resolution does not always occur. Although these adverse events are believed to be related to the ergoline structure of these compounds, whether other, nonergot derived drugs (e.g., entacapone) that increase dopaminergic activity can cause them is unknown. It should be noted that the expected incidence of fibrotic complications is so low that even if entacapone caused these complications at rates similar to those attributable to other dopaminergic therapies, it is unlikely that it would have been detected in a cohort of the size exposed to entacapone. Four cases of pulmonary fibrosis were reported during clinical development of entacapone; three of these patients were also treated with pergolide and one with bromocriptine. The duration of treatment with entacapone ranged from 7-17 months.

Melanoma: Epidemiological studies have shown that patients with Parkinson's disease have a higher risk (2- to approximately 6-fold higher) of developing melanoma than the general population. Whether the increased risk observed was due to Parkinson's disease or other factors, such as drugs used to treat Parkinson's disease, is unclear.

For the reasons stated above, patients and providers are advised to monitor for melanomas frequently and on a regular basis when using Comtan for *any* indication. Ideally, periodic skin examination should be performed by appropriately qualified individuals (e.g., dermatologists).

Renal Toxicity
In a 1 year toxicity study, entacapone (plasma exposure 20 times that in humans receiving the maximum recommended daily dose of 1600 mg) caused an increased incidence in male rats of nephrotoxicity that was characterized by regenerative tubules, thickening of basement membranes, infiltration of mononuclear cells and tubular protein casts. These effects were not associated with changes in clinical chemistry parameters, and there is no established method for monitoring for the possible occurrence of these lesions in humans. Although this toxicity could represent a species-specific effect, there is not yet evidence that this is so.

Hepatic Impairment
Patients with hepatic impairment should be treated with caution. The AUC and C_{max} of entacapone approximately doubled in patients with documented liver disease compared to controls. *(See CLINICAL PHARMACOLOGY, Pharmacokinetics of Entacapone and DOSAGE AND ADMINISTRATION).*

Information for Patients
Patients should be instructed to take Comtan only as prescribed.

Patients should be informed that hallucinations can occur. Patients should be advised that they may develop postural (orthostatic) hypotension with or without symptoms such as dizziness, nausea, syncope, and sweating. Hypotension may occur more frequently during initial therapy. Accordingly, patients should be cautioned against rising rapidly after sitting or lying down, especially if they have been doing so for prolonged periods, and especially at the initiation of treatment with Comtan.

Patients should be advised that they should neither drive a car nor operate other complex machinery until they have gained sufficient experience on Comtan to gauge whether or not it affects their mental and/or motor performance adversely. Because of the possible additive sedative effects, caution should be used when patients are taking other CNS depressants in combination with Comtan.

Patients should be informed that nausea may occur, especially at the initiation of treatment with Comtan.

Patients should be advised of the possibility of an increase in dyskinesia.

Patients should be advised that treatment with entacapone may cause a change in the color of their urine (a brownish orange discoloration) that is not clinically relevant. In controlled trials, 10% of patients treated with Comtan reported urine discoloration compared to 0% of placebo patients.

Although Comtan has not been shown to be teratogenic in animals, it is always given in conjunction with levodopa/carbidopa, which is known to cause visceral and skeletal malformations in the rabbit. Accordingly, patients should be advised to notify their physicians if they become pregnant or intend to become pregnant during therapy *(see PRECAUTIONS, Pregnancy).*

Entacapone is excreted into maternal milk in rats. Because of the possibility that entacapone may be excreted into human maternal milk, patients should be advised to notify their physicians if they intend to breastfeed or are breastfeeding an infant.

There have been reports of patients experiencing intense urges to gamble, increased sexual urges, and other intense urges and the inability to control these urges while taking one or more of the medications that increase central dopaminergic tone, that are generally used for the treatment of Parkinson's disease, including Comtan. Although it is not proven that the medications caused these events, these urges were reported to have stopped in some cases when the dose was reduced or the medication was stopped. Prescribers should ask patients about the development of new or increased gambling urges, sexual urges or other urges while being treated with Comtan. Patients should inform their physician if they experience new or increased gambling urges, increased sexual urges or other intense urges while taking Comtan. Physicians should consider dose reduction or stopping the medication if a patient develops such urges while taking Comtan.

Laboratory Tests
Comtan is a chelator of iron. The impact of entacapone on the body's iron stores is unknown; however, a tendency towards decreasing serum iron concentrations was noted in clinical trials. In a controlled clinical study serum ferritin levels (as marker of iron deficiency and subclinical anemia) were not changed with entacapone compared to placebo after one year of treatment and there was no difference in rates of anemia or decreased hemoglobin levels.

Special Populations
Patients with hepatic impairment should be treated with caution *(see INDICATIONS, DOSAGE AND ADMINISTRATION).*

Drug Interactions
In vitro studies of human CYP enzymes showed that entacapone inhibited the CYP enzymes 1A2, 2A6, 2C9, 2C19, 2D6, 2E1 and 3A only at very high concentrations (IC50 from 200 to over 1000 µM; an oral 200 mg dose achieves a highest level of approximately 5 µM in people); these enzymes would therefore not be expected to be inhibited in clinical use.

Protein Binding
Entacapone is highly protein bound (98%). *In vitro* studies have shown no binding displacement between entacapone and other highly bound drugs, such as warfarin, salicylic acid, phenylbutazone, and diazepam.

Drugs Metabolized by Catechol-O-methyltransferase (COMT)
See WARNINGS.

Hormone Levels
Levodopa is known to depress prolactin secretion and increase growth hormone levels. Treatment with entacapone coadministered with levodopa/dopa decarboxylase inhibitor does not change these effects.

Effect of Entacapone on the Metabolism of Other Drugs
See WARNINGS regarding concomitant use of Comtan and non-selective MAO inhibitors.

Table 3. German-Austrian Study

Primary Measures

	Baseline	Change from Baseline at Month 6	p-value vs. placebo (LOCF)
UPDRS ADL*			
Placebo	12.0	+0.5	–
Comtan	12.4	-0.4	<0.05
UPDRS Motor*			
Placebo	24.1	+0.1	–
Comtan	24.9	-2.5	<0.05
Hours of Awake Time "On" (Home diary)**			
Placebo	10.1	+0.5	–
Comtan	10.2	+1.1	N.S.‡

Secondary Measures

	Baseline	Change from Baseline at Month 6	p-value vs. placebo
UPDRS Total*			
Placebo	37.7	+0.6	–
Comtan	39.0	-3.4	<0.05
Percent of Awake Time "On" (Home diary)**			
Placebo	59.8	+3.5	–
Comtan	62.0	+6.5	N.S.‡
Hours of Awake Time "Off" (Home diary)**			
Placebo	6.8	-0.6	–
Comtan	6.3	-1.2	0.07
Levodopa Total Daily Dose (mg)*			
Placebo	572	+4	–
Comtan	566	-35	N.S.‡
Frequency of Levodopa Daily Intake*			
Placebo	5.6	+0.2	–
Comtan	5.4	0.0	<0.01
Global (overall) % Improved***			
Placebo	–	34	–
Comtan	–	38	N.S.‡

* Total population; score change at endpoint.
** Fluctuating population, with 5-10 doses; score change at endpoint.
*** Total population; at least one category change at endpoint.
‡ Not significant.

No interaction was noted with the MAO-B inhibitor selegiline in two multiple-dose interaction studies when entacapone was coadministered with a levodopa/dopa decarboxylase inhibitor (n=29). More than 600 Parkinson's Disease patients in clinical trials have used selegiline in combination with entacapone and levodopa/dopa decarboxylase inhibitor.

As most entacapone excretion is via the bile, caution should be exercised when drugs known to interfere with biliary excretion, glucuronidation, and intestinal beta-glucuronidase are given concurrently with entacapone. These include probenecid, cholestyramine, and some antibiotics (e.g., erythromycin, rifampicin, ampicillin and chloramphenicol).

No interaction with the tricyclic antidepressant imipramine was shown in a single-dose study with entacapone without coadministered levodopa/dopa-decarboxylase inhibitor.

Carcinogenesis

Two-year carcinogenicity studies of entacapone were conducted in mice and rats. Rats were treated once daily by oral gavage with entacapone doses of 20, 90, or 400 mg/kg. An increased incidence of renal tubular adenomas and carcinomas was found in male rats treated with the highest dose of entacapone. Plasma exposures (AUC) associated with this dose were approximately 20 times higher than estimated plasma exposures of humans receiving the maximum recommended daily dose of entacapone (MRDD = 1600 mg). Mice were treated once daily by oral gavage with doses of 20, 100 or 600 mg/kg of entacapone (0.05, 0.3, and 2 times the MRDD for humans on a mg/m² basis). Because of a high incidence of premature mortality in mice receiving the highest dose of entacapone, the mouse study is not an adequate assessment of carcinogenicity. Although no treatment related tumors were observed in animals receiving the lower doses, the carcinogenic potential of entacapone has not been fully evaluated. The carcinogenic potential of entacapone administered in combination with levodopa/carbidopa has not been evaluated.

Mutagenesis

Entacapone was mutagenic and clastogenic in the in vitro mouse lymphoma/thymidine kinase assay in the presence and absence of metabolic activation, and was clastogenic in cultured human lymphocytes in the presence of metabolic activation. Entacapone, either alone or in combination with levodopa/carbidopa, was not clastogenic in the in vivo mouse micronucleus test or mutagenic in the bacterial reverse mutation assay (Ames test).

Impairment of Fertility

Entacapone did not impair fertility or general reproductive performance in rats treated with up to 700 mg/kg/day (plasma AUCs 28 times those in humans receiving the MRDD). Delayed mating, but no fertility impairment, was evident in female rats treated with 700 mg/kg/day of entacapone.

Pregnancy

Pregnancy Category C. In embryofetal development studies, entacapone was administered to pregnant animals throughout organogenesis at doses of up to 1000 mg/kg/day in rats and 300 mg/kg/day in rabbits. Increased incidences of fetal variations were evident in litters from rats treated with the highest dose, in the absence of overt signs of maternal toxicity. The maternal plasma drug exposure (AUC) associated with this dose was approximately 34 times the estimated plasma exposure in humans receiving the maximum recommended daily dose (MRDD) of 1600 mg. Increased frequencies of abortions and late/total resorptions and decreased fetal weights were observed in the litters of rabbits treated with maternotoxic doses of 100 mg/kg/day (plasma AUCs 0.4 times those in humans receiving the MRDD) or greater. There was no evidence of teratogenicity in these studies.

However, when entacapone was administered to female rats prior to mating and during early gestation, an increased incidence of fetal eye anomalies (macrophthalmia, microphthalmia, anophthalmia) was observed in the litters of dams treated with doses of 160 mg/kg/day (plasma AUCs 7 times those in humans receiving the MRDD) or greater, in the absence of maternotoxicity. Administration of up to 700 mg/kg/day (plasma AUCs 28 times those in humans receiving the MRDD) to female rats during the latter part of gestation and throughout lactation, produced no evidence of developmental impairment in the offspring.

Entacapone is always given concomitantly with levodopa/carbidopa, which is known to cause visceral and skeletal malformations in rabbits. The teratogenic potential of entacapone in combination with levodopa/carbidopa was not assessed in animals.

There is no experience from clinical studies regarding the use of Comtan in pregnant women. Therefore, Comtan should be used during pregnancy only if the potential benefit justifies the potential risk to the fetus.

Nursing Women

In animal studies, entacapone was excreted into maternal rat milk.

It is not known whether entacapone is excreted in human milk. Because many drugs are excreted in human milk, caution should be exercised when entacapone is administered to a nursing woman.

Pediatric Use

There is no identified potential use of entacapone in pediatric patients.

ADVERSE REACTIONS

During the pre-marketing development of entacapone, 1450 patients with Parkinson's Disease were treated with entacapone. Included were patients with fluctuating symptoms, as well as those with stable responses to levodopa therapy. All patients received concomitant treatment with levodopa preparations, however, and were similar in other clinical aspects.

The most commonly observed adverse events (>5%) in the double-blind, placebo-controlled trials (N=1003) associated with the use of Comtan (entacapone) and not seen at an equivalent frequency among the placebo-treated patients were: dyskinesia/hyperkinesia, nausea, urine discoloration, diarrhea, and abdominal pain.

Approximately 14% of the 603 patients given entacapone in the double-blind, placebo-controlled trials discontinued treatment due to adverse events compared to 9% of the 400 patients who received placebo. The most frequent causes of discontinuation in decreasing order are: psychiatric reasons (2% vs. 1%), diarrhea (2% vs. 0%), dyskinesia/hyperkinesia (2% vs. 1%), nausea (2% vs. 1%), abdominal pain (1% vs. 0%), and aggravation of Parkinson's Disease symptoms (1% vs. 1%).

Adverse Event Incidence in Controlled Clinical Studies

Table 4 lists treatment emergent adverse events that occurred in at least 1% of patients treated with entacapone participating in the double-blind, placebo-controlled studies and that were numerically more common in the entacapone group, compared to placebo. In these studies, either entacapone or placebo was added to levodopa/carbidopa (or levodopa/benserazide).

Table 4
Summary of Patients with Adverse Events after Start of Trial Drug Administration At least 1% in Comtan® (entacapone) group and > Placebo

SYSTEM ORGAN CLASS Preferred term	Comtan (n = 603) % of patients	Placebo (n = 400) % of patients
SKIN AND APPENDAGES DISORDERS		
Sweating increased	2	1
MUSCULOSKELETAL SYSTEM DISORDERS		
Back pain	2	1
CENTRAL & PERIPHERAL NERVOUS SYSTEM DISORDERS		
Dyskinesia	25	15
Hyperkinesia	10	5
Hypokinesia	9	8
Dizziness	8	6
SPECIAL SENSES, OTHER DISORDERS		
Taste perversion	1	0
PSYCHIATRIC DISORDERS		
Anxiety	2	1
Somnolence	2	0
Agitation	1	0
GASTROINTESTINAL SYSTEM DISORDERS		
Nausea	14	8
Diarrhea	10	4
Abdominal pain	8	4
Constipation	6	4
Vomiting	4	1
Mouth dry	3	0
Dyspepsia	2	1
Flatulence	2	0
Gastritis	1	0
Gastrointestinal disorders nos	1	0
RESPIRATORY SYSTEM DISORDERS		
Dyspnea	3	1
PLATELET, BLEEDING & CLOTTING DISORDERS		
Purpura	2	1
URINARY SYSTEM DISORDERS		
Urine discoloration	10	0
BODY AS A WHOLE - GENERAL DISORDERS		
Back pain	4	2
Fatigue	6	4
Asthenia	2	1
RESISTANCE MECHANISM DISORDERS		
Infection bacterial	1	0

The prescriber should be aware that these figures cannot be used to predict the incidence of adverse events in the course of usual medical practice where patient characteristics and other factors differ from those that prevailed in the clinical studies. Similarly, the cited frequencies cannot be compared with figures obtained from other clinical investigations involving different treatments, uses, and investigators. The cited figures do, however, provide the prescriber with some basis for estimating the relative contribution of drug and nondrug factors to the adverse events observed in the population studied.

Effects of Gender and Age on Adverse Reactions

No differences were noted in the rate of adverse events attributable to entacapone by age or gender.

DRUG ABUSE AND DEPENDENCE

Comtan (entacapone) is not a controlled substance. Animal studies to evaluate the drug abuse and potential dependence have not been conducted. Although clinical trials have not revealed any evidence of the potential for abuse, tolerance or physical dependence, systematic studies in humans designed to evaluate these effects have not been performed.

OVERDOSAGE

There have been no reported cases of either accidental or intentional overdose with entacapone tablets. However, COMT inhibition by entacapone treatment is dose-dependent. A massive overdose of Comtan (entacapone) may theoretically produce a 100% inhibition of the COMT enzyme in people, thereby preventing the metabolism of endogenous and exogenous catechols.

The highest single dose of entacapone administered to humans was 800 mg, resulting in a plasma concentration of 14.1 µg/mL. The highest daily dose given to humans was 2400 mg, administered in one study as 400 mg six times daily with levodopa/carbidopa for 14 days in 15 Parkinson's Disease patients, and in another study as 800 mg t.i.d. for 7 days in 8 healthy volunteers. At this daily dose, the peak plasma concentrations of entacapone averaged 2.0 µg/mL (at 45 min., compared to 1.0 and 1.2 µg/mL with 200 mg entacapone at 45 min.). Abdominal pain and loose stools were the most commonly observed adverse events during this study. Daily doses as high as 2000 mg Comtan have been administered as 200 mg 10 times daily with levodopa/carbidopa or levodopa/benserazide for at least 1 year in 10 patients, for at least 2 years in 8 patients and for at least 3 years in 7 patients. Overall, however, clinical experience with daily doses above 1600 mg is limited.

The range of lethal plasma concentrations of entacapone based on animal data was 80-130 µg/mL in mice. Respiratory difficulties, ataxia, hypoactivity, and convulsions were observed in mice after high oral (gavage) doses.

Management of Overdose

Management of Comtan overdose is symptomatic; there is no known antidote to Comtan. Hospitalization is advised, and general supportive care is indicated. There is no experience with hemodialysis or hemoperfusion, but these procedures are unlikely to be of benefit, because Comtan is highly bound to plasma proteins. An immediate gastric lavage and repeated doses of charcoal over time may hasten the elimination of Comtan by decreasing its absorption/reabsorption from the GI tract. The adequacy of the respiratory and circulatory systems should be carefully monitored and appropriate supportive measures employed. The possibility of drug interactions, especially with catechol-structured drugs, should be borne in mind.

DOSAGE AND ADMINISTRATION

The recommended dose of Comtan (entacapone) is one 200 mg tablet administered concomitantly with each levodopa/carbidopa dose to a maximum of 8 times daily (200 mg × 8 = 1600 mg per day). Clinical experience with daily doses above 1600 mg is limited.

Comtan should always be administered in association with levodopa/carbidopa. Entacapone has no antiparkinsonian effect of its own.

In clinical trials, the majority of patients required a decrease in daily levodopa dose if their daily dose of levodopa had been ≥800 mg or if patients had moderate or severe dyskinesias before beginning treatment.

To optimize an individual patient's response, reductions in daily levodopa dose or extending the interval between doses may be necessary. In clinical trials, the average reduction in daily levodopa dose was about 25% in those patients requiring a levodopa dose reduction. (More than 58% of patients with levodopa doses above 800 mg daily required such a reduction.)

Comtan can be combined with both the immediate and sustained-release formulations of levodopa/carbidopa. Comtan may be taken with or without food (see CLINICAL PHARMACOLOGY).

Patients With Impaired Hepatic Function: Patients with hepatic impairment should be treated with caution. The AUC and C_{max} of entacapone approximately doubled in patients with documented liver disease, compared to controls. However, these studies were conducted with single-dose entacapone without levodopa/dopa decarboxylase inhibitor coadministration, and therefore the effects of liver disease on the kinetics of chronically administered entacapone have not been evaluated (see CLINICAL PHARMACOLOGY, Pharmacokinetics of Entacapone).

Withdrawing Patients from Comtan: Rapid withdrawal or abrupt reduction in the Comtan dose could lead to emergence of signs and symptoms of Parkinson's Disease (see CLINICAL PHARMACOLOGY, Clinical Studies), and may lead to Hyperpyrexia and Confusion, a symptom complex resembling the neuroleptic malignant syndrome (see PRECAUTIONS, Other Events Reported with Dopaminergic Therapy). This syndrome should be considered in the differential diagnosis for any patient who develops a high fever or severe rigidity. If a decision is made to discontinue treatment with Comtan, patients should be monitored closely and other dopaminergic treatments should be adjusted as needed. Although tapering Comtan has not been systematically evaluated, it seems prudent to withdraw patients slowly if the decision to discontinue treatment is made.

HOW SUPPLIED

Comtan (entacapone) is supplied as 200-mg film-coated tablets for oral administration. The oval-shaped tablets are brownish-orange, unscored, and embossed "COMTAN" on one side. Tablets are provided in HDPE containers as follows:

Bottles of 100 .... NDC 0078-0327-05
Store at 25°C (77°F) excursions permitted to 15°-30°C (59°-86°F).
[See USP Controlled Room Temperature.]
Comtan (entacapone) tablets are manufactured by Orion Corporation, Orion Pharma (Espoo, Finland) and marketed by Novartis Pharmaceuticals Corporation (East Hanover, N.J. 07936, U.S.A.).

T2009-71

REV: MARCH 2009   Printed in U.S.A.
©Novartis
Shown in Product Identification Guide, page 314

DIOVAN®   ℞
[DYE'-o-van]
(valsartan)
Tablets

The following prescribing information is based on labeling in effect July 2010.
HIGHLIGHTS OF PRESCRIBING INFORMATION
These highlights do not include all the information needed to use Diovan safely and effectively. See full prescribing information for Diovan.
Diovan (valsartan) Tablets
Initial U.S. Approval: 1996

WARNING: USE IN PREGNANCY
When pregnancy is detected, discontinue Diovan as soon as possible. Drugs that act directly on the renin-angiotensin system can cause injury and even death to the developing fetus (5.1)

—————— **RECENT MAJOR CHANGES** ——————
None
—————— **INDICATIONS AND USAGE** ——————
Diovan is an angiotensin II receptor blocker (ARB) indicated for:
• Treatment of **hypertension** (1.1)
• Treatment of **heart failure** (NYHA class II-IV); Diovan significantly reduced hospitalization for heart failure (1.2)
• Reduction of cardiovascular mortality in clinically stable patients with left ventricular failure or left ventricular dysfunction **following myocardial infarction** (1.3)
—————— **DOSAGE AND ADMINISTRATION** ——————
[See table above]
No initial dosage adjustment is required for elderly patients, for patients with mild or moderate renal impairment, or for patients with mild or moderate liver insufficiency. Care should be exercised with dosing of Diovan in patients with hepatic or severe renal impairment. Diovan may be administered with or without food. In **heart failure** patients, consideration should be given to reducing the dose of concomitant diuretics. **Following myocardial infarction,** consideration should be given to a dosage reduction if symptomatic hypotension or renal dysfunction occurs.

Indication	Starting Dose	Dose Range	Target Maintenance Dose*
Adult Hypertension (2.1)	80 or 160 mg once daily	80-320 mg once daily	—
Pediatric Hypertension (6-16 years) (2.1)	1.3 mg/kg once daily (up to 40 mg total)	1.3-2.7 mg/kg once daily (up to 40-160 mg total)	—
Heart Failure (2.2)	40 mg twice daily	40-160 mg twice daily	160 mg twice daily
Post-Myocardial Infarction (2.3)	20 mg twice daily	20-160 mg twice daily	160 mg twice daily

* as tolerated by patient

—————— **DOSAGE FORMS AND STRENGTHS** ——————
Tablets (mg): 40 (scored), 80, 160, 320
—————— **CONTRAINDICATIONS** ——————
None
—————— **WARNINGS AND PRECAUTIONS** ——————
• Avoid fetal or neonatal exposure (5.1)
• Observe for signs and symptoms of hypotension (5.2)
• Use with caution in patients with impaired hepatic (5.3) or renal (5.4) function
—————— **ADVERSE REACTIONS** ——————
Hypertension: Most common adverse reactions are headache, dizziness, viral infection, fatigue and abdominal pain (6.1)
Heart Failure: Most common adverse reactions are dizziness, hypotension, diarrhea, arthralgia, back pain, fatigue and hyperkalemia (6.1)
Post-Myocardial Infarction: Most common adverse reactions which caused patients to discontinue therapy are hypotension, cough and increased blood creatinine (6.1)
To report SUSPECTED ADVERSE REACTIONS, contact Novartis Pharmaceuticals Corporation at 1-888-669-6682 or FDA at 1-800-FDA-1088 or www.fda.gov/medwatch.
—————— **DRUG INTERACTIONS** ——————
Potassium sparing diuretics, potassium supplements or salt substitutes may lead to increases in serum potassium, and in heart failure patients, increases in serum creatinine (7)
—————— **USE IN SPECIFIC POPULATIONS** ——————
Nursing Mothers: Nursing or drug should be discontinued (8.3); **Pediatrics:** Efficacy and safety data support use in 6-16 year old patients (8.4); **Geriatrics:** No overall difference in efficacy or safety vs. younger patients, but greater sensitivity of some older individuals cannot be ruled out (8.5)

See 17 for PATIENT COUNSELING INFORMATION and FDA-approved patient labeling
                                                Revised: 06/2010

FULL PRESCRIBING INFORMATION: CONTENTS*
WARNING: USE IN PREGNANCY
1   **INDICATIONS AND USAGE**
   1.1   Hypertension
   1.2   Heart Failure
   1.3   Post-Myocardial Infarction
2   **DOSAGE AND ADMINISTRATION**
   2.1   Adult Hypertension
   2.2   Pediatric Hypertension 6-16 years of age
   2.3   Heart Failure
   2.4   Post-Myocardial Infarction
3   **DOSAGE FORMS AND STRENGTHS**
4   **CONTRAINDICATIONS**
5   **WARNINGS AND PRECAUTIONS**
   5.1   Fetal/Neonatal Morbidity and Mortality
   5.2   Hypotension
   5.3   Impaired Hepatic Function
   5.4   Impaired Renal Function
6   **ADVERSE REACTIONS**
   6.1   Clinical Studies Experience
   6.2   Post-Marketing Experience
7   **DRUG INTERACTIONS**
   7.1   Clinical Laboratory Test Findings
8   **USE IN SPECIFIC POPULATIONS**
   8.1   Pregnancy
   8.3   Nursing Mothers
   8.4   Pediatric Use
   8.5   Geriatric Use
10 **OVERDOSAGE**
11 **DESCRIPTION**
12 **CLINICAL PHARMACOLOGY**
   12.1 Mechanism of Action
   12.2 Pharmacodynamics
   12.3 Pharmacokinetics
13 **NONCLINICAL TOXICOLOGY**
   13.1 Carcinogenesis, Mutagenesis, Impairment of Fertility
   13.2 Animal Toxicology and/or Pharmacology
14 **CLINICAL STUDIES**
   14.1 Hypertension
   14.2 Heart Failure
   14.3 Post-Myocardial Infarction

16 **HOW SUPPLIED/STORAGE AND HANDLING**
17 **PATIENT COUNSELING INFORMATION**
* Sections or subsections omitted from the full prescribing information are not listed

FULL PRESCRIBING INFORMATION

WARNING: USE IN PREGNANCY
When used in pregnancy, drugs that act directly on the renin-angiotensin system can cause injury and even death to the developing fetus. When pregnancy is detected, Diovan should be discontinued as soon as possible.
See WARNINGS: Fetal/Neonatal Morbidity and Mortality (5.1)

---

1   INDICATIONS AND USAGE
1.1   Hypertension
Diovan® (valsartan) is indicated for the treatment of hypertension. It may be used alone or in combination with other antihypertensive agents.
1.2   Heart Failure
Diovan is indicated for the treatment of heart failure (NYHA class II-IV). In a controlled clinical trial, Diovan significantly reduced hospitalizations for heart failure. There is no evidence that Diovan provides added benefits when it is used with an adequate dose of an ACE inhibitor. *[See Clinical Studies (14.2)]*
1.3   Post-Myocardial Infarction
In clinically stable patients with left ventricular failure or left ventricular dysfunction following myocardial infarction, Diovan is indicated to reduce cardiovascular mortality. *[See Clinical Studies (14.3)]*

2   DOSAGE AND ADMINISTRATION
2.1   Adult Hypertension
The recommended starting dose of Diovan (valsartan) is 80 mg or 160 mg once daily when used as monotherapy in patients who are not volume-depleted. Patients requiring greater reductions may be started at the higher dose. Diovan may be used over a dose range of 80 mg to 320 mg daily, administered once a day.

The antihypertensive effect is substantially present within 2 weeks and maximal reduction is generally attained after 4 weeks. If additional antihypertensive effect is required over the starting dose range, the dose may be increased to a maximum of 320 mg or a diuretic may be added. Addition of a diuretic has a greater effect than dose increases beyond 80 mg.

No initial dosage adjustment is required for elderly patients, for patients with mild or moderate renal impairment, or for patients with mild or moderate liver insufficiency. Care should be exercised with dosing of Diovan in patients with hepatic or severe renal impairment.

Diovan may be administered with other antihypertensive agents.

Diovan may be administered with or without food.

2.2   Pediatric Hypertension 6-16 years of age
For children who can swallow tablets, the usual recommended starting dose is 1.3 mg/kg once daily (up to 40 mg total). The dosage should be adjusted according to blood pressure response. Doses higher than 2.7 mg/kg (up to 160 mg) once daily have not been studied in pediatric patients 6 to 16 years old.

For children who cannot swallow tablets, or children for whom the calculated dosage (mg/kg) does not correspond to the available tablet strengths of Diovan, the use of a suspension is recommended. Follow the suspension preparation instructions below (see **Preparation of Suspension**) to administer valsartan as a suspension. When the suspension is replaced by a tablet, the dose of valsartan may have to be increased. The exposure to valsartan with the suspension is 1.6 times greater than with the tablet.

Diovan is not recommended for treatment of children below the age of 6 years or children of any age with a glomerular filtration rate <30 mL/min/1.73 m^2, as no data are available.

Preparation of Suspension (for 160 mL of a 4 mg/mL suspension)

Add 80 mL of Ora-Plus® oral suspending vehicle to an amber glass bottle containing 8 Diovan 80 mg tablets, and shake for a minimum of 2 minutes. Allow the suspension to stand for a minimum of 1 hour. After the standing time, shake the suspension for a minimum of 1 additional minute. Add 80 mL of Ora-Sweet SF® oral sweetening vehicle to the bottle and shake the suspension for at least 10 seconds to disperse the ingredients. The suspension is homogenous and can be stored for either up to 30 days at room temperature (below 30°C/86°F) or up to 75 days at refrigerated conditions (2-8°C/35-46°F) in the glass bottle with a child-resistant screw-cap closure. Shake the bottle well (at least 10 seconds) prior to dispensing the suspension.

*Ora-Sweet SF® and Ora-Plus® are registered trademarks of Paddock Laboratories, Inc.

2.3   Heart Failure

The recommended starting dose of Diovan is 40 mg twice daily. Uptitration to 80 mg and 160 mg twice daily should be done to the highest dose, as tolerated by the patient. Consideration should be given to reducing the dose of concomitant diuretics. The maximum daily dose administered in clinical trials is 320 mg in divided doses.

2.4   Post-Myocardial Infarction

Diovan may be initiated as early as 12 hours after a myocardial infarction. The recommended starting dose of Diovan is 20 mg twice daily. Patients may be uptitrated within 7 days to 40 mg twice daily, with subsequent titrations to a target maintenance dose of 160 mg twice daily, as tolerated by the patient. If symptomatic hypotension or renal dysfunction occurs, consideration should be given to a dosage reduction. Diovan may be given with other standard post-myocardial infarction treatment, including thrombolytics, aspirin, beta-blockers, and statins.

3   DOSAGE FORMS AND STRENGTHS

40 mg are scored yellow ovaloid tablets with beveled edges, imprinted NVR/DO (Side 1/Side 2)
80 mg are pale red almond-shaped tablets with beveled edges, imprinted NVR/DV
160 mg are grey-orange almond-shaped tablets with beveled edges, imprinted NVR/DX
320 mg are dark grey-violet almond-shaped tablets with beveled edges, imprinted NVR/DXL

4   CONTRAINDICATIONS

None

5   WARNINGS AND PRECAUTIONS

5.1   Fetal/Neonatal Morbidity and Mortality

Diovan can cause fetal harm when administered to a pregnant woman. If this drug is used during pregnancy, or if the patient becomes pregnant while taking this drug, the patient should be apprised of the potential hazard to the fetus. Drugs that act on the renin-angiotensin system can cause fetal and neonatal morbidity and mortality when used in pregnancy. In several dozen published cases, ACE inhibitor use during the second and third trimesters of pregnancy was associated with fetal and neonatal injury, including hypotension, neonatal skull hypoplasia, anuria, reversible or irreversible renal failure, and death. [See Use in Specific Populations (8.1)]

5.2   Hypotension

Excessive hypotension was rarely seen (0.1%) in patients with uncomplicated hypertension treated with Diovan alone. In patients with an activated renin-angiotensin system, such as volume- and/or salt-depleted patients receiving high doses of diuretics, symptomatic hypotension may occur. This condition should be corrected prior to administration of Diovan, or the treatment should start under close medical supervision.

Caution should be observed when initiating therapy in patients with heart failure or post-myocardial infarction patients. Patients with heart failure or post-myocardial infarction patients given Diovan commonly have some reduction in blood pressure, but discontinuation of therapy because of continuing symptomatic hypotension usually is not necessary when dosing instructions are followed. In controlled trials in heart failure patients, the incidence of hypotension in valsartan-treated patients was 5.5% compared to 1.8% in placebo-treated patients. In the Valsartan in Acute Myocardial Infarction Trial (VALIANT), hypotension in post-myocardial infarction patients led to permanent discontinuation of therapy in 1.4% of valsartan-treated patients and 0.8% of captopril-treated patients.

If excessive hypotension occurs, the patient should be placed in the supine position and, if necessary, given an intravenous infusion of normal saline. A transient hypotensive response is not a contraindication to further treatment, which usually can be continued without difficulty once the blood pressure has stabilized.

5.3   Impaired Hepatic Function

As the majority of valsartan is eliminated in the bile, patients with mild-to-moderate hepatic impairment, including

patients with biliary obstructive disorders, showed lower valsartan clearance (higher AUCs). Care should be exercised in administering Diovan to these patients.

5.4   Impaired Renal Function

In studies of ACE inhibitors in hypertensive patients with unilateral or bilateral renal artery stenosis, increases in serum creatinine or blood urea nitrogen have been reported. In a 4-day trial of valsartan in 12 hypertensive patients with unilateral renal artery stenosis, no significant increases in serum creatinine or blood urea nitrogen were observed. There has been no long-term use of Diovan in patients with unilateral or bilateral renal artery stenosis, but an effect similar to that seen with ACE inhibitors should be anticipated.

As a consequence of inhibiting the renin-angiotensin-aldosterone system, changes in renal function may be anticipated in susceptible individuals. In patients with severe heart failure whose renal function may depend on the activity of the renin-angiotensin-aldosterone system, treatment with angiotensin-converting enzyme inhibitors and angiotensin receptor antagonists has been associated with oliguria and/or progressive azotemia and (rarely) with acute renal failure and/or death. Similar outcomes have been reported with Diovan.

Some patients with heart failure have developed increases in blood urea nitrogen, serum creatinine, and potassium. These effects are usually minor and transient, and they are more likely to occur in patients with pre-existing renal impairment. Dosage reduction and/or discontinuation of the diuretic and/or Diovan may be required. In the Valsartan Heart Failure Trial, in which 93% of patients were on concomitant ACE inhibitors, treatment was discontinued for elevations in creatinine or potassium (total of 1.0% on valsartan vs. 0.2% on placebo). In the Valsartan in Acute Myocardial Infarction Trial (VALIANT), discontinuations due to various types of renal dysfunction occurred in 1.1% of valsartan-treated patients and 0.8% of captopril-treated patients. Evaluation of patients with heart failure or post-myocardial infarction should always include assessment of renal function.

6   ADVERSE REACTIONS

6.1   Clinical Studies Experience

Because clinical studies are conducted under widely varying conditions, adverse reactions rates observed in the clinical studies of a drug cannot be directly compared to rates in the clinical studies of another drug and may not reflect the rates observed in practice.

Adult Hypertension

Diovan (valsartan) has been evaluated for safety in more than 4,000 patients, including over 400 treated for over 6 months, and more than 160 for over 1 year. Adverse reactions have generally been mild and transient in nature and have only infrequently required discontinuation of therapy. The overall incidence of adverse reactions with Diovan was similar to placebo.

The overall frequency of adverse reactions was neither dose-related nor related to gender, age, race, or regimen. Discontinuation of therapy due to side effects was required in 2.3% of valsartan patients and 2.0% of placebo patients. The most common reasons for discontinuation of therapy with Diovan were headache and dizziness.

The adverse reactions that occurred in placebo-controlled clinical trials in at least 1% of patients treated with Diovan and at a higher incidence in valsartan (n=2,316) than placebo (n=888) patients included viral infection (3% vs. 2%), fatigue (2% vs. 1%), and abdominal pain (2% vs. 1%).

Headache, dizziness, upper respiratory infection, cough, diarrhea, rhinitis, sinusitis, nausea, pharyngitis, edema, and arthralgia occurred at a more than 1% rate but at about the same incidence in placebo and valsartan patients.

In trials in which valsartan was compared to an ACE inhibitor with or without placebo, the incidence of dry cough was significantly greater in the ACE-inhibitor group (7.9%) than in the groups who received valsartan (2.6%) or placebo (1.5%). In a 129-patient trial limited to patients who had had dry cough when they had previously received ACE inhibitors, the incidences of cough in patients who received valsartan, HCTZ, or lisinopril were 20%, 19%, and 69% respectively (p <0.001).

Dose-related orthostatic effects were seen in less than 1% of patients. An increase in the incidence of dizziness was observed in patients treated with Diovan 320 mg (8%) compared to 10 to 160 mg (2% to 4%).

Diovan has been used concomitantly with hydrochlorothiazide without evidence of clinically important adverse interactions.

Other adverse reactions that occurred in controlled clinical trials of patients treated with Diovan (>0.2% of valsartan patients) are listed below. It cannot be determined whether these events were causally related to Diovan.

Body as a Whole: Allergic reaction and asthenia

Cardiovascular: Palpitations

Dermatologic: Pruritus and rash

Digestive: Constipation, dry mouth, dyspepsia, and flatulence

Musculoskeletal: Back pain, muscle cramps, and myalgia

Neurologic and Psychiatric: Anxiety, insomnia, paresthesia, and somnolence

Respiratory: Dyspnea

Special Senses: Vertigo

Urogenital: Impotence

Other reported events seen less frequently in clinical trials included chest pain, syncope, anorexia, vomiting, and angioedema.

Pediatric Hypertension

No relevant differences were identified between the adverse experience profile for pediatric patients aged 6-16 years and that previously reported for adult patients. Neurocognitive and developmental assessment of pediatric patients aged 6 to 16 years revealed no overall clinically relevant adverse impact after treatment with Diovan for up to one year.

In the one study (n=90) of pediatric patients (1-5 years), two deaths and three cases of on-treatment transaminase elevations were seen in the one-year open-label extension phase. These 5 events occurred in a study population in which patients frequently had significant co-morbidities. A causal relationship to Diovan has not been established.

Heart Failure

The adverse experience profile of Diovan in heart failure patients was consistent with the pharmacology of the drug and the health status of the patients. In the Valsartan Heart Failure Trial, comparing valsartan in total daily doses up to 320 mg (n=2,506) to placebo (n=2,494), 10% of valsartan patients discontinued for adverse reactions vs. 7% of placebo patients.

The table shows adverse reactions in double-blind short-term heart failure trials, including the first 4 months of the Valsartan Heart Failure Trial, with an incidence of at least 2% that were more frequent in valsartan-treated patients than in placebo-treated patients. All patients received standard drug therapy for heart failure, frequently as multiple medications, which could include diuretics, digitalis, beta-blockers, or ACE inhibitors.

	Valsartan (n=3,282)	Placebo (n=2,740)
Dizziness	17%	9%
Hypotension	7%	2%
Diarrhea	5%	4%
Arthralgia	3%	2%
Fatigue	3%	2%
Back Pain	3%	2%
Dizziness, postural	2%	1%
Hyperkalemia	2%	1%
Hypotension, postural	2%	1%

Other adverse reactions with an incidence greater than 1% and greater than placebo included headache NOS, nausea, renal impairment NOS, syncope, blurred vision, upper abdominal pain and vertigo (NOS = not otherwise specified). From the long-term data in the Valsartan Heart Failure Trial, there did not appear to be any significant adverse reactions not previously identified.

Post-Myocardial Infarction

The safety profile of Diovan was consistent with the pharmacology of the drug and the background diseases, cardiovascular risk factors, and clinical course of patients treated in the post-myocardial infarction setting. The table shows the percent of patients discontinued in the valsartan and captopril-treated groups in the Valsartan in Acute Myocardial Infarction Trial (VALIANT) with a rate of at least 0.5% in either of the treatment groups.

	Valsartan (n=4,885)	Captopril (n=4,879)
Discontinuation for adverse reaction	5.8%	7.7%
Adverse reactions		
Hypotension NOS	1.4%	0.8%
Cough	0.6%	2.5%
Blood creatinine increased	0.6%	0.4%
Rash NOS	0.2%	0.6%

6.2   Post-Marketing Experience

The following additional adverse reactions have been reported in post-marketing experience:

Hypersensitivity: There are rare reports of angioedema;

Digestive: Elevated liver enzymes and very rare reports of hepatitis;
Renal: Impaired renal function;
Clinical Laboratory Tests: Hyperkalemia;
Dermatologic: Alopecia;
Blood and Lymphatic: There are very rare reports of thrombocytopenia;
Vascular: Vasculitis.

Rare cases of rhabdomyolysis have been reported in patients receiving angiotensin II receptor blockers.

Because these reactions are reported voluntarily from a population of uncertain size, it is not always possible to reliably estimate their frequency or establish a causal relationship to drug exposure.

7 DRUG INTERACTIONS

No clinically significant pharmacokinetic interactions were observed when Diovan (valsartan) was coadministered with amlodipine, atenolol, cimetidine, digoxin, furosemide, glyburide, hydrochlorothiazide, or indomethacin. The valsartan-atenolol combination was more antihypertensive than either component, but it did not lower the heart rate more than atenolol alone.

Coadministration of valsartan and warfarin did not change the pharmacokinetics of valsartan or the time-course of the anticoagulant properties of warfarin.

CYP 450 Interactions: The enzyme(s) responsible for valsartan metabolism have not been identified but do not seem to be CYP 450 isozymes. The inhibitory or induction potential of valsartan on CYP 450 is also unknown.

Transporters: The results from an *in vitro* study with human liver tissue indicate that valsartan is a substrate of the hepatic uptake transporter OATP1B1 and the hepatic efflux transporter MRP2. Co-administration of inhibitors of the uptake transporter (rifampin, cyclosporine) or efflux transporter (ritonavir) may increase the systemic exposure to valsartan.

As with other drugs that block angiotensin II or its effects, concomitant use of potassium sparing diuretics (e.g., spironolactone, triamterene, amiloride), potassium supplements, or salt substitutes containing potassium may lead to increases in serum potassium and in heart failure patients to increases in serum creatinine.

7.1 Clinical Laboratory Test Findings

In controlled clinical trials, clinically important changes in standard laboratory parameters were rarely associated with administration of Diovan.

Creatinine: Minor elevations in creatinine occurred in 0.8% of patients taking Diovan and 0.6% given placebo in controlled clinical trials of hypertensive patients. In heart failure trials, greater than 50% increases in creatinine were observed in 3.9% of Diovan-treated patients compared to 0.9% of placebo-treated patients. In post-myocardial infarction patients, doubling of serum creatinine was observed in 4.2% of valsartan-treated patients and 3.4% of captopril-treated patients.

Hemoglobin and Hematocrit: Greater than 20% decreases in hemoglobin and hematocrit were observed in 0.4% and 0.8%, respectively, of Diovan patients, compared with 0.1% and 0.1% in placebo-treated patients. One valsartan patient discontinued treatment for microcytic anemia.

Liver Function Tests: Occasional elevations (greater than 150%) of liver chemistries occurred in Diovan-treated patients. Three patients (<0.1%) treated with valsartan discontinued treatment for elevated liver chemistries.

Neutropenia: Neutropenia was observed in 1.9% of patients treated with Diovan and 0.8% of patients treated with placebo.

Serum Potassium: In hypertensive patients, greater than 20% increases in serum potassium were observed in 4.4% of Diovan-treated patients compared to 2.9% of placebo-treated patients. In heart failure patients, greater than 20% increases in serum potassium were observed in 10.0% of Diovan-treated patients compared to 5.1% of placebo-treated patients.

Blood Urea Nitrogen (BUN): In heart failure trials, greater than 50% increases in BUN were observed in 16.6% of Diovan-treated patients compared to 6.3% of placebo-treated patients.

8 USE IN SPECIFIC POPULATIONS

8.1 Pregnancy

Teratogenic Effects: Pregnancy Category D

Diovan, like other drugs that act on the renin-angiotensin system, can cause fetal and neonatal morbidity and death when used during the second or third trimester of pregnancy. Diovan can cause fetal harm when administered to a pregnant woman. If this drug is used during pregnancy, or if the patient becomes pregnant while taking this drug, the patient should be apprised of the potential hazard to the fetus.

Angiotensin II receptor antagonists, like valsartan, and angiotensin converting enzyme (ACE) inhibitors exert similar effects on the renin-angiotensin system. In several dozen published cases, ACE inhibitor use during the second and third trimesters of pregnancy was associated with fetal and neonatal injury, including hypotension, neonatal skull hypoplasia, anuria, reversible or irreversible renal failure, and death. Oligohydramnios was also reported, presumably from decreased fetal renal function. In this setting, oligohydramnios was associated with fetal limb contractures, craniofacial deformation, and hypoplastic lung development. Prematurity, intrauterine growth retardation, and patent ductus arteriosus were also reported, although it is not clear whether these occurrences were due to exposure to the drug. In a retrospective study, first trimester use of ACE inhibitors, a specific class of drugs acting on the renin-angiotensin system, was associated with a potential risk of birth defects.

When pregnancy occurs in a patient using Diovan, the physician should discontinue Diovan treatment as soon as possible. The physician should inform the patient about potential risks to the fetus based on the time of gestational exposure to Diovan (first trimester only or later). If exposure occurs beyond the first trimester, an ultrasound examination should be done.

In rare cases when another antihypertensive agent cannot be used to treat the pregnant patient, serial ultrasound examinations should be performed to assess the intraamniotic environment. Routine fetal testing with non-stress tests, biophysical profiles, and/or contraction stress tests may be appropriate based on gestational age and standards of care in the community. If oligohydramnios occurs in these situations, individualized decisions about continuing or discontinuing Diovan treatment and about pregnancy management should be made by the patient, her physician, and experts in the management of high risk pregnancy. Patients and physicians should be aware that oligohydramnios may not appear until after the fetus has sustained irreversible injury.

Infants with histories of *in utero* exposure to Diovan should be closely observed for hypotension, oliguria, and hyperkalemia. If oliguria occurs, these infants may require blood pressure and renal perfusion support. Exchange transfusion or dialysis may be required to reverse hypotension and/or support decreased renal function.

Healthcare professionals who prescribe drugs acting directly on the renin-angiotensin system should counsel women of childbearing potential about the risks of these agents during pregnancy. *[See Nonclincial Toxicology (13.2)]*

8.3 Nursing Mothers

It is not known whether Diovan is excreted in human milk. Diovan was excreted in the milk of lactating rats; however, animal breast milk drug levels may not accurately reflect human breast milk levels. Because many drugs are excreted into human milk and because of the potential for adverse reactions in nursing infants from Diovan, a decision should be made whether to discontinue nursing or discontinue the drug, taking into account the importance of the drug to the mother.

8.4 Pediatric Use

The antihypertensive effects of Diovan have been evaluated in two randomized, double-blind clinical studies in pediatric patients from 1-5 and 6-16 years of age *[see Clinical Studies (14.1)]*. The pharmacokinetics of Diovan have been evaluated in pediatric patients 1 to 16 years of age *[see Pharmacokinetics, Special Populations, Pediatric (12.3)]*. Diovan was generally well tolerated in children 6-16 years and the adverse experience profile was similar to that described for adults. Diovan is not recommended for pediatric patients under 6 years of age due to safety findings for which a relationship to treatment could not be excluded *[see Adverse Reactions, Pediatric Hypertension (6.1)]*.

Daily oral dosing of neonatal/juvenile rats with valsartan at doses as low as 1 mg/kg/day (about 10% of the maximum recommended pediatric dose on a mg/m^2 basis) from postnatal day 7 to postnatal day 70 produced persistent, irreversible kidney damage. These kidney effects in neonatal rats represent expected exaggerated pharmacological effects that are observed if rats are treated during the first 13 days of life. Since this period coincides with up to 44 weeks after conception in humans, it is not considered to point toward an increased safety concern in 6 to 16 year old children.

Diovan is not recommended for treatment of children with glomerular filtration rates <30 mL/min/1.73 m^2, as no data are available.

8.5 Geriatric Use

In the controlled clinical trials of valsartan, 1,214 (36.2%) of hypertensive patients treated with valsartan were ≥65 years and 265 (7.9%) were ≥75 years. No overall difference in the efficacy or safety of valsartan was observed in this patient population, but greater sensitivity of some older individuals cannot be ruled out.

Of the 2,511 patients with heart failure randomized to valsartan in the Valsartan Heart Failure Trial, 45% (1,141) were 65 years of age or older. In the Valsartan in Acute Myocardial Infarction Trial (VALIANT), 53% (2,596) of the 4,909 patients treated with valsartan and 51% (2,515) of the 4,885 patients treated with valsartan + captopril were 65 years of age or older. There were no notable differences in efficacy or safety between older and younger patients in either trial.

10 OVERDOSAGE

Limited data are available related to overdosage in humans. The most likely manifestations of overdosage would be hypotension and tachycardia; bradycardia could occur from parasympathetic (vagal) stimulation. Depressed level of consciousness, circulatory collapse and shock have been reported. If symptomatic hypotension should occur, supportive treatment should be instituted.

Diovan (valsartan) is not removed from the plasma by hemodialysis.

Valsartan was without grossly observable adverse effects at single oral doses up to 2000 mg/kg in rats and up to 1000 mg/kg in marmosets, except for salivation and diarrhea in the rat and vomiting in the marmoset at the highest dose (60 and 31 times, respectively, the maximum recommended human dose on a mg/m^2 basis). (Calculations assume an oral dose of 320 mg/day and a 60-kg patient.)

11 DESCRIPTION

Diovan (valsartan) is a nonpeptide, orally active, and specific angiotensin II receptor blocker acting on the AT$_1$ receptor subtype.

Valsartan is chemically described as *N*-(1-oxopentyl)-*N*-[[2′-(1*H*-tetrazol-5-yl) [1,1′-biphenyl]-4-yl]methyl]-L-valine. Its empirical formula is $C_{24}H_{29}N_5O_3$, its molecular weight is 435.5, and its structural formula is

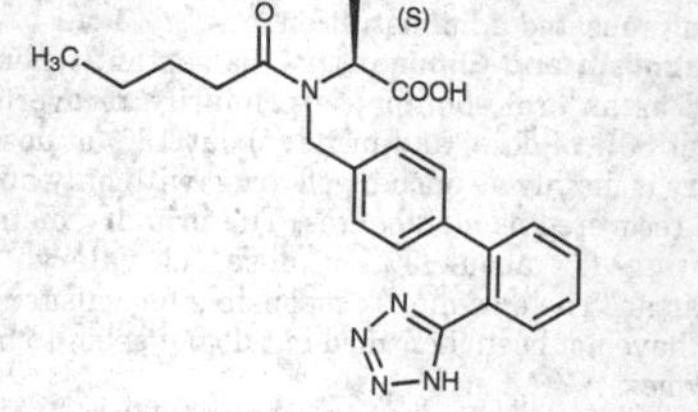

Valsartan is a white to practically white fine powder. It is soluble in ethanol and methanol and slightly soluble in water.

Diovan is available as tablets for oral administration, containing 40 mg, 80 mg, 160 mg or 320 mg of valsartan. The inactive ingredients of the tablets are colloidal silicon dioxide, crospovidone, hydroxypropyl methylcellulose, iron oxides (yellow, black and/or red), magnesium stearate, microcrystalline cellulose, polyethylene glycol 8000, and titanium dioxide.

12 CLINICAL PHARMACOLOGY

12.1 Mechanism of Action

Angiotensin II is formed from angiotensin I in a reaction catalyzed by angiotensin-converting enzyme (ACE, kininase II). Angiotensin II is the principal pressor agent of the renin-angiotensin system, with effects that include vasoconstriction, stimulation of synthesis and release of aldosterone, cardiac stimulation, and renal reabsorption of sodium. Diovan (valsartan) blocks the vasoconstrictor and aldosterone-secreting effects of angiotensin II by selectively blocking the binding of angiotensin II to the AT$_1$ receptor in many tissues, such as vascular smooth muscle and the adrenal gland. Its action is therefore independent of the pathways for angiotensin II synthesis.

There is also an AT$_2$ receptor found in many tissues, but AT$_2$ is not known to be associated with cardiovascular homeostasis. Valsartan has much greater affinity (about 20,000-fold) for the AT$_1$ receptor than for the AT$_2$ receptor. The increased plasma levels of angiotensin II following AT$_1$ receptor blockade with valsartan may stimulate the unblocked AT$_2$ receptor. The primary metabolite of valsartan is essentially inactive with an affinity for the AT$_1$ receptor about one-200th that of valsartan itself.

Blockade of the renin-angiotensin system with ACE inhibitors, which inhibit the biosynthesis of angiotensin II from angiotensin I, is widely used in the treatment of hypertension. ACE inhibitors also inhibit the degradation of bradykinin, a reaction also catalyzed by ACE. Because valsartan does not inhibit ACE (kininase II), it does not affect the response to bradykinin. Whether this difference has clinical relevance is not yet known. Valsartan does not bind to or block other hormone receptors or ion channels known to be important in cardiovascular regulation.

Blockade of the angiotensin II receptor inhibits the negative regulatory feedback of angiotensin II on renin secretion, but the resulting increased plasma renin activity and angiotensin II circulating levels do not overcome the effect of valsartan on blood pressure.

12.2 Pharmacodynamics

Valsartan inhibits the pressor effect of angiotensin II infusions. An oral dose of 80 mg inhibits the pressor effect by about 80% at peak with approximately 30% inhibition persisting for 24 hours. No information on the effect of larger doses is available.

Removal of the negative feedback of angiotensin II causes a 2- to 3-fold rise in plasma renin and consequent rise in angiotensin II plasma concentration in hypertensive patients. Minimal decreases in plasma aldosterone were observed after administration of valsartan; very little effect on serum potassium was observed.

In multiple-dose studies in hypertensive patients with stable renal insufficiency and patients with renovascular hypertension, valsartan had no clinically significant effects on glomerular filtration rate, filtration fraction, creatinine clearance, or renal plasma flow.

In multiple-dose studies in hypertensive patients, valsartan had no notable effects on total cholesterol, fasting triglycerides, fasting serum glucose, or uric acid.

12.3 Pharmacokinetics

Valsartan peak plasma concentration is reached 2 to 4 hours after dosing. Valsartan shows bi-exponential decay kinetics following intravenous administration, with an average elimination half-life of about 6 hours. Absolute bioavailability for Diovan is about 25% (range 10%-35%). The bioavailability of the suspension (see [2.2] Dosage and Administration; Pediatric Hypertension) is 1.6 times greater than with the tablet. With the tablet, food decreases the exposure (as measured by AUC) to valsartan by about 40% and peak plasma concentration (C_{max}) by about 50%. AUC and C_{max} values of valsartan increase approximately linearly with increasing dose over the clinical dosing range. Valsartan does not accumulate appreciably in plasma following repeated administration.

Metabolism and Elimination: Valsartan, when administered as an oral solution, is primarily recovered in feces (about 83% of dose) and urine (about 13% of dose). The recovery is mainly as unchanged drug, with only about 20% of dose recovered as metabolites. The primary metabolite, accounting for about 9% of dose, is valeryl 4-hydroxy valsartan. The enzyme(s) responsible for valsartan metabolism have not been identified but do not seem to be CYP 450 isozymes.

Following intravenous administration, plasma clearance of valsartan is about 2 L/h and its renal clearance is 0.62 L/h (about 30% of total clearance).

Distribution: The steady state volume of distribution of valsartan after intravenous administration is small (17 L), indicating that valsartan does not distribute into tissues extensively. Valsartan is highly bound to serum proteins (95%), mainly serum albumin.

Special Populations:

Pediatric: In a study of pediatric hypertensive patients (n=26, 1-16 years of age) given single doses of a suspension of Diovan (mean: 0.9 to 2 mg/kg), the clearance (L/h/kg) of valsartan for children was similar to that of adults receiving the same formulation.

Geriatric: Exposure (measured by AUC) to valsartan is higher by 70% and the half-life is longer by 35% in the elderly than in the young. No dosage adjustment is necessary [see Dosage and Administration (2.1)].

Gender: Pharmacokinetics of valsartan does not differ significantly between males and females.

Heart Failure: The average time to peak concentration and elimination half-life of valsartan in heart failure patients are similar to that observed in healthy volunteers. AUC and C_{max} values of valsartan increase linearly and are almost proportional with increasing dose over the clinical dosing range (40 to 160 mg twice a day). The average accumulation factor is about 1.7. The apparent clearance of valsartan following oral administration is approximately 4.5 L/h. Age does not affect the apparent clearance in heart failure patients.

Renal Insufficiency: There is no apparent correlation between renal function (measured by creatinine clearance) and exposure (measured by AUC) to valsartan in patients with different degrees of renal impairment. Consequently, dose adjustment is not required in patients with mild-to-moderate renal dysfunction. No studies have been performed in patients with severe impairment of renal function (creatinine clearance <10 mL/min). Valsartan is not removed from the plasma by hemodialysis. In the case of severe renal disease, exercise care with dosing of valsartan [see Dosage and Administration (2.1)].

Hepatic Insufficiency: On average, patients with mild-to-moderate chronic liver disease have twice the exposure (measured by AUC values) to valsartan of healthy volunteers (matched by age, sex and weight). In general, no dosage adjustment is needed in patients with mild-to-moderate liver disease. Care should be exercised in patients with liver disease [see Dosage and Administration (2.1)].

13 NONCLINICAL TOXICOLOGY

13.1 Carcinogenesis, Mutagenesis, Impairment of Fertility

There was no evidence of carcinogenicity when valsartan was administered in the diet to mice and rats for up to 2 years at doses up to 160 and 200 mg/kg/day, respectively. These doses in mice and rats are about 2.6 and 6 times, respectively, the maximum recommended human dose on a mg/m^2 basis. (Calculations assume an oral dose of 320 mg/day and a 60-kg patient.)

Mutagenicity assays did not reveal any valsartan-related effects at either the gene or chromosome level. These assays included bacterial mutagenicity tests with Salmonella (Ames) and E coli; a gene mutation test with Chinese hamster V79 cells; a cytogenetic test with Chinese hamster ovary cells; and a rat micronucleus test.

Valsartan had no adverse effects on the reproductive performance of male or female rats at oral doses up to 200 mg/kg/day. This dose is 6 times the maximum recommended human dose on a mg/m^2 basis. (Calculations assume an oral dose of 320 mg/day and a 60-kg patient.)

13.2 Animal Toxicology and/or Pharmacology Reproductive Toxicology Studies

No teratogenic effects were observed when valsartan was administered to pregnant mice and rats at oral doses up to 600 mg/kg/day and to pregnant rabbits at oral doses up to 10 mg/kg/day. However, significant decreases in fetal weight, pup birth weight, pup survival rate, and slight delays in developmental milestones were observed in studies in which parental rats were treated with valsartan at oral, maternally toxic (reduction in body weight gain and food consumption) doses of 600 mg/kg/day during organogenesis or late gestation and lactation. In rabbits, fetotoxicity (i.e., resorptions, litter loss, abortions, and low body weight) associated with maternal toxicity (mortality) was observed at doses of 5 and 10 mg/kg/day. The no observed adverse effect doses of 600, 200 and 2 mg/kg/day in mice, rats and rabbits represent 9, 6, and 0.1 times, respectively, the maximum recommended human dose on a mg/m^2 basis. Calculations assume an oral dose of 320 mg/day and a 60-kg patient.

14 CLINICAL STUDIES

14.1 Hypertension

Adult Hypertension

The antihypertensive effects of Diovan (valsartan) were demonstrated principally in 7 placebo-controlled, 4- to 12-week trials (one in patients over 65) of dosages from 10 to 320 mg/day in patients with baseline diastolic blood pressures of 95-115. The studies allowed comparison of once-daily and twice-daily regimens of 160 mg/day; comparison of peak and trough effects; comparison (in pooled data) of response by gender, age, and race; and evaluation of incremental effects of hydrochlorothiazide.

Administration of valsartan to patients with essential hypertension results in a significant reduction of sitting, supine, and standing systolic and diastolic blood pressure, usually with little or no orthostatic change.

In most patients, after administration of a single oral dose, onset of antihypertensive activity occurs at approximately 2 hours, and maximum reduction of blood pressure is achieved within 6 hours. The antihypertensive effect persists for 24 hours after dosing, but there is a decrease from peak effect at lower doses (40 mg) presumably reflecting loss of inhibition of angiotensin II. At higher doses, however (160 mg), there is little difference in peak and trough effect. During repeated dosing, the reduction in blood pressure with any dose is substantially present within 2 weeks, and maximal reduction is generally attained after 4 weeks. In long-term follow-up studies (without placebo control), the effect of valsartan appeared to be maintained for up to two years. The antihypertensive effect is independent of age, gender or race. The latter finding regarding race is based on pooled data and should be viewed with caution, because antihypertensive drugs that affect the renin-angiotensin system (that is, ACE inhibitors and angiotensin-II blockers)

have generally been found to be less effective in low-renin hypertensives (frequently blacks) than in high-renin hypertensives (frequently whites). In pooled, randomized, controlled trials of Diovan that included a total of 140 blacks and 830 whites, valsartan and an ACE-inhibitor control were generally at least as effective in blacks as whites. The explanation for this difference from previous findings is unclear.

Abrupt withdrawal of valsartan has not been associated with a rapid increase in blood pressure.

The blood pressure lowering effect of valsartan and thiazide-type diuretics are approximately additive.

The 7 studies of valsartan monotherapy included over 2,000 patients randomized to various doses of valsartan and about 800 patients randomized to placebo. Doses below 80 mg were not consistently distinguished from those of placebo at trough, but doses of 80, 160 and 320 mg produced dose-related decreases in systolic and diastolic blood pressure, with the difference from placebo of approximately 6-9/3-5 mmHg at 80-160 mg and 9/6 mmHg at 320 mg. In a controlled trial the addition of HCTZ to valsartan 80 mg resulted in additional lowering of systolic and diastolic blood pressure by approximately 6/3 and 12/5 mmHg for 12.5 and 25 mg of HCTZ, respectively, compared to valsartan 80 mg alone.

Patients with an inadequate response to 80 mg once daily were titrated to either 160 mg once daily or 80 mg twice daily, which resulted in a comparable response in both groups.

In controlled trials, the antihypertensive effect of once-daily valsartan 80 mg was similar to that of once-daily enalapril 20 mg or once-daily lisinopril 10 mg.

There was essentially no change in heart rate in valsartan-treated patients in controlled trials.

Pediatric Hypertension

The antihypertensive effects of Diovan were evaluated in two randomized, double-blind clinical studies.

In a clinical study involving 261 hypertensive pediatric patients 6 to 16 years of age, patients who weighed <35 kg received 10, 40 or 80 mg of valsartan daily (low, medium and high doses), and patients who weighed ≥35 kg received 20, 80, and 160 mg of valsartan daily (low, medium and high doses). Renal and urinary disorders, and essential hypertension with or without obesity were the most common underlying causes of hypertension in children enrolled in this study. At the end of 2 weeks, valsartan reduced both systolic and diastolic blood pressure in a dose-dependent manner. Overall, the three dose levels of valsartan (low, medium and high) significantly reduced systolic blood pressure by -8, -10, -12 mmHg from the baseline, respectively. Patients were re-randomized to either continue receiving the same dose of valsartan or were switched to placebo. In patients who continued to receive the medium and high doses of valsartan, systolic blood pressure at trough was -4 and -7 mmHg lower than patients who received the placebo treatment. In patients receiving the low dose of valsartan, systolic blood pressure at trough was similar to that of patients who received the placebo treatment. Overall, the dose-dependent antihypertensive effect of valsartan was consistent across all the demographic subgroups.

In a clinical study involving 90 hypertensive pediatric patients 1 to 5 years of age with a similar study design, there was some evidence of effectiveness, but safety findings for which a relationship to treatment could not be excluded mitigate against recommending use in this age group [see Adverse Reactions (6.1)].

14.2 Heart Failure

The Valsartan Heart Failure Trial (Val-HeFT) was a multinational, double-blind study in which 5,010 patients with NYHA class II (62%) to IV (2%) heart failure and LVEF <40%, on baseline therapy chosen by their physicians, were randomized to placebo or valsartan (titrated from 40 mg twice daily to the highest tolerated dose or 160 mg twice daily) and followed for a mean of about 2 years. Although Val-HeFT's primary goal was to examine the effect of valsartan when added to an ACE inhibitor, about 7% were not receiving an ACE inhibitor. Other background therapy included diuretics (86%), digoxin (67%), and beta-blockers (36%). The population studied was 80% male, 46% 65 years or older and 89% Caucasian. At the end of the trial, patients in the valsartan group had a blood pressure that was 4 mmHg systolic and 2 mmHg diastolic lower than the placebo group. There were two primary end points, both assessed as time to first event: all-cause mortality and heart failure morbidity, the latter defined as all-cause mortality, sudden death with resuscitation, hospitalization for heart failure, and the need for intravenous inotropic or vasodilatory drugs for at least 4 hours. These results are summarized in the table below.

[See table at left]

Although the overall morbidity result favored valsartan, this result was largely driven by the 7% of patients not receiving an ACE inhibitor, as shown in the following table.

[See first table at top of next page]

	Placebo (N=2,499)	Valsartan (N=2,511)	Hazard Ratio (95% CI*)	Nominal p-value
All-cause mortality	484 (19.4%)	495 (19.7%)	1.02 (0.90-1.15)	0.8
HF morbidity	801 (32.1%)	723 (28.8%)	0.87 (0.79-0.97)	0.009

*CI = Confidence Interval

The modest favorable trend in the group receiving an ACE inhibitor was largely driven by the patients receiving less than the recommended dose of ACE inhibitor. Thus, there is little evidence of further clinical benefit when valsartan is added to an adequate dose of ACE inhibitor.

Secondary end points in the subgroup not receiving ACE inhibitors were as follows.

[See second table at right]

In patients not receiving an ACE inhibitor, valsartan-treated patients had an increase in ejection fraction and reduction in left ventricular internal diastolic diameter (LVIDD).

Effects were generally consistent across subgroups defined by age and gender for the population of patients not receiving an ACE inhibitor. The number of black patients was small and does not permit a meaningful assessment in this subset of patients.

14.3 Post-Myocardial Infarction

The VALsartan In Acute myocardial iNfarcTion trial (VALIANT) was a randomized, controlled, multinational, double-blind study in 14,703 patients with acute myocardial infarction and either heart failure (signs, symptoms or radiological evidence) or left ventricular systolic dysfunction (ejection fraction ≤40% by radionuclide ventriculography or ≤35% by echocardiography or ventricular contrast angiography). Patients were randomized within 12 hours to 10 days after the onset of myocardial infarction symptoms to one of three treatment groups: valsartan (titrated from 20 or 40 mg twice daily to the highest tolerated dose up to a maximum of 160 mg twice daily), the ACE inhibitor, captopril (titrated from 6.25 mg three times daily to the highest tolerated dose up to a maximum of 50 mg three times daily), or the combination of valsartan plus captopril. In the combination group, the dose of valsartan was titrated from 20 mg twice daily to the highest tolerated dose up to a maximum of 80 mg twice daily; the dose of captopril was the same as for monotherapy. The population studied was 69% male, 94% Caucasian, and 53% were 65 years of age or older. Baseline therapy included aspirin (91%), beta-blockers (70%), ACE inhibitors (40%), thrombolytics (35%) and statins (34%). The mean treatment duration was two years. The mean daily dose of Diovan in the monotherapy group was 217 mg.

The primary endpoint was time to all-cause mortality. Secondary endpoints included (1) time to cardiovascular (CV) mortality, and (2) time to the first event of cardiovascular mortality, reinfarction, or hospitalization for heart failure. The results are summarized in the table below:

[See third table at right]

There was no difference in overall mortality among the three treatment groups. There was thus no evidence that combining the ACE inhibitor captopril and the angiotensin II blocker valsartan was of value.

The data were assessed to see whether the effectiveness of valsartan could be demonstrated by showing in a non-inferiority analysis that it preserved a fraction of the effect of captopril, a drug with a demonstrated survival effect in this setting. A conservative estimate of the effect of captopril (based on a pooled analysis of 3 post-infarction studies of captopril and 2 other ACE inhibitors) was a 14-16% reduction in mortality compared to placebo. Valsartan would be considered effective if it preserved a meaningful fraction of that effect and unequivocally preserved some of that effect. As shown in the table, the upper bound of the CI for the hazard ratio (valsartan/captopril) for overall or CV mortality is 1.09-1.11, a difference of 9-11%, thus making it unlikely that valsartan has less than about half of the estimated effect of captopril and clearly demonstrating an effect of valsartan. The other secondary endpoints were consistent with this conclusion.

Effects on Mortality Amongst Subgroups in VALIANT

Subgroups	Patient (%)
All Patients	100.0
< 65 y	47.0
≥ 65 y	53.0
Male	68.6
Female	31.4
Caucasian	93.7
Non-Caucasian	6.3
US	27.0
Non-US	73.0
Beta-blocker	70.4
Beta-blocker (No)	29.6

0.5 (Favors Valsartan) — 1.0 — 1.5 (Favors Captopril)

Valsartan vs. Captopril

There were no clear differences in all-cause mortality based on age, gender, race, or baseline therapies, as shown in the figure above.

	Without ACE Inhibitor		With ACE Inhibitor	
	Placebo (N=181)	Valsartan (N=185)	Placebo (N=2,318)	Valsartan (N=2,326)
Events (%)	77 (42.5%)	46 (24.9%)	724 (31.2%)	677 (29.1%)
Hazard ratio (95% CI)	0.51 (0.35, 0.73)		0.92 (0.82, 1.02)	
p-value	0.0002		0.0965	

	Placebo (N=181)	Valsartan (N=185)	Hazard Ratio (95% CI)
Components of HF morbidity			
All-cause mortality	49 (27.1%)	32 (17.3%)	0.59 (0.37, 0.91)
Sudden death with resuscitation	2 (1.1%)	1 (0.5%)	0.47 (0.04, 5.20)
CHF therapy	1 (0.6%)	0 (0.0%)	
CHF hospitalization	48 (26.5%)	24 (13.0%)	0.43 (0.27, 0.71)
Cardiovascular mortality	40 (22.1%)	29 (15.7%)	0.65 (0.40, 1.05)
Non-fatal morbidity	49 (27.1%)	24 (13.0%)	0.42 (0.26, 0.69)

	Valsartan vs. Captopril (N=4,909) (N=4,909)			Valsartan + Captopril vs. Captopril (N=4,885) (N=4,909)		
	No. of Deaths Valsartan/Captopril	Hazard Ratio CI	p-value	No. of Deaths Comb/Captopril	Hazard Ratio CI	p-value
All-cause mortality	979 (19.9%)/ 958 (19.5%)	1.001 (0.902, 1.111)	0.98	941 (19.3%)/ 958 (19.5%)	0.984 (0.886, 1.093)	0.73
CV mortality	827 (16.8%)/ 830 (16.9%)	0.976 (0.875, 1.090)				
CV mortality, hospitalization for HF, and recurrent non-fatal MI	1,529 (31.1%)/ 1,567 (31.9%)	0.995 (0.881, 1.035)				

Tablet	Color	Deboss		NDC 0078-####-##					
		Side 1	Side 2	30	90	Bottle of 3500	7000	14000	Blister Packages of 100
40 mg	Yellow	NVR	DO	0423-15	–	–	–	–	0423-06
80 mg	Pale red	NVR	DV	–	0358-34	–	–	0358-33	0358-06
160 mg	Grey-orange	NVR	DX	–	0359-34	–	0359-17	–	0359-06
320 mg	Dark grey-violet	NVR	DXL	–	0360-34	0360-11	–	–	0360-06

16 HOW SUPPLIED/STORAGE AND HANDLING

Diovan (valsartan) is available as tablets containing valsartan 40 mg, 80 mg, 160 mg, or 320 mg. All strengths are packaged in bottles and unit dose blister packages (10 strips of 10 tablets) as described below.

40 mg tablets are scored on one side and ovaloid with bevelled edges. 80 mg, 160 mg, and 320 mg tablets are unscored and almond-shaped with bevelled edges.

[See fourth table above]

Store at 25°C (77°F); excursions permitted to 15-30°C (59-86°F) [see USP Controlled Room Temperature].

Protect from moisture.

Dispense in tight container (USP).

17 PATIENT COUNSELING INFORMATION

Information for Patients

Pregnancy: Female patients of childbearing age should be told that use of drugs like Diovan that act on the renin-angiotensin system during pregnancy can cause serious problems in the fetus and infant including: low blood pressure, poor development of skull bones, kidney failure and death. Women using Diovan who become pregnant should notify their physician as soon as possible.

DIOVAN (DYE′-o-van)

(valsartan) **Tablets**

Read the Patient Information that comes with DIOVAN before you take it and each time you get a refill. There may be new information. This leaflet does not take the place of talking with your doctor about your medical condition or treatment. If you have any questions about DIOVAN, ask your doctor or pharmacist.

What is the most important information I should know about DIOVAN?

Taking DIOVAN during pregnancy can cause injury and even death to your unborn baby. If you get pregnant, stop taking DIOVAN and call your doctor right away. Talk to your doctor about other ways to lower your blood pressure if you plan to become pregnant.

What is DIOVAN?

DIOVAN is a prescription medicine called an angiotensin receptor blocker (ARB). It is used in adults to:

• lower high blood pressure (hypertension) in adults and children, 6 to 16 years of age.

• treat heart failure in adults. In these patients, DIOVAN may lower the need for hospitalization that happens from heart failure.

• improve the chance of living longer after a heart attack (myocardial infarction) in adults.

DIOVAN is not for children under 6 years of age or children with certain kidney problems.

High Blood Pressure (Hypertension). Blood pressure is the force in your blood vessels when your heart beats and when your heart rests. You have high blood pressure when the force is too much. DIOVAN can help your blood vessels relax so your blood pressure is lower.

High blood pressure makes the heart work harder to pump blood throughout the body and causes damage to the blood vessels. If high blood pressure is not treated, it can lead to stroke, heart attack, heart failure, kidney failure and vision problems.

Heart Failure occurs when the heart is weak and cannot pump enough blood to your lungs and the rest of your body. Just walking or moving can make you short of breath, so you may have to rest a lot.

Heart Attack (Myocardial Infarction): A heart attack is caused by a blocked artery that results in damage to the heart muscle.

What should I tell my doctor before taking DIOVAN?

Tell your doctor about all your medical conditions including whether you:

• have any allergies. See the end of this leaflet for a complete list of ingredients in DIOVAN.

• have a heart condition

• have liver problems

• have kidney problems

- **are pregnant or planning to become pregnant.** See "What is the most important information I should know about DIOVAN?"
- **are breast-feeding.** It is not known if DIOVAN passes into your breast milk. You and your doctor should decide if you will take DIOVAN or breast-feed, but not both. Talk with your doctor about the best way to feed your baby if you take DIOVAN.

Tell your doctor about all the medicines you take including prescription and nonprescription medicines, vitamins and herbal supplements. Especially tell your doctor if you take:
- other medicines for high blood pressure or a heart problem
- water pills (also called "diuretics")
- potassium supplements
- a salt substitute

Know the medicines you take. Keep a list of your medicines with you to show to your doctor and pharmacist when a new medicine is prescribed. Talk to your doctor or pharmacist before you start taking any new medicine. Your doctor or pharmacist will know what medicines are safe to take together.

How should I take DIOVAN?
- Take DIOVAN exactly as prescribed by your doctor.
- For treatment of high blood pressure, take DIOVAN one time each day, at the same time each day.
- If your child cannot swallow tablets, or if tablets are not available in the prescribed strength, your pharmacist will mix DIOVAN as a liquid suspension for your child. If your child switches between taking the tablet and the suspension, your doctor will adjust the dose as needed. Shake the bottle of suspension well for at least 10 seconds before pouring the dose of medicine to give to your child.
- For adult patients with heart failure or who have had a heart attack, take DIOVAN two times each day, at the same time each day. Your doctor may start you on a low dose of DIOVAN and may increase the dose during your treatment.
- DIOVAN can be taken with or without food.
- If you miss a dose, take it as soon as you remember. If it is close to your next dose, do not take the missed dose. Take the next dose at your regular time.
- If you take too much DIOVAN, call your doctor or Poison Control Center, or go to the nearest hospital emergency room.

What are the possible side effects of DIOVAN?
DIOVAN may cause the following serious side effects:
Injury or death to an unborn baby. See "What is the most important information I should know about DIOVAN?"
Low Blood Pressure (Hypotension). Low blood pressure is most likely to happen if you also take water pills, are on a low-salt diet, get dialysis treatments, have heart problems, or get sick with vomiting or diarrhea. Lie down, if you feel faint or dizzy. Call your doctor right away.
Kidney problems. Kidney problems may get worse in people that already have kidney disease. Some people will have changes on blood tests for kidney function and may need a lower dose of DIOVAN. Call your doctor if you get swelling in your feet, ankles, or hands, or unexplained weight gain. If you have heart failure, your doctor should check your kidney function before prescribing DIOVAN.
The most common side effects of DIOVAN used to treat people with high blood pressure include:
- headache
- dizziness
- flu symptoms
- tiredness
- stomach (abdominal) pain

Side effects were generally mild and brief. They generally have not caused patients to stop taking DIOVAN.
The most common side effects of DIOVAN used to treat people with heart failure include:
- dizziness
- low blood pressure
- diarrhea
- joint and back pain
- tiredness
- high blood potassium

Common side effects of DIOVAN used to treat people after a heart attack which caused them to stop taking the drug include:
- low blood pressure
- cough
- high blood creatinine (decreased kidney function)
- rash

Tell your doctor if you get any side effect that bothers you or that does not go away.
These are not all the possible side effects of DIOVAN. For a complete list, ask your doctor or pharmacist.

How do I store DIOVAN?
- Store DIOVAN tablets at room temperature between 59° to 86°F (15°C-30°C).
- Keep DIOVAN tablets in a closed container in a dry place.

- Store bottles of DIOVAN suspension at room temperature less than 86°F (30°C) for up to 30 days, or refrigerate between 35°F-46°F (2°C-8°C) for up to 75 days.
- Keep DIOVAN and all medicines out of the reach of children.

General information about DIOVAN
Medicines are sometimes prescribed for conditions that are not mentioned in patient information leaflets. Do not use DIOVAN for a condition for which it was not prescribed. Do not give DIOVAN to other people, even if they have the same symptoms you have. It may harm them.
This leaflet summarizes the most important information about DIOVAN. If you would like more information, talk with your doctor. You can ask your doctor or pharmacist for information about DIOVAN that is written for health professionals.
For more information about DIOVAN, ask your pharmacist or doctor, visit www.DIOVAN.com on the Internet, or call **1-866-404-6361.**

What are the ingredients in DIOVAN?
Active ingredient: valsartan
Inactive ingredients: colloidal silicon dioxide, crospovidone, hydroxypropyl methylcellulose, iron oxides (yellow, black and/or red), magnesium stearate, microcrystalline cellulose, polyethylene glycol 8000, and titanium dioxide
T2010-13/T2007-110

Distributed by:
Novartis Pharmaceuticals Corp.
East Hanover, NJ 07936
©Novartis

Shown in Product Identification Guide, page 314

DIOVAN HCT®   ℞
[*DYE´-o-van HCT*]
(valsartan and hydrochlorothiazide, USP)
Tablets

The following prescribing information is based on official labeling in effect July 2010.
HIGHLIGHTS OF PRESCRIBING INFORMATION
These highlights do not include all the information needed to use Diovan Hct safely and effectively. See full prescribing information for Diovan Hct.
Diovan Hct® *(valsartan and hydrochlorothiazide, USP)*
Tablets
Initial U.S. Approval: 1998

> **WARNING: AVOID USE IN PREGNANCY**
> *See full prescribing information for complete boxed warning.*
> **When pregnancy is detected, discontinue Diovan Hct as soon as possible. Drugs that act directly on the renin-angiotensin system can cause injury and even death to the developing fetus. (5.1)**

————RECENT MAJOR CHANGES————
Indications and Usage (1)   7/2008
Dosage and Administration, Initial Therapy (2.4)   7/2008
Warnings and Precautions: Avoid Use
    in Pregnancy   9/2007
————INDICATIONS AND USAGE————
Diovan Hct is the combination tablet of valsartan (Diovan), an angiotensin II receptor blocker (ARB) and hydrochlorothiazide (HCTZ), a diuretic. Diovan Hct is indicated for the treatment of hypertension:
- In patients not adequately controlled with monotherapy (1)
- As initial therapy in patients likely to need multiple drugs to achieve their blood pressure goals (1)
————DOSAGE AND ADMINISTRATION————
General considerations:
- Maximum effects within 2 to 4 weeks after dose change (2.1)
- Renal impairment: Not recommended for patients with severe renal impairment (creatinine clearance ≤30 mL/min) (2.1, 5.8)
- Diovan Hct may be administered with or without food
Hypertension:
- **Add-on therapy** OR **Initial therapy:** Initiate with 160/12.5 mg. Titrate upwards as needed to a maximum dose of 320/25 mg. One tablet daily (2.2, 2.4)
- **Replacement therapy:** May be substituted for titrated components (2.3)
————DOSAGE FORMS AND STRENGTHS————
Tablets (valsartan/HCTZ mg): 80/12.5, 160/12.5, 160/25, 320/12.5, 320/25
————CONTRAINDICATIONS————
Anuria; Hypersensitivity to any sulfonamide-derived drugs (4)
————WARNINGS AND PRECAUTIONS————
- Avoid fetal or neonatal exposure (5.1)
- Symptomatic hypotension with volume- and/or salt-

depletion. Correct volume-depletion prior to administration. Not recommended as initial therapy in volume-depleted patients (2.4, 5.2)
- Use with caution in patients with impaired hepatic (5.3) or renal (5.8) function
- Observe for signs of fluid or electrolyte imbalance (5.7)
- Thiazide diuretics may cause an exacerbation or activation of systemic lupus erythematosus (5.5)
————ADVERSE REACTIONS————
The most common reasons for discontinuation of therapy with Diovan HCT were headache and dizziness. The only adverse experience that occurred in ≥2% of patients treated with Diovan HCT and at a higher incidence than placebo was nasopharyngitis (2.4% vs. 1.9%) (6.1)
To report SUSPECTED ADVERSE REACTIONS, contact Novartis Pharmaceuticals Corporation at 1-888-669-6682 or FDA at 1-800-FDA-1088 or www.fda.gov/medwatch
————DRUG INTERACTIONS————
Hydrochlorothiazide (7):
- Alcohol, barbiturates, narcotics: Potentiation of orthostatic hypotension
- Antidiabetic drugs: Dosage adjustment of antidiabetic may be required
- Cholestyramine and colestipol: Reduced absorption of thiazides
- Corticosteroids, Adrenocorticotrophic Hormone (ACTH): Hypokalemia, electrolyte depletion
- Lithium: Reduced renal clearance and high risk of lithium toxicity when used with diuretics. Should not be given with diuretics
- Non-Steroidal Anti-Inflammatory Drugs (NSAIDs): Can reduce diuretic, natriuretic and antihypertensive effects of diuretics. Observe patient closely.
————USE IN SPECIFIC POPULATIONS————
Nursing Mothers: Nursing or drug should be discontinued (8.3)
See 17 for PATIENT COUNSELING INFORMATION and FDA-Approved Patient Labeling
Revised: 04/2010

FULL PRESCRIBING INFORMATION: CONTENTS*
WARNING: AVOID USE IN PREGNANCY

*Sections or subsections omitted from the full prescribing information are not listed

FULL PRESCRIBING INFORMATION

> **WARNING: AVOID USE IN PREGNANCY**
> **When pregnancy is detected, discontinue Diovan Hct® as soon as possible. Drugs that act directly on the**

renin-angiotensin system can cause injury and even death to the developing fetus [see *Warnings and Precautions (5.1)*].

1 INDICATIONS AND USAGE

Diovan HCT (valsartan and hydrochlorothiazide, USP) is indicated for the treatment of hypertension.

Diovan HCT may be used in patients whose blood pressure is not adequately controlled on monotherapy.

Diovan HCT may be used as initial therapy in patients who are likely to need multiple drugs to achieve blood pressure goals.

The choice of Diovan HCT as initial therapy for hypertension should be based on an assessment of potential benefits and risks.

Patients with stage 2 hypertension are at a relatively high risk for cardiovascular events (such as strokes, heart attacks, and heart failure), kidney failure, and vision problems, so prompt treatment is clinically relevant. The decision to use a combination as initial therapy should be individualized and should be shaped by considerations such as baseline blood pressure, the target goal and the incremental likelihood of achieving goal with a combination compared to monotherapy. Individual blood pressure goals may vary based upon the patient's risk.

Data from the high dose multifactorial trial [see *Clinical Studies (14.1)*] provide estimates of the probability of reaching a target blood pressure with Diovan HCT compared to valsartan or hydrochlorothiazide monotherapy. The figures below provide estimates of the likelihood of achieving systolic or diastolic blood pressure control with Diovan HCT 320/25 mg, based upon baseline systolic or diastolic blood pressure. The curve of each treatment group was estimated by logistic regression modeling. The estimated likelihood at the right tail of each curve is less reliable due to small numbers of subjects with high baseline blood pressures.

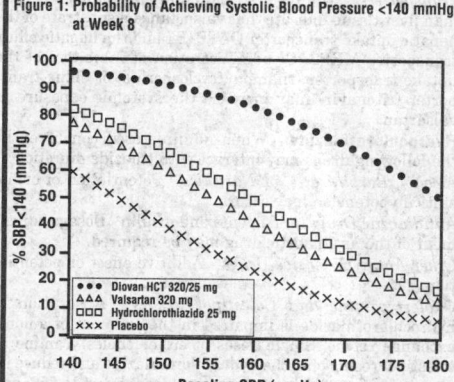

Figure 1: Probability of Achieving Systolic Blood Pressure <140 mmHg at Week 8

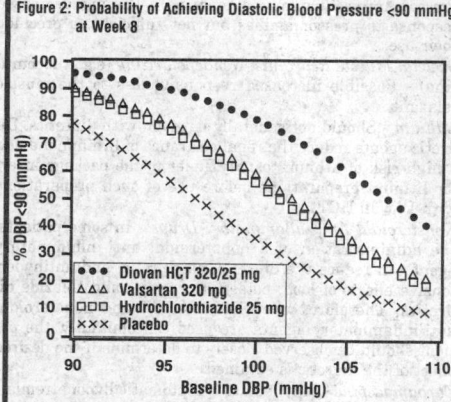

Figure 2: Probability of Achieving Diastolic Blood Pressure <90 mmHg at Week 8

[See figure 3 at top of next column]
[See figure 4 on next column]

For example, a patient with a baseline blood pressure of 160/100 mmHg has about a 41% likelihood of achieving a goal of <140 mmHg (systolic) and 60% likelihood of achieving <90 mmHg (diastolic) on valsartan alone and the likelihood of achieving these goals on HCTZ alone is about 50% (systolic) or 57% (diastolic). The likelihood of achieving these goals on Diovan HCT rises to about 84% (systolic) or 80% (diastolic). The likelihood of achieving these goals on placebo is about 23% (systolic) or 36% (diastolic).

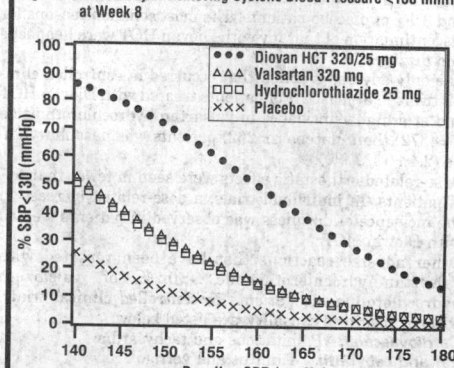

Figure 3: Probability of Achieving Systolic Blood Pressure <130 mmHg at Week 8

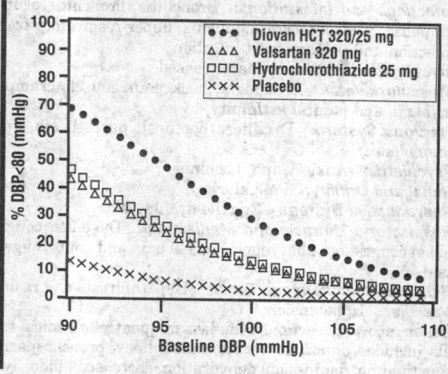

Figure 4: Probability of Achieving Diastolic Blood Pressure <80 mmHg at Week 8

2 DOSAGE AND ADMINISTRATION

2.1 General Considerations

The side effects of valsartan are generally rare and appear independent of dose. Those of hydrochlorothiazide are a mixture of dose-dependent (primarily hypokalemia) and dose-independent phenomena (e.g., pancreatitis), the former much more common than the latter [see *Adverse Reactions (6)*].

Dose once-daily. Maximum antihypertensive effects are attained within 2 to 4 weeks after a change in dose.

Diovan HCT may be administered with or without food.

Diovan HCT may be administered with other antihypertensive agents.

Elderly patients: No initial dosage adjustment is required for elderly patients.

Renal impairment: The usual regimens of therapy with Diovan HCT may be followed as long as the patient's creatinine clearance is >30 mL/min. In patients with more severe renal impairment, loop diuretics are preferred to thiazides, so Diovan HCT is not recommended.

Hepatic impairment: Care should be exercised with dosing of Diovan HCT in patients with hepatic impairment. Start with a low dose and titrate slowly in patients with hepatic impairment [see *Warnings and Precautions (5.3)*].

2.2 Add-On Therapy

A patient whose blood pressure is not adequately controlled with valsartan (or another ARB) alone or hydrochlorothiazide alone may be switched to combination therapy with Diovan HCT.

A patient who experiences dose-limiting adverse reactions on either component alone may be switched to Diovan HCT containing a lower dose of that component in combination with the other to achieve similar blood pressure reductions. The clinical response to Diovan HCT should be subsequently evaluated and if blood pressure remains uncontrolled after 3 to 4 weeks of therapy, the dose may be titrated up to a maximum of 320/25 mg.

2.3 Replacement Therapy

Diovan HCT may be substituted for the titrated components.

2.4 Initial Therapy

The usual starting dose is Diovan HCT 160/12.5 mg once daily. The dosage can be increased after 1 to 2 weeks of therapy to a maximum of one 320/25 mg tablet once daily as needed to control blood pressure [see *Clinical Studies (14.2)*]. Diovan HCT is not recommended as initial therapy in patients with intravascular volume depletion [see *Warnings and Precautions (5.2)*].

3 DOSAGE FORMS AND STRENGTHS

80/12.5 mg tablets, imprinted CG/HGH (Side 1/Side 2)
160/12.5 mg tablets, imprinted CG/HHH
160/25 mg tablets, imprinted NVR/HXH
320/12.5 mg tablets, imprinted NVR/HIL
320/25 mg tablets, imprinted NVR/CTI

4 CONTRAINDICATIONS

Diovan HCT (valsartan and hydrochlorothiazide, USP) is contraindicated in patients who are hypersensitive to any component of this product.

Because of the hydrochlorothiazide component, this product is contraindicated in patients with anuria or hypersensitivity to other sulfonamide-derived drugs.

5 WARNINGS AND PRECAUTIONS

5.1 Fetal/Neonatal Morbidity and Mortality

Diovan HCT can cause fetal harm when administered to a pregnant woman. If this drug is used during pregnancy, or if the patient becomes pregnant while taking this drug, the patient should be apprised of the potential hazard to the fetus.

Drugs that act on the renin-angiotensin system can cause fetal and neonatal morbidity and mortality when used in pregnancy. In several dozen published cases, ACE inhibitor use during the second and third trimesters of pregnancy was associated with fetal and neonatal injury, including hypotension, neonatal skull hypoplasia, anuria, reversible or irreversible renal failure, and death [see *Use in Specific Populations (8.1)*].

Intrauterine exposure to thiazide diuretics is associated with fetal or neonatal jaundice, thrombocytopenia, and possibly other adverse reactions that have occurred in adults.

5.2 Hypotension in Volume- and/or Salt-Depleted Patients

Excessive reduction of blood pressure was rarely seen (0.7%) in patients with uncomplicated hypertension treated with Diovan HCT in controlled trials. In patients with an activated renin-angiotensin system, such as volume- and/or salt-depleted patients receiving high doses of diuretics, symptomatic hypotension may occur. This condition should be corrected prior to administration of Diovan HCT, or the treatment should start under close medical supervision.

If hypotension occurs, the patient should be placed in the supine position and, if necessary, given an intravenous infusion of normal saline. A transient hypotensive response is not a contraindication to further treatment, which usually can be continued without difficulty once the blood pressure has stabilized.

5.3 Impaired Hepatic Function

Hydrochlorothiazide: Thiazide diuretics should be used with caution in patients with impaired hepatic function or progressive liver disease, since minor alterations of fluid and electrolyte balance may precipitate hepatic coma.

Valsartan: As the majority of valsartan is eliminated in the bile, patients with mild-to-moderate hepatic impairment, including patients with biliary obstructive disorders, showed lower valsartan clearance (higher AUCs). Care should be exercised in administering Diovan (valsartan) to these patients.

5.4 Hypersensitivity Reaction

Hydrochlorothiazide: Hypersensitivity reactions to hydrochlorothiazide may occur in patients with or without a history of allergy or bronchial asthma, but are more likely in patients with such a history.

5.5 Systemic Lupus Erythematosus

Hydrochlorothiazide: Thiazide diuretics have been reported to cause exacerbation or activation of systemic lupus erythematosus.

5.6 Lithium Interaction

Hydrochlorothiazide: Lithium generally should not be given with thiazides [see *Drug Interactions (7)*].

5.7 Serum Electrolytes

Valsartan – Hydrochlorothiazide: In the controlled trials of various doses of the combination of valsartan and hydrochlorothiazide the incidence of hypertensive patients who developed hypokalemia (serum potassium <3.5 mEq/L) was 3.0%; the incidence of hyperkalemia (serum potassium >5.7 mEq/L) was 0.4%.

In controlled clinical trials of Diovan HCT (valsartan and hydrochlorothiazide, USP), the average change in serum potassium was near zero in subjects who received Diovan HCT 160/12.5, 320/12.5 or 320/25 mg, but the average subject who received Diovan HCT 80/12.5 mg, 80/25 mg or 160/25 mg experienced a mild reduction in serum potassium.

In clinical trials, the opposite effects of valsartan (80, 160 or 320 mg) and hydrochlorothiazide (12.5 mg) on serum potassium approximately balanced each other in many patients. In other patients, one or the other effect may be dominant. Periodic determinations of serum electrolytes to detect possible electrolyte imbalance should be performed at appropriate intervals.

Hydrochlorothiazide: All patients receiving thiazide therapy should be observed for clinical signs of fluid or electrolyte imbalance: hyponatremia, hypochloremic alkalosis, and hypokalemia. Serum and urine electrolyte determinations are particularly important when the patient is vomiting excessively or receiving parenteral fluids. Warning signs or symptoms of fluid and electrolyte imbalance, irrespective of cause, include dryness of mouth, thirst, weakness, lethargy, drowsiness, restlessness, confusion, seizures, muscle pains or cramps, muscular fatigue, hypotension, oliguria, tachycardia, and gastrointestinal disturbances such as nausea and vomiting.

Hypokalemia may develop, especially with brisk diuresis, when severe cirrhosis is present, or after prolonged therapy. Interference with adequate oral electrolyte intake will also contribute to hypokalemia. Hypokalemia may cause cardiac arrhythmia and may also sensitize or exaggerate the response of the heart to the toxic effects of digitalis (e.g., increased ventricular irritability).

Although any chloride deficit is generally mild and usually does not require specific treatment except under extraordinary circumstances (as in liver disease or renal disease), chloride replacement may be required in the treatment of metabolic alkalosis.

Dilutional hyponatremia may occur in edematous patients in hot weather; appropriate therapy is water restriction, rather than administration of salt except in rare instances when the hyponatremia is life-threatening. In actual salt depletion, appropriate replacement is the therapy of choice.

Hyperuricemia may occur or frank gout may be precipitated in certain patients receiving thiazide therapy.

In diabetic patients, dosage adjustments of insulin or oral hypoglycemic agents may be required. Hyperglycemia may occur with thiazide diuretics. Thus latent diabetes mellitus may become manifest during thiazide therapy.

The antihypertensive effects of the drug may be enhanced in the postsympathectomy patient.

If progressive renal impairment becomes evident, consider withholding or discontinuing diuretic therapy.

Thiazides have been shown to increase the urinary excretion of magnesium; this may result in hypomagnesemia.

Thiazides may decrease urinary calcium excretion. Thiazides may cause intermittent and slight elevation of serum calcium in the absence of known disorders of calcium metabolism. Marked hypercalcemia may be evidence of hidden hyperparathyroidism. Thiazides should be discontinued before carrying out tests for parathyroid function.

Increases in cholesterol and triglyceride levels may be associated with thiazide diuretic therapy.

5.8 Impaired Renal Function

Valsartan: As a consequence of inhibiting the renin-angiotensin-aldosterone system, changes in renal function may be anticipated in susceptible individuals. In patients whose renal function may depend on the activity of the renin-angiotensin-aldosterone system (e.g., patients with severe congestive heart failure), treatment with angiotensin-converting enzyme inhibitors and angiotensin receptor antagonists has been associated with oliguria and/or progressive azotemia and (rarely) with acute renal failure and/or death. Similar outcomes have been reported with Diovan®.

In studies of ACE inhibitors in patients with unilateral or bilateral renal artery stenosis, increases in serum creatinine or blood urea nitrogen have been reported. In a 4-day trial of valsartan in 12 patients with unilateral renal artery stenosis, no significant increases in serum creatinine or blood urea nitrogen were observed. There has been no long-term use of valsartan in patients with unilateral or bilateral renal artery stenosis, but an effect similar to that seen with ACE inhibitors should be anticipated.

Hydrochlorothiazide: Thiazides should be used with caution in severe renal disease. In patients with renal disease, thiazides may precipitate azotemia. Cumulative effects of the drug may develop in patients with impaired renal function.

6 ADVERSE REACTIONS

6.1 Clinical Trials Experience

Because clinical studies are conducted under widely varying conditions, adverse reactions rates observed in the clinical studies of a drug cannot be directly compared to rates in the clinical studies of another drug and may not reflect the rates observed in practice. The adverse reaction information from clinical trials does, however, provide a basis for identifying the adverse events that appear to be related to drug use and for approximating rates.

Hypertension

Diovan HCT (valsartan and hydrochlorothiazide, USP) has been evaluated for safety in more than 5,700 patients, including over 990 treated for over 6 months, and over 370 for over 1 year. Adverse experiences have generally been mild and transient in nature and have only infrequently required discontinuation of therapy. The overall incidence of adverse reactions with Diovan HCT was comparable to placebo.

The overall frequency of adverse reactions was neither dose-related nor related to gender, age, or race. In controlled clin-

ical trials, discontinuation of therapy due to side effects was required in 2.3% of valsartan-hydrochlorothiazide patients and 3.1% of placebo patients. The most common reasons for discontinuation of therapy with Diovan HCT were headache and dizziness.

The only adverse reaction that occurred in controlled clinical trials in at least 2% of patients treated with Diovan HCT and at a higher incidence in valsartan-hydrochlorothiazide (n=4372) than placebo (n=262) patients was nasopharyngitis (2.4% vs. 1.9%).

Dose-related orthostatic effects were seen in fewer than 1% of patients. In individual trials, a dose-related increase in the incidence of dizziness was observed in patients treated with Diovan HCT.

Other adverse reactions that have been reported with valsartan-hydrochlorothiazide (>0.2% of valsartan-hydrochlorothiazide patients in controlled clinical trials) without regard to causality, are listed below:

Cardiovascular: Palpitations and tachycardia

Ear and Labyrinth: Tinnitus and vertigo

Gastrointestinal: Dyspepsia, diarrhea, flatulence, dry mouth, nausea, abdominal pain, abdominal pain upper, and vomiting

General and Administration Site Conditions: Asthenia, chest pain, fatigue, peripheral edema and pyrexia

Infections and Infestations: Bronchitis, bronchitis acute, influenza, gastroenteritis, sinusitis, upper respiratory tract infection and urinary tract infection

Investigations: Blood urea increased

Musculoskeletal: Arthralgia, back pain, muscle cramps, myalgia, and pain in extremity

Nervous System: Dizziness postural, paresthesia, and somnolence

Psychiatric: Anxiety and insomnia

Renal and Urinary: Pollakiuria

Reproductive System: Erectile dysfunction

Respiratory, Thoracic and Mediastinal: Dyspnea, cough, nasal congestion, pharyngolaryngeal pain and sinus congestion

Skin and Subcutaneous Tissue: Hyperhidrosis and rash

Vascular: Hypotension

Other reported reactions seen less frequently in clinical trials included abnormal vision, anaphylaxis, bronchospasm, constipation, depression, dehydration, decreased libido, dysuria, epistaxis, flushing, gout, increased appetite, muscle weakness, pharyngitis, pruritus, sunburn, syncope, and viral infection.

Valsartan: In trials in which valsartan was compared to an ACE inhibitor with or without placebo, the incidence of dry cough was significantly greater in the ACE inhibitor group (7.9%) than in the groups who received valsartan (2.6%) or placebo (1.5%). In a 129-patient trial limited to patients who had had dry cough when they had previously received ACE inhibitors, the incidences of cough in patients who received valsartan, hydrochlorothiazide, or lisinopril were 20%, 19%, 69% respectively (p <0.001).

Other reported reactions seen less frequently in clinical trials included chest pain, syncope, anorexia, vomiting, and angioedema.

Hydrochlorothiazide: Other adverse reactions that have been reported with hydrochlorothiazide, without regard to causality, are listed below:

Body As A Whole: weakness;

Digestive: pancreatitis, jaundice (intrahepatic cholestatic jaundice), sialadenitis, cramping, gastric irritation;

Hematologic: aplastic anemia, agranulocytosis, leukopenia, hemolytic anemia, thrombocytopenia;

Hypersensitivity: purpura, photosensitivity, urticaria, necrotizing angiitis (vasculitis and cutaneous vasculitis), fever, respiratory distress including pneumonitis and pulmonary edema, anaphylactic reactions;

Metabolic: hyperglycemia, glycosuria, hyperuricemia;

Musculoskeletal: muscle spasm;

Nervous System/Psychiatric: restlessness;

Renal: renal failure, renal dysfunction, interstitial nephritis;

Skin: erythema multiforme including Stevens-Johnson syndrome, exfoliative dermatitis including toxic epidermal necrolysis;

Special Senses: transient blurred vision, xanthopsia.

Initial Therapy – Hypertension

In a clinical study in patients with severe hypertension (diastolic blood pressure ≥110 mmHg and systolic blood pressure ≥140 mmHg), the overall pattern of adverse reactions reported through six weeks of follow-up was similar in patients treated with Diovan HCT as initial therapy and in patients treated with valsartan as initial therapy. Comparing the groups treated with Diovan HCT (force-titrated to 320/25 mg) and valsartan (force-titrated to 320 mg), dizziness was observed in 6% and 2% of patients, respectively. Hypotension was observed in 1% of those patients receiving Diovan HCT and 0% of patients receiving valsartan. There were no reported cases of syncope in either treatment group. Laboratory changes with Diovan HCT as initial ther-

apy in patients with severe hypertension were similar to those reported with Diovan HCT in patients with less severe hypertension [see Clinical Studies (14.2) and Drug Interactions (7.3)].

6.2 Postmarketing Experience

The following additional adverse reactions have been reported in valsartan or valsartan/hydrochlorothiazide postmarketing experience:

Hypersensitivity: There are rare reports of angioedema;

Digestive: Elevated liver enzymes and very rare reports of hepatitis;

Renal: Impaired renal function;

Clinical Laboratory Tests: Hyperkalemia;

Dermatologic: Alopecia;

Vascular: Vasculitis;

Nervous System: Syncope.

Rare cases of rhabdomyolysis have been reported in patients receiving angiotensin II receptor blockers.

Because these reactions are reported voluntarily from a population of uncertain size, it is not always possible to reliably estimate their frequency or establish a causal relationship to drug exposure.

7 DRUG INTERACTIONS

Valsartan: No clinically significant pharmacokinetic interactions were observed when valsartan was coadministered with amlodipine, atenolol, cimetidine, digoxin, furosemide, glyburide, hydrochlorothiazide, or indomethacin. The valsartan-atenolol combination was more antihypertensive than either component, but it did not lower the heart rate more than atenolol alone.

Coadministration of valsartan and warfarin did not change the pharmacokinetics of valsartan or the time-course of the anticoagulant properties of warfarin.

CYP 450 Interactions: In vitro metabolism studies indicate that CYP 450 mediated drug interactions between valsartan and co-administered drugs are unlikely because of low extent of metabolism [see Pharmacokinetics (12.3)].

Transporters: The results from an in vitro study with human liver tissue indicate that valsartan is a substrate of the hepatic uptake transporter OATP1B1 and the hepatic efflux transporter MRP2. Co-administration of inhibitors of the uptake transporter (rifampin, cyclosporine) or efflux transporter (ritonavir) may increase the systemic exposure to valsartan.

Hydrochlorothiazide: When administered concurrently, the following drugs may interact with thiazide diuretics:

Alcohol, Barbiturates, or Narcotics - Potentiation of orthostatic hypotension may occur.

Antidiabetic Drugs (oral agents and insulin - Dosage adjustment of the antidiabetic drug may be required.

Other Antihypertensive Drugs - Additive effect or potentiation.

Cholestyramine and Colestipol Resins - Absorption of hydrochlorothiazide is impaired in the presence of anionic exchange resins. Single doses of either cholestyramine or colestipol resins bind the hydrochlorothiazide and reduce its absorption from the gastrointestinal tract by up to 85% and 43% respectively.

Corticosteroids, ACTH - Intensified electrolyte depletion, particularly hypokalemia.

Pressor Amines (e.g., norepinephrine) - Possible decreased response to pressor amines but not sufficient to preclude their use.

Skeletal Muscle Relaxants, Nondepolarizing (e.g., tubocurarine) - Possible increased responsiveness to the muscle relaxant.

Lithium - Should not generally be given with diuretics. Diuretic agents reduce the renal clearance of lithium and add a high risk of lithium toxicity. Refer to the package insert for lithium preparations before use of such preparations with Diovan HCT.

Nonsteroidal Anti-inflammatory Drugs - In some patients, the administration of a nonsteroidal anti-inflammatory agent can reduce the diuretic, natriuretic, and antihypertensive effects of loop, potassium-sparing and thiazide diuretics. Therefore, when Diovan HCT and nonsteroidal anti-inflammatory agents are used concomitantly, the patient should be observed closely to determine if the desired effect of the diuretic is obtained.

Carbamazepine - May lead to symptomatic hyponatremia.

7.3 Clinical Laboratory Test Findings

In controlled clinical trials, clinically important changes in standard laboratory parameters were rarely associated with administration of Diovan HCT.

Creatinine/Blood Urea Nitrogen (BUN): Minor elevations in creatinine and BUN occurred in 2% and 15% respectively, of patients taking Diovan HCT and 0.4% and 6% respectively, given placebo in controlled clinical trials.

Hemoglobin and Hematocrit: Greater than 20% decreases in hemoglobin and hematocrit were observed in less than 0.1% of Diovan HCT patients, compared with 0.0% in placebo-treated patients.

Liver Function Tests: Occasional elevations (greater than 150%) of liver chemistries occurred in Diovan HCT-treated patients.
Neutropenia: Neutropenia was observed in 0.1% of patients treated with Diovan HCT and 0.4% of patients treated with placebo.
Serum Electrolytes: [*see Warnings and Precautions (5.7)*].

8 USE IN SPECIFIC POPULATIONS

8.1 Pregnancy

Pregnancy Category D [*see Warnings and Precautions (5.1)*]
Diovan HCT, like other drugs that act on the renin-angiotensin system, can cause fetal and neonatal morbidity and death when used during the second or third trimester of pregnancy. Diovan HCT can cause fetal harm when administered to a pregnant woman. If this drug is used during pregnancy, or if the patient becomes pregnant while taking this drug, the patient should be apprised of the potential hazard to the fetus.
Angiotensin II receptor antagonists, like valsartan, and angiotensin-converting enzyme (ACE) inhibitors exert similar effects on the renin-angiotensin system. In several dozen published cases, ACE inhibitor use during the second and third trimesters of pregnancy was associated with fetal and neonatal injury, including hypotension, neonatal skull hypoplasia, anuria, reversible or irreversible renal failure, and death. Oligohydramnios was also reported, presumably from decreased fetal renal function. In this setting, oligohydramnios was associated with fetal limb contractures, craniofacial deformation, and hypoplastic lung development. Prematurity, intrauterine growth retardation, and patent ductus arteriosus were also reported, although it is not clear whether these occurrences were due to exposure to the drug. In a retrospective study, first trimester use of ACE inhibitors, a specific class of drugs acting on the renin-angiotensin system, was associated with a potential risk of birth defects.
When pregnancy occurs in a patient using Diovan HCT, the physician should discontinue Diovan HCT treatment as soon as possible. The physician should inform the patient about potential risks to the fetus based on the time of gestational exposure to Diovan HCT (first trimester only or later). If exposure occurs beyond the first trimester, an ultrasound examination should be done.
In rare cases when another antihypertensive agent can not be used to treat the pregnant patient, serial ultrasound examinations should be performed to assess the intraamniotic environment. Routine fetal testing with non-stress tests, biophysical profiles, and/or contraction stress tests may be appropriate based on gestational age and standards of care in the community. If oligohydramnios occurs in these situations, individualized decisions about continuing or discontinuing Diovan HCT treatment and about pregnancy management should be made by the patient, her physician, and experts in the management of high-risk pregnancy. Patients and physicians should be aware that oligohydramnios may not appear until after the fetus has sustained irreversible injury.
Infants with histories of *in utero* exposure to Diovan HCT should be closely observed for hypotension, oliguria, and hyperkalemia. If oliguria occurs, these infants may require blood pressure and renal perfusion support. Exchange transfusion or dialysis may be required to reverse hypotension and/or support decreased renal function.
Healthcare professionals who prescribe drugs acting directly on the renin-angiotensin system should counsel women of childbearing potential about the risks of these agents during pregnancy [*see Nonclinical Toxicology (13)*].

8.3 Nursing Mothers

It is not known whether valsartan is excreted in human milk. Valsartan was excreted into the milk of lactating rats; however, animal breast milk drug levels may not accurately reflect human breast milk levels. Hydrochlorothiazide is excreted in human breast milk. Because many drugs are excreted into human milk and because of the potential for adverse reactions in nursing infants from Diovan HCT, a decision should be made whether to discontinue nursing or discontinue the drug, taking into account the importance of the drug to the mother.

8.4 Pediatric Use

Safety and effectiveness of Diovan HCT in pediatric patients have not been established.

8.5 Geriatric Use

In the controlled clinical trials of Diovan HCT, 764 (17.5%) of patients treated with valsartan-hydrochlorothiazide were ≥65 years and 118 (2.7%) were ≥75 years. No overall difference in the efficacy or safety of valsartan-hydrochlorothiazide was observed between these patients and younger patients, but greater sensitivity of some older individuals cannot be ruled out.

10 OVERDOSAGE

Valsartan-Hydrochlorothiazide: Limited data are available related to overdosage in humans. The most likely manifestations of overdosage would be hypotension and tachycardia; bradycardia could occur from parasympathetic (vagal) stimulation. Depressed level of consciousness, circulatory collapse and shock have been reported. If symptomatic hypotension should occur, supportive treatment should be instituted.
Valsartan is not removed from the plasma by dialysis.
The degree to which hydrochlorothiazide is removed by hemodialysis has not been established. The most common signs and symptoms observed in patients are those caused by electrolyte depletion (hypokalemia, hypochloremia, hyponatremia) and dehydration resulting from excessive diuresis. If digitalis has also been administered, hypokalemia may accentuate cardiac arrhythmias.
In rats and marmosets, single oral doses of valsartan up to 1524 and 762 mg/kg in combination with hydrochlorothiazide at doses up to 476 and 238 mg/kg, respectively, were very well tolerated without any treatment-related effects. These no adverse effect doses in rats and marmosets, respectively, represent 46.5 and 23 times the maximum recommended human dose (MRHD) of valsartan and 188 and 113 times the MRHD of hydrochlorothiazide on a mg/m^2 basis. (Calculations assume an oral dose of 320 mg/day valsartan in combination with 25 mg/day hydrochlorothiazide and a 60-kg patient.)
Valsartan: Valsartan was without grossly observable adverse effects at single oral doses up to 2000 mg/kg in rats and up to 1000 mg/kg in marmosets, except for salivation and diarrhea in the rat and vomiting in the marmoset at the highest dose (60 and 31 times, respectively, the maximum recommended human dose on a mg/m^2 basis). (Calculations assume an oral dose of 320 mg/day and a 60-kg patient.)
Hydrochlorothiazide: The oral LD_{50} of hydrochlorothiazide is greater than 10 g/kg in both mice and rats, which represents 2027 and 4054 times, respectively, the maximum recommended human dose on a mg/m^2 basis. (Calculations assume an oral dose of 25 mg/day and a 60-kg patient.)

11 DESCRIPTION

Diovan HCT (valsartan and hydrochlorothiazide, USP) is a combination of valsartan, an orally active, specific angiotensin II receptor blocker (ARB) acting on the AT_1 receptor subtype, and hydrochlorothiazide, a diuretic.
Valsartan, a nonpeptide molecule, is chemically described as *N*-(1-oxopentyl)-*N*-[[2′-(1*H*-tetrazol-5-yl)[1,1′-biphenyl]-4-yl]methyl]-L-Valine. Its empirical formula is $C_{24}H_{29}N_5O_3$, its molecular weight is 435.5, and its structural formula is

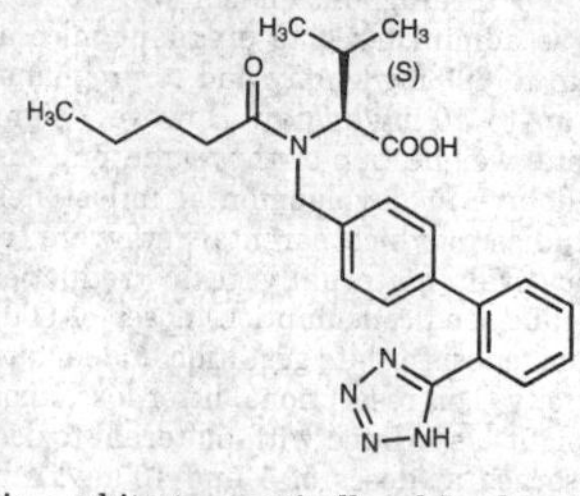

Valsartan is a white to practically white fine powder. It is soluble in ethanol and methanol and slightly soluble in water.
Hydrochlorothiazide USP is a white, or practically white, practically odorless, crystalline powder. It is slightly soluble in water; freely soluble in sodium hydroxide solution, in *n*-butylamine, and in dimethylformamide; sparingly soluble in methanol; and insoluble in ether, in chloroform, and in dilute mineral acids. Hydrochlorothiazide is chemically described as 6-chloro-3,4-dihydro-2*H*-1,2,4-benzothiadiazine-7-sulfonamide 1,1-dioxide.
Hydrochlorothiazide is a thiazide diuretic. Its empirical formula is $C_7H_8ClN_3O_4S_2$, its molecular weight is 297.73, and its structural formula is

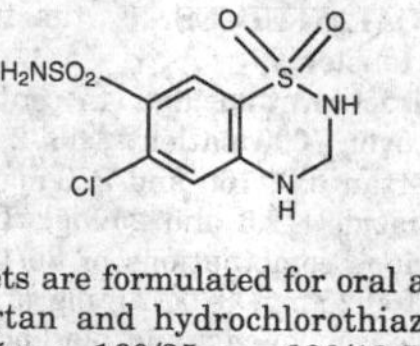

Diovan HCT tablets are formulated for oral administration to contain valsartan and hydrochlorothiazide, USP 80/12.5 mg, 160/12.5 mg, 160/25 mg, 320/12.5 mg and 320/25 mg. The inactive ingredients of the tablets are colloidal silicon dioxide, crospovidone, hydroxypropyl methylcellulose, iron oxides, magnesium stearate, microcrystalline cellulose, polyethylene glycol, talc, and titanium dioxide.

12 CLINICAL PHARMACOLOGY

12.1 Mechanism of Action

Angiotensin II is formed from angiotensin I in a reaction catalyzed by angiotensin-converting enzyme (ACE, kininase II). Angiotensin II is the principal pressor agent of the renin-angiotensin system, with effects that include vasoconstriction, stimulation of synthesis and release of aldosterone, cardiac stimulation, and renal reabsorption of sodium. Valsartan blocks the vasoconstrictor and aldosterone-secreting effects of angiotensin II by selectively blocking the binding of angiotensin II to the AT_1 receptor in many tissues, such as vascular smooth muscle and the adrenal gland. Its action is therefore independent of the pathways for angiotensin II synthesis.
There is also an AT_2 receptor found in many tissues, but AT_2 is not known to be associated with cardiovascular homeostasis. Valsartan has much greater affinity (about 20,000-fold) for the AT_1 receptor than for the AT_2 receptor. The primary metabolite of valsartan is essentially inactive with an affinity for the AT_1 receptor about one 200th that of valsartan itself.
Blockade of the renin-angiotensin system with ACE inhibitors, which inhibit the biosynthesis of angiotensin II from angiotensin I, is widely used in the treatment of hypertension. ACE inhibitors also inhibit the degradation of bradykinin, a reaction also catalyzed by ACE. Because valsartan does not inhibit ACE (kininase II) it does not affect the response to bradykinin. Whether this difference has clinical relevance is not yet known. Valsartan does not bind to or block other hormone receptors or ion channels known to be important in cardiovascular regulation.
Blockade of the angiotensin II receptor inhibits the negative regulatory feedback of angiotensin II on renin secretion, but the resulting increased plasma renin activity and angiotensin II circulating levels do not overcome the effect of valsartan on blood pressure.
Hydrochlorothiazide is a thiazide diuretic. Thiazides affect the renal tubular mechanisms of electrolyte reabsorption, directly increasing excretion of sodium and chloride in approximately equivalent amounts. Indirectly, the diuretic action of hydrochlorothiazide reduces plasma volume, with consequent increases in plasma renin activity, increases in aldosterone secretion, increases in urinary potassium loss, and decreases in serum potassium. The renin-aldosterone link is mediated by angiotensin II, so coadministration of an angiotensin II receptor antagonist tends to reverse the potassium loss associated with these diuretics.
The mechanism of the antihypertensive effect of thiazides is unknown.

12.2 Pharmacodynamics

Valsartan: Valsartan inhibits the pressor effect of angiotensin II infusions. An oral dose of 80 mg inhibits the pressor effect by about 80% at peak with approximately 30% inhibition persisting for 24 hours. No information on the effect of larger doses is available.
Removal of the negative feedback of angiotensin II causes a 2- to 3-fold rise in plasma renin and consequent rise in angiotensin II plasma concentration in hypertensive patients. Minimal decreases in plasma aldosterone were observed after administration of valsartan; very little effect on serum potassium was observed.
In multiple-dose studies in hypertensive patients with stable renal insufficiency and patients with renovascular hypertension, valsartan had no clinically significant effects on glomerular filtration rate, filtration fraction, creatinine clearance, or renal plasma flow.
In multiple-dose studies in hypertensive patients, valsartan had no notable effects on total cholesterol, fasting triglycerides, fasting serum glucose, or uric acid.
Hydrochlorothiazide: After oral administration of hydrochlorothiazide, diuresis begins within 2 hours, peaks in about 4 hours and lasts about 6 to 12 hours.

12.3 Pharmacokinetics

Valsartan: Valsartan peak plasma concentration is reached 2 to 4 hours after dosing. Valsartan shows bi-exponential decay kinetics following intravenous administration, with an average elimination half-life of about 6 hours. Absolute bioavailability for the capsule formulation is about 25% (range 10%-35%). Food decreases the exposure (as measured by AUC) to valsartan by about 40% and peak plasma concentration (C_{max}) by about 50%. AUC and C_{max} values of valsartan increase approximately linearly with increasing dose over the clinical dosing range. Valsartan does not accumulate appreciably in plasma following repeated administration.
Hydrochlorothiazide: Thiazide diuretics are eliminated by the kidney, with a terminal half-life of 5-15 hours.
Geriatric: Exposure (measured by AUC) to valsartan is higher by 70% and the half-life is longer by 35% in the elderly than in the young. No dosage adjustment is necessary [*see Dosage and Administration (2.1)*].
Gender: Pharmacokinetics of valsartan does not differ significantly between males and females.
Race: Pharmacokinetic differences due to race have not been studied.
Renal Insufficiency: There is no apparent correlation between renal function (measured by creatinine clearance) and exposure (measured by AUC) to valsartan in patients with different degrees of renal impairment. Consequently, dose adjustment is not required in patients with mild-to-

moderate renal dysfunction. No studies have been performed in patients with severe impairment of renal function (creatinine clearance <10 mL/min). Valsartan is not removed from the plasma by hemodialysis. In the case of severe renal disease, exercise care with dosing of valsartan [*see Dosage and Administration (2.1)*].

In a study of patients with impaired renal function (mean creatinine clearance of 19 mL/min), the half-life of hydrochlorothiazide elimination was lengthened to 21 hours.

Hepatic Insufficiency: On average, patients with mild-to-moderate chronic liver disease have twice the exposure (measured by AUC values) to valsartan of healthy volunteers (matched by age, sex, and weight). In general, no dosage adjustment is needed in patients with mild-to-moderate liver disease. Care should be exercised in patients with liver disease [*see Dosage and Administration (2.1)*].

Distribution

Valsartan: The steady state volume of distribution of valsartan after intravenous administration is small (17 L), indicating that valsartan does not distribute into tissues extensively. Valsartan is highly bound to serum proteins (95%), mainly serum albumin.

Hydrochlorothiazide: Hydrochlorothiazide crosses the placental but not the blood-brain barrier and is excreted in breast milk.

Metabolism

Valsartan: The primary metabolite, accounting for about 9% of dose, is valeryl 4-hydroxy valsartan. *In vitro* metabolism studies involving recombinant CYP 450 enzymes indicated that the CYP 2C9 isoenzyme is responsible for the formation of valeryl-4-hydroxy valsartan. Valsartan does not inhibit CYP 450 isozymes at clinically relevant concentrations. CYP 450 mediated drug interaction between valsartan and co-administered drugs are unlikely because of the low extent of metabolism.

Hydrochlorothiazide: Is not metabolized.

Excretion

Valsartan: Valsartan, when administered as an oral solution, is primarily recovered in feces (about 83% of dose) and urine (about 13% of dose). The recovery is mainly as unchanged drug, with only about 20% of dose recovered as metabolites.

Following intravenous administration, plasma clearance of valsartan is about 2 L/h and its renal clearance is 0.62 L/h (about 30% of total clearance).

Hydrochlorothiazide: Hydrochlorothiazide is not metabolized but is eliminated rapidly by the kidney. At least 61% of the oral dose is eliminated as unchanged drug within 24 hours. The elimination half-life is between 5.8 and 18.9 hours.

13 NONCLINICAL TOXICOLOGY

13.1 Carcinogenesis, Mutagenesis, Impairment of Fertility

Valsartan-Hydrochlorothiazide: No carcinogenicity, mutagenicity or fertility studies have been conducted with the combination of valsartan and hydrochlorothiazide. However, these studies have been conducted for valsartan as well as hydrochlorothiazide alone. Based on the preclinical safety and human pharmacokinetic studies, there is no indication of any adverse interaction between valsartan and hydrochlorothiazide.

Valsartan: There was no evidence of carcinogenicity when valsartan was administered in the diet to mice and rats for up to 2 years at doses up to 160 and 200 mg/kg/day, respectively. These doses in mice and rats are about 2.6 and 6 times, respectively, the maximum recommended human dose on a mg/m^2 basis. (Calculations assume an oral dose of 320 mg/day and a 60-kg patient.)

Mutagenicity assays did not reveal any valsartan-related effects at either the gene or chromosome level. These assays included bacterial mutagenicity tests with *Salmonella* (Ames) and *E. coli*; a gene mutation test with Chinese hamster V79 cells; a cytogenetic test with Chinese hamster ovary cells; and a rat micronucleus test.

Valsartan had no adverse effects on the reproductive performance of male or female rats at oral doses up to 200 mg/kg/day. This dose is about 6 times the maximum recommended human dose on a mg/m^2 basis. (Calculations assume an oral dose of 320 mg/day and a 60-kg patient.)

Hydrochlorothiazide: Two-year feeding studies in mice and rats conducted under the auspices of the National Toxicology Program (NTP) uncovered no evidence of a carcinogenic potential of hydrochlorothiazide in female mice (at doses of up to approximately 600 mg/kg/day) or in male and female rats (at doses of up to approximately 100 mg/kg/day). The NTP, however, found equivocal evidence for hepatocarcinogenicity in male mice.

Hydrochlorothiazide was not genotoxic *in vitro* in the Ames mutagenicity assay of Salmonella Typhimurium strains TA 98, TA 100, TA 1535, TA 1537, and TA 1538 and in the Chinese Hamster Ovary (CHO) test for chromosomal aberrations, or *in vivo* in assays using mouse germinal cell chromosomes, Chinese hamster bone marrow chromosomes, and the Drosophila sex-linked recessive lethal trait gene. Positive test results were obtained only in the *in vitro* CHO Sister Chromatid Exchange (clastogenicity) and in the Mouse Lymphoma Cell (mutagenicity) assays, using concentrations of hydrochlorothiazide from 43 to 1300 mcgm/mL, and in the Aspergillus Nidulans non-disjunction assay at an unspecified concentration.

Hydrochlorothiazide had no adverse effects on the fertility of mice and rats of either sex in studies wherein these species were exposed, via their diet, to doses of up to 100 and 4 mg/kg, respectively, prior to mating and throughout gestation. These doses of hydrochlorothiazide in mice and rats represent 19 and 1.5 times, respectively, the maximum recommended human dose on a mg/m^2 basis. (Calculations assume an oral dose of 25 mg/day and a 60-kg patient.)

13.3 Developmental Toxicity Studies

Valsartan-Hydrochlorothiazide: There was no evidence of teratogenicity in mice, rats, or rabbits treated orally with valsartan at doses up to 600, 100 and 10 mg/kg/day, respectively, in combination with hydrochlorothiazide at doses up to 188, 31 and 3 mg/kg/day. These non-teratogenic doses in mice, rats and rabbits, respectively, represent 9, 3.5 and 0.5 times the maximum recommended human dose (MRHD) of valsartan and 38, 13 and 2 times the MRHD of hydrochlorothiazide on a mg/m^2 basis. (Calculations assume an oral dose of 320 mg/day valsartan in combination with 25 mg/day hydrochlorothiazide and a 60-kg patient.)

Fetotoxicity was observed in association with maternal toxicity in rats and rabbits at valsartan doses of ≥200 and 10 mg/kg/day, respectively, in combination with hydrochlorothiazide doses of ≥63 and 3 mg/kg/day. Fetotoxicity in rats was considered to be related to decreased fetal weights and included fetal variations of sternebrae, vertebrae, ribs and/or renal papillae. Fetotoxicity in rabbits included increased numbers of late resorptions with resultant increases in total resorptions, postimplantation losses and decreased number of live fetuses. The no observed adverse effect doses in mice, rats and rabbits for valsartan were 600, 100 and 3 mg/kg/day, respectively, in combination with hydrochlorothiazide doses of 188, 31 and 1 mg/kg/day. These no adverse effect doses in mice, rats and rabbits, respectively, represent 9, 3 and 0.18 times the MRHD of valsartan and 38, 13 and 0.5 times the MRHD of hydrochlorothiazide on a mg/m^2 basis. (Calculations assume an oral dose of 320 mg/day valsartan in combination with 25 mg/day hydrochlorothiazide and a 60-kg patient.)

Valsartan: No teratogenic effects were observed when valsartan was administered to pregnant mice and rats at oral doses up to 600 mg/kg/day and to pregnant rabbits at oral doses up to 10 mg/kg/day. However, significant decreases in fetal weight, pup birth weight, pup survival rate, and slight delays in developmental milestones were observed in studies in which parental rats were treated with valsartan at oral, maternally toxic (reduction in body weight gain and food consumption) doses of 600 mg/kg/day during organogenesis or late gestation and lactation. In rabbits, fetotoxicity (i.e., resorptions, litter loss, abortions, and low body weight) associated with maternal toxicity (mortality) was observed at doses of 5 and 10 mg/kg/day. The no observed adverse effect doses of 600, 200 and 2 mg/kg/day in mice, rats and rabbits represent 9, 6 and 0.1 times, respectively, the maximum recommended human dose on a mg/m^2 basis. (Calculations assume an oral dose of 320 mg/day and a 60-kg patient.)

Hydrochlorothiazide: Under the auspices of the National Toxicology Program, pregnant mice and rats that received hydrochlorothiazide via gavage at doses up to 3000 and 1000 mg/kg/day, respectively, on gestation days 6 through 15 showed no evidence of teratogenicity. These doses of hydrochlorothiazide in mice and rats represent 608 and 405 times, respectively, the maximum recommended human dose on a mg/m^2 basis. (Calculations assume an oral dose of 25 mg/day and a 60-kg patient.)

14 CLINICAL STUDIES

14.1 Hypertension

Valsartan-Hydrochlorothiazide: In controlled clinical trials including over 7600 patients, 4372 patients were exposed to valsartan (80, 160 and 320 mg) and concomitant hydrochlorothiazide (12.5 and 25 mg). Two factorial trials compared various combinations of 80/12.5 mg, 80/25 mg, 160/12.5 mg, 160/25 mg, 320/12.5 mg and 320/25 mg with their respective components and placebo. The combination of valsartan and hydrochlorothiazide resulted in additive placebo-adjusted decreases in systolic and diastolic blood pressure at trough of 14-21/8-11 mmHg at 80/12.5 mg to 320/25 mg, compared to 7-10/4-5 mmHg for valsartan 80 mg to 320 mg and 5-11/2-5 mmHg for hydrochlorothiazide 12.5 mg to 25 mg, alone.

Three other controlled trials investigated the addition of hydrochlorothiazide to patients who did not respond adequately to valsartan 80 mg to valsartan 320 mg, resulted in the additional lowering of systolic and diastolic blood pressure by approximately 4-12/2-5 mmHg.

The maximal antihypertensive effect was attained 4 weeks after the initiation of therapy, the first time point at which blood pressure was measured in these trials.

In long-term follow-up studies (without placebo control) the effect of the combination of valsartan and hydrochlorothiazide appeared to be maintained for up to two years. The antihypertensive effect is independent of age or gender. The overall response to the combination was similar for Black and non-Black patients.

There was essentially no change in heart rate in patients treated with the combination of valsartan and hydrochlorothiazide in controlled trials.

Valsartan: The antihypertensive effects of valsartan were demonstrated principally in 7 placebo-controlled, 4- to 12-week trials (one in patients over 65) of dosages from 10 to 320 mg/day in patients with baseline diastolic blood pressures of 95-115. The studies allowed comparison of once-daily and twice-daily regimens of 160 mg/day; comparison of peak and trough effects; comparison (in pooled data) of response by gender, age, and race; and evaluation of incremental effects of hydrochlorothiazide.

Administration of valsartan to patients with essential hypertension results in a significant reduction of sitting, supine, and standing systolic and diastolic blood pressure, usually with little or no orthostatic change.

In most patients, after administration of a single oral dose, onset of antihypertensive activity occurs at approximately 2 hours, and maximum reduction of blood pressure is achieved within 6 hours. The antihypertensive effect persists for 24 hours after dosing, but there is a decrease from peak effect at lower doses (40 mg) presumably reflecting loss of inhibition of angiotensin II. At higher doses, however (160 mg), there is little difference in peak and trough effect. During repeated dosing, the reduction in blood pressure with any dose is substantially present within 2 weeks, and maximal reduction is generally attained after 4 weeks. In long-term follow-up studies (without placebo control) the effect of valsartan appeared to be maintained for up to two years. The antihypertensive effect is independent of age, gender or race. The latter finding regarding race is based on pooled data and should be viewed with caution, because antihypertensive drugs that affect the renin-angiotensin system (that is, ACE inhibitors and angiotensin II blockers) have generally been found to be less effective in low-renin hypertensives (frequently Blacks) than in high-renin hypertensives (frequently Whites). In pooled, randomized, controlled trials of Diovan that included a total of 140 Blacks and 830 Whites, valsartan and an ACE-inhibitor control were generally at least as effective in Blacks as Whites. The explanation for this difference from previous findings is unclear.

Abrupt withdrawal of valsartan has not been associated with a rapid increase in blood pressure.

The 7 studies of valsartan monotherapy included over 2000 patients randomized to various doses of valsartan and about 800 patients randomized to placebo. Doses below 80 mg were not consistently distinguished from those of placebo at trough, but doses of 80, 160 and 320 mg produced dose-related decreases in systolic and diastolic blood pressure, with the difference from placebo of approximately 6-9/3-5 mmHg at 80-160 mg and 9/6 mmHg at 320 mg.

Patients with an inadequate response to 80 mg once daily were titrated to either 160 mg once daily or 80 mg twice daily, which resulted in a comparable response in both groups.

In another 4-week study, 1876 patients randomized to valsartan 320 mg once daily had an incremental blood pressure reduction 3/1 mmHg lower than did 1900 patients randomized to valsartan 160 mg once daily.

In controlled trials, the antihypertensive effect of once daily valsartan 80 mg was similar to that of once daily enalapril 20 mg or once daily lisinopril 10 mg.

There was essentially no change in heart rate in valsartan-treated patients in controlled trials.

14.2 Initial Therapy – Hypertension

The safety and efficacy of Diovan HCT as initial therapy for patients with severe hypertension (defined as a sitting diastolic blood pressure ≥110 mmHg and systolic blood pressure ≥140 mmHg off all antihypertensive therapy) was studied in a 6-week multicenter, randomized, double-blind study. Patients were randomized to either Diovan HCT (valsartan and hydrochlorothiazide 160/12.5 mg once daily) or to valsartan (160 mg once daily) and followed for blood pressure response. Patients were force-titrated at 2-week intervals. Patients on combination therapy were subsequently titrated to 160/25 mg followed by 320/25 mg valsartan/hydrochlorothiazide. Patients on monotherapy were subsequently titrated to 320 mg valsartan followed by a titration to 320 mg valsartan to maintain the blind.

The study randomized 608 patients, including 261 (43%) females, 147 (24%) Blacks, and 75 (12%) ≥65 years of age. The mean blood pressure at baseline for the total population was 168/112 mmHg. The mean age was 52 years. After 4 weeks of therapy, reductions in systolic and diastolic blood pressure were 9/5 mmHg greater in the group treated with Diovan HCT compared to valsartan. Similar trends were seen when the patients were grouped according to gender, race or age.

16 HOW SUPPLIED/STORAGE AND HANDLING

Diovan HCT (valsartan and hydrochlorothiazide, USP) is available as non-scored tablets containing valsartan/hydrochlorothiazide 80/12.5 mg, 160/12.5 mg, 160/25 mg, 320/12.5 mg and 320/25 mg. Strengths are available as follows.

80/12.5 mg Tablet - Light orange, ovaloid with slightly convex faces debossed CG on one side and HGH on the other side.

Bottles of 90	NDC 0078-0314-34
Bottles of 14,000	NDC 0078-0314-33
Unit Dose (blister pack)	NDC 0078-0314-06
Box of 100 (strips of 10)	

160/12.5 mg Tablet - Dark red, ovaloid with slightly convex faces debossed CG on one side and HHH on the other side.

Bottles of 90	NDC 0078-0315-34
Bottles of 7,000	NDC 0078-0315-17
Unit Dose (blister pack)	NDC 0078-0315-06
Box of 100 (strips of 10)	
Unit Dose (blister pack of 30)	NDC 0078-0315-15

160/25 mg Tablet - Brown orange, ovaloid with slightly convex faces debossed NVR on one side and HXH on the other side.

Bottles of 90	NDC 0078-0383-34
Bottles of 7,000	NDC 0078-0383-17
Unit Dose (blister pack)	NDC 0078-0383-06
Box of 100 (strips of 10)	
Unit Dose (blister pack of 30)	NDC 0078-0383-15

320/12.5 mg Tablet - Pink, ovaloid with beveled edge, debossed NVR on one side and HIL on the other side.

Bottles of 90	NDC 0078-0471-34
Bottles of 3,500	NDC 0078-0471-11
Unit Dose (blister pack)	NDC 0078-0471-06
Box of 100 (strips of 10)	
Unit Dose (blister pack of 30)	NDC 0078-0471-15

320/25 mg Tablet - Yellow, ovaloid with beveled edge, debossed NVR on one side and CTI on the other side.

Bottles of 90	NDC 0078-0472-34
Bottles of 3,500	NDC 0078-0472-11
Unit Dose (blister pack)	NDC 0078-0472-06
Box of 100 (strips of 10)	
Unit Dose (blister pack of 30)	NDC 0078-0472-15

Store at 25°C (77°F); excursions permitted to 15-30°C (59-86°F) [see USP Controlled Room Temperature]. Protect from moisture.

Dispense in tight container (USP).

17 PATIENT COUNSELING INFORMATION

17.1 Information for Patients

Pregnancy: Female patients of childbearing age should be told that use of drugs like Diovan HCT that act on the renin-angiotensin system during pregnancy can cause serious problems in the fetus and infant including: low blood pressure, poor development of skull bones, kidney failure and death. Discuss other treatment options with female patients planning to become pregnant. Women using Diovan HCT who become pregnant should notify their physician as soon as possible.

Symptomatic Hypotension: A patient receiving Diovan HCT should be cautioned that lightheadedness can occur, especially during the first days of therapy, and that it should be reported to the prescribing physician. The patients should be told that if syncope occurs, Diovan HCT should be discontinued until the physician has been consulted.

All patients should be cautioned that inadequate fluid intake, excessive perspiration, diarrhea, or vomiting can lead to an excessive fall in blood pressure, with the same consequences of lightheadedness and possible syncope.

Potassium Supplements: A patient receiving Diovan HCT should be told not to use potassium supplements or salt substitutes containing potassium without consulting the prescribing physician.

17.2 FDA-Approved Patient Labeling

PATIENT INFORMATION

DIOVAN HCT (DYE´-o-van HCT)

(valsartan and hydrochlorothiazide)

Tablets

Read the Patient Information that comes with DIOVAN HCT before you start taking it and each time you get a refill. There may be new information. This leaflet does not take the place of talking with your doctor about your condition and treatment. If you have any questions about DIOVAN HCT, ask your doctor or pharmacist.

What is the most important information I should know about DIOVAN HCT?

If you become pregnant, stop taking DIOVAN HCT and call your doctor right away. DIOVAN HCT can harm an unborn baby causing injury and even death. If you plan to become pregnant, talk to your doctor about other treatment options to lower your high blood pressure before taking DIOVAN HCT.

What is DIOVAN HCT?

DIOVAN HCT contains two prescription medicines:
1. valsartan, an angiotensin receptor blocker (ARB)
2. hydrochlorothiazide (HCTZ), a water pill (diuretic)

DIOVAN HCT may be used to lower high blood pressure (hypertension) in adults:
- when one medicine to lower your high blood pressure is not enough
- as the first medicine to lower high blood pressure if your doctor decides you are likely to need more than one medicine.

DIOVAN HCT has not been studied in children under 18 years of age.

Who should not take DIOVAN HCT?

Do not take DIOVAN HCT if you:
- are allergic to any of the ingredients in DIOVAN HCT. See the end of this leaflet for a complete list of ingredients in DIOVAN HCT.
- make less urine due to kidney problems
- are allergic to medicines that contain sulfonamides

What should I tell my doctor before taking DIOVAN HCT?

Tell your doctor about all your medical conditions including if you:
- **are pregnant or plan to become pregnant.** See "What is the most important information I should know about DIOVAN HCT?"
- **are breast-feeding.** DIOVAN HCT passes into breast milk. You should choose either to take DIOVAN HCT or breast-feed, but not both.
- **have liver problems**
- **have kidney problems**
- **have or had gallstones**
- **have Lupus**

Tell your doctor about all the medicines you take including prescription and nonprescription medicines, vitamins and herbal supplements. Some of your other medicines and DIOVAN HCT could affect each other, causing serious side effects. Especially, tell your doctor if you take:
- other medicines for high blood pressure or a heart problem
- water pills (diuretics)
- potassium supplements
- a salt substitute containing potassium
- antidiabetic medicines including insulin
- narcotic pain medicines
- sleeping pills
- lithium, a medicine used in some types of depression (Eskalith®, Lithobid®, Lithium Carbonate, Lithium Citrate)
- aspirin or other medicines called Non-Steroidal Anti-Inflammatory Drugs (NSAIDs)

Ask your doctor if you are not sure if you are taking one of these medicines.

Know the medicines you take. Keep a list of your medicines with you to show to your doctor and pharmacist when a new medicine is prescribed. Talk to your doctor or pharmacist before you start taking any new medicine. Your doctor or pharmacist will know what medicines are safe to take together.

How should I take DIOVAN HCT?
- Take DIOVAN HCT exactly as prescribed by your doctor. Your doctor may change your dose if needed.
- Take DIOVAN HCT once each day.
- DIOVAN HCT can be taken with or without food.
- If you miss a dose, take it as soon as you remember. If it is close to your next dose, do not take the missed dose. Just take the next dose at your regular time.
- If you take too much DIOVAN HCT, call your doctor or Poison Control Center, or go to the nearest hospital emergency room.

What should I avoid while taking DIOVAN HCT?

You should not take DIOVAN HCT during pregnancy. See "What is the most important information I should know about DIOVAN HCT?"

What are the possible side effects of DIOVAN HCT?

DIOVAN HCT may cause serious side effects including:
- **Harm to an unborn baby causing injury and even death.** See "What is the most important information I should know about DIOVAN HCT?"
- **Low blood pressure (hypotension).** Low blood pressure is most likely to happen if you:
  - take water pills
  - are on a low salt diet
  - get dialysis treatments
  - have heart problems
  - get sick with vomiting or diarrhea
  - drink alcohol

Lie down if you feel faint or dizzy. Call your doctor right away.

- **Worsening liver problems.** Liver problems may get worse in people who already have liver problems and take DIOVAN HCT.
- **Allergic reactions.** People with and without allergy problems or asthma who take DIOVAN HCT may get allergic reactions.
- **Worsening of Lupus.** Hydrochlorothiazide, one of the medicines in DIOVAN HCT may cause Lupus to become active or worse.
- **Fluid and electrolyte (salt) problems.** Tell your doctor about any of the following signs and symptoms of fluid and electrolyte problems:
  - dry mouth
  - thirst
  - lack of energy (lethargic)
  - weakness
  - drowsiness
  - restlessness
  - confusion
  - seizures
  - muscle pain or cramps
  - muscle fatigue
  - very low urine output
  - fast heartbeat
  - nausea and vomiting
- **Kidney problems.** Kidney problems may become worse in people that already have kidney disease. Some people will have changes on blood tests for kidney function and may need a lower dose of DIOVAN HCT. Call your doctor if you get swelling in your feet, ankles, or hands, or unexplained weight gain. If you have heart failure, your doctor should check your kidney function before prescribing DIOVAN HCT.
- **Skin rash.** Call your doctor right away if you have an unusual skin rash.

Other side effects were generally mild and brief. They generally have not caused patients to stop taking DIOVAN HCT.

Tell your doctor if you have any side effect that bothers you or that does not go away.

These are not all the possible side effects of DIOVAN HCT. For a complete list, ask your doctor or pharmacist.

Call your doctor for medical advice about side effects. You may report side effects to FDA at 1-800-FDA-1088.

How do I store DIOVAN HCT?
- Store DIOVAN HCT tablets at room temperature between 59°F to 86°F (15°C to 30°C).
- Keep DIOVAN HCT in a closed container in a dry place.

Keep DIOVAN HCT and all medicines out of the reach of children.

General information about DIOVAN HCT

Medicines are sometimes prescribed for conditions that are not mentioned in patient information leaflets. Do not use DIOVAN HCT for a condition for which it was not prescribed. Do not give DIOVAN HCT to other people, even if they have the same symptoms you have. It may harm them. This leaflet summarizes the most important information about DIOVAN HCT. If you would like more information, talk with your doctor. You can ask your doctor or pharmacist for information about DIOVAN HCT that is written for health professionals. For more information about DIOVAN HCT, go to www.DIOVAN.com or call 1-866-404-6359.

What are the ingredients in DIOVAN HCT?

Active ingredients: Valsartan and hydrochlorothiazide

Inactive ingredients: colloidal silicon dioxide, crospovidone, hydroxypropyl methylcellulose, iron oxides, magnesium stearate, microcrystalline cellulose, polyethylene glycol, talc, and titanium dioxide.

What is high blood pressure (hypertension)?

Blood pressure is the force in your blood vessels when your heart beats and when your heart rests. You have high blood pressure when the force is too much. DIOVAN HCT can help your blood vessels relax and reduce the amount of water in your body so your blood pressure is lower. Medicines that lower blood pressure lower your risk of having a stroke or heart attack.

High blood pressure makes the heart work harder to pump blood throughout the body and causes damage to the blood vessels. If high blood pressure is not treated, it can lead to stroke, heart attack, heart failure, kidney failure, and vision problems.

Eskalith® and Lithobid® are registered trademarks of Noven Pharmaceuticals, Inc.

Revised: APRIL 2010 Printed in U.S.A. T2010-06/T2008-20

5002425
5002426
5002475

Distributed by:
Novartis Pharmaceuticals Corporation
East Hanover, New Jersey 07936
©Novartis

Shown in Product Identification Guide, page 315

ELIDEL® ℞

[EL'-ee-del]
(pimecrolimus) Cream 1%
FOR DERMATOLOGIC USE ONLY
NOT FOR OPHTHALMIC USE
Rx only

The following prescribing information is based on official labeling in effect July 2010.
Prescribing Information
See WARNINGS, boxed WARNING concerning long-term safety of topical calcineurin inhibitors.

DESCRIPTION

ELIDEL® (pimecrolimus) Cream 1% contains the compound pimecrolimus, the immunosuppressant 33-epichloro-derivative of the macrolactam ascomycin.
Chemically, pimecrolimus is (1R,9S,12S,13R,14S,17R,18E, 21S,23S,24R,25S,27R)-12-[(1E)-2-[(1R,3R,4S)-4-chloro-3-methoxycyclohexyl]-1-methylvinyl]-17-ethyl-1,14-dihydroxy-23,25-dimethoxy-13,19,21,27-tetramethyl-11,28-dioxa-4-aza-tricyclo[22.3.1.0^{4,9}]octacos-18-ene-2,3,10,16-tetraone.
The compound has the empirical formula $C_{43}H_{68}ClNO_{12}$ and the molecular weight of 810.47. The structural formula is

Pimecrolimus is a white to off-white fine crystalline powder. It is soluble in methanol and ethanol and insoluble in water. Each gram of ELIDEL Cream 1% contains 10 mg of pimecrolimus in a whitish cream base of benzyl alcohol, cetyl alcohol, citric acid, mono- and di-glycerides, oleyl alcohol, propylene glycol, sodium cetostearyl sulphate, sodium hydroxide, stearyl alcohol, triglycerides, and water.

CLINICAL PHARMACOLOGY

Mechanism of Action/Pharmacodynamics

The mechanism of action of pimecrolimus in atopic dermatitis is not known. While the following have been observed, the clinical significance of these observations in atopic dermatitis is not known. It has been demonstrated that pimecrolimus binds with high affinity to macrophilin-12 (FKBP-12) and inhibits the calcium-dependent phosphatase, calcineurin. As a consequence, it inhibits T cell activation by blocking the transcription of early cytokines. In particular, pimecrolimus inhibits at nanomolar concentrations Interleukin-2 and interferon gamma (Th1-type) and Interleukin-4 and Interleukin-10 (Th2-type) cytokine synthesis in human T cells. In addition, pimecrolimus prevents the release of inflammatory cytokines and mediators from mast cells *in vitro* after stimulation by antigen/IgE.

Pharmacokinetics

Absorption

In adult patients (n=52) being treated for atopic dermatitis [13%-62% Body Surface Area (BSA) involvement] for periods up to a year, a maximum pimecrolimus concentration of 1.4 ng/mL was observed among those subjects with detectable blood levels. In the majority of samples in adult (91%; 1,244/1,362) subjects, blood concentrations of pimecrolimus were below 0.5 ng/mL. Data on blood levels of pimecrolimus measured in pediatric patients are described below in **Special Populations, Pediatrics**.

Distribution

Laboratory in vitro plasma protein binding studies using equilibrium gel filtration have shown that 99.5% of pimecrolimus in plasma is bound to proteins over the pimecrolimus concentration range of 2-100 ng/mL tested. The major fraction of pimecrolimus in plasma appears to be bound to various lipoproteins. As with other topical calcineurin inhibitors, it is not known whether pimecrolimus is absorbed into cutaneous lymphatic vessels or in regional lymph nodes.

Metabolism

Following the administration of a single oral radiolabeled dose of pimecrolimus numerous circulating O-demethylation metabolites were seen. Studies with human liver microsomes indicate that pimecrolimus is metabolized *in vitro* by the CYP3A sub-family of metabolizing enzymes. No evidence of skin mediated drug metabolism was identified in vivo using the minipig or in vitro using stripped human skin.

Elimination

Based on the results of the aforementioned radiolabeled study, following a single oral dose of pimecrolimus ~81% of the administered radioactivity was recovered, primarily in the feces (78.4%) as metabolites. Less than 1% of the radioactivity found in the feces was due to unchanged pimecrolimus.

Special Populations

Pediatrics

The systemic exposure to pimecrolimus from ELIDEL® (pimecrolimus) Cream 1% was investigated in 28 pediatric patients with atopic dermatitis (20%-80% BSA involvement) between the ages of 8 months-14 yrs. Following twice daily application for three weeks, blood concentrations of pimecrolimus were <2 ng/mL with 60% (96/161) of the blood samples having blood concentration below the limit of quantification (0.5 ng/mL). However, the children (23 children out of the total 28 children investigated) had at least one detectable blood level as compared to the adults (12 adults out of the total 52 adults investigated) over a 3-week treatment period. Due to the erratic nature of the blood levels observed, no correlation could be made between amount of cream, degree of BSA involvement, and blood concentrations. In general, the blood concentrations measured in adult atopic dermatitis patients were comparable to those seen in the pediatric population.
In a second group of 30 pediatric patients aged 3-23 months with 10%-92% BSA involvement, following twice daily application for three weeks, blood concentrations of pimecrolimus were <2.6 ng/mL with 65% (75/116) of the blood samples having blood concentration below 0.5 ng/mL, and 27% (31/116) below the limit of quantification (0.1 ng/mL) for these studies.
Overall, a higher proportion of detectable blood levels was seen in the pediatric patient population as compared to adult population. This increase in the absolute number of positive blood levels may be due to the larger surface area to body mass ratio seen in these younger subjects. In addition, a higher incidence of upper respiratory symptoms/infections was also seen relative to the older age group in the PK studies. At this time, a causal relationship between these findings and ELIDEL use cannot be ruled out.
ELIDEL Cream is not indicated for use in children less than 2 years of age (see **INDICATIONS AND USAGE, WARNINGS, boxed WARNING,** and **PRECAUTIONS, Pediatric Use**).

Renal Insufficiency

The effect of renal insufficiency on the pharmacokinetics of topically administered pimecrolimus has not been evaluated but dose-adjustment is not expected to be needed as 80% of the drug is excreted in the feces.

Hepatic Insufficiency

The effect of hepatic insufficiency on the pharmacokinetics of topically administered pimecrolimus has not been evaluated but dose-adjustment is not expected to be needed.

CLINICAL STUDIES

Three randomized, double-blind, vehicle-controlled, multi-center, Phase 3 studies were conducted in 589 pediatric patients ages 3 months-17 years old to evaluate ELIDEL® (pimecrolimus) Cream 1% for the treatment of mild to moderate atopic dermatitis. Two of the three trials support the use of ELIDEL Cream in patients 2 years and older with mild to moderate atopic dermatitis (see **PRECAUTIONS, Pediatric Use**). Three other trials in 1,619 pediatric and adult patients provided additional data regarding the safety of ELIDEL Cream in the treatment of atopic dermatitis. Two of these other trials were vehicle-controlled with optional sequential use of a medium potency topical corticosteroid in pediatric patients and one trial was an active comparator trial in adult patients with atopic dermatitis (see **PRECAUTIONS, Pediatric Use** and **ADVERSE REACTIONS**).
Two identical 6-week, randomized, vehicle-controlled, multi-center, Phase 3 trials were conducted to evaluate ELIDEL Cream for the treatment of mild to moderate atopic dermatitis. A total of 403 pediatric patients 2-17 years old were included in the studies. The male/female ratio was approximately 50% and 29% of the patients were African American. At study entry, 59% of patients had moderate disease and the mean body surface area (BSA) affected was 26%. About 75% of patients had atopic dermatitis affecting the face and/or neck region. In these studies, patients applied either ELIDEL Cream or vehicle cream twice daily to 5% to 96% of their BSA for up to 6 weeks. At endpoint, based on the physician's global evaluation of clinical response, 35% of patients treated with ELIDEL Cream were clear or almost clear of signs of atopic dermatitis compared to only 18% of vehicle-treated patients. More ELIDEL patients (57%) had mild or no pruritus at 6 weeks compared to vehicle patients (34%). The improvement in pruritus occurred in conjunction with the improvement of the patients' atopic dermatitis.

In these two 6-week studies of ELIDEL, the combined efficacy results at endpoint are as follows:

	% Patients	
	Elidel® (N= 267)	Vehicle (N= 136)
Global Assessment		
Clear	28 (10%)	5 (4%)
Clear or Almost Clear	93 (35%)	25 (18%)
Clear to Mild Disease	180 (67%)	55 (40%)

In the two pediatric studies that independently support the use of ELIDEL Cream in mild to moderate atopic dermatitis, a significant treatment effect was seen by day 15. Of the key signs of atopic dermatitis, erythema, infiltration/papulation, lichenification, and excoriations, erythema and infiltration/papulation were reduced at day 8 when compared to vehicle.
The following graph depicts the time course of improvement in the percent body surface area affected as a result of treatment with ELIDEL Cream in 2-17 year olds.

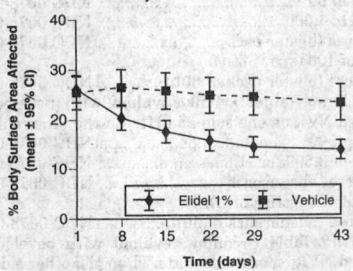

Figure 1
Body Surface Area Over Time

The following graph shows the time course of improvement in erythema as a result of treatment with ELIDEL Cream in 2-17 year olds.

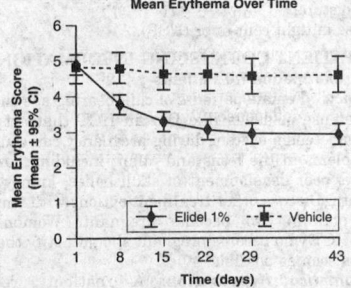

Figure 2
Mean Erythema Over Time

INDICATIONS AND USAGE

ELIDEL® (pimecrolimus) Cream 1% is indicated as *second-line therapy* for the short-term and non-continuous chronic treatment of mild to moderate atopic dermatitis in non-immunocompromised adults and children 2 years of age and older, who have failed to respond adequately to other topical prescription treatments, or when those treatments are not advisable.
ELIDEL Cream is not indicated for use in children less than 2 years of age (see WARNINGS, boxed WARNING, and PRECAUTIONS, Pediatric Use).

CONTRAINDICATIONS

ELIDEL® (pimecrolimus) Cream 1% is contraindicated in individuals with a history of hypersensitivity to pimecrolimus or any of the components of the cream.

WARNINGS

> **WARNING**
> **Long-term Safety of Topical Calcineurin Inhibitors Has Not Been Established**
> Although a causal relationship has not been established, rare cases of malignancy (e.g., skin and lymphoma) have been reported in patients treated with topical calcineurin inhibitors, including ELIDEL Cream.
> Therefore:
> • Continuous long-term use of topical calcineurin inhibitors, including ELIDEL Cream, in any age group should be avoided, and application limited to areas of involvement with atopic dermatitis.

• ELIDEL Cream is not indicated for use in children less than 2 years of age.

Prolonged systemic use of calcineurin inhibitors for sustained immunosuppression in animal studies and transplant patients following systemic administration has been associated with an increased risk of infections, lymphomas, and skin malignancies. These risks are associated with the intensity and duration of immunosuppression.

Based on this information and the mechanism of action, there is a concern about a potential risk with the use of topical calcineurin inhibitors, including ELIDEL Cream. While a causal relationship has not been established, rare cases of skin malignancy and lymphoma have been reported in patients treated with topical calcineurin inhibitors, including ELIDEL Cream. Therefore:

• ELIDEL Cream should not be used in immunocompromised adults and children.
• If signs and symptoms of atopic dermatitis do not improve within 6 weeks, patients should be re-examined by their healthcare provider and their diagnosis be confirmed (see PRECAUTIONS).
• The safety of ELIDEL Cream has not been established beyond one year of non-continuous use.

(See **CLINICAL PHARMACOLOGY, WARNINGS, boxed WARNING, PRECAUTIONS, INDICATIONS AND USAGE,** and **DOSAGE AND ADMINISTRATION**.)

PRECAUTIONS

General

The use of ELIDEL Cream should be avoided on malignant or pre-malignant skin conditions. Malignant or pre-malignant skin conditions, such as cutaneous T-cell lymphoma (CTCL), can present as dermatitis.

ELIDEL Cream should not be used in patients with Netherton's Syndrome or other skin diseases where there is the potential for increased systemic absorption of pimecrolimus. The safety of ELIDEL Cream has not been established in patients with generalized erythroderma.

The use of ELIDEL Cream may cause local symptoms such as skin burning (burning sensation, stinging, soreness) or pruritus. Localized symptoms are most common during the first few days of ELIDEL Cream application and typically improve as the lesions of atopic dermatitis resolve (see ADVERSE REACTIONS).

Bacterial and Viral Skin Infections: Before commencing treatment with ELIDEL Cream, bacterial or viral infections at treatment sites should be resolved. Studies have not evaluated the safety and efficacy of ELIDEL Cream in the treatment of clinically infected atopic dermatitis.

While patients with atopic dermatitis are predisposed to superficial skin infections including eczema herpeticum (Kaposi's varicelliform eruption), treatment with ELIDEL Cream may be independently associated with an increased risk of varicella zoster virus infection (chicken pox or shingles), herpes simplex virus infection, or eczema herpeticum.

In clinical studies, 15/1,544 (1%) cases of skin papilloma (warts) were observed in patients using ELIDEL Cream. The youngest patient was age 2 and the oldest was age 12. In cases where there is worsening of skin papillomas or they do not respond to conventional therapy, discontinuation of ELIDEL Cream should be considered until complete resolution of the warts is achieved.

Patients with Lymphadenopathy: In clinical studies, 14/1,544 (0.9%) cases of lymphadenopathy were reported while using ELIDEL Cream. These cases of lymphadenopathy were usually related to infections and noted to resolve upon appropriate antibiotic therapy. Of these 14 cases, the majority had either a clear etiology or were known to resolve. Patients who receive ELIDEL Cream and who develop lymphadenopathy should have the etiology of their lymphadenopathy investigated. In the absence of a clear etiology for the lymphadenopathy, or in the presence of acute infectious mononucleosis, ELIDEL Cream should be discontinued. Patients who develop lymphadenopathy should be monitored to ensure that the lymphadenopathy resolves.

Sun Exposure: During the course of treatment, it is prudent for patients to minimize or avoid natural or artificial sunlight exposure, even while ELIDEL is not on the skin. The potential effects of ELIDEL Cream on skin response to ultraviolet damage are not known.

Immunocompromised Patients: The safety and efficacy of ELIDEL Cream in immunocompromised patients have not been studied.

Information for Patients

(See Medication Guide.)

Patients using ELIDEL Cream should receive the following information and instructions:

What is the most important information a patient should know about ELIDEL Cream?

The safety of using ELIDEL Cream for a long period of time is not known. A very small number of people who have used

ELIDEL Cream have had cancer (for example, skin or lymphoma). However, a link with ELIDEL Cream use has not been shown. Because of this concern:

• A patient should not use ELIDEL Cream continuously for a long time.
• ELIDEL Cream should be used only on areas of skin that have eczema.
• ELIDEL Cream is not for use on a child under 2 years old.

How should a patient use ELIDEL Cream?

• A patient should use ELIDEL Cream exactly as prescribed.
• A patient should use ELIDEL Cream only on areas of skin that have eczema.
• A patient should use ELIDEL Cream for short periods, and if needed, treatment may be repeated with breaks in between.
• A patient should stop ELIDEL Cream when the signs and symptoms of eczema, such as itching, rash, and redness go away, or as directed by the physician.
• A patient should follow the physician's advice if symptoms of eczema return after a treatment with ELIDEL Cream.
• A patient should contact the physician if:
  • symptoms get worse with ELIDEL Cream
  • the patient gets a skin infection
  • if burning on the skin is severe or lasts for more than one week
  • if eye irritation does not go away
  • symptoms do not improve after 6 weeks of treatment

To apply ELIDEL Cream:

• A patient or caregiver should wash their hands before using ELIDEL Cream. When applying ELIDEL Cream after a bath or shower, the skin should be dry.
• A patient or caregiver should apply a thin layer of ELIDEL Cream only to the affected skin areas, twice a day, as directed by the physician.
• A patient or caregiver should use the smallest amount of ELIDEL Cream needed to control the signs and symptoms of eczema.
• Caregivers applying ELIDEL Cream to a patient, or a patient who is not treating the hands should wash their hands with soap and water after applying ELIDEL Cream. This should remove any cream left on the hands.
• A patient should not bathe, shower or swim right after applying ELIDEL Cream. This could wash off the cream.
• A patient can use moisturizers with ELIDEL Cream. They should be sure to check with the physician first about the products that are right for them. Because the skin of patients with eczema can be very dry, it is important they keep up good skin care practices. If a patient uses moisturizers, he or she should apply them after ELIDEL Cream.

What should a patient avoid while using ELIDEL Cream?

• A patient should not use sun lamps, tanning beds, or get treatment with ultraviolet light therapy during treatment with ELIDEL Cream.
• A patient should limit sun exposure during treatment with ELIDEL Cream even when the medicine is not on the skin. If a patient needs to be outdoors after applying ELIDEL Cream, the patient should wear loose fitting clothing that protects the treated area from the sun. The physician should advise the patient about other types of protection from the sun.
• A patient should not cover the skin being treated with bandages, dressings or wraps. A patient can wear normal clothing.
• ELIDEL Cream is for use on the skin only. Do not get ELIDEL Cream in your eyes, nose, mouth, vagina, or rectum (mucous membranes). If you get ELIDEL Cream in any of these areas, burning or irritation can happen. Wipe off any ELIDEL Cream from the affected area and then rinse the area well with cold water. ELIDEL Cream is for external use only.
• A patient should not swallow ELIDEL Cream and should contact the physician if they do.

Drug Interactions

Potential interactions between ELIDEL and other drugs, including immunizations, have not been systematically evaluated. Due to low blood levels of pimecrolimus detected in some patients after topical application, systemic drug interactions are not expected, but cannot be ruled out. The concomitant administration of known CYP3A family of inhibitors in patients with widespread and/or erythrodermic disease should be done with caution. Some examples of such drugs are erythromycin, itraconazole, ketoconazole, fluconazole, calcium channel blockers and cimetidine.

Carcinogenesis, Mutagenesis, Impairment of Fertility

In a 2-year rat dermal carcinogenicity study using ELIDEL Cream, a statistically significant increase in the incidence of follicular cell adenoma of the thyroid was noted in low, mid and high dose male animals compared to vehicle and saline control male animals. Follicular cell adenoma of the thyroid was noted in the dermal rat carcinogenicity study at the lowest dose of 2 mg/kg/day [0.2% pimecrolimus cream; 1.5× the Maximum Recommended Human Dose (MRHD) based

on AUC comparisons]. No increase in the incidence of follicular cell adenoma of the thyroid was noted in the oral carcinogenicity study in male rats up to 10 mg/kg/day (66× MRHD based on AUC comparisons). However, oral studies may not reflect continuous exposure or the same metabolic profile as by the dermal route. In a mouse dermal carcinogenicity study using pimecrolimus in an ethanolic solution, no increase in incidence of neoplasms was observed in the skin or other organs up to the highest dose of 4 mg/kg/day (0.32% pimecrolimus in ethanol) 27× MRHD based on AUC comparisons. However, lymphoproliferative changes (including lymphoma) were noted in a 13 week repeat dose dermal toxicity study conducted in mice using pimecrolimus in an ethanolic solution at a dose of 25 mg/kg/day (47× MRHD based on AUC comparisons). No lymphoproliferative changes were noted in this study at a dose of 10 mg/kg/day (17× MRHD based on AUC comparison). However, the latency time to lymphoma formation was shortened to 8 weeks after dermal administration of pimecrolimus dissolved in ethanol at a dose of 100 mg/kg/day (179-217× MRHD based on AUC comparisons).

In a mouse oral (gavage) carcinogenicity study, a statistically significant increase in the incidence of lymphoma was noted in high dose male and female animals compared to vehicle control male and female animals. Lymphomas were noted in the oral mouse carcinogenicity study at a dose of 45 mg/kg/day (258-340× MRHD based on AUC comparisons). No drug-related tumors were noted in the mouse oral carcinogenicity study at a dose of 15 mg/kg/day (60-133× MRHD based on AUC comparisons). In an oral (gavage) rat carcinogenicity study, a statistically significant increase in the incidence of benign thymoma was noted in 10 mg/kg/day pimecrolimus treated male and female animals compared to vehicle control treated male and female animals. In addition, a significant increase in the incidence of benign thymoma was noted in another oral (gavage) rat carcinogenicity study in 5 mg/kg/day pimecrolimus treated male animals compared to vehicle control treated male animals. No drug-related tumors were noted in the rat oral carcinogenicity study at a dose of 1 mg/kg/day male animals (1.1× MRHD based on AUC comparisons) and at a dose of 5 mg/kg/day for female animals (21× MRHD based on AUC comparisons).

In a 52-week dermal photo-carcinogenicity study, the median time to onset of skin tumor formation was decreased in hairless mice following chronic topical dosing with concurrent exposure to UV radiation (40 weeks of treatment followed by 12 weeks of observation) with the ELIDEL Cream vehicle alone. No additional effect on tumor development beyond the vehicle effect was noted with the addition of the active ingredient, pimecrolimus, to the vehicle cream.

A 39-week oral monkey toxicology study was conducted with pimecrolimus doses of 15, 45 and 120 mg/kg/day. A dose dependent increase in expression of immunosuppressive-related lymphoproliferative disorder (IRLD) associated with lymphocryptovirus (a monkey strain of virus related to human Epstein Barr virus) was observed. IRLD in monkeys mirrors what has been noted in human transplant patients after chronic systemic immunosuppressive therapy, post transplantation lymphoproliferative disease (PTLD), after treatment with chronic systemic immunosuppressive therapy. Both IRLD and PTLD can progress to lymphoma, which is dependent on the dose and duration of systemic immunosuppressive therapy. A dose dependent increase in opportunistic infections (a signal of systemic immunosuppression) was also noted in this monkey study. A no-observed adverse effect level (NOAEL) for IRLD and opportunistic infections was not established in this study. IRLD occurred at the lowest dose of 15 mg/kg/day for 39 weeks [31× the Maximum Recommended Human Dose (MRHD) of ELIDEL Cream based on AUC comparisons] in this study. A partial recovery from IRLD was noted upon cessation of dosing in this study.

A battery of *in vitro* genotoxicity tests, including Ames assay, mouse lymphoma L5178Y assay, and chromosome aberration test in V79 Chinese hamster cells and an *in vivo* mouse micronucleus test revealed no evidence for a mutagenic or clastogenic potential for the drug.

An oral fertility and embryofetal developmental study in rats revealed estrus cycle disturbances, post-implantation loss and reduction in litter size at the 45 mg/kg/day dose (38× MRHD based on AUC comparisons). No effect on fertility in female rats was noted at 10 mg/kg/day (12× MRHD based on AUC comparisons). No effect on fertility in male rats was noted at 45 mg/kg/day (23× MRHD based on AUC comparisons), which was the highest dose tested in this study.

A second oral fertility and embryofetal developmental study in rats revealed reduced testicular and epididymal weights, reduced testicular sperm counts and motile sperm for males and estrus cycle disturbances, decreased corpora lutea, decreased implantations and viable fetuses for females at

Treatment Emergent Adverse Events (≥1%) in Elidel® Treatment Groups

	Pediatric Patients* Vehicle-Controlled (6 weeks)		Pediatric Patients* Open-Label (20 weeks)	Pediatric Patients* Vehicle-Controlled (1 year)		Adult Active Comparator (1 year)
	Elidel® Cream (N=267) N (%)	Vehicle (N=136) N (%)	Elidel® Cream (N=335) N (%)	Elidel® Cream (N=272) N (%)	Vehicle (N=75) N (%)	Elidel® Cream (N=328) N (%)
At least 1 AE	182 (68.2%)	97 (71.3%)	240 (72.0%)	230 (84.6%)	56 (74.7%)	256 (78.0%)
Infections and Infestations						
Upper Respiratory Tract Infection NOS	38 (14.2%)	18 (13.2%)	65 (19.4%)	13 (4.8%)	6 (8.0%)	14 (4.3%)
Nasopharyngitis	27 (10.1%)	10 (7.4%)	32 (19.6%)	72 (26.5%)	16 (21.3%)	25 (7.6%)
Skin Infection NOS	8 (3.0%)	9 (5.1%)	18 (5.4%)	6 (2.2%)	3 (4.0%)	21 (6.4%)
Influenza	8 (3.0%)	1 (0.7%)	22 (6.6%)	36 (13.2%)	1 (1.3%)	2 (0.6%)
Ear Infection NOS	6 (2.2%)	2 (1.5%)	19 (5.7%)	9 (3.3%)	1 (1.3%)	2 (0.6%)
Otitis Media	6 (2.2%)	1 (0.7%)	10 (3.0%)	8 (2.9%)	4 (5.3%)	2 (0.6%)
Impetigo	5 (1.9%)	3 (2.2%)	12 (3.6%)	11 (4.0%)	4 (5.3%)	8 (2.4%)
Bacterial Infection	4 (1.5%)	3 (2.2%)	4 (1.2%)	3 (1.1%)	0	6 (1.8%)
Folliculitis	3 (1.1%)	1 (0.7%)	3 (0.9%)	6 (2.2%)	3 (4.0%)	20 (6.1%)
Sinusitis	3 (1.1%)	1 (0.7%)	11 (3.3%)	6 (2.2%)	1 (1.3%)	2 (0.6%)
Pneumonia NOS	3 (1.1%)	1 (0.7%)	5 (1.5%)	0	1 (1.3%)	1 (0.3%)
Pharyngitis NOS	2 (0.7%)	2 (1.5%)	3 (0.9%)	22 (8.1%)	2 (2.7%)	3 (0.9%)
Pharyngitis Streptococcal	2 (0.7%)	2 (1.5%)	10 (3.0%)	0	<1%	0
Molluscum Contagiosum	2 (0.7%)	0	4 (1.2%)	5 (1.8%)	0	0
Staphylococcal Infection	1 (0.4%)	5 (3.7%)	7 (2.1%)	0	<1%	3 (0.9%)
Bronchitis NOS	1 (0.4%)	3 (2.2%)	4 (1.2%)	29 (10.7%)	6 (8.0%)	8 (2.4%)
Herpes Simplex	1 (0.4%)	0	4 (1.2%)	9 (3.3%)	2 (2.7%)	13 (4.0%)
Tonsillitis NOS	1 (0.4%)	0	3 (0.9%)	17 (6.3%)	0	2 (0.6%)
Viral Infection NOS	2 (0.7%)	1 (0.7%)	1 (0.3%)	18 (6.6%)	1 (1.3%)	0
Gastroenteritis NOS	0	3 (2.2%)	2 (0.6%)	20 (7.4%)	2 (2.7%)	6 (1.8%)
Chickenpox	2 (0.7%)	0	3 (0.9%)	8 (2.9%)	3 (4.0%)	1 (0.3%)
Skin Papilloma	1 (0.4%)	0	2 (0.6%)	9 (3.3%)	<1%	0
Tonsillitis Acute NOS	0	0	0	7 (2.6%)	0	0
Upper Respiratory Tract Infection Viral NOS	1 (0.4%)	0	3 (0.9%)	4 (1.5%)	0	1 (0.3%)
Herpes Simplex Dermatitis	0	0	1 (0.3%)	4 (1.5%)	0	2 (0.6%)
Bronchitis Acute NOS	0	0	0	4 (1.5%)	0	0
Eye Infection NOS	0	0	0	3 (1.1%)	<1%	1 (0.3%)
General Disorders and Administration Site Conditions						
Application Site Burning	28 (10.4%)	17 (12.5%)	5 (1.5%)	23 (8.5%)	5 (6.7%)	85 (25.9%)
Pyrexia	20 (7.5%)	12 (8.8%)	41 (12.2%)	34 (12.5%)	4 (5.3%)	4 (1.2%)
Application Site Reaction NOS	8 (3.0%)	7 (5.1%)	7 (2.1%)	9 (3.3%)	2 (2.7%)	48 (14.6%)
Application Site Irritation	8 (3.0%)	8 (5.9%)	3 (0.9%)	1 (0.4%)	3 (4.0%)	21 (6.4%)
Influenza Like Illness	1 (0.4%)	0	2 (0.6%)	5 (1.8%)	2 (2.7%)	6 (1.8%)
Application Site Erythema	1 (0.4%)	0	0	6 (2.2%)	0	7 (2.1%)
Application Site Pruritus	3 (1.1%)	2 (1.5%)	2 (0.6%)	5 (1.8%)	0	18 (5.5%)
Respiratory, Thoracic and Mediastinal Disorders						
Cough	31 (11.6%)	11 (8.1%)	31 (9.3%)	43 (15.8%)	8 (10.7%)	8 (2.4%)
Nasal Congestion	7 (2.6%)	2 (1.5%)	6 (1.8%)	4 (1.5%)	1 (1.3%)	2 (0.6%)
Rhinorrhea	5 (1.9%)	1 (0.7%)	3 (0.9%)	1 (0.4%)	1 (1.3%)	0
Asthma Aggravated	4 (1.5%)	3 (2.2%)	13 (3.9%)	3 (1.1%)	1 (1.3%)	0
Sinus Congestion	3 (1.1%)	1 (0.7%)	2 (0.6%)	<1%	<1%	3 (0.9%)
Rhinitis	1 (0.4%)	0	5 (1.5%)	12 (4.4%)	5 (6.7%)	7 (2.1%)
Wheezing	1 (0.4%)	1 (0.7%)	4 (1.2%)	2 (0.7%)	<1%	0
Asthma NOS	2 (0.7%)	1 (0.7%)	11 (3.3%)	10 (3.7%)	2 (2.7%)	8 (2.4%)
Epistaxis	0	1 (0.7%)	0	9 (3.3%)	1 (1.3%)	1 (0.3%)
Dyspnea NOS	0	0	0	5 (1.8%)	1 (1.3%)	2 (0.6%)
Gastrointestinal Disorders						
Abdominal Pain Upper	11 (4.1%)	6 (4.4%)	10 (3.0%)	15 (5.5%)	5 (6.7%)	1 (0.3%)
Sore Throat	9 (3.4%)	5 (3.7%)	15 (5.4%)	22 (8.1%)	4 (5.3%)	12 (3.7%)
Vomiting NOS	8 (3.0%)	6 (4.4%)	14 (4.2%)	18 (6.6%)	6 (8.0%)	2 (0.6%)
Diarrhea NOS	3 (1.1%)	1 (0.7%)	2 (0.6%)	21 (7.7%)	4 (5.3%)	7 (2.1%)
Nausea	1 (0.4%)	3 (2.2%)	4 (1.2%)	11 (4.0%)	5 (6.7%)	6 (1.8%)
Abdominal Pain NOS	1 (0.4%)	1 (0.7%)	5 (1.5%)	12 (4.4%)	3 (4.0%)	1 (0.3%)
Toothache	1 (0.4%)	1 (0.7%)	2 (0.6%)	7 (2.6%)	1 (1.3%)	2 (0.6%)
Constipation	1 (0.4%)	0	2 (0.6%)	10 (3.7%)	<1%	0
Loose Stools	0	1 (0.7%)	4 (1.2%)	<1%	<1%	0

(Table continued on next page)

45 mg/kg/day dose (123× MRHD for males and 192× MRHD for females based on AUC comparisons). No effect on fertility in female rats was noted at 10 mg/kg/day (5× MRHD based on AUC comparisons). No effect on fertility in male rats was noted at 2 mg/kg/day (0.7× MRHD based on AUC comparisons).

Pregnancy
Teratogenic Effects: Pregnancy Category C
There are no adequate and well-controlled studies of topically administered pimecrolimus in pregnant women. The experience with ELIDEL Cream when used by pregnant women is too limited to permit assessment of the safety of its use during pregnancy.

In dermal embryofetal developmental studies, no maternal or fetal toxicity was observed up to the highest practicable doses tested, 10 mg/kg/day (1% pimecrolimus cream) in rats (0.14× MRHD based on body surface area) and 10 mg/kg/day (1% pimecrolimus cream) in rabbits (0.65× MRHD based on AUC comparisons). The 1% pimecrolimus cream was administered topically for 6 hours/day during the period of organogenesis in rats and rabbits (gestational days 6-21 in rats and gestational days 6-20 in rabbits).

A second dermal embryofetal development study was conducted in rats using pimecrolimus cream applied dermally to pregnant rats (1 g cream/kg body weight of 0.2%, 0.6% and 1.0% pimecrolimus cream) from gestation day 6 to 17 at doses of 2, 6, and 10 mg/kg/day with daily exposure of approximately 22 hours. No maternal, reproductive, or embryo-fetal toxicity attributable to pimecrolimus was noted at 10 mg/kg/day (0.66× MRHD based on AUC comparisons), the highest dose evaluated in this study. No teratogenicity was noted in this study at any dose.

A combined oral fertility and embryofetal developmental study was conducted in rats and an oral embryofetal developmental study was conducted in rabbits. Pimecrolimus was administered during the period of organogenesis (2 weeks prior to mating until gestational day 16 in rats, gestational days 6-18 in rabbits) up to dose levels of 45 mg/kg/day in rats and 20 mg/kg/day in rabbits. In the absence of maternal toxicity, indicators of embryofetal toxicity (post-implantation loss and reduction in litter size) were noted at 45 mg/kg/day (38× MRHD based on AUC comparisons) in the oral fertility and embryofetal developmental study conducted in rats. No malformations in the fetuses were noted at 45 mg/kg/day (38× MRHD based on AUC comparisons) in this study. No maternal toxicity, embryotoxicity or teratogenicity were noted in the oral rabbit embryofetal developmental toxicity study at 20 mg/kg/day (3.9× MRHD based on AUC comparisons), which was the highest dose tested in this study.

A second oral embryofetal development study was conducted in rats. Pimecrolimus was administered during the period of organogenesis (gestational days 6-17) at doses of 2, 10 and 45 mg/kg/day. Maternal toxicity, embryolethality and fetotoxicity were noted at 45 mg/kg/day (271× MRHD based on AUC comparisons). A slight increase in skeletal variations that were indicative of delayed skeletal ossification was also noted at this dose. No maternal toxicity, embryolethality or fetotoxicity were noted at 10 mg/kg/day (16× MRHD based on AUC comparisons). No teratogenicity was noted in this study at any dose.

A second oral embryofetal development study was conducted in rabbits. Pimecrolimus was administered during the period of organogenesis (gestational days 7-20) at doses of 2, 6 and 20 mg/kg/day. Maternal toxicity, embryotoxicity and fetotoxicity were noted at 20 mg/kg/day (12× MRHD based on AUC comparisons). A slight increase in skeletal variations that were indicative of delayed skeletal ossification was also noted at this dose. No maternal toxicity, embryotoxicity or fetotoxicity were noted at 6 mg/kg/day (5× MRHD based on AUC comparisons). No teratogenicity was noted in this study at any dose.

An oral peri- and post-natal developmental study was conducted in rats. Pimecrolimus was administered from gestational day 6 through lactational day 21 up to a dose level of 40 mg/kg/day. Only 2 of 22 females delivered live pups at the highest dose of 40 mg/kg/day. Postnatal survival, development of the F1 generation, their subsequent maturation and fertility were not affected at 10 mg/kg/day (12× MRHD based on AUC comparisons), the highest dose evaluated in this study.

Pimecrolimus was transferred across the placenta in oral rat and rabbit embryofetal developmental studies.

There are, however, no adequate and well-controlled studies in pregnant women. Because animal reproduction studies are not always predictive of human response, this drug should be used only if clearly needed during pregnancy.

Nursing Mothers
It is not known whether this drug is excreted in human milk. Because of the potential for serious adverse reactions in nursing infants from pimecrolimus, a decision should be made whether to discontinue nursing or to discontinue the drug, taking into account the importance of the drug to the mother.

Pediatric Use
ELIDEL Cream is not indicated for use in children less than 2 years of age.
The long-term safety and effects of ELIDEL Cream on the developing immune system are unknown (see **WARNINGS, boxed WARNING,** and **INDICATIONS AND USAGE**).
Three Phase 3 pediatric studies were conducted involving 1,114 patients 2-17 years of age. Two studies were 6-week randomized vehicle-controlled studies with a 20-week open-label phase and one was a vehicle-controlled (up to 1 year) safety study with the option for sequential topical corticosteroid use. Of these patients 542 (49%) were 2-6 years of age. In the short-term studies, 11% of ELIDEL patients did not complete these studies and 1.5% of ELIDEL patients discontinued due to adverse events. In the one-year study, 32% of ELIDEL patients did not complete this study and 3% of ELIDEL patients discontinued due to adverse events. Most discontinuations were due to unsatisfactory therapeutic effect.
The most common local adverse event in the short-term studies of ELIDEL Cream in pediatric patients ages 2-17 was application site burning (10% vs. 13% vehicle); the incidence in the long-term study was 9% ELIDEL vs. 7% vehicle (see **ADVERSE REACTIONS**). Adverse events that were more frequent (>5%) in patients treated with ELIDEL Cream compared to vehicle were headache (14% vs. 9%) in

the short-term trial. Nasopharyngitis (26% vs. 21%), influenza (13% vs. 4%), pharyngitis (8% vs. 3%), viral infection (7% vs. 1%), pyrexia (13% vs. 5%), cough (16% vs. 11%), and headache (25% vs. 16%) were increased over vehicle in the 1-year safety study (see **ADVERSE REACTIONS**). In 843 patients ages 2-17 years treated with ELIDEL Cream, 9 (0.8%) developed eczema herpeticum (5 on ELIDEL Cream alone and 4 on ELIDEL Cream used in sequence with corticosteroids). In 211 patients on vehicle alone, there were no cases of eczema herpeticum. The majority of adverse events were mild to moderate in severity.

Two Phase 3 studies were conducted involving 436 infants age 3 months-23 months. One 6-week randomized vehicle-controlled study with a 20-week open-label phase and one safety study, up to one year, were conducted. In the 6-week study, 11% of ELIDEL and 48% of vehicle patients did not complete this study; no patient in either group discontinued due to adverse events. Infants on ELIDEL Cream had an increased incidence of some adverse events compared to vehicle. In the 6-week vehicle-controlled study these adverse events included pyrexia (32% vs. 13% vehicle), URI (24% vs. 14%), nasopharyngitis (15% vs. 8%), gastroenteritis (7% vs. 3%), otitis media (4% vs. 0%), and diarrhea (8% vs. 0%). In the open-label phase of the study, for infants who switched to ELIDEL Cream from vehicle, the incidence of the above-cited adverse events approached or equaled the incidence of those patients who remained on ELIDEL Cream. In the 6 month safety data, 16% of ELIDEL and 35% of vehicle patients discontinued early and 1.5% of ELIDEL and 0% of vehicle patients discontinued due to adverse events. Infants on ELIDEL Cream had a greater incidence of some adverse events as compared to vehicle. These included pyrexia (30% vs. 20%), URI (21% vs. 17%), cough (15% vs. 9%), hypersitivity (8% vs. 2%), teething (27% vs. 22%), vomiting (9% vs. 4%), rhinitis (13% vs. 9%), viral rash (4% vs. 0%), rhinorrhea (4% vs. 0%), and wheezing (4% vs. 0%).

Geriatric Use

Nine (9) patients ≥65 years old received ELIDEL Cream in Phase 3 studies. Clinical studies of ELIDEL did not include sufficient numbers of patients aged 65 and over to assess efficacy and safety.

ADVERSE REACTIONS

No phototoxicity and no photoallergenicity were detected in clinical studies with 24 and 33 normal volunteers, respectively. In human dermal safety studies, ELIDEL® (pimecrolimus) Cream 1% did not induce contact sensitization or cumulative irritation.

In a one-year safety study in pediatric patients age 2-17 years old involving sequential use of ELIDEL Cream and a topical corticosteroid, 43% of ELIDEL patients and 68% of vehicle patients used corticosteroids during the study. Corticosteroids were used for more than 7 days by 34% of ELIDEL patients and 54% of vehicle patients. An increased incidence of impetigo, skin infection, superinfection (infected atopic dermatitis), rhinitis, and urticaria were found in the patients that had used ELIDEL Cream and topical corticosteroid sequentially as compared to ELIDEL Cream alone.

In 3 randomized, double-blind vehicle-controlled pediatric studies and one active-controlled adult study, 843 and 328 patients respectively, were treated with ELIDEL Cream. In these clinical trials, 48 (4%) of the 1,171 ELIDEL patients and 13 (3%) of 408 vehicle-treated patients discontinued therapy due to adverse events. Discontinuations for AEs were primarily due to application site reactions, and cutaneous infections. The most common application site reaction was application site burning, which occurred in 8%-26% of patients treated with ELIDEL Cream.

The following table depicts the incidence of adverse events pooled across the 2 identically designed 6-week studies with their open label extensions and the 1-year safety study for pediatric patients ages 2-17. Data from the adult active-controlled study is also included in this table. Adverse events are listed regardless of relationship to study drug. [See table on previous page and above]

Two cases of septic arthritis have been reported in infants less than one year of age in clinical trials conducted with ELIDEL Cream (n = 2,443). Causality has not been established.

POST-MARKETING EVENTS

The following adverse reactions have been reported in patients using ELIDEL Cream. Because these reactions are reported voluntarily from a population of uncertain size, it is not always possible to reliably estimate their frequency or establish a causal relationship to drug exposure.

General: Anaphylactic reactions, ocular irritation after application of the cream to the eye lids or near the eyes, angioneurotic edema, facial edema, skin flushing associated with alcohol use, skin discoloration.

Hematology/Oncology: Lymphomas, basal cell carcinoma, malignant melanoma, squamous cell carcinoma

	Pediatric Patients* Vehicle-Controlled (6 weeks)		Pediatric Patients* Open-Label (20 weeks)	Pediatric Patients* Vehicle-Controlled (1 year)		Adult Active Comparator (1 year)
	Elidel® Cream (N=267) N (%)	Vehicle (N=136) N (%)	Elidel® Cream (N=335) N (%)	Elidel® Cream (N=272) N (%)	Vehicle (N=75) N (%)	Elidel® Cream (N=328) N (%)
Reproductive System and Breast Disorders						
Dysmenorrhea	3 (1.1%)	0	5 (1.5%)	3 (1.1%)	1 (1.3%)	4 (1.2%)
Eye Disorders						
Conjunctivitis NEC	2 (0.7%)	1 (0.7%)	7 (2.1%)	6 (2.2%)	3 (4.0%)	10 (3.0%)
Skin & Subcutaneous Tissue Disorders						
Urticaria	3 (1.1%)	0	1 (0.3%)	1 (0.4%)	<1%	3 (0.9%)
Acne NOS	0	1 (0.7%)	1 (0.3%)	4 (1.5%)	<1%	6 (1.8%)
Immune System Disorders						
Hypersensitivity NOS	11 (4.1%)	6 (4.4%)	16 (4.8%)	14 (5.1%)	1 (1.3%)	11 (3.4%)
Injury and Poisoning						
Accident NOS	3 (1.1%)	1 (0.7%)	1 (0.3%)	<1%	1 (1.3%)	0
Laceration	2 (0.7%)	1 (0.7%)	5 (1.5%)	<1%	<1%	0
Musculoskeletal, Connective Tissue and Bone Disorders						
Back Pain	1 (0.4%)	2 (1.5%)	1 (0.3%)	<1%	0	6 (1.8%)
Arthralgias	0	0	1 (0.3%)	3 (1.1%)	1 (1.3%)	5 (1.5%)
Ear and Labyrinth Disorders						
Earache	2 (0.7%)	1 (0.7%)	0	8 (2.9%)	2 (2.7%)	
Nervous System Disorders						
Headache	37 (13.9%)	12 (8.8%)	38 (11.3%)	69 (25.4%)	12 (16.0%)	23 (7.0%)

*Ages 2-17 years

OVERDOSAGE

There has been no experience of overdose with ELIDEL® (pimecrolimus) Cream 1%. If oral ingestion occurs, medical advice should be sought.

DOSAGE AND ADMINISTRATION

* The patient or care giver should apply a thin layer of ELIDEL (pimecrolimus) Cream 1% to the affected skin twice daily. The patient or caregiver should stop using when signs and symptoms (e.g., itch, rash and redness) resolve and should be instructed on what actions to take if symptoms recur.
* If signs and symptoms persist beyond 6 weeks, patients should be re-examined by their health care provider to confirm the diagnosis of atopic dermatitis.
* Continuous long-term use of ELIDEL Cream should be avoided, and application should be limited to areas of involvement with atopic dermatitis.

The safety of ELIDEL Cream under occlusion, which may promote systemic exposure, has not been evaluated. ELIDEL Cream should not be used with occlusive dressings.

HOW SUPPLIED

ELIDEL® (pimecrolimus) Cream 1% is available in tubes of 30 grams, 60 grams, and 100 grams.

30 gram tube .... NDC 0078-0375-46
60 gram tube .... NDC 0078-0375-49
100 gram tube .... NDC 0078-0375-63
Store at 25°C (77°F); excursions permitted to 15°C-30°C (59°F-86°F). Do not freeze.

Manufactured by:
Novartis Pharma Produktions GmbH
Wehr, Germany

Distributed by:
Novartis Pharmaceuticals Corp.
East Hanover, NJ 070396

MEDICATION GUIDE

ELIDEL® [EL'-ee-del] (pimecrolimus) Cream 1%

Important Note: ELIDEL Cream is for use on the skin only (topical). Do not get ELIDEL Cream in your eyes, nose, mouth, vagina, or rectum.

Read the Medication Guide that comes with ELIDEL Cream before you or a family member start using it and each time you refill your prescription. There may be new information. This Medication Guide does not take the place of talking with your doctor about your medical condition or treatment. If you have any questions about ELIDEL Cream, ask your doctor or pharmacist for more information.

What is the most important information I should know about ELIDEL Cream?

It is not known if ELIDEL Cream is safe to use for a long period of time. A very small number of people who have used ELIDEL Cream have gotten cancer (for example, skin cancer or lymphoma). But a link that ELIDEL Cream use caused these cancers has not been shown. Because of this concern:

* Do not use ELIDEL Cream continuously for a long time.
* Use ELIDEL Cream only on areas of your skin that have eczema.
* Do not use ELIDEL Cream on a child under 2 years old.

What is ELIDEL Cream?

ELIDEL Cream is a prescription medicine used on the skin (topical) to treat eczema (atopic dermatitis). ELIDEL Cream is in a class of medicines called topical calcineurin inhibitors. ELIDEL Cream is for adults and children age 2 years and older who do not have a weakened immune system. ELIDEL Cream is used on the skin for short periods, and if needed, treatment may be repeated with breaks in between. ELIDEL Cream is for use after other prescription medicines have not worked for you or if your doctor recommends that other prescription medicines should not be used.

It is not known if ELIDEL Cream is safe and effective in people who have a weakened immune system.

ELIDEL Cream is not for use in children under 2 years of age.

Who should not use ELIDEL Cream?

Do not use ELIDEL Cream:

* if you are allergic to ELIDEL Cream or anything in it. See the end of this Medication Guide for a complete list of ingredients in ELIDEL Cream.

What should I tell my doctor before starting ELIDEL Cream?

Before you start using ELIDEL Cream, tell your doctor about all of your medical conditions, including if you:

* have a skin disease called Netherton's syndrome (a rare inherited condition)
* have any infection on your skin including chicken pox or herpes
* have been told you have a weakened immune system
* are pregnant, breastfeeding, or planning to become pregnant

Tell your doctor about all the medicines you take including prescription and nonprescription medicines, vitamins, and herbal supplements. Tell your doctor about all the skin medicines and products you use.

Know the medicines you take. Keep a list of them with you to show your doctor and pharmacist each time you get a new medicine.

How should I use ELIDEL Cream?

* Use ELIDEL Cream exactly as prescribed.
* Use ELIDEL Cream only on areas of your skin that have eczema.
* Use ELIDEL Cream for short periods, and if needed, treatment may be repeated with breaks in between.

- Stop ELIDEL Cream when the signs and symptoms of eczema, such as itching, rash, and redness go away, or as directed by your doctor.
- Follow your doctor's advice if symptoms of eczema return after a treatment with ELIDEL Cream.
- Call your doctor if:
  - your symptoms get worse with ELIDEL Cream
  - you get an infection on your skin
  - your symptoms do not improve after 6 weeks of treatment. Sometimes other skin diseases can look like eczema.

To apply ELIDEL Cream:
Read and carefully follow the directions below.
- Wash your hands before using ELIDEL Cream. If you apply ELIDEL Cream after a bath or shower, make sure your skin is dry.
- Apply a thin layer of ELIDEL Cream only to the affected skin areas, two times each day, as directed by your doctor.
- Use the smallest amount of ELIDEL Cream needed to control the signs and symptoms of eczema.
- If you apply ELIDEL Cream to another person, or if you have eczema and are not treating your hands, it is important for you to wash your hands with soap and water after applying ELIDEL Cream. This should remove any cream left on your hands.
- Do not bathe, shower or swim right after applying ELIDEL Cream. This could wash off the cream.
- You can use moisturizers with ELIDEL Cream. Make sure you check with your doctor first about the products that are right for you. People with eczema can have very dry skin, so it is important to keep up good skin care practices. If you use moisturizers, apply them after ELIDEL Cream.

What should I avoid while using ELIDEL Cream?
- You should not use sun lamps, tanning beds, or get treatment with ultraviolet light therapy during treatment with ELIDEL Cream.
- Limit your time in the sun during treatment with ELIDEL Cream even when the medicine is not on your skin. If you need to be outdoors after applying ELIDEL Cream, wear loose fitting clothing that protects the treated area from the sun. Ask your doctor what other types of protection from the sun you should use. It is not known how ELIDEL Cream may affect your skin with exposure to ultraviolet light.
- Do not cover the skin being treated with bandages, dressings or wraps. You can wear normal clothing.
- ELIDEL Cream is for use on the skin only. Do not get ELIDEL Cream in your eyes, nose, mouth, vagina, or rectum (mucous membranes). If you get ELIDEL Cream in any of these areas, burning or irritation can happen. Wipe off any ELIDEL Cream from the affected area and then rinse the area well with cold water.
- Do not swallow ELIDEL Cream. If you do, call your doctor.
- Avoid using ELIDEL Cream on skin areas that have cancers or pre-cancers.

What are the possible side effects of ELIDEL Cream?
ELIDEL Cream may cause serious side effects. A very small number of people who have used ELIDEL Cream have gotten cancer (for example, skin cancer or lymphoma). But, a link that ELIDEL Cream caused these cancers has not been shown.

The most common side effect at the skin application site is burning or a feeling of warmth. These side effects are usually mild or moderate, happen during the first few days of treatment, and usually clear up in a few days. Call your doctor if the burning feeling is severe or lasts for more than 1 week.

Other side effects include headache, common cold or stuffy nose, sore throat, influenza, fever, viral infection, and cough. Some people may get viral skin infections (like cold sores, chicken pox, shingles, or warts) or swollen lymph nodes (glands).
Tell your doctor if you have a skin infection or if you have any side effect (for example, swollen glands) that bothers you or that does not go away.
These are not all the possible side effects with ELIDEL Cream. Ask your doctor or pharmacist for more information. Call your doctor for medical advice about side effects. You may report side effects to FDA at 1-800-FDA-1088.

How should I store ELIDEL Cream?
- Store ELIDEL Cream at room temperature between 59° to 86°F (15° to 30°C).
- **Keep ELIDEL Cream and all medicines out of the reach of children.**

General advice about ELIDEL Cream
Medicines are sometimes prescribed for purposes other than those listed in a Medication Guide. Use ELIDEL Cream only for the condition for which it was prescribed. Do not give ELIDEL Cream to other people even if they have the same symptoms you have, as it may not be right for them.

This Medication Guide summarizes the most important information about ELIDEL Cream. If you would like more information, talk with your doctor.
Your doctor or pharmacist can give you information about ELIDEL Cream that is written for health care professionals. For more information, you can also visit the Novartis Internet site at www.elidel.com or call the ELIDEL Cream help line at 877-4 ELIDEL (877-435-4335).

What are the ingredients in ELIDEL Cream?
Active ingredient: pimecrolimus
Inactive ingredients: benzyl alcohol, cetyl alcohol, citric acid, mono- and di-glycerides, oleyl alcohol, propylene glycol, sodium cetostearyl sulphate, sodium hydroxide, stearyl alcohol, triglycerides, and water

Manufactured by:
Novartis Pharma Produktions GmbH
Wehr, Germany
Distributed by:
Novartis Pharmaceuticals Corp.
East Hanover, New Jersey 07936
This Medication Guide has been approved by the U.S. Food and Drug Administration
REV. August 2010
T2010-70/T2010-71
© Novartis

ENABLEX®

[en-a-blex]
(darifenacin)
Extended-release Tablets
Rx only

℞

The following prescribing information is based on official labeling in effect July 2010.
Prescribing Information

DESCRIPTION

ENABLEX® (darifenacin) is an extended-release tablet which contains 7.5 mg or 15 mg darifenacin as its hydrobromide salt. The active moiety, darifenacin, is a potent muscarinic receptor antagonist.
Chemically, darifenacin hydrobromide is (S)-2-{1-[2-(2,3-dihydrobenzofuran-5-yl)ethyl]-3-pyrrolidinyl}-2,2-diphenylacetamide hydrobromide. The empirical formula of darifenacin hydrobromide is $C_{28}H_{30}N_2O_2 \cdot HBr$.
The structural formula is

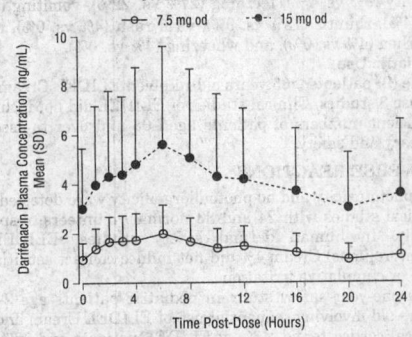

Darifenacin hydrobromide is a white to almost white, crystalline powder, with a molecular weight of 507.5.
ENABLEX is a once-a-day extended-release tablet and contains the following inactive ingredients: dibasic calcium phosphate, hypromellose (hydroxypropyl methylcellulose), magnesium stearate, polyethylene glycol, talc, titanium dioxide. The 15-mg tablet also contains iron oxide red and iron oxide yellow.

CLINICAL PHARMACOLOGY
General
Darifenacin is a competitive muscarinic receptor antagonist. Muscarinic receptors play an important role in several major cholinergically mediated functions, including contractions of the urinary bladder smooth muscle and stimulation of salivary secretion.

In vitro studies using human recombinant muscarinic receptor subtypes show that darifenacin has greater affinity for the M_3 receptor than for the other known muscarinic receptors (9- and 12-fold greater affinity for M_3 compared to M_1 and M_5, respectively, and 59-fold greater affinity for M_3 compared to both M_2 and M_4). M_3 receptors are involved in contraction of human bladder and gastrointestinal smooth muscle, saliva production, and iris sphincter function. Adverse drug effects such as dry mouth, constipation and abnormal vision may be mediated through effects on M_3 receptors in these organs.

Pharmacodynamics
In three cystometric studies performed in patients with involuntary detrusor contractions, increased bladder capacity was demonstrated by an increased volume threshold for unstable contractions and diminished frequency of unstable detrusor contractions after ENABLEX® (darifenacin) extended-release tablet treatment. These findings are consistent with an antimuscarinic action on the urinary bladder.

Pharmacokinetics
Absorption
After oral administration of ENABLEX to healthy volunteers, peak plasma concentrations of darifenacin are reached approximately seven hours after multiple dosing and steady-state plasma concentrations are achieved by the sixth day of dosing. The mean (SD) steady-state time course of ENABLEX 7.5 mg and 15 mg extended-release tablets is depicted in Figure 1.

Figure 1
Mean (SD) Steady-State Darifenacin Plasma Concentration-Time Profiles for ENABLEX® 7.5 mg and 15 mg in Healthy Volunteers Including Both CYP2D6 EMs and PMs*

*Includes 95 EMs and 6 PMs for 7.5 mg; 104 EMs and 10 PMs for 15 mg.

A summary of mean (standard deviation, SD) steady-state pharmacokinetic parameters of ENABLEX 7.5 mg and 15 mg extended-release tablets in extensive (EMs) and poor (PMs) metabolizers of CYP2D6 is provided in Table 1.
[See table below]
The mean oral bioavailability of ENABLEX in EMs at steady state is estimated to be 15% and 19% for 7.5-mg and 15-mg tablets, respectively.

Effect of Food
There is no effect of food on multiple-dose pharmacokinetics from ENABLEX extended-release tablets.

Distribution
Darifenacin is approximately 98% bound to plasma proteins (primarily to alpha-1-acid-glycoprotein). The steady-state volume of distribution (V_{ss}) is estimated to be 163 L.

Table 1
Mean (SD) Steady-State Pharmacokinetic Parameters from ENABLEX® 7.5 mg and 15 mg Extended-Release Tablets Based on Pooled Data by Predicted CYP2D6 Phenotype

	ENABLEX® 7.5 mg (N=68 EM, 5 PM)					ENABLEX® 15 mg (N=102 EM, 17 PM)				
	AUC_{24} (ng.h/mL)	C_{max} (ng/mL)	C_{avg} (ng/mL)	T_{max} (h)	$t_{1/2}$ (h)	AUC_{24} (ng.h/mL)	C_{max} (ng/mL)	C_{avg} (ng/mL)	T_{max} (h)	$t_{1/2}$ (h)
EM	29.24 (15.47)	2.01 (1.04)	1.22 (0.64)	6.49 (4.19)	12.43 (5.64)[a]	88.90 (67.87)	5.76 (4.24)	3.70 (2.83)	7.61 (5.06)	12.05 (12.37)[b]
PM	67.56 (13.13)	4.27 (0.98)	2.81 (0.55)	5.20 (1.79)	19.95[c] —	157.71 (77.08)	9.99 (5.09)	6.58 (3.22)	6.71 (3.58)	7.40[d] —

[a]N=25; [b]N=8; [c]N=2; [d]N=1; AUC_{24} = Area under the plasma concentration versus time curve for 24h; C_{max} = Maximum observed plasma concentration; C_{avg} = Average plasma concentration at steady state; T_{max} = Time of occurrence of C_{max}; $t_{1/2}$ = Terminal elimination half-life. Regarding EM and PM, *see CLINICAL PHARMACOLOGY, Pharmacokinetics, Variability in Metabolism.*

Metabolism

Darifenacin is extensively metabolized by the liver following oral dosing.

Metabolism is mediated by cytochrome P450 enzymes CYP2D6 and CYP3A4. The three main metabolic routes are as follows:

(i) monohydroxylation in the dihydrobenzofuran ring;
(ii) dihydrobenzofuran ring opening;
(iii) N-dealkylation of the pyrrolidine nitrogen.

The initial products of the hydroxylation and N-dealkylation pathways are the major circulating metabolites but they are unlikely to contribute significantly to the overall clinical effect of darifenacin.

Variability in Metabolism

A subset of individuals (approximately 7% Caucasians and 2% African Americans) are poor metabolizers (PMs) of CYP2D6 metabolized drugs. Individuals with normal CYP2D6 activity are referred to as extensive metabolizers (EMs). The metabolism of darifenacin in PMs will be principally mediated via CYP3A4. The darifenacin ratios (PM: EM) for C_{max} and AUC following darifenacin 15 mg once-daily at steady state were 1.9 and 1.7, respectively.

Excretion

Following administration of an oral dose of ^{14}C-darifenacin solution to healthy volunteers, approximately 60% of the radioactivity was recovered in the urine and 40% in the feces. Only a small percentage of the excreted dose was unchanged darifenacin (3%). Estimated darifenacin clearance is 40 L/h for EMs and 32 L/h for PMs. The elimination half-life of darifenacin following chronic dosing is approximately 13-19 hours.

Pharmacokinetics in Special Populations

Age: No dose adjustment is recommended for the elderly. A population pharmacokinetic analysis of patient data indicated a trend for clearance of darifenacin to decrease with age (6% per decade relative to a median age of 44). Following administration of ENABLEX 15 mg once-daily, darifenacin exposure at steady state was approximately 12%-19% higher in volunteers between 45 and 65 years of age compared to younger volunteers aged 18 to 44 years *(see PRECAUTIONS, Geriatric Use).*

Pediatric: The pharmacokinetics of ENABLEX have not been studied in the pediatric population.

Gender: No dose adjustment is recommended based on gender. PK parameters were calculated for 22 male and 25 female healthy volunteers. Darifenacin C_{max} and AUC at steady state were approximately 57%-79% and 61%-73% higher in females than in males, respectively.

Race: The effect of race on the pharmacokinetics of ENABLEX has not been characterized.

Renal Insufficiency: No dose adjustment is recommended for patients with renal impairment. A study of subjects with varying degrees of renal impairment (creatinine clearance between 10 and 136 mL/min) given ENABLEX 15 mg once daily to steady state demonstrated no clear relationship between renal function and darifenacin clearance.

Hepatic Insufficiency: The daily dose of ENABLEX should not exceed 7.5 mg once daily for patients with moderate hepatic impairment (Child Pugh B) *(see PRECAUTIONS and DOSAGE AND ADMINISTRATION).* No dose adjustment is recommended for patients with mild hepatic impairment (Child Pugh A).

ENABLEX pharmacokinetics were investigated in subjects with mild (Child Pugh A) or moderate (Child Pugh B) impairment of hepatic function given ENABLEX 15 mg once daily to steady state. Mild hepatic impairment had no effect on the pharmacokinetics of darifenacin. However, protein binding of darifenacin was affected by moderate hepatic impairment. After adjusting for plasma protein binding, unbound darifenacin exposure was estimated to be 4.7-fold higher in subjects with moderate hepatic impairment than subjects with normal hepatic function.

Subjects with severe hepatic impairment (Child Pugh C) have not been studied, therefore ENABLEX is not recommended for use in these patients *(see PRECAUTIONS and DOSAGE AND ADMINISTRATION).*

Drug-Drug Interactions

Effects of Other Drugs on Darifenacin

Darifenacin metabolism is primarily mediated by the cytochrome P450 enzymes CYP2D6 and CYP3A4. Therefore, inducers of CYP3A4 or inhibitors of either of these enzymes may alter darifenacin pharmacokinetics.

CYP2D6 Inhibitors: No dosing adjustments are recommended in the presence of CYP2D6 inhibitors. Darifenacin exposure following 30 mg once daily at steady state was 33% higher in the presence of the potent CYP2D6 inhibitor paroxetine 20 mg.

CYP3A4 Inhibitors: The daily dose of ENABLEX should not exceed 7.5 mg when coadministered with potent CYP3A4 inhibitors (e.g., ketoconazole, itraconazole, ritonavir, nelfinavir, clarithromycin and nefazodone) *(see PRECAUTIONS and DOSAGE AND ADMINISTRATION).*

In a drug interaction study, when a 7.5 mg once-daily dose of ENABLEX was given to steady state and coadministered with the potent CYP3A4 inhibitor ketoconazole 400 mg, mean darifenacin C_{max} increased to 11.2 ng/mL for EMs (n=10) and 55.4 ng/mL for one PM subject (n=1). Mean AUC increased to 143 and 939 ng.h/mL for EMs and for one PM subject, respectively. When a 15 mg daily dose of ENABLEX was given with ketoconazole, mean darifenacin C_{max} increased to 67.6 ng/mL and 58.9 ng/mL for EMs (n=3) and one PM subject (n=1), respectively. Mean AUC increased to 1110 and 931 ng.h/mL for EMs and for one PM subject, respectively.

No dosing adjustments are recommended in the presence of moderate CYP3A4 inhibitors (e.g., erythromycin, fluconazole, diltiazem and verapamil). The mean C_{max} and AUC of darifenacin following 30 mg once-daily dosing at steady state were 128% and 95% higher, respectively, in the presence of erythromycin. Coadministration of fluconazole and darifenacin 30 mg once daily at steady state increased darifenacin C_{max} and AUC by 88% and 84%, respectively.

The mean C_{max} and AUC of darifenacin following 30 mg once daily at steady state were 42% and 34% higher, respectively, in the presence of cimetidine, a mixed CYP P450 enzyme inhibitor.

Effects of Darifenacin on Other Drugs

In Vitro Studies: Based on *in vitro* human microsomal studies, ENABLEX is not expected to inhibit CYP1A2 or CYP2C9 at clinically relevant concentrations.

In Vivo Studies: The potential for clinical doses of ENABLEX to act as inhibitors of CYP2D6 or CYP3A4 substrates was investigated in specific drug interaction studies.

CYP2D6 Substrates: Caution should be taken when ENABLEX is used concomitantly with medications that are predominantly metabolized by CYP2D6 and which have a narrow therapeutic window, such as flecainide, thioridazine and tricyclic antidepressants *(see PRECAUTIONS, Drug Interactions).*

The mean C_{max} and AUC of imipramine, a CYP2D6 substrate, were increased 57% and 70%, respectively, in the presence of steady-state darifenacin 30 mg once daily. This was accompanied by a 3.6-fold increase in the mean C_{max} and AUC of desipramine, the active metabolite of imipramine.

CYP3A4 Substrates: Darifenacin (30 mg daily) coadministered with a single oral dose of midazolam 7.5 mg resulted in a 17% increase in midazolam exposure.

Darifenacin (10 mg t.i.d.) had no effect on the pharmacokinetics of the combination oral contraceptives containing levonorgestrel and ethinylestradiol.

Other Drugs: Darifenacin had no significant effect on prothrombin time when a single dose of warfarin 30 mg was coadministered with darifenacin (30 mg daily) at steady state. Standard therapeutic prothrombin time monitoring for warfarin should be continued.

Routine therapeutic drug monitoring for digoxin should be continued. Darifenacin (30 mg daily) coadministered with digoxin (0.25 mg) at steady state resulted in a 16% increase in digoxin exposure.

Electrophysiology

The effect of six-day treatment of 15-mg and 75-mg ENABLEX on QT/QTc interval was evaluated in a multiple-dose, double-blind, randomized, placebo- and active-controlled (moxifloxacin 400 mg) parallel-arm design study in 179 healthy adults (44% male, 56% female) aged 18 to 65. Subjects included 18% PMs and 82% EMs. The QT interval was measured over a 24-hour period both predosing and at steady state. The 75-mg ENABLEX dose was chosen because this achieves exposure similar to that observed in CYP2D6 poor metabolizers administered the highest recommended dose (15 mg) of darifenacin in the presence of a potent CYP3A4 inhibitor. At the doses studied, ENABLEX did not result in QT/QTc interval prolongation at any time during the steady state, while moxifloxacin treatment resulted in a mean increase from baseline QTcF of about 7.0 msec when compared to placebo. In this study, darifenacin 15-mg and 75-mg doses demonstrated a mean heart rate change of 3.1 and 1.3 bpm, respectively, when compared to placebo. However, in the Phase II/III clinical studies, the change in median HR following treatment with ENABLEX was no different from placebo.

CLINICAL STUDIES

ENABLEX® (darifenacin) extended-release tablets were evaluated for the treatment of patients with overactive bladder with symptoms of urgency, urge urinary incontinence, and increased urinary frequency in three randomized, fixed-dose, placebo-controlled, multicenter, double-blind, 12-week studies (Studies 1, 2 and 3) and one randomized, double-blind, placebo-controlled, multicenter, dose-titration study (Study 4). For study eligibility in all four studies, patients with symptoms of overactive bladder for at least six months were required to demonstrate at least eight micturitions and at least one episode of urinary urgency per day, and at least five episodes of urge urinary incontinence per week. The majority of patients were white (94%) and female (84%), with a mean age of 58 years, range 19 to 93 years. Thirty-three percent of patients were ≥65 years of age. These characteristics were well balanced across treatment groups. The study population was inclusive of both naïve patients who had not received prior pharmacotherapy for overactive bladder (60%) and those who had (40%).

Table 2 shows the efficacy data collected from 7- or 14-day voiding diaries in the three fixed-dose placebo-controlled studies of 1,059 patients treated with placebo, 7.5 mg or 15 mg once-daily ENABLEX for 12 weeks. A significant decrease in the primary endpoint, change from baseline in average weekly urge urinary incontinence episodes was observed in all three studies. Data is also shown for two secondary endpoints, change from baseline in the average number of micturitions per day (urinary frequency) and change from baseline in the average volume voided per micturition.

[See table 2 above]

Table 2
Difference Between ENABLEX® (7.5 mg, 15 mg) and Placebo for the Week 12 Change from Baseline (Studies 1, 2 and 3)

	Study 1			Study 2			Study 3	
	ENABLEX® 7.5 mg	ENABLEX® 15 mg	Placebo	ENABLEX® 7.5 mg	ENABLEX® 15 mg	Placebo	ENABLEX® 15 mg	Placebo
No. of Patients Entered	229	115	164	108	107	109	112	115
Incontinence Episodes per Week								
Median Baseline	16.3	17.0	16.6	14.0	17.3	16.1	16.2	15.5
Median Change from Baseline	-9.0	-10.4	-7.6	-8.1	-10.4	-5.9	-11.4	-9.0
Median Difference to Placebo	-1.5*	-2.1*	–	-2.8*	-4.3*	–	-2.4*	–
Micturitions per Day								
Median Baseline	10.1	10.1	10.1	10.3	11.0	10.1	10.5	10.4
Median Change from Baseline	-1.6	-1.7	-0.8	-1.7	-1.9	-1.1	-1.9	-1.2
Median Difference to Placebo	-0.8*	-0.9*	–	-0.5	-0.7*	–	-0.5	–
Volume of Urine Passed per Void (mL)								
Median Baseline	160.2	151.8	162.4	161.7	157.3	162.2	155.0	147.1
Median Change from Baseline	14.9	30.9	7.6	16.8	23.6	7.1	26.7	4.6
Median Difference to Placebo	9.1*	20.7*	–	9.2	16.6*	–	20.1*	–

*Indicates statistically significant difference versus placebo ($p<0.05$, Wilcoxon rank-sum test)

Table 3 shows the efficacy data from the dose-titration study in 395 patients who initially received 7.5-mg ENABLEX or placebo daily with the option to increase to 15-mg ENABLEX or placebo daily after two weeks.

[See table 3 at top of next page]

As seen in Figures 2 a, b and c, reductions in the number of incontinence episodes per week were observed within the

Table 3
Difference Between ENABLEX® (7.5 mg/15 mg) and Placebo for the Week 12 Change from Baseline (Study 4)

	ENABLEX® 7.5 mg/15 mg	Placebo
No. of Patients Treated	268	127
Incontinence Episodes per Week		
Median Baseline	16.0	14.0
Median Change from Baseline	-8.2	-6.0
Median Difference to Placebo	-1.4*	–
Micturitions per Day		
Median Baseline	9.9	10.4
Median Change from Baseline	-1.9	-1.0
Median Difference to Placebo	-0.8*	–
Volume of Urine Passed per Void (mL)		
Median Baseline	173.7	177.2
Median Change from Baseline	18.8	6.6
Median Difference to Placebo	13.3*	–

* Indicates statistically significant difference versus placebo (p<0.05, Wilcoxon rank-sum test)

first two weeks in patients treated with ENABLEX 7.5 mg and 15 mg once daily compared to placebo. Further, these effects were sustained throughout the 12-week treatment period.

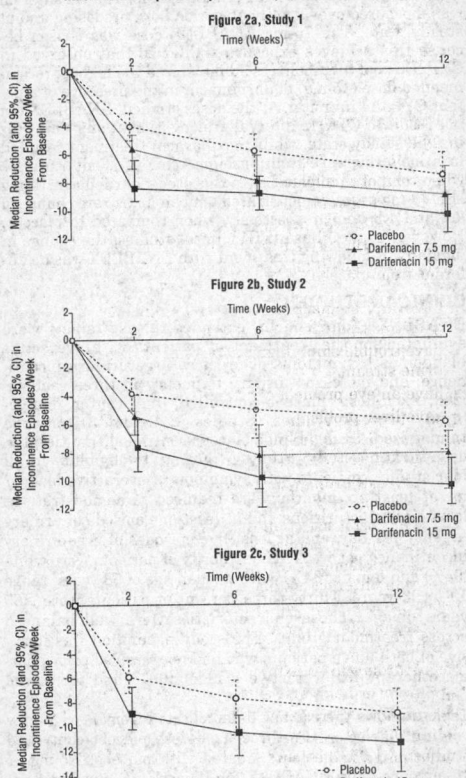

Figures 2 a,b,c
Median Change from Baseline at Weeks 2, 6, 12 for Number of Incontinence Episodes per Week (Studies 1, 2 and 3)

Figure 2a, Study 1

Figure 2b, Study 2

Figure 2c, Study 3

INDICATIONS AND USAGE

ENABLEX® (darifenacin) extended-release tablets are indicated for the treatment of overactive bladder with symptoms of urge urinary incontinence, urgency and frequency.

CONTRAINDICATIONS

ENABLEX® (darifenacin) extended-release tablets are contraindicated in patients with urinary retention, gastric retention or uncontrolled narrow-angle glaucoma and in patients who are at risk for these conditions. ENABLEX is also contraindicated in patients with known hypersensitivity to the drug or its ingredients.

PRECAUTIONS
General
Risk of Urinary Retention
ENABLEX® (darifenacin) extended-release tablets should be administered with caution to patients with clinically significant bladder outflow obstruction because of the risk of urinary retention.

Decreased Gastrointestinal Motility
ENABLEX should be administered with caution to patients with gastrointestinal obstructive disorders because of the risk of gastric retention. ENABLEX, like other anticholinergic drugs, may decrease gastrointestinal motility and should be used with caution in patients with conditions such as severe constipation, ulcerative colitis, and myasthenia gravis.

Controlled Narrow-Angle Glaucoma
ENABLEX should be used with caution in patients being treated for narrow-angle glaucoma and only where the potential benefits outweigh the risks.

Patients with Hepatic Impairment
There are no dosing adjustments for patients with mild hepatic impairment. The daily dose of ENABLEX should not exceed 7.5 mg for patients with moderate hepatic impairment. ENABLEX has not been studied in patients with severe hepatic impairment and therefore is not recommended for use in this patient population *(see CLINICAL PHARMACOLOGY, Pharmacokinetics in Special Populations and DOSAGE AND ADMINISTRATION).*

Information for Patients
Patients should be informed that anticholinergic agents, such as ENABLEX, may produce clinically significant adverse effects related to anticholinergic pharmacological activity including constipation, urinary retention and blurred vision. Heat prostration (due to decreased sweating) can occur when anticholinergics such as ENABLEX are used in a hot environment. Because anticholinergics, such as ENABLEX, may produce dizziness or blurred vision, patients should be advised to exercise caution in decisions to engage in potentially dangerous activities until the drug's effects have been determined. Patients should read the patient information leaflet before starting therapy with ENABLEX.

ENABLEX extended-release tablets should be taken once daily with liquid. They may be taken with or without food, and should be swallowed whole and not chewed, divided or crushed.

Drug Interactions
The daily dose of ENABLEX should not exceed 7.5 mg when coadministered with potent CYP3A4 inhibitors (e.g., ketoconazole, itraconazole, ritonavir, nelfinavir, clarithromycin and nefazadone) *(see CLINICAL PHARMACOLOGY and DOSAGE AND ADMINISTRATION).*

Caution should be taken when ENABLEX is used concomitantly with medications that are predominantly metabolized by CYP2D6 and which have a narrow therapeutic window, such as flecainide, thioridazine and tricyclic antidepressants *(see CLINICAL PHARMACOLOGY).*

The concomitant use of ENABLEX with other anticholinergic agents may increase the frequency and/or severity of dry mouth, constipation, blurred vision and other anticholinergic pharmacological effects. Anticholinergic agents may potentially alter the absorption of some concomitantly administered drugs due to effects on gastrointestinal motility.

Drug Laboratory Test Interactions
Interactions between darifenacin and laboratory tests have not been studied.

Carcinogenesis/Mutagenesis/Impairment of Fertility
Carcinogenicity studies with darifenacin were conducted in mice and rats. No evidence of drug-related carcinogenicity was revealed in a 24-month study in mice at dietary doses up to 100 mg/kg/day or approximately 32 times the estimated human-free AUC_{0-24h} reached with 15 mg, the maximum recommended human dose (AUC at MRHD) and in a 24-month study in rats at doses up to 15 mg/kg/day or up to approximately 12 times the AUC at MRHD in female rats and approximately eight times the AUC at MRHD in male rats.

Darifenacin was not mutagenic in the bacterial mutation assays (Ames test) and the Chinese hamster ovary assay, and not clastogenic in the human lymphocyte assay, and the *in vivo* mouse bone marrow cytogenetics assay.

There was no evidence for effects on fertility in male or female rats treated at oral doses up to 50 mg/kg/day. Exposures in this study correspond to approximately 78 times the AUC at MRHD.

Pregnancy Category C
Darifenacin was not teratogenic in rats and rabbits at doses up to 50 and 30 mg/kg/day, respectively. At the dose of 50 mg/kg in rats, there was a delay in the ossification of the sacral and caudal vertebrae which was not observed at 10 mg/kg (approximately 13 times the AUC of free plasma concentration at MRHD). Exposure in this study at 50 mg/kg corresponds to approximately 59 times the AUC of free plasma concentration at MRHD. Dystocia was observed in dams at 10 mg/kg/day (17 times the AUC of free plasma concentration at MRHD). Slight developmental delays were observed in pups at this dose. At 3 mg/kg/day (five times the AUC of free plasma concentration at MRHD) there were no effects on dams or pups. At the dose of 30 mg/kg in rabbits, darifenacin was shown to increase postimplantation loss but not at 10 mg/kg (nine times the AUC of free plasma concentration at MRHD). Exposure to unbound drug at 30 mg/kg in this study corresponds to approximately 28 times the AUC at MRHD. In rabbits, dilated ureter and/or kidney pelvis was observed in offspring at 30 mg/kg/day and one case was observed at 10 mg/kg/day along with urinary bladder dilation consistent with pharmacological action of darifenacin. No effect was observed at 3 mg/kg/day (2.8 times the AUC of free plasma concentration at MRHD). There are no studies of darifenacin in pregnant women. Because animal reproduction studies are not always predictive of human response, ENABLEX should be used during pregnancy only if the benefit to the mother outweighs the potential risk to the fetus.

Nursing Mothers
Darifenacin is excreted into the milk of rats. It is not known whether darifenacin is excreted into human milk and therefore caution should be exercised before ENABLEX is administered to a nursing woman.

Pediatric Use
The safety and effectiveness of ENABLEX in pediatric patients have not been established.

Geriatric Use
In the Phase III fixed-dose, placebo-controlled, clinical studies, 30% of patients treated with ENABLEX were over 65 years of age. No overall differences in safety or efficacy were observed between these patients (n=207) and younger patients <65 years (n=464). No dose adjustment is recommended for elderly patients *(see CLINICAL PHARMACOLOGY, Pharmacokinetics in Special Populations and CLINICAL STUDIES).*

ADVERSE REACTIONS
During the clinical development of ENABLEX® (darifenacin) extended-release tablets, a total of 7,363 patients and volunteers were treated with doses of darifenacin from 3.75 mg to 75 mg once daily.

The safety of ENABLEX was evaluated in Phase II and III controlled clinical trials in a total of 8,830 patients, 6,001 of whom were treated with ENABLEX. Of this total, 1,069 patients participated in three, 12-week, Phase III, fixed-dose efficacy and safety studies. Of this total, 337 and 334 patients received ENABLEX 7.5 mg daily and 15 mg daily, respectively. In all long-term trials combined, 1,216 and 672 patients received treatment with ENABLEX for at least 24 and 52 weeks, respectively.

In all placebo-controlled trials combined, the incidence of serious adverse events for 7.5 mg, 15 mg and placebo was similar.

In all fixed-dose Phase III studies combined, 3.3% of patients treated with ENABLEX discontinued due to all adverse events versus 2.6% in placebo. Dry mouth leading to study discontinuation occurred in 0%, 0.9%, and 0% of patients treated with ENABLEX 7.5 mg daily, ENABLEX 15 mg daily and placebo, respectively. Constipation leading to study discontinuation occurred in 0.6%, 1.2%, and 0.3% of patients treated with ENABLEX 7.5 mg daily, ENABLEX 15 mg daily and placebo, respectively.

Table 4 lists the adverse events reported (regardless of causality) in 2% or more of patients treated with 7.5-mg or 15-mg ENABLEX extended-release tablets and greater than placebo in the three, fixed-dose, placebo-controlled Phase III studies (Studies 1, 2 and 3). Adverse events were

reported by 54% and 66% of patients receiving 7.5 mg and 15 mg once-daily ENABLEX extended-release tablets, respectively, and by 49% of patients receiving placebo. In these studies, the most frequently reported adverse events were dry mouth and constipation. The majority of adverse events in ENABLEX-treated subjects were mild or moderate in severity and most occurred during the first two weeks of treatment.
[See table 4 at right]
Other adverse events reported, regardless of causality, by ≥1% of ENABLEX patients in either the 7.5 mg or 15 mg once-daily darifenacin-dose groups in these fixed-dose, placebo-controlled Phase III studies include: abnormal vision, accidental injury, back pain, dry skin, flu syndrome, pain, hypertension, vomiting, peripheral edema, weight gain, arthralgia, bronchitis, pharyngitis, rhinitis, sinusitis, rash, pruritus, urinary tract disorder and vaginitis.
Study 4 was a 12-week, placebo-controlled, dose-titration regimen study in which ENABLEX was administered in accordance with dosing recommendations (see DOSAGE AND ADMINISTRATION). All patients initially received placebo or ENABLEX 7.5 mg daily, and after two weeks, patients and physicians were allowed to adjust upward to ENABLEX 15 mg if needed. In this study, the most commonly reported adverse events were also constipation and dry mouth. The incidence of discontinuation due to all adverse events was 3.1% and 6.7% for placebo and for ENABLEX, respectively. Table 5 lists the adverse events (regardless of causality) reported in >3% of patients treated with ENABLEX extended-release tablets and greater than placebo.
[See table 5 at right]
Acute urinary retention (AUR) requiring treatment was reported in a total of 16 patients in the ENABLEX Phase I-III clinical trials. Of these 16 cases, seven were reported as serious adverse events, including one patient with detrusor hyperreflexia secondary to a stroke, one patient with benign prostatic hypertrophy (BPH), one patient with irritable bowel syndrome (IBS) and four overactive bladder (OAB) patients taking darifenacin 30 mg daily. Of the remaining nine cases, none were reported as serious adverse events. Three occurred in OAB patients taking the recommended doses, and two of these required bladder catheterization for 1-2 days.
Constipation was reported as a serious adverse event in six patients in the ENABLEX Phase I-III clinical trials, including one patient with benign prostatic hypertrophy (BPH), one OAB patient taking darifenacin 30 mg daily, and only one OAB patient taking the recommended doses. The latter patient was hospitalized for investigation with colonoscopy after reporting nine months of chronic constipation that was reported as being moderate in severity.

Postmarketing Experience
The following events have been reported in association with darifenacin use in worldwide postmarketing experience. Because these spontaneously reported events are from the worldwide postmarketing experience, the frequency of events and the role of darifenacin in their causation cannot be reliably determined.
General: hypersensitivity reactions, including angioedema.
Central Nervous: confusion and hallucinations.
Cardiovascular: palpitations.

OVERDOSAGE
Overdosage with antimuscarinic agents, including ENABLEX® (darifenacin) extended-release tablets, can result in severe antimuscarinic effects. Treatment should be symptomatic and supportive. In the event of overdosage, ECG monitoring is recommended. ENABLEX has been administered in clinical trials at doses up to 75 mg (five times the maximum therapeutic dose) and signs of overdose were limited to abnormal vision.

DOSAGE AND ADMINISTRATION
The recommended starting dose of ENABLEX® (darifenacin) extended-release tablets is 7.5 mg once daily. Based upon individual response, the dose may be increased to 15 mg once daily, as early as two weeks after starting therapy.
ENABLEX extended-release tablets should be taken once daily with liquid. They may be taken with or without food, and should be swallowed whole and not chewed, divided or crushed.
For patients with moderate hepatic impairment or when co-administered with potent CYP3A4 inhibitors (e.g., ketoconazole, itraconazole, ritonavir, nelfinavir, clarithromycin and nefazodone), the daily dose of ENABLEX should not exceed 7.5 mg. ENABLEX is not recommended for use in patients with severe hepatic impairment (see CLINICAL PHARMACOLOGY and PRECAUTIONS).

HOW SUPPLIED
ENABLEX® 7.5 mg extended-release tablets are round, shallow, convex, white-colored tablets, and are identified with "DF" on one side and "7.5" on the reverse.

Table 4
Incidence of Adverse Events* Reported in ≥2.0% of Patients Treated with ENABLEX® Extended-Release Tablets and More Frequent with ENABLEX® than with Placebo in Three, Fixed-Dose, Placebo-Controlled, Phase III Studies (Studies 1, 2, and 3)

Body System	Adverse Event	Percentage of Subjects with Adverse Event (%)		
		ENABLEX® 7.5 mg N=337	ENABLEX® 15 mg N=334	Placebo N=388
Digestive	Dry Mouth	20.2	35.3	8.2
	Constipation	14.8	21.3	6.2
	Dyspepsia	2.7	8.4	2.6
	Abdominal Pain	2.4	3.9	0.5
	Nausea	2.7	1.5	1.5
	Diarrhea	2.1	0.9	1.8
Urogenital	Urinary Tract Infection	4.7	4.5	2.6
Nervous	Dizziness	0.9	2.1	1.3
Body as a Whole	Asthenia	1.5	2.7	1.3
Eye	Dry Eyes	1.5	2.1	0.5

* Regardless of causality

Table 5
Number (%) of Adverse Events* Reported in >3% of Patients Treated with ENABLEX® Extended-Release Tablets, and More Frequent with ENABLEX® than Placebo, in the Placebo-Controlled, Dose-Titration, Phase III Study (Study 4)

Adverse Event	ENABLEX® 7.5 mg/15 mg N=268	Placebo N=127
Constipation	56 (20.9%)	10 (7.9%)
Dry Mouth	50 (18.7%)	11 (8.7%)
Headache	18 (6.7%)	7 (5.5%)
Dyspepsia	12 (4.5%)	2 (1.6%)
Nausea	11 (4.1%)	2 (1.6%)
Urinary Tract Infection	10 (3.7%)	4 (3.1%)
Accidental Injury	8 (3.0%)	3 (2.4%)
Flu Syndrome	8 (3.0%)	3 (2.4%)

* Regardless of causality

Bottle of 30 .... NDC 0078-0419-15
Bottle of 90 .... NDC 0078-0419-34
ENABLEX® 15 mg extended-release tablets are round, shallow, convex, light peach-colored tablets, and are identified with "DF" on one side and "15" on the reverse.
Bottle of 30 .... NDC 0078-0420-15
Bottle of 90 .... NDC 0078-0420-34
Storage
Store at 25°C (77°F); excursions permitted to 15-30°C (59-86°F) [see USP Controlled Room Temperature]. Protect from light.
Keep this and all drugs out of the reach of children.
REV: JANUARY 2010   T2010-04

INFORMATION FOR PATIENTS
ENABLEX® (ĕn-a-blĕx)
(darifenacin)
Extended-release tablets
7.5 mg or 15 mg
Rx only
Read the Patient Information that comes with ENABLEX® before you start taking it and each time you get a refill. There may be new information. This leaflet does not take the place of talking to your doctor or other healthcare professional about your medical condition or your treatment. Only your doctor or healthcare professional can determine if treatment with ENABLEX is right for you.
What is ENABLEX?
ENABLEX is a prescription medicine used in adults to treat the following symptoms due to a condition called overactive bladder:
• having a strong need to go to the bathroom right away (also called "urgency")
• leaking or wetting accidents (also called "urinary incontinence")
• having to go to the bathroom too often (also called "urinary frequency")
What is overactive bladder?
Overactive bladder happens when you cannot control your bladder contractions. When these muscle contractions happen too often or cannot be controlled, you get symptoms of overactive bladder, which are urinary urgency, urinary incontinence (leakage) and urinary frequency.
Who should not take ENABLEX?
Do not take ENABLEX if you:
• are not able to empty your bladder (also called "urinary retention")
• have delayed or slow emptying of your stomach (also called "gastric retention")

• have an eye problem called "uncontrolled narrow-angle glaucoma"
• are allergic to ENABLEX or to any of its ingredients. See the end of this leaflet for a complete list of ingredients. ENABLEX has not been studied in children.
What should I tell my doctor before starting ENABLEX?
Before starting ENABLEX, tell your doctor or healthcare professional about all of your medical conditions including if you:
• have any stomach or intestinal problems, or problems with constipation
• have trouble emptying your bladder or if you have a weak urine stream
• have an eye problem called narrow-angle glaucoma
• have liver problems
• are pregnant or are planning to become pregnant. It is not known if ENABLEX can harm your unborn baby.
• are breast-feeding. It is not known if ENABLEX passes into breast milk and if it can harm your baby.
Tell your doctor about all the medicines you take, including prescription and nonprescription medicines, vitamins, and herbal supplements. ENABLEX and certain other medicines can interact with each other, causing side effects. Especially tell your doctor if you take:
• ketoconazole (Nizoral®) or itraconazole (Sporanox®), antifungal medicines
• clarithromycin (Biaxin®), an antibiotic medicine
• ritonivir or nelfinavir (Viracept®), antiviral medicines
• nefazodone (Serzone®), a depression medicine
• flecainide (Tambocor™), an abnormal heartbeat (antiarrhythmia) medicine
• thioridazine (Mellaril®), a mental disorder (antipsychotic) medicine
• a medicine called a tricyclic antidepressant
Know all the medicines you take. Keep a list of them with you to show your doctor and pharmacist each time you get a new medicine.
How should I take ENABLEX?
Take ENABLEX exactly as prescribed. Your doctor will prescribe the dose that is right for you. Your doctor may prescribe the lowest dose if you have certain medical conditions such as liver problems.
• You should take ENABLEX once daily with liquid.
• **ENABLEX should be swallowed whole and not chewed, divided or crushed.**
• ENABLEX may be taken with or without food.

- If you miss a dose of ENABLEX, begin taking ENABLEX again the next day. Do not take two doses of ENABLEX in the same day.
- If you take too much ENABLEX, call your local Poison Control Center or emergency room right away.

What are the possible side effects of ENABLEX?

The most common side effects with ENABLEX are:

- dry mouth
- constipation

ENABLEX may cause other less common side effects that include:

- blurred vision. Use caution while driving or doing dangerous activities until you know how ENABLEX affects you.
- heat prostration. Heat prostration (due to decreased sweating) can occur when drugs such as ENABLEX are used in a hot environment.

These are not all the side effects with ENABLEX. For more information, ask your doctor, healthcare professional or pharmacist.

How do I store ENABLEX?

- **Keep ENABLEX and all medicines out of the reach of children.**
- Store ENABLEX at room temperature, 59 to 86°F (15 to 30°C). Protect from light.
- Safely dispose of ENABLEX that is out of date or no longer needed.

General information about ENABLEX

Medicines are sometimes prescribed for conditions that are not mentioned in patient information leaflets. Do not give ENABLEX to other people, even if they have the same symptoms you have. It may harm them.

This leaflet summarizes the most important information about ENABLEX. If you would like more information, talk with your doctor. You can ask your pharmacist or doctor for information about ENABLEX that is written for health professionals. You can also call the product information department at 1-888-44-ENABLEX (1-888-443-6225) or visit the website at www.Enablex.com.

What are the ingredients in ENABLEX?

Active Ingredient: darifenacin

Inactive Ingredients: dibasic calcium phosphate, hypromellose (hydroxypropyl methylcellulose), magnesium stearate, polyethylene glycol, talc, titanium dioxide. The 15-mg tablet also contains iron oxide red and iron oxide yellow.

Appearance:

The 7.5-mg tablet is round and white-colored with "DF" on one side and "7.5" on the other side.

The 15-mg tablet is round and peach-colored with "DF" on one side and "15" on the other side.

*Mellaril® is a registered trademark of Novartis. The other brands listed are the trademarks of their respective owners and are not trademarks of Novartis.

REV: JANUARY 2010 T2010-05

REV: JANUARY 2010 Printed in U.S.A. T2010-04/T2010-05

5002459

5002460

Manufactured by:
Novartis Pharma Stein AG
Stein, Switzerland
Distributed by:
Novartis Pharmaceuticals Corporation
East Hanover, New Jersey 07936
Marketed with:
Warner Chilcott Pharmaceuticals Inc.
Mason, Ohio 45040
©Novartis

Shown in Product Identification Guide, page 315

EXELON® ℞

[ĕx'ə-lŏn]

(rivastigmine tartrate)
Capsules and Oral Solution
Rx only

Prescribing Information

The following prescribing information is based on official labeling in effect July 2008.

DESCRIPTION

Exelon® (rivastigmine tartrate) is a reversible cholinesterase inhibitor and is known chemically as (S)-N-Ethyl-N-methyl - 3 - [1 - (dimethylamino)ethyl] - phenyl carbamate hydrogen - (2R,3R) - tartrate. Rivastigmine tartrate is commonly referred to in the pharmacological literature as SDZ ENA 713 or ENA 713. It has an empirical formula of $C_{14}H_{22}N_2O_2$ • $C_4H_6O_6$ (hydrogen tartrate salt – hta salt) and a molecular weight of 400.43 (hta salt). Rivastigmine tartrate is a white to off-white, fine crystalline powder that is very soluble in water, soluble in ethanol and acetonitrile, slightly soluble in n-octanol and very slightly soluble in ethyl acetate. The distribution coefficient at 37°C in n-octanol/phosphate buffer solution pH 7 is 3.0.

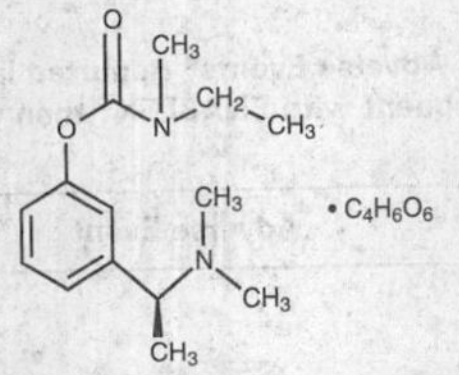

Exelon Capsules contain rivastigmine tartrate, equivalent to 1.5, 3, 4.5 and 6 mg of rivastigmine base for oral administration. Inactive ingredients are hydroxypropyl methylcellulose, magnesium stearate, microcrystalline cellulose, and silicon dioxide. Each hard-gelatin capsule contains gelatin, titanium dioxide and red and/or yellow iron oxides.

Exelon Oral Solution is supplied as a solution containing rivastigmine tartrate, equivalent to 2 mg/mL of rivastigmine base for oral administration. Inactive ingredients are citric acid, D&C yellow #10, purified water, sodium benzoate and sodium citrate.

CLINICAL PHARMACOLOGY

Mechanism of Action

Pathological changes in dementia of the Alzheimer type and dementia associated with Parkinson's disease involve cholinergic neuronal pathways that project from the basal forebrain to the cerebral cortex and hippocampus. These pathways are thought to be intricately involved in memory, attention, learning, and other cognitive processes. While the precise mechanism of rivastigmine's action is unknown, it is postulated to exert its therapeutic effect by enhancing cholinergic function. This is accomplished by increasing the concentration of acetylcholine through reversible inhibition of its hydrolysis by cholinesterase. If this proposed mechanism is correct, Exelon's effect may lessen as the disease process advances and fewer cholinergic neurons remain functionally intact. There is no evidence that rivastigmine alters the course of the underlying dementing process. After a 6-mg dose of rivastigmine, anticholinesterase activity is present in CSF for about 10 hours, with a maximum inhibition of about 60% 5 hours after dosing.

In vitro and *in vivo* studies demonstrate that the inhibition of cholinesterase by rivastigmine is not affected by the concomitant administration of memantine, an N-methyl-D-aspartate receptor antagonist.

Clinical Trial Data

Dementia of the Alzheimer's Type

The effectiveness of Exelon® (rivastigmine tartrate) as a treatment for Alzheimer's disease is demonstrated by the results of 2 randomized, double-blind, placebo-controlled clinical investigations in patients with Alzheimer's disease [diagnosed by NINCDS-ADRDA and DSM-IV criteria, Mini-Mental State Examination (MMSE) ≥10 and ≤26, and the Global Deterioration Scale (GDS)]. The mean age of patients participating in Exelon trials was 73 years with a range of 41-95. Approximately 59% of patients were women and 41% were men. The racial distribution was Caucasian 87%, Black 4% and Other races 9%.

Study Outcome Measures

In each study, the effectiveness of Exelon was evaluated using a dual outcome assessment strategy.

The ability of Exelon to improve cognitive performance was assessed with the cognitive subscale of the Alzheimer's Disease Assessment Scale (ADAS-cog), a multi-item instrument that has been extensively validated in longitudinal cohorts of Alzheimer's disease patients. The ADAS-cog examines selected aspects of cognitive performance including elements of memory, orientation, attention, reasoning, language and praxis. The ADAS-cog scoring range is from 0 to 70, with higher scores indicating greater cognitive impairment. Elderly normal adults may score as low as 0 or 1, but it is not unusual for non-demented adults to score slightly higher.

The patients recruited as participants in each study had mean scores on ADAS-cog of approximately 23 units, with a range from 1 to 61. Experience gained in longitudinal studies of ambulatory patients with mild to moderate Alzheimer's disease suggests that they gain 6-12 units a year on the ADAS-cog. Lesser degrees of change, however, are seen in patients with very mild or very advanced disease because the ADAS-cog is not uniformly sensitive to change over the course of the disease. The annualized rate of decline in the placebo patients participating in Exelon trials was approximately 3-8 units per year.

The ability of Exelon to produce an overall clinical effect was assessed using a Clinician's Interview-Based Impression of Change (CIBIC) that required the use of caregiver information, the CIBIC-Plus. The CIBIC-Plus is not a single instrument and is not a standardized instrument like the ADAS-cog. Clinical trials for investigational drugs have used a variety of CIBIC formats, each different in terms of depth and structure. As such, results from a CIBIC-Plus reflect clinical experience from the trial or trials in which it was used and cannot be compared directly with the results of CIBIC-Plus evaluations from other clinical trials. The CIBIC-Plus used in the Exelon trials was a structured instrument based on a comprehensive evaluation at baseline and subsequent time-points of three domains: patient cognition, behavior and functioning, including assessment of activities of daily living. It represents the assessment of a skilled clinician using validated scales based on his/her observation at interviews conducted separately with the patient and the caregiver familiar with the behavior of the patient over the interval rated. The CIBIC-Plus is scored as a 7-point categorical rating, ranging from a score of 1, indicating "markedly improved," to a score of 4, indicating "no change" to a score of 7, indicating "marked worsening." The CIBIC-Plus has not been systematically compared directly to assessments not using information from caregivers or other global methods.

U.S. 26-Week Study

In a study of 26 weeks duration, 699 patients were randomized to either a dose range of 1-4 mg or 6-12 mg of Exelon per day or to placebo, each given in divided doses. The 26-week study was divided into a 12-week forced-dose titration phase and a 14-week maintenance phase. The patients in the active treatment arms of the study were maintained at their highest tolerated dose within the respective range.

Effects on the ADAS-cog: Figure 1 illustrates the time course for the change from baseline in ADAS-cog scores for all three dose groups over the 26 weeks of the study. At 26 weeks of treatment, the mean differences in the ADAS-cog change scores for the Exelon-treated patients compared to the patients on placebo were 1.9 and 4.9 units for the 1-4 mg and 6-12 mg treatments, respectively. Both treatments were statistically significantly superior to placebo and the 6-12 mg/day range was significantly superior to the 1-4 mg/day range.

Figure 1: Time-course of the Change from Baseline in ADAS-cog Score for Patients Completing 26 Weeks of Treatment

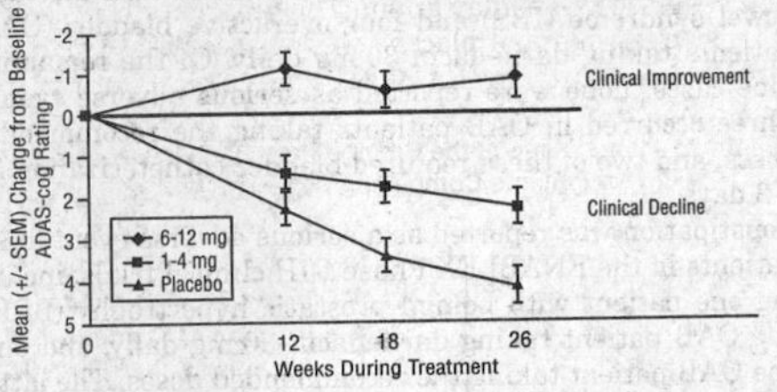

Figure 2 illustrates the cumulative percentages of patients from each of the three treatment groups who had attained at least the measure of improvement in ADAS-cog score shown on the X axis. Three change scores, (7-point and 4-point reductions from baseline or no change in score) have been identified for illustrative purposes, and the percent of patients in each group achieving that result is shown in the inset table.

The curves demonstrate that both patients assigned to Exelon and placebo have a wide range of responses, but that the Exelon groups are more likely to show the greater improvements. A curve for an effective treatment would be shifted to the left of the curve for placebo, while an ineffective or deleterious treatment would be superimposed upon, or shifted to the right of the curve for placebo, respectively.

Figure 2: Cumulative Percentage of Patients Completing 26 Weeks of Double-blind Treatment with Specified Changes from Baseline ADAS-cog Scores. The Percentages of Randomized Patients who Completed the Study were: Placebo 84%, 1-4 mg 85%, and 6-12 mg 65%.

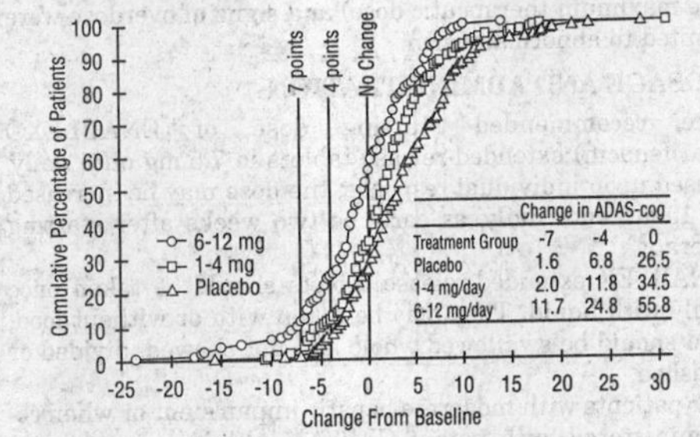

	Change in ADAS-cog		
Treatment Group	-7	-4	0
Placebo	1.6	6.8	26.5
1-4 mg/day	2.0	11.8	34.5
6-12 mg/day	11.7	24.8	55.8

Effects on the CIBIC-Plus: Figure 3 is a histogram of the frequency distribution of CIBIC-Plus scores attained by patients assigned to each of the three treatment groups who completed 26 weeks of treatment. The mean Exelon-placebo differences for these groups of patients in the mean rating of change from baseline were 0.32 units and 0.35 units for 1-4 mg and 6-12 mg of Exelon, respectively. The mean ratings for the 6-12 mg/day and 1-4 mg/day groups were statistically significantly superior to placebo. The differences between the 6-12 mg/day and the1-4 mg/day groups were statistically significant.

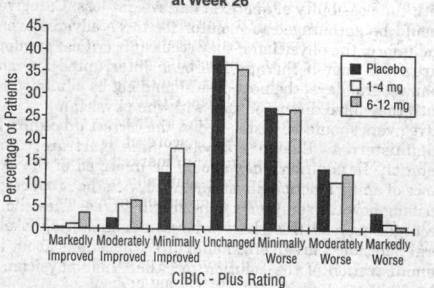

Figure 3: Frequency Distribution of CIBIC-Plus Scores at Week 26

Global 26-Week Study

In a second study of 26 weeks duration, 725 patients were randomized to either a dose range of 1-4 mg or 6-12 mg of Exelon per day or to placebo, each given in divided doses. The 26-week study was divided into a 12-week forced-dose titration phase and a 14-week maintenance phase. The patients in the active treatment arms of the study were maintained at their highest tolerated dose within the respective range.

Effects on the ADAS-cog: Figure 4 illustrates the time course of the change from baseline in ADAS-cog scores for all three dose groups over the 26 weeks of the study. At 26 weeks of treatment, the mean differences in the ADAS-cog change scores for the Exelon-treated patients compared to the patients on placebo were 0.2 and 2.6 units for the 1-4 mg and 6-12 mg treatments, respectively. The 6-12 mg/day group was statistically significantly superior to placebo, as well as to the 1-4 mg/day group. The difference between the 1-4 mg/day group and placebo was not statistically significant.

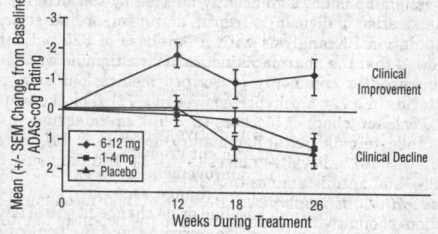

Figure 4: Time-course of the Change from Baseline in ADAS-cog Score for Patients Completing 26 Weeks of Treatment

Figure 5 illustrates the cumulative percentages of patients from each of the three treatment groups who had attained at least the measure of improvement in ADAS-cog score shown on the X axis. Similar to the U.S. 26-week study, the curves demonstrate that both patients assigned to Exelon and placebo have a wide range of responses, but that the 6-12 mg/day Exelon group is more likely to show the greater improvements.

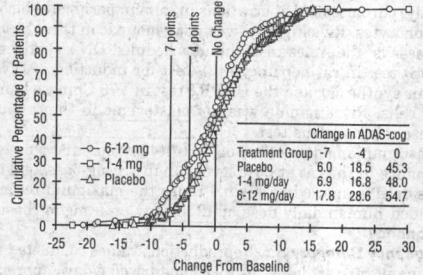

Figure 5: Cumulative Percentage of Patients Completing 26 Weeks of Double-blind Treatment with Specified Changes from Baseline ADAS-cog Scores. The Percentages of Randomized Patients who Completed the Study were: Placebo 87%, 1-4 mg 86%, and 6-12 mg 67%.

Treatment Group	Change in ADAS-cog		
	-7	-4	0
Placebo	6.0	18.5	45.3
1-4 mg/day	6.9	16.8	48.0
6-12 mg/day	17.8	28.6	54.7

Effects on the CIBIC-Plus: Figure 6 is a histogram of the frequency distribution of CIBIC-Plus scores attained by patients assigned to each of the three treatment groups who completed 26 weeks of treatment. The mean Exelon-placebo differences for these groups of patients for the mean rating of change from baseline were 0.14 units and 0.41 units for 1-4 mg and 6-12 mg of Exelon, respectively. The mean ratings for the 6-12 mg/day group were statistically significantly superior to placebo. The comparison of the mean rat-

ings for the 1-4 mg/day group and placebo group was not statistically significant.

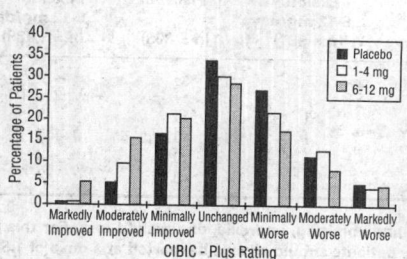

Figure 6: Frequency Distribution of CIBIC-Plus Scores at Week 26

U.S. Fixed-Dose Study

In a study of 26 weeks duration, 702 patients were randomized to doses of 3, 6, or 9 mg/day of Exelon or to placebo, each given in divided doses. The fixed-dose study design, which included a 12-week forced-dose titration phase and a 14-week maintenance phase, led to a high dropout rate in the 9 mg/day group because of poor tolerability. At 26 weeks of treatment, significant differences were observed for the ADAS-cog mean change from baseline for the 9 mg/day and 6 mg/day groups, compared to placebo. No significant differences were observed between any of the Exelon-dose groups and placebo for the analysis of the CIBIC-Plus mean rating of change. Although no significant differences were observed between Exelon treatment groups, there was a trend toward numerical superiority with higher doses.

Dementia Associated with Parkinson's Disease (PDD)
International 24-Week Study

The effectiveness of Exelon as a treatment for dementia associated with Parkinson's disease is demonstrated by the results of one randomized, double-blind, placebo-controlled clinical investigation in patients with mild to moderate dementia, with onset at least 2 years after the initial diagnosis of idiopathic Parkinson's disease. The diagnosis of idiopathic Parkinson's disease was based on the United Kingdom Parkinson's Disease Society Brain Bank clinical criteria. The diagnosis of dementia was based on the criteria stipulated under the DSM-IV category "Dementia Due To Other General Medical Condition" (code 294.1x), but patients were not required to have a distinctive pattern of cognitive deficits as part of the dementia. Alternate causes of dementia were excluded by clinical history, physical and neurological examination, brain imaging, and relevant blood tests. Patients enrolled in the study had a MMSE score $\geq$10 and $\leq$24 at entry. The mean age of patients participating in this trial was 72.7 years with a range of 50-91. Approximately, 35.1% of patients were women and 64.9% of patients were men. The racial distribution was 99.6% Caucasian and Other races 0.4%.

Study Outcome Measures

This study used a dual outcome assessment strategy to evaluate the effectiveness of Exelon.

The ability of Exelon to improve cognitive performance was assessed with the ADAS-cog.

The ability of Exelon to produce an overall clinical effect was assessed using the Alzheimer's Disease Cooperative Study – Clinician's Global Impression of Change (ADCS-CGIC). The ADCS-CGIC is a more standardized form of CIBIC-Plus and is also scored as a 7-point categorical rating, ranging from a score of 1, indicating "markedly improved," to a score of 4, indicating "no change" to a score of 7, indicating "marked worsening."

Study Results

In this study, 541 patients were randomized to a dose range of 3-12 mg of Exelon per day or to placebo in a ratio of 2:1, given in divided doses. The 24-week study was divided into a 16-week titration phase and an 8-week maintenance phase. The patients in the active treatment arm of the study were maintained at their highest tolerated dose within the specified dose range.

Effects on the ADAS-cog: Figure 7 illustrates the time course for the change from baseline in ADAS-cog scores for both treatment groups over the 24-week study. At 24 weeks of treatment, the mean difference in the ADAS-cog change scores for the Exelon-treated patients compared to the patients on placebo was 3.8 points. This treatment difference was statistically significant in favor of Exelon when compared to placebo.

[See figure at top of next column]

Effects on the ADCS-CGIC: Figure 8 is a histogram of the distribution of patients' scores on the ADCS-CGIC (Alzheimer's Disease Cooperative Study – Clinician's Global Impression of Change) at 24 weeks. The mean difference in change scores between the Exelon and placebo groups from

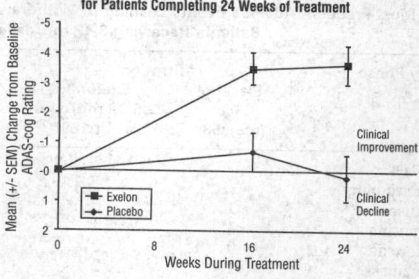

Figure 7: Time Course of the Change from Baseline in ADAS-cog Score for Patients Completing 24 Weeks of Treatment

baseline was 0.5 points. This difference was statistically significant in favor of Exelon treatment.

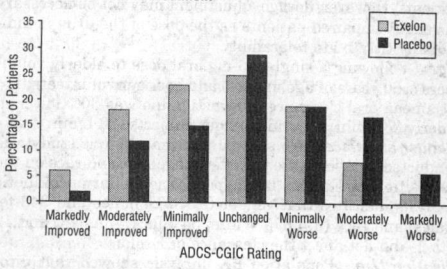

Figure 8: Distribution of ADCS-CGIC Scores for Patients Completing 24 Weeks of Treatment

Age, Gender and Race

Patients' age, gender, or race did not predict clinical outcome of Exelon treatment.

Pharmacokinetics

Rivastigmine is well absorbed with absolute bioavailability of about 40% (3-mg dose). It shows linear pharmacokinetics up to 3 mg BID but is non-linear at higher doses. Doubling the dose from 3 to 6 mg BID results in a 3-fold increase in AUC. The elimination half-life is about 1.5 hours, with most elimination as metabolites via the urine.

Absorption: Rivastigmine is rapidly and completely absorbed. Peak plasma concentrations are reached in approximately 1 hour. Absolute bioavailability after a 3-mg dose is about 36%. Administration of Exelon with food delays absorption (t_{max}) by 90 minutes, lowers C_{max} by approximately 30% and increases AUC by approximately 30%.

Distribution: Rivastigmine is widely distributed throughout the body with a volume of distribution in the range of 1.8-2.7 L/kg. Rivastigmine penetrates the blood brain barrier, reaching CSF peak concentrations in 1.4-2.6 hours. Mean AUC_{1-12hr} ratio of CSF/plasma averaged 40 ± 0.5% following 1-6 mg BID doses.

Rivastigmine is about 40% bound to plasma proteins at concentrations of 1-400 ng/mL, which cover the therapeutic concentration range. Rivastigmine distributes equally between blood and plasma with a blood-to-plasma partition ratio of 0.9 at concentrations ranging from 1-400 ng/mL.

Metabolism: Rivastigmine is rapidly and extensively metabolized, primarily via cholinesterase-mediated hydrolysis to the decarbamylated metabolite. Based on evidence from *in vitro* and animal studies, the major cytochrome P450 isozymes are minimally involved in rivastigmine metabolism. Consistent with these observations is the finding that no drug interactions related to cytochrome P450 have been observed in humans (*see Drug-Drug Interactions*).

Elimination: The major pathway of elimination is via the kidneys. Following administration of ^{14}C-rivastigmine to 6 healthy volunteers, total recovery of radioactivity over 120 hours was 97% in urine and 0.4% in feces. No parent drug was detected in urine. The sulfate conjugate of the decarbamylated metabolite is the major component excreted in urine and represents 40% of the dose. Mean oral clearance of rivastigmine is 1.8 ± 0.6 L/min after 6 mg BID.

Special Populations

Hepatic Disease: Following a single 3-mg dose, mean oral clearance of rivastigmine was 60% lower in hepatically impaired patients (n = 10, biopsy proven) than in healthy subjects (n = 10). After multiple 6-mg BID oral dosing, the mean clearance of rivastigmine was 65% lower in mild (n = 7, Child-Pugh score 5-6) and moderate (n = 3, Child-Pugh score 7-9) hepatically impaired patients (biopsy proven, liver cirrhosis) than in healthy subjects (n = 10). Dosage adjustment is not necessary in hepatically impaired patients as the dose of drug is individually titrated to tolerability.

Renal Disease: Following a single 3-mg dose, mean oral clearance of rivastigmine is 64% lower in moderately impaired renal patients (n = 8, GFR = 10-50 mL/min) than in healthy subjects (n = 10, GFR $\geq$60 mL/min); Cl/F = 1.7 L/min (cv = 45%) and 4.8 L/min (cv = 80%), respectively. In severely impaired renal patients (n = 8, GFR <10 mL/min), mean oral clearance of rivastigmine is 43% higher than in healthy subjects (n = 10, GFR $\geq$60 mL/min);

Table 1
Most Frequent Adverse Events Leading to Withdrawal from Clinical Trials during Titration and Maintenance in Patients Receiving 6-12 mg/day Exelon® Using a Forced-Dose Titration

Study Phase	Titration		Maintenance		Overall	
	Placebo (n = 868)	Exelon® ≥6-12 mg/day (n = 1,189)	Placebo (n = 788)	Exelon® ≥6-12 mg/day (n = 987)	Placebo (n = 868)	Exelon® ≥6-12 mg/day (n = 1,189)
Event/% Discontinuing						
Nausea	<1	8	<1	1	1	8
Vomiting	<1	4	<1	1	<1	5
Anorexia	0	2	<1	1	<1	3
Dizziness	<1	2	<1	1	<1	2

Cl/F = 6.9 L/min and 4.8 L/min, respectively. For unexplained reasons, the severely impaired renal patients had a higher clearance of rivastigmine than moderately impaired patients. However, dosage adjustment may not be necessary in renally impaired patients as the dose of the drug is individually titrated to tolerability.

Age: Following a single 2.5-mg oral dose to elderly volunteers (>60 years of age, n = 24) and younger volunteers (n = 24), mean oral clearance of rivastigmine was 30% lower in elderly (7 L/min) than in younger subjects (10 L/min).

Gender and Race: No specific pharmacokinetic study was conducted to investigate the effect of gender and race on the disposition of Exelon, but a population pharmacokinetic analysis indicates that gender (n = 277 males and 348 females) and race (n = 575 White, 34 Black, 4 Asian, and 12 Other) did not affect the clearance of Exelon.

Nicotine Use: Population PK analysis showed that nicotine use increases the oral clearance of rivastigmine by 23% (n = 75 Smokers and 549 Nonsmokers).

Drug-Drug Interactions

Effect of Exelon on the Metabolism of Other Drugs: Rivastigmine is primarily metabolized through hydrolysis by esterases. Minimal metabolism occurs via the major cytochrome P450 isoenzymes. Based on *in vitro* studies, no pharmacokinetic drug interactions with drugs metabolized by the following isoenzyme systems are expected: CYP1A2, CYP2D6, CYP3A4/5, CYP2E1, CYP2C9, CYP2C8, or CYP2C19.

No pharmacokinetic interaction was observed between rivastigmine and digoxin, warfarin, diazepam, or fluoxetine in studies in healthy volunteers. The elevation of prothrombin time induced by warfarin is not affected by administration of Exelon.

Effect of Other Drugs on the Metabolism of Exelon: Drugs that induce or inhibit CYP450 metabolism are not expected to alter the metabolism of rivastigmine. Single-dose pharmacokinetic studies demonstrated that the metabolism of rivastigmine is not significantly affected by concurrent administration of digoxin, warfarin, diazepam, or fluoxetine.

Population PK analysis with a database of 625 patients showed that the pharmacokinetics of rivastigmine were not influenced by commonly prescribed medications such as antacids (n = 77), antihypertensives (n = 72), ß-blockers (n = 42), calcium channel blockers (n = 75), antidiabetics (n = 21), nonsteroidal antiinflammatory drugs (n = 79), estrogens (n = 70), salicylate analgesics (n = 177), antianginals (n = 35), and antihistamines (n = 15). In addition, in clinical trials, no increased risk of clinically relevant untoward effects was observed in patients treated concomitantly with Exelon and these agents.

INDICATIONS AND USAGE

Exelon® (rivastigmine tartrate) is indicated for the treatment of mild to moderate dementia of the Alzheimer's type. Exelon® (rivastigmine tartrate) is indicated for the treatment of mild to moderate dementia associated with Parkinson's disease.

The dementia of Parkinson's disease is purportedly characterized by impairments in executive function, memory retrieval, and attention in patients with an established diagnosis of Parkinson's disease. The diagnosis of the dementia of Parkinson's disease, however, can reliably be made in patients in whom a progressive dementia syndrome occurs (without the necessity to document the specific deficits described above) at least 2 years after a diagnosis of Parkinson's disease has been made, and in whom other causes of dementia have been ruled out *(see CLINICAL PHARMACOLOGY, Clinical Trial Data)*.

CONTRAINDICATIONS

Exelon® (rivastigmine tartrate) is contraindicated in patients with known hypersensitivity to rivastigmine, other carbamate derivatives or other components of the formulation *(see DESCRIPTION)*.

WARNINGS

Gastrointestinal Adverse Reactions

Exelon® (rivastigmine tartrate) use is associated with significant gastrointestinal adverse reactions, including nausea and vomiting, anorexia, and weight loss. For this reason, patients should always be started at a dose of 1.5 mg BID and titrated to their maintenance dose. If treatment is interrupted for longer than several days, treatment should be reinitiated with the lowest daily dose *(see DOSAGE AND ADMINISTRATION)* to reduce the possibility of severe vomiting and its potentially serious sequelae (e.g., there has been one postmarketing report of severe vomiting with esophageal rupture following inappropriate reinitiation of treatment with a 4.5-mg dose after 8 weeks of treatment interruption).

Nausea and Vomiting: **In the controlled clinical trials, 47% of the patients treated with an Exelon dose in the therapeutic range of 6-12 mg/day (n = 1189) developed nausea (compared with 12% in placebo). A total of 31% of Exelon-treated patients developed at least one episode of vomiting (compared with 6% for placebo). The rate of vomiting was higher during the titration phase (24% vs. 3% for placebo) than in the maintenance phase (14% vs. 3% for placebo). The rates were higher in women than men. Five percent of patients discontinued for vomiting, compared to less than 1% for patients on placebo. Vomiting was severe in 2% of Exelon-treated patients and was rated as mild or moderate each in 14% of patients. The rate of nausea was higher during the titration phase (43% vs. 9% for placebo) than in the maintenance phase (17% vs. 4% for placebo).**

Weight Loss: **In the controlled trials, approximately 26% of women on high doses of Exelon (greater than 9 mg/day) had weight loss equal to or greater than 7% of their baseline weight compared to 6% in the placebo-treated patients. About 18% of the males in the high-dose group experienced a similar degree of weight loss compared to 4% in placebo-treated patients. It is not clear how much of the weight loss was associated with anorexia, nausea, vomiting, and the diarrhea associated with the drug.**

Anorexia: In the controlled clinical trials, of the patients treated with an Exelon dose of 6-12 mg/day, 17% developed anorexia compared to 3% of the placebo patients. Neither the time course nor the severity of the anorexia is known.

Peptic Ulcers/Gastrointestinal Bleeding: Because of their pharmacological action, cholinesterase inhibitors may be expected to increase gastric acid secretion due to increased cholinergic activity. Therefore, patients should be monitored closely for symptoms of active or occult gastrointestinal bleeding, especially those at increased risk for developing ulcers, e.g., those with a history of ulcer disease or those receiving concurrent nonsteroidal antiinflammatory drugs (NSAIDs). Clinical studies of Exelon have shown no significant increase, relative to placebo, in the incidence of either peptic ulcer disease or gastrointestinal bleeding.

Anesthesia

Exelon as a cholinesterase inhibitor, is likely to exaggerate succinylcholine-type muscle relaxation during anesthesia.

Cardiovascular Conditions

Drugs that increase cholinergic activity may have vagotonic effects on heart rate (e.g., bradycardia). The potential for this action may be particularly important to patients with "sick sinus syndrome" or other supraventricular cardiac conduction conditions. In clinical trials, Exelon was not associated with any increased incidence of cardiovascular adverse events, heart rate or blood pressure changes, or ECG abnormalities. Syncopal episodes have been reported in 3% of patients receiving 6-12 mg/day of Exelon, compared to 2% of placebo patients.

Genitourinary

Although this was not observed in clinical trials of Exelon, drugs that increase cholinergic activity may cause urinary obstruction.

Neurological Conditions

Seizures: Drugs that increase cholinergic activity are believed to have some potential for causing seizures. However, seizure activity also may be a manifestation of Alzheimer's disease.

Pulmonary Conditions

Like other drugs that increase cholinergic activity, Exelon should be used with care in patients with a history of asthma or obstructive pulmonary disease.

PRECAUTIONS

Information for Patients and Caregivers

Caregivers should be advised of the high incidence of nausea and vomiting associated with the use of the drug along with the possibility of anorexia and weight loss. Caregivers should be encouraged to monitor for these adverse events and inform the physician if they occur. It is critical to inform caregivers that if therapy has been interrupted for more than several days, the next dose should not be administered until they have discussed this with the physician.

Caregivers should be instructed in the correct procedure for administering Exelon® (rivastigmine tartrate) Oral Solution. In addition, they should be informed of the existence of an Instruction Sheet (included with the product) describing how the solution is to be administered. They should be urged to read this sheet prior to administering Exelon Oral Solution. Caregivers should direct questions about the administration of the solution to either their physician or pharmacist.

Caregivers and patients should be advised that like other cholinomimetics, Exelon® may exacerbate or induce extrapyramidal symptoms. Worsening in patients with Parkinson's disease, including an increased incidence or intensity of tremor, has been observed.

Drug-Drug Interactions

Effect of Exelon on the Metabolism of Other Drugs: Rivastigmine is primarily metabolized through hydrolysis by esterases. Minimal metabolism occurs via the major cytochrome P450 isoenzymes. Based on *in vitro* studies, no pharmacokinetic drug interactions with drugs metabolized by the following isoenzyme systems are expected: CYP1A2, CYP2D6, CYP3A4/5, CYP2E1, CYP2C9, CYP2C8, or CYP2C19.

No pharmacokinetic interaction was observed between rivastigmine and digoxin, warfarin, diazepam, or fluoxetine in studies in healthy volunteers. The elevation of prothrombin time induced by warfarin is not affected by administration of Exelon.

Effect of Other Drugs on the Metabolism of Exelon: Drugs that induce or inhibit CYP450 metabolism are not expected to alter the metabolism of rivastigmine. Single-dose pharmacokinetic studies demonstrated that the metabolism of rivastigmine is not significantly affected by concurrent administration of digoxin, warfarin, diazepam, or fluoxetine.

Population PK analysis with a database of 625 patients showed that the pharmacokinetics of rivastigmine were not influenced by commonly prescribed medications such as antacids (n = 77), antihypertensives (n = 72), ß-blockers (n = 42), calcium channel blockers (n = 75), antidiabetics (n = 21), nonsteroidal antiinflammatory drugs (n = 79), estrogens (n = 70), salicylate analgesics (n = 177), antianginals (n = 35), and antihistamines (n = 15).

Use with Anticholinergics: Because of their mechanism of action, cholinesterase inhibitors have the potential to interfere with the activity of anticholinergic medications.

Use with Cholinomimetics and Other Cholinesterase Inhibitors: A synergistic effect may be expected when cholinesterase inhibitors are given concurrently with succinylcholine, similar neuromuscular blocking agents or cholinergic agonists such as bethanechol.

Carcinogenesis, Mutagenesis, Impairment of Fertility

In carcinogenicity studies conducted at dose levels up to 1.1 mg-base/kg/day in rats and 1.6 mg-base/kg/day in mice, rivastigmine was not carcinogenic. These dose levels are approximately 0.9 times and 0.7 times the maximum recommended human daily dose of 12 mg/day on a mg/m^2 basis.

Rivastigmine was clastogenic in two *in vitro* assays in the presence, but not the absence, of metabolic activation. It caused structural chromosomal aberrations in V79 Chinese hamster lung cells and both structural and numerical (polyploidy) chromosomal aberrations in human peripheral blood lymphocytes. Rivastigmine was not genotoxic in three *in vitro* assays: the Ames test, the unscheduled DNA synthesis (UDS) test in rat hepatocytes (a test for induction of DNA repair synthesis), and the HGPRT test in V79 Chinese hamster cells. Rivastigmine was not clastogenic in the *in vivo* mouse micronucleus test.

Rivastigmine had no effect on fertility or reproductive performance in the rat at dose levels up to 1.1 mg-base/kg/day. This dose is approximately 0.9 times the maximum recommended human daily dose of 12 mg/day on a mg/m^2 basis.

Pregnancy

Pregnancy Category B: Reproduction studies conducted in pregnant rats at doses up to 2.3 mg-base/kg/day (approximately 2 times the maximum recommended human dose on a mg/m^2 basis) and in pregnant rabbits at doses up to 2.3 mg-base/kg/day (approximately 4 times the maximum recommended human dose on a mg/m^2 basis) revealed no evidence of teratogenicity. Studies in rats showed slightly decreased fetal/pup weights, usually at doses causing some maternal toxicity; decreased weights were seen at doses which were several fold lower than the maximum recommended human dose on a mg/m^2 basis. There are no adequate or well-controlled studies in pregnant women.

Table 2
Adverse Events Reported in Controlled Clinical Trials in at Least 2% of Patients Receiving Exelon®
(6-12 mg/day) and at a Higher Frequency than Placebo-treated Patients

Body System/Adverse Event	Placebo (n = 868)	Exelon® (6-12 mg/day) (n = 1,189)
Percent of Patients with any Adverse Event	79	92
Autonomic Nervous System		
Sweating Increased	1	4
Syncope	2	3
Body as a Whole		
Accidental Trauma	9	10
Fatigue	5	9
Asthenia	2	6
Malaise	2	5
Influenza-like Symptoms	2	3
Weight Decrease	<1	3
Cardiovascular Disorders, General		
Hypertension	2	3
Central and Peripheral Nervous System		
Dizziness	11	21
Headache	12	17
Somnolence	3	5
Tremor	1	4
Gastrointestinal System		
Nausea	12	47
Vomiting	6	31
Diarrhea	11	19
Anorexia	3	17
Abdominal Pain	6	13
Dyspepsia	4	9
Constipation	4	5
Flatulence	2	4
Eructation	1	2
Psychiatric Disorders		
Insomnia	7	9
Confusion	7	8
Depression	4	6
Anxiety	3	5
Hallucination	3	4
Aggressive Reaction	2	3
Resistance Mechanism Disorders		
Urinary Tract Infection	6	7
Respiratory System		
Rhinitis	3	4

Because animal reproduction studies are not always predictive of human response, Exelon should be used during pregnancy only if the potential benefit justifies the potential risk to the fetus.

Nursing Mothers
It is not known whether rivastigmine is excreted in human breast milk. Exelon has no indication for use in nursing mothers.

Pediatric Use
There are no adequate and well-controlled trials documenting the safety and efficacy of Exelon in any illness occurring in children.

ADVERSE REACTIONS
Dementia of the Alzheimer's Type
Adverse Events Leading to Discontinuation
The rate of discontinuation due to adverse events in controlled clinical trials of Exelon® (rivastigmine tartrate) was 15% for patients receiving 6-12 mg/day compared to 5% for patients on placebo during forced weekly dose titration. While on a maintenance dose, the rates were 6% for patients on Exelon compared to 4% for those on placebo.
The most common adverse events leading to discontinuation, defined as those occurring in at least 2% of patients and at twice the incidence seen in placebo patients, are shown in Table 1.
[See table at top of previous page]
Most Frequent Adverse Clinical Events Seen in Association with the Use of Exelon
The most common adverse events, defined as those occurring at a frequency of at least 5% and twice the placebo rate, are largely predicted by Exelon's cholinergic effects. These include nausea, vomiting, anorexia, dyspepsia, and asthenia.

Gastrointestinal Adverse Reactions
Exelon use is associated with significant nausea, vomiting, and weight loss (see WARNINGS).
Adverse Events Reported in Controlled Trials
Table 2 lists treatment-emergent signs and symptoms that were reported in at least 2% of patients in placebo-controlled trials and for which the rate of occurrence was greater for patients treated with Exelon doses of 6-12 mg/day than for those treated with placebo. The prescriber

should be aware that these figures cannot be used to predict the frequency of adverse events in the course of usual medical practice when patient characteristics and other factors may differ from those prevailing during clinical studies. Similarly, the cited frequencies cannot be directly compared with figures obtained from other clinical investigations involving different treatments, uses, or investigators. An inspection of these frequencies, however, does provide the prescriber with one basis by which to estimate the relative contribution of drug and non-drug factors to the adverse event incidences in the population studied.
In general, adverse reactions were less frequent later in the course of treatment.
No systematic effect of race or age could be determined from the incidence of adverse events in the controlled studies. Nausea, vomiting and weight loss were more frequent in women than men.
[See table above]
Other adverse events observed at a rate of 2% or more on Exelon 6-12 mg/day but at a greater or equal rate on placebo were chest pain, peripheral edema, vertigo, back pain, arthralgia, pain, bone fracture, agitation, nervousness, delusion, paranoid reaction, upper respiratory tract infection, infection (general), coughing, pharyngitis, bronchitis, rash (general), urinary incontinence.

Dementia Associated with Parkinson's Disease
Adverse Events Leading to Discontinuation
The rate of discontinuation due to adverse events in the single controlled trial of Exelon (rivastigmine tartrate) was 18.2% for patients receiving 3-12 mg/day compared to 11.2% for patients on placebo during the 24-week study.
The most frequent adverse events that led to discontinuation from this study, defined as those occurring in at least 1% of patients receiving Exelon and more frequent than those receiving placebo, were nausea (3.6% Exelon vs. 0.6% placebo), vomiting (1.9% Exelon vs. 0.6% placebo), and tremor (1.7% Exelon vs. 0.0% placebo).
Most Frequent Adverse Clinical Events Seen in Association with the Use of Exelon
The most common adverse events, defined as those occurring at a frequency of at least 5% and twice the placebo rate, are largely predicted by Exelon's cholinergic effects. These include nausea, vomiting, tremor, anorexia, and dizziness.

Adverse Events Reported in Controlled Trials
Table 3 lists treatment-emergent signs and symptoms that were reported in at least 2% of patients in placebo-controlled trials and for which the rate of occurrence was greater for patients treated with Exelon doses of 3-12 mg/day than for those treated with placebo. The prescriber should be aware that these figures cannot be used to predict the frequency of adverse events in the course of usual medical practice when patient characteristics and other factors may differ from those prevailing during clinical studies. Similarly, the cited frequencies cannot be directly compared with figures obtained from other clinical investigations involving different treatments, uses, or investigators. An inspection of these frequencies, however, does provide the prescriber with one basis by which to estimate the relative contribution of drug and non-drug factors to the adverse event incidences in the population studied.
In general, adverse reactions were less frequent later in the course of treatment.

Table 3
Adverse Events Reported in the Single Controlled Clinical Trial in at Least 2% of Patients Receiving Exelon® (3-12 mg/day) and at a Higher Frequency than Placebo-treated Patients

Body System/Adverse Event	Placebo (n = 179)	Exelon® (3-12 mg/day) (n = 362)
Percent of Patients with any Adverse Event	71	84
Gastrointestinal Disorders		
Nausea	11	29
Vomiting	2	17
Diarrhea	4	7
Upper Abdominal Pain	1	4
General Disorders and Administrative Site Conditions		
Fatigue	3	4
Asthenia	1	2
Metabolism and Nutritional Disorders		
Anorexia	3	6
Dehydration	1	2
Nervous System Disorders		
Tremor	4	10
Dizziness	1	6
Headache	3	4
Somnolence	3	4
Parkinson's Disease (worsening)	1	3
Parkinsonism	1	2
Psychiatric Disorders		
Anxiety	1	4
Insomnia	2	3

Other Adverse Events Observed During Clinical Trials
Dementia of the Alzheimer's Type
Exelon has been administered to over 5,297 individuals during clinical trials worldwide. Of these, 4,326 patients have been treated for at least 3 months, 3,407 patients have been treated for at least 6 months, 2,150 patients have been treated for 1 year, 1,250 patients have been treated for 2 years, and 168 patients have been treated for over 3 years. With regard to exposure to the highest dose, 2,809 patients were exposed to doses of 10-12 mg, 2,615 patients treated for 3 months, 2,328 patients treated for 6 months, 1,378 patients treated for 1 year, 917 patients treated for 2 years, and 129 patients treated for over 3 years.
Treatment-emergent signs and symptoms that occurred during 8 controlled clinical trials and 9 open-label trials in North America, Western Europe, Australia, South Africa, and Japan were recorded as adverse events by the clinical investigators using terminology of their own choosing. To provide an overall estimate of the proportion of individuals having similar types of events, the events were grouped into a smaller number of standardized categories using a modified WHO dictionary, and event frequencies were calculated across all studies. These categories are used in the listing below. The frequencies represent the proportion of 5,297 patients from these trials who experienced that event while receiving Exelon. All adverse events occurring in at least 6 patients (approximately 0.1%) are included, except for those already listed elsewhere in labeling, WHO terms too general to be informative, relatively minor events, or events unlikely to be drug-caused. Events are classified by body

system and listed using the following definitions: frequent adverse events – those occurring in at least 1/100 patients; infrequent adverse events – those occurring in 1/100 to 1/1,000 patients. These adverse events are not necessarily related to Exelon treatment and in most cases were observed at a similar frequency in placebo-treated patients in the controlled studies.

Autonomic Nervous System: *Infrequent:* Cold clammy skin, dry mouth, flushing, increased saliva.

Body as a Whole: *Frequent:* Accidental trauma, fever, edema, allergy, hot flushes, rigors. *Infrequent:* Edema periorbital or facial, hypothermia, edema, feeling cold, halitosis.

Cardiovascular System: *Frequent:* Hypotension, postural hypotension, cardiac failure.

Central and Peripheral Nervous System: *Frequent:* Abnormal gait, ataxia, paresthesia, convulsions. *Infrequent:* Paresis, apraxia, aphasia, dysphonia, hyperkinesia, hyperreflexia, hypertonia, hypoesthesia, hypokinesia, migraine, neuralgia, nystagmus, peripheral neuropathy.

Endocrine System: *Infrequent:* Goiter, hypothyroidism.

Gastrointestinal System: *Frequent:* Fecal incontinence, gastritis. *Infrequent:* Dysphagia, esophagitis, gastric ulcer, gastroesophageal reflux, GI hemorrhage, hernia, intestinal obstruction, melena, rectal hemorrhage, gastroenteritis, ulcerative stomatitis, duodenal ulcer, hematemesis, gingivitis, tenesmus, pancreatitis, colitis, glossitis.

Hearing and Vestibular Disorders: *Frequent:* Tinnitus.

Heart Rate and Rhythm Disorders: *Frequent:* Atrial fibrillation, bradycardia, palpitation. *Infrequent:* AV block, bundle branch block, sick sinus syndrome, cardiac arrest, supraventricular tachycardia, extrasystoles, tachycardia.

Liver and Biliary System Disorders: *Infrequent:* Abnormal hepatic function, cholecystitis.

Metabolic and Nutritional Disorders: *Frequent:* Dehydration, hypokalemia. *Infrequent:* Diabetes mellitus, gout, hypercholesterolemia, hyperlipemia, hypoglycemia, cachexia, thirst, hyperglycemia, hyponatremia.

Musculoskeletal Disorders: *Frequent:* Arthritis, leg cramps, myalgia. *Infrequent:* Cramps, hernia, muscle weakness.

Myo-, Endo-, Pericardial and Valve Disorders: *Frequent:* Angina pectoris, myocardial infarction.

Platelet, Bleeding, and Clotting Disorders: *Frequent:* Epistaxis. *Infrequent:* Hematoma, thrombocytopenia, purpura.

Psychiatric Disorders: *Frequent:* Paranoid reaction, confusion. *Infrequent:* Abnormal dreaming, amnesia, apathy, delirium, dementia, depersonalization, emotional lability, impaired concentration, decreased libido, personality disorder, suicide attempt, increased libido, neurosis, suicidal ideation, psychosis.

Red Blood Cell Disorders: *Frequent:* Anemia. *Infrequent:* Hypochromic anemia.

Reproductive Disorders (Female & Male): *Infrequent:* Breast pain, impotence, atrophic vaginitis.

Resistance Mechanism Disorders: *Infrequent:* Cellulitis, cystitis, herpes simplex, otitis media.

Respiratory System: *Infrequent:* Bronchospasm, laryngitis, apnea.

Skin and Appendages: *Frequent:* Rashes of various kinds (maculopapular, eczema, bullous, exfoliative, psoriaform, erythematous). *Infrequent:* Alopecia, skin ulceration, urticaria, contact dermatitis.

Special Senses: *Infrequent:* Perversion of taste, loss of taste.

Urinary System Disorders: *Frequent:* Hematuria. *Infrequent:* Albuminuria, oliguria, acute renal failure, dysuria, micturition urgency, nocturia, polyuria, renal calculus, urinary retention.

Vascular (extracardiac) Disorders: *Infrequent:* Hemorrhoids, peripheral ischemia, pulmonary embolism, thrombosis, deep thrombophlebitis, aneurysm, intracranial hemorrhage.

Vision Disorders: *Frequent:* Cataract. *Infrequent:* Conjunctival hemorrhage, blepharitis, diplopia, eye pain, glaucoma.

White Cell and Resistance Disorders: *Infrequent:* Lymphadenopathy, leukocytosis.

Dementia Associated with Parkinson's Disease

Exelon has been administered to 485 individuals during clinical trials worldwide. Of these, 413 patients have been treated for at least 3 months, 253 patients have been treated for at least 6 months, and 113 patients have been treated for 1 year.

Additional treatment-emergent adverse events in patients with Parkinson's disease dementia occurring in at least 1 patient (approximately 0.3%) are listed below, excluding events that are already listed above for the dementia of the Alzheimer's type or elsewhere in labeling, WHO terms too general to be informative, relatively minor events, or events unlikely to be drug-caused. Events are classified by body system and listed using the following definitions: frequent adverse events – those occurring in at least 1/100 patients; infrequent adverse events – those occurring in 1/100 to 1/1,000 patients. These adverse events are not necessarily related to Exelon treatment and in most cases were observed at a similar frequency in placebo-treated patients in the controlled studies.

Cardiovascular System: *Frequent:* Chest pain. *Infrequent:* Sudden cardiac death.

Central and Peripheral Nervous System: *Frequent:* Dyskinesia, bradykinesia, restlessness, transient ischemic attack. *Infrequent:* Dystonia, hemiparesis, epilepsy, restless leg syndrome.

Endocrine System: *Infrequent:* Elevated prolactin level.

Gastrointestinal System: *Frequent:* Dyspepsia. *Infrequent:* Fecaloma, dysphagia, diverticulitis, peritonitis.

Hearing and Vestibular Disorders: *Frequent:* Vertigo. *Infrequent:* Meniere's disease.

Heart Rate and Rhythm Disorders: *Infrequent:* Adam-Stokes syndrome.

Liver and Biliary System Disorders: *Infrequent:* Elevated alkaline phosphatase level, elevated gamma-glutamyltransferase level.

Musculoskeletal Disorders: *Frequent:* Back pain. *Infrequent:* Muscle stiffness, myoclonus, freezing phenomenon.

Psychiatric Disorders: *Frequent:* Agitation, depression. *Infrequent:* Delusion, insomnia.

Reproductive Disorders (Female & Male): *Infrequent:* endometrial hypertrophy, mastitis, prostatic adenoma.

Respiratory System: *Frequent:* Dyspnea. *Infrequent:* Cough.

Urinary System Disorders: *Infrequent:* Urinary incontinence, neurogenic bladder.

Vascular (extracardiac) Disorders: *Infrequent:* Vasovagal syncope, vasculitis.

Vision Disorders: *Infrequent:* Blurred vision, blepharospasm, conjunctivitis, retinopathy.

Post-Introduction Reports

Voluntary reports of adverse events temporally associated with Exelon that have been received since market introduction that are not listed above, and that may or may not be causally related to the drug include the following:

Skin and Appendages: Stevens-Johnson syndrome.

OVERDOSAGE

Because strategies for the management of overdose are continually evolving, it is advisable to contact a Poison Control Center to determine the latest recommendations for the management of an overdose of any drug.

As Exelon® (rivastigmine tartrate) has a short plasma half-life of about one hour and a moderate duration of acetylcholinesterase inhibition of 8-10 hours, it is recommended that in cases of asymptomatic overdoses, no further dose of Exelon should be administered for the next 24 hours.

As in any case of overdose, general supportive measures should be utilized. Overdosage with cholinesterase inhibitors can result in cholinergic crisis characterized by severe nausea, vomiting, salivation, sweating, bradycardia, hypotension, respiratory depression, collapse and convulsions. Increasing muscle weakness is a possibility and may result in death if respiratory muscles are involved. Atypical responses in blood pressure and heart rate have been reported with other drugs that increase cholinergic activity when co-administered with quaternary anticholinergics such as glycopyrrolate. Due to the short half-life of Exelon, dialysis (hemodialysis, peritoneal dialysis, or hemofiltration) would not be clinically indicated in the event of an overdose.

In overdoses accompanied by severe nausea and vomiting, the use of antiemetics should be considered. In a documented case of a 46-mg overdose with Exelon, the patient experienced vomiting, incontinence, hypertension, psychomotor retardation, and loss of consciousness. The patient fully recovered within 24 hours and conservative management was all that was required for treatment.

DOSAGE AND ADMINISTRATION

Dementia of the Alzheimer's Type

The dosage of Exelon® (rivastigmine tartrate) shown to be effective in controlled clinical trials in Alzheimer's disease is 6-12 mg/day, given as twice-a-day dosing (daily doses of 3 to 6 mg BID). There is evidence from the clinical trials that doses at the higher end of this range may be more beneficial.

The starting dose of Exelon is 1.5 mg twice a day (BID). If this dose is well tolerated, after a minimum of 2 weeks of treatment, the dose may be increased to 3 mg BID. Subsequent increases to 4.5 mg BID and 6 mg BID should be attempted after a minimum of 2 weeks at the previous dose. If adverse effects (e.g., nausea, vomiting, abdominal pain, loss of appetite) cause intolerance during treatment, the patient should be instructed to discontinue treatment for several doses and then restart at the same or next lower dose level. If treatment is interrupted for longer than several days, treatment should be reinitiated with the lowest daily dose and titrated as described above *(see WARNINGS)*. The maximum dose is 6 mg BID (12 mg/day).

Dementia Associated with Parkinson's Disease

The dosage of Exelon shown to be effective in the single controlled clinical trial conducted in dementia associated with Parkinson's disease is 3-12 mg/day, given as twice-a-day dosing (daily doses of 1.5-6 mg BID). In that medical condition, the starting dose of Exelon is 1.5 mg BID; subsequently, the dose may be increased to 3 mg BID and further to 4.5 mg BID and 6 mg BID, based on tolerability, with a minimum of 4 weeks at each dose.

Exelon should be taken with meals in divided doses in the morning and evening.

Recommendations for Administration

Caregivers should be instructed in the correct procedure for administering Exelon Oral Solution. In addition, they should be directed to the Instruction Sheet (included with the product) describing how the solution is to be administered. Caregivers should direct questions about the administration of the solution to either their physician or pharmacist *(see PRECAUTIONS: Information for Patients and Caregivers)*.

Patients should be instructed to remove the oral dosing syringe provided in its protective case, and using the provided syringe, withdraw the prescribed amount of Exelon Oral Solution from the container. Each dose of Exelon Oral Solution may be swallowed directly from the syringe or first mixed with a small glass of water, cold fruit juice or soda. Patients should be instructed to stir and drink the mixture.

Exelon Oral Solution and Exelon Capsules may be interchanged at equal doses.

HOW SUPPLIED

Exelon® (rivastigmine tartrate) Capsules equivalent to 1.5 mg, 3 mg, 4.5 mg, or 6 mg of rivastigmine base are available as follows:

1.5 mg Capsule – yellow, "Exelon 1,5 mg" is printed in red on the body of the capsule.

Bottles of 60	NDC 0078-0323-44
Bottles of 500	NDC 0078-0323-08
Unit Dose (blister pack)	
Box of 100 (strips of 10)	NDC 0078-0323-06
Unit Dose Blister Card of 30	NDC 0078-0323-15

3 mg Capsule – orange, "Exelon 3 mg" is printed in red on the body of the capsule.

Bottles of 60	NDC 0078-0324-44
Bottles of 500	NDC 0078-0324-08
Unit Dose (blister pack)	
Box of 100 (strips of 10)	NDC 0078-0324-06
Unit Dose Blister Card of 30	NDC 0078-0324-15

4.5 mg Capsule – red, "Exelon 4,5 mg" is printed in white on the body of the capsule.

Bottles of 60	NDC 0078-0325-44
Bottles of 500	NDC 0078-0325-08
Unit Dose (blister pack)	
Box of 100 (strips of 10)	NDC 0078-0325-06
Unit Dose Blister Card of 30	NDC 0078-0325-15

6 mg Capsule – orange and red, "Exelon 6 mg" is printed in red on the body of the capsule.

Bottles of 60	NDC 0078-0326-44
Bottles of 500	NDC 0078-0326-08
Unit Dose (blister pack)	
Box of 100 (strips of 10)	NDC 0078-0326-06
Unit Dose Blister Card of 30	NDC 0078-0326-15

Store at 25°C (77°F); excursions permitted to 15-30°C (59-86°F) [see USP Controlled Room Temperature]. Store in a tight container.

Exelon® (rivastigmine tartrate) Oral Solution is supplied as 120 mL of a clear, yellow solution (2 mg/mL base) in a 4-ounce USP Type III amber glass bottle with a child-resistant 28-mm cap, 0.5-mm foam liner, dip tube and self-aligning plug. The oral solution is packaged with a dispenser set which consists of an assembled oral dosing syringe that allows dispensing a maximum volume of 3 mL corresponding to a 6-mg dose, with a plastic tube container.

Bottles of 120 mL .... NDC 0078-0339-31

Store at 25°C (77°F); excursions permitted to 15-30°C (59-86°F) [see USP Controlled Room Temperature]. Store in an upright position and protect from freezing.

When Exelon Oral Solution is combined with cold fruit juice or soda, the mixture is stable at room temperature for up to 4 hours.

Exelon® (rivastigmine tartrate)
Oral Solution
Instructions for Use

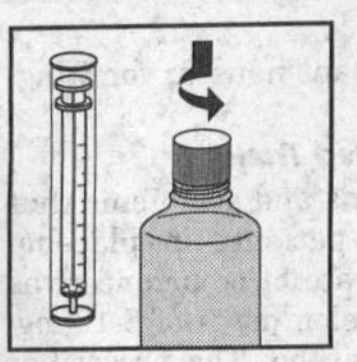

1. Remove oral dosing syringe from its protective case. Push down and twist child-resistant closure to open bottle.

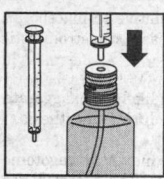

2. Insert tip of syringe into opening of white stopper.

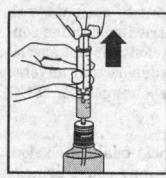

3. While holding the syringe, pull the plunger up to the level (see markings on side of syringe) that equals the dose prescribed by your doctor.

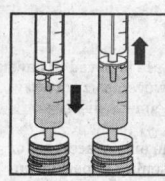

4. Before removing syringe containing prescribed dose from bottle, push out **large** bubbles by moving plunger up and down a few times. After the large bubbles are gone, pull the plunger again to the level that equals the dose prescribed by your doctor. Do not worry about a few tiny bubbles. This will not affect your dose in any way.

Remove the syringe from the bottle.

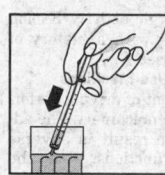

5. You may swallow Exelon Oral Solution directly from the syringe or mix with a small glass of water, cold fruit juice or soda. If mixing with water, juice or soda, be sure to stir completely and to drink the entire mixture. DO NOT MIX WITH OTHER LIQUIDS.

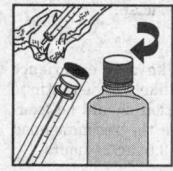

6. After use, wipe outside of syringe with a clean tissue and put it back into its case. Close bottle using child-resistant closure.

Store Exelon Oral Solution at room temperature below 25°C (77°F) in an upright position. Do not place in freezer.

Distributed by:
Novartis Pharmaceuticals Corporation
East Hanover, New Jersey 07936
REV: JUNE 2006   T2006-73
©Novartis

Shown in Product Identification Guide, page 315

EXELON® PATCH   ℞
[ĕx′ ə-lŏn]
(rivastigmine transdermal system)

The following prescribing information is based on official labeling in effect July 2010.

HIGHLIGHTS OF PRESCRIBING INFORMATION
These highlights do not include all the information needed to use Exelon® Patch safely and effectively. See full prescribing information for Exelon Patch.

Exelon® Patch (rivastigmine transdermal system)
Initial U.S. Approval: 2000

──────────**INDICATIONS AND USAGE**──────────
Exelon Patch contains rivastigmine, an acetylcholinesterase inhibitor indicated for the:
- Treatment of mild to moderate dementia of the Alzheimer's type (1.1)
- Treatment of mild to moderate dementia associated with Parkinson's disease (1.2)

──────────**DOSAGE AND ADMINISTRATION**──────────

Initial Dose	one Exelon Patch 4.6 mg/24 hours once daily (2.1)
Maintenance Dose	one Exelon Patch 9.5 mg/24 hours once daily (2.1)

A minimum of 4 weeks of treatment and good tolerability with the previous dose should be observed before increasing the dose (2.1). The patch should be replaced with a new one every 24 hours. Only one patch should be worn at a time. The previous day's patch must be removed before applying a new patch.

──────────**DOSAGE FORMS AND STRENGTHS**──────────
Exelon Patch is a transdermal system.
Exelon Patch 4.6 mg/24 hours: 5 cm² size containing 9 mg rivastigmine
Exelon Patch 9.5 mg/24 hours: 10 cm² size containing 18 mg rivastigmine (3)

──────────**CONTRAINDICATIONS**──────────
Exelon Patch (rivastigmine transdermal system) is contraindicated in patients with known hypersensitivity to rivastigmine, other carbamate derivatives, or other components of the formulation (4.1).

──────────**WARNINGS AND PRECAUTIONS**──────────
• Hospitalization, and rarely death have been reported due to the application of multiple patches at the same time (5.1).
• Gastrointestinal adverse effects including nausea and vomiting can be significant and at times severe at higher than the recommended dose. The dose should be titrated as prescribed and reinitiated at the lowest dose if interrupted for more than a few days (5.2).
• Weight should be monitored during Exelon Patch therapy (5.2).
• As with other cholinomimetics, caution is recommended in patients with sick sinus syndrome, conduction defects (sino-atrial block, atrio-ventricular block), gastroduodenal ulcerative conditions (including those predisposed to such conditions by concomitant medications), asthma or chronic obstructive pulmonary disease, urinary obstruction, and seizures (5.6).
• Extrapyramidal symptoms may appear or be exacerbated (particularly tremor) (5.6).

──────────**ADVERSE REACTIONS**──────────
The most commonly observed adverse events occurring at a frequency of at least 5% and at a frequency at least greater than placebo with administration of 9.5 mg/24 hours were nausea, vomiting and diarrhea. Other less common and sometimes serious adverse events have been reported (6).
To report SUSPECTED ADVERSE REACTIONS, contact Novartis Pharmaceuticals Corporation at 1-888-669-6682 or FDA at 1-800-FDA-1088 or www.fda.gov/medwatch.

──────────**DRUG INTERACTIONS**──────────
Other cholinomimetic drugs, anticholinergic medications, succinylcholine-type muscle relaxants during anesthesia (7).

──────────**USE IN SPECIFIC POPULATIONS**──────────
Caution is advised in patients with body weight below 50 kg (2.1, 5.9, 8.8). The safety of Exelon Patch is not established in pregnant and lactating women (8.2). Not recommended for use in children (8.4).
See 17 for PATIENT COUNSELING INFORMATION and FDA-approved patient labeling
Revised: 08/2010

FULL PRESCRIBING INFORMATION

1   INDICATIONS AND USAGE
1.1   Alzheimer's Disease
Exelon Patch (rivastigmine transdermal system) is indicated for the treatment of mild to moderate dementia of the Alzheimer's type.

1.2   Parkinson's Disease Dementia
Exelon Patch (rivastigmine transdermal system) is indicated for the treatment of mild to moderate dementia associated with Parkinson's disease.

The dementia of Parkinson's disease is purportedly characterized by impairments in executive function, memory retrieval, and attention in patients with an established diagnosis of Parkinson's disease. The diagnosis of dementia of Parkinson's disease can be made reliably in patients in whom a progressive dementia syndrome occurs (without the necessity to document the specific deficits described above) at least 2 years after a diagnosis of Parkinson's disease has been made, and in whom other causes of dementia have been ruled out.

2   DOSAGE AND ADMINISTRATION
2.1   Alzheimer's Disease

Table 1: Patch Size, Drug Content and Nominal Delivery Rate

Rivastigmine Nominal Dose	Rivastigmine Content per Exelon Patch	Exelon Patch Size
4.6 mg/24 hours	9 mg	5 cm²
9.5 mg/24 hours	18 mg	10 cm²

Initial Dose
Treatment is started with Exelon Patch 4.6 mg/24 hours.
After a minimum of 4 weeks of treatment and if well tolerated, this dose should be increased to Exelon Patch 9.5 mg/24 hours, which is the recommended effective dose.
Maintenance Dose
Dose increases should occur only after a minimum of 4 weeks at the previous dose, and only if the previous dose has been well tolerated. The maximum recommended dose is 9.5 mg/24 hours. Higher doses confer no appreciable additional benefit, and are associated with significant increase in the incidence of adverse events [see *Adverse Reactions (6)*].
If adverse effects (e.g., nausea, vomiting, diarrhea, loss of appetite) cause intolerance during treatment, the patient

should be instructed to discontinue treatment for three or more days and then restart at the same or next lower dose level. If treatment is interrupted for longer than three days, treatment should be reinitiated with the lowest daily dose and titrated as described above [also see *Warnings and Precautions (5)*].

Switching from Capsules or Oral Solution
Patients treated with Exelon capsules or oral solution may be switched to Exelon Patch as follows:
A patient who is on a total daily dose of <6 mg of oral rivastigmine can be switched to Exelon Patch 4.6 mg/24 hours.
A patient who is on a total daily dose of 6-12 mg of oral rivastigmine may be directly switched to Exelon Patch 9.5 mg/24 hours.
It is recommended to apply the first patch on the day following the last oral dose.

Method of Administration
Exelon Patch is intended for transdermal use (on intact skin) only. The patch should not be used if the pouch seal is broken or the patch is cut, damaged, or changed in any way. Exelon Patch should be applied once a day to clean, dry, hairless, intact healthy skin in a place that will not be rubbed against by tight clothing. The upper or lower back is recommended as the site of application because the patch is less likely to be removed by the patient; however, when sites on the back are not accessible the patch can be applied to the upper arm or chest. The patch should not be applied to skin that is red, irritated, or cut. It is recommended that the site of patch application be changed daily to avoid potential irritation, although consecutive patches can be applied to the same anatomic site (e.g., another spot on the upper back).
The patch should be pressed down firmly until the edges stick well. The patch can be used in situations that include bathing and hot weather.
The patch should be replaced with a new one every 24 hours. Only one patch should be worn at a time [see *Overdosage (10)*]. Do not apply a new patch to that same spot for at least 14 days. The previous day's patch must be removed before applying a new patch. Patients and caregivers should be instructed accordingly [see *Patient Counseling Information (17)*].
Used patches should be placed in the previously saved pouch and discarded safely in the trash, away from pets or children.

Incompatibilities
To prevent interference with the adhesive properties of the patch, the patch should not be applied to a skin area where cream, lotion or powder has recently been applied.

Special Populations
Hepatic Impairment
Dosage adjustment is not necessary in hepatically impaired patients, as the dose of drug is individually titrated to tolerability.
Renal Impairment
No dose adjustment is necessary for patients with renal impairment.
Low Body Weight
Patients with body weight below 50 kg may experience more adverse events and may be more likely to discontinue due to adverse events. Particular caution should be exercised in titrating these patients above the recommended maintenance dose of Exelon Patch 9.5 mg/24 hours.

2.2 Parkinson's Disease Dementia
See *Dosage and Administration (2.1)*.

3 DOSAGE FORMS AND STRENGTHS
3.1 Dosage Form
Patch.
Each patch is a thin, matrix-type transdermal system consisting of three layers when worn by the patient. A fourth layer, the release liner, covers the adhesive layer prior to use and is removed at the time the system is applied to the skin.
The outside of the backing layer is beige and labeled for each dose as follows:
- "EXELON® PATCH "4.6 mg/24 hours" and "AMCX"
- "EXELON® PATCH "9.5 mg/24 hours" and "BHDI"

3.2 Dosage Strengths
Table 1 summarizes the available strengths and quantity of rivastigmine provided in each patch:
• Each 5 cm² patch contains 9 mg rivastigmine base, with *in-vivo* release rate of 4.6 mg/24 hours.
• Each 10 cm² patch contains 18 mg rivastigmine base, with *in-vivo* release rate of 9.5 mg/24 hours.
For a full list of excipients, see *Description (11)*.

4 CONTRAINDICATIONS
4.1 Hypersensitivity
Exelon Patch (rivastigmine transdermal system) is contraindicated in patients with known hypersensitivity to rivastigmine, other carbamate derivatives, or other components of the formulation [see *Description (11)*].

5 WARNINGS AND PRECAUTIONS
5.1 Medication Errors Resulting in Overdose
Medication errors with Exelon patches have resulted in serious adverse events; some cases have required hospitalization, and rarely, led to death. The majority of medication errors have involved not removing the old patch when putting on a new one and the use of multiple patches at one time. Patients and caregivers must be given proper instruction on the dosage and administration of Exelon patches.

5.2 Gastrointestinal Adverse Reactions
At higher than recommended doses, Exelon Patch (rivastigmine transdermal system) use is associated with significant gastrointestinal adverse reactions, including nausea, vomiting, diarrhea, anorexia/decreased appetite and weight loss. For this reason, patients administered Exelon Patch should always be started at a dose of 4.6 mg/24 hours and titrated to the maintenance dose of 9.5 mg/24 hours. If treatment is interrupted for longer than three days, treatment should be reinitiated with the lowest daily dose [see *Dosage and Administration (2)*] to reduce the possibility of severe vomiting and its potentially serious sequelae (e.g., there has been one post-marketing report of severe vomiting with esophageal rupture following inappropriate reinitiation of treatment with a 4.5-mg dose of an oral formulation after 8 weeks of treatment interruption).
At higher than recommended doses, caregivers should be advised of the high incidence of nausea and vomiting associated with the use of Exelon Patch along with the possibility of anorexia and weight loss. Caregivers should be encouraged to monitor for these adverse events and inform the physician if they occur. It is critical to inform caregivers that if therapy has been interrupted for more than three days, the next dose should not be administered until they have discussed this with the physician.

Nausea and Vomiting
In the controlled clinical trial, 7% of patients treated with Exelon Patch 9.5 mg/24 hours developed nausea, as compared to 23% of patients who received the Exelon capsule at doses up to 6 mg BID and 5% of those who received placebo. In the same clinical trial, 6% of patients treated with Exelon Patch 9.5 mg/24 hours developed vomiting, as compared with 17% of patients who received the Exelon capsule at doses up to 6 mg BID and 3% of those who received placebo. The proportion of patients who discontinued treatment on account of vomiting was 0% of the patients who received Exelon Patch 9.5 mg/24 hours as well as 2% of patients who received the Exelon capsule at doses up to 6 mg BID and 0% of those who received placebo. Vomiting was severe in 0% of patients who received Exelon Patch 9.5 mg/24 hours and 1% of patients who received the Exelon capsule at doses up to 6 mg BID and 0% of those who received placebo.
In the same clinical trial, 21% of patients treated with the higher dose of Exelon Patch 17.4 mg/24 hours developed nausea, 19% developed vomiting, and the proportion of these patients who discontinued treatment on account of vomiting was 2%. Vomiting was severe in 1% of patients treated with Exelon Patch 17.4 mg/24 hours.

Weight Loss
In the controlled clinical trial, the proportion of patients who had weight loss equal to or greater than 7% of their baseline weight was 8% of those treated with Exelon Patch 9.5 mg/24 hours, 11% of patients who received the Exelon capsule at doses up to 6 mg BID and 6% of those who received placebo.
In the same clinical trial, 12% of those treated with 17.4 mg/24 hours had weight loss equal to or greater than 7% of their baseline weight. It is not clear how much of the weight loss was associated with anorexia, nausea, vomiting, and the diarrhea associated with the drug.

Diarrhea
In the controlled clinical trial, 6% of patients treated with Exelon Patch 9.5 mg/24 hours developed diarrhea, as compared with 5% of patients who received the Exelon capsule at doses up to 6 mg BID, 10% of those treated with 17.4 mg/24 hours and 3% of those who received placebo.

Anorexia/Decreased Appetite
In the controlled clinical trial, 3% of patients treated with Exelon Patch 9.5 mg/24 hours were recorded as developing decreased appetite or anorexia, as compared with 9% of patients who received the Exelon capsule at doses up to 6 mg BID, 9% of those treated with Exelon Patch 17.4 mg/24 hours and 2% of those who received placebo.

Peptic Ulcers/Gastrointestinal Bleeding
Because of their pharmacological action, cholinesterase inhibitors may be expected to increase gastric acid secretion due to increased cholinergic activity. Therefore, patients should be monitored closely for symptoms of active or occult gastrointestinal bleeding, especially those at increased risk for developing ulcers, e.g., those with a history of ulcer disease or those receiving concurrent nonsteroidal anti-inflammatory drugs (NSAIDs). Clinical studies of Exelon

have shown no significant increase, relative to placebo, in the incidence of either peptic ulcer disease or gastrointestinal bleeding.

5.3 Anesthesia
Exelon, as a cholinesterase inhibitor, is likely to exaggerate succinylcholine-type muscle relaxation during anesthesia.

5.4 Cardiovascular Conditions
Drugs that increase cholinergic activity may have vagotonic effects on heart rate (e.g., bradycardia). The potential for this action may be particularly important to patients with sick sinus syndrome or other supraventricular cardiac conduction conditions. In clinical trials, Exelon was not associated with any increased incidence of cardiovascular adverse events, heart rate or blood pressure changes, or ECG abnormalities.

5.5 Genitourinary Conditions
Although this was not observed in clinical trials of Exelon, drugs that increase cholinergic activity may cause urinary obstruction.

5.6 Neurological Conditions
Seizures
Drugs that increase cholinergic activity are believed to have some potential for causing seizures. However, seizure activity also may be a manifestation of Alzheimer's disease.
Extrapyramidal Symptoms
Like other cholinomimetics, rivastigmine may exacerbate or induce extrapyramidal symptoms. Worsening of parkinsonian symptoms, particularly tremor, has been observed in patients with dementia associated with Parkinson's disease who were treated with Exelon capsules.

5.7 Pulmonary Conditions
Like other drugs that increase cholinergic activity, Exelon should be used with care in patients with a history of asthma or obstructive pulmonary disease.

5.8 Effects on Ability to Drive and Use Machines
Dementia may cause gradual impairment of driving performance or compromise the ability to use machinery. The administration of rivastigmine may also result in adverse events that are detrimental to these functions. Thus, the ability to continue driving or operating machinery should be routinely evaluated by the treating physician.

5.9 Special Populations
Low Body Weight
Patients with body weight below 50 kg may experience more adverse events and may be more likely to discontinue due to adverse events. Particular caution should be exercised in titrating these patients above the recommended maintenance dose of the Exelon Patch 9.5 mg/24 hours.

6 ADVERSE REACTIONS
Significant gastrointestinal adverse reactions including nausea, vomiting, anorexia, and weight loss have been reported with the Exelon Patch at higher than recommended doses [see *Warnings and Precautions (5.1)*].

6.1 Incidence in Controlled Clinical Trial in Alzheimer's Disease
Associated with Discontinuation of Treatment
In the single controlled clinical trial of Exelon Patch [see *Clinical Studies (14)*], which randomized a total of 1195 patients, the proportions of patients in the Exelon Patch 9.5 mg/24 hours, Exelon Patch 17.4 mg/24 hours, Exelon capsules 6 mg BID, and placebo groups who discontinued treatment due to adverse events were 9.6%, 8.6%, 8.1%, and 5.0%, respectively.
The most common adverse events in the Exelon Patch-treated groups that led to treatment discontinuation in this study were nausea and vomiting. The proportions of patients who discontinued treatment due to nausea were 0.7%, 1.7%, 1.7%, and 1.3% in the Exelon Patch 9.5 mg/24 hours, Exelon Patch 17.4 mg/24 hours, Exelon capsules 6 mg BID, and placebo groups, respectively. The proportions of patients who discontinued treatment due to vomiting were 0%, 1.7%, 2.0%, and 0.3% in the Exelon Patch 9.5 mg/24 hours, Exelon Patch 17.4 mg/24 hours, Exelon capsules 6 mg BID, and placebo groups, respectively.

Most Commonly Observed Adverse Events
The most commonly observed adverse events seen in patients administered Exelon Patch in the controlled clinical trial, defined as those occurring at a frequency of at least 5% in the 9.5 mg/24 hours group and at a frequency at least as high as in the placebo group are largely predicted by the cholinergic effects of Exelon. These are nausea, vomiting, and diarrhea. All these events were more common at the higher Exelon Patch dose of 17.4 mg/24 hours than at a dose of 9.5 mg/24 hours.

Adverse Events Observed at an Incidence of ≥2%
The following table lists treatment-emergent adverse events that were seen at an incidence of ≥2% in either Exelon Patch-treated group in the controlled clinical trial and for which the rate of occurrence was greater for patients treated with that dose of Exelon Patch than for those treated with placebo. The prescriber should be aware that these frequencies cannot be used to predict the frequency of adverse events in the course of usual medical practice when

patient characteristics and other factors may differ from those prevailing during clinical studies. Similarly, the cited frequencies cannot be directly compared with frequencies obtained from other clinical investigations involving different treatments, uses, or investigators. An inspection of these frequencies, however, does provide the prescriber with one basis by which to estimate the relative contribution of drug and non-drug factors to the adverse event incidences in the population studied.

[See table 2 at right]

Incidence of Application Site Reactions

The vast majority of patients participating in the controlled clinical trial had either no observed skin irritation or mild to moderate skin reactions. Among the skin reactions reported were the following: application site reactions, application site dermatitis, application site irritation and application site eczema. The incidence of severe reactions was very low regardless of administered dosage.

6.2 Other Adverse Events Observed During Clinical Trials

Exelon Patch has been administered to 1071 patients with Alzheimer's disease during clinical trials worldwide. Of these, 869 patients have been treated for at least 3 months, 706 patients have been treated for at least 6 months, and 212 patients have been treated for 1 year.

Treatment-emergent signs and symptoms that occurred during 1 controlled and 4 open-label trials in North America, Europe, Latin America, Asia and Japan were recorded as adverse events by the clinical investigators using terminology of their own choosing.

To provide an overall estimate of the proportion of individuals having similar types of events, the events were grouped into a smaller number of standardized categories using the MedDRA dictionary, and event frequencies were calculated across all studies. These categories are used in the listing below. The frequencies represent the proportion of 1071 patients from these trials who experienced that event while receiving Exelon Patch. All patch doses are pooled.

All adverse events occurring in at least 1 patient (approximately 0.1%) are included, except for those already listed elsewhere in labeling, too general to be informative, or relatively minor events.

Events are classified by system organ class and listed using the following definitions: *Frequent* – those occurring in at least 1/100 patients; *Infrequent* – those occurring in 1/100 to 1/1000 patients. These adverse events are not necessarily related to Exelon Patch treatment and in most cases were observed at a similar frequency in placebo-treated patients in the controlled studies.

Blood and Lymphatic System Disorders: *Frequent:* Anemia.

Cardiac Disorders: *Infrequent:* Angina pectoris, cardiac failure, bradycardia, atrial fibrillation, supraventricular extrasystoles, myocardial infarction, tachycardia, arrhythmia, atrioventricular block.

Ear and Labyrinth Disorders: *Infrequent:* Tinnitus.

Eye Disorders: *Infrequent:* Cataract, glaucoma, vision blurred.

Gastrointestinal System: *Frequent:* Constipation, gastritis. *Infrequent:* Gastroesophageal reflux disease, hematochezia, peptic ulcer, hematemesis, pancreatitis, salivary hypersecretion.

General Disorders and Administration Site Conditions: *Infrequent:* Application site dermatitis, application site irritation, peripheral edema, chest pain, application site eczema, hyperpyrexia.

Hepatobiliary Disorders: *Infrequent:* Cholecystitis.

Infections and Infestations: *Frequent:* Nasopharyngitis, pneumonia. *Infrequent:* Diverticulitis.

Injury, Poisoning and Procedural Complications: *Frequent:* Fall. *Infrequent:* Hip fracture, subdural hematoma.

Investigations: *Infrequent:* Blood creatine phosphokinase increased, lipase increased, blood amylase increased, electrocardiogram QT prolonged.

Metabolic and Nutritional Disorders: *Frequent:* Dehydration. *Infrequent:* Hyperlipidemia, hypokalemia, hyponatremia.

Musculoskeletal and Connective Tissue Disorders: *Infrequent:* Arthralgia, muscle spasms, myalgia.

Nervous System Disorders: *Frequent:* Tremor. *Infrequent:* Migraine, parkinsonism, epilepsy.

Psychiatric Disorders: *Infrequent:* Delusion.

Renal and Urinary Disorders: *Frequent:* Urinary incontinence. *Infrequent:* Pollakiuria, hematuria, nocturia, renal failure.

Reproductive System and Breast Disorders: *Infrequent:* Benign prostatic hyperplasia.

Respiratory, Thoracic, and Mediastinal Disorders: *Infrequent:* Dyspnea, bronchospasm, chronic obstructive pulmonary disease.

Skin and Subcutaneous Tissue Disorders: *Frequent:* Pruritus. *Infrequent:* Erythema, eczema, dermatitis, rash erythematous, skin ulcer.

Vascular Disorders: *Infrequent:* Hypotension.

Table 2: Adverse Events Observed with a Frequency of ≥ 2% and Occurring with a Rate Greater Than Placebo

	Exelon Patch 9.5 mg/ 24 hours n (%)	Exelon Patch 17.4 mg/ 24 hours n (%)	Exelon capsule 6 mg BID n (%)	Placebo n (%)
Total Patients Studied	291	303	294	302
Total Number of Patients with AEs	147 (51)	200 (66)	186 (63)	139 (46)
Nausea	21 (7)	64 (21)	68 (23)	15 (5)
Vomiting	18 (6)	57 (19)	50 (17)	10 (3)
Diarrhea	18 (6)	31 (10)	16 (5)	10 (3)
Depression	11 (4)	12 (4)	13 (4)	4 (1)
Headache	10 (3)	13 (4)	18 (6)	5 (2)
Anxiety	9 (3)	8 (3)	5 (2)	4 (1)
Anorexia/Decreased Appetite	9 (3)	27 (9)	26 (9)	6 (2)
Weight Decreased	8 (3)	23 (8)	16 (5)	4 (1)
Dizziness	7 (2)	21 (7)	22 (7)	7 (2)
Abdominal Pain	7 (2)	11 (4)	4 (1)	2 (1)
Urinary Tract Infection	6 (2)	5 (2)	4 (1)	3 (1)
Asthenia	5 (2)	9 (3)	17 (6)	3 (1)
Fatigue	5 (2)	7 (2)	2 (1)	4 (1)
Insomnia	4 (1)	12 (4)	6 (2)	6 (2)
Abdominal Pain Upper	3 (1)	8 (3)	6 (2)	6 (2)
Vertigo	0 (0)	7 (2)	4 (1)	3 (1)

6.3 Post-Introduction Reports

The following additional adverse reactions have been identified based on post-marketing spontaneous reports and are not listed above. Because these reactions are reported voluntarily from a population of uncertain size, it is not always possible to reliably estimate their frequency or establish a causal relationship to drug exposure.

Hypertension, application site hypersensitivity, urticaria, blister, dermatitis allergic, seizure, worsening of Parkinson's disease in patients with Parkinson's disease who were treated with Exelon patches.

6.4 Additional Adverse Reactions Reported

The following additional adverse reactions have been observed with Exelon capsules/oral solution.

Confusion, abnormal liver function tests, duodenal ulcers.

7 DRUG INTERACTIONS

No specific interaction studies have been conducted with Exelon Patch (rivastigmine transdermal system).

7.1 Effect of Exelon on the Metabolism of Other Drugs

Rivastigmine is primarily metabolized through hydrolysis by esterases. Minimal metabolism occurs via the major cytochrome P450 isoenzymes. Based on *in-vitro* studies, no pharmacokinetic drug interactions with drugs metabolized by the following isoenzyme systems are expected: CYP1A2, CYP2D6, CYP3A4/5, CYP2E1, CYP2C9, CYP2C8, or CYP2C19.

No pharmacokinetic interaction was observed between rivastigmine taken orally and digoxin, warfarin, diazepam or fluoxetine in studies in healthy volunteers. The increase in prothrombin time induced by warfarin is not affected by administration of rivastigmine.

7.2 Effect of Other Drugs on the Metabolism of Exelon

Drugs that induce or inhibit CYP450 metabolism are not expected to alter the metabolism of rivastigmine.

Population PK analysis with a database of 625 patients showed that the pharmacokinetics of rivastigmine taken orally were not influenced by commonly prescribed medications such as antacids (n=77), antihypertensives (n=72), β-blockers (n=42), calcium channel blockers (n=75), antidiabetics (n=21), nonsteroidal anti-inflammatory drugs (n=79), estrogens (n=70), salicylate analgesics (n=177), antianginals (n=35) and antihistamines (n=15).

7.3 Use with Anticholinergics, Cholinomimetics and Other Cholinesterase Inhibitors

In view of its pharmacodynamic effects, rivastigmine should not be given concomitantly with other cholinomimetic drugs and might interfere with the activity of anticholinergic medications. A synergistic effect may be expected when cholinesterase inhibitors are given concurrently with succinylcholine, similar neuromuscular blocking agents or cholinergic agonists such as bethanechol.

8 USE IN SPECIFIC POPULATIONS

8.1 Pregnancy

Pregnancy Category B

There are no adequate or well-controlled studies in pregnant women. Because animal reproduction studies are not always predictive of human response, Exelon Patch should be used during pregnancy only if the potential benefit outweighs the potential risk to the fetus. No dermal reproduction studies in animals have been conducted. Oral reproduction studies conducted in pregnant rats at doses up to 2.3 mg base/kg/day and in pregnant rabbits at doses up to 2.3 mg base/kg/day revealed no evidence of teratogenicity. Studies in rats showed slightly decreased fetal/pup weights, usually at doses causing some maternal toxicity.

8.3 Nursing Mothers

Milk transfer studies in animals have not been conducted with dermal rivastigmine. In rats given rivastigmine orally, concentrations of rivastigmine plus metabolites were approximately two times higher in milk than in plasma. It is not known whether rivastigmine is excreted in human breast milk. Exelon Patch (rivastigmine transdermal system) has no indication for use in nursing mothers.

8.4 Pediatric Use

There are no adequate and well-controlled trials documenting the safety and efficacy of Exelon in any illness occurring in children.

8.5 Geriatric Use

Age had no impact on the exposure to rivastigmine in Alzheimer's disease patients treated with Exelon Patch.

8.6 Hepatic Disease

No pharmacokinetic study was conducted with Exelon Patch in subjects with hepatic impairment. Following a single 3-mg dose, mean oral clearance of rivastigmine was 60% lower in hepatically impaired patients (n=10, biopsy proven) than in healthy subjects (n=10). After multiple 6-mg BID oral dosing, the mean clearance of rivastigmine was 65% lower in mild (n=7, Child-Pugh score 5-6) and moderate (n=3, Child-Pugh score 7-9) hepatically impaired patients (biopsy proven, liver cirrhosis) than in healthy subjects (n=10). Dosage adjustment is not necessary in hepatically impaired patients as the dose of drug is individually titrated to tolerability.

8.7 Renal Disease

No study was conducted with Exelon Patch in subjects with renal impairment. Following a single 3-mg dose, mean oral clearance of rivastigmine is 64% lower in moderately impaired renal patients (n=8, GFR=10-50 mL/min) than in healthy subjects (n=10, GFR≥60 mL/min); Cl/F=1.7 L/min (cv=45%) and 4.8 L/min (cv=80%), respectively. In severely impaired renal patients (n=8, GFR<10 mL/min), mean oral clearance of rivastigmine is 43% higher than in healthy subjects (n=10, GFR≥60 mL/min); Cl/F=6.9 L/min and 4.8 L/min, respectively. For unexplained reasons, the severely impaired renal patients had a higher clearance of rivastigmine than moderately impaired patients. However, dosage adjustment may not be necessary in renally impaired patients as the dose of the drug is individually titrated to tolerability.

8.8 Low Body Weight

Rivastigmine exposure is higher in subjects with low body weight. Compared to a patient with a body weight of 65 kg, the rivastigmine steady-state concentrations in a patient with a body weight of 35 kg would be approximately doubled, while for a patient with a body weight of 100 kg the concentrations would be approximately halved. This suggests special attention should be given to patients with very low body weight during up-titration [see *Dosage and Administration (2)*].

8.9 Gender and Race

No specific pharmacokinetic study was conducted to investigate the effect of gender and race on the disposition of Exelon, but a population pharmacokinetic analysis indicates that gender (n=277 males and 348 females) and race (n=575 White, 34 Black, 4 Asian, and 12 Other) did not affect the clearance of Exelon administered orally. Similar results were seen with analyses of pharmacokinetic data obtained after the administration of Exelon Patch.

8.10 Nicotine Use

Population pharmacokinetic analysis showed that nicotine use increases the oral clearance of rivastigmine by 23%

(n=75 Smokers and 549 Nonsmokers). No dose adjustment is necessary as the dose of the drug is individually titrated to tolerability.

10 OVERDOSAGE

Because strategies for the management of overdose are continually evolving, it is advisable to contact a Poison Control Center to determine the latest recommendations for the management of an overdose of any drug. As in any case of overdose, general supportive measures should be utilized.

As rivastigmine has a plasma half-life of about 3.4 hours after patch administration and a duration of acetylcholinesterase inhibition of about 9 hours, it is recommended that in cases of asymptomatic overdose the patch should be immediately removed and no further patch should be applied for the next 24 hours.

As in any case of overdose, general supportive measures should be utilized. Overdosage with cholinesterase inhibitors can result in cholinergic crisis characterized by severe nausea, vomiting, salivation, sweating, bradycardia, hypotension, respiratory depression, collapse and convulsions. Increasing muscle weakness is a possibility and may result in death if respiratory muscles are involved. Atypical responses in blood pressure and heart rate have been reported with other drugs that increase cholinergic activity when co-administered with quaternary anticholinergics such as glycopyrrolate. Due to the short plasma elimination half-life of rivastigmine after patch administration, dialysis (hemodialysis, peritoneal dialysis, or hemofiltration) would not be clinically indicated in the event of an overdose.

In overdose accompanied by severe nausea and vomiting, the use of antiemetics should be considered. In a documented case of an oral 46-mg overdose with Exelon, the patient experienced vomiting, incontinence, hypertension, psychomotor retardation, and loss of consciousness. The patient fully recovered within 24 hours and conservative management was all that was required for treatment.

Overdose with Exelon Patch has been reported in the postmarketing setting. Overdoses have occurred due to application of more than one patch at one time and not removing the previous day's patch before applying a new patch. The symptoms reported in these overdose cases are similar to those seen in cases of overdose associated with Exelon oral formulations.

11 DESCRIPTION

Exelon Patch (rivastigmine transdermal system) is a reversible cholinesterase inhibitor and is known chemically as (S)-3-[1-(dimethylamino) ethyl]phenyl ethylmethylcarbamate. It has an empirical formula of $C_{14}H_{22}N_2O_2$ as the base and a molecular weight of 250.34 (as the base). Rivastigmine is a viscous, clear, and colorless to yellow to very slightly brown liquid that is sparingly soluble in water and very soluble in ethanol, acetonitrile, n-octanol and ethyl acetate.

The distribution coefficient at 37°C in n-octanol/phosphate buffer solution pH 7 is 4.27.

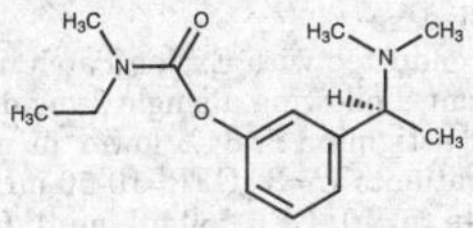

Exelon Patch is for transdermal administration. The patch comprises a four-layer laminate containing the backing layer, drug matrix, adhesive matrix and overlapping release liner. The release liner is removed and discarded prior to use. *See Figure 1 for a detailed illustration.*

Figure 1: Cross Section of the Patch

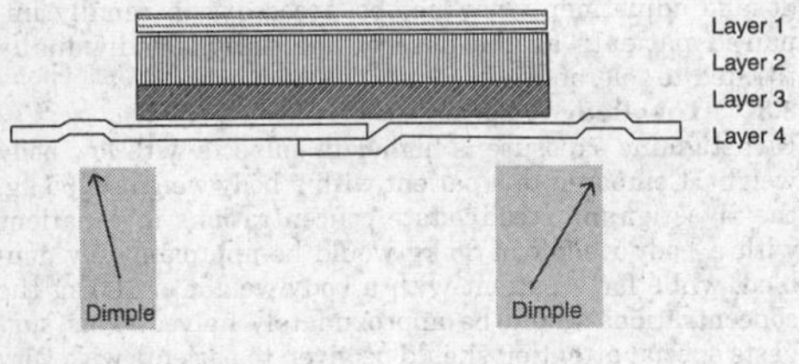

Layer 1 Backing Film
Layer 2 Drug Product (Acrylic) Matrix
Layer 3 Adhesive (Silicone) Matrix
Layer 4 Release Liner (removed at time of use)

Excipients within the formulation include acrylic copolymer, poly(butylmethacrylate, methylmethacrylate), silicone adhesive applied to a flexible polymer backing film, silicone oil, and vitamin E.

12 CLINICAL PHARMACOLOGY

12.1 Mechanism of Action

Pathological changes in dementia of the Alzheimer's type and dementia associated with Parkinson's disease involve cholinergic neuronal pathways that project from the basal forebrain to the cerebral cortex and hippocampus. These pathways are thought to be intricately involved in memory, attention, learning, and other cognitive processes. While the precise mechanism of action for rivastigmine is unknown, it is postulated to exert its therapeutic effect by enhancing cholinergic function. This is accomplished by increasing the concentration of acetylcholine through reversible inhibition of its hydrolysis by cholinesterase. If this proposed mechanism is correct, the effect of rivastigmine may lessen as the disease process advances and fewer cholinergic neurons remain functionally intact. There is no evidence that rivastigmine alters the course of the underlying dementing process.

12.2 Pharmacodynamics

After a 6-mg oral dose of rivastigmine in humans, anticholinesterase activity is present in CSF for about 10 hours, with a maximum inhibition of about 60% 5 hours after dosing.

In-vitro and *in-vivo* studies demonstrate that the inhibition of cholinesterase by rivastigmine is not affected by the concomitant administration of memantine, an N-methyl-D-aspartate receptor antagonist.

12.3 Pharmacokinetics

Absorption

After the first dose, there is a lag time of 0.5-1 hour in the absorption of rivastigmine from Exelon Patch (rivastigmine transdermal system). Concentrations then rise slowly typically reaching a maximum after 8 hours, although maximum values (C_{max}) are often reached at later times as well (10-16 hours). After the peak, plasma concentrations slowly decrease over the remainder of the 24-hour period of application. At steady state, trough levels are approximately 60-80% of peak levels. Fluctuation (between C_{max} and C_{min}) is lower for Exelon Patch than for the oral formulation. Exelon Patch 9.5 mg/24 hours exhibited exposure approximately the same as that provided by an oral dose of 6 mg twice daily (i.e., 12 mg/day).

Figure 2: Rivastigmine Plasma Concentrations Following Dermal 24-Hour Patch Application

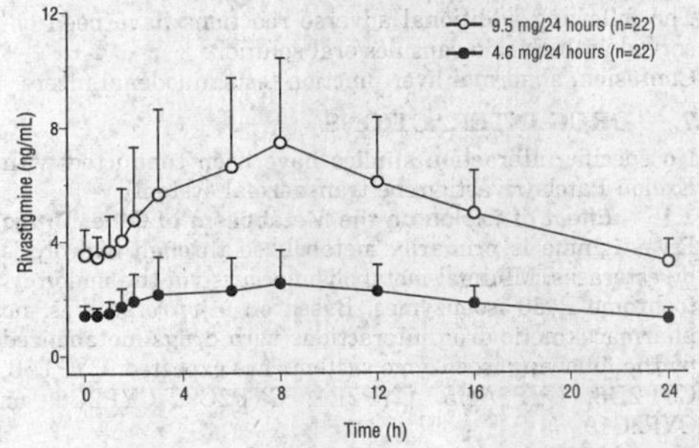

Inter-subject variability in exposure was lower (43-49%) for the Exelon Patch formulation as compared with the oral formulations (73-103%).

A relationship between drug exposure at steady state (rivastigmine and metabolite NAP226-90) and body weight was observed in Alzheimer's dementia patients. Compared to a patient with a body weight of 65 kg, the rivastigmine steady-state concentrations in a patient with a body weight of 35 kg are approximately doubled, while for a patient with a body weight of 100 kg the concentrations are approximately halved. The effect of body weight on drug exposure suggests special attention to patients with very low body weight during up-titration [see *Dosage and Administration (2)*].

Over a 24-hour dermal application, approximately 50% of the drug load is released from the system.

Exposure (AUC_∞) to rivastigmine (and metabolite NAP266-90) was highest when the patch was applied to the upper back, chest, or upper arm. Two other sites (abdomen and thigh) could be used if none of the three other sites is available, but the practitioner should keep in mind that the rivastigmine plasma exposure associated with these sites was approximately 20-30% lower.

There was no relevant accumulation of rivastigmine or the metabolite NAP226-90 in plasma in patients with Alzheimer's disease upon multiple dosing.

Distribution

Rivastigmine is weakly bound to plasma proteins (approximately 40%) over the therapeutic range. It readily crosses the blood-brain barrier, reaching CSF peak concentrations in 1.4-2.6 hours. It has an apparent volume of distribution in the range of 1.8-2.7 L/kg.

Metabolism

Rivastigmine is extensively metabolized primarily via cholinesterase-mediated hydrolysis to the decarbamylated metabolite NAP226-90. *In-vitro*, this metabolite shows minimal inhibition of acetylcholinesterase (<10%). Based on evidence from *in-vitro* and animal studies, the major cytochrome P450 isoenzymes are minimally involved in rivastigmine metabolism.

The metabolite-to-parent AUC_∞ ratio was about 0.7 after Exelon Patch application versus 3.5 after oral administration, indicating that much less metabolism occurred after dermal treatment. Less NAP226-90 is formed following patch application, presumably because of the lack of presystemic (hepatic first pass) metabolism. Based on *in-vitro* studies, no unique metabolic routes were detected in human skin.

Elimination

Renal excretion of the metabolites is the major route of elimination. Unchanged rivastigmine is found in trace amounts in the urine. Following administration of ^{14}C-rivastigmine, renal elimination was rapid and essentially complete (>90%) within 24 hours. Less than 1% of the administered dose is excreted in the feces. The apparent elimination half-life in plasma is approximately 3 hours after patch removal. Renal clearance was approximately 2.1-2.8 L/hr.

13 NONCLINICAL TOXICOLOGY

13.1 Carcinogenesis, Mutagenesis, Impairment of Fertility

In oral carcinogenicity studies conducted at doses up to 1.1 mg base/kg/day in rats and 1.6 mg base/kg/day in mice, rivastigmine was not carcinogenic.

In a dermal carcinogenicity study conducted at doses up to 0.75 mg base/kg/day in mice, rivastigmine was not carcinogenic. The mean rivastigmine plasma exposure (AUC) at this dose was 0.3-0.4 times that observed in Alzheimer's disease patients at the recommended clinical dose (one Exelon Patch 9.5 mg/24 hours).

Rivastigmine was clastogenic in two *in-vitro* assays in the presence, but not the absence, of metabolic activation. It caused structural chromosomal aberrations in V79 Chinese hamster lung cells and both structural and numerical (polyploidy) chromosomal aberrations in human peripheral blood lymphocytes. Rivastigmine was not genotoxic in three *in-vitro* assays: the Ames test, the unscheduled DNA synthesis (UDS) test in rat hepatocytes (a test for induction of DNA repair synthesis), and the HGPRT test in V79 Chinese hamster cells. Rivastigmine was not clastogenic in the *in-vivo* mouse micronucleus test.

No fertility or reproduction studies have been conducted in animals treated with dermal rivastigmine. Rivastigmine had no effect on fertility or reproductive performance in rats at oral doses up to 1.1 mg base/kg/day.

14 CLINICAL STUDIES

The effectiveness of the Exelon Patch (rivastigmine transdermal system) in Alzheimer's disease and dementia associated with Parkinson's disease was based on the results of a single controlled trial in patients with Alzheimer's disease *(see below)* as well as on three controlled trials of the immediate-release capsule in Alzheimer's disease and one controlled trial in dementia associated with Parkinson's disease *(see package insert for the Exelon capsules and oral solution for details)*.

14.1 International 24-Week Study of Exelon Patch (rivastigmine transdermal system)

This was a randomized double-blind clinical investigation in patients with Alzheimer's disease [diagnosed by NINCDS-ADRDA and DSM-IV criteria, Mini-Mental Status Examination (MMSE) score ≥10 and ≤20]. The mean age of patients participating in this trial was 74 years with a range of 50-90 years. Approximately 67% of patients were women and 33% were men. The racial distribution was Caucasian 75%, Black 1%, Oriental 9% and Other Races 15%.

14.2 Study Outcome Measures

The effectiveness of the Exelon Patch (rivastigmine transdermal system) was evaluated in this study using a dual outcome assessment strategy.

The ability of the Exelon Patch to improve cognitive performance was assessed with the cognitive subscale of the Alzheimer's Disease Assessment Scale (ADAS-Cog), a multi-item instrument that has been extensively validated in longitudinal cohorts of Alzheimer's disease patients. The ADAS-Cog examines selected aspects of cognitive performance including elements of memory, orientation, attention, reasoning, language and praxis. The ADAS-Cog scoring range is from 0-70, with higher scores indicating greater cognitive impairment. Elderly normal adults may score as low as 0 or 1, but it is not unusual for non-demented adults to score slightly higher.

The ability of the Exelon Patch to produce an overall clinical effect was assessed using the Alzheimer's Disease Cooperative Study - Clinical Global Impression of Change (ADCS-CGIC). The ADCS-CGIC is a more standardized form of CIBIC-Plus and is also scored as a seven-point categorical rating, ranging from a score of 1, indicating "markedly improved," to a score of 4, indicating "no change" to a score of 7, indicating "marked worsening."

14.3 Study Results

In this study, 1195 patients were randomized to one of the following 4 treatments: Exelon Patch 9.5 mg/24 hours, Exelon Patch 17.4 mg/24 hours, Exelon capsules in a dose of 6 mg BID, or placebo. This 24-week study was divided into a 16-week titration phase followed by an 8-week maintenance phase. In the active treatment arms of this study, doses below the target dose were permitted during the maintenance phase in the event of poor tolerability.

Effects on the ADAS-Cog

Figure 3 illustrates the time course for the change from baseline in ADAS-Cog scores for all 4 treatment groups over the 24-week study. At 24 weeks, the mean differences in the ADAS-Cog change scores for the Exelon-treated patients, compared to the patients on placebo, were 1.8, 2.9, and 1.8 units for the Exelon Patch 9.5 mg/24 hours, Exelon Patch 17.4 mg/24 hours, and Exelon capsule 6 mg BID groups, respectively. The difference between each of these groups and placebo was statistically significant.

Effects on the ADCS-CGIC

Figure 4 is a histogram of the distribution of patients' scores on the ADCS-CGIC for all 4 treatment groups.

At 24 weeks, the mean difference in the ADCS-CGIC scores for the comparison of patients in each of the Exelon-treated groups with the patients on placebo was 0.2 units. The difference between each of these groups and placebo was statistically significant.

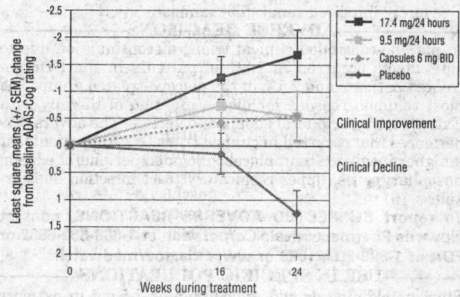

Figure 3: Time Course of the Change from Baseline in ADAS-Cog Score for Patients Observed at Each Time Point

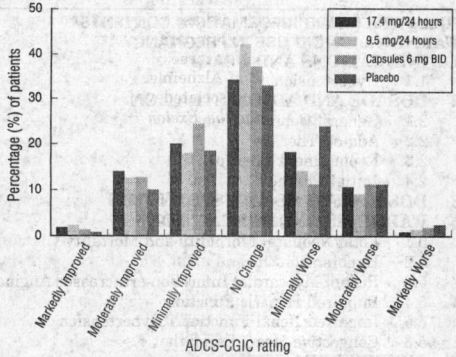

Figure 4: Distribution of ADCS-CGIC Scores for Patients Completing the Study

16 HOW SUPPLIED/STORAGE AND HANDLING

Patch 4.6 mg/24 hours

Each patch of 5 cm^2 contains 9 mg rivastigmine base with in-vivo release rate of 4.6 mg/24 hours.
Carton of 30 .... NDC 0078-0501-15

Patch 9.5 mg/24 hours

Each patch of 10 cm^2 contains 18 mg rivastigmine base with in-vivo release rate of 9.5 mg/24 hours.
Carton of 30 .... NDC 0078-0502-15
Store at 25°C (77°F); excursions permitted to 15-30°C (59-86°F) [see USP Controlled Room Temperature].
Keep Exelon Patch (rivastigmine transdermal system) in the individual sealed pouch until use.
Used systems should be folded, with the adhesive surfaces pressed together, and discarded safely.
Each pouch contains one patch.

17 PATIENT COUNSELING INFORMATION

17.1 General

Patient information is printed in section 17.8. To assure safe and effective use of Exelon Patch, this information and instructions provided in the patient information section should be discussed with patients.

17.2 Importance of Correct Usage

Patients or caregivers should be informed of the importance of applying the correct dose on the correct part of their body. They should be instructed to rotate the application site in order to minimize skin irritation. The same site should not be used within 14 days. The previous day's patch must be removed before applying a new patch to a different skin location. Exelon Patch should be replaced every 24 hours and the time of day should be consistent. It may be helpful for this to be part of a daily routine, such as the daily bath or shower.

Patients or caregivers should be told to avoid exposure of the patch to external heat sources (excessive sunlight, saunas, solariums) for long periods of time.

17.3 Discarding Used Patches

Patients or caregivers should be instructed to fold the patch in half after use. Return the used patch to its original pouch and discard it out of the reach and sight of children and pets. They should also be informed that drug still remains in the patch after 24-hour usage. They should be instructed to avoid eye contact and to wash their hands after handling the patch.

17.4 Concomitant Use of Drugs with Cholinergic Action

Patients or caregivers should be told that while wearing Exelon Patch they should not be taking Exelon capsules or Exelon oral solution or other drugs with cholinergic effects.

17.5 Gastrointestinal Adverse Events

Patients or caregivers should be informed of the potential gastrointestinal adverse events such as nausea, vomiting and diarrhea. Patients and caregivers should be instructed to observe for these adverse reactions at all times, in particular when treatment is initiated or the dose is increased. Patients and caregivers should be instructed to inform their physician if these adverse events persist as a dose adjustment/reduction may be required.

17.6 Monitoring the Patient's Weight

Patients or caregivers should be informed that Exelon Patch may affect the patient's appetite and/or the patient's weight. Any loss of appetite or weight reduction needs to be monitored.

17.7 Missed Doses

If the patient has missed a dose, he/she should be instructed to apply a new patch immediately. They may apply the next patch at the usual time the next day. Patients should not apply two patches to make up for one missed.

If treatment has been missed for three or more days, the patient or caregiver should be informed to restart treatment with the starting patch dose of 4.6 mg/24 hours. Titration to the next patch dose should proceed after 4 weeks [see Dosage and Administration (2.1)].

PATIENT INFORMATION

Exelon Patch [ECS-'el-on]
(rivastigmine transdermal system)
Exelon Patch is for skin use only.

Read this Patient Information leaflet before you start using Exelon Patch and each time you get a refill. There may be new information. This information does not take the place of talking to your healthcare provider about your medical condition or your treatment. If you do not understand the information, or have any questions about Exelon Patch, talk with your healthcare provider or pharmacist.

What is Exelon Patch?

Exelon Patch is a prescription medicine used to treat:
• mild to moderate memory problems (dementia) associated with Alzheimer's disease.
• mild to moderate memory problems (dementia) associated with Parkinson's disease.

It is not known if Exelon Patch is safe or effective in children.

Who should not use Exelon Patch?

Do not use Exelon Patch if you are allergic to rivastigmine, carbamate derivatives, or any of the ingredients in Exelon Patch. See the end of this leaflet for a complete list of ingredients in Exelon Patch.

Ask your healthcare provider if you are not sure.

What should I tell my healthcare provider before using Exelon Patch?

Before you use Exelon Patch, tell your healthcare provider if you:
• have or ever had a stomach ulcer
• are planning to have surgery
• have or ever had problems with your heart
• have problems passing urine
• have or ever had seizures
• have problems with movement (tremors)
• have asthma or breathing problems
• have a loss of appetite or are losing weight
• are pregnant or plan to become pregnant. It is not known if Exelon Patch will harm your unborn baby. Talk to your healthcare provider if you are pregnant or plan to become pregnant.
• are breastfeeding or plan to breastfeed. It is not known if Exelon Patch passes into your breast milk. Talk to your healthcare provider about the best way to feed your baby if you use Exelon Patch.

Tell your healthcare provider about all the medicines you take, including prescription and non-prescription medicines, vitamins, and herbal supplements.

Especially tell your healthcare provider if you take:
• a medicine used to treat inflammation (nonsteroidal anti-inflammatory drugs)
• other medicines used to treat Alzheimer's or Parkinson's disease
• an anticholinergic medicine, such as an allergy or cold medicine, a medicine to treat bladder or bowel spasms, or certain asthma medicines

Ask your healthcare provider if you are not sure if your medicine is one listed above.

Know the medicines you take. Keep a list of them to show to your healthcare provider and pharmacist when you get a new medicine.

How should I use Exelon Patch?
• Use Exelon Patch exactly as your healthcare provider tells you to use it.
• Your healthcare provider may change your dose as needed.
• Wear only 1 Exelon Patch at a time.
• Exelon Patch is for skin use only.
• Apply Exelon Patch to clean, dry, hairless, intact skin.
• Avoid applying Exelon Patch to areas on your body that will be rubbed against tight clothing.
• Do not apply Exelon Patch to skin that is red, irritated, or has cuts.
• Do not apply Exelon Patch to skin that has cream, lotion, or powder on it.
• Change your Exelon Patch every 24 hours at the same time of day. You may write the date and time you put on the Exelon Patch with a ballpoint pen before applying the patch to help you remember when to remove it.
• Change your application site every day to avoid skin irritation. You can use the same area, but do not use the same spot for at least 14 days after your last application.
• Check to see if the patch is loosened when engaging in activities such as bathing, swimming, or showering.
• If your Exelon Patch falls off, put on another patch right away and then replace the new patch the next day at the same time as usual. Do not use overlays, bandages, or tape to secure patches that have loosened or reapply patches that have fallen off.
• If you miss a dose or forget to change your Exelon Patch apply your next Exelon Patch as soon as you remember. Do not apply 2 Exelon Patches to make up for the missed dose.
• If you miss more than three days of applying Exelon Patch, call your healthcare provider before putting on another patch.
• You must remove Exelon Patch from the previous day before applying a new one.
• **Having more than one patch on your body at the same time can cause you to get too much Exelon. If you accidentally use more than one Exelon Patch at a time call your healthcare provider. If you are unable to reach your healthcare provider, contact your local Poison Control Center or go to the nearest hospital emergency room right away.**

Where should I apply Exelon Patch?
• Apply 1 Exelon Patch to **ONLY ONE** of the outlined areas shown in the figures below (See Figure A):
  • upper back, left or right side
  • lower back, left or right side
  • upper arm, left or right
  • chest, left or right side

Figure A

Apply one patch to ONLY ONE of the following possible sites each day.

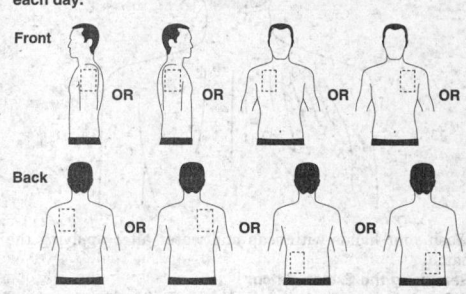

Front

Back

The diagram represents areas on the body where Exelon Patch may be applied. Only one patch should be worn at a time. Do not apply multiple patches to the body.

Apply **ONLY ONE** patch per day to **ONLY ONE** of the following locations (as illustrated above): the upper **or** lower back if it is likely that the patient will remove it. If this is not a concern, the patch can be applied **instead** to the upper arm or chest. Avoid places where the patch can be rubbed off by tight clothing.

Apply Exelon Patch as follows:
The patch is a thin, beige, plastic patch that sticks to the skin. Each patch is sealed in a pouch that protects it until you are ready to put it on. Do not open the pouch or remove a patch until just before you apply it.

1. Cut the pouch along the dotted line to open and remove the patch (See Figure B). Save the pouch for later use. **The patch should not be cut or folded sharply.**

Figure B

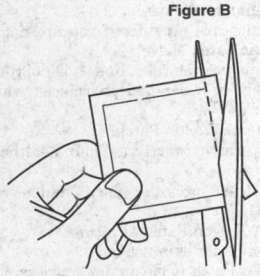

2. A protective liner covers the sticky (adhesive) side of the patch. Peel off one side of the protective cover. Do not touch the sticky part of the patch with your finger (See Figure C).

Figure C

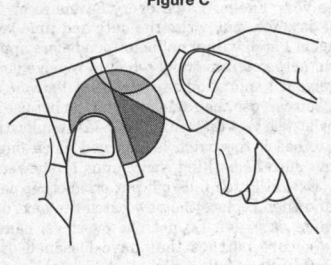

3. Apply the sticky side of the patch onto your chosen skin site.
4. Peel off the other side of the protective cover (See Figure D).

Figure D

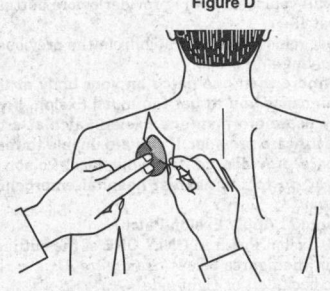

5. Press down on the patch firmly to make sure that the edges stick well (See Figure E).

Figure E

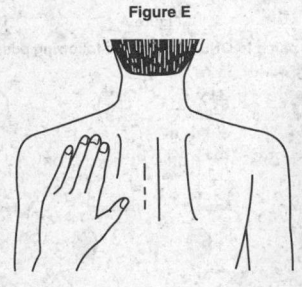

Wash your hands with soap and water after applying the patch.

Removing the Exelon Patch:
• Gently pull on 1 edge of the Exelon Patch to remove it off your skin.
• Fold the Exelon Patch in half and put it back into the pouch that you saved.
• Throw the used Exelon Patch in the trash out of the reach of children and pets.
• Wash your hands with soap and water right away.

What should I avoid while using Exelon Patch?
• Do not touch your eyes after you touch the Exelon Patch.
• Exelon Patch can cause drowsiness, dizziness, weakness, or fainting. Do not drive, operate heavy machinery, or do other dangerous activities until you know how Exelon Patch affects you.
• Avoid exposure to external heat sources such as excessive sunlight, saunas, or solariums for long periods of time.

What are the possible side effects of Exelon Patch?
Exelon Patch may cause serious side effects including:
• **Stomach or bowel (intestinal) problems,** including:
   • nausea
   • vomiting
   • diarrhea
   • loss of appetite
   • weight loss
   • bleeding in your stomach (ulcers)
• **heart problems**
• **seizures**
• **problems with movement (tremors)**
The most common side effects of Exelon Patch include:
• depression
• headache
• anxiety
• dizziness
• stomach pain
• urinary tract infections
• muscle weakness
• tiredness
• trouble sleeping

Tell your healthcare provider if you have any side effect that bothers you or that does not go away.
These are not all the possible side effects of Exelon Patch. For more information, ask your healthcare provider or pharmacist.
Call your doctor for medical advice about side effects. You may report side effects to the FDA at 1-800-FDA-1088.
How should I store Exelon Patch?
• Store Exelon Patch at 59°F to 86°F (15°C to 30°C).
• Keep Exelon Patch in the sealed pouch until ready to use.
Keep Exelon Patch and all medicines out of the reach of children.
General information about the safe and effective use of Exelon Patch.
Medicines are sometimes prescribed for purposes other than those listed in the Patient Information leaflet. Do not use Exelon Patch for a condition for which it was not prescribed. Do not give Exelon Patch to other people, even if they have the same symptoms you have. It may harm them.
This Patient Information leaflet summarizes the most important information about Exelon Patch. If you would like more information, talk with your healthcare provider. You can ask your pharmacist or healthcare provider for information about Exelon Patch that is written for health professionals.
What are the ingredients of Exelon Patch?
Active ingredient: rivastigmine

REV: August 2010   Printed in U.S.A.   T2010-42
                                                5002649

Distributed by:
Novartis Pharmaceuticals Corporation
East Hanover, New Jersey 07936
©Novartis

Shown in Product Identification Guide, page 315

EXFORGE®   ℞
[X-phorj]
(amlodipine and valsartan)
Tablets

The following prescribing information is based on official labeling in effect July 2009.
HIGHLIGHTS OF PRESCRIBING INFORMATION
These highlights do not include all the information needed to use Exforge safely and effectively. See full prescribing information for Exforge.
Exforge® *(amlodipine and valsartan)* **Tablets**
Initial U.S. Approval: 2007

WARNING: AVOID USE IN PREGNANCY
See full prescribing information for complete boxed warning.
When pregnancy is detected, discontinue Exforge as soon as possible. Drugs that act directly on the renin-angiotensin system can cause injury and even death to the developing fetus. (5.1)

———RECENT MAJOR CHANGES———
Indications and Usage (1)   7/2008
Dosage and Administration, Initial Therapy (2.4)   7/2008

———INDICATIONS AND USAGE———
Exforge is the combination tablet of amlodipine, a dihydro-pyridine calcium channel blocker (DHP CCB), and valsartan, an angiotensin II receptor blocker (ARB). Exforge is indicated for the treatment of hypertension:
• In patients not adequately controlled on monotherapy (1)
• As initial therapy in patients likely to need multiple drugs to achieve their blood pressure goals (1)
———DOSAGE AND ADMINISTRATION———
General Considerations:
• Majority of effect attained within 2 weeks (2.1)
• May be administered with other antihypertensive agents (2.1)
Hypertension
• May be used as add-on therapy for patients not controlled on monotherapy (2.2)
• Patients who experience dose-limiting adverse reactions on monotherapy may be switched to Exforge containing a lower dose of that component (2.2)
• May be substituted for titrated components (2.3)
• When used as initial therapy: Initiate with 5/160 mg, then titrate upwards as necessary to a maximum of 10/320 mg once daily (2.4)
———DOSAGE FORMS AND STRENGTHS———
Tablets (amlodipine/valsartan mg): 5/160, 10/160, 5/320, 10/320 (3)
———WARNINGS AND PRECAUTIONS———
• Avoid fetal or neonatal exposure (5.1)
• Assess for hypotension (5.2)
• Warn patients with severe obstructive coronary artery disease about the risk of myocardial infarction or increased angina (5.3)
• Titrate slowly in patients with impaired hepatic (5.4) or severely impaired renal (5.5) function
———ADVERSE REACTIONS———
In placebo-controlled clinical trials, discontinuation due to side effects occurred in 1.8% of patients in the Exforge-treated patients and 2.1% in the placebo-treated group. The most common reasons for discontinuation of therapy with Exforge were peripheral edema and vertigo. The adverse experiences that occurred in clinical trials (≥2% of patients) at a higher incidence than placebo included peripheral edema, nasopharyngitis, upper respiratory tract infection and dizziness. (6)
To report SUSPECTED ADVERSE REACTIONS, contact Novartis Pharmaceuticals Corporation at 1-888-669-6682 or FDA at 1-800-FDA-1088 or www.fda.gov/medwatch
———USE IN SPECIFIC POPULATIONS———
Start amlodipine or add amlodipine at 2.5 mg in patients ≥75 years old or in patients with hepatic impairment. (8.5)
Nursing Mothers: Choose breastfeeding or Exforge therapy, but not both. (8.3)
See 17 for PATIENT COUNSELING INFORMATION and FDA-approved patient labeling.
                                              Revised: 02/2009

FULL PRESCRIBING INFORMATION: CONTENTS*
WARNING: AVOID USE IN PREGNANCY

FULL PRESCRIBING INFORMATION

WARNING: AVOID USE IN PREGNANCY
When pregnancy is detected, discontinue Exforge as soon as possible. Drugs that act directly on the renin-angiotensin system can cause injury and even death to the developing fetus. [*See Warnings and Precautions (5.1)*]

1 INDICATIONS AND USAGE

1.1 Hypertension

Exforge (amlodipine and valsartan) is indicated for the treatment of hypertension.

Exforge may be used in patients whose blood pressure is not adequately controlled on either monotherapy.

Exforge may also be used as initial therapy in patients who are likely to need multiple drugs to achieve their blood pressure goals.

The choice of Exforge as initial therapy for hypertension should be based on an assessment of potential benefits and risks including whether the patient is likely to tolerate the lowest dose of Exforge.

Patients with stage 2 hypertension (moderate or severe) are at a relatively higher risk for cardiovascular events (such as strokes, heart attacks, and heart failure), kidney failure and vision problems, so prompt treatment is clinically relevant. The decision to use a combination as initial therapy should be individualized and should be shaped by considerations such as baseline blood pressure, the target goal and the incremental likelihood of achieving goal with a combination compared to monotherapy. Individual blood pressure goals may vary based upon the patient's risk.

Data from the high-dose multifactorial study [*see Clinical Studies (14)*] provide estimates of the probability of reaching a blood pressure goal with Exforge compared to amlodipine or valsartan monotherapy. The figures below provide estimates of the likelihood of achieving systolic or diastolic blood pressure control with Exforge 10/320 mg, based upon baseline systolic or diastolic blood pressure. The curve of each treatment group was estimated by logistic regression modeling. The estimated likelihood at the right tail of each curve is less reliable due to small numbers of subjects with high baseline blood pressures.

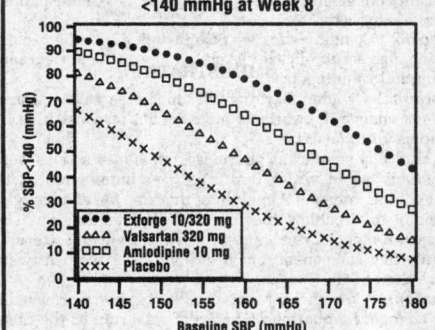

Figure 1: Probability of Achieving Systolic Blood Pressure <140 mmHg at Week 8

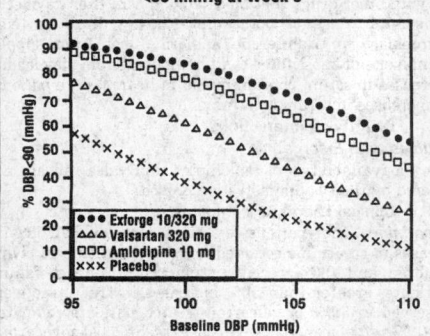

Figure 2: Probability of Achieving Diastolic Blood Pressure <90 mmHg at Week 8

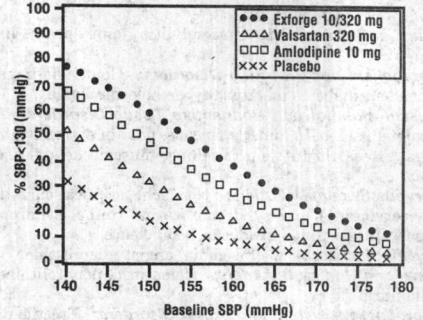

Figure 3: Probability of Achieving Systolic Blood Pressure <130 mmHg at Week 8

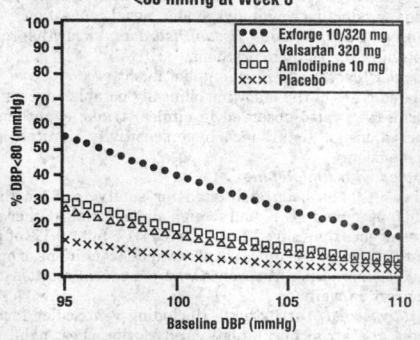

Figure 4: Probability of Achieving Diastolic Blood Pressure <80 mmHg at Week 8

For example, a patient with a baseline blood pressure of 160/100 mmHg has about a 67% likelihood of achieving a goal of <140 mmHg (systolic) and 80% likelihood of achieving <90 mmHg (diastolic) on amlodipine alone, and the likelihood of achieving these goals on valsartan alone is about 47% (systolic) or 62% (diastolic). The likelihood of achieving these goals on Exforge rises to about 80% (systolic) or 85% (diastolic). The likelihood of achieving these goals on placebo is about 28% (systolic) or 37% (diastolic).

2 DOSAGE AND ADMINISTRATION

2.1 General Considerations

Amlodipine is an effective treatment of hypertension in once daily doses of 2.5 mg to 10 mg while valsartan is effective in doses of 80 mg to 320 mg. In clinical trials with once daily Exforge (amlodipine and valsartan) using amlodipine doses of 5 mg to 10 mg and valsartan doses of 160 mg to 320 mg, the antihypertensive effects increased with increasing doses.

The hazards [*see Warnings and Precautions (5)*] of valsartan are generally independent of dose; those of amlodipine are a mixture of dose-dependent phenomena (primarily peripheral edema) and dose-independent phenomena, the former much more common than the latter [*see Adverse Reactions (6)*].

The majority of the antihypertensive effect is attained within 2 weeks after initiation of therapy or a change in dose. The dosage can be increased after 1 to 2 weeks of therapy to a maximum of one 10/320 mg tablet once daily as needed to control blood pressure [*see Clinical Studies (14)*]. Exforge may be administered with or without food.

Exforge may be administered with other antihypertensive agents.

Elderly patients: Because of decreased clearance of amlodipine, therapy should usually be initiated at 2.5 mg.

Renal Impairment: No initial dosage adjustment is required for patients with mild or moderate renal impairment. Titrate slowly in patients with severe renal impairment.

Hepatic Impairment: No initial dosage adjustment is required for patients with mild or moderate liver insufficiency. Titrate slowly in patients with hepatic impairment.

2.2 Add-on Therapy

A patient whose blood pressure is not adequately controlled with amlodipine (or another dihydropyridine calcium-channel blocker) alone or with valsartan (or another angiotensin II receptor blocker) alone may be switched to combination therapy with Exforge.

A patient who experiences dose-limiting adverse reactions on either component alone may be switched to Exforge containing a lower dose of that component in combination with the other to achieve similar blood pressure reductions. The clinical response to Exforge should be subsequently evaluated and if blood pressure remains uncontrolled after 3 to 4 weeks of therapy, the dose may be titrated up to a maximum of 10/320 mg.

2.3 Replacement Therapy

For convenience, patients receiving amlodipine and valsartan from separate tablets may instead wish to receive tablets of Exforge containing the same component doses.

2.4 Initial Therapy

A patient may be initiated on Exforge if it is unlikely that control of blood pressure would be achieved with a single agent. The usual starting dose is Exforge 5/160 mg once daily in patients who are not volume-depleted.

3 DOSAGE FORMS AND STRENGTHS

5/160 mg tablets, debossed with NVR/ECE (side 1/side 2)
10/160 mg tablets, debossed with NVR/UIC
5/320 mg tablets, debossed with NVR/CSF
10/320 mg tablets, debossed with NVR/LUF

5 WARNINGS AND PRECAUTIONS

5.1 Fetal/Neonatal Morbidity and Mortality

Exforge can cause fetal harm when administered to a pregnant woman. If this drug is used during pregnancy, or if the patient becomes pregnant while taking this drug, the patient should be apprised of the potential hazard to the fetus.

Drugs that act on the renin-angiotensin system can cause fetal and neonatal morbidity and mortality when used in pregnancy. In several dozen published cases, ACE inhibitor use during the second and third trimesters of pregnancy was associated with fetal and neonatal injury, including hypotension, neonatal skull hypoplasia, anuria, reversible or irreversible renal failure, and death [*see Use in Specific Populations (8.1)*].

5.2 Hypotension

Excessive hypotension was seen in 0.4% of patients with uncomplicated hypertension treated with Exforge in placebo-controlled studies. In patients with an activated renin-angiotensin system, such as volume- and/or salt-depleted patients receiving high doses of diuretics, symptomatic hypotension may occur in patients receiving angiotensin receptor blockers. Volume depletion should be corrected prior to administration of Exforge. Treatment with Exforge should start under close medical supervision.

Initiate therapy cautiously in patients with heart failure or recent myocardial infarction and in patients undergoing surgery or dialysis. Patients with heart failure or post-myocardial infarction patients given valsartan commonly have some reduction in blood pressure, but discontinuation of therapy because of continuing symptomatic hypotension usually is not necessary when dosing instructions are followed. In controlled trials in heart failure patients, the incidence of hypotension in valsartan-treated patients was 5.5% compared to 1.8% in placebo-treated patients. In the Valsartan in Acute Myocardial Infarction Trial (VALIANT), hypotension in post-myocardial infarction patients led to permanent discontinuation of therapy in 1.4% of valsartan-treated patients and 0.8% of captopril-treated patients.

Since the vasodilation induced by amlodipine is gradual in onset, acute hypotension has rarely been reported after oral administration. Nonetheless, caution, as with any other peripheral vasodilator, should be exercised when administering amlodipine, particularly in patients with severe aortic stenosis.

If excessive hypotension occurs with Exforge, the patient should be placed in a supine position and, if necessary, given an intravenous infusion of normal saline. A transient hypotensive response is not a contraindication to further treatment, which usually can be continued without difficulty once the blood pressure has stabilized.

5.3 Risk of Myocardial Infarction or Increased Angina

Rarely, patients, particularly those with severe obstructive coronary artery disease, have developed documented increased frequency, duration or severity of angina or acute myocardial infarction on starting calcium channel blocker therapy or at the time of dosage increase. The mechanism of this effect has not been elucidated.

5.4 Impaired Hepatic Function

Studies with Amlodipine: Amlodipine is extensively metabolized by the liver and the plasma elimination half-life ($t\frac{1}{2}$) is 56 hours in patients with impaired hepatic function, therefore, caution should be exercised when administering amlodipine to patients with severe hepatic impairment.

Studies with Valsartan: As the majority of valsartan is eliminated in the bile, patients with mild-to-moderate hepatic impairment, including patients with biliary obstructive disorders, showed lower valsartan clearance (higher AUCs). Care should be exercised in administering valsartan to these patients.

5.5 Impaired Renal Function - Hypertension

In studies of ACE inhibitors in hypertensive patients with unilateral or bilateral renal artery stenosis, increases in serum creatinine or blood urea nitrogen have been reported. In a 4-day trial of valsartan in 12 hypertensive patients with unilateral renal artery stenosis, no significant increases in serum creatinine or blood urea nitrogen were observed. There has been no long-term use of valsartan in patients with unilateral or bilateral renal artery stenosis, but an effect similar to that seen with ACE inhibitors should be anticipated.

As a consequence of inhibiting the renin-angiotensin-aldosterone system, changes in renal function may occur particularly in volume depleted patients. In patients with severe heart failure whose renal function may depend on the activity of the renin-angiotensin-aldosterone system, treatment with angiotensin-converting enzyme inhibitors and angiotensin receptor antagonists has been associated with oliguria and/or progressive azotemia and (rarely) with acute renal failure and/or death. Similar outcomes have been reported with valsartan.

5.6 Congestive Heart Failure

Studies with Amlodipine: In general, calcium channel blockers should be used with caution in patients with heart failure. Amlodipine (5-10 mg per day) has been studied in a placebo-controlled trial of 1,153 patients with NYHA Class III or IV heart failure on stable doses of ACE inhibitor, digoxin, and diuretics. Follow-up was at least 6 months, with a mean of about 14 months. There was no overall adverse effect on survival or cardiac morbidity (as defined by life-threatening arrhythmia, acute myocardial infarction, or hospitalization for worsened heart failure). Amlodipine has been compared to placebo in four 8-12 week studies of patients with NYHA class II/III heart failure, involving a total of 697 patients. In these studies, there was no evidence of worsened heart failure based on measures of exercise tolerance, NYHA classification, symptoms, or LVEF.

Studies with Valsartan: Some patients with heart failure have developed increases in blood urea nitrogen, serum creatinine, and potassium on valsartan. These effects are usually minor and transient, and they are more likely to occur in patients with pre-existing renal impairment. Dosage reduction and/or discontinuation of the diuretic and/or valsartan may be required. In the Valsartan Heart Failure Trial, in which 93% of patients were on concomitant ACE inhibitors, treatment was discontinued for elevations in creatinine or potassium (total of 1.0% on valsartan vs. 0.2% on placebo). In the Valsartan in Acute Myocardial Infarction Trial (VALIANT), discontinuation due to various types of renal dysfunction occurred in 1.1% of valsartan-treated patients and 0.8% of captopril-treated patients. Evaluation of patients with heart failure or post-myocardial infarction should always include assessment of renal function.

6 ADVERSE REACTIONS

6.1 Clinical Trials Experience

Because clinical trials are conducted under widely varying conditions, adverse reaction rates observed in the clinical trials of a drug cannot be directly compared to rates in the clinical trials of another drug and may not reflect the rates observed in practice. The adverse reaction information from clinical trials does, however, provide a basis for identifying the adverse events that appear to be related to drug use and for approximating rates.

Studies with Exforge:

Exforge has been evaluated for safety in over 2,600 patients with hypertension; over 1,440 of these patients were treated for at least 6 months and over 540 of these patients were treated for at least one year. Adverse reactions have generally been mild and transient in nature and have only infrequently required discontinuation of therapy.

The overall frequency of adverse reactions was neither dose-related nor related to gender, age, or race. In placebo-controlled clinical trials, discontinuation due to side effects occurred in 1.8% of patients in the Exforge-treated patients and 2.1% in the placebo-treated group. The most common reasons for discontinuation of therapy with Exforge were peripheral edema (0.4%), and vertigo (0.2%).

The adverse reactions that occurred in placebo-controlled clinical trials in at least 2% of patients treated with Exforge but at a higher incidence in amlodipine/valsartan patients (n=1,437) than placebo (n=337) included peripheral edema (5.4% vs. 3.0%), nasopharyngitis (4.3% vs. 1.8%), upper respiratory tract infection (2.9% vs 2.1%) and dizziness (2.1% vs 0.9%).

Orthostatic events (orthostatic hypotension and postural dizziness) were seen in less than 1% of patients.

Other adverse reactions that occurred in placebo-controlled clinical trials with Exforge (≥0.2%) are listed below. It cannot be determined whether these events were causally related to Exforge.

Blood and Lymphatic System Disorders: Lymphadenopathy

Cardiac Disorders: Palpitations, tachycardia

Ear and Labyrinth Disorders: Ear pain

Gastrointestinal Disorders: Diarrhea, nausea, constipation, dyspepsia, abdominal pain, abdominal pain upper, gastritis, vomiting, abdominal discomfort, abdominal distention, dry mouth, colitis

General Disorders and Administration Site Conditions: Fatigue, chest pain, asthenia, pitting edema, pyrexia, edema

Immune System Disorders: Seasonal allergies

Infections and Infestations: Nasopharyngitis, sinusitis, bronchitis, pharyngitis, gastroenteritis, pharyngotonsillitis, bronchitis acute, tonsillitis

Injury and Poisoning: Epicondylitis, joint sprain, limb injury

Metabolism and Nutrition Disorders: Gout, non-insulin dependent diabetes mellitus, hypercholesterolemia

Musculoskeletal and Connective Tissue Disorders: Arthralgia, back pain, muscle spasms, pain in extremity, myalgia, osteoarthritis, joint swelling, musculoskeletal chest pain

Nervous System Disorders: Headache, sciatica, parasthesia, cerviocobrachial syndrome, carpal tunnel syndrome, hypoaesthesia, sinus headache, somnolence

Psychiatric Disorders: Insomnia, anxiety, depression

Renal and Urinary Disorders: Hematuria, nephrolithiasis, pollakiuria

Reproductive System and Breast Disorders: Erectile dysfunction

Respiratory, Thoracic and Mediastinal Disorders: Cough, pharyngolaryngeal pain, sinus congestion, dyspnea, epistaxis, productive cough, dysphonia, nasal congestion

Skin and Subcutaneous Tissue Disorders: Pruritus, rash, hyperhidrosis, eczema, erythema

Vascular Disorders: Flushing, hot flush

Isolated cases of the following clinically notable adverse reactions were also observed in clinical trials: exanthema, syncope, visual disturbance, hypersensitivity, tinnitus, and hypotension.

Studies with Amlodipine:

Norvasc®* has been evaluated for safety in more than 11,000 patients in U.S. and foreign clinical trials. Other adverse events that have been reported <1% but >0.1% of patients in controlled clinical trials or under conditions of open trials or marketing experience where a causal relationship is uncertain were:

Cardiovascular: arrhythmia (including ventricular tachycardia and atrial fibrillation), bradycardia, chest pain, peripheral ischemia, syncope, postural hypotension, vasculitis

Central and Peripheral Nervous System: neuropathy peripheral, tremor

Gastrointestinal: anorexia, dysphagia, pancreatitis, gingival hyperplasia

General: allergic reaction, hot flushes, malaise, rigors, weight gain, weight loss

Musculoskeletal System: arthrosis, muscle cramps

Psychiatric: sexual dysfunction (male and female), nervousness, abnormal dreams, depersonalization

Respiratory System: dyspnea

Skin and Appendages: angioedema, erythema multiforme, rash erythematous, rash maculopapular

Special Senses: abnormal vision, conjunctivitis, diplopia, eye pain, tinnitus

Urinary System: micturation frequency, micturation disorder, nocturia

Autonomic Nervous System: sweating increased

Metabolic and Nutritional: hyperglycemia, thirst

Hemopoietic: leukopenia, purpura, thrombocytopenia

Other events reported with amlodipine at a frequency of ≤0.1% of patients include: cardiac failure, pulse irregularity, extrasystoles, skin discoloration, urticaria, skin dryness, alopecia, dermatitis, muscle weakness, twitching, ataxia, hypertonia, migraine, cold and clammy skin, apathy, agitation, amnesia, gastritis, increased appetite, loose stools, rhinitis, dysuria, polyuria, parosmia, taste perversion, abnormal visual accommodation, and xerophthalmia. Other reactions occurred sporadically and cannot be distinguished from medications or concurrent disease states such as myocardial infarction and angina.

Adverse reactions reported for amlodipine for indications other than hypertension may be found in the prescribing information for Norvasc.

Studies with Valsartan:

Diovan® has been evaluated for safety in more than 4,000 hypertensive patients in clinical trials. In trials in which valsartan was compared to an ACE inhibitor with or without placebo, the incidence of dry cough was significantly greater in the ACE inhibitor group (7.9%) than in the groups who received valsartan (2.6%) or placebo (1.5%). In a 129 patient trial limited to patients who had had dry cough when they had previously received ACE inhibitors, the incidences of cough in patients who received valsartan, HCTZ, or lisinopril were 20%, 19%, and 69% respectively (p<0.001). Other adverse reactions, not listed above, occurring in >0.2% of patients in controlled clinical trials with valsartan are:

Body as a Whole: allergic reaction, asthenia

Musculoskeletal: muscle cramps

Neurologic and Psychiatric: paresthesia

Respiratory: sinusitis, pharyngitis

Urogenital: impotence

Other reported events seen less frequently in clinical trials were: angioedema.

Adverse reactions reported for valsartan for indications other than hypertension may be found in the prescribing information for Diovan.

6.2 Postmarketing Experience

Amlodipine: Gynecomastia has been reported infrequently and a causal relationship is uncertain. Jaundice and hepatic enzyme elevations (mostly consistent with cholestasis or hepatitis), in some cases severe enough to require hospitalization, have been reported in association with use of amlodipine.

Valsartan: The following additional adverse reactions have been reported in post-marketing experience with valsartan:

Blood and Lymphatic: There are very rare reports of thrombocytopenia.

Hypersensitivity: There are rare reports of angioedema.

Digestive: Elevated liver enzymes and very rare reports of hepatitis

Renal: Impaired renal function

Clinical Laboratory Tests: Hyperkalemia

Dermatologic: Alopecia

Vascular: Vasculitis

Rare cases of rhabdomyolysis have been reported in patients receiving angiotensin II receptor blockers.

7 DRUG INTERACTIONS

7.1 Drug/Drug Interactions

No drug interaction studies have been conducted with Exforge and other drugs, although studies have been conducted with the individual amlodipine and valsartan components, as described below:

Studies with Amlodipine

In clinical trials, amlodipine has been safely administered with thiazide diuretics, beta-blockers, angiotensin-converting enzyme inhibitors, long-acting nitrates, sublingual nitroglycerin, digoxin, warfarin, non-steroidal anti-inflammatory drugs, antibiotics, and oral hypoglycemic drugs.

Cimetidine: Co-administration of amlodipine with cimetidine did not alter the pharmacokinetics of amlodipine.

Grapefruit juice: Co-administration of 240 mL of grapefruit juice with a single oral dose of amlodipine 10 mg in 20 healthy volunteers had no significant effect on the pharmacokinetics of amlodipine.

Maalox® (antacid): Co-administration of the antacid Maalox with a single dose of amlodipine had no significant effect on the pharmacokinetics of amlodipine.

Sildenafil: A single 100 mg dose of sildenafil (Viagra®**) in subjects with essential hypertension had no effect on the pharmacokinetic parameters of amlodipine. When amlodipine and sildenafil were used in combination, each agent independently exerted its own blood pressure lowering effect.

Atorvastatin: Co-administration of multiple 10 mg doses of amlodipine with 80 mg of atorvastatin resulted in no significant change in the steady state pharmacokinetic parameters of atorvastatin.

Digoxin: Co-administration of amlodipine with digoxin did not change serum digoxin levels or digoxin renal clearance in normal volunteers.

Warfarin: Co-administration of amlodipine with warfarin did not change the warfarin prothrombin response time.

Studies with Valsartan

No clinically significant pharmacokinetic interactions were observed when valsartan was co-administered with amlodipine, atenolol, cimetidine, digoxin, furosemide, glyburide, hydrochlorothiazide, or indomethacin. The valsartan-atenolol combination was more antihypertensive than either component, but it did not lower the heart rate more than atenolol alone.

Warfarin: Co-administration of valsartan and warfarin did not change the pharmacokinetics of valsartan or the timecourse of the anticoagulant properties of warfarin.

7.2 CYP 450 Interactions

The enzyme(s) responsible for valsartan metabolism have not been identified but do not seem to be CYP 450 isozymes. The inhibitory or induction potential of valsartan on CYP 450 is also unknown.

As with other drugs that block angiotensin II or its effects, concomitant use of potassium sparing diuretics (e.g., spironolactone, triamterene, amiloride), potassium supplements, or salt substitutes containing potassium may lead to increases in serum potassium and in heart failure patients to increases in serum creatinine.

7.3 Drug/Food Interactions

Studies with Exforge

The bioavailabilities of amlodipine and valsartan are not altered by the co-administration of food.

7.4 Clinical Laboratory Findings

Creatinine: In hypertensive patients, greater than 50% increases in creatinine occurred in 0.4% of patients receiving Exforge and 0.6% receiving placebo. In heart failure patients, greater than 50% increases in creatinine were observed in 3.9% of valsartan-treated patients compared to 0.9% of placebo-treated patients. In post-myocardial infarction patients, doubling of serum creatinine was observed in 4.2% of valsartan-treated patients and 3.4% of captopril-treated patients.

Liver Function Tests: Occasional elevations (greater than 150%) of liver chemistries occurred in Exforge-treated patients.

Serum Potassium: In hypertensive patients, greater than 20% increases in serum potassium were observed in 2.8% of Exforge-treated patients compared to 3.4% of placebo-treated patients. In heart failure patients, greater than 20% increases in serum potassium were observed in 10% of valsartan-treated patients compared to 5.1% of placebo-treated patients.

Blood Urea Nitrogen (BUN): In hypertensive patients, greater than 50% increases in BUN were observed in 5.5% of Exforge-treated patients compared to 4.7% of placebo-treated patients. In heart failure patients, greater than 50% increases in BUN were observed in 16.6% of valsartan-treated patients compared to 6.3% of placebo-treated patients.

Neutropenia: Neutropenia was observed in 1.9% of patients treated with Diovan and 0.8% of patients treated with placebo.

8 USE IN SPECIFIC POPULATIONS

8.1 Pregnancy

Pregnancy Category D [*see Warnings and Precautions (5.1)*]

Exforge, like other drugs that act on the renin-angiotensin system, can cause fetal and neonatal morbidity and death when used during the second or third trimester of pregnancy. Exforge can cause fetal harm when administered to a pregnant woman. If this drug is used during pregnancy, or if the patient becomes pregnant while taking this drug, the patient should be apprised of the potential hazard to the fetus.

Angiotensin II receptor antagonists, like valsartan, and angiotensin converting enzyme (ACE) inhibitors exert similar effects on the renin-angiotensin system. In several dozen published cases, ACE inhibitor use during the second and third trimesters of pregnancy was associated with fetal and neonatal injury, including hypotension, neonatal skull hypoplasia, anuria, reversible or irreversible renal failure, and death. Oligohydramnios was also reported, presumably from decreased fetal renal function. In this setting, oligohydramnios was associated with fetal limb contractures, craniofacial deformation, and hypoplastic lung development. Prematurity, intrauterine growth retardation, and patent ductus arteriosus were also reported, although it is not clear whether these occurrences were due to exposure to the drug. In a retrospective study, first trimester use of ACE inhibitors, a specific class of drugs acting on the renin-angiotensin system, was associated with a potential risk of birth defects.

When pregnancy occurs in a patient using Exforge, the physician should discontinue Exforge treatment as soon as possible. The physician should inform the patient about potential risks to the fetus based on the time of gestational exposure to Exforge (first trimester only or later). If exposure occurs beyond the first trimester, an ultrasound examination should be done.

In rare cases when another antihypertensive agent cannot be used to treat the pregnant patient, serial ultrasound examinations should be performed to assess the intraamniotic environment. Routine fetal testing with non-stress tests, biophysical profiles, and/or contraction stress tests may be appropriate based on gestational age and standards of care in the community. If oligohydramnios occurs in these situations, individualized decisions about continuing or discontinuing Exforge treatment and about pregnancy management should be made by the patient, her physician, and experts in the management of high risk pregnancy. Patients and physicians should be aware that oligohydramnios may not appear until after the fetus has sustained irreversible injury.

Infants with histories of *in utero* exposure to Exforge should be closely observed for hypotension, oliguria, and hyperkalemia. If oliguria occurs, these infants may require blood pressure and renal perfusion support. Exchange transfusion or dialysis may be required to reverse hypotension and/or support decreased renal function.

Healthcare professionals who prescribe drugs acting directly on the renin-angiotensin system should counsel women of childbearing potential about the risks of these agents during pregnancy [*see Nonclinical Toxicology (13.2)*].

8.2 Labor and Delivery

The effect of Exforge on labor and delivery has not been studied.

8.3 Nursing Mothers

It is not known whether amlodipine is excreted in human milk. In the absence of this information, it is recommended that nursing be discontinued while amlodipine is administered.

It is not known whether valsartan is excreted in human milk. Valsartan was excreted into the milk of lactating rats; however, animal breast milk drug levels may not accurately reflect human breast milk levels. Because many drugs are excreted into human milk and because of the potential for adverse reactions in nursing infants from Exforge, a decision should be made whether to discontinue nursing or discontinue the drug, taking into account the importance of the drug to the mother.

8.4 Pediatric Use

Safety and effectiveness of Exforge in pediatric patients have not been established.

8.5 Geriatric Use

In controlled clinical trials, 323 (22.5%) hypertensive patients treated with Exforge were ≥65 years and 79 (5.5%) were ≥75 years. No overall differences in the efficacy or safety of Exforge was observed in this patient population, but greater sensitivity of some older individuals cannot be ruled out.

Amlodipine: Clinical studies of amlodipine besylate tablets did not include sufficient numbers of subjects aged 65 and over to determine whether they respond differently from younger subjects. Other reported clinical experience has not identified differences in responses between the elderly and younger patients. In general, dose selection for an elderly patient should be cautious, usually starting at the low end of the dosing range, reflecting the greater frequency of decreased hepatic, renal or cardiac function, and of concomitant disease or other drug therapy. Elderly patients have decreased clearance of amlodipine with a resulting increase of AUC of approximately 40-60%, and a lower initial dose may be required [*see Dosage and Administration (2.1)*].

Valsartan: In the controlled clinical trials of valsartan, 1,214 (36.2%) of hypertensive patients treated with valsartan were ≥65 years and 265 (7.9%) were ≥75 years. No overall difference in the efficacy or safety of valsartan was observed in this patient population, but greater sensitivity of some older individuals cannot be ruled out.

10 OVERDOSAGE

Information on Amlodipine

Single oral doses of amlodipine maleate equivalent to 40 mg/kg and 100 mg/kg amlodipine in mice and rats, respectively, caused deaths. Single oral doses equivalent to 4 or more mg/kg amlodipine in dogs (11 or more times the maximum recommended human dose on a mg/m^2 basis) caused a marked peripheral vasodilation and hypotension.

Overdosage might be expected to cause excessive peripheral vasodilation with marked hypotension. In humans, experience with intentional overdosage of amlodipine is limited. Reports of intentional overdosage include a patient who ingested 250 mg and was asymptomatic and was not hospitalized; another (120 mg) who was hospitalized underwent gastric lavage and remained normotensive; the third (105 mg) was hospitalized and had hypotension (90/50 mmHg) which normalized following plasma expansion. A case of accidental drug overdose has been documented in a 19-month-old male who ingested 30 mg amlodipine (about 2 mg/kg). During the emergency room presentation, vital signs were stable with no evidence of hypotension, but a heart rate of 180 bpm. Ipecac was administered 3.5 hours after ingestion and on subsequent observation (overnight) no sequelae was noted.

If massive overdose should occur, active cardiac and respiratory monitoring should be instituted. Frequent blood pressure measurements are essential. Should hypotension occur, cardiovascular support including elevation of the extremities and the judicious administration of fluids should be initiated. If hypotension remains unresponsive to these conservative measures, administration of vasopressors (such as phenylephrine) should be considered with attention to circulating volume and urine output. Intravenous calcium gluconate may help to reverse the effects of calcium entry blockade. As amlodipine is highly protein bound, hemodialysis is not likely to be of benefit.

Information on Valsartan

Limited data are available related to overdosage in humans. The most likely effect of overdose with valsartan would be peripheral vasodilation, hypotension and tachycardia; bradycardia could occur from parasympathetic (vagal) stimulation. Depressed level of consciousness, circulatory collapse and shock have been reported. If symptomatic hypotension should occur, supportive treatment should be instituted.

Valsartan is not removed from the plasma by hemodialysis. Valsartan was without grossly observable adverse effects at single oral doses up to 2000 mg/kg in rats and up to 1000 mg/kg in marmosets, except for the salivation and diarrhea in the rat and vomiting in the marmoset at the highest dose (60 and 37 times, respectively, the maximum recommended human dose on a mg/m^2 basis). (Calculations assume an oral dose of 320 mg/day and a 60-kg patient.)

11 DESCRIPTION

Exforge is a fixed combination of amlodipine and valsartan. Exforge contains the besylate salt of amlodipine, a dihydropyridine calcium-channel blocker (CCB). Amlodipine besylate is a white to pale yellow crystalline powder, slightly soluble in water and sparingly soluble in ethanol. Amlodipine besylate's chemical name is 3-Ethyl-5-methyl(4RS)-2-[(2-aminoethoxy)methyl]-4-(2-chlorophenyl)-6-methyl-1,4-dihydropyridine-3,5-dicarboxylate benzenesulphonate; its structural formula is

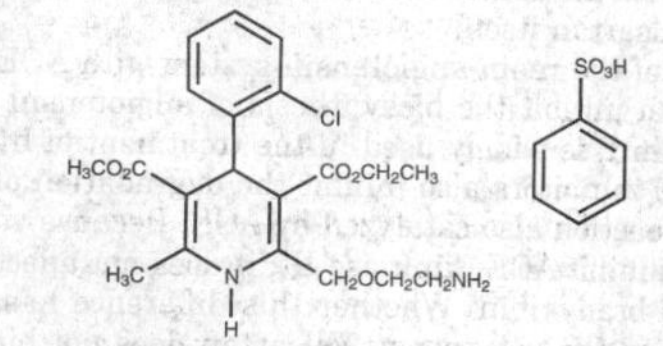

Its empirical formula is $C_{20}H_{25}ClN_2O_5 \bullet C_{66}O_3S$ and its molecular weight is 567.1.

Valsartan is a nonpeptide, orally active, and specific angiotensin II antagonist acting on the AT_1 receptor subtype. Valsartan is a white to practically white fine powder, soluble in ethanol and methanol and slightly soluble in water. Valsartan's chemical name is N-(1-oxopentyl)-N-[[2′-(1H-tetrazol-5-yl) [1,1′-biphenyl]-4-yl]methyl]-L-valine; its structural formula is

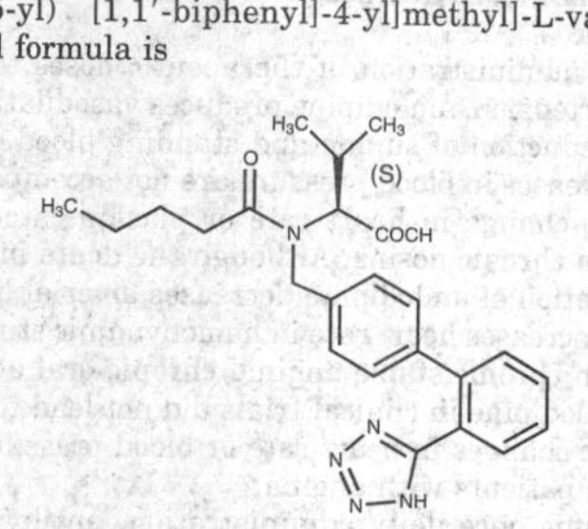

Its empirical formula is $C_{24}H_{29}N_5O_3$ and its molecular weight is 435.5.

Exforge tablets are formulated in four strengths for oral administration with a combination of amlodipine besylate, equivalent to 5 mg or 10 mg of amlodipine free-base, with 160 mg, or 320 mg of valsartan providing for the following available combinations: 5/160 mg, 10/160 mg, 5/320 mg, and 10/320 mg.

The inactive ingredients for all strengths of the tablets are colloidal silicon dioxide, crospovidone, magnesium stearate and microcrystalline cellulose. Additionally the 5/320 mg and 10/320 mg strengths contain iron oxide yellow and sodium starch glycolate. The film coating contains hypromellose, iron oxides, polyethylene glycol, talc and titanium dioxide.

12 CLINICAL PHARMACOLOGY

12.1 Mechanism of Action

Amlodipine

Amlodipine is a dihydropyridine calcium channel blocker that inhibits the transmembrane influx of calcium ions into vascular smooth muscle and cardiac muscle. Experimental data suggest that amlodipine binds to both dihydropyridine and nondihydropyridine binding sites. The contractile processes of cardiac muscle and vascular smooth muscle are dependent upon the movement of extracellular calcium ions into these cells through specific ion channels. Amlodipine inhibits calcium ion influx across cell membranes selectively, with a greater effect on vascular smooth muscle cells than on cardiac muscle cells. Negative inotropic effects can be detected *in vitro* but such effects have not been seen in intact animals at therapeutic doses. Serum calcium concentration is not affected by amlodipine. Within the physiologic pH range, amlodipine is an ionized compound (pKa=8.6), and its kinetic interaction with the calcium channel receptor is characterized by a gradual rate of association and dissociation with the receptor binding site, resulting in a gradual onset of effect.

Amlodipine is a peripheral arterial vasodilator that acts directly on vascular smooth muscle to cause a reduction in peripheral vascular resistance and reduction in blood pressure.

Valsartan

Angiotensin II is formed from angiotensin I in a reaction catalyzed by angiotensin-converting enzyme (ACE, kininase II). Angiotensin II is the principal pressor agent of the renin-angiotensin system, with effects that include vasoconstriction, stimulation of synthesis and release of aldosterone, cardiac stimulation, and renal reabsorption of sodium. Valsartan blocks the vasoconstrictor and aldosterone-secreting effects of angiotensin II by selectively blocking the binding of angiotensin II to the AT_1 receptor in many tissues, such as vascular smooth muscle and the adrenal gland. Its action is therefore independent of the pathways for angiotensin II synthesis.

There is also an AT_2 receptor found in many tissues, but AT_2 is not known to be associated with cardiovascular homeostasis. Valsartan has much greater affinity (about 20,000-fold) for the AT_1 receptor than for the AT_2 receptor. The increased plasma levels of angiotensin following AT_1 receptor blockade with valsartan may stimulate the unblocked AT_2 receptor. The primary metabolite of valsartan is essentially inactive with an affinity for the AT_1 receptor about one-200th that of valsartan itself.

Blockade of the renin-angiotensin system with ACE inhibitors, which inhibit the biosynthesis of angiotensin II from angiotensin I, is widely used in the treatment of hypertension. ACE inhibitors also inhibit the degradation of bradykinin, a reaction also catalyzed by ACE. Because valsartan does not inhibit ACE (kininase II), it does not affect the response to bradykinin. Whether this difference has clinical relevance is not yet known. Valsartan does not bind to or block other hormone receptors or ion channels known to be important in cardiovascular regulation.

Blockade of the angiotensin II receptor inhibits the negative regulatory feedback of angiotensin II on renin secretion, but the resulting increased plasma renin activity and angiotensin II circulating levels do not overcome the effect of valsartan on blood pressure.

12.2 Pharmacodynamics

Amlodipine

Following administration of therapeutic doses to patients with hypertension, amlodipine produces vasodilation resulting in a reduction of supine and standing blood pressures. These decreases in blood pressure are not accompanied by a significant change in heart rate or plasma catecholamine levels with chronic dosing. Although the acute intravenous administration of amlodipine decreases arterial blood pressure and increases heart rate in hemodynamic studies of patients with chronic stable angina, chronic oral administration of amlodipine in clinical trials did not lead to clinically significant changes in heart rate or blood pressures in normotensive patients with angina.

With chronic once daily administration, antihypertensive effectiveness is maintained for at least 24 hours. Plasma concentrations correlate with effect in both young and elderly patients. The magnitude of reduction in blood pressure with amlodipine is also correlated with the height of pretreatment elevation; thus, individuals with moderate hypertension (diastolic pressure 105-114 mmHg) had about a 50% greater response than patients with mild hypertension (diastolic pressure 90-104 mmHg). Normotensive subjects experienced no clinically significant change in blood pressure (+1/-2 mmHg).

In hypertensive patients with normal renal function, therapeutic doses of amlodipine resulted in a decrease in renal vascular resistance and an increase in glomerular filtration rate and effective renal plasma flow without change in filtration fraction or proteinuria.

As with other calcium channel blockers, hemodynamic measurements of cardiac function at rest and during exercise (or pacing) in patients with normal ventricular function treated with amlodipine have generally demonstrated a small increase in cardiac index without significant influence on dP/dt or on left ventricular end diastolic pressure or volume. In hemodynamic studies, amlodipine has not been associated with a negative inotropic effect when administered in the therapeutic dose range to intact animals and man, even when co-administered with beta-blockers to man. Similar findings, however, have been observed in normals or well-compensated patients with heart failure with agents possessing significant negative inotropic effects.

Amlodipine does not change sinoatrial nodal function or atrioventricular conduction in intact animals or man. In patients with chronic stable angina, intravenous administration of 10 mg did not significantly alter A-H and H-V conduction and sinus node recovery time after pacing. Similar results were obtained in patients receiving amlodipine and concomitant beta-blockers. In clinical studies in which amlodipine was administered in combination with beta-blockers to patients with either hypertension or angina, no adverse effects of electrocardiographic parameters were observed. In clinical trials with angina patients alone, amlodipine therapy did not alter electrocardiographic intervals or produce higher degrees of AV blocks.

Amlodipine has indications other than hypertension which can be found in the Norvasc* package insert.

Valsartan

Valsartan inhibits the pressor effect of angiotensin II infusions. An oral dose of 80 mg inhibits the pressor effect by about 80% at peak with approximately 30% inhibition persisting for 24 hours. No information on the effect of larger doses is available.

Removal of the negative feedback of angiotensin II causes a 2- to 3-fold rise in plasma renin and consequent rise in angiotensin II plasma concentration in hypertensive patients. Minimal decreases in plasma aldosterone were observed after administration of valsartan; very little effect on serum potassium was observed.

In multiple dose studies in hypertensive patients with stable renal insufficiency and patients with renovascular hypertension, valsartan had no clinically significant effects on glomerular filtration rate, filtration fraction, creatinine clearance, or renal plasma flow.

Administration of valsartan to patients with essential hypertension results in a significant reduction of sitting, supine, and standing systolic blood pressure, usually with little or no orthostatic change.

Valsartan has indications other than hypertension which can be found in the Diovan package insert.

Exforge

Exforge has been shown to be effective in lowering blood pressure. Both amlodipine and valsartan lower blood pressure by reducing peripheral resistance, but calcium influx blockade and reduction of angiotensin II vasoconstriction are complementary mechanisms.

12.3 Pharmacokinetics

Amlodipine

Peak plasma concentrations of amlodipine are reached 6-12 hours after administration of amlodipine alone. Absolute bioavailability has been estimated to be between 64% and 90%. The bioavailability of amlodipine is not altered by the presence of food.

The apparent volume of distribution of amlodipine is 21 L/kg. Approximately 93% of circulating amlodipine is bound to plasma proteins in hypertensive patients.

Amlodipine is extensively (about 90%) converted to inactive metabolites via hepatic metabolism with 10% of the parent compound and 60% of the metabolites excreted in the urine. Elimination of amlodipine from the plasma is biphasic with a terminal elimination half-life of about 30-50 hours. Steady state plasma levels of amlodipine are reached after 7-8 days of consecutive daily dosing.

Valsartan

Following oral administration of valsartan alone peak plasma concentrations of valsartan are reached in 2-4 hours. Absolute bioavailability is about 25% (range 10%-35%). Food decreases the exposure (as measured by AUC) to valsartan by about 40% and peak plasma concentration (C_{max}) by about 50%.

The steady state volume of distribution of valsartan after intravenous administration is 17 L indicating that valsartan does not distribute into tissues extensively. Valsartan is highly bound to serum proteins (95%), mainly serum albumin.

Valsartan shows bi-exponential decay kinetics following intravenous administration with an average elimination half-life of about 6 hours. The recovery is mainly as unchanged drug, with only about 20% of dose recovered as metabolites. The primary metabolite, accounting for about 9% of dose, is valeryl 4-hydroxy valsartan. The enzyme(s) responsible for valsartan metabolism have not been identified but do not seem to be CYP 450 isoenzymes.

Valsartan, when administered as an oral solution, is primarily recovered in feces (about 83% of dose) and urine (about 13% of dose). Following intravenous administration, plasma clearance of valsartan is about 2 L/h and its renal clearance is 0.62 L/h (about 30% of total clearance).

Exforge

Following oral administration of Exforge in normal healthy adults, peak plasma concentrations of valsartan and amlodipine are reached in 3 and 6-8 hours, respectively. The rate and extent of absorption of valsartan and amlodipine from Exforge are the same as when administered as individual tablets.

Special Populations

Geriatric

Studies with Amlodipine: Elderly patients have decreased clearance of amlodipine with a resulting increase in AUC of approximately 40%-60%; therefore a lower initial dose of amlodipine may be required.

Studies with Valsartan: Exposure (measured by AUC) to valsartan is higher by 70% and the half-life is longer by 35% in the elderly than in the young. No dosage adjustment is necessary.

Gender

Studies with Valsartan: Pharmacokinetics of valsartan does not differ significantly between males and females.

Renal Insufficiency

Studies with Amlodipine: The pharmacokinetics of amlodipine is not significantly influenced by renal impairment. Patients with renal failure may therefore receive the usual initial dose.

Studies with Valsartan: There is no apparent correlation between renal function (measured by creatinine clearance) and exposure (measured by AUC) to valsartan in patients with different degrees of renal impairment. Consequently, dose adjustment is not required in patients with mild-to-moderate renal dysfunction. No studies have been performed in patients with severe impairment of renal function (creatinine clearance <10 mL/min). Valsartan is not removed from the plasma by hemodialysis. In the case of severe renal disease, exercise care with dosing of valsartan.

Hepatic Insufficiency

Studies with Amlodipine: Patients with hepatic insufficiency have decreased clearance of amlodipine with resulting increase in AUC of approximately 40%-60%; therefore, a lower initial dose of amlodipine may be required.

Studies with Valsartan: On average, patients with mild-to-moderate chronic liver disease have twice the exposure (measured by AUC values) to valsartan of healthy volunteers (matched by age, sex and weight). In general, no dosage adjustment is needed in patients with mild-to-moderate liver disease. Care should be exercised in patients with liver disease.

13 NONCLINICAL TOXICOLOGY

13.1 Carcinogenesis, Mutagenesis, Impairment of Fertility

Studies with Amlodipine

Rats and mice treated with amlodipine maleate in the diet for up to two years, at concentrations calculated to provide daily dosage levels of 0.5, 1.25, and 2.5 mg amlodipine/kg/day, showed no evidence of a carcinogenic effect of the drug. For the mouse, the highest dose was, on mg/m^2 basis, similar to the maximum recommended human dose [MRHD] of 10 mg amlodipine/day. For the rat, the highest dose was, on a mg/m^2 basis, about two and a half times the MRHD. (Calculations based on a 60 kg patient.)

Mutagenicity studies conducted with amlodipine maleate revealed no drug-related effects at either the gene or chromosome level.

There was no effect on the fertility of rats treated orally with amlodipine maleate (males for 64 days and females for 14 days prior to mating) at doses of up to 10 mg amlodipine/kg/day (about 10 times the MRHD of 10 mg/day on a mg/m^2 basis).

Studies with Valsartan

There was no evidence of carcinogenicity when valsartan was administered in the diet to mice and rats for up to 2 years at concentrations calculated to provide doses of up to 160 and 200 mg/kg/day, respectively. These doses in mice and rats are about 2.4 and 6 times, respectively, the MRHD of 320 mg/day on a mg/m^2 basis. (Calculations based on a 60 kg patient.)

Mutagenicity assays did not reveal any valsartan-related effects at either the gene or chromosome level. These assays included bacterial mutagenicity tests with Salmonella and *E. coli*, a gene mutation test with Chinese hamster V79 cells, a cytogenetic test with Chinese hamster ovary cells, and a rat micronucleus test.

Valsartan had no adverse effects on the reproductive performance of male or female rats at oral doses of up to 200 mg/kg/day. This dose is about 6 times the maximum recommended human dose on a mg/m^2 basis.

13.3 Developmental Toxicity Studies

Studies with Amlodipine

No evidence of teratogenicity or other embryo/fetal toxicity was found when pregnant rats and rabbits were treated orally with amlodipine maleate at doses of up to 10 mg amlodipine/kg/day (respectively, about 10 and 20 times the maximum recommended human dose [MRHD] of 10 mg amlodipine on a mg/m^2 basis) during their respective periods of major organogenesis. (Calculations based on a patient weight of 60 kg.) However, litter size was significantly decreased (by about 50%) and the number of intrauterine deaths was significantly increased (about 5-fold) for rats receiving amlodipine maleate at a dose equivalent to 10 mg amlodipine/kg/day for 14 days before mating and throughout mating and gestation. Amlodipine maleate has been shown to prolong both the gestation period and the duration of labor in rats at this dose. There are no adequate and well-controlled studies in pregnant women. Amlodipine should be used during pregnancy only if the potential benefit justifies the potential risk to the fetus.

Studies with Valsartan

No teratogenic effects were observed when valsartan was administered to pregnant mice and rats at oral doses of up to 600 mg/kg/day and to pregnant rabbits at oral doses of up to 10 mg/kg/day. However, significant decreases in fetal weight, pup birth weight, pup survival rate, and slight delays in developmental milestones were observed in studies in which parental rats were treated with valsartan at oral, maternally toxic (reduction in body weight gain and food consumption) doses of 600 mg/kg/day during organogenesis or late gestation and lactation. In rabbits, fetotoxicity (i.e., resorptions, litter loss, abortions, and low body weight) associated with maternal toxicity (mortality) was observed at doses of 5 and 10 mg/kg/day. The no observed adverse effect doses of 600, 200 and 2 mg/kg/day in mice, rats and rabbits, respectively, are about 9, 6 and 0.1 times the MRHD of 320 mg/day on a mg/m^2 basis. (Calculations based on a patient weight of 60 kg.)

Studies with Amlodipine Besylate and Valsartan

In the oral embryo-fetal development study in rats using amlodipine besylate plus valsartan at doses equivalent to 5 mg/kg/day amlodipine plus 80 mg/kg/day valsartan,

10 mg/kg/day amlodipine plus 160 mg/kg/day valsartan, and 20 mg/kg/day amlodipine plus 320 mg/kg/day valsartan, treatment-related maternal and fetal effects (developmental delays and alterations noted in the presence of significant maternal toxicity) were noted with the high dose combination. The no-observed-adverse-effect level (NOAEL) for embryo-fetal effects was 10 mg/kg/day amlodipine plus 160 mg/kg/day valsartan. On a systemic exposure [$AUC_{(0-\infty)}$] basis, these doses are, respectively, 4.3 and 2.7 times the systemic exposure [$AUC_{(0-\infty)}$] in humans receiving the MRHD (10/320 mg/60 kg).

14 CLINICAL STUDIES

Exforge was studied in 2 placebo-controlled and 4 active-controlled trials in hypertensive patients. In a double-blind, placebo controlled study, a total of 1,012 patients with mild-to-moderate hypertension received treatments of three combinations of amlodipine and valsartan (5/80, 5/160, 5/320 mg) or amlodipine alone (5 mg), valsartan alone (80, 160, or 320 mg) or placebo. All doses with the exception of the 5/320 mg dose were initiated at the randomized dose. The high dose was titrated to that dose after a week at a dose of 5/160 mg. At week 8, the combination treatments were statistically significantly superior to their monotherapy components in reduction of diastolic and systolic blood pressures.
[See table 1 above]
[See table 2 at right]
In a double-blind, placebo controlled study, a total of 1,246 patients with mild to moderate hypertension received treatments of two combinations of amlodipine and valsartan (10/160, 10/320 mg) or amlodipine alone (10 mg), valsartan alone (160 or 320 mg) or placebo. With the exception of the 10/320 mg dose, treatment was initiated at the randomized dose. The high dose was initiated at a dose of 5/160 mg and titrated to the randomized dose after 1 week. At week 8, the combination treatments were statistically significantly superior to their monotherapy components in reduction of diastolic and systolic blood pressures.
[See table 3 at right]
[See table 4 at right]
In a double-blind, active-controlled study, a total of 947 patients with mild to moderate hypertension who were not adequately controlled on valsartan 160 mg received treatments of two combinations of amlodipine and valsartan (10/160, 5/160 mg), or valsartan alone (160 mg). At week 8, the combination treatments were statistically significantly superior to the monotherapy component in reduction of diastolic and systolic blood pressures.
[See table 5 at top of next page]
In a double-blind, active-controlled study, a total of 944 patients with mild to moderate hypertension who were not adequately controlled on amlodipine 10 mg received a combination of amlodipine and valsartan (10/160 mg), or amlodipine alone (10 mg). At week 8, the combination treatment was statistically significantly superior to the monotherapy component in reduction of diastolic and systolic blood pressures.
[See table 6 on next page]
Exforge was also evaluated for safety in a 6-week, double-blind, active-controlled trial of 130 hypertensive patients with severe hypertension (mean baseline BP of 171/113 mmHg). Adverse events were similar in patients with severe hypertension and mild/moderate hypertension treated with Exforge.
A wide age range of the adult population, including the elderly was studied (range 19-92 years, mean 54.7 years). Women comprised almost half of the studied population (47.3%). Of the patients in the studied Exforge group, 87.6% were Caucasian. Black and Asian patients each represented approximately 4% of the population in the studied Exforge group.
Two additional double-blind, active-controlled studies were conducted in which Exforge was administered as initial therapy. In one study, a total of 572 Black patients with moderate to severe hypertension were randomized to receive either combination amlodipine/valsartan or amlodipine monotherapy for 12 weeks. The initial dose of amlodipine/valsartan was 5/160 mg for 2 weeks with forced titration to 10/160 mg for 2 weeks, followed by optional titration to 10/320 mg for 4 weeks and optional addition of HCTZ 12.5 mg for 4 weeks. The initial dose of amlodipine was 5 mg for 2 weeks with forced titration to 10 mg for 2 weeks, followed by optional titration to 10 mg for 4 weeks and optional addition of HCTZ 12.5 mg for 4 weeks. At the primary endpoint of 8 weeks, the treatment difference between amlodipine/valsartan and amlodipine was 6.7/2.8 mmHg.
In the other study of similar design, a total of 646 patients with moderate to severe hypertension (MSSBP ≥160 mmHg and <200 mmHg) were randomized to receive either combination amlodipine/valsartan or amlodipine

Table 1: Effect of Exforge on Sitting Diastolic Blood Pressure

Amlodipine dosage	Valsartan dosage							
	0 mg		80 mg		160 mg		320 mg	
	Mean Change*	Placebo-subtracted	Mean Change*	Placebo-subtracted	Mean Change*	Placebo-subtracted	Mean Change*	Placebo-subtracted
0 mg	-6.4	—	-9.5	-3.1	-10.9	-4.5	-13.2	-6.7
5 mg	-11.1	-4.7	-14.2	-7.8	-14.0	-7.6	-15.7	-9.3

*Mean Change and Placebo-Subtracted Mean Change from Baseline (mmHg) at Week 8 in Sitting Diastolic Blood Pressure. Mean baseline diastolic BP was 99.3 mmHg.

Table 2: Effect of Exforge on Sitting Systolic Blood Pressure

Amlodipine dosage	Valsartan dosage							
	0 mg		80 mg		160 mg		320 mg	
	Mean Change*	Placebo-subtracted	Mean Change*	Placebo-subtracted	Mean Change*	Placebo-subtracted	Mean Change*	Placebo-subtracted
0 mg	-6.2	—	-12.9	-6.8	-14.3	-8.2	-16.3	-10.1
5 mg	-14.8	-8.6	-20.7	-14.5	-19.4	-13.2	-22.4	-16.2

*Mean Change and Placebo-Subtracted Mean Change from Baseline (mmHg) at Week 8 in Sitting Systolic Blood Pressure. Mean baseline systolic BP was 152.8 mmHg.

Table 3: Effect of Exforge on Sitting Diastolic Blood Pressure

Amlodipine dosage	Valsartan dosage					
	0 mg		160 mg		320 mg	
	Mean Change*	Placebo-subtracted	Mean Change*	Placebo-subtracted	Mean Change*	Placebo-subtracted
0 mg	-8.2	—	-12.8	-4.5	-12.8	-4.5
10 mg	-15.0	-6.7	-17.2	-9.0	-18.1	-9.9

*Mean Change and Placebo-Subtracted Mean Change from Baseline (mmHg) at Week 8 in Sitting Diastolic Blood Pressure. Mean baseline diastolic BP was 99.1 mmHg.

Table 4: Effect of Exforge on Sitting Systolic Blood Pressure

Amlodipine dosage	Valsartan dosage					
	0 mg		160 mg		320 mg	
	Mean Change*	Placebo-subtracted	Mean Change*	Placebo-subtracted	Mean Change*	Placebo-subtracted
0 mg	-11.0	—	-18.1	-7.0	-18.5	-7.5
10 mg	-22.2	-11.2	-26.6	-15.5	-26.9	-15.9

*Mean Change and Placebo-Subtracted Mean Change from Baseline (mmHg) at Week 8 in Sitting Systolic Blood Pressure. Mean baseline systolic BP was 156.7 mmHg.

monotherapy for 8 weeks. The initial dose of amlodipine/valsartan was 5/160 mg for 2 weeks with forced titration to 10/160 mg for 2 weeks, followed by the optional addition of HCTZ 12.5 mg for 4 weeks. The initial dose of amlodipine was 5 mg for 2 weeks with forced titration to 10 mg for 2 weeks, followed by the optional addition of HCTZ 12.5 mg for 4 weeks. At the primary endpoint of 4 weeks, the treatment difference between amlodipine/valsartan and amlodipine was 6.6/3.9 mmHg.

16 HOW SUPPLIED/STORAGE AND HANDLING

Exforge is available as non-scored tablets containing amlodipine besylate equivalent to 5 mg, or 10 mg of amlodipine free-base with valsartan 160 mg or 320 mg, providing for the following available combinations: 5/160 mg, 10/160 mg, 5/320 mg and 10/320 mg.
All strengths are packaged in bottles of 30 and 90 count.
5/160 mg Tablets - dark yellow, ovaloid shaped, film coated tablet with beveled edge, debossed with "NVR" on one side and "ECE" on the other side.
Bottles of 30 .... NDC # 0078-0488-15
Bottles of 90 .... NDC # 0078-0488-34
10/160 mg Tablets - light yellow, ovaloid shaped, film coated tablet with beveled edge, debossed with "NVR" on one side and "UIC" on the other side.

Bottles of 30 .... NDC # 0078-0489-15
Bottles of 90 .... NDC # 0078-0489-34
5/320 mg Tablets - very dark yellow, ovaloid shaped, film coated tablet with beveled edge, debossed with "NVR" on one side and "CSF" on the other side.
Bottles of 30 .... NDC # 0078-0490-15
Bottles of 90 .... NDC # 0078-0490-34
10/320 mg Tablets - dark yellow, ovaloid shaped, film coated tablet with beveled edge, debossed with "NVR" on one side and "LUF" on the other side.
Bottles of 30 .... NDC # 0078-0491-15
Bottles of 90 .... NDC # 0078-0491-34
Store at 25°C (77°F); excursions permitted to 15-30°C (59-86°F). [See USP Controlled Room Temperature.] Protect from moisture.

17 PATIENT COUNSELING INFORMATION
17.1 Information for Patients

Pregnancy: Female patients of childbearing age should be told that use of drugs like valsartan that act on the renin-angiotensin system can cause serious problems in the fetus and infant including: low blood pressure, poor development of skull bones, kidney failure and death. Discuss other treatment options with female patients planning to become pregnant. Women using Exforge who become pregnant should notify their physicians as soon as possible.

Table 5: Effect of Exforge on Sitting Diastolic/Systolic Blood Pressure

Treatment Group	Diastolic BP		Systolic BP	
	Mean change*	Treatment Difference**	Mean change*	Treatment Difference**
Exforge 10/160 mg	-11.4	-4.8	-13.9	-5.7
Exforge 5/160 mg	-9.6	-3.1	-12.0	-3.9
Valsartan 160 mg	-6.6	—	-8.2	—

*Mean Change from Baseline at Week 8 in Sitting Diastolic/Systolic Blood Pressure. Mean baseline BP was 149.5/96.5 (systolic/diastolic) mmHg
**Treatment Difference = difference in mean BP reduction between Exforge and the control group (Valsartan 160 mg)

Table 6: Effect of Exforge on Sitting Diastolic/Systolic Blood Pressure

Treatment Group	Diastolic BP		Systolic BP	
	Mean change*	Treatment Difference**	Mean change*	Treatment Difference**
Exforge 10/160 mg	-11.8	-1.8	-12.7	-1.9
Amlodipine 10 mg	-10.0	—	-10.8	—

*Mean Change from Baseline at Week 8 in Sitting Diastolic/Systolic Blood Pressure. Mean baseline BP was 147.0/95.1 (systolic/diastolic) mmHg
**Treatment Difference = difference in mean BP reduction between Exforge and the control group (Amlodipine 10 mg)

17.2 FDA-Approved Patient Labeling

PATIENT INFORMATION
EXFORGE® (X-phorj)
(amlodipine and valsartan)
Tablets

Read the Patient Information that comes with EXFORGE before you start taking it and each time you get a refill. There may be new information. This leaflet does not take the place of talking with your doctor about your medical condition or treatment. If you have any questions about EXFORGE, ask your doctor or pharmacist.

What is the most important information I should know about EXFORGE?
If you become pregnant, stop taking EXFORGE and call your doctor right away. EXFORGE can harm an unborn baby causing injury and even death. If you plan to become pregnant, talk to your doctor about other treatment options to lower your blood pressure before taking EXFORGE.

What is EXFORGE?
EXFORGE contains two prescription medicines:
1. amlodipine, a calcium channel blocker
2. valsartan, an angiotensin receptor blocker (ARB).
EXFORGE may be used to lower high blood pressure (hypertension) in adults
- when one medicine to lower your high blood pressure is not enough
- as the first medicine to lower high blood pressure if your doctor decides you are likely to need more than one medicine.
EXFORGE has not been studied in children under 18 years of age.

What should I tell my doctor before taking EXFORGE?
Tell your doctor about all of your medical conditions, including if you:
- **are pregnant or plan to become pregnant.** See "What is the most important information I should know about EXFORGE?"
- **are breast-feeding or plan to breast-feed.** EXFORGE may pass into your milk. Do not breast-feed while you are taking EXFORGE.
- have heart problems
- have liver problems
- have kidney problems
- are vomiting or having a lot of diarrhea
Tell your doctor about all the medicines you take, including prescription and nonprescription medicines, vitamins, and herbal supplements. Some of your other medicines and EXFORGE could affect each other, causing serious side effects.
Especially tell your doctor if you take:
- other medicines for high blood pressure or a heart problem
- water pills (diuretics)
- potassium supplements
- a salt substitute

Know the medicines you take. Keep a list of your medicines and show it to your doctor or pharmacist when you get a new medicine. Talk to your doctor or pharmacist before you start taking any new medicine. Your doctor or pharmacist will know what medicines are safe to take together.

How should I take EXFORGE?
- Take EXFORGE exactly as your doctor tells you.
- Take EXFORGE once each day.
- EXFORGE can be taken with or without food.
- If you miss a dose, take it as soon as you remember. If it is close to your next dose, do not take the missed dose. Just take the next dose at your regular time.
- If you take too much EXFORGE, call your doctor or Poison Control Center, or go to the emergency room.
- Tell all your doctors or dentist you are taking EXFORGE if you:
  - are going to have surgery
  - go for kidney dialysis

What should I avoid while taking EXFORGE?
You should not take EXFORGE during pregnancy. See "What is the most important information I should know about EXFORGE?"

What are the possible side effects of EXFORGE?
EXFORGE may cause **serious side effects** including:
- **harm to an unborn baby causing injury and even death.** See "What is the most important information I should know about EXFORGE?"
- **low blood pressure (hypotension).** Low blood pressure is most likely to happen if you:
  - take water pills
  - are on a low salt diet
  - get dialysis treatments
  - have heart problems
  - get sick with vomiting or diarrhea
  - drink alcohol
  Lie down if you feel faint or dizzy. Call your doctor right away.
- **more heart attacks and chest pain (angina)** in people that already have severe heart problems. This may happen when you start EXFORGE or when there is an increase in your dose of EXFORGE. Get emergency help if you get worse chest pain or chest pain that does not go away.
- **kidney problems.** Kidney problems may become worse in people that already have kidney disease. Some people will have changes in blood tests for kidney function and may need a lower dose of EXFORGE. Call your doctor if you have swelling in your feet, ankles, or hands or unexplained weight gain. If you have heart failure, your doctor should check your kidney function before prescribing EXFORGE.
- **laboratory blood test changes in people with congestive heart failure.** Some people with congestive heart failure who take valsartan, one of the medicines in EXFORGE, have changes in blood tests including increased potassium and decreased kidney function.
The most common side effects of EXFORGE include:
- swelling (edema) of the hands, ankles, or feet
- nasal congestion, sore throat and discomfort when swallowing

- upper respiratory tract infection (head or chest cold)
- dizziness
Tell your doctor if you have any side effect that bothers you or that does not go away.
These are not all the possible side effects of EXFORGE. For more information, ask your doctor or pharmacist.
Call your doctor for medical advice about side effects. You may report side effects to FDA at 1-800-FDA-1088.

How should I store EXFORGE?
- Store EXFORGE at room temperature between 59°F to 86°F (15°C to 30°C).
- Keep EXFORGE dry (protect it from moisture).
Keep EXFORGE and all medicines out of the reach of children.

General Information about EXFORGE
Medicines are sometimes prescribed for conditions that are not mentioned in the patient information leaflet. Do not use EXFORGE for a condition for which it was not prescribed. Do not give EXFORGE to other people, even if they have the same symptoms that you have. It may harm them.
This patient information leaflet summarizes the most important information about EXFORGE. If you would like more information about EXFORGE, talk with your doctor. You can ask your doctor or pharmacist for information about EXFORGE that is written for health professionals. For more information go to www.EXFORGE.com or call 1-888-839-3674.

What are the ingredients in EXFORGE?
Active ingredients: Amlodipine besylate and valsartan
The inactive ingredients of all strengths of the tablets are colloidal silicon dioxide, crospovidone, magnesium stearate and microcrystalline cellulose. Additionally, the 5/320 mg and 10/320 mg strengths contain iron oxide yellow and sodium starch glycolate. The film coating contains hypromellose, iron oxides, polyethylene glycol, talc and titanium dioxide.

What is high blood pressure (hypertension)?
Blood pressure is the force of blood in your blood vessels when your heart beats and when your heart rests. You have high blood pressure when the force is too much. EXFORGE can help your blood vessels relax so your blood pressure is lower. Medicines that lower blood pressure lower your chance of having a stroke or heart attack.
High blood pressure makes the heart work harder to pump blood throughout the body and causes damage to blood vessels. If high blood pressure is not treated, it can lead to stroke, heart attack, heart failure, kidney failure and vision problems.
*Norvasc® is a registered trademark of Pfizer, Inc.
**Viagra® is a registered trademark of Pfizer, Inc.

T2009-27/T2008-31
5002237
Revised February 2009   5002238
Distributed by:
Novartis Pharmaceuticals Corporation
East Hanover, New Jersey 07936
©Novartis
Shown in Product Identification Guide, page 315

EXFORGE HCT®   ℞
[X-phorj HCT]
(amlodipine, valsartan, hydrochlorothiazide)
Tablets

The following prescribing information is based on official labeling in effect July 2010.
HIGHLIGHTS OF PRESCRIBING INFORMATION
These highlights do not include all the information needed to use Exforge HCT safely and effectively. See full prescribing information for Exforge HCT.
Exforge HCT *(amlodipine, valsartan, hydrochlorothiazide)* **Tablets**
Initial U.S. Approval: 2009

WARNING: AVOID USE IN PREGNANCY
When pregnancy is detected, discontinue Exforge HCT as soon as possible. Drugs that act directly on the renin-angiotensin system can cause injury or death to the developing fetus. (5.1)

————INDICATIONS AND USAGE————
- Exforge HCT is for the treatment of hypertension (1)
- Not indicated for initial therapy
————DOSAGE AND ADMINISTRATION————
- Dose once-daily.
- Exforge HCT may be used as add-on/switch therapy for patients not adequately controlled on any two of the following antihypertensive classes: calcium channel blockers, angiotensin receptor blockers, and diuretics. (2)
- Exforge HCT may be substituted for its individually titrated components for patients on amlodipine, valsartan and hydrochlorothiazide (2).
- The full blood pressure lowering effect was achieved 2 weeks after being on the maximal dose of Exforge HCT (2).

—DOSAGE FORMS AND STRENGTHS—
Tablets: (amlodipine/valsartan/hydrochlorothiazide mg)
5/160/12.5
10/160/12.5
5/160/25
10/160/25
10/320/25 (3)

—CONTRAINDICATIONS—
• Anuria; Hypersensitivity to sulfonamide-derived drugs (4)

—WARNINGS AND PRECAUTIONS—
• Avoid fetal or neonatal exposure (5.1)
• Symptomatic hypotension with volume- or salt-depletion. Correct volume-depletion prior to administration (5.2)
• Increased angina and/or myocardial infarction (5.3)
• Avoid in patients with severely impaired hepatic (2.1, 5.4) or renal function (creatinine clearance ≤30 mL/min) (2.1, 5.5)
• Observe for signs of fluid or electrolyte imbalance (5.10)
• Thiazide diuretics may cause an exacerbation or activation of systemic lupus erythematosus (5.8)

—ADVERSE REACTIONS—
Most common adverse events (≥2% incidence) are dizziness, peripheral edema, headache, dyspepsia, fatigue, muscle spasms, back pain, nausea and nasopharyngitis. To report SUSPECTED ADVERSE REACTIONS, contact Novartis Pharmaceuticals Corporation at 1-888-669-6682 or FDA at 1-800-FDA-1088 or www.fda.gov/medwatch

—DRUG INTERACTIONS—
Hydrochlorothiazide (7):
• Alcohol, barbiturates, narcotics: Potentiation of orthostatic hypotension
• Antidiabetic drugs: Dosage adjustment of antidiabetic may be required
• Cholestyramine and colestipol: Reduced absorption of thiazides
• Corticosteroids, ACTH: Hypokalemia, electrolyte depletion
• Lithium: Reduced renal clearance and high risk of lithium toxicity when used with diuretics. Should not be given with diuretics.
• NSAIDs: Can reduce diuretic, natriuretic and antihypertensive effects of diuretics.

—USE IN SPECIFIC POPULATIONS—
Pregnancy: Avoid use in pregnancy. (5.1)
Nursing Mothers: Avoid use while nursing – discontinue either nursing or drug. (8.3)
Geriatric Patients: No overall differences in the efficacy or safety of Exforge HCT was observed in this patient population, but greater sensitivity of some older individuals cannot be ruled out. (8.5)

See 17 for PATIENT COUNSELING INFORMATION and FDA-approved patient labeling

Revised: 08/2009

FULL PRESCRIBING INFORMATION

WARNING: AVOID USE IN PREGNANCY
When pregnancy is detected, discontinue Exforge HCT as soon as possible. Drugs that act directly on the renin-angiotensin system can cause injury or death to the developing fetus [see Warnings and Precautions (5.1)].

---

1 INDICATIONS AND USAGE
Exforge HCT (amlodipine, valsartan, hydrochlorothiazide) is indicated for the treatment of hypertension.
This fixed combination drug is not indicated for the initial therapy of hypertension [see Dosage and Administration (2)].

2 DOSAGE AND ADMINISTRATION
2.1 General Considerations
Dose once-daily. The dosage may be increased after two weeks of therapy. The full blood pressure lowering effect was achieved 2 weeks after being on the maximal dose of Exforge HCT. The maximum recommended dose of Exforge HCT is 10/320/25 mg.
Exforge HCT may be administered with or without food.
No initial dosage adjustment is required for elderly patients.
Renal impairment: The usual regimens of therapy with Exforge HCT may be followed if the patient's creatinine clearance is >30 mL/min. In patients with more severe renal impairment, loop diuretics are preferred to thiazides, so avoid use of Exforge HCT [see Impaired Renal Function (5.5)].
Hepatic impairment: Avoid Exforge HCT in patients with severe hepatic impairment. In patients with lesser degrees of hepatic impairment, monitor for worsening of hepatic or renal function and adverse reactions [see Impaired Hepatic Function (5.4)].
2.2 Add-on/Switch Therapy
Exforge HCT may be used for patients not adequately controlled on any two of the following antihypertensive classes: calcium channel blockers, angiotensin receptor blockers, and diuretics.
A patient who experiences dose-limiting adverse reactions to an individual component while on any dual combination of the components of Exforge HCT may be switched to Exforge HCT containing a lower dose of that component to achieve similar blood pressure reductions.
2.3 Replacement Therapy
Exforge HCT may be substituted for the individually titrated components.

3 DOSAGE FORMS AND STRENGTHS
• 5 mg amlodipine/160 mg valsartan/12.5 mg hydrochlorothiazide Tablets – White, non-scored, film-coated tablet, ovaloid, biconvex with beveled edge with debossing "NVR" on one side and "VCL" on the other side.
• 10 mg amlodipine/160 mg valsartan/12.5 mg hydrochlorothiazide Tablets – Pale yellow, non-scored, film-coated tablet, ovaloid, biconvex with beveled edge with debossing "NVR" on one side and "VDL" on the other side.
• 5 mg amlodipine/160 mg valsartan/25 mg hydrochlorothiazide Tablets – Yellow, non-scored, film-coated tablet, ovaloid, biconvex with beveled edge with debossing "NVR" on one side and "VEL" on the other side.
• 10 mg amlodipine/160 mg valsartan/25 mg hydrochlorothiazide Tablets – Brown-yellow, non-scored, film-coated tablet, ovaloid, biconvex with beveled edge with debossing "NVR" on one side and "VHL" on the other side.
• 10 mg amlodipine/320 mg valsartan/25 mg hydrochlorothiazide Tablets – Brown-yellow, non-scored, film-coated tablet, ovaloid, biconvex with beveled edge with debossing "NVR" on one side and "VFL" on the other side.

4 CONTRAINDICATIONS
Because of the hydrochlorothiazide component, Exforge HCT is contraindicated in patients with anuria or hypersensitivity to other sulfonamide-derived drugs.

5 WARNINGS AND PRECAUTIONS
5.1 Fetal/Neonatal Morbidity and Mortality
Exforge HCT can cause harm to the fetus when administered to a pregnant woman. If this drug is used during pregnancy, or if the patient becomes pregnant while taking this drug, the patient should be apprised of the potential hazard to the fetus.
Drugs that act on the renin-angiotensin system can cause fetal and neonatal morbidity and mortality when used in pregnancy. In several dozen published cases, ACE inhibitor use during the second and third trimesters of pregnancy was associated with fetal and neonatal injury, including hypotension, neonatal skull hypoplasia, anuria, reversible or irreversible renal failure, and death [see Use in Specific Populations (8.1)].
5.2 Hypotension in Volume- or Salt-Depleted Patients
Excessive hypotension, including orthostatic hypotension, was seen in 1.7% of patients treated with the maximum dose of Exforge HCT (10/320/25 mg) compared to 1.8% of valsartan/HCTZ (320/25 mg) patients, 0.4% of amlodipine/valsartan (10/320 mg) patients, and 0.2% of HCTZ/amlodipine (25/10 mg) patients in a controlled trial in patients with moderate to severe uncomplicated hypertension. In patients with an activated renin-angiotensin system, such as volume- or salt-depleted patients receiving high doses of diuretics, symptomatic hypotension may occur in patients receiving angiotensin receptor blockers. Correct this condition prior to administration of Exforge HCT.
Exforge HCT has not been studied in patients with heart failure, recent myocardial infarction, or in patients undergoing surgery or dialysis. Patients with heart failure or post-myocardial infarction patients given valsartan commonly have some reduction in blood pressure, but discontinuation of therapy because of continuing symptomatic hypotension usually is not necessary when dosing instructions are followed. In controlled trials in heart failure patients, the incidence of hypotension in valsartan-treated patients was 5.5% compared to 1.8% in placebo-treated patients. In the Valsartan in Acute Myocardial Infarction Trial (VALIANT), hypotension in post-myocardial infarction patients led to permanent discontinuation of therapy in 1.4% of valsartan-treated patients and 0.8% of captopril-treated patients.
Since the vasodilation induced by amlodipine is gradual in onset, acute hypotension has rarely been reported after oral administration. Do not initiate treatment with Exforge HCT in patients with aortic or mitral stenosis or obstructive hypertrophic cardiomyopathy.
If excessive hypotension occurs with Exforge HCT, the patient should be placed in a supine position and, if necessary, given an intravenous infusion of normal saline. A transient hypotensive response is not a contraindication to further treatment, which usually can be continued without difficulty once the blood pressure has stabilized.
5.3 Increased Angina and/or Myocardial Infarction
Rarely, patients, particularly those with severe obstructive coronary artery disease, have developed documented increased frequency, duration or severity of angina or acute myocardial infarction upon starting calcium channel blocker therapy or at the time of dosage increase. The mechanism of this effect has not been elucidated.
5.4 Impaired Hepatic Function
Amlodipine is extensively metabolized by the liver and the plasma elimination half-life ($t_{1/2}$) is 56 hours in patients with impaired hepatic function.
As the majority of valsartan is eliminated in the bile, patients with mild-to-moderate hepatic impairment, including patients with biliary obstructive disorders, showed lower valsartan clearance (higher AUCs).
In patients with impaired hepatic function or progressive liver disease, minor alterations of fluid and electrolyte balance, such as those resulting from diuretic use, may precipitate hepatic coma.
Therefore, avoid the use of Exforge HCT in patients with severe hepatic impairment. When administering Exforge HCT to patients with mild-to-moderate hepatic impairment, including patients with biliary obstructive disorders, monitor for worsening of hepatic or renal function, including fluid status and electrolytes, and adverse reactions.
5.5 Impaired Renal Function
As a consequence of inhibiting the renin-angiotensin-aldosterone system, changes in renal function may be anticipated in susceptible individuals. In patients with severe heart failure whose renal function may depend on the activity of the renin-angiotensin-aldosterone system, treatment with angiotensin-converting enzyme inhibitors and angiotensin receptor antagonists has been associated with oliguria and/or progressive azotemia and (rarely) with acute renal failure and/or death. Similar outcomes have been reported with valsartan.
In studies of ACE inhibitors in hypertensive patients with unilateral or bilateral renal artery stenosis, increases in serum creatinine or blood urea nitrogen have been reported. In a 4-day trial of valsartan in 12 hypertensive patients with unilateral renal artery stenosis, no significant increases in serum creatinine or blood urea nitrogen were observed. There has been no long-term use of valsartan in patients with unilateral or bilateral renal artery stenosis, but an effect similar to that seen with ACE inhibitors should be anticipated.

In patients with renal disease, thiazides may precipitate azotemia. Cumulative effects of the drug may develop in patients with impaired renal function.

Avoid use of Exforge HCT in severe renal disease (creatinine clearance ≤30 mL/min). The usual regimens of therapy with Exforge HCT may be followed if the patient's creatinine clearance is >30 mL/min.

There is no experience in the use of Exforge HCT in patients with a recent kidney transplant.

5.6 Heart Failure

Exforge HCT has not been studied in patients with heart failure.

Studies with amlodipine: In general, calcium channel blockers should be used with close monitoring, including close follow-up of fluid status, electrolytes, renal function, and blood pressure in patients with heart failure. Amlodipine (5-10 mg per day) has been studied in a placebo-controlled trial of 1,153 patients with NYHA Class III or IV heart failure on stable doses of ACE inhibitor, digoxin, and diuretics. Follow-up was at least 6 months, with a mean of about 14 months. There was no overall adverse effect on survival or cardiac morbidity (as defined by life-threatening arrhythmia, acute myocardial infarction, or hospitalization for worsened heart failure). Amlodipine has been compared to placebo in four 8-12 week studies of patients with NYHA Class II/III heart failure, involving a total of 697 patients. In these studies, there was no evidence of worsened heart failure based on measures of exercise tolerance, NYHA classification, symptoms, or LVEF.

Studies with valsartan: Some patients with heart failure have developed increases in blood urea nitrogen, serum creatinine, and potassium on valsartan. These effects are usually minor and transient, and they are more likely to occur in patients with pre-existing renal impairment. Dosage reduction and/or discontinuation of the diuretic and/or valsartan may be required. In the Valsartan Heart Failure Trial, in which 93% of patients were on concomitant ACE inhibitors, treatment was discontinued for elevations in creatinine or potassium (total of 1.0% on valsartan vs. 0.2% on placebo). In the Valsartan in Acute Myocardial Infarction Trial (VALIANT), discontinuation due to various types of renal dysfunction occurred in 1.1% of valsartan-treated patients and 0.8% of captopril-treated patients. Evaluation of patients with heart failure or post-myocardial infarction should always include assessment of renal function.

5.7 Hypersensitivity Reaction

Hypersensitivity reactions to hydrochlorothiazide may occur in patients with or without a history of allergy or bronchial asthma, but are more likely in patients with such a history.

5.8 Systemic Lupus Erythematosus

Thiazide diuretics have been reported to cause exacerbation or activation of systemic lupus erythematosus.

5.9 Lithium Interaction

Lithium generally should not be given with thiazides [see *Drug Interactions, Hydrochlorothiazide, Lithium (7)*].

5.10 Electrolytes and Metabolic Imbalances

Amlodipine-Valsartan-Hydrochlorothiazide

In the controlled trial of Exforge HCT in moderate to severe hypertensive patients, the incidence of hypokalemia (serum potassium <3.5 mEq/L) at any time post-baseline with the maximum dose of Exforge HCT (10/320/25 mg) was 10% compared to 25% with HCTZ/amlodipine (25/10 mg), 7% with valsartan/HCTZ (320/25 mg), and 3% with amlodipine/valsartan (10/320 mg). One patient (0.2%) discontinued therapy due to an adverse event of hypokalemia in each of the Exforge HCT and HCTZ/amlodipine groups. The incidence of hyperkalemia (serum potassium >5.7 mEq/L) was 0.4% with Exforge HCT compared to 0.2-0.7% with the dual therapies. Monitor serum electrolytes periodically based on Exforge HCT use and other factors such as renal function, other medications, or history of prior electrolyte imbalances.

Hydrochlorothiazide

All patients receiving thiazide therapy should be observed for clinical signs of fluid or electrolyte imbalance: hyponatremia, hypochloremic alkalosis, and hypokalemia. Serum and urine electrolyte determinations are particularly important when the patient is vomiting excessively or receiving parenteral fluids. Warning signs or symptoms of fluid and electrolyte imbalance, irrespective of cause, include dryness of mouth, thirst, weakness, lethargy, drowsiness, restlessness, confusion, seizures, muscle pains or cramps, muscular fatigue, hypotension, oliguria, tachycardia, and gastrointestinal disturbances such as nausea and vomiting.

Hypokalemia may develop, especially with brisk diuresis, when severe cirrhosis is present, or after prolonged therapy. Interference with adequate oral electrolyte intake will also contribute to hypokalemia. Hypokalemia may cause cardiac arrhythmia and may also sensitize or exaggerate the response of the heart to the toxic effects of digitalis (e.g., increased ventricular irritability).

Although any chloride deficit is generally mild and usually does not require specific treatment except under extraordinary circumstances (as in liver disease or renal disease), chloride replacement may be required in the treatment of metabolic alkalosis.

Dilutional hyponatremia may occur in edematous patients in hot weather; appropriate therapy is water restriction, rather than administration of salt except in rare instances when the hyponatremia is life-threatening. In actual salt depletion, appropriate replacement is the therapy of choice. Hyperuricemia may occur or frank gout may be precipitated in certain patients receiving thiazide therapy.

In diabetic patients, dosage adjustments of insulin or oral hypoglycemic agents may be required. Hyperglycemia may occur with thiazide diuretics. Thus latent diabetes mellitus may become manifest during thiazide therapy.

The antihypertensive effects of the drug may be enhanced in the postsympathectomy patient.

If progressive renal impairment becomes evident, consider withholding or discontinuing Exforge HCT therapy or substituting other antihypertensive therapy.

Thiazides have been shown to increase the urinary excretion of magnesium; this may result in hypomagnesemia.

Thiazides may decrease urinary calcium excretion. Thiazides may cause intermittent and slight elevation of serum calcium in the absence of known disorders of calcium metabolism. Marked hypercalcemia may be evidence of hidden hyperparathyroidism. Exforge HCT should be discontinued or non-thiazide antihypertensive therapy substituted before carrying out tests for parathyroid function.

Increases in cholesterol and triglyceride levels may be associated with thiazide diuretic therapy.

6 ADVERSE REACTIONS

6.1 Clinical Trials Experience

Because clinical studies are conducted under widely varying conditions, adverse reaction rates observed in the clinical studies of a drug cannot be directly compared to rates in the clinical studies of another drug and may not reflect the rates observed in clinical practice.

In the controlled trial of Exforge HCT, where only the maximum dose (10/320/25 mg) was evaluated, safety data were obtained in 582 patients with hypertension. Adverse reactions have generally been mild and transient in nature and have only infrequently required discontinuation of therapy. The overall frequency of adverse reactions was similar between men and women, younger (<65 years) and older (≥65 years) patients, and black and white patients. In the active controlled clinical trial, discontinuation because of adverse events occurred in 4.0% of patients treated with Exforge HCT 10/320/25 mg compared to 2.9% of patients treated with valsartan/HCTZ 320/25 mg, 1.6% of patients treated with amlodipine/valsartan 10/320 mg, and 3.4% of patients treated with HCTZ/amlodipine 25/10 mg. The most common reasons for discontinuation of therapy with Exforge HCT were dizziness (1.0%) and hypotension (0.7%).

The most frequent adverse events that occurred in the active controlled clinical trial in at least 2% of patients treated with Exforge HCT are presented in the table below:

[See table below]

Orthostatic events (orthostatic hypotension and postural dizziness) were seen in 0.5% of patients. Other adverse reactions that occurred in clinical trials with Exforge HCT (>0.2%) are listed below. It cannot be determined whether these events were causally related to Exforge HCT.

Cardiac Disorders: tachycardia

Ear and Labyrinth Disorders: vertigo, tinnitus

Eye Disorders: vision blurred

Gastrointestinal Disorders: diarrhea, abdominal pain upper, vomiting, abdominal pain, toothache, dry mouth, gastritis, hemorrhoids

General Disorders and Administration Site Conditions: asthenia, non-cardiac chest pain, chills, malaise

Infections and Infestations: upper respiratory tract infection, bronchitis, influenza, pharyngitis, tooth abscess, gastroenteritis viral, respiratory tract infection, rhinitis, urinary tract infection

Injury, Poisoning and Procedural Complications: back injury, contusion, joint sprain, procedural pain

Investigations: blood uric acid increased, blood creatine phosphokinase increased, weight decreased

Metabolism and Nutrition Disorders: hypokalaemia, diabetes mellitus, hyperlipidemia, hyponatremia

Musculoskeletal and Connective Tissue Disorders: pain in extremity, arthralgia, musculoskeletal pain, muscular weakness, musculoskeletal weakness, musculoskeletal stiffness, joint swelling, neck pain, osteoarthritis, tendonitis

Nervous System Disorders: paraesthesia, somnolence, syncope, carpal tunnel syndrome, disturbance in attention, dizziness postural, dysgeusia, head discomfort, lethargy, sinus headache, tremor

Psychiatric Disorders: anxiety, depression, insomnia

Renal and Urinary Disorders: pollakiuria

Reproductive System and Breast Disorders: erectile dysfunction

Respiratory, Thoracic and Mediastinal Disorders: dyspnea, nasal congestion, cough, pharyngolaryngeal pain

Skin and Subcutaneous Tissue Disorders: pruritus, hyperhidrosis, night sweats, rash

Vascular Disorders: hypotension

Isolated cases of the following clinically notable adverse reactions were also observed in clinical trials: anorexia, constipation, dehydration, dysuria, increased appetite, viral infection.

Amlodipine

Amlodipine has been evaluated for safety in more than 11,000 patients in U.S. and foreign clinical trials. Other adverse reactions not listed above that have been reported in <1% but >0.1% of patients in controlled clinical trials or under conditions of open trials or marketing experience where a causal relationship is uncertain were:

Cardiovascular: arrhythmia (including ventricular tachycardia and atrial fibrillation), bradycardia, chest pain, peripheral ischemia, syncope, postural hypotension, vasculitis

Central and Peripheral Nervous System: neuropathy peripheral, tremor

Gastrointestinal: anorexia, dysphagia, pancreatitis, gingival hyperplasia

General: allergic reaction, hot flushes, malaise, rigors, weight gain

Musculoskeletal System: arthrosis, muscle cramps

Psychiatric: sexual dysfunction (male and female), nervousness, abnormal dreams, depersonalization

Skin and Appendages: angioedema, erythema multiforme, rash erythematous, rash maculopapular

Special Senses: abnormal vision, conjunctivitis, diplopia, eye pain, tinnitus

Urinary System: micturation frequency, micturation disorder, nocturia

Autonomic Nervous System: sweating increased

Metabolic and Nutritional: hyperglycemia, thirst

Hemopoietic: leukopenia, purpura, thrombocytopenia

Other adverse reactions reported with amlodipine at a frequency of ≤0.1% of patients include: cardiac failure, pulse irregularity, extrasystoles, skin discoloration, urticaria, skin dryness, alopecia, dermatitis, muscle weakness, twitching, ataxia, hypertonia, migraine, cold and clammy skin, apathy, agitation, amnesia, gastritis, increased appetite, loose stools, rhinitis, dysuria, polyuria, parosmia, taste perversion, abnormal visual accommodation, and xerophthalmia. Other reactions occurred sporadically and cannot be distinguished from medications or concurrent disease states such as myocardial infarction and angina.

Adverse reactions reported for amlodipine for indications other than hypertension may be found in its full prescribing information.

Valsartan

Valsartan has been evaluated for safety in more than 4,000 hypertensive patients in clinical trials. In trials in which valsartan was compared to an ACE inhibitor with or without placebo, the incidence of dry cough was significantly greater in the ACE inhibitor group (7.9%) than in the groups who received valsartan (2.6%) or placebo (1.5%). In a 129 patient trial limited to patients who had had dry cough when they had previously received ACE inhibitors, the incidences of cough in patients who received valsartan, HCTZ, or lisinopril were 20%, 19%, and 69% respectively (p<0.001).

Preferred Term	Aml/Val/HCTZ 10/320/25 mg N=582 n (%)	Val/HCTZ 320/25 mg N=559 n (%)	Aml/Val 10/320 mg N=566 n (%)	HCTZ/Aml 25/10 mg N=561 n (%)
Dizziness	48 (8.2)	40 (7.2)	14 (2.5)	23 (4.1)
Edema	38 (6.5)	8 (1.4)	65 (11.5)	63 (11.2)
Headache	30 (5.2)	31 (5.5)	30 (5.3)	40 (7.1)
Dyspepsia	13 (2.2)	5 (0.9)	6 (1.1)	2 (0.4)
Fatigue	13 (2.2)	15 (2.7)	12 (2.1)	8 (1.4)
Muscle spasms	13 (2.2)	7 (1.3)	7 (1.2)	5 (0.9)
Back pain	12 (2.1)	13 (2.3)	5 (0.9)	12 (2.1)
Nausea	12 (2.1)	7 (1.3)	10 (1.8)	12 (2.1)
Nasopharyngitis	12 (2.1)	13 (2.3)	13 (2.3)	12 (2.1)

Other adverse reactions, not listed above, occurring in >0.2% of patients in controlled clinical trials with valsartan are:

Digestive: flatulence
Respiratory: sinusitis, pharyngitis
Urogenital: impotence

Adverse reactions reported for valsartan for indications other than hypertension may be found in the prescribing information for Diovan.

Hydrochlorothiazide
Other adverse reactions not listed above that have been reported with hydrochlorothiazide, without regard to causality, are listed below:
Body as a Whole: weakness
Digestive: pancreatitis, jaundice (intrahepatic cholestatic jaundice), sialadenitis, cramping, gastric irritation
Hematologic: aplastic anemia, agranulocytosis, hemolytic anemia
Hypersensitivity: photosensitivity, urticaria, necrotizing angiitis (vasculitis and cutaneous vasculitis), fever, respiratory distress including pneumonitis and pulmonary edema, anaphylactic reactions
Metabolic: glycosuria, hyperuricemia
Nervous System/Psychiatric: restlessness
Renal: renal failure, renal dysfunction, interstitial nephritis
Skin: erythema multiforme including Stevens-Johnson syndrome, exfoliative dermatitis including toxic epidermal necrolysis
Special Senses: transient blurred vision, xanthopsia.

6.2   Post-Marketing Experience
Amlodipine
With amlodipine, gynecomastia has been reported infrequently and a causal relationship is uncertain. Jaundice and hepatic enzyme elevations (mostly consistent with cholestasis or hepatitis), in some cases severe enough to require hospitalization, have been reported in association with use of amlodipine.

Valsartan
The following additional adverse reactions have been reported in post-marketing experience with valsartan or valsartan/hydrochlorothiazide:
Blood and Lymphatic: There are very rare reports of thrombocytopenia.
Hypersensitivity: There are rare reports of angioedema.
Digestive: Elevated liver enzymes and very rare reports of hepatitis
Renal: Impaired renal function
Clinical Laboratory Tests: Hyperkalemia
Dermatologic: Alopecia
Vascular: Vasculitis
Nervous System: Syncope
Rare cases of rhabdomyolysis have been reported in patients receiving angiotensin II receptor blockers. Because these reactions are reported voluntarily from a population of uncertain size, it is not always possible to reliably estimate their frequency or establish a causal relationship to drug exposure.

7   DRUG INTERACTIONS
No drug interaction studies have been conducted with Exforge HCT and other drugs, although studies have been conducted with the individual components. A pharmacokinetic drug-drug interaction study has been conducted to address the potential for pharmacokinetic interaction between the triple combination, Exforge HCT, and the corresponding three double combinations. No clinically relevant interaction was observed.

Amlodipine
In clinical trials, amlodipine has been safely administered with thiazide diuretics, beta-blockers, angiotensin-converting enzyme inhibitors, long-acting nitrates, sublingual nitroglycerin, digoxin, warfarin, non-steroidal anti-inflammatory drugs, antibiotics, and oral hypoglycemic drugs.
Cimetidine: Co-administration of amlodipine with cimetidine did not alter the pharmacokinetics of amlodipine.
Grapefruit juice: Co-administration of 240 mL of grapefruit juice with a single oral dose of amlodipine 10 mg in 20 healthy volunteers had no significant effect on the pharmacokinetics of amlodipine.
Magnesium and aluminum hydroxide (antacid): Co-administration of the magnesium and aluminum hydroxide antacid with a single dose of amlodipine had no significant effect on the pharmacokinetics of amlodipine.
Sildenafil: A single 100 mg dose of sildenafil in subjects with essential hypertension had no effect on the pharmacokinetic parameters of amlodipine. When amlodipine and sildenafil were used in combination, each agent independently exerted its own blood pressure lowering effect.
Atorvastatin: Co-administration of multiple 10 mg doses of amlodipine with 80 mg of atorvastatin resulted in no significant change in the steady state pharmacokinetic parameters of atorvastatin.

Digoxin: Co-administration of amlodipine with digoxin did not change serum digoxin levels or digoxin renal clearance in normal volunteers.
Warfarin: Co-administration of amlodipine with warfarin did not change the warfarin prothrombin response time.
Valsartan
No clinically significant pharmacokinetic interactions were observed when valsartan was co-administered with amlodipine, atenolol, cimetidine, digoxin, furosemide, glyburide, hydrochlorothiazide, or indomethacin. The valsartan-atenolol combination was more antihypertensive than either component, but it did not lower the heart rate more than atenolol alone.
In vitro metabolism studies have indicated that CYP450 mediated drug interaction between valsartan and co-administered drugs are unlikely because of the low extent of metabolism [see Pharmacokinetics – Valsartan (12.3)].
Co-administration of valsartan and warfarin did not change the pharmacokinetics of valsartan or the time-course of the anticoagulant properties of warfarin.
As with other drugs that block angiotensin II or its effects, concomitant use of potassium sparing diuretics (e.g., spironolactone, triamterene, amiloride), potassium supplements, or salt substitutes containing potassium may lead to increases in serum potassium and in heart failure patients to increases in serum creatinine.
Hydrochlorothiazide
When administered concurrently the following drugs may interact with thiazide diuretics:
Alcohol, barbiturates, or narcotics: Potentiation of orthostatic hypotension may occur.
Antidiabetic drugs (oral agents and insulin): Dosage adjustment of the antidiabetic drug may be required.
Other antihypertensive drugs: Additive effect or potentiation.
Cholestyramine and colestipol resins: Absorption of hydrochlorothiazide is impaired in the presence of anionic exchange resins. Single doses of either cholestyramine or colestipol resins bind the hydrochlorothiazide and reduce its absorption from the gastrointestinal tract by up to 85% and 43% respectively.
Corticosteroids, ACTH: Intensified electrolyte depletion, particularly hypokalemia.
Pressor amines (e.g., norepinephrine): Possible decreased response to pressor amines but not sufficient to preclude their use.
Skeletal muscle relaxants, nondepolarizing (e.g., tubocurarine): Possible increased responsiveness to the muscle relaxant.
Lithium: Should not generally be given with diuretics. Diuretic agents reduce the renal clearance of lithium and add a high risk of lithium toxicity. Refer to the package insert for lithium preparations before use of such preparations with Exforge HCT.
Non-steroidal anti-inflammatory drugs: In some patients, the administration of a non-steroidal anti-inflammatory agent can reduce the diuretic, natriuretic, and antihypertensive effects of loop, potassium-sparing and thiazide diuretics.
Carbamazepine: May lead to symptomatic hyponatremia.
7.1   Clinical Laboratory Test Findings
Clinical laboratory test findings for Exforge HCT were obtained in a controlled trial of Exforge HCT administered at the maximal dose of 10/320/25 mg compared to maximal doses of dual therapies, i.e., valsartan/HCTZ 320/25 mg, amlodipine/valsartan 10/320 mg, and HCTZ/amlodipine 25/10 mg. Findings for the components of Exforge HCT were obtained from other trials.
Creatinine: In hypertensive patients, greater than 50% increases in creatinine occurred in 2.1% of Exforge HCT patients compared to 2.4% of valsartan/HCTZ patients, 0.7% of amlodipine/valsartan patients, and 1.8% of HCTZ/amlodipine patients.
In heart failure patients, greater than 50% increases in creatinine were observed in 3.9% of valsartan-treated patients compared to 0.9% of placebo-treated patients. In post-myocardial infarction patients, doubling of serum creatinine was observed in 4.2% of valsartan-treated patients and 3.4% of captopril-treated patients.
Liver Function Tests: Occasional elevations (greater than 150%) of liver chemistries occurred in Exforge HCT-treated patients.
Blood Urea Nitrogen (BUN): In hypertensive patients, greater than 50% increases in BUN were observed in 30% of Exforge HCT-treated patients compared to 29% of valsartan/HCTZ patients, 15.8% of amlodipine/valsartan patients, and 18.5% of HCTZ/amlodipine patients. The majority of BUN values remained within normal limits.
In heart failure patients, greater than 50% increases in BUN were observed in 17% of valsartan-treated patients compared to 6% of placebo-treated patients.
Serum Electrolytes (Potassium): In hypertensive patients, greater than 20% decreases in serum potassium were observed in 6.5% of Exforge HCT-treated patients compared to

3.3% of valsartan/HCTZ patients, 0.4% of amlodipine/valsartan patients, and 19.3% of HCTZ/amlodipine patients. Greater than 20% increases in potassium were observed in 3.5% of Exforge HCT-treated patients compared to 2.4% of valsartan/HCTZ patients, 6.2% of amlodipine/valsartan patients, and 2.2% of HCTZ/amlodipine patients. In heart failure patients, greater than 20% increases in serum potassium were observed in 10% of valsartan-treated patients compared to 5.1% of placebo-treated patients [see Warnings and Precautions, Electrolytes and Metabolic Imbalances (5.10)].
Neutropenia: Neutropenia (<1500/L) was observed in 1.9% of patients treated with valsartan and 0.8% of patients treated with placebo.
7.3   Drug/Food Interactions
The bioavailability of amlodipine, valsartan, and HCTZ were not altered when Exforge HCT was administered with food.

8   USE IN SPECIFIC POPULATIONS
8.1   Pregnancy
Pregnancy Category D
Valsartan, like other drugs that act on the renin-angiotensin system, can cause fetal and neonatal morbidity and death when used during the second or third trimester of pregnancy. If Exforge HCT is used during pregnancy, or if the patient becomes pregnant while taking this drug, the patient should be apprised of the potential hazard to the fetus.
Angiotensin II receptor antagonists, like valsartan, and angiotensin-converting enzyme (ACE) inhibitors exert similar effects on the renin-angiotensin system. In several dozen published cases, ACE inhibitor use during the second and third trimesters of pregnancy was associated with fetal and neonatal injury, including hypotension, neonatal skull hypoplasia, anuria, reversible or irreversible renal failure, and death. Oligohydramnios was also reported, presumably from decreased fetal renal function. In this setting, oligohydramnios was associated with fetal limb contractures, craniofacial deformation, and hypoplastic lung development. Prematurity, intrauterine growth retardation, and patent ductus arteriosus were also reported, although it is not clear whether these occurrences were due to exposure to the drug. In a retrospective study, first trimester use of ACE inhibitors, a specific class of drugs acting on the renin-angiotensin system, was associated with a potential risk of birth defects.
When pregnancy occurs in a patient using Exforge HCT, the physician should discontinue Exforge HCT treatment as soon as possible. The physician should inform the patient about potential risks to the fetus based on the time of gestational exposure to Exforge HCT (first trimester only or later). If exposure occurs beyond the first trimester, an ultrasound examination should be done.
In rare cases when another antihypertensive agent cannot be used to treat the pregnant patient, serial ultrasound examinations should be performed to assess the intraamniotic environment. Routine fetal testing with non-stress tests, biophysical profiles, and/or contraction stress tests may be appropriate based on gestational age and standards of care in the community. If oligohydramnios occurs in these situations, individualized decisions about continuing or discontinuing Exforge HCT treatment and about pregnancy management should be made by the patient, her physician, and experts in the management of high risk pregnancy. Patients and physicians should be aware that oligohydramnios may not appear until after the fetus has sustained irreversible injury.
Infants with histories of in utero exposure to Exforge HCT should be closely observed for hypotension, oliguria, and hyperkalemia. If oliguria occurs, these infants may require blood pressure and renal perfusion support. Exchange transfusion or dialysis may be required to reverse hypotension and/or support decreased renal function.
Healthcare professionals who prescribe drugs acting directly on the renin-angiotensin system should counsel women of childbearing potential about the risks of these agents during pregnancy [see Nonclinical Toxicology (13.3)].
8.3   Nursing Mothers
It is not known whether amlodipine and valsartan are excreted in human milk, but thiazides are excreted in human milk and valsartan is excreted in rat milk. Because of the potential for adverse effects on the nursing infant, a decision should be made whether to discontinue nursing or discontinue the drug, taking into account the importance of the drug to the mother.
8.4   Pediatric Use
The safety and effectiveness of Exforge HCT in pediatric patients have not been established.
8.5   Geriatric Use
In controlled clinical trials, 82 hypertensive patients treated with Exforge HCT were ≥65 years and 13 were ≥75 years. No overall differences in the efficacy or safety of Exforge

HCT were observed in this patient population, but greater sensitivity of some older individuals cannot be ruled out.

10 OVERDOSAGE

Limited data are available related to overdosage in humans. The most likely manifestations of overdosage would be hypotension and tachycardia; bradycardia could occur from parasympathetic (vagal) stimulation. If symptomatic hypotension should occur, supportive treatment should be instituted.

Amlodipine

Single oral doses of amlodipine maleate equivalent to 40 mg/kg and 100 mg/kg amlodipine in mice and rats, respectively, caused deaths. Single oral doses equivalent to 4 or more mg/kg amlodipine in dogs (11 or more times the maximum recommended human dose on a mg/m^2 basis) caused a marked peripheral vasodilation and hypotension. Overdosage might be expected to cause excessive peripheral vasodilation with marked hypotension. In humans, experience with intentional overdosage of amlodipine is limited. Reports of intentional overdosage include a patient who ingested 250 mg and was asymptomatic and was not hospitalized; another (120 mg) who was hospitalized underwent gastric lavage and remained normotensive; the third (105 mg) was hospitalized and had hypotension (90/50 mmHg) which normalized following plasma expansion. A case of accidental drug overdose has been documented in a 19-month-old male who ingested 30 mg amlodipine (about 2 mg/kg). During the emergency room presentation, vital signs were stable with no evidence of hypotension, but a heart rate of 180 bpm. Ipecac was administered 3.5 hours after ingestion and on subsequent observation (overnight) no sequelae were noted.

If massive overdose should occur, active cardiac and respiratory monitoring should be instituted. Frequent blood pressure measurements are essential. Should hypotension occur, cardiovascular support including elevation of the extremities and the judicious administration of fluids should be initiated. If hypotension remains unresponsive to these conservative measures, administration of vasopressors (such as phenylephrine) should be considered with attention to circulating volume and urine output. Intravenous calcium gluconate may help to reverse the effects of calcium entry blockade. As amlodipine is highly protein bound, hemodialysis is not likely to be of benefit.

Valsartan

Depressed level of consciousness, circulatory collapse and shock have been reported.

Valsartan is not removed from the plasma by hemodialysis. Valsartan was without grossly observable adverse effects at single oral doses up to 2000 mg/kg in rats and up to 1000 mg/kg in marmosets, except for the salivation and diarrhea in the rat and vomiting in the marmoset at the highest dose (60 and 31 times, respectively, the maximum recommended human dose on a mg/m^2 basis). (Calculations assume an oral dose of 320 mg/day and a 60-kg patient.)

Hydrochlorothiazide

The degree to which hydrochlorothiazide is removed by hemodialysis has not been established. The most common signs and symptoms observed in patients are those caused by electrolyte depletion (hypokalemia, hypochloremia, hyponatremia) and dehydration resulting from excessive diuresis. If digitalis has also been administered, hypokalemia may accentuate cardiac arrhythmias.

The oral LD_{50} of hydrochlorothiazide is greater than 10 g/kg in both mice and rats, 2000 and 4000 times, respectively, the maximum recommended human dose on a mg/m^2 basis. (Calculations assume an oral dose of 25 mg/day and a 60-kg patient.)

Valsartan and Hydrochlorothiazide

In rats and marmosets, single oral doses of valsartan up to 1524 and 762 mg/kg in combination with hydrochlorothiazide at doses up to 476 and 238 mg/kg, respectively, were very well tolerated without any treatment-related effects. These no adverse effect doses in rats and marmosets, respectively, represent 46.5 and 23 times the maximum recommended human dose (MRHD) of valsartan and 188 and 113 times the MRHD of hydrochlorothiazide on a mg/m^2 basis. (Calculations assume an oral dose of 320 mg/day valsartan in combination with 25 mg/day hydrochlorothiazide and a 60-kg patient.)

11 DESCRIPTION

Exforge HCT is a fixed combination of amlodipine, valsartan and hydrochlorothiazide.

Exforge HCT contains the besylate salt of amlodipine, a dihydropyridine calcium channel blocker (CCB). Amlodipine besylate, USP is a white to pale yellow crystalline powder, slightly soluble in water and sparingly soluble in ethanol. Amlodipine besylate's chemical name is 3-Ethyl 5-methyl (±)-2-[(2-aminoethoxy)methyl]-4-(*o*-chlorophenyl)-1,4-dihydro-6-methyl-3,5-pyridinedicarboxylate, monobenzenesulfonate; its structural formula is

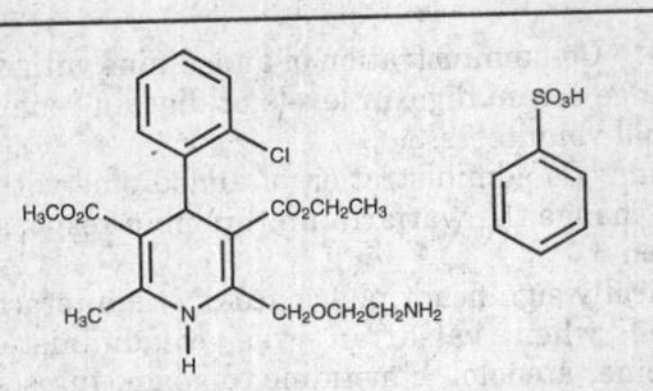

Its empirical formula is $C_{20}H_{25}ClN_2O_5 \bullet C_6H_6O_3S$ and its molecular weight is 567.1.

Valsartan, USP is a nonpeptide, orally active, and specific angiotensin II antagonist acting on the AT_1 receptor subtype. Valsartan is a white to practically white fine powder, soluble in ethanol and methanol and slightly soluble in water. Valsartan's chemical name is N-(1-oxopentyl)-N-[[2'-(1*H*-tetrazol-5-yl) [1,1'-biphenyl]-4-yl]methyl]-L-valine; its structural formula is

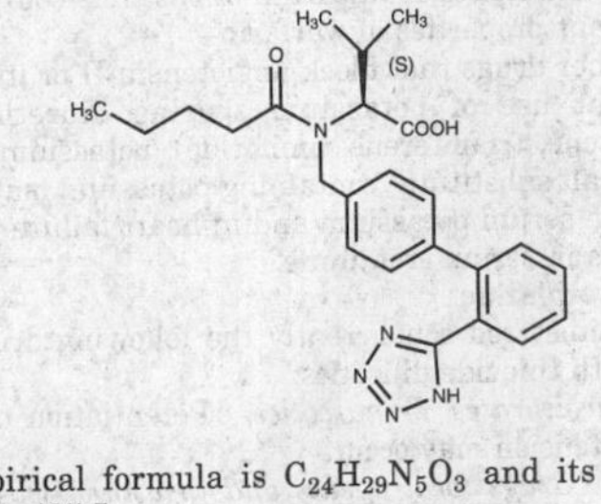

Its empirical formula is $C_{24}H_{29}N_5O_3$ and its molecular weight is 435.5.

Hydrochlorothiazide, USP is a white, or practically white, practically odorless, crystalline powder. It is slightly soluble in water; freely soluble in sodium hydroxide solution, in *n*-butylamine, and in dimethylformamide; sparingly soluble in methanol; and insoluble in ether, in chloroform, and in dilute mineral acids. Hydrochlorothiazide is chemically described as 6-chloro-3,4-dihydro-2*H*-1,2,4-benzothiadiazine-7-sulfonamide 1,1-dioxide.

Hydrochlorothiazide is a thiazide diuretic. Its empirical formula is $C_7H_8ClN_3O_4S_2$, its molecular weight is 297.73, and its structural formula is

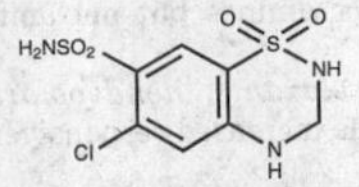

Exforge HCT film-coated tablets are formulated in five strengths for oral administration with a combination of amlodipine besylate, valsartan and hydrochlorothiazide, providing for the following available combinations: 5/160/12.5 mg, 10/160/12.5 mg, 5/160/25 mg, 10/160/25 mg and 10/320/25 mg amlodipine besylate/valsartan/hydrochlorothiazide. The inactive ingredients for all strengths of the tablets include microcrystalline cellulose; crospovidone; colloidal anhydrous silica; magnesium stearate; hypromellose, macrogol 4000 and talc. Additionally, the 5/160/12.5 mg strength contains titanium dioxide; the 10/160/12.5 strength contains titanium dioxide and yellow and red iron oxides; the 5/160/25 mg strength contains titanium dioxide and yellow iron oxide and the 10/160/25 mg and 10/320/25 mg strengths both contain yellow iron oxide.

12 CLINICAL PHARMACOLOGY

12.1 Mechanism of Action

The active ingredients of Exforge HCT target three separate mechanisms involved in blood pressure regulation. Specifically, amlodipine blocks the contractile effects of calcium on cardiac and vascular smooth muscle cells; valsartan blocks the vasoconstriction and sodium retaining effects of angiotensin II on cardiac, vascular smooth muscle, adrenal and renal cells; and hydrochlorothiazide directly promotes the excretion of sodium and chloride in the kidney leading to reductions in intravascular volume. A more detailed description of the mechanism of action of each individual component follows.

Amlodipine

Amlodipine is a dihydropyridine calcium channel blocker that inhibits the transmembrane influx of calcium ions into vascular smooth muscle and cardiac muscle. Experimental data suggest that amlodipine binds to both dihydropyridine and nondihydropyridine binding sites. The contractile processes of cardiac muscle and vascular smooth muscle are dependent upon the movement of extracellular calcium ions into these cells through specific ion channels. Amlodipine inhibits calcium ion influx across cell membranes selectively, with a greater effect on vascular smooth muscle cells than on cardiac muscle cells. Negative inotropic effects can be detected *in vitro* but such effects have not been seen in intact animals at therapeutic doses. Serum calcium concentration is not affected by amlodipine. Within the physiologic pH range, amlodipine is an ionized compound (pKa=8.6), and its kinetic interaction with the calcium channel receptor is characterized by a gradual rate of association and dissociation with the receptor binding site, resulting in a gradual onset of effect.

Amlodipine is a peripheral arterial vasodilator that acts directly on vascular smooth muscle to cause a reduction in peripheral vascular resistance and reduction in blood pressure.

Valsartan

Angiotensin II is formed from angiotensin I in a reaction catalyzed by angiotensin-converting enzyme (ACE, kininase II). Angiotensin II is the principal pressor agent of the renin-angiotensin system, with effects that include vasoconstriction, stimulation of synthesis and release of aldosterone, cardiac stimulation, and renal reabsorption of sodium. Valsartan blocks the vasoconstrictor and aldosterone-secreting effects of angiotensin II by selectively blocking the binding of angiotensin II to the AT_1 receptor in many tissues, such as vascular smooth muscle and the adrenal gland. Its action is therefore independent of the pathways for angiotensin II synthesis.

There is also an AT_2 receptor found in many tissues, but AT_2 is not known to be associated with cardiovascular homeostasis. Valsartan has much greater affinity (about 20,000-fold) for the AT_1 receptor than for the AT_2 receptor. The increased plasma levels of angiotensin following AT_1 receptor blockade with valsartan may stimulate the unblocked AT_2 receptor. The primary metabolite of valsartan is essentially inactive with an affinity for the AT_1 receptor about one-200th that of valsartan itself.

Blockade of the renin-angiotensin system with ACE inhibitors, which inhibit the biosynthesis of angiotensin II from angiotensin I, is widely used in the treatment of hypertension. ACE inhibitors also inhibit the degradation of bradykinin, a reaction also catalyzed by ACE. Because valsartan does not inhibit ACE (kininase II), it does not affect the response to bradykinin. Whether this difference has clinical relevance is not yet known. Valsartan does not bind to or block other hormone receptors or ion channels known to be important in cardiovascular regulation.

Blockade of the angiotensin II receptor inhibits the negative regulatory feedback of angiotensin II on renin secretion, but the resulting increased plasma renin activity and angiotensin II circulating levels do not overcome the effect of valsartan on blood pressure.

Hydrochlorothiazide

Hydrochlorothiazide is a thiazide diuretic. Thiazides affect the renal tubular mechanisms of electrolyte reabsorption, directly increasing excretion of sodium and chloride in approximately equivalent amounts. Indirectly, the diuretic action of hydrochlorothiazide reduces plasma volume, with consequent increases in plasma renin activity, increases in aldosterone secretion, increases in urinary potassium loss, and decreases in serum potassium. The renin-aldosterone link is mediated by angiotensin II, so coadministration of an angiotensin II receptor antagonist tends to reverse the potassium loss associated with these diuretics.

The mechanism of the antihypertensive effect of thiazides is unknown.

12.2 Pharmacodynamics

Exforge HCT has been shown to be effective in lowering blood pressure. The three components of Exforge HCT (amlodipine, valsartan, hydrochlorothiazide) lower the blood pressure through complementary mechanisms, each working at a separate site and blocking different effector pathways. The pharmacodynamics of each individual component is described below.

Exforge HCT has not been studied in indications other than hypertension.

Amlodipine

Following administration of therapeutic doses to patients with hypertension, amlodipine produces vasodilation resulting in a reduction of supine and standing blood pressures. These decreases in blood pressure are not accompanied by a significant change in heart rate or plasma catecholamine levels with chronic dosing. Although the acute intravenous administration of amlodipine decreases arterial blood pressure and increases heart rate in hemodynamic studies of patients with chronic stable angina, chronic oral administration of amlodipine in clinical trials did not lead to clinically significant changes in heart rate or blood pressures in normotensive patients with angina.

With chronic once daily administration, antihypertensive effectiveness is maintained for at least 24 hours. Plasma concentrations correlate with effect in both young and elderly patients. The magnitude of reduction in blood pressure with amlodipine is also correlated with the height of pretreatment elevation; thus, individuals with moderate hypertension (diastolic pressure 105-114 mmHg) had about a 50% greater response than patients with mild hypertension (diastolic pressure 90-104 mmHg). Normotensive subjects experienced no clinically significant change in blood pressure (+1/-2 mmHg).

In hypertensive patients with normal renal function, therapeutic doses of amlodipine resulted in a decrease in renal vascular resistance and an increase in glomerular filtration rate and effective renal plasma flow without change in filtration fraction or proteinuria.

As with other calcium channel blockers, hemodynamic measurements of cardiac function at rest and during exercise (or pacing) in patients with normal ventricular function treated with amlodipine have generally demonstrated a small increase in cardiac index without significant influence on dP/dt or on left ventricular end diastolic pressure or volume. In hemodynamic studies, amlodipine has not been associated with a negative inotropic effect when administered in the therapeutic dose range to intact animals and man, even when co-administered with beta-blockers to man. Similar findings, however, have been observed in normals or well-compensated patients with heart failure with agents possessing significant negative inotropic effects.

Amlodipine does not change sinoatrial nodal function or atrioventricular conduction in intact animals or man. In patients with chronic stable angina, intravenous administration of 10 mg did not significantly alter A-H and H-V conduction and sinus node recovery time after pacing. Similar results were obtained in patients receiving amlodipine and concomitant beta-blockers. In clinical studies in which amlodipine was administered in combination with beta-blockers to patients with either hypertension or angina, no adverse effects of electrocardiographic parameters were observed. In clinical trials with angina patients alone, amlodipine therapy did not alter electrocardiographic intervals or produce higher degrees of AV blocks.

Amlodipine has indications other than hypertension which are described in its full prescribing information.

Valsartan
Valsartan inhibits the pressor effect of angiotensin II infusions. An oral dose of 80 mg inhibits the pressor effect by about 80% at peak with approximately 30% inhibition persisting for 24 hours. No information on the effect of larger doses is available.

Removal of the negative feedback of angiotensin II causes a 2- to 3-fold rise in plasma renin and consequent rise in angiotensin II plasma concentration in hypertensive patients. Minimal decreases in plasma aldosterone were observed after administration of valsartan; very little effect on serum potassium was observed.

In multiple dose studies in hypertensive patients with stable renal insufficiency and patients with renovascular hypertension, valsartan had no clinically significant effects on glomerular filtration rate, filtration fraction, creatinine clearance, or renal plasma flow.

Administration of valsartan to patients with essential hypertension results in a significant reduction of sitting, supine, and standing systolic blood pressure, usually with little or no orthostatic change.

Valsartan has indications other than hypertension which are described in its full prescribing information.

Hydrochlorothiazide
After oral administration of hydrochlorothiazide, diuresis begins within 2 hours, peaks in about 4 hours and lasts about 6 to 12 hours.

12.3   Pharmacokinetics
Exforge HCT
Following oral administration of Exforge HCT in normal healthy adults, peak plasma concentrations of amlodipine, valsartan and HCTZ are reached in about 6 hours, 3 hours, and 2 hours, respectively. The rate and extent of absorption of amlodipine, valsartan and HCTZ from Exforge HCT are the same as when administered as individual dosage forms.

Amlodipine
Peak plasma concentrations of amlodipine are reached 6-12 hours after administration of amlodipine alone. Absolute bioavailability has been estimated to be between 64% and 90%. The apparent volume of distribution of amlodipine is 21 L/kg. Approximately 93% of circulating amlodipine is bound to plasma proteins in hypertensive patients.

Amlodipine is extensively (about 90%) converted to inactive metabolites via hepatic metabolism with 10% of the parent compound and 60% of the metabolites excreted in the urine. Elimination of amlodipine from the plasma is biphasic with a terminal elimination half-life of about 30-50 hours. Steady state plasma levels of amlodipine are reached after 7 to 8 days of consecutive daily dosing.

Valsartan
Following oral administration of valsartan alone peak plasma concentrations of valsartan are reached in 2 to 4 hours. Absolute bioavailability is about 25% (range 10%-35%).

The steady state volume of distribution of valsartan after intravenous administration is 17 L indicating that valsartan does not distribute into tissues extensively. Valsartan is highly bound to serum proteins (95%), mainly serum albumin.

Valsartan shows bi-exponential decay kinetics following intravenous administration with an average elimination half-life of about 6 hours. The recovery is mainly as unchanged drug, with only about 20% of dose recovered as metabolites.

The primary metabolite, accounting for about 9% of dose, is valeryl 4-hydroxy valsartan. *In vitro* metabolism studies involving recombinant CYP450 enzymes indicated that the CYP2C9 isoenzyme is responsible for the formation of valeryl-4-hydroxy valsartan. Valsartan does not inhibit CYP450 isozymes at clinically relevant concentrations. CYP450 mediated drug interaction between valsartan and co-administered drugs are unlikely because of the low extent of metabolism.

Valsartan, when administered as an oral solution, is primarily recovered in feces (about 83% of dose) and urine (about 13% of dose). Following intravenous administration, plasma clearance of valsartan is about 2 L/h and its renal clearance is 0.62 L/h (about 30% of total clearance).

Hydrochlorothiazide
Hydrochlorothiazide is not metabolized but is eliminated rapidly by the kidney. At least 61% of the oral dose is eliminated as unchanged drug within 24 hours. The elimination half-life is between 5.8 and 18.9 hours. Hydrochlorothiazide crosses the placental but not the blood-brain barrier and is excreted in breast milk.

Geriatric
Studies with amlodipine: Elderly patients have decreased clearance of amlodipine with a resulting increase in AUC of approximately 40%-60%; therefore a lower initial dose of amlodipine may be required.

Studies with valsartan: Exposure (measured by AUC) to valsartan is higher by 70% and the half-life is longer by 35% in the elderly than in the young. No dosage adjustment is necessary.

Gender
Studies with valsartan: Pharmacokinetics of valsartan does not differ significantly between males and females.

Renal Insufficiency
Studies with amlodipine: The pharmacokinetics of amlodipine is not significantly influenced by renal impairment. Patients with renal failure may therefore receive the usual initial dose.

Studies with valsartan: There is no apparent correlation between renal function (measured by creatinine clearance) and exposure (measured by AUC) to valsartan in patients with different degrees of renal impairment. Consequently, dose adjustment is not required in patients with mild-to-moderate renal dysfunction. No studies have been performed in patients with severe impairment of renal function (creatinine clearance <10 mL/min). Valsartan is not removed from the plasma by hemodialysis. In the case of severe renal disease, exercise care with dosing of valsartan.

Studies with hydrochlorothiazide: The half-life of hydrochlorothiazide elimination was lengthened to 21 hours in a study of patients with impaired renal function (mean creatinine clearance of 19 mL/min).

Hepatic Insufficiency
Studies with amlodipine: Patients with hepatic insufficiency have decreased clearance of amlodipine with resulting increase in AUC of approximately 40%-60%; therefore, a lower initial dose of amlodipine may be required.

Studies with valsartan: On average, patients with mild-to-moderate chronic liver disease have twice the exposure (measured by AUC values) to valsartan of healthy volunteers (matched by age, sex and weight). In general, no dosage adjustment is needed in patients with mild-to-moderate liver disease. Care should be exercised in patients with liver disease.

13   NONCLINICAL TOXICOLOGY
13.1   Carcinogenesis, Mutagenesis, Impairment of Fertility
Studies with amlodipine/valsartan/hydrochlorothiazide:
No carcinogenicity, mutagenicity or fertility studies have been conducted with this combination. However, these studies have been conducted for amlodipine, valsartan and hydrochlorothiazide alone. Based on the preclinical safety and human pharmacokinetic studies, there is no indication of any toxicologically significant adverse interaction between these components.

Studies with amlodipine: Rats and mice treated with amlodipine maleate in the diet for up to two years, at concentrations calculated to provide daily dosage levels of 0.5, 1.25, and 2.5 mg amlodipine/kg/day, showed no evidence of a carcinogenic effect of the drug. For the mouse, the highest dose was, on mg/m^2 basis, similar to the maximum recommended human dose [MRHD] of 10 mg amlodipine/day. For the rat, the highest dose was, on a mg/m^2 basis, about two and a half times the MRHD. (Calculations based on a 60 kg patient.)

Mutagenicity studies conducted with amlodipine maleate revealed no drug-related effects at either the gene or chromosome level.

There was no effect on the fertility of rats treated orally with amlodipine maleate (males for 64 days and females for 14 days prior to mating) at doses of up to 10 mg amlodipine/kg/day (about 10 times the MRHD of 10 mg/day on a mg/m^2 basis).

Studies with valsartan: There was no evidence of carcinogenicity when valsartan was administered in the diet to mice and rats for up to 2 years at concentrations calculated to provide doses of up to 160 and 200 mg/kg/day, respec-

tively. These doses in mice and rats are about 2.4 and 6 times, respectively, the MRHD of 320 mg/day on a mg/m^2 basis. (Calculations based on a 60 kg patient.)

Mutagenicity assays did not reveal any valsartan-related effects at either the gene or chromosome level. These assays included bacterial mutagenicity tests with Salmonella and E. coli, a gene mutation test with Chinese hamster V79 cells, a cytogenetic test with Chinese hamster ovary cells, and a rat micronucleus test.

Valsartan had no adverse effects on the reproductive performance of male or female rats at oral doses of up to 200 mg/kg/day. This dose is about 6 times the maximum recommended human dose on a mg/m^2 basis.

Studies with hydrochlorothiazide: Two-year feeding studies in mice and rats conducted under the auspices of the National Toxicology Program (NTP) uncovered no evidence of a carcinogenic potential of hydrochlorothiazide in female mice (at doses of up to approximately 600 mg/kg/day) or in male and female rats (at doses of up to approximately 100 mg/kg/day). The NTP, however, found equivocal evidence for hepatocarcinogenicity in male mice.

Hydrochlorothiazide was not genotoxic *in vitro* in the Ames mutagenicity assay of Salmonella Typhimurium strains TA 98, TA 100, TA 1535, TA 1537, and TA 1538 and in the Chinese Hamster Ovary (CHO) test for chromosomal aberrations, or *in vivo* in assays using mouse germinal cell chromosomes, Chinese hamster bone marrow chromosomes, and the Drosophila sex-linked recessive lethal trait gene. Positive test results were obtained in the *in vitro* CHO Sister Chromatid Exchange (clastogenicity) and Mouse Lymphoma Cell (mutagenicity) assays and in the Aspergillus Nidulans non-disjunction assay.

Hydrochlorothiazide had no adverse effects on the fertility of mice and rats of either sex in studies wherein these species were exposed via diet at doses of up to 100 and 4 mg/kg, respectively, prior to mating and throughout gestation. These doses of hydrochlorothiazide in mice and rats are 19 and 1.5 times, respectively, the maximum recommended human dose on a mg/m^2 basis. (Calculations assume an oral dose of 25 mg/day and a 60-kg patient.)

13.3   Developmental Toxicity
Studies with amlodipine: No evidence of teratogenicity or other embryo/fetal toxicity was found when pregnant rats and rabbits were treated orally with amlodipine maleate at doses of up to 10 mg amlodipine/kg/day (respectively, about 10 and 20 times the maximum recommended human dose [MRHD] of 10 mg amlodipine on a mg/m^2 basis) during their respective periods of major organogenesis. (Calculations based on a patient weight of 60 kg.) However, litter size was significantly decreased (by about 50%) and the number of intrauterine deaths was significantly increased (about 5-fold) for rats receiving amlodipine maleate at a dose equivalent to 10 mg amlodipine/kg/day for 14 days before mating and throughout mating and gestation. Amlodipine maleate has been shown to prolong both the gestation period and the duration of labor in rats at this dose. There are no adequate and well-controlled studies in pregnant women.

Studies with valsartan: No teratogenic effects were observed when valsartan was administered to pregnant mice and rats at oral doses of up to 600 mg/kg/day and to pregnant rabbits at oral doses of up to 10 mg/kg/day. However, significant decreases in fetal weight, pup birth weight, pup survival rate, and slight delays in developmental milestones were observed in studies in which parental rats were treated with valsartan at oral, maternally toxic (reduction in body weight gain and food consumption) doses of 600 mg/kg/day during organogenesis or late gestation and lactation. In rabbits, fetotoxicity (i.e., resorptions, litter loss, abortions, and low body weight) associated with maternal toxicity (mortality) was observed at doses of 5 and 10 mg/kg/day. The no observed adverse effect doses of 600, 200 and 2 mg/kg/day in mice, rats and rabbits, respectively, are about 9, 6 and 0.1 times the MRHD of 320 mg/day on a mg/m^2 basis. (Calculations based on a patient weight of 60 kg.)

Studies with hydrochlorothiazide: Under the auspices of the National Toxicology Program, pregnant mice and rats that received hydrochlorothiazide via gavage at doses up to 3000 and 1000 mg/kg/day, respectively, on gestation days 6 through 15 showed no evidence of teratogenicity. These doses of hydrochlorothiazide in mice and rats are 608 and 405 times, respectively, the maximum recommended human dose on a mg/m^2 basis. (Calculations assume an oral dose of 25 mg/day and a 60-kg patient.)

Studies with amlodipine and valsartan: In the oral embryo-fetal development study in rats using amlodipine besylate plus valsartan at doses equivalent to 5 mg/kg/day amlodipine plus 80 mg/kg/day valsartan, 10 mg/kg/day amlodipine plus 160 mg/kg/day valsartan, and 20 mg/kg/day amlodipine plus 320 mg/kg/day valsartan, treatment-related maternal and fetal effects (developmental delays and alterations noted in the presence of significant maternal toxicity) were noted with the high dose combination. The no-observed-adverse-effect level (NOAEL) for embryo-fetal effects was 10 mg/kg/day amlodipine plus 160 mg/kg/day valsartan. On a systemic exposure [AUC$_{(0-\infty)}$] basis, these doses are, respectively, 4.3 and 2.7 times the systemic exposure [AUC$_{(0-\infty)}$] in humans receiving the MRHD (10/320 mg/60 kg).

Studies with valsartan and hydrochlorothiazide: There was no evidence of teratogenicity in mice, rats, or rabbits treated orally with valsartan at doses up to 600, 100 and 10 mg/kg/day, respectively, in combination with hydrochlorothiazide at doses up to 188, 31 and 3 mg/kg/day. These non-teratogenic doses in mice, rats and rabbits are, respectively, 9, 3.5 and 0.5 times the maximum recommended human dose (MRHD) of valsartan and 38, 13 and 2 times the MRHD of hydrochlorothiazide on a mg/m^2 basis. (Calculations assume an oral dose of 320 mg/day valsartan in combination with 25 mg/day hydrochlorothiazide in a 60-kg patient.)

Fetotoxicity was observed in association with maternal toxicity in rats at valsartan/hydrochlorothiazide doses ≥200/63 mg/kg/day and in rabbits at valsartan/hydrochlorothiazide doses of 10/3 mg/kg/day. Evidence of fetotoxicity in rats consisted of decreased fetal weight and fetal variations of sternebrae, vertebrae, ribs and/or renal papillae. Evidence of fetotoxicity in rabbits included increased numbers of late resorptions with resultant increases in total resorptions, postimplantation losses and decreased number of live fetuses. The no observed adverse effect doses of the valsartan/hydrochlorothiazide combination in mice, rats and rabbits were 600/188, 100/31 and 3/1 mg/kg/day, respectively. These doses in mice, rats and rabbits are, respectively, 9, 3 and 0.18 times the MRHD of valsartan and 38, 13 and 0.5 times the MRHD of hydrochlorothiazide on a mg/m^2 basis. (Calculations assume an oral dose of 320 mg/day valsartan in combination with 25 mg/day hydrochlorothiazide in a 60-kg patient.)

14   CLINICAL STUDIES

Exforge HCT was studied in a double-blind, active controlled study in hypertensive patients. A total of 2,271 patients with moderate to severe hypertension (mean baseline systolic/diastolic blood pressure was 170/107 mmHg) received treatments of amlodipine/valsartan/HCTZ 10/320/25 mg, valsartan/HCTZ 320/25 mg, amlodipine/valsartan 10/320 mg, or HCTZ/amlodipine 25/10 mg. At study initiation patients assigned to the two-component arms received lower doses of their treatment combination while patients assigned to the Exforge HCT arm received 160/12.5 mg valsartan/hydrochlorothiazide. After one week, Exforge HCT patients were titrated to 5/160/12.5 mg amlodipine/valsartan/hydrochlorothiazide, while all other patients continued receiving their initial doses. After two weeks, all patients were titrated to their full treatment dose. A total of 55% of patients were male, 14% were 65 years or older, 72% were Caucasian, and 17% were Black.

At week 8, the triple combination therapy produced greater reductions in blood pressure than each of the three dual combination treatments (p<0.0001 for both diastolic and systolic blood pressures reductions). The reductions in systolic/diastolic blood pressure with Exforge HCT were 7.6/5.0 mmHg greater than with valsartan/HCTZ, 6.2/3.3 mmHg greater than with amlodipine/valsartan, and 8.2/5.3 mmHg greater than with amlodipine/HCTZ *(see Figure 1).* The full blood pressure lowering effect was achieved 2 weeks after being on the maximal dose of Exforge HCT *(see Figure 2 and Figure 3).* As the pivotal study was an active controlled trial, the treatment effects shown in Figure 1, 2, and 3 include a placebo effect of unknown size.

Figure 1: Reduction in Mean Blood Pressure at Endpoint

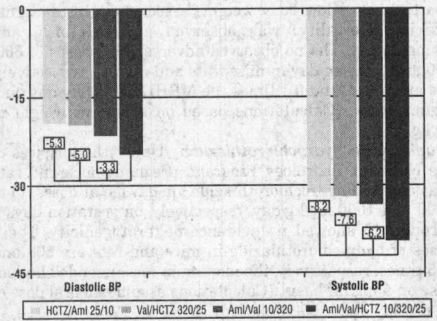

[See figure 2 at top of next column]
[See figure 3 on next column]
A subgroup of 283 patients was studied with ambulatory blood pressure monitoring. The blood pressure lowering effect in the triple therapy group was maintained throughout the 24-hour period *(see Figure 4 and Figure 5).*
[See figure 4 on next column]
[See figure 5 on next column]

16   HOW SUPPLIED/STORAGE AND HANDLING

Exforge HCT (amlodipine, valsartan, hydrochlorothiazide) is available as film-coated tablets containing amlodipine

Figure 2: Mean Sitting Diastolic Blood Pressure by Treatment and Week

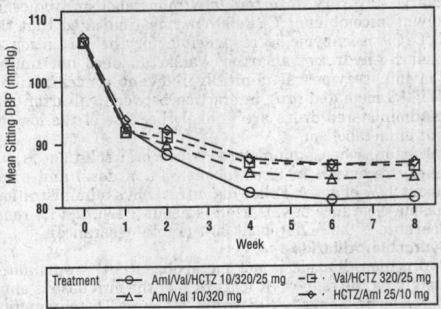

Figure 3: Mean Sitting Systolic Blood Pressure by Treatment and Week

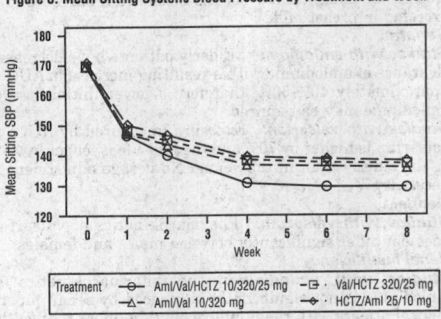

Figure 4: Mean Ambulatory Diastolic Blood Pressure at Endpoint by Treatment and Hour

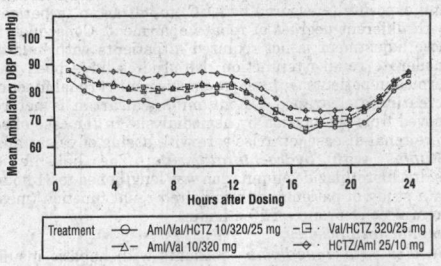

Figure 5: Mean Ambulatory Systolic Blood Pressure at Endpoint by Treatment and Hour

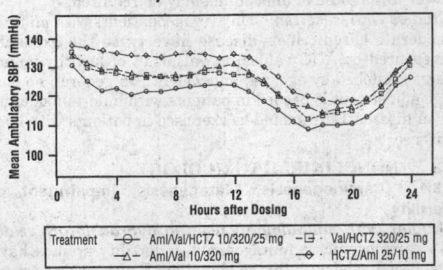

besylate equivalent to 5 mg or 10 mg of amlodipine free-base with valsartan 160 mg or 320 mg and hydrochlorothiazide 12.5 mg or 25 mg, providing for the following available combinations: 5/160/12.5 mg, 10/160/12.5 mg, 5/160/25 mg, 10/160/25 mg and 10/320/25 mg. All strengths are packaged in bottles of 30 and 90 tablets.

5 mg   amlodipine/160 mg   valsartan/12.5 mg hydrochlorothiazide Tablets – White, non-scored, film-coated tablet, ovaloid, biconvex with beveled edge with debossing "NVR" on one side and "VCL" on the other side.
Bottles of 30   NDC 0078-0559-15
Bottles of 90   NDC 0078-0559-34
10 mg   amlodipine/160 mg   valsartan/12.5 mg hydrochlorothiazide Tablets – Pale yellow, non-scored, film-coated tablet, ovaloid, biconvex with beveled edge with debossing "NVR" on one side and "VDL" on the other side.
Bottles of 30   NDC 0078-0561-15
Bottles of 90   NDC 0078-0561-34
5 mg   amlodipine/160 mg   valsartan/25 mg hydrochlorothiazide Tablets – Yellow, non-scored, film-coated tablet, ovaloid, biconvex with beveled edge with debossing "NVR" on one side and "VEL" on the other side.
Bottles of 30   NDC 0078-0560-15
Bottles of 90   NDC 0078-0560-34
10 mg   amlodipine/160 mg   valsartan/25 mg hydrochlorothiazide Tablets – Brown-yellow, non-scored,

film-coated tablet, ovaloid, biconvex with beveled edge with debossing "NVR" on one side and "VHL" on the other side.
Bottles of 30   NDC 0078-0562-15
Bottles of 90   NDC 0078-0562-34
10 mg   amlodipine/320 mg   valsartan/25 mg hydrochlorothiazide Tablets – Brown-yellow, non-scored, film-coated tablet, ovaloid, biconvex with beveled edge with debossing "NVR" on one side and "VFL" on the other side.
Bottles of 30   NDC 0078-0563-15
Bottles of 90   NDC 0078-0563-34
Store at 25°C (77°F); excursions permitted to 15-30°C (59-86°F), [see USP controlled room temperature].
Protect from moisture.
Dispense in tight container (USP).

17   PATIENT COUNSELING INFORMATION

Pregnancy: Female patients of childbearing age should be told that use of drugs like Exforge HCT that act on the renin-angiotensin system during pregnancy can cause serious problems in the fetus and infant including: low blood pressure, poor development of skull bones, kidney failure and death. Discuss other treatment options with female patients planning to become pregnant. Women using Exforge HCT who become pregnant should notify their physician as soon as possible.

Symptomatic Hypotension: A patient receiving Exforge HCT should be cautioned that lightheadedness can occur, especially during the first days of therapy, and that it should be reported to the prescribing physician. The patients should be told that if syncope occurs, Exforge HCT should be discontinued until the physician has been consulted.

All patients should be cautioned that inadequate fluid intake, excessive perspiration, diarrhea, or vomiting can lead to an excessive fall in blood pressure, with the same consequences of lightheadedness and possible syncope.

Potassium Supplements: A patient receiving Exforge HCT should be told not to use potassium supplements or salt substitutes containing potassium without consulting the prescribing physician.

17.1   Information for Patients
Patient Information
Exforge HCT (X-phorj HCT)
(amlodipine and valsartan and hydrochlorothiazide) Tablets
Read the Patient Information that comes with EXFORGE HCT before you start taking it and each time you get a refill. There may be new information. This leaflet does not take the place of talking with your doctor about your medical condition or treatment.
What is the most important information I should know about EXFORGE HCT?
If you become pregnant while taking EXFORGE HCT, stop taking EXFORGE HCT and call your doctor right away. EXFORGE HCT can harm an unborn baby causing injury or death. Talk to your doctor about other treatment options to lower your blood pressure before taking EXFORGE HCT if you plan to become pregnant.
What is EXFORGE HCT?
EXFORGE HCT contains three prescription medicines:
1. amlodipine, a calcium channel blocker
2. valsartan, an angiotensin receptor blocker, and
3. hydrochlorothiazide, a diuretic (water pill)
EXFORGE HCT may be used to lower blood pressure in adults when two medicines to lower your high blood pressure are not enough.
EXFORGE HCT has not been studied in children under 18 years of age.
Who should not take EXFORGE HCT?
Do not take EXFORGE HCT if you have low or no urine output (anuria).
What should I tell my doctor before taking EXFORGE HCT?
Tell your doctor about all of your medical conditions, including if you:
• **are pregnant or plan to become pregnant.** See "What is the most important information I should know about EXFORGE HCT?"
• **are breast-feeding or plan to breast-feed.** EXFORGE HCT may pass into your milk. Do not breast-feed while you are taking EXFORGE HCT.
• **are allergic to any of the ingredients in EXFORGE HCT.** See the end of this leaflet for a list of the ingredients in EXFORGE HCT.
• have heart problems
• have liver problems
• have kidney problems
• are vomiting or having a lot of diarrhea
• have or had gallstones
• have Lupus
Tell your doctor about all the medicines you take, including prescription and nonprescription medicines, vitamins, and herbal supplements. Some of your other medicines and EXFORGE HCT could affect each other, causing serious side effects.

Especially tell your doctor if you take:
- other medicines for high blood pressure or a heart problem
- water pills ("diuretics")
- potassium supplements or using a salt substitute containing potassium
- diabetes medicine including insulin
- narcotic pain medicines
- sleeping pills and anti-seizure medicines called barbiturates
- lithium, a medicine used to treat some types of depression
- aspirin or other medicines called non-steriodal anti-inflammatory drugs (NSAIDs)
- steroids
- cholesterol lowering medicine
- alcohol

Know the medicines you take. Keep a list of your medicines and show it to your doctor or pharmacist when you get a new medicine.

How should I take EXFORGE HCT?
- Take EXFORGE HCT exactly as your doctor tells you.
- Take EXFORGE HCT one time each day.
- EXFORGE HCT can be taken with or without food.
- If you miss a dose, take it as soon as you remember. If it is close to your next dose, do not take the missed dose. Just take the next dose at the regular time.
- If you take too much EXFORGE HCT, call your doctor or Poison Control Center, or go to the emergency room.
- Tell all your doctors and dentist you are taking EXFORGE HCT.
  This is especially important if you:
  - are going to have surgery
  - go for kidney dialysis

What are the possible side effects of EXFORGE HCT?
EXFORGE HCT may cause **serious side effects** including:
- **harm to an unborn baby causing injury or death.** See "What is the most important information I should know about EXFORGE HCT?"
- **low blood pressure** (hypotension). Low blood pressure is most likely to happen if you:
  - take water pills
  - are on a low salt diet
  - have heart problems
  - get dialysis treatments
  - get sick with vomiting or diarrhea
  - drink alcohol

  Lie down if you feel faint or dizzy. If you faint (lose consciousness), stop taking EXFORGE HCT. Call your doctor right away.
- Get emergency help if you get worse chest pain or chest pain that does not go away.
- **kidney problems.** Kidney problems may become worse in people that already have kidney disease. Some people will have changes in blood tests for kidney function and may need a lower dose of EXFORGE HCT. Call your doctor if you have swelling in your feet, ankles, or hands, or unexplained weight gain. If you have heart failure, your doctor should check your kidney function before prescribing EXFORGE HCT.
- **laboratory blood test changes in people with congestive heart failure.** Some people with congestive heart failure who take valsartan, one of the medicines in EXFORGE HCT, have changes in blood tests including increased potassium and decreased kidney function.
- **allergic reactions**
- **skin rash.** Call your doctor right away if you get an unusual skin rash.

The **most common** side effects of EXFORGE HCT include:
- dizziness
- swelling (edema) of the hands, ankles, or feet
- headache
- indigestion
- tiredness
- muscle spasms
- back pain
- nausea

Tell your doctor if you have any side effect that bothers you or that does not go away.
These are not all the possible side effects of EXFORGE HCT. For more information, ask your doctor or pharmacist. Call your doctor for medical advice about side effects. You may report side effects to FDA at 1-800-FDA-1088.

How should I store EXFORGE HCT?
- Store EXFORGE HCT at room temperature between 59°F to 86°F (15°C to 30°C).
- Keep EXFORGE HCT dry (protect it from moisture).

Keep EXFORGE HCT and all medicines out of the reach of children.

General Information about EXFORGE HCT
Medicines are sometimes prescribed for conditions that are not mentioned in the patient information leaflet. Do not use EXFORGE HCT for a condition for which it was not prescribed. Do not give EXFORGE HCT to other people, even if they have the same symptoms that you have. It may harm them.

This patient information leaflet summarizes the most important information about EXFORGE HCT. If you would like more information about EXFORGE HCT, talk with your doctor. You can ask your doctor or pharmacist for information about EXFORGE HCT that is written for health professionals. For more information go to www.EXFORGE.com or call 1-888-839-3674.

What are the ingredients in EXFORGE HCT?
Active ingredients: amlodipine besylate, valsartan and hydrochlorothiazide
The inactive ingredients of all strengths of the tablets are crospovidone, magnesium stearate, microcrystalline cellulose, and colloidal anhydrous silica. The film coating contains hypromellose, talc, macrogol 4000 and may contain titanium dioxide or yellow and red iron oxides.

What is high blood pressure (hypertension)?
Blood pressure is the force of blood in your blood vessels when your heart beats and when your heart rests. You have high blood pressure when the force is too much. EXFORGE HCT can help your blood vessels relax so your blood pressure is lower. Drugs that lower blood pressure lower your chance of having a stroke or heart attack.
High blood pressure makes the heart work harder to pump blood throughout the body and causes damage to blood vessels. If high blood pressure is not treated, it can lead to stroke, heart attack, heart failure, kidney failure and vision problems.

REV: AUGUST 2009   T2009-93/T2009-02
Distributed by:
Novartis Pharmaceuticals Corporation
East Hanover, New Jersey 07936
©Novartis

Shown in Product Identification Guide, page 315

EXJADE®   ℞
[x-jāde]
(deferasirox)
Tablets for Oral Suspension

The following prescribing information is based on official labeling in effect July 2010.
HIGHLIGHTS OF PRESCRIBING INFORMATION
These highlights do not include all the information needed to use Exjade safely and effectively. See full prescribing information for Exjade.
Exjade® *(deferasirox)* **tablets for oral suspension**
Initial U.S. Approval: 2005

WARNING: RENAL, HEPATIC FAILURE AND/OR GASTROINTESTINAL HEMORRHAGE
See full prescribing information for complete boxed warning
Exjade may cause:
• renal impairment, including failure
• hepatic impairment, including failure
• gastrointestinal hemorrhage
In some reported cases, these reactions were fatal. These reactions were more frequently observed in patients with advanced age, high risk myelodysplastic syndromes (MDS), underlying renal or hepatic impairment or low platelet counts (<50 × 10⁹/L). Exjade therapy requires close patient monitoring, including laboratory tests of renal and hepatic function. (4, 5)

---RECENT MAJOR CHANGES---

---INDICATIONS AND USAGE---
Exjade is an iron chelating agent indicated for the treatment of chronic iron overload due to blood transfusions in patients 2 years of age and older. (1)
Individualize the decision to initiate Exjade therapy based on consideration of the anticipated clinical benefit and risks of the therapy, taking into consideration factors such as the life expectancy and comorbidities of the patient. (1)
The safety and efficacy of Exjade when administered with other iron chelation therapy have not been established. (1)

---DOSAGE AND ADMINISTRATION---
- Recommended initial daily dose is 20 mg/kg body weight, taken on an empty stomach at least 30 minutes before food. (2.1)
- Calculate dose to the nearest whole tablet. (2.1)
- Do not chew or swallow the tablets whole. (2.1)
- Disperse tablets by stirring in an appropriate amount of water, orange juice, or apple juice. (2.1)

- Consider increasing the initial dose of Exjade dose to 30 mg/kg when co-administered with potent UGT inducers or with cholestyramine. (2.2)

---DOSAGE FORMS AND STRENGTHS---
Tablets for oral suspension: 125 mg, 250 mg, 500 mg. (3)

---CONTRAINDICATIONS---
- Creatinine clearance <40 mL/min or serum creatinine >2 times the age-appropriate upper limit of normal. (4)
- Poor performance status and high-risk MDS or advanced malignancies. (4, 5.7)
- Platelet counts <50 × 10⁹/L. (4)
- Known hypersensitivity to deferasirox or any component of Exjade. (4)

---WARNINGS AND PRECAUTIONS---
- Fatal and non-fatal gastrointestinal bleeding, ulceration, and irritation may occur during Exjade treatment. Use caution in patients who are taking Exjade in combination with drugs that have known ulcerogenic or hemorrhagic potential, such as NSAIDs, corticosteroids, oral bisphosphonates, and anticoagulants. (5.3)
- Cytopenias, including agranulocytosis, neutropenia and thrombocytopenia have been reported. Monitor blood counts during Exjade therapy. (5.4)
- Serious hypersensitivity reactions have been reported. If reactions are severe, discontinue Exjade and institute appropriate medical intervention. (5.5)
- Reports of serious adverse reactions, some with a fatal outcome, occurred in postmarketing experience, predominantly when the drug was administered to patients with advanced age, advanced disease or co-morbid conditions. Elderly patients have an increased risk of adverse events. (5.7)

---ADVERSE REACTIONS---
The most frequently occurring adverse reactions are diarrhea, vomiting, nausea, abdominal pain, skin rashes, and increases in serum creatinine. (6.1)
To report SUSPECTED ADVERSE REACTIONS, contact Novartis Pharmaceuticals Corporation at 1-888-669-6682 or FDA at 1-800-FDA-1088 or www.fda.gov/medwatch

---DRUG INTERACTIONS---
- Based on Exjade's mechanism of action, do not take Exjade with aluminum-containing antacid preparations. (7)
- Use caution when Exjade is administered with drugs metabolized by CYP3A4. (7.1, 7.2)
- Exjade increases repaglinide exposure. Consider repaglinide dose reduction and carefully monitor blood glucose levels when repaglinide is used concomitantly with Exjade. An interaction between Exjade and other CYP2C8 substrates cannot be excluded. (7.3)

---USE IN SPECIFIC POPULATIONS---
- Pregnancy: Based on animal studies, may cause fetal harm. (8.1)
- Nursing Mothers: Discontinue drug or nursing taking into consideration importance of drug to mother. (8.3)
- Elderly: Closely monitor due to the greater frequency of decreased hepatic, renal, or cardiac function in these patients. These patients may need Exjade dose adjustments based on early signs and/or symptoms of toxicity. (8.5)

See 17 for PATIENT COUNSELING INFORMATION
Revised: 01/2010

*Sections or subsections omitted from the full prescribing information are not listed

FULL PRESCRIBING INFORMATION

WARNING: RENAL, HEPATIC FAILURE AND/OR GASTROINTESTINAL HEMORRHAGE

Exjade may cause:

- **renal impairment, including failure**
- **hepatic impairment, including failure**
- **gastrointestinal hemorrhage**

In some reported cases, these reactions were fatal. These reactions were more frequently observed in patients with advanced age, high risk myelodysplastic syndromes (MDS), underlying renal or hepatic impairment or low platelet counts (<50 × 10^9/L) [*see Contraindications (4), Warnings and Precautions (5.1-5.7)*]. Exjade therapy requires close patient monitoring, including measurement of:

- **serum creatinine and/or creatinine clearance prior to initiation of therapy and monthly thereafter; in patients with underlying renal impairment or risk factors for renal impairment, monitor creatinine and/or creatinine clearance weekly for the first month, then monthly thereafter;**
- **serum transaminases and bilirubin prior to initiation of therapy, every two weeks during the first month and monthly thereafter.**

1 INDICATIONS AND USAGE

Exjade (deferasirox) is indicated for the treatment of chronic iron overload due to blood transfusions (transfusional hemosiderosis) in patients 2 years of age and older. In these patients, Exjade has been shown to reduce liver iron concentration and serum ferritin levels. Clinical trials to demonstrate increased survival or to confirm clinical benefit have not been completed [*see Clinical Studies (14)*].

Individualize the decision to initiate Exjade therapy based on consideration of the anticipated clinical benefit and risks of the therapy, taking into consideration factors such as the life expectancy and comorbidities of the patient [*see Warnings and Precautions (5.1-5.6) and Contraindications (4)*].

The safety and efficacy of Exjade when administered with other iron chelation therapy have not been established.

2 DOSAGE AND ADMINISTRATION

2.1 Dosing Information

Prior to starting therapy, obtain baseline serum ferritin and iron levels. The risk for toxicity may be increased when Exjade is given to patients with low iron burden or with serum ferritin levels that are only slightly elevated [*see Dose Modifications (2.2)*].

The recommended initial daily dose of Exjade is 20 mg/kg body weight.

Take Exjade once daily on an empty stomach at least 30 minutes before food, preferably at the same time each day. Do not chew tablets or swallow them whole. Do not take Exjade with aluminum-containing antacid products. Calculate doses (mg/kg per day) to the nearest whole tablet. Completely disperse tablets by stirring in water, orange juice, or apple juice until a fine suspension is obtained. Disperse doses of <1 g in 3.5 ounces of liquid and doses of ≥1 g in 7.0 ounces of liquid. After swallowing the suspension, resuspend any residue in a small volume of liquid and swallow.

Individualize the decision to remove accumulated iron based on anticipated clinical benefit and risks of Exjade therapy. In patients who are in need of iron chelation therapy, it is recommended that therapy with Exjade (deferasirox) be started when a patient has evidence of chronic iron overload, such as the transfusion of approximately 100 mL/kg of packed red blood cells (approximately 20 units for a 40-kg patient) and a serum ferritin consistently >1000 mcg/L.

2.2 Dose Modifications

Exjade may require dose adjustment, interruption or cessation of the therapy due to toxicity or any of the following [*see Warnings and Precautions (5.1-5.6), Geriatric Use (8.5)*].

Based on Serum Ferritin

After commencing initial therapy, monitor serum ferritin every month and adjust the dose of Exjade if necessary every 3-6 months based on serum ferritin trends. Make dose adjustments in steps of 5 or 10 mg/kg and tailor adjustments to the individual patient's response and therapeutic goals (maintenance or reduction of body iron burden). In patients not adequately controlled with doses of 30 mg/kg (e.g., serum ferritin levels persistently above 2500 mcg/L and not showing a decreasing trend over time), doses of up to 40 mg/kg may be considered. Doses above 40 mg/kg are not recommended.

If the serum ferritin falls consistently below 500 mcg/L, consider temporarily interrupting therapy with Exjade.

Based on Serum Creatinine

For adults, reduce the daily dose of Exjade by 10 mg/kg if a rise in serum creatinine to >33% above the average of the pretreatment measurements is seen at 2 consecutive visits, and cannot be attributed to other causes. For pediatric patients, reduce the dose by 10 mg/kg if serum creatinine levels rise above the age-appropriate upper limit of normal at 2 consecutive visits.

Concomitant UGT Inducers or Cholestyramine

Concomitant use of UGT inducers or cholestyramine decreases deferasirox systemic exposure (AUC). Avoid the concomitant use of cholestyramine or potent UGT inducers (e.g., rifampicin, phenytoin, phenobarbital, ritonavir) with Exjade. If you must co-administer these agents together, consider increasing the initial dose of Exjade to 30 mg/kg, and monitor serum ferritin levels and clinical responses for further dose modification [*see Drug Interactions (7.4, 7.5)*].

3 DOSAGE FORMS AND STRENGTHS

125 mg tablets

Off-white, round, flat tablet with beveled edge and imprinted with "J" and "125" on one side and "NVR" on the other.

250 mg tablets

Off-white, round, flat tablet with beveled edge and imprinted with "J" and "250" on one side and "NVR" on the other.

500 mg tablets

Off-white, round, flat tablet with beveled edge and imprinted with "J" and "500" on one side and "NVR" on the other.

4 CONTRAINDICATIONS

Exjade is contraindicated in patients with:

- creatinine clearance <40 mL/min or serum creatinine >2 times the age-appropriate upper limit of normal;
- poor performance status and high-risk myelodysplastic syndromes or advanced malignancies [*see Warnings and Precautions (5.7)*];
- platelet counts <50 × 10^9/L;
- known hypersensitivity to deferasirox or any component of Exjade.

5 WARNINGS AND PRECAUTIONS

5.1 Renal

Acute renal failure, fatal in some patients and requiring dialysis in others, has been reported following the postmarketing use of Exjade (deferasirox). Most fatalities occurred in patients with multiple comorbidities and who were in advanced stages of their hematological disorders. Monitor serum creatinine and/or creatinine clearance in patients who: are at increased risk of complications, have preexisting renal conditions, are elderly, have comorbid conditions, or are receiving medicinal products that depress renal function. Closely monitor the renal function of patients with creatinine clearances between 40 and less than 60 mL/min, particularly in situations where patients have additional risk factors that may further impair renal function such as concomitant medications, dehydration, or severe infections.

Assess serum creatinine and/or creatinine clearance in duplicate before initiating therapy to establish a reliable pretreatment baseline, due to variations in measurements. Monitor serum creatinine and/or creatinine clearance monthly thereafter. In patients with additional renal risk factors *(see above)*, monitor serum creatinine and/or creatinine clearance weekly during the first month after initiation or modification of therapy and monthly thereafter.

Consider dose reduction, interruption, or discontinuation for increases in serum creatinine. If there is a progressive increase in serum creatinine beyond the age-appropriate upper limit of normal, interrupt Exjade use. Once the creatinine has returned to within the normal range, therapy with Exjade may be reinitiated at a lower dose followed by gradual dose escalation, if the clinical benefit is expected to outweigh potential risks [*see Dose Modifications (2.2)*].

In the clinical studies, for increases of serum creatinine on 2 consecutive measures (>33% in patients >15 years of age or >33% and greater than the age-appropriate upper limit of normal in patients <15 years of age), the daily dose of Exjade was reduced by 10 mg/kg. Patients with baseline serum creatinine above the upper limit of normal were excluded from clinical studies.

In the clinical studies, Exjade-treated patients experienced dose-dependent increases in serum creatinine. These increases occurred at a greater frequency compared to deferoxamine-treated patients (38% vs. 14%, respectively, in Study 1 and 36% vs 22%, respectively, within Study 3). Most of the creatinine elevations remained within the normal range [*see Adverse Reactions (6.1)*]. There have also been reports of renal tubulopathy in patients treated with Exjade. The majority of these patients were children and adolescents with β-thalassemia and serum ferritin levels <1500 mcg/L.

5.2 Hepatic Dysfunction and Failure

In Study 1, 4 patients discontinued Exjade because of hepatic abnormalities (drug-induced hepatitis in 2 patients and increased serum transaminases in 2 additional patients). There have been postmarketing reports of hepatic failure, some with a fatal outcome, in patients treated with Exjade. Most of these events occurred in patients greater than 55 years of age. Most reports of hepatic failure involved patients with significant comorbidities, including liver cirrhosis and multiorgan failure. Serum transaminases and bilirubin should be monitored before the initiation of treatment, every 2 weeks during the first month and monthly thereafter. Consider dose modifications or interruption of treatment for severe or persistent elevations.

5.3 Gastrointestinal

Fatal GI hemorrhages, especially in elderly patients who had advanced hematologic malignancies and/or low platelet counts, have been reported. Non-fatal upper GI irritation, ulceration and hemorrhage have been reported in patients, including children and adolescents, receiving Exjade [*see Adverse Reactions (6.1)*]. Physicians and patients should remain alert for signs and symptoms of GI ulceration and hemorrhage during Exjade therapy and promptly initiate additional evaluation and treatment if a serious GI adverse event is suspected. Use caution when administering Exjade in combination with drugs that have ulcerogenic or hemorrhagic potential, such as non-steroidal anti-inflammatory drugs (NSAIDs), corticosteroids, oral bisphosphonates, or anticoagulants.

5.4 Cytopenias

There have been postmarketing reports (both spontaneous and from clinical trials) of cytopenias, including agranulocytosis, neutropenia and thrombocytopenia, in patients treated with Exjade. Some of these patients died. The relationship of these episodes to treatment with Exjade is uncertain. Most of these patients had preexisting hematologic disorders that are frequently associated with bone marrow failure [*see Adverse Reactions (6.2)*]. Monitor blood counts regularly. Consider interrupting treatment with Exjade in patients who develop unexplained cytopenia. Reintroduction of therapy with Exjade may be considered, once the cause of the cytopenia has been elucidated.

5.5 Hypersensitivity

Serious hypersensitivity reactions (such as anaphylaxis and angioedema) have been reported in patients receiving Exjade, with the onset of the reaction occurring in the majority of cases within the first month of treatment [*see Adverse Reactions (6.2)*]. If reactions are severe, discontinue Exjade and institute appropriate medical intervention.

5.6 Rash

Rashes may occur during Exjade (deferasirox) treatment. For rashes of mild to moderate severity, Exjade may be continued without dose adjustment, since the rash often resolves spontaneously. In severe cases, Exjade may be interrupted. Reintroduction at a lower dose with escalation may be considered in combination with a short period of oral steroid administration. Erythema multiforme has been reported during Exjade treatment.

5.7 Co-morbidities

Clinical trials to demonstrate increased survival or to confirm clinical benefit have not been completed. Exjade has been shown to decrease serum ferritin and liver iron concentration in clinical trials. Consider the importance of these factors as well as individual patient factors and the prognosis associated with any underlying conditions before initiation of Exjade therapy [*see Contraindications (4)*].

In postmarketing experience, there have been reports of serious adverse reactions, some with a fatal outcome, in patients taking Exjade therapy, predominantly when the drug was administered to patients with advanced age, complications from underlying conditions or very advanced disease. Most of these deaths occurred within six months of Exjade initiation and generally involved worsening of the underlying condition. The reports do not rule out the possibility that Exjade may have contributed to the deaths.

5.8 Special Senses

Auditory disturbances (high frequency hearing loss, decreased hearing), and ocular disturbances (lens opacities, cataracts, elevations in intraocular pressure, and retinal disorders) have been reported at a frequency of <1% with Exjade therapy in the clinical studies. Auditory and ophthalmic testing (including slit lamp examinations and dilated fundoscopy) are recommended before starting Exjade treatment and thereafter at regular intervals (every 12 months). If disturbances are noted, consider dose reduction or interruption.

5.9 Laboratory Tests

Measure serum ferritin monthly to assess response to therapy and to evaluate for the possibility of overchelation of iron. If the serum ferritin falls consistently below 500 mcg/L, consider temporarily interrupting therapy with Exjade [see Dosage and Administration (2.2)].

In the clinical studies, the correlation coefficient between the serum ferritin and LIC was 0.63. Therefore, changes in serum ferritin levels may not always reliably reflect changes in LIC.

Perform laboratory monitoring of renal and hepatic function [see Warnings and Precautions (5.1, 5.3)].

6 ADVERSE REACTIONS

6.1 Clinical Trials Experience

The following adverse reactions are also discussed in other sections of the labeling:
Renal Failure [see Warnings and Precautions (5.1)]. Hepatic Failure [see Warnings and Precautions (5.2)]. Fatal and non-fatal Gastrointestinal Bleedings [see Warnings and Precautions (5.3)]. Cytopenias [see Warnings and Precautions (5.4)].

Because clinical trials are conducted under widely varying conditions, adverse reaction rates observed in the clinical trials of a drug cannot be directly compared to rates in the clinical trials of another drug and may not reflect the rates observed in practice.

A total of 700 adult and pediatric patients were treated with Exjade (deferasirox) for 48 weeks in premarketing studies. These included 469 patients with β-thalassemia, 99 with rare anemias, and 132 with sickle cell disease. Of these patients, 45% were male, 70% were Caucasian and 292 patients were <16 years of age. In the sickle cell disease population, 89% of patients were Black. Median treatment duration among the sickle cell patients was 51 weeks. Of the 700 patients treated, 469 (403 β-thalassemia and 66 rare anemias) were entered into extensions of the original clinical protocols. In ongoing extension studies, median durations of treatment were 88-205 weeks.

Table 1 displays adverse reactions occurring in >5% of Exjade-treated β-thalassemia patients (Study 1) and sickle cell disease patients (Study 3) with a suspected relationship to study drug. Abdominal pain, nausea, vomiting, diarrhea, skin rashes, and increases in serum creatinine were the most frequent adverse reactions reported with a suspected relationship to Exjade. Gastrointestinal symptoms, increases in serum creatinine, and skin rash were dose related.

[See table 1 above]

In Study 1, a total of 113 (38%) patients treated with Exjade had increases in serum creatinine >33% above baseline on 2 separate occasions (Table 2) and 25 (8%) patients required dose reductions. Increases in serum creatinine appeared to be dose related [see Warnings and Precautions (5.1)]. In this study, 17 (6%) patients treated with Exjade developed elevations in SGPT/ALT levels >5 times the upper limit of normal at 2 consecutive visits. Of these, 2 patients had liver biopsy proven drug-induced hepatitis and both discontinued Exjade therapy [see Warnings and Precautions (5.2)]. An additional 2 patients, who did not have elevations in SGPT/ALT >5 times the upper limit of normal, discontinued Exjade because of increased SGPT/ALT. Increases in transaminases did not appear to be dose related. Adverse reactions that led to discontinuations included abnormal liver function tests (2 patients) and drug-induced hepatitis (2 patients), skin rash, glycosuria/proteinuria, Henoch Schönlein purpura, hyperactivity/insomnia, drug fever, and cataract (1 patient each).

In Study 3, a total of 48 (36%) patients treated with Exjade had increases in serum creatinine >33% above baseline on 2 separate occasions (Table 2) [see Warnings and Precautions (5.1)]. Of the patients who experienced creatinine increases in Study 3, 8 Exjade-treated patients required dose reductions. In this study, 5 patients in the Exjade group developed elevations in SGPT/ALT levels >5 times the upper limit of normal at 2 consecutive visits and 1 patient subsequently had Exjade permanently discontinued. Four additional patients discontinued Exjade due to adverse reactions with a suspected relationship to study drug, including diarrhea, pancreatitis associated with gallstones, atypical tuberculosis, and skin rash.

[See table 2 above]

Proteinuria

In clinical studies, urine protein was measured monthly. Intermittent proteinuria (urine protein/creatinine ratio >0.6 mg/mg) occurred in 18.6% of Exjade-treated patients compared to 7.2% of deferoxamine-treated patients in

Table 1. Adverse Reactions Occurring in >5% of Exjade-treated Patients in Study 1 and Study 3*

	Study 1 (β-Thalassemia)		Study 3 (Sickle Cell Disease)	
Preferred Term	EXJADE N=296 n (%)	Deferoxamine N=290 n (%)	EXJADE N=132 n (%)	Deferoxamine N=63 n (%)
Abdominal Pain**	63 (21.3)	41 (14.1)	37 (28.0)	9 (14.3)
Diarrhea	35 (11.8)	21 (7.2)	26 (19.7)	3 (4.8)
Creatinine Increased***	33 (11.1)	0 (0)	9 (6.8)	0
Nausea	31 (10.5)	14 (4.8)	30 (22.7)	7 (11.1)
Vomiting	30 (10.1)	28 (9.7)	28 (21.2)	10 (15.9)
Rash	25 (8.4)	9 (3.1)	14 (10.6)	3 (4.8)

* Adverse reaction frequencies are based on adverse events reported regardless of relationship to study drug.
** Includes 'abdominal pain', 'abdominal pain lower', and 'abdominal pain upper' which were reported as adverse events.
*** Includes 'blood creatinine increased' and 'blood creatinine abnormal' which were reported as adverse events. *Also see Table 2.*

Table 2. Number (%) of Patients with Increases in Serum Creatinine or SGPT/ALT in Study 1 and Study 3

	Study 1 (β-Thalassemia)		Study 3 (Sickle Cell Disease)	
Laboratory Parameter	EXJADE N=296 n (%)	Deferoxamine N=290 n (%)	EXJADE N=132 n (%)	Deferoxamine N=63 n (%)
Serum Creatinine				
Creatinine increase >33% and <ULN at 2 consecutive postbaseline visits	113 (38.2)	41 (14.1)	48 (36.4)	14 (22.2)
Creatinine increase >33% and >ULN at 2 consecutive postbaseline visits	7 (2.4)	1 (0.3)	3 (2.3)	2 (3.2)
SGPT/ALT				
SGPT/ALT >5 × ULN at 2 postbaseline visits	25 (8.4)	7 (2.4)	2 (1.5)	0
SGPT/ALT >5 × ULN at 2 consecutive postbaseline visits	17 (5.7)	5 (1.7)	5 (3.8)	0

Study 1. Although no patients were discontinued from Exjade in clinical studies up to 1 year due to proteinuria, monthly monitoring is recommended. The mechanism and clinical significance of the proteinuria are uncertain.

Other Adverse Reactions

In the population of more than 5,000 patients who have been treated with Exjade during clinical trials, adverse reactions occurring in 0.1% to 1% of patients included gastritis, edema, sleep disorder, pigmentation disorder, dizziness, anxiety, maculopathy, cholelithiasis, pyrexia, fatigue, pharyngolaryngeal pain, early cataract, hearing loss, gastrointestinal hemorrhage, gastric ulcer (including multiple ulcers), duodenal ulcer, and renal tubulopathy (Fanconi's syndrome). Adverse reactions occurring in 0.01% to 0.1% of patients included optic neuritis, esophagitis, and erythema multiforme. Adverse reactions which most frequently led to dose interruption or dose adjustment during clinical trials were rash, gastrointestinal disorders, infections, increased serum creatinine, and increased serum transaminases.

6.2 Postmarketing Experience

The following adverse reactions have been spontaneously reported during post-approval use of Exjade. Because these reactions are reported voluntarily from a population of uncertain size, in which patients may have received concomitant medication, it is not always possible to reliably estimate frequency or establish a causal relationship to drug exposure.

Skin and subcutaneous tissue disorders: leukocytoclastic vasculitis, urticaria, alopecia

Immune system disorders: hypersensitivity reactions (including anaphylaxis and angioedema).

7 DRUG INTERACTIONS

The concomitant administration of Exjade and aluminum-containing antacid preparations has not been formally studied. Although deferasirox has a lower affinity for aluminum than for iron, do not administer Exjade with aluminum-containing antacid preparations.

7.1 Effect of Deferasirox on Drug Metabolizing Enzymes

Deferasirox inhibits human CYP3A4, CYP2C8, CYP1A2, CYP2A6, CYP2D6, and CYP2C19 in vitro. The clinical significance of deferasirox inhibition of CYP1A2, CYP2A6, CYP2D6, and CYP2C19 is unknown.

7.2 Interaction with Agents Metabolized by CYP3A4

In healthy volunteers, the concomitant administration of Exjade and midazolam (a CYP3A4 probe substrate) resulted in a decrease of midazolam peak concentration by 23% and exposure by 17%. In the clinical setting, this effect may be more pronounced. Therefore, due to a possible decrease in CYP3A4 substrate concentration and potential loss of effec-

tiveness, use caution when deferasirox is administered with drugs metabolized by CYP3A4 (e.g., cyclosporine, simvastatin, hormonal contraceptive agents).

7.3 Interaction with Agents Metabolized by CYP2C8

In a healthy volunteer study, the concomitant administration of Exjade (30 mg/kg/day for 4 days) and the CYP2C8 probe substrate repaglinide (single dose of 0.5 mg) resulted in an increase in repaglinide systemic exposure (AUC) to 2.3-fold of control and an increase in C_{max} of 62%. If Exjade and repaglinide are used concomitantly, consider decreasing the dose of repaglinide and perform careful monitoring of blood glucose levels. Exercise caution when Exjade and other CYP2C8 substrates like paclitaxel are co-administered.

7.4 Interaction with Agents Inducing UDP-glucuronosyltransferase (UGT) Metabolism

In a healthy volunteer study, the concomitant administration of Exjade (single dose of 30 mg/kg) and the potent UDP-glucuronosyltransferase (UGT) inducer rifampicin (600 mg/day for 9 days) resulted in a decrease of deferasirox systemic exposure (AUC) by 44%. Therefore, the concomitant use of Exjade with potent UGT inducers (e.g., rifampicin, phenytoin, phenobarbital, ritonavir) may result in a decrease in Exjade efficacy.

Avoid the concomitant use of potent UGT inducers with Exjade. If you must co-administer these agents together, consider increasing the initial dose of Exjade to 30 mg/kg and monitor serum ferritin levels and clinical responses for further dose modification [see Dosage and Administration (2.2)].

7.5 Interaction with Cholestyramine

The concomitant use of Exjade with cholestyramine may result in a decrease in Exjade efficacy. In healthy volunteers, the administration of cholestyramine after a single dose of deferasirox resulted in a 45% decrease in deferasirox exposure (AUC). Avoid the concomitant use of cholestyramine with Exjade. If you must co-administer these agents together, consider increasing the initial dose of Exjade to 30 mg/kg and monitor serum ferritin levels and clinical responses for further dose modification [see Dosage and Administration (2.2)].

8 USE IN SPECIFIC POPULATIONS

8.1 Pregnancy

Pregnancy Category C

There are no adequate and well-controlled studies with Exjade in pregnant women. Administration of deferasirox to animals during pregnancy and lactation resulted in decreased offspring viability and an increase in renal anomalies in male offspring at exposures that were less than the recommended human exposure. Exjade should be used during pregnancy only if the potential benefit justifies the potential risk to the fetus.

In embryofetal developmental studies, pregnant rats and rabbits received oral deferasirox during the period of organogenesis at doses up to (100 mg/kg/day in rats and 50 mg/kg/day in rabbits) 0.8 times the MRHD (Maximum Recommended Human Dose) on a mg/m^2 basis. These doses resulted in maternal toxicity but no fetal harm was observed.

In a prenatal and postnatal developmental study, pregnant rats received oral deferasirox daily from organogenesis through lactation day 20 at doses (10, 30, and 90 mg/kg/day) 0.08, 0.2, and 0.7 times the MRHD on a mg/m^2 basis. Maternal toxicity, loss of litters, and decreased offspring viability occurred at 0.7 times the MRHD on a mg/m^2 basis, and increases in renal anomalies in male offspring occurred at 0.2 times the MRHD on a mg/m^2 basis.

8.3 Nursing Mothers

It is not known whether Exjade is excreted in human milk. Deferasirox and its metabolites were excreted in rat milk. Because many drugs are excreted in human milk and because of the potential for serious adverse reactions in nursing infants from deferasirox and its metabolites, a decision should be made whether to discontinue nursing or to discontinue the drug, taking into account the importance of the drug to the mother.

8.4 Pediatric Use

Of the 700 patients who received Exjade during clinical studies, 292 were pediatric patients 2-<16 years of age with various congenital and acquired anemias, including 52 patients age 2-<6 years, 121 patients age 6-<12 years and 119 patients age 12-<16 years. Seventy percent of these patients had β-thalassemia. Children between the ages of 2-<6 years have a systemic exposure to Exjade approximately 50% of that of adults [*see Clinical Pharmacology (12.3)*]. However, the safety and efficacy of Exjade in pediatric patients was similar to that of adult patients, and younger pediatric patients responded similarly to older pediatric patients. The recommended starting dose and dosing modification are the same for children and adults [*see Clinical Studies (14), Indications and Usage (1), and Dosage and Administration (2.1)*].

Growth and development were within normal limits in children followed for up to 5 years in clinical trials.

8.5 Geriatric Use

Four hundred and thirty-one (431) patients ≥65 years of age have been studied in clinical trials of Exjade. The majority of these patients had myelodysplastic syndrome (MDS) (n=393). In these trials, elderly patients experienced a higher frequency of adverse reactions than younger patients. Closely monitor elderly patients for early signs or symptoms of adverse reactions that may require a dose adjustment. Elderly patients are at increased risk for Exjade toxicity due to the greater frequency of decreased hepatic, renal, or cardiac function, and of concomitant disease or other drug therapy.

8.6 Renal Impairment

Exjade has not been studied in patients with renal impairment [*see Warnings and Precautions (5.1)*].

8.7 Hepatic Impairment

Exjade has not been studied in patients with hepatic impairment.

10 OVERDOSAGE

Cases of overdose (2-3 times the prescribed dose for several weeks) have been reported. In one case, this resulted in hepatitis which resolved without long-term consequences after a dose interruption. Single doses up to 80 mg/kg/day in iron overloaded β-thalassemic patients have been tolerated with nausea and diarrhea noted. In healthy volunteers, single doses of up to 40 mg/kg/day were tolerated. There is no specific antidote for Exjade. In case of overdose, induce vomiting and employ gastric lavage.

11 DESCRIPTION

Exjade (deferasirox) is an iron chelating agent. Exjade tablets for oral suspension contain 125 mg, 250 mg, or 500 mg deferasirox. Deferasirox is designated chemically as 4-[3,5-Bis (2-hydroxyphenyl)-1H-1,2,4-triazol-1-yl]-benzoic acid and its structural formula is

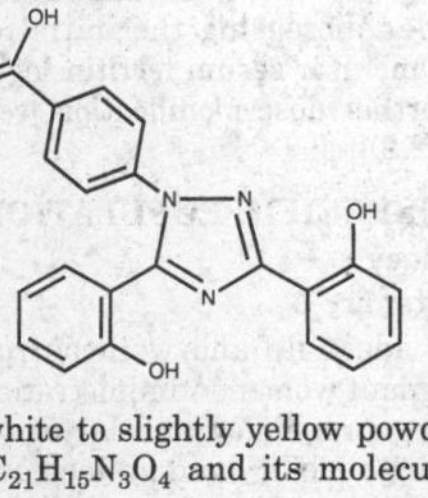

Deferasirox is a white to slightly yellow powder. Its molecular formula is $C_{21}H_{15}N_3O_4$ and its molecular weight is 373.4.

Inactive Ingredients: Lactose monohydrate (NF), crospovidone (NF), povidone (K30) (NF), sodium lauryl sulphate (NF), microcrystalline cellulose (NF), silicon dioxide (NF), and magnesium stearate (NF).

12 CLINICAL PHARMACOLOGY

12.1 Mechanism of Action

Exjade (deferasirox) is an orally active chelator that is selective for iron (as Fe^{3+}). It is a tridentate ligand that binds iron with high affinity in a 2:1 ratio. Although deferasirox has very low affinity for zinc and copper there are variable decreases in the serum concentration of these trace metals after the administration of deferasirox. The clinical significance of these decreases is uncertain.

12.2 Pharmacodynamics

Pharmacodynamic effects tested in an iron balance metabolic study showed that deferasirox (10, 20 and 40 mg/kg per day) was able to induce a mean net iron excretion (0.119, 0.329 and 0.445 mg Fe/kg body weight per day, respectively) within the clinically relevant range (0.1-0.5 mg/kg per day). Iron excretion was predominantly fecal.

12.3 Pharmacokinetics

Absorption

Exjade is absorbed following oral administration with median times to maximum plasma concentration (t_{max}) of about 1.5-4 hours. The C_{max} and AUC of deferasirox increase approximately linearly with dose after both single administration and under steady-state conditions. Exposure to deferasirox increased by an accumulation factor of 1.3-2.3 after multiple doses. The absolute bioavailability (AUC) of deferasirox tablets for oral suspension is 70% compared to an intravenous dose. The bioavailability (AUC) of deferasirox was variably increased when taken with a meal.

Distribution

Deferasirox is highly (~99%) protein bound almost exclusively to serum albumin. The percentage of deferasirox confined to the blood cells was 5% in humans. The volume of distribution at steady state (V_{ss}) of deferasirox is 14.37 ± 2.69 L in adults.

Metabolism

Glucuronidation is the main metabolic pathway for deferasirox, with subsequent biliary excretion. Deconjugation of glucuronidates in the intestine and subsequent reabsorption (enterohepatic recycling) is likely to occur. Deferasirox is mainly glucuronidated by UGT1A1 and to a lesser extent UGT1A3. CYP450-catalyzed (oxidative) metabolism of deferasirox appears to be minor in humans (about 8%). Deconjugation of glucuronide metabolites in the intestine and subsequent reabsorption (enterohepatic recycling) was confirmed in a healthy volunteer study in which the administration of cholestyramine 12 g twice daily (strongly binds to deferasirox and its conjugates) 4 and 10 hours after a single dose of deferasirox resulted in a 45% decrease in deferasirox exposure (AUC) by interfering with the enterohepatic recycling of deferasirox.

Excretion

Deferasirox and metabolites are primarily (84% of the dose) excreted in the feces. Renal excretion of deferasirox and metabolites is minimal (8% of the administered dose). The mean elimination half-life ($t_{1/2}$) ranged from 8-16 hours following oral administration.

Pharmacokinetics in Special Populations

Pediatric: Following oral administration of single or multiple doses, systemic exposure of adolescents and children to deferasirox was less than in adult patients. In children <6 years of age, systemic exposure was about 50% lower than in adults.

Geriatric: The pharmacokinetics of deferasirox have not been studied in geriatric patients (65 years of age or older).

Gender: Females have a moderately lower apparent clearance (by 17.5%) for deferasirox compared to males.

Renal Insufficiency: Deferasirox is minimally (8%) excreted via the kidney.

Hepatic Impairment: Deferasirox is principally excreted by glucuronidation and is minimally (8%) metabolized by oxidative cytochrome P450 enzymes. Exjade treatment has been initiated in patients with baseline liver transaminase levels up to 5 times the upper limit of the normal range. The pharmacokinetics of deferasirox were not influenced by such transaminase levels.

12.6 QT Prolongation

The effect of 20 and 40 mg/kg per day of deferasirox on the QT interval was evaluated in a single-dose, double-blind, randomized, placebo- and active-controlled (moxifloxacin 400 mg), parallel group study in 182 healthy male and female volunteers age 18-65 years. No evidence of prolongation of the QTc interval was observed in this study.

13 NONCLINICAL TOXICOLOGY

13.1 Carcinogenesis, Mutagenesis, Impairment of Fertility

A 104-week oral carcinogenicity study in Wistar rats showed no evidence of carcinogenicity from deferasirox at doses up to 60 mg/kg per day (0.48 times the MRHD (Maximum Recommended Human Dose) on a mg/m^2 basis). A 26-week oral carcinogenicity study in p53 (+/-) transgenic mice has shown no evidence of carcinogenicity from deferasirox at doses up to 200 mg/kg per day (0.81 times the MRHD on a mg/m^2 basis) in males and 300 mg/kg per day (1.21 times the MRHD on a mg/m^2 basis) in females.

Deferasirox was negative in the Ames test and chromosome aberration test with human peripheral blood lymphocytes. It was positive in 1 of 3 *in-vivo* oral rat micronucleus tests. Deferasirox at oral doses up to 75 mg/kg per day (0.6 times the MRHD on a mg/m^2 basis) was found to have no adverse effect on fertility and reproductive performance of male and female rats.

14 CLINICAL STUDIES

The primary efficacy study, Study 1, was a multicenter, open-label, randomized, active comparator control study to compare Exjade (deferasirox) and deferoxamine in patients with β-thalassemia and transfusional hemosiderosis. Patients ≥2 years of age were randomized in a 1:1 ratio to receive either oral Exjade at starting doses of 5, 10, 20 or 30 mg/kg once daily or subcutaneous Desferal (deferoxamine) at starting doses of 20 to 60 mg/kg for at least 5 days per week based on LIC (liver iron concentration) at baseline (2-3, >3-7, >7-14 and >14 mg Fe/g dry weight). Patients randomized to deferoxamine who had LIC values <7 mg Fe/g dry weight were permitted to continue on their prior deferoxamine dose, even though the dose may have been higher than specified in the protocol.

Patients were to have a liver biopsy at baseline and end of study (after 12 months) for LIC. The primary efficacy endpoint was defined as a reduction in LIC of ≥3 mg Fe/g dry weight for baseline values ≥10 mg Fe/g dry weight, reduction of baseline values between 7 and <10 to <7 mg Fe/g dry weight, or maintenance or reduction for baseline values <7 mg Fe/g dry weight.

A total of 586 patients were randomized and treated, 296 with Exjade and 290 with deferoxamine. The mean age was 17.1 years (range, 2-53 years); 52% were females and 88% were Caucasian. The primary efficacy population consisted of 553 patients (Exjade n=276; deferoxamine n=277) who had LIC evaluated at baseline and 12 months or discontinued due to an adverse event. The percentage of patients achieving the primary endpoint was 52.9% for Exjade and 66.4% for deferoxamine. The relative efficacy of Exjade to deferoxamine cannot be determined from this study.

In patients who had an LIC at baseline and at end of study, the mean change in LIC was -2.4 mg Fe/g dry weight in patients treated with Exjade and -2.9 mg Fe/g dry weight in patients treated with deferoxamine.

Reduction of LIC and serum ferritin was observed with Exjade doses of 20 to 30 mg/kg per day. Exjade doses below 20 mg/kg per day failed to provide consistent lowering of LIC and serum ferritin levels (Figure 1). Therefore, a starting dose of 20 mg/kg per day is recommended [*see Dosage and Administration (2.1)*].

Figure 1. Changes in Liver Iron Concentration and Serum Ferritin Following EXJADE (5-30 mg/kg per day) in Study 1

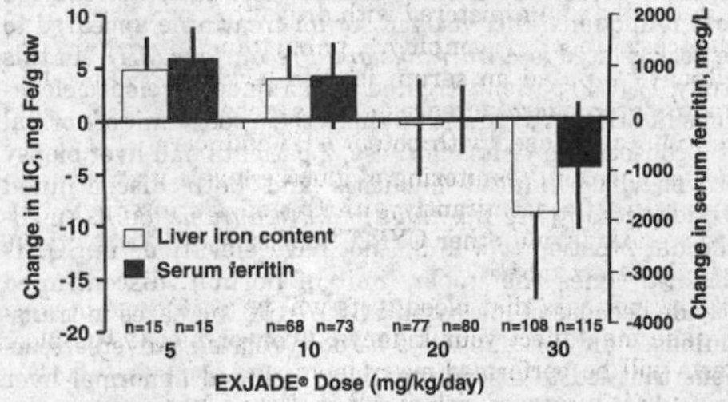

Study 2 was an open-label, noncomparative trial of efficacy and safety of Exjade given for 1 year to patients with chronic anemias and transfusional hemosiderosis. Similar to Study 1, patients received 5, 10, 20, or 30 mg/kg per day of Exjade based on baseline LIC.

A total of 184 patients were treated in this study: 85 patients with β-thalassemia and 99 patients with other congenital or acquired anemias (myelodysplastic syndromes, n=47; Diamond-Blackfan syndrome, n=30; other, n=22). 19% of patients were <16 years of age and 16% were ≥65 years of age. There was a reduction in the absolute LIC from baseline to end of study (-4.2 mg Fe/g dry weight).

Study 3 was a multicenter, open-label, randomized trial of the safety and efficacy of Exjade relative to deferoxamine given for 1 year in patients with sickle cell disease and transfusional hemosiderosis. Patients were randomized to Exjade at doses of 5, 10, 20, or 30 mg/kg per day or subcutaneous deferoxamine at doses of 20-60 mg/kg per day for 5 days per week according to baseline LIC.

A total of 195 patients were treated in this study: 132 with Exjade and 63 with deferoxamine. 44% of patients were <16 years of age and 91% were Black. At end of study, the mean change in LIC (as measured by magnetic susceptometry by a superconducting quantum interference device) in the per protocol-1 (PP-1) population, which consisted of patients who had at least one postbaseline LIC assessment, was -1.3 mg Fe/g dry weight for patients receiving Exjade (n=113) and -0.7 mg Fe/g dry weight for patients receiving deferoxamine (n=54).

16 HOW SUPPLIED/STORAGE AND HANDLING

Exjade is provided as 125 mg, 250 mg, and 500 mg tablets for oral suspension.

125 mg
Off-white, round, flat tablet with beveled edge and imprinted with "J" and "125" on one side and "NVR" on the other.
Bottles of 30 tablets .... (NDC 0078-0468-15)

250 mg
Off-white, round, flat tablet with beveled edge and imprinted with "J" and "250" on one side and "NVR" on the other.
Bottles of 30 tablets .... (NDC 0078-0469-15)

500 mg
Off-white, round, flat tablet with beveled edge and imprinted with "J" and "500" on one side and "NVR" on the other.
Bottles of 30 tablets .... (NDC 0078-0470-15)

Store Exjade tablets at 25°C (77°F); excursions are permitted to 15-30°C (59-86°F) [see USP Controlled Room Temperature]. Protect from moisture.

17 PATIENT COUNSELING INFORMATION

Advise patients to take Exjade once daily on an empty stomach at least 30 minutes prior to food, preferably at the same time every day. Instruct patients to completely disperse the tablets in water, orange juice, or apple juice, and drink the resulting suspension immediately. After the suspension has been swallowed, resuspend any residue in a small volume of the liquid and swallow.

Advise patients not to chew tablets or swallow them whole.

Advise patients who experience diarrhea or vomiting to maintain adequate hydration.

Caution patients not to take aluminum-containing antacids and Exjade simultaneously.

Because auditory and ocular disturbances have been reported with Exjade, conduct auditory testing and ophthalmic testing before starting Exjade treatment and thereafter at regular intervals [see Warnings and Precautions (5.5)].

Caution patients experiencing dizziness to avoid driving or operating machinery [see Adverse Reactions (6.1)].

Caution patients about the potential for the development of GI ulcers or bleeding when taking Exjade in combination with drugs that have ulcerogenic or hemorrhagic potential, such as NSAIDs, corticosteroids, oral bisphosphonates, or anticoagulants.

Caution patients about potential loss of effectiveness of drugs metabolized by CYP3A4 (e.g., cyclosporine, simvastatin, hormonal contraceptive agents) when Exjade is administered with these drugs.

Caution patients about potential loss of effectiveness of Exjade when administered with drugs that are potent UGT inducers (e.g., rifampicin, phenytoin, phenobarbital, ritonavir). Based on serum ferritin levels and clinical response, consider increases in the dose of Exjade when concomitantly used with potent UGT inducers.

Perform careful monitoring of glucose levels when repaglinide is used concomitantly with Exjade. An interaction between Exjade and other CYP2C8 substrates like paclitaxel cannot be excluded.

Advise patients that blood tests will be performed because Exjade may affect your kidneys, liver, or blood. The blood tests will be performed every month or more frequently if you are at increased risk of complications (e.g., pre-existing kidney condition, are elderly, have multiple medical conditions, or are taking medicine that affects your organs). There have been reports of severe kidney and liver problems, blood disorders, stomach bleeds and death in patients taking Exjade.

Skin rashes may occur during Exjade treatment and if severe treatment should be interrupted. Serious allergic reactions (which include swelling of the throat) have been reported in patients taking Exjade, usually within the first month of treatment. If reactions are severe, advise patients to stop taking Exjade and contact their doctor immediately. Certain patients should not receive Exjade. These include patients with creatinine clearance <40 mL/min or serum creatinine >2 times the age-appropriate upper limit of normal, patients with poor performance status and high-risk myelodysplastic syndromes or advanced malignancies, patients with platelet counts <50 × 10⁹/L, and those with hypersensitivity to deferasirox or any component of Exjade.

T2010-22

Manufactured by:
Novartis Pharma Stein AG
Stein, Switzerland

Distributed by:
Novartis Pharmaceuticals Corporation
East Hanover, New Jersey 07936
©Novartis
Shown in Product Identification Guide, page 315

EXTAVIA® ℞
(Interferon beta-1b)
Kit for subcutaneous use

The following prescribing information is based on official labeling in effect July 2009.

HIGHLIGHTS OF PRESCRIBING INFORMATION
These highlights do not include all the information needed to use Extavia safely and effectively. See full prescribing information for Extavia.

Extavia (Interferon beta-1b) Kit for subcutaneous use
Initial U.S. Approval: 1993

──────INDICATIONS AND USAGE──────
EXTAVIA is an interferon beta indicated for the treatment of relapsing forms of multiple sclerosis to reduce the frequency of clinical exacerbations. Patients with multiple sclerosis in whom efficacy has been demonstrated include patients who have experienced a first clinical episode and have MRI features consistent with multiple sclerosis. (1)

──────DOSAGE AND ADMINISTRATION──────
• For subcutaneous use only. (2)
• The recommended dose is 0.25 mg injected subcutaneously every other day. Generally, start at 0.0625 mg (0.25 mL) subcutaneously every other day, and increase over a six week period to 0.25 mg (1 mL) every other day. (2)
• Instruct patients in the use of aseptic technique when administering Extavia. (17.6)

──────DOSAGE FORMS AND STRENGTHS──────
Lyophilized powder containing 0.3 mg of Interferon beta-1b, 15 mg Albumin (Human), USP, and 15 mg Mannitol, USP. (3)

──────CONTRAINDICATIONS──────
History of hypersensitivity to natural or recombinant interferon beta, Albumin (Human), USP, or any other component of the formulation. (4)

──────WARNINGS AND PRECAUTIONS──────
• Depression and suicide: advise patients to immediately report any symptom of depression and/or suicidal ideation; consider discontinuation of Extavia if depression occurs. (5.1)
• Injection site necrosis: do not administer Extavia into affected area until it is fully healed; if multiple lesions occur, therapy should be discontinued until healing occurs. (5.2)
• Injection site reactions. (5.3)
• Anaphylaxis and other allergic reactions. (5.4)
• Flu-Like Symptom Complex. (5.5)
• Leukopenia: monitor CBC. (5.6, 5.8)
• Liver enzymes abnormalities: monitor liver function tests. (5.7, 5.8)
• Monitor thyroid function tests every 6 months in patients with history of thyroid dysfunction. (5.8)

──────ADVERSE REACTIONS──────
In controlled studies with interferon beta-1b, the most common adverse reactions (at least 2% more than placebo) were: Lymphopenia, neutropenia, leukopenia, lymphadenopathy, headache, insomnia, incoordination, hypertension, dyspnea, abdominal pain, increased liver enzymes, rash, skin disorder, hypertonia, myalgia, urinary urgency, metrorrhagia, impotence, injection site reaction, asthenia, flu-like symptom complex, pain, fever, chills, peripheral edema, chest pain, malaise, and injection site necrosis. (6.1)

To report SUSPECTED ADVERSE REACTIONS, contact Novartis Pharmaceuticals Corporation at 1-888-669-6682 or FDA at 1-800-FDA-1088 or www.fda.gov/medwatch

──────DRUG INTERACTIONS──────
No formal drug interaction studies have been conducted. (7)

──────USE IN SPECIFIC POPULATIONS──────
• Pregnancy: Based on animal data, may cause fetal harm. (8.1)
• Nursing Mothers: Use EXTAVIA with caution. (8.3)
• Pediatric Use: Safety and efficacy not established in patients under 18 years of age. (8.3)
• Geriatric Use: Safety and efficacy not established in patients age 65 years or older. (8.4)

See 17 for PATIENT COUNSELING INFORMATION and Medication Guide

Revised: 08/2009

FULL PRESCRIBING INFORMATION

1 INDICATIONS AND USAGE

EXTAVIA (Interferon beta-1b) is indicated for the treatment of relapsing forms of multiple sclerosis to reduce the frequency of clinical exacerbations. Patients with multiple sclerosis in whom efficacy has been demonstrated include patients who have experienced a first clinical episode and have MRI features consistent with multiple sclerosis.

2 DOSAGE AND ADMINISTRATION

The recommended dose of EXTAVIA is 0.25 mg injected subcutaneously every other day.

Generally, patients should be started at 0.0625 mg (0.25 mL) subcutaneously every other day, and increased over a six week period to 0.25 mg (1 mL) every other day (see Table 1).

Table 1. Schedule for Dose Titration

	Recommended Titration	EXTAVIA Dose	Volume
Weeks 1-2	25%	0.0625 mg	0.25 mL
Weeks 3-4	50%	0.125 mg	0.5 mL
Weeks 5-6	75%	0.1875 mg	0.75 mL
Week 7+	100%	0.25 mg	1 mL

To reconstitute lyophilized EXTAVIA for injection, attach the prefilled syringe containing the diluent (Sodium Chloride, 0.54% Solution) to the EXTAVIA vial using the vial adapter. Slowly inject 1.2 mL of diluent into the EXTAVIA vial. Gently swirl the vial to dissolve the drug completely; do not shake. Foaming may occur during reconstitution or if the vial is swirled or shaken too vigorously. If foaming occurs, allow the vial to sit undisturbed until the foam settles. Visually inspect the reconstituted product before use; discard the product if it contains particulate matter or is discolored. Keeping the syringe and vial adapter in place, turn the assembly over so that the vial is on top. Withdraw the appropriate dose of EXTAVIA solution. Remove the vial from the vial adapter before injecting EXTAVIA. One mL of reconstituted EXTAVIA solution contains 0.25 mg of Interferon beta-1b/mL.

EXTAVIA is intended for use under the guidance and supervision of a physician. It is recommended that physicians or qualified medical personnel train patients in the proper technique for self-administering subcutaneous injections. Patients should be advised to rotate sites for subcutaneous injections (see Patient Counseling Information 17.6). Concurrent use of analgesics and/or antipyretics may help ameliorate flu-like symptoms on treatment days. EXTAVIA should be visually inspected for particulate matter and discoloration prior to administration.

3 DOSAGE FORMS AND STRENGTHS

EXTAVIA is supplied as a lyophilized powder containing 0.3 mg of Interferon beta-1b, 15 mg Albumin (Human), USP, and 15 mg Mannitol, USP. Drug is packaged in a clear glass, single-use vial (3 mL capacity). A pre-filled single-use syringe containing 1.2 mL of diluent (Sodium Chloride, 0.54% solution), two alcohol prep pads, and one vial adapter with attached 27 gauge needle are included for each vial of drug. EXTAVIA and the diluent are for single-use only. Unused portions should be discarded. Store at room temperature.

4 CONTRAINDICATIONS

EXTAVIA is contraindicated in patients with a history of hypersensitivity to natural or recombinant interferon beta, Albumin (Human), USP, or any other component of the formulation.

5 WARNINGS AND PRECAUTIONS

5.1 Depression and Suicide

EXTAVIA (Interferon beta-1b) should be used with caution in patients with depression, a condition that is common in people with multiple sclerosis. Depression and suicide have been reported to occur with increased frequency in patients receiving interferon compounds, including Interferon beta-1b. Patients treated with EXTAVIA should be advised to report immediately any symptoms of depression and/or suicidal ideation to their prescribing physicians. If a patient develops depression, cessation of EXTAVIA therapy should be considered.

In the four randomized controlled studies there were three suicides and eight suicide attempts among the 1532 patients in the Interferon beta-1b treated groups compared to one suicide and four suicide attempts among the 965 patients in the placebo groups.

5.2 Injection Site Necrosis

Injection site necrosis (ISN) has been reported in 4% of patients in controlled clinical trials [see Adverse Reactions (6.1)]. Typically, injection site necrosis occurs within the first four months of therapy, although postmarketing reports have been received of ISN occurring over one year after initiation of therapy. Necrosis may occur at a single or multiple injection sites. The necrotic lesions are typically three cm or less in diameter, but larger areas have been reported. Generally the necrosis has extended only to subcutaneous fat. However, there are also reports of necrosis extending to and including fascia overlying muscle. In some lesions where biopsy results are available, vasculitis has been reported. For some lesions debridement and, infrequently, skin grafting have been required.

As with any open lesion, it is important to avoid infection and, if it occurs, to treat the infection. Time to healing was varied depending on the severity of the necrosis at the time treatment was begun. In most cases healing was associated with scarring.

Some patients have experienced healing of necrotic skin lesions while Interferon beta-1b therapy continued; others have not. Whether to discontinue therapy following a single site of necrosis is dependent on the extent of necrosis. For patients who continue therapy with EXTAVIA after injection site necrosis has occurred, EXTAVIA should not be administered into the affected area until it is fully healed. If multiple lesions occur, therapy should be discontinued until healing occurs.

Patient understanding and use of aseptic self-injection techniques and procedures should be periodically reevaluated, particularly if injection site necrosis has occurred.

5.3 Injection Site Reactions

In controlled clinical trials, injection site reactions occurred in 78% of patients receiving Interferon beta-1b with injection site necrosis in 4%. Injection site inflammation (42%), injection site pain (16%), injection site hypersensitivity (4%), injection site necrosis (4%), injection site mass (2%), injection site edema (2%) and non-specific reactions were significantly associated with Interferon beta-1b treatment. The incidence of injection site reactions tended to decrease over time. Approximately 69% of patients experienced the event during the first three months of treatment, compared to approximately 40% at the end of the studies.

5.4 Anaphylaxis

Anaphylaxis has been reported as a rare complication of Interferon beta-1b use. Other allergic reactions have included dyspnea, bronchospasm, tongue edema, skin rash and urticaria [see Adverse Reactions (6.1)].

5.5 Flu-Like Symptom Complex

In controlled clinical trials, the rate of flu-like symptom complex was approximately 57%. The incidence decreased over time, with only 10% of patients reporting flu-like symptom complex at the end of the studies. The median duration of flu-like symptom complex in Study 1 was 7.5 days [see Clinical Studies (14)].

5.6 Leukopenia

In controlled clinical trials, leukopenia was reported in 18% of patients receiving Interferon beta-1b, leading to a reduction of the dose of Interferon beta-1b in some patients [see Adverse Reactions (6.1)]. Monitoring of complete blood and differential white blood cell counts is recommended [see Warnings and Precautions (5.8)].

5.7 Hepatic Enzymes Elevations

In controlled clinical trials, elevations of SGPT to greater than five times baseline value were reported in 12% of patients receiving Interferon beta-1b, and increase of SGOT to greater than five times baseline value were reported in 4% of patients receiving Interferon beta-1b, leading to dose-reduction or discontinuation of treatment in some patients [see Adverse Reactions (6.1)]. Monitoring of liver function tests is recommended [see Warnings and Precautions (5.8)].

5.8 Laboratory Tests

In addition to those laboratory tests normally required for monitoring patients with multiple sclerosis, complete blood and differential white blood cell counts, platelet counts and blood chemistries, including liver function tests, are recommended at regular intervals (one, three, and six months) following introduction of EXTAVIA therapy, and then periodically thereafter in the absence of clinical symptoms. Thyroid function tests are recommended every six months in patients with a history of thyroid dysfunction or as clinically indicated. Patients with myelosuppression may require more intensive monitoring of complete blood cell counts, with differential and platelet counts.

5.9 Albumin (Human), USP

This product contains albumin, a derivative of human blood. Based on effective donor screening and product manufacturing processes, it carries an extremely remote risk for transmission of viral diseases. A theoretical risk for transmission of Creutzfeldt-Jakob disease (CJD) also is considered extremely remote. No cases of transmission of viral diseases or CJD have ever been identified for albumin.

6 ADVERSE REACTIONS

6.1 Clinical Studies Experience

In all studies, the most serious adverse reactions with Interferon beta-1b were depression, suicidal ideation and injection site necrosis (see Warnings and Precautions). The incidence of depression of any severity was approximately 30% in both Interferon beta-1b-treated patients and placebo-treated patients. Anaphylaxis and other allergic reactions have been reported in patients using Interferon beta-1b [see Warnings and Precautions (5.4)]. The most commonly reported adverse reactions were lymphopenia (lymphocytes <1500/mm³), injection site reaction, asthenia, flu-like symptom complex, headache, and pain. The most frequently reported adverse reactions resulting in clinical intervention (e.g., discontinuation of Interferon beta-1b, adjustment in dosage, or the need for concomitant medication to treat an adverse reaction symptom) were depression, flu-like symptom complex, injection site reactions, leukopenia, increased liver enzymes, asthenia, hypertonia, and myasthenia.

Because clinical trials are conducted under widely varying conditions and over varying lengths of time, adverse reaction rates observed in the clinical trials of Interferon beta-1b cannot be directly compared to rates in clinical trials of other drugs, and may not reflect the rates observed in practice. The adverse reaction information from clinical trials does, however, provide a basis for identifying the adverse events that appear to be related to drug use and for approximating rates.

The data described below reflect exposure to Interferon beta-1b in the four placebo controlled trials of 1407 patients with MS treated with 0.25 mg or 0.16 mg/m², including 1261 exposed for greater than one year. The population encompassed an age range from 18-65 years. Sixty-four percent (64%) of the patients were female. The percentages of Caucasian, Black, Asian, and Hispanic patients were 94.8%, 3.5%, 0.1%, and 0.7%, respectively.

The safety profiles for Interferon beta-1b-treated patients with SPMS and RRMS were similar. Clinical experience with Interferon beta-1b in other populations (patients with cancer, HIV positive patients, etc.) provides additional data regarding adverse reactions; however, experience in non-MS populations may not be fully applicable to the MS population.

Table 2 enumerates adverse events and laboratory abnormalities that occurred among all patients treated with 0.25 mg or 0.16 mg/m² Interferon beta-1b every other day for periods of up to three years in the four placebo controlled trials (Study 1-4) at an incidence that was at least 2.0% more than that observed in the placebo patients (System Organ Class, MedDRA v. 8.0).

Table 2. Adverse Reactions and Laboratory Abnormalities

System Organ Class MedDRA v. 8.0[#] Adverse Reaction	Placebo (n=965)	Interferon beta-1b (n=1407)
Blood and lymphatic system disorders		
Lymphocytes count decreased (<1500/mm³)[x]	66%	86%
Absolute neutrophil count decreased (<1500/mm³)[x]	5%	13%
White blood cell count decreased (<3000/mm³)[x]	4%	13%
Lymphadenopathy	3%	6%
Nervous system disorders		
Headache	43%	50%
Insomnia	16%	21%
Incoordination	15%	17%
Vascular disorders		
Hypertension	4%	6%
Respiratory, thoracic and mediastinal disorders		
Dyspnea	3%	6%
Gastrointestinal disorders		
Abdominal pain	11%	16%
Hepatobiliary disorders		
Alanine aminotransferase increased (SGPT >5 times baseline)[x]	4%	12%
Aspartate aminotransferase increased (SGOT >5 times baseline)[x]	1%	4%
Skin and subcutaneous tissue disorders		
Rash	15%	21%
Skin disorder	8%	10%
Musculoskeletal and connective tissue disorders		
Hypertonia	33%	40%
Myalgia	14%	23%
Renal and urinary disorders		
Urinary urgency	8%	11%
Reproductive system and breast disorders		
Metrorrhagia*	7%	9%
Impotence**	6%	8%
General disorders and administration site conditions		
Injection site reaction (various kinds)[0]	26%	78%
Asthenia	48%	53%
Flu-like symptoms (complex)[§]	37%	57%
Pain	35%	42%
Fever	19%	31%
Chills	9%	21%

Peripheral edema	10%	12%
Chest pain	6%	9%
Malaise	3%	6%
Injection site necrosis	0%	4%

[#] except for "injection site reaction (various kinds)[o]" and "flu-like symptom complex[§]" the most appropriate MedDRA term is used to describe a certain reaction and its synonyms and related conditions.
[x] laboratory abnormality
[*] pre-menopausal women
[**] men
[o] "Injection site reaction (various kinds)" comprises all adverse events occurring at the injection site (except injection site necrosis), i.e., the following terms: injection site reaction, injection site hemorrhage, injection site hypersensitivity, injection site inflammation, injection site mass, injection site pain, injection site edema and injection site atrophy.
[§] "Flu-like symptom complex" denotes flu syndrome and/or a combination of at least two AEs from fever, chills, myalgia, malaise, sweating.

Laboratory Abnormalities

In the four clinical trials, leukopenia was reported in 18% and 6% of patients in Interferon beta-1b- and placebo-treated groups, respectively. No patients were withdrawn or dose reduced for neutropenia in Study 1. Three percent (3%) of patients in Studies 2 and 3 experienced leukopenia and were dose-reduced. Monitoring of complete blood and differential white blood cell counts is recommended *[see Warnings and Precautions (5.6, 5.8)]*.

Other abnormalities included increase of SGPT to greater than five times baseline value (12%), and increase of SGOT to greater than five times baseline value (4%). In Study 1, two patients were dose reduced for increased hepatic enzymes; one continued on treatment and one was ultimately withdrawn. In Studies 2 and 3, 1.5% of Interferon beta-1b patients were dose-reduced or interrupted treatment for increased hepatic enzymes. In Study 4, 1.7% of patients were withdrawn from treatment due to increased hepatic enzymes, two of them after a dose reduction. In Studies 1-4, nine (0.6%) patients were withdrawn from treatment with Interferon beta-1b for any laboratory abnormality, including four (0.3%) patients following dose reduction. Monitoring of liver function tests is recommended *[see Warnings and Precautions (5.7, 5.8)]*.

6.2 Postmarketing Experience

The following adverse events have been observed during postmarketing experience with Interferon beta-1b and are classified within body system categories:

Blood and lymphatic system disorders: Anemia, Thrombocytopenia

Endocrine disorders: Hypothyroidism, Hyperthyroidism, Thyroid dysfunction

Metabolism and nutrition disorders: Hypocalcemia, Hyperuricemia, Triglyceride increased, Anorexia, Weight decrease

Psychiatric disorders: Confusion, Depersonalization, Emotional lability

Nervous system disorders: Ataxia, Convulsion, Paresthesia, Psychotic symptoms

Cardiac disorders: Cardiomyopathy

Vascular disorders: Deep vein thrombosis, Pulmonary embolism

Respiratory, thoracic and mediastinal disorders: Bronchospasm, Pneumonia

Gastrointestinal disorders: Pancreatitis, Vomiting

Hepatobiliary disorders: Hepatitis, Gamma GT increased

Skin and subcutaneous tissue disorders: Pruritus, Skin discoloration, Urticaria

Renal and urinary disorders: Urinary tract infection, Urosepsis

General disorders and administration site conditions: Fatal capillary leak syndrome*.

*The administration of cytokines to patients with a preexisting monoclonal gammopathy has been associated with the development of this syndrome.

6.3 Immunogenicity

As with all therapeutic proteins, there is a potential for immunogenicity. Serum samples were monitored for the development of antibodies to Interferon beta-1b during Study 1 *[see Clinical Studies (14)]*. In patients receiving 0.25 mg every other day 56/124 (45%) were found to have serum neutralizing activity at one or more of the time points tested. In Study 4 *[see Clinical Studies (14)]*, neutralizing activity was measured every 6 months and at end of study. At individual visits after start of therapy, activity was observed in 16.5% up to 25.2% of the Interferon beta-1b treated patients. Such neutralizing activity was measured at least once in 75 (29.9%) out of 251 Interferon beta-1b patients who provided samples during treatment phase; of these, 17 (22.7%) converted to negative status later in the study.

Based on all the available evidence, the relationship between antibody formation and clinical safety or efficacy is not known.

These data reflect the percentage of patients whose test results were considered positive for antibodies to Interferon beta-1b using a biological neutralization assay that measures the ability of immune sera to inhibit the production of the interferon-inducible protein, MxA. Neutralization assays are highly dependent on the sensitivity and specificity of the assay. Additionally, the observed incidence of neutralizing activity in an assay may be influenced by several factors including sample handling, timing of sample collection, concomitant medications, and underlying disease. For these reasons, comparison of the incidence of antibodies to Interferon beta-1b with the incidence of antibodies to other products may be misleading.

Anaphylactic reactions have rarely been reported with the use of Interferon beta-1b *[see Warnings and Precautions (5.4)]*.

7 DRUG INTERACTIONS

No formal drug interaction studies have been conducted with Interferon beta-1b. In the placebo controlled studies in MS, corticosteroids or ACTH were administered for treatment of relapses for periods of up to 28 days in patients (N=664) receiving Interferon beta-1b.

8 USE IN SPECIFIC POPULATIONS

8.1 Pregnancy

Pregnancy Category C: There are no adequate and well-controlled studies of Interferon beta-1b in pregnant women; however, spontaneous abortions while on treatment were reported in four patients participating in the Interferon beta-1b RRMS clinical trial. Interferon beta-1b should be used during pregnancy only if the potential benefit justifies the potential risk to the fetus.

When Interferon beta-1b (doses ranging from 0.028 to 0.42 mg/kg) was administered to pregnant rhesus monkeys throughout the period of organogenesis (gestation days 20 to 70), a dose-related abortifacient effect was observed. The low effect dose is approximately 3 times the recommended human dose of 0.25 mg on a body surface are (mg/m^2) basis. A no-effect dose for embryo-fetal developmental toxicity in rhesus monkeys was not established.

8.3 Nursing Mothers

It is not known whether Interferon beta-1b is excreted in human milk. Because many drugs are excreted in human milk and because of the potential for serious adverse reactions in nursing infants from Interferon beta-1b, a decision should be made to either discontinue nursing or discontinue the drug, taking into account the importance of drug to the mother.

8.4 Pediatric Use

Safety and efficacy in pediatric patients have not been established.

8.5 Geriatric Use

Clinical studies of Interferon beta-1b did not include sufficient numbers of patients aged 65 and over to determine whether they respond differently than younger patients.

10 OVERDOSAGE

Safety of doses higher than 0.25 mg every other day has not been adequately evaluated. The maximum amount of Interferon beta-1b that can be safely administered has not been determined.

11 DESCRIPTION

EXTAVIA® (Interferon beta-1b) is a purified, sterile, lyophilized protein product produced by recombinant DNA techniques. Interferon beta-1b is manufactured by bacterial fermentation of a strain of *Escherichia coli* that bears a genetically engineered plasmid containing the gene for human interferon beta$_{ser17}$. The native gene was obtained from human fibroblasts and altered in a way that substitutes serine for the cysteine residue found at position 17. Interferon beta-1b has 165 amino acids and an approximate molecular weight of 18,500 daltons. It does not include the carbohydrate side chains found in the natural material. EXTAVIA contains the same active ingredients as other Interferon beta-1b products. For this reason, these products should not be given concomitantly.

The specific activity of EXTAVIA is approximately 32 million international units (IU)/mg Interferon beta-1b. Each vial contains 0.3 mg of Interferon beta-1b. The unit measurement is derived by comparing the antiviral activity of the product to the World Health Organization (WHO) reference standard of recombinant human interferon beta. Mannitol, USP and Albumin (Human), USP (15 mg each/vial) are added as stabilizers.

Lyophilized EXTAVIA is a sterile, white to off-white powder, for subcutaneous injection after reconstitution with the diluent supplied (Sodium Chloride, 0.54% Solution).

12 CLINICAL PHARMACOLOGY

12.1 Mechanism of Action

The mechanism of action of Interferon beta-1b in patients with multiple sclerosis is unknown.

12.2 Pharmacodynamics

Interferons (IFNs) are a family of naturally occurring proteins, produced by eukaryotic cells in response to viral infection and other biologic agents. Four major groups of interferons have been distinguished: alpha, beta, gamma and lambda. Interferons-alpha and -beta comprise the Type I interferons, interferon-gamma is the sole Type II interferon, and interferon-lambda is designated as Type III interferon. Type I interferons have considerably overlapping but also distinct biologic activities. The bioactivities of IFNs are mediated by their interactions with specific receptors found on the surfaces of human cells. Differences in bioactivities induced by IFNs likely reflect divergences in the signal transduction process induced by IFN-receptor binding.

Interferon beta-1b receptor binding induces the expression of proteins that are responsible for the pleiotropic bioactivities of Interferon beta-1b. A number of these proteins (including neopterin, β_2-microglobulin, MxA protein, and IL-10) have been measured in blood fractions from Interferon beta-1b-treated patients and Interferon beta-1b-treated healthy volunteers. Immunomodulatory effects of Interferon beta-1b include the enhancement of suppressor T cell activity, reduction of pro-inflammatory cytokine production, down-regulation of antigen presentation, and inhibition of lymphocyte trafficking into the central nervous system. It is not known if these effects play an important role in the observed clinical activity of Interferon beta-1b in multiple sclerosis (MS).

12.3 Pharmacokinetics

Because serum concentrations of Interferon beta-1b are low or not detectable following subcutaneous administration of 0.25 mg or less of Interferon beta-1b, pharmacokinetic information in patients with MS receiving the recommended dose of Interferon beta-1b is not available. Following single and multiple daily subcutaneous administrations of 0.5 mg Interferon beta-1b to healthy volunteers (N=12), serum Interferon beta-1b concentrations were generally below 100 IU/mL. Peak serum Interferon beta-1b concentrations occurred between one to eight hours, with a mean peak serum interferon concentration of 40 IU/mL. Bioavailability, based on a total dose of 0.5 mg Interferon beta-1b given as two subcutaneous injections at different sites, was approximately 50%.

After intravenous administration of Interferon beta-1b (0.006 mg to 2.0 mg), similar pharmacokinetic profiles were obtained from healthy volunteers (N=12) and from patients with diseases other than MS (N=142). In patients receiving single intravenous doses up to 2.0 mg, increases in serum concentrations were dose proportional. Mean serum clearance values ranged from 9.4 mL/min•kg^{-1} to 28.9 mL/min•kg^{-1} and were independent of dose.

Mean terminal elimination half-life values ranged from 8.0 minutes to 4.3 hours and mean steady-state volume of distribution values ranged from 0.25 L/kg to 2.88 L/kg. Three-times-a-week intravenous dosing for two weeks resulted in no accumulation of Interferon beta-1b in sera of patients. Pharmacokinetic parameters after single and multiple intravenous doses of Interferon beta-1b were comparable.

Following every other day subcutaneous administration of 0.25 mg Interferon beta-1b in healthy volunteers, biologic response marker levels (neopterin, β_2-microglobulin, MxA protein, and the immunosuppressive cytokine, IL-10) increased significantly above baseline six-twelve hours after the first Interferon beta-1b dose. Biologic response marker levels peaked between 40 and 124 hours and remained elevated above baseline throughout the seven-day (168-hour) study. The relationship between serum Interferon beta-1b levels or induced biologic response marker levels and the clinical effects of Interferon beta-1b in multiple sclerosis is unknown.

13 NONCLINICAL TOXICOLOGY

13.1 Carcinogenesis, Mutagenesis, Impairment of Fertility

Carcinogenesis: Interferon beta-1b has not been tested for its carcinogenic potential in animals.

Mutagenesis: Interferon beta-1b was not genotoxic in the *in vitro* Ames bacterial test or the *in vitro* chromosomal aberration assay in human peripheral blood lymphocytes. Interferon beta-1b treatment of mouse BALBc-3T3 cells did not result in increased transformation frequency in an *in vitro* model of tumor transformation.

Impairment of fertility: Administration of Interferon beta-1b (doses of up to 0.33 mg/kg) to normally cycling female rhesus monkeys had no apparent adverse effects on either menstrual cycle duration or associated hormonal profiles (progesterone and estradiol) when administered over three consecutive menstrual cycles. The highest dose tested is approximately 30 times the recommended human dose of 0.25 mg on a body surface area (mg/m^2) basis. The potential for other effects on fertility or reproductive performance was not evaluated.

14 CLINICAL STUDIES

The clinical effects of Interferon beta-1b were studied in four randomized, multicenter, double-blind, placebo-controlled studies in patients with multiple sclerosis.

The effectiveness of Interferon beta-1b in relapsing-remitting MS (Study 1) was evaluated in a double blind, multiclinic, randomized, parallel, placebo controlled clinical investigation of two years' duration. The study enrolled MS patients, aged 18 to 50, who were ambulatory (EDSS of ≤5.5), exhibited a relapsing-remitting clinical course, met Poser's criteria[1] for clinically definite and/or laboratory supported definite MS and had experienced at least two exacerbations over two years preceding the trial without exacerbation in the preceding month. Patients who had received prior immunosuppressant therapy were excluded.

An exacerbation was defined as the appearance of a new clinical sign/symptom or the clinical worsening of a previous sign/symptom (one that had been stable for at least 30 days) that persisted for a minimum of 24 hours.

Patients selected for study were randomized to treatment with either placebo (N=123), 0.05 mg of Interferon beta-1b (N=125), or 0.25 mg of Interferon beta-1b (N=124) self-administered subcutaneously every other day. Outcome based on the 372 randomized patients was evaluated after two years.

Patients who required more than three 28-day courses of corticosteroids were removed from the study. Minor analgesics (acetaminophen, codeine), antidepressants, and oral baclofen were allowed ad libitum, but chronic nonsteroidal anti-inflammatory drug (NSAID) use was not allowed.

The primary protocol-defined outcome measures were 1) frequency of exacerbations per patient and 2) proportion of exacerbation free patients. A number of secondary clinical and magnetic resonance imaging (MRI) measures were also employed. All patients underwent annual T2 MRI imaging and a subset of 52 patients at one site had MRIs performed every six weeks for assessment of new or expanding lesions. The study results are shown in **Table 3**.

[See table 3 above]

Of the 372 RRMS patients randomized, 72 (19%) failed to complete two full years on their assigned treatments.

Over the two-year period, there were 25 MS-related hospitalizations in the 0.25 mg Interferon beta-1b-treated group compared to 48 hospitalizations in the placebo group. In comparison, non-MS hospitalizations were evenly distributed among the groups, with 16 in the 0.25 mg Interferon beta-1b group and 15 in the placebo group. The average number of days of MS-related steroid use was 41 days in the 0.25 mg Interferon beta-1b group and 55 days in the placebo group (p=0.004).

MRI data were also analyzed for patients in this study. A frequency distribution of the observed percent changes in MRI area at the end of two years was obtained by grouping the percentages in successive intervals of equal width. Figure 1 displays a histogram of the proportions of patients, which fell into each of these intervals. The median percent change in MRI area for the 0.25 mg group was -1.1%, which was significantly smaller than the 16.5% observed for the placebo group (p=0.0001).

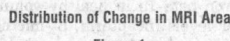

Distribution of Change in MRI Area
Figure 1

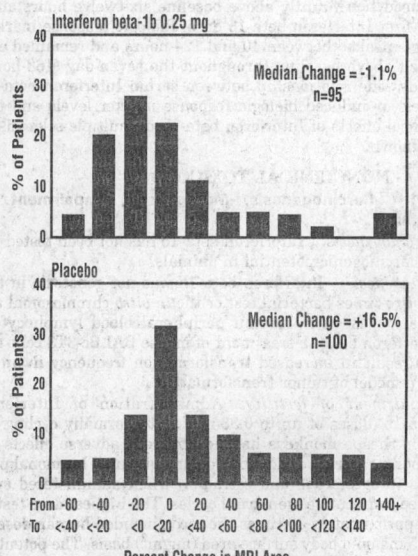

Interferon beta-1b 0.25 mg
Median Change = -1.1%
n=95

Placebo
Median Change = +16.5%
n=100

Percent Change in MRI Area

In an evaluation of frequent MRI scans (every six weeks) on 52 patients at one site, the percent of scans with new or expanding lesions was 29% in the placebo group and 6% in the 0.25 mg treatment group (p=0.006).

Table 3. Two Year RRMS Study Results. Primary and Secondary Clinical Outcomes

Efficacy Parameters		Treatment Groups			Statistical Comparisons p-value		
Primary Endpoints		Placebo N=123	0.05 mg N=125	0.25 mg N=124	Placebo vs 0.05 mg	0.05 mg vs 0.25 mg	Placebo vs 0.25 mg
Annual exacerbation rate		1.31	1.14	0.90	0.005	0.113	**0.0001**
Proportion of exacerbation-free patients[†]		16%	18%	25%	0.609	0.288	**0.094**
Exacerbation frequency per patient	0[†]	20	22	29	0.151	0.077	**0.001**
	1	32	31	39			
	2	20	28	17			
	3	15	15	14			
	4	15	7	9			
	≥5	21	16	8			
Secondary Endpoints[††]							
Median number of months to first on-study exacerbation		5	6	9	0.299	0.097	**0.010**
Rate of moderate or severe exacerbations per year		0.47	0.29	0.23	0.020	0.257	**0.001**
Mean number of moderate or severe exacerbation days per patient		44.1	33.2	19.5	0.229	0.064	**0.001**
Mean change in EDSS score[‡] at endpoint		0.21	0.21	-0.07	0.995	0.108	**0.144**
Mean change in Scripps score[‡‡] at endpoint		-0.53	-0.50	0.66	0.641	0.051	**0.126**
Median duration in days per exacerbation		36	33	35.5	ND	ND	**ND**
% change in mean MRI lesion area at endpoint		21.4%	9.8%	-0.9%	0.015	0.019	**0.0001**

ND Not done
† 14 exacerbation free patients (0 from placebo, six from 0.05 mg, and eight from 0.25 mg) dropped out of the study before completing six months of therapy. These patients are excluded from this analysis.
†† Sequelae and Functional Neurologic Status, both required by protocol, were not analyzed individually but are included as a function of the EDSS.
‡ EDSS scores range from 1-10, with higher scores reflecting greater disability
‡‡ Scripps neurologic rating scores range from 0-100, with smaller scores reflecting greater disability.

The exact relationship between MRI findings and clinical status of patients is unknown. Changes in lesion area often do not correlate with changes in disability progression. The prognostic significance of the MRI findings in this study has not been evaluated.

Studies 2 and 3 were multicenter, randomized, double-blind, placebo controlled trials conducted to assess the effect of Interferon beta-1b in patients with SPMS. Study 2 was conducted in Europe and Study 3 was conducted in North America. Both studies enrolled patients with clinically definite or laboratory-supported MS in the secondary progressive phase, and who had evidence of disability progression (both Study 2 and 3) or two relapses (Study 2 only) within the previous two years. Baseline Kurtzke expanded disability status scale (EDSS) scores ranged from 3.0 to 6.5.[2] Patients in Study 2 were randomized to receive Interferon beta-1b 0.25 mg (n=360) or placebo (n=358). Patients in Study 3 were randomized to Interferon beta-1b 0.25 mg (n=317), Interferon beta-1b 0.16 mg/m² of body surface area (n=314, mean assigned dose 0.30 mg), or placebo (n=308). Test agents were administered subcutaneously, every other day for three years.

The primary outcome measure was progression of disability, defined as a 1.0 point increase in the EDSS score, or a 0.5 point increase for patients with baseline EDSS ≥ 6.0. In Study 2, time to progression in EDSS was longer in the Interferon beta-1b treatment group (p=0.005), with estimated annualized rates of progression of 16% and 19% in the Interferon beta-1b and placebo groups, respectively. In Study 3, the rates of progression did not differ significantly between treatment groups, with estimated annualized rates of progression of 12%, 14%, and 12% in the Interferon beta-1b fixed dose, surface area-adjusted dose, and placebo groups, respectively.

Multiple analyses, including covariate and subset analyses based on sex, age, disease duration, clinical disease activity prior to study enrollment, MRI measures at baseline and early changes in MRI following treatment were evaluated in order to interpret the discordant study results. No demographic or disease-related factors enabled identification of a patient subset where Interferon beta-1b treatment was predictably associated with delayed progression of disability.

In Studies 2 and 3, like Study 1, a statistically significant decrease in the incidence of relapses associated with Interferon beta-1b treatment was demonstrated. In Study 2, the mean annual relapse rate was 0.42 and 0.63 in the Interferon beta-1b and placebo groups, respectively (p<0.001). In Study 3, the mean annual relapse rates were 0.16, 0.20, and 0.28, for the fixed dose, surface area-adjusted dose, and placebo groups, respectively (p<0.02).

MRI endpoints in both Study 2 and Study 3 showed lesser increases in T2 MRI lesion area and decreased number of active MRI lesions in patients in the Interferon beta-1b groups. The exact relationship between MRI findings and the clinical status of patients is unknown. Changes in MRI findings often do not correlate with changes in disability progression. The prognostic significance of the MRI findings in these studies is not known.

In Study 4, 468 patients who had recently (within 60 days) experienced an isolated demyelinating event, and who had lesions typical of multiple sclerosis on brain MRI were randomized to receive either 0.25 mg Interferon beta-1b (n = 292) or placebo (n= 176) subcutaneously every other day (ratio 5:3). The primary outcome measure was time to development of a second exacerbation with involvement of at least two distinct anatomical regions. Secondary outcomes were brain MRI measures, including the cumulative number of newly active lesions, and the absolute change in T2 lesion volume. Patients were followed for up to two years or until they fulfilled the primary endpoint.

Eight percent of subjects on Interferon beta-1b and 6% of subjects on placebo withdrew from the study for a reason other than the development of a second exacerbation. Time to development of a second exacerbation was significantly delayed in patients treated with Interferon beta-1b compared to placebo (p<0.0001). The Kaplan-Meier estimates of the percentage of patients developing an exacerbation within 24 months were 45% in the placebo group and 28% of the Interferon beta-1b group (Figure 2). The risk for developing a second exacerbation in the Interferon beta-1b group was 53% of the risk in the placebo group (Hazard ratio= 0.53; 95% confidence interval 0.39 to 0.73).

Figure 2. Onset of Second Exacerbation by Time on Study (Kaplan-Meier Methodology)

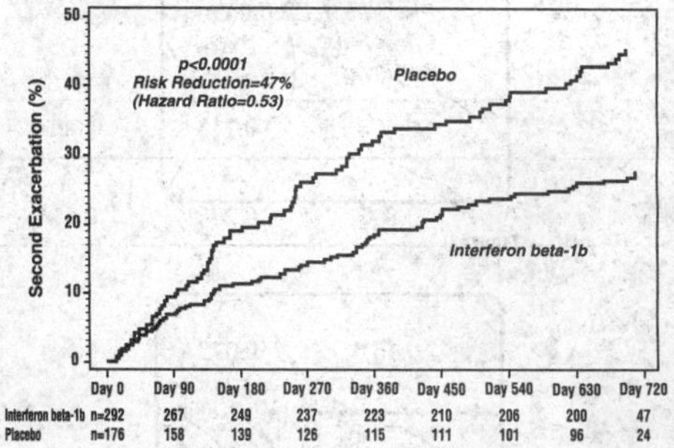
Second Exacerbation (%)
50
40
30
20
10
0
p<0.0001
Risk Reduction=47%
(Hazard Ratio=0.53)
Placebo
Interferon beta-1b
Day 0 Day 90 Day 180 Day 270 Day 360 Day 450 Day 540 Day 630 Day 720
Interferon beta-1b n=292 267 249 237 223 210 206 200 47
Placebo n=176 158 139 126 115 111 101 96 24

Patients treated with Interferon beta-1b demonstrated a lower number of newly active lesions during the course of the study. A significant difference between Interferon beta-1b and placebo was not seen in the absolute change in T2 lesion volume during the course of the study.

Safety and efficacy of treatment with Interferon beta-1b beyond three years are not known.

15 REFERENCES

1. Poser CM, et al. Ann Neurol 1983; 13(3): 227-231.
2. Kurtzke JF. Neurology 1983; 33(11): 1444-1452.

16 HOW SUPPLIED/STORAGE AND HANDLING

The reconstituted product contains no preservative. Before reconstitution with diluent, store EXTAVIA at room temperature 25°C (77°F). Excursions of 15° to 30°C (59° to 86°F) are permitted. After reconstitution, if not used immediately, the product should be refrigerated and used within three hours. Do not freeze.

EXTAVIA is supplied as a lyophilized powder containing 0.3 mg of Interferon beta-1b, 15 mg Albumin (Human), USP, and 15 mg Mannitol, USP. Drug is packaged in a clear glass, single-use vial (3 mL capacity). A pre-filled single-use syringe containing 1.2 mL of diluent (Sodium Chloride, 0.54% solution), two alcohol prep pads, and one vial adapter with attached 27 gauge needle are included for each vial of drug. EXTAVIA and the diluent are for single-use only. Unused portions should be discarded. Store at room temperature.

15 blister units, 0.3 mg/vial .... NDC 0078-0569-12

17 PATIENT COUNSELING INFORMATION

All patients should be instructed to carefully read the supplied EXTAVIA Medication Guide. Patients should be cautioned not to change the dose or schedule of administration without medical consultation.

17.1 Depression

Advise patients that depression and suicidal ideation have been reported during the use of Interferon beta-1b. Advise patients of the symptoms of depression or suicidal ideation, and instruct patients to report them immediately to their physician *[see Warnings and Precautions (5.1)]*.

17.2 Injection Site Reactions, Including Necrosis

Advise patients that injection site reactions occur in most patients treated with Interferon beta-1b, and that injection site necrosis may occur at one or multiple sites. Instruct patients to promptly report any break in the skin, which may be associated with blue-black discoloration, swelling, or drainage of fluid from the injection site, prior to continuing their EXTAVIA therapy *[see Warnings and Precautions (5.2, 5.3)]*.

17.3 Allergic Reactions and Anaphylaxis

Advise patients of the symptoms of allergic reactions and anaphylaxis, and instruct patients to seek immediate medical attention if these symptoms occur *[see Warnings and Precautions (5.4)]*.

17.4 Flu-like Symptoms

Patients should be informed that flu-like symptoms are common following initiation of therapy with Interferon beta-1b. In controlled clinical trials, antipyretics and analgesics were permitted for relief of these symptoms. In addition, gradual dose titration during initiation of Interferon beta-1b treatment may reduce flu-like symptoms *[see Warnings and Precautions (5.5) and Dosage And Administration (2)]*.

17.5 Pregnancy

Advise patients that EXTAVIA should not be used during pregnancy unless the potential benefit justifies the potential risk to the fetus *[see Use in Special Population (8.1)]*.

17.6 Instruction on Self-injection Technique and Procedures

Patients should be instructed in the use of aseptic technique when administering EXTAVIA. Appropriate instruction for reconstitution of EXTAVIA and methods of self-injection should be provided, including careful review of the EXTAVIA Medication Guide. The first injection should be performed under the supervision of an appropriately qualified health care professional.

Patients should be cautioned against the re-use of needles or syringes and instructed in safe disposal procedures. A puncture resistant container for disposal of used needles and syringes should be supplied to the patient along with instructions for safe disposal of full containers.

Patients should be advised of the importance of rotating areas of injection with each dose, to minimize the likelihood of severe injection site reactions, including necrosis or localized infection *(see Choose an Injection Site section of the Medication Guide)*.

REV: AUGUST 2009 T2009-97

Manufactured by:
Bayer HealthCare Pharmaceuticals Inc.
Montville, NJ 07045
For
Novartis Pharmaceuticals Corporation
East Hanover, NJ 07936
Distributed by:
Novartis Pharmaceuticals Corporation
East Hanover, NJ 07936
U.S. License No. 1244

MEDICATION GUIDE

EXTAVIA *(ex tā vee uh)* Interferon beta-1b

Read the Medication Guide that comes with EXTAVIA before you start taking it and each time you get a refill. There may be new information. This Medication Guide does not take the place of talking with your doctor about your medical condition or your treatment.

What is the most important information I should know about EXTAVIA?

EXTAVIA and other Interferon beta-1b medicines will not cure multiple sclerosis (MS) but have been shown to decrease the number of flare-ups of the disease. Interferon beta-1b medicines, including EXTAVIA, can cause serious side effects. Before you start to take EXTAVIA, you should talk to your doctor about the possible risks and benefits of EXTAVIA.

Possible serious side effects with EXTAVIA include:

Depression. Some people who take interferon medicines, including EXTAVIA, become seriously depressed (feeling sad or sinking spirits). Some people have thoughts about killing themselves (suicidal thoughts) or try to kill themselves. Depression is not uncommon in people with multiple sclerosis.

- Before you start to take EXTAVIA, tell your doctor if you ever had any mental illness, including depression, or if you take any medicines for depression.
- While you take EXTAVIA, if you feel noticeably sadder or helpless, or feel like hurting yourself or others, you should tell a family member or friend right away and call your doctor as soon as possible. You may need to stop taking EXTAVIA.

Risk to pregnancy. If you become pregnant while you take EXTAVIA, stop taking EXTAVIA and call your doctor right away. Interferon beta-1b medicines, including EXTAVIA, may cause you to lose your pregnancy (miscarriage) or may cause harm to your unborn child. You and your doctor will need to decide whether the possible benefit of taking EXTAVIA is more important than the possible risks to your unborn child.

Allergic reactions. Some people who take Interferon beta-1b medicines, including EXTAVIA, have severe allergic reactions which can lead to trouble breathing and swallowing. Significant swelling of the mouth and tongue may occur with these severe allergic reactions. These reactions can happen quickly. Allergic reactions can happen after your first dose of EXTAVIA or may not happen until after you have taken EXTAVIA many times. Less severe allergic reactions such as rash, itching, skin bumps or minor swelling of the mouth and tongue can also happen. If you think you are having an allergic reaction, stop taking EXTAVIA right away and call your doctor.

Injection site problems. Interferon beta-1b medicines, including EXTAVIA, may cause redness, pain or swelling at the place where an injection was given (injection site). Serious skin reactions can happen in some people, including skin infections or areas of severe damage to skin and tissue below the skin (necrosis). These reactions can happen anywhere you inject EXTAVIA.

Call your doctor right away if you have any of these signs of a serious problem at any of your injection sites:

- the area is swollen and painful
- the area looks infected, and does not heal within a few days
- the area has fluid draining from it
- you notice any breaks in your skin or blue-black skin discoloration of your skin along with a break in your skin.

Most skin reactions are not serious, but you may need medical treatment if you develop a serious skin reaction. In most cases healing was associated with scarring.

If multiple lesions occur, therapy should be discontinued until healing occurs.

What is EXTAVIA?

EXTAVIA is a man-made form of a protein called beta interferon. EXTAVIA is similar to certain interferon proteins that are produced in the body.

EXTAVIA is used to treat relapsing forms of multiple sclerosis (MS). It will not cure your MS but may decrease the number of flare-ups of the disease. MS is a life-long disease that affects your nervous system by destroying the protective covering (myelin) that surrounds your nerve fibers. The way EXTAVIA works in MS is not known.

Who should not take EXTAVIA?

Do not take EXTAVIA if you:

- have had an allergic reaction such as trouble breathing, skin flushing, or hives, with another interferon beta product, or to human albumin.
- are allergic to any of the ingredients in EXTAVIA. See the end of this Medication Guide for a list of the ingredients in EXTAVIA.

What should I tell my doctor before taking EXTAVIA?

Tell your doctor about all your medical conditions, including if you have:

- or had depression, anxiety (feeling uneasy, nervous, or fearful), or trouble sleeping
- liver problems
- thyroid problems
- blood problems, such as bleeding or bruising easily, and low red blood cells (anemia) or low white blood cells
- are pregnant, breastfeeding, or planning to become pregnant. **See "What is the most important information I should know about EXTAVIA?"**
- are breastfeeding or plan to breastfeed. It is not known if EXTAVIA passes into your milk. You and your doctor should decide if you will breastfeed or take EXTAVIA. You should not do both without talking with your doctor.

Tell your doctor about all the medicines you take, including prescription and non-prescription medicines, vitamins, and herbal supplements.

Know the medicines you take. Keep a list of them and show it to your doctor and pharmacist when you get a new medicine.

How should I take EXTAVIA?

- Take EXTAVIA exactly as prescribed by your doctor. Do not change your dose unless told to by your doctor.
- If your doctor decides that you or a caregiver may be able to give your injections of EXTAVIA at home, your doctor or nurse should instruct you on the right way to prepare and inject EXTAVIA. Do not try to inject EXTAVIA yourself until you have been instructed by your doctor or nurse the right way to prepare and give the injections.
- EXTAVIA is given by injection under the skin (subcutaneous injection) every other day.
- If you miss a dose of EXTAVIA, take your next dose as soon as you remember or are able to take it. Take your next injection about 2 days after that dose. If you are not sure when you should take your next dose, call your doctor.
- **Do not take EXTAVIA two days in a row (consecutive days).**
- Call your doctor right away if you take more than your prescribed dose of EXTAVIA, or take it two days in a row.
- **Always use a new, unopened, vial of EXTAVIA and syringe for each injection. Throw away any unused medicine. Do not reuse any vials, syringes, or needles.**
- It is important for you to change your injection site each time you inject EXTAVIA. This will lessen the chance of you having a serious skin reaction at the site where you inject EXTAVIA.
- Avoid injecting EXTAVIA into an area of skin that is sore, red, infected or has other problems.
- See the end of this Medication Guide for detailed Patient Instructions for Use for information about how to mix and inject EXTAVIA the right way.

What are the possible side effects of EXTAVIA?

EXTAVIA can cause serious side effects. See "What is the most important information I should know about EXTAVIA?"

Common side effects of EXTAVIA include:

- **Flu-like symptoms.** Most people have flu-like symptoms (fever, chills, sweating, muscle aches and tiredness) when taking EXTAVIA. These symptoms may lessen or go away over time. Talk to your doctor about whether you should take a non-prescription medicine for pain, or to lower fever before or after you take your dose of EXTAVIA.
- **Liver problems.** EXTAVIA may affect your liver function. Your doctor will do blood tests to check for these problems while you take EXTAVIA. Tell your doctor if you have any of these symptoms of a liver problem:
  - yellowing of the skin and whites of the eyes

- easy bruising
- right-sided stomach area (abdominal) pain
- **Blood problems.** You may have a decrease in the amount of certain blood cells, including white blood cells (blood cells that fight infection), red blood cells (blood cells that carry oxygen to body tissues), or platelets (blood cells that help you form blood clots). If this decrease is severe, your body may be less able to fight infections, you may feel tired or sluggish, or you may bruise or bleed easily.
- **Thyroid problems.** Your thyroid function may change. Symptoms of changes in the function of your thyroid include feeling cold or hot much of the time, or change in your weight (gain or loss) without a change in your diet or amount of exercise you are getting.
- **Asthenia.** You may feel excessively or unusually fatigued. Talk to your doctor about your fatigue if it is persistent and bothersome to you.
- **Headache.** You may develop headaches. You should tell your doctor if you experience headaches while taking EXTAVIA, and you should make a plan with your doctor for monitoring your headaches. Talk to your doctor about whether you should take an additional medicine for the headaches.
- **Pain.** You may experience pain while taking EXTAVIA. Talk to your doctor about whether you should take a non-prescription medicine for pain and keep your doctor informed about any changes in the pain you experience.

You should discuss with your doctor the need for blood testing to monitor for these problems. Your doctor will arrange for testing your blood at regular intervals to help detect blood, thyroid, liver, or other problems that may develop. These blood tests will be needed even if you do not have any symptoms.

Tell your doctor if you have any side effect that bothers you or that does not go away. These are not all the possible side effects of EXTAVIA. For more information ask your doctor or pharmacist.

Call your doctor for medical advice about side effects. You may report side effects to FDA at 1-800-FDA-1088.

How should I store EXTAVIA?
- Before mixing, store EXTAVIA at room temperature 25°C (77°F). Storage at temperatures between 15° to 30°C (59° to 86°F) for brief periods of time are acceptable.
- After mixing, if you can not inject EXTAVIA right away, refrigerate the medicine and inject it **within 3 hours.** If you can not inject the mixed medicine within 3 hours, do not use it. Follow the information in the Patient Instructions for Use section "Dispose of used needles, syringes, and vials" for the right way to throw away the syringe with the unused medicine, and needle.
- Do not freeze EXTAVIA.

Keep EXTAVIA and all medicines out of the reach of children.

General information about EXTAVIA
Medicines are sometimes prescribed for purposes other than those listed in a Medication Guide. Do not use EXTAVIA for a condition for which it has not been prescribed. Do not give EXTAVIA to other people even if they have the same symptoms that you have. It may harm them.

This Medication Guide summarizes the most important information about EXTAVIA. If you would like more information, talk with your doctor. You can ask your doctor or pharmacist for information about EXTAVIA that is written for health professionals. For more information go to the web site www.EXTAVIA.com or call the EXTAVIA toll-free medical information line at 1-888-669-6682.

What are the ingredients in EXTAVIA?
Active ingredient: interferon beta-1b
Inactive ingredients: mannitol, albumin (human).
The diluent contains sodium chloride solution.

EXTAVIA Patient Instructions for Use
If your doctor decides that you or a caregiver may be able to give your injections of EXTAVIA at home, your doctor or nurse should instruct you on the right way to prepare and inject EXTAVIA. To lower your risk of infection, it is important that you follow the technique that your doctor or nurse discussed with you to prepare and inject EXTAVIA. Do not try to inject EXTAVIA yourself until you have been shown by your doctor or nurse the right way to prepare and give the injections.

It is important for you to read, understand, and follow these instructions. Call your doctor if you or your caregiver has any questions about the right way to prepare or inject EXTAVIA.

Important safety information
- Do not leave the blister pack containing EXTAVIA where others might tamper with it.
- Keep the blister pack containing EXTAVIA out of the reach of children.
- Do not open the blister pack or take out any of the items until right before you are ready to use them.
- Do not use EXTAVIA if the seal on the vial is broken. If the seal is broken, the product may not be safe for you to use.

- Do not use EXTAVIA after the expiration date shown on the blister pack label or box (Figure 1). If it has expired, return the entire pack to the pharmacy.

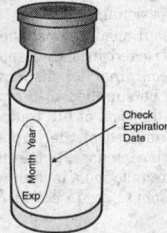

Figure 1

- Do not use any of the items in the blister pack more than one time. See the section at the end of this leaflet, "Dispose of used syringes, needles, and vials." Throw away any open and unused medicine.

Gather your supplies
You will need the following supplies to get ready to give your injection of EXTAVIA:
- **A blister pack containing the following items (Figure 2)**
  - a vial of EXTAVIA
  - a prefilled syringe of diluent (Sodium Chloride, 0.54% solution)
  - a vial adapter with a 27-gauge needle attached (in its own container)
  - two (2) alcohol wipes

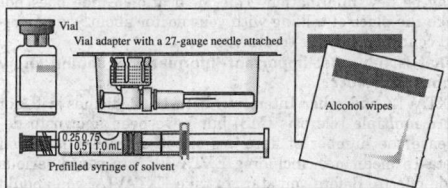

Figure 2

- a dry cotton ball and gauze
- a sharps disposal container (Figure 3). See the section "Dispose of used syringes, needles, and vials."

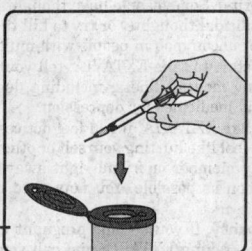

Figure 3

Prepare for self-injection
1. Wash your hands well with soap and water.
2. Open the blister pack by peeling off the label and take out all the items. Make sure the blister pack containing the vial adapter is sealed. Check to make sure the rubber cap on the diluent syringe is firmly attached.
3. Turn the blister pack over, and place the vial in the well (vial holder) and place the prefilled syringe in the U-shaped trough (Figure 4).

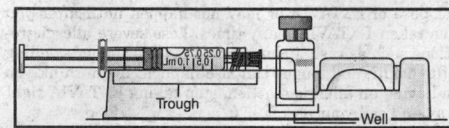

Figure 4

Mix EXTAVIA
4. Remove the EXTAVIA vial from the well and take the cap off the vial (Figure 5).
[See figure 5 at top of next column]
5. Place the vial back in the vial holder.
6. Use an alcohol wipe to clean the top of the vial (Figure 6). Wipe in one direction only.
[See figure 6 on next column]
7. Leave the alcohol wipe on top of the vial until step 9 below.
8. Peel the label off the container with the vial adapter in it, but do not remove the vial adapter. The vial adapter is sterile, so do not touch it.

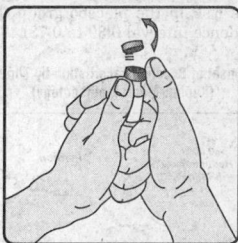

Figure 5

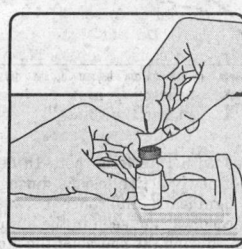

Figure 6

9. Remove the alcohol wipe from the top of the vial. Pick up the container that holds the vial adapter. Turn over the container keeping the vial adaptor inside. Put the adapter on top of the vial. Push down on the adapter until it pierces the rubber top of the vial and snaps in place (Figure 7). Lift the container off the vial adapter.

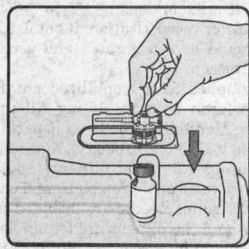

Figure 7

10. Remove the rubber cap from the prefilled syringe using a twist and pull motion (Figure 8). Throw away the rubber cap.

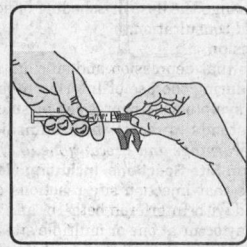

Figure 8

11. Remove the vial from the vial holder by grasping the vial. Do not touch any part of the vial adapter. Be careful not to pull the vial adapter off the top of the vial.
12. Connect the prefilled syringe of diluent to the vial adapter by turning clockwise and tighten carefully (Figure 9).

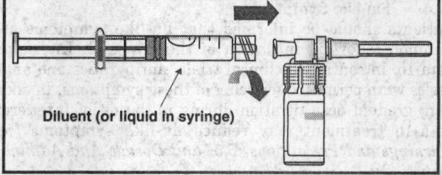

Figure 9

13. Slowly push the plunger of the prefilled syringe all the way in. This will push all of the liquid from the syringe into the vial (Figure 10). Continue to hold the plunger while you mix EXTAVIA with the liquid from the syringe. If you do not hold the plunger in it may return to its original position after you let go.

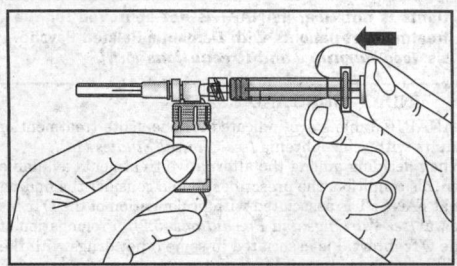

Figure 10

14. Gently swirl the vial to completely dissolve the white powder (EXTAVIA). **Do not shake.** Shaking and even gentle mixing can cause foaming of the medicine. If there is foam, let the vial sit until the foam settles.
15. After the powder dissolves, look closely at the solution in the vial. Do not use the solution if it is not clear or colorless, or if it contains particles.

The injection should be given right away after you mix EXTAVIA and let any foam in the solution settle. If you must wait for any reason before giving yourself the injection, you may refrigerate the medicine after you mix it. But you should use it within three hours.

16. With your thumb still pushing the plunger, turn the syringe and vial, so that the vial is on top (Figure 11).
17. Slowly pull the plunger back to withdraw the entire contents of the vial into the syringe.

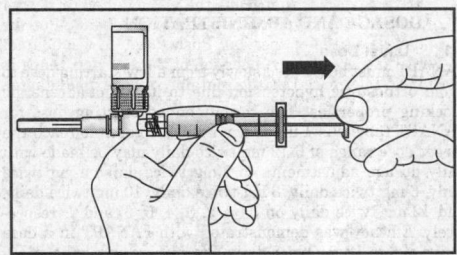

Figure 11

18. Turn the syringe so that the needle end is pointing up. Remove any air bubbles by tapping the outside of the syringe with your fingers (Figure 12). Slowly push the plunger to the 1 mL mark on the syringe or to the mark that matches the amount of EXTAVIA prescribed by your doctor. If too much solution is pushed back into the vial, return to step 16.

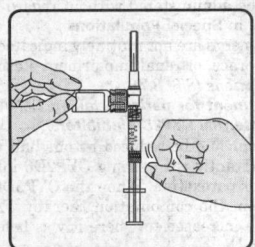

Figure 12

19. Remove the vial adapter and the vial from the syringe by twisting the vial adapter (Figure 13).

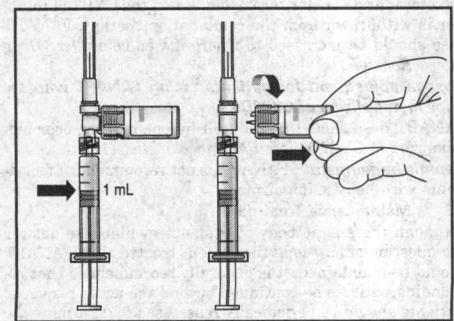

1 mL

Figure 13

Choose an Injection Site

• EXTAVIA is injected under the skin and into the fat layer between the skin and the muscles (subcutaneous tissue). The best areas for injection are where the skin is loose and soft and away from the joints, nerves, and bones. Do

not use the area near your navel (belly button) or waist-line. If you are very thin, use only the thigh or outer surface of the arm for injection.
• Choose a different site each time you give yourself an injection. Figure 14 shows different areas for giving injections. Do not inject in the same area for two injections in a row. Keep a record of your injections to help make sure you change (rotate) your injection sites. If there are any sites that are difficult for you to reach, you can ask someone who has been trained to give the injection to you.

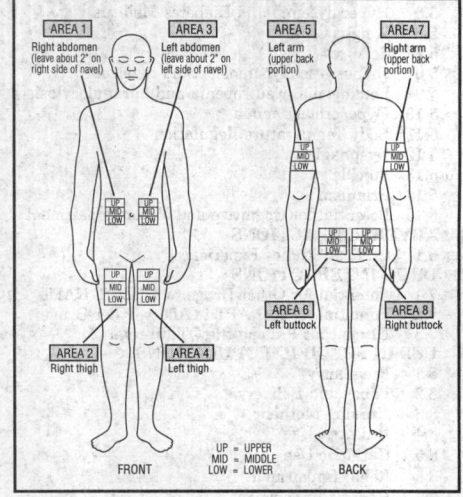

Figure 14

• Do not inject EXTAVIA in a site where the skin is red, bruised, infected, or scabbed, has broken open, or has lumps, bumps, or pain. Tell your doctor if you find skin conditions like the ones mentioned here or any other unusual looking areas where you have been given injections.

Injecting EXTAVIA

20. Using a circular motion, clean the injection site with an alcohol wipe, starting at the injection site and moving outward (Figure 15). Let the skin area air dry.

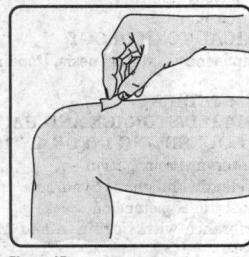

Figure 15

21. Remove the cap from the needle (Figure 16).

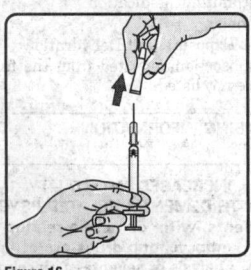

Figure 16

22. Gently pinch the skin around the site with your thumb and forefinger of the other hand (Figure 17). Insert the needle straight up and down into your skin at a 90° angle with a quick, dart-like motion.

[See figure at top of next column]

23. Once the needle is in your skin, slowly pull back on the plunger. If blood appears in the syringe it means that you have entered a blood vessel. Do not inject EXTAVIA. Withdraw the needle. Throw away the syringe and needle in your puncture-proof container. Do not use the same syringe or any of the other supplies that you used for this injection. Repeat the above steps to prepare your dose using a new blister pack. Choose and clean a new injection site.
24. If no blood appears in the syringe, slowly push the plunger all the way in until the syringe is empty (Fig-

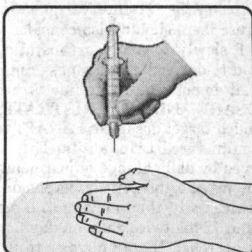

Figure 17

ure 18). Remove the needle from the skin; then place a dry cotton ball or gauze pad over the injection site. Gently massage the injection site for a few minutes with the dry cotton ball or gauze pad. Throw away the syringe in your puncture-proof disposal container.

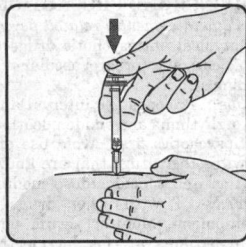

Figure 18

Dispose of used syringes, needles, and vials

• To prevent needle-stick injury and spread of infection, do not try to re-cap the needle.
• Place used needles, syringes, and vials in a closeable, puncture-resistant container. You may use a sharps container (such as a red biohazard container), a hard plastic container (such as a detergent bottle), or a metal container (such as an empty coffee can). Do not use glass or clear plastic containers. Ask your doctor for instructions on the right way to throw away (dispose of) the container. There may be state and local laws about how you should throw away used needles and syringes.
• **Do not throw used needles, syringes, or vials in your household trash or recycle.** Throw away any unused medicine. Do not save any unused EXTAVIA for a future dose.

Keep the disposal container, needles, syringes, and vials of EXTAVIA out of the reach of children.

This Medication Guide has been approved by the U.S. Food and Drug Administration.

T2009-98
REV: AUGUST 2009   T2009-97/T2009-98
Manufactured by:
Bayer HealthCare Pharmaceuticals Inc.
Montville, NJ 07045
For
Novartis Pharmaceuticals Corporation
East Hanover, NJ 07936
Distributed by:
Novartis Pharmaceuticals Corporation
East Hanover, NJ 07936
U.S. License No. 1244
©Novartis
Shown in Product Identification Guide, page 315

FANAPT®   ℞
[fan-apt]
(iloperidone)
Tablets

The following prescribing information is based on official labeling in effect July 2010.
HIGHLIGHTS OF PRESCRIBING INFORMATION
These highlights do not include all the information needed to use FANAPT safely and effectively. See full prescribing information for FANAPT.
FANAPT® *(iloperidone)* tablets
Initial U.S. Approval: 2009

> **WARNING: INCREASED MORTALITY IN ELDERLY PATIENTS WITH DEMENTIA-RELATED PSYCHOSIS**
> *See full prescribing information for complete boxed warning.*
> Elderly patients with dementia-related psychosis treated with antipsychotic drugs are at an increased risk of death. FANAPT is not approved for use in patients with dementia-related psychosis. (5.1)

———————INDICATIONS AND USAGE———————
FANAPT is an atypical antipsychotic agent indicated for the acute treatment of schizophrenia in adults. (1) In choosing among treatments, prescribers should consider the ability of

FANAPT to prolong the QT interval and the use of other drugs first. Prescribers should also consider the need to titrate FANAPT slowly to avoid orthostatic hypotension, which may lead to delayed effectiveness compared to some other drugs that do not require similar titration.

DOSAGE AND ADMINISTRATION
The recommended target dosage of FANAPT tablets is 12 to 24 mg/day administered twice daily. This target dosage range is achieved by daily dosage adjustments, alerting patients to symptoms of orthostatic hypotension, starting at a dose of 1 mg twice daily, then moving to 2 mg, 4 mg, 6 mg, 8 mg, 10 mg, and 12 mg twice daily on days 2, 3, 4, 5, 6, and 7 respectively, to reach the 12 mg/day to 24 mg/day dose range. FANAPT can be administered without regard to meals. (2.1)

DOSAGE FORMS AND STRENGTHS
1 mg, 2 mg, 4 mg, 6 mg, 8 mg, 10 mg and 12 mg tablets. (3)

CONTRAINDICATIONS
Known hypersensitivity to FANAPT or to any components in the formulation. (4)

WARNINGS AND PRECAUTIONS
• *Elderly patients with dementia-related psychosis* who are treated with atypical antipsychotic drugs are at an increased risk of death and cerebrovascular-related adverse events, including stroke. (5.1)
• *QT prolongation:* Prolongs QT interval and may be associated with arrhythmia and sudden death—consider using other antipsychotics first. Avoid use of FANAPT in combination with other drugs that are known to prolong QTc; use caution and consider dose modification when prescribing FANAPT with other drugs that inhibit FANAPT metabolism. Monitor serum potassium and magnesium in patients at risk for electrolyte disturbances. (1, 5.2, 7.1, 7.3, 12.3)
• *Neuroleptic Malignant Syndrome:* Manage with immediate discontinuation of drug and close monitoring. (5.3)
• *Tardive dyskinesia:* Discontinue if clinically appropriate. (5.4)
• *Hyperglycemia and diabetes mellitus:* Monitor glucose regularly in patients at risk for diabetes. (5.5)
• *Seizures:* Use cautiously in patients with a history of seizures or with conditions that lower seizure threshold. (5.7)
• *Orthostatic hypotension:* Dizziness, tachycardia, and syncope can occur with standing. (5.8)
• *Leukopenia, Neutropenia, and Agranulocytosis* have been reported with antipsychotics. Patients with a pre-existing low white blood cell count (WBC) or a history of leukopenia/neutropenia should have their complete blood count (CBC) monitored frequently during the first few months of therapy and should discontinue FANAPT at the first sign of a decline in WBC in the absence of other causative factors. (5.9)
• *Suicide:* Close supervision of high risk patients. (5.13)
• *Priapism:* Cases have been reported in association with FANAPT treatment. (5.14)
• *Potential for cognitive and motor impairment:* Use caution when operating machinery. (5.15)
• See Full Prescribing Information for additional *WARNINGS and PRECAUTIONS.*

ADVERSE REACTIONS
Commonly observed adverse reactions (incidence ≥5% and two-fold greater than placebo) were: dizziness, dry mouth, fatigue, nasal congestion, orthostatic hypotension, somnolence, tachycardia, and weight increased. (6.1)

To report SUSPECTED ADVERSE REACTIONS, contact Vanda Pharmaceuticals at 1-888-49VANDA (1-888-498-2632) or FDA at 1-800-FDA-1088 or www.fda.gov/medwatch.

DRUG INTERACTIONS
• The dose of FANAPT should be reduced in patients co-administered a strong CYP2D6 or CYP3A4 inhibitor. (2.2, 7.1)

USE IN SPECIFIC POPULATIONS
• Pregnancy: No human or animal data. Use only if clearly needed. (8.1)
• Nursing Mothers: Should not breast feed. (8.3)
• Pediatric Use: Safety and effectiveness not established in children and adolescents. (8.4)
• Hepatic Impairment: Not recommended for patients with hepatic impairment. (8.7)
• The dose of FANAPT should be reduced in patients who are poor metabolizers of CYP2D6. (12.3)

See 17 for PATIENT COUNSELING INFORMATION

Revised: 8/2010

FULL PRESCRIBING INFORMATION: CONTENTS*
WARNING: INCREASED MORTALITY IN ELDERLY PATIENTS WITH DEMENTIA-RELATED PSYCHOSIS

*Sections or subsections omitted from the full prescribing information are not listed.

FULL PRESCRIBING INFORMATION

> **WARNING: INCREASED MORTALITY IN ELDERLY PATIENTS WITH DEMENTIA-RELATED PSYCHOSIS**
> Elderly patients with dementia-related psychosis treated with antipsychotic drugs are at an increased risk of death. Analysis of seventeen placebo-controlled trials (modal duration 10 weeks), largely in patients taking atypical antipsychotic drugs, revealed a risk of death in the drug-treated patients of between 1.6 to 1.7 times the risk of death in placebo-treated patients. Over the course of a typical 10-week controlled trial, the rate of death in drug-treated patients was about 4.5%, compared to a rate of about 2.6% in the placebo group. Although the causes of death were varied, most of the deaths appeared to be either cardiovascular (e.g., heart failure, sudden death) or infectious (e.g., pneumonia) in nature.
> Observational studies suggest that, similar to atypical antipsychotic drugs, treatment with conventional antipsychotic drugs may increase mortality. The extent to which the findings of increased mortality in observational studies may be attributed to the antipsychotic drug as opposed to some characteristic(s) of the patients is not clear. FANAPT is not approved for the treatment of patients with Dementia-Related Psychosis. *[see Warnings and Precautions (5.1)]*

1   INDICATIONS AND USAGE
FANAPT® tablets are indicated for the acute treatment of adults with schizophrenia *[see Clinical Studies (14)].*
When deciding among the alternative treatments available for this condition, the prescriber should consider the finding that FANAPT is associated with prolongation of the QTc interval *[see Warnings and Precautions (5.2)].* Prolongation of the QTc interval is associated in some other drugs with the ability to cause torsade de pointes-type arrhythmia, a potentially fatal polymorphic ventricular tachycardia which can result in sudden death. In many cases this would lead to the conclusion that other drugs should be tried first. Whether FANAPT will cause torsade de pointes or increase the rate of sudden death is not yet known.
Patients must be titrated to an effective dose of FANAPT. Thus, control of symptoms may be delayed during the first 1 to 2 weeks of treatment compared to some other antipsychotic drugs that do not require a similar titration. Prescribers should be mindful of this delay when selecting an antipsychotic drug for the acute treatment of schizophrenia *[see Dosage and Administration (2.1) and Clinical Studies (14)].* The effectiveness of FANAPT in long-term use, that is, for more than 6 weeks, has not been systematically evaluated in controlled trials. Therefore, the physician who elects to use FANAPT for extended periods should periodically re-evaluate the long-term usefulness of the drug for the individual patient *[see Dosage and Administration (2.3)].*

2   DOSAGE AND ADMINISTRATION

2.1   Usual Dose
FANAPT must be titrated slowly from a low starting dose to avoid orthostatic hypotension due to its alpha-adrenergic blocking properties. The recommended starting dose for FANAPT tablets is 1 mg twice daily. Increases to reach the target dose range of 6-12 mg twice daily may be made with daily dosage adjustments to 2 mg twice daily, 4 mg twice daily, 6 mg twice daily, 8 mg twice daily, 10 mg twice daily, and 12 mg twice daily on days 2, 3, 4, 5, 6, and 7, respectively. Efficacy was demonstrated with FANAPT in a dose range of 6 to 12 mg twice daily. Prescribers should be mindful of the fact that patients need to be titrated to an effective dose of FANAPT. Thus, control of symptoms may be delayed during the first 1 to 2 weeks of treatment compared to some other antipsychotic drugs that do not require similar titration. Prescribers should also be aware that some adverse effects associated with FANAPT use are dose related.
The maximum recommended dose is 12 mg twice daily (24 mg/day); FANAPT doses above 24 mg/day have not been systematically evaluated in the clinical trials.
FANAPT can be administered without regard to meals.

2.2   Dosage in Special Populations
Dosage adjustments are not routinely indicated on the basis of age, gender, race, or renal impairment status *[see Use in Specific Populations (8.6, 8.7)].*
Dosage adjustment for patients taking FANAPT concomitantly with potential CYP2D6 inhibitors:
FANAPT dose should be reduced by one-half when administered concomitantly with strong CYP2D6 inhibitors such as fluoxetine or paroxetine. When the CYP2D6 inhibitor is withdrawn from the combination therapy, FANAPT dose should then be increased to where it was before *[see Drug Interactions (7.1)].*
Dosage adjustment for patients taking FANAPT concomitantly with potential CYP3A4 inhibitors:
FANAPT dose should be reduced by one-half when administered concomitantly with strong CYP3A4 inhibitors such as ketoconazole or clarithromycin. When the CYP3A4 inhibitor is withdrawn from the combination therapy, FANAPT dose should be increased to where it was before *[see Drug Interactions (7.1)].*
Dosage adjustment for patients taking FANAPT who are poor metabolizers of CYP2D6:
FANAPT dose should be reduced by one-half for poor metabolizers of CYP2D6 *[see Pharmacokinetics (12.3)].*
Hepatic Impairment: FANAPT is not recommended for patients with hepatic impairment.

2.3   Maintenance Treatment
Although there is no body of evidence available to answer the question of how long the patient treated with FANAPT should be maintained, it is generally recommended that responding patients be continued beyond the acute response. Patients should be periodically reassessed to determine the need for maintenance treatment.

2.4   Reinitiation of Treatment in Patients Previously Discontinued
Although there are no data to specifically address reinitiation of treatment, it is recommended that the initiation titration schedule be followed whenever patients have had an interval off FANAPT of more than 3 days.

2.5 Switching from Other Antipsychotics

There are no specific data to address how patients with schizophrenia can be switched from other antipsychotics to FANAPT or how FANAPT can be used concomitantly with other antipsychotics. Although immediate discontinuation of the previous antipsychotic treatment may be acceptable for some patients with schizophrenia, more gradual discontinuation may be most appropriate for others. In all cases, the period of overlapping antipsychotic administration should be minimized.

3 DOSAGE FORMS AND STRENGTHS

FANAPT tablets are available in the following strengths: 1 mg, 2 mg, 4 mg, 6 mg, 8 mg, 10 mg and 12 mg.

The tablets are white, round, flat, beveled-edged and identified with a logo "⊕" debossed on one side and tablet strength "1", "2", "4", "6", "8", "10", or "12" debossed on the other side.

4 CONTRAINDICATIONS

FANAPT is contraindicated in individuals with a known hypersensitivity reaction to the product. Reactions have included pruritus and urticaria.

5 WARNINGS AND PRECAUTIONS

5.1 Increased Risks in Elderly Patients with Dementia-Related Psychosis

Increased Mortality

Elderly patients with dementia-related psychosis treated with atypical antipsychotic drugs are at an increased risk of death compared to placebo. FANAPT is not approved for the treatment of patients with dementia-related psychosis *[see Boxed Warning].*

Cerebrovascular Adverse Events, Including Stroke

In placebo-controlled trials with risperidone, aripiprazole, and olanzapine in elderly patients with dementia, there was a higher incidence of cerebrovascular adverse events (cerebrovascular accidents and transient ischemic attacks) including fatalities compared to placebo-treated patients. FANAPT is not approved for the treatment of patients with dementia-related psychosis *[see Boxed Warning].*

5.2 QT Prolongation

In an open-label QTc study in patients with schizophrenia or schizoaffective disorder (n=160), FANAPT was associated with QTc prolongation of 9 msec at an iloperidone dose of 12 mg twice daily. The effect of FANAPT on the QT interval was augmented by the presence of CYP450 2D6 or 3A4 metabolic inhibition (paroxetine 20 mg once daily and ketoconazole 200 mg twice daily, respectively). Under conditions of metabolic inhibition for both 2D6 and 3A4, FANAPT 12 mg twice daily was associated with a mean QTcF increase from baseline of about 19 msec.

No cases of torsade de pointes or other severe cardiac arrhythmias were observed during the pre-marketing clinical program.

The use of FANAPT should be avoided in combination with other drugs that are known to prolong QTc including Class 1A (e.g., quinidine, procainamide) or Class III (e.g., amiodarone, sotalol) antiarrhythmic medications, antipsychotic medications (e.g., chlorpromazine, thioridazine), antibiotics (e.g., gatifloxacin, moxifloxacin), or any other class of medications known to prolong the QTc interval (e.g., pentamidine, levomethadyl acetate, methadone). FANAPT should also be avoided in patients with congenital long QT syndrome and in patients with a history of cardiac arrhythmias.

Certain circumstances may increase the risk of torsade de pointes and/or sudden death in association with the use of drugs that prolong the QTc interval, including (1) bradycardia; (2) hypokalemia or hypomagnesemia; (3) concomitant use of other drugs that prolong the QTc interval; and (4) presence of congenital prolongation of the QT interval; (5) recent acute myocardial infarction; and/or (6) uncompensated heart failure.

Caution is warranted when prescribing FANAPT with drugs that inhibit FANAPT metabolism *[see Drug Interaction (7.1)],* and in patients with reduced activity of CYP2D6 *[see Clinical Pharmacology (12.3)].*

It is recommended that patients being considered for FANAPT treatment who are at risk for significant electrolyte disturbances have baseline serum potassium and magnesium measurements with periodic monitoring. Hypokalemia (and/or hypomagnesemia) may increase the risk of QT prolongation and arrhythmia. FANAPT should be avoided in patients with histories of significant cardiovascular illness, e.g., QT prolongation, recent acute myocardial infarction, uncompensated heart failure, or cardiac arrhythmia. FANAPT should be discontinued in patients who are found to have persistent QTc measurements >500 ms.

If patients taking FANAPT experience symptoms that could indicate the occurrence of cardiac arrhythmias, e.g., dizziness, palpitations, or syncope, the prescriber should initiate further evaluation, including cardiac monitoring.

5.3 Neuroleptic Malignant Syndrome (NMS)

A potentially fatal symptom complex sometimes referred to as Neuroleptic Malignant Syndrome (NMS) has been reported in association with administration of antipsychotic drugs. Clinical manifestations include hyperpyrexia, muscle rigidity, altered mental status (including catatonic signs) and evidence of autonomic instability (irregular pulse or blood pressure, tachycardia, diaphoresis, and cardiac dysarrhythmia). Additional signs may include elevated creatine phosphokinase, myoglobinuria (rhabdomyolysis), and acute renal failure.

The diagnostic evaluation of patients with this syndrome is complicated. In arriving at a diagnosis, it is important to identify cases in which the clinical presentation includes both serious medical illness (e.g., pneumonia, systemic infection, etc.) and untreated or inadequately treated extrapyramidal signs and symptoms (EPS). Other important considerations in the differential diagnosis include central anticholinergic toxicity, heat stroke, drug fever, and primary central nervous system (CNS) pathology.

The management of this syndrome should include: (1) immediate discontinuation of the antipsychotic drugs and other drugs not essential to concurrent therapy, (2) intensive symptomatic treatment and medical monitoring, and (3) treatment of any concomitant serious medical problems for which specific treatments are available. There is no general agreement about specific pharmacological treatment regimens for NMS.

If a patient requires antipsychotic drug treatment after recovery from NMS, the potential reintroduction of drug therapy should be carefully considered. The patient should be carefully monitored, since recurrences of NMS have been reported.

5.4 Tardive Dyskinesia

Tardive dyskinesia is a syndrome consisting of potentially irreversible, involuntary, dyskinetic movements, which may develop in patients treated with antipsychotic drugs. Although the prevalence of the syndrome appears to be highest among the elderly, especially elderly women, it is impossible to rely on prevalence estimates to predict, at the inception of antipsychotic treatment, which patients are likely to develop the syndrome. Whether antipsychotic drug products differ in their potential to cause tardive dyskinesia is unknown.

The risk of developing tardive dyskinesia and the likelihood that it will become irreversible are believed to increase as the duration of treatment and the total cumulative dose of antipsychotic administered increases. However, the syndrome can develop, although much less commonly, after relatively brief treatment periods at low doses.

There is no known treatment for established cases of tardive dyskinesia, although the syndrome may remit, partially or completely, if antipsychotic treatment is withdrawn. Antipsychotic treatment itself, however, may suppress (or partially suppress) the signs and symptoms of the syndrome and thereby may possibly mask the underlying process. The effect that symptomatic suppression has upon the long-term course of the syndrome is unknown.

Given these considerations, FANAPT should be prescribed in a manner that is most likely to minimize the occurrence of tardive dyskinesia. Chronic antipsychotic treatment should generally be reserved for patients who suffer from a chronic illness that (1) is known to respond to antipsychotic drugs, and (2) for whom alternative, equally effective, but potentially less harmful treatments are not available or appropriate. In patients who do require chronic treatment, the smallest dose and the shortest duration of treatment producing a satisfactory clinical response should be sought. The need for continued treatment should be reassessed periodically.

If signs and symptoms of tardive dyskinesia appear in a patient on FANAPT, drug discontinuation should be considered. However, some patients may require treatment with FANAPT despite the presence of the syndrome.

5.5 Hyperglycemia and Diabetes Mellitus

Hyperglycemia, in some cases extreme and associated with ketoacidosis or hyperosmolar coma or death, has been reported in patients treated with atypical antipsychotics including FANAPT. Assessment of the relationship between atypical antipsychotic use and glucose abnormalities is complicated by the possibility of an increased background risk of diabetes mellitus in patients with schizophrenia and the increasing incidence of diabetes mellitus in the general population. Given these confounders, the relationship between atypical antipsychotic use and hyperglycemia-related adverse events is not completely understood. However, epidemiological studies suggest an increased risk of treatment-emergent hyperglycemia-related adverse events in patients treated with the atypical antipsychotics included in these studies. Because FANAPT was not marketed at the time these studies were performed, it is not known if FANAPT is associated with this increased risk. Precise risk estimates for hyperglycemia-related adverse events in patients treated with atypical antipsychotics are not available.

Patients with an established diagnosis of diabetes mellitus who are started on atypical antipsychotics should be monitored regularly for worsening of glucose control. Patients with risk factors for diabetes mellitus (e.g., obesity, family history of diabetes) who are starting treatment with atypical antipsychotics should undergo fasting blood glucose testing at the beginning of treatment and periodically during treatment. Any patient treated with atypical antipsychotics should be monitored for symptoms of hyperglycemia including polydipsia, polyuria, polyphagia, and weakness. Patients who develop symptoms of hyperglycemia during treatment with atypical antipsychotics should undergo fasting blood glucose testing. In some cases, hyperglycemia has resolved when the atypical antipsychotic was discontinued; however, some patients required continuation of antidiabetic treatment despite discontinuation of the suspect drug.

5.6 Weight Gain

Based on the pooled data from the four placebo-controlled, 4- or 6-week, fixed- or flexible-dose studies, the proportions of patients having a weight gain of ≥7% body weight was 12% for FANAPT 10-16 mg/day, 18% for FANAPT 20-24 mg/day, and 13% for FANAPT (combined doses) versus 4% for placebo. The mean weight change from baseline to endpoint in the short-term studies was -0.1 kg for placebo versus 2.0 kg for FANAPT-treated patients. Across all short- and long-term studies, the overall mean change from baseline at endpoint was 2.1 kg.

5.7 Seizures

In short-term placebo-controlled trials (4- to 6-weeks), seizures occurred in 0.1% (1/1344) of patients treated with FANAPT compared to 0.3% (2/587) on placebo. As with other antipsychotics, FANAPT should be used cautiously in patients with a history of seizures or with conditions that potentially lower the seizure threshold, e.g., Alzheimer's dementia. Conditions that lower the seizure threshold may be more prevalent in a population of 65 years or older.

5.8 Orthostatic Hypotension and Syncope

FANAPT can induce orthostatic hypotension associated with dizziness, tachycardia, and syncope. This reflects its alpha1-adrenergic antagonist properties. In double-blind placebo-controlled short-term studies, where the dose was increased slowly, as recommended above, syncope was reported in 0.4% (5/1344) of patients treated with FANAPT, compared with 0.2% (1/587) on placebo. Orthostatic hypotension was reported in 5% of patients given 20-24 mg/day, 3% of patients given 10-16 mg/day, and 1% of patients given placebo. More rapid titration would be expected to increase the rate of orthostatic hypotension and syncope.

FANAPT should be used with caution in patients with known cardiovascular disease (e.g., heart failure, history of myocardial infarction, ischemia, or conduction abnormalities), cerebrovascular disease, or conditions that predispose the patient to hypotension (dehydration, hypovolemia, and treatment with antihypertensive medications). Monitoring of orthostatic vital signs should be considered in patients who are vulnerable to hypotension.

5.9 Leukopenia, Neutropenia and Agranulocytosis

In clinical trial and postmarketing experience, events of leukopenia/neutropenia have been reported temporally related to antipsychotic agents. Agranulocytosis (including fatal cases) has also been reported.

Possible risk factors for leukopenia/neutropenia include preexisting low white blood cell count (WBC) and history of drug induced leukopenia/neutropenia. Patients with a preexisting low WBC or a history of drug induced leukopenia/neutropenia should have their complete blood count (CBC) monitored frequently during the first few months of therapy and should discontinue FANAPT at the first sign of a decline in WBC in the absence of other causative factors.

Patients with neutropenia should be carefully monitored for fever or other symptoms or signs of infection and treated promptly if such symptoms or signs occur. Patients with severe neutropenia (absolute neutrophil count <1000/mm^3) should discontinue FANAPT and have their WBC followed until recovery.

5.10 Hyperprolactinemia

As with other drugs that antagonize dopamine D_2 receptors, FANAPT elevates prolactin levels.

Hyperprolactinemia may suppress hypothalamic GnRH, resulting in reduced pituitary gonadotropin secretion. This, in turn, may inhibit reproductive function by impairing gonadalsteroidogenesis in both female and male patients. Galactorrhea, amenorrhea, gynecomastia, and impotence have been reported with prolactin-elevating compounds. Longstanding hyperprolactinemia when associated with hypogonadism may lead to decreased bone density in both female and male patients.

Tissue culture experiments indicate that approximately one-third of human breast cancers are prolactin-dependent *in vitro*, a factor of potential importance if the prescription of these drugs is contemplated in a patient with previously detected breast cancer. Mammary gland proliferative changes and increases in serum prolactin were seen in mice and rats treated with FANAPT *[see Nonclinical Toxicology*

(13.1)]. Neither clinical studies nor epidemiologic studies conducted to date have shown an association between chronic administration of this class of drugs and tumorigenesis in humans; the available evidence is considered too limited to be conclusive at this time.

In a short-term placebo-controlled trial (4-weeks), the mean change from baseline to endpoint in plasma prolactin levels for the FANAPT 24 mg/day-treated group was an increase of 2.6 ng/mL compared to a decrease of 6.3 ng/mL in the placebo-group. In this trial, elevated plasma prolactin levels were observed in 26% of adults treated with FANAPT compared to 12% in the placebo group. In the short-term trials, FANAPT was associated with modest levels of prolactin elevation compared to greater prolactin elevations observed with some other antipsychotic agents. In pooled analysis from clinical studies including longer term trials, in 3210 adults treated with iloperidone, gynecomastia was reported in 2 male subjects (0.1%) compared to 0% in placebo-treated patients, and galactorrhea was reported in 8 female subjects (0.2%) compared to 3 female subjects (0.5%) in placebo-treated patients.

5.11   Body Temperature Regulation
Disruption of the body's ability to reduce core body temperature has been attributed to antipsychotic agents. Appropriate care is advised when prescribing FANAPT for patients who will be experiencing conditions which may contribute to an elevation in core body temperature, e.g., exercising strenuously, exposure to extreme heat, receiving concomitant medication with anticholinergic activity, or being subject to dehydration.

5.12   Dysphagia
Esophageal dysmotility and aspiration have been associated with antipsychotic drug use. Aspiration pneumonia is a common cause of morbidity and mortality in elderly patients, in particular those with advanced Alzheimer's dementia. FANAPT and other antipsychotic drugs should be used cautiously in patients at risk for aspiration pneumonia *[see Boxed Warning].*

5.13   Suicide
The possibility of a suicide attempt is inherent in psychotic illness, and close supervision of high-risk patients should accompany drug therapy. Prescriptions for FANAPT should be written for the smallest quantity of tablets consistent with good patient management in order to reduce the risk of overdose.

5.14   Priapism
Three cases of priapism were reported in the pre-marketing FANAPT program. Drugs with alpha-adrenergic blocking effects have been reported to induce priapism. FANAPT shares this pharmacologic activity. Severe priapism may require surgical intervention.

5.15   Potential for Cognitive and Motor Impairment
FANAPT, like other antipsychotics, has the potential to impair judgment, thinking or motor skills. In short-term, placebo-controlled trials, somnolence (including sedation) was reported in 11.9% (104/874) of adult patients treated with FANAPT at doses of 10 mg/day or greater versus 5.3% (31/587) treated with placebo. Patients should be cautioned about operating hazardous machinery, including automobiles, until they are reasonably certain that therapy with FANAPT does not affect them adversely.

6   ADVERSE REACTIONS
6.1   Clinical Studies Experience
Because clinical trials are conducted under widely varying conditions, adverse reaction rates observed in the clinical trial of a drug cannot be directly compared to rates in the clinical trials of another drug and may not reflect the rates observed in clinical practice. The information below is derived from a clinical trial database for FANAPT consisting of 2070 patients exposed to FANAPT at doses of 10 mg/day or greater, for the treatment of schizophrenia. All of these patients who received FANAPT were participating in multiple-dose clinical trials. The conditions and duration of treatment with FANAPT varied greatly and included (in overlapping categories), open-label and double-blind phases of studies, inpatients and outpatients, fixed-dose and flexible-dose studies, and short-term and longer-term exposure.

Adverse reactions during exposure were obtained by general inquiry and recorded by clinical investigators using their own terminology. Consequently, to provide a meaningful estimate of the proportion of individuals experiencing adverse reactions, reactions were grouped in standardized categories using MedDRA terminology.

The stated frequencies of adverse reactions represent the proportions of individuals who experienced a treatment-emergent adverse reaction of the type listed. A reaction was considered treatment emergent if it occurred for the first time or worsened while receiving therapy following baseline evaluation.

The information presented in these sections was derived from pooled data from four placebo-controlled, 4- or 6-week, fixed- or flexible-dose studies in patients who received FANAPT at daily doses within a range of 10 to 24 mg (n=874).

Adverse Reactions Occurring at an Incidence of 2% or More among FANAPT-Treated Patients and More Frequent than Placebo
Table 1 enumerates the pooled incidences of treatment-emergent adverse reactions that were spontaneously reported in four placebo-controlled, 4- or 6-week, fixed- or flexible-dose studies, listing those reactions that occurred in 2% or more of patients treated with FANAPT in any of the dose groups, and for which the incidence in FANAPT-treated patients in any dose group was greater than the incidence in patients treated with placebo.
[See table 1 below]

Dose-Related Adverse Reactions in Clinical Trials
Based on the pooled data from four placebo-controlled, 4- or 6-week, fixed- or flexible-dose studies, adverse reactions that occurred with a greater than 2% incidence in the patients treated with FANAPT, and for which the incidence in patients treated with FANAPT 20-24 mg/day were twice than the incidence in patients treated FANAPT 10-16 mg/day were: abdominal discomfort, dizziness, hypotension, musculoskeletal stiffness, tachycardia, and weight increased.

Common and Drug-Related Adverse Reactions in Clinical Trials
Based on the pooled data from four placebo-controlled, 4- or 6-week, fixed- or flexible-dose studies, the following adverse reactions occurred in ≥5% incidence in the patients treated with FANAPT and at least twice the placebo rate for at least one dose: dizziness, dry mouth, fatigue, nasal congestion, somnolence, tachycardia, orthostatic hypotension, and weight increased. Dizziness, tachycardia, and weight increased were at least twice as common on 20-24 mg/day as on 10-16 mg/day.

Extrapyramidal Symptoms (EPS) in Clinical Trials
Pooled data from the four placebo-controlled, 4- or 6-week, fixed- or flexible-dose studies provided information regarding treatment-emergent EPS. Adverse event data collected from those trials showed the following rates of EPS-related adverse events as shown in Table 3.

Table 3:   Percentage of EPS Compared to Placebo

Adverse Event Term	Placebo (%) (N=587)	FANAPT 10-16 mg/ day (%) (N=483)	FANAPT 20-24 mg/ day (%) (N=391)
All EPS events	11.6	13.5	15.1
Akathisia	2.7	1.7	2.3
Bradykinesia	0	0.6	0.5
Dyskinesia	1.5	1.7	1.0
Dystonia	0.7	1.0	0.8
Parkinsonism	0	0.2	0.3
Tremor	1.9	2.5	3.1

Adverse Reactions Associated with Discontinuation of Treatment in Clinical Trials
Based on the pooled data from four placebo-controlled, 4- or 6-week, fixed- or flexible-dose studies, there was no difference in the incidence of discontinuation due to adverse events between FANAPT-treated (5%) and placebo-treated (5%) patients. The types of adverse events that led to discontinuation were similar for the FANAPT- and placebo-treated patients.

Demographic Differences in Adverse Reactions in Clinical Trials
An examination of population subgroups in the four placebo-controlled, 4- or 6-week, fixed- or flexible-dose studies did not reveal any evidence of differences in safety on the basis of age, gender or race *[see Warnings and Precautions (5.1)].*

Laboratory Test Abnormalities in Clinical Trials
A between-group comparison of the pooled data from four placebo-controlled, 4- or 6-week studies, revealed no medically important differences between FANAPT and placebo in mean change from baseline to endpoint in routine hematology, urinalysis, or serum chemistry, including glucose. Similarly, there were no medically important changes in triglyceride and total cholesterol measurements (Table 3). There were no differences between FANAPT and placebo in the incidence of discontinuation due to changes in hematology, urinalysis, or serum chemistry.

Table 3:   Change in Lipids Compared to Placebo

Mean change from baseline (mg/dL)	Placebo (N=587)	FANAPT 10-16 mg/ day (N=483)	FANAPT 20-24 mg/ day (N=391)
Triglycerides	-26.5	-26.5	-8.8
Total Cholesterol	-7.7	-3.9	3.9

Table 1:   Treatment-Emergent Adverse Reactions in Short-Term, Fixed- or Flexible-Dose, Placebo-Controlled Trials in Adult Patients*

Body System or Organ Class Dictionary-derived Term	Placebo (N=587)	FANAPT 10-16 mg/day (N=483)	FANAPT 20-24 mg/day (N=391)
Body as a Whole			
Arthralgia	2	3	3
Fatigue	3	4	6
Musculoskeletal Stiffness	1	1	3
Weight Increased	1	1	9
Cardiac Disorders			
Tachycardia	1	3	12
Eye Disorders			
Vision Blurred	2	3	1
Gastrointestinal Disorders			
Nausea	8	7	10
Dry Mouth	1	8	10
Diarrhea	4	5	7
Abdominal Discomfort	1	1	3
Infections			
Nasopharyngitis	3	4	3
Upper Respiratory Tract Infection	1	2	3
Nervous System Disorders			
Dizziness	7	10	20
Somnolence	5	9	15
Extrapyramidal Disorder	4	5	4
Tremor	2	3	3
Lethargy	1	3	1
Reproductive System			
Ejaculation Failure	<1	2	2
Respiratory			
Nasal Congestion	2	5	8
Dyspnea	<1	2	2
Skin			
Rash	2	3	2
Vascular Disorders			
Orthostatic Hypotension	1	3	5
Hypotension	<1	<1	3

* Table includes adverse reactions that were reported in 2% or more of patients in any of the FANAPT dose groups and which occurred at greater incidence than in the placebo group. Figures rounded to the nearest integer.

In short-term placebo-controlled trials (4- to 6-weeks), there were 1.0% (13/1342) iloperidone-treated patients with hematocrit at least one time below the extended normal range during post-randomization treatment, compared to 0.3% (2/585) on placebo. The extended normal range for lowered hematocrit was defined in each of these trials as the value 15% below the normal range for the centralized laboratory that was used in the trial.

Other Reactions During the Pre-marketing Evaluation of FANAPT

The following is a list of MedDRA terms that reflect treatment-emergent adverse reactions in patients treated with FANAPT at multiple doses ≥4 mg/day during any phase of a trial with the database of 3210 FANAPT-treated patients. All reported reactions are included except those already listed in Table 1, or other parts of the *Adverse Reactions (6)* section, those considered in the *Warnings and Precautions (5)*, those reaction terms which were so general as to be uninformative, reactions reported in fewer than 3 patients and which were neither serious nor life-threatening, reactions that are otherwise common as background reactions, and reactions considered unlikely to be drug related. It is important to emphasize that, although the reactions reported occurred during treatment with FANAPT, they were not necessarily caused by it.

Reactions are further categorized by MedDRA system organ class and listed in order of decreasing frequency according to the following definitions: frequent adverse events are those occurring in at least 1/100 patients (only those not listed in Table 1 appear in this listing); infrequent adverse reactions are those occurring in 1/100 to 1/1000 patients; rare events are those occurring in fewer than 1/1000 patients.

Blood and Lymphatic Disorders: Infrequent – anemia, iron deficiency anemia; *Rare* – leukopenia

Cardiac Disorders: Frequent – palpitations; *Rare* – arrhythmia, atrioventricular block first degree, cardiac failure (including congestive and acute)

Ear and Labyrinth Disorders: Infrequent – vertigo, tinnitus

Endocrine Disorders: Infrequent – hypothyroidism

Eye Disorders: Frequent - conjunctivitis (including allergic); *Infrequent* – dry eye, blepharitis, eyelid edema, eye swelling, lenticular opacities, cataract, hyperemia (including conjunctival)

Gastrointestinal Disorders: Infrequent – gastritis, salivary hypersecretion, fecal incontinence, mouth ulceration; *Rare* – aphthous stomatitis, duodenal ulcer, hiatus hernia, hyperchlorhydria, lip ulceration, reflux esophagitis, stomatitis

General Disorders and Administrative Site Conditions: Infrequent – edema (general, pitting, due to cardiac disease), difficulty in walking, thirst; *Rare* – hyperthermia

Hepatobiliary Disorders: Infrequent – cholelithiasis

Investigations: Frequent: weight decreased; *Infrequent* – hemoglobin decreased, neutrophil count increased, hematocrit decreased

Metabolism and Nutrition Disorders: Infrequent – increased appetite, dehydration, hypokalemia, fluid retention

Musculoskeletal and Connective Tissue Disorders: Frequent – myalgia, muscle spasms; *Rare* – torticollis

Nervous System Disorders: Infrequent – paraesthesia, psychomotor hyperactivity, restlessness, amnesia, nystagmus; *Rare* – restless legs syndrome

Psychiatric Disorders: Frequent – restlessness, aggression, delusion; *Infrequent* – hostility, libido decreased, paranoia, anorgasmia, confusional state, mania, catatonia, mood swings, panic attack, obsessive-compulsive disorder, bulimia nervosa, delirium, polydipsia psychogenic, impulse-control disorder, major depression

Renal and Urinary Disorders: Frequent – urinary incontinence; *Infrequent* – dysuria, pollakiuria, enuresis, nephrolithiasis; *Rare* – urinary retention, renal failure acute

Reproductive System and Breast Disorders: Frequent – erectile dysfunction; *Infrequent* – testicular pain, amenorrhea, breast pain; *Rare* – menstruation irregular, gynecomastia, menorrhagia, metrorrhagia, postmenopausal hemorrhage, prostatitis.

Respiratory, Thoracic and Mediastinal Disorders: Infrequent – epistaxis, asthma, rhinorrhea, sinus congestion, nasal dryness; *Rare* – dry throat, sleep apnea syndrome, dyspnea exertional

7 DRUG INTERACTIONS

Given the primary CNS effects of FANAPT, caution should be used when it is taken in combination with other centrally acting drugs and alcohol. Due to its α1-adrenergic receptor antagonism, FANAPT has the potential to enhance the effect of certain antihypertensive agents.

7.1 Potential for Other Drugs to Affect FANAPT

Iloperidone is not a substrate for CYP1A1, CYP1A2, CYP2A6, CYP2B6, CYP2C8, CYP2C9, CYP2C19, or CYP2E1 enzymes. This suggests that an interaction of iloperidone with inhibitors or inducers of these enzymes, or other factors, like smoking, is unlikely.

Both CYP3A4 and CYP2D6 are responsible for iloperidone metabolism. Inhibitors of CYP3A4 (e.g., ketoconazole) or CYP2D6 (e.g., fluoxetine, paroxetine) can inhibit iloperidone elimination and cause increased blood levels.

Ketoconazole: Co-administration of ketoconazole (200 mg twice daily for 4 days), a potent inhibitor of CYP3A4, with a 3 mg single dose of iloperidone to 19 healthy volunteers, ages 18-45, increased the AUC of iloperidone and its metabolites P88 and P95 by 57%, 55% and 35%, respectively. Iloperidone doses should be reduced by about one-half when administered with ketoconazole or other strong inhibitors of CYP3A4 (e.g., itraconazole). Weaker inhibitors (e.g., erythromycin, grapefruit juice) have not been studied. When the CYP3A4 inhibitor is withdrawn from the combination therapy, the iloperidone dose should be returned to the previous level.

Fluoxetine: Co-administration of fluoxetine (20 mg twice daily for 21 days), a potent inhibitor of CYP2D6, with a single 3 mg dose of iloperidone to 23 healthy volunteers, ages 29-44, who were classified as CYP2D6 extensive metabolizers, increased the AUC of iloperidone and its metabolite P88, by about 2-3 fold, and decreased the AUC of its metabolite P95 by one-half. Iloperidone doses should be reduced by one-half when administered with fluoxetine. When fluoxetine is withdrawn from the combination therapy, the iloperidone dose should be returned to the previous level. Other strong inhibitors of CYP2D6 would be expected to have similar effects and would need appropriate dose reductions. When the CYP2D6 inhibitor is withdrawn from the combination therapy, iloperidone dose could then be increased to the previous level.

Paroxetine: Co-administration of paroxetine (20 mg/day for 5-8 days), a potent inhibitor of CYP2D6, with multiple doses of iloperidone (8 or 12 mg twice daily) to patients with schizophrenia ages 18-65 resulted in increased mean steady-state peak concentrations of iloperidone and its metabolite P88, by about 1.6 fold, and decreased mean steady-state peak concentrations of its metabolite P95 by one-half. Iloperidone doses should be reduced by one-half when administered with paroxetine. When paroxetine is withdrawn from the combination therapy, the iloperidone dose should be returned to the previous level. Other strong inhibitors of CYP2D6 would be expected to have similar effects and would need appropriate dose reductions. When the CYP2D6 inhibitor is withdrawn from the combination therapy, iloperidone dose could then be increased to previous levels.

Paroxetine and Ketoconazole: Co-administration of paroxetine (20 mg once daily for 10 days), a CYP2D6 inhibitor, and ketoconazole (200 mg twice daily) with multiple doses of iloperidone (8 or 12 mg twice daily) to patients with schizophrenia ages 18-65 resulted in a 1.4 fold increase in steady-state concentrations of iloperidone and its metabolite P88 and a 1.4 fold decrease in the P95 in the presence of paroxetine. So giving iloperidone with inhibitors of both of its metabolic pathways did not add to the effect of either inhibitor given alone. Iloperidone doses should therefore be reduced by about one-half if administered concomitantly with both a CYP2D6 and CYP3A4 inhibitor.

7.2 Potential for FANAPT to Affect Other Drugs

In vitro studies in human liver microsomes showed that iloperidone does not substantially inhibit the metabolism of drugs metabolized by the following cytochrome P450 isozymes: CYP1A1, CYP1A2, CYP2A6, CYP2B6, CYP2C8, CYP2C9, or CYP2E1. Furthermore, *in vitro* studies in human liver microsomes showed that iloperidone does not have enzyme inducing properties, specifically for the following cytochrome P450 isozymes: CYP1A2, CYP2C8, CYP2C9, CYP2C19, CYP3A4 and CYP3A5.

Dextromethorphan: A study in healthy volunteers showed that changes in the pharmacokinetics of dextromethorphan (80 mg dose) when a 3 mg dose of iloperidone was co-administered resulted in a 17% increase in total exposure and a 26% increase in C_{max} of dextromethorphan. Thus, an interaction between iloperidone and other CYP2D6 substrates is unlikely.

Fluoxetine: A single 3 mg dose of iloperidone had no effect on the pharmacokinetics of fluoxetine (20 mg twice daily).

7.3 Drugs that Prolong the QT Interval

FANAPT should not be used with any other drugs that prolong the QT interval *[see Warnings and Precautions (5.2)]*.

8 USE IN SPECIFIC POPULATIONS

8.1 Pregnancy

Pregnancy Category C

FANAPT caused developmental toxicity, but was not teratogenic, in rats and rabbits.

In an embryo-fetal development study, pregnant rats were given 4, 16, or 64 mg/kg/day (1.6, 6.5, and 26 times the maximum recommended human dose [MRHD] of 24 mg/day on a mg/m^2 basis) of iloperidone orally during the period of organogenesis. The highest dose caused increased early intrauterine deaths, decreased fetal weight and length, decreased fetal skeletal ossification, and an increased incidence of minor fetal skeletal anomalies and variations; this dose also caused decreased maternal food consumption and weight gain.

In an embryo-fetal development study, pregnant rabbits were given 4, 10, or 25 mg/kg/day (3, 8, and 20 times the MRHD on a mg/m^2 basis) of iloperidone during the period of organogenesis. The highest dose caused increased early intrauterine deaths and decreased fetal viability at term; this dose also caused maternal toxicity.

In additional studies in which rats were given iloperidone at doses similar to the above beginning from either pre-conception or from day 17 of gestation and continuing through weaning, adverse reproductive effects included prolonged pregnancy and parturition, increased stillbirth rates, increased incidence of fetal visceral variations, decreased fetal and pup weights, and decreased post-partum pup survival. There were no drug effects on the neurobehavioral or reproductive development of the surviving pups. No-effect doses ranged from 4 to 12 mg/kg except for the increase in stillbirth rates which occurred at the lowest dose tested of 4 mg/kg, which is 1.6 times the MRHD on a mg/m^2 basis. Maternal toxicity was seen at the higher doses in these studies.

The iloperidone metabolite P95, which is a major circulating metabolite of iloperidone in humans but is not present in significant amounts in rats, was given to pregnant rats during the period of organogenesis at oral doses of 20, 80, or 200 mg/kg/day. No teratogenic effects were seen. Delayed skeletal ossification occurred at all doses. No significant maternal toxicity was produced. Plasma levels of P95 (AUC) at the highest dose tested were 2 times those in humans receiving the MRHD of iloperidone.

There are no adequate and well-controlled studies in pregnant women. FANAPT should be used during pregnancy only if the potential benefit justifies the potential risk to the fetus.

8.2 Labor and Delivery

The effect of FANAPT on labor and delivery in humans is unknown.

8.3 Nursing Mothers

FANAPT was excreted in milk of rats during lactation. It is not known whether FANAPT or its metabolites are excreted in human milk. It is recommended that women receiving FANAPT should not breast feed.

8.4 Pediatric Use

Safety and effectiveness in pediatric and adolescent patients have not been established.

8.5 Geriatric Use

Clinical Studies of FANAPT in the treatment of schizophrenia did not include sufficient numbers of patients aged 65 years and over to determine whether or not they respond differently than younger adult patients. Of the 3210 patients treated with FANAPT in pre-marketing trials, 25 (0.5%) were ≥65 years old and there were no patients ≥75 years old.

Studies of elderly patients with psychosis associated with Alzheimer's disease have suggested that there may be a different tolerability profile (i.e., increased risk in mortality and cerebrovascular events including stroke) in this population compared to younger patients with schizophrenia *[see Boxed Warning and Warnings and Precautions (5.1)]*. The safety and efficacy of FANAPT in the treatment of patients with psychosis associated with Alzheimer's disease has not been established. If the prescriber elects to treat such patients with FANAPT, vigilance should be exercised.

8.6 Renal Impairment

Because FANAPT is highly metabolized, with less than 1% of the drug excreted unchanged, renal impairment alone is unlikely to have a significant impact on the pharmacokinetics of FANAPT. Renal impairment (creatinine clearance <30 mL/min) had minimal effect on maximum plasma concentrations (C_{max}) of iloperidone (given in a single dose of 3 mg) and its metabolites P88 and P95 any of the three analytes measured. $AUC_{0-\infty}$ was increased by 24%, decreased by 6%, and increased by 52% for iloperidone, P88 and P95, respectively, in subjects with renal impairment.

8.7 Hepatic Impairment

A study in mild and moderate liver impairment has not been conducted. FANAPT is not recommended for patients with hepatic impairment.

8.8 Smoking Status

Based on *in vitro* studies utilizing human liver enzymes, FANAPT is not a substrate for CYP1A2; smoking should therefore not have an effect on the pharmacokinetics of FANAPT.

9 DRUG ABUSE AND DEPENDENCE

9.1 Controlled Substance

FANAPT is not a controlled substance.

9.2 Abuse

FANAPT has not been systematically studied in animals or humans for its potential for abuse, tolerance, or physical dependence. While the clinical trials did not reveal any tendency for drug-seeking behavior, these observations were not systematic and it is not possible to predict on the basis of this experience the extent to which a CNS active drug, FANAPT, will be misused, diverted, and/or abused once marketed. Consequently, patients should be evaluated carefully for a history of drug abuse, and such patients should be observed closely for signs of FANAPT misuse or abuse (e.g. development of tolerance, increases in dose, drug-seeking behavior).

10 OVERDOSAGE

10.1 Human Experience

In pre-marketing trials involving over 3210 patients, accidental or intentional overdose of FANAPT was documented in eight patients ranging from 48 mg to 576 mg taken at once and 292 mg taken over a three-day period. No fatalities were reported from these cases. The largest confirmed single ingestion of FANAPT was 576 mg; no adverse physical effects were noted for this patient. The next largest confirmed ingestion of FANAPT was 438 mg over a four-day period; extrapyramidal symptoms and a QTc interval of 507 msec were reported for this patient with no cardiac sequelae. This patient resumed FANAPT treatment for an additional 11 months. In general, reported signs and symptoms where those resulting from an exaggeration of the known pharmacological effects (e.g., drowsiness and sedation, tachycardia and hypotension) of FANAPT.

10.2 Management of Overdose

There is no specific antidote for FANAPT. Therefore appropriate supportive measures should be instituted. In case of acute overdose, the physician should establish and maintain an airway and ensure adequate oxygenation and ventilation. Gastric lavage (after intubation, if patient is unconscious) and administration of activated charcoal together with a laxative should be considered. The possibility of obtundation, seizures or dystonic reaction of the head and neck following overdose may create a risk of aspiration with induced emesis. Cardiovascular monitoring should commence immediately and should include continuous ECG monitoring to detect possible arrhythmias. If antiarrhythmic therapy is administered, disopyramide, procainamide and quinidine should not be used, as they have the potential for QT-prolonging effects that might be additive to those of FANAPT. Similarly, it is reasonable to expect that the alpha-blocking properties of bretylium might be additive to those of FANAPT, resulting in problematic hypotension. Hypotension and circulatory collapse should be treated with appropriate measures such as intravenous fluids or sympathomimetic agents (epinephrine and dopamine should not be used, since beta stimulation may worsen hypotension in the setting of FANAPT-induced alpha blockade). In cases of severe extrapyramidal symptoms, anticholinergic medication should be administered. Close medical supervision should continue until the patient recovers.

11 DESCRIPTION

FANAPT is a psychotropic agent belonging to the chemical class of piperidinyl-benzisoxazole derivatives. Its chemical name is 4′-[3-[4-(6-Fluoro-1,2-benzisoxazol-3-yl)piperidino] propoxy]-3′-methoxyacetophenone. Its molecular formula is $C_{24}H_{27}FN_2O_4$ and its molecular weight is 426.48. The structural formula is:

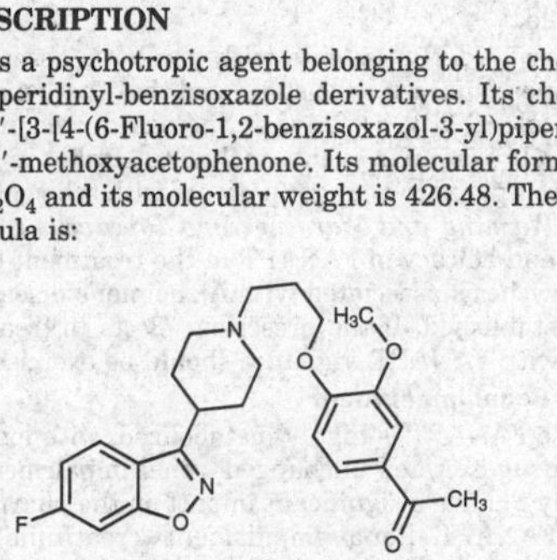

Iloperidone is a white to off-white finely crystalline powder. It is practically insoluble in water, very slightly soluble in 0.1 N HCl and freely soluble in chloroform, ethanol, methanol, and acetonitrile.

FANAPT tablets are intended for oral administration only. Each round, uncoated tablet contains 1 mg, 2 mg, 4 mg, 6 mg, 8 mg, 10 mg, or 12 mg of iloperidone. Inactive ingredients are: lactose monohydrate, microcrystalline cellulose, hydroxypropylmethylcellulose, crospovidone, magnesium stearate, colloidal silicon dioxide, and purified water (removed during processing). The tablets are white, round, flat, beveled-edged and identified with a logo "⊛" debossed on one side and tablet strength "1", "2", "4", "6", "8", "10", or "12" debossed on the other side.

12 CLINICAL PHARMACOLOGY

12.1 Mechanism of Action

The mechanism of action of FANAPT, as with other drugs having efficacy in schizophrenia, is unknown. However it is proposed that the efficacy of FANAPT is mediated through a combination of dopamine type 2 (D_2) and serotonin type 2 ($5\text{-}HT_2$) antagonisms.

12.2 Pharmacodynamics

FANAPT exhibits high (nM) affinity binding to serotonin $5\text{-}HT_{2A}$ and dopamine D_2 and D_3 receptors (K_i values of 5.6, 6.3, 7.1 nM, respectively). FANAPT has moderate affinity for dopamine D_4, serotonin $5\text{-}HT_6$ and $5\text{-}HT_7$, and norepinephrine $NE\alpha_1$ receptors (K_i values of 25, 43, 22, and 36 nM respectively), and low affinity for the serotonin $5\text{-}HT_{1A}$, dopamine D_1, and histamine H_1 receptors (K_i values of 168, 216 and 473 nM, respectively). FANAPT has no appreciable affinity (K_i>1000 nM) for cholinergic muscarinic receptors. FANAPT functions as an antagonist at the dopamine D_2, D_3, serotonin $5\text{-}HT_{1A}$ and norepinephrine α_1/α_{2C} receptors. The affinity of the FANAPT metabolite P88 is generally equal or less than that of the parent compound. In contrast, the metabolite P95 only shows affinity for $5\text{-}HT_{2A}$ (K_i value of 3.91) and the $NE\alpha_{1A}$, $NE\alpha_{1B}$, $NE\alpha_{1D}$, and $NE\alpha_{2C}$ receptors (K_i values of 4.7, 2.7, 8.8 and 4.7 nM respectively).

12.3 Pharmacokinetics

The observed mean elimination half-lives for iloperidone, P88 and P95 in CYP2D6 extensive metabolizers (EM) are 18, 26 and 23 hours, respectively, and in poor metabolizers (PM) are 33, 37 and 31 hours, respectively. Steady-state concentrations are attained within 3-4 days of dosing. Iloperidone accumulation is predictable from single-dose pharmacokinetics. The pharmacokinetics of iloperidone is more than dose proportional. Elimination of iloperidone is mainly through hepatic metabolism involving two P450 isozymes, CYP2D6 and CYP3A4.

Absorption: Iloperidone is well absorbed after administration of the tablet with peak plasma concentrations occurring within 2 to 4 hours; while the relative bioavailability of the tablet formulation compared to oral solution is 96%. Administration of iloperidone with a standard high-fat meal did not significantly affect the C_{max} or AUC of iloperidone, P88, or P95, but delayed T_{max} by 1 hour for iloperidone, 2 hours for P88 and 6 hours for P95. FANAPT can be administered without regard to meals.

Distribution: Iloperidone has an apparent clearance (clearance/bioavailability) of 47 to 102 L/h, with an apparent volume of distribution of 1340-2800 L. At therapeutic concentrations, iloperidone and its metabolites are ~95% bound to serum proteins.

Metabolism and Elimination: Iloperidone is metabolized primarily by three biotransformation pathways: carbonyl reduction, hydroxylation (mediated by CYP2D6) and *O*-demethylation (mediated by CYP3A4). There are two predominant iloperidone metabolites, P95 and P88. The iloperidone metabolite P95 represents 47.9% of the AUC of iloperidone and its metabolites in plasma at steady-state for extensive metabolizers (EM) and 25% for poor metabolizers (PM). The active metabolite P88 accounts for 19.5% and 34.0% of total plasma exposure in EM and PM, respectively. Approximately 7-10% of Caucasians and 3-8% of Black/African Americans lack the capacity to metabolize CYP2D6 substrates and are classified as poor metabolizers (PM), whereas the rest are intermediate, extensive or ultrarapid metabolizers. Co-administration of FANAPT with known strong inhibitors of CYP2D6 like fluoxetine results in a 2.3 fold increase in iloperidone plasma exposure, and therefore one-half of the FANAPT dose should be administered.

Similarly, PMs of CYP2D6 have higher exposure to iloperidone compared with EMs and PMs should have their dose reduced by one-half. Laboratory tests are available to identify CYP2D6 PMs.

The bulk of the radioactive materials were recovered in the urine (mean 58.2% and 45.1% in EM and PM, respectively), with feces accounting for 19.9% (EM) to 22.1% (PM) of the dosed radioactivity.

13 NONCLINICAL TOXICOLOGY

13.1 Carcinogenesis, Mutagenesis, Impairment of Fertility

Carcinogenesis: Lifetime carcinogenicity studies were conducted in CD-1 mice and Sprague Dawley rats. Iloperidone was administered orally at doses of 2.5, 5.0 and 10 mg/kg/day to CD-1 mice and 4, 8 and 16 mg/kg/day to Sprague Dawley rats (0.5, 1.0 and 2.0 times and 1.6, 3.2 and 6.5 times, respectively, the maximum recommended human dose [MRHD] of 24 mg/day on a mg/m² basis). There was an increased incidence of malignant mammary gland tumors in female mice treated with the lowest dose (2.5 mg/kg/day) only. There were no treatment-related increases in neoplasia in rats.

Proliferative and/or neoplastic changes in the mammary gland of rodents have been observed following the chronic administration of antipsychotic drugs and are considered to be prolactin mediated. Mammary gland proliferative changes and increases in serum prolactin were seen in mice and rats treated with iloperidone.

The iloperidone metabolite P95, which is a major circulating metabolite of iloperidone in humans but is not present in significant amounts in mice or rats, was given orally to Wistar rats for 26 weeks at doses of 50 or 500 mg/kg/day. Although this study was not adequate for assessment of carcinogenic potential, proliferative responses were seen in several organs: mammary gland hyperplasia in males and females, thyroid follicular hyperplasia in females, ovarian interstitial cell hyperplasia, pituitary cell proliferation in males, and endocrine pancreas proliferation in males and females. The above were seen at both doses except for the ovarian and pancreas effects which were seen at the higher dose only. Plasma levels of P95 (AUC) at the lower dose were 2.5 times those in humans receiving the MRHD of iloperidone, but as indicated above a no-effect dose for the proliferative responses was not determined. It is not known if these proliferative responses will progress to neoplasia with longer term treatment.

Mutagenesis: Iloperidone was negative in the Ames test and in the *in vivo* mouse bone marrow and rat liver micronucleus tests. Iloperidone induced chromosomal aberrations in Chinese Hamster Ovary (CHO) cells *in vitro* at concentrations which also caused some cytotoxicity.

The iloperidone metabolite P95 was negative in the Ames test, the V79 chromosome aberration test, and an *in vivo* mouse bone marrow micronucleus test.

Impairment of Fertility: Iloperidone decreased fertility at 12 and 36 mg/kg in a study in which both male and female rats were treated. The no-effect dose was 4 mg/kg, which is 1.6 times the maximum recommended human dose of 24 mg/day on a mg/m² basis.

14 CLINICAL STUDIES

The efficacy of FANAPT in the treatment of schizophrenia was supported by two placebo- and active-controlled short-term (4- and 6-week) trials. Both trials enrolled patients who met the DSM-III/IV criteria for schizophrenia.

Two instruments were used for assessing psychiatric signs and symptoms in these studies. The Positive and Negative Syndrome Scale (PANSS) and Brief Psychiatric Rating Scale (BPRS) are both multi-item inventories of general psychopathology usually used to evaluate the effects of drug treatment in schizophrenia.

A 6-week, placebo-controlled trial (n=706) involved two dose ranges of FANAPT (12-16 mg/day or 20-24 mg/day) compared to placebo and an active control. This study involved titration of FANAPT starting at 1 mg twice daily on day 1 and increasing to 2, 4, 6, 8, 10 and 12 mg twice daily on days 2, 3, 4, 5, 6, and 7, as needed. The primary endpoint was change from baseline on the BPRS total score at the end of treatment (Day 42). Both the 12-16 mg/day and the 20-24 mg/day dose ranges of FANAPT were superior to placebo on the BPRS total score. The active control antipsychotic drug appeared to be superior to FANAPT in this trial within the first 2 weeks, a finding that may in part be explained by the more rapid titration that was possible for that drug.

A 4-week, placebo-controlled trial (n=604) involved one fixed dose of FANAPT (24 mg/day) compared to placebo and an active control. The titration schedule for this study was similar to that for the 6-week study. This study involved titration of FANAPT starting at 1 mg twice daily on day 1 and increasing to 2, 4, 6, 8, 10 and 12 mg twice daily on days 2, 3, 4, 5, 6, and 7. The primary endpoint was change from baseline on the PANSS total score at the end of treatment (Day 28). The 24 mg/day FANAPT dose was superior to placebo in the PANSS total score. FANAPT appeared to have similar efficacy to the active control drug which also needed a slow titration to the target dose.

16 HOW SUPPLIED/STORAGE AND HANDLING

FANAPT tablets are white, round and identified with a logo "⊛" debossed on one side and tablet strength "1", "2", "4", "6", "8", "10", or "12" debossed on the other side. Tablets are supplied in the following strengths and package configurations:

Package Configuration	Tablet Strength (mg)	NDC Code
Bottles of 60	1 mg	43068-101-02
Bottles of 60	2 mg	43068-102-02
Bottles of 60	4 mg	43068-104-02
Bottles of 60	6 mg	43068-106-02
Bottles of 60	8 mg	43068-108-02
Bottles of 60	10 mg	43068-110-02
Bottles of 60	12 mg	43068-112-02
Titration Pack	2×1 mg, 2×2 mg, 2×4 mg, 2×6 mg (Total of 8 tablets)	43068-113-04

Storage

Store FANAPT tablets at controlled room temperature, 25°C (77°F); excursions permitted to 15°-30°C (59°-86°F)

[See USP Controlled Room Temperature]. Protect FANAPT tablets from exposure to light and moisture.

17 PATIENT COUNSELING INFORMATION

Physicians are advised to discuss the following issues with patients for whom they prescribe FANAPT:

17.1 QT Interval Prolongation

Patients should be advised to consult their physician immediately if they feel faint, lose consciousness or have heart palpitations. Patients should be counseled not to take FANAPT with other drugs that cause QT interval prolongation *[see Warnings and Precautions (5.2)]*. Patients should be told to inform physicians that they are taking FANAPT before any new drug is taken.

17.2 Neuroleptic Malignant Syndrome

Patients and caregivers should be counseled that a potentially fatal symptom complex sometimes referred to as NMS has been reported in association with administration of antipsychotic drugs. Signs and symptoms of NMS include hyperpyrexia, muscle rigidity, altered mental status, and evidence of autonomic instability (irregular pulse or blood pressure, tachycardia, diaphoresis, and cardiac dysrhythmia) *[see Warnings and Precautions (5.3)]*.

17.3 Orthostatic Hypotension

Patients should be advised of the risk of orthostatic hypotension, particularly at the time of initiating treatment, re-initiating treatment, or increasing the dose *[see Warnings and Precautions (5.8)]*.

17.4 Interference with Cognitive and Motor Performance

Because FANAPT may have the potential to impair judgment, thinking, or motor skills, patients should be cautioned about operating hazardous machinery, including automobiles, until they are reasonably certain that FANAPT therapy does not affect them adversely *[see Warnings and Precautions (5.15)]*.

17.5 Pregnancy

Patients should be advised to notify their physician if they become pregnant or intend to become pregnant during therapy with FANAPT *[see Use in Specific Populations (8.1)]*.

17.6 Nursing

Patients should be advised not to breast-feed an infant if they are taking FANAPT *[see Use in Specific Populations (8.3)]*.

17.7 Concomitant Medication

Patients should be advised to inform their physicians if they are taking, or plan to take, any prescription or over-the-counter drugs, since there is a potential for interactions *[see Drug Interactions (7)]*.

17.8 Alcohol

Patients should be advised to avoid alcohol while taking FANAPT.

17.9 Heat Exposure and Dehydration

Patients should be advised regarding appropriate care in avoiding overheating and dehydration.

FANAPT is a trademark of Vanda Pharmaceuticals Inc. Distributed by Vanda Pharmaceuticals Inc. Rockville, MD 20850

Shown in Product Identification Guide, page 315

FEMARA®   ℞

[fĕm-ara]
(letrozole)
Tablets

The following prescribing information is based on official labeling in effect July 2010.

HIGHLIGHTS OF PRESCRIBING INFORMATION
These highlights do not include all the information needed to use Femara safely and effectively. See full prescribing information for Femara.
Femara *(letrozole)* **tablets**
Initial U.S. Approval: 1997

——————RECENT MAJOR CHANGES——————

Adjuvant Treatment of Early Breast Cancer
(1.1, 2.2)   04/2010

——————INDICATIONS AND USAGE——————

Femara is an aromatase inhibitor indicated for:
- Adjuvant treatment of postmenopausal women with hormone receptor positive early breast cancer (1.1)
- Extended adjuvant treatment of postmenopausal women with early breast cancer who have received prior standard adjuvant tamoxifen therapy (1.2)
- First and second-line treatment of postmenopausal women with hormone receptor positive or unknown advanced breast cancer (1.3)

——————DOSAGE AND ADMINISTRATION——————

Femara tablets are taken orally without regard to meals (2):
- Recommended dose: 2.5 mg once daily (2.1)
- Patients with cirrhosis or severe hepatic impairment: 2.5 mg every other day (2.5, 5.3)

——————DOSAGE FORMS AND STRENGTHS——————

2.5 milligram tablets (3)

——————CONTRAINDICATIONS——————

Women of premenopausal endocrine status, including pregnant women (4)

——————WARNINGS AND PRECAUTIONS——————

- Decreases in bone mineral density may occur. Consider bone mineral density monitoring (5.1)
- Increases in total cholesterol may occur. Consider cholesterol monitoring (5.2)
- Fatigue, dizziness and somnolence may occur. Exercise caution when operating machinery (5.4)

——————ADVERSE REACTIONS——————

The most common adverse reactions (>20%) were hot flashes, arthralgia (6.1); flushing, asthenia, edema, arthralgia, headache, dizziness, hypercholesterolemia, sweating increased, bone pain (6.2, 6.3); and musculoskeletal (6.4).

To report SUSPECTED ADVERSE REACTIONS, contact NOVARTIS PHARMACEUTICALS CORPORATION at 1-888-669-6682 or FDA at 1-800-FDA-1088 or www.fda.gov/medwatch.

See 17 for PATIENT COUNSELING INFORMATION

Revised: 06/2010

FULL PRESCRIBING INFORMATION: CONTENTS*

*Sections or subsections omitted from the full prescribing information are not listed

FULL PRESCRIBING INFORMATION

1 INDICATIONS AND USAGE

1.1 Adjuvant Treatment of Early Breast Cancer

Femara (letrozole) is indicated for the adjuvant treatment of postmenopausal women with hormone receptor positive early breast cancer.

1.2 Extended Adjuvant Treatment of Early Breast Cancer

Femara is indicated for the extended adjuvant treatment of early breast cancer in postmenopausal women, who have received 5 years of adjuvant tamoxifen therapy. The effectiveness of Femara in extended adjuvant treatment of early breast cancer is based on an analysis of disease-free survival in patients treated with Femara for a median of 60 months *[see Clinical Studies (14.2, 14.3)]*.

1.3 First and Second-Line Treatment of Advanced Breast Cancer

Femara is indicated for first-line treatment of postmenopausal women with hormone receptor positive or unknown, locally advanced or metastatic breast cancer. Femara is also indicated for the treatment of advanced breast cancer in postmenopausal women with disease progression following antiestrogen therapy *[see Clinical Studies (14.4, 14.5)]*.

2 DOSAGE AND ADMINISTRATION

2.1 Recommended Dose

The recommended dose of Femara is one 2.5 mg tablet administered once a day, without regard to meals.

2.2 Use in Adjuvant Treatment of Early Breast Cancer

In the adjuvant setting, the optimal duration of treatment with letrozole is unknown. The planned duration of treatment in the study was 5 years with 73% of the patients having completed adjuvant therapy. Treatment should be discontinued at relapse *[see Clinical Studies (14.1)]*.

2.3 Use in Extended Adjuvant Treatment of Early Breast Cancer

In the extended adjuvant setting, the optimal treatment duration with Femara is not known. The planned duration of treatment in the study was 5 years. In the final updated analysis, conducted at a median follow-up of 62 months, the median treatment duration was 60 months. Seventy-one percent of patients were treated for at least 3 years and 58% of patients completed at least 4.5 years of extended adjuvant treatment. The treatment should be discontinued at tumor relapse *[see Clinical Studies (14.2)]*.

2.4 Use in First and Second-Line Treatment of Advanced Breast Cancer

In patients with advanced disease, treatment with Femara should continue until tumor progression is evident *[see Clinical Studies (14.4, 14.5)]*.

2.5 Use in Hepatic Impairment

No dosage adjustment is recommended for patients with mild to moderate hepatic impairment, although Femara blood concentrations were modestly increased in subjects with moderate hepatic impairment due to cirrhosis. The dose of Femara in patients with cirrhosis and severe hepatic dysfunction should be reduced by 50% *[see Warnings and Precautions (5.3)]*. The recommended dose of Femara for such patients is 2.5 mg administered every other day. The effect of hepatic impairment on Femara exposure in noncirrhotic cancer patients with elevated bilirubin levels has not been determined.

2.6 Use in Renal Impairment

No dosage adjustment is required for patients with renal impairment if creatinine clearance is ≥10 mL/min *[see Clinical Pharmacology (12.3)]*.

3 DOSAGE FORMS AND STRENGTHS

2.5 mg tablets: dark yellow, film-coated, round, slightly biconvex, with beveled edges (imprinted with the letters FV on one side and CG on the other side).

4 CONTRAINDICATIONS

Femara may cause fetal harm when administered to a pregnant woman and the clinical benefit to premenopausal women with breast cancer has not been demonstrated. Femara is contraindicated in women who are or may become pregnant. If Femara is used during pregnancy, or if the patient becomes pregnant while taking this drug, the patient should be apprised of the potential hazard to a fetus *[see Use in Specific Populations (8.1)]*.

5 WARNINGS AND PRECAUTIONS

5.1 Bone Effects

Use of Femara may cause decreases in bone mineral density (BMD). Consideration should be given to monitoring BMD. Results of a substudy to evaluate safety in the adjuvant setting comparing the effect on lumbar spine (L2-L4) bone mineral density (BMD) of adjuvant treatment with letrozole to that with tamoxifen showed at 24 months a median decrease in lumbar spine BMD of 4.1% in the letrozole arm compared to a median increase of 0.3% in the tamoxifen arm (difference = 4.4%) (P<0.0001) *[see Adverse Reactions (6.1)]*. Updated results from the BMD sub-study in the extended adjuvant setting demonstrated that at 2 years

Table 1
Patients with Adverse Reactions (CTC Grades 1-4, Irrespective of Relationship to Study Drug) in the Adjuvant Study – Monotherapy Arms Analysis (Median Follow-up 73 Months; Median Treatment 60 Months)

Adverse Reaction	Grades 1-4		Grades 3-4	
	Femara N=2448 n (%)	tamoxifen N=2447 n (%)	Femara N=2448 n (%)	tamoxifen N=2447 n (%)
Pts with Any Adverse Event	2310 (94.4)	2214 (90.5)	635 (25.9)	604 (24.7)
Hypercholesterolemia	1280 (52.3)	700 (28.6)	11 (0.4)	6 (0.2)
Hot Flashes/Flushes	821 (33.5)	929 (38.0)	0 -	0 -
Arthralgia/Arthritis	618 (25.2)	501 (20.4)	85 (3.5)	50 (2.0)
Night Sweats	357 (14.6)	426 (17.4)	0 -	0 -
Bone Fractures[2]	338 (13.8)	257 (10.5)	-	-
Weight Increase	317 (12.9)	378 (15.4)	27 (1.1)	39 (1.6)
Nausea	283 (11.6)	277 (11.3)	6 (0.2)	9 (0.4)
Bone Fractures[1]	247 (10.1)	174 (7.1)	-	-
Fatigue (Lethargy, Malaise, Asthenia)	235 (9.6)	250 (10.2)	6 (0.2)	7 (0.3)
Myalgia	217 (8.9)	212 (8.7)	18 (0.7)	14 (0.6)
Edema	164 (6.7)	160 (6.5)	3 (0.1)	1 (<0.1)
Weight Decrease	140 (5.7)	129 (5.3)	8 (0.3)	5 (0.2)
Vaginal Bleeding	128 (5.2)	320 (13.1)	1 (<0.1)	8 (0.3)
Back Pain	125 (5.1)	136 (5.6)	7 (0.3)	11 (0.4)
Osteoporosis NOS	124 (5.1)	66 (2.7)	10 (0.4)	5 (0.2)
Bone Pain	123 (5.0)	109 (4.5)	6 (0.2)	4 (0.2)
Depression	119 (4.9)	114 (4.7)	16 (0.7)	14 (0.6)
Vaginal Irritation	111 (4.5)	77 (3.1)	2 (<0.1)	2 (<0.1)
Headache	105 (4.3)	94 (3.8)	9 (0.4)	5 (0.2)
Pain in Extremity	103 (4.2)	79 (3.2)	6 (0.2)	4 (0.2)
Osteopenia	87 (3.6)	74 (3.0)	0 -	2 (<0.1)
Dizziness/Light-Headedness	84 (3.4)	84 (3.4)	1 (<0.1)	6 (0.2)
Alopecia	83 (3.4)	84 (3.4)	0 -	0 -
Vomiting	80 (3.3)	80 (3.3)	3 (0.1)	5 (0.2)
Cataract	49 (2.0)	54 (2.2)	16 (0.7)	17 (0.7)
Constipation	49 (2.0)	71 (2.9)	3 (0.1)	1 (<0.1)
Breast Pain	37 (1.5)	43 (1.8)	1 (<0.1)	0 -
Anorexia	20 (0.8)	20 (0.8)	1 (<0.1)	1 (<0.1)
Endometrial Hyperplasia/Cancer[2,3]	11/1909 (0.6)	70/1943 (3.6)	-	-
Endometrial Proliferation Disorders	10 (0.3)	71 (1.8)	0 -	14 (0.6)
Endometrial Hyperplasia/Cancer[1,3]	6/1909 (0.3)	57/1943 (2.9)	-	-
Other Endometrial Disorders	2 (<0.1)	3 (0.1)	0 -	0 -
Myocardial Infarction[1]	24 (1.0)	12 (0.5)	-	-
Myocardial Infarction[2]	37 (1.5)	25 (1.0)	-	-
Myocardial Ischemia	6 (0.2)	9 (0.4)	-	-
Cerebrovascular Accident[1]	52 (2.1)	46 (1.9)	-	-
Cerebrovascular Accident[2]	70 (2.9)	63 (2.6)	-	-
Angina[1]	26 (1.1)	24 (1.0)	-	-
Angina[2]	32 (1.3)	31 (1.3)	-	-
Thromboembolic Event[1]	51 (2.1)	89 (3.6)	-	-
Thromboembolic Event[2]	71 (2.9)	111 (4.5)	-	-
Other Cardiovascular[1]	260 (10.6)	256 (10.5)	-	-
Other Cardiovascular[2]	312 (12.7)	337 (13.8)	-	-
Second Malignancies[1]	53 (2.2)	78 (3.2)	-	-
Second Malignancies[2]	102 (4.2)	119 (4.9)	-	-

[1] During study treatment, based on Safety Monotherapy population
[2] Any time after randomization, including post treatment follow-up
[3] Excluding women who had undergone hysterectomy before study entry
Note: Cardiovascular (including cerebrovascular and thromboembolic), skeletal and urogenital/endometrial events and second malignancies were collected life-long. All of these events were assumed to be of CTC grade 3-5 and were not individually graded.

patients receiving letrozole had a median decrease from baseline of 3.8% in hip BMD compared to a median decrease of 2.0% in the placebo group. The changes from baseline in lumbar spine BMD in letrozole and placebo treated groups were not significantly different [see *Adverse Reactions (6.2)*]. In the adjuvant trial the incidence of bone fractures at any time after randomization was 13.8% for letrozole and 10.5% for tamoxifen. The incidence of osteoporosis was 5.1% for letrozole and 2.7% for tamoxifen [see *Adverse Reactions (6.1)*]. In the extended adjuvant trial the incidence of bone fractures at any time after randomization was 13.3% for letrozole and 7.8% for placebo. The incidence of new osteoporosis was 14.5% for letrozole and 7.8% for placebo [see *Adverse Reactions (6.3)*].

5.2 Cholesterol
Consideration should be given to monitoring serum cholesterol. In the adjuvant trial hypercholesterolemia was reported in 52.3% of letrozole patients and 28.6% of tamoxifen patients. CTC grade 3-4 hypercholesterolemia was reported in 0.4% of letrozole patients and 0.1% of tamoxifen patients. Also in the adjuvant setting, an increase of ≥1.5 × ULN in total cholesterol (generally non-fasting) was observed in patients on monotherapy who had baseline total serum cholesterol within the normal range (i.e., <=1.5 × ULN) in 151/1843 (8.2%) on letrozole vs 57/1840 (3.2%). Lipid lowering medications were required for 25% of patients on letrozole and 16% on tamoxifen [see *Adverse Reactions (6.1)*].

5.3 Hepatic Impairment
Subjects with cirrhosis and severe hepatic impairment who were dosed with 2.5 mg of Femara experienced approximately twice the exposure to Femara as healthy volunteers with normal liver function. Therefore, a dose reduction is recommended for this patient population. The effect of hepatic impairment on Femara exposure in cancer patients with elevated bilirubin levels has not been determined [see *Dosage and Administration (2.5)*].

5.4 Fatigue and Dizziness
Because fatigue, dizziness, and somnolence have been reported with the use of Femara, caution is advised when driving or using machinery until it is known how the patient reacts to Femara use.

5.5 Laboratory Test Abnormalities
No dose-related effect of Femara on any hematologic or clinical chemistry parameter was evident. Moderate decreases in lymphocyte counts, of uncertain clinical significance, were observed in some patients receiving Femara 2.5 mg. This depression was transient in about half of those affected. Two patients on Femara developed thrombocytopenia; relationship to the study drug was unclear. Patient withdrawal due to laboratory abnormalities, whether related to study treatment or not, was infrequent.

6 ADVERSE REACTIONS
The most serious adverse reactions from the use of Femara are:

- Bone effects [see *Warnings and Precautions (5.1)*]
- Increases in cholesterol [see *Warnings and Precautions (5.2)*]

Because clinical trials are conducted under widely varying conditions, adverse reactions rates observed in the clinical trials of a drug cannot be directly compared to rates in the clinical trials of another drug and may not reflect the rates observed in practice.

6.1 Adjuvant Treatment of Early Breast Cancer
The median treatment duration of adjuvant treatment was 60 months and the median duration of follow-up for safety was 73 months for patients receiving Femara and tamoxifen.

Certain adverse reactions were prospectively specified for analysis, based on the known pharmacologic properties and side effect profiles of the two drugs.

Adverse reactions were analyzed irrespective of whether a symptom was present or absent at baseline. Most adverse reactions reported (approximately 75% of patients reporting 1 or more AE) were Grade 1 or Grade 2 applying the Common Toxicity Criteria Version 2.0/Common Terminology Criteria for Adverse Events, version 3.0. Table 1 describes adverse reactions (Grades 1-4) irrespective of relationship to study treatment in the adjuvant trial for the monotherapy arms analysis (safety population).

[See table 1 at left]

When considering all grades during study treatment, a higher incidence of events was seen for Femara regarding fractures (10.1% vs 7.1%), myocardial infarctions (1.0% vs 0.5%), and arthralgia (25.2% vs 20.4%) (Femara vs tamoxifen respectively). A higher incidence was seen for tamoxifen regarding thromboembolic events (2.1% vs 3.6%), endometrial hyperplasia/cancer (0.3% vs 2.9%), and endometrial proliferation disorders (0.3% vs 1.8%) (Femara vs tamoxifen respectively).

At a median follow up of 73 months, a higher incidence of events was seen for Femara (13.8%) than for tamoxifen (10.5%) regarding fractures. A higher incidence was seen for tamoxifen compared to Femara regarding thromboembolic events (4.5% vs 2.9%), and endometrial hyperplasia or cancer (2.9% vs 0.4%) (tamoxifen vs Femara, respectively).

Bone Study: Results of a phase 3 safety trial in 262 postmenopausal women with resected receptor positive early breast cancer in the adjuvant setting comparing the effect on lumbar spine (L2-L4) bone mineral density (BMD) of adjuvant treatment with letrozole to that with tamoxifen showed at 24 months a median decrease in lumbar spine BMD of 4.1% in the letrozole arm compared to a median increase of 0.3% in the tamoxifen arm (difference = 4.4%) (P<0.0001). No patients with a normal BMD at baseline became osteoporotic over the 2 years and only 1 patient with osteopenia at baseline (T score of -1.9) developed osteoporosis during the treatment period (assessment by central review). The results for total hip BMD were similar, although the differences between the two treatments were less pronounced. During the 2 year period, fractures were reported by 4 of 103 patients (4%) in the letrozole arm, and 6 of 97 patients (6%) in the tamoxifen arm.

Lipid Study: In a phase 3 safety trial in 262 postmenopausal women with resected receptor positive early breast cancer at 24 months comparing the effects on lipid profiles of adjuvant letrozole to tamoxifen, 12% of patients on letrozole had at least one total cholesterol value of a higher CTCAE grade than at baseline compared with 4% of patients on tamoxifen.

6.2 Extended Adjuvant Treatment of Early Breast Cancer, Median Treatment Duration of 24 Months
The median duration of extended adjuvant treatment was 24 months and the median duration of follow-up for safety was 28 months for patients receiving Femara and placebo. Table 2 describes the adverse reactions occurring at a frequency of at least 5% in any treatment group during treatment. Most adverse reactions reported were Grade 1 and Grade 2 based on the Common Toxicity Criteria Version 2.0. In the extended adjuvant setting, the reported drug-related adverse reactions that were significantly different from placebo were hot flashes, arthralgia/arthritis, and myalgia.

[See table 2 at top of next page]

Based on a median follow-up of patients for 28 months, the incidence of clinical fractures from the core randomized study in patients who received Femara was 5.9% (152) and placebo was 5.5% (142). The incidence of self-reported osteoporosis was higher in patients who received Femara 6.9% (176) than in patients who received placebo 5.5% (141). Bisphosphonates were administered to 21.1% of the patients who received Femara and 18.7% of the patients who received placebo.

The incidence of cardiovascular ischemic events from the core randomized study was comparable between patients who received Femara 6.8% (175) and placebo 6.5% (167).

A patient-reported measure that captures treatment impact on important symptoms associated with estrogen deficiency demonstrated a difference in favor of placebo for vasomotor and sexual symptom domains.

Bone Sub-study: [see Warnings and Precautions (5.1)].

Lipid Sub-study: In the extended adjuvant setting, based on a median duration of follow-up of 62 months, there was no significant difference between Femara and placebo in total cholesterol or in any lipid fraction at any time over 5 years. Use of lipid lowering drugs or dietary management of elevated lipids was allowed [see Warnings and Precautions (5.2)].

6.3 Updated Analysis, Extended Adjuvant Treatment of Early Breast Cancer, Median Treatment Duration of 60 Months

The extended adjuvant treatment trial was unblinded early [see Adverse Reactions (6.2)]. At the updated (final analysis), overall the side effects seen were consistent to those seen at a median treatment duration of 24 months.

During treatment or within 30 days of stopping treatment (median duration of treatment 60 months) a higher rate of fractures was observed for Femara (10.4%) compared to placebo (5.8%), as also a higher rate of osteoporosis (Femara 12.2% vs placebo 6.4%).

Based on 62 months median duration of follow-up in the randomized letrozole arm in the Safety population the incidence of new fractures at any time after randomization was 13.3% for letrozole and 7.8% for placebo. The incidence of new osteoporosis was 14.5% for letrozole and 7.8% for placebo.

During treatment or within 30 days of stopping treatment (median duration of treatment 60 months) the incidence of cardiovascular events was 9.8% for Femara and 7.0% for placebo.

Based on 62 months median duration of follow-up in the randomized letrozole arm in the Safety population the incidence of cardiovascular disease at any time after randomization was 14.4% for letrozole and 9.8% for placebo.

Lipid sub-study: In the extended adjuvant setting, based on a median duration of follow-up of 62 months, there was no significant difference between Femara and placebo in total cholesterol or in any lipid fraction over 5 years. Use of lipid lowering drugs or dietary management of elevated lipids was allowed [see Warnings and Precautions (5.2)].

6.4 First-Line Treatment of Advanced Breast Cancer

A total of 455 patients were treated for a median time of exposure of 11 months. The incidence of adverse reactions was similar for Femara and tamoxifen. The most frequently reported adverse reactions were bone pain, hot flushes, back pain, nausea, arthralgia and dyspnea. Discontinuations for adverse reactions other than progression of tumor occurred in 10/455 (2%) of patients on Femara and in 15/455 (3%) of patients on tamoxifen.

Adverse reactions, regardless of relationship to study drug, that were reported in at least 5% of the patients treated with Femara 2.5 mg or tamoxifen 20 mg in the first-line treatment study are shown in Table 3.

Table 3
Percentage (%) of Patients with Adverse Reactions

Adverse Reaction	Femara 2.5 mg (N=455) %	tamoxifen 20 mg (N=455) %
General Disorders		
Fatigue	13	13
Chest Pain	8	9
Edema Peripheral	5	6
Pain NOS	5	7
Weakness	6	4
Investigations		
Weight Decreased	7	5
Vascular Disorders		
Hot Flushes	19	16
Hypertension	8	4
Gastrointestinal Disorders		
Nausea	17	17
Constipation	10	11
Diarrhea	8	4
Vomiting	7	8
Infections/Infestations		
Influenza	6	4
Urinary Tract Infection NOS	6	3
Injury, Poisoning and Procedural Complications		
Post-Mastectomy Lymphedema	7	7
Metabolism and Nutrition Disorders		
Anorexia	4	6
Musculoskeletal and Connective Tissue Disorders		
Bone Pain	22	21
Back Pain	18	19
Arthralgia	16	15
Pain in Limb	10	8
Nervous System Disorders		
Headache NOS	8	7

Table 2
Percentage of Patients with Adverse Reactions

	Number (%) of Patients with Grade 1-4 Adverse Reaction		Number (%) of Patients with Grade 3-4 Adverse Reaction	
	Femara N=2563	Placebo N=2573	Femara N=2563	Placebo N=2573
Any Adverse Reaction	2232 (87.1)	2174 (84.5)	419 (16.3)	389 (15.1)
Vascular Disorders	1375 (53.6)	1230 (47.8)	59 (2.3)	74 (2.9)
Flushing	1273 (49.7)	1114 (43.3)	3 (0.1)	0 -
General Disorders	1154 (45)	1090 (42.4)	30 (1.2)	28 (1.1)
Asthenia	862 (33.6)	826 (32.1)	16 (0.6)	7 (0.3)
Edema NOS	471 (18.4)	416 (16.2)	4 (0.2)	3 (0.1)
Musculoskeletal Disorders	978 (38.2)	836 (32.5)	71 (2.8)	50 (1.9)
Arthralgia	565 (22)	465 (18.1)	25 (1)	20 (0.8)
Arthritis NOS	173 (6.7)	124 (4.8)	10 (0.4)	5 (0.2)
Myalgia	171 (6.7)	122 (4.7)	8 (0.3)	6 (0.2)
Back Pain	129 (5)	112 (4.4)	8 (0.3)	7 (0.3)
Nervous System Disorders	863 (33.7)	819 (31.8)	65 (2.5)	58 (2.3)
Headache	516 (20.1)	508 (19.7)	18 (0.7)	17 (0.7)
Dizziness	363 (14.2)	342 (13.3)	9 (0.4)	6 (0.2)
Skin Disorders	830 (32.4)	787 (30.6)	17 (0.7)	16 (0.6)
Sweating Increased	619 (24.2)	577 (22.4)	1 (<0.1)	0 -
Gastrointestinal Disorders	725 (28.3)	731 (28.4)	43 (1.7)	42 (1.6)
Constipation	290 (11.3)	304 (11.8)	6 (0.2)	2 (<0.1)
Nausea	221 (8.6)	212 (8.2)	3 (0.1)	10 (0.4)
Diarrhea NOS	128 (5)	143 (5.6)	12 (0.5)	8 (0.3)
Metabolic Disorders	551 (21.5)	537 (20.9)	24 (0.9)	32 (1.2)
Hypercholesterolemia	401 (15.6)	398 (15.5)	2 (<0.1)	5 (0.2)
Reproductive Disorders	303 (11.8)	357 (13.9)	9 (0.4)	8 (0.3)
Vaginal Hemorrhage	123 (4.8)	171 (6.6)	2 (<0.1)	5 (0.2)
Vulvovaginal Dryness	137 (5.3)	127 (4.9)	0 -	0 -
Psychiatric Disorders	320 (12.5)	276 (10.7)	21 (0.8)	16 (0.6)
Insomnia	149 (5.8)	120 (4.7)	2 (<0.1)	2 (<0.1)
Respiratory Disorders	279 (10.9)	260 (10.1)	30 (1.2)	28 (1.1)
Dyspnea	140 (5.5)	137 (5.3)	21 (0.8)	18 (0.7)
Investigations	184 (7.2)	147 (5.7)	13 (0.5)	13 (0.5)
Infections and Infestations	166 (6.5)	163 (6.3)	40 (1.6)	33 (1.3)
Renal Disorders	130 (5.1)	100 (3.9)	12 (0.5)	6 (0.2)

Psychiatric Disorders		
Insomnia	7	4
Reproductive System and Breast Disorders		
Breast Pain	7	7
Respiratory, Thoracic and Mediastinal Disorders		
Dyspnea	18	17
Cough	13	13
Chest Wall Pain	6	6

Other less frequent (≤2%) adverse reactions considered consequential for both treatment groups, included peripheral thromboembolic events, cardiovascular events, and cerebrovascular events. Peripheral thromboembolic events included venous thrombosis, thrombophlebitis, portal vein thrombosis and pulmonary embolism. Cardiovascular events included angina, myocardial infarction, myocardial ischemia, and coronary heart disease. Cerebrovascular events included transient ischemic attacks, thrombotic or hemorrhagic strokes and development of hemiparesis.

6.5 Second-Line Treatment of Advanced Breast Cancer

Study discontinuations in the megestrol acetate comparison study for adverse reactions other than progression of tumor were 5/188 (2.7%) on Femara 0.5 mg, in 4/174 (2.3%) on Femara 2.5 mg, and in 15/190 (7.9%) on megestrol acetate. There were fewer thromboembolic events at both Femara doses than on the megestrol acetate arm (0.6% vs 4.7%). There was also less vaginal bleeding (0.3% vs 3.2%) on Femara than on megestrol acetate. In the aminoglutethimide comparison study, discontinuations for reasons other than progression occurred in 6/193 (3.1%) on 0.5 mg Femara, 7/185 (3.8%) on 2.5 mg Femara, and 7/178 (3.9%) of patients on aminoglutethimide.

Comparisons of the incidence of adverse reactions revealed no significant differences between the high and low dose Femara groups in either study. Most of the adverse reactions observed in all treatment groups were mild to moderate in severity and it was generally not possible to distinguish adverse reactions due to treatment from the consequences of the patient's metastatic breast cancer, the effects of estrogen deprivation, or intercurrent illness.

Adverse reactions, regardless of relationship to study drug, that were reported in at least 5% of the patients treated with Femara 0.5 mg, Femara 2.5 mg, megestrol acetate, or aminoglutethimide in the two controlled trials are shown in Table 4.

[See table 4 at top of next page]

Other less frequent (<5%) adverse reactions considered consequential and reported in at least 3 patients treated with Femara, included hypercalcemia, fracture, depression, anxiety, pleural effusion, alopecia, increased sweating and vertigo.

6.6 First and Second-Line Treatment of Advanced Breast Cancer

In the combined analysis of the first- and second-line metastatic trials and post-marketing experiences other adverse reactions that were reported were cataract, eye irritation, palpitations, cardiac failure, tachycardia, dysesthesia (including hypesthesia/paresthesia), arterial thrombosis, memory impairment, irritability, nervousness, urticaria, increased urinary frequency, leukopenia, stomatitis cancer pain, pyrexia, vaginal discharge, appetite increase, dryness of skin and mucosa (including dry mouth), and disturbances of taste and thirst.

6.7 Postmarketing Experience

Cases of blurred vision, increased hepatic enzymes, angioedema, anaphylactic reactions, toxic epidermal necrolysis, erythema multiforme, and hepatitis have been reported.

7 DRUG INTERACTIONS

Tamoxifen

Coadministration of Femara and tamoxifen 20 mg daily resulted in a reduction of letrozole plasma levels of 38% on average. Clinical experience in the second-line breast cancer trials indicates that the therapeutic effect of Femara therapy is not impaired if Femara is administered immediately after tamoxifen.

Cimetidine

A pharmacokinetic interaction study with cimetidine showed no clinically significant effect on letrozole pharmacokinetics.

Warfarin

An interaction study with warfarin showed no clinically significant effect of letrozole on warfarin pharmacokinetics.

Other anticancer agents

There is no clinical experience to date on the use of Femara in combination with other anticancer agents.

8 USE IN SPECIFIC POPULATIONS

8.1 Pregnancy

Pregnancy Category X [see Contraindications (4)]. Femara may cause fetal harm when administered to a pregnant woman and the clinical benefit to premenopausal women with breast cancer has not been demonstrated. Femara is contraindicated in women who are or may become pregnant. If this drug is used during pregnancy, or if the patient becomes pregnant while taking this drug, the patient should be apprised of the potential hazard to a fetus.

Femara caused adverse pregnancy outcomes, including congenital malformations, in rats and rabbits at doses much smaller than the daily maximum recommended human dose (MRHD) on a mg/m^2 basis. Effects included increased postimplantation pregnancy loss and resorptions, fewer live fetuses, and fetal malformations affecting the renal and skeletal systems. Animal data and letrozole's mechanism of action raise concerns that letrozole could be a human teratogen as well.

Reproduction studies in rats showed embryo and fetal toxicity at letrozole doses during organogenesis equal to or greater than 1/100 the daily maximum recommended human dose (MHRD) (mg/m^2 basis). Adverse effects included: intrauterine mortality; increased resorptions and postimplantation loss; decreased numbers of live fetuses; and fetal anomalies including absence and shortening of renal papilla, dilation of ureter, edema and incomplete ossification of frontal skull and metatarsals. Letrozole doses 1/10 the daily MHRD (mg/m^2 basis) caused fetal domed head and cervical/centrum vertebral fusion. In rabbits, letrozole caused embryo and fetal toxicity at doses about 1/100,000 and 1/10,000 the daily MHRD respectively (mg/m^2 basis). Fetal anomalies included incomplete ossification of the skull, sternebrae, and fore- and hind legs [see Nonclinical Toxicology (13.2)]. Physicians should discuss the need for adequate contraception with women who are recently menopausal. Contraception should be used until postmenopausal status is clinically well established.

8.3 Nursing Mothers
It is not known if letrozole is excreted in human milk. Because many drugs are excreted in human milk and because of the potential for serious adverse reactions in nursing infants from letrozole, a decision should be made whether to discontinue nursing or to discontinue the drug, taking into account the importance of the drug to the mother.

8.4 Pediatric Use
The safety and effectiveness in pediatric patients have not been established.

8.5 Geriatric Use
The median age of patients in all studies of first-line and second-line treatment of metastatic breast cancer was 64-65 years. About 1/3 of the patients were ≥70 years old. In the first-line study, patients ≥70 years of age experienced longer time to tumor progression and higher response rates than patients <70.

For the extended adjuvant setting, more than 5,100 postmenopausal women were enrolled in the clinical study. In total, 41% of patients were aged 65 years or older at enrollment, while 12% were 75 or older. In the extended adjuvant setting, no overall differences in safety or efficacy were observed between these older patients and younger patients, and other reported clinical experience has not identified differences in responses between the elderly and younger patients, but greater sensitivity of some older individuals cannot be ruled out.

In the adjuvant setting, more than 8,000 postmenopausal women were enrolled in the clinical study. In total, 36% of patients were aged 65 years or older at enrollment, while 12% were 75 or older. More adverse reactions were generally reported in elderly patients irrespective of study treatment allocation. However, in comparison to tamoxifen, no overall differences with regards to the safety and efficacy profiles were observed between elderly patients and younger patients.

10 OVERDOSAGE
Isolated cases of Femara overdose have been reported. In these instances, the highest single dose ingested was 62.5 mg or 25 tablets. While no serious adverse reactions were reported in these cases, because of the limited data available, no firm recommendations for treatment can be made. However, emesis could be induced if the patient is alert. In general, supportive care and frequent monitoring of vital signs are also appropriate. In single-dose studies, the highest dose used was 30 mg, which was well tolerated; in multiple-dose trials, the largest dose of 10 mg was well tolerated.

Lethality was observed in mice and rats following single oral doses that were equal to or greater than 2,000 mg/kg (about 4,000 to 8,000 times the daily maximum recommended human dose on a mg/m^2 basis); death was associated with reduced motor activity, ataxia and dyspnea. Lethality was observed in cats following single IV doses that were equal to or greater than 10 mg/kg (about 50 times the daily maximum recommended human dose on a mg/m^2 basis); death was preceded by depressed blood pressure and arrhythmias.

11 DESCRIPTION
Femara tablets for oral administration contains 2.5 mg of letrozole, a nonsteroidal aromatase inhibitor (inhibitor of estrogen synthesis). It is chemically described as 4,4′-(1H-1,2,4-Triazol-1-ylmethylene)dibenzonitrile, and its structural formula is

Letrozole is a white to yellowish crystalline powder, practically odorless, freely soluble in dichloromethane, slightly soluble in ethanol, and practically insoluble in water. It has a molecular weight of 285.31, empirical formula $C_{17}H_{11}N_5$, and a melting range of 184°C-185°C.

Femara is available as 2.5 mg tablets for oral administration.

Inactive Ingredients: Colloidal silicon dioxide, ferric oxide, hydroxypropyl methylcellulose, lactose monohydrate, magnesium stearate, maize starch, microcrystalline cellulose, polyethylene glycol, sodium starch glycolate, talc, and titanium dioxide.

12 CLINICAL PHARMACOLOGY
12.1 Mechanism of Action
The growth of some cancers of the breast is stimulated or maintained by estrogens. Treatment of breast cancer thought to be hormonally responsive (i.e., estrogen and/or progesterone receptor positive or receptor unknown) has included a variety of efforts to decrease estrogen levels (ovariectomy, adrenalectomy, hypophysectomy) or inhibit estrogen effects (antiestrogens and progestational agents). These interventions lead to decreased tumor mass or delayed progression of tumor growth in some women.

In postmenopausal women, estrogens are mainly derived from the action of the aromatase enzyme, which converts adrenal androgens (primarily androstenedione and testosterone) to estrone and estradiol. The suppression of estrogen biosynthesis in peripheral tissues and in the cancer tissue itself can therefore be achieved by specifically inhibiting the aromatase enzyme.

Letrozole is a nonsteroidal competitive inhibitor of the aromatase enzyme system; it inhibits the conversion of androgens to estrogens. In adult nontumor- and tumor-bearing female animals, letrozole is as effective as ovariectomy in reducing uterine weight, elevating serum LH, and causing the regression of estrogen-dependent tumors. In contrast to ovariectomy, treatment with letrozole does not lead to an increase in serum FSH. Letrozole selectively inhibits gonadal steroidogenesis but has no significant effect on adrenal mineralocorticoid or glucocorticoid synthesis.

Letrozole inhibits the aromatase enzyme by competitively binding to the heme of the cytochrome P450 subunit of the enzyme, resulting in a reduction of estrogen biosynthesis in all tissues. Treatment of women with letrozole significantly lowers serum estrone, estradiol and estrone sulfate and has not been shown to significantly affect adrenal corticosteroid synthesis, aldosterone synthesis, or synthesis of thyroid hormones.

12.2 Pharmacodynamics
In postmenopausal patients with advanced breast cancer, daily doses of 0.1 mg to 5 mg Femara (letrozole) suppress plasma concentrations of estradiol, estrone, and estrone sulfate by 75%-95% from baseline with maximal suppression achieved within two-three days. Suppression is dose-related, with doses of 0.5 mg and higher giving many values of estrone and estrone sulfate that were below the limit of detection in the assays. Estrogen suppression was maintained throughout treatment in all patients treated at 0.5 mg or higher.

Letrozole is highly specific in inhibiting aromatase activity. There is no impairment of adrenal steroidogenesis. No clinically-relevant changes were found in the plasma concentrations of cortisol, aldosterone, 11-deoxycortisol, 17-hydroxy-progesterone, ACTH or in plasma renin activity among postmenopausal patients treated with a daily dose of Femara 0.1 mg to 5 mg. The ACTH stimulation test performed after 6 and 12 weeks of treatment with daily doses of 0.1, 0.25, 0.5, 1, 2.5, and 5 mg did not indicate any attenuation of aldosterone or cortisol production. Glucocorticoid or mineralocorticoid supplementation is, therefore, not necessary.

No changes were noted in plasma concentrations of androgens (androstenedione and testosterone) among healthy postmenopausal women after 0.1, 0.5, and 2.5 mg single doses of Femara or in plasma concentrations of androstenedione among postmenopausal patients treated with daily doses of 0.1 mg to 5 mg. This indicates that the blockade of estrogen biosynthesis does not lead to accumulation of androgenic precursors. Plasma levels of LH and FSH were not affected by letrozole in patients, nor was thyroid function as evaluated by TSH levels, T3 uptake, and T4 levels.

12.3 Pharmacokinetics
Absorption and Distribution: Letrozole is rapidly and completely absorbed from the gastrointestinal tract and

Table 4
Percentage (%) of Patients with Adverse Reactions

Adverse Reaction	Pooled Femara 2.5 mg (N=359) %	Pooled Femara 0.5 mg (N=380) %	megestrol acetate 160 mg (N=189) %	aminoglutethimide 500 mg (N=178) %
Body as a Whole				
Fatigue	8	6	11	3
Chest Pain	6	3	7	3
Peripheral Edema[1]	5	5	8	3
Asthenia	4	5	4	5
Weight Increase	2	2	9	3
Cardiovascular				
Hypertension	5	7	5	6
Digestive System				
Nausea	13	15	9	14
Vomiting	7	7	5	9
Constipation	6	7	9	7
Diarrhea	6	5	3	4
Pain-Abdominal	6	5	9	8
Anorexia	5	3	5	5
Dyspepsia	3	4	6	5
Infections/Infestations				
Viral Infection	6	6	6	3
Lab Abnormality				
Hypercholesterolemia	3	3	0	6
Musculoskeletal System				
Musculoskeletal[2]	21	22	30	14
Arthralgia	8	8	8	3
Nervous System				
Headache	9	12	9	7
Somnolence	3	2	2	9
Dizziness	3	5	7	3
Respiratory System				
Dyspnea	7	9	16	5
Coughing	6	5	7	5
Skin and Appendages				
Hot Flushes	6	5	4	3
Rash[3]	5	4	3	12
Pruritus	1	2	5	3

[1] Includes peripheral edema, leg edema, dependent edema, edema
[2] Includes musculoskeletal pain, skeletal pain, back pain, arm pain, leg pain
[3] Includes rash, erythematous rash, maculopapular rash, psoriasiform rash, vesicular rash

absorption is not affected by food. It is metabolized slowly to an inactive metabolite whose glucuronide conjugate is excreted renally, representing the major clearance pathway. About 90% of radiolabeled letrozole is recovered in urine. Letrozole's terminal elimination half-life is about 2 days and steady-state plasma concentration after daily 2.5 mg dosing is reached in 2-6 weeks. Plasma concentrations at steady state are 1.5 to 2 times higher than predicted from the concentrations measured after a single dose, indicating a slight non-linearity in the pharmacokinetics of letrozole upon daily administration of 2.5 mg. These steady-state levels are maintained over extended periods, however, and continuous accumulation of letrozole does not occur. Letrozole is weakly protein bound and has a large volume of distribution (approximately 1.9 L/kg).

Metabolism and Excretion: Metabolism to a pharmacologically-inactive carbinol metabolite (4,4'-methanol-bisbenzonitrile) and renal excretion of the glucuronide conjugate of this metabolite is the major pathway of letrozole clearance. Of the radiolabel recovered in urine, at least 75% was the glucuronide of the carbinol metabolite, about 9% was two unidentified metabolites, and 6% was unchanged letrozole.

In human microsomes with specific CYP isozyme activity, CYP3A4 metabolized letrozole to the carbinol metabolite while CYP2A6 formed both this metabolite and its ketone analog. In human liver microsomes, letrozole strongly inhibited CYP2A6 and moderately inhibited CYP2C19.

Pediatric, Geriatric and Race: In the study populations (adults ranging in age from 35 to >80 years), no change in pharmacokinetic parameters was observed with increasing age. Differences in letrozole pharmacokinetics between adult and pediatric populations have not been studied. Differences in letrozole pharmacokinetics due to race have not been studied.

Renal Impairment: In a study of volunteers with varying renal function (24-hour creatinine clearance: 9-116 mL/min), no effect of renal function on the pharmacokinetics of single doses of 2.5 mg of Femara was found. In addition, in a study of 347 patients with advanced breast cancer, about half of whom received 2.5 mg Femara and half 0.5 mg Femara, renal impairment (calculated creatinine clearance: 20-50 mL/min) did not affect steady-state plasma letrozole concentrations.

Hepatic Impairment: In a study of subjects with mild to moderate non-metastatic hepatic dysfunction (e.g., cirrhosis, Child-Pugh classification A and B), the mean AUC values of the volunteers with moderate hepatic impairment were 37% higher than in normal subjects, but still within the range seen in subjects without impaired function.

In a pharmacokinetic study, subjects with liver cirrhosis and severe hepatic impairment (Child-Pugh classification C, which included bilirubins about 2-11 times ULN with minimal to severe ascites) had two-fold increase in exposure (AUC) and 47% reduction in systemic clearance. Breast cancer patients with severe hepatic impairment are thus expected to be exposed to higher levels of letrozole than patients with normal liver function receiving similar doses of this drug [see Dosage and Administration (2.5)].

13 NONCLINICAL TOXICOLOGY

13.1 Carcinogenesis, Mutagenesis, Impairment of Fertility

A conventional carcinogenesis study in mice at doses of 0.6 to 60 mg/kg/day (about 1 to 100 times the daily maximum recommended human dose on a mg/m^2 basis) administered by oral gavage for up to 2 years revealed a dose-related increase in the incidence of benign ovarian stromal tumors. The incidence of combined hepatocellular adenoma and carcinoma showed a significant trend in females when the high dose group was excluded due to low survival. In a separate study, plasma AUC_{0-12hr} levels in mice at 60 mg/kg/day were 55 times higher than the AUC_{0-24hr} level in breast cancer patients at the recommended dose. The carcinogenicity study in rats at oral doses of 0.1 to 10 mg/kg/day (about 0.4 to 40 times the daily maximum recommended human dose on a mg/m^2 basis) for up to 2 years also produced an increase in the incidence of benign ovarian stromal tumors at 10 mg/kg/day. Ovarian hyperplasia was observed in females at doses equal to or greater than 0.1 mg/kg/day. At 10 mg/kg/day, plasma AUC_{0-24hr} levels in rats were 80 times higher than the level in breast cancer patients at the recommended dose.

Femara (letrozole) was not mutagenic in in vitro tests (Ames and E. coli bacterial tests) but was observed to be a potential clastogen in in vitro assays (CHO K1 and CCL 61 Chinese hamster ovary cells). Letrozole was not clastogenic in vivo (micronucleus test in rats).

Studies to investigate the effect of letrozole on fertility have not been conducted; however, repeated dosing caused sexual inactivity in females and atrophy of the reproductive tract in males and females at doses of 0.6, 0.1 and 0.03 mg/kg in mice, rats and dogs, respectively (about one, 0.4 and 0.4 the daily maximum recommended human dose on a mg/m^2 basis, respectively).

Letrozole administered to young (postnatal day 7) rats for 12 weeks duration at 0.003, 0.03, 0.3 mg/kg/day by oral gavage, resulted in adverse skeletal/growth effects (bone maturation, bone mineral density) and neuroendocrine and reproductive developmental perturbations of the hypothalamic-pituitary axis at exposures less than exposure anticipated at the clinical dose of 2.5 mg/day. Decreased fertility was accompanied by hypertrophy of the hypophysis and testicular changes that included degeneration of the seminiferous tubular epithelium and atrophy of the female reproductive tract. Young rats in this study were allowed to recover following discontinuation of letrozole treatment for 42 days. Histopathological changes were not reversible at clinically relevant exposures.

13.2 Animal Toxicology and/or Pharmacology

Reproductive Toxicology: Reproduction studies in rats at letrozole doses equal to or greater than 0.003 mg/kg (about 1/100 the daily maximum recommended human dose on a mg/m^2 basis) administered during the period of organogenesis, have shown that letrozole is embryotoxic and fetotoxic, as indicated by intrauterine mortality, increased resorption, increased postimplantation loss, decreased numbers of live fetuses and fetal anomalies including absence and shortening of renal papilla, dilation of ureter, edema and incomplete ossification of frontal skull and metatarsals. Letrozole was teratogenic in rats. A 0.03 mg/kg dose (about 1/10 the daily maximum recommended human dose on a mg/m^2 basis) caused fetal domed head and cervical/centrum vertebral fusion.

Letrozole is embryotoxic at doses equal to or greater than 0.002 mg/kg and fetotoxic when administered to rabbits at 0.02 mg/kg (about 1/100,000 and 1/10,000 the daily maximum recommended human dose on a mg/m^2 basis, respectively). Fetal anomalies included incomplete ossification of the skull, sternebrae, and fore- and hind legs.

14 CLINICAL STUDIES

14.1 Updated Adjuvant Treatment of Early Breast Cancer

In a multicenter study enrolling over 8,000 postmenopausal women with resected, receptor-positive early breast cancer, one of the following treatments was randomized in a double-blind manner:

Option 1:
A. tamoxifen for 5 years
B. Femara for 5 years
C. tamoxifen for 2 years followed by Femara for 3 years
D. Femara for 2 years followed by tamoxifen for 3 years

Option 2:
A. tamoxifen for 5 years
B. Femara for 5 years

The study in the adjuvant setting, BIG 1-98 was designed to answer two primary questions: whether Femara for 5 years was superior to tamoxifen for 5 years (Primary Core Analysis) and whether switching endocrine treatments at 2 years was superior to continuing the same agent for a total of 5 years (Sequential Treatments Analysis). Selected baseline characteristics for the study population are shown in Table 5.

The primary endpoint of this trial was disease-free survival (DFS) (i.e., interval between randomization and earliest occurrence of a local, regional, or distant recurrence, or invasive contralateral breast cancer, or death from any cause). The secondary endpoints were overall survival (OS),

Table 5
Adjuvant Study - Patient and Disease Characteristics (ITT Population)

Characteristic	Primary Core Analysis (PCA) Femara N=4003 n (%)	tamoxifen N=4007 n (%)	Monotherapy Arms Analysis (MAA) Femara N=2463 n (%)	tamoxifen N=2459 n (%)
Age (median, years)	61	61	61	61
Age range (years)	38-89	39-90	38-88	39-90
Hormone receptor status (%)				
ER+ and/or PgR+	99.7	99.7	99.7	99.7
Both unknown	0.3	0.3	0.3	0.3
Nodal status (%)				
Node negative	52	52	50	52
Node positive	41	41	43	41
Nodal status unknown	7	7	7	7
Prior adjuvant chemotherapy (%)	24	24	24	24

Table 6
Updated Adjuvant Study Results - Monotherapy Arms Analysis (Median Follow-up 73 Months)

		Femara N=2463 Events (%)	5-year rate	tamoxifen N=2459 Events (%)	5-year rate	Hazard ratio (95% CI)	P
Disease-free survival[1]	ITT	445 (18.1)	87.4	500 (20.3)	84.7	0.87 (0.76, 0.99)	0.03
	Censor	445	87.4	483	84.2	0.84 (0.73, 0.95)	
0 positive nodes	ITT	165	92.2	189	90.3	0.88 (0.72, 1.09)	
1-3 positive nodes	ITT	151	85.6	163	83.0	0.85 (0.68, 1.06)	
>=4 positive nodes	ITT	123	71.2	142	62.6	0.81 (0.64, 1.03)	
Adjuvant chemotherapy	ITT	119	86.4	150	80.6	0.77 (0.60, 0.98)	
No chemotherapy	ITT	326	87.8	350	86.1	0.91 (0.78, 1.06)	
Systemic DFS[2]	ITT	401	88.5	446	86.6	0.88 (0.77, 1.01)	
Time to distant metastasis[3]	ITT	257	92.4	298	90.1	0.85 (0.72, 1.00)	
Adjuvant chemotherapy	ITT	84	-	109	-	0.75 (0.56, 1.00)	
No chemotherapy	ITT	173	-	189	-	0.90 (0.73, 1.11)	
Distant DFS[4]	ITT	385	89.0	432	87.1	0.87 (0.76, 1.00)	
Contralateral breast cancer	ITT	34	99.2	44	98.6	0.76 (0.49, 1.19)	
Overall survival	ITT	303	91.8	343	90.9	0.87 (0.75, 1.02)	
	Censor	303	91.8	338	90.1	0.82 (0.70, 0.96)	
0 positive nodes	ITT	107	95.2	121	94.8	0.90 (0.69, 1.16)	
1-3 positive nodes	ITT	99	90.8	114	90.6	0.81 (0.62, 1.06)	
>=4 positive nodes	ITT	92	80.2	104	73.6	0.86 (0.65, 1.14)	
Adjuvant chemotherapy	ITT	76	91.5	96	88.4	0.79 (0.58, 1.06)	
No chemotherapy	ITT	227	91.9	247	91.8	0.91 (0.76, 1.08)	

Definition of:
[1] Disease-free survival: Interval from randomization to earliest event of invasive loco-regional recurrence, distant metastasis, invasive contralateral breast cancer, or death without a prior event
[2] Systemic disease-free survival: Interval from randomization to invasive regional recurrence, distant metastasis, or death without a prior cancer event
[3] Time to distant metastasis: Interval from randomization to distant metastasis
[4] Distant disease-free survival: Interval from randomization to earlier event of relapse in a distant site or death from any cause
ITT analysis ignores selective crossover in tamoxifen arms
Censored analysis censors follow-up at the date of selective crossover in 632 patients who crossed to Femara or another aromatase inhibitor after the tamoxifen arms were unblinded in 2005

Table 8
Extended Adjuvant Study Results

	Femara N=2582	Placebo N=2586	Hazard Ratio (95% CI)	P-Value
Disease Free Survival (DFS)[1] Events	122 (4.7%)	193 (7.5%)	0.62 (0.49, 0.78)[2]	0.00003
Local Breast Recurrence	9	22		
Local Chest Wall Recurrence	2	8		
Regional Recurrence	7	4		
Distant Recurrence	55	92	0.61 (0.44-0.84)	0.003
Contralateral Breast Cancer	19	29		
Deaths Without Recurrence or Contralateral Breast Cancer	30	38		

CI = confidence interval for hazard ratio. Hazard ratio of less than 1.0 indicates difference in favor of Femara (lesser risk of recurrence); hazard ratio greater than 1.0 indicates difference in favor of placebo (higher risk of recurrence with Femara).
[1] First event of loco-regional recurrence, distant relapse, contralateral breast cancer or death from any cause
[2] Analysis stratified by receptor status, nodal status and prior adjuvant chemotherapy (stratification factors as at randomization). P-value based on stratified logrank test.

Table 9
Update of Extended Adjuvant Study Results

	Femara N=2582 (%)	Placebo N=2586 (%)	Hazard Ratio[1] (95% CI)	P-Value[2]
Disease Free Survival (DFS) Events[3]	344 (13.3)	402 (15.5)	0.89 (0.77, 1.03)	0.12
Breast Cancer Recurrence (Protocol definition of DFS events[4])	209	286	0.75 (0.63, 0.89)	0.001
Local Breast Recurrence	15	44		
Local Chest Wall Recurrence	6	14		
Regional Recurrence	10	8		
Distant Recurrence	140	167		
Distant Recurrence (first or subsequent events)	142	169	0.88 (0.70, 1.10)	0.246
Contralateral Breast Cancer	37	53		
Deaths Without Recurrence or Contralateral Breast Cancer	135	116		

[1] Adjusted by receptor status, nodal status and prior chemotherapy
[2] Stratified logrank test, stratified by receptor status, nodal status and prior chemotherapy
[3] DFS events defined as earliest of loco-regional recurrence, distant metastasis, contralateral breast cancer or death from any cause, and ignoring switches to Femara in 60% of the placebo arm
[4] Protocol definition does not include deaths from any cause

systemic disease-free survival (SDFS), invasive contralateral breast cancer, time to breast cancer recurrence (TBR) and time to distant metastasis (TDM).

The Primary Core Analysis (PCA) included all patients and all follow-up in the monotherapy arms in both randomization options, but follow-up in the two sequential treatments arms was truncated 30 days after switching treatments. The PCA was conducted at a median treatment duration of 24 months and a median follow-up of 26 months. Femara was superior to tamoxifen in all endpoints except overall survival and contralateral breast cancer [e.g., DFS: hazard ratio, HR 0.79; 95% CI (0.68, 0.92); P=0.002; SDFS: HR 0.83; 95% CI (0.70, 0.97); TDM: HR 0.73; 95% CI (0.60, 0.88); OS: HR 0.86; 95% CI (0.70, 1.06).

In 2005, based on recommendations by the independent Data Monitoring Committee, the tamoxifen arms were unblinded and patients were allowed to complete initial adjuvant therapy with Femara (if they had received tamoxifen for at least 2 years) or to start extended adjuvant treatment with Femara (if they had received tamoxifen for at least 4.5 years) if they remained alive and disease-free. In total, 632 patients crossed to Femara or another aromatase inhibitor. Approximately 70% (448) of these 632 patients crossed to Femara to complete initial adjuvant therapy and most of these crossed in years 3 to 4. All of these patients were in Option 1. A total of 184 patients started extended adjuvant therapy with Femara (172 patients) or with another aromatase inhibitor (12 patients). To explore the impact of this selective crossover, results from analyses censoring follow-up at the date of the selective crossover (in the tamoxifen arm) are presented for the Monotherapy Arms Analysis (MAA).

The PCA allowed the results of Femara for 5 years compared with tamoxifen for 5 years to be reported in 2005 after a median follow-up of only 26 months. The design of the PCA is not optimal to evaluate the effect of Femara after a longer time (because follow-up was truncated in two arms at around 25 months). The Monotherapy Arms Analysis (ignoring the two sequential treatment arms) provided follow-up equally as long in each treatment and did not over-emphasize early recurrences as the PCA did. The MAA thus

provides the clinically appropriate updated efficacy results in answer to the first primary question, despite the confounding of the tamoxifen reference arm by the selective crossover to Femara. The updated results for the MAA are summarized in Table 6. Median follow-up for this analysis is 73 months.

The Sequential Treatments Analysis (STA) addresses the second primary question of the study. The primary analysis for the Sequential Treatments Analysis (STA) was from switch (or equivalent time-point in monotherapy arms) + 30 days (STA-S) with a two-sided test applied to each pair-wise comparison at the 2.5% level. Additional analyses were conducted from randomization (STA-R) but these comparisons (added in light of changing medical practice) were underpowered for efficacy.

[See table 5 at top of previous page]
[See table 6 on previous page]
Figure 1 shows the Kaplan-Meier curves for Disease-Free Survival Monotherapy Analysis.

Figure 1
Disease-Free Survival (Median follow-up 73 months, ITT Approach)

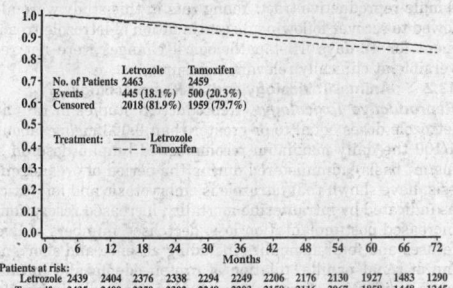

DFS events defined as loco-regional recurrence, distant metastasis, invasive contralateral breast cancer, or death from any cause (i.e., definition excludes second non-breast primary cancers).

The medians of overall survival for both arms were not reached for the Monotherapy Arms Analysis (MAA). There was no statistically significant difference in overall survival.

The hazard ratio for survival in the Femara arm compared to the tamoxifen arm was 0.87, with 95% CI (0.75, 1.02) (see Table 6).

There were no significant differences in DFS, OS, SDFS, and Distant DFS from switch in the Sequential Treatments Analysis with respect to either monotherapy (e.g., [Tamoxifen 2 years followed by] Femara 3 years versus tamoxifen beyond 2 years, DFS HR 0.89; 97.5% CI 0.68, 1.15 and [Femara 2 years followed by] tamoxifen 3 years versus Femara beyond 2 years, DFS HR 0.93; 97.5% CI 0.71, 1.22). There were no significant differences in DFS, OS, SDFS, and Distant DFS from randomization in the Sequential Treatments Analyses.

14.2 Extended Adjuvant Treatment of Early Breast Cancer, Median Treatment Duration of 24 Months
A double-blind, randomized, placebo-controlled trial of Femara was performed in over 5,100 postmenopausal women with receptor-positive or unknown primary breast cancer who were disease free after 5 years of adjuvant treatment with tamoxifen.

The planned duration of treatment for patients in the study was 5 years, but the trial was terminated early because of an interim analysis showing a favorable Femara effect on time without recurrence or contralateral breast cancer. At the time of unblinding, women had been followed for a median of 28 months, 30% of patients had completed 3 or more years of follow-up and less than 1% of patients had completed 5 years of follow-up.

Selected baseline characteristics for the study population are shown in Table 7.

Table 7
Selected Study Population Demographics (Modified ITT Population)

Baseline Status	Femara N=2582	Placebo N=2586
Hormone Receptor Status (%)		
ER+ and/or PgR+	98	98
Both Unknown	2	2
Nodal Status (%)		
Node Negative	50	50
Node Positive	46	46
Nodal Status Unknown	4	4
Chemotherapy	46	46

Table 8 shows the study results. Disease-free survival was measured as the time from randomization to the earliest event of loco-regional or distant recurrence of the primary disease or development of contralateral breast cancer or death. DFS by hormone receptor status, nodal status and adjuvant chemotherapy were similar to the overall results. Data were premature for an analysis of survival.
[See table 8 above]

14.3 Updated Analyses of Extended Adjuvant Treatment of Early Breast Cancer, Median Treatment Duration of 60 Months
[See table 9 above]

Updated analyses were conducted at a median follow-up of 62 months. In the Femara arm, 71% of the patients were treated for at least 3 years and 58% of patients completed at least 4.5 years of extended adjuvant treatment. After the unblinding of the study at a median follow-up of 28 months, approximately 60% of the selected patients in the placebo arm opted to switch to Femara.

In this updated analysis shown in Table 9, Femara significantly reduced the risk of breast cancer recurrence or contralateral breast cancer compared with placebo (HR 0.75; 95% CI 0.63, 0.89; P=0.001). However, in the updated DFS analysis (interval between randomization and earliest event of loco-regional recurrence, distant metastasis, contralateral breast cancer, or death from any cause) the treatment difference was heavily diluted by 60% of the patients in the placebo arm switching to Femara and accounting for 64% of the total placebo patient-years of follow-up. Ignoring these switches, the risk of a DFS event was reduced by a non-significant 11% (HR 0.89; 95% CI 0.77, 1.03). There was no significant difference in distant disease-free survival or overall survival.

14.4 First-Line Treatment of Advanced Breast Cancer
A randomized, double-blind, multinational trial compared Femara 2.5 mg with tamoxifen 20 mg in 916 postmenopausal patients with locally advanced (Stage IIIB or loco-regional recurrence not amenable to treatment with surgery or radiation) or metastatic breast cancer. Time to progression (TTP) was the primary endpoint of the trial. Selected baseline characteristics for this study are shown in Table 10.

Table 10
Selected Study Population Demographics

Baseline Status	Femara N=458	tamoxifen N=458
Stage of Disease		
IIIB	6%	7%
IV	93%	92%
Receptor Status		
ER and PgR Positive	38%	41%
ER or PgR Positive	26%	26%
Both Unknown	34%	33%
ER or PgR/Other Unknown	<1%	0
Previous Antiestrogen Therapy		
Adjuvant	19%	18%
None	81%	82%
Dominant Site of Disease		
Soft Tissue	25%	25%
Bone	32%	29%
Viscera	43%	46%

Femara was superior to tamoxifen in TTP and rate of objective tumor response (*see Table 11*).
Table 11 summarizes the results of the trial, with a total median follow-up of approximately 32 months. (All analyses are unadjusted and use 2-sided *P*-values.)
[See table 11 above]
Figure 2 shows the Kaplan-Meier curves for TTP.

Figure 2
Kaplan-Meier Estimates of Time to Progression (Tamoxifen Study)

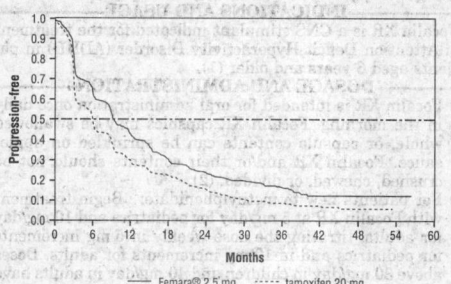

Table 12 shows results in the subgroup of women who had received prior antiestrogen adjuvant therapy, Table 13, results by disease site and Table 14, the results by receptor status.
[See table 12 above]
[See table 13 at right]
[See table 14 at right]
Figure 3 shows the Kaplan-Meier curves for survival.

Figure 3
Survival by Randomized Treatment Arm

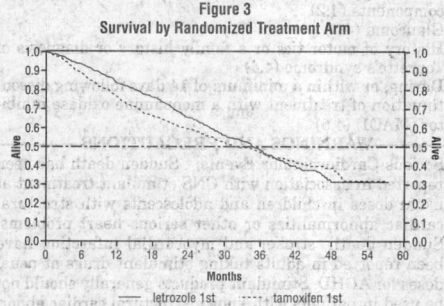

Legend: Randomized Femara: n=458, events 57%, median overall survival 35 months (95% CI 32 to 38 months)
Randomized tamoxifen: n=458, events 57%, median overall survival 32 months (95% CI 28 to 37 months)
Overall logrank *P*=0.5136 (i.e., there was no significant difference between treatment arms in overall survival).
The median overall survival was 35 months for the Femara group and 32 months for the tamoxifen group, with a *P*-value 0.5136. Study design allowed patients to cross over upon progression to the other therapy. Approximately 50% of patients crossed over to the opposite treatment arm and almost all patients who crossed over had done so by 36 months. The median time to crossover was 17 months (Femara to tamoxifen) and 13 months (tamoxifen to Femara). In patients who did not cross over to the opposite treatment arm, median survival was 35 months with Femara (n=219, 95% CI 29 to 43 months) vs 20 months with tamoxifen (n=229, 95% CI 16 to 26 months).

Table 11
Results of First-Line Treatment of Advanced Breast Cancer

	Femara 2.5 mg N=453	tamoxifen 20 mg N=454	Hazard or Odds Ratio (95% CI) *P*-Value (2-Sided)
Median Time to Progression	9.4 months	6.0 months	0.72 (0.62, 0.83)[1] P<0.0001
Objective Response Rate			
(CR + PR)	145 (32%)	95 (21%)	1.77 (1.31, 2.39)[2] P=0.0002
(CR)	42 (9%)	15 (3%)	2.99 (1.63, 5.47)[2] P=0.0004
Duration of Objective Response			
Median	18 months (N=145)	16 months (N=95)	
Overall Survival	35 months (N=458)	32 months (N=458)	P=0.5136[3]

[1] Hazard ratio
[2] Odds ratio
[3] Overall logrank test

Table 12
Efficacy in Patients Who Received Prior Antiestrogen Therapy

Variable	Femara 2.5 mg N=84	tamoxifen 20 mg N=83
Median Time to Progression (95% CI)	8.9 months (6.2, 12.5)	5.9 months (3.2, 6.2)
Hazard Ratio for TTP (95% CI)	0.60 (0.43, 0.84)	
Objective Response Rate		
(CR + PR)	22 (26%)	7 (8%)
Odds Ratio for Response (95% CI)	3.85 (1.50, 9.60)	

Hazard ratio less than 1 or odds ratio greater than 1 favors Femara; hazard ratio greater than 1 or odds ratio less than 1 favors tamoxifen.

Table 13
Efficacy by Disease Site

	Femara 2.5 mg	tamoxifen 20 mg
Dominant Disease Site		
Soft Tissue:	N=113	N=115
Median TTP	12.1 months	6.4 months
Objective Response Rate	50%	34%
Bone:	N=145	N=131
Median TTP	9.5 months	6.3 months
Objective Response Rate	23%	15%
Viscera:	N=195	N=208
Median TTP	8.3 months	4.6 months
Objective Response Rate	28%	17%

Table 14
Efficacy by Receptor Status

Variable	Femara 2.5 mg	tamoxifen 20 mg
Receptor Positive	N=294	N=305
Median Time to Progression (95% CI)	9.4 months (8.9, 11.8)	6.0 months (5.1, 8.5)
Hazard Ratio for TTP (95% CI)	0.69 (0.58, 0.83)	
Objective Response Rate (CR+PR)	97 (33%)	66 (22%)
Odds Ratio for Response (95% CI)	1.78 (1.20, 2.60)	
Receptor Unknown	N=159	N=149
Median Time to Progression (95% CI)	9.2 months (6.1, 12.3)	6.0 months (4.1, 6.4)
Hazard Ratio for TTP (95% CI)	0.77 (0.60, 0.99)	
Objective Response Rate (CR+PR)	48 (30%)	29 (20%)
Odds Ratio for Response (95% CI)	1.79 (1.10, 3.00)	

Hazard ratio less than 1 or odds ratio greater than 1 favors Femara; hazard ratio greater than 1 or odds ratio less than 1 favors tamoxifen.

14.5 Second-Line Treatment of Advanced Breast Cancer
Femara was initially studied at doses of 0.1 mg to 5.0 mg daily in six non-comparative Phase I/II trials in 181 postmenopausal estrogen/progesterone receptor positive or unknown advanced breast cancer patients previously treated with at least antiestrogen therapy. Patients had received other hormonal therapies and also may have received cytotoxic therapy. Eight (20%) of forty patients treated with Femara 2.5 mg daily in Phase I/II trials achieved an objective tumor response (complete or partial response).

Two large randomized, controlled, multinational (predominantly European) trials were conducted in patients with advanced breast cancer who had progressed despite antiestrogen therapy. Patients were randomized to Femara 0.5 mg daily, Femara 2.5 mg daily, or a comparator (megestrol acetate 160 mg daily in one study; and aminoglutethimide 250 mg b.i.d. with corticosteroid supplementation in the other study). In each study over 60% of the patients had received therapeutic antiestrogens, and about one-fifth of these patients had an objective response. The megestrol

Table 16
Megestrol Acetate Study Results

	Femara 0.5 mg N=188	Femara 2.5 mg N=174	megestrol acetate N=190
Objective Response (CR + PR)	22 (11.7%)	41 (23.6%)	31 (16.3%)
Median Duration of Response	552 days	(Not reached)	561 days
Median Time to Progression	154 days	170 days	168 days
Median Survival	633 days	730 days	659 days
Odds Ratio for Response	Femara 2.5: Femara 0.5=2.33 (95% CI: 1.32, 4.17); P=0.004*		Femara 2.5: megestrol=1.58 (95% CI: 0.94, 2.66); P=0.08*
Relative Risk of Progression	Femara 2.5: Femara 0.5=0.81 (95% CI: 0.63, 1.03); P=0.09*		Femara 2.5: megestrol=0.77 (95% CI: 0.60, 0.98); P=0.03*

*two-sided P-value

Table 17
Aminoglutethimide Study Results

	Femara 0.5 mg N=193	Femara 2.5 mg N=185	aminoglutethimide N=179
Objective Response (CR + PR)	34 (17.6%)	34 (18.4%)	22 (12.3%)
Median Duration of Response	619 days	706 days	450 days
Median Time to Progression	103 days	123 days	112 days
Median Survival	636 days	792 days	592 days
Odds Ratio for Response	Femara 2.5: Femara 0.5=1.05 (95% CI: 0.62, 1.79); P=0.85*		Femara 2.5: aminoglutethimide=1.61 (95% CI: 0.90, 2.87); P=0.11*
Relative Risk of Progression	Femara 2.5: Femara 0.5=0.86 (95% CI: 0.68, 1.11); P=0.25*		Femara 2.5: aminoglutethimide=0.74 (95% CI: 0.57, 0.94); P=0.02*

*two-sided P-value

acetate controlled study was double-blind; the other study was open label. Selected baseline characteristics for each study are shown in Table 15.

Table 15
Selected Study Population Demographics

Parameter	megestrol acetate study	aminoglutethimide study
No. of Participants	552	557
Receptor Status		
ER/PR Positive	57%	56%
ER/PR Unknown	43%	44%
Previous Therapy		
Adjuvant Only	33%	38%
Therapeutic +/- Adj.	66%	62%
Sites of Disease		
Soft Tissue	56%	50%
Bone	50%	55%
Viscera	40%	44%

Confirmed objective tumor response (complete response plus partial response) was the primary endpoint of the trials. Responses were measured according to the Union Internationale Contre le Cancer (UICC) criteria and verified by independent, blinded review. All responses were confirmed by a second evaluation 4-12 weeks after the documentation of the initial response.

Table 16 shows the results for the first trial, with a minimum follow-up of 15 months, that compared Femara 0.5 mg, Femara 2.5 mg, and megestrol acetate 160 mg daily. (All analyses are unadjusted.)
[See table 16 above]
The Kaplan-Meier curves for progression for the megestrol acetate study are shown in Figure 4.
[See figure 4 at top of next column]
The results for the study comparing Femara to aminoglutethimide, with a minimum follow-up of 9 months, are shown in Table 17. (Unadjusted analyses are used.)
[See table 17 above]
The Kaplan-Meier curves for progression for the aminoglutethimide study is shown in Figure 5.
[See figure 5 on next column]

16 HOW SUPPLIED/STORAGE AND HANDLING
Packaged in HDPE bottles with a safety screw cap.
2.5 milligram tablets
Bottles of 30 tablets .... NDC 0078-0249-15
Store at 25°C (77°F); excursions permitted to 15-30°C (59-86°F) [see USP Controlled Room Temperature].

Figure 4
Kaplan-Meier Estimates of Time to Progression (Megestrol Acetate Study)

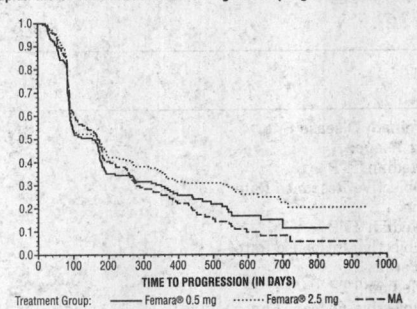

Treatment Group: —— Femara® 0.5 mg ----- Femara® 2.5 mg — — — MA

Figure 5
Kaplan-Meier Estimates of Time to Progression (Aminoglutethimide Study)

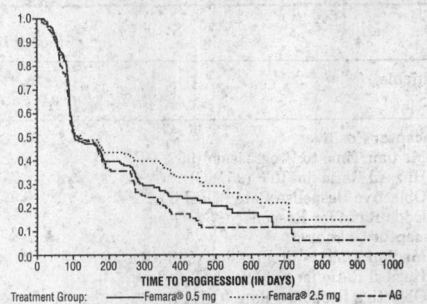

Treatment Group: —— Femara® 0.5 mg ----- Femara® 2.5 mg — — — AG

17 PATIENT COUNSELING INFORMATION
Information for Patients
Pregnancy: Femara is contraindicated in women of premenopausal endocrine status. The physician needs to discuss the necessity of adequate contraception with women who have the potential to become pregnant including women who are perimenopausal or who recently became postmenopausal, until their postmenopausal status is fully established.
Fatigue and Dizziness: Since fatigue and dizziness have been observed with the use of Femara and somnolence was uncommonly reported, caution is advised when driving or using machinery.
Bone Effects: Consideration should be given to monitoring bone mineral density.

T2010-58

Novartis Pharmaceuticals Corporation
East Hanover, New Jersey 07936
©Novartis
Shown in Product Identification Guide, page 315

FOCALIN® XR   C R
[fŏk' ă-lĭn X-R]
(dexmethylphenidate hydrochloride)
Extended-Release Capsules CII for Oral Use

The following prescribing information is based on official labeling in effect July 2010.
HIGHLIGHTS OF PRESCRIBING INFORMATION
These highlights do not include all the information needed to use FOCALIN XR safely and effectively. See full prescribing information for FOCALIN XR.
FOCALIN XR (dexmethylphenidate hydrochloride)
Extended-Release Capsules CII for oral use
Initial U.S. Approval: 2005

WARNING: DRUG DEPENDENCE
See full prescribing information for complete boxed warning
Focalin XR should be given cautiously to patients with a history of drug dependence or alcoholism. Chronic abusive use can lead to marked tolerance and psychological dependence, with varying degrees of abnormal behavior.

RECENT MAJOR CHANGES

Dosage and Administration (2)	10/2009
Dosage and Administration: Patients new to methylphenidate (2.1)	10/2009
Dosage and Administration: Patients currently using methylphenidate (2.1)	10/2009

INDICATIONS AND USAGE
Focalin XR is a CNS stimulant indicated for the treatment of Attention Deficit Hyperactivity Disorder (ADHD) in patients aged 6 years and older (1)

DOSAGE AND ADMINISTRATION
- Focalin XR is intended for oral administration once daily in the morning. Focalin XR capsules may be swallowed whole, or capsule contents can be sprinkled on applesauce. Focalin XR and/or their contents should not be crushed, chewed, or divided. (2)
- For patients new to methylphenidate: Begin treatment with Focalin XR at 5 mg/day for pediatrics and 10 mg/day for adults, titrating the dose weekly in 5 mg increments for pediatrics and in 10 mg increments for adults. Doses above 30 mg/day in children and 40 mg/day in adults have not been studied. (2.1)
- For patients already using methylphenidate: Initiate Focalin XR therapy with half (1/2) the current total daily dose of methylphenidate. (2.2)
- Patients already using Focalin (dexmethylphenidate) immediate release: Switch to the same daily dose of Focalin XR. (2.2)

DOSAGE FORMS AND STRENGTHS
Extended-release capsules: 5, 10, 15, 20, 30, and 40 mg

CONTRAINDICATIONS
- Agitation, marked anxiety, and tension (4.1)
- Known hypersensitivity to methylphenidate or product components (4.2)
- Glaucoma (4.3)
- History of motor tics or a family history or diagnosis of Tourette's syndrome (4.4)
- During, or within a minimum of 14 days following discontinuation of treatment with a monoamine oxidase inhibitor (MAOI) (4.5)

WARNINGS AND PRECAUTIONS
- Serious Cardiovascular Events: Sudden death has been reported in association with CNS stimulant treatment at usual doses in children and adolescents with structural cardiac abnormalities or other serious heart problems. Sudden death, stroke, and myocardial infarction have been reported in adults taking stimulant drugs at usual doses for ADHD. Stimulant products generally should not be used in patients with known structural cardiac abnormalities, cardiomyopathy, serious heart rhythm abnormalities, coronary artery disease, or other serious heart problems. (5.1)
- Increased Blood Pressure and Heart Rate: have been reported. Monitor patients for changes in blood pressure and heart rate. Caution should be exercised in treating patients whose underlying medical conditions might be compromised by increases in blood pressure or heart rate. (5.2)
- Assess Cardiovascular Status: prior to stimulant treatment, assess for cardiac disease with history and exam and, if suggested by findings, conduct further cardiac evaluation. Patients with emerging symptoms suggestive of cardiac disease should undergo a prompt cardiac evaluation. (5.3)
- Psychotic Symptoms: may be exacerbated in patients with psychotic disorders. (5.4)
- Bipolar Disorder: Use with particular care in ADHD patients with comorbid Bipolar Disorder. Before initiating

stimulant therapy, obtain a detailed psychiatric history for patients with comorbid depressive symptoms, in order to determine risk for Bipolar Disorder. (5.5)
- Emergence of New Psychotic or Manic Symptoms: Treatment-emergent psychotic or manic symptoms without a prior history can be caused by stimulants at usual doses. Discontinuation of stimulant therapy may be indicated. (5.6)
- Aggression: Monitor for appearance of or worsening of aggressive behavior or hostility. (5.7)
- Long-Term Suppression of Growth: monitor height and weight in pediatric patients at appropriate intervals. Patients who are not growing or gaining weight as expected may need to have their treatment interrupted. (5.8)
- Seizures: The threshold for seizures may be lowered. In the presence of seizure, discontinue treatment. (5.9)
- Visual Disturbance: difficulties with accommodation and blurring of vision have been reported with stimulant treatment. (5.10)
- Hematologic Monitoring: periodic monitoring of CBC with differential is advised during prolonged therapy. (5.12)

ADVERSE REACTIONS
Most common adverse reactions (at least 5% and twice the incidence among placebo-treated patients) are dyspepsia, decreased appetite, headache, and anxiety for pediatric patients and dry mouth, dyspepsia, headache, and anxiety for adult patients. (6)

To report SUSPECTED ADVERSE REACTIONS, contact Novartis Pharmaceuticals Corporation at 1-888-669-6682 or FDA at 1-800-FDA-1088 or www.fda.gov/medwatch.

DRUG INTERACTIONS
- Focalin XR should not be used in patients being treated (currently or within the preceding two weeks) with MAO Inhibitors (4.5)
- Focalin XR should be used cautiously with pressor agents (7)
- Antacids or acid suppressants could alter the release of Focalin XR (7)
- Racemic methylphenidate may inhibit the metabolism of coumarin anticoagulants, anticonvulsants, and tricyclic drugs (7)
- Serious adverse events have been reported in concomitant use with clonidine, no causality has been established (7)

USE IN SPECIFIC POPULATIONS
- Focalin XR should not be used in **children under 6 years of age**. (5.11)
- Pregnancy: Limited human data. Based on animal data, may cause fetal harm. (8.1)
- Nursing Mothers: Caution should be exercised when administered to a nursing woman. (8.3)

See 17 for PATIENT COUNSELING INFORMATION and Medication Guide

Revised: 08/2010

FULL PRESCRIBING INFORMATION

WARNING: DRUG DEPENDENCE
Focalin XR should be given cautiously to patients with a history of drug dependence or alcoholism. Chronic abusive use can lead to marked tolerance and psychological dependence with varying degrees of abnormal behavior. Frank psychotic episodes can occur, especially with parenteral abuse. Careful supervision is required during withdrawal from abusive use, since severe depression may occur. Withdrawal following chronic therapeutic use may unmask symptoms of the underlying disorder that may require follow-up.

1 INDICATIONS AND USAGE
Focalin XR is indicated for the treatment of Attention Deficit Hyperactivity Disorder (ADHD) in patients aged 6 years and older.
The effectiveness of Focalin XR in the treatment of ADHD in patients aged 6 years and older was established in two placebo-controlled studies in patients meeting DSM-IV criteria for ADHD [see Clinical Studies (14)].
A diagnosis of Attention Deficit Hyperactivity Disorder (ADHD; DSM-IV) implies the presence of hyperactive-impulsive or inattentive symptoms that caused impairment and were present before age 7 years. The symptoms must cause clinically significant impairment, e.g., in social, academic, or occupational functioning, and be present in two or more settings, e.g., school (or work) and at home. The symptoms must not be better accounted for by another mental disorder. For the Inattentive Type, at least six of the following symptoms must have persisted for at least 6 months: lack of attention to details/careless mistakes; lack of sustained attention; poor listener; failure to follow through on tasks; poor organization; avoids tasks requiring sustained mental effort; loses things; easily distracted; forgetful. For the Hyperactive-Impulsive Type, at least six of the following symptoms must have persisted for at least 6 months: fidgeting/squirming; leaving seat; inappropriate running/climbing; difficulty with quiet activities; "on the go"; excessive talking; blurting answers; can't wait turn; intrusive. The Combined Types requires both inattentive and hyperactive-impulsive criteria to be met.
Special Diagnostic Considerations
Specific etiology of this syndrome is unknown, and there is no single diagnostic test. Adequate diagnosis requires the use not only of medical but of special psychological, educational, and social resources. Learning may or may not be impaired. The diagnosis must be based upon a complete history and evaluation of the child and not solely on the presence of the required number of DSM-IV characteristics.
Need for Comprehensive Treatment Program
Focalin XR is indicated as an integral part of a total treatment program for ADHD that may include other measures (psychological, educational, social) for patients with this syndrome. Drug treatment may not be indicated for all children with this syndrome. Stimulants are not intended for use in the child who exhibits symptoms secondary to environmental factors and/or other primary psychiatric disorders, including psychosis. Appropriate educational placement is essential and psychosocial intervention is often helpful. When remedial measures alone are insufficient, the decision to prescribe stimulant medication will depend upon the physician's assessment of the chronicity and severity of the child's symptoms.
Long-Term Use
The effectiveness of Focalin XR for long-term use, i.e., for more than 7 weeks, has not been systematically evaluated in controlled trials. Therefore, the physician who elects to use Focalin XR for extended periods should periodically re-evaluate the long-term usefulness of the drug for the individual patient [see Dosage and Administration (2.3)].

2 DOSAGE AND ADMINISTRATION
Focalin XR is for oral administration once daily in the morning.
Focalin XR may be swallowed as whole capsules or alternatively may be administered by sprinkling the capsule contents on a small amount of applesauce (see specific instructions below). Focalin XR and/or their contents should not be crushed, chewed, or divided.
The capsules may be carefully opened and the beads sprinkled over a spoonful of applesauce. The mixture of drug and applesauce should be consumed immediately in its entirety. The drug and applesauce mixture should not be stored for future use.
Dosage should be individualized according to the needs and responses of the patient.

2.1 Patients New to Methylphenidate
The recommended starting dose of Focalin XR for patients who are not currently taking dexmethylphenidate or racemic methylphenidate, or for patients who are on stimulants other than methylphenidate, is 5 mg/day for pediatric patients and 10 mg/day for adult patients.
Dosage may be adjusted in 5 mg increments for pediatric patients and in 10 mg increments for adult patients. In general, dosage adjustments may proceed at approximately weekly intervals. The patient should be observed for a sufficient duration at a given dose to ensure that a maximal benefit has been achieved before a dose increase is considered. In dose-response (fixed-dose) studies (pediatric from 10 to 30 mg/day and adult from 20 to 40 mg/day), all doses were effective vs. placebo. There was no clear finding, however, of greater average benefits for the higher doses compared to the lower doses. Adverse events and discontinuations, however, were dose-related. Doses above 30 mg/day in pediatrics and 40 mg/day in adults have not been studied and are not recommended.

2.2 Patients Currently Using Methylphenidate
For patients currently using methylphenidate, the recommended starting dose of Focalin XR is half the total daily dose of racemic methylphenidate. Patients currently using Focalin (dexmethylphenidate) may be switched to the same daily dose of Focalin XR.

2.3 Maintenance/Extended Treatment
There is no body of evidence available from controlled trials to indicate how long the patient with ADHD should be treated with Focalin XR. It is generally agreed, however, that pharmacological treatment of ADHD may be needed for extended periods. Nevertheless, the physician who elects to use Focalin XR for extended periods in patients with ADHD should periodically reevaluate the long-term usefulness of the drug for the individual patient with periods off medication to assess the patient's functioning without pharmacotherapy. Improvement may be sustained when the drug is either temporarily or permanently discontinued.

2.4 Dose Reduction and Discontinuation
If paradoxical aggravation of symptoms or other adverse events occur, the dosage should be reduced, or, if necessary, the drug should be discontinued.
If improvement is not observed after appropriate dosage adjustment over a 1-month period, the drug should be discontinued.

3 DOSAGE FORMS AND STRENGTHS
5 mg extended-release capsules
10 mg extended-release capsules
15 mg extended-release capsules
20 mg extended-release capsules
30 mg extended-release capsules
40 mg extended-release capsules

4 CONTRAINDICATIONS
4.1 Agitation
Focalin XR is contraindicated in patients with marked anxiety, tension, and agitation, since the drug may aggravate these symptoms.

4.2 Hypersensitivity to Methylphenidate

Focalin XR is contraindicated in patients known to be hypersensitive to methylphenidate, or other components of the product.

4.3 Glaucoma

Focalin XR is contraindicated in patients with glaucoma.

4.4 Tics

Focalin XR is contraindicated in patients with motor tics or with a family history or diagnosis of Tourette's syndrome [*see Adverse Reactions (6.1)*].

4.5 Monoamine Oxidase Inhibitors

Focalin XR is contraindicated during treatment with monoamine oxidase inhibitors, and also within a minimum of 14 days following discontinuation of treatment with a monoamine oxidase inhibitor (hypertensive crises may result).

5 WARNINGS AND PRECAUTIONS

5.1 Sudden Death and Pre-Existing Structural Cardiac Abnormalities or Other Serious Heart Problems

Children and Adolescents

Sudden death has been reported in association with CNS stimulant treatment at usual doses in children and adolescents with structural cardiac abnormalities or other serious heart problems. Although some serious heart problems alone carry an increased risk of sudden death, stimulant products generally should not be used in children or adolescents with known serious structural cardiac abnormalities, cardiomyopathy, serious heart rhythm abnormalities, or other serious cardiac problems that may place them at increased vulnerability to the sympathomimetic effects of a stimulant drug.

Adults

Sudden death, stroke, and myocardial infarction have been reported in adults taking stimulant drugs at usual doses for ADHD. Although the role of stimulants in these adult cases is also unknown, adults have a greater likelihood than children of having serious structural cardiac abnormalities, cardiomyopathy, serious heart rhythm abnormalities, coronary artery disease, or other serious cardiac problems. Adults with such abnormalities should also generally not be treated with stimulant drugs.

5.2 Hypertension and Other Cardiovascular Conditions

Stimulant medications cause a modest increase in average blood pressure (about 2-4 mmHg) and average heart rate (about 3-6 bpm), and individuals may have larger increases. While the mean changes alone would not be expected to have short-term consequences, all patients should be monitored for larger changes in heart rate and blood pressure. Caution is indicated in treating patients whose underlying medical conditions might be compromised by increases in blood pressure or heart rate, e.g., those with pre-existing hypertension, heart failure, recent myocardial infarction, or ventricular arrhythmia.

5.3 Assessing Cardiovascular Status in Patients being Treated with Stimulant Medications

Children, adolescents, or adults who are being considered for treatment with stimulant medications should have a careful history (including assessment for a family history of sudden death or ventricular arrhythmia) and physical exam to assess for the presence of cardiac disease, and should receive further cardiac evaluation if findings suggest such disease (e.g., electrocardiogram and echocardiogram). Patients who develop symptoms such as exertional chest pain, unexplained syncope, or other symptoms suggestive of cardiac disease during stimulant treatment should undergo a prompt cardiac evaluation.

5.4 Pre-Existing Psychosis

Administration of stimulants may exacerbate symptoms of behavior disturbance and thought disorder in patients with a pre-existing psychotic disorder.

5.5 Bipolar Illness

Particular care should be taken in using stimulants to treat ADHD in patients with comorbid bipolar disorder because of concern for possible induction of a mixed/manic episode in such patients. Prior to initiating treatment with a stimulant, patients with comorbid depressive symptoms should be adequately screened to determine if they are at risk for bipolar disorder; such screening should include a detailed psychiatric history, including a family history of suicide, bipolar disorder, and depression.

5.6 Emergence of New Psychotic or Manic Symptoms

Treatment emergent psychotic or manic symptoms, e.g., hallucinations, delusional thinking, or mania in children and adolescents without a prior history of psychotic illness or mania can be caused by stimulants at usual doses. If such symptoms occur, consideration should be given to a possible causal role of the stimulant, and discontinuation of treatment may be appropriate. In a pooled analysis of multiple short-term, placebo-controlled studies, such symptoms occurred in about 0.1% (4 patients with events out of 3,482 exposed to methylphenidate or amphetamine for several weeks at usual doses) of stimulant-treated patients compared to 0 in placebo-treated patients.

5.7 Aggression

Aggressive behavior or hostility is often observed in children and adolescents with ADHD, and has been reported in clinical trials and the post marketing experience of some medications indicated for the treatment of ADHD. Although there is no systematic evidence that stimulants cause aggressive behavior or hostility, patients beginning treatment for ADHD should be monitored for the appearance of or worsening of aggressive behavior or hostility.

5.8 Long-Term Suppression of Growth

Careful follow-up of weight and height in children ages 7 to 10 years who were randomized to either methylphenidate or non-medication treatment groups over 14 months, as well as in naturalistic subgroups of newly methylphenidate-treated and non-medication treated children over 36 months (to the ages of 10 to 13 years), suggests that consistently medicated children (i.e., treatment for 7 days per week throughout the year) have a temporary slowing in growth rate (on average, a total of about 2 cm less growth in height and 2.7 kg less growth in weight over 3 years), without evidence of growth rebound during this period of development. In the 7-week double-blind placebo-controlled study of Focalin XR, the mean weight gain was greater for patients receiving placebo (+0.4 kg) than for patients receiving Focalin XR (-0.5 kg). Published data are inadequate to determine whether chronic use of amphetamines may cause a similar suppression of growth, however, it is anticipated that they likely have this effect as well. Therefore, growth should be monitored during treatment with stimulants, and patients who are not growing or gaining height or weight as expected may need to have their treatment interrupted.

5.9 Seizures

There is some clinical evidence that stimulants may lower the convulsive threshold in patients with prior history of seizures, in patients with prior EEG abnormalities in absence of seizures, and, very rarely, in patients without a history of seizures and no prior EEG evidence of seizures. In the presence of seizures, the drug should be discontinued.

5.10 Visual Disturbance

Difficulties with accommodation and blurring of vision have been reported with stimulant treatment.

5.11 Use in Children Under Six Years of Age

Focalin XR should not be used in children under 6 years of age, since safety and efficacy in this age group have not been established.

5.12 Hematologic Monitoring

Periodic CBC, differential, and platelet counts are advised during prolonged therapy.

6 ADVERSE REACTIONS

Focalin XR was administered to 46 children and 7 adolescents with ADHD for up to 7 weeks and 206 adults with ADHD in clinical studies. During the clinical studies, 101 adult patients were treated for at least 6 months.

Adverse events during exposure were obtained primarily by general inquiry and recorded by clinical investigators using terminology of their own choosing. Consequently, it is not possible to provide a meaningful estimate of the proportion of individuals experiencing adverse events without first grouping similar types of events into a smaller number of standardized event categories. In the tables and listings that follow, MedDRA terminology has been used to classify reported adverse events. The stated frequencies of adverse events represent the proportion of individuals who experienced, at least once, a treatment-emergent adverse event of the type listed. An event was considered treatment emergent if it occurred for the first time or worsened while receiving therapy following baseline evaluation.

6.1 Adverse Events Associated with Discontinuation of Treatment in Acute Clinical Studies with Focalin XR - Children

Overall, 50 of 684 children treated with Focalin immediate-release formulation (7.3%) experienced an adverse event that resulted in discontinuation. The most common reasons for discontinuation were twitching (described as motor or vocal tics), anorexia, insomnia, and tachycardia (approximately 1% each). None of the 53 Focalin XR-treated pediatric patients discontinued treatment due to adverse events in the 7-week placebo-controlled study.

6.2 Adverse Events Occurring at an Incidence of 5% or More Among Focalin XR-Treated Treated Patients - Children

Table 1 enumerates treatment-emergent adverse events for the placebo-controlled, parallel-group study in children and adolescents with ADHD at flexible Focalin XR doses of 5-30 mg/day. The table includes only those events that occurred in 5% or more of patients treated with Focalin XR and for which the incidence in patients treated with Focalin XR was at least twice the incidence in placebo-treated patients. The prescriber should be aware that these figures cannot be used to predict the incidence of adverse events in the course of usual medical practice where patient characteristics and other factors differ from those which prevailed in the clinical trials. Similarly, the cited frequencies cannot be compared with figures obtained from other clinical investigations involving different treatments, uses, and investigators. The cited figures, however, do provide the prescribing physician with some basis for estimating the relative contribution of drug and non-drug factors to the adverse event incidence rate in the population studied.

Table 1. Treatment-Emergent Adverse Events[1] Occurring During Double-Blind Treatment – Pediatric Patients

	Focalin XR N=53	Placebo N=47
No. of Patients with AEs		
Total	76%	57%
Primary System Organ Class/ Adverse Event Preferred Term		
Gastrointestinal Disorders	38%	19%
Dyspepsia	8%	4%
Metabolism and Nutrition Disorders	34%	11%
Decreased Appetite	30%	9%
Nervous System Disorders	30%	13%
Headache	25%	11%
Psychiatric Disorders	26%	15%
Anxiety	6%	0%

[1] Events, regardless of causality, for which the incidence for patients treated with Focalin XR was at least 5% and twice the incidence among placebo-treated patients. Incidence has been rounded to the nearest whole number.

Table 2 below enumerates the incidence of dose-related adverse events that occurred during a fixed-dose, double-blind, placebo controlled trial of Focalin XR up to 30 mg/day versus placebo in children and adolescents with ADHD.

[See table 2 at left]

Table 2. Dose-related Adverse Events from a Fixed-dose Study of Double-Blind Treatment in Pediatric Patients By Organ-System and Preferred Term

ADVERSE EVENT	Focalin XR 10 mg/d N=64	Focalin XR 20 mg/d N=60	Focalin XR 30 mg/d N=58	Placebo N=63
Gastrointestinal Disorders	22%	23%	29%	24%
Vomiting	2%	8%	9%	0
Metabolism and Nutritional Disorders	16%	17%	22%	5%
Anorexia	5%	5%	7%	0
Psychiatric Disorders	19%	20%	38%	8%
Insomnia	5%	8%	17%	3%
Depression	0	0	3%	0
Mood Swings	0	0	3%	2%
Other Adverse Events				
Irritability	0	2%	5%	0
Nasal Congestion	0	0	5%	0
Pruritus	0	0	3%	0

6.3 Adverse Events Associated with Discontinuation of Treatment in Clinical Studies with Focalin XR - Adults

In the adult placebo-controlled study, 10.7% of the Focalin XR-treated patients and 7.5% of the placebo-treated patients discontinued for adverse events. Among Focalin XR-treated patients, insomnia (1.8%, n=3), feeling jittery (1.8%, n=3), anorexia (1.2%, n=2), and anxiety (1.2%, n=2) were the reasons for discontinuation reported by more than 1 patient.

6.4 Adverse Events Occurring at an Incidence of 5% or More Among Focalin XR-Treated Patients - Adults

Table 3 enumerates treatment-emergent adverse events for the placebo-controlled, parallel-group study in adults with ADHD at fixed Focalin XR doses of 20, 30, and 40 mg/day. The table includes only those events that occurred in 5% or more of patients in a Focalin XR dose group and for which the incidences in patients treated with Focalin XR appeared to increase with dose. The prescriber should be aware that these figures cannot be used to predict the incidence of adverse events in the course of usual medical practice where patient characteristics and other factors differ from those which prevailed in the clinical trials. Similarly, the cited frequencies cannot be compared with figures obtained from other clinical investigations involving different treatments, uses, and investigators. The cited figures, however, do provide the prescribing physician with some basis for estimating the relative contribution of drug and non-drug factors to the adverse event incidence rate in the population studied. [See table 3 at right]

Two other adverse reactions occurring in clinical trials with Focalin XR at a frequency greater than placebo, but which were not dose related were: Feeling jittery (12% and 2%, respectively) and Dizziness (6% and 2%, respectively).

Table 4 summarizes changes in vital signs and weight that were recorded in the adult study (N=218) of Focalin XR in the treatment of ADHD.

[See table 4 at right]

6.5 Adverse Events with Other Methylphenidate HCl Dosage Forms

Nervousness and insomnia are the most common adverse reactions reported with other methylphenidate products. In children, loss of appetite, abdominal pain, weight loss during prolonged therapy, insomnia, and tachycardia may occur more frequently; however, any of the other adverse reactions listed below may also occur.

Other reactions include:

Cardiac: angina, arrhythmia, palpitations, pulse increased or decreased, tachycardia

Gastrointestinal: abdominal pain, nausea

Immune: hypersensitivity reactions including skin rash, urticaria, fever, arthralgia, exfoliative dermatitis, erythema multiforme with histopathological findings of necrotizing vasculitis, and thrombocytopenic purpura

Metabolism/Nutrition: anorexia, weight loss during prolonged therapy

Nervous System: dizziness, drowsiness, dyskinesia, headache, rare reports of Tourette's syndrome, toxic psychosis

Vascular: blood pressure increased or decreased, cerebral arteritis and/or occlusion

Although a definite causal relationship has not been established, the following have been reported in patients taking methylphenidate:

Blood/Lymphatic: leukopenia and/or anemia

Hepatobiliary: abnormal liver function, ranging from transaminase elevation to hepatic coma

Psychiatric: transient depressed mood, aggressive behavior

Skin/Subcutaneous: scalp hair loss

Very rare reports of neuroleptic malignant syndrome (NMS) have been received, and, in most of these, patients were concurrently receiving therapies associated with NMS. In a single report, a ten-year-old boy who had been taking methylphenidate for approximately 18 months experienced an NMS-like event within 45 minutes of ingesting his first dose of venlafaxine. It is uncertain whether this case represented a drug-drug interaction, a response to either drug alone, or some other cause.

7 DRUG INTERACTIONS

Focalin XR should not be used in patients being treated (currently or within the preceding two weeks) with MAO Inhibitors [see *Contraindications (4.5)*].

Because of possible effects on blood pressure, Focalin XR should be used cautiously with pressor agents.

Methylphenidate may decrease the effectiveness of drugs used to treat hypertension.

Dexmethylphenidate is metabolized primarily to *d*-ritalinic acid by de-esterification and not through oxidative pathways.

The effects of gastrointestinal pH alterations on the absorption of dexmethylphenidate from Focalin XR have not been studied. Since the modified release characteristics of Focalin XR are pH dependent, the coadministration of antacids or acid suppressants could alter the release of dexmethylphenidate.

Human pharmacologic studies have shown that racemic methylphenidate may inhibit the metabolism of coumarin anticoagulants, anticonvulsants (e.g., phenobarbital, phenytoin, primidone), and tricyclic drugs (e.g., imipramine, clomipramine, desipramine). Downward dose adjustments of these drugs may be required when given concomitantly with methylphenidate. It may be necessary to adjust the dosage and monitor plasma drug concentration (or, in the case of coumarin, coagulation times), when initiating or discontinuing methylphenidate.

Serious adverse events have been reported in concomitant use with clonidine, although no causality for the combination has been established. The safety of using methylphenidate in combination with clonidine or other centrally-acting alpha-2-agonists has not been systematically evaluated.

8 USE IN SPECIFIC POPULATIONS

8.1 Pregnancy

Pregnancy Category C:

There are no adequate and well controlled studies of Focalin in pregnant women. Dexmethylphenidate did not cause major malformations in rats or rabbits; however, it did cause delayed skeletal ossification and decreased postweaning weight gain in rats. Focalin XR should be used during pregnancy only if the potential benefit justifies the potential risk to the fetus.

In studies conducted in rats and rabbits, dexmethylphenidate was administered orally at doses of up to 20 and 100 mg/kg/day, respectively, during the period of organogenesis. No evidence of teratogenic activity was found in either the rat or rabbit study; however, delayed fetal skeletal ossification was observed at the highest dose level in rats. When dexmethylphenidate was administered to rats throughout pregnancy and lactation at doses of up to 20 mg/kg/day, postweaning body weight gain was decreased in male offspring at the highest dose, but no other effects on postnatal development were observed. At the highest doses tested, plasma levels (AUCs) of dexmethylphenidate in pregnant rats and rabbits were approximately 5 and 1 times, respectively, those in adults dosed with 20 mg/day. Racemic methylphenidate has been shown to have teratogenic effects in rabbits when given in doses of 200 mg/kg/day throughout organogenesis.

8.2 Labor and Delivery

Focalin XR has not been studied in labor and delivery.

8.3 Nursing Mothers

It is not known whether dexmethylphenidate is excreted in human milk. Because many drugs are excreted in human milk, caution should be exercised if Focalin XR is administered to a nursing woman. Information from 4 published case reports on the use of racemic methylphenidate during breastfeeding suggest that at maternal doses of 35-80 mg/day, milk concentrations of methylphenidate range from undetectable to 15.4 ng/mL. Based on these limited data, the calculated infant daily dose for an exclusively breastfed infant would be about 0.4-2.9 µg/kg/day or about 0.2-0.7% of the maternal weight adjusted dose.

8.4 Pediatric Use

The safety and efficacy of Focalin XR in children under 6 years old have not been established. Long-term effects of Focalin in children have not been well established [see *Warnings and Precautions (5.11)*].

In a study conducted in young rats, racemic methylphenidate was administered orally at doses of up to 100 mg/kg/day for 9 weeks, starting early in the postnatal period (Postnatal Day 7) and continuing through sexual maturity (Postnatal Week 10). When these animals were tested as adults (Postnatal Weeks 13-14), decreased spontaneous locomotor activity was observed in males and females previously treated with 50 mg/kg/day (approximately 6 times the maximum recommended human dose [MRHD] of racemic methylphenidate on a mg/m² basis) or greater, and a deficit in the acquisition of a specific learning task was seen in females exposed to the highest dose (12 times the racemic MRHD on a mg/m² basis). The no effect level for juvenile neurobehavioral development in rats was 5 mg/kg/day (half the racemic MRHD on a mg/m² basis). The clinical significance of the long-term behavioral effects observed in rats is unknown.

8.5 Geriatric Use

Focalin XR has not been studied in the geriatric population.

9 DRUG ABUSE AND DEPENDENCE

9.1 Controlled Substance Class

Focalin XR, like other methylphenidate products, is classified as a Schedule II controlled substance by Federal regulation.

9.2 Abuse, Dependence, Tolerance

See complete boxed warning for drug abuse and dependence information at the beginning of *Full Prescribing Information.*

10 OVERDOSAGE

10.1 Signs and Symptoms

Signs and symptoms of acute methylphenidate overdosage, resulting principally from overstimulation of the CNS and from excessive sympathomimetic effects, may include the following: vomiting, agitation, tremors, hyperreflexia, muscle twitching, convulsions (may be followed by coma), euphoria, confusion, hallucinations, delirium, sweating, flushing, headache, hyperpyrexia, tachycardia, palpitations, cardiac arrhythmias, hypertension, mydriasis, and dryness of mucous membranes.

10.2 Poison Control Center

The physician may wish to consider contacting a poison control center for up-to-date information on the management of overdosage with methylphenidate.

10.3 Recommended Treatment

As with the management of all overdosage, the possibility of multiple drug ingestion should be considered.

When treating overdose, practitioners should bear in mind that there is a prolonged release of dexmethylphenidate from Focalin XR.

Treatment consists of appropriate supportive measures. The patient must be protected against self-injury and against external stimuli that would aggravate overstimulation already present. Gastric contents may be evacuated by gastric lavage as indicated. Before performing gastric lavage, control agitation and seizures if present and protect the airway. Other measures to detoxify the gut include administration of activated charcoal and a cathartic. Intensive care must be provided to maintain adequate circulation and respiratory exchange; external cooling procedures may be required for hyperpyrexia.

Efficacy of peritoneal dialysis for Focalin overdosage has not been established.

11 DESCRIPTION

Focalin XR is an extended-release formulation of dexmethylphenidate with a bi-modal release profile.

Table 3. Treatment-Emergent Adverse Events[1] Occurring During Double-Blind Treatment – Adults

	Focalin XR 20 mg N=57	Focalin XR 30 mg N=54	Focalin XR 40 mg N=54	Placebo N=53
No. of Patients with AEs				
Total	84%	94%	85%	68%
Primary System Organ Class/ Adverse Event Preferred Term				
Gastrointestinal Disorders	28%	32%	44%	19%
Dry Mouth	7%	20%	20%	4%
Dyspepsia	5%	9%	9%	2%
Nervous System Disorders	37%	39%	50%	28%
Headache	26%	30%	39%	19%
Psychiatric Disorders	40%	43%	46%	30%
Anxiety	5%	11%	11%	2%
Respiratory, Thoracic and Mediastinal Disorders	16%	9%	15%	8%
Pharyngolaryngeal Pain	4%	4%	7%	2%

[1] Events, regardless of causality, for which the incidence was at least 5% in a Focalin XR group and which appeared to increase with randomized dose. Incidence has been rounded to the nearest whole number.

Table 4. Changes (Mean ± SD) in Vital Signs and Weight by Randomized Dose During Double-Blind Treatment – Adults

	Focalin XR 20 mg (N=57)	Focalin XR 30 mg (N=54)	Focalin XR 40 mg (N=54)	Placebo (N=53)
Pulse (bpm)	3.1 ± 11.1	4.3 ± 11.7	6.0 ± 10.1	-1.4 ± 9.3
Diastolic BP (mmHg)	-0.2 ± 8.2	1.2 ± 8.9	2.1 ± 8.0	0.3 ± 7.8
Weight (kg)	-1.4 ± 2.0	-1.2 ± 1.9	-1.7 ± 2.3	-0.1 ± 3.9

Focalin XR uses the proprietary SODAS (Spheroidal Oral Drug Absorption System) technology. Each bead-filled Focalin XR capsule contains half the dose as immediate-release beads and half as enteric-coated, delayed-release beads, thus providing an immediate release of dexmethylphenidate and a second delayed release of dexmethylphenidate. Focalin XR is available as 5, 10, 15, 20, 30, and 40 mg extended-release capsules. Focalin XR 5, 10, 15, 20, 30, and 40 mg extended-release capsules provide in a single dose the same amount of dexmethylphenidate as dosages of 2.5, 5, 7.5, 10, 15 or 20 mg of Focalin given b.i.d. as tablets.

Dexmethylphenidate hydrochloride, the *d-threo* enantiomer of racemic methylphenidate hydrochloride, is a central nervous system (CNS) stimulant.

Dexmethylphenidate hydrochloride is methyl α-phenyl-2-piperidineacetate hydrochloride, (R,R′)-(+)-. Its empirical formula is $C_{14}H_{19}NO_2 \cdot HCl$. Its molecular weight is 269.77 and its structural formula is

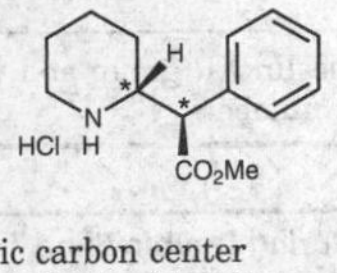

Note* = asymmetric carbon center

Dexmethylphenidate hydrochloride is a white to off white powder. Its solutions are acid to litmus. It is freely soluble in water and in methanol, soluble in alcohol, and slightly soluble in chloroform and in acetone.

Inactive ingredients: ammonio methacrylate copolymer, FD&C Blue #2 (5 mg, 15 mg and 40 mg strengths), FDA/E172 yellow iron oxide (10 mg, 15 mg, 30 mg, and 40 mg strengths), gelatin, ink Tan SW-8010, methacrylic acid copolymer, polyethylene glycol, sugar spheres, talc, titanium dioxide, and triethyl citrate.

12 CLINICAL PHARMACOLOGY

12.1 Mechanism of Action

Dexmethylphenidate hydrochloride, the active ingredient in Focalin XR, is a central nervous system stimulant. Dexmethylphenidate, the more pharmacologically active *d*-enantiomer of racemic methylphenidate, is thought to block the reuptake of norepinephrine and dopamine into the presynaptic neuron and increase the release of these monoamines into the extraneuronal space. The mode of therapeutic action in Attention Deficit Hyperactivity Disorder (ADHD) is not known.

12.2 Pharmacodynamics

Effects on QT Interval

The effect of Focalin® XR on the QT interval was evaluated in a double-blind, placebo- and open label active (moxifloxacin)-controlled study following single doses of Focalin® XR 40 mg in 75 healthy volunteers. ECGs were collected up to 12 h post-dose. Frederica's method for heart rate correction was employed to derive the corrected QT interval (QTcF). The maximum mean prolongation of QTcF intervals was <5 ms, and the upper limit of the 90% confidence interval was below 10 ms for all time matched comparisons versus placebo. This was below the threshold of clinical concern and there was no evident-exposure response relationship.

12.3 Pharmacokinetics

Absorption

Focalin XR produces a bi-modal plasma concentration-time profile (i.e., two distinct peaks approximately 4 hours apart) when orally administered to healthy adults. The initial rate of absorption for Focalin XR is similar to that of Focalin tablets as shown by the similar rate parameters between the two formulations, i.e., first peak concentration (C_{max1}), and time to the first peak (t_{max1}), which is reached in 1½ hours (typical range 1-4 hours). The mean time to the interpeak minimum (t_{minip}) is slightly shorter, and time to the second peak (t_{max2}) is slightly longer for Focalin XR given once daily (about 6.5 hours, range 4.5-7 hours) compared to Focalin tablets given in two doses 4 hours apart *(see Figure 1)*, although the ranges observed are greater for Focalin XR.

Focalin XR given once daily exhibits a lower second peak concentration (C_{max2}), higher interpeak minimum concentrations (C_{minip}), and less peak and trough fluctuations than Focalin tablets given in two doses given 4 hours apart. This is due to an earlier onset and more prolonged absorption from the delayed-release beads *(see Figure 1)*.

The AUC (exposure) after administration of Focalin XR given once daily is equivalent to the same total dose of Focalin tablets given in two doses 4 hours apart. The variability in C_{max}, C_{min}, and AUC is similar between Focalin XR and Focalin IR with approximately a three-fold range in each.

Radiolabeled racemic methylphenidate is well absorbed after oral administration with approximately 90% of the radioactivity recovered in urine. However, due to first pass metabolism the mean absolute bioavailability of dexmethylphenidate when administered in various formulations was 22-25%.

Figure 1. Mean Dexmethylphenidate Plasma Concentration-Time Profiles After Administration of 1 x 20 mg Focalin XR (n=24) Capsules and 2 x 10 mg Focalin Immediate-Release Tablets (n=25)

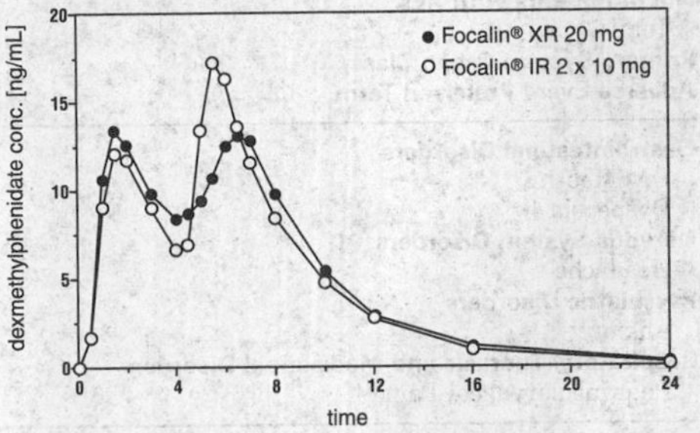

Dose Proportionality

Dose proportionality of Focalin XR was evaluated in a randomized, single-dose, five-period, cross-over study with administration of single doses of 5, 10, 20, 30 and 40 mg to healthy adults. Results confirmed dose proportionality within this dose range.

Food Effects

Administration times relative to meals and meal composition may need to be individually titrated.

No food effect study was performed with Focalin XR. However, the effect of food has been studied in adults with racemic methylphenidate in the same type of extended-release formulation. The findings of that study are considered applicable to Focalin XR. After a high fat breakfast, there was a longer lag time until absorption began and variable delays in the time until the first peak concentration, the time until the interpeak minimum, and the time until the second peak. The first peak concentration and the extent of absorption were unchanged after food relative to the fasting state, although the second peak was approximately 25% lower. The effect of a high fat lunch was not examined. There is no evidence of dose dumping in the presence or absence of food. There were no differences in the plasma concentration-time profile, when administered with applesauce, compared to administration in the fasting condition. The results are expected not to differ for Focalin XR.

For patients unable to swallow the capsule, the contents may be sprinkled on applesauce and administered [*see Dosage and Administration (2)*].

Distribution

The plasma protein binding of dexmethylphenidate is not known; racemic methylphenidate is bound to plasma proteins by 12-15%, independent of concentration. Dexmethylphenidate shows a volume of distribution of 2.65±1.11 L/kg. Plasma dexmethylphenidate concentrations decline monophasically following oral administration of Focalin XR.

Metabolism and Excretion

In humans, dexmethylphenidate is metabolized primarily to *d*-α-phenyl-piperidine acetic acid (also known as *d*-ritalinic acid) by de-esterification. This metabolite has little or no pharmacological activity. There is no *in vivo* interconversion to the *l-threo*-enantiomer, based on a finding of no levels of *l-threo*-methylphenidate being detectable after administration of up to 40 mg dexmethylphenidate in adults. After oral dosing of radiolabeled racemic methylphenidate in humans, about 90% of the radioactivity was recovered in urine. The main urinary metabolite of racemic (*d,l*-) methylphenidate was *d,l*-ritalinic acid, accountable for approximately 80% of the dose. Urinary excretion of parent compound accounted for 0.5% of an intravenous dose.

In vitro studies showed that dexmethylphenidate did not inhibit cytochrome P450 isoenzymes at concentrations observed after therapeutic doses.

Intravenous dexmethylphenidate was eliminated with a mean clearance of 0.40±0.12 $L/kg.h^{-1}$ corresponding to 0.56±0.18 L/min. The mean terminal elimination half-life of dexmethylphenidate was just over 3 hours in healthy adults and typically varied between 2 and 4.5 hours with an occasional subject exhibiting a terminal half-life between 5 and 7 hours. Children tend to have slightly shorter half-lives with means of 2-3 hours.

Special Populations

Gender

After administration of Focalin XR the first peak, (C_{max1}), was on average 45% higher in women. The interpeak minimum and the second peak also tended to be slightly higher in women although the difference was not statistically significant, and these patterns remained even after weight normalization. Pharmacokinetic parameters for dexmethylphenidate after Focalin immediate-release tablets were similar for boys and girls.

Race

There is insufficient experience with the use of Focalin XR to detect ethnic variations in pharmacokinetics.

Age

The pharmacokinetics of dexmethylphenidate after Focalin XR administration have not been studied in children less than 18 years of age. When a similar formulation of racemic methylphenidate was examined in 15 children between 10 and 12 years of age and 3 children with ADHD between 7 and 9 years of age, the time to the first peak was similar, although the time until the between peak minimum, and the time until the second peak were delayed and more variable in children compared to adults. After administration of the same dose to children and adults, concentrations in children were approximately twice the concentrations observed in adults. This higher exposure is almost completely due to smaller body size as no relevant age-related differences in dexmethylphenidate pharmacokinetic parameters (i.e., clearance and volume of distribution) are observed after normalization to dose and weight.

Renal Insufficiency

There is no experience with the use of Focalin XR in patients with renal insufficiency. After oral administration of radiolabeled racemic methylphenidate in humans, methylphenidate was extensively metabolized and approximately 80% of the radioactivity was excreted in the urine in the form of racemic ritalinic acid which is pharmacologically inactive. Very little unchanged drug is excreted in the urine, thus renal insufficiency is expected to have little effect on the pharmacokinetics of Focalin XR.

Hepatic Insufficiency

There is no experience with the use of Focalin XR in patients with hepatic insufficiency [*see Drug Interactions (7)*].

13 NONCLINICAL TOXICOLOGY

13.1 Carcinogenesis, Mutagenesis, and Impairment of Fertility

Carcinogenesis

Lifetime carcinogenicity studies have not been carried out with dexmethylphenidate. In a lifetime carcinogenicity study carried out in B6C3F1 mice, racemic methylphenidate caused an increase in hepatocellular adenomas, and in males only, an increase in hepatoblastomas at a daily dose of approximately 60 mg/kg/day. Hepatoblastoma is a relatively rare rodent malignant tumor type. There was no increase in total malignant hepatic tumors. The mouse strain used is sensitive to the development of hepatic tumors, and the significance of these results to humans is unknown.

Racemic methylphenidate did not cause any increase in tumors in a lifetime carcinogenicity study carried out in F344 rats; the highest dose used was approximately 45 mg/kg/day.

In a 24-week study of racemic methylphenidate in the transgenic mouse strain p53+/-, which is sensitive to genotoxic carcinogens, there was no evidence of carcinogenicity. Mice were fed diets containing the same concentrations as in the lifetime carcinogenicity study; the high-dose group was exposed to 60-74 mg/kg/day of racemic methylphenidate.

Mutagenesis

Dexmethylphenidate was not mutagenic in the *in vitro* Ames reverse mutation assay, the *in vitro* mouse lymphoma cell forward mutation assay, or the *in vivo* mouse bone marrow micronucleus test.

Racemic methylphenidate was not mutagenic in the *in vitro* Ames reverse mutation assay or the *in vitro* mouse lymphoma cell forward mutation assay, and was negative *in vivo* in the mouse bone marrow micronucleus assay. However, sister chromatid exchanges and chromosome aberrations were increased, indicative of a weak clastogenic response, in an *in vitro* assay of racemic methylphenidate in cultured Chinese Hamster Ovary (CHO) cells.

Impairment of Fertility

Racemic methylphenidate did not impair fertility in male or female mice that were fed diets containing the drug in an 18-week Continuous Breeding study. The study was conducted at doses of up to 160 mg/kg/day.

14 CLINICAL STUDIES

The effectiveness of Focalin XR in the treatment of ADHD was established in randomized, double-blind, placebo-controlled studies in children and adolescents and in adults who met Diagnostic and Statistical Manual 4th edition (DSM-IV) criteria for ADHD [*see Indications and Usage (1)*].

14.1 Children and Adolescents

The effectiveness of Focalin XR was established in a randomized, double-blind, placebo-controlled, parallel-group study in 103 pediatric patients (ages 6 to 12, n=86; ages 13 to 17, n=17) who met DSM-IV criteria for ADHD. Patients were randomized to receive either a flexible dose of Focalin XR (5 to 30 mg/day) or placebo once daily for 7 weeks. During the first 5 weeks of treatment patients were titrated to their optimal dose and in the last 2 weeks of the study patients remained on their optimal dose without dose changes or interruption.

Signs and symptoms of ADHD were evaluated by comparing the mean change from baseline to endpoint for Focalin XR- and placebo-treated patients using an intent-to-treat analysis of the primary efficacy outcome measure, the DSM-IV total subscale score of the Conners ADHD/DSM-IV Scales for Teachers (CADS-T).

There was a statistically significant treatment effect in favor of Focalin XR. There were insufficient adolescents enrolled in this study to assess the efficacy for Focalin XR in the adolescent population. However, pharmacokinetic considerations and evidence of effectiveness of immediate-release Focalin in adolescents support the effectiveness of Focalin XR in this population.

In two additional studies in pediatric patients aged 6-12 years who received 20 mg Focalin XR or placebo in a cross-over design, Focalin XR was found to have a statistically significant treatment effect versus placebo on the Swanson, Kotkin, Agler, M-Flynn & Pelham (SKAMP) rating scale combined score at all time points after dosing in each study (0.5, 1, 3, 4, 5, 7, 9, 10, 11 and 12 hours in one study and 1, 2, 4, 6, 8, 9, 10, 11 and 12 hours in the other study). A treatment effect was also observed 0.5 hours after administration of Focalin XR 20 mg in an additional study of ADHD patients aged 6-12 years. The SKAMP is a reliable and validated scale that assesses specific classroom behaviors related to attention (e.g., getting started, sticking with activities, completing work, and stopping for transition) and deportment or behavior (e.g., remaining quiet, remaining seated, interacting with other students, and interacting with the teacher). Each item is rated on a 7-point impairment scale, and an average rating per item is calculated for the subscales of Attention and Deportment.

14.2 Adults

The effectiveness of Focalin XR was established in a randomized, double-blind, placebo-controlled, parallel-group study in 221 adult patients (ages 18 to 60) who met DSM-IV criteria for ADHD. Patients were randomized to receive either a fixed dose of Focalin XR (20, 30, or 40 mg/day) or placebo once daily for 5 weeks. Patients randomized to Focalin XR were initiated on a 10 mg/day starting dose and titrated in increments of 10 mg/week to the randomly assigned fixed dose. Patients were maintained on their fixed dose (20, 30 or 40 mg/day) for a minimum of 2 weeks.

Signs and symptoms of ADHD were evaluated by comparing the mean change from baseline to endpoint for Focalin XR- and placebo-treated patients using an intent-to-treat analysis of the primary efficacy outcome measure, the investigator-administered DSM-IV Attention-Deficit/Hyperactivity Disorder Rating Scale (DSM-IV ADHD RS). All three Focalin XR doses were statistically significantly superior to placebo. There was no obvious increase in effectiveness with increasing dose.

15 REFERENCES

American Psychiatric Association. Diagnosis and Statistical Manual of Mental Disorders. 4th ed. Washington DC: American Psychiatric Association 1994.

16 HOW SUPPLIED/STORAGE AND HANDLING

5 mg Extended-Release Capsules (NDC 0078-0430-05) light-blue, (imprinted NVR D5) supplied in bottles of 100

10 mg Extended-Release Capsules (NDC 0078-0431-05) light caramel (imprinted NVR D10) supplied in bottles of 100

15 mg Extended-Release Capsules (NDC 0078-0493-05) green (imprinted NVR D15) supplied in bottles of 100

20 mg Extended-Release Capsules (NDC 0078-0432-05) white (imprinted NVR D20) supplied in bottles of 100

30 mg Extended-Release Capsules (NDC 0078-0433-05) light caramel and white (imprinted NVR D30) supplied in bottles of 100

40 mg Extended-Release Capsules (NDC 0078-0434-05) green and white (imprinted NVR D40) supplied in bottles of 100

Store Focalin XR at 25°C (77°F), excursions permitted 15°-30°C (59°-86°F).

[See USP Controlled Room Temperature.]

Dispense in tight container (USP).

17 PATIENT COUNSELING INFORMATION

INFORMATION FOR PATIENTS

Prescribers or other health professionals should inform patients, their families, and their caregivers about the benefits and risks associated with treatment with dexmethylphenidate and should counsel them in its appropriate use. A patient Medication Guide is available for Focalin XR. The prescriber or health professional should instruct patients, their families, and their caregivers to read the Medication Guide and should assist them in understanding its contents. Patients should be given the opportunity to discuss the contents of the Medication Guide and to obtain answers to any questions they may have. The complete text of the Medication Guide is reprinted at the end of this document.

MEDICATION GUIDE
FOCALIN XR
(dexmethylphenidate hydrochloride)
extended-release capsules CII

Read the Medication Guide that comes with FOCALIN XR before you or your child starts taking it and each time you get a refill. There may be new information. This Medication Guide does not take the place of talking to your doctor about your or your child's treatment with FOCALIN XR.

What is the most important information I should know about FOCALIN XR?

The following have been reported with use of dexmethylphenidate hydrochloride and other stimulant medicines.

1. Heart-related problems:

- **sudden death in patients who have heart problems or heart defects**
- **stroke and heart attack in adults**
- **increased blood pressure and heart rate**

Tell your doctor if you or your child have any heart problems, heart defects, high blood pressure, or a family history of these problems.

Your doctor should check you or your child carefully for heart problems before starting FOCALIN XR.

Your doctor should check your or your child's blood pressure and heart rate regularly during treatment with FOCALIN XR.

Call your doctor right away if you or your child has any signs of heart problems such as chest pain, shortness of breath, or fainting while taking FOCALIN XR.

2. Mental (Psychiatric) problems:

All Patients

- **new or worse behavior and thought problems**
- **new or worse bipolar illness**
- **new or worse aggressive behavior or hostility**

Children and Teenagers

- **new psychotic symptoms (such as hearing voices, believing things that are not true, are suspicious) or new manic symptoms**

Tell your doctor about any mental problems you or your child have, or about a family history of suicide, bipolar illness, or depression.

Call your doctor right away if you or your child have any new or worsening mental symptoms or problems while taking FOCALIN XR, especially seeing or hearing things that are not real, believing things that are not real, or are suspicious.

What Is FOCALIN XR?

FOCALIN XR is a central nervous system stimulant prescription medicine. **It is used for the treatment of attention deficit and hyperactivity disorder (ADHD).** FOCALIN XR may help increase attention and decrease impulsiveness and hyperactivity in patients with ADHD.

FOCALIN XR should be used as a part of a total treatment program for ADHD that may include counseling or other therapies.

FOCALIN XR is a federally controlled substance (CII) because it can be abused or lead to dependence. Keep FOCALIN XR in a safe place to prevent misuse and abuse. Selling or giving away FOCALIN XR may harm others, and is against the law.

Tell your doctor if you or your child have (or have a family history of) ever abused or been dependent on alcohol, prescription medicines or street drugs.

Who should not take FOCALIN XR?

FOCALIN XR should not be taken if you or your child:

- are very anxious, tense, or agitated
- have an eye problem called glaucoma
- have tics or Tourette's syndrome, or a family history of Tourette's syndrome. Tics are hard to control repeated movements or sounds.
- are taking or have taken within the past 14 days an anti-depression medicine called a monoamine oxidase inhibitor or MAOI.
- are allergic to anything in FOCALIN XR. See the end of this Medication Guide for a complete list of ingredients.

FOCALIN XR should not be used in children less than 6 years old because it has not been studied in this age group.

FOCALIN XR may not be right for you or your child. Before starting FOCALIN XR tell your or your child's doctor about all health conditions (or a family history of) including:

- heart problems, heart defects, high blood pressure
- mental problems including psychosis, mania, bipolar illness, or depression
- tics or Tourette's syndrome
- seizures or have had an abnormal brain wave test (EEG)

Tell your doctor if you or your child is pregnant, planning to become pregnant, or breast-feeding.

Can FOCALIN XR be taken with other medicines?

Tell your doctor about all of the medicines that you or your child take including prescription and nonprescription medicines, vitamins, and herbal supplements. FOCALIN XR and some medicines may interact with each other and cause serious side effects. Sometimes the doses of other medicines will need to be adjusted while taking FOCALIN XR.

Your doctor will decide whether FOCALIN XR can be taken with other medicines.

Especially tell your doctor if you or your child takes:

- anti-depression medicines including MAOIs
- seizure medicines
- blood thinner medicines
- blood pressure medicines
- antacids
- cold or allergy medicines that contain decongestants

Know the medicines that you or your child takes. Keep a list of your medicines with you to show your doctor and pharmacist.

Do not start any new medicine while taking FOCALIN XR without talking to your doctor first.

How should FOCALIN XR be taken?

- **Take FOCALIN XR exactly as prescribed.** Your doctor may adjust the dose until it is right for you or your child.
- Take FOCALIN XR once each day in the morning. FOCALIN XR is an extended-release capsule. It releases medicine into your body throughout the day.
- FOCALIN XR can be taken with or without food. Taking FOCALIN XR with food may slow the time it takes for the medicine to start working.
- Swallow FOCALIN XR capsules whole with water or other liquids. **Do not chew, crush, or divide the capsules or the beads in the capsule.** If you or your child cannot swallow the capsule, open it and sprinkle the small beads of medicine over a spoonful of applesauce and swallow it right away without chewing.
- From time to time, your doctor may stop FOCALIN XR treatment for a while to check ADHD symptoms.
- Your doctor may do regular checks of the blood, heart, and blood pressure while taking FOCALIN XR. Children should have their height and weight checked often while taking FOCALIN XR. FOCALIN XR treatment may be stopped if a problem is found during these check-ups.
- **If you or your child takes too much FOCALIN XR or overdoses, call your doctor or poison control center right away, or get emergency treatment.**

What are possible side effects of FOCALIN XR?

See **"What is the most important information I should know about FOCALIN XR?"** for information on reported heart and mental problems.

Other serious side effects include:

- slowing of growth (height and weight) in children
- seizures, mainly in patients with a history of seizures
- eyesight changes or blurred vision

Common side effects include:

- headache
- upset stomach
- trouble sleeping
- anxiety
- decreased appetite
- dry mouth
- dizziness
- nervousness

Talk to your doctor if you or your child has side effects that are bothersome or do not go away.

This is not a complete list of possible side effects. Ask your doctor or pharmacist for more information.

How should I store FOCALIN XR?

- Store FOCALIN XR in a safe place at room temperature, 59 to 86° F (15 to 30° C).
- **Keep FOCALIN XR and all medicines out of the reach of children.**

General information about FOCALIN XR

Medicines are sometimes prescribed for purposes other than those listed in a Medication Guide. Do not use FOCALIN XR for a condition for which it was not prescribed. Do not give FOCALIN XR to other people, even if they have the same condition. It may harm them and it is against the law.

This Medication Guide summarizes the most important information about FOCALIN XR. If you would like more information, talk with your doctor. You can ask your doctor or pharmacist for information about FOCALIN XR that was written for healthcare professionals. For more information about FOCALIN XR call 1-888-669-6682.

What are the ingredients in FOCALIN XR?

Active Ingredient: dexmethylphenidate hydrochloride

Inactive Ingredients: ammonio methacrylate copolymer, FD&C Blue #2 (5 mg, 15 mg and 40 mg strengths), FDA/E172 yellow iron oxide (10 mg, 15 mg, 30 mg and 40 mg strengths), gelatin, ink Tan SW-8010, methacrylic acid copolymer, polyethylene glycol, sugar spheres, talc, titanium dioxide, and triethyl citrate.

This Medication Guide has been approved by the U.S. Food and Drug Administration.

Focalin XR is a trademark of Novartis AG.

SODAS® is a registered trademark of Elan Pharma International Ltd.
This product is covered by US patents including 5,837,284, 5,908,850, 6,228,398, 6,355,656, and 6,635,284.
REV: AUGUST 2010 T2010-72/T2010-73
Manufactured for
Novartis Pharmaceuticals Corporation
East Hanover, New Jersey 07936
By ELAN HOLDINGS INC.
Pharmaceutical Division
Gainesville, GA 30504

Shown in Product Identification Guide, page 315

GILENYA™ ℞
[je-LEN-yah]
(fingolimod)
capsules

The following prescribing information is based on official labeling in effect July 2010.

HIGHLIGHTS OF PRESCRIBING INFORMATION
These highlights do not include all the information needed to use GILENYA™ safely and effectively. See full prescribing information for GILENYA.
GILENYA™ (fingolimod) capsules
Initial U.S. Approval: 2010

INDICATIONS AND USAGE

GILENYA is a sphingosine 1-phosphate receptor modulator indicated for the treatment of patients with relapsing forms of multiple sclerosis to reduce the frequency of clinical exacerbations and to delay the accumulation of physical disability. (1)

DOSAGE AND ADMINISTRATION

Recommended dose: 0.5 mg orally once daily, with or without food. (2)

DOSAGE FORMS AND STRENGTHS

0.5 mg hard capsules. (3)

CONTRAINDICATIONS

None. (4)

WARNINGS AND PRECAUTIONS

- Decrease in heart rate and/or atrioventricular conduction after first dose of GILENYA: Observe all patients for signs and symptoms of bradycardia for 6 hours after first dose. Obtain baseline ECG before first dose if not recently available in those at higher risk of bradyarrhythmia. Patients receiving Class Ia or Class III antiarrhythmic drugs, beta blockers, calcium channel blockers, those with a low heart rate, history of syncope, sick sinus syndrome, 2nd degree or higher conduction block, ischemic heart disease, or congestive heart failure are at increased risk of developing bradycardia or heart blocks. (5.1)
- Infections: GILENYA may increase the risk of infections. A recent CBC should be available before initiating treatment with GILENYA. Monitor for signs and symptoms of infection during treatment and for two months after discontinuation. Do not start GILENYA treatment in patients with active acute or chronic infections. (5.2)
- Macular edema: Can occur with or without visual symptoms. An ophthalmologic evaluation should be performed before starting GILENYA and at 3-4 months after treatment initiation. Monitor visual acuity at baseline and during routine evaluations of patients. Patients with diabetes mellitus or a history of uveitis are at increased risk and should have regular ophthalmologic evaluations. (5.3)
- Decrease in pulmonary function tests with GILENYA: Obtain spirometry and diffusion lung capacity for carbon monoxide (DLCO) when clinically indicated. (5.4)
- Hepatic effects: GILENYA may increase liver transaminases. Recent liver enzyme results should be available before initiating treatment with GILENYA. Assess liver enzymes if symptoms suggestive of hepatic injury develop. Discontinue GILENYA if significant liver injury is confirmed. (5.5)
- Fetal risk: Women of childbearing potential should use effective contraception during and for two months after stopping GILENYA treatment. (5.6)

ADVERSE REACTIONS

Most common adverse reactions (incidence ≥10% and > placebo): Headache, influenza, diarrhea, back pain, liver transaminase elevations and cough. (6.1)

To report SUSPECTED ADVERSE REACTIONS, contact Novartis Pharmaceuticals Corporation at 1-888-669-6682 or FDA at 1-800-332-1088 or www.fda.gov/medwatch.

DRUG INTERACTIONS

- Class Ia or Class III antiarrhythmic drugs: Because of a risk of serious rhythm disturbances, carefully monitor patients on Class Ia or Class III antiarrhythmic drugs during initiation of therapy. (5.1, 7)
- Beta blockers: Because of a risk of additive effect on heart rate, carefully monitor patients on beta blockers during initiation of therapy. (5.1, 7)
- Ketoconazole: Monitor patients closely, as GILENYA exposure is increased by 70% during concomitant use with systemic ketoconazole, and risk of adverse reactions is greater. (7, 12.3)
- Vaccines: Avoid live attenuated vaccines during, and for 2 months after stopping GILENYA treatment, due to risk of infection. (5.2, 7)

USE IN SPECIFIC POPULATIONS

- Pregnancy: Based on animal data, may cause fetal harm. Pregnancy registry available. (8.1)
- Pediatric patients: Safety and effectiveness have not been established. (8.4)
- Hepatic impairment: Monitor patients with severe hepatic impairment closely, as GILENYA exposure is doubled, and risk of adverse reactions is greater. (5.5, 8.5, 12.3)

See 17 for PATIENT COUNSELING INFORMATION and Medication Guide

Revised: 09/2010

FULL PRESCRIBING INFORMATION: CONTENTS*

1 INDICATIONS AND USAGE
2 DOSAGE AND ADMINISTRATION
3 DOSAGE FORMS AND STRENGTHS
4 CONTRAINDICATIONS
5 WARNINGS AND PRECAUTIONS
5.1 Bradyarrhythmia and Atrioventricular Blocks
5.2 Infections
5.3 Macular Edema
5.4 Respiratory Effects
5.5 Hepatic Effects
5.6 Fetal Risk
5.7 Blood Pressure Effects
5.8 Immune System Effects Following GILENYA Discontinuation
6 ADVERSE REACTIONS
6.1 Clinical Trials Experience
7 DRUG INTERACTIONS
8 USE IN SPECIFIC POPULATIONS
8.1 Pregnancy
8.2 Labor and Delivery
8.3 Nursing Mothers
8.4 Pediatric Use
8.5 Geriatric Use
8.6 Hepatic Impairment
8.7 Renal Impairment
10 OVERDOSAGE
11 DESCRIPTION
12 CLINICAL PHARMACOLOGY
12.1 Mechanism of Action
12.2 Pharmacodynamics
12.3 Pharmacokinetics
13 NONCLINICAL TOXICOLOGY
13.1 Carcinogenesis, Mutagenesis, Impairment of Fertility
13.2 Animal Toxicology and/or Pharmacology
14 CLINICAL STUDIES
16 HOW SUPPLIED/STORAGE AND HANDLING
17 PATIENT COUNSELING INFORMATION
17.1 Benefits and Risks
17.2 Cardiac Effects
17.3 Risk of Infections
17.4 Macular Edema
17.5 Respiratory Effects
17.6 Hepatic Effects
17.7 Fetal Risk
17.8 Persistence of GILENYA Effects After Drug Discontinuation

* Sections or subsections omitted from the full prescribing information are not listed

FULL PRESCRIBING INFORMATION

1 INDICATIONS AND USAGE

GILENYA is indicated for the treatment of patients with relapsing forms of multiple sclerosis (MS) to reduce the frequency of clinical exacerbations and to delay the accumulation of physical disability.

2 DOSAGE AND ADMINISTRATION

The recommended dose of GILENYA is 0.5 mg orally once daily. Patients should be observed for 6 hours after the first dose to monitor for signs and symptoms of bradycardia [*see Warnings and Precautions (5.1)*]. Fingolimod doses higher than 0.5 mg are associated with a greater incidence of adverse reactions without additional benefit.
GILENYA can be taken with or without food.

3 DOSAGE FORMS AND STRENGTHS

GILENYA is available as 0.5 mg hard capsules with a white opaque body and bright yellow cap imprinted with "FTY 0.5 mg" on the cap and two radial bands imprinted on the capsule body with yellow ink.

4 CONTRAINDICATIONS

None

5 WARNINGS AND PRECAUTIONS

5.1 Bradyarrhythmia and Atrioventricular Blocks

Reduction in heart rate

Initiation of GILENYA treatment results in a decrease in heart rate [*see Clinical Pharmacology (12.2)*]. Observe all patients for a period of 6 hours for signs and symptoms of bradycardia. Should post-dose bradyarrhythmia-related symptoms occur, initiate appropriate management and continue observation until the symptoms have resolved.

To identify underlying risk factors for bradycardia and atrioventricular (AV) block, if a recent electrocardiogram (i.e., within 6 months) is not available, obtain one in patients using anti-arrhythmics including beta-blockers and calcium channel blockers, those with cardiac risk factors, as described below, and those who on examination have a slow or irregular heart beat prior to starting GILENYA.

Experience with GILENYA in patients receiving concurrent therapy with beta blockers or in those with a history of syncope is limited. GILENYA has not been studied in patients with sitting heart rate less than 55 bpm. GILENYA has not been studied in patients with second degree or higher AV block, sick sinus syndrome, prolonged QT interval, ischemic cardiac disease, or congestive heart failure. GILENYA has not been studied in patients with arrhythmias requiring treatment with Class Ia (e.g., quinidine, procainamide) or Class III (e.g., amiodarone, sotalol) antiarrhythmic drugs. Class Ia and Class III antiarrhythmic drugs have been associated with cases of torsades de pointes in patients with bradycardia.

After the first dose of GILENYA, the heart rate decrease starts within an hour and the Day 1 decline is maximal at approximately 6 hours. Following the second dose a further decrease in heart rate may occur when compared to the heart rate prior to the second dose, but this change is of a smaller magnitude than that observed following the first dose. With continued dosing, the heart rate returns to baseline within one month of chronic treatment. The mean decrease in heart rate in patients on GILENYA 0.5 mg at 6 hours after the first dose was approximately 13 beats per minute (bpm). Heart rates below 40 bpm were rarely observed. Adverse reactions of bradycardia following the first dose were reported in 0.5% of patients receiving GILENYA 0.5 mg, but in no patient on placebo. Patients who experienced bradycardia were generally asymptomatic, but some patients experienced mild to moderate dizziness, fatigue, palpitations, and chest pain that resolved within the first 24 hours on treatment.

Atrioventricular blocks

Initiation of GILENYA treatment has resulted in transient AV conduction delays. In controlled clinical trials, adverse reactions of first degree AV block (prolonged PR interval on ECG) following the first dose were reported in 0.1% of patients receiving GILENYA 0.5 mg, but in no patient on placebo. Second degree AV blocks following the first dose were also identified in 0.1% of patients receiving GILENYA 0.5 mg, but in no patient on placebo. In a study of 698 patients with available 24-hour Holter monitoring data after their first dose (N=351 on GILENYA 0.5 mg and N=347 on placebo), second degree AV blocks, usually Mobitz type I (Wenckebach) were reported in 3.7% (N=13) of patients receiving GILENYA 0.5 mg and 2% (N=7) of patients on placebo. The conduction abnormalities were usually transient and asymptomatic, and resolved within the first 24 hours on treatment, but they occasionally required treatment with atropine or isoproterenol. One patient developed syncope and complete AV block following the first dose of fingolimod 1.25 mg (a dose higher than recommended) in an uncontrolled study.

Re-initiation of therapy following discontinuation

If GILENYA therapy is discontinued for more than two weeks the effects on heart rate and AV conduction may recur on reintroduction of GILENYA treatment and the same precautions as for initial dosing should apply.

5.2 Infections

Risk of infections

GILENYA causes a dose-dependent reduction in peripheral lymphocyte count to 20-30% of baseline values because of reversible sequestration of lymphocytes in lymphoid tissues. GILENYA may therefore increase the risk of infections, some serious in nature [*see Clinical Pharmacology (12.2)*].

Before initiating treatment with GILENYA, a recent CBC (i.e. within 6 months) should be available. Consider suspending treatment with GILENYA if a patient develops a serious infection, and reassess the benefits and risks prior to re-initiation of therapy. Because the elimination of fingolimod after discontinuation may take up to two months, continue monitoring for infections throughout this period. Instruct patients receiving GILENYA to report symptoms of infections to a physician. Patients with active acute or chronic infections should not start treatment until the infection(s) is resolved.

Two patients died of herpetic infections during GILENYA controlled studies in the premarketing database (one disseminated primary herpes zoster and one herpes simplex encephalitis). In both cases, the patients were receiving a fingolimod dose (1.25 mg) higher than recommended for the treatment of MS (0.5 mg), and had received high dose corticosteroid therapy for suspected MS relapse. No deaths due to viral infections occurred in patients treated with GILENYA 0.5 mg in the premarketing database.

In MS controlled studies, the overall rate of infections (72%) and serious infections (2%) with GILENYA 0.5 mg was similar to placebo. However, bronchitis and, to a lesser extent, pneumonia were more common in GILENYA-treated patients.

Concomitant use with antineoplastic, immunosuppressive or immune modulating therapies

GILENYA has not been administered concomitantly with antineoplastic, immunosuppressive or immune modulating therapies used for treatment of MS. Concomitant use of GILENYA with any of these therapies would be expected to increase the risk of immunosuppression [*see Drug Interactions (7)*].

Varicella zoster virus antibody testing/vaccination

As for any immune modulating drug, before initiating GILENYA therapy, patients without a history of chickenpox or without vaccination against varicella zoster virus (VZV) should be tested for antibodies to VZV. VZV vaccination of antibody-negative patients should be considered prior to commencing treatment with GILENYA, following which initiation of treatment with GILENYA should be postponed for 1 month to allow the full effect of vaccination to occur.

5.3 Macular Edema

In patients receiving GILENYA 0.5 mg, macular edema occurred in 0.4% of patients. An adequate ophthalmologic evaluation should be performed at baseline and 3-4 months after treatment initiation. If patients report visual disturbances at any time while on GILENYA therapy, additional ophthalmologic evaluation should be undertaken.

In MS controlled studies involving 1204 patients treated with GILENYA 0.5 mg and 861 patients treated with placebo, macular edema with or without visual symptoms was reported in 0.4% of patients treated with GILENYA 0.5 mg and 0.1% of patients treated with placebo; it occurred predominantly in the first 3-4 months of therapy. Some patients presented with blurred vision or decreased visual acuity, but others were asymptomatic and diagnosed on routine ophthalmologic examination. Macular edema generally improved or resolved with or without treatment after drug discontinuation, but some patients had residual visual acuity loss even after resolution of macular edema.

Continuation of GILENYA in patients who develop macular edema has not been evaluated. A decision on whether or not to discontinue GILENYA therapy should include an assessment of the potential benefits and risks for the individual patient. The risk of recurrence after rechallenge has not been evaluated.

Macular edema in patients with history of uveitis or diabetes mellitus

Patients with a history of uveitis and patients with diabetes mellitus are at increased risk of macular edema during GILENYA therapy. The incidence of macular edema is also increased in MS patients with a history of uveitis. The rate was approximately 20% in patients with a history of uveitis vs. 0.6% in those without a history of uveitis, in the combined experience with all doses of fingolimod. MS patients with diabetes mellitus or a history of uveitis should undergo an ophthalmologic evaluation prior to initiating GILENYA therapy and have regular follow-up ophthalmologic evaluations while receiving GILENYA therapy. GILENYA has not been tested in MS patients with diabetes mellitus.

5.4 Respiratory Effects

Dose-dependent reductions in forced expiratory volume over 1 second (FEV1) and diffusion lung capacity for carbon monoxide (DLCO) were observed in patients treated with GILENYA as early as 1 month after treatment initiation. At Month 24, the reduction from baseline in the percent of predicted values for FEV1 was 3.1% for GILENYA 0.5 mg and 2% for placebo. For DLCO, the reductions from baseline in percent of predicted values at Month 24 were 3.8% for GILENYA 0.5 mg and 2.7% for placebo. The changes in FEV1 appear to be reversible after treatment discontinuation. There is insufficient information to determine the reversibility of the decrease of DLCO after drug discontinuation. In MS controlled trials, dyspnea was reported in 5% of patients receiving GILENYA 0.5 mg and 4% of patients receiving placebo. Several patients discontinued GILENYA because of unexplained dyspnea during the extension (uncontrolled) studies. GILENYA has not been tested in MS patients with compromised respiratory function.

Spirometric evaluation of respiratory function and evaluation of DLCO should be performed during therapy with GILENYA if clinically indicated.

5.5 Hepatic Effects

Elevations of liver enzymes may occur in patients receiving GILENYA. Recent (i.e., within last 6 months) transaminase and bilirubin levels should be available before initiation of GILENYA therapy.

During clinical trials, 3-fold the upper limit of normal (ULN) or greater elevation in liver transaminases occurred in 8% of patients treated with GILENYA 0.5 mg, as compared to 2% of patients on placebo. Elevations 5-fold the ULN occurred in 2% of patients on GILENYA and 1% of patients on placebo. In clinical trials, GILENYA was discontinued if the elevation exceeded 5 times the ULN. Recurrence of liver transaminase elevations occurred with rechallenge in some patients, supporting a relationship to drug. The majority of elevations occurred within 3-4 months. Serum transaminase levels returned to normal within approximately 2 months after discontinuation of GILENYA.

Liver enzymes should be monitored in patients who develop symptoms suggestive of hepatic dysfunction, such as unexplained nausea, vomiting, abdominal pain, fatigue, anorexia, or jaundice and/or dark urine. GILENYA should be discontinued if significant liver injury is confirmed. Patients with pre-existing liver disease may be at increased risk of developing elevated liver enzymes when taking GILENYA. Because GILENYA exposure is doubled in patients with severe hepatic impairment, these patients should be closely monitored, as the risk of adverse reactions is greater [*see Use in Specific Populations (8.5) and Clinical Pharmacology (12.3)*].

5.6 Fetal Risk

Based on animal studies, GILENYA may cause fetal harm. Because it takes approximately 2 months to eliminate GILENYA from the body, women of childbearing potential should use effective contraception to avoid pregnancy during and for 2 months after stopping GILENYA treatment.

5.7 Blood Pressure Effects

In MS clinical trials, patients treated with GILENYA 0.5 mg had an average increase of approximately 2 mmHg in systolic pressure, and approximately 1 mmHg in diastolic pressure, first detected after approximately 2 months of treatment initiation, and persisting with continued treatment. In controlled studies involving 854 MS patients on GILENYA 0.5 mg and 511 MS patients on placebo, hypertension was reported as an adverse reaction in 5% of patients on GILENYA 0.5 mg and in 3% of patients on placebo. Blood pressure should be monitored during treatment with GILENYA.

5.8 Immune System Effects Following GILENYA Discontinuation

Fingolimod remains in the blood and has pharmacodynamic effects, including decreased lymphocyte counts, for up to 2 months following the last dose of GILENYA. Lymphocyte counts generally return to the normal range within 1-2 months of stopping therapy [*see Clinical Pharmacology (12.2)*].

Because of the continuing pharmacodynamic effects of fingolimod, initiating other drugs during this period warrants the same considerations needed for concomitant administration (e.g., risk of additive immunosuppressant effects) [*see Drug Interactions (7)*].

6 ADVERSE REACTIONS

The following serious adverse reactions are described elsewhere in labeling:

- Bradyarrhythmia and atrioventricular blocks [*see Warnings and Precautions (5.1)*]
- Infections [*see Warnings and Precautions (5.2)*]
- Macular edema [*see Warnings and Precautions (5.3)*]
- Respiratory effects [*see Warnings and Precautions (5.4)*]
- Hepatic effects [*see Warnings and Precautions (5.5)*]

The most frequent adverse reactions (incidence ≥10% and > placebo) for GILENYA 0.5 mg were headache, influenza, diarrhea, back pain, liver enzyme elevations, and cough. The only adverse event leading to treatment interruption reported at an incidence >1% for GILENYA 0.5 mg was serum transaminase elevations (3.8%).

6.1 Clinical Trials Experience

A total of 1703 patients on GILENYA (0.5 or 1.25 mg once daily) constituted the safety population in the 2 controlled studies in patients with relapsing remitting MS (RRMS) [*see Clinical Studies (14)*].

Study 1 was a 2-year placebo-controlled clinical study in 1272 MS patients treated with GILENYA 0.5 mg (n=425), GILENYA 1.25 mg (n=429) or placebo (n=418).

Table 1 Adverse Reactions in Study 1 (occurring in ≥1% of patients, and reported for GILENYA 0.5 mg at ≥1% higher rate than for placebo)

Primary System Organ Class Preferred Term	GILENYA 0.5 mg N=425 %	Placebo N=418 %
Infections		
Influenza viral infections	13	10
Herpes viral infections	9	8
Bronchitis	8	4
Sinusitis	7	5
Gastroenteritis	5	3
Tinea infections	4	1
Cardiac disorders		
Bradycardia	4	1
Nervous system disorders		
Headache	25	23
Dizziness	7	6
Paresthesia	5	4
Migraine	5	1
Gastrointestinal disorders		
Diarrhea	12	7
General disorders and administration site conditions		
Asthenia	3	1
Musculoskeletal and connective tissue disorders		
Back pain	12	7
Skin and subcutaneous tissue disorders		
Alopecia	4	2
Eczema	3	2
Pruritus	3	1
Investigations		
ALT/AST increased	14	5
GGT increased	5	1
Weight decreased	5	3
Blood triglycerides increased	3	1
Respiratory, thoracic and mediastinal disorders		
Cough	10	8
Dyspnea	8	5
Psychiatric disorders		
Depression	8	7
Eye disorders		
Vision blurred	4	1
Eye pain	3	1
Vascular disorders		
Hypertension	6	4
Blood and lymphatic system disorders		
Lymphopenia	4	1
Leukopenia	3	<1

Adverse reactions in Study 2, a 1-year active-controlled (vs. interferon beta-1a, n=431) study including 849 patients with MS treated with fingolimod, were generally similar to those in Study 1.

Vascular Events

Vascular events, including ischemic and hemorrhagic strokes, peripheral arterial occlusive disease and posterior reversible encephalopathy syndrome were reported in premarketing clinical trials in patients who received GILENYA doses (1.25-5 mg) higher than recommended for use in MS. No vascular events were observed with GILENYA 0.5 mg in the premarketing database.

Lymphomas

Cases of lymphoma (cutaneous T-cell lymphoproliferative disorders or diffuse B-cell lymphoma) were reported in premarketing clinical trials in MS patients receiving GILENYA at, or above, the recommended dose of 0.5 mg. Based on the small number of cases and short duration of exposure, the relationship to GILENYA remains uncertain.

7 DRUG INTERACTIONS

Class Ia or Class III antiarrhythmic drugs

GILENYA has not been studied in patients with arrhythmias requiring treatment with Class Ia (e.g., quinidine, procainamide) or Class III (e.g., amiodarone, sotalol) antiarrhythmic drugs. Class Ia and Class III antiarrhythmic drugs have been associated with cases of torsades de pointes in patients with bradycardia. Since initiation of GILENYA treatment results in decreased heart rate, patients on Class Ia or Class III antiarrhythmic drugs should be closely monitored [*see Warnings and Precautions (5.1)*].

Ketoconazole

The blood levels of fingolimod and fingolimod-phosphate are increased by 1.7-fold when coadministered with ketoconazole. Patients who use GILENYA and systemic ketoconazole concomitantly should be closely monitored, as the risk of adverse reactions is greater.

Vaccines

Vaccination may be less effective during and for up to 2 months after discontinuation of treatment with GILENYA [*see Clinical Pharmacology (12.2)*]. The use of live attenuated vaccines should be avoided during and for 2 months after treatment with GILENYA because of the risk of infection.

Antineoplastic, immunosuppressive or immunomodulating therapies

Antineoplastic, immunosuppressive or immune modulating therapies are expected to increase the risk of immunosuppression. Use caution when switching patients from long-acting therapies with immune effects such as natalizumab or mitoxantrone.

Heart rate-lowering drugs (e.g., beta blockers or diltiazem)
Experience with GILENYA in patients receiving concurrent therapy with beta blockers is limited. These patients should be carefully monitored during initiation of therapy. When GILENYA is used with atenolol, there is an additional 15% reduction of heart rate upon GILENYA initiation, an effect not seen with diltiazem [*see Warnings and Precautions* (*5.1*)].

Laboratory test interaction
Because GILENYA reduces blood lymphocyte counts via re-distribution in secondary lymphoid organs, peripheral blood lymphocyte counts cannot be utilized to evaluate the lymphocyte subset status of a patient treated with GILENYA. A recent CBC should be available before initiating treatment with GILENYA.

8 USE IN SPECIFIC POPULATIONS

8.1 Pregnancy

Pregnancy Category C
There are no adequate and well-controlled studies in pregnant women. In oral studies conducted in rats and rabbits, fingolimod demonstrated developmental toxicity, including teratogenicity (rats) and embryolethality, when given to pregnant animals. In rats, the highest no-effect dose was less than the recommended human dose (RHD) of 0.5 mg/day on a body surface area (mg/m^2) basis. The most common fetal visceral malformations in rats included persistent truncus arteriosus and ventricular septal defect. The receptor affected by fingolimod (sphingosine 1-phosphate receptor) is known to be involved in vascular formation during embryogenesis. Because it takes approximately 2 months to eliminate fingolimod from the body, potential risks to the fetus may persist after treatment ends [*see Warnings and Precautions* (*5.7, 5.8*)]. GILENYA should be used during pregnancy only if the potential benefit justifies the potential risk to the fetus.

Pregnancy Registry
A pregnancy registry has been established to collect information about the effect of GILENYA use during pregnancy. Physicians are encouraged to enroll pregnant patients, or pregnant women may enroll themselves in the GILENYA pregnancy registry by calling 1-877-598-7237.

Animal Data
When fingolimod was orally administered to pregnant rats during the period of organogenesis (0, 0.03, 0.1, and 0.3 mg/kg/day or 0, 1, 3, and 10 mg/kg/day), increased incidences of fetal malformations and embryo-fetal deaths were observed at all but the lowest dose tested (0.03 mg/kg/day), which is less than the RHD on a mg/m^2 basis. Oral administration to pregnant rabbits during organogenesis (0, 0.5, 1.5, and 5 mg/kg/day) resulted in increased incidences of embryo-fetal mortality and fetal growth retardation at the mid and high doses. The no-effect dose for these effects in rabbits (0.5 mg/kg/day) is approximately 20 times the RHD on a mg/m^2 basis.
When fingolimod was orally administered to female rats during pregnancy and lactation (0, 0.05, 0.15, and 0.5 mg/kg/day), pup survival was decreased at all doses and a neurobehavioral (learning) deficit was seen in offspring at the high dose. The low-effect dose of 0.05 mg/kg/day is similar to the RHD on a mg/m^2 basis.

8.2 Labor and Delivery

The effects of GILENYA on labor and delivery are unknown.

8.3 Nursing Mothers

Fingolimod is excreted in the milk of treated rats. It is not known whether this drug is excreted in human milk. Because many drugs are excreted in human milk and because of the potential for serious adverse reactions in nursing infants from GILENYA, a decision should be made whether to discontinue nursing or to discontinue the drug, taking into account the importance of the drug to the mother.

8.4 Pediatric Use

The safety and effectiveness of GILENYA in pediatric patients with MS below the age of 18 have not been established.

8.5 Geriatric Use

Clinical MS studies of GILENYA did not include sufficient numbers of patients aged 65 years and over to determine whether they respond differently than younger patients. GILENYA should be used with caution in patients aged 65 years and over, reflecting the greater frequency of decreased hepatic, or renal, function and of concomitant disease or other drug therapy.

8.6 Hepatic Impairment

Because fingolimod, but not fingolimod-phosphate, exposure is doubled in patients with severe hepatic impairment, patients with severe hepatic impairment should be closely monitored, as the risk of adverse reactions may be greater [*see Warnings and Precautions* (*5.5*) and *Clinical Pharmacology* (*12.3*)].
No dose adjustment is needed in patients with mild or moderate hepatic impairment.

8.7 Renal Impairment

The blood level of some GILENYA metabolites is increased (up to 13-fold) in patients with severe renal impairment [*see Clinical Pharmacology* (*12.3*)]. The toxicity of these metabolites has not been fully explored. The blood level of these metabolites has not been assessed in patients with mild or moderate renal impairment.

10 OVERDOSAGE

No cases of overdosage have been reported. However, single doses up to 80-fold the recommended dose (0.5 mg) resulted in no clinically significant adverse reactions. At 40 mg, 5 of 6 subjects reported mild chest tightness or discomfort which was clinically consistent with small airway reactivity.
Neither dialysis nor plasma exchange results in removal of fingolimod from the body.

11 DESCRIPTION

Fingolimod is a sphingosine 1-phosphate receptor modulator.
Chemically, fingolimod is 2-amino-2-[2-(4-octylphenyl)ethyl]propan-1,3-diol hydrochloride. Its structure is shown below:

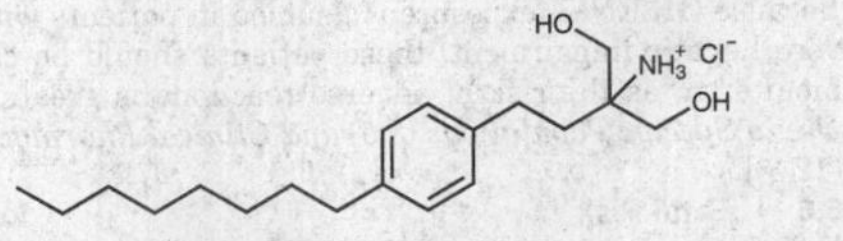

Fingolimod hydrochloride is a white to practically white powder that is freely soluble in water and alcohol and soluble in propylene glycol. It has a molecular weight of 343.93.
GILENYA is provided as 0.5 mg hard gelatin capsules for oral use. Each capsule contains 0.56 mg of fingolimod hydrochloride, equivalent to 0.5 mg of fingolimod.
Each GILENYA 0.5 mg capsule contains the following inactive ingredients: gelatin, magnesium stearate, mannitol, titanium dioxide, yellow iron oxide.

12 CLINICAL PHARMACOLOGY

12.1 Mechanism of Action

Fingolimod is metabolized by sphingosine kinase to the active metabolite, fingolimod-phosphate. Fingolimod-phosphate is a sphingosine 1-phosphate receptor modulator, and binds with high affinity to sphingosine 1-phosphate receptors 1, 3, 4, and 5. Fingolimod-phosphate blocks the capacity of lymphocytes to egress from lymph nodes, reducing the number of lymphocytes in peripheral blood. The mechanism by which fingolimod exerts therapeutic effects in multiple sclerosis is unknown, but may involve reduction of lymphocyte migration into the central nervous system.

12.2 Pharmacodynamics

Heart rate and rhythm
Fingolimod causes a transient reduction in heart rate and AV conduction at treatment initiation [*see Warnings and Precautions* (*5.1*)]. The maximal decline of heart rate is seen in the first 6 hours post-dose, with 70% of the negative chronotropic effect achieved on the first day. Heart rate progressively increases after the first day, returning to baseline values within 1 month of the start of chronic treatment.
Autonomic responses of the heart, including diurnal variation of heart rate and response to exercise, are not affected by fingolimod treatment.
Fingolimod treatment is not associated with a decrease in cardiac output.

Potential to prolong the QT interval
In a thorough QT interval study of doses of 1.25 or 2.5 mg fingolimod at steady-state, when a negative chronotropic effect of fingolimod was still present, fingolimod treatment resulted in a prolongation of QTc, with the upper bound of the 90% confidence interval (CI) of 14.0 ms. There is no consistent signal of increased incidence of QTc outliers, either absolute or change from baseline, associated with fingolimod treatment. In MS studies, there was no clinically relevant prolongation of QT interval, but patients at risk for QT prolongation were not included in clinical studies.

Immune system
Effects on immune cell numbers in the blood
In a study in which 12 subjects received GILENYA 0.5 mg daily, the lymphocyte count decreased to approximately 60% of baseline within 4-6 hours after the first dose. With continued daily dosing, the lymphocyte count continued to decrease over a 2-week period, reaching a nadir count of approximately 500 cells/μL or approximately 30% of baseline. In a placebo-controlled study in 1272 MS patients (of whom 425 received fingolimod 0.5 mg daily and 418 received placebo), 18% (N=78) of patients on fingolimod 0.5 mg reached a nadir of <200 cells/μL on at least one occasion. No patient on placebo reached a nadir of <200 cells/μL. Low lymphocyte counts are maintained with chronic daily dosing of GILENYA 0.5 mg daily.
Chronic fingolimod dosing leads to a mild decrease in the neutrophil count to approximately 80% of baseline. Monocytes are unaffected by fingolimod.
Peripheral lymphocyte count increases are evident within days of stopping fingolimod treatment and typically normal counts are reached within 1 to 2 months.

Effect on antibody response
The immunogenicity of keyhole limpet Hemocyanin (KLH) and pneumococcal polysaccharide vaccine (PPV-23) immunization were assessed by IgM and IgG titers in a steady-state, randomized, placebo-controlled study in healthy volunteers. Compared to placebo, antigen-specific IgM titers were decreased by 91% and 25% in response to KLH and PPV, respectively, in subjects on GILENYA 0.5 mg. Similarly, IgG titers were decreased by 45% and 50%, in response to KLH and PPV, respectively, in subjects on GILENYA 0.5 mg daily compared to placebo. The responder rate for GILENYA 0.5 mg as measured by the number of subjects with a >4-fold increase in KLH IgG was comparable to placebo and 25% lower for PPV-23 IgG, while the number of subjects with a >4-fold increase in KLH and PPV-23 IgM was 75% and 40% lower, respectively, compared to placebo. The capacity to mount a skin delayed-type hypersensitivity reaction to Candida and tetanus toxoid was decreased by approximately 30% in subjects on GILENYA 0.5 mg daily, compared to placebo. Immunologic responses were further decreased with fingolimod 1.25 mg (a dose higher than recommended in MS) [*see Warnings and Precautions* (*5.2*)].

Pulmonary function
Single fingolimod doses ≥5 mg (10-fold the recommended dose) are associated with a dose-dependent increase in airway resistance. In a 14-day study of 0.5, 1.25, or 5 mg/day, fingolimod was not associated with impaired oxygenation or oxygen desaturation with exercise or an increase in airway responsiveness to methacholine. Subjects on fingolimod treatment had a normal bronchodilator response to inhaled beta-agonists.
In a 14-day placebo-controlled study of patients with moderate asthma, no effect was seen for GILENYA 0.5 mg (recommended dose in MS). A 10% reduction in mean FEV1 at 6 hours after dosing was observed in patients receiving fingolimod 1.25 mg (a dose higher than recommended for use in MS) on Day 10 of treatment. Fingolimod 1.25 mg was associated with a 5-fold increase in the use of rescue short acting beta-agonists.

12.3 Pharmacokinetics

Absorption
The T_{max} of fingolimod is 12-16 hours. The apparent absolute oral bioavailability is 93%.
Food intake does not alter C_{max} or exposure (AUC) of fingolimod or fingolimod-phosphate. Therefore GILENYA may be taken without regard to meals.
Steady-state blood concentrations are reached within 1 to 2 months following once-daily administration and steady-state levels are approximately 10-fold greater than with the initial dose.

Distribution
Fingolimod highly (86%) distributes in red blood cells. Fingolimod-phosphate has a smaller uptake in blood cells of <17%. Fingolimod and fingolimod-phosphate are >99.7% protein bound. Fingolimod and fingolimod-phosphate protein binding is not altered by renal or hepatic impairment.
Fingolimod is extensively distributed to body tissues with a volume of distribution of about 1200±260 L.

Metabolism
The biotransformation of fingolimod in humans occurs by three main pathways: by reversible stereoselective phosphorylation to the pharmacologically active *(S)*-enantiomer of fingolimod-phosphate, by oxidative biotransformation mainly via the cytochrome P450 4F2 isoenzyme and subsequent fatty acid-like degradation to inactive metabolites, and by formation of pharmacologically inactive non-polar ceramide analogs of fingolimod.
Fingolimod is primarily metabolized via human CYP4F2 with a minor contribution of CYP2D6, 2E1, 3A4, and 4F12. Inhibitors or inducers of these isozymes might alter the exposure of fingolimod or fingolimod-phosphate. The involvement of multiple CYP isoenzymes in the oxidation of fingolimod suggests that the metabolism of fingolimod will not be subject to substantial inhibition in the presence of an inhibitor of a single specific CYP isozyme.
Following single oral administration of [^{14}C] fingolimod, the major fingolimod-related components in blood, as judged from their contribution to the AUC up to 816 hours post-dose of total radiolabeled components, are fingolimod itself (23.3%), fingolimod-phosphate (10.3%), and inactive metabolites [M3 carboxylic acid metabolite (8.3%), M29 ceramide metabolite (8.9%), and M30 ceramide metabolite (7.3%)].

Elimination
Fingolimod blood clearance is 6.3±2.3 L/h, and the average apparent terminal half-life ($t_{1/2}$) is 6-9 days. Blood levels of fingolimod-phosphate decline in parallel with those of fingolimod in the terminal phase, yielding similar half-lives for both.
After oral administration, about 81% of the dose is slowly excreted in the urine as inactive metabolites. Fingolimod and fingolimod-phosphate are not excreted intact in urine but are the major components in the feces with amounts of each representing less than 2.5% of the dose.

Special Populations

Renal Impairment

In patients with severe renal impairment, fingolimod C_{max} and AUC are increased by 32% and 43%, respectively, and fingolimod-phosphate C_{max} and AUC are increased by 25% and 14%, respectively, with no change in apparent elimination half-life. Based on these findings, the GILENYA 0.5 mg dose is appropriate for use in patients with renal impairment. The systemic exposure of two metabolites (M2 and M3) is increased by 3- and 13-fold, respectively. The toxicity of these metabolites has not been fully characterized.

A study in patients with mild or moderate renal impairment has not been conducted.

Hepatic Impairment

In subjects with mild, moderate, or severe hepatic impairment, no change in fingolimod C_{max} was observed, but fingolimod AUC was increased respectively by 12%, 44%, and 103%. In patients with severe hepatic impairment, fingolimod-phosphate C_{max} was decreased by 22% and AUC was not substantially changed. The pharmacokinetics of fingolimod-phosphate were not evaluated in patients with mild or moderate hepatic impairment. The apparent elimination half-life of fingolimod is unchanged in subjects with mild hepatic impairment, but is prolonged by about 50% in patients with moderate or severe hepatic impairment.

Patients with severe hepatic impairment should be closely monitored, as the risk of adverse reactions is greater [*See Warnings and Precautions (5.5)*].

No dose adjustment is needed in patients with mild or moderate hepatic impairment.

Race

The effects of race on fingolimod and fingolimod-phosphate pharmacokinetics cannot be adequately assessed due to a low number of non-white patients in the clinical program.

Gender

Gender has no clinically significant influence on fingolimod and fingolimod-phosphate pharmacokinetics.

Geriatric patients

The mechanism for elimination and results from population pharmacokinetics suggest that dose adjustment would not be necessary in elderly patients. However, clinical experience in patients aged above 65 years is limited.

Pharmacokinetic interactions

Ketoconazole

The coadministration of ketoconazole (a potent inhibitor of CYP3A and CYP4F) 200 mg twice daily at steady-state and a single dose of fingolimod 5 mg led to a 70% increase in AUC of fingolimod and fingolimod-phosphate. Patients who use GILENYA and systemic ketoconazole concomitantly should be closely monitored, as the risk of adverse reactions is greater. [*see Drug Interactions (7)*].

Potential of fingolimod and fingolimod-phosphate to inhibit the metabolism of co-medications

In vitro inhibition studies in pooled human liver microsomes and specific metabolic probe substrates demonstrate that fingolimod has little or no capacity to inhibit the activity of the following CYP450 enzymes: CYP1A2, CYP2A6, CYP2B6, CYP2C9, CYP2C19, CYP2D6, CYP2E1, CYP3A4/5, or CYP4A9/11, and similarly fingolimod-phosphate has little or no capacity to inhibit the activity of CYP1A2, CYP2A6, CYP2C8, CYP2C9, CYP2C19, CYP2D6, CYP2E1, or CYP3A4 at concentrations up to three orders of magnitude of therapeutic concentrations. Therefore, fingolimod and fingolimod-phosphate are unlikely to reduce the clearance of drugs that are mainly cleared through metabolism by the major cytochrome P450 isoenzymes described above. The potential of fingolimod to inhibit CYP2C8 and fingolimod-phosphate to inhibit CYP2B6 is unknown.

Potential of fingolimod and fingolimod-phosphate to induce its own and/or the metabolism of co-medications

Fingolimod was examined for its potential to induce human CYP3A4, CYP1A2, CYP4F2, and MDR1 (P-glycoprotein) mRNA and CYP3A, CYP1A2, CYP2B6, CYP2C8, CYP2C9, CYP2C19, and CYP4F2 activity in primary human hepatocytes. Fingolimod did not induce mRNA or activity of the different CYP450 enzymes and MDR1 with respect to the vehicle control; therefore, no clinically relevant induction of the tested CYP450 enzymes or MDR1 by fingolimod are expected at therapeutic concentrations. The potential of fingolimod-phosphate to induce CYP450 isoenzymes is unknown.

Transporters

Fingolimod as well as fingolimod-phosphate are not expected to inhibit the uptake of co-medications and/or biologics transported by OATP1B1, OATP1B3, or NTCP. Similarly, they are not expected to inhibit the efflux of co-medications and/or biologics transported by the breast cancer resistant protein (MXR), the bile salt export pump (BSEP), the multidrug resistance-associated protein 2 (MRP2), and MDR1-mediated transport at therapeutic concentrations.

Table 2. Clinical and MRI Results of Study 1

	GILENYA 0.5 mg N=425	Placebo N=418	p-value
Clinical Endpoints			
Annualized relapse rate (primary endpoint)	0.18	0.40	<0.001
Percentage of patients without relapse	70%	46%	<0.001
Hazard ratio‡ of disability progression (95% CI)	0.70 (0.52, 0.96)		0.02
MRI Endpoint			
Mean (median) number of new or newly enlarging T2 lesions over 24 months	2.5 (0)	9.8 (5.0)	<0.001

All analyses of clinical endpoints were intent-to-treat. MRI analysis used evaluable dataset.

‡ Hazard ratio is an estimate of relative risk of having the event of disability progression on GILENYA as compared to placebo.

Cyclosporine

The pharmacokinetics of single-dose fingolimod were not altered during coadministration with cyclosporine at steady-state, nor was cyclosporine steady-state pharmacokinetics altered by fingolimod. These data indicate that GILENYA is unlikely to reduce the clearance of drugs mainly cleared by CYP3A4 and show that the potent inhibition of transporters MDR1, MRP2, and OATP-C does not influence fingolimod disposition.

Isoproterenol, atropine, atenolol, and diltiazem

Single-dose fingolimod and fingolimod-phosphate exposure was not altered by coadministered isoproterenol or atropine. Likewise, the single-dose pharmacokinetics of fingolimod and fingolimod-phosphate and the steady-state pharmacokinetics of both atenolol and diltiazem were unchanged during the coadministration of the latter two drugs individually with fingolimod.

Population pharmacokinetics analysis

A population pharmacokinetics evaluation performed in MS patients did not provide evidence for a significant effect of fluoxetine and paroxetine (strong CYP2D6 inhibitors) and carbamazepine (potent enzyme inducer) on fingolimod or fingolimod-phosphate pre-dose concentrations. In addition, the following commonly co-prescribed substances had no clinically relevant effect (<20%) on fingolimod or fingolimod-phosphate pre-dose concentrations: baclofen, gabapentin, oxybutynin, amantadine, modafinil, amitriptyline, pregabalin, and corticosteroids.

13 NONCLINICAL TOXICOLOGY

13.1 Carcinogenesis, Mutagenesis, Impairment of Fertility

Oral carcinogenicity studies of fingolimod were conducted in mice and rats. In mice, fingolimod was administered at oral doses of 0, 0.025, 0.25, and 2.5 mg/kg/day for up to 2 years. The incidence of malignant lymphoma was increased in males and females at the mid and high dose. The lowest dose tested (0.025 mg/kg/day) is less than the recommended human dose (RHD) of 0.5 mg/day on a body surface area (mg/m^2) basis. In rats, fingolimod was administered at oral doses of 0, 0.05, 0.15, 0.5, and 2.5 mg/kg/day. No increase in tumors was observed. The highest dose tested (2.5 mg/kg/day) is approximately 50 times the RHD on a mg/m^2 basis.

Fingolimod was negative in a battery of *in vitro* (Ames, mouse lymphoma thymidine kinase, chromosomal aberration in mammalian cells) and *in vivo* (micronucleus in mouse and rat) assays.

When fingolimod was administered orally (0, 1, 3, and 10 mg/kg/day) to male and female rats prior to and during mating, and continuing to Day 7 of gestation in females, no effect on fertility was observed up to the highest dose tested (10 mg/kg), which is approximately 200 times the RHD on a mg/m^2 basis.

13.2 Animal Toxicology and/or Pharmacology

Lung toxicity was observed in two different strains of rat and in dog and monkey. The primary findings included increase in lung weight, associated with smooth muscle hypertrophy, hyperdistension of the alveoli, and/or increased collagen. Insufficient or lack of pulmonary collapse at necropsy, generally correlated with microscopic changes, was observed in all species. In rat and monkey, lung toxicity was observed at all oral doses tested in chronic studies. The lowest doses tested in rat (0.05 mg/kg/day in the 2-year carcinogenicity study) and monkey (0.5 mg/kg/day in the 39-week toxicity study) are similar to and approximately 20 times the RHD on a mg/m^2 basis, respectively.

In the 52-week oral study in monkey, respiratory distress associated with ketamine administration was observed at doses of 3 and 10 mg/kg/day; the most affected animal became hypoxic and required oxygenation. As ketamine is not generally associated with respiratory depression, this effect was attributed to fingolimod. In a subsequent study in rat, ketamine was shown to potentiate the bronchoconstrictive effects of fingolimod. The relevance of these findings to humans is unknown.

14 CLINICAL STUDIES

The efficacy of GILENYA was demonstrated in 2 studies that evaluated once-daily doses of GILENYA 0.5 mg and 1.25 mg in patients with relapsing remitting MS (RRMS). Both studies included patients who had experienced at least 2 clinical relapses during the 2 years prior to randomization or at least 1 clinical relapse during the 1 year prior to randomization, and had an Expanded Disability Status Scale (EDSS) score from 0 to 5.5. Study 1 was a 2-year randomized, double-blind, placebo-controlled study in patients with RRMS who had not received any interferon-beta or glatiramer acetate for at least the previous 3 months and had not received any natalizumab for at least the previous 6 months. Neurological evaluations were performed at screening, every 3 months and at time of suspected relapse. MRI evaluations were performed at screening, month 6, month 12, and month 24. The primary endpoint was the annualized relapse rate.

Median age was 37 years, median disease duration was 6.7 years and median EDSS score at baseline was 2.0. Patients were randomized to receive GILENYA 0.5 mg (n=425), 1.25 mg (n=429), or placebo (n=418) for up to 24 months. Median time on study drug was 717 days on 0.5 mg, 715 days on 1.25 mg and 719 days on placebo.

The annualized relapse rate was significantly lower in patients treated with GILENYA than in patients who received placebo. The secondary endpoint was the time to 3-month confirmed disability progression as measured by at least a 1-point increase from baseline in EDSS (0.5 point increase for patients with baseline EDSS of 5.5) sustained for 3 months. Time to onset of 3-month confirmed disability progression was significantly delayed with GILENYA treatment compared to placebo. The 1.25 mg dose resulted in no additional benefit over the GILENYA 0.5 mg dose. The results for this study are shown in Table 2 and Figure 1.

[See table 2 above]

Figure 1 Time to 3-month Confirmed Disability Progression – Study 1 (ITT population)

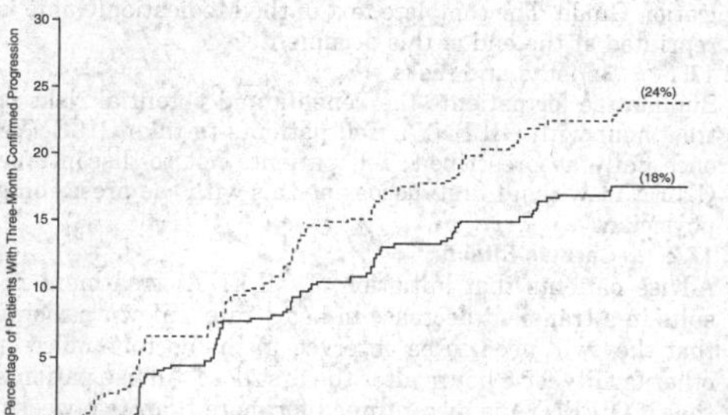

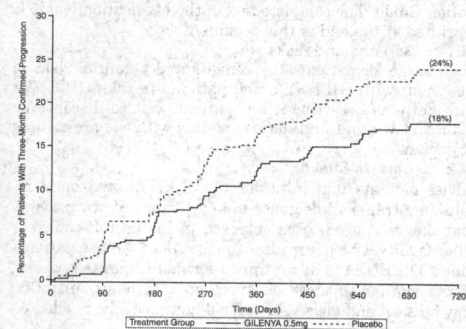

Study 2 was a 1-year randomized, double-blind, double-dummy, active-controlled study in patients with RRMS who had not received any natalizumab in the previous 6 months. Prior therapy with interferon-beta or glatiramer acetate up to the time of randomization was permitted.

Neurological evaluations were performed at screening, every 3 months, and at the time of suspected relapses. MRI evaluations were performed at screening and at month 12. The primary endpoint was the annualized relapse rate.

Median age was 36 years, median disease duration was 5.9 years, and median EDSS score at baseline was 2.0. Patients were randomized to receive GILENYA 0.5 mg (n=431), 1.25 mg (n=426), or interferon beta-1a, 30 micrograms via the intramuscular route (IM) once weekly (n=435) for up to 12 months. Median time on study drug was 365 days on GILENYA 0.5 mg, 354 days on 1.25 mg, and 361 days on interferon beta-1a IM.

Table 3 Clinical and MRI Results of Study 2

	GILENYA 0.5 mg N=429	Interferon beta-1a IM 30 µg N=431	p-value
Clinical Endpoints			
Annualized relapse rate (primary endpoint)	0.16	0.33	<0.001
Percentage of patients without relapse	83%	70%	<0.001
Hazard ratio‡ of disability progression (95% CI)	0.71 (0.42, 1.21)		0.21
MRI Endpoint			
Mean (median) number of new or newly enlarging T2 lesions over 12 months	1.6 (0)	2.6 (1.0)	0.002

All analyses of clinical endpoints were intent-to-treat. MRI analysis used evaluable dataset.

‡ Hazard ratio is an estimate of the relative risk of having the event of disability progression on GILENYA as compared to control.

The annualized relapse rate was significantly lower in patients treated with GILENYA 0.5 mg than in patients who received interferon beta-1a IM. The key secondary endpoints were number of new and newly enlarging T2 lesions and time to onset of 3-month confirmed disability progression as measured by at least a 1-point increase from baseline in EDSS (0.5 point increase for those with baseline EDSS of 5.5) sustained for 3 months. The number of new and newly enlarging T2 lesions was significantly lower in patients treated with GILENYA than in patients who received interferon beta-1a IM. There was no significant difference in the time to 3-month confirmed disability progression between GILENYA and interferon beta-1a-treated patients at 1 year. The 1.25 mg dose resulted in no additional benefit over the GILENYA 0.5 mg dose. The results for this study are shown in Table 3.

[See table 3 above]

Pooled results of study 1 and study 2 showed a consistent and statistically significant reduction of annualized relapse rate compared to comparator in subgroups defined by gender, age, prior MS therapy, and disease activity.

16 HOW SUPPLIED/STORAGE AND HANDLING

0.5 mg GILENYA capsules are hard gelatin capsules with a white opaque body and bright yellow cap imprinted with "FTY 0.5 mg" on the cap and two radial bands imprinted on the capsule body with yellow ink.

GILENYA capsules are supplied in blister packs.

Carton of 28 capsules containing 2 folded blister cards of 14 capsules per blister card .... NDC 0078-0607-51

Carton of 7 capsules containing 1 blister card of 7 capsules per blister card .... NDC 0078-0607-89

GILENYA capsules should be stored at 25°C (77°F); excursions permitted to 15-30°C (59-86°F).

Protect from moisture.

17 PATIENT COUNSELING INFORMATION

See Medication Guide.

A Medication Guide is required for distribution with GILENYA. Encourage patients to read the GILENYA Medication Guide. The complete text of the Medication Guide is reprinted at the end of this document.

17.1 Benefits and Risks

Summarize for patients the benefits and potential risks of treatment with GILENYA. Tell patients to take GILENYA once daily as prescribed. Tell patients not to discontinue GILENYA without first discussing this with the prescribing physician.

17.2 Cardiac Effects

Advise patients that initiation of GILENYA treatment results in a transient decrease in heart rate. Inform patients that they will need to be observed in the doctor's office or other facility for 6 hours after the first dose. Advise patients that if GILENYA is discontinued for more than two weeks, effects similar to those observed on treatment initiation may be seen and observation for 6 hours will be needed on treatment re-initiation.

17.3 Risk of Infections

Inform patients that they may be more likely to get infections when taking GILENYA, and that they should contact their physician if they develop symptoms of infection. Advise patients that the use of some vaccines should be avoided during treatment with GILENYA and for 2 months after discontinuation. Advise patients who have not had chickenpox or vaccination to consider VZV vaccination prior to commencing treatment with GILENYA.

17.4 Macular Edema

Advise patients that GILENYA may cause macular edema, and that they should contact their physician if they experience any changes in their vision. Inform patients with diabetes mellitus or a history of uveitis that their risk of macular edema is increased.

17.5 Respiratory Effects

Advise patients that they should contact their physician if they experience new onset or worsening of dyspnea.

17.6 Hepatic Effects

Inform patients that GILENYA may increase liver enzymes. Advise patients that they should contact their physician if they have any unexplained nausea, vomiting, abdominal pain, fatigue, anorexia, or jaundice and/or dark urine.

17.7 Fetal Risk

Inform patients that, based on animal studies, GILENYA may cause fetal harm. Discuss with women of childbearing age whether they are pregnant, might be pregnant or are trying to become pregnant. Advise women of childbearing age of the need for effective contraception during GILENYA treatment and for two months after stopping GILENYA. Advise the patient that if she should nevertheless become pregnant, she should immediately inform her physician.

17.8 Persistence of GILENYA Effects After Drug Discontinuation

Advise patients that GILENYA remains in the blood and continues to have effects, including decreased blood lymphocyte counts, for up to two months following the last dose.

MEDICATION GUIDE

GILENYA™ (je-LEN-yah)

(fingolimod)

capsules

Read this Medication Guide before you start using GILENYA and each time you get a refill. There may be new information. This information does not take the place of talking with your doctor about your medical condition or your treatment.

What is the most important information I should know about GILENYA?

GILENYA may cause serious side effects, including:

1. **Slow Heart Rate (bradycardia or bradyarrhythmia) when you start taking GILENYA.** GILENYA can cause your heart rate to slow down, especially after you take the first dose. Your heart rate will usually slow down the most about 6 hours after you take your first dose of GILENYA. You might feel dizzy or tired or be aware of a slow or irregular heartbeat if your heart rate slows down. Usually, if you experience these types of symptoms due to the slowing down of your heart rate, they will occur during the first 6 hours after the first dose. Your doctor will watch you for the first 6 hours after you take the first dose to see if you have any serious side effects. Your slow heart rate will usually return to normal within 1 month after you start taking GILENYA.

Call your doctor if at any time you have:
- dizziness
- tiredness
- a slow or irregular heartbeat

2. **Infections.** GILENYA can increase your risk of serious infections. GILENYA lowers the number of white blood cells (lymphocytes) in your blood. This will usually go back to normal within 2 months of stopping treatment. Your doctor may do a blood test before you start taking GILENYA. Call your doctor right away if you have any of these symptoms of an infection:
- fever
- tiredness
- body aches
- chills
- nausea
- vomiting

3. **A problem with your vision called macular edema.** Macular edema can cause some of the same vision symptoms as an MS attack (optic neuritis). You may not notice any symptoms with macular edema. Macular edema usually starts in the first 3 to 4 months after you start taking GILENYA. Your doctor should test your vision before you start taking GILENYA and 3 to 4 months after you start taking GILENYA, or any time you notice vision changes during treatment with GILENYA. Your risk of macular edema may be higher if you have diabetes or have had an inflammation of your eye called uveitis.

Call your doctor right away if you have any of the following:
- blurriness or shadows in the center of your vision
- a blind spot in the center of your vision
- sensitivity to light
- unusually colored (tinted) vision

What is GILENYA?

GILENYA is a prescription medicine used to treat relapsing forms of multiple sclerosis (MS) in adults. GILENYA can decrease the number of MS flare-ups (relapses). GILENYA does not cure MS, but it can help slow down the physical problems that MS causes.

It is not known if GILENYA is safe and effective in children under age 18.

What should I tell my doctor before taking GILENYA?

Before you take GILENYA, tell your doctor about all your medical conditions, including if you had or now have:
- an irregular or abnormal heartbeat (arrhythmia)
- a heart rate less than 55 beats a minute
- heart problems
- a history of fainting (syncope)
- a fever or infection, or you are unable to fight infections. Tell your doctor if you have had chicken pox or have received the vaccine for chicken pox. Your doctor may do a blood test for chicken pox virus. You may need to get the vaccine for chicken pox and then wait 1 month before you start taking GILENYA.
- eye problems, especially an inflammation of the eye called uveitis
- diabetes
- breathing problems
- liver problems
- high blood pressure
- Are pregnant or plan to become pregnant. GILENYA may harm your unborn baby. Talk to your doctor if you are pregnant or are planning to become pregnant.
  - Tell your doctor right away if you become pregnant while taking GILENYA or if you become pregnant within 2 months after you stop taking GILENYA.
  - If you are a female who can become pregnant, you should use effective birth control during your treatment with GILENYA and for at least 2 months after you stop taking GILENYA.

Pregnancy Registry: There is a registry for women who become pregnant during treatment with GILENYA. If you become pregnant while taking GILENYA, talk to your doctor about registering with the GILENYA Pregnancy Registry. The purpose of this registry is to collect information about your health and your baby's health.

For more information, you can call the GILENYA Pregnancy Registry at 1-877-598-7237.
- Are breastfeeding or plan to breastfeed. It is not known if GILENYA passes into your breast milk. You and your doctor should decide if you will take GILENYA or breastfeed. You should not do both.

Tell your doctor about all the medicines you take, including prescription and non-prescription medicines, vitamins, and herbal supplements.

Know the medicines you take. Keep a list of your medicines with you to show your doctor and pharmacist when you get a new medicine.

Using GILENYA and other medicines together may affect each other causing serious side effects.

Especially tell your doctor if you take:
- Medicines for heart problems or high blood pressure
- Vaccines. Tell your doctor if you have been vaccinated within 1 month before you start taking GILENYA. You should not get certain vaccines while you take GILENYA and for at least 2 months after you stop taking GILENYA. If you take certain vaccines, you may get the infection the vaccine should have prevented. Vaccines may not work as well when given during GILENYA treatment.
- Medicines that could raise your chance of getting infections, such as medicines to treat cancer or to control your immune system.
- ketoconazole (an antifungal drug) by mouth

Ask your doctor or pharmacist for a list of these medicines if you are not sure.

How should I take GILENYA?
- Your first dose of GILENYA will be given in a doctor's office or clinic, where you will be observed for 6 hours after your first dose of GILENYA.
- Take GILENYA exactly as your doctor tells you to take it.
- Take GILENYA 1 time each day.
- Take GILENYA with or without food.
- Do not stop taking GILENYA without talking with your doctor first.
- If you start GILENYA again after stopping for 2 weeks or more, you will start taking GILENYA again in your doctor's office or clinic.

What are possible side effects of GILENYA?

GILENYA can cause serious side effects.

See "What is the most important information I should know about GILENYA?"

Serious side effects include:
- **Breathing Problems.** Some people who take GILENYA have shortness of breath. Call your doctor right away if you have trouble breathing.
- **Liver problems.** GILENYA may cause liver problems. Your doctor should do blood tests to check your liver before you start taking GILENYA. Call your doctor right away if you have any of the following symptoms of liver problems:
  - nausea
  - vomiting
  - stomach pain
  - loss of appetite
  - tiredness
  - your skin or the whites of your eyes turn yellow
  - dark urine

The most common side effects of GILENYA include:
- headache
- flu
- diarrhea
- back pain
- abnormal liver tests
- cough

Tell your doctor if you have any side effect that bothers you or that does not go away.

These are not all of the possible side effects of GILENYA. For more information, ask your doctor or pharmacist. Call your doctor for medical advice about side effects. You may report side effects to FDA at 1-800-332-1088.

How do I store GILENYA?
- Store GILENYA in the original blister pack in a dry place.
- Store GILENYA at room temperature between 59°F to 86°F (15°C to 30°C).
- Keep GILENYA and all medicines out of the reach of children.

General information about GILENYA

Medicines are sometimes prescribed for purposes other than those listed in a Medication Guide. Do not use GILENYA for a condition for which it was not prescribed. Do not give GILENYA to other people, even if they have the same symptoms you have. It may harm them.

This Medication Guide summarizes the most important information about GILENYA. If you would like more information, talk with your doctor. You can ask your doctor or pharmacist for information about GILENYA that is written for healthcare professionals.

For more information, go to www.pharma.US.Novartis.com or call 1-888-669-6682.

What are the ingredients in GILENYA?
Active ingredient: fingolimod
Inactive ingredients: gelatin, magnesium stearate, mannitol, titanium dioxide, yellow iron oxide.

This Medication Guide has been approved by the U.S. Food and Drug Administration.

GILENYA is a trademark of Novartis AG.

Issued September 2010

T2010-81/T2010-82
5002679
Printed in the USA

Manufactured by:
Novartis Pharma Stein AG
Stein, Switzerland
Distributed by:
Novartis Pharmaceuticals Corporation
East Hanover, New Jersey 07936
© Novartis

GLEEVEC® ℞

[glē-věk]
(imatinib mesylate)
Tablets for Oral Use

The following prescribing information is based on labeling in effect July 2010.

HIGHLIGHTS OF PRESCRIBING INFORMATION
These highlights do not include all the information needed to use Gleevec safely and effectively. See full prescribing information for Gleevec.

GLEEVEC (imatinib mesylate) **tablets for oral use**
Initial U.S. Approval: 2001

RECENT MAJOR CHANGES

Indications and Usage: Newly Diagnosed
Ph+ CML (1.1)   05/2009

INDICATIONS AND USAGE

Gleevec is a kinase inhibitor indicated for the treatment of:
- Newly diagnosed adult patients with Philadelphia chromosome positive chronic myeloid leukemia (Ph+ CML) in chronic phase
- Patients with Philadelphia chromosome positive chronic myeloid leukemia (Ph+ CML) in blast crisis (BC), accelerated phase (AP), or in chronic phase (CP) after failure of interferon-alpha therapy (1.2)
- Pediatric patients with Ph+ CML in chronic phase who are newly diagnosed or whose disease has recurred after stem cell transplant or who are resistant to interferon-

alpha therapy. There are no controlled trials in pediatric patients demonstrating a clinical benefit, such as improvement in disease-related symptoms or increased survival (1.3)
- Adult patients with relapsed or refractory Philadelphia chromosome positive acute lymphoblastic leukemia (Ph+ ALL) (1.4)
- Adult patients with myelodysplastic/myeloproliferative diseases (MDS/MPD) associated with PDGFR (platelet-derived growth factor receptor) gene re-arrangements (1.5)
- Adult patients with aggressive systemic mastocytosis (ASM) without the D816V c-Kit mutation or with c-Kit mutational status unknown (1.6)
- Adult patients with hypereosinophilic syndrome (HES) and/or chronic eosinophilic leukemia (CEL) who have the FIP1L1-PDGFRα fusion kinase (mutational analysis or FISH demonstration of CHIC2 allele deletion) and for patients with HES and/or CEL who are FIP1L1-PDGFRα fusion kinase negative or unknown (1.7)
- Adult patients with unresectable, recurrent and/or metastatic dermatofibrosarcoma protuberans (DFSP) (1.8)
- Patients with Kit (CD117) positive unresectable and/or metastatic malignant gastrointestinal stromal tumors (GIST) (1.9)
- Adjuvant treatment of adult patients following resection of Kit (CD117) positive GIST (1.10)

DOSAGE AND ADMINISTRATION

- Adults with Ph+ CML CP (2.1): 400 mg/day
- Adults with Ph+ CML AP or BC (2.1): 600 mg/day
- Pediatrics with Ph+ CML (2.2): 340 mg/m²/day or 260 mg/m²/day
- Adults with Ph+ ALL (2.3): 600 mg/day
- Adults with MDS/MPD (2.4): 400 mg/day
- Adults with ASM (2.5): 100 mg/day or 400 mg/day
- Adults with HES/CEL (2.6): 100 mg/day or 400 mg/day
- Adults with DFSP (2.7): 800 mg/day
- Adults with metastatic and/or unresectable GIST (2.8): 400 mg/day
- Adjuvant treatment of adults with GIST (2.8): 400 mg/day
- Patients with mild to moderate hepatic impairment (2.9): 400 mg/day
- Patients with severe hepatic impairment (2.9): 300 mg/day

All doses of Gleevec should be taken with a meal and a large glass of water. Doses of 400 mg or 600 mg should be administered once daily, whereas a dose of 800 mg should be administered as 400 mg twice a day. Gleevec can be dissolved in water or apple juice for patients having difficulty swallowing. Daily dosing of 800 mg and above should be accomplished using the 400 mg tablet to reduce exposure to iron.

DOSAGE FORMS AND STRENGTHS

Tablets (scored): 100 mg and 400 mg (3)

CONTRAINDICATIONS

None (4)

WARNINGS AND PRECAUTIONS

- Edema and severe fluid retention have occurred. Weigh patients regularly and manage unexpected rapid weight gain by drug interruption and diuretics (5.1, 6.1, 6.11)
- Cytopenias, particularly anemia, neutropenia, and thrombocytopenia, have occurred. Manage with dose reduction or dose interruption and in rare cases discontinuation of treatment. Perform complete blood counts weekly for the first month, biweekly for the second month, and periodically thereafter (5.2)
- Severe congestive heart failure and left ventricular dysfunction have been reported, particularly in patients with comorbidities and risk factors. Patients with cardiac disease or risk factors for cardiac failure should be monitored and treated (5.3)
- Severe hepatotoxicity may occur. Assess liver function before initiation of treatment and monthly thereafter or as clinically indicated. Monitor liver function when combined with chemotherapy known to be associated with liver dysfunction (5.4)
- Grade 3/4 hemorrhage has been reported in clinical studies in patients with newly diagnosed CML and with GIST. GI tumor sites may be the source of GI bleeds in GIST (5.5)
- Gastrointestinal perforations, some fatal, have been reported (5.6)
- Cardiogenic shock/left ventricular dysfunction has been associated with the initiation of Gleevec in patients with conditions associated with high eosinophil levels (e.g., HES, MDS/MPD and ASM) (5.7)
- Bullous dermatologic reactions (e.g., erythema multiforme and Stevens-Johnson syndrome) have been reported with the use of Gleevec (5.8)
- Hypothyroidism has been reported in thyroidectomy patients undergoing levothyroxine replacement. Closely monitor TSH levels in such patients (5.9)

- Consider potential toxicities, specifically, liver, kidney, and cardiac toxicity, and immunosuppression from long-term use (5.10)
- Fetal harm can occur when administered to a pregnant woman. Women should be apprised of the potential harm to the fetus (5.11, 8.1)

ADVERSE REACTIONS

The most frequently reported adverse reactions (≥30%) were edema, nausea, vomiting, muscle cramps, musculoskeletal pain, diarrhea, rash, fatigue and abdominal pain (6.1, 6.11)

To report SUSPECTED ADVERSE REACTIONS, contact Novartis Pharmaceuticals Corporation at 1-888-669-6682 or FDA at 1-800-FDA-1088 or www.fda.gov/medwatch.

DRUG INTERACTIONS

- CYP3A4 inducers may decrease Gleevec C_{max} and AUC (2.9, 7.1)
- CYP3A4 inhibitors may increase Gleevec C_{max} and AUC (7.2)
- Gleevec is an inhibitor of CYP3A4 and CYP2D6 which may increase the C_{max} and AUC of other drugs (7.3, 7.4)
- Patients who require anticoagulation should receive low-molecular weight or standard heparin and not warfarin (7.3)
- Systemic exposure to acetaminophen is expected to increase when co-administered with Gleevec (7.5)

USE IN SPECIFIC POPULATIONS

- There is no experience in children less than 2 years of age (8.4)

See 17 for PATIENT COUNSELING INFORMATION
Revised: 02/2010

FULL PRESCRIBING INFORMATION

1 INDICATIONS AND USAGE

1.1 Newly Diagnosed Philadelphia Positive Chronic Myeloid Leukemia (Ph+ CML)

Newly diagnosed adult patients with Philadelphia chromosome positive chronic myeloid leukemia in chronic phase.

1.2 Ph+ CML in Blast Crisis (BC), Accelerated Phase (AP) or Chronic Phase (CP) After Interferon-alpha (IFN) Therapy

Patients with Philadelphia chromosome positive chronic myeloid leukemia in blast crisis, accelerated phase, or in chronic phase after failure of interferon-alpha therapy.

1.3 Pediatric Patients with Ph+ CML in Chronic Phase

Pediatric patients with Ph+ CML in chronic phase who are newly diagnosed or whose disease has recurred after stem cell transplant or who are resistant to interferon-alpha therapy. There are no controlled trials in pediatric patients demonstrating a clinical benefit, such as improvement in disease-related symptoms or increased survival.

1.4 Ph+ Acute Lymphoblastic Leukemia (ALL)

Adult patients with relapsed or refractory Philadelphia chromosome positive acute lymphoblastic leukemia.

1.5 Myelodysplastic/Myeloproliferative Diseases (MDS/MPD)

Adult patients with myelodysplastic/myeloproliferative diseases associated with PDGFR (platelet-derived growth factor receptor) gene re-arrangements.

1.6 Aggressive Systemic Mastocytosis (ASM)

Adult patients with aggressive systemic mastocytosis without the D816V c-Kit mutation or with c-Kit mutational status unknown.

1.7 Hypereosinophilic Syndrome (HES) and/or Chronic Eosinophilic Leukemia (CEL)

Adult patients with hypereosinophilic syndrome and/or chronic eosinophilic leukemia who have the FIP1L1-PDGFRα fusion kinase (mutational analysis or FISH demonstration of CHIC2 allele deletion) and for patients with HES and/or CEL who are FIP1L1-PDGFRα fusion kinase negative or unknown.

1.8 Dermatofibrosarcoma Protuberans (DFSP)

Adult patients with unresectable, recurrent and/or metastatic dermatofibrosarcoma protuberans.

1.9 Kit+ Gastrointestinal Stromal Tumors (GIST)

Patients with Kit (CD117) positive unresectable and/or metastatic malignant gastrointestinal stromal tumors.

1.10 Adjuvant Treatment of GIST

Adjuvant treatment of adult patients following complete gross resection of Kit (CD117) positive GIST.

2 DOSAGE AND ADMINISTRATION

Therapy should be initiated by a physician experienced in the treatment of patients with hematological malignancies or malignant sarcomas, as appropriate. The prescribed dose should be administered orally, with a meal and a large glass of water. Doses of 400 mg or 600 mg should be administered once daily, whereas a dose of 800 mg should be administered as 400 mg twice a day.

In children, Gleevec treatment can be given as a once-daily dose or alternatively the daily dose may be split into two - once in the morning and once in the evening. There is no experience with Gleevec treatment in children under 2 years of age.

For patients unable to swallow the film-coated tablets, the tablets may be dispersed in a glass of water or apple juice. The required number of tablets should be placed in the appropriate volume of beverage (approximately 50 mL for a 100 mg tablet, and 200 mL for a 400 mg tablet) and stirred with a spoon. The suspension should be administered immediately after complete disintegration of the tablet(s).

For daily dosing of 800 mg and above, dosing should be accomplished using the 400 mg tablet to reduce exposure to iron.

Treatment may be continued as long as there is no evidence of progressive disease or unacceptable toxicity.

2.1 Adult Patients with Ph+ CML CP, AP and BC

The recommended dose of Gleevec is 400 mg/day for adult patients in chronic phase CML and 600 mg/day for adult patients in accelerated phase or blast crisis.

In CML, a dose increase from 400 mg to 600 mg in adult patients with chronic phase disease, or from 600 mg to 800 mg (given as 400 mg twice daily) in adult patients in accelerated phase or blast crisis may be considered in the absence of severe adverse drug reaction and severe non-leukemia related neutropenia or thrombocytopenia in the following circumstances: disease progression (at any time), failure to achieve a satisfactory hematologic response after at least 3 months of treatment, failure to achieve a cytogenetic response after 6-12 months of treatment, or loss of a previously achieved hematologic or cytogenetic response.

2.2 Pediatric Patients with Ph+ CML

The recommended dose of Gleevec for children with newly diagnosed Ph+ CML is 340 mg/m²/day (not to exceed 600 mg). The recommended Gleevec dose is 260 mg/m²/day for children with Ph+ chronic phase CML recurrent after stem cell transplant or who are resistant to interferon-alpha therapy.

2.3 Ph+ ALL

The recommended dose of Gleevec is 600 mg/day for adult patients with relapsed/refractory Ph+ ALL.

2.4 MDS/MPD

The recommended dose of Gleevec is 400 mg/day for adult patients with MDS/MPD.

2.5 ASM

The recommended dose of Gleevec is 400 mg/day for adult patients with ASM without the D816V c-Kit mutation. If c-Kit mutational status is not known or unavailable, treatment with Gleevec 400 mg/day may be considered for patients with ASM not responding satisfactorily to other therapies. For patients with ASM associated with eosinophilia, a clonal hematological disease related to the fusion kinase FIP1L1-PDGFRα, a starting dose of 100 mg/day is recommended. Dose increase from 100 mg to 400 mg for these patients may be considered in the absence of adverse drug reactions if assessments demonstrate an insufficient response to therapy.

2.6 HES/CEL

The recommended dose of Gleevec is 400 mg/day for adult patients with HES/CEL. For HES/CEL patients with demonstrated FIP1L1-PDGFRα fusion kinase, a starting dose of 100 mg/day is recommended. Dose increase from 100 mg to 400 mg for these patients may be considered in the absence of adverse drug reactions if assessments demonstrate an insufficient response to therapy.

2.7 DFSP

The recommended dose of Gleevec is 800 mg/day for adult patients with DFSP.

2.8 GIST

The recommended dose of Gleevec is 400 mg/day for adult patients with unresectable and/or metastatic, malignant GIST. A dose increase up to 800 mg daily (given as 400 mg twice daily) may be considered, as clinically indicated, in

Table 1: Dose Adjustments for Neutropenia and Thrombocytopenia

ASM associated with eosinophilia (starting dose 100 mg)	ANC <1.0 × 10⁹/L and/or platelets <50 × 10⁹/L	1. Stop Gleevec until ANC ≥1.5 × 10⁹/L and platelets ≥75 × 10⁹/L 2. Resume treatment with Gleevec at previous dose (i.e., dose before severe adverse reaction)
HES/CEL with FIP1L1-PDGFRα fusion kinase (starting dose 100 mg)	ANC <1.0 × 10⁹/L and/or platelets <50 × 10⁹/L	1. Stop Gleevec until ANC ≥1.5 × 10⁹/L and platelets ≥75 × 10⁹/L 2. Resume treatment with Gleevec at previous dose (i.e., dose before severe adverse reaction)
Chronic Phase CML (starting dose 400 mg) MDS/MPD, ASM and HES/CEL (starting dose 400 mg) GIST (starting dose 400 mg)	ANC <1.0 × 10⁹/L and/or platelets <50 × 10⁹/L	1. Stop Gleevec until ANC ≥1.5 × 10⁹/L and platelets ≥75 × 10⁹/L 2. Resume treatment with Gleevec at the original starting dose of 400 mg 3. If recurrence of ANC <1.0 × 10⁹/L and/or platelets <50 × 10⁹/L, repeat step 1 and resume Gleevec at a reduced dose of 300 mg
Ph+ CML: Accelerated Phase and Blast Crisis (starting dose 600 mg) Ph+ ALL (starting dose 600 mg)	ANC <0.5 × 10⁹/L and/or platelets <10 × 10⁹/L	1. Check if cytopenia is related to leukemia (marrow aspirate or biopsy) 2. If cytopenia is unrelated to leukemia, reduce dose of Gleevec to 400 mg 3. If cytopenia persists 2 weeks, reduce further to 300 mg 4. If cytopenia persists 4 weeks and is still unrelated to leukemia, stop Gleevec until ANC ≥1 × 10⁹/L and platelets ≥20 × 10⁹/L and then resume treatment at 300 mg
DFSP (starting dose 800 mg)	ANC <1.0 × 10⁹/L and/or platelets <50 × 10⁹/L	1. Stop Gleevec until ANC ≥1.5 × 10⁹/L and platelets ≥75 × 10⁹/L 2. Resume treatment with Gleevec at 600 mg 3. In the event of recurrence of ANC <1.0 × 10⁹L and/or platelets <50 × 10⁹L, repeat step 1 and resume Gleevec at reduced dose of 400 mg
Pediatric newly diagnosed chronic phase CML (starting dose 340 mg/m²)	ANC <1.0 × 10⁹/L and/or platelets <50 × 10⁹/L	1. Stop Gleevec until ANC ≥1.5 × 10⁹/L and platelets ≥75 × 10⁹/L 2. Resume treatment with Gleevec at previous dose (i.e., dose before severe adverse reaction) 3. In the event of recurrence of ANC <1.0 × 10⁹L and/or platelets <50 × 10⁹/L, repeat step 1 and resume Gleevec at reduced dose of 260 mg/m²
Pediatric patients with chronic phase CML recurring after transplant or resistant to Interferon (starting dose 260 mg/m²)	ANC <1.0 × 10⁹/L and/or platelets <50 × 10⁹/L	1. Stop Gleevec until ANC ≥1.5 × 10⁹/L and platelets ≥75 × 10⁹/L 2. Resume treatment with Gleevec at previous dose (i.e., dose before severe adverse reaction) 3. In the event of recurrence of ANC <1.0 × 10⁹/L and/or platelets <50 × 10⁹/L, repeat step 1 and resume Gleevec at reduced dose of 200 mg/m²

patients showing clear signs or symptoms of disease progression at a lower dose and in the absence of severe adverse drug reactions.

The recommended dose of Gleevec is 400 mg/day for the adjuvant treatment of adult patients following complete gross resection of GIST. In the clinical study, Gleevec was administered for one year. The optimal treatment duration with Gleevec is not known.

2.9 Dose Modification Guidelines

Concomitant Strong CYP3A4 Inducers: The use of concomitant strong CYP3A4 inducers should be avoided (e.g., dexamethasone, phenytoin, carbamazepine, rifampin, rifabutin, rifampacin, phenobarbital). If patients must be co-administered a strong CYP3A4 inducer, based on pharmacokinetic studies, the dosage of Gleevec should be increased by at least 50%, and clinical response should be carefully monitored [see Drug Interactions (7.1)].

Hepatic Impairment: Patients with mild and moderate hepatic impairment do not require a dose adjustment and should be treated per the recommended dose. A 25% decrease in the recommended dose should be used for patients with severe hepatic impairment [see Use in Specific Populations (8.6)].

Renal Impairment: Patients with moderate renal impairment (CrCL = 20-39 mL/min) should receive a 50% decrease in the recommended starting dose and future doses can be increased as tolerated. Doses greater than 600 mg are not recommended in patients with mild renal impairment (CrCL = 40-59 mL/min). For patients with moderate renal impairment doses greater than 400 mg are not recommended.

Imatinib should be used with caution in patients with severe renal impairment. A dose of 100 mg/day was tolerated in two patients with severe renal impairment. [See Use in Specific Populations (8.7)]

2.10 Dose Adjustment for Hepatotoxicity and Non-Hematologic Adverse Reactions

If elevations in bilirubin >3 × institutional upper limit of normal (IULN) or in liver transaminases >5 × IULN occur, Gleevec should be withheld until bilirubin levels have returned to a <1.5 × IULN and transaminase levels to <2.5 × IULN. In adults, treatment with Gleevec may then be continued at a reduced daily dose (i.e., 400 mg to 300 mg, 600 mg to 400 mg or 800 mg to 600 mg). In children, daily doses can be reduced under the same circumstances from 340 mg/m^2/day to 260 mg/m^2/day or from 260 mg/m^2/day to 200 mg/m^2/day, respectively.

If a severe non-hematologic adverse reaction develops (such as severe hepatotoxicity or severe fluid retention), Gleevec should be withheld until the event has resolved. Thereafter, treatment can be resumed as appropriate depending on the initial severity of the event.

2.11 Dose Adjustment for Hematologic Adverse Reactions

Dose reduction or treatment interruptions for severe neutropenia and thrombocytopenia are recommended as indicated in Table 1.

[See table 1 at top of previous page]

3 DOSAGE FORMS AND STRENGTHS

100 mg film-coated tablets
Very dark yellow to brownish orange, film-coated tablets, round, biconvex with bevelled edges, debossed with "NVR" on one side, and "SA" with score on the other side
400 mg film-coated tablets
Very dark yellow to brownish orange, film-coated tablets, ovaloid, biconvex with bevelled edges, debossed with "400" on one side with score on the other side, and "SL" on each side of the score

4 CONTRAINDICATIONS

None

5 WARNINGS AND PRECAUTIONS

5.1 Fluid Retention and Edema

Gleevec is often associated with edema and occasionally serious fluid retention [see Adverse Reactions (6.1)]. Patients should be weighed and monitored regularly for signs and symptoms of fluid retention. An unexpected rapid weight gain should be carefully investigated and appropriate treatment provided. The probability of edema was increased with higher Gleevec dose and age >65 years in the CML studies. Severe superficial edema was reported in 1.5% of newly diagnosed CML patients taking Gleevec, and in 2%-6% of other adult CML patients taking Gleevec. In addition, other severe fluid retention (e.g., pleural effusion, pericardial effusion, pulmonary edema, and ascites) reactions were reported in 1.3% of newly diagnosed CML patients taking Gleevec, and in 2%-6% of other adult CML patients taking Gleevec. Severe fluid retention was reported in 9% to 13.1% of patients taking Gleevec for GIST [see Adverse Reactions (6.11)].

5.2 Hematologic Toxicity

Treatment with Gleevec is associated with anemia, neutropenia, and thrombocytopenia. Complete blood counts should

Table 2: Adverse Reactions Reported in Newly Diagnosed CML Clinical Trial (≥10% of Gleevec Treated Patients)[1]

Preferred Term	All Grades		CTC Grades 3/4	
	Gleevec N=551 (%)	IFN+Ara-C N=533 (%)	Gleevec N=551 (%)	IFN+Ara-C N=533 (%)
Fluid Retention	61.7	11.1	2.5	0.9
– Superficial Edema	59.9	9.6	1.5	0.4
– Other Fluid Retention Reactions[2]	6.9	1.9	1.3	0.6
Nausea	49.5	61.5	1.3	5.1
Muscle Cramps	49.2	11.8	2.2	0.2
Musculoskeletal Pain	47.0	44.8	5.4	8.6
Diarrhea	45.4	43.3	3.3	3.2
Rash and Related Terms	40.1	26.1	2.9	2.4
Fatigue	38.8	67.0	1.8	25.1
Headache	37.0	43.3	0.5	3.8
Joint Pain	31.4	38.1	2.5	7.7
Abdominal Pain	36.5	25.9	4.2	3.9
Nasopharyngitis	30.5	8.8	0	0.4
Hemorrhage	28.9	21.2	1.8	1.7
– GI Hemorrhage	1.6	1.1	0.5	0.2
– CNS Hemorrhage	0.2	0.4	0	0.4
Myalgia	24.1	38.8	1.5	8.3
Vomiting	22.5	27.8	2.0	3.4
Dyspepsia	18.9	8.3	0	0.8
Cough	20.0	23.1	0.2	0.6
Pharyngolaryngeal Pain	18.1	11.4	0.2	0
Upper Respiratory Tract Infection	21.2	8.4	0.2	0.4
Dizziness	19.4	24.4	0.9	3.8
Pyrexia	17.8	42.6	0.9	3.0
Weight Increased	15.6	2.6	2.0	0.4
Insomnia	14.7	18.6	0	0
Depression	14.9	35.8	0.5	13.1
Influenza	13.8	6.2	0.2	0.2
Bone Pain	11.3	15.6	1.6	3.4
Constipation	11.4	14.4	0.7	0.2
Sinusitis	11.4	6.0	0.2	0.2

[1] All adverse reactions occurring in ≥10% of Gleevec treated patients are listed regardless of suspected relationship to treatment.

[2] Other fluid retention reactions include pleural effusion, ascites, pulmonary edema, pericardial effusion, anasarca, edema aggravated, and fluid retention not otherwise specified.

be performed weekly for the first month, biweekly for the second month, and periodically thereafter as clinically indicated (for example, every 2-3 months). In CML, the occurrence of these cytopenias is dependent on the stage of disease and is more frequent in patients with accelerated phase CML or blast crisis than in patients with chronic phase CML. In pediatric CML patients the most frequent toxicities observed were Grade 3 or 4 cytopenias including neutropenia, thrombocytopenia and anemia. These generally occur within the first several months of therapy [see Dosage and Administration (2.11)].

5.3 Severe Congestive Heart Failure and Left Ventricular Dysfunction

Severe congestive heart failure and left ventricular dysfunction have occasionally been reported in patients taking Gleevec. Most of the patients with reported cardiac reactions have had other co-morbidities and risk factors, including advanced age and previous medical history of cardiac disease. In an international randomized phase 3 study in 1,106 patients with newly diagnosed Ph+ CML in chronic phase, severe cardiac failure and left ventricular dysfunction were observed in 0.7% of patients taking Gleevec compared to 0.9% of patients taking IFN + Ara-C. Patients with cardiac disease or risk factors for cardiac failure should be monitored carefully and any patient with signs or symptoms consistent with cardiac failure should be evaluated and treated.

5.4 Hepatotoxicity

Hepatotoxicity, occasionally severe, may occur with Gleevec [see Adverse Reactions (6.3)]. Liver function (transaminases, bilirubin, and alkaline phosphatase) should be monitored before initiation of treatment and monthly, or as clinically indicated. Laboratory abnormalities should be managed with interruption and/or dose reduction of the treatment with Gleevec [see Dosage and Administration (2.10)].

When Gleevec is combined with chemotherapy, liver toxicity in the form of transaminase elevation and hyperbilirubinemia has been observed. Additionally, there have been reports of acute liver failure. Monitoring of hepatic function is recommended.

5.5 Hemorrhage

In the newly diagnosed CML trial, 1.8% of patients had Grade 3/4 hemorrhage. In the Phase 3 unresectable or metastatic GIST studies 211 patients (12.9%) reported Grade 3/4 hemorrhage at any site. In the Phase 2 unresectable or metastatic GIST study 7 patients (5%) had a total of 8 CTC Grade 3/4 hemorrhages; gastrointestinal (GI) (3 pa-

tients), intra-tumoral (3 patients) or both (1 patient). Gastrointestinal tumor sites may have been the source of GI hemorrhages.

5.6 Gastrointestinal Disorders

Gleevec is sometimes associated with GI irritation. Gleevec should be taken with food and a large glass of water to minimize this problem. There have been rare reports, including fatalities, of gastrointestinal perforation.

5.7 Hypereosinophilic Cardiac Toxicity

In patients with hypereosinophilic syndrome and cardiac involvement, cases of cardiogenic shock/left ventricular dysfunction have been associated with the initiation of Gleevec therapy. The condition was reported to be reversible with the administration of systemic steroids, circulatory support measures and temporarily withholding Gleevec. Myelodysplastic/myeloproliferative disease and systemic mastocytosis may be associated with high eosinophil levels. Performance of an echocardiogram and determination of serum troponin should therefore be considered in patients with HES/CEL, and in patients with MDS/MPD or ASM associated with high eosinophil levels. If either is abnormal, the prophylactic use of systemic steroids (1-2 mg/kg) for one to two weeks concomitantly with Gleevec should be considered at the initiation of therapy.

5.8 Dermatologic Toxicities

Bullous dermatologic reactions, including erythema multiforme and Stevens-Johnson syndrome, have been reported with use of Gleevec.

5.9 Hypothyroidism

Clinical cases of hypothyroidism have been reported in thyroidectomy patients undergoing levothyroxine replacement during treatment with Gleevec. TSH levels should be closely monitored in such patients.

5.10 Toxicities from Long-Term Use

It is important to consider potential toxicities suggested by animal studies, specifically, liver, kidney and cardiac toxicity and immunosuppression. Severe liver toxicity was observed in dogs treated for 2 weeks, with elevated liver enzymes, hepatocellular necrosis, bile duct necrosis, and bile duct hyperplasia. Renal toxicity was observed in monkeys treated for 2 weeks, with focal mineralization and dilation of the renal tubules and tubular nephrosis. Increased BUN and creatinine were observed in several of these animals. An increased rate of opportunistic infections was observed with chronic imatinib treatment in laboratory animal studies. In a 39-week monkey study, treatment with imatinib resulted in worsening of normally suppressed malarial infections in

Table 3: Adverse Reactions Reported in Other CML Clinical Trials (≥10% of All Patients in any Trial)[1]

Preferred Term	Myeloid Blast Crisis (n=260) % All Grades	Myeloid Blast Crisis (n=260) % Grade 3/4	Accelerated Phase (n=235) % All Grades	Accelerated Phase (n=235) % Grade 3/4	Chronic Phase, IFN Failure (n=532) % All Grades	Chronic Phase, IFN Failure (n=532) % Grade 3/4
Fluid Retention	72	11	76	6	69	4
– Superficial Edema	66	6	74	3	67	2
– Other Fluid Retention Reactions[2]	22	6	15	4	7	2
Nausea	71	5	73	5	63	3
Muscle Cramps	28	1	47	0.4	62	2
Vomiting	54	4	58	3	36	2
Diarrhea	43	4	57	5	48	3
Hemorrhage	53	19	49	11	30	2
– CNS Hemorrhage	9	7	3	3	2	1
– GI Hemorrhage	8	4	6	5	2	0.4
Musculoskeletal Pain	42	9	49	9	38	2
Fatigue	30	4	46	4	48	1
Skin Rash	36	5	47	5	47	3
Pyrexia	41	7	41	8	21	2
Arthralgia	25	5	34	6	40	1
Headache	27	5	32	2	36	0.6
Abdominal Pain	30	6	33	4	32	1
Weight Increased	5	1	17	5	32	7
Cough	14	0.8	27	0.9	20	0
Dyspepsia	12	0	22	0	27	0
Myalgia	9	0	24	2	27	0.2
Nasopharyngitis	10	0	17	0	22	0
Asthenia	18	5	21	5	15	0.2
Dyspnea	15	4	21	7	12	0.9
Upper Respiratory Tract Infection	3	0	12	0.4	19	0
Anorexia	14	2	17	2	7	0
Night Sweats	13	0.8	17	1	14	0.2
Constipation	16	2	16	0.9	9	0.4
Dizziness	12	0.4	13	0	16	0.2
Pharyngitis	10	0	12	0	15	0
Insomnia	10	0	14	0	14	0.2
Pruritus	8	1	14	0.9	14	0.8
Hypokalemia	13	4	9	2	6	0.8
Pneumonia	13	7	10	7	4	1
Anxiety	8	0.8	12	0	8	0.4
Liver Toxicity	10	5	12	6	6	3
Rigors	10	0	12	0.4	10	0
Chest Pain	7	2	10	0.4	11	0.8
Influenza	0.8	0.4	6	0	11	0.2
Sinusitis	4	0.4	11	0.4	9	0.4

[1] All adverse reactions occurring in ≥10% of patients are listed regardless of suspected relationship to treatment.
[2] Other fluid retention reactions include pleural effusion, ascites, pulmonary edema, pericardial effusion, anasarca, edema aggravated, and fluid retention not otherwise specified.

Table 4: Lab Abnormalities in Newly Diagnosed CML Clinical Trial

CTC Grades	Gleevec N=551 % Grade 3	Gleevec N=551 % Grade 4	IFN+Ara-C N=533 % Grade 3	IFN+Ara-C N=533 % Grade 4
Hematology Parameters*				
– Neutropenia*	13.1	3.6	20.8	4.5
– Thrombocytopenia*	8.5	0.4	15.9	0.6
– Anemia	3.3	1.1	4.1	0.2
Biochemistry Parameters				
– Elevated Creatinine	0	0	0.4	0
– Elevated Bilirubin	0.9	0.2	0.2	0
– Elevated Alkaline Phosphatase	0.2	0	0.8	0
– Elevated SGOT/SGPT	4.7	0.5	7.1	0.4

* $p < 0.001$ (difference in Grade 3 plus 4 abnormalities between the two treatment groups)

these animals. Lymphopenia was observed in animals (as in humans). Additional long-term toxicities were identified in a 2-year rat study. Histopathological examination of the treated rats that died on study revealed cardiomyopathy (both sexes), chronic progressive nephropathy (females) and preputial gland papilloma as principal causes of death or reasons for sacrifice. Non-neoplastic lesions seen in this 2-year study which were not identified in earlier preclinical studies were the cardiovascular system, pancreas, endocrine organs and teeth. The most important changes included cardiac hypertrophy and dilatation, leading to signs of cardiac insufficiency in some animals.

5.11 Use in Pregnancy
Pregnancy Category D
Women of childbearing potential should be advised to avoid becoming pregnant while taking Gleevec. Sexually active female patients taking Gleevec should use adequate contraception. Imatinib mesylate was teratogenic in rats when ad-

ministered during organogenesis at doses approximately equal to the maximum human dose of 800 mg/day based on body surface area. Significant post-implantation loss was seen in female rats administered imatinib mesylate at doses approximately one-half the maximum human dose of 800 mg/day based on body surface area [see Use in Specific Populations (8.1)].

6 ADVERSE REACTIONS
Because clinical trials are conducted under widely varying conditions, the adverse reaction rates observed cannot be directly compared to rates on other clinical trials and may not reflect the rates observed in clinical practice.

6.1 Chronic Myeloid Leukemia
The majority of Gleevec-treated patients experienced adverse reactions at some time. Most reactions were of mild-to-moderate grade, but drug was discontinued for drug-related adverse reactions in 2.4% of newly diagnosed

patients, 4% of patients in chronic phase after failure of interferon-alpha therapy, 4% in accelerated phase and 5% in blast crisis.

The most frequently reported drug-related adverse reactions were edema, nausea and vomiting, muscle cramps, musculoskeletal pain, diarrhea and rash (Table 2 for newly diagnosed CML, Table 3 for other CML patients). Edema was most frequently periorbital or in lower limbs and was managed with diuretics, other supportive measures, or by reducing the dose of Gleevec [see Dosage and Administration (2.10)]. The frequency of severe superficial edema was 1.5%-6%.

A variety of adverse reactions represent local or general fluid retention including pleural effusion, ascites, pulmonary edema and rapid weight gain with or without superficial edema. These reactions appear to be dose related, were more common in the blast crisis and accelerated phase studies (where the dose was 600 mg/day), and are more common in the elderly. These reactions were usually managed by interrupting Gleevec treatment and using diuretics or other appropriate supportive care measures. A few of these reactions may be serious or life threatening, and one patient with blast crisis died with pleural effusion, congestive heart failure, and renal failure.

Adverse reactions, regardless of relationship to study drug, that were reported in at least 10% of the Gleevec treated patients are shown in Tables 2 and 3.
[See table 2 at top of previous page]
[See table 3 at left]

6.2 Hematologic Toxicity
Cytopenias, and particularly neutropenia and thrombocytopenia, were a consistent finding in all studies, with a higher frequency at doses ≥750 mg (Phase 1 study). The occurrence of cytopenias in CML patients was also dependent on the stage of the disease.

In patients with newly diagnosed CML, cytopenias were less frequent than in the other CML patients (see Tables 4 and 5). The frequency of Grade 3 or 4 neutropenia and thrombocytopenia was between 2- and 3-fold higher in blast crisis and accelerated phase compared to chronic phase (see Tables 4 and 5). The median duration of the neutropenic and thrombocytopenic episodes varied from 2 to 3 weeks, and from 2 to 4 weeks, respectively.

These reactions can usually be managed with either a reduction of the dose or an interruption of treatment with Gleevec, but in rare cases require permanent discontinuation of treatment.
[See table 4 at left]
[See table 5 at top of next page]

6.3 Hepatotoxicity
Severe elevation of transaminases or bilirubin occurred in approximately 5% of CML patients (see Tables 4 and 5) and were usually managed with dose reduction or interruption (the median duration of these episodes was approximately 1 week). Treatment was discontinued permanently because of liver laboratory abnormalities in less than 1.0% of CML patients. One patient, who was taking acetaminophen regularly for fever, died of acute liver failure. In the Phase 2 GIST trial, Grade 3 or 4 SGPT (ALT) elevations were observed in 6.8% of patients and Grade 3 or 4 SGOT (AST) elevations were observed in 4.8% of patients. Bilirubin elevation was observed in 2.7% of patients.

6.4 Adverse Reactions in Pediatric Population
The overall safety profile of pediatric patients treated with Gleevec in 93 children studied was similar to that found in studies with adult patients, except that musculoskeletal pain was less frequent (20.5%) and peripheral edema was not reported. Nausea and vomiting were the most commonly reported individual adverse reactions with an incidence similar to that seen in adult patients. Although most patients experienced adverse reactions at some time during the study, the incidence of Grade 3/4 adverse reactions was low.

6.5 Adverse Reactions in Other Subpopulations
In older patients (≥65 years old), with the exception of edema, where it was more frequent, there was no evidence of an increase in the incidence or severity of adverse reactions. In women there was an increase in the frequency of neutropenia, as well as Grade 1/2 superficial edema, headache, nausea, rigors, vomiting, rash, and fatigue. No differences were seen that were related to race but the subsets were too small for proper evaluation.

6.6 Acute Lymphoblastic Leukemia
The adverse reactions were similar for Ph+ ALL as for Ph+ CML. The most frequently reported drug-related adverse reactions reported in the Ph+ ALL studies were mild nausea and vomiting, diarrhea, myalgia, muscle cramps and rash, which were easily manageable. Superficial edema was a common finding in all studies and were described primarily as periorbital or lower limb edemas. These edemas were rarely severe and may be managed with diuretics, other supportive measures, or in some patients by reducing the dose of Gleevec.

6.7 Myelodysplastic/Myeloproliferative Diseases
Adverse reactions, regardless of relationship to study drug, that were reported in at least 10% of the patients treated

with Gleevec for MDS/MPD in the phase 2 study, are shown in Table 6.

Table 6: Adverse Reactions Reported (More than One Patient) in MPD Patients in the Phase 2 Study (≥10% All Patients) All Grades

Preferred Term	N=7 n (%)
Nausea	4 (57.1)
Diarrhea	3 (42.9)
Anemia	2 (28.6)
Fatigue	2 (28.6)
Muscle Cramp	3 (42.9)
Arthralgia	2 (28.6)
Periorbital Edema	2 (28.6)

6.8 Aggressive Systemic Mastocytosis

All ASM patients experienced at least one adverse reaction at some time. The most frequently reported adverse reactions were diarrhea, nausea, ascites, muscle cramps, dyspnea, fatigue, peripheral edema, anemia, pruritus, rash and lower respiratory tract infection. None of the 5 patients in the phase 2 study with ASM discontinued Gleevec due to drug-related adverse reactions or abnormal laboratory values.

6.9 Hypereosinophilic Syndrome and Chronic Eosinophilic Leukemia

The safety profile in the HES/CEL patient population does not appear to be different from the safety profile of Gleevec observed in other hematologic malignancy populations, such as Ph+ CML. All patients experienced at least one adverse reaction, the most common being gastrointestinal, cutaneous and musculoskeletal disorders. Hematological abnormalities were also frequent, with instances of CTC Grade 3 leukopenia, neutropenia, lymphopenia and anemia.

6.10 Dermatofibrosarcoma Protuberans

Adverse reactions, regardless of relationship to study drug, that were reported in at least 10% of the 12 patients treated with Gleevec for DFSP in the phase 2 study are shown in Table 7.

Table 7: Adverse Reactions Reported in DFSP Patients in the Phase 2 Study (≥10% All Patients) All Grades

Preferred Term	N=12 n (%)
Nausea	5 (41.7)
Diarrhea	3 (25.0)
Vomiting	3 (25.0)
Periorbital Edema	4 (33.3)
Face Edema	2 (16.7)
Rash	3 (25.0)
Fatigue	5 (41.7)
Edema Peripheral	4 (33.3)
Pyrexia	2 (16.7)
Eye Edema	4 (33.3)
Lacrimation Increased	3 (25.0)
Dyspnea Exertional	2 (16.7)
Anemia	3 (25.0)
Rhinitis	2 (16.7)
Anorexia	2 (16.7)

Clinically relevant or severe laboratory abnormalities in the 12 patients treated with Gleevec for DFSP in the phase 2 study are presented in Table 8.

Table 8: Laboratory Abnormalities Reported in DFSP Patients in the Phase 2 Study

CTC Grades[1]	N=12 Grade 3	Grade 4
Hematology Parameters		
– Anemia	17%	0%
– Thrombocytopenia	17%	0%
– Neutropenia	0%	8%
Biochemistry Parameters		
– Elevated Creatinine	0%	8%

[1] CTC Grades: neutropenia (Grade 3 ≥0.5-1.0 × 10^9/L, Grade 4 <0.5 × 10^9/L), thrombocytopenia (Grade 3 ≥10-50 × 10^9/L, Grade 4 <10 × 10^9/L), anemia (Grade 3 ≥65-80 g/L, Grade 4 <65 g/L), elevated creatinine (Grade 3 >3-6 × upper limit normal range [ULN], Grade 4 >6 × ULN)

6.11 Gastrointestinal Stromal Tumors

Unresectable and/or Malignant Metastatic GIST

In the Phase 3 trials the majority of Gleevec-treated patients experienced adverse reactions at some time. The most

Table 5: Lab Abnormalities in Other CML Clinical Trials

	Myeloid Blast Crisis (n=260) 600 mg n=223 400 mg n=37 %		Accelerated Phase (n=235) 600 mg n=158 400 mg n=77 %		Chronic Phase, IFN Failure (n=532) 400 mg %	
CTC Grades[1]	Grade 3	Grade 4	Grade 3	Grade 4	Grade 3	Grade 4
Hematology Parameters						
– Neutropenia	16	48	23	36	27	9
– Thrombocytopenia	30	33	31	13	21	<1
– Anemia	42	11	34	7	6	1
Biochemistry Parameters						
– Elevated Creatinine	1.5	0	1.3	0	0.2	0
– Elevated Bilirubin	3.8	0	2.1	0	0.6	0
– Elevated Alkaline Phosphatase	4.6	0	5.5	0.4	0.2	0
– Elevated SGOT (AST)	1.9	0	3.0	0	2.3	0
– Elevated SGPT (ALT)	2.3	0.4	4.3	0	2.1	0

[1] CTC Grades: neutropenia (Grade 3 ≥0.5-1.0 × 10^9/L, Grade 4 <0.5 × 10^9/L), thrombocytopenia (Grade 3 ≥10-50 × 10^9/L, Grade 4 <10 × 10^9/L), anemia (hemoglobin ≥65-80 g/L, Grade 4 <65 g/L), elevated creatinine (Grade 3 >3-6 × upper limit normal range [ULN], Grade 4 >6 × ULN), elevated bilirubin (Grade 3 >3-10 × ULN, Grade 4 >10 × ULN), elevated alkaline phosphatase (Grade 3 >5-20 × ULN, Grade 4 >20 × ULN), elevated SGOT or SGPT (Grade 3 >5-20 × ULN, Grade 4 >20 × ULN)

Table 9: Number (%) of Patients with Adverse Reactions where Frequency is ≥10% in any One Group (Full Analysis Set) in the Phase 3 Unresectable and/or Malignant Metastatic GIST Clinical Trials

	Imatinib 400 mg N=818		Imatinib 800 mg N=822	
Reported or Specified Term	All Grades %	Grades 3/4/5 %	All Grades %	Grades 3/4/5 %
Edema	76.7	9.0	86.1	13.1
Fatigue/lethargy, malaise, asthenia	69.3	11.7	74.9	12.2
Nausea	58.1	9.0	64.5	7.8
Abdominal pain/cramping	57.2	13.8	55.2	11.8
Diarrhea	56.2	8.1	58.2	8.6
Rash/desquamation	38.1	7.6	49.8	8.9
Vomiting	37.4	9.2	40.6	7.5
Myalgia	32.2	5.6	30.2	3.8
Anemia	32.0	4.9	34.8	6.4
Anorexia	31.1	6.6	35.8	4.7
Other GI toxicity	25.2	8.1	28.1	6.6
Headache	22.0	5.7	19.7	3.6
Other pain (excluding tumor related pain)	20.4	5.9	20.8	5.0
Other dermatology/skin toxicity	17.6	5.9	20.1	5.7
Leukopenia	17.0	0.7	19.6	1.6
Other constitutional symptoms	16.7	6.4	15.2	4.4
Cough	16.1	4.5	14.5	3.2
Infection (without neutropenia)	15.5	6.6	16.5	5.6
Pruritus	15.4	5.4	18.9	4.3
Other neurological toxicity	15.0	6.4	15.2	4.9
Constipation	14.8	5.1	14.4	4.1
Other renal/genitourinary toxicity	14.2	6.5	13.6	5.2
Arthralgia (joint pain)	13.6	4.8	12.3	3.0
Dyspnea (shortness of breath)	13.6	6.8	14.2	5.6
Fever in absence of neutropenia (ANC <1.0 × 10^9/L)	13.2	4.9	12.9	3.4
Sweating	12.7	4.6	8.5	2.8
Other hemorrhage	12.3	6.7	13.3	6.1
Weight gain	12.0	1.0	10.6	0.6
Alopecia	11.9	4.3	14.8	3.2
Dyspepsia/heartburn	11.5	0.6	10.9	0.5
Neutropenia/granulocytopenia	11.5	3.1	16.1	4.1
Rigors/chills	11.0	4.6	10.2	3.0
Dizziness/lightheadedness	11.0	4.8	10.0	2.8
Creatinine increase	10.8	0.4	10.1	0.6
Flatulence	10.0	0.2	10.1	0.1
Stomatitis/pharyngitis (oral/pharyngeal mucositis)	9.2	5.4	10.0	4.3
Lymphopenia	6.0	0.7	10.1	1.9

frequently reported adverse reactions were edema, fatigue, nausea, abdominal pain, diarrhea, rash, vomiting, myalgia, anemia and anorexia. Drug was discontinued for adverse reactions in a total of 89 patients (5.4%). Superficial edema, most frequently periorbital or lower extremity edema was managed with diuretics, other supportive measures, or by reducing the dose of Gleevec [see *Dosage and Administration (2.10)*]. Severe (CTC Grade 3/4) edema was observed in 182 patients (11.1%).

Adverse reactions, regardless of relationship to study drug, that were reported in at least 10% of the patients treated with Gleevec are shown in Table 9.

Overall the incidence of all grades of adverse reactions and the incidence of severe adverse reactions (CTC Grade 3 and above) were similar between the two treatment arms except for edema, which was reported more frequently in the 800 mg group.

[See table 9 above]

Clinically relevant or severe abnormalities of routine hematologic or biochemistry laboratory values were not reported or evaluated in the Phase 3 GIST trials. Severe abnormal laboratory values reported in the Phase 2 GIST trial are presented in Table 10.

[See table 10 at top of next page]

Adjuvant Treatment of GIST

The majority of both Gleevec and placebo treated patients experienced at least one adverse reaction at some time. The most frequently reported adverse reactions were similar to

Table 10: Laboratory Abnormalities in the Phase 2 Unresectable and/or Malignant Metastatic GIST Trial

CTC Grades[1]	400 mg (n=73) %		600 mg (n=74) %	
	Grade 3	Grade 4	Grade 3	Grade 4
Hematology Parameters				
– Anemia	3	0	8	1
– Thrombocytopenia	0	0	1	0
– Neutropenia	7	3	8	3
Biochemistry Parameters				
– Elevated Creatinine	0	0	3	0
– Reduced Albumin	3	0	4	0
– Elevated Bilirubin	1	0	1	3
– Elevated Alkaline Phosphatase	0	0	3	0
– Elevated SGOT (AST)	4	0	3	3
– Elevated SGPT (ALT)	6	0	7	1

[1] CTC Grades: neutropenia (Grade 3 ≥0.5-1.0 × 10⁹/L, Grade 4 <0.5 × 10⁹/L), thrombocytopenia (Grade 3 ≥10-50 × 10⁹/L, Grade 4 <10 × 10⁹/L), anemia (Grade 3 ≥65-80 g/L, Grade 4 <65 g/L), elevated creatinine (Grade 3 >3-6 × upper limit normal range [ULN], Grade 4 >6 × ULN), elevated bilirubin (Grade 3 >3-10 × ULN, Grade 4 >10 × ULN), elevated alkaline phosphatase, SGOT or SGPT (Grade 3 >5-20 × ULN, Grade 4 >20 × ULN), albumin (Grade 3 <20 g/L)

Table 11: Adverse Reactions Reported in the Adjuvant GIST Trial (≥5% of Gleevec Treated Patients)[1]

Preferred Term	All CTC Grades		CTC Grade 3 and above	
	Gleevec (n=337) %	Placebo (n=345) %	Gleevec (n=337) %	Placebo (n=345) %
Diarrhea	59.3	29.3	3.0	1.4
Fatigue	57.0	40.9	2.1	1.2
Nausea	53.1	27.8	2.4	1.2
Periorbital Edema	47.2	14.5	1.2	0
Hemoglobin Decreased	46.9	27.0	0.6	0
Peripheral Edema	26.7	14.8	0.3	0
Rash (Exfoliative)	26.1	12.8	2.7	0
Vomiting	25.5	13.9	2.4	0.6
Abdominal Pain	21.1	22.3	3.0	1.4
Headache	19.3	20.3	0.6	0
Dyspepsia	17.2	13.0	0.9	0
Anorexia	16.9	8.7	0.3	0
Weight Increased	16.9	11.6	0.3	0
Liver Enzymes (ALT) Increased	16.6	13.0	2.7	0
Muscle Spasms	16.3	3.3	0	0
Neutrophil Count Decreased	16.0	6.1	3.3	0.9
Arthralgia	15.1	14.5	0	0.3
White Blood Cell Count Decreased	14.5	4.3	0.6	0.3
Constipation	12.8	17.7	0	0.3
Dizziness	12.5	10.7	0	0.3
Liver Enzymes (AST) Increased	12.2	7.5	2.1	0
Myalgia	12.2	11.6	0	0.3
Blood Creatinine Increased	11.6	5.8	0	0.3
Cough	11.0	11.3	0	0
Pruritus	11.0	7.8	0.9	0
Weight Decreased	10.1	5.2	0	0
Hyperglycemia	9.8	11.3	0.6	1.7
Insomnia	9.8	7.2	0.9	0
Lacrimation Increased	9.8	3.8	0	0
Alopecia	9.5	6.7	0	0
Flatulence	8.9	9.6	0	0
Rash	8.9	5.2	0.9	0
Abdominal Distension	7.4	6.4	0.3	0.3
Back Pain	7.4	8.1	0.6	0
Pain in Extremity	7.4	7.2	0.3	0
Hypokalemia	7.1	2.0	0.9	0.6
Depression	6.8	6.4	0.9	0.6
Facial Edema	6.8	1.2	0.3	0
Blood Alkaline Phosphatase Increased	6.5	7.5	0	0
Dry Skin	6.5	5.2	0	0
Dysgeusia	6.5	2.9	0	0
Abdominal Pain Upper	6.2	6.4	0.3	0
Neuropathy Peripheral	5.9	6.4	0	0
Hypocalcemia	5.6	1.7	0.3	0
Leukopenia	5.0	2.6	0.3	0
Platelet Count Decreased	5.0	3.5	0	0
Stomatitis	5.0	1.7	0.6	0
Upper Respiratory Tract Infection	5.0	3.5	0	0
Vision Blurred	5.0	2.3	0	0

[1] All adverse reactions occurring in ≥5% of patients are listed regardless of suspected relationship to treatment. A patient with multiple occurrences of an adverse reaction is counted only once in the adverse reaction category.

those reported in other clinical studies in other patient populations and include diarrhea, fatigue, nausea, edema, decreased hemoglobin, rash, vomiting and abdominal pain. No new adverse reactions were reported in the adjuvant GIST treatment setting that had not been previously re-

ported in other patient populations including patients with unresectable and/or malignant metastatic GIST. Drug was discontinued for adverse reactions in 57 patients (17%) and 11 patients (3%) of the Gleevec and placebo treated patients respectively. Edema, gastrointestinal disturbances (nausea,

vomiting, abdominal distention and diarrhea), fatigue, low hemoglobin and rash were the most frequently reported adverse reactions at the time of discontinuation.

Adverse reactions, regardless of relationship to study drug, that were reported in at least 5% of the patients treated with Gleevec are shown in Table 11.

[See table 11 at left]

6.12 Additional Data from Multiple Clinical Trials

The following adverse reactions have been reported during clinical trials of Gleevec.

Cardiac Disorders:

Estimated 0.1%-1%: congestive cardiac failure, tachycardia, palpitations, pulmonary edema

Estimated 0.01%-0.1%: arrhythmia, atrial fibrillation, cardiac arrest, myocardial infarction, angina pectoris, pericardial effusion

Vascular Disorders:

Estimated 1%-10%: flushing, hemorrhage

Estimated 0.1%-1%: hypertension, hypotension, peripheral coldness, Raynauds phenomenon, hematoma

Clinical Laboratory Tests:

Estimated 0.1%-1%: blood CPK increased, blood LDH increased

Estimated 0.01%-0.1%: blood amylase increased

Dermatologic:

Estimated 1%-10%: dry skin, alopecia, face edema, erythema, photosensitivity reaction

Estimated 0.1%-1%: exfoliative dermatitis, bullous eruption, nail disorder, purpura, psoriasis, rash pustular, contusion, sweating increased, urticaria, ecchymosis, increased tendency to bruise, hypotrichosis, skin hypopigmentation, skin hyperpigmentation, onychoclasis, folliculitis, petechiae

Estimated 0.01%-0.1%: vesicular rash, Stevens-Johnson syndrome, acute generalized exanthematous pustulosis, acute febrile neutrophilic dermatosis (Sweet's syndrome), nail discoloration, angioneurotic edema, erythema multiforme, leucocytoclastic vasculitis

Digestive:

Estimated 1%-10%: abdominal distention, gastroesophageal reflux, dry mouth, gastritis

Estimated 0.1%-1%: gastric ulcer, stomatitis, mouth ulceration, eructation, melena, esophagitis, ascites, hematemesis, chelitis, dysphagia, pancreatitis

Estimated 0.01%-0.1%: colitis, ileus, inflammatory bowel disease

General Disorders and Administration Site Conditions:

Estimated 1%-10%: weakness, anasarca, chills

Estimated 0.1%-1%: malaise

Hematologic:

Estimated 1%-10%: pancytopenia, febrile neutropenia

Estimated 0.1%-1%: thrombocythemia, lymphopenia, bone marrow depression, eosinophilia, lymphadenopathy

Estimated 0.01%-0.1%: hemolytic anemia, aplastic anemia

Hepatobiliary:

Estimated 0.1%-1%: hepatitis, jaundice

Estimated 0.01%-0.1%: hepatic failure and hepatic necrosis[1]

Hypersensitivity:

Estimated 0.01%-0.1%: angioedema

Infections:

Estimated 0.1%-1%: sepsis, herpes simplex, herpes zoster, cellulitis, urinary tract infection, gastroenteritis

Estimated 0.01%-0.1%: fungal infection

Metabolic and Nutritional:

Estimated 1%-10%: weight decreased

Estimated 0.1%-1%: hypophosphatemia, dehydration, gout, increased appetite, decreased appetite, hyperuricemia, hypercalcemia, hyperglycemia, hyponatremia

Estimated 0.01%-0.1%: hyperkalemia, hypomagnesemia

Musculoskeletal:

Estimated 1%-10%: joint swelling

Estimated 0.1%-1%: joint and muscle stiffness

Estimated 0.01%-0.1%: muscular weakness, arthritis

Nervous System/Psychiatric:

Estimated 1%-10%: paresthesia, hypesthesia

Estimated 0.1%-1%: syncope, peripheral neuropathy, somnolence, migraine, memory impairment, libido decreased, sciatica, restless leg syndrome, tremor

Estimated 0.01%-0.1%: increased intracranial pressure[1], confusional state, convulsions, optic neuritis

Renal:

Estimated 0.1%-1%: renal failure acute, urinary frequency increased, hematuria, renal pain

Reproductive:

Estimated 0.1%-1%: breast enlargement, menorrhagia, sexual dysfunction, gynecomastia, erectile dysfunction, menstruation irregular, nipple pain, scrotal edema

Respiratory:

Estimated 1%-10%: epistaxis

Estimated 0.1%-1%: pleural effusion

Estimated 0.01%-0.1%: interstitial pneumonitis, pulmonary fibrosis, pleuritic pain, pulmonary hypertension, pulmonary hemorrhage

Special Senses:

Estimated 1%-10%: conjunctivitis, vision blurred, eyelid edema, conjunctival hemorrhage, dry eye

Estimated 0.1%-1%: vertigo, tinnitus, eye irritation, eye pain, orbital edema, scleral hemorrhage, retinal hemorrhage, blepharitis, macular edema, hearing loss

Estimated 0.01%-0.1%: papilledema[1], glaucoma, cataract

[1]Including some fatalities

6.13 Postmarketing Experience

The following additional adverse reactions have been identified during post approval use of Gleevec. Because these reactions are reported voluntarily from a population of uncertain size, it is not always possible to reliably estimate their frequency or establish a causal relationship to drug exposure.

Nervous system disorders: cerebral edema[1]

Eye disorders: vitreous hemorrhage

Cardiac disorders: pericarditis, cardiac tamponade[1]

Vascular disorders: thrombosis/embolism, anaphylactic shock

Respiratory, thoracic and mediastinal disorders: acute respiratory failure[1], interstitial lung disease

Gastrointestinal disorders: ileus/intestinal obstruction, tumor hemorrhage/tumor necrosis, gastrointestinal perforation[1] [*see Warnings and Precautions (5.6)*], diverticulitis

Skin and subcutaneous tissue disorders: lichenoid keratosis, lichen planus, toxic epidermal necrolysis, palmar-plantar erythrodysesthesia syndrome

Musculoskeletal and connective tissue disorders: avascular necrosis/hip osteonecrosis, rhabdomyolysis/myopathy

Reproduction disorders: hemorrhagic corpus luteum/ hemorrhagic ovarian cyst

[1]Including some fatalities

In some cases of bullous dermatologic reactions, including erythema multiforme and Stevens-Johnson syndrome reported during postmarketing surveillance, a recurrent dermatologic reaction was observed upon rechallenge. Several foreign post-marketing reports have described cases in which patients tolerated the reintroduction of Gleevec therapy after resolution or improvement of the bullous reaction. In these instances, Gleevec was resumed at a dose lower than that at which the reaction occurred and some patients also received concomitant treatment with corticosteroids or antihistamines.

7 DRUG INTERACTIONS

7.1 Agents Inducing CYP3A Metabolism

Pretreatment of healthy volunteers with multiple doses of rifampin followed by a single dose of Gleevec, increased Gleevec oral-dose clearance by 3.8-fold, which significantly ($p<0.05$) decreased mean C_{max} and AUC.

Similar findings were observed in patients receiving 400-1200 mg/day Gleevec concomitantly with enzyme-inducing anti-epileptic drugs (EIAED) (e.g., carbamazepine, oxcarbamazepine, phenytoin, fosphenytoin, phenobarbital, and primidone). The mean dose normalized AUC for imatinib in the patients receiving EIAEDs decreased by 73% compared to patients not receiving EIAED.

Concomitant administration of Gleevec and St. John's Wort led to a 30% reduction in the AUC of imatinib.

Consider alternative therapeutic agents with less enzyme induction potential in patients when rifampin or other CYP3A4 inducers are indicated. Gleevec doses up to 1200 mg/day (600 mg BID) have been given to patients receiving concomitant strong CYP3A4 inducers [*see Dosage and Administration (2.9)*].

7.2 Agents Inhibiting CYP3A Metabolism

There was a significant increase in exposure to imatinib (mean C_{max} and AUC increased by 26% and 40%, respectively) in healthy subjects when Gleevec was co-administered with a single dose of ketoconazole (a CYP3A4 inhibitor). Caution is recommended when administering Gleevec with strong CYP3A4 inhibitors (e.g., ketoconazole, itraconazole, clarithromycin, atazanavir, indinavir, nefazodone, nelfinavir, ritonavir, saquinavir, telithromycin, and voriconazole). Grapefruit juice may also increase plasma concentrations of imatinib and should be avoided. Substances that inhibit the cytochrome P450 isoenzyme (CYP3A4) activity may decrease metabolism and increase imatinib concentrations.

7.3 Interactions with Drugs Metabolized by CYP3A4

Gleevec increases the mean C_{max} and AUC of simvastatin (CYP3A4 substrate) 2- and 3.5-fold, respectively, suggesting an inhibition of the CYP3A4 by Gleevec. Particular caution is recommended when administering Gleevec with CYP3A4 substrates that have a narrow therapeutic window (e.g., alfentanil, cyclosporine, diergotamine, ergotamine, fentanyl, pimozide, quinidine, sirolimus or tacrolimus).

Table 12: Liver Function Classification

Liver Function Test	Normal (n=14)	Mild (n=30)	Moderate (n=20)	Severe (n=20)
Total Bilirubin	≤ULN	>1.0-1.5× ULN	>1.5-3× ULN	>3-10× ULN
SGOT	≤ULN	>ULN (can be normal if Total Bilirubin is >ULN)	Any	Any

ULN=upper limit of normal for the institution

Gleevec will increase plasma concentration of other CYP3A4 metabolized drugs (e.g., triazolo-benzodiazepines, dihydropyridine calcium channel blockers, certain HMG-CoA reductase inhibitors, etc.).

Because warfarin is metabolized by CYP2C9 and CYP3A4, patients who require anticoagulation should receive low-molecular weight or standard heparin instead of warfarin.

7.4 Interactions with Drugs Metabolized by CYP2D6

Gleevec increased the mean C_{max} and AUC of metoprolol by approximately 23% suggesting that Gleevec has a weak inhibitory effect on CYP2D6-mediated metabolism. No dose adjustment is necessary, however, caution is recommended when administering Gleevec with CYP2D6 substrates that have a narrow therapeutic window.

7.5 Interaction with Acetaminophen

In vitro, Gleevec inhibits acetaminophen O-glucuronidation (K_i value of 58.5 μM) at therapeutic levels. Systemic exposure to acetaminophen is expected to be increased when co-administered with Gleevec. No specific studies in humans have been performed and caution is recommended.

8 USE IN SPECIFIC POPULATIONS

8.1 Pregnancy

Pregnancy Category D [*see Warnings and Precautions (5.11)*].

Gleevec can cause fetal harm when administered to a pregnant woman. Imatinib mesylate was teratogenic in rats when administered during organogenesis at doses ≥100 mg/kg (approximately equal to the maximum human dose of 800 mg/day based on body surface area). Teratogenic effects included exencephaly or encephalocele, absent/ reduced frontal and absent parietal bones. Female rats administered doses ≥45 mg/kg (approximately one-half the maximum human dose of 800 mg/day based on body surface area) also experienced significant post-implantation loss as evidenced by either early fetal resorption or stillbirths, non-viable pups and early pup mortality between postpartum Days 0 and 4. At doses higher than 100 mg/kg, total fetal loss was noted in all animals. Fetal loss was not seen at doses ≤30 mg/kg (one-third the maximum human dose of 800 mg).

There are no adequate and well-controlled studies with Gleevec in pregnant women. Women should be advised not to become pregnant when taking Gleevec. If this drug is used during pregnancy, or if the patient becomes pregnant while taking this drug, the patient should be apprised of the potential hazard to the fetus.

8.3 Nursing Mothers

Imatinib and its active metabolite are excreted into human milk. Based on data from three breastfeeding women taking Gleevec, the milk:plasma ratio is about 0.5 for imatinib and about 0.9 for the active metabolite. Considering the combined concentration of imatinib and active metabolite, a breastfed infant could receive up to 10% of the maternal therapeutic dose based on body weight. Because of the potential for serious adverse reactions in nursing infants from Gleevec, a decision should be made whether to discontinue nursing or to discontinue the drug, taking into account the importance of the drug to the mother.

8.4 Pediatric Use

Gleevec safety and efficacy have been demonstrated in children with newly diagnosed Ph+ chronic phase CML and in children with Ph+ chronic phase CML with recurrence after stem cell transplantation or resistance to interferon-alpha therapy. There are no data in children under 2 years of age. Follow-up in children with newly diagnosed Ph+ chronic phase CML is limited.

As in adult patients, imatinib was rapidly absorbed after oral administration in pediatric patients, with a C_{max} of 2-4 hours. Apparent oral clearance was similar to adult values (11.0 L/hr/m^2 in children vs. 10.0 L/hr/m^2 in adults), as was the half-life (14.8 hours in children vs. 17.1 hours in adults). Dosing in children at both 260 mg/m^2 and 340 mg/m^2 achieved an AUC similar to the 400 mg dose in adults. The comparison of AUC on Day 8 vs. Day 1 at 260 mg/m^2 and 340 mg/m^2 dose levels revealed a 1.5- and 2.2-fold drug accumulation, respectively, after repeated once-daily dosing. Mean imatinib AUC did not increase proportionally with increasing dose.

8.5 Geriatric Use

In the CML clinical studies, approximately 20% of patients were older than 65 years. In the study of patients with newly diagnosed CML, 6% of patients were older than 65 years. No difference was observed in the safety profile in patients older than 65 years as compared to younger patients, with the exception of a higher frequency of edema [*see Warnings and Precautions (5.1)*]. The efficacy of Gleevec was similar in older and younger patients.

In the unresectable or metastatic GIST study, 16% of patients were older than 65 years. No obvious differences in the safety or efficacy profile were noted in patients older than 65 years as compared to younger patients, but the small number of patients does not allow a formal analysis. In the adjuvant GIST study, 221 patients (31%) were older than 65 years. No difference was observed in the safety profile in patients older than 65 years as compared to younger patients, with the exception of a higher frequency of edema. The efficacy of Gleevec was similar in patients older than 65 years and younger patients.

8.6 Hepatic Impairment

The effect of hepatic impairment on the pharmacokinetics of both imatinib and its major metabolite, CGP74588, was assessed in 84 cancer patients with varying degrees of hepatic impairment (Table 12) at imatinib doses ranging from 100-800 mg. Exposure to both imatinib and CGP74588 was comparable between each of the mildly and moderately hepatically-impaired groups and the normal group. Patients with severe hepatic impairment tend to have higher exposure to both imatinib and its metabolite than patients with normal hepatic function. At steady state, the mean C_{max}/dose and AUC/dose for imatinib increased by about 63% and 45%, respectively, in patients with severe hepatic impairment compared to patients with normal hepatic function. The mean C_{max}/dose and AUC/dose for CGP74588 increased by about 56% and 55%, respectively, in patients with severe hepatic impairment compared to patients with normal hepatic function [*see Dosage and Administration (2.10)*].

[See table 12 above]

8.7 Renal Impairment

The effect of renal impairment on the pharmacokinetics of imatinib was assessed in 59 cancer patients with varying degrees of renal impairment (Table 13) at single and steady state imatinib doses ranging from 100 to 800 mg/day. The mean exposure to imatinib (dose normalized AUC) in patients with mild and moderate renal impairment increased 1.5- to 2-fold compared to patients with normal renal function. The AUCs did not increase for doses greater than 600 mg in patients with mild renal impairment. The AUCs did not increase for doses greater than 400 mg in patients with moderate renal impairment. Two patients with severe renal impairment were dosed with 100 mg/day and their exposures were similar to those seen in patients with normal renal function receiving 400 mg/day. Dose reductions are necessary for patients with moderate and severe renal impairment [*see Dosage and Administration (2.9)*].

Table 13: Renal Function Classification

Renal Dysfunction	Renal Function Tests
Mild	CrCL = 40-59 mL/min
Moderate	CrCL = 20-39 mL/min
Severe	CrCL = <20 mL/min

CrCL = Creatinine Clearance

10 OVERDOSAGE

Experience with doses greater than 800 mg is limited. Isolated cases of Gleevec overdose have been reported. In the event of overdosage, the patient should be observed and appropriate supportive treatment given.

Adult Overdose

1,200 to 1,600 mg (duration varying between 1 to 10 days): Nausea, vomiting, diarrhea, rash erythema, edema, swelling, fatigue, muscle spasms, thrombocytopenia, pancytopenia, abdominal pain, headache, decreased appetite.

1,800 to 3,200 mg (as high as 3,200 mg daily for 6 days): Weakness, myalgia, increased CPK, increased bilirubin, gastrointestinal pain.

6,400 mg (single dose): One case in the literature reported one patient who experienced nausea, vomiting, abdominal pain, pyrexia, facial swelling, neutrophil count decreased, increase transaminases.

8 to 10 g (single dose): Vomiting and gastrointestinal pain have been reported.

A patient with myeloid blast crisis experienced Grade 1 elevations of serum creatinine, Grade 2 ascites and elevated liver transaminase levels, and Grade 3 elevations of bilirubin after inadvertently taking 1,200 mg of Gleevec daily for 6 days. Therapy was temporarily interrupted and complete reversal of all abnormalities occurred within 1 week. Treatment was resumed at a dose of 400 mg daily without recurrence of adverse reactions. Another patient developed severe muscle cramps after taking 1,600 mg of Gleevec daily for 6 days. Complete resolution of muscle cramps occurred following interruption of therapy and treatment was subsequently resumed. Another patient that was prescribed 400 mg daily, took 800 mg of Gleevec on Day 1 and 1,200 mg on Day 2. Therapy was interrupted, no adverse reactions occurred and the patient resumed therapy.

Pediatric Overdose

One 3-year-old male exposed to a single dose of 400 mg experienced vomiting, diarrhea and anorexia and another 3-year-old male exposed to a single dose of 980 mg experienced decreased white blood cell count and diarrhea.

11 DESCRIPTION

Imatinib is a small molecule kinase inhibitor. Gleevec film-coated tablets contain imatinib mesylate equivalent to 100 mg or 400 mg of imatinib free base. Imatinib mesylate is designated chemically as 4-[(4-Methyl-1-piperazinyl)-methyl]-N-[4-methyl-3-[[4-(3-pyridinyl)-2-pyrimidinyl]amino]-phenyl]benzamide methanesulfonate and its structural formula is

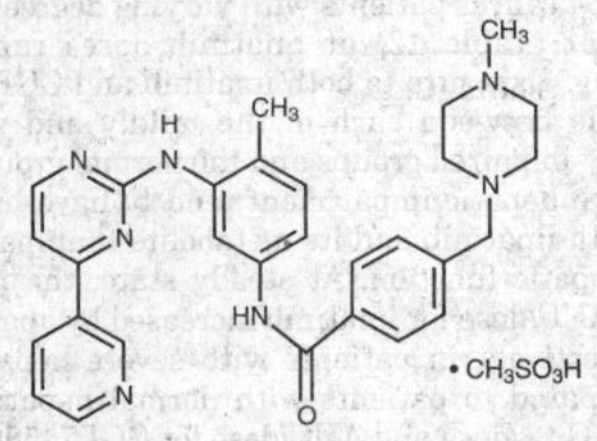

Imatinib mesylate is a white to off-white to brownish or yellowish tinged crystalline powder. Its molecular formula is $C_{29}H_{31}N_7O \cdot CH_4SO_3$ and its molecular weight is 589.7. Imatinib mesylate is soluble in aqueous buffers ≤pH 5.5 but is very slightly soluble to insoluble in neutral/alkaline aqueous buffers. In non-aqueous solvents, the drug substance is freely soluble to very slightly soluble in dimethyl sulfoxide, methanol and ethanol, but is insoluble in n-octanol, acetone and acetonitrile.

Inactive Ingredients: colloidal silicon dioxide (NF); crospovidone (NF); hydroxypropyl methylcellulose (USP); magnesium stearate (NF); and microcrystalline cellulose (NF). Tablet coating: ferric oxide, red (NF); ferric oxide, yellow (NF); hydroxypropyl methylcellulose (USP); polyethylene glycol (NF) and talc (USP).

12 CLINICAL PHARMACOLOGY

12.1 Mechanism of Action

Imatinib mesylate is a protein-tyrosine kinase inhibitor that inhibits the bcr-abl tyrosine kinase, the constitutive abnormal tyrosine kinase created by the Philadelphia chromosome abnormality in CML. Imatinib inhibits proliferation and induces apoptosis in bcr-abl positive cell lines as well as fresh leukemic cells from Philadelphia chromosome positive chronic myeloid leukemia. Imatinib inhibits colony formation in assays using *ex vivo* peripheral blood and bone marrow samples from CML patients.

In vivo, imatinib inhibits tumor growth of bcr-abl transfected murine myeloid cells as well as bcr-abl positive leukemia lines derived from CML patients in blast crisis.

Imatinib is also an inhibitor of the receptor tyrosine kinases for platelet-derived growth factor (PDGF) and stem cell factor (SCF), c-kit, and inhibits PDGF- and SCF-mediated cellular events. *In vitro*, imatinib inhibits proliferation and induces apoptosis in GIST cells, which express an activating c-kit mutation.

12.3 Pharmacokinetics

The pharmacokinetics of Gleevec have been evaluated in studies in healthy subjects and in population pharmacokinetic studies in over 900 patients. The pharmacokinetics of Gleevec are similar in CML and GIST patients. Imatinib is well absorbed after oral administration with C_{max} achieved within 2-4 hours post-dose. Mean absolute bioavailability is 98%. Following oral administration in healthy volunteers, the elimination half-lives of imatinib and its major active metabolite, the N-demethyl derivative (CGP74588), are approximately 18 and 40 hours, respectively. Mean imatinib AUC increases proportionally with increasing doses ranging from 25 mg-1,000 mg. There is no significant change in the pharmacokinetics of imatinib on repeated dosing, and accumulation is 1.5- to 2.5-fold at steady state when Gleevec is dosed once daily. At clinically relevant concentrations of imatinib, binding to plasma proteins in *in vitro* experiments is approximately 95%, mostly to albumin and α1-acid glycoprotein.

CYP3A4 is the major enzyme responsible for metabolism of imatinib. Other cytochrome P450 enzymes, such as CYP1A2, CYP2D6, CYP2C9, and CYP2C19, play a minor role in its metabolism. The main circulating active metabolite in humans is the N-demethylated piperazine derivative, formed predominantly by CYP3A4. It shows *in vitro* potency similar to the parent imatinib. The plasma AUC for this metabolite is about 15% of the AUC for imatinib. The plasma protein binding of N-demethylated metabolite CGP74588 is similar to that of the parent compound. Human liver microsome studies demonstrated that Gleevec is a potent competitive inhibitor of CYP2C9, CYP2D6, and CYP3A4/5 with K_i values of 27, 7.5 and 8 μM, respectively.

Imatinib elimination is predominately in the feces, mostly as metabolites. Based on the recovery of compound(s) after an oral ^{14}C-labeled dose of imatinib, approximately 81% of the dose was eliminated within 7 days, in feces (68% of dose) and urine (13% of dose). Unchanged imatinib accounted for 25% of the dose (5% urine, 20% feces), the remainder being metabolites.

Typically, clearance of imatinib in a 50-year-old patient weighing 50 kg is expected to be 8 L/h, while for a 50-year-old patient weighing 100 kg the clearance will increase to 14 L/h. The inter-patient variability of 40% in clearance does not warrant initial dose adjustment based on body weight and/or age but indicates the need for close monitoring for treatment-related toxicity.

13 NONCLINICAL TOXICOLOGY

13.1 Carcinogenesis, Mutagenesis, Impairment of Fertility

In the 2-year rat carcinogenicity study administration of imatinib at 15, 30 and 60 mg/kg/day resulted in a statistically significant reduction in the longevity of males at 60 mg/kg/day and females at ≥30 mg/kg/day. Target organs for neoplastic changes were the kidneys (renal tubule and renal pelvis), urinary bladder, urethra, preputial and clitoral gland, small intestine, parathyroid glands, adrenal glands and non-glandular stomach. Neoplastic lesions were not seen at: 30 mg/kg/day for the kidneys, urinary bladder, urethra, small intestine, parathyroid glands, adrenal glands and non-glandular stomach, and 15 mg/kg/day for the preputial and clitoral gland. The papilloma/carcinoma of the preputial/clitoral gland were noted at 30 and 60 mg/kg/day, representing approximately 0.5 to 4 or 0.3 to 2.4 times the human daily exposure (based on AUC) at 400 mg/day or 800 mg/day, respectively, and 0.4 to 3.0 times the daily exposure in children (based on AUC) at 340 mg/m^2. The renal tubule adenoma/carcinoma, renal pelvis transitional cell neoplasms, the urinary bladder and urethra transitional cell papillomas, the small intestine adenocarcinomas, the parathyroid glands adenomas, the benign and malignant medullary tumors of the adrenal glands and the non-glandular stomach papillomas/carcinomas were noted at 60 mg/kg/day. The relevance of these findings in the rat carcinogenicity study for humans is not known.

Positive genotoxic effects were obtained for imatinib in an *in vitro* mammalian cell assay (Chinese hamster ovary) for clastogenicity (chromosome aberrations) in the presence of metabolic activation. Two intermediates of the manufacturing process, which are also present in the final product, are positive for mutagenesis in the Ames assay. One of these intermediates was also positive in the mouse lymphoma assay. Imatinib was not genotoxic when tested in an *in vitro* bacterial cell assay (Ames test), an *in vitro* mammalian cell assay (mouse lymphoma) and an *in vivo* rat micronucleus assay.

In a study of fertility, male rats were dosed for 70 days prior to mating and female rats were dosed 14 days prior to mating and through to gestational Day 6. Testicular and epididymal weights and percent motile sperm were decreased at 60 mg/kg, approximately three-fourths the maximum clinical dose of 800 mg/day based on body surface area. This was not seen at doses ≤20 mg/kg (one-fourth the maximum human dose of 800 mg). The fertility of male and female rats was not affected.

In a pre- and post-natal development study in female rats dosed with imatinib mesylate at 45 mg/kg (approximately one-half the maximum human dose of 800 mg/day, based on body surface area) from gestational Day 6 until the end of lactation, red vaginal discharge was noted on either gestational Day 14 or 15. In the first generation offspring at this same dose level, mean body weights were reduced from birth until terminal sacrifice. First generation offspring fertility was not affected but reproductive effects were noted at 45 mg/kg/day including an increased number of resorptions and a decreased number of viable fetuses.

Fertility was not affected in the preclinical fertility and early embryonic development study although lower testes and epididymal weights as well as a reduced number of motile sperm were observed in the high dose male rats. In the preclinical pre- and postnatal study in rats, fertility in the first generation offspring was also not affected by Gleevec. Human studies on male patients receiving Gleevec and its affect on male fertility and spermatogenesis have not been performed. Male patients concerned about their fertility on Gleevec treatment should consult with their physician.

14 CLINICAL STUDIES

14.1 Chronic Myeloid Leukemia

Chronic Phase, Newly Diagnosed: An open-label, multicenter, international randomized Phase 3 study has been conducted in patients with newly diagnosed Philadelphia chromosome positive (Ph+) chronic myeloid leukemia (CML) in chronic phase. This study compared treatment with either single-agent Gleevec or a combination of interferon-alpha (IFN) plus cytarabine (Ara-C). Patients were allowed to cross over to the alternative treatment arm if they failed to show a complete hematologic response (CHR) at 6 months, a major cytogenetic response (MCyR) at 12 months, or if they lost a CHR or MCyR. Patients with increasing WBC or severe intolerance to treatment were also allowed to cross over to the alternative treatment arm with the permission of the study monitoring committee (SMC). In the Gleevec arm, patients were treated initially with 400 mg daily. Dose escalations were allowed from 400 mg daily to 600 mg daily, then from 600 mg daily to 800 mg daily. In the IFN arm, patients were treated with a target dose of IFN of 5 MIU/m^2/day subcutaneously in combination with subcutaneous Ara-C 20 mg/m^2/day for 10 days/month.

A total of 1,106 patients were randomized from 177 centers in 16 countries, 553 to each arm. Baseline characteristics were well balanced between the two arms. Median age was 51 years (range 18-70 years), with 21.9% of patients ≥60 years of age. There were 59% males and 41% females; 89.9% Caucasian and 4.7% Black patients. At the cut-off for this analysis (7 years after last patient had been recruited), the median duration of first-line treatment was 82 and 8 months in the Gleevec and IFN arm, respectively. The median duration of second-line treatment with Gleevec was 64 months. Sixty percent of patients randomized to Gleevec are still receiving first-line treatment. In these patients, the average dose of Gleevec was 403 mg ± 57 mg. Overall, in patients receiving first line Gleevec, the average daily dose delivered was 406 mg ± 76 mg. Due to discontinuations and cross-overs, only 2% of patients randomized to IFN were still on first-line treatment. In the IFN arm, withdrawal of consent (14%) was the most frequent reason for discontinuation of first-line therapy, and the most frequent reason for cross over to the Gleevec arm was severe intolerance to treatment (26%) and progression (14%).

The primary efficacy endpoint of the study was progression-free survival (PFS). Progression was defined as any of the following events: progression to accelerated phase or blast crisis (AP/BC), death, loss of CHR or MCyR, or in patients not achieving a CHR an increasing WBC despite appropriate therapeutic management. The protocol specified that the progression analysis would compare the intent to treat (ITT) population: patients randomized to receive Gleevec were compared with patients randomized to receive IFN. Patients that crossed over prior to progression were not censored at the time of cross-over, and events that occurred in these patients following cross-over were attributed to the original randomized treatment. The estimated rate of progression-free survival at 84 months in the ITT population was 81.2% [95% CI: 78, 85] in the Gleevec arm and 60.6% [56, 65] in the IFN arm (p<0.0001, log-rank test), (Figure 1). With 7 years follow up there were 93 (16.8%) progression events in the Gleevec arm: 37 (6.7%) progression to AP/BC, 31 (5.6%) loss of MCyR, 15 (2.7%) loss of CHR or increase in WBC and 10 (1.8%) CML unrelated deaths. In contrast, there were 165 (29.8%) events in the IFN+Ara-C arm of which 130 occurred during first-line treatment with IFN-Ara-C. The estimated rate of patients free of progression to accelerated phase (AP) or blast crisis (BC) at 84 months was 92.5% [90, 95] in the Gleevec arm compared to the 85.1%, [82, 89] (p≤0.001) in the IFN arm, (Figure 2). The annual rates of any progression events have decreased with time on therapy. The probability of remaining progression free at 60 months was 95% for patients who were in complete cytogenetic response (CCyR) with molecular response (≥3 log reduction in Bcr-Abl transcripts as measured by quantitative reverse transcriptase polymerase chain reaction) at 12 months, compared to 89% for patients in complete cytogenetic response but without a major molecular response and 70% in patients who were not in complete cytogenetic response at this time point (p<0.001).

[See figure 1 at top of next column]

[See figure 2 on next column]

A total of 71 (12.8%) and 85 (15.4%) patients died in the Gleevec and IFN+Ara-C group, respectively. At 84 months the estimated overall survival is 86.4% (83, 90) vs. 83.3% (80, 87) in the randomized Gleevec and the IFN+Ara-C group, respectively (p=0.073 log-rank test). The hazard ratio

Figure 1: Progression-Free Survival (ITT Principle)

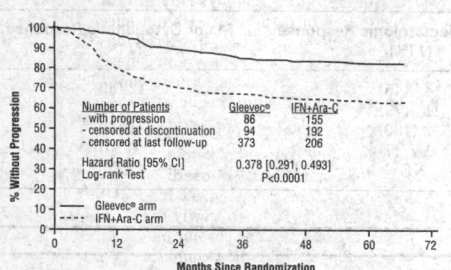

Figure 2: Time to Progression to AP or BC (ITT Principle)

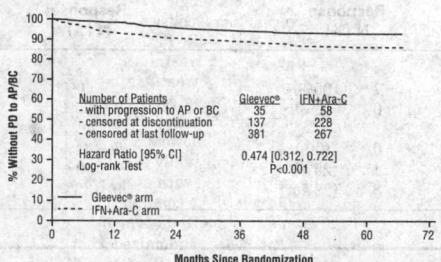

Table 14: Response in Newly Diagnosed CML Study (84-Month Data)

(Best Response Rate)	Gleevec n=553	IFN+Ara–C n=553
Hematologic Response[1]		
CHR Rate n (%)	534 (96.6%)*	313 (56.6%)*
[95% CI]	[94.7%, 97.9%]	[52.4%, 60.8%]
Cytogenetic Response[2]		
Major Cytogenetic Response n (%)	472 (85.4%)*	93 (16.8%)*
[95% CI]	[82.1%, 88.2%]	[13.8%, 20.2%]
Unconfirmed[3]	88.6%*	23.3%*
Complete Cytogenetic Response n (%)	413 (74.7%)*	36 (6.5%)*
[95% CI]	[70.8, 78.3]	[4.6, 8.9]
Unconfirmed[3]	82.5%*	11.6%*

* p<0.001, Fischer's exact test
[1] **Hematologic response criteria** (all responses to be confirmed after ≥4 weeks): WBC <10 × 10⁹/L, platelet <450 × 10⁹/L, myelocyte + metamyelocyte <5% in blood, no blasts and promyelocytes in blood, no extramedullary involvement.
[2] **Cytogenetic response criteria** (confirmed after ≥4 weeks): complete (0% Ph+ metaphases) or partial (1%-35%). A major response (0%-35%) combines both complete and partial responses.
[3] **Unconfirmed cytogenetic response** is based on a single bone marrow cytogenetic evaluation, therefore unconfirmed complete or partial cytogenetic responses might have had a lesser cytogenetic response on a subsequent bone marrow evaluation.

Table 15: Response in CML Studies

	Chronic Phase IFN Failure (n=532) 400 mg	Accelerated Phase (n=235) 600 mg n=158 400 mg n=77	Myeloid Blast Crisis (n=260) 600 mg n=223 400 mg n=37
		% of patients [CI₉₅%]	
Hematologic Response[1]	95% [92.3-96.3]	71% [64.8-76.8]	31% [25.2-36.8]
Complete Hematologic Response (CHR)	95%	38%	7%
No Evidence of Leukemia (NEL)	Not applicable	13%	5%
Return to Chronic Phase (RTC)	Not applicable	20%	18%
Major Cytogenetic Response[2]	60% [55.3-63.8]	21% [16.2-27.1]	7% [4.5-11.2]
(Unconfirmed[3])	(65%)	(27%)	(15%)
Complete[4] (Unconfirmed[3])	39% (47%)	16% (20%)	2% (7%)

[1] **Hematologic response criteria** (all responses to be confirmed after ≥4 weeks):
CHR: Chronic phase study [WBC <10 × 10⁹/L, platelet <450 × 10⁹/L, myelocytes + metamyelocytes <5% in blood, no blasts and promyelocytes in blood, basophils <20%, no extramedullary involvement] and in the accelerated and blast crisis studies [ANC ≥1.5 × 10⁹/L, platelets ≥100 × 10⁹/L, no blood blasts, BM blasts <5% and no extramedullary disease]
NEL: Same criteria as for CHR but ANC ≥1 × 10⁹/L and platelets ≥20 × 10⁹/L (accelerated and blast crisis studies)
RTC: <15% blasts BM and PB, <30% blasts + promyelocytes in BM and PB, <20% basophils in PB, no extramedullary disease other than spleen and liver (accelerated and blast crisis studies)
BM=bone marrow, PB=peripheral blood
[2] **Cytogenetic response criteria** (confirmed after ≥4 weeks): complete (0% Ph+ metaphases) or partial (1%-35%). A major response (0%-35%) combines both complete and partial responses.
[3] **Unconfirmed cytogenetic response** is based on a single bone marrow cytogenetic evaluation, therefore unconfirmed complete or partial cytogenetic responses might have had a lesser cytogenetic response on a subsequent bone marrow evaluation.
[4] **Complete cytogenetic response** confirmed by a second bone marrow cytogenetic evaluation performed at least 1 month after the initial bone marrow study.

is 0.750 with 95% CI 0.547-1.028. This time-to-event endpoint may be affected by the high crossover rate from IFN+Ara-C to Gleevec. Major cytogenetic response, hematologic response, evaluation of minimal residual disease (molecular response), time to accelerated phase or blast crisis and survival were main secondary endpoints. Response data are shown in Table 14. Complete hematologic response, major cytogenetic response and complete cytogenetic response were also statistically significantly higher in the Gleevec arm compared to the IFN+Ara-C arm (no cross-over data considered for evaluation of responses). Median time to CCyR in the 454 responders was 6 months (range 2-64 months, 25th to 75th percentiles = 3 to 11 months) with 10% of responses seen only after 22 months of therapy.
[See table 14 above]

Molecular response was defined as follows: in the peripheral blood, after 12 months of therapy, reduction of ≥3 logarithms in the amount of bcr-abl transcripts (measured by real-time quantitative reverse transcriptase PCR assay) over a standardized baseline. Molecular response was only evaluated in a subset of patients who had a complete cytogenetic response by 12 months or later (N=333). The molecular response rate in patients who had a complete cytogenetic response in the Gleevec arm was 59% at 12 months and 72% at 24 months.

Physical, functional, and treatment-specific biologic response modifier scales from the FACT-BRM (Functional Assessment of Cancer Therapy - Biologic Response Modifier) instrument were used to assess patient-reported general effects of interferon toxicity in 1,067 patients with CML in chronic phase. After one month of therapy to six months of therapy, there was a 13%-21% decrease in median index from baseline in patients treated with IFN, consistent with increased symptoms of IFN toxicity. There was no apparent change from baseline in median index for patients treated with Gleevec.

Late Chronic Phase CML and Advanced Stage CML: Three international, open-label, single-arm phase 2 studies were conducted to determine the safety and efficacy of Gleevec in patients with Ph+ CML: 1) in the chronic phase after failure of IFN therapy, 2) in accelerated phase disease, or 3) in myeloid blast crisis. About 45% of patients were women and 6% were Black. In clinical studies 38%-40% of patients were ≥60 years of age and 10%-12% of patients were ≥70 years of age.

Chronic Phase, Prior Interferon-Alpha Treatment: 532 patients were treated at a starting dose of 400 mg; dose escalation to 600 mg was allowed. The patients were distributed in three main categories according to their response to prior interferon: failure to achieve (within 6 months), or loss of a complete hematologic response (29%), failure to achieve (within 1 year) or loss of a major cytogenetic response (35%), or intolerance to interferon (36%). Patients had received a median of 14 months of prior IFN therapy at doses ≥25 × 10⁶ IU/week and were all in late chronic phase, with a median time from diagnosis of 32 months. Effectiveness was evaluated on the basis of the rate of hematologic response and by bone marrow exams to assess the rate of major cytogenetic response (up to 35% Ph+ metaphases) or complete cytogenetic response (0% Ph+ metaphases). Median dura-

tion of treatment was 29 months with 81% of patients treated for ≥24 months (maximum = 31.5 months). Efficacy results are reported in Table 15. Confirmed major cytogenetic response rates were higher in patients with IFN intolerance (66%) and cytogenetic failure (64%), than in patients with hematologic failure (47%). Hematologic response was achieved in 98% of patients with cytogenetic failure, 94% of patients with hematologic failure, and 92% of IFN-intolerant patients.

Accelerated Phase: 235 patients with accelerated phase disease were enrolled. These patients met one or more of the following criteria: ≥15%-<30% blasts in PB or BM; ≥30% blasts + promyelocytes in PB or BM; ≥20% basophils in PB; and <100 × 10⁹/L platelets. The first 77 patients were started at 400 mg, with the remaining 158 patients starting at 600 mg.
Effectiveness was evaluated primarily on the basis of the rate of hematologic response, reported as either complete hematologic response, no evidence of leukemia (i.e., clearance of blasts from the marrow and the blood, but without a full peripheral blood recovery as for complete responses), or return to chronic phase CML. Cytogenetic responses were also evaluated. Median duration of treatment was 18 months with 45% of patients treated for ≥24 months (maximum=35 months). Efficacy results are reported in Table 15. Response rates in accelerated phase CML were higher for the 600 mg dose group than for the 400 mg group: hematologic response (75% vs. 64%), confirmed and unconfirmed major cytogenetic response (31% vs. 19%).

Myeloid Blast Crisis: 260 patients with myeloid blast crisis were enrolled. These patients had ≥30% blasts in PB or BM

and/or extramedullary involvement other than spleen or liver; 95 (37%) had received prior chemotherapy for treatment of either accelerated phase or blast crisis ("pretreated patients") whereas 165 (63%) had not ("untreated patients"). The first 37 patients were started at 400 mg; the remaining 223 were started at 600 mg.
Effectiveness was evaluated primarily on the basis of rate of hematologic response, reported as either complete hematologic response, no evidence of leukemia, or return to chronic phase CML using the same criteria as for the study in accelerated phase. Cytogenetic responses were also assessed. Median duration of treatment was 4 months with 21% of patients treated for ≥12 months and 10% for ≥24 months (maximum=35 months). Efficacy results are reported in Table 15. The hematologic response rate was higher in untreated patients than in treated patients (36% vs. 22%, respectively) and in the group receiving an initial dose of 600 mg rather than 400 mg (33% vs. 16%). The confirmed and unconfirmed major cytogenetic response rate was also higher for the 600 mg dose group than for the 400 mg dose group (17% vs. 8%).
[See table 15 above]

The median time to hematologic response was 1 month. In late chronic phase CML, with a median time from diagnosis of 32 months, an estimated 87.8% of patients who achieved MCyR maintained their response 2 years after achieving their initial response. After 2 years of treatment, an estimated 85.4% of patients were free of progression to AP or BC, and estimated overall survival was 90.8% [88.3, 93.2]. In accelerated phase, median duration of hematologic response was 28.8 months for patients with an initial dose of

600 mg (16.5 months for 400 mg). An estimated 63.8% of patients who achieved MCyR were still in response 2 years after achieving initial response. The median survival was 20.9 [13.1, 34.4] months for the 400 mg group and was not yet reached for the 600 mg group (p=0.0097). An estimated 46.2% [34.7, 57.7] vs. 65.8% [58.4, 73.3] of patients were still alive after 2 years of treatment in the 400 mg vs. 600 mg dose groups, respectively. In blast crisis, the estimated median duration of hematologic response is 10 months. An estimated 27.2% [16.8, 37.7] of hematologic responders maintained their response 2 years after achieving their initial response. Median survival was 6.9 [5.8, 8.6] months, and an estimated 18.3% [13.4, 23.3] of all patients with blast crisis were alive 2 years after start of study.

Efficacy results were similar in men and women and in patients younger and older than age 65. Responses were seen in Black patients, but there were too few Black patients to allow a quantitative comparison.

14.2 Pediatric CML

A total of 51 pediatric patients with newly diagnosed and untreated CML in chronic phase were enrolled in an open-label, multicenter, single arm phase 2 trial. Patients were treated with Gleevec 340 mg/m²/day, with no interruptions in the absence of dose limiting toxicity. Complete hematologic response (CHR) was observed in 78% of patients after 8 weeks of therapy. The complete cytogenetic response rate (CCyR) was 65%, comparable to the results observed in adults. Additionally, partial cytogenetic response (PCyR) was observed in 16%. The majority of patients who achieved a CCyR developed the CCyR between months 3 and 10 with a median time to response based on the Kaplan-Meier estimate of 6.74 months.

One open-label, single-arm study enrolled 14 pediatric patients with Ph+ chronic phase CML recurrent after stem cell transplant or resistant to interferon-alpha therapy. Patients ranged in age from 3-20 years old; 3 were 3-11 years old, 9 were 12-18 years old, and 2 were >18 years old. Patients were treated at doses of 260 mg/m²/day (n=3), 340 mg/m²/day (n=4), 440 mg/m²/day (n=5) and 570 mg/m²/day (n=2). In the 13 patients for whom cytogenetic data are available, 4 achieved a major cytogenetic response, 7 achieved a complete cytogenetic response, and 2 had a minimal cytogenetic response.

In a second study, 2 of 3 patients with Ph+ chronic phase CML resistant to interferon-alpha therapy achieved a complete cytogenetic response at doses of 242 and 257 mg/m²/day.

14.3 Acute Lymphoblastic Leukemia

A total of 48 Philadelphia chromosome positive acute lymphoblastic leukemia (Ph+ ALL) patients with relapsed/refractory disease were studied, 43 of whom received the recommended Gleevec dose of 600 mg/day. In addition 2 patients with relapsed/refractory Ph+ ALL received Gleevec 600 mg/day in a phase 1 study.

Confirmed and unconfirmed hematologic and cytogenetic response rates for the 43 relapsed/refractory Ph+ ALL phase 2 study patients and for the 2 phase 1 patients are shown in Table 16. The median duration of hematologic response was 3.4 months and the median duration of MCyR was 2.3 months.

Table 16: Effect of Gleevec on Relapsed/Refractory Ph+ ALL

	Phase 2 Study (N=43)	Phase 1 Study (N=2)
CHR	8 (19%)	2 (100%)
NEL	5 (12%)	
RTC/PHR	11 (26%)	
MCyR	15 (35%)	
CCyR	9 (21%)	
PCyR	6 (14%)	

14.4 Myelodysplastic/Myeloproliferative Diseases

An open-label, multicenter, phase 2 clinical trial was conducted testing Gleevec in diverse populations of patients suffering from life-threatening diseases associated with Abl, Kit or PDGFR protein tyrosine kinases. This study included 7 patients with MDS/MPD. These patients were treated with Gleevec 400 mg daily. The ages of the enrolled patients ranged from 20 to 86 years. A further 24 patients with MDS/MPD aged 2 to 79 years were reported in 12 published case reports and a clinical study. These patients also received Gleevec at a dose of 400 mg daily with the exception of three patients who received lower doses. Of the total population of 31 patients treated for MDS/MPD, 14 (45%) achieved a complete hematological response and 12 (39%) a major cytogenetic response (including 10 with a complete cytogenetic response). Sixteen patients had a translocation, involving chromosome 5q33 or 4q12, resulting in a PDGFR gene rearrangement. All of these patients responded hematologically (13 completely). Cytogenetic response was evaluated

Table 17: Response in MDS/MPD

	N	Complete Hematologic Response N (%)	Major Cytogenetic Response N (%)
Overall Population	31	14 (45)	12 (39)
Chromosome 5 Translocation	14	11 (79)	11 (79)
Chromosome 4 Translocation	2	2 (100)	1 (50)
Others/no Translocation	14	1 (7)	0 (0)
Molecular Relapse	1	NE[1]	NE[1]

[1] NE: Not Evaluable

Table 18: Response in ASM

Cytogenetic Abnormality	Number of Patients	Complete Hematologic Response N (%)	Partial Hematologic Response N (%)
FIP1L1-PDGFRα Fusion Kinase (or CHIC2 Deletion)	7	7 (100%)	0%
Juxtamembrane Mutation	2	0 (0%)	2 (100%)
Unknown or No Cytogenetic Abnormality Detected	15	0 (0%)	7 (44%)
D816V Mutation	4	1* (25%)	0%
Total	28	8 (29%)	9 (32%)

*Patient had concomitant CML and ASM

Table 19: Response in HES/CEL

Cytogenetic Abnormality	Number of Patients	Complete Hematologic Response N (%)	Partial Hematologic Response N (%)
Positive FIP1L1-PDGFRα Fusion Kinase	61	61 (100%)	0%
Negative FIP1L1-PDGFRα Fusion Kinase	56	12 (21%)	9 (16%)
Unknown Cytogenetic Abnormality	59	34 (58%)	7 (12%)
Total	176	107 (61%)	23 (13%)

in 12 out of 14 patients, all of whom responded (10 patients completely). Only 1 (7%) out of the 14 patients without a translocation associated with PDGFR gene re-arrangement achieved a complete hematological response and none achieved a major cytogenetic response. A further patient with a PDGFR gene re-arrangement in molecular relapse after bone marrow transplant responded molecularly. Median duration of therapy was 12.9 months (0.8-26.7) in the 7 patients treated within the phase 2 study and ranged between 1 week and more than 18 months in responding patients in the published literature. Results are provided in Table 17. Response durations of phase 2 study patients ranged from 141+ days to 457+ days.
[See table 17 above]

14.5 Aggressive Systemic Mastocytosis

One open-label, multicenter, phase 2 study was conducted testing Gleevec in diverse populations of patients with life-threatening diseases associated with Abl, Kit or PDGFR protein tyrosine kinases. This study included 5 patients with aggressive systemic mastocytosis (ASM) treated with 100 mg to 400 mg of Gleevec daily. These 5 patients ranged from 49 to 74 years of age. In addition to these 5 patients, 10 published case reports and case series describe the use of Gleevec in 23 additional patients with ASM aged 26 to 85 years who also received 100 mg to 400 mg of Gleevec daily. Cytogenetic abnormalities were evaluated in 20 of the 28 ASM patients treated with Gleevec from the published reports and in the phase 2 study. Seven of these 20 patients had the FIP1L1-PDGFRα fusion kinase (or CHIC2 deletion). Patients with this cytogenetic abnormality were predominantly males and had eosinophilia associated with their systemic mast cell disease. Two patients had a Kit mutation in the juxtamembrane region (one Phe522Cys and one K509I) and four patients had a D816V c-Kit mutation (not considered sensitive to Gleevec), one with concomitant CML.

Of the 28 patients treated for ASM, 8 (29%) achieved a complete hematologic response and 9 (32%) a partial hematologic response (61% overall response rate). Median duration of Gleevec therapy for the 5 ASM patients in the phase 2 study was 13 months (range 1.4-22.3 months) and between 1 month and more than 30 months in the responding patients described in the published medical literature. A summary of the response rates to Gleevec in ASM is provided in Table 18. Response durations of literature patients ranged from 1+ to 30+ months.
[See table 18 above]
Gleevec has not been shown to be effective in patients with less aggressive forms of systemic mastocytosis (SM).

Gleevec is therefore not recommended for use in patients with cutaneous mastocytosis, indolent systemic mastocytosis (smoldering SM or isolated bone marrow mastocytosis), SM with an associated clonal hematological non-mast cell lineage disease, mast cell leukemia, mast cell sarcoma or extracutaneous mastocytoma. Patients that harbor the D816V mutation of c-Kit are not sensitive to Gleevec and should not receive Gleevec.

14.6 Hypereosinophilic Syndrome/Chronic Eosinophilic Leukemia

One open-label, multicenter, phase 2 study was conducted testing Gleevec in diverse populations of patients with life-threatening diseases associated with Abl, Kit or PDGFR protein tyrosine kinases. This study included 14 patients with Hypereosinophilic Syndrome/Chronic Eosinophilic Leukemia (HES/CEL). HES patients were treated with 100 mg to 1000 mg of Gleevec daily. The ages of these patients ranged from 16 to 64 years. A further 162 patients with HES/CEL aged 11 to 78 years were reported in 35 published case reports and case series. These patients received Gleevec at doses of 75 mg to 800 mg daily. Hematologic response rates are summarized in Table 19. Response durations for literature patients ranged from 6+ weeks to 44 months.
[See table 19 above]

14.7 Dermatofibrosarcoma Protuberans

Dermatofibrosarcoma Protuberans (DFSP) is a cutaneous soft tissue sarcoma. It is characterized by a translocation of chromosomes 17 and 22 that results in the fusion of the collagen type 1 alpha 1 gene and the PDGF B gene.

An open-label, multicenter, phase 2 study was conducted testing Gleevec in a diverse population of patients with life-threatening diseases associated with Abl, Kit or PDGFR protein tyrosine kinases. This study included 12 patients with DFSP who were treated with Gleevec 800 mg daily (age range 23 to 75 years). DFSP was metastatic, locally recurrent following initial surgical resection and not considered amenable to further surgery at the time of study entry. A further 6 DFSP patients treated with Gleevec are reported in 5 published case reports, their ages ranging from 18 months to 49 years. The total population treated for DFSP therefore comprises 18 patients, 8 of them with metastatic disease. The adult patients reported in the published literature were treated with either 400 mg (4 cases) or 800 mg (1 case) Gleevec daily. A single pediatric patient received 400 mg/m²/daily, subsequently increased to 520 mg/m²/daily. Ten patients had the PDGF B gene rearrangement, 5 had no available cytogenetics and 3 had complex cytogenetic abnormalities. Responses to treatment are described in Table 20.

Table 20: Response in DFSP

	Number of Patients (n=18)	%
Complete Response	7	39
Partial Response*	8	44
Total Responders	15	83

*5 patients made disease free by surgery

Twelve of these 18 patients either achieved a complete response (7 patients) or were made disease free by surgery after a partial response (5 patients, including one child) for a total complete response rate of 67%. A further 3 patients achieved a partial response, for an overall response rate of 83%. Of the 8 patients with metastatic disease, five responded (62%), three of them completely (37%). For the 10 study patients with the PDGF B gene rearrangement there were 4 complete and 6 partial responses. The median duration of response in the phase 2 study was 6.2 months, with a maximum duration of 24.3 months, while in the published literature it ranged between 4 weeks and more than 20 months.

14.8 Gastrointestinal Stromal Tumors

Unresectable and/or Malignant Metastatic GIST

Two open-label, randomized, multinational Phase 3 studies were conducted in patients with unresectable or metastatic malignant gastrointestinal stromal tumors (GIST). The two study designs were similar allowing a predefined combined analysis of safety and efficacy. A total of 1640 patients were enrolled into the two studies and randomized 1:1 to receive either 400 mg or 800 mg orally daily continuously until disease progression or unacceptable toxicity. Patients in the 400 mg daily treatment group who experienced disease progression were permitted to crossover to receive treatment with 800 mg daily. The studies were designed to compare response rates, progression-free survival and overall survival between the dose groups. Median age at patient entry was 60 years. Males comprised 58% of the patients enrolled. All patients had a pathologic diagnosis of CD117 positive unresectable and/or metastatic malignant GIST.

The primary objective of the two studies was to evaluate either progression-free survival (PFS) with a secondary objective of overall survival (OS) in one study or overall survival with a secondary objective of PFS in the other study. A planned analysis of both OS and PFS from the combined datasets from these two studies was conducted. Results from this combined analysis are shown in Table 21.

Table 21: Overall Survival, Progression-Free Survival and Tumor Response Rates in the Phase 3 GIST Trials

	Gleevec 400 mg N=818	Gleevec 800 mg N=822
Progression-Free Survival (months)		
Median	18.9	23.2
95% CI	17.4-21.2	20.8-24.9
Overall Survival (months)	49.0	48.7
95% CI	45.3-60.0	45.3-51.6
Best Overall Tumor Response		
Complete Response (CR)	43 (5.3%)	41 (5.0%)
Partial Response (PR)	377 (46.1%)	402 (48.9%)

Median follow up for the combined studies was 37.5 months. There were no observed differences in overall survival between the treatment groups (p=0.98). Patients who crossed over following disease progression from the 400 mg/day treatment group to the 800 mg/day treatment group (n=347) had a 3.4 month median and a 7.7 month mean exposure to Gleevec following crossover.

One open-label, multinational Phase 2 study was conducted in patients with Kit (CD117) positive unresectable or metastatic malignant GIST. In this study, 147 patients were enrolled and randomized to receive either 400 mg or 600 mg orally q.d. for up to 36 months. The primary outcome of the study was objective response rate. Tumors were required to be measurable at entry in at least one site of disease, and response characterization was based on Southwestern Oncology Group (SWOG) criteria. There were no differences in response rates between the 2 dose groups. The response rate was 68.5% for the 400 mg group and 67.6% for the 600 mg group. The median time to response was 12 weeks (range was 3-98 weeks) and the estimated median duration of response is 118 weeks (95% CI: 86, not reached).

Adjuvant Treatment of GIST

In the adjuvant setting, Gleevec was investigated in a multicenter, double-blind, placebo-controlled, randomized study involving 713 patients. After complete gross resection of primary GIST, patients were randomized to one of the two arms: Gleevec at 400 mg/day or matching placebo for one year. The ages of these patients ranged from 18 to 91 years. Patients were included who had a histologic diagnosis of primary GIST expressing KIT protein by immunochemistry and a tumor size ≥3 cm in maximum dimension, with complete gross resection of primary GIST within 14 to 70 days prior to registration.

The efficacy endpoint of the study was recurrence free survival (RFS) defined as the time from date of randomization to the date of recurrence or death from any cause. At a median follow up of 14.0 months, there were 30 RFS events in the Gleevec arm compared to 70 RFS events in the placebo arm (hazard ratio=0.398 [95% CI: 0.259, 0.610], p<0.0001). Based on an interim analysis, patients still receiving placebo were allowed to cross over to Gleevec. The current follow-up is too short to evaluate survival.

Figure 3: Recurrence Free Survival

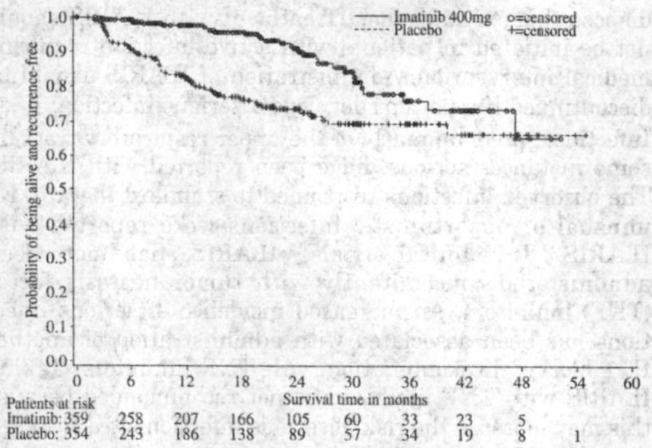
Imatinib 400mg o=censored
Placebo +=censored
Probability of being alive and recurrence-free
1.0
0.9
0.8
0.7
0.6
0.5
0.4
0.3
0.2
0.1
0.0
0 6 12 18 24 30 36 42 48 54 60
Survival time in months
Patients at risk
Imatinib: 359 258 207 166 105 60 33 23 5
Placebo: 354 243 186 138 89 57 34 19 8 1

15 REFERENCES

1. Preventing Occupational Exposures to Antineoplastic and Other Hazardous Drugs in Health Care Settings. NIOSH Alert 2004-165.
2. OSHA Technical Manual, TED 1-0.15A, Section VI: Chapter 2. Controlling Occupational Exposure to Hazardous Drugs. OSHA, 1999. http://www.osha.gov/dts/osta/otm/otm_vi/otm_vi_2.html
3. American Society of Health-System Pharmacists. ASHP guidelines on handling hazardous drugs. *Am J Health-Syst Pharm*. 2006;63:1172-1193.
4. Polovich, M., White, J. M., & Kelleher, L.O. (eds.) 2005. Chemotherapy and biotherapy guidelines and recommendations for practice (2nd. ed.) Pittsburgh, PA: Oncology Nursing Society.

16 HOW SUPPLIED/STORAGE AND HANDLING

Each film-coated tablet contains 100 mg or 400 mg of imatinib free base.

100 mg Tablets

Very dark yellow to brownish orange, film-coated tablets, round, biconvex with bevelled edges, debossed with "NVR" on one side, and "SA" with score on the other side.

Bottles of 90 tablets .... NDC 0078-0401-34

400 mg Tablets

Very dark yellow to brownish orange, film-coated tablets, ovaloid, biconvex with bevelled edges, debossed with "400" on one side with score on the other side, and "SL" on each side of the score.

Bottles of 30 tablets .... NDC 0078-0438-15

Storage and Handling

Store at 25°C (77°F); excursions permitted to 15-30°C (59-86°F) [see USP Controlled Room Temperature]. Protect from moisture.

Dispense in a tight container, USP.

Procedures for proper handling and disposal of anticancer drugs should be considered. Several guidelines on this subject have been published.[1-4]

Gleevec tablets should not be crushed. Direct contact of crushed tablets with the skin or mucous membranes should be avoided. If such contact occurs, wash thoroughly as outlined in the references. Personnel should avoid exposure to crushed tablets [*see Nonclinical Toxicology (13.1)*].

17 PATIENT COUNSELING INFORMATION

17.1 Dosing and Administration

Patients should be informed to take Gleevec exactly as prescribed, not to change their dose or to stop taking Gleevec unless they are told to do so by their doctor. If patients miss a dose they should be advised to take their dose as soon as possible unless it is almost time for their next dose in which case the missed dose should not be taken. A double dose should not be taken to make up for any missed dose. Patients should be advised to take Gleevec with a meal and a large glass of water.

17.2 Pregnancy and Breast-Feeding

Patients should be advised to inform their doctor if they are or think they may be pregnant. Patients should also be advised not to breast feed while taking Gleevec.

17.3 Adverse Reactions

Patients should be advised to tell their doctor if they experience side effects during Gleevec therapy including fever, shortness of breath, blood in their stools, jaundice, sudden weight gain, symptoms of cardiac failure, or if they have a history of cardiac disease or risk factors for cardiac failure.

17.4 Drug Interactions

Patients should be advised not to take any other medications, including over-the-counter medications such as acetaminophen or herbal products without talking to their doctor or pharmacist first. Examples of other medications that should not be taken with Gleevec are warfarin, erythromycin, and phenytoin. Patients should also be advised to tell their doctor if they are taking or plan to take iron supplements. Patients should also avoid grapefruit juice and other foods known to inhibit CYP3A4 while taking Gleevec.

T2010-21

Distributed by:
Novartis Pharmaceuticals Corporation
East Hanover, New Jersey 07936
©Novartis

Shown in Product Identification Guide, page 315

ILARIS® ℞

(canakinumab)
Injection for Subcutaneous use

The following prescribing information is based on official labeling in effect July 2009.

HIGHLIGHTS OF PRESCRIBING INFORMATION

These highlights do not include all the information needed to use ILARIS safely and effectively. See full prescribing information for ILARIS.

ILARIS *(canakinumab)* **Injection for Subcutaneous use**
Initial U.S. Approval: 2009

INDICATIONS AND USAGE

ILARIS is an interleukin-1β blocker indicated for the treatment of Cryopyrin-Associated Periodic Syndromes (CAPS), in adults and children 4 years of age and older including:
- Familial Cold Autoinflammatory Syndrome (FCAS)
- Muckle-Wells Syndrome (MWS) (1)

DOSAGE AND ADMINISTRATION

150 mg for CAPS patients with body weight greater than 40 kg and 2 mg/kg for CAPS patients with body weight greater than or equal to 15 kg and less than or equal to 40 kg. For children 15 to 40 kg with an inadequate response, the dose can be increased to 3 mg/kg. (2.2)

DOSAGE FORMS AND STRENGTHS

Sterile, single-use 6-mL, glass vial containing 180 mg of ILARIS as a lyophilized powder for reconstitution. (3)

CONTRAINDICATIONS

None. (4)

WARNINGS AND PRECAUTIONS

- Interleukin-1 blockade may interfere with immune response to infections. Treatment with medications that work through inhibition of IL-1 has been associated with an increased risk of serious infections. ILARIS has been associated with an increased incidence of serious infections. Physicians should exercise caution when administering ILARIS to patients with infections, a history of recurring infections or underlying conditions which may predispose them to infections. Discontinue treatment with ILARIS if a patient develops a serious infection. Do not initiate treatment with ILARIS in patients with active infection requiring medical intervention. (5.1)
- Live vaccines should not be given concurrently with ILARIS. Prior to initiation of therapy with ILARIS, patients should receive all recommended vaccinations. (5.3)

ADVERSE REACTIONS

The most common adverse reactions reported by patients with CAPS treated with ILARIS are nasopharyngitis, diarrhea, influenza, headache and nausea. (6)

To report SUSPECTED ADVERSE REACTIONS, contact Novartis Pharmaceuticals Corporation at 1-888-669-6682 or FDA at 1-800-FDA-1088 or www.fda.gov/medwatch

DRUG INTERACTIONS

No formal drug interaction studies have been conducted with ILARIS.

USE IN SPECIFIC POPULATIONS

- Pregnancy: No Human data. Because animal reproduction studies are not always predictive of human response, this drug should be used during pregnancy only if clearly needed. (8.1)
- Nursing Mothers: Caution should be exercised when administered to a nursing woman. (8.3)

See 17 for PATIENT COUNSELING INFORMATION and FDA-approved patient labeling

Revised: 06/2009

FULL PRESCRIBING INFORMATION: CONTENTS*

FULL PRESCRIBING INFORMATION

1   INDICATIONS AND USAGE

ILARIS (canakinumab) is an interleukin-1β blocker indicated for the treatment of Cryopyrin-Associated Periodic Syndromes (CAPS), in adults and children 4 years of age and older including:
• Familial Cold Autoinflammatory Syndrome (FCAS)
• Muckle-Wells Syndrome (MWS)

2   DOSAGE AND ADMINISTRATION

2.1   General Dosing Information
INJECTION FOR SUBCUTANEOUS USE ONLY.

2.2   Recommended Dose
The recommended dose of ILARIS is 150 mg for CAPS patients with body weight greater than 40 kg. For CAPS patients with body weight between 15 kg and 40 kg, the recommended dose is 2 mg/kg. For children 15 to 40 kg with an inadequate response, the dose can be increased to 3 mg/kg. ILARIS is administered every eight weeks as a single dose via subcutaneous injection.

2.3   Preparation for Administration
Using aseptic technique, reconstitute each vial of ILARIS by slowly injecting 1 mL of preservative-free Sterile Water for Injection with a 1 mL syringe and an 18 G × 2″ needle. Swirl the vial slowly at an angle of about 45° for approximately 1 minute and allow to stand for 5 minutes. Then gently turn the vial upside down and back again ten times. Avoid touching the rubber stopper with your fingers. Allow to stand for about 15 minutes at room temperature to obtain a clear solution. Do not shake. Do not use if particulate matter is present in the solution. Tap the side of the vial to remove any residual liquid from the stopper. The reconstituted solution should be essentially free from particulates, and clear to opalescent. The solution should be colorless or may have a slight brownish-yellow tint. If the solution has a distinctly brown discoloration it should not be used. If not used within 60 minutes of reconstitution, the solution should be stored in the refrigerator at 2 to 8°C (36 to 46°F) and used within 4 hours. Slight foaming of the product upon reconstitution is not unusual.

Using a sterile syringe and needle carefully withdraw the required volume depending on the dose to be administered (0.2 mL to 1 mL) and subcutaneously inject using a 27 G × 0.5″ needle.

Injection into scar tissue should be avoided as this may result in insufficient exposure to ILARIS.

ILARIS 180-mg powder for solution for injection is supplied in a single-use vial. Any unused product or waste material should be disposed of in accordance with local requirements.

3   DOSAGE FORMS AND STRENGTHS

ILARIS is supplied as a 180 mg white lyophilized powder for solution for subcutaneous injection. Reconstitution with 1 mL of preservative-free Sterile Water for Injection is required prior to subcutaneous administration of the drug, resulting in a total volume of 1.2 mL reconstituted solution. The reconstituted ILARIS is a clear to slightly opalescent, colorless to a slight brownish yellow tint, essentially free from particulates, 150 mg/mL solution.

4   CONTRAINDICATIONS
None

5   WARNINGS AND PRECAUTIONS

5.1   Serious Infections
ILARIS may be associated with an increased risk of serious infections. Physicians should exercise caution when administering ILARIS to patients with infections, a history of recurring infections or underlying conditions which may predispose them to infections. Treatment with ILARIS should not be initiated in patients with active infection requiring medical intervention. Administration of ILARIS should be discontinued if a patient develops a serious infection.

Infections, predominantly of the upper respiratory tract, in some instances serious, have been reported with ILARIS. The observed infections responded to standard therapy. No unusual or opportunistic infections were reported with ILARIS. In clinical trials, ILARIS has not been administered concomitantly with tumor necrosis factor (TNF) inhibitors. An increased incidence of serious infections has been associated with administration of another IL-1 blocker in combination with TNF inhibitors. Taking ILARIS with TNF inhibitors is not recommended because this may increase the risk of serious infections [see Drug Interactions (7.1)].

Drugs that affect the immune system by blocking TNF have been associated with an increased risk of reactivation of latent tuberculosis (TB). It is possible that taking drugs such as ILARIS that block IL-1 increases the risk of TB or other atypical or opportunistic infections.

Prior to initiating immunomodulatory therapies, including ILARIS, patients should be tested for latent tuberculosis infection. ILARIS has not been studied in patients with a positive tuberculosis screen, and the safety of ILARIS in individuals with latent tuberculosis infection is unknown. Patients testing positive in tuberculosis screening should be treated by standard medical practice prior to therapy with ILARIS.

Healthcare providers should follow current CDC guidelines both to evaluate for and to treat possible latent tuberculosis infections before initiating therapy with ILARIS.

5.2   Immunosuppression
The impact of treatment with anti-interleukin-1 (IL-1) therapy on the development of malignancies is not known. However, treatment with immunosuppressants, including ILARIS, may result in an increase in the risk of malignancies.

5.3   Immunizations
Live vaccines should not be given concurrently with ILARIS [see Drug Interactions (7.2)]. Since no data are available on either the efficacy or on the risks of secondary transmission of infection by live vaccines in patients receiving ILARIS, live vaccines should not be given concurrently with ILARIS. In addition, because ILARIS may interfere with normal immune response to new antigens, vaccinations may not be effective in patients receiving ILARIS. No data are available on the effectiveness of vaccinations with inactivated (killed) antigens in patients receiving ILARIS [see Drug Interactions (7.2)].

Because IL-1 blockade may interfere with immune response to infections, it is recommended that prior to initiation of therapy with ILARIS, adult and pediatric patients receive all recommended vaccinations, as appropriate, including pneumococcal vaccine and inactivated influenza vaccine. (See current recommended immunization schedules at the website of the Centers for Disease Control, http://www.cdc.gov/vaccines/recs/schedules/).

6   ADVERSE REACTIONS

The data described herein reflect exposure to ILARIS in 104 adult and pediatric CAPS patients (including 20 FCAS, 72 MWS, 10 MWS/NOMID (Neonatal Onset Multisystem Inflammatory Disorder) overlap, 1 non-FCAS non-MWS, and 1 mis-diagnosed in placebo-controlled (35 patients) and uncontrolled) trials). Sixty-two patients were exposed to ILARIS for at least 6 months, 56 for at least 1 year and 4 for at least 3 years. A total of 9 serious adverse reactions were reported for CAPS patients. Among these were vertigo (2 patients), infections (3 patients), including intra-abdominal abscess following appendectomy (1 patient). The most commonly reported adverse reactions associated with ILARIS treatment in the CAPS patients were nasopharyngitis, diarrhea, influenza, headache, and nausea. No impact on the

type or frequency of adverse drug reactions was seen with longer-term treatment. One patient discontinued treatment due to potential infection.

Because clinical trials are conducted under widely varying conditions, adverse reaction rates observed in the clinical trials of a drug cannot be directly compared to rates in the clinical trials of another drug and may not reflect the rates observed in practice.

6.1   Clinical Trial Experience
Approximately 833 subjects have been treated with ILARIS in blinded and open-label clinical trials in CAPS and other diseases, and healthy volunteers. A total of 15 patients reported serious adverse reactions during the clinical program.

Study 1 investigated the safety of ILARIS in an 8-week, open-label period (Part 1), followed by a 24-week, randomized withdrawal period (Part 2), followed by a 16-week, open-label period (Part 3). All patients were treated with ILARIS 150 mg subcutaneously or 2 mg/kg if body weight was greater than or equal to 15 kg and less than or equal to 40 kg (see Table 1).

Since all CAPS patients received ILARIS in Part 1, there are no controlled data on adverse events (AEs). Data in Table 1 are for all AEs for all CAPS patients receiving canakinumab. In study 1, no pattern was observed for any type or frequency of adverse events throughout the three study periods.

Table 1. Number (%) of Patients with AEs by Preferred Terms, in > 10% of Patients in Parts 1 to 3 of the Phase 3 Trial for CAPS Patients

Preferred Term	ILARIS N=35 n (%)
n % of Patients with Adverse Events	35 (100)
Nasopharyngitis	12 (34)
Diarrhea	7 (20)
Influenza	6 (17)
Rhinitis	6 (17)
Nausea	5 (14)
Headache	5 (14)
Bronchitis	4 (11)
Gastroenteritis	4 (11)
Pharyngitis	4 (11)
Weight increased	4 (11)
Musculoskeletal pain	4 (11)
Vertigo	4 (11)

6.2   Vertigo
Vertigo has been reported in 9 to 14% of patients in CAPS studies, exclusively in MWS patients, and reported as a serious adverse event in two cases. All events resolved with continued treatment with ILARIS.

6.3   Injection Site Reactions
In Study 1, subcutaneous injection site reactions were observed in 9% of patients in Part 1 with mild tolerability reactions; in Part 2, one patient each (7%) had a mild or a moderate tolerability reaction and, in Part 3, one patient had a mild local tolerability reaction. No severe injection-site reactions were reported and none led to discontinuation of treatment.

6.4   Immunogenicity
A specific biosensor binding assay was used to detect antibodies directed against canakinumab in patients who received ILARIS. None of the 60 CAPS patients who had received ILARIS tested positive for treatment-emergent binding antibodies at the time points tested. Thirty-one of 60 CAPS patients had a duration of exposure to canakinumab >48 weeks. The data obtained in an assay is highly dependent on several factors including assay sensitivity and specificity, assay methodology, sample handling, timing of sample collection, concomitant medications, underlying disease, and the number of patients tested. For these reasons, comparison of the incidence of antibodies to canakinumab with the incidence of antibodies to other products may be misleading.

7   DRUG INTERACTIONS

Interactions between ILARIS and other medicinal products have not been investigated in formal studies.

7.1   TNF-Blocker and IL-1 Blocking Agent
An increased incidence of serious infections and an increased risk of neutropenia have been associated with administration of another IL-1 blocker in combination with TNF inhibitors in another patient population. Use of ILARIS with TNF inhibitors may also result in similar toxicities and is not recommended because this may increase the risk of serious infections [see Warnings and Precautions (5.1)].

The concomitant administration of ILARIS with other drugs that block IL-1 has not been studied. Based upon the potential for pharmacological interactions between ILARIS and a recombinant IL-1ra, concomitant administration of ILARIS and other agents that block IL-1 or its receptors is not recommended.

7.2 Immunization

No data are available on either the effects of live vaccination or the secondary transmission of infection by live vaccines in patients receiving ILARIS. Therefore, live vaccines should not be given concurrently with ILARIS. It is recommended that, if possible, pediatric and adult patients should complete all immunizations in accordance with current immunization guidelines prior to initiating ILARIS therapy [*see Warnings and Precautions (5.3)*].

7.3 Cytochrome P450 Substrates

The formation of CYP450 enzymes is suppressed by increased levels of cytokines (e.g., IL-1) during chronic inflammation. Thus it is expected that for a molecule that binds to IL-1, such as canakinumab, the formation of CYP450 enzymes could be normalized. This is clinically relevant for CYP450 substrates with a narrow therapeutic index, where the dose is individually adjusted (e.g., warfarin). Upon initiation of canakinumab, in patients being treated with these types of medicinal products, therapeutic monitoring of the effect or drug concentration should be performed and the individual dose of the medicinal product may need to be adjusted as needed.

8 USE IN SPECIFIC POPULATIONS

8.1 Pregnancy

Pregnancy Category C

Canakinumab has been shown to produce delays in fetal skeletal development when evaluated in marmoset monkeys using doses 23-fold the maximum recommended human dose (MRHD) and greater (based on a plasma area under the time-concentration curve [AUC] comparison). Doses producing exposures within the clinical exposure range at the MRHD were not evaluated. Similar delays in fetal skeletal development were observed in mice administered a murine analog of canakinumab. There are no adequate and well-controlled studies of ILARIS in pregnant women. Because animal reproduction studies are not always predictive of human response, this drug should be used during pregnancy only if clearly needed.

Embryofetal developmental toxicity studies were performed in marmoset monkeys and mice. Pregnant marmoset monkeys were administered canakinumab subcutaneously twice weekly at doses of 15, 50 or 150 mg/kg (representing 23- to 230-fold the human dose based on a plasma AUC comparison at the MRHD) from gestation days 25 to 109 which revealed no evidence of embryotoxicity or fetal malformations. There were increases in the incidence of incomplete ossification of the terminal caudal vertebra and misaligned and/or bipartite vertebra in fetuses at all dose levels when compared to concurrent controls suggestive of delay in skeletal development in the marmoset. Since canakinumab does not cross-react with mouse or rat IL-1, pregnant mice were subcutaneously administered a murine analog of canakinumab at doses of 15, 50, or 150 mg/kg on gestation days 6, 11 and 17. The incidence of incomplete ossification of the parietal and frontal skull bones of fetuses was increased in a dose-dependent manner at all dose levels tested.

8.3 Nursing Mothers

It is not known whether canakinumab is excreted in human milk. Because many drugs are excreted in human milk, caution should be exercised when ILARIS is administered to a nursing woman.

8.4 Pediatric Use

The CAPS trials with ILARIS included a total of 23 pediatric patients with an age range from 4 years to 17 years (11 adolescents were treated subcutaneously with 150 mg, and 12 children were treated with 2 mg/kg based on body weight greater than or equal to 15 kg and less than or equal to 40 kg). The majority of patients achieved improvement in clinical symptoms and objective markers of inflammation (e.g., Serum Amyloid A and C-Reactive Protein). Overall, the efficacy and safety of ILARIS in pediatric and adult patients were comparable. Infections of the upper respiratory tract were the most frequently reported infection. The safety and effectiveness of ILARIS in patients under 4 years of age has not been established [*see Pharmacokinetics (12.3)*].

8.5 Geriatric Use

Clinical studies of ILARIS did not include sufficient numbers of subjects aged 65 and over to determine whether they respond differently from younger subjects.

8.6 Patients with Renal Impairment

No formal studies have been conducted to examine the pharmacokinetics of ILARIS administered subcutaneously in patients with renal impairment.

8.7 Patients with Hepatic Impairment

No formal studies have been conducted to examine the pharmacokinetics of ILARIS administered subcutaneously in patients with hepatic impairment.

Table 2. Physician's Global Assessment of Auto-Inflammatory Disease Activity and Assessment of Skin Disease: Frequency Table and Treatment Comparison in Part 2 (Using LOCF, ITT Population)

		ILARIS N=15		Placebo N=16	
	Baseline	Start of Part 2 (Week 8)	End of Part 2	Start of Part 2 (Week 8)	End of Part 2
Physician's Global Assessment of Auto-Inflammatory Disease Activity – n (%)					
Absent	0/31 (0)	9/15 (60)	8/15 (53)	8/16 (50)	0/16 (0)
Minimal	1/31 (3)	4/15 (27)	7/15 (47)	8/16 (50)	4/16 (25)
Mild	7/31 (23)	2/15 (13)	0/15 (0)	0/16 (0)	8/16 (50)
Moderate	19/31 (61)	0/15 (0)	0/15 (0)	0/16 (0)	4/16 (25)
Severe	4/31 (13)	0/15 (0)	0/15 (0)	0/16 (0)	0/16 (0)
Assessment of Skin Disease – n (%)					
Absent	3/31 (10)	13/15 (87)	14/15 (93)	13/16 (81)	5/16 (31)
Minimal	6/31 (19)	2/15 (13)	1/15 (7)	3/16 (19)	3/16 (19)
Mild	9/31 (29)	0/15 (0)	0/15 (0)	0/16 (0)	5/16 (31)
Moderate	12/31 (39)	0/15 (0)	0/15 (0)	0/16 (0)	3/16 (19)
Severe	1/32 (3)	0/15 (0)	0/15 (0)	0/16 (0)	0/16 (0)

10 OVERDOSAGE

No case of overdose has been reported. In the case of overdose, it is recommended that the subject be monitored for any signs and symptoms of adverse reactions or effects, and appropriate symptomatic treatment be instituted immediately.

11 DESCRIPTION

Canakinumab is a recombinant, human anti-human-IL-1β monoclonal antibody that belongs to the IgG1/κ isotype subclass. It is expressed in a murine Sp2/0-Ag14 cell line and comprised of two 447- (or 448-) residue heavy chains and two 214-residue light chains, with a molecular mass of 145157 Daltons when deglycosylated. Both heavy chains of canakinumab contain oligosaccharide chains linked to the protein backbone at asparagine 298 (Asn 298).

The biological activity of canakinumab is measured by comparing its inhibition of IL-1β-dependent expression of the reporter gene luciferase to that of a canakinumab internal reference standard, using a stably transfected cell line.

ILARIS is supplied in a sterile, single-use, colorless, 6 mL glass vial with coated stopper and aluminum flip-off cap. Each vial contains 180 mg of canakinumab as a white, preservative-free, lyophilized powder. Reconstitution with 1 mL of preservative-free Sterile Water for Injection is required prior to subcutaneous administration of the drug. The reconstituted canakinumab is a 150 mg/mL solution essentially free of particulates, clear to slightly opalescent, and is colorless or may have a slightly brownish-yellow tint. A volume of up to 1 mL can be withdrawn for delivery of 150 mg/mL canakinumab for subcutaneous administration. Each reconstituted vial contains 180 mg canakinumab, sucrose, L-histidine, L-histidine HCl monohydrate, polysorbate 80 and Sterile Water for Injection. No preservatives are present.

12 CLINICAL PHARMACOLOGY

12.1 Mechanism of Action

CAPS refer to rare genetic syndromes generally caused by mutations in the NLRP-3 [nucleotide-binding domain, leucine rich family (NLR), pyrin domain containing 3] gene (also known as Cold-Induced Auto-inflammatory Syndrome-1 [CIAS1]). CAPS disorders are inherited in an autosomal dominant pattern with male and female offspring equally affected. Features common to all disorders include fever, urticaria-like rash, arthralgia, myalgia, fatigue, and conjunctivitis.

The NLRP-3 gene encodes the protein cryopyrin, an important component of the inflammasome. Cryopyrin regulates the protease caspase-1 and controls the activation of interleukin-1 beta (IL-1β). Mutations in NLRP-3 result in an overactive inflammasome resulting in excessive release of activated IL-1β that drives inflammation.

Canakinumab is a human monoclonal anti-human IL-1β antibody of the IgG1/κ isotype. Canakinumab binds to human IL-1β and neutralizes its activity by blocking its interaction with IL-1 receptors, but it does not bind IL-1α or IL-1 receptor antagonist (IL-1ra).

12.2 Pharmacodynamics

C-reactive protein and Serum Amyloid A (SAA) are indicators of inflammatory disease activity that are elevated in patients with CAPS. Elevated SAA has been associated with the development of systemic amyloidosis in patients with CAPS. Following ILARIS treatment, CRP and SAA levels normalize within 8 days.

12.3 Pharmacokinetics

Absorption

The peak serum canakinumab concentration (C_{max}) of 16 ± 3.5 μg/mL occurred approximately 7 days after subcutaneous administration of a single, 150-mg dose subcutaneously to adult CAPS patients. The mean terminal half-life was 26 days. The absolute bioavailability of subcutaneous canakinumab was estimated to be 70%. Exposure parameters (such as AUC and C_{max}) increased in proportion to dose over the dose range of 0.30 to 10 mg/kg given as intravenous infusion or from 150 to 300 mg as subcutaneous injection.

Distribution

Canakinumab binds to serum IL-1β. Canakinumab volume of distribution (V_{ss}) varied according to body weight and was estimated to be 6.01 liters in a typical CAPS patient weighing 70 kg. The expected accumulation ratio was 1.3-fold following 6 months of subcutaneous dosing of 150 mg ILARIS every 8 weeks.

Elimination

Clearance (CL) of canakinumab varied according to body weight and was estimated to be 0.174 L/day in a typical CAPS patient weighing 70 kg. There was no indication of accelerated clearance or time-dependent change in the pharmacokinetic properties of canakinumab following repeated administration. No gender- or age-related pharmacokinetic differences were observed after correction for body weight.

Pediatrics

Peak concentrations of canakinumab occurred between 2 to 7 days following single subcutaneous administration of ILARIS 150 mg or 2 mg/kg in pediatric patients. The terminal half-life ranged from 22.9 to 25.7 days, similar to the pharmacokinetic properties observed in adults.

13 NONCLINICAL TOXICOLOGY

13.1 Carcinogenesis, Mutagenesis, Impairment of Fertility

Long-term animal studies have not been performed to evaluate the carcinogenic potential of canakinumab.

The mutagenic potential of canakinumab was not evaluated.

As canakinumab does not cross-react with rodent IL-1β, male and female fertility was evaluated in a mouse model using a murine analog of canakinumab. Male mice were treated weekly beginning 4 weeks prior to mating and continuing through 3 weeks after mating. Female mice were treated weekly for 2 weeks prior to mating through gestation day 3 or 4. The murine analog of canakinumab did not alter either male or female fertility parameters at subcutaneous doses up to 150 mg/kg.

14 CLINICAL STUDIES

The efficacy and safety of ILARIS for the treatment of CAPS was demonstrated in Study 1, a 3-part trial in patients 9 to 74 years of age with the MWS phenotype of CAPS. Throughout the trial, patients weighing more than 40 kg received ILARIS 150 mg and patients weighing 15 to 40 kg received 2 mg/kg. Part 1 was an 8-week open-label, single-dose period where all patients received ILARIS. Patients who achieved a complete clinical response and did not relapse by Week 8 were randomized into Part 2, a 24-week randomized, double-blind, placebo-controlled withdrawal period. Patients who completed Part 2 or experienced a disease flare entered Part 3, a 16-week open-label active treatment phase. A complete response was defined as ratings of minimal or better for physician's assessment of disease activity (PHY) and assessment of skin disease (SKD) and had serum levels of C-Reactive Protein (CRP) and Serum Amyloid A (SAA) less than 10 mg/L. A disease flare was defined as a CRP and/or SAA values greater than 30 mg/L and either a score of mild or worse for PHY or a score of minimal or worse for PHY and SKD.

In Part 1, a complete clinical response was observed in 71% of patients one week following initiation of treatment and in 97% of patients by Week 8 (*see Figure 1 and Table 2*). In the randomized withdrawal period, a total of 81% of the patients randomized to placebo flared as compared to none (0%) of the patients randomized to ILARIS. The 95%

confidence interval for treatment difference in the proportion of flares was 53% to 96%. At the end of Part 2, all 15 patients treated with ILARIS had absent or minimal disease activity and skin disease (*see Table 2*).

In a second trial, patients 4 to 74 years of age with both MWS and FCAS phenotypes of CAPS were treated in an open-label manner. Treatment with ILARIS resulted in clinically significant improvement of signs and symptoms and in normalization of high CRP and SAA in a majority of patients within 1 week.

[See table 2 at top of previous page]

Markers of inflammation CRP and SAA normalized within 8 days of treatment in the majority of patients. Normal mean CRP (Figure 1) and SAA values were sustained throughout Study 1 in patients continuously treated with canakinumab. After withdrawal of canakinumab in Part 2 CRP (Figure 1) and SAA values again returned to abnormal values and subsequently normalized after reintroduction of canakinumab in Part 3. The pattern of normalization of CRP and SAA was similar.

Figure 1. Mean C-Reactive Protein Levels at the End of Parts 1, 2 and 3 of Study 1

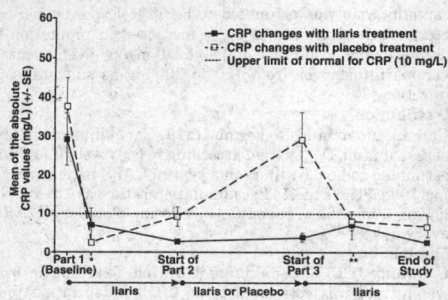

*1 week after the start of Part 1; **8 weeks after the start of Part 3

16   HOW SUPPLIED/STORAGE AND HANDLING

Carton of 1 vial .... NDC 0078-0582-61
Each 6 mL single-use vial of ILARIS contains a sterile, preservative free, white lyophilized powder containing 180 mg of canakinumab. Each vial is to be reconstituted with 1 mL of preservative-free Sterile Water for Injection in a 150 mg/mL solution.

Special Precautions for Storage

The unopened vial must be stored refrigerated at 2 to 8°C (36 to 46°F). Do not freeze. Store in the original carton to protect from light. Do not use beyond the date stamped on the label. After reconstitution, ILARIS should be kept from light, and can be kept at room temperature if used within 60 minutes of reconstitution. Otherwise, it should be refrigerated at 2 to 8°C (36 to 46°F) and used within 4 hours of reconstitution. ILARIS does not contain preservatives. Unused portions of ILARIS should be discarded.
Keep this and all drugs out of the reach of children.

17   PATIENT COUNSELING INFORMATION

See FDA-approved Patient Labeling.

Patients should be provided the opportunity to read the Patient Information for ILARIS prior to the first treatment and any questions resulting from the patient's reading of the guide should be discussed.

17.1   Drug Administration

Healthcare providers should perform administration of ILARIS by the subcutaneous injection route.

17.2   Infections

Patients should be cautioned that ILARIS use has been associated with serious infections. Patients should be counseled to contact their healthcare professional immediately if they develop an infection after starting ILARIS. Treatment with ILARIS should be discontinued if a patient develops a serious infection. Patients should be counseled not to take any IL-1 blocking drug, if they are also taking a drug that blocks TNF such as etanercept, infliximab, or adalimumab. Use of ILARIS with other IL-1 blocking agents, such as rilonacept and anakinra is not recommended. Patients should be cautioned not to initiate treatment with ILARIS if they have a chronic or active infection, including HIV, Hepatitis B or C.

17.3   Vaccinations

Prior to initiation of therapy with ILARIS, physicians should review with adult and pediatric patients their vaccination history relative to current medical guidelines for vaccine use, including taking into account the potential of increased risk of infection during treatment with ILARIS.

17.4   Injection-site Reactions

Physicians should explain to patients that a very small number of patients in the clinical trials experienced a reaction at the subcutaneous injection site. Injection-site reactions may include pain, erythema, swelling, pruritus, bruising, mass, inflammation, dermatitis, edema, urticaria,

vesicles, warmth, and hemorrhage. Healthcare providers should be cautioned to avoid injecting into an area that is already swollen or red. Any persistent reaction should be brought to the attention of the prescribing physician.

INFORMATION FOR PATIENTS

See patient information leaflet.

Patient Information

ILARIS® (i-LAHR-us)
(canakinumab)

Read the Patient Information that comes with ILARIS before you start taking it and each time you get a refill. There may be new information. This leaflet does not take the place of talking with your doctor about your medical condition or treatment.

What is ILARIS?

ILARIS is a prescription medicine injected just below the skin (subcutaneous) used in adults and children 4 years and older to treat auto-inflammatory diseases known as Cryopyrin-Associated Periodic Syndromes (CAPS), including:
• Familial Cold Autoinflammatory Syndrome (FCAS)
• Muckle-Wells Syndrome (MWS)
It is not known if ILARIS is safe or effective in children under 4 years of age.

What should I tell my healthcare provider before taking ILARIS?

Before you take ILARIS, tell your healthcare provider if you:
• think you have an infection
• are being treated for an infection
• have signs of an infection, such as fever, cough, or flu-like symptoms
• have a history of infections that keep coming back
• have or have had HIV, Hepatitis B, or Hepatitis C
• have an immune system problem. People with these conditions have a higher chance for infections.
• have tuberculosis (TB), or if you have been in close contact with someone who has or has had tuberculosis
• are scheduled to receive any immunizations (vaccines). You should not get 'live vaccines' if you take ILARIS.
• are pregnant or planning to become pregnant. It is not known if ILARIS will harm your unborn baby. Tell your healthcare provider right away if you become pregnant while taking ILARIS.
• are breastfeeding or planning to breastfeed. It is not known if ILARIS passes into your breast milk. You and your healthcare provider should decide if you will take ILARIS or breastfeed. You should not do both.

Tell your healthcare provider about all the medicines you take, including prescription and non-prescription medicines, vitamins and herbal supplements. Especially tell your healthcare provider if you take:
• medicines that affect your immune system
• IL-1 blocking agents such as Kineret® (anakinra), Arcalyst® (rilonacept)
• Tumor Necrosis Factor (TNF) inhibitors such as Enbrel® (etanercept)
• Humira® (adalimumab), or Remicade® (infliximab)
• medicines that can affect enzyme metabolism. Ask your healthcare provider if you are not sure.
Ask your healthcare provider or pharmacist for a list of these medicines, if you are not sure.
Know the medicines you take. Keep a list of them and show it to your healthcare provider and pharmacist when you get a new medicine.

How will I receive ILARIS?

• Do not receive ILARIS if you have an infection.
• ILARIS is given by your healthcare provider every 8 weeks.
• Your healthcare provider may change your dose if needed.

What are the possible side effects of ILARIS?

ILARIS can cause serious side effects including:
• serious infections
• decrease your body's ability to fight infections (immunosuppression)
• feeling like you are spinning (vertigo)
Call your healthcare provider right away if you have any of these signs of an infection:
• a fever lasting longer than 3 days
• a cough that does not go away
• redness in one part of your body
• warm feeling or swelling of your skin

The most common side effects include:
• cold symptoms
• diarrhea
• flu (influenza)
• runny nose
• nausea
• headache
• injection site reaction (such as redness, swelling, warmth, itching)
Tell your healthcare provider if you have any side effect that bothers you or that does not go away.

These are not all the possible side effects of ILARIS. For more information, ask your healthcare provider or pharmacist.
Call your doctor for medical advice about side effects.
You may report side effects to FDA at 1-800-FDA-1088.

General information about the safe and effective use of ILARIS

Medicines are sometimes prescribed for purposes other than those listed in patient information leaflets. Do not use ILARIS for a condition for which it was not prescribed.
This leaflet summarizes the most important information about ILARIS. If you would like more information, talk with your healthcare provider. You can ask your healthcare provider or pharmacist for information about ILARIS that was written for health professionals. For more information about ILARIS, call 1-877-452-7471 or visit www.ILARIS.com.

What are the ingredients in ILARIS?

Active ingredients: canakinumab
Inactive ingredients: sucrose, L-histidine, L-histidine HCl monohydrate, polysorbate 80, preservative-free Sterile Water for Injection.

What is CAPS Disease?

In patients with CAPS, the body produces excessive amounts of a chemical messenger called interleukin-1 beta (IL-1β). This may lead to symptoms such as fever, headache, fatigue, skin rash, painful joints and muscles. In some patients, more severe outcomes such as hearing impairment are observed.
Kineret®, Arcalyst®, Enbrel®, Humira®, Remicade® are trademarks of Amgen, Regeneron, Immunex Corporation, Abbott Laboratories, Centocor Ortho Biotech Inc., respectively.
REV: JUNE 2009   T2009-82

Manufactured By:
Novartis Pharma Stein AG
Stein, Switzerland

Distributed By:
Novartis Pharmaceuticals Corporation
East Hanover, New Jersey 07936
©Novartis

Shown in Product Identification Guide, page 315

MYFORTIC®   ℞

[*mi-for-tic*]
(mycophenolic acid*)
delayed-release tablets
***as mycophenolate sodium**
Rx only

Prescribing Information

The following prescribing information is based on official labeling in effect July 2010.

WARNING
Immunosuppression may lead to increased susceptibility to infection and possible development of lymphoma and other neoplasms. Only physicians experienced in immunosuppressive therapy and management of organ transplant recipients should use Myfortic® (mycophenolic acid). Patients receiving Myfortic should be managed in facilities equipped and staffed with adequate laboratory and supportive medical resources. The physician responsible for maintenance therapy should have complete information requisite for the follow-up of the patient.
Female users of childbearing potential must use contraception. Use of Myfortic® during pregnancy is associated with increased risks of pregnancy loss and congenital malformations.

DESCRIPTION

Myfortic® (mycophenolic acid) delayed-release tablets are an enteric formulation of mycophenolate sodium that delivers the active moiety mycophenolic acid (MPA). Myfortic is an immunosuppressive agent. As the sodium salt, MPA is chemically designated as (E)-6-(4-hydroxy-6-methoxy-7-methyl-3-oxo-1,3-dihydroisobenzofuran-5-yl)-4-methylhex-4-enoic acid sodium salt.
Its empirical formula is $C_{17}H_{19}O_6$ Na. The molecular weight is 342.32 and the structural formula is

Myfortic, as the sodium salt, is a white to off-white, crystalline powder and is highly soluble in aqueous media at physiological pH and practically insoluble in 0.1 N hydrochloric acid.

Myfortic is available for oral use as delayed-release tablets containing either 180 mg or 360 mg of mycophenolic acid. Inactive ingredients include colloidal silicon dioxide, crospovidone, lactose anhydrous, magnesium stearate, povidone (K-30), and starch. The enteric coating of the tablet consists of hypromellose phthalate, titanium dioxide, iron oxide yellow, and indigotine (180 mg) or iron oxide red (360 mg).

CLINICAL PHARMACOLOGY
Mechanism of Action
MPA is an uncompetitive and reversible inhibitor of inosine monophosphate dehydrogenase (IMPDH), and therefore inhibits the *de novo* pathway of guanosine nucleotide synthesis without incorporation to DNA. Because T- and B-lymphocytes are critically dependent for their proliferation on *de novo* synthesis of purines, whereas other cell types can utilize salvage pathways, MPA has potent cytostatic effects on lymphocytes.

Mycophenolate sodium has been shown to prevent the occurrence of acute rejection in rat models of kidney and heart allotransplantation. Mycophenolate sodium also decreases antibody production in mice.

Pharmacokinetics
Absorption
In vitro studies demonstrated that the enteric-coated Myfortic® (mycophenolic acid) tablet does not release MPA under acidic conditions (pH <5) as in the stomach but is highly soluble in neutral pH conditions as in the intestine. Following Myfortic oral administration without food in several pharmacokinetic studies conducted in renal transplant patients, consistent with its enteric-coated formulation, the median delay (T_{lag}) in the rise of MPA concentration ranged between 0.25 and 1.25 hours and the median time to maximum concentration (T_{max}) of MPA ranged between 1.5 and 2.75 hours. In comparison, following the administration of mycophenolate mofetil, the median T_{max} ranged between 0.5 and 1.0 hours. In stable renal transplant patients on cyclosporine, USP (MODIFIED) based immunosuppression, gastrointestinal absorption and absolute bioavailability of MPA following the administration of Myfortic delayed-release tablet was 93% and 72%, respectively. Myfortic pharmacokinetics is dose proportional over the dose range of 360 to 2160 mg.

Distribution
The mean (± SD) volume of distribution at steady state and elimination phase for MPA is 54 (± 25) L and 112 (± 48) L, respectively. MPA is highly protein bound to albumin, >98%. The protein binding of mycophenolic acid glucuronide (MPAG) is 82%. The free MPA concentration may increase under conditions of decreased protein binding (uremia, hepatic failure, and hypoalbuminemia).

Metabolism
MPA is metabolized principally by glucuronyl transferase to glucuronidated metabolites. The phenolic glucuronide of MPA, mycophenolic acid glucuronide (MPAG), is the predominant metabolite of MPA and does not manifest pharmacological activity. The acyl glucuronide is a minor metabolite and has comparable pharmacological activity to MPA. In stable renal transplant patients on cyclosporine, USP (MODIFIED) based immunosuppression, approximately 28% of the oral Myfortic dose was converted to MPAG by pre-systemic metabolism. The AUC ratio of MPA:MPAG:acyl glucuronide is approximately 1:24:0.28 at steady state. The mean clearance of MPA was 140 (± 30) mL/min.

Elimination
The majority of MPA dose administered is eliminated in the urine primarily as MPAG (>60%) and approximately 3% as unchanged MPA following Myfortic administration to stable renal transplant patients. The mean renal clearance of MPAG was 15.5 (± 5.9) mL/min. MPAG is also secreted in the bile and available for deconjugation by gut flora. MPA resulting from the deconjugation may then be reabsorbed and produce a second peak of MPA approximately 6-8 hours after Myfortic dosing. The mean elimination half-life of MPA and MPAG ranged between 8 and 16 hours, and 13 and 17 hours, respectively.

Food Effect
Compared to the fasting state, administration of Myfortic 720 mg with a high-fat meal (55 g fat, 1000 calories) had no effect on the systemic exposure (AUC) of MPA. However, there was a 33% decrease in the maximal concentration (C_{max}), a 3.5-hour delay in the T_{lag} (range, -6 to 18 hours), and 5.0-hour delay in the T_{max} (range, -9 to 20 hours) of MPA. To avoid the variability in MPA absorption between doses, Myfortic should be taken on an empty stomach (*see DOSAGE AND ADMINISTRATION and PRECAUTIONS, Information for Patients*).

Pharmacokinetics in Renal Transplant Patients
The mean pharmacokinetic parameters for MPA following the administration of Myfortic in renal transplant patients on cyclosporine, USP (MODIFIED) based immunosuppression are shown in Table 1. Single-dose Myfortic pharmaco-

kinetics predicts multiple-dose pharmacokinetics. However, in the early post-transplant period, mean MPA AUC and C_{max} were approximately one-half of those measured 6 months post-transplant.

After near equimolar dosing of Myfortic 720 mg BID and mycophenolate mofetil 1000 mg BID (739 mg as MPA) in both the single- and multiple-dose cross-over trials, mean systemic MPA exposure (AUC) was similar.
[See table 1 above]

Special Populations
Renal Insufficiency: No specific pharmacokinetic studies in individuals with renal impairment were conducted with Myfortic. However, based on studies of renal impairment with mycophenolate mofetil, MPA exposure is not expected to be appreciably increased over the range of normal to severely-impaired renal function following Myfortic administration. In contrast, MPAG exposure would be increased markedly with decreased renal function; MPAG exposure being approximately 8-fold higher in the setting of anuria. Although dialysis may be used to remove the inactive metabolite MPAG, it would not be expected to remove clinically significant amounts of the active moiety MPA. This is in large part due to the high plasma protein binding of MPA.

Hepatic Insufficiency: No specific pharmacokinetic studies in individuals with hepatic impairment were conducted with Myfortic. In a single dose (mycophenolate mofetil 1000 mg) study of 18 volunteers with alcoholic cirrhosis and 6 healthy volunteers, hepatic MPA glucuronidation processes appeared to be relatively unaffected by hepatic parenchymal disease when the pharmacokinetic parameters of healthy volunteers and alcoholic cirrhosis patients within this study were compared. However, it should be noted that for unexplained reasons, the healthy volunteers in this study had about a 50% lower AUC compared to healthy volunteers in other studies, thus making comparison between volunteers with alcoholic cirrhosis and healthy volunteers difficult. Effects of hepatic disease on this process probably depend on the particular disease. Hepatic disease, such as primary biliary cirrhosis, with other etiologies may show a different effect.

Pediatrics: Limited data are available on the use of Myfortic at a dose of 450 mg/m² body surface area in children. The mean MPA pharmacokinetic parameters for stable pediatric renal transplant patients, 5-16 years, on cyclosporine, USP (MODIFIED) are shown in Table 1. At the same dose administered based on body surface area, the respective mean C_{max} and AUC of MPA determined in children were higher by 33% and 18% than those determined for adults. The clinical impact of the increase in MPA exposure is not known.

Gender: There are no significant gender differences in Myfortic pharmacokinetics.

Elderly: Pharmacokinetics in the elderly have not been formally studied.

CLINICAL STUDIES
The safety and efficacy of Myfortic® (mycophenolic acid) in combination with cyclosporine, USP (MODIFIED) and corticosteroids for the prevention of organ rejection was assessed in two multicenter, randomized, double-blind trials in *de novo* and maintenance renal transplant patients compared to mycophenolate mofetil.

The *de novo* study was conducted in 423 renal transplant patients (ages 18-75 years) in Austria, Canada, Germany, Hungary, Italy, Norway, Spain, UK and USA. Cadaveric donor specimens accounted for 84% of randomized patients. Patients were administered either Myfortic 1.44 g/day or mycophenolate mofetil 2 g/day within 48 hours post-transplant for 12 months in combination with cyclosporine, USP (MODIFIED) and corticosteroids. Forty-one percent of patients received antibody therapy as induction treatment. Treatment failure was defined as the first occurrence of biopsy-proven acute rejection, graft loss, death or lost to follow-up at 6 months. The incidence of treatment failure was similar in Myfortic- and mycophenolate mofetil-treated patients at 6 and 12 months (Table 2). The cumulative incidence of graft loss, death and lost to follow-up at 12 months is also given in Table 2.
[See table 2 above]
The maintenance study was conducted in 322 renal transplant patients (ages 18-75 years), who were at least 6

Table 1
Mean ± SD Pharmacokinetic Parameters for MPA Following the Oral Administration of Myfortic® to Renal Transplant Patients on Cyclosporine, USP (MODIFIED) Based Immunosuppression

Study Patient	Myfortic® Dosing	n	Dose (mg)	T_{max}* (hr)	C_{max} (μg/mL)	AUC_{0-12hr} (μg*hr/mL)
Adult	Single	24	720	2 (0.8-8)	26.1 ± 12.0	66.5 ± 22.6**
Pediatric***	Single	10	450/m²	2.5 (1.5-24)	36.3 ± 20.9	74.3 ± 22.5**
Adult	Multiple × 6 days, BID	10	720	2 (1.5-3.0)	37.0 ± 13.3	67.9 ± 20.3
Adult	Multiple × 28 days, BID	36	720	2.5 (1.5-8)	31.2 ± 18.1	71.2 ± 26.3
Adult	Chronic, multiple dose, BID					
	2 weeks post-transplant	12	720	1.8 (1.0-5.3)	15.0 ± 10.7	28.6 ± 11.5
	3 months post-transplant	12	720	2 (0.5-2.5)	26.2 ± 12.7	52.3 ± 17.4
	6 months post-transplant	12	720	2 (0-3)	24.1 ± 9.6	57.2 ± 15.3
Adult	Chronic, multiple dose, BID	18	720	1.5 (0-6)	18.9 ± 7.9	57.4 ± 15.0

* median (range), ** $AUC_{0-∞}$, *** age range of 5-16 years

Table 2
Treatment Failure in *de novo* Renal Transplant Patients (Percent of Patients) at 6- and 12-Months of Treatment when Administered in Combination with Cyclosporine* and Corticosteroids

	Myfortic® 1.44 g/day (n=213)	mycophenolate mofetil 2 g/day (n=210)
6 Months	n (%)	n (%)
Treatment failure#	55 (25.8)	55 (26.2)
Biopsy-proven acute rejection	46 (21.6)	48 (22.9)
Graft loss	7 (3.3)	9 (4.3)
Death	1 (0.5)	2 (1.0)
Lost to follow-up**	3 (1.4)	0
12 Months	n (%)	n (%)
Graft loss or death or lost to follow-up***	20 (9.4)	18 (8.6)
Treatment failure	61 (28.6)	59 (28.1)
Biopsy-proven acute rejection	48 (22.5)	51 (24.3)
Graft loss	9 (4.2)	9 (4.3)
Death	2 (0.9)	5 (2.4)
Lost to follow-up**	5 (2.3)	0

* USP (MODIFIED)

** Lost to follow-up indicates patients who were lost to follow-up without prior biopsy-proven acute rejection, graft loss or death

*** Lost to follow-up indicates patients who were lost to follow-up without prior graft loss or death (9 Myfortic patients and 4 mycophenolate mofetil patients)

\# 95% confidence interval of the difference in treatment failure at 6 months (Myfortic – mycophenolate mofetil) is (-8.7%, 8.0%).

months post-transplant receiving 2 g/day mycophenolate mofetil in combination with cyclosporine, USP (MODIFIED), with or without corticosteroids for at least two weeks prior to entry in the study. Patients were randomized to Myfortic 1.44 g/day or mycophenolate mofetil 2 g/day for 12 months. The study was conducted in Austria, Belgium, Canada, Germany, Italy, Spain, and USA. Treatment failure was defined as the first occurrence of biopsy-proven acute rejection, graft loss, death, or lost to follow-up at 6 and 12 months. The incidences of treatment failure at 6 and 12 months were similar between Myfortic- and mycophenolate mofetil-treated patients (Table 3). The cumulative incidence of graft loss, death and lost to follow-up at 12 months is also given in Table 3.
[See table 3 below]
The safety and efficacy of Myfortic has not been studied in hepatic or cardiac transplant trials.

INDICATIONS AND USAGE
Myfortic® (mycophenolic acid) delayed-release tablets are indicated for the prophylaxis of organ rejection in patients receiving allogeneic renal transplants, administered in combination with cyclosporine and corticosteroids.

CONTRAINDICATIONS
Myfortic® (mycophenolic acid) is contraindicated in patients with a hypersensitivity to mycophenolate sodium, mycophenolic acid, mycophenolate mofetil, or to any of its excipients.

WARNINGS (SEE BOXED WARNING)
Lymphoma and Other Malignancies
Patients receiving immunosuppressive regimens involving combinations of drugs, including Myfortic® (mycophenolic acid), as part of an immunosuppressive regimen are at increased risk of developing lymphomas and other malignancies, particularly of the skin (see ADVERSE REACTIONS). The risk appears to be related to the intensity and duration of immunosuppression rather than to the use of any specific agent.
The rates for lymphoproliferative disease or lymphoma in Myfortic-treated patients were comparable to the mycophenolate mofetil group in the de novo and maintenance studies (see ADVERSE REACTIONS). As usual for patients with increased risk for skin cancer, exposure to sunlight and UV light should be limited by wearing protective clothing and using a sunscreen with a high protection factor.

Infections
Oversuppression of the immune system can also increase susceptibility to infection, including opportunistic infections, fatal infections, and sepsis. Fatal infections can occur in patients receiving immunosuppressive therapy (see ADVERSE REACTIONS).

Latent Viral Infections
Immunosuppressed patients are at increased risk for opportunistic infections, including activation of latent viral infections. These include cases of progressive multifocal leukoencephalopathy (PML) and BK virus-associated nephropathy (BKVAN) which have been observed in patients receiving immunosuppressants, including Myfortic. Cases of progressive multifocal leukoencephalopathy (PML), sometimes fatal, have been reported in patients

treated with mycophenolate mofetil (MMF). Hemiparesis, apathy, confusion, cognitive deficiencies and ataxia were the most frequent clinical features observed. Mycophenolate mofetil (MMF) is metabolized to mycophenolic acid (MPA), the active ingredient in Myfortic and the active form of the drug. The reported cases generally had risk factors for PML, including treatment with immunosuppressant therapies and impairment of immune functions. In immunosuppressed patients, physicians should consider PML in the differential diagnosis in patients reporting neurological symptoms and consultation with a neurologist should be considered as clinically indicated. Consideration should be given to reducing the amount of immunosuppression in patients who develop PML. In transplant patients, physicians should also consider the risk that reduced immunosuppression represents to the graft.
BKVAN is associated with serious outcomes, including deteriorating renal function and renal graft loss (see ADVERSE REACTIONS, Postmarketing Experience). Patient monitoring may help detect patients at risk for BK virus-associated nephropathy. Reduction in immunosuppression should be considered for patients who develop evidence of BK virus-associated nephropathy.

Pure Red Cell Aplasia
Cases of pure red cell aplasia (PRCA) have been reported in patients treated with mycophenolate mofetil (MMF) in combination with other immunosuppressive agents. MMF is metabolized to mycophenolic acid (MPA), the active ingredient in Myfortic and the active form of the drug. The mechanism for MMF induced PRCA is unknown; the relative contribution of other immunosuppressants and their combinations in an immunosuppressive regimen are also unknown. In some cases PRCA was found to be reversible with dose reduction or cessation of MMF therapy. In transplant patients, however, reduced immunosuppression may place the graft at risk. Changes to Myfortic therapy should only be undertaken under appropriate supervision in transplant recipients in order to minimize the risk of graft rejection (see ADVERSE REACTIONS, Postmarketing Experience).

Concomitant Use
Myfortic has been administered in combination with the following agents in clinical trials: antithymocyte/lymphocyte immunoglobulin, muromonab-CD3, basiliximab, daclizumab, cyclosporine, and corticosteroids. The efficacy and safety of Myfortic in combination with other immunosuppression agents have not been determined.

Pregnancy: *Teratogenic Effects:* Pregnancy Category D Mycophenolate mofetil (MMF) can cause fetal harm when administered to a pregnant woman. Following oral or IV administration, MMF is metabolized to mycophenolic acid (MPA), the active ingredient in Myfortic and the active form of the drug. Use of Myfortic during pregnancy is associated with an increased risk of first trimester pregnancy loss and an increased risk of congenital malformations, especially external ear and other facial abnormalities including cleft lip and palate, and anomalies of the distal limbs, heart, esophagus, and kidney. In the National Transplantation Pregnancy Registry (NTPR), there were data on 33 MMF-exposed pregnancies in 24 transplant patients; there were 15 spontaneous abortions (45%) and 18 live-born infants.

Four of these 18 infants had structural malformations (22%). In postmarketing data (collected from 1995 to 2007) on 77 women exposed to systemic MMF during pregnancy, 25 had spontaneous abortions and 14 had a malformed infant or fetus. Six of 14 malformed offspring had ear abnormalities. Because these postmarketing data are reported voluntarily, it is not always possible to reliably estimate the frequency of particular adverse outcomes. These malformations are similar to findings in animal reproductive toxicology studies. For comparison, the background rate for congenital anomalies in the United States is about 3%, and NTPR data show a rate of 4-5% among babies born to organ transplant patients using other immunosuppressive drugs. In a teratology study performed with mycophenolate sodium in rats, at a dose as low as 1 mg/kg, malformations in the offspring were observed, including anophthalmia, exencephaly and umbilical hernia. The systemic exposure at this dose represents 0.05 times the clinical exposure at the dose of 1.44 g/day Myfortic. In teratology studies in rabbits, fetal resorptions and malformations occurred from 80 mg/kg/day, in the absence of maternal toxicity (dose levels are equivalent to about 0.8 times the recommended clinical dose, corrected for BSA). There are no relevant qualitative or quantitative differences in the teratogenic potential of mycophenolate sodium and mycophenolate mofetil.
If this drug is used during pregnancy, or if the patient becomes pregnant while taking this drug, the patient should be apprised of the potential hazard to the fetus. In certain situations, the patient and her healthcare practitioner may decide that the maternal benefits outweigh the risks to the fetus. Women using Myfortic at any time during pregnancy should be encouraged to enroll in the National Transplantation Pregnancy Registry.

Pregnancy Exposure Prevention
Women of childbearing potential should have a negative serum or urine pregnancy test with a sensitivity of at least 25 mIU/mL within 1 week prior to beginning therapy. Myfortic therapy should not be initiated until a negative pregnancy test report is obtained.
Women of childbearing potential (including pubertal girls and peri-menopausal women) taking Myfortic must receive contraceptive counseling and use effective contraception. The patient should begin using her two chosen methods of contraception 4 weeks prior to starting Myfortic therapy, unless abstinence is the chosen method. She should continue contraceptive use during therapy and for 6 weeks after stopping Myfortic. Patients should be aware that Myfortic reduces blood levels of the hormones in the oral contraceptive pill and could theoretically reduce its effectiveness (see PRECAUTIONS, Information for Patients and PRECAUTIONS, Drug Interactions, Oral Contraceptives).
Patients receiving Myfortic should be monitored for neutropenia (see PRECAUTIONS, Laboratory Tests). The development of neutropenia may be related to Myfortic itself, concomitant medications, viral infections, or some combination of these events. If neutropenia develops (ANC $<1.3\times10^3/\mu L$), dosing with Myfortic should be interrupted or the dose reduced, appropriate diagnostic tests performed, and the patient managed appropriately (see DOSAGE AND ADMINISTRATION).
Patients receiving Myfortic should be instructed to immediately report any evidence of infection, unexpected bruising, bleeding, or any other manifestation of bone marrow suppression.

PRECAUTIONS
General
Gastrointestinal bleeding (requiring hospitalization) has been reported in de novo renal transplant patients (1.0%) and maintenance patients (1.3%) treated with Myfortic® (mycophenolic acid) (up to 12 months). Intestinal perforations, gastrointestinal hemorrhage, gastric ulcers and duodenal ulcers have rarely been observed. Most patients receiving Myfortic were also receiving other drugs known to be associated with these complications. Patients with active peptic ulcer disease were excluded from enrollment in studies with Myfortic. Because MPA derivatives have been associated with an increased incidence of digestive system adverse events, including infrequent cases of gastrointestinal tract ulceration, hemorrhage, and perforation, Myfortic should be administered with caution in patients with active serious digestive system disease (see ADVERSE REACTIONS).
Subjects with severe chronic renal impairment (GFR <25 mL/min/1.73 m^2) may present higher plasma MPA and MPAG AUCs relative to subjects with lesser degrees of renal impairment or normal healthy volunteers. No data are available on the safety of long-term exposure to these levels of MPAG.
In the de novo study, 18.3% of Myfortic patients versus 16.7% in the mycophenolate mofetil group experienced

Table 3
Treatment Failure in Maintenance Transplant Patients (Percent of Patients) at 6- and 12-Months of Treatment when Administered in Combination with Cyclosporine* and with or without Corticosteroids

	Myfortic® 1.44 g/day (n=159)	mycophenolate mofetil 2 g/day (n=163)
6 Months	n (%)	n (%)
Treatment failure#	7 (4.4)	11 (6.7)
Biopsy-proven acute rejection	2 (1.3)	2 (1.2)
Graft loss	0	1 (0.6)
Death	0	1 (0.6)
Lost to follow-up**	5 (3.1)	7 (4.3)
12 Months	n (%)	n (%)
Graft loss or death or lost to follow-up***	10 (6.3)	17 (10.4)
Treatment failure	12 (7.5)	20 (12.3)
Biopsy-proven acute rejection	2 (1.3)	5 (3.1)
Graft loss	0	1 (0.6)
Death	2 (1.3)	4 (2.5)
Lost to follow-up**	8 (5.0)	10 (6.1)

* USP (MODIFIED)
** Lost to follow-up indicates patients who were lost to follow-up without prior biopsy-proven acute rejection, graft loss, or death
*** Lost to follow-up indicates patients who were lost to follow-up without prior graft loss or death (8 Myfortic patients and 12 mycophenolate mofetil patients)
# 95% confidence interval of the difference in treatment failure at 6 months (Myfortic – mycophenolate mofetil) is (-7.4%, 2.7%).

delayed graft function (DGF). Although patients with DGF experienced a higher incidence of certain adverse events (anemia, leukopenia, and hyperkalemia) than patients without DGF, these events in DGF patients were not more frequent in patients receiving Myfortic compared to mycophenolate mofetil. No dose adjustment is recommended for these patients; however, such patients should be carefully observed (see CLINICAL PHARMACOLOGY and DOSAGE AND ADMINISTRATION).

In view of the significant reduction in the AUC of MPA by cholestyramine when administered with mycophenolate mofetil, caution should be used in the concomitant administration of Myfortic with drugs that interfere with enterohepatic recirculation because of the potential to reduce the efficacy (see PRECAUTIONS, Drug Interactions).

On theoretical grounds, because Myfortic is an IMPDH Inhibitor, it should be avoided in patients with rare hereditary deficiency of hypoxanthine-guanine phosphoribosyltransferase (HGPRT) such as Lesch-Nyhan and Kelley-Seegmiller syndrome.

During treatment with Myfortic, the use of live attenuated vaccines should be avoided and patients should be advised that vaccinations may be less effective (see PRECAUTIONS, Drug Interactions, Live Vaccines).

Information for Patients

- It is recommended that Myfortic be administered on an empty stomach, one hour before or two hours after food intake (see DOSAGE AND ADMINISTRATION).
- In order to maintain the integrity of the enteric coating of the tablet, patients should be instructed not to crush, chew, or cut Myfortic tablets and to swallow the tablets whole.
- Give patients complete dosage instructions and inform them about the increased risk of lymphoproliferative disease and certain other malignancies.
- Inform patients that they need repeated appropriate laboratory tests while they are taking Myfortic.
- Inform women of childbearing potential that use of Myfortic in pregnancy is associated with an increased risk of first trimester pregnancy loss and an increased risk of birth defects, and that they must use effective contraception.
- Discuss pregnancy plans with female patients of childbearing potential.
- Any female of childbearing potential must use highly effective (two methods) contraception 4 weeks prior to starting Myfortic therapy and continue contraception until 6 weeks after stopping Myfortic treatment, unless abstinence is the chosen method (see WARNINGS, Pregnancy).
- A patient who is planning a pregnancy should not use Myfortic unless she can not be successfully treated with other immunosuppressant drugs. Risks and benefits of Myfortic and alternative immunosuppressants should be discussed with the patient.

Laboratory Tests

Complete blood count should be performed weekly during the first month, twice monthly for the second and the third month of treatment, then monthly through the first year. If neutropenia develops (ANC $<1.3\times10^3/\mu L$), dosing with Myfortic should be interrupted or the dose reduced, appropriate tests performed, and the patient managed accordingly (see WARNINGS).

Drug Interactions

The following drug interaction studies have been conducted with Myfortic:

Antacids: Absorption of a single dose of Myfortic was decreased when administered to 12 stable renal transplant patients also taking magnesium-aluminum-containing antacids (30 mL): the mean C_{max} and $AUC_{(0-t)}$ values for MPA were 25% and 37% lower, respectively, than when Myfortic was administered alone under fasting conditions. It is recommended that Myfortic and antacids not be administered simultaneously.

Cyclosporine: When studied in stable renal transplant patients, cyclosporine, USP (MODIFIED) pharmacokinetics were unaffected by steady-state dosing of Myfortic.

The following recommendations are derived from drug interaction studies conducted following the administration of mycophenolate mofetil:

Acyclovir/Ganciclovir: May be taken with Myfortic; however, during the period of treatment, physicians should monitor blood cell counts. Both acyclovir/ganciclovir and MPAG concentrations are increased in the presence of renal impairment, their coexistence may compete for tubular secretion and further increase in the concentrations of the two.

Azathioprine/Mycophenolate Mofetil: Given that azathioprine and mycophenolate mofetil inhibit purine metabolism, it is recommended that Myfortic not be administered concomitantly with azathioprine or mycophenolate mofetil.

Cholestyramine and Drugs that Bind Bile Acids: These drugs interrupt enterohepatic recirculation and reduce MPA exposure when coadministered with mycophenolate

mofetil. Therefore, do not administer Myfortic with cholestyramine or other agents that may interfere with enterohepatic recirculation or drugs that may bind bile acids, for example bile acid sequestrates or oral activated charcoal, because of the potential to reduce the efficacy of Myfortic.

Oral Contraceptives: Given the different metabolism of Myfortic and oral contraceptives, no drug interaction between these two classes of drug is expected. However, in a drug-drug interaction study, mean levonorgesterol AUC was decreased by 15% when coadministered with mycophenolate mofetil. Therefore, it is recommended that oral contraceptives are coadministered with Myfortic with caution and additional birth control methods be considered (see PRECAUTIONS, Pregnancy).

Live Vaccines: During treatment with Myfortic, the use of live attenuated vaccines should be avoided and patients should be advised that vaccinations may be less effective. Influenza vaccination may be of value. Prescribers should refer to national guidelines for influenza vaccination (see PRECAUTIONS, General).

Drugs that alter the gastrointestinal flora may interact with Myfortic by disrupting enterohepatic recirculation. Interference of MPAG hydrolysis may lead to less MPA available for absorption.

Carcinogenesis, Mutagenesis, Impairment of Fertility

In a 104-week oral carcinogenicity study in rats, mycophenolate sodium was not tumorigenic at daily doses up to 9 mg/kg, the highest dose tested. This dose resulted in approximately 0.6-1.2 times the systemic exposure (based upon plasma AUC) observed in renal transplant patients at the recommended dose of 1.44 g/day. Similar results were observed in a parallel study in rats performed with mycophenolate mofetil. In a 104-week oral carcinogenicity study in mice, mycophenolate mofetil was not tumorigenic at a daily dose level as high as 180 mg/kg (which corresponds to 0.6 times the proposed mycophenolate sodium therapeutic dose based upon body surface area).

The genotoxic potential of mycophenolate sodium was determined in five assays. Mycophenolate sodium was genotoxic in the mouse lymphoma/thymidine kinase assay, the micronucleus test in V79 Chinese hamster cells, and the in vivo mouse micronucleus assay. Mycophenolate sodium was not genotoxic in the bacterial mutation assay (Salmonella typhimurium TA 1535, 97a, 98, 100, & 102) or the chromosomal aberration assay in human lymphocytes.

Mycophenolate mofetil generated similar genotoxic activity. The genotoxic activity of MPA is probably due to the depletion of the nucleotide pool required for DNA synthesis as a result of the pharmacodynamic mode of action of MPA (inhibition of nucleotide synthesis).

Mycophenolate sodium had no effect on male rat fertility at daily oral doses as high as 18 mg/kg and exhibited no testicular or spermatogenic effects at daily oral doses of 20 mg/kg for 13 weeks (approximately two-fold the therapeutic systemic exposure of MPA). No effects on female fertility were seen up to a daily dose of 20 mg/kg, which was approximately three-fold higher than the recommended therapeutic dose based upon systemic exposure.

Pregnancy

Teratogenic Effects: Pregnancy Category D. (See WARNINGS.)

Nursing Mothers

It is not known whether MPA is excreted in human milk. Because of the potential for serious adverse reactions in nursing infants from MPA, a decision should be made whether to discontinue the drug or to discontinue nursing while on treatment or within 6 weeks after stopping therapy, taking into account the importance of the drug to the mother.

Pediatric Use

De novo Renal Transplant

The safety and effectiveness of Myfortic in de novo pediatric renal transplant patients have not been established.

Stable Renal Transplant

There are no pharmacokinetic data available for pediatric patients <5 years. The safety and effectiveness of Myfortic have been established in the age group 5-16 years in stable pediatric renal transplant patients. Use of Myfortic in this age group is supported by evidence from adequate and well-controlled studies of Myfortic in stable adult renal transplant patients. Limited pharmacokinetic data are available for stable pediatric renal transplant patients in the age group 5-16 years. Pediatric doses for patients with BSA <1.19 m² cannot be accurately administered using currently available formulations of Myfortic tablets (see CLINICAL PHARMACOLOGY, Special Populations, and DOSAGE AND ADMINISTRATION).

Geriatric Use

Patients ≥65 years may generally be at increased risk of adverse drug reactions due to immunosuppression. Clinical studies of Myfortic did not include sufficient numbers of

Table 4
Adverse Events (%) in Controlled de novo and Maintenance Renal Studies Reported in ≥20% of Patients

	de novo Renal Study		Maintenance Renal Study	
	Myfortic® 1.44 g/day (n=213)	mycophenolate mofetil 2 g/day (n=210)	Myfortic® 1.44 g/day (n=159)	mycophenolate mofetil 2 g/day (n=163)
Blood and Lymphatic System Disorders				
Anemia	21.6	21.9	–	–
Leukopenia	19.2	20.5	–	–
Gastrointestinal System Disorders				
Constipation	38.0	39.5	–	–
Nausea	29.1	27.1	24.5	19.0
Diarrhea	23.5	24.8	21.4	24.5
Vomiting	23.0	20.0	–	–
Dyspepsia	22.5	19.0	–	–
Infections and Infestations				
Urinary Tract Infection	29.1	33.3	–	–
CMV Infection	20.2	18.1	–	–
Nervous System Disorder				
Insomnia	23.5	23.8	–	–
Surgical and Medical Procedure				
Post-Operative Pain	23.9	18.6	–	–

Table 5
Viral and Fungal Infections (%) Reported Over 0-12 Months

	de novo Renal Study		Maintenance Renal Study	
	Myfortic® 1.44 g/day (n=213)	mycophenolate mofetil 2 g/day (n=210)	Myfortic® 1.44 g/day (n=159)	mycophenolate mofetil 2 g/day (n=163)
	(%)	(%)	(%)	(%)
Any Cytomegalovirus	21.6	20.5	1.9	1.8
- Cytomegalovirus Disease	4.7	4.3	0	0.6
Herpes Simplex	8.0	6.2	1.3	2.5
Herpes Zoster	4.7	3.8	1.9	3.1
Any Fungal Infection	10.8	11.9	2.5	1.8
- Candida NOS	5.6	6.2	0	1.8
- Candida Albicans	2.3	3.8	0.6	0

Table 6
Adverse Events Reported in 3% to <20% of Patients Treated with Myfortic®
in Combination with Cyclosporine* and Corticosteroids

	de novo Renal Study	Maintenance Renal Study
Blood and Lymphatic Disorders	Lymphocele, thrombocytopenia	Leukopenia, anemia
Cardiac Disorder	Tachycardia	–
Eye Disorder	Vision blurred	–
Endocrine Disorders	Cushingoid, hirsutism	–
Gastrointestinal Disorders	Abdominal pain upper, flatulence, abdominal distension, sore throat, abdominal pain lower, abdominal pain, gingival hyperplasia, loose stool	Vomiting, dyspepsia, abdominal pain, constipation, gastroesophageal reflux disease, loose stool, flatulence, abdominal pain upper
General Disorders and Administration Site Conditions	Edema, edema lower limb, pyrexia, pain, fatigue, edema peripheral, chest pain	Fatigue, pyrexia, edema, chest pain, peripheral edema
Infections and Infestations	Nasopharyngitis, herpes simplex, upper respiratory tract infection, oral candidiasis, herpes zoster, sinusitis, wound infection, implant infection, pneumonia	Nasopharyngitis, upper respiratory tract infection, urinary tract infection, influenza, sinusitis
Injury, Poisoning, and Procedural Complications	Drug toxicity	Postprocedural pain
Investigations	Blood creatinine increased, hemoglobin decrease, blood pressure increased, liver function tests abnormal	Blood creatinine increase, weight increase
Metabolism and Nutrition Disorders	Hypocalcemia, hyperuricemia, hyperlipidemia, hypokalemia, hypophosphatemia, hypercholesterolemia, hyperkalemia, hypomagnesemia, diabetes mellitus, hyperphosphatemia, dehydration, fluid overload, hyperglycemia, hypercalcemia	Dehydration, hypokalemia, hypercholesterolemia
Musculoskeletal and Connective Tissue Disorders	Back pain, arthralgia, pain in limb, muscle cramps, myalgia	Arthralgia, pain in limb, back pain, muscle cramps, peripheral swelling, myalgia
Nervous System Disorders	Tremor, headache, dizziness (excluding vertigo)	Headache, dizziness
Psychiatric Disorders	Anxiety	Insomnia, depression
Renal and Urinary Disorders	Renal tubular necrosis, renal impairment, dysuria, hematuria, hydronephrosis, bladder spasm, urinary retention	–
Respiratory, Thoracic and Mediastinal Disorders	Cough, dyspnea, dyspnea exertional	Cough, dyspnea, pharyngolaryngeal pain, sinus congestion
Skin and Subcutaneous Tissue Disorders	Acne, pruritus	Rash, contusion
Surgical and Medical Procedures	Complications of transplant surgery, postoperative complications, postoperative wound complication	–
Vascular Disorders	Hypertension, hypertension aggravated, hypotension	Hypertension

* USP (MODIFIED)

subjects aged 65 and over to determine whether they respond differently from younger subjects. Other reported clinical experience has not identified differences in responses between the elderly and younger patients. In general, dose selection for an elderly patient should be cautious, reflecting the greater frequency of decreased hepatic, renal, or cardiac function, and of concomitant disease or other drug therapy.

ADVERSE REACTIONS
The incidence of adverse events for Myfortic® (mycophenolic acid) was determined in randomized, comparative, active-controlled, double-blind, double-dummy trials in prevention of acute rejection in *de novo* and maintenance kidney transplant patients.
The principal adverse reactions associated with the administration of Myfortic include constipation, nausea, and urinary tract infection in *de novo* patients and nausea, diarrhea and nasopharyngitis in maintenance patients.
Adverse events reported in ≥20% of patients receiving Myfortic or mycophenolate mofetil in the 12-month *de novo*

renal study and maintenance renal study, when used in combination with cyclosporine, USP (MODIFIED) and corticosteroids, are listed in Table 4. Adverse event rates were similar between Myfortic and mycophenolate mofetil in both *de novo* and maintenance patients.
[See table 4 at top of previous page]
Table 5 summarizes the incidence of opportunistic infections in *de novo* and maintenance transplant patients, which were similar in both treatment groups.
[See table 5 on previous page]
The following opportunistic infections occurred rarely in the above controlled trials: aspergillus and cryptococcus.
The incidence of malignancies and lymphoma is consistent with that reported in the literature for this patient population. Lymphoma developed in 2 *de novo* patients (0.9%), (one diagnosed 9 days after treatment initiation) and in 2 maintenance patients (1.3%) (one was AIDS-related), receiving Myfortic with other immunosuppressive agents in the 12-month controlled clinical trials. Non-melanoma skin carcinoma occurred in 0.9% *de novo* and 1.8% maintenance patients. Other types of malignancy occurred in 0.5% *de novo* and 0.6% maintenance patients.

The following adverse events were reported between 3% to <20% incidence in *de novo* and maintenance patients treated with Myfortic in combination with cyclosporine and corticosteroids are listed in Table 6.
[See table 6 at left]
The following additional adverse reactions have been associated with the exposure to MPA when administered as a sodium salt or as mofetil ester:
Gastrointestinal: Colitis (sometimes caused by CMV), pancreatitis, esophagitis, intestinal perforation, gastrointestinal hemorrhage, gastric ulcers, duodenal ulcers, and ileus (see *PRECAUTIONS*).
Resistance Mechanism Disorders: Serious life-threatening infections such as meningitis and infectious endocarditis have been reported occasionally and there is evidence of a higher frequency of certain types of serious infections such as tuberculosis and atypical mycobacterial infection.
Respiratory: Interstitial lung disorders, including fatal pulmonary fibrosis, have been reported rarely with MPA administration and should be considered in the differential diagnosis of pulmonary symptoms ranging from dyspnea to respiratory failure in post-transplant patients receiving MPA derivatives.

Postmarketing Experience
- Cases of progressive multifocal leukoencephalopathy (PML), sometimes fatal, have been reported in patients treated with mycophenolate mofetil (MMF). Mycophenolate mofetil (MMF) is metabolized to mycophenolic acid (MPA), the active ingredient in Myfortic and the active form of the drug (see *WARNINGS, Latent Viral Infections*).
- BK virus-associated nephropathy has been observed in patients receiving immunosuppressants, including Myfortic. This infection is associated with serious outcomes, including deteriorating renal function and renal graft loss (see *WARNINGS, Latent Viral Infections*).
- Congenital malformations have been reported in offspring of patients exposed to mycophenolate mofetil (MMF) during pregnancy (see *WARNINGS, Pregnancy*).
- Cases of pure red cell aplasia (PRCA) have been reported in patients treated with mycophenolate mofetil in combination with other immunosuppressive agents (see *WARNINGS*).

OVERDOSAGE
Signs and Symptoms
There has been no reported experience of acute overdose of Myfortic® (mycophenolic acid) in humans.
Possible signs and symptoms of acute overdose could include the following: hematological abnormalities such as leukopenia and neutropenia, and gastrointestinal symptoms such as abdominal pain, diarrhea, nausea and vomiting, and dyspepsia.

Treatment and Management
General supportive measures and symptomatic treatment should be followed in all cases of overdosage. Although dialysis may be used to remove the inactive metabolite MPAG, it would not be expected to remove clinically significant amounts of the active moiety MPA due to the 98% plasma protein binding of MPA. By interfering with enterohepatic circulation of MPA, activated charcoal or bile acid sequestrants, such as cholestyramine, may reduce the systemic MPA exposure.

DOSAGE AND ADMINISTRATION
The recommended dose of Myfortic® (mycophenolic acid) is 720 mg administered twice daily (1440 mg total daily dose) on an empty stomach, one hour before or two hours after food intake (see *CLINICAL PHARMACOLOGY, Food Effect*).
Myfortic delayed-release tablets and mycophenolate mofetil tablets and capsules should not be used interchangeably without physician supervision because the rate of absorption following the administration of these two products is not equivalent.
Patients are to be instructed that Myfortic tablets should not be crushed, chewed, or cut prior to ingesting. The tablets should be swallowed whole in order to maintain the integrity of the enteric coating.
Pediatric: Based on a pharmacokinetic study conducted in stable renal pediatric transplant patients, the recommended dose of Myfortic in stable pediatric patients is 400 mg/m² body surface area (BSA) administered twice daily (up to a maximum dose of 720 mg administered twice daily). Patients with a BSA of 1.19 to 1.58 m² may be dosed either with three Myfortic 180 mg tablets or one 180 mg tablet plus one 360 mg tablet twice daily (1080 mg daily dose). Patients with a BSA of >1.58 m² may be dosed either with four Myfortic 180 mg tablets or two Myfortic 360 mg tablets twice daily (1440 mg daily dose). Pediatric doses for patients with BSA <1.19 m² cannot be accurately administered using currently available formulations of Myfortic tablets.

Geriatrics: The maximum recommended dose is 720 mg administered twice daily.

Treatment During Rejection Episodes

Renal transplant rejection does not lead to changes in MPA pharmacokinetics; dosage reduction or interruption of Myfortic is not required.

Patients with Renal Impairment

No dose adjustments are needed in patients experiencing delayed renal graft function post-operatively. Patients with severe chronic renal impairment (GFR <25 mL/min/1.73 m² BSA) should be carefully followed for potential adverse reactions due to increase in free MPA and total MPAG concentrations (*see CLINICAL PHARMACOLOGY, Pharmacokinetics, Special Populations*).

Patients with Hepatic Impairment

No dose adjustments are needed for renal transplant patients with hepatic parenchymal disease. However, it is not known whether dosage adjustments are needed for hepatic disease with other etiologies (*see CLINICAL PHARMACOLOGY, Pharmacokinetics*).

HOW SUPPLIED

Myfortic® (mycophenolic acid) delayed-released tablets
360 mg tablet: Pale orange-red film-coated ovaloid tablet with imprint (debossing) "CT" on one side, containing 360 mg mycophenolic acid formulated as a sodium salt.
Bottles of 120 .... NDC 0078-0386-66
180 mg tablet: Lime green film-coated round tablet with bevelled edges and the imprint (debossing) "C" on one side, containing 180 mg mycophenolic acid formulated as a sodium salt.
Bottles of 120 .... NDC 0078-0385-66

Storage

Store at 25°C (77°F); excursions permitted to 15-30°C (59-86°F) [see USP Controlled Room Temperature]. Protect from moisture.

Dispense in a tight container (USP).

Handling

Tablets should not be crushed or cut.
REV: OCTOBER 2009   T2009-106
Manufactured by:
Novartis Pharma Stein AG
Stein, Switzerland
Distributed by:
Novartis Pharmaceuticals Corporation
East Hanover, New Jersey 07936
©Novartis

MEDICATION GUIDE

Myfortic® (my-for-tic)
(mycophenolic acid)
delayed-release tablets
Read the Medication Guide that comes with Myfortic before you start taking it and each time you get a refill. There may be new information. This Medication Guide does not take the place of talking with your healthcare provider about your medical condition or treatment. If you have any questions about Myfortic, ask your healthcare provider.

What is the most important information I should know about Myfortic?

Myfortic can cause serious side effects including:
- **Possible loss of pregnancy and higher risk of birth defects.** Women who take Myfortic during pregnancy, have a higher risk of losing a pregnancy (miscarriage) during the first three months (first trimester), and a higher risk that their baby will be born with birth defects.
If you are a female and are able to become pregnant:
  - Your healthcare provider must talk with you about effective birth control methods (contraceptive counseling).
  - You should have a negative pregnancy test within 1 week before starting Myfortic therapy.
  - You must use two different types of effective birth control at the same time, for 4 weeks before you start taking Myfortic, during your entire Myfortic therapy, and for 6 weeks after stopping Myfortic, unless you choose to avoid sexual intercourse completely (abstinence). Myfortic decreases blood levels of the hormones in the birth control pills that you take by mouth. Birth control pills may not work as well while you are taking Myfortic, and you could get pregnant.
  - If you plan to become pregnant, talk with your healthcare provider. Your healthcare provider will decide if other medicines to prevent rejection may be right for you. In certain situations, you and your doctor may decide that taking Myfortic is more important to your health than the possible risks to your unborn baby.
  - **If you get pregnant while taking Myfortic, <u>do not stop</u> taking Myfortic.** Call your healthcare provider right away. You and your healthcare provider should report any cases of pregnancy to:
    - Novartis Drug Safety at 1-888-669-6682
    - FDA MedWatch at 1-800-FDA-1088
Talk to your healthcare provider about joining the National Transplantation Pregnancy Registry at: 1-877-955-6877.

- **Increased risk of getting serious infections.** Myfortic weakens the body's immune system and affects your ability to fight infections. Serious infections can happen with Myfortic and can lead to death.
Types of infections can include:
- **Viral infections.** Certain viruses can live in your body and cause active infections when your immune system is weak. Viral infections that can happen with Myfortic include:
  - Shingles, other herpes infections, and cytomegalovirus (CMV). CMV can cause serious tissue and blood infections.
  - BK virus. BK virus can affect how your kidney works and cause your transplanted kidney to fail.
- **A brain infection called Progressive Multifocal Leukoencephalopathy (PML).** In some patients Myfortic may cause an infection of the brain that may cause death. You are at risk for this brain infection because you have a weakened immune system. You should tell your healthcare provider right away if you have any of the following symptoms:
  - You do not care about things that you usually care about (apathy)
  - You are confused or have problems thinking
  - Weakness on one side of the body
  - You cannot control your muscles
- **Fungal infections.** Yeast and other types of fungal infections can happen with Myfortic and cause serious tissue and blood infections. See "What are the possible side effects of Myfortic?"

Call your healthcare provider right away if you have any of these signs and symptoms of infection:
- Temperature of 100.5°F or greater
- Cold symptoms, such as a runny nose or sore throat
- Flu symptoms, such as an upset stomach, stomach pain, vomiting or diarrhea
- Earache or headache
- Pain during urination or you need to urinate often
- White patches in the mouth or throat
- Unexpected bruising or bleeding
- Cuts, scrapes or incisions that are red, warm and oozing pus

Increased risk of getting certain cancers. People who take Myfortic have a higher risk of getting lymphoma, and other cancers, especially skin cancer. Tell your healthcare provider if you have:
- unexplained fever, tiredness that does not go away, weight loss, or lymph node swelling
- a brown or black skin lesion with uneven borders, or one part of the lesion does not look like other parts
- a change in the size or color of a mole
- a new skin lesion or bump
- any other changes to your health

See the section "What are the possible side effects of Myfortic?" for other serious side effects.

What is Myfortic?

Myfortic is a prescription medicine given to prevent rejection (antirejection medicine) in people who have received a kidney transplant. Rejection is when the body's immune system senses the new organ as "foreign" and attacks it.
Myfortic is used with other medicines containing cyclosporine (Sandimmune®, Gengraf®, and Neoral®) and corticosteroids. These medicines work together to help prevent rejection to your transplanted kidney.
Myfortic can be used to prevent rejection in children who are 5 years or older and are stable after having a kidney transplant. It is not known if Myfortic is safe and works in children younger than 5 years. It is not known how Myfortic works in children who have just received a new kidney transplant.

Who should not take Myfortic?

Do not take Myfortic if you are allergic to mycophenolic acid, mycophenolate sodium, mycophenolate mofetil, or any of the ingredients in Myfortic. See the end of this Medication Guide for a complete list of ingredients in Myfortic.

What should I tell my healthcare provider before I start taking Myfortic?

Tell your healthcare provider about all of your medical conditions, including if you:
- **have any digestive problems, such as ulcers**
- **plan to receive any vaccines.** You should not receive live vaccines while you take Myfortic. Some vaccines may not work as well during treatment with Myfortic.
- **have Lesch-Nyhan or Kelley-Seegmiller syndrome or another rare inherited deficiency of hypoxanthine-guanine phosphoribosyl-transferase (HGPRT).** You should not take Myfortic if you have one of these disorders.
- **are pregnant or planning to become pregnant.** See "What is the most important information I should know about Myfortic?"
- **are breastfeeding.** It is not known if Myfortic passes into breast milk. You and your healthcare provider will decide if you will stop taking Myfortic or breast-feed. You should not do both without first talking to your healthcare provider.

Tell your healthcare provider about all the medicines you take, including prescription and nonprescription medicines, vitamins, and herbal supplements. Some medicines may affect the way Myfortic works and Myfortic may affect how some medicines work. Especially tell your doctor if you take:
- birth control pills (oral contraceptives). See "What is the most important information I should know about Myfortic?"
- antacids that contain aluminum or magnesium. Myfortic and antacids should not be taken at the same time.
- acyclovir (Zovirax®), Ganciclovir (Cytovene® IV, Valcyte®)
- azathioprine (Azasan®, Imuran®)
- cholestyramine (Questran® Light, Questran®, Locholest Light, Prevalite®)

Know the medicines you take. Keep a list of your medicines with you to show your healthcare provider and pharmacist when you get a new medicine. Do not take any new medicine without talking to your healthcare provider.

How should I take Myfortic?
- Take Myfortic exactly as prescribed. Your healthcare provider will tell you how much Myfortic to take.
- Do not stop taking or change your dose of Myfortic without talking to your healthcare provider.
- Take Myfortic on an empty stomach, either 1 hour before or 2 hours after a meal.
- Swallow Myfortic whole. Do not crush, chew, or cut Myfortic. The Myfortic tablets have a coating so that the medicine will pass through your stomach and dissolve in your intestine.
- **If you forget to take Myfortic,** take it as soon as you remember and then take your next dose at its regular time. If it is almost time for your next dose, skip the missed dose. Do not take two doses at the same time. Call your healthcare provider or pharmacist if you are not sure what to do.
- **If you take more than the prescribed dose of Myfortic,** call your healthcare provider right away.
- **Do not change (substitute) between using Myfortic delayed-release tablets and mycophenolate mofetil tablets, capsules, or oral suspension for one another unless your healthcare provider tells you to.** These medicines are absorbed differently. This may affect the amount of medicine in your blood.
- Be sure to keep all appointments at your transplant clinic. During these visits, your healthcare provider may perform regular blood tests.

What should I avoid while taking Myfortic?

Avoid pregnancy. See "What is the most important information I should know about Myfortic?"
- Limit the amount of time you spend in sunlight. Avoid using tanning beds and sunlamps. People who take Myfortic have a higher risk of getting skin cancer. **See "What is the most important information I should know about Myfortic?"** Wear protective clothing when you are in the sun and use a sunscreen with a high sun protection factor (SPF 30 and above). This is especially important if your skin is fair (light colored) or you have a family history of skin cancer.
- Elderly patients 65 years of age or older may have more side effects with Myfortic because of a weaker immune system.

What are the possible side effects of Myfortic?

Myfortic can cause serious side effects.
See "What is the most important information I should know about Myfortic?"
Stomach and intestinal bleeding can happen in people who take Myfortic. Bleeding can be severe and you may have to be hospitalized for treatment.
The most common side effects of taking Myfortic include:
In people with a new transplant:
- low blood cell counts
  - red blood cells
  - white blood cells
  - platelets
- constipation
- nausea
- diarrhea
- vomiting
- urinary tract infections
- stomach upset
In people who take Myfortic for a long time (long-term) after transplant:
- low blood cell counts
  - red blood cells
  - white blood cells
- nausea
- diarrhea
- sore throat

Your healthcare provider will do blood tests before you start taking Myfortic and during treatment with Myfortic to check your blood cell counts. Tell your healthcare provider right away if you have any signs of infection (see "**What is**

the most important information I should know about Myfortic?"), or any unexpected bruising or bleeding. Also, tell your healthcare provider if you have unusual tiredness, dizziness or fainting.

These are not all the possible side effects of Myfortic. Your healthcare provider may be able to help you manage these side effects.

Call your doctor for medical advice about side effects. You may report side effects to FDA at 1-800-FDA-1088.

How should I store Myfortic?

- Store Myfortic tablets at room temperature, 59° to 86°F (15° to 30°C). Myfortic does not need to be refrigerated.
- Keep the container tightly closed. Store Myfortic in a dry place.
- **Keep Myfortic and all medicines out of the reach of children.**

General information about Myfortic

Medicines are sometimes prescribed for purposes other than those listed in a Medication Guide. Do not use Myfortic for a condition for which it was not prescribed. Do not give Myfortic to other people, even if they have the same symptoms you have. It may harm them.

This Medication Guide summarizes the most important information about Myfortic. If you would like more information, talk with your doctor. You can ask your doctor or pharmacist for information about Myfortic that is written for healthcare professionals. You can also call 1-888-669-6682 or visit the Myfortic website at www.myfortic.com.

What are the ingredients in Myfortic?

Active ingredient: mycophenolic acid (as mycophenolate sodium)

Inactive ingredients: colloidal silicon dioxide, crospovidone, lactose anhydrous, magnesium stearate, povidone (K-30), and starch. The enteric coating of the tablet consists of hypromellose phthalate, titanium dioxide, iron oxide yellow, and indigotine (for the 180-mg tablet) or iron oxide red (for the 360-mg tablet)

This Medication Guide has been approved by the U.S. Food and Drug Administration.

Sandimmune and Neoral are registered trademarks of Novartis Pharmaceuticals Corporation.

Any other trademarks in this document are the property of their respective owners.

REV: OCTOBER 2009 T2009-107

T2009-106/T2009-107

5002411

Manufactured by:
Novartis Pharma Stein AG
Stein, Switzerland
Distributed by: Novartis Pharmaceuticals Corporation
East Hanover, New Jersey 07936
©Novartis

Shown in Product Identification Guide, page 315

NEORAL® SOFT GELATIN CAPSULES ℞

[*nē ō 'ral*]

(cyclosporine capsules, USP)

MODIFIED

NEORAL® ORAL SOLUTION

(cyclosporine oral solution, USP)

MODIFIED

Rx only

The following prescribing information is based on official labeling in effect July 2010.

Prescribing Information

WARNING

Only physicians experienced in management of systemic immunosuppressive therapy for the indicated disease should prescribe Neoral®. At doses used in solid organ transplantation, only physicians experienced in immunosuppressive therapy and management of organ transplant recipients should prescribe Neoral®. Patients receiving the drug should be managed in facilities equipped and staffed with adequate laboratory and supportive medical resources. The physician responsible for maintenance therapy should have complete information requisite for the follow-up of the patient.

Neoral®, a systemic immunosuppressant, may increase the susceptibility to infection and the development of neoplasia. In kidney, liver, and heart transplant patients Neoral® may be administered with other immunosuppressive agents. Increased susceptibility to infection and the possible development of lymphoma and other neoplasms may result from the increase in the degree of immunosuppression in transplant patients.

Neoral® Soft Gelatin Capsules (cyclosporine capsules, USP) MODIFIED and Neoral® Oral Solution (cyclosporine oral solution, USP) MODIFIED have increased bioavailability in comparison to Sandimmune® Soft Gelatin Capsules (cyclosporine capsules, USP) and Sandimmune® Oral Solution (cyclosporine oral solution, USP). Neoral® and Sandimmune® are not bioequivalent and cannot be used interchangeably without physician supervision. For a given trough concentration, cyclosporine exposure will be greater with Neoral® than with Sandimmune®. If a patient who is receiving exceptionally high doses of Sandimmune® is converted to Neoral®, particular caution should be exercised. Cyclosporine blood concentrations should be monitored in transplant and rheumatoid arthritis patients taking Neoral® to avoid toxicity due to high concentrations. Dose adjustments should be made in transplant patients to minimize possible organ rejection due to low concentrations. Comparison of blood concentrations in the published literature with blood concentrations obtained using current assays must be done with detailed knowledge of the assay methods employed.

For Psoriasis Patients ***(See also Boxed WARNINGS above)***

Psoriasis patients previously treated with PUVA and to a lesser extent, methotrexate or other immunosuppressive agents, UVB, coal tar, or radiation therapy, are at an increased risk of developing skin malignancies when taking Neoral®.

Cyclosporine, the active ingredient in Neoral®, in recommended dosages, can cause systemic hypertension and nephrotoxicity. The risk increases with increasing dose and duration of cyclosporine therapy. Renal dysfunction, including structural kidney damage, is a potential consequence of cyclosporine, and therefore, renal function must be monitored during therapy.

DESCRIPTION

Neoral® is an oral formulation of cyclosporine that immediately forms a microemulsion in an aqueous environment.

Cyclosporine, the active principle in Neoral®, is a cyclic polypeptide immunosuppressant agent consisting of 11 amino acids. It is produced as a metabolite by the fungus species *Beauveria nivea.*

Chemically, cyclosporine is designated as [*R*-[*R**,*R**-(*E*)]]-cyclic-(L-alanyl-D-alanyl-*N*-methyl-L-leucyl-*N*-methyl-L-leucyl-*N*-methyl-L-valyl-3-hydroxy-*N*,4-dimethyl-L-2-amino-6-octenoyl-L-α-aminobutyryl-*N*-methylglycyl-*N*-methyl-L-leucyl-L-valyl-*N*-methyl-L-leucyl).

Neoral® Soft Gelatin Capsules

(cyclosporine capsules, USP) MODIFIED are available in 25 mg and 100 mg strengths.

Each 25 mg capsule contains:

cyclosporine	25 mg
alcohol, USP dehydrated	11.9% v/v (9.5% wt/vol.)

Each 100 mg capsule contains:

cyclosporine	100 mg
alcohol, USP dehydrated	11.9% v/v (9.5% wt/vol.)

Inactive Ingredients: Corn oil-mono-di-triglycerides, polyoxyl 40 hydrogenated castor oil NF, DL-α-tocopherol USP, gelatin NF, glycerol, iron oxide black, propylene glycol USP, titanium dioxide USP, carmine, and other ingredients.

Neoral® Oral Solution

(cyclosporine oral solution, USP) MODIFIED is available in 50 mL bottles.

Each mL contains:

cyclosporine	100 mg/mL
alcohol, USP dehydrated	11.9% v/v (9.5% wt/vol.)

Inactive Ingredients: Corn oil-mono-di-triglycerides, polyoxyl 40 hydrogenated castor oil NF, DL-α-tocopherol USP, propylene glycol USP.

The chemical structure of cyclosporine (also known as cyclosporin A) is:

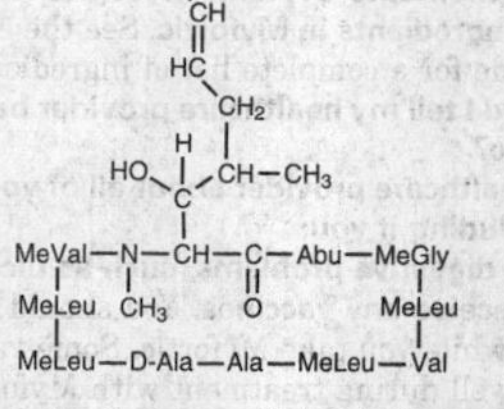

$C_{62}H_{111}N_{11}O_{12}$ Mol. Wt. 1202.63

CLINICAL PHARMACOLOGY

Cyclosporine is a potent immunosuppressive agent that in animals prolongs survival of allogeneic transplants involving skin, kidney, liver, heart, pancreas, bone marrow, small intestine, and lung. Cyclosporine has been demonstrated to suppress some humoral immunity and to a greater extent, cell-mediated immune reactions such as allograft rejection, delayed hypersensitivity, experimental allergic encephalomyelitis, Freund's adjuvant arthritis, and graft vs. host disease in many animal species for a variety of organs.

The effectiveness of cyclosporine results from specific and reversible inhibition of immunocompetent lymphocytes in the G_0- and G_1-phase of the cell cycle. T-lymphocytes are preferentially inhibited. The T-helper cell is the main target, although the T-suppressor cell may also be suppressed. Cyclosporine also inhibits lymphokine production and release including interleukin-2.

No effects on phagocytic function (changes in enzyme secretions, chemotactic migration of granulocytes, macrophage migration, carbon clearance *in vivo*) have been detected in animals. Cyclosporine does not cause bone marrow suppression in animal models or man.

Pharmacokinetics

The immunosuppressive activity of cyclosporine is primarily due to parent drug. Following oral administration, absorption of cyclosporine is incomplete. The extent of absorption of cyclosporine is dependent on the individual patient, the patient population, and the formulation. Elimination of cyclosporine is primarily biliary with only 6% of the dose (parent drug and metabolites) excreted in urine. The disposition of cyclosporine from blood is generally biphasic, with a terminal half-life of approximately 8.4 hours (range 5-18 hours). Following intravenous administration, the blood clearance of cyclosporine (assay: HPLC) is approximately 5-7 mL/min/kg in adult recipients of renal or liver allografts. Blood cyclosporine clearance appears to be slightly slower in cardiac transplant patients.

The Neoral® Soft Gelatin Capsules (cyclosporine capsules, USP) MODIFIED and Neoral® Oral Solution (cyclosporine oral solution, USP) MODIFIED are bioequivalent. Neoral® Oral Solution diluted with orange juice or apple juice is bioequivalent to Neoral Oral Solution diluted with water. The effect of milk on the bioavailability of cyclosporine when administered as Neoral Oral Solution has not been evaluated.

The relationship between administered dose and exposure (area under the concentration versus time curve, AUC) is linear within the therapeutic dose range. The intersubject variability (total, %CV) of cyclosporine exposure (AUC) when Neoral® or Sandimmune® is administered ranges from approximately 20% to 50% in renal transplant patients. This intersubject variability contributes to the need for individualization of the dosing regimen for optimal therapy *(see DOSAGE AND ADMINISTRATION)*. Intrasubject variability of AUC in renal transplant recipients (%CV) was 9%-21% for Neoral® and 19%-26% for Sandimmune®. In the same studies, intrasubject variability of trough concentrations (%CV) was 17%-30% for Neoral® and 16%-38% for Sandimmune®.

Absorption

Neoral® has increased bioavailability compared to Sandimmune®. The absolute bioavailability of cyclosporine administered as Sandimmune® is dependent on the patient population, estimated to be less than 10% in liver transplant patients and as great as 89% in some renal transplant patients. The absolute bioavailability of cyclosporine administered as Neoral® has not been determined in adults. In studies of renal transplant, rheumatoid arthritis and psoriasis patients, the mean cyclosporine AUC was approximately 20% to 50% greater and the peak blood cyclosporine concentration (C_{max}) was approximately 40% to 106% greater following administration of Neoral® compared to following administration of Sandimmune®. The dose normalized AUC in *de novo* liver transplant patients administered Neoral® 28 days after transplantation was 50% greater and C_{max} was 90% greater than in those patients administered Sandimmune®. AUC and C_{max} are also increased (Neoral® relative to Sandimmune®) in heart transplant patients, but data are very limited. Although the AUC and C_{max} values are higher on Neoral® relative to Sandimmune®, the pre-dose trough concentrations (dose-normalized) are similar for the two formulations.

Following oral administration of Neoral®, the time to peak blood cyclosporine concentrations (T_{max}) ranged from 1.5-2.0 hours. The administration of food with Neoral® decreases the cyclosporine AUC and C_{max}. A high fat meal (669 kcal, 45 grams fat) consumed within one-half hour before Neoral® administration decreased the AUC by 13% and C_{max} by 33%. The effects of a low fat meal (667 kcal, 15 grams fat) were similar.

The effect of T-tube diversion of bile on the absorption of cyclosporine from Neoral® was investigated in eleven *de novo* liver transplant patients. When the patients were administered Neoral® with and without T-tube diversion of bile, very little difference in absorption was observed, as measured by the change in maximal cyclosporine blood concentrations from pre-dose values with the T-tube closed relative to when it was open: 6.9±41% (range -55% to 68%).

[See first table at top of next page]

Distribution

Cyclosporine is distributed largely outside the blood volume. The steady state volume of distribution during intravenous dosing has been reported as 3-5 L/kg in solid organ transplant recipients. In blood, the distribution is concentration dependent. Approximately 33%-47% is in plasma, 4%-9% in lymphocytes, 5%-12% in granulocytes, and 41%-58% in erythrocytes. At high concentrations, the binding capacity of leukocytes and erythrocytes becomes saturated. In plasma, approximately 90% is bound to proteins, primarily lipoproteins. Cyclosporine is excreted in human milk. (See PRECAUTIONS, Nursing Mothers)

Metabolism
Cyclosporine is extensively metabolized by the cytochrome P-450 3A enzyme system in the liver, and to a lesser degree in the gastrointestinal tract, and the kidney. The metabolism of cyclosporine can be altered by the co-administration of a variety of agents. (See PRECAUTIONS, Drug Interactions) At least 25 metabolites have been identified from human bile, feces, blood, and urine. The biological activity of the metabolites and their contributions to toxicity are considerably less than those of the parent compound. The major metabolites (M1, M9, and M4N) result from oxidation at the 1-beta, 9-gamma, and 4-N-demethylated positions, respectively. At steady state following the oral administration of Sandimmune®, the mean AUCs for blood concentrations of M1, M9, and M4N are about 70%, 21%, and 7.5% of the AUC for blood cyclosporine concentrations, respectively. Based on blood concentration data from stable renal transplant patients (13 patients administered Neoral® and Sandimmune® in a crossover study), and bile concentration data from de novo liver transplant patients (4 administered Neoral®, 3 administered Sandimmune®), the percentage of dose present as M1, M9, and M4N metabolites is similar when either Neoral® or Sandimmune® is administered.

Excretion
Only 0.1% of a cyclosporine dose is excreted unchanged in the urine. Elimination is primarily biliary with only 6% of the dose (parent drug and metabolites) excreted in the urine. Neither dialysis nor renal failure alter cyclosporine clearance significantly.

Drug Interactions
(See PRECAUTIONS, Drug Interactions) When diclofenac or methotrexate was co-administered with cyclosporine in rheumatoid arthritis patients, the AUC of diclofenac and methotrexate, each was significantly increased. (See PRECAUTIONS, Drug Interactions) No clinically significant pharmacokinetic interactions occurred between cyclosporine and aspirin, ketoprofen, piroxicam, or indomethacin.

Special Populations
Pediatric Population
Pharmacokinetic data from pediatric patients administered Neoral® or Sandimmune® are very limited. In 15 renal transplant patients aged 3-16 years, cyclosporine whole blood clearance after IV administration of Sandimmune® was 10.6±3.7 mL/min/kg (assay: Cyclo-trac specific RIA). In a study of 7 renal transplant patients aged 2-16, the cyclosporine clearance ranged from 9.8-15.5 mL/min/kg. In 9 liver transplant patients aged 0.6-5.6 years, clearance was 9.3±5.4 mL/min/kg (assay: HPLC).
In the pediatric population, Neoral® also demonstrates an increased bioavailability as compared to Sandimmune®. In 7 liver de novo transplant patients aged 1.4-10 years, the absolute bioavailability of Neoral® was 43% (range 30%-68%) and for Sandimmune® in the same individuals absolute bioavailability was 28% (range 17%-42%).
[See second table above]

Geriatric Population
Comparison of single dose data from both normal elderly volunteers (N=18, mean age 69 years) and elderly rheumatoid arthritis patients (N=16, mean age 68 years) to single dose data in young adult volunteers (N=16, mean age 26 years) showed no significant difference in the pharmacokinetic parameters.

CLINICAL TRIALS
Rheumatoid Arthritis
The effectiveness of Sandimmune® and Neoral® in the treatment of severe rheumatoid arthritis was evaluated in 5 clinical studies involving a total of 728 cyclosporine treated patients and 273 placebo treated patients.
A summary of the results is presented for the "responder" rates per treatment group, with a responder being defined as a patient having *completed* the trial with a 20% improvement in the tender and the swollen joint count and a 20% improvement in 2 of 4 of investigator global, patient global, disability, and erythrocyte sedimentation rates (ESR) for the Studies 651 and 652 and 3 of 5 of investigator global, patient global, disability, visual analog pain, and ESR for Studies 2008, 654 and 302.
Study 651 enrolled 264 patients with active rheumatoid arthritis with at least 20 involved joints, who had failed at least one major RA drug, using a 3:3:3 randomization to one of the following three groups: (1) cyclosporine dosed at 2.5-5 mg/kg/day, (2) methotrexate at 7.5-15 mg/week, or (3) placebo. Treatment duration was 24 weeks. The mean

cyclosporine dose at the last visit was 3.1 mg/kg/day. See Graph below.
Study 652 enrolled 250 patients with active RA with >6 active painful or tender joints who had failed at least one major RA drug. Patients were randomized using a 3:3:2 randomization to 1 of 3 treatment arms: (1) 1.5-5 mg/kg/day of cyclosporine, (2) 2.5-5 mg/kg/day of cyclosporine, and (3) placebo. Treatment duration was 16 weeks. The mean cyclosporine dose for group 2 at the last visit was 2.92 mg/kg/day. See Graph below.
Study 2008 enrolled 144 patients with active RA and >6 active joints who had unsuccessful treatment courses of aspirin and gold or Penicillamine. Patients were randomized to 1 of 2 treatment groups: (1) cyclosporine 2.5-5 mg/kg/day with adjustments after the first month to achieve a target trough level and (2) placebo. Treatment duration was 24 weeks. The mean cyclosporine dose at the last visit was 3.63 mg/kg/day. See Graph below.
Study 654 enrolled 148 patients who remained with active joint counts of 6 or more despite treatment with maximally tolerated methotrexate doses for at least three months. Patients continued to take their current dose of methotrexate and were randomized to receive, in addition, one of the following medications: (1) cyclosporine 2.5 mg/kg/day with dose increases of 0.5 mg/kg/day at weeks 2 and 4 if there was no evidence of toxicity and further increases of 0.5 mg/kg/day at weeks 8 and 16 if a <30% decrease in active joint count occurred without any significant toxicity; dose decreases could be made at any time for toxicity or (2) placebo. Treatment duration was 24 weeks. The mean cyclosporine dose at the last visit was 2.8 mg/kg/day (range: 1.3-4.1). See Graph below.
Study 302 enrolled 299 patients with severe active RA, 99% of whom were unresponsive or intolerant to at least one prior major RA drug. Patients were randomized to 1 of 2 treatment groups: (1) Neoral® and (2) cyclosporine, both of which were started at 2.5 mg/kg/day and increased after 4 weeks for inefficacy in increments of 0.5 mg/kg/day to a maximum of 5 mg/kg/day and decreased at any time for toxicity. Treatment duration was 24 weeks. The mean cyclosporine dose at the last visit was 2.91 mg/kg/day

(range: 0.72-5.17) for Neoral® and 3.27 mg/kg/day (range: 0.73-5.68) for cyclosporine. See Graph below.
[See figure at top of next page]

INDICATIONS AND USAGE
Kidney, Liver, and Heart Transplantation
Neoral® is indicated for the prophylaxis of organ rejection in kidney, liver, and heart allogeneic transplants. Neoral® has been used in combination with azathioprine and corticosteroids.

Rheumatoid Arthritis
Neoral® is indicated for the treatment of patients with severe active, rheumatoid arthritis where the disease has not adequately responded to methotrexate. Neoral® can be used in combination with methotrexate in rheumatoid arthritis patients who do not respond adequately to methotrexate alone.

Psoriasis
Neoral® is indicated for the treatment of *adult, nonimmunocompromised* patients with severe (i.e., extensive and/or disabling), recalcitrant, plaque psoriasis who have failed to respond to at least one systemic therapy (eg., PUVA, retinoids, or methotrexate) or in patients for whom other systemic therapies are contraindicated, or cannot be tolerated. While rebound rarely occurs, most patients will experience relapse with Neoral® as with other therapies upon cessation of treatment.

CONTRAINDICATIONS
General
Neoral® is contraindicated in patients with a hypersensitivity to cyclosporine or to any of the ingredients of the formulation.

Rheumatoid Arthritis
Rheumatoid arthritis patients with abnormal renal function, uncontrolled hypertension, or malignancies should not receive Neoral®.

Psoriasis
Psoriasis patients who are treated with Neoral® should not receive concomitant PUVA or UVB therapy, methotrexate or other immunosuppressive agents, coal tar or radiation therapy. Psoriasis patients with abnormal renal function, uncontrolled hypertension, or malignancies should not receive Neoral®.

Pharmacokinetic Parameters (mean ± SD)							
Patient Population	Dose/day[1] (mg/d)	Dose/weight) (mg/kg/d)	AUC[2] (ng·hr/mL)	C_{max} (ng/mL)	Trough[3] (ng/mL)	CL/F (mL/min)	CL/F (mL/min/kg)
De novo renal transplant[4] Week 4 (N=37)	597±174	7.95±2.81	8772±2089	1802±428	361±129	593±204	7.8±2.9
Stable renal transplant[4] (N=55)	344±122	4.10±1.58	6035±2194	1333±469	251±116	492±140	5.9±2.1
De novo liver transplant[5] Week 4 (N=18)	458±190	6.89±3.68	7187±2816	1555±740	268±101	577±309	8.6±5.7
De novo rheumatoid arthritis[6] (N=23)	182±55.6	2.37±0.36	2641±877	728±263	96.4±37.7	613±196	8.3±2.8
De novo psoriasis[6] Week 4 (N=18)	189±69.8	2.48±0.65	2324±1048	655±186	74.9±46.7	723±186	10.2±3.9

[1] Total daily dose was divided into two doses administered every 12 hours
[2] AUC was measured over one dosing interval
[3] Trough concentration was measured just prior to the morning Neoral® dose, approximately 12 hours after the previous dose
[4] Assay: TDx specific monoclonal fluorescence polarization immunoassay
[5] Assay: Cyclo-trac specific monoclonal radioimmunoassay
[6] Assay: INCSTAR specific monoclonal radioimmunoassay

Pediatric Pharmacokinetic Parameters (mean ± SD)						
Patient Population	Dose/day (mg/d)	Dose/weight (mg/kg/d)	AUC[1] (ng·hr/mL)	C_{max} (ng/mL)	CL/F (mL/min)	CL/F (mL/min/kg)
Stable liver transplant[2] Age 2-8, Dosed TID (N=9)	101±25	5.95±1.32	2163±801	629±219	285±94	16.6±4.3
Age 8-15, Dosed BID (N=8)	188±55	4.96±2.09	4272±1462	975±281	378±80	10.2±4.0
Stable liver transplant[3] Age 3, Dosed BID (N=1)	120	8.33	5832	1050	171	11.9
Age 8-15, Dosed BID (N=5)	158±55	5.51±1.91	4452±2475	1013±635	328±121	11.0±1.9
Stable renal transplant[3] Age 7-15, Dosed BID (N=5)	328±83	7.37±4.11	6922±1988	1827±487	418±143	8.7±2.9

[1] AUC was measured over one dosing interval
[2] Assay: Cyclo-trac specific monoclonal radioimmunoassay
[3] Assay: TDx specific monoclonal fluorescence polarization immunoassay

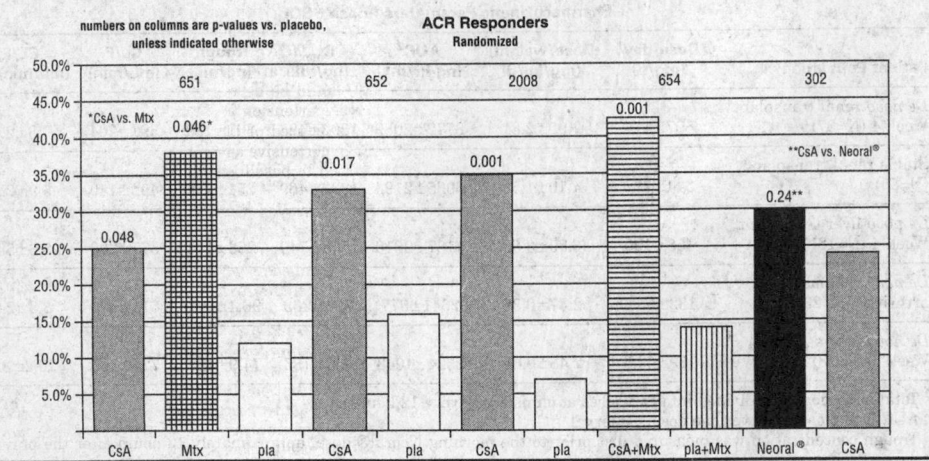

numbers on columns are p-values vs. placebo, unless indicated otherwise

ACR Responders Randomized

Nephrotoxicity vs. Rejection

Parameter	Nephrotoxicity	Rejection
History	Donor >50 years old or hypotensive Prolonged kidney preservation Prolonged anastomosis time Concomitant nephrotoxic drugs	Anti-donor immune response Retransplant patient
Clinical	Often >6 weeks postop[b] Prolonged initial nonfunction (acute tubular necrosis)	Often <4 weeks postop[b] Fever >37.5°C Weight gain >0.5 kg Graft swelling and tenderness Decrease in daily urine volume >500 mL (or 50%)
Laboratory	CyA serum trough level >200 ng/mL Gradual rise in Cr (<0.15 mg/dL/day)[a] Cr plateau <25% above baseline BUN/Cr ≥ 20	CyA serum trough level <150 ng/mL Rapid rise in Cr (>0.3 mg/dL/day)[a] Cr >25% above baseline BUN/Cr <20
Biopsy	Arteriolopathy (medial hypertrophy[a], hyalinosis, nodular deposits, intimal thickening, endothelial vacuolization, progressive scarring) Tubular atrophy, isometric vacuolization, isolated calcifications Minimal edema Mild focal infiltrates[c]	Endovasculitis[c] (proliferation[a], intimal arteritis[b], necrosis, sclerosis) Tubulitis with RBC[b] and WBC[b] casts, some irregular vacuolization Interstitial edema[c] and hemorrhage[b] Diffuse moderate to severe mononuclear infiltrates[d]
Aspiration Cytology	Diffuse interstitial fibrosis, often striped form CyA deposits in tubular and endothelial cells Fine isometric vacuolization of tubular cells	Glomerulitis (mononuclear cells)[c] Inflammatory infiltrate with mononuclear phagocytes, macrophages, lymphoblastoid cells, and activated T-cells These strongly express HLA-DR antigens
Urine Cytology	Tubular cells with vacuolization and granularization	Degenerative tubular cells, plasma cells, and lymphocyturia >20% of sediment
Manometry	Intracapsular pressure <40 mm Hg[b]	Intracapsular pressure >40 mm Hg[b]
Ultrasonography	Unchanged graft cross sectional area	Increase in graft cross sectional area AP diameter ≥ Transverse diameter
Magnetic Resonance Imagery	Normal appearance	Loss of distinct corticomedullary junction, swelling image intensity of parachyma approaching that of psoas, loss of hilar fat
Radionuclide Scan	Normal or generally decreased perfusion Decrease in tubular function (^{131}I-hippuran) > decrease in perfusion (^{99m}Tc DTPA)	Patchy arterial flow Decrease in perfusion > decrease in tubular function Increased uptake of Indium 111 labeled platelets or Tc-99m in colloid
Therapy	Responds to decreased cyclosporine	Responds to increased steroids or antilymphocyte globulin

[a]p < 0.05, [b]p < 0.01, [c]p < 0.001, [d]p < 0.0001

WARNINGS
(See also Boxed WARNING)
All Patients
Cyclosporine, the active ingredient of Neoral®, can cause nephrotoxicity and hepatotoxicity. The risk increases with increasing doses of cyclosporine. Renal dysfunction including structural kidney damage is a potential consequence of Neoral® and therefore renal function must be monitored during therapy. **Care should be taken in using cyclosporine with nephrotoxic drugs.** *(See PRECAUTIONS)*
Patients receiving Neoral® require frequent monitoring of serum creatinine. *(See Special Monitoring under DOSAGE AND ADMINISTRATION)* Elderly patients should be monitored with particular care, since decreases in renal function also occur with age. If patients are not properly monitored and doses are not properly adjusted, cyclosporine therapy can be associated with the occurrence of structural kidney damage and persistent renal dysfunction.

An increase in serum creatinine and BUN may occur during Neoral® therapy and reflect a reduction in the glomerular filtration rate. Impaired renal function at any time requires close monitoring, and frequent dosage adjustment may be indicated. The frequency and severity of serum creatinine elevations increase with dose and duration of cyclosporine therapy. These elevations are likely to become more pronounced without dose reduction or discontinuation.
Because Neoral® is not bioequivalent to Sandimmune®, conversion from Neoral® to Sandimmune® using a 1:1 ratio (mg/kg/day) may result in lower cyclosporine blood concentrations. Conversion from Neoral® to Sandimmune® should be made with increased monitoring to avoid the potential of underdosing.
Kidney, Liver, and Heart Transplant
Cyclosporine, the active ingredient of Neoral®, can cause nephrotoxicity and hepatotoxicity when used in high doses. It is not unusual for serum creatinine and BUN levels to be

elevated during cyclosporine therapy. These elevations in renal transplant patients do not necessarily indicate rejection, and each patient must be fully evaluated before dosage adjustment is initiated.
Based on the historical Sandimmune® experience with oral solution, nephrotoxicity associated with cyclosporine had been noted in 25% of cases of renal transplantation, 38% of cases of cardiac transplantation, and 37% of cases of liver transplantation. Mild nephrotoxicity was generally noted 2-3 months after renal transplant and consisted of an arrest in the fall of the pre-operative elevations of BUN and creatinine at a range of 35-45 mg/dL and 2.0-2.5 mg/dL respectively. These elevations were often responsive to cyclosporine dosage reduction.
More overt nephrotoxicity was seen early after transplantation and was characterized by a rapidly rising BUN and creatinine. Since these events are similar to renal rejection episodes, care must be taken to differentiate between them. This form of nephrotoxicity is usually responsive to cyclosporine dosage reduction.
Although specific diagnostic criteria which reliably differentiate renal graft rejection from drug toxicity have not been found, a number of parameters have been significantly associated with one or the other. It should be noted however, that up to 20% of patients may have simultaneous nephrotoxicity and rejection.
[See table at left]
A form of a cyclosporine-associated nephropathy is characterized by serial deterioration in renal function and morphologic changes in the kidneys. From 5%-15% of transplant recipients who have received cyclosporine will fail to show a reduction in rising serum creatinine despite a decrease or discontinuation of cyclosporine therapy. Renal biopsies from these patients will demonstrate one or several of the following alterations: tubular vacuolization, tubular microcalcifications, peritubular capillary congestion, arteriolopathy, and a striped form of interstitial fibrosis with tubular atrophy. Though none of these morphologic changes is entirely specific, a diagnosis of cyclosporine-associated structural nephrotoxicity requires evidence of these findings.
When considering the development of cyclosporine-associated nephropathy, it is noteworthy that several authors have reported an association between the appearance of interstitial fibrosis and higher cumulative doses or persistently high circulating trough levels of cyclosporine. This is particularly true during the first 6 post-transplant months when the dosage tends to be highest and when, in kidney recipients, the organ appears to be most vulnerable to the toxic effects of cyclosporine. Among other contributing factors to the development of interstitial fibrosis in these patients are prolonged perfusion time, warm ischemia time, as well as episodes of acute toxicity, and acute and chronic rejection. The reversibility of interstitial fibrosis and its correlation to renal function have not yet been determined. Reversibility of arteriolopathy has been reported after stopping cyclosporine or lowering the dosage.
Impaired renal function at any time requires close monitoring, and frequent dosage adjustment may be indicated.
In the event of severe and unremitting rejection, when rescue therapy with pulse steroids and monoclonal antibodies fail to reverse the rejection episode, it may be preferable to switch to alternative immunosuppressive therapy rather than increase the Neoral® dose to excessive levels.
Occasionally patients have developed a syndrome of thrombocytopenia and microangiopathic hemolytic anemia which may result in graft failure. The vasculopathy can occur in the absence of rejection and is accompanied by avid platelet consumption within the graft as demonstrated by Indium 111 labeled platelet studies. Neither the pathogenesis nor the management of this syndrome is clear. Though resolution has occurred after reduction or discontinuation of cyclosporine and 1) administration of streptokinase and heparin or 2) plasmapheresis, this appears to depend upon early detection with Indium 111 labeled platelet scans. *(See ADVERSE REACTIONS)*
Significant hyperkalemia (sometimes associated with hyperchloremic metabolic acidosis) and hyperuricemia have been seen occasionally in individual patients.
Hepatotoxicity associated with cyclosporine use had been noted in 4% of cases of renal transplantation, 7% of cases of cardiac transplantation, and 4% of cases of liver transplantation. This was usually noted during the first month of therapy when high doses of cyclosporine were used and consisted of elevations of hepatic enzymes and bilirubin. The chemistry elevations usually decreased with a reduction in dosage.
As in patients receiving other immunosuppressants, those patients receiving cyclosporine are at increased risk for development of lymphomas and other malignancies, particularly those of the skin. Patients taking cyclosporine should be warned to avoid excess ultraviolet light exposure. The increased risk appears related to the intensity and duration of immunosuppression rather than to the use of specific

agents. Because of the danger of oversuppression of the immune system resulting in increased risk of infection or malignancy, a treatment regimen containing multiple immunosuppressants should be used with caution. Some malignancies may be fatal. Transplant patients receiving cyclosporine are at increased risk for serious infection with fatal outcome.

Latent Viral Infections

Immunosuppressed patients are at increased risk for opportunistic infections, including activation of latent viral infections. These include BK virus-associated nephropathy which has been observed in patients receiving immunosuppressants, including Neoral. This infection is associated with serious outcomes, including deteriorating renal function and renal graft loss. Patient monitoring may help detect patients at risk for BK virus-associated nephropathy. Reduction in immunosuppression should be considered for patients who develop evidence of BK virus-associated nephropathy.

There have been reports of convulsions in adult and pediatric patients receiving cyclosporine, particularly in combination with high dose methylprednisolone.

Encephalopathy has been described both in post-marketing reports and in the literature. Manifestations include impaired consciousness, convulsions, visual disturbances (including blindness), loss of motor function, movement disorders and psychiatric disturbances. In many cases, changes in the white matter have been detected using imaging techniques and pathologic specimens. Predisposing factors such as hypertension, hypomagnesemia, hypocholesterolemia, high-dose corticosteroids, high cyclosporine blood concentrations, and graft-versus-host disease have been noted in many but not all of the reported cases. The changes in most cases have been reversible upon discontinuation of cyclosporine, and in some cases improvement was noted after reduction of dose. It appears that patients receiving liver transplant are more susceptible to encephalopathy than those receiving kidney transplant. Another rare manifestation of cyclosporine-induced neurotoxicity, occurring in transplant patients more frequently than in other indications, is optic disc edema including papilloedema, with possible visual impairment, secondary to benign intracranial hypertension.

Care should be taken in using cyclosporine with nephrotoxic drugs. *(See PRECAUTIONS)*

Rheumatoid Arthritis

Cyclosporine nephropathy was detected in renal biopsies of 6 out of 60 (10%) rheumatoid arthritis patients after the average treatment duration of 19 months. Only one patient, out of these 6 patients, was treated with a dose ≤ 4 mg/kg/day. Serum creatinine improved in all but one patient after discontinuation of cyclosporine. The "maximal creatinine increase" appears to be a factor in predicting cyclosporine nephropathy.

There is a potential, as with other immunosuppressive agents, for an increase in the occurrence of malignant lymphomas with cyclosporine. It is not clear whether the risk with cyclosporine is greater than that in rheumatoid arthritis patients or in rheumatoid arthritis patients on cytotoxic treatment for this indication. Five cases of lymphoma were detected: four in a survey of approximately 2,300 patients treated with cyclosporine for rheumatoid arthritis, and another case of lymphoma was reported in a clinical trial. Although other tumors (12 skin cancers, 24 solid tumors of diverse types, and 1 multiple myeloma) were also reported in this survey, epidemiologic analyses did not support a relationship to cyclosporine other than for malignant lymphomas.

Patients should be thoroughly evaluated before and during Neoral® treatment for the development of malignancies. Moreover, use of Neoral® therapy with other immunosuppressive agents may induce an excessive immunosuppression which is known to increase the risk of malignancy.

Psoriasis

(See also Boxed WARNINGS for Psoriasis)

Since cyclosporine is a potent immunosuppressive agent with a number of potentially serious side effects, the risks and benefits of using Neoral® should be considered before treatment of patients with psoriasis. Cyclosporine, the active ingredient in Neoral®, can cause nephrotoxicity and hypertension *(see PRECAUTIONS)* and the risk increases with increasing dose and duration of therapy. Patients who may be at increased risk such as those with abnormal renal function, uncontrolled hypertension or malignancies, should not receive Neoral®.

Renal dysfunction is a potential consequence of Neoral® therefore renal function must be monitored during therapy. Patients receiving Neoral® require frequent monitoring of serum creatinine. *(See Special Monitoring under DOSAGE AND ADMINISTRATION)* Elderly patients should be monitored with particular care, since decreases in renal function also occur with age. If patients are not properly monitored and doses are not properly adjusted, cyclosporine therapy can cause structural kidney damage and persistent renal dysfunction.

An increase in serum creatinine and BUN may occur during Neoral® therapy and reflects a reduction in the glomerular filtration rate.

Kidney biopsies from 86 psoriasis patients treated for a mean duration of 23 months with 1.2-7.6 mg/kg/day of cyclosporine showed evidence of cyclosporine nephropathy in 18/86 (21%) of the patients. The pathology consisted of renal tubular atrophy and interstitial fibrosis. On repeat biopsy of 13 of these patients maintained on various dosages of cyclosporine for a mean of 2 additional years, the number with cyclosporine induced nephropathy rose to 26/86 (30%). The majority of patients (19/26) were on a dose of ≥ 5.0 mg/kg/day (the highest recommended dose is 4 mg/kg/day). The patients were also on cyclosporine for greater than 15 months (18/26) and/or had a clinically significant increase in serum creatinine for greater than 1 month (21/26). Creatinine levels returned to normal range in 7 of 11 patients in whom cyclosporine therapy was discontinued.

There is an increased risk for the development of skin and lymphoproliferative malignancies in cyclosporine-treated psoriasis patients. The relative risk of malignancies is comparable to that observed in psoriasis patients treated with other immunosuppressive agents.

Tumors were reported in 32 (2.2%) of 1439 psoriasis patients treated with cyclosporine worldwide from clinical trials. Additional tumors have been reported in 7 patients in cyclosporine postmarketing experience. Skin malignancies were reported in 16 (1.1%) of these patients; all but 2 of them had previously received PUVA therapy. Methotrexate was received by 7 patients. UVB and coal tar had been used by 2 and 3 patients, respectively. Seven patients had either a history of previous skin cancer or a potentially predisposing lesion was present prior to cyclosporine exposure. Of the 16 patients with skin cancer, 11 patients had 18 squamous cell carcinomas and 7 patients had 10 basal cell carcinomas. There were two lymphoproliferative malignancies; one case of non-Hodgkin's lymphoma which required chemotherapy, and one case of mycosis fungoides which regressed spontaneously upon discontinuation of cyclosporine. There were four cases of benign lymphocytic infiltration: 3 regressed spontaneously upon discontinuation of cyclosporine, while the fourth regressed despite continuation of the drug. The remainder of the malignancies, 13 cases (0.9%), involved various organs.

Patients should not be treated concurrently with cyclosporine and PUVA or UVB, other radiation therapy, or other immunosuppressive agents, because of the possibility of excessive immunosuppression and the subsequent risk of malignancies. *(See CONTRAINDICATIONS)* Patients should also be warned to protect themselves appropriately when in the sun, and to avoid excessive sun exposure. Patients should be thoroughly evaluated before and during treatment for the presence of malignancies remembering that malignant lesions may be hidden by psoriatic plaques. Skin lesions not typical of psoriasis should be biopsied before starting treatment. Patients should be treated with Neoral® only after complete resolution of suspicious lesions, and only if there are no other treatment options. *(See Special Monitoring for Psoriasis Patients)*

PRECAUTIONS

General

Hypertension

Cyclosporine is the active ingredient of Neoral®. Hypertension is a common side effect of cyclosporine therapy which may persist. *(See ADVERSE REACTIONS and DOSAGE AND ADMINISTRATION for monitoring recommendations)* Mild or moderate hypertension is encountered more frequently than severe hypertension and the incidence decreases over time. In recipients of kidney, liver, and heart allografts treated with cyclosporine, antihypertensive therapy may be required. *(See Special Monitoring of Rheumatoid Arthritis and Psoriasis Patients)* However, since cyclosporine may cause hyperkalemia, potassium-sparing diuretics should not be used. While calcium antagonists can be effective agents in treating cyclosporine-associated hypertension, they can interfere with cyclosporine metabolism. *(See Drug Interactions)*

Vaccination

During treatment with cyclosporine, vaccination may be less effective; and the use of live attenuated vaccines should be avoided.

Special Monitoring of Rheumatoid Arthritis Patients

Before initiating treatment, a careful physical examination, including blood pressure measurements (on at least two occasions) and two creatinine levels to estimate baseline should be performed. Blood pressure and serum creatinine should be evaluated every 2 weeks during the initial 3 months and then monthly if the patient is stable. It is advisable to monitor serum creatinine and blood pressure always after an increase of the dose of nonsteroidal anti-inflammatory drugs and after initiation of new nonsteroidal anti-inflammatory drug therapy during Neoral® treatment.

If co-administered with methotrexate, CBC and liver function tests are recommended to be monitored monthly. *(See also PRECAUTIONS, General, Hypertension)*

In patients who are receiving cyclosporine, the dose of Neoral® should be decreased by 25%-50% if hypertension occurs. If hypertension persists, the dose of Neoral® should be further reduced or blood pressure should be controlled with antihypertensive agents. In most cases, blood pressure has returned to baseline when cyclosporine was discontinued.

In placebo-controlled trials of rheumatoid arthritis patients, systolic hypertension (defined as an occurrence of two systolic blood pressure readings >140 mmHg) and diastolic hypertension (defined as two diastolic blood pressure readings >90 mmHg) occurred in 33% and 19% of patients treated with cyclosporine, respectively. The corresponding placebo rates were 22% and 8%.

Special Monitoring for Psoriasis Patients

Before initiating treatment, a careful dermatological and physical examination, including blood pressure measurements (on at least two occasions) should be performed. Since Neoral® is an immunosuppressive agent, patients should be evaluated for the presence of occult infection on their first physical examination and for the presence of tumors initially, and throughout treatment with Neoral®. Skin lesions not typical for psoriasis should be biopsied before starting Neoral®. Patients with malignant or premalignant changes of the skin should be treated with Neoral® only after appropriate treatment of such lesions and if no other treatment option exists.

Baseline laboratories should include serum creatinine (on two occasions), BUN, CBC, serum magnesium, potassium, uric acid, and lipids.

The risk of cyclosporine nephropathy is reduced when the starting dose is low (2.5 mg/kg/day), the maximum dose does not exceed 4.0 mg/kg/day, serum creatinine is monitored regularly while cyclosporine is administered, and the dose of Neoral® is decreased when the rise in creatinine is greater than or equal to 25% above the patient's pretreatment level. The increase in creatinine is generally reversible upon timely decrease of the dose of Neoral® or its discontinuation.

Serum creatinine and BUN should be evaluated every 2 weeks during the initial 3 months of therapy and then monthly if the patient is stable. If the serum creatinine is greater than or equal to 25% above the patient's pretreatment level, serum creatinine should be repeated within two weeks. If the change in serum creatinine remains greater than or equal to 25% above baseline, Neoral® should be reduced by 25%-50%. If at **any time** the serum creatinine increases by greater than or equal to 50% above pretreatment level, Neoral® should be reduced by 25%-50%. Neoral® should be discontinued if reversibility (within 25% of baseline) of serum creatinine is not achievable after two dosage modifications. It is advisable to monitor serum creatinine after an increase of the dose of nonsteroidal anti-inflammatory drug and after initiation of new nonsteroidal anti-inflammatory therapy during Neoral® treatment.

Blood pressure should be evaluated every 2 weeks during the initial 3 months of therapy and then monthly if the patient is stable, or more frequently when dosage adjustments are made. Patients without a history of previous hypertension before initiation of treatment with Neoral®, should have the drug reduced by 25%-50% if found to have sustained hypertension. If the patient continues to be hypertensive despite multiple reductions of Neoral®, then Neoral® should be discontinued. For patients with treated hypertension, before the initiation of Neoral® therapy, their medication should be adjusted to control hypertension while on Neoral®. Neoral® should be discontinued if a change in hypertension management is not effective or tolerable.

CBC, uric acid, potassium, lipids, and magnesium should also be monitored every 2 weeks for the first 3 months of therapy, and then monthly if the patient is stable or more frequently when dosage adjustments are made. Neoral® dosage should be reduced by 25%-50% for any abnormality of clinical concern.

In controlled trials of cyclosporine in psoriasis patients, cyclosporine blood concentrations did not correlate well with either improvement or with side effects such as renal dysfunction.

Information for Patients: Patients should be advised that any change of cyclosporine formulation should be made cautiously and only under physician supervision because it may result in the need for a change in dosage.

Patients should be informed of the necessity of repeated laboratory tests while they are receiving cyclosporine. Patients should be advised of the potential risks during pregnancy and informed of the increased risk of neoplasia. Patients should also be informed of the risk of hypertension and renal dysfunction.

Patients should be advised that during treatment with cyclosporine, vaccination may be less effective and the use of live attenuated vaccines should be avoided.

Antibiotics	Antineoplastics	Anti-inflammatory Drugs	Gastrointestinal Agents	Other Drugs
ciprofloxacin	melphalan	azapropazon	cimetidine	fiber acid derivatives
gentamicin		colchicine	ranitidine	(e.g., bezofibrate,
tobramycin	Antifungals	diclofenac		fenofibrate)
vancomycin	amphotericin B	naproxen	Immunosuppressives	methotrexate
trimethoprim	ketoconazole	sulindac	tacrolimus	
with sulfamethoxazole				

Calcium Channel Blockers	Antifungals	Antibiotics	Glucocorticoids	Other Drugs
diltiazem	fluconazole	azithromycin	methylprednisolone	allopurinol
nicardipine	itraconazole	clarithromycin		amiodarone
verapamil	ketoconazole	erythromycin		bromocriptine
	voriconazole	quinupristin/		colchicine
		dalfopristin		danazol
				imatinib
				metoclopramide
				nefazodone
				oral contraceptives

Antibiotics	Anticonvulsants	Other Drugs/Dietary Supplements		
nafcillin	carbamazepine	bosentan	octreotide	terbinafine
rifampin	oxcarbazepine	octreotide		ticlopidine
	phenobarbital	orlistat		St. John's Wort
	phenytoin	sulfinpyrazone		

		Randomized Kidney Patients		Cyclosporine Patients (Sandimmune®)		
Body System	Adverse Reactions	Sandimmune® (N=227)%	Azathioprine (N=228)%	Kidney (N=705)%	Heart (N=112)%	Liver (N=75)%
Genitourinary	Renal Dysfunction	32	6	25	38	37
Cardiovascular	Hypertension	26	18	13	53	27
	Cramps	4	<1	2	<1	0
Skin	Hirsutism	21	<1	21	28	45
	Acne	6	8	2	2	1
Central Nervous System	Tremor	12	0	21	31	55
	Convulsions	3	1	1	4	5
	Headache	2	<1	2	15	4
Gastrointestinal	Gum Hyperplasia	4	0	9	5	16
	Diarrhea	3	<1	3	4	8
	Nausea/Vomiting	2	<1	4	10	4
	Hepatotoxicity	<1	<1	4	7	4
	Abdominal Discomfort	<1	0	<1	7	0
Autonomic Nervous System	Paresthesia	3	0	1	2	1
	Flushing	<1	0	4	0	4
Hematopoietic	Leukopenia	2	19	<1	6	0
	Lymphoma	<1	0	1	6	1
Respiratory	Sinusitis	<1	0	4	3	7
Miscellaneous	Gynecomastia	<1	0	<1	4	3

Patients should be given careful dosage instructions. Neoral® Oral Solution (cyclosporine oral solution, USP) MODIFIED should be diluted, preferably with orange or apple juice that is at room temperature. The combination of Neoral® Oral Solution (cyclosporine oral solution, USP) MODIFIED with milk can be unpalatable.

Patients should be advised to take Neoral® on a consistent schedule with regard to time of day and relation to meals. Grapefruit and grapefruit juice affect metabolism, increasing blood concentration of cyclosporine, thus should be avoided.

Laboratory Tests

In all patients treated with cyclosporine, renal and liver functions should be assessed repeatedly by measurement of serum creatinine, BUN, serum bilirubin, and liver enzymes. Serum lipids, magnesium, and potassium should also be monitored. Cyclosporine blood concentrations should be routinely monitored in transplant patients (see DOSAGE AND ADMINISTRATION, Blood Concentration Monitoring in Transplant Patients), and periodically monitored in rheumatoid arthritis patients.

Drug Interactions

All of the individual drugs cited below are well substantiated to interact with cyclosporine. In addition, concomitant nonsteroidal anti-inflammatory drugs, particularly in the setting of dehydration, may potentiate renal dysfunction.

Drugs That May Potentiate Renal Dysfunction

[See first table above]

Drugs That Alter Cyclosporine Concentrations

Cyclosporine is extensively metabolized by CYP 3A isoenzymes, in particular CYP3A4, and is a substrate of the multidrug efflux transporter P-glycoprotein. Various agents are known to either increase or decrease plasma or whole blood of cyclosporine levels usually by inhibition or induction of CYP3A4 or P-glycoprotein transporter or both. Compounds that decrease cyclosporine absorption such as orlistat should be avoided. Monitoring of circulating cyclosporine concentrations and appropriate Neoral® dosage adjustment are essential when these drugs are used concomitantly. (See Blood Concentration Monitoring)

Drugs That Increase Cyclosporine Concentrations

[See second table above]

The HIV protease inhibitors (e.g., indinavir, nelfinavir, ritonavir, and saquinavir) are known to inhibit cytochrome P-450 3A and thus could potentially increase the concentrations of cyclosporine, however no formal studies of the interaction are available. Care should be exercised when these drugs are administered concomitantly.

Grapefruit and grapefruit juice affect metabolism, increasing blood concentrations of cyclosporine, thus should be avoided.

Drugs/Dietary Supplements That Decrease Cyclosporine Concentrations

[See third table above]

There have been reports of a serious drug interaction between cyclosporine and the herbal dietary supplement, St. John's Wort. This interaction has been reported to produce a marked reduction in the blood concentrations of cyclosporine, resulting in subtherapeutic levels, rejection of transplanted organs, and graft loss.

Rifabutin is known to increase the metabolism of other drugs metabolized by the cytochrome P-450 system. The interaction between rifabutin and cyclosporine has not been studied. Care should be exercised when these two drugs are administered concomitantly.

Nonsteroidal Anti-inflammatory Drug (NSAID) Interactions

Clinical status and serum creatinine should be closely monitored when cyclosporine is used with nonsteroidal anti-inflammatory agents in rheumatoid arthritis patients. (See WARNINGS)

Pharmacodynamic interactions have been reported to occur between cyclosporine and both naproxen and sulindac, in that concomitant use is associated with additive decreases in renal function, as determined by ^{99m}Tc-diethylenetriaminepentaacetic acid (DTPA) and (p-aminohippuric acid) PAH clearances. Although concomitant administration of diclofenac does not affect blood levels of cyclosporine, it has been associated with approximate doubling of diclofenac blood levels and occasional reports of reversible decreases in renal function. Consequently, the dose of diclofenac should be in the lower end of the therapeutic range.

Methotrexate Interaction

Preliminary data indicate that when methotrexate and cyclosporine were co-administered to rheumatoid arthritis patients (N=20), methotrexate concentrations (AUCs) were increased approximately 30% and the concentrations (AUCs) of its metabolite, 7-hydroxy methotrexate, were decreased by approximately 80%. The clinical significance of this interaction is not known. Cyclosporine concentrations do not appear to have been altered (N=6).

Other Drug Interactions

Cyclosporine is an inhibitor of CYP3A4 and of the multidrug efflux transporter P-glycoprotein and may increase plasma concentrations of comedications that are substrates of CYP3A4 or P-glycoprotein or both.

Cyclosporine may reduce the clearance of digoxin, colchicine, prednisolone, HMG-CoA reductase inhibitors (statins) and etoposide. Severe digitalis toxicity has been seen within days of starting cyclosporine in several patients taking digoxin. There are also reports on the potential of cyclosporine to enhance the toxic effects of colchicine such as myopathy and neuropathy, especially in patients with renal dysfunction. If digoxin or colchicine are used concurrently with cyclosporine, close clinical observation is required in order to enable early detection of toxic manifestations of digoxin or colchicine, followed by reduction of dosage or its withdrawal.

Literature and postmarketing cases of myotoxicity, including muscle pain and weakness, myositis, and rhabdomyolysis, have been reported with concomitant administration of cyclosporine with lovastatin, simvastatin, atorvastatin, pravastatin, and, rarely fluvastatin. When concurrently administered with cyclosporine, the dosage of these statins should be reduced according to label recommendations. Statin therapy needs to be temporarily withheld or discontinued in patients with signs and symptoms of myopathy or those with risk factors predisposing to severe renal injury, including renal failure, secondary to rhabdomyolysis.

Cyclosporine may increase the plasma concentrations of repaglinide and thereby increase the risk of hypoglycemia. In 12 healthy male subjects who received two doses of 100 mg cyclosporine capsule orally 12 hours apart with a single dose of 0.25 mg repaglinide tablet (one half of a 0.5 mg tablet) orally 13 hours after the cyclosporine initial dose, the repaglinide mean C_{max} and AUC were increased 1.8 fold (range: 0.6-3.7 fold) and 2.4 fold (range 1.2-5.3 fold), respectively. Close monitoring of blood glucose level is advisable for a patient taking cyclosporine and repaglinide concomitantly.

Cyclosporine should not be used with potassium-sparing diuretics because hyperkalemia can occur. Caution is also required when cyclosporine is co-administered with potassium sparing drugs (e.g., angiotensin converting enzyme inhibitors, angiotensin II receptor antagonists), potassium containing drugs as well as in patients on a potassium rich diet. Control of potassium levels in these situations is advisable.

Elevations in serum creatinine were observed in studies using sirolimus in combination with full-dose cyclosporine. This effect is often reversible with cyclosporine dose reduction. Simultaneous co-administration of cyclosporine significantly increases blood levels of sirolimus. To minimize increases in sirolimus concentrations, it is recommended that sirolimus be given 4 hours after cyclosporine administration.

During treatment with cyclosporine, vaccination may be less effective. The use of live vaccines should be avoided. Frequent gingival hyperplasia with nifedipine, and convulsions with high dose methylprednisolone have been reported.

Psoriasis patients receiving other immunosuppressive agents or radiation therapy (including PUVA and UVB) should not receive concurrent cyclosporine because of the possibility of excessive immunosuppression.

For additional information on Cyclosporine Drug Interactions please contact Novartis Medical Affairs Department at 888-NOW-NOVA [888-669-6682].

Carcinogenesis, Mutagenesis, and Impairment of Fertility

Carcinogenicity studies were carried out in male and female rats and mice. In the 78-week mouse study, evidence of a statistically significant trend was found for lymphocytic lymphomas in females, and the incidence of hepatocellular carcinomas in mid-dose males significantly exceeded the control value. In the 24-month rat study, pancreatic islet cell adenomas significantly exceeded the control rate in the low dose level. Doses used in the mouse and rat studies were 0.01 to 0.16 times the clinical maintenance dose (6 mg/kg). The hepatocellular carcinomas and pancreatic islet cell adenomas were not dose related. Published reports indicate that co-treatment of hairless mice with UV irradiation and cyclosporine or other immunosuppressive agents shorten the time to skin tumor formation compared to UV irradiation alone.

Cyclosporine was not mutagenic in appropriate test systems. Cyclosporine has not been found to be mutagenic/genotoxic in the Ames Test, the V79-HGPRT Test, the micronucleus test in mice and Chinese hamsters, the chromosome-aberration tests in Chinese hamster bone-marrow, the mouse dominant lethal assay, and the DNA-repair test in sperm from treated mice. A recent study analyzing sister chromatid exchange (SCE) induction by cyclosporine using human lymphocytes *in vitro* gave indication of a positive effect (i.e., induction of SCE), at high concentrations in this system. In two published research studies, rabbits exposed to cyclosporine *in utero* (10 mg/kg/day subcutaneously) demonstrated reduced numbers of nephrons, renal hypertrophy, systemic hypertension and progressive renal insufficiency up to 35 weeks of age. Pregnant rats which received 12 mg/kg/day of cyclosporine intravenously (twice the recommended human intravenous dose) had fetuses with an increased incidence of ventricular septal defect. These findings have not been demonstrated in other species and their relevance for humans is unknown. No impairment in fertility was demonstrated in studies in male and female rats.

Widely distributed papillomatosis of the skin was observed after chronic treatment of dogs with cyclosporine at 9 times the human initial psoriasis treatment dose of 2.5 mg/kg, where doses are expressed on a body surface area basis. This papillomatosis showed a spontaneous regression upon discontinuation of cyclosporine.

An increased incidence of malignancy is a recognized complication of immunosuppression in recipients of organ transplants and patients with rheumatoid arthritis and psoriasis. The most common forms of neoplasms are non-Hodgkin's lymphoma and carcinomas of the skin. The risk of malignancies in cyclosporine recipients is higher than in the normal, healthy population but similar to that in patients receiving other immunosuppressive therapies. Reduction or discontinuance of immunosuppression may cause the lesions to regress.

In psoriasis patients on cyclosporine, development of malignancies, especially those of the skin has been reported. *(See WARNINGS)* Skin lesions not typical for psoriasis should be biopsied before starting cyclosporine treatment. Patients with malignant or premalignant changes of the skin should be treated with cyclosporine only after appropriate treatment of such lesions and if no other treatment option exists.

Pregnancy:

Pregnancy Category C

Animal studies have shown reproductive toxicity in rats and rabbits. Cyclosporine gave no evidence of mutagenic or teratogenic effects in the standard test systems with oral application (rats up to 17 mg/kg and rabbits up to 30 mg/kg per day orally). Only at dose levels toxic to dams, were adverse effects seen in reproduction studies in rats. Cyclosporine has been shown to be embryo- and fetotoxic in rats and rabbits following oral administration at maternally toxic doses. Fetal toxicity was noted in rats at 0.8 and rabbits at 5.4 times the transplant doses in humans of 6.0 mg/kg, where dose corrections are based on body surface area. Cyclosporine was embryo- and fetotoxic as indicated by increased pre- and postnatal mortality and reduced fetal weight together with related skeletal retardation.

There are no adequate and well-controlled studies in pregnant women therefore, Neoral® should not be used during pregnancy unless the potential benefit to the mother justifies the potential risk to the fetus.

In pregnant transplant recipients who are being treated with immunosuppressants the risk of premature birth is increased. The following data represent the reported outcomes of 116 pregnancies in women receiving cyclosporine during pregnancy, 90% of whom were transplant patients, and most of whom received cyclosporine throughout the entire gestational period. The only consistent patterns of abnormality were premature birth (gestational period of 28 to 36 weeks) and low birth weight for gestational age. Sixteen fetal losses occurred. Most of the pregnancies (85 of 100) were complicated by disorders; including, pre-eclampsia, eclampsia, premature labor, abruptio placentae, oligohydramnios, Rh incompatibility, and fetoplacental dysfunction. Pre-term delivery occurred in 47%. Seven malformations were reported in 5 viable infants and in 2 cases of fetal loss. Twenty-eight percent of the infants were small for gestational age. Neonatal complications occurred in 27%. Therefore, the risks and benefits of using Neoral® during pregnancy should be carefully weighed.

Infectious Complications in Historical Randomized Studies in Renal Transplant Patients Using Sandimmune®

Complication	Cyclosporine Treatment (N=227) % of Complications	Azathioprine with Steroids* (N=228) % of Complications
Septicemia	5.3	4.8
Abscesses	4.4	5.3
Systemic Fungal Infection	2.2	3.9
Local Fungal Infection	7.5	9.6
Cytomegalovirus	4.8	12.3
Other Viral Infections	15.9	18.4
Urinary Tract Infections	21.1	20.2
Wound and Skin Infections	7.0	10.1
Pneumonia	6.2	9.2

*Some patients also received ALG.

A limited number of observations in children exposed to cyclosporine *in utero* are available, up to an age of approximately 7 years. Renal function and blood pressure in these children were normal.

Because of the possible disruption of maternal-fetal interaction, the risk/benefit ratio of using Neoral® in psoriasis patients during pregnancy should carefully be weighed with serious consideration for discontinuation of Neoral®.

Nursing Mothers

Cyclosporine passes into breast milk. Mothers receiving treatment with Neoral® should not breast-feed.

Pediatric Use

Although no adequate and well-controlled studies have been completed in children, transplant recipients as young as one year of age have received Neoral® with no unusual adverse effects. The safety and efficacy of Neoral® treatment in children with juvenile rheumatoid arthritis or psoriasis below the age of 18 have not been established.

Geriatric Use

In rheumatoid arthritis clinical trials with cyclosporine, 17.5% of patients were age 65 or older. These patients were more likely to develop systolic hypertension on therapy, and more likely to show serum creatinine rises ≥50% above the baseline after 3-4 months of therapy.

Clinical studies of Neoral® in transplant and psoriasis patients did not include a sufficient number of subjects aged 65 and over to determine whether they respond differently from younger subjects. Other reported clinical experiences have not identified differences in response between the elderly and younger patients. In general, dose selection for an elderly patient should be cautious, usually starting at the low end of the dosing range, reflecting the greater frequency of decreased hepatic, renal, or cardiac function, and of concomitant disease or other drug therapy.

ADVERSE REACTIONS

Kidney, Liver, and Heart Transplantation

The principal adverse reactions of cyclosporine therapy are renal dysfunction, tremor, hirsutism, hypertension, and gum hyperplasia.

Hypertension, which is usually mild to moderate, may occur in approximately 50% of patients following renal transplantation and in most cardiac transplant patients.

Glomerular capillary thrombosis has been found in patients treated with cyclosporine and may progress to graft failure. The pathologic changes resembled those seen in the hemolytic-uremic syndrome and included thrombosis of the renal microvasculature, with platelet-fibrin thrombi occluding glomerular capillaries and afferent arterioles, microangiopathic hemolytic anemia, thrombocytopenia, and decreased renal function. Similar findings have been observed when other immunosuppressives have been employed post-transplantation.

Hypomagnesemia has been reported in some, but not all, patients exhibiting convulsions while on cyclosporine therapy. Although magnesium-depletion studies in normal subjects suggest that hypomagnesemia is associated with neurologic disorders, multiple factors, including hypertension, high dose methylprednisolone, hypocholesterolemia, and nephrotoxicity associated with high plasma concentrations of cyclosporine appear to be related to the neurological manifestations of cyclosporine toxicity.

In controlled studies, the nature, severity, and incidence of the adverse events that were observed in 493 transplanted patients treated with Neoral® were comparable with those observed in 208 transplanted patients who received Sandimmune® in these same studies when the dosage of the two drugs was adjusted to achieve the same cyclosporine blood trough concentrations.

Based on the historical experience with Sandimmune®, the following reactions occurred in 3% or greater of 892 patients involved in clinical trials of kidney, heart, and liver transplants.

[See fourth table on previous page]

Among 705 kidney transplant patients treated with cyclosporine oral solution (Sandimmune®) in clinical trials, the reason for treatment discontinuation was renal toxicity in 5.4%, infection in 0.9%, lack of efficacy in 1.4%, acute tubular necrosis in 1.0%, lymphoproliferative disorders in 0.3%, hypertension in 0.3%, and other reasons in 0.7% of the patients.

The following reactions occurred in 2% or less of Sandimmune®-treated patients: allergic reactions, anemia, anorexia, confusion, conjunctivitis, edema, fever, brittle fingernails, gastritis, hearing loss, hiccups, hyperglycemia, muscle pain, peptic ulcer, thrombocytopenia, tinnitus.

The following reactions occurred rarely: anxiety, chest pain, constipation, depression, hair breaking, hematuria, joint pain, lethargy, mouth sores, myocardial infarction, night sweats, pancreatitis, pruritus, swallowing difficulty, tingling, upper GI bleeding, visual disturbance, weakness, weight loss.

Patients receiving immunosuppressive therapies, including cyclosporine and cyclosporine-containing regimens, are at increased risk of infections (viral, bacterial, fungal, parasitic). Both generalized and localized infections can occur. Pre-existing infections may also be aggravated. Fatal outcomes have been reported. *(See Warnings)*

[See table above]

Postmarketing Experience, Kidney, Liver and Heart Transplantation

BK virus associated nephropathy has been observed in patients receiving immunosuppressants, including Neoral. This infection is associated with serious outcomes, including deteriorating renal function and renal graft loss. *(See WARNINGS, Kidney, Liver, and Heart Transplant)*

Rheumatoid Arthritis

The principal adverse reactions associated with the use of cyclosporine in rheumatoid arthritis are renal dysfunction *(see WARNINGS)*, hypertension *(see PRECAUTIONS)*, headache, gastrointestinal disturbances, and hirsutism/hypertrichosis.

In rheumatoid arthritis patients treated in clinical trials within the recommended dose range, cyclosporine therapy was discontinued in 5.3% of the patients because of hypertension and in 7% of the patients because of increased creatinine. These changes are usually reversible with timely dose decrease or drug discontinuation. The frequency and severity of serum creatinine elevations increase with dose and duration of cyclosporine therapy. These elevations are likely to become more pronounced without dose reduction or discontinuation.

The following adverse events occurred in controlled clinical trials:

[See table on pages 2566 and 2567]

In addition, the following adverse events have been reported in 1% to <3% of the rheumatoid arthritis patients in the cyclosporine treatment group in controlled clinical trials.

Autonomic Nervous System: dry mouth, increased sweating;

Body as a Whole: allergy, asthenia, hot flushes, malaise, overdose, procedure NOS*, tumor NOS*, weight decrease, weight increase;

Cardiovascular: abnormal heart sounds, cardiac failure, myocardial infarction, peripheral ischemia;

Central and Peripheral Nervous System: hypoesthesia, neuropathy, vertigo;

Endocrine: goiter;

Gastrointestinal: constipation, dysphagia, enanthema, eructation, esophagitis, gastric ulcer, gastritis, gastroenteritis, gingival bleeding, glossitis, peptic ulcer, salivary gland enlargement, tongue disorder, tooth disorder;

Infection: abscess, bacterial infection, cellulitis, folliculitis, fungal infection, herpes simplex, herpes zoster, renal abscess, moniliasis, tonsillitis, viral infection;

Hematologic: anemia, epistaxis, leukopenia, lymphadenopathy;

Liver and Biliary System: bilirubinemia;

Metabolic and Nutritional: diabetes mellitus, hyperkalemia, hyperuricemia, hypoglycemia;

Musculoskeletal System: arthralgia, bone fracture, bursitis, joint dislocation, myalgia, stiffness, synovial cyst, tendon disorder;

Neoplasms: breast fibroadenosis, carcinoma;

Psychiatric: anxiety, confusion, decreased libido, emotional lability, impaired concentration, increased libido, nervousness, paroniria, somnolence;

Reproductive (Female): breast pain, uterine hemorrhage;

Respiratory System: abnormal chest sounds, bronchospasm;

Skin and Appendages: abnormal pigmentation, angioedema, dermatitis, dry skin, eczema, nail disorder, pruritus, skin disorder, urticaria;

Special Senses: abnormal vision, cataract, conjunctivitis, deafness, eye pain, taste perversion, tinnitus, vestibular disorder;

Urinary System: abnormal urine, hematuria, increased BUN, micturition urgency, nocturia, polyuria, pyelonephritis, urinary incontinence.

*NOS = Not Otherwise Specified.

Psoriasis

The principal adverse reactions associated with the use of cyclosporine in patients with psoriasis are renal dysfunction, headache, hypertension, hypertriglyceridemia, hirsutism/hypertrichosis, paresthesia or hyperesthesia, influenza-like symptoms, nausea/vomiting, diarrhea, abdominal discomfort, lethargy, and musculoskeletal or joint pain.

In psoriasis patients treated in US controlled clinical studies within the recommended dose range, cyclosporine therapy was discontinued in 1.0% of the patients because of hypertension and in 5.4% of the patients because of increased creatinine. In the majority of cases, these changes were reversible after dose reduction or discontinuation of cyclosporine.

There has been one reported death associated with the use of cyclosporine in psoriasis. A 27-year-old male developed renal deterioration and was continued on cyclosporine. He had progressive renal failure leading to death.

Frequency and severity of serum creatinine increases with dose and duration of cyclosporine therapy. These elevations are likely to become more pronounced and may result in irreversible renal damage without dose reduction or discontinuation.

[See first table on next page]

The following events occurred in 1% to less than 3% of psoriasis patients treated with cyclosporine:

Body as a Whole: fever, flushes, hot flushes;

Cardiovascular: chest pain;

Central and Peripheral Nervous System: appetite increased, insomnia, dizziness, nervousness, vertigo;

Gastrointestinal: abdominal distention, constipation, gingival bleeding;

Liver and Biliary System: hyperbilirubinemia;

Neoplasms: skin malignancies [squamous cell (0.9%) and basal cell (0.4%) carcinomas];

Reticuloendothelial: platelet, bleeding, and clotting disorders, red blood cell disorder;

Respiratory: infection, viral and other infection;

Skin and Appendages: acne, folliculitis, keratosis, pruritus, rash, dry skin;

Urinary System: micturition frequency;

Vision: abnormal vision.

Mild hypomagnesemia and hyperkalemia may occur but are asymptomatic. Increases in uric acid may occur and attacks of gout have been rarely reported. A minor and dose related hyperbilirubinemia has been observed in the absence of hepatocellular damage. Cyclosporine therapy may be associated with a modest increase of serum triglycerides or cholesterol. Elevations of triglycerides (>750 mg/dL) occur in about 15% of psoriasis patients; elevations of cholesterol (>300 mg/dL) are observed in less than 3% of psoriasis patients. Generally these laboratory abnormalities are reversible upon dose reduction or discontinuation of cyclosporine.

OVERDOSAGE

There is a minimal experience with cyclosporine overdosage. Forced emesis and gastric lavage can be of value up to 2 hours after administration of Neoral®. Transient hepatotoxicity and nephrotoxicity may occur which should resolve following drug withdrawal. Oral doses of cyclosporine up to 10 g (about 150 mg/kg) have been tolerated with relatively minor clinical consequences, such as vomiting, drowsiness, headache, tachycardia, and, in a few patients, moderately severe, reversible impairment of renal function. However, serious symptoms of intoxication have been reported following accidental parenteral overdosage with cyclosporine in premature neonates. General supportive measures and symptomatic treatment should be followed in all cases of overdosage. Cyclosporine is not dialyzable to any great ex-

tent, nor is it cleared well by charcoal hemoperfusion. The oral dosage at which half of experimental animals are estimated to die is 31 times, 39 times, and >54 times the human maintenance dose for transplant patients (6 mg/kg; corrections based on body surface area) in mice, rats, and rabbits.

DOSAGE AND ADMINISTRATION

Neoral® Soft Gelatin Capsules (cyclosporine capsules, USP) MODIFIED and Neoral® Oral Solution (cyclosporine oral solution, USP) MODIFIED

Neoral® has increased bioavailability in comparison to Sandimmune®. Neoral® and Sandimmune® are not bioequivalent and cannot be used interchangeably without physician supervision.

The daily dose of Neoral® should always be given in two divided doses (BID). It is recommended that Neoral® be administered on a consistent schedule with regard to time of day and relation to meals. Grapefruit and grapefruit juice affect metabolism, increasing blood concentration of cyclosporine, thus should be avoided.

Newly Transplanted Patients

The initial oral dose of Neoral® can be given 4-12 hours prior to transplantation or be given postoperatively. The initial dose of Neoral® varies depending on the transplanted organ and the other immunosuppressive agents included in the immunosuppressive protocol. In newly transplanted patients, the initial oral dose of Neoral® is the same as the initial oral dose of Sandimmune®. Suggested initial doses

Neoral®/Sandimmune® Rheumatoid Arthritis
Percentage of Patients with Adverse Events ≥3% in any Cyclosporine Treated Group

Body System / Preferred Term	Studies 651+652+2008 Sandimmune®† (N=269)	Study 302 Sandimmune® (N=155)	Study 654 Methotrexate & Sandimmune® (N=74)	Study 654 Methotrexate & Placebo (N=73)	Study 302 Neoral® (N=143)	Studies 651+652+2008 Placebo (N=201)
Autonomic Nervous System Disorders						
Flushing	2%	2%	3%	0%	5%	2%
Body As A Whole–General Disorders						
Accidental Trauma	0%	1%	10%	4%	4%	0%
Edema NOS*	5%	14%	12%	4%	10%	<1%
Fatigue	6%	3%	8%	12%	3%	7%
Fever	2%	3%	0%	0%	2%	4%
Influenza-like symptoms	<1%	6%	1%	0%	3%	2%
Pain	6%	9%	10%	15%	13%	4%
Rigors	1%	1%	4%	0%	3%	1%
Cardiovascular Disorders						
Arrhythmia	2%	5%	5%	6%	2%	1%
Chest Pain	4%	5%	1%	1%	6%	1%
Hypertension	8%	26%	16%	12%	25%	2%
Central and Peripheral Nervous System Disorders						
Dizziness	8%	6%	7%	3%	8%	3%
Headache	17%	23%	22%	11%	25%	9%
Migraine	2%	3%	0%	0%	3%	1%
Paresthesia	8%	7%	8%	4%	11%	1%
Tremor	8%	7%	7%	3%	13%	4%
Gastrointestinal System Disorders						
Abdominal Pain	15%	15%	15%	7%	15%	10%
Anorexia	3%	3%	1%	0%	3%	3%
Diarrhea	12%	12%	18%	15%	13%	8%
Dyspepsia	12%	12%	10%	8%	8%	4%
Flatulence	5%	5%	5%	4%	4%	1%
Gastrointestinal Disorder NOS*	0%	2%	1%	4%	4%	0%
Gingivitis	4%	3%	0%	0%	0%	1%
Gum Hyperplasia	2%	4%	1%	3%	4%	1%
Nausea	23%	14%	24%	15%	18%	14%
Rectal Hemorrhage	0%	3%	0%	0%	1%	1%
Stomatitis	7%	5%	16%	12%	6%	8%
Vomiting	9%	8%	14%	7%	6%	5%
Hearing and Vestibular Disorders						
Ear Disorder NOS*	0%	5%	0%	0%	1%	0%
Metabolic and Nutritional Disorders						
Hypomagnesemia	0%	4%	0%	0%	6%	0%
Musculoskeletal System Disorders						
Arthropathy	0%	5%	0%	1%	4%	0%
Leg Cramps/ Involuntary Muscle Contractions	2%	11%	11%	3%	12%	1%
Psychiatric Disorders						
Depression	3%	6%	3%	1%	1%	2%
Insomnia	4%	1%	1%	0%	3%	2%
Renal						
Creatinine Elevations ≥30%	43%	39%	55%	19%	48%	13%
Creatinine Elevations ≥50%	24%	18%	26%	8%	18%	3%
Reproductive Disorders, Female						
Leukorrhea	1%	0%	4%	0%	1%	0%
Menstrual Disorder	3%	2%	1%	0%	1%	1%

(Table continued on next page)

are available from the results of a 1994 survey of the use of Sandimmune® in US transplant centers. The mean ± SD initial doses were 9±3 mg/kg/day for renal transplant patients (75 centers), 8±4 mg/kg/day for liver transplant patients (30 centers), and 7±3 mg/kg/day for heart transplant patients (24 centers). Total daily doses were divided into two equal daily doses. The Neoral® dose is subsequently adjusted to achieve a pre-defined cyclosporine blood concentration. (See Blood Concentration Monitoring in Transplant Patients, below) If cyclosporine trough blood concentrations are used, the target range is the same for Neoral® as for Sandimmune®. Using the same trough concentration target range for Neoral® as for Sandimmune® results in greater cyclosporine exposure when Neoral® is administered. (See Pharmacokinetics, Absorption) Dosing should be titrated based on clinical assessments of rejection and tolerability. Lower Neoral® doses may be sufficient as maintenance therapy.

Adjunct therapy with adrenal corticosteroids is recommended initially. Different tapering dosage schedules of prednisone appear to achieve similar results. A representative dosage schedule based on the patient's weight started with 2.0 mg/kg/day for the first 4 days tapered to 1.0 mg/kg/day by 1 week, 0.6 mg/kg/day by 2 weeks, 0.3 mg/kg/day by 1 month, and 0.15 mg/kg/day by 2 months and thereafter as a maintenance dose. Steroid doses may be further tapered on an individualized basis depending on status of patient and function of graft. Adjustments in dosage of prednisone must be made according to the clinical situation.

Conversion from Sandimmune® to Neoral® in Transplant Patients

In transplanted patients who are considered for conversion to Neoral® from Sandimmune®, Neoral® should be started with the same daily dose as was previously used with Sandimmune® (1:1 dose conversion). The Neoral® dose should subsequently be adjusted to attain the pre-conversion cyclosporine blood trough concentration. Using the same trough concentration target range for Neoral® as for Sandimmune® results in greater cyclosporine exposure when Neoral® is administered. (See Pharmacokinetics, Absorption) Patients with suspected poor absorption of Sandimmune® require different dosing strategies. (See Transplant Patients with Poor Absorption of Sandimmune®, below) In some patients, the increase in blood trough concentration is more pronounced and may be of clinical significance.

Until the blood trough concentration attains the pre-conversion value, it is strongly recommended that the cyclosporine blood trough concentration be monitored every 4 to 7 days after conversion to Neoral®. In addition, clinical safety parameters such as serum creatinine and blood pressure should be monitored every two weeks during the first two months after conversion. If the blood trough concentrations are outside the desired range and/or if the clinical safety parameters worsen, the dosage of Neoral® must be adjusted accordingly.

Transplant Patients with Poor Absorption of Sandimmune®

Patients with lower than expected cyclosporine blood trough concentrations in relation to the oral dose of Sandimmune® may have poor or inconsistent absorption of cyclosporine from Sandimmune®. After conversion to Neoral®, patients tend to have higher cyclosporine concentrations. **Due to the increase in bioavailability of cyclosporine following conversion to Neoral®, the cyclosporine blood trough concentration may exceed the target range. Particular caution should be exercised when converting patients to Neoral® at doses greater than 10 mg/kg/day.** The dose of Neoral® should be titrated individually based on cyclosporine trough concentrations, tolerability, and clinical response. In this population the cyclosporine blood trough concentration should be measured more frequently, at least twice a week (daily, if initial dose exceeds 10 mg/kg/day) until the concentration stabilizes within the desired range.

Rheumatoid Arthritis

The initial dose of Neoral® is 2.5 mg/kg/day, taken twice daily as a divided (BID) oral dose. Salicylates, nonsteroidal anti-inflammatory agents, and oral corticosteroids may be continued. (See WARNINGS and PRECAUTIONS, Drug Interactions) Onset of action generally occurs between 4 and 8 weeks. If insufficient clinical benefit is seen and tolerability is good (including serum creatinine less than 30% above baseline), the dose may be increased by 0.5-0.75 mg/kg/day after 8 weeks and again after 12 weeks to a maximum of 4 mg/kg/day. If no benefit is seen by 16 weeks of therapy, Neoral® therapy should be discontinued.

Dose decreases by 25%-50% should be made at any time to control adverse events, e.g., hypertension elevations in serum creatinine (30% above patient's pretreatment level) or clinically significant laboratory abnormalities. (See WARNINGS and PRECAUTIONS)

If dose reduction is not effective in controlling abnormalities or if the adverse event or abnormality is severe, Neoral® should be discontinued. The same initial dose and dosage range should be used if Neoral® is combined with the rec-

Neoral®/Sandimmune® Rheumatoid Arthritis
Percentage of Patients with Adverse Events ≥3% in any Cyclosporine Treated Group (cont.)

Body System	Preferred Term	Studies 651+652+2008 Sandimmune®† (N=269)	Study 302 Sandimmune® (N=155)	Study 654 Methotrexate & Sandimmune® (N=74)	Study 654 Methotrexate & Placebo (N=73)	Study 302 Neoral® (N=143)	Studies 651+652+2008 Placebo (N=201)
Respiratory System Disorders							
	Bronchitis	1%	3%	1%	0%	1%	3%
	Coughing	5%	3%	5%	7%	4%	4%
	Dyspnea	5%	1%	3%	3%	1%	2%
	Infection NOS*	9%	5%	0%	7%	3%	10%
	Pharyngitis	3%	5%	5%	6%	4%	4%
	Pneumonia	1%	0%	4%	0%	1%	1%
	Rhinitis	0%	3%	11%	10%	1%	0%
	Sinusitis	4%	4%	8%	4%	3%	3%
	Upper Respiratory Tract	0%	14%	23%	15%	13%	0%
Skin and Appendages Disorders							
	Alopecia	3%	0%	1%	1%	4%	4%
	Bullous Eruption	1%	0%	4%	1%	1%	1%
	Hypertrichosis	19%	17%	12%	0%	15%	3%
	Rash	7%	12%	10%	7%	8%	10%
	Skin Ulceration	1%	1%	3%	4%	0%	2%
Urinary System Disorders							
	Dysuria	0%	0%	11%	3%	1%	2%
	Micturition Frequency	2%	4%	3%	1%	2%	2%
	NPN, Increased	0%	19%	12%	0%	18%	0%
	Urinary Tract Infection	0%	3%	5%	4%	3%	0%
Vascular (Extracardiac) Disorders							
	Purpura	3%	4%	1%	1%	2%	0%

† Includes patients in 2.5 mg/kg/day dose group only. *NOS = Not Otherwise Specified.

Adverse Events Occurring in 3% or More of Psoriasis Patients in Controlled Clinical Trials

Body System*	Preferred Term	Neoral® (N=182)	Sandimmune® (N=185)
Infection or Potential Infection		24.7%	24.3%
	Influenza-Like Symptoms	9.9%	8.1%
	Upper Respiratory Tract Infections	7.7%	11.3%
Cardiovascular System		28.0%	25.4%
	Hypertension**	27.5%	25.4%
Urinary System		24.2%	16.2%
	Increased Creatinine	19.8%	15.7%
Central and Peripheral Nervous System		26.4%	20.5%
	Headache	15.9%	14.0%
	Paresthesia	7.1%	4.8%
Musculoskeletal System		13.2%	8.7%
	Arthralgia	6.0%	1.1%
Body As a Whole–General		29.1%	22.2%
	Pain	4.4%	3.2%
Metabolic and Nutritional		9.3%	9.7%
Reproductive, Female		8.5% (4 of 47 females)	11.5% (6 of 52 females)
Resistance Mechanism		18.7%	21.1%
Skin and Appendages		17.6%	15.1%
	Hypertrichosis	6.6%	5.4%
Respiratory System		5.0%	6.5%
	Bronchospasm, Coughing, Dyspnea, Rhinitis	5.0%	4.9%
Psychiatric		5.0%	3.8%
Gastrointestinal System		19.8%	28.7%
	Abdominal Pain	2.7%	6.0%
	Diarrhea	5.0%	5.9%
	Dyspepsia	2.2%	3.2%
	Gum Hyperplasia	3.8%	6.0%
	Nausea	5.5%	5.9%
White Cell and RES		4.4%	2.7%

* Total percentage of events within the system
** Newly occurring hypertension = SBP ≥160 mm Hg and/or DBP ≥90 mm Hg

ommended dose of methotrexate. Most patients can be treated with Neoral® doses of 3 mg/kg/day or below when combined with methotrexate doses of up to 15 mg/week. (See CLINICAL PHARMACOLOGY, Clinical Trials) There is limited long-term treatment data. Recurrence of rheumatoid arthritis disease activity is generally apparent within 4 weeks after stopping cyclosporine.

Psoriasis

The initial dose of Neoral® should be 2.5 mg/kg/day. Neoral® should be taken twice daily, as a divided (1.25 mg/kg BID) oral dose. Patients should be kept at that dose for at least 4 weeks, barring adverse events. If significant clinical improvement has not occurred in patients by that time, the patient's dosage should be increased at 2-week intervals. Based on patient response, dose increases of approximately 0.5 mg/kg/day should be made to a maximum of 4.0 mg/kg/day.

Dose decreases by 25%-50% should be made at any time to control adverse events, e.g., hypertension, elevations in serum creatinine (≥25% above the patient's pretreatment level), or clinically significant laboratory abnormalities. If dose reduction is not effective in controlling abnormalities, or if the adverse event or abnormality is severe, Neoral® should be discontinued. *(See Special Monitoring of Psoriasis Patients)*

Patients generally show some improvement in the clinical manifestations of psoriasis in 2 weeks. Satisfactory control and stabilization of the disease may take 12-16 weeks to achieve. Results of a dose-titration clinical trial with Neoral® indicate that an improvement of psoriasis by 75% or more (based on PASI) was achieved in 51% of the patients after 8 weeks and in 79% of the patients after 16 weeks. Treatment should be discontinued if satisfactory response cannot be achieved after 6 weeks at 4 mg/kg/day or the patient's maximum tolerated dose. Once a patient is adequately controlled and appears stable the dose of Neoral® should be lowered, and the patient treated with the lowest dose that maintains an adequate response (this should not necessarily be total clearing of the patient). In clinical trials, cyclosporine doses at the lower end of the recommended dosage range were effective in maintaining a satisfactory response in 60% of the patients. Doses below 2.5 mg/kg/day may also be equally effective.

Upon stopping treatment with cyclosporine, relapse will occur in approximately 6 weeks (50% of the patients) to 16 weeks (75% of the patients). In the majority of patients rebound does not occur after cessation of treatment with cyclosporine. Thirteen cases of transformation of chronic plaque psoriasis to more severe forms of psoriasis have been reported. There were 9 cases of pustular and 4 cases of erythrodermic psoriasis. Long term experience with Neoral® in psoriasis patients is limited and continuous treatment for extended periods greater than one year is not recommended. Alternation with other forms of treatment should be considered in the long term management of patients with this life long disease.

Neoral® Oral Solution (cyclosporine oral solution, USP) MODIFIED – Recommendations for Administration

To make Neoral® Oral Solution (cyclosporine oral solution, USP) MODIFIED more palatable, it should be diluted with orange or apple juice that is at room temperature. Patients should avoid switching diluents frequently. Grapefruit juice affects metabolism of cyclosporine and should be avoided. The combination of Neoral® solution with milk can be unpalatable. The effect of milk on the bioavailability of cyclosporine when administered as Neoral Oral Solution has not been evaluated.

Take the prescribed amount of Neoral® Oral Solution (cyclosporine oral solution, USP) MODIFIED from the container using the dosing syringe supplied, after removal of the protective cover, and transfer the solution to a glass of orange or apple juice. Stir well and drink at once. Do not allow diluted oral solution to stand before drinking. Use a glass container (not plastic). Rinse the glass with more diluent to ensure that the total dose is consumed. After use, dry the outside of the dosing syringe with a clean towel and replace the protective cover. Do not rinse the dosing syringe with water or other cleaning agents. If the syringe requires cleaning, it must be completely dry before reuse.

Blood Concentration Monitoring in Transplant Patients

Transplant centers have found blood concentration monitoring of cyclosporine to be an essential component of patient management. Of importance to blood concentration analysis are the type of assay used, the transplanted organ, and other immunosuppressant agents being administered. While no fixed relationship has been established, blood concentration monitoring may assist in the clinical evaluation of rejection and toxicity, dose adjustments, and the assessment of compliance.

Various assays have been used to measure blood concentrations of cyclosporine. Older studies using a nonspecific assay often cited concentrations that were roughly twice those of the specific assays. Therefore, comparison between concentrations in the published literature and an individual patient concentration using current assays must be made with detailed knowledge of the assay methods employed. Current assay results are also not interchangeable and their use should be guided by their approved labeling. A discussion of the different assay methods is contained in *Annals of Clinical Biochemistry* 1994;31:420-446. While several assays and assay matrices are available, there is a consensus that parent-compound-specific assays correlate best with clinical events. Of these, HPLC is the standard reference, but the monoclonal antibody RIAs and the monoclonal antibody FPIA offer sensitivity, reproducibility, and convenience. Most clinicians base their monitoring on trough concentrations. *Applied Pharmacokinetics, Principles of Therapeutic Drug Monitoring* (1992) contains a broad discussion of cyclosporine pharmacokinetics and drug monitoring techniques. Blood concentration monitoring is not a replacement for renal function monitoring or tissue biopsies.

HOW SUPPLIED

Neoral® Soft Gelatin Capsules (cyclosporine capsules, USP) MODIFIED

25 mg
Oval, blue-gray imprinted in red, "Neoral" over "25 mg."
Packages of 30 unit-dose blisters (NDC 0078-0246-15).

100 mg
Oblong, blue-gray imprinted in red, "NEORAL" over "100 mg."
Packages of 30 unit-dose blisters (NDC 0078-0248-15).

Store and Dispense
In the original unit-dose container at controlled room temperature 68°-77°F (20°-25°C).

Neoral® Oral Solution (cyclosporine oral solution, USP) MODIFIED

A clear, yellow liquid supplied in 50 mL bottles containing 100 mg/mL (NDC 0078-0274-22).

Store and Dispense
In the original container at controlled room temperature 68°-77°F (20°-25°C). Do not store in the refrigerator. Once opened, the contents must be used within two months. At temperatures below 68°F (20°C) the solution may gel; light flocculation or the formation of a light sediment may also occur. There is no impact on product performance or dosing using the syringe provided. Allow to warm to room temperature 77°F (25°C) to reverse these changes.

Neoral® Soft Gelatin Capsules (cyclosporine capsules, USP) MODIFIED

Neoral® Oral Solution (cyclosporine oral solution, USP) MODIFIED

REV: OCTOBER 2009   T2009-104
Distributed by:
Novartis Pharmaceuticals Corporation
East Hanover, New Jersey 07936
©Novartis

Shown in Product Identification Guide, page 315

RECLAST®   ℞
[*RE-klast*]
(zoledronic acid)
Injection

The following prescribing information is based on official labeling in effect July 2010.

HIGHLIGHTS OF PRESCRIBING INFORMATION

These highlights do not include all the information needed to use Reclast safely and effectively. See full prescribing information for Reclast.

Reclast® *(zoledronic acid)* **Injection**
Initial U.S. Approval: 2001

RECENT MAJOR CHANGES

Indications and Usage, Prevention of Postmenopausal Osteoporosis (1.2)	5/2009
Indications and Usage, Glucocorticoid Osteoporosis (1.4)	3/2009
Dosage and Administration, Prevention of Postmenopausal Osteoporosis (2.2)	5/2009
Dosage and Administration, Glucocorticoid-Induced Osteoporosis (2.4)	3/2009
Warnings and Precautions, Renal Impairment (5.3)	3/2009

INDICATIONS AND USAGE

Reclast is a bisphosphonate indicated for:
• Treatment of osteoporosis in postmenopausal women (1.1)
• Prevention of osteoporosis in postmenopausal women (1.2)
• Treatment to increase bone mass in men with osteoporosis (1.3)
• Treatment and prevention of glucocorticoid-induced osteoporosis in patients expected to be on glucocorticoids for at least 12 months (1.4)
• Treatment of Paget's disease of bone in men and women (1.5)

DOSAGE AND ADMINISTRATION

• Treatment of osteoporosis in postmenopausal women (2.1); treatment to increase bone mass in men with osteoporosis (2.3): treatment and prevention of glucocorticoid-induced osteoporosis (2.4): a 5 mg infusion once a year given intravenously over no less than 15 minutes
• Prevention of osteoporosis in postmenopausal women: a 5 mg infusion given once every 2 years intravenously over no less than 15 minutes (2.2)
• Treatment of Paget's disease of bone: a single 5 mg infusion given intravenously over no less than 15 minutes (2.5)
• Patients with Paget's disease should receive 1500 mg elemental calcium and 800 IU vitamin D daily, particularly during the 2 weeks after dosing (2.5)
• Administer through a separate vented infusion line and do not allow to come in contact with any calcium or divalent cation-containing solutions (2.6)

DOSAGE FORMS AND STRENGTHS

5 mg in a 100 mL ready-to-infuse solution (3)

CONTRAINDICATIONS

• Hypocalcemia (4.1)
• Hypersensitivity to any component of Reclast (4.2, 6.2)

WARNINGS AND PRECAUTIONS

• Reclast and Zometa contain the same active ingredient. Patients receiving Zometa should not receive Reclast (5.1)
• Patients must be adequately supplemented with calcium and vitamin D (5.2)
• A single dose should not exceed 5 mg and the duration of infusion should be no less than 15 minutes (2.1, 2.2, 5.3)
• Renal toxicity may be greater in patients with underlying renal impairment or with other risk factors such as dehydration that may occur in the post-dosing period. Patients with severe renal impairment (creatinine clearance <35 mL/min) should not receive Reclast. Monitor serum creatinine before each dose (5.3)
• Osteonecrosis of the jaw has been reported rarely in postmenopausal osteoporosis patients treated with bisphosphonates, including zoledronic acid. All patients should have a routine oral exam by the prescriber prior to treatment (5.4)
• Reclast can cause fetal harm. Women of childbearing potential should be advised of the potential hazard to the fetus and to avoid becoming pregnant (5.5, 8.1)
• Severe incapacitating bone, joint, and/or muscle pain may occur. Withhold future doses of Reclast if severe symptoms occur (5.6)

ADVERSE REACTIONS

The most common adverse reactions (>10%) were pyrexia, myalgia, headache, arthralgia, pain in extremity (6.1). Other clinically important adverse reactions were flu-like illness, nausea, vomiting, diarrhea (6.2), and eye inflammation (6.1).

To report SUSPECTED ADVERSE REACTIONS, contact Novartis Pharmaceuticals Corporation at 1-888-669-6682 or FDA at 1-800-FDA-1088 or www.fda.gov/medwatch.

DRUG INTERACTIONS

• Aminoglycosides: May have an additive effect to lower serum calcium for prolonged periods (7.1)
• Loop diuretics: Concomitant use with Reclast may increase risk of hypocalcemia (7.2)
• Nephrotoxic drugs: Use with caution (7.3)
• Drugs primarily excreted by the kidney: Exposure may be increased in the presence of renal impairment. Consider monitoring serum creatinine in patients at risk for renal impairment (7.4)

USE IN SPECIFIC POPULATIONS

Nursing Mothers: Reclast should not be given to nursing women (8.3)
Pediatric Use: Not indicated for use in pediatric patients (8.4)
Geriatric Use: Special care to monitor renal function (8.5)

See 17 for PATIENT COUNSELING INFORMATION and FDA-approved patient labeling

Revised: 01/2010

FULL PRESCRIBING INFORMATION: CONTENTS*

*Sections or subsections omitted from the full prescribing information are not listed

FULL PRESCRIBING INFORMATION

1 INDICATIONS AND USAGE

1.1 Treatment of Osteoporosis in Postmenopausal Women

Reclast is indicated for treatment of osteoporosis in postmenopausal women. In postmenopausal women with osteoporosis, diagnosed by bone mineral density (BMD) or prevalent vertebral fracture, Reclast reduces the incidence of fractures (hip, vertebral and non-vertebral osteoporosis-related fractures). In patients at high risk of fracture, defined as a recent low-trauma hip fracture, Reclast reduces the incidence of new clinical fractures [*see Clinical Studies (14.1)*].

1.2 Prevention of Osteoporosis in Postmenopausal Women

Reclast is indicated for prevention of osteoporosis in postmenopausal women [*see Clinical Studies (14.2)*].

1.3 Osteoporosis in Men

Reclast is indicated for treatment to increase bone mass in men with osteoporosis [*see Clinical Studies (14.3)*].

1.4 Glucocorticoid-Induced Osteoporosis

Reclast is indicated for the treatment and prevention of glucocorticoid-induced osteoporosis in men and women who are either initiating or continuing systemic glucocorticoids in a daily dosage equivalent to 7.5 mg or greater of prednisone and who are expected to remain on glucocorticoids for at least 12 months [*see Clinical Studies (14.4)*].

1.5 Paget's Disease of Bone

Reclast is indicated for treatment of Paget's disease of bone in men and women. Treatment is indicated in patients with Paget's disease of bone with elevations in serum alkaline phosphatase of two times or higher than the upper limit of the age-specific normal reference range, or those who are symptomatic, or those at risk for complications from their disease [*see Clinical Studies (14.5)*].

2 DOSAGE AND ADMINISTRATION

Parenteral drug products should be inspected visually for particulate matter and discoloration prior to administration, whenever solution and container permit.

Patients must be appropriately hydrated prior to administration of Reclast [*see Warnings and Precautions (5.3)*].

Administration of acetaminophen following Reclast administration may reduce the incidence of acute-phase reaction symptoms.

A 5 mg dose of Reclast administered intravenously is recommended for patients with creatinine clearance ≥35 mL/min [*see Warnings and Precautions (5.3)*].

2.1 Treatment of Osteoporosis in Postmenopausal Women

The recommended regimen is a 5 mg infusion once a year given intravenously over no less than 15 minutes. For osteoporosis treatment, and to reduce the risk of hypocalcemia, patients must be adequately supplemented with calcium and vitamin D if dietary intake is not sufficient. Postmenopausal women require an average of at least 1200 mg calcium and 800-1000 IU vitamin D daily.

2.2 Prevention of Osteoporosis in Postmenopausal Women

The recommended regimen is a 5 mg infusion given once every 2 years intravenously over no less than 15 minutes. Patients must be adequately supplemented with calcium and vitamin D if dietary intake is not sufficient. Postmenopausal women require an average of 1200 mg calcium and 800-1000 IU vitamin D daily.

2.3 Osteoporosis in Men

The recommended regimen is a 5 mg infusion once a year given intravenously over no less than 15 minutes. Patients must be adequately supplemented with calcium and vitamin D if dietary intake is not sufficient. An average of at least 1200 mg calcium and 800-1000 IU vitamin D daily is recommended.

2.4 Treatment and Prevention of Glucocorticoid-Induced Osteoporosis

The recommended regimen is a 5 mg infusion once a year given intravenously over no less than 15 minutes. Patients must be adequately supplemented with calcium and vitamin D if dietary intake is not sufficient. An average of at least 1200 mg calcium and 800-1000 IU vitamin D daily is recommended.

2.5 Treatment of Paget's Disease of Bone

The recommended dose is a 5 mg infusion. The infusion time must not be less than 15 minutes given over a constant infusion rate.

To reduce the risk of hypocalcemia, all patients with Paget's disease should receive 1500 mg elemental calcium daily in divided doses (750 mg two times a day, or 500 mg three times a day) and 800 IU vitamin D daily, particularly in the 2 weeks following Reclast administration. All patients should be instructed on the importance of calcium and vitamin D supplementation in maintaining serum calcium levels, and on the symptoms of hypocalcemia [*see Warnings and Precautions (5.2)*].

Re-treatment of Paget's Disease

After a single treatment with Reclast in Paget's disease an extended remission period is observed. Specific re-treatment data are not available. However, re-treatment with Reclast may be considered in patients who have relapsed, based on increases in serum alkaline phosphatase, or in those patients who failed to achieve normalization of their serum alkaline phosphatase, or in those patients with symptoms, as dictated by medical practice.

2.6 Method of Administration

The Reclast infusion time must not be less than 15 minutes given over a constant infusion rate.

Reclast solution for infusion must not be allowed to come in contact with any calcium or other divalent cation-containing solutions, and should be administered as a single intravenous solution through a separate vented infusion line.

If refrigerated, allow the refrigerated solution to reach room temperature before administration. After opening, the solution is stable for 24 hours at 2°C-8°C (36°F-46°F) [*see How Supplied/Storage and Handling (16)*].

3 DOSAGE FORMS AND STRENGTHS

5 mg in a 100 mL ready to infuse solution.

4 CONTRAINDICATIONS

4.1 Hypocalcemia

[*See Warnings and Precautions (5.2)*].

4.2 Hypersensitivity to Zoledronic Acid or Any Components of Reclast

Hypersensitivity reactions including rare cases of urticaria, angioedema, and anaphylactic reaction/shock have been reported [*see Post-Marketing Experience (6.2)*].

5 WARNINGS AND PRECAUTIONS

5.1 Drug Products with Same Active Ingredient

Reclast contains the same active ingredient found in Zometa, used for oncology indications, and a patient being treated with Zometa should not be treated with Reclast.

5.2 Hypocalcemia and Mineral Metabolism

Pre-existing hypocalcemia and disturbances of mineral metabolism (e.g., hypoparathyroidism, thyroid surgery, parathyroid surgery; malabsorption syndromes, excision of small intestine) must be effectively treated before initiating therapy with Reclast. Clinical monitoring of calcium and mineral levels (phosphorus and magnesium) is highly recommended for these patients [*see Contraindications (4)*].

Hypocalcemia following Reclast administration is a significant risk in Paget's disease. All patients should be instructed about the symptoms of hypocalcemia and the importance of calcium and vitamin D supplementation in maintaining serum calcium levels [*see Dosage and Administration (2), Adverse Reactions (6.1), Information for Patients (17.1)*].

All osteoporosis patients should be instructed on the importance of calcium and vitamin D supplementation in maintaining serum calcium levels [*see Dosage and Administration (2), Adverse Reactions (6.1), Information for Patients (17.1)*].

5.3 Renal Impairment

A single dose of Reclast should not exceed 5 mg and the duration of infusion should be no less than 15 minutes [*see Dosage and Administration (2.1)*].

Reclast should not be used in patients with severe renal impairment (creatinine clearance <35 mL/min) due to lack of adequate clinical experience in this population [*see Adverse Reactions (6.1)*].

Renal impairment has been observed following the administration of zoledronic acid, especially in patients with pre-existing renal compromise or other risk factors including concomitant nephrotoxic medications, concomitant diuretic therapy, or severe dehydration occurring before or after Reclast administration. Renal impairment has been observed in patients after a single administration. Rare reports of hospitalization and/or dialysis occurred in patients with underlying moderate to severe renal impairment [*see Post-Marketing Experience (6.2)*]. Renal impairment may lead to increased exposure of concomitant medications that are primarily renally excreted [*see Drug Interactions (7.4)*]. Serum creatinine should be measured before each Reclast dose. Transient increase in serum creatinine may be greater in patients with impaired renal function; consider interim monitoring of serum creatinine in at-risk patients. Patients, especially those receiving diuretic therapy, should be appropriately hydrated prior to administration of Reclast. Reclast should be used with caution with other nephrotoxic drugs [*see Drug Interactions (7.3)*]. Consider monitoring serum creatinine in patients at risk for renal impairment who are taking concomitant medications that are primarily excreted by the kidney [*see Drug Interactions (7.4)*].

5.4 Osteonecrosis of the Jaw

Osteonecrosis of the jaw (ONJ) has been reported in patients treated with bisphosphonates, including zoledronic acid. Most cases have been in cancer patients treated with intravenous bisphosphonates undergoing dental procedures. Some cases have occurred in patients with postmenopausal osteoporosis treated with either oral or intravenous bisphosphonates. A routine oral examination should be performed by the prescriber prior to initiation of bisphosphonate treatment. A dental examination with appropriate preventive dentistry should be considered prior to treatment with bisphosphonates in patients with a history of concomitant risk factors (e.g., cancer, chemotherapy, radiotherapy, corticosteroids, poor oral hygiene, pre-existing dental disease or infection, anemia, coagulopathy).

While on treatment, patients with concomitant risk factors should avoid invasive dental procedures if possible. For patients who develop ONJ while on bisphosphonate therapy, dental surgery may exacerbate the condition. For patients requiring dental procedures, there are no data available to suggest whether discontinuation of bisphosphonate treatment reduces the risk of ONJ. The clinical judgment of the treating physician should guide the management plan of each patient based on individual benefit/risk assessment [*see Adverse Reactions (6.1)*].

5.5 Pregnancy

RECLAST SHOULD NOT BE USED DURING PREGNANCY. Reclast may cause fetal harm when administered to a pregnant woman. If the patient becomes pregnant while taking this drug, the patient should be apprised of the potential harm to the fetus. Women of childbearing potential should be advised to avoid becoming pregnant while on Reclast therapy [*see Use in Specific Populations (8.1)*].

5.6 Musculoskeletal Pain

In post-marketing experience, severe and occasionally incapacitating bone, joint, and/or muscle pain have been infrequently reported in patients taking bisphosphonates, including Reclast. The time to onset of symptoms varied from one day to several months after starting the drug. Consider withholding future Reclast treatment if severe symptoms develop. Most patients had relief of symptoms after stopping. A subset had recurrence of symptoms when rechallenged with the same drug or another bisphosphonate [*see Adverse Reactions (6.2)*].

5.7 Patients with Asthma

While not observed in clinical trials with Reclast, there have been reports of bronchoconstriction in aspirin-sensitive patients receiving bisphosphonates. Use Reclast with caution in aspirin-sensitive patients.

6 ADVERSE REACTIONS

6.1 Clinical Studies Experience

Because clinical trials are conducted under widely varying conditions, adverse reaction rates observed in the clinical trials of a drug cannot be directly compared to rates in the clinical trials of another drug and may not reflect the rates observed in practice.

Treatment of Osteoporosis in Postmenopausal Women

The safety of Reclast in the treatment of postmenopausal osteoporosis was assessed in Study 1, a large, randomized, double-blind, placebo-controlled, multinational study of 7736 postmenopausal women aged 65-89 years with osteoporosis, diagnosed by bone mineral density or the presence of a prevalent vertebral fracture. The duration of the trial was three years with 3862 patients exposed to Reclast and 3852 patients exposed to placebo administered once annually as a single 5 mg dose in 100 mL solution infused over at

Table 1. Adverse Reactions Occurring in ≥2.0% of Patients with Osteoporosis and More Frequently than in Placebo-Treated Patients

	Study 1		Study 2	
System Organ Class	5 mg IV Reclast once per year % (N=3862)	Placebo once per year % (N=3852)	5 mg IV Reclast once per year % (N=1054)	Placebo once per year % (N=1057)
Blood and the Lymphatic System Disorders				
Anemia	4.4	3.6	5.3	5.2
Metabolism and Nutrition Disorders				
Dehydration	0.6	0.6	2.5	2.3
Anorexia	2.0	1.1	1.0	1.0
Nervous System Disorders				
Headache	12.4	8.1	3.9	2.5
Dizziness	7.6	6.7	2.0	4.0
Ear and Labyrinth Disorders				
Vertigo	4.3	4.0	1.3	1.7
Cardiac Disorders				
Atrial Fibrillation	2.4	1.9	2.8	2.6
Vascular Disorders				
Hypertension	12.7	12.4	6.8	5.4
Gastrointestinal Disorders				
Nausea	8.5	5.2	4.5	4.5
Diarrhea	6.0	5.6	5.2	4.7
Vomiting	4.6	3.2	3.4	3.4
Abdominal Pain Upper	4.6	3.1	0.9	1.5
Dyspepsia	4.3	4.0	1.7	1.6
Musculoskeletal, Connective Tissue and Bone Disorders				
Arthralgia	23.8	20.4	17.9	18.3
Myalgia	11.7	3.7	4.9	2.7
Pain in Extremity	11.3	9.9	5.9	4.8
Shoulder Pain	6.9	5.6	0.0	0.0
Bone Pain	5.8	2.3	3.2	1.0
Neck Pain	4.4	3.8	1.4	1.1
Muscle Spasms	3.7	3.4	1.5	1.7
Osteoarthritis	9.1	9.7	5.7	4.5
Musculoskeletal Pain	0.4	0.3	3.1	1.2
General Disorders and Administrative Site Conditions				
Pyrexia	17.9	4.6	8.7	3.1
Influenza-like Illness	8.8	2.7	0.8	0.4
Fatigue	5.4	3.5	2.1	1.2
Chills	5.4	1.0	1.5	0.5
Asthenia	5.3	2.9	3.2	3.0
Peripheral Edema	4.6	4.2	5.5	5.3
Pain	3.3	1.3	1.5	0.5
Malaise	2.0	1.0	1.1	0.3
Hyperthermia	0.3	<0.1	2.3	0.5
Chest Pain	1.3	1.1	2.4	1.8
Investigations				
Creatinine Renal Clearance Decreased	2.0	2.4	2.1	1.7

least 15 minutes, for a total of three doses. All women received 1000 to 1500 mg of elemental calcium plus 400 to 1200 IU of vitamin D supplementation per day.

The incidence of all-cause mortality was similar between groups: 3.4% in the Reclast group and 2.9% in the placebo group. The incidence of serious adverse events was 29.2% in the Reclast group and 30.1% in the placebo group. The percentage of patients who withdrew from the study due to adverse events was 5.4% and 4.8% for the Reclast and placebo groups, respectively.

The safety of Reclast in the treatment of osteoporosis patients with a recent (within 90 days) low-trauma hip fracture was assessed in Study 2, a randomized, double-blind, placebo-controlled, multinational endpoint-driven study of 2127 men and women aged 50-95 years; 1065 patients were randomized to Reclast and 1062 patients were randomized to placebo. Reclast was administered once annually as a single 5 mg dose in 100 mL solution infused over at least 15 minutes. The study continued until at least 211 patients had a confirmed clinical fracture in the study population who were followed for an average of approximately 2 years on study drug. Vitamin D levels were not routinely measured but a loading dose of vitamin D (50,000 to 125,000 IU orally or IM) was given to patients and they were started on 1000 to 1500 mg of elemental calcium plus 800 to 1200 IU of vitamin D supplementation per day for at least 14 days prior to the study drug infusions.

The incidence of all-cause mortality was 9.6% in the Reclast group and 13.3% in the placebo group. The incidence of serious adverse events was 38.3% in the Reclast group and 41.3% in the placebo group. The percentage of patients who withdrew from the study due to adverse events was 5.3% and 4.7% for the Reclast and placebo groups, respectively. Adverse reactions reported in at least 2% of patients with osteoporosis and more frequently in the Reclast-treated patients than placebo-treated patients in either osteoporosis trial are shown below in Table 1.
[See table 1 above]

Renal Impairment

Treatment with intravenous bisphosphonates, including zoledronic acid, has been associated with renal impairment manifested as deterioration in renal function (i.e., increased serum creatinine) and in rare cases, acute renal failure. In the clinical trial for postmenopausal osteoporosis, patients with baseline creatinine clearance <30 mL/min, urine dipstick ≥2+ protein or increase in serum creatinine of >0.5 mg/dL during the screening visits were excluded. The change in creatinine clearance (measured annually prior to dosing) and the incidence of renal failure and impairment was comparable for both the Reclast and placebo treatment groups over 3 years, including patients with mild to moderate renal impairment (creatinine clearance between 30-60 mL/min) at baseline. Overall, there was a transient increase in serum creatinine observed within 10 days of dosing in 1.8% of Reclast-treated patients versus 0.8% of placebo-treated patients which resolved without specific therapy [see Warnings and Precautions (5.3)].

Acute Phase Reaction

The signs and symptoms of acute phase reaction occurred in Study 1 following Reclast infusion including, fever (18%), myalgia (9%), and flu-like symptoms (8%), headache (7%), and arthralgia (7%). The majority of these symptoms occurred within the first 3 days following the dose of Reclast and usually resolved within 3 days of onset but resolution could take up to 7-14 days. In Study 2, patients without a contraindication to acetaminophen were provided with a standard oral dose at the time of the IV infusion and instructed to use additional acetaminophen at home for the next 72 hours as needed. Reclast was associated with fewer signs and symptoms of a transient acute phase reaction in this trial: fever (7%) and arthralgia (3%). The incidence of these symptoms decreased with subsequent doses of Reclast.

Laboratory Findings

In Study 1, in women with postmenopausal osteoporosis, approximately 0.2% of patients had notable declines of serum calcium levels (less than 7.5 mg/dL) following Reclast administration. No symptomatic cases of hypocalcemia were observed. In Study 2, following pre-treatment with vitamin D, no patients had treatment emergent serum calcium levels below 7.5 mg/dL.

Injection Site Reactions

In the osteoporosis trials, local reactions at the infusion site such as itching, redness and/or pain have been reported in 0 to 0.7% of patients following the administration of Reclast and 0 to 0.5% of patients following administration of placebo.

Osteonecrosis of the Jaw

In the postmenopausal osteoporosis trial, Study 1, in 7736 patients, after initiation of therapy, symptoms consistent with ONJ occurred in one patient treated with placebo and one patient treated with Reclast. Both cases resolved after appropriate treatment [see Warnings and Precautions (5.4)]. No reports of osteonecrosis of the jaw were reported in either treatment group in Study 2.

Atrial Fibrillation

In the postmenopausal osteoporosis trial, Study 1, adjudicated serious adverse events of atrial fibrillation in the zoledronic acid treatment group occurred in 1.3% of patients (50 out of 3862) compared to 0.4% (17 out of 3852) in the placebo group. The overall incidence of all atrial fibrillation adverse events in the zoledronic acid treatment group was reported in 2.5% of patients (96 out of 3862) in the Reclast group vs. 1.9% of patients (75 out of 3852) in the placebo group. Over 90% of these events in both treatment groups occurred more than a month after the infusion. In an ECG sub-study, ECG measurements were performed on a subset of 559 patients before and 9 to 11 days after treatment. There was no difference in the incidence of atrial fibrillation between treatment groups suggesting these events were not related to the acute infusions. In Study 2, adjudicated serious adverse events of atrial fibrillation in the zoledronic acid treatment group occurred in 1.0% of patients (11 out of 1054) compared to 1.2% (13 out of 1057) in the placebo group demonstrating no difference between treatment groups.

Ocular Adverse Events

Cases of iritis/uveitis/episcleritis/conjunctivitis have been reported in patients treated with bisphosphonates, including zoledronic acid. In the osteoporosis trials, 1 (<0.1%) to 9 (0.2%) patients treated with Reclast and 0 (0%) to 1 (<0.1%) patient treated with placebo developed iritis/uveitis/episcleritis.

Prevention of Osteoporosis in Postmenopausal Women

The safety of Reclast in postmenopausal women with osteopenia (low bone mass) was assessed in a 2-year randomized, multi-center, double-blind, placebo-controlled study of 581 postmenopausal women aged ≥45 years. Patients were randomized to one of three treatment groups: (1) Reclast given at randomization and Month 12 (n=198); (2) Reclast given at randomization and placebo at Month 12 (n=181); and (3) placebo given at randomization and Month 12 (n=202). Reclast was administered as a single 5 mg dose in 100 mL solution infused over at least 15 minutes. All women received 500 to 1200 mg elemental calcium plus 400 to 800 IU vitamin D supplementation per day.

The incidence of serious adverse events was similar for subjects given (1) Reclast at randomization and at Month 12 (10.6%), (2) Reclast at randomization and placebo given at Month 12 (9.4%), and (3) placebo at randomization and at Month 12 (11.4%). The percentages of patients who withdrew from the study due to adverse events were 7.1%, 7.2%, and 3.0% in the two Reclast groups and placebo group, respectively. Adverse reactions reported in at least 2% of patients with osteopenia and more frequently in the Reclast-treated patients than placebo-treated patients are shown in Table 2.

Table 2. Adverse Reactions Occurring in ≥ 2% of Patients with Osteopenia and More Frequently than in Placebo-Treated Patients

System Organ Class	5 mg IV Reclast Once Per Year % (N=198)	5 mg IV Reclast Once % (N=181)	Placebo once per year % (N=202)
Metabolism and nutrition disorders			
Anorexia	2.0	0.6	0.0
Nervous system disorders			
Headache	14.6	20.4	11.4
Dizziness	7.6	6.1	3.5
Hypoesthesia	5.6	2.2	2.0
Ear and labyrinth disorders			
Vertigo	2.0	1.7	1.0
Vascular disorders			
Hypertension	5.1	8.3	6.9

Gastrointestinal disorders

Nausea	17.7	11.6	7.9
Diarrhea	8.1	6.6	7.9
Vomiting	7.6	5.0	4.5
Dyspepsia	7.1	6.6	5.0
Abdominal pain*	8.6	6.6	7.9
Constipation	6.6	7.2	6.9
Abdominal discomfort	2.0	1.1	0.5
Abdominal distension	2.0	0.6	0.0

Skin and subcutaneous tissue disorders

Rash	3.0	2.2	2.5

Musculoskeletal and connective tissue disorders

Arthralgia	27.3	18.8	19.3
Myalgia	19.2	22.7	6.9
Back pain	18.2	16.6	11.9
Pain in extremity	11.1	16.0	9.9
Muscle spasms	5.6	2.8	5.0
Musculoskeletal pain**	8.1	7.2	7.9
Bone pain	5.1	3.3	1.0
Neck pain	5.1	6.6	5.0
Arthritis	4.0	2.2	1.5
Joint stiffness	3.5	1.1	2.0
Joint swelling	3.0	0.6	0.0
Flank pain	2.0	0.6	0.0
Pain in jaw	2.0	3.9	2.5

General disorders and administration site conditions

Pain	24.2	14.9	3.5
Pyrexia	21.7	21.0	4.5
Chills	18.2	18.2	3.0
Fatigue	14.6	9.9	4.0
Asthenia	6.1	2.8	1.0
Peripheral edema	5.6	3.9	3.5
Non-cardiac chest pain	3.5	7.7	3.0
Influenza-like illness	1.5	3.3	2.0
Malaise	1.0	2.2	0.5

* Combined abdominal pain, abdominal pain upper, and abdominal pain lower as one ADR
** Combined musculoskeletal pain and musculoskeletal chest pain as one ADR

Ocular Adverse Events
Cases of iritis/uveitis/episcleritis/conjunctivitis have been reported in patients treated with bisphosphonates, including zoledronic acid. In the osteoporosis prevention trial, 4 (1.1%) patients treated with Reclast and 0 (0%) patients treated with placebo developed iritis/uveitis.

Acute Phase Reaction
In patients given Reclast at randomization and placebo at Month 12, Reclast was associated with signs and symptoms of an acute phase reaction: Myalgia (20.4%), fever (19.3%), chills (18.2%), pain (13.8%), headache (13.3%), fatigue (8.3%), arthralgia (6.1%), pain in extremity (3.9%), influenza-like illness (3.3%), and back pain (1.7%), which occurred within the first 3 days following the dose of Reclast. The majority of these symptoms were mild to moderate and resolved within 3 days of the event onset but resolution could take up to 7-14 days.

Osteoporosis in Men
The safety of Reclast in men with osteoporosis or osteoporosis secondary to hypogonadism, was assessed in a two year randomized, multicenter, double-blind, active controlled group study of 302 men aged 25-86 years. One hundred fifty three (153) patients were exposed to Reclast administered once annually with a 5 mg dose in 100 mL infused over 15 minutes for up to a total of two doses, and 148 patients were exposed to a commercially-available oral weekly bisphosphonate (active control) for up to two years. All participants received 1000 mg of elemental calcium plus 800 to 1000 IU of vitamin D supplementation per day.

The incidence of all-cause mortality (one in each group) and serious adverse events were similar between the Reclast and active control treatment groups. The percentage of patients experiencing at least one adverse event was comparable between the Reclast and active control groups, with the exception of a higher incidence of post-dose symptoms in the Reclast group that occurred within 3 days after infusion. The overall safety and tolerability of Reclast was similar to the active control.

Adverse reactions reported in at least 2% of men with osteoporosis and more frequently in the Reclast-treated patients than the active control-treated patients and either (1) not reported in the postmenopausal osteoporosis treatment trial or (2) reported more frequently in the trial of osteoporosis in men are presented in Table 3. Therefore, Table 3 should be viewed in conjunction with Table 1.

Table 3. Adverse Reactions Occurring in ≥ 2% of Men with Osteoporosis and More Frequently in the Reclast-Treated Patients than the Active Control-Treated Patients and either (1) Not Reported in the Postmenopausal Osteoporosis Treatment Trial or (2) Reported More Frequently in this Trial

System Organ Class	5 mg IV Reclast once per year % (N=153)	Active Control once weekly % (N=148)
Nervous System Disorders		
Headache	15.0	6.1
Lethargy	3.3	1.4
Eye Disorders		
Eye pain	2.0	0.0
Cardiac Disorders		
Atrial fibrillation	3.3	2.0
Palpitations	2.6	0.0
Respiratory, Thoracic and Mediastinal Disorders		
Dyspnea	6.5	4.7
Abdominal pain*	7.9	4.1
Skin and Subcutaneous Tissue Disorders		
Hyperhidrosis	2.6	2.0
Musculoskeletal, Connective Tissue and Bone Disorders		
Myalgia	19.6	6.8
Musculoskeletal pain**	12.4	10.8
Musculoskeletal stiffness	4.6	0.0
Renal and Urinary Disorders		
Blood creatinine increased	2.0	0.7
General Disorders and Administrative Site Conditions		
Fatigue	17.6	6.1
Pain	11.8	4.1
Chills	9.8	2.7
Influenza-like illness	9.2	2.0
Malaise	7.2	0.7
Acute phase reaction	3.9	0.0
Investigations		
C-reactive protein increased	4.6	1.4

* Combined abdominal pain, abdominal pain upper, and abdominal pain lower as one ADR
** Combined musculoskeletal pain and musculoskeletal chest pain as one ADR

Renal Impairment
Creatinine clearance was measured annually prior to dosing and changes in long-term renal function over 24 months was comparable in the Reclast and active control groups. [See Warnings and Precautions (5.3)].

Acute Phase Reaction
Reclast was associated with signs and symptoms of an acute phase reaction: Myalgia (17.1%), fever (15.7%), fatigue (12.4%), arthralgia (11.1%), pain (10.5%), chills (9.8%), headache (9.8%), influenza-like illness (8.5%), malaise (5.2%), and back pain (3.3%), which occurred within the first 3 days following the dose of Reclast. The majority of these symptoms were mild to moderate and resolved within 3 days of the event onset but resolution could take up to 7-14 days. The incidence of these symptoms decreased with subsequent doses of Reclast.

Atrial Fibrillation
The incidence of all atrial fibrillation adverse events in the Reclast treatment group was 3.3% (5 out of 153) compared to 2.0% (3 out of 148) in the active control group. However, there were no patients with adjudicated serious adverse events of atrial fibrillation in the Reclast treatment group.

Laboratory Findings
There were no patients who had treatment emergent serum calcium levels below 7.5 mg/dL.

Injection Site Reactions
There were 4 patients (2.6%) on Reclast vs. 2 patients (1.4%) on active control with local site reactions.

Osteonecrosis of the Jaw
In this trial there were no cases of osteonecrosis of the jaw. [See Warnings and Precautions (5.4)].

Glucocorticoid-Induced Osteoporosis
The safety of Reclast in men and women in the treatment and prevention of glucocorticoid-induced osteoporosis was assessed in a randomized, multicenter, double-blind, active controlled, stratified study of 833 men and women aged 18-85 years treated with ≥7.5 mg/day oral prednisone (or equivalent). Patients were stratified according to the duration of their pre-study corticosteroid therapy: ≤3 months prior to randomization (prevention subpopulation), and >3 months prior to randomization (treatment subpopulation). The duration of the trial was one year with 416 patients exposed to Reclast administered once as a single 5 mg dose in 100 mL infused over 15 minutes, and 417 patients exposed to a commercially-available oral daily bisphosphonate

(active control) for one year. All participants received 1000 mg of elemental calcium plus 400 to 1000 IU of vitamin D supplementation per day.

The incidence of all-cause mortality was similar between treatment groups: 0.9% in the Reclast group and 0.7% in the active control group. The incidence of serious adverse events was similar between the Reclast treatment and prevention groups, 18.4% and 18.1%, respectively, and the active control treatment and prevention groups, 19.8% and 16.0%, respectively. The percentage of subjects who withdrew from the study due to adverse events was 2.2% in the Reclast group vs. 1.4% in the active control group. The overall safety and tolerability were similar between Reclast and active control groups with the exception of a higher incidence of post-dose symptoms in the Reclast group that occurred within 3 days after infusion. The overall safety and tolerability profile of Reclast in glucocorticoid-induced osteoporosis was similar to the adverse events reported in the Reclast postmenopausal osteoporosis clinical trial.

Adverse reactions reported in at least 2% of patients that were either not reported in the postmenopausal osteoporosis treatment trial or reported more frequently in the treatment and prevention of glucocorticoid-induced osteoporosis trial included the following: abdominal pain (Reclast 7.5%; active control 5.0%), and musculoskeletal pain (Reclast 3.1%; active control 1.7%). Other musculoskeletal events included back pain (Reclast 4.3%, active control 6.2%), bone pain (Reclast 3.1%, active control 2.2%), and pain in the extremity (Reclast 3.1%, active control 1.2%). In addition, the following adverse events occurred more frequently than in the postmenopausal osteoporosis trial: nausea (Reclast 9.6%; active control 8.4%), and dyspepsia (Reclast 5.5%; active control 4.3%).

Renal Impairment
Renal function measured prior to dosing and at the end of the 12 month study was comparable in the Reclast and active control groups. [See Warnings and Precautions (5.3)].

Acute Phase Reaction
Reclast was associated with signs and symptoms of a transient acute phase reaction that was similar to that seen in the Reclast postmenopausal osteoporosis clinical trial.

Atrial Fibrillation
The incidence of atrial fibrillation adverse events was 0.7% (3 of 416) in the Reclast group compared to no adverse events in the active control group. All subjects had a prior history of atrial fibrillation and no cases were adjudicated as serious adverse events. One patient had atrial flutter in the active control group.

Laboratory Findings
There were no patients who had treatment emergent serum calcium levels below 7.5 mg/dL.

Injection Site Reactions
There were no local reactions at the infusion site.

Osteonecrosis of the Jaw
In this trial there were no cases of osteonecrosis of the jaw. [See Warnings and Precautions (5.4)].

Paget's Disease of Bone
In the Paget's disease trials, two 6-month, double-blind, comparative, multinational studies of 349 men and women aged >30 years with moderate to severe disease and with confirmed Paget's disease of bone, 177 patients were exposed to Reclast and 172 patients exposed to risedronate. Reclast was administered once as a single 5 mg dose in 100 mL solution infused over at least 15 minutes. Risedronate was given as an oral daily dose of 30 mg for 2 months.

The incidence of serious adverse events was 5.1% in the Reclast group and 6.4% in the risedronate group. The percentage of patients who withdrew from the study due to adverse events was 1.7% and 1.2% for the Reclast and risedronate groups, respectively.

Adverse reactions occurring in at least 2% of the Paget's patients receiving Reclast (single 5 mg IV infusion) or risedronate (30 mg oral daily dose for 2 months) over a 6-month study period are listed by system organ class in Table 4.

Table 4. Adverse Reactions Reported in at Least 2% of Paget's Patients Receiving Reclast (Single 5 mg IV Infusion) or Risedronate (Oral 30 mg Daily for 2 Months) Over a 6-Month Follow-Up Period

System Organ Class	5 mg IV Reclast % (N=177)	30 mg/day × 2 Months risedronate % (N=172)
Infections and Infestations		
Influenza	7	5
Metabolism and Nutrition Disorders		
Hypocalcemia	3	1
Anorexia	2	2

Nervous System Disorders		
Headache	11	10
Dizziness	9	4
Lethargy	5	1
Paraesthesia	2	0
Respiratory, Thoracic and Mediastinal Disorders		
Dyspnea	5	1
Gastrointestinal Disorders		
Nausea	9	6
Diarrhea	6	6
Constipation	6	5
Dyspepsia	5	4
Abdominal Distension	2	1
Abdominal Pain	2	2
Vomiting	2	2
Abdominal Pain Upper	1	2
Skin and Subcutaneous Tissue Disorders		
Rash	3	2
Musculoskeletal, Connective Tissue and Bone Disorders		
Arthralgia	9	11
Bone Pain	9	5
Myalgia	7	4
Back Pain	4	7
Musculoskeletal Stiffness	2	1
General Disorders and Administrative Site Conditions		
Influenza-like Illness	11	6
Pyrexia	9	2
Fatigue	8	4
Rigors	8	1
Pain	5	4
Peripheral Edema	3	1
Asthenia	2	1

Laboratory Findings

In the Paget's disease trials, early, transient decreases in serum calcium and phosphate levels were observed. Approximately 21% of patients had serum calcium levels <8.4 mg/dL 9-11 days following Reclast administration.

Renal Impairment

In clinical trials in Paget's disease there were no cases of renal deterioration following a single 5 mg 15-minute infusion [*see Warnings and Precautions (5.3)*].

Acute Phase Reaction

The signs and symptoms of acute phase reaction (influenza-like illness, pyrexia, myalgia, arthralgia, and bone pain) were reported in 25% of patients in the Reclast-treated group compared to 8% in the risedronate-treated group. Symptoms usually occur within the first 3 days following Reclast administration. The majority of these symptoms resolved within 4 days of onset.

Osteonecrosis of the Jaw

Osteonecrosis of the jaw has been reported with zoledronic acid [*see Warnings and Precautions (5.4)*].

6.2 Post-Marketing Experience

Because these reactions are reported voluntarily from a population of uncertain size, it is not always possible to reliably estimate their frequency or establish a causal relationship to drug exposure.

The following adverse reactions have been identified during post approval use of Reclast:

Acute Phase Reactions

Fever, headache, flu-like symptoms, nausea, vomiting, diarrhea, arthralgia, and myalgia. Symptoms may be significant and lead to dehydration.

Acute Renal Impairment

Transient rise in serum creatinine correctable with intravenous fluids; acute renal failure requiring hospitalization and/or dialysis. Increased serum creatinine was reported in patients with underlying renal disease and 1) dehydration secondary to fever, gastrointestinal losses, diuretic therapy or 2) other risk factors such as concomitant nephrotoxic drugs in the post-infusion period.

Allergic Reactions

There have been rare reports of allergic reaction with intravenous zoledronic acid including urticaria, angioedema, and bronchoconstriction. Rare cases of anaphylactic reaction/shock have also been reported.

Other

Rare cases of the following events have been reported: hypocalcemia, hypotension in patients with underlying risk factors, osteonecrosis of the jaw, scleritis and orbital inflammation.

7 DRUG INTERACTIONS

No *in vivo* drug interaction studies have been performed for Reclast. *In vitro* and *ex vivo* studies showed low affinity of zoledronic acid for the cellular components of human blood. *In vitro* mean zoledronic acid protein binding in human plasma ranged from 28% at 200 ng/mL to 53% at 50 ng/mL. *In vivo* studies showed that zoledronic acid is not metabolized, and is excreted into the urine as the intact drug.

7.1 Aminoglycosides

Caution is advised when bisphosphonates, including zoledronic acid, are administered with aminoglycosides, since these agents may have an additive effect to lower serum calcium level for prolonged periods. This effect has not been reported in zoledronic acid clinical trials.

7.2 Loop Diuretics

Caution should also be exercised when Reclast is used in combination with loop diuretics due to an increased risk of hypocalcemia.

7.3 Nephrotoxic Drugs

Caution is indicated when Reclast is used with other potentially nephrotoxic drugs such as nonsteroidal anti-inflammatory drugs.

7.4 Drugs Primarily Excreted by the Kidney

Renal impairment has been observed following the administration of zoledronic acid in patients with pre-existing renal compromise or other risk factors [*see Warnings and Precautions (5.3)*]. In patients with renal impairment, the exposure to concomitant medications that are primarily renally excreted (e.g., digoxin) may increase. Consider monitoring serum creatinine in patients at risk for renal impairment who are taking concomitant medications that are primarily excreted by the kidney.

8 USE IN SPECIFIC POPULATIONS

8.1 Pregnancy

Pregnancy Category D [*see Warnings and Precautions (5.5)*]. RECLAST SHOULD NOT BE USED DURING PREGNANCY. If the patient becomes pregnant while taking this drug, the patient should be apprised of the potential harm to the fetus. Women of childbearing potential should be advised to avoid becoming pregnant while receiving Reclast.

Bisphosphonates are incorporated into the bone matrix, from where they are gradually released over periods of weeks to years. The extent of bisphosphonate incorporation into adult bone, and hence, the amount available for release back into the systemic circulation, is directly related to the total dose and duration of bisphosphonate use. Although there are no data on fetal risk in humans, bisphosphonates do cause fetal harm in animals, and animal data suggest that uptake of bisphosphonates into fetal bone is greater than into maternal bone. Therefore, there is a theoretical risk of fetal harm (e.g., skeletal and other abnormalities) if a woman becomes pregnant after completing a course of bisphosphonate therapy. The impact of variables such as time between cessation of bisphosphonate therapy to conception space, the particular bisphosphonate used, and the route of administration (intravenous versus oral) on this risk has not been established.

In female rats given daily subcutaneous doses of zoledronic acid beginning 15 days before mating and continuing through gestation, the number of stillbirths was increased and survival of neonates was decreased at approximately ≥0.3 times the anticipated human systemic exposure following a 5 mg intravenous dose (based on an AUC comparison). Adverse maternal effects were observed in all dose groups at ≥0.1 times the human systemic exposure following a 5 mg intravenous dose (based on an AUC comparison) and included dystocia and periparturient mortality in pregnant rats allowed to deliver. Maternal mortality was considered related to drug-induced inhibition of skeletal calcium mobilization, resulting in periparturient hypocalcemia. This appears to be a bisphosphonate class effect.

In pregnant rats given daily subcutaneous dose of zoledronic acid during gestation, adverse fetal effects were observed at about 2 and 4 times human systemic exposure following a 5 mg intravenous dose (based on an AUC comparison). These adverse effects included increases in pre- and post-implantation losses, decreases in viable fetuses, and fetal skeletal, visceral, and external malformations.

In pregnant rabbits given daily subcutaneous doses of zoledronic acid during gestation at doses ≤0.4 times the anticipated human systemic exposure following a 5 mg intravenous dose (based on a mg/m^2 comparison) no adverse fetal effects were observed. Maternal mortality and abortion occurred in all treatment groups (at doses ≥0.04 times the human 5 mg intravenous dose, based on a mg/m^2 comparison). Adverse maternal effects were associated with, and may have been caused by, drug-induced hypocalcemia [*see Nonclinical Toxicology (13.3)*].

8.3 Nursing Mothers

It is not known whether Reclast is excreted in human milk. Because many drugs are excreted in human milk, and because Reclast binds to bone long-term, Reclast should not be administered to a nursing woman.

8.4 Pediatric Use

Reclast is not indicated for use in children.

The safety and effectiveness of zoledronic acid was studied in a one-year active controlled trial of 152 pediatric subjects (74 receiving zoledronic acid). The enrolled population was subjects with severe osteogenesis imperfecta, aged 1-17 years, 55% male, 84% Caucasian, with a mean lumbar spine BMD of 0.431 gm/cm^2, which is 2.7 standard deviations below the mean for age-matched controls (BMD Z-score of -2.7). At one year, increases in BMD were observed in the zoledronic acid treatment group. However, changes in BMD in individual patients with severe osteogenesis imperfecta did not necessarily correlate with the risk for fracture or the incidence or severity of chronic bone pain. The adverse events observed with zoledronic acid use in children did not raise any new safety findings beyond those previously seen in adults treated for Paget's disease of bone and treatment of osteoporosis including osteonecrosis of the jaw (ONJ) and renal impairment. However, adverse reactions seen more commonly in pediatric patients included pyrexia (61%), arthralgia (26%), hypocalcemia (22%) and headache (22%). These reactions, excluding arthralgia, occurred most frequently within three days after the first infusion and became less common with repeat dosing. No cases of ONJ or renal impairment were observed in this study. Because of long-term retention in bone, Reclast should only be used in children if the potential benefit outweighs the potential risk.

Plasma zoledronic acid concentration data was obtained from 10 patients with severe osteogenesis imperfecta (4 in the age group of 3-8 years and 6 in the age group of 9-17 years) infused with 0.05 mg/kg dose over 30 minutes. Mean C_{max} and $AUC_{(0\text{-last})}$ was 167 ng/mL and 220 ng•h/mL respectively. The plasma concentration time profile of zoledronic acid in pediatric patients represent a multi-exponential decline, as observed in adult cancer patients at an approximately equivalent mg/kg dose.

8.5 Geriatric Use

The combined osteoporosis trials included 4863 Reclast-treated patients who were at least 65 years of age, while 2101 patients were at least 75 years old. No overall differences in efficacy or safety were observed between patients under 75 years of age with those at least 75 years of age, except that the acute phase reactions occurred less frequently in the older patients.

Of the patients receiving Reclast in the osteoporosis study in men, glucocorticoid-induced osteoporosis, and Paget's disease studies, 83, 116, and 132 patients, respectively were 65 years of age or over, while 24, 29, and 68 patients, respectively were at least 75 years of age.

However, because decreased renal function occurs more commonly in the elderly, special care should be taken to monitor renal function.

8.6 Renal Impairment

Reclast should not be used in patients with severe renal impairment (creatinine clearance <35 mL/min) due to lack of adequate clinical experience in this population. No dosage adjustment is required in patients with a creatinine clearance of ≥35 mL/min [*see Warnings and Precautions (5.3), Clinical Pharmacology (12.3)*]. Risk of renal impairment may increase with underlying renal disease and dehydration secondary to fever, gastrointestinal losses, diuretic therapy, etc. [*see Post-Marketing Experience (6.2)*].

8.7 Hepatic Impairment

Reclast is not metabolized in the liver. No clinical data are available for use of Reclast in patients with hepatic impairment.

10 OVERDOSAGE

Clinical experience with acute overdosage of zoledronic acid (Reclast) solution for intravenous infusion is limited. Patients who have received doses higher than those recommended should be carefully monitored. Overdosage may cause clinically significant renal impairment, hypocalcemia, hypophosphatemia, and hypomagnesemia. Clinically relevant reductions in serum levels of calcium, phosphorus, and magnesium should be corrected by intravenous administration of calcium gluconate, potassium or sodium phosphate, and magnesium sulfate, respectively.

Single doses of Reclast should not exceed 5 mg and the duration of the intravenous infusion should be no less than 15 minutes [*see Dosage and Administration (2)*].

11 DESCRIPTION

Reclast contains zoledronic acid, a bisphosphonic acid which is an inhibitor of osteoclastic bone resorption. Zoledronic acid is designated chemically as (1-Hydroxy-2-imidazol-1-yl-phosphonoethyl) phosphonic acid monohydrate and its structural formula is:

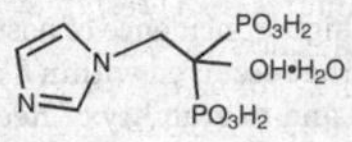

Zoledronic acid monohydrate is a white crystalline powder. Its molecular formula is $C_5H_{10}N_2O_7P_2$ • H_2O and a molar mass of 290.1 g/Mol. Zoledronic acid monohydrate is highly soluble in 0.1N sodium hydroxide solution, sparingly soluble in water and 0.1N hydrochloric acid, and practically insoluble in organic solvents. The pH of the Reclast solution for infusion is approximately 6.0-7.0.

Reclast Injection is available as a sterile solution in bottles for intravenous infusion. One bottle with 100 mL solution contains 5.330 mg of zoledronic acid monohydrate, equivalent to 5 mg zoledronic acid on an anhydrous basis.
Inactive Ingredients: 4950 mg of mannitol, USP; and 30 mg of sodium citrate, USP.

12 CLINICAL PHARMACOLOGY

12.1 Mechanism of Action

Reclast is a bisphosphonate and acts primarily on bone. It is an inhibitor of osteoclast-mediated bone resorption.
The selective action of bisphosphonates on bone is based on their high affinity for mineralized bone. Intravenously administered zoledronic acid rapidly partitions to bone and localizes preferentially at sites of high bone turnover. The main molecular target of zoledronic acid in the osteoclast is the enzyme farnesyl pyrophosphate synthase. The relatively long duration of action of zoledronic acid is attributable to its high binding affinity to bone mineral.

12.2 Pharmacodynamics

In the osteoporosis treatment trial, the effect of Reclast treatment on markers of bone resorption (serum beta-C-telopeptides (b-CTx)) and bone formation (bone specific alkaline phosphatase (BSAP)), serum N-terminal propeptide of type I collagen (P1NP)) was evaluated in patients (subsets ranging from 517 to 1246 patients) at periodic intervals. Treatment with a 5 mg annual dose of Reclast reduces bone turnover markers to the pre-menopausal range with an approximate 55% reduction in b-CTx, a 29% reduction in BSAP and a 52% reduction in P1NP over 36 months. There was no progressive reduction of bone turnover markers with repeated annual dosing.

12.3 Pharmacokinetics

Pharmacokinetic data in patients with osteoporosis and Paget's disease of bone are not available.
Distribution: Single or multiple (q 28 days) 5-minute or 15-minute infusions of 2, 4, 8 or 16 mg zoledronic acid were given to 64 patients with cancer and bone metastases. The post-infusion decline of zoledronic acid concentrations in plasma was consistent with a triphasic process showing a rapid decrease from peak concentrations at end-of-infusion to <1% of C_{max} 24 hours post infusion with population half-lives of $t_{1/2\alpha}$ 0.24 hours and $t_{1/2\beta}$ 1.87 hours for the early disposition phases of the drug. The terminal elimination phase of zoledronic acid was prolonged, with very low concentrations in plasma between Days 2 and 28 post infusion, and a terminal elimination half-life $t_{1/2\gamma}$ of 146 hours. The area under the plasma concentration versus time curve ($AUC_{0\text{-}24h}$) of zoledronic acid was dose proportional from 2 to 16 mg. The accumulation of zoledronic acid measured over three cycles was low, with mean $AUC_{0\text{-}24h}$ ratios for cycles 2 and 3 versus 1 of 1.13 ± 0.30 and 1.16 ± 0.36, respectively.
In vitro and *ex vivo* studies showed low affinity of zoledronic acid for the cellular components of human blood. *In vitro* mean zoledronic acid protein binding in human plasma ranged from 28% at 200 ng/mL to 53% at 50 ng/mL.
Metabolism: Zoledronic acid does not inhibit human P450 enzymes *in vitro*. Zoledronic acid does not undergo biotransformation *in vivo*. In animal studies, <3% of the administered intravenous dose was found in the feces, with the balance either recovered in the urine or taken up by bone, indicating that the drug is eliminated intact via the kidney. Following an intravenous dose of 20 nCi ^{14}C-zoledronic acid in a patient with cancer and bone metastases, only a single radioactive species with chromatographic properties identical to those of parent drug was recovered in urine, which suggests that zoledronic acid is not metabolized.
Excretion: In 64 patients with cancer and bone metastases on average (± s.d.) 39 ± 16% of the administered zoledronic acid dose was recovered in the urine within 24 hours, with only trace amounts of drug found in urine post Day 2. The cumulative percent of drug excreted in the urine over 0-24 hours was independent of dose. The balance of drug not recovered in urine over 0-24 hours, representing drug presumably bound to bone, is slowly released back into the systemic circulation, giving rise to the observed prolonged low plasma concentrations. The 0-24 hour renal clearance of zoledronic acid was 3.7 ± 2.0 L/h.
Zoledronic acid clearance was independent of dose but dependent upon the patient's creatinine clearance. In a study in patients with cancer and bone metastases, increasing the infusion time of a 4 mg dose of zoledronic acid from 5 minutes (n=5) to 15 minutes (n=7) resulted in a 34% decrease in the zoledronic acid concentration at the end of the infusion ([mean ± SD] 403 ± 118 ng/mL vs. 264 ± 86 ng/mL) and a 10% increase in the total AUC (378 ± 116 ng × h/mL vs. 420 ± 218 ng × h/mL). The difference between the AUC means was not statistically significant.
Special Populations
Pediatrics: Reclast is not indicated for use in children [*see Pediatric Use (8.4)*].
Geriatrics: The pharmacokinetics of zoledronic acid was not affected by age in patients with cancer and bone metastases whose age ranged from 38 years to 84 years.

Table 5. Proportion of Patients with New Morphometric Vertebral Fractures

Outcome	Reclast (%)	Placebo (%)	Absolute Reduction in Fracture Incidence % (95% CI)	Relative Reduction in Fracture Incidence % (95% CI)
At least one new vertebral fracture (0-1 year)	1.5	3.7	2.2 (1.4, 3.1)	60 (43, 72)**
At least one new vertebral fracture (0-2 years)	2.2	7.7	5.5 (4.4, 6.6)	71 (62, 78)**
At least one new vertebral fracture (0-3 years)	3.3	10.9	7.6 (6.3, 9.0)	70 (62, 76)**

** p <0.0001

Race: The pharmacokinetics of zoledronic acid was not affected by race in patients with cancer and bone metastases.
Hepatic Impairment: No clinical studies were conducted to evaluate the effect of hepatic impairment on the pharmacokinetics of zoledronic acid.
Renal Impairment: The pharmacokinetic studies conducted in 64 cancer patients represented typical clinical populations with normal to moderately-impaired renal function. Compared to patients with normal renal function (creatinine clearance >80 mL/min, N=37), patients with mild renal impairment (creatinine clearance = 50-80 mL/min, N=15) showed an average increase in plasma AUC of 15%, whereas patients with moderate renal impairment (creatinine clearance = 30-50 mL/min, N=11) showed an average increase in plasma AUC of 43%. No dosage adjustment is required in patients with a creatinine clearance of ≥35 mL/min. Reclast is not recommended for patients with severe renal impairment (creatinine clearance <35 mL/min) due to lack of clinical experience in this population [*see Warnings and Precautions (5.3), Use in Specific Populations (8.6)*].

13 NONCLINICAL TOXICOLOGY

13.1 Carcinogenesis, Mutagenesis, Impairment of Fertility

Carcinogenesis: Standard lifetime carcinogenicity bioassays were conducted in mice and rats. Mice were given daily oral doses of zoledronic acid of 0.1, 0.5, or 2.0 mg/kg/day. There was an increased incidence of Harderian gland adenomas in males and females in all treatment groups (at doses ≥0.002 times the human intravenous dose of 5 mg, based on a mg/m^2 comparison). Rats were given daily oral doses of zoledronic acid of 0.1, 0.5, or 2.0 mg/kg/day. No increased incidence of tumors was observed (at doses ≤0.1 times the human intravenous dose of 5 mg, based on a mg/m^2 comparison).
Mutagenesis: Zoledronic acid was not genotoxic in the Ames bacterial mutagenicity assay, in the Chinese hamster ovary cell assay, or in the Chinese hamster gene mutation assay, with or without metabolic activation. Zoledronic acid was not genotoxic in the *in vivo* rat micronucleus assay.
Impairment of Fertility: Female rats were given daily subcutaneous doses of zoledronic acid of 0.01, 0.03, or 0.1 mg/kg beginning 15 days before mating and continuing through gestation. Effects observed in the high-dose group (equivalent to human systemic exposure following a 5 mg intravenous dose, based on an AUC comparison) included inhibition of ovulation and a decrease in the number of pregnant rats. Effects observed in both the mid-dose group and high-dose group (0.3 to 1 times human systemic exposure following a 5 mg intravenous dose, based on an AUC comparison) included an increase in pre-implantation losses and a decrease in the number of implantations and live fetuses.

13.2 Animal Pharmacology

Bone Safety Studies: Zoledronic acid is a potent inhibitor of osteoclastic bone resorption. In the ovariectomized rat, single IV doses of zoledronic acid of 4-500 μg/kg (<0.1 to 3.5 times human exposure at the 5 mg intravenous dose, based on a mg/m^2 comparison) suppressed bone turnover and protected against trabecular bone loss, cortical thinning and the reduction in vertebral and femoral bone strength in a dose-dependent manner. At a dose equivalent to human exposure at the 5 mg intravenous dose, the effect persisted for 8 months, which corresponds to approximately 8 remodeling cycles or 3 years in humans.
In ovariectomized rats and monkeys, weekly treatment with zoledronic acid dose-dependently suppressed bone turnover and prevented the decrease in cancellous and cortical BMD and bone strength, at yearly cumulative doses up to 3.5 times the intravenous human dose of 5 mg, based on a mg/m^2 comparison. Bone tissue was normal and there was no evidence of a mineralization defect, no accumulation of osteoid, and no woven bone.

13.3 Reproductive and Developmental Toxicology

In female rats given subcutaneous doses of zoledronic acid of 0.01, 0.03, or 0.1 mg/kg/day beginning 15 days before mating and continuing through gestation, the number of stillbirths was increased and survival of neonates was decreased in the mid- and high-dose groups (≥0.3 times the anticipated human systemic exposure following a 5 mg intravenous dose, based on an AUC comparison). Adverse maternal effects were observed in all dose groups (≥0.1 times the human systemic exposure following a 5 mg intravenous dose, based on an AUC comparison) and included dystocia and periparturient mortality in pregnant rats allowed to deliver. Maternal mortality was considered related to drug-induced inhibition of skeletal calcium mobilization, resulting in periparturient hypocalcemia. This appears to be a bisphosphonate class effect.
In pregnant rats given daily subcutaneous dose of zoledronic acid of 0.1, 0.2, or 0.4 mg/kg during gestation, adverse fetal effects were observed in the mid- and high-dose groups (about 2 and 4 times human systemic exposure following a 5 mg intravenous dose, based on an AUC comparison). These adverse effects included increases in pre- and post-implantation losses, decreases in viable fetuses, and fetal skeletal, visceral, and external malformations. Fetal skeletal effects observed in the high-dose group included unossified or incompletely ossified bones, thickened, curved or shortened bones, wavy ribs, and shortened jaw. Other adverse fetal effects observed in the high-dose group included reduced lens, rudimentary cerebellum, reduction or absence of liver lobes, reduction of lung lobes, vessel dilation, cleft palate, and edema. Skeletal variations were also observed in the low-dose group (about 1.2 times the anticipated human systemic exposure, based on an AUC comparison). Signs of maternal toxicity were observed in the high-dose group and included reduced body weights and food consumption, indicating that maximal exposure levels were achieved in this study.
In pregnant rabbits given subcutaneous doses of zoledronic acid of 0.01, 0.03, or 0.1 mg/kg/day during gestation (at doses ≤0.4 times the anticipated human systemic exposure following a 5 mg intravenous dose, based on a mg/m^2 comparison) no adverse fetal effects were observed. Maternal mortality and abortion occurred in all treatment groups (at doses ≥0.04 times the human 5 mg intravenous dose, based on a mg/m^2 comparison). Adverse maternal effects were associated with, and may have been caused by, drug-induced hypocalcemia.

14 CLINICAL STUDIES

14.1 Treatment of Postmenopausal Osteoporosis

Study 1: The efficacy and safety of Reclast in the treatment of postmenopausal osteoporosis was demonstrated in Study 1, a randomized, double-blind, placebo-controlled, multinational study of 7736 women aged 65-89 years (mean age of 73) with either: a femoral neck BMD T-score less than or equal to -1.5 and at least two mild or one moderate existing vertebral fracture(s); or a femoral neck BMD T-score less than or equal to -2.5 with or without evidence of an existing vertebral fracture(s). Women were stratified into two groups: Stratum I: no concomitant use of osteoporosis therapy or Stratum II: baseline concomitant use of osteoporosis therapies which included calcitonin, raloxifene, tamoxifen, hormone replacement therapy; but excluded other bisphosphonates.
Women enrolled in Stratum I (n= 5661) were evaluated annually for incidence of vertebral fractures. All women (Strata I and II) were evaluated for the incidence of hip and other clinical fractures. Reclast was administered once a year for three consecutive years, as a single 5 mg dose in 100 mL solution infused over at least 15 minutes, for a total of three doses. All women received 1000 to 1500 mg of elemental calcium plus 400 to 1200 IU of vitamin D supplementation per day.
The two primary efficacy variables were the incidence of morphometric vertebral fractures at 3 years and the incidence of hip fractures over a median duration of 3 years. The diagnosis of an incident vertebral fracture was based on both qualitative diagnosis by the radiologist and quantitative morphometric criterion. The morphometric criterion required the dual occurrence of 2 events: a relative height ratio or relative height reduction in a vertebral body of at least 20%, together with at least a 4 mm absolute decrease in height.
Effect on Vertebral Fractures
Reclast significantly decreased the incidence of new vertebral fractures at one, two, and three years as shown in Table 5.
[See table 5 above]

Table 6. Between–Treatment Comparisons of the Incidence of Clinical Fracture Variables Over 3 Years

Outcome	Reclast (N=3875) Event Rate n (%)+	Placebo (N=3861) Event Rate n (%)+	Absolute Reduction in Fracture Incidence % (95% CI)+	Relative Risk Reduction in Fracture Incidence % (95% CI)
Any clinical fracture (1)	308 (8.4)	456 (12.8)	4.4 (3.0, 5.8)	33 (23, 42)**
Clinical vertebral fracture (2)	19 (0.5)	84 (2.6)	2.1 (1.5, 2.7)	77 (63, 86)**
Non-vertebral fracture (3)	292 (8.0)	388 (10.7)	2.7 (1.4, 4.0)	25 (13, 36)*

* p-value <0.001, **p-value <0.0001
\+ Event rates based on Kaplan-Meier estimates at 36 months
(1) Excluding finger, toe, and facial fractures
(2) Includes clinical thoracic and clinical lumbar vertebral fractures
(3) Excluding finger, toe, facial, and clinical thoracic and lumbar vertebral fractures

Table 7. Between-Treatment Comparisons of the Incidence of Key Clinical Fracture Variables

Outcome	Reclast (N=1065) Event Rate n (%)+	Placebo (N=1062) Event Rate n (%)+	Absolute Reduction in Fracture Incidence % (95% CI)+	Relative Risk Reduction in Fracture Incidence % (95% CI)
Any clinical fracture (1)	92 (8.6)	139 (13.9)	5.3 (2.3, 8.3)	35 (16, 50)**
Clinical vertebral fracture (2)	21 (1.7)	39 (3.8)	2.1 (0.5, 3.7)	46 (8, 68)*

* p-value <0.05, **p-value <0.005
\+ Event rates based on Kaplan-Meier estimates at 24 months
(1) Excluding finger, toe, and facial fractures
(2) Including clinical thoracic and clinical lumbar vertebral fractures

The reductions in vertebral fractures over three years were consistent (including new/worsening and multiple vertebral fractures) and significantly greater than placebo regardless of age, geographical region, baseline body mass index, number of baseline vertebral fractures, femoral neck BMD T-score, or prior bisphosphonate usage.

Effect on Hip Fracture over 3 years

Reclast demonstrated a 1.1% absolute reduction and 41% relative reduction in the risk of hip fractures over a median duration of follow-up of 3 years. The hip fracture event rate was 1.4% for Reclast-treated patients compared to 2.5% for placebo-treated patients.

Figure 1. Cumulative Incidence of Hip Fracture Over 3 Years

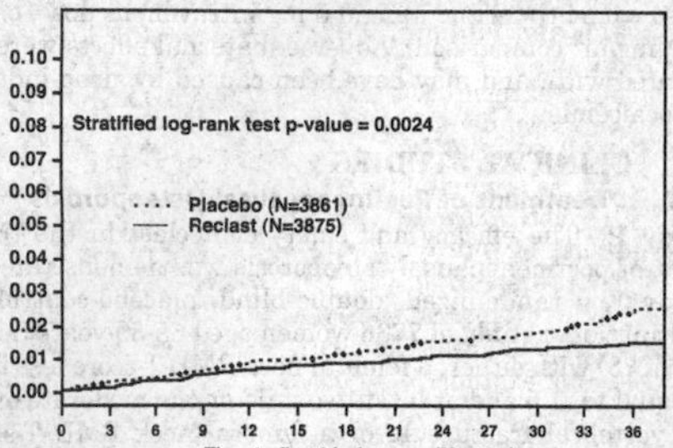

The reductions in hip fractures over three years were greater for Reclast than placebo regardless of femoral neck BMD T-score.

Effect on All Clinical Fractures

Reclast demonstrated superiority to placebo in reducing the incidence of all clinical fractures, clinical (symptomatic) vertebral and non-vertebral fractures (excluding finger, toe, facial, and clinical thoracic and lumbar vertebral fractures). All clinical fractures were verified based on the radiographic and/or clinical evidence. A summary of results is presented in Table 6.

[See table 6 above]

Effect on Bone Mineral Density (BMD)

Reclast significantly increased BMD at the lumbar spine, total hip and femoral neck, relative to treatment with placebo at time points 12, 24, and 36 months. Treatment with Reclast resulted in a 6.7% increase in BMD at the lumbar spine, 6.0% at the total hip, and 5.1% at the femoral neck, over 3 years as compared to placebo.

Bone Histology

Bone biopsy specimens were obtained between Months 33 and 36 from 82 postmenopausal patients with osteoporosis treated with 3 annual doses of Reclast. Of the biopsies obtained, 81 were adequate for qualitative histomorphometry assessment, 59 were adequate for partial quantitative histomorphometry assessment, and 38 were adequate for full quantitative histomorphometry assessment. Micro CT analysis was performed on 76 specimens. Qualitative, quantitative and micro CT assessments showed bone of normal architecture and quality without mineralization defects.

Effect on Height

In the 3-year osteoporosis study standing height was measured annually using a stadiometer. The Reclast group revealed less height loss compared to placebo (4.2 mm vs. 7.0 mm, respectively (p<0.001)).

Study 2: The efficacy and safety of Reclast in the treatment of patients with osteoporosis who suffered a recent low-trauma hip fracture was demonstrated in Study 2, a randomized, double-blind, placebo-controlled, multinational endpoint study of 2127 men and women aged 50-95 years (mean age of 74.5). Concomitant osteoporosis therapies excluding other bisphosphonates and parathyroid hormone were allowed. Reclast was administered once a year as a single 5 mg dose in 100 mL solution, infused over at least 15 minutes. The study continued until at least 211 patients had confirmed clinical fractures in the study population. Vitamin D levels were not routinely measured but a loading dose of vitamin D (50,000 to 125,000 IU orally or IM) was given to patients and they were started on 1000 to 1500 mg of elemental calcium plus 800 to 1200 IU of vitamin D supplementation per day for at least 14 days prior to the study drug infusions. The primary efficacy variable was the incidence of clinical fractures over the duration of the study.

Reclast significantly reduced the incidence of any clinical fracture by 35%. There was also a 46% reduction in the risk of a clinical vertebral fracture (Table 7).

[See table 7 above]

Effect on Bone Mineral Density (BMD)

Reclast significantly increased BMD relative to placebo at the hip and femoral neck at all timepoints (12, 24, and 36 months). Treatment with Reclast resulted in a 6.4% increase in BMD at the total hip and a 4.3% increase at the femoral neck over 36 months as compared to placebo.

14.2 Prevention of Postmenopausal Osteoporosis

The efficacy and safety of Reclast in postmenopausal women with osteopenia (low bone mass) was assessed in a 2-year randomized, multi-center, double-blind, placebo-controlled study of 581 postmenopausal women aged ≥45 years, who were stratified by years since menopause: Stratum I women <5 years from menopause (n=224); Stratum II women ≥5 years from menopause (n= 357). Patients within Stratum I and II were randomized to one of three treatment groups: (1) Reclast given at randomization and at Month 12 (n=77) in Stratum I and (n=121) in Stratum II; (2) Reclast given at randomization and placebo at Month 12 (n=70) in Stratum I and (n=111) in Stratum II; and (3) Placebo given at randomization and Month 12 (n=202). Reclast was administered as a single 5 mg dose in 100 mL solution infused over at least 15 minutes. All women received 500 to 1200 mg elemental calcium plus 400 to 800 IU vitamin D supplementation per day. The primary efficacy variable was the percent change of BMD at 24 months relative to baseline.

Effect on Bone Mineral Density (BMD)

Reclast significantly increased lumbar spine BMD relative to placebo at Month 24 across both strata. Reclast given once at randomization (and placebo given at Month 12) resulted in 4.0% increase in BMD in Stratum I patients and 4.8% increase in Stratum II patients over 24 months. Placebo given at randomization and at Month 12 resulted in 2.2% decrease in BMD in Stratum I patients and 0.7% decrease in BMD in Stratum II patients over 24 months. Therefore, Reclast given once at randomization (and placebo given at Month 12) resulted in a 6.3% increase in BMD in Stratum I patients and 5.4% increase in Stratum II patients over 24 months as compared to placebo (both p<0.0001).

Reclast also significantly increased total hip BMD relative to placebo at Month 24 across both strata. Reclast given once at randomization (and placebo given at Month 12) resulted in 2.6% increase in BMD in Stratum I patients and 2.1% in Stratum II patients over 24 months. Placebo given at randomization and at Month 12 resulted in 2.1% decrease in BMD in Stratum I patients and 1.0% decrease in BMD in Stratum II patients over 24 months. Therefore, Reclast given once at randomization (and placebo given at Month 12) resulted in a 4.7% increase in BMD in Stratum I patients and 3.2% increase in Stratum II patients over 24 months as compared to placebo (both p<0.0001).

14.3 Osteoporosis in Men

The efficacy and safety of Reclast in men with osteoporosis or significant osteoporosis secondary to hypogonadism, was assessed in a randomized, multicenter, double-blind, active controlled, study of 302 men aged 25-86 years (mean age of 64). The duration of the trial was two years. Patients were randomized to either Reclast which was administered once annually as a 5 mg dose in 100 mL infused over 15 minutes for a total of up to two doses, or to an oral weekly bisphosphonate (active control) for up to two years. All participants received 1000 mg of elemental calcium plus 800 to 1000 IU of vitamin D supplementation per day.

Effect on Bone Mineral Density (BMD)

An annual infusion of Reclast was non-inferior to the oral weekly bisphosphonate active control based on the percentage change in lumbar spine BMD at Month 24 relative to baseline (Reclast: 6.1% increase; active control: 6.2% increase).

14.4 Treatment and Prevention of Glucocorticoid-Induced Osteoporosis

The efficacy and safety of Reclast to prevent and treat glucocorticoid-induced osteoporosis (GIO) was assessed in a randomized, multicenter, double-blind, stratified, active controlled study of 833 men and women aged 18-85 years (mean age of 54.4 years) treated with ≥7.5 mg/day oral prednisone (or equivalent). Patients were stratified according to the duration of their pre-study corticosteroid therapy: ≤3 months prior to randomization (prevention subpopulation), and >3 months prior to randomization (treatment subpopulation). The duration of the trial was one year. Patients were randomized to either Reclast which was administered once as a 5 mg dose in 100 mL infused over 15 minutes, or to an oral daily bisphosphonate (active control) for one year. All participants received 1000 mg of elemental calcium plus 400 to 1000 IU of vitamin D supplementation per day.

Effect on Bone Mineral Density (BMD)

In the GIO treatment subpopulation, Reclast demonstrated a significant mean increase in lumbar spine BMD compared to the active control at one year (Reclast 4.1%, active control 2.7%) with a treatment difference of 1.4% (p<0.001). In the GIO prevention subpopulation, Reclast demonstrated a significant mean increase in lumbar spine BMD compared to active control at one year (Reclast 2.6%, active control 0.6%) with a treatment difference of 2.0% (p<0.001).

Bone Histology

Bone biopsy specimens were obtained from 23 patients (12 in the Reclast treatment group and 11 in the active control treatment group) at Month 12 treated with an annual dose of Reclast or daily oral active control. Qualitative assessments showed bone of normal architecture and quality without mineralization defects. Apparent reductions in activation frequency and remodeling rates were seen when compared with the histomorphometry results seen with Reclast in the postmenopausal osteoporosis population. The long-term consequences of this degree of suppression of bone remodeling in glucocorticoid-treated patients is unknown.

14.5 Treatment of Paget's Disease of Bone

Reclast was studied in male and female patients with moderate to severe Paget's disease of bone, defined as serum alkaline phosphatase level at least twice the upper limit of the age-specific normal reference range at the time of study entry. Diagnosis was confirmed by radiographic evidence.

The efficacy of one infusion of 5 mg Reclast vs. oral daily doses of 30 mg risedronate for 2 months was demonstrated in two identically designed 6-month randomized, double-blind trials. The mean age of patients in the two trials was 70. Ninety-three percent (93%) of patients were Caucasian. Therapeutic response was defined as either normalization of serum alkaline phosphatase (SAP) or a reduction of at least 75% from baseline in total SAP excess at the end of 6 months. SAP excess was defined as the difference between the measured level and midpoint of normal range.

In both trials Reclast demonstrated a superior and more rapid therapeutic response compared with risedronate and returned more patients to normal levels of bone turnover, as evidenced by biochemical markers of formation (SAP, serum N-terminal propeptide of type I collagen [P1NP]) and resorption (serum CTx 1 [cross-linked C-telopeptides of type I collagen] and urine α-CTx).

The 6-month combined data from both trials showed that 96% (169/176) of Reclast-treated patients achieved a therapeutic response as compared with 74% (127/171) of patients treated with risedronate. Most Reclast patients achieved a therapeutic response by the Day 63 visit. In addition, at 6 months, 89% (156/176) of Reclast-treated patients achieved normalization of SAP levels, compared to 58% (99/171) of patients treated with risedronate ($p<0.0001$) *(see Figure 2)*.

Figure 2. Therapeutic Response/Serum Alkaline Phosphatase (SAP) Normalization Over Time

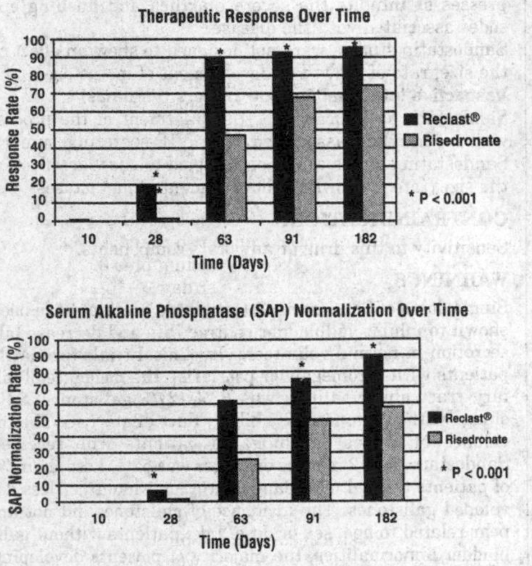

The therapeutic response to Reclast was similar across demographic and disease-severity groups defined by gender, age, previous bisphosphonate use, and disease severity. At 6 months, the percentage of Reclast-treated patients who achieved therapeutic response was 97% and 95%, respectively, in each of the baseline disease severity subgroups (baseline SAP <3×ULN, ≥3×ULN) compared to 75% and 74%, respectively, for the same disease severity subgroups of risedronate-treated patients.

In patients who had previously received treatment with oral bisphosphonates, therapeutic response rates were 96% and 55% for Reclast and risedronate, respectively. The comparatively low risedronate response was due to the low response rate (7/23, 30%) in patients previously treated with risedronate. In patients naïve to previous treatment, a greater therapeutic response was also observed with Reclast (98%) relative to risedronate (86%). In patients with symptomatic pain at screening, therapeutic response rates were 94% and 70% for Reclast and risedronate respectively. For patients without pain at screening, therapeutic response rates were 100% and 82% for Reclast and risedronate respectively.

Bone histology was evaluated in 7 patients with Paget's disease 6 months after being treated with Reclast 5 mg. Bone biopsy results showed bone of normal quality with no evidence of impaired bone remodeling and no evidence of mineralization defect.

16 HOW SUPPLIED/STORAGE AND HANDLING

Each bottle contains 5 mg/100 mL. NDC 0078-0435-61

Handling

After opening the solution, it is stable for 24 hours at 2°C-8°C (36°F-46°F).

If refrigerated, allow the refrigerated solution to reach room temperature before administration.

Storage

Store at 25°C (77°F); excursions permitted to 15°C-30°C (59°F-86°F) [see USP Controlled Room Temperature].

17 PATIENT COUNSELING INFORMATION

See FDA-Approved Patient Labeling.

Information for Patients

Patients should be made aware that Reclast contains the same active ingredient (zoledronic acid) found in Zometa®, and that patients being treated with Zometa should not be treated with Reclast.

Before being given Reclast patients should tell their doctor if they have kidney problems and what medications they are taking.

Reclast should not be given if the patient is pregnant or plans to become pregnant, or if she is breast-feeding [*see Warnings and Precautions (5.5)*].

There have been reports of bronchoconstriction in aspirin-sensitive patients receiving bisphosphonates, including Reclast. Before being given Reclast, patients should tell their doctor if they are aspirin-sensitive.

If the patient had surgery to remove some or all of the parathyroid glands in their neck, or had sections of their intestine removed, or are unable to take calcium supplements they should tell their doctor.

Reclast is given as an infusion into a vein by a nurse or a doctor, and the infusion time must not be less than 15 minutes.

On the day of treatment the patient should eat and drink normally, which includes drinking at least 2 glasses of fluid such as water within a few hours prior to the infusion, as directed by their doctor, before receiving Reclast.

After getting Reclast it is strongly recommended patients with Paget's disease take calcium in divided doses (for example, 2 to 4 times a day) for a total of 1500 mg calcium a day to prevent low blood calcium levels. This is especially important for the two weeks after getting Reclast [*see Warnings and Precautions (5.2)*].

Adequate calcium and vitamin D intake is important in patients with osteoporosis and the current recommended daily intake of calcium is 1200 mg and vitamin D is 800 IU-1000 IU daily. All patients should be instructed on the importance of calcium and vitamin D supplementation in maintaining serum calcium levels.

Patients should be aware of the most commonly associated side effects of therapy. Patients may experience one or more side effects that could include: fever, flu-like symptoms, myalgia, arthralgia, and headache. Most of these side effects occur within the first 3 days following the dose of Reclast. They usually resolve within 3 days of onset but may last for up to 7 to 14 days. Patients should consult their physician if they have questions or if these symptoms persist. The incidence of these symptoms decreased markedly with subsequent doses of Reclast.

Administration of acetaminophen following Reclast administration may reduce the incidence of these symptoms.

Physicians should inform their patients that there have been reports of persistent pain and/or a non-healing sore of the mouth or jaw, primarily in patients treated with bisphosphonates for other illnesses. If they experience these symptoms, they should inform their physician or dentist.

Severe and occasionally incapacitating bone, joint, and/or muscle pain have been infrequently reported in patients taking bisphosphonates, including Reclast. Consider withholding future Reclast treatment if severe symptoms develop.

FDA-APPROVED PATIENT LABELING

Reclast® (pronounced RE-klast)

(zoledronic acid)

Injection

> **IMPORTANT: You should not receive Reclast if you are already receiving Zometa. Reclast and Zometa are the same medicine. They both contain zoledronic acid.**

Read this leaflet carefully before your first infusion of Reclast and before each infusion. There may be new information. This leaflet does not replace talking with your healthcare professional.

What is the most important information I should know about Reclast?

Patients with severe kidney problems should not receive Reclast Injection.

Low blood calcium should be corrected prior to receiving Reclast. If you are being treated for Paget's disease of the bone it is important to take 1500 mg of calcium and 800 IU of vitamin D daily, especially during the first 2 weeks after getting Reclast. You should take calcium and vitamin D daily as recommended by your healthcare professional.

What is Reclast?

Reclast is a prescription medicine used to:

- Treat osteoporosis in women after menopause, and in patients after a recent hip fracture
- Prevent osteoporosis in women after menopause
- Increase bone mass in men with osteoporosis
- Treat and prevent osteoporosis in men and women caused by treatment with steroid medicines such as prednisone
- Treat men and women with Paget's disease of the bone

Reclast strengthens your bones by increasing bone mass and lowers the chance of breaking bones (fractures).

Who should not get Reclast?

You should not get Reclast if:

- Your blood calcium level is too low.
- You are allergic to zoledronic acid or any other ingredient in Reclast. See section "What are the ingredients in Reclast?" for a complete list of ingredients.

Talk to your healthcare provider before taking this medication if you have any of these conditions.

What should I tell my doctor before getting Reclast?

Reclast may not be right for you. Tell your doctor about all your medical conditions, including if you:

- have kidney problems
- have or have had low blood calcium
- are not able to take daily calcium and vitamin D supplements
- had parathyroid or thyroid surgery (these glands are located in your neck)
- have trouble absorbing minerals in your stomach or intestines ("malabsorption syndrome")
- had sections of your intestine removed
- have asthma (wheezing) from taking aspirin
- have a planned dental surgery such as tooth extraction
- are pregnant or plan to become pregnant; Reclast may harm your unborn baby
- are breast-feeding or planning to breast-feed. It is not known if Reclast passes into breast milk.
- have recent vomiting, diarrhea or decreased appetite

Tell your doctor about all the medicines you take, including prescription and nonprescription drugs, vitamins and minerals, and herbal supplements. Some medicines may increase your chance for low blood calcium levels or kidney problems when used with Reclast. **Especially tell your doctor if you are taking:**

- Zometa
- A diuretic or "water pill"
- Non-steroidal anti-inflammatory medicines (NSAIDs)
- An antibiotic. Certain antibiotics called aminoglycosides may increase the effect of Reclast in lowering your blood calcium for a long period of time.

Ask your healthcare provider or pharmacist to learn if your medicine is one that is listed above.

Know the medicines you take. Keep a list of your medicines and show it to your healthcare provider and pharmacist each time you get a new medicine.

How will I receive Reclast?

- Reclast is always given to you by a healthcare provider. Reclast is given by infusion into a vein (IV) that should take at least 15 minutes.
- Before you receive Reclast, drink at least 2 glasses of fluid (such as water) within a few hours as directed by your healthcare provider. You may eat normally before your infusion.

For Osteoporosis:

- To treat osteoporosis Reclast is given once a year
- To prevent osteoporosis Reclast is given once every 2 years
- In patients with osteoporosis, the current recommended daily intake of calcium is 1200 mg and vitamin D 800 IU to 1000 IU daily. If you have osteoporosis you should take calcium and vitamin D daily as recommended by your doctor.
- During treatment with Reclast, your doctor may order a bone mineral density test to check your osteoporosis.

For Paget's Disease:

- Is given as a single treatment or your doctor may choose to give you more Reclast infusions based on signs or symptoms of your disease.
- To prevent low blood calcium, it is important to take calcium and vitamin D supplements. If you have Paget's disease you should take 1500 mg of calcium a day in divided doses (for example, 750 mg two times a day, or 500 mg three times a day) and 800 IU vitamin D a day. It is especially important to take the calcium and vitamin D supplements during the first 2 weeks after getting Reclast.
- During treatment with Reclast, your doctor may order a blood test to check your Paget's disease.

What are the possible side effects of Reclast?

Reclast may cause serious side effects. Call your healthcare provider right away if you have any of these symptoms after receiving Reclast:

- **Low blood calcium (hypocalcemia).** Symptoms may include numbness or tingling feeling (especially in the area around the mouth) or muscle spasms. Call your doctor right away if you notice any of these symptoms after receiving Reclast.
- **Kidney problems.** Your doctor may do a blood test to check your kidneys before each dose of Reclast. It is important for you to drink at least 2 glasses of fluid (such as water), within a few hours before receiving Reclast, as directed by your healthcare provider.
- **Jaw-bone problems (Osteonecrosis of the jaw).** Jaw-bone problems may occur in some people and include: infection, slower healing after teeth are pulled.
- **Severe muscle, bone and joint pain.** Tell your doctor if you have severe muscle, bone, or joint pain after receiving Reclast.

The most common side effects of Reclast include: flu-like illness, fever, pain in your muscles or joints, and headache that can happen over several days after you get Reclast. Ask your healthcare provider how to lessen these symptoms. Acetaminophen (a mild pain reliever) may reduce these symptoms. The side effects lessen each time you receive Reclast.

Tell your healthcare provider about any side effect that bothers you or does not go away. These are not all the possible side effects of Reclast. If you have questions, talk to your healthcare provider.

Call your healthcare provider for medical advice about side effects. You may report side effects to FDA at 1-800-FDA-1088.

General Information about Reclast

Medicines are sometimes prescribed for conditions that are not mentioned in patient information leaflets.

This leaflet is a summary of the most important information about Reclast. If you would like more information, talk with your healthcare provider. You can ask your healthcare provider or pharmacist for information about Reclast that is written for healthcare professionals. For more information, go to www.reclast.com or call 1-866-732-5278.

What are the ingredients in Reclast?

Active ingredient: zoledronic acid. **Inactive ingredients:** mannitol, USP; sodium citrate, USP; and water for injection, USP.

What is Osteoporosis?

Osteoporosis is a disease that involves a thinning and weakening of bones. Weaker bone can break more easily. Throughout life your body keeps your bones strong and healthy by replacing old bone with new bone. In osteoporosis, however, the body removes bone faster than it is formed. This causes loss of bone mass and weakening of bones. Weak bones are more likely to break. Osteoporosis is common in women after menopause, with increasing age, and may also occur in men. People who have an increased risk of osteoporosis: 1) are Caucasian (white) or Asian; 2) are thin; 3) have a family member with osteoporosis; 4) do not get enough calcium or vitamin D; 5) do not exercise; 6) smoke or drink alcohol often or 7) take medicines that cause bone loss (like prednisone – a steroid) over a long period of time.

At first, osteoporosis usually has no symptoms, but people with osteoporosis are more likely to break (fracture) their bones. Fractures most often occur at the hip, back (spine), or wrist bones. Fractures of the spine may not be painful, but over time they can make you shorter. Over time fractures can lead to pain, severe disability, or loss of ability to move around. Reclast strengthens your bones and therefore makes them less likely to break.

What is Paget's disease of bone?

Normally bone breaks down and is replaced by new bone. In Paget's disease, bone breaks down too much and the new bone made is not normal. Bones affected by Paget's disease like the skull, spine, and legs, become deformed and weaker than normal. This can cause problems like bone pain and the bones can bend or break.

REV: JANUARY 2010   T2010-11

Manufactured by:
Novartis Pharma Stein AG
Stein, Switzerland
Distributed by:
Novartis Pharmaceuticals Corporation
East Hanover, New Jersey 07936
©Novartis
Shown in Product Identification Guide, page 315

SANDOSTATIN®   ℞

[săn-dō-stă-tĭn]
octreotide acetate
Injection
Rx Only
Prescribing Information

The following prescribing information is based on official labeling in effect July 2010.

DESCRIPTION

Sandostatin® (octreotide acetate) Injection, a cyclic octapeptide prepared as a clear sterile solution of octreotide, acetate salt, in a buffered lactic acid solution for administration by deep subcutaneous (intrafat) or intravenous injection. Octreotide acetate, known chemically as L-Cysteinamide, D-phenylalanyl-L-cysteinyl-L-phenylalanyl-D-tryptophyl-L-lysyl-L-threonyl-N-[2-hydroxy-1-(hydroxymethyl)propyl]-, cyclic (2→7)-disulfide; [R-(R*, R*)] acetate salt, is a long-acting octapeptide with pharmacologic actions mimicking those of the natural hormone somatostatin.

Sandostatin Injection is available as: sterile 1-mL ampuls in 3 strengths, containing 50, 100, or 500 mcg octreotide (as acetate), and sterile 5-mL multi-dose vials in 2 strengths, containing 200 and 1000 mcg/mL of octreotide (as acetate).

Each ampul also contains:

lactic acid, USP	3.4 mg
mannitol, USP	45 mg
sodium bicarbonate, USP	qs to pH 4.2 ± 0.3
water for injection, USP	qs to 1 mL

Each mL of the multi-dose vials also contains:

lactic acid, USP	3.4 mg
mannitol, USP	45 mg
phenol, USP	5.0 mg
sodium bicarbonate, USP	qs to pH 4.2 ± 0.3
water for injection, USP	qs to 1 mL

Lactic acid and sodium bicarbonate are added to provide a buffered solution, pH to 4.2 ± 0.3.

The molecular weight of octreotide acetate is 1019.3 (free peptide, $C_{49}H_{66}N_{10}O_{10}S_2$) and its amino acid sequence is:

H-D-Phe-Cys-Phe-D-Trp-Lys-Thr-Cys-Thr-ol,
xCH₃COOH   where x = 1.4 to 2.5

CLINICAL PHARMACOLOGY

Sandostatin® (octreotide acetate) exerts pharmacologic actions similar to the natural hormone, somatostatin. It is an even more potent inhibitor of growth hormone, glucagon, and insulin than somatostatin. Like somatostatin, it also suppresses LH response to GnRH, decreases splanchnic blood flow, and inhibits release of serotonin, gastrin, vasoactive intestinal peptide, secretin, motilin, and pancreatic polypeptide.

By virtue of these pharmacological actions, Sandostatin has been used to treat the symptoms associated with metastatic carcinoid tumors (flushing and diarrhea), and Vasoactive Intestinal Peptide (VIP) secreting adenomas (watery diarrhea).

Sandostatin substantially reduces growth hormone and/or IGF-I (somatomedin C) levels in patients with acromegaly. Single doses of Sandostatin have been shown to inhibit gallbladder contractility and to decrease bile secretion in normal volunteers. In controlled clinical trials the incidence of gallstone or biliary sludge formation was markedly increased (see WARNINGS).

Sandostatin suppresses secretion of thyroid stimulating hormone (TSH).

Pharmacokinetics

After subcutaneous injection, octreotide is absorbed rapidly and completely from the injection site. Peak concentrations of 5.2 ng/mL (100-mcg dose) were reached 0.4 hours after dosing. Using a specific radioimmunoassay, intravenous and subcutaneous doses were found to be bioequivalent. Peak concentrations and area under the curve values were dose proportional after intravenous single doses up to 200 mcg and subcutaneous single doses up to 500 mcg and after subcutaneous multiple doses up to 500 mcg t.i.d. (1500 mcg/day).

In healthy volunteers the distribution of octreotide from plasma was rapid ($t\alpha 1/2 = 0.2$ h), the volume of distribution (Vdss) was estimated to be 13.6 L, and the total body clearance ranged from 7 L/hr to 10 L/hr. In blood, the distribution into the erythrocytes was found to be negligible and about 65% was bound in the plasma in a concentration-independent manner. Binding was mainly to lipoprotein and, to a lesser extent, to albumin.

The elimination of octreotide from plasma had an apparent half-life of 1.7 to 1.9 hours compared with 1-3 minutes with the natural hormone. The duration of action of Sandostatin is variable but extends up to 12 hours depending upon the type of tumor. About 32% of the dose is excreted unchanged into the urine. In an elderly population, dose adjustments may be necessary due to a significant increase in the half-life (46%) and a significant decrease in the clearance (26%) of the drug.

In patients with acromegaly, the pharmacokinetics differ somewhat from those in healthy volunteers. A mean peak concentration of 2.8 ng/mL (100-mcg dose) was reached in 0.7 hours after subcutaneous dosing. The volume of distribution (Vdss) was estimated to be 21.6 ± 8.5 L and the total body clearance was increased to 18 L/h. The mean percent of the drug bound was 41.2%. The disposition and elimination half-lives were similar to normals.

In patients with renal impairment the elimination of octreotide from plasma was prolonged and total body clearance reduced. In mild renal impairment (Cl_{CR} 40-60 mL/min) octreotide $t_{1/2}$ was 2.4 hours and total body clearance was 8.8 L/hr, in moderate impairment (Cl_{CR} 10-39 mL/min) $t_{1/2}$ was 3.0 hours and total body clearance 7.3 L/hr, and in severely renally impaired patients not requiring dialysis (Cl_{CR} <10 mL/min) $t_{1/2}$ was 3.1 hours and total body clearance was 7.6 L/hr. In patients with severe renal failure requiring dialysis, total body clearance was reduced to about half that found in healthy subjects (from approximately 10 L/hr to 4.5 L/hr).

Patients with liver cirrhosis showed prolonged elimination of drug, with octreotide $t_{1/2}$ increasing to 3.7 hr and total body clearance decreasing to 5.9 L/hr, whereas patients with fatty liver disease showed $t_{1/2}$ increased to 3.4 hr and total body clearance of 8.2 L/hr.

INDICATIONS AND USAGE

Acromegaly

Sandostatin® (octreotide acetate) is indicated to reduce blood levels of growth hormone and IGF-I (somatomedin C) in acromegaly patients who have had inadequate response to or cannot be treated with surgical resection, pituitary irradiation, and bromocriptine mesylate at maximally tolerated doses. The goal is to achieve normalization of growth hormone and IGF-I (somatomedin C) levels (see DOSAGE AND ADMINISTRATION). In patients with acromegaly, Sandostatin reduces growth hormone to within normal ranges in 50% of patients and reduces IGF-I (somatomedin C) to within normal ranges in 50%-60% of patients. Since the effects of pituitary irradiation may not become maximal for several years, adjunctive therapy with Sandostatin to reduce blood levels of growth hormone and IGF-I (somatomedin C) offers potential benefit before the effects of irradiation are manifested.

Improvement in clinical signs and symptoms or reduction in tumor size or rate of growth were not shown in clinical trials performed with Sandostatin; these trials were not optimally designed to detect such effects.

Carcinoid Tumors

Sandostatin is indicated for the symptomatic treatment of patients with metastatic carcinoid tumors where it suppresses or inhibits the severe diarrhea and flushing episodes associated with the disease.

Sandostatin studies were not designed to show an effect on the size, rate of growth or development of metastases.

Vasoactive Intestinal Peptide Tumors (VIPomas)

Sandostatin is indicated for the treatment of the profuse watery diarrhea associated with VIP-secreting tumors. Sandostatin studies were not designed to show an effect on the size, rate of growth or development of metastases.

CONTRAINDICATIONS

Sensitivity to this drug or any of its components.

WARNINGS

Single doses of Sandostatin® (octreotide acetate) have been shown to inhibit gallbladder contractility and decrease bile secretion in normal volunteers. In clinical trials (primarily patients with acromegaly or psoriasis), the incidence of biliary tract abnormalities was 63% (27% gallstones 24% sludge without stones, 12% biliary duct dilatation). The incidence of stones or sludge in patients who received Sandostatin for 12 months or longer was 52%. Less than 2% of patients treated with Sandostatin for 1 month or less developed gallstones. The incidence of gallstones did not appear related to age, sex or dose. Like patients without gallbladder abnormalities, the majority of patients developing gallbladder abnormalities on ultrasound had gastrointestinal symptoms. The symptoms were not specific for gallbladder disease. A few patients developed acute cholecystitis, ascending cholangitis, biliary obstruction, cholestatic hepatitis, or pancreatitis during Sandostatin therapy or following its withdrawal. One patient developed ascending cholangitis during Sandostatin therapy and died.

PRECAUTIONS

General

Sandostatin® (octreotide acetate) alters the balance between the counter-regulatory hormones, insulin, glucagon and growth hormone, which may result in hypoglycemia or hyperglycemia. Sandostatin also suppresses secretion of thyroid stimulating hormone, which may result in hypothyroidism. Cardiac conduction abnormalities have also occurred during treatment with Sandostatin. However, the incidence of these adverse events during long-term therapy was determined vigorously only in acromegaly patients who, due to their underlying disease and/or the subsequent treatment they receive, are at an increased risk for the development of diabetes mellitus, hypothyroidism, and cardiovascular disease. Although the degree to which these abnormalities are related to Sandostatin therapy is not clear, new abnormalities of glycemic control, thyroid function and ECG developed during Sandostatin therapy as described below.

Risk of Pregnancy with Normalization of IGF-1 and GH

Although acromegaly may lead to infertility, there are reports of pregnancy in acromegalic women. In women with active acromegaly who have been unable to become pregnant, normalization of GH and IGF-1 may restore fertility. Female patients of childbearing potential should be advised to use adequate contraception during treatment with octreotide.

The hypoglycemia or hyperglycemia which occurs during Sandostatin therapy is usually mild, but may result in overt diabetes mellitus or necessitate dose changes in insulin or other hypoglycemic agents. Hypoglycemia and hyperglycemia occurred on Sandostatin in 3% and 16% of acromegalic patients, respectively. Severe hyperglycemia, subsequent pneumonia, and death following initiation of Sandostatin therapy was reported in one patient with no history of hyperglycemia.

In patients with concomitant Type I diabetes mellitus, Sandostatin Injection and Sandostatin LAR® Depot (octreotide acetate for injectable suspension) are likely to affect glucose regulation, and insulin requirements may be reduced. Symptomatic hypoglycemia, which may be severe, has been reported in these patients. In non-diabetics and Type II diabetics with partially intact insulin reserves,

Sandostatin Injection or Sandostatin LAR Depot administration may result in decreases in plasma insulin levels and hyperglycemia. It is therefore recommended that glucose tolerance and antidiabetic treatment be periodically monitored during therapy with these drugs.

In acromegalic patients, 12% developed biochemical hypothyroidism only, 8% developed goiter, and 4% required initiation of thyroid replacement therapy while receiving Sandostatin. Baseline and periodic assessment of thyroid function (TSH, total and/or free T_4) is recommended during chronic therapy.

In acromegalics, bradycardia (<50 bpm) developed in 25%; conduction abnormalities occurred in 10% and arrhythmias occurred in 9% of patients during Sandostatin therapy. Other EKG changes observed included QT prolongation, axis shifts, early repolarization, low voltage, R/S transition, and early R wave progression. These ECG changes are not uncommon in acromegalic patients. Dose adjustments in drugs such as beta-blockers that have bradycardia effects may be necessary. In one acromegalic patient with severe congestive heart failure, initiation of Sandostatin therapy resulted in worsening of CHF with improvement when drug was discontinued. Confirmation of a drug effect was obtained with a positive rechallenge.

Several cases of pancreatitis have been reported in patients receiving Sandostatin therapy.

Sandostatin may alter absorption of dietary fats in some patients.

In patients with severe renal failure requiring dialysis, the half-life of Sandostatin may be increased, necessitating adjustment of the maintenance dosage.

Depressed vitamin B_{12} levels and abnormal Schilling's tests have been observed in some patients receiving Sandostatin therapy, and monitoring of vitamin B_{12} levels is recommended during chronic Sandostatin therapy.

Information for Patients

Careful instruction in sterile subcutaneous injection technique should be given to the patients and to other persons who may administer Sandostatin Injection.

Laboratory Tests

Laboratory tests that may be helpful as biochemical markers in determining and following patient response depend on the specific tumor. Based on diagnosis, measurement of the following substances may be useful in monitoring the progress of therapy:

Acromegaly:	Growth Hormone, IGF-I (somatomedin C) Responsiveness to Sandostatin may be evaluated by determining growth hormone levels at 1-4 hour intervals for 8-12 hours post dose. Alternatively, a single measurement of IGF-I (somatomedin C) level may be made two weeks after drug initiation or dosage change.
Carcinoid:	5-HIAA (urinary 5-hydroxyindole acetic acid), plasma serotonin, plasma Substance P
VIPoma:	VIP (plasma vasoactive intestinal peptide)

Baseline and periodic total and/or free T_4 measurements should be performed during chronic therapy (*see PRECAUTIONS – General*).

Drug Interactions

Sandostatin has been associated with alterations in nutrient absorption, so it may have an effect on absorption of orally administered drugs. Concomitant administration of Sandostatin with cyclosporine may decrease blood levels of cyclosporine and result in transplant rejection.

Patients receiving insulin, oral hypoglycemic agents, beta blockers, calcium channel blockers, or agents to control fluid and electrolyte balance, may require dose adjustments of these therapeutic agents.

Concomitant administration of octreotide and bromocriptine increases the availability of bromocriptine. Limited published data indicate that somatostatin analogs might decrease the metabolic clearance of compounds known to be metabolized by cytochrome P450 enzymes, which may be due to the suppression of growth hormones. Since it cannot be excluded that octreotide may have this effect, other drugs mainly metabolized by CYP3A4 and which have a low therapeutic index (e.g., quinidine, terfenadine) should therefore be used with caution.

Drug Laboratory Test Interactions

No known interference exists with clinical laboratory tests, including amine or peptide determinations.

Carcinogenesis/Mutagenesis/Impairment of Fertility

Studies in laboratory animals have demonstrated no mutagenic potential of Sandostatin.

No carcinogenic potential was demonstrated in mice treated subcutaneously for 85-99 weeks at doses up to 2000 mcg/kg/day (8× the human exposure based on body surface area). In a 116-week subcutaneous study in rats, a 27% and 12% incidence of injection site sarcomas or squamous cell carcinomas was observed in males and females, respectively, at the highest dose level of 1250 mcg/kg/day (10× the human exposure based on body surface area) compared to an incidence of 8%-10% in the vehicle-control groups. The increased incidence of injection site tumors was most probably caused by irritation and the high sensitivity of the rat to repeated subcutaneous injections at the same site. Rotating injection sites would prevent chronic irritation in humans. There have been no reports of injection site tumors in patients treated with Sandostatin for up to 5 years. There was also a 15% incidence of uterine adenocarcinomas in the 1250 mcg/kg/day females compared to 7% in the saline-control females and 0% in the vehicle-control females. The presence of endometritis coupled with the absence of corpora lutea, the reduction in mammary fibroadenomas, and the presence of uterine dilatation suggest that the uterine tumors were associated with estrogen dominance in the aged female rats which does not occur in humans.

Sandostatin did not impair fertility in rats at doses up to 1000 mcg/kg/day, which represents 7× the human exposure based on body surface area.

Pregnancy Category B

There are no adequate and well-controlled studies of octreotide use in pregnant women. Reproduction studies have been performed in rats and rabbits at doses up to 16 times the highest recommended human dose based on body surface area and revealed no evidence of harm to the fetus due to octreotide. However, because animal reproduction studies are not always predictive of human response, this drug should be used during pregnancy only if clearly needed.

In postmarketing data, a limited number of exposed pregnancies have been reported in patients with acromegaly. Most women were exposed to octreotide during the first trimester of pregnancy at doses ranging from 100-300 mcg/day of Sandostatin s.c. or 20-30 mg/month of Sandostatin LAR, however some women elected to continue octreotide therapy throughout pregnancy. In cases with a known outcome, no congenital malformations were reported.

Nursing Mothers

It is not known whether octreotide is excreted into human milk. Because many drugs are excreted in human milk, caution should be exercised when octreotide is administered to a nursing woman.

Pediatric Use

Safety and efficacy of Sandostatin Injection in the pediatric population have not been demonstrated.

No formal controlled clinical trials have been performed to evaluate the safety and effectiveness of Sandostatin in pediatric under age 6 years. In post-marketing reports, serious adverse events, including hypoxia, necrotizing enterocolitis, and death, have been reported with Sandostatin use in children, most notably in children under 2 years of age. The relationship of these events to octreotide has not been established as the majority of these pediatric patients had serious underlying co-morbid conditions.

The efficacy and safety of Sandostatin using the Sandostatin LAR Depot formulation was examined in a single randomized, double-blind, placebo-controlled, six–month pharmacokinetics study in 60 pediatric patients age 6-17 years with hypothalamic obesity resulting from cranial insult. The mean octreotide concentration after 6 doses of 40 mg Sandostatin LAR Depot administered by IM injection every four weeks was approximately 3 ng/mL. Steady-state concentrations was achieved after 3 injections of a 40 mg dose. Mean BMI increased 0.1 kg/m^2 in Sandostatin LAR Depot-treated subjects compared to 0.0 kg/m^2 in saline control-treated subjects. Efficacy was not demonstrated. Diarrhea occurred in 11 of 30 (37%) patients treated with Sandostatin LAR Depot. No unexpected adverse events were observed. However, with Sandostatin LAR Depot 40 mg once a month, the incidence of new cholelithiasis in this pediatric population (33%) was higher than that seen in other adults indications such as acromegaly (22%) or malignant carcinoid syndrome (24%), where Sandostatin LAR Depot was 10 to 30 mg once a month.

Geriatric Use

Clinical studies of Sandostatin did not include sufficient numbers of subjects aged 65 and over to determine whether they respond differently from younger subjects. Other reported clinical experience has not identified differences in responses between the elderly and younger patients. In general, dose selection for an elderly patient should be cautious, usually starting at the low end of the dosing range, reflecting the greater frequency of decreased hepatic, renal, or cardiac function, and of concomitant disease or other drug therapy.

ADVERSE REACTIONS

Gallbladder Abnormalities

Gallbladder abnormalities, especially stones and/or biliary sludge, frequently develop in patients on chronic Sandostatin® (octreotide acetate) therapy (*see WARNINGS*).

Cardiac

In acromegalics, sinus bradycardia (<50 bpm) developed in 25%; conduction abnormalities occurred in 10% and arrhythmias developed in 9% of patients during Sandostatin therapy (*see PRECAUTIONS – General*).

Gastrointestinal

Diarrhea, loose stools, nausea and abdominal discomfort were each seen in 34%-61% of acromegalic patients in U.S. studies although only 2.6% of the patients discontinued therapy due to these symptoms. These symptoms were seen in 5%-10% of patients with other disorders.

The frequency of these symptoms was not dose-related, but diarrhea and abdominal discomfort generally resolved more quickly in patients treated with 300 mcg/day than in those treated with 750 mcg/day. Vomiting, flatulence, abnormal stools, abdominal distention, and constipation were each seen in less than 10% of patients.

In rare instances, gastrointestinal side effects may resemble acute intestinal obstruction, with progressive abdominal distension, severe epigastric pain, abdominal tenderness and guarding.

Hypo/Hyperglycemia

Hypoglycemia and hyperglycemia occurred in 3% and 16% of acromegalic patients, respectively, but only in about 1.5% of other patients. Symptoms of hypoglycemia were noted in approximately 2% of patients.

Hypothyroidism

In acromegalics, biochemical hypothyroidism alone occurred in 12% while goiter occurred in 6% during Sandostatin therapy (*see PRECAUTIONS – General*). In patients without acromegaly, hypothyroidism has only been reported in several isolated patients and goiter has not been reported.

Other Adverse Events

Pain on injection was reported in 7.7%, headache in 6% and dizziness in 5%. Pancreatitis was also observed (*see WARNINGS and PRECAUTIONS*).

Other Adverse Events 1%-4%

Other events (relationship to drug not established), each observed in 1%-4% of patients, included fatigue, weakness, pruritus, joint pain, backache, urinary tract infection, cold symptoms, flu symptoms, injection site hematoma, bruise, edema, flushing, blurred vision, pollakiuria, fat malabsorption, hair loss, visual disturbance and depression.

Other Adverse Events <1%

Events reported in less than 1% of patients and for which relationship to drug is not established are listed: *Gastrointestinal:* hepatitis, jaundice, increase in liver enzymes, GI bleeding, hemorrhoids, appendicitis, gastric/peptic ulcer, gallbladder polyp; *Integumentary:* rash, cellulitis, petechiae, urticaria, basal cell carcinoma; *Musculoskeletal:* arthritis, joint effusion, muscle pain, Raynaud's phenomenon; *Cardiovascular:* chest pain, shortness of breath, thrombophlebitis, ischemia, congestive heart failure, hypertension, hypertensive reaction, palpitations, orthostatic BP decrease, tachycardia; *CNS:* anxiety, libido decrease, syncope, tremor, seizure, vertigo, Bell's Palsy, paranoia, pituitary apoplexy, increased intraocular pressure, amnesia, hearing loss, neuritis; *Respiratory:* pneumonia, pulmonary nodule, status asthmaticus; *Endocrine:* galactorrhea, hypoadrenalism, diabetes insipidus, gynecomastia, amenorrhea, polymenorrhea, oligomenorrhea, vaginitis; *Urogenital:* nephrolithiasis, hematuria; *Hematologic:* anemia, iron deficiency, epistaxis; *Miscellaneous:* otitis, allergic reaction, increased CK, weight loss.

Evaluation of 20 patients treated for at least 6 months has failed to demonstrate titers of antibodies exceeding background levels. However, antibody titers to Sandostatin were subsequently reported in three patients and resulted in prolonged duration of drug action in two patients. Anaphylactoid reactions, including anaphylactic shock, have been reported in several patients receiving Sandostatin.

OVERDOSAGE

A limited number of accidental overdoses of Sandostatin® in adults have been reported. In adults, the doses ranged from 2,400-6,000 micrograms/day administered by continuous infusion (100-250 micrograms/hour) or subcutaneously (1,500 micrograms t.i.d.). Adverse events in some patients included arrhythmia, hypotension, cardiac arrest, brain hypoxia, pancreatitis, hepatitis steatosis, hepatomegaly, lactic acidosis, flushing, diarrhea, lethargy, weakness, and weight loss.

Sandostatin Injection given in intravenous boluses of 1 mg (1000 mcg) to healthy volunteers did not result in serious ill effects, nor did doses of 30 mg (30,000 mcg) given intravenously over 20 minutes and of 120 mg (120,000 mcg) given intravenously over 8 hours to research patients.

If overdose occurs, symptomatic management is indicated. Up-to-date information about the treatment of overdose can often be obtained from the National Poison Control Center at 1-800-222-1222.

Drug Abuse and Dependence

There is no indication that Sandostatin has potential for drug abuse or dependence. Sandostatin levels in the central nervous system are negligible, even after doses up to 30,000 mcg.

DOSAGE AND ADMINISTRATION

Sandostatin® (octreotide acetate) may be administered subcutaneously or intravenously. Subcutaneous injection is the usual route of administration of Sandostatin for control of symptoms. Pain with subcutaneous administration may be reduced by using the smallest volume that will deliver the desired dose. Multiple subcutaneous injections at the same site within short periods of time should be avoided. Sites should be rotated in a systematic manner.

Parenteral drug products should be inspected visually for particulate matter and discoloration prior to administration. **Do not use if particulates and/or discoloration are observed.** Proper sterile technique should be used in the preparation of parenteral admixtures to minimize the possibility of microbial contamination. **Sandostatin is not compatible in Total Parenteral Nutrition (TPN) solutions because of the formation of a glycosyl octreotide conjugate which may decrease the efficacy of the product.**

Sandostatin is stable in sterile isotonic saline solutions or sterile solutions of dextrose 5% in water for 24 hours. It may be diluted in volumes of 50-200 mL and infused intravenously over 15-30 minutes or administered by IV push over 3 minutes. In emergency situations (e.g., carcinoid crisis) it may be given by rapid bolus.

The initial dosage is usually 50 mcg administered twice or three times daily. Upward dose titration is frequently required. Dosage information for patients with specific tumors follows.

Acromegaly

Dosage may be initiated at 50 mcg t.i.d. Beginning with this low dose may permit adaptation to adverse gastrointestinal effects for patients who will require higher doses. IGF-I (somatomedin C) levels every 2 weeks can be used to guide titration. Alternatively, multiple growth hormone levels at 0-8 hours after Sandostatin® (octreotide acetate) administration permit more rapid titration of dose. The goal is to achieve growth hormone levels less than 5 ng/mL or IGF-I (somatomedin C) levels less than 1.9 U/mL in males and less than 2.2 U/mL in females. The dose most commonly found to be effective is 100 mcg t.i.d., but some patients require up to 500 mcg t.i.d. for maximum effectiveness. Doses greater than 300 mcg/day seldom result in additional biochemical benefit, and if an increase in dose fails to provide additional benefit, the dose should be reduced. IGF-I (somatomedin C) or growth hormone levels should be re-evaluated at 6-month intervals.

Sandostatin should be withdrawn yearly for approximately 4 weeks from patients who have received irradiation to assess disease activity. If growth hormone or IGF-I (somatomedin C) levels increase and signs and symptoms recur, Sandostatin therapy may be resumed.

Carcinoid Tumors

The suggested daily dosage of Sandostatin during the first 2 weeks of therapy ranges from 100-600 mcg/day in 2-4 divided doses (mean daily dosage is 300 mcg). In the clinical studies, the **median** daily maintenance dosage was approximately 450 mcg, but clinical and biochemical benefits were obtained in some patients with as little as 50 mcg, while others required doses up to 1500 mcg/day. However, experience with doses above 750 mcg/day is limited.

VIPomas

Daily dosages of 200-300 mcg in 2-4 divided doses are recommended during the initial 2 weeks of therapy (range 150-750 mcg) to control symptoms of the disease. On an individual basis, dosage may be adjusted to achieve a therapeutic response, but usually doses above 450 mcg/day are not required.

HOW SUPPLIED

Sandostatin® (octreotide acetate) Injection is available in 1-mL ampuls and 5-mL multi-dose vials as follows:

Ampuls

50 mcg/mL octreotide (as acetate)
Package of 10 ampuls .... NDC 0078-0180-01
100 mcg/mL octreotide (as acetate)
Package of 10 ampuls .... NDC 0078-0181-01
500 mcg/mL octreotide (as acetate)
Package of 10 ampuls .... NDC 0078-0182-01

Multi-Dose Vials

200 mcg/mL octreotide (as acetate)
Box of one .... NDC 0078-0183-25
1000 mcg/mL octreotide (as acetate)
Box of one .... NDC 0078-0184-25

Storage

For prolonged storage, Sandostatin ampuls and multi-dose vials should be stored at refrigerated temperatures 2°C-8°C (36°F-46°F) and store in outer carton in order to protect from light. At room temperature, (20°C-30°C or 70°F-86°F), Sandostatin is stable for 14 days if protected from light. The solution can be allowed to come to room temperature prior to administration. Do not warm artificially. After initial use, multiple-dose vials should be discarded within 14 days. Ampuls should be opened just prior to administration and the unused portion discarded. Dispose unused product or waste properly.

*Thomson Healthcare, Inc.
REV: JANUARY 2010   T2010-24

Manufactured by:
Novartis Pharma Stein AG
Stein, Switzerland
Distributed by:
Novartis Pharmaceuticals Corporation
East Hanover, NJ 07936
© Novartis
Shown in Product Identification Guide, page 315

SANDOSTATIN LAR® DEPOT   ℞

[săn-dō-stă-tĭn]
(octreotide acetate for injectable suspension)

The following prescribing information is based on official labeling in effect July 2010.

HIGHLIGHTS OF PRESCRIBING INFORMATION
These highlights do not include all the information needed to use Sandostatin LAR safely and effectively. See full prescribing information for Sandostatin LAR.
Sandostatin LAR® Depot *(octreotide acetate for injectable suspension)*
Initial U.S. Approval: 1988

————————INDICATIONS AND USAGE————————
Sandostatin LAR is a somatostatin analogue indicated for: Treatment in patients who have responded to and tolerated Sandostatin Injection subcutaneous injection for:
• Acromegaly (1.1)
• Severe diarrhea/flushing episodes associated with metastatic carcinoid tumors (1.2)
• Profuse watery diarrhea associated with VIP-secreting tumors (1.3)

————————DOSAGE AND ADMINISTRATION————————
Patients not currently receiving Sandostatin Injection subcutaneously:
• Acromegaly: 50 mcg three times daily Sandostatin Injection subcutaneously for 2 weeks followed by Sandostatin LAR 20 mg intragluteally every 4 weeks for 3 months (2.1)
• Carcinoid Tumors and VIPomas: Sandostatin Injection subcutaneously 100-600 mcg/day in 2-4 divided doses for 2 weeks followed by Sandostatin LAR 20 mg every 4 weeks for 2 months (2.2)
Patients currently receiving Sandostatin Injection subcutaneously:
• Acromegaly: 20 mg every 4 weeks for 3 months (2.1)
• Carcinoid Tumors and VIPomas: 20 mg every 4 weeks for 2 months (2.2)
Renal Impairment, patients on dialysis: 10 mg every 4 weeks (2.3)
Hepatic Impairment, patients with cirrhosis: 10 mg every 4 weeks (2.4)

————————DOSAGE FORMS AND STRENGTHS————————
Vials: 10 mg per 5 mL, 20 mg per 5 mL or 30 mg per 5 mL (3)

————————CONTRAINDICATIONS————————
None (4)

————————WARNINGS AND PRECAUTIONS————————
• Gallbladder abnormalities may occur. Monitor periodically. (5.1)
• Glucose Metabolism: Hypoglycemia or hyperglycemia may occur. Glucose monitoring is recommended and antidiabetic treatment may need adjustment. (5.2)
• Thyroid Function: Hypothyroidism may occur. Monitor thyroid levels periodically. (5.3)
• Cardiac Function: Bradycardia, arrhythmia or conduction abnormalities may occur. Use with caution in at-risk patients. (5.4)

————————ADVERSE REACTIONS————————
The most common adverse reactions, occurring in ≥20% of patients are:
• Acromegaly: diarrhea, cholelithiasis, abdominal pain, flatulence (6.1)
• Carcinoid Syndrome: back pain, fatigue, headache, abdominal pain, nausea, dizziness (6.1)
To report SUSPECTED ADVERSE REACTIONS, contact Novartis Pharmaceuticals Corporation at 1-888-669-6682 or FDA at 1-800-FDA-1088 or www.fda.gov/medwatch.

————————DRUG INTERACTIONS————————
The following drugs require monitoring and possible dose adjustment when used with Sandostatin LAR: cyclosporine, insulin, oral hypoglycemic agents, beta-blockers, bromocriptine (7)

See 17 for PATIENT COUNSELING INFORMATION
Revised: 01/2010

FULL PRESCRIBING INFORMATION: CONTENTS*

FULL PRESCRIBING INFORMATION

1   INDICATIONS AND USAGE

Sandostatin LAR Depot 10 mg, 20 mg and 30 mg is indicated in patients in whom initial treatment with Sandostatin Injection has been shown to be effective and tolerated.

1.1   Acromegaly

Long-term maintenance therapy in acromegalic patients who have had an inadequate response to surgery and/or radiotherapy, or for whom surgery and/or radiotherapy is not an option. The goal of treatment in acromegaly is to reduce GH and IGF-1 levels to normal [see *Clinical Studies (14) and Dosage and Administration (2)*].

1.2   Carcinoid Tumors

Long-term treatment of the severe diarrhea and flushing episodes associated with metastatic carcinoid tumors.

1.3   Vasoactive Intestinal Peptide Tumors (VIPomas)

Long-term treatment of the profuse watery diarrhea associated with VIP-secreting tumors.

1.4   Important Limitations of Use

In patients with carcinoid syndrome and VIPomas, the effect of Sandostatin Injection and Sandostatin LAR Depot on tumor size, rate of growth and development of metastases, has not been determined.

2   DOSAGE AND ADMINISTRATION

• Sandostatin LAR Depot should be administered by a trained health care provider. It is important to closely follow the mixing instructions included in the packaging. Sandostatin LAR Depot must be administered immediately after mixing.
• **Do not directly inject diluent without preparing suspension.**
• Sandostatin LAR Depot should be administered intragluteally at 4-week intervals. Administration of Sandostatin LAR Depot at intervals greater than 4 weeks is not recommended.
• Injection sites should be rotated in a systematic manner to avoid irritation. Deltoid injections should be avoided due to significant discomfort at the injection site when given in that area.
• **Sandostatin LAR Depot should never be administered intravenously or subcutaneously.**

The following dosage regimens are recommended.

2.1 Acromegaly

Patients Not Currently Receiving Octreotide Acetate

Patients not currently receiving octreotide acetate should begin therapy with Sandostatin Injection given subcutaneously in an initial dose of 50 mcg three times daily which may be titrated. Most patients require doses of 100 mcg to 200 mcg three times daily for maximum effect but some patients require up to 500 mcg three times daily.

Patients should be maintained on Sandostatin Injection subcutaneous for at least 2 weeks to determine tolerance to octreotide. Patients who are considered to be "responders" to the drug, based on GH and IGF-1 levels and who tolerate the drug can then be switched to Sandostatin LAR Depot in the dosage scheme described below (Patients Currently Receiving Sandostatin Injection).

Patients Currently Receiving Sandostatin Injection

Patients currently receiving Sandostatin Injection can be switched directly to Sandostatin LAR Depot in a dose of 20 mg given IM intragluteally at 4-week intervals for 3 months. After 3 months, dosage may be adjusted as follows:

- GH ≤2.5 ng/mL, IGF-1 normal and clinical symptoms controlled: maintain Sandostatin LAR Depot dosage at 20 mg every 4 weeks.
- GH >2.5 ng/mL, IGF-1 elevated, and/or clinical symptoms uncontrolled, increase Sandostatin LAR Depot dosage to 30 mg every 4 weeks.
- GH ≤1 ng/mL, IGF-1 normal and clinical symptoms controlled, reduce Sandostatin LAR Depot dosage to 10 mg every 4 weeks.
- If GH, IGF-1, or symptoms are not adequately controlled at a dose of 30 mg, the dose may be increased to 40 mg every 4 weeks. Doses higher than 40 mg are not recommended.

In patients who have received pituitary irradiation, Sandostatin LAR Depot should be withdrawn yearly for approximately 8 weeks to assess disease activity. If GH or IGF-1 levels increase and signs and symptoms recur, Sandostatin LAR Depot therapy may be resumed.

2.2 Carcinoid Tumors and VIPomas

Patients Not Currently Receiving Octreotide Acetate

Patients not currently receiving octreotide acetate should begin therapy with Sandostatin Injection given subcutaneously. The suggested daily dosage for carcinoid tumors during the first 2 weeks of therapy ranges from 100-600 mcg/day in 2-4 divided doses (mean daily dosage is 300 mcg). Some patients may require doses up to 1500 mcg/day. The suggested daily dosage for VIPomas is 200-300 mcg in 2-4 divided doses (range 150-750 mcg); dosage may be adjusted on an individual basis to control symptoms but usually doses above 450 mcg/day are not required.

Sandostatin Injection should be continued for at least 2 weeks. Thereafter, patients who are considered "responders" to octreotide acetate and who tolerate the drug may be switched to Sandostatin LAR Depot in the dosage regimen as described below (Patients Currently Receiving Sandostatin Injection).

Patients Currently Receiving Sandostatin Injection

Patients currently receiving Sandostatin Injection can be switched to Sandostatin LAR Depot in a dosage of 20 mg given IM intragluteally at 4-week intervals for 2 months. Because of the need for serum octreotide to reach therapeutically effective levels following initial injection of Sandostatin LAR Depot, carcinoid tumor and VIPoma patients should continue to receive Sandostatin Injection subcutaneously for at least 2 weeks in the same dosage they were taking before the switch. Failure to continue subcutaneous injections for this period may result in exacerbation of symptoms. (Some patients may require 3 or 4 weeks of such therapy.)

After 2 months, dosage may be adjusted as follows:

- If symptoms are adequately controlled, consider a dose reduction to 10 mg for a trial period. If symptoms recur, dosage should then be increased to 20 mg every 4 weeks. Many patients can, however, be satisfactorily maintained at a 10-mg dosage every 4 weeks.
- If symptoms are not adequately controlled, increase Sandostatin LAR Depot to 30 mg every 4 weeks if symptoms are not adequately controlled. Patients who achieve good control on a 20-mg dose may have their dose lowered to 10 mg for a trial period. If symptoms recur, dosage should then be increased to 20 mg every 4 weeks.
- Dosages higher than 30 mg are not recommended.

Despite good overall control of symptoms, patients with carcinoid tumors and VIPomas often experience periodic exacerbation of symptoms (regardless of whether they are being maintained on Sandostatin Injection or Sandostatin LAR Depot). During these periods they may be given Sandostatin Injection subcutaneously for a few days at the dosage they were receiving prior to switching to Sandostatin LAR Depot. When symptoms are again controlled, the Sandostatin Injection subcutaneous can be discontinued.

2.3 Special Populations: Renal Impairment

In patients with renal failure requiring dialysis, the starting dose should be 10 mg every 4 weeks. In other patients with renal impairment, the starting dose should be similar to a nonrenal patient (i.e., 20 mg every 4 weeks) [*see Clinical Pharmacology (12)*].

2.4 Special Populations: Hepatic Impairment – Cirrhotic Patients

In patients with established cirrhosis of the liver, the starting dose should be 10 mg every 4 weeks [*see Clinical Pharmacology (12)*].

3 DOSAGE FORMS AND STRENGTHS

Sandostatin LAR Depot is available in single-use kits containing a 5-mL vial of 10 mg, 20 mg, or 30 mg strength, a syringe containing 2.5 mL of diluent, two sterile 1½" 19 gauge needles, and two alcohol wipes. An instruction booklet for the preparation of drug suspension for injection is also included with each kit.

4 CONTRAINDICATIONS

None

5 WARNINGS AND PRECAUTIONS

5.1 Cholelithiasis and Gallbladder Sludge

Sandostatin may inhibit gallbladder contractility and decrease bile secretion, which may lead to gallbladder abnormalities or sludge. Patients should be monitored periodically [*see Adverse Reactions (6)*].

5.2 Hyperglycemia and Hypoglycemia

Octreotide alters the balance between the counter-regulatory hormones, insulin, glucagon, and growth hormone, which may result in hypoglycemia or hyperglycemia. Blood glucose levels should be monitored when Sandostatin LAR treatment is initiated, or when the dose is altered. Antidiabetic treatment should be adjusted accordingly [*see Adverse Reactions (6)*].

5.3 Thyroid Function Abnormalities

Octreotide suppresses the secretion of thyroid-stimulating hormone, which may result in hypothyroidism. Baseline and periodic assessment of thyroid function (TSH, total and/or free T_4) is recommended during chronic octreotide therapy [*see Adverse Reactions (6)*].

5.4 Cardiac Function Abnormalities

In both acromegalic and carcinoid syndrome patients, bradycardia, arrhythmias and conduction abnormalities have been reported during octreotide therapy. Other EKG changes were observed such as QT prolongation, axis shifts, early repolarization, low voltage, R/S transition, early R wave progression, and nonspecific ST-T wave changes. The relationship of these events to octreotide acetate is not established because many of these patients have underlying cardiac disease. Dose adjustments in drugs such as beta-blockers that have bradycardia effects may be necessary. In one acromegalic patient with severe congestive heart failure, initiation of Sandostatin Injection therapy resulted in worsening of CHF with improvement when drug was discontinued. Confirmation of a drug effect was obtained with a positive rechallenge [*see Adverse Reactions (6)*].

5.5 Nutrition

Octreotide may alter absorption of dietary fats.

Depressed vitamin B_{12} levels and abnormal Schilling tests have been observed in some patients receiving octreotide therapy, and monitoring of vitamin B_{12} levels is recommended during therapy with Sandostatin LAR Depot.

Octreotide has been investigated for the reduction of excessive fluid loss from the G.I. tract in patients with conditions producing such a loss. If such patients are receiving total parenteral nutrition (TPN), serum zinc may rise excessively when the fluid loss is reversed. Patients on TPN and octreotide should have periodic monitoring of zinc levels.

5.6 Monitoring: Laboratory Tests

Laboratory tests that may be helpful as biochemical markers in determining and following patient response depend on the specific tumor. Based on diagnosis, measurement of the following substances may be useful in monitoring the progress of therapy [*see Dosage and Administration (2.0)*].

Acromegaly: Growth Hormone, IGF-1 (somatomedin C)

Carcinoid: 5-HIAA (urinary 5-hydroxyindole acetic acid), plasma serotonin, plasma Substance P

VIPoma: VIP (plasma vasoactive intestinal peptide) baseline and periodic total and/or free T_4 measurements should be performed during chronic therapy

5.7 Drug Interactions

Octreotide has been associated with alterations in nutrient absorption, so it may have an effect on absorption of orally administered drugs. Concomitant administration of octreotide injection with cyclosporine may decrease blood levels of cyclosporine [*see Drug Interactions (7.2)*].

6 ADVERSE REACTIONS

6.1 Clinical Studies Experience

Because clinical trials are conducted under widely varying conditions, adverse reaction rates observed in the clinical trials of a drug cannot be directly compared to rates in the clinical trial of another drug and may not reflect the rates observed in practice.

6.1.1 Acromegaly

The safety of Sandostatin LAR in the treatment of acromegaly has been evaluated in three phase 3 studies in 261 patients, including 209 exposed for 48 weeks and 96 exposed for greater than 108 weeks. Sandostatin LAR was studied primarily in a double-blind, cross-over manner. Patients on subcutaneous Sandostatin Injection were switched to the LAR formulation followed by an open-label extension. The population age range was 14-81 years old and 53% were female. Approximately 35% of these acromegaly patients had not been treated with surgery and/or radiation. Most patients received a starting dose of 20 mg every 4 weeks intramuscularly. Dose was up or down titrated based on efficacy and tolerability to a final dose between 10-60 mg every 4 weeks. Table 1 below reflects adverse events from these studies regardless of presumed causality to study drug.

Table 1. Adverse Events Occurring in ≥10% of Acromegalic Patients in the Phase 3 Studies

WHO Preferred Term	Phase 3 Studies (Pooled) Number (%) of Subjects with AE's 10 mg/20 mg/30 mg (n=261) n (%)
Diarrhea	93 (35.6)
Abdominal Pain	75 (28.7)
Flatulence	66 (25.3)
Influenza-Like Symptoms	52 (19.9)
Constipation	46 (17.6)
Headache	40 (15.3)
Anemia	40 (15.3)
Injection Site Pain	36 (13.8)
Cholelithiasis	35 (13.4)
Hypertension	33 (12.6)
Dizziness	30 (11.5)
Fatigue	29 (11.1)

The safety of Sandostatin LAR in the treatment of acromegaly was also evaluated in a postmarketing randomized phase 4 study. 104 patients were randomized to either pituitary surgery or 20 mg of Sandostatin LAR. All the patients were treatment naïve ('de novo'). Crossover was allowed according to treatment response and a total of 76 patients were exposed to Sandostatin LAR. Approximately half of the patients initially randomized to Sandostatin LAR were exposed to Sandostatin LAR up to 1 year. The population age range was between 20-76 years old and 45% were female, 93% were Caucasian, and 1% Black. The majority of these patients were exposed to 30 mg every 4 weeks. Table 2 below reflects the adverse events occurring in this study regardless of presumed causality to study drug.

Table 2. Adverse Events Occurring in ≥10% of Acromegalic Patients in Phase 4 Study

WHO Preferred Term	Phase 4 Study SAS LAR N=76 n (%)	Phase 4 Study Surgery N=64 n (%)
Diarrhea	36 (47.4)	2 (3.1)
Cholelithiasis	29 (38.2)	3 (4.7)
Abdominal Pain	19 (25.0)	2 (3.1)
Nausea	12 (15.8)	5 (7.8)
Alopecia	10 (13.2)	5 (7.8)
Injection Site Pain	9 (11.8)	0
Abdominal Pain Upper	8 (10.5)	0
Headache	8 (10.5)	6 (9.4)
Epistaxis	0	7 (10.9)

Gallbladder Abnormalities

Single doses of Sandostatin Injection have been shown to inhibit gallbladder contractility and decrease bile secretion in normal volunteers. In clinical trials with Sandostatin Injection (primarily patients with acromegaly or psoriasis) in patients who had not previously received octreotide, the incidence of biliary tract abnormalities was 63% (27% gallstones, 24% sludge without stones, 12% biliary duct dilatation). The incidence of stones or sludge in patients who received Sandostatin Injection for 12 months or longer was 52%. The incidence of gallbladder abnormalities did not appear to be related to age, sex, or dose but was related to duration of exposure.

In clinical trials 52% of acromegalic patients, most of whom received Sandostatin LAR Depot for 12 months or longer, developed new biliary abnormalities including gallstones, microlithiasis, sediment, sludge, and dilatation. The incidence of new cholelithiasis was 22%, of which 7% were microstones.

Across all trials, a few patients developed acute cholecystitis, ascending cholangitis, biliary obstruction, cholestatic hepatitis, or pancreatitis during octreotide therapy or following its withdrawal. One patient developed ascending cholangitis during Sandostatin Injection therapy and died. Despite the high incidence of new gallstones in patients receiving octreotide, 1% of patients developed acute symptoms requiring cholecystectomy.

Glucose Metabolism – Hypoglycemia/Hyperglycemia
In acromegaly patients treated with either Sandostatin Injection or Sandostatin LAR Depot, hypoglycemia occurred in approximately 2% and hyperglycemia in approximately 15% of patients [see Warnings and Precautions (5)].

Hypothyroidism
In acromegaly patients receiving Sandostatin Injection, 12% developed biochemical hypothyroidism, 8% developed goiter, and 4% required initiation of thyroid replacement therapy while receiving Sandostatin Injection. In acromegalics treated with Sandostatin LAR Depot, hypothyroidism was reported as an adverse event in 2% and goiter in 2%. Two patients receiving Sandostatin LAR Depot required initiation of thyroid hormone replacement therapy [see Warnings and Precautions (5)].

Cardiac
In acromegalics, sinus bradycardia (<50 bpm) developed in 25%; conduction abnormalities occurred in 10% and arrhythmias developed in 9% of patients during Sandostatin Injection therapy. The relationship of these events to octreotide acetate is not established because many of these patients have underlying cardiac disease [see Warnings and Precautions (5)].

Gastrointestinal
The most common symptoms are gastrointestinal. The overall incidence of the most frequent of these symptoms in clinical trials of acromegalic patients treated for approximately 1 to 4 years is shown in Table 3.

Table 3. Number (%) of Acromegalic Patients with Common G.I. Adverse Events

Adverse Event	Sandostatin Injection S.C. Three Times Daily n=114		Sandostatin LAR Depot Every 28 Days n=261	
	n	%	n	%
Diarrhea	66	(57.9)	95	(36.4)
Abdominal Pain or Discomfort	50	(43.9)	76	(29.1)
Nausea	34	(29.8)	27	(10.3)
Flatulence	15	(13.2)	67	(25.7)
Constipation	10	(8.8)	49	(18.8)
Vomiting	5	(4.4)	17	(6.5)

Only 2.6% of the patients on Sandostatin Injection in U.S. clinical trials discontinued therapy due to these symptoms. No acromegalic patient receiving Sandostatin LAR Depot discontinued therapy for a G.I. event.

In patients receiving Sandostatin LAR Depot, the incidence of diarrhea was dose related. Diarrhea, abdominal pain, and nausea developed primarily during the first month of treatment with Sandostatin LAR Depot. Thereafter, new cases of these events were uncommon. The vast majority of these events were mild-to-moderate in severity.

In rare instances, gastrointestinal adverse effects may resemble acute intestinal obstruction, with progressive abdominal distention, severe epigastric pain, abdominal tenderness, and guarding.

Dyspepsia, steatorrhea, discoloration of feces, and tenesmus were reported in 4%-6% of patients.

In a clinical trial of carcinoid syndrome, nausea, abdominal pain, and flatulence were reported in 27%-38% and constipation or vomiting in 15%-21% of patients treated with Sandostatin LAR Depot. Diarrhea was reported as an adverse event in 14% of patients but since most of the patients had diarrhea as a symptom of carcinoid syndrome, it is difficult to assess the actual incidence of drug-related diarrhea.

Pain at the Injection Site
Pain on injection, which is generally mild-to-moderate, and short-lived (usually about 1 hour) is dose related, being reported by 2%, 9%, and 11% of acromegalics receiving doses of 10 mg, 20 mg, and 30 mg, respectively, of Sandostatin LAR Depot. In carcinoid patients, where a diary was kept, pain at the injection site was reported by about 20%-25% at a 10-mg dose and about 30%-50% at the 20-mg and 30-mg dose.

Antibodies to Octreotide
Studies to date have shown that antibodies to octreotide develop in up to 25% of patients treated with octreotide acetate. These antibodies do not influence the degree of efficacy response to octreotide; however, in two acromegalic patients who received Sandostatin Injection, the duration of GH suppression following each injection was about twice as long as in patients without antibodies. It has not been determined whether octreotide antibodies will also prolong the duration of GH suppression in patients being treated with Sandostatin LAR Depot.

6.1.2 Carcinoid and VIPomas
The safety of Sandostatin LAR in the treatment of carcinoid tumors and VIPomas has been evaluated in one phase 3 study. Study 1 randomized 93 patients with carcinoid syndrome to Sandostatin LAR 10 mg, 20 mg, or 30 mg in a blind fashion or to open-label Sandostatin Injection subcutaneously. The population age range was between 25-78 years old and 44% were female, 95% were Caucasian, and 3% Black. All the patients had symptom control on their previous Sandostatin subcutaneous treatment. 80 patients finished the initial 24 weeks of Sandostatin exposure in Study 1. In Study 1, comparable numbers of patients were randomized to each dose. Table 4 below reflects the adverse events occurring in >15% of patients regardless of presumed causality to study drug.

[See table 4 below]

Gallbladder Abnormalities
In clinical trials, 62% of malignant carcinoid patients who received Sandostatin LAR Depot for up to 18 months developed new biliary abnormalities including jaundice, gallstones, sludge, and dilatation. New gallstones occurred in a total of 24% of patients.

Glucose Metabolism – Hypoglycemia/Hyperglycemia
In carcinoid patients, hypoglycemia occurred in 4% and hyperglycemia in 27% of patients treated with Sandostatin LAR Depot [see Warnings and Precautions (5)].

Hypothyroidism
In carcinoid patients, hypothyroidism has only been reported in isolated patients and goiter has not been reported [see Warnings and Precautions (5)].

Cardiac
Electrocardiograms were performed only in carcinoid patients receiving Sandostatin LAR Depot. In carcinoid syndrome patients, sinus bradycardia developed in 19%, con-

duction abnormalities occurred in 9%, and arrhythmias developed in 3%. The relationship of these events to octreotide acetate is not established because many of these patients have underlying cardiac disease [see Warnings and Precautions (5)].

Other Clinical Studies Adverse Events
Other clinically significant adverse events (relationship to drug not established) in acromegalic and/or carcinoid syndrome patients receiving Sandostatin LAR Depot were malignant hyperpyrexia, cerebral vascular disorder, rectal bleeding, ascites, pulmonary embolism, pneumonia and pleural effusion.

6.2 Postmarketing Experience
The following adverse reactions have been identified during the postapproval use of Sandostatin. Because these reactions are reported voluntarily from a population of uncertain size, it is not always possible to reliably estimate their frequency or establish a causal relationship to drug exposure.

Myocardial infarction has been observed in the postmarketing setting, mainly in patients with cardiovascular risk factors. Hypoadrenalism has been reported in some reports in patients 18 months of age and under.

Additional events reported in the postmarketing setting include anaphylactoid reactions, including anaphylactic shock, cardiac arrest, renal failure, renal insufficiency, convulsions, atrial fibrillation, aneurysm, hepatitis, increased liver enzymes, gastrointestinal hemorrhage, pancreatitis, pancytopenia, thrombocytopenia, arterial thrombosis of the arm, retinal vein thrombosis, intracranial hemorrhage, hemiparesis, paresis, deafness, visual field defect, aphasia, scotoma, status asthmaticus, pulmonary hypertension, diabetes mellitus, intestinal obstruction, peptic/gastric ulcer, appendicitis, creatinine increased, CK increased, arthritis, joint effusion, pituitary apoplexy, breast carcinoma, suicide attempt, paranoia, migraines, urticaria, facial edema, generalized edema, hematuria, orthostatic hypotension, Raynaud's syndrome, glaucoma, pulmonary nodule, pneumothorax aggravated, cellulitis, Bell's palsy, diabetes insipidus, gynecomastia, galactorrhea, gallbladder polyp, fatty liver, abdomen enlarged, libido decrease, and petechiae.

7 DRUG INTERACTIONS
7.1 Cyclosporine
Concomitant administration of octreotide injection with cyclosporine may decrease blood levels of cyclosporine and result in transplant rejection.

7.2 Insulin and Oral Hypoglycemic Drugs
Octreotide inhibits the secretion of insulin and glucagon. Therefore, blood glucose levels should be monitored when Sandostatin LAR treatment is initiated or when the dose is altered and antidiabetic treatment should be adjusted accordingly.

7.3 Bromocriptine
Concomitant administration of octreotide and bromocriptine increases the availability of bromocriptine.

7.4 Other Concomitant Drug Therapy
Concomitant administration of bradycardia-inducing drugs (e.g., beta-blockers) may have an additive effect on the reduction of heart rate associated with octreotide. Dose adjustments of concomitant medication may be necessary. Octreotide has been associated with alterations in nutrient absorption, so it may have an effect on absorption of orally administered drugs.

7.5 Drug Metabolism Interactions
Limited published data indicate that somatostatin analogs may decrease the metabolic clearance of compounds known to be metabolized by cytochrome P450 enzymes, which may be due to the suppression of growth hormone. Since it cannot be excluded that octreotide may have this effect, other drugs mainly metabolized by CYP3A4 and which have a low therapeutic index (e.g., quinidine, terfenadine) should therefore be used with caution.

8 USE IN SPECIFIC POPULATIONS
8.1 Pregnancy
Pregnancy Category B
There are no adequate and well-controlled studies in pregnant women. Reproduction studies have been performed in rats and rabbits at doses up to 16× the highest recommended human dose and have revealed no evidence of harm to the fetus due to octreotide. However, because animal reproduction studies are not always predictive of human response, this drug should be used during pregnancy only if clearly needed [see Nonclinical Toxicology (13.2)].

8.3 Nursing Mothers
It is not known whether octreotide is excreted into human milk. Because many drugs are excreted in human milk, caution should be exercised when Sandostatin LAR Depot is administered to a nursing woman.

8.4 Pediatric Use
Safety and efficacy of Sandostatin LAR Depot in the pediatric population have not been demonstrated.

No formal controlled clinical trials have been performed to evaluate the safety and effectiveness of Sandostatin LAR

Table 4. Adverse Events Occurring in ≥15% of Carcinoid Tumor and VIPoma Patients in Study 1

WHO Preferred Term	Number (%) of Subjects with AE's (n=93)			
	Sc N=26	10 mg N=22	20 mg N=20	30 mg N=25
Abdominal Pain	8 (30.8)	8 (35.4)	2 (10.0)	5 (20.0)
Arthropathy	5 (19.2)	2 (9.1)	3 (15.0)	2 (8.0)
Back Pain	7 (26.9)	6 (27.3)	2 (10.0)	2 (8.0)
Dizziness	4 (15.4)	4 (18.2)	4 (20.0)	5 (20.0)
Fatigue	3 (11.5)	7 (31.8)	2 (10.0)	2 (8.0)
Flatulence	3 (11.5)	2 (9.1)	2 (10.0)	4 (16.0)
Generalized Pain	4 (15.4)	2 (9.1)	3 (15.0)	1 (4.0)
Headache	5 (19.2)	4 (18.2)	6 (30.0)	4 (16.0)
Musculoskeletal Pain	4 (15.4)	0	1 (5.0)	0
Myalgia	0	4 (18.2)	1 (5.0)	1 (4.0)
Nausea	8 (30.8)	9 (40.9)	6 (30.0)	6 (24.0)
Pruritus	0	4 (18.2)	0	0
Rash	1 (3.8)	0	3 (15.0)	0
Sinusitis	4 (15.4)	0	1 (5.0)	3 (12.0)
URTI	6 (23.1)	4 (18.2)	2 (10.0)	3 (12.0)
Vomiting	3 (11.5)	0	0	4 (16.0)

Depot in pediatric under 6 years of age. In post-marketing reports, serious adverse events, including hypoxia, necrotizing enterocolitis, and death, have been reported with Sandostatin use in children, most notably in children under 2 years of age. The relationship of these events to octreotide has not been established as the majority of these pediatric patients had serious underlying co-morbid conditions.

The efficacy and safety of Sandostatin LAR Depot was examined in a single randomized, double-blind, placebo-controlled, six-month pharmacokinetics study in 60 pediatric patients age 6-17 years with hypothalamic obesity resulting from cranial insult. The mean octreotide concentration after 6 doses of 40 mg Sandostatin LAR Depot administered by IM injection every four weeks was approximately 3 ng/mL. Steady-state concentrations was achieved after 3 injections of a 40 mg dose. Mean BMI increased 0.1 kg/m^2 in Sandostatin LAR Depot-treated subjects compared to 0.0 kg/m^2 in saline control-treated subjects. Efficacy was not demonstrated. Diarrhea occurred in 11 of 30 (37%) patients treated with Sandostatin LAR Depot. No unexpected adverse events were observed. However, with Sandostatin LAR Depot 40 mg once a month, the incidence of new cholelithiasis in this pediatric population (33%) was higher than that seen in other adults indications such as acromegaly (22%) or malignant carcinoid syndrome (24%), where Sandostatin LAR Depot was 10 to 30 mg once a month.

8.5 Geriatric Use

Clinical studies of Sandostatin did not include sufficient numbers of subjects age 65 and over to determine whether they respond differently from younger subjects. Other reported clinical experience has not identified differences in responses between the elderly and younger patients. In general, dose selection for an elderly patient should be cautious, usually starting at the low end of the dosing range, reflecting the greater frequency of decreased hepatic, renal, or cardiac function, and of concomitant disease or other drug therapy.

8.6 Renal Impairment

In patients with renal failure requiring dialysis, the starting dose should be 10 mg. This dose should be up titrated based on clinical response and speed of response as deemed necessary by the physician. In patients with mild, moderate, or severe renal impairment there is no need to adjust the starting dose of Sandostatin. The maintenance dose should be adjusted thereafter based on clinical response and tolerability as in nonrenal patients [see Clinical Pharmacology (12)].

8.7 Hepatic Impairment – Cirrhotic Patients

In patients with established liver cirrhosis, the starting dose should be 10 mg. This dose should be up titrated based on clinical response and speed of response as deemed necessary by the physician. Once at a higher dose, patient should be maintained or dose adjusted based on response and tolerability as in any noncirrhotic patients [see Clinical Pharmacology (12)].

10 OVERDOSAGE

No frank overdose has occurred in any patient to date. Sandostatin Injection given in intravenous bolus doses of 1 mg (1000 mcg) to healthy volunteers did not result in serious ill effects, nor did doses of 30 mg (30,000 mcg) given intravenously over 20 minutes and of 120 mg (120,000 mcg) given intravenously over 8 hours to research patients. Doses of 2.5 mg (2500 mcg) of Sandostatin Injection subcutaneously have, however, caused hypoglycemia, flushing, dizziness, and nausea.

Up-to-date information about the treatment of overdose can often be obtained from a certified Regional Poison Control Center. Telephone numbers of certified Regional Poison Control Centers are listed in the Physicians' Desk Reference®**.

Mortality occurred in mice and rats given 72 mg/kg and 18 mg/kg intravenously, respectively, of octreotide.

11 DESCRIPTION

Octreotide is the acetate salt of a cyclic octapeptide. It is a long-acting octapeptide with pharmacologic properties mimicking those of the natural hormone somatostatin. Octreotide is known chemically as L-Cysteinamide, D-phenylalanyl-L-cysteinyl-L-phenylalanyl-D-tryptophyl-L-lysyl-L-threonyl-N-[2-hydroxy-1-(hydroxy-methyl) propyl]-, cyclic (2→7)-disulfide; [R-(R*,R*)].

Sandostatin LAR Depot is available in a vial containing the sterile drug product, which when mixed with diluent, becomes a suspension that is given as a monthly intragluteal injection. The octreotide is uniformly distributed within the microspheres which are made of a biodegradable glucose star polymer, D,L-lactic and glycolic acids copolymer. Sterile mannitol is added to the microspheres to improve suspendability.

Sandostatin LAR Depot is available as: sterile 5-mL vials in 3 strengths delivering 10 mg, 20 mg, or 30 mg octreotide-free peptide. Each vial of Sandostatin LAR Depot delivers:

Name of Ingredient	10 mg	20 mg	30 mg
octreotide acetate	11.2 mg*	22.4 mg*	33.6 mg*
D,L-lactic and glycolic acids copolymer	188.8 mg	377.6 mg	566.4 mg
mannitol	41.0 mg	81.9 mg	122.9 mg

* Equivalent to 10/20/30 mg octreotide base.

[See table above]

Each syringe of diluent contains:

carboxymethylcellulose sodium	12.5 mg
mannitol	15.0 mg
water for injection	2.5 mL

The molecular weight of octreotide is 1019.3 (free peptide, $C_{49}H_{66}N_{10}O_{10}S_2$) and its amino acid sequence is

H-D-Phe-Cys-Phe-D-Trp-Lys-Thr-Cys-Thr-ol•xCH$_3$COOH
where x = 1.4 to 2.5

12 CLINICAL PHARMACOLOGY

Sandostatin LAR Depot is a long-acting dosage form consisting of microspheres of the biodegradable glucose star polymer, D,L-lactic and glycolic acids copolymer, containing octreotide. It maintains all of the clinical and pharmacological characteristics of the immediate-release dosage form Sandostatin Injection with the added feature of slow release of octreotide from the site of injection, reducing the need for frequent administration. This slow release occurs as the polymer biodegrades, primarily through hydrolysis. Sandostatin LAR Depot is designed to be injected intramuscularly (intragluteally) once every 4 weeks.

12.1 Mechanism of Action

Octreotide exerts pharmacologic actions similar to the natural hormone, somatostatin. It is an even more potent inhibitor of growth hormone, glucagon, and insulin than somatostatin. Like somatostatin, it also suppresses LH response to GnRH, decreases splanchnic blood flow, and inhibits release of serotonin, gastrin, vasoactive intestinal peptide, secretin, motilin, and pancreatic polypeptide.

By virtue of these pharmacological actions, octreotide has been used to treat the symptoms associated with metastatic carcinoid tumors (flushing and diarrhea), and Vasoactive Intestinal Peptide (VIP) secreting adenomas (watery diarrhea).

12.2 Pharmacodynamics

Octreotide substantially reduces and in many cases can normalize growth hormone and/or IGF-1 (somatomedin C) levels in patients with acromegaly.

Single doses of Sandostatin Injection given subcutaneously have been shown to inhibit gallbladder contractility and to decrease bile secretion in normal volunteers. In controlled clinical trials, the incidence of gallstone or biliary sludge formation was markedly increased [see Warnings and Precautions (5)].

Octreotide may cause clinically significant suppression of thyroid-stimulating hormone (TSH).

12.3 Pharmacokinetics

Sandostatin Injection

According to data obtained with the immediate-release formulation, Sandostatin Injection solution, after subcutaneous injection, octreotide is absorbed rapidly and completely from the injection site. Peak concentrations of 5.2 ng/mL (100-mcg dose) were reached 0.4 hours after dosing. Using a specific radioimmunoassay, intravenous and subcutaneous doses were found to be bioequivalent. Peak concentrations and area-under-the-curve values were dose proportional both after subcutaneous or intravenous single doses up to 400 mcg and with multiple doses of 200 mcg three times daily (600 mcg/day). Clearance was reduced by about 66% suggesting nonlinear kinetics of the drug at daily doses of 600 mcg/day compared to 150 mcg/day. The relative decrease in clearance with doses above 600 mcg/day is not defined.

In healthy volunteers, the distribution of octreotide from plasma was rapid (t$\alpha_{1/2}$ = 0.2 h), the volume of distribution (Vdss) was estimated to be 13.6 L and the total body clearance was 10 L/h.

In blood, the distribution of octreotide into the erythrocytes was found to be negligible and about 65% was bound in the plasma in a concentration-independent manner. Binding was mainly to lipoprotein and, to a lesser extent, to albumin.

The elimination of octreotide from plasma had an apparent half-life of 1.7 hours, compared with the 1-3 minutes with the natural hormone, somatostatin. The duration of action of subcutaneously administered Sandostatin Injection solution is variable but extends up to 12 hours depending upon the type of tumor, necessitating multiple daily dosing with this immediate-release dosage form. About 32% of the dose is excreted unchanged into the urine. In an elderly popula-

tion, dose adjustments may be necessary due to a significant increase in the half-life (46%) and a significant decrease in the clearance (26%) of the drug.

In patients with acromegaly, the pharmacokinetics differ somewhat from those in healthy volunteers. A mean peak concentration of 2.8 ng/mL (100-mcg dose) was reached in 0.7 hours after subcutaneous dosing. The volume of distribution (Vdss) was estimated to be 21.6 ± 8.5 L and the total body clearance was increased to 18 L/h. The mean percent of the drug bound was 41.2%. The disposition and elimination half-lives were similar to normals.

The half-life in renal-impaired patients was slightly longer than normal subjects (2.4-3.1 h versus 1.9 h). The clearance in renal-impaired patients was 7.3-8.8 L/h as compared to 8.3 L/h in healthy subjects. In patients with severe renal failure requiring dialysis, clearance was reduced to about half that found in healthy subjects (from approximately 10 L/h to 4.5 L/h).

Patients with liver cirrhosis showed prolonged elimination of drug, with octreotide half-life increasing to 3.7 h and total body clearance decreasing to 5.9 L/h, whereas patients with fatty liver disease showed half-life increasing to 3.4 h and total body clearance of 8.4 L/h. In normal subjects, octreotide half-life is 1.9 h and the clearance is 8.3 L/h which is comparable with the clearance in fatty-liver patients.

Sandostatin LAR Depot

The magnitude and duration of octreotide serum concentrations after an intramuscular injection of the long-acting depot formulation Sandostatin LAR Depot reflect the release of drug from the microsphere polymer matrix. Drug release is governed by the slow biodegration of the microspheres in the muscle, but once present in the systemic circulation, octreotide distributes and is eliminated according to its known pharmacokinetic properties which are as follows.

After a single IM injection of the long-acting depot dosage form Sandostatin LAR Depot in healthy volunteer subjects, the serum octreotide concentration reached a transient initial peak of about 0.03 ng/mL/mg within 1 hour after administration progressively declining over the following 3-5 days to a nadir of <0.01 ng/mL/mg, then slowly increasing and reaching a plateau about 2-3 weeks postinjection. Plateau concentrations were maintained over a period of nearly 2-3 weeks, showing dose proportional peak concentrations of about 0.07 ng/mL/mg. After about 6 weeks postinjection, octreotide concentration slowly decreased, to <0.01 ng/mL/mg by Weeks 12 to 13, concomitant with the terminal degradation phase of the polymer matrix of the dosage form. The relative bioavailability of the long-acting release Sandostatin LAR Depot compared to immediate-release Sandostatin Injection solution given subcutaneously was 60%-63%.

In patients with acromegaly, the octreotide concentrations after single doses of 10 mg, 20 mg, and 30 mg Sandostatin LAR Depot were dose proportional. The transient Day 1 peak, amounting to 0.3 ng/mL, 0.8 ng/mL, and 1.3 ng/mL, respectively, was followed by plateau concentrations of 0.5 ng/mL, 1.3 ng/mL, and 2.0 ng/mL, respectively, achieved about 3 weeks postinjection. These plateau concentrations were maintained for nearly 2 weeks.

Following multiple doses of Sandostatin LAR Depot given every 4 weeks, steady-state octreotide serum concentrations were achieved after the third injection. Concentrations were dose proportional and higher by a factor of approximately 1.6 to 2.0 compared to the concentrations after a single dose. The steady-state octreotide concentrations were 1.2 ng/mL and 2.1 ng/mL, respectively, at trough and 1.6 ng/mL and 2.6 ng/mL, respectively, at peak with 20 mg and 30 mg Sandostatin LAR Depot given every 4 weeks. No accumulation of octreotide beyond that expected from the overlapping release profiles occurred over a duration of up to 28 monthly injections of Sandostatin LAR Depot. With the long-acting depot formulation Sandostatin LAR Depot administered IM every 4 weeks the peak-to-trough variation in octreotide concentrations ranged from 44%-68%, compared to the 163%-209% variation encountered with the daily subcutaneous three times daily regimen of Sandostatin Injection solution.

In patients with carcinoid tumors, the mean octreotide concentrations after 6 doses of 10 mg, 20 mg, and 30 mg Sandostatin LAR Depot administered by IM injection every 4 weeks were 1.2 ng/mL, 2.5 ng/mL, and 4.2 ng/mL, respectively. Concentrations were dose proportional and steady-state concentrations were reached after 2 injections of 20 mg and 30 mg and after 3 injections of 10 mg.

Table 5. Hormonal Response in Acromegalic Patients Receiving 27 to 28 Injections During[1] Treatment with Sandostatin LAR Depot

Mean Hormone Level	Sandostatin Injection S.C.		Sandostatin LAR Depot	
	n	%	n	%
GH <5.0 ng/mL	69/88	78	73/88	83
<2.5 ng/mL	44/88	50	41/88	47
<1.0 ng/mL	6/88	7	10/88	11
IGF-1 normalized	36/88	41	45/88	51
GH <5.0 ng/mL + IGF-1 normalized	36/88	41	45/88	51
<2.5 ng/mL + IGF-1 normalized	30/88	34	37/88	42
<1.0 ng/mL + IGF-1 normalized	5/88	6	10/88	11

[1]Average of monthly levels of GH and IGF-1 over the course of the trials

Table 6. Hormonal Response in Acromegalic Patients Receiving 12 Injections During[1] Treatment with Sandostatin LAR Depot

Mean Hormone Level	Sandostatin Injection S.C.		Sandostatin LAR Depot	
	n	%	n	%
GH <5.0 ng/mL	116/122	95	118/122	97
<2.5 ng/mL	84/122	69	80/122	66
<1.0 ng/mL	25/122	21	28/122	23
IGF-1 normalized	82/122	67	82/122	67
GH <5.0 ng/mL + IGF-1 normalized	80/122	66	82/122	67
<2.5 ng/mL + IGF-1 normalized	65/122	53	70/122	57
<1.0 ng/mL + IGF-1 normalized	23/122	19	27/122	22

[1]Average of monthly levels of GH and IGF-1 over the course of the trial

Table 7. Average No. of Daily Stools and Flushing Episodes in Patients with Malignant Carcinoid Syndrome

Treatment		Daily Stools (Average No.)		Daily Flushing Episodes (Average No.)	
	n	Baseline	Last Visit	Baseline	Last Visit
Sandostatin Injection S.C.	26	3.7	2.6	3.0	0.5
Sandostatin LAR Depot					
10 mg	22	4.6	2.8	3.0	0.9
20 mg	20	4.0	2.1	5.9	0.6
30 mg	24	4.9	2.8	6.1	1.0

Sandostatin LAR Depot has not been studied in patients with renal impairment.
Sandostatin LAR Depot has not been studied in patients with hepatic impairment.

13 NONCLINICAL TOXICOLOGY

13.1 Carcinogenesis, Mutagenesis, Impairment of Fertility

Studies in laboratory animals have demonstrated no mutagenic potential of Sandostatin. No mutagenic potential of the polymeric carrier in Sandostatin LAR Depot, D,L-lactic and glycolic acids copolymer, was observed in the Ames mutagenicity test.

No carcinogenic potential was demonstrated in mice treated subcutaneously with octreotide for 85-99 weeks at doses up to 2000 mcg/kg/day (8× the human exposure based on body surface area). In a 116-week subcutaneous study in rats administered octreotide, a 27% and 12% incidence of injection site sarcomas or squamous cell carcinomas was observed in males and females, respectively, at the highest dose level of 1250 mcg/kg/day (10× the human exposure based on body surface area) compared to an incidence of 8%-10% in the vehicle-control groups. The increased incidence of injection site tumors was most probably caused by irritation and the high sensitivity of the rat to repeated subcutaneous injections at the same site. Rotating injection sites would prevent chronic irritation in humans. There have been no reports of injection site tumors in patients treated with Sandostatin Injection for at least 5 years. There was also a 15% incidence of uterine adenocarcinomas in the 1250 mcg/kg/day females compared to 7% in the saline-control females and 0% in the vehicle-control females. The presence of endometritis coupled with the absence of corpora lutea, the reduction in mammary fibroadenomas, and the presence of uterine dilatation suggest that the uterine tumors were associated with estrogen dominance in the aged female rats which does not occur in humans.

Octreotide did not impair fertility in rats at doses up to 1000 mcg/kg/day, which represents 7× the human exposure based on body surface area.

13.2 Reproductive Toxicology Studies

Reproduction studies have been performed in rats and rabbits at doses up to 16× the highest recommended human dose based on body surface area and have revealed no evidence of harm to the fetus due to octreotide.

14 CLINICAL STUDIES

14.1 Acromegaly

The clinical trials of Sandostatin LAR Depot were performed in patients who had been receiving Sandostatin Injection for a period of weeks to as long as 10 years. The acromegaly studies with Sandostatin LAR Depot described below were performed in patients who achieved GH levels of <10 ng/mL (and, in most cases <5 ng/mL) while on subcutaneous Sandostatin Injection. However, some patients enrolled were partial responders to subcutaneous Sandostatin Injection, i.e., GH levels were reduced by >50% on subcutaneous Sandostatin Injection compared to the untreated state, although not suppressed to <5 ng/mL.

Sandostatin LAR Depot was evaluated in three clinical trials in acromegalic patients.

In two of the clinical trials, a total of 101 patients were entered who had, in most cases, achieved a GH level <5 ng/mL on Sandostatin Injection given in doses of 100 mcg or 200 mcg three times daily. Most patients were switched to 20 mg or 30 mg doses of Sandostatin LAR Depot given once every 4 weeks for up to 27 to 28 injections. A few patients received doses of 10 mg and a few required doses of 40 mg. Growth hormone and IGF-1 levels were at least as well controlled with Sandostatin LAR Depot as they had been on Sandostatin Injection and this level of control remained for the entire duration of the trials.

A third trial was a 12-month study that enrolled 151 patients who had a GH level <10 ng/mL after treatment with Sandostatin Injection (most had levels <5 ng/mL). The starting dose of Sandostatin LAR Depot was 20 mg every 4 weeks for 3 doses. Thereafter, patients received 10 mg, 20 mg or 30 mg every 4 weeks, depending upon the degree of GH suppression [see Dosage and Administration (2)]. Growth hormone and IGF-1 were at least as well controlled on Sandostatin LAR Depot as they had been on Sandostatin Injection.

Table 5 summarizes the data on hormonal control (GH and IGF-1) for those patients in the first two clinical trials who received all 27 to 28 injections of Sandostatin LAR Depot.
[See table 5 above]

For the 88 patients in Table 5, a mean GH level of <2.5 ng/mL was observed in 47% receiving Sandostatin LAR Depot. Over the course of the trials, 42% of patients maintained mean growth hormone levels of <2.5 ng/mL and mean normal IGF-1 levels.

Table 6 summarizes the data on hormonal control (GH and IGF-1) for those patients in the third clinical trial who received all 12 injections of Sandostatin LAR Depot.
[See table 6 at left]

For the 122 patients in Table 6, who received all 12 injections in the third trial, a mean GH level of <2.5 ng/mL was observed in 66% receiving Sandostatin LAR Depot. Over the course of the trial, 57% of patients maintained mean growth hormone levels of <2.5 ng/mL and mean normal IGF-1 levels. In comparing the hormonal response in these trials, note that a higher percentage of patients in the third trial suppressed their mean GH to <5 ng/mL on subcutaneous Sandostatin Injection, 95%, compared to 78% across the two previous trials.

In all three trials, GH, IGF-1, and clinical symptoms were similarly controlled on Sandostatin LAR Depot as they had been on Sandostatin Injection.

Of the 25 patients who completed the trials and were partial responders to Sandostatin Injection (GH >5.0 ng/mL but reduced by >50% relative to untreated levels), 1 patient (4%) responded to Sandostatin LAR Depot with a reduction of GH to <2.5 ng/mL and 8 patients (32%) responded with a reduction of GH to <5.0 ng/mL.

Two open-label clinical studies investigated a 48-week treatment with Sandostatin LAR Depot in 143 untreated (de novo) acromegalic patients. The median reduction in tumor volume was 20.6% in Study 1 (49 patients) at 24 weeks and 24.5% in Study 2 (94 patients) at 24 weeks and 36.2% at 48 weeks.

14.2 Carcinoid Syndrome

A 6-month clinical trial of malignant carcinoid syndrome was performed in 93 patients who had previously been shown to be responsive to Sandostatin Injection. 67 patients were randomized at baseline to receive, double-blind, doses of 10 mg, 20 mg or 30 mg Sandostatin LAR Depot every 28 days and 26 patients continued, unblinded, on their previous Sandostatin Injection regimen (100-300 mcg three times daily).

In any given month after steady-state levels of octreotide were reached, approximately 35%-40% of the patients who received Sandostatin LAR Depot required supplemental subcutaneous Sandostatin Injection therapy usually for a few days, to control exacerbation of carcinoid symptoms. In any given month, the percentage of patients randomized to subcutaneous Sandostatin Injection who required supplemental treatment with an increased dose of Sandostatin Injection was similar to the percentage of patients randomized to Sandostatin LAR Depot. Over the 6-month treatment period, approximately 50%-70% of patients who completed the trial on Sandostatin LAR Depot required subcutaneous Sandostatin Injection supplemental therapy to control exacerbation of carcinoid symptoms although steady-state serum Sandostatin LAR Depot levels had been reached.

Table 7 presents the average number of daily stools and flushing episodes in malignant carcinoid patients.
[See table 7 at left]

Overall, mean daily stool frequency was as well controlled on Sandostatin LAR Depot as on Sandostatin Injection (approximately 2-2.5 stools/day).

Mean daily flushing episodes were similar at all doses of Sandostatin LAR Depot and on Sandostatin Injection (approximately 0.5-1 episode/day).

In a subset of patients with variable severity of disease, median 24 hour urinary 5-HIAA (5-hydroxyindole acetic acid) levels were reduced by 38%-50% in the groups randomized to Sandostatin LAR Depot.

The reductions are within the range reported in the published literature for patients treated with octreotide (about 10%-50%).

78 patients with malignant carcinoid syndrome who had participated in this 6-month trial, subsequently participated in a 12-month extension study in which they received 12 injections of Sandostatin LAR Depot at 4-week intervals. For those who remained in the extension trial, diarrhea and flushing were as well controlled as during the 6-month trial. Because malignant carcinoid disease is progressive, as expected, a number of deaths (8 patients: 10%) occurred due to disease progression or complications from the underlying disease. An additional 22% of patients prematurely discontinued Sandostatin LAR Depot due to disease progression or worsening of carcinoid symptoms.

16 HOW SUPPLIED/STORAGE AND HANDLING

Sandostatin LAR Depot is available in single-use kits containing a 5-mL vial of 10 mg, 20 mg or 30 mg strength, a syringe containing 2.5 mL of diluent, two sterile 1½" 19 gauge needles, and two alcohol wipes. An instruction booklet for the preparation of drug suspension for injection is also included with each kit.

Drug Product Kits

10 mg kit	NDC 0078-0340-61
20 mg kit	NDC 0078-0341-61
30 mg kit	NDC 0078-0342-61
Demonstration kit	NDC 0078-9342-61

For prolonged storage, Sandostatin LAR Depot should be stored at refrigerated temperatures between 2°C-8°C (36°F-46°F) and protected from light until the time of use. Sandostatin LAR Depot drug product kit should remain at room temperature for 30-60 minutes prior to preparation of the drug suspension. However, after preparation the drug suspension must be administered immediately.

17 PATIENT COUNSELING INFORMATION

Patients with carcinoid tumors and VIPomas should be advised to adhere closely to their scheduled return visits for reinjection in order to minimize exacerbation of symptoms. Patients with acromegaly should also be urged to adhere to their return visit schedule to help assure steady control of GH and IGF-1 levels.

**Trademark of Thomson Healthcare, Inc.

T2010-23

Sandostatin LAR® Depot vials are manufactured by:
Sandoz GmbH, Schaftenau, Austria
(Subsidiary of Novartis Pharma AG, Basle, Switzerland)
The diluent syringes are manufactured by:
Solvay Pharmaceuticals B.V.
Olst, The Netherlands
Distributed by:
Novartis Pharmaceuticals Corporation
East Hanover, New Jersey 07936
©Novartis

Shown in Product Identification Guide, page 316

SIMULECT®

℞

[*sĭm ew lĕkt*]
(basiliximab)
For Injection
Rx only

Prescribing Information

The following prescribing information is based on official labeling in effect July 2008.

WARNING

Only physicians experienced in immunosuppression therapy and management of organ transplantation patients should prescribe Simulect® (basiliximab). The physician responsible for Simulect administration should have complete information requisite for the follow-up of the patient. Patients receiving the drug should be managed in facilities equipped and staffed with adequate laboratory and supportive medical resources.

DESCRIPTION

Simulect® (basiliximab) is a chimeric (murine/human) monoclonal antibody (IgG_{1k}), produced by recombinant DNA technology, that functions as an immunosuppressive agent, specifically binding to and blocking the interleukin 2 receptor α-chain (IL 2Rα, also known as CD25 antigen) on the surface of activated T-lymphocytes. Based on the amino acid sequence, the calculated molecular weight of the protein is 144 kilodaltons. It is a glycoprotein obtained from fermentation of an established mouse myeloma cell line genetically engineered to express plasmids containing the human heavy and light chain constant region genes and mouse heavy and light chain variable region genes encoding the RFT5 antibody that binds selectively to the IL 2Rα.

The active ingredient, basiliximab, is water soluble. The drug product, Simulect, is a sterile lyophilisate which is available in 6 mL colorless glass vials and is available in 10 mg and 20 mg strengths.

Each 10-mg vial contains 10 mg basiliximab, 3.61 mg monobasic potassium phosphate, 0.50 mg disodium hydrogen phosphate (anhydrous), 0.80 mg sodium chloride, 10 mg sucrose, 40 mg mannitol and 20 mg glycine, to be reconstituted in 2.5 mL of Sterile Water for Injection, USP. No preservatives are added.

Each 20-mg vial contains 20 mg basiliximab, 7.21 mg monobasic potassium phosphate, 0.99 mg disodium hydrogen phosphate (anhydrous), 1.61 mg sodium chloride, 20 mg sucrose, 80 mg mannitol and 40 mg glycine, to be reconstituted in 5 mL of Sterile Water for Injection, USP. No preservatives are added.

CLINICAL PHARMACOLOGY

General

Mechanism of Action: Basiliximab functions as an IL 2 receptor antagonist by binding with high affinity ($K_a = 1 \times 10^{10}$ M^{-1}) to the alpha chain of the high affinity IL 2 receptor complex and inhibiting IL 2 binding. Basiliximab is specifically targeted against IL 2Rα, which is selectively expressed on the surface of activated T-lymphocytes. This specific high affinity binding of Simulect® (basiliximab) to IL 2Rα competitively inhibits IL 2-mediated activation of lymphocytes, a critical pathway in the cellular immune response involved in allograft rejection.

While in the circulation, Simulect impairs the response of the immune system to antigenic challenges. Whether the ability to respond to repeated or ongoing challenges with those antigens returns to normal after Simulect is cleared is unknown *(see PRECAUTIONS)*.

Pharmacokinetics

Adults: Single-dose and multiple-dose pharmacokinetic studies have been conducted in patients undergoing first kidney transplantation. Cumulative doses ranged from 15 mg up to 150 mg. Peak mean ± SD serum concentration following intravenous infusion of 20 mg over 30 minutes is 7.1 ± 5.1 mg/L. There is a dose-proportional increase in C_{max} and AUC up to the highest tested single dose of 60 mg. The volume of distribution at steady state is 8.6 ± 4.1 L. The extent and degree of distribution to various body compartments have not been fully studied. The terminal half-life is 7.2 ± 3.2 days. Total body clearance is 41 ± 19 mL/h. No clinically relevant influence of body weight or gender on distribution volume or clearance has been observed in adult patients. Elimination half-life was not influenced by age (20-69 years), gender or race *(see DOSAGE AND ADMINISTRATION)*.

Pediatric: The pharmacokinetics of Simulect have been assessed in 39 pediatric patients undergoing renal transplantation. In infants and children (1-11 years of age, n = 25), the distribution volume and clearance were reduced by about 50% compared to adult renal transplantation patients. The volume of distribution at steady state was 4.8 ± 2.1 L, half-life was 9.5 ± 4.5 days and clearance was 17 ± 6 mL/h. Disposition parameters were not influenced to a clinically relevant extent by age (1-11 years of age), body weight (9-37 kg) or body surface area (0.44-1.20 m^2) in this age group. In adolescents (12-16 years of age, n = 14), disposition was similar to that in adult renal transplantation patients. The volume of distribution at steady state was 7.8 ± 5.1 L, half-life was 9.1 ± 3.9 days and clearance was 31 ± 19 mL/h *(see DOSAGE AND ADMINISTRATION)*.

Pharmacodynamics

Complete and consistent binding to IL 2Rα in adults is maintained as long as serum Simulect levels exceed 0.2 μg/mL. As concentrations fall below this threshold, the IL 2Rα sites are no longer fully bound and the number of T cells expressing unbound IL 2Rα returns to pretherapy values within 1-2 weeks. The relationship between serum concentration and receptor saturation was assessed in 13 pediatric patients and was similar to that characterized in adult renal transplantation patients. *In vitro* studies using human tissues indicate that Simulect binds only to lymphocytes.

The duration of clinically relevant IL 2 receptor blockade after the recommended course of Simulect is not known. When basiliximab was added to a regimen of cyclosporine, USP (MODIFIED) and corticosteroids in adult patients, the duration of IL 2α saturation was 36 ± 14 days (mean ± SD), similar to that observed in pediatric patients (36 ± 14 days) *(see DOSAGE AND ADMINISTRATION)*. When basiliximab was added to a triple therapy regimen consisting of cyclosporine, USP (MODIFIED), corticosteroids, and azathioprine in adults, the duration was 50 ± 20 days and when added to cyclosporine, USP (MODIFIED), corticosteroids, and mycophenolate mofetil in adults, the duration was 59 ± 17 days *(see PRECAUTIONS, Drug Interactions)*. No significant changes to circulating lymphocyte numbers or cell phenotypes were observed by flow cytometry.

CLINICAL STUDIES

The safety and efficacy of Simulect® (basiliximab) for the prophylaxis of acute organ rejection in adults following cadaveric- or living-donor renal transplantation were assessed in four randomized, double-blind, placebo-controlled clinical studies (1,184 patients). Of these four, two studies (Study 1 [EU/CAN] and Study 2 [US Study]) compared two 20-mg doses of Simulect with placebo, each administered intravenously as an infusion, as part of a standard immunosuppressive regimen comprised of cyclosporine, USP (MODIFIED) and corticosteroids. The other two controlled studies compared two 20-mg doses of Simulect with placebo, each administered intravenously as a bolus injection, as part of a standard triple-immunosuppressive regimen comprised of cyclosporine, USP (MODIFIED), corticosteroids and either azathioprine or mycophenolate mofetil (Study 3 and Study 4, respectively). The first dose of Simulect or placebo was administered within 2 hours prior to transplantation surgery (Day 0) and the second dose administered on Day 4 post-transplantation. The regimen of Simulect was chosen to provide 30-45 days of IL 2Rα saturation.

729 patients were enrolled in the two studies using a dual maintenance immunosuppressive regimen comprised of cyclosporine, USP (MODIFIED) and corticosteroids, of which 363 patients were treated with Simulect and 358 patients were placebo-treated. Study 1 was conducted at 21 sites in Europe and Canada (EU/CAN Study); Study 2 was conducted at 21 sites in the USA (US Study). Patients 18-75 years of age undergoing first cadaveric- (Study 1 and Study 2) or living-donor (Study 2 only) renal transplantation, with ≥1 HLA mismatch, were enrolled.[1,2]

The primary efficacy endpoint in both studies was the incidence of death, graft loss or an episode of acute rejection during the first 6 months post-transplantation. Secondary efficacy endpoints included the primary efficacy variable measured during the first 12 months post-transplantation, the incidence of biopsy-confirmed acute rejection during the first 6 and 12 months post-transplantation, and patient survival and graft survival, each measured at 12 months post-transplantation. Table 1 summarizes the results of these studies. Figure 1 displays the Kaplan-Meier estimates of the percentage of patients by treatment group experiencing the primary efficacy endpoint during the first 12 months post-transplantation for Study 2. Patients in both studies receiving Simulect experienced a significantly lower incidence of biopsy-confirmed rejection episodes at both 6 and 12 months post-transplantation. There was no difference in the rate of delayed graft function, patient survival, or graft survival between Simulect-treated patients and placebo-treated patients in either study.

There was no evidence that the clinical benefit of Simulect was limited to specific subpopulations based on age, gender, race, donor type (cadaveric or living donor allograft) or history of diabetes mellitus.

Table 1
Efficacy Parameters (Percentage of Patients)

	Dual-therapy Regimen (cyclosporine* and corticosteroids)					
	Study 1			Study 2		
	Placebo (N = 185)	Simulect® (N = 190)	p-value	Placebo (N = 173)	Simulect® (N = 173)	p-value
Primary endpoint						
Death, graft loss or acute rejection episode (0-6 months)	57%	42%	0.003	55%	38%	0.002
Secondary endpoints						
Death, graft loss or acute rejection episode (0-12 months)	60%	46%	0.007	58%	41%	0.001
Biopsy-confirmed rejection episode (0-6 months)	44%	30%	0.007	46%	33%	0.015
Biopsy-confirmed rejection episode (0-12 months)	46%	32%	0.005	49%	35%	0.009
Patient survival (12 months)	97%	95%	0.29	96%	97%	0.56
Patients with functioning graft (12 months)	87%	88%	0.70	93%	95%	0.50

*USP (MODIFIED)

[See table 1 above]
[See figure 1 at top of next column]

Two double-blind, randomized, placebo-controlled studies (Study 3 and Study 4) assessed the safety and efficacy of Simulect for the prophylaxis of acute renal transplant rejection in adults when used in combination with a triple immunosuppressive regimen. In Study 3, 340 patients were concomitantly treated with cyclosporine, USP (MODIFIED), corticosteroids and azathioprine (AZA), of which 168 patients were treated with Simulect and 172 patients were treated with placebo. In Study 4, 123 patients were concomitantly treated with cyclosporine, USP (MODIFIED), corticosteroids and mycophenolate mofetil (MMF), of which 59 patients were treated with Simulect and 64 patients were treated with placebo. Patients 18-70 years of age undergoing first or second cadaveric or living donor (related or unrelated) renal transplantation were enrolled in both studies.

Table 2
Efficacy Parameters (Percentage of Patients)

Study 3: Triple-therapy Regimen (cyclosporine*, corticosteroids, and azathioprine)	Placebo (N = 172)	Simulect® (N = 168)	p-value
Primary endpoint			
Acute rejection episode (0-6 months)	35%	21%	0.005
Secondary endpoints			
Death, graft loss or acute rejection episode (0-6 months)	40%	26%	0.008
Biopsy-confirmed rejection episode (0-6 months)	29%	18%	0.023
Patient survival (12 months)	97%	98%	1.000
Patients with functioning graft (12 months)	88%	90%	0.599

*USP (MODIFIED)

Figure 1
Kaplan-Meier Estimate of the Percentage of Subjects with Death, Graft Loss or First Rejection Episode (Dual Therapy)
Month: 0 – 12

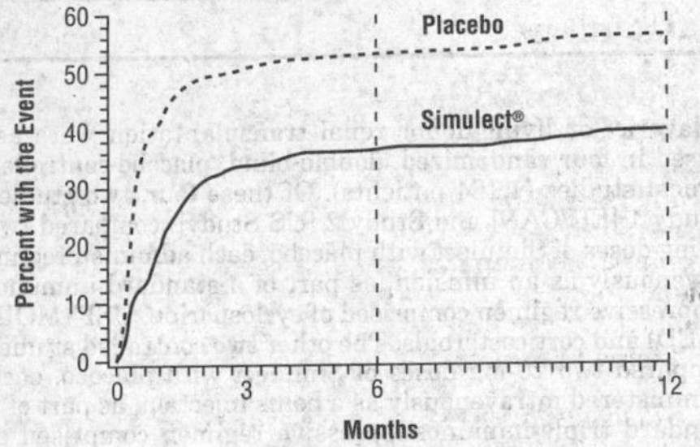

The results of Study 3 are shown in Table 2. These results are consistent with the findings from Study 1 and Study 2. [See table 2 above]

In Study 4, the percentage of patients experiencing biopsy-proven acute rejection by 6 months was 15% (9 of 59 patients) in the Simulect group and 27% (17 of 64 patients) in the placebo group. Although numerically lower, the difference in acute rejection was not significant.

In a multicenter, randomized, double-blind, placebo-controlled trial of Simulect for the prevention of allograft rejection in liver transplant recipients (n = 381) receiving concomitant cyclosporine, USP (MODIFIED) and steroids, the incidence of the combined endpoint of death, graft loss, or first biopsy-confirmed rejection episode at either 6 or 12 months was similar between patients randomized to receive Simulect and those randomized to receive placebo.

The efficacy of Simulect for the prophylaxis of acute rejection in recipients of a second renal allograft has not been demonstrated.

Long Term Follow-up

Five-year patient survival and graft survival data were provided by 71% and 58% of the original subjects of Study 1 and Study 2, respectively. Subjects in both studies continued to receive a dual-therapy regimen with cyclosporine, USP (MODIFIED) and corticosteroid. No difference was observed between groups in the 5-year graft survival in either Study 1 (91% Simulect group, 92% placebo group) or Study 2 (85% Simulect group, 86% placebo group). In Study 1, patient survival was lower in the Simulect-treated patients compared to the placebo-treated patients (142/163 [87%] vs. 156/164 [95%], respectively). The cause of this difference in survival is unknown. The data do not indicate an increase in malignancy- or infection-related mortality. In Study 2, patient survival in the placebo group (90%) was the same compared to Simulect group (90%).

INDICATIONS AND USAGE

Simulect® (basiliximab) is indicated for the prophylaxis of acute organ rejection in patients receiving renal transplantation when used as part of an immunosuppressive regimen that includes cyclosporine, USP (MODIFIED) and corticosteroids.

The efficacy of Simulect for the prophylaxis of acute rejection in recipients of other solid organ allografts has not been demonstrated.

CONTRAINDICATIONS

Simulect® (basiliximab) is contraindicated in patients with known hypersensitivity to basiliximab or any other component of the formulation. *See composition of Simulect under DESCRIPTION.*

WARNINGS. *See Boxed WARNING.*

General

Simulect® (basiliximab) should be administered under qualified medical supervision. Patients should be informed of the potential benefits of therapy and the risks associated with administration of immunosuppressive therapy.

While neither the incidence of lymphoproliferative disorders nor opportunistic infections was higher in Simulect-treated patients than in placebo-treated patients, patients on immunosuppressive therapy are at increased risk for developing these complications and should be monitored accordingly.

Hypersensitivity

Severe acute (onset within 24 hours) hypersensitivity reactions including anaphylaxis have been observed both on initial exposure to Simulect and/or following re-exposure after several months. These reactions may include hypotension, tachycardia, cardiac failure, dyspnea, wheezing, bronchospasm, pulmonary edema, respiratory failure, urticaria, rash, pruritus, and/or sneezing. Extreme caution should be exercised in all patients previously given Simulect when being administered a subsequent course of Simulect. A subgroup of patients may be particularly at risk of developing severe hypersensitivity reactions on re-administration. These are patients in whom concomitant immunosuppression was discontinued prematurely (e.g., due to abandoned transplantation or early loss of the graft) following the initial administration of Simulect. If a severe hypersensitivity reaction occurs, therapy with Simulect should be permanently discontinued. Medications for the treatment of severe hypersensitivity reactions including anaphylaxis should be available for immediate use.

PRECAUTIONS

General

It is not known whether Simulect® (basiliximab) use will have a long-term effect on the ability of the immune system to respond to antigens first encountered during Simulect-induced immunosuppression.

Immunogenicity

Of renal transplantation patients treated with Simulect and tested for anti-idiotype antibodies, 4/339 developed an anti-idiotype antibody response, with no deleterious clinical effect upon the patient. In none of these cases was there evidence that the presence of anti-idiotype antibody accelerated Simulect clearance or decreased the period of receptor saturation. In Study 2, the incidence of human anti-murine antibody (HAMA) in renal transplantation patients treated with Simulect was 2/138 in patients not exposed to muromonab-CD3 and 4/34 in patients who subsequently received muromonab-CD3. The available clinical data on the use of muromonab-CD3 in patients previously treated with Simulect suggest that subsequent use of muromonab-CD3 or other murine anti-lymphocytic antibody preparations is not precluded.

These data reflect the percentage of patients whose test results were considered positive for antibodies to Simulect in an ELISA assay, and are highly dependent on the sensitivity and specificity of the assay. Additionally the observed incidence of antibody positivity in an assay may be influenced by several factors including sample handling, concomitant medications, and underlying disease. For these reasons, comparison of the incidence of antibodies to Simulect with the incidence of antibodies to other products may be misleading.

Drug Interactions

No dose adjustment is necessary when Simulect is added to triple-immunosuppression regimens including cyclosporine, corticosteroids, and either azathioprine or mycophenolate mofetil. Three clinical trials have investigated Simulect use in combination with triple-therapy regimens. Pharmacokinetics were assessed in two of these trials. Total body clearance of Simulect was reduced by an average 22% and 51% when azathioprine and mycophenolate mofetil, respectively, were added to a regimen consisting of cyclosporine, USP (MODIFIED) and corticosteroids. Nonetheless, the range of individual Simulect clearance values in the presence of azathioprine (12-57 mL/h) or mycophenolate mofetil (7-54 mL/h) did not extend outside the range observed with dual therapy (10-78 mL/h). The following medications have been administered in clinical trials with Simulect with no increase in adverse reactions: ATG/ALG, azathioprine, corticosteroids, cyclosporine, mycophenolate mofetil, and muromonab-CD3.

Carcinogenesis/Mutagenesis/Impairment of Fertility

No mutagenic potential of Simulect was observed in the *in vitro* assays with Salmonella (Ames) and V79 Chinese hamster cells. No long-term or fertility studies in laboratory animals have been performed to evaluate the potential of Simulect to produce carcinogenicity or fertility impairment, respectively.

Pregnancy Category B

There are no adequate and well-controlled studies in pregnant women. No maternal toxicity, embryotoxicity, or teratogenicity was observed in cynomolgus monkeys 100 days post coitum following dosing with basiliximab during the organogenesis period; blood levels in pregnant monkeys were 13-fold higher than those seen in human patients. Immunotoxicology studies have not been performed in the offspring. Because IgG molecules are known to cross the placental barrier, because the IL 2 receptor may play an important role in development of the immune system, and because animal reproduction studies are not always predictive of human response, Simulect should only be used in pregnant women when the potential benefit justifies the potential risk to the fetus. Women of childbearing potential should use effective contraception before beginning Simulect therapy, during therapy, and for 4 months after completion of Simulect therapy.

Nursing Mothers

It is not known whether Simulect is excreted in human milk. Because many drugs including human antibodies are excreted in human milk, and because of the potential for adverse reactions, a decision should be made to discontinue nursing or to discontinue the drug, taking into account the importance of the drug to the mother.

Pediatric Use

No randomized, placebo-controlled studies have been completed in pediatric patients. In a safety and pharmacokinetic study, 41 pediatric patients (1-11 years of age [n = 27], 12-16 years of age [n = 14], median age 8.1 years) were treated with Simulect via intravenous bolus injection in addition to standard immunosuppressive agents including cyclosporine, USP (MODIFIED), corticosteroids, azathioprine, and mycophenolate mofetil. The acute rejection rate at 6 months was comparable to that in adults in the triple-therapy trials. The most frequently reported adverse events were hypertension, hypertrichosis, and rhinitis (49% each), urinary tract infections (46%), and fever (39%). Overall, the adverse event profile was consistent with general clinical experience in the pediatric renal transplantation population and with the profile in the controlled adult renal transplantation studies. The available pharmacokinetic data in children and adolescents are described in CLINICAL PHARMACOLOGY and DOSAGE AND ADMINISTRATION.

It is not known whether the immune response to vaccines, infection, and other antigenic stimuli administered or encountered during Simulect therapy is impaired or whether such response will remain impaired after Simulect therapy.

Geriatric Use

Controlled clinical studies of Simulect have included a small number of patients 65 years and older (Simulect 28; placebo 32). From the available data comparing Simulect and placebo-treated patients, the adverse event profile in patients ≥65 years of age is not different from patients <65 years of age and no age-related dosing adjustment is required. Caution must be used in giving immunosuppressive drugs to elderly patients.

ADVERSE REACTIONS

Because clinical trials are conducted under widely varying conditions, adverse reaction rates observed in the clinical trials of a drug cannot be directly compared to rates in the clinical trials of another drug and may not reflect the rates observed in practice. The adverse reaction information from clinical trials does, however, provide a basis for identifying the adverse events that appear to be related to drug use and for approximating rates.

The incidence of adverse events for Simulect® (basiliximab) was determined in four randomized, double-blind, placebo-controlled clinical trials for the prevention of renal allograft rejection. Two of the studies (Study 1 and Study 2), used a dual maintenance immunosuppressive regimen comprised of cyclosporine, USP (MODIFIED) and corticosteroids, whereas the other two studies (Study 3 and Study 4) used a triple-immunosuppressive regimen comprised of cyclosporine, USP (MODIFIED), corticosteroids, and either azathioprine or mycophenolate mofetil.

Simulect did not appear to add to the background of adverse events seen in organ transplantation patients as a consequence of their underlying disease and the concurrent administration of immunosuppressants and other medications. Adverse events were reported by 96% of the patients in the placebo-treated group and 96% of the patients in the Simulect-treated group. In the four placebo-controlled studies, the pattern of adverse events in 590 patients treated with the recommended dose of Simulect was similar to that in 594 patients treated with placebo. Simulect did not increase the incidence of serious adverse events observed compared with placebo.

The most frequently reported adverse events were gastrointestinal disorders, reported in 69% of Simulect-treated patients and 67% of placebo-treated patients.

The incidence and types of adverse events were similar in Simulect-treated and placebo-treated patients. The following adverse events occurred in ≥10% of Simulect-treated patients:

Gastrointestinal System: constipation, nausea, abdominal pain, vomiting, diarrhea, dyspepsia;
Body as a Whole-General: pain, peripheral edema, fever, viral infection;
Metabolic and Nutritional: hyperkalemia, hypokalemia, hyperglycemia, hypercholesterolemia, hypophosphatemia, hyperuricemia;
Urinary System: urinary tract infection;
Respiratory System: dyspnea, upper respiratory tract infection;
Skin and Appendages: surgical wound complications, acne;
Cardiovascular Disorders-General: hypertension;
Central and Peripheral Nervous System: headache, tremor;
Psychiatric: insomnia;
Red Blood Cell: anemia.

The following adverse events, not mentioned above, were reported with an incidence of ≥ 3% and <10% in pooled analysis of patients treated with Simulect in the four controlled clinical trials, or in an analysis of the two dual-therapy trials:

Body as a Whole-General: accidental trauma, asthenia, chest pain, increased drug level, infection, face edema, fatigue, dependent edema, generalized edema, leg edema, malaise, rigors, sepsis;
Cardiovascular: abnormal heart sounds, aggravated hypertension, angina pectoris, cardiac failure, chest pain, hypotension;
Endocrine: increased glucocorticoids;
Gastrointestinal: enlarged abdomen, esophagitis, flatulence, gastrointestinal disorder, gastroenteritis, GI hemorrhage, gum hyperplasia, melena, moniliasis, ulcerative stomatitis;
Heart Rate and Rhythm: arrhythmia, atrial fibrillation, tachycardia;
Metabolic and Nutritional: acidosis, dehydration, diabetes mellitus, fluid overload, hypercalcemia, hyperlipemia, hyper-triglyceridemia, hypocalcemia, hypoglycemia, hypomagnesemia, hypoproteinemia, weight increase;
Musculoskeletal: arthralgia, arthropathy, back pain, bone fracture, cramps, hernia, myalgia, leg pain;
Nervous System: dizziness, neuropathy, paraesthesia, hypoesthesia;
Platelet and Bleeding: hematoma, hemorrhage, purpura, thrombocytopenia, thrombosis;
Psychiatric: agitation, anxiety, depression;
Red Blood Cell: polycythemia;
Reproductive Disorders, Male: genital edema, impotence;
Respiratory: bronchitis, bronchospasm, abnormal chest sounds, coughing, pharyngitis, pneumonia, pulmonary disorder, pulmonary edema, rhinitis, sinusitis;
Skin and Appendages: cyst, herpes simplex, herpes zoster, hypertrichosis, pruritus, rash, skin disorder, skin ulceration;
Urinary: albuminuria, bladder disorder, dysuria, frequent micturition, hematuria, increased non-protein nitrogen, oliguria, abnormal renal function, renal tubular necrosis, surgery, ureteral disorder, urinary retention;
Vascular Disorders: vascular disorder;
Vision Disorders: cataract, conjunctivitis, abnormal vision;
White Blood Cell: leucopenia. Among these events, leucopenia and hypertriglyceridemia occurred more frequently in the two triple-therapy studies using azathioprine and mycophenolate mofetil than in the dual-therapy studies.

Malignancies
The incidence of malignancies in the controlled clinical trials of renal transplant was not significantly different between groups at 1 year (9/590 Simulect-treated patients vs. 12/594 placebo-treated patients) or among patients with 5-year follow-up from Studies 1 and 2 (21/295 Simulect-treated patients vs. 21/291 placebo-treated patients). The incidence of lymphoproliferative disease was not significantly different between groups, and less than 1% in the Simulect-treated patients.

Infections
The overall incidence of cytomegalovirus infection was similar in Simulect- and placebo-treated patients (15% vs. 17%) receiving a dual- or triple-immunosuppression regimen. However, in patients receiving a triple-immunosuppression regimen, the incidence of serious cytomegalovirus infection was higher in Simulect-treated patients compared to placebo-treated patients (11% vs. 5%). The rates of infections, serious infections, and infectious organisms were similar in the Simulect- and placebo-treatment groups among dual- and triple-therapy treated patients.

Post Marketing Experience
Severe acute hypersensitivity reactions including anaphylaxis characterized by hypotension, tachycardia, cardiac failure, dyspnea, wheezing, bronchospasm, pulmonary edema, respiratory failure, urticaria, rash, pruritus, and/or sneezing, as well as capillary leak syndrome and cytokine release syndrome, have been reported during post-marketing experience with Simulect.

OVERDOSAGE
A maximum tolerated dose of Simulect® (basiliximab) has not been determined in patients. During the course of clinical studies, Simulect has been administered to adult renal transplantation patients in single doses of up to 60 mg, or in divided doses over 3-5 days of up to 120 mg, without any associated serious adverse events. There has been one spontaneous report of a pediatric renal transplantation patient who received a single 20-mg dose (2.3 mg/kg) without adverse events.

DOSAGE AND ADMINISTRATION
Simulect® (basiliximab) is used as part of an immunosuppressive regimen that includes cyclosporine, USP (MODIFIED) and corticosteroids. Simulect is for central or peripheral intravenous administration only. Reconstituted Simulect should be given either as a bolus injection or diluted to a volume of 25 mL (10-mg vial) or 50 mL (20-mg vial) with normal saline or dextrose 5% and administered as an intravenous infusion over 20 to 30 minutes. Bolus administration may be associated with nausea, vomiting and local reactions, including pain.

Simulect should only be administered once it has been determined that the patient will receive the graft and concomitant immunosuppression. Patients previously administered Simulect should only be re-exposed to a subsequent course of therapy with extreme caution due to the potential risk of hypersensitivity (see WARNINGS).

Parenteral drug products should be inspected visually for particulate matter and discoloration before administration. After reconstitution, Simulect should be a clear-to-opalescent, colorless solution. If particulate matter is present or the solution is colored, do not use.

Care must be taken to assure sterility of the prepared solution because the drug product does not contain any antimicrobial preservatives or bacteriostatic agents.

It is recommended that after reconstitution, the solution should be used immediately. If not used immediately, it can be stored at 2°C to 8°C for 24 hours or at room temperature for 4 hours. Discard the reconstituted solution if not used within 24 hours.

No incompatibility between Simulect and polyvinyl chloride bags or infusion sets has been observed. No data are available on the compatibility of Simulect with other intravenous substances. Other drug substances should not be added or infused simultaneously through the same intravenous line.

Adults
In adult patients, the recommended regimen is two doses of 20 mg each. The first 20-mg dose should be given within 2 hours prior to transplantation surgery. The recommended second 20-mg dose should be given 4 days after transplantation. The second dose should be withheld if complications such as severe hypersensitivity reactions to Simulect or graft loss occur.

Pediatric
In pediatric patients weighing less than 35 kg, the recommended regimen is two doses of 10 mg each. In pediatric patients weighing 35 kg or more, the recommended regimen is two doses of 20 mg each. The first dose should be given within 2 hours prior to transplantation surgery. The recommended second dose should be given 4 days after transplantation. The second dose should be withheld if complications such as severe hypersensitivity reactions to Simulect or graft loss occur.

Reconstitution of 10 mg Simulect® Vial
To prepare the reconstituted solution, add 2.5 mL of Sterile Water for Injection, USP, using aseptic technique, to the vial containing the Simulect powder. Shake the vial gently to dissolve the powder.

The reconstituted solution is isotonic and may be given either as a bolus injection or diluted to a volume of 25 mL with normal saline or dextrose 5% for infusion. When mixing the solution, gently invert the bag in order to avoid foaming; DO NOT SHAKE.

Reconstitution of 20 mg Simulect® Vial
To prepare the reconstituted solution, add 5 mL of Sterile Water for Injection, USP, using aseptic technique, to the vial containing the Simulect powder. Shake the vial gently to dissolve the powder.

The reconstituted solution is isotonic and may be given either as a bolus injection or diluted to a volume of 50 mL with normal saline or dextrose 5% for infusion. When mixing the solution, gently invert the bag in order to avoid foaming; DO NOT SHAKE.

HOW SUPPLIED
Simulect® (basiliximab) is supplied in a single use glass vial.
Each carton contains one of the following:
1 Simulect 10 mg vial .... NDC 0078-0393-61
1 Simulect 20 mg vial .... NDC 0078-0331-84
Store lyophilized Simulect under refrigerated conditions (2°C to 8°C; 36°F to 46°F).
Do not use beyond the expiration date stamped on the vial.

REFERENCES
1. Kahan, B.D., Rajagopalan P.R. and Hall M., Transplantation, 67, 276-284 (1999).
2. Nashan, B., Moore R., Amlot P., Schmidt A.-G., Abeywickrama K. and Soulillou J.-P., Lancet 350, 1193-1198 (1997).
US License No. 1244

REV: SEPTEMBER 2005
T2005-28
2027722
Novartis Pharmaceuticals Corporation
East Hanover, New Jersey 07936
©Novartis
Shown in Product Identification Guide, page 316

STALEVO® 50 ℞
STALEVO® 75
STALEVO® 100
STALEVO® 125
STALEVO® 150
STALEVO® 200
[sta-lee-vō]
(carbidopa, levodopa and entacapone)
Tablets
Rx only
Prescribing Information

The following prescribing information is based on official labeling in effect July 2009.

DESCRIPTION
Stalevo® (carbidopa, levodopa and entacapone) is a combination of carbidopa, levodopa and entacapone for the treatment of Parkinson's disease.

Carbidopa, an inhibitor of aromatic amino acid decarboxylation, is a white, crystalline compound, slightly soluble in water, with a molecular weight of 244.3. It is designated chemically as (-)-L-α-hydrazino-α-methyl-β-(3,4-dihydroxybenzene) propanoic acid monohydrate. Its empirical formula is $C_{10}H_{14}N_2O_4 \cdot H_2O$, and its structural formula is

Tablet content is expressed in terms of anhydrous carbidopa, which has a molecular weight of 226.3.

Levodopa, an aromatic amino acid, is a white, crystalline compound, slightly soluble in water, with a molecular weight of 197.2. It is designated chemically as (-)-L-α-amino-β-(3,4-dihydroxybenzene) propanoic acid. Its empirical formula is $C_9H_{11}NO_4$, and its structural formula is

Entacapone, an inhibitor of catechol-O-methyltransferase (COMT), is a nitro-catechol-structured compound with a molecular weight of 305.3. The chemical name of entacapone is (E)-2-cyano-3-(3,4-dihydroxy-5-nitrophenyl)-N,N-diethyl-2-propenamide. Its empirical formula is $C_{14}H_{15}N_3O_5$ and its structural formula is

Stalevo® (carbidopa, levodopa and entacapone) is supplied as tablets in six strengths:
Stalevo 50, containing 12.5 mg of carbidopa, 50 mg of levodopa and 200 mg of entacapone;
Stalevo 75, containing 18.75 mg of carbidopa, 75 mg of levodopa and 200 mg of entacapone;
Stalevo 100, containing 25 mg of carbidopa, 100 mg of levodopa and 200 mg of entacapone;

Stalevo 125, containing 31.25 mg of carbidopa, 125 mg of levodopa and 200 mg of entacapone;
Stalevo 150, containing 37.5 mg of carbidopa, 150 mg of levodopa and 200 mg of entacapone;
Stalevo 200, containing 50 mg of carbidopa, 200 mg of levodopa and 200 mg of entacapone.
The inactive ingredients of the Stalevo tablet are corn starch, croscarmellose sodium, glycerol 85%, hypromellose, magnesium stearate, mannitol, polysorbate 80, povidone, sucrose, red iron oxide, and titanium dioxide. Stalevo 50, Stalevo 100, and Stalevo 150 also contain yellow iron oxide.

CLINICAL PHARMACOLOGY

Parkinson's disease is a progressive, neurodegenerative disorder of the extrapyramidal nervous system affecting the mobility and control of the skeletal muscular system. Its characteristic features include resting tremor, rigidity, and bradykinetic movements.

Mechanism of Action

Levodopa

Current evidence indicates that symptoms of Parkinson's disease are related to depletion of dopamine in the corpus striatum. Administration of dopamine is ineffective in the treatment of Parkinson's disease apparently because it does not cross the blood-brain barrier. However, levodopa, the metabolic precursor of dopamine, does cross the blood-brain barrier, and presumably is converted to dopamine in the brain. This is thought to be the mechanism whereby levodopa relieves symptoms of Parkinson's disease.

Carbidopa

When levodopa is administered orally it is rapidly decarboxylated to dopamine in extracerebral tissues so that only a small portion of a given dose is transported unchanged to the central nervous system. Carbidopa inhibits the decarboxylation of peripheral levodopa, making more levodopa available for transport to the brain. When coadministered with levodopa, carbidopa increases plasma levels of levodopa and reduces the amount of levodopa required to produce a given response by about 75%. Carbidopa prolongs the plasma half-life of levodopa from 50 minutes to 1.5 hours and decreases plasma and urinary dopamine and its major metabolite, homovanillic acid. The T_{max} of levodopa, however, was unaffected by the coadministration.

Entacapone

Entacapone is a selective and reversible inhibitor of catechol-O-methyltransferase (COMT).
In mammals, COMT is distributed throughout various organs with the highest activities in the liver and kidney. COMT also occurs in neuronal tissues, especially in glial cells. COMT catalyzes the transfer of the methyl group of S-adenosyl-L-methionine to the phenolic group of substrates that contain a catechol structure. Physiological substrates of COMT include DOPA, catecholamines (dopamine, norepinephrine, and epinephrine) and their hydroxylated metabolites. The function of COMT is the elimination of biologically active catechols and some other hydroxylated metabolites. When decarboxylation of levodopa is prevented by carbidopa, COMT becomes the major metabolizing enzyme for levodopa, catalyzing its metabolism to 3-methoxy-4-hydroxy-L-phenylalanine (3-OMD).
When entacapone is given in conjunction with levodopa and carbidopa, plasma levels of levodopa are greater and more sustained than after administration of levodopa and carbidopa alone. It is believed that at a given frequency of levodopa administration, these more sustained plasma levels of levodopa result in more constant dopaminergic stimulation in the brain, leading to greater effects on the signs and symptoms of Parkinson's disease. The higher levodopa levels may also lead to increased levodopa adverse effects, sometimes requiring a decrease in the dose of levodopa.
When 200 mg entacapone is coadministered with levodopa/carbidopa, it increases levodopa plasma exposure (AUC) by 35%-40% and prolongs its elimination half-life in Parkinson's disease patients from 1.3 to 2.4 hours. Plasma levels of the major COMT-mediated dopamine metabolite, 3-methoxy-4-hydroxy-L-phenylalanine (3-OMD), are also markedly decreased proportionally with increasing dose of entacapone.
In animals, while entacapone enters the CNS to a minimal extent, it has been shown to inhibit central COMT activity. In humans, entacapone inhibits the COMT enzyme in peripheral tissues. The effects of entacapone on central COMT activity in humans have not been studied.

Pharmacokinetics

The pharmacokinetics of Stalevo® (carbidopa, levodopa and entacapone) tablets have been studied in healthy subjects (age 45-75 years old). Overall, following administration of corresponding doses of levodopa, carbidopa and entacapone as Stalevo or as carbidopa/levodopa product plus Comtan® (entacapone) tablets, the mean plasma concentrations of levodopa, carbidopa, and entacapone are comparable.

Absorption/Distribution:

Both levodopa and entacapone are rapidly absorbed and eliminated, and their distribution volume is moderately small. Carbidopa is absorbed and eliminated slightly more slowly compared with levodopa and entacapone. There are substantial inter- and intra-individual variations in the absorption of levodopa, carbidopa and entacapone, particularly concerning its C_{max}.
The food-effect on the Stalevo tablet has not been evaluated.

Levodopa

The pharmacokinetic properties of levodopa following the administration of single-dose Stalevo® (carbidopa, levodopa and entacapone) tablets are summarized in Table 1.
[See table 1 below]
Since levodopa competes with certain amino acids for transport across the gut wall, the absorption of levodopa may be impaired in some patients on a high protein diet. Meals rich in large neutral amino acids may delay and reduce the absorption of levodopa *(see PRECAUTIONS)*.
Levodopa is bound to plasma protein only to a minor extent (about 10%-30%).

Carbidopa

Following administration of Stalevo as a single dose to healthy male and female subjects, the peak concentration of carbidopa was reached within 2.5 to 3.4 hours on average. The mean C_{max} ranged from about 40 to 225 ng/mL and the mean AUC from 170 to 1200 ng•h/mL, with different Stalevo strengths providing 12.5 mg, 25 mg, 37.5 mg or 50 mg of carbidopa.
Carbidopa is approximately 36% bound to plasma protein.

Entacapone

Following administration of Stalevo as a single dose to healthy male and female subjects, the peak concentration of entacapone in plasma was reached within 0.8 to 1.2 hours on average. The mean C_{max} of entacapone was about 1200 to 1500 ng/mL and the AUC 1250 to 1750 ng•h/mL after administration of different Stalevo strengths all providing 200 mg of entacapone.
The plasma protein binding of entacapone is 98% over the concentration range of 0.4-50 μg/mL. Entacapone binds mainly to serum albumin.

Metabolism and Elimination:

Levodopa

The elimination half-life of levodopa, the active moiety of antiparkinsonian activity, was 1.7 hours (range 1.1-3.2 hours).
Levodopa is extensively metabolized to various metabolites. Two major pathways are decarboxylation by dopa decarboxylase (DDC) and O-methylation by catechol-O-methyltransferase (COMT).

Carbidopa

The elimination half-life of carbidopa was on average 1.6 to 2 hours (range 0.7-4.0 hours).
Carbidopa is metabolized to two main metabolites (α-methyl-3-methoxy-4-hydroxyphenylpropionic acid and α-methyl-3,4-dihydroxyphenylpropionic acid). These 2 metabolites are primarily eliminated in the urine unchanged or as glucuronide conjugates. Unchanged carbidopa accounts for 30% of the total urinary excretion.

Entacapone

The elimination half-life of entacapone was on average 0.8 to 1 hour (0.3-4.5 hours).
Entacapone is almost completely metabolized prior to excretion with only a very small amount (0.2% of dose) found unchanged in urine. The main metabolic pathway is isomerization to the *cis*-isomer, the only active metabolite. Entacapone and the *cis*-isomer are eliminated in the urine as glucuronide conjugates. The glucuronides account for 95% of all urinary metabolites (70% as parent and 25% as *cis*-isomer glucuronides). The glucuronide conjugate of the *cis*-isomer is inactive. After oral administration of a ^{14}C-labeled dose of entacapone, 10% of labeled parent and metabolite is excreted in urine and 90% in feces.
Due to short elimination half-lives, no true accumulation of levodopa or entacapone occurs when they are administered repeatedly.

Special Populations:

Hepatic Impairment:

Stalevo® (carbidopa, levodopa and entacapone)

While there are no studies on the pharmacokinetics of carbidopa and levodopa in patients with hepatic impairment, Stalevo should be administered cautiously to patients with biliary obstruction or hepatic disease since biliary excretion appears to be the major route of excretion of entacapone and hepatic impairment had a significant effect on the pharmacokinetics of entacapone when 200 mg entacapone was administered alone.

Entacapone

Hepatic impairment had a significant effect on the pharmacokinetics of entacapone when 200 mg entacapone was administered alone. A single 200 mg dose of entacapone, without levodopa/dopa decarboxylase inhibitor coadministration, showed approximately two-fold higher AUC and C_{max} values in patients with a history of alcoholism and hepatic impairment (n=10) compared to normal subjects (n=10). All patients had biopsy-proven liver cirrhosis caused by alcohol. According to Child-Pugh grading 7 patients with liver disease had mild hepatic impairment and 3 patients had moderate hepatic impairment. As only about 10% of the entacapone dose is excreted in urine, as parent compound and conjugated glucuronide, biliary excretion appears to be the major route of excretion of this drug. Consequently, Stalevo should be administered with care to patients with biliary obstruction or hepatic disease.

Renal Impairment:

Stalevo® (carbidopa, levodopa and entacapone)

Stalevo should be administered cautiously to patients with severe renal disease. There are no studies on the pharmacokinetics of levodopa and carbidopa in patients with renal impairment.

Entacapone

No important effects of renal function on the pharmacokinetics of entacapone were found. The pharmacokinetics of entacapone have been investigated after a single 200 mg entacapone dose, without levodopa/dopa decarboxylase inhibitor coadministration, in a specific renal impairment study. There were three groups: normal subjects (n=7; creatinine clearance >1.12 mL/sec/1.73 m^2), moderate impairment (n=10; creatinine clearance ranging from 0.60-0.89 mL/sec/1.73 m^2), and severe impairment (n=7; creatinine clearance ranging from 0.20-0.44 mL/sec/1.73 m^2).

Concurrent Diseases:

Stalevo should be administered cautiously to patients with biliary obstruction, hepatic disease, severe cardiovascular or pulmonary disease, bronchial asthma, renal, or endocrine disease.

Elderly:

Stalevo tablets have not been studied in Parkinson's disease patients or in healthy volunteers older than 75 years old. In the pharmacokinetics studies conducted in healthy volunteers following single dose of carbidopa/levodopa/entacapone (as Stalevo or as separate carbidopa/levodopa and Comtan tablets):

Levodopa

The AUC of levodopa is significantly (on average 10%-20%) higher in elderly (60-75 years) than younger subjects (45-60 years). There is no significant difference in the C_{max} of levodopa between younger (45-60 years) and elderly subjects (60-75 years).

Carbidopa

There is no significant difference in the C_{max} and AUC of carbidopa, between younger (45-60 years) and elderly subjects (60-75 years).

Entacapone

The AUC of entacapone is significantly (on average, 15%) higher in elderly (60-75 years) than younger subjects (45-60 years). There is no significant difference in the C_{max} of entacapone between younger (45-60 years) and elderly subjects (60-75 years).

Gender:

The bioavailability of levodopa is significantly higher in females when given with or without carbidopa and/or entacapone. Following a single dose of carbidopa, levodopa and entacapone together, either as Stalevo or as separate carbidopa/levodopa and Comtan tablets in healthy volunteers (age range 45-74 years):

Levodopa

The plasma exposure (AUC and C_{max}) of levodopa is significantly higher in females than males (on average, 40% for AUC and 30% for C_{max}). These differences are primarily explained by body weight. Other published literature showed significant gender effect (higher concentrations in females) even after correction for body weight.

Carbidopa

There is no gender difference in the pharmacokinetics of carbidopa.

Table 1
Pharmacokinetic Characteristics of Levodopa With Different Tablet Strengths of Stalevo® (mean ± SD)

Tablet Strength	$AUC_{0-\infty}$ (ng•h/mL)	C_{max} (ng/mL)	T_{max} (h)
12.5 - 50 - 200 mg	1040 ± 314	470 ± 154	1.1 ± 0.5
25 - 100 - 200 mg	2910 ± 715	975 ± 247	1.4 ± 0.6
37.5 - 150 - 200 mg	3770 ± 1120	1270 ± 329	1.5 ± 0.9
50 - 200 - 200 mg	6115 ± 1536	1859 ± 455	1.76 ± 0.7

Entacapone
There is no gender difference in the pharmacokinetics of entacapone.

Drug Interactions: *See PRECAUTIONS, Drug Interactions.*

Clinical Studies
Each Stalevo tablet, provided in six single dose strengths, contains carbidopa and levodopa in ratio 1:4 and a 200 mg dose of entacapone. Four Stalevo tablet strengths 12.5/50/200 mg, 25/100/200 mg, 37.5/150/200 mg and 50/200/200 mg have been shown to be bioequivalent to the corresponding doses of standard release carbidopa/levodopa 25/100 mg tablets and Comtan 200 mg tablets.

The effectiveness of entacapone as an adjunct to levodopa in the treatment of Parkinson's disease was established in three 24-week multicenter, randomized, double-blind placebo-controlled trials in patients with Parkinson's disease. In two of these trials, the patients' disease was "fluctuating," i.e., was characterized by documented periods of "On" (periods of relatively good functioning) and "Off" (periods of relatively poor functioning), despite optimum levodopa therapy. There was also a withdrawal period following 6 months of treatment. In the third trial patients were not required to have been experiencing fluctuations. Prior to the controlled part of these trials, patients were stabilized on levodopa for 2-4 weeks.

There is limited experience of using entacapone in patients who do not experience fluctuations.

In the first two studies to be described, patients were randomized to receive placebo or entacapone 200 mg administered concomitantly with each dose of carbidopa-levodopa (up to 10 times daily, but averaging 4-6 doses per day). The formal double-blind portion of both trials was 6 months long. Patients recorded the time spent in the "On" and "Off" states in home diaries periodically throughout the duration of the trial. In one study, conducted in the Nordic countries, the primary outcome measure was the total mean time spent in the "On" state during an 18-hour diary recorded day (6 a.m. to midnight). In the other study, the primary outcome measure was the proportion of awake time spent over 24 hours in the "On" state.

In addition to the primary outcome measure, the amount of time spent in the "Off" state was evaluated, and patients were also evaluated by subparts of the Unified Parkinson's Disease Rating Scale (UPDRS), a frequently used multi-item rating scale intended to assess mentation (Part I), activities of daily living (Part II), motor function (Part III), complications of therapy (Part IV), and disease staging (Part V & VI); an investigator's and patient's global assessment of clinical condition, a 7-point subjective scale designed to assess global functioning in Parkinson's disease; and the change in daily carbidopa-levodopa dose.

In one of the studies, 171 patients were randomized in 16 centers in Finland, Norway, Sweden, and Denmark (Nordic Study), all of whom received concomitant levodopa plus dopa-decarboxylase inhibitor (either carbidopa-levodopa or benserazide-levodopa). In the second trial, 205 patients were randomized in 17 centers in North America (US and Canada); all patients received concomitant carbidopa-levodopa.

The following tables display the results of these two trials:
[See table 2 above]
[See table 3 at top of next page]

Effects on "On" time did not differ by age, sex, weight, disease severity at baseline, levodopa dose and concurrent treatment with dopamine agonists or selegiline.

Withdrawal of entacapone:
In the North American Study, abrupt withdrawal of entacapone, without alteration of the dose of carbidopa-levodopa, resulted in a significant worsening of fluctuations, compared to placebo. In some cases, symptoms were slightly worse than at baseline, but returned to approximately baseline severity within two weeks following levodopa dose increase on average by 80 mg. In the Nordic Study, similarly, a significant worsening of parkinsonian symptoms was observed after entacapone withdrawal, as assessed two weeks after drug withdrawal. At this phase, the symptoms were approximately at baseline severity following levodopa dose increase by about 50 mg.

In the third placebo-controlled trial, a total of 301 patients were randomized in 32 centers in Germany and Austria. In this trial, as in the other two trials, entacapone 200 mg was administered with each dose of levodopa/dopa decarboxylase inhibitor (up to 10 times daily) and UPDRS Parts II and III and total daily "On" time were the primary measures of effectiveness. The following results were seen for the primary measures, as well as for some secondary measures:
[See table 4 at top of page 2589]

INDICATIONS
Stalevo® (carbidopa, levodopa and entacapone) is indicated to treat patients with idiopathic Parkinson's disease:

1. To substitute (with equivalent strength of each of the three components) for immediate-release carbidopa/levodopa and entacapone previously administered as individual products.
2. To replace immediate-release carbidopa/levodopa therapy (without entacapone) when patients experience the signs and symptoms of end-of-dose "wearing-off" (only for patients taking a total daily dose of levodopa of 600 mg or less and not experiencing dyskinesias, *see DOSAGE AND ADMINISTRATION*).

CONTRAINDICATIONS
Stalevo® (carbidopa, levodopa and entacapone) tablets are contraindicated in patients who have demonstrated hypersensitivity to any component (carbidopa, levodopa, or entacapone) of the drug or its excipients.

Monoamine oxidase (MAO) and COMT are the two major enzyme systems involved in the metabolism of catecholamines. It is theoretically possible, therefore, that the combination of entacapone and a non-selective MAO inhibitor (e.g., phenelzine and tranylcypromine) would result in inhibition of the majority of the pathways responsible for normal catecholamine metabolism. As with carbidopa-levodopa, nonselective monoamine oxidase (MAO) inhibitors are contraindicated for use with Stalevo. These inhibitors must be discontinued at least two weeks prior to initiating therapy with Stalevo. Stalevo may be administered concomitantly with the manufacturer's recommended dose of MAO inhibitors with selectivity for MAO type B (e.g., selegiline HCl). (*See PRECAUTIONS, Drug Interactions.*)

Stalevo is contraindicated in patients with narrow-angle glaucoma.

Because levodopa may activate malignant melanoma, Stalevo should not be used in patients with suspicious, undiagnosed skin lesions or a history of melanoma.

WARNINGS
The addition of carbidopa to levodopa reduces the peripheral effects (nausea, vomiting) due to decarboxylation of levodopa; however, carbidopa does not decrease the adverse reactions due to the central effects of levodopa. Because carbidopa as well as entacapone permits more levodopa to reach the brain and more dopamine to be formed, certain adverse CNS effects, e.g., dyskinesia (involuntary movements) may occur at lower dosages and sooner with levodopa preparations containing carbidopa and entacapone than with levodopa alone.

The occurrence of dyskinesias may require dosage reduction (*see PRECAUTIONS, Dyskinesia*).

Stalevo® (carbidopa, levodopa and entacapone) may cause mental disturbances. These reactions are thought to be due to increased brain dopamine following administration of levodopa. All patients should be observed carefully for the development of depression with concomitant suicidal tendencies. Patients with past or current psychoses should be treated with caution.

Stalevo should be administered cautiously to patients with severe cardiovascular or pulmonary disease, bronchial asthma, renal, hepatic or endocrine disease.

As with levodopa, care should be exercised in administering Stalevo to patients with a history of myocardial infarction who have residual atrial, nodal, or ventricular arrhythmias. In such patients, cardiac function should be monitored carefully during the period of initial dosage adjustment, in a facility with provisions for intensive cardiac care.

As with levodopa, treatment with Stalevo may increase the possibility of upper gastrointestinal hemorrhage in patients with a history of peptic ulcer.

Neuroleptic Malignant Syndrome (NMS)
Sporadic cases of a symptom complex resembling NMS have been reported in association with dose reductions or

Table 2
Nordic Study

Primary Measure from Home Diary (from an 18-hour Diary Day)

	Baseline	Change from Baseline at Month 6*	p-value vs. placebo
Hours of Awake Time "On"			
Placebo	9.2	+0.1	—
Entacapone	9.3	+1.5	<0.001
Duration of "On" Time After First AM Dose (Hrs)			
Placebo	2.2	0.0	—
Entacapone	2.1	+0.2	<0.05

Secondary Measures from Home Diary (from an 18-hour Diary Day)

	Baseline	Change from Baseline at Month 6*	p-value vs. placebo
Hours of Awake Time "Off"			
Placebo	5.3	0.0	—
Entacapone	5.5	-1.3	<0.001
Proportion of Awake Time "On"*(%)**			
Placebo	63.8	+0.6	—
Entacapone	62.7	+9.3	<0.001
Levodopa Total Daily Dose (mg)			
Placebo	705	+14	—
Entacapone	701	-87	<0.001
Frequency of Levodopa Daily Intakes			
Placebo	6.1	+0.1	—
Entacapone	6.2	-0.4	<0.001

Other Secondary Measures

	Baseline	Change from Baseline at Month 6	p-value vs. placebo
Investigator's Global (overall) % Improved**			
Placebo	—	28	—
Entacapone	—	56	<0.01
Patient's Global (overall) % Improved**			
Placebo	—	22	—
Entacapone	—	39	N.S.‡
UPDRS Total			
Placebo	37.4	-1.1	—
Entacapone	38.5	-4.8	<0.01
UPDRS Motor			
Placebo	24.6	-0.7	—
Entacapone	25.5	-3.3	<0.05
UPDRS ADL			
Placebo	11.0	-0.4	—
Entacapone	11.2	-1.8	<0.05

* Mean; the month 6 values represent the average of weeks 8, 16, and 24, by protocol-defined outcome measure.
** At least one category change at endpoint.
*** Not an endpoint for this study but primary endpoint in the North American Study.
‡ Not significant.

Table 3
North American Study

Primary Measure from Home Diary (for a 24-hour Diary Day)

	Baseline	Change from Baseline at Month 6*	p-value vs. placebo
Percent of Awake Time "On"			
Placebo	60.8	+2.0	—
Entacapone	60.0	+6.7	<0.05

Secondary Measures from Home Diary (for a 24-hour Diary Day)

	Baseline	Change from Baseline at Month 6*	p-value vs. placebo
Hours of Awake Time "Off"			
Placebo	6.6	-0.3	—
Entacapone	6.8	-1.2	<0.01
Hours of Awake Time "On"			
Placebo	10.3	+0.4	—
Entacapone	10.2	+1.0	N.S.‡
Levodopa Total Daily Dose (mg)			
Placebo	758	+19	—
Entacapone	804	-93	<0.001
Frequency of Levodopa Daily Intakes			
Placebo	6.0	+0.2	—
Entacapone	6.2	0.0	N.S.‡

Other Secondary Measures

	Baseline	Change from Baseline at Month 6	p-value vs. placebo
Investigator's Global (overall) % Improved**			
Placebo	—	21	—
Entacapone	—	34	<0.05
Patient's Global (overall) % Improved**			
Placebo	—	20	—
Entacapone	—	31	<0.05
UPDRS Total**			
Placebo	35.6	+2.8	—
Entacapone	35.1	-0.6	<0.05
UPDRS Motor**			
Placebo	22.6	+1.2	—
Entacapone	22.0	-0.9	<0.05
UPDRS ADL**			
Placebo	11.7	+1.1	—
Entacapone	11.9	0.0	<0.05

* Mean; the month 6 values represent the average of weeks 8, 16, and 24, by protocol-defined outcome measure.
** At least one category change at endpoint.
*** Score change at endpoint similarly to the Nordic Study.
‡ Not significant.

withdrawal of therapy with carbidopa-levodopa. Therefore, patients should be observed carefully when the dosage of Stalevo is reduced abruptly or discontinued, especially if the patient is receiving neuroleptics. NMS is an uncommon but life-threatening syndrome characterized by fever or hyperthermia. Neurological findings, including muscle rigidity, involuntary movements, altered consciousness, mental status changes; other disturbances, such as autonomic dysfunction, tachycardia, tachypnea, sweating, hyper- or hypotension; laboratory findings, such as creatine phosphokinase elevation, leukocytosis, myoglobinuria, and increased serum myoglobin have been reported.

The early diagnosis of this condition is important for the appropriate management of these patients. Considering NMS as a possible diagnosis and ruling out other acute illnesses (e.g., pneumonia, systemic infection, etc.) is essential. This may be especially complex if the clinical presentation includes both serious medical illness and untreated or inadequately treated extrapyramidal signs and symptoms (EPS). Other important considerations in the differential diagnosis include central anticholinergic toxicity, heat stroke, drug fever, and primary central nervous system (CNS) pathology. The management of NMS should include: 1) intensive symptomatic treatment and medical monitoring and 2) treatment of any concomitant serious medical problems for which specific treatments are available. Dopamine agonists, such as bromocriptine, and muscle relaxants, such as dantrolene, are often used in the treatment of NMS, however, their effectiveness has not been demonstrated in controlled studies.

Drugs Metabolized By Catechol-O-Methyltransferase (COMT)
When a single 400 mg dose of entacapone was given together with intravenous isoprenaline (isoproterenol) and epinephrine without coadministered levodopa/dopa decarboxylase inhibitor, the overall mean maximal changes in heart rate during infusion were about 50% and 80% higher than with placebo, for isoprenaline and epinephrine, respectively.

Therefore, drugs known to be metabolized by COMT, such as isoproterenol, epinephrine, norepinephrine, dopamine, dobutamine, alpha-methyldopa, apomorphine, isoetherine, and bitolterol should be administered with caution in patients receiving entacapone regardless of the route of administration (including inhalation), as their interaction may result in increased heart rates, possibly arrhythmias, and excessive changes in blood pressure.

Ventricular tachycardia was noted in one 32-year-old healthy male volunteer in an interaction study after epinephrine infusion and oral entacapone administration. Treatment with propranolol was required. A causal relationship to entacapone administration appears probable but cannot be attributed with certainty.

PRECAUTIONS
General
As with levodopa, periodic evaluations of hepatic, hematopoietic, cardiovascular, and renal function are recommended during extended therapy.

Patients with chronic wide-angle glaucoma may be treated cautiously with Stalevo® (carbidopa, levodopa and entacapone) provided the intraocular pressure is well controlled and the patient is monitored carefully for changes in intraocular pressure during therapy.

Hypotension/Syncope
In the large controlled trials of entacapone, approximately 1.2% and 0.8% of 200 mg entacapone and placebo patients treated also with levodopa/dopa decarboxylase inhibitor, respectively, reported at least one episode of syncope. Reports of syncope were generally more frequent in patients in both treatment groups who had an episode of documented hypotension (although the episodes of syncope, obtained by history, were themselves not documented with vital sign measurement).

Diarrhea
In clinical trials of entacapone, diarrhea developed in 60 of 603 (10.0%) and 16 of 400 (4.0%) of patients treated with 200 mg of entacapone or placebo in combination with levodopa/dopa decarboxylase inhibitor, respectively. In pa-

tients treated with entacapone, diarrhea was generally mild to moderate in severity (8.6%) but was regarded as severe in 1.3%. Diarrhea resulted in withdrawal in 10 of 603 (1.7%) patients, 7 (1.2%) with mild and moderate diarrhea and 3 (0.5%) with severe diarrhea. Diarrhea generally resolved after discontinuation of entacapone. Two patients with diarrhea were hospitalized. Typically, diarrhea presents within 4-12 weeks after entacapone is started, but it may appear as early as the first week and as late as many months after the initiation of treatment.

Hallucinations
Dopaminergic therapy in Parkinson's disease patients has been associated with hallucinations. In clinical trials of entacapone, hallucinations developed in approximately 4.0% of patients treated with 200 mg entacapone or placebo in combination with levodopa/dopa decarboxylase inhibitor. Hallucinations led to drug discontinuation and premature withdrawal from clinical trials in 0.8% and 0% of patients treated with 200 mg entacapone and placebo, respectively. Hallucinations led to hospitalization in 1.0% and 0.3% of patients in the 200 mg entacapone and placebo groups, respectively.

Dyskinesia
Entacapone may potentiate the dopaminergic side effects of levodopa and may therefore cause and/or exacerbate pre-existing dyskinesia. Although decreasing the dose of levodopa may ameliorate this side effect, many patients in controlled trials continued to experience frequent dyskinesias despite a reduction in their dose of levodopa. The rates of withdrawal for dyskinesia were 1.5% and 0.8% for 200 mg entacapone and placebo, respectively.

Other Events Reported With Dopaminergic Therapy
The events listed below are rare events known to be associated with the use of drugs that increase dopaminergic activity, although they are most often associated with the use of direct dopamine agonists.

Rhabdomyolysis: Cases of severe rhabdomyolysis have been reported with entacapone when used in combination with levodopa. The complicated nature of these cases makes it impossible to determine what role, if any, entacapone played in their pathogenesis. Severe prolonged motor activity including dyskinesia may account for rhabdomyolysis. One case, however, included fever and alteration of consciousness. It is therefore possible that the rhabdomyolysis may be a result of the syndrome described in Hyperpyrexia and Confusion (see PRECAUTIONS, Other Events Reported With Dopaminergic Therapy).

Hyperpyrexia and Confusion: Cases of a symptom complex resembling the neuroleptic malignant syndrome characterized by elevated temperature, muscular rigidity, altered consciousness, and elevated CPK have been reported in association with the rapid dose reduction or withdrawal of other dopaminergic drugs. No cases have been reported following the abrupt withdrawal or dose reduction of entacapone treatment during clinical studies.

Prescribers should exercise caution when discontinuing carbidopa, levodopa and entacapone combination treatment. When considered necessary, withdrawal should proceed slowly. If a decision is made to discontinue treatment with Stalevo, recommendations include monitoring the patient closely and adjusting other dopaminergic treatments as needed. This syndrome should be considered in the differential diagnosis for any patient who develops a high fever or severe rigidity. Tapering entacapone has not been systematically evaluated.

Fibrotic Complications: Cases of retroperitoneal fibrosis, pulmonary infiltrates, pleural effusion, and pleural thickening have been reported in some patients treated with ergot derived dopaminergic agents. These complications may resolve when the drug is discontinued, but complete resolution does not always occur. Although these adverse events are believed to be related to the ergoline structure of these compounds, whether other, nonergot derived drugs (e.g., entacapone, levodopa) that increase dopaminergic activity can cause them is unknown. It should be noted that the expected incidence of fibrotic complications is so low that even if entacapone caused these complications at rates similar to those attributable to other dopaminergic therapies, it is unlikely that it would have been detected in a cohort of the size exposed to entacapone. Four cases of pulmonary fibrosis were reported during clinical development of entacapone; three of these patients were also treated with pergolide and one with bromocriptine. The duration of treatment with entacapone ranged from 7-17 months.

Melanoma: Epidemiological studies have shown that patients with Parkinson's disease have a higher risk (2- to approximately 6-fold higher) of developing melanoma than the general population. Whether the increased risk observed was due to Parkinson's disease or other factors, such as drugs used to treat Parkinson's disease, is unclear.

For the reasons stated above, patients and providers are advised to monitor for melanomas frequently and on a regular basis when using Stalevo for *any* indication. Ideally, periodic skin examination should be performed by appropriately qualified individuals (e.g., dermatologists).

Renal Toxicity

In a one-year toxicity study, entacapone (plasma exposure 20 times that in humans receiving the maximum recommended daily dose of 1600 mg) caused an increased incidence of nephrotoxicity in male rats that was characterized by regenerative tubules, thickening of basement membranes, infiltration of mononuclear cells and tubular protein casts. These effects were not associated with changes in clinical chemistry parameters, and there is no established method for monitoring for the possible occurrence of these lesions in humans. Although this toxicity could represent a species-specific effect, there is not yet evidence that this is so.

Hepatic Impairment

Patients with hepatic impairment should be treated with caution. The AUC and C_{max} of entacapone approximately doubled in patients with documented liver disease compared to controls. (See CLINICAL PHARMACOLOGY, Pharmacokinetics, and DOSAGE AND ADMINISTRATION.)

Biliary Obstruction

Caution should be exercised when administering Stalevo to patients with biliary obstruction, as entacapone is excreted mostly via the bile.

Information for Patients

The patient should be instructed to take Stalevo only as prescribed. The patient should be informed that Stalevo is a standard-release formulation of carbidopa-levodopa combined with entacapone that is designed to begin release of ingredients within 30 minutes after ingestion. It is important that Stalevo be taken at regular intervals according to the schedule outlined by the physician. The patient should be cautioned not to change the prescribed dosage regimen and not to add any additional antiparkinsonian medications, including other carbidopa-levodopa preparations, without first consulting the physician.

Patients should be advised that sometimes a "wearing-off" effect may occur at the end of the dosing interval. The physician should be notified for possible treatment adjustments if such response poses a problem to patient's everyday life.

Patients should be advised that occasionally, dark color (red, brown, or black) may appear in saliva, urine, or sweat after ingestion of Stalevo. Although the color appears to be clinically insignificant, garments may become discolored.

The patient should be advised that a change in diet to foods that are high in protein may delay the absorption of levodopa and may reduce the amount taken up in the circulation. Excessive acidity also delays stomach emptying, thus delaying the absorption of levodopa. Iron salts (such as in multi-vitamin tablets) may also reduce the amount of levodopa available to the body. The above factors may reduce the clinical effectiveness of the levodopa, carbidopa-levodopa and Stalevo therapy.

NOTE: The suggested advice to patients being treated with Stalevo is intended to aid in the safe and effective use of this medication. It is not a disclosure of all possible adverse or intended effects.

Patients should be informed that hallucinations can occur. Patients should be advised that they may develop postural (orthostatic) hypotension with or without symptoms such as dizziness, nausea, syncope, and sweating. Hypotension may occur more frequently during initial therapy or when total daily levodopa dosage is increased. Accordingly, patients should be cautioned against rising rapidly after sitting or lying down, especially if they have been doing so for prolonged periods, and especially at the initiation of treatment with Stalevo.

Patients should be advised that they should neither drive a car nor operate other complex machinery until they have gained sufficient experience on Stalevo to gauge whether or not it affects their mental and/or motor performance adversely. Because of the possible additive sedative effects, caution should be used when patients are taking other CNS depressants in combination with Stalevo.

Patients should be informed that nausea may occur, especially at the initiation of treatment with Stalevo.

Patients should be advised of the possibility of an increase in dyskinesia.

Carbidopa-levodopa combination and entacapone are known to affect embryo-fetal development in the rabbit and in the rat, respectively. Accordingly, patients should be advised to notify their physicians if they become pregnant or intend to become pregnant during therapy (see PRECAUTIONS, Pregnancy).

Carbidopa and entacapone are known to be excreted into maternal milk in rats. Because of the possibility that carbidopa, levodopa and entacapone may be excreted into human maternal milk, patients should be advised to notify their physicians if they intend to breast-feed or are breast-feeding an infant.

There have been reports of patients experiencing intense urges to gamble, increased sexual urges, and other intense urges and the inability to control these urges while taking one or more of the medications that increase central dopaminergic tone, that are generally used for the treatment of Parkinson's disease, including Stalevo. Although it is not proven that the medications caused these events, these urges were reported to have stopped in some cases when the dose was reduced or the medication was stopped. Prescribers should ask patients about the development of new or increased gambling urges, sexual urges or other urges while being treated with Stalevo. Patients should inform their physician if they experience new or increased gambling urges, increased sexual urges or other intense urges while taking Stalevo. Physicians should consider dose reduction or stopping the medication if a patient develops such urges while taking Stalevo.

Laboratory Tests

Abnormalities in laboratory tests may include elevations of liver function tests such as alkaline phosphatase, SGOT (AST), SGPT (ALT), lactic dehydrogenase, and bilirubin. Abnormalities in blood urea nitrogen and positive Coombs' test have also been reported. Commonly, levels of blood urea nitrogen, creatinine, and uric acid are lower during administration of Stalevo than with levodopa.

Stalevo may cause a false-positive reaction for urinary ketone bodies when a test tape is used for determination of ketonuria. This reaction will not be altered by boiling the urine specimen. False-negative tests may result with the use of glucose-oxidase methods of testing for glucosuria.

Cases of falsely diagnosed pheochromocytoma in patients on carbidopa-levodopa therapy have been reported very rarely. Caution should be exercised when interpreting the plasma and urine levels of catecholamines and their metabolites in patients on carbidopa-levodopa therapy.

Entacapone is a chelator of iron. The impact of entacapone on the body's iron stores is unknown; however, a tendency towards decreasing serum iron concentrations was noted in clinical trials. In a controlled clinical study serum ferritin levels (as marker of iron deficiency and subclinical anemia) were not changed with entacapone compared to placebo after one year of treatment and there was no difference in rates of anemia or decreased hemoglobin levels.

Drug Interactions

Caution should be exercised when the following drugs are administered concomitantly with Stalevo.

Anti-hypertensive agents: Symptomatic postural hypotension has occurred when carbidopa-levodopa was added to the treatment of patients receiving antihypertensive drugs. Therefore, when therapy with Stalevo is started, dosage adjustment of the antihypertensive drug may be required.

MAO inhibitors: For patients receiving nonselective MAO inhibitors, see CONTRAINDICATIONS. Concomitant therapy with selegiline and carbidopa-levodopa may be associated with severe orthostatic hypotension not attributable to carbidopa-levodopa alone.

Tricyclic antidepressants: There have been rare reports of adverse reactions, including hypertension and dyskinesia, resulting from the concomitant use of tricyclic antidepressants and carbidopa-levodopa.

Dopamine D2 receptor antagonists (e.g., phenothiazines, butyrophenones, risperidone) and isoniazid: Dopamine D2 receptor antagonists (e.g., phenothiazines, butyrophenones, risperidone) and isoniazid may reduce the therapeutic effects of levodopa.

Phenytoin and papaverine: The beneficial effects of levodopa in Parkinson's disease have been reported to be reversed by phenytoin and papaverine. Patients taking these drugs with carbidopa-levodopa should be carefully observed for loss of therapeutic response.

Iron salts: Iron salts may reduce the bioavailability of levodopa, carbidopa and entacapone. The clinical relevance is unclear.

Metoclopramide: Although metoclopramide may increase the bioavailability of levodopa by increasing gastric emptying, metoclopramide may also adversely affect disease control by its dopamine receptor antagonistic properties.

Drugs known to interfere with biliary excretion, glucuronidation, and intestinal beta-glucuronidase (probenecid, cholestyramine, erythromycin, rifampicin, ampicillin and chloramphenicol): As most entacapone excretion is via the bile, caution should be exercised when drugs known to interfere with biliary excretion, glucuronidation, and intestinal beta-glucuronidase are given concurrently with entacapone. These include probenecid, cholestyramine, and some antibiotics (e.g., erythromycin, rifampicin, ampicillin and chloramphenicol).

Pyridoxine: Stalevo can be given to patients receiving supplemental pyridoxine. Oral coadministration of 10-25 mg of pyridoxine hydrochloride (vitamin B6) with levodopa may reverse the effects of levodopa by increasing the rate of aromatic amino acid decarboxylation. Carbidopa inhibits this action of pyridoxine; therefore, Stalevo can be given to patients receiving supplemental pyridoxine.

Effect of levodopa and carbidopa in Stalevo on the metabolism of other drugs: Inhibition or induction effect of levodopa and carbidopa has not been investigated.

Table 4
German-Austrian Study

Primary Measures

	Baseline	Change from Baseline at Month 6	p-value vs. placebo (LOCF)
UPDRS ADL*			
Placebo	12.0	+0.5	—
Entacapone	12.4	-0.4	<0.05
UPDRS Motor*			
Placebo	24.1	+0.1	—
Entacapone	24.9	-2.5	<0.05
Hours of Awake Time "On" (Home Diary)**			
Placebo	10.1	+0.5	—
Entacapone	10.2	+1.1	N.S.‡

Secondary Measures

	Baseline	Change from Baseline at Month 6	p-value vs. placebo
UPDRS Total*			
Placebo	37.7	+0.6	—
Entacapone	39.0	-3.4	<0.05
Percent of Awake Time "On" (Home Diary)**			
Placebo	59.8	+3.5	—
Entacapone	62.0	+6.5	N.S.‡
Hours of Awake Time "Off" (Home Diary)**			
Placebo	6.8	-0.6	—
Entacapone	6.3	-1.2	0.07
Levodopa Total Daily Dose (mg)*			
Placebo	572	+4	—
Entacapone	566	-35	N.S.‡
Frequency of Levodopa Daily Intake*			
Placebo	5.6	+0.2	—
Entacapone	5.4	0.0	<0.01
Global (overall) % Improved**			
Placebo	—	34	—
Entacapone	—	38	N.S.‡

* Total population; score change at endpoint.
** Fluctuating population, with 5-10 doses; score change at endpoint.
*** Total population; at least one category change at endpoint.
‡ Not significant.

Effect of entacapone in Stalevo on the metabolism of other drugs: Entacapone is unlikely to inhibit the metabolism of other drugs that are metabolized by major P450s including CYP1A2, CYP2A6, CYP2C9, CYP2C19, CYP2D6, CYP2E1 and CYP3A. *In vitro* studies of human CYP enzymes showed that entacapone inhibited the CYP enzymes 1A2, 2A6, 2C9, 2C19, 2D6, 2E1 and 3A only at very high concentrations (IC50 from 200 to over 1000 µM; an oral 200 mg dose achieves a highest level of approximately 5 µM in people); these enzymes would therefore not be expected to be inhibited in clinical use. However, no information is available regarding the induction effect from entacapone.

Drugs that are highly protein bound (such as warfarin, salicylic acid, phenylbutazone, and diazepam):

Levodopa

Levodopa is bound to plasma protein only to a minor extent (about 10%-30%).

Carbidopa

Carbidopa is approximately 36% bound to plasma protein.

Entacapone

Entacapone is highly protein bound (98%). *In vitro* studies have shown no binding displacement between entacapone and other highly bound drugs, such as warfarin, salicylic acid, phenylbutazone, and diazepam.

Hormone Levels

Of the ingredients in Stalevo, levodopa is known to depress prolactin secretion and increase growth hormone levels.

Carcinogenesis

In a two-year bioassay of carbidopa-levodopa, no evidence of carcinogenicity was found in rats receiving doses of approximately two times the maximum daily human dose of carbidopa and four times the maximum daily human dose of levodopa.

Two-year carcinogenicity studies of entacapone were conducted in mice and rats. Rats were treated once daily by oral gavage with entacapone doses of 20, 90, or 400 mg/kg. An increased incidence of renal tubular adenomas and carcinomas was found in male rats treated with the highest dose of entacapone. Plasma exposures (AUC) associated with this dose were approximately 20 times higher than estimated plasma exposures of humans receiving the maximum recommended daily dose of entacapone (MRDD = 1600 mg). Mice were treated once daily by oral gavage with doses of 20, 100 or 600 mg/kg of entacapone (0.05, 0.3, and two times the MRDD for humans on a mg/m^2 basis). Because of a high incidence of premature mortality in mice receiving the highest dose of entacapone, the mouse study is not an adequate assessment of carcinogenicity. Although no treatment related tumors were observed in animals receiving the lower doses, the carcinogenic potential of entacapone has not been fully evaluated. The carcinogenic potential of entacapone administered in combination with carbidopa-levodopa has not been evaluated.

Mutagenesis

Carbidopa was positive in the Ames test in the presence and absence of metabolic activation, was mutagenic in the *in vitro* mouse lymphoma/thymidine kinase assay in the absence of metabolic activation, and was negative in the *in vivo* mouse micronucleus test.

Entacapone was mutagenic and clastogenic in the *in vitro* mouse lymphoma/thymidine kinase assay in the presence and absence of metabolic activation, and was clastogenic in cultured human lymphocytes in the presence of metabolic activation. Entacapone, either alone or in combination with carbidopa-levodopa, was not clastogenic in the *in vivo* mouse micronucleus test or mutagenic in the bacterial reverse mutation assay (Ames test).

Impairment of Fertility

In reproduction studies with carbidopa-levodopa, no effects on fertility were found in rats receiving doses of approximately two times the maximum daily human dose of carbidopa and four times the maximum daily human dose of levodopa.

Entacapone did not impair fertility or general reproductive performance in rats treated with up to 700 mg/kg/day (plasma AUCs 28 times those in humans receiving the MRDD). Delayed mating, but no fertility impairment, was evident in female rats treated with 700 mg/kg/day of entacapone.

Pregnancy

Pregnancy Category C

Carbidopa-levodopa caused both visceral and skeletal malformations in rabbits at all doses and ratios of carbidopa-levodopa tested, which ranged from 10 times/5 times the maximum recommended human dose of carbidopa-levodopa to 20 times/10 times the maximum recommended human dose of carbidopa-levodopa. There was a decrease in the number of live pups delivered by rats receiving approximately two times the maximum recommended human dose of carbidopa and approximately five times the maximum recommended human dose of levodopa during organogenesis. No teratogenic effects were observed in mice receiving up to 20 times the maximum recommended human dose of carbidopa-levodopa.

It has been reported from individual cases that levodopa crosses the human placental barrier, enters the fetus, and is metabolized. Carbidopa concentrations in fetal tissue appeared to be minimal.

In embryo-fetal development studies, entacapone was administered to pregnant animals throughout organogenesis at doses of up to 1000 mg/kg/day in rats and 300 mg/kg/day in rabbits. Increased incidences of fetal variations were evident in litters from rats treated with the highest dose, in the absence of overt signs of maternal toxicity. The maternal plasma drug exposure (AUC) associated with this dose was approximately 34 times the estimated plasma exposure in humans receiving the maximum recommended daily dose (MRDD) of 1600 mg. Increased frequencies of abortions and late/total resorptions and decreased fetal weights were observed in the litters of rabbits treated with maternotoxic doses of 100 mg/kg/day (plasma AUCs 0.4 times those in humans receiving the MRDD) or greater. There was no evidence of teratogenicity in these studies.

However, when entacapone was administered to female rats prior to mating and during early gestation, an increased incidence of fetal eye anomalies (macrophthalmia, microphthalmia, anophthalmia) was observed in the litters of dams treated with doses of 160 mg/kg/day (plasma AUCs seven times those in humans receiving the MRDD) or greater, in the absence of maternotoxicity. Administration of up to 700 mg/kg/day (plasma AUCs 28 times those in humans receiving the MRDD) to female rats during the latter part of gestation and throughout lactation, produced no evidence of developmental impairment in the offspring.

There is no experience from clinical studies regarding the use of Stalevo in pregnant women. Therefore, Stalevo should be used during pregnancy only if the potential benefit justifies the potential risk to the fetus.

Nursing Women

In animal studies, carbidopa and entacapone were excreted into maternal rat milk. It is not known whether entacapone or carbidopa-levodopa are excreted in human milk. Because many drugs are excreted in human milk, caution should be exercised when Stalevo is administered to a nursing woman.

Pediatric Use

Safety and effectiveness in pediatric patients have not been established.

ADVERSE REACTIONS

Carbidopa-levodopa

The most common adverse reactions reported with carbidopa-levodopa have included dyskinesias, such as choreiform, dystonic, and other involuntary movements and nausea.

The following other adverse reactions have been reported with carbidopa-levodopa:

Body as a Whole: Chest pain, asthenia.

Cardiovascular: Cardiac irregularities, hypotension, orthostatic effects including orthostatic hypotension, hypertension, syncope, phlebitis, palpitation.

Gastrointestinal: Dark saliva, gastrointestinal bleeding, development of duodenal ulcer, anorexia, vomiting, diarrhea, constipation, dyspepsia, dry mouth, taste alterations.

Hematologic: Agranulocytosis, hemolytic and nonhemolytic anemia, thrombocytopenia, leukopenia.

Hypersensitivity: Angioedema, urticaria, pruritus, Henoch-Schönlein purpura, bullous lesions (including pemphigus-like reactions).

Musculoskeletal: Back pain, shoulder pain, muscle cramps.

Nervous System/Psychiatric: Psychotic episodes including delusions, hallucinations, and paranoid ideation, neuroleptic malignant syndrome *(see WARNINGS)*, bradykinetic episodes ("on-off" phenomenon), confusion, agitation, dizziness, somnolence, dream abnormalities including nightmares, insomnia, paresthesia, headache, depression with or without development of suicidal tendencies, dementia, increased libido. Convulsions also have occurred; however, a causal relationship with carbidopa-levodopa has not been established.

Respiratory: Dyspnea, upper respiratory infection.

Skin: Rash, increased sweating, alopecia, dark sweat.

Urogenital: Urinary tract infection, urinary frequency, dark urine.

Laboratory Tests: Decreased hemoglobin and hematocrit; abnormalities in alkaline phosphatase, SGOT (AST), SGPT (ALT), lactic dehydrogenase, bilirubin, blood urea nitrogen (BUN), Coombs' test; elevated serum glucose; white blood cells, bacteria, and blood in the urine.

Other adverse reactions that have been reported with levodopa alone and with various carbidopa-levodopa formulations, and may occur with Stalevo® (carbidopa, levodopa and entacapone) are:

Body as a Whole: Abdominal pain and distress, fatigue.

Cardiovascular: Myocardial infarction.

Gastrointestinal: Gastrointestinal pain, dysphagia, sialorrhea, flatulence, bruxism, burning sensation of the tongue, heartburn, hiccups.

Metabolic: Edema, weight gain, weight loss.

Musculoskeletal: Leg pain.

Nervous System/Psychiatric: Ataxia, extrapyramidal disorder, failing, anxiety, gait abnormalities, nervousness, decreased mental acuity, memory impairment, disorientation, euphoria, blepharospasm (which may be taken as an early sign of excess dosage; consideration of dosage reduction may be made at this time), trismus, increased tremor, numbness, muscle twitching, activation of latent Horner's syndrome, peripheral neuropathy.

Respiratory: Pharyngeal pain, cough.

Skin: Malignant melanoma *(see also CONTRAINDICATIONS)*, flushing.

Special Senses: Oculogyric crisis, diplopia, blurred vision, dilated pupils.

Urogenital: Urinary retention, urinary incontinence, priapism.

Miscellaneous: Bizarre breathing patterns, faintness, hoarseness, malaise, hot flashes, sense of stimulation.

Laboratory Tests: Decreased white blood cell count and serum potassium; increased serum creatinine and uric acid; protein and glucose in urine.

Entacapone

The most commonly observed adverse events (>5%) in the double-blind, placebo-controlled trials of entacapone (n=1003) associated with the use of entacapone alone and not seen at an equivalent frequency among the placebo-treated patients were: dyskinesia/hyperkinesia, nausea, urine discoloration, diarrhea, and abdominal pain.

Approximately 14% of the 603 patients given entacapone in the double-blind, placebo-controlled trials discontinued treatment due to adverse events compared to 9% of the 400 patients who received placebo. The most frequent causes of discontinuation in decreasing order are: psychiatric reasons (2% vs. 1%), diarrhea (2% vs. 0%), dyskinesia/hyperkinesia (2% vs. 1%), nausea (2% vs. 1%), abdominal pain (1% vs. 0%), and aggravation of Parkinson's disease symptoms (1% vs. 1%).

Adverse Event Incidence in Controlled Clinical Studies of Entacapone

Table 5 lists treatment emergent adverse events that occurred in at least 1% of patients treated with entacapone participating in the double-blind, placebo-controlled studies and that were numerically more common in the entacapone group, compared to placebo. In these studies, either entacapone or placebo was added to carbidopa-levodopa (or benserazide-levodopa).

[See table 5 at top of next page]

The prescriber should be aware that these figures cannot be used to predict the incidence of adverse events in the course of usual medical practice where patient characteristics and other factors differ from those that prevailed in the clinical studies. Similarly, the cited frequencies cannot be compared with figures obtained from other clinical investigations involving different treatments, uses, and investigators. The cited figures do, however, provide the prescriber with some basis for estimating the relative contribution of drug and nondrug factors to the adverse events observed in the population studied.

Effects of Gender and Age on Adverse Reactions

No differences were noted in the rate of adverse events attributable to entacapone alone by age or gender.

DRUG ABUSE AND DEPENDENCE

Controlled substance class: Stalevo® (carbidopa, levodopa and entacapone) is not a controlled substance.

Physical and psychological dependence: Stalevo has not been systematically studied, in animal or humans, for its potential for abuse, tolerance or physical dependence. In premarketing clinical experience, carbidopa-levodopa did not reveal any tendency for a withdrawal syndrome or any drug-seeking behavior. However, there are rare post-marketing reports of abuse and dependence of medications containing levodopa. In general, these reports consist of patients taking increasing doses of medication in order to achieve a euphoric state.

OVERDOSAGE

Management of acute overdosage with Stalevo® (carbidopa, levodopa and entacapone) is the same as management of acute overdosage with levodopa and entacapone. Pyridoxine is not effective in reversing the actions of Stalevo.

Hospitalization is advised, and general supportive measures should be employed, along with immediate gastric lavage and repeated doses of charcoal over time. This may hasten the elimination of entacapone in particular, by decreasing its absorption/reabsorption from the GI tract. Intravenous fluids should be administered judiciously and an adequate airway maintained.

The adequacy of the respiratory, circulatory and renal systems should be carefully monitored and appropriate supportive measures employed. Electrocardiographic monitoring should be instituted and the patient carefully observed for the development of arrhythmias; if required, appropriate antiarrhythmic therapy should be given. The possibility that the patient may have taken other drugs, increasing the risk of drug interactions (especially catechol-structured drugs) should be taken into consideration. To date, no experience has been reported with dialysis; hence, its value in overdosage is not known. Hemodialysis or hemoperfusion is unlikely to reduce entacapone levels due to its high binding to plasma proteins.

There are very few cases of overdosage with levodopa reported in the published literature. Based on the limited available information, the acute symptoms of levodopa/dopa decarboxylase inhibitor overdosage can be expected to arise from dopaminergic overstimulation. Doses of a few grams may result in CNS disturbances, with an increasing likelihood of cardiovascular disturbance (e.g., hypotension, tachycardia) and more severe psychiatric problems at higher doses. An isolated report of rhabdomyolysis and another of transient renal insufficiency suggest that levodopa overdosage may give rise to systemic complications, secondary to dopaminergic overstimulation.

There have been no reported cases of either accidental or intentional overdose with entacapone tablets. However, COMT inhibition by entacapone treatment is dose-dependent. A massive overdose of entacapone may theoretically produce a 100% inhibition of the COMT enzyme in people, thereby preventing the O-methylation of endogenous and exogenous catechols.

The highest single dose of entacapone administered to humans was 800 mg, resulting in a plasma concentration of 14.1 µg/mL. The highest daily dose given to humans was 2400 mg, administered in one study as 400 mg six times daily with carbidopa-levopoda for 14 days in 15 Parkinson's disease patients, and in another study as 800 mg t.i.d. for 7 days in 8 healthy volunteers. At this daily dose, the peak plasma concentrations of entacapone averaged 2.0 µg/mL (at 45 min., compared to 1.0 and 1.2 µg/mL with 200 mg entacapone at 45 min.). Abdominal pain and loose stools were the most commonly observed adverse events during this study. Daily doses as high as 2000 mg entacapone have been administered as 200 mg 10 times daily with carbidopa-levodopa or benserazide-levodopa for at least 1 year in 10 patients, for at least 2 years in 8 patients and for at least 3 years in 7 patients. Overall, however, clinical experience with daily doses above 1600 mg is limited.

The range of lethal plasma concentrations of entacapone based on animal data was 80-130 µg/mL in mice. Respiratory difficulties, ataxia, hypoactivity, and convulsions were observed in mice after high oral (gavage) doses.

DOSAGE AND ADMINISTRATION

Individual tablets should not be fractionated and only one tablet should be administered at each dosing interval.

Generally speaking, Stalevo® (carbidopa, levodopa and entacapone) should be used as a substitute for patients already stabilized on equivalent doses of carbidopa-levodopa and entacapone. However, some patients who have been stabilized on a given dose of carbidopa-levodopa may be treated with Stalevo if a decision has been made to add entacapone (see below).

The optimum daily dosage of Stalevo must be determined by careful titration in each patient. Stalevo tablets are available in six strengths, each in a 1:4 ratio of carbidopa to levodopa and combined with 200 mg of entacapone in a standard release formulation (Stalevo 50 containing 12.5 mg of carbidopa, 50 mg of levodopa and 200 mg of entacapone; Stalevo 75, containing 18.75 mg of carbidopa, 75 mg of levodopa and 200 mg of entacapone; Stalevo 100 containing 25 mg of carbidopa, 100 mg of levodopa and 200 mg of entacapone; Stalevo 125, containing 31.25 mg of carbidopa, 125 mg of levodopa and 200 mg of entacapone; Stalevo 150 containing 37.5 mg of carbidopa, 150 mg of levodopa and 200 mg of entacapone; and Stalevo 200 containing 50 mg of carbidopa, 200 mg of levodopa and 200 mg of entacapone).

Therapy should be individualized and adjusted according to the desired therapeutic response.

Studies show that peripheral dopa decarboxylase is saturated by carbidopa at approximately 70 mg to 100 mg a day. Patients receiving less than this amount of carbidopa are more likely to experience nausea and vomiting.

Clinical experience with daily doses above 1600 mg of entacapone is limited. It is recommended that no more than one Stalevo tablet be taken at each dosing administration. Thus the maximum recommended daily dose of Stalevo 50, Stalevo 75, Stalevo 100, Stalevo 125 and Stalevo 150, defined by the maximum daily dose of entacapone, is eight tablets per day. Because there is limited experience with total daily doses of carbidopa greater than 300 mg, the maximum recommended daily dose of Stalevo 200 is six tablets per day.

How to transfer patients taking carbidopa-levodopa preparations and Comtan® (entacapone) tablets to Stalevo® (carbidopa, levodopa and entacapone) tablets

There is no experience in transferring patients currently treated with formulations of carbidopa-levodopa other than

immediate-release carbidopa-levodopa with a 1:4 ratio (controlled-release formulations, or standard-release presentations with a 1:10 ratio of carbidopa-levodopa) and entacapone to Stalevo.

Patients who are currently treated with Comtan 200 mg tablet with each dose of standard-release carbidopa-levodopa, can be directly switched to the corresponding strength of Stalevo containing the same amounts of levodopa and carbidopa. For example, patients receiving one tablet of standard-release carbidopa-levodopa 25/100 mg and one tablet of Comtan 200 mg at each administration can be switched to a single Stalevo 100 tablet (containing 25 mg of carbidopa, 100 mg of levodopa and 200 mg of entacapone).

How to transfer patients not currently treated with Comtan® (entacapone) tablets from carbidopa-levodopa to Stalevo® (carbidopa, levodopa and entacapone) tablets

In patients with Parkinson's disease who experience the signs and symptoms of end-of-dose "wearing-off" on their current standard-release carbidopa-levodopa treatment, clinical experience shows that patients with a history of moderate or severe dyskinesias or taking more than 600 mg of levodopa per day are likely to require a reduction in daily levodopa dose when entacapone is added to their treatment. Since dose adjustment of the individual components is impossible with fixed-dose products, it is recommended that patients first be titrated individually with a carbidopa-levodopa product (ratio 1:4) and an entacapone product, and then transferred to a corresponding dose of Stalevo once the patient's status has stabilized.

In patients who take a total daily levodopa dose up to 600 mg, and who do not have dyskinesias, an attempt can be made to transfer to the corresponding daily dose of Stalevo. Even in these patients, a reduction of carbidopa-levodopa or entacapone may be necessary however, the provider is reminded that this may not be possible with Stalevo. Since entacapone prolongs and enhances the effects of levodopa, therapy should be individualized and adjusted if necessary according to the desired therapeutic response.

Maintenance of Stalevo® Treatment

Therapy should be individualized and adjusted for each patient according to the desired therapeutic response.

When less levodopa is required, the total daily dosage of carbidopa-levodopa should be reduced by either decreasing

the strength of Stalevo at each administration or by decreasing the frequency of administration by extending the time between doses.

When more levodopa is required, the next higher strength of Stalevo should be taken and/or the frequency of doses should be increased, up to a maximum of 8 times daily of Stalevo 50, Stalevo 75, Stalevo 100, Stalevo 125, and Stalevo 150, and maximum of 6 times daily of Stalevo 200.

Addition of Other Antiparkinsonian Medications

Standard drugs for Parkinson's disease may be used concomitantly while Stalevo is being administered, although dosage adjustments may be required.

Interruption of Therapy

Sporadic cases of a symptom complex resembling Neuroleptic Malignant Syndrome (NMS) have been associated with dose reductions and withdrawal of Stalevo preparations. Patients should be observed carefully if abrupt reduction or discontinuation of Stalevo is required, especially if the patient is receiving neuroleptics. (See WARNINGS.)

If general anesthesia is required, Stalevo may be continued as long as the patient is permitted to take fluids and medication by mouth. If therapy is interrupted temporarily, the patient should be observed for symptoms resembling NMS, and the usual daily dosage may be administered as soon as the patient is able to take oral medication.

Special Populations

Patients With Impaired Hepatic Function:

Patients with hepatic impairment should be treated with caution. The AUC and C_{max} of entacapone approximately doubled in patients with documented liver disease, compared to controls. However, these studies were conducted with single-dose entacapone without levodopa/dopa decarboxylase inhibitor coadministration, and therefore the effects of liver disease on the kinetics of chronically administered entacapone have not been evaluated (see CLINICAL PHARMACOLOGY, Pharmacokinetics of Entacapone).

HOW SUPPLIED

Stalevo® (carbidopa, levodopa and entacapone) is supplied as film-coated tablets for oral administration in the following six strengths:

Stalevo 50 film-coated tablets containing 12.5 mg of carbidopa, 50 mg of levodopa and 200 mg of entacapone. The round, bi-convex shaped tablets are brownish- or greyish-red, unscored, and embossed "LCE 50" on one side.

Table 5
Summary of Patients with Adverse Events After Start of Trial Drug Administration
At Least 1% in Entacapone Group and >Placebo

SYSTEM ORGAN CLASS Preferred Term	Entacapone (n = 603) % of patients	Placebo (n = 400) % of patients
SKIN AND APPENDAGES DISORDERS		
Sweating Increased	2	1
MUSCULOSKELETAL SYSTEM DISORDERS		
Back Pain	2	1
CENTRAL & PERIPHERAL NERVOUS SYSTEM DISORDERS		
Dyskinesia	25	15
Hyperkinesia	10	5
Hypokinesia	9	8
Dizziness	8	6
SPECIAL SENSES, OTHER DISORDERS		
Taste Perversion	1	0
PSYCHIATRIC DISORDERS		
Anxiety	2	1
Somnolence	2	0
Agitation	1	0
GASTROINTESTINAL SYSTEM DISORDERS		
Nausea	14	8
Diarrhea	10	4
Abdominal Pain	8	4
Constipation	6	4
Vomiting	4	1
Mouth Dry	3	0
Dyspepsia	2	1
Flatulence	2	0
Gastritis	1	0
Gastrointestinal Disorders NOS	1	0
RESPIRATORY SYSTEM DISORDERS		
Dyspnea	3	1
PLATELET, BLEEDING & CLOTTING DISORDERS		
Purpura	2	1
URINARY SYSTEM DISORDERS		
Urine Discoloration	10	0
BODY AS A WHOLE - GENERAL DISORDERS		
Back Pain	4	2
Fatigue	6	4
Asthenia	2	1
RESISTANCE MECHANISM DISORDERS		
Infection Bacterial	1	0

HDPE bottle of 100 tablets .... NDC 0078-0407-05
HDPE bottle of 250 tablets .... NDC 0078-0407-28
Stalevo 75 film-coated tablets containing 18.75 mg of carbidopa, 75 mg of levodopa and 200 mg of entacapone. The oval-shaped tablets are light brownish red, unscored, and embossed with code "LCE 75" on one side.
HDPE bottle of 100 tablets .... NDC 0078-0544-05
Stalevo 100 film-coated tablets containing 25 mg of carbidopa, 100 mg of levodopa and 200 mg of entacapone. The oval-shaped tablets are brownish- or greyish-red, unscored, and embossed "LCE 100" on one side.
HDPE bottle of 100 tablets .... NDC 0078-0408-05
HDPE bottle of 250 tablets .... NDC 0078-0408-28
Stalevo 125 film-coated tablets containing 31.25 mg of carbidopa, 125 mg of levodopa and 200 mg of entacapone. The oval-shaped tablets are light brownish red, unscored, and embossed with code "LCE 125" on one side.
HDPE bottle of 100 tablets .... NDC 0078-0545-05
Stalevo 150 film-coated tablets containing 37.5 mg of carbidopa, 150 mg of levodopa and 200 mg of entacapone The elongated-ellipse shaped tablets are brownish- or greyish-red, unscored, and embossed "LCE 150" on one side.
HDPE bottle of 100 tablets .... NDC 0078-0409-05
HDPE bottle of 250 tablets .... NDC 0078-0409-28
Stalevo 200 film-coated tablets containing 50 mg of carbidopa, 200 mg of levodopa and 200 mg of entacapone The oval shaped tablets are dark brownish red, unscored, and embossed "LCE 200" on one side.
HDPE bottle of 100 tablets .... NDC 0078-0527-05
Store at 25°C (77°F); excursions permitted to 15°-30°C (59°-86°F). [see USP Controlled Room Temperature.] Dispense in tight container (USP).

T2009-37

REV. MARCH 2009   Printed in U.S.A.
Manufactured by: Orion Corporation, ORION PHARMA, Orionintie 1, FIN-02200 Espoo, Finland
Marketed by: Novartis Pharmaceuticals Corporation, East Hanover, New Jersey 07936
©Novartis
Shown in Product Identification Guide, page 316

TASIGNA®   ℞
[ta-sig-na]
(nilotinib)
Capsules

The following prescribing information is based on official labeling in effect July 2010.
HIGHLIGHTS OF PRESCRIBING INFORMATION
These highlights do not include all the information needed to use Tasigna safely and effectively. See full prescribing information for Tasigna.
Tasigna® *(nilotinib)* **Capsules**
Initial U.S. Approval: 2007

WARNING: QT PROLONGATION AND SUDDEN DEATHS
See full prescribing information for complete boxed warning.
Tasigna prolongs the QT interval (5.2). Sudden deaths have been reported in patients receiving nilotinib (5.3). Tasigna should not be used in patients with hypokalemia, hypomagnesemia, or long QT syndrome (4). Hypokalemia or hypomagnesemia must be corrected prior to Tasigna administration and should be periodically monitored (5.2). Drugs known to prolong the QT interval and strong CYP3A4 inhibitors should be avoided (5.7). Patients should avoid food 2 hours before and 1 hour after taking dose (5.8). A dose reduction is recommended in patients with hepatic impairment (5.9). ECGs should be obtained to monitor the QTc at baseline, seven days after initiation, and periodically thereafter, as well as following any dose adjustments (5.2, 5.3, 5.6, 5.12).

———RECENT MAJOR CHANGES———
Indications and Usage: Newly diagnosed Ph+ CML-CP (1.1)   06/2010
Dosage and Administration: Recommended Dosing (2.1), Dose Adjustments or Modifications (2.2)   06/2010
Warnings and Precautions: Myelosuppression (5.1), Sudden Deaths (5.3), Elevated Serum Lipase (5.4), Total Gastrectomy (5.10)   06/2010

———INDICATIONS AND USAGE———
Treatment of newly diagnosed adult patients with Philadelphia chromosome positive chronic myeloid leukemia (Ph+ CML) in chronic phase. The study is ongoing and further data will be required to determine long-term outcome. (1.1)
Treatment of chronic phase (CP) and accelerated phase (AP) Ph+ CML in adult patients resistant to or intolerant to prior

therapy that included imatinib. Clinical benefit, such as improvement in disease-related symptoms or increased survival, has not been demonstrated. (1.2)

———DOSAGE AND ADMINISTRATION———
• Recommended Dose: Newly diagnosed Ph+ CML-CP: 300 mg orally twice daily. Resistant or intolerant Ph+ CML-CP and CML-AP: 400 mg orally twice daily. (2.1)
• Administer Tasigna approximately 12 hours apart and must not take with food. (2.1)
• Swallow the capsules whole with water. Do not consume food for at least 2 hours before the dose is taken and for at least one hour after. (2.1)
• Dose adjustment may be required for hematologic and non-hematologic toxicities, and drug interactions. (2.2)
• A lower starting dose is recommended in patients with hepatic impairment (at baseline). (2.2)

———DOSAGE FORMS AND STRENGTHS———
150 mg and 200 mg hard capsules (3)

———CONTRAINDICATIONS———
Do not use in patients with hypokalemia, hypomagnesemia, or long QT syndrome. (4)

———WARNINGS AND PRECAUTIONS———
• Myelosuppression: Associated with neutropenia, thrombocytopenia and anemia. CBC should be done every 2 weeks for the first 2 months, then monthly. Reversible by withholding dose. Dose reduction may be required. (5.1)
• QT Prolongation: Tasigna prolongs the QT interval. Correct hypokalemia or hypomagnesemia prior to administration and monitor periodically. (5.2) Avoid drugs known to prolong the QT interval and strong CYP3A4 inhibitors. (5.7) Use with caution in patients with hepatic impairment. (5.9) Obtain ECGs at baseline, seven days after initiation, and periodically thereafter, as well as following any dose adjustments. (5.2, 5.3, 5.6, 5.12)
• Sudden deaths: Sudden deaths have been reported in patients with resistant or intolerant Ph+ CML receiving nilotinib. Ventricular repolarization abnormalities may have contributed to their occurrence. (5.3)
• Elevated serum lipase: Check serum lipase periodically. In case lipase elevations are accompanied by abdominal symptoms, interrupt doses and consider appropriate diagnostics to exclude pancreatitis. Caution is recommended in patients with history of pancreatitis. (5.4)
• Liver function abnormality: Tasigna may result in elevations in bilirubin, AST/ALT, and alkaline phosphatase. Check hepatic function tests periodically. (5.5)
• Electrolyte abnormalities: Tasigna can cause hypophosphatemia, hypokalemia, hyperkalemia, hypocalcemia, and hyponatremia. Correct electrolyte abnormalities prior to initiating Tasigna and monitor periodically during therapy. (5.6, 5.12)
• Hepatic impairment: Nilotinib exposure is increased in patients with impaired hepatic function (at baseline). A dose reduction is recommended in these patients and QT interval should be monitored closely. (5.9)
• Drug interactions: Avoid concomitant use of strong inhibitors or inducers of CYP3A4. If patients must be co-administered a strong CYP3A4 inhibitor, dose reduction should be considered and the QT interval should be monitored closely. (5.7)
• Food Effects: Food increases blood levels of Tasigna.
• Avoid food 2 hours before and 1 hour after a dose. (5.8)
• Total gastrectomy: More frequent follow-up of these patients should be considered. If necessary, dose increase may be considered. (5.10)
• Pregnancy: Fetal harm can occur when administered to a pregnant woman. Women should be advised not to become pregnant when taking Tasigna. (5.13, 8.1)

———ADVERSE REACTIONS———
The most commonly reported non-hematologic adverse reactions (≥10%) in patients with newly diagnosed Ph+ CML-CP, resistant or intolerant Ph+ CML-CP, or resistant or intolerant Ph+ CML-AP were rash, pruritus, headache, nausea, fatigue, myalgia, nasopharyngitis, constipation, diarrhea, abdominal pain, vomiting, arthralgia, pyrexia, upper urinary tract infection, back pain, cough, and asthenia. Hematologic adverse drug reactions include myelosuppression: thrombocytopenia, neutropenia and anemia. (6.1)
To report SUSPECTED ADVERSE REACTIONS, contact Novartis Pharmaceuticals Corporation at 1-888-669-6682 or FDA at 1-800-FDA-1088 or www.fda.gov/medwatch

———DRUG INTERACTIONS———
• Tasigna is an inhibitor of CYP3A4, CYP2C8, CYP2C9, and CYP2D6. It may also induce CYP2B6, CYP2C8 and CYP2C9. Therefore, Tasigna may alter serum concentration of other drugs (7.1)
• CYP3A4 inhibitors may affect serum concentration (7.2)
• CYP3A4 inducers may affect serum concentration (7.2)

———USE IN SPECIFIC POPULATIONS———
• Sexually active female patients should use effective contraception during treatment (8.1)
• Should not breast-feed (8.3)
• No data to support use in pediatrics (8.4)

• A lower starting dose is recommended in patients with hepatic impairment (at baseline) (2.2, 8.7)

See 17 for PATIENT COUNSELING INFORMATION and Medication Guide

Revised: 06/2010

FULL PRESCRIBING INFORMATION

WARNING: QT PROLONGATION AND SUDDEN DEATHS
Tasigna prolongs the QT interval (5.2). Sudden deaths have been reported in patients receiving nilotinib (5.3). Tasigna should not be used in patients with hypokalemia, hypomagnesemia, or long QT syndrome (4). Hypokalemia or hypomagnesemia must be corrected prior to Tasigna administration and should be periodically monitored (5.2). Drugs known to prolong the QT interval and strong CYP3A4 inhibitors should be avoided (5.7). Patients should avoid food 2 hours before and 1 hour after taking dose (5.8). A dose reduction is recommended in patients with hepatic impairment (5.9). ECGs should be obtained to monitor the QTc at

baseline, seven days after initiation, and periodically thereafter, as well as following any dose adjustments (5.2, 5.3, 5.6, 5.12).

1 INDICATIONS AND USAGE

1.1 Newly Diagnosed Ph+ CML-CP

Tasigna (nilotinib) is indicated for the treatment of adult patients with newly diagnosed Philadelphia chromosome positive chronic myeloid leukemia (Ph+ CML) in chronic phase. The effectiveness of Tasigna is based on major molecular response and cytogenetic response rates [see Clinical Studies (14.1)]. The study is ongoing and further data will be required to determine long-term outcome.

1.2 Resistant or Intolerant Ph+ CML-CP and CML-AP

Tasigna is indicated for the treatment of chronic phase and accelerated phase Philadelphia chromosome positive chronic myelogenous leukemia (Ph+ CML) in adult patients resistant or intolerant to prior therapy that included imatinib. The effectiveness of Tasigna is based on hematologic and cytogenetic response rates [see Clinical Studies (14.2)]. There are no controlled trials demonstrating a clinical benefit, such as improvement in disease-related symptoms or increased survival.

2 DOSAGE AND ADMINISTRATION

2.1 Recommended Dosing

Newly Diagnosed Ph+ CML-CP

The recommended dose of Tasigna is 300 mg orally twice daily [see Clinical Pharmacology (12.3)].

Resistant or Intolerant Ph+ CML-CP and CML-AP

The recommended dose of Tasigna (nilotinib) is 400 mg orally twice daily [see Clinical Pharmacology (12.3)]. Tasigna should be taken twice daily at approximately 12 hour intervals and must not be taken with food. The capsules should be swallowed whole with water. No food should be consumed for at least 2 hours before the dose is taken and no food should be consumed for at least one hour after the dose is taken [see Boxed Warning, Warnings and Precautions (5.8), Clinical Pharmacology (12.3)].

If a dose is missed, the patient should not take a make-up dose, but should resume taking the next prescribed daily dose.

Tasigna may be given in combination with hematopoietic growth factors such as erythropoietin or G-CSF if clinically indicated. Tasigna may be given with hydroxyurea or anagrelide if clinically indicated.

2.2 Dose Adjustments or Modifications

QT interval prolongation:

Table 1. Dose Adjustments for QT Prolongation

ECGs with a QTc >480 msec	1. Withhold Tasigna, and perform an analysis of serum potassium and magnesium, and if below lower limit of normal, correct with supplements to within normal limits. Concomitant medication usage must be reviewed. 2. Resume within 2 weeks at prior dose if QTcF returns to <450 msec and to within 20 msec of baseline. 3. If QTcF is between 450 msec and 480 msec after 2 weeks reduce the dose to 400 mg once daily. 4. If, following dose-reduction to 400 mg once daily, QTcF returns to >480 msec, Tasigna should be discontinued. 5. An ECG should be repeated approximately 7 days after any dose adjustment.

Myelosuppression: Tasigna may need to be withheld and/or dose reduced for hematological toxicities (neutropenia, thrombocytopenia) that are not related to underlying leukemia (Table 2).

[See table 2 above]

See Table 3 for dose adjustments for elevations of lipase, amylase, bilirubin, and/or hepatic transaminases [see Adverse Reactions (6.1)].

Table 3. Dose Adjustments for Selected Non-hematologic Laboratory Abnormalities

Elevated serum lipase or amylase ≥Grade 3	1. Withhold Tasigna, and monitor serum lipase or amylase 2. Resume treatment at 400 mg once daily if serum lipase or amylase return to ≤Grade 1

Elevated bilirubin ≥Grade 3	1. Withhold Tasigna, and monitor bilirubin 2. Resume treatment at 400 mg once daily if bilirubin return to ≤Grade 1
Elevated hepatic transaminases ≥Grade 3	1. Withhold Tasigna, and monitor hepatic transaminases 2. Resume treatment at 400 mg once daily if hepatic transaminases return to ≤Grade 1

Other Non-hematologic Toxicities: If other clinically significant moderate or severe non-hematologic toxicity develops, withhold dosing, and resume at 400 mg once daily when the toxicity has resolved. If clinically appropriate, escalation of the dose back to 300 mg (newly diagnosed Ph+ CML-CP) or 400 mg (resistant or intolerant Ph+ CML-CP and CML-AP) twice daily should be considered. For Grade 3 to 4 lipase elevations, dosing should be withheld, and may be resumed at 400 mg once daily. Test serum lipase levels monthly or as clinically indicated. For Grade 3 to 4 bilirubin or hepatic transaminase elevations, dosing should be withheld, and may be resumed at 400 mg once daily. Test bilirubin and hepatic transaminases levels monthly or as clinically indicated [see Warnings and Precautions (5.4, 5.5), Use in Specific Populations (8.7)].

Hepatic Impairment: If possible, consider alternative therapies. If Tasigna must be administered to patients with hepatic impairment, consider the following dose reduction: [See table 4 above]

Concomitant Strong CYP3A4 Inhibitors: Avoid the concomitant use of strong CYP3A4 inhibitors (e.g., ketoconazole, itraconazole, clarithromycin, atazanavir, indinavir, nefazodone, nelfinavir, ritonavir, saquinavir, telithromycin, voriconazole). Grapefruit products may also increase serum concentrations of nilotinib and should be avoided. Should treatment with any of these agents be required, it is recommended that therapy with Tasigna be interrupted. If patients must be co-administered a strong CYP3A4 inhibitor, based on pharmacokinetic studies, consider a dose reduction to 300 mg once daily in patients with resistant or intolerant Ph+ CML or to 200 mg once daily in patients with newly diagnosed Ph+ CML-CP. However, there are no clinical data with this dose adjustment in patients receiving strong CYP3A4 inhibitors. If the strong inhibitor is discontinued, a washout period should be allowed before the Tasigna dose is adjusted upward to the indicated dose. Close monitoring for prolongation of the QT interval is indicated for patients who cannot avoid strong CYP3A4 inhibitors [see Boxed Warning, Warnings and Precautions (5.2, 5.7), Drug Interactions (7.2)].

Concomitant Strong CYP3A4 Inducers: Avoid the concomitant use of strong CYP3A4 inducers (e.g., dexamethasone, phenytoin, carbamazepine, rifampin, rifabutin, rifapentine, phenobarbital). Patients should also refrain from taking St. John's Wort. Based on the nonlinear pharmacokinetic profile of nilotinib, increasing the dose of Tasigna when co-administered with such agents is unlikely to compensate for the loss of exposure [see Drug Interactions (7.2)].

Table 2. Dose Adjustments for Neutropenia and Thrombocytopenia

Newly diagnosed Ph+ CML in chronic phase at 300 mg twice daily Resistant or intolerant Ph+ CML in chronic phase or accelerated phase at 400 mg twice daily	ANC* <1.0 × 10⁹/L and/or platelet counts <50 × 10⁹/L	1. Stop Tasigna, and monitor blood counts 2. Resume within 2 weeks at prior dose if ANC >1.0 × 10⁹/L and platelets >50 × 10⁹/L 3. If blood counts remain low for >2 weeks, reduce the dose to 400 mg once daily

*ANC = absolute neutrophil count

Table 4. Dose Adjustments for Hepatic Impairment (At Baseline)

Newly diagnosed Ph+ CML in chronic phase at 300 mg twice daily	Mild, Moderate or Severe*	An initial dosing regimen of 200 mg twice daily followed by dose escalation to 300 mg twice daily based on tolerability
Resistant or intolerant Ph+ CML in chronic phase or accelerated phase at 400 mg twice daily	Mild or Moderate*	An initial dosing regimen of 300 mg twice daily followed by dose escalation to 400 mg twice daily based on tolerability
	Severe*	A starting dose of 200 mg twice daily followed by a sequential dose escalation to 300 mg twice daily and then to 400 mg twice daily based on tolerability

*Mild = mild hepatic impairment (Child-Pugh Class A); Moderate = moderate hepatic impairment (Child-Pugh Class B); Severe = severe hepatic impairment (Child-Pugh Class C) [see Boxed Warning, Warnings and Precautions (5.9), Use in Specific Populations (8.7)].

3 DOSAGE FORMS AND STRENGTHS

150 mg red opaque hard gelatin capsules with black axial imprint "NVR/BCR".
200 mg light yellow opaque hard gelatin capsules with a red axial imprint "NVR/TKI".

4 CONTRAINDICATIONS

Do not use in patients with hypokalemia, hypomagnesemia, or long QT syndrome [see Boxed Warning].

5 WARNINGS AND PRECAUTIONS

5.1 Myelosuppression

Treatment with Tasigna can cause Grade 3/4 thrombocytopenia, neutropenia and anemia. Perform complete blood counts every two weeks for the first 2 months and then monthly thereafter, or as clinically indicated. Myelosuppression was generally reversible and usually managed by withholding Tasigna temporarily or dose reduction [see Dosage and Administration (2.2)].

5.2 QT Prolongation

Tasigna has been shown to prolong cardiac ventricular repolarization as measured by the QT interval on the surface ECG in a concentration-dependent manner [see Adverse Reactions (6.1), Clinical Pharmacology (12.4)]. Prolongation of the QT interval can result in a type of ventricular tachycardia called Torsade de pointes, which may result in syncope, seizure, and/or death. ECGs should be performed at baseline, seven days after initiation, periodically as clinically indicated and following dose adjustments [see Warnings and Precautions (5.12)].

Tasigna should not be used in patients who have hypokalemia, hypomagnesemia or long QT syndrome. Hypokalemia or hypomagnesemia must be corrected prior to initiating Tasigna and these electrolytes should be monitored periodically during therapy [see Warnings and Precautions (5.12)].

Significant prolongation of the QT interval may occur when Tasigna is inappropriately taken with food, and/or strong CYP3A4 inhibitors and/or medicinal products with a known potential to prolong QT. Therefore, co-administration with food must be avoided and concomitant use with strong CYP3A4 inhibitors and/or medicinal products with a known potential to prolong QT should be avoided [see Warnings and Precautions (5.7, 5.8)]. The presence of hypokalemia and hypomagnesemia may further enhance this effect [see Warnings and Precautions (5.6, 5.12)].

5.3 Sudden Deaths

Sudden deaths have been reported in patients with resistant or intolerant Ph+ CML receiving nilotinib (n=867; 0.6%). A similar incidence was also reported in the expanded access program for patients with resistance or intolerant Ph+ CML. The relative early occurrence of some of these deaths relative to the initiation of nilotinib suggests the possibility that ventricular repolarization abnormalities may have contributed to their occurrence.

5.4 Elevated Serum Lipase

The use of Tasigna can cause increases in serum lipase. Caution is recommended in patients with a previous history of pancreatitis. If lipase elevations are accompanied by abdominal symptoms, interrupt dosing and consider appropriate diagnostics to exclude pancreatitis. Test serum lipase levels monthly or as clinically indicated.

5.5 Hepatotoxicity
The use of Tasigna may result in elevations in bilirubin, AST/ALT, and alkaline phosphatase. Hepatic function tests should be checked monthly or as clinically indicated [see Warnings and Precautions (5.12)].

5.6 Electrolyte Abnormalities
The use of Tasigna can cause hypophosphatemia, hypokalemia, hyperkalemia, hypocalcemia, and hyponatremia. Electrolyte abnormalities must be corrected prior to initiating Tasigna and these electrolytes should be monitored periodically during therapy [see Warnings and Precautions (5.6)].

5.7 Drug Interactions
The administration of Tasigna with agents that are strong CYP3A4 inhibitors or anti-arrhythmic drugs (including, but not limited to amiodarone, disopyramide, procainamide, quinidine and sotalol) and other drugs that may prolong QT interval (including, but not limited to chloroquine, clarithromycin, haloperidol, methadone, moxifloxacin and pimozide) should be avoided. Should treatment with any of these agents be required, it is recommended that therapy with Tasigna be interrupted. If interruption of treatment with Tasigna is not possible, patients who require treatment with a drug that prolongs QT or strongly inhibits CYP3A4 should be closely monitored for prolongation of the QT interval [see Boxed Warning, Dosage and Administration (2.2), Drug Interactions (7.2)].

5.8 Food Effects
The bioavailability of nilotinib is increased with food. Tasigna must not be taken with food. No food should be taken at least 2 hours before and at least one hour after the dose is taken. Grapefruit products and other foods that are known to inhibit CYP3A4 should be avoided [see Boxed Warning, Drug Interactions (7.2) and Clinical Pharmacology (12.3)].

5.9 Hepatic Impairment
Nilotinib exposure is increased in patients with impaired hepatic function. A lower starting dose is recommended for patients with mild to severe hepatic impairment (at baseline) and QT interval should be monitored closely [see Boxed Warning, Dosage and Administration (2.2) and Use in Specific Populations (8.7)].

5.10 Total Gastrectomy
The exposure of nilotinib is reduced in patients with total gastrectomy. More frequent follow-up of these patients should be considered. Dose increase or alternative therapy may be considered in patients with total gastrectomy [see Clinical Pharmacology (12.3)].

5.11 Lactose
Since the capsules contain lactose, Tasigna is not recommended for patients with rare hereditary problems of galactose intolerance, severe lactase deficiency with a severe degree of intolerance to lactose-containing products or of glucose-galactose malabsorption.

5.12 Monitoring Laboratory Tests
Complete blood counts should be performed every two weeks for the first two months and then monthly thereafter. Chemistry panels, including the lipid profile, should be checked periodically. ECGs should be obtained at baseline, seven days after initiation and periodically thereafter, as well as following dose adjustments [see Warnings and Precautions (5.2)]. Laboratory monitoring for patients receiving Tasigna may need to be performed more or less frequently at the physician's discretion.

5.13 Use in Pregnancy
There are no adequate and well controlled studies of Tasigna in pregnant women. However, Tasigna may cause fetal harm when administered to a pregnant woman. Nilotinib caused embryo-fetal toxicities in animals at maternal exposures that were lower than the expected human exposure at the recommended doses of nilotinib. If this drug is used during pregnancy, or if the patient becomes pregnant while taking this drug, the patient should be apprised of the potential hazard to the fetus. Women of child-bearing potential should avoid becoming pregnant while taking Tasigna [see Use in Specific Populations (8.1)].

6 ADVERSE REACTIONS
The following serious adverse reactions can occur with Tasigna and are discussed in greater detail in other sections of the package insert [see Boxed Warning, Warnings and Precautions (5)].
Myelosuppression [see Warnings and Precautions (5.1)]
QT prolongation [see Boxed Warning, Warnings and Precautions (5.2)]

Sudden deaths [see Boxed Warning, Warnings and Precautions (5.3)]
Elevated serum lipase [see Warnings and Precautions (5.4)]
Hepatotoxicity [see Warnings and Precautions (5.5)]
Electrolyte abnormalities [see Boxed Warning, Warnings and Precautions (5.6)]

6.1 Clinical Trials Experience
Because clinical trials are conducted under widely varying conditions, adverse reaction rates observed in the clinical trials of a drug cannot be directly compared to rates in the clinical trials of another drug and may not reflect the rates observed in practice.

Newly Diagnosed Ph+ CML-CP
The data below reflect exposure to Tasigna from a randomized trial in newly diagnosed patients with Ph+ CML in chronic phase treated at the recommended dose of 300 mg twice daily (n=279). The median time on treatment in the nilotinib 300 mg twice daily group was 18.6 months. The median actual dose intensity was 593 mg/day in the nilotinib 300 mg twice daily group.

The most common (>10%) non-hematologic adverse drug reactions were rash, pruritus, headache, nausea, fatigue and myalgia. Upper abdominal pain, alopecia, constipation, diarrhea, dry skin, muscle spasms, arthralgia, abdominal pain, peripheral edema and asthenia were observed less commonly (≤10% and >5%) and have been of mild to moderate severity, manageable and generally did not require dose reduction. Pleural and pericardial effusions occurred in 1% of patients. Gastrointestinal hemorrhage was reported in 0.4% of patients.

Increase in QTcF >60 msec from baseline was observed in 1 patient (0.4%) in the 300 mg twice daily treatment group. No patient had an absolute QTcF of >500 msec.

The most common hematologic adverse drug reactions (all grades) were myelosuppression including: thrombocytopenia (17%), neutropenia (15%) and anemia (7%) See Table 7 for Grade 3/4 laboratory abnormalities.

Discontinuation for adverse events regardless of causality was observed in 7% of patients.

Resistant or Intolerant Ph+ CML-CP and CML-AP
In the single open-label multicenter clinical trial, a total of 438 patients with Ph+ CML-CP and CML-AP resistant to or intolerant to at least one prior therapy including imatinib were treated (CML-CP=318; CML-AP=120) at the recommended dose of 400 mg twice daily.

The median duration of exposure in days for CML-CP and CML-AP patients is 245 (range 1-502) and 138 (range 2-503), respectively. The median dose intensity was 797 mg/day (range 145-1149) was similar for both the chronic and accelerated phase patients and corresponded to the planned 400 mg twice daily dosing.

The median cumulative duration in days of dose interruptions for the CML-CP patients was 18 (range 1-185), and the median duration in days of dose interruptions for the CML-AP patients was 22 (range 1-163).

In CML-CP patients, the most commonly reported adverse drug reactions (>10%) were rash, pruritus, nausea, fatigue, headache, constipation, diarrhea and vomiting. The common serious drug-related adverse reactions were thrombocytopenia and neutropenia.

In CML-AP patients, the most commonly reported adverse drug reactions (>10%) were rash, pruritus and constipation. The common serious adverse drug reactions were thrombocytopenia, neutropenia, pneumonia, febrile neutropenia, leukopenia, intracranial hemorrhage, elevated lipase and pyrexia.

Sudden deaths and QT prolongation were reported. The maximum mean QTcF change from baseline at steady-state was 10 msec. Increase in QTcF >60 msec from baseline was observed in 2.1% of the patients and QTcF of >500 msec was observed in 3 patients (<1%) [see Boxed Warning, Warnings and Precautions (5.2, 5.3), Clinical Pharmacology (12.4)].

Discontinuation for drug-related adverse reactions was observed in 11% of CML-CP and 8% of CML-AP patients.

Most Frequently Reported Adverse Reactions
Tables 5 and 6 show the percentage of patients experiencing treatment-emergent adverse reactions (excluding laboratory abnormalities) regardless of relationship to study drug. Adverse reactions reported in greater than 10% of patients who received at least one dose of Tasigna are listed.
[See table 5 at left]
[See table 6 at top of next page]

Laboratory Abnormalities
Table 7 shows the percentage of patients experiencing treatment-emergent Grade 3/4 laboratory abnormalities in patients who received at least one dose of Tasigna.
[See table 7 on next page]

6.2 Additional Data from Clinical Trials
The following adverse drug reactions were reported in patients in the Tasigna clinical studies at the recommended doses. These adverse drug reactions are ranked under a heading of frequency, the most frequent first using the following convention: common (1%-10%), uncommon (0.1%-1%), and unknown frequency (single events). For adverse

Table 5. Most Frequently Reported Non-hematologic Adverse Reactions (Regardless of Relationship to Study Drug) in Patients with Newly Diagnosed Ph+ CML-CP (≥10% in Tasigna 300 mg twice daily or Gleevec 400 mg once daily groups)[a]

Body System and Preferred Term		TASIGNA 300 mg twice daily	GLEEVEC 400 mg once daily	TASIGNA 300 mg twice daily	GLEEVEC 400 mg once daily
		N=279	N=280	N=279	N=280
		All Grades		CTC Grades[b] 3/4 (%)	
Skin and subcutaneous tissue disorders	Rash	36	16	<1	1
	Pruritus	19	7	<1	0
	Alopecia	10	5	0	0
Gastrointestinal disorders	Nausea	19	38	1	1
	Constipation	15	4	0	0
	Diarrhea	14	37	<1	2
	Vomiting	9	22	0	<1
	Abdominal pain upper	15	10	<1	<1
	Abdominal pain	12	9	1	<1
Nervous system disorders	Headache	28	16	3	<1
General disorders and administration site conditions	Fatigue	19	14	<1	1
	Pyrexia	10	12	0	0
	Asthenia	11	9	<1	0
	Edema, peripheral	8	17	0	0
Musculoskeletal and connective tissue disorders	Myalgia	14	16	<1	0
	Arthralgia	15	13	<1	0
	Muscle spasms	10	29	0	<1
	Pain in extremity	9	13	0	<1
	Back pain	12	10	<1	1
Respiratory, thoracic and mediastinal disorders	Cough	12	9	0	0
Infections and infestations	Nasopharyngitis	19	15	0	0
	Upper respiratory tract infection	13	9	0	0
Eye disorders	Eyelid edema	1	14	0	<1

[a] Excluding laboratory abnormalities
[b] NCI Common Terminology Criteria for Adverse Events, Version 3.0

drug reactions listed under "Investigations," very common events (≥10%), which were not included in Tables 5 and 6, are also reported. These adverse reactions are included based on clinical relevance and ranked in order of decreasing seriousness within each category.

Infections and Infestations: Common: folliculitis. Uncommon: upper respiratory tract infection (including pharyngitis, nasopharyngitis, rhinitis), pneumonia, urinary tract infection, gastroenteritis. Unknown frequency: sepsis, bronchitis, herpes virus infection, candidiasis, subcutaneous abscess, anal abscess, furuncle, tinea pedis.

Neoplasms Benign, Malignant and Unspecified: Common: Skin papilloma. Unknown frequency: papilloma.

Blood and Lymphatic System Disorders: Common: febrile neutropenia, pancytopenia, lymphopenia. Unknown frequency: thrombocytosis, leukocytosis.

Immune System Disorders: Unknown frequency: hypersensitivity.

Endocrine Disorders: Uncommon: hyperthyroidism. Unknown frequency: hypothyroidism, hyperparathyroidism secondary, thyroiditis.

Metabolism and Nutrition Disorders: Common: electrolyte imbalance (including hypomagnesemia, hyperkalemia, hypokalemia, hyponatremia, hypocalcemia, hypophosphatemia, hypercalcemia, hyperphosphatemia), diabetes mellitus, hyperglycemia, hypercholesterolemia, hyperlipidemia. Uncommon: dehydration, decreased appetite, increased appetite. Unknown frequency: hyperuricemia, gout, hypoglycemia, dyslipidemia.

Psychiatric Disorders: Common: depression, insomnia. Uncommon: anxiety. Unknown frequency: disorientation, confusional state, amnesia, dysphoria.

Nervous System Disorders: Common: dizziness, hypoaesthesia, paresthesia. Uncommon: intracranial hemorrhage, migraine, loss of consciousness (including syncope), tremor, disturbance in attention, hyperesthesia. Unknown frequency: brain edema, optic neuritis, peripheral neuropathy, lethargy, dysaesthesia.

Eye Disorders: Common: eye hemorrhage, periorbital edema, eye pruritus, conjunctivitis, dry eye. Uncommon: vision impairment, vision blurred, visual acuity reduced, photopsia, eye irritation. Unknown frequency: papilloedema, diplopia, photophobia, eye swelling, blepharitis, eye pain, chorioretinopathy, conjunctival hemorrhage, conjunctivitis allergic, conjunctival hyperaemia, ocular hyperaemia, ocular surface disease, scleral hyperaemia.

Ear and Labyrinth Disorders: Common: vertigo. Unknown frequency: hearing impaired, ear pain, tinnitus.

Cardiac Disorders: Common: angina pectoris, arrhythmia (including atrioventricular block, cardiac flutter, extrasystoles, atrial fibrillation, bradycardia), palpitations, electrocardiogram QT prolonged. Uncommon: cardiac failure, pericardial effusion, coronary artery disease, cyanosis, cardiac murmur. Unknown frequency: myocardial infarction, ventricular dysfunction, pericarditis, ejection fraction decrease.

Vascular Disorders: Common: hypertension, flushing. Uncommon: hypertensive crisis, hematoma. Unknown frequency: shock hemorrhagic, hypotension, thrombosis.

Respiratory, Thoracic and Mediastinal Disorders: Common: dyspnea, dyspnea exertional, epistaxis, cough, dysphonia. Uncommon: pulmonary edema, pleural effusion, interstitial lung disease, pleuritic pain, pleurisy, pharyngolaryngeal pain, throat irritation. Unknown frequency: pulmonary hypertension, wheezing.

Gastrointestinal Disorders: Common: pancreatitis, abdominal discomfort, abdominal distension, dyspepsia, flatulence. Uncommon: gastrointestinal hemorrhage, melena, mouth ulceration, gastroesophageal reflux, stomatitis, esophageal pain, dysgeusia, dry mouth. Unknown frequency: gastrointestinal ulcer perforation, retroperitoneal hemorrhage, hematemesis, gastric ulcer, esophagitis ulcerative, subileus, gastritis, hemorrhoids, hiatus hernia, rectal hemorrhage, sensitivity of teeth, gingivitis.

Hepatobiliary Disorders: Common: hepatic function abnormal. Uncommon: hepatitis, jaundice. Unknown frequency: cholestasis, hepatotoxicity, hepatomegaly.

Skin and Subcutaneous Tissue Disorders: Common: night sweats, eczema, urticaria, erythema, hyperhidrosis, contusion, acne, dermatitis, dry skin. Uncommon: exfoliative rash, drug eruption, pain of skin, ecchymosis, swelling face. Unknown frequency: erythema nodosum, skin ulcer, palmar-plantar erythrodysasthesia syndrome, petechiae, photosensitivity, blister, dermal cyst, sebaceous hyperplasia, skin atrophy, skin discoloration, skin exfoliation, skin hyperpigmentation, skin hypertrophy.

Musculoskeletal and Connective Tissue Disorders: Common: bone pain, musculoskeletal chest pain, musculoskeletal pain, flank pain. Uncommon: musculoskeletal stiffness, muscular weakness, joint swelling. Unknown frequency: arthritis.

Renal and Urinary Disorders: Common: pollakiuria. Uncommon: dysuria, micturition urgency, nocturia. Unknown frequency: renal failure, hematuria, urinary incontinence, chromaturia.

Table 6. Most Frequently Reported Non-hematologic Adverse Reactions in Patients with Resistant or Intolerant Ph+ CML receiving Tasigna 400 mg twice daily (Regardless of Relationship to Study Drug) (≥10% in any Group)[a]

Body System and Preferred Term		CML-CP N=318 All Grades (%)	CML-CP N=318 CTC Grades[b] 3/4 (%)	CML-AP N=120 All Grades (%)	CML-AP N=120 CTC Grades[b] 3/4 (%)
Skin and subcutaneous tissue disorders	Rash	33	2	28	0
	Pruritus	29	<1	20	0
Gastrointestinal disorders	Nausea	31	1	18	<1
	Constipation	21	<1	18	0
	Diarrhea	22	3	19	2
	Vomiting	21	<1	10	0
	Abdominal pain	11	1	13	3
Nervous system disorders	Headache	31	3	21	2
General disorders and administration site conditions	Fatigue	28	1	16	<1
	Pyrexia	14	1	24	2
	Asthenia	14	0	12	2
	Edema, peripheral	11	0	11	
Musculoskeletal and connective tissue disorders	Myalgia	14	2	14	<1
	Arthralgia	18	2	16	0
	Muscle spasms	11	<1	14	0
	Bone pain	11	<1	13	<1
	Pain in extremity	13	1	16	2
	Back pain	10	<1	13	<1
Respiratory, thoracic and mediastinal disorders	Cough	17	<1	13	0
	Dyspnea	11	1	8	3
Infections and infestations	Nasopharyngitis	16	<1	11	0

[a] Excluding laboratory abnormalities
[b] NCI Common Terminology Criteria for Adverse Events, Version 3.0

Table 7. Percent Incidence of Clinically Relevant Grade 3/4* Laboratory Abnormalities

	Patient Population			
	Newly Diagnosed Ph+ CML-CP		Resistant or Intolerant Ph+	
			CML-CP	CML-AP
	TASIGNA 300 mg twice daily N=279 (%)	GLEEVEC 400 mg once daily N=280 (%)	TASIGNA 400 mg twice daily N=318 (%)	TASIGNA 400 mg twice daily N=120 (%)
Hematologic Parameters				
Thrombocytopenia	10	9	28[1]	37[2]
Neutropenia	12	20	28	37[3]
Anemia	4	5	8	23
Biochemistry Parameters				
Elevated lipase	7	3	15	17
Hyperglycemia	6	0	11	4
Hypophosphatemia	5	8	10	10
Elevated bilirubin (total)	4	<1	9	10
Elevated SGPT (ALT)	4	3	4	2
Hyperkalemia	2	1	4	3
Hyponatremia	<1	<1	3	1
Hypokalemia	<1	1	3	5
Elevated SGOT (AST)	1	1	1	1
Decreased albumin	0	1	1	1
Hypocalcemia	<1	0	1	4
Elevated alkaline phosphatase	0	<1	0	3
Elevated creatinine	0	<1	<1	0

* NCI Common Terminology Criteria for Adverse Events, version 3.0
[1] CML-CP: Thrombocytopenia: 11% were Grade 3, 17% were Grade 4
[2] CML-AP: Thrombocytopenia: 7% were Grade 3, 30% were Grade 4
[3] CML-AP: Neutropenia: 12% were Grade 3, 25% were Grade 4

Reproductive System and Breast Disorders: Uncommon: breast pain, gynecomastia, erectile dysfunction. Unknown frequency: breast induration, menorrhagia, nipple swelling.

General Disorders and Administration Site Conditions: Common: pyrexia, chest pain, pain (including neck pain and back pain), chest discomfort. Uncommon: face edema, gravitational edema, influenza-like illness, chills, malaise. Unknown frequency: feeling hot, localized edema.

Investigations: Common: blood amylase increased, gamma-glutamyltransferase increased, blood creatinine phosphokinase increased, weight decreased, weight increased. Uncommon: hemoglobin decreased, blood lactate dehydrogenase increased, blood urea increased. Unknown frequency: troponin increased, blood bilirubin unconjugated increased, blood insulin increased, very low density lipoprotein increased, blood parathyroid hormone increased, blood pressure increased.

6.3 Postmarketing Experience

The following additional adverse reactions have been reported during post approval use of Tasigna. Because these reactions are reported voluntarily from a population of uncertain size, it is not always possible to reliably estimate their frequency or establish a causal relationship to drug exposure.

Cases of tumor lysis syndrome have been reported in Tasigna treated patients with resistant or intolerant CML. Malignant disease progression, high WBC counts and/or dehydration were present in majority of these cases.

7 DRUG INTERACTIONS

7.1 Effects of Nilotinib on Drug Metabolizing Enzymes and Drug Transport Systems

Nilotinib is a competitive inhibitor of CYP3A4, CYP2C8, CYP2C9, CYP2D6 and UGT1A1 *in vitro*, potentially increasing the concentrations of drugs eliminated by these enzymes. *In vitro* studies also suggest that nilotinib may induce CYP2B6, CYP2C8 and CYP2C9, and decrease the concentrations of drugs which are eliminated by these enzymes.

Single-dose administration of Tasigna with midazolam (a CYP3A4 substrate) to healthy subjects increased midazolam exposure by 30%. Single-dose administration of Tasigna to healthy subjects did not change the pharmacokinetics and pharmacodynamics of warfarin (a CYP2C9 substrate). The ability of Tasigna to induce metabolism has not been determined *in vivo*. Exercise caution when co-administering Tasigna with substrates for these enzymes that have a narrow therapeutic index.

Nilotinib inhibits human P-glycoprotein. If Tasigna is administered with drugs that are substrates of P-gp, increased concentrations of the substrate drug are likely, and caution should be exercised.

7.2 Drugs that Inhibit or Induce Cytochrome P450 3A4 Enzymes

Nilotinib undergoes metabolism by CYP3A4, and concomitant administration of strong inhibitors or inducers of CYP3A4 can increase or decrease nilotinib concentrations significantly. The administration of Tasigna with agents that are strong CYP3A4 inhibitors should be avoided *[see Boxed Warning, Dosage and Administration (2.2), Warnings and Precautions (5.2, 5.7)]*. Concomitant use of Tasigna with medicinal products and herbal preparations that are potent inducers of CYP3A4 is likely to reduce exposure to nilotinib to a clinically relevant extent. Therefore, in patients receiving Tasigna, concomitant use of alternative therapeutic agents with less potential for CYP3A4 induction should be selected.

Ketoconazole: In healthy subjects receiving ketoconazole, a CYP3A4 inhibitor, at 400 mg once daily for 6 days, systemic exposure (AUC) to nilotinib was increased approximately 3-fold.

Rifampicin: In healthy subjects receiving the CYP3A4 inducer, rifampicin, at 600 mg daily for 12 days, systemic exposure (AUC) to nilotinib was decreased approximately 80%.

7.3 Drugs that Affect Gastric pH

Nilotinib has pH-dependent solubility, with decreased solubility at higher pH. Drugs such as proton pump inhibitors that inhibit gastric acid secretion to elevate the gastric pH may decrease the solubility of nilotinib and reduce its bioavailability. In healthy subjects, co-administration of a single 400 mg dose of Tasigna with multiple doses of esomeprazole (a proton pump inhibitor) at 40 mg daily decreased the nilotinib AUC by 34%. Increasing the dose of Tasigna when co-administered with such agents is not likely to compensate for the loss of exposure. Since proton pump inhibitors affect pH of the upper GI tract for an extended period, separation of doses may not eliminate the interaction. The concomitant use of proton pump inhibitors with Tasigna should be used with caution. If a H2 blocker or an antacid is necessary, the doses between the H2 blocker and Tasigna or the doses between the antacid and Tasigna should be separated at least by several hours. However, no clinical study has been conducted to evaluate the effect of H2 blockers or antacids on nilotinib pharmacokinetics.

7.4 Drugs that Inhibit Drug Transport Systems

Nilotinib is a substrate of the efflux transporter P-glycoprotein (P-gp, ABCB1). If Tasigna is administered with drugs that inhibit P-gp, increased concentrations of nilotinib are likely, and caution should be exercised.

7.5 Drugs that May Prolong the QT Interval

The administration of Tasigna with agents that may prolong the QT interval such as anti-arrhythmic medicines should be avoided *[see Boxed Warning, Dosage and Administration (2.2), Warnings and Precautions (5.2, 5.7)]*.

8 USE IN SPECIFIC POPULATIONS

8.1 Pregnancy

Pregnancy Category D *[see Warnings and Precautions (5.13)]*.

Based on its mechanism of action and findings in animals, Tasigna may cause fetal harm when administered to a pregnant woman. There are no adequate and well controlled studies with Tasigna in pregnant women. Women should be advised to avoid becoming pregnant while on Tasigna. If this drug is used during pregnancy, or if the patient becomes pregnant while taking this drug, the patient should be apprised of the potential hazard to the fetus.

Nilotinib was studied for effects on embryo-fetal development in pregnant rats and rabbits given oral doses of 10, 30, 100 mg/kg/day, and 30, 100, 300 mg/kg/day, respectively, during organogenesis. In rats, nilotinib at doses of 100 mg/kg/day (approximately 5.7 times the AUC in patients at the dose of 400 mg twice daily) was associated with maternal toxicity (decreased gestation weight, gravid uterine weight, net weight gain, and food consumption). Nilotinib at doses ≥30 mg/kg/day (approximately 2 times the AUC in patients at the dose of 400 mg twice daily) resulted in embryo-fetal toxicity as shown by increased resorption and post-implantation loss, and at 100 mg/kg/day a decrease in viable fetuses. In rabbits, maternal toxicity at 300 mg/kg/day (approximately one-half the human exposure based on AUC) was associated with mortality, abortion, decreased gestation weights and decreased food consumption. Embryonic toxicity (increased resorption) and minor skeletal anomalies were observed at a dose of 300 mg/kg/day. Nilotinib is not considered teratogenic.

When pregnant rats were dosed with nilotinib during organogenesis and through lactation, the adverse effects included a longer gestational period, lower pup body weights until weaning and decreased fertility indices in the pups when they reached maturity, all at a maternal dose of 360 mg/m^2 (approximately 0.7 times the clinical dose of 400 mg twice daily based on body surface area). At doses up to 120 mg/m^2 (approximately 0.25 times the clinical dose of 400 mg twice daily based on body surface area) no adverse effects were seen in the maternal animals or the pups.

8.3 Nursing Mothers

It is not known whether nilotinib is excreted in human milk. One study in lactating rats demonstrates that nilotinib is excreted into milk. Because many drugs are excreted in human milk and because of the potential for serious adverse reactions in nursing infants from Tasigna, a decision should be made whether to discontinue nursing or to discontinue the drug taking into account the importance of the drug to the mother.

8.4 Pediatric Use

The safety and effectiveness of Tasigna in pediatric patients have not been established.

8.5 Geriatric Use

In the clinical trials of Tasigna (patients with newly diagnosed Ph+ CML-CP and resistant or intolerant Ph+ CML-CP and CML-AP), approximately 12% and 30% of patients were 65 or over.

- Patients with newly diagnosed Ph+ CML-CP: There was no difference in major molecular response between patients aged <65 years and those ≥65 years.
- Patients with resistant or intolerant CML-CP: There was no difference in major cytogenetic response rate between patients aged <65 years and those ≥65 years.
- Patients with resistant or intolerant CML-AP: The major hematologic response rate was 31% in patients <65 years of age and 15% in patients ≥65 years.

No major differences were observed for safety in patients ≥65 years of age as compared to patients <65 years.

8.6 Cardiac Disorders

In the clinical trials, patients with a history of uncontrolled or significant cardiovascular disease, including recent myocardial infarction, congestive heart failure, unstable angina or clinically significant bradycardia were excluded. Caution should be exercised in patients with relevant cardiac disorders *[see Boxed Warning, Warnings and Precautions (5.2)]*.

8.7 Hepatic Impairment

Nilotinib exposure is increased in patients with impaired hepatic function. In a study of subjects with mild to severe hepatic impairment following a single dose administration of 200 mg of Tasigna, the mean AUC values were increased on average of 35%, 35% and 56% in subjects with mild (Child-Pugh class A, score 5-6), moderate (Child-Pugh class B, score 7-9) and severe hepatic impairment (Child-Pugh class C, score 10-15), respectively, compared to a control group of subjects with normal hepatic function. Table 8 summarizes the Child-Pugh Liver Function Classification applied in this study. A lower starting dose is recommended in patients with hepatic impairment and the QT interval should be monitored closely in these patients *[see Boxed Warning, Dosage and Administration (2.2), Warnings and Precautions (5.9)]*.

Table 8. Child-Pugh Liver Function Classification

Assessment	Degree of Abnormality	Score
Encephalopathy Grade	None 1 or 2 3 or 4	1 2 3
Ascites	Absent Slight Moderate	1 2 3
Total Bilirubin (mg/dL)	<2 2-3 >3	1 2 3
Serum Albumin (g/dL)	>3.5 2.8-3.5 <2.8	1 2 3
Prothrombin Time (seconds prolonged)	<4 4-6 >6	1 2 3

8.8 Renal Impairment

Clinical studies have not been performed in patients with impaired renal function. Clinical studies have excluded patients with serum creatinine concentration >1.5 times the upper limit of the normal range.

Since nilotinib and its metabolites are not renally excreted, a decrease in total body clearance is not anticipated in patients with renal impairment.

10 OVERDOSAGE

Overdose with nilotinib has been reported, where an unspecified number of Tasigna capsules were ingested in combination with alcohol and other drugs. Events included neutropenia, vomiting, and drowsiness. In the event of overdose, the patient should be observed and appropriate supportive treatment given.

11 DESCRIPTION

Tasigna (nilotinib) belongs to a pharmacologic class of drugs known as kinase inhibitors.

Nilotinib drug substance, a monohydrate monohydrochloride, is a white to slightly yellowish to slightly greenish yellow powder with the anhydrous molecular formula and weight, respectively, of $C_{28}H_{22}F_3N_7O \cdot HCl \cdot H_2O$ and 584. The solubility of nilotinib in aqueous solutions decreases with increasing pH. Nilotinib is not optically active. The pK$_a$1 was determined to be 2.1; pK$_a$2 was estimated to be 5.4.

The chemical name of nilotinib is 4-methyl-N-[3-(4-methyl-1H-imidazol-1-yl)-5-(trifluoromethyl)phenyl]-3-[[4-(3-pyridinyl)-2-pyrimidinyl]amino]-benzamide, monohydrochloride, monohydrate. Its structure is shown below:

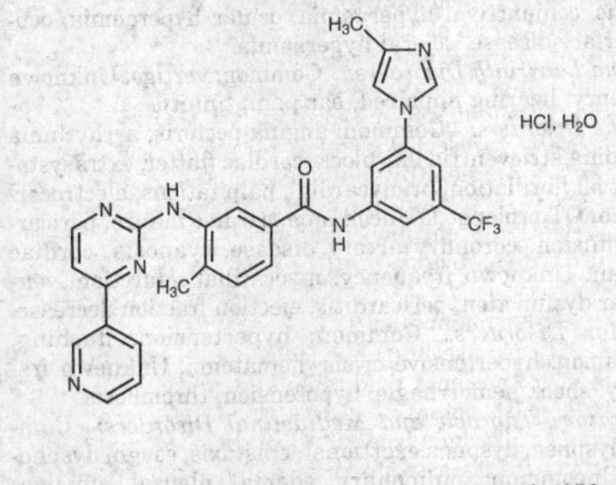

Tasigna (nilotinib) capsules, for oral use, contain 150 mg or 200 mg nilotinib base, anhydrous (as hydrochloride, monohydrate) with the following inactive ingredients: colloidal silicon dioxide, crospovidone, lactose monohydrate, magnesium stearate and polyoxamer 188. The capsules contain gelatin, iron oxide (red), iron oxide (yellow), iron oxide (black) and titanium dioxide.

12 CLINICAL PHARMACOLOGY

12.1 Mechanism of Action

Nilotinib is an inhibitor of the Bcr-Abl kinase. Nilotinib binds to and stabilizes the inactive conformation of the kinase domain of Abl protein. *In vitro*, nilotinib inhibited Bcr-Abl mediated proliferation of murine leukemic cell lines and human cell lines derived from patients with Ph+ CML. Under the conditions of the assays, nilotinib was able to overcome imatinib resistance resulting from Bcr-Abl kinase mutations, in 32 out of 33 mutations tested. *In vivo*, nilotinib reduced the tumor size in a murine Bcr-Abl xenograft model. Nilotinib inhibited the autophosphorylation of the following kinases at IC$_{50}$ values as indicated: Bcr-Abl (20-60 nM), PDGFR (69 nM), c-Kit (210 nM), CSF-1R (125-250 nM) and DDR (3.7 nM).

12.3 Pharmacokinetics

Absorption and Distribution:

Peak concentrations of nilotinib are reached 3 hours after oral administration.

Steady-state nilotinib exposure was dose-dependent with less than dose-proportional increases in systemic exposure at dose levels higher than 400 mg given as once daily dosing. Daily serum exposure to nilotinib following 400 mg twice daily dosing at steady state was 35% higher than with 800 mg once daily dosing. Steady state exposure (AUC) of nilotinib with 400 mg twice daily dosing was 13% higher than with 300 mg twice daily dosing. The average steady state nilotinib trough and peak concentrations did not change over 12 months. There was no relevant increase in exposure to nilotinib when the dose was increased with 400 mg twice daily to 600 mg twice daily.

The bioavailability of nilotinib was increased when given with a meal. Compared to the fasted state, the systemic exposure (AUC) increased by 82% when the dose was given 30 minutes after a high fat meal.

The blood-to-serum ratio of nilotinib is 0.68. Serum protein binding is approximately 98% on the basis of *in vitro* experiments.

Median steady-state trough concentration of nilotinib was decreased by 53% in patients with total gastrectomy compared to patients who had not undergone surgeries *[see Warnings and Precautions (5.10)]*.

Pharmacokinetics, Metabolism and Excretion:

The apparent elimination half-life estimated from the multiple dose pharmacokinetic studies with daily dosing was approximately 17 hours. Inter-patient variability in nilotinib AUC was 32% to 64%. Steady state conditions were achieved by Day 8. An increase in serum exposure to nilotinib between the first dose and steady state was approximately 2-fold for daily dosing and 3.8-fold for twice-daily dosing.

Main metabolic pathways identified in healthy subjects are oxidation and hydroxylation. Nilotinib is the main circulating component in the serum. None of the metabolites contribute significantly to the pharmacological activity of nilotinib.

After a single dose of radiolabeled nilotinib in healthy subjects, more than 90% of the administered dose was eliminated within 7 days mainly in feces (93% of the dose). Parent drug accounted for 69% of the dose.

Age, body weight, gender, or ethnic origin did not significantly affect the pharmacokinetics of nilotinib.

Drug-Drug Interactions:

In a Phase 1 trial of nilotinib 400 mg twice daily in combination with imatinib 400 mg daily or 400 mg twice daily, the AUC increased 30%-50% for nilotinib and approximately 20% for imatinib.

12.4 QT/QTc Prolongation

In a placebo-controlled study in healthy volunteers designed to assess the effects of Tasigna on the QT interval, administration of Tasigna was associated with concentration-dependent QT prolongation; the maximum mean placebo-adjusted QTcF change from baseline was 18 msec (1-sided 95% Upper CI: 26 msec). A positive control was not included in the QT study of healthy volunteers. Peak plasma concentrations in the QT study were 26% lower than those observed in patients enrolled in the single-arm study *[see Boxed Warning, Warnings and Precautions (5.2) and Adverse Reactions (6.1)]*.

12.5 Pharmacogenomics

Tasigna can increase bilirubin levels. A pharmacogenetic analysis of 97 patients evaluated the polymorphisms of UGT1A1 and its potential association with hyperbilirubinemia during Tasigna treatment. In this study, the (TA)7/(TA)7 genotype was associated with a statistically significant increase in the risk of hyperbilirubinemia relative to the (TA)6/(TA)6 and (TA)6/(TA)7 genotypes. However, the largest increases in bilirubin were observed in the (TA)7/(TA)7 genotype (UGT1A1*28) patients *[see Warnings and Precautions (5.5)]*.

13 NONCLINICAL TOXICOLOGY

13.1 Carcinogenesis, Mutagenesis, Impairment of Fertility

Carcinogenicity studies with nilotinib have not been performed.

Nilotinib was not mutagenic in a bacterial mutagenesis (Ames) assay, was not clastogenic in a chromosome aberration assay in human lymphocytes, did not induce DNA damage (comet assay) in L5178Y mouse lymphoma cells, nor was it clastogenic in an *in vivo* rat bone marrow micronucleus assay with two oral treatments at doses up to 2000 mg/kg/dose.

There were no effects on male or female rat and female rabbit mating or fertility at doses up to 180 mg/kg in rats (approximately 4-7 fold for males and females, respectively, the AUC in patients at the dose of 400 mg twice daily) or 300 mg/kg in rabbits (approximately one-half the AUC in patients at the dose of 400 mg twice daily). The effect of Tasigna on human fertility is unknown. In a study where male and female rats were treated with nilotinib at oral doses of 20-180 mg/kg/day (approximately 1-6.6 fold the AUC in patients at the dose of 400 mg twice daily) during the pre-mating and mating periods and then mated, and dosing of pregnant rats continued through gestation Day 6, nilotinib increased post-implantation loss and early resorption, and decreased the number of viable fetuses and litter size at all doses tested.

14 CLINICAL STUDIES

14.1 Newly Diagnosed Ph+ CML-CP

An open label, multicenter, randomized trial was conducted to determine the efficacy of Tasigna versus Gleevec® (imatinib mesylate) Tablets in adult patients with cytogenetically confirmed newly diagnosed Ph+ CML-CP. Patients were within six months of diagnosis and were previously untreated for CML-CP, except for hydroxyurea and/or anagrelide. Efficacy was based on a total of 846 patients: 283 patients in the imatinib 400 mg once daily group, 282 patients in the nilotinib 300 mg twice daily group, 281 patients in the nilotinib 400 mg twice daily group.

Median age was 46 years in the imatinib group and 47 years in both nilotinib groups, with 12%, 13% and 10% of patients ≥65 years of age in imatinib 400 mg once daily, nilotinib 300 mg twice daily and nilotinib 400 mg twice daily treatment groups, respectively. There were slightly more male than female patients in all groups (56%, 56% and 62% in imatinib 400 mg once daily, nilotinib 300 mg twice daily and nilotinib 400 mg twice daily treatment groups, respectively). More than 60% of all patients were Caucasian, and 25% were Asian.

The primary data analysis was performed when all 846 patients completed 12 months of treatment (or discontinued earlier). The median time on treatment was 18.6 months in all three treatment groups. This study is on-going.

The primary efficacy endpoint was major molecular response (MMR) at 12 months after the start of study medication. MMR was defined as ≤0.1% BCR-ABL/ABL % by international scale measured by RQ-PCR, which corresponds to a ≥3 log reduction of BCR-ABL transcript from standardized baseline. Efficacy endpoints are summarized in Table 9 below.

Two patients on the nilotinib arm progressed to either accelerated phase or blast crisis while 17 patients on the imatinib arm progressed to either accelerated phase or blast crisis.

Table 9. Efficacy of TASIGNA Compared to GLEEVEC in Newly Diagnosed Ph+ CML-CP

	TASIGNA 300 mg twice daily	GLEEVEC 400 mg once daily
	N=282	N=283
MMR at 12 months (95% CI)	44% (38.4, 50.3)	22% (17.6, 27.6)
P-Value[a]	<0.0001	
CCyR[b] by 12 months (95% CI)	80% (75.0, 84.6)	65% (59.2, 70.6)

[a] CMH test stratified by Sokal risk group

[b] CCyR: 0% Ph+ metaphases. Cytogenetic responses were based on the percentage of Ph-positive metaphases among ≥20 metaphase cells in each bone marrow sample.

14.2 Patients with Resistant or Intolerant Ph+ CML-CP and CML-AP

A single arm, open label, multicenter study was conducted to evaluate the efficacy and safety of Tasigna (400 mg twice daily) in patients with imatinib-resistant or -intolerant CML with separate cohorts for chronic and accelerated phase disease. The definition of imatinib resistance included failure to achieve a complete hematologic response (by 3 months), cytogenetic response (by 6 months) or major cytogenetic response (by 12 months) or progression of disease after a previous cytogenetic or hematologic response. Imatinib intolerance was defined as discontinuation of treatment due to toxicity and lack of a major cytogenetic response at time of study entry. At the time of data cut-off, 280 CML-CP patients with a minimum follow-up of 6 months and 105 CML-AP patients with a minimum follow-up of 4 months were enrolled. Of these, 232 patients with CML-CP and all patients with CML-AP were evaluable for efficacy. In this study, about 50% of CML-CP and CML-AP patients were males, over 80% were Caucasian, and approximately 30% were age 65 years or older.

Overall, 73% of patients were imatinib resistant while 27% were imatinib intolerant. The median time of prior imatinib treatment was approximately 31 months. Prior therapy included hydroxyurea in 85% of patients, interferon in 62% and stem cell or bone marrow transplant in 8%. The median highest prior imatinib dose was 600 mg/day for CML-CP patients and 800 mg/day for CML-AP patients, and the highest prior imatinib dose was ≥600 mg/day in 77% of all patients with 44% of patients receiving imatinib doses ≥800 mg/day.

Median duration of nilotinib treatment was 8.7 months in CML-CP patients and 5.6 months in CML-AP patients.

The efficacy endpoint in chronic phase CML was unconfirmed major cytogenetic response (MCyR) which included complete and partial cytogenetic responses.

The efficacy endpoint in accelerated phase CML was confirmed hematologic response (HR), defined as either a complete hematologic response (CHR) or no evidence of leukemia (NEL). The rates of response for CML-CP and CML-AP patients are reported in Table 10.

Table 10. Efficacy of Tasigna in Resistant or Intolerant Ph+ CML-CP and CML-AP

Cytogenetic Response Rate (Unconfirmed) (%)[a]	Chronic Phase n=232
Major (95% CI)	40% (33,46)
Complete (95% CI)	28% (22,34)
Partial (95% CI)	12% (8,16)
	Accelerated Phase n=105
Hematologic Response Rate (95% CI)[b]	26% (18,35)
Complete Hematologic Response Rate (95% CI)	18% (11,27)
No Evidence of Leukemia (95% CI)	8% (3,15)

[a] Cytogenetic response criteria: Complete (0% Ph+ metaphases) or partial (1%-35%). Cytogenetic responses were based on the percentage of Ph-positive metaphases among ≥20 metaphase cells in each bone marrow sample.

[b] Hematologic response = CHR + NEL (all responses confirmed after 4 weeks).

CHR (CML-CP): WBC <10 × 10⁹/L, platelets <450,000/mm³, no blasts or promyelocytes in peripheral blood, <5% myelocytes + metamyelocytes in bone marrow, <20% basophils in peripheral blood, and no extramedullary involvement.

CHR (CML-AP): neutrophils ≥1.5 × 10⁹/L, platelets ≥100 × 10⁹/L, no myeloblasts in peripheral blood, myeloblasts <5% in bone marrow, and no extramedullary involvement.

NEL: same criteria as for CHR but neutrophils ≥1.0 × 10⁹/L and platelets >20 × 10⁹/L without transfusions or bleeding.

The median duration of response has not been reached for CML-CP and CML-AP. Based on current follow-up, 59% of CML-CP patients with a major cytogenetic response had a duration of response of at least 6 months. Based on current follow-up, 63% of CML-AP patients with a confirmed hematologic response had a duration of response of at least 6 months.

After imatinib failure, 24 different BCR-ABL mutations were noted in 19% of chronic phase and 25% of accelerated phase CML patients who were evaluated for mutations. Patients harboring a variety of BCR-ABL mutations associated with imatinib resistance, except T315I, responded to Tasigna.

16 HOW SUPPLIED/STORAGE AND HANDLING

Tasigna (nilotinib) 150 mg capsules are red opaque hard gelatin capsules, size 1 with black axial imprint "NVR/BCR." Tasigna (nilotinib) 200 mg capsules are light yellow opaque hard gelatin capsules, size 0 with the red axial imprint "NVR/TKI." Tasigna capsules are supplied in blister packs.

150 mg
Carton of 4 blister packs of (4×28) ...... NDC 0078-0592-87
Blisters of 28 capsules .... NDC 0078-0592-51

200 mg
Carton of 4 blister packs of (4×28) .... NDC 0078-0526-87
Blisters of 28 capsules .... NDC 0078-0526-51

Each blister pack contains one folded blister card of 28 capsules each, for dosing two in the morning and two in the evening at 12 hour intervals over a 7 day period.

Tasigna (nilotinib) capsules should be stored at 25°C (77°F); excursions permitted between 15°-30°C (59°-86°F) *[see USP Controlled Room Temperature]*.

17 PATIENT COUNSELING INFORMATION

See Medication Guide

A Medication Guide is required for distribution with Tasigna. Encourage patients to read the Tasigna Medication Guide. The complete text of the Medication Guide is reprinted at the end of this document.

17.1 Taking Tasigna

Tasigna doses should be taken twice daily approximately 12 hours apart and should not be taken with food. The capsules should be swallowed whole with water.

Patients should be advised to take Tasigna on an empty stomach. Tasigna should be taken at least 2 hours after a meal. No food should be consumed for at least one hour after the dose is taken. Patients should not consume grapefruit products and other foods that are known to inhibit CYP3A4 at all times during Tasigna treatment [see Dosage and Administration (2.1), Warnings and Precautions (5.7, 5.8) and Medication Guide].

17.2   Drug Interactions
Tasigna, and certain other medicines, including over the counter medications or herbal supplements (such as St. John's Wort) can interact with each other [see Warnings and Precautions (5.7) and Drug Interactions (7)].

17.3   Pregnancy
Patients should be advised that the use of Tasigna during pregnancy may cause harm to the fetus and should not be taken during pregnancy, unless necessary. Women of childbearing potential should use effective contraceptives if taking Tasigna. Sexually active female patients taking Tasigna should use adequate contraception [see Warnings and Precautions (5.13) and Use in Specific Populations (8.1)].

17.4   Compliance
Patients should be advised of the following:
• Continue taking Tasigna every day for as long as their doctor tells them.
• This is a long-term treatment.
• Do not change dose or stop taking Tasigna without first consulting their doctor.
• If a dose is missed, take the next dose as scheduled. Do not take a double dose to make up for the forgotten capsules.

MEDICATION GUIDE
TASIGNA® (ta-sig-na)
(nilotinib)
Capsules
Read this Medication Guide before you start taking Tasigna® and each time you get a refill. There may be new information. This information does not take the place of talking to your doctor about your medical condition or treatment.

What is the most important information I should know about Tasigna?
Tasigna can cause a possible life-threatening heart problem called QTc prolongation. QTc prolongation causes an irregular heartbeat, which can lead to sudden death.
Your doctor should check the electrical activity of your heart with a test called an electrocardiogram (ECG):
• before starting Tasigna
• 7 days after starting Tasigna
• with any dose changes
• regularly during Tasigna treatment
You may lower your chances for having QTc prolongation with Tasigna if you:
• Take Tasigna:
  • on an empty stomach. Do not take Tasigna with food.
  • at least 2 hours after eating any food, and
  • wait at least 1 hour before eating any food
• Avoid grapefruit, grapefruit juice, and any supplement containing grapefruit extract while taking Tasigna. Food and grapefruit products increase the amount of Tasigna in your body.
• Avoid taking other medicines or supplements with Tasigna that can also cause QTc prolongation.
• Tasigna can interact with many medicines and supplements and increase your chance for serious and life-threatening side effects.
• Do not take any other medicine while taking Tasigna unless your doctor tells you it is okay to do so.
Call your doctor right away if you feel lightheaded, faint or have an irregular heartbeat while taking Tasigna. These can be symptoms of QTc prolongation.
What is Tasigna?
Tasigna is a prescription medicine used to treat a type of leukemia called Philadelphia chromosome positive chronic myeloid leukemia (Ph+ CML) in adults who:
• are newly diagnosed, **or**
• are no longer benefiting from previous other treatments, including treatment with imatinib (Gleevec®), **or**
• have taken other treatments, including imatinib (Gleevec®), and cannot tolerate them.
It is not known if Tasigna is safe or effective in children.
Who should not take Tasigna?
Do not take if you have:
• low levels of potassium or magnesium in your blood
• long QTc syndrome
What should I tell my doctor before starting Tasigna?
Tasigna may not be right for you. Before taking Tasigna, tell your doctor about all of your medical conditions, including if you have:
• heart problems
• irregular heartbeat
• QTc prolongation or a family history of it
• liver problems
• had pancreatitis
• low blood levels of potassium or magnesium in your blood

• a severe problem with lactose (milk sugar) or other sugars. The Tasigna capsules contain lactose. Most patients who have mild or moderate lactose intolerance can take Tasigna.
• had a surgical procedure involving the removal of the entire stomach (total gastrectomy)
• are pregnant or plan to become pregnant. Tasigna may harm your unborn baby. If you are able to become pregnant, you should use effective birth control during treatment with Tasigna. Talk to your doctor about the best birth control methods to prevent pregnancy while you are taking Tasigna.
• are breastfeeding or plan to breastfeed. It is not known if Tasigna passes into your breast milk. You and your doctor should decide if you will take Tasigna or breastfeed. You should not do both.
Tell your doctor about all the medicines you take, including prescription and non prescription medicines, vitamins and herbal supplements.
Tasigna can interact with many medicines and supplements and increase your chance for serious and life-threatening side effects. See "What is the most important information I should know about Tasigna?"
Know the medicines you take. Keep a list of them and show it to your doctor and pharmacist when you get a new medicine.
How should I take Tasigna?
• Take Tasigna exactly as your doctor tells you to take it. Do not change your dose or stop taking Tasigna unless your doctor tells you.
• Tasigna is a long-term treatment.
• Your doctor will tell you how many Tasigna capsules to take and when to take them.
• **Do not take Tasigna with food. Take Tasigna at least 2 hours after you eat and at least 1 hour before you eat.**
• Swallow Tasigna capsules whole with water. If you cannot swallow Tasigna capsules whole, tell your doctor.
• Do not drink grapefruit juice, eat grapefruit, or take supplements containing grapefruit extract at any time during treatment. See "What is the most important information I should know about Tasigna?"
• If you miss a dose, just take your next dose as scheduled. Do not make up for a missed dose.
• If you take too much Tasigna, call your doctor or poison control center right away. Symptoms may include vomiting and drowsiness. During treatment with Tasigna your doctor will do tests to check for side effects and to see how well Tasigna is working for you. The tests will check your:
  • heart
  • blood cells (white blood cells, red blood cells, and platelets). Your blood cells should be checked every two weeks for the first two months and then monthly.
  • electrolytes (potassium, magnesium)
  • pancreas and liver function
  • bone marrow samples
• Your doctor may change your dose. Your doctor may have you stop Tasigna for some time or lower your dose if you have side effects with it.
What are the possible side effects of Tasigna?
Tasigna may cause serious side effects including:
• See "What is the most important information I should know about Tasigna?"
• **Low blood counts.** Low blood counts are common with Tasigna. Your doctor will check your blood counts regularly during treatment with Tasigna. Symptoms of low blood counts include:
  • unexplained bleeding or bruising
  • blood in urine or stool
  • unexplained weakness
• **Liver damage.** Symptoms include yellow skin and eyes.
• **Pancreas inflammation (pancreatitis).** Symptoms include sudden stomach area pain with nausea and vomiting.
• **Bleeding in the brain.** Symptoms include sudden headache, changes in your eyesight, not being aware of what is going on around you and becoming unconscious.
The most common side effects of Tasigna include:
• low blood count
• rash
• nausea
• fever
• headache
• itching
• tiredness
• stomach (abdominal) pain
• diarrhea
• constipation
• muscle and joint pain
• back pain
• muscle spasms
• weakness
• hair loss
• runny or stuffy nose, sneezing, sore throat
• cough

Tell your doctor if you have any side effect that bothers you or does not go away.
These are not all of the possible side effects of Tasigna. For more information, ask your doctor or pharmacist.
Call your doctor for medical advice about side effects. You may report side effects to FDA at 1-800-FDA-1088.
How should I store Tasigna?
• Store Tasigna at room temperature, 59° to 86°F (15° to 30°C).
• Safely throw away medicine that is out of date or no longer needed.
• **Keep Tasigna and all medicines out of the reach of children.**
General information about Tasigna
Medicines are sometimes prescribed for purposes other than those listed in a Medication Guide. Do not use Tasigna for a condition for which it was not prescribed. Do not give Tasigna to other people, even if they have the same problem you have. It may harm them.
This Medication Guide summarizes the most important information about Tasigna. If you would like more information, talk with your doctor. You can ask your doctor or pharmacist for information about Tasigna that is written for healthcare professionals.
For more information, go to www.us.tasigna.com or call 1-866-411-8274.
What are the ingredients in Tasigna?
Active ingredient: nilotinib
Inactive ingredients: colloidal silicon dioxide, crospovidone, lactose monohydrate, magnesium stearate and poloxamer 188.
The capsule shell contains gelatin, titanium dioxide (E171), iron oxide yellow (E172) and iron oxide black or iron oxide red for stamping of the imprint (E172).
This Medication Guide has been approved by the U.S. Food and Drug Administration.

T2010-34/T2010-35

Manufactured by:
Novartis Pharma Stein AG
Stein, Switzerland
Distributed by:
Novartis Pharmaceuticals Corporation
East Hanover, New Jersey 07936
©Novartis

Shown in Product Identification Guide, page 316

TEKAMLO™   ℞
[těk'-ăm-lō]
(aliskiren and amlodipine)
tablets

The following prescribing information is based on official labeling in effect September 2010.
HIGHLIGHTS OF PRESCRIBING INFORMATION
These highlights do not include all the information needed to use TEKAMLO safely and effectively. See full prescribing information for TEKAMLO.
Tekamlo *(aliskiren and amlodipine)* tablets
Initial U.S. Approval: 2010

WARNING: AVOID USE IN PREGNANCY
See full prescribing information for complete boxed warning.
When pregnancy is detected, discontinue Tekamlo as soon as possible. Drugs that act directly on the renin-angiotensin-aldosterone system can cause injury and even death to the developing fetus. (5.1, 8.1)

————INDICATIONS AND USAGE————
Tekamlo is a combination of aliskiren, a renin inhibitor, and amlodipine, a dihydropyridine calcium channel blocker, indicated for the treatment of hypertension:
• As initial therapy in patients likely to need multiple drugs to achieve their blood pressure goals. (1)
• In patients not adequately controlled with monotherapy. (1)
• As a substitute for its titrated components. (1)
————DOSAGE AND ADMINISTRATION————
• Add-on therapy or initial therapy: Initiate with 150 mg/5 mg. Titrate as needed up to a maximum of 300 mg/10 mg. (2.1, 2.3, 2.5)
• The blood pressure lowering effect is largely attained within 1-2 weeks. (2.2)
• Replacement therapy: May substitute for titrated components. (2.4)
• Administer one tablet daily with a routine pattern with regard to meals. (2.7)
• May administer with other antihypertensive agents. (2.7)
• Additive effects with ACE inhibitors at maximal doses have not been studied.

DOSAGE FORMS AND STRENGTHS

Tablets (aliskiren/amlodipine): 150 mg/5 mg, 150 mg/10 mg, 300 mg/5 mg, 300 mg/10 mg. (3)

WARNINGS AND PRECAUTIONS

- Avoid fetal and neonatal exposure. (5.1)
- Head and neck angioedema: Discontinue Tekamlo and monitor until signs and symptoms resolve. (5.2)
- Hypotension in volume- and/or salt-depleted patients: Correct imbalances before initiating therapy with Tekamlo. (5.3)
- Increased angina or myocardial infarction with calcium channel blockers may occur upon dosage initiation or increase. (5.4)
- Patients with renal impairment: Decrease in renal function may be anticipated with susceptible individuals. (5.5)
- Patients with hepatic impairment: Titrate slowly. (5.6)
- Patients with heart failure: Titrate slowly. (5.7)
- Hyperkalemia: Monitor serum potassium when co-administering with ACEI, potassium-sparing diuretics, potassium supplements, or other potassium-containing salt substitutes.

ADVERSE REACTIONS

The most common adverse event (incidence ≥2% and more common than with placebo) is peripheral edema. (6.1)

To report SUSPECTED ADVERSE REACTIONS, contact Novartis Pharmaceuticals Corporation at 1-888-669-6682 or FDA at 1-800-FDA-1088 or www.fda.gov/medwatch.

DRUG INTERACTIONS

Aliskiren:
- Cyclosporine: Concomitant use is not recommended. (7)

USE IN SPECIFIC POPULATIONS

Nursing Mothers: Discontinue drug or nursing. (8.3)

See 17 for PATIENT COUNSELING INFORMATION and FDA-approved patient labeling

Revised 08/2010

FULL PRESCRIBING INFORMATION

WARNING: AVOID USE IN PREGNANCY
When pregnancy is detected, discontinue Tekamlo as soon as possible. Drugs that act directly on the renin-angiotensin-aldosterone system can cause injury and even death to the developing fetus. [See Warnings and Precautions (5.1) and Use in Specific Populations (8.1)].

1   INDICATIONS AND USAGE

Tekamlo is indicated for the treatment of hypertension, alone or with other antihypertensive agents.

Initial Therapy
Use Tekamlo as initial therapy in patients who are likely to need multiple drugs to achieve their blood pressure goals. Base the choice of Tekamlo as initial therapy on an assessment of potential benefits and risks.

Add-On Therapy
Switch a patient whose blood pressure is not adequately controlled with aliskiren alone or amlodipine besylate (or another dihydropyridine calcium channel blocker) to combination therapy with Tekamlo.

Replacement Therapy
Tekamlo may be substituted for its titrated components. Patients with moderate or severe hypertension are at a relatively high risk for cardiovascular events (such as strokes, heart attacks, and heart failure), kidney failure, and vision problems, so prompt treatment is clinically relevant. Individualize the decision to use a combination as initial therapy by weighing factors such as baseline blood pressure, the target goal, and the incremental likelihood of achieving goal with a combination compared to monotherapy. Individual blood pressure goals may vary based upon the patient's risk. Data from the high-dose multifactorial study [see Clinical Studies (14)] provide estimates of the probability of reaching a target blood pressure with Tekamlo compared to aliskiren or amlodipine monotherapy. The figures below provide estimates of the likelihood of achieving systolic or diastolic blood pressure control with Tekamlo 300 mg/10 mg, based upon baseline systolic or diastolic blood pressure. The curve of each treatment group was estimated by logistic regression modeling. The estimated likelihood at the right tail of each curve is less reliable because of a small number of subjects with high baseline blood pressures.

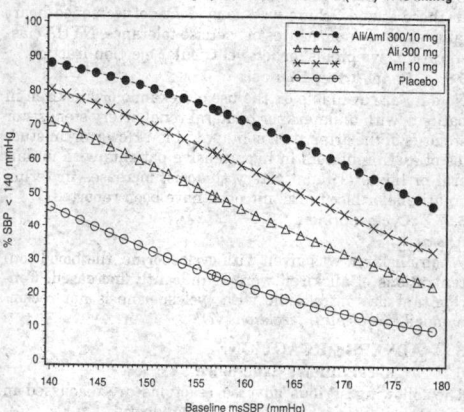

Figure 1: Probability of Achieving Systolic Blood Pressure (SBP) <140 mmHg

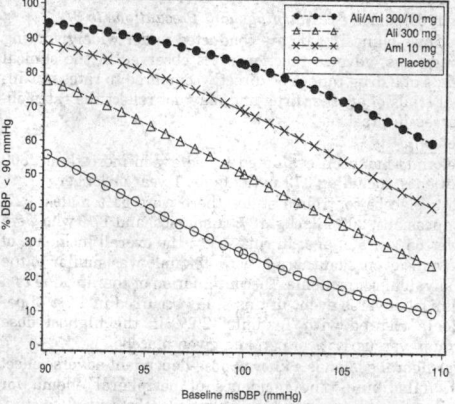

Figure 2: Probability of Achieving Diastolic Blood Pressure (DBP) <90 mmHg

[See figure 3 at top of next column]
[See figure 4 on next column]

The figures above provide an approximation of the likelihood of reaching a targeted blood pressure goal (e.g. SBP

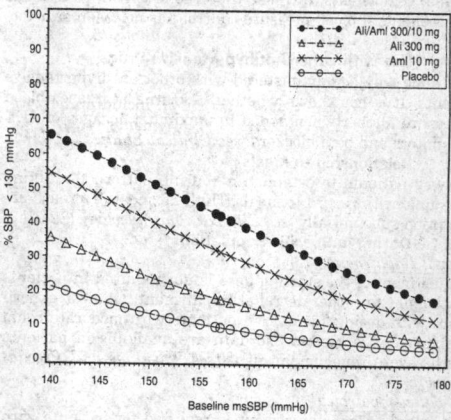

Figure 3: Probability of Achieving Systolic Blood Pressure (SBP) <130 mmHg

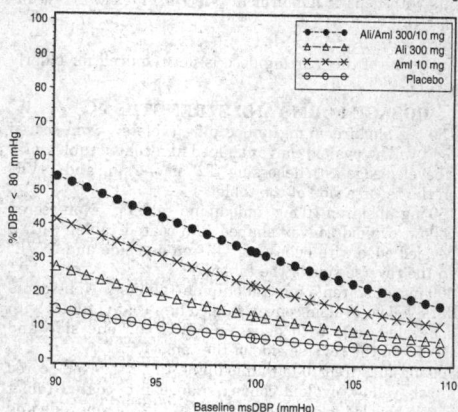

Figure 4: Probability of Achieving Diastolic Blood Pressure (DBP) <80 mmHg

<140 mmHg or <130 mmHg) for the high dose groups evaluated in the study. At all levels of baseline blood pressure, the probability of achieving any given diastolic or systolic goal is greater with the combination than for either monotherapy. For example, the mean baseline SBP/DBP for patients participating in this multifactorial study was 157/100 mmHg. A patient with a baseline blood pressure of 157/100 mmHg has about a 49% likelihood of achieving a goal of <140 mmHg (systolic) and 50% likelihood of achieving <90 mmHg (diastolic) on aliskiren alone, and the likelihood of achieving these goals on amlodipine alone is about 62% (systolic) and 69% (diastolic). The likelihood of achieving these goals on Tekamlo rises to about 74% (systolic) and 83% (diastolic). The likelihood of achieving these goals on placebo is about 25% (systolic) and 27% (diastolic) [see Dosage and Administration (2) and Clinical Studies (14)].

2   DOSAGE AND ADMINISTRATION

2.1   General Considerations

The blood pressure lowering effects are largely attained within 1-2 weeks.

2.2   Dose Selection

The recommended initial once-daily dose of Tekamlo is 150 mg/5 mg. Titrate as needed to a maximum of 300 mg/10 mg.

2.3   Dose Titration

If blood pressure remains uncontrolled after 2 to 4 weeks of therapy, titrate the dose to a maximum of Tekamlo 300 mg/10 mg once daily.

2.4   Initial Therapy

The usual recommended starting dose of Tekamlo is 150 mg/5 mg once daily as needed to control blood pressure. Titrate the dose to a maximum of 300 mg/10 mg once daily. Tekamlo is not recommended for use as initial therapy in patients with intravascular volume depletion [see Warnings and Precautions (5.3)].

2.5   Add-on Therapy

Use Tekamlo for patients not adequately controlled with aliskiren alone or amlodipine besylate (or another dihydropyridine calcium channel blocker) alone.

Switch a patient who experiences dose-limiting adverse reactions on either component alone to Tekamlo containing a lower dose of that component in combination with the other to achieve similar blood pressure reductions.

2.6   Replacement Therapy

Switch patients receiving aliskiren and amlodipine besylate from separate tablets to a single tablet of Tekamlo containing the same component doses. When substituting for individual components, increase the dose of one or both of the components if blood pressure control has not been satisfactory.

2.7 Use with Other Antihypertensive Drugs

Tekamlo may be administered with other antihypertensive agents. It is not known whether Tekturna decreases blood pressure further when added to maximum dosages of ACE inhibitors and beta blockers *[see Clinical Studies (14)]*.

2.8 Relationship to Meals

Advise patients to establish a routine pattern for taking Tekamlo with regard to meals. High-fat meals decrease absorption substantially *[see Clinical Pharmacology (12.3)]*.

2.9 Dosing in Specific Populations

Renal Impairment

Adjustment of the starting dose is not required in patients with mild to moderate renal impairment. Clinical experience with dosing Tekamlo in patients with moderate renal impairment is limited. No data are available in patients with severe renal impairment *[see Warnings and Precautions (5.5)]*.

Hepatic Impairment

No initial dosage adjustment is required for patients with mild or moderate liver insufficiency. Titrate slowly in patients with hepatic impairment *[see Warnings and Precautions (5.6)]*.

Elderly Patients

Adjustment of the starting dose is not required for elderly patients.

3 DOSAGE FORMS AND STRENGTHS

- 150 mg aliskiren/5 mg amlodipine tablets: Non-scored light yellow, ovaloid convex shaped film-coated tablet with a beveled edge with debossing "T2" on one side and "NVR" on the reverse side of the tablet.
- 150 mg aliskiren/10 mg amlodipine tablets: Non-scored yellow, ovaloid convex shaped film-coated tablet with a beveled edge with debossing "T7" on one side and "NVR" on the reverse side of the tablet.
- 300 mg aliskiren/5 mg amlodipine tablets: Non-scored dark yellow, ovaloid convex shaped film-coated tablet with a beveled edge with debossing "T11" on one side and "NVR" on the reverse side of the tablet.
- 300 mg aliskiren/10 mg amlodipine tablets: Non-scored brown yellow, ovaloid convex shaped film-coated tablet with a beveled edge with debossing "T12" on one side and "NVR" on the reverse side of the tablet.

4 CONTRAINDICATIONS

None.

5 WARNINGS AND PRECAUTIONS

5.1 Fetal/Neonatal Morbidity and Mortality

The use of drugs that act directly on the renin-angiotensin-aldosterone system during pregnancy can cause fetal and neonatal morbidity and death. No animal studies were conducted with Tekamlo; however, decreased fetal birth weight was observed in animal studies with aliskiren and intrauterine deaths were observed in animal studies with amlodipine. Tekamlo can cause fetal harm when administered to a pregnant woman. When pregnancy is detected, discontinue Tekamlo as soon as possible. If Tekamlo is used during pregnancy, or if a patient becomes pregnant while taking this drug, apprise the patient of the potential hazard to the fetus *[see Use in Specific Populations (8.1)]*.

5.2 Head and Neck Angioedema

Aliskiren

Angioedema of the face, extremities, lips, tongue, glottis and/or larynx has been reported in patients treated with aliskiren and has necessitated hospitalization and intubation. This may occur at any time during treatment and has occurred in patients with and without a history of angioedema with ACE inhibitors or angiotensin receptor antagonists. If angioedema involves the throat, tongue, glottis or larynx, or if the patient has a history of upper respiratory surgery, airway obstruction may occur and be fatal. Patients who experience these effects, even without respiratory distress, require prolonged observation, since treatment with antihistamines and corticosteroids may not be sufficient to prevent respiratory involvement. Prompt administration of subcutaneous epinephrine solution 1:1000 (0.3 to 0.5 mL) and measures to ensure a patent airway may be necessary. Discontinue Tekamlo immediately in patients who develop angioedema and do not readminister.

5.3 Hypotension

An excessive fall in blood pressure (hypotension) was rarely seen (0.2%) in patients with uncomplicated hypertension treated with Tekamlo in controlled trials.

In patients with an activated renin-angiotensin-aldosterone system, such as volume- and/or salt-depleted patients receiving high doses of diuretics, symptomatic hypotension may occur in patients receiving renin-angiotensin-aldosterone system (RAAS) blockers. Correct these conditions prior to administration of Tekamlo, or start the treatment under close medical supervision.

If an excessive fall in blood pressure occurs with Tekamlo, place the patient in the supine position and, if necessary, give an intravenous infusion of normal saline. A transient hypotensive response is not a contraindication to further treatment, which usually can be continued without difficulty once the blood pressure has stabilized.

5.4 Risk of Myocardial Infarction or Increased Angina

Rarely, initiation or change to the dose of a calcium channel blocker has resulted in the development of documented increased frequency, duration or severity of angina or acute myocardial infarction, particularly in patients with severe obstructive coronary artery disease. The mechanism of this effect has not been elucidated.

5.5 Impaired Renal Function

Tekamlo

Clinical trials with Tekamlo in hypertension excluded patients with severe renal impairment.

Aliskiren

Clinical trials of aliskiren in hypertension excluded patients with severe renal dysfunction (creatinine 1.7 mg/dL for women and 2.0 mg/dL for men and/or estimated GFR <30 mL/min), a history of dialysis, nephrotic syndrome, or renovascular hypertension. Consider periodic determinations of serum electrolytes to detect possible electrolyte imbalances.

5.6 Patients with Hepatic Impairment

Amlodipine besylate

Amlodipine is extensively metabolized by the liver and the plasma elimination half-life is 56 hours in patients with impaired hepatic function, therefore, caution should be exercised when administering Tekamlo to patients with severe hepatic impairment.

5.7 Patients with Congestive Heart Failure

Amlodipine besylate

Amlodipine (5-10 mg per day) has been studied in a placebo-controlled trial of 1153 patients with NYHA Class III or IV heart failure on stable doses of ACE inhibitor, digoxin, and diuretics. Follow-up was at least 6 months, with a mean of about 14 months. There was no overall adverse effect on survival or cardiac morbidity (as defined by life-threatening arrhythmia, acute myocardial infarction, or hospitalization for worsened heart failure). Amlodipine has been compared to placebo in four 8-12 week studies of patients with NYHA Class II/III heart failure, involving a total of 697 patients. In these studies, there was no evidence of worsened heart failure based on measures of exercise tolerance, NYHA classification, symptoms, or left ventricular ejection fraction.

5.8 Renal Artery Stenosis

No data are available on the use of Tekamlo or aliskiren in patients with unilateral or bilateral renal artery stenosis or stenosis of the artery to a solitary kidney. However, in studies of ACE inhibitors in hypertensive patients with unilateral or bilateral renal artery stenosis, increases in serum creatinine or blood urea nitrogen have been reported.

5.9 Cyclosporine

Aliskiren

When aliskiren was given with cyclosporine, the blood concentrations of aliskiren were significantly increased. Concomitant use of Tekamlo with cyclosporine is not recommended *[see Drug Interactions (7)]*.

6 ADVERSE REACTIONS

6.1 Clinical Studies Experience

The following serious adverse reactions are discussed in greater detail in other sections of the label:

- Risk of fetal/neonatal morbidity and mortality *[see Warnings and Precautions (5.1)]*
- Head and neck angioedema *[see Warnings and Precautions (5.2)]*
- Hypotension *[see Warnings and Precautions (5.3)]*

Because clinical trials are conducted under widely varying conditions, adverse reaction rates observed in the clinical trials of a drug cannot be directly compared to rates in clinical trials of another drug and may not reflect the rates observed in practice.

Tekamlo

Tekamlo has been evaluated for safety in more than 2800 patients, including 372 patients for 1 year or longer.

In a placebo-controlled study, there were 51% males, 62% Caucasians, 20% Blacks, 18% Hispanics, and 17% who were over 65 years of age. In this study, the overall incidence of adverse events on therapy with Tekamlo was similar to the individual components. Discontinuation of therapy due to a clinical adverse event in this study occurred in 1.7% of patients treated with Tekamlo (2.2% in the highest dose group) versus 1.5% of patients given placebo.

Peripheral edema is a known, dose-dependent adverse effect of amlodipine. The incidence of peripheral edema for Tekamlo in short-term double-blind placebo-controlled studies was lower than or equal to that of the corresponding amlodipine doses.

The adverse event in a placebo-controlled trial that occurred in at least 2% of patients treated with Tekamlo and at a higher incidence than placebo was peripheral edema (6.2% versus 1.0%). The incidence rate of peripheral edema at high dose was 8.9%.

In a long-term safety trial, the safety profile of adverse events was similar to that seen in the short-term controlled trials.

Aliskiren

Aliskiren has been evaluated for safety in 6460 patients, including 1740 treated for longer than 6 months, and 1250 for longer than 1 year. In placebo-controlled clinical trials, discontinuation of therapy because of a clinical adverse event, including uncontrolled hypertension, occurred in 2.2% of patients treated with aliskiren, versus 3.5% of patients given placebo.

Two cases of angioedema with respiratory symptoms were reported with aliskiren use in the clinical studies. Two other cases of periorbital edema without respiratory symptoms were reported as possible angioedema and resulted in discontinuation. The rate of these angioedema cases in the completed studies was 0.06%.

In addition, 26 other cases of edema involving the face, hands, or whole body were reported with aliskiren use, including 4 leading to discontinuation.

In the placebo-controlled studies, however, the incidence of edema involving the face, hands, or whole body was 0.4% with aliskiren compared with 0.5% with placebo. In a long-term active-controlled study with aliskiren and HCTZ arms, the incidence of edema involving the face, hands, or whole body was 0.4% in both treatment arms.

Aliskiren produces dose-related gastrointestinal (GI) adverse reactions. Diarrhea was reported by 2.3% of patients at 300 mg, compared to 1.2% in placebo patients. In women and the elderly (age ≥65) increases in diarrhea rates were evident starting at a dose of 150 mg daily, with rates for these subgroups at 150 mg similar to those seen at 300 mg for men or younger patients (all rates about 2%). Other GI symptoms included abdominal pain, dyspepsia, and gastroesophageal reflux, although increased rates for abdominal pain and dyspepsia were distinguished from placebo only at 600 mg daily. Diarrhea and other GI symptoms were typically mild and rarely led to discontinuation.

Aliskiren was associated with a slight increase in cough in the placebo-controlled studies (1.1% for any aliskiren use versus 0.6% for placebo). In active-controlled trials with ACE inhibitor (ramipril, lisinopril) arms, the rates of cough for the aliskiren arms were about one-third to one-half the rates in the ACE inhibitor arms.

Other adverse reactions with increased rates for aliskiren compared to placebo included rash (1% versus 0.3%), elevated uric acid (0.4% versus 0.1%), gout (0.2% versus 0.1%), and renal stones (0.2% versus 0%).

Single episodes of tonic-clonic seizures with loss of consciousness were reported in two patients treated with aliskiren in the clinical trials. One patient had predisposing causes for seizures and had a negative electroencephalogram (EEG) and cerebral imaging following the seizures; for the other patient, EEG and imaging results were not reported. Aliskiren was discontinued and there was no rechallenge in either case.

No clinically meaningful changes in vital signs or in ECG (including QTc interval) were observed in patients treated with aliskiren.

Amlodipine besylate

Amlodipine (Norvasc®) has been evaluated for safety in more than 11,000 patients in U.S. and foreign clinical trials. Other adverse events that have been reported <1% but >0.1% of patients in controlled clinical trials or under conditions of open trials or marketing experience where a causal relationship is uncertain were:

Cardiovascular: arrhythmia (including ventricular tachycardia and atrial fibrillation), bradycardia, chest pain, peripheral ischemia, syncope, postural hypotension, vasculitis

Central and Peripheral Nervous System: neuropathy peripheral, paresthesia, tremor, vertigo

Gastrointestinal: anorexia, constipation, dyspepsia,** dysphagia, diarrhea, flatulence, pancreatitis, vomiting, gingival hyperplasia

General: allergic reaction, asthenia,** back pain, hot flushes, malaise, pain, rigors, weight gain, weight decrease

Musculoskeletal System: arthralgia, arthrosis, muscle cramps,** myalgia

Psychiatric: sexual dysfunction (male** and female), insomnia, nervousness, depression, abnormal dreams, anxiety, depersonalization

Respiratory System: dyspnea, epistaxis

Skin and Appendages: angioedema, erythema multiforme, pruritus,** rash,** rash erythematous, rash maculopapular

**These events occurred in less than 1% in placebo-controlled trials, but the incidence of these side effects was between 1% and 2% in all multiple dose studies.

Special Senses: abnormal vision, conjunctivitis, diplopia, eye pain, tinnitus

Urinary System: micturation frequency, micturation disorder, nocturia

IMPORTANT NOTICE: Updated drug information is sent bi-monthly via the PDR® Update Insert. For *monthly* email updates, register at PDR.net.

Autonomic Nervous System: dry mouth, sweating increased
Metabolic and Nutritional: hyperglycemia, thirst
Hemopoietic: leukopenia, purpura, thrombocytopenia
Other events reported with amlodipine at a frequency of ≤0.1% of patients include: cardiac failure, pulse irregularity, extrasystoles, skin discoloration, urticaria, skin dryness, alopecia, dermatitis, muscle weakness, twitching, ataxia, hypertonia, migraine, cold and clammy skin, apathy, agitation, amnesia, gastritis, increased appetite, loose stools, rhinitis, dysuria, polyuria, parosmia, taste perversion, abnormal visual accommodation, and xerophthalmia. Other reactions occurred sporadically and cannot be distinguished from medications or concurrent disease states such as myocardial infarction and angina.

6.2 Clinical Laboratory Test Abnormalities
RBC Count, Hemoglobin and Hematocrit: Small mean changes from baseline were seen in RBC count, hemoglobin and hematocrit in patients treated with both Tekamlo and aliskiren monotherapy. This effect is also seen with other agents acting on the renin-angiotensin system. In aliskiren monotherapy trials these decreases led to slight increases in rates of anemia compared to placebo (0.1% for any aliskiren use, 0.3% for aliskiren 600 mg daily, vs. 0% for placebo). No patients discontinued due to anemia.
Blood Urea Nitrogen (BUN)/Creatinine: Elevations in BUN (>40 mg/dL) and creatinine (>2.0 mg/dL) in patients treated with Tekamlo were less than <1.0%.
Serum Potassium: Increases in serum potassium >5.5 mEq/L were infrequent in patients with essential hypertension treated with both Tekamlo and aliskiren monotherapy (0.9% compared to 0.6% with placebo). However, when aliskiren was used in combination with an angiotensin-converting enzyme inhibitor (ACEI) in a diabetic population, increases in serum potassium were more frequent (5.5%). Monitor electrolytes and renal function in this population.

6.3 Post-marketing Experience
The following adverse reactions have been identified during postapproval use of either aliskiren or amlodipine. Because these reactions are reported voluntarily from a population of uncertain size, it is not always possible to reliably estimate their frequency or establish a causal relationship to drug exposure:
Hypersensitivity: angioedema requiring airway management and hospitalization
Aliskiren: peripheral edema
Amlodipine: The following postmarketing event has been reported infrequently where a causal relationship is uncertain: gynecomastia. In postmarketing experience, jaundice and hepatic enzyme elevations (mostly consistent with cholestasis or hepatitis), in some cases severe enough to require hospitalization, have been reported in association with use of amlodipine.

7 DRUG INTERACTIONS
No drug interaction studies have been conducted with Tekamlo and other drugs, although studies with the individual aliskiren and amlodipine besylate components are described below.

Aliskiren

Effects of Other Drugs on Aliskiren
Based on _in vitro_ studies, aliskiren is metabolized by CYP 3A4.
Irbesartan: Coadministration of irbesartan reduced aliskiren C_{max} up to 50% after multiple dosing.
P-glycoprotein Effects: Pgp (MDR1/Mdr1a/1b) was found to be the major efflux system involved in absorption and disposition of aliskiren in preclinical studies. The potential for drug interactions at the Pgp site will likely depend on the degree of inhibition of this transporter.
Atorvastatin: Coadministration of atorvastatin resulted in about a 50% increase in aliskiren C_{max} and AUC after multiple dosing.
Ketoconazole: Coadministration of 200 mg twice-daily ketoconazole with aliskiren resulted in an approximate 80% increase in plasma levels of aliskiren. A 400-mg once-daily dose was not studied but would be expected to increase aliskiren blood levels further.
Verapamil: Coadministration of a single oral dose of 300 mg aliskiren with 240 mg verapamil increased AUC and C_{max} of aliskiren by ~2-fold. However, no dosage adjustment is necessary.
Cyclosporine: Coadministration of 200 mg and 600 mg cyclosporine with 75 mg aliskiren resulted in an approximately 2.5-fold increase in C_{max} and 5-fold increase in AUC of aliskiren. Concomitant use of aliskiren with cyclosporine is not recommended.
Drugs with no clinically significant effects: Coadministration of lovastatin, atenolol, warfarin, furosemide, digoxin, celecoxib, hydrochlorothiazide, ramipril, amlodipine besylate, metformin and amlodipine did not result in clinically significant increases in aliskiren exposure.

Effects of Aliskiren on Other Drugs
Aliskiren does not inhibit the CYP450 isoenzymes (CYP1A2, 2C8, 2C9, 2C19, 2D6, 2E1, and CYP 3A) or induce CYP 3A4.
Furosemide: When aliskiren was coadministered with furosemide, the AUC and C_{max} of furosemide were reduced by about 30% and 50%, respectively. Patients receiving furosemide could find its effect diminished after starting aliskiren.
Drugs with no clinically significant effects: Coadministration of aliskiren did not significantly affect the pharmacokinetics of lovastatin, digoxin, valsartan, amlodipine, metformin, celecoxib, atenolol, atorvastatin, ramipril or hydrochlorothiazide.
Warfarin: The effects of aliskiren on warfarin pharmacokinetics have not been evaluated.

Amlodipine besylate
In clinical trials, amlodipine has been safely administered with thiazide diuretics, beta-blockers, angiotensin-converting enzyme inhibitors, long-acting nitrates, sublingual nitroglycerin, digoxin, warfarin, non-steroidal antiinflammatory drugs, antibiotics, and oral hypoglycemic drugs.
Cimetidine: Co-administration of amlodipine with cimetidine did not alter the pharmacokinetics of amlodipine.
Grapefruit juice: Co-administration of 240 mL of grapefruit juice with a single oral dose of amlodipine 10 mg in 20 healthy volunteers had no significant effect on the pharmacokinetics of amlodipine.
Maalox® (antacid): Co-administration of the antacid Maalox with a single dose of amlodipine had no significant effect on the pharmacokinetics of amlodipine.
Sildenafil: A single 100 mg dose of sildenafil in subjects with essential hypertension had no effect on the pharmacokinetic parameters of amlodipine. When amlodipine and sildenafil were used in combination, each agent independently exerted its own blood pressure lowering effect.
Atorvastatin: Co-administration of multiple 10 mg doses of amlodipine with 80 mg of atorvastatin resulted in no significant change in the steady-state pharmacokinetic parameters of atorvastatin.
Digoxin: Co-administration of amlodipine with digoxin did not change serum digoxin levels or digoxin renal clearance in normal volunteers.
Ethanol (alcohol): Single and multiple 10 mg doses of amlodipine had no significant effect on the pharmacokinetics of ethanol.
Warfarin: Co-administration of amlodipine with warfarin did not change the warfarin prothrombin response time.

8 USE IN SPECIFIC POPULATIONS
8.1 Pregnancy
Pregnancy Category D _[See Warnings and Precautions Section]_
The use of drugs that act directly on the renin-angiotensin-aldosterone system during the second and third trimesters of pregnancy can cause fetal and neonatal morbidity and death. In addition, first trimester use of ACE inhibitors has been associated with birth defects in retrospective data. No animal studies were conducted with Tekamlo; however, decreased fetal birth weight was observed in animal studies with aliskiren and intrauterine deaths were observed in animal studies with amlodipine. Tekamlo can cause fetal harm when administered to a pregnant woman. When pregnancy is detected, discontinue Tekamlo as soon as possible. If Tekamlo is used during pregnancy, or if the patient becomes pregnant while taking this drug, the patient should be apprised of the potential hazard to the fetus.
Human Data and Clinical Considerations
Maternal hypertension is associated with increased risks for preterm delivery, intrauterine growth restriction, placental abruption, preeclampsia, and perinatal mortality. Appropriate management of maternal hypertension during pregnancy is important to optimize outcomes for both mother and fetus. Renin inhibitors (like aliskiren), angiotensin II receptor antagonists and angiotensin converting enzyme (ACE) inhibitors exert similar effects on the renin-angiotensin-aldosterone system. Based on several dozen published cases, ACE inhibitor use during the second and third trimesters of pregnancy is associated with fetal and neonatal injury, including hypotension, neonatal skull hypoplasia, anuria, reversible or irreversible renal failure, and death. Decreased fetal renal function may result in oligohydramnios and associated with fetal limb contractures, craniofacial deformation, and hypoplastic lung development. Prematurity, intrauterine growth retardation, and patent ductus arteriosus have been reported in women using these drugs, but it is not clear whether these occurrences were due to drug exposure. Limited data are conflicting about whether first trimester use of ACE inhibitors is associated with an increased risk of birth defects, but the drugs' mechanism of action raises a theoretical concern.
When pregnancy occurs in a patient using Tekamlo, the physician should discontinue Tekamlo treatment as soon as

possible. Inform the patient about potential risks to the fetus based on the time of gestational exposure to Tekamlo (first trimester only or later). If exposure occurs beyond the first trimester, perform an ultrasound examination.
In rare cases when another antihypertensive agent cannot be used to treat the pregnant patient, serial ultrasound examinations should be used to assess the intraamniotic environment. Routine fetal testing with non-stress tests, biophysical profiles, and/or contraction stress tests may be appropriate based on gestational age and standards of care in the community. If oligohydramnios occurs in these situations, individualized decisions about continuing or discontinuing Tekamlo treatment and about pregnancy management should be made by the patient and her physicians. Patients and physicians should be aware that oligohydramnios may not appear until after the fetus has sustained irreversible injury.
Infants exposed to Tekamlo _in-utero_ should be closely observed for hypotension, oliguria, and hyperkalemia. If oliguria occurs, these infants may require blood pressure and renal perfusion support. Exchange transfusion or dialysis may be required to reverse hypotension and/or support decreased renal function.
Animal Data
No reproductive toxicity studies have been conducted with the combination of aliskiren and amlodipine besylate. However, these studies have been conducted for aliskiren and amlodipine besylate alone.
Aliskiren
In developmental toxicity studies, pregnant rats and rabbits received oral aliskiren hemifumarate during organogenesis at doses up to 20 and 7 times the maximum recommended human dose (MRHD) based on body surface area (mg/m²), respectively, in rats and rabbits. (Actual animal doses were up to 600 mg/kg/day in rats and up to 100 mg/kg/day in rabbits.) No teratogenicity was observed; however, fetal birth weight was decreased in rabbits at doses 3.2 times the MRHD based on body surface area (mg/m²). Aliskiren was present in placentas, amniotic fluid and fetuses of pregnant rabbits.
Amlodipine
In developmental toxicity studies, pregnant rats and rabbits received oral amlodipine maleate during organogenesis at doses approximately 10 and 20 times the maximum recommended human dose (MRHD) based on body surface area (mg/m²), respectively, in rats and rabbits. (Actual animal doses were up to 10 mg/kg/day.) No evidence of teratogenicity or other embryofetal toxicity was observed. However, litter size was decreased approximately 50% and the number of intrauterine deaths was increased approximately 5-fold for rats receiving amlodipine maleate at doses approximately 10 times the MRHD based on body surface area (mg/m²) for 14 days before mating and throughout mating and gestation. Amlodipine maleate has been shown to prolong both the gestation period and the duration of labor in rats at this dose.

8.3 Nursing Mothers
It is not known whether aliskiren or amlodipine is excreted in human milk. Both aliskiren and amlodipine are secreted in the milk of lactating rats. Because of the potential for serious adverse reactions in human milk-fed infants from Tekamlo, a decision should be made whether to discontinue nursing or discontinue Tekamlo, taking into account the importance of the drug to the mother.

8.4 Pediatric Use
Safety and effectiveness of Tekamlo in pediatric patients have not been established.

8.5 Geriatric Use
Tekamlo
In the short-term controlled clinical trials of Tekamlo, 17% of patients treated with Tekamlo were ≥ 65 years. No overall differences in safety or effectiveness were observed between these subjects and younger subjects. Other reported clinical experience has not identified differences in responses between the elderly and younger patients, but greater sensitivity of some older individuals cannot be ruled out.
Aliskiren
Impact of aging on aliskiren pharmacokinetics has been assessed, when compared to young adults (18-40 years), aliskiren mean AUC and C_{max} in elderly subjects (> 65 years) are increased by 57% and 28%, respectively. However, differences in efficacy and safety between the elderly and younger populations were minor, indicating that differences in exposure due to age do not significantly alter the clinical effect of the drug. Therefore, no starting dose adjustment in geriatric population is required.
Amlodipine
Other reported clinical experience has not identified differences in responses between the elderly and younger patients. However, elderly patients have decreased clearance of amlodipine with a resulting increase of AUC of approximately 40-60%. In general dose selection for an elderly patient should be cautious, usually starting at the low end of

the dosing range, reflecting the greater frequency of decreased hepatic, renal or cardiac function, and of concomitant disease or other drug therapy.

10 OVERDOSAGE

Aliskiren

Limited data are available related to overdosage in humans. The most likely manifestation of overdosage would be hypotension. If symptomatic hypotension should occur, provide supportive treatment.

Amlodipine besylate

Single oral doses of amlodipine maleate equivalent to 40 mg amlodipine/kg and 100 mg amlodipine/kg in mice and rats, respectively, caused deaths. Single oral amlodipine maleate doses equivalent to 4 or more mg amlodipine/kg or higher in dogs (11 or more times the maximum recommended human dose on a mg/m^2 basis) caused a marked peripheral vasodilation and hypotension.

Overdosage might be expected to cause excessive peripheral vasodilation with marked hypotension and possibly a reflex tachycardia. In humans, experience with intentional overdosage of amlodipine is limited. Reports of intentional overdosage include a patient who ingested 250 mg and was asymptomatic and was not hospitalized; another (120 mg) was hospitalized, underwent gastric lavage and remained normotensive; the third (105 mg) was hospitalized and had hypotension (90/50 mmHg) which normalized following plasma expansion. A case of accidental drug overdose has been documented in a 19-month-old male who ingested 30 mg amlodipine (about 2 mg/kg). During the emergency room presentation, vital signs were stable with no evidence of hypotension, but a heart rate of 180 bpm. Ipecac was administered 3.5 hours after ingestion and on subsequent observation (overnight) no sequelae were noted.

If massive overdose should occur, active cardiac and respiratory monitoring should be instituted. Frequent blood pressure measurements are essential. Should hypotension occur, cardiovascular support including elevation of the extremities and the judicious administration of fluids should be initiated. If hypotension remains unresponsive to these conservative measures, administration of vasopressors (such as phenylephrine) should be considered with attention to circulating volume and urine output. Intravenous calcium gluconate may help to reverse the effects of calcium entry blockade. As amlodipine is highly protein bound, hemodialysis is not likely to be of benefit.

11 DESCRIPTION

Tekamlo is a single tablet of aliskiren hemifumarate (an orally active, nonpeptide, potent direct renin inhibitor) and amlodipine besylate (a dihydropyridine calcium channel blocker).

Aliskiren hemifumarate

Aliskiren hemifumarate is chemically described as (2*S*, 4*S*,5*S*,7*S*)-N-(2-Carbamoyl-2-methylpropyl)-5-amino-4-hydroxy-2,7-diisopropyl-8-[4-methoxy-3-(3-methoxy-propoxy) phenyl]-octanamide hemifumarate and its structural formula is:

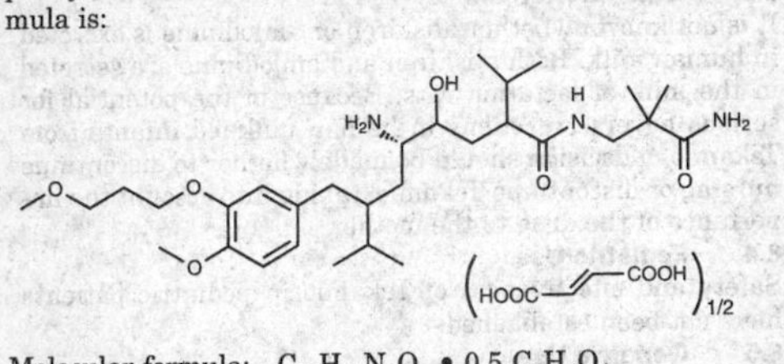

Molecular formula: $C_{30}H_{53}N_3O_6 \bullet 0.5\ C_4H_4O_4$

Aliskiren hemifumarate is a white to slightly yellowish powder with a molecular weight of 609.8 (free base-551.8). It is highly soluble in water, and freely soluble in methanol, ethanol and isopropanol.

Amlodipine besylate

Amlodipine besylate, USP is chemically described as 3-Ethyl 5-methyl (±)-2-[(2-aminoethoxy)methyl]-4-(o-chlorophenyl)-1,4-dihydro-6-methyl-3,5-pyridinedicarboxylate, monobenzenesulfonate, and its structural formula is:

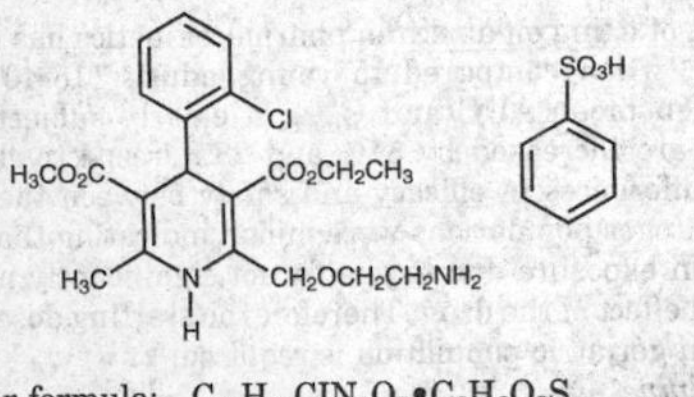

Molecular formula: $C_{20}H_{25}ClN_2O_5 \bullet C_6H_6O_3S$

Amlodipine besylate is a white to pale yellow crystalline powder with a molecular weight of 567.1. It is slightly soluble in water and sparingly soluble in ethanol.

Tekamlo tablets are formulated for oral administration to contain aliskiren hemifumarate and amlodipine besylate providing for the following available combinations: 150 mg/5 mg, 150 mg/10 mg, 300 mg/5 mg and 300 mg/10 mg aliskiren/amlodipine. The inactive ingredients for all strengths of the tablets may contain colloidal silicon dioxide, crospovidone, hypromellose, iron oxide red, iron oxide yellow, magnesium stearate, microcrystalline cellulose, polyethylene glycol, povidone, talc, and titanium dioxide.

12 CLINICAL PHARMACOLOGY

12.1 Mechanism of Action

Aliskiren

Renin is secreted by the kidney in response to decreases in blood volume and renal perfusion. Renin cleaves angiotensinogen to form the inactive decapeptide angiotensin I (Ang I). Ang I is converted to the active octapeptide angiotensin II (Ang II) by angiotensin-converting enzyme (ACE) and non-ACE pathways. Ang II is a powerful vasoconstrictor and leads to the release of catecholamines from the adrenal medulla and prejunctional nerve endings. It also promotes aldosterone secretion and sodium reabsorption. Together, these effects increase blood pressure. Ang II also inhibits renin release, thus providing a negative feedback to the system. This cycle, from renin through angiotensin to aldosterone and its associated negative feedback loop, is known as the renin-angiotensin-aldosterone system (RAAS). Aliskiren is a direct renin inhibitor, decreasing plasma renin activity (PRA) and inhibiting the conversion of angiotensinogen to Ang I. Whether aliskiren affects other RAAS components, e.g., ACE or non-ACE pathways, is not known.

All agents that inhibit the RAAS, including renin inhibitors, suppress the negative feedback loop, leading to a compensatory rise in plasma renin concentration. When this rise occurs during treatment with ACE inhibitors and ARBs, the result is increased levels of PRA. During treatment with aliskiren, however, the effect of increased renin levels is blocked, so that PRA, Ang I and Ang II are all reduced, whether aliskiren is used as monotherapy or in combination with other antihypertensive agents.

Amlodipine besylate

Amlodipine is a dihydropyridine calcium channel blocker that inhibits the transmembrane influx of calcium ions into vascular smooth muscle and cardiac muscle. Experimental data suggest that amlodipine binds to both dihydropyridine and nondihydropyridine binding sites. The contractile processes of cardiac muscle and vascular smooth muscle are dependent upon the movement of extracellular calcium ions into these cells through specific ion channels. Amlodipine inhibits calcium ion influx across cell membranes selectively, with a greater effect on vascular smooth muscle cells than on cardiac muscle cells. Negative inotropic effects can be detected *in vitro* but such effects have not been seen in intact animals at therapeutic doses. Serum calcium concentration is not affected by amlodipine. Within the physiologic pH range, amlodipine is an ionized compound (pKa=8.6), and its kinetic interaction with the calcium channel receptor is characterized by a gradual rate of association and dissociation with the receptor binding site, resulting in a gradual onset of effect.

Amlodipine is a peripheral arterial vasodilator that acts directly on vascular smooth muscle to cause a reduction in peripheral vascular resistance and reduction in blood pressure.

Tekamlo

The effects of combined treatment of aliskiren and amlodipine arise from the actions of these two agents on different, but complementary mechanisms that regulate blood pressure, calcium channel-mediated vasoconstriction and RAAS-mediated effects on vascular tone and sodium excretion.

12.2 Pharmacodynamics

Aliskiren

PRA reductions in clinical trials ranged from approximately 50% to 80%, were not dose-related and did not correlate with blood pressure reductions. The clinical implications of the differences in effect on PRA are not known.

Amlodipine besylate

Following administration of therapeutic doses to patients with hypertension, amlodipine produces vasodilation resulting in a reduction of supine and standing blood pressures. These decreases in blood pressure are not accompanied by a significant change in heart rate or plasma catecholamine levels with chronic dosing. Although the acute intravenous administration of amlodipine decreases arterial blood pressure and increase heart rate in hemodynamic studies of patients with chronic stable angina, chronic oral administration of amlodipine in clinical trials did not lead to clinically significant changes in heart rate or blood pressures in normotensive patients with angina.

With chronic once daily administration, antihypertensive effectiveness is maintained for at least 24 hours. Plasma concentrations correlate with effect in both young and elderly patients. The magnitude of reduction in blood pressure with amlodipine is also correlated with the height of pretreatment elevation; thus, individuals with moderate hypertension (diastolic pressure 105-114 mmHg) had about 50% greater response than patients with mild hypertension (diastolic pressure 90-104 mmHg). Normotensive subjects experienced no clinically significant change in blood pressure (+1/-2 mmHg).

In hypertensive patients with normal renal function, therapeutic doses of amlodipine resulted in a decrease in renal vascular resistance and an increase in glomerular filtration rate and effective renal plasma flow without change in filtration fraction or proteinuria.

As with other calcium channel blockers, hemodynamic measurements of cardiac function at rest and during exercise (or pacing) in patients with normal ventricular function treated with amlodipine have generally demonstrated a small increase in cardiac index without significant influence on dP/dt or on left ventricular end diastolic pressure or volume. In hemodynamic studies, amlodipine has not been associated with a negative inotropic effect when administered in therapeutic dose range to intact animals and man, even when co-administered with beta-blockers to man. Similar findings, however, have been observed in normal or well-compensated patients with heart failure with agents possessing significant negative inotropic effects.

Amlodipine does not change sinoatrial nodal function or atrioventricular conduction in intact animals or man. In patients with chronic stable angina, intravenous administration of 10 mg did not significantly alter A-H and H-V conduction and sinus node recovery time after pacing. Similar results were obtained in patients receiving amlodipine and concomitant beta-blockers. In clinical studies in which amlodipine was administered in combination with beta-blockers to patients with either hypertension or angina, no adverse effects of electrocardiographic parameters were observed. In clinical trials with angina patients alone, amlodipine therapy did not alter electrocardiographic intervals or produce higher degrees of AV blocks.

Amlodipine has indications other than hypertension which can be found in the Norvasc® package insert.

Tekamlo

In a placebo-controlled study in hypertensive patients, amlodipine was associated with an increase in PRA (59-73% increase) whereas aliskiren monotherapy was associated with a 61-68% reduction in PRA. Aliskiren in combination with amlodipine reduced PRA (55-68% reduction).

12.3 Pharmacokinetics

Absorption and Distribution

Tekamlo

Following oral administration of the aliskiren/amlodipine combination tablets, the median peak plasma concentration times are within 3.0 hours for aliskiren and 8.0 hours for amlodipine. The rate and extent of absorption of aliskiren and amlodipine from Tekamlo are the same as when administered as individual tablets. When taken with food, mean AUC and C_{max} of aliskiren are decreased by 79% and 90%, respectively, while there is no impact of food on the AUC and C_{max} of amlodipine.

Aliskiren

Aliskiren is poorly absorbed (bioavailability about 2.5%) with an accumulation half life of about 24 hours. Steady state blood levels are reached in about 7-8 days. Following oral administration, peak plasma concentrations of aliskiren are reached within 1-3 hours. When taken with a high fat meal, mean AUC and C_{max} of aliskiren are decreased by 71% and 85% respectively. In the clinical trials, aliskiren was administered without a fixed relation to meals.

Amlodipine besylate

Peak plasma concentrations of amlodipine are reached 6-12 hours after an oral administration of amlodipine. Absolute bioavailability has been estimated to be between 64% and 90%. The bioavailability of amlodipine is not altered by the presence of food. Steady state plasma levels of amlodipine are reached after 7 to 8 days of consecutive daily dosing. Approximately 93% of circulating amlodipine is bound to plasma proteins in hypertensive patients.

Metabolism and Elimination

Aliskiren

About one-fourth of the absorbed dose appears in the urine as parent drug. How much of the absorbed dose is metabolized is unknown. Based on the *in vitro* studies, the major enzyme responsible for aliskiren metabolism appears to be CYP 3A4.

Amlodipine besylate

Amlodipine is extensively (about 90%) converted to inactive metabolites via hepatic metabolism with 10% of the parent compound and 60% of the metabolites excreted in the urine. Elimination of amlodipine from the plasma is biphasic with a terminal elimination half-life of about 30-50 hours.

Special Populations

Pediatric Patients

The pharmacokinetics of Tekamlo have not been investigated in patients <18 years of age.

Geriatric Patients

The pharmacokinetics of aliskiren were studied in the elderly (≥65 years). Exposure (measured by AUC) is increased in elderly patients. Adjustment of the starting dose is not required in these patients.

Elderly patients have decreased clearance of amlodipine with a resulting increase in AUC of approximately 40%-60%; therefore, a lower initial dose of amlodipine may be required [see Dosage and Administration (2.9)].

Race

With Tekamlo, pharmacokinetic differences due to race have not been studied. The pharmacokinetic differences among Blacks, Caucasians, and Japanese are minimal with aliskiren therapy.

Renal Impairment

Aliskiren

The pharmacokinetics of aliskiren were evaluated in patients with varying degrees of renal impairment. Rate and extent of exposure (AUC and C_{max}) of aliskiren in subjects with renal impairment did not show a consistent correlation with the severity of renal impairment. Adjustment of the starting dose is not required in these patients [see Dosage and Administration (2.8)].

Amlodipine besylate

The pharmacokinetics of amlodipine is not significantly influenced by renal impairment. Patients with renal failure may therefore receive the usual initial dose [see Dosage and Administration (2.8)].

Hepatic Impairment

Aliskiren

The pharmacokinetics of aliskiren were not significantly affected in patients with mild-to-severe liver disease. Consequently, adjustment of the starting dose is not required in these patients [see Dosage and Administration (2.8)].

Amlodipine besylate

Patients with hepatic insufficiency have decreased clearance of amlodipine with resulting increase in AUC of approximately 40%-60%; therefore, a lower initial dose of amlodipine may be required [see Dosage and Administration (2.8)].

Drug Interactions

Aliskiren exposure is increased slightly (AUC increased 29%) when aliskiren is co-administered with amlodipine, while amlodipine exposure remains unchanged when co-administered with aliskiren. The slight exposure increase of aliskiren in the presence of amlodipine is not clinically relevant.

13   NONCLINICAL TOXICOLOGY

13.1   Carcinogenesis, Mutagenesis, Impairment of Fertility

Studies with Aliskiren hemifumarate and Amlodipine besylate

No carcinogenicity, mutagenicity or fertility studies have been conducted with the combination of aliskiren hemifumarate and amlodipine besylate. However, these studies have been conducted for aliskiren hemifumarate and amlodipine besylate alone.

Studies with Aliskiren hemifumarate

Carcinogenic potential was assessed in a 2-year rat study and a 6-month transgenic (rasH2) mouse study with aliskiren hemifumarate at oral doses of up to 1500 mg aliskiren/kg/day. Although there were no statistically significant increases in tumor incidence associated with exposure to aliskiren, mucosal epithelial hyperplasia (with or without erosion/ulceration) was observed in the lower gastrointestinal tract at doses of 750 or more mg/kg/day in both species, with a colonic adenoma identified in one rat and a cecal adenocarcinoma identified in another, rare tumors in the strain of rat studied. On a systemic exposure (AUC_{0-24hr}) basis, 1500 mg/kg/day in the rat is about 4 times and in the mouse about 1.5 times the maximum recommended human dose (300 mg aliskiren/day). Mucosal hyperplasia in the cecum or colon of rats was also observed at doses of 250 mg/kg/day (the lowest tested dose) as well as at higher doses in 4- and 13-week studies.

Aliskiren hemifumarate was devoid of genotoxic potential in the Ames reverse mutation assay with *S. typhimurium* and *E. coli*, the *in vitro* Chinese hamster ovary cell chromosomal aberration assay, the *in vitro* Chinese hamster V79 cell gene mutation test and the *in vivo* rat bone marrow micronucleus assay.

Fertility of male and female rats was unaffected at doses of up to aliskiren 250 mg/kg/day (8 times the maximum recommended human dose of aliskiren 300 mg/60 kg on a mg/m² basis).

Studies with Amlodipine besylate

Rats and mice treated with amlodipine maleate in the diet for up to two years, at concentrations calculated to provide daily dosage levels of 0.5, 1.25, and 2.5 mg amlodipine/kg/day, showed no evidence of a carcinogenic effect of the drug. For the mouse, the highest dose was, on mg/m² basis, similar to the maximum recommended human dose (MRHD) of 10 mg amlodipine/day. For the rat, the

highest dose was, on a mg/m² basis, about two and a half times the MRHD. (Calculations based on a 60 kg patient.) Mutagenicity studies conducted with amlodipine maleate revealed no drug-related effects at either the gene or chromosome level.

There was no effect on the fertility of rats treated orally with amlodipine maleate (males for 64 days and females for 14 days prior to mating) at doses of up to 10 mg amlodipine/kg/day (about 10 times the MRHD of 10 mg/day on a mg/m² basis).

13.2   Animal Toxicology and/or Pharmacology

Preclinical safety studies have demonstrated that the combination of aliskiren hemifumarate and amlodipine besylate was well tolerated in rats. The findings from the 2- and 13-week oral toxicity studies in rats were consistent with those of aliskiren hemifumarate and amlodipine besylate when both drugs were administered alone. There were no new toxicities or increased severity of the toxicities which were associated with either component.

Animal reproductive and developmental toxicology findings are described elsewhere [see Use in Specific Populations (8.1)].

14   CLINICAL STUDIES

Tekamlo

Tekamlo was studied in a total of 5549 patients with mild to moderate hypertension (diastolic blood pressure between 90 mmHg and 109 mmHg).

Aliskiren 150 mg and 300 mg and amlodipine besylate 5 mg and 10 mg were studied alone and in combination in an 8-week, randomized, double-blind, placebo-controlled, multifactorial study comparing the combinations 150 mg/5 mg, 150 mg/10 mg, 300 mg/5 mg and 300 mg/10 mg of aliskiren and amlodipine with their components and placebo. The combination of aliskiren and amlodipine resulted in placebo-adjusted decreases in systolic/diastolic blood pressure at trough of 14-17/9-11 mmHg compared to 4-9/3-5 mmHg for aliskiren alone and 9-14/6-8 mmHg for amlodipine alone.

Treatment with Tekamlo resulted overall in significantly greater reductions in diastolic and systolic blood pressure compared to the respective monotherapy components.

The antihypertensive effect of Tekamlo was similar in patients with and without diabetes, obese and non-obese patients, in patients ≥65 years of age and <65 years of age, and in women and men.

A subgroup of 819 patients was studied with ambulatory blood pressure monitoring. The blood pressure lowering effect in the aliskiren/amlodipine group was maintained throughout the 24-hour period (see Figure 5 and Figure 6).

Figure 5: Mean Ambulatory Diastolic Blood Pressure at Endpoint by Treatment and Hour

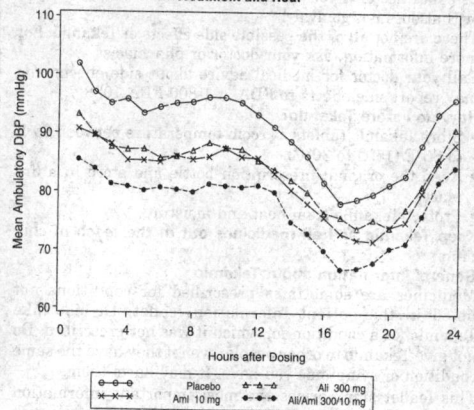

[See figure 6 at top of next column]

Two additional double-blind, active-controlled studies of similar design were conducted in which Tekamlo was administered as initial therapy in patients with moderate to severe hypertension (SBP 160-200 mmHg). Patients were randomized to receive either combination aliskiren/amlodipine or amlodipine monotherapy. The initial dose of aliskiren/amlodipine was 150 mg/5 mg for 1 week with forced titration to 300 mg/10 mg for 7 weeks. The initial dose of amlodipine was 5 mg for 1 week with forced titration to 10 mg for 7 weeks. In one study of 443 Black patients, at the primary endpoint of 8 weeks, the treatment difference between aliskiren/amlodipine and amlodipine was 5.2/3.8 mmHg. In the other study of 484 patients, at the primary endpoint of 8 weeks, the treatment difference between aliskiren/amlodipine and amlodipine was 7.1/3.8 mmHg. The blood pressure lowering effects of Tekamlo are largely attained within 1-2 weeks.

Figure 6: Mean Ambulatory Systolic Blood Pressure at Endpoint by Treatment and Hour

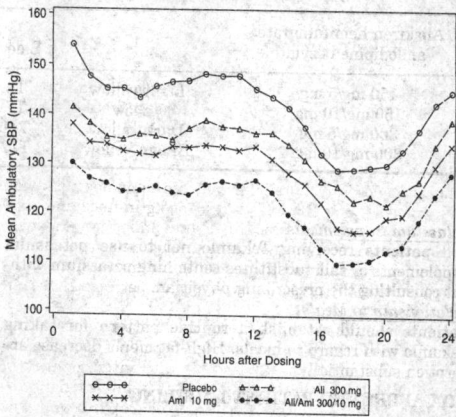

16   HOW SUPPLIED/STORAGE AND HANDLING

Tekamlo (aliskiren and amlodipine) is supplied as follows:

150 mg aliskiren/5 mg amlodipine Tablets—Non-scored light yellow, ovaloid convex-shaped, film-coated tablet with a beveled edge with debossing "T2" on one side and "NVR" on the reverse side of the tablet. The tablet dimensions are approximately 16 × 6.3 mm.

150 mg aliskiren/10 mg amlodipine Tablets—Non-scored yellow, ovaloid convex-shaped, film-coated tablet with a beveled edge with debossing "T7" on one side and "NVR" on the reverse side of the tablet. The tablet dimensions are approximately 16 × 6.3 mm.

300 mg aliskiren/5 mg amlodipine Tablets—Non-scored dark yellow, ovaloid convex-shaped, film-coated tablet with a beveled edge with debossing "T11" on one side and "NVR" on the reverse side of the tablet. The tablet dimensions are approximately 21 × 8.3 mm.

300 mg aliskiren/10 mg amlodipine Tablets—Non-scored brown yellow, ovaloid convex-shaped, film-coated tablet with a beveled edge with debossing "T12" on one side and "NVR" on the reverse side of the tablet. The tablet dimensions are approximately 21 × 8.3 mm.

All strengths are packaged in bottles and unit-dose blister packages (10 strips of 10 tablets) as described below.

[See table 1 at top of next page]

Storage

Store at 25°C (77°F); excursions permitted to 15-30°C (59-86°F) in original container.

Protect from heat and moisture.

Dispense in tight container (USP).

17   PATIENT COUNSELING INFORMATION

See FDA-Approved Patient Labeling

Healthcare professionals should instruct their patients to read the Patient Package Insert before starting Tekamlo and to reread each time the prescription is renewed. Patients should be instructed to inform their doctor or pharmacist if they develop any unusual symptom, or if any known symptom persists or worsens.

Pregnancy

Inform pregnant patients that use of drugs that act on the renin-angiotensin-aldosterone system during pregnancy is associated with fetal and neonatal injury, including hypotension, neonatal skull hypoplasia, anuria, reversible or irreversible renal failure, and death. Decreased fetal renal function may result in oligohydramnios and associated with fetal limb contractures, craniofacial deformation, and hypoplastic lung development.

Female Patients of Childbearing Potential

Female patients of childbearing potential should be told about the consequences of pregnancy exposure to drugs that act on the renin-angiotensin-aldosterone system. Discuss other treatment options with female patients planning to become pregnant. These patients should be asked to report pregnancies to their physicians as soon as possible.

Symptomatic Hypotension

Caution patients receiving Tekamlo that lightheadedness can occur, especially during the first days of therapy, and that it should be reported to the prescribing physician. Tell patients that if syncope occurs, discontinue Tekamlo until the physician has been consulted.

Caution all patients that inadequate fluid intake, excessive perspiration, diarrhea, or vomiting can lead to an excessive fall in blood pressure, with the same consequences of lightheadedness and possible syncope.

Angioedema

Patients should be advised and told to report immediately any signs or symptoms suggesting angioedema (swelling of face, extremities, eyes, lips, tongue, difficulty in swallowing or breathing) and to take no more drug until they have consulted with the prescribing physician.

Table 1: Tekamlo Tablets Supply

Tablet	Color	Debossed Side 1	Debossed Side 2	NDC 0078-XXXX-XX Bottle of 30	Bottle of 90	Blister Packages of 100
Aliskiren hemifumarate/ amlodipine besylate						
150 mg/5 mg	Light yellow	T2	NVR	0603-15	0603-34	0603-35
150 mg/10 mg	Yellow	T7	NVR	0604-15	0604-34	0604-35
300 mg/5 mg	Dark yellow	T11	NVR	0605-15	0605-34	0605-35
300 mg/10 mg	Brown yellow	T12	NVR	0606-15	0606-34	0606-35

Potassium Supplements

Tell patients receiving Tekamlo not to use potassium supplements or salt substitutes containing potassium without consulting the prescribing physician.

Relationship to Meals

Patients should establish a routine pattern for taking Tekamlo with regard to meals. High-fat meals decrease absorption substantially.

FDA-APPROVED PATIENT LABELING

Patient Information

Tekamlo™ (tĕk'-ăm-lō)

Tekamlo

(aliskiren and amlodipine)

Tablets

Read the Patient Information that comes with Tekamlo before you start taking it and each time you get a refill. There may be new information. This information does not take the place of talking with your doctor about your condition and treatment. If you have any questions about Tekamlo, ask your doctor or pharmacist.

What is the most important information I should know about Tekamlo?

If you become pregnant while taking Tekamlo, stop taking Tekamlo and call your doctor right away. Tekamlo may harm an unborn baby, causing injury or death. Talk to your doctor about other medicines to treat your high blood pressure if you plan to become pregnant.

What is Tekamlo?

Tekamlo is a prescription medicine that may be used:

- as the first medicine to lower your high blood pressure if your doctor decides that you are likely to need more than one medicine.
- to treat your high blood pressure when one medicine to lower your high blood pressure has not worked well enough.
- if you are already taking the medicines aliskiren and amlodipine to treat your high blood pressure.

Tekamlo contains:

- aliskiren, a direct renin inhibitor (DRI)
- amlodipine, a calcium channel blocker (CCB)

Your doctor may prescribe other medicines for you to take along with Tekamlo to treat your high blood pressure.

It is not known if Tekamlo is safe and works in children under 18 years of age.

What should I tell my doctor before taking Tekamlo?

Before taking Tekamlo, tell your doctor if you:

- have kidney problems
- have liver problems
- have ever had an allergic reaction to another blood pressure medicine. Symptoms may include: swelling of the face, lips, tongue, throat, arms and legs, and trouble breathing.
- have any other medical problems
- are pregnant or planning to become pregnant. **See "What is the most important information I should know about Tekamlo?"**
- are breastfeeding. It is not known if Tekamlo passes into your breast milk and if it can harm your baby. You and your doctor should decide if you will take Tekamlo or breastfeed. You should not do both.

Tell your doctor about all the medicines you take including prescription and nonprescription medicines, vitamins and herbal supplements. Tekamlo and certain other medicines may affect each other and cause side effects.

Especially tell your doctor if you take:

- other medicines for high blood pressure or a heart problem
- water pills (also called "diuretics")
- medicines for treating fungus or fungal infections
- cyclosporine (Gengraf®, Neoral, Sandimmune), a medicine used to suppress the immune system
- potassium-containing medicines, potassium supplements, or salt substitutes containing potassium
- atorvastatin (Lipitor®)

Know your medicines. Keep a list of all your medicines. Show this list to your doctor or pharmacist when you get a new medicine. Your doctor or pharmacist will know what medicines are safe to take together.

How should I take Tekamlo?

- Take Tekamlo exactly as prescribed by your doctor. It is important to take Tekamlo every day to control your blood pressure.
- Take Tekamlo one time a day, about the same time each day.
- Take Tekamlo the same way every day, either with or without a meal.
- Your doctor may change your dose of Tekamlo if needed. Do not change the amount of Tekamlo you take without talking to your doctor.
- If you miss a dose of Tekamlo, take it as soon as you remember. If it is close to your next dose, do not take the missed dose. Just take the next dose at your regular time.
- If you take too much Tekamlo, call your doctor or a Poison Control Center, or go to the nearest hospital emergency room.

What are the possible side effects of Tekamlo?

Tekamlo may cause serious side effects:

- **Harm to an unborn baby, causing injury or death. See "What is the most important information I should know about Tekamlo?"**
- Aliskiren, one of the medicines in Tekamlo, can cause swelling of your face, lips, tongue, throat, arms and legs, or the whole body. Get medical help right away and tell your doctor if you get any one or more of these symptoms. Serious allergic reactions can happen at any time while you are taking Tekamlo.
- **Low blood pressure (hypotension).** Your blood pressure may get too low if you also take water pills, are on a low-salt diet, get dialysis treatments, have heart problems, or get sick with vomiting or diarrhea. Lie down if you feel faint or get dizzy. Call your doctor right away.
- **Possible increased chest pain or risk of heart attack.** It is rare, but when you first start taking Tekamlo or increase your dose, you may have a heart attack or your angina may get worse. If that happens, call your doctor right away or go directly to a hospital emergency room.

The most common side effects of Tekamlo include:

- Swelling of your lower legs

Tell your doctor if you have any side effect that bothers you or that does not go away.

These are not all of the possible side effects of Tekamlo. For more information, ask your doctor or pharmacist.

Call your doctor for medical advice about side effects. You may report side effects to FDA at 1-800-FDA-1088.

How do I store Tekamlo?

- Store Tekamlo tablets at room temperature between 59°F to 86°F (15°C to 30°C).
- Keep the original prescription bottle and store in a dry place.
- Protect Tekamlo from heat and moisture.

Keep Tekamlo and all medicines out of the reach of children.

General information about Tekamlo

Medicines are sometimes prescribed for conditions not listed in the patient information leaflet. Do not take Tekamlo for a condition for which it was not prescribed. Do not give Tekamlo to other people, even if they have the same condition or symptoms you have. It may harm them.

This leaflet summarizes the most important information about Tekamlo. If you have questions about Tekamlo talk with your doctor. You can ask your doctor or pharmacist for information that is written for healthcare professionals.

For more information about Tekamlo, visit www.Tekamlo.com, or call 1-888-NOW-NOVA (1-888-669-6682).

What are the ingredients in Tekamlo?

Active Ingredients: Aliskiren hemifumarate and amlodipine

Inactive ingredients: Colloidal silicon dioxide, crospovidone, hypromellose, iron oxide red, iron oxide yellow, magnesium stearate, microcrystalline cellulose, polyethylene glycol, povidone, talc, and titanium dioxide.

What is high blood pressure (hypertension)?

Blood pressure is the force of blood in your blood vessels when your heart beats and when your heart rests. You have high blood pressure when the force is too much.

High blood pressure makes the heart work harder to pump blood through the body and causes damage to blood vessels. Tekamlo can help your blood vessels relax so your blood pressure is lower. Medicines that lower your blood pressure may lower your chance of having a stroke or heart attack.

T2010-69

Distributed by:
Novartis Pharmaceuticals Corporation
East Hanover, New Jersey 07936
©Novartis

TEKTURNA® ℞

[tek-turn-a]

(aliskiren)

Tablets, Oral

The following prescribing information is based on official labeling in effect September 2010.

HIGHLIGHTS OF PRESCRIBING INFORMATION

These highlights do not include all the information needed to use Tekturna® safely and effectively. See full prescribing information for Tekturna®.

TEKTURNA® (aliskiren) Tablets, Oral

Initial U.S. Approval: 2007

WARNING: AVOID USE IN PREGNANCY

See full prescribing information for complete boxed warning

When pregnancy is detected, discontinue Tekturna as soon as possible. Drugs that act directly on the renin-angiotensin system can cause injury and death to the developing fetus. (5.1)

——INDICATIONS AND USAGE——

Tekturna is a direct renin inhibitor (DRI) indicated for:

- The treatment of hypertension (1.1)

——DOSAGE AND ADMINISTRATION——

General Considerations

- Majority of effect of given dose substantially attained in 2 weeks (2.1)
- May be administered with other anti-hypertensive agents (2.2)
- Additive effects with ACEI at maximal doses have not been studied (2.2)

Hypertension

- Starting dose: 150 mg once daily with a routine pattern with regard to meals.* If blood pressure remains uncontrolled titrate up to 300 mg daily (2.1, 2.3)
- *No initial dosage adjustment required in the elderly, in patients with mild to severe renal or hepatic impairment. (2.4, 12.3)

——DOSAGE FORMS AND STRENGTHS——

Tablets: 150 mg, 300 mg (3)

——WARNINGS AND PRECAUTIONS——

- Avoid neonatal/fetal exposure (5.1)
- Head and neck angioedema. Discontinue use of Tekturna and monitor until signs and symptoms resolve (5.2)
- Hypotension in volume- and/or salt-depleted patients: Correct imbalances before initiating therapy with Tekturna (5.3)
- Patients with severe renal dysfunction: Consider periodic determinations of serum electrolytes to detect possible electrolyte imbalances (5.4)
- Hyperkalemia: Caution should be exercised when co-administered with ACEI, potassium-sparing diuretics, potassium supplements or other potassium containing salt substitutes (5.5)

——ADVERSE REACTIONS——

Most common adverse reaction: diarrhea (incidence 2.3%) (6.1)

To report SUSPECTED ADVERSE REACTIONS, contact Novartis Pharmaceuticals Corporation at 1-888-669-6682 or FDA at 1-800-FDA-1088 or www.fda.gov/medwatch.

——DRUG INTERACTIONS——

- Concomitant use with cyclosporine or itraconazole is not recommended (7.1)

——USE IN SPECIFIC POPULATIONS——

Nursing Mothers: Adverse reactions may occur in nursing infants (8.3)

See 17 for PATIENT COUNSELING INFORMATION and FDA-approved patient labeling

Revised: 08/2010

FULL PRESCRIBING INFORMATION: CONTENTS*

WARNING: AVOID USE IN PREGNANCY

1 INDICATIONS AND USAGE
    1.1 Hypertension

2 DOSAGE AND ADMINISTRATION
    2.1 Hypertension
    2.2 Use with Other Antihypertensives
    2.3 Relationship to Meals
    2.4 Dosing in Special Populations

3 DOSAGE FORMS AND STRENGTHS

4 CONTRAINDICATIONS

5 WARNINGS AND PRECAUTIONS
    5.1 Fetal/Neonatal Morbidity and Mortality
    5.2 Head and Neck Angioedema
    5.3 Hypotension
    5.4 Impaired Renal Function

*Sections or subsections omitted from the full prescribing information are not listed

FULL PRESCRIBING INFORMATION

WARNING: AVOID USE IN PREGNANCY
When pregnancy is detected, discontinue Tekturna as soon as possible. Drugs that act directly on the renin-angiotensin system can cause injury and death to the developing fetus. ***[See Warnings and Precautions (5.1)]***

1 INDICATIONS AND USAGE

1.1 Hypertension

Tekturna is indicated for the treatment of hypertension. It may be used alone or in combination with other antihypertensive agents. Use with maximal doses of ACE inhibitors has not been adequately studied.

2 DOSAGE AND ADMINISTRATION

2.1 Hypertension

The usual recommended starting dose of Tekturna is 150 mg once daily. In patients whose blood pressure is not adequately controlled, the daily dose may be increased to 300 mg. Doses above 300 mg did not give an increased blood pressure response but resulted in an increased rate of diarrhea. The antihypertensive effect of a given dose is substantially attained (85-90%) by 2 weeks.

2.2 Use with Other Antihypertensives

Tekturna may be administered with other antihypertensive agents. Most exposure to date is with diuretics and an angiotensin receptor blocker (valsartan) and the drugs together have a greater effect at their maximum recommended doses than either drug alone. It is not known whether additive effects are present when Tekturna is used with angiotensin-converting enzyme inhibitors (ACEI) or beta blockers (BB).

2.3 Relationship to Meals

Patients should establish a routine pattern for taking Tekturna with regard to meals. High fat meals decrease absorption substantially. *[See Clinical Pharmacology (12.3)]*

2.4 Dosing in Special Populations

No adjustment of the starting dose is required in elderly patients, patients with mild-to-severe renal impairment or mild-to-severe hepatic insufficiency. However, care should be taken when dosing Tekturna in patients with severe renal impairment, as clinical experience with such patients is limited. *[See Clinical Pharmacology (12.3) and Warnings and Precautions (5.4)]*

3 DOSAGE FORMS AND STRENGTHS

150 mg light pink biconvex round tablet, imprinted NVR/IL (Side 1/Side 2)

300 mg light red biconvex ovaloid round tablet, imprinted NVR/IU (Side 1/Side 2)

4 CONTRAINDICATIONS

None.

5 WARNINGS AND PRECAUTIONS

5.1 Fetal/Neonatal Morbidity and Mortality

Drugs that act directly on the renin-angiotensin system can cause fetal and neonatal morbidity and death when administered to pregnant women. If this drug is used during pregnancy, or if the patient becomes pregnant while taking this drug, the patient should be apprised of the potential hazard to the fetus. *[See Use in Specific Populations (8.1)]* In several dozen published cases, ACE inhibitor use during the second and third trimesters of pregnancy was associated with fetal and neonatal injury, including hypotension, neonatal skull hypoplasia, anuria, reversible or irreversible renal failure, and death. In addition, first trimester use of ACE inhibitors has been associated with birth defects in retrospective data.

5.2 Head and Neck Angioedema

Angioedema of the face, extremities, lips, tongue, glottis and/or larynx has been reported in patients treated with Tekturna and has necessitated hospitalization and intubation. This may occur at any time during treatment and has occurred in patients with and without a history of angioedema with ACE inhibitors or angiotensin receptor antagonists. If angioedema involves the throat, tongue, glottis or larynx, or if the patient has a history of upper respiratory surgery, airway obstruction may occur and be fatal. Patients who experience these effects, even without respiratory distress, require prolonged observation since treatment with antihistamines and corticosteroids may not be sufficient to prevent respiratory involvement. Prompt administration of subcutaneous epinephrine solution 1:1000 (0.3 to 0.5 mL) and measures to ensure a patient airway may be necessary. Discontinue Tekturna immediately in patients who develop angioedema, and do not readminister.

5.3 Hypotension

An excessive fall in blood pressure was rarely seen (0.1%) in patients with uncomplicated hypertension treated with Tekturna alone in controlled trials and in <1% during combination therapy with other antihypertensive agents. In patients with an activated renin-angiotensin system, such as volume- and/or salt-depleted patients (e.g., those receiving high doses of diuretics), symptomatic hypotension may occur after initiation of treatment with Tekturna. This condition should be corrected prior to administration of Tekturna, or the treatment should start under close medical supervision.

If an excessive fall in blood pressure occurs, the patient should be placed in the supine position and, if necessary, given an intravenous infusion of normal saline. A transient hypotensive response is not a contraindication to further treatment, which usually can be continued without difficulty once the blood pressure has stabilized.

5.4 Impaired Renal Function

Patients with greater than moderate renal dysfunction (creatinine 1.7 mg/dL for women and 2.0 mg/dL for men and/or estimated GFR <30 mL/min), a history of dialysis, nephrotic syndrome, or renovascular hypertension were excluded from clinical trials of Tekturna in hypertension. Consider periodic determinations of serum electrolytes to detect possible electrolyte imbalances particularly in patients with severe renal impairment.

5.5 Hyperkalemia

Increases in serum potassium >5.5 mEq/L were infrequent with Tekturna alone (0.9% compared to 0.6% with placebo). However, when used in combination with an ACE inhibitor in a diabetic population, increases in serum potassium were more frequent (5.5%). Routine monitoring of electrolytes and renal function is indicated in this population. Concomitant use of Tekturna with potassium-sparing diuretics, potassium supplements, salt substitutes containing potassium, or other drugs that increase potassium levels may lead to increases in serum potassium. If concomitant use is considered necessary, caution should be exercised.

5.6 Renal Artery Stenosis

No data are available on the use of Tekturna in patients with unilateral or bilateral renal artery stenosis or stenosis of the artery to a solitary kidney.

5.7 Cyclosporine or Itraconazole

When aliskiren was given with cyclosporine or itraconazole, the blood concentra- tions of aliskiren were significantly increased. Concomitant use of aliskiren with cyclosporine or itraconazole is not recommended. *[See Drug Interactions (7)]*

6 ADVERSE REACTIONS

6.1 Clinical Trials Experience

Because clinical trials are conducted under widely varying conditions, adverse reaction rates observed in the clinical trials of a drug cannot be directly compared to rates in clinical trials of another drug and may not reflect the rates observed in practice.

Data described below reflect the evaluation of the safety of Tekturna in more than 6,460 patients, including over 1,740 treated for longer than 6 months, and more than 1,250 patients for longer than 1 year. In placebo controlled clinical trials, discontinuation of therapy due to a clinical adverse event, including uncontrolled hypertension occurred in 2.2% of patients treated with Tekturna vs. 3.5% of patients given placebo.

Angioedema: Two cases of angioedema with respiratory symptoms were reported with Tekturna use in the clinical studies. Two other cases of periorbital edema without respiratory symptoms were reported as possible angioedema and resulted in discontinuation. The rate of these angioedema cases in the completed studies was 0.06%. In addition, 26 other cases of edema involving the face, hands, or whole body were reported with Tekturna use including 4 leading to discontinuation. In the placebo controlled studies, however, the incidence of edema involved the face, hands or whole body was 0.4% with Tekturna compared with 0.5% with placebo. In a long term active control study with Tekturna and HCTZ arms, the incidence of edema involving the face, hand or whole body was 0.4% in both treatment arms. *[See Warnings and Precautions (5.2)]*

Gastrointestinal: Tekturna produces dose-related gastrointestinal (GI) adverse effects. Diarrhea was reported by 2.3% of patients at 300 mg, compared to 1.2% in placebo patients. In women and the elderly (age ≥65) increases in diarrhea rates were evident starting at a dose of 150 mg daily, with rates for these subgroups at 150 mg comparable to those seen at 300 mg for men or younger patients (all rates about 2.0-2.3%). Other GI symptoms included abdominal pain, dyspepsia, and gastroesophageal reflux, although increased rates for abdominal pain and dyspepsia were distinguished from placebo only at 600 mg daily. Diarrhea and other GI symptoms were typically mild and rarely led to discontinuation.

Cough: Tekturna was associated with a slight increase in cough in the placebo-controlled studies (1.1% for any Tekturna use vs. 0.6% for placebo). In active-controlled trials with ACE inhibitor (ramipril, lisinopril) arms the rates of cough for the Tekturna arms were about one-third to one-half the rates in the ACE inhibitor arms.

Seizures: Single episodes of tonic-clonic seizures with loss of consciousness were reported in two patients treated with Tekturna in the clinical trials. One of these patients did have predisposing causes for seizures and had a negative electroencephalogram (EEG) and cerebral imaging following the seizures (for the other patient EEG and imaging results were not reported). Tekturna was discontinued and there was no re-challenge.

The following adverse events occurred in placebo-controlled clinical trials at an incidence of more than 1% of patients treated with Tekturna, but also occurred at about the same or greater incidence in patients receiving placebo: headache, nasopharyngitis, dizziness, fatigue, upper respiratory tract infection, back pain and cough.

Other adverse effects with increased rates for Tekturna compared to placebo included rash (1% vs. 0.3%), elevated uric acid (0.4% vs. 0.1%), gout (0.2% vs. 0.1%) and renal stones (0.2% vs. 0%).

Aliskiren's effect on ECG intervals was studied in a randomized, double-blind, placebo and active-controlled (moxifloxacin), 7-day repeat dosing study with Holter-monitoring and 12 lead ECGs throughout the interdosing interval. No effect of aliskiren on QT interval was seen.

6.2 Clinical Laboratory Findings

In controlled clinical trials, clinically relevant changes in standard laboratory parameters were rarely associated with the administration of Tekturna. In multiple-dose studies in hypertensive patients, Tekturna had no clinically important effects on total cholesterol, HDL, fasting triglycerides, fasting glucose, or uric acid.

Blood Urea Nitrogen, Creatinine: Minor increases in blood urea nitrogen (BUN) or serum creatinine were observed in less than 7% of patients with essential hypertension treated with Tekturna alone vs. 6% on placebo.

Hemoglobin and Hematocrit: Small decreases in hemoglobin and hematocrit (mean decreases of approximately 0.08 g/dL and 0.16 volume percent, respectively, for all aliskiren monotherapy) were observed. The decreases were dose-related and were 0.24 g/dL and 0.79 volume percent for 600 mg daily. This effect is also seen with other agents acting on the renin-angiotensin system, such as angiotensin inhibitors and angiotensin receptor blockers and may be mediated by reduction of angiotensin II which stimulates erythropoetin production via the AT1 receptor. These decreases led to slight increases in rates of anemia with aliskiren compared to placebo were observed (0.1% for any aliskiren use, 0.3% for aliskiren 600 mg daily, vs 0% for placebo). No patients discontinued therapy due to anemia.

Serum Potassium: Increases in serum potassium >5.5 mEq/L were infrequent in patients with essential hypertension treated with Tekturna alone (0.9% compared to 0.6% with placebo). However, when used in combination with an angiotensin-converting enzyme inhibitor (ACEI) in a diabetic population increases in serum potassium were more frequent (5.5%) and routine monitoring of electrolytes and renal function is indicated in this population.

Serum Uric Acid: Aliskiren monotherapy produced small median increases in serum uric acid levels (about 6 μmol/L) while HCTZ produced larger increases (about 30 μmol/L). The combination of aliskiren with HCTZ appears to be additive (about 40 μmol/L increase). The increases in uric acid appear to lead to slight increases in uric acid-related AEs:

elevated uric acid (0.4% vs. 0.1%), gout (0.2% vs. 0.1%), and renal stones (0.2% vs. 0%).

Creatine Kinase: Increases in creatine kinase of >300% were recorded in about 1% of aliskiren monotherapy patients vs. 0.5% of placebo patients. Five cases of creatine kinase rises, three leading to discontinuation and one diagnosed as subclinical rhabdomyolysis, and another as myositis, were reported as adverse events with aliskiren use in the clinical trials. No cases were associated with renal dysfunction.

6.3 Post-marketing Experience

The following adverse reactions have been reported in aliskiren post-marketing experience. Because these reactions are reported voluntarily from a population of uncertain size, it is not always possible to estimate their frequency or establish a causal relationship to drug exposure.

Hypersensitivity: angioedema requiring airway management and hospitalization

Peripheral edema

Blood creatinine increased

7 DRUG INTERACTIONS

7.1 Effects of Other Drugs on Aliskiren

Based on *in vitro* studies, aliskiren is metabolized by CYP 3A4.

Irbesartan: Coadministration of irbesartan reduced aliskiren C_{max} up to 50% after multiple dosing.

P-glycoprotein Effects: Pgp (MDR1/Mdr1a/1b) was found to be the major efflux system involved in absorption and disposition of aliskiren in preclinical studies. The potential for drug interactions at the Pgp site will likely depend on the degree of inhibition of this transporter.

Atorvastatin: Coadministration of atorvastatin resulted in about a 50% increase in aliskiren C_{max} and AUC after multiple dosing.

Ketoconazole: Coadministration of 200 mg twice-daily ketoconazole with aliskiren resulted in an approximate 80% increase in plasma levels of aliskiren. A 400-mg once-daily dose was not studied but would be expected to increase aliskiren blood levels further.

Itraconazole: Coadministration of 100 mg itraconazole with 150 mg aliskiren resulted in approximately 5.8-fold increase in C_{max} and 6.5-fold increase in AUC of aliskiren. Concomitant use of aliskiren with itraconazole is not recommended.

Cyclosporine: Coadministration of 200 mg and 600 mg cyclosporine with 75 mg aliskiren resulted in an approximately 2.5-fold increase in C_{max} and 5-fold increase in AUC of aliskiren. Concomitant use of aliskiren with cyclosporine is not recommended.

Verapamil: Coadministration of 240 mg of verapamil with 300 mg aliskiren resulted in an approximately 2-fold increase in C_{max} and AUC of aliskiren. However, no dosage adjustment is necessary.

Drugs with no clinically significant effects: Coadministration of lovastatin, atenolol, warfarin, furosemide, digoxin, celecoxib, hydrochlorothiazide, ramipril, valsartan, metformin and amlodipine did not result in clinically significant increases in aliskiren exposure.

7.2 Effects of Aliskiren on Other Drugs

Aliskiren does not inhibit the CYP450 isoenzymes (CYP1A2, 2C8, 2C9, 2C19, 2D6, 2E1, and 3A) or induce CYP 3A4.

Furosemide: When aliskiren was coadministered with furosemide, the AUC and C_{max} of furosemide were reduced by about 30% and 50%, respectively. Patients receiving furosemide could find its effect diminished after starting aliskiren.

Drugs with no clinically significant effects: Coadministration of aliskiren did not significantly affect the pharmacokinetics of lovastatin, digoxin, valsartan, amlodipine, metformin, celecoxib, atenolol, atorvastatin, ramipril or hydrochlorothiazide.

Warfarin: The effects of aliskiren on warfarin pharmacokinetics have not been evaluated.

8 USE IN SPECIFIC POPULATIONS

8.1 Pregnancy

Pregnancy Categories C (first trimester) and D (second and third trimesters) *[See Warnings and Precautions (5.1)]*

There is no clinical experience with the use of Tekturna in pregnant women.

Drugs that act directly on the renin-angiotensin system can cause fetal and neonatal morbidity and death when administered to pregnant women. Several dozen cases have been reported in the world literature in patients who were taking angiotensin-converting enzyme inhibitors. When pregnancy is detected, Tekturna should be discontinued as soon as possible. The use of drugs that act directly on the renin-angiotensin system during the second and third trimesters of pregnancy has been associated with fetal and neonatal injury, including hypotension, neonatal skull hypoplasia, anuria, reversible or irreversible renal failure, and death. Oligohydramnios has also been reported, presumably resulting from decreased fetal renal function; oligohydramnios in this setting has been associated with fetal contractures, craniofacial deformation, and hypoplastic lung development. Prematurity, intrauterine growth retardation, and patent ductus arteriosus have also been reported, although it is not clear whether these occurrences were due to exposure to the drug.

In addition, first trimester use of ACE inhibitors, a specific class of drugs acting on the renin-angiotensin system, has been associated with a potential risk of birth defects in retrospective data. Healthcare professionals that prescribe drugs acting directly on the renin-angiotensin system should counsel women of childbearing potential about the potential risks of these agents during pregnancy. Rarely (probably less often than once in every thousand pregnancies), no alternative to a drug acting on the renin-angiotensin system will be found. In these rare cases, the mothers should be apprised of the potential hazards to their fetuses and serial ultrasound examination should be performed to assess the intra-amniotic environment. If oligohydramnios is observed, Tekturna should be discontinued unless it is considered life-saving for the mother. Contraction stress testing (CST), a nonstress test (NST) or biophysical profiling (BPP) may be appropriate, depending upon the week of pregnancy. Patients and physicians should be aware, however, that oligohydramnios may not appear until after the fetus has sustained irreversible injury.

Infants with histories of *in-utero* exposure to a renin inhibitor should be closely observed for hypotension, oliguria, and hyperkalemia. If oliguria occurs, attention should be directed toward support of blood pressure and renal perfusion. Exchange transfusion or dialysis may be required as means of reversing hypotension and/or substituting for disordered renal function. *[See Nonclinical Toxicology (13)]*

8.3 Nursing Mothers

It is not known whether aliskiren is excreted in human breast milk. Aliskiren was secreted in the milk of lactating rats. Because of the potential for adverse effects on the nursing infant, a decision should be made whether to discontinue nursing or discontinue the drug, taking into account the importance of the drug to the mother.

8.4 Pediatric Use

Safety and effectiveness of aliskiren in pediatric patients <18 years have not been established.

8.5 Geriatric Use

Of the total number of patients receiving aliskiren in clinical studies, 1,275 (19%) were 65 years or older and 231 (3.4%) were 75 years or older. Blood pressure response and adverse effects were generally similar to those in younger patients.

10 OVERDOSAGE

Limited data area available related to overdosage in humans. The most likely manifestation of overdosage would be hypotension. If symptomatic hypotension occurs, supportive treatment should be initiated.

11 DESCRIPTION

Aliskiren hemifumarate is chemically described as (2S,4S,5S,7S)-N-(2-Carbamoyl-2-methylpropyl)-5-amino-4-hydroxy-2,7-diisopropyl-8-[4-methoxy-3-(3-methoxypropoxy)phenyl]-octanamide hemifumarate and its structural formula is

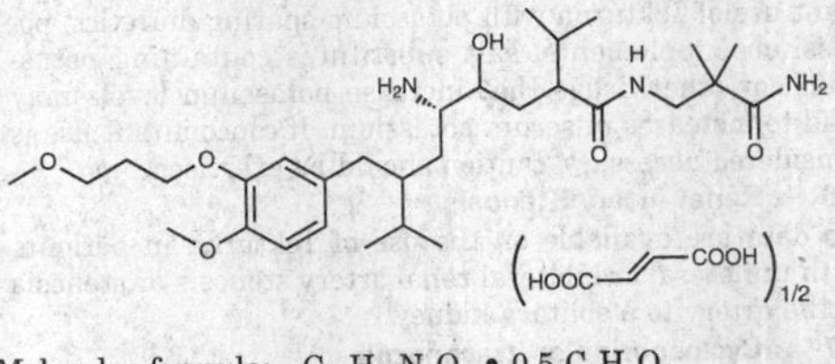

Molecular formula: $C_{30}H_{53}N_3O_6 \cdot 0.5\ C_4H_4O_4$

Aliskiren hemifumarate is a white to slightly yellowish crystalline powder with a molecular weight of 609.8 (free base- 551.8). It is soluble in phosphate buffer, n-Octanol, and highly soluble in water.

12 CLINICAL PHARMACOLOGY

12.1 Mechanism of Action

Renin is secreted by the kidney in response to decreases in blood volume and renal perfusion. Renin cleaves angiotensinogen to form the inactive decapeptide angiotensin I (Ang I). Ang I is converted to the active octapeptide angiotensin II (Ang II) by angiotensin-converting enzyme (ACE) and non-ACE pathways. Ang II is a powerful vasoconstrictor and leads to the release of catecholamines from the adrenal medulla and prejunctional nerve endings. It also promotes aldosterone secretion and sodium reabsorption. Together, these effects increase blood pressure. Ang II also inhibits renin release, thus providing a negative feedback to the system. This cycle, from renin through angiotensin to aldosterone and its associated negative feedback loop, is known as the renin-angiotensin-aldosterone system (RAAS). Aliskiren is a direct renin inhibitor, decreasing plasma renin activity (PRA) and inhibiting the conversion of angiotensinogen to Ang I. Whether aliskiren affects other RAAS components, e.g., ACE or non-ACE pathways, is not known.

All agents that inhibit the RAAS, including renin inhibitors, suppress the negative feedback loop, leading to a compensatory rise in plasma renin concentration. When this rise occurs during treatment with ACE inhibitors and ARBs, the result is increased levels of PRA. During treatment with aliskiren, however, the effect of increased renin levels is blocked so that PRA, Ang I and Ang II are all reduced, whether aliskiren is used as monotherapy or in combination with other antihypertensive agents.

12.2 Pharmacodynamics

In placebo controlled clinical trials, plasma renin activity (PRA) was decreased in a range of 50-80%. This reduction in PRA was not dose-related and did not correlate with blood pressure reductions. The clinical implications of the differences in effect on PRA are not known.

12.3 Pharmacokinetics

Aliskiren is poorly absorbed (bioavailability about 2.5%) with an approximate accumulation half life of 24 hours. Steady state blood levels are reached in about 7-8 days.

Absorption and Distribution

Following oral administration, peak plasma concentrations of aliskiren are reached within 1-3 hours. When taken with a high fat meal, mean AUC and C_{max} of aliskiren are decreased by 71% and 85% respectively. In the clinical trials of aliskiren, it was administered without requiring a fixed relation of administration to meals.

Metabolism and Elimination

About one fourth of the absorbed dose appears in the urine as parent drug. How much of the absorbed dose is metabolized is unknown. Based on the *in vitro* studies, the major enzyme responsible for aliskiren metabolism appears to be CYP3A4.

Renally Impaired Patients: Aliskiren was evaluated in patients with varying degrees of renal insufficiency. The rate and extent of exposure (AUC and C_{max}) of aliskiren in subjects with renal impairment did not show a consistent correlation with the severity of renal impairment. Adjustment of the starting dose is not required in these patients. *[See Dosage and Administration (2.4)]*

Hepatically Impaired Patients: The pharmacokinetics of aliskiren were not significantly affected in patients with mild to severe liver disease. Consequently, adjustment of the starting dose is not required in these patients. *[See Dosage and Administration (2.4)]*

Pediatric Patients: The pharmacokinetics of aliskiren have not been investigated in patients <18 years of age. *[See Dosage and Administration (2.4)]*

Geriatric Patients: Exposure (measured by AUC) is increased in elderly patients ≥65 years. Adjustment of the starting dose is not required in these patients. *[See Dosage and Administration (2.4)]*

Race: The pharmacokinetic differences between Blacks, Caucasians, and the Japanese are minimal.

13 NONCLINICAL TOXICOLOGY

13.1 Carcinogenesis, Mutagenesis, Impairment of Fertility

Carcinogenic potential was assessed in a 2-year rat study and a 6-month transgenic (rasH2) mouse study with aliskiren hemifumarate at oral doses of up to 1500 mg aliskiren/kg/day. Although there were no statistically significant increases in tumor incidence associated with exposure to aliskiren, mucosal epithelial hyperplasia (with or without erosion/ulceration) was observed in the lower gastrointestinal tract at doses of 750 or more mg/kg/day in both species, with a colonic adenoma identified in one rat and a cecal adenocarcinoma identified in another, rare tumors in the strain of rat studied. On a systemic exposure (AUC_{0-24hr}) basis, 1500 mg/kg/day in the rat is about 4 times and in the mouse about 1.5 times the maximum recommended human dose (300 mg aliskiren/day). Mucosal hyperplasia in the cecum or colon of rats was also observed at doses of 250 mg/kg/day (the lowest tested dose) as well as at higher doses in 4- and 13-week studies.

Aliskiren hemifumarate was devoid of genotoxic potential in the Ames reverse mutation assay with *S. typhimurium* and *E. coli*, the *in vitro* Chinese hamster ovary cell chromosomal aberration assay, the *in vitro* Chinese hamster V79 cell gene mutation test and the *in vivo* mouse bone marrow micronucleus assay.

Fertility of male and female rats was unaffected at doses of up to 250 mg aliskiren/kg/day (8 times the maximum recommended human dose of 300 mg Tekturna/60 kg on a mg/m^2 basis).

13.2 Animal Toxicology and/or Pharmacology

Reproductive Toxicology Studies: Reproductive toxicity studies of aliskiren hemifumarate did not reveal any evidence of teratogenicity at oral doses up to 600 mg aliskiren/kg/day (20 times the maximum recommended human dose (MHRD) of 300 mg/day on a mg/m^2 basis) in pregnant rats or up to 100 mg aliskiren/kg/day (7 times the MRHD on a mg/m² basis) in pregnant rabbits. Fetal birth weight was adversely affected in rabbits at 50 mg/kg/day (3.2 times the MRHD on a mg/m² basis). Aliskiren was present in placenta, amniotic fluid and fetuses of pregnant rabbits.

14 CLINICAL STUDIES

14.1 Aliskiren Monotherapy

The antihypertensive effects of Tekturna have been demonstrated in six randomized, double-blind, placebo-controlled 8-week clinical trials in patients with mild-to-moderate hypertension. The placebo response and placebo-subtracted changes from baseline in seated trough cuff blood pressure are shown in Table 1.
[See table 1 at right]

The studies included approximately 2,730 patients given doses of 75-600 mg of aliskiren and 1,231 patients given placebo. As shown in Table 1, there is some increase in response with administered dose in all studies, with reasonable effects seen at 150-300 mg, and no clear further increased at 600 mg. A substantial proportion (85%-90%) of the blood pressure lowering effect was observed within 2 weeks of treatment studies with ambulatory blood pressure monitoring showed reasonable control throughout the interdosing interval; the ratios of mean daytime to mean nighttime ambulatory BP range from 0.6 to 0.9.

Patients in the placebo-controlled trials continued open-label aliskiren for up to one year. A persistent blood pressure lowering effect was demonstrated by a randomized withdrawal study (patients randomized to continue drug or placebo), which showed a statistically significant difference between patients kept on aliskiren and those randomized to placebo. With cessation of treatment, blood pressure gradually returned toward baseline levels over a period of several weeks. There was no evidence of rebound hypertension after abrupt cessation of therapy.

Aliskiren lowered blood pressure in all demographic subgroups, although Black patients tended to have smaller reduction than Caucasians and Asians, as has been seen with ACE inhibitors and ARBs.

There are no studies of Tekturna or members of the direct renin inhibitors demonstrating reductions in cardiovascular risk in patients with hypertension.

14.2 Aliskiren in Combination with Other Antihypertensives

Hydrochlorothiazide

Aliskiren 75, 150, and 300 mg and hydrochlorothiazide 6.25, 12.5, and 25 mg were studied alone and in combination in an 8-week, 2,776-patient, randomized, double-blind, placebo-controlled, parallel-group, 15-arm factorial study. Blood pressure reductions with the combinations were greater than the reductions with the monotherapies as shown in Table 2.
[See table 2 above]

Valsartan

Aliskiren 150 and 300 mg and valsartan 160 and 320 mg were studied alone and in combination in an 8-week, 1,797-patient, randomized, double-blind, placebo-controlled, parallel-group, 4-arm, dose-escalation study. The dosages of aliskiren and valsartan were started at 150 and 160 mg, respectively, and increased at four weeks to 300 mg and 320 mg, respectively. Seated trough cuff blood pressure was measured at baseline, 4, and 8 weeks. Blood pressure reductions with the combinations were greater than the reductions with the monotherapies as shown in Table 3.

Table 1
Reductions in Seated Trough Cuff Blood Pressure in the Placebo-Controlled Studies

| Study | Placebo mean change | Aliskiren daily dose, mg | | | |
| | | 75 | 150 | 300 | 600 |
		Placebo-subtracted	Placebo-subtracted	Placebo-subtracted	Placebo-subtracted
1	2.9/3.3	5.7/4*	5.9/4.5*	11.2/7.5*	—
2	5.3/6.3	—	6.1/2.9*	10.5/5.4*	—
3	10/8.6	2.2/1.7	2.1/1.7	5.1/3.7*	10.4/5.2*
4	7.5/6.9	1.9/1.8	4.8/2*	8.3/3.3*	—
5	3.8/4.9	—	9.3/5.4*	10.9/6.2*	12.1/7.6*
6	4.6/4.1	—	—	8.4/4.9†	—

* p<0.05 vs. placebo by ANCOVA with Dunnett's procedure for multiple comparisons
† p<0.05 vs. placebo by ANCOVA for the pairwise comparison.

Table 2
Placebo-Subtracted Reductions in Seated Trough Cuff Blood Pressure in Combination with Hydrochlorothiazide

| Aliskiren, mg | Placebo mean change | Hydrochlorothiazide, mg | | | |
| | | 0 | 6.25 | 12.5 | 25 |
		Placebo-subtracted	Placebo-subtracted	Placebo-subtracted	Placebo-subtracted
0	7.5/6.9	—	3.5/2.1	6.4/3.2	6.8/2.4
75		1.9/1.8	6.8/3.8	8.2/4.2	9.8/4.5
150		4.8/2	7.8/3.4	10.1/5	12/5.7
300		8.3/3.3	—	12.3/7	13.7/7.3

Table 4
Tekturna Tablets Supply

| Tablet | Color | Imprint Side 1 | Imprint Side 2 | NDC 0078-XXXX-XX | | |
				Bottle of 30	Bottle of 90	Blister Packages of 100
150 mg	Light-Pink	NVR	IL	0485-15	0485-34	0485-35
300 mg	Light-Red	NVR	IU	0486-15	0486-34	0486-35

Table 3
Placebo-Subtracted Reductions in Seated Trough Cuff Blood Pressure in Combination with Valsartan

| Aliskiren, mg | Placebo mean change | Valsartan, mg | | |
		0	160	320
0	4.6/4.1*	—	5.6/3.9	8.2/5.6
150		5.4/2.7	10.0/5.7	12.6/8.1
300		8.4/4.9	—	12.6/8.1

*The placebo change is 5.2/4.8 for week 4 endpoint which was used for the dose groups containing Aliskiren 150 mg or Valsartan 160 mg.

ACE Inhibitors and Amlodipine

Aliskiren has not been studied when added to maximal doses of ACE inhibitors to determine whether aliskiren produces additional blood pressure reduction with a maximal dose of an ACE inhibitor. Aliskiren 150 mg provided additional blood pressure reduction when co-administered with amlodipine 5 mg in one study, but the combination was not statistically significantly better than amlodipine 10 mg.

16 HOW SUPPLIED/STORAGE AND HANDLING

Tekturna is supplied as a light-pink, biconvex round tablet containing 150 mg of aliskiren, and as a light-red biconvex ovaloid tablet containing 300 mg of aliskiren. Tablets are imprinted with NVR on one side and IL, IU, on the other side of the 150 and 300 mg tablets, respectively.
All strengths are packaged in bottles and unit-dose blister packages (10 strips or 10 tablets) as described below in Table 4.
[See table 4 above]
Store at 25°C (77°F); excursions permitted to 15-30°C (59-86°F) [See USP Controlled Room Temperature]. Protect from moisture. Dispense in a tight container (USP).

17 PATIENT COUNSELING INFORMATION

Information for Patients

Pregnancy: Female patients of child bearing age should be told about the consequences of exposure to drugs that act on the renin-angiotensin system. Discuss other treatment options with female patients planning to become pregnant. Patients should be asked to report pregnancies to their physicians as soon as possible.

Angioedema: Angioedema, including laryngeal edema, may occur at any time during treatment with Tekturna. Patients should be advised and told to report immediately any signs or symptoms suggesting angioedema (swelling of face, extremities, eyes, lips, tongue, difficulty in swallowing or breathing) and to take no more drug until they have consulted with the prescribing physicians.

Symptomatic Hypotension: A patient receiving Tekturna should be cautioned that lightheadedness can occur, especially during the first days of therapy, and that it should be reported to the prescribing physician. The patients should be told that if syncope occurs, Tekturna should be discontinued until the physician has been consulted.
All patients should be cautioned that inadequate fluid intake, excessive perspiration, diarrhea, or vomiting can lead to an excessive fall in blood pressure, with the same consequences of lightheadedness and possible syncope.

Potassium Supplements: A patient receiving Tekturna should be told not to use potassium supplements or salt substitutes containing potassium without consulting the prescribing physician.

Relationship to Meals: Patients should establish a routine pattern for taking Tekturna with regard to meals. High-fat meals decrease absorption substantially.

FDA-APPROVED PATIENT LABELING
PATIENT INFORMATION
Tekturna (pronounced tek-turn-a)
(aliskiren)
Tablets
Dosing Strengths:
150 mg tablets
300 mg tablets
Available by Prescription Only
Read the patient information that comes with Tekturna before you start taking it and each time you get a refill. There may be new information. This leaflet does not replace talking to your doctor about your condition or treatment. If you have any questions about Tekturna, ask your doctor or pharmacist.

IMPORTANT WARNING: If you get pregnant, stop taking Tekturna and call your doctor right away. Tekturna may harm an unborn baby, causing injury and even death. If you plan to become pregnant, talk to your doctor about other treatment options before taking Tekturna.

What Is Tekturna?
Tekturna can help your blood vessels relax and widen so blood pressure is lower. Tekturna is a type of prescription medicine called a direct renin inhibitor. By reducing renin, it helps to reduce blood pressure.

What Is High Blood Pressure (Hypertension)?
Blood pressure is the force that pushes the blood through your blood vessels to all the organs of your body. You have high blood pressure when the force of your blood moving through your blood vessels is too great. Renin (pronounced REE-nin) is a chemical in the body that starts a process that makes blood vessels narrow, leading to high blood pressure. Drugs that lower blood pressure lower your risk of having a stroke or heart attack.
High blood pressure makes the heart work harder to pump blood throughout the body and causes damage to the blood vessels. If high blood pressure is not treated, it can lead to stroke, heart attack, heart failure, kidney failure, and vision problems.

Who Should Not Take Tekturna?
• If you get pregnant, stop taking Tekturna and call your doctor right away. If you plan to become pregnant, talk to your doctor about other treatment options for your high blood pressure.
• Do not take Tekturna if you are allergic to any of its ingredients. See the end of this leaflet for a complete list of the ingredients in Tekturna.

- Tekturna has not been studied in children under 18 years of age.

What Should I Tell My Doctor Before Taking Tekturna?

Tell your doctor about all your medical conditions, including whether you:

- are pregnant or planning to become pregnant, see IMPORTANT WARNING.
- are breast-feeding. It is not known if Tekturna passes into your breast milk. You should choose either to take Tekturna or breast-feed, but not both.
- have kidney problems.
- are allergic to any of the ingredients in Tekturna, see "What are the ingredients in Tekturna?"
- have ever had a reaction called angioedema, to an ACE inhibitor medicine. Angioedema causes swelling of the face, lips, tongue, throat, arms, and legs, and may cause difficulty breathing.

Tell your doctor about all the medicines you take including prescription and nonprescription medicines, vitamins and herbal supplements. Especially tell your doctor if you are taking:

- other medicines for high blood pressure or a heart problem.
- Atorvastatin (medicine to lower cholesterol in your blood).
- water pills (also called "diuretics").
- medicines for treating fungus or fungal infections.
- cyclosporine (a medicine used to suppress the immune system).
- potassium-containing medicines, potassium supplements, or salt substitutes containing potassium.

Your doctor or pharmacist will know what medicines are safe to take together.

How Should I Take Tekturna?

- Take Tekturna once a day, at the same time each day. As with any blood pressure medication, it is important to take Tekturna on a regular daily basis exactly as prescribed by your doctor.
- Tekturna can be taken by itself or safely in combination with other medicines to lower high blood pressure. Your doctor may change your dose if needed.
- Tekturna can be taken with or without food.
- If you miss a dose, take it as soon as you remember. If it is close to your next dose, do not take the missed dose. Just take the next dose at your regular time.
- If you take too much Tekturna, call your doctor or Poison Control Center, or go to the nearest hospital emergency room.

What Are Possible Side Effects Of Tekturna?

Tekturna may cause serious side effects:

- **Injury or death to an unborn baby. See IMPORTANT WARNING.**
- **Low blood pressure (hypotension).** Your blood pressure may get too low if you also take water pills, are on a low-salt diet, get dialysis treatments, have heart problems, or get sick with vomiting or diarrhea. Lie down if you feel faint or dizzy. Call your doctor right away.
- **Angioedema:** Aliskiren can cause swelling of the face, lips, tongue, throat, arms and legs or the whole body. Get medical help right away and tell your doctor if you get any one or more of these symptoms. Angioedema can happen at any time while you are taking Tekturna.

Common side effects of Tekturna include:

diarrhea
cough
dizziness
headache
flu-like symptoms
back pain
tiredness

Less common side effects include rash.

Tell your doctor if you have any side effect that bothers you or that does not go away. These are not all of the possible side effects of Tekturna. For a complete list of side effects, ask your doctor or pharmacist.

How Do I Store Tekturna?

- Store Tekturna tablets at room temperature between 59° to 86°F (15°-30°C).
- Keep Tekturna in the original prescription bottle in a dry place. Do not remove the desiccant (drying agent) from the bottle.
- Keep Tekturna and all medicines out of the reach of children.

General Information About Tekturna

Medicines are sometimes prescribed for conditions not listed in the patient information leaflet. Do not take Tekturna for a condition for which it was not prescribed. Do not give Tekturna to other people, even if they have the same condition or symptoms you have. It may harm them. This leaflet summarizes the most important information about Tekturna. If you have more questions about Tekturna talk with your doctor. You can ask your doctor or pharmacist for information that is written for healthcare professionals.

For more information about Tekturna, ask your doctor or pharmacist, visit www.Tekturna.com, or call 1-888-Tekturna (1-888-835-8876).

What are the ingredients in Tekturna?

Active Ingredients: Aliskiren (Tekturna)

Inactive Ingredients: colloidal silicone dioxide, crospovidone, hypromellose, iron oxide colorants, magnesium stearate, microcrystalline cellulose, polyethylene glycol, talc, and titanium dioxide.

T2010-66/T2009-52

Manufactured by:
Novartis Pharma AG, Stein, Switzerland
Novartis Pharma Produktions GmbH, Wehr, Germany
Distributed by:
Novartis Pharmaceuticals Corporation
East Hanover, NJ 07936
©Novartis

Shown in Product Identification Guide, page 316

TEKTURNA HCT®   ℞
[tek-turn-a HCT]
(aliskiren and hydrochlorothiazide)
Tablets

The following prescribing information is based on official labeling in effect September 2010.

HIGHLIGHTS OF PRESCRIBING INFORMATION
These highlights do not include all the information needed to use Tekturna HCT safely and effectively. See full prescribing information for Tekturna HCT.

Tekturna HCT *(aliskiren and hydrochlorothiazide)* **Tablets**
Initial U.S. Approval: 2008

> **WARNING: AVOID USE IN PREGNANCY**
> **When pregnancy is detected, discontinue Tekturna HCT as soon as possible.**
> **Drugs that act directly on the renin-angiotensin system can cause injury and death to the developing fetus. (5.1)**

———————RECENT MAJOR CHANGES———————

Indications and Usage (1)	07/2009
Dosage and Administration	
Add-On Therapy (2.3)	07/2009
Replacement Therapy (2.4)	07/2009
Initial Therapy (2.5)	07/2009

———————INDICATIONS AND USAGE———————
Tekturna HCT is a combination of aliskiren, a direct renin inhibitor, and hydrochlorothiazide (HCTZ), a thiazide diuretic, indicated for the treatment of hypertension:

- In patients not adequately controlled with monotherapy
- As initial therapy in patients likely to need multiple drugs to achieve their blood pressure goals (1)

———————DOSAGE AND ADMINISTRATION———————

- The antihypertensive effect is largely manifested within 1 week, with maximal effects seen at around 4 weeks. If blood pressure remains uncontrolled after 2 to 4 weeks of therapy, titrate up to a maximum of 300/25 mg. (2.2)
- Order of increasing mean effect: 150/12.5 mg, 150/25 mg or 300/12.5 mg, and 300/25 mg. (2.1)
- One tablet daily, with a routine pattern with regard to meals. (2.7)
- May be administered with other antihypertensive agents. (2.6)
- Add-on or Initial therapy: Initiate with 150/12.5 mg. Titrate as needed up to a maximum of 300/25 mg. (2.3, 2.5)
- Replacement therapy: May be substituted for titrated components. (2.4)

———————DOSAGE FORMS AND STRENGTHS———————
Tablets (mg aliskiren/mg HCTZ): 150/12.5, 150/25, 300/12.5, 300/25 (3)

———————CONTRAINDICATIONS———————
Anuria (4)
Hypersensitivity to sulfonamide-derived drugs (4)

———————WARNINGS AND PRECAUTIONS———————

- Head and Neck Angioedema: Discontinue Tekturna HCT and monitor until signs and symptoms resolve. (5.2)
- Hypotension in Volume- and/or Salt-Depleted Patients: Correct imbalances before initiating therapy with Tekturna HCT. (5.3)
- Patients with Severe Renal Impairment: Not recommended if GFR <30 mL/min. (5.4)
- Patients with Hepatic Impairment: Titrate slowly. (5.5)
- Hypersensitivity Reactions: May occur from HCTZ component. (5.6)

———————ADVERSE REACTIONS———————
The most common adverse reactions (incidence ≥1.5% and more common than with placebo) are: dizziness and diarrhea. (6.1)
To report SUSPECTED ADVERSE REACTIONS, contact Novartis Pharmaceuticals Corporation at 1-888-669-6682 or FDA at 1-800-FDA-1088 or www.fda.gov/medwatch.

———————DRUG INTERACTIONS———————
Aliskiren:
- Cyclosporine or Itraconazole: Concomitant use is not recommended. (7)

Hydrochlorothiazide:
- Alcohol, Barbiturates, Narcotics: Potentiation of orthostatic hypotension
- Antidiabetic Drugs: Dosage adjustment of antidiabetic may be required
- Cholestyramine and Colestipol: Reduced absorption of thiazides
- Corticosteroids, ACTH: Hypokalemia, electrolyte depletion
- Lithium: Reduced renal clearance and high risk of lithium toxicity when used with diuretics. Should not be given with diuretics.
- NSAIDs: Can reduce diuretic, natriuretic, and antihypertensive effects of diuretics. Observe patient closely.

———————USE IN SPECIFIC POPULATIONS———————
Nursing Mothers: Nursing or drug should be discontinued. (8.3)

See 17 for PATIENT COUNSELING INFORMATION and FDA-approved patient labeling

Revised: 08/2010

FULL PRESCRIBING INFORMATION: CONTENTS*
WARNING: AVOID USE IN PREGNANCY

FULL PRESCRIBING INFORMATION

> **WARNING: AVOID USE IN PREGNANCY**
> **When pregnancy is detected, discontinue Tekturna HCT as soon as possible.**
> **Drugs that act directly on the renin-angiotensin system can cause injury and death to the developing fetus.**
> **[See Warnings and Precautions (5.1)]**

1   INDICATIONS AND USAGE
Tekturna HCT is indicated for the treatment of hypertension.

Add-On Therapy
A patient whose blood pressure is not adequately controlled with aliskiren alone or hydrochlorothiazide alone may be switched to combination therapy with Tekturna HCT.

A patient whose blood pressure is controlled with hydrochlorothiazide alone but who experiences hypokalemia may be switched to combination therapy with Tekturna HCT.

A patient who experiences dose-limiting adverse reactions on either component alone may be switched to Tekturna

HCT containing a lower dose of that component in combination with the other to achieve similar blood pressure reductions.

Replacement Therapy
Tekturna HCT may be substituted for the titrated components.

Initial Therapy
Tekturna HCT may be used as initial therapy in patients who are likely to need multiple drugs to achieve their blood pressure goals.

The choice of Tekturna HCT as initial therapy should be based on an assessment of potential benefits and risks. Patients with Stage 2 hypertension are at a relatively high risk for cardiovascular events (such as strokes, heart attacks, and heart failure), kidney failure, and vision problems, so prompt treatment is clinically relevant. The decision to use a combination as initial therapy should be individualized and should be shaped by considerations such as baseline blood pressure, the target goal, and the incremental likelihood of achieving goal with a combination compared to monotherapy. Individual blood pressure goals may vary based upon the patient's risk.

Data from the high-dose multifactorial study [see *Clinical Studies (14)*] provides estimates of the probability of reaching a target blood pressure with Tekturna HCT compared to aliskiren or hydrochlorothiazide monotherapy. The figures below provide estimates of the likelihood of achieving systolic or diastolic blood pressure control with Tekturna HCT 300/25 mg, based upon baseline systolic or diastolic blood pressure. The curve of each treatment group was estimated by logistic regression modeling. The estimated likelihood at the right tail of each curve is less reliable because of small numbers of subjects with high baseline blood pressures.

Figure 1: Probability of Achieving Systolic Blood Pressure (SBP) <140 mmHg

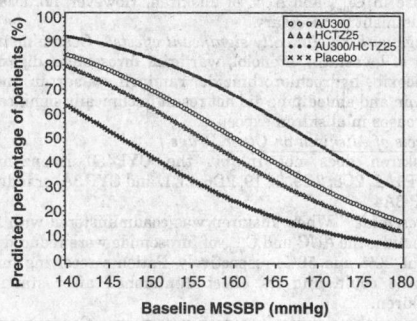

Figure 2: Probability of Achieving Systolic Blood Pressure (SBP) <130 mmHg

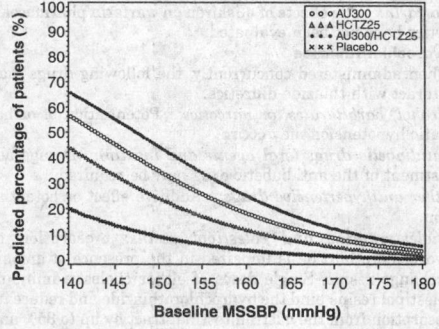

Figure 3: Probability of Achieving Diastolic Blood Pressure (DBP) <90 mmHg

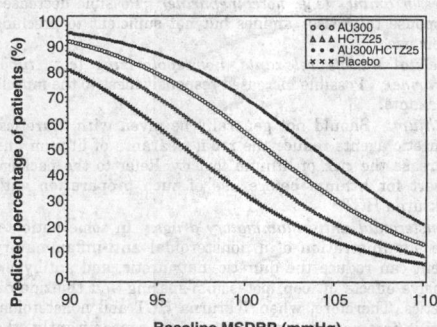

Figure 4: Probability of Achieving Diastolic Blood Pressure (DBP) <80 mmHg

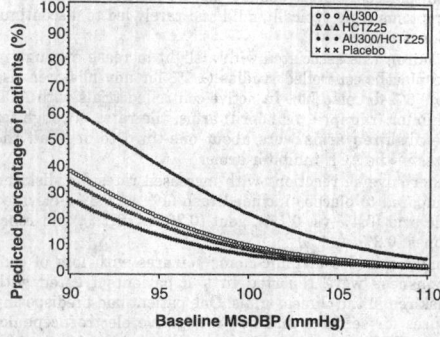

At all levels of baseline blood pressure, the probability of achieving any given diastolic or systolic goal is greater with the combination than for either monotherapy. For example, the mean baseline msSBP/msDBP for patients participating in this multifactorial study was 154/99 mmHg. A patient with a baseline blood pressure of 154/99 mmHg has about a 62% chance of achieving a goal of <140 mmHg (systolic) and 61% chance of achieving <90 mmHg (diastolic) on aliskiren alone, and the chance of achieving these goals on hydrochlorothiazide alone is about 54% (systolic) and 49% (diastolic). The chance of achieving these goals on Tekturna HCT rises to about 77% (systolic) and 74% (diastolic). The chance of achieving these goals on placebo is about 34% (systolic) and 37% (diastolic). [*See Dosage and Administration (2) and Clinical Studies (14).*]

2   DOSAGE AND ADMINISTRATION

2.1   Dose Selection
The recommended once-daily doses of Tekturna HCT in order of increasing mean effect are 150/12.5 mg, 150/25 mg or 300/12.5 mg, and 300/25 mg.

2.2   Dose Titration
The antihypertensive effect of Tekturna HCT is largely manifested within 1 week, with maximal effects generally seen at around 4 weeks. If blood pressure remains uncontrolled after 2 to 4 weeks of therapy, the dose may be titrated up to a maximum of aliskiren 300 mg/ hydrochlorothiazide 25 mg.

2.3   Add-On Therapy
A patient whose blood pressure is not adequately controlled with aliskiren alone or hydrochlorothiazide alone may be switched to combination therapy with Tekturna HCT. The usual recommended starting dose is 150/12.5 mg once daily as needed to control blood pressure. The dose may be titrated up to a maximum of aliskiren 300 mg/ hydrochlorothiazide 25 mg once daily.

2.4   Replacement Therapy
Tekturna HCT may be substituted for the individually titrated components.

2.5   Initial Therapy
The usual recommended starting dose is 150/12.5 mg once daily as needed to control blood pressure. The dose may be titrated up to a maximum of aliskiren 300 mg/ hydrochlorothiazide 25 mg once daily. Tekturna HCT is not recommended for use as initial therapy in patients with intravascular volume depletion. [*See Warnings and Precautions (5.3)*].

2.6   Use with Other Antihypertensive Drugs
Tekturna HCT may be administered with other antihypertensive agents. There are no data available with use of Tekturna HCT with angiotensin-converting enzyme inhibitors or beta blockers [see *Clinical Studies (14)*].

2.7   Relationship to Meals
Patients should establish a routine pattern for taking Tekturna HCT with regard to meals. High-fat meals decrease absorption substantially [see *Clinical Pharmacology (12.3)*].

2.8   Dosing in Specific Populations
Renal Impairment
The usual regimens of Tekturna HCT may be followed as long as the patient's creatinine clearance is >30 mL/min. In patients with more severe renal impairment, loop diuretics are preferred to thiazides, so Tekturna HCT is not recommended.
Hepatic Impairment
Adjustment of the starting dose is not necessary with hepatic impairment.
Elderly Patients
Adjustment of the starting dose is not required for elderly patients.

3   DOSAGE FORMS AND STRENGTHS
- 150 mg/12.5 mg tablets: white, biconvex ovaloid, film-coated tablets imprinted with NVR/LCI
- 150 mg/25 mg tablets: pale yellow, biconvex ovaloid, film-coated tablets imprinted with NVR/CLL

- 300 mg/12.5 mg tablets: violet white, biconvex ovaloid, film-coated tablets imprinted with NVR/CVI
- 300 mg/25 mg tablets: light yellow, biconvex ovaloid, film-coated tablets imprinted with NVR/CVV

4   CONTRAINDICATIONS
Because of the hydrochlorothiazide component, Tekturna HCT is contraindicated in patients with anuria or hypersensitivity to sulfonamide-derived drugs [see *Warnings and Precautions (5.6) and Adverse Reactions (6.1)*]. Hypersensitivity reactions may range from urticaria to anaphylaxis [see *Adverse Reactions (6.1)*].

5   WARNINGS AND PRECAUTIONS
5.1   Fetal/Neonatal Morbidity and Mortality
Tekturna HCT can cause fetal harm when administered to a pregnant woman. If this drug is used during pregnancy, or if the patient becomes pregnant while taking this drug, the patient should be apprised of the potential hazard to the fetus.

Drugs that act directly on the renin-angiotensin system can cause fetal and neonatal morbidity and death when administered to pregnant women. If this drug is used during pregnancy, or if the patient becomes pregnant while taking this drug, apprise the patient of the potential hazard to the fetus [see *Use in Specific Populations (8.1)*]. In several dozen published cases, ACE inhibitors use during the second and third trimesters of pregnancy was associated with fetal and neonatal injury, including hypotension, neonatal skull hypoplasia, anuria, reversible or irreversible renal failure, and death. In addition, first trimester use of ACE inhibitors has been associated with birth defects. Thiazides cross the placenta, and use of thiazides during pregnancy is associated with a risk of fetal or neonatal jaundice, thrombocytopenia, and possible other adverse reactions that have occurred in adults.

5.2   Head and Neck Angioedema
Aliskiren
Angioedema of the face, extremities, lips, tongue, glottis and/or larynx has been reported in patients treated with Tekturna and has necessitated hospitalization and intubation. This may occur at any time during treatment and has occurred in patients with and without a history of angioedema with ACE inhibitors or angiotensin receptor antagonists. If angioedema involves the throat, tongue, glottis or larynx, or if the patient has a history of upper respiratory surgery, airway obstruction may occur and be fatal. Patients who experience these effects, even without respiratory distress, require prolonged observation since treatment with antihistamines and corticosteroids may not be sufficient to prevent respiratory involvement. Prompt administration of subcutaneous epinephrine solution 1:1000 (0.3 to 0.5 mL) and measures to ensure a patient airway may be necessary. Discontinue Tekturna immediately in patients who develop angioedema, and do not readminister.

5.3   Hypotension in Volume- and/or Salt-Depleted Patients
An excessive fall in blood pressure (hypotension) was rarely seen (<1%) in patients with uncomplicated hypertension treated with Tekturna HCT in controlled trials. In patients with an activated renin-angiotensin system, such as volume- and/or salt-depleted patients receiving high doses of diuretics, symptomatic hypotension may occur. Correct these conditions prior to administration of Tekturna HCT, or the treatment should start under close medical supervision.

If an excessive fall in blood pressure occurs, place the patient in the supine position and, if necessary, given an intravenous infusion of normal saline. A transient hypotensive response is not a contraindication to further treatment, which usually can be continued without difficulty once the blood pressure has stabilized.

5.4   Patients with Severe Renal Impairment
Tekturna HCT
In patients with severe renal impairment (GFR <30 mL/ min), loop diuretics are preferred to thiazides, so Tekturna HCT is not recommended.
Hydrochlorothiazide
Uptitrate slowly; in patients with renal disease, thiazides may precipitate azotemia. Cumulative effects of the drug may develop in patients with impaired renal function.

5.5   Patients with Hepatic Impairment
Hydrochlorothiazide
Uptitrate slowly; minor alterations of fluid and electrolyte balance may precipitate hepatic coma.

5.6   Hypersensitivity Reactions
Hydrochlorothiazide
Hypersensitivity reactions to hydrochlorothiazide may occur in patients with or without a history of allergy or bronchial asthma, but are more likely in patients with such a history.

5.7   Systemic Lupus Erythematosus
Hydrochlorothiazide
Thiazide diuretics have been reported to cause exacerbation or activation of systemic lupus erythematosus.

5.8 Lithium Interaction

Hydrochlorothiazide

Lithium generally should not be given with thiazides [*see Drug Interactions (7)*].

5.9 Serum Electrolyte Abnormalities

Tekturna HCT

In the short-term controlled trials of various doses of Tekturna HCT the incidence of hypertensive patients who developed hypokalemia (serum potassium <3.5 mEq/L) was 2.2%; the incidence of hyperkalemia (serum potassium >5.5 mEq/L) was 0.8%. No patients discontinued due to increase or decrease of serum potassium.

Periodic determinations of serum electrolytes to detect possible electrolyte imbalance should be performed at appropriate intervals. The intervals should be based on the history of electrolyte abnormalities in patients with aliskiren or hydrochlorothiazide monotherapy.

Based on experience with the use of other substances that affect the renin-angiotensin system (RAS), concomitant use of Tekturna HCT with potassium-sparing diuretics, potassium supplements, salt substitutes containing potassium, or other drugs that increase potassium levels may lead to increases in serum potassium.

5.10 Renal Artery Stenosis

No data are available on the use of Tekturna HCT in patients with unilateral or bilateral renal artery stenosis or stenosis of the artery to a solitary kidney.

5.11 Cyclosporine or Itraconazole

Aliskiren

When aliskiren was given with cyclosporine or itraconazole, the blood concentrations of aliskiren were significantly increased. Concomitant use of aliskiren with cyclosporine or itraconazole is not recommended [*see Drug Interactions (7)*].

6 ADVERSE REACTIONS

6.1 Clinical Studies Experience

The following serious adverse reactions are discussed in greater detail in other sections of the label:

• Risk of fetal/neonatal morbidity and mortality [*see Warnings and Precautions (5.1)*]
• Head and neck angioedema [*see Warnings and Precautions (5.2)*]
• Hypotension in volume- and/or salt-depleted patients [*see Warnings and Precautions (5.3)*]

Because clinical trials are conducted under widely varying conditions, adverse reaction rates observed in the clinical trials of a drug cannot be directly compared to rates in clinical trials of another drug and may not reflect the rates observed in practice.

Tekturna HCT

Tekturna HCT has been evaluated for safety in more than 2,700 patients, including over 700 treated for 6 months and 190 for over 1 year. In placebo-controlled clinical trials, discontinuation of therapy due to a clinical adverse event (including uncontrolled hypertension) occurred in 2.7% of patients treated with Tekturna HCT versus 3.6% of patients given placebo.

Adverse events in placebo-controlled trials that occurred in at least 1% of patients treated with Tekturna HCT and at a higher incidence than placebo included dizziness (2.3% vs. 1%), influenza (2.3% vs. 1.6%), diarrhea (1.6% vs. 0.5%), cough (1.3% vs. 0.5%), vertigo (1.2% vs. 0.5%), asthenia (1.2% vs. 0%), and arthralgia (1% vs. 0.5%).

Aliskiren

Aliskiren has been evaluated for safety in 6,460 patients, including 1,740 treated for longer than 6 months, and 1,250 for longer than 1 year. In placebo-controlled clinical trials, discontinuation of therapy due to a clinical adverse event, including uncontrolled hypertension occurred in 2.2% of patients treated with aliskiren, versus 3.5% of patients given placebo.

Two cases of angioedema with respiratory symptoms were reported with aliskiren use in the clinical studies. Two other cases of periorbital edema without respiratory symptoms were reported as possible angioedema and resulted in discontinuation. The rate of these angioedema cases in the completed studies was 0.06%.

In addition, 26 other cases of edema involving the face, hands, or whole body were reported with aliskiren use, including 4 leading to discontinuation.

In the placebo-controlled studies, however, the incidence of edema involving the face, hands, or whole body was 0.4% with aliskiren compared with 0.5% with placebo. In a long-term active-controlled study with aliskiren and HCTZ arms, the incidence of edema involving the face, hands, or whole body was 0.4% in both treatment arms.

Aliskiren produces dose-related gastrointestinal (GI) adverse reactions. Diarrhea was reported by 2.3% of patients at 300 mg, compared to 1.2% in placebo patients. In women and the elderly (age ≥65) increases in diarrhea rates were evident starting at a dose of 150 mg daily, with rates for these subgroups at 150 mg comparable to those seen at 300 mg for men or younger patients (all rates about 2% to 2.3%). Other GI symptoms included abdominal pain, dys-

pepsia, and gastroesophageal reflux, although increased rates for abdominal pain and dyspepsia were distinguished from placebo only at 600 mg daily. Diarrhea and other GI symptoms were typically mild and rarely led to discontinuation.

Aliskiren was associated with a slight increase in cough in the placebo-controlled studies (1.1% for any aliskiren use vs. 0.6% for placebo). In active-controlled trials with ACE inhibitor (ramipril, lisinopril) arms, the rates of cough for the aliskiren arms were about one-third to one-half the rates in the ACE inhibitor arms.

Other adverse reactions with increased rates for aliskiren compared to placebo included rash (1% vs. 0.3%), elevated uric acid (0.4% vs. 0.1%), gout (0.2% vs. 0.1%), and renal stones (0.2% vs. 0%).

Single episodes of tonic-clonic seizures with loss of consciousness were reported in two patients treated with aliskiren in the clinical trials. One patient had predisposing causes for seizures and had a negative electroencephalogram (EEG) and cerebral imaging following the seizures; for the other patient, EEG and imaging results were not reported. Aliskiren was discontinued and there was no rechallenge in either case.

The following adverse events occurred in placebo-controlled clinical trials at an incidence of more than 1% of patients treated with aliskiren, but also occurred at about the same or greater incidence in patients receiving placebo: headache, nasopharyngitis, dizziness, fatigue, upper respiratory tract infection, back pain and cough.

No clinically meaningful changes in vital signs or in ECG (including QTc interval) were observed in patients treated with aliskiren.

Hydrochlorothiazide

Other adverse reactions that have been reported with hydrochlorothiazide, without regard to causality, are listed below:

Body As A Whole: weakness

Digestive: pancreatitis, jaundice (intrahepatic cholestatic jaundice), sialadenitis, cramping, gastric irritation

Hematologic: aplastic anemia, agranulocytosis, leukopenia, hemolytic anemia, thrombocytopenia

Hypersensitivity: purpura, photosensitivity, urticaria, necrotizing angiitis (vasculitis and cutaneous vasculitis), fever, respiratory distress including pneumonitis and pulmonary edema, anaphylactic reactions

Metabolic: hyperglycemia, glycosuria, hyperuricemia

Musculoskeletal: muscle spasm

Nervous System/Psychiatric: restlessness

Renal: renal failure, renal dysfunction, interstitial nephritis

Skin: erythema multiforme including Stevens-Johnson syndrome, exfoliative dermatitis including toxic epidermal necrolysis

Special Senses: transient blurred vision, xanthopsia

6.2 Clinical Laboratory Test Abnormalities

In controlled clinical trials, clinically important changes in standard laboratory parameters were rarely associated with administration of Tekturna HCT.

Blood Urea Nitrogen (BUN)/Creatinine: Elevations (greater than 50% increase) in BUN and creatinine occurred in 11.8% and 0.9%, respectively, of patients taking Tekturna HCT, and 7% and 1.1%, respectively, of patients given placebo in short-term controlled clinical trials. No patients were discontinued due to an increase in either BUN or creatinine.

Hemoglobin and Hematocrit: A greater than 20% decrease in hemoglobin and hematocrit were observed in <0.1% and 0.1%, respectively, of patients treated with Tekturna HCT, compared with 0% in placebo-treated patients. No patients were discontinued due to anemia.

Liver Function Tests: Occasional elevations (greater than 150%) in ALT (SGPT) were observed in 1.2% of patients treated with Tekturna HCT, compared with 0% in placebo-treated patients. No patients were discontinued due to abnormal liver function tests.

Serum Uric Acid: Uric acid related abnormalities were more commonly observed in patients treated with Tekturna HCT, compared with placebo; 2.2% versus 0% had a uric acid increase >50% from baseline; gout and renal stones were less commonly observed.

Serum Electrolytes: [*See Warnings and Precautions (5.8).*]

6.3 Post-Marketing Experience

The following adverse reactions have been reported in aliskiren post-marketing experience. Because these reactions are reported voluntarily from a population of uncertain size, it is not always possible to estimate their frequency or establish a causal relationship to drug exposure.

Hypersensitivity: angioedema requiring airway management and hospitalization

Peripheral edema

Blood creatinine increased

7 DRUG INTERACTIONS

No drug interaction studies have been conducted with Tekturna HCT and other drugs, although studies with the individual aliskiren and hydrochlorothiazide components are described below.

Aliskiren

Effects of Other Drugs on Aliskiren

Based on *in vitro* studies, aliskiren is metabolized by CYP 3A4.

Irbesartan: Coadministration of irbesartan reduced aliskiren C_{max} up to 50% after multiple dosing.

P-glycoprotein Effects: Pgp (MDR1/Mdr1a/1b) was found to be the major efflux system involved in absorption and disposition of aliskiren in preclinical studies. The potential for drug interactions at the Pgp site will likely depend on the degree of inhibition of this transporter.

Atorvastatin: Coadministration of atorvastatin resulted in about a 50% increase in aliskiren C_{max} and AUC after multiple dosing.

Ketoconazole: Coadministration of 200 mg twice-daily ketoconazole with aliskiren resulted in an approximate 80% increase in plasma levels of aliskiren. A 400-mg once-daily dose was not studied but would be expected to increase aliskiren blood levels further.

Itraconazole: Coadministration of 100 mg itraconazole with 150 mg aliskiren resulted in approximately 5.8-fold increase in C_{max} and 6.5-fold increase in AUC of aliskiren. Concomitant use of aliskiren with itraconazole is not recommended.

Cyclosporine: Coadministration of 200 mg and 600 mg cyclosporine with 75 mg aliskiren resulted in an approximately 2.5-fold increase in C_{max} and 5-fold increase in AUC of aliskiren. Concomitant use of aliskiren with cyclosporine is not recommended.

Verapamil: Coadministration of 240 mg of verapamil with 300 mg aliskiren resulted in an approximately 2-fold increase in C_{max} and AUC of aliskiren. However, no dosage adjustment is necessary.

Drugs with no clinically significant effects: Coadministration of lovastatin, atenolol, warfarin, furosemide, digoxin, celecoxib, hydrochlorothiazide, ramipril, valsartan, metformin and amlodipine did not result in clinically significant increases in aliskiren exposure.

Effects of Aliskiren on Other Drugs

Aliskiren does not inhibit the CYP450 isoenzymes (CYP1A2, 2C8, 2C9, 2C19, 2D6, 2E1, and CYP 3A) or induce CYP 3A4.

Furosemide: When aliskiren was coadministered with furosemide, the AUC and C_{max} of furosemide were reduced by about 30% and 50%, respectively. Patients receiving furosemide could find its effect diminished after starting aliskiren.

Drugs with no clinically significant effects: Coadministration of aliskiren did not significantly affect the pharmacokinetics of lovastatin, digoxin, valsartan, amlodipine, metformin, celecoxib, atenolol, atorvastatin, ramipril or hydrochlorothiazide.

Warfarin: The effects of aliskiren on warfarin pharmacokinetics have not been evaluated.

Hydrochlorothiazide

When administered concurrently, the following drugs may interact with thiazide diuretics.

Alcohol, barbiturates, or narcotics: Potentiation of orthostatic hypotension may occur.

Antidiabetic drugs (oral agents and insulin): Dosage adjustment of the antidiabetic drug may be required.

Other antihypertensive drugs: Additive effect or potentiation.

Cholestyramine and colestipol resins: Absorption of hydrochlorothiazide is impaired in the presence of anionic exchange resins. Single doses of either cholestyramine or colestipol resins bind the hydrochlorothiazide and reduce its absorption from the gastrointestinal tract by up to 85% and 43%, respectively.

Corticosteroids, ACTH: Intensified electrolyte depletion, particularly hypokalemia.

Pressor amines (e.g., norepinephrine): Possible decreased response to pressor amines but not sufficient to preclude their use.

Skeletal muscle relaxants, nondepolarizing (e.g., tubocurarine): Possible increased responsiveness to the muscle relaxants.

Lithium: Should not generally be given with diuretics. Diuretic agents reduce the renal clearance of lithium and increase the risk of lithium toxicity. Refer to the package insert for lithium before use of such preparation with Tekturna HCT.

Nonsteroidal anti-inflammatory drugs: In some patients, the administration of a nonsteroidal anti-inflammatory agent can reduce the diuretic, natriuretic, and antihypertensive effects of loop, potassium-sparing and thiazide diuretics. Therefore, when Tekturna HCT and nonsteroidal anti-inflammatory agents are used concomitantly, the patient should be observed closely to determine if the desired effect of the diuretic is obtained.

8 USE IN SPECIFIC POPULATIONS

8.1 Pregnancy

Pregnancy Category D [*See Warnings and Precautions (5.1).*]

Tekturna HCT contains both aliskiren (a direct renin inhibitor) and hydrochlorothiazide (a thiazide diuretic). When administered during the second or third trimester of pregnancy, drugs that act directly on the renin-angiotensin system can cause fetal and neonatal morbidity and death.

Thiazides can cross the placenta, and use of thiazides during pregnancy is associated with a risk of fetal or neonatal jaundice, thrombocytopenia, and possibly other adverse reactions that have occurred in adults. Tekturna HCT can cause fetal harm when administered to a pregnant woman. If this drug is used during pregnancy, or if the patient becomes pregnant while taking this drug, apprise the patient of the potential hazard to the fetus.

In several dozen published cases, ACE inhibitor use during the second and third trimesters of pregnancy was associated with fetal and neonatal injury, including hypotension, neonatal skull hypoplasia, anuria, reversible or irreversible renal failure, and death. Oligohydramnios was also reported, presumably from decreased fetal renal function. In this setting, oligohydramnios was associated with fetal limb contractures, craniofacial deformation, and hypoplastic lung development. Prematurity, intrauterine growth retardation, and patent ductus arteriosus were also reported, although it is not clear whether these occurrences were due to exposure to the drug. In addition, first trimester use of ACE inhibitors, a specific class of drugs acting on the renin-angiotensin system, has been associated with a potential risk of birth defects in retrospective data.

When pregnancy occurs in a patient using Tekturna HCT, the physician should discontinue Tekturna HCT treatment as soon as possible. The physician should inform the patient about potential risks to the fetus based on the time of gestational exposure to Tekturna HCT (first trimester only or later). If exposure occurs beyond the first trimester, an ultrasound examination should be done.

In rare cases when another antihypertensive agent cannot be used to treat the pregnant patient, serial ultrasound examinations should be performed to assess the intraamniotic environment. Routine fetal testing with non-stress tests, biophysical profiles, and/or contraction stress tests may be appropriate based on gestational age and standards of care in the community. If oligohydramnios occurs in these situations, individualized decisions about continuing or discontinuing Tekturna HCT treatment and about pregnancy management should be made by the patient, her physician, and experts in the management of high risk pregnancy. Patients and physicians should be aware that oligohydramnios may not appear until after the fetus has sustained irreversible injury. Infants with histories of *in utero* exposure to Tekturna HCT should be closely observed for hypotension, oliguria, and hyperkalemia. If oliguria occurs, these infants may require blood pressure and renal perfusion support. Exchange transfusion or dialysis may be required to reverse hypotension and/or support decreased renal function.

No reproductive toxicity studies have been conducted with the combination of aliskiren and hydrochlorothiazide. However, these studies have been conducted for aliskiren as well as hydrochlorothiazide alone.

Reproductive toxicity studies of aliskiren hemifumarate did not reveal any evidence of teratogenicity at oral doses up to 600 mg aliskiren/kg/day (20 times the maximum recommended human dose [MRHD] of 300 mg/day on a mg/m^2 basis) in pregnant rats or up to 100 mg aliskiren/kg/day (seven times the MRHD on a mg/m^2 basis) in pregnant rabbits. Fetal birth weight was adversely affected in rabbits at 50 mg/kg/day (3.2 times the MRHD on a mg/m^2 basis). Aliskiren was present in placenta, amniotic fluid and fetuses of pregnant rabbits.

When pregnant mice and rats were given hydrochlorothiazide at doses up to 3000 and 1000 mg/kg/day, respectively (about 600 and 400 times the MRHD) during their respective periods of major organogenesis, there was no evidence of fetal harm.

8.3 Nursing Mothers

It is not known whether aliskiren is excreted in human milk, but aliskiren was secreted in the milk of lactating rats. Thiazides appear in human milk. Because of the potential for adverse effects on the nursing infant, a decision should be made whether to discontinue nursing or discontinue the drug, taking into account the importance of the drug to the mother.

8.4 Pediatric Use

Safety and effectiveness in pediatric patients have not been established.

8.5 Geriatric Use

In the short-term controlled clinical trials of Tekturna HCT, 325 (19.6%) patients treated with Tekturna HCT were ≥65 years and 53 (3.2%) were ≥75 years. No overall differences in safety or effectiveness were observed between these subjects and younger subjects, and other reported clinical experience has not identified differences in responses between the elderly and younger patients, but greater sensitivity of some older individuals cannot be ruled out.

10 OVERDOSAGE

Aliskiren

Limited data are available related to overdosage in humans. The most likely manifestation of overdosage would be hypotension. If symptomatic hypotension should occur, supportive treatment should be initiated.

Hydrochlorothiazide

The most common signs and symptoms of overdose observed in humans are those caused by electrolyte depletion (hypokalemia, hypochloremia, hyponatremia) and dehydration resulting from excessive diuresis. If digitalis has also been administered, hypokalemia may accentuate cardiac arrhythmias. The degree to which hydrochlorothiazide is removed by hemodialysis has not been established. The oral LD_{50} of hydrochlorothiazide is greater than 10 g/kg in both mice and rats.

11 DESCRIPTION

Tekturna HCT is a fixed combination of aliskiren, an orally active, nonpeptide, direct renin inhibitor, and hydrochlorothiazide, a thiazide diuretic.

Aliskiren

Aliskiren hemifumarate is chemically described as (2S,4S,5S,7S)-N-(2-Carbamoyl-2-methylpropyl)-5-amino-4-hydroxy-2,7-diisopropyl-8-[4-methoxy-3-(3-methoxypropoxy)phenyl]-octanamide hemifumarate and its structural formula is

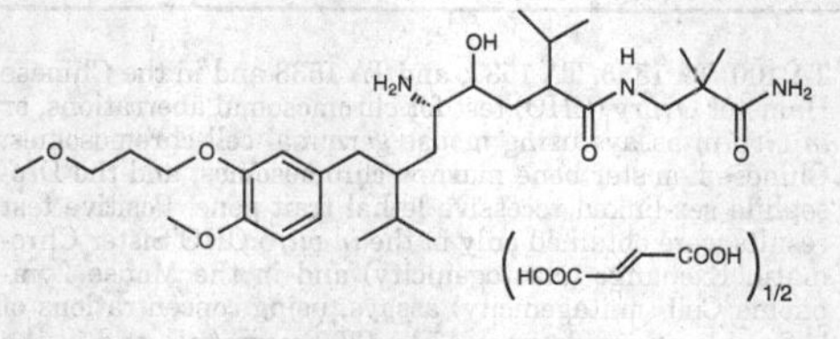

Molecular formula: $C_{30}H_{53}N_3O_6 \bullet 0.5\ C_4H_4O_4$

Aliskiren hemifumarate is a white to slightly yellowish crystalline powder with a molecular weight of 609.8 (free base- 551.8). It is soluble in phosphate buffer, n-Octanol, and highly soluble in water.

Hydrochlorothiazide

Hydrochlorothiazide USP is a white, or practically white, practically odorless, crystalline powder. It is slightly soluble in water; freely soluble in sodium hydroxide solution, in *n*-butylamine, and in dimethylformamide; sparingly soluble in methanol; and insoluble in ether, in chloroform, and in dilute mineral acids. Hydrochlorothiazide is chemically described as 6-chloro-3,4-dihydro-2*H*-1,2,4-benzothiadiazine-7-sulfonamide 1,1-dioxide.

Hydrochlorothiazide is a thiazide diuretic. Its empirical formula is $C_7H_8ClN_3O_4S_2$, its molecular weight is 297.73, and its structural formula is

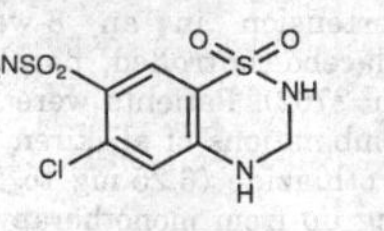

Tekturna HCT tablets are formulated for oral administration to contain aliskiren and hydrochlorothiazide, USP 150/12.5 mg, 150/25 mg, 300/12.5 mg and 300/25 mg. The inactive ingredients for all strengths of the tablets are colloidal silicon dioxide, crospovidone, hydroxypropyl methylcellulose, iron oxide colorants, lactose, magnesium stearate, microcrystalline cellulose, polyethylene glycol, povidone, talc, titanium dioxide, and wheat starch.

12 CLINICAL PHARMACOLOGY

12.1 Mechanism of Action

Aliskiren

Renin is secreted by the kidney in response to decreases in blood volume and renal perfusion. Renin cleaves angiotensinogen to form the inactive decapeptide angiotensin I (Ang I). Ang I is converted to the active octapeptide angiotensin II (Ang II) by angiotensin-converting enzyme (ACE) and non-ACE pathways. Ang II is a powerful vasoconstrictor and leads to the release of catecholamines from the adrenal medulla and prejunctional nerve endings. It also promotes aldosterone secretion and sodium reabsorption. Together, these effects increase blood pressure. Ang II also inhibits renin release, thus providing a negative feedback to the system. This cycle, from renin through angiotensin to aldosterone and its associated negative feedback loop, is known as the renin-angiotensin-aldosterone system (RAAS). Aliskiren is a direct renin inhibitor, decreasing plasma renin activity (PRA) and inhibiting the conversion of angiotensinogen to Ang I. Whether aliskiren affects other RAAS components, e.g., ACE or non-ACE pathways, is not known.

All agents that inhibit the RAAS, including renin inhibitors, suppress the negative feedback loop, leading to a compensatory rise in plasma renin concentration. When this rise occurs during treatment with ACE inhibitors and ARBs, the result is increased levels of PRA. During treatment with aliskiren, however, the effect of increased renin levels is blocked, so that PRA, Ang I and Ang II are all reduced, whether aliskiren is used as monotherapy or in combination with other antihypertensive agents.

Hydrochlorothiazide

Hydrochlorothiazide is a thiazide diuretic. Thiazides affect the renal tubular mechanisms of electrolyte reabsorption, directly increasing excretion of sodium and chloride in approximately equivalent amounts. Indirectly, the diuretic action of hydrochlorothiazide reduces plasma volume, with consequent increases in plasma renin activity, increases in aldosterone secretion, increases in urinary potassium loss, and decreases in serum potassium. The renin-aldosterone link is mediated by angiotensin II, so coadministration of agents that block the production or function of angiotensin II tends to reverse the potassium loss associated with these diuretics.

The mechanism of action of the antihypertensive effect of thiazides is unknown.

12.2 Pharmacodynamics

Tekturna HCT

In placebo-controlled clinical trials, PRA was decreased with aliskiren monotherapy (ranging from 54% to 65%) and increased with hydrochlorothiazide monotherapy (ranging from 4% to 72%). Treatment with Tekturna HCT resulted in PRA reductions ranging from approximately 46% to 63% in various doses despite the increase in PRA with hydrochlorothiazide treatment. The clinical implications of the differences in effect on PRA are not known.

Aliskiren

PRA reductions in clinical trials ranged from approximately 50% to 80%, were not dose-related and did not correlate with blood pressure reductions. The clinical implications of the differences in effect on PRA are not known.

Hydrochlorothiazide

After oral administration of hydrochlorothiazide, diuresis begins within 2 hours, peaks in about 4 hours, and lasts about 6 to 12 hours.

12.3 Pharmacokinetics

Absorption and Distribution

Tekturna HCT

Following oral administration of Tekturna HCT combination tablets, the median peak plasma concentration time are within 1 hour for aliskiren and 2.5 hours for hydrochlorothiazide. When taken with food, mean AUC and C_{max} of aliskiren are decreased by 60% and 82%, respectively; mean AUC and C_{max} of hydrochlorothiazide increased by 13% and 10%, respectively. As a result, patients should establish a routine pattern for taking Tekturna HCT with regard to meals and should be advised that high-fat meals decrease absorption of aliskiren substantially.

Hydrochlorothiazide

Hydrochlorothiazide crosses the placental but not the blood-brain barrier and is excreted in breast milk.

Metabolism and Elimination

Aliskiren

About one-fourth of the absorbed dose appears in the urine as parent drug. How much of the absorbed dose is metabolized is unknown. Based on the *in vitro* studies, the major enzyme responsible for aliskiren metabolism appears to be CYP 3A4.

Hydrochlorothiazide

Hydrochlorothiazide is not metabolized but is eliminated rapidly by the kidney. At least 61% of the oral dose is eliminated as unchanged drug within 24 hours. The elimination half-life is between 5.8 and 18.9 hours.

Special Populations

Pediatric Patients

The pharmacokinetics of aliskiren have not been investigated in patients <18 years of age.

Geriatric Patients

The pharmacokinetics of aliskiren were studied in the elderly (≥65 years). Exposure (measured by AUC) is increased in elderly patients. Adjustment of the starting dose is not required in these patients [*see Dosage and Administration (2)*].

Race

Too few non-Caucasians have been studied with Tekturna HCT to assess pharmacokinetic differences among races. The pharmacokinetic differences among Blacks, Caucasians, and Japanese are minimal with aliskiren therapy.

Renal Impairment

The pharmacokinetics of aliskiren were evaluated in patients with varying degrees of renal impairment. Rate and extent of exposure (AUC and C_{max}) of aliskiren in subjects with renal impairment did not show a consistent correlation

Table 1: Placebo-Subtracted Reductions in Seated Trough Cuff Blood Pressure in Combination with Hydrochlorothiazide

Aliskiren, mg	Placebo Mean Change	Hydrochlorothiazide, mg			
		0	6.25	12.5	25
		Placebo-subtracted	Placebo-subtracted	Placebo-subtracted	Placebo-subtracted
0	7.5/6.9	—	3.5/2.1	6.4/3.2	6.8/2.4
75	—	1.9/1.8	6.8/3.8	8.2/4.2	9.8/4.5
150	—	4.8/2	7.8/3.4	10.1/5	12/5.7
300	—	8.3/3.3		12.3/7	13.7/7.3

Table 2: Reductions in Seated Trough Cuff Blood Pressure in the Placebo-Controlled Studies of Aliskiren Monotherapy

Study	Placebo Mean Change	Aliskiren Daily Dose, mg			
		75	150	300	600
		Placebo-subtracted	Placebo-subtracted	Placebo-subtracted	Placebo-subtracted
1	2.9/3.3	5.7/4*	5.9/4.5*	11.2/7.5*	—
2	5.3/6.3	—	6.1/2.9*	10.5/5.4*	10.4/5.2*
3	10/8.6	2.2/1.7	2.1/1.7	5.1/3.7*	—
4	7.5/6.9	1.9/1.8	4.8/2*	8.3/3.3*	—
5	3.8/4.9	—	9.3/5.4*	10.9/6.2*	12.1/7.6*
6	4.6/4.1	—	—	8.4/4.9†	—

* $p<0.05$ vs. placebo by ANCOVA with Dunnett's procedure for multiple comparisons.
$\dagger$ $p<0.05$ vs. placebo by ANCOVA for the pairwise comparison.

with the severity of renal impairment. Adjustment of the starting dose is not required in patients with mild or moderate renal impairment, but Tekturna HCT is not recommended in patients with severe renal impairment [see Dosage and Administration (2) and Warnings and Precautions (5.4)].

Hepatic Impairment
The pharmacokinetics of aliskiren were not significantly affected in patients with mild-to-severe liver disease. Consequently, adjustment of the starting dose is not required in these patients [see Dosage and Administration (2)].

13 NONCLINICAL TOXICOLOGY

13.1 Carcinogenesis, Mutagenesis, Impairment of Fertility

Tekturna HCT
No carcinogenicity, mutagenicity or fertility studies have been conducted with Tekturna HCT. However, these studies have been conducted for aliskiren as well as hydrochlorothiazide alone.

Aliskiren
Carcinogenic potential was assessed in a 2-year rat study and a 6-month transgenic (rasH2) mouse study with aliskiren hemifumarate at oral doses of up to 1500 mg aliskiren/kg/day. Although there were no statistically significant increases in tumor incidence associated with exposure to aliskiren, mucosal epithelial hyperplasia (with or without erosion/ulceration) was observed in the lower gastrointestinal tract at doses of 750 or more mg/kg/day in both species, with a colonic adenoma identified in one rat and a cecal adenocarcinoma identified in another, rare tumors in the strain of rat studied. On a systemic exposure (AUC_{0-24hr}) basis, 1500 mg/kg/day in the rat is about 4 times and in the mouse about 1.5 times the maximum recommended human dose (300 mg aliskiren/day). Mucosal hyperplasia in the cecum or colon of rats was also observed at doses of 250 mg/kg/day (the lowest tested dose) as well as at higher doses in 4- and 13-week studies.

Aliskiren hemifumarate was devoid of genotoxic potential in the Ames reverse mutation assay with *S. typhimurium* and *E. coli*, the *in vitro* Chinese hamster ovary cell chromosomal aberration assay, the *in vitro* Chinese hamster V79 cell gene mutation test and the *in vivo* mouse bone marrow micronucleus assay.

Fertility of male and female rats was unaffected at doses of up to 250 mg aliskiren/kg/day (8 times the maximum recommended human dose of 300 mg Tekturna/60 kg on a mg/m^2 basis).

Hydrochlorothiazide
Two-year feeding studies in mice and rats conducted under the auspices of the National Toxicology Program (NTP) uncovered no evidence of a carcinogenic potential of hydrochlorothiazide in female mice (at doses of up to approximately 600 mg/kg/day) or in male and female rats (at doses of up to approximately 100 mg/kg/day). The NTP, however, found equivocal evidence for hepatocarcinogenicity in male mice.

Hydrochlorothiazide was not genotoxic *in vitro* in the Ames mutagenicity assay of *S. typhimurium* strains TA 98,

TA 100, TA 1535, TA 1537, and TA 1538 and in the Chinese Hamster Ovary (CHO) test for chromosomal aberrations, or *in vivo* in assays using mouse germinal cell chromosomes, Chinese hamster bone marrow chromosomes, and the Drosophila sex-linked recessive lethal trait gene. Positive test results were obtained only in the *in vitro* CHO Sister Chromatid Exchange (clastogenicity) and in the Mouse Lymphoma Cell (mutagenicity) assays, using concentrations of hydrochlorothiazide from 43 to 1300 mcgm/mL, and in the Aspergillums Nidulans nondisjunction assay at an unspecified concentration.

Hydrochlorothiazide had no adverse effects on the fertility of mice and rats of either sex in studies wherein these species were exposed, via their diet, to doses of up to 100 and 4 mg/kg, respectively, prior to mating and throughout gestation. These doses of hydrochlorothiazide in mice and rats represent 19 and 1.5 times, respectively, the maximum recommended human dose on an mg/m^2 basis. (Calculations assume an oral dose of 25 mg/day and a 60-kg patient.)

14 CLINICAL STUDIES

Tekturna HCT
In all clinical trials including over 6,200 patients, more than 2,700 patients were exposed to combinations of aliskiren and hydrochlorothiazide. The safety and efficacy of Tekturna HCT were evaluated in patients with mild-to-moderate hypertension in an 8-week, randomized, double-blind, placebo-controlled, parallel-group, 15-arm factorial trial (n=2762). Patients were randomized to receive various combinations of aliskiren (75 mg to 300 mg) plus hydrochlorothiazide (6.25 mg to 25 mg) once daily (without titrating up from monotherapy) and followed for blood pressure response. The combination of aliskiren and hydrochlorothiazide resulted in additive placebo-adjusted decreases in systolic and diastolic blood pressure at trough of 10-14/5-7 mmHg at doses of 150-300 mg/12.5-25 mg, compared to 5-8/2-3 mmHg for aliskiren 150 mg to 300 mg and 6-7/2-3 mmHg for hydrochlorothiazide 12.5 mg to 25 mg, alone. Blood pressure reductions with the combinations were greater than the reductions with the monotherapies as shown in Table 1.
[See table 1 above]
The safety and efficacy of Tekturna HCT as initial therapy was evaluated in this trial. All patients randomized to the combination groups received the combination treatment of Tekturna HCT at assigned doses as initial therapy without titration from monotherapy. The figures [see Indications and Usage (1)] display the probability that a patient will achieve systolic or diastolic blood pressure goal with Tekturna HCT 300/25 mg, based upon their baseline systolic or diastolic blood pressure. At all levels of baseline blood pressure, the probability of achieving any given diastolic or systolic goal is greater with the combination than for either monotherapy.
The antihypertensive effect of Tekturna HCT was largely manifested within 1 week. The maximum antihypertensive effect was generally attained after about 4 weeks of therapy. One active-controlled trial investigated the addition of 300 mg aliskiren in obese hypertensive patients who did not

respond adequately to hydrochlorothiazide 25 mg, and showed incremental decreases of systolic and diastolic blood pressure of approximately 7/4 mmHg.
In long-term follow-up studies (without placebo control) the effect of the combination of aliskiren and hydrochlorothiazide was maintained for over 1 year.
The antihypertensive effect was independent of age and gender. There were too few non-Caucasians to assess differences in blood pressure effects by race.

Aliskiren Monotherapy
The antihypertensive effects of aliskiren have been demonstrated in six randomized, double-blind, placebo-controlled, 8-week clinical trials in patients with mild-to-moderate hypertension. The placebo response and placebo-subtracted changes from baseline in seated trough cuff blood pressure are shown in Table 2.
[See table 2 at left]
The studies included approximately 2,730 patients given doses of 75 mg to 600 mg of aliskiren and 1,231 patients given placebo. As shown in Table 2, there is some increase in response with administered dose in all studies, with reasonable effects seen at 150 mg to 300 mg, and no clear further increase at 600 mg. A substantial proportion (85% to 90%) of the blood pressure lowering effect was observed within 2 weeks of treatment. Studies with ambulatory blood pressure monitoring showed reasonable control throughout the interdosing interval, e.g., the ratios of mean daytime to mean nighttime ambulatory BP ranged from 0.6 to 0.9. Patients in the placebo-controlled trials continued open-label aliskiren for up to one year. A persistent blood pressure lowering effect was demonstrated by a randomized withdrawal study (patients randomized to continued drug or placebo), which showed a statistically significant difference between patients kept on aliskiren and those randomized to placebo. With cessation of treatment, blood pressure gradually returned toward baseline levels over a period of several weeks. There was no evidence of rebound hypertension after abrupt cessation of therapy.
The effectiveness of aliskiren was demonstrated across all demographic subgroups, although Black patients tended to have smaller reductions in blood pressure than Caucasians and Asians, as has been seen with ACE inhibitors and ARBs.

Aliskiren in Combination with Other Antihypertensives
Valsartan
Aliskiren 150 mg and 300 mg and valsartan 160 mg and 320 mg were studied alone and in combination in an 8-week, 1,797-patient, randomized, double-blind, placebo-controlled, parallel-group, 4-arm, dose-escalation study. The dosages of aliskiren and valsartan were started at 150 mg and 160 mg, respectively, and increased at four weeks to 300 mg and 320 mg, respectively. Seated trough cuff blood pressure was measured at baseline, 4, and 8 weeks. Blood pressure reductions with the combinations were greater than the reductions with the monotherapies as shown in Table 3.

Table 3: Placebo-Subtracted Reductions in Seated Trough Cuff Blood Pressure of Aliskiren in Combination with Valsartan

Aliskiren, mg	Placebo Mean Change	Valsartan, mg		
		0	160	320
0	4.6/4.1*	—	5.6/3.9	8.2/5.6
150	—	5.4/2.7	10.0/5.7	—
300	—	8.4/4.9	—	12.6/8.1

* The placebo change is 5.2/4.8 for Week 4 endpoint which was used for the dose groups containing aliskiren 150 mg or valsartan 160 mg.

ACE inhibitors and Amlodipine
Aliskiren has not been studied when added to maximal doses of ACE inhibitors to determine whether aliskiren produces additional blood pressure reduction with a maximal dose of an ACE inhibitor. Aliskiren 150 mg provided additional blood pressure reduction when coadministered with amlodipine 5 mg in one study, but the combination was not statistically significantly better than amlodipine 10 mg.

16 HOW SUPPLIED/STORAGE AND HANDLING
Tekturna HCT is supplied as biconvex, ovaloid film-coated tablets.
All strengths are packaged in bottles and unit-dose blister packages (10 strips of 10 tablets) as described below.
[See table 4 at top of next page]
Storage
Store at 25°C (77°F); excursions permitted to 15-30°C (59-86°F) [see USP Controlled Room Temperature].
Protect from moisture.
Dispense in tight container (USP).

Table 4: Tekturna HCT Tablets Supply

Tablet	Color	Imprint	Imprint	NDC 0078-XXXX-XX		
Aliskiren/HCTZ		Side 1	Side 2	Bottle of 30	Bottle of 90	Blister Packages of 100
150 mg/12.5 mg	White	NVR	LCI	0521-15	0521-34	0521-35
150 mg/25 mg	Pale Yellow	NVR	CLL	0522-15	0522-34	0522-35
300 mg/12.5 mg	Violet White	NVR	CVI	0523-15	0523-34	0523-35
300 mg/25 mg	Light Yellow	NVR	CVV	0524-15	0524-34	0524-35

17   PATIENT COUNSELING INFORMATION

Healthcare professionals should instruct their patients to read the Patient Package Insert before starting Tekturna HCT and to reread each time the prescription is renewed. Patients should be instructed to inform their doctor or pharmacist if they develop any unusual symptom, or if any known symptom persists or worsens.

Pregnancy
Female patients of childbearing age should be told about the consequences of exposure to drugs that act on the renin-angiotensin system. Discuss other treatment options with female patients planning to become pregnant. These patients should be asked to report pregnancies to their physicians as soon as possible.

Symptomatic Hypotension
A patient receiving Tekturna HCT should be cautioned that lightheadedness can occur, especially during the first days of therapy, and that it should be reported to the prescribing physician. The patients should be told that if syncope occurs, Tekturna HCT should be discontinued until the physician has been consulted.

All patients should be cautioned that inadequate fluid intake, excessive perspiration, diarrhea, or vomiting can lead to an excessive fall in blood pressure, with the same consequences of lightheadedness and possible syncope.

Potassium Supplements
A patient receiving Tekturna HCT should be told not to use potassium supplements or salt substitutes containing potassium without consulting the prescribing physician.

Relationship to Meals
Patients should establish a routine pattern for taking Tekturna HCT with regard to meals. High-fat meals decrease absorption substantially.

PATIENT INFORMATION

Tekturna HCT® (tek-turn-a HCT)
(aliskiren and hydrochlorothiazide, USP)
Combination Tablets
Read the Patient Information that comes with Tekturna HCT before you start taking it and each time you get a refill. There may be new information. This leaflet does not take the place of talking with your doctor about your condition and treatment.

IMPORTANT WARNING: Tekturna HCT may harm an unborn baby, causing injury and even death. If you get pregnant, stop taking Tekturna HCT and call your doctor right away. If you plan to become pregnant, talk to your doctor about other medicines to treat your high blood pressure before taking Tekturna HCT.

What is Tekturna HCT?
Tekturna HCT contains two prescription medicines in one tablet that work together to lower blood pressure. It contains:
• aliskiren (Tekturna), a direct renin inhibitor (DRI)
• hydrochlorothiazide, a diuretic (water pill)
Aliskiren (Tekturna) reduces the effect of renin, and the harmful process that narrows blood vessels. Aliskiren also helps blood vessels relax and widen so blood pressure is lower. Hydrochlorothiazide reduces the amount of salt and water in your body so your blood pressure is lower.
Tekturna HCT may be used to lower high blood pressure in adults
• when one medicine to lower high blood pressure is not enough
• as the first medicine to lower high blood pressure if your doctor decides that you are likely to need more than one medicine
Tekturna HCT has not been studied in children under 18 years of age.
Your doctor may prescribe other medicines for you to take along with Tekturna HCT to treat your high blood pressure.

What is high blood pressure (hypertension)?
Blood pressure is the force that pushes the blood through your blood vessels to all the organs of your body. You have high blood pressure when the force of your blood moving through your blood vessels is too great. One cause of high blood pressure is renin, a chemical in the body that starts a process that makes blood vessels narrow, leading to high blood pressure.
Tekturna HCT reduces high blood pressure. Medicines that lower your blood pressure lower your chance of having a stroke or heart attack. High blood pressure makes the heart work harder to pump blood throughout the body and causes damage to the blood vessels. If high blood pressure is not treated, it can lead to stroke, heart attack, heart failure, kidney failure, and vision problems.

Who should not take Tekturna HCT?
• If you get pregnant, stop taking Tekturna HCT and call your doctor right away. If you plan to become pregnant, talk to your doctor about other treatment options for your high blood pressure.
• Do not take Tekturna HCT if you make very little or no urine due to kidney problems.
• Do not take Tekturna HCT if you are allergic to any of its ingredients. See the end of this leaflet for a complete list of the ingredients in Tekturna HCT.

What should I tell my doctor before taking Tekturna HCT?
Tell your doctor about all your medical conditions, including whether you:
• are pregnant or planning to become pregnant. See IMPORTANT WARNING.
• have any allergies or asthma
• have kidney problems
• have liver problems
• have systemic lupus erythematosus (SLE). Tekturna HCT can make your SLE active or worse.
• have ever had a reaction called angioedema, to an ACE inhibitor medicine. Angioedema causes swelling of the face, lips, tongue, throat, arms and legs, and may cause difficulty breathing.
• are breast-feeding. It is not known if Tekturna HCT passes into your breast milk.

Tell your doctor about all the medicines you take including prescription and nonprescription medicines, vitamins and herbal supplements. Especially tell your doctor if you are taking:
• other medicines for high blood pressure or a heart problem
• atorvastatin (medicine to lower cholesterol in your blood)
• water pills (also called "diuretics")
• medicines for treating fungus or fungal infections
• cyclosporine (a medicine used to suppress the immune system)
• potassium-containing medicines, potassium supplements, or salt substitutes containing potassium
• cholestyramine (for example, Questran, Questran Light, Cholestyramine Light, Locholest Light, Locholest, Prevalite) (medicines to lower the cholesterol in your blood)
• colestipol (for example, Colestipol hydrochloride, Colestid, Flavored Colestid) (medicines to lower the cholesterol in your blood)
• potassium supplements
• medicines to treat diabetes, including insulin
• lithium, a medicine used in some types of depression. Do not take Tekturna HCT if you are taking lithium.
• Nonsteroidal anti-inflammatory (NSAIDs) medicines. Ask your doctor if you are not sure if you are taking one of these medicines.
• blood thinners
• barbiturate or narcotic medicines. Ask your doctor if you are not sure if you are taking one of these medicines.
Your doctor or pharmacist will know what medicines are safe to take together. Know your medicines. Keep a list of your medicines and show it to your doctor or pharmacist when you get a new medicine.

How should I take Tekturna HCT?
• Take Tekturna HCT exactly as prescribed by your doctor. It is important to take Tekturna HCT every day to control your blood pressure.
• Take Tekturna HCT once each day, about the same time each day.
• Take Tekturna HCT the same way every day, either with or without a meal.
• Your doctor may change your dose of Tekturna HCT if needed.
• If you miss a dose of Tekturna HCT, take it as soon as you remember. If it is close to your next dose, do not take the missed dose. Just take the next dose at your regular time.
• If you take too much Tekturna HCT, call your doctor or a Poison Control Center, or go to the nearest hospital emergency room.

What are the possible side effects of Tekturna HCT?
Tekturna HCT may cause serious side effects:
• **Injury or death to an unborn baby.** See IMPORTANT WARNING.
• **Low blood pressure (hypotension).** Your blood pressure may get too low if you also take water pills, are on a low-salt diet, get dialysis treatments, have heart problems, or get sick with vomiting or diarrhea. Drinking alcohol and taking certain medicines (barbiturates or narcotics) can cause low blood pressure to get worse. Lie down if you feel faint or dizzy, and call your doctor right away.
• **Angioedema.** Aliskiren in Tekturna HCT can cause swelling of the face, lips, tongue, throat, arms and legs, or the whole body. Get medical help right away and tell your doctor if you get any one or more of these symptoms. Angioedema can happen at any time while you are taking Tekturna HCT.
• **Active or worsened Systemic Lupus Erythematosus (SLE).** If you have SLE, tell your doctor right away if you get any new or worse symptoms.
Common side effects of Tekturna HCT include:
• dizziness
• flu-like symptoms
• diarrhea
• cough
• tiredness
Other less common side effects include skin rash.
Tell your doctor if you have any side effect that bothers you or that does not go away. These are not all of the possible side effects of Tekturna HCT. For a complete list of side effects, ask your doctor or pharmacist.

How do I store Tekturna HCT?
• Store Tekturna HCT tablets at room temperature between 59°F-86°F (15°C-30°C).
• Keep Tekturna HCT in the original prescription bottle in a dry place. Do not remove the desiccant (drying agent) from the bottle.
Keep Tekturna HCT and all medicines out of the reach of children.
General information about Tekturna HCT
Medicines are sometimes prescribed for conditions not listed in the patient information leaflet. Do not take Tekturna HCT for a condition for which it was not prescribed. Do not give Tekturna HCT to other people, even if they have the same condition or symptoms you have. It may harm them.
This leaflet summarizes the most important information about Tekturna HCT. If you have questions about Tekturna HCT talk with your doctor. You can ask your doctor or pharmacist for information that is written for healthcare professionals.
For more information about Tekturna HCT, visit www.TekturnaHCT.com, or call 1-888-669-6682.
What are the ingredients in Tekturna HCT?
Active ingredients: Aliskiren and hydrochlorothiazide
Inactive ingredients: Colloidal silicon dioxide, crospovidone, hydroxypropyl methylcellulose, iron oxide colorants, lactose, magnesium stearate, microcrystalline cellulose, polyethylene glycol, povidone, talc, titanium dioxide, and wheat starch
Call your doctor for medical advice about side effects. You may report side effects to FDA at 1-800-FDA-1088.

T2010-67/T2010-17

Manufactured by:
Novartis Pharma Produktions GmbH
Wehr, Germany
Distributed by:
Novartis Pharmaceuticals Corporation
East Hanover, New Jersey 07936
©Novartis

Shown in Product Identification Guide, page 316

TOBI®   ℞
[toe-bye]
(tobramycin inhalation solution, USP)
Nebulizer Solution—For Inhalation Use Only
Rx only
Prescribing Information

The following prescribing information is based on official labeling in effect July 2010.

DESCRIPTION

TOBI® is a tobramycin solution for inhalation. It is a sterile, clear, slightly yellow, non-pyrogenic, aqueous solution with the pH and salinity adjusted specifically for administration by a compressed air driven reusable nebulizer. The chemical formula for tobramycin is $C_{18}H_{37}N_5O_9$ and the molecular weight is 467.52. Tobramycin is O-3-amino-3-deoxy-α-D-glucopyranosyl-(1→4)-O-[2,6-diamino-2,3,6-trideoxy-α-D-*ribo*-hexopyranosyl-(1→6)]-2-deoxy-L-streptamine. The structural formula for tobramycin is:

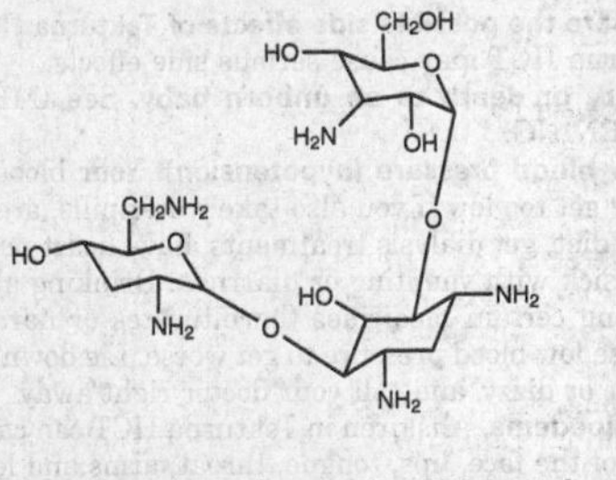

Each single-use 5 mL ampule contains 300 mg tobramycin and 11.25 mg sodium chloride in sterile water for injection. Sulfuric acid and sodium hydroxide are added to adjust the pH to 6.0. Nitrogen is used for sparging. All ingredients meet USP requirements. The formulation contains no preservatives.

CLINICAL PHARMACOLOGY

TOBI® is specifically formulated for administration by inhalation. When inhaled, tobramycin is concentrated in the airways.

Pharmacokinetics

TOBI® contains tobramycin, a cationic polar molecule that does not readily cross epithelial membranes.[1] The bioavailability of TOBI® may vary because of individual differences in nebulizer performance and airway pathology.[2] Following administration of TOBI®, tobramycin remains concentrated primarily in the airways.

Sputum Concentrations: Ten minutes after inhalation of the first 300-mg dose of TOBI®, the average concentration of tobramycin was 1237 µg/g (ranging from 35 to 7414 µg/g) in sputum. Tobramycin does not accumulate in sputum; after 20 weeks of therapy with the TOBI® regimen, the average concentration of tobramycin at ten minutes after inhalation was 1154 µg/g (ranging from 39 to 8085 µg/g) in sputum. High variability of tobramycin concentration in sputum was observed. Two hours after inhalation, sputum concentrations declined to approximately 14% of tobramycin levels at ten minutes after inhalation.

Serum Concentrations: The average serum concentration of tobramycin one hour after inhalation of a single 300-mg dose of TOBI® by cystic fibrosis patients was 0.95 µg/mL. After 20 weeks of therapy on the TOBI® regimen, the average serum tobramycin concentration one hour after dosing was 1.05 µg/mL.

Elimination: The elimination half-life of tobramycin from serum is approximately 2 hours after intravenous (IV) administration. Assuming tobramycin absorbed following inhalation behaves similarly to tobramycin following IV administration, systemically absorbed tobramycin is eliminated principally by glomerular filtration. Unabsorbed tobramycin, following TOBI® administration, is probably eliminated primarily in expectorated sputum.

Microbiology

Tobramycin is an aminoglycoside antibiotic produced by *Streptomyces tenebrarius*.[1] It acts primarily by disrupting protein synthesis, leading to altered cell membrane permeability, progressive disruption of the cell envelope, and eventual cell death.[3]

Tobramycin has *in-vitro* activity against a wide range of gram-negative organisms including *Pseudomonas aeruginosa*. It is bactericidal at concentrations equal to or slightly greater than inhibitory concentrations.

Susceptibility Testing

A single sputum sample from a cystic fibrosis patient may contain multiple morphotypes of *Pseudomonas aeruginosa* and each morphotype may have a different level of *in-vitro* susceptibility to tobramycin. Treatment for 6 months with TOBI® in two clinical studies did not affect the susceptibility of the majority of *P. aeruginosa* isolates tested; however, increased minimum inhibitory concentrations (MICs) were noted in some patients. The clinical significance of this information has not been clearly established in the treatment of *P. aeruginosa* in cystic fibrosis patients. For additional information regarding the effects of TOBI® on *P. aeruginosa* MIC values and bacterial sputum density, please refer to the CLINICAL STUDIES section.

The *in-vitro* antimicrobial susceptibility test methods used for parenteral tobramycin therapy can be used to monitor the susceptibility of *P. aeruginosa* isolated from cystic fibrosis patients. If decreased susceptibility is noted, the results should be reported to the clinician.

Susceptibility breakpoints established for parenteral administration of tobramycin do not apply to aerosolized administration of TOBI®. The relationship between *in-vitro* susceptibility test results and clinical outcome with TOBI® therapy is not clear.

INDICATIONS AND USAGE

TOBI® is indicated for the management of cystic fibrosis patients with *P. aeruginosa*.

Safety and efficacy have not been demonstrated in patients under the age of 6 years, patients with FEV_1 <25% or >75% predicted, or patients colonized with *Burkholderia cepacia* (*see CLINICAL STUDIES*).

CONTRAINDICATIONS

TOBI® is contraindicated in patients with a known hypersensitivity to any aminoglycoside.

WARNINGS

Caution should be exercised when prescribing TOBI® to patients with known or suspected renal, auditory, vestibular, or neuromuscular dysfunction. Patients receiving concomitant parenteral aminoglycoside therapy should be monitored as clinically appropriate.

Aminoglycosides can cause fetal harm when administered to a pregnant woman. Aminoglycosides cross the placenta, and streptomycin has been associated with several reports of total, irreversible, bilateral congenital deafness in pediatric patients exposed *in utero*. Patients who use TOBI® during pregnancy, or become pregnant while taking TOBI® should be apprised of the potential hazard to the fetus.

Ototoxicity

Ototoxicity, as measured by complaints of hearing loss or by audiometric evaluations, did not occur with TOBI® therapy during clinical studies. However, transient tinnitus occurred in eight TOBI®-treated patients versus no placebo patients in the clinical studies. Tinnitus may be a sentinel symptom of ototoxicity, and therefore the onset of this symptom warrants caution (*see ADVERSE REACTIONS*). Ototoxicity, manifested as both auditory and vestibular toxicity, has been reported with parenteral aminoglycosides. Vestibular toxicity may be manifested by vertigo, ataxia or dizziness.

In postmarketing experience, patients receiving TOBI® have reported hearing loss. Some of these reports occurred in patients with previous or concomitant treatment with systemic aminoglycosides. Patients with hearing loss frequently reported tinnitus.

Nephrotoxicity

Nephrotoxicity was not seen during TOBI® clinical studies but has been associated with aminoglycosides as a class. If nephrotoxicity occurs in a patient receiving TOBI®, tobramycin therapy should be discontinued until serum concentrations fall below 2 µg/mL.

Muscular Disorders

TOBI® should be used cautiously in patients with muscular disorders, such as myasthenia gravis or Parkinson's disease, since aminoglycosides may aggravate muscle weakness because of a potential curare-like effect on neuromuscular function.

Bronchospasm

Bronchospasm can occur with inhalation of TOBI®. In clinical studies of TOBI®, changes in FEV_1 measured after the inhaled dose were similar in the TOBI® and placebo groups. Bronchospasm should be treated as medically appropriate.

PRECAUTIONS

Information for Patients

NOTE: In addition to information provided below, a Patient Medication Guide providing instructions for proper use of TOBI® is contained inside the package.

Safety Information

TOBI® is in a class of antibiotics that have caused hearing loss, dizziness, kidney damage, and harm to a fetus. Ringing in the ears and hoarseness were two symptoms that were seen in more patients taking TOBI® than placebo in research studies. Patients with cystic fibrosis can have many symptoms. Some of these symptoms may be related to your medications. If you have new or worsening symptoms, you should tell your doctor.

Hearing: You should tell your doctor if you have ringing in the ears, dizziness, or any changes in hearing.

Kidney Damage: Inform your doctor if you have any history of kidney problems.

Pregnancy: If you want to become pregnant or are pregnant while on TOBI®, you should talk with your doctor about the possibility of TOBI® causing any harm.

Nursing Mothers: If you are nursing a baby, you should talk with your doctor before using TOBI®.

TOBI® Packaging

TOBI® comes in a single dose, ready-to-use ampule containing 300 mg tobramycin. Each foil pouch contains 4 ampules, for 2 days of TOBI® therapy.

Dosage

The 300 mg dose of TOBI® is the same for patients regardless of age or weight. TOBI® has not been studied in patients less than 6 years old. Doses should be inhaled as close to 12 hours apart as possible and not less than 6 hours apart.

You should not mix TOBI® with dornase alfa (PULMOZYME®, Genentech) in the nebulizer.

If you are taking several medications the recommended order is as follows: bronchodilator first, followed by chest physiotherapy, then other inhaled medications and, finally, TOBI®.

Treatment Schedule

You should take TOBI® in repeated cycles of 28 days on drug followed by 28 days off drug. You should take TOBI® twice a day during the 28-day period on drug.

How To Administer TOBI®

THIS INFORMATION IS NOT INTENDED TO REPLACE CONSULTATION WITH YOUR PHYSICIAN AND CF CARE TEAM ABOUT PROPERLY TAKING MEDICATION OR USING INHALATION EQUIPMENT.

TOBI® is specifically formulated for inhalation using a PARI LC PLUS™ Reusable Nebulizer and a DeVilbiss® Pulmo-Aide® air compressor. TOBI® can be taken at home, school, or at work. The following are instructions on how to use the DeVilbiss® Pulmo-Aide® air compressor and PARI LC PLUS™ Reusable Nebulizer to administer TOBI®.

You will need the following supplies:

- TOBI® plastic ampule (vial)
- DeVilbiss® Pulmo-Aide® air compressor
- PARI LC PLUS™ Reusable Nebulizer
- Tubing to connect the nebulizer and compressor
- Clean paper or cloth towels
- Nose clips (optional)

It is important that your nebulizer and compressor function properly before starting your TOBI® therapy.

Note: Please refer to the manufacturers' care and use instructions for important information.

Preparing Your TOBI® for Inhalation

1. Wash your hands thoroughly with soap and water.

2a. TOBI® is packaged with 4 ampules per foil pouch.

2b. Separate one ampule by gently pulling apart at the bottom tabs. Store all remaining ampules in the refrigerator as directed.

3. Lay out the contents of a PARI LC PLUS™ Reusable Nebulizer package on a clean, dry paper or cloth towel. You should have the following parts:
   - Nebulizer Top and Bottom (Nebulizer Cup) Assembly
   - Inspiratory Valve Cap
   - Mouthpiece with Valve
   - Tubing
4. Remove the Nebulizer Top from the Nebulizer Cup by twisting the Nebulizer Top counter-clockwise, and then lifting. Place the Nebulizer Top on the clean paper or cloth towel. Stand the Nebulizer Cup upright on the towel.
5. Connect one end of the tubing to the compressor air outlet. The tubing should fit snugly. Plug in your compressor to an electrical outlet.
6. Open the TOBI® ampule by holding the bottom tab with one hand and twisting off the top of the ampule with the other hand. Be careful not to squeeze the ampule until you are ready to empty its contents into the Nebulizer Cup.
7. Squeeze **all** the contents of the ampule into the Nebulizer Cup.
8. Replace the Nebulizer Top. Note: In order to insert the Nebulizer Top into the Nebulizer Cup, the semi-circle halfway down the stem of the Nebulizer Top should face the Nebulizer Outlet.
9. Attach the Mouthpiece to the Nebulizer Outlet. Then firmly push the Inspiratory Valve Cap in place on the Nebulizer Top. Note: the Inspiratory Valve Cap will fit snugly.
10. Connect the free end of the tubing to the Air Intake on the bottom of the nebulizer, making sure to keep the nebulizer upright. Press the tubing on the Air Intake firmly.

TOBI® Treatment

1. Turn on the compressor.
2. Check for a steady mist from the Mouthpiece. If there is no mist, check all tubing connections and confirm that the compressor is working properly.
3. Sit or stand in an upright position that will allow you to breathe normally.
4. Place Mouthpiece between your teeth and on top of your tongue and breathe normally only through your mouth. Nose clips may help you breathe through your mouth and not through your nose. Do not block airflow with your tongue.
5. Continue treatment until all your TOBI® is gone, and there is no longer any mist being produced. You may hear a sputtering sound when the Nebulizer Cup is empty. The entire TOBI® treatment should take approximately 15 minutes to complete. Note: if you are interrupted, need to cough or rest during your TOBI® treatment, turn off the compressor to save your medication. Turn the compressor back on when you are ready to resume your therapy.
6. Follow the nebulizer cleaning and disinfecting instructions after completing therapy.

Cleaning Your Nebulizer

To reduce the risk of infection, illness or injury from contamination, you must thoroughly clean all parts of the nebulizer as instructed after each treatment. Never use a nebulizer with a clogged nozzle. If the nozzle is clogged, no aerosol mist is produced, which will alter the effectiveness of the treatment. Replace the nebulizer if clogging occurs.

1. Remove tubing from nebulizer and disassemble nebulizer parts.
2. Wash all parts (except tubing) with warm water and liquid dish soap.
3. Rinse thoroughly with warm water and shake out water.
4. Air dry or hand dry nebulizer parts on a clean, lint-free cloth. Reassemble nebulizer when dry, and store.
5. You can also wash all parts of the nebulizer in a dishwasher (except tubing). Place the nebulizer parts in a dishwasher basket, then place on the top rack of the dishwasher. Remove and dry the parts when the cycle is complete.

Disinfecting Your Nebulizer

Your nebulizer is for your use only - Do not share your nebulizer with other people. You must regularly disinfect the nebulizer. Failure to do so could lead to serious or fatal illness.

Clean the nebulizer as described above. Every other treatment day, disinfect the nebulizer parts (except tubing) by boiling them in water for a full 10 minutes. Dry parts on a clean, lint-free cloth.

Care and Use of Your Pulmo-Aide® Compressor

Follow the manufacturer's instructions for care and use of your compressor.

Filter Change:
1. DeVilbiss® Compressor filters should be changed every six months or sooner if filter turns completely gray in color.

Compressor Cleaning:
1. With power switch in the "Off" position, unplug power cord from wall outlet.
2. Wipe outside of the compressor cabinet with a clean, damp cloth every few days to keep dust free.
Caution: Do not submerge in water; doing so will result in compressor damage.

Storage Instructions

You should store TOBI® ampules in a refrigerator (2-8°C or 36-46°F). However, when you don't have a refrigerator available (e.g., transporting your TOBI®), you may store the foil pouches (opened or unopened) at room temperature (up to 25°C/77°F) for up to 28 days.

Avoid exposing TOBI® ampules to intense light.

Unrefrigerated TOBI®, which is normally slightly yellow, may darken with age; however, the color change does not indicate any change in the quality of the product.

You should not use TOBI® if it is cloudy, if there are particles in the solution, or if it has been stored at room temperature for more than 28 days. You should not use TOBI® beyond the expiration date stamped on the ampule.

Additional Information

Nebulizer: 1-800-327-8632
Compressor: 1-800-338-1988
TOBI®: 1-888-NOW-NOVA (1-888-669-6682)

Laboratory Tests

Audiograms

Clinical studies of TOBI® did not identify hearing loss using audiometric tests which evaluated hearing up to 8000 Hz. **Physicians should consider an audiogram for patients who show any evidence of auditory dysfunction, or who are at increased risk for auditory dysfunction.** Tinnitus may be a sentinel symptom of ototoxicity, and therefore the onset of this symptom warrants caution.

Serum Concentrations

In patients with normal renal function treated with TOBI®, serum tobramycin concentrations are approximately 1 μg/mL 1 hour after dose administration and do not require routine monitoring. Serum concentrations of tobramycin in patients with renal dysfunction or patients treated with concomitant parenteral tobramycin should be monitored at the discretion of the treating physician.

Renal Function

The clinical studies of TOBI® did not reveal any imbalance in the percentage of patients in the TOBI® and placebo groups who experienced at least a 50% rise in serum creatinine from baseline (see ADVERSE REACTIONS). Laboratory tests of urine and renal function should be conducted at the discretion of the treating physician.

Drug Interactions

In clinical studies of TOBI®, patients taking TOBI® concomitantly with dornase alfa (PULMOZYME®, Genentech), β-agonists, inhaled corticosteroids, other anti-pseudomonal antibiotics, or parenteral aminoglycosides demonstrated adverse experience profiles similar to the study population as a whole.

Concurrent and/or sequential use of TOBI® with other drugs with neurotoxic or ototoxic potential should be avoided. Some diuretics can enhance aminoglycoside toxicity by altering antibiotic concentrations in serum and tissue. TOBI® should not be administered concomitantly with ethacrynic acid, furosemide, urea, or mannitol.

Carcinogenesis, Mutagenesis, Impairment of Fertility

A two-year rat inhalation toxicology study to assess carcinogenic potential of TOBI® has been completed. Rats were exposed to TOBI® for up to 1.5 hours per day for 95 weeks. The clinical formulation of the drug was used for this carcinogenicity study. Serum levels of tobramycin of up to 35 mcg/mL were measured in rats, in contrast to the average 1 mcg/mL levels observed in cystic fibrosis patients in clinical trials. There was no drug-related increase in the incidence of any variety of tumor.

Additionally, TOBI® has been evaluated for genotoxicity in a battery of in-vitro and in-vivo tests. The Ames bacterial reversion test, conducted with 5 tester strains, failed to show a significant increase in revertants with or without metabolic activation in all strains. Tobramycin was negative in the mouse lymphoma forward mutation assay, did not induce chromosomal aberrations in Chinese hamster ovary cells, and was negative in the mouse micronucleus test. Subcutaneous administration of up to 100 mg/kg of tobramycin did not affect mating behavior or cause impairment of fertility in male or female rats.

Pregnancy

Teratogenic Effects—Pregnancy Category D
(See WARNINGS.)

No reproduction toxicology studies have been conducted with TOBI®. However, subcutaneous administration of tobramycin at doses of 100 or 20 mg/kg/day during organogenesis was not teratogenic in rats or rabbits, respectively. Doses of tobramycin ≥40 mg/kg/day were severely maternally toxic to rabbits and precluded the evaluation of teratogenicity. Aminoglycosides can cause fetal harm (e.g., congenital deafness) when administered to a pregnant woman. Ototoxicity was not evaluated in offspring during nonclinical reproduction toxicity studies with tobramycin. If TOBI® is used during pregnancy, or if the patient becomes pregnant while taking TOBI®, the patient should be apprised of the potential hazard to the fetus.

Nursing Mothers

It is not known if TOBI® will reach sufficient concentrations after administration by inhalation to be excreted in human breast milk. Because of the potential for ototoxicity and nephrotoxicity in infants, a decision should be made whether to terminate nursing or discontinue TOBI®.

Pediatric Use

The safety and efficacy of TOBI® have not been studied in pediatric patients under 6 years of age.

ADVERSE REACTIONS

TOBI® was generally well tolerated during two clinical studies in 258 cystic fibrosis patients ranging in age from 6 to 48 years. Patients received TOBI® in alternating periods of 28 days on and 28 days off drug in addition to their standard cystic fibrosis therapy for a total of 24 weeks.

Voice alteration and tinnitus were the only adverse experiences reported by significantly more TOBI®-treated patients. Thirty-three patients (13%) treated with TOBI® complained of voice alteration compared to 17 (7%) placebo patients. Voice alteration was more common in the on-drug periods.

Eight patients from the TOBI® group (3%) reported tinnitus compared to no placebo patients. All episodes were transient, resolved without discontinuation of the TOBI® treatment regimen, and were not associated with loss of hearing in audiograms. Tinnitus is one of the sentinel symptoms of cochlear toxicity, and patients with this symptom should be carefully monitored for high frequency hearing loss. The numbers of patients reporting vestibular adverse experiences such as dizziness were similar in the TOBI® and placebo groups.

Nine (3%) patients in the TOBI® group and nine (3%) patients in the placebo group had increases in serum creatinine of at least 50% over baseline. In all nine patients in the TOBI® group, creatinine decreased at the next visit.

Table 1 lists the percent of patients with treatment-emergent adverse experiences (spontaneously reported and solicited) that occurred in >5% of TOBI® patients during the two Phase III studies.

Table 1: Percent of Patients With Treatment Emergent Adverse Experiences Occurring in >5% of TOBI® Patients

Adverse Event	TOBI® (n=258) %	Placebo (n=262) %
Cough Increased	46.1	47.3
Pharyngitis	38.0	39.3
Sputum Increased	37.6	39.7
Asthenia	35.7	39.3
Rhinitis	34.5	33.6
Dyspnea	33.7	38.5
Fever[1]	32.9	43.5
Lung Disorder	31.4	31.3
Headache	26.7	32.1
Chest Pain	26.0	29.8
Sputum Discoloration	21.3	19.8
Hemoptysis	19.4	23.7
Anorexia	18.6	27.9
Lung Function Decreased[2]	16.3	15.3
Asthma	15.9	20.2
Vomiting	14.0	22.1
Abdominal Pain	12.8	23.7
Voice Alteration	12.8	6.5
Nausea	11.2	16.0
Weight Loss	10.1	15.3
Pain	8.1	12.6
Sinusitis	8.1	9.2
Ear Pain	7.4	8.8
Back Pain	7.0	8.0
Epistaxis	7.0	6.5
Taste Perversion	6.6	6.9
Diarrhea	6.2	10.3
Malaise	6.2	5.3
Lower Respiratory Tract Infection	5.8	8.0
Dizziness	5.8	7.6
Hyperventilation	5.4	9.9
Rash	5.4	6.1

[1] Includes subjective complaints of fever.
[2] Includes reported decreases in pulmonary function tests or decreased lung volume on chest radiograph associated with intercurrent illness or study drug administration.

OVERDOSAGE

Signs and symptoms of acute toxicity from overdosage of IV tobramycin might include dizziness, tinnitus, vertigo, loss of high-tone hearing acuity, respiratory failure, and neuromuscular blockade. Administration by inhalation results in low systemic bioavailability of tobramycin. Tobramycin is not significantly absorbed following oral administration. Tobramycin serum concentrations may be helpful in monitoring overdosage.

In all cases of suspected overdosage, physicians should contact the Regional Poison Control Center for information about effective treatment. In the case of any overdosage, the possibility of drug interactions with alterations in drug disposition should be considered.

DOSAGE AND ADMINISTRATION

The recommended dosage for both adults and pediatric patients 6 years of age and older is 1 single-use ampule (300 mg) administered BID for 28 days. Dosage is not adjusted by weight. All patients should be administered 300 mg BID. The doses should be taken as close to 12 hours apart as possible; they should not be taken less than 6 hours apart.

TOBI® is inhaled while the patient is sitting or standing upright and breathing normally through the mouthpiece of the nebulizer. Nose clips may help the patient breathe through the mouth.

TOBI® is administered BID in alternating periods of 28 days. After 28 days of therapy, patients should stop TOBI® therapy for the next 28 days, and then resume therapy for the next 28 day on/28 day off cycle.

TOBI® is supplied as a single-use ampule and is administered by inhalation, using a hand-held PARI LC PLUS™ Reusable Nebulizer with a DeVilbiss® Pulmo-Aide® compressor. TOBI® is not for subcutaneous, intravenous or intrathecal administration.

Usage

TOBI® is administered by inhalation over an approximately 15-minute period, using a hand-held PARI LC PLUS™ Reusable Nebulizer with a DeVilbiss® Pulmo-Aide® compressor. TOBI® should not be diluted or mixed with dornase alfa (PULMOZYME®, Genentech) in the nebulizer.

During clinical studies, patients on multiple therapies were instructed to take them first, followed by TOBI®.

HOW SUPPLIED

TOBI® 300 mg is available as follows:
NDC 0078-0494-71
5 mL single-dose ampule (carton of 56)

Storage

TOBI® should be stored under refrigeration at 2-8°C/36-46°F. Upon removal from the refrigerator, or if refrigeration is unavailable, TOBI® pouches (opened or unopened) may be stored at room temperature (up to 25°C/77°F) for up to 28 days. TOBI® should not be used beyond the expiration date stamped on the ampule when stored under refrigeration (2-8°C/36-46°F) or beyond 28 days when stored at room temperature (25°C/77°F).

Table 2: Dosing Regimens in Clinical Studies

	Cycle 1		Cycle 2		Cycle 3	
	28 days	28 days	28 days	28 days	28 days	28 days
TOBI® regimen n=258	TOBI® 300 mg BID	No drug	TOBI® 300 mg BID	No drug	TOBI® 300 mg BID	No drug
Placebo regimen n=262	placebo BID	No drug	placebo BID	No drug	placebo BID	No drug

TOBI® ampules should not be exposed to intense light. The solution in the ampule is slightly yellow, but may darken with age if not stored in the refrigerator; however, the color change does not indicate any change in the quality of the product as long as it is stored within the recommended storage conditions.

Clinical Studies

Two identically designed, double-blind, randomized, placebo-controlled, parallel group, 24-week clinical studies (Study 1 and Study 2) at a total of 69 cystic fibrosis centers in the United States were conducted in cystic fibrosis patients with *P. aeruginosa*. Subjects who were less than 6 years of age, had a baseline creatinine of >2 mg/dL, or had *Burkholderia cepacia* isolated from sputum were excluded. All subjects had baseline FEV$_1$% predicted between 25% and 75%. In these clinical studies, 258 patients received TOBI® therapy on an outpatient basis *(see Table 2)* using a hand-held PARI LC PLUS™ Reusable Nebulizer with a DeVilbiss® Pulmo-Aide® compressor.

[See table above]

All patients received either TOBI® or placebo (saline with 1.25 mg quinine for flavoring) in addition to standard treatment recommended for cystic fibrosis patients, which included oral and parenteral anti-pseudomonal therapy, β$_2$-agonists, cromolyn, inhaled steroids, and airway clearance techniques. In addition, approximately 77% of patients were concurrently treated with dornase alfa (PULMOZYME®, Genentech).

In each study, TOBI®-treated patients experienced significant improvement in pulmonary function. Improvement was demonstrated in the TOBI® group in Study 1 by an average increase in FEV$_1$% predicted of about 11% relative to baseline (Week 0) during 24 weeks compared to no average change in placebo patients. In Study 2, TOBI®-treated patients had an average increase of about 7% compared to an average decrease of about 1% in placebo patients. Figure 1 shows the average relative change in FEV$_1$% predicted over 24 weeks for both studies.

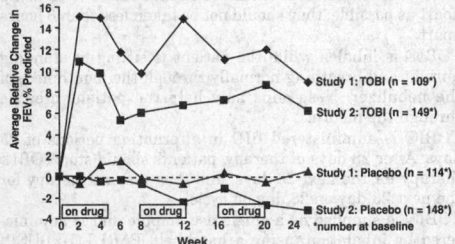

Figure 1: Relative Change From Baseline in FEV$_1$% Predicted

In each study, TOBI® therapy resulted in a significant reduction in the number of *P. aeruginosa* colony forming units (CFUs) in sputum during the on-drug periods. Sputum bacterial density returned to baseline during the off-drug periods. Reductions in sputum bacterial density were smaller in each successive cycle. *(see Figure 2)*.

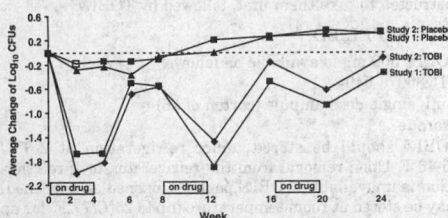

Figure 2: Absolute Change From Baseline in Log$_{10}$ CFUs

Patients treated with TOBI® were hospitalized for an average of 5.1 days compared to 8.1 days for placebo patients.

Patients treated with TOBI® required an average of 9.6 days of parenteral anti-pseudomonal antibiotic treatment compared to 14.1 days for placebo patients. During the 6 months of treatment, 40% of TOBI® patients and 53% of placebo patients were treated with parenteral anti-pseudomonal antibiotics.

The relationship between *in-vitro* susceptibility test results and clinical outcome with TOBI® therapy is not clear. However, 4 TOBI® patients who began the clinical trial with *P. aeruginosa* isolates having MIC values ≥128 μg/mL did not experience an improvement in FEV$_1$ or a decrease in sputum bacterial density.

Treatment with TOBI® did not affect the susceptibility of the majority of *P. aeruginosa* isolates during the 6-month studies. However, some *P. aeruginosa* isolates did exhibit increased tobramycin MICs. The percentage of patients with *P. aeruginosa* isolates with tobramycin MICs ≥ 16 μg/mL was 13% at the beginning, and 23% at the end of 6 months of the TOBI® regimen.

REFERENCES

1. Neu HC. Tobramycin: an overview. [Review]. J Infect Dis 1976; Suppl 134:S3-19.
2. Weber A, Smith A, Williams-Warren J et al. Nebulizer delivery of tobramycin to the lower respiratory tract. Pediatr Pulmonol 1994; 17 (5):331-9.
3. Bryan LE. Aminoglycoside resistance. Bryan LE, Ed. Antimicrobial drug resistance. Orlando, FL: Academic Press, 1984: 241-77.

U.S. Patent 5,508,269; other patents pending.

T2009-119

REV: NOVEMBER 2009   5002443

Distributed by:
Novartis Pharmaceuticals Corporation
East Hanover, New Jersey 07936
© Novartis

INFORMATION FOR PATIENTS

Safety Information

TOBI® is in a class of antibiotics that have caused hearing loss, dizziness, kidney damage, and harm to a fetus. Ringing in the ears and hoarseness were two symptoms that were seen in more patients taking TOBI® than placebo in research studies. Patients with cystic fibrosis can have many symptoms. Some of these symptoms may be related to your medications. If you have new or worsening symptoms, you should tell your doctor.

Hearing: You should tell your doctor if you have ringing in the ears, dizziness, or any changes in hearing.

Kidney Damage: Inform your doctor if you have any history of kidney problems.

Pregnancy: If you want to become pregnant or are pregnant while on TOBI®, you should talk with your doctor about the possibility of TOBI® causing any harm.

Nursing Mothers: If you are nursing a baby, you should talk with your doctor before using TOBI®.

TOBI® Packaging

TOBI® comes in a single dose, ready-to-use ampule containing 300 mg tobramycin. Each foil pouch contains 4 ampules, for 2 days of TOBI® therapy.

Dosage

The 300 mg dose of TOBI® is the same for patients regardless of age or weight. TOBI® has not been studied in patients less than 6 years old. Doses should be inhaled as close to 12 hours apart as possible and not less than 6 hours apart.

You should not mix TOBI® with dornase alfa (PULMOZYME®, Genentech) in the nebulizer.

If you are taking several medications the recommended order is as follows: bronchodilator first, followed by chest physiotherapy, then other inhaled medications and, finally, TOBI®.

Treatment Schedule

You should take TOBI® in repeated cycles of 28 days on drug followed by 28 days off drug. You should take TOBI® twice a day during the 28-day period on drug.

How To Administer TOBI®

THIS INFORMATION IS NOT INTENDED TO REPLACE CONSULTATION WITH YOUR PHYSICIAN AND CF CARE TEAM ABOUT PROPERLY TAKING MEDICATION OR USING INHALATION EQUIPMENT.

TOBI® is specifically formulated for inhalation using a PARI LC PLUS™ Reusable Nebulizer and a DeVilbiss® Pulmo-Aide® air compressor. TOBI® can be taken at home, school, or at work. The following are instructions on how to use the DeVilbiss® Pulmo-Aide® air compressor and PARILC PLUS™ Reusable Nebulizer to administer TOBI®. You will need the following supplies:

• TOBI® plastic ampule (vial)
• DeVilbiss® Pulmo-Aide® air compressor
• PARI LC PLUS™ Reusable Nebulizer
• Tubing to connect the nebulizer and compressor
• Clean paper or cloth towels
• Nose clips (optional)

It is important that your nebulizer and compressor function properly before starting your TOBI® therapy.

Note: Please refer to the manufacturers' care and use instructions for important information.

Preparing Your TOBI® for Inhalation

1. Wash your hands thoroughly with soap and water.

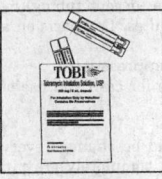

2a. TOBI® is packaged with 4 ampules per foil pouch.

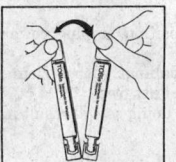

2b. Separate one ampule by gently pulling apart at the bottom tabs. Store all remaining ampules in the refrigerator as directed.

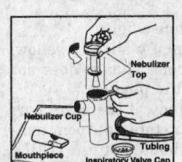

3. Lay out the contents of a PARILC PLUS™ Reusable Nebulizer package on a clean, dry paper or cloth towel. You should have the following parts:
   • Nebulizer Top and Bottom (Nebulizer Cup) Assembly
   • Inspiratory Valve Cap
   • Mouthpiece with Valve
   • Tubing

4. Remove the Nebulizer Top from the Nebulizer Cup by twisting the Nebulizer Top counterclockwise, and then lifting. Place the Nebulizer Top on the clean paper or cloth towel. Stand the Nebulizer Cup upright on the towel.

5. Connect one end of the tubing to the compressor air outlet. The tubing should fit snugly. Plug in your compressor to an electrical outlet.

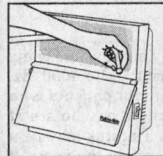

6. Open the TOBI ampule by holding the bottom tab with one hand and twisting off the top of the ampule with the other hand. Be careful not to squeeze the ampule until you are ready to empty its contents into the Nebulizer Cup.

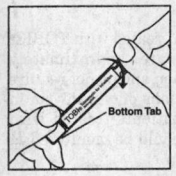

7. Squeeze all the contents of the ampule into the Nebulizer Cup.

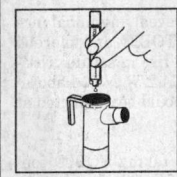

8. Replace the Nebulizer Top. Note: In order to insert the Nebulizer Top into the Nebulizer Cup, the semi-circle halfway down the stem of the Nebulizer Top should face the Nebulizer Outlet (see illustration). Turn the Nebulizer Top clockwise until securely fastened to the Nebulizer Cup.

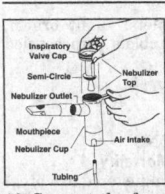

9. Attach the Mouthpiece to the Nebulizer Outlet. Then firmly push the Inspiratory Valve Cap in place on the Nebulizer Top. Note: The Inspiratory Valve Cap will fit snugly.

10. Connect the free end of the tubing to the Air Intake on the bottom of the nebulizer, making sure to keep the nebulizer upright. Press the tubing on the Air Intake firmly.

TOBI® Treatment

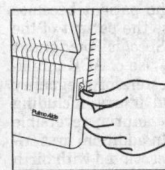

1. Turn on the compressor.

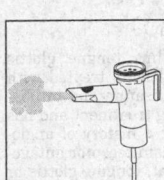

2. Check for a steady mist from the Mouthpiece. If there is no mist, check all tubing connections and confirm that the compressor is working properly.

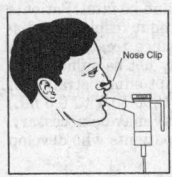

3. Sit or stand in an upright position that will allow you to breathe normally.

4. Place Mouthpiece between your teeth and on top of your tongue and breathe normally only through your mouth. Nose clips may help you breathe through your mouth and not through your nose. Do not block airflow with your tongue.

5. Continue treatment until all of your TOBI® is gone, and there is no longer any mist being produced. You may hear a sputtering sound when the Nebulizer Cup is empty. The entire TOBI® treatment should take approximately 15 minutes to complete. Note: If you are interrupted, need to cough or rest during your TOBI® treatment, turn off the compressor to save your medication. Turn the compressor back on when you are ready to resume your therapy.

6. Follow the nebulizer cleaning and disinfecting instructions after completing therapy.

Cleaning Your Nebulizer

To reduce the risk of infection, illness or injury from contamination, you must thoroughly clean all parts of the nebulizer as instructed after each treatment. Never use a nebulizer with a clogged nozzle. If the nozzle is clogged, no aerosol mist is produced which will alter the effectiveness of the treatment. Replace the nebulizer if clogging occurs.

1. Remove tubing from nebulizer and disassemble nebulizer parts.

2. Wash all parts (except tubing) with warm water and liquid dish soap.

3. Rinse thoroughly with warm water and shake out water.

4. Air dry or hand dry nebulizer parts on a clean, lint-free cloth. Reassemble nebulizer when dry, and store.

5. You can also wash all parts of the nebulizer in a dishwasher (except tubing). Place the nebulizer parts in a dishwasher basket, then place on the top rack of the dishwasher. Remove and dry the parts when the cycle is complete.

Disinfecting Your Nebulizer

Your nebulizer is for your use only—Do not share your nebulizer with other people. You must regularly disinfect the nebulizer. Failure to do so could lead to serious or fatal illness.

Clean the nebulizer as described above. Every other treatment day, disinfect the nebulizer parts (except tubing) by boiling them in water for a full 10 minutes. Dry parts on a clean, lint-free cloth.

Care and Use of Your Pulmo-Aide® Compressor

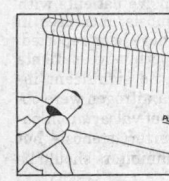

Follow the manufacturer's instructions for care and use of your compressor.

Filter Change:

1. DeVilbiss® Compressor filters should be changed every six months or sooner if filter turns completely gray in color.

Compressor Cleaning:

1. With power switch in the "Off" position, unplug power cord from wall outlet.

2. Wipe outside of the compressor cabinet with a clean, damp cloth every few days to keep dust free.

Caution: Do not submerge in water; doing so will result in compressor damage.

Storage Instructions

You should store TOBI® ampules in a refrigerator (2-8°C or 36–46°F). However, when you don't have a refrigerator available (e.g., transporting your TOBI®), you may store the foil pouches (opened or unopened) at room temperature (up to 25°C/77°F) for up to 28 days.

Avoid exposing TOBI® ampules to intense light.

Unrefrigerated TOBI®, which is normally slightly yellow, may darken with age; however, the color change does not indicate any change in the quality of the product.

You should not use TOBI® if it is cloudy, if there are particles in the solution, or if it has been stored at room temperature for more than 28 days. You should not use TOBI® beyond the expiration date stamped on the ampule.

Additional Information
Nebulizer: 1-800-327-8632
Compressor: 1-800-338-1988
TOBI®: 1-888-NOW-NOVA (1-888-669-6682)

REV: NOVEMBER 2009   Printed in USA   T2009-120
                                        5002444
Distributed by:
Novartis Pharmaceuticals Corporation
East Hanover, New Jersey 07936
©Novartis

Shown in Product Identification Guide, page 316

VALTURNA®   ℞
[*val-tur-na*]
(aliskiren and valsartan, USP)
Tablets

The following prescribing information is based on official labeling in effect September 2010.

HIGHLIGHTS OF PRESCRIBING INFORMATION
These highlights do not include all the information needed to use Valturna safely and effectively. See full prescribing information for Valturna.

Valturna *(aliskiren and valsartan, USP)* **Tablets**
Initial U.S. Approval: 2009

> **WARNING: AVOID USE IN PREGNANCY**
> *See full prescribing information for complete boxed warning.*
> **When pregnancy is detected, discontinue Valturna as soon as possible. When used in pregnancy during the second and third trimester, drugs that act directly on the renin-angiotensin system can cause injury and death to the developing fetus. (5.1)**

———INDICATIONS AND USAGE———
Valturna is a combination of aliskiren, a direct renin inhibitor, and valsartan, an angiotensin II receptor blocker (ARB), indicated for the treatment of hypertension:
• In patients not adequately controlled with monotherapy. (1)
• May be substituted for titrated components. (1)
• As initial therapy in patients likely to need multiple drugs to achieve their blood pressure goals. (1)

———DOSAGE AND ADMINISTRATION———
• Add-on therapy or initial therapy: Initiate with 150/160 mg. Titrate as needed up to a maximum of 300/320 mg. (2.1, 2.3, 2.5)
• Majority of effect attained within 2 weeks. (2.2)
• Replacement therapy: may be substituted for titrated components. (2.4)
• One tablet daily, with a routine pattern with regard to meals. (2.7)

———DOSAGE FORMS AND STRENGTHS———
Tablets (mg aliskiren/mg valsartan): 150/160, 300/320. (3)

———WARNINGS AND PRECAUTIONS———
• Avoid fetal or neonatal exposure. (5.1)
• Head and neck angioedema: Discontinue Valturna and monitor until signs and symptoms resolve. (5.2)
• Hypotension in volume- or salt-depleted patients: Correct imbalances before initiating therapy with Valturna. (5.3)
• Patients with renal impairment: Decreases in renal function may be anticipated in susceptible individuals. (5.4)
• Patients with hepatic impairment: Slower clearance may occur. (5.5)
• Hyperkalemia: Consider periodic determinations of serum electrolytes to detect possible electrolyte imbalances, particularly in patients at risk. (5.7)

———ADVERSE REACTIONS———
The most common adverse events (incidence ≥1.5% and more common than with placebo) are: Fatigue and nasopharyngitis. (6.1)

To report SUSPECTED ADVERSE REACTIONS, contact Novartis Pharmaceuticals Corporation at 1-888-669-6682 or FDA at 1-800-FDA-1088 or www.fda.gov/medwatch.

———DRUG INTERACTIONS———
Aliskiren:
• Cyclosporine or itraconazole: Concomitant use is not recommended. (7)
Valsartan:
• Potassium sparing diuretics, potassium supplements or salt substitutes may lead to increases in serum potassium, and in heart failure patients, increases in serum creatinine. (7)

———USE IN SPECIFIC POPULATIONS———
Nursing Mothers: Nursing or drug should be discontinued. (8.3)

See 17 for PATIENT COUNSELING INFORMATION and FDA-approved patient labeling

Revised: 08/2010

FULL PRESCRIBING INFORMATION: CONTENTS*
WARNING: AVOID USE IN PREGNANCY
1   INDICATIONS AND USAGE
2   DOSAGE AND ADMINISTRATION
   2.1   Dose Selection
   2.2   Dose Titration
   2.3   Add-on Therapy
   2.4   Replacement Therapy
   2.5   Initial Therapy
   2.6   Use with Other Antihypertensive Drugs
   2.7   Relationship to Meals
   2.8   Dosing in Specific Populations
3   DOSAGE FORMS AND STRENGTHS
4   CONTRAINDICATIONS
5   WARNINGS AND PRECAUTIONS
   5.1   Fetal/Neonatal Morbidity and Mortality
   5.2   Head and Neck Angioedema
   5.3   Hypotension
   5.4   Patients with Severe Renal Impairment
   5.5   Patients with Hepatic Impairment
   5.6   Patients with Congestive Heart Failure and Post-Myocardial Infarction
   5.7   Serum Electrolyte Abnormalities
   5.8   Renal Artery Stenosis
   5.9   Cyclosporine or Itraconazole
6   ADVERSE REACTIONS
   6.1   Clinical Studies Experience
   6.2   Clinical Laboratory Test Abnormalities
   6.3   Post-Marketing Experience
7   DRUG INTERACTIONS
8   USE IN SPECIFIC POPULATIONS
   8.1   Pregnancy
   8.3   Nursing Mothers
   8.4   Pediatric Use
   8.5   Geriatric Use
10 OVERDOSAGE
11 DESCRIPTION
12 CLINICAL PHARMACOLOGY
   12.1 Mechanism of Action
   12.2 Pharmacodynamics
   12.3 Pharmacokinetics
13 NONCLINICAL TOXICOLOGY
   13.1 Carcinogenesis, Mutagenesis, Impairment of Fertility
   13.2 Animal Toxicology and/or Pharmacology
14 CLINICAL STUDIES
16 HOW SUPPLIED/STORAGE AND HANDLING
17 PATIENT COUNSELING INFORMATION
*Sections or subsections omitted from the full prescribing information are not listed

---

FULL PRESCRIBING INFORMATION

> **WARNING: AVOID USE IN PREGNANCY**
> **When pregnancy is detected, discontinue Valturna as soon as possible. When used in pregnancy during the second and third trimesters, drugs that act directly on the renin-angiotensin-aldosterone system can cause injury and death to the developing fetus. [See Warnings and Precautions (5.1)].**

1   INDICATIONS AND USAGE
Valturna is indicated for the treatment of hypertension.
Add-on Therapy
A patient whose blood pressure is not adequately controlled with aliskiren alone or valsartan (or another angiotensin receptor blocker) alone may be switched to combination therapy with Valturna.
Replacement Therapy
Valturna may be substituted for the titrated components.

Initial Therapy

Valturna may be used as initial therapy in patients who are likely to need multiple drugs to achieve their blood pressure goals.

The choice of Valturna as initial therapy should be based on an assessment of potential benefits and risks.

Patients with Stage 2 hypertension are at a relatively high risk for cardiovascular events (such as strokes, heart attacks, and heart failure), kidney failure, and vision problems, so prompt treatment is clinically relevant. The decision to use a combination as initial therapy should be individualized and should be shaped by considerations such as baseline blood pressure, the target goal, and the incremental likelihood of achieving goal with a combination compared to monotherapy. Individual blood pressure goals may vary based upon the patient's risk.

Data from the high-dose multifactorial study *[see Clinical Studies (14)]* provide estimates of the probability of reaching a target blood pressure with Valturna compared to aliskiren or valsartan monotherapy. The figures below provide estimates of the likelihood of achieving systolic or diastolic blood pressure control with Valturna 300/320 mg, based upon baseline systolic or diastolic blood pressure. The curve of each treatment group was estimated by logistic regression modeling. The estimated likelihood at the right tail of each curve is less reliable because of a small number of subjects with high baseline blood pressures.

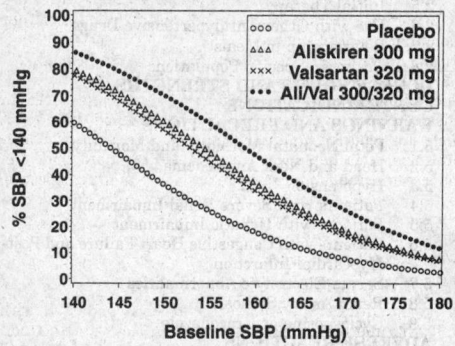

Figure 1: Probability of Achieving Systolic Blood Pressure (SBP) <140 mmHg in Patients at Endpoint

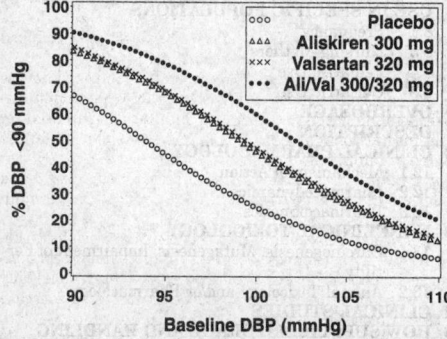

Figure 2: Probability of Achieving Diastolic Blood Pressure (DBP) <90 mmHg in Patients at Endpoint

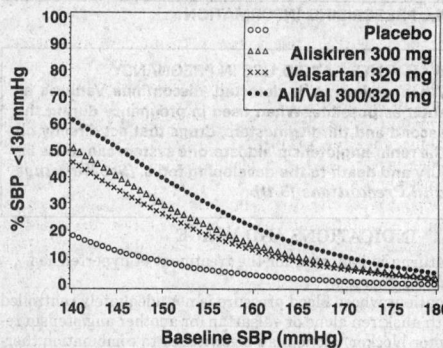

Figure 3: Probability of Achieving Systolic Blood Pressure (SBP) <130 mmHg in Patients at Endpoint

[See figure 4 at top of next column]

At all levels of baseline blood pressure, the probability of achieving any given diastolic or systolic goal is greater with

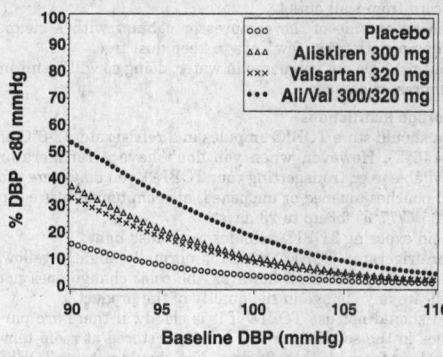

Figure 4: Probability of Achieving Diastolic Blood Pressure (DBP) <80 mmHg in Patients at Endpoint

the combination than for either monotherapy. For example, the mean baseline SBP/DBP for patients participating in this multifactorial study was 154/100 mmHg. A patient with a baseline blood pressure of 154/100 mmHg has about a 51% likelihood of achieving a goal of <140 mmHg (systolic) and 46% likelihood of achieving <90 mmHg (diastolic) on aliskiren alone, and the likelihood of achieving these goals on valsartan alone is about 47% (systolic) and 47% (diastolic). The likelihood of achieving these goals on Valturna rises to about 62% (systolic) and 60% (diastolic). The likelihood of achieving these goals on placebo is about 28% (systolic) and 25% (diastolic) *[see Dosage and Administration (2) and Clinical Studies (14)]*.

2   DOSAGE AND ADMINISTRATION

2.1   Dose Selection

The recommended once-daily dose of Valturna is 150/160 mg or 300/320 mg. The recommended initial once-daily dose of Valturna is 150/160 mg. Titrate as needed to a maximum of 300/320 mg.

Patients switched from monotherapy to Valturna on average experience greater blood pressure reductions with use of the combination product.

2.2   Dose Titration

The antihypertensive effect of Valturna is largely attained within 2 weeks. If blood pressure remains uncontrolled after 2 to 4 weeks of therapy, the dose may be titrated up to a maximum of 300/320 mg.

2.3   Add-on Therapy

A patient whose blood pressure is not adequately controlled with aliskiren alone or valsartan (or another angiotensin receptor blocker) alone may be switched to combination therapy with Valturna. The usual recommended starting dose is 150/160 mg once daily as needed to control blood pressure.

2.4   Replacement Therapy

For convenience, patients receiving aliskiren and valsartan from separate tablets may instead wish to receive a single tablet of Valturna containing the same component doses.

2.5   Initial Therapy

The usual recommended starting dose of Valturna is 150/160 mg once daily as needed to control blood pressure. The dose may be titrated up to a maximum of 300/320 mg once daily.

Valturna is not recommended for use as initial therapy in patients with intravascular volume depletion *[see Warnings and Precautions (5.3)]*.

2.6   Use with Other Antihypertensive Drugs

Valturna may be administered with other antihypertensive agents. There are no data available with use of Valturna with angiotensin-converting enzyme inhibitors or other renin-angiotensin-aldosterone blockers.

2.7   Relationship to Meals

Patients should establish a routine pattern for taking Valturna with regard to meals. High-fat meals decrease absorption substantially *[see Clinical Pharmacology (12.3)]*.

2.8   Dosing in Specific Populations

Renal Impairment

Adjustment of the starting dose is not required in patients with mild-to-moderate renal impairment. Clinical experience with dosing Valturna in patients with moderate renal impairment is limited. No data are available in patients with severe renal impairment *[see Warnings and Precautions (5.4)]*.

Hepatic Impairment

Adjustment of the starting dose is not necessary with mild or moderate hepatic impairment. Clinical experience with dosing Valturna in patients with severe hepatic impairment is limited *[see Warnings and Precautions (5.5)]*.

Elderly Patients

Adjustment of the starting dose is not required for elderly patients.

3   DOSAGE FORMS AND STRENGTHS

- 150/160 mg aliskiren/valsartan tablets: light red, standard convex ovaloid, film-coated tablets with beveled edges debossed with NVR/HDU

- 300/320 mg aliskiren/valsartan tablets: light brown, shallow convex ovaloid, film-coated tablets with beveled edges debossed with NVR/SNB

4   CONTRAINDICATIONS

None.

5   WARNINGS AND PRECAUTIONS

5.1   Fetal/Neonatal Morbidity and Mortality

Valturna can cause fetal harm when administered to a pregnant woman. If this drug is used during pregnancy, or if a patient becomes pregnant while taking this drug, apprise the patient of the potential hazard to the fetus.

Drugs that act directly on the renin-angiotensin-aldosterone system can cause fetal and neonatal morbidity and death when administered to pregnant women. If this drug is used during pregnancy, or if the patient becomes pregnant while taking this drug, apprise the patient of the potential hazard to the fetus *[see Use in Specific Populations (8.1)]*. In several dozen published cases, use of ACE inhibitors during the second and third trimesters of pregnancy was associated with fetal and neonatal injury, including hypotension, neonatal skull hypoplasia, anuria, reversible or irreversible renal failure, and death. In addition, first trimester use of ACE inhibitors has been associated with birth defects in retrospective data.

5.2   Head and Neck Angioedema

Aliskiren

Angioedema of the face, extremities, lips, tongue, glottis and/or larynx has been reported in patients treated with aliskiren and has necessitated hospitalization and intubation. This may occur at any time during treatment and has occurred in patients with and without a history of angioedema with ACE inhibitors or angiotensin receptor antagonists. If angioedema involves the throat, tongue, glottis or larynx, or if the patient has a history of upper respiratory surgery, airway obstruction may occur and be fatal. Patients who experience these effects, even without respiratory distress, require prolonged observation since treatment with antihistamines and corticosteroids may not be sufficient to prevent respiratory involvement. Prompt administration of subcutaneous epinephrine solution 1:1000 (0.3 to 0.5 mL) and measures to ensure a patent airway may be necessary. Discontinue aliskiren immediately in patients who develop angioedema and do not readminister.

5.3   Hypotension

An excessive fall in blood pressure (hypotension) was rarely seen (<0.5%) in patients with uncomplicated hypertension treated with Valturna in controlled trials.

In patients with an activated renin-angiotensin-aldosterone system, such as volume- or salt-depleted patients receiving high doses of diuretics, symptomatic hypotension may occur in patients receiving renin-angiotensin-aldosterone system (RAAS) blockers. Correct these conditions prior to the administration of Valturna, or start the treatment under close medical supervision.

Initiate therapy cautiously in patients with heart failure or recent myocardial infarction and in patients undergoing surgery or dialysis. Patients with heart failure or post-myocardial infarction patients given valsartan commonly have some reduction in blood pressure, but discontinuation of therapy because of continuing symptomatic hypotension usually is not necessary when dosing instructions are followed. In controlled trials in heart failure patients, the incidence of hypotension in valsartan-treated patients was 5.5% compared to 1.8% in placebo-treated patients. In the Valsartan in Acute Myocardial Infarction Trial (VALIANT), hypotension in post-myocardial infarction patients led to permanent discontinuation of therapy in 1.4% of valsartan-treated patients and 0.8% of captopril-treated patients.

If an excessive fall in blood pressure occurs with Valturna, place the patient in the supine position and, if necessary, give an intravenous infusion of normal saline. A transient hypotensive response is not a contraindication to further treatment, which usually can be continued without difficulty once the blood pressure has stabilized.

5.4   Patients with Severe Renal Impairment

Valturna

Patients with severe renal impairment were excluded from clinical trials with Valturna in hypertension.

Aliskiren

Patients with severe renal dysfunction (creatinine 1.7 mg/dL for women and 2.0 mg/dL for men and/or estimated GFR <30 mL/min), a history of dialysis, nephrotic syndrome, or renovascular hypertension were excluded from clinical trials of aliskiren in hypertension. Safety information with aliskiren and the potential for other drugs acting on the renin-angiotensin-aldosterone system to increase serum creatinine and blood urea nitrogen are not available.

Valsartan

In studies of ACE inhibitors in hypertensive patients with unilateral or bilateral renal artery stenosis, increases in serum creatinine or blood urea nitrogen have been reported. In a 4-day trial of valsartan in 12 hypertensive patients with unilateral renal artery stenosis, no significant increases in serum creatinine or blood urea nitrogen were observed. There has been no long-term use of valsartan in patients with unilateral or bilateral renal artery stenosis, but an effect similar to that seen with ACE inhibitors should be anticipated.

As a consequence of inhibiting the renin-angiotensin-aldosterone system, changes in renal function may occur particularly in volume depleted patients. In patients with severe heart failure whose renal function may depend on the activity of the renin-angiotensin-aldosterone system, treatment with angiotensin-converting enzyme inhibitors and angiotensin receptor antagonists has been associated with oliguria or progressive azotemia and (rarely) with acute renal failure or death. Similar outcomes have been reported with valsartan.

5.5 Patients with Hepatic Impairment
Valsartan
As the majority of valsartan is eliminated in the bile, patients with mild-to-moderate hepatic impairment, including patients with biliary obstructive disorders, showed lower valsartan clearance (higher AUCs).

5.6 Patients with Congestive Heart Failure and Post-Myocardial Infarction
Valsartan
Some patients with heart failure have developed increases in blood urea nitrogen, serum creatinine, and potassium on valsartan. These effects are usually minor and transient, and they are more likely to occur in patients with pre-existing renal impairment. Dosage reduction and/or discontinuation of the diuretic and/or valsartan may be required. In the Valsartan Heart Failure Trial, in which 93% of patients were on concomitant ACE inhibitors, treatment was discontinued for elevations in creatinine or potassium (total of 1.0% on valsartan vs. 0.2% on placebo). In the Valsartan in Acute Myocardial Infarction Trial (VALIANT), discontinuation due to various types of renal dysfunction occurred in 1.1% of valsartan-treated patients and 0.8% of captopril-treated patients. Include assessment of renal function when evaluating patients with heart failure or post-myocardial infarction.

5.7 Serum Electrolyte Abnormalities
Valturna
In the short-term controlled trials of various doses of Valturna, the incidence of hyperkalemia (serum potassium >5.5 mEq/L) was about 1%-2% higher in the combination treatment group compared with the monotherapies aliskiren and valsartan, or with placebo.
In a long-term, uncontrolled study with median treatment duration of about one year, about 4% of the patients had at least one serum potassium >5.5 mEq/L at some time during the study; about 0.8% of patients discontinued study treatment and had a high serum potassium at some point during the study. Patients with hyperkalemia were older (median age 65 vs. 55) with slightly lower mean baseline estimated creatinine clearance compared to patients without hyperkalemia. While about 25% of the hyperkalemic episodes occurred in the first two months, other initial episodes were reported throughout the study.
Periodic determinations of serum electrolytes to detect possible electrolyte imbalances is advised, particularly in patients at risk for hyperkalemia such as those with renal impairment.
Caution is advised with concomitant use of Valturna with potassium-sparing diuretics, potassium supplements, salt substitutes containing potassium, or other drugs that increase potassium levels may lead to increases in serum potassium.

5.8 Renal Artery Stenosis
Aliskiren
No data are available on the use of aliskiren in patients with unilateral or bilateral renal artery stenosis or stenosis of the artery to a solitary kidney.
Valsartan
In studies of ACE inhibitors in hypertensive patients with unilateral or bilateral renal artery stenosis, increases in serum creatinine or blood urea nitrogen have been reported. In a 4-day trial of valsartan in 12 hypertensive patients with unilateral renal artery stenosis, no significant increases in serum creatinine or blood urea nitrogen were observed. There has been no long-term use of valsartan in patients with unilateral or bilateral renal artery stenosis, but an effect similar to that seen with ACE inhibitors should be anticipated.

5.9 Cyclosporine or Itraconazole
Aliskiren
When aliskiren was given with cyclosporine or itraconazole, the blood concentrations of aliskiren were significantly increased. Concomitant use of aliskiren with cyclosporine or itraconazole is not recommended [see Drug Interactions (7)].

6 ADVERSE REACTIONS
6.1 Clinical Studies Experience
The following serious adverse reactions are discussed in greater detail in other sections of the label:
- Risk of fetal/neonatal morbidity and mortality [see Warnings and Precautions (5.1)]
- Head and neck angioedema [see Warnings and Precautions (5.2)]
- Hypotension [see Warnings and Precautions (5.3)]

Because clinical trials are conducted under widely varying conditions, adverse reaction rates observed in the clinical trials of a drug cannot be directly compared to rates in clinical trials of another drug and may not reflect the rates observed in practice.
Valturna
Valturna has been evaluated for safety in more than 1,225 patients, including over 316 patients for over 1 year. In placebo-controlled clinical trials, discontinuation of therapy because of a clinical adverse event (including uncontrolled hypertension) occurred in 1.4% of patients treated with Valturna versus 2.7% of patients given placebo.
Adverse events in placebo-controlled trials that occurred in at least 1% of patients treated with Valturna and at a higher incidence than placebo included fatigue (2.6% vs. 1.4%), nasopharyngitis (2.6% vs. 2.2%), diarrhea (1.4% vs 0.9%), upper respiratory tract infection (1.4% vs. 1.1%), urinary tract infection (1.4% vs. 0.6%), influenza (1.1% vs. 0.2%), and vertigo (1.1% vs. 0.3%).
Hyperkalemia has been observed as a serum electrolyte abnormality in Valturna clinical trials [see Warnings and Precautions (5.7)].
Aliskiren
Aliskiren has been evaluated for safety in 6,460 patients, including 1,740 treated for longer than 6 months, and 1,250 for longer than 1 year. In placebo-controlled clinical trials, discontinuation of therapy because of a clinical adverse event, including uncontrolled hypertension occurred in 2.2% of patients treated with aliskiren, versus 3.5% of patients given placebo.
Two cases of angioedema with respiratory symptoms were reported with aliskiren use in the clinical studies. Two other cases of periorbital edema without respiratory symptoms were reported as possible angioedema and resulted in discontinuation. The rate of these angioedema cases in the completed studies was 0.06%.
In addition, 26 other cases of edema involving the face, hands, or whole body were reported with aliskiren use, including 4 leading to discontinuation.
In the placebo-controlled studies, however, the incidence of edema involving the face, hands, or whole body was 0.4% with aliskiren compared with 0.5% with placebo. In a long-term active-controlled study with aliskiren and HCTZ arms, the incidence of edema involving the face, hands, or whole body was 0.4% in both treatment arms.
Aliskiren produces dose-related gastrointestinal (GI) adverse reactions. Diarrhea was reported by 2.3% of patients at 300 mg, compared to 1.2% in placebo patients. In women and the elderly (age ≥65) increases in diarrhea rates were evident starting at a dose of 150 mg daily, with rates for these subgroups at 150 mg similar to those seen at 300 mg for men or younger patients (all rates about 2%). Other GI symptoms included abdominal pain, dyspepsia, and gastroesophageal reflux, although increased rates for abdominal pain and dyspepsia were distinguished from placebo only at 600 mg daily. Diarrhea and other GI symptoms were typically mild and rarely led to discontinuation.
Aliskiren was associated with a slight increase in cough in the placebo-controlled studies (1.1% for any aliskiren use vs. 0.6% for placebo). In active-controlled trials with ACE inhibitor (ramipril, lisinopril) arms, the rates of cough for the aliskiren arms were about one-third to one-half the rates in the ACE inhibitor arms.
Other adverse reactions with increased rates for aliskiren compared to placebo included rash (1% vs. 0.3%), elevated uric acid (0.4% vs. 0.1%), gout (0.2% vs. 0.1%), and renal stones (0.2% vs. 0%).
Single episodes of tonic-clonic seizures with loss of consciousness were reported in two patients treated with aliskiren in the clinical trials. One patient had predisposing causes for seizures and had a negative electroencephalogram (EEG) and cerebral imaging following the seizures; for the other patient, EEG and imaging results were not reported. Aliskiren was discontinued and there was no rechallenge in either case.
The following adverse events occurred in placebo-controlled clinical trials at an incidence of more than 1% of patients treated with aliskiren, but also occurred at about the same or greater incidence in patients receiving placebo: headache, nasopharyngitis, dizziness, fatigue, upper respiratory tract infection, back pain and cough.
No clinically meaningful changes in vital signs or in ECG (including QTc interval) were observed in patients treated with aliskiren.
Valsartan
Valsartan has been evaluated for safety in more than 4,000 hypertensive patients in clinical trials, including over 400 treated for over 6 months, and more than 160 for over 1 year.
In trials in which valsartan was compared to an ACE inhibitor with or without placebo, the incidence of dry cough was significantly greater in the ACE inhibitor group (7.9%) than in the groups who received valsartan (2.6%) or placebo (1.5%). In a 129 patient trial limited to patients who had

had dry cough when they had previously received ACE inhibitors, the incidences of cough in patients who received valsartan, HCTZ, or lisinopril were 20%, 19%, and 69% respectively (p<0.001).
Other adverse reactions, not listed above, occurring in >0.2% of patients in controlled clinical trials with valsartan are:
Body as a Whole: allergic reaction, asthenia
Musculoskeletal: muscle cramps
Neurologic and Psychiatric: paresthesia
Respiratory: sinusitis, pharyngitis
Urogenital: impotence
Other reported events seen less frequently in clinical trials were: angioedema.
Adverse reactions reported for valsartan for indications other than hypertension may be found in the prescribing information for Diovan.

6.2 Clinical Laboratory Test Abnormalities
RBC count, hemoglobin and hematocrit:
Small mean decreases from baseline were seen in RBC count, hemoglobin and hematocrit in both monotherapies and combination therapy. These changes were small, but changes in hemoglobin were slightly more pronounced with the combination therapy (-0.26 g/dL) than with monotherapy regimens (-0.04 g/dL in aliskiren or -0.13 g/dL in valsartan) or placebo (+0.07 g/dL).
Blood Urea Nitrogen (BUN)/Creatinine:
Elevations in BUN (>40 mg/dL) and creatinine (>2.0 mg/dL) in any treatment group were less than 1.0%. For creatinine, 0.5% (3/599) of patients on combination treatment had a creatinine level >1.5 mg/dL at the end of the study and a 30% increase from baseline compared to none in either monotherapy or placebo.
Serum Electrolytes: See Warnings and Precautions (5.7)

6.3 Post-Marketing Experience
The following adverse reactions have been reported in aliskiren post-marketing experience. Because these reactions are reported voluntarily from a population of uncertain size, it is not always possible to estimate their frequency or establish a causal relationship to drug exposure.
Hypersensitivity: angioedema requiring airway management and hospitalization
Peripheral edema
Blood creatinine increased

7 DRUG INTERACTIONS
No drug interaction studies have been conducted with Valturna and other drugs, although studies with the individual aliskiren and valsartan components are described below.
Aliskiren
Effects of Other Drugs on Aliskiren
Based on *in vitro* studies, aliskiren is metabolized by CYP 3A4.
Irbesartan: Coadministration of irbesartan reduced aliskiren C_{max} up to 50% after multiple dosing.
P-glycoprotein Effects: Pgp (MDR1/Mdr1a/1b) was found to be the major efflux system involved in absorption and disposition of aliskiren in preclinical studies. The potential for drug interactions at the Pgp site will likely depend on the degree of inhibition of this transporter.
Atorvastatin: Coadministration of atorvastatin resulted in about a 50% increase in aliskiren C_{max} and AUC after multiple dosing.
Ketoconazole: Coadministration of 200 mg twice-daily ketoconazole with aliskiren resulted in approximate 80% increase in plasma levels of aliskiren. A 400-mg once-daily dose was not studied but would be expected to increase aliskiren blood levels further.
Itraconazole: Coadministration of 100 mg itraconazole with 150 mg aliskiren resulted in approximately 5.8-fold increase in C_{max} and 6.5-fold increase in AUC of aliskiren. Concomitant use of aliskiren with itraconazole is not recommended.
Cyclosporine: Coadministration of 200 mg and 600 mg cyclosporine with 75 mg aliskiren resulted in an approximately 2.5-fold increase in C_{max} and 5-fold increase in AUC of aliskiren. Concomitant use of aliskiren with cyclosporine is not recommended.
Verapamil: Coadministration of 240 mg of verapamil with 300 mg aliskiren resulted in an approximately 2-fold increase in C_{max} and AUC of aliskiren. However, no dosage adjustment is necessary.
Drugs with no clinically significant effects: Coadministration of lovastatin, atenolol, warfarin, furosemide, digoxin, celecoxib, hydrochlorothiazide, ramipril, valsartan, metformin and amlodipine did not result in clinically significant increases in aliskiren exposure.
Effects of Aliskiren on Other Drugs
Aliskiren does not inhibit the CYP450 isoenzymes (CYP1A2, 2C8, 2C9, 2C19, 2D6, 2E1, and CYP 3A) or induce CYP 3A4.
Furosemide: When aliskiren was coadministered with furosemide, the AUC and C_{max} of furosemide were reduced by

about 30% and 50%, respectively. Patients receiving furosemide could find its effect diminished after starting aliskiren.

Drugs with no clinically significant effects: Coadministration of aliskiren did not significantly affect the pharmacokinetics of lovastatin, digoxin, valsartan, amlodipine, metformin, celecoxib, atenolol, atorvastatin, ramipril or hydrochlorothiazide.

Warfarin: The effects of aliskiren on warfarin pharmacokinetics have not been evaluated.

Valsartan

No clinically significant pharmacokinetic interactions were observed when valsartan was coadministered with aliskiren, amlodipine, atenolol, cimetidine, digoxin, furosemide, glyburide, hydrochlorothiazide, or indomethacin. The valsartan-atenolol combination was more antihypertensive than either component, but it did not lower the heart rate more than atenolol alone.

Warfarin: Coadministration of valsartan and warfarin did not change the pharmacokinetics of valsartan or the time-course of the anticoagulant properties of warfarin.

CYP 450 Interactions: In vitro metabolism studies have indicated that CYP450 mediated drug interactions between valsartan and coadministered drugs are unlikely because of low extent of metabolism *[see Pharmacokinetics – Valsartan (12.3)]*.

Transporters: The results from an *in vitro* study with human liver tissue indicate that valsartan is a substrate of the hepatic uptake transporter OATP1B1 and the hepatic efflux transporter MRP2. Coadministration of inhibitors of the uptake transporter (rifampin, cyclosporine) or efflux transporter (ritonavir) may increase the systemic exposure to valsartan.

As with other drugs that block angiotensin II or its effects, concomitant use of potassium sparing diuretics (e.g., spironolactone, triamterene, amiloride), potassium supplements, or salt substitutes containing potassium may lead to increases in serum potassium and in heart failure patients to increases in serum creatinine.

8 USE IN SPECIFIC POPULATIONS

8.1 Pregnancy

Pregnancy Category D *[see Warnings and Precautions (5.1)]*.

Valturna contains both aliskiren (a direct renin inhibitor) and valsartan (an angiotensin II receptor blocker). When administered during the second or third trimester of pregnancy, drugs that act directly on the renin-angiotensin-aldosterone system can cause fetal and neonatal morbidity and death. Valturna can cause fetal harm when administered to a pregnant woman. If this drug is used during pregnancy, or if the patient becomes pregnant while taking this drug, apprise the patient of the potential hazard to the fetus.

Angiotensin II receptor antagonists, like valsartan, and angiotensin-converting enzyme (ACE) inhibitors exert similar effects on the renin-angiotensin-aldosterone system. In several dozen published cases, ACE inhibitor use during the second and third trimesters of pregnancy was associated with fetal and neonatal injury, including hypotension, neonatal skull hypoplasia, anuria, reversible or irreversible renal failure, and death. Oligohydramnios was also reported, presumably from decreased fetal renal function. In this setting, oligohydramnios was associated with fetal limb contractures, craniofacial deformation, and hypoplastic lung development. Prematurity, intrauterine growth retardation, and patent ductus arteriosus were also reported, although it is not clear whether these occurrences were due to exposure to the drug. In addition, first trimester use of ACE inhibitors, a specific class of drugs acting on the renin-angiotensin-aldosterone system, has been associated with a potential risk of birth defects in retrospective data.

When pregnancy occurs in a patient using Valturna, discontinue Valturna treatment as soon as possible. Inform the patient about potential risks to the fetus based on the time of gestational exposure to Valturna (first trimester only or later). If exposure occurs beyond the first trimester, perform an ultrasound examination.

In rare cases when another antihypertensive agent cannot be used to treat the pregnant patient, perform serial ultrasound examinations to assess the intraamniotic environment. Routine fetal testing with non-stress tests, biophysical profiles, and/or contraction stress tests may be appropriate based on gestational age and standards of care in the community. If oligohydramnios occurs in these situations, individualized decisions about continuing or discontinuing Valturna treatment and about pregnancy management should be made by the patient, her physician, and experts in the management of high risk pregnancy. Patients and physicians should be aware that oligohydramnios may not appear until after the fetus has sustained irreversible injury.

Closely observe infants with histories of *in utero* exposure to Valturna for hypotension, oliguria, and hyperkalemia. If oliguria occurs, these infants may require blood pressure and renal perfusion support. Exchange transfusion or dialysis may be required to reverse hypotension or support decreased renal function.

No reproductive toxicity studies have been conducted with the combination of aliskiren and valsartan. However, these studies have been conducted for aliskiren as well as valsartan alone *[see Nonclinical Toxicology (13)]*.

8.3 Nursing Mothers

It is not known whether aliskiren is excreted in human milk, but aliskiren was secreted in the milk of lactating rats. It is not known whether valsartan is excreted in human milk. Valsartan was excreted into the milk of lactating rats; however, animal breast milk drug levels may not accurately reflect human breast milk levels. Because of the potential for adverse effects on the nursing infant, a decision should be made whether to discontinue nursing or discontinue the drug, taking into account the importance of the drug to the mother.

8.4 Pediatric Use

Safety and effectiveness of Valturna in pediatric patients have not been established.

8.5 Geriatric Use

In the short-term controlled clinical trials of Valturna, 99 (15.9%) patients treated with Valturna were ≥65 years and 14 (2.2%) were ≥75 years.

No overall differences in safety or effectiveness were observed between these subjects and younger subjects, and other reported clinical experience has not identified differences in responses between the elderly and younger patients, but greater sensitivity of some older individuals cannot be ruled out.

10 OVERDOSAGE

Aliskiren

Limited data are available related to overdosage in humans. The most likely manifestation of overdosage would be hypotension. If symptomatic hypotension occurs, provide supportive treatment.

Valsartan

Limited data are available related to overdosage in humans. The most likely effect of overdose with valsartan would be hypotension and tachycardia; bradycardia could occur from parasympathetic (vagal) stimulation. Depressed level of consciousness, circulatory collapse and shock have been reported. If symptomatic hypotension occurs, provide supportive treatment.

Valsartan is not removed from the plasma by hemodialysis. Valsartan was without grossly observable adverse effects at single oral doses up to 2000 mg/kg in rats and up to 1000 mg/kg in marmosets, except for the salivation and diarrhea in the rat and vomiting in the marmoset at the highest dose (60 and 31 times, respectively, the maximum recommended human dose on a mg/m^2 basis). (Calculations assume an oral dose of 320 mg/day and a 60-kg patient.)

11 DESCRIPTION

Valturna is a single tablet of aliskiren (an orally active, nonpeptide, potent direct renin inhibitor) and valsartan (an orally active, nonpeptide, specific angiotensin II antagonist acting on the AT_1 receptor subtype).

Aliskiren

Aliskiren hemifumarate is chemically described as (2S,4S,5S,7S)-N-(2-Carbamoyl-2-methylpropyl)-5-amino-4-hydroxy-2,7-diisopropyl-8-[4-methoxy-3-(3-methoxypropoxy)phenyl]-octanamide hemifumarate and its structural formula is

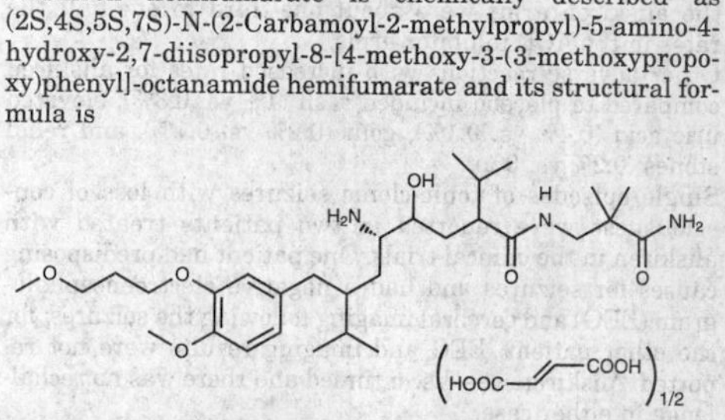

Molecular formula: $C_{30}H_{53}N_3O_6 \bullet 0.5\ C_4H_4O_4$

Aliskiren hemifumarate is a white to slightly yellowish crystalline powder with a molecular weight of 609.8 (free base- 551.8). It is soluble in phosphate buffer, n-octanol, and highly soluble in water.

Valsartan

Valsartan is a white to practically white fine powder, soluble in ethanol and methanol and slightly soluble in water. Valsartan's chemical name is N-(1-oxopentyl)-N-[[2'-(1H-tetrazol-5-yl) [1,1'-biphenyl]-4-yl]methyl]-L-valine; its structural formula is

[See chemical structure at top of next column]

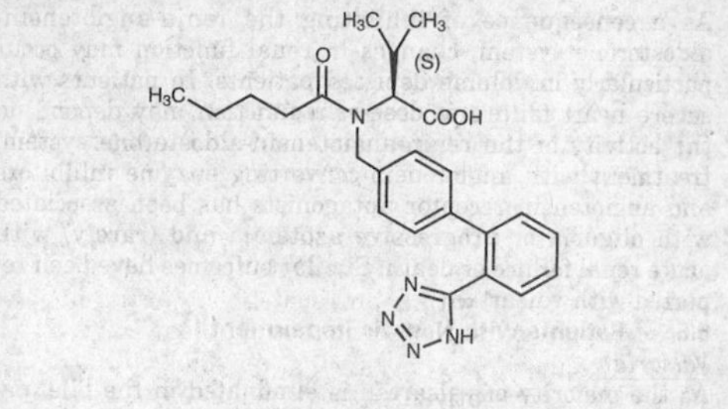

Its empirical formula is $C_{24}H_{29}N_5O_3$ and its molecular weight is 435.5.

Valturna tablets are formulated for oral administration to contain aliskiren hemifumarate and valsartan, USP 150/160 mg, and 300/320 mg. The inactive ingredients for all strengths of the tablets are colloidal silicon dioxide, crospovidone, hydroxypropylcellulose, indigotin blue lake, iron oxide black, iron oxide red, iron oxide yellow, magnesium stearate, microcrystalline cellulose, polyethylene glycol, talc, titanium dioxide and hypromellose.

12 CLINICAL PHARMACOLOGY

12.1 Mechanism of Action

Aliskiren

Renin is secreted by the kidney in response to decreases in blood volume and renal perfusion. Renin cleaves angiotensinogen to form the inactive decapeptide angiotensin I (Ang I). Ang I is converted to the active octapeptide angiotensin II (Ang II) by angiotensin-converting enzyme (ACE) and non-ACE pathways. Ang II is a powerful vasoconstrictor and leads to the release of catecholamines from the adrenal medulla and prejunctional nerve endings. It also promotes aldosterone secretion and sodium reabsorption. Together, these effects increase blood pressure. Ang II also inhibits renin release, thus providing a negative feedback to the system. This cycle, from renin through angiotensin to aldosterone and its associated negative feedback loop, is known as the renin-angiotensin-aldosterone system (RAAS). Aliskiren is a direct renin inhibitor, decreasing plasma renin activity (PRA) and inhibiting the conversion of angiotensinogen to Ang I. Whether aliskiren affects other RAAS components, e.g., ACE or non-ACE pathways, is not known.

All agents that inhibit the RAAS, including renin inhibitors, suppress the negative feedback loop, leading to a compensatory rise in plasma renin concentration. When this rise occurs during treatment with ACE inhibitors and ARBs, the result is increased levels of PRA. During treatment with aliskiren, however, the effect of increased renin levels is blocked, so that PRA, Ang I and Ang II are all reduced, whether aliskiren is used as monotherapy or in combination with other antihypertensive agents.

Valsartan

Ang II is formed from Ang I in a reaction catalyzed by angiotensin-converting enzyme (ACE, kininase II). Ang II is the principal pressor agent of the renin-angiotensin-aldosterone system, with effects that include vasoconstriction, stimulation of synthesis and release of aldosterone, cardiac stimulation, and renal reabsorption of sodium. Valsartan blocks the vasoconstrictor and aldosterone-secreting effects of Ang II by selectively blocking the binding of Ang II to the AT_1 receptor in many tissues, such as vascular smooth muscle and the adrenal gland. Its action is therefore independent of the pathways for Ang II synthesis. There is also an AT_2 receptor found in many tissues, but AT_2 is not known to be associated with cardiovascular homeostasis. Valsartan has much greater affinity (about 20,000-fold) for the AT_1 receptor than for the AT_2 receptor. The increased plasma levels of angiotensin following AT_1 receptor blockade with valsartan may stimulate the unblocked AT_2 receptor. The primary metabolite of valsartan is essentially inactive with an affinity for the AT_1 receptor about one-200th that of valsartan itself.

Blockade of the renin-angiotensin-aldosterone system with ACE inhibitors, which inhibit the biosynthesis of Ang II from Ang I, is widely used in the treatment of hypertension. ACE inhibitors also inhibit the degradation of bradykinin, a reaction also catalyzed by ACE. Because valsartan does not inhibit ACE (kininase II), it does not affect the response to bradykinin. Whether this difference has clinical relevance is not yet known. Valsartan does not bind to or block other hormone receptors or ion channels known to be important in cardiovascular regulation.

Blockade of the Ang II receptor inhibits the negative regulatory feedback of Ang II on renin secretion, but the resulting increased PRA and Ang II circulating levels do not overcome the effect of valsartan on blood pressure.

Valsartan has indications other than hypertension which can be found in the Diovan® package insert.

Valturna

Since aliskiren and valsartan block the RAAS at different sites (inhibition of plasma renin activity and antagonism of the AT_1 receptor), their combination provides a complementary mechanism to achieve a pharmacologic inhibition of the RAAS. Such RAAS inhibition with Valturna is associated with significant reductions in PRA, Ang I, Ang II and aldosterone.

12.2 Pharmacodynamics

Aliskiren

PRA reductions in clinical trials ranged from approximately 50% to 80%, were not dose-related and did not correlate with blood pressure reductions. The clinical implications of the differences in effect on PRA are not known.

Valsartan

Valsartan inhibits the pressor effect of angiotensin II infusions. An oral dose of 80 mg inhibits the pressor effect by about 80% at peak with approximately 30% inhibition persisting for 24 hours. No information on the effect of larger doses is available.

Removal of the negative feedback of angiotensin II causes a 2- to 3-fold rise in plasma renin and consequent rise in angiotensin II plasma concentration in hypertensive patients. Minimal decreases in plasma aldosterone were observed after administration of valsartan; very little effect on serum potassium was observed.

In multiple-dose studies in hypertensive patients with stable renal insufficiency and patients with renovascular hypertension, valsartan had no clinically significant effects on glomerular filtration rate, filtration fraction, creatinine clearance, or renal plasma flow.

In multiple-dose studies in hypertensive patients, valsartan had no notable effects on total cholesterol, fasting triglycerides, fasting serum glucose, or uric acid.

Administration of valsartan to patients with essential hypertension results in a significant reduction of sitting, supine, and standing systolic blood pressure, usually with little or no orthostatic change.

Valturna

In normotensive subjects receiving sodium supplementation, a single oral dose of 320 mg valsartan increased PRA, angiotensin I and angiotensin II, whereas 300 mg of aliskiren decreased them for 48 hours. In combination, 150 mg of aliskiren neutralized the 160 mg valsartan-induced increase in PRA, plasma angiotensin I and angiotensin II for 48 hours. The reduction in urinary aldosterone excretion with the 150/160 mg aliskiren/valsartan combination was similar to 300 mg of aliskiren and greater than that of 320 mg of valsartan and placebo.

12.3 Pharmacokinetics

Absorption and Distribution

Valturna

Following oral administration of Valturna combination tablets, the median peak plasma concentration times are within 1 hour for aliskiren and 3 hours for valsartan. The mean half-lives of aliskiren and valsartan are 34 hours and 12 hours, respectively. The rate and extent of absorption of aliskiren and valsartan from Valturna are the same as when administered as individual tablets. When taken with food, mean AUC and C_{max} of aliskiren are decreased by 76% and 88%, respectively; mean AUC and C_{max} of valsartan were not significantly affected. In clinical trials of Valturna, it was administered without requiring a fixed relation of administration to meals.

Valsartan

The steady state volume of distribution of valsartan after intravenous administration is 17 L indicating that valsartan does not distribute into tissues extensively. Valsartan is highly bound to serum proteins (95%), mainly serum albumin.

Metabolism and Elimination

Aliskiren

About one-fourth of the absorbed dose appears in the urine as parent drug. How much of the absorbed dose is metabolized is unknown. Based on the *in vitro* studies, the major enzyme responsible for aliskiren metabolism appears to be CYP 3A4.

Valsartan

Valsartan shows bi-exponential decay kinetics following intravenous administration with an average elimination half-life of about 6 hours. The recovery is mainly as unchanged drug, with only about 20% of dose recovered as metabolites. The primary metabolite, accounting for about 9% of dose, is valeryl 4-hydroxy valsartan. *In vitro* metabolism studies involving recombinant CYP450 enzymes indicated that the CYP2C9 isozyme is responsible for the formation of valeryl-4-hydroxy valsartan. It has also been shown that valsartan does not inhibit CYP450 isozymes at clinically relevant concentrations. CYP450 mediated drug interactions between valsartan and coadministered drugs are unlikely because of the low extent of metabolism.

Valsartan, when administered as an oral solution, is primarily recovered in feces (about 83% of dose) and urine (about 13% of dose). Following intravenous administration, plasma clearance of valsartan is about 2 L/h and its renal clearance is 0.62 L/h (about 30% of total clearance).

Special Populations

Pediatric Patients

The pharmacokinetics of Valturna have not been investigated in patients <18 years of age.

Table 1: Reductions in Seated Trough Cuff Blood Pressure of Aliskiren in Combination with Valsartan

Aliskiren, mg	(mmHg)	Valsartan, mg 0	160	320
0	Mean Change	4.6/4.1*	10.9/8.7	12.8/9.7
	Placebo-Subtracted Mean Change	—	5.6/3.9p	8.2/5.6p
150	Mean Change	10.7/7.5	15.3/10.5	—
	Placebo-Subtracted Mean Change	5.4/2.7p	10.0/5.7pav	—
300	Mean Change	13.0/9.0	—	17.2/12.2
	Placebo-Subtracted Mean Change	8.4/4.9p	—	12.6/8.1pav

* The placebo change is 5.2/4.8 for Week 4 endpoint which was used for the dose groups containing aliskiren 150 mg or valsartan 160 mg.

p p<0.05 vs. placebo by ANCOVA for the pairwise comparison.

a p<0.05 vs. respective aliskiren monotherapy by ANCOVA for the pairwise comparison.

v p<0.05 vs. respective valsartan monotherapy by ANCOVA for the pairwise comparison.

Geriatric Patients

The pharmacokinetics of aliskiren were studied in the elderly (≥65 years). Exposure (measured by AUC) is increased in elderly patients. Adjustment of the starting dose is not required in these patients. Exposure (measured by AUC) to valsartan is higher by 70% and the half-life is longer by 35% in the elderly than in the young. No dosage adjustment is necessary *[see Dosage and Administration (2.8)]*.

Race

With Valturna, pharmacokinetic differences due to race have not been studied. The pharmacokinetic differences among Blacks, Caucasians, and Japanese are minimal with aliskiren therapy.

Renal Impairment

Aliskiren

The pharmacokinetics of aliskiren were evaluated in patients with varying degrees of renal impairment. Rate and extent of exposure (AUC and C_{max}) of aliskiren in subjects with renal impairment did not show a consistent correlation with the severity of renal impairment. Adjustment of the starting dose is not required in these patients *[see Dosage and Administration (2.8)]*.

Valsartan

There is no apparent correlation between renal function (measured by creatinine clearance) and exposure (measured by AUC) to valsartan in patients with different degrees of renal impairment. Consequently, dose adjustment is not required in patients with mild-to-moderate renal dysfunction. No studies have been performed in patients with severe impairment of renal function (creatinine clearance <10 mL/min). Valsartan is not removed from the plasma by hemodialysis *[see Dosage and Administration (2.8)]*.

Hepatic Impairment

Aliskiren

The pharmacokinetics of aliskiren were not significantly affected in patients with mild-to-severe liver disease. Consequently, adjustment of the starting dose is not required in these patients *[see Dosage and Administration (2.8)]*.

Valsartan

On average, patients with mild-to-moderate chronic liver disease have twice the exposure (measured by AUC values) to valsartan of healthy volunteers (matched by age, sex and weight). In general, no dosage adjustment is needed in patients with mild-to-moderate liver disease *[see Dosage and Administration (2.8)]*.

13 NONCLINICAL TOXICOLOGY

13.1 Carcinogenesis, Mutagenesis, Impairment of Fertility

Valturna

No carcinogenicity, mutagenicity or fertility studies have been conducted for Valturna alone as these studies have been conducted for each individual component. Valturna has been studied in 2- and 13-week toxicity studies and was generally well-tolerated. Findings were primarily attributable to the exaggerated pharmacological effects of each component.

Aliskiren

Carcinogenic potential was assessed in a 2-year rat study and a 6-month transgenic (rasH2) mouse study with aliskiren hemifumarate at oral doses of up to 1500 mg aliskiren/kg/day. Although there were no statistically significant increases in tumor incidence associated with exposure to aliskiren, mucosal epithelial hyperplasia (with or without erosion/ulceration) was observed in the lower gastrointestinal tract at doses of 750 or more mg/kg/day in both species, with a colonic adenoma identified in one rat and a cecal adenocarcinoma identified in another, rare tumors in the strain of rat studied. On a systemic exposure ($AUC_{0\text{-}24hr}$) basis, 1500 mg/kg/day in the rat is about 4 times and in the mouse about 1.5 times the maximum recommended human dose (300 mg aliskiren/day). Mucosal hyperplasia in the cecum or colon of rats was also observed at doses of 250 mg/kg/day (the lowest tested dose) as well as at higher doses in 4- and 13-week studies.

Aliskiren hemifumarate was devoid of genotoxic potential in the Ames reverse mutation assay with *S. typhimurium* and *E. coli*, the *in vitro* Chinese hamster ovary cell chromosomal aberration assay, the *in vitro* Chinese hamster V79 cell gene mutation test and the *in vivo* mouse bone marrow micronucleus assay.

Fertility of male and female rats was unaffected at doses of up to 250 mg aliskiren/kg/day (8 times the maximum recommended human dose of 300 mg Tekturna/60 kg on a mg/m^2 basis).

Valsartan

There was no evidence of carcinogenicity when valsartan was administered in the diet to mice and rats for up to 2 years at concentrations calculated to provide doses of up to 160 and 200 mg/kg/day, respectively. These doses in mice and rats are about 2.4 and 6 times, respectively, the MRHD of 320 mg/day on a mg/m^2 basis. (Calculations based on a 60 kg patient.)

Mutagenicity assays did not reveal any valsartan-related effects at either the gene or chromosome level. These assays included bacterial mutagenicity tests with *Salmonella* and *E. coli*, a gene mutation test with Chinese hamster V79 cells, a cytogenetic test with Chinese hamster ovary cells, and a rat micronucleus test.

13.2 Animal Toxicology and/or Pharmacology

Reproductive Toxicology Studies

Aliskiren

Reproductive toxicity studies of aliskiren hemifumarate did not reveal any evidence of teratogenicity at oral doses up to 600 mg aliskiren/kg/day (20 times the maximum recommended human dose [MRHD] of 300 mg/day on a mg/m^2 basis) in pregnant rats or up to 100 mg aliskiren/kg/day (seven times the MRHD on a mg/m^2 basis) in pregnant rabbits. Fetal birth weight was adversely affected in rabbits at 50 mg/kg/day (3.2 times the MRHD on a mg/m^2 basis). Aliskiren was present in placenta, amniotic fluid and fetuses of pregnant rabbits.

Valsartan

No teratogenic effects were observed when valsartan was administered to pregnant mice and rats at oral doses up at 600 mg/kg/day and to pregnant rabbits at oral doses up to 10 mg/kg/day. However, significant decreases in fetal weight, pup birth weight, pup survival rate, and slight delays in developmental milestones were observed in studies in which parental rats were treated with valsartan at oral, maternally toxic (reduction in body weight gain and food consumption) doses of 600 mg/kg/day during organogenesis or late gestation and lactation. In rabbits, fetotoxicity (i.e., resorptions, litter loss, abortions, and low body weight) associated with maternal toxicity (mortality) was observed at doses of 5 and 10 mg/kg/day. The no observed adverse effect doses of 600, 200 and 2 mg/kg/day in mice, rats and rabbits represent 9, 6, and 0.1 times, respectively, the maximum recommended human dose on a mg/m^2 basis. Calculations assume an oral dose of 320 mg/day and a 60-kg patient.

14 CLINICAL STUDIES

Valturna

Aliskiren 150 mg and 300 mg and valsartan 160 mg and 320 mg were studied alone and in combination in an 8-week, 1,797-patient, randomized, double-blind, placebo-controlled, parallel-group, 4-arm, dose-escalation study. The dosages of aliskiren and valsartan were started at 150 mg and 160 mg, respectively, and increased at four weeks to 300 mg and 320 mg, respectively. Seated trough cuff blood pressure was measured at baseline, 4, and 8 weeks. Blood pressure reductions with the combinations were statistically significantly (p<0.05) greater than the reductions with the monotherapies as shown in Table 1.

[See table 1 above]

Table 2: Valturna Tablets Supply

Tablet	Color	Debossed Side 1	Debossed Side 2	NDC 0078-XXXX-XX Bottle of 30	Bottle of 90	Blister Packages of 100
Aliskiren/valsartan						
150 mg/160 mg	Light Red	NVR	HDU	0572-15	0572-34	0572-35
300 mg/320 mg	Light Brown	NVR	SNB	0574-15	0574-34	0574-35

The safety and efficacy of Valturna as initial therapy were evaluated. The figures *[see Indications and Usage (1)]* display the probability that a patient will achieve systolic or diastolic blood pressure goal with Valturna 300/320 mg, based upon their baseline systolic or diastolic blood pressure. At all levels of baseline blood pressure, the probability of achieving any given diastolic or systolic goal is greater with the combination than for either monotherapy.

The antihypertensive effect of Valturna was attained within 2 weeks.

One active-controlled trial investigated the addition of aliskiren 300 mg plus valsartan 320 mg in hypertensive patients who did not respond adequately to HCTZ 25 mg, and showed decreases from baseline in systolic and diastolic blood pressure of approximately 22/16 mmHg compared with approximately 6/6 mmHg with continuation of HCTZ 25 mg alone.

The antihypertensive effect was similar in patients with or without diabetes, in patients ≥65 years of age and <65 years of age, and in women and men. The effects of aliskiren, valsartan, and the combination were diminished in Blacks compared to Caucasians as has been seen with ACE inhibitors, other angiotensin receptor blockers, and beta blockers.

16   HOW SUPPLIED/STORAGE AND HANDLING

Valturna is supplied as convex, beveled edged, ovaloid film-coated tablets.

All strengths are packaged in bottles and unit-dose blister packages (10 strips of 10 tablets) as described below.
[See table 2 above]

Storage
Store at 25°C (77°F); excursions permitted to 15-30°C (59-86°F) in original container. [See USP Controlled Room Temperature.]
Protect from moisture.
Dispense in tight container (USP).

17   PATIENT COUNSELING INFORMATION

Healthcare professionals should instruct their patients to read the Patient Package Insert before starting Valturna and to reread each time the prescription is renewed. Patients should be instructed to inform their doctor or pharmacist if they develop any unusual symptom, or if any known symptom persists or worsens.

Pregnancy
Tell female patients of childbearing age about the consequences of exposure to drugs that act on the renin-angiotensin-aldosterone system. Discuss other treatment options with female patients planning to become pregnant. Ask these patients to report pregnancies to their physicians as soon as possible.

Symptomatic Hypotension
Caution patients receiving Valturna that lightheadedness can occur, especially during the first days of therapy, and that it should be reported to the prescribing physician. Tell the patients that if syncope occurs, discontinue Valturna until the physician has been consulted.
Caution all patients that inadequate fluid intake, excessive perspiration, diarrhea, or vomiting can lead to an excessive fall in blood pressure, with the same consequences of lightheadedness and possible syncope.

Potassium Supplements
Tell patients receiving Valturna not to use potassium supplements or salt substitutes containing potassium without consulting the prescribing physician.

Relationship to Meals
Patients should establish a routine pattern for taking Valturna with regard to meals. High-fat meals decrease absorption substantially.

FDA-APPROVED PATIENT LABELING
Patient Information
Valturna® (val-tur-na)
(aliskiren and valsartan, USP) Tablets
Read the Patient Information that comes with Valturna before you start taking it and each time you get a refill. There may be new information. This leaflet does not take the place of talking with your doctor about your condition and treatment.
IMPORTANT WARNING: Valturna may harm an unborn baby, causing injury and death. If you get pregnant, stop taking Valturna and call your doctor right away. If you plan
to become pregnant, talk to your doctor about other medicines to treat your high blood pressure before taking Valturna.

What is Valturna?
Valturna contains two prescription medicines in one tablet that work together to lower blood pressure. It contains:
• aliskiren (Tekturna), a direct renin inhibitor (DRI)
• valsartan (Diovan), an angiotensin receptor blocker (ARB)
Aliskiren (Tekturna) reduces the effect of renin, and the harmful process that narrows blood vessels. Aliskiren also helps blood vessels relax and widen so blood pressure is lower. Valsartan (Diovan) can help lower your blood pressure by blocking a potent chemical, angiotensin II, that leads to blood vessel constriction and narrowing.
Valturna may be used to lower high blood pressure in adults:
• when one medicine to lower high blood pressure is not enough
• as the first medicine to lower high blood pressure if your doctor decides that you are likely to need more than one medicine
Valturna has not been studied in children under 18 years of age.
Your doctor may prescribe other medicines for you to take along with Valturna to treat your high blood pressure.

What is high blood pressure (hypertension)?
Blood pressure is the force that pushes the blood through your blood vessels to all the organs of your body. You have high blood pressure when the force of your blood moving through your blood vessels is too great. One cause of high blood pressure is renin, a chemical in the body that starts a process that makes blood vessels narrow, leading to high blood pressure.
Valturna reduces high blood pressure. Medicines that lower your blood pressure lower your chance of having a stroke or heart attack. High blood pressure makes the heart work harder to pump blood throughout the body and causes damage to the blood vessels. If high blood pressure is not treated, it can lead to stroke, heart attack, heart failure, kidney failure, and vision problems.
Blood pressure is reduced more with Valturna than when either Tekturna or Diovan is taken by itself.

Who should not take Valturna?
• If you get pregnant, stop taking Valturna and call your doctor right away. If you plan to become pregnant, talk to your doctor about other treatment options for your high blood pressure.
• Do not take Valturna if you are allergic to any of its ingredients. See the end of this leaflet for a complete list of the ingredients in Valturna.

What should I tell my doctor before taking Valturna?
Tell your doctor about all your medical conditions, including whether you:
• have kidney problems
• have liver problems
• have ever had a reaction called angioedema, to another blood pressure medicine. Angioedema causes swelling of the face, lips, tongue, throat, arms and legs, and may cause difficulty breathing.
• are pregnant or planning to become pregnant. See IMPORTANT WARNING.
• are breast-feeding. It is not known if Valturna passes into your breast milk.
Tell your doctor about all the medicines you take including prescription and nonprescription medicines, vitamins and herbal supplements. Especially tell your doctor if you are taking:
• other medicines for high blood pressure or a heart problem
• water pills (also called "diuretics")
• medicines for treating fungus or fungal infections
• cyclosporine (a medicine used to suppress the immune system)
• potassium-containing medicines, potassium supplements, or salt substitutes containing potassium
• atorvastatin
Your doctor or pharmacist will know what medicines are safe to take together. Know your medicines. Keep a list of your medicines and show it to your doctor or pharmacist when you get a new medicine.

How should I take Valturna?
• Take Valturna exactly as prescribed by your doctor. It is important to take Valturna every day to control your blood pressure.
• Take Valturna once each day, about the same time each day.
• Take Valturna the same way every day, either with or without a meal.
• Your doctor may change your dose of Valturna if needed.
• If you miss a dose of Valturna, take it as soon as you remember. If it is close to your next dose, do not take the missed dose. Just take the next dose at your regular time.
• If you take too much Valturna, call your doctor or a Poison Control Center, or go to the nearest hospital emergency room.

What are the possible side effects of Valturna?
Valturna may cause serious side effects:
• **Injury or death to an unborn baby.** See IMPORTANT WARNING.
• **Low blood pressure (hypotension).** Your blood pressure may get too low if you also take water pills, are on a low-salt diet, get dialysis treatments, have heart problems, or get sick with vomiting or diarrhea. Drinking alcohol and taking certain medicines (barbiturates or narcotics) can cause low blood pressure to get worse. Lie down if you feel faint or dizzy, and call your doctor right away.
• **Angioedema.** Aliskiren, a component in Valturna, can cause swelling of the face, lips, tongue, throat, arms and legs, or the whole body. Get medical help right away and tell your doctor if you get any one or more of these symptoms. Angioedema can happen at any time while you are taking Valturna.

Common side effects of Valturna include:
• Tiredness
• Sore throat
• Runny nose
• Diarrhea
• Upper respiratory tract infection
• Urinary tract infection
• Flu or flu-like symptoms
• Dizziness
Tell your doctor if you have any side effect that bothers you or that does not go away. These are not all of the possible side effects of Valturna. For a complete list of side effects, ask your doctor or pharmacist.

How do I store Valturna?
• Store Valturna tablets at room temperature between 59°F-86°F (15°C-30°C).
• Keep Valturna in the original prescription bottle in a dry place. Do not remove the desiccant (drying agent) from the bottle.
Keep Valturna and all medicines out of the reach of children.

General information about Valturna
Medicines are sometimes prescribed for conditions not listed in the patient information leaflet. Do not take Valturna for a condition for which it was not prescribed. Do not give Valturna to other people, even if they have the same condition or symptoms you have. It may harm them. This leaflet summarizes the most important information about Valturna. If you have questions about Valturna talk with your doctor. You can ask your doctor or pharmacist for information that is written for healthcare professionals.
For more information about Valturna, visit www.valturna.com or call 1-877-282-5887.

What are the ingredients in Valturna?
Active ingredients: Aliskiren and valsartan
Inactive ingredients: The inactive ingredients for all strengths of the tablets are colloidal silicon dioxide, crospovidone, hydroxypropylcellulose, indigotin blue lake, iron oxide black, iron oxide red, iron oxide yellow, magnesium stearate, microcrystalline cellulose, polyethylene glycol, talc, titanium dioxide, and hypromellose.
Call your doctor for medical advice about side effects. You may report side effects to FDA at 1-800-FDA-1088.

T2010-68/T2009-04

Manufactured by:
Novartis Pharma Stein AG
Stein, Switzerland
Distributed by:
Novartis Pharmaceuticals Corporation
East Hanover, New Jersey 07936
©Novartis
Shown in Product Identification Guide, page 316

XOLAIR®   ℞
[zō-lar]
(omalizumab)
For injection, for subcutaneous use

The following prescribing information is based on official labeling in effect July 2010.
HIGHLIGHTS OF PRESCRIBING INFORMATION
These highlights do not include all the information needed to use Xolair safely and effectively. See full prescribing information for Xolair.

XOLAIR® [omalizumab]
For injection, for subcutaneous use
Initial U.S. Approval: 2003

WARNING: ANAPHYLAXIS
See full prescribing information for complete boxed warning.
Anaphylaxis, presenting as bronchospasm, hypotension, syncope, urticaria, and/or angioedema of the throat or tongue, has been reported to occur after administration of Xolair. Anaphylaxis has occurred after the first dose of Xolair but also has occurred beyond 1 year after beginning treatment. Closely observe patients for an appropriate period of time after Xolair administration and be prepared to manage anaphylaxis that can be life-threatening. Inform patients of the signs and symptoms of anaphylaxis and have them seek immediate medical care should symptoms occur.

————————RECENT MAJOR CHANGES————————

Indications and Usage, Pediatric Patients (Age 0 to <12) (1)	01/2010
Use in Specific Populations, Pediatric Use (Age 0 to <12) (8.4)	01/2010
Warnings and Precautions, Fever, Arthralgia, and Rash (5.6)	07/10
Adverse Reactions, Postmarketing Experience (6.2)	07/10

————————INDICATIONS AND USAGE————————

Xolair is indicated for:
• Moderate to severe persistent asthma in patients with a positive skin test or in vitro reactivity to a perennial aeroallergen and symptoms that are inadequately controlled with inhaled corticosteroids.

Important Limitations of Use:
• Not indicated for other allergic conditions. (1)
• Not indicated for acute bronchospasm or status asthmaticus (1, 5.3)
• Not indicated for pediatric patients less than 12 years of age (1, 8.4)

————————DOSAGE AND ADMINISTRATION————————

For subcutaneous (SC) administration only.
Administer Xolair 150 to 375 mg SC every 2 or 4 weeks. (2.1)
• Determine dose (mg) and dosing frequency by serum total IgE level (IU/mL), measured before the start of treatment, and body weight (kg). See the dose determination charts (2.1)
• Divide doses of more than 150 mg among more than one injection site to limit injections to not more than 150 mg per site. (2.3)

————————DOSAGE FORMS AND STRENGTHS————————

• Lyophilized, sterile powder in a single-use 5 mL vial, 150 mg (3)

————————CONTRAINDICATIONS————————

• Severe hypersensitivity reaction to Xolair or any ingredient of Xolair. (4, 5.1)

————————WARNINGS AND PRECAUTIONS————————

• Anaphylaxis—Administer only in a healthcare setting prepared to manage anaphylaxis that can be life-threatening and observe patients for an appropriate period of time after administration. (5.1)
• Malignancy—Malignancies have been observed in clinical studies. (5.2)
• Acute Asthma Symptoms—Do not use for the treatment of acute bronchospasm or status asthmaticus. (5.3)
• Corticosteroid Reductions—Do not abruptly discontinue corticosteroids upon initiation of Xolair therapy. (5.4)
• Fever, Arthralgia, and Rash—Stop Xolair if patients develop signs and symptoms similar to serum sickness (5.6)
• Eosinophilic Conditions—Be alert to eosinophilia, vasculitic rash, worsening pulmonary symptoms, cardiac complications, and/or neuropathy, especially upon reduction of oral corticosteroids. (5.5)

————————ADVERSE REACTIONS————————

In the adult and adolescent patients (≥12 years of age), the most commonly observed adverse reactions in clinical studies (≥1% more frequent in Xolair-treated patients) were arthralgia, pain (general), leg pain, fatigue, dizziness, fracture, arm pain, pruritus, dermatitis, and earache. (6.1)
To report SUSPECTED ADVERSE REACTIONS, contact Genentech at 1-888-835-2555 or FDA at 1-800-FDA-1088 or www.fda.gov/medwatch.

————————DRUG INTERACTIONS————————

• No formal drug interaction studies have been performed. (7)

————————USE IN SPECIFIC POPULATIONS————————

• Pregnancy: No adequate data in humans. Xolair Pregnancy Exposure Registry available (1-866-496-5247) (8.1)

See 17 for PATIENT COUNSELING INFORMATION and Medication Guide.

Revised: *07/2010*

FULL PRESCRIBING INFORMATION: CONTENTS*
WARNING: ANAPHYLAXIS
1 INDICATIONS AND USAGE
2 DOSAGE AND ADMINISTRATION
  2.1 Dosing
  2.2 Dosing Adjustments
  2.3 Preparation and Administration
3 DOSAGE FORMS AND STRENGTHS
4 CONTRAINDICATIONS
5 WARNINGS AND PRECAUTIONS
  5.1 Anaphylaxis
  5.2 Malignancy
  5.3 Acute Asthma Symptoms
  5.4 Corticosteroid Reductions
  5.5 Eosinophilic Conditions
  5.6 Fever, Arthralgia, and Rash
  5.7 Parasitic (Helminth) Infection
  5.8 Laboratory Tests
6 ADVERSE REACTIONS
  6.1 Clinical Trials Experience
  6.2 Postmarketing Experience
7 DRUG INTERACTIONS
8 USE IN SPECIFIC POPULATIONS
  8.1 Pregnancy
  8.3 Nursing Mothers
  8.4 Pediatric Use
  8.5 Geriatric Use
10 OVERDOSAGE
11 DESCRIPTION
12 CLINICAL PHARMACOLOGY
  12.1 Mechanism of Action
  12.2 Pharmacodynamics
  12.3 Pharmacokinetics
13 NONCLINICAL TOXICOLOGY
  13.1 Carcinogenesis, Mutagenesis, Impairment of Fertility
  13.2 Animal Toxicology and/or Pharmacology
14 CLINICAL STUDIES
16 HOW SUPPLIED/STORAGE AND HANDLING
17 PATIENT COUNSELING INFORMATION
  17.1 Information for Patients
* Sections or subsections omitted from the full prescribing information are not listed.

FULL PRESCRIBING INFORMATION

WARNING: Anaphylaxis
Anaphylaxis presenting as bronchospasm, hypotension, syncope, urticaria, and/or angioedema of the throat or tongue, has been reported to occur after administration of Xolair. Anaphylaxis has occurred as early after the first dose of Xolair, but also has occurred beyond 1 year after beginning regularly administered treatment. Because of the risk of anaphylaxis, observe patients closely for an appropriate period of time after Xolair administration. Health care providers administering Xolair should be prepared to manage anaphylaxis that can be life-threatening. Inform patients of the signs and symptoms of anaphylaxis and instruct them to seek immediate medical care should symptoms occur [*see Warnings and Precautions (5.1)*].

---

1 INDICATIONS AND USAGE

Xolair (omalizumab) is indicated for adults and adolescents (12 years of age and above) with moderate to severe persistent asthma who have a positive skin test or in vitro reactivity to a perennial aeroallergen and whose symptoms are inadequately controlled with inhaled corticosteroids.
Xolair has been shown to decrease the incidence of asthma exacerbations in these patients.
Important Limitations of Use
Xolair is not indicated for treatment of other allergic conditions.
Xolair is not indicated for the relief of acute bronchospasm or status asthmaticus.
Xolair is not indicated for use in pediatric patients less than 12 years of age.

2 DOSAGE AND ADMINISTRATION

2.1 Dosing
Administer Xolair (omalizumab) 150 to 375 mg by subcutaneous (SC) injection every 2 or 4 weeks. Determine doses (mg) and dosing frequency by serum total IgE level (IU/mL), measured before the start of treatment, and body weight (kg). *See the dose determination charts below (Table 1 and Table 2) for appropriate dose assignment.*

Periodically reassess the need for continued therapy based upon the patient's disease severity and level of asthma control.

Table 1
Administration Every 4 Weeks
Xolair Doses (milligrams) Administered by Subcutaneous Injection Every 4 Weeks for Adults and Adolescents 12 Years of Age and Older

Pre-treatment Serum IgE (IU/mL)	Body Weight (kg)			
	30-60	> 60-70	> 70-90	> 90-150
≥30-100	150	150	150	300
>100-200	300	300	300	
>200-300	300			
>300-400		SEE TABLE 2		
>400-500				
>500-600				

Table 2
Administration Every 2 Weeks
Xolair Doses (milligrams) Administered by Subcutaneous Injection Every 2 Weeks for Adults and Adolescents 12 Years of Age and Older

Pre-treatment Serum IgE (IU/mL)	Body Weight (kg)			
	30-60	> 60-70	> 70-90	> 90-150
≥30-100		SEE TABLE 1		
>100-200				225
>200-300		225	225	300
>300-400	225	225	300	
>400-500	300	300	375	
>500-600	300	375	DO NOT DOSE	
>600-700	375			

2.2 Dosing Adjustments
Adjust doses for significant changes in body weight (*see Table 1 and Table 2*).
Total IgE levels are elevated during treatment and remain elevated for up to one year after the discontinuation of treatment. Therefore, re-testing of IgE levels during Xolair treatment cannot be used as a guide for dose determination.
• Interruptions lasting less than one year: Dose based on serum IgE levels obtained at the initial dose determination.
• Interruptions lasting one year or more: Re-test total serum IgE levels for dose determination.

2.3 Preparation and Administration
Prepare Xolair for subcutaneous injection using Sterile Water for Injection (SWFI), USP, ONLY. Each vial of Xolair is for single use only and contains no preservatives.
Reconstitution
The lyophilized product takes 15-20 minutes to dissolve. The fully reconstituted product will appear clear or slightly opalescent and it is acceptable if there are a few small bubbles or foam around the edge of the vial. The reconstituted product is somewhat viscous; in order to obtain the full 1.2 mL dose, ALL OF THE PRODUCT MUST BE WITHDRAWN from the vial before expelling any air or excess solution from the syringe.
Use the solution within 8 hours following reconstitution when stored in the vial at 2-8°C (36-46°F), or within 4 hours of reconstitution when stored at room temperature. Reconstituted Xolair vials should be protected from sunlight.
Preparation
STEP 1: Draw 1.4 mL of SWFI, USP into a 3 mL syringe equipped with a 1-inch, 18-gauge needle.
STEP 2: Place the vial upright on a flat surface and using standard aseptic technique, insert the needle and inject the SWFI, USP directly onto the product.
STEP 3: Keeping the vial upright, gently swirl the upright vial for approximately 1 minute to evenly wet the powder. Do not shake.
STEP 4: After completing STEP 3, gently swirl the vial for 5-10 seconds approximately every 5 minutes in order to dissolve any remaining solids. There should be no visible gel-like particles in the solution. Do not use if foreign particles are present.

Note: If it takes longer than 20 minutes to dissolve completely, repeat STEP 4 until there are no visible gel-like particles in the solution. Do not use if the contents of the vial do not dissolve completely by 40 minutes.

STEP 5: Invert the vial for 15 seconds in order to allow the solution to drain toward the stopper. Using a new 3 mL syringe equipped with a 1-inch, 18-gauge needle, insert the needle into the inverted vial. Position the needle tip at the very bottom of the solution in the vial stopper when drawing the solution into the syringe. Before removing the needle from the vial, pull the plunger all the way back to the end of the syringe barrel in order to remove all of the solution from the inverted vial.

STEP 6: Replace the 18-gauge needle with a 25-gauge needle for subcutaneous injection.

STEP 7: Expel air, large bubbles, and any excess solution in order to obtain the required 1.2 mL dose. A thin layer of small bubbles may remain at the top of the solution in the syringe.

Administration

Administer Xolair by subcutaneous injection. The injection may take 5-10 seconds to administer because the solution is slightly viscous. Each vial delivers 1.2 mL (150 mg) of Xolair. Do not administer more than 150 mg per injection site. Divide doses of more than 150 mg among two or more injection sites. (Table 3).

Table 3
Number of Injections and Total Injection Volumes

Xolair Dose (mg)	Number of Injections	Total Volume Injected (mL)
150	1	1.2
225	2	1.8
300	2	2.4
375	3	3.0

3 DOSAGE FORMS AND STRENGTHS

150 mg of omalizumab as lyophilized, sterile powder in a single-use 5 mL vial.

4 CONTRAINDICATIONS

The use of Xolair is contraindicated in the following:
Severe hypersensitivity reaction to Xolair or any ingredient of Xolair [*see Warnings and Precautions (5.1)*].

5 WARNINGS AND PRECAUTIONS

5.1 Anaphylaxis

Anaphylaxis has been reported to occur after administration of Xolair in premarketing clinical trials and in postmarketing spontaneous reports. Signs and symptoms in these reported cases have included bronchospasm, hypotension, syncope, urticaria, and/or angioedema of the throat or tongue. Some of these events have been life-threatening. In premarketing clinical trials the frequency of anaphylaxis attributed to Xolair use was estimated to be 0.1%. In postmarketing spontaneous reports, the frequency of anaphylaxis attributed to Xolair use was estimated to be at least 0.2% of patients based on an estimated exposure of about 57,300 patients from June 2003 through December 2006. Anaphylaxis has occurred as early as after the first dose of Xolair, but also has occurred beyond one year after beginning regularly scheduled treatment.

Administer Xolair only in a healthcare setting by healthcare providers prepared to manage anaphylaxis that can be life-threatening. Observe patients closely for an appropriate period of time after administration of Xolair, taking into account the time to onset of anaphylaxis seen in premarketing clinical trials and postmarketing spontaneous reports [*see Adverse Reactions (6)*]. Inform patients of the signs and symptoms of anaphylaxis, and instruct them to seek immediate medical care should signs or symptoms occur.

Discontinue Xolair in patients who experience a severe hypersensitivity reaction [*see Contraindications (4)*].

5.2 Malignancy

Malignant neoplasms were observed in 20 of 4127 (0.5%) Xolair-treated patients compared with 5 of 2236 (0.2%) control patients in clinical studies of adults and adolescents (≥12 years of age) with asthma and other allergic disorders. The observed malignancies in Xolair-treated patients were a variety of types, with breast, non-melanoma skin, prostate, melanoma, and parotid occurring more than once, and five other types occurring once each. The majority of patients were observed for less than 1 year. The impact of longer exposure to Xolair or use in patients at higher risk for malignancy (e.g., elderly, current smokers) is not known [*see Adverse Reactions (6)*].

5.3 Acute Asthma Symptoms

Xolair has not been shown to alleviate asthma exacerbations acutely. Do not use Xolair to treat acute bronchospasm or status asthmaticus.

5.4 Corticosteroid Reduction

Do not discontinue systemic or inhaled corticosteroids abruptly upon initiation of Xolair therapy. Decrease corticosteroids gradually under the direct supervision of a physician.

5.5 Eosinophilic Conditions

In rare cases, patients with asthma on therapy with Xolair may present with serious systemic eosinophilia sometimes presenting with clinical features of vasculitis consistent with Churg-Strauss syndrome, a condition which is often treated with systemic corticosteroid therapy. These events usually, but not always, have been associated with the reduction of oral corticosteroid therapy. Physicians should be alert to eosinophilia, vasculitic rash, worsening pulmonary symptoms, cardiac complications, and/or neuropathy presenting in their patients. A causal association between Xolair and these underlying conditions has not been established.

5.6 Fever, Arthralgia, and Rash

In post-approval use, some patients have experienced a constellation of signs and symptoms including arthritis/arthralgia, rash (urticaria or other forms), fever and lymphadenopathy with an onset 1 to 5 days after the first or subsequent injections of Xolair. These signs and symptoms have recurred after additional doses in some patients. Although circulating immune complexes or a skin biopsy consistent with a Type III reaction were not seen with these cases, these signs and symptoms are similar to those seen in patients with serum sickness. Physicians should stop Xolair if a patient develops this constellation of signs and symptoms. [*see Adverse Reactions, Postmarketing Experience (6.2)*]

5.7 Parasitic (Helminth) Infection

Monitor patients at high risk of geohelminth infection while on Xolair therapy. Insufficient data are available to determine the length of monitoring required for geohelminth infections after stopping Xolair treatment.

In a one-year clinical trial conducted in Brazil in patients at high risk for geohelminthic infections (roundworm, hookworm, whipworm, threadworm), 53% (36/68) of Xolair-treated patients experienced an infection, as diagnosed by standard stool examination, compared to 42% (29/69) of placebo controls. The point estimate of the odds ratio for infection was 1.96, with a 95% confidence interval (0.88, 4.36) indicating that in this study a patient who had an infection was anywhere from 0.88 to 4.36 times as likely to have received Xolair than a patient who did not have an infection. Response to appropriate anti-geohelminth treatment of infection as measured by stool egg counts was not different between treatment groups.

5.8 Laboratory Tests

Serum total IgE levels increase following administration of Xolair due to formation of Xolair:IgE complexes [*see Clinical Pharmacology (12.2)*]. Elevated serum total IgE levels may persist for up to 1 year following discontinuation of Xolair. Do not use serum total IgE levels obtained less than 1 year following discontinuation to reassess the dosing regimen because these levels may not reflect steady state free IgE levels.

6 ADVERSE REACTIONS

Use of Xolair has been associated with:
- Anaphylaxis [*see Boxed Warning and Warning and Precautions (5.1)*]
- Malignancies [*see Warnings and Precautions (5.2)*]

Anaphylaxis was reported in 3 of 3507 (0.1%) patients in clinical trials. Anaphylaxis occurred with the first dose of Xolair in two patients and with the fourth dose in one patient. The time to onset of anaphylaxis was 90 minutes after administration in two patients and 2 hours after administration in one patient. In clinical trials the observed incidence of malignancy among Xolair-treated patients (0.5%) was numerically higher than among patients in control groups (0.2%).

6.1 Clinical Trials Experience

Adult and Adolescent Patients 12 years of Age and Older
The data described below reflect Xolair exposure for 2076 adult and adolescent patients ages 12 and older, including 1687 patients exposed for six months and 555 exposed for one year or more, in either placebo-controlled or other controlled asthma studies. The mean age of patients receiving Xolair was 42 years, with 134 patients 65 years of age or older; 60% were women, and 85% Caucasian. Patients received Xolair 150 to 375 mg every 2 or 4 weeks or, for patients assigned to control groups, standard therapy with or without a placebo. Because clinical studies are conducted under widely varying conditions, adverse reaction rates observed in the clinical studies of one drug cannot be directly compared with rates in the clinical studies of another drug and may not reflect the rates observed in medical practice. The adverse events most frequently resulting in clinical intervention (e.g., discontinuation of Xolair, or the need for concomitant medication to treat an adverse event) were injection site reaction (45%), viral infections (23%), upper res-

piratory tract infection (20%), sinusitis (16%), headache (15%), and pharyngitis (11%). These events were observed at similar rates in Xolair-treated patients and control patients.

Table 4 shows adverse reactions from four placebo-controlled asthma studies that occurred ≥1% and more frequently in patients receiving Xolair than in those receiving placebo. Adverse events were classified using preferred terms from the International Medical Nomenclature (IMN) dictionary. Injection site reactions were recorded separately from the reporting of other adverse events and are described following Table 4.

Table 4
Adverse Reactions ≥1% More Frequent in Xolair-Treated Adult or Adolescent Patients 12 Years of Age and Older Four placebo-controlled asthma studies

Adverse reaction	Xolair n=738 (%)	Placebo n=717 (%)
Body as a whole		
Pain	7	5
Fatigue	3	2
Musculoskeletal system		
Arthralgia	8	6
Fracture	2	1
Leg pain	4	2
Arm pain	2	1
Nervous system		
Dizziness	3	2
Skin and appendages		
Pruritus	2	1
Dermatitis	2	1
Special senses		
Earache	2	1

There were no differences in the incidence of adverse reactions based on age (among patients under 65), gender or race.

Injection Site Reactions

Injection site reactions of any severity occurred at a rate of 45% in Xolair-treated patients compared with 43% in placebo-treated patients. The types of injection site reactions included: bruising, redness, warmth, burning, stinging, itching, hive formation, pain, indurations, mass, and inflammation.

Severe injection site reactions occurred more frequently in Xolair-treated patients compared with patients in the placebo group (12% versus 9%).

The majority of injection site reactions occurred within 1 hour-post injection, lasted less than 8 days, and generally decreased in frequency at subsequent dosing visits.

Immunogenicity

Antibodies to Xolair were detected in approximately 1/1723 (<0.1%) of patients treated with Xolair. The data reflect the percentage of patients whose test results were considered positive for antibodies to Xolair in an ELISA assay and are highly dependent on the sensitivity and specificity of the assay. Additionally, the observed incidence of antibody positivity in the assay may be influenced by several factors including sample handling, timing of sample collection, concomitant medications, and underlying disease. Therefore, comparison of the incidence of antibodies to Xolair with the incidence of antibodies to other products may be misleading.

6.2 Postmarketing Experience

The following adverse reactions have been identified during postapproval use of Xolair in adult and adolescent patients 12 years of age and older. Because these reactions are reported voluntarily from a population of uncertain size, it is not always possible to reliably estimate their frequency or establish a causal relationship to drug exposure.

Anaphylaxis: Based on spontaneous reports and an estimated exposure of about 57,300 patients from June 2003 through December 2006, the frequency of anaphylaxis attributed to Xolair use was estimated to be at least 0.2% of patients. Diagnostic criteria of anaphylaxis were skin or mucosal tissue involvement, and, either airway compromise, and/or reduced blood pressure with or without associated symptoms, and a temporal relationship to Xolair administration with no other identifiable cause. Signs and symptoms in these reported cases included bronchospasm, hypotension, syncope, urticaria, angioedema of the throat or tongue, dyspnea, cough, chest tightness, and/or cutaneous angioedema. Pulmonary involvement was reported in 89% of the cases. Hypotension or syncope was reported in 14% of cases. Fifteen percent of the reported cases resulted in hospitalization. A previous history of anaphylaxis unrelated to Xolair was reported in 24% of the cases.

Of the reported cases of anaphylaxis attributed to Xolair, 39% occurred with the first dose, 19% occurred with the second dose, 10% occurred with the third dose, and the rest after subsequent doses. One case occurred after 39 doses (after 19 months of continuous therapy, anaphylaxis occurred when treatment was restarted following a 3 month gap). The time to onset of anaphylaxis in these cases was up to 30 minutes in 35%, greater than 30 and up to 60 minutes in 16%, greater than 60 and up to 90 minutes in 2%, greater than 90 and up to 120 minutes in 6%, greater than 2 hours and up to 6 hours in 5%, greater than 6 hours and up to 12 hours in 14%, greater than 12 hours and up to 24 hours in 8%, and greater than 24 hours and up to 4 days in 5%. In 9% of cases the times to onset were unknown.

Twenty-three patients who experienced anaphylaxis were rechallenged with Xolair and 18 patients had a recurrence of similar symptoms of anaphylaxis. In addition, anaphylaxis occurred upon rechallenge with Xolair in 4 patients who previously experienced urticaria only.

Eosinophilic Conditions: Eosinophilic conditions have been reported [see *Warnings and Precautions (5.5)*].

Fever, Arthralgia, and Rash: A constellation of signs and symptoms including arthritis/arthralgia, rash (urticaria or other forms), fever and lymphadenopathy similar to serum sickness have been reported in postapproval use of Xolair [see *Warnings and Precautions (5.6)*]

Hematologic: Severe thrombocytopenia has been reported.

Skin: Hair loss has been reported.

7 DRUG INTERACTIONS

No formal drug interaction studies have been performed with Xolair. The concomitant use of Xolair and allergen immunotherapy has not been evaluated.

8 USE IN SPECIFIC POPULATIONS

8.1 Pregnancy

Teratogenic Effects: Pregnancy Category B

There are no adequate and well-controlled studies of Xolair in pregnant women. Reproduction studies have been performed in Cynomolgus monkeys at subcutaneous doses up to 10 times the maximum recommended human dose on a mg/kg basis and have revealed no evidence of impaired fertility or harm to the fetus due to Xolair. Because animal reproduction studies are not always predictive of human response, administer Xolair during pregnancy only if clearly needed [see *Nonclinical Toxicology (13.2)*].

Pregnancy Exposure Registry

To monitor outcomes of pregnant women exposed to Xolair, including women who are exposed to at least one dose of Xolair within 8 weeks prior to conception or any time during pregnancy, a pregnancy exposure registry has been established. Encourage patients to call 1-866-4XOLAIR (1-866-496-5247) to enroll in the Xolair Pregnancy Exposure Registry. Call this number to obtain further information about this registry.

8.3 Nursing Mothers

There are no data from controlled clinical trials on the use of Xolair by nursing mothers. It is not known whether Xolair is excreted in human breast milk. However, IgG is excreted in human breast milk and therefore it is expected that Xolair will be excreted in human breast milk. The potential for Xolair absorption or harm to the infant is unknown; therefore caution should be exercised when Xolair is administered to a nursing woman.

The excretion of omalizumab in milk was evaluated in female Cynomolgus monkeys at a subcutaneous dose approximately 10 times the maximum recommended human dose on a mg/kg basis. Neonatal plasma levels of omalizumab after in utero exposure and 28 days of nursing were between 11% and 94% of the maternal plasma level. Milk levels of omalizumab were 1.5% of maternal blood concentration [see *Nonclinical Toxicology (13.2)*].

8.4 Pediatric Use

Safety and effectiveness of Xolair were evaluated in 2 studies in 926 (Xolair 624; placebo 302) asthma patients 6 to <12 years of age. One study was a pivotal study of similar design and conduct to that of adult and adolescent studies 1 and 2 [see *Clinical Trials (14)*]. The other study was primarily a safety study and included evaluation of efficacy as a secondary outcome. In the pivotal study, Xolair-treated patients had a statistically significant reduction in the rate of exacerbations (exacerbation was defined as worsening of asthma that required treatment with systemic corticosteroids or a doubling of the baseline ICS dose), but other efficacy variables such as nocturnal symptom scores, beta-agonist use, and measures of airflow (FEV$_1$) were not significantly different in Xolair-treated patients compared to placebo. Considering the risk of anaphylaxis and malignancy seen in Xolair-treated patients ≥12 years old and the modest efficacy of Xolair in the pivotal pediatric study, the risk-benefit assessment does not support the use of Xolair in patients 6 to <12 years of age. Although patients treated with Xolair in these two studies did not develop anaphylaxis or malignancy, the studies are not adequate to address these concerns because patients with a history of anaphylaxis or malignancy were excluded, and the duration of exposure and sample size were not large enough to exclude these risks in

patients 6 to <12 years of age. Furthermore, there is no reason to expect that younger pediatric patients would not be at risk of anaphylaxis and malignancy seen in adult and adolescent patients with Xolair. [see *Warnings and Precautions (5.1) (5.2); and Adverse Reactions (6)*].

Studies in patients 0-5 years of age were not required because of the safety concerns of anaphylaxis and malignancy associated with the use of Xolair in adults and adolescents.

8.5 Geriatric Use

In clinical trials 134 patients 65 years of age or older were treated with Xolair. Although there were no apparent age-related differences observed in these studies, the number of patients aged 65 and over is not sufficient to determine whether they respond differently from younger patients.

10 OVERDOSAGE

The maximum tolerated dose of Xolair has not been determined. Single intravenous doses of up to 4000 mg have been administered to patients without evidence of dose limiting toxicities. The highest cumulative dose administered to patients was 44,000 mg over a 20 week period, which was not associated with toxicities.

11 DESCRIPTION

Xolair (omalizumab) is a recombinant DNA-derived humanized IgG1κ monoclonal antibody that selectively binds to human immunoglobulin E (IgE). The antibody has a molecular weight of approximately 149 kiloDaltons. Xolair is produced by a Chinese hamster ovary cell suspension culture in a nutrient medium containing the antibiotic gentamicin. Gentamicin is not detectable in the final product.

Xolair is a sterile, white, preservative free, lyophilized powder contained in a single use vial that is reconstituted with Sterile Water for Injection (SWFI), USP, and administered as a subcutaneous (SC) injection. Each 202.5 mg vial of omalizumab also contains L-histidine (1.8 mg), L-histidine hydrochloride monohydrate (2.8 mg), polysorbate 20 (0.5 mg) and sucrose (145.5 mg) and is designed to deliver 150 mg of omalizumab in 1.2 mL after reconstitution with 1.4 mL SWFI, USP.

12 CLINICAL PHARMACOLOGY

12.1 Mechanism of Action

Omalizumab inhibits the binding of IgE to the high-affinity IgE receptor (FcεRI) on the surface of mast cells and basophils. Reduction in surface-bound IgE on FcεRI-bearing cells limits the degree of release of mediators of the allergic response. Treatment with Xolair also reduces the number of FcεRI receptors on basophils in atopic patients.

12.2 Pharmacodynamics

In clinical studies, serum free IgE levels were reduced in a dose dependent manner within 1 hour following the first dose and maintained between doses. Mean serum free IgE decrease was greater than 96% using recommended doses. Serum total IgE levels (i.e., bound and unbound) increased after the first dose due to the formation of omalizumab:IgE complexes, which have a slower elimination rate compared with free IgE. At 16 weeks after the first dose, average serum total IgE levels were five-fold higher compared with pre-treatment when using standard assays. After discontinuation of Xolair dosing, the Xolair-induced increase in total IgE and decrease in free IgE were reversible, with no observed rebound in IgE levels after drug washout. Total IgE levels did not return to pre-treatment levels for up to one year after discontinuation of Xolair.

12.3 Pharmacokinetics

After SC administration, omalizumab is absorbed with an average absolute bioavailability of 62%. Following a single SC dose in adult and adolescent patients with asthma, omalizumab was absorbed slowly, reaching peak serum concentrations after an average of 7-8 days. The pharmacokinetics of omalizumab are linear at doses greater than 0.5 mg/kg. Following multiple doses of Xolair, areas under the serum concentration-time curve from Day 0 to Day 14 at steady state were up to 6-fold of those after the first dose.

In vitro, omalizumab forms complexes of limited size with IgE. Precipitating complexes and complexes larger than 1 million daltons in molecular weight are not observed in vitro or in vivo. Tissue distribution studies in Cynomolgus monkeys showed no specific uptake of ^{125}I-omalizumab by any organ or tissue. The apparent volume of distribution in patients following SC administration was 78 ± 32 mL/kg. Clearance of omalizumab involves IgG clearance processes as well as clearance via specific binding and complex formation with its target ligand, IgE. Liver elimination of IgG includes degradation in the liver reticuloendothelial system (RES) and endothelial cells. Intact IgG is also excreted in bile. In studies with mice and monkeys, omalizumab:IgE complexes were eliminated by interactions with Fcγ receptors within the RES at rates that were generally faster than IgG clearance. In asthma patients omalizumab serum elimination half-life averaged 26 days, with apparent clearance averaging 2.4 ± 1.1 mL/kg/day. In addition, doubling body weight approximately doubled apparent clearance.

Special Populations

The population pharmacokinetics of omalizumab were analyzed to evaluate the effects of demographic characteristics. Analyses of these data suggest that no dose adjustments are necessary for age (12-76 years), race, ethnicity, or gender.

13 NONCLINICAL TOXICOLOGY

13.1 Carcinogenesis, Mutagenesis, Impairment of Fertility

No long-term studies have been performed in animals to evaluate the carcinogenic potential of Xolair.

No evidence of mutagenic activity was observed in Ames tests using six different strains of bacteria with and without metabolic activation at omalizumab concentrations up to 5000 µg/mL.

There were no effects on fertility and reproductive performance in male and female Cynomolgus monkeys that received Xolair at subcutaneous doses up to 75 mg/kg/week (approximately 5 times the maximum recommended human dose on an AUC basis).

13.2 Animal Toxicology and/or Pharmacology

Reproductive Toxicology Studies:

Reproductive studies have been performed in Cynomolgus monkeys at subcutaneous doses up to 75 mg/kg (approximately 10 times the maximum recommended human dose on a mg/kg basis) and have revealed no evidence of maternal toxicity, embryotoxicity, or teratogenicity when administered throughout organogenesis and did not elicit adverse effects on fetal or neonatal growth when administered throughout late gestation, delivery and nursing. IgG molecules are known to cross the placental barrier [see *Use in Specific Populations (8.1)*].

Lactation Studies:

The excretion of omalizumab in milk was evaluated in female Cynomolgus monkeys receiving a subcutaneous dose of 75 mg/kg/week (approximately 10 times the maximum recommended human dose on a mg/kg basis). Neonatal plasma levels of omalizumab after in utero exposure and 28 days of nursing were between 11% and 94% of the maternal plasma level. Milk levels of Xolair were 1.5% of maternal blood concentration. [see *Use in Specific Population (8.3)*].

14 CLINICAL STUDIES

Adult and Adolescent Patients 12 Years of Age and Older

The safety and efficacy of Xolair were evaluated in three randomized, double-blind, placebo-controlled, multicenter trials.

The trials enrolled patients 12 to 76 years old, with moderate to severe persistent (NHLBI criteria) asthma for at least one year, and a positive skin test reaction to a perennial aeroallergen. In all trials, Xolair dosing was based on body weight and baseline serum total IgE concentration. All patients were required to have a baseline IgE between 30 and 700 IU/mL and body weight not more than 150 kg. Patients were treated according to a dosing table to administer at least 0.016 mg/kg/IU (IgE/mL) of Xolair or a matching volume of placebo over each 4-week period. The maximum Xolair dose per 4 weeks was 750 mg.

In all three studies an exacerbation was defined as a worsening of asthma that required treatment with systemic corticosteroids or a doubling of the baseline ICS dose. Most exacerbations were managed in the out-patient setting and the majority were treated with systemic steroids. Hospitalization rates were not significantly different between Xolair and placebo-treated patients; however, the overall hospitalization rate was small. Among those patients who experienced an exacerbation, the distribution of exacerbation severity was similar between treatment groups.

Studies 1 and 2

At screening, patients in Studies 1 and 2 had a forced expiratory volume in one second (FEV$_1$) between 40% and 80% predicted. All patients had a FEV1 improvement of at least 12% following beta$_2$-agonist administration. All patients were symptomatic and were being treated with inhaled corticosteroids (ICS) and short acting beta$_2$-agonists. Patients receiving other concomitant controller medications were excluded, and initiation of additional controller medications while on study was prohibited. Patients currently smoking were excluded.

Each study was comprised of a run-in period to achieve a stable conversion to a common ICS (beclomethasone dipropionate), followed by randomization to Xolair or placebo. Patients received Xolair for 16 weeks with an unchanged corticosteroid dose unless an acute exacerbation necessitated an increase. Patients then entered an ICS reduction phase of 12 weeks during which ICS dose reduction was attempted in a step-wise manner.

The distribution of the number of asthma exacerbations per patient in each group during a study was analyzed separately for the stable steroid and steroid-reduction periods.

In both Studies 1 and 2 the number of exacerbations per patient was reduced in patients treated with Xolair compared with placebo (Table 5).

Measures of airflow (FEV$_1$) and asthma symptoms were also evaluated in these studies. The clinical relevance of the treatment-associated differences is unknown. Results from the stable steroid phase Study 1 are shown in Table 6. Results from the stable steroid phase of Study 2 and the steroid reduction phases of both Studies 1 and 2 were similar to those presented in Table 6.

Table 5
Frequency of Asthma Exacerbations per Patient by Phase in Studies 1 and 2

	Stable Steroid Phase (16 wks)			
	Study 1		Study 2	
Exacerbations per patient	Xolair N=268 (%)	Placebo N=257 (%)	Xolair N=274 (%)	Placebo N=272 (%)
0	85.8	76.7	87.6	69.9
1	11.9	16.7	11.3	25.0
≥2	2.2	6.6	1.1	5.1
p-Value	0.005		<0.001	
Mean number exacerbations/patient	0.2	0.3	0.1	0.4

	Steroid Reduction Phase (12 wks)			
	Study 1		Study 2	
Exacerbations per patient	Xolair N=268 (%)	Placebo N=257 (%)	Xolair N=274 (%)	Placebo N=272 (%)
0	78.7	67.7	83.9	70.2
1	19.0	28.4	14.2	26.1
≥2	2.2	3.9	1.8	3.7
p-Value	0.004		<0.001	
Mean number exacerbations/patient	0.2	0.4	0.2	0.3

[See table below]

Study 3

In Study 3, there was no restriction on screening FEV_1, and unlike Studies 1 and 2, long-acting beta₂-agonists were allowed. Patients were receiving at least 1000 µg/day fluticasone propionate and a subset was also receiving oral corticosteroids. Patients receiving other concomitant controller medications were excluded, and initiation of additional controller medications while on study was prohibited. Patients currently smoking were excluded.

The study was comprised of a run-in period to achieve a stable conversion to a common ICS (fluticasone propionate), followed by randomization to Xolair or placebo. Patients were stratified by use of ICS-only or ICS with concomitant use of oral steroids. Patients received Xolair for 16 weeks with an unchanged corticosteroid dose unless an acute exacerbation necessitated an increase. Patients then entered an ICS reduction phase of 16 weeks during which ICS or oral steroid dose reduction was attempted in a step-wise manner.

The number of exacerbations in patients treated with Xolair was similar to that in placebo-treated patients (Table 7). The absence of an observed treatment effect may be related to differences in the patient population compared with Studies 1 and 2, study sample size, or other factors.

Table 7
Percentage of Patients with Asthma Exacerbations by Subgroup and Phase in Study 3

	Stable Steroid Phase (16 wks)			
	Inhaled Only		Oral + Inhaled	
	Xolair N=126	Placebo N=120	Xolair N=50	Placebo N=45
% Patients with ≥1 exacerbations	15.9	15.0	32.0	22.2
Difference (95% CI)	0.9 (-9.7, 13.7)		9.8 (-10.5, 31.4)	

	Steroid Reduction Phase (16 wks)			
	Inhaled Only		Oral + Inhaled	
	Xolair N=126	Placebo N=120	Xolair N=50	Placebo N=45
% Patients with ≥1 exacerbations	22.2	26.7	42.0	42.2
Difference (95% CI)	-4.4 (-17.6, 7.4)		-0.2 (-22.4, 20.1)	

In all three of the studies, a reduction of asthma exacerbations was not observed in the Xolair-treated patients who had FEV_1 >80% at the time of randomization. Reductions in exacerbations were not seen in patients who required oral steroids as maintenance therapy.

Pediatric Patients 6 to <12 Years of Age
Clinical studies with Xolair in pediatric patients 6 to 11 years of age have been conducted [*see Use in Specific Populations (8.4)*].

Pediatric Patients <6 Years of Age
Clinical studies with Xolair in pediatric patients less than 6 years of age have not been conducted [*see Use in Specific Populations (8.4)*]

16 HOW SUPPLIED/STORAGE AND HANDLING
Xolair (omalizumab) is supplied as a lyophilized, sterile powder in a single-use, 5 mL vial without preservatives. Each vial delivers 150 mg of Xolair upon reconstitution with 1.4 mL SWFI, USP. Each carton contains one single-use vial of Xolair® (omalizumab) NDC 50242-040-62.
Xolair should be shipped at controlled ambient temperature (≤30°C [≤86°F]). Store Xolair under refrigerated conditions 2-8°C (36-46°F). Do not use beyond the expiration date stamped on carton.
Use the solution for subcutaneous administration within 8 hours following reconstitution when stored in the vial at 2-8°C (36-46°F), or within 4 hours of reconstitution when stored at room temperature.
Reconstituted Xolair vials should be protected from direct sunlight.

17 PATIENT COUNSELING INFORMATION
[*See Medication Guide*]
17.1 Information for Patients
Provide and instruct patients to read the accompanying Medication Guide before starting treatment and before each subsequent treatment. The complete text of the Medication Guide is reprinted at the end of this document.
Inform patients of the risk of life-threatening anaphylaxis with Xolair including the following points [*see Warnings and Precautions (5.1)*]:
• There have been reports of anaphylaxis up to 4 days after administration of Xolair

• Xolair should only be administered in a healthcare setting by healthcare providers.
• Patients should be closely observed following administration
• Patients should be informed of the signs and symptoms of anaphylaxis
• Patients should be instructed to seek immediate medical care should such signs or symptoms occur
Instruct patients receiving Xolair not to decrease the dose of, or stop taking any other asthma medications unless otherwise instructed by their physician. Inform patients that they may not see immediate improvement in their asthma after beginning Xolair therapy.

Pregnancy Exposure Registry
Encourage pregnant women exposed to Xolair to enroll in the Xolair Pregnancy Exposure Registry [1-866-4XOLAIR (1-866-496-5247)] (8.1)

MEDICATION GUIDE
XOLAIR®
(omalizumab)
IMPORTANT: XOLAIR SHOULD ALWAYS BE INJECTED IN YOUR DOCTOR'S OFFICE.

WHAT IS THE MOST IMPORTANT INFORMATION I SHOULD KNOW ABOUT XOLAIR?
A severe allergic reaction called anaphylaxis has happened in some patients after they received Xolair. Anaphylaxis is a life-threatening condition and can lead to death so get emergency medical treatment right away if symptoms occur.

Signs and Symptoms of anaphylaxis include:
• wheezing, shortness of breath, cough, chest tightness, or trouble breathing
• low blood pressure, dizziness, fainting, rapid or weak heartbeat, anxiety, or feeling of "impending doom"
• flushing, itching, hives, or feeling warm
• swelling of the throat or tongue, throat tightness, hoarse voice, or trouble swallowing
Get emergency medical treatment right away if you have signs or symptoms of anaphylaxis after receiving Xolair.

Anaphylaxis from Xolair can happen:
• right after receiving a Xolair injection or hours later
• after any Xolair injection. Anaphylaxis has occurred after the first Xolair injection or after many Xolair injections.
Your healthcare provider should watch you for some time in the office for signs or symptoms of anaphylaxis after injecting Xolair. If you have signs or symptoms of anaphylaxis, tell your healthcare provider right away.
Your healthcare provider should instruct you about getting emergency medical treatment and further medical care if you have signs or symptoms of anaphylaxis after leaving the doctor's office.

WHAT IS XOLAIR?
Xolair is an injectable medicine for patients 12 years of age and older with moderate to severe persistent allergic asthma whose asthma symptoms are not controlled by asthma medicines called inhaled corticosteroids. A skin or blood test is done to see if you have allergic asthma.

WHAT ELSE SHOULD I KNOW ABOUT XOLAIR?
• You should not receive Xolair if you have ever had an allergic reaction to a Xolair injection.
• Do not change or stop taking any of your other asthma medicines unless your healthcare provider tells you to do so.
• There are other possible side effects with Xolair. Talk to your doctor for more information. You can also go to www.xolair.com or call 1-866-496-5247).
• You may report side effects to FDA at 1-800-FDA-1088.

This Medication Guide has been approved by the U.S. Food and Drug Administration.

Manufactured by:
Genentech, Inc.
A Member of the Roche Group
1 DNA Way
South San Francisco, CA 94080-4990
Jointly marketed by:
Genentech USA, Inc.
A Member of the Roche Group
1 DNA Way
South San Francisco, CA 94080-4990
Novartis Pharmaceuticals Corporation
One Health Plaza
East Hanover, NJ 07936-1080
7390209/XOL-400050
LX1331
4855302
Initial US Approval: June 2003
Revision Date: July 2010
Xolair® is a registered trademark of Novartis AG Corporation.
©2010 Genentech USA, Inc.
©Novartis

Table 6
Asthma Symptoms and Pulmonary Function During Stable Steroid Phase of Study 1

Endpoint	Xolair N=268[a]		Placebo N=257[a]	
	Mean Baseline	Median Change (Baseline to Wk 16)	Mean Baseline	Median Change (Baseline to Wk 16)
Total asthma symptom score	4.3	-1.5[b]	4.2	-1.1[b]
Nocturnal asthma score	1.2	-0.4[b]	1.1	-0.2[b]
Daytime asthma score	2.3	-0.9[b]	2.3	-0.6[b]
FEV_1 % predicted	68	3[b]	68	0[b]

Asthma symptom scale: total score from 0 (least) to 9 (most); nocturnal and daytime scores from 0 (least) to 4 (most symptoms).
[a] Number of patients available for analysis ranges 255-258 in the Xolair group and 238-239 in the placebo group.
[b] Comparison of Xolair versus placebo (p<0.05).

ZOMETA® ℞
[zō-mĕ-ta]
(zoledronic acid)
Injection
Concentrate for Intravenous Infusion

The following prescribing information is based on official labeling in effect July 2010.

HIGHLIGHTS OF PRESCRIBING INFORMATION
These highlights do not include all the information needed to use Zometa safely and effectively. See full prescribing information for Zometa.

ZOMETA® *(zoledronic acid)* **Injection**
Concentrate for Intravenous Infusion
Initial U.S. Approval: 2001

────────**INDICATIONS AND USAGE**────────
Zometa is a bisphosphonate indicated for the treatment of:
• Hypercalcemia of malignancy (1.1)
• Patients with multiple myeloma and patients with documented bone metastases from solid tumors, in conjunction with standard antineoplastic therapy. Prostate cancer should have progressed after treatment with at least one hormonal therapy (1.2)
Important limitation of use: The safety and efficacy of Zometa has not been established for use in hyperparathyroidism or nontumor-related hypercalcemia (1.3)

──────**DOSAGE AND ADMINISTRATION**──────
Hypercalcemia of malignancy (2.1)
• 4 mg as a single-dose intravenous infusion over no less than 15 minutes
• 4 mg as retreatment after a minimum of 7 days
Multiple myeloma and bone metastasis from solid tumors (2.2)
• 4 mg as a single-dose intravenous infusion over no less than 15 minutes every 3-4 weeks for patients with creatinine clearance of >60 mL/min
• Reduce the dose for patients with renal impairment
• Coadminister oral calcium supplements of 500 mg and a multiple vitamin containing 400 IU of Vitamin D daily.
Administer through a separate vented infusion line and do not allow to come in contact with any calcium or divalent cation-containing solutions (2.3)

─────**DOSAGE FORMS AND STRENGTHS**─────
4 mg/5 mL single dose vials (3)

────────**CONTRAINDICATIONS**────────
Hypersensitivity to any component of Zometa (4)

──────**WARNINGS AND PRECAUTIONS**──────
• Patients being treated with Zometa should not be treated with Reclast® (5.1)
• Adequately rehydrate patients with hypercalcemia of malignancy prior to administration of Zometa and monitor electrolytes during treatment (5.2)
• Renal toxicity may be greater in patients with renal impairment. Do not use doses greater than 4 mg. Treatment in patients with severe renal impairment is not recommended. Monitor serum creatinine before each dose (5.3)
• Osteonecrosis of the jaw has been reported. Preventive dental exams should be performed before starting Zometa. Avoid invasive dental procedures (5.4)
• Zometa can cause fetal harm. Women of childbearing potential should be advised of the potential hazard to the fetus and to avoid becoming pregnant (5.5, 8.1)
• Severe incapacitating bone, joint, muscle pain may occur. Discontinue Zometa if severe symptoms occur (5.6)

────────**ADVERSE REACTIONS**────────
The most common adverse events (>25%) were nausea, fatigue, anemia, bone pain, constipation, fever, vomiting, and dyspnea (6.1)

To report SUSPECTED ADVERSE REACTIONS, contact Novartis Pharmaceuticals Corporation at 1-888-669-6682 or FDA at 1-800-FDA-1088 or www.fda.gov/medwatch

────────**DRUG INTERACTIONS**────────
• Aminoglycosides: May have an additive effect to lower serum calcium for prolonged periods (7.1)
• Loop diuretics: Concomitant use with Zometa may increase risk of hypocalcemia (7.2)
• Nephrotoxic drugs: Use with caution (7.3)
• Thalidomide: Combination use in patients with multiple myeloma may increase the risk of renal dysfunction (7.4)

──────**USE IN SPECIFIC POPULATIONS**──────
• Nursing Mothers: Zometa should not be given to nursing women (8.2)
• Pediatric Use: Not indicated for use in pediatric patients (8.4)
• Geriatric Use: Special care to monitor renal function (8.5)

See 17 for PATIENT COUNSELING INFORMATION

Revised: 10/2009

────────────────────────────

FULL PRESCRIBING INFORMATION: CONTENTS*
*Sections or subsections omitted from the full prescribing information are not listed

────────────────────────────

FULL PRESCRIBING INFORMATION

1 INDICATIONS AND USAGE

1.1 Hypercalcemia of Malignancy
Zometa is indicated for the treatment of hypercalcemia of malignancy defined as an albumin-corrected calcium (cCa) of >12 mg/dL [3.0 mmol/L] using the formula: cCa in mg/dL=Ca in mg/dL + 0.8 (mid-range of measured albumin in mg/dL).

1.2 Multiple Myeloma and Bone Metastases of Solid Tumors
Zometa is indicated for the treatment of patients with multiple myeloma and patients with documented bone metastases from solid tumors, in conjunction with standard antineoplastic therapy. Prostate cancer should have progressed after treatment with at least one hormonal therapy.

1.3 Important Limitation of Use
The safety and efficacy of Zometa in the treatment of hypercalcemia associated with hyperparathyroidism or with other nontumor-related conditions has not been established.

2 DOSAGE AND ADMINISTRATION

Parenteral drug products should be inspected visually for particulate matter and discoloration prior to administration, whenever solution and container permit.

2.1 Hypercalcemia of Malignancy
The maximum recommended dose of Zometa in hypercalcemia of malignancy (albumin-corrected serum calcium ≥12 mg/dL [3.0 mmol/L]) is 4 mg. The 4-mg dose must be given as a single-dose intravenous infusion over **no less than 15 minutes**. Patients who receive Zometa should have serum creatinine assessed prior to each treatment.
Dose adjustments of Zometa are not necessary in treating patients for hypercalcemia of malignancy presenting with mild-to-moderate renal impairment prior to initiation of therapy (serum creatinine <400 µmol/L or <4.5 mg/dL).
Patients should be adequately rehydrated prior to administration of Zometa [see Warnings And Precautions (5.2)].
Consideration should be given to the severity of, as well as the symptoms of, tumor-induced hypercalcemia when considering use of Zometa. Vigorous saline hydration, an integral part of hypercalcemia therapy, should be initiated promptly and an attempt should be made to restore the urine output to about 2 L/day throughout treatment. Mild or asymptomatic hypercalcemia may be treated with conservative measures (i.e., saline hydration, with or without loop diuretics). Patients should be hydrated adequately throughout the treatment, but overhydration, especially in those patients who have cardiac failure, must be avoided. Diuretic therapy should not be employed prior to correction of hypovolemia.
Retreatment with Zometa 4 mg may be considered if serum calcium does not return to normal or remain normal after initial treatment. It is recommended that a minimum of 7 days elapse before retreatment, to allow for full response to the initial dose. Renal function must be carefully monitored in all patients receiving Zometa and serum creatinine must be assessed prior to retreatment with Zometa [see Warnings And Precautions (5.2)].

2.2 Multiple Myeloma and Metastatic Bone Lesions of Solid Tumors
The recommended dose of Zometa in patients with multiple myeloma and metastatic bone lesions from solid tumors for patients with creatinine clearance >60 mL/min is 4 mg infused over **no less than 15 minutes** every 3-4 weeks. The optimal duration of therapy is not known.
Upon treatment initiation, the recommended Zometa doses for patients with reduced renal function (mild and moderate renal impairment) are listed in Table 1. These doses are calculated to achieve the same AUC as that achieved in patients with creatinine clearance of 75 mL/min. Creatinine clearance (CrCl) is calculated using the Cockcroft-Gault formula [see Warnings And Precautions (5.2)].

Table 1. Reduced Doses for Patients with Baseline CrCl ≤60 mL/min

Baseline Creatinine Clearance (mL/min)	Zometa Recommended Dose*
>60	4 mg
50-60	3.5 mg
40-49	3.3 mg
30-39	3 mg

*Doses calculated assuming target AUC of 0.66 (mg•hr/L) (CrCl = 75 mL/min)

During treatment, serum creatinine should be measured before each Zometa dose and treatment should be withheld for renal deterioration. In the clinical studies, renal deterioration was defined as follows:
For patients with normal baseline creatinine, increase of 0.5 mg/dL
For patients with abnormal baseline creatinine, increase of 1.0 mg/dL
In the clinical studies, Zometa treatment was resumed only when the creatinine returned to within 10% of the baseline value. Zometa should be reinitiated at the same dose as that prior to treatment interruption.
Patients should also be administered an oral calcium supplement of 500 mg and a multiple vitamin containing 400 IU of Vitamin D daily.

2.3 Preparation of Solution
4 mg Dose
Vials of Zometa concentrate for infusion contain overfill allowing for the withdrawal of 5 mL of concentrate (equivalent to 4 mg zoledronic acid). This concentrate should immediately be diluted in 100 mL of sterile 0.9% Sodium Chloride, USP, or 5% Dextrose Injection, USP. Do not store undiluted concentrate in a syringe, to avoid inadvertent injection.

Preparing Reduced Doses for Patients with Baseline CrCl ≤60 mL/min
Withdraw the appropriate volume of the Zometa concentrate from the vial for the dose required (see Table 2).

Table 2. Preparation of Reduced Doses

Zometa Volume (mL)	Dose (mg)
4.4	3.5
4.1	3.3
3.8	3.0

The withdrawn concentrate must be diluted in 100 mL of sterile 0.9% Sodium Chloride, USP, or 5% Dextrose Injection, USP.

For All Prepared Doses
If not used immediately after dilution with infusion media, for microbiological integrity, the solution should be refrigerated at 2°C-8°C (36°F-46°F). The refrigerated solution should then be equilibrated to room temperature prior to administration. The total time between dilution, storage in the refrigerator, and end of administration must not exceed 24 hours.

Zometa must not be mixed with calcium or other divalent cation-containing infusion solutions, such as Lactated Ringer's solution, and should be administered as a single intravenous solution in a line separate from all other drugs.

2.4 Method of Administration

Due to the risk of clinically significant deterioration in renal function, which may progress to renal failure, single doses of Zometa should not exceed 4 mg and the duration of infusion should be no less than 15 minutes [*see Warnings And Precautions (5.2)*]. In the trials and in postmarketing experience, renal deterioration, progression to renal failure and dialysis, have occurred in patients, including those treated with the approved dose of 4 mg infused over 15 minutes. There have been instances of this occurring after the initial Zometa dose.

3 DOSAGE FORMS AND STRENGTHS

4 mg/5 mL single-dose vial

4 CONTRAINDICATIONS

4.1 Hypersensitivity to Zoledronic Acid or Any Components of Zometa

Hypersensitivity reactions including rare cases of urticaria and angioedema, and very rare cases of anaphylactic reaction/shock have been reported [*see Adverse Reactions (6.2)*].

5 WARNINGS AND PRECAUTIONS

5.1 Drugs with Same Active Ingredient

Zometa contains the same active ingredient as found in Reclast® (zoledronic acid). Patients being treated with Zometa should not be treated with Reclast.

5.2 Hydration and Electrolyte Monitoring

Patients with hypercalcemia of malignancy must be adequately rehydrated prior to administration of Zometa. Loop diuretics should not be used until the patient is adequately rehydrated and should be used with caution in combination with Zometa in order to avoid hypocalcemia. Zometa should be used with caution with other nephrotoxic drugs.

Standard hypercalcemia-related metabolic parameters, such as serum levels of calcium, phosphate, and magnesium, as well as serum creatinine, should be carefully monitored following initiation of therapy with Zometa. If hypocalcemia, hypophosphatemia, or hypomagnesemia occur, short-term supplemental therapy may be necessary.

5.3 Renal Impairment

Zometa is excreted intact primarily via the kidney, and the risk of adverse reactions, in particular renal adverse reactions, may be greater in patients with impaired renal function. Safety and pharmacokinetic data are limited in patients with severe renal impairment and the risk of renal deterioration is increased [*see Adverse Reactions (6.1)*]. Preexisting renal insufficiency and multiple cycles of Zometa and other bisphosphonates are risk factors for subsequent renal deterioration with Zometa. Factors predisposing to renal deterioration, such as dehydration or the use of other nephrotoxic drugs, should be identified and managed, if possible.

Zometa treatment in patients with hypercalcemia of malignancy with severe renal impairment should be considered only after evaluating the risks and benefits of treatment. In the clinical studies, patients with serum creatinine >400 µmol/L or >4.5 mg/dL were excluded.

Zometa treatment is not recommended in patients with bone metastases with severe renal impairment. In the clinical studies, patients with serum creatinine >265 µmol/L or >3.0 mg/dL were excluded and there were only 8 of 564 patients treated with Zometa 4 mg by 15-minute infusion with a baseline creatinine >2 mg/dL. Limited pharmacokinetic data exists in patients with creatinine clearance <30 mL/min [*see Clinical Pharmacology (12.3)*].

5.4 Osteonecrosis of the Jaw

Osteonecrosis of the jaw (ONJ) has been reported predominantly in cancer patients treated with intravenous bisphosphonates, including Zometa. Many of these patients were also receiving chemotherapy and corticosteroids which may be risk factors for ONJ. Postmarketing experience and the literature suggest a greater frequency of reports of ONJ based on tumor type (advanced breast cancer, multiple myeloma), and dental status (dental extraction, periodontal disease, local trauma including poorly fitting dentures). Many reports of ONJ involved patients with signs of local infection including osteomyelitis.

Cancer patients should maintain good oral hygiene and should have a dental examination with preventive dentistry prior to treatment with bisphosphonates.

While on treatment, these patients should avoid invasive dental procedures if possible. For patients who develop ONJ while on bisphosphonate therapy, dental surgery may exacerbate the condition. For patients requiring dental procedures, there are no data available to suggest whether discontinuation of bisphosphonate treatment reduces the risk of ONJ. Clinical judgment of the treating physician should guide the management plan of each patient based on individual benefit/risk assessment [*see Adverse Reactions (6.2)*].

5.5 Pregnancy

ZOMETA SHOULD NOT BE USED DURING PREGNANCY. Zometa may cause fetal harm when administered to a pregnant woman. In reproductive studies in the pregnant rat, subcutaneous doses equivalent to 2.4 or 4.8 times the human systemic exposure (an IV dose of 4 mg based on an AUC comparison) resulted in pre- and postimplantation losses, decreases in viable fetuses and fetal skeletal, visceral, and external malformations. If this drug is used during pregnancy, or if the patient becomes pregnant while taking this drug, the patient should be apprised of the potential hazard to a fetus [*see Use In Specific Populations (8.1)*].

5.6 Musculoskeletal Pain

In postmarketing experience, severe and occasionally incapacitating bone, joint, and/or muscle pain has been reported in patients taking bisphosphonates. This category of drugs includes Zometa. The time to onset of symptoms varied from one day to several months after starting the drug. Discontinue use if severe symptoms develop. Most patients had relief of symptoms after stopping. A subset had recurrence of symptoms when rechallenged with the same drug or another bisphosphonate [*see Adverse Reactions (6.2)*].

5.7 Patients with Asthma

While not observed in clinical trials with Zometa, there have been reports of bronchoconstriction in aspirin sensitive patients receiving bisphosphonates.

5.8 Hepatic Impairment

Only limited clinical data are available for use of Zometa to treat hypercalcemia of malignancy in patients with hepatic insufficiency, and these data are not adequate to provide guidance on dosage selection or how to safely use Zometa in these patients.

6 ADVERSE REACTIONS

6.1 Clinical Studies Experience

Because clinical trials are conducted under widely varying conditions, adverse reaction rates observed in the clinical trials of a drug cannot be directly compared to rates in the clinical trials of another drug and may not reflect the rates observed in practice.

Hypercalcemia of Malignancy

The safety of Zometa was studied in 185 patients with hypercalcemia of malignancy (HCM) who received either Zometa 4 mg given as a 5-minute intravenous infusion (n=86) or pamidronate 90 mg given as a 2-hour intravenous infusion (n=103). The population was aged 33-84 years, 60% male and 81% Caucasian, with breast, lung, head and neck, and renal cancer as the most common forms of malignancy. NOTE: pamidronate 90 mg was given as a 2-hour intravenous infusion. The relative safety of pamidronate 90 mg given as a 2-hour intravenous infusion compared to the same dose given as a 24-hour intravenous infusion has not been adequately studied in controlled clinical trials.

Renal Toxicity

Administration of Zometa 4 mg given as a 5-minute intravenous infusion has been shown to result in an increased risk of renal toxicity, as measured by increases in serum creatinine, which can progress to renal failure. The incidence of renal toxicity and renal failure has been shown to be reduced when Zometa 4 mg is given as a 15-minute intravenous infusion. Zometa should be administered by intravenous infusion over no less than 15 minutes [*see Warnings And Precautions (5) and Dosage And Administration (2)*].

The most frequently observed adverse events were fever, nausea, constipation, anemia, and dyspnea (*see Table 3*).

Table 3 provides adverse events that were reported by 10% or more of the 189 patients treated with Zometa 4 mg or Pamidronate 90 mg from the two HCM trials. Adverse events are listed regardless of presumed causality to study drug.

Table 3. Percentage of Patients with Adverse Events ≥10% Reported in Hypercalcemia of Malignancy Clinical Trials by Body System

	Zometa 4 mg n	(%)	Pamidronate 90 mg n	(%)
Patients Studied				
Total No. of Patients Studied	86	(100)	103	(100)
Total No. of Patients with any AE	81	(94)	95	(92)
Body as a Whole				
Fever	38	(44)	34	(33)
Progression of Cancer	14	(16)	21	(20)
Cardiovascular				
Hypotension	9	(11)	2	(2)
Digestive				
Nausea	25	(29)	28	(27)
Constipation	23	(27)	13	(13)
Diarrhea	15	(17)	17	(17)
Abdominal Pain	14	(16)	13	(13)
Vomiting	12	(14)	17	(17)
Anorexia	8	(9)	14	(14)
Hemic and Lymphatic System				
Anemia	19	(22)	18	(18)
Infections				
Moniliasis	10	(12)	4	(4)
Laboratory Abnormalities				
Hypophosphatemia	11	(13)	2	(2)
Hypokalemia	10	(12)	16	(16)
Hypomagnesemia	9	(11)	5	(5)
Musculoskeletal				
Skeletal Pain	10	(12)	10	(10)
Nervous				
Insomnia	13	(15)	10	(10)
Anxiety	12	(14)	8	(8)
Confusion	11	(13)	13	(13)
Agitation	11	(13)	8	(8)
Respiratory				
Dyspnea	19	(22)	20	(19)
Coughing	10	(12)	12	(12)
Urogenital				
Urinary Tract Infection	12	(14)	15	(15)

The following adverse events from the two controlled multicenter HCM trials (n=189) were reported by a greater percentage of patients treated with Zometa 4 mg than with pamidronate 90 mg and occurred with a frequency of greater than or equal to 5% but less than 10%. Adverse events are listed regardless of presumed causality to study drug: Asthenia, chest pain, leg edema, mucositis, dysphagia, granulocytopenia, thrombocytopenia, pancytopenia, nonspecific infection, hypocalcemia, dehydration, arthralgias, headache and somnolence.

Rare cases of rash, pruritus, and chest pain have been reported following treatment with Zometa.

Acute Phase Reaction-like Events

Symptoms consistent with acute phase reaction (APR) can occur with intravenous bisphosphonate use. Fever has been the most commonly associated symptom, occurring in 44% of patients treated with Zometa 4 mg and 33% of patients treated with Pamidronate 90 mg. Occasionally, patients experience a flu-like syndrome consisting of fever, chills, flushing, bone pain and/or arthralgias, and myalgias.

Mineral and Electrolyte Abnormalities

Electrolyte abnormalities, most commonly hypocalcemia, hypophosphatemia and hypomagnesemia, can occur with bisphosphonate use.

Grade 3 and Grade 4 laboratory abnormalities for serum creatinine, serum calcium, serum phosphorus, and serum magnesium observed in two clinical trials of Zometa in patients with HCM are shown in Table 4 and 5.

Table 4. Grade 3 Laboratory Abnormalities for Serum Creatinine, Serum Calcium, Serum Phosphorus, and Serum Magnesium in Two Clinical Trials in Patients with HCM

Laboratory Parameter	Grade 3 Zometa 4 mg n/N	(%)	Pamidronate 90 mg n/N	(%)
Serum Creatinine[1]	2/86	(2%)	3/100	(3%)
Hypocalcemia[2]	1/86	(1%)	2/100	(2%)
Hypophosphatemia[3]	36/70	(51%)	27/81	(33%)
Hypomagnesemia[4]	0/71	—	0/84	—

Table 5. Grade 4 Laboratory Abnormalities for Serum Creatinine, Serum Calcium, Serum Phosphorus, and Serum Magnesium in Two Clinical Trials in Patients with HCM

Laboratory Parameter	Grade 4 Zometa 4 mg n/N	(%)	Pamidronate 90 mg n/N	(%)
Serum Creatinine[1]	0/86	—	1/100	(1%)
Hypocalcemia[2]	0/86	—	0/100	—
Hypophosphatemia[3]	1/70	(1%)	4/81	(5%)
Hypomagnesemia[4]	0/71	—	1/84	(1%)

[1] Grade 3 (>3× Upper Limit of Normal); Grade 4 (>6× Upper Limit of Normal)
[2] Grade 3 (<7 mg/dL); Grade 4 (<6 mg/dL)
[3] Grade 3 (<2 mg/dL); Grade 4 (<1 mg/dL)
[4] Grade 3 (<0.8 mEq/L); Grade 4 (<0.5 mEq/L)

Table 6. Percentage of Patients with Adverse Events ≥10% Reported in Three Bone Metastases Clinical Trials by Body System

	Zometa 4 mg n (%)		Pamidronate 90 mg n (%)		Placebo n (%)	
Patients Studied						
Total No. of Patients	1031	(100)	556	(100)	455	(100)
Total No. of Patients with any AE	1015	(98)	548	(99)	445	(98)
Blood and Lymphatic						
Anemia	344	(33)	175	(32)	128	(28)
Neutropenia	124	(12)	83	(15)	35	(8)
Thrombocytopenia	102	(10)	53	(10)	20	(4)
Gastrointestinal						
Nausea	476	(46)	266	(48)	171	(38)
Vomiting	333	(32)	183	(33)	122	(27)
Constipation	320	(31)	162	(29)	174	(38)
Diarrhea	249	(24)	162	(29)	83	(18)
Abdominal Pain	143	(14)	81	(15)	48	(11)
Dyspepsia	105	(10)	74	(13)	31	(7)
Stomatitis	86	(8)	65	(12)	14	(3)
Sore Throat	82	(8)	61	(11)	17	(4)
General Disorders and Administration Site						
Fatigue	398	(39)	240	(43)	130	(29)
Pyrexia	328	(32)	172	(31)	89	(20)
Weakness	252	(24)	108	(19)	114	(25)
Edema Lower Limb	215	(21)	126	(23)	84	(19)
Rigors	112	(11)	62	(11)	28	(6)
Infections						
Urinary Tract Infection	124	(12)	50	(9)	41	(9)
Upper Respiratory Tract Infection	101	(10)	82	(15)	30	(7)
Metabolism						
Anorexia	231	(22)	81	(15)	105	(23)
Weight Decreased	164	(16)	50	(9)	61	(13)
Dehydration	145	(14)	60	(11)	59	(13)
Appetite Decreased	130	(13)	48	(9)	45	(10)
Musculoskeletal						
Bone Pain	569	(55)	316	(57)	284	(62)
Myalgia	239	(23)	143	(26)	74	(16)
Arthralgia	216	(21)	131	(24)	73	(16)
Back Pain	156	(15)	106	(19)	40	(9)
Pain in Limb	143	(14)	84	(15)	52	(11)
Neoplasms						
Malignant Neoplasm Aggravated	205	(20)	97	(17)	89	(20)
Nervous						
Headache	191	(19)	149	(27)	50	(11)
Dizziness (excluding vertigo)	180	(18)	91	(16)	58	(13)
Insomnia	166	(16)	111	(20)	73	(16)
Paresthesia	149	(14)	85	(15)	35	(8)
Hypoesthesia	127	(12)	65	(12)	43	(10)
Psychiatric						
Depression	146	(14)	95	(17)	49	(11)
Anxiety	112	(11)	73	(13)	37	(8)
Confusion	74	(7)	39	(7)	47	(10)
Respiratory						
Dyspnea	282	(27)	155	(28)	107	(24)
Cough	224	(22)	129	(23)	65	(14)
Skin						
Alopecia	125	(12)	80	(14)	36	(8)
Dermatitis	114	(11)	74	(13)	38	(8)

Table 7. Grade 3 Laboratory Abnormalities for Serum Creatinine, Serum Calcium, Serum Phosphorus, and Serum Magnesium in Three Clinical Trials in Patients with Bone Metastases

	Grade 3					
Laboratory Parameter	Zometa 4 mg		Pamidronate 90 mg		Placebo	
	n/N	(%)	n/N	(%)	n/N	(%)
Serum Creatinine[1]*	7/529	(1%)	4/268	(2%)	4/241	(2%)
Hypocalcemia[2]	6/973	(<1%)	4/536	(<1%)	0/415	—
Hypophosphatemia[3]	115/973	(12%)	38/537	(7%)	14/415	(3%)
Hypermagnesemia[4]	19/971	(2%)	2/535	(<1%)	8/415	(2%)
Hypomagnesemia[5]	1/971	(<1%)	0/535	—	1/415	(<1%)

[1] Grade 3 (>3× Upper Limit of Normal); Grade 4 (>6× Upper Limit of Normal)
*Serum creatinine data for all patients randomized after the 15-minute infusion amendment
[2] Grade 3 (<7 mg/dL); Grade 4 (<6 mg/dL)
[3] Grade 3 (<2 mg/dL); Grade 4 (<1 mg/dL)
[4] Grade 3 (>3 mEq/L); Grade 4 (>8 mEq/L)
[5] Grade 3 (<0.9 mEq/L); Grade 4 (<0.7 mEq/L)

Injection Site Reactions

Local reactions at the infusion site, such as redness or swelling, were observed infrequently. In most cases, no specific treatment is required and the symptoms subside after 24-48 hours.

Ocular Adverse Events

Ocular inflammation such as uveitis and scleritis can occur with bisphosphonate use, including Zometa. No cases of iritis, scleritis or uveitis were reported during these clinical

trials. However, cases have been seen in postmarketing use [see Adverse Reactions (6.2)].

Multiple Myeloma and Bone Metastases of Solid Tumors

The safety analysis includes patients treated in the core and extension phases of the trials. The analysis includes the 2,042 patients treated with Zometa 4 mg, pamidronate 90 mg, or placebo in the three controlled multicenter bone metastases trials, including 969 patients completing the efficacy phase of the trial, and 619 patients that continued in the safety extension phase. Only 347 patients completed the extension phases and were followed for 2 years (or 21 months for the other solid tumor patients). The median duration of exposure for safety analysis for Zometa 4 mg (core plus extension phases) was 12.8 months for breast cancer and multiple myeloma, 10.8 months for prostate cancer, and 4.0 months for other solid tumors.

Table 6 describes adverse events that were reported by ≥10% of patients. Adverse events are listed regardless of presumed causality to study drug.

[See table 6 at left]

Grade 3 and Grade 4 laboratory abnormalities for serum creatinine, serum calcium, serum phosphorus, and serum magnesium observed in three clinical trials of Zometa in patients with bone metastases are shown in Tables 7 and 8.

[See table 7 at left]

[See table 8 at top of next page]

Among the less frequently occurring adverse events (<15% of patients), rigors, hypokalemia, influenza-like illness, and hypocalcemia showed a trend for more events with bisphosphonate administration (Zometa 4 mg and pamidronate groups) compared to the placebo group.

Less common adverse events reported more often with Zometa 4 mg than pamidronate included decreased weight, which was reported in 16% of patients in the Zometa 4 mg group compared with 9% in the pamidronate group. Decreased appetite was reported in slightly more patients in the Zometa 4 mg group (13%) compared with the pamidronate (9%) and placebo (10%) groups, but the clinical significance of these small differences is not clear.

Renal Toxicity

In the bone metastases trials, renal deterioration was defined as an increase of 0.5 mg/dL for patients with normal baseline creatinine (<1.4 mg/dL) or an increase of 1.0 mg/dL for patients with an abnormal baseline creatinine (≥1.4 mg/dL). The following are data on the incidence of renal deterioration in patients receiving Zometa 4 mg over 15 minutes in these trials (see Table 9).

Table 9. Percentage of Patients with Treatment Emergent Renal Function Deterioration by Baseline Serum Creatinine*

Patient Population/Baseline Creatinine				
Multiple Myeloma and Breast Cancer	Zometa 4 mg		Pamidronate 90 mg	
	n/N	(%)	n/N	(%)
Normal	27/246	(11%)	23/246	(9%)
Abnormal	2/26	(8%)	2/22	(9%)
Total	29/272	(11%)	25/268	(9%)
Solid Tumors	Zometa 4 mg		Placebo	
	n/N	(%)	n/N	(%)
Normal	17/154	(11%)	10/143	(7%)
Abnormal	1/11	(9%)	1/20	(5%)
Total	18/165	(11%)	11/163	(7%)
Prostate Cancer	Zometa 4 mg		Placebo	
	n/N	(%)	n/N	(%)
Normal	12/82	(15%)	8/68	(12%)
Abnormal	4/10	(40%)	2/10	(20%)
Total	16/92	(17%)	10/78	(13%)

*Table includes only patients who were randomized to the trial after a protocol amendment that lengthened the infusion duration of Zometa to 15 minutes.

The risk of deterioration in renal function appeared to be related to time on study, whether patients were receiving Zometa (4 mg over 15 minutes), placebo, or pamidronate. In the trials and in postmarketing experience, renal deterioration, progression to renal failure and dialysis have occurred in patients with normal and abnormal baseline renal function, including patients treated with 4 mg infused over a 15-minute period. There have been instances of this occurring after the initial Zometa dose.

Table 8. Grade 4 Laboratory Abnormalities for Serum Creatinine, Serum Calcium, Serum Phosphorus, and Serum Magnesium in Three Clinical Trials in Patients with Bone Metastases

Laboratory Parameter	Grade 4					
	Zometa 4 mg		Pamidronate 90 mg		Placebo	
	n/N	(%)	n/N	(%)	n/N	(%)
Serum Creatinine[1]*	2/529	(<1%)	1/268	(<1%)	0/241	—
Hypocalcemia[2]	7/973	(<1%)	3/536	(<1%)	2/415	(<1%)
Hypophosphatemia[3]	5/973	(<1%)	0/537	—	1/415	(<1%)
Hypermagnesemia[4]	0/971	—	0/535	—	2/415	(<1%)
Hypomagnesemia[5]	2/971	(<1%)	1/535	(<1%)	0/415	—

[1] Grade 3 (>3× Upper Limit of Normal); Grade 4 (>6× Upper Limit of Normal)
* Serum creatinine data for all patients randomized after the 15-minute infusion amendment
[2] Grade 3 (<7 mg/dL); Grade 4 (<6 mg/dL)
[3] Grade 3 (<2 mg/dL); Grade 4 (<1 mg/dL)
[4] Grade 3 (>3 mEq/L); Grade 4 (>8 mEq/L)
[5] Grade 3 (<0.9 mEq/L); Grade 4 (<0.7 mEq/L)

6.2 Postmarketing Experience

The following adverse reactions have been reported during postapproval use of Zometa. Because these reports are from a population of uncertain size and are subject to confounding factors, it is not possible to reliably estimate their frequency or establish a causal relationship to drug exposure.

Osteonecrosis of the Jaw
Cases of osteonecrosis (primarily involving the jaws) have been reported predominantly in cancer patients treated with intravenous bisphosphonates including Zometa. Many of these patients were also receiving chemotherapy and corticosteroids which may be a risk factor for ONJ. Data suggests a greater frequency of reports of ONJ in certain cancers, such as advanced breast cancer and multiple myeloma. The majority of the reported cases are in cancer patients following invasive dental procedures, such as tooth extraction. It is therefore prudent to avoid invasive dental procedures as recovery may be prolonged [see Warnings And Precautions (5)].

Musculoskeletal Pain
Severe and occasionally incapacitating bone, joint, and/or muscle pain has been reported with bisphosphonate use [see Warnings And Precautions (5)].

Ocular Adverse Events
Cases of uveitis, scleritis, episcleritis, conjunctivitis, iritis, and orbital inflammation including orbital edema have been reported during postmarketing use. In some cases, symptoms resolved with topical steroids.

Hypersensitivity Reactions
There have been rare reports of allergic reaction with intravenous zoledronic acid including angioedema, and bronchoconstriction. Very rare cases of anaphylactic reaction/shock have also been reported.
Additional adverse reactions reported in postmarketing use include:
CNS: taste disturbance, hyperesthesia, tremor; **Special Senses:** blurred vision; **Gastrointestinal:** dry mouth; **Skin:** increased sweating; **Musculoskeletal:** muscle cramps; **Cardiovascular:** hypertension, bradycardia, hypotension (associated with syncope or circulatory collapse primarily in patients with underlying risk factors); **Respiratory:** bronchoconstriction; **Renal:** hematuria, proteinuria; **General Disorders and Administration Site:** weight increase; **Laboratory Abnormalities:** hyperkalemia, hypernatremia.

7 DRUG INTERACTIONS

In-vitro studies indicate that zoledronic acid is approximately 22% bound to plasma proteins. In-vitro studies also indicate that zoledronic acid does not inhibit microsomal CYP450 enzymes. In-vivo studies showed that zoledronic acid is not metabolized, and is excreted into the urine as the intact drug. However, no in-vivo drug interaction studies have been performed.

7.1 Aminoglycosides
Caution is advised when bisphosphonates are administered with aminoglycosides, since these agents may have an additive effect to lower serum calcium level for prolonged periods. This effect has not been reported in Zometa clinical trials.

7.2 Loop Diuretics
Caution should also be exercised when Zometa is used in combination with loop diuretics due to an increased risk of hypocalcemia.

7.3 Nephrotoxic Drugs
Caution is indicated when Zometa is used with other potentially nephrotoxic drugs.

7.4 Thalidomide
In multiple myeloma patients, the risk of renal dysfunction may be increased when Zometa is used in combination with thalidomide.

8 USE IN SPECIFIC POPULATIONS

8.1 Pregnancy
ZOMETA SHOULD NOT BE USED DURING PREGNANCY. There are no studies in pregnant women using Zometa. If the patient becomes pregnant while taking this drug, the patient should be apprised of the potential harm to the fetus. Women of childbearing potential should be advised to avoid becoming pregnant [see Warnings And Precautions (5.4)].

Pregnancy Category D
Bisphosphonates are incorporated into the bone matrix, from where they are gradually released over periods of weeks to years. The extent of bisphosphonate incorporation into adult bone, and hence, the amount available for release back into the systemic circulation, is directly related to the total dose and duration of bisphosphonate use. Although there are no data on fetal risk in humans, bisphosphonates do cause fetal harm in animals, and animal data suggest that uptake of bisphosphonates into fetal bone is greater than into maternal bone. Therefore, there is a theoretical risk of fetal harm (e.g., skeletal and other abnormalities) if a woman becomes pregnant after completing a course of bisphosphonate therapy. The impact of variables such as time between cessation of bisphosphonate therapy to conception, the particular bisphosphonate used, and the route of administration (intravenous versus oral) on this risk has not been established.

In female rats given subcutaneous doses of zoledronic acid of 0.01, 0.03, or 0.1 mg/kg/day beginning 15 days before mating and continuing through gestation, the number of stillbirths was increased and survival of neonates was decreased in the mid- and high-dose groups (≥0.2 times the human systemic exposure following an intravenous dose of 4 mg, based on an AUC comparison). Adverse maternal effects were observed in all dose groups (with a systemic exposure of ≥0.07 times the human systemic exposure following an intravenous dose of 4 mg, based on an AUC comparison) and included dystocia and periparturient mortality in pregnant rats allowed to deliver. Maternal mortality may have been related to drug-induced inhibition of skeletal calcium mobilization, resulting in periparturient hypocalcemia. This appears to be a bisphosphonate-class effect.

In pregnant rats given a subcutaneous dose of zoledronic acid of 0.1, 0.2, or 0.4 mg/kg/day during gestation, adverse fetal effects were observed in the mid- and high-dose groups (with systemic exposures of 2.4 and 4.8 times, respectively, the human systemic exposure following an intravenous dose of 4 mg, based on an AUC comparison). These adverse effects included increases in pre- and postimplantation losses, decreases in viable fetuses, and fetal skeletal, visceral, and external malformations. Fetal skeletal effects observed in the high-dose group included unossified or incompletely ossified bones, thickened, curved or shortened bones, wavy ribs, and shortened jaw. Other adverse fetal effects observed in the high-dose group included reduced lens, rudimentary cerebellum, reduction or absence of liver lobes, reduction of lung lobes, vessel dilation, cleft palate, and edema. Skeletal variations were also observed in the low-dose group (with systemic exposure of 1.2 times the human systemic exposure following an intravenous dose of 4 mg, based on an AUC comparison). Signs of maternal toxicity were observed in the high-dose group and included reduced body weights and food consumption, indicating that maximal exposure levels were achieved in this study.

In pregnant rabbits given subcutaneous doses of zoledronic acid of 0.01, 0.03, or 0.1 mg/kg/day during gestation (≤0.5 times the human intravenous dose of 4 mg, based on a comparison of relative body surface areas), no adverse fetal effects were observed. Maternal mortality and abortion occurred in all treatment groups (at doses ≥0.05 times the human intravenous dose of 4 mg, based on a comparison of relative body surface areas). Adverse maternal effects were associated with, and may have been caused by, drug-induced hypocalcemia.

8.3 Nursing Mothers
It is not known whether Zometa is excreted in human milk. Because many drugs are excreted in human milk, and because Zometa binds to bone long term, Zometa should not be administered to a nursing woman.

8.4 Pediatric Use
Zometa is not indicated for use in children.
The safety and effectiveness of zoledronic acid was studied in a one-year active-controlled trial of 152 pediatric subjects (74 receiving zoledronic acid). The enrolled population was subjects with severe osteogenesis imperfecta, aged 1-17 years, 55% male, 84% Caucasian, with a mean lumbar spine BMD of 0.431 gm/cm², which is 2.7 standard deviations below the mean for age-matched controls (BMD Z-score of -2.7). At one year, increases in BMD were observed in the zoledronic acid treatment group. However, changes in BMD in individual patients with severe osteogenesis imperfecta did not necessarily correlate with the risk for fracture or the incidence or severity of chronic bone pain. The adverse events observed with Zometa use in children did not raise any new safety findings beyond those previously seen in adults treated for hypercalcemia of malignancy or bone metastases.
However, adverse reactions seen more commonly in pediatric patients included pyrexia (61%), arthralgia (26%), hypocalcemia (22%) and headache (22%). These reactions, excluding arthralgia, occurred most frequently within 3 days after the first infusion and became less common with repeat dosing. Because of long-term retention in bone, Zometa should only be used in children if the potential benefit outweighs the potential risk.
Plasma zoledronic acid concentration data was obtained from 10 patients with severe osteogenesis imperfecta (4 in the age group of 3-8 years and 6 in the age group of 9-17 years) infused with 0.05 mg/kg dose over 30 min. Mean C_{max} and $AUC_{(0-last)}$ was 167 ng/mL and 220 ng.h/mL, respectively. The plasma concentration time profile of zoledronic acid in pediatric patients represent a multi-exponential decline, as observed in adult cancer patients at an approximately equivalent mg/kg dose.

8.5 Geriatric Use
Clinical studies of Zometa in hypercalcemia of malignancy included 34 patients who were 65 years of age or older. No significant differences in response rate or adverse reactions were seen in geriatric patients receiving Zometa as compared to younger patients. Controlled clinical studies of Zometa in the treatment of multiple myeloma and bone metastases of solid tumors in patients over age 65 revealed similar efficacy and safety in older and younger patients. Because decreased renal function occurs more commonly in the elderly, special care should be taken to monitor renal function.

10 OVERDOSAGE

Clinical experience with acute overdosage of Zometa is limited. Two patients received Zometa 32 mg over 5 minutes in clinical trials. Neither patient experienced any clinical or laboratory toxicity. Overdosage may cause clinically significant hypocalcemia, hypophosphatemia, and hypomagnesemia. Clinically relevant reductions in serum levels of calcium, phosphorus, and magnesium should be corrected by intravenous administration of calcium gluconate, potassium or sodium phosphate, and magnesium sulfate, respectively. In an open-label study of zoledronic acid 4 mg in breast cancer patients, a female patient received a single 48-mg dose of zoledronic acid in error. Two days after the overdose, the patient experienced a single episode of hyperthermia (38°C), which resolved after treatment. All other evaluations were normal, and the patient was discharged seven days after the overdose.
A patient with non-Hodgkin's lymphoma received zoledronic acid 4 mg daily on four successive days for a total dose of 16 mg. The patient developed paresthesia and abnormal liver function tests with increased GGT (nearly 100U/L, each value unknown). The outcome of this case is not known.
In controlled clinical trials, administration of Zometa 4 mg as an intravenous infusion over 5 minutes has been shown to increase the risk of renal toxicity compared to the same dose administered as a 15-minute intravenous infusion. In controlled clinical trials, Zometa 8 mg has been shown to be associated with an increased risk of renal toxicity compared to Zometa 4 mg, even when given as a 15-minute intravenous infusion, and was not associated with added benefit in patients with hypercalcemia of malignancy [see Dosage And Administration (2.4)].

11 DESCRIPTION

Zometa contains zoledronic acid, a bisphosphonic acid which is an inhibitor of osteoclastic bone resorption. Zoledronic acid is designated chemically as (1-Hydroxy-2-imidazol-1-yl-phosphonoethyl) phosphonic acid monohydrate and its structural formula is

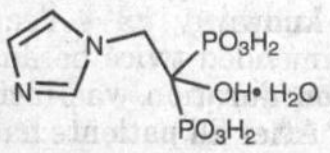

Zoledronic acid is a white crystalline powder. Its molecular formula is $C_5H_{10}N_2O_7P_2 \bullet H_2O$ and its molar mass is 290.1 g/Mol. Zoledronic acid is highly soluble in 0.1N sodium hydroxide solution, sparingly soluble in water and 0.1N hydrochloric acid, and practically insoluble in organic solvents. The pH of a 0.7% solution of zoledronic acid in water is approximately 2.0.

Zometa is available in vials as a sterile liquid concentrate solution for intravenous infusion. Each 5-mL vial contains 4.264 mg of zoledronic acid monohydrate, corresponding to 4 mg zoledronic acid on an anhydrous basis.

Inactive Ingredients: mannitol, USP, as bulking agent, water for injection and sodium citrate, USP, as buffering agent.

12 CLINICAL PHARMACOLOGY

12.1 Mechanism of Action

The principal pharmacologic action of zoledronic acid is inhibition of bone resorption. Although the antiresorptive mechanism is not completely understood, several factors are thought to contribute to this action. *In vitro*, zoledronic acid inhibits osteoclastic activity and induces osteoclast apoptosis. Zoledronic acid also blocks the osteoclastic resorption of mineralized bone and cartilage through its binding to bone. Zoledronic acid inhibits the increased osteoclastic activity and skeletal calcium release induced by various stimulatory factors released by tumors.

12.2 Pharmacodynamics

Clinical studies in patients with hypercalcemia of malignancy (HCM) showed that single-dose infusions of Zometa are associated with decreases in serum calcium and phosphorus and increases in urinary calcium and phosphorus excretion.

Osteoclastic hyperactivity resulting in excessive bone resorption is the underlying pathophysiologic derangement in hypercalcemia of malignancy (HCM, tumor-induced hypercalcemia) and metastatic bone disease. Excessive release of calcium into the blood as bone is resorbed results in polyuria and gastrointestinal disturbances, with progressive dehydration and decreasing glomerular filtration rate. This, in turn, results in increased renal resorption of calcium, setting up a cycle of worsening systemic hypercalcemia. Reducing excessive bone resorption and maintaining adequate fluid administration are, therefore, essential to the management of hypercalcemia of malignancy.

Patients who have hypercalcemia of malignancy can generally be divided into two groups according to the pathophysiologic mechanism involved: humoral hypercalcemia and hypercalcemia due to tumor invasion of bone. In humoral hypercalcemia, osteoclasts are activated and bone resorption is stimulated by factors such as parathyroid hormone-related protein, which are elaborated by the tumor and circulate systemically. Humoral hypercalcemia usually occurs in squamous cell malignancies of the lung or head and neck or in genitourinary tumors such as renal cell carcinoma or ovarian cancer. Skeletal metastases may be absent or minimal in these patients.

Extensive invasion of bone by tumor cells can also result in hypercalcemia due to local tumor products that stimulate bone resorption by osteoclasts. Tumors commonly associated with locally mediated hypercalcemia include breast cancer and multiple myeloma.

Total serum calcium levels in patients who have hypercalcemia of malignancy may not reflect the severity of hypercalcemia, since concomitant hypoalbuminemia is commonly present. Ideally, ionized calcium levels should be used to diagnose and follow hypercalcemic conditions; however, these are not commonly or rapidly available in many clinical situations. Therefore, adjustment of the total serum calcium value for differences in albumin levels (corrected serum calcium, CSC) is often used in place of measurement of ionized calcium; several nomograms are in use for this type of calculation [*see Dosage And Administration (2)*].

12.3 Pharmacokinetics

Pharmacokinetic data in patients with hypercalcemia are not available.

Distribution

Single or multiple (q 28 days) 5-minute or 15-minute infusions of 2, 4, 8 or 16 mg Zometa were given to 64 patients with cancer and bone metastases. The postinfusion decline of zoledronic acid concentrations in plasma was consistent with a triphasic process showing a rapid decrease from peak concentrations at end of infusion to <1% of C_{max} 24 hours postinfusion with population half-lives of $t_{1/2\alpha}$ 0.24 hours and $t_{1/2\beta}$ 1.87 hours for the early disposition phases of the drug. The terminal elimination phase of zoledronic acid was prolonged, with very low concentrations in plasma between

$$CrCl = \frac{[140\text{-age (years)}] \times \text{weight (kg)}}{[72 \times \text{serum creatinine (mg/dL)}]} \quad \{\times\ 0.85 \text{ for female patients}\}$$

Days 2 and 28 postinfusion, and a terminal elimination half-life $t_{1/2\gamma}$ of 146 hours. The area under the plasma concentration versus time curve ($AUC_{0\text{-}24h}$) of zoledronic acid was dose proportional from 2-16 mg. The accumulation of zoledronic acid measured over three cycles was low, with mean $AUC_{0\text{-}24h}$ ratios for cycles 2 and 3 versus 1 of 1.13 ± 0.30 and 1.16 ± 0.36, respectively.

In-vitro and *ex-vivo* studies showed low affinity of zoledronic acid for the cellular components of human blood. *In vitro*, mean zoledronic acid protein binding in human plasma ranged from 28% at 200 ng/mL to 53% at 50 ng/mL.

Metabolism

Zoledronic acid does not inhibit human P450 enzymes *in vitro*. Zoledronic acid does not undergo biotransformation *in vivo*. In animal studies, <3% of the administered intravenous dose was found in the feces, with the balance either recovered in the urine or taken up by bone, indicating that the drug is eliminated intact via the kidney. Following an intravenous dose of 20 nCi ^{14}C-zoledronic acid in a patient with cancer and bone metastases, only a single radioactive species with chromatographic properties identical to those of parent drug was recovered in urine, which suggests that zoledronic acid is not metabolized.

Excretion

In 64 patients with cancer and bone metastases, on average (± s.d.) 39 ± 16% of the administered zoledronic acid dose was recovered in the urine within 24 hours, with only trace amounts of drug found in urine post-Day 2. The cumulative percent of drug excreted in the urine over 0-24 hours was independent of dose. The balance of drug not recovered in urine over 0-24 hours, representing drug presumably bound to bone, is slowly released back into the systemic circulation, giving rise to the observed prolonged low plasma concentrations. The 0-24 hour renal clearance of zoledronic acid was 3.7 ± 2.0 L/h.

Zoledronic acid clearance was independent of dose but dependent upon the patient's creatinine clearance. In a study in patients with cancer and bone metastases, increasing the infusion time of a 4-mg dose of zoledronic acid from 5 minutes (n=5) to 15 minutes (n=7) resulted in a 34% decrease in the zoledronic acid concentration at the end of the infusion ([mean ± SD] 403 ± 118 ng/mL versus 264 ± 86 ng/mL) and a 10% increase in the total AUC (378 ± 116 ng x h/mL versus 420 ± 218 ng x h/mL). The difference between the AUC means was not statistically significant.

Special Populations

Pediatrics

Zometa is not indicated for use in children [*see Pediatric Use (8.4)*].

Geriatrics

The pharmacokinetics of zoledronic acid were not affected by age in patients with cancer and bone metastases who ranged in age from 38 years to 84 years.

Race

Population pharmacokinetic analyses did not indicate any differences in pharmacokinetics among Japanese and North American (Caucasian and African American) patients with cancer and bone metastases.

Hepatic Insufficiency

No clinical studies were conducted to evaluate the effect of hepatic impairment on the pharmacokinetics of zoledronic acid.

Renal Insufficiency

The pharmacokinetic studies conducted in 64 cancer patients represented typical clinical populations with normal to moderately impaired renal function. Compared to patients with normal renal function (N=37), patients with mild renal impairment (N=15) showed an average increase in plasma AUC of 15%, whereas patients with moderate renal impairment (N=11) showed an average increase in plasma AUC of 43%. Limited pharmacokinetic data are available for Zometa in patients with severe renal impairment (creatinine clearance <30 mL/min). Based on population PK/PD modeling, the risk of renal deterioration appears to increase with AUC, which is doubled at a creatinine clearance of 10 mL/min. Creatinine clearance is calculated by the Cockcroft-Gault formula:

[See table above]

Zometa systemic clearance in individual patients can be calculated from the population clearance of Zometa, CL (L/h)=$6.5(CL_{cr}/90)^{0.4}$. These formulae can be used to predict the Zometa AUC in patients, where CL = Dose/$AUC_{0\text{-}\infty}$. The average $AUC_{0\text{-}24}$ in patients with normal renal function was 0.42 mg•h/L and the calculated $AUC_{0\text{-}\infty}$ for a patient with creatinine clearance of 75 mL/min was 0.66 mg•h/L following a 4-mg dose of Zometa. However, efficacy and safety of adjusted dosing based on these formulae have not been prospectively assessed [*see Warnings And Precautions (5.2)*].

13 NONCLINICAL TOXICOLOGY

13.1 Carcinogenesis, Mutagenesis, Impairment of Fertility

Carcinogenesis

Standard lifetime carcinogenicity bioassays were conducted in mice and rats. Mice were given oral doses of zoledronic acid of 0.1, 0.5, or 2.0 mg/kg/day. There was an increased incidence of Harderian gland adenomas in males and females in all treatment groups (at doses ≥0.002 times a human intravenous dose of 4 mg, based on a comparison of relative body surface areas). Rats were given oral doses of zoledronic acid of 0.1, 0.5, or 2.0 mg/kg/day. No increased incidence of tumors was observed (at doses ≤0.2 times the human intravenous dose of 4 mg, based on a comparison of relative body surface areas).

Mutagenesis

Zoledronic acid was not genotoxic in the Ames bacterial mutagenicity assay, in the Chinese hamster ovary cell assay, or in the Chinese hamster gene mutation assay, with or without metabolic activation. Zoledronic acid was not genotoxic in the *in-vivo* rat micronucleus assay.

Impairment of Fertility

Female rats were given subcutaneous doses of zoledronic acid of 0.01, 0.03, or 0.1 mg/kg/day beginning 15 days before mating and continuing through gestation. Effects observed in the high-dose group (with systemic exposure of 1.2 times the human systemic exposure following an intravenous dose of 4 mg, based on AUC comparison) included inhibition of ovulation and a decrease in the number of pregnant rats. Effects observed in both the mid-dose group (with systemic exposure of 0.2 times the human systemic exposure following an intravenous dose of 4 mg, based on an AUC comparison) and high-dose group included an increase in preimplantation losses and a decrease in the number of implantations and live fetuses.

14 CLINICAL STUDIES

14.1 Hypercalcemia of Malignancy

Two identical multicenter, randomized, double-blind, double-dummy studies of Zometa 4 mg given as a 5-minute intravenous infusion or pamidronate 90 mg given as a 2-hour intravenous infusion were conducted in 185 patients with hypercalcemia of malignancy (HCM). **NOTE: Administration of Zometa 4 mg given as a 5-minute intravenous infusion has been shown to result in an increased risk of renal toxicity, as measured by increases in serum creatinine, which can progress to renal failure. The incidence of renal toxicity and renal failure has been shown to be reduced when Zometa 4 mg is given as a 15-minute intravenous infusion. Zometa should be administered by intravenous infusion over no less than 15 minutes [*see Warnings And Precautions (5.1, 5.2) and Dosage And Administration (2.4)*].** The treatment groups in the clinical studies were generally well balanced with regards to age, sex, race, and tumor types. The mean age of the study population was 59 years; 81% were Caucasian, 15% were Black, and 4% were of other races. 60% of the patients were male. The most common tumor types were lung, breast, head and neck, and renal.

In these studies, HCM was defined as a corrected serum calcium (CSC) concentration of ≥12.0 mg/dL (3.00 mmol/L). The primary efficacy variable was the proportion of patients having a complete response, defined as the lowering of the CSC to ≤10.8 mg/dL (2.70 mmol/L) within 10 days after drug infusion.

To assess the effects of Zometa versus those of pamidronate, the two multicenter HCM studies were combined in a preplanned analysis. The results of the primary analysis revealed that the proportion of patients that had normalization of corrected serum calcium by Day 10 were 88% and 70% for Zometa 4 mg and pamidronate 90 mg, respectively (P=0.002) (*see Figure 1*). **In these studies, no additional benefit was seen for Zometa 8 mg over Zometa 4 mg; however, the risk of renal toxicity of Zometa 8 mg was significantly greater than that seen with Zometa 4 mg.**

Figure 1. Proportion of Complete Responders by Day 10 in Pooled HCM Studies

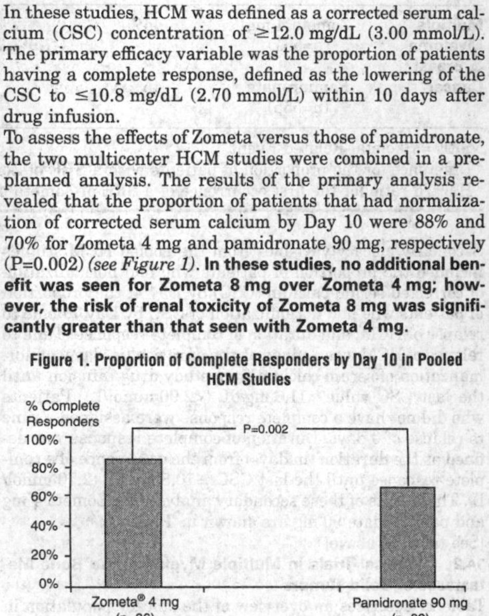

Table 10. Secondary Efficacy Variables in Pooled HCM Studies

Complete Response	Zometa 4 mg		Pamidronate 90 mg	
	N	Response Rate	N	Response Rate
By Day 4	86	45.3%	99	33.3%
By Day 7	86	82.6%*	99	63.6%
Duration of Response	N	Median Duration (Days)	N	Median Duration (Days)
Time to Relapse	86	30*	99	17
Duration of Complete Response	76	32	69	18

*P less than 0.05 versus pamidronate 90 mg.

Table 11. Overview of Efficacy Population for Phase III Studies

Patient Population	No. of Patients	Zometa Dose	Control	Median Duration (Planned Duration) Zometa 4 mg
Multiple myeloma or metastatic breast cancer	1,648	4 and 8* mg Q3-4 weeks	Pamidronate 90 mg Q3-4 weeks	12.0 months (13 months)
Metastatic prostate cancer	643	4 and 8* mg Q3 weeks	Placebo	10.5 months (15 months)
Metastatic solid tumor other than breast or prostate cancer	773	4 and 8* mg Q3 weeks	Placebo	3.8 months (9 months)

*Patients who were randomized to the 8 mg Zometa group are not included in any of the analyses in this package insert.

Table 12. Zometa Compared to Placebo in Patients with Bone Metastases from Prostate Cancer or Other Solid Tumors

Study	I. Analysis of Proportion of Patients with a SRE[1]				II. Analysis of Time to the First SRE		
	Study Arm & Patient Number	Proportion	Difference[2] & 95% CI	P-value	Median (Days)	Hazard Ratio[3] & 95% CI	P-value
Prostate Cancer	Zometa 4 mg (n=214)	33%	-11% (-20%, -1%)	0.02	Not Reached	0.67 (0.49, 0.91)	0.011
	Placebo (n=208)	44%			321		
Solid Tumors	Zometa 4 mg (n=257)	38%	-7% (-15%, 2%)	0.13	230	0.73 (0.55, 0.96)	0.023
	Placebo (n=250)	44%			163		

[1] SRE=Skeletal-Related Event
[2] Difference for the proportion of patients with a SRE of Zometa 4 mg versus placebo.
[3] Hazard ratio for the first occurrence of a SRE of Zometa 4 mg versus placebo.

Table 13. Zometa Compared to Pamidronate in Patients with Multiple Myeloma or Bone Metastases from Breast Cancer

Study	I. Analysis of Proportion of Patients with a SRE[1]				II. Analysis of Time to the First SRE		
	Study Arm & Patient Number	Proportion	Difference[2] & 95% CI	P-value	Median (Days)	Hazard Ratio[3] & 95% CI	P-value
Multiple Myeloma & Breast Cancer	Zometa 4 mg (n=561)	44%	-2% (-7.9%, 3.7%)	0.46	373	0.92 (0.77, 1.09)	0.32
	Pamidronate (n=555)	46%			363		

[1] SRE = Skeletal-Related Event
[2] Difference for the proportion of patients with a SRE of Zometa 4 mg versus pamidronate 90 mg.
[3] Hazard ratio for the first occurrence of a SRE of Zometa 4 mg versus pamidronate 90 mg.

Secondary efficacy variables from the pooled HCM studies included the proportion of patients who had normalization of corrected serum calcium (CSC) by Day 4; the proportion of patients who had normalization of CSC by Day 7; time to relapse of HCM; and duration of complete response. Time to relapse of HCM was defined as the duration (in days) of normalization of serum calcium from study drug infusion until the last CSC value <11.6 mg/dL (<2.90 mmol/L). Patients who did not have a complete response were assigned a time to relapse of 0 days. Duration of complete response was defined as the duration (in days) from the occurrence of a complete response until the last CSC ≤10.8 mg/dL (2.70 mmol/L). The results of these secondary analyses for Zometa 4 mg and pamidronate 90 mg are shown in Table 10.
[See table 10 above]

14.2   Clinical Trials in Multiple Myeloma and Bone Metastases of Solid Tumors
Table 11 describes an overview of the efficacy population in three randomized Zometa trials in patients with multiple myeloma and bone metastases of solid tumors. These trials included a pamidronate-controlled study in breast cancer and multiple myeloma, a placebo-controlled study in prostate cancer, and a placebo-controlled study in other solid tumors. The prostate cancer study required documentation of previous bone metastases and 3 consecutive rising PSAs while on hormonal therapy. The other placebo-controlled solid tumor study included patients with bone metastases from malignancies other than breast cancer and prostate cancer, including NSCLC, renal cell cancer, small cell lung cancer, colorectal cancer, bladder cancer, GI/genitourinary cancer, head and neck cancer, and others. These trials were comprised of a core phase and an extension phase. In the solid tumor, breast cancer and multiple myeloma trials, only the core phase was evaluated for efficacy as a high percentage of patients did not choose to participate in the extension phase. In the prostate cancer trials, both the core and extension phases were evaluated for efficacy showing the Zometa effect during the first 15 months was maintained

without decrement or improvement for another 9 months. The design of these clinical trials does not permit assessment of whether more than one-year administration of Zometa is beneficial. The optimal duration of Zometa administration is not known.

The studies were amended twice because of renal toxicity. The Zometa infusion duration was increased from 5 minutes to 15 minutes. After all patients had been accrued, but while dosing and follow-up continued, patients in the 8 mg Zometa treatment arm were switched to 4 mg due to toxicity. Patients who were randomized to the Zometa 8 mg group are not included in these analyses.
[See table 11 at left]

Each study evaluated skeletal-related events (SREs), defined as any of the following: pathologic fracture, radiation therapy to bone, surgery to bone, or spinal cord compression. Change in antineoplastic therapy due to increased pain was a SRE in the prostate cancer study only. Planned analyses included the proportion of patients with a SRE during the study and time to the first SRE. Results for the two Zometa placebo-controlled studies are given in Table 12.
[See table 12 at left]

In the breast cancer and myeloma trial, efficacy was determined by a noninferiority analysis comparing Zometa to pamidronate 90 mg for the proportion of patients with a SRE. This analysis required an estimation of pamidronate efficacy. Historical data from 1,128 patients in three pamidronate placebo-controlled trials demonstrated that pamidronate decreased the proportion of patients with a SRE by 13.1% (95% CI = 7.3%, 18.9%). Results of the comparison of treatment with Zometa compared to pamidronate are given in Table 13.
[See table 13 at left]

16   HOW SUPPLIED/STORAGE AND HANDLING
Each 5 mL vial contains 4.264 mg zoledronic acid monohydrate, corresponding to 4 mg zoledronic acid on an anhydrous basis, 220 mg of mannitol, USP, water for injection, and 24 mg of sodium citrate, USP.
Carton of 1 vial .... NDC 0078-0387-25
Store at 25°C (77°F); excursions permitted to 15-30°C (59-86°F) [see USP Controlled Room Temperature].

17   PATIENT COUNSELING INFORMATION
• Patients should be instructed to tell their doctor if they have kidney problems before being given Zometa.
• Patients should be informed of the importance of getting their blood tests (serum creatinine) during the course of their Zometa therapy.
• Zometa should not be given if the patient is pregnant or plans to become pregnant, or if she is breast-feeding.
• Patients should be advised to have a dental examination prior to treatment with Zometa and should avoid invasive dental procedures during treatment.
• Patients should be informed of the importance of good dental hygiene and routine dental care.
• Patients with multiple myeloma and bone metastasis of solid tumors should be advised to take an oral calcium supplement of 500 mg and a multiple vitamin containing 400 IU of Vitamin D daily.
• Patients should be aware of the most common side effects including: anemia, nausea, vomiting, constipation, diarrhea, fatigue, pyrexia, weakness, lower limb edema, anorexia, decreased weight, bone pain, myalgia, arthralgia, back pain, malignant neoplasm aggravated, headache, dizziness, insomnia, paresthesia, dyspnea, cough, and abdominal pain.

REV: OCTOBER 2009   T2009-101
Manufactured by
Novartis Pharma Stein AG
Stein, Switzerland for
Novartis Pharmaceuticals Corporation
East Hanover, New Jersey 07936
©Novartis
Shown in Product Identification Guide, page 316

ZORTRESS®   ℞
[ZOR-tres]
(everolimus)
Tablets

The following prescribing information is based on official labeling in effect September 2010.
HIGHLIGHTS OF PRESCRIBING INFORMATION
These highlights do not include all the information needed to use Zortress (everolimus) safely and effectively. See full prescribing information for Zortress.
Zortress® *(everolimus)* Tablets
Tablets for oral administration
Initial U.S. Approval: 2010

WARNING: IMMUNOSUPPRESSION AND RENAL FUNCTION
See Full Prescribing Information For Complete Boxed Warning

- Only physicians experienced in immunosuppressive therapy and management of transplant patients should use everolimus. (5.1)
- Increased susceptibility to infection and the possible development of malignancies may result from immunosuppression. (5.2, 5.3)
- Reduced doses of cyclosporine are required for use in combination with everolimus in order to reduce nephrotoxicity. (5.8)
- Increased incidence of kidney graft thrombosis. (5.5)

──────INDICATIONS AND USAGE──────
- Prophylaxis of organ rejection in adult patients at low-moderate immunologic risk receiving a kidney transplant.
- Use in combination with basiliximab and concurrently with reduced doses of cyclosporine and corticosteroids. (1.1)
- Use in patients at high immunologic risk is not established. (1.2)
- Use for prophylaxis in organs other than kidney is not established. (1.2)
- Safety and efficacy in pediatric patients (<18 years) have not been established. (1.2)

──────DOSAGE AND ADMINISTRATION──────
- Starting oral dose of 0.75 mg twice daily. Adjust maintenance dose to achieve everolimus trough concentrations within the 3-8 ng/mL target range. (2.1) Administer as soon as possible after transplantation.
- Routine everolimus and cyclosporine therapeutic drug concentration monitoring is recommended. (2.2, 2.3)
- Administer consistently with or without food (12) at the same time as cyclosporine. (2.4)
- Moderate hepatic impairment: Reduce daily dose by half and monitor blood concentrations. (2.5)

──────DOSAGE FORMS AND STRENGTHS──────
Zortress is available as 0.25 mg, 0.5 mg, and 0.75 mg tablets. (3)

──────CONTRAINDICATIONS──────
- Patients with known hypersensitivity to everolimus, sirolimus, or to components of the drug product. (4)

──────WARNINGS AND PRECAUTIONS──────
- Lymphoma and Other Malignancies: Increased risk with all immunosuppressants; appears related to intensity and duration of use. Avoid prolonged exposure to UV light and sunlight. (5.2)
- Serious Infections: Increased risk of bacterial, viral, fungal and protozoal infections, including opportunistic infections; combination immunosuppression should be used with caution. (5.3)
- Angioedema: Increased risk with concomitant ACE inhibitors; monitor for symptoms and treat promptly. (5.4)
- Wound Healing/Fluid Accumulation: Increased risk for delayed wound healing. Monitor symptoms; treat promptly to minimize complications. (5.6)
- Hyperlipidemia: Elevations of serum cholesterol and triglycerides are common. Monitoring is recommended; consider intervention including anti-lipid therapy. (5.7)
- Proteinuria: Increased risk with higher trough concentrations; monitor urine protein. (5.9)
- Polyoma Virus Infections: Risk of activation of latent viral infections; BK-virus associated nephropathy has been observed; consider reducing immunosuppression. (5.10)
- Interactions with Strong Inhibitors and Inducers of CYP3A4: Closely monitor everolimus trough concentrations with concomitant use. (5.11)
- Non-Infectious Pneumonitis: Monitor for clinical symptoms or radiologic changes; fatal cases have occurred. Manage by dose reduction or discontinuation until symptoms resolve; consider use of corticosteroids. (5.12)
- TMA/TTP/HUS: Concomitant use with cyclosporine may increase risk. Monitor for hematological changes or clinical symptoms. (5.13)
- New Onset Diabetes After Transplantation: Blood glucose elevations may occur in dose related manner. Monitor serum glucose. (5.14)
- Male Infertility: Azospermia or oligospermia may occur. (5.15, 13.1)
- Immunizations: Live vaccines should be avoided. (5.16)

──────ADVERSE REACTIONS──────
The most common (incidence ≥20%) adverse events are: peripheral edema, constipation, hypertension, nausea, anemia, UTI, and hyperlipidemia. (6.2)
To report SUSPECTED ADVERSE REACTIONS, contact Novartis Pharmaceuticals Corporation at 1-888-669-6682 or FDA at 1-800-FDA-1088 or www.fda.gov/medwatch.

──────DRUG INTERACTIONS──────
CYP3A4 inhibitors and inducers: Strong-moderate inhibitors (e.g., cyclosporine, ketoconazole, erythromycin, verapamil) and inducers (e.g., rifampin) may affect everolimus concentrations. Blood concentration monitoring is recommended; consider dose adjustment of everolimus. (7)

──────USE IN SPECIFIC POPULATIONS──────
- Pregnancy: Based on animal data may cause fetal harm. (8.1)

- Nursing Mothers: Discontinue drug or nursing taking into consideration importance of drug to mother. (8.3)

See 17 for PATIENT COUNSELING INFORMATION

Revised: 03/2010

FULL PRESCRIBING INFORMATION: CONTENTS*
WARNING: IMMUNOSUPPRESSION AND RENAL FUNCTION
See Full Prescribing Information For Complete Boxed Warning
WARNING: IMMUNOSUPPRESSION, RENAL FUNCTION, AND GRAFT THROMBOSIS

──────
FULL PRESCRIBING INFORMATION

WARNING: IMMUNOSUPPRESSION, RENAL FUNCTION, AND GRAFT THROMBOSIS
- Increased susceptibility to infection and the possible development of malignancies such as lymphoma and skin cancer may result from immunosuppression. [*See Warnings and Precautions (5.2)*]
- Only physicians experienced in immunosuppressive therapy and management of transplant patients should prescribe Zortress. Patients receiving the drug should be managed in facilities equipped and staffed with adequate laboratory and supportive medical resources. The physician responsible for maintenance therapy should have complete information requisite for the follow-up of the patient. [*See Warnings and Precautions (5.1)*]
- Increased nephrotoxicity can occur with use of standard doses of cyclosporine in combination with everolimus. Therefore reduced doses of cyclosporine should be used in combination with everolimus in order to reduce renal dysfunction. It is important to monitor the cyclosporine and everolimus whole blood trough concentrations. [*See Dosage and Administration (2.2 and 2.3) and Warnings and Precautions (5.8) and Clinical Pharmacology (12.5 and 12.6)*]
- An increased risk of kidney arterial and venous thrombosis, resulting in graft loss, was reported, mostly within the first 30 days post-transplantation. [*See Warnings and Precautions (5.5)*]

1 INDICATIONS AND USAGE

1.1 Prophylaxis of Organ Rejection in Renal Transplantation
Zortress is indicated for the prophylaxis of organ rejection in adult patients at low-moderate immunologic risk receiving a kidney transplant. [*See Clinical Studies (14.1)*] Zortress is to be administered in combination with basiliximab induction and concurrently with reduced doses of cyclosporine and corticosteroids. Therapeutic drug monitoring of everolimus and cyclosporine is recommended for all patients receiving these products. [*See Dosage and Administration (2.2 and 2.3)*]

1.2 Limitations of Use
- In patients at high immunologic risk, the safety and efficacy of everolimus has not been established.
- Use of everolimus for the prophylaxis of organ rejection in transplanted organs other than kidney has not been established.
- Standard doses of cyclosporine should be avoided with everolimus in order to reduce the risk of nephrotoxicity. [*See Warnings and Precautions (5), and Adverse Reactions (6.2)*]
- The safety and efficacy of Zortress have not been established in pediatric patients (<18 years).

2 DOSAGE AND ADMINISTRATION
2.1 Dosage in Adult Kidney Transplant Patients
An initial everolimus dose of 0.75 mg orally twice daily (1.5 mg/day) is recommended for adult kidney transplant patients in combination with reduced dose cyclosporine, administered as soon as possible after transplantation. [*See Therapeutic Drug Monitoring (2.2 and 2.3), Clinical Studies (14.1)*] Patients receiving everolimus may require dose adjustments based on everolimus blood concentrations achieved, tolerability, individual response, change in concomitant medications and the clinical situation. Dose adjustments can be made at 4-5 day intervals. [*See Therapeutic Drug Monitoring (2.2)*]
Oral prednisone should be initiated once oral medication is tolerated. Steroid doses may be further tapered on an individualized basis depending on the clinical status of patient and function of graft.

2.2 Therapeutic Drug Monitoring – Everolimus
Routine everolimus whole blood therapeutic drug concentration monitoring is recommended for all patients using appropriate assay methodology. The recommended everolimus therapeutic range is 3 to 8 ng/mL. [*See Clinical Pharmacology (12.5)*] Careful attention should be made to clinical signs and symptoms, tissue biopsies, and laboratory parameters.

Description of Zortress (everolimus) Tablets

Dosage Strength	0.25 mg	0.5 mg	0.75 mg
Appearance	White to yellowish, marbled, round, flat tablets with bevelled edge		
Imprint	"C" on one side and "NVR" on the other	"CH" on one side and "NVR" on the other	"CL" on one side and "NVR" on the other

It is important to monitor everolimus blood concentrations, in patients with hepatic impairment, during concomitant administration of CYP3A4 inducers or inhibitors, when switching cyclosporine formulations and/or when cyclosporine dosing is reduced according to recommended target concentrations. [*See Clinical Pharmacology (12.5 and 12.6)*]

Optimally, dose adjustments of everolimus should be based on trough concentrations obtained 4 or 5 days after a previous dosing change. There is an interaction of cyclosporine on everolimus, and consequently, everolimus concentrations may decrease if cyclosporine exposure is reduced. [*See Drug Interactions (7.2)*]

2.3 Therapeutic Drug Monitoring – Cyclosporine

Both cyclosporine doses and the target range for whole blood trough concentrations should be reduced, when given in a regimen with everolimus, in order to minimize the risk of nephrotoxicity. [*See Warnings and Precautions (5.8) and Drug Interactions (7.2), Clinical Pharmacology (12.6)*]

The recommended cyclosporine therapeutic range when administered with everolimus are 100 to 200 ng/mL through Month 1 post-transplant, 75 to 150 ng/mL at Months 2 and 3 post-transplant, 50 to 100 ng/mL at Month 4 post-transplant, and 25 to 50 ng/mL from Month 6 through Month 12 post-transplant. The median trough concentrations observed in the clinical trial ranged between 161 to 185 ng/mL through Month 1 post-transplant and between 111 to 140 ng/mL at Months 2 and 3 post-transplant. The median trough concentration was 99 ng/mL at Month 4 post-transplant and ranged between 46 to 75 ng/mL from Months 6 through Month 12 post-transplant. [*See Clinical Pharmacology (12.6) and Clinical Studies (14.1)*]

Cyclosporine, USP Modified is to be administered as oral capsules twice daily unless cyclosporine oral solution or i.v. administration of cyclosporine cannot be avoided. Cyclosporine, USP Modified should be initiated as soon as possible – and no later than 48 hours – after reperfusion of the graft and dose adjusted to target concentrations from Day 5 onwards.

If impairment of renal function is progressive the treatment regimen should be adjusted. In renal transplant patients, the cyclosporine dose should be based on cyclosporine whole blood trough concentrations. [*See Clinical Pharmacology (12.6)*]

In renal transplantation, there are limited data regarding dosing everolimus with reduced cyclosporine trough concentrations of 25 to 50 ng/mL after 12 months. Everolimus has not been evaluated in clinical trials with other formulations of cyclosporine. Prior to dose reduction of cyclosporine it should be ascertained that steady-state everolimus whole blood trough concentration is at least 3 ng/mL. There is an interaction of cyclosporine on everolimus, and consequently, everolimus concentrations may decrease if cyclosporine exposure is reduced. [*See Drug Interactions (7.2)*]

2.4 Administration

Everolimus tablets should be swallowed whole with a glass of water and not crushed before use.

Administer everolimus consistently approximately 12 hours apart with or without food to minimize variability in absorption and at the same time as cyclosporine. [*See Clinical Pharmacology (12.3)*]

2.5 Hepatic Impairment

No dose adjustment is needed for patients with mild hepatic impairment (Child-Pugh Class A). In patients with moderate hepatic impairment (Child-Pugh Class B), the daily dose needs to be reduced by one-half the recommended initial daily dose and blood concentrations should be monitored to make further adjustments as necessary. There is no information on the effects of severe hepatic impairment (Child-Pugh Class C) on everolimus pharmacokinetics. [*See Clinical Pharmacology (12.3)*]

3 DOSAGE FORMS AND STRENGTHS

Zortress is available as 0.25 mg, 0.5 mg, and 0.75 mg tablets.
[See table above]

4 CONTRAINDICATIONS

4.1 Hypersensitivity Reactions

Zortress is contraindicated in patients with known hypersensitivity to everolimus, sirolimus, or to components of the drug product.

5 WARNINGS AND PRECAUTIONS

5.1 Management of Immunosuppression

Only physicians experienced in management of systemic immunosuppressant therapy in transplantation should prescribe Zortress. Patients receiving the drug should be managed in facilities equipped and staffed with adequate laboratory and supportive medical resources. The physician responsible for the maintenance therapy should have complete information requisite for the follow-up of the patient. [*See Boxed Warning*]

5.2 Lymphomas and Other Malignancies

Patients receiving immunosuppressants, including everolimus, are at increased risk of developing lymphomas and other malignancies, particularly of the skin. [*See Boxed Warning*] The risk appears to be related to the intensity and duration of immunosuppression rather than to the use of any specific agent.

As usual for patients with increased risk for skin cancer, exposure to sunlight and ultraviolet light should be limited by wearing protective clothing and using a sunscreen with a high protection factor.

5.3 Serious Infections

Patients receiving immunosuppressants, including everolimus, are at increased risk of developing bacterial, viral, fungal, and protozoal infections, including opportunistic infections. [*See Warnings and Precautions (5.10) and Adverse Reactions (6.2)*] These infections may lead to serious, including fatal, outcomes. Because of the danger of over immunosuppression of the immune system which can cause increased susceptibility to infection, combination immunosuppressant therapy should be used with caution.

5.4 Angioedema

Zortress has been associated with the development of angioedema. The concomitant use of everolimus with other drugs known to cause angioedema, such as angiotensin converting enzyme (ACE) inhibitors may increase the risk of developing angioedema.

5.5 Graft Thrombosis

An increased risk of kidney arterial and venous thrombosis, resulting in graft loss, has been reported, usually within the first 30 days post-transplantation. [*See Boxed Warning*]

5.6 Wound Healing and Fluid Accumulation

Everolimus delays wound healing and increases the occurrence of wound-related complications like wound dehiscence, wound infection, incisional hernia, lymphocele and seroma. These wound-related complications may require more surgical intervention. Generalized fluid accumulation, including peripheral edema (e.g., lymphoedema) and other types of localized fluid collection, such as pericardial and pleural effusions and ascites have also been reported.

5.7 Hyperlipidemia

Increased serum cholesterol and triglycerides, requiring the need for anti-lipid therapy, have been reported to occur following initiation of everolimus and the risk of hyperlipidemia is increased with higher everolimus whole blood trough concentrations. [*See Adverse Reactions (6.2)*] Use of anti-lipid therapy may not normalize lipid levels in patients receiving Zortress.

Any patient who is administered everolimus should be monitored for hyperlipidemia. If detected, interventions, such as diet, exercise, and lipid-lowering agents should be initiated as outlined by the National Cholesterol Education Program guidelines. The risk/benefit should be considered in patients with established hyperlipidemia before initiating an immunosuppressive regimen containing everolimus. Similarly, the risk/benefit of continued everolimus therapy should be re-evaluated in patients with severe refractory hyperlipidemia. Everolimus has not been studied in patients with baseline cholesterol levels >350 mg/dL.

Due to an interaction with cyclosporine, clinical trials of everolimus and cyclosporine in kidney transplant patients strongly discouraged patients from receiving the HMG-CoA reductase inhibitors simvastatin and lovastatin. During everolimus therapy with cyclosporine, patients administered an HMG-CoA reductase inhibitor and/or fibrate should be monitored for the possible development of rhabdomyolysis and other adverse effects, as described in the respective labeling for these agents. [*See Drug Interactions (7.6)*]

5.8 Nephrotoxicity

Everolimus with standard dose cyclosporine increases the risk of nephrotoxicity resulting in a lower glomerular filtration rate. Reduced doses of cyclosporine are required for use in combination with everolimus in order to reduce renal dysfunction. [*See Boxed Warning, Indications and Usage (1.2), Clinical Pharmacology (12.6)*] Renal function should be monitored during the administration of everolimus in combination with cyclosporine. Consider switching to other immunosuppressive therapies if renal function does not improve after dose adjustments or if the dysfunction is thought to be drug related. Caution should be exercised when using other drugs which are known to impair renal function.

5.9 Proteinuria

The use of everolimus with cyclosporine in transplant patients has been associated with increased proteinuria. The risk of proteinuria increased with higher everolimus whole blood trough concentrations. Patients receiving everolimus should be monitored for proteinuria. [*See Adverse Reactions (6.2)*]

5.10 Polyoma Virus Infections

Patients receiving immunosuppressants, including everolimus, are at increased risk for opportunistic infections; including polyoma virus infections. [*See Boxed Warning*] BK virus-associated nephropathy (BKVAN) has been observed in patients receiving everolimus. BKVAN is associated with serious outcomes; including deteriorating renal function and renal graft loss. [*See Adverse Reactions (6.2)*] Patient monitoring may help detect patients at risk for BK virus-associated nephropathy. Reductions in immunosuppression should be considered for patients who develop evidence of BK virus-associated nephropathy.

5.11 Interaction with Strong Inhibitors and Inducers of CYP3A4

Co-administration with strong CYP3A4-inhibitors (e.g., ketoconazole, itraconazole, voriconazole, clarithromycin, telithromycin, ritonavir) and strong inducers (e.g., rifampin, rifabutin) is not recommended without close monitoring of everolimus whole blood trough concentrations. [*See Drug Interactions (7)*]

5.12 Non-Infectious Pneumonitis

A diagnosis of non-infectious pneumonitis should be considered in patients presenting with symptoms consistent with infectious pneumonia or radiologic changes in whom infectious, neoplastic and other non-drug causes have been ruled out through appropriate investigations. Fatal cases have been reported. Non-infectious pneumonitis may respond to drug interruption with or without glucocorticoid therapy. [*See Adverse Reactions (6.2)*]

5.13 Thrombotic Microangiopathy/Thrombotic Thrombocytopenic Purpura/Hemolytic Uremic Syndrome (TMA/TTP/HUS)

The concomitant use of everolimus with cyclosporine may increase the risk of thrombotic microangiopathy/thrombotic thrombocytopenic purpura/hemolytic uremic syndrome. Monitor hematologic parameters. [*See Adverse Reactions (6.2)*]

5.14 New Onset Diabetes After Transplant

Everolimus has been shown to increase the risk of new onset diabetes mellitus after transplant. Blood glucose concentrations should be monitored closely in patients using everolimus.

5.15 Male Infertility

Azospermia or oligospermia may be observed. [*See Adverse Reactions (6.3) and Carcinogenesis, Mutagenesis, Impairment of Fertility (13.1)*] Everolimus is an anti-proliferative drug and affects rapidly dividing cells like the germ cells.

5.16 Immunizations

The use of live vaccines should be avoided during treatment with everolimus; examples include (not limited to) the following: intranasal influenza, measles, mumps, rubella, oral polio, BCG, yellow fever, varicella, and TY21a typhoid vaccines.

5.17 Interaction with Grapefruit Juice

Grapefruit and grapefruit juice inhibit cytochrome P450 3A4 and P-gp activity and should therefore be avoided with concomitant use of everolimus and cyclosporine.

5.18 Patients with Hereditary Disorders/Other

Patients with rare hereditary problems of galactose intolerance, the Lapp lactase deficiency or glucose-galactose malabsorption should not take everolimus as this may result in diarrhea and malabsorption.

6 ADVERSE REACTIONS

6.1 Serious and Otherwise Important Adverse Reactions

The following adverse reactions are discussed in greater detail in other sections of the label.

- Hypersensitivity reactions [*See Contraindications (4.1)*]
- Lymphomas and Other Malignancies [*See Boxed Warning, Warnings and Precautions (5.2)*]
- Serious Infections [*See Warnings and Precautions (5.3)*]
- Angioedema [*See Warnings and Precautions (5.4)*]
- Graft Thrombosis [*See Warnings and Precautions (5.5)*]
- Wound Healing and Fluid Accumulation [*See Warnings and Precautions (5.6)*]
- Hyperlipidemia [*See Warnings and Precautions (5.7)*]
- Nephrotoxicity [*See Warnings and Precautions (5.8)*]
- Proteinuria [*See Warnings and Precautions (5.9)*]
- Polyoma Virus Infections [*See Warnings and Precautions (5.10)*]
- Non-infectious Pneumonitis [*See Warnings and Precautions (5.12)*]

- Thrombotic Microangiopathy/Thrombotic Thrombocytopenic Purpura/Hemolytic Uremic Syndrome (TMA/TTP/HUS) [See Warnings and Precautions (5.13)]
- New Onset Diabetes After Transplant [See Warnings and Precautions (5.14)]
- Male Infertility [See Warnings and Precautions (5.15)]

6.2   Clinical Studies Experience

Because clinical trials are conducted under widely varying conditions, the adverse reaction rates observed cannot be directly compared to rates in other trials and may not reflect the rates observed in clinical practice.

The data described below reflect exposure to everolimus in an open-label, randomized trial of de novo kidney transplant patients of concentration-controlled everolimus at an initial starting dose of 1.5 mg per day [target trough concentrations 3 to 8 ng/mL with reduced doses of cyclosporine (n=274) compared to mycophenolic acid (n=273) with standard doses of cyclosporine]. All patients received basiliximab induction therapy and corticosteroids. The population was between 18 and 70 years; more than 43% were 50 years of age or older, 63% of all recipients were male and 64% were Caucasian. Demographic characteristics were comparable between treatment groups. The most frequent diseases leading to transplantation were balanced between groups and included hypertension/nephrosclerosis, glomerulonephritis/glomerular disease and diabetes mellitus.

Adverse reactions were systematically collected in this trial. In this clinical trial, significantly more patients discontinued everolimus 1.5 mg/day treatment (83/277, 30%) than discontinued the control regimen (60/277, 22%). Of those patients who prematurely discontinued treatment, most discontinuations were due to adverse reactions: 18% in the everolimus group compared to 9% in the control group (p-value = 0.004). This difference was more prominent between treatment groups among female patients. In those patients discontinuing study medication, adverse reactions were collected up to 7 days after study medication discontinuation and serious adverse reactions up to 30 days after study medication discontinuation.

Discontinuation of everolimus at a higher dose (3 mg/day) was 95/279, 34%, including 20% due to adverse reactions, and this regimen is not recommended (see below).

The overall incidences of serious adverse events were 57% (159/278) in the everolimus group and 52% (141/273) in the mycophenolic acid group. Infections and infestations reported as serious adverse reactions had the highest incidence in both groups [20% (54/274) in the everolimus group and 25% (69/273) in the control group]. The difference was mainly due to the higher incidence of viral infections in the Myfortic group, mainly CMV and BK virus infections. Injury, poisoning and procedural complications reported as serious adverse reactions had the second highest incidence in both groups [14% (39/274) in the everolimus group and 12% (32/273) in the control group] followed by renal and urinary disorders [10% (28/274) in the everolimus group and 13% (36/273) in the control group] and vascular disorders [10% (26/274) in the everolimus group and 7% (20/273) in the control group].

A total of 13 patients died during the first 12 months of study; 7 (3%) in the everolimus group and 6 (2%) in the control group. The most common causes of death across the study groups were related to cardiac conditions and infections.

There were 12 (4%) graft losses in the everolimus group and 8 (3%) in the control group over the 12 month study period. Of the graft losses, 4 were due to renal artery and two due to renal vein thrombosis in the everolimus group (2%) compared to two renal artery thromboses in the control group (1%). [See Boxed Warning and Warnings and Precautions (5.5)]

The most common (≥20%) adverse reactions observed in the everolimus group were: peripheral edema, constipation, hypertension, nausea, anemia, urinary tract infection, and hyperlipidemia.

Infections

The overall incidence of bacterial, fungal and viral infections reported as adverse reactions was higher in the control group (68%) compared to the everolimus group (64%) and was primarily due to an increased number of viral infections (21% in the control group and 10% in the everolimus group). The incidence of cytomegalovirus (CMV) infections reported as adverse reactions was 8% in the control group compared to 1% in the everolimus group; and 3% of the serious CMV infections in the control group versus 0% in the everolimus group were considered serious. [See Warnings and Precautions (5.3)]

BK Virus

BK virus infections were lower in incidence in the everolimus group (2 patients, 1%) compared to the control group (11 patients, 4%). One of the two BK virus infections in the everolimus group and two of the 11 BK virus infections in the control group were also reported as serious adverse events. BK virus infections did not result in graft loss in any of the groups in the clinical trial.

Table 1
Incidence Rates of Frequent (≥10% in Any Treatment Group) Adverse Reactions by Primary System Organ Class and Preferred Term

Primary System Organ Class Preferred Term	Zortress (everolimus) 1.5 mg With reduced dose cyclosporine N=274/n (%)	Myfortic (mycophenolic acid) 1.44 g With standard dose cyclosporine N=273/n (%)
Any Adverse Events*	271 (99)	270 (99)
Blood lymphatic system disorders	93 (34)	111 (41)
Anemia	70 (26)	68 (25)
Leukopenia	8 (3)	33 (12)
Gastrointestinal disorders	196 (72)	207 (76)
Constipation	105 (38)	117 (43)
Nausea	79 (29)	85 (31)
Diarrhea	51 (19)	54 (20)
Vomiting	40 (15)	60 (22)
Abdominal pain	36 (13)	42 (15)
Dyspepsia	12 (4)	31 (11)
Abdominal pain upper	9 (3)	30 (11)
General disorders and administrative site conditions	181 (66)	160 (59)
Edema peripheral	123 (45)	108 (40)
Pyrexia	51 (19)	40 (15)
Fatigue	25 (9)	28 (10)
Infections and infestations	169 (62)	185 (68)
Urinary tract infection	60 (22)	63 (23)
Upper respiratory tract infection	44 (16)	49 (18)
Injury, poisoning and procedural complications	163 (60)	163 (60)
Incision site pain	45 (16)	47 (17)
Procedural pain	40 (15)	37 (14)
Investigations	137 (50)	133 (49)
Blood creatinine increased	48 (18)	59 (22)
Metabolism and nutrition disorders	222 (81)	199 (73)
Hyperlipidemia	57 (21)	43 (16)
Hyperkalemia	49 (18)	48 (18)
Hypercholesterolemia	47 (17)	34 (13)
Dyslipidemia	41 (15)	24 (9)
Hypomagnesemia	37 (14)	40 (15)
Hypophosphatemia	35 (13)	35 (13)
Hyperglycemia	34 (12)	38 (14)
Hypokalemia	32 (12)	32 (12)
Musculoskeletal and connective tissue disorders	112 (41)	105 (39)
Pain in extremity	32 (12)	29 (11)
Back pain	30 (11)	28 (10)
Nervous system disorders	92 (34)	109 (40)
Headache	49 (18)	40 (15)
Tremor	23 (8)	38 (14)
Psychiatric disorders	90 (33)	72 (26)
Insomnia	47 (17)	43 (16)
Renal and urinary disorders	112 (41)	124 (45)
Hematuria	33 (12)	33 (12)
Dysuria	29 (11)	28 (10)
Respiratory, thoracic and mediastinal disorders	86 (31)	93 (34)
Cough	20 (7)	30 (11)
Vascular disorders	122 (45)	124 (45)
Hypertension	81 (30)	82 (30)

*As reported in the safety analysis population defined as all randomized patients who received at least one dose of treatment and had at least one post-baseline safety assessment.

Wound Healing and Fluid Collections

Wound healing-related reactions were identified through a retrospective search and request for additional data. The overall incidence of wound-related events, including lymphocele, seroma, hematoma, dehiscence, incisional hernia, and infections was 35% in the everolimus group compared to 26% in the control group. More patients required intraoperative repair debridement or drainage of incisional wound complications and more required drainage of lymphoceles and seromas in the everolimus group compared to control.

Adverse reactions due to major fluid collections such as edema and other types of fluid collections was 45% in the everolimus group and 40% in the control group. [See Warnings and Precautions (5.6)]

Neoplasms

Adverse events due to malignant and benign neoplasms were reported in 3% of patients in the everolimus group and 6% in the control group. The most frequently reported neoplasms in the control group were basal cell carcinoma, squamous cell carcinoma, skin papilloma and seborrhoeic keratosis. One patient in the everolimus group who underwent a melanoma excision prior to transplantation died due to metastatic melanoma. [See Boxed Warning and Warnings and Precautions (5.2)]

New Onset Diabetes Mellitus (NODM)

NODM reported based on adverse reactions and random serum glucose values, was 9% in the everolimus group compared to 7% in the control group.

Endocrine Effects in Males

In the everolimus group, serum testosterone levels significantly decreased while the FSH levels significantly increased without significant changes being observed in the control group. In both the everolimus and the control groups mean testosterone and FSH levels remained within the normal range with the mean FSH level in the everolimus group being at the upper limit of the normal range (11.1 U/L). More patients were reported with erectile dysfunction in the everolimus treatment group compared to the control group (5% compared to 2%, respectively).

Table 1 compares the incidence of treatment-emergent adverse reactions reported with an incidence of ≥10% for patients receiving everolimus with reduced dose cyclosporine or mycophenolic acid with standard dose cyclosporine. Within each MedDRA system organ class, the adverse reactions are presented in order of decreasing frequency.

[See table 1 above]

Adverse events that occurred with at least a 5% higher frequency in the everolimus 1.5 mg group compared to the control group were: peripheral edema (45% compared to 40%), hyperlipidemia (21% compared to 16%), dyslipidemia (15% compared to 9%), and stomatitis/mouth ulceration (8% compared to 3%).

A third treatment group of everolimus 3.0 mg per day (1.5 mg twice daily; target trough concentrations 6 to 12 ng/mL) with reduced-dose cyclosporine was included in the study described above. Although as effective as the lower dose everolimus group, the overall safety was worse and consequently higher doses of everolimus cannot be recommended. Out of 279 patients, 95 (34%) discontinued the study medication with 57 (20%) doing so because of adverse reactions. The most frequent adverse reactions leading to discontinuation of everolimus when used at this higher dose were injury, poisoning and procedural complications (everolimus 1.5 mg: 5%, everolimus 3.0 mg: 7%, and control: 2%), infections (2%, 6%, and 3%, respectively), renal and urinary disorders (4%, 7%, and 4%, respectively) and gastrointestinal disorders (1%, 3%, and 2%).

Less common adverse reactions, occurring in ≥1% to <10% of patients treated with everolimus include:

Blood and Lymphatic System Disorders: leukocytosis, leucopenia, lymphadenopathy, thrombocythemia, thrombocytopenia

Cardiac and Vascular Disorders: angina pectoris, atrial fibrillation, cardiac failure congestive, palpitations, tachycardia, hypertension including hypertensive crisis, hypotension, deep vein thrombosis

Endocrine Disorders: Cushingoid, hyperparathyroidism

Eye Disorders: cataract, conjunctivitis, vision blurred

Gastrointestinal Disorders: abdominal pain, abdominal distention, dyspepsia, dysphagia, epigastric discomfort, flatulence, gastroesophageal reflux disease, gingival hypertrophy, hematemesis, hemorrhoids, ileus, mouth ulceration, peritonitis, stomatitis

General Disorders and Administrative Site Conditions: chest discomfort, chest pain, chills, fatigue, malaise, edema including generalized edema

Hepatobiliary Disorders: hepatic enzyme increased, bilirubin increased

Infections and Infestations: BK virus infection [See Warnings and Precautions (5.10)], bacteremia, bronchitis, candidiasis, cellulitis, folliculitis, gastroenteritis, influenza, nasopharyngitis, onychomycosis, oral candidiasis, osteomyelitis, pneumonia, pyelonephritis, sinusitis, tinea pedis, urethritis, wound infection, herpes infections [See Boxed Warning and Warnings and Precautions (5.2)]

Injury Poisoning and Procedural Complications: incision site complications including infections, perinephric collection, seroma, wound dehiscence, incisional hernia, perinephric hematoma, localized intraabdominal fluid collection, impaired healing, lymophocele, lymphorrhea

Metabolism and Nutrition Disorders: blood urea increased, acidosis, anorexia, dehydration, diabetes mellitus [See Warnings and Precautions (5.14)], fluid retention, gout, hypercalcemia, hypercholesterolemia [See Warnings and Precautions (5.7)], hyperphosphatemia, hypertriglyceridemia, hyperuricemia, hypocalcemia, hypoglycemia, hyponatremia, iron deficiency, vitamin B12 deficiency

Musculoskeletal and Connective Tissues Disorders: arthralgia, joint swelling, muscle spasms, muscular weakness, musculoskeletal pain, myalgia, osteonecrosis, osteopenia, osteoporosis, spondylitis

Nervous System Disorders: dizziness, hemiparesis, hypoaesthesia, paresthesia, somnolence, syncope, tremor

Psychiatric Disorders: agitation, anxiety, depression, hallucination

Renal and Urinary Disorders: bladder spasm, hydronephrosis, micturition urgency, nephritis interstitial, pollakiuria, polyuria, proteinuria [See Warnings and Precautions (5.9)], pyuria, renal artery thrombosis [See Boxed Warning and Warnings and Precautions (5.5)], acute renal failure, renal impairment [See Warnings and Precautions (5.8)], urinary retention

Reproductive System and Breast Disorders: erectile dysfunction, ovarian cyst, scrotal edema

Respiratory, Thoracic, Mediastinal Disorders: atelectasis, cough, dyspnea, epistaxis, nasal congestion, pleural effusions, pulmonary edema, rhinorrhea, sinus congestion, wheezing

Skin and Subcutaneous Tissue Disorders: alopecia, dermatitis acneiform, hirsutism, hyperhydrosis, hypertrichosis, night sweats, pruritus, rash

Less common, serious adverse reactions include:
- Non-infectious Pneumonitis [See Warnings and Precautions (5.12) and Adverse Reactions (6.2)]
- Thrombotic Microangiopathy (TMA), Thrombotic Thrombocytopenic Purpura (TTP), and Hemolytic Uremic Syndrome (HUS) [See Warnings and Precautions (5.13)]

The combination of fixed dose everolimus and standard doses cyclosporine in previous clinical trials resulted in frequent elevations of serum creatinine with higher mean and median serum creatinine values was observed than in the current study with reduced doses of cyclosporine. These results indicate that everolimus increases the cyclosporine-induced nephrotoxicity; and therefore should only be used in a concentration-controlled regimen with reduced doses of cyclosporine. [See Boxed Warnings, Indications and Usage (1.2) and Warnings and Precautions (5.8)]

6.3 Post Marketing Experience

Adverse reactions identified from the post-marketing use of the combination regimen of everolimus and cyclosporine that are not specific to any one transplant indication include angioedema [See Warnings and Precautions (5.4)] and pancreatitis. There have also been reports of male infertility with mTOR inhibitors including everolimus. [See Warnings and Precautions (5.15)]

7 DRUG INTERACTIONS

7.1 Interactions with Strong Inhibitors or Inducers of CYP3A4 and P-glycoprotein

Everolimus is mainly metabolized by CYP3A4 in the liver and to some extent in the intestinal wall and is a substrate for the multidrug efflux pump, P-glycoprotein. Therefore, absorption and subsequent elimination of systemically absorbed everolimus may be influenced by medicinal products that affect CYP3A4 and/or P-glycoprotein. Concurrent treatment with strong inhibitors (e.g., ketoconazole, itraconazole, voriconazole, clarithromycin, telithromycin, ritonavir) and inducers (e.g., rifampin, rifabutin) of CYP3A4 is not recommended. Inhibitors of P-glycoprotein (e.g., digoxin, cyclosporine) may decrease the efflux of everolimus from intestinal cells and increase everolimus blood concentrations. In vitro, everolimus was a competitive inhibitor of CYP3A4 and of CYP2D6, potentially increasing the concentrations of medicinal products eliminated by these enzymes. Thus, caution should be exercised when co-administering everolimus with CYP3A4 and CYP2D6 substrates with a narrow therapeutic index. [See Therapeutic Drug Monitoring (2.2)]

All in vivo interaction studies were conducted without concomitant cyclosporine. Pharmacokinetic interactions between everolimus and concomitantly administered drugs are discussed below. Drug interaction studies have not been conducted with drugs other than those described below.

7.2 Cyclosporine (CYP3A4/P-gp Inhibitor and CYP3A4 Substrate)

The steady-state C_{max} and AUC estimates of everolimus were significantly increased by co-administration of single dose cyclosporine. [See Clinical Pharmacology (12.3)] Dose adjustment of everolimus might be needed if the cyclosporine dose is altered. [See Dosage and Administration (2.3)] Everolimus had a clinically minor influence on cyclosporine pharmacokinetics in transplant patients receiving cyclosporine (Neoral).

7.3 Ketoconazole (Strong CYP3A4 Inhibitor)

Multiple-dose ketoconazole administration to healthy volunteers significantly increased single dose estimates of everolimus C_{max}, AUC, and half-life. It is recommended that strong inhibitors of CYP3A4 (e.g., ketoconazole, itraconazole, voriconazole, clarithromycin, telithromycin, ritonavir) not be co-administered with everolimus. [See Warnings and Precautions (5.11), and Clinical Pharmacology (12.3)]

7.4 Erythromycin (Moderate CYP3A4 Inhibitor)

Multiple-dose erythromycin administration to healthy volunteers significantly increased single dose estimates of everolimus C_{max}, AUC, and half-life. If erythromycin is co-administered, everolimus blood concentrations should be monitored and a dose adjustment made as necessary. [See Clinical Pharmacology (12.3)]

7.5 Verapamil (CYP3A4 and P-gp Substrate)

Multiple-dose verapamil administration to healthy volunteers significantly increased single dose estimates of everolimus C_{max} and AUC. Everolimus half-life was not changed. If verapamil is co-administered, everolimus blood concentrations should be monitored and a dose adjustment made as necessary. [See Clinical Pharmacology (12.3)]

7.6 Atorvastatin (CYP3A4 Substrate) and Pravastatin (P-gp Substrate)

Single-dose administration of everolimus with either atorvastatin or pravastatin to healthy subjects did not influence the pharmacokinetics of atorvastatin, pravastatin and everolimus, as well as total HMG-CoA reductase bioreactivity in plasma to a clinically relevant extent. However, these results cannot be extrapolated to other HMG-CoA reductase inhibitors. Patients should be monitored for the development of rhabdomyolysis and other adverse events as described in the respective labeling for these products.

7.7 Simvastatin and Lovastatin

Due to an interaction with cyclosporine, clinical studies of everolimus with cyclosporine conducted in kidney transplant patients strongly discouraged patients with receiving HMG-CoA reductase inhibitors such as simvastatin and lovastatin. [See Warnings and Precautions (5.7)]

7.8 Rifampin (Strong CYP3A4) Inducers

Pre-treatment of healthy subjects with multiple-dose rifampin followed by a single dose of everolimus increased everolimus clearance and decreased the everolimus C_{max} and AUC estimates. Combination with rifampin is not recommended. [See Warnings and Precautions (5.1) and Clinical Pharmacology (12.3)]

7.9 Other Possible Interactions

Moderate inhibitors of CYP3A4 and P-gp may increase everolimus blood concentrations (e.g., fluconazole; macrolide antibiotics; nicardipine, diltiazem; nelfinavir, indinavir, amprenavir). Inducers of CYP3A4 may increase the metabolism of everolimus and decrease everolimus blood concentrations (e.g., St. John's Wort [Hypericum perforatum]; anticonvulsants: carbamazepine, phenobarbital, phenytoin; efavirenz, nevirapine).

8 USE IN SPECIFIC POPULATIONS

8.1 Pregnancy

Pregnancy Category C

There are no adequate and well-controlled studies of everolimus in pregnant women. In rats and rabbits, everolimus crossed the placenta and was toxic to the conceptus. The potential risk for humans is unknown. Everolimus should be given to pregnant women only if the potential benefit to the mother justifies the potential risk to the fetus. Women of childbearing potential should be advised to use effective contraception methods while they are receiving everolimus and up to 8 weeks after treatment has been stopped.

Everolimus administered daily to pregnant rats by oral gavage at 0.1 mg/kg from before mating through organogenesis resulted in increased preimplantation loss and early resorptions of fetal implants. AUCs in rats at this dose were approximately one-third those in humans administered the starting dose (0.75 mg twice daily). Everolimus administered daily by oral gavage at 0.8 mg/kg to pregnant rabbits during organogenesis resulted in increased late resorptions of fetal implants. At this dose, AUCs in rabbits were slightly less than the AUCs in humans administered the starting clinical dose.

8.3 Nursing Mothers

It is not known whether everolimus is excreted in human milk. Everolimus and/or its metabolites readily transferred into milk of lactating rats at a concentration 3.5 times higher than in maternal serum. Because many drugs are excreted in human milk and because of the potential for serious adverse reactions in nursing infants from everolimus, women should avoid breast-feeding during treatment with Zortress.

8.4 Pediatric Use

The safe and effective use of Zortress in kidney transplant patients younger than 18 years of age has not been established. [See Clinical Pharmacology (12.4)]

8.5 Geriatric Use

There is limited clinical experience on the use of Zortress in patients of age 65 or older. There is no evidence to suggest that elderly patients will require a different dosage recommendation from younger adult patients. [See Clinical Pharmacology (12.4)]

8.6 Hepatic Impairment

No dosage adjustment is needed for patients with mild hepatic impairment (Child-Pugh Class A). In patients with moderate hepatic impairment (Child-Pugh Class B), the daily dose needs to be reduced by one-half recommended initial daily dose. There is no information on the effects of severe hepatic impairment (Child-Pugh Class C) on everolimus pharmacokinetics. [See Clinical Pharmacology (12.3)]

8.7 Renal Impairment

No dose adjustment is needed in patients with renal impairment. [See Clinical Pharmacology (12.3)]

10 OVERDOSAGE

Reported experience with overdose in humans is very limited. There is a single case of an accidental ingestion of 1.5 mg everolimus in a two-year-old child where no adverse reactions were observed. Single doses up to 25 mg have been administered to transplant patients with acceptable acute tolerability. Single doses up to 70 mg (without cyclosporine) have been given with acceptable acute tolerability. General supportive measures should be followed in all cases of overdose. Everolimus is not considered dialyzable to any relevant degree (<10% of everolimus removed within 6 hours of hemodialysis). In animal studies, everolimus showed a low acute toxic potential. No lethality or severe toxicity was observed after single oral doses of 2000 mg/kg (limit test) in either mice or rats.

11 DESCRIPTION

Zortress (everolimus) is a macrolide immunosuppressant. The chemical name of everolimus is (1R, 9S, 12S, 15R, 16E, 18R, 19R, 21R, 23S, 24E, 26E, 28E, 30S, 32S, 35R)-1, 18-dihydroxy-12-[(1R)-2-[(1S,3R,4R)-4-(2-hydroxyethoxy)-3-methoxycyclohexyl]-1-methylethyl-19,30-dimethoxy-15, 17, 21, 23, 29, 35-hexamethyl-11, 36-dioxa-4-aza-tricyclo[30.3.1.0^{4,9}] hexatriaconta-16,24,26,28-tetraene-2,3,10,14,20-pentaone.

The molecular formula is $C_{53}H_{83}NO_{14}$ and the molecular weight is 958.25. The structural formula is

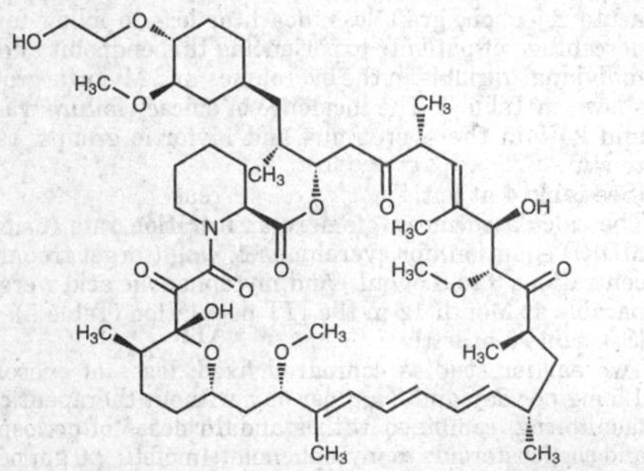

Everolimus is supplied as tablets for oral administration containing 0.25 mg, 0.5 mg and 0.75 mg of everolimus together with butylated hydroxytoluene, magnesium stearate, lactose monohydrate, hypromellose, crospovidone and lactose anhydrous as inactive ingredients.

12 CLINICAL PHARMACOLOGY

12.1 Mechanism of Action

Everolimus inhibits antigenic and interleukin (IL-2 and IL-15) stimulated activation and proliferation of T and B lymphocytes.

In cells, everolimus binds to a cytoplasmic protein, the FK506 Binding Protein-12 (FKBP-12), to form an immunosuppressive complex (everolimus: FKBP-12) that binds to and inhibits the mammalian Target Of Rapamycin (mTOR), a key regulatory kinase. In the presence of everolimus phosphorylation of p70 S6 ribosomal protein kinase (p70S6K), a substrate of mTOR, is inhibited. Consequently, phosphorylation of the ribosomal S6 protein and subsequent protein synthesis and cell proliferation are inhibited. The everolimus:FKBP-12 complex has no effect on calcineurin activity.

In rats and non-human primate models, everolimus effectively reduces kidney allograft rejection resulting in prolonged graft survival.

12.3 Pharmacokinetics

Everolimus pharmacokinetics have been characterized after oral administration of single and multiple doses to adult kidney transplant patients, hepatically-impaired patients, and healthy subjects.

Absorption

After oral dosing, peak everolimus concentrations occur 1 to 2 h post dose. Over the dose range of 0.5 mg to 2 mg twice daily, everolimus C_{max} and AUC are dose proportional in transplant patients at steady-state.

Food Effect

In 24 healthy subjects, a high-fat breakfast (44.5 g fat) reduced everolimus C_{max} by 60%, delayed t_{max} by a median 1.3 hours, and reduced AUC by 16% compared with a fasting administration. To minimize variability, everolimus should be taken consistently with or without food. [*See Dosage and Administration (2.4)*]

Distribution

The blood-to-plasma ratio of everolimus is concentration dependent ranging from 17% to 73% over the range of 5 ng/mL to 5000 ng/mL. Plasma protein binding is approximately 74% in healthy subjects and in patients with moderate hepatic impairment. The apparent distribution volume associated with the terminal phase (Vz/F) from a single-dose pharmacokinetic study in maintenance kidney transplant patients is 342 to 107 L (range 128 to 589 L).

Metabolism

Everolimus is a substrate of CYP3A4 and P-glycoprotein. The main metabolic pathways identified in man were monohydroxylations and O-dealkylations. Two main metabolites were formed by hydrolysis of the cyclic lactone. Everolimus was the main circulating component in blood. None of the main metabolites contribute significantly to the immunosuppressive activity of everolimus.

Excretion

After a single dose of radiolabeled everolimus was given to transplant patients receiving cyclosporine, the majority (80%) of radioactivity was recovered from the feces and only a minor amount (5%) was excreted in urine. Parent drug was not detected in urine and feces.

Pharmacokinetics in Kidney Transplant Patients

Steady-state is reached by Day 4 with an accumulation in blood levels of 2- to 3-fold compared with the exposure after the first dose.

[See table 2 above]

Table 2
Pharmacokinetic Parameters (mean +/- SD)
Following the Administration of 0.75 mg Twice Daily

C_{max}	T_{max}	AUC	CL/F[1]	Vc/F[1]	Half-life ($T_{1/2}$)
11.1 + 4.6 ng/mL	1-2 h	75 + 31 ng.h/mL	8.8 L/h	110 L	30 ± 11 h

[1] population pharmacokinetic analysis

The half-life estimates from 12 maintenance renal transplant patients who received single doses of everolimus capsules at 0.75 mg or 2.5 mg with their maintenance cyclosporine regimen indicate that the pharmacokinetics of everolimus are linear over the clinically-relevant dose range. Results indicate the half-life of everolimus in maintenance renal transplant patients receiving single doses of 0.75 mg or 2.5 mg everolimus during steady-state cyclosporine treatment was 30 ± 11 hours (range 19 to 53 hours).

Drug-Drug Interactions

Everolimus is known to be a substrate for both cytochrome CYP3A4 and P-gp. The pharmacokinetic interaction between everolimus and concomitantly administered drugs is discussed below. Drug interaction studies have not been conducted with drugs other than those described below. [*See Warnings and Precautions (5.11), and Drug Interactions (7)*]

Cyclosporine (CYP3A4/P-gp Inhibitor and CYP3A4 Substrate): Everolimus should be taken concomitantly with cyclosporine. Everolimus concentrations may decrease when doses of cyclosporine are reduced, unless the everolimus dose is increased. [*See Dosage and Administration (2.1), Drug Interactions (7.1)*]

In a single-dose study in healthy subjects, cyclosporine (Neoral) administered at a dose of 175 mg increased everolimus AUC by 168% (range, 46% to 365%) and C_{max} by 82% (range, 25% to 158%) when administered with 2 mg everolimus compared with administration of everolimus alone. [*See Drug Interactions (7.2)*]

Ketoconazole *(Strong CYP3A4 Inhibitor):* Multiple-dose administration of 200 mg ketoconazole twice daily for 5 days to 12 healthy volunteers significantly increased everolimus C_{max}, AUC, and half-life by 3.9-fold, 15-fold, and 89%, respectively, when co-administered with 2 mg everolimus. It is recommended that strong inhibitors of CYP3A4 (e.g., ketoconazole, itraconazole, voriconazole, clarithromycin, telithromycin, ritonavir) not be co-administered with everolimus. [*See Warnings and Precautions (5.11) and Drug Interactions (7.3)*]

Erythromycin *(Moderate CYP3A4 Inhibitor):* Multiple-dose administration of 500 mg erythromycin three times daily for 5 days to 16 healthy volunteers significantly increased everolimus C_{max}, AUC, and half-life by 2.0-fold, 4.4-fold, and 39%, respectively, when co-administered with 2 mg everolimus. If erythromycin is co-administered, everolimus blood concentrations should be monitored and a dose adjustment made as necessary. [*See Drug Interactions (7.4)*]

Verapamil *(CYP3A4 Inhibitor and P-gp Substrate):* Multiple-dose administration of 80 mg verapamil three times daily for 5 days to 16 healthy volunteers significantly increased everolimus C_{max} and AUC by 2.3-fold and 3.5-fold, respectively, when co-administered with 2 mg everolimus. Everolimus half-life was not changed. If verapamil is co-administered, everolimus blood concentrations should be monitored and a dose adjustment made as necessary. [*See Drug Interactions (7.5)*]

Atorvastatin *(CYP3A4 Substrate) and* ***Pravastatin*** *(P-gp Substrate):* Following administration of a single dose of 2 mg everolimus to 12 healthy subjects, the concomitant administration of a single oral dose administration of atorvastatin 20 mg or pravastatin 20 mg only slightly decreased everolimus C_{max} and AUC by 9% and 10%, respectively. There was no apparent change in the mean $T_{1/2}$ or median T_{max}. In the same study, the concomitant everolimus dose slightly increased the mean C_{max} of atorvastatin by 11% and slightly decreased the AUC by 7%. The concomitant everolimus dose decreased the mean C_{max} and AUC of pravastatin by 10% and 5%, respectively. No dosage adjustments are needed for concomitant administration of everolimus and atorvastatin and pravastatin. [*See Drug Interactions (7.6)*]

Rifampin *(Strong CYP3A4/P-gp Inducer):* Pre-treatment of 12 healthy subjects with multiple-dose rifampin (600 mg once-daily for 8 days) followed by a single dose of 4 mg everolimus increased everolimus clearance nearly 3-fold, and decreased C_{max} by 58% and AUC by 63%. Combination with rifampin is not recommended. [*See Drug Interactions (7.7)*]

Special Populations

Hepatic Impairment

Everolimus AUC was increased an average 2-fold in 8 patients with moderate hepatic impairment (Child-Pugh Class B) compared with 8 healthy subjects. AUC was positively correlated with serum bilirubin concentration and with prolongation in prothrombin time and negatively correlated with serum albumin concentration. The AUC of everolimus tended to be greater than that of healthy subjects if bilirubin was >34 µmol/L, prothrombin time was >1.3 INR >4 sec prolongation, and/or albumin concentration was <35 g/L. The impact of severe hepatic impairment (Child-Pugh Class C) on everolimus pharmacokinetics has not been assessed but the effect on everolimus AUC is likely to be as large or larger compared with moderate impairment. [*See Dosage and Administration (2.5)*] No dosing adjustment is needed for patients with mild hepatic impairment. In patients with moderate hepatic impairment (Child-Pugh Class B), the daily dose needs to be reduced by one-half the recommended initial daily dose and blood concentrations should be monitored to make further adjustments as needed.

Renal Impairment

No pharmacokinetic studies in patients with renal impairment were conducted. Post-transplant renal function (creatinine clearance range 11 to 107 mL/min) did not affect the pharmacokinetics of everolimus, therefore, no dosage adjustments are needed in patients with renal impairment.

Pediatrics

The safety and efficacy of everolimus have not been established in pediatric patients.

Geriatrics

A limited reduction in everolimus oral CL of 0.33% per year was estimated in adults (age range studied was 16 to 70 years). There is no evidence to suggest that elderly patients will require a different dosage recommendation from younger adult patients.

Race

Based on analysis of population pharmacokinetics, oral clearance (CL/F) is, on average, 20% higher in Black transplant patients.

12.5 Everolimus Whole Blood Concentrations Observed in Kidney Transplant Patients

Based on exposure-efficacy and exposure-safety analyses of clinical trials, kidney transplant patients achieving everolimus whole blood trough concentrations ≥3.0 ng/mL have been found to have a lower incidence of treated biopsy-proven acute rejection compared with patients whose trough concentrations were below 3.0 ng/mL. Patients who attained everolimus trough concentrations within the range of 6 to 12 ng/mL had similar efficacy and more adverse events than patients who attained lower trough concentrations between 3 to 8 ng/mL. [*See Dosage and Administration (2.2)*]

In the clinical trial [*See Clinical Studies (14.1)*], everolimus whole blood trough concentrations were measured at Days 3, 7, and 14 and Months 1, 2, 3, 4, 6, 7, 9, and 12. The proportion of patients receiving 0.75 mg twice daily everolimus treatment regimen who had everolimus whole blood trough concentrations within the protocol specified target range of 3 to 8 ng/mL at Days 3, 7, and 14 were 55%, 71% and 69%, respectively. Approximately 80% of patients had everolimus whole blood trough concentrations within the 3 to 8 ng/mL target range by Month 1 and remained stable within range through Month 12. The median everolimus trough concentration for the 0.75 mg twice daily treatment group was between 3 and 8 ng/mL throughout the study duration.

12.6 Cyclosporine Concentrations Observed in Kidney Transplant Patients

In the clinical trial [*See Clinical Studies (14.1)*], the target cyclosporine whole blood trough concentration for the everolimus treatment arm of 0.75 mg twice daily were 100 to 200 ng/mL through Month 1 post-transplant, 75 to 150 ng/mL at Months 2 and 3 post-transplant, 50 to 100 ng/mL at Month 4 post-transplant, and 25 to 50 ng/mL from Month 6 through Month 12 post-transplant. Table 3 below provides a summary of the observed cyclosporine whole blood trough concentrations during the study.

[See table 3 at top of next page]

13 NONCLINICAL TOXICOLOGY

13.1 Carcinogenesis, Mutagenesis, Impairment of Fertility

Everolimus was not carcinogenic in mice or rats when administered daily by oral gavage for 2 years at doses of 0.9 mg/kg. In these studies, AUCs in mice were much higher (at least 20 times) than those in humans receiving 0.75 mg twice daily, and AUCs in rats were in the same range as those in humans receiving 0.75 mg twice daily.

Everolimus was not mutagenic in the bacterial reverse mutation, the mouse lymphoma thymidine kinase assay, or the chromosome aberration assay using V79 Chinese hamster cells, or *in vivo* following two daily doses of 500 mg/kg in the mouse micronucleus assay.

In a 13-week male fertility oral gavage study in rats, testicular morphology was affected at 0.5 mg/kg and above, and

Table 3
Cyclosporine Trough Concentrations Over 12 Months – Renal Study A2309 Median Values (ng/mL)
with 10th and 90th Percentiles

Treatment group	Visit	N	Target (ng/mL)	Median	10th Percentile	90th Percentile
Everolimus 0.75 mg twice daily	Day 3	242	100-200	172	46	388
	Day 7	265	100-200	185	75	337
	Day 14	243	100-200	182	97	309
	Month 1	245	100-200	161	85	274
	Month 2	232	75-150	140	84	213
	Month 3	220	75-150	111	68	187
	Month 4	208	50-100	99	56	156
	Month 6	200	25-50	75	43	142
	Month 7	199	25-50	59	36	117
	Month 9	194	25-50	49	28	91
	Month 12	186	25-50	46	25	100

Table 4
Efficacy Failure by Treatment Group (ITT Population) at 12 Months

	Zortress (everolimus) 1.5 mg/day With reduced dose CsA N=277 n (%)	Mycophenolic Acid 1.44 gm/day With standard dose CsA N=277 n (%)
Efficacy Endpoints[3]		
Primary Efficacy Failure Endpoint[1]	70 (25.3)	67 (24.2)
Treated Biopsy Proven Acute Rejection	45 (16.2)	47 (17.0)
Death	7 (2.5)	6 (2.2)
Graft Loss	12 (4.3)	9 (3.2)
Loss to Follow-up	12 (4.3)	9 (3.2)
Graft Loss or Death or Loss to Follow-up[2]	32 (11.6)	26 (9.4)
Graft Loss or Death	18 (6.5)	15 (5.4)
Loss to Follow-up[2]	14 (5.1)	11 (4.0)

[1] Includes treated BPAR, graft loss, death or loss to follow-up by Month 12 where loss to follow-up represents patient who did not experience treated BPAR, graft loss or death and whose last contact date is prior to 12 month visit
[2] Loss to follow-up (for Graft Loss, Death, or Loss to Follow-up) represents patient who did not experience death or graft loss and whose last contact date is prior to 12 month visit
[3] The difference in rates (everolimus – mycophenolic acid) with 95% CI for primary efficacy failure endpoint is 1.1% (-6.1%, 8.3%); and for the graft loss, death or loss to follow-up endpoint is 2.2% (-2.9%, 7.3%).

Table 5
Calculated Glomerular Filtration Rates (mL/min/1.73m^2)
by MDRD At 12 Months Post-Transplant*

Month 12 GFR (MDRD)	Zortress (everolimus) 1.5 mg/day with reduced dose CsA n=276	Mycophenolic Acid 1.44 gm/day with standard dose CsA n=277
Mean (SD)**	54.6 (21.7)	52.3 (26.5)
Median (Range)	55.0 (0-140.9)	50.1 (0.0-366.4)

* Analysis based on using a subject's last observation carried forward for missing data at 12 months due to death or lost to follow-up data, a value of zero is used for subjects who experienced a graft loss.
**SD=standard deviation

sperm motility, sperm head count and plasma testosterone concentrations were diminished at 5 mg/kg which caused a decrease in male fertility. There was evidence of reversibility of these findings in animals examined after 13 weeks post-dosing. The 0.5 mg/kg dose in male rats resulted in AUCs in the range of clinical exposures, and the 5 mg/kg dose resulted in AUCs approximately 5 times the AUCs in humans receiving 0.75 mg twice daily. Everolimus did not affect female fertility in nonclinical studies, but everolimus crossed the placenta and was toxic to the conceptus. [See Pregnancy (8.1)]

14 CLINICAL STUDIES
14.1 Prevention of Organ Rejection after Renal Transplantation
A 24-month, multi-national, open-label, randomized (1:1:1) trial was conducted comparing two concentration-controlled everolimus regimens of 1.5 mg per day starting dose (targeting 3 to 8 ng/mL) and 3.0 mg per day starting dose (targeting 6 to 12 ng/mL) with reduced doses of cyclosporine and corticosteroids, to 1.44 gm per day of mycophenolic acid with standard doses of cyclosporine and corticosteroids. The mean cyclosporine starting dose was 5.2, 5.0 and 5.7 mg/kg body weight/day in the everolimus 1.5 mg, 3.0 mg and in mycophenolic acid groups, respectively. The cyclosporine dose in the everolimus group was then adjusted to the blood trough concentration ranges indicated in Table 3, whereas

in the Myfortic group the target ranges were 200-300 ng/mL starting Day 5: 200-300 ng/mL, and 100-250 ng/mL from Month 2 to Month 12.
All patients received basiliximab induction therapy. The study population consisted of 18 to 70 year old male and female low to moderate risk renal transplant recipients undergoing their first transplant. Low to moderate immunologic risk was defined in the study as an ABO blood type compatible first organ or tissue transplant recipient with anti-HLA Class I PRA <20% by a complement dependant cytotoxicity-based assay, or <50% by a flow cytometry or ELISA-based assay, and with a negative T-cell cross match. Eight hundred thirty-three (833) patients were randomized after transplantation; 277 randomized to the everolimus 1.5 mg per day group, 279 to the everolimus 3.0 mg per day group and 277 to the Myfortic 1.44 gm per day group. The study was conducted at 79 renal transplant centers across Europe, South Africa, North and South America, and Asia-Pacific. There were no major baseline differences between treatment groups with regard to recipient or donor disease characteristics. The majority of transplant recipients in all groups (70% to 76%) had three or more HLA mismatches; mean percentage of panel reactive antibodies ranged from 1% to 2%. The rate of premature treatment discontinuation at 12 months was 30% and 22% in the everolimus 1.5 mg and Myfortic groups, respectively, (p=0.03, Fisher's exact test) and was more prominent between groups among

female patients. Results at 12 months indicated that everolimus 1.5 mg per day is comparable to Myfortic with respect to efficacy failure, defined as treated biopsy-proven acute rejection, graft loss, death or loss to follow-up. The percentage of patients experiencing this endpoint and each individual variable in the everolimus and Myfortic groups is shown in Table 4. The incidence of efficacy failure was 25% and 24% in the everolimus and Myfortic groups, respectively.
[See table 4 at left]
The calculated mean glomerular filtration rate (using the MDRD equation) for everolimus 1.5 mg (target trough concentrations 3 to 8 ng/mL) and mycophenolic acid were comparable at Month 12 in the ITT population (Table 5).
[See table 5 at left]
Two earlier studies compared fixed doses of everolimus 1.5 mg per day and 3 mg per day, without therapeutic drug monitoring, combined with standard doses of cyclosporine and corticosteroids to mycophenolate mofetil 2.0 gm per day and corticosteroids. Antilymphocyte antibody induction was prohibited in both studies. Both were multicenter, double-blind (for first 12 months), randomized trials (1:1:1) of 588 and 583 de novo renal transplant patients, respectively. The 12 month analysis of GFR showed increased rates of renal impairment in both the everolimus groups compared to the mycophenolate mofetil group in both studies. Therefore, reduced doses of cyclosporine should be used in combination with everolimus in order to avoid renal dysfunction and everolimus trough concentrations should be adjusted using therapeutic drug monitoring to maintain trough concentrations between 3 to 8 ng/mL. [See Boxed Warning, Dosage and Administration (2.3) and Warnings and Precautions (5.8)]

16 HOW SUPPLIED/STORAGE AND HANDLING
Zortress (everolimus) Tablets are packed in child-resistant blisters.
[See table at top of next page]
Each strength is available in boxes of 60 tablets (6 blister strips of 10 tablets each).
Storage
Store at 25°C (77°F); excursions permitted to 15-30°C (59-86°F). [see USP Controlled Room Temperature] Protect from light and moisture.

17 PATIENT COUNSELING INFORMATION
17.1 Administration
Inform patients that Zortress should be taken orally twice a day approximately 12 hours apart consistently either with or without food.
Inform patients to avoid grapefruit and grapefruit juice which increase blood drug concentrations of Zortress. [See Warnings and Precautions (5.17)]
Advise patients that Zortress should be used concurrently with reduced doses of cyclosporine and that any change of cyclosporine dose should be made under physician supervision and may also require a change in the dosage of Zortress.
Inform patients of the necessity of repeated laboratory tests according to physician recommendations while they are taking Zortress.

17.2 Development of Lymphomas and Other Malignancies
Inform patients they are at risk of developing lymphomas and other malignancies, particularly of the skin, due to immunosuppression. Advise patients to limit exposure to sunlight and ultraviolet (UV) light by wearing protective clothing and using a sunscreen with a high protection factor. [See Warnings and Precautions (5.2)]

17.3 Increased Risk of Infection
Inform patients they are at increased risk of developing a variety of infections, including opportunistic infections, due to immunosuppression. Advise patients to contact their physician if they develop any symptoms of infection. [See Warnings and Precautions (5.3, 5.10)]

17.4 Nephrotoxicity
Advise patients of the risks of impaired kidney function with the combination of Zortress and cyclosporine as well as the need for routine blood concentration monitoring for both drugs. Advise patients of the importance of serum creatinine monitoring. [See Boxed Warning and Warnings and Precautions (5.8)]

17.5 Graft Thrombosis
Inform patients that Zortress has been associated with an increased risk of kidney arterial and venous thrombosis, resulting in graft loss, usually within the first 30 days post-transplantation. [See Boxed Warning and Warnings and Precautions (5.5)]

17.6 Pregnancy
Advise women of childbearing age to avoid becoming pregnant throughout treatment and for 8 weeks after Zortress therapy has stopped.

17.7 Angioedema
Inform patients of the risk of angioedema and that concomitant use of angiotensin converting enzyme (ACE) inhibitors may increase this risk. Advise patients to seek prompt medical attention if symptoms occur. [See Warnings and Precautions (5.4)]

17.8 Wound Healing Complications and Fluid Accumulation

Inform patients the use of Zortress has been associated with impaired or delayed wound healing, fluid accumulation and the need for careful observation of their incision site. [*See Warnings and Precautions (5.6)*]

17.9 Hyperlipidemia

Inform patients the use of Zortress has been associated with increased serum cholesterol and triglycerides that may require treatment and the need for monitoring of blood lipid concentrations. [*See Warnings and Precautions (5.7)*]

17.10 Proteinuria

Inform patients the use of Zortress has been associated with an increased risk of proteinuria. [*See Warnings and Precautions (5.9)*]

17.11 Medications that Interfere with Zortress

Some medications can increase or decrease blood concentrations of Zortress. Advise patients to inform their physician if they are taking any of the following: antifungals, antibiotics, anti-epileptic medicines including carbamazepine, phenytoin and barbiturates, herbal/dietary supplements (St. John's Wort), and/or rifampin. [*See Warnings and Precautions (5.11)*]

17.12 Non-Infectious Pneumonitis

Inform patients the use of Zortress may increase the risk of non-infectious pneumonitis. Advise patients to seek medical attention if they develop clinical symptoms consistent with pneumonia. [*See Warnings and Precautions (5.12)*]

17.13 New Onset Diabetes

Inform patients the use of Zortress may increase the risk of diabetes mellitus and to contact their physician if they develop symptoms. [*See Warnings and Precautions (5.14)*]

17.14 Immunizations

Inform patients that vaccinations may be less effective while they are being treated with Zortress. Advise patients live vaccines should be avoided. [*See Warnings and Precautions (5.16)*]

17.15 Patient with Hereditary Disorders

Advise patients to inform their physicians that if they have hereditary disorders of galactose intolerance (Lapp-lactase deficiency or glucose-galactose malabsorption) not to take Zortress. [*See Warnings and Precautions (5.18)*]

MARCH 2010   T2010-25

MEDICATION GUIDE
ZORTRESS (ZOR-tres) Tablets
(everolimus)

Read this Medication Guide before you start using ZORTRESS and each time you get a refill. There may be new information. This information does not take the place of talking with your doctor about your medical condition or treatment.

What is the most important information I should know about ZORTRESS?

ZORTRESS can cause serious side effects, including:

- **Increased risk of getting certain cancers.** People who take ZORTRESS have a higher chance of getting lymphoma and other cancers, especially skin cancer. Talk to your doctor about your risk for cancer.
- **Increased risk of serious infections.** ZORTRESS weakens the body's immune system and affects your ability to fight infections. Serious infections can happen with ZORTRESS that may lead to death. People taking ZORTRESS have a higher chance of getting infections caused by viruses, bacteria, and fungi (yeast).
  - Call your doctor if you have symptoms of infection including fever or chills.
- **Serious problems with your transplanted kidney (nephrotoxicity).** You will need to start with a lower dose of cyclosporine.
- **Blood clot in the blood vessels of your transplanted kidney.** If this happens, it usually occurs within the first 30 days after your kidney transplant. Tell your doctor right away if you:
  - have pain in your groin, lower back, side or stomach (abdomen)
  - make less urine or you do not pass any urine
  - have blood in your urine or dark colored urine (tea-colored)
  - have fever, nausea, or vomiting

See the section "What are the possible side effects of ZORTRESS?" for information about other serious side effects.

What Is ZORTRESS?

ZORTRESS is a prescription medicine used to prevent transplant rejection (antirejection medicine) in people who have received a kidney transplant. Transplant rejection happens when the body's immune system perceives the new transplanted kidney as "foreign" and attacks it.

ZORTRESS is used with other medicines called cyclosporine, corticosteroids and certain other transplant medicines to prevent rejection of your transplanted kidney.

It is not known if ZORTRESS is safe and effective in children.

Description of Zortress (everolimus) Tablets			
Dosage Strength	0.25 mg	0.5 mg	0.75 mg
Appearance	White to yellowish, marbled, round, flat tablets with beveled edge		
Imprint	"C" on one side and "NVR" on the other	"CH" on one side and "NVR" on the other	"CL" on one side and "NVR" on the other
NDC Number	0078-0417-20	0078-0414-20	0078-0415-20

Who should not take ZORTRESS?

Do not take ZORTRESS if you are allergic to:
- everolimus (AFINITOR®) or any of the ingredients in ZORTRESS. See the end of this Medication Guide for a complete list of ingredients in ZORTRESS.
- sirolimus (Rapamune®)

What should I tell my doctor before taking ZORTRESS?

Before taking ZORTRESS, tell your doctor if you:
- have liver problems
- have skin cancer or it runs in your family
- have high cholesterol or triglycerides (fat in your blood)
- have Lapp lactase deficiency or glucose-galactose malabsorption. You should not take ZORTRESS if you have this disorder.
- have any other medical conditions
- are pregnant or plan to become pregnant. It is not known if ZORTRESS will harm your unborn baby. Talk with your doctor if you are pregnant or plan to become pregnant.
  - Women who may become pregnant should use effective birth control (contraception) while taking ZORTRESS and for 8 weeks after stopping ZORTRESS.
- are breastfeeding or plan to breastfeed. It is not known if ZORTRESS passes into your breast milk. You and your doctor should decide if you will take ZORTRESS or breastfeed. You should not do both.

Tell your doctor about all the medicines you take, including prescription and non-prescription medicines, vitamins, and herbal supplements. ZORTRESS may affect the way other medicines work, and other medicines may affect how ZORTRESS works.

Especially tell your doctor if you take:
- antifungal medicine
- antibiotic medicine
- heart medicine
- high blood pressure medicine
- a medicine to lower cholesterol or triglycerides
- cyclosporine (Sandimmune, Gengraf, Neoral)
- tuberculosis (TB) medicine
- HIV medicine
- St. John's Wort
- seizure (anticonvulsant) medicine

Know the medicines you take. Keep a list of them to show your doctor and pharmacist when you get a new medicine. Do not take any new medicine without talking with your doctor first.

How should I take ZORTRESS?

- Take ZORTRESS exactly as your doctor tells you.
- **Do not** stop taking ZORTRESS or change your dose unless your doctor tells you to.
- Take ZORTRESS at the same time as your dose of cyclosporine medicine. **Do not** stop taking or change your dose of cyclosporine medicine unless your doctor tells you to.
- Take ZORTRESS 2 times a day about 12 hours apart.
- Swallow ZORTRESS tablets whole with a glass of water. Do not crush or chew ZORTRESS tablets.
- Take ZORTRESS tablets with or without food. If you take ZORTRESS tablets **with food**, always take ZORTRESS tablets **with food.** If you take ZORTRESS tablets **without food**, always take ZORTRESS tablets **without food.**
- **Your doctor will do regular blood tests to check your kidney function while you take ZORTRESS. It is important that you get these tests done when your doctor tells you to. Blood tests will monitor how your kidneys are working and make sure you are getting the right dose of ZORTRESS.**
- If you take too much ZORTRESS, call your doctor or go to the nearest hospital emergency room right away.

What should I avoid while taking ZORTRESS?

- Avoid receiving any live vaccines while taking ZORTRESS. Some vaccines may not work as well while you are taking ZORTRESS.
- Do not eat grapefruit or drink grapefruit juice while you are taking ZORTRESS. Grapefruit may change your blood level of ZORTRESS.
- Limit the amount of time you spend in the sunlight. Avoid using tanning beds or sunlamps. People who take ZORTRESS have a higher risk of getting skin cancer. See the section "What is the most important information I should know about ZORTRESS?" Wear protective clothing when you are in the sun and use a sunscreen with a high

protection factor (SPF 30 and above). This is especially important if you have fair skin or if you have a family history of skin cancer.
- Avoid becoming pregnant. See the section "What should I tell my doctor before taking ZORTRESS?"

What are possible side effects of ZORTRESS?

ZORTRESS can cause serious side effects, including:
- See **"What is the most important information I should know about ZORTRESS?"**
- **swelling under your skin especially around your mouth, eyes and in your throat (angioedema).** Your chance of having swelling under your skin is higher if you take ZORTRESS along with certain other medicines. Tell your doctor right away or go to the nearest emergency room if you have any of these symptoms of angioedema:
  - sudden swelling of your face, mouth, throat, tongue or hands
  - hives or welts
  - itchy or painful swollen skin
  - trouble breathing
- **delayed wound healing.** ZORTRESS can cause your incision to heal slowly or not heal well. Call your doctor right away if you have any of the following symptoms:
  - your incision is red, warm or painful
  - blood, fluid, or pus in your incision
  - your incision opens up
  - swelling of your incision
- **increased cholesterol and triglycerides (fat in your blood).** If your cholesterol and triglyceride levels are high, your doctor may want to lower them with diet, exercise and certain medicines.
- **change in kidney function.** ZORTRESS may cause kidney problems when taken along with a standard dose of cyclosporine medicine instead of a lower dose.
- **protein in your urine (proteinuria). Your doctor should do blood and urine tests to monitor your cholesterol, triglycerides and kidney function.**
- **viral infections.** Certain viruses can live in your body and cause active infections when your immune system is weak. Viral infections that can happen with ZORTRESS include BK virus-associated nephropathy. BK virus can affect how your kidney works and cause your transplanted kidney to fail.
- **lung or breathing problems.** Tell your doctor right away if you have new or worsening cough, shortness of breath, difficulty breathing or wheezing. In some patients lung or breathing problems have been severe, and can even lead to death. Your doctor may need to stop ZORTRESS or lower your dose.
- **blood clotting problems.**
- **diabetes.** Tell your doctor if you have frequent urination, increased thirst or hunger.
- **male infertility (low or no sperm count).**

The most common side effects of ZORTRESS include:
- swelling of the lower legs, ankles and feet
- constipation
- nausea
- high blood pressure
- low red blood cell count (anemia)
- urinary tract infection
- increased fat in the blood (cholesterol and triglycerides)

These are not all of the possible side effects of ZORTRESS. Tell your doctor about any side effect that bothers you or that does not go away.

Call your doctor for medical advice about side effects. You may report side effects to the FDA at 1-800-FDA-1088.

How do I store ZORTRESS?
- Store ZORTRESS tablets between 59°F to 86°F (15°C to 30°C).
- Keep ZORTRESS out of the light.
- Keep ZORTRESS tablets dry.

Keep ZORTRESS and all medicines out of the reach of children.

General information about the safe and effective use of ZORTRESS

Medicines are sometimes prescribed for purposes other than those listed in a Medication Guide. Do not use ZORTRESS for a condition for which it was not prescribed. Do not give ZORTRESS to other people, even if they have the same symptoms you have. It may harm them.

This Medication Guide summarizes the most important information about ZORTRESS. For more information, talk with your doctor. You can ask your doctor or pharmacist for information about ZORTRESS that is written for healthcare professionals. For more information, call 1-888-669-6682 or visit www.zortress.com.

What are the ingredients in ZORTRESS?
Active ingredient: everolimus
Inactive ingredients: butylated hydroxytoluene, magnesium stearate, lactose monohydrate, hypromellose, crospovidone and lactose anhydrous.
This Medication Guide has been approved by the U.S. Food and Drug Administration.
Any other trademarks in this document are the property of their respective owners.

T2010-26

MARCH 2010   Printed in U.S.A.   T2010-25/T2010-26
                                    5001535

Manufactured by:
Novartis Pharma Stein AG
Stein, Switzerland
Distributed by:
Novartis Pharmaceuticals Corporation
East Hanover, New Jersey 07936
©Novartis
Rapamune® is a registered trademark of Pfizer Inc
Gengraf® is a registered trademark of Abbott Laboratories
Shown in Product Identification Guide, page 316

Novo Nordisk Inc.
100 COLLEGE ROAD WEST
PRINCETON, NJ 08540

Direct Inquiries to:
Novo Nordisk Inc.
(800) 727-6500
8:30 AM - 6 PM EST M–F
In Emergencies after hours and weekends:
609-987-5800

LEVEMIR®
[lev'e-mīr]
(insulin detemir [rDNA origin] injection)   R

DESCRIPTION
LEVEMIR® (insulin detemir [rDNA origin] injection) is a sterile solution of insulin detemir for use as an injection. Insulin detemir is a long-acting basal insulin analog, with up to 24 hours duration of action, produced by a process that includes expression of recombinant DNA in *Saccharomyces cerevisiae* followed by chemical modification.
Insulin detemir differs from human insulin in that the amino acid threonine in position B30 has been omitted, and a C14 fatty acid chain has been attached to the amino acid B29. Insulin detemir has a molecular formula of $C_{267}H_{402}O_{76}N_{64}S_6$ and a molecular weight of 5916.9. It has the following structure:
[See chemical structure above]
LEVEMIR is a clear, colorless, aqueous, neutral sterile solution. Each milliliter of LEVEMIR contains 100 U (14.2 mg/mL) insulin detemir, 65.4 mcg zinc, 2.06 mg m-cresol, 16.0 mg glycerol, 1.80 mg phenol, 0.89 mg disodium phosphate dihydrate, 1.17 mg sodium chloride, and water for injection. Hydrochloric acid and/or sodium hydroxide may be added to adjust pH. LEVEMIR has a pH of approximately 7.4.

CLINICAL PHARMACOLOGY
Mechanism of Action
The primary activity of insulin detemir is the regulation of glucose metabolism. Insulins, including insulin detemir, exert their specific action through binding to insulin receptors. Receptor-bound insulin lowers blood glucose by facilitating cellular uptake of glucose into skeletal muscle and fat and by inhibiting the output of glucose from the liver. Insulin inhibits lipolysis in the adipocyte, inhibits proteolysis, and enhances protein synthesis.
Pharmacodynamics
Insulin detemir is a soluble, long-acting basal human insulin analog with a relatively flat action profile. The mean duration of action of insulin detemir ranged from 5.7 hours at the lowest dose to 23.2 hours at the highest dose (sampling period 24 hours).
The prolonged action of LEVEMIR is mediated by the slow systemic absorption of insulin detemir molecules from the injection site due to strong self-association of the drug molecules and albumin binding. Insulin detemir is distributed more slowly to peripheral target tissues since insulin detemir in the bloodstream is highly bound to albumin.
Figure 1 shows glucose infusion rate results from a glucose clamp study in patients with type 1 diabetes.

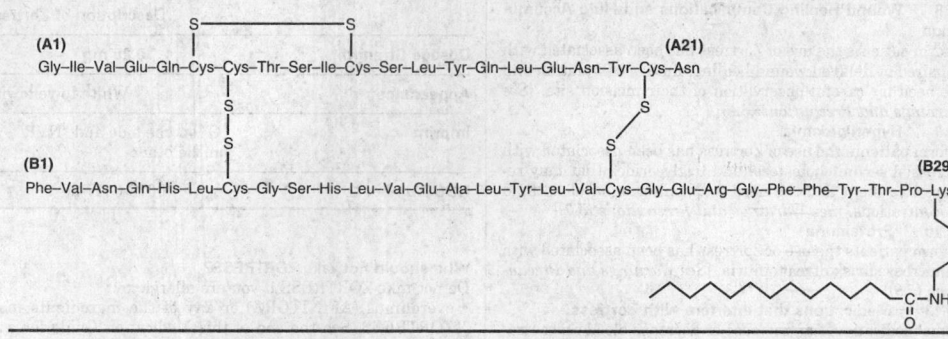

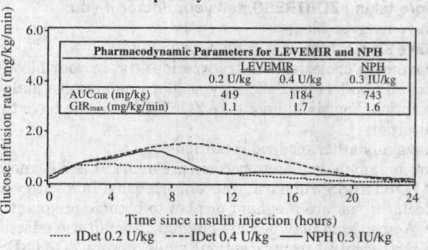

Figure 1: Activity Profiles in Patients with Type 1 Diabetes in a 24-hour Glucose Clamp Study

Pharmacodynamic Parameters for LEVEMIR and NPH			
	LEVEMIR		NPH
	0.2 U/kg	0.4 U/kg	0.3 IU/kg
AUC$_{GIR}$ (mg/kg)	419	1184	743
GIR$_{max}$ (mg/kg/min)	1.1	1.7	1.6

----- IDet 0.2 U/kg ----IDet 0.4 U/kg —— NPH 0.3 IU/kg

Figure 2 shows glucose infusion rate results from a 16-hour glucose clamp study in patients with type 2 diabetes. The clamp study was terminated at 16 hours according to protocol.

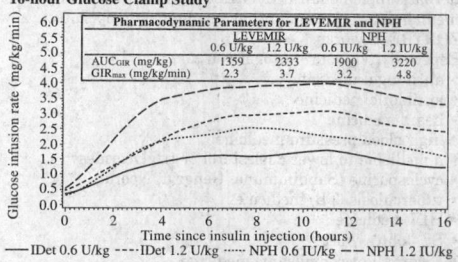

Figure 2: Activity Profiles in Patients with Type 2 Diabetes in a 16-hour Glucose Clamp Study

Pharmacodynamic Parameters for LEVEMIR and NPH			
	LEVEMIR		NPH	
	0.6 U/kg	1.2 U/kg	0.6 U/kg	1.2 IU/kg
AUC$_{GIR}$ (mg/kg)	1359	2333	1900	3220
GIR$_{max}$ (mg/kg/min)	3.0	3.9	3.2	4.8

—— IDet 0.6 U/kg --- IDet 1.2 U/kg ···· NPH 0.6 U/kg — — NPH 1.2 IU/kg

For doses in the interval of 0.2 to 0.4 U/kg, LEVEMIR exerts more than 50% of its maximum effect from 3 to 4 hours up to approximately 14 hours after dose administration.
In a glucose clamp study, the overall glucodynamic effect (AUC$_{GIR\ 0-24h}$) [mean mg/kg ± SD (CV)] of four separate subcutaneous injections in the thigh was 1702.6 ± 489 mg/kg (29%) in the LEVEMIR group and 1922.8 ± 765 mg/kg (40%) for NPH. The clinical significance of this difference has not been established.
Pharmacokinetics
Absorption
After subcutaneous injection of insulin detemir in healthy subjects and in patients with diabetes, insulin detemir serum concentrations indicated a slower, more prolonged absorption over 24 hours in comparison to NPH human insulin.
Maximum serum concentration (C$_{max}$) is reached between 6 and 8 hours after administration.
The absolute bioavailability of insulin detemir is approximately 60%.
Distribution and Elimination
More than 98% insulin detemir in the bloodstream is bound to albumin. LEVEMIR has a small apparent volume of distribution of approximately 0.1 L/kg. LEVEMIR, after subcutaneous administration, has a terminal half-life of 5 to 7 hours depending on dose.
Special Populations
Children and Adolescents-The pharmacokinetic properties of LEVEMIR were investigated in children (6 to 12 years) and adolescents (13 to 17 years) and adults with type 1 diabetes. Similar to NPH human insulin, slightly higher plasma Area Under the Curve (AUC) and C$_{max}$ were observed in children by 10% and 24%, respectively, compared to adolescents and adults. There was no difference in pharmacokinetics between adolescents and adults.
Geriatrics-In a clinical trial investigating differences in pharmacokinetics of a single subcutaneous dose of LEVEMIR in young (25 to 35 years) versus elderly (≥68 years) healthy subjects, higher insulin AUC levels (up to

35%) were found in elderly subjects due to a reduced clearance. As with other insulin preparations, LEVEMIR should always be titrated according to individual requirements.
Gender-In controlled clinical trials, no clinically relevant difference between genders is seen in pharmacokinetic parameters based on subgroup analyses.
Race-In two trials in healthy Japanese and Caucasian subjects, there were no clinically relevant differences seen in pharmacokinetic parameters. Pharmacokinetics and pharmacodynamics of LEVEMIR were investigated in a clamp trial comparing patients with type 2 diabetes of Caucasian, African-American, and Latino origin. Dose-response relationships were comparable for LEVEMIR in these three populations.
Renal impairment-Individuals with renal impairment showed no difference in pharmacokinetic parameters as compared to healthy volunteers. However, literature reports have shown that clearance of human insulin is decreased in renally impaired patients. Careful glucose monitoring and dose adjustments of insulin, including LEVEMIR, may be necessary in patients with renal dysfunction (see PRECAUTIONS, Renal Impairment).
Hepatic impairment-Individuals with severe hepatic dysfunction, without diabetes, were observed to have lower AUCs as compared to healthy volunteers. Careful glucose monitoring and dose adjustments of insulin, including LEVEMIR, may be necessary in patients with hepatic dysfunction (see PRECAUTIONS, Hepatic Impairment).
Pregnancy-The effect of pregnancy on the pharmacokinetics and pharmacodynamics of LEVEMIR has not been studied (see PRECAUTIONS, Pregnancy).
Smoking-The effect of smoking on the pharmacokinetics and pharmacodynamics of LEVEMIR has not been studied.

CLINICAL STUDIES
The efficacy and safety of LEVEMIR given once-daily at bedtime or twice-daily (before breakfast and at bedtime, before breakfast and with the evening meal, or at 12-hour intervals) was compared to that of once-daily or twice-daily NPH human insulin or once-daily insulin glargine in non-blinded, randomized, parallel studies of 6004 patients with diabetes (3724 with type 1, and 2280 with type 2). In general, patients treated with LEVEMIR achieved levels of glycemic control similar to those treated with NPH human insulin or insulin glargine, as measured by glycosylated hemoglobin (HbA$_{1c}$).
Type 1 Diabetes – Adult
In one non-blinded clinical study (Study A, n=409), adult patients with type 1 diabetes were randomized to treatment with either LEVEMIR at 12-hour intervals, LEVEMIR morning and bedtime or NPH human insulin morning and bedtime. Insulin aspart was also administered before each meal. At 16 weeks of treatment, the combined LEVEMIR-treated patients had similar HbA$_{1c}$ and fasting plasma glucose (FPG) reductions to NPH-treated patients (Table 1). Differences in timing of LEVEMIR administration (or flexible dosing) had no effect on HbA$_{1c}$, FPG, body weight, or risk of having hypoglycemic episodes.
Overall glycemic control achieved with LEVEMIR was compared to that achieved with insulin glargine in a randomized, non-blinded, clinical study (Study B, n=320) in which patients with type 1 diabetes were treated for 26 weeks with either twice-daily (morning and bedtime) LEVEMIR or once-daily (bedtime) insulin glargine. Insulin aspart was administered before each meal. LEVEMIR-treated patients had a decrease in HbA$_{1c}$ similar to that of insulin glargine-treated patients.
In a randomized, controlled clinical study (Study C, n=749), patients with type 1 diabetes were treated with once-daily (bedtime) LEVEMIR or NPH human insulin, both in combination with human soluble insulin before each meal for 6 months. LEVEMIR and NPH human insulin had a similar effect on HbA$_{1c}$.

Table 1: Efficacy and Insulin Dosage in Type 1 Diabetes Mellitus - Adult

	Study A	
Treatment duration	16 weeks	
Treatment in combination with	NovoLog® (insulin aspart)	
	LEVEMIR	NPH
Number of subjects treated	276	133
HbA$_{1c}$ (%)		
Baseline	8.64	8.51
End of study adjusted mean	7.76	7.94
Mean change from baseline	-0.82	-0.60
Fasting Plasma Glucose (mg/dL)		
End of study adjusted mean	168	202
Mean change from baseline	-42.48	-10.80
Daily Basal Insulin Dose (U/kg)		
Prestudy mean	0.36	0.39
End of study mean	0.49	0.45
Daily Bolus Insulin Dose (U/kg)		
Prestudy mean	0.40	0.40
End of study mean	0.38	0.38

Baseline values were included as covariates in an ANCOVA analysis.

Type 1 Diabetes - Pediatric

In a non-blinded, randomized, controlled clinical study (Study D, n=347), pediatric patients (age range 6 to 17) with type 1 diabetes were treated for 26 weeks with a basal-bolus insulin regimen. LEVEMIR and NPH human insulin were administered once- or twice-daily (bedtime or morning and bedtime) according to pretrial dose regimen. Bolus insulin aspart was administered before each meal. LEVEMIR-treated patients had a decrease in HbA$_{1c}$ similar to that of NPH human insulin.

Table 2: Efficacy and Insulin Dosage in Type 1 Diabetes Mellitus - Pediatric

	Study D	
Treatment duration	26 weeks	
Treatment in combination with	NovoLog® (insulin aspart)	
	LEVEMIR	NPH
Number of subjects treated	232	115
HbA$_{1c}$ (%)		
Baseline	8.75	8.77
End of study adjusted mean	8.02	7.93
Mean change from baseline	-0.72	-0.80
Fasting Plasma Glucose (mg/dL)		
End of study adjusted mean	151.92	172.44
Mean change from baseline	-45.00	-19.98
Daily Basal Insulin Dose (U/kg)		
Prestudy mean	0.48	0.49
End of study mean	0.67	0.64
Daily Bolus Insulin Dose (U/kg)		
Prestudy mean	0.52	0.47
End of study mean	0.52	0.51

Type 2 Diabetes – Adult

In a 24-week, non-blinded, randomized, clinical study (Study E, n=476), LEVEMIR administered twice-daily (before breakfast and evening) was compared to a similar regimen of NPH human insulin as part of a regimen of combination therapy with one or two of the following oral antidiabetes agents (metformin, insulin secretagogue, or α–glucosidase inhibitor). LEVEMIR and NPH similarly lowered HbA$_{1c}$ from baseline (Table 3).

Table 3: Efficacy and Insulin Dosage in Type 2 Diabetes Mellitus

	Study E	
Treatment duration	24 weeks	
Treatment in combination with	OAD	
	LEVEMIR	NPH
Number of subjects treated	237	239
HbA$_{1c}$ (%)		
Baseline	8.61	8.51
End of study adjusted mean	6.58	6.46
Mean change from baseline	-1.84	-1.90
Proportion achieving HbA$_{1c}$ ≤7%	70%	74%
Fasting Plasma Glucose (mg/dL)		
End of study adjusted mean	119.16	113.40
Mean change from baseline	-75.96	-74.34
Daily Insulin Dose (U/kg)		
End of study mean	0.77	0.52

In a 22-week, non-blinded, randomized, clinical study (Study F, n=395) in adults with Type 2 diabetes, LEVEMIR and NPH human insulin were given once- or twice-daily as part of a basal-bolus regimen. As measured by HbA$_{1c}$ or FPG, LEVEMIR had efficacy similar to NPH human insulin.

INDICATIONS AND USAGE

LEVEMIR is indicated for once- or twice-daily subcutaneous administration for the treatment of adult and pediatric patients with type 1 diabetes mellitus or adult patients with type 2 diabetes mellitus who require basal (long acting) insulin for the control of hyperglycemia.

CONTRAINDICATIONS

LEVEMIR is contraindicated in patients hypersensitive to insulin detemir or one of its excipients.

WARNINGS

Hypoglycemia is the most common adverse effect of insulin therapy, including LEVEMIR. As with all insulins, the timing of hypoglycemia may differ among various insulin formulations.
Glucose monitoring is recommended for all patients with diabetes.
LEVEMIR is not to be used in insulin infusion pumps.
Any change of insulin dose should be made cautiously and only under medical supervision. Changes in insulin strength, timing of dosing, manufacturer, type (e.g., regular, NPH, or insulin analogs), species (animal, human), or method of manufacture (rDNA versus animal-source insulin) may result in the need for a change in dosage. Concomitant oral antidiabetic treatment may need to be adjusted.
Needles and Levemir FlexPen must not be shared.

PRECAUTIONS
General

Inadequate dosing or discontinuation of treatment may lead to hyperglycemia and, in patients with type 1 diabetes, diabetic ketoacidosis. The first symptoms of hyperglycemia usually occur gradually over a period of hours or days. They include nausea, vomiting, drowsiness, flushed dry skin, dry mouth, increased urination, thirst and loss of appetite as well as acetone breath. Untreated hyperglycemic events are potentially fatal.

LEVEMIR is not intended for intravenous or intramuscular administration. The prolonged duration of activity of insulin detemir is dependent on injection into subcutaneous tissue. Intravenous administration of the usual subcutaneous dose could result in severe hypoglycemia. Absorption after intramuscular administration is both faster and more extensive than absorption after subcutaneous administration.
LEVEMIR should not be diluted or mixed with any other insulin preparations (see PRECAUTIONS, Mixing of Insulins).
Insulin may cause sodium retention and edema, particularly if previously poor metabolic control is improved by intensified insulin therapy.
Lipodystrophy and hypersensitivity are among potential clinical adverse effects associated with the use of all insulins.
As with all insulin preparations, the time course of LEVEMIR action may vary in different individuals or at different times in the same individual and is dependent on site of injection, blood supply, temperature, and physical activity.
Adjustment of dosage of any insulin may be necessary if patients change their physical activity or their usual meal plan.
Hypoglycemia
As with all insulin preparations, hypoglycemic reactions may be associated with the administration of LEVEMIR. Hypoglycemia is the most common adverse effect of insulins. Early warning symptoms of hypoglycemia may be different or less pronounced under certain conditions, such as long duration of diabetes, diabetic nerve disease, use of medications such as beta-blockers, or intensified diabetes control (see PRECAUTIONS, Drug Interactions). Such situations may result in severe hypoglycemia (and, possibly, loss of consciousness) prior to patients' awareness of hypoglycemia.
The time of occurrence of hypoglycemia depends on the action profile of the insulins used and may, therefore, change when the treatment regimen or timing of dosing is changed. In patients being switched from other intermediate or long-acting insulin preparations to once- or twice-daily LEVEMIR, dosages can be prescribed on a unit-to-unit basis; however, as with all insulin preparations, dose and timing of administration may need to be adjusted to reduce the risk of hypoglycemia (see DOSAGE AND ADMINISTRATION, Changeover to LEVEMIR).
Renal Impairment
As with other insulins, the requirements for LEVEMIR may need to be adjusted in patients with renal impairment (see CLINICAL PHARMACOLOGY, Pharmacokinetics).
Hepatic Impairment
As with other insulins, the requirements for LEVEMIR may need to be adjusted in patients with hepatic impairment (see CLINICAL PHARMACOLOGY, Pharmacokinetics).
Injection Site and Allergic Reactions
As with any insulin therapy, lipodystrophy may occur at the injection site and delay insulin absorption. Other injection site reactions with insulin therapy may include redness, pain, itching, hives, swelling, and inflammation. Continuous rotation of the injection site within a given area may help to reduce or prevent these reactions. Reactions usually resolve in a few days to a few weeks. On rare occasions, injection site reactions may require discontinuation of LEVEMIR.
In some instances, these reactions may be related to factors other than insulin, such as irritants in a skin cleansing agent or poor injection technique.
Systemic allergy: Generalized allergy to insulin, which is less common but potentially more serious, may cause rash (including pruritus) over the whole body, shortness of breath, wheezing, reduction in blood pressure, rapid pulse, or sweating. Severe cases of generalized allergy, including anaphylactic reaction, may be life-threatening.
Intercurrent Conditions
Insulin requirements may be altered during intercurrent conditions such as illness, emotional disturbances, or other stresses.
Information for Patients
LEVEMIR must only be used if the solution appears clear and colorless with no visible particles (see DOSAGE AND ADMINISTRATION, Preparation and Handling). Patients should be informed about potential risks and advantages of LEVEMIR therapy, including the possible side effects. Patients should be offered continued education and advice on insulin therapies, injection technique, life-style management, regular glucose monitoring, periodic glycosylated hemoglobin testing, recognition and management of hypo- and hyperglycemia, adherence to meal planning, complications of insulin therapy, timing of dosage, instruction for use of injection devices and proper storage of insulin. Patients should be informed that frequent, patient-performed blood glucose measurements are needed to achieve effective glycemic control to avoid both hyperglycemia and hypoglycemia. Patients must be instructed on handling of special situations such as intercurrent conditions (illness, stress, or emotional disturbances), an inadequate or skipped insulin dose, inadvertent administration of an increased insulin dose, inadequate food intake, or skipped meals. Refer patients to the LEVEMIR "Patient Information" circular for additional information.
As with all patients who have diabetes, the ability to concentrate and/or react may be impaired as a result of hypoglycemia or hyperglycemia.

Patients with diabetes should be advised to inform their health care professional if they are pregnant or are contemplating pregnancy (see PRECAUTIONS, Pregnancy).

Laboratory Tests

As with all insulin therapy, the therapeutic response to LEVEMIR should be monitored by periodic blood glucose tests. Periodic measurement of HbA$_{1c}$ is recommended for the monitoring of long-term glycemic control.

Drug Interactions

A number of substances affect glucose metabolism and may require insulin dose adjustment and particularly close monitoring.

The following are examples of substances that may reduce the blood-glucose-lowering effect of insulin: corticosteroids, danazol, diuretics, sympathomimetic agents (e.g., epinephrine, albuterol, terbutaline), isoniazid, phenothiazine derivatives, somatropin, thyroid hormones, estrogens, progestogens (e.g., in oral contraceptives).

The following are examples of substances that may increase the blood-glucose-lowering effect of insulin and susceptibility to hypoglycemia: oral antidiabetic drugs, ACE inhibitors, disopyramide, fibrates, fluoxetine, MAO inhibitors, propoxyphene, salicylates, somatostatin analog (e.g., octreotide), and sulfonamide antibiotics.

Beta-blockers, clonidine, lithium salts, and alcohol may either potentiate or weaken the blood-glucose-lowering effect of insulin. Pentamidine may cause hypoglycemia, which may sometimes be followed by hyperglycemia. In addition, under the influence of sympatholytic medicinal products such as beta-blockers, clonidine, guanethidine, and reserpine, the signs of hypoglycemia may be reduced or absent. The results of in-vitro and in-vivo protein binding studies demonstrate that there is no clinically relevant interaction between insulin detemir and fatty acids or other protein bound drugs.

Mixing of Insulins

If LEVEMIR is mixed with other insulin preparations, the profile of action of one or both individual components may change. Mixing LEVEMIR with insulin aspart, a rapid acting insulin analog, resulted in about 40% reduction in AUC$_{(0-2h)}$ and C$_{max}$ for insulin aspart compared to separate injections when the ratio of insulin aspart to LEVEMIR was less than 50%.

LEVEMIR should NOT be mixed or diluted with any other insulin preparations.

Carcinogenesis, Mutagenesis, Impairment of Fertility

Standard 2-year carcinogenicity studies in animals have not been performed. Insulin detemir tested negative for genotoxic potential in the in-vitro reverse mutation study in bacteria, human peripheral blood lymphocyte chromosome aberration test, and the in-vivo mouse micronucleus test.

Pregnancy

Pregnancy Category C

Teratogenic effects

In a fertility and embryonic development study, insulin detemir was administered to female rats before mating, during mating, and throughout pregnancy at doses up to 300 nmol/kg/day (3 times the recommended human dose, based on plasma Area Under the Curve (AUC) ratio). Doses of 150 and 300 nmol/kg/day produced numbers of litters with visceral anomalies. Doses up to 900 nmol/kg/day (approximately 135 times the recommended human dose based on AUC ratio) were given to rabbits during organogenesis. Drug-dose related increases in the incidence of fetuses with gall bladder abnormalities such as small, bilobed, bifurcated and missing gall bladders were observed at a dose of 900 nmol/kg/day. The rat and rabbit embryofetal development studies that included concurrent human insulin control groups indicated that insulin detemir and human insulin had similar effects regarding embryotoxicity and teratogenicity.

Nursing mothers

It is unknown whether LEVEMIR is excreted in significant amounts in human milk. For this reason, caution should be exercised when LEVEMIR is administered to a nursing mother. Patients with diabetes who are lactating may require adjustments in insulin dose, meal plan, or both.

Pediatric use

In a controlled clinical study, HbA$_{1c}$ concentrations and rates of hypoglycemia were similar among patients treated with LEVEMIR and patients treated with NPH human insulin.

Geriatric use

Of the total number of subjects in intermediate and long-term clinical studies of LEVEMIR, 85 (type 1 studies) and 363 (type 2 studies) were 65 years and older. No overall differences in safety or effectiveness were observed between these subjects and younger subjects, and other reported clinical experience has not identified differences in responses between the elderly and younger patients, but greater sensitivity of some older individuals cannot be ruled out. In elderly patients with diabetes, the initial dosing, dose increments, and maintenance dosage should be conservative to avoid hypoglycemic reactions. Hypoglycemia may be difficult to recognize in the elderly.

ADVERSE REACTIONS

Adverse events commonly associated with human insulin therapy include the following:

Body as Whole: allergic reactions (see PRECAUTIONS, Allergy).

Skin and Appendages: lipodystrophy, pruritus, rash. Mild injection site reactions occurred more frequently with LEVEMIR than with NPH human insulin and usually resolved in a few days to a few weeks (see PRECAUTIONS, Allergy).

Other:

Hypoglycemia: (see WARNINGS and PRECAUTIONS).

In trials of up to 6 months duration in patients with type 1 and type 2 diabetes, the incidence of severe hypoglycemia with LEVEMIR was comparable to the incidence with NPH, and, as expected, greater overall in patients with type 1 diabetes (Table 4).

Weight gain:

In trials of up to 6 months duration in patients with type 1 and type 2 diabetes, LEVEMIR was associated with somewhat less weight gain than NPH (Table 4). Whether these observed differences represent true differences in the effects of LEVEMIR and NPH insulin is not known, since these trials were not blinded and the protocols (e.g., diet and exercise instructions and monitoring) were not specifically directed at exploring hypotheses related to weight effects of the treatments compared. The clinical significance of the observed differences has not been established.

[See table below]

OVERDOSAGE

Hypoglycemia may occur as a result of an excess of insulin relative to food intake, energy expenditure, or both. Mild episodes of hypoglycemia usually can be treated with oral glucose. Adjustments in drug dosage, meal patterns, or exercise may be needed. More severe episodes with coma, seizure, or neurologic impairment may be treated with intramuscular/subcutaneous glucagon or concentrated intravenous glucose. After apparent clinical recovery from hypoglycemia, continued observation and additional carbohydrate intake may be necessary to avoid reoccurrence of hypoglycemia.

DOSAGE AND ADMINISTRATION

LEVEMIR can be administered once- or twice-daily. The dose of LEVEMIR should be adjusted according to blood glucose measurements. The dosage of LEVEMIR should be individualized based on the physician's advice, in accordance with the needs of the patient.

- For patients treated with Levemir once-daily, the dose should be administered with the evening meal or at bedtime.
- For patients who require twice-daily dosing for effective blood glucose control, the evening dose can be administered either with the evening meal, at bedtime, or 12 hours after the morning dose.

LEVEMIR should be administered by subcutaneous injection in the thigh, abdominal wall, or upper arm. Injection sites should be rotated within the same region. As with all insulins, the duration of action will vary according to the dose, injection site, blood flow, temperature, and level of physical activity.

Dose Determination for LEVEMIR

- For patients with type 1 or type 2 diabetes on basal-bolus treatment, changing the basal insulin to LEVEMIR can be done on a unit-to-unit basis. The dose of LEVEMIR should then be adjusted to achieve glycemic targets. In some patients with type 2 diabetes, more LEVEMIR may be required than NPH insulin. In a clinical study, the mean dose at end of treatment was 0.77 U/kg for LEVEMIR and 0.52 IU/kg for NPH human insulin (see Table 3).
- For patients currently receiving only basal insulin, changing the basal insulin to LEVEMIR can be done on a unit-to-unit basis.
- For insulin-naïve patients with type 2 diabetes who are inadequately controlled on oral antidiabetic drugs, LEVEMIR should be started at a dose of 0.1 to 0.2 U/kg once-daily in the evening or 10 units once- or twice-daily, and the dose adjusted to achieve glycemic targets.
- As with all insulins, close glucose monitoring is recommended during the transition and in the initial weeks thereafter. Dose and timing of concurrent short-acting insulins or other concomitant antidiabetic treatment may need to be adjusted.

Preparation and Handling

LEVEMIR should be inspected visually prior to administration and should only be used if the solution appears clear and colorless.

LEVEMIR should not be mixed or diluted with any other insulin preparations.

After each injection, patients must **remove the needle without recapping** and dispose of it in a puncture-resistant container. Used syringes, needles, or lancets should be placed in "sharps" containers (such as red biohazard containers), hard plastic containers (such as detergent bottles), or metal containers (such as an empty coffee can). Such containers should be sealed and disposed of properly.

HOW SUPPLIED

LEVEMIR is available in the following package sizes: each presentation containing 100 Units of insulin detemir per mL (U-100).

10 mL vial	NDC 0169-3687-12
3 mL PenFill® cartridges*	NDC 0169-3305-11
3 mL InnoLet®	NDC 0169-2312-11
3 mL FlexPen®	NDC 0169-6439-10

*LEVEMIR PenFill® cartridges are for use with Novo Nordisk 3 mL PenFill® cartridge compatible insulin delivery devices and NovoFine® disposable needles.

Table 4: Safety Information on Clinical Studies*

	Treatment	# of subjects	Weight (kg) Baseline	Weight (kg) End of treatment	Hypoglycemia (events/subject/month) Major†	Hypoglycemia (events/subject/month) Minor‡
Type 1						
Study A	LEVEMIR	N=276	75.0	75.1	0.045	2.184
	NPH	N=133	75.7	76.4	0.035	3.063
Study C	LEVEMIR	N=492	76.5	76.3	0.029	2.397
	NPH	N=257	76.1	76.5	0.027	2.564
Study D Pediatric	LEVEMIR	N=232	N/A	N/A	0.076	2.677
	NPH	N=115	N/A	N/A	0.083	3.203
Type 2						
Study E	LEVEMIR	N=237	82.7	83.7	0.001	0.306
	NPH	N=239	82.4	85.2	0.006	0.595
Study F	LEVEMIR	N=195	81.8	82.3	0.003	0.193
	NPH	N=200	79.6	80.9	0.006	0.235

* See CLINICAL STUDIES section for description of individual studies
† Major = requires assistance of another individual because of neurologic impairment
‡ Minor = plasma glucose <56 mg/dl, subject able to deal with the episode him/herself

RECOMMENDED STORAGE

Unused LEVEMIR should be stored between 2° and 8°C (36° to 46° F). *Do not freeze.* **Do not use LEVEMIR if it has been frozen.**

Vials:
After initial use, vials should be stored in a refrigerator, never in a freezer. If refrigeration is not possible, the in-use vial can be kept unrefrigerated at room temperature, below 30°C (86°F), for up to 42 days, as long as it is kept as cool as possible and away from direct heat and light.

Unpunctured vials can be used until the expiration date printed on the label if they are stored in a refrigerator. Keep unused vials in the carton so they will stay clean and protected from light.

PenFill® cartridges, FlexPen® or InnoLet®:
After initial use, a cartridge (PenFill®) or a prefilled syringe (including FlexPen® or InnoLet®) may be used for up to 42 days if it is kept at room temperature, below 30°C (86°F). In-use cartridges and prefilled syringes in-use must NOT be stored in a refrigerator and must NOT be stored with the needle in place. Keep all cartridges and prefilled syringes away from direct heat and sunlight.

Not in-use (unopened) LEVEMIR PenFill®, FlexPen® or InnoLet® can be used until the expiration date printed on the label if they are stored in a refrigerator. Keep unused cartridges and prefilled syringes in the carton so they will stay clean and protected from light.

The storage conditions are summarized in the following table:
[See table above]

Date of issue: July 15, 2009
Version: 5

Novo Nordisk®, Levemir®, NovoLog®, FlexPen®, InnoLet®, PenFill®, and NovoFine® are registered trademarks owned by Novo Nordisk A/S.

© 2005/2009 Novo Nordisk Inc.
Levemir® is covered by US Patent Nos. 5,750,497; 5,866,538; 6,011,007; 6,869,930 and other patents pending. FlexPen® is covered by US Patent Nos. 6,004,297; 6,235,004; 6,582,404 and other patents pending.

Manufactured for:
Novo Nordisk Inc.
Princeton, NJ 08540
www.novonordisk-us.com
Manufactured by:
Novo Nordisk A/S
DK-2880 Bagsvaerd, Denmark

PATIENT INFORMATION

Levemir® (LEV-uh-mere)
(insulin detemir [rDNA origin] injection)

Important:
Know your insulin. Do not change the type of insulin you use unless told to do so by your healthcare provider. The amount of insulin you take as well as the best time for you to take your insulin may need to change if you take a different type of insulin.

Make sure you know the type and strength of insulin prescribed for you.

Read the Patient Information that comes with Levemir before you start taking it and each time you get a refill. There may be new information. This leaflet does not take the place of talking with your healthcare provider about your diabetes or your treatment. Make sure that you know how to manage your diabetes. Ask your healthcare provider if you have any questions about managing your diabetes.

What is Levemir?
Levemir is a man-made long-acting insulin that is used to control high blood sugar in adults and children with diabetes mellitus.

Who should not use Levemir?
Do not take Levemir if:
• Your blood sugar is too low (hypoglycemia).
• You are allergic to anything in Levemir. See the end of this leaflet for a complete list of ingredients in Levemir. Check with your healthcare provider if you are not sure.

Tell your healthcare provider:
• **about all of your medical conditions.** Medical conditions can affect your insulin needs and your dose of Levemir.
• **if you are pregnant or breast-feeding.** You and your healthcare provider should talk about the best way to manage your diabetes while you are pregnant or breast-feeding. Levemir has not been studied in pregnant or nursing women.
• **about all medicines you take,** including prescriptions and non-prescription medicines, vitamins and herbal supplements. Your Levemir dose may change if you take other medicines.

Know the medicines you take. Keep a list of your medicines with you to show your healthcare provider when you get a new medicine.

	Not in-use (unopened) Room Temperature (below 30°C)	Not in-use (unopened) Refrigerated	In-use (opened) Room Temperature (below 30°C)
10 mL vial	42 days	Until expiration date	42 days refrigerated/room temperature
3 mL PenFill® cartridges	42 days	Until expiration date	42 days **(Do not refrigerate)**
3 mL InnoLet®	42 days	Until expiration date	42 days **(Do not refrigerate)**
3 mL FlexPen®	42 days	Until expiration date	42 days **(Do not refrigerate)**

How should I take Levemir?
Only use Levemir if it appears clear and colorless. There may be air bubbles. This is normal. If it looks cloudy, thickened, or colored, or if it contains solid particles do not use it and call Novo Nordisk at 1-800-727-6500.

Levemir comes in:
• 10 mL vials (small bottles) for use with a syringe
• 3 mL PenFill® cartridges for use with the Novo Nordisk 3 mL PenFill cartridge compatible insulin delivery devices and NovoFine® disposable needles. The cartridge delivery device can be used with a NovoPen® 3 PenMate®)
• 3 mL Levemir FlexPen®
• 3 mL Levemir InnoLet®

Read the instructions for use that come with your Levemir product. Talk to your healthcare provider if you have any questions. Your healthcare provider should show you how to inject Levemir before you start taking it.

• **Take Levemir exactly as prescribed.**
• **Levemir is a long-acting insulin.** The effect of Levemir may last up to 24 hours after injection.
• **Inject Levemir into the skin of your stomach area, upper arms, or thighs.** Levemir may affect your blood sugar levels sooner if you inject it into the skin of your stomach area or upper arm. **Never inject Levemir into a vein or into a muscle.**
• **Change (rotate) your injection site within the chosen area (for example, stomach or upper arm) with each dose. Do not inject into the exact same spot for each injection.**
• **If you take too much Levemir, your blood sugar may fall low (hypoglycemia).** You can treat mild low blood sugar (hypoglycemia) by drinking or eating something sugary right away (fruit juice, sugar candies, or glucose tablets). It is important to treat low blood sugar (hypoglycemia) right away because it could get worse and you could pass out (become unconscious). If you pass out you will need help from another person or emergency medical services right away, and will need treatment with a glucagon injection or treatment at a hospital. See "What are the possible side effects of Levemir?" for more information on low blood sugar (hypoglycemia).
• **If you forget to take your dose of Levemir, your blood sugar may go too high (hyperglycemia).** If high blood sugar (hyperglycemia) is not treated it can lead to serious problems, like loss of consciousness (passing out), coma or even death. Follow your healthcare provider's instructions for treating high blood sugar. Know your symptoms of high blood sugar which may include:

• increased thirst	• a hard time breathing
• frequent urination	• fruity smell on the breath
• drowsiness	• high amounts of sugar and ketones in your urine
• loss of appetite	• nausea, vomiting (throwing up) or stomach pain

• **Check your blood sugar levels.** Ask your healthcare provider what your blood sugar levels should be and when you should check your blood sugar levels.
• **Never mix Levemir with other insulin products.**
• **Never use Levemir in an insulin pump.**

Your insulin dosage may need to change because of:

• illness	• change in diet
• stress	• change in physical activity or exercise
• other medicines you take	

What should I avoid while using Levemir?
• **Alcohol.** Alcohol, including beer and wine, may affect your blood sugar when you take Levemir.
• **Driving and operating machinery.** You may have difficulty concentrating or reacting if you have low blood sugar (hy-

poglycemia). Be careful when you drive a car or operate machinery. Ask your healthcare provider if it is alright to drive if you often have:
• low blood sugar
• decreased or no warning signs of low blood sugar

What are the possible side effects of Levemir?
• **low blood sugar (hypoglycemia).** Symptoms of low blood sugar may include:

• sweating	• trouble concentrating or confusion
• dizziness or lightheadedness	• blurred vision
• shakiness	• slurred speech
• hunger	• anxiety, irritability or mood changes
• fast heart beat	• headache
• tingling of lips and tongue	

Severe low blood sugar can cause unconsciousness (passing out), seizures, and death. Know your symptoms of low blood sugar. Follow your healthcare provider's instructions for treating low blood sugar. Talk to your healthcare provider if low blood sugar is a problem for you.
• **Serious allergic reaction (whole body reaction). Get medical help right away, if you develop** a rash over your whole body, have trouble breathing, a fast heartbeat, or sweating.
• **Reactions at the injection site (local allergic reaction).** You may get redness, swelling, and itching at the injection site. If you keep having skin reactions or they are serious, talk to your healthcare provider. You may need to stop using Levemir and use a different insulin. Do not inject insulin into skin that is red, swollen, or itchy.
• **Skin thickens or pits at the injection site (lipodystrophy).** Change (rotate) where you inject your insulin to help to prevent these skin changes from happening. Do not inject insulin into this type of skin.
• **Swelling of your hands and feet.**
• **Vision changes.**
• **Low potassium in your blood (hypokalemia)**

These are not all of the possible side effects from Levemir. Ask your healthcare provider or pharmacist for more information.

Call your healthcare provider for medical advice about side effects.

You may report side effects to FDA at 1-800-FDA-1088.

How should I store Levemir?
All Unopened Levemir:
• **Keep all unopened Levemir in the refrigerator between 36° to 46°F (2° to 8°C).**
• Do not freeze. Do not use Levemir if it has been frozen.
• Keep unopened Levemir in the carton to protect from light.

Levemir in use:
• **Vials:**
 • Keep in the refrigerator or at room temperature below 86°F (30°C) for up to 42 days.
 • Keep vials away from direct heat or light.
 • Throw away an opened vial after 42 days of use, even if there is insulin left in the vial.
 • Unopened vials can be used until the expiration date on the Levemir label, if the medicine has been stored in a refrigerator.
• **Levemir FlexPen:**
 • Keep at room temperature below 86°F (30°C) for up to 42 days.
 • Do not store a Levemir FlexPen that you are using in the refrigerator.
 • Keep Levemir FlexPen away from direct heat or light.
 • Throw away a used Levemir FlexPen after 42 days, even if there is insulin left in the syringe.

General advice about Levemir

Medicines are sometimes prescribed for conditions that are not mentioned in the patient leaflet. Do not use Levemir for a condition for which it was not prescribed. Do not give Levemir to other people, even if they have the same symptoms you have. It may harm them. This leaflet summarizes the most important information about Levemir. If you would like more information about Levemir or diabetes, talk with your healthcare provider. You can ask your healthcare provider or pharmacist for information about Levemir that is written for healthcare professionals. Call 1-800-727-6500 or visit www.novonordisk-us.com for more information.

Helpful information for people with diabetes is published by the American Diabetes Association, 1701 N Beauregard Street, Alexandria, VA 22311 and on www.diabetes.org. Levemir ingredients include:

• Insulin detemir	• Zinc
• Glycerol	• Disodium hydrogen phosphate dihydrate
• Phenol	• Sodium chloride
• Metacresol	• Water for injection
	• Hydrochloric acid or sodium hydroxide

All Levemir vials and Levemir FlexPen are latex free.
Date of Issue: May 22, 2009
Version: 4
Levemir®, PenFill®, FlexPen®, NovoPen®, NovoFine®, PenMate®, are trademarks of Novo Nordisk A/S.
Levemir® is covered by US Patent Nos. 5,750,497, 5,866,538, 6,011,007, 6,869,930, and other patents pending. FlexPen® is covered by US Patent Nos. 6,582,404, 6,004,297, 6,235,004, and other patents pending. PenFill® is covered by US Patent Nos. 6,126,646, 5,693,027, DES 347894, and other patents pending.
© 2005-2009 Novo Nordisk Inc.
Manufactured by:
Novo Nordisk A/S
DK-2880 Bagsvaerd, Denmark
For information about Levemir® contact:
Novo Nordisk Inc.
100 College Road West,
Princeton, New Jersey 08540

INSTRUCTIONS FOR USE

Levemir® 10 mL vial (100 units/mL, U-100)
Levemir® 3 mL PenFill® cartridge (100 units/mL, U-100)
How should I prepare and deliver the injection using different delivery devices?
Using the 10 mL vial:
1. At your first use, remove the tamper-resistant cap from the vial. If the cap has already been removed, do not use this vial and return it to your pharmacy.
2. Wipe the rubber membrane with an alcohol swab.
3. Do not roll or shake the vial. Vigorous shaking right before the dose is drawn into the syringe may cause bubbles or froth, which could cause dosage errors. The insulin should be used only if it is clear and colorless.
4. Pull back the plunger on your syringe until the black tip reaches the marking for the number of units you will inject.
5. Push the needle through the rubber membrane into the vial.
6. Push the plunger all the way in. This inserts air into the vial.
7. Turn the vial and syringe upside down together and slowly pull the plunger back to a few units beyond the correct dose.
8. If there are air bubbles, tap the syringe gently with your finger to raise the air bubbles to the needle. Then slowly push the plunger to the correct unit marking.
9. Lift the vial off the syringe.
10. Inject right away.
11. The syringe and vial should be disposed of properly without recapping the needle. After each injection, patients must **remove the needle without recapping** and dispose of it in a puncture-resistant container. Used syringes, needles, or lancets should be placed in sharps containers (such as red biohazard containers), hard plastic containers (such as detergent bottles), or metal containers (such as an empty coffee can). Such containers should be sealed and disposed of properly.

Using the **LEVEMIR 3 mL PenFill® cartridge in 3 mL PenFill® cartridge delivery devices* (*see 3 mL PenFill® cartridge compatible delivery devices section):**
1. Read the instruction manuals for the 3 mL PenFill® cartridge compatible delivery device* before the device is used.

2. The insulin should be used only if it is clear and colorless. Insert the PenFill® cartridge into the 3 mL PenFill® cartridge compatible delivery device*.
3. Place the needle onto the 3 mL PenFill® cartridge compatible delivery device* immediately before use
4. Airshots should be done prior to each injection. Directions for performing an airshot and setting the dose are provided in your insulin delivery device instruction manual.
5. Discard needle after each dose. The needle should not be recapped to avoid needlesticks. After each injection, patients must **remove the needle without recapping** and dispose of it in a puncture-resistant container. Used syringes, needles, or lancets should be placed in sharps containers (such as red biohazard containers), hard plastic containers (such as detergent bottles), or metal containers (such as an empty coffee can). Such containers should be sealed and disposed of properly.

After the first use of PenFill® cartridge:
1. Airshots should be done prior to each injection. Directions for performing an airshot and setting the dose are provided in your insulin delivery device instruction manual.
2. To avoid needle sticks, **do not recap** the needle. Throw away the needle safely after each injection

How should I inject LEVEMIR insulin with a syringe or 3 mL PenFill® cartridge compatible delivery device*?
1. Pinch your skin between two fingers, push the needle into the skinfold, and push the plunger to inject the insulin under your skin. The needle should be perpendicular to the skin. This means the needle will be straight in.
2. Keep the needle under your skin for at least 6 seconds to make sure you have injected all the insulin.
3. If blood appears after you pull the needle from your skin, press the injection site lightly with a finger. Do not rub the area.

* LEVEMIR PenFill® cartridges are for use with Novo Nordisk 3 mL PenFill® cartridge compatible insulin delivery devices and NovoFine® disposable needles.

INSTRUCTIONS FOR USE

Levemir® 3 mL InnoLet (100 units/mL, U-100)
LEVEMIR InnoLet (3 mL) directions for use
LEVEMIR InnoLet is a disposable dial-a-dose insulin delivery system able to deliver 1 to a maximum of 50 units. The dose can be adjusted in increments of 1 unit. LEVEMIR InnoLet is designed for use with NovoFine® single-use needles. LEVEMIR InnoLet is not recommended for the blind or severely visually impaired patients without the assistance of a sighted individual trained in the proper use of the product.

Please read and follow these instructions completely each time you use this device. If you do not follow these instructions completely, you may get too much or too little insulin.
Every time you give an injection using LEVEMIR InnoLet:
• **Use a new needle**
• **Prime to make sure the InnoLet is ready to dose**
• **Make sure you got your full dose**

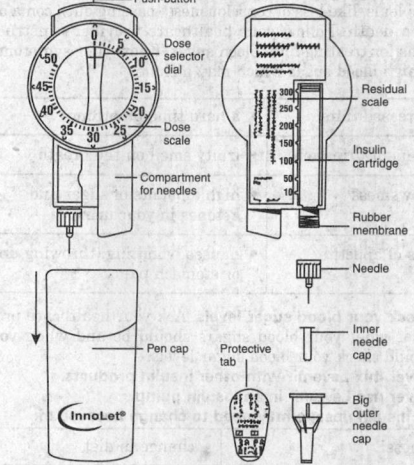

1. PREPARING THE LEVEMIR INNOLET
a. Pull off the cap.
b. Wipe the rubber membrane with an alcohol swab.
[See figure at top of next column]
c. Remove the protective tab from the disposable needle and screw the needle onto the InnoLet (see diagram **1A**). Never place a disposable needle on your InnoLet until you are ready to give an injection. Remove the needle from InnoLet immediately after the use. If the needle is not removed, some liquid may leak from the LEVEMIR InnoLet.
d. **Giving the air shot before each injection**

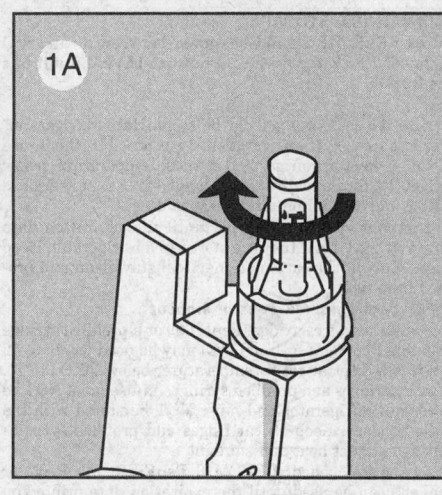

Small amounts of air may collect in the needle and insulin reservoir during normal use. **To avoid injecting air and to ensure proper dosing**, dial 2 units by turning the dose selector clockwise. Hold the LEVEMIR InnoLet with the needle pointing up and tap the LEVEMIR InnoLet gently with your finger so any air bubbles collect in the top of the reservoir. Remove both the plastic outer and inner needle cap.

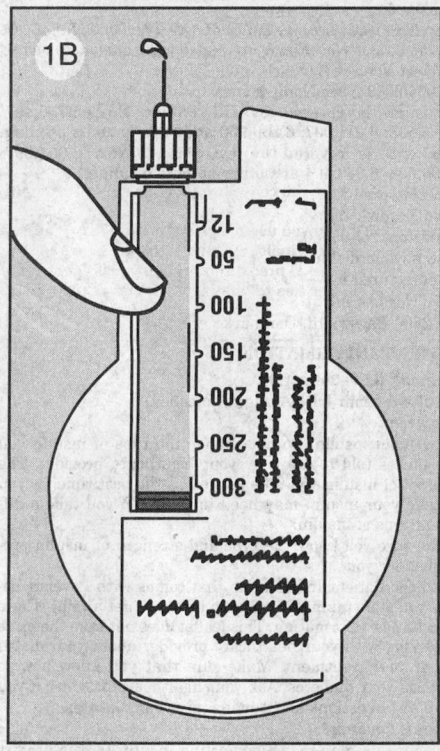

With the needle pointing up, press the push button as far as it will go and the dose selector returns to zero. See if a drop of insulin appears at the needle tip (see Figure **1B**). If not, repeat the procedure until insulin appears.
1. Before the first use of LEVEMIR InnoLet, you may need to perform up to 6 airshots to get a droplet of insulin at the needle tip. If you need to make more than 6 airshots, do not use the LEVEMIR InnoLet, and contact Novo Nordisk® at 1-800-727-6500. A small air bubble may remain but it will not be injected because the operating mechanism prevents the reservoir from being completely emptied.

2. SETTING THE DOSE
[See figure at top of next column]
Always check that the push button is fully depressed and the dose selector is set at 0. Hold the LEVEMIR InnoLet® in front of you and dial the dose selector clockwise to set the required dose. Do not put your hand over the push button when dialing the dose. If the button is not allowed to rise freely, insulin will be pushed out of the needle. You will hear a click for every single unit dialed. Do not rely on the clicking sound as a means for setting your dose. If you have set a wrong dose, simply dial the dose selector forward or backwards until the right number of dose has been set.

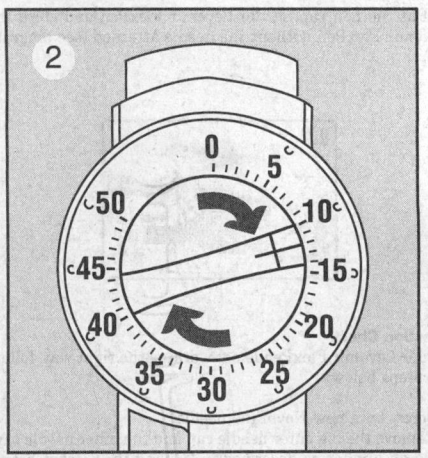

50 units is the maximum dose.

3. GIVING THE INJECTION

Use the injection technique recommended by your doctor or health care professionals.

a. Check that you have set the proper dose and depress the push button as far as it will go. Make sure not to block the dose selector while injecting, as the dose selector must be allowed to return to zero when you press the push button. When depressing the push button, you may hear a clicking sound. Do not rely on this clicking sound as a means of confirming delivery of your dose.

After making the injection, unscrew the needle and discard appropriately. After each injection, you must **remove the needle before replacing the device cap** and dispose of the needle in a puncture-resistant container. Used syringes, needles, or lancets should be placed in "sharps" containers (such as red biohazard containers), hard plastic containers (such as detergent bottles), or metal containers (such as an empty coffee can). Such containers should be sealed and disposed of properly.

It is important that you use a new needle for each injection. Health care professionals, relatives, and other caregivers, should follow general precautionary measures for removal and disposal of needles to eliminate the risk of unintended needlestick.

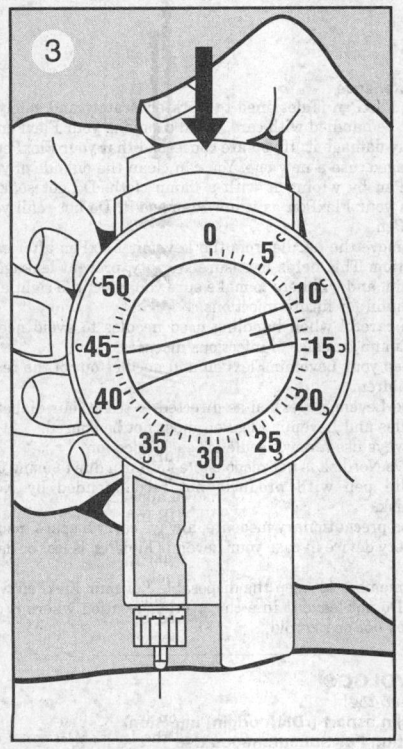

4. LATER (SUBSEQUENT) INJECTIONS

Always check that the push button is fully depressed before using the LEVEMIR InnoLet® again. If not, turn the dose selector until the push button is completely down. Then proceed as stated in steps 1-3.

The numbers on the insulin reservoir can be used to estimate the amount of insulin left in the LEVEMIR InnoLet.

Do not use these numbers to measure the insulin dose. You cannot set a dose greater than the number of units remaining in the reservoir.

5. FUNCTION CHECK

If you think that your LEVEMIR InnoLet is not working properly, follow this procedure:

a. Screw on a new NovoFine needle
b. Perform air shot as described in *1. PREPARING THE LEVEMIR INNOLET®*, *steps (d) through (e) and Figure 1B*
c. Put the outer needle cap onto the needle
d. Dispense 20 units into the needle cap.

The insulin will fill the lower part of the cap (as shown in the figure above).

If the LEVEMIR InnoLet has released too much or too little insulin, repeat the test. If it happens again, do not use your LEVEMIR InnoLet and contact Novo Nordisk at 1-800-727-6500.

6. IMPORTANT NOTES

- If you need to perform more than 6 air shots before the first use of the disposable LEVEMIR InnoLet to get a droplet of insulin at the needle tip, do not use your LEVEMIR InnoLet and contact Novo Nordisk at 1-800-727-6500.
- Remember to perform an air shot before each injection. See figure **1B**.
- Do not drop, damage, or crush the disposable LEVEMIR InnoLet.
- Remember to keep the disposable LEVEMIR InnoLet with you. Don't leave it in a car or other location where it can get too hot or too cold.
- LEVEMIR InnoLet is not supplied with needles. NovoFine® disposable needles are designed and recommended for use with Novo Nordisk® insulin delivery devices, including LEVEMIR InnoLet.
- Never place a disposable needle on the LEVEMIR InnoLet until you are ready to use it. Remove the needle right after the use without recapping.
- **Discard the needle after each injection. After each injection, remove the needle before replacing the device cap and dispose the needle in a puncture-resistant container. Used syringes, needles, or lancets should be placed in "sharps" containers (such as red biohazard containers), hard plastic containers (such as detergent bottles), or metal containers (such as an empty coffee can). Such containers should be sealed and disposed of properly.**
- Throw away the empty LEVEMIR InnoLet without the needle attached.
- Always carry an extra LEVEMIR InnoLet with you in case your LEVEMIR InnoLet you are using is damaged or lost.
- To avoid possible transmission of disease, do not share your LEVEMIR InnoLet with anyone, even if you attach a new needle.
- **Novo Nordisk is not responsible for harm due to using this insulin delivery system with products not recommended by Novo Nordisk.**
- Keep this disposable LEVEMIR InnoLet out of the reach of children.

INSTRUCTIONS FOR USE
LEVEMIR® FlexPen®
Introduction

Please read the following instructions carefully before using your Levemir® FlexPen®.

Levemir FlexPen is a disposable dial-a-dose insulin pen. You can select doses from 1 to 60 units in increments of 1 unit. Levemir FlexPen is designed to be used with NovoFine® needles.

Δ Levemir FlexPen should not be used by people who are blind or have severe visual problems without the help of a person who has good eyesight and who is trained to use the Levemir FlexPen the right way.

Getting ready

Make sure you have the following items:
- Levemir FlexPen
- New NovoFine needle
- Alcohol swab

[See figure below]

Preparing your Levemir FlexPen

Wash your hands with soap and water. Before you start to prepare your injection, check the label to make sure that you are taking the right type of insulin. This is especially important if you take more than 1 type of insulin. Levemir should look clear.

A. Pull off the pen cap (see diagram A).

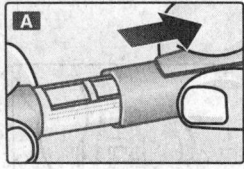

Wipe the rubber stopper with an alcohol swab.

B. Attaching the needle

Remove the protective tab from a disposable needle. Screw the needle tightly onto your FlexPen. It is important that the needle is put on straight (see diagram B).

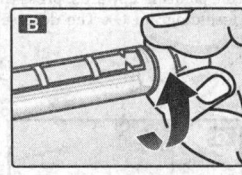

Never place a disposable needle on your Levemir FlexPen until you are ready to take your injection.

C. Pull off the big outer needle cap (see diagram C).

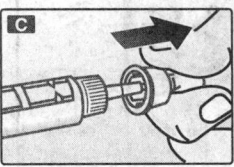

D. Pull off the inner needle cap and dispose of it (see diagram D).

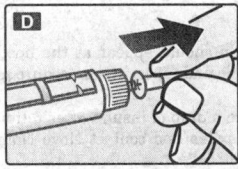

Δ Always use a new needle for each injection to help ensure sterility and prevent blocked needles.

Δ Be careful not to bend or damage the needle before use.

Δ To reduce the risk of unexpected needle sticks, never put the inner needle cap back on the needle.

Giving the airshot before each injection

Before each injection small amounts of air may collect in the cartridge during normal use. To avoid injecting air and to ensure proper dosing:

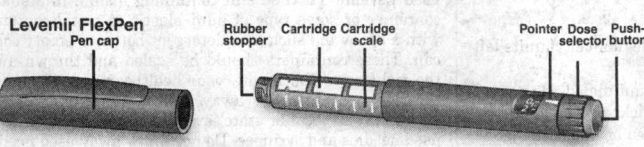

Levemir FlexPen — Pen cap — Rubber stopper — Cartridge — Cartridge scale — Pointer — Dose selector — Push-button — NovoFine needle — Big outer needle cap — Inner needle cap — Needle — Protective tab

E. Turn the dose selector to select 2 units (see diagram E).

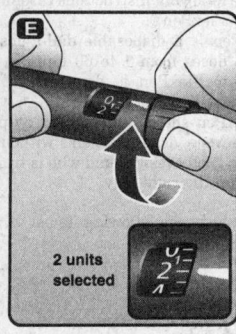

2 units selected

F. Hold your Levemir FlexPen with the needle pointing up. Tap the cartridge gently with your finger a few times to make any air bubbles collect at the top of the cartridge (see diagram F).

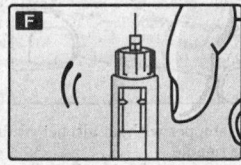

G. Keep the needle pointing upwards, press the push-button all the way in (see diagram G). The dose selector returns to 0.

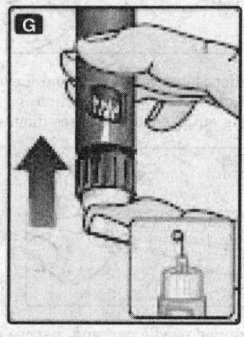

A drop of insulin should appear at the needle tip. If not, change the needle and repeat the procedure no more than 6 times.

If you do not see a drop of insulin after 6 times, do not use the Levemir FlexPen and contact Novo Nordisk at 1-800-727-6500.

A small air bubble may remain at the needle tip, but it will not be injected.

Selecting your dose

Check and make sure that the dose selector is set at 0.

H. Turn the dose selector to the number of units you need to inject. The pointer should line up with your dose.

The dose can be corrected either up or down by turning the dose selector in either direction until the correct dose lines up with the pointer (see diagram H). When turning the dose selector, be careful not to press the push-button as insulin will come out.

[See figure at top of next column]

You cannot select a dose larger than the number of units left in the cartridge.

You will hear a click for every single unit dialed. Do not set the dose by counting the number of clicks you hear.

Δ Do not use the cartridge scale printed on the cartridge to measure your dose of insulin.

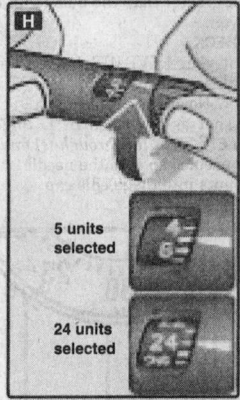

5 units selected

24 units selected

Giving the injection

Do the injection exactly as shown to you by your healthcare provider. Your healthcare provider should tell you if you need to pinch the skin before injecting.

I. Insert the needle into your skin.

Inject the dose by pressing the push-button all the way in until the 0 lines up with the pointer (see diagram I). Be careful only to push the button when injecting.

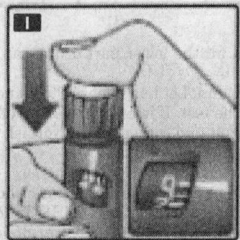

Turning the dose selector will not inject insulin.

J. Keep the needle in the skin for at least 6 seconds, and keep the push-button pressed all the way in until the needle has been pulled out from the skin (see diagram J).

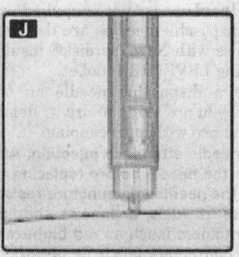

This will make sure that the full dose has been given. You may see a drop of Levemir at the needle tip. This is normal and has no effect on the dose you just received. If blood appears after you take the needle out of your skin, press the injection site lightly with a finger. **Do not rub the area.**

After the injection

Do not recap the needle. Recapping can lead to a needle stick injury. Remove the needle from the Levemir FlexPen after each injection. This helps to prevent infection, leakage of insulin, and will help to make sure you inject the right dose of insulin. The Levemir FlexPen prevents the cartridge from being completely emptied. It is designed to deliver 300 units.

Δ Put the needle and any empty Levemir FlexPen or any used Levemir FlexPen still containing insulin in a sharps container or some type of hard plastic or metal container with a screw top such as a detergent bottle or empty coffee can. These containers should be sealed and thrown away the right way. Check with your healthcare provider about the right way to throw away used syringes and needles. There may be local or state laws about how to throw away used needles and syringes. Do not throw away used needles and syringes in household trash or recycling bins.

K. Put the pen cap on the Levemir FlexPen and store the Levemir FlexPen without the needle attached (see diagram K).

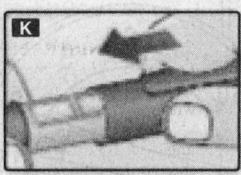

Function Check

If your Levemir FlexPen is not working the right way, follow the steps below:

L.

• Screw on a new NovoFine needle.
• Remove the big outer needle cap and the inner needle cap.
• Do an airshot as described in "Giving the airshot before each injection".
• Put the big outer needle cap onto the needle. Do not put on the inner needle cap.
• Turn the dose selector so the dose indicator window shows 20 units.
• Hold the Levemir FlexPen so the needle is pointing down.
• Press the push-button all the way in.

The insulin should fill the lower part of the big outer needle cap (see diagram L). If Levemir FlexPen has released too much or too little insulin, do the function check again. If the same problem happens again, do not use your Levemir FlexPen and contact Novo Nordisk at 1-800-727-6500.

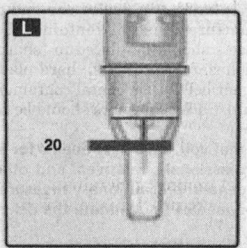

20

Maintenance

Your FlexPen is designed to work accurately and safely. It must be handled with care. Avoid dropping your FlexPen as it may damage it. If you are concerned that your FlexPen is damaged, use a new one. You can clean the outside of your FlexPen by wiping it with a damp cloth. Do not soak or wash your FlexPen as it may damage it. Do not refill your FlexPen.

Δ Remove the needle from the Levemir FlexPen after each injection. This helps to ensure sterility, prevent leakage of insulin, and will help to make sure you inject the right dose of insulin for future injections.

Δ Be careful when handling used needles to avoid needle sticks and transfer of infectious diseases.

Δ Keep your Levemir FlexPen and needles out of the reach of children.

Δ Use Levemir FlexPen as directed to treat your diabetes. Needles and Levemir FlexPen must not be shared.

Δ Always use a new needle for each injection.

Δ Novo Nordisk is not responsible for harm due to using this insulin pen with products not recommended by Novo Nordisk.

Δ As a precautionary measure, always carry a spare insulin delivery device in case your Levemir FlexPen is lost or damaged.

Δ Remember to keep the disposable Levemir FlexPen with you. Do not leave it in a car or other location where it can get too hot or too cold.

NOVOLOG® ℞
[NO-vō-log]
(insulin aspart [rDNA origin] injection)
Solution For Subcutaneous Use

HIGHLIGHTS OF PRESCRIBING INFORMATION
These highlights do not include all the information needed to use NovoLog safely and effectively.
See full prescribing information for NovoLog.
NovoLog® (insulin aspart [rDNA origin] injection) solution for subcutaneous use
Initial U.S. Approval: 2000

———RECENT MAJOR CHANGES———
- Dosage and Administration (2.3) 7/2009
- Warnings and Precautions, Administration (5.1) 10/2009

———INDICATIONS AND USAGE———
- NovoLog is an insulin analog indicated to improve glycemic control in adults and children with diabetes mellitus (1.1).

———DOSAGE AND ADMINISTRATION———
- The dosage of NovoLog must be individualized.
- *Subcutaneous injection:* NovoLog should generally be given immediately (within 5-10 minutes) prior to the start of a meal (2.2).
- *Use in pumps:* Change the NovoLog in the reservoir at least every 6 days, change the infusion set, and the infusion set insertion site at least every 3 days. NovoLog should not be mixed with other insulins or with a diluent when it is used in the pump (2.3).
- *Intravenous use:* NovoLog should be used at concentrations from 0.05 U/mL to 1.0 U/mL insulin aspart in infusion systems using polypropylene infusion bags. NovoLog has been shown to be stable in infusion fluids such as 0.9% sodium chloride (2.4).

———DOSAGE FORMS AND STRENGTHS———
Each presentation contains 100 Units of insulin aspart per mL (U-100)
- 10 mL vials (3)
- 3 mL PenFill® cartridges for the 3 mL PenFill cartridge device (3)
- 3 mL NovoLog FlexPen (3)

———CONTRAINDICATIONS———
- Do not use during episodes of hypoglycemia (4).
- Do not use in patients with hypersensitivity to NovoLog or one of its excipients.

———WARNINGS AND PRECAUTIONS———
- Hypoglycemia is the most common adverse effect of insulin therapy. Glucose monitoring is recommended for all patients with diabetes. Any change of insulin dose should be made cautiously and only under medical supervision (5.1, 5.2).
- Insulin, particularly when given intravenously or in settings of poor glycemic control, can cause hypokalemia. Use caution in patients predisposed to hypokalemia (5.3).
- Like all insulins, NovoLog requirements may be reduced in patients with renal impairment or hepatic impairment (5.4, 5.5).
- Severe, life-threatening, generalized allergy, including anaphylaxis, may occur with insulin products, including NovoLog (5.6).

———ADVERSE REACTIONS———
Adverse reactions observed with NovoLog include hypoglycemia, allergic reactions, local injection site reactions, lipodystrophy, rash and pruritus (6).

To report SUSPECTED ADVERSE REACTIONS, contact Novo Nordisk Inc. at 1-800-727-6500 or FDA at 1-800-FDA-1088 or www.fda.gov/medwatch.

———DRUG INTERACTIONS———
- The following may increase the blood-glucose-lowering effect and susceptibility to hypoglycemia: oral antidiabetic products, pramlintide, ACE inhibitors, disopyramide, fibrates, fluoxetine, monoamine oxidase inhibitors, propoxyphene, salicylates, somatostatin analogs, sulfonamide antibiotics (7).
- The following may reduce the blood-glucose-lowering effect: corticosteroids, niacin, danazol, diuretics, sympathomimetic agents (e.g., epinephrine, salbutamol, terbutaline), isoniazid, phenothiazine derivatives, somatropin, thyroid hormones, estrogens, progestogens (e.g., in oral contraceptives), atypical antipsychotics (7).
- Beta-blockers, clonidine, lithium salts, and alcohol may either potentiate or weaken the blood-glucose-lowering effect of insulin (7).
- Pentamidine may cause hypoglycemia, which may sometimes be followed by hyperglycemia (7).
- The signs of hypoglycemia may be reduced or absent in patients taking sympatholytic products such as beta-blockers, clonidine, guanethidine, and reserpine (7).

———USE IN SPECIFIC POPULATIONS———
- Pediatric: Has not been studied in children with type 2 diabetes. Has not been studied in children with type 1 diabetes <2 years of age (8.4).

See 17 for PATIENT COUNSELING INFORMATION and FDA-approved patient labeling

Revised: 03/2010

———

PATIENT INFORMATION
* Sections or subsections omitted from the full prescribing information are not listed

———

FULL PRESCRIBING INFORMATION

1 INDICATIONS AND USAGE
1.1 Treatment of Diabetes Mellitus
NovoLog is an insulin analog indicated to improve glycemic control in adults and children with diabetes mellitus.

2 DOSAGE AND ADMINISTRATION
2.1 Dosing
NovoLog is an insulin analog with an earlier onset of action than regular human insulin. The dosage of NovoLog must be individualized. NovoLog given by subcutaneous injection should generally be used in regimens with an intermediate or long-acting insulin [*see Warnings and Precautions (5), How Supplied/Storage and Handling (16.2)*]. The total daily insulin requirement may vary and is usually between 0.5 to 1.0 units/kg/day. When used in a meal-related subcutaneous injection treatment regimen, 50 to 70% of total insulin requirements may be provided by NovoLog and the remainder provided by an intermediate-acting or long-acting insulin. Because of NovoLog's comparatively rapid onset and short duration of glucose lowering activity, some patients may require more basal insulin and more total insulin to prevent pre-meal hyperglycemia when using NovoLog than when using human regular insulin.

Do not use NovoLog that is viscous (thickened) or cloudy; use only if it is clear and colorless. NovoLog should not be used after the printed expiration date.

2.2 Subcutaneous Injection
NovoLog should be administered by subcutaneous injection in the abdominal region, buttocks, thigh, or upper arm. Because NovoLog has a more rapid onset and a shorter duration of activity than human regular insulin, it should be injected immediately (within 5-10 minutes) before a meal. Injection sites should be rotated within the same region to reduce the risk of lipodystrophy. As with all insulins, the duration of action of NovoLog will vary according to the dose, injection site, blood flow, temperature, and level of physical activity.

NovoLog may be diluted with Insulin Diluting Medium for NovoLog for subcutaneous injection. Diluting one part NovoLog to nine parts diluent will yield a concentration one-tenth that of NovoLog (equivalent to U-10). Diluting one part NovoLog to one part diluent will yield a concentration one-half that of NovoLog (equivalent to U-50).

2.3 Continuous Subcutaneous Insulin Infusion (CSII) by External Pump
NovoLog can also be infused subcutaneously by an external insulin pump [*see Warnings and Precautions (5.8, 5.9), How Supplied/Storage and Handling (16.2)*]. Diluted insulin

should not be used in external insulin pumps. Because NovoLog has a more rapid onset and a shorter duration of activity than human regular insulin, pre-meal boluses of NovoLog should be infused immediately (within 5-10 minutes) before a meal. Infusion sites should be rotated within the same region to reduce the risk of lipodystrophy. The initial programming of the external insulin infusion pump should be based on the total daily insulin dose of the previous regimen. Although there is significant interpatient variability, approximately 50% of the total dose is usually given as meal-related boluses of NovoLog and the remainder is given as a basal infusion. **Change the NovoLog in the reservoir at least every 6 days, change the infusion sets and the infusion set insertion site at least every 3 days.**

The following insulin pumps† have been used in NovoLog clinical or *in vitro* studies conducted by Novo Nordisk, the manufacturer of NovoLog:
- Medtronic Paradigm® 512 and 712
- MiniMed 508
- Disetronic® D-TRON® and H-TRON®

Before using a different insulin pump with NovoLog, read the pump label to make sure the pump has been evaluated with NovoLog.

2.4 Intravenous Use
NovoLog can be administered intravenously under medical supervision for glycemic control with close monitoring of blood glucose and potassium levels to avoid hypoglycemia and hypokalemia [*see Warnings and Precautions (5), How Supplied/Storage and Handling (16.2)*]. For intravenous use, NovoLog should be used at concentrations from 0.05 U/mL to 1.0 U/mL insulin aspart in infusion systems using polypropylene infusion bags. NovoLog has been shown to be stable in infusion fluids such as 0.9% sodium chloride.

Inspect NovoLog for particulate matter and discoloration prior to parenteral administration.

3 DOSAGE FORMS AND STRENGTHS
NovoLog is available in the following package sizes: each presentation contains 100 units of insulin aspart per mL (U-100).
- 10 mL vials
- 3 mL PenFill cartridges for the 3 mL PenFill cartridge delivery device (with or without the addition of a NovoPen® 3 PenMate®) with NovoFine® disposable needles
- 3 mL NovoLog FlexPen

4 CONTRAINDICATIONS
NovoLog is contraindicated
- during episodes of hypoglycemia
- in patients with hypersensitivity to NovoLog or one of its excipients.

5 WARNINGS AND PRECAUTIONS
5.1 Administration
NovoLog has a more rapid onset of action and a shorter duration of activity than regular human insulin. An injection of NovoLog should immediately be followed by a meal within 5-10 minutes. Because of NovoLog's short duration of action, a longer acting insulin should also be used in patients with type 1 diabetes and may also be needed in patients with type 2 diabetes. Glucose monitoring is recommended for all patients with diabetes and is particularly important for patients using external pump infusion therapy.

Any change of insulin dose should be made cautiously and only under medical supervision. Changing from one insulin product to another or changing the insulin strength may result in the need for a change in dosage. As with all insulin preparations, the time course of NovoLog action may vary in different individuals or at different times in the same individual and is dependent on many conditions, including the site of injection, local blood supply, temperature, and physical activity. Patients who change their level of physical activity or meal plan may require adjustment of insulin dosages. Insulin requirements may be altered during illness, emotional disturbances, or other stresses.

Patients using continuous subcutaneous insulin infusion pump therapy must be trained to administer insulin by injection and have alternate insulin therapy available in case of pump failure.

Needles and NovoLog FlexPen must not be shared.
5.2 Hypoglycemia
Hypoglycemia is the most common adverse effect of all insulin therapies, including NovoLog. Severe hypoglycemia may lead to unconsciousness and/or convulsions and may result in temporary or permanent impairment of brain function or death. Severe hypoglycemia requiring the assistance of another person and/or parenteral glucose infusion or glucagon administration has been observed in clinical trials with insulin, including trials with NovoLog.

The timing of hypoglycemia usually reflects the time-action profile of the administered insulin formulations [*see Clinical Pharmacology (12)*]. Other factors such as changes in food

Table 1: Treatment-Emergent Adverse Events in Patients with Type 1 Diabetes Mellitus (Adverse events with frequency ≥ 5% and occurring more frequently with NovoLog compared to human regular insulin are listed)

Preferred Term	NovoLog + NPH N= 596		Human Regular Insulin + NPH N= 286	
	N	(%)	N	(%)
Hypoglycemia*	448	75%	205	72%
Headache	70	12%	28	10%
Injury accidental	65	11%	29	10%
Nausea	43	7%	13	5%
Diarrhea	28	5%	9	3%

* Hypoglycemia is defined as an episode of blood glucose concentration <45 mg/dL with or without symptoms. See Section 14 for the incidence of serious hypoglycemia in the individual clinical trials.

Table 2: Treatment-Emergent Adverse Events in Patients with Type 2 Diabetes Mellitus (except for hypoglycemia, adverse events with frequency ≥ 5% and occurring more frequently with NovoLog compared to human regular insulin are listed)

	NovoLog + NPH N= 91		Human Regular Insulin + NPH N= 91	
	N	(%)	N	(%)
Hypoglycemia*	25	27%	33	36%
Hyporeflexia	10	11%	6	7%
Onychomycosis	9	10%	5	5%
Sensory disturbance	8	9%	6	7%
Urinary tract infection	7	8%	6	7%
Chest pain	5	5%	3	3%
Headache	5	5%	3	3%
Skin disorder	5	5%	2	2%
Abdominal pain	5	5%	1	1%
Sinusitis	5	5%	1	1%

* Hypoglycemia is defined as an episode of blood glucose concentration <45 mg/dL, with or without symptoms. See Section 14 for the incidence of serious hypoglycemia in the individual clinical trials.

intake (e.g., amount of food or timing of meals), injection site, exercise, and concomitant medications may also alter the risk of hypoglycemia [see Drug Interactions (7)]. As with all insulins, use caution in patients with hypoglycemia unawareness and in patients who may be predisposed to hypoglycemia (e.g., patients who are fasting or have erratic food intake). The patient's ability to concentrate and react may be impaired as a result of hypoglycemia. This may present a risk in situations where these abilities are especially important, such as driving or operating other machinery.

Rapid changes in serum glucose levels may induce symptoms of hypoglycemia in persons with diabetes, regardless of the glucose value. Early warning symptoms of hypoglycemia may be different or less pronounced under certain conditions, such as longstanding diabetes, diabetic nerve disease, use of medications such as beta-blockers, or intensified diabetes control [see Drug Interactions (7)]. These situations may result in severe hypoglycemia (and, possibly, loss of consciousness) prior to the patient's awareness of hypoglycemia. Intravenously administered insulin has a more rapid onset of action than subcutaneously administered insulin, requiring more close monitoring for hypoglycemia.

5.3 Hypokalemia
All insulin products, including NovoLog, cause a shift in potassium from the extracellular to intracellular space, possibly leading to hypokalemia that, if left untreated, may cause respiratory paralysis, ventricular arrhythmia, and death. Use caution in patients who may be at risk for hypokalemia (e.g., patients using potassium-lowering medications, patients taking medications sensitive to serum potassium concentrations, and patients receiving intravenously administered insulin).

5.4 Renal Impairment
As with other insulins, the dose requirements for NovoLog may be reduced in patients with renal impairment [see Clinical Pharmacology (12.3)].

5.5 Hepatic Impairment
As with other insulins, the dose requirements for NovoLog may be reduced in patients with hepatic impairment [see Clinical Pharmacology (12.3)].

5.6 Hypersensitivity and Allergic Reactions
Local Reactions—As with other insulin therapy, patients may experience redness, swelling, or itching at the site of NovoLog injection. These reactions usually resolve in a few days to a few weeks, but in some occasions, may require discontinuation of NovoLog. In some instances, these reactions may be related to factors other than insulin, such as irritants in a skin cleansing agent or poor injection technique. Localized reactions and generalized myalgias have been reported with injected metacresol, which is an excipient in NovoLog.

Systemic Reactions—Severe, life-threatening, generalized allergy, including anaphylaxis, may occur with any insulin product, including NovoLog. Anaphylactic reactions with NovoLog have been reported post-approval. Generalized allergy to insulin may also cause whole body rash (including pruritus), dyspnea, wheezing, hypotension, tachycardia, or diaphoresis. In controlled clinical trials, allergic reactions were reported in 3 of 735 patients (0.4%) treated with regular human insulin and 10 of 1394 patients (0.7%) treated with NovoLog. In controlled and uncontrolled clinical trials, 3 of 2341 (0.1%) NovoLog-treated patients discontinued due to allergic reactions.

5.7 Antibody Production
Increases in anti-insulin antibody titers that react with both human insulin and insulin aspart have been observed in patients treated with NovoLog. Increases in anti-insulin antibodies are observed more frequently with NovoLog than with regular human insulin. Data from a 12-month controlled trial in patients with type 1 diabetes suggest that the increase in these antibodies is transient, and the differences in antibody levels between the regular human insulin and insulin aspart treatment groups observed at 3 and 6

months were no longer evident at 12 months. The clinical significance of these antibodies is not known. These antibodies do not appear to cause deterioration in glycemic control or necessitate increases in insulin dose.

5.8 Mixing of Insulins
• Mixing NovoLog with NPH human insulin immediately before injection attenuates the peak concentration of NovoLog, without significantly affecting the time to peak concentration or total bioavailability of NovoLog. If NovoLog is mixed with NPH human insulin, NovoLog should be drawn into the syringe first, and the mixture should be injected immediately after mixing.
• The efficacy and safety of mixing NovoLog with insulin preparations produced by other manufacturers have not been studied.
• Insulin mixtures should not be administered intravenously.

5.9 Continuous Subcutaneous Insulin Infusion by External Pump
When used in an external subcutaneous insulin infusion pump, NovoLog should not be mixed with any other insulin or diluent. When using NovoLog in an external insulin pump, the NovoLog-specific information should be followed (e.g., in-use time, frequency of changing infusion sets) because NovoLog-specific information may differ from general pump manual instructions.

Pump or infusion set malfunctions or insulin degradation can lead to a rapid onset of hyperglycemia and ketosis because of the small subcutaneous depot of insulin. This is especially pertinent for rapid-acting insulin analogs that are more rapidly absorbed through skin and have a shorter duration of action. Prompt identification and correction of the cause of hyperglycemia or ketosis is necessary. Interim therapy with subcutaneous injection may be required [see Dosage and Administration (2.3), Warnings and Precautions (5.8, 5.9), How Supplied/Storage and Handling (16.2), and Patient Counseling Information (17.2)].

NovoLog should not be exposed to temperatures greater than 37°C (98.6°F). **NovoLog that will be used in a pump should not be mixed with other insulin or with a diluent** [see Dosage and Administration (2.3), Warnings and Precautions (5.8, 5.9), How Supplied/Storage and Handling (16.2), and Patient Counseling Information (17.2)].

6 ADVERSE REACTIONS
Clinical Trial Experience
Because clinical trials are conducted under widely varying designs, the adverse reaction rates reported in one clinical trial may not be easily compared to those rates reported in another clinical trial, and may not reflect the rates actually observed in clinical practice.

• *Hypoglycemia*
Hypoglycemia is the most commonly observed adverse reaction in patients using insulin, including NovoLog [see Warnings and Precautions (5)].

• *Insulin initiation and glucose control intensification*
Intensification or rapid improvement in glucose control has been associated with a transitory, reversible ophthalmologic refraction disorder, worsening of diabetic retinopathy, and acute painful peripheral neuropathy. However, long-term glycemic control decreases the risk of diabetic retinopathy and neuropathy.

• *Lipodystrophy*
Long-term use of insulin, including NovoLog, can cause lipodystrophy at the site of repeated insulin injections or infusion. Lipodystrophy includes lipohypertrophy (thickening of adipose tissue) and lipoatrophy (thinning of adipose tissue), and may affect insulin absorption. Rotate insulin injection or infusion sites within the same region to reduce the risk of lipodystrophy.

• *Weight gain*
Weight gain can occur with some insulin therapies, including NovoLog, and has been attributed to the anabolic effects of insulin and the decrease in glucosuria.

• *Peripheral Edema*
Insulin may cause sodium retention and edema, particularly if previously poor metabolic control is improved by intensified insulin therapy.

• *Frequencies of adverse drug reactions*
The frequencies of adverse drug reactions during NovoLog clinical trials in patients with type 1 diabetes mellitus and type 2 diabetes mellitus are listed in the tables below.
[See table 1 above]
[See table 2 above]

Postmarketing Data
The following additional adverse reactions have been identified during postapproval use of NovoLog. Because these adverse reactions are reported voluntarily from a population of uncertain size, it is generally not possible to reliably estimate their frequency. Medication errors in which other insulins have been accidentally substituted for NovoLog have been identified during postapproval use [see Patient Counseling Information (17)].

7 DRUG INTERACTIONS

A number of substances affect glucose metabolism and may require insulin dose adjustment and particularly close monitoring.

- The following are examples of substances that may increase the blood-glucose-lowering effect and susceptibility to hypoglycemia: oral antidiabetic products, pramlintide, ACE inhibitors, disopyramide, fibrates, fluoxetine, monoamine oxidase (MAO) inhibitors, propoxyphene, salicylates, somatostatin analog (e.g., octreotide), sulfonamide antibiotics.
- The following are examples of substances that may reduce the blood-glucose-lowering effect: corticosteroids, niacin, danazol, diuretics, sympathomimetic agents (e.g., epinephrine, salbutamol, terbutaline), isoniazid, phenothiazine derivatives, somatropin, thyroid hormones, estrogens, progestogens (e.g., in oral contraceptives), atypical antipsychotics.
- Beta-blockers, clonidine, lithium salts, and alcohol may either potentiate or weaken the blood-glucose-lowering effect of insulin.
- Pentamidine may cause hypoglycemia, which may sometimes be followed by hyperglycemia.
- The signs of hypoglycemia may be reduced or absent in patients taking sympatholytic products such as beta-blockers, clonidine, guanethidine, and reserpine.

8 USE IN SPECIFIC POPULATIONS

8.1 Pregnancy

Pregnancy Category B. All pregnancies have a background risk of birth defects, loss, or other adverse outcome regardless of drug exposure. This background risk is increased in pregnancies complicated by hyperglycemia and may be decreased with good metabolic control. It is essential for patients with diabetes or history of gestational diabetes to maintain good metabolic control before conception and throughout pregnancy. Insulin requirements may decrease during the first trimester, generally increase during the second and third trimesters, and rapidly decline after delivery. Careful monitoring of glucose control is essential in these patients. Therefore, female patients should be advised to tell their physician if they intend to become, or if they become pregnant while taking NovoLog.

An open-label, randomized study compared the safety and efficacy of NovoLog (n=157) versus regular human insulin (n=165) in 322 pregnant women with type 1 diabetes. Two-thirds of the enrolled patients were already pregnant when they entered the study. Because only one-third of the patients enrolled before conception, the study was not large enough to evaluate the risk of congenital malformations. Both groups achieved a mean HbA_{1c} of ~ 6% during pregnancy, and there was no significant difference in the incidence of maternal hypoglycemia.

Subcutaneous reproduction and teratology studies have been performed with NovoLog and regular human insulin in rats and rabbits. In these studies, NovoLog was given to female rats before mating, during mating, and throughout pregnancy, and to rabbits during organogenesis. The effects of NovoLog did not differ from those observed with subcutaneous regular human insulin. NovoLog, like human insulin, caused pre- and post-implantation losses and visceral/skeletal abnormalities in rats at a dose of 200 U/kg/day (approximately 32 times the human subcutaneous dose of 1.0 U/kg/day, based on U/body surface area) and in rabbits at a dose of 10 U/kg/day (approximately three times the human subcutaneous dose of 1.0 U/kg/day, based on U/body surface area). The effects are probably secondary to maternal hypoglycemia at high doses. No significant effects were observed in rats at a dose of 50 U/kg/day and in rabbits at a dose of 3 U/kg/day. These doses are approximately 8 times the human subcutaneous dose of 1.0 U/kg/day for rats and equal to the human subcutaneous dose of 1.0 U/kg/day for rabbits, based on U/body surface area.

8.3 Nursing Mothers

It is unknown whether insulin aspart is excreted in human milk. Use of NovoLog is compatible with breastfeeding, but women with diabetes who are lactating may require adjustments of their insulin doses.

8.4 Pediatric Use

NovoLog is approved for use in children for subcutaneous daily injections and for subcutaneous continuous infusion by external insulin pump. NovoLog has not been studied in pediatric patients younger than 2 years of age. NovoLog has not been studied in pediatric patients with type 2 diabetes. Please see *Section 14* ***CLINICAL STUDIES*** for summaries of clinical studies.

8.5 Geriatric Use

Of the total number of patients (n= 1,375) treated with NovoLog in 3 controlled clinical studies, 2.6% (n=36) were 65 years of age or over. One-half of these patients had type 1 diabetes (18/1285) and the other half had type 2 diabetes (18/90). The HbA_{1c} response to NovoLog, as compared to human insulin, did not differ by age, particularly in patients with type 2 diabetes. Additional studies in larger populations of patients 65 years of age or over are needed to permit conclusions regarding the safety of NovoLog in elderly compared to younger patients. Pharmacokinetic/pharmacodynamic studies to assess the effect of age on the onset of NovoLog action have not been performed.

10 OVERDOSAGE

Excess insulin administration may cause hypoglycemia and, particularly when given intravenously, hypokalemia. Mild episodes of hypoglycemia usually can be treated with oral glucose. Adjustments in drug dosage, meal patterns, or exercise, may be needed. More severe episodes with coma, seizure, or neurologic impairment may be treated with intramuscular/subcutaneous glucagon or concentrated intravenous glucose. Sustained carbohydrate intake and observation may be necessary because hypoglycemia may recur after apparent clinical recovery. Hypokalemia must be corrected appropriately.

11 DESCRIPTION

NovoLog (insulin aspart [rDNA origin] injection) is a rapid-acting human insulin analog used to lower blood glucose. NovoLog is homologous with regular human insulin with the exception of a single substitution of the amino acid proline by aspartic acid in position B28, and is produced by recombinant DNA technology utilizing *Saccharomyces cerevisiae* (baker's yeast). Insulin aspart has the empirical formula $C_{256}H_{381}N_{65}O_{79}S_6$ and a molecular weight of 5825.8.

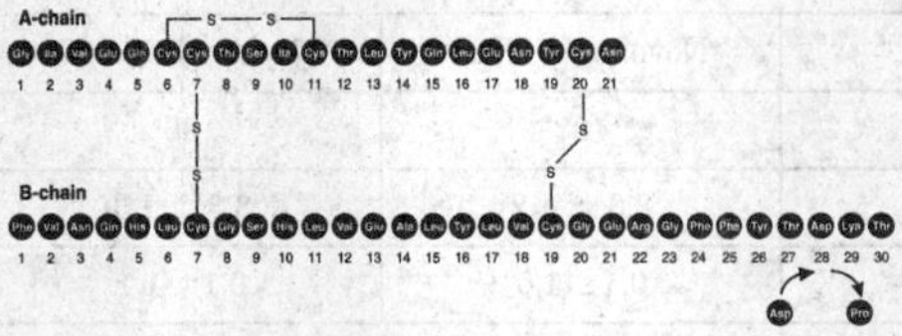

Figure 1. Structural formula of insulin aspart.

NovoLog is a sterile, aqueous, clear, and colorless solution, that contains insulin aspart 100 Units/mL, glycerin 16 mg/mL, phenol 1.50 mg/mL, metacresol 1.72 mg/mL, zinc 19.6 mcg/mL, disodium hydrogen phosphate dihydrate 1.25 mg/mL, sodium chloride 0.58 mg/mL and water for injection. NovoLog has a pH of 7.2-7.6. Hydrochloric acid 10% and/or sodium hydroxide 10% may be added to adjust pH.

12 CLINICAL PHARMACOLOGY

12.1 Mechanism of Action

The primary activity of NovoLog is the regulation of glucose metabolism. Insulins, including NovoLog, bind to the insulin receptors on muscle and fat cells and lower blood glucose by facilitating the cellular uptake of glucose and simultaneously inhibiting the output of glucose from the liver.

12.2 Pharmacodynamics

Studies in normal volunteers and patients with diabetes demonstrated that subcutaneous administration of NovoLog has a more rapid onset of action than regular human insulin.

In a study in patients with type 1 diabetes (n=22), the maximum glucose-lowering effect of NovoLog occurred between 1 and 3 hours after subcutaneous injection (see Figure 2). The duration of action for NovoLog is 3 to 5 hours. The time course of action of insulin and insulin analogs such as NovoLog may vary considerably in different individuals or within the same individual. The parameters of NovoLog activity (time of onset, peak time and duration) as designated in Figure 2 should be considered only as general guidelines. The rate of insulin absorption and onset of activity is affected by the site of injection, exercise, and other variables [*see Warnings and Precautions (5.1)*].

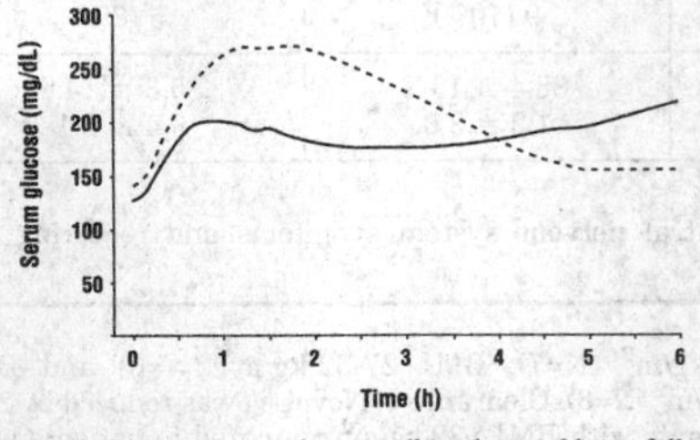

Figure 2. Serial mean serum glucose collected up to 6 hours following a single pre-meal dose of NovoLog (solid curve) or regular human insulin (hatched curve) injected immediately before a meal in 22 patients with type 1 diabetes.

A double-blind, randomized, two-way cross-over study in 16 patients with type 1 diabetes demonstrated that intravenous infusion of NovoLog resulted in a blood glucose profile that was similar to that after intravenous infusion with regular human insulin. NovoLog or human insulin was infused until the patient's blood glucose decreased to 36 mg/dL, or until the patient demonstrated signs of hypoglycemia (rise in heart rate and onset of sweating), defined as the time of autonomic reaction (R) (see Figure 3).

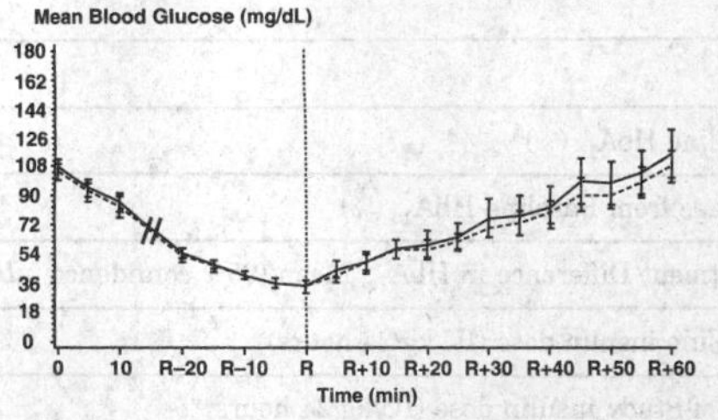

Note: The slashes on the mean profile indicate a jump on the time axis

Figure 3. Mean blood glucose profiles following intravenous infusion of NovoLog (hatched curve) and regular human insulin (solid curve) in 16 patients with type 1 diabetes. R represents the time of autonomic reaction.

12.3 Pharmacokinetics

The single substitution of the amino acid proline with aspartic acid at position B28 in NovoLog reduces the molecule's tendency to form hexamers as observed with regular human insulin. NovoLog is, therefore, more rapidly absorbed after subcutaneous injection compared to regular human insulin.

In a randomized, double-blind, crossover study 17 healthy Caucasian male subjects between 18 and 40 years of age received an intravenous infusion of either NovoLog or regular human insulin at 1.5 mU/kg/min for 120 minutes. The mean insulin clearance was similar for the two groups with mean values of 1.2 l/h/kg for the NovoLog group and 1.2 l/h/kg for the regular human insulin group.

Bioavailability and Absorption—NovoLog has a faster absorption, a faster onset of action, and a shorter duration of action than regular human insulin after subcutaneous injection (see Figure 2 and Figure 4). The relative bioavailability of NovoLog compared to regular human insulin indicates that the two insulins are absorbed to a similar extent.

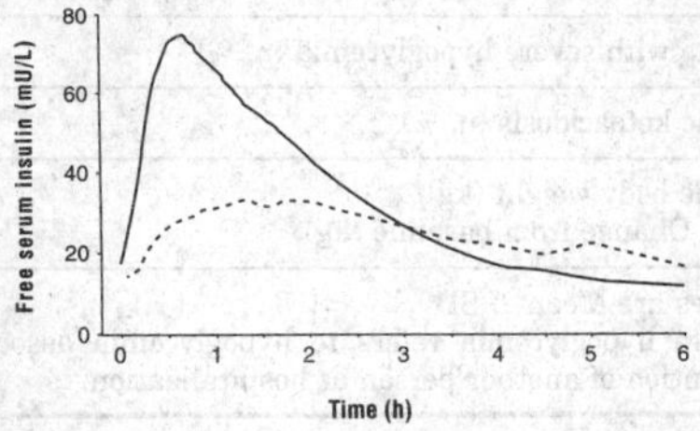

Figure 4. Serial mean serum free insulin concentration collected up to 6 hours following a single pre-meal dose of NovoLog (solid curve) or regular human insulin (hatched curve) injected immediately before a meal in 22 patients with type 1 diabetes.

In studies in healthy volunteers (total n=l07) and patients with type 1 diabetes (total n=40), NovoLog consistently reached peak serum concentrations approximately twice as fast as regular human insulin. The median time to maximum concentration in these trials was 40 to 50 minutes for NovoLog versus 80 to 120 minutes for regular human insulin. In a clinical trial in patients with type 1 diabetes, NovoLog and regular human insulin, both administered subcutaneously at a dose of 0.15 U/kg body weight, reached mean maximum concentrations of 82 and 36 mU/L, respectively. Pharmacokinetic/pharmacodynamic characteristics of insulin aspart have not been established in patients with type 2 diabetes.

The intra-individual variability in time to maximum serum insulin concentration for healthy male volunteers was significantly less for NovoLog than for regular human insulin. The clinical significance of this observation has not been established.

In a clinical study in healthy non-obese subjects, the pharmacokinetic differences between NovoLog and regular human insulin described above, were observed independent of the site of injection (abdomen, thigh, or upper arm).

Distribution and Elimination—NovoLog has low binding to plasma proteins (<10%), similar to that seen with regular human insulin. After subcutaneous administration in normal male volunteers (n=24), NovoLog was more rapidly eliminated than regular human insulin with an average apparent half-life of 81 minutes compared to 141 minutes for regular human insulin.

Specific Populations

Children and Adolescents—The pharmacokinetic and pharmacodynamic properties of NovoLog and regular human insulin were evaluated in a single dose study in 18 children (6-12 years, n=9) and adolescents (13-17 years [Tanner grade ≥ 2], n=9) with type 1 diabetes. The relative differences in pharmacokinetics and pharmacodynamics in

Table 3. Subcutaneous NovoLog Administration in Type 1 Diabetes (24 weeks; n=882)

	NovoLog + NPH	Novolin R + NPH
N	596	286
Baseline HbA$_{1c}$ (%)*	7.9 ±1.1	8.0 ± 1.2
Change from Baseline HbA$_{1c}$ (%)	-0.1 ± 0.8	0.0 ± 0.8
Treatment Difference in HbA$_{1c}$, Mean (95% confidence interval)	-0.2 (-0.3, -0.1)	
Baseline insulin dose (IU/kg/24 hours)*	0.7 ± 0.2	0.7 ± 0.2
End-of-Study insulin dose (IU/kg/24 hours)*	0.7 ± 0.2	0.7 ± 0.2
Patients with severe hypoglycemia (n, %)†	104 (17%)	54 (19%)
Baseline body weight (kg)*	75.3 ± 14.5	75.9 ± 13.1
Weight Change from baseline (kg)*	0.5 ± 3.3	0.9 ± 2.9

* Values are Mean ± SD
† Severe hypoglycemia refers to hypoglycemia associated with central nervous system symptoms and requiring the intervention of another person or hospitalization.

Table 4. Pediatric Subcutaneous Administration of NovoLog in Type 1 Diabetes (24 weeks; n=283)

	NovoLog + NPH	Novolin R + NPH
N	187	96
Baseline HbA$_{1c}$ (%)*	8.3 ± 1.2	8.3 ± 1.3
Change from Baseline HbA$_{1c}$ (%)	0.1± 1.0	0.1± 1.1
Treatment Difference in HbA$_{1c}$, Mean (95% confidence interval)	0.1 (-0.5, 0.1)	
Baseline insulin dose (IU/kg/24 hours)*	0.4 ± 0.2	0.6 ± 0.2
End-of-Study insulin dose (IU/kg/24 hours)*	0.4 ± 0.2	0.7 ± 0.2
Patients with severe hypoglycemia (n, %)†	11 (6%)	9 (9%)
Diabetic ketoacidosis (n, %)	10 (5%)	2 (2%)
Baseline body weight (kg)*	50.6 ± 19.6	48.7 ± 15.8
Weight Change from baseline (kg)*	2.7 ± 3.5	2.4 ± 2.6

* Values are Mean ± SD
† Severe hypoglycemia refers to hypoglycemia associated with central nervous system symptoms and requiring the intervention of another person or hospitalization.

Table 5. Subcutaneous NovoLog Administration in Type 2 Diabetes (6 months; n=176)

	NovoLog + NPH	Novolin R + NPH
N	90	86
Baseline HbA$_{1c}$ (%)*	8.1 ± 1.2	7.8 ± 1.1
Change from Baseline HbA$_{1c}$ (%)	-0.3 ± 1.0	-0.1 ± 0.8
Treatment Difference in HbA$_{1c}$, Mean (95% confidence interval)	-0.1 (-0.4, -0.1)	
Baseline insulin dose (IU/kg/24 hours)*	0.6 ± 0.3	0.6 ± 0.3
End-of-Study insulin dose (IU/kg/24 hours)*	0.7 ± 0.3	0.7 ± 0.3
Patients with severe hypoglycemia (n, %)†	9 (10%)	5 (8%)
Baseline body weight (kg)*	88.4 ± 13.3	85.8 ± 14.8
Weight Change from baseline (kg)*	1.2 ± 3.0	0.4 ± 3.1

* Values are Mean ± SD
† Severe hypoglycemia refers to hypoglycemia associated with central nervous system symptoms and requiring the intervention of another person or hospitalization.

children and adolescents with type 1 diabetes between NovoLog and regular human insulin were similar to those in healthy adult subjects and adults with type 1 diabetes.
Gender—In healthy volunteers, no difference in insulin aspart levels was seen between men and women when body weight differences were taken into account. There was no significant difference in efficacy noted (as assessed by HbA$_{1c}$) between genders in a trial in patients with type 1 diabetes.
Obesity—A single subcutaneous dose of 0.1 U/kg NovoLog was administered in a study of 23 patients with type 1 diabetes and a wide range of body mass index (BMI, 22-39 kg/m^2). The pharmacokinetic parameters, AUC and C$_{max}$, of NovoLog were generally unaffected by BMI in the different groups – BMI 19-23 kg/m^2 (N=4); BMI

23-27 kg/m^2 (N=7); BMI 27-32 kg/m^2 (N=6) and BMI >32 kg/m^2 (N=6). Clearance of NovoLog was reduced by 28% in patients with BMI >32 kg/m^2 compared to patients with BMI <23 kg/m^2.
Renal Impairment—Some studies with human insulin have shown increased circulating levels of insulin in patients with renal failure. A single subcutaneous dose of 0.08 U/kg NovoLog was administered in a study to subjects with either normal (N=6) creatinine clearance (CLcr) (> 80 ml/min) or mild (N=7; CLcr = 50-80 ml/min), moderate (N=3; CLcr = 30-50 ml/min) or severe (but not requiring hemodialysis) (N=2; CLcr = <30 ml/min) renal impairment. In this small study, there was no apparent effect of creatinine clearance values on AUC and C$_{max}$ of NovoLog. Careful glucose mon-

itoring and dose adjustments of insulin, including NovoLog, may be necessary in patients with renal dysfunction [*see Warnings and Precautions (5.4)*].
Hepatic Impairment—Some studies with human insulin have shown increased circulating levels of insulin in patients with liver failure. A single subcutaneous dose of 0.06 U/kg NovoLog was administered in an open-label, single-dose study of 24 subjects (N=6/group) with different degree of hepatic impairment (mild, moderate and severe) having Child-Pugh Scores ranging from 0 (healthy volunteers) to 12 (severe hepatic impairment). In this small study, there was no correlation between the degree of hepatic failure and any NovoLog pharmacokinetic parameter. Careful glucose monitoring and dose adjustments of insulin, including NovoLog, may be necessary in patients with hepatic dysfunction [*see Warnings and Precautions (5.5)*].
The effect of age, ethnic origin, pregnancy and smoking on the pharmacokinetics and pharmacodynamics of NovoLog has not been studied.

13 NONCLINICAL TOXICOLOGY
13.1 Carcinogenesis, Mutagenesis, Impairment of Fertility
Standard 2-year carcinogenicity studies in animals have not been performed to evaluate the carcinogenic potential of NovoLog. In 52-week studies, Sprague-Dawley rats were dosed subcutaneously with NovoLog at 10, 50, and 200 U/kg/day (approximately 2, 8, and 32 times the human subcutaneous dose of 1.0 U/kg/day, based on U/body surface area, respectively). At a dose of 200 U/kg/day, NovoLog increased the incidence of mammary gland tumors in females when compared to untreated controls. The incidence of mammary tumors for NovoLog was not significantly different than for regular human insulin. The relevance of these findings to humans is not known. NovoLog was not genotoxic in the following tests: Ames test, mouse lymphoma cell forward gene mutation test, human peripheral blood lymphocyte chromosome aberration test, *in vivo* micronucleus test in mice, and in *ex vivo* UDS test in rat liver hepatocytes. In fertility studies in male and female rats, at subcutaneous doses up to 200 U/kg/day (approximately 32 times the human subcutaneous dose, based on U/body surface area), no direct adverse effects on male and female fertility, or general reproductive performance of animals was observed.
13.2 Animal Toxicology and/or Pharmacology
In standard biological assays in mice and rabbits, one unit of NovoLog has the same glucose-lowering effect as one unit of regular human insulin. In humans, the effect of NovoLog is more rapid in onset and of shorter duration, compared to regular human insulin, due to its faster absorption after subcutaneous injection (see *Section 12 CLINICAL PHARMACOLOGY* Figure 2 and Figure 4).

14 CLINICAL STUDIES
14.1 Subcutaneous Daily Injections
Two six-month, open-label, active-controlled studies were conducted to compare the safety and efficacy of NovoLog to Novolin R in adult patients with type 1 diabetes. Because the two study designs and results were similar, data are shown for only one study (see Table 3). NovoLog was administered by subcutaneous injection immediately prior to meals and regular human insulin was administered by subcutaneous injection 30 minutes before meals. NPH insulin was administered as the basal insulin in either single or divided daily doses. Changes in HbA$_{1c}$ and the incidence rates of severe hypoglycemia (as determined from the number of events requiring intervention from a third party) were comparable for the two treatment regimens in this study (Table 3) as well as in the other clinical studies that are cited in this section. Diabetic ketoacidosis was not reported in any of the adult studies in either treatment group.
[See table 3 above]
A 24-week, parallel-group study of children and adolescents with type 1 diabetes (n = 283) aged 6 to 18 years compared two subcutaneous multiple-dose treatment regimens: NovoLog (n = 187) or Novolin R (n = 96). NPH insulin was administered as the basal insulin. NovoLog achieved glycemic control comparable to Novolin R, as measured by change in HbA$_{1c}$ (Table 4) and both treatment groups had a comparable incidence of hypoglycemia. Subcutaneous administration of NovoLog and regular human insulin have also been compared in children with type 1 diabetes (n=26) aged 2 to 6 years with similar effects on HbA$_{1c}$ and hypoglycemia.
[See table 4 above]
One six-month, open-label, active-controlled study was conducted to compare the safety and efficacy of NovoLog to Novolin R in patients with type 2 diabetes (Table 5). NovoLog was administered by subcutaneous injection immediately prior to meals and regular human insulin was administered by subcutaneous injection 30 minutes before meals. NPH insulin was administered as the basal insulin in either single or divided daily doses. Changes in HbA$_{1c}$ and the rates of severe hypoglycemia (as determined from the number of events requiring intervention from a third party) were comparable for the two treatment regimens.
[See table 5 above]

14.2 Continuous Subcutaneous Insulin Infusion (CSII) by External Pump

Two open-label, parallel design studies (6 weeks [n=29] and 16 weeks [n=118]) compared NovoLog to buffered regular human insulin (Velosulin) in adults with type 1 diabetes receiving a subcutaneous infusion with an external insulin pump. The two treatment regimens had comparable changes in HbA_{1c} and rates of severe hypoglycemia.

[See table 6 at right]

A randomized, 16-week, open-label, parallel design study of children and adolescents with type 1 diabetes (n=298) aged 4-18 years compared two subcutaneous infusion regimens administered via an external insulin pump: NovoLog (n=198) or insulin lispro (n=100). These two treatments resulted in comparable changes from baseline in HbA_{1c} and comparable rates of hypoglycemia after 16 weeks of treatment (see Table 7).

[See table 7 at right]

An open-label, 16-week parallel design trial compared preprandial NovoLog injection in conjunction with NPH injections to NovoLog administered by continuous subcutaneous infusion in 127 adults with type 2 diabetes. The two treatment groups had similar reductions in HbA_{1c} and rates of severe hypoglycemia (Table 8) [see *Indications and Usage (1), Dosage and Administration (2), Warnings and Precautions (5) and How Supplied/Storage and Handling (16.2)*].

[See table 8 at right]

14.3 Intravenous Administration of NovoLog

See Section 12.2 *CLINICAL PHARMACOLOGY/Pharmacodynamics.*

16 HOW SUPPLIED/STORAGE AND HANDLING

16.1 How Supplied

NovoLog is available in the following package sizes: each presentation containing 100 Units of insulin aspart per mL (U-100).

10 mL vials	NDC 0169-7501-11
3 mL PenFill cartridges*	NDC 0169-3303-12
3 mL NovoLog FlexPen	NDC 0169-6339-10

* NovoLog PenFill cartridges are designed for use with Novo Nordisk 3 mL PenFill cartridge compatible insulin delivery devices (with or without the addition of a NovoPen 3 PenMate) with NovoFine disposable needles.

16.2 Recommended Storage

Unused NovoLog should be stored in a refrigerator between 2° and 8°C (36° to 46°F). Do not store in the freezer or directly adjacent to the refrigerator cooling element. **Do not freeze NovoLog and do not use NovoLog if it has been frozen.** NovoLog should not be drawn into a syringe and stored for later use.

Vials: After initial use a vial may be kept at temperatures below 30°C (86°F) for up to 28 days, but should not be exposed to excessive heat or sunlight. Opened vials may be refrigerated.

Unpunctured vials can be used until the expiration date printed on the label if they are stored in a refrigerator. Keep unused vials in the carton so they will stay clean and protected from light.

PenFill cartridges or NovoLog FlexPen:

Once a cartridge or a NovoLog FlexPen is punctured, it should be kept at temperatures below 30°C (86°F) for up to 28 days, but should not be exposed to excessive heat or sunlight. A NovoLog FlexPen or cartridge in use must NOT be stored in the refrigerator. Keep the NovoLog FlexPen and all PenFill cartridges away from direct heat and sunlight. Unpunctured NovoLog FlexPen and PenFill cartridges can be used until the expiration date printed on the label if they are stored in a refrigerator. Keep unused NovoLog FlexPen and PenFill cartridges in the carton so they will stay clean and protected from light.

Always remove the needle after each injection and store the 3 mL PenFill cartridge delivery device or NovoLog FlexPen without a needle attached. This prevents contamination and/or infection, or leakage of insulin, and will ensure accurate dosing. Always use a new needle for each injection to prevent contamination.

Pump:

NovoLog in the pump reservoir should be discarded after at least every 6 days of use or after exposure to temperatures that exceed 37°C (98.6°F). The infusion set and the infusion set insertion site should be changed at least every 3 days.

Summary of Storage Conditions:

The storage conditions are summarized in the following table:

[See table 9 at top of next page]

Table 6. Adult Insulin Pump Study in Type 1 Diabetes (16 weeks; n=118)

	NovoLog	Buffered human insulin
N	59	59
Baseline HbA$_{1c}$ (%)*	7.3 ± 0.7	7.5 ± 0.8
Change from Baseline HbA$_{1c}$ (%)	0.0 ± 0.5	0.2 ± 0.6
Treatment Difference in HbA$_{1c}$, Mean (95% confidence interval)	0.3 (-0.1, 0.4)	
Baseline insulin dose (IU/kg/24 hours)*	0.7 ± 0.8	0.6 ± 0.2
End-of-Study insulin dose (IU/kg/24 hours)*	0.7 ± 0.7	0.6 ± 0.2
Patients with severe hypoglycemia (n, %)†	1 (2%)	2 (3%)
Baseline body weight (kg)*	77.4 ± 16.1	74.8 ± 13.8
Weight Change from baseline (kg)*	0.1 ± 3.5	-0.0 ± 1.7

* Values are Mean ± SD
† Severe hypoglycemia refers to hypoglycemia associated with central nervous system symptoms and requiring the intervention of another person or hospitalization.

Table 7. Pediatric Insulin Pump Study in Type 1 Diabetes (16 weeks; n=298)

	NovoLog	Lispro
N	198	100
Baseline HbA$_{1c}$ (%)*	8.0 ± 0.9	8.2 ± 0.8
Change from Baseline HbA$_{1c}$ (%)	-0.1 ± 0.8	-0.1 ± 0.7
Treatment Difference in HbA$_{1c}$, Mean (95% confidence interval)	-0.1 (-0.3, 0.1)	
Baseline insulin dose (IU/kg/24 hours)*	0.9 ± 0.3	0.9 ± 0.3
End-of-Study insulin dose (IU/kg/24 hours)*	0.9 ± 0.2	0.9 ± 0.2
Patients with severe hypoglycemia (n, %)†	19 (10%)	8 (8%)
Diabetic ketoacidosis (n, %)	1 (0.5%)	0 (0)
Baseline body weight (kg)*	54.1 ± 19.7	55.5 ± 19.0
Weight Change from baseline (kg)*	1.8 ± 2.1	1.6 ± 2.1

* Values are Mean ± SD
† Severe hypoglycemia refers to hypoglycemia associated with central nervous system symptoms and requiring the intervention of another person or hospitalization.

Table 8. Pump Therapy in Type 2 Diabetes (16 weeks; n=127)

	NovoLog pump	NovoLog + NPH
N	66	61
Baseline HbA$_{1c}$ (%)*	8.2 ± 1.4	8.0 ± 1.1
Change from Baseline HbA$_{1c}$ (%)	-0.6 ± 1.1	-0.5 ± 0.9
Treatment Difference in HbA$_{1c}$, Mean (95% confidence interval)	0.1 (0.4, 0.3)	
Baseline insulin dose (IU/kg/24 hours)*	0.7 ± 0.3	0.8 ± 0.5
End-of-Study insulin dose (IU/kg/24 hours)*	0.9 ± 0.4	0.9 ± 0.5
Baseline body weight (kg)*	96.4 ± 17.0	96.9 ± 17.9
Weight Change from baseline (kg)*	1.7 ± 3.7	0.7 ± 4.1

* Values are Mean ± SD

Storage of Diluted NovoLog

NovoLog diluted with Insulin Diluting Medium for NovoLog to a concentration equivalent to U-10 or equivalent to U-50 may remain in patient use at temperatures below 30°C (86°F) for 28 days.

Storage of NovoLog in Infusion Fluids

Infusion bags prepared as indicated under *Dosage and Administration (2)* are stable at room temperature for 24 hours. Some insulin will be initially adsorbed to the material of the infusion bag.

17 PATIENT COUNSELING INFORMATION

[See *FDA-Approved Patient Labeling (17.3)*]

17.1 Physician Instructions

Maintenance of normal or near-normal glucose control is a treatment goal in diabetes mellitus and has been associated with a reduction in diabetic complications. Patients should be informed about potential risks and benefits of NovoLog therapy including the possible adverse reactions. Patients should also be offered continued education and advice on insulin therapies, injection technique, life-style management, regular glucose monitoring, periodic glycosylated hemoglobin testing, recognition and management of hypo- and hyperglycemia, adherence to meal planning, complications of insulin therapy, timing of dose, instruction in the use of injection or subcutaneous infusion devices, and proper storage of insulin. Patients should be informed that frequent, patient-performed blood glucose measurements are needed to achieve optimal glycemic control and avoid both hyper- and hypoglycemia.

The patient's ability to concentrate and react may be impaired as a result of hypoglycemia. This may present a risk in situations where these abilities are especially important, such as driving or operating other machinery. Patients who have frequent hypoglycemia or reduced or absent warning signs of hypoglycemia should be advised to use caution when driving or operating machinery.

Table 9. Storage conditions for vial, PenFill cartridges and NovoLog FlexPen

NovoLog presentation	Not in-use (unopened) Room Temperature (below 30°C)	Not in-use (unopened) Refrigerated	In-use (opened) Room Temperature (below 30°C)
10 mL vial	28 days	Until expiration date	28 days (refrigerated/room temperature)
3 mL PenFill cartridges	28 days	Until expiration date	28 days (Do not refrigerate)
3 mL NovoLog FlexPen	28 days	Until expiration date	28 days (Do not refrigerate)

Accidental substitutions between NovoLog and other insulin products have been reported. Patients should be instructed to always carefully check that they are administering the appropriate insulin to avoid medication errors between NovoLog and any other insulin. **The written prescription for NovoLog should be written clearly, to avoid confusion with other insulin products, for example, NovoLog Mix 70/30.**

17.2   Patients Using Pumps
Patients using external pump infusion therapy should be trained in intensive insulin therapy with multiple injections and in the function of their pump and pump accessories. The following insulin pumps† have been used in NovoLog clinical or *in vitro* studies conducted by Novo Nordisk, the manufacturer of NovoLog:
- Medtronic Paradigm® 512 and 712
- MiniMed 508
- Disetronic® D-TRON® and H-TRON®

Before using another insulin pump with NovoLog, read the pump label to make sure the pump has been evaluated with NovoLog.
NovoLog is recommended for use in any reservoir and infusion sets that are compatible with insulin and the specific pump. Please see recommended reservoir and infusion sets in the pump manual.
To avoid insulin degradation, infusion set occlusion, and loss of the preservative (metacresol), insulin in the reservoir should be replaced at least every 6 days; infusion sets and infusion set insertion sites should be changed at least every 3 days.
Insulin exposed to temperatures higher than 37°C (98.6°F) should be discarded. The temperature of the insulin may exceed ambient temperature when the pump housing, cover, tubing, or sport case is exposed to sunlight or radiant heat. Infusion sites that are erythematous, pruritic, or thickened should be reported to medical personnel, and a new site selected because continued infusion may increase the skin reaction and/or alter the absorption of NovoLog. Pump or infusion set malfunctions or insulin degradation can lead to hyperglycemia and ketosis in a short time because of the small subcutaneous depot of insulin. This is especially pertinent for rapid-acting insulin analogs that are more rapidly absorbed through skin and have shorter duration of action. These differences are particularly relevant when patients are switched from multiple injection therapy. Prompt identification and correction of the cause of hyperglycemia or ketosis is necessary. Problems include pump malfunction, infusion set occlusion, leakage, disconnection or kinking, and degraded insulin. Less commonly, hypoglycemia from pump malfunction may occur. If these problems cannot be promptly corrected, patients should resume therapy with subcutaneous insulin injection and contact their physician [*see Dosage and Administration (2), Warnings and Precautions (5) and How Supplied/Storage and Handling (16.2)*].

17.3   FDA Approved Patient Labeling
Date of Issue: March 17, 2010
Version: 17
NovoLog®, NovoPen® 3, PenFill®, Novolin®, FlexPen®, PenMate®, and NovoFine® are registered trademarks of Novo Nordisk A/S.
NovoLog® is covered by US Patent Nos. 5,618,913, 5,866,538, and other patents pending.
FlexPen® is covered by US Patent Nos. 6,582,404, 6,004,297, 6,235,004, and other patents pending.
PenFill® is covered by US Patent No. 5,693,027
†*The brands listed are the registered trademarks of their respective owners and are not trademarks of Novo Nordisk A/S.*
© 2002-2010 Novo Nordisk A/S
Manufactured by:
Novo Nordisk A/S
DK-2880 Bagsvaerd, Denmark
For information about NovoLog contact:
Novo Nordisk Inc.
Princeton, New Jersey 08540
1-800-727-6500
www.novonordisk-us.com

PATIENT INFORMATION
NovoLog® (NŌ-vō-log)
(insulin aspart [rDNA origin] Injection)
Important:
Know your insulin. Do not change the type of insulin you use unless told to do so by your healthcare provider. The amount of insulin you take as well as the best time for you to take your insulin may need to change if you take a different type of insulin.
Make sure you know the type and strength of insulin prescribed for you.
Read the Patient Information that comes with NovoLog before you start taking it and each time you get a refill. There may be new information. This leaflet does not take the place of talking with your healthcare provider about your diabetes or your treatment. Make sure you know how to manage your diabetes. Ask your healthcare provider if you have any questions about managing your diabetes.

What is NovoLog?
NovoLog is a man-made insulin that is used to control high blood sugar in adults and children with diabetes mellitus.

Who should not use NovoLog?
Do not take NovoLog if:
- Your blood sugar is too low (hypoglycemia).
- You are allergic to anything in NovoLog. See the end of this leaflet for a complete list of ingredients in NovoLog. Check with your healthcare provider if you are not sure.

Tell your healthcare provider:
- **about all of your medical conditions.** Medical conditions can affect your insulin needs and your dose of NovoLog.
- **if you are pregnant or breastfeeding.** You and your healthcare provider should talk about the best way to manage your diabetes while you are pregnant or breastfeeding. NovoLog has not been studied in nursing women.
- **about all medicines you take,** including prescriptions and non-prescription medicines, vitamins and herbal supplements. Your NovoLog dose may change if you take other medicines.

Know the medicines you take. Keep a list of your medicines with you to show your healthcare providers when you get a new medicine.

How should I take NovoLog?
Only use NovoLog if it appears clear and colorless. There may be air bubbles. This is normal. If it looks cloudy, thickened, or colored, or if it contains solid particles do not use it and call Novo Nordisk at 1-800-727-6500.
NovoLog comes in:
- 10 mL vials (small bottles) for use with syringe
- 3 mL PenFill® cartridges for use with the Novo Nordisk 3 mL PenFill cartridge compatible insulin delivery devices and NovoFine® disposable needles. The cartridge delivery device can be used with a NovoPen® 3 PenMate®
- 3 mL NovoLog FlexPen®

Read the instructions for use that come with your NovoLog product. Talk to your healthcare provider if you have any questions. Your healthcare provider should show you how to inject NovoLog before you start taking it.
- **Take NovoLog exactly as prescribed.** You should eat a meal within 5 to 10 minutes after using NovoLog to avoid low blood sugar.
- **NovoLog is a fast-acting insulin.** The effects of NovoLog start working 10 to 20 minutes after injection or bolus pump infusion.
- **Do not inject NovoLog if you do not plan to eat right after your injection or bolus pump infusion.**
- The greatest blood sugar lowering effect is between 1 and 3 hours after the injection or infusion. This blood sugar lowering lasts for 3 to 5 hours.
- **While using NovoLog you may have to change** your total dose of insulin, your dose of longer-acting insulin, or the number of injections of longer-acting insulin you use. Pump users given NovoLog may need to change the amount of total insulin given as a basal infusion.
- **Do not mix NovoLog:**
  - with any other insulins when used in a pump
  - with any insulins other than NPH when used with injections by syringe

If your healthcare provider recommends diluting NovoLog, follow your healthcare provider's instructions exactly so that you know:
- **How to make NovoLog more dilute** (that is, a smaller number of units of NovoLog for a given amount of liquid) and
- **How to use this more dilute form of NovoLog. Do not use dilute insulin in a pump.**
- **Inject NovoLog into the skin of your stomach area, upper arms, buttocks or upper legs.** NovoLog may affect your blood sugar levels sooner if you inject it into the skin of your stomach area. **Never inject NovoLog into a vein or into a muscle.**
- **Change (rotate) your injection site within the chosen area (for example, stomach or upper arm) with each dose. Do not inject into the exact same spot for each injection.**
- **If you take too much NovoLog, your blood sugar may fall low (hypoglycemia).** You can treat mild low blood sugar (hypoglycemia) by drinking or eating something sugary right away (fruit juice, sugar candies, or glucose tablets). It is important to treat low blood sugar (hypoglycemia) right away because it could get worse and you could pass out (become unconscious). If you pass out you will need help from another person or emergency medical services right away, and will need treatment with a glucagon injection or treatment at a hospital. See "What are the possible side effects of NovoLog?" for more information on low blood sugar (hypoglycemia).
- **If you forget to take your dose of NovoLog, your blood sugar may go too high (hyperglycemia).** If high blood sugar (hyperglycemia) is not treated it can lead to serious problems, like loss of consciousness (passing out), coma or even death. Follow your healthcare provider's instructions for treating high blood sugar. Know your symptoms of high blood sugar which may include:

• increased thirst	• fruity smell on the breath
• frequent urination	• high amounts of sugar
• drowsiness	and ketones in your urine
• loss of appetite	• nausea, vomiting (throwing up)
• a hard time	or stomach pain
breathing	

- **Check your blood sugar levels.** Ask your healthcare provider what your blood sugars should be and when you should check your blood sugar levels.

Your insulin dosage may need to change because of:

• illness	• change in diet
• stress	• change in physical
• other medicines you take	activity or exercise

What should I avoid while using NovoLog?
- **Alcohol.** Alcohol, including beer and wine, may affect your blood sugar when you take NovoLog.
- **Driving and operating machinery.** You may have difficulty concentrating or reacting if you have low blood sugar (hypoglycemia). Be careful when you drive a car or operate machinery. Ask your healthcare provider if it is alright to drive if you often have:
  - low blood sugar
  - decreased or no warning signs of low blood sugar

What are the possible side effects of NovoLog?
- **Low blood sugar (hypoglycemia).** Symptoms of low blood sugar may include:

• sweating	• trouble concentrating or confusion
• dizziness or lightheadedness	• blurred vision
• shakiness	• slurred speech
• hunger	• anxiety, irritability or mood changes
• fast heart beat	• headache
• tingling of lips and tongue	

Severe low blood sugar can cause unconsciousness (passing out), seizures, and death. Know your symptoms of low blood sugar. Follow your healthcare provider's instructions for treating low blood sugar. Talk to your healthcare provider if low blood sugar is a problem for you.
- **Serious allergic reaction (whole body reaction). Get medical help right away, if you develop** a rash over your whole body, have trouble breathing, a fast heartbeat, or sweating.

- **Reactions at the injection site (local allergic reaction).** You may get redness, swelling, and itching at the injection site. If you keep having skin reactions or they are serious talk to your healthcare provider. You may need to stop using NovoLog and use a different insulin. Do not inject insulin into skin that is red, swollen, or itchy.
- **Skin thickens or pits at the injection site (lipodystrophy).** Change (rotate) where you inject your insulin to help to prevent these skin changes from happening. Do not inject insulin into this type of skin.
- **Swelling of your hands and feet**
- **Vision changes**
- **Low potassium in your blood (hypokalemia)**
- **Weight gain**

These are not all of the possible side effects from NovoLog. Ask your healthcare provider or pharmacist for more information.

Call your healthcare provider for medical advice about side effects. You may report side effects to FDA at 1-800-FDA-1088.

How should I store NovoLog?

All Unopened NovoLog:

- **Keep all unopened NovoLog in the refrigerator between 36° to 46°F (2° to 8°C).**
- Do not freeze. Do not use NovoLog if it has been frozen.
- Keep unopened NovoLog in the carton to protect from light.

NovoLog in use:

- **Vials**
  - Keep in the refrigerator or at room temperature below 86°F (30°C) for up to 28 days.
  - Keep vials away from direct heat or light.
  - Throw away an opened vial after 28 days of use, even if there is insulin left in the vial.
  - Do not draw up NovoLog into a syringe and store for later use.
  - Unopened vials can be used until the expiration date on the NovoLog label, if the medicine has been stored in a refrigerator.
- **PenFill Cartridges or NovoLog FlexPen**
  - Keep at room temperature below 86°F (30°C) for up to 28 days.
  - Do not store a PenFill cartridge or NovoLog FlexPen that you are using in the refrigerator.
  - Keep PenFill cartridges and NovoLog FlexPen away from direct heat or light.
  - Throw away a used PenFill cartridge or NovoLog FlexPen after 28 days, even if there is insulin left in the cartridge or syringe.
- **NovoLog in the pump reservoir and the complete external pump infusion set**
  - The infusion set and the infusion site should be changed **at least every 3 days**. The insulin in the reservoir should be changed **at least every 6 days** even if you have not used all of the insulin. Change the infusion set and the infusion site more often than every 3 days if you have high blood sugar (hyperglycemia), the pump alarm sounds, or the insulin flow is blocked (occlusion).

General advice about NovoLog

Medicines are sometimes prescribed for conditions that are not mentioned in the patient leaflet. Do not use NovoLog for a condition for which it was not prescribed. Do not give NovoLog to other people, even if they have the same symptoms you have. It may harm them.

This leaflet summarizes the most important information about NovoLog. If you would like more information about NovoLog or diabetes, talk with your healthcare provider. You can ask your healthcare provider or pharmacist for information about NovoLog that is written for healthcare professionals. Call 1-800-727-6500 or visit www.novonordisk-us.com for more information.

Helpful information for people with diabetes is published by the American Diabetes Association, 1701 N Beauregard Street, Alexandria, VA 22311 and on www.diabetes.org.

NovoLog ingredients include:

• insulin aspart	• zinc
• glycerin	• disodium hydrogen phosphate dihydrate
• phenol	• sodium chloride
• metacresol	• water for injection

All NovoLog vials, PenFill cartridges and NovoLog FlexPen are latex free.

Date of Issue: March 17, 2010

Version: 9

NovoLog®, *PenFill*®, *FlexPen*®, *NovoPen*®, *NovoFine*®, *PenMate*®, are registered trademarks of Novo Nordisk A/S.
NovoLog® is covered by US Patent Nos. 5,618,913, 5,866,538, and other patents pending.
FlexPen® is covered by US Patent Nos. 6,582,404, 6,004,297, 6,235,004, and other patents pending.
PenFill® is covered by US Patent No. 5,693,027
© 2002-2010 Novo Nordisk A/S

Manufactured by:
Novo Nordisk A/S
DK-2880 Bagsvaerd, Denmark

For information about NovoLog® contact:
Novo Nordisk Inc.
100 College Road West
Princeton, New Jersey 08540

PATIENT INSTRUCTIONS FOR USE

NovoLog® 10 mL vial (100 Units/mL, U-100)

Before starting, gather all of the supplies that you will need to use for preparing and giving your insulin injection. Never re-use syringes and needles.

How should I use the NovoLog vial?

1. Check to make sure that you have the correct type of insulin. This is especially important if you use different types of insulin.
2. Look at the vial and the insulin. The insulin should be clear and colorless. The tamper-resistant cap should be in place before the first use. If the cap had been removed before your first use of the vial, or if the insulin is cloudy or colored, do not use it and call Novo Nordisk at 1-800-727-6500.
3. Wash your hands with soap and water. If you clean your injection site with an alcohol swab, let the injection site dry before you inject. Talk with your healthcare provider about how to rotate injection sites and how to give an injection.
4. If you are using a new vial, pull off the tamper-resistant cap. Wipe the rubber stopper with an alcohol wipe.
5. Do not roll or shake the vial. Shaking right before the dose is drawn into the syringe may cause bubbles or froth. This can cause you to draw up the wrong dose of insulin.
6. Pull back the plunger on the syringe until the black tip reaches the marking for the number of units you will inject.
7. Push the needle through the rubber stopper of the vial, and push the plunger all the way in to force air into the vial.
8. Turn the vial and syringe upside down and slowly pull the plunger back to a few units beyond correct dose.
9. If there are any air bubbles, tap the syringe gently with your finger to raise the air bubbles to the top. Then slowly push the plunger to the marking for your correct dose. This process should move any air bubbles present in the syringe back into the vial.
10. Check to make sure you have the right dose of NovoLog in the syringe.
11. Pull the syringe out of the vial's rubber stopper.
12. Your doctor should tell you if you need to pinch the skin before inserting the needle. This can vary from patient to patient so it is important to ask your doctor if you did not receive instructions on pinching the skin. Insert the needle into the pinched skin. Press the plunger of the syringe to inject the insulin. When you are finished injecting the insulin, pull the needle out of your skin. You may see a drop of NovoLog at the needle tip. This is normal and has no effect on the dose you just received. If you see blood after you take the needle out of your skin, press the injection site lightly with a piece of gauze or an alcohol wipe. **Do not rub the area.**
13. After your injection, do not recap the needle. Place used syringes, needles and used insulin vials in a disposable puncture-resistant sharps container, or some type of hard plastic or metal container with a screw on cap such as a detergent bottle or coffee can.
14. Ask your healthcare provider about the right way to throw away used syringes and needles. There may be state or local laws about the right way to throw away used syringes and needles. Do not throw away used needles and syringes in household trash or recycle.

How should I mix insulins?

NovoLog should be mixed only when injections with syringes are used. NovoLog can be mixed with NPH human insulin right before use. The NovoLog should be drawn into the syringe before you draw up the NPH insulin. **NovoLog should not be mixed with any other insulin except NPH.**

1. Add together the doses (total number of units) of NPH and NovoLog that you need to inject. The total dose will determine the final amount (volume) in the syringe after drawing up both insulins into the syringe. For example, if you need 5 units of NPH and 2 units of NovoLog, the total dose of insulin in the syringe would be 7 units.
2. Roll the NPH vial between your hands until the liquid is equally cloudy throughout.
3. Draw into the syringe the same amount of air as the NPH dose. Inject this air into the NPH vial and then remove the needle from the vial but do not withdraw any of the NPH insulin. (Transferring NPH to the NovoLog vial will contaminate the NovoLog vial and may change how quickly it works.)
4. Draw into the syringe the same amount of air as the NovoLog dose. Inject this air into the NovoLog vial. With the needle in place, turn the vial upside down and withdraw the correct dose of NovoLog. The tip of the needle must be in the NovoLog to get the full dose and not an air dose.
5. After withdrawing the needle from the NovoLog vial, insert the needle into the NPH vial. Turn the NPH vial upside down with the syringe and needle still in it. Withdraw the correct dose of NPH.
6. Inject right away to avoid changes in how quickly the insulin works.

How do I use NovoLog in a pump?

- Checking your blood sugar is very important for patients using pumps. Pump or infusion set problems can result in you not getting enough insulin. This can quickly cause you to have high blood sugar and diabetic ketoacidosis.
- Use insulin from a new vial of NovoLog if unexplained high blood sugar or pump alarms do not respond to all of the following:
  - a repeat dose (injection or bolus) of NovoLog
  - a change in the infusion set, including the NovoLog in the reservoir
  - a change in the infusion site
- If these measures do not work, you may need to go back to injecting NovoLog with syringes, or insulin pens. Continue to monitor your blood sugars and ketones. If problems continue, you must contact your healthcare provider.
- When NovoLog is used in pumps, **use only pumps that are recommended by your healthcare provider.** The infusion set and infusion site should be changed at least every 3 days. The insulin in the reservoir should be changed at least every 6 days even if you have not used all of the insulin. The reservoir, the infusion set, and infusion site should also be changed:
  - with unexpected high blood sugar
  - when the alarm sounds (see your pump manual)
  - if the insulin or pump has been exposed to temperatures over 98.6°F (37°C), such as in a sauna, with long showers, or on an unusually hot day.
  - if the insulin or pump could have absorbed heat, for example from sunlight, that would heat the insulin to over 98.6°F (37°C). Dark colored pump cases or sport covers can increase this type of heat. The location where the pump is worn may also affect the temperature

Patients who develop local skin reactions may need to change infusion sites more often than every 3 days.

Use only insulin pumps that have been specially tested with NovoLog. Follow your healthcare provider or pharmacist instructions for which insulin pumps may be used.

Check with your healthcare provider or pharmacist to see if your pump and infusion set can be used with NovoLog.

1. Check to make sure that you have the right type of insulin.
2. Look at the vial and insulin. The insulin should be clear and colorless. The tamper-resistant cap should be in place before the first use. If the cap had been removed before your first use, or if the insulin is cloudy or colored, do not use it and call Novo Nordisk at 1-800-727-6500.
3. Wash your hands with soap and water.
4. Fill the reservoir-syringe with 2 days worth of NovoLog plus about 25 extra units to prime the pump and the infusion tubing.
5. Remove air bubbles from the reservoir by following the pump manufacturers' instructions.
6. Attach the infusion set to the reservoir. Make sure the connection is tight. Prime the infusion set until you see a drop of insulin coming out of the infusion needle-catheter. Follow the pump manufacturers' instructions for priming and removing air bubbles.
7. Clean your insertion site with an alcohol swab and let the site dry before you insert the needle-catheter. Talk with your healthcare provider about how to rotate insertion sites and how to insert the needle-catheter into the skin.
8. Insert the needle-catheter into the skin, remove the needle and prime the catheter according to the pump manufacturers' instructions. Do not insert the needle-catheter into skin that is reddened, itchy, bumpy, or thickened.
9. Program the pump for mealtime NovoLog boluses and NovoLog basal insulin infusion according to instructions from your healthcare provider and the manufacturer of your pump equipment.
10. Change the infusion site and infusion set at least every 3 days, and change the insulin in the reservoir at least every 6 days even if you have not used all of the insulin. This will help ensure that NovoLog and the pump work well.
11. Change the infusion site, the infusion set, the insulin reservoir and the insulin if you experience a pump alarm, catheter blockage, high blood sugars, or if your pump insulin has been exposed to heat greater than 98.6° F (37° C).
12. If you have high blood sugar (hyperglycemia) when you check your blood sugar, this may be the first sign of a problem with the pump, infusion set, or NovoLog. If you have high blood sugar without a pump alarm, you must still check the pump because alarms may not detect all the changes to NovoLog that could result in high blood sugar. You may need to start insulin injections with syringes if the

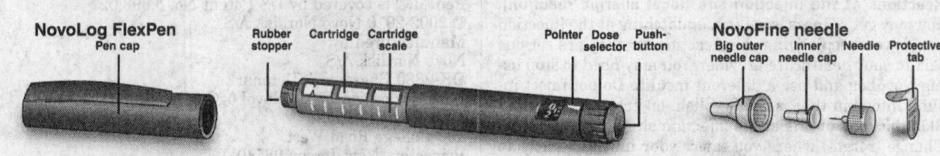

NovoLog FlexPen — Pen cap · Rubber stopper · Cartridge · Cartridge scale · Pointer · Dose selector · Push-button

NovoFine needle — Big outer needle cap · Inner needle cap · Needle · Protective tab

cause of the problem cannot be found quickly or fixed. Long lengths of infusion-set tubing increase the risk for kinking and expose the insulin in the tubing to more changes in temperature.

PATIENT INSTRUCTIONS FOR USE
NovoLog® 3 mL PenFill® cartridge (100 Units/mL, U-100)
Before using the NovoLog cartridge

1. Talk with your healthcare provider for information about where to inject NovoLog (injection sites) and how to give an injection with your insulin delivery device.
2. Read the instruction manual that comes with your insulin delivery device for complete instructions on how to use the PenFill cartridge with the device.

How to use the NovoLog cartridge

1. **Check your insulin.** Just before using your NovoLog cartridge, check to make sure that you have the right type of insulin. This is especially important if you use different types of insulin.
2. **Carefully look at the cartridge and the insulin inside it.** The insulin should be clear and colorless. The tamper-resistant foil should be in place before the first use. If the foil has been broken or removed before your first use of the cartridge, or if the insulin is cloudy or colored, do not use it. Call Novo Nordisk at 1-800-727-6500.
3. **Wash your hands** well with soap and water. If you clean your injection site with an alcohol swab, let the injection site dry before you inject. Talk with your healthcare provider for guidance on injection sites and how to give an injection with your insulin delivery device.
4. Gather your supplies for injecting NovoLog.
5. Insert a 3 mL cartridge into your Novo Nordisk 3 mL PenFill cartridge compatible insulin delivery device. Wipe the front rubber stopper of the 3 mL PenFill cartridge with an alcohol swab, then screw on a new needle. For NovoFine needles, remove the big outer needle cap and the inner needle cap. Always use a new needle for each injection to prevent infection.

Giving the airshot before each injection:

To prevent the injection of air and to make sure insulin is delivered, you must do an air shot before each injection. Hold the device with the needle pointing up and gently tap the PenFill® cartridge holder with your finger a few times to raise any air bubbles to the top of the cartridge. Do the air shot as described in the device instruction manual.

Giving the injection

6. Dial the number of units on the insulin delivery device that you need to inject. Inject the right way as shown to you by your healthcare provider.
7. Insert the needle into the skin. Inject the dose by pressing the push button all the way in. Keep the needle in the skin for at least 6 seconds, and keep the push button pressed all the way in until the needle has been pulled out from the skin. This will make sure that the full dose has been given. You may see a drop of NovoLog at the needle tip. This is normal and has no effect on the dose you just received. If blood appears after you take the needle out of your skin, press the injection site lightly with a finger. **Do not rub the area.**

After the injection

8. **Do not recap the needle.** Recapping can lead to a needle stick injury.
9. Remove the needle from the PenFill cartridge after each injection. Keep the 3 mL PenFill cartridge in the insulin delivery device. The needle should not be attached to the 3 mL PenFill cartridge during storage. This will prevent infection or leakage of insulin and will help ensure that you receive the right dose of NovoLog.
10. Put the used needle and cartridge in a sharps container, or some type of hard plastic or metal container with a screw on top such as a detergent bottle or coffee can. Check with your doctor about the right way to throw away used needles and cartridges. There may be local or state laws about how to throw away used needles and syringes. Do not throw used needles and cartridges in household trash or recycling bins.
11. Put the pen cap back on the Novo Nordisk 3 mL PenFill cartridge compatible insulin delivery device.

PATIENT INSTRUCTIONS FOR USE
NovoLog® FlexPen®
Introduction

Please read the following instructions carefully before using your NovoLog® FlexPen®.

NovoLog FlexPen is a disposable dial-a-dose insulin pen. You can select doses from 1 to 60 units in increments of 1 unit. NovoLog FlexPen is designed to be used with NovoFine® needles.

Δ NovoLog FlexPen should not be used by people who are blind or have severe visual problems without the help of a person who has good eyesight and who is trained to use the NovoLog FlexPen the right way.

Getting ready

Make sure you have the following items:
• NovoLog FlexPen
• New NovoFine needle
• Alcohol swab

[See figure above]
Preparing Your NovoLog FlexPen

Wash your hands with soap and water. Before you start to prepare your injection, check the label to make sure that you are taking the right type of insulin. This is especially important if you take more than 1 type of insulin. NovoLog should look clear.

A. Pull off the pen cap (see diagram A).

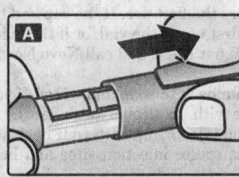

Wipe the rubber stopper with an alcohol swab.
B. Attaching the needle

Remove the protective tab from a disposable needle. Screw the needle tightly onto your FlexPen. It is important that the needle is put on straight (see diagram B).

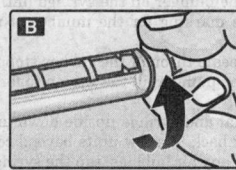

Never place a disposable needle on your NovoLog FlexPen until you are ready to take your injection.
C. Pull off the big outer needle cap (see diagram C).

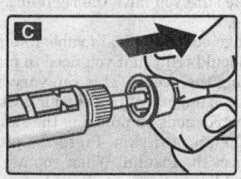

D. Pull off the inner needle cap and dispose of it (see diagram D).
Δ Always use a new needle for each injection to help ensure sterility and prevent blocked needles.
Δ Be careful not to bend or damage the needle before use.
Δ To reduce the risk of unexpected needle sticks, never put the inner needle cap back on the needle.

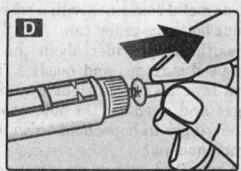

Giving the airshot before each injection

Before each injection small amounts of air may collect in the cartridge during normal use. To avoid injecting air and to ensure proper dosing:
E. Turn the dose selector to select 2 units (see diagram E).
[See figure at top of next column]
F. Hold your NovoLog FlexPen with the needle pointing up. Tap the cartridge gently with your finger a few times to make any air bubbles collect at the top of the cartridge (see diagram F).

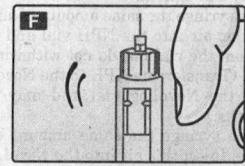

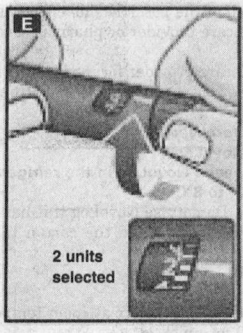

2 units selected

G. Keep the needle pointing upwards, press the push-button all the way in (see diagram G). The dose selector returns to 0.

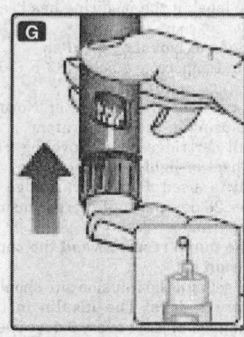

A drop of insulin should appear at the needle tip. If not, change the needle and repeat the procedure no more than 6 times.

If you do not see a drop of insulin after 6 times, do not use the NovoLog FlexPen and contact Novo Nordisk at 1-800-727-6500.

A small air bubble may remain at the needle tip, but it will not be injected.

Selecting your dose

Check and make sure that the dose selector is set at 0.
H. Turn the dose selector to the number of units you need to inject. The pointer should line up with your dose.

The dose can be corrected either up or down by turning the dose selector in either direction until the correct dose lines up with the pointer (see diagram H). When turning the dose selector, be careful not to press the push-button as insulin will come out.
[See figure at top of next column]
You cannot select a dose larger than the number of units left in the cartridge.

You will hear a click for every single unit dialed. Do not set the dose by counting the number of clicks you hear.
Δ Do not use the cartridge scale printed on the cartridge to measure your dose of insulin.

Giving the injection

Do the injection exactly as shown to you by your healthcare provider. Your healthcare provider should tell you if you need to pinch the skin before injecting.
I. Insert the needle into your skin.
Inject the dose by pressing the push-button all the way in until the 0 lines up with the pointer (see diagram I). Be careful only to push the button when injecting.
[See figure H on next column]
Turning the dose selector will not inject insulin.
J. Keep the needle in the skin for at least 6 seconds, and keep the push-button pressed all the way in until the needle has been pulled out from the skin (see diagram J). This will make sure that the full dose has been given.

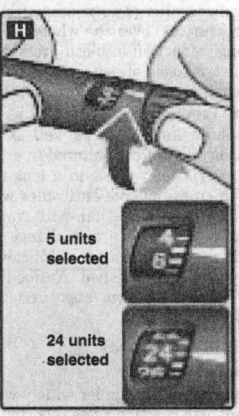

5 units selected

24 units selected

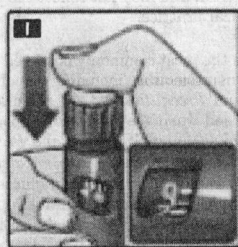

You may see a drop of NovoLog at the needle tip. This is normal and has no effect on the dose you just received. If blood appears after you take the needle out of your skin, press the injection site lightly with a finger. **Do not rub the area.**

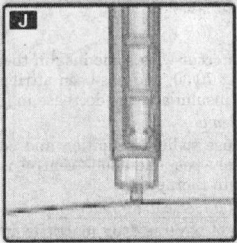

After the injection
Do not recap the needle. Recapping can lead to a needle stick injury. Remove the needle from the NovoLog FlexPen after each injection. This helps to prevent infection, leakage of insulin, and will help to make sure you inject the right dose of insulin.
Δ Put the needle and any empty NovoLog FlexPen or any used NovoLog FlexPen still containing insulin in a sharps container or some type of hard plastic or metal container with a screw top such as a detergent bottle or empty coffee can. These containers should be sealed and thrown away the right way. Check with your healthcare provider about the right way to throw away used syringes and needles. There may be local or state laws about how to throw away used needles and syringes. Do not throw away used needles and syringes in household trash or recycling bins.
The NovoLog FlexPen prevents the cartridge from being completely emptied. It is designed to deliver 300 units.
K. Put the pen cap on the NovoLog FlexPen and store the NovoLog FlexPen without the needle attached (see diagram K).

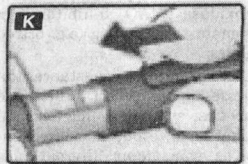

Function Check
L. If your NovoLog FlexPen is not working the right way, follow the steps below:
• Screw on a new NovoFine needle.
• Remove the big outer needle cap and the inner needle cap.
• Do an airshot as described in "Giving the airshot before each injection".
• Put the big outer needle cap onto the needle. Do not put on the inner needle cap.
• Turn the dose selector so the dose indicator window shows 20 units.
• Hold the NovoLog FlexPen so the needle is pointing down.
• Press the push-button all the way in.
The insulin should fill the lower part of the big outer needle cap (see diagram L). If the NovoLog FlexPen has released too much or too little insulin, do the function check again. If the same problem happens again, do not use your NovoLog FlexPen and contact Novo Nordisk at 1-800-727-6500.

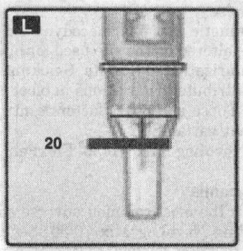

20

Maintenance
Your FlexPen is designed to work accurately and safely. It must be handled with care. Avoid dropping your FlexPen as it may damage it. If you are concerned that your FlexPen is damaged, use a new one. You can clean the outside of your FlexPen by wiping it with a damp cloth. Do not soak or wash your FlexPen as it may damage it. Do not refill your FlexPen.
Δ Remove the needle from the NovoLog FlexPen after each injection. This helps to ensure sterility, prevent leakage of insulin, and will help to make sure you inject the right dose of insulin for future injections.
Δ Be careful when handling used needles to avoid needle sticks and transfer of infectious diseases.
Δ Keep your NovoLog FlexPen and needles out of the reach of children.
Δ Use NovoLog FlexPen as directed to treat your diabetes. Needles and NovoLog FlexPen must not be shared.
Δ Always use a new needle for each injection.
Δ Novo Nordisk is not responsible for harm due to using this insulin pen with products not recommended by Novo Nordisk.
Δ As a precautionary measure, always carry a spare insulin delivery device in case your NovoLog FlexPen is lost or damaged.
Δ Remember to keep the disposable NovoLog FlexPen with you. Do not leave it in a car or other location where it can get too hot or too cold.

NOVOLOG® MIX 70/30   ℞
[*NO-vō-log-MIX-SEV-en-tee-THIR-tee*]
(70% insulin aspart protaminesuspension and 30% insulin aspart injection, [rDNA origin])
Suspension for subcutaneous injection

HIGHLIGHTS OF PRESCRIBING INFORMATION
These highlights do not include all the information needed to use NovoLog Mix 70/30 safely and effectively. See full prescribing information for NovoLog Mix 70/30.
NovoLog® Mix 70/30 **(70% insulin aspart protamine suspension and 30% insulin aspart injection, [rDNA origin]) Suspension for subcutaneous injection**
Initial U.S. Approval: 2001
————————RECENT MAJOR CHANGES————————
• Indications and Usage (1) 5/2010
• Dosage and Administration (2.1) 5/2010
————————INDICATIONS AND USAGE————————
NovoLog Mix 70/30 is an insulin analog indicated to improve glycemic control in patients with diabetes mellitus.
Important Limitations of Use: In premix insulins, such as NovoLog Mix 70/30, the proportions of rapid acting and long acting insulins are fixed and do not allow for basal versus prandial dose adjustments (1).
————————DOSAGE AND ADMINISTRATION————————
• Only for subcutaneous injection (2.1)
Type 1 DM: dose within 15 minutes before meal initiation.

Type 2 DM: dose within 15 minutes before or after starting a meal.
• Do not administer intravenously (2.1).
• Do not use in insulin infusion pumps (2.1).
• Must be resuspended immediately before use (2.2).
————————DOSAGE FORMS AND STRENGTHS————————
Each presentation contains 100 Units of insulin aspart per mL (U-100) (3)
• 10 mL vials
• 3 mL NovoLog Mix 70/30 FlexPen
————————CONTRAINDICATIONS————————
• Do not use during episodes of hypoglycemia (4).
• Do not use in patients with hypersensitivity to NovoLog Mix 70/30 or one of its excipients (4).
————————WARNINGS AND PRECAUTIONS————————
• NovoLog Mix 70/30 should not be mixed with any other insulin product (5.1).
• Hypoglycemia is the most common adverse effect of insulin therapy. Glucose monitoring is recommended for all patients with diabetes. Any change of insulin dose should be made cautiously and only under medical supervision (5.1,5.2).
• Insulin, particularly when given in settings of poor glycemic control, can cause hypokalemia. Use caution in patients predisposed to hypokalemia (5.3).
• Like all insulins, NovoLog Mix 70/30 requirements may be reduced in patients with renal impairment or hepatic impairment (5.4, 5.5).
• Severe, life-threatening, generalized allergy, including anaphylaxis, may occur with insulin products, including NovoLog Mix 70/30 (5.6).
————————ADVERSE REACTIONS————————
Adverse reactions observed with insulin therapy include hypoglycemia, allergic reactions, local injection site reactions, lipodystrophy, rash and pruritus (6).
To report SUSPECTED ADVERSE REACTIONS, contact Novo Nordisk Inc. at 1-800-727-6500 or FDA at 1-800-FDA-1088 or www.fda.gov/medwatch
————————DRUG INTERACTIONS————————
• The following may increase the blood glucose lowering effect and susceptibility to hypoglycemia: oral antidiabetic products, pramlintide, ACE inhibitors, disopyramide, fibrates, fluoxetine, monoamine oxidase (MAO) inhibitors, propoxyphene, salicylates, somatostatin analog (e.g. octreotide), sulfonamide antibiotics (7).
• The following may reduce the blood-glucose-lowering effect: corticosteroids, niacin, danazol, diuretics, sympathomimetic agents (e.g., epinephrine, salbutamol, terbutaline), isoniazid, phenothiazine derivatives, somatropin, thyroid hormones, estrogens, progestogens (e.g., in oral contraceptives), atypical antipsychotics (7).
• Beta-blockers, clonidine, lithium salts, and alcohol may either potentiate or weaken the blood-glucose-lowering effect of insulin (7).
• Pentamidine may cause hypoglycemia, which may be followed by hyperglycemia (7).
• The signs of hypoglycemia may be reduced or absent in patients taking sympatholytic products such as beta-blockers, clonidine, guanethidine, and reserpine (7).
See 17 for PATIENT COUNSELING INFORMATION and FDA-approved patient labeling

Revised: 05/2010

15 REFERENCES
16 HOW SUPPLIED/STORAGE AND HANDLING
 16.1 How Supplied
 16.2 Recommended Storage
17 PATIENT COUNSELING INFORMATION
 17.1 Physician Instructions
PATIENT INFORMATION
 General advice about NovoLog® Mix 70/30
* Sections or subsections omitted from the full prescribing information are not listed

---

FULL PRESCRIBING INFORMATION

1 INDICATIONS AND USAGE

NovoLog Mix 70/30 is an insulin analog indicated to improve glycemic control in patients with diabetes mellitus.
Important Limitations of Use:
In premix insulins, such as Novolog Mix 70/30, the proportions of rapid acting and long acting insulins are fixed and do not allow for basal versus prandial dose adjustments.

2 DOSAGE AND ADMINISTRATION
2.1 Dosing
NovoLog Mix 70/30 is an insulin analog with an earlier onset and intermediate duration of action in comparison to the basal human insulin premix. The addition of protamine to the rapid-acting aspart insulin analog (NovoLog) results in insulin activity that is 30% short-acting and 70% long-acting. NovoLog Mix 70/30 is typically dosed on a twice-daily basis (with each dose intended to cover 2 meals or a meal and a snack). The dosage of NovoLog Mix 70/30 must be individualized. The written prescription for NovoLog Mix 70/30 should include the full name, to avoid confusion with NovoLog (insulin aspart) and Novolin 70/30 (human premix).
NovoLog Mix 70/30 should appear uniformly white and cloudy. Do not use it if it looks clear or if it contains solid particles. NovoLog Mix 70/30 should not be used after the printed expiration date.
NovoLog Mix 70/30 should be administered by subcutaneous injection in the abdominal region, buttocks, thigh, or upper arm. NovoLog Mix 70/30 has a faster onset of action than human insulin premix 70/30 and should be dosed within 15 minutes before meal initiation for patients with type 1 diabetes. For patients with type 2 diabetes, dosing should occur within 15 minutes before or after meal initiation. Injection sites should be rotated within the same region to reduce the risk of lipodystrophy. As with all insulins, the duration of action may vary according to the dose, injection site, blood flow, temperature, and level of physical activity.
NovoLog Mix 70/30 should not be administered intravenously or used in insulin infusion pumps. Dose regimens of NovoLog Mix 70/30 will vary among patients and should be determined by the health care professional familiar with the patient's recommended glucose treatment goals, metabolic needs, eating habits, and other lifestyle variables.

2.2 Resuspension
NovoLog Mix 70/30 is a suspension that must be visually inspected and resuspended immediately before use. The NovoLog Mix 70/30 vial should be rolled gently in your hands in a horizontal position 10 times to mix it. The rolling procedure must be repeated until the suspension appears uniformly white and cloudy. Inject immediately. Resuspension is easier when the insulin has reached room temperature.
The NovoLog Mix 70/30 FlexPen should be rolled 10 times gently between your hands in a horizontal position. Thereafter, turn the NovoLog Mix 70/30 FlexPen upside down so that the glass ball moves from one end of the reservoir to the other. Do this at least 10 times. The rolling and turning procedure must be repeated until the suspension appears uniformly white and cloudy. Inject immediately. Before each subsequent injection, turn the disposable NovoLog Mix 70/30 FlexPen upside down so that the glass ball moves from one end of the reservoir to the other at least 10 times and until the suspension appears uniformly white and cloudy. Inject immediately.

3 DOSAGE FORMS AND STRENGTHS
NovoLog Mix 70/30 is available in the following package sizes: each presentation contains 100 units of insulin aspart per mL (U-100).
• 10 mL vials
• 3 mL NovoLog Mix 70/30 FlexPen

4 CONTRAINDICATIONS
NovoLog Mix 70/30 is contraindicated
• during episodes of hypoglycemia
• in patients with hypersensitivity to NovoLog Mix 70/30 or one of its excipients

5 WARNINGS AND PRECAUTIONS
5.1 Administration
The short and long-acting components of insulin mixes, including NovoLog Mix 70/30, cannot be titrated independently. Because NovoLog Mix 70/30 has peak pharmacodynamic activity between 1-4 hours after injection, it should be administered within 15 minutes of meal initiation [see Clinical Pharmacology (12)]. The dose of insulin required to provide adequate glycemic control for one of the meals may result in hyper- or hypoglycemia for the other meal. The pharmacodynamic profile may also be inadequate for patients who require more frequent meals.
NovoLog Mix 70/30 should not be mixed with any other insulin product.
NovoLog Mix 70/30 should not be used intravenously.
NovoLog Mix 70/30 should not be used in insulin infusion pumps.
Glucose monitoring is recommended for all patients with diabetes. Any change of insulin dose should be made cautiously and only under medical supervision. Changing from one insulin product to another or changing the insulin strength may result in the need for a change in dosage. Changes may also be necessary during illness, emotional stress, and other physiologic stress in addition to changes in meals and exercise.
The pharmacokinetic and pharmacodynamic profiles of all insulins may be altered by the site used for injection and the degree of vascularization of the site. Smoking, temperature, and exercise contribute to variations in blood flow and insulin absorption. These and other factors contribute to inter- and intra-patient variability.
Needles and NovoLog Mix 70/30 FlexPen must not be shared.

5.2 Hypoglycemia
Hypoglycemia is the most common adverse effect of insulin therapy, including NovoLog Mix 70/30. Severe hypoglycemia may lead to unconsciousness and/or convulsions and may result in temporary or permanent impairment of brain function or even death. Severe hypoglycemia requiring the assistance of another person and/or parenteral glucose infusion or glucagon administration has been observed in clinical trials with insulin, including trials with NovoLog Mix 70/30.
The timing of hypoglycemia may reflect the time-action profile of the insulin formulation [see Clinical Pharmacology (12)]. Other factors, such as changes in dietary intake (e.g., amount of food or timing of meals), injection site, exercise, and concomitant medications may also alter the risk of hypoglycemia [see Drug Interactions (7)]. As with all insulins, use caution in patients with hypoglycemia unawareness and in patients who may be predisposed to hypoglycemia (e.g. patients who are fasting or have erratic food intake). The patient's ability to concentrate and react may be impaired as a result of hypoglycemia. This may present a risk in situations where these abilities are especially important, such as driving or operating machinery.
Rapid changes in serum glucose levels may induce symptoms of hypoglycemia in persons with diabetes, regardless of the glucose value. Early warning symptoms of hypoglycemia may be different or less pronounced under certain conditions, such as long duration of diabetes, diabetic nerve disease, use of medications such as beta-blockers, or intensified diabetes control [see Drug Interactions (7)].

5.3 Hypokalemia
All insulin products, including NovoLog Mix 70/30, cause a shift in potassium from the extracellular to intracellular space, possibly leading to hypokalemia that, if left untreated, may cause respiratory paralysis, ventricular arrhythmia, and death. Use caution in patients who may be at risk for hypokalemia (e.g. patients using potassium-lowering medications or patients taking medications sensitive to potassium concentrations).

5.4 Renal Impairment
Clinical or pharmacology studies with NovoLog Mix 70/30 in diabetic patients with various degrees of renal impairment have not been conducted. As with other insulins, the requirements for NovoLog Mix 70/30 may be reduced in patients with renal impairment [see Clinical Pharmacology (12.3)].

5.5 Hepatic Impairment
Clinical or pharmacology studies with NovoLog Mix 70/30 in diabetic patients with various degrees of hepatic impairment have not been conducted. As with other insulins, the requirements for NovoLog Mix 70/30 may be reduced in patients with hepatic impairment [see Clinical Pharmacology (12.3)].

5.6 Hypersensitivity and Allergic Reactions
Local Reactions—As with other insulin therapy, patients may experience reactions such as erythema, edema or pruritus at the site of NovoLog Mix 70/30 injection. These reactions usually resolve in a few days to a few weeks, but in some occasions, may require discontinuation of NovoLog Mix 70/30. In some instances, these reactions may be related to the insulin molecule, other components in the insulin preparation including protamine and cresol, components in skin cleansing agents, or injection techniques. Localized reactions and generalized myalgias have been reported with the use of cresol as an injectable excipient.

Systemic Reactions—Less common, but potentially more serious, is generalized allergy to insulin, which may cause rash (including pruritus) over the whole body, shortness of breath, wheezing, reduction in blood pressure, rapid pulse, or sweating. Severe cases of generalized allergy, including anaphylactic reaction, may be life threatening.

5.7 Antibody Production
Specific anti-insulin antibodies as well as cross-reacting anti-insulin antibodies were monitored in a 3-month, open-label comparator trial as well as in a long-term extension trial. Changes in cross-reactive antibodies were more common after NovoLog Mix 70/30 than with Novolin 70/30 but these changes did not correlate with change in HbA$_{1c}$ or increase in insulin dose. The clinical significance of these antibodies has not been established. Antibodies did not increase further after long-term exposure (>6 months) to NovoLog Mix 70/30.

6 ADVERSE REACTIONS
Clinical Trial Experience
Clinical trials are conducted under widely varying designs, therefore, the adverse reaction rates reported in one clinical trial may not be easily compared to those rates reported in another clinical trial, and may not reflect the rates actually observed in clinical practice.
• *Hypoglycemia*
Hypoglycemia is the most commonly observed adverse reaction in patients using insulin, including NovoLog Mix 70/30 [see Warnings and Precautions (5.2)]. NovoLog Mix 70/30 should not be used during episodes of hypoglycemia [see Contraindications (4)] and [Warnings and Precautions (5)].
• *Insulin initiation and glucose control intensification*
Intensification or rapid improvement in glucose control has been associated with transitory, reversible ophthalmologic refraction disorder, worsening of diabetic retinopathy, and acute painful peripheral neuropathy. However, long-term glycemic control decreases the risk of diabetic retinopathy and neuropathy.
• *Lipodystrophy*
Long-term use of insulin, including NovoLog Mix 70/30, can cause lipodystrophy at the site of repeated insulin injections. Lipodystrophy includes lipohypertrophy (thickening of adipose tissue) and lipoatrophy (thinning of adipose tissue), and may affect insulin absorption. Rotate insulin injection sites within the same region to reduce the risk of lipodystrophy.
• *Weight gain*
Weight gain can occur with some insulin therapies, including NovoLog Mix 70/30, and has been attributed to the anabolic effects of insulin and the decrease in glycosuria.
• *Peripheral Edema*
Insulin may cause sodium retention and edema, particularly if previously poor metabolic control is improved by intensified insulin therapy.
• *Frequencies of adverse drug reactions*
The frequencies of adverse drug reactions during a clinical trial with NovoLog Mix 70/30 in patients with type 1 diabetes mellitus and type 2 diabetes mellitus are listed in the tables below. The trial was a three-month, open-label trial in patients with Type 1 or Type 2 diabetes who were treated twice daily (before breakfast and before supper) with NovoLog Mix 70/30.

[See table 1 at top of next page]
[See table 2 on next page]

Postmarketing Data
Additional adverse reactions have been identified during post-approval use of NovoLog Mix 70/30. Because these adverse reactions are reported voluntarily from a population of uncertain size, it is generally not possible to reliably estimate their frequency. They include medication errors in which other insulins have been accidentally substituted for NovoLog Mix 70/30 [see Patient Counseling Information (17)].

7 DRUG INTERACTIONS
A number of substances affect glucose metabolism and may require insulin dose adjustment and particularly close monitoring.
• The following are examples of substances that may increase the blood-glucose-lowering effect and susceptibility to hypoglycemia: oral antidiabetic products, pramlintide, ACE inhibitors, disopyramide, fibrates, fluoxetine, monoamine oxidase (MAO) inhibitors, propoxyphene, salicylates, somatostatin analog (e.g. octreotide), sulfonamide antibiotics.
• The following are examples of substances that may reduce the blood-glucose-lowering effect: corticosteroids, niacin, danazol, diuretics, sympathomimetic agents (e.g. epinephrine, salbutamol, terbutaline), isoniazid, phenothiazine derivatives, somatropin, thyroid hormones, estrogens, progestogens (e.g., in oral contraceptives), atypical antipsychotics.

- Beta-blockers, clonidine, lithium salts, and alcohol may either potentiate or weaken the blood-glucose-lowering effect of insulin.
- Pentamidine may cause hypoglycemia, which may sometimes be followed by hyperglycemia.
- The signs of hypoglycemia may be reduced or absent in patients taking sympatholytic products such as beta-blockers, clonidine, guanethidine, and reserpine.

8 USE IN SPECIFIC POPULATIONS

8.1 Pregnancy

Pregnancy Category B.

All pregnancies have a background risk of birth defects, loss, or other adverse outcome regardless of drug exposure. This background risk is increased in pregnancies complicated by hyperglycemia and may be decreased with good metabolic control. It is essential for patients with diabetes or history of gestational diabetes to maintain good metabolic control before conception and throughout pregnancy. Insulin requirements may decrease during the first trimester, generally increase during the second and third trimesters, and rapidly decline after delivery. Careful monitoring of glucose control is essential in such patients.

An open-label, randomized study compared the safety and efficacy of NovoLog (the rapid-acting component of NovoLog Mix 70/30) versus human insulin in the treatment of pregnant women with Type 1 diabetes (322 exposed pregnancies (NovoLog: 157, human insulin: 165)). Two-thirds of the enrolled patients were already pregnant when they entered the study. Since only one-third of the patients enrolled before conception, the study was not large enough to evaluate the risk of congenital malformations. Mean HbA$_{1c}$ of $\sim$ 6% was observed in both groups during pregnancy, and there was no significant difference in the incidence of maternal hypoglycemia.

Animal reproduction studies have not been conducted with NovoLog Mix 70/30. However, subcutaneous reproduction and teratology studies have been performed with NovoLog (the rapid-acting component of NovoLog Mix 70/30) and regular human insulin in rats and rabbits. In these studies, NovoLog was given to female rats before mating, during mating, and throughout pregnancy, and to rabbits during organogenesis. The effects of NovoLog did not differ from those observed with subcutaneous regular human insulin. NovoLog, like human insulin, caused pre- and post-implantation losses and visceral/skeletal abnormalities in rats at a dose of 200 U/kg/day (approximately 32-times the human subcutaneous dose of 1.0 U/kg/day, based on U/body surface area), and in rabbits at a dose of 10 U/kg/day (approximately three times the human subcutaneous dose of 1.0 U/kg/day, based on U/body surface area). The effects are probably secondary to maternal hypoglycemia at high doses. No significant effects were observed in rats at a dose of 50 U/kg/day and rabbits at a dose of 3 U/kg/day. These doses are approximately 8 times the human subcutaneous dose of 1.0 U/kg/day for rats and equal to the human subcutaneous dose of 1.0 U/kg/day for rabbits based on U/body surface area.

Female patients should be advised to discuss with their physician if they intend to, or if they become pregnant. There are no adequate and well-controlled studies of the use of NovoLog Mix 70/30 in pregnant women.

8.3 Nursing Mothers

It is unknown whether insulin aspart is excreted in human milk as occurs with human insulin. There are no adequate and well-controlled studies of the use of NovoLog Mix 70/30 or NovoLog in lactating women. Women with diabetes who are lactating may require adjustments of their insulin doses.

8.4 Pediatric Use

Safety and effectiveness of NovoLog Mix 70/30 have not been established in pediatric patients.

8.5 Geriatric Use

Clinical studies of NovoLog Mix 70/30 did not include sufficient numbers of patients aged 65 and over to determine whether they respond differently than younger patients. In general, dose selection for an elderly patient should be cautious, usually starting at the low end of the dosing range reflecting the greater frequency of decreased hepatic, renal, or cardiac function, and of concomitant disease or other drug therapy in this population.

10 OVERDOSAGE

Hypoglycemia may occur as a result of an excess of insulin relative to food intake, energy expenditure, or both. Mild episodes of hypoglycemia usually can be treated with oral glucose. Adjustments in drug dosage, meal patterns, or exercise, may be needed. More severe episodes of hypoglycemia with coma, seizure, or neurologic impairment may be treated with intramuscular/subcutaneous glucagon or concentrated intravenous glucose. Sustained carbohydrate intake and observation may be necessary because hypoglycemia may recur after apparent clinical recovery.

Table 1: Treatment-Emergent Adverse Events in Patients with Type 1 diabetes mellitus (Adverse events with frequency ≥ 5% are included.)

Preferred Term	NovoLog Mix 70/30 (N=55)		Novolin 70/30 (N=49)	
	N	%	N	%
Hypoglycemia	38	69	37	76
Headache	19	35	6	12
Influenza-like symptoms	7	13	1	2
Dyspepsia	5	9	3	6
Back pain	4	7	2	4
Diarrhea	4	7	3	6
Pharyngitis	4	7	1	2
Rhinitis	3	5	6	12
Skeletal pain	3	5	2	4
Upper respiratory tract infection	3	5	1	2

Table 2: Treatment-Emergent Adverse Events in Patients with Type 2 diabetes mellitus (Adverse events with frequency ≥ 5% are included.)

Preferred Term	NovoLog Mix 70/30 (N=85)		Novolin 70/30 (N=102)	
	N	%	N	%
Hypoglycemia	40	47	51	50
Upper respiratory tract infection	10	12	6	6
Headache	8	9	8	8
Diarrhea	7	8	2	2
Neuropathy	7	8	2	2
Pharyngitis	5	6	4	4
Abdominal pain	4	5	0	0
Rhinitis	4	5	2	2

11 DESCRIPTION

NovoLog Mix 70/30 (70% insulin aspart protamine suspension and 30% insulin aspart injection, [rDNA origin]) is a human insulin analog suspension containing 70% insulin aspart protamine crystals and 30% soluble insulin aspart. NovoLog Mix 70/30 is a blood glucose-lowering agent with an earlier onset and an intermediate duration of action. Insulin aspart is homologous with regular human insulin with the exception of a single substitution of the amino acid proline by aspartic acid in position B28, and is produced by recombinant DNA technology utilizing *Saccharomyces cerevisiae* (baker's yeast). Insulin aspart (NovoLog) has the empirical formula $C_{256}H_{381}N_{65}O_{79}S_6$ and a molecular weight of 5825.8 Da.

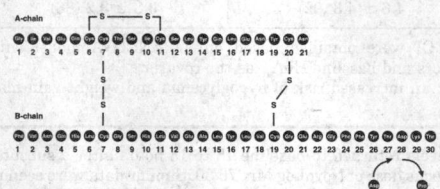

Figure 1. Structural formula of insulin aspart

NovoLog Mix 70/30 is a uniform, white, sterile suspension that contains insulin aspart 100 Units/mL.

Inactive ingredients for the 10 mL vial are mannitol 36.4 mg/mL, phenol 1.50 mg/mL, metacresol 1.72 mg/mL, zinc 19.6 µg/mL, disodium hydrogen phosphate dihydrate 1.25 mg/mL, sodium chloride 0.58 mg/mL, and protamine sulfate 0.32 mg/mL.

Inactive ingredients for the NovoLog Mix 70/30 FlexPen are glycerol 16.0 mg/mL, phenol 1.50 mg/mL, metacresol 1.72 mg/mL, zinc 19.6 µg/mL, disodium hydrogen phosphate dihydrate 1.25 mg/mL, sodium chloride 0.877 mg/mL, and protamine sulfate 0.32 mg/mL. NovoLog Mix 70/30 has a pH of 7.20 - 7.44. Hydrochloric acid or sodium hydroxide may be added to adjust pH.

12 CLINICAL PHARMACOLOGY

12.1 Mechanism of Action

The primary activity of NovoLog Mix 70/30 is the regulation of glucose metabolism. Insulins, including NovoLog Mix 70/30, bind to the insulin receptors on muscle, liver and fat cells and lower blood glucose by facilitating the cellular uptake of glucose and simultaneously inhibiting the output of glucose from the liver.

12.2 Pharmacodynamics

The two euglycemic clamp studies described below *[see Clinical Pharmacology (12.3)]* assessed glucose utilization after dosing of healthy volunteers. NovoLog Mix 70/30 has an earlier onset of action than human premix 70/30 in studies of normal volunteers and patients with diabetes. The onset of action is between 10-20 minutes for NovoLog Mix 70/30 compared to 30 minutes for Novolin 70/30. The mean ± SD time to peak activity for NovoLog Mix 70/30 is 2.4 hr ± 0.8hr compared to 4.2 hr ± 0.4 hr for Novolin 70/30. The duration of action may be as long as 24 hours (see Figure 2).

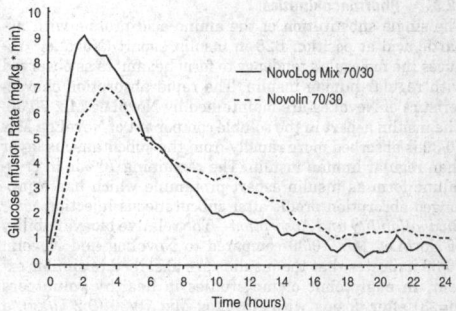

Figure 2. Pharmacodynamic Activity Profile of NovoLog Mix 70/30 and Novolin 70/30 in healthy subjects.

Table 3: Glycemic Parameters at the End of Treatment [Mean ± SD (N subjects)]

	NovoLog Mix 70/30	Novolin 70/30
Type 1, N=104		
Fasting Blood Glucose (mg/dL)	174 ± 64 (48)	142 ± 59 (44)
1.5 Hour Post Breakfast (mg/dL)	187 ± 82 (48)	200 ± 82 (42)
1.5 Hour Post Dinner (mg/dL)	162 ± 77 (47)	171 ± 66 (41)
HbA$_{1c}$ (%) Baseline	8.4 ± 1.2 (51)	8.5 ± 1.1 (46)
HbA$_{1c}$ (%) Week 12	8.4 ± 1.1 (51)	8.3 ± 1.0 (47)
Type 2, N=187		
Fasting Blood Glucose (mg/dL)	153 ± 40 (76)	152 ± 69 (93)
1.5 Hour Post Breakfast (mg/dL)	182 ± 65 (75)	200 ± 80 (92)
1.5 Hour Post Dinner (mg/dL)	168 ± 51 (75)	191 ± 65 (93)
HbA$_{1c}$ (%) Baseline	8.1 ± 1.2 (82)	8.2 ± 1.3 (98)
HbA$_{1c}$ (%) Week 12	7.9 ± 1.0 (81)	8.1 ± 1.1 (96)

Table 4: Combination Therapy with Oral Agents and Insulin in Patients with Type 2 Diabetes Mellitus [Mean (SD)]

Treatment duration 24-weeks	NovoLog Mix 70/30 + Metformin + Pioglitazone	Metformin + Pioglitazone
HbA$_{1c}$		
Baseline mean ± SD (n)	8.1 ± 1.0 (102)	8.1 ± 1.0 (98)
End-of-study mean ± SD (n) - LOCF	6.6 ± 1.0 (93)	7.8 ± 1.2 (87)
Adjusted Mean change from baseline ± SE (n)*	-1.6 ± 0.1 (93)	-0.3 ± 0.1 (87)
Treatment difference mean ± SE* 95% CI*	-1.3 ± 0.1 (-1.6, -1.0)	
Percentage of subjects reaching HbA$_{1c}$ <7.0%	76%	24%
Percentage of subjects reaching HbA$_{1c}$ ≤6.5%	59%	12%
Fasting Blood Glucose (mg/dL)		
Baseline Mean ± SD (n)	173 ± 39.8 (93)	163 ± 35.4 (88)
End of Study Mean ± SD (n) - LOCF	130 ± 50.0 (90)	162 ± 40.8 (84)
Adjusted Mean change from baseline ± SE (n)*	-43.0 ± 5.3 (90)	-3.9 ± 5.3 (84)
End-of-Study Blood Glucose (Plasma) (mg/dL)		
2 Hour Post Breakfast	138 ± 42.8 (86)	188 ± 57.7 (74)
2 Hour Post Lunch	150 ± 41.5 (86)	176 ± 56.5 (74)
2 Hour Post Dinner	141 ± 57.8 (86)	195 ± 60.1 (74)
% of patients with severe hypoglycemia**	3	0
% of patients with minor hypoglycemia**	52	3
Weight gain at end of study (kg)**	4.6 ± 4.3 (92)	0.8 ± 3.2 (86)

*Adjusted mean per group, treatment difference, and 95% CI were obtained based on an ANCOVA model with treatment, FPG stratum, and secretagogue stratum as fixed factors and baseline HbA$_{1c}$ as the covariate.
**If metabolic control is improved by intensified insulin therapy, an increased risk of hypoglycemia and weight gain may occur.

12.3   Pharmacokinetics
The single substitution of the amino acid proline with aspartic acid at position B28 in insulin aspart (NovoLog) reduces the molecule's tendency to form hexamers as observed with regular human insulin. The rapid absorption characteristics of NovoLog are maintained by NovoLog Mix 70/30. The insulin aspart in the soluble component of NovoLog Mix 70/30 is absorbed more rapidly from the subcutaneous layer than regular human insulin. The remaining 70% is in crystalline form as insulin aspart protamine which has a prolonged absorption profile after subcutaneous injection.
Bioavailability and Absorption—The relative bioavailability of NovoLog Mix 70/30 compared to NovoLog and Novolin 70/30 indicates that the insulins are absorbed to similar extent. In euglycemic clamp studies in healthy volunteers (n=23) after dosing with NovoLog Mix 70/30 (0.2 U/kg), a mean maximum serum concentration (C$_{max}$) of 23.4 ± 5.3 mU/L was reached after 60 minutes. The mean half-life (t$_{1/2}$) of NovoLog Mix 70/30 was about 8 to 9 hours. Serum insulin

levels returned to baseline 15 to 18 hours after a subcutaneous dose of NovoLog Mix 70/30. Similar data were seen in a separate euglycemic clamp study in healthy volunteers (n=24) after dosing with NovoLog Mix 70/30 (0.3 U/kg). A C$_{max}$ of 61.3 ± 20.1 mU/L was reached after 85 minutes. Serum insulin levels returned to baseline 12 hours after a subcutaneous dose.
The C$_{max}$ and the area under the insulin concentration-time curve (AUC) after administration of NovoLog Mix 70/30 was approximately 20% greater than those after administration of Novolin 70/30, (see Fig. 3 for pharmacokinetic profiles).
[See figure at top of next column]
Distribution and Elimination—NovoLog has a low binding to plasma proteins, 0 to 9%, similar to regular human insulin. After subcutaneous administration in normal male volunteers (n=24), NovoLog was more rapidly eliminated than regular human insulin with an average apparent half-life of 81 minutes compared to 141 minutes for regular human insulin.

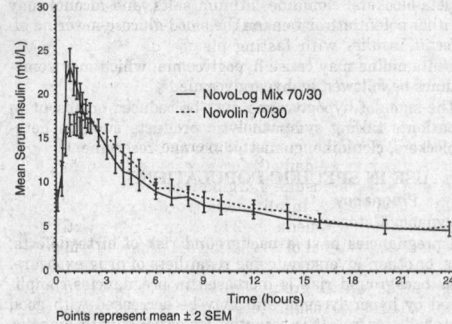

Figure 3. Pharmacokinetic Profiles of NovoLog Mix 70/30 and Novolin 70/30

The effect of sex, age, obesity, ethnic origin, renal and hepatic impairment, pregnancy, or smoking, on the pharmacodynamics and pharmacokinetics of NovoLog Mix 70/30 has not been studied.

13   NONCLINICAL TOXICOLOGY
13.1   Carcinogenesis, Mutagenesis, Impairment of Fertility
Standard 2-year carcinogenicity studies in animals have not been performed to evaluate the carcinogenic potential of NovoLog Mix 70/30. In 52-week studies, Sprague-Dawley rats were dosed subcutaneously with NovoLog, the rapid-acting component of NovoLog Mix 70/30, at 10, 50, and 200 U/kg/day (approximately 2, 8, and 32 times the human subcutaneous dose of 1.0 U/kg/day, based on U/body surface area, respectively). At a dose of 200 U/kg/day, NovoLog increased the incidence of mammary gland tumors in females when compared to untreated controls. The incidence of mammary tumors found with NovoLog was not significantly different from that found with regular human insulin. The relevance of these findings to humans is not known.
NovoLog was not genotoxic in the following tests: Ames test, mouse lymphoma cell forward gene mutation test, human peripheral blood lymphocyte chromosome aberration test, *in vivo* micronucleus test in mice, and in *ex vivo* UDS test in rat liver hepatocytes.
In fertility studies in male and female rats, NovoLog at subcutaneous doses up to 200 U/kg/day (approximately 32 times the human subcutaneous dose, based on U/body surface area) had no direct adverse effects on male and female fertility, or on general reproductive performance of animals.
13.2   Animal Toxicology and/or Pharmacology
In standard biological assays in mice and rabbits, one unit of NovoLog has the same glucose-lowering effect as one unit of regular human insulin. However, the effect of NovoLog Mix 70/30 is more rapid in onset compared to Novolin (human insulin) 70/30 due to its faster absorption after subcutaneous injection.

14   CLINICAL STUDIES
14.1   NovoLog Mix 70/30 versus Novolin 70/30
In a three-month, open-label trial, patients with Type 1 (n=104) or Type 2 (n=187) diabetes were treated twice daily (before breakfast and before supper) with NovoLog Mix 70/30 or Novolin 70/30. Patients had received insulin for at least 24 months before the study. Oral hypoglycemic agents were not allowed within 1 month prior to the study or during the study. The small changes in HbA$_{1c}$ were comparable across the treatment groups (see Table 3).
[See table 3 above]
The significance, with respect to the long-term clinical sequelae of diabetes, of the differences in postprandial hyperglycemia between treatment groups has not been established.
Specific anti-insulin antibodies as well as cross-reacting anti-insulin antibodies were monitored in the 3-month, open-label comparator trial as well as in a long-term extension trial.
14.2   Combination Therapy: Insulin and Oral Agents in Patients with Type 2 Diabetes
Trial 1:
In a 34-week, open-label trial, insulin-naïve patients with type 2 diabetes currently treated with 2 oral antidiabetic agents were switched to treatment with metformin and pioglitazone. During an 8-week optimization period metformin and pioglitazone were increased to 2500 mg per day and 30 or 45 mg per day, respectively. After the optimization period, subjects were randomized to receive either NovoLog Mix 70/30 twice daily added on to the metformin and pioglitazone regimen or continue the current optimized metformin and pioglitazone therapy. NovoLog Mix 70/30 was started at a dose of 6 IU twice daily (before breakfast and before supper). Insulin doses were titrated to a pre-meal glucose goal of 80-110 mg/dL. The total daily insulin dose at the end of the study was 56.9 ± 30.5 IU.
[See table 4 above]

Trial 2:

In a 28-week, open-label trial, insulin-naïve patients with type 2 diabetes with fasting plasma glucose above 140 mg/dL currently treated with metformin ± thiazolidinedione therapy were randomized to receive either NovoLog Mix 70/30 twice daily [before breakfast and before supper] or insulin glargine once daily[1] (see Table 5). NovoLog Mix 70/30 was started at an average dose of 5-6 IU (0.07 ± 0.03 IU/kg) twice daily (before breakfast and before supper), and bedtime insulin glargine was started at 10-12 IU (0.13 ± 0.03 IU/kg). Insulin doses were titrated weekly by decrements or increments of -2 to +6 units per injection to a pre-meal glucose goal of 80-110 mg/dL. The metformin dose was adjusted to 2550 mg/day. Approximately one-third of the patients in each group were also treated with pioglitazone (30 mg/day). Insulin secretagogues were discontinued in order to reduce the risk of hypoglycemia. Most patients were Caucasian (53%), and the mean initial weight was 90 kg.

[See table 5 at right]

15   REFERENCES

1. Raskin R, Allen E, Hollander P, et al. Initiating insulin therapy in type 2 diabetes: a comparison of biphasic and basal insulin analogs. *Diabetes Care.* 2005; 28:260-265.

16   HOW SUPPLIED/STORAGE AND HANDLING

16.1   How Supplied

NovoLog Mix 70/30 is available in the following package sizes: each presentation contains 100 Units of insulin aspart per mL (U-100).

10 mL vials	NDC 0169-3685-12
3 mL NovoLog Mix 70/30 FlexPen	NDC 0169-3696-19

NovoLog Mix 70/30 vials and NovoLog Mix 70/30 FlexPen are latex free.

16.2   Recommended Storage

Unused NovoLog Mix 70/30 should be stored in a refrigerator between 2°C and 8°C (36°F to 46°F). Do not store in the freezer or directly adjacent to the refrigerator cooling element. **Do not freeze NovoLog Mix 70/30 or use NovoLog Mix 70/30 if it has been frozen.**

Vials: After initial use, a vial may be kept at temperatures below 30°C (86°F) for up to 28 days, but should not be exposed to excessive heat or sunlight. Open vials may be refrigerated.

Unpunctured vials can be used until the expiration date printed on the label if they are stored in a refrigerator. Keep unused vials in the carton so they will stay clean and protected from light.

NovoLog Mix 70/30 FlexPen: Once a NovoLog Mix 70/30 FlexPen is punctured, it should be kept at temperatures below 30°C (86°F) for up to 14 days, but should not be exposed to excessive heat or sunlight. A NovoLog Mix 70/30 FlexPen in use must NOT be stored in the refrigerator. Keep the disposable NovoLog Mix 70/30 FlexPen away from direct heat and sunlight. An unpunctured NovoLog Mix 70/30 FlexPen can be used until the expiration date printed on the label if they are stored in a refrigerator. Keep any unused NovoLog Mix 70/30 FlexPen in the carton so it will stay clean and protected from light.

These storage conditions are summarized in the following table:

[See second table above]

17   PATIENT COUNSELING INFORMATION

[see FDA-Approved Patient Labeling]

17.1   Physician Instructions

Maintenance of normal or near-normal glucose control is a treatment goal in diabetes mellitus and has been associated with a reduction in diabetic complications. Patients should be informed about potential risks and advantages of NovoLog Mix 70/30 therapy including the possible adverse reactions. Patients should also be offered continued education and advice on insulin therapies, injection technique, life-style management, regular glucose monitoring, periodic glycosylated hemoglobin testing, recognition and management of hypo- and hyperglycemia, adherence to meal planning, complications of insulin therapy, timing of dose, instruction for use of injection devices, and proper storage of insulin. See Patient Information supplied with the product. Patients should be informed that frequent, patient-performed blood glucose measurements are needed to achieve optimal glycemic control and avoid both hyper- and hypoglycemia, and diabetic ketoacidosis.

The patient's ability to concentrate and react may be impaired as a result of hypoglycemia. This may present a risk in situations where these abilities are especially important, such as driving or operating other machinery. Patients who

Table 5: Combination Therapy with Oral Agents and Two Types of Insulin in Patients with Type 2 Diabetes Mellitus [Mean (SD)]

Treatment duration 28-weeks	NovoLog Mix 70/30 + Metformin ± Pioglitazone	Insulin Glargine + Metformin ± Pioglitazone
Number of patients	117	116
HbA$_{1c}$		
Baseline mean (%)	9.7 ± 1.5 (117)	9.8 ± 1.4 (114)
End-of-study mean (± SD)	6.9 ± 1.2 (108)	7.4 ± 1.2 (114)
Mean change from baseline	-2.7 ± 1.6 (108)	-2.4 ± 1.5 (114)
Percentage of subjects reaching HbA$_{1c}$ <7.0%	66%	40%
Total Daily Insulin Dose at end of study (U)	78 ± 40 (117)	51 ± 27 (116)
% of patients with severe hypoglycemia	0	0
% of minor hypoglycemia	43	16
Weight gain at end of study	5.4 ± 4.8 (117)	3.5 ± 4.5 (116)

	Not in-use (unopened) Room Temperature (below 30°C[86°F])	Not in-use (unopened) Refrigerated (2°C-8°C [36°F-46°F])	In-use (opened) Room Temperature (below 30°C[86°F])
10 mL vial	**28 days**	**Until expiration date**	**28 days (refrigerated/room temperature)**
3mL NovoLog Mix 70/30 FlexPen	**14 days**	**Until expiration date**	**14 days (Do not refrigerate)**

have frequent hypoglycemia or reduced or absent warning signs of hypoglycemia should be advised to use caution when driving or operating machinery.

Accidental substitutions between NovoLog Mix 70/30 and other insulin products have been reported. Patients should be instructed to always carefully check that they are administering the appropriate insulin to avoid medication errors between NovoLog Mix 70/30 and any other insulin. **The prescription for NovoLog Mix 70/30 should be written clearly in order to avoid confusion with other insulin products, for example, NovoLog or Novolin 70/30. In addition, the written prescription should clearly indicate the presentation, for example FlexPen or vial.**

Date of Issue: May 7, 2010
Version: 9

Novo Nordisk®, NovoLog®, FlexPen®, and Novolin®, are trademarks owned by Novo Nordisk® A/S.

NovoLog® Mix 70/30 is covered by US Patent Nos. 5,547,930, 5,618,913, 5,834,422, 5,840,680, 5,866,538 and other patents pending.

FlexPen® is covered by US Patent Nos. 6,582,404, 6,004,297, 6,235,004 and other patents pending.

© 2002–2010 Novo Nordisk A/S

Manufactured by:
Novo Nordisk A/S
DK-2880 Bagsvaerd, Denmark

For information about NovoLog Mix 70/30 contact:
Novo Nordisk Inc.
Princeton, New Jersey 08540
1-800-727-6500
www.novonordisk-us.com

PATIENT INFORMATION

NovoLog® Mix 70/30
(NŌ-vō-log-MIX-SEV-en-tee-THIR-tee)
(70% insulin aspart protamine suspension and 30% insulin aspart injection, [rDNA origin])

Read the Patient Information leaflet that comes with NovoLog® Mix 70/30 before you start taking it and each time you get a refill. There may be new information. This leaflet does not take the place of talking with your healthcare provider about your diabetes or your treatment. Make sure you know how to manage your diabetes. Ask your healthcare provider if you have any questions about managing your diabetes.

What is NovoLog® Mix 70/30?

NovoLog® Mix 70/30 is a man-made insulin that is used to control high blood sugar in adults with diabetes mellitus. It is not known if NovoLog® Mix 70/30 is safe or effective in children.

Who should not use NovoLog® Mix 70/30?

Do not take NovoLog® Mix 70/30 if:

- Your blood sugar is too low (hypoglycemia)
- You are allergic to any of the ingredients in NovoLog®

Mix 70/30. See the end of this leaflet for a complete list of ingredients in NovoLog® Mix 70/30. Check with your healthcare provider if you are not sure.

What should I tell my healthcare provider before taking NovoLog® Mix 70/30?

Before you use NovoLog® Mix 70/30, tell your healthcare provider if you:

- have kidney or liver problems
- **have any other medical conditions.** Medical conditions can affect your insulin needs and your dose of NovoLog® Mix 70/30.
- **are pregnant or plan to become pregnant.** It is not known if NovoLog® Mix 70/30 will harm your unborn baby. Talk to your healthcare provider if you are pregnant or plan to become pregnant. You and your healthcare provider should decide about the best way to manage your diabetes while you are pregnant.
- **are breastfeeding or plan to breastfeed.** It is not known if NovoLog® Mix 70/30 passes into your breast milk. You and your healthcare provider should decide if you will take NovoLog® Mix 70/30 while you breastfeed.

Tell your healthcare provider about all medicines you take, including prescriptions and non-prescription medicines, vitamins and herbal supplements.

NovoLog® Mix 70/30 may affect the way other medicines work, and other medicines may affect how NovoLog® Mix 70/30 works. Your NovoLog® Mix 70/30 dose may change if you take other medicines.

Know the medicines you take. Keep a list of your medicines with you to show your healthcare providers and pharmacist when you get a new medicine.

How should I take NovoLog® Mix 70/30?

- Take NovoLog® Mix 70/30 exactly as your healthcare provider tells you to take it.
- Your healthcare provider will tell you how much NovoLog® Mix 70/30 to take and when to take it.
- Do not make any changes to your dose or type of insulin unless your healthcare provider tells you to.
- **NovoLog Mix 70/30 starts acting fast. If you have Type 1 diabetes, inject it up to 15 minutes before you eat a meal.** Do not inject NovoLog® Mix 70/30 if you are not planning to eat within 15 minutes.
- **If you have Type 2 diabetes, you may inject NovoLog® Mix 70/30 up to 15 minutes before or after starting your meal.**
- **Do Not** mix NovoLog® Mix 70/30 with other insulin products.
- **Do Not** use NovoLog® Mix 70/30 in an insulin pump.
- **Inject NovoLog® Mix 70/30 under the skin (subcutaneously) of your stomach area, upper arms, buttocks or upper legs.** NovoLog® Mix 70/30 may affect your blood sugar levels faster if you inject it under the skin of your stomach area. Never inject NovoLog® Mix 70/30 into a vein or into a muscle.

- **Change (rotate) injection sites** within the area you choose with each dose. **Do not** inject into the exact same spot for each injection.
- **Read the instructions for use that come with your NovoLog® Mix 70/30.** Talk to your healthcare provider if you have any questions. Your healthcare provider should show you how to inject NovoLog® Mix 70/30 before you start using it.
- NovoLog® Mix 70/30 comes in:
  - 10 mL vials for use with a syringe
  - 3 mL NovoLog® Mix 70/30 FlexPen®
- **If you take too much NovoLog® Mix 70/30, your blood sugar may fall too low (hypoglycemia).** You can treat mild low blood sugar (hypoglycemia) by drinking or eating something sugary right away (fruit juice, sugar candies, or glucose tablets). It is important to treat low blood sugar (hypoglycemia) right away because it could get worse and you could pass out (loss of consciousness).
- **If you forget to take your dose of NovoLog® Mix 70/30, your blood sugar may go too high (hyperglycemia).** If high blood sugar (hyperglycemia) is not treated it can lead to serious problems, like passing out (loss of consciousness), coma or even death. Follow your healthcare provider's instructions for treating high blood sugar. Know your symptoms of high blood sugar which may include:

• increased thirst	• a hard time breathing
• frequent urination	• fruity smell on the breath
• drowsiness	• high amounts of sugar
• loss of appetite	and ketones in your urine
	• nausea, vomiting
	(throwing up) or stomach
	pain

- Do not share needles, insulin pens or syringes with others.
- **Check your blood sugar levels.** Ask your healthcare provider what your blood sugars should be and when you should check your blood sugar levels.

Your insulin dosage may need to change because of:

• illness	• change in diet
• stress	• change in physical
• other medicines you take	activity or exercise

See the end of this patient information for instructions about preparing and giving your injection.

What should I consider while using NovoLog® Mix 70/30?
- **Alcohol.** Drinking alcohol may affect your blood sugar when you take NovoLog® Mix 70/30.
- **Driving and operating machinery.** You may have trouble paying attention or reacting if you have low blood sugar (hypoglycemia). Be careful when you drive a car or operate machinery. Ask your healthcare provider if it is alright for you to drive if you often have:
  - low blood sugar
  - decreased or no warning signs of low blood sugar

What are the possible side effects of NovoLog® Mix 70/30?
NovoLog® Mix 70/30 may cause serious side effects, including:
- **low blood sugar (hypoglycemia).** Symptoms of low blood sugar may include:

• sweating	• trouble concentrating or
• dizziness or	confusion
lightheadedness	• blurred vision
• shakiness	• slurred speech
• hunger	• anxiety, irritability or
• fast heart beat	mood changes
• tingling of lips and tongue	• headache

Very low blood sugar can cause you to pass out (loss of consciousness), seizures, and death. Talk to your healthcare provider about how to tell if you have low blood sugar and what to do if this happens while taking NovoLog® Mix 70/30. Know your symptoms of low blood sugar. Follow your healthcare provider's instructions for treating low blood sugar.
Talk to your healthcare provider if low blood sugar is a problem for you. Your dose of NovoLog® Mix 70/30 may need to be changed.
- **Low potassium in your blood (hypokalemia)**
- **Reactions at the injection site (local allergic reaction).** You may get redness, swelling, and itching at the injection site. If you keep having skin reactions or they are serious talk to your healthcare provider.
- **Serious allergic reaction (whole body reaction).** Get medical help right away, if you have any of these symptoms of an allergic reaction:

- a rash over your whole body
- have trouble breathing
- a fast heartbeat
- sweating
- feel faint

The most common side effects of NovoLog® Mix 70/30 include:
- **Skin thickening or pits at the injection site (lipodystrophy).** Change (rotate) where you inject your insulin to help to prevent these skin changes from happening. Do not inject insulin into this type of skin.
- **Weight gain**
- **Swelling of your hands and feet**
- **Vision changes**

These are not all of the possible side effects from NovoLog® Mix 70/30. Ask your healthcare provider or pharmacist for more information.
Call your doctor for medical advice about side effects. You may report side effects to FDA at 1-800-FDA-1088.

How should I store NovoLog® Mix 70/30?
All Unopened NovoLog® Mix 70/30:
- Keep all unopened NovoLog® Mix 70/30 in the refrigerator between 36°F to 46°F (2°C to 8°C).
- **Do not freeze or store next to the refrigerator cooling element.** Do not use NovoLog® Mix 70/30 if it has been frozen.
- Keep unopened NovoLog® Mix 70/30 in the carton to protect from light.
- Unopened vials can be used until the expiration date on the NovoLog® Mix 70/30 label, if the medicine has been stored in a refrigerator.
- Unused NovoLog® Mix 70/30 FlexPen® can be used until the expiration date on the NovoLog® Mix 70/30 FlexPen® label, if the medicine has been stored in a refrigerator.

After NovoLog® Mix 70/30 has been opened:
- **Vials**
  - Keep in the refrigerator or at room temperature below 86°F (30°C) for up to 28 days.
  - Keep vials away from direct heat or light.
  - Throw away an opened vial after 28 days of use, even if there is insulin left in the vial.
- **NovoLog® Mix 70/30 FlexPen®**
  - Keep at room temperature below 86°F (30°C) for up to 14 days.
  - **Do not** store a NovoLog® Mix 70/30 FlexPen® that you are using in the refrigerator.
  - Keep NovoLog® Mix 70/30 FlexPen® away from direct heat or light.
  - Throw away a used NovoLog® Mix 70/30 FlexPen® after 14 days, even if there is insulin left in the syringe.

Never use insulin after the expiration date that is printed on the label and carton.
Keep NovoLog® Mix 70/30 and all medicines out of the reach of children.

General advice about NovoLog® Mix 70/30
Medicines are sometimes prescribed for conditions that are not mentioned in the patient leaflet. Do not use NovoLog® Mix 70/30 for a condition for which it was not prescribed. Do not give NovoLog® Mix 70/30 to other people, even if they have the same symptoms you have. It may harm them.
This leaflet summarizes the most important information about NovoLog® Mix 70/30. If you would like more information about NovoLog® Mix 70/30 or diabetes, talk with your healthcare provider. You can ask your healthcare provider or pharmacist for information about NovoLog® Mix 70/30 that is written for healthcare professionals. For more information call 1-800-727-6500 or go to www.novonordisk-us.com.

What are the ingredients in NovoLog® Mix 70/30?
- **Active Ingredients NovoLog® Mix 70/30 FlexPen® and Vial:** 70% Insulin aspart protamine suspension and 30% insulin aspart injection (rDNA origin).
- **Inactive Ingredients NovoLog® Mix 70/30 FlexPen®:** glycerol, phenol, metacresol, zinc, disodium hydrogen phosphate dihydrate, sodium chloride, protamine sulfate, water for injection, hydrochloric acid or sodium hydroxide.
- **Inactive Ingredients NovoLog® Mix 70/30 Vial:** mannitol, phenol, metacresol, zinc, disodium hydrogen phosphate dihydrate, sodium chloride, protamine sulfate, water for injection, hydrochloric acid or sodium hydroxide.

All NovoLog® Mix 70/30 vials and NovoLog® Mix 70/30 FlexPen® are latex free.
Helpful information for people with diabetes is published by the American Diabetes Association, 1701 N Beauregard Street, Alexandria, VA 22311 and is available www.diabetes.org.
Date of Issue: May 7, 2010
Version: 7
NovoLog®, FlexPen®, NovoFine®, are trademarks of Novo Nordisk A/S.
NovoLog® is covered by US Patent Nos. 5,547,930, 5,618,913, 5,834,422, 5,840,680, 5,866,538 and other patents pending.

FlexPen® is covered by US Patent Nos. 6,582,404, 6,004,297, 6,235,004 and other patents pending.
© 2002-2010 Novo Nordisk A/S
Manufactured by:
Novo Nordisk A/S
DK-2880 Bagsvaerd, Denmark
For information about NovoLog Mix 70/30® contact:
Novo Nordisk Inc.
100 College Road West
Princeton, New Jersey 08540
PATIENT INSTRUCTIONS FOR USE
NovoLog® Mix 70/30 10 mL vial (100 Units/mL, U-100)
Read the following Patient Instructions for Use carefully before you start using your NovoLog® Mix 70/30 10mL vial and each time you get a refill. There may be new information. You should read the instructions even if you have used NovoLog® Mix 70/30 10mL vials before.
Before starting, gather all of the supplies that you will need to use for preparing and giving your insulin injection.
Never re-use syringes and needles.
How should I prepare and deliver the injection using the NovoLog® Mix 70/30 10 mL vial?
1. Check to make sure you have the correct type of insulin. This is especially important if you use different types of insulin.
2. Look at the vial and the insulin. The insulin should be white and cloudy after mixing. The tamper-resistant cap should be on the vial before the first use. If the cap has already been removed before your first use of the vial, or if the insulin looks clear or contains any particles, do not use it and return it to your pharmacy.
3. Wash your hands with soap and water. Clean your injection site with an alcohol swab and let the injection site dry before you inject. Talk with your healthcare provider about how to rotate injection sites and how to give an injection.
4. If you are using a new vial, pull off the tamper-resistant cap. Wipe the rubber stopper with an alcohol swab.
5. Roll the vial gently 10 times in your hands to mix it. This should be done with the vial in a horizontal (flat) position between your palms. **Do not** shake the vial. Shaking right before the dose is drawn into the syringe may cause bubbles or foam. This can cause you to draw up the wrong dose of insulin. The insulin should be used only if it looks white and cloudy.
6. Pull back the plunger on the syringe until the black tip reaches the marking for the number of units you will inject.
7. Push the needle through the rubber stopper into the vial, and push the plunger all the way in to force air into the vial.
8. Turn the vial and syringe upside down and slowly pull the plunger back to a few units beyond the correct dose needed.
9. If there are air bubbles in the syringe, tap the syringe gently with your finger to raise the air bubbles to the top. Slowly push the plunger to the marking for your dose. This should move any air bubbles in the syringe back into the vial.
10. Check to make sure you have the right dose of NovoLog® Mix 70/30 in the syringe.
11. Pull the syringe out of the vial's rubber stopper.
12. If there is a delay after you rolled the vial, you will have to roll it again to remix the insulin and redraw your medicine. Your healthcare provider should tell you if you need to pinch the skin before inserting the needle. This can be different from person to person so it is important to ask your doctor if you did not receive instructions on pinching the skin. Insert the needle into the skin right away. Push the plunger to inject the insulin under your skin. Keep the needle under your skin for at least 6 seconds to make sure you have injected all the insulin. When you are finished injecting the insulin, pull the needle out of your skin.
13. Your may see a drop of NovoLog® Mix 70/30 at the needle tip. This is normal and has no effect on the dose you just received. If blood appears after you pull the needle from your skin, press the injection site lightly with an alcohol swab. **Do not** rub the area. **Do not** recap the needle.
14. **After the injection, dispose of the needle and syringe in a puncture-resistant container.** Place used syringes, needles, and insulin vials in a disposable puncture-resistant sharps container, or some type of hard plastic or metal container with a screw on cap such as a detergent bottle or coffee can.
15. Ask your healthcare provider about the right way to throw away used syringes and needles. There may be state or local laws about the right way to throw away used syringes and needles. **Do not** throw away used needles and syringes in household trash or recycling bins.

Helpful information for people with diabetes is published by the American Diabetes Association, 1701 N. Beauregard Street, Alexandria, VA 22311.
Date of Issue: May 7, 2010

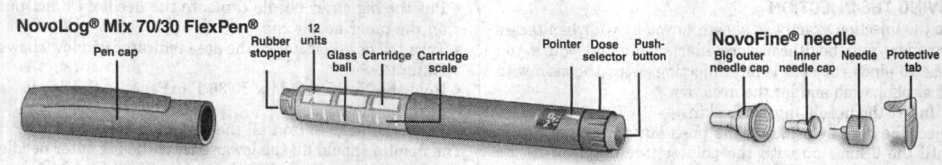

NovoLog® Mix 70/30 FlexPen® — Pen cap · Rubber stopper · 12 units · Glass ball · Cartridge · Cartridge scale · Pointer · Dose selector · Push-button

NovoFine® needle — Big outer needle cap · Inner needle cap · Needle · Protective tab

Version: 6

Novo Nordisk®, NovoLog®, FlexPen® and NovoFine® are trademarks owned by Novo Nordisk A/S.

© 2002–2010 Novo Nordisk A/S

NovoLog® Mix 70/30 is covered by US Patent Nos. 5,547,930, 5,618,913, 5,834,422, 5,840,680, 5,866,538 and other patents pending.

For information about NovoLog® Mix 70/30 contact:

Novo Nordisk Inc.

100 College Road West

Princeton, New Jersey 08540

1-800-727-6500

www.novonordisk-us.com

Manufactured by:

Novo Nordisk A/S

DK-2880 Bagsvaerd, Denmark

PATIENT INSTRUCTIONS FOR USE

NovoLog® Mix 70/30 FlexPen®

Read the following instructions carefully before you start using your NovoLog® Mix 70/30 FlexPen® and each time you get a refill. There may be new information. You should read the instructions even if you have used NovoLog® Mix 70/30 FlexPen® before.

NovoLog® Mix 70/30 FlexPen® is a disposable dial-a-dose insulin pen. You can select doses from 1 to 60 units in increments of 1 unit. NovoLog® Mix 70/30 FlexPen® is designed to be used with NovoFine® needles.

NovoLog Mix® 70/30 FlexPen® should not be used by people who are blind or have severe visual problems without the help of a person who has good eyesight and who is trained to use the NovoLog® Mix 70/30 FlexPen® the right way.

Getting ready

Make sure you have the following items:

• NovoLog® Mix 70/30 FlexPen®

• New NovoFine® needle

• Alcohol swab

[See figure above]

PREPARING YOUR NOVOLOG® MIX 70/30 FLEXPEN®

• Wash your hands with soap and water.

• Before you start to prepare your injection, check the label to make sure that you are taking the right type of insulin. This is especially important if you take more than 1 type of insulin. NovoLog® Mix 70/30 should look cloudy after mixing.

Before your first injection with a new NovoLog® Mix 70/30 FlexPen® you must mix the insulin:

A. Let the insulin reach room temperature before you use it. This makes it easier to mix. Pull off the pen cap (see diagram A).

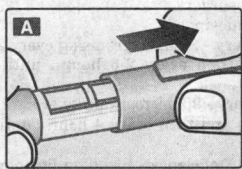

B. Roll the pen between your palms 10 times - it is important that the pen is kept horizontal (see diagram B).

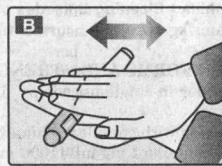

C. Then gently move the pen up and down ten times between position **1** and **2** as shown, so the glass ball moves from one end of the cartridge to the other (see diagram C).

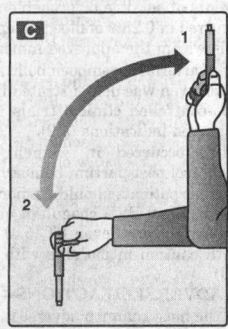

Repeat rolling and moving the pen until the liquid appears white and cloudy.

For every following injection move the pen up and down between positions 1 and 2 at least ten times until the liquid appears white and cloudy.

After mixing, complete all the following steps of the injection right away. If there is a delay, the insulin will need to be mixed again.

Wipe the rubber stopper with an alcohol swab.

Δ Before you inject, there must be at least 12 units of insulin left in the cartridge to make sure the remaining insulin is evenly mixed. If there are less than 12 units left, use a new NovoLog® Mix 70/30 FlexPen®.

Attaching the needle

D. Remove the protective tab from a disposable needle. Screw the needle tightly onto your NovoLog® Mix 70/30 FlexPen®. It is important that the needle is put on straight (see diagram D).

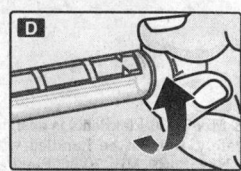

Never place a disposable needle on your NovoLog® Mix 70/30 FlexPen® until you are ready to take your injection.

E. Pull off the big outer needle cap (see diagram E).

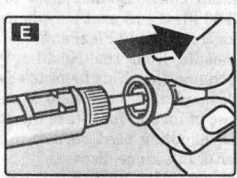

F. Pull off the inner needle cap and dispose of it (see diagram F).

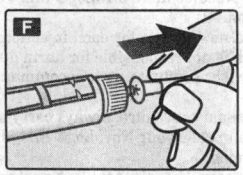

Δ Always use a new needle for each injection to help ensure sterility and prevent blocked needles.

Δ Be careful not to bend or damage the needle before use.

Δ To reduce the risk of a needle stick, **never put the inner needle cap back on the needle.**

Giving the airshot before each injection

Before each injection small amounts of air may collect in the cartridge during normal use. **To avoid injecting air and to make sure you take the right dose of insulin:**

G. Turn the dose selector to select 2 units (see diagram G).

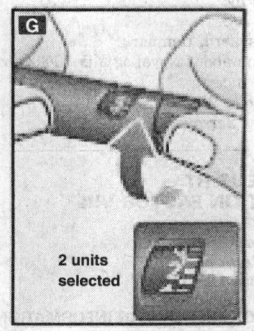

2 units selected

H. Hold your NovoLog® Mix 70/30 FlexPen® with the needle pointing up. Tap the cartridge gently with your finger a few times to make any air bubbles collect at the top of the cartridge (see diagram H).

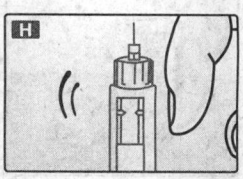

I. Keep the needle pointing upwards, press the push-button all the way in (see diagram I). The dose selector returns to 0.

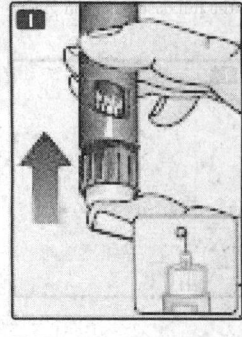

A drop of insulin should appear at the needle tip. If not, change the needle and repeat the procedure no more than 6 times.

If you do not see a drop of insulin after 6 times, do not use the NovoLog Mix® 70/30 FlexPen® and contact Novo Nordisk at 1-800-727-6500.

A small air bubble may remain at the needle tip, but it will not be injected.

SELECTING YOUR DOSE

Check and make sure that the dose selector is set at 0.

J. Turn the dose selector to the number of units you need to inject. The pointer should line up with your dose.

The dose can be corrected either up or down by turning the dose selector in either direction until the correct dose lines up with the pointer (see diagram J). When turning the dose selector, be careful not to press the push-button as insulin will come out.

You cannot select a dose larger than the number of units left in the cartridge.

You will hear a click for every single unit dialed. Do not set the dose by counting the number of clicks you hear.

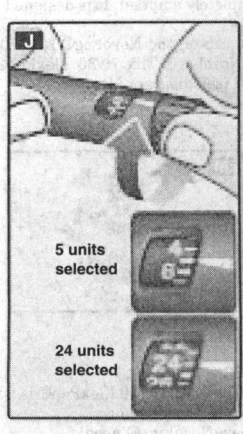

5 units selected

24 units selected

Δ Do not use the cartridge scale printed on the cartridge to measure your dose of insulin.

GIVING THE INJECTION

Do the injection exactly as shown to you by your healthcare provider. Your healthcare provider should tell you if you need to pinch the skin before injecting. Wipe the skin with an alcohol swab and let the area dry.

K. Insert the needle into your skin.

Inject the dose by pressing the push-button all the way in until the 0 lines up with the pointer (see diagram K). Be careful only to push the button when injecting.

Turning the dose selector will not inject insulin.

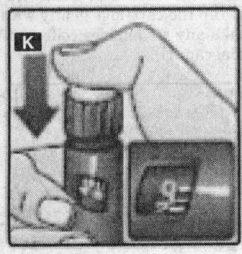

L. Keep the needle in the skin for at least 6 seconds, and keep the push-button pressed all the way in until the needle has been pulled out from the skin (see diagram L). This will make sure that the full dose has been given.

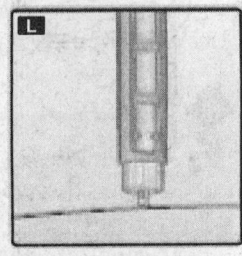

You may see a drop of NovoLog® Mix 70/30 at the needle tip. This is normal and has no effect on the dose you just received. If blood appears after you take the needle out of your skin, press the injection site lightly with an alcohol swab. **Do not rub the area.**

After the injection

Do not recap the needle. Recapping can lead to a needle stick injury. Remove the needle from the NovoLog® Mix 70/30 FlexPen® after each injection. This helps to prevent infection, leakage of insulin, and will help to make sure you inject the right dose of insulin.

Δ Put the needle and any empty NovoLog® Mix 70/30 FlexPen® or any used NovoLog® Mix 70/30 FlexPen® still containing insulin in a sharps container or some type of hard plastic or metal container with a screw top such as a detergent bottle or empty coffee can. These containers should be sealed and thrown away the right way. Check with your healthcare provider about the right way to throw away used syringes and needles. There may be local or state laws about how to throw away used needles and syringes. Do not throw away used needles and syringes in household trash or recycling bins.

The NovoLog® Mix 70/30 FlexPen® prevents the cartridge from being completely emptied. It is designed to deliver 300 units.

M. Put the pen cap on the NovoLog® Mix 70/30 FlexPen® and store the NovoLog® Mix 70/30 FlexPen® without the needle attached (see diagram M).

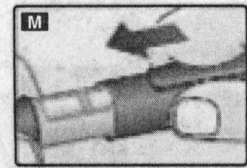

FUNCTION CHECK

N. If your NovoLog® Mix 70/30 FlexPen® is not working the right way, follow the steps below:
• Screw on a new NovoFine® needle.
• Remove the big outer needle cap and the inner needle cap.
• Do an airshot as described in "Giving the airshot before each injection".

• Put the big outer needle cap onto the needle. Do not put on the inner needle cap.
• Turn the dose selector so the dose indicator window shows 20 units.
• Hold the NovoLog® Mix 70/30 FlexPen® so the needle is pointing down.
• Press the push-button all the way in.

The insulin should fill the lower part of the big outer needle cap (see diagram N). If NovoLog® Mix 70/30 FlexPen® has released too much or too little insulin, do the function check again. If the same problem happens again, do not use your NovoLog® Mix 70/30 FlexPen® and contact Novo Nordisk at 1-800-727-6500.

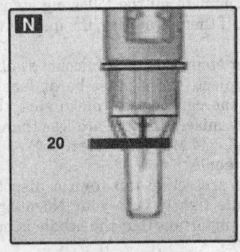

Maintenance

Your NovoLog® Mix 70/30 FlexPen® is designed to work accurately and safely. It must be handled with care. Avoid dropping your NovoLog® Mix 70/30 FlexPen® as it may damage it. If you are concerned that your NovoLog® Mix 70/30 FlexPen® is damaged, use a new one. You can clean the outside of your NovoLog® Mix 70/30 FlexPen® by wiping it with a damp cloth. Do not soak or wash your NovoLog® Mix 70/30 FlexPen® as it may damage it. Do not refill your NovoLog® Mix 70/30 FlexPen®.

Δ Remove the needle from the NovoLog® Mix 70/30 FlexPen® after each injection. This helps to ensure sterility, prevent leakage of insulin, and will help to make sure you inject the right dose of insulin for future injections.

Δ Be careful when handling used needles to avoid needle sticks and transfer of infectious diseases.

Δ Keep your NovoLog® Mix 70/30 FlexPen® and needles out of the reach of children.

Δ Use NovoLog® Mix 70/30 FlexPen® as directed to treat your diabetes. Needles and NovoLog® Mix 70/30 FlexPen® must not be shared.

Δ Always use a new needle for each injection.

Δ Novo Nordisk is not responsible for harm due to using this insulin pen with products not recommended by Novo Nordisk.

Δ As a precautionary measure, always carry a spare insulin delivery device in case your NovoLog® Mix 70/30 FlexPen® is lost or damaged.

Remember to keep the disposable NovoLog® Mix 70/30 FlexPen® with you. Do not leave it in a car or other location where it can get too hot or too cold.

Date of Issue: May 7, 2010

Version: 8

NovoLog®, FlexPen®, NovoFine®, are trademarks of Novo Nordisk A/S.

NovoLog® is covered by US Patent Nos. 5,547,930, 5,618,913, 5,834,422, 5,840,680, 5,866,538 and other patents pending.

FlexPen® is covered by US Patent Nos. 6,582,404, 6,004,297, 6,235,004 and other patents pending.

© 2002-2010 Novo Nordisk A/S

Manufactured by:

Novo Nordisk A/S

DK-2880 Bagsvaerd, Denmark

For information about NovoLog Mix 70/30® contact:

Novo Nordisk Inc.

100 College Road West,

Princeton, New Jersey 08540

NOVOSEVEN® RT
COAGULATION FACTOR VIIa
(Recombinant)
Room Temperature Stable,
Lyophilized Powder
For Intravenous Use Only

B/

HIGHLIGHTS OF PRESCRIBING INFORMATION

These highlights do not include all the information needed to use NovoSeven RT safely and effectively. See full prescribing information for NovoSeven RT.

NovoSeven® RT Coagulation Factor VIIa (Recombinant)
Room Temperature Stable, Lyophilized Powder

For Intravenous Use Only
Initial U.S. Approval: 1999

> **Warning:** **Serious thrombotic adverse events are associated with the use of NovoSeven RT outside labeled indications**
> Arterial and venous thrombotic and thromboembolic events following administration of NovoSeven have been reported during postmarketing surveillance. Clinical studies have shown an increased risk of arterial thromboembolic adverse events with NovoSeven RT when administered outside the current approved indications. Fatal and non-fatal thrombotic events have been reported. Discuss the risks and explain the signs and symptoms of thrombotic and thromboembolic events to patients who will receive NovoSeven RT. Monitor patients for signs or symptoms of activation of the coagulation system and for thrombosis. **See WARNINGS AND PRECAUTIONS section of prescribing information.**
> **Safety and efficacy of NovoSeven RT has not been established outside the approved indications.**

---RECENT MAJOR CHANGES---

Boxed Warning
Warnings and Precautions (5) 1/2010

---INDICATIONS AND USAGE---

• Treatment of bleeding episodes in hemophilia A or B with inhibitors and in acquired hemophilia (1.1)
• Prevention of bleeding in surgical interventions or invasive procedures in hemophilia A or B with inhibitors and in acquired hemophilia (1.2)
• Treatment of bleeding episodes in congenital FVII deficiency (1.3)
• Prevention of bleeding in surgical interventions or invasive procedures in congenital FVII deficiency (1.4)

---DOSAGE AND ADMINISTRATION---

• For intravenous bolus injection only. After reconstitution, administer within 3 hours; do not freeze or store in syringes (2.6)
• NovoSeven RT should be administered to patients only under the supervision of a physician experienced in the treatment of bleeding disorders (2.1)

Hemophilia A or B with Inhibitors - Bleeding Episodes (2.2)
• 90 micrograms/kg bolus injection every 2 hours until hemostasis is achieved
• Post-hemostatic dosing every 3-6 hours for severe bleeds

Hemophilia A or B with Inhibitors - Surgery (2.2)
• 90 micrograms/kg immediately before surgery and every 2 hours during surgery
• Post-surgical dosing:
  • Minor surgery - 90 micrograms/kg every 2 hours for 48 hours and then every 2-6 hours, until healing has occurred
  • Major surgery - 90 micrograms/kg every 2 hours for the first 5 days and then every 4 hours, until healing has occurred

Congenital FVII Deficiency - Bleeding Episodes or Surgery (2.3)
• 15-30 micrograms/kg every 4-6 hours until hemostasis is achieved

Acquired Hemophilia - Bleeding Episodes or Surgery (2.4)
• 70-90 micrograms/kg every 2-3 hours until hemostasis is achieved

---DOSAGE FORMS AND STRENGTHS---

• Lyophilized powder in single-use vials: 1, 2, 5, or 8 mg rFVIIa (3)
• After reconstitution with specified volume of histidine diluent, each vial contains 1 mg/mL (1000 micrograms/mL) of recombinant FVIIa (3)

---CONTRAINDICATIONS---

None (4)

---WARNINGS AND PRECAUTIONS---

• Thrombotic events of possible or probable relationship to NovoSeven occurred in 0.28% of bleeding episodes treated in clinical trials within the approved indications (5.1)
• Increased risk of arterial thromboembolic adverse events with use of NovoSeven was demonstrated in 2 meta analyses of placebo-controlled clinical trials in populations outside the approved indications (5.2)
• Thrombosis has occurred in women treated with NovoSeven to control post-partum hemorrhage (5.2)
• Factor VII deficient patients should be monitored for prothrombin time (PT) and FVII coagulant activity, and for antibody formation to NovoSeven RT (5.4)
• Administer with caution in patients with known hypersensitivity (5.5)

---ADVERSE REACTIONS---

In clinical trials, the most common adverse reactions are pyrexia, hemorrhage, injection site reaction, arthralgia, headache, hypertension, hypotension, nausea, vomiting, pain, edema and rash (6.1)

To report SUSPECTED ADVERSE REACTIONS, contact Novo Nordisk Inc. at 1-877-668-6777 or FDA at 1-800-FDA-1088 or www.fda.gov/medwatch.

―――DRUG INTERACTIONS―――

• Avoid simultaneous use of NovoSeven RT and PCCs/aPCCs (7.1)
• NovoSeven RT should not be mixed with infusion solutions (7.2)

See 17 for PATIENT COUNSELING INFORMATION

Revised: 08/2010

FULL PRESCRIBING INFORMATION: CONTENTS*

WARNING: SERIOUS THROMBOTIC ADVERSE EVENTS ARE ASSOCIATED WITH THE USE OF NOVOSEVEN RT OUTSIDE LABELED INDICATIONS

FULL PRESCRIBING INFORMATION

Warning: Serious thrombotic adverse events are associated with the use of NovoSeven RT outside labeled indications

Arterial and venous thrombotic and thromboembolic events following administration of NovoSeven have been reported during postmarketing surveillance. Clinical studies have shown an increased risk of arterial thromboembolic adverse events with NovoSeven RT when administered outside the current approved indications. Fatal and non-fatal thrombotic events have been reported. Discuss the risks and explain the signs and symptoms of thrombotic and thromboembolic

---

events to patients who will receive NovoSeven RT. Monitor patients for signs or symptoms of activation of the coagulation system and for thrombosis. **See WARNINGS AND PRECAUTIONS section of prescribing information.**

Safety and efficacy of NovoSeven RT has not been established outside the approved indications.

1 INDICATIONS AND USAGE

NovoSeven RT Coagulation Factor VIIa (Recombinant) Room Temperature Stable is indicated for:

1.1 Treatment of bleeding episodes in hemophilia A or B patients with inhibitors to Factor VIII or Factor IX and in patients with acquired hemophilia

1.2 Prevention of bleeding in surgical interventions or invasive procedures in hemophilia A or B patients with inhibitors to Factor VIII or Factor IX and in patients with acquired hemophilia

1.3 Treatment of bleeding episodes in patients with congenital FVII deficiency

1.4 Prevention of bleeding in surgical interventions or invasive procedures in patients with congenital FVII deficiency

2 DOSAGE AND ADMINISTRATION

2.1 General

• NovoSeven RT is intended for intravenous bolus administration only.
• Evaluation of hemostasis should be used to determine the effectiveness of NovoSeven RT and to provide a basis for modification of the NovoSeven RT treatment schedule.
• Coagulation parameters do not necessarily correlate with or predict the effectiveness of NovoSeven RT.
• NovoSeven RT should be administered to patients only under the supervision of a physician experienced in the treatment of bleeding disorders.

2.2 Hemophilia A or B with Inhibitors

Treatment of Acute Bleeding Episodes

Hemostatic Dosing

• 90 micrograms/kg given every two hours by bolus infusion until hemostasis is achieved, or until the treatment has been judged to be inadequate.
• Doses between 35 and 120 micrograms/kg have been used successfully in clinical trials for hemophilia A or B patients with inhibitors, and both the dose and administration interval may be adjusted based on the severity of the bleeding and degree of hemostasis achieved.[1]
• The minimum effective dose has not been established. For patients treated for joint or muscle bleeds, a decision on outcome was reached for a majority of patients within eight doses although more doses were required for severe bleeds.
• A majority of patients who reported adverse experiences received more than twelve doses.

Post-hemostatic Dosing

• The appropriate duration of post-hemostatic dosing has not been studied.
• For severe bleeds, dosing should continue at 3-6 hour intervals after hemostasis is achieved, to maintain the hemostatic plug.
• The biological and clinical effects of prolonged elevated levels of Factor VIIa have not been studied; therefore, the duration of post-hemostatic dosing should be minimized.
• Patients should be appropriately monitored by a physician experienced in the treatment of hemophilia during this time period.

Dosing for Surgical Interventions

Minor Surgery

• An initial dose of 90 micrograms per kg body weight should be given immediately before the intervention and repeated at 2-hour intervals for the duration of the surgery.
• For minor surgery, post-surgical dosing by bolus injection should occur at 2-hour intervals for the first 48 hours and then at 2- to 6-hour intervals until healing has occurred.

Major Surgery

• An initial dose of 90 micrograms per kg body weight should be given immediately before the intervention and repeated at 2-hour intervals for the duration of the surgery.
• For major surgery, post-surgical dosing by bolus injection should occur at 2 hour intervals for 5 days, followed by 4 hour intervals until healing has occurred. Additional bolus doses should be administered if required.

2.3 Congenital Factor VII deficiency

• The recommended dose range for treatment of bleeding episodes or for prevention of bleeding in surgical interven-

tions or invasive procedures in congenital Factor VII deficient patients is 15-30 micrograms per kg body weight every 4-6 hours until hemostasis is achieved.

• Effective treatment has been achieved with doses as low as 10 micrograms/kg.
• Dose and frequency of injections should be adjusted to each individual.
• The minimum effective dose has not been determined.

2.4 Acquired Hemophilia

• The recommended dose range for the treatment of patients with acquired hemophilia is 70-90 micrograms/kg repeated every 2-3 hours until hemostasis is achieved.
• The minimum effective dose in acquired hemophilia has not been determined.
• The majority of the effective outcomes were observed with treatment in the recommended dose range. The largest number of treatments with any single dose was 90 micrograms/kg; of the 15 treated, 10 (67%) were effective and 2 (13%) were partially effective.

2.5 Reconstitution

Calculate the NovoSeven RT dosage you will need and select the appropriate NovoSeven RT vial package. The selected package contains 1 vial of NovoSeven RT powder and 1 vial of histidine diluent required to prepare reconstituted NovoSeven RT solution. Reconstitute only with the histidine diluent provided with NovoSeven RT. Do not reconstitute with sterile water or other diluent. Reconstitution should be performed using the following procedures:

1. Always use aseptic technique.
2. Bring NovoSeven RT (white, lyophilized powder) and the specified volume of histidine (diluent) to room temperature, but not above 37° C (98.6° F). The specified volume of diluent corresponding to the amount of NovoSeven RT is as follows:

1 mg (1000 micrograms) vial + 1.1 mL Histidine diluent
2 mg (2000 micrograms) vial + 2.1 mL Histidine diluent
5 mg (5000 micrograms) vial + 5.2 mL Histidine diluent
8 mg (8000 micrograms) vial + 8.1 mL Histidine diluent

After reconstitution with the specified volume of diluent, each vial contains approximately 1 mg/mL NovoSeven RT (1000 micrograms/mL).

3. Remove caps from the NovoSeven RT vials to expose the central portion of the rubber stopper. Cleanse the rubber stoppers with an alcohol swab and allow to dry prior to use.
4. Draw back the plunger of a sterile syringe (attached to sterile needle) and admit air into the syringe. It is recommended to use syringe needles of gauge size 20-26.
5. Insert the needle of the syringe into the Histidine diluent vial. Inject air into the vial and withdraw the quantity required for reconstitution.
6. Insert the syringe needle containing the diluent into the NovoSeven RT vial through the center of the rubber stopper, aiming the needle against the side so that the stream of liquid runs down the vial wall (the NovoSeven RT vial does not contain a vacuum). **Do not inject the diluent directly on the NovoSeven RT powder.**
7. Gently swirl the vial until all the material is dissolved. The reconstituted solution is a clear, colorless solution which may be stored either at room temperature or refrigerated for up to 3 hours after reconstitution.

2.6 Administration

• NovoSeven RT is intended for intravenous bolus injection only and should not be mixed with infusion solutions.
• Reconstituted NovoSeven RT should be inspected visually for particulate matter and discoloration prior to administration, whenever solution and container permit. Do not use if particulate matter or discoloration is observed.
• Administration should take place within 3 hours after reconstitution.
• Any unused solution should be discarded. Do not freeze reconstituted NovoSeven RT or store it in syringes.

Administration should be performed using the following procedures:

1. Always use aseptic technique.
2. Draw back the plunger of a sterile syringe (attached to sterile needle) and admit air into the syringe.
3. Insert needle into the vial of reconstituted NovoSeven RT. Inject air into the vial and then withdraw the appropriate amount of reconstituted NovoSeven RT into the syringe.
4. Remove and discard the needle from the syringe.
5. Administer as a slow bolus injection over 2 to 5 minutes, depending on the dose administered.
6. If line needs to be flushed before or after NovoSeven RT administration, use 0.9% Sodium Chloride Injection, USP.
7. Discard any unused reconstituted NovoSeven RT after 3 hours.

3 DOSAGE FORMS AND STRENGTHS

NovoSeven RT is supplied as a white lyophilized powder in single-use vials containing 1 mg (1000 micrograms), 2 mg (2000 micrograms), 5 mg (5000 micrograms), or 8 mg

(8000 micrograms) rFVIIa per vial. The diluent for reconstitution of NovoSeven RT is a 10 mmol solution of L-histidine in water for injection and is supplied as a clear colorless solution and is referred to as the histidine diluent. After reconstitution with the histidine diluent, each vial contains approximately 1 mg/mL NovoSeven RT (1000 micrograms/mL).

4 CONTRAINDICATIONS

None

5 WARNINGS AND PRECAUTIONS

5.1 Thrombotic Events within the Licensed Indications

Clinical trials within the approved indications revealed that thrombotic events of possible or probable relationship to NovoSeven occurred in 0.28% of bleeding episodes treated, with the incidence within hemophilia patients with inhibitors to be 0.20%, and in acquired hemophilia an incidence of 4%. Thrombotic events have been identified through postmarketing surveillance following NovoSeven RT use for each of the approved indications[2]. The incidence of thrombotic events can not be determined from postmarketing data. Patients with disseminated intravascular coagulation (DIC), advanced atherosclerotic disease, crush injury, septicemia, or concomitant treatment with aPCCs/PCCs (activated or nonactivated prothrombin complex concentrates) have an increased risk of developing thrombotic events due to circulating tissue factor (TF) or predisposing coagulopathy *[See Adverse Reactions (6.1) and Drug Interactions (7.1)]*. Caution should be exercised when administering NovoSeven RT to patients with an increased risk of thromboembolic complications. These include, but are not limited to, patients with a history of coronary heart disease, liver disease, disseminated intravascular coagulation, postoperative immobilization, elderly patients and neonates. In each of these situations, the potential benefit of treatment with NovoSeven RT should be weighed against the risk of these complications.

Patients who receive NovoSeven RT should be monitored for development of signs or symptoms of activation of the coagulation system or thrombosis. When there is laboratory confirmation of intravascular coagulation or presence of clinical thrombosis, the NovoSeven RT dosage should be reduced or the treatment stopped, depending on the patient's symptoms.

5.2 Thrombotic Events outside the Licensed Indications

NovoSeven has been studied in placebo controlled trials outside the approved indications to control bleeding in intracerebral hemorrhage, advanced liver disease, trauma, cardiac surgery, spinal surgery, and other therapeutic areas. Safety and effectiveness has not been established in these settings and the use is not approved by FDA. Two meta analyses of these pooled data indicate an increased risk of thrombotic events (10.0% in patients treated with NovoSeven versus 7.5% in placebo-treated patients). Arterial thromboembolic adverse events including myocardial infarction, myocardial ischemia, cerebral infarction and cerebral ischemia were statistically significantly increased with the use of NovoSeven compared to placebo (5.3 to 5.6% in subjects treated with NovoSeven versus 2.8 to 3.0% in placebo-treated patients). Other arterial thromboembolic events (such as retinal artery embolism, renal artery thrombosis, arterial thrombosis of limb, bowel infarction and intestinal infarction) have also been reported.[3,4,5,6,7] While venous thromboembolic events such as deep venous thrombosis, portal vein thrombosis and pulmonary embolism have been reported in clinical trials, the meta analysis of these pooled data from placebo-controlled trials performed outside the currently approved indications did not suggest an increased risk of venous thromboembolic events in patients treated with NovoSeven versus placebo (4.8% in patients treated with NovoSeven versus 4.7% in placebo-treated patients).

In spontaneous reports of women without a prior diagnosis of bleeding disorders receiving NovoSeven for uncontrolled post-partum hemorrhage, thrombotic events were observed. During this period, patients are at increased risk for thrombotic complications.

5.3 Post-Hemostatic Dosing

Precautions should be exercised when NovoSeven RT is used for prolonged dosing *[See Dosage and Administration (2.2)]*.

5.4 Antibody Formation in Factor VII Deficient Patients

Factor VII deficient patients should be monitored for prothrombin time (PT) and factor VII coagulant activity before and after administration of NovoSeven RT. If the factor VIIa activity fails to reach the expected level, or prothrombin time is not corrected, or bleeding is not controlled after treatment with the recommended doses, antibody formation may be suspected and analysis for antibodies should be performed.

5.5 Hypersensitivity Reactions

NovoSeven RT should be administered with caution in patients with known hypersensitivity to NovoSeven RT or any of its components, or in patients with known hypersensitivity to mouse, hamster, or bovine proteins.

5.6 Laboratory Tests

Laboratory coagulation parameters (PT/INR, aPTT, FVII:C) have shown no direct correlation to achieving hemostasis. Assays of prothrombin time (PT/INR), activated partial thromboplastin time (aPTT), and plasma FVII clotting activity (FVII:C), may give different results with different reagents. Treatment with NovoSeven has been shown to produce the following characteristics:

PT: As shown below, in patients with hemophilia A/B with inhibitors, the PT shortened to about a 7-second plateau at a FVII:C level of approximately 5 U/mL. For FVII:C levels > 5 U/mL, there is no further change in PT. The clinical relevance of prothrombin time shortening following NovoSeven RT administration is unknown.

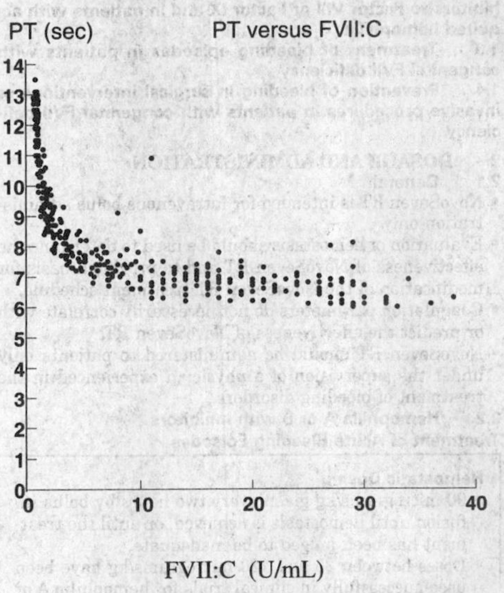

INR: NovoSeven has demonstrated the ability to normalize INR. However, INR values have not been shown to directly predict bleeding outcomes, nor has it been possible to demonstrate the impact of NovoSeven on bleeding times/volume in models of clinically-induced bleeding in healthy volunteers who had received Warfarin, when laboratory parameters (PT/INR, aPTT, thromboelastogram) have normalized.

aPTT: While administration of NovoSeven shortens the prolonged aPTT in hemophilia A/B patients with inhibitors, normalization has usually not been observed in doses shown to induce clinical improvement. Data indicate that clinical improvement was associated with a shortening of aPTT of 15 to 20 seconds.

FVIIa:C: FVIIa:C levels were measured two hours after NovoSeven administration of 35 micrograms/kg and 90 micrograms/kg following two days of dosing at two hour intervals. Average steady state levels were 11 and 28 U/mL for the two dose levels, respectively.

6 ADVERSE REACTIONS

Because clinical studies are conducted under widely varying conditions, adverse reaction rates observed in the clinical trials of a drug product cannot be directly compared to rates in clinical trials of another drug, and may not reflect rates observed in practice.

6.1 Clinical Trials Experience

Thrombotic events following the administration of NovoSeven occurred in 0.28% of bleeding episodes treated, with the incidence in acquired hemophilia of 4% and in hemophilia patients of 0.20% in clinical trials within the approved indications *[See Warnings and Precautions (5.1)]*.

Adverse reactions observed in clinical trials for all labeled indications of NovoSeven included pyrexia, hemorrhage, injection site reaction, arthralgia, headache, hypertension, hypotension, nausea, vomiting, pain, edema, rash (including allergic dermatitis and rash erythematous), pruritus, urticaria, hypersensitivity, cerebral artery occlusion, cerebrovascular accident, pulmonary embolism, deep vein thrombosis, angina pectoris, increased levels of fibrin degradation products, disseminated intravascular coagulation and related laboratory findings including elevated levels of D-dimer and AT-III, thrombosis at i.v. site, non-specified thrombosis, thrombophlebitis, superficial thrombophlebitis. The following sections describe the adverse event profile observed during clinical studies for each of the labeled indications.

Hemophilia A or B Patients with Inhibitors

Two studies (Studies 1 and 2) are described for hemophilia A or B patients with inhibitors treated for bleeding episodes *[See Clinical Studies (14.1)]*. The table below lists adverse events that were reported in ≥2% of the 298 patients with hemophilia A or B with inhibitors that were treated with NovoSeven for 1,939 bleeding episodes. The events listed are considered to be at least possibly related or of unknown relationship to NovoSeven administration.

Body System Event	**# of episodes reported** (n=1,939 treatments)	**# of unique patients** (n=298 patients)
Body as a whole		
Fever	16	13
Platelets, Bleeding, and Clotting		
Hemorrhage NOS	15	8
Fibrinogen plasma decreased	10	5
Skin and Musculoskeletal		
Hemarthrosis	14	8
Cardiovascular		
Hypertension	9	6

Events which were reported in 1% of patients and were considered to be at least possibly or of unknown relationship to NovoSeven administration were: allergic reaction, arthrosis, bradycardia, coagulation disorder, DIC, edema, fibrinolysis increased, headache, hypotension, injection site reaction, pain, pneumonia, prothrombin decreased, pruritus, purpura, rash, renal function abnormal, therapeutic response decreased, and vomiting.

Serious adverse events that were probably or possibly related, or where the relationship to NovoSeven was not specified, occurred in 14 of the 298 patients (4.7%). Six of the 14 patients died of the following conditions: worsening of chronic renal failure, anesthesia complications during proctoscopy, renal failure complicating a retroperitoneal bleed, ruptured abscess leading to sepsis and DIC, pneumonia, and splenic hematoma and gastrointestinal bleeding. Thrombosis was reported in two of the 298 patients with hemophilia.

Surgery Studies

Two clinical trials (Studies 3 and 4) were conducted to evaluate the safety and efficacy of NovoSeven administration during and after surgery in hemophilia A or B patients with inhibitors *[See Clinical Studies (14.1)]*.

In Study 3, six patients experienced serious adverse events: two of these patients had events which were considered probably or possibly related to study medication (acute postoperative hemarthrosis, internal jugular thrombosis). No deaths occurred during the study.

In Study 4, seven of 24 patients had serious adverse events (4 for bolus injection, 3 for continuous infusion). There were 4 serious adverse events which were considered probably or possibly related to NovoSeven treatment (2 events of decreased therapeutic response in each treatment arm). No deaths occurred during the study period.

Congenital Factor VII Deficiency

Data collected from the compassionate/emergency use programs, the published literature, a pharmacokinetics study, and the Hemophilia and Thrombosis Research Society (HTRS) registry showed that at least 75 patients with Factor VII deficiency had received NovoSeven - 70 patients for 124 bleeding episodes, surgeries, or prophylaxis regimens; 5 patients in the pharmacokinetics trial.

In the compassionate/emergency use programs, 28 adverse events in 13 patients and 10 serious adverse events in 9 patients were reported. Non-serious adverse events in the compassionate/emergency use programs were single events in one patient, except for fever (3 patients), intracranial hemorrhage (3 patients), and pain (2 patients). The most common serious adverse event in the compassionate/emergency programs was serious bleeding in critically ill patients. All nine patients with serious adverse events died. One adverse event (localized phlebitis) was reported in the literature. No adverse events were reported in the pharmacokinetics reports or for the HTRS registry. No thromboembolic complications were reported for the 75 patients included here.

As with all therapeutic proteins, there is a potential for immunogenicity. Isolated cases of factor VII deficient patients developing antibodies against factor VII were reported after treatment with NovoSeven. These patients had previously been treated with human plasma and/or plasma-derived factor VII. In some cases the antibodies showed inhibitory effect *in vitro*. The incidence of antibody formation is highly dependent on the sensitivity and specificity of the assay. Additionally, the observed incidence of antibody (including neutralizing antibody) positivity in an assay may be influenced by several factors including assay methodology, sample handling, timing of sample collection, concomitant medications, and underlying disease. For these reasons, comparison of the incidence of antibodies to NovoSeven RT with the incidence of antibodies to other products may be misleading.

Acquired Hemophilia

Data collected from four compassionate use programs, the HTRS registry, and the published literature showed that 139 patients with acquired hemophilia received NovoSeven for 204 bleeding episodes, surgeries and traumatic injuries. Of these 139 patients, 10 experienced 12 serious adverse events that were of possible, probable, or unknown relationship to treatment with NovoSeven. Thrombotic serious adverse events included cerebral infarction, cerebral ischemia, angina pectoris, myocardial infarction, pulmonary embolism and deep vein thrombosis. Additional serious adverse events included shock and subdural hematoma.

Data collected for mortality in the compassionate use programs, the HTRS registry and the publications spanning a 10 year period, was overall 32/139 (23%). Deaths due to hemorrhage were 10, cardiovascular failure 4, neoplasia 4, unknown causes 4, respiratory failure 3, thrombotic events 2, sepsis 2, arrhythmia 2 and trauma 1.

6.2 Postmarketing Experience

The following adverse reactions have been identified during post approval use of NovoSeven. Because these reactions are reported voluntarily from a population of uncertain size, it is not always possible to reliably estimate their frequency or establish a causal relationship.

The following additional adverse events were reported following the use of NovoSeven in labeled and unlabeled indications that included individuals with and without coagulopathy: high D-dimer levels and consumptive coagulopathy, thrombosis, thrombophlebitis, arterial thrombosis, and thromboembolic events including myocardial ischemia, myocardial infarction, bowel infarction, cerebral ischemia, cerebral infarction, hepatic artery thrombosis, renal artery thrombosis, portal vein thrombosis, phlebitis, peripheral ischemia, deep vein thrombosis and related pulmonary embolism, injection site pain and isolated cases of hypersensitivity/allergic reactions including anaphylactic shock, flushing, urticaria, rash, and angioedema *[See Warnings and Precautions (5.1)]*.

Fatal and non-fatal thromboembolic events have been reported with use of NovoSeven when used for off-label or labeled indications.

The Hemophilia and Thrombosis Research Society (HTRS) Registry surveillance program is designed to collect data on the treatment of congenital and acquired bleeding disorders.[8] All prescribers can obtain information regarding contribution of patient data to this program by calling 1-877-362-7355 or at www.novosevensurveillance.com.

7 DRUG INTERACTIONS

7.1 Coagulation Factor Concentrates

The risk of a potential interaction between NovoSeven RT and coagulation factor concentrates has not been adequately evaluated in preclinical or clinical studies. Simultaneous use of activated prothrombin complex concentrates or prothrombin complex concentrates should be avoided.

7.2 Infusion Solutions

NovoSeven RT should not be mixed with infusion solutions.

8 USE IN SPECIFIC POPULATIONS

8.1 Pregnancy

Pregnancy Category C. There are no adequate and well-controlled studies in pregnant women. NovoSeven RT should be used during pregnancy only if the potential benefit justifies the potential risk to the fetus.

Treatment of rats and rabbits with NovoSeven in reproduction studies has been associated with mortality at doses up to 6 mg/kg and 5 mg/kg. At 6 mg/kg in rats, the abortion rate was 0 out of 25 litters; in rabbits at 5 mg/kg, the abortion rate was 2 out of 25 litters. Twenty-three out of 25 female rats given 6 mg/kg of NovoSeven gave birth successfully, however, two of the 23 litters died during the early period of lactation. No evidence of teratogenicity was observed after dosing with NovoSeven.

8.2 Labor and Delivery

NovoSeven was administered to a FVII deficient patient (25 years of age, 66 kg) during a vaginal delivery (36 micrograms/kg) and during a tubal ligation (90 micrograms/kg). No adverse reactions were reported during labor, vaginal delivery, or the tubal ligation.

There are no adequate and well-controlled studies in labor, delivery, and postpartum periods. In spontaneous reports of women without a prior diagnosis of bleeding disorders receiving NovoSeven for uncontrolled post-partum hemor-

Contents	1 mg Vial	2 mg Vial	5 mg Vial	8 mg Vial
rFVIIa	1000 micrograms	2000 micrograms	5000 micrograms	8000 micrograms
sodium chloride*	2.34 mg	4.68 mg	11.7 mg	18.72 mg
calcium chloride dihydrate*	1.47 mg	2.94 mg	7.35 mg	11.76 mg
glycylglycine	1.32 mg	2.64 mg	6.60 mg	10.56 mg
polysorbate 80	0.07 mg	0.14 mg	0.35 mg	0.56 mg
mannitol	25 mg	50 mg	125 mg	200 mg
Sucrose	10 mg	20 mg	50 mg	80 mg
Methionine	0.5 mg	1.0 mg	2.5 mg	4 mg

*per mg of rFVIIa: 0.4 mEq sodium, 0.01 mEq calcium

rhage, thrombotic events were observed. During this period, patients are at increased risk for thrombotic complications. It is not known to what extent NovoSeven contributed to the occurrence of these events.

8.3 Nursing Mothers

It is not known whether NovoSeven RT is excreted in human milk. Because many drugs are excreted in human milk, and because of the potential for serious adverse reactions in nursing infants, a decision should be made whether to discontinue nursing or to discontinue the drug, taking into account the importance of the drug to the mother.

8.4 Pediatric Use

Clinical trials enrolling pediatric patients were conducted with dosing determined according to body weight and not according to age. The safety and effectiveness of NovoSeven RT has not been studied to determine if there are differences among various age groups, from infants to adolescents (0 to 16 years of age).

8.5 Geriatric Use

Clinical studies of NovoSeven in congenital factor deficiencies did not include sufficient numbers of subjects aged 65 and over to determine whether they respond differently from younger subjects.

10 OVERDOSAGE

There are no adequate and well controlled studies to support the safety or efficacy of using higher than labeled doses in the indicated populations.

Dose limiting toxicities of NovoSeven RT have not been investigated in clinical trials. The following are examples of accidental overdose.

Congenital Factor VII Deficiency

A newborn female with congenital factor VII deficiency was administered an overdose of NovoSeven (single dose: 800 micrograms/kg). Following additional administration of NovoSeven and various plasma products, antibodies against rFVIIa were detected, but no thrombotic complications were reported. A Factor VII deficient male (83 years of age, 111.1 kg) received two doses of 324 micrograms/kg (10-20 times the recommended dose) and experienced a thrombotic event (occipital stroke).

Hemophilia A or B with Inhibitors

One hemophilia B patient (16 years of age, 68 kg) received a single dose of 352 micrograms/kg and one hemophilia A patient (2 years of age, 14.6 kg) received doses ranging from 246 micrograms/kg to 986 micrograms/kg on five consecutive days. There were no reported complications in either case.

11 DESCRIPTION

NovoSeven RT is recombinant human coagulation Factor VIIa (rFVIIa), intended for promoting hemostasis by activating the extrinsic pathway of the coagulation cascade.[9] NovoSeven RT is a vitamin K-dependent glycoprotein consisting of 406 amino acid residues (MW 50 K Dalton). NovoSeven RT is structurally similar to human plasma-derived Factor VIIa.

The gene for human Factor VII is cloned and expressed in baby hamster kidney cells (BHK cells). Recombinant FVII is secreted into the culture media (containing newborn calf serum) in its single-chain form and then proteolytically converted by autocatalysis to the active two-chain form, rFVIIa, during a chromatographic purification process. The purification process has been demonstrated to remove exogenous viruses (MuLV, SV40, Pox virus, Reovirus, BEV, IBR virus). No human serum or other proteins are used in the production or formulation of NovoSeven RT.

NovoSeven RT is supplied as a sterile, white lyophilized powder of rFVIIa in single-use vials. Each vial of lyophilized drug contains the following:

[See table above]

The diluent for reconstitution of NovoSeven RT is a 10 mmol solution of histidine in water for injection and is supplied as a clear colorless solution.

After reconstitution with the appropriate volume of **histidine** diluent, each vial contains approximately 1 mg/mL NovoSeven RT (corresponding to 1000 micrograms/mL). The reconstituted vials have a pH of approximately 6.0 in sodium chloride (2.3 mg/mL), calcium chloride dihydrate (1.5 mg/mL), glycylglycine (1.3 mg/mL), polysorbate 80 (0.1 mg/mL), mannitol (25 mg/mL), sucrose (10 mg/mL), methionine (0.5 mg/mL), and histidine (1.6 mg/mL).

The reconstituted product is a clear colorless solution which contains no preservatives. NovoSeven RT contains trace amounts of proteins derived from the manufacturing and purification processes such as mouse IgG (maximum of 1.2 ng/mg), bovine IgG (maximum of 30 ng/mg), and protein from BHK-cells and media (maximum of 19 ng/mg).

12 CLINICAL PHARMACOLOGY

12.1 Mechanism of Action

NovoSeven RT is recombinant Factor VIIa and, when complexed with tissue factor can activate coagulation Factor X to Factor Xa, as well as coagulation Factor IX to Factor IXa. Factor Xa, in complex with other factors, then converts prothrombin to thrombin, which leads to the formation of a hemostatic plug by converting fibrinogen to fibrin and thereby inducing local hemostasis. This process may also occur on the surface of activated platelets.

12.2 Pharmacodynamics

The effect of NovoSeven RT upon coagulation in patients with or without hemophilia has been assessed in different model systems. In an *in vitro* model of tissue-factor-initiated blood coagulation (Figure A)[10], the addition of rFVIIa increased both the rate and level of thrombin generation in normal and hemophilia A blood, with an effect shown at rFVIIa concentrations as low as 10 nM. In this model, fresh human blood was treated with corn trypsin inhibitor (CTI) to block the contact pathway of blood coagulation. Tissue factor (TF) was added to initiate clotting in the presence and absence of rFVIIa for both types of blood.

In a separate model, and in line with previous reports[11], escalating doses of rFVIIa in hemophilia plasma demonstrate a dose-dependent increase in thrombin generation (Figure B). In this model, platelet rich normal and hemophilia plasma was adjusted with autologous plasma to 200,000 platelets/microliter. Coagulation was initiated by addition of tissue factor and $CaCl_2$. Thrombin generation was measured in the presence of a thrombin substrate and various added concentrations of rFVIIa.

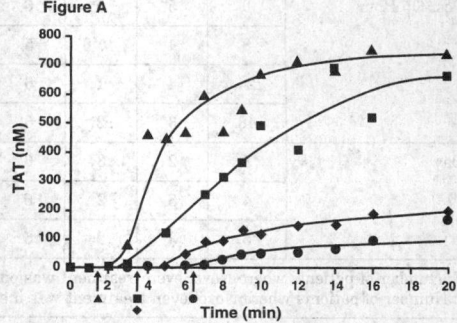

Figure A

TF-initiated clotting of normal blood and congenital hemophilia A blood in the presence of factor VIIa. Clotting of CTI-inhibited (0.1 mg/mL) normal blood initiated with 12.5 pM TF (■) and addition of 10 nM factor VIIa (▲) and of hemophilia A blood with (♦) and without (●) addition of 10 nM factor VIIa. Figure A shows Thrombin Anti-Thrombin generation over time. Arrows indicate clotting times.

Figure B

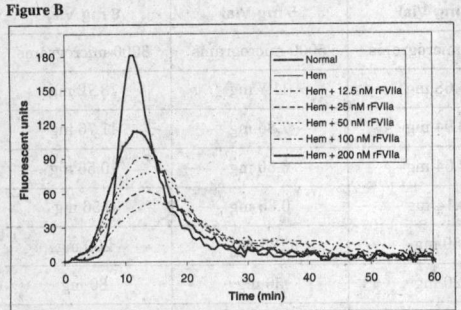

TF-initiated clotting of normal and hemophilia A platelet rich plasma in the presence of rFVIIa.

12.3 Pharmacokinetics

Healthy Subjects

The pharmacokinetics of NovoSeven was investigated in 35 healthy Caucasian and Japanese subjects in a dose-escalation study. Subjects were stratified according to gender and ethnic group and dosed with 40, 80 and 160 micrograms/kg NovoSeven[12]. The pharmacokinetics of rFVII were linear over the dose range of 40 to 180 micrograms/kg. Pharmacokinetics were similar across gender and ethnic groups. Mean steady state volume of distribution ranged from 130 to 165 mL/kg, mean values of clearance ranged from 33 to 37 mL/h × kg, and mean terminal half-life ranged from 3.9 to 6.0 hours.

Hemophilia A or B

Single-dose pharmacokinetics of NovoSeven (17.5, 35, and 70 micrograms/kg) exhibited dose-proportional behavior in 15 subjects with hemophilia A or B.[13] Factor VII clotting activities were measured in plasma drawn prior to and during a 24-hour period after NovoSeven administration. The median apparent volume of distribution at steady state was 103 mL/kg (range 78-139). The median clearance was 33 mL/kg/hr (range 27-49). The median residence time was 3.0 hours (range 2.4-3.3), and the $t_{1/2}$ was 2.3 hours (range 1.7-2.7). The median in vivo plasma recovery was 44% (30-71%). The products NovoSeven RT and NovoSeven are pharmacokinetically equivalent.[14]

In a bolus single-dose pharmacokinetic study, 5 male adults (90 micrograms/kg) and 10 male pediatric (2-12 years) patients (crossover, 90 and 180 micrograms/kg) with severe hemophilia A (10 of 18 subjects had inhibitors) received NovoSeven[15]. The PK of rFVII following 90 and 180 micrograms/kg IV dose in children indicated dose linearity. Based on the FVII:C assay, the terminal half-life of NovoSeven was 2.6 hrs in pediatric patients and 3.1 hrs in adults. Based on the 90 microgram/kg dose, the total clearance of NovoSeven in adults and children was 2767 ± 385 mL/hr (37.6 ± 13.1 mL/hr/kg) and 1375 ± 396 mL/hr

(57.3 ± 9.5 mL/hr/kg), respectively. The volume of distribution at steady state (V_{ss}) in adults and children was 121 ± 30 and 153 ± 29 mL/kg, respectively.

Congenital Factor VII deficiency

Single dose pharmacokinetics of NovoSeven in congenital Factor VII deficiency, at doses of 15 and 30 micrograms per kg body weight, showed no significant difference between the two doses used with regard to dose-independent parameters: total body clearance (70.8-79.1 mL/hr × kg), volume of distribution at steady state (280-290 mL/kg), mean residence time (3.75-3.80 hr), and half-life (2.82-3.11 hr). The mean in vivo plasma recovery was approximately 20% (18.9%-22.2%).

The normal Factor VII plasma concentration is 0.5 micrograms/mL. Factor VII levels of 15-25% (0.075–0.125 micrograms/mL) are generally sufficient to achieve normal hemostasis.[16] For example, a 70 kg individual with FVII deficiency (plasma volume of approximately 3000 mL) would thus require 3.2-5.4 micrograms/kg of NovoSeven RT to secure hemostasis, assuming 100% recovery but, since the mean plasma recovery for NovoSeven is 20% for FVII-deficient patients, a NovoSeven RT dose range of 16-27 micrograms/kg would be required to achieve sufficient FVII plasma levels for hemostasis, which is consistent with the recommended dose range.

13 NONCLINICAL TOXICOLOGY

13.1 Carcinogenesis, Mutagenesis, Impairment of Fertility

Two mutagenicity studies have given no indication of carcinogenic potential for NovoSeven. The clastogenic activity of NovoSeven was evaluated in both in vitro studies (i.e., cultured human lymphocytes) and in vivo studies (i.e., mouse micronucleus test). Neither of these studies indicated clastogenic activity of NovoSeven. Other gene mutation studies have not been performed with NovoSeven RT (e.g., Ames test). No chronic carcinogenicity studies have been performed with NovoSeven RT.

A reproductive study in male and female rats at dose levels up to 3.0 mg/kg/day had no effect on mating performance, fertility, or litter characteristics.

Treatment of rats and rabbits with NovoSeven in reproduction studies has been associated with mortality at doses up to 6 mg/kg and higher. At 6 mg/kg in rats, the abortion rate was 0 out of 25 litters; in rabbits at 5 mg/kg, the abortion rate was 2 out of 25 litters. Twenty-three out of 25 female rats given 6 mg/kg of NovoSeven gave birth successfully, however, two of the 23 litters died during the early period of lactation. No evidence of teratogenicity was observed after dosing with NovoSeven.

14 CLINICAL STUDIES

No direct comparisons to other coagulation products have been conducted, therefore no conclusions regarding the comparative safety or efficacy can be made.

14.1 Hemophilia A or B with Inhibitors

Open Protocol Use

The largest number of patients who received NovoSeven during the investigational phase of product development

were in an open protocol study (Study 1)[17,18,19] that began enrollment in 1988, shortly after the completion of the pharmacokinetic study. These patients included persons with hemophilia types A or B (with or without inhibitors), persons with acquired inhibitors to Factor VIII or Factor IX, and a few FVII deficient patients. The clinical situations were diverse and included muscle/joint bleeds, mucocutaneous bleeds, surgical prophylaxis, intracerebral bleeds, and other emergent situations. Dose schedules were suggested by Novo Nordisk, but they were subject to the option of the investigator. Clinical outcomes were not reported in a standardized manner. Therefore, the clinical data from Study 1 are problematic for the evaluation of the safety and efficacy of the product by statistical methods.

Dosing Study

Study 2[20] was a double-blind, randomized comparison trial of two dose levels of NovoSeven in the treatment of joint, muscle and mucocutaneous hemorrhages in hemophilia A and B patients with and without inhibitors. Patients received NovoSeven as soon as they could be evaluated in the treatment centers (4 to 18 hours after experiencing a bleed). Thirty-five patients were treated at the 35 micrograms/kg dose (59 joint, 15 muscle and 5 mucocutaneous bleeding episodes) and 43 patients were treated at the 70 micrograms/kg dose (85 joint and 14 muscle bleeding episodes). Dosing was to be repeated at 2.5 hour intervals but ranged up to four hours for some patients. Efficacy was assessed at 12 ± 2 hours or at end of treatment, whichever occurred first. Based on a subjective evaluation by the investigator, the respective efficacy rates for the 35 and 70 micrograms/kg groups were: excellent 59% and 60%, effective 12% and 11%, and partially effective 17% and 20%. The average number of injections required to achieve hemostasis was 2.8 and 3.2 for the 35 and 70 micrograms/kg groups, respectively.

One patient in the 35 micrograms/kg group and three in the 70 micrograms/kg group experienced serious adverse events that were not considered related to NovoSeven. Two unrelated deaths occurred; one patient died of AIDS and the other of intracranial hemorrhage secondary to trauma.

Surgery Studies

Two clinical trials (Studies 3 and 4) were conducted to evaluate the safety and efficacy of NovoSeven administration during and after surgery in hemophilia A or B patients with inhibitors.

Study 3 was a randomized, double-blind, parallel group clinical trial (29 patients with hemophilia A or B and inhibitors or acquired inhibitors to FVIII/FIX, undergoing major or minor surgical procedures).[21] Patients received bolus intravenous NovoSeven (either 35 micrograms/kg, N=15; or 90 micrograms/kg, N=14) prior to surgery, intra-operatively as required, then every 2 hours for the following 48 hours beginning at closure of the wound. Additional doses were administered every 2 to 6 hours up to an additional 3 days to maintain hemostasis. After a maximum of 5 days of double-blind treatment, therapy could be continued in an open-label manner if necessary (90 micrograms/kg NovoSeven every 2-6 hours). Efficacy was assessed during the intra-operative period, and post-operatively from the time of wound closure (Hour 0) through Day 5.

When efficacy assessments at each time point were tabulated by a last value carried forward approach (patients who completed the study early having achieved effective hemostasis were counted as "effective" and those who discontinued due to treatment failure or adverse events were counted as "ineffective" at each time point thereafter), the results at the end of the 5-day double-blind treatment period were as summarized in the table below. Twenty-three patients successfully completed the entire study (including the open-label period after the 5-day double blind period) with satisfactory hemostasis.

[See study 3 at left]
[See study 3 at top of next page]

Study 4 was an open-label, randomized, parallel trial conducted to compare the safety and efficacy of IV bolus (N=12) and IV continuous infusion (N=12) administration of NovoSeven in hemophilia A or B patients with inhibitors who were undergoing elective major surgery. The types of surgeries that were performed included knee (N=13), hip (N=3), abdomen/lower pelvis (N=2), groin/inguinal area (N=2), circumcision (N=1), eye (N=1), frontal/temporal region of cranium (N=1), and oral cavity (N=1). Prior to surgery, a 90 micrograms/kg bolus dose of NovoSeven was administered to both bolus and continuous infusion groups. The bolus injection group then received 90 micrograms/kg NovoSeven by IV bolus injection every 2 hours during the procedure and for the first 5 days, then every 4 hours from Day 6 to Day 10. The continuous infusion group received 50 micrograms/kg/h NovoSeven by IV continuous infusion for the first 5 days, and infusion of 25 micrograms/kg/h from Day 6 to Day 10. For both NovoSeven-treated groups, two bolus rescue doses of 90 micrograms/kg were permitted during any 24-hour period.

Study 3: Dose Comparison of Efficacy in Major and Minor Surgery - Last Value Carried Forward*

	Number of effective (E)/ineffective (I) responses in each dose group									
	Major Surgery				**Minor Surgery**					
	35 µg/kg[†] (n = 5)		90 µg/kg (n = 6)		35 µg/kg (n = 10)		90 µg/kg (n = 8)		Total (n = 29)	
	E	I	E	I	E	I	E	I	E	I
Intraoperative	5	0	6	0	10	0	7	1	28	1
Post-Op Hour 0	5	0	6	0	8	2	6	2	25	4
8	4	1	5	1	9	1	7	1	25	4
24	4	1	6	0	9	1	6	2	25	4
48	3	2	6	0	8	2	8	0	25	4
Day 3	2	3	6	0	8	2	8	0	24	5
4	3	2	6	0	8	2	8	0	25	4
5	3	2	5	1	8	2	8	0	24	5

E: Number of patients where NovoSeven treatment was effective
I: Number of patients where NovoSeven treatment was ineffective

* Patients who completed the study early having achieved effective hemostasis were counted as effective at subsequent time-points, and patients who discontinued due to treatment failure or adverse events were counted as ineffective at subsequent time-points. Only effective ratings were counted as successful hemostasis (ratings of "partially effective" were not counted). Ten patients completed the study by Day 5 because their bleeding had resolved and they were discharged from the hospital. Three patients dropped out of the study due to ineffective therapy and 1 patient left the study due to an adverse event.

† µg/kg = micrograms/kg

The bolus injection (90 micrograms/kg) and continuous infusion (50 micrograms/kg/h) treatment groups showed comparable efficacy in achieving and maintaining hemostasis in major surgery from wound closure through Day 10. For the Global Hemostasis Treatment Evaluation for overall success in achieving and maintaining hemostasis at the end of the study period, treatment was rated as being effective in 9 patients (75%) and ineffective in 3 patients (25%) for both treatment groups.

When efficacy assessments at each time point were tabulated by a last value carried forward approach (patients who completed the study early having achieved effective hemostasis were counted as "effective" at each time point, and those who discontinued due to treatment failure counted as "ineffective" at each time point thereafter), the results were as summarized in the table below.

[See study 4 at right]

[See study 4 at top of next page]

14.2 Congenital Factor VII Deficiency

Data were collected from the published literature and internal sources for 70 patients with Factor VII deficiency treated with NovoSeven for 124 bleeding episodes, surgeries, or prophylaxis regimens. Thirty-two of these patients were enrolled in emergency and compassionate use trials conducted by Novo Nordisk (43 non-surgical bleeding episodes, 26 surgeries); 35 were reported in the published literature (20 surgeries, 10 non-surgical bleeding episodes, 4 cases of caesarean section or vaginal birth, and 10 cases of long-term prophylaxis, and 1 case of on-demand therapy); and 3 were from a registry maintained by the Hemophilia and Thrombosis Research Society (9 bleeding episodes, 1 surgery). Dosing ranged from 6-98 micrograms/kg administered every 2-12 hours (except for prophylaxis, where doses were administered from 2 times per day up to 2 times per week). Patients were treated with an average of 1-10 doses. Treatment was effective (bleeding stopped or treatment was rated as effective by the physician) in 93% of episodes (90% for trial patients, 98% for published patients, 90% for HTRS registry patients).

14.3 Acquired Hemophilia

Data were collected from four studies in the compassionate use program conducted by Novo Nordisk and the Hemophilia and Thrombosis Research Society (HTRS) registry. A total of 70 patients with acquired hemophilia were treated with NovoSeven for 113 bleeding episodes, surgeries, or traumatic injuries. Sixty-one of these patients were from the compassionate use program with 100 bleeding episodes (68 non-surgical and 32 surgical bleeding episodes) and 9 patients were from the HTRS registry with 13 bleeding episodes (8 non-surgical, 3 surgical and 2 episodes classified as other). Concomitant use of other hemostatic agents occurred in 29/70 (41%); 13 (19%) received more than one hemostatic agent. The most common hemostatic agents used were antifibrinolytics, Factor VIII and activated prothrombin complex concentrates.

The compassionate use programs and the HTRS registry were not designed to select doses or compare first-line efficacy or efficacy when used after failure of other hemostatic agents (salvage treatment). A dose response was not seen in doses ranging from 70-90 micrograms/kg.

The mean dose of NovoSeven administered was 90 micrograms/kg (range: 31 to 197 micrograms/kg); the mean number of injections per day was 6 (range: 1 to 10 injections per day). Overall efficacy i.e., effective and partially effective outcomes, was 87/112 (78%); with 77/100 (77%) efficacy in the compassionate use programs and 10/12 (83%) efficacy in the HTRS registry. In the compassionate use programs, overall efficacy for the first-line treatment was 38/44 (86%) compared to 39/56 (70%) when used as salvage treatment.

[See second table on next page]

15 REFERENCES

1. Hedner, U.: Dosing and Monitoring NovoSeven® Treatment, Haemostasis 1996; 26 (suppl 1): 102-108.

2. Girolami, B., et al.: Arterial and venous thrombosis in rare congenital bleeding disorders: a critical review, Haemophilia (2006); 12, 345-351.

3. Mayer, S.A., et al.: Recombinant Activated Factor VII for Acute Intracerebral Hemorrhage, New England Journal of Medicine 2005; 352: 777-785.

4. Mayer, S.A., et al.: Efficacy and Safety of Recombinant Activated Factor VII for Acute Intracerebral Hemorrhage, New England Journal of Medicine 2008; 358:2127-37.

5. Thomas, R, et al: Thromboembolic complications associated with Factor VIIa administration, J Trauma 2007; 62:564-569.

6. Hsia, Cyrus C., et al., "Use of Recombinant Activated Factor VII in Patients Without Hemophilia, A Meta-Analysis of Randomized Control Trials," Annals of Surgery, Vol 248, No. 1, July 2008.

7. Hardy, Jean-Francois, et al, "Efficacy and Safety of Recombinant Activated Factor VII to Control Bleeding in Nonhemophiliac Patients: A Review of 17 Randomized Controlled Trials," Ann Thorac Surg 2008; 86: 1038-48.

8. Parameswaran, R., et al.: Dose effect and efficacy of rFVIIa in the treatment of haemophilia patients with inhibitors: analysis from the Hemophilia and Thrombosis Research Society Registry, Haemophilia 2005; 11: 100-106.

9. Roberts, H.R.: Thoughts on the mechanism of action of FVIIa, 2nd Symposium on New Aspects of Hemophilia Treatment, Copenhagen, Denmark, 1991, pgs. 153-156.

10. Butenas, S., et al.: Mechanism of factor VIIa-dependent coagulation in hemophilia blood, Blood 2002; 99: 923-930. Figure A Copyright American Society of Hematology, used with permission.

11. Allen, G.A., et al.: The effect of factor X level on thrombin generation and the procoagulant effect of activated factor VII in a cell-based model of coagulation, Blood Coagulation and Fibrinolysis 2000; 11 (suppl 1): 3-7.

12. Fridberg M.J., et al.: A study of the pharmacokinetics and safety of recombinant activated factor VII in healthy Caucasian and Japanese subjects, Blood Coagulation and Fibrinolysis 2005, 16 (4): 259-266.

13. Lindley, C.M., et al.: Pharmacokinetics and pharmacodynamics of recombinant Factor VIIa, Clinical Pharmacology & Therapeutics 1994; 55 (6): 638-648.

14. Bysted B.V., et al.: A randomized double-blind trial demonstrating bioequivalence of the current recombinant activated factor VII formulation and a new robust 25°C stable formulation, Haemophilia 2007, 13, 527-532.

15. Villar, A., et al.: Pharmacokinetics of activated recombinant coagulation factor VIIa (NovoSeven®) in children vs. adults with haemophilia A, Haemophilia 2004; 10 (4):352-359.

16. Bauer, K.A.: Treatment of Factor VII deficiency with recombinant Factor VIIa, Haemostasis 1996; 26 (suppl 1): 155-158.

17. Lusher, J., et al.: Clinical experience with recombinant Factor VIIa, Blood Coagulation and Fibrinolysis 1998; 9: 119-128.

18. Bech, M.R.: Recombinant Factor VIIa in Joint and Muscle Bleeding Episodes, Haemostasis 1996; 26 (suppl 1): 135-138.

19. Lusher, J.M.: Recombinant Factor VIIa (NovoSeven®) in the Treatment of Internal Bleeding in Patients with Factor VIII and IX Inhibitors, Haemostasis 1996; 26 (suppl 1): 124-130.

20. Lusher, J.M., et al.: A randomized, double-blind comparison of two dosage levels of recombinant factor VIIa in the treatment of joint, muscle and mucocutaneous haemorrhages in persons with hemophilia A and B, with and without inhibitor, Haemophilia 1998; 4: 790-798.

21. Shapiro A.D., et al: Prospective, Randomised Trial of Two Doses of rFVIIa in Haemophilia Patients with Inhibitors Undergoing Surgery, Thrombosis and Haemostasis 1998; 80: 773-778.

16 HOW SUPPLIED/STORAGE AND HANDLING

NovoSeven RT Coagulation Factor VIIa (Recombinant) Room Temperature Stable is supplied as a white, lyophilized powder in single-use vials, one vial per carton. The vials are made of glass, closed with a latex-free, chlorobutyl rubber stopper, and sealed with an aluminum cap. The vials are equipped with a snap-off polypropylene cap. The amount of rFVIIa in milligrams and in micrograms is stated on the label as follows:

1 mg per vial (1000 micrograms/vial) NDC 0169-7010-01
2 mg per vial (2000 micrograms/vial) NDC 0169-7020-01
5 mg per vial (5000 micrograms/vial) NDC 0169-7050-01
8 mg per vial (8000 micrograms/vial) NDC 0169-7040-01

Study 3: Dosing by Surgery Category

	Major Surgery		Minor Surgery	
	35 µg/kg* (n = 5)	90 µg/kg (n = 6)	35 µg/kg (n = 10)	90 µg/kg (n = 8)
Days of dosing, median (range)	15 (2-26)	9.5 (8-17)	4 (3-6)	6 (3-13)
No. injections, median (range)	135 (11-186)	81 (71-128)	29.5 (24-44)	39.5 (26-98)
Median total dose, mg (range)	656 (31-839)	569 (107-698)	45.5 (14-171)	67 (31-122)

*µg/kg = micrograms/kg

Study 4: Efficacy of Bolus Dosing vs. Continuous Infusion in Major Surgery - Last Value Carried Forward*

		Number of effective (E)/ineffective (I) responses in each dose group			
		Bolus Injection (NovoSeven 90 micrograms/kg) n = 12		Continuous Infusion (NovoSeven 50 micrograms/kg/h) n = 12	
		E	I	E	I
Post-Op Hour	0	12	0	12	0
	8	12	0	11	1
	24	12	0	10	2
	48	10	2	11	1
	72	9	3	11	1
Day	4	11	1	10	2
	5	11	1	10	2
	6	11	1	10	2
	7	9	3	10	2
	8	10	2	10	2
	9	9	3	10	2
	10	9	3	10	2

E: Number of patients where NovoSeven treatment was effective
I: Number of patients where NovoSeven treatment was ineffective

* Patients who completed the study early having achieved hemostasis counted as effective at subsequent time-points, and patients who discontinued due to treatment failure counted as ineffective at subsequent time-points. Eight patients completed the study early because their bleeding had resolved and they were discharged from the hospital. Four patients dropped out of the study due to ineffective therapy and 1 patient left the study due to a hemarthrosis that was described as an adverse event.

Study 4: Dosing by Treatment Group

	Bolus Injection 90 micrograms/kg (n = 12)	Continuous Infusion 50 micrograms/kg/h (n = 12)
Days of dosing, median (range)	10 (4-15)*	10 (2-116)
No. bolus injections, median (range)	38 (36-42)	1.5 (0-7)
No. of additional bolus injections, median (range)	0 (0-3)	0 (0-4)
Mean total dose, mg	237.5	292.2

*Includes dosing during the follow-up period after the 10-day study period.

Efficacy by Dose Group, for Patients Receiving Doses Ranging from <61 to >90 micrograms/kg NovoSeven, Compassionate Use Programs and HTRS Registry

Outcome*	Unknown	<61	61-69	70-80	81-89	90	>90	Total
Effective N (%)	1 (33)	3 (75)	5 (63)	10 (63)	12 (57)	10 (67)	26 (58)	67
Partial N (%)	1 (33)	0 (0)	0 (0)	3 (19)	3 (14)	2 (13)	11 (24)	20
Ineffective N (%)	0 (0)	1 (25)	3 (38)	2 (13)	2 (10)	2 (13)	7 (16)	17
Unknown N (%)	1 (33)	0 (0)	0 (0)	1 (6)	4 (19)	1 (7)	1 (2)	8
No. of Bleeding Episodes†	3	4	8	16	21	15	45	112‡

* Outcome assessed at end of treatment, last observation carried forward.
† N (%) do not add up to 100 due to rounding.
‡ One patient in the HTRS registry was excluded from efficacy analysis since NovoSeven was used to maintain hemostasis after bleeding had been controlled.

The diluent for reconstitution of NovoSeven RT is a 10 mmol solution of L-histidine in water for injection and is supplied as a clear colorless solution, and referred to as the histidine diluent. The vials are made of glass closed with a latex-free, chlorobutyl rubber disc, and covered with an aluminum cap. The closed vials are equipped with a tamper-evident snap-off cap which is made of polypropylene.
Prior to reconstitution, keep refrigerated or store between 2-25°C/36-77°F. Do not freeze. Store protected from light. Do not use past the expiration date.
After reconstitution, NovoSeven RT may be stored either at room temperature or refrigerated for up to 3 hours. Do not freeze reconstituted NovoSeven RT or store it in syringes.

17   PATIENT COUNSELING INFORMATION
Patients receiving NovoSeven RT should be informed of the benefits and risks associated with treatment. Patients should be warned about the early signs of hypersensitivity reactions, including hives, urticaria, tightness of the chest, wheezing, hypotension, and anaphylaxis. Patients should also be warned about the signs of thrombosis, including new onset swelling and pain in the limbs or abdomen, new onset chest pain, shortness of breath, loss of sensation or motor power, or altered consciousness or speech. Patients should be told to immediately seek medical help if any of the above signs or symptoms occur.
Date of issue: August 6, 2010
Version: 4
License Number: 1261
Novo Nordisk® is a registered trademark of Novo Nordisk A/S.
NovoSeven® is a registered trademark of Novo Nordisk Health Care AG.
© 1998-2010 Novo Nordisk A/S
For information contact:
Novo Nordisk Inc.
100 College Road West
Princeton, NJ 08540, USA
1-877-NOVO-777
www.NovoSevenRT.com
Manufactured by:
Novo Nordisk A/S
2880 Bagsvaerd, Denmark

VICTOZA®
[VIC-tow-za]
(liraglutide (rDNA origin) injection)
Solution for Subcutaneous Use

HIGHLIGHTS OF PRESCRIBING INFORMATION
These highlights do not include all the information needed to use Victoza safely and effectively. See full prescribing information for Victoza.
Victoza® (liraglutide (rDNA origin) injection)

℞

solution for subcutaneous use
Initial U.S. Approval: 2010

WARNING: RISK OF THYROID C-CELL TUMORS
See full prescribing information for complete boxed warning.
- **Liraglutide causes thyroid C-cell tumors at clinically relevant exposures in rodents. It is unknown whether Victoza causes thyroid C-cell tumors, including medullary thyroid carcinoma (MTC), in humans, as human relevance could not be determined by clinical or nonclinical studies (5.1).**
- **Victoza is contraindicated in patients with a personal or family history of MTC or in patients with Multiple Endocrine Neoplasia syndrome type 2 (MEN 2) (5.1).**

INDICATIONS AND USAGE
Victoza is a glucagon-like peptide-1 (GLP-1) receptor agonist indicated as an adjunct to diet and exercise to improve glycemic control in adults with type 2 diabetes mellitus (1).
Important Limitations of Use (1.1):
- Not recommended as first-line therapy for patients inadequately controlled on diet and exercise (5.1).
- Has not been studied sufficiently in patients with a history of pancreatitis. Use caution (5.2).
- Not for treatment of type 1 diabetes mellitus or diabetic ketoacidosis.
- Has not been studied in combination with insulin.

DOSAGE AND ADMINISTRATION
- Administer once daily at any time of day, independently of meals (2).
- Inject subcutaneously in the abdomen, thigh or upper arm (2).
- The injection site and timing can be changed without dose adjustment (2).
- Initiate at 0.6 mg per day for one week. This dose is intended to reduce gastrointestinal symptoms during initial titration, and is not effective for glycemic control. After one week, increase the dose to 1.2 mg. If the 1.2 mg dose does not result in acceptable glycemic control, the dose can be increased to 1.8 mg (2).
- When initiating Victoza, consider reducing the dose of concomitantly-administered insulin secretagogues to reduce the risk of hypoglycemia (2).

DOSAGE FORMS AND STRENGTHS
- Solution for subcutaneous injection, pre-filled, multi-dose pen that delivers doses of 0.6 mg, 1.2 mg, or 1.8 mg (6 mg/mL, 3 mL) (3).

CONTRAINDICATIONS
Do not use in patients with a personal or family history of medullary thyroid carcinoma or in patients with Multiple Endocrine Neoplasia syndrome type 2 (4).

WARNINGS AND PRECAUTIONS
- Thyroid C-cell tumors in animals: Human relevance unknown. Counsel patients regarding the risk of medullary thyroid carcinoma and the symptoms of thyroid tumors (5.1).
- Pancreatitis: In clinical trials, there were more cases of pancreatitis among Victoza-treated patients than among comparator-treated patients. If pancreatitis is suspected, Victoza and other potentially suspect drugs should be discontinued. Victoza should not be restarted if pancreatitis is confirmed. Use with caution in patients with a history of pancreatitis (5.2).
- Serious hypoglycemia: Can occur when Victoza is used with an insulin secretagogue (e.g. a sulfonylurea). Consider lowering the dose of the insulin secretagogue to reduce the risk of hypoglycemia (5.3).
- Macrovascular outcomes: There have been no studies establishing conclusive evidence of macrovascular risk reduction with Victoza or any other antidiabetic drug (5.4).

ADVERSE REACTIONS
- The most common adverse reactions, reported in ≥5% of patients treated with Victoza and more commonly than in patients treated with placebo are: headache, nausea, diarrhea and anti-liraglutide antibody formation (6).
- Immunogenicity-related events, including urticaria, were more common among Victoza-treated patients (0.8%) than among comparator-treated patients (0.4%) in clinical trials (6).

To report SUSPECTED ADVERSE REACTIONS, contact Novo Nordisk Inc. at 1-877-484-2869 or FDA at 1-800-FDA-1088 or www.fda.gov/medwatch.

DRUG INTERACTIONS
- Victoza delays gastric emptying. May impact absorption of concomitantly administered oral medications. Use caution (7).

USE IN SPECIFIC POPULATIONS
- There are no data in patients below 18 years of age (8.4).
- Use with caution in patients with renal or hepatic impairment. Limited data (8.6, 8.7).

See 17 for PATIENT COUNSELING INFORMATION and Medication Guide

Revised: 04/2010

FULL PRESCRIBING INFORMATION: CONTENTS*
WARNING: RISK OF THYROID C-CELL TUMORS
1   INDICATIONS AND USAGE
    1.1   Important Limitations of Use
2   DOSAGE AND ADMINISTRATION
3   DOSAGE FORMS AND STRENGTHS
4   CONTRAINDICATIONS
5   WARNINGS AND PRECAUTIONS
    5.1   Risk of Thyroid C-cell Tumors
    5.2   Pancreatitis
    5.3   Use with Medications Known to Cause Hypoglycemia
    5.4   Macrovascular Outcomes
6   ADVERSE REACTIONS
    6.1   Clinical Trials Experience
7   DRUG INTERACTIONS
    7.1   Oral Medications
8   USE IN SPECIFIC POPULATIONS
    8.1   Pregnancy
    8.3   Nursing Mothers
    8.4   Pediatric Use
    8.5   Geriatric Use
    8.6   Renal Impairment
    8.7   Hepatic Impairment
    8.8   Gastroparesis
10   OVERDOSAGE
11   DESCRIPTION
12   CLINICAL PHARMACOLOGY
    12.1   Mechanism of Action
    12.2   Pharmacodynamics
    12.3   Pharmacokinetics
13   NONCLINICAL TOXICOLOGY
    13.1   Carcinogenesis, Mutagenesis, Impairment of Fertility
14   CLINICAL STUDIES
    14.1   Monotherapy
    14.2   Combination Therapy
16   HOW SUPPLIED/STORAGE AND HANDLING
    16.1   How Supplied
    16.2   Recommended Storage
17   PATIENT COUNSELING INFORMATION
    17.1   Risk of Thyroid C-cell Tumors
    17.2   Pancreatitis
    17.3   Never Share a Victoza Pen Between Patients
    17.4   Instructions
    17.5   Laboratory Tests
    17.6   FDA-Approved Medication Guide

MEDICATION GUIDE
*** Sections or subsections omitted from the full prescribing information are not listed**

FULL PRESCRIBING INFORMATION

WARNING: RISK OF THYROID C-CELL TUMORS
Liraglutide causes dose-dependent and treatment-duration-dependent thyroid C-cell tumors at clinically relevant exposures in both genders of rats and mice. It is unknown whether Victoza causes thyroid C-cell tumors, including medullary thyroid carcinoma (MTC), in humans, as human relevance could not be ruled out by clinical or nonclinical studies. Victoza is contraindicated in patients with a personal or family history of MTC and in patients with Multiple Endocrine Neoplasia syndrome type 2 (MEN 2). Based on the findings in rodents, monitoring with serum calcitonin or thyroid ultrasound was performed during clinical trials, but this may have increased the number of unnecessary thyroid surgeries. It is unknown whether monitoring with serum calcitonin or thyroid ultrasound will mitigate human risk of thyroid C-cell tumors. Patients should be counseled regarding the risk and symptoms of thyroid tumors *[see Contraindications (4), Warnings and Precautions (5.1) and Nonclinical Toxicology (13.1)]*.

1 INDICATIONS AND USAGE
Victoza is indicated as an adjunct to diet and exercise to improve glycemic control in adults with type 2 diabetes mellitus.

1.1 Important Limitations of Use
- Because of the uncertain relevance of the rodent thyroid C-cell tumor findings to humans, prescribe Victoza only to patients for whom the potential benefits are considered to outweigh the potential risk. Victoza is not recommended as first-line therapy for patients who have inadequate glycemic control on diet and exercise.
- In clinical trials of Victoza, there were more cases of pancreatitis with Victoza than with comparators. Victoza has not been studied sufficiently in patients with a history of pancreatitis to determine whether these patients are at increased risk for pancreatitis while using Victoza. Use with caution in patients with a history of pancreatitis.
- Victoza is not a substitute for insulin. Victoza should not be used in patients with type 1 diabetes mellitus or for the treatment of diabetic ketoacidosis, as it would not be effective in these settings.
- The concurrent use of Victoza and insulin has not been studied.

2 DOSAGE AND ADMINISTRATION
Victoza can be administered once daily at any time of day, independently of meals, and can be injected subcutaneously in the abdomen, thigh or upper arm. The injection site and timing can be changed without dose adjustment.
For all patients, Victoza should be initiated with a dose of 0.6 mg per day for one week. The 0.6 mg dose is a starting dose intended to reduce gastrointestinal symptoms during initial titration, and is not effective for glycemic control. After one week at 0.6 mg per day, the dose should be increased to 1.2 mg. If the 1.2 mg dose does not result in acceptable glycemic control, the dose can be increased to 1.8 mg.
When initiating Victoza, consider reducing the dose of concomitantly administered insulin secretagogues (such as sulfonylureas) to reduce the risk of hypoglycemia *[see Warnings and Precautions (5.3) and Adverse Reactions (6)]*.
Victoza solution should be inspected prior to each injection, and the solution should be used only if it is clear, colorless, and contains no particles.

3 DOSAGE FORMS AND STRENGTHS
Solution for subcutaneous injection, pre-filled, multi-dose pen that delivers doses of 0.6 mg, 1.2 mg, or 1.8 mg (6 mg/mL, 3 mL).

4 CONTRAINDICATIONS
Victoza is contraindicated in patients with a personal or family history of medullary thyroid carcinoma (MTC) or in patients with Multiple Endocrine Neoplasia syndrome type 2 (MEN 2).

5 WARNINGS AND PRECAUTIONS
5.1 Risk of Thyroid C-cell Tumors
Liraglutide causes dose-dependent and treatment-duration-dependent thyroid C-cell tumors (adenomas and/or carcinomas) at clinically relevant exposures in both genders of rats and mice *[see Nonclinical Toxicology (13.1)]*. Malignant thyroid C-cell carcinomas were detected in rats and mice. A statistically significant increase in cancer was observed in rats receiving liraglutide at 8-times clinical exposure compared to controls. It is unknown whether Victoza will cause thyroid C-cell tumors, including medullary thyroid carcinoma (MTC), in humans, as the human relevance of liraglutide-induced rodent thyroid C-cell tumors could not be determined by clinical or nonclinical studies *[see Boxed Warning, Contraindications (4)]*.
In the clinical trials, there have been 4 reported cases of thyroid C-cell hyperplasia among Victoza-treated patients and 1 case in a comparator-treated patient (1.3 vs. 0.6 cases per 1000 patient-years). One additional case of thyroid C-cell hyperplasia in a Victoza-treated patient and 1 case of MTC in a comparator-treated patient have subsequently been reported. This comparator-treated patient with MTC had pre-treatment serum calcitonin concentrations >1000 ng/L suggesting pre-existing disease. All of these cases were diagnosed after thyroidectomy, which was prompted by abnormal results on routine, protocol-specified measurements of serum calcitonin. Four of the five liraglutide-treated patients had elevated calcitonin concentrations at baseline and throughout the trial. One liraglutide and one non-liraglutide-treated patient developed elevated calcitonin concentrations while on treatment.
Calcitonin, a biological marker of MTC, was measured throughout the clinical development program. The serum calcitonin assay used in the Victoza clinical trials had a lower limit of quantification (LLOQ) of 0.7 ng/L and the upper limit of the reference range was 5.0 ng/L for women and 8.4 ng/L for men. At Weeks 26 and 52 in the clinical trials, adjusted mean serum calcitonin concentrations were higher in Victoza-treated patients compared to placebo-treated patients but not compared to patients receiving active comparator. At these timepoints, the adjusted mean serum calcitonin values (~ 1.0 ng/L) were just above the LLOQ with between-group differences in adjusted mean serum calcitonin values of approximately 0.1 ng/L or less. Among patients with pre-treatment serum calcitonin below the upper limit of the reference range, shifts to above the upper limit of the reference range which persisted in subsequent measurements occurred most frequently among patients treated with Victoza 1.8 mg/day. In trials with on-treatment serum calcitonin measurements out to 5-6 months, 1.9% of patients treated with Victoza 1.8 mg/day developed new and persistent calcitonin elevations above the upper limit of the reference range compared to 0.8-1.1% of patients treated with control medication or the 0.6 and 1.2 mg doses of Victoza. In trials with on-treatment serum calcitonin measurements out to 12 months, 1.3% of patients treated with Victoza 1.8 mg/day had new and persistent elevations of calcitonin from below or within the reference range to above the upper limit of the reference range, compared to 0.6%, 0% and 1.0% of patients treated with Victoza 1.2 mg, placebo and active control, respectively.
Otherwise, Victoza did not produce consistent dose-dependent or time-dependent increases in serum calcitonin.
Patients with MTC usually have calcitonin values >50 ng/L. In Victoza clinical trials, among patients with pre-treatment serum calcitonin <50 ng/L, one Victoza-treated patient and no comparator-treated patients developed serum calcitonin >50 ng/L. The Victoza-treated patient who developed serum calcitonin >50 ng/L had an elevated pre-treatment serum calcitonin of 10.7 ng/L that increased to 30.7 ng/L at Week 12 and 53.5 ng/L at the end of the 6-month trial. Follow-up serum calcitonin was 22.3 ng/L more than 2.5 years after the last dose of Victoza. The largest increase in serum calcitonin in a comparator-treated patient was seen with glimepiride in a patient whose serum calcitonin increased from 19.3 ng/L at baseline to 44.8 ng/L at Week 65 and 38.1 ng/L at Week 104. Among patients who began with serum calcitonin <20 ng/L, calcitonin elevations to >20 ng/L occurred in 0.7% of Victoza-treated patients, 0.3% of placebo-treated patients, and 0.5% of active-comparator-treated patients, with an incidence of 1.1% among patients treated with 1.8 mg/day of Victoza. The clinical significance of these findings is unknown.
Counsel patients regarding the risk for MTC and the symptoms of thyroid tumors (e.g. a mass in the neck, dysphagia, dyspnea or persistent hoarseness). It is unknown whether monitoring with serum calcitonin or thyroid ultrasound will mitigate the potential risk of MTC, and such monitoring may increase the risk of unnecessary procedures, due to low test specificity for serum calcitonin and a high background incidence of thyroid disease. Patients with thyroid nodules noted on physical examination or neck imaging obtained for other reasons should be referred to an endocrinologist for further evaluation. Although routine monitoring of serum calcitonin is of uncertain value in patients treated with Victoza, if serum calcitonin is measured and found to be elevated, the patient should be referred to an endocrinologist for further evaluation.

5.2 Pancreatitis
In clinical trials of Victoza, there were 7 cases of pancreatitis among Victoza-treated patients and 1 case among comparator-treated patients (2.2 vs. 0.6 cases per 1000 patient-years). Five cases with Victoza were reported as acute pancreatitis and two cases with Victoza were reported as chronic pancreatitis. In one case in a Victoza-treated patient, pancreatitis, with necrosis, was observed and led to death; however clinical causality could not be established. One additional case of pancreatitis has subsequently been reported in a Victoza-treated patient. Some patients had other risk factors for pancreatitis, such as a history of cholelithiasis or alcohol abuse. There are no conclusive data establishing a risk of pancreatitis with Victoza treatment. After initiation of Victoza, and after dose increases, observe patients carefully for signs and symptoms of pancreatitis (including persistent severe abdominal pain, sometimes radiating to the back and which may or may not be accompanied by vomiting). If pancreatitis is suspected, Victoza and other potentially suspect medications should be discontinued promptly, confirmatory tests should be performed and appropriate management should be initiated. If pancreatitis is confirmed, Victoza should not be restarted. Use with caution in patients with a history of pancreatitis.

5.3 Use with Medications Known to Cause Hypoglycemia
Patients receiving Victoza in combination with an insulin secretagogue (e.g., sulfonylurea) may have an increased risk of hypoglycemia. In the clinical trials of at least 26 weeks duration, hypoglycemia requiring the assistance of another person for treatment occurred in 7 Victoza-treated patients and in no comparator-treated patients. Six of these 7 patients treated with Victoza were also taking a sulfonylurea. The risk of hypoglycemia may be lowered by a reduction in the dose of sulfonylurea or other insulin secretagogues *[see Adverse Reactions (6.1)]*.

5.4 Macrovascular Outcomes
There have been no clinical studies establishing conclusive evidence of macrovascular risk reduction with Victoza or any other antidiabetic drug.

6 ADVERSE REACTIONS
6.1 Clinical Trials Experience
Because clinical trials are conducted under widely varying conditions, adverse reaction rates observed in the clinical trials of a drug cannot be directly compared to rates in the clinical trials of another drug and may not reflect the rates observed in practice.
The safety of Victoza was evaluated in a 52-week monotherapy trial and in four 26-week, add-on combination therapy trials. In the monotherapy trial, patients were treated with Victoza 1.2 mg daily, Victoza 1.8 mg daily, or glimepiride 8 mg daily. In the add-on to metformin trial, patients were treated with Victoza 0.6 mg, Victoza 1.2 mg, Victoza 1.8 mg, placebo, or glimepiride 4 mg. In the add-on to glimepiride trial, patients were treated with Victoza 0.6 mg, Victoza 1.2 mg, Victoza 1.8 mg, placebo, or rosiglitazone 4 mg. In the add-on to metformin + glimepiride trial, patients were treated with Victoza 1.8 mg, placebo, or insulin glargine. In the add-on to metformin + rosiglitazone trial, patients were treated with Victoza 1.2 mg, Victoza 1.8 mg or placebo *[see Clinical Studies (14)]*.
Withdrawals
The incidence of withdrawal due to adverse events was 7.8% for Victoza-treated patients and 3.4% for comparator-treated patients in the five controlled trials of 26 weeks duration or longer. This difference was driven by withdrawals due to gastrointestinal adverse reactions, which occurred in 5.0% of Victoza-treated patients and 0.5% of comparator-treated patients. The most common adverse reactions leading to withdrawal for Victoza-treated patients were nausea (2.8% versus 0% for comparator) and vomiting (1.5% versus 0.1% for comparator). Withdrawal due to gastrointestinal adverse events mainly occurred during the first 2-3 months of the trials.
Tables 1 and 2 summarize the adverse events reported in ≥5% of Victoza-treated patients in the five controlled trials of 26 weeks duration or longer.

Table 1 Adverse events reported in ≥5% of Victoza-treated patients or ≥5% of glimepiride-treated patients: 52-week monotherapy trial

	All Victoza N = 497	Glimepiride N = 248
Adverse Event Term	(%)	(%)
Nausea	28.4	8.5
Diarrhea	17.1	8.9
Vomiting	10.9	3.6
Constipation	9.9	4.8
Upper Respiratory Tract Infection	9.5	5.6
Headache	9.1	9.3
Influenza	7.4	3.6
Urinary Tract Infection	6.0	4.0

Dizziness	5.8	5.2
Sinusitis	5.6	6.0
Nasopharyngitis	5.2	5.2
Back Pain	5.0	4.4
Hypertension	3.0	6.0

[See table 2 at right]

Gastrointestinal adverse events

In the five clinical trials of 26 weeks duration or longer, gastrointestinal adverse events were reported in 41% of Victoza-treated patients and were dose-related. Gastrointestinal adverse events occurred in 17% of comparator-treated patients. Events that occurred more commonly among Victoza-treated patients included nausea, vomiting, diarrhea, dyspepsia and constipation. In clinical trials of 26 weeks duration or longer, the percentage of patients who reported nausea declined over time. Approximately 13% of Victoza-treated patients and 2% of comparator-treated patients reported nausea during the first 2 weeks of treatment.

Immunogenicity

Consistent with the potentially immunogenic properties of protein and peptide pharmaceuticals, patients treated with Victoza may develop anti-liraglutide antibodies. Approximately 50-70% of Victoza-treated patients in the five clinical trials of 26 weeks duration or longer were tested for the presence of anti-liraglutide antibodies at the end of treatment. Low titers (concentrations not requiring dilution of serum) of anti-liraglutide antibodies were detected in 8.6% of these Victoza-treated patients. Sampling was not performed uniformly across all patients in the clinical trials, and this may have resulted in an underestimate of the actual percentage of patients who developed antibodies. Cross-reacting anti-liraglutide antibodies to native glucagon-like peptide-1 (GLP-1) occurred in 6.9% of the Victoza-treated patients in the 52-week monotherapy trial and in 4.8% of the Victoza-treated patients in the 26-week add-on combination therapy trials. These cross-reacting antibodies were not tested for neutralizing effect against native GLP-1, and thus the potential for clinically significant neutralization of native GLP-1 was not assessed. Antibodies that had a neutralizing effect on liraglutide in an *in vitro* assay occurred in 2.3% of the Victoza-treated patients in the 52-week monotherapy trial and in 1.0% of the Victoza-treated patients in the 26-week add-on combination therapy trials.

Among Victoza-treated patients who developed anti-liraglutide antibodies, the most common category of adverse events was that of infections, which occurred among 40% of these patients compared to 36%, 34% and 35% of antibody-negative Victoza-treated, placebo-treated and active-control-treated patients, respectively. The specific infections which occurred with greater frequency among Victoza-treated antibody-positive patients were primarily nonserious upper respiratory tract infections, which occurred among 11% of Victoza-treated antibody-positive patients; and among 7%, 7% and 5% of antibody-negative Victoza-treated, placebo-treated and active-control-treated patients, respectively. Among Victoza-treated antibody-negative patients, the most common category of adverse events was that of gastrointestinal events, which occurred in 43%, 18% and 19% of antibody-negative Victoza-treated, placebo-treated and active-control-treated patients, respectively. Antibody formation was not associated with reduced efficacy of Victoza when comparing mean HbA$_{1c}$ of all antibody-positive and all antibody-negative patients. However, the 3 patients with the highest titers of anti-liraglutide antibodies had no reduction in HbA$_{1c}$ with Victoza treatment.

In clinical trials of Victoza, events from a composite of adverse events potentially related to immunogenicity (e.g. urticaria, angioedema) occurred among 0.8% of Victoza-treated patients and among 0.4% of comparator-treated patients. Urticaria accounted for approximately one-half of the events in this composite for Victoza-treated patients. Patients who developed anti-liraglutide antibodies were not more likely to develop events from the immunogenicity events composite than were patients who did not develop anti-liraglutide antibodies.

Injection site reactions

Injection site reactions (e.g., injection site rash, erythema) were reported in approximately 2% of Victoza-treated patients in the five clinical trials of at least 26 weeks duration. Less than 0.2% of Victoza-treated patients discontinued due to injection site reactions.

Papillary thyroid carcinoma

In clinical trials of Victoza, there were 6 reported cases of papillary thyroid carcinoma in patients treated with Victoza and 1 case in a comparator-treated patient (1.9 vs. 0.6 cases per 1000 patient-years). Most of these papillary thyroid carcinomas were <1 cm in greatest diameter and were diagnosed in surgical pathology specimens after thyroidectomy prompted by findings on protocol-specified screening with serum calcitonin or thyroid ultrasound.

Hypoglycemia

In the clinical trials of at least 26 weeks duration, hypoglycemia requiring the assistance of another person for treatment occurred in 7 Victoza-treated patients (2.6 cases per 1000 patient-years) and in no comparator-treated patients. Six of these 7 patients treated with Victoza were also taking a sulfonylurea. One other patient was taking Victoza in combination with metformin but had another likely explanation for the hypoglycemia (this event occurred during hospitalization and after insulin infusion) (Table 3). Two additional cases of hypoglycemia requiring the assistance of another person for treatment have subsequently been reported in patients who were not taking a concomitant sul-

fonylurea. Both patients were receiving Victoza, one as monotherapy and the other in combination with metformin. Both patients had another likely explanation for the hypoglycemia (one received insulin during a frequently-sampled intravenous glucose tolerance test, and the other had intracranial hemorrhage and uncertain food intake).

[See table 3 at top of next page]

In a pooled analysis of clinical trials, the incidence rate (per 1,000 patient-years) for malignant neoplasms (based on investigator-reported events, medical history, pathology reports, and surgical reports from both blinded and open-label study periods) was 10.9 for Victoza, 6.3 for placebo, and 7.2 for active comparator. After excluding papillary thyroid carcinoma events *[see Adverse Reactions (6.1)]*, no particular cancer cell type predominated. Seven malignant neoplasm events were reported beyond 1 year of exposure to study medication, six events among Victoza-treated patients

Table 2 Adverse events reported in ≥5% of Victoza-treated patients and occurring more frequently with Victoza compared to placebo: 26-week combination therapy trials

Add-on to Metformin Trial

Adverse Event Term	All Victoza + Metformin N = 724	Placebo + Metformin N = 121	Glimepiride + Metformin N = 242
	(%)	(%)	(%)
Nausea	15.2	4.1	3.3
Diarrhea	10.9	4.1	3.7
Headache	9.0	6.6	9.5
Vomiting	6.5	0.8	0.4

Add-on to Glimepiride Trial

Adverse Event Term	All Victoza + Glimepiride N = 695	Placebo + Glimepiride N = 114	Rosiglitazone + Glimepiride N = 231
	(%)	(%)	(%)
Nausea	7.5	1.8	2.6
Diarrhea	7.2	1.8	2.2
Constipation	5.3	0.9	1.7
Dyspepsia	5.2	0.9	2.6

Add-on to Metformin + Glimepiride

Adverse Event Term	Victoza 1.8 + Metformin + Glimepiride N = 230	Placebo + Metformin + Glimepiride N = 114	Glargine + Metformin + Glimepiride N = 232
	(%)	(%)	(%)
Nausea	13.9	3.5	1.3
Diarrhea	10.0	5.3	1.3
Headache	9.6	7.9	5.6
Dyspepsia	6.5	0.9	1.7
Vomiting	6.5	3.5	0.4

Add-on to Metformin + Rosiglitazone

Adverse Event Term	All Victoza + Metformin + Rosiglitazone N = 355	Placebo + Metformin + Rosiglitazone N = 175
	(%)	(%)
Nausea	34.6	8.6
Diarrhea	14.1	6.3
Vomiting	12.4	2.9
Decreased Appetite	9.3	1.1
Anorexia	9.0	0.0
Headache	8.2	4.6
Constipation	5.1	1.1
Fatigue	5.1	1.7

(4 colon, 1 prostate and 1 nasopharyngeal), no events with placebo and one event with active comparator (colon). Causality has not been established.

Laboratory Tests
In the five clinical trials of at least 26 weeks duration, mildly elevated serum bilirubin concentrations (elevations to no more than twice the upper limit of the reference range) occurred in 4.0% of Victoza-treated patients, 2.1% of placebo-treated patients and 3.5% of active-comparator-treated patients. This finding was not accompanied by abnormalities in other liver tests. The significance of this isolated finding is unknown.

7   DRUG INTERACTIONS
7.1   Oral Medications
Victoza causes a delay of gastric emptying, and thereby has the potential to impact the absorption of concomitantly administered oral medications. In clinical pharmacology trials, Victoza did not affect the absorption of the tested orally administered medications to any clinically relevant degree. Nonetheless, caution should be exercised when oral medications are concomitantly administered with Victoza.

8   USE IN SPECIFIC POPULATIONS
8.1   Pregnancy
Pregnancy Category C.
There are no adequate and well-controlled studies of Victoza in pregnant women. Victoza should be used during pregnancy only if the potential benefit justifies the potential risk to the fetus. Liraglutide has been shown to be teratogenic in rats at or above 0.8 times the human systemic exposures resulting from the maximum recommended human dose (MRHD) of 1.8 mg/day based on plasma area under the time-concentration curve (AUC). Liraglutide has been shown to cause reduced growth and increased total major abnormalities in rabbits at systemic exposures below human exposure at the MRHD based on plasma AUC.
Female rats given subcutaneous doses of 0.1, 0.25 and 1.0 mg/kg/day liraglutide beginning 2 weeks before mating through gestation day 17 had estimated systemic exposures 0.8-, 3-, and 11-times the human exposure at the MRHD based on plasma AUC comparison. The number of early embryonic deaths in the 1 mg/kg/day group increased slightly. Fetal abnormalities and variations in kidneys and blood vessels, irregular ossification of the skull, and a more complete state of ossification occurred at all doses. Mottled liver and minimally kinked ribs occurred at the highest dose. The incidence of fetal malformations in liraglutide-treated groups exceeding concurrent and historical controls were misshapen oropharynx and/or narrowed opening into larynx at 0.1 mg/kg/day and umbilical hernia at 0.1 and 0.25 mg/kg/day.
Pregnant rabbits given subcutaneous doses of 0.01, 0.025 and 0.05 mg/kg/day liraglutide from gestation day 6 through day 18 inclusive, had estimated systemic exposures less than the human exposure at the MRHD of 1.8 mg/day at all doses, based on plasma AUC. Liraglutide decreased fetal weight and dose-dependently increased the incidence of total major fetal abnormalities at all doses. The incidence of malformations exceeded concurrent and historical controls at 0.01 mg/kg/day (kidneys, scapula), ≥ 0.01 mg/kg/day (eyes, forelimb), 0.025 mg/kg/day (brain, tail and sacral vertebrae, major blood vessels and heart, umbilicus), ≥ 0.025 mg/kg/day (sternum) and at 0.05 mg/kg/day (parietal bones, major blood vessels). Irregular ossification and/or skeletal abnormalities occurred in the skull and jaw, vertebrae and ribs, sternum, pelvis, tail, and scapula; and dose-dependent minor skeletal variations were observed. Visceral abnormalities occurred in blood vessels, lung, liver, and esophagus. Bilobed or bifurcated gallbladder was seen in all treatment groups, but not in the control group.
In pregnant female rats given subcutaneous doses of 0.1, 0.25 and 1.0 mg/kg/day liraglutide from gestation day 6 through weaning or termination of nursing on lactation day 24, estimated systemic exposures were 0.8-, 3-, and 11-times human exposure at the MRHD of 1.8 mg/day, based on plasma AUC. A slight delay in parturition was observed in the majority of treated rats. Group mean body weight of neonatal rats from liraglutide-treated dams was lower than neonatal rats from control group dams. Bloody scabs and agitated behavior occurred in male rats descended from dams treated with 1 mg/kg/day liraglutide. Group mean body weight from birth to postpartum day 14 trended lower in F_2 generation rats descended from liraglutide-treated rats compared to F_2 generation rats descended from controls, but differences did not reach statistical significance for any group.

8.3   Nursing Mothers
It is not known whether Victoza is excreted in human milk. Because many drugs are excreted in human milk and because of the potential for tumorigenicity shown for liraglutide in animal studies, a decision should be made whether to discontinue nursing or to discontinue Victoza, taking into account the importance of the drug to the

Table 3 Incidence (%) and Rate (episodes/patient year) of Hypoglycemia in the 52-Week Monotherapy Trial and in the 26-Week Combination Therapy Trials

	Victoza Treatment	Active Comparator	Placebo Comparator
Monotherapy	Victoza (N = 497)	Glimepiride (N = 248)	None
Patient not able to self-treat	0	0	-
Patient able to self-treat	9.7 (0.24)	25.0 (1.66)	-
Not classified	1.2 (0.03)	2.4 (0.04)	-
Add-on to Metformin	Victoza + Metformin (N = 724)	Glimepiride + Metformin (N = 242)	Placebo + Metformin (N = 121)
Patient not able to self-treat	0.1 (0.001)	0	0
Patient able to self-treat	3.6 (0.05)	22.3 (0.87)	2.5 (0.06)
Add-on to Glimepiride	Victoza + Glimepiride (N = 695)	Rosiglitazone + Glimepiride (N = 231)	Placebo + Glimepiride (N = 114)
Patient not able to self-treat	0.1 (0.003)	0	0
Patient able to self-treat	7.5 (0.38)	4.3 (0.12)	2.6 (0.17)
Not classified	0.9 (0.05)	0.9 (0.02)	0
Add-on to Metformin + Rosiglitazone	Victoza + Metformin + Rosiglitazone (N = 355)	None	Placebo + Metformin + Rosiglitazone (N = 175)
Patient not able to self-treat	0	-	0
Patient able to self-treat	7.9 (0.49)	-	4.6 (0.15)
Not classified	0.6 (0.01)	-	1.1 (0.03)
Add-on to Metformin + Glimepiride	Victoza + Metformin + Glimepiride (N = 230)	Insulin glargine + Metformin + Glimepiride (N = 232)	Placebo + Metformin + Glimepiride (N = 114)
Patient not able to self-treat	2.2 (0.06)	0	0
Patient able to self-treat	27.4 (1.16)	28.9 (1.29)	16.7 (0.95)
Not classified	0	1.7 (0.04)	0

mother. In lactating rats, liraglutide was excreted unchanged in milk at concentrations approximately 50% of maternal plasma concentrations.

8.4   Pediatric Use
Safety and effectiveness of Victoza have not been established in pediatric patients. Victoza is not recommended for use in pediatric patients.

8.5   Geriatric Use
In the Victoza clinical trials, a total of 797 (20%) of the patients were 65 years of age and over and 113 (2.8%) were 75 years of age and over. No overall differences in safety or effectiveness were observed between these patients and younger patients, but greater sensitivity of some older individuals cannot be ruled out.

8.6   Renal Impairment
There is limited experience in patients with mild, moderate, and severe renal impairment, including end-stage renal disease. Therefore, Victoza should be used with caution in this patient population. No dose adjustment of Victoza is recommended for patients with renal impairment [see Clinical Pharmacology (12.3)].

8.7   Hepatic Impairment
There is limited experience in patients with mild, moderate or severe hepatic impairment. Therefore, Victoza should be used with caution in this patient population. No dose adjustment of Victoza is recommended for patients with hepatic impairment [see Clinical Pharmacology (12.3)].

8.8   Gastroparesis
Victoza slows gastric emptying. Victoza has not been studied in patients with pre-existing gastroparesis.

10   OVERDOSAGE
In a clinical trial, one patient with type 2 diabetes experienced a single overdose of Victoza 17.4 mg subcutaneous (10 times the maximum recommended dose). Effects of the overdose included severe nausea and vomiting requiring hospitalization. No hypoglycemia was reported. The patient recovered without complications. In the event of overdosage, appropriate supportive treatment should be initiated according to the patient's clinical signs and symptoms.

11   DESCRIPTION
Victoza contains liraglutide, an analog of human GLP-1 and acts as a GLP-1 receptor agonist. The peptide precursor of liraglutide, produced by a process that includes expression of recombinant DNA in *Saccharomyces cerevisiae*, has been engineered to be 97% homologous to native human GLP-1 by substituting arginine for lysine at position 34. Liraglutide is made by attaching a C-16 fatty acid (palmitic acid) with a glutamic acid spacer on the remaining lysine residue at position 26 of the peptide precursor. The molecular formula of liraglutide is $C_{172}H_{265}N_{43}O_{51}$ and the molecular weight is 3751.2 Daltons. The structural formula (Figure 1) is:

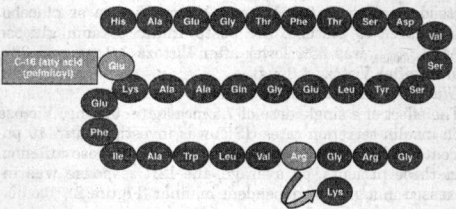

Figure 1: Structural Formula of liraglutide. Each 1 mL of Victoza solution contains 6 mg of liraglutide. Each pre-filled pen contains a 3 mL solution of Victoza equivalent to 18 mg liraglutide (free-base, anhydrous) and the following inactive ingredients: disodium phosphate dihydrate, 1.42 mg; propylene glycol, 14 mg; phenol, 5.5 mg; and water for injection.

12   CLINICAL PHARMACOLOGY
12.1   Mechanism of Action
Liraglutide is an acylated human Glucagon-Like Peptide-1 (GLP-1) receptor agonist with 97% amino acid sequence homology to endogenous human GLP-1(7-37). GLP-1(7-37) represents <20% of total circulating endogenous GLP-1. Like GLP-1(7-37), liraglutide activates the GLP-1 receptor,

Table 4 Results of a 52-week monotherapy trial*

	Victoza 1.8 mg	Victoza 1.2 mg	Glimepiride 8 mg
Intent-to-Treat Population (N)	246	251	248
HbA₁c (%) (Mean)			
Baseline	8.2	8.2	8.2
Change from baseline (adjusted mean)[†]	-1.1	-0.8	-0.5
Difference from glimepiride arm (adjusted mean)[†]	-0.6[‡]	-0.3[§]	
95% Confidence Interval	(-0.8, -0.4)	(-0.5, -0.1)	
Patients (%) achieving A₁c <7%	51	43	28
Fasting Plasma Glucose (mg/dL) (Mean)			
Baseline	172	168	172
Change from baseline (adjusted mean)[†]	-26	-15	-5
Difference from glimepiride arm (adjusted mean)[†]	-20[‡]	-10[§]	
95% Confidence Interval	(-29, -12)	(-19, -1)	
Body Weight (kg) (Mean)			
Baseline	92.6	92.1	93.3
Change from baseline (adjusted mean)[†]	-2.5	-2.1	+1.1
Difference from glimepiride arm (adjusted mean)[†]	-3.6[‡]	-3.2[‡]	
95% Confidence Interval	(-4.3, -2.9)	(-3.9, -2.5)	

* Intent-to-treat population using last observation on study
† Least squares mean adjusted for baseline value
‡ p-value <0.0001
§ p-value <0.05

a membrane-bound cell-surface receptor coupled to adenylyl cyclase by the stimulatory G-protein, Gs, in pancreatic beta cells. Liraglutide increases intracellular cyclic AMP (cAMP) leading to insulin release in the presence of elevated glucose concentrations. This insulin secretion subsides as blood glucose concentrations decrease and approach euglycemia. Liraglutide also decreases glucagon secretion in a glucose-dependent manner. The mechanism of blood glucose lowering also involves a delay in gastric emptying.

GLP-1(7-37) has a half-life of 1.5-2 minutes due to degradation by the ubiquitous endogenous enzymes, dipeptidyl peptidase IV (DPP-IV) and neutral endopeptidases (NEP). Unlike native GLP-1, liraglutide is stable against metabolic degradation by both peptidases and has a plasma half-life of 13 hours after subcutaneous administration. The pharmacokinetic profile of liraglutide, which makes it suitable for once daily administration, is a result of self-association that delays absorption, plasma protein binding and stability against metabolic degradation by DPP-IV and NEP.

12.2 Pharmacodynamics
Victoza's pharmacodynamic profile is consistent with its pharmacokinetic profile observed after single subcutaneous administration as Victoza lowered fasting, premeal and postprandial glucose throughout the day [see Clinical Pharmacology (12.3)].

Fasting and postprandial glucose was measured before and up to 5 hours after a standardized meal after treatment to steady state with 0.6, 1.2 and 1.8 mg Victoza or placebo. Compared to placebo, the postprandial plasma glucose AUC₀₋₃₀₀min was 35% lower after Victoza 1.2 mg and 38% lower after Victoza 1.8 mg.

Glucose-dependent insulin secretion
The effect of a single dose of 7.5 mcg/kg (~ 0.7 mg) Victoza on insulin secretion rates (ISR) was investigated in 10 patients with type 2 diabetes during graded glucose infusion. In these patients, on average, the ISR response was increased in a glucose-dependent manner (Figure 2).
[See figure at top of next column]

Glucagon secretion
Victoza lowered blood glucose by stimulating insulin secretion and lowering glucagon secretion. A single dose of Victoza 7.5 mcg/kg (~ 0.7 mg) did not impair glucagon response to low glucose concentrations.

Gastric emptying
Victoza causes a delay of gastric emptying, thereby reducing the rate at which postprandial glucose appears in the circulation.

Cardiac Electrophysiology (QTc)
The effect of Victoza on cardiac repolarization was tested in a QTc study. Victoza at steady state concentrations with daily doses up to 1.8 mg did not produce QTc prolongation.

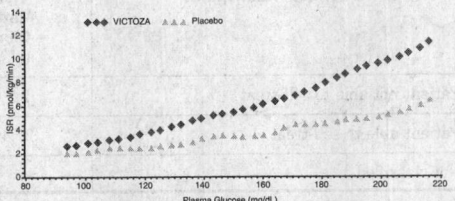

Figure 2 Mean Insulin Secretion Rate (ISR) versus Glucose Concentration Following Single-Dose Victoza 7.5 mcg/kg (~0.7 mg) or Placebo in Patients with Type 2 Diabetes (N=10) During Graded Glucose Infusion

12.3 Pharmacokinetics
Absorption—Following subcutaneous administration, maximum concentrations of liraglutide are achieved at 8-12 hours post dosing. The mean peak (Cₘₐₓ) and total (AUC) exposures of liraglutide were 35 ng/mL and 960 ng·h/mL, respectively, for a subcutaneous single dose of 0.6 mg. After subcutaneous single dose administrations, Cₘₐₓ and AUC of liraglutide increased proportionally over the therapeutic dose range of 0.6 mg to 1.8 mg. At 1.8 mg Victoza, the average steady state concentration of liraglutide over 24 hours was approximately 128 ng/mL. AUC₀₋∞ was equivalent between upper arm and abdomen, and between upper arm and thigh. AUC₀₋∞ from thigh was 22% lower than that from abdomen. However, liraglutide exposures were considered comparable among these three subcutaneous injection sites. Absolute bioavailability of liraglutide following subcutaneous administration is approximately 55%.

Distribution—The mean apparent volume of distribution after subcutaneous administration of Victoza 0.6 mg is approximately 13 L. The mean volume of distribution after intravenous administration of Victoza is 0.07 L/kg. Liraglutide is extensively bound to plasma protein (>98%).

Metabolism—During the initial 24 hours following administration of a single [³H]-liraglutide dose to healthy subjects, the major component in plasma was intact liraglutide. Liraglutide is endogenously metabolized in a similar manner to large proteins without a specific organ as a major route of elimination.

Elimination—Following a [³H]-liraglutide dose, intact liraglutide was not detected in urine or feces. Only a minor part of the administered radioactivity was excreted as liraglutide-related metabolites in urine or feces (6% and 5%, respectively). The majority of urine and feces radioactivity was excreted during the first 6-8 days. The mean apparent clearance following subcutaneous administration of a single dose of liraglutide is approximately 1.2 L/h with an elimi-

nation half-life of approximately 13 hours, making Victoza suitable for once daily administration.

Specific Populations
Elderly—Age had no effect on the pharmacokinetics of Victoza based on a pharmacokinetic study in healthy elderly subjects (65 to 83 years) and population pharmacokinetic analyses of patients 18 to 80 years of age [see Use in Specific Populations (8.5)].

Gender—Based on the results of population pharmacokinetic analyses, females have 34% lower weight-adjusted clearance of Victoza compared to males. Based on the exposure response data, no dose adjustment is necessary based on gender.

Race and Ethnicity—Race and ethnicity had no effect on the pharmacokinetics of Victoza based on the results of population pharmacokinetic analyses that included Caucasian, Black, Asian and Hispanic/Non-Hispanic subjects.

Body Weight—Body weight significantly affects the pharmacokinetics of Victoza based on results of population pharmacokinetic analyses. The exposure of liraglutide decreases with an increase in baseline body weight. However, the 1.2 mg and 1.8 mg daily doses of Victoza provided adequate systemic exposures over the body weight range of 40–160 kg evaluated in the clinical trials. Liraglutide was not studied in patients with body weight >160 kg.

Pediatric—Victoza has not been studied in pediatric patients [see Use in Specific Populations (8.4)].

Renal Impairment—The single-dose pharmacokinetics of Victoza were evaluated in subjects with varying degrees of renal impairment. Subjects with mild (estimated creatinine clearance 50-80 mL/min) to severe (estimated creatinine clearance <30 mL/min) renal impairment and subjects with end-stage renal disease requiring dialysis were included in the trial. Compared to healthy subjects, liraglutide AUC in mild, moderate, and severe renal impairment and in end-stage renal disease was on average 35%, 19%, 29% and 30% lower, respectively [see Use in Specific Populations (8.6)].

Hepatic Impairment—The single-dose pharmacokinetics of Victoza were evaluated in subjects with varying degrees of hepatic impairment. Subjects with mild (Child Pugh score 5-6) to severe (Child Pugh score > 9) hepatic impairment were included in the trial. Compared to healthy subjects, liraglutide AUC in subjects with mild, moderate and severe hepatic impairment was on average 11%, 14% and 42% lower, respectively [see Use in Specific Populations (8.7)].

Drug Interactions
In vitro assessment of drug-drug interactions
Victoza has low potential for pharmacokinetic drug-drug interactions related to cytochrome P450 (CYP) and plasma protein binding.

In vivo assessment of drug-drug interactions
The drug-drug interaction studies were performed at steady state with Victoza 1.8 mg/day. Before administration of concomitant treatment, subjects underwent a 0.6 mg weekly dose increase to reach the maximum dose of 1.8 mg/day. Administration of the interacting drugs was timed so that Cₘₐₓ of Victoza (8-12 h) would coincide with the absorption peak of the co-administered drugs.

Digoxin
A single dose of digoxin 1 mg was administered 7 hours after the dose of Victoza at steady state. The concomitant administration with Victoza resulted in a reduction of digoxin AUC by 16%; Cₘₐₓ decreased by 31%. Digoxin median time to maximal concentration (Tₘₐₓ) was delayed from 1 h to 1.5 h.

Lisinopril
A single dose of lisinopril 20 mg was administered 5 minutes after the dose of Victoza at steady state. The co-administration with Victoza resulted in a reduction of lisinopril AUC by 15%; Cₘₐₓ decreased by 27%. Lisinopril median Tₘₐₓ was delayed from 6 h to 8 h with Victoza.

Atorvastatin
Victoza did not change the overall exposure (AUC) of atorvastatin following a single dose of atorvastatin 40 mg, administered 5 hours after the dose of Victoza at steady state. Atorvastatin Cₘₐₓ was decreased by 38% and median Tₘₐₓ was delayed from 1 h to 3 h with Victoza.

Acetaminophen
Victoza did not change the overall exposure (AUC) of acetaminophen following a single dose of acetaminophen 1000 mg, administered 8 hours after the dose of Victoza at steady state. Acetaminophen Cₘₐₓ was decreased by 31% and median Tₘₐₓ was delayed up to 15 minutes.

Griseofulvin
Victoza did not change the overall exposure (AUC) of griseofulvin following co-administration of a single dose of griseofulvin 500 mg with Victoza at steady state. Griseofulvin Cₘₐₓ increased by 37% while median Tₘₐₓ did not change.

Oral Contraceptives
A single dose of an oral contraceptive combination product containing 0.03 mg ethinylestradiol and 0.15 mg levonorgestrel was administered under fed conditions and 7 hours after the dose of Victoza at steady state. Victoza lowered ethinylestradiol and levonorgestrel Cₘₐₓ by 12% and 13%,

Table 5 Results of a 26 Week Trial of Victoza as add-on to Metformin*

	Victoza 1.8 mg + Metformin	Victoza 1.2 mg + Metformin	Placebo + Metformin	Glimepiride 4 mg[†]+ Metformin
Intent-to-Treat Population (N)	242	240	121	242
HbA$_{1c}$ (%) (Mean)				
Baseline	8.4	8.3	8.4	8.4
Change from baseline (adjusted mean)[‡]	-1.0	-1.0	+0.1	-1.0
Difference from placebo + metformin arm (adjusted mean)[‡]	-1.1[§]	-1.1[§]		
95% Confidence Interval	(-1.3, -0.9)	(-1.3, -0.9)		
Difference from glimepiride + metformin arm (adjusted mean)[‡]	0.0	0.0		
95% Confidence Interval	(-0.2, 0.2)	(-0.2, 0.2)		
Patients (%) achieving A$_{1c}$ <7%	42	35	11	36
Fasting Plasma Glucose (mg/dL) (Mean)				
Baseline	181	179	182	180
Change from baseline (adjusted mean)[‡]	-30	-30	+7	-24
Difference from placebo + metformin arm (adjusted mean)[‡]	-38[§]	-37[§]		
95% Confidence Interval	(-48, -27)	(-47, -26)		
Difference from glimepiride + metformin arm (adjusted mean)[‡]	-7	-6		
95% Confidence Interval	(-16, 2)	(-15, 3)		
Body Weight (kg) (Mean)				
Baseline	88.0	88.5	91.0	89.0
Change from baseline (adjusted mean)[‡]	-2.8	-2.6	-1.5	+1.0
Difference from placebo + metformin arm (adjusted mean)[‡]	-1.3[¶]	-1.1[¶]		
95% Confidence Interval	(-2.2, -0.4)	(-2.0, -0.2)		
Difference from glimepiride + metformin arm (adjusted mean)[‡]	-3.8[§]	-3.5[§]		
95% Confidence Interval	(-4.5, -3.0)	(-4.3, -2.8)		

* Intent-to-treat population using last observation on study
† For glimepiride, one-half of the maximal approved United States dose.
‡ Least squares mean adjusted for baseline value
§ p-value <0.0001
¶ p-value <0.05

respectively. There was no effect of Victoza on the overall exposure (AUC) of ethinylestradiol. Victoza increased the levonorgestrel AUC$_{0-\infty}$ by 18%. Victoza delayed T$_{max}$ for both ethinylestradiol and levonorgestrel by 1.5 h.

13 NONCLINICAL TOXICOLOGY
13.1 Carcinogenesis, Mutagenesis, Impairment of Fertility
A 104-week carcinogenicity study was conducted in male and female CD-1 mice at doses of 0.03, 0.2, 1.0, and 3.0 mg/kg/day liraglutide administered by bolus subcutaneous injection yielding systemic exposures 0.2-, 2-, 10- and 45-times the human exposure, respectively, at the MRHD of 1.8 mg/day based on plasma AUC comparison. A dose-related increase in benign thyroid C-cell adenomas was seen in the 1.0 and the 3.0 mg/kg/day groups with incidences of 13% and 19% in males and 6% and 20% in females, respectively. C-cell adenomas did not occur in control groups or 0.03 and 0.2 mg/kg/day groups. Treatment-related malignant C-cell carcinomas occurred in 3% of females in the 3.0 mg/kg/day group. Thyroid C-cell tumors are rare findings during carcinogenicity testing in mice. A treatment-related increase in fibrosarcomas was seen on the dorsal skin and subcutis, the body surface used for drug injection, in males in the 3 mg/kg/day group. These fibrosarcomas were attributed to the high local concentration of drug near the injection site. The liraglutide concentration in the clinical formulation (6 mg/mL) is 10-times higher than the concentration in the formulation used to administer 3 mg/kg/day liraglutide to mice in the carcinogenicity study (0.6 mg/mL).

A 104-week carcinogenicity study was conducted in male and female Sprague Dawley rats at doses of 0.075, 0.25 and 0.75 mg/kg/day liraglutide administered by bolus subcutaneous injection with exposures 0.5-, 2- and 8-times the human exposure, respectively, resulting from the MRHD based on plasma AUC comparison. A treatment-related increase in benign thyroid C-cell adenomas was seen in males in 0.25 and 0.75 mg/kg/day liraglutide groups with incidences of 12%, 16%, 42%, and 46% and in all female liraglutide-treated groups with incidences of 10%, 27%, 33%, and 56% in 0 (control), 0.075, 0.25, and 0.75 mg/kg/day groups, respectively. A treatment-related increase in malignant thyroid C-cell carcinomas was observed in all male liraglutide-treated groups with incidences of 2%, 8%, 6%, and 14% and in females at 0.25 and 0.75 mg/kg/day with incidences of 0%, 0%, 4%, and 6% in 0 (control), 0.075, 0.25, and 0.75 mg/kg/day groups, respectively. Thyroid C-cell carcinomas are rare findings during carcinogenicity testing in rats.
Human relevance of thyroid C-cell tumors in mice and rats is unknown and could not be determined by clinical studies or nonclinical studies [see Boxed Warning and Warnings and Precautions (5.1)].
Liraglutide was negative with and without metabolic activation in the Ames test for mutagenicity and in a human peripheral blood lymphocyte chromosome aberration test for clastogenicity. Liraglutide was negative in repeat-dose in vivo micronucleus tests in rats.
In rat fertility studies using subcutaneous doses of 0.1, 0.25 and 1.0 mg/kg/day liraglutide, males were treated for 4 weeks prior to and throughout mating and females were treated 2 weeks prior to and throughout mating until ges-

tation day 17. No direct adverse effects on male fertility was observed at doses up to 1.0 mg/kg/day, a high dose yielding an estimated systemic exposure 11- times the human exposure at the MRHD, based on plasma AUC. In female rats, an increase in early embryonic deaths occurred at 1.0 mg/kg/day. Reduced body weight gain and food consumption were observed in females at the 1.0 mg/kg/day dose.

14 CLINICAL STUDIES
A total of 3978 patients with type 2 diabetes participated in 5 double-blind (one of these trials had an open-label active control insulin glargine arm), randomized, controlled clinical trials, one of 52 weeks duration and four of 26 weeks duration. These multinational trials were conducted to evaluate the glycemic efficacy and safety of Victoza in type 2 diabetes as monotherapy and in combination with one or two oral anti-diabetic medications. The 4 add-on combination therapy trials enrolled patients who were previously treated with anti-diabetic therapy, and approximately two-thirds of patients in the monotherapy trial also were previously treated with anti-diabetic therapy. In total, 272 (7%) of the 3978 patients in these 5 trials were new to anti-diabetic therapy. In these 5 clinical trials, patients ranged in age from 19-80 years old and 54% were men. Approximately 77% of patients were Caucasian, and 6% were Black. In the 2 trials where ethnicity was captured, 27% of patients were Hispanic/Latino and 73% were Non-Hispanic/Latino. In each of these trials, treatment with Victoza produced clinically and statistically significant improvements in hemoglobin A$_{1c}$ and fasting plasma glucose (FPG) compared to placebo. Victoza did not have adverse effects on blood pressure. All Victoza-treated patients started at 0.6 mg/day. The dose was increased in weekly intervals by 0.6 mg to reach 1.2 mg or 1.8 mg for patients randomized to these higher doses. Victoza 0.6 mg is not effective for glycemic control and is intended only as a starting dose to reduce gastrointestinal intolerance [see Dosage and Administration (2)].

14.1 Monotherapy
In this 52-week trial, 746 patients were randomized to Victoza 1.2 mg, Victoza 1.8 mg, or glimepiride 8 mg. Patients who were randomized to glimepiride were initially treated with 2 mg daily for two weeks, increasing to 4 mg daily for another two weeks, and finally increasing to 8 mg daily.
Treatment with Victoza 1.8 mg and 1.2 mg resulted in a statistically significant reduction in HbA$_{1c}$ compared to glimepiride (Table 4). The percentage of patients who discontinued due to ineffective therapy was 3.6% in the Victoza 1.8 mg treatment group, 6.0% in the Victoza 1.2 mg treatment group, and 10.1% in the glimepiride-treatment group.
[See table 4 at top of previous page]

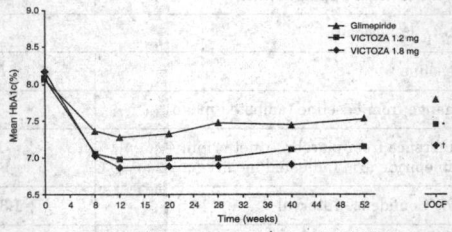

*p-value = 0.0014 for VICTOZA 1.2 mg compared to glimepiride.   †p-value < 0.0001 for VICTOZA 1.8 mg compared
P values derived from change from baseline ANCOVA model.   to glimepiride.

Figure 3 Mean HbA$_{1c}$ for patients who completed the 52-week trial and for the Last Observation Carried Forward (LOCF, intent-to-treat) data at Week 52 (Monotherapy)

14.2 Combination Therapy
Add-on to Metformin
In this 26-week trial, 1091 patients were randomized to Victoza 0.6 mg, Victoza 1.2 mg, Victoza 1.8 mg, placebo, or glimepiride 4 mg (one-half of the maximal approved dose in the United States), all as add-on to metformin. Randomization occurred after a 6-week run-in period consisting of a 3-week initial forced metformin titration period followed by a maintenance period of another 3 weeks. During the titration period, doses of metformin were increased up to 2000 mg/day.
Treatment with Victoza 1.2 mg and 1.8 mg as add-on to metformin resulted in an adjusted mean HbA$_{1c}$ reduction relative to placebo add-on to metformin and resulted in a similar mean HbA$_{1c}$ reduction relative to glimepiride 4 mg add-on to metformin (Table 5). The percentage of patients who discontinued due to ineffective therapy was 5.4% in the Victoza 1.8 mg + metformin treatment group, 3.3% in the Victoza 1.2 mg + metformin treatment group, 23.8% in the placebo + metformin treatment group, and 3.7% in the glimepiride + metformin treated group.

Table 6 Results of a 26-week trial of Victoza as add-on to sulfonylurea*

	Victoza 1.8 mg + Glimepiride	Victoza 1.2 mg + Glimepiride	Placebo + Glimepiride	Rosiglitazone 4 mg[†] + Glimepiride
Intent-to-Treat Population (N)	234	228	114	231
HbA$_{1c}$ (%) (Mean)				
Baseline	8.5	8.5	8.4	8.4
Change from baseline (adjusted mean)[‡]	-1.1	-1.1	+0.2	-0.4
Difference from placebo + glimepiride arm (adjusted mean)[‡]	-1.4[§]	-1.3[§]		
95% Confidence Interval	(-1.6, -1.1)	(-1.5, -1.1)		
Patients (%) achieving A$_{1c}$ <7%	42	35	7	22
Fasting Plasma Glucose (mg/dL) (Mean)				
Baseline	174	177	171	179
Change from baseline (adjusted mean)[‡]	-29	-28	+18	-16
Difference from placebo + glimepiride arm (adjusted mean)[‡]	-47[§]	-46[§]		
95% Confidence Interval	(-58, -35)	(-58, -35)		
Body Weight (kg) (Mean)				
Baseline	83.0	80.0	81.9	80.6
Change from baseline (adjusted mean)[‡]	-0.2	+0.3	-0.1	+2.1
Difference from placebo + glimepiride arm (adjusted mean)[‡]	-0.1	0.4		
95% Confidence Interval	(-0.9, 0.6)	(-0.4, 1.2)		

* Intent-to-treat population using last observation on study
† For rosiglitazone, one-half of the maximal approved United States dose.
‡ Least squares mean adjusted for baseline value
§ p-value <0.0001

Table 7 Results of a 26-week trial of Victoza as add-on to metformin and sulfonylurea*

	Victoza 1.8 mg + Metformin + Glimepiride	Placebo + Metformin + Glimepiride	Insulin glargine[†] + Metformin + Glimepiride
Intent-to-Treat Population (N)	230	114	232
HbA$_{1c}$ (%) (Mean)			
Baseline	8.3	8.3	8.1
Change from baseline (adjusted mean)[‡]	-1.3	-0.2	-1.1
Difference from placebo + metformin + glimepiride arm (adjusted mean)[‡]	-1.1[§]		
95% Confidence Interval	(-1.3, -0.9)		
Patients (%) achieving A$_{1c}$ <7%	53	15	46
Fasting Plasma Glucose (mg/dL) (Mean)			
Baseline	165	170	164
Change from baseline (adjusted mean)[‡]	-28	+10	-32
Difference from placebo + metformin + glimepiride arm (adjusted mean)[‡]	-38[§]		
95% Confidence Interval	(-46, -30)		
Body Weight (kg) (Mean)			
Baseline	85.8	85.4	85.2
Change from baseline (adjusted mean)[‡]	-1.8	-0.4	1.6
Difference from placebo + metformin + glimepiride arm (adjusted mean)[‡]	-1.4[¶]		
95% Confidence Interval	(-2.1, -0.7)		

* Intent-to-treat population using last observation on study
† For insulin glargine, optimal titration regimen was not achieved for 80% of patients.
‡ Least squares mean adjusted for baseline value
§ p-value <0.0001
¶ p-value <0.05

[See table 5 at top of previous page]
Add-on to Sulfonylurea
In this 26-week trial, 1041 patients were randomized to Victoza 0.6 mg, Victoza 1.2 mg, Victoza 1.8 mg, placebo, or rosiglitazone 4 mg (one-half of the maximal approved dose in the United States), all as add-on to glimepiride. Randomization occurred after a 4-week run-in period consisting of an initial, 2-week, forced-glimepiride titration period followed by a maintenance period of another 2 weeks. During the titration period, doses of glimepiride were increased to 4 mg/day. The doses of glimepiride could be reduced (at the discretion of the investigator) from 4 mg/day to 3 mg/day or 2 mg/day (minimum) after randomization, in the event of unacceptable hypoglycemia or other adverse events.
Treatment with Victoza 1.2 mg and 1.8 mg as add-on to glimepiride resulted in a statistically significant reduction in mean HbA$_{1c}$ compared to placebo add-on to glimepiride (Table 6). The percentage of patients who discontinued due to ineffective therapy was 3.0% in the Victoza 1.8 mg + glimepiride treatment group, 3.5% in the Victoza 1.2 mg + glimepiride treatment group, 17.5% in the placebo + glimepiride treatment group, and 6.9% in the rosiglitazone + glimepiride treatment group.
[See table 6 at left]
Add-on to Metformin and Sulfonylurea
In this 26-week trial, 581 patients were randomized to Victoza 1.8 mg, placebo, or insulin glargine, all as add-on to metformin and glimepiride. Randomization took place after a 6-week run-in period consisting of a 3-week forced metformin and glimepiride titration period followed by a maintenance period of another 3 weeks. During the titration period, doses of metformin and glimepiride were to be increased up to 2000 mg/day and 4 mg/day, respectively. After randomization, patients randomized to Victoza 1.8 mg underwent a 2 week period of titration with Victoza. During the trial, the Victoza and metformin doses were fixed, although glimepiride and insulin glargine doses could be adjusted. Patients titrated glargine twice-weekly during the first 8 weeks of treatment based on self-measured fasting plasma glucose on the day of titration. After Week 8, the frequency of insulin glargine titration was left to the discretion of the investigator, but, at a minimum, the glargine dose was to be revised, if necessary, at Weeks 12 and 18. Only 20% of glargine-treated patients achieved the pre-specified target fasting plasma glucose of ≤100 mg/dL. Therefore, optimal titration of the insulin glargine dose was not achieved in most patients.
Treatment with Victoza as add-on to glimepiride and metformin resulted in a statistically significant mean reduction in HbA$_{1c}$ compared to placebo add-on to glimepiride and metformin (Table 7). The percentage of patients who discontinued due to ineffective therapy was 0.9% in the Victoza 1.8 mg + metformin + glimepiride treatment group, 0.4% in the insulin glargine + metformin + glimepiride treatment group, and 11.3% in the placebo + metformin + glimepiride treatment group.
[See table 7 at left]
Add-on to Metformin and Thiazolidinedione
In this 26-week trial, 533 patients were randomized to Victoza 1.2 mg, Victoza 1.8 mg or placebo, all as add-on to rosiglitazone (8 mg) plus metformin (2000 mg). Patients underwent a 9 week run-in period (3-week forced dose escalation followed by a 6-week dose maintenance phase) with rosiglitazone (starting at 4 mg and increasing to 8 mg/day within 2 weeks) and metformin (starting at 500 mg with increasing weekly increments of 500 mg to a final dose of 2000 mg/day). Only patients who tolerated the final dose of rosiglitazone (8 mg/day) and metformin (2000 mg/day) and completed the 6-week dose maintenance phase were eligible for randomization into the trial.
Treatment with Victoza as add-on to metformin and rosiglitazone produced a statistically significant reduction in mean HbA$_{1c}$ compared to placebo add-on to metformin and rosiglitazone (Table 8). The percentage of patients who discontinued due to ineffective therapy was 1.7% in the Victoza 1.8 mg + metformin + rosiglitazone treatment group, 1.7% in the Victoza 1.2 mg + metformin + rosiglitazone treatment group, and 16.4% in the placebo + metformin + rosiglitazone treatment group.
[See table 8 at top of next page]

16   HOW SUPPLIED/STORAGE AND HANDLING
16.1   How Supplied
Victoza is available in the following package sizes containing disposable, pre-filled, multi-dose pens. Each individual pen delivers doses of 0.6 mg, 1.2 mg, or 1.8 mg (6 mg/mL, 3 mL).
2 × Victoza pen NDC 0169-4060-12
3 × Victoza pen NDC 0169-4060-13
Each Victoza pen is for use by a single patient. A Victoza pen should never be shared between patients, even if the needle is changed.
16.2   Recommended Storage
Prior to first use, Victoza should be stored in a refrigerator between 36°F to 46°F (2°C to 8°C) (Table 9). Do not store in

the freezer or directly adjacent to the refrigerator cooling element. Do not freeze Victoza and do not use Victoza if it has been frozen.

After initial use of the Victoza pen, the pen can be stored for 30 days at controlled room temperature (59°F to 86°F; 15°C to 30°C) or in a refrigerator (36°F to 46°F; 2°C to 8°C). Keep the pen cap on when not in use. Victoza should be protected from excessive heat and sunlight. Always remove and safely discard the needle after each injection and store the Victoza pen without an injection needle attached. This will reduce the potential for contamination, infection, and leakage while also ensuring dosing accuracy.

Table 9 Recommended Storage Conditions for the Victoza Pen

Prior to first use	After first use	
Refrigerated	Room Temperature	Refrigerated
36°F to 46°F (2°C to 8°C)	59°F to 86°F (15°C to 30°C)	36°F to 46°F (2°C to 8°C)
Until expiration date	30 days	

17 PATIENT COUNSELING INFORMATION

17.1 Risk of Thyroid C-cell Tumors
Patients should be informed that liraglutide causes benign and malignant thyroid C-cell tumors in mice and rats and that the human relevance of this finding is unknown. Patients should be counseled to report symptoms of thyroid tumors (e.g., a lump in the neck, hoarseness, dysphagia or dyspnea) to their physician.

17.2 Pancreatitis
Patients should be informed that persistent severe abdominal pain, that may radiate to the back and which may (or may not) be accompanied by vomiting, is the hallmark symptom of acute pancreatitis. Patients should be instructed to discontinue Victoza promptly, and to contact their physician, if persistent severe abdominal pain occurs [see Warnings and Precautions (5.2)].

17.3 Never Share a Victoza Pen Between Patients
Counsel patients that they should never share a Victoza pen with another person, even if the needle is changed. Sharing of the pen between patients may pose a risk of transmission of infection.

17.4 Instructions
Patients should be informed of the potential risks and benefits of Victoza and of alternative modes of therapy. Patients should also be informed about the importance of adherence to dietary instructions, regular physical activity, periodic blood glucose monitoring and A_{1c} testing, recognition and management of hypoglycemia and hyperglycemia, and assessment for diabetes complications. During periods of stress such as fever, trauma, infection, or surgery, medication requirements may change and patients should be advised to seek medical advice promptly.

Patients should be advised that the most common side effects of Victoza are headache, nausea and diarrhea. Nausea is most common when first starting Victoza, but decreases over time in the majority of patients and does not typically require discontinuation of Victoza.

Physicians should instruct their patients to read the Patient Medication Guide before starting Victoza therapy and to re-read each time the prescription is renewed. Patients should be instructed to inform their doctor or pharmacist if they develop any unusual symptom, or if any known symptom persists or worsens.

17.5 Laboratory Tests
Patients should be informed that response to all diabetic therapies should be monitored by periodic measurements of blood glucose and A_{1c} levels, with a goal of decreasing these levels towards the normal range. A_{1c} is especially useful for evaluating long-term glycemic control.

17.6 FDA-Approved Medication Guide
See separate leaflet.
Date of Issue: January 2010
Version: 1
Victoza® is a registered trademark of Novo Nordisk A/S.
Victoza® is covered by US Patent Nos. 6,268,343, 6,458,924 and 7,235,627 and other patents pending.
Victoza® Pen is covered by US Patent Nos. 6,004,297, 6,235,004, 6,582,404 and other patents pending.
© 2010 Novo Nordisk A/S
Manufactured by:
Novo Nordisk A/S
DK-2880 Bagsvaerd, Denmark
For information about Victoza contact:
Novo Nordisk Inc.
100 College Road West
Princeton, NJ 08540
1-877-484-2869

Table 8 Results of a 26-week trial of Victoza as add-on to metformin and thiazolidinedione*

	Victoza 1.8 mg + Metformin + Rosiglitazone	Victoza 1.2 mg + Metformin + Rosiglitazone	Placebo + Metformin + Rosiglitazone
Intent-to-Treat Population (N)	178	177	175
HbA₁c (%) (Mean)			
Baseline	8.6	8.5	8.4
Change from baseline (adjusted mean)†	-1.5	-1.5	-0.5
Difference from placebo + metformin + rosiglitazone arm (adjusted mean)†	-0.9‡	-0.9‡	
95% Confidence Interval	(-1.1, -0.8)	(-1.1, -0.8)	
Patients (%) achieving A₁c <7%	54	57	28
Fasting Plasma Glucose (mg/dL) (Mean)			
Baseline	185	181	179
Change from baseline (adjusted mean)†	-44	-40	-8
Difference from placebo + metformin + rosiglitazone arm (adjusted mean)†	-36‡	-32‡	
95% Confidence Interval	(-44, -27)	(-41, -23)	
Body Weight (kg) (Mean)			
Baseline	94.9	95.3	98.5
Change from baseline (adjusted mean)†	-2.0	-1.0	+0.6
Difference from placebo + metformin + rosiglitazone arm (adjusted mean)†	-2.6‡	-1.6‡	
95% Confidence Interval	(-3.4, -1.8)	(-2.4, -1.0)	

* Intent-to-treat population using last observation on study
† Least squares mean adjusted for baseline value
‡ p-value <0.0001

Medication Guide
Victoza® (VIC-tow-za)
(liraglutide [rDNA origin]) Injection
Read this Medication Guide and Patient Instructions for Use that come with Victoza before you start using Victoza and each time you get a refill. There may be new information. This Medication Guide does not take the place of talking with your healthcare provider about your medical condition or your treatment. If you have questions about Victoza after reading this information, ask your healthcare provider or pharmacist.

What is the most important information I should know about Victoza?
Serious side effects may happen in people who take Victoza, including:
1. **Possible thyroid tumors, including cancer.** During the drug testing process, the medicine in Victoza caused rats and mice to develop tumors of the thyroid gland. Some of these tumors were cancers. It is not known if Victoza will cause thyroid tumors or a type of thyroid cancer called medullary thyroid cancer in people. If medullary thyroid cancer occurs, it may lead to death if not detected and treated early. If you develop tumors or cancer of the thyroid, your thyroid may have to be surgically removed.
• Before you start taking Victoza, tell your healthcare provider if you or any of your family members have had thyroid cancer, especially medullary thyroid cancer, or Multiple Endocrine Neoplasia syndrome type 2. Do not take Victoza if you or any of your family members have medullary thyroid cancer, or if you have Multiple Endocrine Neoplasia syndrome type 2. People with these conditions already have a higher chance of developing medullary thyroid cancer in general and should not take Victoza.
• While taking Victoza, tell your healthcare provider if you get a lump or swelling in your neck, hoarseness, trouble swallowing, or shortness of breath. These may be symptoms of thyroid cancer.
2. **Inflammation of the pancreas (pancreatitis)**, which may be severe and lead to death.
Before taking Victoza, tell your healthcare provider if you have had:
• pancreatitis
• stones in your gallbladder (gallstones)
• a history of alcoholism
• high blood triglyceride levels

These medical conditions can make you more likely to get pancreatitis in general. It is not known if having these conditions will lead to a higher chance of getting pancreatitis while taking Victoza.
While taking Victoza:
Stop taking Victoza and call your healthcare provider right away if you have pain in your stomach area (abdomen) that is severe and will not go away. The pain may happen with or without vomiting. The pain may be felt going from your abdomen through to your back. This type of pain may be a symptom of pancreatitis.
What is Victoza?
• Victoza is an injectable prescription medicine that may improve blood sugar (glucose) in adults with type 2 diabetes mellitus, and should be used along with diet and exercise.
• Victoza is not recommended as the first choice of medication for treating diabetes.
• Victoza is not insulin.
• It is not known if Victoza is safe and effective when used with insulin.
• Victoza is not for use in people with type 1 diabetes or people with diabetic ketoacidosis.
• It is not known if Victoza is safe and effective in children. Victoza is not recommended for use in children.
Who should not use Victoza?
Do not use Victoza if:
• you or any of your family members have a history of medullary thyroid cancer.
• you have Multiple Endocrine Neoplasia syndrome type 2 (MEN 2). This is a disease where people have tumors in more than one gland in their body.
Talk with your healthcare provider if you are not sure if you have any of these conditions.
What should I tell my healthcare provider before using Victoza?
Before taking Victoza, tell your healthcare provider if you:
• have any of the conditions listed in the section "What is the most important information I should know about Victoza?"
• are allergic to liraglutide or any of the other ingredients in Victoza. See the end of this Medication Guide for a list of ingredients in Victoza.
• have severe problems with your stomach, such as slowed emptying of your stomach (gastroparesis) or problems with digesting food.

- have or have had kidney or liver problems.
- have any other medical conditions.
- are pregnant or plan to become pregnant. It is not known if Victoza will harm your unborn baby. Tell your healthcare provider if you become pregnant while taking Victoza.
- are breastfeeding or plan to breastfeed. It is not known if Victoza passes into your breast milk. You and your healthcare provider should decide if you will take Victoza or breastfeed. You should not do both without talking with your healthcare provider first.

Tell your healthcare provider about all the medicines you take including prescription and non-prescription medicines, vitamins, and herbal supplements. Victoza slows stomach emptying and can affect medicines that need to pass through the stomach quickly. Victoza may affect the way some medicines work and some other medicines may affect the way Victoza works. Tell your healthcare provider if you take other diabetes medicines, especially sulfonylurea medicines or insulin.

Know the medicines you take. Keep a list of them with you to show your healthcare provider and pharmacist each time you get a new medicine.

How should I use Victoza?

- Use Victoza exactly as prescribed by your healthcare provider. Your dose should be increased after using Victoza for one week. After that, do not change your dose unless your healthcare provider tells you to.
- Victoza is injected 1 time each day, at any time during the day.
- You can take Victoza with or without food.
- Victoza comes in a prefilled pen.
- Your healthcare provider must teach you how to inject Victoza before you use it for the first time. If you have questions or do not understand the instructions, talk to your healthcare provider or pharmacist. See the Patient Instructions for Use that come with this Medication Guide for detailed information about the right way to use your Victoza pen.
- Pen needles are not included. You may need a prescription to get pen needles from your pharmacist. Ask your healthcare provider which needle size is best for you.
- When starting a new prefilled Victoza pen, you must follow the "First Time Use for Each New Pen" (see the detailed Patient Instructions for Use that comes with this Medication Guide). You only need to do this 1 time with each new pen. You should also do this if you drop your pen. If you do the "First Time Use for Each New Pen" before each injection, you will run out of medicine too soon.
- Inject your dose of Victoza under the skin (subcutaneous injection) in your stomach area (abdomen), upper leg (thigh), or upper arm, as instructed by your healthcare provider. **Do not inject into a vein or muscle.**
- If you take too much Victoza, call your healthcare provider right away. Too much Victoza may cause severe nausea and vomiting.
- Follow your healthcare provider's instructions for diet, exercise, how often to test your blood sugar, and when to get your HbA₁c checked. If you stop using Victoza your blood sugar levels may increase. First talk to your healthcare provider if you want to stop taking Victoza.
- Your dose of diabetes medicines may need to be changed if your body is under certain types of stress. Tell your healthcare provider if you:
  - have fever
  - have trauma
  - have an infection
  - plan to have or have had surgery
- Never share your Victoza pen or needles with another person. You may give an infection to them, or get an infection from them.

What are the possible side effects of Victoza?

Victoza may cause serious side effects, including:

- See "What is the most important information I should know about Victoza?"
- **Low blood sugar (hypoglycemia).** Your risk for getting low blood sugar is higher if you take Victoza with another medicine that can cause low blood sugar, such as a sulfonylurea. In some people, the blood sugar may get so low that they need another person to help them. The dose of your sulfonylurea medicine may need to be lowered while you use Victoza. Signs and symptoms of low blood sugar may include:
- shakiness
- sweating
- headache
- drowsiness
- weakness
- dizziness
- confusion
- irritability
- hunger
- fast heartbeat
- feeling jittery

Talk to your healthcare provider about how to recognize and treat low blood sugar. Make sure that your family and other people who are around you a lot know how to recognize and treat low blood sugar.

Common side effects of Victoza include:

- headache
- nausea
- diarrhea

Nausea is most common when first starting Victoza, but decreases over time in most people as their body gets used to the medicine. Tell your healthcare provider if you have any side effect that bothers you or that does not go away.

These are not all the side effects with Victoza. For more information, ask your healthcare provider or pharmacist.

Call your doctor for medical advice about side effects. You may report side effects to FDA at 1-800-FDA-1088.

How should I store Victoza?

Before use:

- Store your new, unused Victoza pen in the refrigerator at 36°F to 46°F (2°C to 8°C).
- Do not freeze Victoza or use Victoza if it has been frozen. Do not store Victoza near the refrigerator cooling element.

Pen in use:

- Store your Victoza pen for 30 days either at 59°F to 86°F (15°C to 30°C), or in a refrigerator at 36°F to 46°F (2°C to 8°C).
- When carrying the pen away from home, store the pen at a temperature between 59°F to 86°F (15°C to 30°C) and keep it dry.
- If Victoza has been exposed to temperatures above 86°F (30°C), it should be thrown away.
- Protect your Victoza pen from heat and sunlight.
- Keep the pen cap on when your Victoza pen is not in use.
- Use your Victoza pen within 30 days after the first day it is stored outside the refrigerator. After these 30 days, throw away your Victoza pen even if some medicine is left in the pen.
- Do not use Victoza after the expiration date printed on the carton.

Do not store the Victoza pen with the needle attached. Always safely remove and safely throw away the needle after each injection. This may help prevent contamination, infection and leakage. It also helps to make sure that you get the correct dose of Victoza. See the Patient Instructions for Use for information about how to dispose of used pen needles and used Victoza pens.

Keep your Victoza pen, pen needles, and all medicines out of the reach of children.

General information about Victoza

Medicines are sometimes prescribed for purposes other than those listed in a Medication Guide. Do not use Victoza for a condition for which it was not prescribed. Do not give Victoza to other people, even if they have the same symptoms you have. It may harm them.

This Medication Guide summarizes the most important information you should know about using Victoza. If you would like more information, talk with your healthcare provider. You can ask your pharmacist or healthcare provider for information about Victoza that is written for health professionals.

For more information, go to victoza.com or call 1-877-484-2869.

What are the ingredients in Victoza?

Active Ingredient: liraglutide

Inactive Ingredients: disodium phosphate dihydrate, propylene glycol, phenol and water for injection

Manufactured by:
Novo Nordisk A/S
DK-2880 Bagsvaerd, Denmark
For information about Victoza contact:
Novo Nordisk Inc.
100 College Road West
Princeton, NJ 08540
1-877-484-2869
Issued: January 2010
Version: 1

This Medication Guide has been approved by the U.S. Food and Drug Administration.

Victoza® is a registered trademark of Novo Nordisk A/S.
Victoza® is covered by US Patent Nos. 6,268,343, 6,458,924 and 7,235,627 and other patents pending.
Victoza® pen is covered by US Patent Nos. 6,004,297, 6,235,004, 6,582,404 and other patents pending.
© 2010 Novo Nordisk A/S

PATIENT INSTRUCTIONS FOR USE
Victoza (liraglutide [rDNA origin]) injection
[See figure at top of next column]

First read the Medication Guide that comes with your Victoza pen and then read these Patient Instructions for Use for information about how to use your Victoza pen the right way.

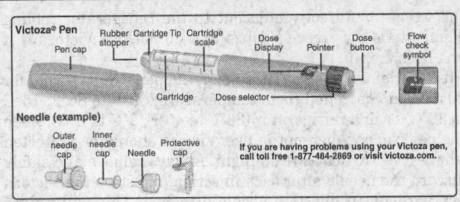

These instructions do not take the place of talking with your healthcare provider about your medical condition or your treatment.

Your Victoza pen contains 3 mL of Victoza and will deliver doses of 0.6 mg, 1.2 mg or 1.8 mg. The number of doses that you can take with a Victoza pen depends on the dose of medicine that is prescribed for you. Your healthcare provider will tell you how much Victoza to take.

Victoza pen should be used with Novo Nordisk disposable needles. Talk to your healthcare provider or pharmacist for more information about needles for your Victoza pen.

Important Information

- Do not share your Victoza pen or needles with anyone else. You may give an infection to them or get an infection from them.
- Always use a new needle for each injection.
- Keep your Victoza pen and all medicines out of the reach of children.
- If you drop your Victoza pen, repeat "First Time Use For Each New Pen" (steps A through D).
- Be careful not to bend or damage the needle.
- Do not use the cartridge scale to measure how much Victoza to inject.
- Be careful when handling used needles to avoid needle stick injuries.
- You can use your Victoza pen for up to 30 days after you use it the first time.

Caring for your Victoza pen

- After removing the needle, put the pen cap on your Victoza pen and store your Victoza pen without the needle attached.

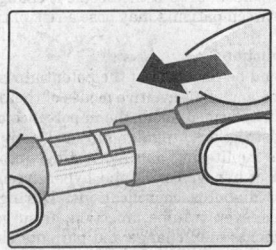

- Do not try to refill your Victoza pen - it is prefilled and is disposable.
- Do not try to repair your pen or pull it apart.
- Keep your Victoza pen away from dust, dirt and liquids.
- If cleaning is needed, wipe the outside of the pen with a clean, damp cloth.

How should I store Victoza?

Before use:

- Store your new, unused Victoza pen in the refrigerator at 36°F to 46°F (2°C to 8°C).
- If Victoza is stored outside of refrigeration (by mistake) prior to first use, it should be used or thrown away within 30 days.
- Do not freeze Victoza or use Victoza if it has been frozen. Do not store Victoza near the refrigerator cooling element.

Pen in use:

- Store your Victoza pen for 30 days at 59°F to 86°F (15°C to 30°C), or in a refrigerator at 36°F to 46°F (2°C to 8°C).
- When carrying the pen away from home, store the pen at a temperature between 59°F to 86°F (15°C to 30°C).
- If Victoza has been exposed to temperatures above 86°F (30°C), it should be thrown away.
- Protect your Victoza pen from heat and sunlight.
- Keep the pen cap on when your Victoza pen is not in use.
- Use a Victoza pen for only 30 days. Throw away a used Victoza pen after 30 days, even if some medicine is left in the pen.

First Time Use for Each New Pen
Step A. Check the Pen

- Take your new Victoza pen out of the refrigerator.
- Wash hands with soap and water before use.
- Check pen label before each use to make sure it is your Victoza pen.

• Pull off pen cap.

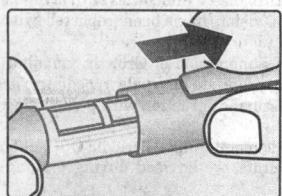

• Check Victoza in the cartridge. The liquid should be clear, colorless and free of particles. If not, do not use.
• Wipe the rubber stopper with an alcohol swab.

Step B. Attach the Needle
• Remove protective tab from outer needle cap.
• Push outer needle cap containing the needle straight onto the pen, then screw needle on until secure.

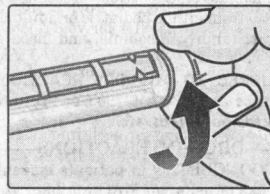

• Pull off outer needle cap. Do not throw away.

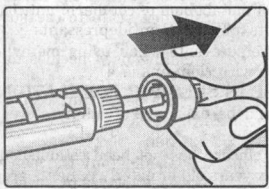

• Pull off inner needle cap and throw away. A small drop of liquid may appear. This is normal.

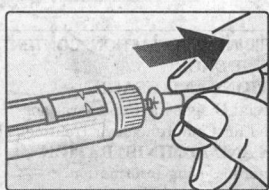

Step C. Dial to the Flow Check Symbol
• Turn dose selector until flow check symbol (--) lines up with pointer.

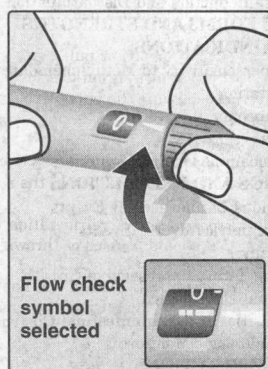

Flow check symbol selected

Step D. Prepare the Pen
• Hold pen with needle pointing up.
• Tap cartridge gently with your finger a few times to bring any air bubbles to the top of the cartridge.

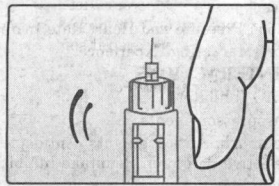

• Keep needle pointing up and press dose button until 0 mg lines up with pointer. Repeat steps C and D, up to 6 times, until a drop of Victoza appears at the needle tip.

If you still see no drop of Victoza, use a new pen and contact Novo Nordisk at 1-877-484-2869.

Continue to Step G under "Routine Use" →

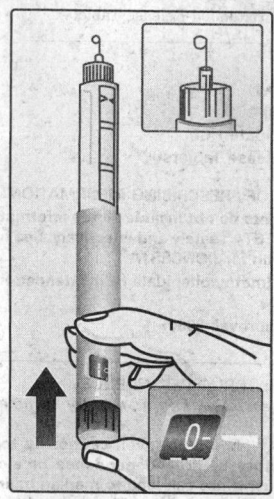

Routine Use
Step E. Check the Pen
• Take your Victoza pen from where it is stored.
• Wash hands with soap and water before use.
• Check pen label before each use to make sure it is your Victoza pen.
• Pull off pen cap.

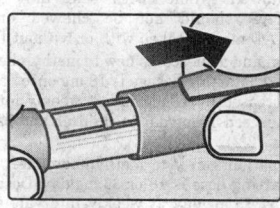

• Check Victoza in the cartridge. The liquid should be clear, colorless and free of particles. If not, do not use.
• Wipe the rubber stopper with an alcohol swab.

Step F. Attach the Needle
• Remove protective tab from outer needle cap.
• Push outer needle cap containing the needle straight onto the pen, then screw needle on until secure.

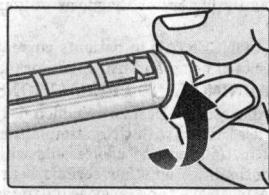

• Pull off outer needle cap. Do not throw away.

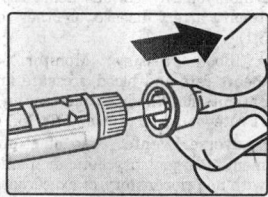

• Pull off inner needle cap and throw away. A small drop of liquid may appear. This is normal.

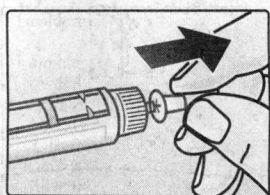

Step G. Dial the Dose
• Victoza pen can give a dose of 0.6 mg (starting dose), 1.2 mg or 1.8 mg. Be sure that you know the dose of Victoza that is prescribed for you.

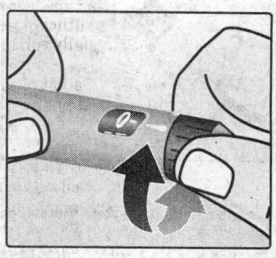

• Turn the dose selector until your needed dose lines up with the pointer (0.6 mg, 1.2 mg or 1.8 mg).

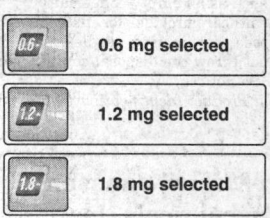

0.6	0.6 mg selected
1.2	1.2 mg selected
1.8	1.8 mg selected

• You will hear a "click" every time you turn the dose selector. **Do not set the dose by counting the number of clicks you hear.**
• If you select a wrong dose, change it by turning the dose selector backwards or forwards until the correct dose lines up with the pointer. Be careful not to press the dose button when turning the dose selector. This may cause Victoza to come out.

Step H. Injecting the Dose
• Insert needle into your skin in the stomach, thigh or upper arm. Use the injection technique shown to you by your healthcare provider. **Do not inject Victoza into a vein or muscle.**
• Press down on the center of the dose button to inject until 0 mg lines up with the pointer.
• Be careful not to touch the dose display with your other fingers. This may block the injection.
• Keep the dose button pressed down and make sure that you keep the needle under the skin for a full count of 6 seconds to make sure the full dose is injected. Keep your thumb on the injection button until you remove the needle from your skin.

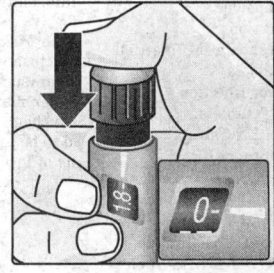

Step I. Withdraw Needle
• You may see a drop of Victoza at the needle tip. This is normal and it does not affect the dose you just received. If blood appears after you take the needle out of your skin, apply light pressure, but **do not rub the area.**

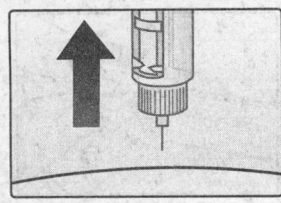

Step J. Remove and Dispose of the Needle
- Carefully put the outer needle cap over the needle. Unscrew the needle.

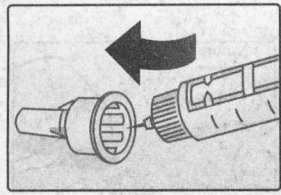

- Safely remove the needle from your Victoza pen after each use.
- Place used needles in a closeable, puncture-resistant container. If your Victoza pen is empty or if you have been using it for 30 days (even if it is not empty), throw away the used pen. You may use a sharps container (such as a red biohazard container), a hard plastic container (such as an empty detergent bottle), or metal container with a screw top (such as an empty coffee can).
- Ask your healthcare provider for instructions on the right way to dispose of your used needles, pens, and the container. Do not throw the disposal container in the household trash. Do not recycle.

Shown in Product Identification Guide, page 316

Ortho-McNeil-Janssen Pharmaceuticals, Inc.
RARITAN, NJ 08869-0602 and TITUSVILLE, NJ 08560-0200

www.ortho-mcneil.com
www.pricara.com
www.janssen.com
www.mcneilpediatrics.net
www.ortho-mcneilneurologics.com
For Medical Information Contact:
(800) 682-6532
In Emergencies:
(908) 218-7325
For Patient Education Materials Contact:
877-323-2200
For Customer Service (Sales and Ordering):
800-631-5273

To obtain Prescribing Information on the following products, please contact:
Ortho-McNeil-Janssen Pharmaceuticals, Inc.
1000 Route 202 South
PO Box 300
Raritan, NJ 08869-0602

AXERT Tablets
DORIBAX Injection
ELMIRON Capsules
HALDOL Injection
HALDOL Decanoate IM Injection
MODICON Tablets
NATRECOR for Injection
ORTHO-CEPT Tablets
ORTHO-CYCLEN Tablets
ORTHO Diaphragm Kits
ORTHO MICRONOR Tablets
ORTHO-NOVUM 1/50 Tablets
ORTHO-NOVUM Tablets
ORTHO TRI-CYCLEN Tablets
ORTHO TRI-CYCLEN LO Tablets
PARAFON FORTE DSC
RAZADYNE Oral Solution
RAZADYNE Tablets
RAZADYNE ER Extended-Release Capsules
RISPERDAL Tablets, Oral Solution, M-Tab
TERAZOL 3 Vaginal Cream

TERAZOL 3 Vaginal Suppositories
TERAZOL 7 Vaginal Cream
TOLECTIN 200/400/600
TOPAMAX Sprinkle Capsules
TOPAMAX Tablets
TYLOX Capsules
ULTRACET Tablets
ULTRAM Tablets
ULTRAM ER Extended-Release Tablets

CONCERTA® Ⓒ ℞
[kon SER-ta]
(methylphenidate HCl)
Extended-Release Tablets Ⓒ

HIGHLIGHTS OF PRESCRIBING INFORMATION
These highlights do not include all the information needed to use CONCERTA® safely and effectively. See full prescribing information for CONCERTA®.
CONCERTA® (methylphenidate HCl) Extended-Release Tablets CII
Initial U.S. Approval: 2000

> **WARNING: DRUG DEPENDENCE**
> *See full prescribing information for complete boxed warning.*
> CONCERTA® should be given cautiously to patients with a history of drug dependence or alcoholism. Chronic abusive use can lead to marked tolerance and psychological dependence, with varying degrees of abnormal behavior.

——INDICATIONS AND USAGE——
CONCERTA® is a CNS stimulant indicated for the treatment of Attention Deficit Hyperactivity Disorder (ADHD) in children 6 years of age and older, adolescents, and adults up to the age of 65. (1)

——DOSAGE AND ADMINISTRATION——
- CONCERTA® should be taken once daily in the morning and swallowed whole with the aid of liquids. CONCERTA® should not be chewed or crushed. CONCERTA® may be taken with or without food. (2.1)
- For children and adolescents new to methylphenidate, the recommended starting dosage is 18 mg once daily. Dosage may be increased by 18 mg/day at weekly intervals and should not exceed 54 mg/day in children and 72 mg/day in adolescents. (2.2)
- For adult patients new to methylphenidate, the recommended starting dose is 18 or 36 mg/day. Dosage may be increased by 18 mg/day at weekly intervals and should not exceed 72 mg/day for adults. (2.2)
- For patients currently using methylphenidate, dosing is based on current dose regimen and clinical judgment. (2.3)

——DOSAGE FORMS AND STRENGTHS——
Tablets: 18, 27, 36, and 54 mg (3)

——CONTRAINDICATIONS——
Known hypersensitivity to the product (4.1)
Marked anxiety, tension, or agitation (4.2)
- Glaucoma (4.3)
- Tics or a family history or diagnosis of Tourette's syndrome (4.4)
- Do not use CONCERTA® in patients currently using or within 2 weeks of using an MAO inhibitor (4.5)

——WARNINGS AND PRECAUTIONS——
- Serious Cardiovascular Events: Sudden death has been reported in association with CNS stimulant treatment at usual doses in children and adolescents with structural cardiac abnormalities or other serious heart problems. Sudden death, stroke, and myocardial infarction have been reported in adults taking stimulant drugs at usual doses for ADHD. Stimulant products generally should not be used in patients with known structural cardiac abnormalities, cardiomyopathy, serious heart rhythm abnormalities, coronary artery disease, or other serious heart problems. (5.1)
- Increase in Blood Pressure: Monitor patients for changes in heart rate and blood pressure and use with caution in patients for whom an increase in blood pressure or heart rate would be problematic. (5.1)
- Psychiatric Adverse Events: Use of stimulants may cause treatment-emergent psychotic or manic symptoms in patients with no prior history, or exacerbation of symptoms in patients with pre-existing psychiatric illness. Clinical evaluation for Bipolar Disorder is recommended prior to stimulant use. Monitor for aggressive behavior. (5.2)

- Seizures: Stimulants may lower the convulsive threshold. Discontinue in the presence of seizures. (5.3)
- Visual Disturbance: difficulties with accommodation and blurring of vision have been reported with stimulant treatment. (5.5)
- Long-Term Suppression of Growth: monitor height and weight at appropriate intervals in pediatric patients. (5.4)
- Gastrointestinal obstruction with pre-existing GI narrowing. (5.6)
- Hematologic monitoring: Periodic CBC, differential, and platelet counts are advised during prolonged therapy. (5.7)

——ADVERSE REACTIONS——
The most common adverse reaction in double-blind clinical trials (>5%) in children and adolescents was abdominal pain upper. The most common adverse reactions in double-blind clinical trials (>5%) in adult patients were decreased appetite, headache, dry mouth, nausea, insomnia, anxiety, dizziness, weight decreased, irritability, and hyperhidrosis. (6.1 and 6.2)
The most common adverse reactions associated with discontinuation (≥1%) from either pediatric or adult clinical trials were anxiety, irritability, insomnia, and blood pressure increased. (6.3)
To report SUSPECTED ADVERSE REACTIONS, contact McNeil Pediatrics at 1-888-440-7903 or FDA at 1-800-FDA-1088 or www.fda.gov/medwatch.

——DRUG INTERACTIONS——
- Do not use CONCERTA® in patients currently using or within 2 weeks of using an MAO inhibitor (7.1)
- CONCERTA® may increase blood pressure; use cautiously with vasopressors (7.2)
- Inhibition of metabolism of coumarin anticoagulants, anticonvulsants, and some antidepressants (7.3)
- Serious adverse events when using methylphenidate in combination with clonidine (7.4)

——USE IN SPECIFIC POPULATIONS——
Caution should be exercised if administered to nursing mothers (8.3)
- Safety and efficacy has not been established in children less than six years old or elderly patients greater than 65 years of age (8.4 and 8.5)
See 17 for PATIENT COUNSELING INFORMATION and Medication Guide

Revised: 01/2010

FULL PRESCRIBING INFORMATION: CONTENTS
DRUG DEPENDENCE

FULL PRESCRIBING INFORMATION

DRUG DEPENDENCE

CONCERTA® should be given cautiously to patients with a history of drug dependence or alcoholism. Chronic abusive use can lead to marked tolerance and psychological dependence with varying degrees of abnormal behavior. Frank psychotic episodes can occur, especially with parenteral abuse. Careful supervision is required during withdrawal from abusive use since severe depression may occur. Withdrawal following chronic therapeutic use may unmask symptoms of the underlying disorder that may require follow-up.

---

1   INDICATIONS AND USAGE

CONCERTA® is indicated for the treatment of Attention Deficit Hyperactivity Disorder (ADHD) in children 6 years of age and older, adolescents, and adults up to the age of 65 [see Clinical Studies (14)].

A diagnosis of Attention Deficit Hyperactivity Disorder (ADHD; DSM-IV) implies the presence of hyperactive-impulsive or inattentive symptoms that caused impairment and were present before age 7 years. The symptoms must cause clinically significant impairment, e.g., in social, academic, or occupational functioning, and be present in two or more settings, e.g., school (or work) and at home. The symptoms must not be better accounted for by another mental disorder. For the Inattentive Type, at least six of the following symptoms must have persisted for at least 6 months: lack of attention to details/careless mistakes; lack of sustained attention; poor listener; failure to follow through on tasks; poor organization; avoids tasks requiring sustained mental effort; loses things; easily distracted; forgetful. For the Hyperactive-Impulsive Type, at least six of the following symptoms must have persisted for at least 6 months: fidgeting/squirming; leaving seat; inappropriate running/climbing; difficulty with quiet activities; "on the go;" excessive talking; blurting answers; can't wait turn; intrusive. The Combined Type requires both inattentive and hyperactive-impulsive criteria to be met.

1.1   Special Diagnostic Considerations

Specific etiology of this syndrome is unknown, and there is no single diagnostic test. Adequate diagnosis requires the use of medical and special psychological, educational, and social resources. Learning may or may not be impaired. The diagnosis must be based upon a complete history and evaluation of the patient and not solely on the presence of the required number of DSM-IV characteristics.

1.2   Need for Comprehensive Treatment Program

CONCERTA® is indicated as an integral part of a total treatment program for ADHD that may include other measures (psychological, educational, social). Drug treatment may not be indicated for all patients with ADHD. Stimulants are not intended for use in patients who exhibit symptoms secondary to environmental factors and/or other primary psychiatric disorders, including psychosis. Appropriate educational placement is essential and psychosocial intervention is often helpful. When remedial measures alone are insufficient, the decision to prescribe stimulant medication will depend upon the physician's assessment of the chronicity and severity of the patient's symptoms.

2   DOSAGE AND ADMINISTRATION

2.1   General Dosing Information

CONCERTA® should be administered orally once daily in the morning with or without food.

CONCERTA® must be swallowed whole with the aid of liquids, and must not be chewed, divided, or crushed [see Patient Counseling Information (17)].

2.2   Patients New to Methylphenidate

The recommended starting dose of CONCERTA® for patients who are not currently taking methylphenidate or stimulants other than methylphenidate is 18 mg once daily for children and adolescents and 18 or 36 mg once daily for adults (see Table 1).

[See table 1 above]

2.3   Patients Currently Using Methylphenidate

The recommended dose of CONCERTA® for patients who are currently taking methylphenidate twice daily or three times daily, at doses of 10 to 60 mg/day is provided in Table 2. Dosing recommendations are based on current dose regimen and clinical judgment. Conversion dosage should not exceed 72 mg daily.

[See table 2 above]

Other methylphenidate regimens: Clinical judgment should be used when selecting the starting dose.

2.4   Dose Titration

Doses may be increased in 18 mg increments at weekly intervals for patients who have not achieved an optimal response at a lower dose. Daily dosages above 54 mg in children and 72 mg in adolescents have not been studied and are not recommended. Daily dosages above 72 mg in adults are not recommended.

A 27 mg dosage strength is available for physicians who wish to prescribe between the 18 mg and 36 mg dosages.

2.5   Maintenance/Extended Treatment

There is no body of evidence available from controlled trials to indicate how long the patient with ADHD should be treated with CONCERTA®. It is generally agreed, however, that pharmacological treatment of ADHD may be needed for extended periods.

The effectiveness of CONCERTA® for long-term use, i.e., for more than 7 weeks, has not been systematically evaluated in controlled trials. The physician who elects to use CONCERTA® for extended periods in patients with ADHD should periodically re-evaluate the long-term usefulness of the drug for the individual patient with trials off medication to assess the patient's functioning without pharmacotherapy. Improvement may be sustained when the drug is either temporarily or permanently discontinued.

2.6   Dose Reduction and Discontinuation

If paradoxical aggravation of symptoms or other adverse events occur, the dosage should be reduced, or, if necessary, the drug should be discontinued.

If improvement is not observed after appropriate dosage adjustment over a one-month period, the drug should be discontinued.

3   DOSAGE FORMS AND STRENGTHS

CONCERTA® (methylphenidate HCl) Extended-Release Tablets are available in the following dosage strengths: 18 mg tablets are yellow and imprinted with "alza 18," 27 mg tablets are gray and imprinted with "alza 27," 36 mg tablets are white and imprinted with "alza 36," and 54 mg tablets are brownish-red and imprinted with "alza 54."

4   CONTRAINDICATIONS

4.1   Hypersensitivity to Methylphenidate

Hypersensitivity reactions, such as angioedema and anaphylactic reactions, have been observed in patients treated with CONCERTA®. Therefore, CONCERTA® is contraindicated in patients known to be hypersensitive to methylphenidate or other components of the product [see Adverse Reactions (6.6)].

4.2   Agitation

CONCERTA® is contraindicated in patients with marked anxiety, tension, and agitation, since the drug may aggravate these symptoms.

4.3   Glaucoma

CONCERTA® is contraindicated in patients with glaucoma.

4.4   Tics

CONCERTA® is contraindicated in patients with motor tics or with a family history or diagnosis of Tourette's syndrome [see Adverse Reactions (6.4)].

4.5   Monoamine Oxidase Inhibitors

CONCERTA® is contraindicated during treatment with monoamine oxidase (MAO) inhibitors, and also within a minimum of 14 days following discontinuation of a MAO-inhibitor (hypertensive crises may result) [see Drug Interactions (7.1)].

5   WARNINGS AND PRECAUTIONS

5.1   Serious Cardiovascular Events

Sudden Death and Pre-existing Structural Cardiac Abnormalities or Other Serious Heart Problems

Children and Adolescents

Sudden death has been reported in association with CNS stimulant treatment at usual doses in children and adolescents with structural cardiac abnormalities or other serious heart problems. Although some serious heart problems alone carry an increased risk of sudden death, stimulant products generally should not be used in children or adolescents with known serious structural cardiac abnormalities, cardiomyopathy, serious heart rhythm abnormalities, or other serious cardiac problems that may place them at increased vulnerability to the sympathomimetic effects of a stimulant drug.

Adults

Sudden deaths, stroke, and myocardial infarction have been reported in adults taking stimulant drugs at usual doses for ADHD. Although the role of stimulants in these adult cases is also unknown, adults have a greater likelihood than children of having serious structural cardiac abnormalities, cardiomyopathy, serious heart rhythm abnormalities, coronary artery disease, or other serious cardiac problems. Adults with such abnormalities should also generally not be treated with stimulant drugs.

Hypertension and other Cardiovascular Conditions

Stimulant medications cause a modest increase in average blood pressure (about 2 to 4 mmHg) and average heart rate (about 3 to 6 bpm) [see Adverse Reactions (6.5)], and individuals may have larger increases. While the mean changes alone would not be expected to have short-term consequences, all patients should be monitored for larger changes in heart rate and blood pressure. Caution is indicated in treating patients whose underlying medical conditions might be compromised by increases in blood pressure or heart rate, e.g., those with pre-existing hypertension, heart failure, recent myocardial infarction, or ventricular arrhythmia.

TABLE 1. CONCERTA® Recommended Starting Doses and Dose Ranges

Patient Age	Recommended Starting Dose	Dose Range
Children 6–12 years of age	18 mg/day	18 mg–54 mg/day
Adolescents 13–17 years of age	18 mg/day	18 mg–72 mg/day not to exceed 2 mg/kg/day
Adults 18–65 years of age	18 or 36 mg/day	18 mg–72 mg/day

TABLE 2. Recommended Dose Conversion from Methylphenidate Regimens to CONCERTA®

Previous Methylphenidate Daily Dose	Recommended CONCERTA® Starting Dose
5 mg Methylphenidate twice daily or three times daily	18 mg every morning
10 mg Methylphenidate twice daily or three times daily	36 mg every morning
15 mg Methylphenidate twice daily or three times daily	54 mg every morning
20 mg Methylphenidate twice daily or three times daily	72 mg every morning

Assessing Cardiovascular Status in Patients being Treated with Stimulant Medications

Children, adolescents, or adults who are being considered for treatment with stimulant medications, should have a careful history (including assessment for a family history of sudden death or ventricular arrhythmia) and physical exam to assess for the presence of cardiac disease, and should receive further cardiac evaluation if findings suggest such disease (e.g., electrocardiogram and echocardiogram). Patients who develop symptoms such as exertional chest pain, unexplained syncope, or other symptoms suggestive of cardiac disease during stimulant treatment should undergo a prompt cardiac evaluation.

5.2 Psychiatric Adverse Events

Pre-Existing Psychosis

Administration of stimulants may exacerbate symptoms of behavior disturbance and thought disorder in patients with a pre-existing psychotic disorder.

Bipolar Illness

Particular care should be taken in using stimulants to treat ADHD in patients with comorbid bipolar disorder because of concern for possible induction of a mixed/manic episode in such patients. Prior to initiating treatment with a stimulant, patients with comorbid depressive symptoms should be adequately screened to determine if they are at risk for bipolar disorder; such screening should include a detailed psychiatric history, including a family history of suicide, bipolar disorder, and depression.

Emergence of New Psychotic or Manic Symptoms

Treatment-emergent psychotic or manic symptoms, e.g., hallucinations, delusional thinking, or mania in patients without a prior history of psychotic illness or mania can be caused by stimulants at usual doses. If such symptoms occur, consideration should be given to a possible causal role of the stimulant, and discontinuation of treatment may be appropriate. In a pooled analysis of multiple short-term, placebo-controlled studies, such symptoms occurred in about 0.1% (4 patients with events out of 3482 exposed to methylphenidate or amphetamine for several weeks at usual doses) of stimulant-treated patients compared to 0 in placebo-treated patients.

Aggression

Aggressive behavior or hostility is often observed in patients with ADHD, and has been reported in clinical trials and the postmarketing experience of some medications indicated for the treatment of ADHD. Although there is no systematic evidence that stimulants cause aggressive behavior or hostility, patients beginning treatment for ADHD should be monitored for the appearance of or worsening of aggressive behavior or hostility.

5.3 Seizures

There is some clinical evidence that stimulants may lower the convulsive threshold in patients with prior history of seizures, in patients with prior EEG abnormalities in absence of seizures, and, very rarely, in patients without a history of seizures and no prior EEG evidence of seizures. In the presence of seizures, the drug should be discontinued.

5.4 Long-Term Suppression of Growth

Careful follow-up of weight and height in children ages 7 to 10 years who were randomized to either methylphenidate or non-medication treatment groups over 14 months, as well as in naturalistic subgroups of newly methylphenidate-treated and non-medication treated children over 36 months (to the ages of 10 to 13 years), suggests that consistently medicated children (i.e., treatment for 7 days per week throughout the year) have a temporary slowing in growth rate (on average, a total of about 2 cm less growth in height and 2.7 kg less growth in weight over 3 years), without evidence of growth rebound during this period of development. Published data are inadequate to determine whether chronic use of amphetamines may cause similar suppression of growth, however, it is anticipated that they likely have this effect as well. Therefore, growth should be monitored during treatment with stimulants, and patients who are not growing or gaining height or weight as expected may need to have their treatment interrupted.

5.5 Visual Disturbance

Difficulties with accommodation and blurring of vision have been reported with stimulant treatment.

5.6 Potential for Gastrointestinal Obstruction

Because the CONCERTA® tablet is nondeformable and does not appreciably change in shape in the GI tract, CONCERTA® should not ordinarily be administered to patients with preexisting severe gastrointestinal narrowing (pathologic or iatrogenic, for example: esophageal motility disorders, small bowel inflammatory disease, "short gut" syndrome due to adhesions or decreased transit time, past history of peritonitis, cystic fibrosis, chronic intestinal pseudoobstruction, or Meckel's diverticulum). There have been rare reports of obstructive symptoms in patients with known strictures in association with the ingestion of drugs in nondeformable controlled-release formulations. Due to the controlled-release design of the tablet, CONCERTA® should only be used in patients who are able to swallow the tablet whole [see Patient Counseling Information (17)].

5.7 Hematologic Monitoring

Periodic CBC, differential, and platelet counts are advised during prolonged therapy.

6 ADVERSE REACTIONS

The following are discussed in more detail in other sections of the labeling:

- Drug Dependence [see Box Warning]
- Hypersensitivity to Methylphenidate [see Contraindications (4.1)]
- Agitation [see Contraindications (4.2)]
- Glaucoma [see Contraindications (4.3)]
- Tics [see Contraindications (4.4)]
- Monoamine Oxidase Inhibitors [see Contraindications (4.5) and Drug Interactions (7.1)]
- Serious Cardiovascular Events [see Warnings and Precautions (5.1)]
- Psychiatric Adverse Events [see Warnings and Precautions (5.2)]
- Seizures [see Warnings and Precautions (5.3)]
- Long-Term Suppression of Growth [see Warnings and Precautions (5.4)]
- Visual Disturbance [see Warnings and Precautions (5.5)]
- Potential for Gastrointestinal Obstruction [see Warnings and Precautions (5.6)]
- Hematologic Monitoring [see Warnings and Precautions (5.7)]

The most common adverse reaction in double-blind clinical trials (>5%) in pediatric patients (children and adolescents) was abdominal pain upper. The most common adverse reactions in double-blind clinical trials (>5%) in adult patients were decreased appetite, headache, dry mouth, nausea, insomnia, anxiety, dizziness, weight decreased, irritability, and hyperhidrosis [see Adverse Reactions (6.1)].

The most common adverse reactions associated with discontinuation (≥1%) from either pediatric or adult clinical trials were anxiety, irritability, insomnia, and blood pressure increased [see Adverse Reactions (6.3)].

The development program for CONCERTA® included exposures in a total of 3733 participants in clinical trials. Children, adolescents, and adults with ADHD were evaluated in 6 controlled clinical studies and 11 open-label clinical studies (see Table 3). Safety was assessed by collecting adverse events, vital signs, weights, ECGs, and by performing physical examinations and laboratory analyses.

Table 3. CONCERTA® Exposure in Double-Blind and Open-Label Clinical Studies

Patient Population	N	Dose Range
Children	2216	18 to 54 mg once daily
Adolescents	502	18 to 72 mg once daily
Adults	1015	18 to 108 mg once daily

Adverse events during exposure were obtained primarily by general inquiry and recorded by clinical investigators using their own terminology. Consequently, to provide a meaningful estimate of the proportion of individuals experiencing adverse events, events were grouped in standardized categories using MedDRA terminology.

The stated frequencies of adverse events represent the proportion of individuals who experienced, at least once, a treatment-emergent adverse event of the type listed. An event was considered treatment-emergent if it occurred for the first time or worsened while receiving therapy following baseline evaluation.

Throughout this section, adverse reactions are reported. Adverse reactions are adverse events that were considered to be reasonably associated with the use of CONCERTA® based on the comprehensive assessment of the available adverse event information. A causal association for CONCERTA® often cannot be reliably established in individual cases. Further, because clinical trials are conducted under widely varying conditions, adverse reaction rates observed in the clinical trials of a drug cannot be directly compared to rates in clinical trials of another drug and may not reflect the rates observed in clinical practice.

The majority of adverse reactions were mild to moderate in severity.

6.1 Commonly-Observed Adverse Reactions in Double-Blind, Placebo-Controlled Clinical Trials

Adverse reactions in either the pediatric or adult double-blind adverse reactions tables may be relevant for both patient populations.

Children and Adolescents

Table 4 lists the adverse reactions reported in 1% or more of CONCERTA®-treated children and adolescent patients in 4 placebo-controlled, double-blind clinical trials.

Table 4. Adverse Reactions Reported by ≥1% of CONCERTA®-Treated Children and Adolescent Patients in 4 Placebo-Controlled, Double-Blind Clinical Trials of CONCERTA®

System/Organ Class Adverse Reaction	CONCERTA® (n=321) %	Placebo (n=318) %
Gastrointestinal Disorders		
Abdominal pain upper	5.9	3.8
Vomiting	2.8	1.6
General Disorders		
Pyrexia	2.2	0.9
Infections and Infestations		
Nasopharyngitis	2.8	2.2
Nervous System Disorders		
Dizziness	1.9	0
Psychiatric Disorders		
Insomnia	2.8	0.3
Respiratory, Thoracic and Mediastinal Disorders		
Cough	1.9	0.3
Pharyngolaryngeal pain	1.2	0.9

The majority of adverse reactions were mild to moderate in severity.

Adults

Table 5 lists the adverse reactions reported in 1% or more of CONCERTA®-treated adults in 2 placebo-controlled, double-blind clinical trials.

Table 5. Adverse Reactions Reported by ≥1% of CONCERTA®-Treated Adult Patients in 2 Placebo-Controlled, Double-Blind Clinical Trials*

System/Organ Class Adverse Reaction	CONCERTA® (n=415) %	Placebo (n=212) %
Cardiac Disorders		
Tachycardia	4.8	0
Palpitations	3.1	0.9
Ear and Labyrinth Disorders		
Vertigo	1.7	0
Eye Disorders		
Vision blurred	1.7	0.5
Gastrointestinal Disorders		
Dry mouth	14.0	3.8
Nausea	12.8	3.3
Dyspepsia	2.2	0.9
Vomiting	1.7	0.5
Constipation	1.4	0.9
General Disorders and Administration Site Conditions		
Irritability	5.8	1.4
Infections and Infestations		
Upper respiratory tract infection	2.2	0.9
Investigations		
Weight decreased	6.5	3.3
Metabolism and Nutrition Disorders		
Decreased appetite	25.3	6.6
Anorexia	1.7	0
Musculoskeletal and Connective Tissue Disorders		
Muscle tightness	1.9	0
Nervous System Disorder		
Headache	22.2	15.6
Dizziness	6.7	5.2
Tremor	2.7	0.5
Paresthesia	1.2	0
Sedation	1.2	0
Tension headache	1.2	0.5
Psychiatric Disorders		
Insomnia	12.3	6.1
Anxiety	8.2	2.4
Initial insomnia	4.3	2.8
Depressed mood	3.9	1.4
Nervousness	3.1	0.5
Restlessness	3.1	0
Agitation	2.2	0.5
Aggression	1.7	0.5
Bruxism	1.7	0.5

Depression	1.7	0.9
Libido decreased	1.7	0.5
Affect lability	1.4	0.9
Confusional state	1.2	0.5
Tension	1.2	0.5
Respiratory, Thoracic and Mediastinal Disorders		
Pharyngolaryngeal pain	1.7	1.4
Skin and Subcutaneous Tissue Disorders		
Hyperhidrosis	5.1	0.9

*Included doses up to 108 mg.

The majority of ADRs were mild to moderate in severity.

6.2 Other Adverse Reactions Observed in CONCERTA® Clinical Trials

The following adverse reactions occurred in <1% of all patients in the above double-blind, placebo-controlled clinical trial data sets. In addition, the following also includes all adverse reactions reported in CONCERTA®-treated subjects who participated in open-label studies. Adverse reactions listed in Tables 4 and 5 above are not included below.

Blood and Lymphatic System Disorders: Leukopenia

Eye Disorders: Dry eyes

Gastrointestinal Disorders: Abdominal pain, Diarrhea, Stomach discomfort

General Disorders and Administrative Site Conditions: Fatigue, Feeling jittery

Investigations: Blood pressure increased, Cardiac murmur, Heart rate increased

Nervous System Disorders: Lethargy, Psychomotor hyperactivity, Somnolence

Psychiatric Disorders: Anger, Hypervigilance, Mood altered, Mood swings, Sleep disorder, Tearfulness, Tic

Reproductive System and Breast Disorders: Erectile dysfunction

Respiratory, Thoracic and Mediastinal Disorders: Dyspnea

Skin and Subcutaneous Tissue Disorders: Rash, Rash-Macular

Vascular Disorders: Hypertension

6.3 Discontinuation Due to Adverse Reactions

In the 4 placebo-controlled studies of children and adolescents, 2 CONCERTA® patients (0.6%) discontinued due to adverse reactions of depressed mood (1, 0.3%) and headache and insomnia (1, 0.3%) and 4 placebo subjects (1.3%) discontinued due to adverse reactions of headache and insomnia, irritability, psychomotor hyperactivity, and tic (1 each, 0.3%).

In the 2 placebo-controlled studies of adults, 24 CONCERTA® patients (5.8%) and 4 placebo patients (1.9%) discontinued due to an adverse reaction. Those events with an incidence of >0.5% in the CONCERTA® patients included anxiety (1.7%), irritability (1.4%), blood pressure increased (1.0%), and nervousness (0.7%). In placebo patients, blood pressure increased and depressed mood had an incidence of >0.5% (0.9%).

In the 11 open-label studies of children, adolescents and adults, 265 CONCERTA® patients (7.4%) discontinued due to an adverse reaction. Those events with an incidence of >0.5% included insomnia (1.3%), irritability (0.8%), anxiety (0.8%), decreased appetite (0.7%), headache (0.6%), and tic (0.6%).

6.4 Tics

In a long-term uncontrolled study (n=432 children), the cumulative incidence of new onset of tics was 9% after 27 months of treatment with CONCERTA®.

In a second uncontrolled study (n=682 children) the cumulative incidence of new onset tics was 1% (9/682 children). The treatment period was up to 9 months with mean treatment duration of 7.2 months.

6.5 Blood Pressure and Heart Rate Increases

In the laboratory classroom clinical trials in children (Studies 1 and 2), both CONCERTA® once daily and methylphenidate three times daily increased resting pulse by an average of 2 to 6 bpm and produced average increases of systolic and diastolic blood pressure of roughly 1 to 4 mm Hg during the day, relative to placebo. In the placebo-controlled adolescent trial (Study 4), mean increases from baseline in resting pulse rate were observed with CONCERTA® and placebo at the end of the double-blind phase (5 and 3 beats/minute, respectively). Mean increases from baseline in blood pressure at the end of the double-blind phase for CONCERTA® and placebo-treated patients were 0.7 and 0.7 mm Hg (systolic) and 2.6 and 1.4 mm Hg (diastolic), respectively. In one placebo-controlled study in adults (Study 6), dose-dependent mean increases of 3.9 to 9.8 bpm from baseline in standing pulse rate were observed with CONCERTA® at the end of the double-blind treatment vs. an increase of 2.7 beats/minute with placebo. Mean changes from baseline in standing blood pressure at the end of double-blind treatment ranged from 0.1 to 2.2 mm Hg (systolic) and -0.7 to 2.2 mm Hg (diastolic) for CONCERTA® and was 1.1 mm Hg (systolic) and -1.8 mm Hg (diastolic) for placebo. In a second placebo-controlled study in adults (Study 5), mean changes from baseline in resting pulse rate were observed for CONCERTA® and placebo at the end of the double-blind treatment (3.6 and –1.6 beats/minute, respectively). Mean changes from baseline in blood pressure at the end of the double–blind treatment for CONCERTA® and placebo-treated patients were –1.2 and –0.5 mm Hg (systolic) and 1.1 and 0.4 mm Hg (diastolic), respectively *[see Warnings and Precautions (5.1)]*.

6.6 Post-Marketing Experience

The following additional adverse reactions have been identified during post-approval use of CONCERTA®. Because these reactions are reported voluntarily from a population of uncertain size, it is not always possible to reliably estimate their frequency:

Blood and Lymphatic System Disorders: Pancytopenia, Thrombocytopenia, Thrombocytopenic purpura

Cardiac Disorders: Angina pectoris, Bradycardia, Extrasystoles, Supraventricular tachycardia, Ventricular extrasystoles

Eye Disorders: Diplopia, Mydriasis, Visual disturbance

General Disorders: Chest pain, Chest discomfort, Drug effect decreased, Hyperpyrexia, Therapeutic response decreased

Immune System Disorders: Hypersensitivity reactions such as Angioedema, Anaphylactic reactions, Auricular swelling, Bullous conditions, Exfoliative conditions, Urticarias, Pruritus NEC, Rashes, Eruptions, and Exanthemas NEC

Investigations: Blood alkaline phosphatase increased, Blood bilirubin increased, Hepatic enzyme increased, Platelet count decreased, White blood cell count abnormal

Musculoskeletal, Connective Tissue and Bone Disorders: Arthralgia, Myalgia, Muscle twitching

Nervous System Disorders: Convulsions, Grand mal convulsions, Dyskinesia

Psychiatric Disorders: Disorientation, Hallucinations, Hallucinations auditory, Hallucinations visual, Mania

Skin and Subcutaneous Tissue Disorders: Alopecia, Erythema

Vascular Disorders: Raynaud's phenomenon

7 DRUG INTERACTIONS

7.1 MAO Inhibitors

CONCERTA® should not be used in patients being treated (currently or within the proceeding 2 weeks) with MAO inhibitors *[see Contraindications (4.5)]*.

7.2 Vasopressor Agents

Because of possible increases in blood pressure, CONCERTA® should be used cautiously with vasopressor agents *[see Warnings and Precautions (5.1)]*.

7.3 Coumarin Anticoagulants, Antidepressants, and Selective Serotonin Reuptake Inhibitors

Human pharmacologic studies have shown that methylphenidate may inhibit the metabolism of coumarin anticoagulants, anticonvulsants (eg, phenobarbital, phenytoin, primidone), and some antidepressants (tricyclics and selective serotonin reuptake inhibitors). Downward dose adjustment of these drugs may be required when given concomitantly with methylphenidate. It may be necessary to adjust the dosage and monitor plasma drug concentrations (or, in the case of coumarin, coagulation times), when initiating or discontinuing concomitant methylphenidate.

7.4 Clonidine

Serious adverse events have been reported in concomitant use with clonidine, although no causality for the combination has been established. The safety of using methylphenidate in combination with clonidine or other centrally acting alpha-2 agonists has not been systematically evaluated.

8 USE IN SPECIFIC POPULATIONS

8.1 Pregnancy

Pregnancy Category C

Methylphenidate has been shown to have teratogenic effects in rabbits when given in doses of 200 mg/kg/day, which is approximately 100 times and 40 times the maximum recommended human dose on a mg/kg and mg/m^2 basis, respectively.

A reproduction study in rats revealed no evidence of harm to the fetus at oral doses up to 30 mg/kg/day, approximately 15-fold and 3-fold the maximum recommended human dose of CONCERTA® on a mg/kg and mg/m^2 basis, respectively. The approximate plasma exposure to methylphenidate plus its main metabolite PPAA in pregnant rats was 1–2 times that seen in trials in volunteers and patients with the maximum recommended dose of CONCERTA® based on the AUC.

The safety of methylphenidate for use during human pregnancy has not been established. There are no adequate and well-controlled studies in pregnant women. CONCERTA® should be used during pregnancy only if the potential benefit justifies the potential risk to the fetus.

8.2 Labor and Delivery

The effect of CONCERTA® on labor and delivery in humans is unknown.

8.3 Nursing Mothers

It is not known whether methylphenidate is excreted in human milk. Because many drugs are excreted in human milk, caution should be exercised if CONCERTA® is administered to a nursing woman.

In lactating female rats treated with a single oral dose of 5 mg/kg radiolabeled methylphenidate, radioactivity (representing methylphenidate and/or its metabolites) was observed in milk and levels were generally similar to those in plasma.

8.4 Pediatric Use

CONCERTA® should not be used in children under six years, since safety and efficacy in this age group have not been established. Long-term effects of methylphenidate in children have not been well established.

8.5 Geriatric Use

CONCERTA® has not been studied in patients greater than 65 years of age.

9 DRUG ABUSE AND DEPENDENCE

9.1 Controlled Substance

Methylphenidate is a Schedule II controlled substance under the Controlled Substances Act.

9.2 Abuse

As noted in the *Box Warning*, CONCERTA® should be given cautiously to patients with a history of drug dependence or alcoholism. Chronic abusive use can lead to marked tolerance and psychological dependence with varying degrees of abnormal behavior. Frank psychotic episodes can occur, especially with parenteral abuse.

In two placebo-controlled human abuse potential studies, single oral doses of CONCERTA® were compared to single oral doses of immediate-release methylphenidate (IR MPH) and placebo in subjects with a history of recreational stimulant use to assess relative abuse potential. For the purpose of this assessment, the response for each of the subjective measures was defined as the maximum effect within the first 8 hours after dose administration.

In one study (n=40), both CONCERTA® (108 mg) and 60 mg IR MPH compared to placebo produced statistically significantly greater responses on the five subjective measures suggestive of abuse potential. In comparisons between the two active treatments, however, CONCERTA® (108 mg) produced variable responses on positive subjective measures that were either statistically indistinguishable from (Abuse Potential, Drug Liking, Amphetamine, and Morphine Benzedrine Group [Euphoria]) or statistically less than (Stimulation – Euphoria) responses produced by 60 mg IR MPH.

In another study (n=49), both doses of CONCERTA® (54 mg and 108 mg) and both doses of IR MPH (50 mg and 90 mg) produced statistically significantly greater responses compared to placebo on the two primary scales used in the study (Drug Liking, Euphoria). When doses of CONCERTA® (54 mg and 108 mg) were compared to IR MPH (50 mg and 90 mg), respectively, CONCERTA® produced statistically significantly lower subjective responses on these two scales than IR MPH. CONCERTA® (108 mg) produced responses that were statistically indistinguishable from the responses on these two scales produced by IR MPH (50 mg). Differences in subjective responses to the respective doses should be considered in the context that only 22% of the total amount of methylphenidate in CONCERTA® tablets is available for immediate release from the drug overcoat *[see System Components and Performance (11.1)]*.

Although these findings reveal a relatively lower response to CONCERTA® on subjective measures suggestive of abuse potential compared to IR MPH at roughly equivalent total MPH doses, the relevance of these findings to the abuse potential of CONCERTA® in the community is unknown.

9.3 Dependence

As noted in the *Box Warning*, careful supervision is required during withdrawal from abusive use since severe depression may occur. Withdrawal following chronic therapeutic use may unmask symptoms of the underlying disorder that may require follow up.

10 OVERDOSAGE

10.1 Signs and Symptoms

Signs and symptoms of CONCERTA® overdosage, resulting principally from overstimulation of the CNS and from excessive sympathomimetic effects, may include the following: vomiting, agitation, muscle twitching, convulsion, grand mal convulsion, confusional state, hallucinations (auditory and/or visual), hyperhidrosis, headache, pyrexia, tachycardia, palpitations, heart rate increased, sinus arrhythmia, hypertension, mydriasis, and dry mouth.

10.2 Recommended Treatment

Treatment consists of appropriate supportive measures. The patient must be protected against self-injury and against external stimuli that would aggravate overstimulation already present. Gastric contents may be evacuated by gastric lavage as indicated. Before performing gastric lavage, control agitation and seizures if present and protect the airway. Other measures to detoxify the gut include administration of activated charcoal and a cathartic. Intensive care must be provided to maintain adequate circulation and respiratory exchange; external cooling procedures may be required for pyrexia.

Efficacy of peritoneal dialysis or extracorporeal hemodialysis for CONCERTA® overdosage has not been established. The prolonged release of methylphenidate from CONCERTA® should be considered when treating patients with overdose.

10.3 Poison Control Center

As with the management of all overdosage, the possibility of multiple drug ingestion should be considered. The physician may wish to consider contacting a poison control center for up-to-date information on the management of overdosage with methylphenidate.

11 DESCRIPTION

CONCERTA® is a central nervous system (CNS) stimulant. CONCERTA® is available in four tablet strengths. Each extended-release tablet for once-a-day oral administration contains 18, 27, 36, or 54 mg of methylphenidate HCl USP and is designed to have a 12-hour duration of effect. Chemically, methylphenidate HCl is d,l (racemic) methyl α-phenyl-2-piperidineacetate hydrochloride. Its empirical formula is $C_{14}H_{19}NO_2 \cdot HCl$. Its structural formula is:

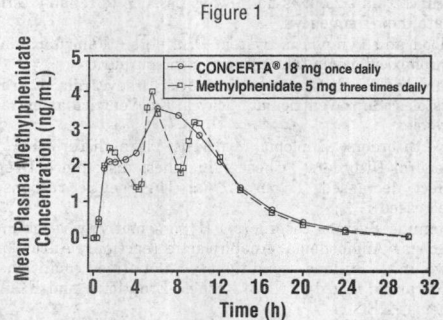

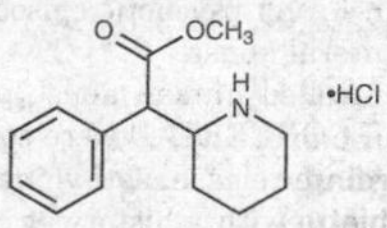

Methylphenidate HCl USP is a white, odorless crystalline powder. Its solutions are acid to litmus. It is freely soluble in water and in methanol, soluble in alcohol, and slightly soluble in chloroform and in acetone. Its molecular weight is 269.77.

CONCERTA® also contains the following inert ingredients: butylated hydroxytoluene, carnauba wax, cellulose acetate, hypromellose, lactose, phosphoric acid, poloxamer, polyethylene glycol, polyethylene oxides, povidone, propylene glycol, sodium chloride, stearic acid, succinic acid, synthetic iron oxides, titanium dioxide, and triacetin.

11.1 System Components and Performance

CONCERTA® uses osmotic pressure to deliver methylphenidate HCl at a controlled rate. The system, which resembles a conventional tablet in appearance, comprises an osmotically active trilayer core surrounded by a semipermeable membrane with an immediate-release drug overcoat. The trilayer core is composed of two drug layers containing the drug and excipients, and a push layer containing osmotically active components. There is a precision-laser drilled orifice on the drug-layer end of the tablet. In an aqueous environment, such as the gastrointestinal tract, the drug overcoat dissolves within one hour, providing an initial dose of methylphenidate. Water permeates through the membrane into the tablet core. As the osmotically active polymer excipients expand, methylphenidate is released through the orifice. The membrane controls the rate at which water enters the tablet core, which in turn controls drug delivery. Furthermore, the drug release rate from the system increases with time over a period of 6 to 7 hours due to the drug concentration gradient incorporated into the two drug layers of CONCERTA®. The biologically inert components of the tablet remain intact during gastrointestinal transit and are eliminated in the stool as a tablet shell along with insoluble core components. It is possible that CONCERTA® extended-release tablets may be visible on abdominal x-rays under certain circumstances, especially when digital enhancing techniques are utilized.

12 CLINICAL PHARMACOLOGY

12.1 Mechanism of Action

Methylphenidate HCl is a central nervous system (CNS) stimulant. The mode of therapeutic action in Attention Deficit Hyperactivity Disorder (ADHD) is not known. Methylphenidate is thought to block the reuptake of norepinephrine and dopamine into the presynaptic neuron and increase the release of these monoamines into the extraneuronal space.

12.2 Pharmacodynamics

Methylphenidate is a racemic mixture comprised of the d- and l-isomers. The d-isomer is more pharmacologically active than the l-isomer.

12.3 Pharmacokinetics

Absorption

Methylphenidate is readily absorbed. Following oral administration of CONCERTA®, plasma methylphenidate concentrations increase rapidly reaching an initial maximum at about 1 hour, followed by gradual ascending concentrations over the next 5 to 9 hours after which a gradual decrease begins. Mean times to reach peak plasma concentrations across all doses of CONCERTA® occurred between 6 to 10 hours.

CONCERTA® once daily minimizes the fluctuations between peak and trough concentrations associated with immediate-release methylphenidate three times daily (see Figure 1). The relative bioavailability of CONCERTA® once daily and methylphenidate three times daily in adults is comparable.

Figure 1

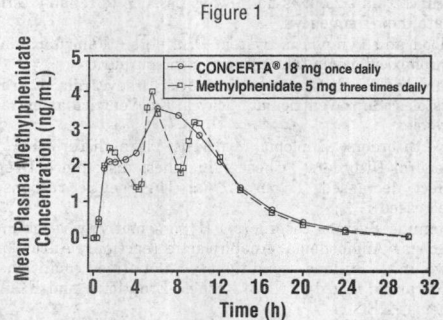

Figure 1. Mean methylphenidate plasma concentrations in 36 adults, following a single dose of CONCERTA® 18 mg once daily and immediate-release methylphenidate 5 mg three times daily administered every 4 hours.

The mean single dose pharmacokinetic parameters in 36 healthy adults following the administration of CONCERTA® 18 mg once daily and methylphenidate 5 mg three times daily are summarized in Table 6.

TABLE 6. Pharmacokinetic Parameters (Mean ± SD) After Single Dose in Healthy Adults

Parameters	CONCERTA® (18 mg once daily) (n=36)	Methylphenidate (5 mg three times daily) (n=35)
C_{max} (ng/mL)	3.7 ± 1.0	4.2 ± 1.0
T_{max} (h)	6.8 ± 1.8	6.5 ± 1.8
AUC_{inf} (ng•h/mL)	41.8 ± 13.9	38.0 ± 11.0
$t_{1/2}$ (h)	3.5 ± 0.4	3.0 ± 0.5

The pharmacokinetics of CONCERTA® were evaluated in healthy adults following single and multiple dose administration (steady-state) of doses up to 144 mg/day. The mean half-life was about 3.6 hours. No differences in the pharmacokinetics of CONCERTA® were noted following single and repeated once-daily dosing indicating no significant drug accumulation. The AUC and $t_{1/2}$ following repeated once-daily dosing are similar to those following the first dose of CONCERTA® in a dose range of 18 to 144 mg.

Dose Proportionality

Following administration of CONCERTA® in single doses of 18, 36, and 54 mg/day to healthy adults, C_{max} and $AUC_{(0-inf)}$ of d-methylphenidate were proportional to dose, whereas l-methylphenidate C_{max} and $AUC_{(0-inf)}$ increased disproportionately with respect to dose. Following administration of CONCERTA®, plasma concentrations of the l-isomer were approximately 1/40th the plasma concentrations of the d-isomer.

In healthy adults, single and multiple dosing of once daily CONCERTA® doses from 54 to 144 mg/day resulted in linear and dose proportional increases in C_{max} and AUC_{inf} for total methylphenidate (MPH) and its major metabolite, α-phenyl-piperidine acetic acid (PPAA). There was no time dependency in the pharmacokinetics of methylphenidate. The ratio of metabolite (PPAA) to parent drug (MPH) was constant across doses from 54 to 144 mg/day, both after single dose and upon multiple dosing.

In a multiple-dose study in adolescent ADHD patients aged 13 to 16 administered their prescribed dose (18 to 72 mg/day) of CONCERTA®, mean C_{max} and AUC_{TAU} of d- and total methylphenidate increased proportionally with respect to dose.

Distribution

Plasma methylphenidate concentrations in adults and adolescents decline biexponentially following oral administration. The half-life of methylphenidate in adults and adolescents following oral administration of CONCERTA® was approximately 3.5 hours.

Metabolism and Excretion

In humans, methylphenidate is metabolized primarily by de-esterification to PPAA, which has little or no pharmacologic activity. In adults the metabolism of CONCERTA® once daily as evaluated by metabolism to PPAA is similar to that of methylphenidate three times daily. The metabolism of single and repeated once-daily doses of CONCERTA® is similar.

After oral dosing of radiolabeled methylphenidate in humans, about 90% of the radioactivity was recovered in urine. The main urinary metabolite was PPAA, accounting for approximately 80% of the dose.

Food Effects

In patients, there were no differences in either the pharmacokinetics or the pharmacodynamic performance of CONCERTA® when administered after a high fat breakfast. There is no evidence of dose dumping in the presence or absence of food.

Special Populations

Gender

In healthy adults, the mean dose-adjusted $AUC_{(0-inf)}$ values for CONCERTA® were 36.7 ng•h/mL in men and 37.1 ng•h/mL in women, with no differences noted between the two groups.

Race

In adults receiving CONCERTA®, dose-adjusted $AUC_{(0-inf)}$ was consistent across ethnic groups; however, the sample size may have been insufficient to detect ethnic variations in pharmacokinetics.

Age

Increase in age resulted in increased apparent oral clearance (CL/F) (58% increase in adolescents compared to children). Some of these differences could be explained by body weight differences among these populations. This suggests that subjects with higher body weight may have lower exposures of total methylphenidate at similar doses.

The pharmacokinetics of CONCERTA® has not been studied in children less than 6 years of age.

Renal Insufficiency

There is no experience with the use of CONCERTA® in patients with renal insufficiency. After oral administration of radiolabeled methylphenidate in humans, methylphenidate was extensively metabolized and approximately 80% of the radioactivity was excreted in the urine in the form of PPAA. Since renal clearance is not an important route of methylphenidate clearance, renal insufficiency is expected to have little effect on the pharmacokinetics of CONCERTA®.

Hepatic Insufficiency

There is no experience with the use of CONCERTA® in patients with hepatic insufficiency.

13 NON-CLINICAL TOXICOLOGY

13.1 Carcinogenesis, Mutagenesis, and Impairment of Fertility

Carcinogenesis

In a lifetime carcinogenicity study carried out in B6C3F1 mice, methylphenidate caused an increase in hepatocellular adenomas and, in males only, an increase in hepatoblastomas at a daily dose of approximately 60 mg/kg/day. This dose is approximately 30 times and 4 times the maximum recommended human dose of CONCERTA® on a mg/kg and mg/m^2 basis, respectively. Hepatoblastoma is a relatively rare rodent malignant tumor type. There was no increase in total malignant hepatic tumors. The mouse strain used is sensitive to the development of hepatic tumors, and the significance of these results to humans is unknown.

Methylphenidate did not cause any increases in tumors in a lifetime carcinogenicity study carried out in F344 rats; the highest dose used was approximately 45 mg/kg/day, which is approximately 22 times and 5 times the maximum recommended human dose of CONCERTA® on a mg/kg and mg/m^2 basis, respectively.

In a 24-week carcinogenicity study in the transgenic mouse strain p53+/-, which is sensitive to genotoxic carcinogens, there was no evidence of carcinogenicity. Male and female mice were fed diets containing the same concentration of methylphenidate as in the lifetime carcinogenicity study; the high-dose groups were exposed to 60 to 74 mg/kg/day of methylphenidate.

Mutagenesis

Methylphenidate was not mutagenic in the *in vitro* Ames reverse mutation assay or the *in vitro* mouse lymphoma cell forward mutation assay. Sister chromatid exchanges and chromosome aberrations were increased, indicative of a weak clastogenic response, in an *in vitro* assay in cultured Chinese Hamster Ovary cells. Methylphenidate was negative *in vivo* in males and females in the mouse bone marrow micronucleus assay.

Impairment of Fertility

Methylphenidate did not impair fertility in male or female mice that were fed diets containing the drug in an 18-week Continuous Breeding study. The study was conducted at doses up to 160 mg/kg/day, approximately 80-fold and 8-fold the highest recommended human dose of CONCERTA® on a mg/kg and mg/m^2 basis, respectively.

14 CLINICAL STUDIES

CONCERTA® was demonstrated to be effective in the treatment of Attention Deficit Hyperactivity Disorder (ADHD) in 4 randomized, double-blind, placebo-controlled studies in children and adolescents and 2 double-blind placebo-controlled studies in adults who met the Diagnostic and Statistical Manual 4th edition (DSM-IV) criteria for ADHD.

14.1 Children

Three double-blind, active- and placebo-controlled studies were conducted in 416 children aged 6 to 12 years. The controlled studies compared CONCERTA® given once daily (18, 36, or 54 mg), methylphenidate given three times daily over 12 hours (15, 30, or 45 mg total daily dose), and placebo in two single-center, 3-week crossover studies (Studies 1 and 2) and in a multicenter, 4-week, parallel-group comparison (Study 3). The primary comparison of interest in all three trials was CONCERTA® versus placebo.

Symptoms of ADHD were evaluated by community schoolteachers using the Inattention/Overactivity with Aggression (IOWA) Conners scale. Statistically significant reduction in the Inattention/Overactivity subscale versus placebo was shown consistently across all three controlled studies for CONCERTA®. The scores for CONCERTA® and placebo for the three studies are presented in Figure 2.

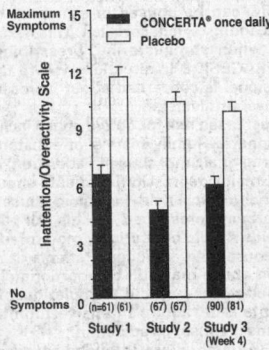

Figure 2: Mean Community School Teacher IOWA Conners Inattention/Overactivity Scores with CONCERTA® once-daily (18, 36, or 54 mg) and placebo. Studies 1 and 2 involved a 3-way crossover of 1 week per treatment arm. Study 3 involved 4 weeks of parallel group treatments with a Last Observation Carried Forward analysis at week 4. Error bars represent the mean plus standard error of the mean.

In Studies 1 and 2, symptoms of ADHD were evaluated by laboratory schoolteachers using the SKAMP[1] laboratory school rating scale. The combined results from these two studies demonstrated statistically significant improvements in attention and behavior in patients treated with CONCERTA® versus placebo that were maintained through 12 hours after dosing. Figure 3 presents the laboratory schoolteacher SKAMP ratings for CONCERTA® and placebo.

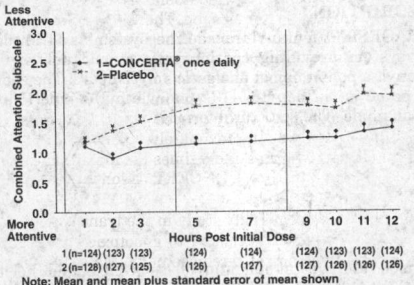

Figure 3: Laboratory School Teacher SKAMP Ratings: Mean (SEM) of Combined Attention (Studies 1 and 2)

[1]Swanson, Kotkin, Agler, M-Fynn and Pelham

14.2 Adolescents

In a randomized, double-blind, multi-center, placebo-controlled trial (Study 4) involving 177 patients, CONCERTA® was demonstrated to be effective in the treatment of ADHD in adolescents aged 13 to 18 years at doses up to 72 mg/day (1.4 mg/kg/day). Of 220 patients who entered an open 4-week titration phase, 177 were titrated to an individualized dose (maximum of 72 mg/day) based on meeting specific improvement criteria on the ADHD Rating Scale and the Global Assessment of Effectiveness with acceptable tolerability. Patients who met these criteria were then randomized to receive either their individualized dose of CONCERTA® (18–72 mg/day, n=87) or placebo (n=90) during a two-week double-blind phase. At the end of this phase, mean scores for the investigator rating on the ADHD Rating Scale demonstrated that CONCERTA® was statistically significantly superior to placebo.

14.3 Adults

Two double-blind, placebo-controlled studies were conducted in 627 adults aged 18 to 65 years. The controlled studies compared CONCERTA® administered once daily and placebo in a multicenter, parallel group, 7-week dose-titration study (Study 5) (36 to 108 mg/day) and in a multicenter, parallel group, 5-week, fixed-dose study (Study 6) (18, 36, and 72 mg/day).

Study 5 demonstrated the effectiveness of CONCERTA® in the treatment of ADHD in adults aged 18 to 65 years at doses from 36 mg/day to 108 mg/day based on the change from baseline to final study visit on the Adult ADHD Investigator Rating Scale (AISRS). Of 226 patients who entered the 7-week trial, 110 were randomized to CONCERTA® and 116 were randomized to placebo. Treatment was initiated at 36 mg/day and patients continued with incremental increases of 18 mg/day (36 to 108 mg/day) based on meeting specific improvement criteria with acceptable tolerability. At the final study visit, mean change scores (LS Mean, SEM) for the investigator rating on the AISRS demonstrated that CONCERTA® was statistically significantly superior to placebo.

Study 6 was a multicenter, double-blind, randomized, placebo-controlled, parallel group, dose-response study (5-week duration) with 3 fixed dose groups (18, 36, and 72 mg). Patients were randomized to receive CONCERTA® administered at doses of 18 mg (n=101), 36 mg (n=102), 72 mg/day (n=102), or placebo (n=96). All three doses of CONCERTA® were statistically significantly more effective than placebo in improving CAARS (Conners' Adult ADHD Rating Scale) total scores at double-blind end point in adult subjects with ADHD.

15 REFERENCES

American Psychiatric Association. Diagnosis and Statistical Manual of Mental Disorders. 4th ed. Washington DC: American Psychiatric Association 1994.

16 HOW SUPPLIED/STORAGE AND HANDLING

CONCERTA® (methylphenidate HCl) Extended-release Tablets are available in 18 mg, 27 mg, 36 mg, and 54 mg dosage strengths. The 18 mg tablets are yellow and imprinted with "alza 18". The 27 mg tablets are gray and imprinted with "alza 27". The 36 mg tablets are white and imprinted with "alza 36". The 54 mg tablets are brownish-red and imprinted with "alza 54". All four dosage strengths are supplied in bottles containing 100 tablets.

18 mg	100 count bottle	NDC 50458-585-01
27 mg	100 count bottle	NDC 50458-588-01
36 mg	100 count bottle	NDC 50458-586-01
54 mg	100 count bottle	NDC 50458-587-01

Storage and Handling

Store at 25°C (77°F); excursions permitted to 15–30°C (59–86°F) [see USP Controlled Room Temperature]. Protect from humidity.

17 PATIENT COUNSELING INFORMATION

See Medication Guide

17.1 Information for Patients

Prescribers or other health professionals should inform patients, their families, and their caregivers about the benefits and risks associated with treatment with methylphenidate and should counsel them in its appropriate use. A patient Medication Guide is available for CONCERTA®. The prescriber or health professional should instruct patients, their families, and their caregivers to read the Medication Guide and should assist them in understanding its contents. Patients should be given the opportunity to discuss the contents of the Medication Guide and to obtain answers to any questions they may have. The complete text of the Medication Guide is reprinted at the end of this document.

Patients should be informed that CONCERTA® should be swallowed whole with the aid of liquids. Tablets should not be chewed, divided, or crushed. The medication is contained within a nonabsorbable shell designed to release the drug at a controlled rate. The tablet shell, along with insoluble core components, is eliminated from the body; patients should not be concerned if they occasionally notice in their stool something that looks like a tablet.

Stimulants may impair the ability of the patient to operate potentially hazardous machinery or vehicles. Patients should be cautioned accordingly until they are reasonably certain that CONCERTA® does not adversely affect their ability to engage in such activities.

For more information call 1-888-440-7903.

Manufactured by:
Janssen-Cilag Manufacturing, LLC
Gurabo, Puerto Rico 00778 or

Alza Corp.
Vacaville, CA 95688
Manufactured for:
McNeil Pediatrics, Division of Ortho-McNeil-Janssen Pharmaceuticals, Inc.
Titusville, NJ 08560
10180603
Revised: January 2010

MEDICATION GUIDE

CONCERTA® (kon SER-ta)
(methylphenidate HCl) Extended-release Tablets CII
Read the Medication Guide that comes with CONCERTA® before you or your child starts taking it and each time you get a refill. There may be new information. This Medication Guide does not take the place of talking to your doctor about you or your child's treatment with CONCERTA®.

What is the most important information I should know about CONCERTA®?
The following have been reported with use of methylphenidate HCl and other stimulant medicines:
1. Heart-related problems:
- sudden death in patients who have heart problems or heart defects
- stroke and heart attack in adults
- increased blood pressure and heart rate
Tell your doctor if you or your child have any heart problems, heart defects, high blood pressure, or a family history of these problems.
Your doctor should check you or your child carefully for heart problems before starting CONCERTA®.
Your doctor should check you or your child's blood pressure and heart rate regularly during treatment with CONCERTA®.
Call your doctor right away if you or your child has any signs of heart problems such as chest pain, shortness of breath, or fainting while taking CONCERTA®.
2. Mental (Psychiatric) problems:
All Patients
- new or worse behavior and thought problems
- new or worse bipolar illness
- new or worse aggressive behavior or hostility
Children and Teenagers
- new psychotic symptoms (such as hearing voices, believing things that are not true, are suspicious) or new manic symptoms
Tell your doctor about any mental problems you or your child have, or about a family history of suicide, bipolar illness, or depression.
Call your doctor right away if you or your child have any new or worsening mental symptoms or problems while taking CONCERTA®, especially seeing or hearing things that are not real, believing things that are not real, or are suspicious.

What is CONCERTA®?
CONCERTA® is a central nervous system stimulant prescription medicine. It is used for the treatment of attention deficit and hyperactivity disorder (ADHD). CONCERTA® may help increase attention and decrease impulsiveness and hyperactivity in patients with ADHD.
CONCERTA® should be used as a part of a total treatment program for ADHD that may include counseling or other therapies.

CONCERTA® is a federally controlled substance (CII) because it can be abused or lead to dependence. Keep CONCERTA® in a safe place to prevent misuse and abuse. Selling or giving away CONCERTA® may harm others, and is against the law.
Tell your doctor if you or your child have (or have a family history of) ever abused or been dependent on alcohol, prescription medicines or street drugs.

Who should not take CONCERTA®?
CONCERTA® should not be taken if you or your child:
- are very anxious, tense, or agitated
- have an eye problem called glaucoma
- have tics or Tourette's syndrome, or a family history of Tourette's syndrome. Tics are hard to control repeated movements or sounds.
- are taking or have taken within the past 14 days an anti-depression medicine called a monoamine oxidase inhibitor or MAOI.
- are allergic to anything in CONCERTA®. See the end of this Medication Guide for a complete list of ingredients.
CONCERTA® should not be used in children less than 6 years old because it has not been studied in this age group.
CONCERTA® may not be right for you or your child. Before starting CONCERTA® tell your or your child's doctor about all health conditions (or a family history of) including:
- heart problems, heart defects, or high blood pressure

- mental problems including psychosis, mania, bipolar illness, or depression
- tics or Tourette's syndrome
- seizures or have had an abnormal brain wave test (EEG)
- esophagus, stomach, or small or large intestine problems

Tell your doctor if you or your child is pregnant, planning to become pregnant, or breastfeeding.

Can CONCERTA® be taken with other medicines?

Tell your doctor about all of the medicines that you or your child take including prescription and nonprescription medicines, vitamins, and herbal supplements. CONCERTA® and some medicines may interact with each other and cause serious side effects. Sometimes the doses of other medicines will need to be adjusted while taking CONCERTA®.

Your doctor will decide whether CONCERTA® can be taken with other medicines.

Especially tell your doctor if you or your child takes:

- anti-depression medicines including MAOIs
- seizure medicines
- blood thinner medicines
- blood pressure medicines
- cold or allergy medicines that contain decongestants

Know the medicines that you or your child takes. Keep a list of your medicines with you to show your doctor and pharmacist.

Do not start any new medicine while taking CONCERTA® without talking to your doctor first.

How should CONCERTA® be taken?

- **Take CONCERTA® exactly as prescribed.** Your doctor may adjust the dose until it is right for you or your child.
- **Do not chew, crush, or divide the tablets.** Swallow CONCERTA® tablets whole with water or other liquids. Tell your doctor if you or your child cannot swallow CONCERTA® whole. A different medicine may need to be prescribed.
- CONCERTA® can be taken with or without food.
- Take CONCERTA® once each day in the morning. CONCERTA® is an extended release tablet. It releases medication into your/your child's body throughout the day.
- The CONCERTA® tablet does not dissolve completely in the body after all the medicine has been released. You or your child may sometimes notice the empty tablet in a bowel movement. This is normal.
- From time to time, your doctor may stop CONCERTA® treatment for a while to check ADHD symptoms.
- Your doctor may do regular checks of the blood, heart, and blood pressure while taking CONCERTA®. Children should have their height and weight checked often while taking CONCERTA®. CONCERTA® treatment may be stopped if a problem is found during these check-ups.
- **If you or your child takes too much CONCERTA® or overdoses, call your doctor or poison control center right away, or get emergency treatment.**

What are possible side effects of CONCERTA®?

See "What is the most important information I should know about CONCERTA®?" for information on reported heart and mental problems.

Other serious side effects include:

- slowing of growth (height and weight) in children
- seizures, mainly in patients with a history of seizures
- eyesight changes or blurred vision
- blockage of the esophagus, stomach, small or large intestine in patients who already have a narrowing in any of these organs

Common side effects include:

• decreased appetite	• headache
• dry mouth	• nausea
• trouble sleeping	• anxiety
• dizziness	• weight loss
• stomach ache	• irritability
• increased sweating	

Stimulants may impair the ability of you or your child to operate potentially hazardous machinery or vehicles. You or your child should exercise caution until you/your child is reasonably certain that CONCERTA® does not adversely affect your/your child's ability to engage in such activities.

Talk to your doctor if you or your child has side effects that are bothersome or do not go away.

This is not a complete list of possible side effects. Ask your doctor or pharmacist for more information.

Call your doctor for medical advice about side effects. You may report side effects to FDA at 1-800-FDA-1088.

You may also report side effects to McNeil Pediatrics at 1-888-440-7903.

How should I store CONCERTA®?

- Store CONCERTA® in a safe place at room temperature, 59 to 86° F (15 to 30° C). Protect from moisture.
- **Keep CONCERTA® and all medicines out of the reach of children.**

General information about CONCERTA®

Medicines are sometimes prescribed for purposes other than those listed in a Medication Guide. Do not use CONCERTA® for a condition for which it was not prescribed. Do not give CONCERTA® to other people, even if they have the same condition. It may harm them and it is against the law.

This Medication Guide summarizes the most important information about CONCERTA®. If you would like more information, talk with your doctor. You can ask your doctor or pharmacist for information about CONCERTA® that was written for healthcare professionals. For more information about CONCERTA® call 1-888-440-7903.

What are the ingredients in CONCERTA®?

Active Ingredient: methylphenidate HCl

Inactive Ingredients: butylated hydroxytoluene, carnuba wax, cellulose acetate, hypromellose, lactose, phosphoric acid, poloxamer, polyethylene glycol, polyethylene oxides, povidone, propylene glycol, sodium chloride, stearic acid, succinic acid, synthetic iron oxides, titanium dioxide, and triacetin.

This Medication Guide has been approved by the U.S. Food and Drug Administration.

Manufactured by:
Janssen-Cilag Manufacturing, LLC
Gurabo, Puerto Rico 00778 or
Alza Corp.
Vacaville, CA 95688
Manufactured for:
McNeil Pediatrics
Division of Ortho-McNeil-Janssen Pharmaceuticals, Inc.,
Titusville, NJ 08560
10180603
Revised: January 2010

Shown in Product Identification Guide, page 316

DURAGESIC® CII ℞

[dər 'ă-jēsĭk]

(Fentanyl Transdermal System)

Full Prescribing Information

FOR USE IN OPIOID-TOLERANT PATIENTS ONLY

DURAGESIC® contains a high concentration of a potent Schedule II opioid agonist, fentanyl. Schedule II opioid substances which include fentanyl, hydromorphone, methadone, morphine, oxycodone, and oxymorphone have the highest potential for abuse and associated risk of fatal overdose due to respiratory depression. Fentanyl can be abused and is subject to criminal diversion. The high content of fentanyl in the patches (DURAGESIC®) may be a particular target for abuse and diversion.

DURAGESIC® is indicated for management of persistent, moderate to severe chronic pain that:

- **requires continuous, around-the-clock opioid administration for an extended period of time, and**
- **cannot be managed by other means such as non-steroidal analgesics, opioid combination products, or immediate-release opioids**

DURAGESIC® should ONLY be used in patients who are already receiving opioid therapy, who have demonstrated opioid tolerance, and who require a total daily dose at least equivalent to DURAGESIC® 25 mcg/h. Patients who are considered opioid-tolerant are those who have been taking, for a week or longer, at least 60 mg of morphine daily, or at least 30 mg of oral oxycodone daily, or at least 8 mg of oral hydromorphone daily or an equianalgesic dose of another opioid.

Because serious or life-threatening hypoventilation could occur, DURAGESIC® (fentanyl transdermal system) is contraindicated:

- **in patients who are not opioid-tolerant**
- **in the management of acute pain or in patients who require opioid analgesia for a short period of time**
- **in the management of post-operative pain, including use after out-patient or day surgeries (e.g., tonsillectomies)**
- **in the management of mild pain**
- **in the management of intermittent pain (e.g., use on an as needed basis [prn])**

(See CONTRAINDICATIONS for further information.)

Since the peak fentanyl concentrations generally occur between 20 and 72 hours of treatment, prescribers should be aware that serious or life threatening hypoventilation may occur, even in opioid-tolerant patients, during the initial application period.

The concomitant use of DURAGESIC® with all cytochrome P450 3A4 inhibitors (such as ritonavir, ketoconazole, itraconazole, troleandomycin, clarithromycin, nelfinavir, nefazodone, amiodarone, amprenavir, aprepitant, diltiazem, erythromycin, fluconazole, fosamprenavir, grapefruit juice, and verapamil) may result in an increase in fentanyl plasma concentrations, which could increase or prolong adverse drug effects and may cause potentially fatal respiratory depression. Patients receiving DURAGESIC® and any CYP3A4 inhibitor should be carefully monitored for an extended period of time and dosage adjustments should be made if warranted (see CLINICAL PHARMACOLOGY – Drug Interactions, WARNINGS, PRECAUTIONS, and DOSAGE AND ADMINISTRATION for further information).

The safety of DURAGESIC® has not been established in children under 2 years of age. DURAGESIC® should be administered to children only if they are opioid-tolerant and 2 years of age or older (see PRECAUTIONS-Pediatric Use).

DURAGESIC® is ONLY for use in patients who are already tolerant to opioid therapy of comparable potency. Use in non-opioid tolerant patients may lead to fatal respiratory depression. Overestimating the DURAGESIC® dose when converting patients from another opioid medication can result in fatal overdose with the first dose (see DOSAGE AND ADMINISTRATION – Initial DURAGESIC® Dose Selection). Due to the mean half-life of approximately 20-27 hours, patients who are thought to have had a serious adverse event, including overdose, will require monitoring and treatment for at least 24 hours.

DURAGESIC® can be abused in a manner similar to other opioid agonists, legal or illicit. This risk should be considered when administering, prescribing, or dispensing DURAGESIC® in situations where the healthcare professional is concerned about increased risk of misuse, abuse, or diversion.

Persons at increased risk for opioid abuse include those with a personal or family history of substance abuse (including drug or alcohol abuse or addiction) or mental illness (e.g., major depression). Patients should be assessed for their clinical risks for opioid abuse or addiction prior to being prescribed opioids. All patients receiving opioids should be routinely monitored for signs of misuse, abuse, and addiction. Patients at increased risk of opioid abuse may still be appropriately treated with modified-release opioid formulations; however, these patients will require intensive monitoring for signs of misuse, abuse, or addiction.

DURAGESIC® patches are intended for transdermal use (on intact skin) only. Do not use a DURAGESIC® patch if the pouch seal is broken or the patch is cut, damaged, or changed in any way.

Avoid exposing the DURAGESIC® application site and surrounding area to direct external heat sources, such as heating pads or electric blankets, heat or tanning lamps, saunas, hot tubs, and heated water beds, while wearing the system. Avoid taking hot baths or sunbathing. There is a potential for temperature-dependent increases in fentanyl released from the system resulting in possible overdose and death. Patients wearing DURAGESIC® systems who develop fever or increased core body temperature due to strenuous exertion should be monitored for opioid side effects and the DURAGESIC® dose should be adjusted if necessary.

DESCRIPTION

DURAGESIC® (fentanyl transdermal system) is a transdermal system providing continuous systemic delivery of fentanyl, a potent opioid analgesic, for 72 hours. The chemical name is N-Phenyl-N-(1-(2-phenylethyl)-4-piperidinyl) propanamide. The structural formula is:

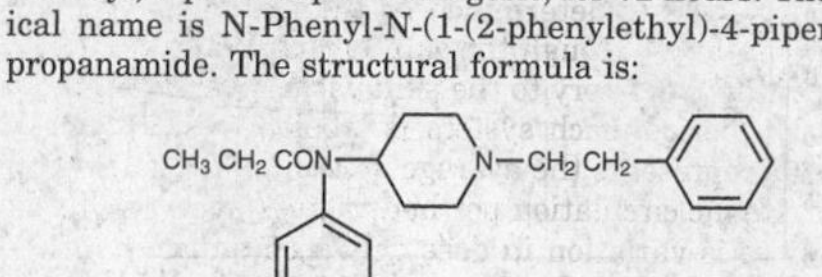

The molecular weight of fentanyl base is 336.5, and the empirical formula is $C_{22}H_{28}N_2O$. The n-octanol:water partition coefficient is 860:1. The pKa is 8.4.

System Components and Structure

The amount of fentanyl released from each system per hour is proportional to the surface area (25 mcg/h per 10.5 cm^2). The composition per unit area of all system sizes is identical.

Dose* (mcg/h)	Size (cm^2)	Fentanyl Content (mg)
12**	5.25	2.1
25	10.5	4.2
50	21	8.4
75	31.5	12.6
100	42	16.8

*Nominal delivery rate per hour
**Nominal delivery rate is 12.5 mcg/hr

DURAGESIC® is a rectangular transparent unit comprising a protective liner and two functional layers. Proceeding from the outer surface toward the surface adhering to skin, these layers are:
1) a backing layer of polyester/ethyl vinyl acetate film; 2) a drug-in-adhesive layer. Before use, a protective liner covering the adhesive layer is removed and discarded.

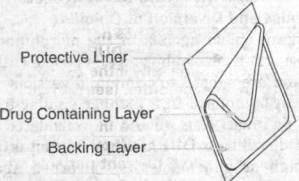

Protective Liner

Drug Containing Layer

Backing Layer

The active component of the system is fentanyl. The remaining components are pharmacologically inactive.

CLINICAL PHARMACOLOGY

Pharmacology

Fentanyl is an opioid analgesic. Fentanyl interacts predominately with the opioid mu-receptor. These mu-binding sites are discretely distributed in the human brain, spinal cord, and other tissues. In clinical settings, fentanyl exerts its principal pharmacologic effects on the central nervous system.

In addition to analgesia, alterations in mood, euphoria, dysphoria, and drowsiness commonly occur. Fentanyl depresses the respiratory centers, depresses the cough reflex, and constricts the pupils. Analgesic blood concentrations of fentanyl may cause nausea and vomiting directly by stimulating the chemoreceptor trigger zone, but nausea and vomiting are significantly more common in ambulatory than in recumbent patients, as is postural syncope.

Opioids increase the tone and decrease the propulsive contractions of the smooth muscle of the gastrointestinal tract. The resultant prolongation in gastrointestinal transit time may be responsible for the constipating effect of fentanyl. Because opioids may increase biliary tract pressure, some patients with biliary colic may experience worsening rather than relief of pain.

While opioids generally increase the tone of urinary tract smooth muscle, the net effect tends to be variable, in some cases producing urinary urgency, in others, difficulty in urination. At therapeutic dosages, fentanyl usually does not exert major effects on the cardiovascular system. However, some patients may exhibit orthostatic hypotension and fainting.

Histamine assays and skin wheal testing in clinical studies indicate that clinically significant histamine release rarely occurs with fentanyl administration. Clinical assays show no clinically significant histamine release in dosages up to 50 mcg/kg.

Pharmacokinetics

(see graph and tables)

The DURAGESIC® (fentanyl transdermal system) is a drug-in-adhesive matrix designed formulation. Fentanyl is released from the matrix at a nearly constant amount per unit time. The concentration gradient existing between the matrix and the lower concentration in the skin drives drug release. Fentanyl moves in the direction of the lower concentration at a rate determined by the matrix and the diffusion of fentanyl through the skin layers. While the actual rate of fentanyl delivery to the skin varies over the 72-hour application period, each system is labeled with a nominal flux which represents the average amount of drug delivered to the systemic circulation per hour across average skin.

While there is variation in dose delivered among patients, the nominal flux of the systems (12.5, 25, 50, 75, and 100 mcg of fentanyl per hour) is sufficiently accurate as to allow individual titration of dosage for a given patient.

Following DURAGESIC® application, the skin under the system absorbs fentanyl, and a depot of fentanyl concentrates in the upper skin layers. Fentanyl then becomes available to the systemic circulation. Serum fentanyl concentrations increase gradually following initial DURAGESIC® application, generally leveling off between 12 and 24 hours and remaining relatively constant, with some fluctuation, for the remainder of the 72-hour application period. Peak serum concentrations of fentanyl generally occurred between 20 and 72 hours after initial application (see Table A). Serum fentanyl concentrations achieved are proportional to the DURAGESIC® delivery rate. With continuous use, serum fentanyl concentrations continue to rise for the first two system applications. By the end of the second 72-hour application, a steady-state serum concentration is reached and is maintained during subsequent applications of a patch of the same size. Patients reach and maintain a steady-state serum concentration that is determined by individual variation in skin permeability and body clearance of fentanyl.

TABLE A
FENTANYL PHARMACOKINETIC PARAMETERS FOLLOWING FIRST 72-HOUR APPLICATION OF DURAGESIC®

	Mean (SD) Time to Maximal Concentration T_{max} (h)	Mean (SD) Maximal Concentration C_{max} (ng/mL)
DURAGESIC® 12 mcg/h	28.8 (13.7)	0.38 (0.13)*
DURAGESIC® 25 mcg/h	31.7 (16.5)	0.85 (0.26)
DURAGESIC® 50 mcg/h	32.8 (15.6)	1.72 (0.53)
DURAGESIC® 75 mcg/h	35.8 (14.1)	2.32 (0.86)
DURAGESIC® 100 mcg/h	29.9 (13.3)	3.36 (1.28)

* Cmax values dose normalized from 4 × 12.5 mcg/h

TABLE B
RANGE OF PHARMACOKINETIC PARAMETERS OF INTRAVENOUS FENTANYL IN PATIENTS

	Clearance (L/h) Range [70 kg]	Volume of Distribution V_{ss} (L/kg) Range	Half-Life $t_{1/2}$ (h) Range
Surgical Patients	27-75	3-8	3-12
Hepatically Impaired Patients	3-80+	0.8-8+	4-12+
Renally Impaired Patients	30-78	–	–

+ Estimated

After system removal, serum fentanyl concentrations decline gradually, falling about 50% in approximately 20-27 hours. Continued absorption of fentanyl from the skin accounts for a slower disappearance of the drug from the serum than is seen after an IV infusion, where the apparent half-life is approximately 7 (range 3-12) hours.

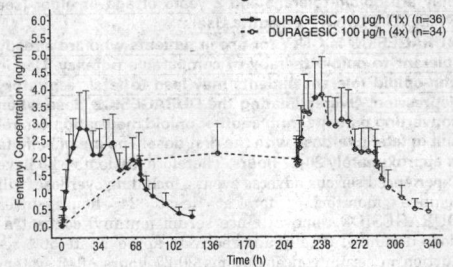

**Serum Fentanyl Concentrations
Following Single and Multiple Applications of DURAGESIC®
100 mcg/h**

— DURAGESIC 100 µg/h (1x) (n=36)
-◦- DURAGESIC 100 µg/h (4x) (n=34)

[See table A above]

NOTE: After system removal there is continued systemic absorption from residual fentanyl in the skin so that serum concentrations fall 50%, on average, in approximately 20-27 hours.

[See table B above]

NOTE: Information on volume of distribution and half-life not available for renally impaired patients.

Fentanyl plasma protein binding capacity decreases with increasing ionization of the drug. Alterations in pH may affect its distribution between plasma and the central nervous system. Fentanyl accumulates in the skeletal muscle and fat and is released slowly into the blood. The average volume of distribution for fentanyl is 6 L/kg (range 3-8; N=8). Fentanyl is metabolized primarily via human cytochrome P450 3A4 isoenzyme system. In humans, the drug appears to be metabolized primarily by oxidative N-dealkylation to norfentanyl and other inactive metabolites that do not contribute materially to the observed activity of the drug. Within 72 hours of IV fentanyl administration, approximately 75% of the dose is excreted in urine, mostly as metabolites with less than 10% representing unchanged drug. Approximately 9% of the dose is recovered in the feces, primarily as metabolites. Mean values for unbound fractions of fentanyl in plasma are estimated to be between 13 and 21%. Skin does not appear to metabolize fentanyl delivered transdermally. This was determined in a human keratinocyte cell assay and in clinical studies in which 92% of the dose delivered from the system was accounted for as unchanged fentanyl that appeared in the systemic circulation.

Special Populations
Hepatic or Renal Disease

Insufficient information exists to make recommendations regarding the use of DURAGESIC® in patients with impaired renal or hepatic function. Fentanyl is metabolized primarily via human cytochrome P450 3A4 isoenzyme system and mostly eliminated in urine. If the drug is used in these patients, it should be used with caution because of the hepatic metabolism and renal excretion of fentanyl.

Pediatric Use

In 1.5 to 5 year old, non-opioid-tolerant pediatric patients, the fentanyl plasma concentrations were approximately twice as high as that of adult patients. In older pediatric patients, the pharmacokinetic parameters were similar to that of adults. However, these findings have been taken into consideration in determining the dosing recommendations for opioid-tolerant pediatric patients (2 years of age and older). For pediatric dosing information, refer to **DOSAGE AND ADMINISTRATION** section.

Geriatric Use

Data from intravenous studies with fentanyl suggest that the elderly patients may have reduced clearance and a prolonged half-life. Moreover elderly patients may be more sensitive to the active substance than younger patients. A study conducted with the DURAGESIC® fentanyl transdermal patch in elderly patients demonstrated that fentanyl pharmacokinetics did not differ significantly from young adult subjects, although peak serum concentrations tended to be lower and mean half-life values were prolonged to approximately 34 hours.

Respiratory depression is the chief hazard in elderly or debilitated patients, usually following large initial doses in non-tolerant patients or when opioids are given in conjunction with other agents that depress respiration.

DURAGESIC® should be used with caution in elderly, cachectic or debilitated patients as they may have altered pharmacokinetics due to poor fat stores, muscle wasting, or altered clearance (see **DOSAGE AND ADMINISTRATION**).

Drug Interactions

The interaction between ritonavir, a CPY3A4 inhibitor, and fentanyl was investigated in eleven healthy volunteers in a randomized crossover study. Subjects received oral ritonavir or placebo for 3 days. The ritonavir dose was 200 mg tid on Day 1 and 300 mg tid on Day 2 followed by one morning dose of 300 mg on Day 3. On Day 2, fentanyl was given as a single IV dose at 5 mcg/kg two hours after the afternoon dose of oral ritonavir or placebo. Naloxone was administered to counteract the side effects of fentanyl. The results suggested that ritonavir might decrease the clearance of fentanyl by 67%, resulting in a 174% (range 52%-420%) increase in fentanyl AUC$_{0-\infty}$. Coadministration of ritonavir in patients receiving DURAGESIC® has not been studied; however, an increase in fentanyl AUC is expected (see **BOX WARNING, WARNINGS, PRECAUTIONS** and **DOSAGE AND ADMINISTRATION**).

Fentanyl is metabolized mainly via the human cytochrome P450 3A4 isoenzyme system (CYP3A4), therefore, potential interactions may occur when DURAGESIC® is given concurrently with agents that affect CYP3A4 activity. Coadminstration with agents that induce CYP3A4 activity may reduce the efficacy of DURAGESIC®. The concomitant use of transdermal fentanyl with all CYP3A4 inhibitors (such as ritonavir, ketoconazole, itraconazole, troleandomycin, clarithromycin, nelfinavir, nefazadone, amiodarone, amprenavir, aprepitant, diltiazem, erythromycin, fluconazole, fosamprenavir, grapefruit juice, and verapamil) may result in an increase in fentanyl plasma concentrations, which could increase or prolong adverse drug effects and may cause potentially fatal respiratory depression. Patients receiving DURAGESIC® and any CYP3A4 inhibitor should be carefully monitored for an extended period of time and dosage adjustments should be made if warranted (see **BOX WARNING, WARNINGS, PRECAUTIONS,** and **DOSAGE AND ADMINISTRATION** for further information).

PHARMACODYNAMICS
Ventilatory Effects
Because of the risk for serious or life-threatening hypoventilation, DURAGESIC® is CONTRAINDICATED in the treatment of post-operative and acute pain and in patients who are not opioid-tolerant. In clinical trials of 357 patients with acute pain treated with DURAGESIC®, 13 patients experienced hypoventilation. Hypoventilation was manifested by respiratory rates of less than 8 breaths/minute or a pCO_2 greater than 55 mm Hg. In these studies, the incidence of hypoventilation was higher in nontolerant women (10) than in men (3) and in patients weighing less than 63 kg (9 of 13). Although patients with impaired respiration were not common in the trials, they had higher rates of hypoventilation. In addition, post-marketing reports have been received that describe opioid-naive post-operative patients who have experienced clinically significant hypoventilation and death with DURAGESIC®.

While most adult and pediatric patients using DURAGESIC® chronically develop tolerance to fentanyl induced hypoventilation, episodes of slowed respirations may occur at any time during therapy.

Hypoventilation can occur throughout the therapeutic range of fentanyl serum concentrations, especially for patients who have an underlying pulmonary condition or who receive usual doses of opioids or other CNS drugs associated with hypoventilation in addition to DURAGESIC®. The use of DURAGESIC® is contraindicated in patients who are not tolerant to opioid therapy.

The use of DURAGESIC® should be monitored by clinical evaluation, especially within the initial 24-72 hours when serum concentrations from the initial patch will peak, and following increases in dosage. DURAGESIC® should be administered to children only if they are opioid-tolerant and 2 years of age or older.

See **BOX WARNING, CONTRAINDICATIONS, WARNINGS, PRECAUTIONS, ADVERSE REACTIONS,** and **OVERDOSAGE** for additional information on hypoventilation.

Cardiovascular Effects
Fentanyl may infrequently produce bradycardia. The incidence of bradycardia in clinical trials with DURAGESIC® was less than 1%.

CNS Effects
Central nervous system effects increase with increasing serum fentanyl concentrations.

INDICATIONS AND USAGE
DURAGESIC® is indicated for management of persistent, moderate to severe chronic pain that:
• requires continuous, around-the-clock opioid administration for an extended period of time, and
• cannot be managed by other means such as non-steroidal analgesics, opioid combination products, or immediate-release opioids.

DURAGESIC® should ONLY be used in patients who are already receiving opioid therapy, who have demonstrated opioid tolerance, and who require a total daily dose at least equivalent to DURAGESIC® 25 mcg/h (see **DOSAGE AND ADMINISTRATION**). Patients who are considered opioid-tolerant are those who have been taking, for a week or longer, at least 60 mg of morphine daily, or at least 30 mg of oral oxycodone daily, or at least 8 mg of oral hydromorphone daily, or an equianalgesic dose of another opioid.

Because serious or life-threatening hypoventilation could result, DURAGESIC® is contraindicated for use on an as needed basis (i.e., prn), for the management of post-operative or acute pain, or in patients who are not opioid-tolerant or who require opioid analgesia for a short period of time (see **BOX WARNING** and **CONTRAINDICATIONS**).

An evaluation of the appropriateness and adequacy of treating with immediate-release opioids is advisable prior to initiating therapy with any modified-release opioid. Prescribers should individualize treatment in every case, initiating therapy at the appropriate point along a progression from

non-opioid analgesics, such as non-steroidal anti-inflammatory drugs and acetaminophen, to opioids, in a plan of pain management such as outlined by the World Health Organization, the Agency for Health Research and Quality, the Federation of State Medical Boards Model Policy, or the American Pain Society.

Patients should be assessed for their clinical risks for opioid abuse or addiction prior to being prescribed opioids. Patients receiving opioids should be routinely monitored for signs of misuse, abuse, and addiction. Persons at increased risk for opioid abuse include those with a personal or family history of substance abuse (including drug or alcohol abuse or addiction) or mental illness (e.g., major depression). Patients at increased risk may still be appropriately treated with modified-release opioid formulations; however these patients will require intensive monitoring for signs of misuse, abuse, or addiction.

CONTRAINDICATIONS
Because serious or life-threatening hypoventilation could occur, DURAGESIC® (fentanyl transdermal system) is contraindicated:
• **in patients who are not opioid-tolerant**
• **in the management of acute pain or in patients who require opioid analgesia for a short period of time**
• **in the management of post-operative pain, including use after out-patient or day surgeries, (e.g., tonsillectomies)**
• **in the management of mild pain**
• **in the management of intermittent pain (e.g., use on an as needed basis [prn])**
• **in situations of significant respiratory depression, especially in unmonitored settings where there is a lack of resuscitative equipment**
• **in patients who have acute or severe bronchial asthma**
DURAGESIC® (fentanyl transdermal system) is contraindicated in patients who have or are suspected of having paralytic ileus.

DURAGESIC® (fentanyl transdermal system) is contraindicated in patients with known hypersensitivity to fentanyl or any components of this product.

WARNINGS
DURAGESIC® patches are intended for transdermal use (on intact skin) only. Do not use a DURAGESIC® patch if the pouch seal is broken or the patch is cut, damaged, or changed in any way.

The safety of DURAGESIC® (fentanyl transdermal system) has not been established in children under 2 years of age. DURAGESIC® should be administered to children only if they are opioid-tolerant and 2 years of age or older (see PRECAUTIONS – Pediatric Use).

DURAGESIC® is ONLY for use in patients who are already tolerant to opioid therapy of comparable potency. Use in non-opioid tolerant patients may lead to fatal respiratory depression. Overestimating the DURAGESIC® dose when converting patients from another opioid medication can result in fatal overdose with the first dose. The mean half-life is approximately 20-27 hours. Therefore, patients who have experienced serious adverse events, including overdose, will require monitoring for at least 24 hours after DURAGESIC® removal since serum fentanyl concentrations decline gradually and reach an approximate 50% reduction in serum concentrations 20-27 hours after system removal.

DURAGESIC® should be prescribed only by persons knowledgeable in the continuous administration of potent opioids, in the management of patients receiving potent opioids for treatment of pain, and in the detection and management of hypoventilation including the use of opioid antagonists.

All patients and their caregivers should be advised to avoid exposing the DURAGESIC® application site and surrounding area to direct external heat sources, such as heating pads or electric blankets, heat or tanning lamps, saunas, hot tubs, and heated water beds, etc., while wearing the system. Patients should be advised against taking hot baths or sunbathing. There is a potential for temperature-dependent increases in fentanyl released from the system resulting in possible overdose and death. A clinical pharmacology trial conducted in healthy adult subjects has shown that the application of heat over the DURAGESIC® system increased mean fentanyl AUC values by 120% and mean C_{max} values by 61%.

Based on a pharmacokinetic model, serum fentanyl concentrations could theoretically increase by approximately one-third for patients with a body temperature of 40°C (104°F) due to temperature-dependent increases in fentanyl released from the system and increased skin permeability. **Patients wearing DURAGESIC® systems who develop fever or increased core body temperature due to strenuous exertion should be monitored for opioid side effects and the DURAGESIC® dose should be adjusted if necessary.**

Death and other serious medical problems have occurred when people were accidentally exposed to DURAGESIC®. Examples of accidental exposure include transfer of a

DURAGESIC® patch from an adult's body to a child while hugging, accidental sitting on a patch and possible accidental exposure of a caregiver's skin to the medication in the patch while the caregiver was applying or removing the patch.

Placing DURAGESIC® in the mouth, chewing it, swallowing it, or using it in ways other than indicated may cause choking or overdose that could result in death.

Misuse, Abuse and Diversion of Opioids
Fentanyl is an opioid agonist of the morphine-type. Such drugs are sought by drug abusers and people with addiction disorders and are subject to criminal diversion.

Fentanyl can be abused in a manner similar to other opioids, legal or illicit. This should be considered when prescribing or dispensing DURAGESIC® in situations where the physician or pharmacist is concerned about an increased risk of misuse, abuse, or diversion.

DURAGESIC® has been reported as being abused by other methods and routes of administration. These practices will result in uncontrolled delivery of the opioid and pose a significant risk to the abuser that could result in overdose and death (see **WARNINGS** and **DRUG ABUSE AND ADDICTION**).

Concerns about abuse, addiction, and diversion should not prevent the proper management of pain. However, all patients treated with opioids require careful monitoring for signs of abuse and addiction, since use of opioid analgesic products carries the risk of addiction even under appropriate medical use.

Healthcare professionals should contact their state professional licensing board or state controlled substances authority for information on how to prevent and detect abuse or diversion of this product.

Hypoventilation (Respiratory Depression)
Serious or life-threatening hypoventilation may occur at any time during the use of DURAGESIC® especially during the initial 24-72 hours following initiation of therapy and following increases in dose.

Because significant amounts of fentanyl continue to be absorbed from the skin for 20-27 hours or more after the patch is removed, hypoventilation may persist beyond the removal of DURAGESIC®. Consequently, patients with hypoventilation should be carefully observed for degree of sedation and their respiratory rate monitored until respiration has stabilized.

The use of concomitant CNS active drugs requires special patient care and observation.

Respiratory depression is the chief hazard of opioid agonists, including fentanyl the active ingredient in DURAGESIC®. Respiratory depression is more likely to occur in elderly or debilitated patients, usually following large initial doses in non-tolerant patients, or when opioids are given in conjunction with other drugs that depress respiration.

Respiratory depression from opioids is manifested by a reduced urge to breathe and a decreased rate of respiration, often associated with the "sighing" pattern of breathing (deep breaths separated by abnormally long pauses). Carbon dioxide retention from opioid-induced respiratory depression can exacerbate the sedating effects of opioids. This makes overdoses involving drugs with sedative properties and opioids especially dangerous.

DURAGESIC® should be used with extreme caution in patients with significant chronic obstructive pulmonary disease or cor pulmonale, and in patients having a substantially decreased respiratory reserve, hypoxia, hypercapnia, or pre-existing respiratory depression. In such patients, even usual therapeutic doses of DURAGESIC® may decrease respiratory drive to the point of apnea. In these patients, alternative non-opioid analgesics should be considered, and opioids should be employed only under careful medical supervision at the lowest effective dose.

Chronic Pulmonary Disease
Because potent opioids can cause serious or life-threatening hypoventilation, DURAGESIC® should be administered with caution to patients with pre-existing medical conditions predisposing them to hypoventilation. In such patients, normal analgesic doses of opioids may further decrease respiratory drive to the point of respiratory failure.

Head Injuries and Increased Intracranial Pressure
DURAGESIC® should not be used in patients who may be particularly susceptible to the intracranial effects of CO_2 retention such as those with evidence of increased intracranial pressure, impaired consciousness, or coma. Opioids may obscure the clinical course of patients with head injury. DURAGESIC® should be used with caution in patients with brain tumors.

Interactions with Other CNS Depressants
The concomitant use of DURAGESIC® (fentanyl transdermal system) with other central nervous system depressants, including but not limited to other opioids,

sedatives, hypnotics, tranquilizers (e.g., benzodiazepines), general anesthetics, phenothiazines, skeletal muscle relaxants, and alcohol, may cause respiratory depression, hypotension, and profound sedation or potentially result in coma. When such combined therapy is contemplated, the dose of one or both agents should be significantly reduced.

Interactions with Alcohol and Drugs of Abuse
Fentanyl may be expected to have additive CNS depressant effects when used in conjunction with alcohol, other opioids, or illicit drugs that cause central nervous system depression.

Interactions with CYP3A4 Inhibitors
The concomitant use of transdermal fentanyl with all CYP3A4 inhibitors (such as ritonavir, ketoconazole, itraconazole, troleandomycin, clarithromycin, nelfinavir, nefazadone, amiodarone, amprenavir, aprepitant, diltiazem, erythromycin, fluconazole, fosamprenavir, grapefruit juice, and verapamil) may result in an increase in fentanyl plasma concentrations, which could increase or prolong adverse drug effects and may cause potentially fatal respiratory depression. Patients receiving DURAGESIC® and any CYP3A4 inhibitor should be carefully monitored for an extended period of time, and dosage adjustments should be made if warranted (see BOX WARNING, CLINICAL PHARMACOLOGY – Drug Interactions, PRECAUTIONS, and DOSAGE AND ADMINISTRATION for further information).

PRECAUTIONS
General
DURAGESIC® (fentanyl transdermal system) should not be used to initiate opioid therapy in patients who are not opioid-tolerant. Children converting to DURAGESIC® should be opioid-tolerant and 2 years of age or older (see BOX WARNING).
Patients, family members, and caregivers should be instructed to keep patches (new and used) out of the reach of children and others for whom DURAGESIC® was not prescribed. A considerable amount of active fentanyl remains in DURAGESIC® even after use as directed. Accidental or deliberate application or ingestion by a child or adolescent will cause respiratory depression that could result in death.

Cardiac Disease
Fentanyl may produce bradycardia. Fentanyl should be administered with caution to patients with bradyarrhythmias.

Hepatic or Renal Disease
Insufficient information exists to make recommendations regarding the use of DURAGESIC® in patients with impaired renal or hepatic function. If the drug is used in these patients, it should be used with caution because of the hepatic metabolism and renal excretion of fentanyl.

Use in Pancreatic/Biliary Tract Disease
DURAGESIC® may cause spasm of the sphincter of Oddi and should be used with caution in patients with biliary tract disease, including acute pancreatitis. Opioids like DURAGESIC® may cause increases in the serum amylase concentration.

Tolerance
Tolerance is a state of adaptation in which exposure to a drug induces changes that result in a diminution of one or more of the drug's effects over time. Tolerance may occur to both the desired and undesired effects of drugs, and may develop at different rates for different effects.

Physical Dependence
Physical dependence is a state of adaptation that is manifested by an opioid specific withdrawal syndrome that can be produced by abrupt cessation, rapid dose reduction, decreasing blood concentration of the drug, and/or administration of an antagonist. The opioid abstinence or withdrawal syndrome is characterized by some or all of the following: restlessness, lacrimation, rhinorrhea, yawning, perspiration, chills, piloerection, myalgia, mydriasis, irritability, anxiety, backache, joint pain, weakness, abdominal cramps, insomnia, nausea, anorexia, vomiting, diarrhea, or increased blood pressure, respiratory rate, or heart rate. In general, opioids should not be abruptly discontinued (see DOSAGE AND ADMINISTRATION – Discontinuation of DURAGESIC®).

Ambulatory Patients
Strong opioid analgesics impair the mental or physical abilities required for the performance of potentially dangerous tasks, such as driving a car or operating machinery. Patients who have been given DURAGESIC® should not drive or operate dangerous machinery unless they are tolerant to the effects of the drug.

Information for Patients
Patients and their caregivers should be provided with a Medication Guide each time DURAGESIC® is dispensed because new information may be available.
Patients receiving DURAGESIC® patches should be given the following instructions by the physician:
1. Patients should be advised that DURAGESIC® patches contain fentanyl, an opioid pain medicine similar to

morphine, hydromorphone, methadone, oxycodone, and oxymorphone.
2. Patients should be advised that each DURAGESIC® patch may be worn continuously for 72 hours, and that each patch should be applied to a different skin site after removal of the previous transdermal patch.
3. Patients should be advised that DURAGESIC® patches should be applied to intact, non-irritated, and non-irradiated skin on a flat surface such as the chest, back, flank, or upper arm. Additionally, patients should be advised of the following:
 • In young children or persons with cognitive impairment, the patch should be put on the upper back to lower the chances that the patch will be removed and placed in the mouth.
 • Hair at the application site should be clipped (not shaved) prior to patch application.
 • If the site of DURAGESIC® application must be cleansed prior to application of the patch, do so with clear water.
 • Do not use soaps, oils, lotions, alcohol, or any other agents that might irritate the skin or alter its characteristics.
 • Allow the skin to dry completely prior to patch application.
4. Patients should be advised that DURAGESIC® should be applied immediately upon removal from the sealed pouch and after removal of the protective liner. Additionally the patient should be advised of the following:
 • The DURAGESIC® patch should not be used if the pouch seal is broken, or if the patch is cut, damaged, or changed in any way.
 • The transdermal patch should be pressed firmly in place with the palm of the hand for 30 seconds, making sure the contact is complete, especially around the edges.
 • The patch should not be folded so that only part of the patch is exposed.
5. Patients should be advised that the dose of DURAGESIC® or the number of patches applied to the skin should NEVER be adjusted without the prescribing healthcare professional's instruction.
6. Patients should be advised that while wearing the patch, they should avoid exposing the DURAGESIC® application site and surrounding area to direct external heat sources, such as:
 • heating pads,
 • electric blankets,
 • sunbathing,
 • heat or tanning lamps,
 • saunas,
 • hot tubs or hot baths, and
 • heated water beds, etc.
7. Patients should also be advised of a potential for temperature-dependent increases in fentanyl release from the patch that could result in an overdose of fentanyl; therefore, patients who develop a high fever or increased body temperature due to strenuous exertion while wearing the patch should contact their physician.
8. Patients should be advised that if they experience problems with adhesion of the DURAGESIC® patch, they may tape the edges of the patch with first aid tape. If problems with adhesion persist, patients may overlay the patch with a transparent adhesive film dressing (e.g., Bioclusive™ or Tegaderm™).
9. Patients should be advised that if the patch falls off before 72 hours a new patch may be applied to a different skin site.
10. Patients should be advised to fold (so that the adhesive side adheres to itself) and immediately flush down the toilet used DURAGESIC® patches after removal from the skin.
11. Patients should be advised that DURAGESIC® may impair mental and/or physical ability required for the performance of potentially hazardous tasks (e.g., driving, operating machinery).
12. Patients should be advised to refrain from any potentially dangerous activity when starting on DURAGESIC® or when their dose is being adjusted, until it is established that they have not been adversely affected.
13. Patients should be advised that DURAGESIC® should not be combined with alcohol or other CNS depressants (e.g. sleep medications, tranquilizers) because dangerous additive effects may occur, resulting in serious injury or death.
14. Patients should be advised to consult their physician or pharmacist if other medications are being or will be used with DURAGESIC®.
15. Patients should be advised of the potential for severe constipation.
16. Patients should be advised that if they have been receiving treatment with DURAGESIC® and cessation of

therapy is indicated, it may be appropriate to taper the DURAGESIC® dose, rather than abruptly discontinue it, due to the risk of precipitating withdrawal symptoms.
17. Patients should be advised that DURAGESIC® contains fentanyl, a drug with high potential for abuse.
18. Patients, family members, and caregivers should be advised to protect DURAGESIC® from theft or misuse in the work or home environment.
19. Patients should be instructed to keep DURAGESIC® in a secure place out of the reach of children due to the high risk of fatal respiratory depression.
20. Patients should be advised that DURAGESIC® should never be given to anyone other than the individual for whom it was prescribed because of the risk of death or other serious medical problems to that person for whom it was not intended.
21. Patients should be informed that, if the patch dislodges and accidentally sticks to the skin of another person, they should immediately take the patch off, wash the exposed area with water and seek medical attention for the accidentally exposed individual.
22. When DURAGESIC® is no longer needed, the unused patches should be removed from their pouches, folded so that the adhesive side of the patch adheres to itself, and flushed down the toilet.
23. Women of childbearing potential who become, or are planning to become pregnant, should be advised to consult a physician prior to initiating or continuing therapy with DURAGESIC®.
24. Patients should be informed that accidental exposure or misuse may lead to death or other serious medical problems.

Drug Interactions
Agents Affecting Cytochrome P450 3A4 Isoenzyme System
Fentanyl is metabolized mainly via the human cytochrome P450 3A4 isoenzyme system (CYP3A4), therefore potential interactions may occur when DURAGESIC® is given concurrently with agents that affect CYP3A4 activity. Coadminstration with agents that induce CYP3A4 activity may reduce the efficacy of DURAGESIC®. The concomitant use of transdermal fentanyl with all CYP3A4 inhibitors (such as ritonavir, ketoconazole, itraconazole, troleandomycin, clarithromycin, nelfanivir, nefazadone, amiodarone, amprenavir, aprepitant, diltiazem, erythromycin, fluconazole, fosamprenavir, grapefruit juice, and verapamil) may result in an increase in fentanyl plasma concentrations, which could increase or prolong adverse drug effects and may cause fatal respiratory depression. Patients receiving DURAGESIC® and any CYP3A4 inhibitor should be carefully monitored for an extended period of time, and dosage adjustments should be made if warranted (see BOX WARNING, CLINICAL PHARMACOLOGY – Drug Interactions, WARNINGS, and DOSAGE AND ADMINISTRATION for further information).

Central Nervous System Depressants
The concomitant use of DURAGESIC® (fentanyl transdermal system) with other central nervous system depressants, including but not limited to other opioids, sedatives, hypnotics, tranquilizers (e.g., benzodiazepines), general anesthetics, phenothiazines, skeletal muscle relaxants, and alcohol, may cause respiratory depression, hypotension, and profound sedation, or potentially result in coma or death. When such combined therapy is contemplated, the dose of one or both agents should be significantly reduced.

MAO Inhibitors
DURAGESIC® is not recommended for use in patients who have received MAOI within 14 days because severe and unpredictable potentiation by MAO inhibitors has been reported with opioid analgesics.

Carcinogenesis, Mutagenesis, and Impairment of Fertility
In a two-year carcinogenicity study conducted in rats, fentanyl was not associated with an increased incidence of tumors at subcutaneous doses up to 33 μg/kg/day in males or 100 μg/kg/day in females (0.16 and 0.39 times the human daily exposure obtained via the 100 mcg/h patch based on AUC_{0-24h} comparison). There was no evidence of mutagenicity in the Ames Salmonella mutagenicity assay, the primary rat hepatocyte unscheduled DNA synthesis assay, the BALB/c 3T3 transformation test, and the human lymphocyte and CHO chromosomal aberration in-vitro assays.
The potential effects of fentanyl on male and female fertility were examined in the rat model via two separate experiments. In the male fertility study, male rats were treated with fentanyl (0, 0.025, 0.1 or 0.4 mg/kg/day) via continuous intravenous infusion for 28 days prior to mating; female rats were not treated. In the female fertility study, female rats were treated with fentanyl (0, 0.025, 0.1 or 0.4 mg/kg/day) via continuous intravenous infusion for 14 days prior to mating until day 16 of pregnancy; male rats were not treated. Analysis of fertility parameters in both studies indicated that an intravenous dose of fentanyl up to 0.4 mg/kg/day to either the male or the female alone produced no effects on fertility (this dose is approximately 1.6 times the

TABLE 1: ADVERSE EVENTS (at rate of ≥ 1%)
Adult (N=380) and Pediatric (N=291) Clinical Trial Experience

Body System	Adults	Pediatrics
Body as a Whole	Abdominal pain*, headache*, fatigue*, back pain, influenza-like symptoms*, fever, accidental injury, rigors	Pain*, headache*, fever, syncope, abdominal pain, allergic reaction, flushing
Cardiovascular	Arrhythmia, chest pain	Hypertension, tachycardia
Digestive	Nausea**, vomiting**, constipation**, dry mouth**, anorexia*, diarrhea*, dyspepsia*, flatulence	Nausea**, vomiting**, constipation*, dry mouth, diarrhea
Nervous	Somnolence**, insomnia, confusion**, asthenia**, dizziness*, nervousness*, hallucinations*, anxiety*, depression*, euphoria*, tremor, abnormal coordination, speech disorder, abnormal thinking, abnormal gait, abnormal dreams, agitation, paresthesia, amnesia, syncope, paranoid reaction	Somnolence*, nervousness*, insomnia*, asthenia*, hallucinations, anxiety, depression, convulsions, dizziness, tremor, speech disorder, agitation, stupor, confusion, paranoid reaction
Respiratory	Dyspnea*, hypoventilation*, apnea*, hemoptysis*, pharyngitis*, hiccups, bronchitis, rhinitis, sinusitis, upper respiratory tract infection*	Dyspnea, respiratory depression, rhinitis, coughing
Skin and Appendages	Sweating**, pruritus*, rash, application site reaction – erythema, papules, itching, edema	Pruritus*, application site reaction*, sweating increased, rash, rash erythematous, skin reaction localized
Urogenital	Urinary retention*, Micturition disorder	Urinary retention

* Reactions occurring in 3%-10% of DURAGESIC® patients
**Reactions occurring in 10% or more of DURAGESIC® patients

daily human dose administered by a 100 mcg/hr patch on a mg/m² basis. In a separate study, a single daily bolus dose of fentanyl was shown to impair fertility in rats when given in intravenous doses of 0.3 times the human dose for a period of 12 days.

Pregnancy – Pregnancy Category C
No epidemiological studies of congenital anomalies in infants born to women treated with fentanyl during pregnancy have been reported.

The potential effects of fentanyl on embryo-fetal development were studied in the rat, mouse, and rabbit models. Published literature reports that administration of fentanyl (0, 10, 100, or 500 µg/kg/day) to pregnant female Sprague-Dawley rats from day 7 to 21 via implanted microosmotic minipumps did not produce any evidence of teratogenicity (the high dose is approximately 2 times the daily human dose administered by a 100 mcg/hr patch on a mg/m² basis). In contrast, the intravenous administration of fentanyl (0, 0.01, or 0.03 mg/kg) to bred female rats from gestation day 6 to 18 suggested evidence of embryotoxicity and a slight increase in mean delivery time in the 0.03 mg/kg/day group. There was no clear evidence of teratogenicity noted. Pregnant female New Zealand White rabbits were treated with fentanyl (0, 0.025, 0.1, 0.4 mg/kg) via intravenous infusion from day 6 to day 18 of pregnancy. Fentanyl produced a slight decrease in the body weight of the live fetuses at the high dose, which may be attributed to maternal toxicity. Under the conditions of the assay, there was no evidence for fentanyl induced adverse effects on embryo-fetal development at doses up to 0.4 mg/kg (approximately 3 times the daily human dose administered by a 100 mcg/hr patch on a mg/m² basis).

There are no adequate and well-controlled studies in pregnant women. DURAGESIC® should be used during pregnancy only if the potential benefit justifies the potential risk to the fetus.

Nonteratogenic Effects
Chronic maternal treatment with fentanyl during pregnancy has been associated with transient respiratory depression, behavioral changes, or seizures characteristic of neonatal abstinence syndrome in newborn infants. Symptoms of neonatal respiratory or neurological depression were no more frequent than expected in most studies of infants born to women treated acutely during labor with intravenous or epidural fentanyl. Transient neonatal muscular rigidity has been observed in infants whose mothers were treated with intravenous fentanyl.

The potential effects of fentanyl on prenatal and postnatal development were examined in the rat model. Female Wistar rats were treated with 0, 0.025, 0.1, or 0.4 mg/kg/day fentanyl via intravenous infusion from day 6 of pregnancy through 3 weeks of lactation. Fentanyl treatment (0.4 mg/kg/day) significantly decreased body weight in male and female pups and also decreased survival in pups at day 4. Both the mid-dose and high-dose of fentanyl animals demonstrated alterations in some physical landmarks of devel-

opment (delayed incisor eruption and eye opening) and transient behavioral development (decreased locomotor activity at day 28 which recovered by day 50). The mid-dose and the high-dose are 0.4 and 1.6 times the daily human dose administered by a 100 mcg/hr patch on a mg/m² basis.

Labor and Delivery
Fentanyl readily passes across the placenta to the fetus; therefore, DURAGESIC® is not recommended for analgesia during labor and delivery.

Nursing Mothers
Fentanyl is excreted in human milk; therefore, DURAGESIC® is not recommended for use in nursing women because of the possibility of effects in their infants.

Pediatric Use
The safety of DURAGESIC® was evaluated in three open-label trials in 291 pediatric patients with chronic pain, 2 years of age through 18 years of age. Starting doses of 25 mcg/h and higher were used by 181 patients who had been on prior daily opioid doses of at least 45 mg/day of oral morphine or an equianalgesic dose of another opioid. Initiation of DURAGESIC® therapy in pediatric patients taking less than 60 mg/day of oral morphine or an equianalgesic dose of another opioid has not been evaluated in controlled clinical trials. Approximately 90% of the total daily opioid requirement (DURAGESIC® plus rescue medication) was provided by DURAGESIC®.

DURAGESIC® was not studied in children under 2 years of age.

DURAGESIC® should be administered to children only if they are opioid-tolerant and 2 years of age or older (see **DOSAGE AND ADMINISTRATION** and **BOX WARNING**).

To guard against accidental ingestion by children, use caution when choosing the application site for DURAGESIC® (see **DOSAGE AND ADMINISTRATION**) and monitor adhesion of the system closely.

Geriatric Use
Data from intravenous studies with fentanyl suggest that the elderly patients may have reduced clearance and a prolonged half-life. Moreover elderly patients may be more sensitive to the active substance than younger patients. A study conducted with the DURAGESIC® fentanyl transdermal patch in elderly patients demonstrated that fentanyl pharmacokinetics did not differ significantly from young adult subjects, although peak serum concentrations tended to be lower and mean half-life values were prolonged to approximately 34 hours.

Respiratory depression is the chief hazard in elderly or debilitated patients, usually following large initial doses in non-tolerant patients, or when opioids are given in conjunction with other agents that depress respiration.

DURAGESIC® should be used with caution in elderly, cachectic, or debilitated patients as they may have altered pharmacokinetics due to poor fat stores, muscle wasting or altered clearance (see **DOSAGE AND ADMINISTRATION**).

ADVERSE REACTIONS
In post-marketing experience, deaths from hypoventilation due to use of DURAGESIC® (fentanyl transdermal system) have been reported (see BOX WARNING and CONTRAINDICATIONS).

Pre-Marketing Clinical Trial Experience
Although DURAGESIC® use in post-operative or acute pain and in patients who are not opioid-tolerant is CONTRAINDICATED, the safety of DURAGESIC® was originally evaluated in 357 post-operative adult patients for 1 to 3 days and 153 cancer patients for a total of 510 patients. The duration of DURAGESIC® use varied in cancer patients; 56% of patients used DURAGESIC® for over 30 days, 28% continued treatment for more than 4 months, and 10% used DURAGESIC® for more than 1 year.

Hypoventilation was the most serious adverse reaction observed in 13 (4%) post-operative patients and in 3 (2%) of the cancer patients. Hypotension and hypertension were observed in 11 (3%) and 4 (1%) of the opioid-naive patients. Various adverse events were reported; a causal relationship to DURAGESIC® was not always determined. The frequencies presented here reflect the actual frequency of each adverse effect in patients who received DURAGESIC®. There has been no attempt to correct for a placebo effect, concomitant use of other opioids, or to subtract the frequencies reported by placebo-treated patients in controlled trials.

Adverse reactions reported in 153 cancer patients at a frequency of 1% or greater are presented in Table 1; similar reactions were seen in the 357 post-operative patients.

In the pediatric population, the safety of DURAGESIC® has been evaluated in 291 patients with chronic pain 2-18 years of age. The duration of DURAGESIC® use varied; 20% of pediatric patients were treated for ≤ 15 days; 46% for 16-30 days; 16% for 31-60 days; and 17% for at least 61 days. Twenty-five patients were treated with DURAGESIC® for at least 4 months and 9 patients for more than 9 months. There was no apparent pediatric-specific risk associated with DURAGESIC® use in children as young as 2 years old when used as directed. The most common adverse events were fever (35%), vomiting (33%), and nausea (24%).

Adverse events reported in pediatric patients at a rate of ≥ 1% are presented in Table 1.

[See table 1 above]

The following adverse effects have been reported in less than 1% of the 510 adult post-operative and cancer patients studied:

Cardiovascular: bradycardia
Digestive: abdominal distention
Nervous: aphasia, hypertonia, vertigo, stupor, hypotonia, depersonalization, hostility
Respiratory: stertorous breathing, asthma, respiratory disorder
Skin and Appendages, General: exfoliative dermatitis, pustules
Special Senses: amblyopia
Urogenital: bladder pain, oliguria, urinary frequency

Post-Marketing Experience - Adults
The following adverse reactions have been reported in association with the use of DURAGESIC® and not reported in the pre-marketing adverse reactions section above.

Body as a Whole: edema
Cardiovascular: tachycardia
Metabolic and Nutritional: weight loss
Special Senses: blurred vision
Urogenital: decreased libido, anorgasmia, ejaculatory difficulty

DRUG ABUSE AND ADDICTION
DURAGESIC® contains a high concentration of fentanyl, a potent Schedule II opioid agonist. Schedule II opioid substances, which include hydromorphone, methadone, morphine, oxycodone, and oxymorphone, have the highest potential for abuse and risk of fatal overdose due to respiratory depression. Fentanyl, like morphine and other opioids used in analgesia, can be abused and is subject to criminal diversion.

The high content of fentanyl in the patches (DURAGESIC®) may be a particular target for abuse and diversion.

Addiction is a primary, chronic, neurobiologic disease, with genetic, psychosocial, and environmental factors influencing its development and manifestations. It is characterized by behaviors that include one or more of the following: impaired control over drug use, compulsive use, continued use despite harm, and craving. Drug addiction is a treatable disease, utilizing a multidisciplinary approach, but relapse is common.

"Drug seeking" behavior is very common in addicts and drug abusers. Drug-seeking tactics include emergency calls or visits near the end of office hours, refusal to undergo appropriate examination, testing or referral, repeated "loss" of prescriptions, tampering with prescriptions and reluctance to provide prior medical records or contact information for other treating physician(s). "Doctor shopping" to obtain additional prescriptions is common among drug abusers and people suffering from untreated addiction.

Abuse and addiction are separate and distinct from physical dependence and tolerance. Physicians should be aware that addiction may be accompanied by concurrent tolerance and symptoms of physical dependence. In addition, abuse of opioids can occur in the absence of true addiction and is characterized by misuse for non-medical purposes, often in combination with other psychoactive substances. Since DURAGESIC® may be diverted for non-medical use, careful record keeping of prescribing information, including quantity, frequency, and renewal requests is strongly advised. Proper assessment of the patient, proper prescribing practices, periodic re-evaluation of therapy, and proper dispensing and storage are appropriate measures that help to limit abuse of opioid drugs.

DURAGESIC® patches are intended for transdermal use (to be applied on the skin) only. Do not use a DURAGESIC® patch if the pouch seal is broken or the patch is cut, damaged, or changed in any way.

OVERDOSAGE
Clinical Presentation
The manifestations of fentanyl overdosage are an extension of its pharmacologic actions with the most serious significant effect being hypoventilation.

Treatment
For the management of hypoventilation, immediate countermeasures include removing the DURAGESIC® (fentanyl transdermal system) system and physically or verbally stimulating the patient. These actions can be followed by administration of a specific narcotic antagonist such as naloxone. The duration of hypoventilation following an overdose may be longer than the effects of the narcotic antagonist's action (the half-life of naloxone ranges from 30 to 81 minutes). The interval between IV antagonist doses should be carefully chosen because of the possibility of renarcotization after system removal; repeated administration of naloxone may be necessary. Reversal of the narcotic effect may result in acute onset of pain and the release of catecholamines.

Always ensure a patent airway is established and maintained, administer oxygen and assist or control respiration as indicated and use an oropharyngeal airway or endotracheal tube if necessary. Adequate body temperature and fluid intake should be maintained.

If severe or persistent hypotension occurs, the possibility of hypovolemia should be considered and managed with appropriate parenteral fluid therapy.

DOSAGE AND ADMINISTRATION
Special Precautions
DURAGESIC® contains a high concentration of a potent Schedule II opioid agonist, fentanyl. Schedule II opioid substances which include fentanyl, hydromorphone, methadone, morphine, oxycodone, and oxymorphone have the highest potential for abuse and associated risk of fatal overdose due to respiratory depression. Fentanyl can be abused and is subject to criminal diversion. The high content of fentanyl in the patches (DURAGESIC®) may be a particular target for abuse and diversion.

DURAGESIC® patches are intended for transdermal use (on intact skin) only. The DURAGESIC® patch should not be used if the pouch seal is broken, or the patch is cut, damaged, or changed in any way.

Each DURAGESIC® patch may be worn continuously for 72 hours. The next patch should be applied to a different skin site after removal of the previous transdermal system.

If problems with adhesion of the DURAGESIC® patch occur, the edges of the patch may be taped with first aid tape. If problems with adhesion persist, the patch may be overlayed with a transparent adhesive film dressing (e.g., Bioclusive™ or Tegaderm™).

If the patch falls off before 72 hours, dispose of it by folding in half and flushing down the toilet. A new patch may be applied to a different skin site.

DURAGESIC® is ONLY for use in patients who are already tolerant to opioid therapy of comparable potency. Use in non-opioid tolerant patients may lead to fatal respiratory depression. Overestimating the DURAGESIC® dose when converting patients from another opioid medication can result in fatal overdose with the first dose. Due to the mean half-life of approximately 20-27 hours, patients who are thought to have had a serious adverse event, including overdose, will require monitoring and treatment for at least 24 hours.

The concomitant use of DURAGESIC® with all cytochrome P450 3A4 inhibitors (such as ritonavir, ketoconazole, itraconazole, troleandomycin, clarithromycin, nelfinavir, nefazodone, amiodarone, amprenavir, aprepitant, diltiazem, erythromycin, fluconazole, fosamprenavir, grapefruit juice, and verapamil) may result in an increase in fentanyl plasma concentrations, which could increase or prolong adverse drug effects and may cause potentially fatal respiratory depression. Patients receiving DURAGESIC® and any CYP3A4 inhibitor should be carefully monitored for an extended period of time and dosage adjustments should be made if warranted (see BOX WARNING, CLINICAL PHARMACOLOGY – Drug Interactions, WARNINGS and PRECAUTIONS for further information).

TABLE C[1]
DOSE CONVERSION GUIDELINES

Current Analgesic	Daily Dosage (mg/d)			
Oral morphine	60-134	135-224	225-314	315-404
IM/IV morphine	10-22	23-37	38-52	53-67
Oral oxycodone	30-67	67.5-112	112.5-157	157.5-202
IM/IV oxycodone	15-33	33.1-56	56.1-78	78.1-101
Oral codeine	150-447	448-747	748-1047	1048-1347
Oral hydromorphone	8-17	17.1-28	28.1-39	39.1-51
IV hydromorphone	1.5-3.4	3.5-5.6	5.7-7.9	8-10
IM meperidine	75-165	166-278	279-390	391-503
Oral methadone	20-44	45-74	75-104	105-134
IM methadone	10-22	23-37	38-52	53-67
	↓	↓	↓	↓
Recommended DURAGESIC® Dose	25 mcg/h	50 mcg/h	75 mcg/h	100 mcg/h

Alternatively, for adult and pediatric patients taking opioids or doses not listed in Table C, use the conversion methodology outlined above with Table D.

[1] Table C should not be used to convert from DURAGESIC® to other therapies because this conversion to DURAGESIC® is conservative. Use of table C for conversion to other analgesic therapies can overestimate the dose of the new agent. Overdosage of the new analgesic agent is possible (see DOSAGE AND ADMINISTRATION - Discontinuation of DURAGESIC®).

Pediatric patients converting to DURAGESIC® with a 25 mcg/h patch should be opioid-tolerant and receiving at least 60 mg of oral morphine or the equivalent per day. The dose conversion schedule described in Table C, and method of titration described below are recommended in opioid-tolerant pediatric patients over 2 years of age with chronic pain (see PRECAUTIONS – Pediatric Use).

Respiratory depression is the chief hazard in elderly or debilitated patients, usually following large initial doses in non-tolerant patients, or when opioids are given in conjunction with other agents that depress respiration.

DURAGESIC® should be used with caution in elderly, cachectic, or debilitated patients as they may have altered pharmacokinetics due to poor fat stores, muscle wasting, or altered clearance (see CLINICAL PHARMACOLOGY – Special Populations, Geriatric Use).

General Principles
DURAGESIC® is indicated for management of persistent, moderate to severe chronic pain that:

• requires continuous, around-the-clock opioid administration for an extended period of time
• cannot be managed by other means such as non-steroidal analgesics, opioid combination products, or immediate-release opioids.

DURAGESIC® should be used ONLY in patients who are already receiving opioid therapy, who have demonstrated opioid tolerance, and who require a total daily dose at least equivalent to DURAGESIC® 25 mcg/h. Patients who are considered opioid-tolerant are those who have been taking, for a week or longer, at least 60 mg of morphine daily, or at least 30 mg of oral oxycodone daily, or at least 8 mg oral hydromorphone daily, or an equianalgesic dose of another opioid.

Because serious or life-threatening hypoventilation could occur, DURAGESIC® (fentanyl transdermal system) is contraindicated:

• in patients who are not opioid-tolerant
• in the management of acute pain or in patients who require opioid analgesia for a short period of time.
• in the management of post-operative pain, including use after out-patient or day surgeries (e.g., tonsillectomies)
• in the management of mild pain
• in the management of intermittent pain (e.g., use on an as needed basis [prn])

(See CONTRAINDICATIONS for further information.)

Safety of DURAGESIC® has not been established in children under 2 years of age. DURAGESIC® should be administered to children only if they are opioid-tolerant and 2 years of age or older (see PRECAUTIONS - Pediatric Use).

Prescribers should individualize treatment using a progressive plan of pain management such as outlined by the World Health Organization, the Agency for Health Research and Quality, the Federation of State Medical Boards Model Policy, or the American Pain Society.

With all opioids, the safety of patients using the products is dependent on health care practitioners prescribing them in strict conformity with their approved labeling with respect to patient selection, dosing, and proper conditions for use. As with all opioids, dosage should be individualized. The most important factor to be considered in determining the appropriate dose is the extent of pre-existing opioid-tolerance (see BOX WARNING and CONTRAINDICATIONS). Initial doses should be reduced in elderly or debilitated patients (see PRECAUTIONS).

DURAGESIC® (fentanyl transdermal system) should be applied to intact, non-irritated and non-irradiated skin on a flat surface such as the chest, back, flank, or upper arm. In young children and persons with cognitive impairment, adhesion should be monitored and the upper back is the preferred location to minimize the potential of inappropriate patch removal. Hair at the application site should be clipped (not shaved) prior to system application. If the site of DURAGESIC® application must be cleansed prior to application of the patch, do so with clear water. Do not use soaps, oils, lotions, alcohol, or any other agents that might irritate the skin or alter its characteristics. Allow the skin to dry completely prior to patch application.

DURAGESIC® should be applied immediately upon removal from the sealed package. Do not use if the pouch seal is broken. Do not alter the patch (e.g., cut) in any way prior to application and do not use cut or damaged patches.

The transdermal system should be pressed firmly in place with the palm of the hand for 30 seconds, making sure the contact is complete, especially around the edges.

DURAGESIC® should be kept out of the reach of children. Used patches should be folded so that the adhesive side of the patch adheres to itself, then the patch should be flushed down the toilet immediately upon removal. Patients should dispose of any patches remaining from a prescription as soon as they are no longer needed. Unused patches should be removed from their pouches, folded so that the adhesive side of the patch adheres to itself, and flushed down the toilet.

Dose Selection
Doses must be individualized based upon the status of each patient and should be assessed at regular intervals after DURAGESIC® application. Reduced doses of DURAGESIC® are suggested for the elderly and other groups discussed in PRECAUTIONS.

DURAGESIC® is ONLY for use in patients who are already tolerant to opioid therapy of comparable potency. Use in non-opioid tolerant patients may lead to fatal respiratory depression.

In selecting an initial DURAGESIC® dose, attention should be given to 1) the daily dose, potency, and characteristics of the opioid the patient has been taking previously (e.g., whether it is a pure agonist or mixed agonist-antagonist), 2) the reliability of the relative potency estimates used to calculate the DURAGESIC® dose needed (potency estimates may vary with the route of administration), 3) the degree of opioid tolerance and 4) the general condition and medical status of the patient. Each patient should be maintained at the lowest dose providing acceptable pain control.

Initial DURAGESIC® Dose Selection

Overestimating the DURAGESIC® dose when converting patients from another opioid medication can result in fatal overdose with the first dose. Due to the mean half-life of approximately 20-27 hours, patients who are thought to have had a serious adverse event, including overdose, will require monitoring and treatment for at least 24 hours.

There has been no systematic evaluation of DURAGESIC® as an initial opioid analgesic in the management of chronic pain, since most patients in the clinical trials were converted to DURAGESIC® from other narcotics. The efficacy of DURAGESIC® 12 mcg/h as an initiating dose has not been determined. In addition, patients who are not opioid-tolerant have experienced hypoventilation and death during use of DURAGESIC®. Therefore, DURAGESIC® should be used only in patients who are opioid-tolerant.

To convert adult and pediatric patients from oral or parenteral opioids to DURAGESIC®, use Table C:

Alternatively, for adult and pediatric patients taking opioids or doses not listed in Table C, use the following methodology:

1. Calculate the previous 24-hour analgesic requirement.
2. Convert this amount to the equianalgesic oral morphine dose using Table D.
3. Table E displays the range of 24-hour oral morphine doses that are recommended for conversion to each DURAGESIC® dose. Use this table to find the calculated 24-hour morphine dose and the corresponding DURAGESIC® dose. Initiate DURAGESIC® treatment using the recommended dose and titrate patients upwards (no more frequently than every 3 days after the initial dose or than every 6 days thereafter) until analgesic efficacy is attained. The recommended starting dose when converting from other opioids to DURAGESIC® is likely too low for 50% of patients. This starting dose is recommended to minimize the potential for overdosing patients with the first dose. For delivery rates in excess of 100 mcg/h, multiple systems may be used.

[See table C at top of previous page]

TABLE D[1a]
EQUIANALGESIC POTENCY CONVERSION

Name	Equianalgesic Dose (mg)	
	IM[b,c]	PO
Morphine	10	60 (30)[d]
Hydromorphone (Dilaudid®)	1.5	7.5
Methadone (Dolophine®)	10	20
Oxycodone	15	30
Levorphanol (Levo-Dromoran®)	2	4
Oxymorphone (Numorphan®)	1	10 (PR)
Meperidine (Demerol®)	75	—
Codeine	130	200

[1] Table D should not be used to convert from DURAGESIC® to other therapies because this conversion to DURAGESIC® is conservative. Use of Table D for conversion to other therapies can overestimate the dose of the new agent. Overdosage of the new analgesic agent is possible (see Dosage And Administration - Discontinuation of DURAGESIC®).

[a] All IM and PO doses in this chart are considered equivalent to 10 mg of IM morphine in analgesic effect. IM denotes intramuscular, PO oral, and PR rectal.

[b] Based on single-dose studies in which an intramuscular dose of each drug listed was compared with morphine to establish the relative potency. Oral doses are those recommended when changing from parenteral to an oral route. Reference: Foley, K.M. (1985) The treatment of cancer pain. NEJM 313(2):84-95.

[c] Although controlled studies are not available, in clinical practice it is customary to consider the doses of opioid given IM, IV, or subcutaneously to be equivalent. There may be some differences in pharmacokinetic parameters such as C_{max} and T_{max}.

[d] The conversion ratio of 10 mg parenteral morphine = 30 mg oral morphine is based on clinical experience in patients with chronic pain. The conversion ratio of 10 mg parenteral morphine = 60 mg oral morphine is based on a potency study in acute pain. Reference: Ashburn and Lipman (1993) Management of pain in the cancer patient. Anesth Analg 76:402-416.

TABLE E[1]
RECOMMENDED INITIAL DURAGESIC® DOSE BASED UPON DAILY ORAL MORPHINE DOSE

Oral 24-hour Morphine (mg/day)	DURAGESIC® Dose (mcg/h)
60-134	25
135-224	50
225-314	75
315-404	100
405-494	125
495-584	150
585-674	175
675-764	200
765-854	225
855-944	250
945-1034	275
1035-1124	300

NOTE: In clinical trials, these ranges of daily oral morphine doses were used as a basis for conversion to DURAGESIC®.

[1] Table E should not be used to convert from DURAGESIC® to other therapies because this conversion to DURAGESIC® is conservative. Use of Table E for conversion to other analgesic therapies can overestimate the dose of the new agent. Overdosage of the new analgesic agent is possible (see DOSAGE AND ADMINISTRATION - Discontinuation of DURAGESIC®).

The majority of patients are adequately maintained with DURAGESIC® administered every 72 hours. Some patients may not achieve adequate analgesia using this dosing interval and may require systems to be applied every 48 hours rather than every 72 hours. An increase in the DURAGESIC® dose should be evaluated before changing dosing intervals in order to maintain patients on a 72-hour regimen. Dosing intervals less than every 72 hours were not studied in children and adolescents and are not recommended.

Because of the increase in serum fentanyl concentration over the first 24 hours following initial system application, the initial evaluation of the maximum analgesic effect of DURAGESIC® cannot be made before 24 hours of wearing. The initial DURAGESIC® dose may be increased after 3 days (see **DOSAGE AND ADMINISTRATION - Dose Titration**).

During the initial application of DURAGESIC®, patients should use short-acting analgesics as needed until analgesic efficacy with DURAGESIC® is attained. Thereafter, some patients still may require periodic supplemental doses of other short-acting analgesics for "breakthrough" pain.

Dose Titration

The recommended initial DURAGESIC® dose based upon the daily oral morphine dose is conservative, and 50% of patients are likely to require a dose increase after initial application of DURAGESIC®. The initial DURAGESIC® dose may be increased after 3 days based on the daily dose of supplemental opioid analgesics required by the patient in the second or third day of the initial application.

Physicians are advised that it may take up to 6 days after increasing the dose of DURAGESIC® for the patient to reach equilibrium on the new dose (see graph in **CLINICAL PHARMACOLOGY**). Therefore, patients should wear a higher dose through two applications before any further increase in dosage is made on the basis of the average daily use of a supplemental analgesic.

Appropriate dosage increments should be based on the daily dose of supplementary opioids, using the ratio of 45 mg/24 hours of oral morphine to a 12.5 mcg/h increase in DURAGESIC® dose. DURAGESIC®-12 delivers 12.5 mcg/h of fentanyl.

Discontinuation of DURAGESIC®

To convert patients to another opioid, remove DURAGESIC® and titrate the dose of the new analgesic based upon the patient's report of pain until adequate analgesia has been attained. Upon system removal, 17 hours or more are required for a 50% decrease in serum fentanyl concentrations. Opioid withdrawal symptoms (such as nausea, vomiting, diarrhea, anxiety, and shivering) are possible in some patients after conversion or dose adjustment. For patients requiring discontinuation of opioids, a gradual downward titration is recommended since it is not known at what dose level the opioid may be discontinued without producing the signs and symptoms of abrupt withdrawal.

Tables C, D, and E should not be used to convert to other therapies. Because the conversion to DURAGESIC® is conservative, use of Tables C, D, and E for conversion to other analgesic therapies can overestimate the dose of the new agent. Overdosage of the new analgesic agent is possible.

HOW SUPPLIED

DURAGESIC® (fentanyl transdermal system) is supplied in cartons containing 5 individually packaged systems. See chart for information regarding individual systems.

DURAGESIC® Dose (mcg/h)	System Size (cm²)	Fentanyl Content (mg)	NDC Number
DURAGESIC®-12	5.25	2.1	50458-090-05
DURAGESIC®-25	10.5	4.2	50458-091-05
DURAGESIC®-50	21	8.4	50458-092-05
DURAGESIC®-75	31.5	12.6	50458-093-05
DURAGESIC®-100	42	16.8	50458-094-05

Safety and Handling

DURAGESIC® is supplied in sealed transdermal systems which pose little risk of exposure to health care workers. Do not use a DURAGESIC® patch if the pouch seal is broken or the patch is cut, damaged, or changed in any way.

KEEP DURAGESIC® OUT OF THE REACH OF CHILDREN AND PETS.

Store in original unopened pouch. Store up to 25°C (77°F); excursions permitted to 15-30°C (59-86°F). Apply immediately after removal from individually sealed pouch. Do not use if the pouch seal is broken. **For transdermal use only.**

Bioclusive™ is a trademark of Ethicon, Inc.

Tegaderm™ is a trademark of 3M

A schedule CII narcotic. DEA order form required.

Manufactured by:
ALZA Corporation
Vacaville, CA 95688

Manufactured for:
PriCara®, Division of Ortho-McNeil-Janssen Pharmaceuticals, Inc.
Raritan, NJ 08869
Revised July 2009
© Ortho-McNeil-Janssen Pharmaceuticals, Inc. 2009
0017974-1

MEDICATION GUIDE

DURAGESIC® (Dur-ah-GEE-zik)
(FENTANYL TRANSDERMAL SYSTEM)

IMPORTANT:
- **Keep DURAGESIC® in a safe place away from children and pets.** Accidental use by a child or pet is a medical emergency and may result in death. If a child or pet accidentally uses DURAGESIC®, get emergency help right away.
- **Make sure you read the separate "Instructions for Applying a DURAGESIC® Patch."** Always use a DURAGESIC® Patch the right way. DURAGESIC® can cause serious breathing problems and death, especially if it is used the wrong way.
- **DURAGESIC® is a federally controlled substance (C-II)** because it can be abused. Keep DURAGESIC® in a safe place to prevent theft. Selling or giving away DURAGESIC® may harm others, and is against the law.
- **Tell your doctor if you (or a family member) have ever abused or been dependent on alcohol, prescription medicines or street drugs.**

Read the Medication Guide that comes with DURAGESIC® before you start using it and each time you get a new prescription. There may be new information. This Medication Guide does not take the place of talking to your healthcare provider about your medical condition or your treatment. Make sure you read and understand all the instructions for using DURAGESIC® . Do not use DURAGESIC® unless you understand everything. Talk to your healthcare provider if you have questions.

What is the most important information I should know about DURAGESIC®?

DURAGESIC® is a skin patch that contains fentanyl. Fentanyl is a very strong opioid narcotic pain medicine that can cause serious and life-threatening breathing problems. Serious and life-threatening breathing problems can happen because of an overdose or if the dose you are using is too high for you. Call your doctor right away or get emergency medical help if you:
- have trouble breathing, or have slow or shallow breathing
- have a slow heartbeat
- have severe sleepiness
- have cold, clammy skin
- feel faint, dizzy, confused, or cannot think, walk, or talk normally
- have a seizure
- have hallucinations

DURAGESIC® is only for adults and children over the age of two with persistent, moderate to severe chronic pain and who:

- are already using another strong opioid narcotic pain medicine around-the-clock, and have been using the medicine regularly for a week or longer. This is called being opioid-tolerant.
- have pain that cannot be controlled with other medicines

Do not use DURAGESIC®:

- if you are not already using another opioid narcotic medicine and are not opioid tolerant
- if you need opioid pain medicines for only a short time
- for pain from surgery, medical or dental procedures
- if your pain can be taken care of by occasional use of other pain medicines
- in children who are less than 2 years of age
- if you have asthma symptoms or have severe asthma

A DURAGESIC® patch must be used only on the skin of the person for whom it was prescribed. If the patch comes off and accidentally sticks to the skin of another person, take the patch off of that person right away, wash the area with water, and get medical care for them right away.

DURAGESIC® patch is not safe for everyone. Tell your doctor about all of your medical conditions.

Tell your doctor if you are planning to become pregnant, are pregnant, or breastfeeding. DURAGESIC® may cause serious harm to a baby.

Tell your doctor about all the medicines you take. Some medicines may cause serious or life-threatening side effects when used with DURAGESIC®. Your doctor will tell you if it is safe to take other medicines while you are using DURAGESIC®.

Know the medicines you take. Keep a list of your medicines to show to your doctor and pharmacist.

How should I use DURAGESIC®?

Read the separate "Instructions for Applying a DURAGESIC® Patch".

- **You must** always use DURAGESIC® patches the right way:
  - **Do not** use a DURAGESIC® patch if the pouch seal is broken, or the patch is cut, damaged, or changed in any way.
  - **Do not** use heat sources such as heating pads, electric blankets, heat lamps, tanning lamps, saunas, hot tubs, or heated waterbeds while wearing a DURAGESIC® patch.
  - **Do not** take hot baths or sunbathe while wearing a DURAGESIC® patch.
- **If you have problems with the DURAGESIC® patch not sticking:**
  1. Apply first aid tape only to the edges of the patch.
  2. If problems with the patch not sticking persist, cover the patch with Bioclusive™ or Tegaderm™. These are special see-through adhesive dressings. **Never cover a DURAGESIC® patch with any other bandage or tape.**
- **If your DURAGESIC® patch falls off before 3 days or 72 hours, fold the sticky side together and flush down a toilet. Put a new one on at a different skin site.**
- **Do not change your dose unless your doctor tells you to.** Your doctor may change your dose after seeing how the medicine affects you. Do not use DURAGESIC® more often than prescribed. Call your doctor if your pain is not well controlled while using DURAGESIC®.
- **Do not stop using DURAGESIC® suddenly.** Stopping DURAGESIC® suddenly can make you sick with withdrawal symptoms (for example, nausea, vomiting, diarrhea, anxiety, and shivering). Your body can develop a physical dependence on DURAGESIC®. If your doctor decides you no longer need DURAGESIC®, ask how to slowly reduce this medicine so you don't have withdrawal symptoms. Do not stop taking DURAGESIC® without talking to your doctor.
- **Do not wear more than one DURAGESIC® patch at a time,** unless your doctor tells you to do so.
- **Call your doctor right away if**
  - **You get a fever higher than 102°F**
  - Your body temperature increases from exercise

A fever or increase in body temperature may cause too much of the medicine in DURAGESIC® to pass into your body.

- **If you use more DURAGESIC® than your doctor has prescribed, get emergency medical help right away.**
- **Do not drink any alcohol while using DURAGESIC®.** Alcohol can increase your chances of having serious side effects.
- **Do not drive, operate heavy machinery, or do other possibly dangerous activities** until you know how DURAGESIC® affects you. DURAGESIC® can make you sleepy. Ask your doctor to tell you when it is okay to do these activities.
- When you remove your DURAGESIC® patch, fold the sticky sides of a used DURAGESIC® patch together and flush it down the toilet. **Do not put used DURAGESIC® patches in a trash can.**

What are the possible side effects of DURAGESIC®?
Serious side effects include:

- **Life-threatening breathing problems.** See "What is the most important information I should know about DURAGESIC®?"
- **Low blood pressure.** This can make you feel dizzy if you get up too fast from sitting or lying down.

The common side effects with DURAGESIC® are nausea, vomiting, constipation, dry mouth, sleepiness, confusion, weakness, sweating, and pain and redness where the patch was applied.

Constipation is a very common side effect of all opioid medicines. Talk to your doctor about the use of laxatives and stool softeners to prevent or treat constipation while taking DURAGESIC®.

Talk to your doctor about any side effect that concerns you. These are not all the possible side effects of DURAGESIC®. For a complete list, ask your doctor or pharmacist.

Call your doctor for medical advice about side effects. You may report side effects to FDA at 1-800-FDA-1088.

How should I store DURAGESIC®?

- Store in original unopened pouch at room temperature.
- Keep a DURAGESIC® patch in its protective pouch until you are ready to use it.
- **Keep DURAGESIC® in a safe place out of the reach of children and pets.**
- Dispose of DURAGESIC® patches you no longer need. Open the unused packages, fold the sticky sides of the patches together, and flush them down the toilet.

General information about the safe and effective use of DURAGESIC®

- Do not use DURAGESIC® for a condition for which it was not prescribed.
- **Do not give DURAGESIC® to other people, even if they have the same symptoms you have. DURAGESIC® can harm other people and even cause death. Sharing DURAGESIC® is against the law.**

This Medication Guide summarizes the most important information about DURAGESIC®. If you would like more information, talk with your doctor. You can ask your doctor or pharmacist for information about DURAGESIC® that is written for doctors.

For questions about DURAGESIC®, call the Ortho-McNeil Janssen Scientific Affairs Customer Communications Center at 1-800-526-7736. If this is a medical emergency, please call 911.

What are the ingredients of DURAGESIC®?
Active Ingredient: fentanyl
Inactive ingredients: polyester/ethyl vinyl acetate film backing, polyacrylate adhesive.

This Medication Guide has been approved by the United States Food and Drug Administration.

Bioclusive™ is a trademark of Ethicon, Inc.
Tegaderm™ is a trademark of 3M

Manufactured by:
ALZA Corporation, Vacaville, CA 95688
Manufactured for:
PriCara®, Division of Ortho-McNeil-Janssen Pharmaceuticals, Inc.
Raritan, NJ 08869
July 2009
© Ortho-McNeil-Janssen Pharmaceuticals, Inc. 2009
0017974-1MG

Shown in Product Identification Guide, page 316

INVEGA® ℞
[*in-ve-ga*]
(paliperidone)
Extended-Release Tablets

HIGHLIGHTS OF PRESCRIBING INFORMATION
These highlights do not include all the information needed to use INVEGA® safely and effectively. See full prescribing information for INVEGA®.
INVEGA® (paliperidone) Extended-Release Tablets
Initial U.S. Approval: 2006

> **WARNING: INCREASED MORTALITY IN ELDERLY PATIENTS WITH DEMENTIA-RELATED PSYCHOSIS**
> *See full prescribing information for complete boxed warning.*
> **Elderly patients with dementia-related psychosis treated with antipsychotic drugs are at an increased risk of death. INVEGA® is not approved for use in patients with dementia-related psychosis. (5.1)**

———RECENT MAJOR CHANGES———

Indications and Usage, Schizoaffective
Disorder (1.2)   July 2009

Dosage and Administration,
Schizoaffective Disorder (2.2)   July 2009
Dosage and Administration, Dosage in
Special Populations, Renal Impairment
(2.5)   July 2009
Warnings and Precautions, Leukopenia,
Neutropenia, and Agranulocytosis (5.10)   July 2009

———INDICATIONS AND USAGE———
INVEGA® is an atypical antipsychotic agent indicated for the

- acute and maintenance treatment of schizophrenia (1.1)
- acute treatment of schizoaffective disorder as monotherapy (1.2)
- acute treatment of schizoaffective disorder as an adjunct to mood stabilizers and/or antidepressants (1.2)

———DOSAGE AND ADMINISTRATION———
- For schizophrenia: 6 mg extended-release tablet administered in the morning with or without food. Initial dose titration is not required. Some patients may benefit from either higher doses up to 12 mg/day, or a lower dose of 3 mg/day. If clinical assessment warrants, increase the dose at increments of 3 mg/day at intervals of more than 5 days. Maximum recommended dose is 12 mg/day. (2.1)
- For schizoaffective disorder: 6 mg extended-release tablet administered in the morning with or without food. Initial dose titration is not required. Some patients may benefit from lower or higher doses within the recommended dose range of 3 to 12 mg once daily. If clinical assessment warrants, increase the dose at increments of 3 mg/day at intervals of more than 4 days. Maximum recommended dose is 12 mg/day. (2.2)
- Tablet should be swallowed whole and should not be chewed, divided, or crushed. (2.3)
- Patients may notice tablet-shaped shell in their stool. (2.3)

———DOSAGE FORMS AND STRENGTHS———
Tablets: 1.5 mg, 3 mg, 6 mg, and 9 mg (3)

———CONTRAINDICATIONS———
Known hypersensitivity to paliperidone, risperidone, or to any components in the formulation (4)

———WARNINGS AND PRECAUTIONS———
- *Cerebrovascular Adverse Reactions, Including Stroke, in Elderly Patients with Dementia-Related Psychosis:* Increased incidence of cerebrovascular adverse reactions (e.g. stroke, transient ischemic attack, including fatalities). INVEGA® is not approved for use in patients with dementia-related psychosis (5.2)
- *Neuroleptic Malignant Syndrome:* Manage with immediate discontinuation of drug and close monitoring (5.3)
- *QT Prolongation:* Increase in QT interval, avoid use with drugs that also increase QT interval and in patients with risk factors for prolonged QT interval (5.4)
- *Tardive Dyskinesia:* Discontinue drug if clinically appropriate (5.5)
- *Hyperglycemia and Diabetes Mellitus:* Monitor glucose regularly in patients with and at risk for diabetes (5.6)
- *Hyperprolactinemia:* Prolactin elevations occur and persist during chronic administration (5.7)
- *Gastrointestinal Narrowing:* Obstructive symptoms may result in patients with gastrointestinal disease (5.8)
- *Orthostatic Hypotension and Syncope:* Use with caution in patients with known cardiovascular or cerebrovascular disease and patients predisposed to hypotension (5.9)
- *Leukopenia, Neutropenia, and Agranulocytosis:* has been reported with antipsychotics, including INVEGA®. Patients with a history of a clinically significant low white blood cell count (WBC) or a drug-induced leukopenia/neutropenia should have their complete blood count (CBC) monitored frequently during the first few months of therapy and discontinuation of INVEGA® should be considered at the first sign of a clinically significant decline in WBC in the absence of other causative factors. (5.10)
- *Potential for Cognitive and Motor Impairment:* Use caution when operating machinery (5.11)
- *Seizures:* Use cautiously in patients with a history of seizures or with conditions that lower the seizure threshold (5.12)
- *Suicide:* Closely supervise high-risk patients (5.14)

———ADVERSE REACTIONS———
The most common adverse reactions (incidence ≥ 5% and at least twice that for placebo) were extrapyramidal symptoms, tachycardia, and akathisia in the schizophrenia trials, and extrapyramidal symptoms, somnolence, dyspepsia, constipation, weight increased, and nasopharyngitis in the schizoaffective disorder trials. (6)

To report SUSPECTED ADVERSE REACTIONS, contact Janssen, Division of Ortho-McNeil-Janssen Pharmaceuticals, Inc. at 1-800-JANSSEN (1-800-526-7736) or FDA at 1-800-FDA-1088 or www.fda.gov/medwatch

DRUG INTERACTIONS

- Centrally-acting drugs: Due to CNS effects, use caution in combination. Avoid alcohol. (7.1)
- Drugs that may cause orthostatic hypotension: An additive effect may be observed when co-administered with INVEGA®. (7.1)
- Co-administration with carbamazepine decreased mean steady-state Cmax and AUC of paliperidone by approximately 37%. Adjust dose of INVEGA® if necessary based on clinical assessment. (7.2)
- Co-administration of divalproex sodium increased Cmax and AUC of paliperidone by approximately 50%. Adjust dose of INVEGA® if necessary based on clinical assessment. (7.2)

USE IN SPECIFIC POPULATIONS

- Renal impairment: Dosing must be individualized according to renal function status. For mild renal impairment (creatinine clearance ≥50 mL/min to < 80 mL/min), the recommended initial dose is 3 mg/day, which may be increased to a maximum of 6 mg/day based on clinical response and tolerability. For moderate to severe renal impairment (creatinine clearance ≥10 mL/min to <50 mL/min), the recommended initial dose is 1.5 mg/day, which may be increased to a maximum of 3 mg/day after clinical reassessment. As INVEGA® has not been studied in patients with creatinine clearance < 10 mL/min, use is not recommended in such patients. (2.5)
- Elderly: same as for younger adults (adjust dose according to renal function status). (2.4)
- Nursing Mothers: Limited data. (8.3)
- Pediatric Use: safety and effectiveness not established in patients less than 18 years of age. (8.4)

See 17 for PATIENT COUNSELING INFORMATION

Revised: 01/2010

FULL PRESCRIBING INFORMATION: CONTENTS*

WARNING: INCREASED MORTALITY IN ELDERLY PATIENTS WITH DEMENTIA-RELATED PSYCHOSIS

*** Sections or subsections omitted from the full prescribing information are not listed**

FULL PRESCRIBING INFORMATION

> **WARNING: INCREASED MORTALITY IN ELDERLY PATIENTS WITH DEMENTIA-RELATED PSYCHOSIS**
> Elderly patients with dementia-related psychosis treated with antipsychotic drugs are at an increased risk of death. Analyses of 17 placebo-controlled trials (modal duration of 10 weeks), largely in patients taking atypical antipsychotic drugs, revealed a risk of death in drug-treated patients of between 1.6 to 1.7 times the risk of death in placebo-treated patients. Over the course of a typical 10-week controlled trial, the rate of death in drug-treated patients was about 4.5%, compared to a rate of about 2.6% in the placebo group. Although the causes of death were varied, most of the deaths appeared to be either cardiovascular (e.g., heart failure, sudden death) or infectious (e.g., pneumonia) in nature. Observational studies suggest that, similar to atypical antipsychotic drugs, treatment with conventional antipsychotic drugs may increase mortality. The extent to which the findings of increased mortality in observational studies may be attributed to the antipsychotic drug as opposed to some characteristic(s) of the patients is not clear. INVEGA® (paliperidone) Extended-Release Tablets is not approved for the treatment of patients with dementia-related psychosis. *[see Warnings and Precautions (5.1)]*

1 INDICATIONS AND USAGE

1.1 Schizophrenia

INVEGA® (paliperidone) Extended-Release Tablets are indicated for the acute and maintenance treatment of schizophrenia *[see Clinical Studies (14)]*.

1.2 Schizoaffective Disorder

Monotherapy

INVEGA® (paliperidone) Extended-Release Tablets are indicated for the acute treatment of schizoaffective disorder as monotherapy.

Adjunctive Therapy

INVEGA® (paliperidone) Extended-Release Tablets are indicated for the acute treatment of schizoaffective disorder as an adjunct to mood stabilizers and/or antidepressants.

2 DOSAGE AND ADMINISTRATION

2.1 Schizophrenia

The recommended dose of INVEGA® (paliperidone) Extended-Release Tablets for the treatment of schizophrenia is 6 mg once daily, administered in the morning. Initial dose titration is not required. Although it has not been systematically established that doses above 6 mg have additional benefit, there was a general trend for greater effects with higher doses. This must be weighed against the dose-related increase in adverse reactions. Thus, some patients may benefit from higher doses, up to 12 mg/day, and for some patients, a lower dose of 3 mg/day may be sufficient. Dose increases above 6 mg/day should be made only after clinical reassessment and generally should occur at intervals of more than 5 days. When dose increases are indicated, increments of 3 mg/day are recommended. The maximum recommended dose is 12 mg/day.

In a longer-term study, INVEGA® has been shown to be effective in delaying time to relapse in patients with schizophrenia who were stabilized on INVEGA® for 6 weeks *[see Clinical Studies (14)]*. INVEGA® should be prescribed at the lowest effective dose for maintaining clinical stability and the physician should periodically reevaluate the long-term usefulness of the drug in individual patients.

2.2 Schizoaffective Disorder

The recommended dose of INVEGA® (paliperidone) Extended-Release Tablets for the treatment of schizoaffective disorder is 6 mg once daily, administered in the morning. Initial dose titration is not required. Some patients may benefit from lower or higher doses within the recommended dose range of 3 to 12 mg once daily. A general trend for greater effects was seen with higher doses. This trend must be weighed against dose-related increase in adverse reactions. Dosage adjustment, if indicated, should occur only after clinical reassessment. Dose increases, if indicated, generally should occur at intervals of more than 4 days. When dose increases are indicated, increments of 3 mg/day are recommended. The maximum recommended dose is 12 mg/day.

2.3 Administration Instructions

INVEGA® can be taken with or without food. Clinical trials establishing the safety and efficacy of INVEGA® were carried out in patients without regard to food intake.

INVEGA® must be swallowed whole with the aid of liquids. Tablets should not be chewed, divided, or crushed. The medication is contained within a nonabsorbable shell designed to release the drug at a controlled rate. The tablet shell, along with insoluble core components, is eliminated from the body; patients should not be concerned if they occasionally notice in their stool something that looks like a tablet.

2.4 Use with Risperidone

Concomitant use of INVEGA® with risperidone has not been studied. Since paliperidone is the major active metabolite of risperidone, consideration should be given to the additive paliperidone exposure if risperidone is coadministered with INVEGA®.

2.5 Dosage in Special Populations

Renal Impairment

Dosing must be individualized according to the patient's renal function status. For patients with mild renal impairment (creatinine clearance ≥ 50 mL/min to < 80 mL/min), the recommended initial dose of INVEGA® is 3 mg once daily. The dose may then be increased to a maximum of 6 mg once daily based on clinical response and tolerability. For patients with moderate to severe renal impairment (creatinine clearance ≥ 10 mL/min to < 50 mL/min), the recommended initial dose of INVEGA® is 1.5 mg once daily, which may be increased to a maximum of 3 mg once daily after clinical reassessment. As INVEGA® has not been studied in patients with creatinine clearance below 10 mL/min, use is not recommended in such patients. *[See Clinical Pharmacology (12.3)]*

Hepatic Impairment

For patients with mild to moderate hepatic impairment, (Child-Pugh Classification A and B), no dose adjustment is recommended *[see Clinical Pharmacology (12.3)]*. INVEGA® has not been studied in patients with severe hepatic impairment.

Elderly

Because elderly patients may have diminished renal function, dose adjustments may be required according to their renal function status. In general, recommended dosing for elderly patients with normal renal function is the same as for younger adult patients with normal renal function. For patients with moderate to severe renal impairment (creatinine clearance 10 mL/min to < 50 mL/min), the maximum recommended dose of INVEGA® is 3 mg once daily *[see Renal Impairment above]*.

3 DOSAGE FORMS AND STRENGTHS

INVEGA® Extended-Release Tablets are available in the following strengths and colors: 1.5 mg (orange-brown), 3 mg (white), 6 mg (beige), and 9 mg (pink). All tablets are capsule shaped and are imprinted with either "PAL 1.5", "PAL 3", "PAL 6", or "PAL 9".

4 CONTRAINDICATIONS

Hypersensitivity reactions, including anaphylactic reactions and angioedema, have been observed in patients treated with risperidone and paliperidone. INVEGA® (paliperidone) is a metabolite of risperidone and is therefore contraindicated in patients with a known hypersensitivity to either paliperidone or risperidone, or to any of the excipients in INVEGA®.

5 WARNINGS AND PRECAUTIONS

5.1 Increased Mortality in Elderly Patients with Dementia-Related Psychosis

Elderly patients with dementia-related psychosis treated with antipsychotic drugs are at an increased risk of death. INVEGA® (paliperidone) is not approved for the treatment of dementia-related psychosis [see Boxed Warning].

5.2 Cerebrovascular Adverse Reactions, Including Stroke, in Elderly Patients With Dementia-Related Psychosis

In placebo-controlled trials with risperidone, aripiprazole, and olanzapine in elderly subjects with dementia, there was a higher incidence of cerebrovascular adverse reactions (cerebrovascular accidents and transient ischemic attacks) including fatalities compared to placebo-treated subjects. INVEGA® was not marketed at the time these studies were performed. INVEGA® is not approved for the treatment of patients with dementia-related psychosis [see also Boxed Warning and Warnings and Precautions (5.1)].

5.3 Neuroleptic Malignant Syndrome

A potentially fatal symptom complex sometimes referred to as Neuroleptic Malignant Syndrome (NMS) has been reported in association with antipsychotic drugs, including paliperidone. Clinical manifestations of NMS are hyperpyrexia, muscle rigidity, altered mental status, and evidence of autonomic instability (irregular pulse or blood pressure, tachycardia, diaphoresis, and cardiac dysrhythmia). Additional signs may include elevated creatine phosphokinase, myoglobinuria (rhabdomyolysis), and acute renal failure.

The diagnostic evaluation of patients with this syndrome is complicated. In arriving at a diagnosis, it is important to identify cases in which the clinical presentation includes both serious medical illness (e.g., pneumonia, systemic infection, etc.) and untreated or inadequately treated extrapyramidal signs and symptoms (EPS). Other important considerations in the differential diagnosis include central anticholinergic toxicity, heat stroke, drug fever, and primary central nervous system pathology.

The management of NMS should include: (1) immediate discontinuation of antipsychotic drugs and other drugs not essential to concurrent therapy; (2) intensive symptomatic treatment and medical monitoring; and (3) treatment of any concomitant serious medical problems for which specific treatments are available. There is no general agreement about specific pharmacological treatment regimens for uncomplicated NMS.

If a patient appears to require antipsychotic drug treatment after recovery from NMS, reintroduction of drug therapy should be closely monitored, since recurrences of NMS have been reported.

5.4 QT Prolongation

Paliperidone causes a modest increase in the corrected QT (QTc) interval. The use of paliperidone should be avoided in combination with other drugs that are known to prolong QTc including Class 1A (e.g., quinidine, procainamide) or Class III (e.g., amiodarone, sotalol) antiarrhythmic medications, antipsychotic medications (e.g., chlorpromazine, thioridazine), antibiotics (e.g., gatifloxacin, moxifloxacin), or any other class of medications known to prolong the QTc interval. Paliperidone should also be avoided in patients with congenital long QT syndrome and in patients with a history of cardiac arrhythmias.

Certain circumstances may increase the risk of the occurrence of torsade de pointes and/or sudden death in association with the use of drugs that prolong the QTc interval, including (1) bradycardia; (2) hypokalemia or hypomagnesemia; (3) concomitant use of other drugs that prolong the QTc interval; and (4) presence of congenital prolongation of the QT interval.

The effects of paliperidone on the QT interval were evaluated in a double-blind, active-controlled (moxifloxacin 400 mg single dose), multicenter QT study in adults with schizophrenia and schizoaffective disorder, and in three placebo- and active-controlled 6-week, fixed-dose efficacy trials in adults with schizophrenia.

In the QT study (n = 141), the 8 mg dose of immediate-release oral paliperidone (n=50) showed a mean placebo-subtracted increase from baseline in QTcLD of 12.3 msec (90% CI: 8.9; 15.6) on day 8 at 1.5 hours post-dose. The mean steady-state peak plasma concentration for this 8 mg dose of paliperidone immediate-release was more than twice the exposure observed with the maximum recommended 12 mg dose of INVEGA® (C_{max} ss = 113 ng/mL and 45 ng/mL, respectively, when administered with a standard breakfast). In this same study, a 4 mg dose of the immediate-release oral formulation of paliperidone, for which C_{max} ss = 35 ng/mL, showed an increased placebo-subtracted QTcLD of 6.8 msec (90% CI: 3.6; 10.1) on day 2 at 1.5 hours post-dose. None of the subjects had a change exceeding 60 msec or a QTcLD exceeding 500 msec at any time during this study.

For the three fixed-dose efficacy studies in subjects with schizophrenia, electrocardiogram (ECG) measurements taken at various time points showed only one subject in the INVEGA® 12 mg group had a change exceeding 60 msec at one time-point on Day 6 (increase of 62 msec). No subject receiving INVEGA® had a QtcLD exceeding 500 msec at any time in any of these three studies.

5.5 Tardive Dyskinesia

A syndrome of potentially irreversible, involuntary, dyskinetic movements may develop in patients treated with antipsychotic drugs. Although the prevalence of the syndrome appears to be highest among the elderly, especially elderly women, it is impossible to predict which patients will develop the syndrome. Whether antipsychotic drug products differ in their potential to cause tardive dyskinesia is unknown.

The risk of developing tardive dyskinesia and the likelihood that it will become irreversible appear to increase as the duration of treatment and the total cumulative dose of antipsychotic drugs administered to the patient increase, but the syndrome can develop after relatively brief treatment periods at low doses, although this is uncommon.

There is no known treatment for established tardive dyskinesia, although the syndrome may remit, partially or completely, if antipsychotic treatment is withdrawn. Antipsychotic treatment itself may suppress (or partially suppress) the signs and symptoms of the syndrome and may thus mask the underlying process. The effect of symptomatic suppression on the long-term course of the syndrome is unknown.

Given these considerations, INVEGA® should be prescribed in a manner that is most likely to minimize the occurrence of tardive dyskinesia. Chronic antipsychotic treatment should generally be reserved for patients who suffer from a chronic illness that is known to respond to antipsychotic drugs. In patients who do require chronic treatment, the smallest dose and the shortest duration of treatment producing a satisfactory clinical response should be sought. The need for continued treatment should be reassessed periodically.

If signs and symptoms of tardive dyskinesia appear in a patient treated with INVEGA®, drug discontinuation should be considered. However, some patients may require treatment with INVEGA® despite the presence of the syndrome.

5.6 Hyperglycemia and Diabetes Mellitus

Hyperglycemia, in some cases extreme and associated with ketoacidosis or hyperosmolar coma or death, has been reported in patients treated with all atypical antipsychotics. These cases were, for the most part, seen in post-marketing clinical use and epidemiologic studies, not in clinical trials, and there have been few reports of hyperglycemia or diabetes in trial subjects treated with INVEGA®. Assessment of the relationship between atypical antipsychotic use and glucose abnormalities is complicated by the possibility of an increased background risk of diabetes mellitus in patients with schizophrenia and the increasing incidence of diabetes mellitus in the general population. Given these confounders, the relationship between atypical antipsychotic use and hyperglycemia-related adverse events is not completely understood. However, epidemiological studies suggest an increased risk of treatment-emergent hyperglycemia-related adverse events in patients treated with the atypical antipsychotics. Because INVEGA® was not marketed at the time these studies were performed, it is not known if INVEGA® is associated with this increased risk.

Patients with an established diagnosis of diabetes mellitus who are started on atypical antipsychotics should be monitored regularly for worsening of glucose control. Patients with risk factors for diabetes mellitus (e.g., obesity, family history of diabetes) who are starting treatment with atypical antipsychotics should undergo fasting blood glucose testing at the beginning of treatment and periodically during treatment. Any patient treated with atypical antipsychotics should be monitored for symptoms of hyperglycemia including polydipsia, polyuria, polyphagia, and weakness. Patients who develop symptoms of hyperglycemia during treatment with atypical antipsychotics should undergo fasting blood glucose testing. In some cases, hyperglycemia has resolved when the atypical antipsychotic was discontinued; however, some patients required continuation of anti-diabetic treatment despite discontinuation of the suspect drug.

5.7 Hyperprolactinemia

Like other drugs that antagonize dopamine D_2 receptors, paliperidone elevates prolactin levels and the elevation persists during chronic administration. Paliperidone has a prolactin-elevating effect similar to that seen with risperidone, a drug that is associated with higher levels of prolactin than other antipsychotic drugs.

Hyperprolactinemia, regardless of etiology, may suppress hypothalamic GnRH, resulting in reduced pituitary gonadotrophin secretion. This, in turn, may inhibit reproductive function by impairing gonadal steroidogenesis in both female and male patients. Galactorrhea, amenorrhea, gynecomastia, and impotence have been reported in patients receiving prolactin-elevating compounds. Long-standing hyperprolactinemia when associated with hypogonadism may lead to decreased bone density in both female and male subjects.

Tissue culture experiments indicate that approximately one-third of human breast cancers are prolactin dependent in vitro, a factor of potential importance if the prescription of these drugs is considered in a patient with previously detected breast cancer. An increase in the incidence of pituitary gland, mammary gland, and pancreatic islet cell neoplasia (mammary adenocarcinomas, pituitary and pancreatic adenomas) was observed in the risperidone carcinogenicity studies conducted in mice and rats [see Nonclinical Toxicology (13.1)]. Neither clinical studies nor epidemiologic studies conducted to date have shown an association between chronic administration of this class of drugs and tumorigenesis in humans, but the available evidence is too limited to be conclusive.

5.8 Potential for Gastrointestinal Obstruction

Because the INVEGA® tablet is non-deformable and does not appreciably change in shape in the gastrointestinal tract, INVEGA® should ordinarily not be administered to patients with pre-existing severe gastrointestinal narrowing (pathologic or iatrogenic, for example: esophageal motility disorders, small bowel inflammatory disease, "short gut" syndrome due to adhesions or decreased transit time, past history of peritonitis, cystic fibrosis, chronic intestinal pseudo-obstruction, or Meckel's diverticulum). There have been rare reports of obstructive symptoms in patients with known strictures in association with the ingestion of drugs in non-deformable controlled-release formulations. Because of the controlled-release design of the tablet, INVEGA® should only be used in patients who are able to swallow the tablet whole [see Dosage and Administration (2.3) and Patient Counseling Information (17.8)].

A decrease in transit time, e.g., as seen with diarrhea, would be expected to decrease bioavailability and an increase in transit time, e.g., as seen with gastrointestinal neuropathy, diabetic gastroparesis, or other causes, would be expected to increase bioavailability. These changes in bioavailability are more likely when the changes in transit time occur in the upper GI tract.

5.9 Orthostatic Hypotension and Syncope

Paliperidone can induce orthostatic hypotension and syncope in some patients because of its alpha-blocking activity. In pooled results of the three placebo-controlled, 6-week, fixed-dose trials in subjects with schizophrenia, syncope was reported in 0.8% (7/850) of subjects treated with INVEGA® (3 mg, 6 mg, 9 mg, 12 mg) compared to 0.3% (1/355) of subjects treated with placebo. INVEGA® should be used with caution in patients with known cardiovascular disease (e.g., heart failure, history of myocardial infarction or ischemia, conduction abnormalities), cerebrovascular disease, or conditions that predispose the patient to hypotension (e.g., dehydration, hypovolemia, and treatment with antihypertensive medications). Monitoring of orthostatic vital signs should be considered in patients who are vulnerable to hypotension.

5.10 Leukopenia, Neutropenia, and Agranulocytosis

Class Effect: In clinical trial and/or postmarketing experience, events of leukopenia/neutropenia have been reported temporally related to antipsychotic agents, including INVEGA®. Agranulocytosis has also been reported. Possible risk factors for leukopenia/neutropenia include pre-existing low white blood cell count (WBC) and history of drug-induced leukopenia/neutropenia. Patients with a history of a clinically significant low WBC or a drug-induced leukopenia/neutropenia should have their complete blood count (CBC) monitored frequently during the first few months of therapy and discontinuation of INVEGA® should be considered at the first sign of a clinically significant decline in WBC in the absence of other causative factors. Patients with clinically significant neutropenia should be carefully monitored for fever or other symptoms or signs of infection and treated promptly if such symptoms or signs occur. Patients with severe neutropenia (absolute neutrophil count <1000/mm³) should discontinue INVEGA® and have their WBC followed until recovery.

5.11 Potential for Cognitive and Motor Impairment

Somnolence was reported in subjects treated with INVEGA® [see Adverse Reactions (6.1, 6.2)]. Antipsychotics, including INVEGA®, have the potential to impair judgment, thinking, or motor skills. Patients should be cautioned about performing activities requiring mental alertness, such as operating hazardous machinery or operating a motor vehicle, until they are reasonably certain that paliperidone therapy does not adversely affect them.

5.12 Seizures

During premarketing clinical trials in subjects with schizophrenia (the three placebo-controlled, 6-week, fixed-dose studies and a study conducted in elderly schizophrenic subjects), seizures occurred in 0.22% of subjects treated with INVEGA® (3 mg, 6 mg, 9 mg, 12 mg) and 0.25% of subjects treated with placebo. Like other antipsychotic drugs, INVEGA® should be used cautiously in patients with a history of seizures or other conditions that potentially lower the seizure threshold. Conditions that lower the seizure threshold may be more prevalent in patients 65 years or older.

5.13 Dysphagia

Esophageal dysmotility and aspiration have been associated with antipsychotic drug use. Aspiration pneumonia is a common cause of morbidity and mortality in patients with advanced Alzheimer's dementia. INVEGA® and other antipsychotic drugs should be used cautiously in patients at risk for aspiration pneumonia.

5.14 Suicide

The possibility of suicide attempt is inherent in psychotic illnesses, and close supervision of high-risk patients should accompany drug therapy. Prescriptions for INVEGA® should be written for the smallest quantity of tablets consistent with good patient management in order to reduce the risk of overdose.

5.15 Priapism

Drugs with alpha-adrenergic blocking effects have been reported to induce priapism. Priapism has been reported with INVEGA® during postmarketing surveillance. Severe priapism may require surgical intervention.

5.16 Thrombotic Thrombocytopenic Purpura (TTP)

No cases of TTP were observed during clinical studies with paliperidone. Although cases of TTP have been reported in association with risperidone administration, the relationship to risperidone therapy is unknown.

5.17 Body Temperature Regulation

Disruption of the body's ability to reduce core body temperature has been attributed to antipsychotic agents. Appropriate care is advised when prescribing INVEGA® to patients who will be experiencing conditions which may contribute to an elevation in core body temperature, e.g., exercising strenuously, exposure to extreme heat, receiving concomitant medication with anticholinergic activity, or being subject to dehydration.

5.18 Antiemetic Effect

An antiemetic effect was observed in preclinical studies with paliperidone. This effect, if it occurs in humans, may mask the signs and symptoms of overdosage with certain drugs or of conditions such as intestinal obstruction, Reye's syndrome, and brain tumor.

5.19 Use in Patients with Concomitant Illness

Clinical experience with INVEGA® in patients with certain concomitant illnesses is limited *[see Clinical Pharmacology (12.3)]*.

Patients with Parkinson's Disease or Dementia with Lewy Bodies are reported to have an increased sensitivity to antipsychotic medication. Manifestations of this increased sensitivity include confusion, obtundation, postural instability with frequent falls, extrapyramidal symptoms, and clinical features consistent with the neuroleptic malignant syndrome.

INVEGA® has not been evaluated or used to any appreciable extent in patients with a recent history of myocardial infarction or unstable heart disease. Patients with these diagnoses were excluded from premarketing clinical trials. Because of the risk of orthostatic hypotension with INVEGA®, caution should be observed in patients with known cardiovascular disease *[see Warnings and Precautions (5.9)]*.

5.20 Monitoring: Laboratory Tests

No specific laboratory tests are recommended.

6 ADVERSE REACTIONS

The following are discussed in more detail in other sections of the labeling:

- Increased mortality in elderly patients with dementia-related psychosis *[see Boxed Warning and Warnings and Precautions (5.1)]*
- Cerebrovascular adverse events, including stroke, in elderly patients with dementia-related psychosis *[see Warnings and Precautions (5.2)]*
- Neuroleptic malignant syndrome *[see Warnings and Precautions (5.3)]*
- QT prolongation *[see Warnings and Precautions (5.4)]*
- Tardive dyskinesia *[see Warnings and Precautions (5.5)]*
- Hyperglycemia and diabetes mellitus *[see Warnings and Precautions (5.6)]*
- Hyperprolactinemia *[see Warnings and Precautions (5.7)]*
- Potential for Gastrointestinal Obstruction *[see Warnings and Precautions (5.8)]*
- Orthostatic hypotension and syncope *[see Warnings and Precautions (5.9)]*
- Leukopenia, neutropenia, and agranulocytosis *[see Warnings and Precautions (5.10)]*
- Potential for cognitive and motor impairment *[see Warnings and Precautions (5.11)]*
- Seizures *[see Warnings and Precautions (5.12)]*
- Dysphagia *[see Warnings and Precautions (5.13)]*
- Suicide *[see Warnings and Precautions (5.14)]*
- Priapism *[see Warnings and Precautions (5.15)]*
- Thrombotic thrombocytopenic purpura (TTP) *[see Warnings and Precautions (5.16)]*
- Disruption of body temperature regulation *[see Warnings and Precautions (5.17)]*
- Antiemetic effect *[see Warnings and Precautions (5.18)]*
- Increased sensitivity in patients with Parkinson's disease or those with dementia with Lewy bodies *[see Warnings and Precautions (5.19)]*

Table 1. Adverse Reactions Reported by ≥ 2% of INVEGA®-Treated Subjects with Schizophrenia in Three Short-Term, Fixed-Dose, Placebo-Controlled Clinical Trials*

Body System or Organ Class / Dictionary-Derived Term	Percent of Patients Reporting Event				
		INVEGA®			
	Placebo (N=355)	3 mg once daily (N=127)	6 mg once daily (N=235)	9 mg once daily (N=246)	12 mg once daily (N=242)
Total percentage of subjects with adverse reactions	37	48	47	53	59
Cardiac disorders					
Atrioventricular block first degree	1	2	0	2	1
Bundle branch block	2	3	1	3	<1
Sinus arrhythmia	0	2	1	1	<1
Tachycardia	7	14	12	12	14
Gastrointestinal disorders					
Abdominal pain upper	1	1	3	2	2
Dry mouth	1	2	3	1	3
Salivary hypersecretion	<1	0	<1	1	4
General disorders					
Asthenia	1	2	<1	2	2
Fatigue	1	2	1	2	2
Nervous system disorders					
Akathisia	4	4	3	8	10
Dizziness	4	6	5	4	5
Extrapyramidal symptoms	8	10	7	20	18
Headache	12	11	12	14	14
Somnolence	7	6	9	10	11
Vascular disorders					
Orthostatic hypotension	1	2	1	2	4

* Table includes adverse reactions that were reported in 2% or more of subjects in any of the INVEGA® dose groups and which occurred at greater incidence than in the placebo group. Data are pooled from three studies; one study included once-daily INVEGA® doses of 3 mg and 9 mg, the second study included 6 mg, 9 mg, and 12 mg, and the third study included 6 mg and 12 mg *[see Clinical Studies (14)]*. Extrapyramidal symptoms includes the terms dyskinesia, dystonia, extrapyramidal disorder, hypertonia, muscle rigidity, oculogyration, parkinsonism, and tremor. Somnolence includes the terms sedation and somnolence. Tachycardia includes the terms tachycardia, sinus tachycardia, and heart rate increased. Adverse reactions for which the INVEGA® incidence was equal to or less than placebo are not listed in the table, but included the following: vomiting.

- Diseases or conditions that could affect metabolism or hemodynamic responses *[see Warnings and Precautions (5.19)]*

The most common adverse reactions in clinical trials in subjects with schizophrenia (reported in 5% or more of subjects treated with INVEGA® and at least twice the placebo rate in any of the dose groups) were extrapyramidal symptoms, tachycardia, and akathisia. The most common adverse reactions in clinical trials in patients with schizoaffective disorder (reported in 5% or more of subjects treated with INVEGA® and at least twice the placebo rate) were extrapyramidal symptoms, somnolence, dyspepsia, constipation, weight increased, and nasopharyngitis.

The most common adverse reactions that were associated with discontinuation from clinical trials in subjects with schizophrenia (causing discontinuation in 2% of INVEGA®-treated subjects) were nervous system disorders. The most common adverse reactions that were associated with discontinuation from clinical trials in subjects with schizoaffective disorder were gastrointestinal disorders, which resulted in discontinuation in 1% of INVEGA®-treated subjects. *[See Adverse Reactions (6.4)]*.

The safety of INVEGA® was evaluated in 1205 adult subjects with schizophrenia who participated in three placebo-controlled, 6-week, double-blind trials, of whom 850 subjects received INVEGA® at fixed doses ranging from 3 mg to 12 mg once daily. The information presented in this section was derived from pooled data from these three trials. Additional safety information from the placebo-controlled phase of the long-term maintenance study, in which subjects received INVEGA® at daily doses within the range of 3 mg to 15 mg (n=104), is also included.

The safety of INVEGA® was also evaluated in 622 adult subjects with schizoaffective disorder who participated in two placebo-controlled, 6-week, double-blind trials. In one of these trials, 206 subjects were assigned to one of two dose levels of INVEGA®: 6 mg with the option to reduce to 3 mg (n = 108) or 12 mg with the option to reduce to 9 mg (n = 98) once daily. In the other study, 214 subjects received flexible doses of INVEGA® (3–12 mg once daily). Both studies included subjects who received INVEGA® either as monotherapy or as an adjunct to mood stabilizers and/or antidepressants. Adverse events during exposure to study treatment were obtained by general inquiry and recorded by clinical investigators using their own terminology. Consequently, to provide a meaningful estimate of the proportion of individuals experiencing adverse events, events were grouped in standardized categories using MedDRA terminology.

Throughout this section, adverse reactions are reported. Adverse reactions are adverse events that were considered to be reasonably associated with the use of INVEGA® (adverse drug reactions) based on the comprehensive assessment of the available adverse event information. A causal association for INVEGA® often cannot be reliably established in individual cases. Further, because clinical trials are conducted under widely varying conditions, adverse reaction rates observed in the clinical trials of a drug cannot be directly compared to rates in the clinical trials of another drug and may not reflect the rates observed in clinical practice.

6.1 Commonly-Observed Adverse Reactions in Double-Blind, Placebo-Controlled Clinical Trials - Schizophrenia

Table 1 enumerates the pooled incidences of adverse reactions reported in the three placebo-controlled, 6-week, fixed-dose studies, listing those that occurred in 2% or more of subjects treated with INVEGA® in any of the dose groups, and for which the incidence in INVEGA®-treated subjects in any of the dose groups was greater than the incidence in subjects treated with placebo.

[See table 1 at left]

6.2 Commonly-Observed Adverse Reactions in Double-Blind, Placebo-Controlled Clinical Trials – Schizoaffective Disorder

Table 2 enumerates the pooled incidences of adverse reactions reported in the two placebo-controlled 6-week studies, listing those that occurred in 2% or more of subjects treated with INVEGA® and for which the incidence in INVEGA®-treated subjects was greater than the incidence in subjects treated with placebo.

[See table 2 at top of next page]

Monotherapy versus Adjunctive Therapy

The designs of the two placebo-controlled, 6-week, double-blind trials in subjects with schizoaffective disorder included the option for subjects to receive antidepressants (except monoamine oxidase inhibitors) and/or mood stabilizers (lithium, valproate, or lamotrigine). In the subject population evaluated for safety, 230 (55%) subjects received INVEGA® as monotherapy and 190 (45%) subjects received INVEGA® as an adjunct to mood stabilizers and/or antidepressants. When comparing these 2 subpopulations, only nausea occurred at a greater frequency (≥ 3% difference) in subjects receiving INVEGA® as monotherapy.

6.3 Other Adverse Reactions Observed During Premarketing Evaluation of INVEGA®

The following additional adverse reactions occurred in < 2% of INVEGA®-treated subjects in the above schizophrenia and schizoaffective disorder clinical trial datasets. The following also includes additional adverse reactions reported at any frequency by INVEGA®-treated subjects who participated in other clinical studies.

Cardiac disorders: bradycardia, bundle branch block left, palpitations

Endocrine disorders: hyperprolactinemia

Eye disorders: vision blurred

Gastrointestinal disorders: abdominal pain, flatulence, small intestinal obstruction, swollen tongue

General disorders: edema, edema peripheral

Immune system disorders: anaphylactic reaction

Infections and infestations: urinary tract infection

Investigations: electrocardiogram abnormal

Musculoskeletal and connective tissue disorders: arthralgia, pain in extremity

Nervous system disorders: cerebrovascular accident, convulsion, dizziness postural, grand mal convulsion, lethargy, syncope, transient ischemic attack, additional extrapyramidal symptoms (cogwheel rigidity, muscle spasms, musculoskeletal pain, torticollis, trismus)

Psychiatric disorders: agitation, nightmare

Reproductive system and breast disorders: amenorrhea, breast discharge, breast engorgement, breast tenderness, breast pain, erectile dysfunction, galactorrhea, gynecomastia, menstruation irregular, retrograde ejaculation

Respiratory, thoracic and mediastinal disorders: nasal congestion, pneumonia aspiration

Skin and subcutaneous tissue disorders: pruritus, rash, rash papular

Vascular disorders: hypotension, ischemia

6.4 Discontinuations Due to Adverse Reactions

Schizophrenia Trials

The percentages of subjects who discontinued due to adverse reactions in the three schizophrenia placebo-controlled, 6-week, fixed-dose studies were 3% and 1% in INVEGA®- and placebo-treated subjects, respectively. The most common reasons for discontinuation were nervous system disorders (2% and 0% in INVEGA®- and placebo-treated subjects, respectively).

Schizoaffective Disorder Trials

The percentages of subjects who discontinued due to adverse reactions in the two schizoaffective disorder placebo-controlled 6-week studies were 1% and <1% in INVEGA®- and placebo-treated subjects, respectively. The most common reasons for discontinuation were gastrointestinal disorders (1% and 0% in INVEGA®- and placebo-treated subjects, respectively).

6.5 Dose-Related Adverse Reactions

Schizophrenia Trials

Based on the pooled data from the three placebo-controlled, 6-week, fixed-dose studies in subjects with schizophrenia, among the adverse reactions that occurred with a greater than 2% incidence in the subjects treated with INVEGA®, the incidences of the following adverse reactions increased with dose: somnolence, orthostatic hypotension, akathisia, dystonia, extrapyramidal disorder, hypertonia, parkinsonism, and salivary hypersecretion. For most of these, the increased incidence was seen primarily at the 12 mg dose, and, in some cases, the 9 mg dose.

Schizoaffective Disorder Trials

In a placebo-controlled, 6-week, high- and low-dose study in subjects with schizoaffective disorder, akathisia, dystonia, dysarthria, myalgia, nasopharyngitis, rhinitis, cough, and pharyngolaryngeal pain occurred more frequently (i.e., a difference of at least 2%) in subjects who received higher doses of INVEGA® compared with subjects who received lower doses.

6.6 Demographic Differences

An examination of population subgroups in the three placebo-controlled, 6-week, fixed-dose studies in subjects with schizophrenia and in the two placebo-controlled, 6-week studies in subjects with schizoaffective disorder did not reveal any evidence of clinically relevant differences in safety on the basis of gender or race alone; there was also no difference on the basis of age [see Use in Specific Populations (8.5)].

6.7 Extrapyramidal Symptoms (EPS)

Pooled data from the three placebo-controlled, 6-week, fixed-dose studies in subjects with schizophrenia provided information regarding treatment-emergent EPS. Several methods were used to measure EPS: (1) the Simpson-Angus global score (mean change from baseline) which broadly evaluates Parkinsonism, (2) the Barnes Akathisia Rating Scale global clinical rating score (mean change from baseline) which evaluates akathisia, (3) use of anticholinergic medications to treat emergent EPS (Table 3), and (4) incidence of spontaneous reports of EPS (Table 4). For the Simpson-Angus Scale, spontaneous EPS reports and use of anticholinergic medications, there was a dose-related increase observed for the 9 mg and 12 mg doses. There was no difference observed between placebo and INVEGA® 3 mg and 6 mg doses for any of these EPS measures.
[See table 3 above]
[See table 4 at top of next page]

Table 2. Adverse Drug Reactions Reported by ≥ 2% of INVEGA®-Treated Subjects with Schizoaffective Disorder in Two Double-Blind, Placebo-Controlled Clinical Trials*

Body System or Organ Class Dictionary-Derived Term	Placebo (N=202)	INVEGA® 3–6 mg once-daily fixed-dose range (N=108)	INVEGA® 9–12 mg once-daily fixed-dose range (N=98)	INVEGA® 3–12 mg once-daily flexible dose (N=214)
Total percentage of subjects with adverse reactions	32	48	50	43
Cardiac disorders				
Tachycardia	2	3	1	2
Gastrointestinal disorders				
Abdominal discomfort/Abdominal pain upper	1	1	0	3
Constipation	2	4	5	4
Dyspepsia	2	5	6	6
Nausea	6	8	8	5
Stomach discomfort	1	0	1	2
General disorders				
Asthenia	1	3	4	<1
Infections and Infestations				
Nasopharyngitis	1	2	5	3
Rhinitis	0	1	3	1
Upper respiratory tract infection	1	2	2	2
Investigations				
Weight increased	1	5	4	4
Metabolism and nutrition disorders				
Decreased appetite	<1	1	0	2
Increased appetite	<1	3	2	2
Musculoskeletal and connective tissue disorders				
Back pain	1	1	1	3
Myalgia	<1	2	4	1
Nervous system disorders				
Akathisia	4	4	6	6
Dysarthria	0	1	4	2
Extrapyramidal symptoms	8	20	17	12
Somnolence	5	12	12	8
Psychiatric disorders				
Sleep disorder	<1	2	3	0
Respiratory, thoracic and mediastinal disorders				
Cough	1	1	3	1
Pharyngolaryngeal pain	<1	0	2	1

*Table includes adverse reactions that were reported in 2% or more of subjects in any of the INVEGA® dose groups and which occurred at greater incidence than in the placebo group. Data are pooled from two studies. One study included once-daily INVEGA® doses of 6 mg (with the option to reduce to 3 mg) and 12 mg (with the option to reduce to 9 mg). The second study included flexible once-daily doses of 3 to 12 mg. Among the 420 subjects treated with INVEGA®, 230 (55%) received INVEGA® as monotherapy and 190 (45%) received INVEGA® as an adjunct to mood stabilizers and/or antidepressants. Extrapyramidal symptoms includes the terms bradykinesia, drooling, dyskinesia, dystonia, hypertonia, muscle rigidity, muscle twitching, oculogyration, parkinsonian gait, parkinsonism, restlessness, and tremor. Somnolence includes the terms sedation and somnolence. Tachycardia includes the terms tachycardia, sinus tachycardia, and heart rate increased.

Table 3. Treatment-Emergent Extrapyramidal Symptoms (EPS) Assessed by Incidence of Ratings Scales and Use of Anticholinergic Medication – Schizophrenia Studies

EPS Group	Placebo (N=355)	INVEGA® 3 mg once daily (N=127)	INVEGA® 6 mg once daily (N=235)	INVEGA® 9 mg once daily (N=246)	INVEGA® 12 mg once daily (N=242)
Parkinsonism*	9	11	3	15	14
Akathisia†	6	6	4	7	9
Use of anticholinergic medications‡	10	10	9	22	22

*For Parkinsonism, percent of patients with Simpson-Angus global score > 0.3 (Global score defined as total sum of items score divided by the number of items)
†For Akathisia, percent of patients with Barnes Akathisia Rating Scale global score ≥ 2
‡Percent of patients who received anticholinergic medications to treat emergent EPS

Compared to data from the studies in schizophrenia, pooled data from the two placebo-controlled 6-week studies in subjects with schizoaffective disorder showed similar types and frequencies of EPS as measured by rating scales, anticholinergic medication use, and spontaneous reports of EPS-related adverse events. For subjects with schizoaffective disorder, there was no dose-related increase in EPS observed for parkinsonism with the Simpson-Angus scale or akathisia with the Barnes Akathisia Rating Scale. There was a dose-related increase observed with spontaneous EPS reports of hyperkinesia and dystonia and in the use of anticholinergic medications.

Table 5 shows the EPS data from the pooled schizoaffective disorder trials.
[See table 5 on next page]

Dystonia

Class Effect: Symptoms of dystonia, prolonged abnormal contractions of muscle groups, may occur in susceptible individuals during the first few days of treatment. Dystonic symptoms include: spasm of the neck muscles, sometimes progressing to tightness of the throat, swallowing difficulty, difficulty breathing, and/or protrusion of the tongue. While these symptoms can occur at low doses, they occur more frequently and with greater severity with high potency and at higher doses of first generation antipsychotic drugs. An elevated risk of acute dystonia is observed in males and younger age groups.

6.8 Laboratory Test Abnormalities

In the pooled data from the three placebo-controlled, 6-week, fixed-dose studies in subjects with schizophrenia and from the two placebo-controlled, 6-week studies in subjects with schizoaffective disorder, between-group comparisons revealed no medically important differences between INVEGA® and placebo in the proportions of subjects experiencing potentially clinically significant changes in routine serum chemistry, hematology, or urinalysis parameters. Similarly, there were no differences between INVEGA® and placebo in the incidence of discontinuations due to changes in hematology, urinalysis, or serum chemistry,

Table 4. Treatment-Emergent Extrapyramidal Symptoms (EPS)-Related Adverse Events by MedDRA Preferred Term – Schizophrenia Studies

EPS Group	Placebo (N=355)	INVEGA® 3 mg once daily (N=127)	INVEGA® 6 mg once daily (N=235)	INVEGA® 9 mg once daily (N=246)	INVEGA® 12 mg once daily (N=242)
		Percentage of Patients			
Overall percentage of patients with EPS-related AE	11	13	10	25	26
Dyskinesia	3	5	3	8	9
Dystonia	1	1	1	5	5
Hyperkinesia	4	4	3	8	10
Parkinsonism	2	3	3	7	6
Tremor	3	3	3	4	3

Dyskinesia group includes: Dyskinesia, extrapyramidal disorder, muscle twitching, tardive dyskinesia
Dystonia group includes: Dystonia, muscle spasms, oculogyration, trismus
Hyperkinesia group includes: Akathisia, hyperkinesia
Parkinsonism group includes: Bradykinesia, cogwheel rigidity, drooling, hypertonia, hypokinesia, muscle rigidity, musculoskeletal stiffness, parkinsonism
Tremor group includes: Tremor

Table 5. Treatment-Emergent Extrapyramidal Symptoms (EPS)-Related Adverse Events by MedDRA Preferred Term – Schizoaffective Disorder Studies

EPS Group	Placebo (N=202)	INVEGA® 3–6 mg once-daily fixed-dose range (N=108)	INVEGA® 9–12 mg once-daily fixed-dose range (N=98)	INVEGA® 3–12 mg once-daily flexible dose (N=214)
		Percentage of Patients		
Overall percentage of patients with EPS-related AE	11	23	22	17
Dyskinesia	1	3	1	1
Dystonia	1	2	3	2
Hyperkinesia	5	5	8	7
Parkinsonism	3	14	7	7
Tremor	3	12	11	5

Dyskinesia group includes: Dyskinesia, muscle twitching
Dystonia group includes: Dystonia, muscle spasms, oculogyration
Hyperkinesia group includes: Akathisia, hyperkinesia, restlessness
Parkinsonism group includes: Bradykinesia, drooling, hypertonia, muscle rigidity, muscle tightness, musculoskeletal stiffness, parkinsonian gait, parkinsonism
Tremor group includes: Tremor

including mean changes from baseline in fasting glucose, insulin, c-peptide, triglyceride, HDL, LDL, and total cholesterol measurements. However, INVEGA® was associated with increases in serum prolactin [see Warnings and Precautions (5.7)].

6.9 Weight Gain
Schizophrenia Trials
In the pooled data from the three placebo-controlled, 6-week, fixed-dose studies in subjects with schizophrenia, the proportions of subjects meeting a weight gain criterion of ≥ 7% of body weight were compared, revealing a similar incidence of weight gain for INVEGA® 3 mg and 6 mg (7% and 6%, respectively) compared with placebo (5%), and a higher incidence of weight gain for INVEGA® 9 mg and 12 mg (9% and 9%, respectively).
Schizoaffective Disorder Trials
In the pooled data from the two placebo-controlled, 6-week studies in subjects with schizoaffective disorder, a higher percentage of INVEGA®-treated subjects (5%) had an increase in body weight of ≥ 7% compared with placebo-treated subjects (1%). In the study that examined high- and low-dose groups, the increase in body weight of ≥ 7% was 3% in the low-dose group, 7% in the high-dose group, and 1% in the placebo group.

6.10 Other Findings Observed During Clinical Trials
The safety of INVEGA® was also evaluated in a long-term trial designed to assess the maintenance of effect with INVEGA® in adults with schizophrenia [see Clinical Studies (14)]. In general, adverse reaction types, frequencies, and severities during the initial 14-week open-label phase of this study were comparable to those observed in the 6-week, placebo-controlled, fixed-dose studies. Adverse reactions reported during the long-term double-blind phase of this study were similar in type and severity to those observed in the initial 14-week open-label phase.

6.11 Postmarketing Experience
The following adverse reactions have been identified during postapproval use of INVEGA®; because these reactions were reported voluntarily from a population of uncertain size, it is not possible to reliably estimate their frequency: angioedema, priapism, swollen tongue, tardive dyskinesia, urinary incontinence, urinary retention.

6.12 Adverse Reactions Reported With Risperidone
Paliperidone is the major active metabolite of risperidone. Adverse reactions reported with risperidone can be found in the ADVERSE REACTIONS section of the risperidone package insert.

7 DRUG INTERACTIONS
7.1 Potential for INVEGA® to Affect Other Drugs
Given the primary CNS effects of paliperidone [see Adverse Reactions (6.1, 6.2)], INVEGA® should be used with caution in combination with other centrally acting drugs and alcohol. Paliperidone may antagonize the effect of levodopa and other dopamine agonists.
Because of its potential for inducing orthostatic hypotension, an additive effect may be observed when INVEGA® is administered with other therapeutic agents that have this potential [see Warnings and Precautions (5.9)].
Paliperidone is not expected to cause clinically important pharmacokinetic interactions with drugs that are metabolized by cytochrome P450 isozymes. In vitro studies in human liver microsomes showed that paliperidone does not substantially inhibit the metabolism of drugs metabolized by cytochrome P450 isozymes, including CYP1A2, CYP2A6, CYP2C8/9/10, CYP2D6, CYP2E1, CYP3A4, and CYP3A5. Therefore, paliperidone is not expected to inhibit clearance of drugs that are metabolized by these metabolic pathways in a clinically relevant manner. Paliperidone is also not expected to have enzyme inducing properties.
Paliperidone is a weak inhibitor of P-glycoprotein (P-gp) at high concentrations. No in vivo data are available and the clinical relevance is unknown.
Pharmacokinetic interaction between lithium and INVEGA® is unlikely.
In a clinical study, subjects on a stable dose of valproate showed comparable valproate average plasma concentrations when 3–15 mg of INVEGA® was added to their existing valproate treatment.

7.2 Potential for Other Drugs to Affect INVEGA®
Paliperidone is not a substrate of CYP1A2, CYP2A6, CYP2C9, and CYP2C19, so that an interaction with inhibitors or inducers of these isozymes is unlikely. While in vitro studies indicate that CYP2D6 and CYP3A4 may be mini-

mally involved in paliperidone metabolism, in vivo studies do not show decreased elimination by these isozymes and they contribute to only a small fraction of total body clearance. In vitro studies have shown that paliperidone is a P-gp substrate.
Co-administration of INVEGA® 6 mg once daily with carbamazepine 200 mg twice daily caused a decrease of approximately 37% in the mean steady-state C_{max} and AUC of paliperidone. This decrease is caused, to a substantial degree, by a 35% increase in renal clearance of paliperidone. A minor decrease in the amount of drug excreted unchanged in the urine suggests that there was little effect on the CYP metabolism or bioavailability of paliperidone during carbamazepine co-administration. On initiation of carbamazepine, the dose of INVEGA® should be re-evaluated and increased if necessary. Conversely, on discontinuation of carbamazepine, the dose of INVEGA® should be re-evaluated and decreased if necessary.
Paliperidone is metabolized to a limited extent by CYP2D6 [see Clinical Pharmacology (12.3)]. In an interaction study in healthy subjects in which a single 3 mg dose of INVEGA® was administered concomitantly with 20 mg per day of paroxetine (a potent CYP2D6 inhibitor), paliperidone exposures were on average 16% (90% CI: 4, 30) higher in CYP2D6 extensive metabolizers. Higher doses of paroxetine have not been studied. The clinical relevance is unknown.
Co-administration of a single dose of INVEGA® 12 mg with divalproex sodium extended-release tablets (two 500 mg tablets once daily) resulted in an increase of approximately 50% in the C_{max} and AUC of paliperidone. Dosage reduction for INVEGA® should be considered when INVEGA® is co-administered with valproate after clinical assessment.
Pharmacokinetic interaction between lithium and INVEGA® is unlikely.

8 USE IN SPECIFIC POPULATIONS
8.1 Pregnancy
Pregnancy Category C.
There are no adequate and well controlled studies of INVEGA® in pregnant women. INVEGA® should be used during pregnancy only if the potential benefit justifies the potential risk to the fetus.
Use of first generation antipsychotic drugs during the last trimester of pregnancy has been associated with extrapyramidal symptoms in the neonate. These symptoms are usually self-limited. It is not known whether paliperidone, when taken near the end of pregnancy, will lead to similar neonatal signs and symptoms.
In animal reproduction studies, there were no increases in fetal abnormalities when pregnant rats and rabbits were treated during the period of organogenesis with up to 8 times the maximum recommended human dose of paliperidone (on a mg/m² basis).
In rat reproduction studies with risperidone, which is extensively converted to paliperidone in rats and humans, there were increases in pup deaths seen at oral doses which are less than the maximum recommended human dose of risperidone on a mg/m² basis (see risperidone package insert).

8.3 Nursing Mothers
Paliperidone is 9-hydroxyrisperidone, the active metabolite of risperidone. In animal studies, risperidone and 9-hydroxyrisperidone were excreted in milk. Risperidone and 9-hydroxyrisperidone are also excreted in human breast milk. Caution should be exercised when INVEGA® is administered to a nursing woman. The known benefits of breastfeeding should be weighed against the unknown risks of infant exposure to paliperidone.

8.4 Pediatric Use
Safety and effectiveness of INVEGA® in patients < 18 years of age have not been established.

8.5 Geriatric Use
The safety, tolerability, and efficacy of INVEGA® were evaluated in a 6-week placebo-controlled study of 114 elderly subjects with schizophrenia (65 years of age and older, of whom 21 were 75 years of age and older). In this study, subjects received flexible doses of INVEGA® (3 mg to 12 mg once daily). In addition, a small number of subjects 65 years of age and older were included in the 6-week placebo-controlled studies in which adult schizophrenic subjects received fixed doses of INVEGA® (3 mg to 15 mg once daily) [see Clinical Studies (14)]. There were no subjects ≥ 65 years of age in the schizoaffective disorder studies.
Overall, of the total number of subjects in schizophrenia clinical studies of INVEGA® (n = 1796), including those who received INVEGA® or placebo, 125 (7.0%) were 65 years of age and older and 22 (1.2%) were 75 years of age and older. No overall differences in safety or effectiveness were observed between these subjects and younger subjects, and other reported clinical experience has not identified differences in response between the elderly and younger patients, but greater sensitivity of some older individuals cannot be ruled out.
This drug is known to be substantially excreted by the kidney and clearance is decreased in patients with moderate to severe renal impairment [see Clinical Pharmacology (12.3)],

who should be given reduced doses. Because elderly patients are more likely to have decreased renal function, care should be taken in dose selection, and it may be useful to monitor renal function *[see Dosage and Administration (2.5)]*.

8.6 Renal Impairment

Dosing must be individualized according to the patient's renal function status *[see Dosage and Administration (2.5)]*.

8.7 Hepatic Impairment

No dosage adjustment is required in patients with mild to moderate hepatic impairment. INVEGA® has not been studied in patients with severe hepatic impairment.

9 DRUG ABUSE AND DEPENDENCE

9.1 Controlled Substance

INVEGA® (paliperidone) is not a controlled substance.

9.2 Abuse

Paliperidone has not been systematically studied in animals or humans for its potential for abuse. It is not possible to predict the extent to which a CNS-active drug will be misused, diverted, and/or abused once marketed. Consequently, patients should be evaluated carefully for a history of drug abuse, and such patients should be observed closely for signs of INVEGA® misuse or abuse (e.g., development of tolerance, increases in dose, drug-seeking behavior).

9.3 Dependence

Paliperidone has not been systematically studied in animals or humans for its potential for tolerance or physical dependence.

10 OVERDOSAGE

10.1 Human Experience

While experience with paliperidone overdose is limited, among the few cases of overdose reported in pre-marketing trials, the highest estimated ingestion of INVEGA® was 405 mg. Observed signs and symptoms included extrapyramidal symptoms and gait unsteadiness. Other potential signs and symptoms include those resulting from an exaggeration of paliperidone's known pharmacological effects, i.e., drowsiness and somnolence, tachycardia and hypotension, and QT prolongation. Torsade de pointes and ventricular fibrillation have been reported in a patient in the setting of overdose.

Paliperidone is the major active metabolite of risperidone. Overdose experience reported with risperidone can be found in the OVERDOSAGE section of the risperidone package insert.

10.2 Management of Overdosage

There is no specific antidote to paliperidone, therefore, appropriate supportive measures should be instituted and close medical supervision and monitoring should continue until the patient recovers. Consideration should be given to the extended-release nature of the product when assessing treatment needs and recovery. Multiple drug involvement should also be considered.

In case of acute overdose, establish and maintain an airway and ensure adequate oxygenation and ventilation. Gastric lavage (after intubation if patient is unconscious) and administration of activated charcoal together with a laxative should be considered.

The possibility of obtundation, seizures, or dystonic reaction of the head and neck following overdose may create a risk of aspiration with induced emesis.

Cardiovascular monitoring should commence immediately, including continuous electrocardiographic monitoring for possible arrhythmias. If antiarrhythmic therapy is administered, disopyramide, procainamide, and quinidine carry a theoretical hazard of additive QT-prolonging effects when administered in patients with an acute overdose of paliperidone. Similarly the alpha-blocking properties of bretylium might be additive to those of paliperidone, resulting in problematic hypotension.

Hypotension and circulatory collapse should be treated with appropriate measures, such as intravenous fluids and/or sympathomimetic agents (epinephrine and dopamine should not be used, since beta stimulation may worsen hypotension in the setting of paliperidone-induced alpha blockade). In cases of severe extrapyramidal symptoms, anticholinergic medication should be administered.

11 DESCRIPTION

Paliperidone, the active ingredient in INVEGA® Extended-Release Tablets, is a psychotropic agent belonging to the chemical class of benzisoxazole derivatives. INVEGA® contains a racemic mixture of (+)- and (-)- paliperidone. The chemical name is (±)-3-[2-[4-(6-fluoro-1,2-benzisoxazol-3-yl)-1-piperidinyl]ethyl]-6,7,8,9-tetrahydro-9-hydroxy-2-methyl-4H-pyrido[1,2-a]pyrimidin-4-one. Its molecular formula is $C_{23}H_{27}FN_4O_3$ and its molecular weight is 426.49. The structural formula is:

[See chemical structure at top of next column]

Paliperidone is sparingly soluble in 0.1N HCl and methylene chloride; practically insoluble in water, 0.1N NaOH, and hexane; and slightly soluble in N,N-dimethylformamide.

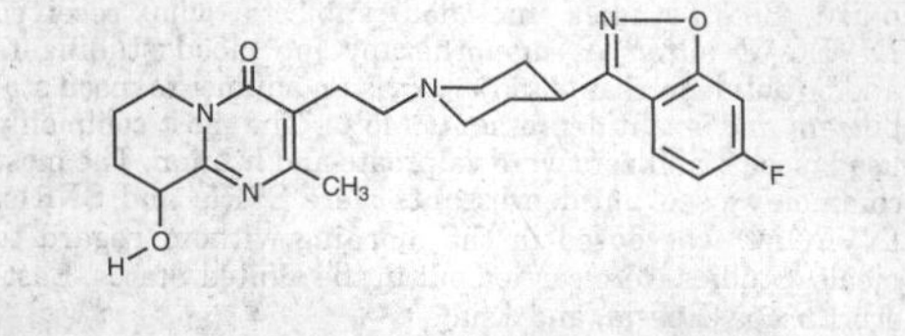

INVEGA® (paliperidone) Extended-Release Tablets are available in 1.5 mg (orange-brown), 3 mg (white), 6 mg (beige), and 9 mg (pink) strengths. INVEGA® utilizes OROS® osmotic drug-release technology *[see Description (11.1)]*.

Inactive ingredients are carnauba wax, cellulose acetate, hydroxyethyl cellulose, propylene glycol, polyethylene glycol, polyethylene oxides, povidone, sodium chloride, stearic acid, butylated hydroxytoluene, hypromellose, titanium dioxide, and iron oxides. The 3 mg tablets also contain lactose monohydrate and triacetin.

11.1 Delivery System Components and Performance

INVEGA® uses osmotic pressure to deliver paliperidone at a controlled rate. The delivery system, which resembles a capsule-shaped tablet in appearance, consists of an osmotically active trilayer core surrounded by a subcoat and semipermeable membrane. The trilayer core is composed of two drug layers containing the drug and excipients, and a push layer containing osmotically active components. There are two precision laser-drilled orifices on the drug-layer dome of the tablet. Each tablet strength has a different colored water-dispersible overcoat and print markings. In an aqueous environment, such as the gastrointestinal tract, the water-dispersible color overcoat erodes quickly. Water then enters the tablet through the semipermeable membrane that controls the rate at which water enters the tablet core, which, in turn, determines the rate of drug delivery. The hydrophilic polymers of the core hydrate and swell, creating a gel containing paliperidone that is then pushed out through the tablet orifices. The biologically inert components of the tablet remain intact during gastrointestinal transit and are eliminated in the stool as a tablet shell, along with insoluble core components.

12 CLINICAL PHARMACOLOGY

12.1 Mechanism of Action

Paliperidone is the major active metabolite of risperidone. The mechanism of action of paliperidone, as with other drugs having efficacy in schizophrenia, is unknown, but it has been proposed that the drug's therapeutic activity in schizophrenia is mediated through a combination of central dopamine Type 2 (D_2) and serotonin Type 2 ($5HT_{2A}$) receptor antagonism.

12.2 Pharmacodynamics

Paliperidone is a centrally active dopamine Type 2 (D_2) antagonist and with predominant serotonin Type 2 ($5HT_{2A}$) activity. Paliperidone is also active as an antagonist at α_1 and α_2 adrenergic receptors and H_1 histaminergic receptors, which may explain some of the other effects of the drug. Paliperidone has no affinity for cholinergic muscarinic or β_1- and β_2-adrenergic receptors. The pharmacological activity of the (+)- and (-)- paliperidone enantiomers is qualitatively and quantitatively similar *in vitro*.

12.3 Pharmacokinetics

Following a single dose, the plasma concentrations of paliperidone gradually rise to reach peak plasma concentration (C_{max}) approximately 24 hours after dosing. The pharmacokinetics of paliperidone following INVEGA® administration are dose-proportional within the available dose range. The terminal elimination half-life of paliperidone is approximately 23 hours.

Steady-state concentrations of paliperidone are attained within 4–5 days of dosing with INVEGA® in most subjects. The mean steady-state peak:trough ratio for an INVEGA® dose of 9 mg was 1.7 with a range of 1.2–3.1.

Following administration of INVEGA®, the (+) and (-) enantiomers of paliperidone interconvert, reaching an AUC (+) to (-) ratio of approximately 1.6 at steady state.

Absorption and Distribution

The absolute oral bioavailability of paliperidone following INVEGA® administration is 28%.

Administration of a 12 mg paliperidone extended-release tablet to healthy ambulatory subjects with a standard high-fat/high-caloric meal gave mean C_{max} and AUC values of paliperidone that were increased by 60% and 54%, respectively, compared with administration under fasting conditions. Clinical trials establishing the safety and efficacy of INVEGA® were carried out in subjects without regard to the timing of meals. While INVEGA® can be taken without regard to food, the presence of food at the time of INVEGA® administration may increase exposure to paliperidone *[see Dosage and Administration (2.3)]*.

Based on a population analysis, the apparent volume of distribution of paliperidone is 487 L. The plasma protein binding of racemic paliperidone is 74%.

Metabolism and Elimination

Although *in vitro* studies suggested a role for CYP2D6 and CYP3A4 in the metabolism of paliperidone, *in vivo* results indicate that these isozymes play a limited role in the overall elimination of paliperidone *[see Drug Interactions (7)]*.

One week following administration of a single oral dose of 1 mg immediate-release ^{14}C-paliperidone to 5 healthy volunteers, 59% (range 51%–67%) of the dose was excreted unchanged into urine, 32% (26%–41%) of the dose was recovered as metabolites, and 6%–12% of the dose was not recovered. Approximately 80% of the administered radioactivity was recovered in urine and 11% in the feces. Four primary metabolic pathways have been identified *in vivo*, none of which could be shown to account for more than 10% of the dose: dealkylation, hydroxylation, dehydrogenation, and benzisoxazole scission.

Population pharmacokinetic analyses found no difference in exposure or clearance of paliperidone between extensive metabolizers and poor metabolizers of CYP2D6 substrates.

Special Populations

Renal Impairment

The dose of INVEGA® should be reduced in patients with moderate or severe renal impairment *[see Dosage and Administration (2.5)]*. The disposition of a single dose paliperidone 3 mg extended-release tablet was studied in subjects with varying degrees of renal function. Elimination of paliperidone decreased with decreasing estimated creatinine clearance. Total clearance of paliperidone was reduced in subjects with impaired renal function by 32% on average in mild (CrCl = 50 mL/min to < 80 mL/min), 64% in moderate (CrCl = 30 mL/min to < 50 mL/min), and 71% in severe (CrCl = 10 mL/min to < 30 mL/min) renal impairment, corresponding to an average increase in exposure (AUCinf) of 1.5 fold, 2.6 fold, and 4.8 fold, respectively, compared to healthy subjects. The mean terminal elimination half-life of paliperidone was 24 hours, 40 hours, and 51 hours in subjects with mild, moderate, and severe renal impairment, respectively, compared with 23 hours in subjects with normal renal function (CrCl ≥ 80 mL/min).

Hepatic Impairment

In a study in subjects with moderate hepatic impairment (Child-Pugh class B), the plasma concentrations of free paliperidone were similar to those of healthy subjects, although total paliperidone exposure decreased because of a decrease in protein binding. Consequently, no dose adjustment is required in patients with mild or moderate hepatic impairment. INVEGA® has not been studied in patients with severe hepatic impairment.

Elderly

No dosage adjustment is recommended based on age alone. However, dose adjustment may be required because of age-related decreases in creatinine clearance *[see Renal Impairment above and Dosage and Administration (2.1, 2.5)]*.

Race

No dosage adjustment is recommended based on race. No differences in pharmacokinetics were observed in a pharmacokinetic study conducted in Japanese and Caucasians.

Gender

No dosage adjustment is recommended based on gender. No differences in pharmacokinetics were observed in a pharmacokinetic study conducted in men and women.

Smoking

No dosage adjustment is recommended based on smoking status. Based on in vitro studies utilizing human liver enzymes, paliperidone is not a substrate for CYP1A2; smoking should, therefore, not have an effect on the pharmacokinetics of paliperidone.

13 NONCLINICAL TOXICOLOGY

13.1 Carcinogenesis, Mutagenesis, Impairment of Fertility

Carcinogenesis

Carcinogenicity studies of paliperidone have not been performed.

Carcinogenicity studies of risperidone, which is extensively converted to paliperidone in rats, mice, and humans, were conducted in Swiss albino mice and Wistar rats. Risperidone was administered in the diet at daily doses of 0.63 mg/kg, 2.5 mg/kg, and 10 mg/kg for 18 months to mice and for 25 months to rats. A maximum tolerated dose was not achieved in male mice. There were statistically significant increases in pituitary gland adenomas, endocrine pancreas adenomas, and mammary gland adenocarcinomas. The no-effect dose for these tumors was less than or equal to the maximum recommended human dose of risperidone on a mg/m^2 basis (see risperidone package insert). An increase in mammary, pituitary, and endocrine pancreas neoplasms has been found in rodents after chronic administration of other antipsychotic drugs and is considered to be mediated by prolonged dopamine D2 antagonism and hyperprolactinemia. The relevance of these tumor findings in rodents in terms of human risk is unknown *[see Warnings and Precautions (5.7)]*.

Mutagenesis

No evidence of genotoxic potential for paliperidone was found in the Ames reverse mutation test, the mouse lymphoma assay, or the *in vivo* rat micronucleus test.

Impairment of Fertility

In a study of fertility, the percentage of treated female rats that became pregnant was not affected at oral doses of paliperidone of up to 2.5 mg/kg/day. However, pre- and post-implantation loss was increased, and the number of live embryos was slightly decreased, at 2.5 mg/kg, a dose that also caused slight maternal toxicity. These parameters were not affected at a dose of 0.63 mg/kg, which is half of the maximum recommended human dose on a mg/m² basis.

The fertility of male rats was not affected at oral doses of paliperidone of up to 2.5 mg/kg/day, although sperm count and sperm viability studies were not conducted with paliperidone. In a subchronic study in Beagle dogs with risperidone, which is extensively converted to paliperidone in dogs and humans, all doses tested (0.31 mg/kg–5.0 mg/kg) resulted in decreases in serum testosterone and in sperm motility and concentration. Serum testosterone and sperm parameters partially recovered, but remained decreased after the last observation (two months after treatment was discontinued).

14 CLINICAL STUDIES

14.1 Schizophrenia

The acute efficacy of INVEGA® (3 mg to 15 mg once daily) was established in three placebo-controlled and active-controlled (olanzapine), 6-week, fixed-dose trials in non-elderly adult subjects (mean age of 37) who met DSM-IV criteria for schizophrenia. Studies were carried out in North America, Eastern Europe, Western Europe, and Asia. The doses studied among these three trials included 3 mg/day, 6 mg/day, 9 mg/day, 12 mg/day, and 15 mg/day. Dosing was in the morning without regard to meals.

Efficacy was evaluated using the Positive and Negative Syndrome Scale (PANSS), a validated multi-item inventory composed of five factors to evaluate positive symptoms, negative symptoms, disorganized thoughts, uncontrolled hostility/excitement, and anxiety/depression. Efficacy was also evaluated using the Personal and Social Performance (PSP) scale. The PSP is a validated clinician-rated scale that measures personal and social functioning in the domains of socially useful activities (e.g., work and study), personal and social relationships, self-care, and disturbing and aggressive behaviors.

In all 3 studies (n = 1665), INVEGA® was superior to placebo on the PANSS at all doses. Mean effects at all doses were fairly similar, although the higher doses in all studies were numerically superior. INVEGA® was also superior to placebo on the PSP in these trials.

An examination of population subgroups did not reveal any evidence of differential responsiveness on the basis of gender, age (there were few patients over 65), or geographic region. There were insufficient data to explore differential effects based on race.

In a longer-term trial, adult outpatients meeting DSM-IV criteria for schizophrenia who had clinically responded (defined as PANSS score ≤ 70 or ≤ 4 on pre-defined PANSS subscales, as well as having been on a stable fixed dose of INVEGA® for the last two weeks of an 8-week run-in phase) were entered into a 6-week open-label stabilization phase where they received INVEGA® (doses ranging from 3 mg to 15 mg once daily). After the stabilization phase, patients were randomized in a double-blind manner to either continue on INVEGA® at their achieved stable dose, or to placebo, until they experienced a relapse of schizophrenia symptoms. Relapse was pre-defined as significant increase in PANSS (or pre-defined PANSS subscales), hospitalization, clinically significant suicidal or homicidal ideation, or deliberate injury to self or others. An interim analysis of the data showed a significantly longer time to relapse in patients treated with INVEGA® compared to placebo, and the trial was stopped early because maintenance of efficacy was demonstrated.

14.2 Schizoaffective Disorder

The acute efficacy of INVEGA® (3 mg to 12 mg once daily) in the treatment of schizoaffective disorder was established in two placebo-controlled, 6–week trials in non-elderly adult subjects. Enrolled subjects 1) met DSM-IV criteria for schizoaffective disorder, as confirmed by the Structured Clinical Interview for DSM-IV Disorders, 2) had a Positive and Negative Syndrome Scale (PANSS) total score of at least 60, and 3) had prominent mood symptoms as confirmed by a score of at least 16 on the Young Mania Rating Scale and/or Hamilton Rating Scale for Depression. The population included subjects with schizoaffective bipolar and depressive types. In one of these trials, efficacy was assessed in 211 subjects who received flexible doses of INVEGA® (3-12 mg once daily). In the other study, efficacy was assessed in 203 subjects who were assigned to one of two dose levels of INVEGA®: 6 mg with the option to reduce to 3 mg (n = 105) or 12 mg with the option to reduce to 9 mg (n = 98) once

daily. Both studies included subjects who received INVEGA® either as monotherapy [no mood stabilizers and/or antidepressants (55%)] or as an adjunct to mood stabilizers and/or antidepressants (45%). The most commonly used mood stabilizers were valproate and lithium. The most commonly used antidepressants were SSRIs and SNRIs. INVEGA® was dosed in the morning without regard to meals. Studies were carried out in the United States, Eastern Europe, Russia, and Asia.

Efficacy was evaluated using the PANSS, a validated multi-item inventory composed of five factors to evaluate positive symptoms, negative symptoms, disorganized thoughts, uncontrolled hostility/excitement, and anxiety/depression. As secondary outcomes, mood symptoms were evaluated using the Hamilton Depression Rating Scale (HAM-D-21) and the Young Mania Rating Scale (YMRS).

The INVEGA® group in the flexible-dose study (dosed between 3 and 12 mg/day, mean modal dose of 8.6 mg/day) and the higher dose group of INVEGA® in the 2 dose-level study (12 mg/day with option to reduce to 9 mg/day) were each superior to placebo in the PANSS. Numerical improvements in mood symptoms were also observed, as measured by the HAM-D-21 and YMRS. In the lower dose group of the 2 dose-level study (6 mg/day with option to reduce to 3 mg/day), INVEGA® was not significantly different from placebo as measured by the PANSS.

Taking the results of both studies together, INVEGA® improved the symptoms of schizoaffective disorder at endpoint relative to placebo when administered either as monotherapy or as an adjunct to mood stabilizers and/or antidepressants. An examination of population subgroups did not reveal any evidence of differential responsiveness on the basis of gender, age, or geographic region. There were insufficient data to explore differential effects based on race.

16 HOW SUPPLIED/STORAGE AND HANDLING

INVEGA® (paliperidone) Extended-Release Tablets are available in the following strengths and packages. All tablets are capsule-shaped.

1.5 mg tablets are orange-brown and imprinted with "PAL 1.5", and are available in bottles of 30 (NDC 50458-554-01).

3 mg tablets are white and imprinted with "PAL 3", and are available in bottles of 30 (NDC 50458-550-01) and hospital unit dose packs of 100 (NDC 50458-550-10).

6 mg tablets are beige and imprinted with "PAL 6", and are available in bottles of 30 (NDC 50458-551-01) and hospital unit dose packs of 100 (NDC 50458-551-10).

9 mg tablets are pink and imprinted with "PAL 9", and are available in bottles of 30 (NDC 50458-552-01) and hospital unit dose packs of 100 (NDC 50458-552-10).

Storage and Handling

Store up to 25°C (77°F); excursions permitted to 15–30°C (59–86°F) [see USP Controlled Room Temperature]. Protect from moisture.

Keep out of reach of children.

17 PATIENT COUNSELING INFORMATION

Physicians are advised to discuss the following issues with patients for whom they prescribe INVEGA®.

17.1 Orthostatic Hypotension

Patients should be advised that there is risk of orthostatic hypotension, particularly at the time of initiating treatment, re-initiating treatment, or increasing the dose [see Warnings and Precautions (5.9)].

17.2 Interference with Cognitive and Motor Performance

As INVEGA® has the potential to impair judgment, thinking, or motor skills, patients should be cautioned about operating hazardous machinery, including automobiles, until they are reasonably certain that INVEGA® therapy does not affect them adversely [see Warnings and Precautions (5.11)].

17.3 Pregnancy

Patients should be advised to notify their physician if they become pregnant or intend to become pregnant during treatment with INVEGA® [see Use in Specific Populations (8.1)].

17.4 Nursing

Caution should be exercised when INVEGA® is administered to a nursing woman. The known benefits of breast-feeding should be weighed against the unknown risks of infant exposure to paliperidone. [See Use in Specific Populations (8.3)].

17.5 Concomitant Medication

Patients should be advised to inform their physicians if they are taking, or plan to take, any prescription or over-the-counter drugs, as there is a potential for interactions [see Drug Interactions (7)].

17.6 Alcohol

Patients should be advised to avoid alcohol while taking INVEGA® [see Drug Interactions (7.1)].

17.7 Heat Exposure and Dehydration

Patients should be advised regarding appropriate care in avoiding overheating and dehydration [see Warnings and Precautions (5.17)].

17.8 Administration

Patients should be informed that INVEGA® should be swallowed whole with the aid of liquids. Tablets should not be chewed, divided, or crushed. The medication is contained within a nonabsorbable shell designed to release the drug at a controlled rate. The tablet shell, along with insoluble core components, is eliminated from the body; patients should not be concerned if they occasionally notice something that looks like a tablet in their stool [see Dosage and Administration (2.3)].

INVEGA® (paliperidone) Extended-Release Tablets

Manufactured by:

ALZA Corporation
Vacaville, CA 95688

OR

Janssen Cilag Manufacturing, LLC
Gurabo, Puerto Rico 00778

Manufactured for:

Janssen, Division of Ortho-McNeil-Janssen Pharmaceuticals, Inc.
Titusville, NJ 08560

OROS is a registered trademark of ALZA Corporation

Revised: January 2010

©Ortho-McNeil-Janssen Pharmaceuticals, Inc. 2007

Shown in Product Identification Guide, page 316

INVEGA® SUSTENNA® ℞

[in-ve-ga su-sten-na]
(paliperidone palmitate)
Extended-Release Injectable Suspension

HIGHLIGHTS OF PRESCRIBING INFORMATION

These highlights do not include all the information needed to use INVEGA® SUSTENNA® safely and effectively. See full prescribing information for INVEGA® SUSTENNA®.

INVEGA® SUSTENNA® (paliperidone palmitate)
Extended-Release Injectable Suspension
Initial U.S. Approval: 2006

WARNING: INCREASED MORTALITY IN ELDERLY PATIENTS WITH DEMENTIA-RELATED PSYCHOSIS
See full prescribing information for complete boxed warning.
Elderly patients with dementia-related psychosis treated with antipsychotic drugs are at an increased risk of death. INVEGA® SUSTENNA® is not approved for use in patients with dementia-related psychosis. (5.1)

———INDICATIONS AND USAGE———

INVEGA® SUSTENNA® is an atypical antipsychotic agent indicated for the acute and maintenance treatment of schizophrenia in adults (1)

———DOSAGE AND ADMINISTRATION———

- For patients who have never taken oral paliperidone or oral or injectable risperidone, tolerability should be established with oral paliperidone or oral risperidone prior to initiating treatment with INVEGA® SUSTENNA®. (2.1)
- Initiate INVEGA® SUSTENNA® with a dose of 234 mg on treatment day 1 and 156 mg one week later, both administered in the deltoid muscle. The recommended monthly maintenance dose is 117 mg; some patients may benefit from lower or higher maintenance doses within the recommended range of 39 mg to 234 mg based on individual patient tolerability and/or efficacy. Following the second dose, monthly maintenance doses can be administered in either the deltoid or gluteal muscle. (2.1)
- Administer by intramuscular injection only, using appropriate needle sizes. For deltoid injection, use 1 ½-inch 22G needle for patients ≥ 90 kg (≥ 200 lb) or 1-inch 23G needle for patients < 90 kg (< 200 lb). For gluteal injection, use 1 ½-inch 22G needle regardless of patient weight. (2.3)

———DOSAGE FORMS AND STRENGTHS———

Prefilled syringes containing 39 mg, 78 mg, 117 mg, 156 mg, or 234 mg paliperidone palmitate. (3)

———CONTRAINDICATIONS———

Known hypersensitivity to paliperidone, risperidone, or to any components in the formulation (4)

———WARNINGS AND PRECAUTIONS———

- *Cerebrovascular Adverse Reactions, Including Stroke, in Elderly Patients with Dementia-Related Psychosis:* Increased incidence of cerebrovascular adverse reactions (e.g. stroke, transient ischemic attack, including fatalities). INVEGA® SUSTENNA® is not approved for use in patients with dementia-related psychosis (5.2)
- *Neuroleptic Malignant Syndrome:* Manage with immediate discontinuation of drug and close monitoring (5.3)
- *QT Prolongation:* Increase in QT interval, avoid use with drugs that also increase QT interval and in patients with risk factors for prolonged QT interval (5.4)
- *Tardive Dyskinesia:* Discontinue drug if clinically appropriate (5.5)

- *Hyperglycemia and Diabetes Mellitus:* Monitor glucose regularly in patients with and at risk for diabetes (5.6)
- *Weight Gain:* Significant weight gain has been reported. Monitor weight gain. (5.7)
- *Hyperprolactinemia:* Prolactin elevations occur and persist during chronic administration (5.8)
- *Orthostatic Hypotension and Syncope:* Use with caution in patients with known cardiovascular or cerebrovascular disease and patients predisposed to hypotension (5.9)
- *Leukopenia, Neutropenia, and Agranulocytosis:* has been reported with antipsychotics, including INVEGA®, an oral form of paliperidone. Patients with a history of a clinically significant low white blood cell count (WBC) or a drug-induced leukopenia/neutropenia should have their complete blood count (CBC) monitored frequently during the first few months of therapy and discontinuation of INVEGA® SUSTENNA® should be considered at the first sign of a clinically significant decline in WBC in the absence of other causative factors. (5.10)
- *Potential for Cognitive and Motor Impairment:* Use caution when operating machinery (5.11)
- *Seizures:* Use cautiously in patients with a history of seizures or with conditions that lower the seizure threshold (5.12)
- *Suicide:* Closely supervise high-risk patients (5.14)
- *Administration:* For intramuscular injection only. Avoid inadvertent injection into a blood vessel. (5.18)

————————ADVERSE REACTIONS————————

The most common adverse reactions (incidence ≥ 5% and occurring at least twice as often as placebo) were injection site reactions, somnolence/sedation, dizziness, akathisia, and extrapyramidal disorder. (6)

To report SUSPECTED ADVERSE REACTIONS, contact Janssen, Division of Ortho-McNeil-Janssen Pharmaceuticals, Inc. at 1-800-JANSSEN (1-800-526-7736) or FDA at 1-800-FDA-1088 or www.fda.gov/medwatch

————————DRUG INTERACTIONS————————

- Centrally-acting drugs: Due to CNS effects, use caution in combination. Avoid alcohol. (7.1)
- Drugs that may cause orthostatic hypotension: An additive effect may be observed when co-administered with INVEGA® SUSTENNA®. (7.1)
- Co-administration of oral paliperidone extended release with carbamazepine decreased mean steady-state C_{max} and AUC of paliperidone by approximately 37%. Adjust dose of INVEGA® SUSTENNA® if necessary. (7.2)

————————USE IN SPECIFIC POPULATIONS————————

- Renal impairment: INVEGA® SUSTENNA® has not been systematically studied in patients with renal impairment. For mild renal impairment (creatinine clearance ≥ 50 mL/min to < 80 mL/min), administer 156 mg on treatment day 1 and 117 mg one week later, both administered in the deltoid muscle. Thereafter, follow with monthly injections of 78 mg. in either the deltoid or gluteal muscle. INVEGA® SUSTENNA® is not recommended for use in patients with moderate to severe renal impairment (creatinine clearance < 50 mL/min). (2.5)
- Elderly: same as for younger adults (adjust dose according to renal function status). (2.5)
- Nursing Mothers: should not breastfeed. (8.3)
- Pediatric Use: safety and effectiveness not established in patients less than 18 years of age. (8.4)

See 17 for PATIENT COUNSELING INFORMATION

Revised: 03/2010

———————————————————————

FULL PRESCRIBING INFORMATION: CONTENTS*
WARNING: INCREASED MORTALITY IN ELDERLY PATIENTS WITH DEMENTIA-RELATED PSYCHOSIS

———————————————————————

FULL PRESCRIBING INFORMATION

———————————————————————

WARNING: INCREASED MORTALITY IN ELDERLY PATIENTS WITH DEMENTIA-RELATED PSYCHOSIS
Elderly patients with dementia-related psychosis treated with antipsychotic drugs are at an increased risk of death. Analyses of 17 placebo-controlled trials (modal duration of 10 weeks), largely in patients taking atypical antipsychotic drugs, revealed a risk of death in drug-treated patients of between 1.6 to 1.7 times the risk of death in placebo-treated patients. Over the course of a typical 10-week controlled trial, the rate of death in drug-treated patients was about 4.5%, compared to a rate of about 2.6% in the placebo group. Although the causes of death were varied, most of the deaths appeared to be either cardiovascular (e.g., heart failure, sudden death) or infectious (e.g., pneumonia) in nature. Observational studies suggest that, similar to atypical antipsychotic drugs, treatment with conventional antipsychotic drugs may increase mortality. The extent to which the findings of increased mortality in observational studies may be attributed to the antipsychotic drug as opposed to some characteristic(s) of

the patients is not clear. INVEGA® SUSTENNA® (paliperidone palmitate) is not approved for the treatment of patients with dementia-related psychosis. *[See Warnings and Precautions (5.1)]*

1 INDICATIONS AND USAGE
INVEGA® SUSTENNA® (paliperidone palmitate) is indicated for the acute and maintenance treatment of schizophrenia in adults *[see Clinical Studies (14)]*.

2 DOSAGE AND ADMINISTRATION
2.1 Recommended Dosing
For patients who have never taken oral paliperidone or oral or injectable risperidone, it is recommended to establish tolerability with oral paliperidone or oral risperidone prior to initiating treatment with INVEGA® SUSTENNA®.
Recommended initiation of INVEGA® SUSTENNA® is with a dose of 234 mg on treatment day 1 and 156 mg one week later, both administered in the deltoid muscle. The recommended monthly maintenance dose is 117 mg; some patients may benefit from lower or higher maintenance doses within the recommended range of 39 to 234 mg based on individual patient tolerability and/or efficacy. Following the second dose, monthly maintenance doses can be administered in either the deltoid or gluteal muscle.
Adjustment of the maintenance dose may be made monthly. When making dose adjustments, the prolonged-release characteristics of INVEGA® SUSTENNA® should be considered *[see Clinical Pharmacology (12.3)]*, as the full effect of the dose adjustment may not be evident for several months.
2.2 Missed Doses
Avoiding Missed Doses
It is recommended that the second initiation dose of INVEGA® SUSTENNA® be given one week after the first dose. To avoid a missed dose, patients may be given the second dose 2 days before or after the one-week timepoint. Similarly, the third and subsequent injections after the initiation regimen are recommended to be given monthly. To avoid a missed monthly dose, patients may be given the injection up to 7 days before or after the monthly timepoint.
Missed Dose (1 Month to 6 Weeks)
After initiation, the recommended injection cycle of INVEGA® SUSTENNA® is monthly. If less than 6 weeks have elapsed since the last injection, then the previously stabilized dose should be administered as soon as possible, followed by injections at monthly intervals.
Missed Dose (> 6 Weeks to 6 Months)
If more than 6 weeks have elapsed since the last injection of INVEGA® SUSTENNA®, **resume the same dose the patient was previously stabilized on (unless the patient was stabilized on a dose of 234 mg, then the first two injections should each be 156 mg)** in the following manner: 1) a deltoid injection as soon as practically possible, followed by 2) another deltoid injection (same dose) one week later, and 3) resumption of either deltoid or gluteal dosing at monthly intervals.
Missed Dose (> 6 Months)
If more than 6 months have elapsed since the last injection of INVEGA® SUSTENNA®, initiate dosing as described in Section 2.1 above.
2.3 Administration Instructions
INVEGA® SUSTENNA® is intended for intramuscular use only. Inject slowly, deep into the muscle. Care should be taken to avoid inadvertent injection into a blood vessel. Each injection should be administered by a health care professional. Administration should be in a single injection. Do not administer the dose in divided injections. Do not administer intravascularly or subcutaneously.
The recommended needle size for administration of INVEGA® SUSTENNA® into the deltoid muscle is determined by the patient's weight. For those ≥ 90 kg (≥ 200 lb), the 1½-inch, 22 gauge needle is recommended. For those < 90 kg (< 200 lb), the 1-inch, 23 gauge needle is recommended. Deltoid injections should be alternated between the two deltoid muscles.
The recommended needle size for administration of INVEGA® SUSTENNA® into the gluteal muscle is the 1½-inch, 22 gauge needle. Administration should be made into the upper-outer quadrant of the gluteal area. Gluteal injections should be alternated between the two gluteal muscles.
2.4 Use with Oral Paliperidone or with Risperidone
Concomitant use of INVEGA® SUSTENNA® with oral paliperidone or oral or injectable risperidone has not been studied. Since paliperidone is the major active metabolite of risperidone, consideration should be given to the additive paliperidone exposure if any of these medications are coadministered with INVEGA® SUSTENNA®.
2.5 Dosage in Special Populations
Renal Impairment
INVEGA® SUSTENNA® has not been systematically studied in patients with renal impairment *[see Clinical Pharmacology (12.3)]*. For patients with mild renal impairment

(creatinine clearance ≥ 50 mL/min to < 80 mL/min), recommended initiation of INVEGA® SUSTENNA® is with a dose of 156 mg on treatment day 1 and 117 mg one week later, both administered in the deltoid muscle. Thereafter, follow with monthly injections of 78 mg in either the deltoid or gluteal muscle.

INVEGA® SUSTENNA® is not recommended in patients with moderate or severe renal impairment (creatinine clearance < 50 mL/min).

Hepatic Impairment

INVEGA® SUSTENNA® has not been studied in patients with hepatic impairment. Based on a study with oral paliperidone, no dose adjustment is required in patients with mild or moderate hepatic impairment. Paliperidone has not been studied in patients with severe hepatic impairment. [See Clinical Pharmacology (12.3)]

Elderly

In general, recommended dosing of INVEGA® SUSTENNA® for elderly patients with normal renal function is the same as for younger adult patients with normal renal function. As elderly patients may have reduced renal function, see *Renal Impairment* above for dosing recommendations in patients with renal impairment.

2.6 Maintenance Therapy

INVEGA® SUSTENNA® has been shown to be effective in delaying time to relapse of symptoms of schizophrenia in long-term use. It is recommended that responding patients be continued on treatment at the lowest dose needed. Patients should be periodically reassessed to determine the need for continued treatment.

2.7 Switching from Other Antipsychotics

There are no systematically collected data to specifically address switching patients with schizophrenia from other antipsychotics to INVEGA® SUSTENNA®, or concerning concomitant administration with other antipsychotics.

Switching from Oral Antipsychotics

For patients who have never taken oral paliperidone or oral or injectable risperidone, tolerability should be established with oral paliperidone or oral risperidone prior to initiating treatment with INVEGA® SUSTENNA®.

Previous oral antipsychotics can be discontinued at the time of initiation of treatment with INVEGA® SUSTENNA®. INVEGA® SUSTENNA® should be initiated as described in Section 2.1. Patients previously stabilized on different doses of INVEGA® Extended-Release tablets can attain similar paliperidone steady-state exposure during maintenance treatment with INVEGA® SUSTENNA® monthly doses as depicted in Table 1.

Table 1. Doses of INVEGA® and INVEGA® SUSTENNA® needed to attain similar paliperidone exposure at steady-state

Formulation	INVEGA® Extended-Release Tablet	INVEGA® SUSTENNA® Injection
Dosing Frequency	Once Daily	Once every 4 weeks
Dose (mg)	12	234
	6	117
	3	39–78

Switching from Long-Acting Injectable Antipsychotics

For patients who have never taken oral paliperidone or oral or injectable risperidone, tolerability should be established with oral paliperidone or oral risperidone prior to initiating treatment with INVEGA® SUSTENNA®.

When switching patients from previous long-acting injectable antipsychotics, initiate INVEGA® SUSTENNA® therapy in place of the next scheduled injection. INVEGA® SUSTENNA® should then be continued at monthly intervals. The one-week initiation dosing regimen as described in Section 2.1 is not required.

If INVEGA® SUSTENNA® is discontinued, its prolonged-release characteristics must be considered. As recommended with other antipsychotic medications, the need for continuing existing extrapyramidal symptoms (EPS) medication should be re-evaluated periodically.

2.8 Instructions for Use

The kit contains a prefilled syringe and 2 safety needles (a 1 ½-inch 22 gauge needle and a 1-inch 23 gauge needle) for intramuscular injection.

[See first figure at top of next column]

INVEGA® SUSTENNA® is for single use only.

- 1. Shake the syringe vigorously for a minimum of 10 seconds to ensure a homogeneous suspension.

[See second figure in next column]

- 2. Select the appropriate needle.

For DELTOID injection, if the patient weighs < 200 lb (< 90 kg), use the 1-inch **23** gauge needle (needle with **blue** colored hub); if the patient weighs ≥ 200 lb

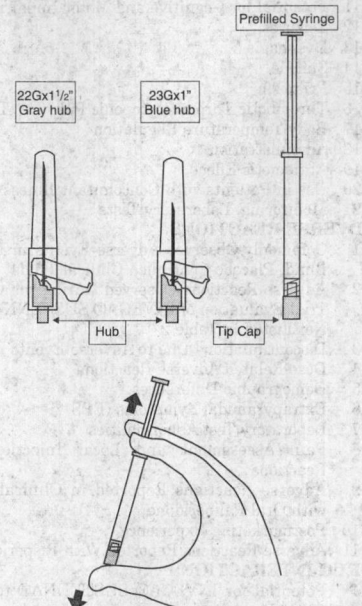

Prefilled Syringe

22Gx1½" Gray hub   23Gx1" Blue hub

Hub   Tip Cap

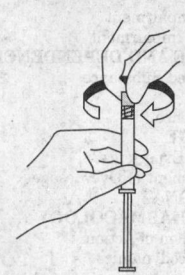

(≥ 90 kg), use the 1 ½-inch **22** gauge needle (needle with **gray** colored hub).

For GLUTEAL injection, use the 1 ½-inch **22** gauge needle (needle with **gray** colored hub).

- 3. While holding the syringe upright, remove the rubber tip cap with an easy clockwise twisting motion.

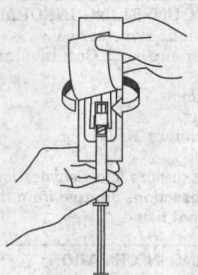

- 4. Peel the safety needle pouch half way open. Grasp the needle sheath using the plastic peel pouch. Attach the safety needle to the luer connection of the syringe with an easy clockwise twisting motion.

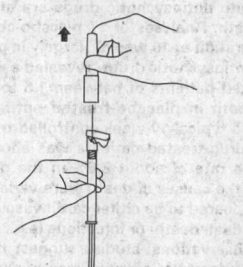

- 5. Pull the needle sheath away from the needle with a straight pull. Do not twist the sheath as the needle may be loosened from the syringe.

- 6. Bring the syringe with the attached needle in upright position to de-aerate. De-aerate the syringe by moving the plunger rod carefully forward.

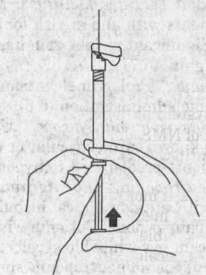

- 7. Inject the entire contents intramuscularly into the selected deltoid or gluteal muscle of the patient. **Do not administer intravascularly or subcutaneously.**
- 8. After the injection is complete, use either thumb or finger of one hand (8a, 8b) or a flat surface (8c) to activate the needle protection system. The needle protection system is fully activated when a 'click' is heard. Discard the syringe with needle appropriately.

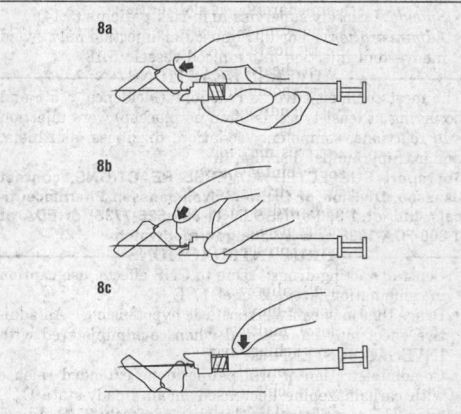

8a

8b

8c

3 DOSAGE FORMS AND STRENGTHS

INVEGA® SUSTENNA® is available as a white to off-white aqueous extended-release suspension for intramuscular injection in dose strengths of 39 mg, 78 mg, 117 mg, 156 mg, and 234 mg paliperidone palmitate.

4 CONTRAINDICATIONS

Hypersensitivity reactions, including anaphylactic reactions and angioedema, have been observed in patients treated with risperidone and paliperidone. Paliperidone palmitate is converted to paliperidone, which is a metabolite of risperidone and is therefore contraindicated in patients with a known hypersensitivity to either paliperidone or risperidone, or to any of the excipients in the INVEGA® SUSTENNA® formulation.

5 WARNINGS AND PRECAUTIONS

5.1 Increased Mortality in Elderly Patients with Dementia-Related Psychosis

Elderly patients with dementia-related psychosis treated with atypical antipsychotic drugs are at an increased risk of death compared to placebo. INVEGA® SUSTENNA® (paliperidone palmitate) is not approved for the treatment of dementia-related psychosis [see Boxed Warning].

5.2 Cerebrovascular Adverse Events, Including Stroke, in Elderly Patients With Dementia-Related Psychosis

In placebo-controlled trials with risperidone, aripiprazole, and olanzapine in elderly subjects with dementia, there was a higher incidence of cerebrovascular adverse events (cerebrovascular accidents and transient ischemic attacks) including fatalities compared to placebo-treated subjects. Oral paliperidone and INVEGA® SUSTENNA® were not marketed at the time these studies were performed and are not approved for the treatment of patients with dementia-related psychosis [see also Boxed Warning and Warnings and Precautions (5.1)].

5.3 Neuroleptic Malignant Syndrome

A potentially fatal symptom complex sometimes referred to as Neuroleptic Malignant Syndrome (NMS) has been reported in association with antipsychotic drugs, including paliperidone. Clinical manifestations of NMS are hyperpyrexia, muscle rigidity, altered mental status, and evidence of autonomic instability (irregular pulse or blood pressure, tachycardia, diaphoresis, and cardiac dysrhythmia). Additional signs may include elevated creatine phosphokinase, myoglobinuria (rhabdomyolysis), and acute renal failure. The diagnostic evaluation of patients with this syndrome is complicated. In arriving at a diagnosis, it is important to identify cases in which the clinical presentation includes both serious medical illness (e.g., pneumonia, systemic infection, etc.) and untreated or inadequately treated extrapyramidal signs and symptoms (EPS). Other important considerations in the differential diagnosis include central anticholinergic toxicity, heat stroke, drug fever, and primary central nervous system pathology.

The management of NMS should include: (1) immediate discontinuation of antipsychotic drugs and other drugs not essential to concurrent therapy; (2) intensive symptomatic treatment and medical monitoring; and (3) treatment of any concomitant serious medical problems for which specific treatments are available. There is no general agreement about specific pharmacological treatment regimens for uncomplicated NMS.

If a patient appears to require antipsychotic drug treatment after recovery from NMS, reintroduction of drug therapy should be closely monitored, since recurrences of NMS have been reported.

5.4 QT Prolongation

Paliperidone causes a modest increase in the corrected QT (QTc) interval. The use of paliperidone should be avoided in combination with other drugs that are known to prolong QTc including Class 1A (e.g., quinidine, procainamide) or Class III (e.g., amiodarone, sotalol) antiarrhythmic medications, antipsychotic medications (e.g., chlorpromazine, thioridazine), antibiotics (e.g., gatifloxacin, moxifloxacin), or any other class of medications known to prolong the QTc interval. Paliperidone should also be avoided in patients with congenital long QT syndrome and in patients with a history of cardiac arrhythmias.

Certain circumstances may increase the risk of the occurrence of torsade de pointes and/or sudden death in association with the use of drugs that prolong the QTc interval, including (1) bradycardia; (2) hypokalemia or hypomagnesemia; (3) concomitant use of other drugs that prolong the QTc interval; and (4) presence of congenital prolongation of the QT interval.

The effects of oral paliperidone on the QT interval were evaluated in a double-blind, active-controlled (moxifloxacin 400 mg single dose), multicenter QT study in adults with schizophrenia and schizoaffective disorder, and in three placebo- and active-controlled 6-week, fixed-dose efficacy trials in adults with schizophrenia.

In the QT study (n = 141), the 8 mg dose of immediate-release oral paliperidone (n=50) showed a mean placebo-subtracted increase from baseline in QTcLD of 12.3 msec (90% CI: 8.9; 15.6) on day 8 at 1.5 hours post-dose. The mean steady-state peak plasma concentration for this 8 mg dose of paliperidone immediate release ($C_{max\ ss}$ = 113 ng/mL) was more than 2-fold the exposure observed with the maximum recommended 234 mg dose of INVEGA® SUSTENNA® administered in the deltoid muscle (predicted median $C_{max\ ss}$ = 50 ng/mL). In this same study, a 4 mg dose of the immediate-release oral formulation of paliperidone, for which $C_{max\ ss}$ = 35 ng/mL, showed an increased placebo-subtracted QTcLD of 6.8 msec (90% CI: 3.6; 10.1) on day 2 at 1.5 hours post-dose.

In the three fixed-dose efficacy studies of oral paliperidone extended release, electrocardiogram (ECG) measurements taken at various time points showed only one subject in the oral paliperidone 12 mg group had a change exceeding 60 msec at one time-point on Day 6 (increase of 62 msec). In the four fixed-dose efficacy studies of INVEGA® SUSTENNA®, no subject experienced a change in QTcLD exceeding 60 msec and no subject had a QTcLD value of > 500 msec at any time point. In the maintenance study, no subject had a QTcLD change > 60 msec, and one subject had a QTcLD value of 507 msec (Bazett's QT corrected interval [QTcB] value of 483 msec); this latter subject also had a heart rate of 45 beats per minute.

5.5 Tardive Dyskinesia

A syndrome of potentially irreversible, involuntary, dyskinetic movements may develop in patients treated with antipsychotic drugs. Although the prevalence of the syndrome appears to be highest among the elderly, especially elderly women, it is impossible to predict which patients will develop the syndrome. Whether antipsychotic drug products differ in their potential to cause tardive dyskinesia is unknown.

The risk of developing tardive dyskinesia and the likelihood that it will become irreversible appear to increase as the duration of treatment and the total cumulative dose of antipsychotic drugs administered to the patient increase, but the syndrome can develop after relatively brief treatment periods at low doses, although this is uncommon.

There is no known treatment for established tardive dyskinesia, although the syndrome may remit, partially or completely, if antipsychotic treatment is withdrawn. Antipsychotic treatment itself may suppress (or partially suppress) the signs and symptoms of the syndrome and may thus mask the underlying process. The effect of symptomatic suppression on the long-term course of the syndrome is unknown.

Given these considerations, INVEGA® SUSTENNA® should be prescribed in a manner that is most likely to minimize the occurrence of tardive dyskinesia. Chronic antipsychotic treatment should generally be reserved for patients who suffer from a chronic illness that is known to respond to antipsychotic drugs. In patients who do require chronic treatment, the smallest dose and the shortest duration of treatment producing a satisfactory clinical response should be sought. The need for continued treatment should be reassessed periodically.

If signs and symptoms of tardive dyskinesia appear in a patient treated with INVEGA® SUSTENNA®, drug discontinuation should be considered. However, some patients may require treatment with INVEGA® SUSTENNA® despite the presence of the syndrome.

5.6 Hyperglycemia and Diabetes Mellitus

Hyperglycemia, in some cases extreme and associated with ketoacidosis or hyperosmolar coma or death, has been reported in patients treated with all atypical antipsychotics. These cases were, for the most part, seen in post-marketing clinical use and epidemiologic studies, not in clinical trials, and there have been few reports of hyperglycemia or diabetes in trial subjects treated with INVEGA® SUSTENNA®. Assessment of the relationship between atypical antipsychotic use and glucose abnormalities is complicated by the possibility of an increased background risk of diabetes mellitus in patients with schizophrenia and the increasing incidence of diabetes mellitus in the general population. Given these confounders, the relationship between atypical antipsychotic use and hyperglycemia-related adverse events is not completely understood. However, epidemiological studies suggest an increased risk of treatment-emergent hyperglycemia-related adverse events in patients treated with the atypical antipsychotics.

Patients with an established diagnosis of diabetes mellitus who are started on atypical antipsychotics should be monitored regularly for worsening of glucose control. Patients with risk factors for diabetes mellitus (e.g., obesity, family history of diabetes) who are starting treatment with atypical antipsychotics should undergo fasting blood glucose testing at the beginning of treatment and periodically during treatment. Any patient treated with atypical antipsychotics should be monitored for symptoms of hyperglycemia including polydipsia, polyuria, polyphagia, and weakness. Patients who develop symptoms of hyperglycemia during treatment with atypical antipsychotics should undergo fasting blood glucose testing. In some cases, hyperglycemia has resolved when the atypical antipsychotic was discontinued; however, some patients required continuation of antidiabetic treatment despite discontinuation of the suspect drug.

5.7 Weight Gain

Weight gain has been observed with INVEGA® SUSTENNA® and other atypical antipsychotics. In the 13-week study involving 234 mg initiation dosing, the proportion of subjects with an abnormal weight increase ≥ 7% showed a dose-related trend, with a 5% incidence rate in the placebo group compared with rates of 6%, 8%, and 13% in the INVEGA® SUSTENNA® 39 mg, 156 mg, and 234 mg groups, respectively. In the two 13-week, fixed-dose, double-blind, placebo-controlled trials (pooled data), the proportions of subjects meeting a weight gain criterion of ≥ 7% of body weight were 6%, 9%, and 10% in the INVEGA® SUSTENNA® 39 mg, 78 mg, and 156 mg groups, respectively, compared with 2% in the placebo group. In the 9-week, fixed-dose, double-blind, placebo-controlled trial, 8% and 6% in the INVEGA® SUSTENNA® 78 mg and 156 mg groups, respectively, met this criterion compared with 4% in the placebo group.

During the 33-week open-label period (9-week flexible-dose transition phase followed by a 24-week maintenance phase flexible-dose and minimum 12-week fixed dose) of the maintenance trial, 12% of INVEGA® SUSTENNA®-treated subjects met this criterion; the mean (SD) weight change from open-label baseline was +0.7 (4.79) kg. In the variable length double-blind phase, this criterion (weight gain of ≥ 7% from double-blind phase to endpoint) was met by 6% of INVEGA® SUSTENNA®-treated subjects compared with 3% of placebo-treated subjects; the mean weight change from double-blind baseline was +0.5 kg for INVEGA® SUSTENNA® compared with –1.0 kg for placebo. Similar results were observed in the open-label extension phase of this study.

5.8 Hyperprolactinemia

Like other drugs that antagonize dopamine D_2 receptors, paliperidone elevates prolactin levels and the elevation persists during chronic administration. Paliperidone has a prolactin-elevating effect similar to that seen with risperidone, a drug that is associated with higher levels of prolactin than other antipsychotic drugs.

Hyperprolactinemia, regardless of etiology, may suppress hypothalamic GnRH, resulting in reduced pituitary gonadotrophin secretion. This, in turn, may inhibit reproductive function by impairing gonadal steroidogenesis in both fe-

male and male patients. Galactorrhea, amenorrhea, gynecomastia, and impotence have been reported in patients receiving prolactin-elevating compounds. Long-standing hyperprolactinemia when associated with hypogonadism may lead to decreased bone density in both female and male subjects.

Tissue culture experiments indicate that approximately one-third of human breast cancers are prolactin dependent in vitro, a factor of potential importance if the prescription of these drugs is considered in a patient with previously detected breast cancer. An increase in the incidence of pituitary gland, mammary gland, and pancreatic islet cell neoplasia (mammary adenocarcinomas, pituitary and pancreatic adenomas) was observed in the risperidone carcinogenicity studies conducted in mice and rats [see Nonclinical Toxicology (13.1)]. Neither clinical studies nor epidemiologic studies conducted to date have shown an association between chronic administration of this class of drugs and tumorigenesis in humans, but the available evidence is too limited to be conclusive.

5.9 Orthostatic Hypotension and Syncope

Paliperidone can induce orthostatic hypotension and syncope in some patients because of its alpha-blocking activity. Syncope was reported in < 1% (4/1293) of subjects treated with INVEGA® SUSTENNA® in the recommended dose range of 39 mg to 234 mg in the four fixed-dose, double-blind, placebo-controlled trials compared with 0% (0/510) of subjects treated with placebo. In the four fixed-dose efficacy studies, orthostatic hypotension was reported as an adverse event by < 1% (2/1293) of INVEGA® SUSTENNA®-treated subjects compared to 0% (0/510) with placebo. Incidences of orthostatic hypotension and syncope in the long-term studies were similar to those observed in the short-term studies. INVEGA® SUSTENNA® should be used with caution in patients with known cardiovascular disease (e.g., heart failure, history of myocardial infarction or ischemia, conduction abnormalities), cerebrovascular disease, or conditions that predispose the patient to hypotension (e.g., dehydration, hypovolemia, and treatment with antihypertensive medications). Monitoring of orthostatic vital signs should be considered in patients who are vulnerable to hypotension.

5.10 Leukopenia, Neutropenia, and Agranulocytosis

Class Effect: In clinical trial and/or postmarketing experience, events of leukopenia/neutropenia have been reported temporally related to antipsychotic agents, including INVEGA®, an oral form of paliperidone. Agranulocytosis has also been reported.

Possible risk factors for leukopenia/neutropenia include pre-existing low white blood cell count (WBC) and history of drug-induced leukopenia/neutropenia. Patients with a history of a clinically significant low WBC or a drug-induced leukopenia/neutropenia should have their complete blood count (CBC) monitored frequently during the first few months of therapy and discontinuation of INVEGA® SUSTENNA® should be considered at the first sign of a clinically significant decline in WBC in the absence of other causative factors.

Patients with clinically significant neutropenia should be carefully monitored for fever or other symptoms or signs of infection and treated promptly if such symptoms or signs occur. Patients with severe neutropenia (absolute neutrophil count <1000/mm³) should discontinue INVEGA® SUSTENNA® and have their WBC followed until recovery.

5.11 Potential for Cognitive and Motor Impairment

Somnolence, sedation, and dizziness were reported as adverse reactions in subjects treated with INVEGA® SUSTENNA® [see Adverse Reactions (6.1)]. Antipsychotics, including INVEGA® SUSTENNA®, have the potential to impair judgment, thinking, or motor skills. Patients should be cautioned about performing activities requiring mental alertness, such as operating hazardous machinery or operating a motor vehicle, until they are reasonably certain that paliperidone therapy does not adversely affect them.

5.12 Seizures

In the four fixed-dose double-blind placebo-controlled studies, <1% (1/1293) of subjects treated with INVEGA® SUSTENNA® in the recommended dose range of 39 mg to 234 mg experienced an adverse event of convulsion compared with <1% (1/510) of placebo-treated subjects who experienced an adverse event of grand mal convulsion.

Like other antipsychotic drugs, INVEGA® SUSTENNA® should be used cautiously in patients with a history of seizures or other conditions that potentially lower the seizure threshold. Conditions that lower the seizure threshold may be more prevalent in patients 65 years or older.

5.13 Dysphagia

Esophageal dysmotility and aspiration have been associated with antipsychotic drug use. Aspiration pneumonia is a common cause of morbidity and mortality in patients with advanced Alzheimer's dementia. INVEGA® SUSTENNA® and other antipsychotic drugs should be used cautiously in patients at risk for aspiration pneumonia.

Table 2. Incidence of Treatment Emergent Adverse Events in ≥ 2% of INVEGA® SUSTENNA®-Treated Subjects with Schizophrenia in Four Fixed-Dose, Double-Blind, Placebo-Controlled Trials

System Organ Class Adverse Event	Placebo* (N=510)	39 mg (N=130)	78 mg (N=302)	156 mg (N=312)	234/39 mg[†] (N=160)	234/156 mg[†] (N=165)	234/234 mg[†] (N=163)
Total percentage of subjects with adverse event	70	75	68	69	63	60	63
Gastrointestinal disorders							
Abdominal discomfort/ abdominal pain upper	2	2	4	4	1	2	4
Constipation	5	3	5	5	2	4	1
Diarrhea	2	0	3	2	1	2	2
Dry mouth	1	3	1	0	1	1	1
Nausea	3	4	4	3	2	2	2
Toothache	1	1	1	3	1	2	3
Vomiting	4	5	4	2	3	2	2
General disorders and administration site conditions							
Asthenia	0	2	1	<1	0	1	1
Fatigue	1	1	2	2	1	2	1
Injection site reactions	2	0	4	6	9	7	10
Infections and infestations							
Nasopharyngitis	2	0	2	2	4	2	2
Upper respiratory tract infection	2	2	2	2	1	2	4
Urinary tract infection	1	0	1	<1	1	1	2
Injury, poisoning and procedural complications							
Skin laceration	<1	2	<1	0	1	0	0
Investigations							
Alanine aminotransferase increased	2	0	2	1	1	1	1
Weight increased	1	4	4	1	1	1	2
Musculoskeletal and connective tissue disorders							
Back pain	2	2	1	3	1	1	1
Musculoskeletal stiffness	1	1	<1	<1	1	1	2
Myalgia	1	2	1	<1	1	0	2
Pain in extremity	1	0	2	2	2	3	0
Nervous system disorders							
Akathisia	3	2	2	3	1	5	6
Dizziness	1	6	2	2	1	4	2
Extrapyramidal disorder	1	5	2	3	1	0	0
Headache	12	11	11	15	11	7	6
Somnolence/sedation	3	5	7	4	1	5	5
Psychiatric disorders							
Agitation	7	10	5	9	8	5	4
Anxiety	7	8	5	3	5	6	6
Insomnia	15	15	15	13	12	10	13
Nightmare	<1	2	0	0	0	0	0
Suicidal ideation	2	0	1	2	2	2	1
Respiratory, thoracic and mediastinal disorders							
Cough	1	2	3	1	0	1	1
Vascular disorders							
Hypertension	1	2	1	1	1	1	0

Percentages are rounded to whole numbers. Table includes adverse events that were reported in 2% or more of subjects in any of the INVEGA® SUSTENNA® dose groups and which occurred at greater incidence than in the placebo group.
* Placebo group is pooled from all studies and included either deltoid or gluteal injection depending on study design.
† Initial deltoid injection of 234 mg followed by either 39 mg, 156 mg, or 234 mg every 4 weeks by deltoid or gluteal injection. Other dose groups (39 mg, 78 mg, and 156 mg) are from studies involving only gluteal injection. [See Clinical Studies (14)]
Adverse events for which the INVEGA® SUSTENNA® incidence was equal to or less than placebo are not listed in the table, but included the following: dyspepsia, psychotic disorder, schizophrenia, and tremor. The following terms were combined: somnolence/sedation, breast tenderness/breast pain, abdominal discomfort/abdominal pain upper/stomach discomfort, and tachycardia/sinus tachycardia/heart rate increased. All injection site reaction-related adverse events were collapsed and are grouped under "Injection site reactions".

5.14 Suicide
The possibility of suicide attempt is inherent in psychotic illnesses, and close supervision of high-risk patients should accompany drug therapy.

5.15 Priapism
Drugs with alpha-adrenergic blocking effects have been reported to induce priapism. Although no cases of priapism have been reported in clinical trials with INVEGA® SUSTENNA®, priapism has been reported with oral paliperidone during postmarketing surveillance. Severe priapism may require surgical intervention.

5.16 Thrombotic Thrombocytopenic Purpura (TTP)
No cases of TTP were observed during clinical studies with oral paliperidone or INVEGA® SUSTENNA®. Although cases of TTP have been reported in association with risperidone administration, the relationship to risperidone therapy is unknown.

5.17 Body Temperature Regulation
Disruption of the body's ability to reduce core body temperature has been attributed to antipsychotic agents. Appropriate care is advised when prescribing INVEGA® SUSTENNA® to patients who will be experiencing conditions which may contribute to an elevation in core body temperature, e.g., exercising strenuously, exposure to extreme heat, receiving concomitant medication with anticholinergic activity, or being subject to dehydration.

5.18 Administration
INVEGA® SUSTENNA® is intended for intramuscular injection, and care must be taken to avoid inadvertent injection into a blood vessel [see Dosage and Administration (2.3)].

5.19 Antiemetic Effect
An antiemetic effect was observed in preclinical studies with paliperidone. This effect, if it occurs in humans, may mask the signs and symptoms of overdosage with certain drugs or of conditions such as intestinal obstruction, Reye's syndrome, and brain tumor.

5.20 Use in Patients with Concomitant Illness
Clinical experience with INVEGA® SUSTENNA® in patients with certain concomitant illnesses is limited [see Clinical Pharmacology (12.3)].
Patients with Parkinson's Disease or Dementia with Lewy Bodies are reported to have an increased sensitivity to antipsychotic medication. Manifestations of this increased sensitivity include confusion, obtundation, postural instability with frequent falls, extrapyramidal symptoms, and clinical features consistent with the neuroleptic malignant syndrome.
INVEGA® SUSTENNA® has not been evaluated or used to any appreciable extent in patients with a recent history of myocardial infarction or unstable heart disease. Patients with these diagnoses were excluded from premarketing clin-

ical trials. Because of the risk of orthostatic hypotension with INVEGA® SUSTENNA®, caution should be observed in patients with known cardiovascular disease [see Warnings and Precautions (5.9)].

5.21 Monitoring: Laboratory Tests
No specific laboratory tests are recommended.

6 ADVERSE REACTIONS
The following are discussed in more detail in other sections of the labeling:
• Increased mortality in elderly patients with dementia-related psychosis [see Boxed Warning and Warnings and Precautions (5.1)]
• Cerebrovascular adverse events, including stroke, in elderly patients with dementia-related psychosis [see Warnings and Precautions (5.2)]
• Neuroleptic malignant syndrome [see Warnings and Precautions (5.3)]
• QT prolongation [see Warnings and Precautions (5.4)]
• Tardive dyskinesia [see Warnings and Precautions (5.5)]
• Hyperglycemia and diabetes mellitus [see Warnings and Precautions (5.6)]
• Weight gain [see Warnings and Precautions (5.7)]
• Hyperprolactinemia [see Warnings and Precautions (5.8)]
• Orthostatic hypotension and syncope [see Warnings and Precautions (5.9)]
• Leukopenia, neutropenia, and agranulocytosis [see Warnings and Precautions (5.10)]
• Potential for cognitive and motor impairment [see Warnings and Precautions (5.11)]
• Seizures [see Warnings and Precautions (5.12)]
• Dysphagia [see Warnings and Precautions (5.13)]
• Suicide [see Warnings and Precautions (5.14)]
• Priapism [see Warnings and Precautions (5.15)]
• Thrombotic Thrombocytopenic Purpura [see Warnings and Precautions (5.16)]
• Disruption of body temperature regulation [see Warnings and Precautions (5.17)]
• Avoidance of inadvertent injection into a blood vessel [see Warnings and Precautions (5.18)]
• Antiemetic effect [see Warnings and Precautions (5.19)]
• Increased sensitivity in patients with Parkinson's disease or those with dementia with Lewy bodies [see Warnings and Precautions (5.20)]
• Diseases or conditions that could affect metabolism or hemodynamic responses [see Warnings and Precautions (5.20)]

Throughout this section, a distinction is made between adverse events and adverse reactions. Adverse events are events reported by the clinician investigator and there is no attempt to assign causality to the study drug. Adverse reactions are adverse events that are considered to be reasonably associated with the use of INVEGA® SUSTENNA® (adverse drug reactions) based on a predetermined method of assessment, e.g., a comparison of adverse event rates for drug and placebo groups for the event of interest. It is not possible to reliably establish causality by considering individual adverse event reports for drug-treated patients. Thus, the section overall is labeled Adverse Reactions, however, individual subsections are labeled adverse reactions or adverse events, depending on what is included in the subsection.

Because clinical trials are conducted under widely varying conditions, adverse reaction rates observed in the clinical trials of a drug cannot be directly compared to rates in the clinical trials of another drug and may not reflect the rates observed in clinical practice.

The most common (at least 5% in any INVEGA® SUSTENNA® group) and likely drug-related (adverse events for which the drug rate is at least twice the placebo rate) adverse reactions from the double-blind, placebo-controlled trials were injection site reactions, somnolence/sedation, dizziness, akathisia, and extrapyramidal disorder.

The data described in this section are derived from a clinical trial database consisting of a total of 3817 subjects with schizophrenia who received at least one dose of INVEGA® SUSTENNA® in the recommended dose range of 39 mg to 234 mg and a total of 510 subjects with schizophrenia who received placebo. Among the 3817 INVEGA® SUSTENNA®-treated subjects, 1293 received INVEGA® SUSTENNA® in four fixed-dose, double-blind, placebo-controlled trials (one 9-week and three 13-week studies), 849 received INVEGA® SUSTENNA® in the maintenance trial (of whom 205 continued to receive INVEGA® SUSTENNA® during the double-blind placebo-controlled phase of this study), and 1675 received INVEGA® SUSTENNA® in five non-placebo controlled trials (three noninferiority active-comparator trials, one long-term open-label pharmacokinetic and safety study, and an injection site [deltoid-gluteal] cross-over trial). One of the 13-week studies included a 234 mg INVEGA® SUSTENNA® initiation dose followed by treatment with either 39 mg, 156 mg, or 234 mg every 4 weeks.

Adverse events during exposure to study treatment were obtained by general inquiry and recorded by clinical investigators using their own terminology. Consequently, to provide a meaningful estimate of the proportion of individuals experiencing adverse events, events were grouped in standardized categories using MedDRA terminology.

The majority of all adverse reactions were mild to moderate in severity.

6.1 Commonly-Observed Adverse Events in Double-Blind, Placebo-Controlled Clinical Trials

Table 2 lists the adverse events reported in 2% or more of INVEGA® SUSTENNA®-treated subjects with schizophrenia in the four fixed-dose, double-blind, placebo-controlled trials.

[See table at top of previous page]

6.2 Adverse Reactions Observed During the Clinical Trial Evaluation of INVEGA® SUSTENNA® and Not Listed in Table 2

The following additional adverse reactions occurred in INVEGA® SUSTENNA®-treated subjects in the above four fixed-dose, double-blind, placebo-controlled trials, in the double-blind phase of the maintenance trial, or in INVEGA® SUSTENNA®-treated subjects with schizophrenia who participated in other clinical trials, and were not reported in Table 2. They were determined to be adverse reactions based upon reasons to suspect causality such as timing of onset or termination with respect to drug use, plausibility in light of the drug's known pharmacology, occurrence at a frequency above that expected in the treated population or occurrence of an event typical of drug-induced adverse reactions.

Cardiac disorders: atrioventricular block first degree, bradycardia, bundle branch block, electrocardiogram QT prolonged, palpitations, postural orthostatic tachycardia syndrome, tachycardia

Ear and labyrinth disorders: vertigo

Endocrine disorders: hyperprolactinemia

Eye disorders: eye movement disorder, eye rolling, oculogyric crisis, vision blurred

Gastrointestinal disorders: salivary hypersecretion

Immune system disorders: hypersensitivity

Investigations: blood cholesterol increased, blood glucose increased, blood triglycerides increased, electrocardiogram abnormal

Metabolism and nutrition disorders: decreased appetite, hyperglycemia, hyperinsulinemia, increased appetite

Musculoskeletal and connective tissue disorders: joint stiffness, muscle rigidity, muscle spasms, muscle tightness, muscle twitching, nuchal rigidity

Nervous system disorders: bradykinesia, cerebrovascular accident, convulsion, dizziness postural, drooling, dysarthria, dyskinesia, dystonia, hypertonia, lethargy, neuroleptic malignant syndrome, oromandibular dystonia, parkinsonism, psychomotor hyperactivity, syncope, tardive dyskinesia

Psychiatric disorders: restlessness

Reproductive system and breast disorders: amenorrhea, breast discharge, erectile dysfunction, galactorrhea, gynecomastia, menstrual disorder, menstruation delayed, menstruation irregular, sexual dysfunction

Skin and subcutaneous tissue disorders: drug eruption, pruritus, pruritus generalized, rash, urticaria

Vascular disorders: orthostatic hypotension

6.3 Discontinuations Due to Adverse Events

The percentages of subjects who discontinued due to adverse events in the four fixed-dose, double-blind, placebo-controlled trials were 5.0% and 7.8% in INVEGA® SUSTENNA®- and placebo-treated subjects, respectively.

6.4 Dose-Related Adverse Reactions

Based on the pooled data from the four fixed-dose, double-blind, placebo-controlled trials, among the adverse reactions that occurred at ≥ 2% incidence in the subjects treated with INVEGA® SUSTENNA®, only akathisia increased with dose. Hyperprolactinemia also exhibited a dose relationship, but did not occur at ≥ 2% incidence in INVEGA® SUSTENNA®-treated subjects from the four fixed-dose studies.

6.5 Demographic Differences

An examination of population subgroups in the double-blind placebo-controlled trials did not reveal any evidence of differences in safety on the basis of age, gender, or race alone; however, there were few subjects ≥ 65 years of age.

6.6 Extrapyramidal Symptoms (EPS)

Pooled data from the two double-blind, placebo-controlled, 13-week, fixed-dose trials provided information regarding treatment-emergent EPS. Several methods were used to measure EPS: (1) the Simpson-Angus global score (mean change from baseline or score at the end of trial) which broadly evaluates Parkinsonism, (2) the Barnes Akathisia Rating Scale global clinical rating score (mean change from baseline or score at the end of trial) which evaluates akathisia, (3) use of anticholinergic medications to treat emergent EPS, (4) the Abnormal Involuntary Movement Scale scores (mean change from baseline or scores at the end of trial) *(Table 3)*, and (5) incidence of spontaneous reports of EPS *(Table 4)*.

Table 3. Treatment-Emergent Extrapyramidal Symptoms (EPS) Assessed by Incidence of Rating Scales and Use of Anticholinergic Medication

	Percentage of Subjects			
		INVEGA® SUSTENNA®		
Scale	Placebo (N=262)	39 mg (N=130)	78 mg (N=223)	156 mg (N=228)
Parkinsonism*	9	12	10	6
Akathisia†	5	5	6	5
Dyskinesia‡	3	4	6	4
Use of Anticholinergic Medications§	12	10	12	11

*For Parkinsonism, percent of subjects with Simpson-Angus Total score > 0.3 at endpoint (Total score defined as total sum of items score divided by the number of items)

†For Akathisia, percent of subjects with Barnes Akathisia Rating Scale global score ≥ 2 at endpoint

‡For Dyskinesia, percent of subjects with a score ≥ 3 on any of the first 7 items or a score ≥ 2 on two or more of any of the first 7 items of the Abnormal Involuntary Movement Scale at endpoint

§Percent of subjects who received anticholinergic medications to treat emergent EPS

Table 4. Treatment-Emergent Extrapyramidal Symptoms (EPS)-Related Adverse Events by MedDRA Preferred Term

	Percentage of Subjects			
		INVEGA® SUSTENNA®		
EPS Group	Placebo (N=262)	39 mg (N=130)	78 mg (N=223)	156 mg (N=228)
Overall percentage of subjects with EPS-related adverse events	10	12	11	11
Parkinsonism	5	6	6	4
Hyperkinesia	2	2	2	4
Tremor	3	2	2	3
Dyskinesia	1	2	3	1
Dystonia	0	1	1	2

Parkinsonism group includes: Extrapyramidal disorder, hypertonia, musculoskeletal stiffness, parkinsonism, drooling, masked facies, muscle tightness, hypokinesia

Hyperkinesia group includes: Akathisia, restless legs syndrome, restlessness

Dyskinesia group includes: Dyskinesia, choreoathetosis, muscle twitching, myoclonus, tardive dyskinesia

Dystonia group includes: Dystonia, muscle spasms

The results across all phases of the maintenance trial exhibited comparable findings. In the 9-week, fixed-dose, double-blind, placebo-controlled trial, the proportions of Parkinsonism and akathisia assessed by incidence of rating scales were higher in the INVEGA® SUSTENNA® 156 mg group (18% and 11%, respectively) than in the INVEGA® SUSTENNA® 78 mg group (9% and 5%, respectively) and placebo group (7% and 4%, respectively).

In the 13-week study involving 234 mg initiation dosing, the incidence of any treatment-emergent EPS-related adverse events was similar to that of the placebo group (8%), but exhibited a dose-related pattern with 6%, 10%, and 11% in the INVEGA® SUSTENNA® 234/39 mg, 234/156 mg, and 234/234 mg groups, respectively. Hyperkinesia was the most frequent category of EPS-related adverse events in this study, and was reported at a similar rate between the placebo (4.9%) and INVEGA® SUSTENNA® 234/156 mg (4.8%) and 234/234 mg (5.5%) groups, but at a lower rate in the 234/39 mg group (1.3%).

Dystonia

Class Effect: Symptoms of dystonia, prolonged abnormal contractions of muscle groups, may occur in susceptible individuals during the first few days of treatment. Dystonic symptoms include: spasm of the neck muscles, sometimes progressing to tightness of the throat, swallowing difficulty, difficulty breathing, and/or protrusion of the tongue. While these symptoms can occur at low doses, they occur more frequently and with greater severity with high potency and at higher doses of first generation antipsychotic drugs. An elevated risk of acute dystonia is observed in males and younger age groups.

6.7 Laboratory Test Abnormalities

In the pooled data from the two double-blind, placebo-controlled, 13-week, fixed-dose trials, a between-group comparison revealed no medically important differences between INVEGA® SUSTENNA® and placebo in the proportions of subjects experiencing potentially clinically significant changes in routine serum chemistry, hematology, or urinalysis parameters. Similarly, there were no differences between INVEGA® SUSTENNA® and placebo in the incidence of discontinuations due to changes in hematology, urinalysis, or serum chemistry, including mean changes from baseline in fasting glucose, insulin, c-peptide, triglyceride, HDL, LDL, and total cholesterol measurements. However, INVEGA® SUSTENNA® was associated with increases in serum prolactin *[see Warnings and Precautions (5.8)]*. The results from the 13-week study involving 234 mg initiation dosing, the 9-week, fixed-dose, double-blind, placebo-controlled trial, and the double-blind phase of the maintenance trial exhibited comparable findings.

6.8 Pain Assessment and Local Injection Site Reactions

In the pooled data from the two 13-week, fixed-dose, double-blind, placebo-controlled trials, the mean intensity of injection pain reported by subjects using a visual analog scale (0 = no pain to 100 = unbearably painful) decreased in all treatment groups from the first to the last injection (placebo: 10.9 to 9.8; 39 mg: 10.3 to 7.7; 78 mg: 10.0 to 9.2; 156 mg: 11.1 to 8.8). The results from both the 9-week, fixed-dose, double-blind, placebo-controlled trial and the double-blind phase of the maintenance trial exhibited comparable findings.

In the 13-week study involving 234 mg initiation dosing, occurrences of induration, redness, or swelling, as assessed by blinded study personnel, were infrequent, generally mild, decreased over time, and similar in incidence between the INVEGA® SUSTENNA® and placebo groups. Investigator ratings of injection pain were similar for the placebo and INVEGA® SUSTENNA® groups. Investigator evaluations of the injection site after the first injection for redness, swelling, induration, and pain were rated as absent for 69–100% of subjects in both the INVEGA® SUSTENNA® and placebo groups. At Day 92, investigators rated absence of redness, swelling, induration, and pain in 95–100% of subjects in both the INVEGA® SUSTENNA® and placebo groups.

6.9 Adverse Reactions Reported in Clinical Trials with Oral Paliperidone

The following is a list of additional adverse reactions that have been reported in clinical trials with oral paliperidone:

Cardiac disorders: bundle branch block left, sinus arrhythmia

Gastrointestinal disorders: abdominal pain, flatulence, small intestinal obstruction

General disorders and administration site conditions: edema, edema peripheral

Immune system disorders: anaphylactic reaction

Infections and infestations: rhinitis

Musculoskeletal and connective tissue disorders: arthralgia, musculoskeletal pain, torticollis, trismus

Nervous system disorders: cogwheel rigidity, grand mal convulsion, parkinsonian gait, transient ischemic attack

Psychiatric disorders: sleep disorder

Reproductive system and breast disorders: breast engorgement, breast tenderness/breast pain, retrograde ejaculation

Respiratory, thoracic and mediastinal disorders: nasal congestion, pharyngolaryngeal pain, pneumonia aspiration

Skin and subcutaneous tissue disorders: rash papular

Vascular disorders: hypotension, ischemia

6.10 Postmarketing Experience

The following adverse reactions have been identified during postapproval use of paliperidone; because these reactions were reported voluntarily from a population of uncertain size, it is not possible to reliably estimate their frequency: angioedema, priapism, swollen tongue, urinary incontinence, urinary retention.

6.11 Adverse Reactions Reported With Risperidone

Paliperidone is the major active metabolite of risperidone. Adverse reactions reported with oral risperidone and risperidone long-acting injection can be found in the ADVERSE REACTIONS sections of the package inserts for those products.

7 DRUG INTERACTIONS

Since paliperidone palmitate is hydrolyzed to paliperidone *[see Clinical Pharmacology (12.3)]*, results from studies with oral paliperidone should be taken into consideration when assessing drug-drug interaction potential.

7.1 Potential for INVEGA® SUSTENNA® to Affect Other Drugs

Given the primary CNS effects of paliperidone *[see Adverse Reactions (6.1)]*, INVEGA® SUSTENNA® should be used with caution in combination with other centrally acting drugs and alcohol. Paliperidone may antagonize the effect of levodopa and other dopamine agonists.

Because of its potential for inducing orthostatic hypotension, an additive effect may be observed when INVEGA® SUSTENNA® is administered with other therapeutic agents that have this potential *[see Warnings and Precautions (5.9)]*.

Paliperidone is not expected to cause clinically important pharmacokinetic interactions with drugs that are metabolized by cytochrome P450 isozymes. *In vitro* studies in human liver microsomes showed that paliperidone does not substantially inhibit the metabolism of drugs metabolized by cytochrome P450 isozymes, including CYP1A2, CYP2A6, CYP2C8/9/10, CYP2D6, CYP2E1, CYP3A4, and CYP3A5. Therefore, paliperidone is not expected to inhibit clearance of drugs that are metabolized by these metabolic pathways in a clinically relevant manner. Paliperidone is also not expected to have enzyme inducing properties.

Paliperidone is a weak inhibitor of P-glycoprotein (P-gp) at high concentrations. No *in vivo* data are available and the clinical relevance is unknown.

7.2 Potential for Other Drugs to Affect INVEGA® SUSTENNA®

Paliperidone is not a substrate of CYP1A2, CYP2A6, CYP2C9, and CYP2C19, so that an interaction with inhibitors or inducers of these isozymes is unlikely. While *in vitro* studies indicate that CYP2D6 and CYP3A4 may be minimally involved in paliperidone metabolism, *in vivo* studies do not show decreased elimination by these isozymes and they contribute to only a small fraction of total body clearance. *In vitro* studies have shown that paliperidone is a P-gp substrate.

Co-administration of oral paliperidone extended release once daily with carbamazepine 200 mg twice daily caused a decrease of approximately 37% in the mean steady-state C_{max} and AUC of paliperidone. This decrease is caused, to a substantial degree, by a 35% increase in renal clearance of paliperidone. A minor decrease in the amount of drug excreted unchanged in the urine suggests that there was little effect on the CYP metabolism or bioavailability of paliperidone during carbamazepine co-administration. On initiation of carbamazepine, the dose of INVEGA® SUSTENNA® should be re-evaluated and increased if necessary. Conversely, on discontinuation of carbamazepine, the dose of INVEGA® SUSTENNA® should be re-evaluated and decreased if necessary.

Paliperidone is metabolized to a limited extent by CYP2D6 *[see Clinical Pharmacology (12.3)]*. In an interaction study in healthy subjects in which a single 3 mg dose of oral paliperidone extended release was administered concomitantly with 20 mg per day of paroxetine (a potent CYP2D6 inhibitor), paliperidone exposures were on average 16% (90% CI: 4, 30) higher in CYP2D6 extensive metabolizers. Higher doses of paroxetine have not been studied. The clinical relevance is unknown.

Co-administration of a single dose of an oral paliperidone extended-release 12 mg tablet with divalproex sodium extended-release tablets (two 500 mg tablets once daily at steady-state) resulted in an increase of approximately 50% in the C_{max} and AUC of paliperidone. Although this interaction has not been studied with INVEGA® SUSTENNA®, a clinically significant interaction would not be expected between divalproex sodium and INVEGA® SUSTENNA® intramuscular injection.

8 USE IN SPECIFIC POPULATIONS

8.1 Pregnancy

Pregnancy Category C.

There were no treatment-related effects on the offspring when pregnant rats were injected intramuscularly with paliperidone palmitate during the period of organogenesis at doses up to 160 mg/kg, which is 10 times the maximum recommended human 234 mg dose of INVEGA® SUSTENNA® on a mg/m^2 basis.

In studies in pregnant rats and rabbits in which paliperidone was given orally during the period of organogenesis, there were no increases in fetal abnormalities up to the highest doses tested (10 mg/kg/day in rats and 5 mg/kg/day in rabbits, which are each 8 times the maximum recommended human dose [12 mg/day] of orally administered paliperidone [INVEGA®] on a mg/m^2 basis).

In rat reproduction studies with risperidone, which is extensively converted to paliperidone in rats and humans, increases in pup deaths were seen at oral doses which are less than the maximum recommended human dose of risperidone on a mg/m^2 basis (see RISPERDAL® package insert).

There are no adequate and well controlled studies of INVEGA® SUSTENNA® in pregnant women. INVEGA® SUSTENNA® should be used during pregnancy only if the potential benefit justifies the potential risk to the fetus.

Use of first generation antipsychotic drugs during the last trimester of pregnancy has been associated with extrapyramidal symptoms in the neonate. These symptoms are usually self-limited. It is not known whether paliperidone, when taken near the end of pregnancy, will lead to similar neonatal signs and symptoms.

8.2 Labor and Delivery

The effect of INVEGA® SUSTENNA® on labor and delivery in humans is unknown.

8.3 Nursing Mothers

In animal studies with paliperidone and in human studies with risperidone, paliperidone was excreted in the milk. Therefore, women receiving INVEGA® SUSTENNA® should not breast feed infants.

8.4 Pediatric Use

Safety and effectiveness of INVEGA® SUSTENNA® in patients < 18 years of age have not been established.

8.5 Geriatric Use

Clinical studies of INVEGA® SUSTENNA® did not include sufficient numbers of subjects aged 65 and over to determine whether they respond differently from younger subjects. Other reported clinical experience has not identified differences in responses between the elderly and younger patients.

This drug is known to be substantially excreted by the kidney and clearance is decreased in patients with renal impairment *[see Clinical Pharmacology (12.3)]*, who should be given reduced doses. Because elderly patients are more likely to have decreased renal function, care should be taken in dose selection, and it may be useful to monitor renal function *[see Dosage and Administration (2.5)]*.

8.6 Renal Impairment

INVEGA® SUSTENNA® has not been systematically studied in patients with renal impairment *[see Clinical Pharmacology (12.3)]*. For patients with mild renal impairment (creatinine clearance ≥ 50 mL/min to < 80 mL/min), recommended initiation of INVEGA® SUSTENNA® is with a dose of 156 mg on treatment day 1 and 117 mg one week later, both administered in the deltoid muscle. Thereafter, follow with monthly injections of 78 mg in either the deltoid or gluteal muscle.

INVEGA® SUSTENNA® is not recommended in patients with moderate or severe renal impairment (creatinine clearance < 50 mL/min).

8.7 Hepatic Impairment

INVEGA® SUSTENNA® has not been studied in patients with hepatic impairment. Based on a study with oral paliperidone, no dose adjustment is required in patients with mild or moderate hepatic impairment. Paliperidone has not been studied in patients with severe hepatic impairment.

9 DRUG ABUSE AND DEPENDENCE

9.1 Controlled Substance

INVEGA® SUSTENNA® (paliperidone) is not a controlled substance.

9.2 Abuse

Paliperidone has not been systematically studied in animals or humans for its potential for abuse.

9.3 Dependence

Paliperidone has not been systematically studied in animals or humans for its potential for tolerance or physical dependence.

10 OVERDOSAGE

10.1 Human Experience

No cases of overdose were reported in premarketing studies with INVEGA® SUSTENNA®. Because INVEGA® SUSTENNA® is to be administered by health care professionals, the potential for overdosage by patients is low.

While experience with paliperidone overdose is limited, among the few cases of overdose reported in premarketing trials with oral paliperidone, the highest estimated ingestion was 405 mg. Observed signs and symptoms included extrapyramidal symptoms and gait unsteadiness. Other potential signs and symptoms include those resulting from an exaggeration of paliperidone's known pharmacological effects, i.e., drowsiness and sedation, tachycardia and hypotension, and QT prolongation. Torsade de pointes and ventricular fibrillation have been reported in a patient in the setting of overdose with oral paliperidone.

Paliperidone is the major active metabolite of risperidone. Overdose experience reported with risperidone can be found in the OVERDOSAGE section of the risperidone package insert.

10.2 Management of Overdosage

There is no specific antidote to paliperidone, therefore, appropriate supportive measures should be instituted and close medical supervision and monitoring should continue until the patient recovers. Consideration should be given to the prolonged-release characteristics of INVEGA® SUSTENNA® and the long apparent half-life of paliperidone when assessing treatment needs and recovery. Multiple drug involvement should also be considered.

In case of acute overdose, establish and maintain an airway and ensure adequate oxygenation and ventilation. The possibility of obtundation, seizures, or dystonic reaction of the head and neck following overdose may create a risk of aspiration with induced emesis.

Cardiovascular monitoring should commence immediately, including continuous electrocardiographic monitoring for possible arrhythmias. If antiarrhythmic therapy is administered, disopyramide, procainamide, and quinidine carry a theoretical hazard of additive QT-prolonging effects when administered in patients with an acute overdose of paliperidone. Similarly the alpha-blocking properties of bretylium might be additive to those of paliperidone, resulting in problematic hypotension.

Hypotension and circulatory collapse should be treated with appropriate measures, such as intravenous fluids and/or sympathomimetic agents (epinephrine and dopamine should not be used, since beta stimulation may worsen hypotension in the setting of paliperidone-induced alpha blockade). In cases of severe extrapyramidal symptoms, anticholinergic medication should be administered.

11 DESCRIPTION

INVEGA® SUSTENNA® contains paliperidone palmitate. The active ingredient, paliperidone palmitate, is a psychotropic agent belonging to the chemical class of benzisoxazole derivatives. INVEGA® SUSTENNA® contains a racemic mixture of (+)- and (-)- paliperidone palmitate. The chemical name is (9*RS*)-3-[2-[4-(6-Fluoro-1,2-benzisoxazol-3-yl)piperidin-1-yl]ethyl]-2-methyl-4-oxo-6,7,8,9-tetrahydro-4*H*-pyrido[1,2-*a*]pyrimadin-9-yl hexadecanoate. Its molecular formula is $C_{39}H_{57}FN_4O_4$ and its molecular weight is 664.89. The structural formula is:

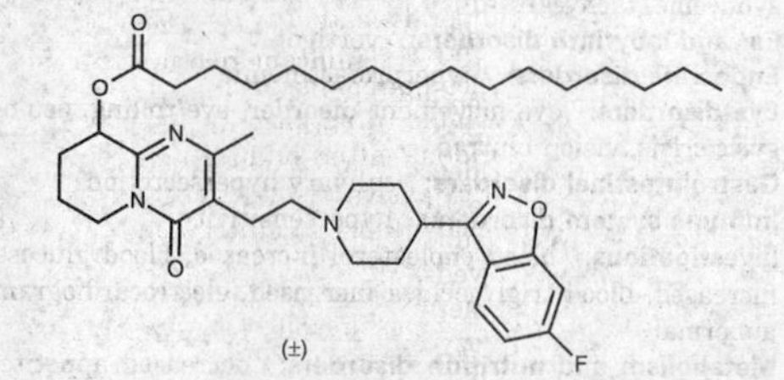

Paliperidone palmitate is very slightly soluble in ethanol and methanol, practically insoluble in polyethylene glycol 400 and propylene glycol, and slightly soluble in ethyl acetate.

INVEGA® SUSTENNA® is available as a white to off-white sterile aqueous extended-release suspension for intramuscular injection in dose strengths of 39 mg, 78 mg, 117 mg, 156 mg, and 234 mg paliperidone palmitate. The drug product hydrolyzes to the active moiety, paliperidone, resulting in dose strengths of 25 mg, 50 mg, 75 mg, 100 mg, and 150 mg of paliperidone, respectively. The inactive ingredients are polysorbate 20, polyethylene glycol 4000, citric acid monohydrate, disodium hydrogen phosphate anhydrous, sodium dihydrogen phosphate monohydrate, sodium hydroxide, and water for injection.

INVEGA® SUSTENNA® is provided in a prefilled syringe (cyclic-olefin-copolymer) with a plunger stopper and tip cap (bromobutyl rubber). The kit also contains 2 safety needles (a 1 ½-inch 22 gauge safety needle and a 1-inch 23 gauge safety needle).

12 CLINICAL PHARMACOLOGY

12.1 Mechanism of Action

Paliperidone palmitate is hydrolyzed to paliperidone *[see Clinical Pharmacology (12.3)]*. Paliperidone is the major active metabolite of risperidone. The mechanism of action of paliperidone, as with other drugs having efficacy in schizophrenia, is unknown, but it has been proposed that the drug's therapeutic activity in schizophrenia is mediated through a combination of central dopamine Type 2 (D_2) and serotonin Type 2 ($5HT_{2A}$) receptor antagonism.

12.2 Pharmacodynamics

Paliperidone is a centrally active dopamine Type 2 (D_2) receptor antagonist and a serotonin Type 2 ($5HT_{2A}$) receptor antagonist. Paliperidone is also active as an antagonist at α_1 and α_2 adrenergic receptors and H_1 histaminergic receptors, which may explain some of the other effects of the drug. Paliperidone has no affinity for cholinergic muscarinic or β_1- and β_2-adrenergic receptors. The pharmacological activity of the (+)- and (-)- paliperidone enantiomers is qualitatively and quantitatively similar *in vitro*.

12.3 Pharmacokinetics

Absorption and Distribution

Due to its extremely low water solubility, paliperidone palmitate dissolves slowly after intramuscular injection before being hydrolyzed to paliperidone and absorbed into the systemic circulation. Following a single intramuscular dose, the plasma concentrations of paliperidone gradually rise to reach maximum plasma concentrations at a median T_{max} of 13 days. The release of the drug starts as early as day 1 and lasts for as long as 126 days.

Following intramuscular injection of single doses (39 mg–234 mg) in the deltoid muscle, on average, a 28% higher C_{max} was observed compared with injection in the gluteal muscle. The two initial deltoid intramuscular injections of 234 mg on day 1 and 156 mg on day 8 help attain therapeutic concentrations rapidly. The release profile and dosing regimen of INVEGA® SUSTENNA® results in sustained therapeutic concentrations. The AUC of paliperidone following INVEGA® SUSTENNA® administration was dose-proportional over a 39 mg–234 mg dose range, and less than dose-proportional for C_{max} for doses exceeding 78 mg. The mean steady-state peak:trough ratio for a INVEGA® SUSTENNA® dose of 156 mg was 1.8 following gluteal administration and 2.2 following deltoid administration.

Following administration of paliperidone palmitate the (+) and (-) enantiomers of paliperidone interconvert, reaching an AUC (+) to (-) ratio of approximately 1.6–1.8.

Based on a population analysis, the apparent volume of distribution of paliperidone is 391 L. The plasma protein binding of racemic paliperidone is 74%.

Metabolism and Elimination

In a study with oral immediate-release ^{14}C-paliperidone, one week following administration of a single oral dose of 1 mg immediate-release ^{14}C-paliperidone, 59% of the dose was excreted unchanged into urine, indicating that paliperidone is not extensively metabolized in the liver. Approximately 80% of the administered radioactivity was recovered in urine and 11% in the feces. Four metabolic pathways have been identified *in vivo*, none of which accounted for more than 10% of the dose: dealkylation, hydroxylation, dehydrogenation, and benzisoxazole scission. Although *in vitro* studies suggested a role for CYP2D6 and CYP3A4 in the metabolism of paliperidone, there is no evidence *in vivo* that these isozymes play a significant role in the metabolism of paliperidone. Population pharmacokinetics analyses indicated no discernable difference on the apparent clearance of paliperidone after administration of oral paliperidone between extensive metabolizers and poor metabolizers of CYP2D6 substrates. *In vitro* studies in human liver microsomes showed that paliperidone does not substantially inhibit the metabolism of medicines metabolized by cytochrome P450 isozymes, including CYP1A2, CYP2A6, CYP2C8/9/10, CYP2D6, CYP2E1, CYP3A4, and CYP3A5.

In vitro studies have shown that paliperidone is a P-gp substrate and a weak inhibitor of P-gp at high concentrations. No *in vivo* data are available and the clinical relevance is unknown.

The median apparent half-life of paliperidone following INVEGA® SUSTENNA® single-dose administration over the dose range of 39 mg–234 mg ranged from 25 days–49 days.

Long-Acting Paliperidone Palmitate Injection versus Oral Extended-Release Paliperidone

INVEGA® SUSTENNA® is designed to deliver paliperidone over a monthly period while extended-release oral paliperidone is administered on a daily basis. The initiation regimen for INVEGA® SUSTENNA® (234 mg/156 mg in the deltoid muscle on Day 1/Day 8) was designed to rapidly attain steady-state paliperidone concentrations when initiating therapy without the use of oral supplementation.

In general, overall initiation plasma levels with INVEGA® SUSTENNA® were within the exposure range observed with 6–12 mg extended-release oral paliperidone. The use of the INVEGA® SUSTENNA® initiation regimen allowed patients to stay in this exposure window of 6–12 mg extended-release oral paliperidone even on trough pre-dose days (Day 8 and Day 36). The intersubject variability for paliperidone pharmacokinetics following delivery from INVEGA® SUSTENNA® was lower relative to the variability determined from extended-release oral paliperidone tablets. Because of the difference in median pharmacokinetic profiles between the two products, caution should be exercised when making a direct comparison of their pharmacokinetic properties.

Special Populations

Renal Impairment

INVEGA® SUSTENNA® has not been systematically studied in patients with renal impairment. Based on a limited number of observations with INVEGA® SUSTENNA® in subjects with mild renal impairment and pharmacokinetic simulations, the dose of INVEGA® SUSTENNA® should be reduced in patients with mild renal impairment; INVEGA® SUSTENNA® is not recommended in patients with moderate or severe renal impairment *[see Dosage and Administration (2.5)]*. Although INVEGA® SUSTENNA® was not studied in patients with moderate or severe renal impairment, the disposition of a single oral dose paliperidone 3 mg extended-release tablet was studied in subjects with varying degrees of renal function. Elimination of paliperidone decreased with decreasing estimated creatinine clearance. Total clearance of paliperidone was reduced in subjects with impaired renal function by 32% on average in mild (CrCl = 50 mL/min to < 80 mL/min), 64% in moderate (CrCl = 30 mL/min to < 50 mL/min), and 71% in severe (CrCl = 10 mL/min to < 30 mL/min) renal impairment, corresponding to an average increase in exposure (AUC_{inf}) of 1.5 fold, 2.6 fold, and 4.8 fold, respectively, compared to healthy subjects. Based on a limited number of observations with INVEGA® SUSTENNA® in subjects with mild renal impairment and pharmacokinetic simulations, the recommended initiation of INVEGA® SUSTENNA® for patients with mild renal impairment is with a dose of 156 mg on treatment day 1 and 117 mg on treatment day 8; thereafter, follow with monthly injections of 78 mg *[see Dosage and Administration (2.5)]*.

Hepatic Impairment

INVEGA® SUSTENNA® has not been studied in patients with hepatic impairment. Based on a study with oral paliperidone in subjects with moderate hepatic impairment (Child-Pugh class B), no dose adjustment is required in patients with mild or moderate hepatic impairment *[see Dosage and Administration (2.5)]*. In the study with oral paliperidone in subjects with moderate hepatic impairment (Child-Pugh class B), the plasma concentrations of free paliperidone were similar to those of healthy subjects, although total paliperidone exposure decreased because of a decrease in protein binding. Paliperidone has not been studied in patients with severe hepatic impairment.

Elderly

No dosage adjustment is recommended based on age alone. However, dose adjustment may be required because of age-related decreases in creatinine clearance *[see Renal Impairment above and Dosage and Administration (2.5)]*.

Race

No dosage adjustment is recommended based on race. No differences in pharmacokinetics were observed between Japanese and Caucasians.

Gender

No dosage adjustment is recommended based on gender, although slower absorption was observed in females in a population pharmacokinetic analysis.

Smoking

No dosage adjustment is recommended based on smoking status. Based on *in vitro* studies utilizing human liver enzymes, paliperidone is not a substrate for CYP1A2; smoking should, therefore, not have an effect on the pharmacokinetics of paliperidone.

13 NONCLINICAL TOXICOLOGY

13.1 Carcinogenesis, Mutagenesis, Impairment of Fertility

Carcinogenesis

The carcinogenic potential of intramuscularly injected paliperidone palmitate was assessed in rats. There was an increase in mammary gland adenocarcinomas in female rats at 16, 47, and 94 mg/kg/month, which is 0.6, 2, and 4 times, respectively, the maximum recommended human 234 mg dose of INVEGA® SUSTENNA® on a mg/m^2 basis. A no-effect dose was not established. Male rats showed an increase in mammary gland adenomas, fibroadenomas, and carcinomas at 47 mg and 94 mg/kg/month. A carcinogenicity study in mice has not been conducted with paliperidone palmitate.

Carcinogenicity studies of risperidone, which is extensively converted to paliperidone in rats, mice, and humans, were conducted in Swiss albino mice and Wistar rats. Risperidone was administered in the diet at daily doses of 0.63, 2.5, and 10 mg/kg for 18 months to mice and for 25 months to rats. A maximum tolerated dose was not achieved in male mice. There were statistically significant increases in pituitary gland adenomas, endocrine pancreas adenomas, and mammary gland adenocarcinomas. The no-effect dose for these tumors was less than or equal to the maximum recommended human dose of risperidone on a mg/m^2 basis (see RISPERDAL® package insert). An increase in mammary, pituitary, and endocrine pancreas neoplasms has been found in rodents after chronic administration of other antipsychotic drugs and is considered to be mediated by prolonged dopamine D_2-receptor antagonism and hyperprolactinemia. The relevance of these tumor findings in rodents in terms of human risk is unknown *[see Warnings and Precautions (5.8)]*.

Mutagenesis

Paliperidone palmitate showed no genotoxic potential in the Ames reverse mutation test or the mouse lymphoma assay. No evidence of genotoxic potential for paliperidone was found in the Ames reverse mutation test, the mouse lymphoma assay, or the *in vivo* rat micronucleus test.

Impairment of Fertility

Fertility studies of paliperidone palmitate have not been performed.

In a study of fertility conducted with orally administered paliperidone, the percentage of treated female rats that became pregnant was not affected at doses of paliperidone of up to 2.5 mg/kg/day. However, pre- and post-implantation loss were increased, and the number of live embryos was slightly decreased, at 2.5 mg/kg, a dose that also caused slight maternal toxicity. These parameters were not affected at a dose of 0.63 mg/kg, which is half of the maximum recommended human dose (12 mg/day) of orally administered paliperidone (INVEGA®) on a mg/m^2 basis.

The fertility of male rats was not affected at oral doses of paliperidone of up to 2.5 mg/kg/day, although sperm count and sperm viability studies were not conducted with paliperidone. In a subchronic study in Beagle dogs with risperidone, which is extensively converted to paliperidone in dogs and humans, all doses tested (0.31 mg/kg–5.0 mg/kg) resulted in decreases in serum testosterone and in sperm motility and concentration. Serum testosterone and sperm parameters partially recovered, but remained decreased after the last observation (two months after treatment was discontinued).

14 CLINICAL STUDIES

The efficacy of INVEGA® SUSTENNA® in the acute treatment of schizophrenia was evaluated in four short-term (one 9-week and three 13-week) double-blind, randomized, placebo-controlled, fixed-dose studies of acutely relapsed adult inpatients who met DSM-IV criteria for schizophrenia. The fixed doses of INVEGA® SUSTENNA® in these studies were given on days 1, 8, and 36 in the 9-week study, and additionally on day 64 of the 13-week studies, i.e., at a weekly interval for the initial two doses and then every 4 weeks for maintenance.

Efficacy was evaluated using the Positive and Negative Syndrome Scale (PANSS), a validated multi-item inventory composed of five factors to evaluate positive symptoms, negative symptoms, disorganized thoughts, uncontrolled hostility/excitement, and anxiety/depression.

In a 13-week study (n=636) comparing three fixed doses of INVEGA® SUSTENNA® (initial deltoid injection of 234 mg followed by 3 gluteal or deltoid doses of either 39 mg/4 weeks, 156 mg/4 weeks or 234 mg/4 weeks) to placebo, all three doses of INVEGA® SUSTENNA® were superior to placebo in improving the PANSS total score.

In another 13-week study (n=349) comparing three fixed doses of INVEGA® SUSTENNA® (78 mg/4 weeks, 156 mg/4 weeks, and 234 mg/4 weeks) to placebo, only 156 mg/4 weeks of INVEGA® SUSTENNA® was superior to placebo in improving the PANSS total score.

In a third 13-week study (n=513) comparing three fixed doses of INVEGA® SUSTENNA® (39 mg/4 weeks, 78 mg/4 weeks, and 156 mg/4 weeks) to placebo, all three doses of INVEGA® SUSTENNA® were superior to placebo in improving the PANSS total score.

In the 9-week study (n=197) comparing two fixed doses of INVEGA® SUSTENNA® (78 mg/4 weeks and 156 mg/4 weeks) to placebo, both doses of INVEGA® SUSTENNA® were superior to placebo in improving PANSS total score.

The efficacy of INVEGA® SUSTENNA® in maintaining symptomatic control in schizophrenia was established in a longer-term double-blind, placebo-controlled, flexible-dose study involving adult subjects who met DSM-IV criteria for schizophrenia. This study included a minimum 12-week fixed-dose stabilization phase, and a randomized, placebo-controlled phase to observe for relapse. During the double-blind phase, patients were randomized to either the same dose of INVEGA® SUSTENNA® they received during the stabilization phase, i.e., 39 mg, 78 mg, or 156 mg administered every 4 weeks, or to placebo. A total of 410 stabilized patients were randomized to either INVEGA® SUSTENNA® or to placebo until they experienced a relapse of schizophrenia symptoms. Relapse was pre-defined as time to first emergence of one or more of the following: psychiatric hospitalization, ≥ 25% increase (if the baseline score was > 40) or a 10-point increase (if the baseline score was ≤ 40) in total PANSS score on two consecutive assessments, deliberate self-injury, violent behavior, suicidal/homicidal ideation, or a score of ≥ 5 (if the maximum baseline score was ≤ 3) or ≥ 6 (if the maximum baseline score was 4) on two consecutive assessments of the individual PANSS items P1 (Delusions), P2 (Conceptual disorganization), P3 (Hallucinatory behavior), P6 (Suspiciousness/persecution), P7 (Hostility), or G8 (Uncooperativeness). The primary efficacy variable was time to relapse. A pre-planned interim analysis showed a statistically significantly longer time to relapse in patients treated with INVEGA® SUSTENNA® compared to placebo, and the study was stopped early because maintenance of efficacy was demonstrated.

An examination of population subgroups did not reveal any clinically significant differences in responsiveness on the basis of gender, age, or race.

16 HOW SUPPLIED/STORAGE AND HANDLING

INVEGA® SUSTENNA® is available as a white to off-white sterile aqueous extended-release suspension for intramuscular injection in dose strengths of 39 mg, 78 mg, 117 mg, 156 mg, and 234 mg paliperidone palmitate. The kit contains a prefilled syringe and 2 safety needles (a 1 ½-inch 22 gauge safety needle and a 1-inch 23 gauge safety needle).

39 mg paliperidone palmitate kit (NDC 50458-560-01)
78 mg paliperidone palmitate kit (NDC 50458-561-01)
117 mg paliperidone palmitate kit (NDC 50458-562-01)
156 mg paliperidone palmitate kit (NDC 50458-563-01)
234 mg paliperidone palmitate kit (NDC 50458-564-01)

Storage and Handling
Store at room temperature (25°C, 77°F); excursions between 15°C and 30°C (between 59°F and 86°F) are permitted.
Keep out of reach of children.

17 PATIENT COUNSELING INFORMATION

Physicians are advised to discuss the following issues with patients for whom they prescribe INVEGA SUSTENNA®. See FDA-approved patient labeling.

17.1 Orthostatic Hypotension
Patients should be advised that there is risk of orthostatic hypotension, particularly at the time of initiating treatment, re-initiating treatment, or increasing the dose [see Warnings and Precautions (5.9)].

17.2 Interference with Cognitive and Motor Performance
As INVEGA® SUSTENNA® has the potential to impair judgment, thinking, or motor skills, patients should be cautioned about operating hazardous machinery, including automobiles, until they are reasonably certain that INVEGA® SUSTENNA® therapy does not affect them adversely [see Warnings and Precautions (5.11)].

17.3 Pregnancy
Patients should be advised to notify their physician if they become pregnant or intend to become pregnant during treatment with INVEGA® SUSTENNA® [see Use in Specific Populations (8.1)].

17.4 Nursing
Patients should be advised not to breast-feed an infant during treatment with INVEGA® SUSTENNA® [see Use in Specific Populations (8.3)].

17.5 Concomitant Medication
Patients should be advised to inform their physicians if they are taking, or plan to take, any prescription or over-the-counter drugs, as there is a potential for interactions [see Drug Interactions (7)].

17.6 Alcohol
Patients should be advised to avoid alcohol while taking INVEGA® SUSTENNA® [see Drug Interactions (7.1)].

17.7 Heat Exposure and Dehydration
Patients should be advised regarding appropriate care in avoiding overheating and dehydration [see Warnings and Precautions (5.17)].

INVEGA® SUSTENNA® (paliperidone palmitate) Extended-Release Injectable Suspension
Manufactured by:
Janssen Pharmaceutica N.V.
Beerse, Belgium
Manufactured for:
Janssen, Division of Ortho-McNeil-Janssen Pharmaceuticals, Inc.
Titusville, NJ 08560
Revised: March 2010
©Ortho-McNeil-Janssen Pharmaceuticals, Inc. 2009

INFORMATION FOR PATIENTS AND CAREGIVERS
INVEGA® SUSTENNA® (paliperidone palmitate)
Extended-Release Injectable Suspension
Important Information
This summary contains important information about INVEGA® SUSTENNA® for patients and caregivers and has been reviewed by the U.S. Food and Drug Administration.

Read this information carefully and talk to your doctor or treatment team if you have any questions about INVEGA® SUSTENNA®. Keep this information handy so that you can refer to it later if you have any questions. Ask your doctor or treatment team if there is any new information that you need to know about INVEGA® SUSTENNA®.
This summary does not contain all the information about INVEGA® SUSTENNA®. It does not take the place of talking with your doctor.

What is INVEGA® SUSTENNA®?
INVEGA® SUSTENNA® is a type of prescription medicine called an atypical antipsychotic given as an injection by a healthcare provider.
INVEGA® SUSTENNA® is used to treat symptoms of schizophrenia. INVEGA® SUSTENNA® can also be used to lessen the chance of your schizophrenia symptoms from coming back.

How does INVEGA® SUSTENNA® work?
Schizophrenia is believed to be caused when certain chemicals in the brain are not in balance. Not all people with schizophrenia have the same symptoms. Some of the most common symptoms of schizophrenia may include:

- Seeing, hearing, or sensing things that are not there (hallucinations)
- Believing that what other people say are not true (delusions)
- Not trusting others and feeling very suspicious (paranoia)
- Avoiding family and friends and wanting to be alone

The exact way INVEGA® SUSTENNA® works is not known. INVEGA® SUSTENNA® is thought to help restore the balance of these chemicals in the brain, and has been shown to help many people manage their symptoms of schizophrenia.
It may take some time before your symptoms of schizophrenia start to improve. Remember that INVEGA® SUSTENNA® is one part of your overall treatment plan. It is important to keep all your appointments so you can get your treatments on time and your treatment team can check your progress.

What is the most important safety information I need to know about INVEGA® SUSTENNA®?
INVEGA® SUSTENNA® is not approved for the treatment of dementia-related psychosis in elderly patients. Elderly patients who were given oral antipsychotics like INVEGA® SUSTENNA® in clinical studies for psychosis caused by dementia (memory problems) had a higher risk of death.
Who should not use INVEGA® SUSTENNA®?
INVEGA® SUSTENNA® is not approved for the treatment of elderly patients who have a diagnosis of psychosis related to dementia.
Do not take INVEGA® SUSTENNA® if you:
- Are allergic to paliperidone (INVEGA® Extended-release Tablets) or any other ingredient in INVEGA® SUSTENNA®. Ask your doctor or pharmacist for a list of these ingredients.
- Are allergic to risperidone (RISPERDAL®).

What should I tell my doctor before starting INVEGA® SUSTENNA®?
Only your doctor can decide if INVEGA® SUSTENNA® is right for you. Before you start INVEGA® SUSTENNA®, be sure to tell your doctor or treatment team if you:
- Have a history of heart problems, any problems with the way your heart beats, or are being treated for high blood pressure.
- Have diabetes or a family history of diabetes.
- Have a history of low white blood cell counts.
- Have low levels of potassium or magnesium in your blood.
- Are being treated for seizures (fits or convulsions), have had seizures in the past, or have conditions that increase the risk of having seizures.
- Have kidney or liver problems.
- Have ever had any conditions that cause dizziness or fainting.
- Are pregnant or plan to become pregnant during treatment.
- Are breast-feeding. Women should not breast-feed a baby during treatment.
- Are taking or plan to take any prescription medicines or over-the-counter medicines such as vitamins, herbal products, or dietary supplements.

How often is INVEGA® SUSTENNA® given?
INVEGA® SUSTENNA® is a long-acting medicine that a healthcare professional will give you by injection. This means that you do not have to take this medicine every day. When you receive your first dose of INVEGA® SUSTENNA® you will need to get a second dose one week later. After that you will only need to get a dose once a month.
Your doctor or healthcare provider will give you the injection into the upper arm or buttocks. People usually feel some pain or discomfort. In clinical studies, most patients reported the injections became less painful over time.

What if I miss an injection of INVEGA® SUSTENNA®?
It is very important to keep all your appointments and get your injections on time. If you think you are going to miss your appointment, call your doctor or treatment team as soon as you can. Your doctor or treatment team will decide what you should do next.

What if I stop receiving INVEGA® SUSTENNA®?
If you stop coming for your injections, your symptoms may return. You should not stop receiving injections of this medicine unless you have discussed this with your doctor.

What are the possible side effects of INVEGA® SUSTENNA®?
As with any medicine, INVEGA® SUSTENNA® may cause side effects in some people. If you think you are developing a side effect, always discuss this with your doctor or treatment team.
Common side effects of INVEGA® SUSTENNA® include:
- Reactions at the injection site
- Sleepiness
- Dizziness
- Feeling of inner restlessness
- Abnormal muscle movements, including tremor (shaking), shuffling, uncontrolled involuntary movements, and abnormal movements of the eyes

Other important safety information
Neuroleptic Malignant Syndrome (NMS) is a rare, but serious side effect that could be fatal and has been reported with INVEGA® SUSTENNA® and similar medicines. Call the doctor right away if you develop symptoms such as a high fever, rigid muscles, shaking, confusion, sweating more than usual, increased heart rate or blood pressure, or muscle pain or weakness. Treatment should be stopped if you are being treated for NMS.
Tardive Dyskinesia (TD) is a rare, but serious and sometimes permanent side effect reported with INVEGA® SUSTENNA® and similar medicines. Call your doctor right away if you start to develop twitching or jerking movements that you cannot control in your face, tongue, or other parts of your body. The risk of developing TD and the chance that it will become permanent is thought to increase with the length of therapy and the total dose received. This condition can also develop after a short period of treatment at low doses but this is less common. There is no known treatment for TD but it may go away partially or completely if the medicine is stopped.
One risk of INVEGA® SUSTENNA® is that it may change your heart rhythm. This effect is potentially serious. You should talk to your doctor about any current or past heart problems. Because these problems could mean you're having a heart rhythm abnormality, contact your doctor IMMEDIATELY if you feel faint or feel a change in the way that your heart beats (palpitations).
High blood sugar and diabetes have been reported with INVEGA® SUSTENNA® and similar medicines. If you already have diabetes or have risk factors such as being overweight or a family history of diabetes, blood sugar testing should be done at the beginning and during the treatment. The complications of diabetes can be serious and even life-threatening. Call your doctor if you develop signs of high blood sugar or diabetes, such as being thirsty all the time, having to urinate or "pass urine" more often than usual, or feeling weak or hungry.
Weight gain has been observed with INVEGA® SUSTENNA® and other atypical antipsychotic medications. If you notice that you are gaining weight, please notify your doctor.
Some people may feel faint, dizzy, or may pass out when they stand up or sit up suddenly. Be careful not to get up too quickly. It may help if you get up slowly and sit on the edge of the bed or chair for a few minutes before you stand up. These symptoms may decrease or go away after your body becomes used to the medicine.
INVEGA® SUSTENNA® and similar medicines have been associated with decreases in the counts of white cells in circulating blood. If you have a history of low white blood cell counts or have unexplained fever or infection, then please contact your doctor right away.
INVEGA® SUSTENNA® and similar medicines can raise the blood levels of a hormone called prolactin and blood levels of prolactin remain high with continued use. This may result in some side effects including menstrual periods, leakage of milk from the breasts, development of breasts in men, or problems with erection.
If you have a prolonged or painful erection lasting more than 4 hours, seek immediate medical help to avoid long-term injury.
Call your doctor right away if you start thinking about suicide or wanting to hurt yourself.
INVEGA® SUSTENNA® can make some people feel dizzy, sleepy, or less alert. Until you know how you are going to respond to INVEGA® SUSTENNA®, be careful driving a car, operating machines, or doing things that require you to be alert.
This medicine may make you more sensitive to heat. You may have trouble cooling off or be more likely to become dehydrated. Be careful when you exercise or spend time doing things that make you warm.
Do not drink alcohol while you are taking INVEGA® SUSTENNA®.
This is not a complete list of all possible side effects. Ask your doctor or treatment team if you have any questions or want more information.

How can I get the most benefit from my INVEGA® SUSTENNA® treatment?
- **Remember to keep all your appointments.** You need to receive your INVEGA® SUSTENNA® treatments on time and your treatment team needs to check your progress. If you are going to miss an appointment, call your doctor's office right away so you can get your next dose as soon as possible.
- **Keep a list of questions.** Discuss this list with your treatment team at your next visit. Your treatment team wants to know how the medicine is working so they can give you the best care possible.
- **Be patient.** It may take some time before your symptoms of schizophrenia start to improve.

- **Follow the plan developed by you and your treatment team.** Remember that INVEGA® SUSTENNA® is one part of your overall treatment plan.

Where can I find more information about INVEGA® SUSTENNA®?

This is a summary of important information about INVEGA® SUSTENNA®. If you have any questions about this information, talk with your doctor or treatment team. You can also visit the website at www.invegasustenna.com or call the toll-free number at 1-800-JANSSEN (1-800-526-7736) for more information about INVEGA® SUSTENNA®. Janssen, Division of Ortho-McNeil-Janssen Pharmaceuticals, Inc.

© Ortho-McNeil-Janssen Pharmaceuticals, Inc. 2009
Revised: March 2010
976781MG

Shown in Product Identification Guide, page 316

LEVAQUIN®   ℞
[lĕv-ă-kwĭn]
(levofloxacin)
Tablet, Film Coated for Oral use
LEVAQUIN®
(levofloxacin)
Solution for Oral use
LEVAQUIN®
(levofloxacin)
Injection, Solution, Concentrate for Intravenous use
LEVAQUIN®
(levofloxacin)
Injection, Solution for Intravenous use

HIGHLIGHTS OF PRESCRIBING INFORMATION
These highlights do not include all the information needed to use LEVAQUIN safely and effectively. See full prescribing information for LEVAQUIN.

LEVAQUIN (levofloxacin) Tablet, Film Coated for Oral use
LEVAQUIN (levofloxacin) Solution for Oral use
LEVAQUIN (levofloxacin) Injection, Solution, Concentrate for Intravenous use
LEVAQUIN (levofloxacin) Injection, Solution for Intravenous use
Initial U.S. Approval: 1996

> **WARNING:**
> Fluoroquinolones, including LEVAQUIN®, are associated with an increased risk of tendinitis and tendon rupture in all ages. This risk is further increased in older patients usually over 60 years of age, in patients taking corticosteroid drugs, and in patients with kidney, heart or lung transplants [*See Warnings and Precautions (5.1)*].

To reduce the development of drug-resistant bacteria and maintain the effectiveness of LEVAQUIN® and other antibacterial drugs, LEVAQUIN® should be used only to treat or prevent infections that are proven or strongly suspected to be caused by bacteria.

─────RECENT MAJOR CHANGES─────
Warnings and Precautions
- Tendinopathy and Tendon Rupture (5.1)   9/2008

─────INDICATIONS AND USAGE─────
LEVAQUIN® is a fluoroquinolone antibacterial indicated in adults (≥18 years of age) with infections caused by designated, susceptible bacteria (1, 12.4).
- Pneumonia: nosocomial (1.1) and community acquired (1.2, 1.3)
- Acute bacterial sinusitis (1.4)
- Acute bacterial exacerbation of chronic bronchitis (1.5)
- Skin and skin structure infections: complicated (1.6) and uncomplicated (1.7)
- Chronic bacterial prostatitis (1.8)
- Urinary tract infections: complicated (1.9, 1.10) and uncomplicated (1.12)
- Acute pyelonephritis (1.11)
- Inhalational anthrax, post-exposure (1.13). Not tested in humans for post-exposure prevention of inhalational anthrax; plasma concentrations are likely to predict efficacy (14.9)

─────DOSAGE AND ADMINISTRATION─────
- Dosage in patients with normal renal function (2.1)

Type of Infection	Dose Every 24 hours	Duration (days)
Nosocomial Pneumonia (1.1)	750 mg	7–14
Community Acquired Pneumonia (1.2)	500 mg	7–14
Community Acquired Pneumonia (1.3)	750 mg	5
Acute Bacterial Sinusitis (1.4)	750 mg	5
	500 mg	10–14
Acute Bacterial Exacerbation of Chronic Bronchitis (1.5)	500 mg	7
Complicated Skin and Skin Structure Infections (SSSI) (1.6)	750 mg	7–14
Uncomplicated SSSI (1.7)	500 mg	7–10
Chronic Bacterial Prostatitis (1.8)	500 mg	28
Complicated Urinary Tract Infection (1.9) or Acute Pyelonephritis (1.11)	750 mg	5
Complicated Urinary Tract Infection (1.10) or Acute Pyelonephritis (1.11)	250 mg	10
Uncomplicated Urinary Tract Infection (1.12)	250 mg	3
Inhalational Anthrax (Post-Exposure) (1.13) Adults and Pediatric Patients > 50 kg and ≥ 6 months of age	500 mg	60
Pediatric Patients < 50 kg and ≥ 6 months of age	8 mg/kg BID (not to exceed 250 mg/dose)	60

- Adjust dose for creatinine clearance < 50 mL/min (2.3, 8.6, 12.3)
- IV Injection, Single-Use or Premix: Slow IV infusion only, over 60 or 90 minutes depending on dose. Avoid rapid or bolus IV (2.5)
- Dilute single-use vials to 5 mg/mL prior to IV infusion (2.6)
- Do not mix with other medications in vial or IV line (2.6)

─────DOSAGE FORMS AND STRENGTHS─────

Formulation (3)	Strength
Tablets	250 mg, 500 mg, and 750 mg
Oral Solution	25 mg/mL
Injection: single-use vials for dilution	500 mg in 20 mL 750 mg in 30 mL
Injection: premix single-use flexible containers	250 mg in 50 mL 500 mg in 100 mL 750 mg in 150 mL

─────CONTRAINDICATIONS─────
Known hypersensitivity to LEVAQUIN® or other quinolones (4, 5.2)

─────WARNINGS AND PRECAUTIONS─────
- Risk of tendinitis and tendon rupture is increased. This risk is further increased in older patients usually over 60 years of age, in patients taking corticosteroids, and in patients with kidney, heart or lung transplants. Discontinue if pain or inflammation in a tendon occurs (5.1, 8.5)
- Anaphylactic reactions and allergic skin reactions, serious, occasionally fatal, may occur after first dose (4, 5.2)
- Hematologic (including agranulocytosis, thrombocytopenia), and renal toxicities may occur after multiple doses (5.3)
- Hepatotoxicity: Severe, and sometimes fatal, hepatotoxicity has been reported. Discontinue immediately if signs and symptoms of hepatitis occur (5.4)
- Central nervous system effects, including convulsions, anxiety, confusion, depression, and insomnia may occur after the first dose. Use with caution in patients with known or suspected disorders that may predispose them to seizures or lower the seizure threshold (5.5)
- *Clostridium difficile*-associated colitis: evaluate if diarrhea occurs (5.6)
- Peripheral neuropathy: discontinue if symptoms occur in order to prevent irreversibility (5.7)
- Prolongation of the QT interval and isolated cases of torsade de pointes have been reported. Avoid use in patients with known prolongation, those with hypokalemia, and with other drugs that prolong the QT interval (5.8, 8.5)

─────ADVERSE REACTIONS─────
The most common reactions (≥3%) were nausea, headache, diarrhea, insomnia, constipation and dizziness (6.2).

To report SUSPECTED ADVERSE REACTIONS, contact Ortho-McNeil-Janssen Scientific Affairs Customer Communications Center at 1-800-526-7736 or FDA at 1-800-FDA-1088 or www.fda.gov/medwatch.

─────DRUG INTERACTIONS─────

Interacting Drug	Interaction
Multivalent cation-containing products including antacids, metal cations or didanosine	Absorption of levofloxacin is decreased when the tablet or oral solution formulation is taken within 2 hours of these products. Do not co-administer the intravenous formulation in the same IV line with a multivalent cation, e.g., magnesium (2.4, 7.1)
Warfarin	Effect may be enhanced. Monitor prothrombin time, INR, watch for bleeding (7.2)
Antidiabetic agents	Carefully monitor blood glucose (5.10, 7.3)

─────USE IN SPECIFIC POPULATIONS─────
- **Geriatrics:** Severe hepatotoxicity has been reported. The majority of reports describe patients 65 years of age or older (5.4, 8.5, 17). May have increased risk of tendinopathy (including rupture), especially with concomitant corticosteroid use (5.1, 8.5, 17). May be more susceptible to prolongation of the QT interval. (5.8, 8.5, 17).
- **Pediatrics:** Musculoskeletal disorders (arthralgia, arthritis, tendonopathy, and gait abnormality) seen in more LEVAQUIN®-treated patients than in comparator. Shown to cause arthropathy and osteochondrosis in juvenile animals (5.9, 8.4, 13.2). Safety in pediatric patients treated for more than 14 days has not been studied. Risk-benefit appropriate only for the treatment of inhalational anthrax (post-exposure) (1.13, 2.2, 8.4, 14.9)

See 17 for PATIENT COUNSELING INFORMATION and Medication Guide

Revised: 07/2009

FULL PRESCRIBING INFORMATION: CONTENTS*
WARNING:
1 INDICATIONS AND USAGE
  1.1   Nosocomial Pneumonia
  1.2   Community-Acquired Pneumonia: 7–14 day Treatment Regimen
  1.3   Community-Acquired Pneumonia: 5-day Treatment Regimen
  1.4   Acute Bacterial Sinusitis: 5-day and 10–14 day Treatment Regimens
  1.5   Acute Bacterial Exacerbation of Chronic Bronchitis
  1.6   Complicated Skin and Skin Structure Infections
  1.7   Uncomplicated Skin and Skin Structure Infections
  1.8   Chronic Bacterial Prostatitis
  1.9   Complicated Urinary Tract Infections: 5-day Treatment Regimen
  1.10   Complicated Urinary Tract Infections: 10-day Treatment Regimen
  1.11   Acute Pyelonephritis: 5 or 10-day Treatment Regimen
  1.12   Uncomplicated Urinary Tract Infections
  1.13   Inhalational Anthrax (Post-Exposure)
2 DOSAGE AND ADMINISTRATION
  2.1   Dosage in Adult Patients with Normal Renal Function
  2.2   Dosage in Pediatric Patients
  2.3   Dosage Adjustment in Adults with Renal Impairment
  2.4   Drug Interaction With Chelation Agents: Antacids, Sucralfate, Metal Cations, Multivitamins
  2.5   Administration Instructions
  2.6   Preparation of Intravenous Product
3 DOSAGE FORMS AND STRENGTHS
4 CONTRAINDICATIONS
5 WARNINGS AND PRECAUTIONS
  5.1   Tendinopathy and Tendon Rupture
  5.2   Hypersensitivity Reactions
  5.3   Other Serious and Sometimes Fatal Reactions
  5.4   Hepatotoxicity
  5.5   Central Nervous System Effects
  5.6   Clostridium difficile-Associated Diarrhea
  5.7   Peripheral Neuropathy
  5.8   Prolongation of the QT Interval

FULL PRESCRIBING INFORMATION

WARNING:
Fluoroquinolones, including LEVAQUIN®, are associated with an increased risk of tendinitis and tendon rupture in all ages. This risk is further increased in older patients usually over 60 years of age, in patients taking corticosteroid drugs, and in patients with kidney, heart or lung transplants [*See Warnings and Precautions (5.1)*].

---

1   INDICATIONS AND USAGE

To reduce the development of drug-resistant bacteria and maintain the effectiveness of LEVAQUIN® and other antibacterial drugs, LEVAQUIN® should be used only to treat or prevent infections that are proven or strongly suspected to be caused by susceptible bacteria. When culture and susceptibility information are available, they should be considered in selecting or modifying antibacterial therapy. In the

Table 1: Dosage in Adult Patients with Normal Renal Function (creatinine clearance ≥ 50 mL/min)

Type of Infection*	Dosed Every 24 hours	Duration (days)[†]
Nosocomial Pneumonia	750 mg	7–14
Community Acquired Pneumonia[‡]	500 mg	7–14
Community Acquired Pneumonia[§]	750 mg	5
Acute Bacterial Sinusitis	750 mg	5
	500 mg	10–14
Acute Bacterial Exacerbation of Chronic Bronchitis	500 mg	7
Complicated Skin and Skin Structure Infections (SSSI)	750 mg	7–14
Uncomplicated SSSI	500 mg	7–10
Chronic Bacterial Prostatitis	500 mg	28
Complicated Urinary Tract Infection (cUTI) or Acute Pyelonephritis (AP)[¶]	750 mg	5
Complicated Urinary Tract Infection (cUTI) or Acute Pyelonephritis (AP)[#]	250 mg	10
Uncomplicated Urinary Tract Infection	250 mg	3
Inhalational Anthrax (Post-Exposure), adult and pediatric patients > 50 kg and ≥ 6 months of age[Þ,ß]	500 mg	60[ß]
Pediatric patients < 50 kg and ≥ 6 months of age[Þ,ß]	see Table 2 below (2.2)	60[ß]

* Due to the designated pathogens [*see Indications and Usage (1)*].
† Sequential therapy (intravenous to oral) may be instituted at the discretion of the physician.
‡ Due to methicillin-susceptible *Staphylococcus aureus, Streptococcus pneumoniae* (including multi-drug-resistant strains [MDRSP]), *Haemophilus influenzae, Haemophilus parainfluenzae, Klebsiella pneumoniae, Moraxella catarrhalis, Chlamydophila pneumoniae, Legionella pneumophila,* or *Mycoplasma pneumoniae* [*see Indications and Usage (1.2)*].
§ Due to *Streptococcus pneumoniae* (excluding multi-drug-resistant strains [MDRSP]), *Haemophilus influenzae, Haemophilus parainfluenzae, Mycoplasma pneumoniae,* or *Chlamydophila pneumoniae* [*see Indications and Usage (1.3)*].
¶ This regimen is indicated for cUTI due to *Escherichia coli, Klebsiella pneumoniae, Proteus mirabilis* and AP due to *E. coli,* including cases with concurrent bacteremia.
# This regimen is indicated for cUTI due to *Enterococcus faecalis, Enterococcus cloacae, Escherichia coli, Klebsiella pneumoniae, Proteus mirabilis, Pseudomonas aeruginosa;* and for AP due to *E. coli.*
Þ Drug administration should begin as soon as possible after suspected or confirmed exposure to aerosolized *B. anthracis.* This indication is based on a surrogate endpoint. Levofloxacin plasma concentrations achieved in humans are reasonably likely to predict clinical benefit [*see Clinical Studies (14.9)*].
ß The safety of LEVAQUIN® in adults for durations of therapy beyond 28 days or in pediatric patients for durations beyond 14 days has not been studied. An increased incidence of musculoskeletal adverse events compared to controls has been observed in pediatric patients [*see Warnings and Precautions (5.9), Use in Specific Populations (8.4), and Clinical Studies (14.9)*]. Prolonged LEVAQUIN® therapy in adults should only be used when the benefit outweighs the risk.

absence of such data, local epidemiology and susceptibility patterns may contribute to the empiric selection of therapy. LEVAQUIN® Tablets/Injection and Oral Solution are indicated for the treatment of adults (≥18 years of age) with mild, moderate, and severe infections caused by susceptible strains of the designated microorganisms in the conditions listed in this section. LEVAQUIN® Injection is indicated when intravenous administration offers a route of administration advantageous to the patient (e.g., patient cannot tolerate an oral dosage form).

Culture and susceptibility testing

Appropriate culture and susceptibility tests should be performed before treatment in order to isolate and identify organisms causing the infection and to determine their susceptibility to levofloxacin [*see Clinical Pharmacology (12.4)*]. Therapy with LEVAQUIN® may be initiated before results of these tests are known; once results become available, appropriate therapy should be selected.

As with other drugs in this class, some strains of *Pseudomonas aeruginosa* may develop resistance fairly rapidly during treatment with LEVAQUIN®. Culture and susceptibility testing performed periodically during therapy will provide information about the continued susceptibility of the pathogens to the antimicrobial agent and also the possible emergence of bacterial resistance.

1.1   Nosocomial Pneumonia

LEVAQUIN® is indicated for the treatment of nosocomial pneumonia due to methicillin-susceptible *Staphylococcus aureus, Pseudomonas aeruginosa, Serratia marcescens, Escherichia coli, Klebsiella pneumoniae, Haemophilus influenzae,* or *Streptococcus pneumoniae.* Adjunctive therapy should be used as clinically indicated. Where *Pseudomonas aeruginosa* is a documented or presumptive pathogen, combination therapy with an anti-pseudomonal β-lactam is recommended [*see Clinical Studies (14.1)*].

1.2   Community-Acquired Pneumonia: 7–14 day Treatment Regimen

LEVAQUIN® is indicated for the treatment of community-acquired pneumonia due to methicillin-susceptible *Staphy-* *lococcus aureus, Streptococcus pneumoniae* (including multi-drug-resistant *Streptococcus pneumoniae* [MDRSP]), *Haemophilus influenzae, Haemophilus parainfluenzae, Klebsiella pneumoniae, Moraxella catarrhalis, Chlamydophila pneumoniae, Legionella pneumophila,* or *Mycoplasma pneumoniae* [*see Dosage and Administration (2.1) and Clinical Studies (14.2)*].

MDRSP isolates are strains resistant to two or more of the following antibacterials: penicillin (MIC ≥2mcg/mL), 2nd generation cephalosporins, e.g., cefuroxime, macrolides, tetracyclines and trimethoprim/sulfamethoxazole.

1.3   Community-Acquired Pneumonia: 5-day Treatment Regimen

LEVAQUIN® is indicated for the treatment of community-acquired pneumonia due to *Streptococcus pneumoniae* (excluding multi-drug-resistant strains [MDRSP]), *Haemophilus influenzae, Haemophilus parainfluenzae, Mycoplasma pneumoniae,* or *Chlamydophila pneumoniae* [*see Dosage and Administration (2.1) and Clinical Studies (14.3)*].

1.4   Acute Bacterial Sinusitis: 5-day and 10–14 day Treatment Regimens

LEVAQUIN® is indicated for the treatment of acute bacterial sinusitis due to *Streptococcus pneumoniae, Haemophilus influenzae,* or *Moraxella catarrhalis* [*see Clinical Studies (14.4)*].

1.5   Acute Bacterial Exacerbation of Chronic Bronchitis

LEVAQUIN® is indicated for the treatment of acute bacterial exacerbation of chronic bronchitis due to methicillin-susceptible *Staphylococcus aureus, Streptococcus pneumoniae, Haemophilus influenzae, Haemophilus parainfluenzae,* or *Moraxella catarrhalis.*

1.6   Complicated Skin and Skin Structure Infections

LEVAQUIN® is indicated for the treatment of complicated skin and skin structure infections due to methicillin-susceptible *Staphylococcus aureus, Enterococcus faecalis, Streptococcus pyogenes,* or *Proteus mirabilis* [*see Clinical Studies (14.5)*].

1.7 Uncomplicated Skin and Skin Structure Infections

LEVAQUIN® is indicated for the treatment of uncomplicated skin and skin structure infections (mild to moderate) including abscesses, cellulitis, furuncles, impetigo, pyoderma, wound infections, due to methicillin-susceptible *Staphylococcus aureus*, or *Streptococcus pyogenes*.

1.8 Chronic Bacterial Prostatitis

LEVAQUIN® is indicated for the treatment of chronic bacterial prostatitis due to *Escherichia coli*, *Enterococcus faecalis*, or methicillin-susceptible *Staphylococcus epidermidis* *[see Clinical Studies (14.6)]*.

1.9 Complicated Urinary Tract Infections: 5-day Treatment Regimen

LEVAQUIN® is indicated for the treatment of complicated urinary tract infections due to *Escherichia coli*, *Klebsiella pneumoniae*, or *Proteus mirabilis* *[see Clinical Studies (14.7)]*.

1.10 Complicated Urinary Tract Infections: 10-day Treatment Regimen

LEVAQUIN® is indicated for the treatment of complicated urinary tract infections (mild to moderate) due to *Enterococcus faecalis*, *Enterobacter cloacae*, *Escherichia coli*, *Klebsiella pneumoniae*, *Proteus mirabilis*, or *Pseudomonas aeruginosa* *[see Clinical Studies (14.8)]*.

1.11 Acute Pyelonephritis: 5 or 10-day Treatment Regimen

LEVAQUIN® is indicated for the treatment of acute pyelonephritis caused by *Escherichia coli*, including cases with concurrent bacteremia *[see Clinical Studies (14.7, 14.8)]*.

1.12 Uncomplicated Urinary Tract Infections

LEVAQUIN® is indicated for the treatment of uncomplicated urinary tract infections (mild to moderate) due to *Escherichia coli*, *Klebsiella pneumoniae*, or *Staphylococcus saprophyticus*.

1.13 Inhalational Anthrax (Post-Exposure)

LEVAQUIN® is indicated for inhalational anthrax (post-exposure) to reduce the incidence or progression of disease following exposure to aerosolized *Bacillus anthracis*. The effectiveness of LEVAQUIN® is based on plasma concentrations achieved in humans, a surrogate endpoint reasonably likely to predict clinical benefit. LEVAQUIN® has not been tested in humans for the post-exposure prevention of inhalation anthrax. The safety of LEVAQUIN® in adults for durations of therapy beyond 28 days or in pediatric patients for durations of therapy beyond 14 days has not been studied. Prolonged LEVAQUIN® therapy should only be used when the benefit outweighs the risk *[see Dosage and Administration (2.1), (2.2) and Clinical Studies (14.9)]*.

2 DOSAGE AND ADMINISTRATION

2.1 Dosage in Adult Patients with Normal Renal Function

The usual dose of LEVAQUIN® Tablets or Oral Solution is 250 mg, 500 mg, or 750 mg administered orally every 24 hours, as indicated by infection and described in Table 1. The usual dose of LEVAQUIN® Injection is 250 mg or 500 mg administered by slow infusion over 60 minutes every 24 hours or 750 mg administered by slow infusion over 90 minutes every 24 hours, as indicated by infection and described in Table 1.

These recommendations apply to patients with creatinine clearance ≥ 50 mL/min. For patients with creatinine clearance <50 mL/min, adjustments to the dosing regimen are required *[see Dosage and Administration (2.3)]*.

[See table 1 at top of previous page]

2.2 Dosage in Pediatric Patients

The dosage in pediatric patients ≥ 6 months of age is described below in Table 2.

[See table 2 above]

2.3 Dosage Adjustment in Adults with Renal Impairment

Administer LEVAQUIN® with caution in the presence of renal insufficiency. Careful clinical observation and appropriate laboratory studies should be performed prior to and during therapy since elimination of levofloxacin may be reduced.

No adjustment is necessary for patients with a creatinine clearance ≥ 50 mL/min.

In patients with impaired renal function (creatinine clearance <50 mL/min), adjustment of the dosage regimen is necessary to avoid the accumulation of levofloxacin due to decreased clearance *[see Use in Specific Populations (8.6)]*. Table 3 shows how to adjust dose based on creatinine clearance.

[See table 3 above]

2.4 Drug Interaction With Chelation Agents: Antacids, Sucralfate, Metal Cations, Multivitamins

LEVAQUIN® Tablets and Oral Solution

LEVAQUIN® Tablets and Oral Solution should be administered at least two hours before or two hours after antacids containing magnesium, aluminum, as well as sucralfate, metal cations such as iron, and multivitamin preparations with zinc or didanosine chewable/buffered tablets or the pediatric powder for oral solution *[see Drug Interactions (7.1) and Patient Counseling Information (17.2)]*.

LEVAQUIN® Injection

LEVAQUIN® Injection should not be co-administered with any solution containing multivalent cations, e.g., magnesium, through the same intravenous line *[see Dosage and Administration (2.6)]*.

2.5 Administration Instructions

Food and LEVAQUIN® Tablets and Oral Solution

LEVAQUIN® Tablets can be administered without regard to food. It is recommended that LEVAQUIN® Oral Solution be taken 1 hour before or 2 hours after eating.

LEVAQUIN® Injection

Caution: Rapid or bolus intravenous infusion of LEVAQUIN® has been associated with hypotension and must be avoided. LEVAQUIN® Injection should be infused intravenously slowly over a period of not less than 60 or 90 minutes, depending on the dosage. LEVAQUIN® Injection should be administered only by intravenous infusion. It is not for intramuscular, intrathecal, intraperitoneal, or subcutaneous administration.

Hydration for Patients Receiving LEVAQUIN® Tablets, Oral Solution, and Injection

Adequate hydration of patients receiving oral or intravenous LEVAQUIN® should be maintained to prevent the formation of highly concentrated urine. Crystalluria and cylindruria have been reported with quinolones *[see Adverse Reactions (6.1) and Patient Counseling Information (17.2)]*.

2.6 Preparation of Intravenous Product

Parenteral drug products should be inspected visually for particulate matter and discoloration prior to administration, whenever solution and container permit.

Because only limited data are available on the compatibility of LEVAQUIN® Injection with other intravenous substances, additives or other medications should not be added to LEVAQUIN® Injection Premix in Single-Use Flexible Containers and LEVAQUIN® Injection in Single-Use Vials, or infused simultaneously through the same intravenous line. If the same intravenous line is used for sequential infusion of several different drugs, the line should be flushed before and after infusion of LEVAQUIN® Injection with an infusion solution compatible with LEVAQUIN® Injection and with any other drug(s) administered via this common line.

LEVAQUIN® Injection in Single-Use Vials

Single-use vials require dilution prior to administration. LEVAQUIN® Injection is supplied in single-use vials containing a concentrated levofloxacin solution with the equivalent of 500 mg (20 mL vial) and 750 mg (30 mL vial) of levofloxacin in Water for Injection, USP. The 20 mL and 30 mL vials each contain 25 mg of levofloxacin/mL. These LEVAQUIN® Injection single-use vials must be further diluted with an appropriate solution prior to intravenous administration *[see Table 4]*. The concentration of the resulting diluted solution should be 5 mg/mL prior to administration.

Compatible Intravenous Solutions: Any of the following intravenous solutions may be used to prepare a 5 mg/mL levofloxacin solution with the approximate pH values:

Table 4: Compatible Intravenous Solutions

Intravenous Fluids	Final pH of LEVAQUIN® Solution
0.9% Sodium Chloride Injection, USP	4.71
5% Dextrose Injection, USP	4.58
5% Dextrose/0.9% NaCl Injection	4.62
5% Dextrose in Lactated Ringers	4.92
Plasma-Lyte® 56/5% Dextrose Injection	5.03
5% Dextrose, 0.45% Sodium Chloride, and 0.15% Potassium Chloride Injection	4.61
Sodium Lactate Injection (M/6)	5.54

Since no preservative or bacteriostatic agent is present in this product, aseptic technique must be used in preparation of the final intravenous solution. Since the vials are for single-use only, any unused portion remaining in the vial should be discarded. When used to prepare two 250 mg doses from the 20 mL vial containing 500 mg of levofloxacin, the full content of the vial should be withdrawn at once using a single-entry procedure, and a second dose should be prepared and stored for subsequent use *[see Stability of LEVAQUIN® Injection Following Dilution]*.

Prepare the desired dosage of levofloxacin according to Table 5:

Table 5: Preparation of LEVAQUIN® Intravenous Solution

Desired Dosage Strength	From Appropriate Vial, Withdraw Volume	Volume of Diluent	Infusion Time
250 mg	10 mL (20 mL Vial)	40 mL	60 min
500 mg	20 mL (20 mL Vial)	80 mL	60 min
750 mg	30 mL (30 mL Vial)	120 mL	90 min

Table 2: Dosage in Pediatric Patients ≥ 6 months of age

Type of Infection*	Dose	Freq. Once every	Duration†
Inhalational Anthrax (post-exposure)‡,§			
Pediatric patients > 50 kg and ≥ 6 months of age	500 mg	24 hr	60 days§
Pediatric patients < 50 kg and ≥ 6 months of age	8 mg/kg (not to exceed 250 mg per dose)	12 hr	60 days§

* Due to *Bacillus anthracis* *[see Indications and Usage (1.13)]*
† Sequential therapy (intravenous to oral) may be instituted at the discretion of the physician.
‡ Drug administration should begin as soon as possible after suspected or confirmed exposure to aerosolized *B. anthracis*. This indication is based on a surrogate endpoint. Levofloxacin plasma concentrations achieved in humans are reasonably likely to predict clinical benefit *[see Clinical Studies (14.9)]*
§ The safety of LEVAQUIN® in pediatric patients for durations of therapy beyond 14 days has not been studied. An increased incidence of musculoskeletal adverse events compared to controls has been observed in pediatric patients *[see Warnings and Precautions (5.9), Use in Specific Populations (8.4), and Clinical Studies (14.9)]*. Prolonged LEVAQUIN® therapy should only be used when the benefit outweighs the risk.

Table 3: Dosage Adjustment in Adult Patients with Renal Impairment (creatinine clearance < 50 mL/min)

Dosage in Normal Renal Function Every 24 hours	Creatinine Clearance 20 to 49 mL/min	Creatinine Clearance 10 to 19 mL/min	Hemodialysis or Chronic Ambulatory Peritoneal Dialysis (CAPD)
750 mg	750 mg every 48 hours	750 mg initial dose, then 500 mg every 48 hours	750 mg initial dose, then 500 mg every 48 hours
500 mg	500 mg initial dose, then 250 mg every 24 hours	500 mg initial dose, then 250 mg every 48 hours	500 mg initial dose, then 250 mg every 48 hours
250 mg	No dosage adjustment required	250 mg every 48 hours. If treating uncomplicated UTI, then no dosage adjustment is required	No information on dosing adjustment is available

For example, to prepare a 500 mg dose using the 20 mL vial (25 mg/mL), withdraw 20 mL and dilute with a compatible intravenous solution to a total volume of 100 mL.

This intravenous drug product should be inspected visually for particulate matter prior to administration. Samples containing visible particles should be discarded.

Stability of LEVAQUIN® Injection Following Dilution: LEVAQUIN® Injection, when diluted in a compatible intravenous fluid to a concentration of 5 mg/mL, is stable for 72 hours when stored at or below 25°C (77°F) and for 14 days when stored under refrigeration at 5°C (41°F) in plastic intravenous containers. Solutions that are diluted in a compatible intravenous solution and frozen in glass bottles or plastic intravenous containers are stable for 6 months when stored at -20°C (-4°F). Thaw frozen solutions at room temperature 25°C (77°F) or in a refrigerator 8°C (46°F). Do not force thaw by microwave irradiation or water bath immersion. Do not refreeze after initial thawing.

LEVAQUIN® Injection Premix in Single-Use Flexible Containers (5 mg/mL)

LEVAQUIN® Injection is also supplied in flexible containers within a foil overwrap. These contain a premixed, ready to use levofloxacin solution in 5% dextrose (D5W) for single-use. The 100 mL premixed flexible containers contain either 250 mg/50 mL or 500 mg/100 mL of levofloxacin solution. The 150 mL flexible container contains 750 mg/150 mL of levofloxacin solution. The concentration of each container is 5 mg/mL. No further dilution of these preparations is necessary. Because the premix flexible containers are for single-use only, any unused portion should be discarded.

Instructions for the Use of LEVAQUIN® Injection Premix in Flexible Containers:

1. Tear outer wrap at the notch and remove solution container.
2. Check the container for minute leaks by squeezing the inner bag firmly. If leaks are found, or if the seal is not intact, discard the solution, as the sterility may be compromised.
3. Do not use if the solution is cloudy or a precipitate is present.
4. Use sterile equipment.
5. **WARNING: Do not use flexible containers in series connections.** Such use could result in air embolism due to residual air being drawn from the primary container before administration of the fluid from the secondary container is complete.

Preparation for Administration:

1. Close flow control clamp of administration set.
2. Remove cover from port at bottom of container.
3. Insert piercing pin of administration set into port with a twisting motion until the pin is firmly seated. **NOTE: See full directions on administration set carton.**
4. Suspend container from hanger.
5. Squeeze and release drip chamber to establish proper fluid level in chamber during infusion of LEVAQUIN® Injection Premix in Flexible Containers.
6. Open flow control clamp to expel air from set. Close clamp.
7. Regulate rate of administration with flow control clamp.

3 DOSAGE FORMS AND STRENGTHS

TABLETS, Film-coated, capsule-shaped

- 250 mg terra cotta pink tablets, imprinted with "250" on one side and "LEVAQUIN" on the other
- 500 mg peach tablets, imprinted with "500" on one side and "LEVAQUIN" on the other
- 750 mg white tablets, imprinted with "750" on one side and "LEVAQUIN" on the other

ORAL SOLUTION, 25mg/mL, clear yellow to clear greenish-yellow color

INJECTION, Single-Use Vials of concentrated solution for dilution for intravenous infusion, clear yellow to clear greenish-yellow in appearance

- 20 mL vial of 25 mg/mL levofloxacin solution, equivalent to 500 mg of levofloxacin
- 30 mL vial of 25 mg/mL levofloxacin solution, equivalent to 750 mg of levofloxacin

INJECTION (5 mg/mL in 5% Dextrose) Premix in Single-Use Flexible Containers, for intravenous infusion

- 100 mL container, fill volume 50 mL (equivalent to 250 mg levofloxacin)
- 100 mL container, fill volume 100 mL (equivalent to 500 mg levofloxacin)
- 150 mL container, fill volume 150 mL (equivalent to 750 mg levofloxacin)

4 CONTRAINDICATIONS

LEVAQUIN® is contraindicated in persons with known hypersensitivity to levofloxacin, or other quinolone antibacterials *[see Warnings and Precautions (5.2)]*.

5 WARNINGS AND PRECAUTIONS

5.1 Tendinopathy and Tendon Rupture

Fluoroquinolones, including LEVAQUIN®, are associated with an increased risk of tendinitis and tendon rupture in all ages. This adverse reaction most frequently involves the Achilles tendon, and rupture of the Achilles tendon may require surgical repair. Tendinitis and tendon rupture in the rotator cuff (the shoulder), the hand, the biceps, the thumb, and other tendon sites have also been reported. The risk of developing fluoroquinolone-associated tendinitis and tendon rupture is further increased in older patients usually over 60 years of age, in those taking corticosteroid drugs, and in patients with kidney, heart or lung transplants. Factors, in addition to age and corticosteroid use, that may independently increase the risk of tendon rupture include strenuous physical activity, renal failure, and previous tendon disorders such as rheumatoid arthritis. Tendinitis and tendon rupture have been reported in patients taking fluoroquinolones who do not have the above risk factors. Tendon rupture can occur during or after completion of therapy; cases occurring up to several months after completion of therapy have been reported. LEVAQUIN® should be discontinued if the patient experiences pain, swelling, inflammation or rupture of a tendon. Patients should be advised to rest at the first sign of tendinitis or tendon rupture, and to contact their healthcare provider regarding changing to a non-quinolone antimicrobial drug. *[see Adverse Reactions (6.3); Patient Counseling Information (17.3)]*.

5.2 Hypersensitivity Reactions

Serious and occasionally fatal hypersensitivity and/or anaphylactic reactions have been reported in patients receiving therapy with fluoroquinolones, including LEVAQUIN®. These reactions often occur following the first dose. Some reactions have been accompanied by cardiovascular collapse, hypotension/shock, seizure, loss of consciousness, tingling, angioedema (including tongue, laryngeal, throat, or facial edema/swelling), airway obstruction (including bronchospasm, shortness of breath, and acute respiratory distress), dyspnea, urticaria, itching, and other serious skin reactions. LEVAQUIN® should be discontinued immediately at the first appearance of a skin rash or any other sign of hypersensitivity. Serious acute hypersensitivity reactions may require treatment with epinephrine and other resuscitative measures, including oxygen, intravenous fluids, antihistamines, corticosteroids, pressor amines, and airway management, as clinically indicated *[see Adverse Reactions (6); Patient Counseling Information (17.3)]*.

5.3 Other Serious and Sometimes Fatal Reactions

Other serious and sometimes fatal events, some due to hypersensitivity, and some due to uncertain etiology, have been reported rarely in patients receiving therapy with fluoroquinolones, including LEVAQUIN®. These events may be severe and generally occur following the administration of multiple doses. Clinical manifestations may include one or more of the following:

- fever, rash, or severe dermatologic reactions (e.g., toxic epidermal necrolysis, Stevens-Johnson Syndrome);
- vasculitis; arthralgia; myalgia; serum sickness;
- allergic pneumonitis;
- interstitial nephritis; acute renal insufficiency or failure;
- hepatitis; jaundice; acute hepatic necrosis or failure;
- anemia, including hemolytic and aplastic; thrombocytopenia, including thrombotic thrombocytopenic purpura; leukopenia; agranulocytosis; pancytopenia; and/or other hematologic abnormalities.

The drug should be discontinued immediately at the first appearance of skin rash, jaundice, or any other sign of hypersensitivity and supportive measures instituted *[see Adverse Reactions (6); Patient Counseling Information (17.3)]*.

5.4 Hepatotoxicity

Post-marketing reports of severe hepatotoxicity (including acute hepatitis and fatal events) have been received for patients treated with LEVAQUIN®. No evidence of serious drug-associated hepatotoxicity was detected in clinical trials of over 7,000 patients. Severe hepatotoxicity generally occurred within 14 days of initiation of therapy and most cases occurred within 6 days. Most cases of severe hepatotoxicity were not associated with hypersensitivity *[see Warnings and Precautions (5.3)]*. The majority of fatal hepatotoxicity reports occurred in patients 65 years of age or older and most were not associated with hypersensitivity. LEVAQUIN® should be discontinued immediately if the patient develops signs and symptoms of hepatitis *[see Adverse Reactions (6); Patient Counseling Information (17.3)]*.

5.5 Central Nervous System Effects

Convulsions and toxic psychoses have been reported in patients receiving fluoroquinolones, including LEVAQUIN®. Fluoroquinolones may also cause increased intracranial pressure and central nervous system stimulation which may lead to tremors, restlessness, anxiety, lightheadedness, confusion, hallucinations, paranoia, depression, nightmares, insomnia, and, rarely, suicidal thoughts or acts. These reactions may occur following the first dose. If these reactions occur in patients receiving LEVAQUIN®, the drug should be discontinued and appropriate measures instituted. As with other fluoroquinolones, LEVAQUIN® should be used with caution in patients with a known or suspected central nervous system (CNS) disorder that may predispose them to seizures or lower the seizure threshold (e.g., severe cerebral arteriosclerosis, epilepsy) or in the presence of other risk factors that may predispose them to seizures or lower the seizure threshold (e.g., certain drug therapy, renal dysfunction.) *[see Adverse Reactions (6); Drug Interactions (7.4, 7.5); Patient Counseling Information (17.3)]*.

5.6 Clostridium difficile-Associated Diarrhea

Clostridium difficile-associated diarrhea (CDAD) has been reported with use of nearly all antibacterial agents, including LEVAQUIN®, and may range in severity from mild diarrhea to fatal colitis. Treatment with antibacterial agents alters the normal flora of the colon leading to overgrowth of *C. difficile*.

C. difficile produces toxins A and B which contribute to the development of CDAD. Hypertoxin producing strains of *C. difficile* cause increased morbidity and mortality, as these infections can be refractory to antimicrobial therapy and may require colectomy. CDAD must be considered in all patients who present with diarrhea following antibiotic use. Careful medical history is necessary since CDAD has been reported to occur over two months after the administration of antibacterial agents.

If CDAD is suspected or confirmed, ongoing antibiotic use not directed against *C. difficile* may need to be discontinued. Appropriate fluid and electrolyte management, protein supplementation, antibiotic treatment of *C. difficile*, and surgical evaluation should be instituted as clinically indicated *[see Adverse Reactions (6.2), Patient Counseling Information (17.3)]*.

5.7 Peripheral Neuropathy

Rare cases of sensory or sensorimotor axonal polyneuropathy affecting small and/or large axons resulting in paresthesias, hypoesthesias, dysesthesias and weakness have been reported in patients receiving fluoroquinolones, including LEVAQUIN®. LEVAQUIN® should be discontinued if the patient experiences symptoms of neuropathy including pain, burning, tingling, numbness, and/or weakness or other alterations of sensation including light touch, pain, temperature, position sense, and vibratory sensation in order to prevent the development of an irreversible condition *[see Adverse Reactions (6), Patient Counseling Information (17.3)]*.

5.8 Prolongation of the QT Interval

Some fluoroquinolones, including LEVAQUIN®, have been associated with prolongation of the QT interval on the electrocardiogram and infrequent cases of arrhythmia. Rare cases of torsade de pointes have been spontaneously reported during postmarketing surveillance in patients receiving fluoroquinolones, including LEVAQUIN®. LEVAQUIN® should be avoided in patients with known prolongation of the QT interval, patients with uncorrected hypokalemia, and patients receiving Class IA (quinidine, procainamide), or Class III (amiodarone, sotalol) antiarrhythmic agents. Elderly patients may be more susceptible to drug-associated effects on the QT interval *[see Adverse Reactions (6.3), Use in Specific Populations (8.5), and Patient Counseling Information (17.3)]*.

5.9 Musculoskeletal Disorders in Pediatric Patients and Arthropathic Effects in Animals

LEVAQUIN® is indicated in pediatric patients (≥6 months of age) only for the prevention of inhalational anthrax (post-exposure) *[see Indications and Usage (1.13)]*. An increased incidence of musculoskeletal disorders (arthralgia, arthritis, tendonopathy, and gait abnormality) compared to controls has been observed in pediatric patients receiving LEVAQUIN® *[see Use in Specific Populations (8.4)]*.

In immature rats and dogs, the oral and intravenous administration of levofloxacin resulted in increased osteochondrosis. Histopathological examination of the weight-bearing joints of immature dogs dosed with levofloxacin revealed persistent lesions of the cartilage. Other fluoroquinolones also produce similar erosions in the weight-bearing joints and other signs of arthropathy in immature animals of various species *[see Animal Toxicology and/or Pharmacology (13.2)]*.

5.10 Blood Glucose Disturbances

As with other fluoroquinolones, disturbances of blood glucose, including symptomatic hyper- and hypoglycemia, have been reported with LEVAQUIN®, usually in diabetic patients receiving concomitant treatment with an oral hypoglycemic agent (e.g., glyburide) or with insulin. In these patients, careful monitoring of blood glucose is recommended. If a hypoglycemic reaction occurs in a patient being treated with LEVAQUIN®, LEVAQUIN® should be discontinued and appropriate therapy should be initiated immediately *[see Adverse Reactions (6.2); Drug Interactions (7.3); Patient Counseling Information (17.4)]*.

5.11 Photosensitivity/Phototoxicity

Moderate to severe photosensitivity/phototoxicity reactions, the latter of which may manifest as exaggerated sunburn reactions (e.g., burning, erythema, exudation, vesicles, blistering, edema) involving areas exposed to light (typically the face, "V" area of the neck, extensor surfaces of the forearms, dorsa of the hands), can be associated with the use of fluoroquinolones after sun or UV light exposure. Therefore, excessive exposure to these sources of light should be avoided. Drug therapy should be discontinued if photosensitivity/phototoxicity occurs [see Adverse Reactions (6.3); Patient Counseling Information (17.3)].

5.12 Development of Drug Resistant Bacteria

Prescribing LEVAQUIN® in the absence of a proven or strongly suspected bacterial infection or a prophylactic indication is unlikely to provide benefit to the patient and increases the risk of the development of drug-resistant bacteria [see Patient Counseling Information (17.1)].

6 ADVERSE REACTIONS

6.1 Serious and Otherwise Important Adverse Reactions

The following serious and otherwise important adverse drug reactions are discussed in greater detail in other sections of labeling:

- Tendon Effects [see Warnings and Precautions (5.1)]
- Hypersensitivity Reactions [see Warnings and Precautions (5.2)]
- Other Serious and Sometimes Fatal Reactions [see Warnings and Precautions (5.3)]
- Hepatotoxicity [see Warnings and Precautions (5.4)]
- Central Nervous System Effects [see Warnings and Precautions (5.5)]
- Clostridium difficile-Associated Diarrhea [see Warnings and Precautions (5.6)]
- Peripheral Neuropathy [see Warnings and Precautions (5.7)]
- Prolongation of the QT Interval [see Warnings and Precautions (5.8)]
- Musculoskeletal Disorders in Pediatric Patients [see Warnings and Precautions (5.9)]
- Blood Glucose Disturbances [see Warnings and Precautions (5.10)]
- Photosensitivity/Phototoxicity [see Warnings and Precautions (5.11)]
- Development of Drug Resistant Bacteria [see Warnings and Precautions (5.12)]

Hypotension has been associated with rapid or bolus intravenous infusion of LEVAQUIN®. LEVAQUIN® should be infused slowly over 60 to 90 minutes, depending on dosage [see Dosage and Administration (2.5)].

Crystalluria and cylindruria have been reported with quinolones, including LEVAQUIN®. Therefore, adequate hydration of patients receiving LEVAQUIN® should be maintained to prevent the formation of a highly concentrated urine [see Dosage and Administration (2.5)].

6.2 Clinical Trial Experience

Because clinical trials are conducted under widely varying conditions, adverse reaction rates observed in the clinical trials of a drug cannot be directly compared to rates in the clinical trials of another drug and may not reflect the rates observed in practice.

The data described below reflect exposure to LEVAQUIN® in 7537 patients in 29 pooled Phase 3 clinical trials. The population studied had a mean age of 50 years (approximately 74% of the population was < 65 years of age), 50% were male, 71% were Caucasian, 19% were Black. Patients were treated with LEVAQUIN® for a wide variety of infectious diseases [see Indications and Usage (1)]. Patients received LEVAQUIN® doses of 750 mg once daily, 250 mg once daily, or 500 mg once or twice daily. Treatment duration was usually 3–14 days, and the mean number of days on therapy was 10 days.

The overall incidence, type and distribution of adverse reactions was similar in patients receiving LEVAQUIN® doses of 750 mg once daily, 250 mg once daily, and 500 mg once or twice daily. Discontinuation of LEVAQUIN® due to adverse drug reactions occurred in 4.3% of patients overall. 3.8% of patients treated with the 250 mg and 500 mg doses and 5.4% of patients treated with the 750 mg dose. The most common adverse drug reactions leading to discontinuation with the 250 and 500 mg doses were gastrointestinal (1.4%), primarily nausea (0.6%); vomiting (0.4%); dizziness (0.3%); and headache (0.2%). The most common adverse drug reactions leading to discontinuation with the 750 mg dose were gastrointestinal (1.2%), primarily nausea (0.6%); vomiting (0.5%); dizziness (0.3%); and headache (0.3%).

Adverse reactions occurring in ≥1% of LEVAQUIN®-treated patients and less common adverse reactions, occurring in 0.1 to <1% of LEVAQUIN®-treated patients, are shown in Table 6 and Table 7, respectively. The most common adverse drug reactions (≥3%) are nausea, headache, diarrhea, insomnia, constipation, and dizziness.

Table 6: Common (≥1%) Adverse Reactions Reported in Clinical Trials with LEVAQUIN®

System/Organ Class	Adverse Reaction	% (N=7537)
Infections and Infestations	moniliasis	1
Psychiatric Disorders	insomnia* [see Warnings and Precautions (5.5)]	4
Nervous System Disorders	headache	6
	dizziness [see Warnings and Precautions (5.5)]	3
Respiratory, Thoracic and Mediastinal Disorders	dyspnea [see Warnings and Precautions (5.2)]	1
Gastrointestinal Disorders	nausea	7
	diarrhea	5
	constipation	3
	abdominal pain	2
	vomiting	2
	dyspepsia	2
Skin and Subcutaneous Tissue Disorders	rash [see Warnings and Precautions (5.2)]	2
	pruritus	1
Reproductive System and Breast Disorders	vaginitis	1†
General Disorders and Administration Site Conditions	edema	1
	injection site reaction	1
	chest pain	1

* N=7274
† N=3758 (women)

Table 7: Less Common (0.1 to 1%) Adverse Reactions Reported in Clinical Trials with LEVAQUIN® (N=7537)

System/Organ Class	Adverse Reaction
Infections and Infestations	genital moniliasis
Blood and Lymphatic System Disorders	anemia thrombocytopenia granulocytopenia [see Warnings and Precautions (5.3)]
Immune System Disorders	allergic reaction [See Warnings and Precautions (5.2, 5.3)]
Metabolism and Nutrition Disorders	hyperglycemia hypoglycemia [see Warnings and Precautions (5.10)] hyperkalemia
Psychiatric Disorders	anxiety agitation confusion depression hallucination nightmare* [see Warnings and Precautions (5.5)] sleep disorder* anorexia abnormal dreaming*
Nervous System Disorders	tremor convulsions [see Warnings and Precautions (5.5)] paresthesia [see Warnings and Precautions (5.7)] vertigo hypertonia hyperkinesias abnormal gait somnolence* syncope

Respiratory, Thoracic and Mediastinal Disorders	epistaxis
Cardiac Disorders	cardiac arrest palpitation ventricular tachycardia ventricular arrhythmia
Vascular Disorders	phlebitis
Gastrointestinal Disorders	gastritis stomatitis pancreatitis esophagitis gastroenteritis glossitis pseudomembraneous/C. difficile colitis [see Warnings and Precautions (5.6)]
Hepatobiliary Disorders	abnormal hepatic function increased hepatic enzymes increased alkaline phosphatase
Skin and Subcutaneous Tissue Disorders	urticaria [see Warnings and Precautions (5.2)]
Musculoskeletal and Connective Tissue Disorders	arthralgia tendonitis [see Warnings and Precautions (5.1)] myalgia skeletal pain
Renal and Urinary Disorders	abnormal renal function acute renal failure [see Warnings and Precautions (5.3)]

*N = 7274

In clinical trials using multiple-dose therapy, ophthalmologic abnormalities, including cataracts and multiple punctate lenticular opacities, have been noted in patients undergoing treatment with quinolones, including LEVAQUIN®. The relationship of the drugs to these events is not presently established.

6.3 Postmarketing Experience

Table 8 lists adverse reactions that have been identified during post-approval use of LEVAQUIN®. Because these reactions are reported voluntarily from a population of uncertain size, reliably estimating their frequency or establishing a causal relationship to drug exposure is not always possible.

Table 8: Postmarketing Reports Of Adverse Drug Reactions

System/Organ Class	Adverse Reaction
Blood and Lymphatic System Disorders	pancytopenia aplastic anemia leukopenia hemolytic anemia [see Warnings and Precautions (5.3)] eosinophilia
Immune System Disorders	hypersensitivity reactions, sometimes fatal including: anaphylactic/anaphylactoid reactions anaphylactic shock angioneurotic edema serum sickness [see Warnings and Precautions (5.2, 5.3)]
Psychiatric Disorders	psychosis paranoia isolated reports of suicide attempt and suicidal ideation [see Warnings and Precautions (5.5)]
Nervous System Disorders	anosmia ageusia parosmia dysgeusia peripheral neuropathy [see Warnings and Precautions (5.7)]

	isolated reports of encephalopathy abnormal electroencephalogram (EEG) dysphonia
Eye Disorders	vision disturbance, including diplopia visual acuity reduced vision blurred scotoma
Ear and Labyrinth Disorders	hypoacusis tinnitus
Cardiac Disorders	isolated reports of torsade de pointes electrocardiogram QT prolonged *[see Warnings and Precautions (5.8)]* tachycardia
Vascular Disorders	vasodilatation
Respiratory, Thoracic and Mediastinal Disorders	isolated reports of allergic pneumonitis *[see Warnings and Precautions (5.3)]*
Hepatobiliary Disorders	hepatic failure (including fatal cases) hepatitis jaundice *[see Warnings and Precautions (5.3, 5.4)]*
Skin and Subcutaneous Tissue Disorders	bullous eruptions to include: Stevens-Johnson Syndrome toxic epidermal necrolysis erythema multiforme *[see Warnings and Precautions (5.3)]* photosensitivity/photoxicity reaction *[see Warnings and Precautions (5.11)]* leukocytoclastic vasculitis
Musculoskeletal and Connective Tissue Disorders	tendon rupture *[see Warnings and Precautions (5.1)]* muscle injury, including rupture rhabdomyolysis
Renal and Urinary Disorders	interstitial nephritis *[see Warnings and Precautions (5.3)]*
General Disorders and Administration Site Conditions	multi-organ failure pyrexia
Investigations	prothrombin time prolonged international normalized ratio prolonged muscle enzymes increased

7 DRUG INTERACTIONS

7.1 Chelation Agents: Antacids, Sucralfate, Metal Cations, Multivitamins

LEVAQUIN® Tablets and Oral Solution

While the chelation by divalent cations is less marked than with other fluoroquinolones, concurrent administration of LEVAQUIN® Tablets and Oral Solution with antacids containing magnesium, or aluminum, as well as sucralfate, metal cations such as iron, and multivitamin preparations with zinc may interfere with the gastrointestinal absorption of levofloxacin, resulting in systemic levels considerably lower than desired. Tablets with antacids containing magnesium, aluminum, as well as sucralfate, metal cations such as iron, and multivitamins preparations with zinc or didanosine may substantially interfere with the gastrointestinal absorption of levofloxacin, resulting in systemic levels considerably lower than desired. These agents should be taken at least two hours before or two hours after oral LEVAQUIN® administration.

LEVAQUIN® Injection

There are no data concerning an interaction of intravenous fluoroquinolones with oral antacids, sucralfate, multivitamins, didanosine, or metal cations. However, no fluoroquinolone should be co-administered with any solution containing multivalent cations, e.g., magnesium, through the same intravenous line *[see Dosage and Administration (2.5)]*.

7.2 Warfarin

No significant effect of LEVAQUIN® on the peak plasma concentrations, AUC, and other disposition parameters for R- and S-warfarin was detected in a clinical study involving healthy volunteers. Similarly, no apparent effect of warfarin on levofloxacin absorption and disposition was observed. However, there have been reports during the postmarketing experience in patients that LEVAQUIN® enhances the effects of warfarin. Elevations of the prothrombin time in the setting of concurrent warfarin and LEVAQUIN® use have been associated with episodes of bleeding. Prothrombin time, International Normalized Ratio (INR), or other suitable anticoagulation tests should be closely monitored if LEVAQUIN® is administered concomitantly with warfarin. Patients should also be monitored for evidence of bleeding *[see Adverse Reactions (6.3); Patient Counseling Information (17.4)]*.

7.3 Antidiabetic Agents

Disturbances of blood glucose, including hyperglycemia and hypoglycemia, have been reported in patients treated concomitantly with fluoroquinolones and an antidiabetic agent. Therefore, careful monitoring of blood glucose is recommended when these agents are co-administered *[see Warnings and Precautions (5.10); Adverse Reactions (6.2), Patient Counseling Information (17.4)]*.

7.4 Non-Steroidal Anti-Inflammatory Drugs

The concomitant administration of a non-steroidal anti-inflammatory drug with a fluoroquinolone, including LEVAQUIN®, may increase the risk of CNS stimulation and convulsive seizures *[see Warnings and Precautions (5.5)]*.

7.5 Theophylline

No significant effect of LEVAQUIN® on the plasma concentrations, AUC, and other disposition parameters for theophylline was detected in a clinical study involving healthy volunteers. Similarly, no apparent effect of theophylline on levofloxacin absorption and disposition was observed. However, concomitant administration of other fluoroquinolones with theophylline has resulted in prolonged elimination half-life, elevated serum theophylline levels, and a subsequent increase in the risk of theophylline-related adverse reactions in the patient population. Therefore, theophylline levels should be closely monitored and appropriate dosage adjustments made when LEVAQUIN® is co-administered. Adverse reactions, including seizures, may occur with or without an elevation in serum theophylline levels *[see Warnings and Precautions (5.5)]*.

7.6 Cyclosporine

No significant effect of LEVAQUIN® on the peak plasma concentrations, AUC, and other disposition parameters for cyclosporine was detected in a clinical study involving healthy volunteers. However, elevated serum levels of cyclosporine have been reported in the patient population when co-administered with some other fluoroquinolones. Levofloxacin C_{max} and k_e were slightly lower while T_{max} and $t_{1/2}$ were slightly longer in the presence of cyclosporine than those observed in other studies without concomitant medication. The differences, however, are not considered to be clinically significant. Therefore, no dosage adjustment is required for LEVAQUIN® or cyclosporine when administered concomitantly.

7.7 Digoxin

No significant effect of LEVAQUIN® on the peak plasma concentrations, AUC, and other disposition parameters for digoxin was detected in a clinical study involving healthy volunteers. Levofloxacin absorption and disposition kinetics were similar in the presence or absence of digoxin. Therefore, no dosage adjustment for LEVAQUIN® or digoxin is required when administered concomitantly.

7.8 Probenecid and Cimetidine

No significant effect of probenecid or cimetidine on the C_{max} of levofloxacin was observed in a clinical study involving healthy volunteers. The AUC and $t_{1/2}$ of levofloxacin were higher while CL/F and CL_R were lower during concomitant treatment of LEVAQUIN® with probenecid or cimetidine compared to LEVAQUIN® alone. However, these changes do not warrant dosage adjustment for LEVAQUIN® when probenecid or cimetidine is co-administered.

7.9 Interactions with Laboratory or Diagnostic Testing

Some fluoroquinolones, including LEVAQUIN®, may produce false-positive urine screening results for opiates using commercially available immunoassay kits. Confirmation of positive opiate screens by more specific methods may be necessary.

8 USE IN SPECIFIC POPULATIONS

8.1 Pregnancy

Pregnancy Category C. Levofloxacin was not teratogenic in rats at oral doses as high as 810 mg/kg/day which corresponds to 9.4 times the highest recommended human dose based upon relative body surface area, or at intravenous doses as high as 160 mg/kg/day corresponding to 1.9 times the highest recommended human dose based upon relative body surface area. The oral dose of 810 mg/kg/day to rats caused decreased fetal body weight and increased fetal mortality. No teratogenicity was observed when rabbits were dosed orally as high as 50 mg/kg/day which corresponds to 1.1 times the highest recommended human dose based upon relative body surface area, or when dosed intravenously as high as 25 mg/kg/day, corresponding to 0.5 times the highest recommended human dose based upon relative body surface area.

There are, however, no adequate and well-controlled studies in pregnant women. LEVAQUIN® should be used during pregnancy only if the potential benefit justifies the potential risk to the fetus.

8.3 Nursing Mothers

Based on data on other fluoroquinolones and very limited data on LEVAQUIN®, it can be presumed that levofloxacin will be excreted in human milk. Because of the potential for serious adverse reactions from LEVAQUIN® in nursing infants, a decision should be made whether to discontinue nursing or to discontinue the drug, taking into account the importance of the drug to the mother.

8.4 Pediatric Use

Quinolones, including levofloxacin, cause arthropathy and osteochondrosis in juvenile animals of several species. *[see Warnings and Precautions (5.9) and Animal Toxicology and/or Pharmacology (13.2)]*.

Inhalational Anthrax (Post-Exposure)

Levofloxacin is indicated in pediatric patients for inhalational anthrax (post-exposure). The risk-benefit assessment indicates that administration of levofloxacin to pediatric patients is appropriate. The safety of levofloxacin in pediatric patients treated for more than 14 days has not been studied. The pharmacokinetics of levofloxacin following a single intravenous dose were investigated in pediatric patients ranging in age from six months to 16 years. Pediatric patients cleared levofloxacin faster than adult patients resulting in lower plasma exposures than adults for a given mg/kg dose *[see Indications and Usage (1.13), Dosage and Administration (2.2), Clinical Pharmacology (12.3) and Clinical Studies (14.9)]*.

Adverse Events

In clinical trials, 1534 children (6 months to 16 years of age) were treated with oral and intravenous LEVAQUIN®. Children 6 months to 5 years of age received LEVAQUIN® 10 mg/kg twice a day and children greater than 5 years of age received 10 mg/kg once a day (maximum 500 mg per day) for approximately 10 days.

A subset of children in the clinical trials (1340 LEVAQUIN®-treated and 893 non-fluoroquinolone-treated) enrolled in a prospective, long-term surveillance study to assess the incidence of protocol-defined musculoskeletal disorders (arthralgia, arthritis, tendonopathy, gait abnormality) during 60 days and 1 year following the first dose of study drug. Children treated with LEVAQUIN® had a significantly higher incidence of musculoskeletal disorders when compared to the non-fluoroquinolone-treated children as illustrated in Table 9.

Table 9: Incidence of Musculoskeletal Disorders in Pediatric Clinical Trial

Follow-up Period	LEVAQUIN® N = 1340	Non-Fluoroquinolone* N = 893	p-value†
60 days	28 (2.1%)	8 (0.9%)	p = 0.038
1 year‡	46 (3.4%)	16 (1.8%)	p = 0.025

* Non-Fluoroquinolone: ceftriaxone, amoxicillin/clavulanate, clarithromycin

† 2-sided Fisher's Exact Test

‡ There were 1199 LEVAQUIN®-treated and 804 non-fluoroquinolone-treated children who had a one-year evaluation visit. However, the incidence of musculoskeletal disorders were calculated using all reported events during the specified period for all children enrolled regardless of whether they completed the 1-year evaluation visit.

Arthralgia was the most frequently occurring musculoskeletal disorder in both treatment groups. Most of the musculoskeletal disorders in both groups involved multiple weight-bearing joints. Disorders were moderate in 8/46 (17%) children and mild in 35/46 (76%) LEVAQUIN®-treated children and most were treated with analgesics. The median time to resolution was 7 days for LEVAQUIN®-treated children and 9 for non-fluoroquinolone-treated children (approximately 80% resolved within 2 months in both groups). No child had a severe or serious disorder and all musculoskeletal disorders resolved without sequelae.

Vomiting and diarrhea were the most frequently reported adverse events, occurring in similar frequency in the LEVAQUIN®-treated and non-fluoroquinolone-treated children.

In addition to the events reported in pediatric patients in clinical trials, events reported in adults during clinical trials or post-marketing experience *[see Adverse Reactions (6)]* may also be expected to occur in pediatric patients.

8.5 Geriatric Use

Geriatric patients are at increased risk for developing severe tendon disorders including tendon rupture when being treated with a fluoroquinolone such as LEVAQUIN®. This risk is further increased in patients receiving concomitant corticosteroid therapy. Tendinitis or tendon rupture can involve the Achilles, hand, shoulder, or other tendon sites and can occur during or after completion of therapy; cases occurring up to several months after fluoroquinolone treatment have been reported. Caution should be used when prescribing LEVAQUIN® to elderly patients especially those on corticosteroids. Patients should be informed of this potential side effect and advised to discontinue LEVAQUIN® and contact their healthcare provider if any symptoms of tendinitis or tendon rupture occur [see Boxed Warning; Warnings and Precautions (5.1); and Adverse Reactions (6.3)].

In phase 3 clinical trials, 1,945 LEVAQUIN®-treated patients (26%) were ≥ 65 years of age. Of these, 1,081 patients (14%) were between the ages of 65 and 74 and 864 patients (12%) were 75 years or older. No overall differences in safety or effectiveness were observed between these subjects and younger subjects, but greater sensitivity of some older individuals cannot be ruled out.

Severe, and sometimes fatal, cases of hepatotoxicity have been reported post-marketing in association with LEVAQUIN®. The majority of fatal hepatotoxicity reports occurred in patients 65 years of age or older and most were not associated with hypersensitivity. LEVAQUIN® should be discontinued immediately if the patient develops signs and symptoms of hepatitis [see Warnings and Precautions (5.4)].

Elderly patients may be more susceptible to drug-associated effects on the QT interval. Therefore, precaution should be taken when using LEVAQUIN® with concomitant drugs that can result in prolongation of the QT interval (e.g., Class IA or Class III antiarrhythmics) or in patients with risk factors for torsade de pointes (e.g., known QT prolongation, uncorrected hypokalemia) [see Warnings and Precautions (5.8)].

The pharmacokinetic properties of levofloxacin in younger adults and elderly adults do not differ significantly when creatinine clearance is taken into consideration. However, since the drug is known to be substantially excreted by the kidney, the risk of toxic reactions to this drug may be greater in patients with impaired renal function. Because elderly patients are more likely to have decreased renal function, care should be taken in dose selection, and it may be useful to monitor renal function [see Clinical Pharmacology (12.3)].

8.6 Renal Impairment

Clearance of levofloxacin is substantially reduced and plasma elimination half-life is substantially prolonged in patients with impaired renal function (creatinine clearance < 50 mL/min), requiring dosage adjustment in such patients to avoid accumulation. Neither hemodialysis nor continuous ambulatory peritoneal dialysis (CAPD) is effective in removal of levofloxacin from the body, indicating that supplemental doses of LEVAQUIN® are not required following hemodialysis or CAPD [see Dosage and Administration (2.3)].

8.7 Hepatic Impairment

Pharmacokinetic studies in hepatically impaired patients have not been conducted. Due to the limited extent of levofloxacin metabolism, the pharmacokinetics of levofloxacin are not expected to be affected by hepatic impairment.

10 OVERDOSAGE

In the event of an acute overdosage, the stomach should be emptied. The patient should be observed and appropriate hydration maintained. Levofloxacin is not efficiently removed by hemodialysis or peritoneal dialysis.

LEVAQUIN® exhibits a low potential for acute toxicity. Mice, rats, dogs and monkeys exhibited the following clinical signs after receiving a single high dose of LEVAQUIN®: ataxia, ptosis, decreased locomotor activity, dyspnea, prostration, tremors, and convulsions. Doses in excess of 1500 mg/kg orally and 250 mg/kg IV produced significant mortality in rodents.

11 DESCRIPTION

LEVAQUIN® is a synthetic broad-spectrum antibacterial agent for oral and intravenous administration. Chemically, levofloxacin, a chiral fluorinated carboxyquinolone, is the pure (-)-(S)-enantiomer of the racemic drug substance ofloxacin. The chemical name is (-)-(S)-9-fluoro-2,3-dihydro-3-methyl-10-(4-methyl-1-piperazinyl)-7-oxo-7H-pyrido[1,2,3-de]-1,4-benzoxazine-6-carboxylic acid hemihydrate.
[See figure 1 at top of next column]

The empirical formula is $C_{18}H_{20}FN_3O_4 \cdot \frac{1}{2} H_2O$ and the molecular weight is 370.38. Levofloxacin is a light yellowish-white to yellow-white crystal or crystalline powder. The molecule exists as a zwitterion at the pH conditions in the small intestine.

Table 10: Mean ± SD Levofloxacin PK Parameters

Regimen	C_{max} (mcg/mL)	T_{max} (h)	AUC (mcg·h/mL)	CL/F[1] (mL/min)	Vd/F[2] (L)	$t_{1/2}$ (h)	CL_R (mL/min)
Single dose							
250 mg oral tablet[3]	2.8 ± 0.4	1.6 ± 1.0	27.2 ± 3.9	156 ± 20	ND	7.3 ± 0.9	142 ± 21
500 mg oral tablet[3]*	5.1 ± 0.8	1.3 ± 0.6	47.9 ± 6.8	178 ± 28	ND	6.3 ± 0.6	103 ± 30
500 mg oral solution[12]	5.8 ± 1.8	0.8 ± 0.7	47.8 ± 10.8	183 ± 40	112 ± 37.2	7.0 ± 1.4	ND
500 mg IV[3]	6.2 ± 1.0	1.0 ± 0.1	48.3 ± 5.4	175 ± 20	90 ± 11	6.4 ± 0.7	112 ± 25
750 mg oral tablet[5]*	9.3 ± 1.6	1.6 ± 0.8	101 ± 20	129 ± 24	83 ± 17	7.5 ± 0.9	ND
750 mg IV[5]	11.5 ± 4.0[4]	ND	110 ± 40	126 ± 39	75 ± 13	7.5 ± 1.6	ND
Multiple dose							
500 mg every 24h oral tablet[3]	5.7 ± 1.4	1.1 ± 0.4	47.5 ± 6.7	175 ± 25	102 ± 22	7.6 ± 1.6	116 ± 31
500 mg every 24h IV[3]	6.4 ± 0.8	ND	54.6 ± 11.1	158 ± 29	91 ± 12	7.0 ± 1.4	99 ± 28
500 mg or 250 mg every 24h IV, patients with bacterial infection[6]	8.7 ± 4.0[7]	ND	72.5 ± 51.2[7]	154 ± 72	111 ± 58	ND	ND
750 mg every 24h oral tablet[5]	8.6 ± 1.9	1.4 ± 0.5	90.7 ± 17.6	143 ± 29	100 ± 16	8.8 ± 1.5	116 ± 28
750 mg every 24h IV[5]	12.1 ± 4.1[4]	ND	108 ± 34	126 ± 37	80 ± 27	7.9 ± 1.9	ND
500 mg oral tablet single dose, effects of gender and age:							
Male[8]	5.5 ± 1.1	1.2 ± 0.4	54.4 ± 18.9	166 ± 44	89 ± 13	7.5 ± 2.1	126 ± 38
Female[9]	7.0 ± 1.6	1.7 ± 0.5	67.7 ± 24.2	136 ± 44	62 ± 16	6.1 ± 0.8	106 ± 40
Young[10]	5.5 ± 1.0	1.5 ± 0.6	47.5 ± 9.8	182 ± 35	83 ± 18	6.0 ± 0.9	140 ± 33
Elderly[11]	7.0 ± 1.6	1.4 ± 0.5	74.7 ± 23.3	121 ± 33	67 ± 19	7.6 ± 2.0	91 ± 29
500 mg oral single dose tablet, patients with renal insufficiency:							
CLCR 50–80 mL/min	7.5 ± 1.8	1.5 ± 0.5	95.6 ± 11.8	88 ± 10	ND	9.1 ± 0.9	57 ± 8
CLCR 20–49 mL/min	7.1 ± 3.1	2.1 ± 1.3	182.1 ± 62.6	51 ± 19	ND	27 ± 10	26 ± 13
CLCR <20 mL/min	8.2 ± 2.6	1.1 ± 1.0	263.5 ± 72.5	33 ± 8	ND	35 ± 5	13 ± 3
Hemodialysis	5.7 ± 1.0	2.8 ± 2.2	ND	ND	ND	76 ± 42	ND
CAPD	6.9 ± 2.3	1.4 ± 1.1	ND	ND	ND	51 ± 24	ND

[1] clearance/bioavailability
[2] volume of distribution/bioavailability
[3] healthy males 18–53 years of age
[4] 60 min infusion for 250 mg and 500 mg doses, 90 min infusion for 750 mg dose
[5] healthy male and female subjects 18–54 years of age
[6] 500 mg every 48h for patients with moderate renal impairment (CLCR 20–50 mL/min) and infections of the respiratory tract or skin
[7] dose-normalized values (to 500 mg dose), estimated by population pharmacokinetic modeling
[8] healthy males 22–75 years of age
[9] healthy females 18–80 years of age
[10] young healthy male and female subjects 18–36 years of age
[11] healthy elderly male and female subjects 66–80 years of age
[12] healthy males and females 19–55 years of age.
*Absolute bioavailability; F=0.99 ± 0.08 from a 500 mg tablet and F=0.99 ± 0.06 from a 750 mg tablet;
ND=not determined.

Figure 1: The Chemical Structure of Levofloxacin

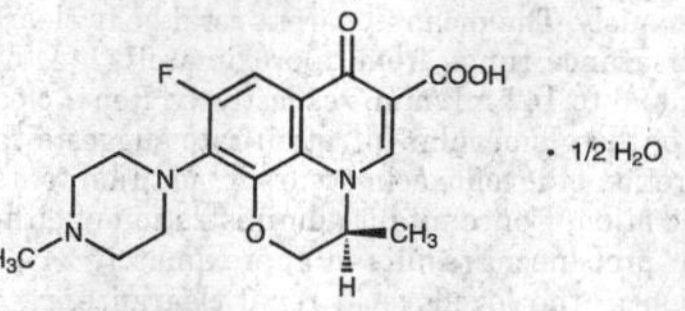

The data demonstrate that from pH 0.6 to 5.8, the solubility of levofloxacin is essentially constant (approximately 100 mg/mL). Levofloxacin is considered soluble to freely soluble in this pH range, as defined by USP nomenclature. Above pH 5.8, the solubility increases rapidly to its maximum at pH 6.7 (272 mg/mL) and is considered freely soluble in this range. Above pH 6.7, the solubility decreases and reaches a minimum value (about 50 mg/mL) at a pH of approximately 6.9.

Levofloxacin has the potential to form stable coordination compounds with many metal ions. This in vitro chelation potential has the following formation order: $Al^{+3} > Cu^{+2} > Zn^{+2} > Mg^{+2} > Ca^{+2}$.

Excipients and Description of Dosage Forms

LEVAQUIN® Tablets

LEVAQUIN® Tablets are available as film-coated tablets and contain the following inactive ingredients:

- 250 mg (as expressed in the anhydrous form): hypromellose, crospovidone, microcrystalline cellulose, magnesium stearate, polyethylene glycol, titanium dioxide, polysorbate 80 and synthetic red iron oxide.
- 500 mg (as expressed in the anhydrous form): hypromellose, crospovidone, microcrystalline cellulose, magnesium stearate, polyethylene glycol, titanium dioxide, polysorbate 80 and synthetic red and yellow iron oxides.
- 750 mg (as expressed in the anhydrous form): hypromellose, crospovidone, microcrystalline cellulose, magnesium stearate, polyethylene glycol, titanium dioxide, polysorbate 80.

LEVAQUIN® Oral Solution

LEVAQUIN® Oral Solution, 25 mg/mL, is a multi-use self-preserving aqueous solution of levofloxacin with pH ranging from 5.0–6.0. The appearance of LEVAQUIN® Oral Solution may range from clear yellow to clear greenish-yellow. This does not adversely affect product potency.

LEVAQUIN® Oral Solution contains the following inactive ingredients: sucrose, glycerin, sucralose, hydrochloric acid, purified water, propylene glycol, artificial and natural flavors, benzyl alcohol, ascorbic acid, and caramel color. It may also contain a solution of sodium hydroxide for pH adjustment.

LEVAQUIN® Injection

The appearance of LEVAQUIN® Injection may range from a clear yellow to a clear greenish-yellow solution. This does not adversely affect product potency.

LEVAQUIN® Injection in Single-Use Vials is a sterile, preservative-free aqueous solution of levofloxacin in Water for Injection, with pH ranging from 3.8 to 5.8.

LEVAQUIN® Injection Premix in Single-Use Flexible Containers is a sterile, preservative-free aqueous solution of levofloxacin with pH ranging from 3.8 to 5.8. This is a dilute, non-pyrogenic, nearly isotonic premixed solution that contains levofloxacin in 5% Dextrose (D_5W). Solutions of hydrochloric acid and sodium hydroxide may have been added to adjust the pH.

The flexible container is fabricated from a specially formulated non-plasticized, thermoplastic copolyester (CR3). The amount of water that can permeate from the container into the overwrap is insufficient to affect the solution significantly. Solutions in contact with the flexible container can leach out certain of the container's chemical components in very small amounts within the expiration period. The suitability of the container material has been confirmed by tests in animals according to USP biological tests for plastic containers.

12 CLINICAL PHARMACOLOGY

12.1 Mechanism of Action

Levofloxacin is a member of the fluoroquinolone class of antibacterial agents *[see Clinical Pharmacology (12.4)]*.

12.3 Pharmacokinetics

The mean ±SD pharmacokinetic parameters of levofloxacin determined under single and steady-state conditions following oral tablet, oral solution, or intravenous (IV) doses of LEVAQUIN® are summarized in Table 10.

[See table 10 at top of previous page]

Absorption

Levofloxacin is rapidly and essentially completely absorbed after oral administration. Peak plasma concentrations are usually attained one to two hours after oral dosing. The absolute bioavailability of levofloxacin from a 500 mg tablet and a 750 mg tablet of LEVAQUIN® are both approximately 99%, demonstrating complete oral absorption of levofloxacin. Following a single intravenous dose of LEVAQUIN® to healthy volunteers, the mean ±SD peak plasma concentration attained was 6.2 ±1.0 mcg/mL after a 500 mg dose infused over 60 minutes and 11.5 ±4.0 mcg/mL after a 750 mg dose infused over 90 minutes. LEVAQUIN® Oral Solution and Tablet formulations are bioequivalent.

Levofloxacin pharmacokinetics are linear and predictable after single and multiple oral or IV dosing regimens. Steady-state conditions are reached within 48 hours following a 500 mg or 750 mg once-daily dosage regimen. The mean ±SD peak and trough plasma concentrations attained following multiple once-daily oral dosage regimens were approximately 5.7 ±1.4 and 0.5 ±0.2 mcg/mL after the 500 mg doses, and 8.6 ±1.9 and 1.1 ±0.4 mcg/mL after the 750 mg doses, respectively. The mean ±SD peak and trough plasma concentrations attained following multiple once-daily IV regimens were approximately 6.4 ±0.8 and 0.6 ±0.2 mcg/mL after the 500 mg doses, and 12.1 ±4.1 and 1.3 ±0.71 mcg/mL after the 750 mg doses, respectively. Oral administration of a 500 mg dose of LEVAQUIN® with food prolongs the time to peak concentration by approximately 1 hour and decreases the peak concentration by approximately 14% following tablet and approximately 25% following oral solution administration. Therefore, LEVAQUIN® Tablets can be administered without regard to food. It is recommended that LEVAQUIN® Oral Solution be taken 1 hour before, or 2 hours after eating.

The plasma concentration profile of levofloxacin after IV administration is similar and comparable in extent of exposure (AUC) to that observed for LEVAQUIN® Tablets when equal doses (mg/mg) are administered. Therefore, the oral and IV routes of administration can be considered interchangeable *(see Figure 2 and Figure 3)*.

[See figure 2 at top of next column]
[See figure 3 in next column]

Distribution

The mean volume of distribution of levofloxacin generally ranges from 74 to 112 L after single and multiple 500 mg or 750 mg doses, indicating widespread distribution into body tissues. Levofloxacin reaches its peak levels in skin tissues

Figure 2: Mean Levofloxacin Plasma Concentration vs. Time Profile: 750 mg

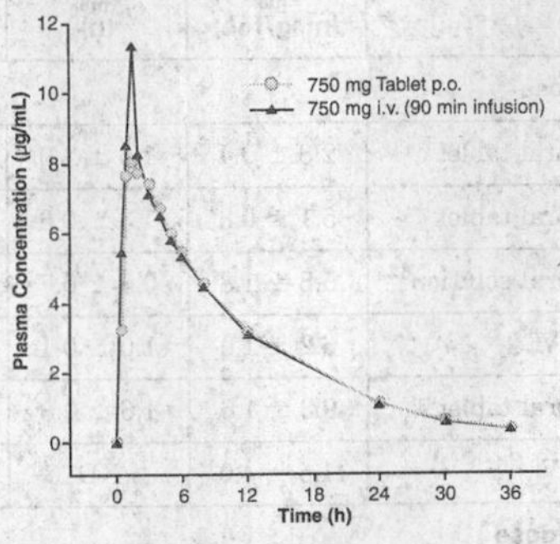

Figure 3: Mean Levofloxacin Plasma Concentration vs. Time Profile: 500 mg

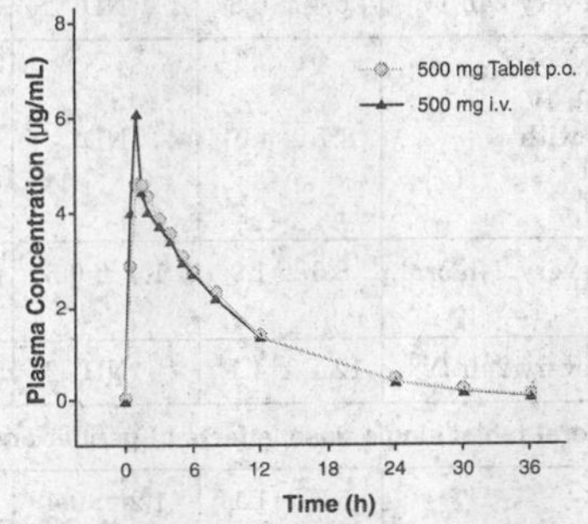

and in blister fluid of healthy subjects at approximately 3 hours after dosing. The skin tissue biopsy to plasma AUC ratio is approximately 2 and the blister fluid to plasma AUC ratio is approximately 1 following multiple once-daily oral administration of 750 mg and 500 mg doses of LEVAQUIN®, respectively, to healthy subjects. Levofloxacin also penetrates well into lung tissues. Lung tissue concentrations were generally 2- to 5-fold higher than plasma concentrations and ranged from approximately 2.4 to 11.3 mcg/g over a 24-hour period after a single 500 mg oral dose.

In vitro, over a clinically relevant range (1 to 10 mcg/mL) of serum/plasma levofloxacin concentrations, levofloxacin is approximately 24 to 38% bound to serum proteins across all species studied, as determined by the equilibrium dialysis method. Levofloxacin is mainly bound to serum albumin in humans. Levofloxacin binding to serum proteins is independent of the drug concentration.

Metabolism

Levofloxacin is stereochemically stable in plasma and urine and does not invert metabolically to its enantiomer, D-ofloxacin. Levofloxacin undergoes limited metabolism in humans and is primarily excreted as unchanged drug in the urine. Following oral administration, approximately 87% of an administered dose was recovered as unchanged drug in urine within 48 hours, whereas less than 4% of the dose was recovered in feces in 72 hours. Less than 5% of an administered dose was recovered in the urine as the desmethyl and N-oxide metabolites, the only metabolites identified in humans. These metabolites have little relevant pharmacological activity.

Excretion

Levofloxacin is excreted largely as unchanged drug in the urine. The mean terminal plasma elimination half-life of levofloxacin ranges from approximately 6 to 8 hours following single or multiple doses of levofloxacin given orally or intravenously. The mean apparent total body clearance and renal clearance range from approximately 144 to 226 mL/min and 96 to 142 mL/min, respectively. Renal clearance in excess of the glomerular filtration rate suggests that tubular secretion of levofloxacin occurs in addition to its glomerular filtration. Concomitant administration of either cimetidine or probenecid results in approximately 24% and 35% reduction in the levofloxacin renal clearance, respectively, indicating that secretion of levofloxacin occurs in the renal proximal tubule. No levofloxacin crystals were found in any of the urine samples freshly collected from subjects receiving LEVAQUIN®.

Geriatric

There are no significant differences in levofloxacin pharmacokinetics between young and elderly subjects when the subjects' differences in creatinine clearance are taken into consideration. Following a 500 mg oral dose of LEVAQUIN® to healthy elderly subjects (66–80 years of age), the mean terminal plasma elimination half-life of levofloxacin was about 7.6 hours, as compared to approximately 6 hours in younger adults. The difference was attributable to the variation in renal function status of the subjects and was not believed to be clinically significant. Drug absorption appears to be unaffected by age. LEVAQUIN® dose adjustment based on age alone is not necessary *[See Use in Specific Populations (8.5)]*.

Pediatrics

The pharmacokinetics of levofloxacin following a single 7 mg/kg intravenous dose were investigated in pediatric patients ranging in age from 6 months to 16 years. Pediatric patients cleared levofloxacin faster than adult patients, resulting in lower plasma exposures than adults for a given mg/kg dose. Subsequent pharmacokinetic analyses predicted that a dosage regimen of 8 mg/kg every 12 hours (not to exceed 250 mg per dose) for pediatric patients 6 months to 17 years of age would achieve comparable steady state plasma exposures (AUC_{0-24} and C_{max}) to those observed in adult patients administered 500 mg of levofloxacin once every 24 hours.

Gender

There are no significant differences in levofloxacin pharmacokinetics between male and female subjects when subjects' differences in creatinine clearance are taken into consideration. Following a 500 mg oral dose of LEVAQUIN® to healthy male subjects, the mean terminal plasma elimination half-life of levofloxacin was about 7.5 hours, as compared to approximately 6.1 hours in female subjects. This difference was attributable to the variation in renal function status of the male and female subjects and was not believed to be clinically significant. Drug absorption appears to be unaffected by the gender of the subjects. Dose adjustment based on gender alone is not necessary.

Race

The effect of race on levofloxacin pharmacokinetics was examined through a covariate analysis performed on data from 72 subjects: 48 white and 24 non-white. The apparent total body clearance and apparent volume of distribution were not affected by the race of the subjects.

Renal Impairment

Clearance of levofloxacin is substantially reduced and plasma elimination half-life is substantially prolonged in adult patients with impaired renal function (creatinine clearance < 50 mL/min), requiring dosage adjustment in such patients to avoid accumulation. Neither hemodialysis nor continuous ambulatory peritoneal dialysis (CAPD) is effective in removal of levofloxacin from the body, indicating that supplemental doses of LEVAQUIN® are not required following hemodialysis or CAPD *[see Dosage and Administration (2.3), Use in Specific Populations (8.6)]*.

Hepatic Impairment

Pharmacokinetic studies in hepatically impaired patients have not been conducted. Due to the limited extent of levofloxacin metabolism, the pharmacokinetics of levofloxacin are not expected to be affected by hepatic impairment *[See Use in Specific Populations (8.7)]*.

Bacterial Infection

The pharmacokinetics of levofloxacin in patients with serious community-acquired bacterial infections are comparable to those observed in healthy subjects.

Drug-Drug Interactions

The potential for pharmacokinetic drug interactions between LEVAQUIN® and antacids warfarin, theophylline, cyclosporine, digoxin, probenecid, and cimetidine has been evaluated *[see Drug Interactions (7)]*.

12.4 Microbiology

Mechanism of Action

Levofloxacin is the L-isomer of the racemate, ofloxacin, a quinolone antimicrobial agent. The antibacterial activity of ofloxacin resides primarily in the L-isomer. The mechanism of action of levofloxacin and other fluoroquinolone antimicrobials involves inhibition of bacterial topoisomerase IV and DNA gyrase (both of which are type II topoisomerases), enzymes required for DNA replication, transcription, repair and recombination.

Drug Resistance

Fluoroquinolone resistance can arise through mutations in defined regions of DNA gyrase or topoisomerase IV, termed the Quinolone-Resistance Determining Regions (QRDRs), or through altered efflux.

Fluoroquinolones, including levofloxacin, differ in chemical structure and mode of action from aminoglycosides, macrolides and β-lactam antibiotics, including penicillins. Fluoroquinolones may, therefore, be active against bacteria resistant to these antimicrobials.

Resistance to levofloxacin due to spontaneous mutation *in vitro* is a rare occurrence (range: 10^{-9} to 10^{-10}). Although cross-resistance has been observed between levofloxacin and some other fluoroquinolones, some microorganisms resistant to other fluoroquinolones may be susceptible to levofloxacin.

Activity in vitro and in vivo

Levofloxacin has in vitro activity against a wide range of Gram-negative and Gram-positive microorganisms. Levofloxacin is often bactericidal at concentrations equal to or slightly greater than inhibitory concentrations.

Levofloxacin has been shown to be active against most strains of the following microorganisms both in vitro and in clinical infections as described in Indications and Usage (1):

Aerobic Gram-Positive Microorganisms

Enterococcus faecalis (many strains are only moderately susceptible)
Staphylococcus aureus (methicillin-susceptible strains)
Staphylococcus epidermidis (methicillin-susceptible strains)
Staphylococcus saprophyticus
Streptococcus pneumoniae (including multi-drug resistant strains [MDRSP])[1]
Streptococcus pyogenes

---

[1] MDRSP (Multi-drug resistant Streptococcus pneumoniae) isolates are strains resistant to two or more of the following antibiotics: penicillin (MIC ≥2 mcg/mL), 2nd generation cephalosporins, e.g., cefuroxime; macrolides, tetracyclines and trimethoprim/sulfamethoxazole.

Aerobic Gram-Negative Microorganisms

Enterobacter cloacae
Escherichia coli
Haemophilus influenzae
Haemophilus parainfluenzae
Klebsiella pneumoniae
Legionella pneumophila
Moraxella catarrhalis
Proteus mirabilis
Pseudomonas aeruginosa[2]
Serratia marcescens

---

[2] As with other drugs in this class, some strains of Pseudomonas aeruginosa may develop resistance fairly rapidly during treatment with LEVAQUIN®.

Other Microorganisms

Chlamydophila pneumoniae
Mycoplasma pneumoniae

Levofloxacin has been shown to be active against Bacillus anthracis both in vitro and by use of plasma levels as a surrogate marker in a rhesus monkey model for anthrax (post-exposure) [see Indications and Usage (1.13), Clinical Studies (14.9)].

The following in vitro data are available, but their clinical significance is unknown: Levofloxacin exhibits in vitro minimum inhibitory concentrations (MIC values) of 2 mcg/mL or less against most (≥90%) strains of the following microorganisms; however, the safety and effectiveness of LEVAQUIN® in treating clinical infections due to these microorganisms have not been established in adequate and well-controlled trials.

Aerobic Gram-Positive Microorganisms

Staphylococcus haemolyticus
β-hemolytic Streptococcus (Group C/F)
β-hemolytic Streptococcus (Group G)
Streptococcus agalactiae
Streptococcus milleri
Viridans group streptococci

Aerobic Gram-Negative Microorganisms

Acinetobacter baumannii
Acinetobacter lwoffii
Bordetella pertussis
Citrobacter koseri
Citrobacter freundii
Enterobacter aerogenes
Enterobacter sakazakii
Klebsiella oxytoca
Morganella morganii
Pantoea agglomerans
Proteus vulgaris
Providencia rettgeri
Providencia stuartii
Pseudomonas fluorescens

Anaerobic Gram-Positive Microorganisms

Clostridium perfringens

Susceptibility Tests

Susceptibility testing for levofloxacin should be performed, as it is the optimal predictor of activity.

• Dilution techniques:

Quantitative methods are used to determine antimicrobial minimal inhibitory concentrations (MIC values). These MIC values provide estimates of the susceptibility of bacteria to antimicrobial compounds. The MIC values should be determined using a standardized procedure. Standardized procedures are based on a dilution method[1] (broth or agar) or equivalent with standardized inoculum concentrations and standardized concentrations of levofloxacin powder. The MIC values should be interpreted according to the criteria outlined in Table 11.

• Diffusion techniques:

Quantitative methods that require measurement of zone diameters also provide reproducible estimates of the susceptibility of bacteria to antimicrobial compounds. One such standardized procedure[2] requires the use of standardized inoculum concentrations. This procedure uses paper disks impregnated with 5 mcg levofloxacin to test the susceptibility of microorganisms to levofloxacin.

Reports from the laboratory providing results of the standard single-disk susceptibility test with a 5 mcg levofloxacin disk should be interpreted according to the criteria outlined in Table 11. Interpretation involves correlation of the diameter obtained in the disk test with the MIC for levofloxacin.
[See table 11 above]

A report of Susceptible indicates that the pathogen is likely to be inhibited if the antimicrobial compound in the blood reaches the concentrations usually achievable. A report of Intermediate indicates that the result should be considered equivocal, and, if the microorganism is not fully susceptible to alternative, clinically feasible drugs, the test should be repeated. This category implies possible clinical applicability in body sites where the drug is physiologically concentrated or in situations where a high dosage of drug can be used. This category also provides a buffer zone which prevents small uncontrolled technical factors from causing major discrepancies in interpretation. A report of Resistant indicates that the pathogen is not likely to be inhibited if the antimicrobial compound in the blood reaches the concentrations usually achievable; other therapy should be selected.

• Quality Control:

Standardized susceptibility test procedures require the use of laboratory control microorganisms to control the technical aspects of the laboratory procedures. For dilution technique, standard levofloxacin powder should give the MIC values provided in Table 12. For diffusion technique, the 5 mcg levofloxacin disk should provide zone diameters provided in Table 12.
[See table 12 above]

13 NONCLINICAL TOXICOLOGY

13.1 Carcinogenesis, Mutagenesis, Impairment of Fertility

In a lifetime bioassay in rats, levofloxacin exhibited no carcinogenic potential following daily dietary administration for 2 years; the highest dose (100 mg/kg/day) was 1.4 times the highest recommended human dose (750 mg) based upon relative body surface area. Levofloxacin did not shorten the time to tumor development of UV-induced skin tumors in hairless albino (Skh-1) mice at any levofloxacin dose level

---

Table 11: Susceptibility Interpretive Criteria for LEVAQUIN®

Pathogen	Minimum Inhibitory Concentrations (mcg/mL)			Disk Diffusion (zone diameter in mm)		
	S	I	R	S	I	R
Enterobacteriaceae	≤2	4	≥8	≥17	14–16	≤13
Enterococcus faecalis	≤2	4	≥8	≥17	14–16	≤13
Methicillin-susceptible Staphylococcus species	≤2	4	≥8	≥17	14–16	≤13
Pseudomonas aeruginosa	≤2	4	≥8	≥17	14–16	≤13
Haemophilus influenzae	≤2*	—†	—†	≥17‡	—†	—†
Haemophilus parainfluenzae	≤2*	—†	—†	≥17‡	—†	—†
Streptococcus pneumoniae	≤2§	4§	≥8§	≥17¶	14–16¶	≤13¶
Streptococcus pyogenes	≤2	4	≥8	≥17	14–16	≤13

S = Susceptible, I = Intermediate, R = Resistant
* These interpretive standards are applicable only to broth microdilution susceptibility testing with Haemophilus influenzae and Haemophilus parainfluenzae using Haemophilus Test Medium.[1]
† The current absence of data on resistant strains precludes defining any categories other than "Susceptible." Strains yielding MIC/zone diameter results suggestive of a "nonsusceptible" category should be submitted to a reference laboratory for further testing.
‡ These interpretive standards are applicable only to disk diffusion susceptibility testing with Haemophilus influenzae and Haemophilus parainfluenzae using Haemophilus Test Medium.[2]
§ These interpretive standards are applicable only to broth microdilution susceptibility tests using cation-adjusted Mueller-Hinton broth with 2–5% lysed horse blood.
¶ These zone diameter standards for Streptococcus spp. including S. pneumoniae apply only to tests performed using Mueller-Hinton agar supplemented with 5% sheep blood and incubated in 5% CO_2.

Table 12: Quality Control for Susceptibility Testing

Microorganism	Microorganism QC Number	MIC (mcg/mL)	Disk Diffusion (zone diameter in mm)
Enterococcus faecalis	ATCC 29212	0.25–2	Not applicable
Escherichia coli	ATCC 25922	0.008–0.06	29–37
Escherichia coli	ATCC 35218	0.015–0.06	Not applicable
Haemophilus influenzae	ATCC 49247	0.008–0.03*	32–40†
Pseudomonas aeruginosa	ATCC 27853	0.5–4	19–26
Staphylococcus aureus	ATCC 29213	0.06–0.5	Not applicable
Staphylococcus aureus	ATCC 25923	Not applicable	25–30
Streptococcus pneumoniae	ATCC 49619	0.5–2‡	20–25§

* This quality control range is applicable to only H. influenzae ATCC 49247 tested by a broth microdilution procedure using Haemophilus Test Medium (HTM).[1]
† This quality control range is applicable to only H. influenzae ATCC 49247 tested by a disk diffusion procedure using Haemophilus Test Medium (HTM).[2]
‡ This quality control range is applicable to only S. pneumoniae ATCC 49619 tested by a broth microdilution procedure using cation-adjusted Mueller-Hinton broth with 2–5% lysed horse blood.
§ This quality control range is applicable to only S. pneumoniae ATCC 49619 tested by a disk diffusion procedure using Mueller-Hinton agar supplemented with 5% sheep blood and incubated in 5% CO_2.

Table 13: Clinical Success Rates and Microbiological Eradication Rates (Nosocomial Pneumonia)

Pathogen	N	LEVAQUIN® No. (%) of Patients Microbiologic/ Clinical Outcomes	N	Imipenem/Cilastatin No. (%) of Patients Microbiologic/ Clinical Outcomes
MSSA*	21	14 (66.7)/13 (61.9)	19	13 (68.4)/15 (78.9)
P. aeruginosa†	17	10 (58.8)/11 (64.7)	17	5 (29.4)/7 (41.2)
S. marcescens	11	9 (81.8)/7 (63.6)	7	2 (28.6)/3 (42.9)
E. coli	12	10 (83.3)/7 (58.3)	11	7 (63.6)/8 (72.7)
K. pneumoniae‡	11	9 (81.8)/5 (45.5)	7	6 (85.7)/3 (42.9)
H. influenzae	16	13 (81.3)/10 (62.5)	15	14 (93.3)/11 (73.3)
S. pneumoniae	4	3 (75.0)/3 (75.0)	7	5 (71.4)/4 (57.1)

* Methicillin-susceptible *S. aureus*
† See above text for use of combination therapy
‡ The observed differences in rates for the clinical and microbiological outcomes may reflect other factors that were not accounted for in the study

Table 15: Clinical and Bacterial Success Rates for LEVAQUIN®-Treated MDRSP in Community Acquired Pneumonia Patients (Population Valid for Efficacy)

Screening Susceptibility	Clinical Success		Bacteriological Success*	
	n/N†	%	n/N‡	%
Penicillin-resistant	16/17	94.1	16/17	94.1
2nd generation Cephalosporin resistant	31/32	96.9	31/32	96.9
Macrolide-resistant	28/29	96.6	28/29	96.6
Trimethoprim/Sulfamethoxazole resistant	17/19	89.5	17/19	89.5
Tetracycline-resistant	12/12	100	12/12	100

* One patient had a respiratory isolate that was resistant to tetracycline, cefuroxime, macrolides and TMP/SMX and intermediate to penicillin and a blood isolate that was intermediate to penicillin and cefuroxime and resistant to the other classes. The patient is included in the database based on respiratory isolate.
† n=the number of microbiologically evaluable patients who were clinical successes; N=number of microbiologically evaluable patients in the designated resistance group.
‡ n=the number of MDRSP isolates eradicated or presumed eradicated in microbiologically evaluable patients; N=number of MDRSP isolates in a designated resistance group.

and was therefore not photo-carcinogenic under conditions of this study. Dermal levofloxacin concentrations in the hairless mice ranged from 25 to 42 mcg/g at the highest levofloxacin dose level (300 mg/kg/day) used in the photo-carcinogenicity study. By comparison, dermal levofloxacin concentrations in human subjects receiving 750 mg of LEVAQUIN® averaged approximately 11.8 mcg/g at C_{max}.

Levofloxacin was not mutagenic in the following assays: Ames bacterial mutation assay (*S. typhimurium* and *E. coli*), CHO/HGPRT forward mutation assay, mouse micronucleus test, mouse dominant lethal test, rat unscheduled DNA synthesis assay, and the mouse sister chromatid exchange assay. It was positive in the in vitro chromosomal aberration (CHL cell line) and sister chromatid exchange (CHL/IU cell line) assays.

Levofloxacin caused no impairment of fertility or reproductive performance in rats at oral doses as high as 360 mg/kg/day, corresponding to 4.2 times the highest recommended human dose based upon relative body surface area and intravenous doses as high as 100 mg/kg/day, corresponding to 1.2 times the highest recommended human dose based upon relative body surface area.

13.2 Animal Toxicology and/or Pharmacology
Levofloxacin and other quinolones have been shown to cause arthropathy in immature animals of most species tested [see Warnings and Precautions (5.9)]. In immature dogs (4–5 months old), oral doses of 10 mg/kg/day for 7 days and intravenous doses of 4 mg/kg/day for 14 days of levofloxacin resulted in arthropathic lesions. Administration at oral doses of 300 mg/kg/day for 7 days and intravenous doses of 60 mg/kg/day for 4 weeks produced arthropathy in juvenile rats. Three-month old beagle dogs dosed orally with levofloxacin at 40 mg/kg/day exhibited clinically severe arthrotoxicity resulting in the termination of dosing at Day 8 of a 14-day dosing routine. Slight musculoskeletal clinical effects, in the absence of gross pathological or histopathological effects, resulted from the lowest dose level of 2.5 mg/kg/day (approximately 0.2-fold the pediatric dose based upon AUC comparisons). Synovitis and articular cartilage lesions were observed at the 10 and 40 mg/kg dose levels (approximately 0.7-fold and 2.4-fold the pediatric dose, respectively, based on AUC comparisons). Articular cartilage gross pathology and histopathology persisted to the end of the 18-week recovery period for those dogs from the 10 and 40 mg/kg/day dose levels.

When tested in a mouse ear swelling bioassay, levofloxacin exhibited phototoxicity similar in magnitude to ofloxacin, but less phototoxicity than other quinolones.

While crystalluria has been observed in some intravenous rat studies, urinary crystals are not formed in the bladder, being present only after micturition and are not associated with nephrotoxicity.

In mice, the CNS stimulatory effect of quinolones is enhanced by concomitant administration of non-steroidal anti-inflammatory drugs.

In dogs, levofloxacin administered at 6 mg/kg or higher by rapid intravenous injection produced hypotensive effects. These effects were considered to be related to histamine release.

In vitro and *in vivo* studies in animals indicate that levofloxacin is neither an enzyme inducer nor inhibitor in the human therapeutic plasma concentration range; therefore, no drug metabolizing enzyme-related interactions with other drugs or agents are anticipated.

14 CLINICAL STUDIES
14.1 Nosocomial Pneumonia
Adult patients with clinically and radiologically documented nosocomial pneumonia were enrolled in a multicenter, randomized, open-label study comparing intravenous LEVAQUIN® (750 mg once daily) followed by oral LEVAQUIN® (750 mg once daily) for a total of 7–15 days to intravenous imipenem/cilastatin (500–1000 mg every 6–8 hours daily) followed by oral ciprofloxacin (750 mg every 12 hours daily) for a total of 7–15 days. LEVAQUIN®-treated patients received an average of 7 days of intravenous therapy (range: 1–16 days); comparator-treated patients received an average of 8 days of intravenous therapy (range: 1–19 days).

Overall, in the clinically and microbiologically evaluable population, adjunctive therapy was empirically initiated at study entry in 56 of 93 (60.2%) patients in the LEVAQUIN® arm and 53 of 94 (56.4%) patients in the comparator arm. The average duration of adjunctive therapy was 7 days in the LEVAQUIN® arm and 7 days in the comparator. In clinically and microbiologically evaluable patients with documented *Pseudomonas aeruginosa* infection, 15 of 17 (88.2%) received ceftazidime (N=11) or piperacillin/tazobactam (N=4) in the LEVAQUIN® arm and 16 of 17 (94.1%) received an aminoglycoside in the comparator arm. Overall, in clinically and microbiologically evaluable patients, vancomycin was added to the treatment regimen of 37 of 93 (39.8%) patients in the LEVAQUIN® arm and 28 of 94 (29.8%) patients in the comparator arm for suspected methicillin-resistant *S. aureus* infection.

Clinical success rates in clinically and microbiologically evaluable patients at the posttherapy visit (primary study endpoint assessed on day 3–15 after completing therapy) were 58.1% for LEVAQUIN® and 60.6% for comparator. The 95% CI for the difference of response rates (LEVAQUIN® minus comparator) was [-17.2, 12.0]. The microbiological eradication rates at the posttherapy visit were 66.7% for LEVAQUIN® and 60.6% for comparator. The 95% CI for the difference of eradication rates (LEVAQUIN® minus comparator) was [-8.3, 20.3]. Clinical success and microbiological eradication rates by pathogen are detailed in Table 13.
[See table 13 at left]

14.2 Community-Acquired Pneumonia: 7–14 day Treatment Regimen
Adult inpatients and outpatients with a diagnosis of community-acquired bacterial pneumonia were evaluated in 2 pivotal clinical studies. In the first study, 590 patients were enrolled in a prospective, multi-center, unblinded randomized trial comparing LEVAQUIN® 500 mg once daily orally or intravenously for 7 to 14 days to ceftriaxone 1 to 2 grams intravenously once or in equally divided doses twice daily followed by cefuroxime axetil 500 mg orally twice daily for a total of 7 to 14 days. Patients assigned to treatment with the control regimen were allowed to receive erythromycin (or doxycycline if intolerant of erythromycin) if an infection due to atypical pathogens was suspected or proven. Clinical and microbiologic evaluations were performed during treatment, 5 to 7 days posttherapy, and 3 to 4 weeks posttherapy. Clinical success (cure plus improvement) with LEVAQUIN® at 5 to 7 days posttherapy, the primary efficacy variable in this study, was superior (95%) to the control group (83%). The 95% CI for the difference of response rates (LEVAQUIN® minus comparator) was [-6, 19]. In the second study, 264 patients were enrolled in a prospective, multi-center, non-comparative trial of 500 mg LEVAQUIN® administered orally or intravenously once daily for 7 to 14 days. Clinical success for clinically evaluable patients was 93%. For both studies, the clinical success rate in patients with atypical pneumonia due to *Chlamydophila pneumoniae*, *Mycoplasma pneumoniae*, and *Legionella pneumophila* were 96%, 96%, and 70%, respectively. Microbiologic eradication rates across both studies are presented in Table 14.

Table 14: Microbiologic Eradication Rates Across 2 Community Acquired Pneumonia Clinical Studies

Pathogen	No. Pathogens	Microbiologic Eradication Rate (%)
H. influenzae	55	98
S. pneumoniae	83	95
S. aureus	17	88
M. catarrhalis	18	94
H. parainfluenzae	19	95
K. pneumoniae	10	100.0

Community-Acquired Pneumonia Due to Multi-Drug Resistant *Streptococcus pneumoniae*
LEVAQUIN® was effective for the treatment of community-acquired pneumonia caused by multi-drug resistant *Streptococcus pneumoniae* (MDRSP). MDRSP isolates are strains resistant to two or more of the following antibacterials: penicillin (MIC ≥2 mcg/ml), 2nd generation cephalosporins (e.g., cefuroxime, macrolides, tetracyclines and trimethoprim/sulfamethoxazole). Of 40 microbiologically evaluable patients with MDRSP isolates, 38 patients (95.0%) achieved clinical and bacteriologic success at posttherapy. The clinical and bacterial success rates are shown in Table 15.

Table 20: Bacteriologic Eradication at Test-of-Cure

	LEVAQUIN® 750 mg orally or IV once daily for 5 days		Ciprofloxacin 400 mg IV/ 500 mg orally twice daily for 10 days		Overall Difference [95% CI]
	n/N	%	n/N	%	LEVAQUIN®- Ciprofloxacin
mITT Population*					
Overall (cUTI or AP)	252/333	75.7	239/318	75.2	0.5 (-6.1, 7.1)
cUTI	168/230	73.0	157/213	73.7	
AP	84/103	81.6	82/105	78.1	
Microbiologically Evaluable Population†					
Overall (cUTI or AP)	228/265	86.0	215/241	89.2	-3.2 [-8.9, 2.5]
cUTI	154/185	83.2	144/165	87.3	
AP	74/80	92.5	71/76	93.4	

* The mITT population included patients who received study medication and who had a positive ($\geq 10^5$ CFU/mL) urine culture with no more than 2 uropathogens at baseline. Patients with missing response were counted as failures in this analysis.

† The Microbiologically Evaluable population included patients with a confirmed diagnosis of cUTI or AP, a causative organism(s) at baseline present at $\geq 10^5$ CFU/mL, a valid test-of-cure urine culture, no pathogen isolated from blood resistant to study drug, no premature discontinuation or loss to follow-up, and compliance with treatment (among other criteria).

[See table 15 on previous page]
Not all isolates were resistant to all antimicrobial classes tested. Success and eradication rates are summarized in Table 16.

Table 16: Clinical Success and Bacteriologic Eradication Rates for Resistant Streptococcus pneumoniae (Community Acquired Pneumonia)

Type of Resistance	Clinical Success	Bacteriologic Eradication
Resistant to 2 antibacterials	17/18 (94.4%)	17/18 (94.4%)
Resistant to 3 antibacterials	14/15 (93.3%)	14/15 (93.3%)
Resistant to 4 antibacterials	7/7 (100%)	7/7 (100%)
Resistant to 5 antibacterials	0	0
Bacteremia with MDRSP	8/9 (89%)	8/9 (89%)

14.3 Community-Acquired Pneumonia: 5-Day Treatment Regimen

To evaluate the safety and efficacy of higher dose and shorter course of LEVAQUIN®, 528 outpatient and hospitalized adults with clinically and radiologically determined mild to severe community-acquired pneumonia were evaluated in a double-blind, randomized, prospective, multicenter study comparing LEVAQUIN® 750 mg, IV or orally, every day for five days or LEVAQUIN® 500 mg IV or orally, every day for 10 days.

Clinical success rates (cure plus improvement) in the clinically evaluable population were 90.9% in the LEVAQUIN® 750 mg group and 91.1% in the LEVAQUIN® 500 mg group. The 95% CI for the difference of response rates (LEVAQUIN® 750 minus LEVAQUIN® 500) was [-5.9, 5.4]. In the clinically evaluable population (31–38 days after enrollment) pneumonia was observed in 7 out of 151 patients in the LEVAQUIN® 750 mg group and 2 out of 147 patients in the LEVAQUIN® 500 mg group. Given the small numbers observed, the significance of this finding cannot be determined statistically. The microbiological efficacy of the 5-day regimen was documented for infections listed in Table 17.

Table 17: Microbiological Eradication Rates (Community-Acquired Pneumonia)

Penicillin susceptible *S. pneumoniae*	19/20
Haemophilus influenzae	12/12
Haemophilus parainfluenzae	10/10
Mycoplasma pneumoniae	26/27
Chlamydophila pneumoniae	13/15

14.4 Acute Bacterial Sinusitis: 5-day and 10–14 day Treatment Regimens

LEVAQUIN® is approved for the treatment of acute bacterial sinusitis (ABS) using either 750 mg by mouth × 5 days or 500 mg by mouth once daily × 10–14 days. To evaluate the safety and efficacy of a high dose short course of LEVAQUIN®, 780 outpatient adults with clinically and radiologically determined acute bacterial sinusitis were evaluated in a double-blind, randomized, prospective, multicenter study comparing LEVAQUIN® 750 mg by mouth once daily for five days to LEVAQUIN® 500 mg by mouth once daily for 10 days.

Clinical success rates (defined as complete or partial resolution of the pre-treatment signs and symptoms of ABS to such an extent that no further antibiotic treatment was deemed necessary) in the microbiologically evaluable population were 91.4% (139/152) in the LEVAQUIN® 750 mg group and 88.6% (132/149) in the LEVAQUIN® 500 mg group at the test-of-cure (TOC) visit (95% CI [-4.2, 10.0] for LEVAQUIN® 750 mg minus LEVAQUIN® 500 mg).

Rates of clinical success by pathogen in the microbiologically evaluable population who had specimens obtained by antral tap at study entry showed comparable results for the five- and ten-day regimens at the test-of-cure visit 22 days post treatment.

Table 18: Clinical Success Rate by Pathogen at the TOC in Microbiologically Evaluable Subjects Who Underwent Antral Puncture (Acute Bacterial Sinusitis)

Pathogen	LEVAQUIN® 750 mg × 5 days	LEVAQUIN® 500 mg × 10 days
Streptococcus pneumoniae*	25/27 (92.6%)	26/27 (96.3%)
Haemophilus influenzae*	19/21 (90.5%)	25/27 (92.6%)
Moraxella catarrhalis*	10/11 (90.9%)	13/13 (100%)

*Note: Forty percent of the subjects in this trial had specimens obtained by sinus endoscopy. The efficacy data for subjects whose specimen was obtained endoscopically were comparable to those presented in the above table

14.5 Complicated Skin and Skin Structure Infections

Three hundred ninety-nine patients were enrolled in an open-label, randomized, comparative study for complicated skin and skin structure infections. The patients were randomized to receive either LEVAQUIN® 750 mg once daily (IV followed by oral), or an approved comparator for a median of 10 ± 4.7 days. As is expected in complicated skin and skin structure infections, surgical procedures were performed in the LEVAQUIN® and comparator groups. Surgery (incision and drainage or debridement) was performed on 45% of the LEVAQUIN®-treated patients and 44% of the comparator treated patients, either shortly before or during antibiotic treatment and formed an integral part of therapy for this indication.

Among those who could be evaluated clinically 2–5 days after completion of study drug, overall success rates (improved or cured) were 116/138 (84.1%) for patients treated with LEVAQUIN® and 106/132 (80.3%) for patients treated with the comparator.

Success rates varied with the type of diagnosis ranging from 68% in patients with infected ulcers to 90% in patients with infected wounds and abscesses. These rates were equivalent to those seen with comparator drugs.

14.6 Chronic Bacterial Prostatitis

Adult patients with a clinical diagnosis of prostatitis and microbiological culture results from urine sample collected after prostatic massage (VB$_3$) or expressed prostatic secretion (EPS) specimens obtained via the Meares-Stamey procedure were enrolled in a multicenter, randomized, double-blind study comparing oral LEVAQUIN® 500 mg, once daily for a total of 28 days to oral ciprofloxacin 500 mg, twice daily for a total of 28 days. The primary efficacy endpoint was microbiologic efficacy in microbiologically evaluable patients. A total of 136 and 125 microbiologically evaluable patients were enrolled in the LEVAQUIN® and ciprofloxacin groups, respectively. The microbiologic eradication rate by patient infection at 5–18 days after completion of therapy was 75.0% in the LEVAQUIN® group and 76.8% in the ciprofloxacin group (95% CI [-12.58, 8.98] for LEVAQUIN® minus ciprofloxacin). The overall eradication rates for pathogens of interest are presented in Table 19.

Table 19: Microbiological Eradication Rates (Chronic Bacterial Prostatitis)

Pathogen	LEVAQUIN® (N=136)		Ciprofloxacin (N=125)	
	N	Eradication	N	Eradication
E. coli	15	14 (93.3%)	11	9 (81.8%)
E. faecalis	54	39 (72.2%)	44	33 (75.0%)
S. epidermidis*	11	9 (81.8%)	14	11 (78.6%)

*Eradication rates shown are for patients who had a sole pathogen only; mixed cultures were excluded.

Eradication rates for *S. epidermidis* when found with other co-pathogens are consistent with rates seen in pure isolates. Clinical success (cure + improvement with no need for further antibiotic therapy) rates in microbiologically evaluable population 5–18 days after completion of therapy were 75.0% for LEVAQUIN®-treated patients and 72.8% for ciprofloxacin-treated patients (95% CI [-8.87, 13.27] for LEVAQUIN® minus ciprofloxacin). Clinical long-term success (24–45 days after completion of therapy) rates were 66.7% for the LEVAQUIN®-treated patients and 76.9% for the ciprofloxacin-treated patients (95% CI [-23.40, 2.89] for LEVAQUIN® minus ciprofloxacin).

14.7 Complicated Urinary Tract Infections and Acute Pyelonephritis: 5-day Treatment Regimen

To evaluate the safety and efficacy of the higher dose and shorter course of LEVAQUIN®, 1109 patients with cUTI and AP were enrolled in a randomized, double-blind, multicenter clinical trial conducted in the US from November 2004 to April 2006 comparing LEVAQUIN® 750 mg IV or orally once daily for 5 days (546 patients) with ciprofloxacin 400 mg IV or 500 mg orally twice daily for 10 days (563 patients). Patients with AP complicated by underlying renal diseases or conditions such as complete obstruction, surgery, transplantation, concurrent infection or congenital malformation were excluded. Efficacy was measured by bacteriologic eradication of the baseline organism(s) at the post-therapy visit in patients with a pathogen identified at baseline. The post-therapy (test-of-cure) visit occurred 10 to 14 days after the last active dose of LEVAQUIN® and 5 to 9 days after the last dose of active ciprofloxacin.

The bacteriologic cure rates overall for LEVAQUIN® and control at the test-of-cure (TOC) visit for the group of all patients with a documented pathogen at baseline (modified intent to treat or mITT) and the group of patients in the mITT population who closely followed the protocol (Microbiologically Evaluable) are summarized in Table 20.

[See table 20 above]

Microbiologic eradication rates in the Microbiologically Evaluable population at TOC for individual pathogens recovered from patients randomized to LEVAQUIN® treatment are presented in Table 21.

Table 21: Microbiological Eradication Rates for Individual Pathogens Recovered From Patients Randomized to LEVAQUIN® 750 mg QD for 5 Days Treatment

Pathogen	Microbiologic Eradication Rate (n/N)	%
*Escherichia coli**	155/172	90
Klebsiella pneumoniae	20/23	87
Proteus mirabilis	12/12	100

*The predominant organism isolated from patients with AP was *E. coli*: 91% (63/69) eradication in AP and 89% (92/103) in patients with cUTI.

14.8 Complicated Urinary Tract Infections and Acute Pyelonephritis: 10-day Treatment Regimen

To evaluate the safety and efficacy of the 250 mg dose, 10 day regimen of LEVAQUIN®, 567 patients with uncomplicated UTI, mild-to-moderate cUTI, and mild-to-moderate AP were enrolled in a randomized, double-blind, multicenter clinical trial conducted in the US from June 1993 to January 1995 comparing LEVAQUIN® 250 orally once daily for 10 days (285 patients) with ciprofloxacin 500 mg orally twice daily for 10 days (282 patients). Patients with a resistant pathogen, recurrent UTI, women over age 55 years, and with an indwelling catheter were initially excluded, prior to protocol amendment which took place after 30% of enrollment. Microbiological efficacy was measured by bacteriologic eradication of the baseline organism(s) at 1–12 days post-therapy in patients with a pathogen identified at baseline.

The bacteriologic cure rates overall for LEVAQUIN® and control at the test-of-cure (TOC) visit for the group of all patients with a documented pathogen at baseline (modified intent to treat or mITT) and the group of patients in the mITT population who closely followed the protocol (Microbiologically Evaluable) are summarized in Table 22.

[See table 22 below]

14.9 Inhalational Anthrax (Post-Exposure)

The effectiveness of LEVAQUIN® for this indication is based on plasma concentrations achieved in humans, a surrogate endpoint reasonably likely to predict clinical benefit. LEVAQUIN® has not been tested in humans for the post-exposure prevention of inhalation anthrax. The mean plasma concentrations of LEVAQUIN® associated with a statistically significant improvement in survival over placebo in the rhesus monkey model of inhalational anthrax are reached or exceeded in adult and pediatric patients receiving the recommended oral and intravenous dosage regimens [see Indications and Usage (1.13); Dosage and Administration (2.1, 2.2)].

Levofloxacin pharmacokinetics have been evaluated in adult and pediatric patients. The mean ($\pm$ SD) steady state peak plasma concentration in human adults receiving 500 mg orally or intravenously once daily is 5.7 $\pm$ 1.4 and 6.4 $\pm$ 0.8 mcg/mL, respectively; and the corresponding total plasma exposure (AUC$_{0-24}$) is 47.5 $\pm$ 6.7 and 54.6 $\pm$ 11.1 mcg.h/mL, respectively. The predicted steady-state pharmacokinetic parameters in pediatric patients ranging in age from 6 months to 17 years receiving 8 mg/kg orally every 12 hours (not to exceed 250 mg per dose) were calculated to be comparable to those observed in adults receiving 500 mg orally once daily [see Clinical Pharmacology (12.3)]. In adults, the safety of LEVAQUIN® for treatment durations of up to 28 days is well characterized. However, information pertaining to extended use at 500 mg daily up to 60 days is limited. Prolonged LEVAQUIN® therapy in adults should only be used when the benefit outweighs the risk.

In pediatric patients, the safety of levofloxacin for treatment durations of more than 14 days has not been studied.

An increased incidence of musculoskeletal adverse events (arthralgia, arthritis, tendonopathy, gait abnormality) compared to controls has been observed in clinical studies with treatment duration of up to 14 days. Long-term safety data, including effects on cartilage, following the administration of levofloxacin to pediatric patients is limited [see Warnings and Precautions (5.9), Use in Specific Populations (8.4)].

A placebo-controlled animal study in rhesus monkeys exposed to an inhaled mean dose of 49 LD$_{50}$ ($\sim$2.7 $\times$ 10^6) spores (range 17–118 LD$_{50}$) of *B. anthracis* (Ames strain) was conducted. The minimal inhibitory concentration (MIC) of levofloxacin for the anthrax strain used in this study was 0.125 mcg/mL. In the animals studied, mean plasma concentrations of levofloxacin achieved at expected T$_{max}$ (1 hour post-dose) following oral dosing to steady state ranged from 2.79 to 4.87 mcg/mL. Steady state trough concentrations at 24 hours post-dose ranged from 0.107 to 0.164 mcg/mL. Mean (SD) steady state AUC$_{0-24}$ was 33.4 $\pm$ 3.2 mcg.h/mL (range 30.4 to 36.0 mcg.h/mL). Mortality due to anthrax for animals that received a 30 day regimen of oral LEVAQUIN® beginning 24 hrs post exposure was significantly lower (1/10), compared to the placebo group (9/10) [P=0.0011, 2-sided Fisher's Exact Test]. The one levofloxacin treated animal that died of anthrax did so following the 30-day drug administration period.

15 REFERENCES

1. Clinical and Laboratory Standards Institute. Methods for Dilution Antimicrobial Susceptibility Tests for Bacteria That Grow Aerobically Approved Standard – Seventh Edition. Clinical and Laboratory Standards Institute document M7-A7, Vol. 26, No. 2, CLSI, Wayne, PA, January 2006.
2. Clinical and Laboratory Standards Institute. Performance Standards for Antimicrobial Disk Susceptibility Tests. Approved Standard – Ninth Edition. Clinical and Laboratory Standards Institute document M2-A9, Vol. 26, No. 1, CLSI, Wayne, PA, January 2006.

16 HOW SUPPLIED/STORAGE AND HANDLING

16.1 LEVAQUIN® Tablets

LEVAQUIN® Tablets are supplied as 250, 500, and 750 mg capsule-shaped, coated tablets. LEVAQUIN® Tablets are packaged in bottles and in unit-dose blister strips in the following configurations:

- 250 mg tablets are terra cotta pink and are imprinted: "LEVAQUIN" on one side and "250" on the other side.
  - bottles of 50 (NDC 50458-920-50)
  - unit-dose/100 tablets (NDC 50458-920-10)
- 500 mg tablets are peach and are imprinted: "LEVAQUIN" on one side and "500" on the other side
  - bottles of 50 (NDC 50458-925-50)
  - unit-dose/100 tablets (NDC 50458-925-10)
- 750 mg tablets are white and are imprinted "LEVAQUIN" on one side and "750" on the other side
  - bottles of 20 (NDC 50458-930-20)
  - unit-dose/100 tablets (NDC 50458-930-10)

LEVAQUIN® Tablets should be stored at 15° to 30°C (59° to 86°F) in well-closed containers.

LEVAQUIN® Tablets are manufactured for PriCara, Division of Ortho-McNeil-Janssen Pharmaceuticals, Inc. Raritan, NJ 08869 by Janssen Ortho LLC, Gurabo, Puerto Rico 00778.

16.2 LEVAQUIN® Oral Solution

LEVAQUIN® Oral Solution is supplied in a 16 oz. multi-use bottle (NDC 50458-170-01). Each bottle contains 480 mL of the 25 mg/mL levofloxacin oral solution

LEVAQUIN® Oral Solution should be stored at 25°C (77°F); excursions permitted to 15°–30°C 30° C (59° to 86°F) [refer to USP controlled room temperature].

LEVAQUIN® Oral Solution is manufactured for PriCara, Division of Ortho-McNeil-Janssen Pharmaceuticals, Inc. Raritan, NJ 08869 by Janssen Pharmaceutica N.V, Beerse, Belgium.

16.3 LEVAQUIN® Injection, Single-Use Vials

LEVAQUIN® Injection is supplied in single-use vials. Each vial contains a concentrated solution with the equivalent of 500 mg of levofloxacin in 20 mL vials and 750 mg of levofloxacin in 30 mL vials.

- 25 mg/mL, 20 mL vials (NDC 50458-164-20)
- 25 mg/mL, 30 mL vials (NDC 50458-165-30)

LEVAQUIN® Injection in Single-Use Vials should be stored at controlled room temperature and protected from light. LEVAQUIN® Injection in Single-Use Vials is manufactured for Ortho-McNeil, Division of Ortho-McNeil-Janssen Pharmaceuticals, Inc. Raritan, NJ 08869 by Janssen Pharmaceutica N.V., Beerse, Belgium.

16.4 LEVAQUIN® Injection Pre-Mixed Solution, Single-Use in Flexible Container

LEVAQUIN® (levofloxacin in 5% dextrose) Injection is supplied as a single-use, premixed solution in flexible containers. Each bag contains a dilute solution with the equivalent of 250, 500, or 750 mg of levofloxacin, respectively, in 5% Dextrose (D5W).

- 5 mg/mL (250 mg), 100 mL flexible container, 50 mL fill (NDC 50458-167-01)
- 5 mg/mL (500 mg), 100 mL flexible container, 100 mL fill (NDC 50458-168-01)
- 5 mg/mL (750 mg), 150 mL flexible container, 150 mL fill (NDC 50458-166-01)

LEVAQUIN® Injection Premix in Flexible Containers should be stored at or below 25°C (77°F); however, brief exposure up to 40°C (104°F) does not adversely affect the product. Avoid excessive heat and protect from freezing and light.

LEVAQUIN® Injection Premix in Flexible Containers is manufactured for Ortho-McNeil, Division of Ortho-McNeil-Janssen Pharmaceuticals, Inc. Raritan, NJ 08869 by Hospira, Inc., Lake Forest, IL 60045.

17 PATIENT COUNSELING INFORMATION

See FDA-Approved Medication Guide (17.5)

17.1 Antibacterial Resistance

Antibacterial drugs including LEVAQUIN® should only be used to treat bacterial infections. They do not treat viral infections (e.g., the common cold). When LEVAQUIN® is prescribed to treat a bacterial infection, patients should be told that although it is common to feel better early in the course of therapy, the medication should be taken exactly as directed. Skipping doses or not completing the full course of therapy may (1) decrease the effectiveness of the immediate treatment and (2) increase the likelihood that bacteria will develop resistance and will not be treatable by LEVAQUIN® or other antibacterial drugs in the future.

17.2 Administration with Food, Fluids, and Concomitant Medications

Patients should be informed that LEVAQUIN® Tablets may be taken with or without food. LEVAQUIN® Oral Solution should be taken 1 hour before or 2 hours after eating. The tablet and oral solution should be taken at the same time each day.

Patients should drink fluids liberally while taking LEVAQUIN® to avoid formation of a highly concentrated urine and crystal formation in the urine.

Antacids containing magnesium, or aluminum, as well as sucralfate, metal cations such as iron, and multivitamin preparations with zinc or didanosine should be taken at least two hours before or two hours after oral LEVAQUIN® administration.

17.3 Serious and Potentially Serious Adverse Reactions

Patients should be informed of the following serious adverse reactions that have been associated with LEVAQUIN® or other fluoroquinolone use:

- **Tendon Disorders:** Patients should contact their healthcare provider if they experience pain, swelling, or inflammation of a tendon, or weakness or inability to use one of their joints; rest and refrain from exercise; and discontinue LEVAQUIN® treatment. The risk of severe tendon disorders with fluoroquinolones is higher in older patients usually over 60 years of age, in patients taking corticosteroid drugs, and in patients with kidney, heart or lung transplants.

- **Hypersensitivity Reactions:** Patients should be informed that LEVAQUIN® can cause hypersensitivity reactions, even following the first dose. Patients should discontinue the drug at the first sign of a skin rash, hives or other skin reactions, a rapid heartbeat, difficulty in swallowing or breathing, any swelling suggesting angioedema (e.g., swelling of the lips, tongue, face, tightness of the throat, hoarseness), or other symptoms of an allergic reaction.

- **Hepatotoxicity:** Severe hepatotoxicity (including acute hepatitis and fatal events) has been reported in patients taking LEVAQUIN®. Patients should inform their physician and be instructed to discontinue LEVAQUIN® treatment immediately if they experience any signs or symptoms of liver injury including: loss of appetite, nausea, vomiting, fever, weakness, tiredness, right upper quadrant tenderness, itching, yellowing of the skin and eyes, light colored bowel movements or dark colored urine.

- **Convulsions:** Convulsions have been reported in patients taking fluoroquinolones, including LEVAQUIN®. Patients should notify their physician before taking this drug if they have a history of convulsions.

Table 22. Bacteriologic Eradication Overall (cUTI or AP) at Test-Of-Cure*

	LEVAQUIN® 250 mg once daily for 10 days		Ciprofloxacin 500 mg twice daily for 10 days	
	n/N	%	n/N	%
mITT Population[†]	174/209	83.3	184/219	84.0
Microbiologically Evaluable Population[‡]	164/177	92.7	159/171	93.0

* 1–9 days posttherapy for 30% of subjects enrolled prior to a protocol amendment; 5–12 days posttherapy for 70% of subjects.
† The mITT population included patients who had a pathogen isolated at baseline. Patients with missing response were counted as failures in this analysis.
‡ The Microbiologically Evaluable population included mITT patients who met protocol-specified evaluability criteria.

- **Neurologic Adverse Effects (e.g., dizziness, lightheadedness):** Patients should know how they react to LEVAQUIN® before they operate an automobile or machinery or engage in other activities requiring mental alertness and coordination.
- **Diarrhea:** Diarrhea is a common problem caused by antibiotics which usually ends when the antibiotic is discontinued. Sometimes after starting treatment with antibiotics, patients can develop watery and bloody stools (with or without stomach cramps and fever) even as late as two or more months after having taken the last dose of the antibiotic. If this occurs, patients should contact their physician as soon as possible.
- **Peripheral Neuropathies:** If symptoms of peripheral neuropathy including pain, burning, tingling, numbness, and/or weakness develop, patients should discontinue treatment and contact their physician.
- **Prolongation of the QT Interval:** Patients should inform their physician of any personal or family history of QT prolongation or proarrhythmic conditions such as hypokalemia, bradycardia, or recent myocardial ischemia; if they are taking any Class IA (quinidine, procainamide), or Class III (amiodarone, sotalol) antiarrhythmic agents. Patients should notify their physicians if they have any symptoms of prolongation of the QT interval, including prolonged heart palpitations or a loss of consciousness.
- **Musculoskeletal Disorders in Pediatric Patients:** Parents should inform their child's physician if their child has a history of joint-related problems before taking this drug. Parents of pediatric patients should also notify their child's physician of any tendon or joint-related problems that occur during or following LEVAQUIN® therapy *[see Warnings and Precautions (5.9) and Use in Specific Populations (8.4)]*.
- **Photosensitivity/Phototoxicity:** Patients should be advised that photosensitivity/phototoxicity has been reported in patients receiving fluoroquinolone antibiotics. Patients should minimize or avoid exposure to natural or artificial sunlight (tanning beds or UVA/B treatment) while taking fluoroquinolones. If patients need to be outdoors when taking fluoroquinolones, they should wear loose-fitting clothes that protect skin from sun exposure and discuss other sun protection measures with their physician. If a sunburn like reaction or skin eruption occurs, patients should contact their physician.

17.4 Drug Interactions with Insulin, Oral Hypoglycemic Agents, and Warfarin

Patients should be informed that if they are diabetic and are being treated with insulin or an oral hypoglycemic agent and a hypoglycemic reaction occurs, they should discontinue LEVAQUIN® and consult a physician.

Patients should be informed that concurrent administration of warfarin and LEVAQUIN® has been associated with increases of the International Normalized Ratio (INR) or prothrombin time and clinical episodes of bleeding. Patients should notify their physician if they are taking warfarin, be monitored for evidence of bleeding, and also have their anticoagulation tests closely monitored while taking warfarin concomitantly.

Manufactured by:
- Janssen Ortho LLC, Gurabo, Puerto Rico 00778 (for the Tablets).
- Janssen Pharmaceutica N.V., Beerse, Belgium (for the Oral Solution and Injection, Single-Use Vials).
- Hospira, Inc., Lake Forest, IL 60045 (for the Injection Pre-Mixed Solution Single-Use in Flexible Container).

Manufactured for:
- PriCara, Division of Ortho-McNeil-Janssen Pharmaceuticals, Inc. Raritan, NJ 08869 (for the Tablets and Oral Solution)
- Ortho-McNeil, Division of Ortho-McNeil-Janssen Pharmaceuticals, Inc. Raritan, NJ 08869 (for the Injection, Single-Use Vials and Injection Pre-Mixed Solution Single-Use in Flexible Container)

©Ortho-McNeil-Janssen Pharmaceuticals, Inc
U.S. Patent No. 5,053,407.
Issued July 2009

17.5 FDA-Approved Medication Guide

MEDICATION GUIDE
LEVAQUIN® [Leave ah kwin]
(levofloxacin)
250 mg Tablets, 500 mg Tablets, and 750 mg Tablets
And
LEVAQUIN® (levofloxacin) Oral Solution, 25 mg/mL
And
LEVAQUIN® (levofloxacin) Injection, for Intravenous Use
And
LEVAQUIN® (levofloxacin in 5% dextrose) Injection, for Intravenous Use

Read the Medication Guide that comes with LEVAQUIN® before you start taking it and each time you get a refill. There may be new information. This Medication Guide does not take the place of talking to your healthcare provider about your medical condition or your treatment.

What is the most important information I should know about LEVAQUIN®?
LEVAQUIN® belongs to a class of antibiotics called fluoroquinolones. LEVAQUIN® can cause side effects that may be serious or even cause death. If you get any of the following serious side effects, get medical help right away. Talk with your healthcare provider about whether you should continue to take LEVAQUIN®.

- **Tendon rupture or swelling of the tendon (tendinitis).**
  - Tendons are tough cords of tissue that connect muscles to bones.
  - Pain, swelling, tears, and inflammation of tendons including the back of the ankle (Achilles), shoulder, hand, or other tendon sites can happen in people of all ages who take fluoroquinolone antibiotics, including LEVAQUIN®. The risk of getting tendon problems is higher if you:
    - are over 60 years of age
    - are taking steroids (corticosteroids)
    - have had a kidney, heart or lung transplant.
  - Swelling of the tendon (tendinitis) and tendon rupture (breakage) have also happened in patients who take fluoroquinolones who do not have the above risk factors.
  - Other reasons for tendon ruptures can include:
    - physical activity or exercise
    - kidney failure
    - tendon problems in the past, such as in people with rheumatoid arthritis (RA).
  - Call your healthcare provider right away at the first sign of tendon pain, swelling or inflammation. Stop taking LEVAQUIN® until tendinitis or tendon rupture has been ruled out by your healthcare provider. Avoid exercise and using the affected area. The most common area of pain and swelling is the Achilles tendon at the back of your ankle. This can also happen with other tendons. Talk to your healthcare provider about the risk of tendon rupture with continued use of LEVAQUIN®. You may need a different antibiotic that is not a fluoroquinolone to treat your infection.
  - Tendon rupture can happen while you are taking or after you have finished taking LEVAQUIN®. Tendon ruptures have happened up to several months after patients have finished taking their fluoroquinolone.
  - Get medical help right away if you get any of the following signs or symptoms of a tendon rupture:
    - hear or feel a snap or pop in a tendon area
    - bruising right after an injury in a tendon area
    - unable to move the affected area or bear weight

See the section **"What are the possible side effects of LEVAQUIN®?"** for more information about side effects

What is LEVAQUIN®?
LEVAQUIN® is a fluoroquinolone antibiotic medicine used in adults, 18 years or older, to treat certain infections caused by certain germs called bacteria.
Children have a higher chance of getting bone, joint, or tendon (musculoskeletal) problems such as pain or swelling while taking LEVAQUIN®.
In children 6 months and older who have breathed the anthrax bacteria germ:
- LEVAQUIN® is used to prevent anthrax disease (inhalation anthrax).
- It is not known if it is safe to use LEVAQUIN® in children for more than 14 days.
It is not known if LEVAQUIN® is safe and works in children under the age of 6 months.
Sometimes infections are caused by viruses rather than by bacteria. Examples include viral infections in the sinuses and lungs, such as the common cold or flu. Antibiotics, including LEVAQUIN®, do not kill viruses.
Call your healthcare provider if you think your condition is not getting better while you are taking LEVAQUIN®.

Who should not take LEVAQUIN®?
Do not take LEVAQUIN® if you have ever had a severe allergic reaction to an antibiotic known as a fluoroquinolone, or if you are allergic to any of the ingredients in LEVAQUIN®. Ask your healthcare provider if you are not sure. See the list of the ingredients in LEVAQUIN® at end of this Medication Guide.

What should I tell my healthcare provider before taking LEVAQUIN®?
See "What is the most important information I should know about LEVAQUIN®?"
Tell your healthcare provider about all your medical conditions, including if you:
- have tendon problems
- have central nervous system problems (such as epilepsy)
- have nerve problems
- have or anyone in your family has an irregular heartbeat, especially a condition called "QT prolongation."
- have low blood potassium (hypokalemia)
- have a history of seizures
- have bone and joint problems
- have kidney problems. You may need a lower dose of LEVAQUIN® if your kidneys do not work well.

- have liver problems
- have rheumatoid arthritis (RA) or other history of joint problems
- are pregnant or planning to become pregnant. It is not known if LEVAQUIN® will harm your unborn child.
- are breast-feeding or planning to breast-feed. LEVAQUIN® is thought to pass into breast milk. You and your healthcare provider should decide whether you will take LEVAQUIN® or breast-feed.

Tell your healthcare provider about all the medicines you take, including prescription and non-prescription medicines, vitamins, herbal and dietary supplements. LEVAQUIN® and other medicines can affect each other causing side effects. Especially tell your healthcare provider if you take:
- an NSAID (Non-Steroidal Anti-Inflammatory Drug). Many common medicines for pain relief are NSAIDs. Taking an NSAID while you take LEVAQUIN® or other fluoroquinolones may increase your risk of central nervous system effects and seizures. See **"What are the possible side effects of LEVAQUIN®?"**
- an oral anti-diabetes medicine or insulin
- a blood thinner (warfarin, Coumadin, Jantoven)
- a medicine to control your heart rate or rhythm (antiarrhythmics). See **"What are the possible side effects of LEVAQUIN®?"**.
- an anti-psychotic medicine
- a tricyclic antidepressant
- a water pill (diuretic)
- a steroid medicine. Corticosteroids taken by mouth or by injection may increase the chance of tendon injury. See **"What is the most important information I should know about LEVAQUIN®?"**
- theophylline (Theo-24®, Elixophyllin®, Theochron®, Uniphyl®, Theolair®)
- Certain medicines may keep LEVAQUIN® from working correctly. Take LEVAQUIN® Tablets or Oral Solution either 2 hours before or 2 hours after taking these products:
  - an antacid, multivitamin, or other product that has magnesium, aluminum, iron, or zinc.
  - sucralfate (Carafate®)
  - didanosine (Videx®, Videx® EC)

Ask your healthcare provider if you are not sure if any of your medicines are listed above.
Know the medicines you take. Keep a list of your medicines and show it to your healthcare provider and pharmacist when you get a new medicine.

How should I take LEVAQUIN®?
- Take LEVAQUIN® exactly as prescribed by your healthcare provider.
- Take LEVAQUIN® at about the same time each day.
- Drink plenty of fluids while taking LEVAQUIN®.
- LEVAQUIN® Tablets can be taken with or without food.
- Take LEVAQUIN® Oral Solution 1 hour before or 2 hours after eating.
- If you miss a dose of LEVAQUIN®, take it as soon as you remember. Do not take more than one dose in one day.
- LEVAQUIN® for Injection is given to you by intravenous (I.V.) infusion into your vein, slowly, over 60 or 90 minutes, as prescribed by your healthcare provider. See "What are the possible side effects of LEVAQUIN®?"
- Do not skip any doses, or stop taking LEVAQUIN® even if you begin to feel better, until you finish your prescribed treatment, unless:
  - you have tendon effects (see "What is the most important information I should know about LEVAQUIN®?"),
  - you have a serious allergic reaction (see "What are the possible side effects of LEVAQUIN®?"), or
  - your healthcare provider tells you to stop.
- This will help make sure that all of the bacteria are killed and lower the chance that the bacteria will become resistant to LEVAQUIN®. If this happens, LEVAQUIN® and other antibiotic medicines may not work in the future.

If you take too much, call your healthcare provider or get medical help immediately.

If you have been prescribed LEVAQUIN® after being exposed to anthrax:
- LEVAQUIN® has been approved to lessen the chance of getting anthrax disease or worsening of the disease after you are exposed to the anthrax bacteria germ.
- Take LEVAQUIN® exactly as prescribed by your healthcare provider. Do not stop taking LEVAQUIN® without talking with your healthcare provider. If you stop taking LEVAQUIN® too soon, it may not keep you from getting the anthrax disease.
- Side effects may happen while you are taking LEVAQUIN®. When taking LEVAQUIN® to prevent anthrax infection, you and your healthcare provider should talk about whether the risks of stopping your medicine too soon are more important than the risks of side effects with LEVAQUIN®. It is not known if it is safe to use LEVAQUIN® for more than 28 days in adults and for more than 14 days in children 6 months of age and older.
- If you are pregnant, or plan to become pregnant while taking LEVAQUIN®, you and your healthcare provider should decide whether the benefits of taking LEVAQUIN® for anthrax are more important than the risks.

What should I avoid while taking LEVAQUIN®?

- LEVAQUIN® can make you feel dizzy and lightheaded. Do not drive, operate machinery, or do other activities that require mental alertness or coordination until you know how LEVAQUIN® affects you.
- Avoid sunlamps, tanning beds, and try to limit your time in the sun. LEVAQUIN® can make your skin sensitive to the sun (photosensitivity) and the light from sunlamps and tanning beds. You could get severe sunburn, blisters or swelling of your skin. If you get any of these symptoms while taking LEVAQUIN®, call your healthcare provider right away. You should use a sunscreen and wear a hat and clothes that cover your skin if you have to be in sunlight.

What are the possible side effects of LEVAQUIN®?

LEVAQUIN® can cause side effects that may be serious or even cause death. See "What is the most important information I should know about LEVAQUIN®?"

Other serious side effects of LEVAQUIN®; include:

- **Liver damage (hepatotoxicity):** Liver damage (hepatotoxicity) can happen in people who take LEVAQUIN®. Call your healthcare provider right away if you have unexplained symptoms such as:
  - nausea or vomiting,
  - stomach pain,
  - fever,
  - weakness,
  - abdominal pain or tenderness,
  - itching,
  - unusual tiredness,
  - loss of appetite,
  - light colored bowel movements,
  - dark colored urine or yellowing of your skin or the whites of your eyes.
- **Central Nervous System Effects.** Seizures have been reported in people who take fluoroquinolone antibiotics including LEVAQUIN®. Tell your healthcare provider if you have a history of seizures. Ask your healthcare provider whether taking LEVAQUIN® will change your risk of having a seizure.
  Central Nervous System (CNS) side effects may happen as soon as after taking the first dose of LEVAQUIN®. Talk to your healthcare provider right away if you get any of these side effects, or other changes in mood or behavior:
  - seizures
  - hear voices, see things, or sense things that are not there (hallucinations)
  - feel restless
  - tremors
  - feel anxious or nervous
  - confusion
  - depression
  - trouble sleeping
  - nightmares
  - feel lightheaded
  - feel more suspicious (paranoia)
  - suicidal thoughts or acts
- **Serious allergic reactions.**
  Allergic reactions can happen in people taking fluoroquinolones, including LEVAQUIN®, even after only one dose. Stop taking LEVAQUIN® and get emergency medical help right away if you get any of the following symptoms of a severe allergic reaction:
  - hives
  - trouble breathing or swallowing
  - swelling of the lips, tongue, face
  - throat tightness, hoarseness
  - rapid heartbeat
  - faint
  - Yellowing of the skin or eyes. Stop taking LEVAQUIN® and tell your healthcare provider right away if you get yellowing of your skin or white part of your eyes, or if you have dark urine. These can be signs of a serious reaction to LEVAQUIN® (a liver problem).
- **Skin rash**
  Skin rash may happen in people taking LEVAQUIN®, even after only one dose. Stop taking LEVAQUIN® at the first sign of a skin rash and call your healthcare provider. Skin rash may be a sign of a more serious reaction to LEVAQUIN®.
- **Intestine infection (Pseudomembranous colitis)**
  Pseudomembranous colitis can happen with most antibiotics, including LEVAQUIN®. Call your healthcare provider right away if you get watery diarrhea, diarrhea that does not go away, or bloody stools. You may have stomach cramps and a fever. Pseudomembranous colitis can happen 2 or more months after you have finished your antibiotic.
- **Changes in sensation and possible nerve damage (Peripheral Neuropathy)**
  Damage to the nerves in arms, hands, legs, or feet can happen in people taking fluoroquinolones, including LEVAQUIN®. Talk with your healthcare provider right

away if you get any of the following symptoms of peripheral neuropathy in your arms, hands, legs, or feet:.
  - pain
  - burning
  - tingling
  - numbness
  - weakness
  LEVAQUIN® may need to be stopped to prevent permanent nerve damage
- **Serious heart rhythm changes** (QT prolongation and torsades de pointes)
  Tell your healthcare provider right away if you have a change in your heart beat (a fast or irregular heartbeat), or if you faint. LEVAQUIN® may cause a rare heart problem known as prolongation of the QT interval. This condition can cause an abnormal heartbeat and can be very dangerous. The chances of this happening are higher in people:
  - who are elderly
  - with a family history of prolonged QT interval
  - with low blood potassium (hypokalemia)
  - who take certain medicines to control heart rhythm (antiarrhythmics)
- **Changes in blood sugar [low blood sugar (hypoglycemia) and high blood sugar (hyperglycemia)]**
  People who take LEVAQUIN® and other fluoroquinolone medicines with oral anti-diabetes medicines or with insulin can get low blood sugar (hypoglycemia) and high blood sugar (hyperglycemia). Follow your healthcare provider's instructions for how often to check your blood sugar. If you have diabetes and you get low blood sugar while taking LEVAQUIN®, stop taking LEVAQUIN® and call your healthcare provider right away. Your antibiotic medicine may need to be changed.
- **Sensitivity to sunlight (photosensitivity)**
  See "What should I avoid while taking LEVAQUIN®?"
- **Joint Problems**
  Increased chance of problems with joints and tissues around joints in children. Tell your child's healthcare provider if your child has any joint problems during or after treatment with LEVAQUIN®.

The most common side effects of LEVAQUIN® include:
- dizziness
- headache
- constipation
- nausea
- diarrhea

In children 6 months and older who take LEVAQUIN® to prevent anthrax disease, vomiting is also common. Low blood pressure can happen with LEVAQUIN® given by IV injection if it is given too fast. Tell your healthcare provider if you feel dizzy, or faint during a treatment with LEVAQUIN®.

LEVAQUIN® may cause false-positive urine screening results for opiates when testing is done with some commercially available kits. A positive result should be confirmed using a more specific test.

These are not all the possible side effects of LEVAQUIN®. Tell your healthcare provider about any side effect that bothers you or that does not go away.

Call your doctor for medical advice about side effects. You may report side effects to FDA at 1 800-FDA-1088.

How should I store LEVAQUIN®?

Store LEVAQUIN® Film-Coated Tablets at 59° to 86° F (15°C to 30°C). Keep the container closed tightly.
Store LEVAQUIN® Oral Solution at 59° to 86° F (15°C to 30°C).
Keep LEVAQUIN® and all medicines out of the reach of children.

General Information about LEVAQUIN®

Medicines are sometimes prescribed for purposes other than those listed in a Medication Guide. Do not use LEVAQUIN® for a condition for which it is not prescribed. Do not give LEVAQUIN® to other people, even if they have the same symptoms that you have. It may harm them.
This Medication Guide summarizes the most important information about LEVAQUIN®. If you would like more information about LEVAQUIN®, talk with your healthcare provider. You can ask your healthcare provider or pharmacist for information about LEVAQUIN® that is written for healthcare professionals. For more information go to www.levaquin.com or call 1-800-526-7736.

What are the ingredients in LEVAQUIN®?

- 250 mg LEVAQUIN® Film-Coated Tablets:
  - Active ingredient: levofloxacin.
  - Inactive ingredients: hypromellose, crospovidone, microcrystalline cellulose, magnesium stearate, polyethylene glycol, titanium dioxide, polysorbate 80 and synthetic red iron oxide.

- 500 mg LEVAQUIN® Film-Coated Tablets:
  - Active ingredient: levofloxacin.
  - Inactive ingredients: hypromellose, crospovidone, microcrystalline cellulose, magnesium stearate, polyethylene glycol, titanium dioxide, polysorbate 80 and synthetic red and yellow iron oxides.
- 750 mg LEVAQUIN® Film-Coated Tablets:
  - Active ingredient: levofloxacin.
  - Inactive ingredients: hypromellose, crospovidone, microcrystalline cellulose, magnesium stearate, polyethylene glycol, titanium dioxide, polysorbate 80.
- LEVAQUIN® Oral Solution (25 mg/mL):
  - Active ingredient: levofloxacin.
  - Inactive ingredients: sucrose, glycerin, sucralose, hydrochloric acid, purified water, propylene glycol, artificial and natural flavors, benzyl alcohol, ascorbic acid, and caramel color. It may also contain a solution of sodium hydroxide for pH adjustment.
    - LEVAQUIN® Oral Solution may look clear yellow to clear greenish-yellow in color.
- LEVAQUIN® Injection in Single-Use Vials:
  - Active ingredient: levofloxacin.
  - Inactive ingredients: water for injection. LEVAQUIN® for Injection Single Use Vials do not contain any preservatives.
- LEVAQUIN® Injection Premix in Single-Use Flexible Containers:
  - Active ingredient: levofloxacin.
  - Inactive ingredients: Dextrose (D_5W). Solutions of hydrochloric acid and sodium hydroxide may have been added to adjust the pH.

Revised July 2009
Manufactured by:
Janssen Ortho LLC, Gurabo, Puerto Rico 00778 (Tablets).
Janssen Pharmaceutica N.V., Beerse, Belgium (Oral Solution, Injection Single-Use Vials).
Hospira, Inc., Lake Forest, IL 60045 (Injection Premix).
Manufactured for:
PriCara, Division of Ortho-McNeil-Janssen Pharmaceuticals, Inc. Raritan, NJ 08869 (Tablets, Oral Solution)
Ortho-McNeil, Division of Ortho-McNeil-Janssen Pharmaceuticals, Inc. Raritan, NJ 08869 (Injection Single-Use Vials, Injection Premix)
©Ortho-McNeil-Janssen Pharmaceuticals, Inc.
U.S. Patent No. 5,053,407.
This Medication Guide has been approved by the U.S. Food and Drug Administration.
10185902

Shown in Product Identification Guide, page 316

NUCYNTA®   ℂ ℞
[new-sinn'-tah]
(tapentadol)
immediate-release oral tablets C-II

HIGHLIGHTS OF PRESCRIBING INFORMATION
These highlights do not include all the information needed to use NUCYNTA® safely and effectively. See full prescribing information for NUCYNTA®.
NUCYNTA® (tapentadol) immediate-release oral tablets C-II
Initial U.S. Approval: 2008
————————INDICATIONS AND USAGE————————
NUCYNTA® is an opioid analgesic indicated for the relief of moderate to severe acute pain in patients 18 years of age or older. (1)
————DOSAGE AND ADMINISTRATION————
- As with many centrally-acting analgesic medications, the dosing regimen of NUCYNTA® should be individualized according to the severity of pain being treated, the previous experience with similar drugs and the ability to monitor the patient. (2)
- Initiate NUCYNTA® with or without food at a dose of 50 mg, 75 mg, or 100 mg every 4 to 6 hours depending upon pain intensity. On the first day of dosing, the second dose may be administered as soon as one hour after the first dose, if adequate pain relief is not attained with the first dose. Subsequent dosing is 50 mg, 75 mg, or 100 mg every 4 to 6 hours and should be adjusted to maintain adequate analgesia with acceptable tolerability. Daily doses greater than 700 mg on the first day of therapy and 600 mg on subsequent days have not been studied and are, therefore, not recommended. (2)
————DOSAGE FORMS AND STRENGTHS————
Tablets: 50 mg, 75 mg, 100 mg (3)
————————CONTRAINDICATIONS————————
- Impaired pulmonary function (significant respiratory depression, acute or severe bronchial asthma or hypercapnia in unmonitored settings or the absence of resuscitative equipment) (4.1)
- Paralytic ileus (4.2)
- Concomitant use with monoamine oxidase inhibitors (MAOI) or use within 14 days (4.3)

—WARNINGS AND PRECAUTIONS—

- Respiratory depression: Increased risk in elderly, debilitated patients, those suffering from conditions accompanied by hypoxia, hypercapnia, or upper airway obstruction. (5.1)
- CNS effects: Additive CNS depressive effects when used in conjunction with alcohol, other opioids, or illicit drugs. (5.2)
- Elevation of intracranial pressure: May be markedly exaggerated in the presence of head injury, other intracranial lesions. (5.3)
- Abuse potential may occur. Monitor patients closely for signs of abuse and addiction. (5.4)
- Impaired mental/physical abilities: Caution must be used with potentially hazardous activities. (5.5)
- Seizures: Use with caution in patients with a history of seizures. (5.7)
- Serotonin Syndrome: Potentially life-threatening condition could result from concomitant serotonergic administration. (5.8)

—ADVERSE REACTIONS—

The most common adverse events were nausea, dizziness, vomiting and somnolence. (6)

To report SUSPECTED ADVERSE REACTIONS, contact PriCara, Division of Ortho-McNeil-Janssen Pharmaceuticals, Inc. at 1-800-526-7736 or FDA at 1-800-FDA-1088 or www.fda.gov/medwatch

—DRUG INTERACTIONS—

- Use NUCYNTA® with caution in patients currently using specified centrally-acting drugs or alcohol. (7.3)
- Do not use NUCYNTA® in patients currently using or within 14 days of using a monoamine oxidase inhibitor (MAOI). (7.4)

—USE IN SPECIFIC POPULATIONS—

- Labor and delivery: should not use during and immediately prior to labor and delivery. Monitor neonates, whose mothers have been taking NUCYNTA®, for respiratory depression. (8.2)
- Nursing mothers: should not breast-feed. (8.3)
- Pediatric use: safety and effectiveness not established in patients less than 18 years of age. (8.4)
- Renal or hepatic impairment: not recommended in patients with severe renal or hepatic impairment. Use with caution in patients with moderate hepatic impairment. (8.6, 8.7)
- Elderly: care should be taken when selecting an initial dose. (2.3)

See 17 for PATIENT COUNSELING INFORMATION and Medication Guide

Revised: 06/2010

FULL PRESCRIBING INFORMATION

1   INDICATIONS AND USAGE

NUCYNTA® (tapentadol) is indicated for the relief of moderate to severe acute pain in patients 18 years of age or older.

2   DOSAGE AND ADMINISTRATION

As with many centrally-acting analgesic medications, the dosing regimen should be individualized according to the severity of pain being treated, the previous experience with similar drugs and the ability to monitor the patient.

The dose is 50 mg, 75 mg, or 100 mg every 4 to 6 hours depending upon pain intensity.

On the first day of dosing, the second dose may be administered as soon as one hour after the first dose, if adequate pain relief is not attained with the first dose. Subsequent dosing is 50 mg, 75 mg, or 100 mg every 4 to 6 hours and should be adjusted to maintain adequate analgesia with acceptable tolerability.

Daily doses greater than 700 mg on the first day of therapy and 600 mg on subsequent days have not been studied and are not recommended.

NUCYNTA® may be given with or without food [see Clinical Pharmacology (12.3)].

2.1   Renal Impairment

No dosage adjustment is recommended in patients with mild or moderate renal impairment [see Clinical Pharmacology (12.3)].

NUCYNTA® has not been studied in patients with severe renal impairment. The use in this population is not recommended.

2.2   Hepatic Impairment

No dosage adjustment is recommended in patients with mild hepatic impairment [see Clinical Pharmacology (12.3)].

NUCYNTA® should be used with caution in patients with moderate hepatic impairment. Treatment in these patients should be initiated at 50 mg with the interval between doses no less than every 8 hours (maximum of three doses in 24 hours). Further treatment should reflect maintenance of analgesia with acceptable tolerability, to be achieved by either shortening or lengthening the dosing interval [see Clinical Pharmacology (12.3)].

NUCYNTA® has not been studied in patients with severe hepatic impairment and use in this population is not recommended [see Warnings and Precautions (5.10)].

2.3   Elderly Patients

In general, recommended dosing for elderly patients with normal renal and hepatic function is the same as for younger adult patients with normal renal and hepatic function. Because elderly patients are more likely to have decreased renal and hepatic function, consideration should be given to starting elderly patients with the lower range of recommended doses.

3   DOSAGE FORMS AND STRENGTHS

NUCYNTA® Tablets are round, biconvex and film-coated and are available in the following strengths, colors, and debossings: 50 mg of tapentadol (yellow with "O-M" on one side and "50" on the other side), 75 mg of tapentadol (yellow-orange with "O-M" on one side and "75" on the other side), and 100 mg of tapentadol (orange with "O-M" on one side and "100" on the other side).

4   CONTRAINDICATIONS

4.1   Impaired Pulmonary Function

Like other drugs with mu-opioid agonist activity, NUCYNTA® is contraindicated in patients with significant respiratory depression in unmonitored settings or the absence of resuscitative equipment. NUCYNTA® is also contraindicated in patients with acute or severe bronchial asthma or hypercapnia in unmonitored settings or the absence of resuscitative equipment [see Warnings and Precautions (5.1)].

4.2   Paralytic Ileus

Like drugs with mu-opioid agonist activity, NUCYNTA® is contraindicated in any patient who has or is suspected of having paralytic ileus.

4.3   Monoamine Oxidase Inhibitors

NUCYNTA® is contraindicated in patients who are receiving monoamine oxidase (MAO) inhibitors or who have taken them within the last 14 days due to potential additive effects on norepinephrine levels which may result in adverse cardiovascular events [see Drug Interactions (7.4)].

5   WARNINGS AND PRECAUTIONS

5.1   Respiratory Depression

Respiratory depression is the primary risk of mu-opioid agonists. Respiratory depression occurs more frequently in elderly or debilitated patients and in those suffering from conditions accompanied by hypoxia, hypercapnia, or upper airway obstruction, in whom even moderate therapeutic doses may significantly decrease pulmonary ventilation.

NUCYNTA® should be administered with caution to patients with conditions accompanied by hypoxia, hypercapnia or decreased respiratory reserve such as: asthma, chronic obstructive pulmonary disease or cor pulmonale, severe obesity, sleep apnea syndrome, myxedema, kyphoscoliosis, central nervous system (CNS) depression, or coma. In such patients, even usual therapeutic doses of NUCYNTA® may increase airway resistance and decrease respiratory drive to the point of apnea. Alternative non-mu-opioid agonist analgesics should be considered and NUCYNTA® should be employed only under careful medical supervision at the lowest effective dose in such patients. If respiratory depression occurs, it should be treated as any mu-opioid agonist-induced respiratory depression [see Overdosage (10.2)].

5.2   CNS Depression

Patients receiving other mu-opioid agonist analgesics, general anesthetics, phenothiazines, other tranquilizers, sedatives, hypnotics, or other CNS depressants (including alcohol) concomitantly with NUCYNTA® may exhibit additive CNS depression. Interactive effects resulting in respiratory depression, hypotension, profound sedation, coma or death may result if these drugs are taken in combination with NUCYNTA®. When such combined therapy is contemplated, a dose reduction of one or both agents should be considered.

5.3   Head Injury and Increased Intracranial Pressure

Opioid analgesics can raise cerebrospinal fluid pressure as a result of respiratory depression with carbon dioxide retention. Therefore, NUCYNTA® should not be used in patients who may be susceptible to the effects of raised cerebrospinal fluid pressure such as those with evidence of head injury and increased intracranial pressure. Opioid analgesics may obscure the clinical course of patients with head injury due to effects on pupillary response and consciousness. NUCYNTA® should be used with caution in patients with head injury, intracranial lesions, or other sources of preexisting increased intracranial pressure.

5.4   Misuse and Abuse

Tapentadol is a mu-opioid agonist and is a Schedule II controlled substance. Such drugs are sought by drug abusers and people with addiction disorders. Diversion of Schedule II products is an act subject to criminal penalty. NUCYNTA® can be abused in a manner similar to other opioid agonists, legal or illicit. This should be considered when prescribing or dispensing NUCYNTA® in situations where the physician or pharmacist is concerned about an increased risk of misuse and abuse. Concerns about abuse and addiction should not prevent the proper management of pain. However, all patients treated with mu-opioid agonists require careful monitoring for signs of abuse and addiction, since use of mu-opioid agonist analgesic products carry the risk of addiction even under appropriate medical use [see Drug Abuse and Dependence (9.2)].

NUCYNTA® may be abused by crushing, chewing, snorting or injecting the product. These practices pose a significant risk to the abuser that could result in overdose and death [see Drug Abuse and Dependence (9)].

5.5 Driving and Operating Machinery

Patients should be cautioned that NUCYNTA® may impair the mental and/or physical abilities required for the performance of potentially hazardous tasks such as driving a car or operating machinery. This is to be expected especially at the beginning of treatment, at any change of dosage as well as in combination with alcohol or tranquilizers [see Drug Interactions (7.3)].

5.6 Interactions with Alcohol and Drugs of Abuse

Due to its mu-opioid agonist activity, NUCYNTA® may be expected to have additive effects when used in conjunction with alcohol, opioids, or illicit drugs that cause central nervous system depression, respiratory depression, hypotension, and profound sedation, coma or death [see Drug Interactions (7.3)].

5.7 Seizures

NUCYNTA® has not been systematically evaluated in patients with a seizure disorder, and such patients were excluded from clinical studies. NUCYNTA® should be prescribed with care in patients with a history of a seizure disorder or any condition that would put the patient at risk of seizures.

5.8 Serotonin Syndrome Risk

The development of a potentially life-threatening serotonin syndrome may occur with use of Serotonin and Norepinephrine Reuptake Inhibitor (SNRI) products, including NUCYNTA®, particularly with concomitant use of serotonergic drugs such as Selective Serotonin Reuptake Inhibitors (SSRIs), SNRIs, tricyclic antidepressants (TCAs), MAOIs and triptans, and with drugs that impair metabolism of serotonin (including MAOIs). This may occur within the recommended dose. Serotonin syndrome may include mental-status changes (e.g., agitation, hallucinations, coma), autonomic instability (e.g., tachycardia, labile blood pressure, hyperthermia), neuromuscular aberrations (e.g., hyperreflexia, incoordination) and/or gastrointestinal symptoms (e.g., nausea, vomiting, diarrhea).

5.9 Withdrawal

Withdrawal symptoms may occur if NUCYNTA® is discontinued abruptly. These symptoms may include: anxiety, sweating, insomnia, rigors, pain, nausea, tremors, diarrhea, upper respiratory symptoms, piloerection, and rarely, hallucinations. Withdrawal symptoms may be reduced by tapering NUCYNTA® [see Drug Abuse and Dependence (9.3)].

5.10 Hepatic Impairment

A study of NUCYNTA® in subjects with hepatic impairment showed higher serum concentrations than in those with normal hepatic function. NUCYNTA® should be used with caution in patients with moderate hepatic impairment [see Dosage and Administration (2.2) and Clinical Pharmacology (12.3)].

NUCYNTA® has not been studied in patients with severe hepatic impairment and, therefore, use in this population is not recommended.

5.11 Use in Pancreatic/Biliary Tract Disease

Like other drugs with mu-opioid agonist activity, NUCYNTA® may cause spasm of the sphincter of Oddi and should be used with caution in patients with biliary tract disease, including acute pancreatitis.

6 ADVERSE REACTIONS

The following treatment-emergent adverse events are discussed in more detail in other sections of the labeling:
- Respiratory Depression [see Contraindications (4.1) and Warnings and Precautions (5.1)]
- CNS Depression [see Warnings and Precautions (5.2)]

Because clinical studies are conducted under widely varying conditions, adverse event rates observed in the clinical studies of a drug cannot be directly compared to rates in the clinical studies of another drug and may not reflect the rates observed in clinical practice. A treatment-emergent adverse event refers to any untoward medical event associated with the use of the drug in humans, whether or not considered drug-related.

Based on data from nine Phase 2/3 studies that administered multiple doses (seven placebo- and/or active-controlled, one noncontrolled and one Phase 3 active-controlled safety study) the most common adverse events (reported by ≥10% in any NUCYNTA® dose group) were: nausea, dizziness, vomiting and somnolence.

The most common reasons for discontinuation due to adverse events in the studies described above (reported by ≥1% in any NUCYNTA® dose group) were dizziness (2.6% vs. 0.5%), nausea (2.3% vs. 0.6%), vomiting (1.4% vs. 0.2%), somnolence (1.3% vs. 0.2%) and headache (0.9% vs. 0.2%) for NUCYNTA®- and placebo-treated patients, respectively. Seventy-six percent of NUCYNTA®-treated patients from the nine studies experienced adverse events.

NUCYNTA® was studied in multiple-dose, active- or placebo-controlled studies, or noncontrolled studies (n = 2178), in single-dose studies (n = 870), in open-label study extension (n = 483) and in Phase 1 studies (n = 597). Of these, 2034 patients were treated with doses of 50 mg to 100 mg of NUCYNTA® dosed every 4 to 6 hours.

The data described below reflect exposure to NUCYNTA® in 3161 patients, including 449 exposed for 45 days. NUCYNTA® was studied primarily in placebo- and active-controlled studies (n = 2266, and n = 2944, respectively). The population was 18 to 85 years old (mean age 46 years), 68% were female, 75% white and 67% were postoperative. Most patients received NUCYNTA® doses of 50 mg, 75 mg, or 100 mg every 4 to 6 hours.

6.1 Commonly-Observed Treatment-Emergent Adverse Events in Double-Blind Controlled Clinical Trials

Table 1 lists the adverse events reported in ≥1% or more of NUCYNTA®-treated patients with acute moderate to severe pain in the pooled safety data from nine Phase 2/3 studies that administered multiple doses (seven placebo-and/or active-controlled, one noncontrolled, and one Phase 3 active-controlled safety study).

Table 1 Treatment-Emergent Adverse Events* Reported by ≥ 1% of NUCYNTA®-Treated Patients In Seven Phase 2/3 Placebo- and/or Oxycodone-Controlled, One Noncontrolled, and One Phase 3 Oxycodone-Controlled Safety, Multiple-Dose Clinical Studies

System/Organ Class MedDRA Preferred Term	NUCYNTA® 21 mg–120 mg (n=2178) %	Placebo (n=619) %
Gastrointestinal disorders		
Nausea	30	13
Vomiting	18	4
Constipation	8	3
Dry mouth	4	<1
Dyspepsia	2	<1
General disorders and administration site conditions		
Fatigue	3	<1
Feeling hot	1	<1
Infections and infestations		
Nasopharyngitis	1	<1
Upper respiratory tract infection	1	<1
Urinary tract infection	1	<1
Metabolism and nutrition disorders		
Decreased appetite	2	0
Musculoskeletal and connective tissue disorders		
Arthralgia	1	<1
Nervous system disorders		
Dizziness	24	8
Somnolence	15	3
Tremor	1	<1
Lethargy	1	<1
Psychiatric disorders		
Insomnia	2	<1
Confusional state	1	0
Abnormal dreams	1	<1
Anxiety	1	<1
Skin and subcutaneous tissue disorders		
Pruritus	5	1
Hyperhidrosis	3	<1
Pruritus generalized	3	<1
Rash	1	<1
Vascular disorders		
Hot flush	1	<1

*A treatment-emergent adverse event refers to any untoward medical event associated with the use of the drug in humans, whether or not considered drug-related.

6.2 Other Adverse Reactions Observed During the Pre-marketing Evaluation of NUCYNTA®

The following adverse drug reactions occurred in <1% of NUCYNTA®-treated patients in the pooled safety data from nine Phase 2/3 studies that administered multiple doses (seven were placebo- and/or active-controlled, one noncontrolled, and one Phase 3 active-controlled safety study):

Cardiac disorders: heart rate increased, heart rate decreased

Eye disorders: visual disturbance

Gastrointestinal disorders: abdominal discomfort, impaired gastric emptying

General disorders and administration site conditions: irritability, edema, drug withdrawal syndrome, feeling drunk

Immune system disorders: hypersensitivity

Investigations: gamma-glutamyltransferase increased, alanine aminotransferase increased, aspartate aminotransferase increased

Musculoskeletal and connective tissue disorders: involuntary muscle contractions, sensation of heaviness

Nervous system disorders: hypoesthesia, paresthesia, disturbance in attention, sedation, dysarthria, depressed level of consciousness, memory impairment, ataxia, presyncope, syncope, coordination abnormal, seizure

Psychiatric disorders: euphoric mood, disorientation, restlessness, agitation, nervousness, thinking abnormal

Renal and urinary disorders: urinary hesitation, pollakiuria

Respiratory, thoracic and mediastinal disorders: oxygen saturation decreased, cough, dyspnea, respiratory depression

Skin and subcutaneous tissue disorders: urticaria

Vascular disorders: blood pressure decreased

In the pooled safety data, the overall incidence of adverse reactions increased with increased dose of NUCYNTA®, as did the percentage of patients with adverse reactions of nausea, dizziness, vomiting, somnolence, and pruritus.

6.3 Post-marketing Experience

The following additional adverse reactions have been identified during post-approval use of NUCYNTA®. Because these reactions are reported voluntarily from a population of uncertain size, it is not always possible to estimate their frequency reliably.

Nervous system disorders: headache
Psychiatric disorders: hallucination

7 DRUG INTERACTIONS

NUCYNTA® is mainly metabolized by glucuronidation. The following substances have been included in a set of interaction studies without any clinically significant finding: acetaminophen, acetylsalicylic acid, naproxen and probenecid [see Clinical Pharmacology (12.3)].

The pharmacokinetics of tapentadol were not affected when gastric pH or gastrointestinal motility were increased by omeprazole and metoclopramide, respectively [see Clinical Pharmacology (12.3)].

7.1 Drugs Metabolized by Cytochrome P450 Enzymes

In vitro investigations indicate that NUCYNTA® does not inhibit or induce P450 enzymes. Thus, clinically relevant interactions mediated by the cytochrome P450 system are unlikely to occur [see Clinical Pharmacology (12.3)].

7.2 Drugs That Inhibit or Induce Cytochrome P450 Enzymes

The major pathway of tapentadol metabolism is conjugation with glucuronic acid to produce glucuronides. To a lesser extent, tapentadol is additionally metabolized to N-desmethyl tapentadol (13%) by CYP2C9 and CYP2C19 to hydroxy tapentadol (2%) by CYP2D6, which are further metabolized by conjugation. Since only a minor amount of NUCYNTA® is metabolized via the oxidative pathway clinically relevant interactions mediated by the cytochrome P450 system are unlikely to occur [see Clinical Pharmacology (12.3)].

7.3 Centrally-Acting Drugs and Alcohol

Patients receiving other opioid agonist analgesics, general anesthetics, phenothiazines, antiemetics, other tranquilizers, sedatives, hypnotics, or other CNS depressants (including alcohol) concomitantly with NUCYNTA® may exhibit an additive CNS depression. Interactive effects resulting in respiratory depression, hypotension, profound sedation, or coma may result if these drugs are taken in combination with NUCYNTA®. When such combined therapy is contemplated, a dose reduction of one or both agents should be considered [see Warnings and Precautions (5.2) and (5.6)].

7.4 Monoamine Oxidase Inhibitors

NUCYNTA® is contraindicated in patients who are receiving monoamine oxidase (MAO) inhibitors or who have taken them within the last 14 days due to potential additive effects on norepinephrine levels which may result in adverse cardiovascular events *[see Contraindications (4.3)]*.

8 USE IN SPECIFIC POPULATIONS

8.1 Pregnancy

Pregnancy Category C.

Tapentadol HCl was evaluated for teratogenic effects in pregnant rats and rabbits following intravenous and subcutaneous exposure during the period of embryofetal organogenesis. When tapentadol was administered twice daily by the subcutaneous route in rats at dose levels of 10, 20, or 40 mg/kg/day [producing up to 1 times the plasma exposure at the maximum recommended human dose (MRHD) of 700 mg/day based on an area under the time-curve (AUC) comparison], no teratogenic effects were observed. Evidence of embryofetal toxicity included transient delays in skeletal maturation (i.e. reduced ossification) at the 40 mg/kg/day dose which was associated with significant maternal toxicity. Administration of tapentadol HCl in rabbits at doses of 4, 10, or 24 mg/kg/day by subcutaneous injection [producing 0.2, 0.6, and 1.85 times the plasma exposure at the MRHD based on an AUC comparison] revealed embryofetal toxicity at doses ≥ 10 mg/kg/day. Findings included reduced fetal viability, skeletal delays and other variations. In addition, there were multiple malformations including gastroschisis/thoracogastroschisis, amelia/phocomelia, and cleft palate at doses ≥ 10 mg/kg/day and above, and ablepharia, encephalopathy, and spina bifida at the high dose of 24 mg/kg/day. Embryofetal toxicity, including malformations, may be secondary to the significant maternal toxicity observed in the study.

In a study of pre- and postnatal development in rats, oral administration of tapentadol at doses of 20, 50, 150, or 300 mg/kg/day to pregnant and lactating rats during the late gestation and early postnatal period [resulting in up to 1.7 times the plasma exposure at the MRHD on an AUC basis] did not influence physical or reflex development, the outcome of neurobehavioral tests or reproductive parameters. Treatment-related developmental delay was observed, including incomplete ossification, and significant reductions in pup body weights and body weight gains at doses associated with maternal toxicity (150 mg/kg/day and above). At maternal tapentadol doses ≥ 150 mg/kg/day, a dose-related increase in pup mortality was observed through postnatal Day 4.

There are no adequate and well controlled studies of NUCYNTA® in pregnant women. NUCYNTA® should be used during pregnancy only if the potential benefit justifies the potential risk to the fetus.

8.2 Labor and Delivery

The effect of tapentadol on labor and delivery in humans is unknown. NUCYNTA® is not recommended for use in women during and immediately prior to labor and delivery. Due to the mu-opioid receptor agonist activity of NUCYNTA®, neonates whose mothers have been taking NUCYNTA® should be monitored for respiratory depression. A specific opioid antagonist, such as naloxone, should be available for reversal of opioid induced respiratory depression in the neonate.

8.3 Nursing Mothers

There is insufficient/limited information on the excretion of tapentadol in human or animal breast milk. Physicochemical and available pharmacodynamic/toxicological data on tapentadol point to excretion in breast milk and risk to the suckling child cannot be excluded. NUCYNTA® should not be used during breast-feeding.

8.4 Pediatric Use

The safety and effectiveness of NUCYNTA® in pediatric patients less than 18 years of age have not been established. NUCYNTA® is not recommended in this population.

8.5 Geriatric Use

Of the total number of patients in Phase 2/3 double-blind, multiple-dose clinical studies of NUCYNTA®, 19% were 65 and over, while 5% were 75 and over. No overall differences in effectiveness were observed between these patients and younger patients. The rate of constipation was higher in subjects greater than or equal to 65 years than those less than 65 years (12% vs. 7%).

In general, recommended dosing for elderly patients with normal renal and hepatic function is the same as for younger adult patients with normal renal and hepatic function. Because elderly patients are more likely to have decreased renal and hepatic function, consideration should be given to starting elderly patients with the lower range of recommended doses *[see Clinical Pharmacology (12.3)]*.

8.6 Renal Impairment

In patients with severe renal impairment, the safety and effectiveness of NUCYNTA® has not been established. NUCYNTA® is not recommended in this population *[see Dosage and Administration (2.1)]*.

8.7 Hepatic Impairment

Administration of NUCYNTA® resulted in higher exposures and serum levels to tapentadol in subjects with impaired hepatic function compared to subjects with normal hepatic function *[see Clinical Pharmacology (12.3)]*. NUCYNTA® should be used with caution in patients with moderate hepatic impairment *[see Dosage and Administration (2.2)]*.

NUCYNTA® has not been studied in patients with severe hepatic impairment, therefore, use of NUCYNTA® is not recommended in this population *[see Warnings and Precautions (5.10)]*.

9 DRUG ABUSE AND DEPENDENCE

9.1 Controlled Substance

NUCYNTA® contains tapentadol, a mu-opioid agonist and is a Schedule II controlled substance. NUCYNTA® has an abuse potential similar to hydromorphone, can be abused and is subject to criminal diversion.

9.2 Abuse

Addiction is a primary, chronic, neurobiologic disease, with genetic, psychosocial, and environmental factors influencing its development and manifestations. It is characterized by behaviors that include one or more of the following: impaired control over drug use, compulsive use, continued use despite harm, and craving. Drug addiction is a treatable disease, utilizing a multidisciplinary approach, but relapse is common.

Concerns about abuse and addiction should not prevent the proper management of pain. However, all patients treated with opioids require careful monitoring for signs of abuse and addiction, because use of opioid analgesic products carries the risk of addiction even under appropriate medical use.

"Drug seeking" behavior is very common in addicts, and drug abusers. Drug-seeking tactics include emergency calls or visits near the end of office hours, refusal to undergo appropriate examination, testing or referral, repeated claims of loss of prescriptions, tampering with prescriptions and reluctance to provide prior medical records or contact information for other treating physician(s). "Doctor shopping" (visiting multiple prescribers) to obtain additional prescriptions is common among drug abusers and people suffering from untreated addiction. Preoccupation with achieving adequate pain relief can be appropriate behavior in a patient with poor pain control.

Abuse and addiction are separate and distinct from physical dependence and tolerance. Physicians should be aware that addiction may not be accompanied by concurrent tolerance and symptoms of physical dependence in all addicts. In addition, abuse of mu-opioid agonists can occur in the absence of true addiction and is characterized by misuse for non-medical purposes, often in combination with other psychoactive substances. Careful recordkeeping of prescribing information, including quantity, frequency, and renewal requests is strongly advised.

Abuse of NUCYNTA® poses a risk of overdose and death. This risk is increased with concurrent abuse of NUCYNTA® with alcohol and other substances. In addition, parenteral drug abuse is commonly associated with transmission of infectious diseases such as hepatitis and HIV.

Proper assessment of the patient, proper prescribing practices, periodic re-evaluation of therapy, and proper dispensing and storage are appropriate measures that help to limit abuse of drugs with mu-opioid agonist properties.

Infants born to mothers physically dependent on opioids will also be physically dependent and may exhibit respiratory difficulties and withdrawal symptoms *[see Warnings and Precautions (5.1)]*. Use of NUCYNTA® in this population has not been characterized. As NUCYNTA® has mu-opioid agonist activity, infants whose mothers have taken NUCYNTA®, should be carefully monitored.

9.3 Dependence

Tolerance is the need for increasing doses of opioids to maintain a defined effect such as analgesia (in the absence of disease progression or other external factors). Physical dependence is manifested by withdrawal symptoms after abrupt discontinuation of a drug or upon administration of an antagonist.

The opioid abstinence or withdrawal syndrome is characterized by some or all of the following: restlessness, lacrimation, rhinorrhea, yawning, perspiration, chills, myalgia, and mydriasis. Other symptoms also may develop, including irritability, anxiety, backache, joint pain, weakness, abdominal cramps, insomnia, nausea, anorexia, vomiting, diarrhea, increased blood pressure, respiratory rate, or heart rate.

Generally, tolerance and/or withdrawal are more likely to occur the longer a patient is on continuous opioid therapy. In a safety study where drug was administered up to 90 days, 82.7% of patients taking NUCYNTA® who stopped abruptly without initiating alternative therapy and were assessed 2 to 4 days after discontinuation, did not have objective signs of opioid withdrawal using the Clinical Opiate Withdrawal Scale. Moderate withdrawal symptoms were seen in 0.3% of patients with the rest (17%) experiencing mild symptoms. Withdrawal symptoms may be reduced by tapering NUCYNTA®.

10 OVERDOSAGE

10.1 Human Experience

Experience with NUCYNTA® overdose is very limited. Preclinical data suggest that symptoms similar to those of other centrally acting analgesics with mu-opioid agonist activity are to be expected upon intoxication with tapentadol. In principle, these symptoms may particularly appear in the clinical setting: miosis, vomiting, cardiovascular collapse, consciousness disorders up to coma, convulsions and respiratory depression up to respiratory arrest.

10.2 Management of Overdose

Management of overdose should be focused on treating symptoms of mu-opioid agonism. Primary attention should be given to re-establishment of a patent airway and institution of assisted or controlled ventilation when overdose of NUCYNTA® is suspected. Supportive measures (including oxygen and vasopressors) should be employed in the management of circulatory shock and pulmonary edema accompanying overdose as indicated. Cardiac arrest or arrhythmias may require cardiac massage or defibrillation.

Pure opioid antagonists, such as naloxone, are specific antidotes to respiratory depression resulting from opioid overdose. Respiratory depression following an overdose may outlast the duration of action of the opioid antagonist. Administration of an opioid antagonist is not a substitute for continuous monitoring of airway, breathing, and circulation following an opioid overdose. If the response to opioid antagonists is suboptimal or only brief in nature, an additional antagonist should be administered as directed by the manufacturer of the product.

Gastrointestinal decontamination may be considered in order to eliminate unabsorbed drug. Gastrointestinal decontamination with activated charcoal or by gastric lavage is only recommended within 2 hours after intake. Gastrointestinal decontamination at a later time point may be useful in case of intoxication with exceptionally large quantities. Before attempting gastrointestinal decontamination, care should be taken to secure the airway.

11 DESCRIPTION

NUCYNTA® (tapentadol) Tablets are immediate-release film-coated tablets for oral administration. The chemical name is 3-[(1*R*,2*R*)-3-(dimethylamino)-1-ethyl-2-methyl-propyl]phenol monohydrochloride. The structural formula is:

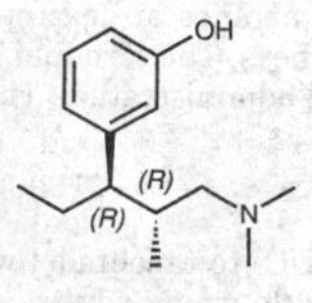

The molecular weight of tapentadol HCl is 257.80, and the molecular formula is $C_{14}H_{23}NO \bullet HCl$. The n-octanol:water partition coefficient log P value is 2.87. The pKa values are 9.34 and 10.45. In addition to the active ingredient tapentadol HCl, tablets also contain the following inactive ingredients: microcrystalline cellulose, lactose monohydrate, croscarmellose sodium, povidone, magnesium stearate, and Opadry® II, a proprietary film-coating mixture containing polyvinyl alcohol, titanium dioxide, polyethylene glycol, talc, and aluminum lake coloring.

12 CLINICAL PHARMACOLOGY

12.1 Mechanism of Action

Tapentadol is a centrally-acting synthetic analgesic. Although its exact mechanism is unknown, analgesic efficacy is thought to be due to mu-opioid agonist activity and the inhibition of norepinephrine reuptake.

12.2 Pharmacodynamics

Tapentadol is a centrally-acting synthetic analgesic. It is 18 times less potent than morphine in binding to the human mu-opioid receptor and is 2–3 times less potent in producing analgesia in animal models. Tapentadol has been shown to inhibit norepinephrine reuptake in the brains of rats resulting in increased norepinephrine concentrations. In preclinical models, the analgesic activity due to the mu-opioid receptor agonist activity of tapentadol can be antagonized by selective mu-opioid antagonists (e.g., naloxone), whereas the norepinephrine reuptake inhibition is sensitive to norepinephrine modulators. Tapentadol exerts its analgesic effects without a pharmacologically active metabolite.

Effects on the cardiovascular system: There was no effect of therapeutic and supratherapeutic doses of tapentadol on the QT interval. In a randomized, double-blind, placebo-

and positive-controlled crossover study, healthy subjects were administered five consecutive doses of NUCYNTA® 100 mg every 6 hours, NUCYNTA® 150 mg every 6 hours, placebo and a single oral dose of moxifloxacin. Similarly, NUCYNTA® had no relevant effect on other ECG parameters (heart rate, PR interval, QRS duration, T-wave or U-wave morphology).

12.3 Pharmacokinetics

Absorption

Mean absolute bioavailability after single-dose administration (fasting) is approximately 32% due to extensive first-pass metabolism. Maximum serum concentrations of tapentadol are typically observed at around 1.25 hours after dosing.

Dose-proportional increases in the C_{max} and AUC values of tapentadol have been observed over the 50 to 150 mg dose range.

A multiple (every 6 hour) dose study with doses ranging from 75 to 175 mg tapentadol showed a mean accumulation factor of 1.6 for the parent drug and 1.8 for the major metabolite tapentadol-O-glucuronide, which are primarily determined by the dosing interval and apparent half-life of tapentadol and its metabolite.

Food Effect

The AUC and C_{max} increased by 25% and 16%, respectively, when NUCYNTA® was administered after a high-fat, high-calorie breakfast. NUCYNTA® may be given with or without food.

Distribution

Tapentadol is widely distributed throughout the body. Following intravenous administration, the volume of distribution (Vz) for tapentadol is 540 +/- 98 L. The plasma protein binding is low and amounts to approximately 20%.

Metabolism and Elimination

In humans, the metabolism of tapentadol is extensive. About 97% of the parent compound is metabolized. Tapentadol is mainly metabolized via Phase 2 pathways, and only a small amount is metabolized by Phase 1 oxidative pathways. The major pathway of tapentadol metabolism is conjugation with glucuronic acid to produce glucuronides. After oral administration approximately 70% (55% O-glucuronide and 15% sulfate of tapentadol) of the dose is excreted in urine in the conjugated form. A total of 3% of drug was excreted in urine as unchanged drug. Tapentadol is additionally metabolized to N-desmethyl tapentadol (13%) by CYP2C9 and CYP2C19 and to hydroxy tapentadol (2%) by CYP2D6, which are further metabolized by conjugation. Therefore, drug metabolism mediated by cytochrome P450 system is of less importance than phase 2 conjugation. None of the metabolites contributes to the analgesic activity.

Tapentadol and its metabolites are excreted almost exclusively (99%) via the kidneys. The terminal half-life is on average 4 hours after oral administration. The total clearance is 1530 +/- 177 ml/min.

Special Populations

Elderly

The mean exposure (AUC) to tapentadol was similar in elderly subjects compared to young adults, with a 16% lower mean C_{max} observed in the elderly subject group compared to young adult subjects.

Renal Impairment

AUC and C_{max} of tapentadol were comparable in subjects with varying degrees of renal function (from normal to severely impaired). In contrast, increasing exposure (AUC) to tapentadol-O-glucuronide was observed with increasing degree of renal impairment. In subjects with mild, moderate, and severe renal impairment, the AUC of tapentadol-O-glucuronide are 1.5-, 2.5-, and 5.5-fold higher compared with normal renal function, respectively.

Hepatic Impairment

Administration of NUCYNTA® resulted in higher exposures and serum levels to tapentadol in subjects with impaired hepatic function compared to subjects with normal hepatic function. The ratio of tapentadol pharmacokinetic parameters for the mild and moderate hepatic impairment groups in comparison to the normal hepatic function group were 1.7 and 4.2, respectively, for AUC; 1.4 and 2.5, respectively, for C_{max}; and 1.2 and 1.4, respectively, for $t_{1/2}$. The rate of formation of tapentadol-O-glucuronide was lower in subjects with increased liver impairment.

Pharmacokinetic Drug Interactions

Tapentadol is mainly metabolized by Phase 2 glucuronidation, a high capacity/low affinity system, therefore, clinically relevant interactions caused by Phase 2 metabolism are unlikely to occur. Naproxen and probenecid increased the AUC of tapentadol by 17% and 57%, respectively. These changes are not considered clinically relevant and no change in dose is required.

No changes in the pharmacokinetic parameters of tapentadol were observed when acetaminophen and acetylsalicylic acid were given concomitantly.

In vitro studies did not reveal any potential of tapentadol to either inhibit or induce cytochrome P450 enzymes. Thus, clinically relevant interactions mediated by the cytochrome P450 system are unlikely to occur.

The pharmacokinetics of tapentadol were not affected when gastric pH or gastrointestinal motility were increased by omeprazole and metoclopramide, respectively.

Plasma protein binding of tapentadol is low (approximately 20%). Therefore, the likelihood of pharmacokinetic drug-drug interactions by displacement from the protein binding site is low.

13   NON-CLINICAL TOXICOLOGY

13.1   Carcinogenesis, Mutagenesis, Impairment of Fertility

Carcinogenesis

Tapentadol was administered to rats (diet) and mice (oral gavage) for two years.

In mice, tapentadol HCl was administered by oral gavage at dosages of 50, 100 and 200 mg/kg/day for 2 years (up to 0.2 times the plasma exposure at the maximum recommended human dose [MRHD] on an area under the time-curve [AUC] basis). No increase in tumor incidence was observed at any dose level.

In rats, tapentadol HCl was administered in diet at dosages of 10, 50, 125 and 250 mg/kg/day for two years (up to 0.2 times in the male rats and 0.6 times in the female rats the MRHD on an AUC basis). No increase in tumor incidence was observed at any dose level.

Mutagenesis

Tapentadol did not induce gene mutations in bacteria, but was clastogenic with metabolic activation in a chromosomal aberration test in V79 cells. The test was repeated and was negative in the presence and absence of metabolic activation. The one positive result for tapentadol was not confirmed *in vivo* in rats, using the two endpoints of chromosomal aberration and unscheduled DNA synthesis, when tested up to the maximum tolerated dose.

Impairment of Fertility

Tapentadol HCl was administered intravenously to male or female rats at dosages of 3, 6, or 12 mg/kg/day (representing exposures of up to approximately 0.4 times the exposure at the MRHD on an AUC basis, based on extrapolation from toxicokinetic analyses in a separate 4-week intravenous study in rats). Tapentadol did not alter fertility at any dose level. Maternal toxicity and adverse effects on embryonic development, including decreased number of implantations, decreased numbers of live conceptuses, and increased pre- and post-implantation losses occurred at dosages ≥6 mg/kg/day.

13.2   Animal Toxicology and/or Pharmacology

In toxicological studies with tapentadol, the most common systemic effects of tapentadol were related to the mu-opioid receptor agonist and norepinephrine reuptake inhibition pharmacodynamic properties of the compound. Transient, dose-dependent and predominantly CNS-related findings were observed, including impaired respiratory function and convulsions, the latter occurring in the dog at plasma levels (C_{max}) which are in the range associated with the maximum recommended human dose (MRHD).

14   CLINICAL STUDIES

The efficacy and safety of NUCYNTA® in the treatment of moderate to severe acute pain has been established in two randomized, double-blind, placebo- and active-controlled studies of moderate to severe pain from first metatarsal bunionectomy and end-stage degenerative joint disease.

14.1   Orthopedic Surgery – Bunionectomy

A randomized, double-blind, parallel-group, active- and placebo-controlled, multiple-dose study demonstrated the efficacy of 50 mg, 75 mg, and 100 mg NUCYNTA® given every 4 to 6 hours for 72 hours in patients aged 18 to 80 years experiencing moderate to severe pain following unilateral, first metatarsal bunionectomy surgery. Patients who qualified for the study with a baseline pain score of ≥4 on an 11-point rating scale ranging from 0 to 10 were randomized to 1 of 5 treatments. Patients were allowed to take a second dose of study medication as soon as 1 hour after the first dose on study Day 1, with subsequent dosing every 4 to 6 hours. If rescue analgesics were required, the patients were discontinued for lack of efficacy. Efficacy was evaluated by comparing the sum of pain intensity difference over the first 48 hours (SPID48) versus placebo. NUCYNTA® at each dose provided a greater reduction in pain compared to placebo based on SPID48 values.

For various degrees of improvement from baseline to the 48-hour endpoint, Figure 1 shows the fraction of patients achieving that level of improvement. The figures are cumulative, such that every patient that achieves a 50% reduction in pain from baseline is included in every level of improvement below 50%. Patients who did not complete the 48-hour observation period in the study were assigned 0% improvement.

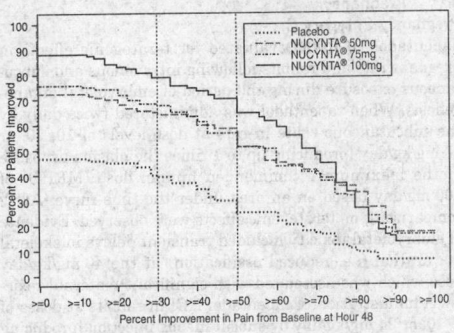

Figure 1: Percentage of Patients Achieving Various Levels of Pain Relief as Measured by Pain Severity at 48 Hours Compared to Baseline- Post Operative Bunionectomy

The proportions of patients who showed reduction in pain intensity at 48 hours of 30% or greater, or 50% or greater were significantly higher in patients treated with NUCYNTA® at each dose versus placebo.

14.2   End-Stage Degenerative Joint Disease

A randomized, double-blind, parallel-group, active- and placebo-controlled, multiple-dose study evaluated the efficacy and safety of 50 mg and 75 mg NUCYNTA® given every 4 to 6 hours during waking hours for 10 days in patients aged 18 to 80 years, experiencing moderate to severe pain from end stage degenerative joint disease of the hip or knee, defined as a 3-day mean pain score of ≥5 on an 11-point pain intensity scale, ranging from 0 to 10. Pain scores were assessed twice daily and assessed the pain the patient had experienced over the previous 12 hours. Patients were allowed to continue non-opioid analgesic therapy for which they had been on a stable regimen before screening throughout the study. Eighty-three percent (83%) of patients in the tapentadol treatment groups and the placebo group took such analgesia during the study. The 75 mg treatment group was dosed at 50 mg for the first day of the study, followed by 75 mg for the remaining nine days. Patients requiring rescue analgesics other than study medication were discontinued for lack of efficacy. Efficacy was evaluated by comparing the sum of pain intensity difference (SPID) versus placebo over the first five days of treatment. NUCYNTA® 50 mg and 75 mg provided improvement in pain compared with placebo based on the 5-Day SPID.

For various degrees of improvement from baseline to the Day 5 endpoint, Figure 2 shows the fraction of patients achieving that level of improvement. The figures are cumulative, such that every patient that achieves a 50% reduction in pain from baseline is included in every level of improvement below 50%. Patients who did not complete the 5-day observation period in the study were assigned 0% improvement.

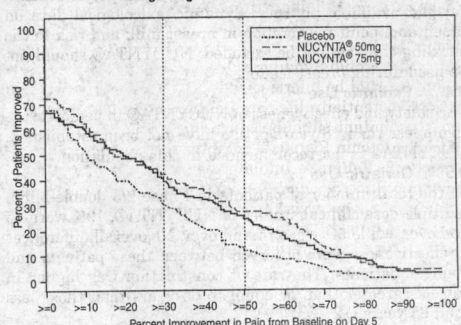

Figure 2: Percentage of Patients Achieving Various Levels of Pain Relief as Measured by Average Pain Severity for the Previous 12 hours, Measured on Study Day 5 Compared to Baseline — End Stage Degenerative Joint Disease

The proportions of patients who showed reduction in pain intensity at 5 days of 30% or greater, or 50% or greater were significantly higher in patients treated with NUCYNTA® at each dose versus placebo.

16   HOW SUPPLIED/STORAGE AND HANDLING

NUCYNTA® Tablets are available in the following strengths and packages. All tablets are round and biconvex-shaped.

50 mg tablets are yellow and debossed with "O-M" on one side and "50" on the other side, and are available in bottles of 100 (NDC 50458-820-04) and hospital unit dose blister packs of 10 (NDC 50458-820-02).

75 mg tablets are yellow-orange and debossed with "O-M" on one side and "75" on the other side, and are available in bottles of 100 (NDC 50458-830-04) and hospital unit dose blister packs of 10 (NDC 50458-830-02).

100 mg tablets are orange and debossed with "O-M" on one side and "100" on the other side, and are available in bottles of 100 (NDC 50458-840-04) and hospital unit dose blister packs of 10 (NDC 50458-840-02).

Store up to 25°C (77°F); excursions permitted to 15°–30°C (59°–86°F) [see USP Controlled Room Temperature]. Protect from moisture.

Keep out of reach of children.

17 PATIENT COUNSELING INFORMATION

Physicians are advised to discuss the following issues with patients for whom they prescribe NUCYNTA®:

17.1 Instructions for Use

Patients should be advised NUCYNTA® should be taken only as directed and to report episodes of breakthrough pain and adverse experiences occurring during therapy to their physician. Individualization of dosage is essential to make optimal use of this medication. Patients should be advised not to adjust the dose of NUCYNTA® without consulting their physician [see Dosage and Administration (2)]. Patients should be advised that it may be appropriate to taper dosing when discontinuing treatment with NUCYNTA® as withdrawal symptoms may occur [see Drug Abuse and Dependence (9.3)]. The physician can provide a dose schedule to accomplish a gradual discontinuation of the medication.

17.2 Misuse and Abuse

Patients should be advised that NUCYNTA® is a potential drug of abuse. Patients should protect NUCYNTA® from theft, and NUCYNTA® should never be given to anyone other than the individual for whom NUCYNTA® was prescribed [see Warnings and Precautions (5.4)].

17.3 Interference with Cognitive and Motor Performance

As NUCYNTA® has the potential to impair judgment, thinking, or motor skills, patients should be cautioned about operating hazardous machinery, including automobiles [see Warnings and Precautions (5.5)].

17.4 Pregnancy

Patients should be advised to notify their physician if they become pregnant or intend to become pregnant during treatment with NUCYNTA® [see Use in Specific Populations (8.1)].

17.5 Nursing

Patients should be advised not to breast-feed an infant during treatment with NUCYNTA® [see Use in Specific Populations (8.3)].

17.6 Monoamine Oxidase Inhibitors

Patients should be informed not to take NUCYNTA® while using any drugs that inhibit monoamine oxidase. Patients should not start any new medications while taking NUCYNTA® until they are assured by their healthcare provider that the new medication is not a monoamine oxidase inhibitor.

17.7 Seizures

Patients should be informed that NUCYNTA® could cause seizures if they are at risk for seizures or have epilepsy. Such patients should be advised to use NUCYNTA® with care [see Warnings and Precautions (5.7)]. Patients should be advised to stop taking NUCYNTA® if they have a seizure while taking NUCYNTA® and call their healthcare provider right away.

17.8 Serotonin Syndrome

Patients should be informed that NUCYNTA® could cause rare but potentially life-threatening conditions resulting from concomitant administration of serotonergic drugs (including Serotonin Reuptake Inhibitors, Serotonin and Norepinephrine Reuptake Inhibitors and tricyclic antidepressants) [see Warnings and Precautions (5.8)].

Patients should be advised to inform their physicians if they are taking, or plan to take, any prescription or over-the-counter drugs as there is a potential for interactions [see Drug Interactions (7)].

17.9 Alcohol

Patients should be advised to avoid alcohol while taking NUCYNTA® [see Drug Interactions (7.3)].

17.10 Medication Guide

See Medication Guide.

Revised: June 2010

Manufactured by:
Janssen Ortho, LLC
Gurabo, PR 00778

Manufactured for:
PriCara®, Division of Ortho-McNeil-Janssen Pharmaceuticals, Inc.
Raritan, NJ 08869

© Ortho-McNeil-Janssen Pharmaceuticals, Inc. 2009

MEDICATION GUIDE

NUCYNTA® (new-SINN-tah)
(tapentadol)
immediate-release oral tablets C-II

> • **NUCYNTA® is a federally controlled substance (C-II) because it can be abused. Keep NUCYNTA® in a safe place to prevent theft. Selling or giving away NUCYNTA® may harm others, and is against the law.**
> • **Tell your doctor if you (or a family member) have ever abused or been dependent on alcohol, prescription medicines, or street drugs.**

Read the Medication Guide that comes with NUCYNTA® before you start taking it and each time you get a new prescription. There may be new information. This Medication Guide does not take the place of talking to your doctor about your medical condition or your treatment. Talk to your doctor if you have any questions.

What is the most important information I should know about NUCYNTA®?
NUCYNTA® is a tablet that contains tapentadol, a strong medicine that is a pain medicine.
Use NUCYNTA® exactly how your doctor tells you to. Do not use NUCYNTA® if it has not been prescribed for you. You should not take NUCYNTA® if your pain is mild and can be controlled with other pain medicines such as nonsteroidal anti-inflammatory medicines (NSAIDS) or acetaminophen.

What is NUCYNTA®?
• NUCYNTA® is a prescription medicine that is used in adults 18 years of age or older to treat moderate to severe pain that is expected to last a short time.
NUCYNTA® is for short-term use only because the risks for withdrawal symptoms, abuse and addiction are higher when NUCYNTA® is used longer.

Who should not take NUCYNTA®?
Do not take NUCYNTA® if you:
• have severe lung problems
• have a gastrointestinal problem called paralytic ileus in which the intestines are not working normally.
• take a monoamine oxidase inhibitor (MAOI) medicine or have taken an MAOI within the last 14 days. Ask your doctor or pharmacist if any of your medicines is an MAOI.

What should I tell my doctor before taking NUCYNTA®?
NUCYNTA® may not be right for you. Tell your doctor about all your medical conditions, including if you have:
• trouble breathing or lung problems
• or had a head injury
• liver or kidney problems
• convulsions or seizures
• dependency problems with alcohol
• pancreas or gall bladder problems
• past or present substance abuse or drug addiction. There is a risk of abuse or addiction with narcotic pain medicines. If you have abused drugs in the past, you may have a higher chance of developing abuse or addiction again while using NUCYNTA®.
• are pregnant or plan to become pregnant
• are breast-feeding. You should not breast-feed while taking NUCYNTA®.

Tell your doctor about all the medicines you take, including prescription and nonprescription medicines, vitamins, and herbal supplements. Using NUCYNTA® with other medicines can cause serious side effects. The doses of some other medicines may need to be changed. Your doctor can tell you what medicines can be safely taken with NUCYNTA®. Especially tell your doctor if you take:
• **Monoamine Oxidase Inhibitors (MAOIs).** See "Who should not take NUCYNTA®."
• **any medicine that makes you sleepy.** NUCYNTA® can make you sleepy and affect your breathing. Taking these medicines together can be dangerous.

How should I take NUCYNTA®?
• Do not take NUCYNTA® unless it has been prescribed for you by your doctor.
• Take NUCYNTA® exactly as prescribed by your doctor.
• **Do not change the dose of NUCYNTA® unless your doctor tells you to.** Your doctor may change your dose after seeing how the medicine affects you. Do not use NUCYNTA® more often than prescribed. Call your doctor if your pain is not well controlled while taking NUCYNTA®.
• Follow your doctor's instructions about how to slowly stop taking NUCYNTA® to help lessen withdrawal symptoms.
• NUCYNTA® can be taken with or without food.

What should I avoid while taking NUCYNTA®?
• Do not drive, operate machinery, or participate in any other possibly dangerous activities until you know how you react to this medicine. NUCYNTA® can make you sleepy.
• You should not drink alcohol while using NUCYNTA®. Alcohol increases your chance of having dangerous side effects.

What are the possible side effects of NUCYNTA®?
NUCYNTA® can cause serious side effects including:
• **Life-threatening breathing problems.** Call your doctor right away or get emergency medical help if you:
  • have trouble breathing, or have slow or shallow breathing

---

• have a slow heartbeat
• have severe sleepiness
• have cold, clammy skin
• feel faint, dizzy, confused, or can not think, walk or talk normally
• have a seizure
• have hallucinations
• **Physical Dependence.** NUCYNTA® can cause physical dependence. Talk to your doctor about slowly stopping NUCYNTA® to avoid getting sick with withdrawal symptoms. You could become sick with uncomfortable symptoms because your body has become used to the medicine. Tell your doctor if you have any of these symptoms of withdrawal: feeling anxious, sweating, sleep problems, shivering, pain, nausea, tremors, diarrhea, upper respiratory symptoms, hallucinations, hair "standing on end." Physical dependence is not the same as drug addiction. Your doctor can tell you more about the differences between physical dependence and drug addiction.
• **Serotonin syndrome.** Serotonin syndrome is a rare, life-threatening problem that could happen if you take NUCYNTA® with Selective Serotonin Reuptake Inhibitors (SSRIs), Serotonin and Norepinephrine Reuptake Inhibitors (SNRIs), Monoamine Oxidase Inhibitors (MAOIs), triptans or certain other medicines. Call your doctor or get medical help right away if you have any one or more of the these symptoms: you feel agitated, have hallucinations, coma, rapid heart beat, feel overheated, loss of coordination, over active reflexes, nausea, vomiting, or diarrhea.
• **Seizures.** NUCYNTA® can cause seizures in people who are at risk for seizures or who have epilepsy. Tell your doctor right away if you have a seizure and stop taking NUCYNTA®.
• **Low blood pressure.** This can make you feel dizzy if you get up too fast from sitting or lying down.

The common side effects with NUCYNTA® are nausea, dizziness, vomiting, sleepiness, and itching.

Constipation is a common side effect of all opioid medicines. Talk to your doctor about the use of laxatives and stool softeners to prevent or treat constipation while taking NUCYNTA®.

Tell your doctor about any side effect that bothers you or that does not go away. These are not all the possible side effects of NUCYNTA®. For a complete list, ask your doctor or pharmacist.

Call your doctor for medical advice about side effects. You may report side effects to FDA at 1-800-FDA-1088.

How should I store NUCYNTA®?
• Store NUCYNTA® at 59°F to 86°F (15°C to 30°C). Keep NUCYNTA® tablets dry.
• Dispose of NUCYNTA® tablets you no longer need.

Keep NUCYNTA® in a safe place out of the reach of children.

General information about NUCYNTA®
Medicines are sometimes prescribed for purposes other than those listed in a Medication Guide. Do not use NUCYNTA® for a condition for which it was not prescribed. **Do not give NUCYNTA® to other people, even if they have the same symptoms you have. Sharing NUCYNTA® could be harmful and is against the law.**

This Medication Guide summarizes the most important information about NUCYNTA®. If you would like more information, talk with your doctor. You can ask your doctor or pharmacist for information about NUCYNTA® that is written for doctors. For more information about NUCYNTA® call 1-800-526-7736.

What are the ingredients in NUCYNTA®?

Active Ingredient: tapentadol
Inactive ingredients: microcrystalline cellulose, lactose monohydrate, croscarmellose sodium, povidone, magnesium stearate, and Opadry® II, a proprietary film-coating mixture containing polyvinyl alcohol, titanium dioxide, polyethylene glycol, talc, and aluminum lake coloring.

This Medication Guide has been approved by the U.S. Food and Drug Administration.
Revised: June 2010
Manufactured by:
Janssen Ortho, LLC
Gurabo, PR 00778
Manufactured for:
PriCara®, Division of Ortho-McNeil-Janssen Pharmaceuticals, Inc.
Raritan, NJ 08869
© Ortho-McNeil-Janssen Pharmaceuticals, Inc. 2009
Shown in Product Identification Guide, page 317

ORTHO EVRA®   ℞

[ōr'-thōō 'evō-ră]
(norelgestromin / ethinyl estradiol
TRANSDERMAL SYSTEM)

Patients should be counseled that this product does not protect against HIV infection (AIDS) and other sexually transmitted diseases.

DESCRIPTION

ORTHO EVRA® is a combination transdermal contraceptive patch with a contact surface area of 20 cm². It contains 6.00 mg norelgestromin (NGMN) and 0.75 mg ethinyl estradiol (EE). Systemic exposures (as measured by area under the curve [AUC] and steady state concentration [C_{ss}]) of NGMN and EE during use of ORTHO EVRA® are higher and peak concentrations (C_{max}) are lower than those produced by an oral contraceptive containing norgestimate 250 mcg / EE 35 mcg. (See BOLDED WARNING; CLINICAL PHARMACOLOGY, Transdermal versus Oral Contraceptives).

ORTHO EVRA® is a thin, matrix-type transdermal contraceptive patch consisting of three layers. The backing layer is composed of a beige flexible film consisting of a low-density pigmented polyethylene outer layer and a polyester inner layer. It provides structural support and protects the middle adhesive layer from the environment. The middle layer contains polyisobutylene/polybutene adhesive, crospovidone, non-woven polyester fabric and lauryl lactate as inactive components. The active components in this layer are the hormones, norelgestromin and ethinyl estradiol. The third layer is the release liner, which protects the adhesive layer during storage and is removed just prior to application. It is a transparent polyethylene terephthalate (PET) film with a polydimethylsiloxane coating on the side that is in contact with the middle adhesive layer.

The outside of the backing layer is heat-stamped "ORTHO EVRA®."

The structural formulas of the components are:

norelgestromin   ethinyl estradiol

Molecular weight, norelgestromin: 327.47
Molecular weight, ethinyl estradiol: 296.41
Chemical name for norelgestromin: 18, 19-dinorpregn-4-en-20-yn-3-one, 13-ethyl-17-hydroxy-, 3-oxime, (17α)
Chemical name for ethinyl estradiol: 19-Norpregna-1, 3, 5 (10)-trien-20-yne-3, 17-diol, (17α)

CLINICAL PHARMACOLOGY

Pharmacodynamics

Norelgestromin is the active progestin largely responsible for the progestational activity that occurs in women following application of ORTHO EVRA®. Norelgestromin is also the primary active metabolite produced following oral administration of norgestimate (NGM), the progestin component of the oral contraceptive products ORTHO-CYCLEN® and ORTHO TRI-CYCLEN®.

Combination oral contraceptives act by suppression of gonadotropins. Although the primary mechanism of this action is inhibition of ovulation, other alterations include changes in the cervical mucus (which increase the difficulty of sperm entry into the uterus) and the endometrium (which reduce the likelihood of implantation).

Receptor and human sex hormone-binding globulin (SHBG) binding studies, as well as studies in animals and humans, have shown that both NGM and NGMN exhibit high progestational activity with minimal intrinsic androgenicity[90–93]. Transdermally-administered norelgestromin, in combination with ethinyl estradiol, does not counteract the estrogen-induced increases in SHBG, resulting in lower levels of free testosterone in serum compared to baseline. One clinical trial assessed the return of hypothalamic-pituitary-ovarian axis function post-therapy and found that FSH, LH, and Estradiol mean values, though suppressed during therapy, returned to near baseline values during the 6 weeks post therapy.

Pharmacokinetics

Absorption

Following a single application of ORTHO EVRA®, both NGMN and EE reach a plateau by approximately 48 hours. Pooled data from the 3 clinical studies have demonstrated that steady state is reached within 2 weeks of application. The mean steady state C_{ss} concentrations ranged from 0.305–1.53 ng/mL for NGMN and from 11.2–137 pg/mL for EE.

Absorption of NGMN and EE following application of ORTHO EVRA® to the buttock, upper outer arm, abdomen and upper torso (excluding breast) was examined. While absorption from the abdomen was slightly lower than from other sites, absorption from these anatomic sites was considered to be therapeutically equivalent.

The mean (%CV) pharmacokinetic parameters C_{ss} and $AUC_{0–168}$ for NGMN and EE following a single buttock application of ORTHO EVRA® are summarized in Table 1.

In multiple dose studies, $AUC_{0–168}$ for NGMN and EE was found to increase over time (Table 1). In a three-cycle study, these pharmacokinetic parameters reached steady state conditions during Cycle 3 (Figures 1 and 2). Upon removal of the patch, serum levels of EE and NGMN reach very low or non-measurable levels within 3 days.

[See table 1 below]

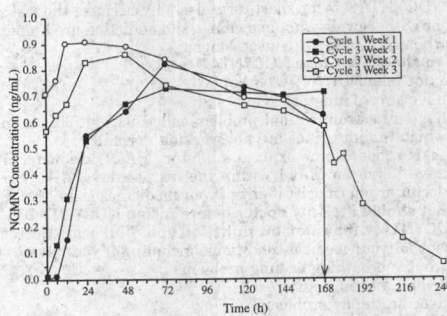

Figure 1: Mean Serum NGMN Concentrations (ng/mL) in Healthy Female Volunteers Following Application of ORTHO EVRA® on the Buttock for Three Consecutive Cycles (Vertical arrow indicates time of patch removal)

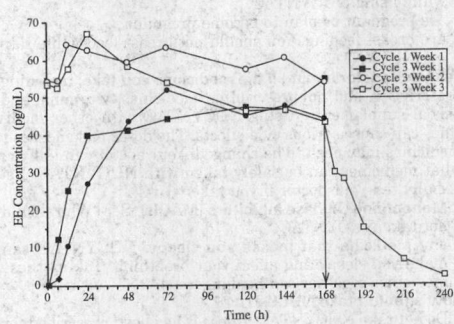

Figure 2: Mean Serum EE Concentrations (pg/mL) in Healthy Female Volunteers Following Application of ORTHO EVRA® on the Buttock for Three Consecutive Cycles (Vertical arrow indicates time of patch removal.)

The absorption of NGMN and EE following application of ORTHO EVRA® was studied under conditions encountered in a health club (sauna, whirlpool and treadmill) and in a cold water bath. The results indicated that for NGMN there were no significant treatment effects on C_{ss} or AUC when compared to normal wear. For EE, increased exposures were observed due to sauna, whirlpool and treadmill. There was no significant effect of cold water on these parameters. Results from a study of consecutive ORTHO EVRA® wear for 7 days and 10 days indicated that serum concentrations of NGMN and EE dropped slightly during the first 6 hours after the patch replacement, and recovered within 12 hours. By Day 10 of patch administration, both NGMN and EE concentrations had decreased by approximately 25% when compared to Day 7 concentrations.

Metabolism

Since ORTHO EVRA® is applied transdermally, first-pass metabolism (via the gastrointestinal tract and/or liver) of NGMN and EE that would be expected with oral administration is avoided. Hepatic metabolism of NGMN occurs and metabolites include norgestrel, which is highly bound to SHBG, and various hydroxylated and conjugated metabolites. Ethinyl estradiol is also metabolized to various hydroxylated products and their glucuronide and sulfate conjugates.

Distribution

NGMN and norgestrel (a serum metabolite of NGMN) are highly bound (>97%) to serum proteins. NGMN is bound to albumin and not to SHBG, while norgestrel is bound primarily to SHBG, which limits its biological activity. Ethinyl estradiol is extensively bound to serum albumin and induces an increase in the serum concentrations of SHBG (See CLINICAL PHARMACOLOGY, Transdermal versus Oral Contraceptives, Table 3).

Elimination

Following removal of patches, the elimination kinetics of NGMN and EE were consistent for all studies with half-life values of approximately 28 hours and 17 hours, respectively. The metabolites of NGMN and EE are eliminated by renal and fecal pathways.

Transdermal versus Oral Contraceptives

The ORTHO EVRA® transdermal patch was designed to deliver EE and NGMN over a seven-day period while oral contraceptives (containing NGM 250 mcg / EE 35 mcg) are administered on a daily basis. Figures 3 and 4 present mean pharmacokinetic (PK) profiles for EE and NGMN following administration of an oral contraceptive (containing NGM 250 mcg / EE 35 mcg) compared to the 7-day transdermal ORTHO EVRA® patch (containing NGMN 6.0 mg / EE 0.75 mg) during cycle 2 in 32 healthy female volunteers.

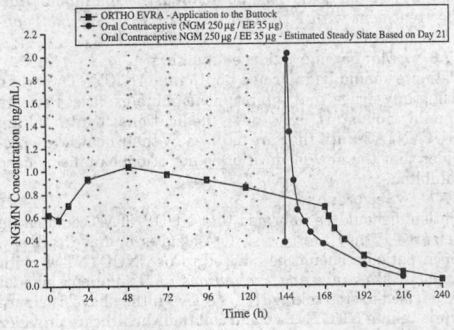

Figure 3: Mean Serum Concentration-Time Profiles of NGMN Following Once-Daily Administration of an Oral Contraceptive for 2 cycles or Application of ORTHO EVRA® for 2 cycles to the Buttock in Healthy Female Volunteers. [Oral contraceptive: Cycle 2, Days 15–21, ORTHO EVRA® : Cycle 2, week 3]

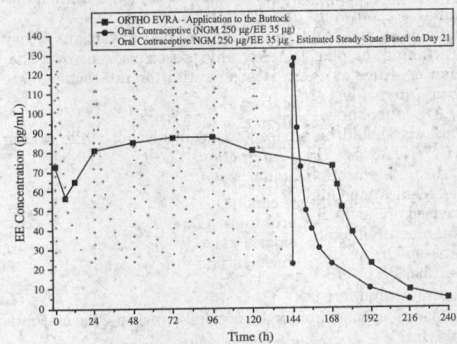

Figure 4: Mean Serum Concentration-Time Profiles of EE Following Once-Daily Administration of an Oral Contraceptive for 2 cycles or Application of ORTHO EVRA® for 2 cycles to the Buttock in Healthy Female Volunteers. [Oral contraceptive: Cycle 2, Days 15–21, ORTHO EVRA® : Cycle 2, week 3]

Table 2 provides the mean (%CV) for NGMN and EE pharmacokinetic (PK) parameters.

Table 1: Mean (%CV*) Pharmacokinetic Parameters of Norelgestromin (NGMN) and Ethinyl Estradiol (EE) Following 3 Consecutive Cycles of ORTHO EVRA® Wear on the Buttock

Analyte	Parameter	Cycle 1 Week 1	Cycle 3 Week 1	Cycle 3 Week 2	Cycle 3 Week 3
NGMN	C_{ss} (ng/mL)	0.70 (39.4)	0.70 (41.8)	0.80 (28.7)	0.70 (45.3)
	$AUC_{0–168}$ (ng·h/mL)	107 (44.2)	105 (43.2)	132 (43.4)	120 (43.9)
	$t_{1/2}$ (h)	nc	nc	nc	32.1 (40.3)
EE	C_{ss} (pg/mL)	46.4 (38.5)	47.6 (36.4)	59.0 (42.5)	49.6 (54.4)
	$AUC_{0–168}$ (pg·h/mL)	6796 (39.3)	7160 (40.4)	10054 (41.8)	8840 (58.6)
	$t_{1/2}$ (h)	nc	nc	nc	21.0 (43.2)

nc = not calculated,
* %CV is % of Coefficient of variation = 100 (standard deviation/mean)

Table 2: Mean (%CV) NGMN and EE Steady State Pharmacokinetic Parameters Following Application of ORTHO EVRA® and Once-daily Administration of an Oral Contraceptive (containing NGM 250 mcg / EE 35 mcg) in Healthy Female Volunteers

Parameter	ORTHO EVRA*	ORAL CONTRACEPTIVE[†]
NGMN[‡]		
C_{max} (ng/mL)	1.12 (33.6)	2.16 (25.2)
AUC_{0-168} (ng·h/mL)	145 (36.8)	123 (30.2)[§]
C_{ss} (ng/mL)	0.888 (36.6)	0.732 (30.2)[¶]
EE		
C_{max} (pg/mL)	97.4 (31.6)	133 (27.7)
AUC_{0-168} (pg·h/mL)	12,971 (33.1)	8,281 (26.9)[§]
C_{ss} (pg/mL)	80.0 (33.5)	49.3 (26.9)[¶]

*Cycle 2, Week 3
†Cycle 2, Day 21
‡NGM is rapidly metabolized to NGMN following oral administration
§Average weekly exposure, calculated as $AUC_{24} \times 7$
¶C_{avg}

In general, overall exposure for NGMN and EE (AUC and C_{ss}) was higher in subjects treated with ORTHO EVRA® for both Cycle 1 and Cycle 2, compared to that for the oral contraceptive, while C_{max} values were higher in subjects administered the oral contraceptive. Under steady state conditions, AUC_{0-168} and C_{ss} for EE were approximately 55% and 60% higher, respectively, for the transdermal patch, and the C_{max} was about 35% higher for the oral contraceptive, respectively. Inter-subject variability (%CV) for the PK parameters following delivery from ORTHO EVRA® was higher relative to the variability determined from the oral contraceptive. The mean pharmacokinetic profiles are different between the two products and caution should be exercised when making a direct comparison of these PK parameters.

In Table 3, percent change in concentrations (%CV) of markers of systemic estrogenic activity (Sex Hormone Binding Globulin [SHBG] and Corticosteroid Binding Globulin [CBG]) from Cycle 1 Day 1 to Cycle 1 Day 22 is presented. Percent change in SHBG concentrations was higher for ORTHO EVRA® users compared to women taking the oral contraceptive; percent change in CBG concentrations were similar for ORTHO EVRA® and oral contraceptive users. Within each group, the absolute values for SHBG were similar for Cycle 1, Day 22 and Cycle 2, Day 22.

Table 3: Mean Percent Change (%CV) in SHBG and CBG Concentrations Following Once-daily Administration of an Oral Contraceptive (containing NGM 250 mcg / EE 35 mcg) for One Cycle and Application of ORTHO EVRA® for One Cycle in Healthy Female Volunteers

Parameter	ORTHO EVRA® (% change from Day 1 to Day 22)	ORAL CONTRACEPTIVE (% change from Day 1 to Day 22)
SHBG	334 (39.3)	200 (43.2)
CBG	153 (40.2)	157 (33.4)

Special Populations
Effects of Age, Body Weight, Body Surface Area and Race
The effects of age, body weight, body surface area and race on the pharmacokinetics of NGMN and EE were evaluated in 230 healthy women from nine pharmacokinetic studies of single 7-day applications of ORTHO EVRA®. For both NGMN and EE, increasing age, body weight and body surface area each were associated with slight decreases in C_{ss} and AUC values. However, only a small fraction (10–25%) of the overall variability in the pharmacokinetics of NGMN and EE following application of ORTHO EVRA® may be associated with any or all of the above demographic parameters. There was no significant effect of race with respect to Caucasians, Hispanics and Blacks.
Renal and Hepatic Impairment
No formal studies were conducted with ORTHO EVRA® to evaluate the pharmacokinetics, safety, and efficacy in women with renal or hepatic impairment. Steroid hormones may be poorly metabolized in patients with impaired liver function (see PRECAUTIONS).
Patch Adhesion
In the clinical trials with ORTHO EVRA®, approximately 2% of the cumulative number of patches completely detached. The proportion of subjects with at least 1 patch that completely detached ranged from 2% to 6%, with a reduc-

tion from Cycle 1 (6%) to Cycle 13 (2%). For instructions on how to manage detachment of patches, refer to the DOSAGE AND ADMINISTRATION section.
INDICATIONS AND USAGE
ORTHO EVRA® is indicated for the prevention of pregnancy in women who elect to use a transdermal patch as a method of contraception.
The pharmacokinetic profile for the ORTHO EVRA® transdermal patch is different from that of an oral contraceptive. Healthcare professionals should balance the higher estrogen exposure and the possible increased risk of venous thromboembolism with ORTHO EVRA® against the chance of pregnancy if a contraceptive pill is not taken daily. (See BOLDED WARNING; WARNINGS; CLINICAL PHARMACOLOGY, Transdermal versus Oral Contraceptives).
Like oral contraceptives, ORTHO EVRA® is highly effective if used as recommended in this label.
In 3 large clinical trials in North America, Europe and South Africa, 3,330 women (ages 18–45) completed 22,155 cycles of ORTHO EVRA® use, pregnancy rates were approximately 1 per 100 women-years of ORTHO EVRA® use. The racial distribution was 91% Caucasian, 4.9% Black, 1.6% Asian, and 2.4% Other.

Table 4: Percentage of Women Experiencing an Unintended Pregnancy During the First Year of Typical Use and the First Year of Perfect Use of Contraception and the Percentage Continuing Use at the End of the First Year. United States.

Method (1)	% of Women Experiencing an Unintended Pregnancy within the First Year of Use		% of Women Continuing Use at One Year* (4)
	Typical Use[†] (2)	Perfect Use[‡] (3)	
Chance[#]	85	85	
Spermicides[b]	26	6	40
Periodic abstinence	25		63
Calendar		9	
Ovulation Method		3	
Sympto-Thermal[ß]		2	
Post-Ovulation		1	
Cap[a]			
Parous Women	40	26	42
Nulliparous Women	20	9	56
Sponge			
Parous Women	40	20	42
Nulliparous Women	20	9	56
Diaphragm[a]	20	6	56
Withdrawal	19	4	
Condom[e]			
Female (Reality®)	21	5	56
Male	14	3	61
Pill	5		71
Progestin Only		0.5	
Combined		0.1	
IUD			
Progesterone T	2.0	1.5	81
Copper T380A	0.8	0.6	78
LNG 20	0.1	0.1	81
Depo-Provera®	0.3	0.3	70
Norplant® and Norplant-2®	0.05	0.05	88
Female Sterilization	0.5	0.5	100
Male Sterilization	0.15	0.10	100

Hatcher et al, 1998, Ref. # 1.
Emergency Contraceptive Pills:
Treatment initiated within 72 hours after unprotected intercourse reduces the risk of pregnancy by at least 75%.[§]
Lactational Amenorrhea Method:
LAM is highly effective, *temporary* method of contraception.[¶]
Source: Trussell J, Contraceptive efficacy. In Hatcher RA, Trussell J, Stewart F, Cates W, Stewart GK, Kowal D, Guest F, Contraceptive Technology: Seventeenth Revised Edition. New York NY: Irvington Publishers, 1998.
*Among couples attempting to avoid pregnancy, the percentage who continue to use a method for one year.
†Among *typical* couples who initiate use of a method (not necessarily for the first time), the percentage who experience an accidental pregnancy during the first year if they do not stop use for any other reason.
‡Among couples who initiate use of a method (not necessarily for the first time) and who use it *perfectly* (both consistently and correctly), the percentage who experience an accidental pregnancy during the first year if they do not stop use for any other reason.
§The treatment schedule is one dose within 72 hours after unprotected intercourse, and a second dose 12 hours after the first dose. The Food and Drug Administration has declared the following brands of oral contraceptives to be safe and effective for emergency contraception: Ovral® (1 dose is 2 white pills), Alesse® (1 dose is 5 pink pills), Nordette® or Levlen® (1 dose is 2 light-orange pills), Lo/Ovral® (1 dose is 4 white pills), Triphasil® or Tri-Levlen® (1 dose is 4 yellow pills).
¶However, to maintain effective protection against pregnancy, another method of contraception must be used as soon as menstruation resumes, the frequency or duration of breastfeeds is reduced, bottle feeds are introduced, or the baby reaches six months of age.
#The percents becoming pregnant in columns (2) and (3) are based on data from populations where contraception is not used and from women who cease using contraception in order to become pregnant. Among such populations, about 89% become pregnant within one year. This estimate was lowered slightly (to 85%) to represent the percent who would become pregnant within one year among women now relying on reversible methods of contraception if they abandoned contraception altogether.
ßFoams, creams, gels, vaginal suppositories, and vaginal film.
ßCervical mucus (ovulation) method supplemented by calendar in the pre-ovulatory and basal body temperature in the post-ovulatory phases.
aWith spermicidal cream or jelly.
eWithout spermicides.

With respect to weight, 5 of the 15 pregnancies reported with ORTHO EVRA® use were among women with a baseline body weight ≥ 198 lbs. (90kg), which constituted < 3% of the study population. The greater proportion of pregnancies among women at or above 198 lbs. was statistically significant and suggests that ORTHO EVRA® may be less effective in these women.
Healthcare professionals who consider ORTHO EVRA® for women at or above 198 lbs. should discuss the patient's individual needs in choosing the most appropriate contraceptive option.
Table 4 lists the accidental pregnancy rates for users of various methods of contraception. The efficacy of these contraceptive methods, except sterilization, IUD, and Norplant® depends upon the reliability with which they are used. Correct and consistent use of methods can result in lower failure rates.
[See table 4 above]
ORTHO EVRA® has not been studied for and is not indicated for use in emergency contraception.
CONTRAINDICATIONS
ORTHO EVRA® should not be used in women who currently have the following conditions:

Table 5: Estimates (Odds Ratios) of Venous Thromboembolism Risk in Current Users of ORTHO EVRA® Compared to Oral Contraceptive Users

Epidemiologic Study	Comparator Product	Odds Ratio (95% C.I.)
i3 Ingenix NGM Study in Ingenix Research Datamart[107,113,,114,115]	NGM/35 mcg EE*	2.2[†] (1.2–4.0)[‡]
BCDSP[§] NGM Study in Pharmetrics database[108,109,111]	NGM/35 mcg EE	1.2 (0.9–1.8)[¶]
BCDSP LNG Study in Pharmetrics database[110]	LNG[#]/30 mcg EE	2.0 (0.9–4.1)[Þ]
BCDSP LNG Study in Marketscan database[110]	LNG/30 mcg EE	1.3 (0.8–2.0)[ß]

*NGM = norgestimate; EE = ethinyl estradiol
†Increase in risk of VTE is statistically significant
‡Pooled odds ratio from references 107 and 113. [Initial 33 months of data: Odds Ratio (95% CI) = 2.5* (1.1–5.5); Separate estimate from 24 months of data on new cases not included in the previous estimate: Odds Ratio (95% CI) = 1.4 (0.5–3.7)]
§BCDSP = Boston Collaborative Drug Surveillance Program
¶Pooled odds ratio from references 108, 109 and 111. [Initial 36 months of data: Odds Ratio (95% CI) = 0.9 (0.5–1.6); Separate estimate from 17 months of data on new cases not included in the previous estimate: Odds Ratio (95% CI) = 1.1 (0.6–2.1); Separate estimate from 14 months of data on new cases not included in the previous estimates: Odds Ratio (95% CI) = 2.4* (1.2–5.0)]
#LNG = levonorgestrel
Þ48 months of data.
ß69 months of data.

- Thrombophlebitis, thromboembolic disorders
- A past history of deep vein thrombophlebitis or thromboembolic disorders
- Known thrombophilic conditions
- Cerebrovascular or coronary artery disease (current or past history)
- Valvular heart disease with complications[103]
- Persistent blood pressure values of ≥ 160 mm Hg systolic or ≥ 100 mg Hg diastolic[103, 112]
- Diabetes with vascular involvement[103]
- Headaches with focal neurological symptoms
- Major surgery with prolonged immobilization
- Known or suspected carcinoma of the breast or personal history of breast cancer
- Carcinoma of the endometrium or other known or suspected estrogen-dependent neoplasia
- Undiagnosed abnormal genital bleeding
- Cholestatic jaundice of pregnancy or jaundice with prior hormonal contraceptive use
- Acute or chronic hepatocellular disease with abnormal liver function[103]
- Hepatic adenomas or carcinomas
- Known or suspected pregnancy
- Hypersensitivity to any component of this product

WARNINGS

> **Cigarette smoking increases the risk of serious cardiovascular side effects from hormonal contraceptive use. This risk increases with age and with heavy smoking (15 or more cigarettes per day) and is quite marked in women over 35 years of age. Women who use hormonal contraceptives, including ORTHO EVRA®, should be strongly advised not to smoke.**

The pharmacokinetic (PK) profile for the ORTHO EVRA® patch is different from the PK profile for oral contraceptives in that it has higher steady state concentrations and lower peak concentrations. AUC and average concentration at steady state for ethinyl estradiol (EE) are approximately 60% higher in women using ORTHO EVRA® compared with women using an oral contraceptive containing EE 35 mcg. In contrast, peak concentrations for EE are approximately 25% lower in women using ORTHO EVRA®. Inter-subject variability results in increased exposure to EE in some women using either ORTHO EVRA® or oral contraceptives. However, inter-subject variability in women using ORTHO EVRA® is higher. It is not known whether there are changes in the risk of serious adverse events based on the differences in pharmacokinetic profiles of EE in women using ORTHO EVRA® compared with women using oral contraceptives containing 35 mcg of EE. Increased estrogen exposure may increase the risk of adverse events, including venous thromboembolism. (See CLINICAL PHARMACOLOGY, Transdermal versus Oral Contraceptives).

Four epidemiologic, case-control studies[107–111,113–115] were conducted in the U.S. using electronic healthcare claims data to evaluate the risk of venous thromboembolism (VTE) among women aged 15–44 who used ORTHO EVRA® compared to women who used oral contraceptives containing 30–35 mcg of ethinyl estradiol (EE) and either norgestimate (NGM) or levonorgestrel (LNG). NGM is the prodrug for norelgestromin, the progestin in ORTHO EVRA®.

These studies (see Table 5) used slightly different designs and reported odds ratios ranging from 1.2 to 2.2. The interpretations of these odds ratios range from no increase in risk to an approximate doubling of risk. Only one study (i3 Ingenix) included patient chart review to confirm the VTE occurrence.

The four studies are:

- The i3 Ingenix study with NGM-containing oral contraceptives as the comparator, including a 24 month extension, based on the Ingenix Research Datamart
- The Boston Collaborative Drug Surveillance Program (BCDSP) with NGM-containing oral contraceptives as the comparator (BCDSP NGM), including two extensions of 17 and 14 months, respectively, based on the Pharmetrics database
- BCDSP with LNG-containing oral contraceptives as the comparator, based on the Pharmetrics database
- BCDSP with LNG-containing oral contraceptives as the comparator, based on the Marketscan database

The i3 Ingenix and BCDSP NGM studies have provided data on additional cases identified in study extensions; however, each study extension was not powered to provide independent estimates of risk. The pooled estimates provide the most reliable estimates of VTE risk. Odds ratios from the original and various extensions of the i3 Ingenix and BCDSP NGM studies are provided in the footnotes to Table 5.

[See table 5 above]

In 3 large clinical trials (N= 3,330 with 1,704 women-years of exposure), one case of non-fatal pulmonary embolism occurred during ORTHO EVRA® use, and one case of postoperative non-fatal pulmonary embolism was reported following ORTHO EVRA® use.

ORTHO EVRA® and other contraceptives that contain both an estrogen and a progestin are called combination hormonal contraceptives. As with any combination hormonal contraceptive, the clinician should be alert to the earliest manifestations of thromboembolic disorders (thrombophlebitis, VTE including pulmonary embolism, cerebrovascular disorders, and retinal thrombosis). Should any of these occur or be suspected, ORTHO EVRA® should be discontinued immediately.

Practitioners prescribing ORTHO EVRA® should be familiar with the following information relating to risks:

The use of combination hormonal contraceptives is associated with increased risks of several serious conditions including myocardial infarction, thromboembolism, stroke, hepatic neoplasia, and gallbladder disease, although the risk of serious morbidity or mortality is very small in healthy women without underlying risk factors. The risk of morbidity and mortality increases significantly in the presence of other underlying risk factors such as hypertension, hyperlipidemias, obesity and diabetes.

The information that follows in this section of the package insert is principally based on studies carried out in women who used combination oral contraceptives with higher formulations of estrogens and progestins than those in common use today. The effect of long-term use of combination hormonal contraceptives with lower doses of both estrogen and progestin administered by any route remains to be determined.

Throughout this labeling, epidemiological studies reported are of two types: retrospective or case control studies and cohort studies. Case control studies provide an estimate of the relative risk or odds for developing a disease, namely, a ratio of the disease among oral contraceptive users to that among nonusers or users of a comparator drug product. The odds ratio does not provide information on the actual clinical occurrence of a disease. Cohort studies provide a measure of the incidence of a disease in an exposed population. The relative risk is the ratio of the incidence density in the exposed population relative to the incidence density in a comparator population. Cohort studies also provide a measure of attributable risk, which is the *difference* in the incidence of disease between hormonal contraceptive users and nonusers or comparator drug products. The attributable risk does provide information about the actual occurrence of a disease in the population (adapted from refs. 2 and 3 with the author's permission). For further information, the reader is referred to a text on epidemiological methods.

1. Thromboembolic Disorders and Other Vascular Problems
a. Thromboembolism

An increased risk of thromboembolic and thrombotic disease associated with the use of hormonal contraceptives is well established. Case control studies have found the relative risk of users compared to nonusers to be 3 for the first episode of superficial venous thrombosis, 4 to 11 for deep vein thrombosis or pulmonary embolism, and 1.5 to 6 for women with predisposing conditions for venous thromboembolic disease[2,3,19–24]. Cohort studies have shown the relative risk to be somewhat lower, about 3 for new cases and about 4.5 for new cases requiring hospitalization[25]. The risk of thromboembolic disease associated with hormonal contraceptives is not related to length of use and disappears after hormonal contraceptive use is stopped[2]. A two- to four-fold increase in relative risk of post-operative thromboembolic complications has been reported with the use of hormonal contraceptives[9,26]. The relative risk of venous thrombosis in women who have predisposing conditions is twice that of women without such medical conditions[9,26]. If feasible, hormonal contraceptives should be discontinued at least four weeks prior to and for two weeks after elective surgery of a type associated with an increase in risk of thromboembolism and during and following prolonged immobilization. Since the immediate postpartum period is also associated with an increased risk of thromboembolism, hormonal contraceptives should be started no earlier than four weeks after delivery in women who elect not to breastfeed.

b. Myocardial Infarction

An increased risk of myocardial infarction has been attributed to hormonal contraceptive use. This risk is primarily in smokers or women with other underlying risk factors for coronary artery disease such as hypertension, hypercholesterolemia, morbid obesity, and diabetes. The relative risk of heart attack for current hormonal contraceptive users has been estimated to be two to six[4–10] compared to non-users. The risk is very low under the age of 30.

Smoking in combination with oral contraceptive use has been shown to contribute substantially to the incidence of myocardial infarctions in women in their mid-thirties or older with smoking accounting for the majority of excess cases[11]. Mortality rates associated with circulatory disease have been shown to increase substantially in smokers, especially in those 35 years of age and older among women who use oral contraceptives. (See Figure 5)

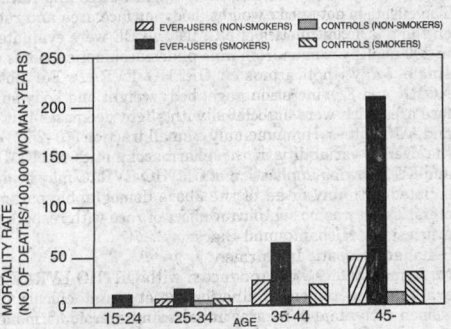

Figure 5: Circulatory Disease Mortality Rates Per 100,000 Women-Years by Age, Smoking Status and Oral Contraceptive Use

Hormonal contraceptives may compound the effects of well-known risk factors, such as hypertension, diabetes, hyperlipidemias, age and obesity[13]. In particular, some progestins are known to decrease HDL cholesterol and cause glucose intolerance, while estrogens may create a state of hyperinsulinism[14–18]. Hormonal contraceptives have been shown to increase blood pressure among some users (see Section 9 in WARNINGS). Similar effects on risk factors have been associated with an increased risk of heart disease. Hormonal contraceptives, including ORTHO EVRA®, must be used with caution in women with cardiovascular disease risk factors.

Norgestimate and norelgestromin have minimal androgenic activity (see CLINICAL PHARMACOLOGY). There is some evidence that the risk of myocardial infarction associated with hormonal contraceptives is lower when the progestin has minimal androgenic activity than when the activity is greater[97].

c. Cerebrovascular Diseases

Hormonal contraceptives have been shown to increase both the relative and attributable risks of cerebrovascular events (thrombotic and hemorrhagic strokes), although, in general, the risk is greatest among older (>35 years), hypertensive women who also smoke. Hypertension was found to be a risk factor for both users and nonusers, for both types of strokes, and smoking interacted to increase the risk of stroke[27–29].

In a large study, the relative risk of thrombotic strokes has been shown to range from 3 for normotensive users to 14 for users with severe hypertension[30]. The relative risk of hemorrhagic stroke is reported to be 1.2 for non-smokers who used hormonal contraceptives, 2.6 for smokers who did not use hormonal contraceptives, 7.6 for smokers who used hormonal contraceptives, 1.8 for normotensive users and 25.7 for users with severe hypertension[30]. The attributable risk is also greater in older women[3].

d. Dose-Related Risk of Vascular Disease from Hormonal Contraceptives

A positive association has been observed between the amount of estrogen and progestin in hormonal contraceptives and the risk of vascular disease[31–33]. A decline in serum high-density lipoproteins (HDL) has been reported with many progestational agents[14–16]. A decline in serum high-density lipoproteins has been associated with an increased incidence of ischemic heart disease. Because estrogens increase HDL cholesterol, the net effect of a hormonal contraceptive depends on a balance achieved between doses of estrogen and progestin and the activity of the progestin used in the contraceptives. The activity and amount of both hormones should be considered in the choice of a hormonal contraceptive.

e. Persistence of Risk of Vascular Disease

There are two studies that have shown persistence of risk of vascular disease for ever-users of combination hormonal contraceptives. In a study in the United States, the risk of developing myocardial infarction after discontinuing combination hormonal contraceptives persists for at least 9 years for women 40–49 years who had used combination hormonal contraceptives for five or more years, but this increased risk was not demonstrated in other age groups[8]. In another study in Great Britain, the risk of developing cerebrovascular disease persisted for at least 6 years after discontinuation of combination hormonal contraceptives, although excess risk was very small[34]. However, both studies were performed with combination hormonal contraceptive formulations containing 50 micrograms or higher of estrogens.

2. Estimates of Mortality from Combination Hormonal Contraceptive Use

One study gathered data from a variety of sources that have estimated the mortality rate associated with different methods of contraception at different ages (Table 6). These estimates include the combined risk of death associated with contraceptive methods plus the risk attributable to pregnancy in the event of method failure. Each method of contraception has its specific benefits and risks. The study concluded that with the exception of combination oral contraceptive users 35 and older who smoke, and 40 and older who do not smoke, mortality associated with all methods of birth control is low and below that associated with childbirth.

The observation of a possible increase in risk of mortality with age for combination oral contraceptive users is based on data gathered in the 1970's but not reported until 1983[35]. Current clinical recommendation involves the use of lower estrogen dose formulations and a careful consideration of risk factors. In 1989, the Fertility and Maternal Health Drugs Advisory Committee was asked to review the use of combination hormonal contraceptives in women 40 years of age and over. The Committee concluded that although cardiovascular disease risks may be increased with combination hormonal contraceptive use after age 40 in healthy non-smoking women (even with the newer low-dose formulations), there are also greater potential health risks associated with pregnancy in older women and with the alternative surgical and medical procedures that may be necessary if such women do not have access to effective and acceptable means of contraception. The Committee recommended that the benefits of low-dose combination hormonal contraceptive use by healthy non-smoking women over 40 may outweigh the possible risks[36, 37].

Table 6: Annual Number of Birth-Related or Method-Related Deaths Associated with Control of Fertility per 100,000 Non-Sterile Women, by Fertility Control Method According to Age

Method of control and outcome	15–19	20–24	25–29	30–34	35–39	40–44
No fertility control methods*	7.0	7.4	9.1	14.8	25.7	28.2
Oral contraceptives, non-smoker†	0.3	0.5	0.9	1.9	13.8	31.6
Oral contraceptives, smoker†	2.2	3.4	6.6	13.5	51.1	117.2
IUD†	0.8	0.8	1.0	1.0	1.4	1.4
Condom*	1.1	1.6	0.7	0.2	0.3	0.4
Diaphragm/spermicide*	1.9	1.2	1.2	1.3	2.2	2.8
Periodic abstinence*	2.5	1.6	1.6	1.7	2.9	3.6

Adapted from H.W. Ory, ref. # 35.
*Deaths are birth-related
†Deaths are method-related

Although the data are mainly obtained with oral contraceptives, this is likely to apply to ORTHO EVRA® as well. Women of all ages who use combination hormonal contraceptives, should use the lowest possible dose formulation that is effective and meets the individual patient needs. [See table 6 above]

3. Carcinoma of the Reproductive Organs and Breasts

Numerous epidemiological studies give conflicting reports on the relationship between breast cancer and COC use. The risk of having breast cancer diagnosed may be slightly increased among current and recent users of combination oral contraceptives. However, this excess risk appears to decrease over time after COC discontinuation and by 10 years after cessation the increased risk disappears. Some studies report an increased risk with duration of use while other studies do not and no consistent relationships have been found with dose or type of steroid. Some studies have found a small increase in risk for women who first use COCs before age 20. Most studies show a similar pattern of risk with COC use regardless of a woman's reproductive history or her family breast cancer history.

In addition, breast cancers diagnosed in current or ever oral contraceptive users may be less clinically advanced than in never-users.

Women who currently have or have had breast cancer should not use hormonal contraceptives because breast cancer is usually a hormonally sensitive tumor.

Some studies suggest that combination oral contraceptive use has been associated with an increase in the risk of cervical intraepithelial neoplasia in some populations of women[45–48]. However, there continues to be controversy about the extent to which such findings may be due to differences in sexual behavior and other factors.

In spite of many studies of the relationship between oral contraceptive use and breast and cervical cancers, a cause-and-effect relationship has not been established. It is not known whether ORTHO EVRA® is distinct from oral contraceptives with regard to the above statements.

4. Hepatic Neoplasia

Benign hepatic adenomas are associated with hormonal contraceptive use, although the incidence of benign tumors is rare in the United States. Indirect calculations have estimated the attributable risk to be in the range of 3.3 cases/100,000 for users, a risk that increases after four or more years of use, especially with hormonal contraceptives containing 50 micrograms or more of estrogen[49]. Rupture of benign, hepatic adenomas may cause death through intra-abdominal hemorrhage[50,51].

Studies from Britain and the U.S. have shown an increased risk of developing hepatocellular carcinoma in long term (≥ 8 years)[52–54,96] oral contraceptive users. However, these cancers are extremely rare in the U.S. and the attributable risk (the excess incidence) of liver cancers in oral contraceptive users approaches less than one per million users. It is unknown whether ORTHO EVRA® is distinct from oral contraceptives in this regard.

5. Ocular Lesions

There have been clinical case reports of retinal thrombosis associated with the use of hormonal contraceptives. ORTHO EVRA® should be discontinued if there is unexplained partial or complete loss of vision; onset of proptosis or diplopia; papilledema; or retinal vascular lesions. Appropriate diagnostic and therapeutic measures should be undertaken immediately.

6. Hormonal Contraceptive Use Before or During Early Pregnancy

Extensive epidemiological studies have revealed no increased risk of birth defects in women who have used oral contraceptives prior to pregnancy[56,57]. Studies also do not indicate a teratogenic effect, particularly in so far as cardiac anomalies and limb reduction defects are concerned[55,56,58,59], when oral contraceptives are taken inadvertently during early pregnancy.

Combination hormonal contraceptives such as ORTHO EVRA® should not be used to induce withdrawal bleeding as a test for pregnancy. ORTHO EVRA® should not be used during pregnancy to treat threatened or habitual abortion. It is recommended that for any patient who has missed two consecutive periods, pregnancy should be ruled out. If the patient has not adhered to the prescribed schedule for the use of ORTHO EVRA® the possibility of pregnancy should be considered at the time of the first missed period. Hormonal contraceptive use should be discontinued if pregnancy is confirmed.

7. Gallbladder Disease

Earlier studies have reported an increased lifetime relative risk of gallbladder surgery in users of hormonal contraceptives and estrogens[60,61]. More recent studies, however, have shown that the relative risk of developing gallbladder disease among hormonal contraceptive users may be minimal[62–64]. The recent findings of minimal risk may be related to the use of hormonal contraceptive formulations containing lower hormonal doses of estrogens and progestins. Combination hormonal contraceptives such as ORTHO EVRA® may worsen existing gallbladder disease and may accelerate the development of this disease in previously asymptomatic women. Women with a history of combination hormonal contraceptive-related cholestasis are more likely to have the condition recur with subsequent combination hormonal contraceptive use.

8. Carbohydrate and Lipid Metabolic Effects

Hormonal contraceptives have been shown to cause a decrease in glucose tolerance in some users[17]. However, in the non-diabetic woman, combination hormonal contraceptives appear to have no effect on fasting blood glucose[67]. Prediabetic and diabetic women in particular should be carefully monitored while taking combination hormonal contraceptives such as ORTHO EVRA®.

In clinical trials with oral contraceptives containing ethinyl estradiol and norgestimate there were no clinically significant changes in fasting blood glucose levels. There were no clinically significant changes in glucose levels over 24 cycles of use. Moreover, glucose tolerance tests showed no clinically significant changes from baseline to cycles 3, 12 and 24. In a 6-cycle clinical trial with ORTHO EVRA® there were no clinically significant changes in fasting blood glucose from baseline to end of treatment.

A small proportion of women will have persistent hypertriglyceridemia while taking hormonal contraceptives. As discussed earlier (see WARNINGS 1a and 1d), changes in serum triglycerides and lipoprotein levels have been reported in hormonal contraceptive users.

9. Elevated Blood Pressure

Women with significant hypertension should not be started on hormonal contraception[103]. Women with a history of hypertension or hypertension-related diseases, or renal disease[70] should be encouraged to use another method of contraception. If these women elect to use ORTHO EVRA®, they should be monitored closely and if a clinically significant persistent elevation of blood pressure (BP) occurs (≥ 160 mm Hg systolic or ≥ 100 mm Hg diastolic) and cannot be adequately controlled, ORTHO EVRA® should be discontinued. In general, women who develop hypertension during hormonal contraceptive therapy should be switched to a non-hormonal contraceptive. If other contraceptive methods are not suitable, hormonal contraceptive therapy may continue combined with antihypertensive therapy. Regular monitoring of BP throughout hormonal contraceptive therapy is recommended.[112] For most women, elevated blood pressure will return to normal after stopping hormonal contraceptives, and there is no difference in the occurrence of hypertension between former and never users[68–71].

An increase in blood pressure has been reported in women taking hormonal contraceptives[68] and this increase is more likely in older hormonal contraceptive users[69] and with extended duration of use[61]. Data from the Royal College of General Practitioners[12] and subsequent randomized trials have shown that the incidence of hypertension increases with increasing progestational activity.

10. Headache

The onset or exacerbation of migraine headache or the development of headache with a new pattern that is recurrent, persistent or severe requires discontinuation of ORTHO EVRA® and evaluation of the cause.

11. Bleeding Irregularities

Breakthrough bleeding and spotting are sometimes encountered in women using ORTHO EVRA®. Non-hormonal causes should be considered and adequate diagnostic measures taken to rule out malignancy, other pathology, or pregnancy in the event of breakthrough bleeding, as in the case of any abnormal vaginal bleeding. If pathology has been excluded, time or a change to another contraceptive product may resolve the bleeding. In the event of amenorrhea, pregnancy should be ruled out before initiating use of ORTHO EVRA®.

Some women may encounter amenorrhea or oligomenorrhea after discontinuation of hormonal contraceptive use, especially when such a condition was pre-existent.

Bleeding Patterns

In the clinical trials most women started their withdrawal bleeding on the fourth day of the drug-free interval, and the median duration of withdrawal bleeding was 5 to 6 days. On average 26% of women per cycle had 7 or more total days of bleeding and/or spotting (this includes both withdrawal flow and breakthrough bleeding and/or spotting).

12. Ectopic Pregnancy

Ectopic as well as intrauterine pregnancy may occur in contraceptive failures.

PRECAUTIONS

Women should be counseled that ORTHO EVRA® does not protect against HIV infection (AIDS) and other sexually transmitted infections.

1. Body Weight ≥198 lbs. (90 kg)

Results of clinical trials suggest that ORTHO EVRA® may be less effective in women with body weight ≥198 lbs. (90 kg) than in women with lower body weights.

2. Physical Examination and Follow-Up

It is good medical practice for women using ORTHO EVRA®, as for all women, to have annual medical evaluation and physical examinations. The physical examination, however, may be deferred until after initiation of hormonal contraceptives if requested by the woman and judged appropriate by the clinician. The physical examination should include special reference to blood pressure, breasts, abdomen and pelvic organs, including cervical cytology, and relevant laboratory tests. In case of undiagnosed, persistent or recurrent abnormal vaginal bleeding, appropriate measures should be conducted to rule out malignancy or other pathology. Women with a strong family history of breast cancer or who have breast nodules should be monitored with particular care.

3. Lipid Disorders

Women who are being treated for hyperlipidemias should be followed closely if they elect to use ORTHO EVRA®. Some progestins may elevate LDL levels and may render the control of hyperlipidemias more difficult.

4. Liver Function

If jaundice develops in any woman using ORTHO EVRA®, the medication should be discontinued. The hormones in ORTHO EVRA® may be poorly metabolized in patients with impaired liver function.

5. Fluid Retention

Steroid hormones like those in ORTHO EVRA® may cause some degree of fluid retention. ORTHO EVRA® should be prescribed with caution, and only with careful monitoring, in patients with conditions which might be aggravated by fluid retention.

6. Emotional Disorders

Women who become significantly depressed while using combination hormonal contraceptives such as ORTHO EVRA® should stop the medication and use another method of contraception in an attempt to determine whether the symptom is drug related. Women with a history of depression should be carefully observed and ORTHO EVRA® discontinued if significant depression occurs.

7. Contact Lenses

Contact lens wearers who develop visual changes or changes in lens tolerance should be assessed by an ophthalmologist.

8. Drug Interactions

Changes in Contraceptive Effectiveness Associated With Co-Administration of Other Drugs

If a woman on hormonal contraceptives takes a drug or herbal product that induces enzymes, including CYP3A4, that metabolize contraceptive hormones, counsel her to use additional contraception or a different method of contraception. Drugs or herbal products that induce such enzymes may decrease the plasma concentrations of contraceptive hormones, and may decrease the effectiveness of hormonal contraceptives or increase breakthrough bleeding. Some drugs or herbal products that may decrease the effectiveness of hormonal contraceptives include:

- barbiturates
- bosentan
- carbamazepine
- felbamate
- griseofulvin
- oxcarbazepine
- phenytoin
- rifampin
- St. John's wort
- topiramate

HIV protease inhibitors and non-nucleoside reverse transcriptase inhibitors

Significant changes (increase or decrease) in the plasma levels of the estrogen and progestin have been noted in some cases of co-administration of HIV protease inhibitors and non-nucleoside reverse transcriptase inhibitors.

Antibiotics

There have been reports of pregnancy while taking hormonal contraceptives and antibiotics, but clinical pharmacokinetic studies have not shown consistent effects of antibiotics on plasma concentrations of synthetic steroids. In a pharmacokinetic drug interaction study, oral administration of tetracycline HCl, 500 mg q.i.d. for 3 days prior to and 7 days during wear of ORTHO EVRA® did not significantly affect the pharmacokinetics of norelgestromin or EE.

Consult the labeling of the concurrently-used drug to obtain further information about interactions with hormonal contraceptives or the potential for enzyme alterations.

Increase in Plasma Hormone Levels Associated With Co-Administered Drugs

Some drugs and grapefruit juice may increase the plasma levels of ethinyl estradiol if co-administered. Examples include:

- acetaminophen
- ascorbic acid
- CYP3A4 inhibitors (including itraconazole, ketoconazole, voriconazole, fluconazole and grapefruit juice)
- HMG-CoA reductase inhibitors (including atorvastatin and rosuvastatin)

Changes in Plasma Levels of Co-Administered Drugs

Data from oral combination hormonal contraceptives indicate that they may also affect the pharmacokinetics of some other drugs if used concomitantly.

Examples of drugs whose plasma levels may be increased (due to CYP inhibition) include:

- cyclosporine
- prednisolone
- theophylline

Examples of drugs whose plasma levels may be decreased (due to induction of glucuronidation) include:

- acetaminophen
- clofibric acid
- lamotrigine (see below)
- morphine
- salicylic acid
- temazepam

Combined hormonal contraceptives have been shown to significantly decrease plasma concentrations of lamotrigine when co-administered likely due to induction of lamotrigine glucuronidation. This may reduce seizure control; therefore, dosage adjustments of lamotrigine may be necessary.

Consult the labeling of concurrently-used drugs to obtain further information about interactions with hormonal contraceptives or the potential for enzyme alterations.

9. Interactions with Laboratory Tests

Certain endocrine and liver function tests and blood components may be affected by hormonal contraceptives:

1. Increased prothrombin and factors VII, VIII, IX, and X; decreased antithrombin 3; increased norepinephrine-induced platelet aggregability.
2. Increased thyroid binding globulin (TBG) leading to increased circulating total thyroid hormone, as measured by protein-bound iodine (PBI), T4 by column or by radioimmunoassay. Free T3 resin uptake is decreased, reflecting the elevated TBG, free T4 concentration is unaltered.
3. Other binding proteins may be elevated in serum.
4. Sex hormone binding globulins are increased and result in elevated levels of total circulating endogenous sex steroids and corticoids; however, free or biologically active levels either decrease or remain unchanged.
5. Triglycerides may be increased and levels of various other lipids and lipoproteins may be affected.
6. Glucose tolerance may be decreased.
7. Serum folate levels may be depressed by hormonal contraceptive therapy. This may be of clinical significance if a woman becomes pregnant shortly after discontinuing ORTHO EVRA®.

10. Carcinogenesis

No carcinogenicity studies were conducted with norelgestromin. However, bridging PK studies were conducted using doses of norgestimate (NGM)/EE which were used previously in the 2-year rat carcinogenicity study and 10-year monkey toxicity study to support the approval of ORTHO-CYCLEN® and ORTHO TRI-CYCLEN® under NDAs 19-653 and 19-697, respectively. The PK studies demonstrated that rats and monkeys were exposed to 16 and 8 times the human exposure, respectively, with the proposed ORTHO EVRA® transdermal contraceptive system.

Norelgestromin was tested in in-vitro mutagenicity assays (bacterial plate incorporation mutation assay, CHO/HGPRT mutation assay, chromosomal aberration assay using cultured human peripheral lymphocytes) and in one in-vivo test (rat micronucleus assay) and found to have no genotoxic potential.

See WARNINGS Section.

11. Pregnancy

Pregnancy Category X

See CONTRAINDICATIONS and WARNINGS Sections.

Norelgestromin was tested for its reproductive toxicity in a rabbit developmental toxicity study by the SC route of administration. Doses of 0, 1, 2, 4 and 6 mg/kg body weight, which gave systemic exposure of approximately 25 to 125 times the human exposure with ORTHO EVRA®, were administered daily on gestation days 7–19. Malformations reported were paw hyperflexion at 4 and 6 mg/kg and paw hyperextension and cleft palate at 6 mg/kg.

12. Nursing Mothers

The effects of ORTHO EVRA® in nursing mothers have not been evaluated and are unknown. Small amounts of combination hormonal contraceptive steroids have been identified in the milk of nursing mothers and a few adverse effects on the child have been reported, including jaundice and breast enlargement. In addition, combination hormonal contraceptives given in the postpartum period may interfere with lactation by decreasing the quantity and quality of breast milk. Long-term follow-up of infants whose mothers used combination hormonal contraceptives while breastfeeding has shown no deleterious effects. However, the nursing mother should be advised not to use ORTHO EVRA® but to use other forms of contraception until she has completely weaned her child.

13. Pediatric Use

Safety and efficacy of ORTHO EVRA® have been established in women of reproductive age. Safety and efficacy are expected to be the same for post-pubertal adolescents under the age of 16 and for users 16 years and older. Use of this product before menarche is not indicated.

14. Geriatric Use

This product has not been studied in women over 65 years of age and is not indicated in this population.

15. Sexually Transmitted Diseases

Patients should be counseled that this product does not protect against HIV infection (AIDS) and other sexually transmitted diseases.

16. Patch Adhesion

Experience with more than 70,000 ORTHO EVRA® patches worn for contraception for 6–13 cycles showed that 4.7% of patches were replaced because they either fell off (1.8%) or were partly detached (2.9%). Similarly, in a small study of patch wear under conditions of physical exertion and variable temperature and humidity, less than 2% of patches were replaced for complete or partial detachment.

If the ORTHO EVRA® patch becomes partially or completely detached and remains detached, insufficient drug delivery occurs. A patch should not be re-applied if it is no longer sticky, if it has become stuck to itself or another surface, if it has other material stuck to it, or if it has become loose or fallen off before. If a patch cannot be re-applied, a new patch should be applied immediately. Supplemental adhesives or wraps should not be used to hold the ORTHO EVRA® patch in place.

If a patch is partially or completely detached for more than one day (24 hours or more) OR if the woman is not sure how long the patch has been detached, she may not be protected from pregnancy. She should stop the current contraceptive cycle and start a new cycle immediately by applying a new patch. Back-up contraception, such as condoms, spermicide, or diaphragm, must be used for the first week of the new cycle.

INFORMATION FOR THE PATIENT

See Patient Labeling printed below.

ADVERSE REACTIONS

The following serious adverse reactions with the use of combination hormonal contraceptives, including ORTHO EVRA®, are discussed elsewhere in the labeling:

- Serious cardiovascular events and smoking (see WARNINGS)
- Vascular events, including venous and arterial thromboembolic events (see WARNINGS)
- Liver disease (see WARNINGS and PRECAUTIONS)

Adverse reactions commonly reported by users of combination hormonal contraceptives are:

- Irregular uterine bleeding
- Nausea
- Breast tenderness
- Headache

Clinical Trials Experience

Because clinical trials are conducted under widely varying conditions, adverse reaction rates observed in the clinical trials of a drug cannot be directly compared to rates in the clinical trials of another drug and may not reflect the rates observed in practice.

The data described below reflect exposure to ORTHO EVRA® in 3330 sexually active women (3322 of whom had safety data) who participated in three Phase 3 clinical trials designed to evaluate contraceptive efficacy and safety. These subjects received six or 13 cycles of contraception (ORTHO EVRA® or an oral contraceptive comparator in 2 of the trials). The women ranged in age from 18 to 45 years and were predominantly white (91%).

The most common adverse reactions reported during clinical trials were breast symptoms, headache, application site disorder, nausea, dysmenorrhea and abdominal pain. The most common events leading to discontinuation were application site reaction, breast symptoms (including breast discomfort, engorgement and pain), nausea and/or vomiting, headache and emotional lability.

Adverse drug reactions reported by ≥ 2.5% of ORTHO EVRA®-treated subjects in these trials are shown in Table 7.

Table 7. Adverse Drug Reactions Reported by ≥ 2.5% of ORTHO EVRA®-treated Subjects in Three Phase 3 Clinical Trials

System/Organ Class* Adverse reaction	ORTHO EVRA® (n=3322)
Reproductive system and breast disorders	
Breast symptoms†	22.4%
Dysmenorrhea	7.8%
Vaginal bleeding and menstrual disorders†	6.4%
Gastrointestinal disorders	
Nausea	16.6%
Abdominal pain†	8.1%
Vomiting	5.1%
Diarrhea	4.2%
Nervous system disorders	
Headache	21.0%
Dizziness	3.3%
Migraine	2.7%
General disorders and administration site conditions	
Application site disorder†	17.1%
Fatigue	2.6%
Psychiatric disorders	
Mood, affect and anxiety disorders†	6.3%
Skin and subcutaneous tissue disorders	
Acne	2.9%
Pruritus	2.5%
Infections and infestations	
Vaginal yeast infection†	3.9%
Investigations	
Weight increased	2.7%

*MedDRA version 10.0
†Represents a bundle of similar terms

Additional adverse drug reactions that occurred in < 2.5% of ORTHO EVRA®-treated subjects in the above clinical trials datasets are:
• **Gastrointestinal disorders:** Abdominal distension
• **General disorders and administration site conditions:** Fluid retention[1], malaise
• **Hepatobiliary disorders:** Cholecystitis
• **Investigations:** Blood pressure increased, lipid disorders[1]
• **Musculoskeletal and connective tissue disorders:** Muscle spasms
• **Psychiatric disorders:** Insomnia, libido decreased, libido increased
• **Reproductive system and breast disorders:** Galactorrhea, genital discharge, premenstrual syndrome, uterine spasm, vaginal discharge, vulvovaginal dryness
• **Respiratory, thoracic and mediastinal disorders:** Pulmonary embolism
• **Skin and subcutaneous tissue disorders:** Chloasma, dermatitis contact, erythema, skin irritation

[1]Represents a bundle of similar terms

Postmarketing Experience
The following adverse reactions (Table 8) have been identified during postapproval use of ORTHO EVRA®. Because these reactions are reported voluntarily from a population of uncertain size, it is not always possible to reliably estimate their frequency or establish a causal relationship to drug exposure.
[See table 8 at top of next page]

OVERDOSAGE

Serious ill effects have not been reported following accidental ingestion of large doses of hormonal contraceptives. Overdosage may cause nausea and vomiting, and withdrawal bleeding may occur in females. Given the nature and design of the ORTHO EVRA® patch, it is unlikely that overdosage will occur. Serious ill effects have not been reported following acute ingestion of large doses of oral contraceptives by young children. In case of suspected overdose, all ORTHO EVRA® patches should be removed and symptomatic treatment given.

DOSAGE AND ADMINISTRATION

To achieve maximum contraceptive effectiveness, ORTHO EVRA® must be used exactly as directed.

Complete instructions to facilitate patient counseling on proper system usage may be found in the Detailed Patient Labeling.

Transdermal Contraceptive System Overview
ORTHO EVRA® is a combination transdermal contraceptive that contains 6.00 mg norelgestromin (NGMN) and 0.75 mg ethinyl estradiol (EE). Systemic exposures (as measured by AUC and C_{ss}) of NGMN and EE during use of ORTHO EVRA® are higher and peak concentrations (C_{max}) are lower than those produced by an oral contraceptive containing norgestimate 250 mcg / EE 35 mcg. (See BOLDED WARNING; CLINICAL PHARMACOLOGY, Transdermal versus Oral Contraceptives.)

This system uses a 28-day (four-week) cycle. A new patch is applied each week for three weeks (21 total days). Week Four is patch-free. Withdrawal bleeding is expected during this time.

Every new patch should be applied on the same day of the week. This day is known as the "Patch Change Day." For example, if the first patch is applied on a Monday, all subsequent patches should be applied on a Monday. Only one patch should be worn at a time.

The ORTHO EVRA® patch should not be cut, damaged or altered in any way. If the ORTHO EVRA® patch is cut, damaged or altered in size, contraceptive efficacy may be impaired.

On the day after Week Four ends a new four-week cycle is started by applying a new patch. Under no circumstances should there be more than a seven-day patch-free interval between dosing cycles.

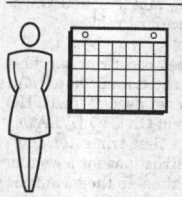

If the woman is starting ORTHO EVRA® for the **first time**, she should **wait until the day she begins her menstrual period.** Either a First Day start or Sunday start may be chosen (see below). The day she applies her first patch will be Day 1. Her "Patch Change Day" will be on this day every week.

CHOOSE ONE OPTION:

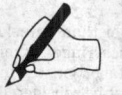

☐ **First Day Start**
or
☐ **Sunday Start**

• for **First Day Start:** the patient should apply her first patch during the first 24 hours of her menstrual period.
If therapy starts after Day 1 of the menstrual cycle, a non-hormonal back-up contraceptive (such as a condoms, spermicide, or diaphragm) should be used concurrently for the first 7 consecutive days of the first treatment cycle.

• for **Sunday Start:** the woman should apply her first patch on the first Sunday after her menstrual period starts. She must use back-up contraception for the first week of her first cycle.

If the menstrual period begins on a Sunday, the first patch should be applied on that day, and no back-up contraception is needed.

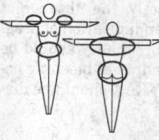

Where to apply the patch. The patch should be applied to clean, dry, intact healthy skin on the buttock, abdomen, upper outer arm or upper torso, in a place where it won't be rubbed by tight clothing. ORTHO EVRA® should not be placed on skin that is red, irritated or cut, nor should it be placed on the breasts.
To prevent interference with the adhesive properties of ORTHO EVRA®, no make-up, creams, lotions, powders or other topical products should be applied to the skin area where the ORTHO EVRA® patch is or will be placed.

Application of the ORTHO EVRA® patch

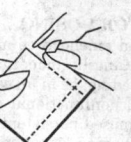

The foil pouch is opened by tearing it along the edge using the fingers.

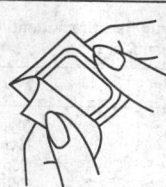

The foil pouch should be peeled apart and open flat.

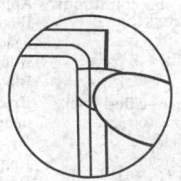

A corner of the patch is grasped firmly and it is gently removed from the foil pouch.

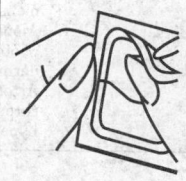

The woman should be instructed to use her fingernail to lift one corner of the patch and peel the patch **and the plastic liner off the foil liner. Sometimes patches can stick to the inside of the pouch – the woman should be careful not to accidentally remove the clear liner as she removes the patch.**
Half of the clear protective liner is to be peeled away. (The woman should avoid touching the sticky surface of the patch.)

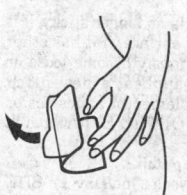

The sticky surface of the patch is applied to the skin and the other half of the liner is removed. The woman should press down firmly on the patch with the palm of her hand for 10 seconds, making sure that the edges stick well. She should check her patch every day to make sure it is sticking.

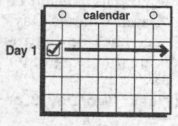

The patch is worn for seven days (one week). On the "Patch Change Day", Day 8, the used patch is removed and a new one is applied immediately. The used patch still contains some active hormones. Used patches should not be flushed down the toilet. For disposal directions, see HOW SUPPLIED: Special Precautions for Storage and Disposal.

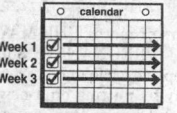

A new patch is applied for Week Two (on Day 8) and again for Week Three (on Day 15), on the usual "Patch Change Day". Patch changes may occur at any time on the Change Day. Each new ORTHO EVRA® patch should be applied to a new spot on the skin to help avoid irritation, although they may be kept within the same anatomic area.

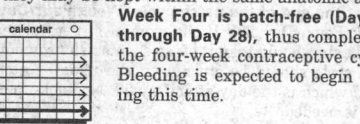

Week Four is patch-free (Day 22 through Day 28), thus completing the four-week contraceptive cycle. Bleeding is expected to begin during this time.

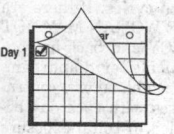

The next four-week cycle is started by applying a new patch on the usual "Patch Change Day," the day after Day 28, no matter when the menstrual period begins or ends. Under no circumstances should there be more than a seven-day patch-free interval between patch cycles.

If the ORTHO EVRA® patch becomes partially or completely detached and remains detached, insufficient drug delivery occurs.
If a patch is partially or completely detached:
• **for less than one day** (up to 24 hours), the woman should try to reapply it to the same place or replace it with a new patch immediately. No back-up contraception is needed. The woman's "Patch Change Day" will remain the same.
• **for more than one day** (24 hours or more) **OR if the woman is not sure how long the patch has been detached, SHE MAY NOT BE PROTECTED FROM PREGNANCY.** She should stop the current contraceptive cycle and start a new cycle immediately by applying a new patch. There is now a new "Day 1" and a new "Patch

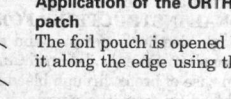

Table 8. Alphabetical List of Adverse Drug Reactions Identified During Postmarketing Experience with ORTHO EVRA®/EVRA® by System Organ Class*

System Organ Class	Adverse Drug Reactions
Cardiac disorders	Myocardial infarction†
Endocrine disorders	Hyperglycemia, insulin resistance
Eye disorders	Contact lens intolerance or complication
Gastrointestinal disorders	Colitis
General disorders and administration site conditions	Application site reaction†, edema†
Hepatobiliary disorders	Blood cholesterol abnormal, cholelithiasis, cholestasis, hepatic lesion, jaundice cholestatic, low density lipoprotein increased
Immune system disorders	Allergic reaction†, urticaria
Investigations	Blood glucose abnormal, blood glucose decreased
Neoplasms benign, malignant and unspecified (Incl cysts and polyps)	Breast cancer†, cervix carcinoma, hepatic adenoma, hepatic neoplasm
Nervous system disorders	Dysgeusia, migraine with aura
Psychiatric disorders	Anger, emotional disorder, frustration, irritability
Reproductive system and breast disorders	Breast mass, cervical dysplasia, fibroadenoma of breast, menstrual disorder†, suppressed lactation, uterine leiomyoma
Skin and subcutaneous tissues disorders	Alopecia, eczema, erythema multiforme, erythema nodosum, photosensitivity reaction, pruritus generalized, rash†, seborrheic dermatitis, skin reaction
Vascular disorders	Arterial thrombosis†, cerebrovascular accident†, deep vein thrombosis†, hemorrhage intracranial†, hypertension, hypertensive crisis, pulmonary embolism†, thrombosis†

*MedDRA version 10.0
†Represents a bundle of similar terms

Change Day." Back-up contraception, such as condoms, spermicide, or diaphragm, must be used for the first week of the new cycle.

A patch should not be re-applied if it is no longer sticky, if it has become stuck to itself or another surface, if it has other material stuck to it or if it has previously become loose or fallen off. If a patch cannot be re-applied, a new patch should be applied immediately. Supplemental adhesives or wraps should not be used to hold the ORTHO EVRA® patch in place.

If the woman forgets to change her patch…

- **at the start of any patch cycle** (Week One/Day 1): SHE MAY NOT BE **PROTECTED** FROM PREGNANCY. She should apply the first patch of her new cycle as soon as she remembers. There is now a new "Patch Change Day" and a new "Day 1." The woman must use back-up contraception, such as condoms, spermicide, or diaphragm, for the first week of the new cycle.
- **in the middle of the patch cycle (Week Two/Day 8 or Week Three/Day 15),**
  - — for **one or two days** (up to 48 hours), she should apply a new patch immediately. The next patch should be applied on the usual "Patch Change Day." No back-up contraception is needed.
  - — for **more than two days** (48 hours or more), SHE MAY NOT BE PROTECTED FROM PREGNANCY. She should stop the current contraceptive cycle and start a new four-week cycle immediately by putting on a new patch. There is now a new "Patch Change Day" and a new "Day 1." The woman must use back-up contraception for one week.
- **at the end of the patch cycle (Week Four/Day 22),**

Week Four (Day 22): If the woman forgets to remove her patch, she should take it off as soon as she remembers. The next cycle should be started on the usual "Patch Change Day," which is the day after Day 28. No back-up contraception is needed.

Under no circumstances should there be more than a seven-day patch-free interval between cycles. If there are more than seven patch-free days, THE WOMAN MAY NOT BE PROTECTED FROM PREGNANCY and back-up contraception, such as condoms, spermicide, or diaphragm, must be used for seven days. As with combined oral contraceptives, the risk of ovulation increases with each day beyond the recommended drug-free period. If coital exposure has occurred during such an extended patch-free interval, the possibility of fertilization should be considered.

Change Day Adjustment

If the woman wishes to change her Patch Change Day she should complete her current cycle, removing the third ORTHO EVRA® patch on the correct day. During the patch-free week, she may select an earlier Patch Day Change by applying a new ORTHO EVRA® patch on the desired day. In no case should there be more than 7 consecutive patch-free days.

Switching From an Oral Contraceptive

Treatment with ORTHO EVRA® should begin on the first day of withdrawal bleeding. If there is no withdrawal bleeding within 5 days of the last active (hormone-containing) tablet, pregnancy must be ruled out. If therapy starts later than the first day of withdrawal bleeding, a non-hormonal contraceptive should be used concurrently for 7 days. If more than 7 days elapse after taking the last active oral contraceptive tablet, the possibility of ovulation and conception should be considered.

Use After Childbirth

Women who elect not to breastfeed should start contraceptive therapy with ORTHO EVRA® no sooner than 4 weeks after childbirth. If a woman begins using ORTHO EVRA® postpartum, and has not yet had a period, the possibility of ovulation and conception occurring prior to use of ORTHO EVRA® should be considered, and she should be instructed to use an additional method of contraception, such as condoms, spermicide, or diaphragm, for the first seven days. (See Precautions: Nursing Mothers, and Warnings: Thromboembolic and Other Vascular Problems.)

Use After Abortion or Miscarriage[106]

After an abortion or miscarriage that occurs in the first trimester, ORTHO EVRA® may be started immediately. An additional method of contraception is not needed if ORTHO EVRA® is started immediately. If use of ORTHO EVRA® is not started within 5 days following a first trimester abortion, the woman should follow the instructions for a woman starting ORTHO EVRA® for the first time. In the meantime she should be advised to use a non-hormonal contraceptive method. Ovulation may occur within 10 days of an abortion or miscarriage.

ORTHO EVRA® should be started no earlier than 4 weeks after a second trimester abortion or miscarriage. When ORTHO EVRA® is used postpartum or postabortion, the increased risk of thromboembolic disease must be considered. (See CONTRAINDICATIONS and WARNINGS concerning thromboembolic disease. See PRECAUTIONS for "Nursing Mothers".)

Breakthrough Bleeding or Spotting

In the event of breakthrough bleeding or spotting (bleeding that occurs on the days that ORTHO EVRA® is worn), treatment should be continued. If breakthrough bleeding persists longer than a few cycles, a cause other than ORTHO EVRA® should be considered.

In the event of no withdrawal bleeding (bleeding that should occur during the patch-free week), treatment should be resumed on the next scheduled Change Day. If ORTHO EVRA® has been used correctly, the absence of withdrawal bleeding is not necessarily an indication of pregnancy. Nevertheless, the possibility of pregnancy should be considered, especially if absence of withdrawal bleeding occurs in 2 consecutive cycles. ORTHO EVRA® should be discontinued if pregnancy is confirmed.

In Case of Vomiting or Diarrhea

Given the nature of transdermal application, dose delivery should be unaffected by vomiting.

In Case of Skin Irritation

If patch use results in uncomfortable irritation, the patch may be removed and a new patch may be applied to a different location until the next Change Day. Only one patch should be worn at a time.

ADDITIONAL INSTRUCTIONS FOR DOSING

Breakthrough bleeding, spotting, and amenorrhea are frequent reasons for patients discontinuing hormonal contraceptives. In case of breakthrough bleeding, as in all cases of irregular bleeding from the vagina, nonfunctional causes should considered. In case of undiagnosed persistent or recurrent abnormal bleeding from the vagina, adequate diagnostic measures are indicated to rule out pregnancy or malignancy. If pathology has been excluded, time or a change to another method of contraception may solve the problem.

Use of Hormonal Contraceptives in the Event of a Missed Menstrual Period

1. If the woman has not adhered to the prescribed schedule, the possibility of pregnancy should be considered at the time of the first missed period. Hormonal contraceptive use should be discontinued if pregnancy is confirmed.
2. If the woman has adhered to the prescribed regimen and misses one period, she should continue using her contraceptive patches.
3. If the woman has adhered to the prescribed regimen and misses two consecutive periods, pregnancy should be ruled out. ORTHO EVRA® use should be discontinued if pregnancy is confirmed.

HOW SUPPLIED

Each beige ORTHO EVRA® patch contains 6.00 mg norelgestromin and 0.75 mg EE.

Each patch surface is heat stamped with ORTHO EVRA®.

Each patch is packaged in a protective pouch.

ORTHO EVRA® is available in folding cartons of 1 cycle each (NDC # 0062-1920-15); each cycle contains 3 patches.

ORTHO EVRA® is available for clinic usage in folding cartons of 1 cycle each (NDC # 0062-1920-24); each cycle contains 3 patches.

ORTHO EVRA® is also available in folding cartons containing a single patch (NDC # 0062-1920-01), intended for use as a replacement in the event that a patch is inadvertently lost or destroyed.

Special Precautions for Storage and Disposal

Store at 25°C (77°F); excursions permitted to 15–30°C (59–86°F).

Store patches in their protective pouches. Apply immediately upon removal from the protective pouch.

Do not store in the refrigerator or freezer.

Used patches still contain some active hormones. The sticky sides of the patch should be folded together and the folded patch placed in a sturdy container, preferably with a child-resistant cap, and the container thrown in the trash. Used patches should not be flushed down the toilet.

REFERENCES

1. Trussell J. Contraceptive efficacy. In Hatcher RA, Trussell J, Stewart F, Cates W, Stewart GK, Kowal D, Guest F. *Contraceptive Technology: Seventeenth Revised Edition.* New York NY: Irvington Publishers, 1998.
2. Stadel BV. Oral contraceptives and cardiovascular disease. (Pt.1). N Engl J Med 1981; 305:612–618.
3. Stadel BV. Oral contraceptives and cardiovascular disease. (Pt.2). N Engl J Med 1981; 305:672–677.
4. Adam SA, Thorogood M. Oral contraception and myocardial infarction revisited: the effects of new preparations and prescribing patterns. Br J Obstet Gynaecol 1981; 88:838–845.
5. Mann J, Inman WH. Oral contraceptives and death from myocardial infarction. Br Med J 1975; 2(5965): 245–248.
6. Mann J, Vessey MP, Thorogood M, Doll R. Myocardial infarction in young women with special reference to oral contraceptive practice. Br Med J 1975; 2(5956): 241–245.
7. Royal College of General Practitioners' Oral Contraception Study: Further analyses of mortality in oral contraceptive users. Lancet 1981; 1:541–546.
8. Slone D, Shapiro S, Kaufman DW, Rosenberg L, Miettinen OS, Stolley PD. Risk of myocardial infarction in relation to current and discontinued use of oral contraceptives. N Engl J Med 1981:305:420–424.
9. Vessey MP. Female hormones and vascular disease-an epidemiological overview. Br J Fam Plann 1980; 6 (Supplement): 1–12.
10. Russell-Briefel RG, Ezzati TM, Fulwood R, Perlman JA, Murphy RS. Cardiovascular risk status and oral contraceptive use, United States, 1976–80. Prevent Med 1986; 15:352–362.
11. Goldbaum GM, Kendrick JS, Hogelin GC, Gentry EM. The relative impact of smoking and oral contraceptive use on women in the United States. JAMA 1987; 258: 1339–1342.
12. Layde PM, Beral V. Further analyses of mortality in oral contraceptive users; Royal College of General Practitioners' Oral Contraception Study. (Table 5) Lancet 1981; 1:541–546.
13. Knopp RH. Arteriosclerosis risk: the roles of oral contraceptives and postmenopausal estrogens. J Reprod Med 1986; 31(9) (Supplement):913–921.
14. Krauss RM, Roy S, Mishell DR, Casagrande J, Pike MC. Effects of two low-dose oral contraceptives on serum lipids and lipoproteins: Differential changes in high-density lipoproteins subclasses. Am J Obstet 1983; 145:446–452.

15. Wahl P, Walden C, Knopp R, Hoover J, Wallace R, Heiss G, Rifkind B. Effect of estrogen/progestin potency on lipid/lipoprotein cholesterol. N Engl J Med 1983; 308:862–867.

16. Wynn V, Niththyananthan R. The effect of progestin in combined oral contraceptives on serum lipids with special reference to high density lipoproteins. Am J Obstet Gynecol 1982;142:766–771.

17. Wynn V, Godsland I. Effects of oral contraceptives on carbohydrate metabolism. J Reprod Med 1986; 31(9)(Supplement):892–897.

18. LaRosa JC. Atherosclerotic risk factors in cardiovascular disease. J Reprod Med 1986;31(9)(Supplement): 906–912.

19. Inman WH, Vessey MP. Investigation of death from pulmonary, coronary, and cerebral thrombosis and embolism in women of child-bearing age. Br Med J 1968;2(5599):193–199.

20. Maguire MG, Tonascia J, Sartwell PE, Stolley PD, Tockman MS. Increased risk of thrombosis due to oral contraceptives: a further report. Am J Epidemiol 1979;110(2):188–195.

21. Petitti DB, Wingerd J, Pellegrin F, Ramacharan S. Risk of vascular disease in women: smoking, oral contraceptives, noncontraceptive estrogens, and other factors. JAMA 1979;242:1150–1154.

22. Vessey MP, Doll R. Investigation of relation between use of oral contraceptives and thromboembolic disease. Br Med J 1968;2(5599):199–205.

23. Vessey MP, Doll R. Investigation of relation between use of oral contraceptives and thromboembolic disease. A further report. Br Med J 1969; 2(5658):651–657.

24. Porter JB, Hunter JR, Danielson DA, Jick H, Stergachis A. Oral contraceptives and non-fatal vascular disease-recent experience. Obstet Gynecol 1982;59(3):299–302.

25. Vessey M, Doll R, Peto R, Johnson B, Wiggins P. A long-term follow-up study of women using different methods of contraception: an interim report. J Biosocial Sci 1976;8:375–427.

26. Royal College of General Practitioners: Oral Contraceptives, venous thrombosis, and varicose veins. J Royal Coll Gen Pract 1978; 28:393–399.

27. Collaborative Group for the Study of Stroke in Young Women: Oral contraception and increased risk of cerebral ischemia or thrombosis. N Engl J Med 1973;288:871–878.

28. Petitti DB, Wingerd J. Use of oral contraceptives, cigarette smoking, and risk of subarachnoid hemorrhage. Lancet 1978;2:234–236.

29. Inman WH. Oral contraceptives and fatal subarachnoid hemorrhage. Br Med J 1979:2(6203):1468–1470.

30. Collaborative Group for the Study of Stroke in Young Women: Oral Contraceptives and stroke in young women: associated risk factors. JAMA 1975; 231: 718–722.

31. Inman WH, Vessey MP, Westerholm B, Engelund A. Thromboembolic disease and the steroidal content of oral contraceptives. A report to the Committee on Safety of Drugs. Br Med J 1970;2:203–209.

32. Meade TW, Greenberg G, Thompson SG. Progestogens and cardiovascular reactions associated with oral contraceptives and a comparison of the safety of 50- and 35-mcg oestrogen preparations. Br Med J 1980;280(6224):1157–1161.

33. Kay CR. Progestogens and arterial disease-evidence from the Royal College of General Practitioners' Study. Am J Obstet Gynecol 1982;142:762–765.

34. Royal College of General Practitioners: Incidence of arterial disease among oral contraceptive users. J Royal Coll Gen Pract 1983;33:75–82.

35. Ory HW. Mortality associated with fertility and fertility control: 1983. Family Planning Perspectives 1983;15:50–56.

36. The Cancer and Steroid Hormone Study of the Centers for Disease Control and the National Institute of Child Health and Human Development: Oral contraceptive use and the risk of breast cancer. N Engl J Med 1986;315:405–411.

37. Pike MC, Henderson BE, Krailo MD, Duke A, Roy S. Breast cancer in young women and use of oral contraceptives: possible modifying effect of formulation and age at use. Lancet 1983;2:926–929.

38. Paul C, Skegg DG, Spears GFS, Kaldor JM. Oral contraceptives and breast cancer: A national study. Br Med J 1986; 293:723–725.

39. Miller DR, Rosenberg L, Kaufman DW, Schottenfeld D, Stolley PD, Shapiro S. Breast cancer risk in relation to early oral contraceptive use. Obstet Gynecol 1986;68: 863–868.

40. Olson H, Olson KL, Moller TR, Ranstam J, Holm P. Oral contraceptive use and breast cancer in young women in Sweden (letter). Lancet 1985; 2:748–749.

41. McPherson K, Vessey M, Neil A, Doll R, Jones L, Roberts M. Early contraceptive use and breast cancer: Results of another case-control study. Br J Cancer 1987; 56:653–660.

42. Huggins GR, Zucker PF. Oral contraceptives and neoplasia; 1987 update. Fertil Steril 1987; 47:733–761.

43. McPherson K, Drife JO. The pill and breast cancer: why the uncertainty? Br Med J 1986; 293:709–710.

44. Shapiro S. Oral contraceptives-time to take stock. N Engl J Med 1987; 315:450–451.

45. Ory H, Naib Z, Conger SB, Hatcher RA, Tyler CW. Contraceptive choice and prevalence of cervical dysplasia and carcinoma in situ. Am J Obstet Gynecol 1976; 124: 573–577.

46. Vessey MP, Lawless M, McPherson K, Yeates D. Neoplasia of the cervix uteri and contraception: a possible adverse effect of the pill. Lancet 1983; 2:930.

47. Brinton LA, Huggins GR, Lehman HF, Malli K, Savitz DA, Trapido E, Rosenthal J, Hoover R. Long term use of oral contraceptives and risk of invasive cervical cancer. Int J Cancer 1986; 38:339–344.

48. WHO Collaborative Study of Neoplasia and Steroid Contraceptives: Invasive cervical cancer and combined oral contraceptives. Br Med J 1985; 290:961–965.

49. Rooks JB, Ory HW, Ishak KG, Strauss LT, Greenspan JR, Hill AP, Tyler CW. Epidemiology of hepatocellular adenoma: the role of oral contraceptive use. JAMA 1979; 242:644–648.

50. Bein NN, Goldsmith HS. Recurrent massive hemorrhage from benign hepatic tumors secondary to oral contraceptives. Br J Surg 1977; 64:433–435.

51. Klatskin G. Hepatic tumors: possible relationship to use of oral contraceptives. Gastroenterology 1977; 73: 386–394.

52. Henderson BE, Preston-Martin S, Edmondson HA, Peters RL, Pike MC. Hepatocellular carcinoma and oral contraceptives. Br J Cancer 1983;48:437–440.

53. Neuberger J, Forman D, Doll R, Williams R. Oral contraceptives and hepatocellular carcinoma. Br Med J 1986; 292:1355–1357.

54. Forman D, Vincent TJ, Doll R. Cancer of the liver and oral contraceptives. Br Med J 1986; 292:1357–1361.

55. Harlap S, Eldor J. Births following oral contraceptive failures. Obstet Gynecol 1980; 55:447–452.

56. Savolainen E, Saksela E, Saxen L. Teratogenic hazards of oral contraceptives analyzed in a national malformation register. Am J Obstet Gynecol 1981; 140:521–524.

57. Janerich DT, Piper JM, Glebatis DM. Oral contraceptives and birth defects. Am J Epidemiol 1980; 112: 73–79.

58. Ferencz C, Matanoski GM, Wilson PD, Rubin JD, Neill CA, Gutberlet R. Maternal hormone therapy and congenital heart disease. Teratology 1980; 21:225–239.

59. Rothman KJ, Fyler DC, Goldblatt A, Kreidberg MB. Exogenous hormones and other drug exposures of children with congenital heart disease. Am J Epidemiol 1979; 109:433–439.

60. Boston Collaborative Drug Surveillance Program: Oral contraceptives and venous thromboembolic disease, surgically confirmed gallbladder disease, and breast tumors. Lancet 1973; 1:1399–1404.

61. Royal College of General Practitioners: Oral contraceptives and health. New York, Pittman 1974.

62. Layde PM, Vessey MP, Yeates D. Risk of gallbladder disease: a cohort study of young women attending family planning clinics. J Epidemiol Community Health 1982; 36:274–278.

63. Rome Group for Epidemiology and Prevention of Cholelithiasis (GREPCO): Prevalence of gallstone disease in an Italian adult female population. Am J Epidemiol 1984; 119:796–805.

64. Strom BL, Tamragouri RT, Morse ML, Lazar EL, West SL, Stolley PD, Jones JK. Oral contraceptives and other risk factors for gallbladder disease. Clin Pharmacol Ther 1986; 39:335–341.

65. Wynn V, Adams PW, Godsland IF, Melrose J, Niththyananthan R, Oakley NW, Seedj A. Comparison of effects of different combined oral contraceptive formulations on carbohydrate and lipid metabolism. Lancet 1979; 1:1045–1049.

66. Wynn V. Effect of progesterone and progestins on carbohydrate metabolism. In: Progesterone and Progestin. Bardin CW, Milgrom E, Mauvis-Jarvis P. eds. New York, Raven Press 1983; pp. 395–410.

67. Perlman JA, Roussell-Briefel RG, Ezzati TM, Lieberknecht G. Oral glucose tolerance and the potency of oral contraceptive progestogens. J Chronic Dis 1985;38:857–864.

68. Royal College of General Practitioners' Oral Contraception Study: Effect on hypertension and benign breast disease of progestogen component in combined oral contraceptives. Lancet 1977; 1:624.

69. Fisch IR, Frank J. Oral contraceptives and blood pressure. JAMA 1977; 237:2499–2503.

70. Laragh AJ. Oral contraceptive induced hypertension-nine years later. Am J Obstet Gynecol 1976; 126: 141–147.

71. Ramcharan S, Peritz E, Pellegrin FA, Williams WT. Incidence of hypertension in the Walnut Creek Contraceptive Drug Study cohort: In: Pharmacology of steroid contraceptive drugs. Garattini S, Berendes HW. Eds. New York, Raven Press, 1977; pp. 277–288, (Monographs of the Mario Negri Institute for Pharmacological Research Milan.)

72. Stockley I. Interactions with oral contraceptives. J Pharm 1976;216:140–143.

73. The Cancer and Steroid Hormone Study of the Centers for Disease Control and the National Institute of Child Health and Human Development: Oral contraceptive use and the risk of ovarian cancer. JAMA 1983; 249: 1596–1599.

74. The Cancer and Steroid Hormone Study of the Centers for Disease Control and the National Institute of Child Health and Human Development: Combination oral contraceptive use and the risk of endometrial cancer. JAMA 1987; 257:796–800.

75. Ory HW. Functional ovarian cysts and oral contraceptives: negative association confirmed surgically. JAMA 1974; 228:68–69.

76. Ory HW, Cole P, MacMahon B, Hoover R. Oral contraceptives and reduced risk of benign breast disease. N Engl J Med 1976; 294:419–422.

77. Ory HW. The noncontraceptive health benefits from oral contraceptive use. Fam Plann Perspect 1982; 14: 182–184.

78. Ory HW, Forrest JD, Lincoln R. Making choices: Evaluating the health risks and benefits of birth control methods. New York, The Alan Guttmacher Institute, 1983; p.1.

79. Schlesselman J, Stadel BV, Murray P, Lai S. Breast cancer in relation to early use of oral contraceptives. JAMA 1988; 259:1828–1833.

80. Hennekens CH, Speizer FE, Lipnick RJ, Rosner B, Bain C, Belanger C, Stampfer MJ, Willett W, Peto R. A case-control study of oral contraceptive use and breast cancer. JNCI 1984; 72:39–42.

81. LaVecchia C, Decarli A, Fasoli M, Franceschi S, Gentile A, Negri E, Parazzini F, Tognoni G. Oral contraceptives and cancers of the breast and of the female genital tract. Interim results from a case-control study. Br J Cancer 1986; 54:311–317.

82. Meirik O, Lund E, Adami H, Bergstrom R, Christoffersen T, Bergsjo P. Oral contraceptive use and breast cancer in young women. A Joint National Case-control study in Sweden and Norway. Lancet 1986; 11: 650–654.

83. Kay CR, Hannaford PC. Breast cancer and the pill-A further report from the Royal College of General Practitioners' oral contraception study. Br J Cancer 1988; 58:675–680.

84. Stadel BV, Lai S, Schlesselman JJ, Murray P. Oral contraceptives and premenopausal breast cancer in nulliparous women. Contraception 1988; 38:287–299.

85. Miller DR, Rosenberg L, Kaufman DW, Stolley P, Warshauer ME, Shapiro S. Breast cancer before age 45 and oral contraceptive use: New Findings. Am J Epidemiol 1989; 129:269–280.

86. The UK National Case-Control Study Group, Oral contraceptive use and breast cancer risk in young women. Lancet 1989; 1:973–982.

87. Schlesselman JJ. Cancer of the breast and reproductive tract in relation to use of oral contraceptives. Contraception 1989; 40:1–38.

88. Vessey MP, McPherson K, Villard-Mackintosh L, Yeates D. Oral contraceptives and breast cancer: latest findings in a large cohort study. Br J Cancer 1989; 59: 613–617.

89. Jick SS, Walker AM, Stergachis A, Jick H. Oral contraceptives and breast cancer. Br J Cancer 1989; 59: 618–621.

90. Anderson FD, Selectivity and minimal androgenicity of norgestimate in monophasic and triphasic oral contraceptives. Acta Obstet Gynecol Scand 1992; 156 (Supplement):15–21.

91. Chapdelaine A, Desmaris J-L, Derman RJ. Clinical evidence of minimal androgenic activity of norgestimate. Int J Fertil 1989; 34(51):347–352.

92. Phillips A, Demarest K, Hahn DW, Wong F, McGuire JL. Progestational and androgenic receptor binding affinities and in vivo activities of norgestimate and other progestins. Contraception 1989; 41(4):399–409.

93. Phillips A, Hahn DW, Klimek S, McGuire JL. A comparison of the potencies and activities of progestogens used in contraceptives. Contraception 1987; 36(2): 181–192.
94. Janaud A, Rouffy J, Upmalis D, Dain M-P. A comparison study of lipid and androgen metabolism with triphasic oral contraceptive formulations containing norgestimate or levonorgestrel Acta Obstet Gynecol Scand 1992; 156 (Supplement):34–38.
95. Collaborative Group on Hormonal Factors in Breast Cancer. Breast cancer and hormonal contraceptives: collaborative reanalysis of individual data on 53 297 women with breast cancer and 100 239 women without breast cancer from 54 epidemiological studies. Lancet 1996; 347:1713–1727.
96. Palmer JR, Rosenberg L, Kaufman DW, Warshauer ME, Stolley P, Shapiro S. Oral Contraceptive Use and Liver Cancer. Am J Epidemiol 1989;130:878–882.
97. Lewis M, Spitzer WO, Heinemann LAJ, MacRae KD, Bruppacher R, Thorogood M on behalf of Transnational Research Group on Oral Contraceptives and Health of Young Women. Third generation oral contraceptives and risk of myocardial infarction: an international case-control study. Br Med J, 1996;312:88–90.
98. Vessey MP, Smith MA, Yeates D. Return of fertility after discontinuation of oral contraceptives: influence of age and parity. Brit J Fam Plan; 1986; 11:120–124.
99. Back DJ, Orme M.L'E. Pharmacokinetic drug interactions with oral contraceptives. Clin Pharmacokinet 1990; 18:472–484.
100. Rosenfeld WE, Doose DR, Walker SA, Nayak RK. Effect of topiramate on the pharmacokinetics of an oral contraceptive containing norethindrone and ethinyl estradiol in patients with epilepsy. Epilepsia 1997 Mar;38(3):317–323.
101. Shenfield GM. Oral Contraceptives. Are drug interaction of clinical significance? Drug Saf 1993 Jul;9(1): 21–37.
102. Ouellet D, Hsu A, Qian J, Locke CS, Eason CJ, Cavanaugh JH, Leonard JM, Granneman GR. Effect of ritonavir on the pharmacokinetics of ethinyl oestradiol in healthy female volunteers. Br J Clin Pharmacol 1998;46(2):111–116.
103. Improving access to quality care in family planning: Medical eligibility criteria for contraceptive use. Geneva, WHO, Family and Reproductive Health, 1996 (WHO/FRH/FPP/96.9).
104. Skolnick JL, Stoler BS, Katz DG, Anderson WH. Rifampicin, oral contraceptives and pregnancy. J Am Med Assoc 1976;236–1382.
105. Henney JE. Risk of drug interactions with St. John's Wort. JAMA 2000;283(13).
106. Lahteennmaki P et al, Coagulation factors in women using oral contraceptives or intrauterine devices immediately after abortion. American Journal of Obstetrics and Gynecology, (1981); 141: 175–179.
107. Cole JA, Norman H, Doherty M, Walker AM. Venous Thromboembolism, Myocardial Infarction, and Stroke Among Transdermal Contraceptive System Users. Obstetrics & Gynecology 2007; 109(2):339–346.
108. Jick SS, Kaye JA, Russmann S, Jick H. Risk of nonfatal venous thromboembolism in women using a contraceptive transdermal patch and oral contraceptives containing norgestimate and 35 mcg of ethinyl estradiol. Contraception 73 (2006): 223–228.
109. Jick S, Kaye JA, Jick H. Further results on the risk of nonfatal venous thromboembolism in users of the contraceptive transdermal patch compared to users of oral contraceptives containing norgestimate and 35 μg of EE. Contraception 2007;76:4–7.
110. Jick S, Hagberg K, Hernandez R, Kaye J. Postmarketing study of ORTHO EVRA® and levonorgestrel oral contraceptives containing hormonal contraceptives with 30 mcg of ethinyl estradiol in relation to nonfatal venous thromboembolism. Contraception 81 (2010): 16–21.
111. Jick S, Hagberg K, Kaye J. ORTHO EVRA® and venous thromboembolism: an update. Letter to the Editor. Contraception 81 (2010): 452–453.
112. Chobanian et al. Seventh report of the joint national committee on prevention, detection, evaluation, and treatment of high blood pressure. Hypertension 2003;42;1206–1252.
113. Dore D, Norman H, Loughlin J, Seeger D. Extended case-control study results on thromboembolic outcomes among transdermal contraceptive users. Contraception 81 (2010): 408–413.
114. Cole JA, Norman H, Doherty M, Walker AM. Venous thromboembolism, myocardial infarction, and stroke among transdermal contraceptive system users [published erratum appears in Obstet Gynecol 2008:111: 1449].
115. Dore D, Norman H, Seeger, J. Eligibility Criteria in Venous Thromboembolism, Myocardial Infarction, and Stroke Among Transdermal Contraceptive System Users. Letter to the Editor. Obstetrics & Gynecology 2009; 114(1):175.

DETAILED PATIENT LABELING

ORTHO EVRA® (norelgestromin/ethinyl estradiol transdermal system)

This product is intended to prevent pregnancy. It does not protect against HIV (AIDS) or other sexually transmitted diseases.

DESCRIPTION

The contraceptive patch ORTHO EVRA® is a thin, beige, plastic patch that sticks to the skin. The sticky part of the patch contains the following hormones: norelgestromin (progestin) and ethinyl estradiol (estrogen). These hormones are absorbed continuously through the skin and into the bloodstream. On average, the amount of estrogen delivered through the skin produces estrogen exposure that is higher than the exposure when taking a birth control pill containing 35 micrograms of estrogen. Each patch is sealed in a pouch that protects it until you are ready to wear it.

INTRODUCTION

Any woman who considers using the contraceptive patch ORTHO EVRA® should understand the benefits and risks of using this form of birth control. This leaflet will give you much of the information you will need to make this decision and will also help you determine if you are at risk of developing any serious side effects. It will tell you how to use the contraceptive patch properly so that it will be as effective as possible. However, this leaflet is not a replacement for a careful discussion between you and your healthcare professional. You should discuss the information provided in this leaflet with him or her, both when you first start using the contraceptive patch ORTHO EVRA® and during your revisits. You should also follow your healthcare professional's advice with regard to regular check-ups while you are using the contraceptive patch.

EFFECTIVENESS OF HORMONAL CONTRACEPTIVE METHODS

Hormonal contraceptives, including ORTHO EVRA®, are used to prevent pregnancy and are more effective than most other non-surgical methods of birth control. When ORTHO EVRA® is used correctly, the chance of becoming pregnant is approximately 1% (1 pregnancy per 100 women per year of use when used correctly), which is comparable to that of the pill. The chance of becoming pregnant increases with incorrect use.

Clinical trials suggested that ORTHO EVRA® may be less effective in women weighing more than 198 lbs. (90 kg). If you weigh more than 198 lbs. (90 kg) you should talk to your healthcare professional about which method of birth control may be best for you.

Typical failure rates for other methods of birth control during the first year of use are as follows:

Implant: <1%
Injection: <1%
IUD: <1–2%
Diaphragm with spermicides: 20%
Spermicides alone: 26%
Female sterilization: <1%
Male sterilization: <1%
Cervical Cap with spermicide: 20 to 40%
Condom alone (male): 14%
Condom alone (female): 21%
Periodic abstinence: 25%
No birth control method: 85%
Withdrawal: 19%

WHO SHOULD NOT USE ORTHO EVRA®

Hormonal contraceptives include birth control pills, injectables, implants, the vaginal ring, and the contraceptive patch. The following information is derived primarily from studies of birth control pills. The contraceptive patch is expected to be associated with similar risks:

Cigarette smoking increases the risk of serious cardiovascular side effects from hormonal contraceptive use. This risk increases with age and with heavy smoking (15 or more cigarettes per day) and is quite marked in women over 35 years of age. Women who use hormonal contraceptives, including ORTHO EVRA®, are strongly advised not to smoke.

Some women should not use the ORTHO EVRA® contraceptive patch. For example, you should not use ORTHO EVRA® if you are pregnant or think you may be pregnant. You should also not use ORTHO EVRA® if you have any of the following conditions:

- A history of heart attack or stroke
- Blood clots in the legs (thrombophlebitis), lungs (pulmonary embolism), or eyes
- A history of blood clots in the deep veins of your legs
- An inherited problem that makes your blood clot more than normal
- Chest pain (angina pectoris)
- Known or suspected breast cancer or cancer of the lining of the uterus, cervix or vagina
- Unexplained vaginal bleeding (until your doctor reaches a diagnosis)
- Hepatitis or yellowing of the whites of your eyes or of the skin (jaundice) during pregnancy or during previous use of hormonal contraceptives such as ORTHO EVRA®, NORPLANT®, or the birth control pill
- Liver tumor (benign or cancerous)
- Known or suspected pregnancy
- Severe high blood pressure
- Diabetes with complications of the kidneys, eyes, nerves, or blood vessels
- Headaches with neurological symptoms
- Use of oral contraceptives (birth control pills)
- Disease of heart valves with complications
- Need for a prolonged period of bed rest following major surgery
- An allergic reaction to any of the components of ORTHO EVRA®

Tell your healthcare professional if you have ever had any of these conditions. Your healthcare professional can recommend a non-hormonal method of birth control.

OTHER CONSIDERATIONS BEFORE USING ORTHO EVRA®

Hormones from ORTHO EVRA® get into the blood stream and are processed by the body differently than hormones from birth control pills. **You will be exposed to about 60% more estrogen if you use ORTHO EVRA® than if you use a typical birth control pill containing 35 micrograms of estrogen.** In general, increased estrogen may increase the risk of side effects.

The risk of venous thromboembolic events (blood clots in the legs and/or the lungs) may be increased with ORTHO EVRA® use compared with use of birth control pills. Studies examined the risk of these serious blood clots in women who used either ORTHO EVRA® or birth control pills containing one of two progestins (levonorgestrel or norgestimate) and 30–35 micrograms of estrogen. Results of these studies ranged from an approximate doubling of risk of serious blood clots to no increase in risk in women using ORTHO EVRA® compared to women using birth control pills.

You should discuss this possible increased risk with your healthcare professional before using ORTHO EVRA®. Call your healthcare professional immediately if any of the adverse side effects listed under "WARNING SIGNALS" occur while you are using ORTHO EVRA®. (See below.)

Also talk to your healthcare professional about using ORTHO EVRA® if:

- you smoke
- you are recovering from the birth of a baby
- you are recovering from a second trimester miscarriage or abortion
- you are breastfeeding
- you weigh 198 pounds or more
- you are taking any other medications

Also, tell your healthcare professional if you have or have had:

- Breast nodules, fibrocystic disease of the breast, an abnormal breast x-ray or mammogram
- A family history of breast cancer
- Diabetes
- Elevated cholesterol or triglycerides
- High blood pressure
- Migraine or other headaches or epilepsy
- Depression
- Gallbladder disease
- Liver disease
- Heart disease
- Kidney disease
- Scanty or irregular menstrual periods

If you have any of these conditions you should be checked often by your healthcare professional if you use the contraceptive patch.

RISKS OF USING HORMONAL CONTRACEPTIVES, INCLUDING ORTHO EVRA®

The following information is derived primarily from studies of birth control pills. Since ORTHO EVRA® contains hormones similar to those found in birth control pills, it is expected to be associated with similar risks:

1. Risk of Developing Blood Clots

Blood clots and blockage of blood vessels that can cause death or serious disability are some of the most serious side effects of using hormonal contraceptives, including the ORTHO EVRA® contraceptive patch. In particular, a clot in the legs can cause thrombophlebitis, and a clot that travels to the lungs can cause sudden blocking of the vessel carrying blood to the lungs. Rarely, clots occur in the blood vessels of the eye and may cause blindness, double vision, or impaired vision.

The risk of venous thromboembolic disease (blood clots in the legs and/or the lungs) may be increased with ORTHO EVRA® compared with that of oral contraceptives containing norgestimate and 35 micrograms of estrogen (see the earlier Section OTHER CONSIDERATIONS BEFORE USING ORTHO EVRA®). You should discuss this possible increased risk with your healthcare professional before using ORTHO EVRA®. Call your healthcare professional immediately should any of the adverse effects listed under "WARNING SIGNALS" occur while you are using ORTHO EVRA®. (See below.)

If you use ORTHO EVRA® and need elective surgery, need to stay in bed for a prolonged illness or injury or have recently delivered a baby, you may be at risk of developing blood clots. You should consult your doctor about stopping ORTHO EVRA® four weeks before surgery and not using it for two weeks after surgery or during bed rest. You should also not use ORTHO EVRA® soon after delivery of a baby. It is advisable to wait for at least four weeks after delivery if you are not breastfeeding. If you are breastfeeding, you should wait until you have weaned your child before using ORTHO EVRA®. (See also the section on Breastfeeding in General Precautions.)

2. Heart Attacks and Strokes

Hormonal contraceptives, including ORTHO EVRA®, may increase the risk of developing strokes (blockage or rupture of blood vessels in the brain) and angina pectoris and heart attacks (blockage of blood vessels in the heart). Any of these conditions can cause death or serious disability.

Smoking and the use of hormonal contraceptives including ORTHO EVRA® greatly increase the chances of developing and dying of heart disease. Smoking also greatly increases the possibility of suffering heart attacks and strokes.

3. Gallbladder Disease

Women who use hormonal contraceptives, including ORTHO EVRA®, probably have a greater risk than nonusers of having gallbladder disease.

4. Liver Tumors

In rare cases, combination oral contraceptives can cause benign but dangerous liver tumors. Since ORTHO EVRA® contains hormones similar to those in birth control pills, this association may also exist with ORTHO EVRA®. These benign liver tumors can rupture and cause fatal internal bleeding. In addition, some studies report an increased risk of developing liver cancer. However, liver cancers are rare.

5. Cancer of the Reproductive Organs and Breasts

Various studies give conflicting reports on the relationship between breast cancer and hormonal contraceptive use. Combination hormonal contraceptives, including ORTHO EVRA®, may slightly increase your chance of having breast cancer diagnosed, particularly after using hormonal contraceptives at a younger age. After you stop using hormonal contraceptives, the chances of having breast cancer diagnosed begin to go back down. You should have regular breast examinations by a healthcare professional and examine your own breasts monthly. Tell your healthcare professional if you have a family history of breast cancer or if you have had breast nodules or an abnormal mammogram.

Women who currently have or have had breast cancer should not use oral contraceptives because breast cancer is usually a hormone-sensitive tumor.

Some studies have found an increase in the incidence of cancer of the cervix in women who use oral contraceptives, although this finding may be related to factors other than the use of oral contraceptives. However, there is insufficient evidence to rule out the possibility that oral contraceptives may cause such cancers.

ESTIMATED RISK OF DEATH FROM A BIRTH CONTROL METHOD OR PREGNANCY

All methods of birth control and pregnancy are associated with a risk of developing certain diseases that may lead to disability or death. An estimate of the number of deaths associated with different methods of birth control and pregnancy has been calculated and is shown in the following table.

ORTHO EVRA® is expected to be associated with similar risks as oral contraceptives:

[See table above]

Annual Number of Birth-Related or Method-Related Deaths Associated With Control of Fertility Per 100,000 Nonsterile Women by Fertility Control Method According to Age

Method of control and outcome	15–19	20–24	25–29	30–34	35–39	40–44
No fertility control methods*	7.0	7.4	9.1	14.8	25.7	28.2
Oral contraceptives non-smoker†	0.3	0.5	0.9	1.9	13.8	31.6
Oral contraceptives smoker†	2.2	3.4	6.6	13.5	51.1	117.2
IUD†	0.8	0.8	1.0	1.0	1.4	1.4
Condom*	1.1	1.6	0.7	0.2	0.3	0.4
Diaphragm / spermicide*	1.9	1.2	1.2	1.3	2.2	2.8
Periodic abstinence*	2.5	1.6	1.6	1.7	2.9	3.6

Adapted from H.W. Ory, ref. #35.
*Deaths are birth-related
†Deaths are method-related

In the above table, the risk of death from any birth control method is less than the risk of childbirth, except for oral contraceptive users over the age of 35 who smoke and pill users over the age of 40 even if they do not smoke. It can be seen in the table that for women aged 15 to 39, the risk of death was highest with pregnancy (7–26 deaths per 100,000 women, depending on age). Among pill users who do not smoke, the risk of death is always lower than that associated with pregnancy for any age group, although over the age of 40, the risk increases to 32 deaths per 100,000 women, compared to 28 associated with pregnancy at that age. However, for pill users who smoke and are over the age of 35, the estimated number of deaths exceeds those for other methods of birth control. If a woman is over the age of 40 and smokes, her estimated risk of death is four times higher (117/100,000 women) than the estimated risk associated with pregnancy (28/100,000 women) in that age group.

In 1989 an Advisory Committee of the FDA concluded that the benefits of low-dose hormonal contraceptive use by healthy, non-smoking women over 40 years of age may outweigh the possible risks.

WARNING SIGNALS

If any of these adverse effects occur while you are using ORTHO EVRA®, call your doctor immediately:

- Sharp chest pain, coughing of blood, or sudden shortness of breath (indicating a possible clot in the lung)
- Pain in the calf (indicating a possible clot in the leg)
- Crushing chest pain or tightness in the chest (indicating a possible heart attack)
- Sudden severe headache or vomiting, dizziness or fainting, disturbances of vision or speech, weakness, or numbness in an arm or leg (indicating a possible stroke)
- Sudden partial or complete loss of vision (indicating a possible clot in the eye)
- Breast lumps (indicating possible breast cancer or fibrocystic disease of the breast; ask your doctor or healthcare professional to show you how to examine your breasts)
- Severe pain or tenderness in the stomach area (indicating a possibly ruptured liver tumor)
- Severe problems with sleeping, weakness, lack of energy, fatigue, or change in mood (possibly indicating severe depression)
- Jaundice or a yellowing of the skin or eyeballs accompanied frequently by fever, fatigue, loss of appetite, dark colored urine, or light colored bowel movements (indicating possible liver problems)

SIDE EFFECTS OF ORTHO EVRA®

1. Most Common Side Effects

The most common side effects of ORTHO EVRA® include nausea, breast symptoms (discomfort, engorgement, or pain), headache, and problems where the patch has been on the skin.

2. Skin Irritation

Skin irritation, redness, pain, swelling, itching or rash may occur at the site of application. If this occurs, the patch may be removed and a new patch may be applied to a new location until the next Change Day. Single replacement patches are available from pharmacies.

3. Vaginal Bleeding

Irregular vaginal bleeding or spotting may occur while you are using ORTHO EVRA®. Irregular bleeding may vary from slight staining between menstrual periods to breakthrough bleeding which is a flow much like a regular period. Irregular bleeding may occur during the first few months of contraceptive patch use but may also occur after you have been using the contraceptive patch for some time. Such bleeding may be temporary and usually does not indicate any serious problems. It is important to continue using your contraceptive patches on schedule. If the bleeding occurs in more than a few cycles or lasts for more than a few days, talk to your healthcare professional.

4. Problems Wearing Contact Lenses

If you wear contact lenses and notice a change in vision or an inability to wear your lenses, contact your healthcare professional.

5. Fluid Retention or Raised Blood Pressure

Edema (fluid retention) with swelling of the fingers or ankles and/or a rise in blood pressure may occur with the use of hormonal contraceptives. If you experience fluid retention, contact your healthcare professional.

6. Melasma

A spotty darkening of the skin is possible, particularly of the face. This may persist after use of hormonal contraceptives is discontinued.

7. Other Side Effects

Other side effects include weight gain, feeling dizzy, migraine, stomach pain or bloating, vomiting, diarrhea, abnormal taste, acne, muscle spasms, vaginal infections, feeling tired or unwell, painful or heavy periods or periods more frequent than normal, uterine cramps, vaginal discharge and mood problems such as depression, mood swings or anxiety.

GENERAL PRECAUTIONS

1. Weight ≥ 198 lbs. (90 kg)

Clinical trials suggest that ORTHO EVRA® may be less effective in women weighing 198 lbs. (90 kg) or more compared with its effectiveness in women with lower body weights. If you weigh 198 lbs. (90 kg) or more you should talk to your healthcare professional about which method of birth control may be best for you.

2. Missed Periods and Use of ORTHO EVRA® Before or During Early Pregnancy

There may be times when you may not menstruate regularly during your patch-free week. If you have used ORTHO EVRA® correctly and miss one menstrual period, continue using your contraceptive patches for the next cycle but be sure to inform your healthcare professional before doing so. If you have not used ORTHO EVRA® as instructed and missed a menstrual period, or if you missed two menstrual periods in a row, you could be pregnant. Check with your healthcare professional immediately to determine whether you are pregnant. Stop using ORTHO EVRA® if you are pregnant.

There is no conclusive evidence that hormonal contraceptive use causes birth defects when taken accidentally during early pregnancy. Previously, a few studies had reported that oral contraceptives might be associated with birth defects, but these findings have not been seen in more recent studies. Nevertheless, hormonal contraceptives, including ORTHO EVRA®, should not be used during pregnancy. You should check with your healthcare professional about risks to your unborn child from any medication taken during pregnancy.

3. While Breastfeeding

If you are breastfeeding, consult your healthcare professional before starting ORTHO EVRA®. Hormonal contraceptives are passed on to the child in the milk. A few adverse effects on the child have been reported, including yellowing of the skin (jaundice) and breast enlargement. In addition, combination hormonal contraceptives may decrease the amount and quality of your milk. If possible, do not use combination hormonal contraceptives such as ORTHO EVRA® while breastfeeding. You should use a barrier method of contraception since breastfeeding provides only partial protection from becoming pregnant and this partial protection decreases significantly as you breastfeed for longer periods of time. You should consider starting ORTHO EVRA® only after you have weaned your child completely.

4. Laboratory Tests

If you are scheduled for any laboratory tests, tell your doctor you are using ORTHO EVRA® since certain blood tests may be affected by hormonal contraceptives.

5. Drug Interactions

Hormonal contraceptives may interact with lamotrigine, an anticonvulsant used for epilepsy. This may increase the risk of seizures so your physician may need to adjust the dose.

Some medicines and herbal products may make your hormonal contraceptive less effective, including:

- barbiturates
- bosentan
- carbamazepine
- felbamate
- griseofulvin
- oxcarbazepine
- phenytoin
- rifampin
- St. John's wort
- topiramate

Blood levels of estrogen from this hormonal contraceptive may be increased if you take certain medicines or drink grapefruit juice. Also, your hormonal contraceptive may make some other medicines less effective. As with all prescription products, you should notify your healthcare professional of any other medications and herbal products you are taking or plan to take. You may need to use a barrier contraceptive when you take medicines or products that can make hormonal contraceptives less effective.

6. Sexually Transmitted Diseases

ORTHO EVRA® is intended to prevent pregnancy. It does not protect against HIV (AIDS) or other sexually transmitted diseases such as chlamydia, genital herpes, genital warts, gonorrhea, hepatitis B, and syphilis.

HOW TO USE ORTHO EVRA®

Instructions for Use

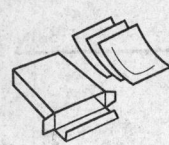

ORTHO EVRA® keeps you from becoming pregnant by transferring hormones to your body through your skin. The patch must stick securely to your skin in order for it to work properly. This method uses a 28 day (four week) cycle. You should apply a new patch each week for three weeks (21 total days). You should not apply a patch during the fourth week. Your menstrual period should start during this patch-free week.

Every new patch should be applied on the same day of the week. This day will be your 'Patch Change Day.' For example, if you apply your first patch on a Monday, all of your patches should be applied on a Monday. You should wear only one patch at a time.

On the day after week four ends, you should begin a new four week cycle by applying a new patch.

Save these instructions.

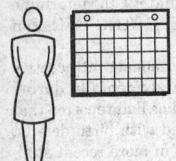

1
If this is the **first time** you are using ORTHO EVRA®, **wait until the day you get your menstrual period.** *The day you apply your first patch will be Day 1. Your 'Patch Change Day' will be on this day every week.*

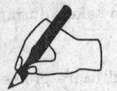

CHOOSE ONE OPTION:

2
You may choose a first day start or Sunday start
• *for First Day* start: apply your first patch during the first 24 hours of your menstrual period

OR

☐ **First Day Start**

or

☐ **Sunday Start**

• *for Sunday* start: apply your first patch on the first Sunday after your menstrual period starts. *You must use back-up contraception, such as a condom, spermicide, or diaphragm for the first week of your first cycle*
• *The day you apply your first patch will be Day 1. Your 'Patch Change Day' will be on this day every week.*

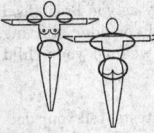

3
Choose a place on your body to put the patch. Put the patch on your buttock, abdomen, upper outer arm or upper torso, in a place where it won't be rubbed by tight clothing. *Never put the patch on your breasts.*
To avoid irritation, apply each new patch to a different place on your skin.

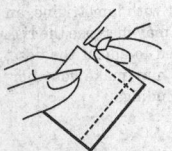

4
Open the foil pouch by tearing it along the top edge **and** one side edge.
Peel the foil pouch apart and open it flat.

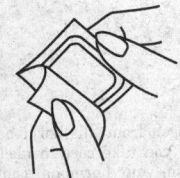

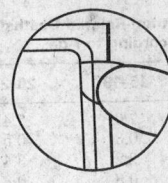

5
You will see that the patch is covered by a layer of clear plastic. It is important to remove the patch **and** the plastic together from the foil pouch.
Using your fingernail, lift one corner of the patch and peel the patch and the plastic off the foil liner.

Sometimes patches can stick to the inside of the pouch – be careful not to accidentally remove the clear liner as you remove the patch.

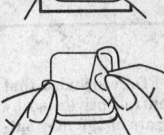

6
Peel away half of the clear plastic and be careful not to touch the exposed sticky surface of the patch with your fingers.

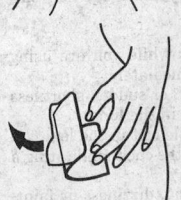

7
Apply the sticky side of the patch to the skin you've cleaned and dried, then remove the other half of the clear plastic.
Press firmly on the patch with the palm of your hand for 10 seconds, making sure the edges stick well. Run your finger around the edge of the patch to make sure it is sticking properly. Check your patch every day to make sure all the edges are sticking.

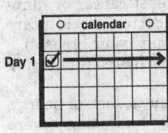

8
Wear the patch for seven days (one week). On your 'Patch Change Day,' Day 8, remove the used patch. Apply a new patch immediately. *The used patch still contains some active hormones. Used patches should not be flushed down the toilet.* For disposal directions, see Special Precautions for Storage and Disposal below.

9

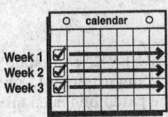

Apply a new patch for week two (on Day 8) and for week three (on Day 15), on your 'Patch Change Day.' *To avoid irritation, do not apply the new patch to the same exact place on your skin.*

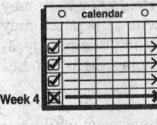

10
Do not wear a patch on week four (Day 22 through Day 28). *Your period should start during this week.*

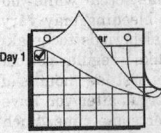

11
Begin your next four week cycle by applying a new patch on your normal 'Patch Change Day,' the day after Day 28 – *no matter when your period begins or ends.*

If your patch has become loose or has fallen off...
• **for less than one day,** try to re-apply it or apply a new patch immediately. No back-up contraception is needed. *Your 'Patch Change Day' will remain the same*

• **for more than one day OR if you are not sure for how long,** YOU MAY BECOME PREGNANT – **Start a new four week cycle immediately** by putting on a new patch. *You now have a new Day 1 and a new 'Patch Change Day.' You must use back-up contraception, such as a condom, spermicide, or diaphragm for the first week of your new cycle.*
• do not try to re-apply a patch if it's no longer sticky, if it has become stuck to itself or another surface, if it has other material stuck to it or if it has previously become loose or fallen off. No tapes or wraps should be used to keep the patch in place. If you cannot re-apply a patch, apply a new patch immediately.

If you forget to change your patch...
• **at the start of any patch cycle,**
Week one (Day 1): If you forget to apply your patch, YOU COULD BECOME PREGNANT – *you must use back-up contraception for one week.* Apply the first patch of your new cycle as soon as you remember. *You now have a new 'Patch Change Day' and new Day 1.*

• **in the middle of your patch cycle,**
Week two or week three: If you forget to change your patch for **one or two days,** apply a new patch as soon as you remember. Apply your next patch on your normal 'Patch Change Day.' No back-up contraception is needed.
Week two or week three: If you forget to change your patch for **more than two days,** YOU COULD BECOME PREGNANT – start a new four week cycle as soon as you remember by putting on a new patch. *You now have a different 'Patch Change Day' and a new Day 1. You must use back-up contraception for the first week of your new cycle.*

• **at the end of your patch cycle,**
Week four: If you forget to remove your patch, take it off as soon as you remember. Start your next cycle on your normal 'Patch Change Day,' the day after Day 28. No back-up contraception is needed.

• **at the start of your next patch cycle,**
Day 1 (week one): If you forget to apply your patch, YOU COULD BECOME PREGNANT – apply the first patch of your new cycle as soon as you remember. *You now have a new 'Patch Change Day' and new Day 1. You must use back-up contraception for the first week of your new cycle.*

• **you should never have the patch off for more than seven days.**

Other information...
• Always apply your patch to clean, dry skin. Avoid skin that is red, irritated or cut. Do not use creams, oils, powder or makeup on your skin where you will put a patch or near a patch you are wearing. It may cause the patch to become loose.
• Do not cut, damage or alter the ORTHO EVRA® patch in any way.
• If patch use results in uncomfortable irritation, the patch may be removed and a new patch may be applied to a new location until the next Change Day. Only one patch should be worn at a time.
• Some medicines may change the way ORTHO EVRA® works. If you are taking any medication, you must talk to your healthcare professional BEFORE you use the patch. *You may need to use back-up contraception.*
• Store at 25°C (77°F); excursions permitted to 15–30°C (59–86°F).
• Single replacement patches are available through your pharmacist.
• For further information log on to www.orthoevra.com or call toll free **1-800-526-7736.**

WHEN YOU SWITCH FROM THE PILL TO ORTHO EVRA®:
If you are switching from the pill to ORTHO EVRA®, wait until you get your menstrual period. If you do not get your period within five days of taking the last active pill, check with your healthcare professional to be sure that you are not pregnant.

IMPORTANT POINTS TO REMEMBER

1. IT IS IMPORTANT TO USE ORTHO EVRA® exactly as directed in this leaflet. Incorrect use increases your chances of becoming pregnant. This includes starting your contraceptive cycle late or missing your scheduled CHANGE DAYS.

2. You should wear one patch per week for three weeks, followed by one week off. **You should never have the patch off for more than seven days in a row.** If you have the patch off for more than seven days in a row and you have had sex during this time, YOU COULD BECOME PREGNANT.

3. **IF YOU ARE NOT SURE WHAT TO DO ABOUT MISTAKES WITH PATCH USE:**
   • Use a BACK-UP METHOD, *such as a condom, spermicide, or diaphragm* anytime you have sex.
   • Contact your healthcare professional for instructions.

4. Do not skip patches even if you do not have sex very often.

5. SOME WOMEN HAVE SPOTTING OR LIGHT BLEEDING, BREAST TENDERNESS OR MAY FEEL SICK TO THEIR STOMACH DURING ORTHO EVRA® USE. If these symptoms occur, do not stop using the contraceptive patch. The problem will usually go away. If it doesn't go away, check with your healthcare professional.

6. MISTAKES IN USING YOUR PATCHES CAN ALSO CAUSE SPOTTING OR LIGHT BLEEDING.

7. If you miss TWO PERIODS IN A ROW contact your healthcare professional because you might be pregnant.

8. The amount of drug you get from the ORTHO EVRA® patch should not be affected by VOMITING OR DIARRHEA.

9. IF YOU TAKE CERTAIN MEDICINES, ORTHO EVRA® may not work as well. Use a non-hormonal back-up method (such as condoms, spermicide, or diaphragm) until you check with your healthcare professional.

IMPORTANT NOTICE: Updated drug information is sent bi-monthly via the PDR® Update Insert. For *monthly* email updates, register at PDR.net.

10. IF YOU WANT TO MOVE YOUR PATCH CHANGE DAY to a different day of the week, finish your current cycle, removing your third ORTHO EVRA® patch on the correct day. **During week four,** the "patch-free week" (Day 22 through Day 28), you may choose an earlier Patch Change Day by applying a new patch on the day you prefer. You now have a new Day 1 and a new Patch Change Day. **You should never have the patch off for more than seven days in a row.**

11. BE SURE YOU HAVE READY AT ALL TIMES:
   • A NON-HORMONAL BIRTH CONTROL method (such as condoms, spermicide, or diaphragm) to use as a back-up in case of dosing errors.

12. IF YOU HAVE TROUBLE REMEMBERING TO CHANGE YOUR CONTRACEPTIVE PATCH, talk to your healthcare professional about how to make patch-changing easier or about using another method of birth control.

13. Single replacement patches are available through your pharmacist.

14. For Patch replacement, see "How to use ORTHO EVRA®" section.

IF YOU HAVE ANY QUESTIONS OR ARE UNSURE ABOUT THE INFORMATION IN THIS LEAFLET, call your healthcare professional.

PREGNANCY DUE TO ORTHO EVRA® FAILURE
The incidence of pregnancy from hormonal contraceptive failure is approximately one percent (i.e., one pregnancy per 100 women per year) if used correctly. The chance of becoming pregnant increases with incorrect use. If contraceptive patch failure does occur, the risk to the fetus is minimal.

PREGNANCY AFTER STOPPING ORTHO EVRA®
There may be some delay in becoming pregnant after you stop using ORTHO EVRA®, especially if you had irregular menstrual cycles before you used hormonal contraceptives. It may be best to postpone conception until you begin menstruation regularly once you have stopped using ORTHO EVRA® and want to become pregnant.
There does not appear to be any increase in birth defects in newborn babies when pregnancy occurs soon after stopping hormonal contraceptives.

OVERDOSAGE
ORTHO EVRA® is unlikely to cause an overdose because the patch releases a steady amount of the hormones. Do not use more than one patch at a time. Serious ill effects have not been reported when large doses of oral contraceptives were accidentally taken by young children. Overdosage may cause nausea and vomiting. Vaginal bleeding may occur in females. In case of overdosage, contact your healthcare professional or pharmacist.

OTHER INFORMATION
Your healthcare professional will take a medical and family history before prescribing ORTHO EVRA® and will examine you. The physical examination may be delayed to another time if you request it and the healthcare professional believes that it is a good medical practice to postpone it. You should be reexamined at least once a year. Be sure to inform your healthcare professional if there is a family history of any of the conditions listed previously in this leaflet. Be sure to keep all appointments with your healthcare professional, because this is a time to determine if there are early signs of side effects of hormonal contraceptive use.
Do not use the drug for any condition other than the one for which it was prescribed. This drug has been prescribed specifically for you; do not give it to others who may want birth control.
If you want more information about ORTHO EVRA®, ask your healthcare professional or pharmacist. They have a more technical leaflet called the Prescribing Information that you may wish to read.

Special Precautions for Storage and Disposal
Store at 25°C (77°F); excursions permitted to 15–30°C (59–86°F).
Store patches in their protective pouches. Apply to the skin immediately upon removal from the protective pouch.
Do not store in the refrigerator or freezer.
Used patches still contain some active hormones. To help protect the environment and help prevent accidental ingestion by children or pets:
   • Fold the sticky sides of the patch together and place it in a sturdy container, preferably with a child-resistant cap or ask your pharmacist for a bottle with a child-resistant cap. Ensure the opening is large enough for a folded patch to go in but small enough that a child's hand cannot enter. If a child-resistant container is unavailable then fold the sticky sides of the patch together and place it in a closable container, such as a sealable bag.
   • Throw the container in the trash. Used patches should not be flushed down the toilet.
   • Return unused, unneeded, or expired patches to your pharmacist.
Mfd. for:
Ortho Women's Health & Urology, Division of Ortho-McNeil-Janssen Pharmaceuticals, Inc.
Raritan, New Jersey 08869

Mfd. by:
Janssen Ortho, LLC
Manati, Puerto Rico 00674
© Ortho-McNeil-Janssen-Pharmaceuticals, Inc. 2001
PRINTED IN U.S.A.
Revised May 2010
10154407
Shown in Product Identification Guide, page 316

PANCREAZE™
[pan-kre-aze]
(pancrelipase)
delayed-release capsules

℞

HIGHLIGHTS OF PRESCRIBING INFORMATION
These highlights do not include all the information needed to use PANCREAZE™ safely and effectively. See full prescribing information for PANCREAZE™.
PANCREAZE™ (pancrelipase) delayed-release capsules
Initial U.S. Approval – 2010

————INDICATIONS AND USAGE————
PANCREAZE™ is a combination of porcine-derived lipases, proteases, and amylases indicated for the treatment of exocrine pancreatic insufficiency due to cystic fibrosis or other conditions (1)

————DOSAGE AND ADMINISTRATION————
Dosage
PANCREAZE™ is not interchangeable with any other pancrelipase product.
Infants (up to 12 months)
• Infants may be given 2,000 to 4,000 lipase units per 120 mL of formula or per breast-feeding. (2.1)
• Do not mix PANCREAZE capsule contents directly into formula or breast milk prior to administration. (2.2)
Children Older than 12 Months and Younger than 4 Years
• Enzyme dosing should begin with 1,000 lipase units/kg of body weight per meal to a maximum of 2,500 lipase units/kg of body weight per meal (or less than or equal to 10,000 lipase units/kg of body weight per day), or less than 4,000 lipase units/g fat ingested per day. (2.1)
Children 4 Years and Older and Adults
• Enzyme dosing should begin with 500 lipase units/kg of body weight per meal to a maximum of 2,500 lipase units/kg of body weight per meal (or less than or equal to 10,000 lipase units/kg of body weight per day), or less than 4,000 lipase units/g fat ingested per day. (2.1)
Limitations on Dosing
• Dosing should not exceed the recommended maximum dosage set forth by the Cystic Fibrosis Foundation Consensus Conferences Guidelines. (2.1)
Administration
• PANCREAZE should be swallowed whole. For infants or patients unable to swallow intact capsules, the contents may be sprinkled on soft acidic food with a pH of 4.5 or less, e.g., applesauce. (2.2)

————DOSAGE FORMS AND STRENGTHS————
• Capsules: 4,200 USP units of lipase; 10,000 USP units of protease; 17,500 USP units of amylase. Capsules have a yellow opaque body and clear cap, printed with "McNEIL" and "MT 4" (3)
• Capsules: 10,500 USP units of lipase; 25,000 USP units of protease; 43,750 USP units of amylase. Capsules have a pink opaque body and clear cap, printed with "McNEIL" and "MT 10" (3)
• Capsules: 16,800 USP units of lipase; 40,000 USP units of protease; 70,000 USP units of amylase. Capsules have a salmon opaque body and clear cap, printed with "McNEIL" and "MT 16" (3)
• Capsules: 21,000 USP units of lipase; 37,000 USP units of protease; 61,000 USP units of amylase. Capsules have a white opaque body and cap, printed with "McNEIL" and "MT 20" (3)

————CONTRAINDICATIONS————
None. (4)

————WARNINGS AND PRECAUTIONS————
• Fibrosing colonopathy is associated with high-dose use of pancreatic enzyme replacement. Exercise caution when doses of PANCREAZE exceed 2,500 lipase units/kg of body weight per meal (or greater than 10,000 lipase units/kg of body weight per day). (5.1)
• To avoid irritation of oral mucosa, do not chew PANCREAZE or retain in the mouth. (5.2)
• Exercise caution when prescribing PANCREAZE to patients with gout, renal impairment, or hyperuricemia. (5.3)
• There is theoretical risk of viral transmission with all pancreatic enzyme products including PANCREAZE. (5.4)
• Exercise caution when administering pancrelipase to a patient with a known allergy to proteins of porcine origin. (5.5)

————ADVERSE REACTIONS————
• Treatment emergent adverse events occurring in at least 2 patients (greater than or equal to 10%) receiving

PANCREAZE or placebo are abdominal pain, abdominal pain upper, flatulence, diarrhea, abnormal feces, and fatigue. (6.1)
To report SUSPECTED ADVERSE REACTIONS, contact McNeil Pediatrics at 1-800-526-7736 or FDA at 1-800-FDA-1088 or www.fda.gov/medwatch

————USE IN SPECIFIC POPULATIONS————
Pediatric Patients
• The safety and effectiveness of PANCREAZE were assessed in pediatric patients, aged 6 to 30 months old and aged 8 to 17 years old. (8.4)
• The safety and efficacy of pancreatic enzyme products with different formulations of pancrelipase in pediatric patients have been described in the medical literature and through clinical experience. (8.4)

See 17 for PATIENT COUNSELING INFORMATION and Medication Guide

Revised: 04/2010

FULL PRESCRIBING INFORMATION

1   INDICATIONS AND USAGE
PANCREAZE (pancrelipase) is indicated for the treatment of exocrine pancreatic insufficiency due to cystic fibrosis or other conditions.

2   DOSAGE AND ADMINISTRATION
2.1   Dosage
PANCREAZE is not interchangeable with other pancrelipase products.
PANCREAZE is orally administered. Therapy should be initiated at the lowest recommended dose and gradually increased. The dosage of PANCREAZE should be individualized based on clinical symptoms, the degree of steatorrhea present, and the fat content of the diet (see Limitations on Dosing below).
Dosage recommendations for pancreatic enzyme replacement therapy were published following the Cystic Fibrosis Foundation Consensus Conferences.[1,2,3] PANCREAZE should be administered in a manner consistent with the recommendations of the Conferences provided in the following paragraphs. Patients may be dosed on a fat ingestion-based or actual body weight-based dosing scheme.
Infants (up to 12 months)
Infants may be given 2,000 to 4,000 lipase units per 120 mL of formula or per breast-feeding. Do not mix PANCREAZE capsule contents directly into formula or breast milk prior to administration *[see Dosage and Administration (2.2)].*
Children Older than 12 Months and Younger than 4 Years
Enzyme dosing should begin with 1,000 lipase units/kg of body weight per meal for children less than age 4 years to a maximum of 2,500 lipase units/kg of body weight per meal

(or less than or equal to 10,000 lipase units/kg of body weight per day), or less than 4,000 lipase units/g fat ingested per day.

Children 4 Years and Older and Adults

Enzyme dosing should begin with 500 lipase units/kg of body weight per meal for those older than age 4 years to a maximum of 2,500 lipase units/kg of body weight per meal (or less than or equal to 10,000 lipase units/kg of body weight per day), or less than 4,000 lipase units/g fat ingested per day.

Usually, half of the prescribed PANCREAZE dose for an individualized full meal should be given with each snack. The total daily dose should reflect approximately three meals plus two or three snacks per day.

Enzyme doses expressed as lipase units/kg of body weight per meal should be decreased in older patients because they weigh more but tend to ingest less fat per kilogram of body weight.

Limitations on Dosing

Dosing should not exceed the recommended maximum dosage set forth by the Cystic Fibrosis Foundation Consensus Conferences Guidelines.[1, 2, 3]

If symptoms and signs of steatorrhea persist, the dosage may be increased by a healthcare professional. Patients should be instructed not to increase the dosage on their own. There is great inter-individual variation in response to enzymes; thus, a range of doses is recommended. Changes in dosage may require an adjustment period of several days. If doses are to exceed 2,500 lipase units/kg of body weight per meal, further investigation is warranted.

Doses greater than 2,500 lipase units/kg of body weight per meal (or greater than 10,000 lipase units/kg of body weight per day) should be used with caution and only if they are documented to be effective by 3-day fecal fat measures that indicate a significantly improved coefficient of fat absorption. Doses greater than 6,000 lipase units/kg of body weight per meal have been associated with colonic strictures, indicative of fibrosing colonopathy, in children with cystic fibrosis less than 12 years of age [see *Warnings and Precautions (5.1)*]. Patients currently receiving higher doses than 6,000 lipase units/kg of body weight per meal should be examined and the dosage either immediately decreased or titrated downward to a lower range.

2.2 Administration

PANCREAZE should always be taken as prescribed by a healthcare professional.

Infants (up to 12 months)

PANCREAZE should be administered to infants immediately prior to each feeding, using a dosage of 2,000 to 4,000 lipase units per 120 mL of formula or per breast-feeding. Contents of the capsule may be sprinkled on small amounts of acidic soft food with a pH of 4.5 or less (e.g., applesauce) and given to the infant within 15 minutes. Contents of the capsule may also be administered directly to the mouth. Administration should be followed by breast milk or formula. Contents of the capsule **should not** be mixed directly into formula or breast milk as this may diminish efficacy. Care should be taken to ensure that PANCREAZE is not crushed or chewed or retained in the mouth, to avoid irritation of the oral mucosa.

Children and Adults

PANCREAZE should be taken during meals or snacks, with sufficient fluid. **PANCREAZE capsules and capsule contents should not be crushed or chewed.** Capsules should be swallowed whole.

For patients who are unable to swallow intact capsules, the capsules may be carefully opened and the contents sprinkled on small amounts of acidic soft food with a pH of 4.5 or less (e.g., applesauce). The PANCREAZE-soft food mixture should be swallowed immediately without crushing or chewing, and followed with water or juice to ensure complete ingestion. Care should be taken to ensure that no drug is retained in the mouth.

3 DOSAGE FORMS AND STRENGTHS

The active ingredient in PANCREAZE evaluated in clinical trials is lipase. PANCREAZE is dosed by lipase units. PANCREAZE is available in 4 color coded capsule strengths.

Other active ingredients include protease and amylase. Each PANCREAZE capsule strength contains the specified amounts of lipase, protease, and amylase as follows:

- 4,200 USP units of lipase; 10,000 USP units of protease; 17,500 USP units of amylase capsules have a yellow opaque body and clear cap, printed with "McNEIL" and "MT 4"
- 10,500 USP units of lipase; 25,000 USP units of protease; 43,750 USP units of amylase capsules have a pink opaque body and clear cap, printed with "McNEIL" and "MT 10"
- 16,800 USP units of lipase; 40,000 USP units of protease; 70,000 USP units of amylase capsules have a salmon opaque body and clear cap, printed with "McNEIL" and "MT 16"

- 21,000 USP units of lipase; 37,000 USP units of protease; 61,000 USP units of amylase capsules have a white opaque body and cap, printed with "McNEIL" and "MT 20"

4 CONTRAINDICATIONS

None.

5 WARNINGS AND PRECAUTIONS

5.1 Fibrosing Colonopathy

Fibrosing colonopathy has been reported following treatment with different pancreatic enzyme products.[4,5] Fibrosing colonopathy is a rare serious adverse reaction initially described in association with high-dose pancreatic enzyme use, usually with use over a prolonged period of time and most commonly reported in pediatric patients with cystic fibrosis. The underlying mechanism of fibrosing colonopathy remains unknown. Doses of pancreatic enzyme products exceeding 6,000 lipase units/kg of body weight per meal have been associated with colonic strictures in children less than 12 years of age.[1] Patients with fibrosing colonopathy should be closely monitored because some patients may be at risk of progressing to stricture formation. It is uncertain whether regression of fibrosing colonopathy occurs.[1] It is generally recommended, unless clinically indicated, that enzyme doses should be less than 2,500 lipase units/kg of body weight per meal (or less than 10,000 lipase units/kg of body weight per day) or less than 4,000 lipase units/g fat ingested per day [see *Dosage and Administration (2.1)*].

Doses greater than 2,500 lipase units/kg of body weight per meal (or greater than 10,000 lipase units/kg of body weight per day) should be used with caution and only if they are documented to be effective by 3-day fecal fat measures that indicate a significantly improved coefficient of fat absorption. Patients receiving higher doses than 6,000 lipase units/kg of body weight per meal should be examined and the dosage either immediately decreased or titrated downward to a lower range.

5.2 Potential for Irritation to Oral Mucosa

Care should be taken to ensure that no drug is retained in the mouth. PANCREAZE should not be crushed or chewed or mixed in foods having a pH greater than 4.5. These actions can disrupt the protective enteric coating resulting in early release of enzymes, irritation of oral mucosa, and/or loss or enzyme activity [see *Dosage and Administration (2.2)* and *Patient Counseling Information (17)*]. For patients who are unable to swallow intact capsules, the capsules may be carefully opened and the contents sprinkled to a small amount of acidic soft food with a pH of 4.5 or less, such as applesauce. The PANCREAZE-soft food mixture should be swallowed immediately and followed with water or juice to ensure complete ingestion.

5.3 Potential for Risk of Hyperuricemia

Caution should be exercised when prescribing PANCREAZE to patients with gout, renal impairment, or hyperuricemia. Porcine- derived pancreatic enzyme products contain purines that may increase blood uric acid levels.

5.4 Potential Viral Exposure from the Product Source

PANCREAZE is sourced from pancreatic tissue from swine used for food consumption. Although the risk that PANCREAZE will transmit an infectious agent to humans has been reduced by testing for certain viruses during manufacturing and by inactivating certain viruses during manufacturing, there is a theoretical risk for transmission of viral disease, including diseases caused by novel or unidentified viruses. Thus, the presence of porcine viruses that might infect humans cannot be definitely excluded. However, no cases of transmission of an infectious illness associated with the use of porcine pancreatic extracts have been reported.

5.5 Allergic Reactions

Caution should be exercised when administering pancrelipase to a patient with a known allergy to proteins of porcine origin. Rarely, severe allergic reactions including anaphylaxis, asthma, hives, and pruritus, have been reported with other pancreatic enzyme products with different formulations of the same active ingredient (pancrelipase). The risks and benefits of continued PANCREAZE treatment in patients with severe allergy should be taken into consideration with the overall clinical needs of the patient.

6 ADVERSE REACTIONS

The most serious adverse reactions reported with different pancreatic enzyme products of the same active ingredient (pancrelipase) include fibrosing colonopathy, hyperuricemia and allergic reactions [see *Warnings and Precautions (5)*]

6.1 Clinical Trials Experience

Because clinical trials are conducted under widely varying conditions, adverse reaction rates observed in the clinical trials of a drug cannot be directly compared to the rates in the clinical trials of another drug and may not reflect the rates observed in clinical practice.

The short-term safety of PANCREAZE was assessed in two clinical trials conducted in 57 patients with exocrine pancreatic insufficiency (EPI) due to CF. Study 1 was conducted

in 40 patients, ages 8 years to 57 years; Study 2 was conducted in 17 patients, ages 6 to 30 months. In Study 1, PANCREAZE was administered in a dose of approximately 6,300 lipase units per kilogram per day for lengths of treatment ranging from 8 to 26 days; in Study 2, PANCREAZE was administered in four treatment arms (doses of 1,375, 2,875, 4,735, and 5,938 lipase units per kilogram per day) for lengths of treatment ranging from 6 to 11 days. The population was nearly evenly distributed in gender, and approximately 96% of patients were Caucasian.

Study 1 was a randomized, double-blind, placebo-controlled, study of 40 patients, ages 8 to 57 years, with EPI due to CF. In this study, patients received PANCREAZE at individually titrated doses (not to exceed 2,500 lipase units per kilogram per meal) for 14 days, followed by randomization to PANCREAZE or matching placebo for 7 days of treatment. The mean exposure to PANCREAZE during this study, including titration period and randomized withdrawal period, was 18 days.

The incidence of adverse events (regardless of causality) was higher during placebo treatment (60%) than during PANCREAZE treatment (40%). The most common adverse events reported during the study were gastrointestinal complaints, which were reported more commonly during placebo treatment (55%) than during PANCREAZE treatment (30%). The type and incidence of adverse events were similar in children (8 to 11 years), adolescents (12 to 17 years), and adults (greater than 18 years).

Table 1 enumerates treatment-emergent adverse events that occurred in at least 2 patients (greater than or equal to 10%) treated with either PANCREAZE or placebo in Study 1. Adverse events were classified by Medical Dictionary for Regulatory Activities (MedDRA) terminology.

Table 1: Treatment-Emergent Adverse Events Occurring in at least 2 Patients (greater than or equal to 10%) in Either Treatment Group of the Placebo-Controlled, Clinical Study of PANCREAZE

MedDRA Primary System Organ Class Preferred Term	PANCREAZE (N=20) n (%)	Placebo (N=20) n (%)
Gastrointestinal Disorders		
Abdominal pain	2 (10%)	3 (15%)
Abdominal pain upper	1 (5%)	3 (15%)
Flatulence	1 (5%)	3 (15%)
Diarrhea	0 (0%)	4 (20%)
Abnormal feces	0 (0%)	3 (15%)
General Disorders And Administration Site Conditions		
Fatigue	0 (0%)	2 (10%)

Study 2 was a randomized, investigator-blinded, dose-ranging study of 17 patients, ages 6 to 30 months, with EPI due to CF. All patients were transitioned from their usual PEP treatment to PANCREAZE at 375 lipase units per kilogram body weight per meal for a 6 day run-in period. Patients were then randomized to receive PANCREAZE at one of four doses (375, 750, 1,125, and 1,500 lipase units per kilogram body weight per meal) for 5 days. Adverse events were collected on patient diary entries and at each study visit.

The most commonly reported adverse events were gastrointestinal, including diarrhea and vomiting, and were similar in type and frequency across treatment arms and to those reported in the double-blind, placebo-controlled trial (Study 1).

6.2 Postmarketing Experience

Post-marketing data for PANCREAZE has been available since 1988. The safety data is similar to that described below.

Delayed- and immediate-release pancreatic enzyme products with different formulations of the same active ingredient (pancrelipase) have been used for the treatment of patients with exocrine pancreatic insufficiency due to cystic fibrosis and other conditions, such as chronic pancreatitis. The long-term safety profile of these products has been described in the medical literature. The most serious adverse events included fibrosing colonopathy, distal intestinal obstruction syndrome (DIOS), recurrence of pre-existing carcinoma, and severe allergic reactions including anaphylaxis, asthma, hives, and pruritus. The most commonly reported adverse events were gastrointestinal disorders, including abdominal pain, diarrhea, flatulence, constipation and nausea, and skin disorders including pruritus, urticaria and rash. In general, these products have a well defined and favorable risk-benefit profile in exocrine pancreatic insufficiency.

Because these reactions are reported voluntarily from a population of uncertain size, it is not always possible to reliably estimate their frequency or establish a causal relationship to drug exposure.

7 DRUG INTERACTIONS

No drug interactions have been identified. No formal interaction studies have been conducted.

8 USE IN SPECIFIC POPULATIONS

8.1 Pregnancy
Teratogenic effects
Pregnancy Category C: Animal reproduction studies have not been conducted with pancrelipase. It is not known whether pancrelipase can cause fetal harm when administered to a pregnant woman or can affect reproduction capacity. PANCREAZE should be given to a pregnant woman only if clearly needed. The risk and benefit of pancrelipase should be considered in the context of the need to provide adequate nutritional support to a pregnant woman with exocrine pancreatic insufficiency. Adequate caloric intake during pregnancy is important for normal maternal weight gain and fetal growth. Reduced maternal weight gain and malnutrition can be associated with adverse pregnancy outcomes.

8.3 Nursing Mothers
It is not known whether this drug is excreted in human milk. Because many drugs are excreted in human milk, caution should be exercised when PANCREAZE is administered to a nursing woman. The risk and benefit of pancrelipase should be considered in the context of the need to provide adequate nutritional support to a nursing mother with exocrine pancreatic insufficiency.

8.4 Pediatric Use
The short-term safety and effectiveness of PANCREAZE were assessed in two clinical studies in pediatric patients with EPI due to CF; one study included patients ages 6 to 30 months, and the other included patients ages 8 years to 17 years.

Study 1 was a randomized, double-blind, placebo-controlled study in 40 patients, 14 of whom were pediatric patients, including 7 children aged 8 to 11 years, and 7 adolescents aged 12 to 17 years. The safety and efficacy in pediatric patients in this study were similar to adult patients [see Adverse Reactions (6.1) and Clinical Studies (14)].

Study 2 was a randomized, investigator-blinded, dose-ranging study in 17 pediatric patients aged 6 to 30 months. When patient regimen was switched from their usual PEP regimen to PANCREAZE, patients showed similar control of their fat malabsorption [see Adverse Reactions (6.1) and Clinical Studies (14)].

The safety and efficacy of pancreatic enzyme products with different formulations of pancrelipase consisting of the same active ingredient (lipases, proteases, and amylases) for treatment of children with exocrine pancreatic insufficiency due to cystic fibrosis has been described in the medical literature and through clinical experience.

Dosing of pediatric patients should be in accordance with recommended guidance from the Cystic Fibrosis Foundation Consensus Conferences [see Dosage and Administration (2.1)]. Doses of other pancreatic enzyme products exceeding 6,000 lipase units/kg of body weight per meal have been associated with fibrosing colonopathy and colonic strictures in children less than 12 years of age [see Warnings and Precautions (5.1)].

10 OVERDOSAGE

In Study 1, a 10 year-old patient was administered a PANCREAZE dose of 12,399 lipase units per kilogram per day for the duration of the open-label and randomized withdrawal periods. The patient experienced mild abdominal pain throughout both study periods. Abnormal chemistry data at the end of the study included mild elevations of aspartate aminotransferase (AST), alanine aminotransferase (ALT), and serum phosphate. Abnormal hematology data at the end of the study included mild elevations of hematocrit. No abnormalities from analyses of urinalysis or uric acid were noted.

Chronic high doses of pancreatic enzyme products have been associated with fibrosing colonopathy and colonic strictures [see Dosage and Administration (2.1) and Warnings and Precautions (5.1)]. High doses of pancreatic enzyme products have been associated with hyperuricosuria and hyperuricemia, and should be used with caution in patients with a history of hyperuricemia, gout, or renal impairment [see Warnings and Precautions (5.3)].

11 DESCRIPTION

PANCREAZE is a pancreatic enzyme preparation consisting of pancrelipase, an extract derived from porcine pancreatic glands. Pancrelipase contains multiple enzyme classes, including porcine-derived lipases, proteases, and amylases.

Each capsule for oral administration contains enteric-coated microtablets that are each approximately 2 mm in diameter.

Table 3. Change in CFA in Study 2 (End of Run-in Period to End of Study)

	375 units lipase/kg/meal n=4	750 units lipase/kg/meal n=4	1,125 units lipase/kg/meal n=4	1,500 units lipase/kg/meal n=4
CFA (%)				
Day 6* (Mean, SD)	93 (2)	90 (5)	81 (11)	93 (3)
Day 11† (Mean, SD)	92 (3)	91 (4)	80 (13)	91 (2)
Change in CFA (%) Day 6 to Day 11 (Mean, SD)	-2 (3)	1 (3)	-1 (3)	-2 (3)

* End of Run-in Period;
† End of Study

The active ingredient evaluated in clinical trials is lipase. PANCREAZE is dosed by lipase units. Other active ingredients include protease and amylase.

Inactive ingredients in PANCREAZE include cellulose, colloidal anhydrous silica, crospovidone, magnesium stearate, methacrylic acid ethyl acrylate copolymer, montan glycol wax, simethicone emulsion, talc and triethyl citrate.

PANCREAZE is available in four color coded strengths. Each PANCREAZE capsule strength contains the specified amounts of lipase, protease, and amylase as follows:

4,200 USP units of lipase; 10,000 USP units of protease; 17,500 USP units of amylase. The hard gelatin capsules have a yellow opaque body and clear cap imprinted with "McNEIL" and "MT 4". The capsule shell contains gelatin, titanium dioxide, sodium lauryl sulfate, sorbitan monolaurate, iron oxide, and gelatin capsule imprint ink.

10,500 USP units of lipase; 25,000 USP units of protease; 43,750 USP units of amylase. The hard gelatin capsules have a pink opaque body and clear cap imprinted with "McNEIL" and "MT 10". The capsule shell contains gelatin, titanium dioxide, sodium lauryl sulfate, sorbitan monolaurate, iron oxide, and gelatin capsule imprint ink.

16,800 USP units of lipase; 40,000 of protease; 70,000 USP units of amylase. The hard gelatin capsules have a salmon opaque body and clear cap imprinted with "McNEIL" and "MT 16". The capsule shell contains gelatin, titanium dioxide, sodium lauryl sulfate, sorbitan monolaurate, iron oxide, and gelatin capsule imprint ink.

21,000 USP units of lipase; 37,000 of protease; 61,000 USP units of amylase. The hard gelatin capsules have a white opaque body and cap imprinted with "McNEIL" and "MT 20". The capsule shell contains gelatin, titanium dioxide, sodium lauryl sulfate, sorbitan monolaurate, and gelatin capsule imprint ink.

12 CLINICAL PHARMACOLOGY

12.1 Mechanism of Action
The pancreatic enzymes in PANCREAZE catalyze the hydrolysis of fats to monoglyceride, glycerol and free fatty acids, proteins into peptides and amino acids, and starches into dextrins and short chain sugars such as maltose and maltriose in the duodenum and proximal small intestine, thereby acting like digestive enzymes physiologically secreted by the pancreas.

12.3 Pharmacokinetics
The pancreatic enzymes in PANCREAZE are enteric-coated to minimize destruction or inactivation in gastric acid. PANCREAZE is expected to release most of the enzymes in vivo at pH greater than 5.5. Pancreatic enzymes are not absorbed from the gastrointestinal tract in appreciable amounts.

13 NONCLINICAL TOXICOLOGY

13.1 Carcinogenesis, Mutagenesis, Impairment of Fertility
Carcinogenicity, genetic toxicology, and animal fertility studies have not been performed with pancrelipase.

14 CLINICAL STUDIES

The short-term safety and efficacy of PANCREAZE were evaluated in two studies conducted in 57 patients with exocrine pancreatic insufficiency (EPI) associated with cystic fibrosis (CF).

Study 1 was a randomized, double-blind, placebo-controlled study of 40 patients, ages 8 to 57 years, with EPI due to CF. In this study, patients received PANCREAZE at individually titrated doses (not to exceed 2,500 lipase units per kilogram per meal) for 14 days (open label period) followed by randomization to PANCREAZE or matching placebo for 7 days of treatment (double-blind withdrawal period). Only patients with coefficient of fat absorption (CFA) ≥80% in the open label period were randomized to the double-blind withdrawal period. The mean dose during the controlled treatment was 6,400 lipase units per kilogram per day. All patients consumed a high-fat diet (greater than or equal to 100 grams of fat per day) during the treatment period.

The primary efficacy endpoint was the change in CFA from the open label period to the end of the double-blind withdrawal period. The CFA was determined by a 72-hour stool collection period during both treatment periods, when both fat excretion and fat ingestion were measured (Table 2).

Table 2. Change in CFA in Study 1 (Open Label Period to End of Double-Blind Withdrawal Period)

	PANCREAZE n=20	Placebo n=20
CFA [%]		
Open Label Period* (Mean, SD)	88 (5)	91 (5)
End of Double-Blind Withdrawal Period† (Mean, SD)	87 (8)	56 (25)
Change in CFA‡ [%]		
Open Label Period to End of Double-Blind Withdrawal Period (Mean, SD)	-2 (6)	-34 (23)
Treatment Difference Point Estimate (95% CI)	33 (25, 40)	

* Minimum of 72 hours from start of open label period.
† Double-blind withdrawal period ranged from 4 to 7 days.
‡ $p < 0.001$

At the end of the double-blind withdrawal period, the mean change in CFA from the open label period to the end of the double-blind withdrawal period was -2% with PANCREAZE treatment compared to -34% with placebo treatment. There were similar responses to PANCREAZE by age and gender.

Study 2 was a randomized, investigator-blinded, dose-ranging study of 17 patients, ages 6 months to 30 months (mean 18 months) with EPI due to CF. The final analysis population was limited to 16 patients; 1 patient was excluded due to withdrawal of consent. All patients were transitioned from their usual PEP treatment to PANCREAZE at 375 lipase units per kilogram body weight per meal for a 6 day run-in period. Patients were then randomized to receive PANCREAZE at one of four doses (375, 750, 1,125, and 1,500 lipase units per kilogram body weight per meal) for 5 days. The CFA was measured at the end of the run-in period and at the end of the randomized period (Table 3).

[See table 3 above]

Overall, patients showed similar CFA at the end of the run-in period (mean PANCREAZE dose of 1,600 lipase units per kilogram body weight per day) as at the end of the study across the four treatment arms.

15 REFERENCES

1. Borowitz DS, Grand RJ, Durie PR, et al. Use of pancreatic enzyme supplements for patients with cystic fibrosis in the context of fibrosing colonopathy. Journal of Pediatrics. 1995; 127: 681–684.

2. Borowitz DS, Baker RD, Stallings V. Consensus report on nutrition for pediatric patients with cystic fibrosis. Journal of Pediatric Gastroenterology Nutrition. 2002 Sep; 35: 246–259.

3. Stallings VA, Start LJ, Robinson KA, et al. Evidence-based practice recommendations for nutrition-related management of children and adults with cystic fibrosis and pancreatic insufficiency: results of a systematic review. Journal of the American Dietetic Association. 2008; 108: 832–839.

4. Smyth RL, Ashby D, O'Hea U, et al. Fibrosing colonopathy in cystic fibrosis: results of a case-control study. Lancet. 1995; 346: 1247–1251.

5. FitzSimmons SC, Burkhart GA, Borowitz DS, et al. High-dose pancreatic-enzyme supplements and fibrosing colonopathy in children with cystic fibrosis. *New England Journal of Medicine.* 1997; 336: 1283–1289.

16 HOW SUPPLIED/STORAGE AND HANDLING

PANCREAZE (pancrelipase) Delayed-Release Capsules
4,200 USP units of lipase; 10,000 USP units of protease; 17,500 USP units of amylase.
PANCREAZE (pancrelipase) is supplied as hard gelatin capsules with a yellow opaque body and clear cap imprinted with "McNEIL" and "MT 4" and packaged in bottles of 100– (NDC 50458-341-60).

PANCREAZE (pancrelipase) Delayed-Release Capsules
10,500 USP units of lipase; 25,000 USP units of protease; 43,750 USP units of amylase.
PANCREAZE (pancrelipase) is supplied as hard gelatin capsules with a pink opaque body and clear cap imprinted with "McNEIL" and "MT 10" and packaged in bottles of 100– (NDC 50458-342-60).

PANCREAZE (pancrelipase) Delayed-Release Capsules
16,800 USP units of lipase; 40,000 USP units of protease; 70,000 USP units of amylase.
PANCREAZE (pancrelipase) is supplied as hard gelatin capsules with a salmon opaque body and clear cap imprinted with "McNEIL" and "MT 16" and packaged in bottles of 100–(NDC 50458-343-60).

PANCREAZE (pancrelipase) Delayed-Release Capsules
21,000 USP units of lipase; 37,000 USP units of protease; 61,000 USP units of amylase.
PANCREAZE (pancrelipase) is supplied as hard gelatin capsules with a white opaque body and cap imprinted with "McNEIL" and "MT 20" and packaged in bottles of 100– (NDC 50458-346-60).

Storage and Handling
Avoid heat. PANCREAZE hard gelatin capsules should be stored in a dry place in the original container. After opening, KEEP THE CONTAINER TIGHTLY CLOSED between uses to PROTECT FROM MOISTURE. Do not store above 25°C (77°F).
The PANCREAZE 4200 USP Units of lipase bottle contains a desiccant packet. DO NOT eat or throw away the packet (desiccant) in your medicine bottle. This packet will protect your medicine from moisture.
Keep out of reach of children.
DO NOT CRUSH PANCREAZE delayed-release capsules or the capsule contents.

17 PATIENT COUNSELING INFORMATION

See Medication Guide
17.1 Dosing and Administration
• Instruct patients and caregivers that PANCREAZE should only be taken as directed by their healthcare professional. Patients should be advised that the total daily dose should not exceed 10,000 lipase units/kg body weight/day unless clinically indicated. This needs to be especially emphasized for patients eating multiple snacks and meals per day. Patients should be informed that if a dose is missed, the next dose should be taken with the next meal or snack as directed. Doses should not be doubled [*see Dosage and Administration (2)*].
• Instruct patients and caregivers that PANCREAZE should always be taken with food. Patients should be advised that PANCREAZE delayed-release capsules and the capsule contents must not be crushed or chewed as doing so could cause early release of enzymes and/or loss of enzymatic activity. Patients should swallow the intact capsules with adequate amounts of liquid at mealtimes. If necessary, the capsules contents can also be sprinkled on soft acidic foods. [*see Dosage and Administration (2)*].
• Instruct patients to notify their healthcare professional if they are pregnant or are thinking of becoming pregnant during treatment with PANCREAZE [*see Use in Specific Populations (8.1)*].
• Instruct patients to notify their healthcare professional if they are breast feeding or are thinking of breast feeding during treatment with PANCREAZE [*see Use in Specific Populations (8.3)*].

17.2 Fibrosing Colonopathy
Advise patients and caregivers to follow dosing instructions carefully, as doses of pancreatic enzyme products exceeding 6,000 lipase units/kg of body weight per meal (10,000 lipase units/kg of body weight/day) have been associated with colonic strictures in children below the age of 12 years [*see Dosage and Administration (2)*].

17.3 Allergic Reactions
Advise patients and caregivers to contact their healthcare professional immediately if allergic reactions to PANCREAZE develop [*see Warnings and Precautions (5.5)*].

Manufactured by:
Nordmark Arzneimittel GmbH & Co. KG
25436 Uetersen, Germany.

Manufactured for:
McNeil Pediatrics, Division of Ortho-McNeil-Janssen Pharmaceuticals, Inc.
Titusville, NJ 08560.
©Ortho-McNeil-Janssen Pharmaceuticals, Inc. 2010

MEDICATION GUIDE

PANCREAZE (pan-kre-aze)
(pancrelipase)
Delayed-Release Capsules
Read this Medication Guide before you start taking PANCREAZE and each time you get a refill. There may be new information. This information does not take the place of talking to your doctor about your medical condition or treatment.

What is the most important information I should know about PANCREAZE?
• PANCREAZE may increase your chance of having a rare bowel disorder called fibrosing colonopathy. This condition is serious and may require surgery. The risk of having this condition may be reduced by following the dosing instructions that your doctor gave you. **Call your doctor right away if you have any unusual or severe:**
  • stomach area (abdominal) pain
  • bloating
  • trouble passing stool (having bowel movements)
  • nausea, vomiting, or diarrhea
Take PANCREAZE exactly as prescribed by your doctor. Do not take more or less PANCREAZE than directed by your doctor.

What is PANCREAZE?
PANCREAZE is a prescription medicine used to treat people who cannot digest food normally because their pancreas does not make enough enzymes due to cystic fibrosis or other conditions. PANCREAZE may help your body use fats, proteins, and sugars from food.
PANCREAZE contains a mixture of digestive enzymes including lipases, proteases, and amylases from pig pancreas. PANCREAZE is safe and effective in children when taken as prescribed by your doctor.

What should I tell my doctor before taking PANCREAZE?
Before taking PANCREAZE, tell your doctor about all your medical conditions, including if you:
• are allergic to pork (pig) products.
• have a history of blockage of your intestines, or scarring or thickening of your bowel wall (fibrosing colonopathy).
• have gout, kidney disease, or high blood uric acid (hyperuricemia)
• have trouble swallowing capsules
• have any other medical condition
• are pregnant or plan to become pregnant. It is not known if PANCREAZE will harm your unborn baby.
• are breast-feeding or plan to breast-feed. It is not known if PANCREAZE passes into your breast milk. You and your doctor should decide if you will take PANCREAZE or breast-feed.
Tell your doctor about all the medicines you take, including prescription and nonprescription medicines, vitamins, or herbal supplements.
Know the medicines you take. Keep a list of them and show it to your doctor and pharmacist when you get a new medicine.

How should I take PANCREAZE?
Take PANCREAZE exactly as your doctor tells you.
• Do not take more capsules in a day than the number your doctor tells you to take (total daily dose).
• Always take PANCREAZE with a meal or snack and plenty of fluid. If you eat a lot of meals or snacks in a day, be careful not to go over your total daily dose.
• Your doctor may change your dose based on the amount of fatty foods you eat or based on your weight.
• **Do not crush or chew the PANCREAZE capsules or their contents, and do not hold the capsule or contents in your mouth.** Crushing, chewing or holding the PANCREAZE Capsules in your mouth may cause irritation in your mouth or change the way PANCREAZE works in your body.

Giving PANCREAZE to infants (children up to 12 months):
1. Give PANCREAZE right before each feeding of formula or breast milk.
2. Do not mix PANCREAZE capsule contents directly into formula or breast milk.
3. Open the capsules and sprinkle the contents directly into your infant's mouth or mix the contents in a small amount of soft food such as applesauce. These foods should be the kind found in baby food jars that you buy at the store, or other food recommended by your doctor.
4. If you sprinkle the PANCREAZE on food, give the PANCREAZE and food mixture to your child right away. Do not store PANCREAZE that is mixed with food.
5. Give your child enough liquid to completely swallow the PANCREAZE contents or the PANCREAZE and food mixture.
6. Look into your child's mouth to make sure that all of the medicine has been swallowed.

Giving PANCREAZE to children and adults
1. Swallow PANCREAZE capsules whole and take them with enough liquid to swallow them right away.
2. If you have trouble swallowing capsules, open the capsules and sprinkle the contents on a small amount of acidic food such as applesauce. Ask your doctor about other foods you can mix with PANCREAZE.
3. If you sprinkle PANCREAZE on food, swallow it right after you mix it and drink plenty of water or juice to make sure the medicine is swallowed completely. Do not store PANCREAZE that is mixed with food.
4. If you forget to take PANCREAZE, call your healthcare provider or wait until your next meal and take your usual number of capsules. Take your next dose at your usual time. Do not make up for missed doses.

What are the possible side effects of PANCREAZE?
PANCREAZE may cause serious side effects, including:
• See "What is the most important information I should know about PANCREAZE?"
• **Irritation of the inside of your mouth.** This can happen if PANCREAZE is not swallowed completely.
• **Increase in blood uric acid levels.** This may cause worsening of swollen, painful joints (gout) caused by an increase in your blood uric acid levels
• **Allergic reactions** including trouble with breathing, skin rashes, or swollen lips.
Call your doctor right away if you have any of these symptoms.

The most common side effects of PANCREAZE include:
• Pain in your stomach (abdominal area)
• Gas

Other Possible Side Effects
PANCREAZE and other pancreatic enzyme products are made from the pancreas of pigs, the same pigs people eat as pork. These pigs may carry viruses. Although it has never been reported, it may be possible for a person to get a viral infection from taking pancreatic enzyme products that come from pigs.
Tell your doctor if you have any side effect that bothers you or does not go away.
These are not all the possible side effects of PANCREAZE. For more information, ask your doctor or pharmacist.
Call your doctor for medical advice about side effects.
You may report side effects to FDA at 1-800-FDA-1088. You may also report side effects to McNeil Pediatrics at 1-800-526-7736.

How do I store PANCREAZE?
• Store PANCREAZE at room temperature below 77°F (25°C). Avoid heat.
• Keep PANCREAZE in a dry place and in the original container.
• After opening the bottle, keep it closed tightly between uses.
• The PANCREAZE 4200 USP Units of lipase bottle contains a desiccant packet. DO NOT eat or throw away the packet (desiccant) in your medicine bottle. This packet will protect your medicine from moisture.
• Store PANCREAZE in a dry place.
Keep PANCREAZE and all medicines out of reach of children.

General information about PANCREAZE
Medicines are sometimes prescribed for purposes other than those listed in a Medication Guide. Do not use PANCREAZE for a condition for which it was not prescribed. Do not give PANCREAZE to other people to take, even if they have the same symptoms you have. It may harm them.
This Medication Guide summarizes the most important information about PANCREAZE. If you would like more information, talk to your doctor. You can ask your pharmacist or doctor for information about PANCREAZE that is written for healthcare providers.
For more information go to *www.RXFORSAFETY.com* or call 1-800-526-7736 (Monday - Friday 9am to 5pm EST).

What are the ingredients in PANCREAZE?
Active Ingredient: lipase, protease, amylase
Inactive Ingredients: cellulose, colloidal anhydrous silica, crospovidone, magnesium stearate, methacrylic acid ethyl acrylate copolymer, montan glycol wax, simethicone emulsion, talc and triethyl citrate. The capsule shell contains gelatin, titanium dioxide, sodium lauryl sulfate, sorbitan monolaurate, and gelatin capsule imprint ink. PANCREAZE 4,200, 10,500, and 16,800 USP Units of lipase also contain iron oxide.

Manufactured by:
Nordmark Arzneimittel GmbH & Co. KG
25436 Uetersen, Germany.

Manufactured for:
McNeil Pediatrics, Division of Ortho-McNeil-Janssen Pharmaceuticals, Inc.
Titusville, NJ 08560.
Revised: April 2010
©Ortho-McNeil-Janssen Pharmaceuticals, Inc. 2010
Shown in Product Identification Guide, page 317

RISPERDAL® CONSTA®
(risperidone)
LONG-ACTING INJECTION

℞

HIGHLIGHTS OF PRESCRIBING INFORMATION
These highlights do not include all the information needed to use RISPERDAL® CONSTA® safely and effectively. See full prescribing information for RISPERDAL® CONSTA®.
RISPERDAL® CONSTA® (risperidone) LONG-ACTING INJECTION
Initial U.S. Approval: 2003

WARNING: INCREASED MORTALITY IN ELDERLY PATIENTS WITH DEMENTIA-RELATED PSYCHOSIS
See full prescribing information for complete boxed warning.
Elderly patients with dementia-related psychosis treated with antipsychotic drugs are at an increased risk of death. RISPERDAL® CONSTA® is not approved for use in patients with dementia-related psychosis. (5.1)

————————RECENT MAJOR CHANGES————————

Indications and Usage, Bipolar Disorder (1.2) Dosage and Administration,	May 2009
Bipolar Disorder (2.2) Warnings and Precautions, Leukopenia,	May 2009
Neutropenia, and Agranulocytosis (5.8)	July 2009
Warnings and Precautions, Suicide (5.17)	May 2009

————————INDICATIONS AND USAGE————————
RISPERDAL® CONSTA® is an atypical antipsychotic indicated:
• for the treatment of schizophrenia. (1.1)
• as monotherapy or as adjunctive therapy to lithium or valproate for the maintenance treatment of Bipolar I Disorder. (1.2)

————————DOSAGE AND ADMINISTRATION————————
• For patients who have never taken oral RISPERDAL®, tolerability should be established with oral RISPERDAL® prior to initiating treatment with RISPERDAL® CONSTA®. (2)
• Administer by deep intramuscular (IM) deltoid or gluteal injection. Each injection should be administered by a health care professional using the appropriate enclosed safety needle (1-inch for deltoid administration alternating injections between the two arms and 2-inch for gluteal administration alternating injections between the two buttocks. Do not administer intravenously. (2)
• 25 mg intramuscular (IM) every 2 weeks. Patients not responding to 25 mg may benefit from a higher dose of 37.5 mg or 50 mg. The maximum dose should not exceed 50 mg every 2 weeks. (2)
• Oral RISPERDAL® (or another antipsychotic medication) should be given with the first injection of RISPERDAL® CONSTA®, and continued for 3 weeks (and then discontinued) to ensure adequate therapeutic plasma concentrations from RISPERDAL® CONSTA®. (2)
• Upward dose adjustment of RISPERDAL® CONSTA® should not be made more frequently than every 4 weeks. Clinical effects of each upward dose adjustment should not be anticipated earlier than 3 weeks after injection. (2)
• Avoid inadvertent administration into a blood vessel. (5.15)
• See Full Prescribing Information Section 2.8 for instructions for use.

————————DOSAGE FORMS AND STRENGTHS————————
Vial kits: 12.5 mg, 25 mg, 37.5 mg, and 50 mg (3)

————————CONTRAINDICATIONS————————
• Known hypersensitivity to the product (4)

————————WARNINGS AND PRECAUTIONS————————
• Cerebrovascular events, including stroke, in elderly patients with dementia-related psychosis. RISPERDAL® CONSTA® is not approved for use in patients with dementia-related psychosis (5.2)
• Neuroleptic Malignant Syndrome: Manage with immediate discontinuation and close monitoring (5.3)
• Tardive Dyskinesia: Discontinue treatment if clinically appropriate (5.4)
• Hyperglycemia and Diabetes Mellitus: in some cases extreme and associated with ketoacidosis or hyperosmolar coma or death, has been reported in patients taking risperidone. Patients with diabetes mellitus should have glucose levels monitored regularly. Patients with risk factors for diabetes mellitus should undergo fasting glucose testing at the beginning of treatment and periodically during treatment. All patients taking risperidone should be monitored for symptoms of hyperglycemia. Symptomatic patients should undergo fasting glucose testing. (5.5)
• Hyperprolactinemia: Risperidone treatment may elevate prolactin levels. Long-standing hyperprolactinemia, when associated with hypogonadism, can lead to decreased bone density in men and women. (5.6)
• Orthostatic hypotension: associated with dizziness, tachycardia, bradycardia, and syncope can occur, espe-

cially during initial dose titration with oral risperidone. Use caution in patients with cardiovascular disease, cerebrovascular disease, and conditions that could affect hemodynamic responses. (5.7)
• Leukopenia, Neutropenia, and Agranulocytosis have been reported with antipsychotics, including RISPERDAL® CONSTA®. Patients with history of a clinically significant low white blood cell count (WBC) or a drug-induced leukopenia/neutropenia should have their complete blood cell count (CBC) monitored frequently during the first few months of therapy and discontinuation of RISPERDAL® CONSTA® should be considered at the first sign of a clinically significant decline in WBC in the absence of other causative factors. (5.8)
• Potential for cognitive and motor impairment: has potential to impair judgment, thinking, and motor skills. Use caution when operating machinery, including automobiles. (5.9)
• Seizures: Use cautiously in patients with a history of seizures or with conditions that potentially lower the seizure threshold. (5.10)
• Dysphagia: Esophageal dysmotility and aspiration can occur. Use cautiously in patients at risk for aspiration pneumonia. (5.11)
• Priapism: has been reported. Severe priapism may require surgical intervention. (5.12)
• Thrombotic Thrombocytopenic Purpura (TTP): has been reported. (5.13)
• Avoid inadvertent administration into a blood vessel (5.15)
• Suicide: There is increased risk of suicide attempt in patients with schizophrenia or bipolar disorder, and close supervision of high-risk patients should accompany drug therapy. (5.17)
• Increased sensitivity in patients with Parkinson's disease or those with dementia with Lewy bodies: has been reported. Manifestations include mental status changes, motor impairment, extrapyramidal symptoms, and features consistent with Neuroleptic Malignant Syndrome. (5.18)
• Diseases or conditions that could affect metabolism or hemodynamic responses: Use with caution in patients with such medical conditions (e.g., recent myocardial infarction or unstable cardiac disease). (5.18)

————————ADVERSE REACTIONS————————
The most common adverse reactions in clinical trials in patients with schizophrenia (≥ 5%) were headache, parkinsonism, dizziness, akathisia, fatigue, constipation, dyspepsia, sedation, weight increased, pain in extremity, and dry mouth. The most common adverse reactions in clinical trials in patients with bipolar disorder were weight increased (5% in monotherapy trial) and tremor and parkinsonism (≥10% in adjunctive therapy trial). (6)
The most common adverse reactions that were associated with discontinuation from clinical trials in patients with schizophrenia were agitation, depression, anxiety, and akathisia. Adverse reactions that were associated with discontinuation from bipolar disorder trials were hyperglycemia (one subject monotherapy trial) and hypokinesia and tardive dyskinesia (one subject each in adjunctive therapy trial). (6)

To report SUSPECTED ADVERSE REACTIONS, contact Janssen, Division of Ortho-McNeil-Janssen Pharmaceuticals, Inc. at 1-800-JANSSEN (1-800-526-7736) or FDA at 1-800-FDA-1088 or www.fda.gov/medwatch

————————DRUG INTERACTIONS————————
• Due to CNS effects, use caution when administering with other centrally-acting drugs. Avoid alcohol. (7.1)
• Due to hypotensive effects, hypotensive effects of other drugs with this potential may be enhanced. (7.2)
• Effects of levodopa and dopamine agonists may be antagonized. (7.3)
• Cimetidine and ranitidine increase the bioavailability of risperidone. (7.5)
• Clozapine may decrease clearance of risperidone. (7.6)
• Fluoxetine and paroxetine increase plasma concentrations of risperidone. (7.11)
• Carbamazepine and other enzyme inducers decrease plasma concentrations of risperidone. (7.12)

————————USE IN SPECIFIC POPULATIONS————————
• Renal or Hepatic Impairment: dose appropriately with oral RISPERDAL® prior to initiating treatment with RISPERDAL® CONSTA®. A lower starting dose of RISPERDAL® CONSTA® of 12.5 mg may be appropriate in some patients. (2.4)
• Nursing Mothers: should not breast feed. (8.3)
• Pediatric Use: safety and effectiveness not established in patients less than 18 years of age. (8.4)
• Elderly: dosing for otherwise healthy elderly patients is the same as for healthy nonelderly. Elderly may be more predisposed to orthostatic effects than nonelderly. (8.5)

See 17 for PATIENT COUNSELING INFORMATION
Revised: 04/2010

*** Sections or subsections omitted from the full prescribing information are not listed**

FULL PRESCRIBING INFORMATION

WARNING: INCREASED MORTALITY IN ELDERLY PATIENTS WITH DEMENTIA-RELATED PSYCHOSIS
Elderly patients with dementia-related psychosis treated with antipsychotic drugs are at an increased risk of death. Analyses of 17 placebo-controlled trials (modal duration of 10 weeks), largely in patients taking atypical antipsychotic drugs, revealed a risk of death in drug-treated patients of between 1.6 to 1.7 times the risk of death in placebo-treated patients. Over the course of a typical 10-week controlled trial, the rate of death in drug-treated patients was about 4.5%, compared to a rate of about 2.6% in the placebo group. Although the causes of death were varied, most of the deaths appeared to be either cardiovascular (e.g., heart failure, sudden death) or infectious (e.g., pneumonia) in nature. Observational studies suggest that, similar to atypical antipsychotic drugs, treatment with conventional antipsychotic drugs may increase mortality. The extent to which the findings of increased mortality in observational studies may be attributed to the antipsychotic drug as opposed to some characteristic(s) of the patients is not clear. RISPERDAL® CONSTA® (risperidone) is not approved for the treatment of patients with dementia-related psychosis. *[See Warnings and Precautions (5.1)]*

1 INDICATIONS AND USAGE

1.1 Schizophrenia

RISPERDAL® CONSTA® (risperidone) is indicated for the treatment of schizophrenia *[see Clinical Studies (14.1)]*.

1.2 Bipolar Disorder

RISPERDAL® CONSTA® is indicated as monotherapy or as adjunctive therapy to lithium or valproate for the maintenance treatment of Bipolar I Disorder *[see Clinical Studies (14.2, 14.3)]*.

2 DOSAGE AND ADMINISTRATION

For patients who have never taken oral RISPERDAL®, it is recommended to establish tolerability with oral RISPERDAL® prior to initiating treatment with RISPERDAL® CONSTA®.

RISPERDAL® CONSTA® should be administered every 2 weeks by deep intramuscular (IM) deltoid or gluteal injection. Each injection should be administered by a health care professional using the appropriate enclosed safety needle *[see Dosage and Administration (2.8)]*. For deltoid administration, use the 1-inch needle alternating injections between the two arms. For gluteal administration, use the 2-inch needle alternating injections between the two buttocks. Do not administer intravenously.

2.1 Schizophrenia

The recommended dose for the treatment of schizophrenia is 25 mg IM every 2 weeks. Although dose response for effectiveness has not been established for RISPERDAL® CONSTA®, some patients not responding to 25 mg may benefit from a higher dose of 37.5 mg or 50 mg. The maximum dose should not exceed 50 mg RISPERDAL® CONSTA® every 2 weeks. No additional benefit was observed with dosages greater than 50 mg RISPERDAL® CONSTA®; however, a higher incidence of adverse effects was observed.

The efficacy of RISPERDAL® CONSTA® in the treatment of schizophrenia has not been evaluated in controlled clinical trials for longer than 12 weeks. Although controlled studies have not been conducted to answer the question of how long patients with schizophrenia should be treated with RISPERDAL® CONSTA®, oral risperidone has been shown to be effective in delaying time to relapse in longer-term use. It is recommended that responding patients be continued on treatment with RISPERDAL® CONSTA® at the lowest dose needed. The physician who elects to use RISPERDAL® CONSTA® for extended periods should periodically re-evaluate the long-term risks and benefits of the drug for the individual patient.

2.2 Bipolar Disorder

The recommended dose for monotherapy or adjunctive therapy to lithium or valproate for the maintenance treatment of Bipolar I Disorder is 25 mg IM every 2 weeks. Some patients may benefit from a higher dose of 37.5 mg or 50 mg. Dosages above 50 mg have not been studied in this population. The physician who elects to use RISPERDAL® CONSTA® for extended periods should periodically re-evaluate the long-term risks and benefits of the drug for the individual patient.

2.3 General Dosing Information

A lower initial dose of 12.5 mg may be appropriate when clinical factors warrant dose adjustment, such as in patients with hepatic or renal impairment, for certain drug interactions that increase risperidone plasma concentrations *[see Drug Interactions (7.11)]* or in patients who have a history of poor tolerability to psychotropic medications. The efficacy of the 12.5 mg dose has not been investigated in clinical trials.

Oral RISPERDAL® (or another antipsychotic medication) should be given with the first injection of RISPERDAL® CONSTA® and continued for 3 weeks (and then discontinued) to ensure that adequate therapeutic plasma concentrations are maintained prior to the main release phase of risperidone from the injection site *[see Clinical Pharmacology (12.3)]*.

Upward dose adjustment should not be made more frequently than every 4 weeks. The clinical effects of this dose adjustment should not be anticipated earlier than 3 weeks after the first injection with the higher dose.

In patients with clinical factors such as hepatic or renal impairment or certain drug interactions that increase risperidone plasma concentrations *[see Drug Interactions (7.11)]*, dose reduction as low as 12.5 mg may be appropriate. The efficacy of the 12.5 mg dose has not been investigated in clinical trials.

Do not combine two different dose strengths of RISPERDAL® CONSTA® in a single administration.

2.4 Dosage in Special Populations

Elderly

For elderly patients treated with RISPERDAL® CONSTA®, the recommended dosage is 25 mg IM every 2 weeks. Oral RISPERDAL® (or another antipsychotic medication) should be given with the first injection of RISPERDAL® CONSTA® and should be continued for 3 weeks to ensure that adequate therapeutic plasma concentrations are maintained prior to the main release phase of risperidone from the injection site *[see Clinical Pharmacology (12.3)]*.

Renal or Hepatic Impairment

Patients with renal or hepatic impairment should be treated with titrated doses of oral RISPERDAL® prior to initiating treatment with RISPERDAL® CONSTA®. The recommended starting dose is 0.5 mg oral RISPERDAL® twice daily during the first week, which can be increased to 1 mg twice daily or 2 mg once daily during the second week. If a total daily dose of at least 2 mg oral RISPERDAL® is well tolerated, an injection of 25 mg RISPERDAL® CONSTA® can be administered every 2 weeks. Oral supplementation should be continued for 3 weeks after the first injection until the main release of risperidone from the injection site has begun. In some patients, slower titration may be medically appropriate. Alternatively, a starting dose of RISPERDAL® CONSTA® of 12.5 mg may be appropriate. The efficacy of the 12.5 mg dose has not been investigated in clinical trials.

Patients with renal impairment may have less ability to eliminate risperidone than normal adults. Patients with impaired hepatic function may have an increase in the free fraction of the risperidone, possibly resulting in an enhanced effect *[see Clinical Pharmacology (12.3)]*. Elderly patients and patients with a predisposition to hypotensive reactions or for whom such reactions would pose a particular risk should be instructed in nonpharmacologic interventions that help to reduce the occurrence of orthostatic hypotension (e.g., sitting on the edge of the bed for several minutes before attempting to stand in the morning and slowly rising from a seated position). These patients should avoid sodium depletion or dehydration, and circumstances that accentuate hypotension (alcohol intake, high ambient temperature, etc.). Monitoring of orthostatic vital signs should be considered *[see Warnings and Precautions (5.7)]*.

2.5 Reinitiation of Treatment in Patients Previously Discontinued

There are no data to specifically address reinitiation of treatment. When restarting patients who have had an interval off treatment with RISPERDAL® CONSTA®, supplementation with oral RISPERDAL® (or another antipsychotic medication) should be administered.

2.6 Switching from Other Antipsychotics

There are no systematically collected data to specifically address switching patients from other antipsychotics to RISPERDAL® CONSTA®, or concerning concomitant administration with other antipsychotics. Previous antipsychotics should be continued for 3 weeks after the first injection of RISPERDAL® CONSTA® to ensure that therapeutic concentrations are maintained until the main release phase of risperidone from the injection site has begun *[see Clinical Pharmacology (12.3)]*. For patients who have never taken oral RISPERDAL®, it is recommended to establish tolerability with oral RISPERDAL® prior to initiating treatment with RISPERDAL® CONSTA®. As recommended with other antipsychotic medications, the need for continuing existing EPS medication should be re-evaluated periodically.

2.7 Co-Administration of RISPERDAL® CONSTA® with Certain Other Medications

Co-administration of carbamazepine and other CYP 3A4 enzyme inducers (e.g., phenytoin, rifampin, phenobarbital) with risperidone would be expected to cause decreases in the plasma concentrations of the sum of risperidone and 9-hydroxyrisperidone combined, which could lead to decreased efficacy of RISPERDAL® CONSTA® treatment. The dose of risperidone needs to be titrated accordingly for patients receiving these enzyme inducers, especially during initiation or discontinuation of therapy with these inducers *[see Drug Interactions (7.11)]*. At the initiation of therapy with carbamazepine or other known CYP 3A4 hepatic enzyme inducers, patients should be closely monitored during the first 4–8 weeks, since the dose of RISPERDAL® CONSTA® may need to be adjusted. A dose increase, or additional oral RISPERDAL®, may need to be considered. On discontinuation of carbamazepine or other CYP 3A4 hepatic enzyme inducers, the dosage of RISPERDAL® CONSTA® should be re-evaluated and, if necessary, decreased. Patients may be placed on a lower dose of RISPERDAL® CONSTA® between 2 to 4 weeks before the planned discontinuation of carbamazepine or other CYP 3A4 inducers to adjust for the expected increase in plasma concentrations of risperidone plus 9-hydroxyrisperidone. For patients treated with the recommended dose of 25 mg RISPERDAL® CONSTA® and discontinuing from carbamazepine or other CYP3A4 enzyme inducers, it is recommended to continue treatment with the 25-mg dose unless clinical judgment necessitates lowering the RISPERDAL® CONSTA® dose to 12.5 mg or necessitates interruption of RISPERDAL® CONSTA® treatment. The efficacy of the12.5 mg dose has not been investigated in clinical trials.

Fluoxetine and paroxetine, CYP 2D6 inhibitors, have been shown to increase the plasma concentration of risperidone 2.5–2.8 fold and 3–9 fold respectively. Fluoxetine did not affect the plasma concentration of 9-hydroxyrisperidone. Paroxetine lowered the concentration of 9-hydroxyrisperidone by about 10%. The dose of risperidone needs to be titrated accordingly when fluoxetine or paroxetine is co-administered. When either concomitant fluoxetine or paroxetine is initiated or discontinued, the physician should re-evaluate the dose of RISPERDAL® CONSTA®. When initiation of fluoxetine or paroxetine is considered, patients may be placed on a lower dose of RISPERDAL® CONSTA® between 2 to 4 weeks before the planned start of fluoxetine or paroxetine therapy to adjust for the expected increase in plasma concentrations of risperidone. When fluoxetine or paroxetine is initiated in patients receiving the recommended dose of 25 mg RISPERDAL® CONSTA®, it is recommended to continue treatment with the 25-mg dose unless clinical judgment necessitates lowering the RISPERDAL® CONSTA® dose to 12.5 mg or necessitates interruption of RISPERDAL® CONSTA® treatment. When RISPERDAL® CONSTA® is initiated in patients already receiving fluoxetine or paroxetine, a starting dose of 12.5 mg can be considered. The efficacy of the 12.5 mg dose has not been investigated in clinical trials. The effects of discontinuation of concomitant fluoxetine or paroxetine therapy on the pharmacokinetics of risperidone and 9-hydroxyrisperidone have not been studied. *[See Drug Interactions (7.11)]*

2.8 Instructions for Use

Dose pack components include:

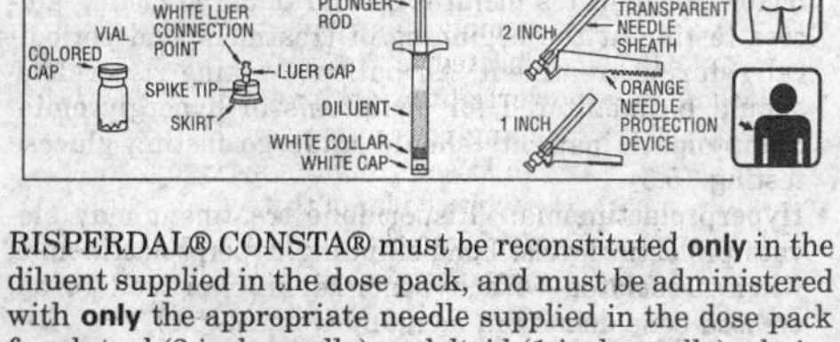

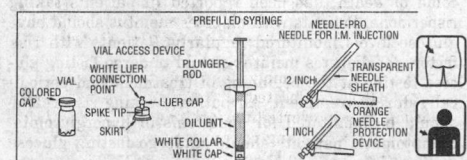

RISPERDAL® CONSTA® must be reconstituted **only** in the diluent supplied in the dose pack, and must be administered with **only** the appropriate needle supplied in the dose pack for gluteal (2-inch needle) or deltoid (1-inch needle) administration. All components are required for administration.

Do not substitute any components of the dose pack. To assure that the intended dose of risperidone is delivered, the full contents from the vial must be administered. Administration of partial contents may not deliver the intended dose of risperidone.

Remove the dose pack of RISPERDAL® CONSTA® from the refrigerator and allow it to come to room temperature prior to reconstitution.

1. Flip off the plastic colored cap from the vial.

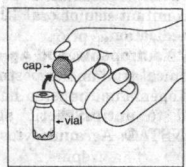

2. Peel back the blister pouch and remove the SmartSite® Needle-Free Vial Access Device by holding the white luer cap. Do not touch the spike tip of the access device at any time.

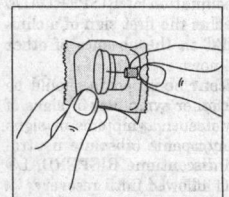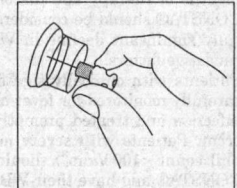

3. Place vial on a hard surface. Hold the base of the vial. Orient the SmartSite® Access Device vertically over the vial so that the spike tip is at the center of the vial's rubber stopper. With a straight downward push, press the spike tip of the SmartSite® Access Device through the center of the vial's rubber stopper until the device securely snaps onto the vial top.

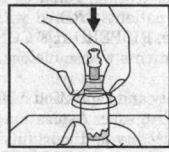

4. Swab the syringe connection point (blue circle) of the SmartSite® Access Device with preferred antiseptic prior to attaching the syringe to the SmartSite® Access Device.

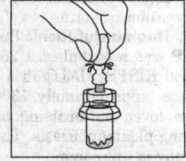

5. The prefilled syringe has a white tip consisting of 2 parts: a white collar and a smooth white cap. To open the syringe, hold the syringe by the white collar and **snap** off the smooth white cap (**DO NOT TWIST OFF THE WHITE CAP**). Remove the white cap together with the rubber tip cap inside.

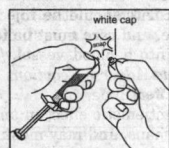

For all syringe assembly steps, hold the syringe only by the white collar located at the tip of the syringe. Be careful to not overtighten components when assembling. Overtightening connections may cause syringe component parts to loosen from the syringe body.

6. While holding the **white collar** of the syringe, insert and **press** the syringe tip into the blue circle of the Smart-Site® Access Device and **twist** in a clockwise motion to secure the connection of the syringe to the SmartSite® Access Device (avoid over-twisting). Hold the skirt of the SmartSite® Access Device during attachment to prevent it from spinning. Keep the syringe and SmartSite® Access Device aligned.

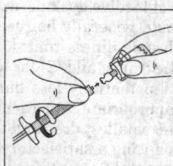

7. Inject the entire contents of the syringe containing the diluent into the vial.

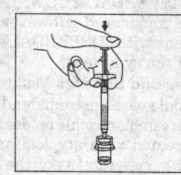

8. Shake the vial vigorously while holding the plunger rod down with the thumb for a minimum of 10 seconds to ensure a homogeneous suspension. When properly mixed, the suspension appears uniform, thick, and milky in color. The microspheres will be visible in liquid, but no dry microspheres remain.

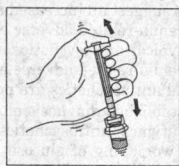

9. Do not store the vial after reconstitution or the suspension may settle. *If 2 minutes pass before injection, re-suspend by shaking vigorously.*

10. Invert the vial completely and slowly withdraw the suspension from the vial into the syringe. Tear section of the vial label at the perforation and apply detached label to syringe for identification purposes.

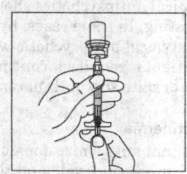

11. While holding the **white collar** of the syringe, unscrew the syringe from the SmartSite® Access Device. Discard both the vial and vial access device appropriately.

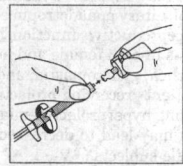

12. Select the appropriate needle:
For GLUTEAL injection, select the **20G TW 2-inch** needle (longer needle with **yellow** colored hub in blister with **yellow** print)
For DELTOID injection, select the **21G UTW 1-inch** needle (shorter needle with **green** colored hub in blister with **green** print)

13. Peel the blister pouch of the Needle-Pro® safety device open halfway. Grasp the transparent needle sheath using the plastic peel pouch. To prevent contamination, be careful not to touch the orange Needle-Pro® safety device's Luer connector. While holding the **white collar** of the syringe, attach the Luer connection of the orange Needle-Pro® safety device to the syringe with an easy clockwise twisting motion.

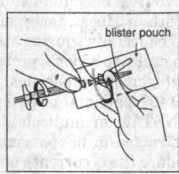

14. While continuing to hold the **white collar** of the syringe, grasp the transparent needle sheath and seat the needle firmly on the orange Needle-Pro® safety device with a push and a clockwise twist.

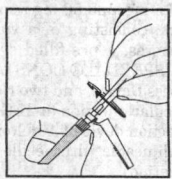

15. *If 2 minutes pass before injection, re-suspend by shaking vigorously.*

16. While holding the **white collar** of the syringe, pull the transparent needle sheath straight away from the needle. DO NOT TWIST the sheath as the Luer connections may be loosened.

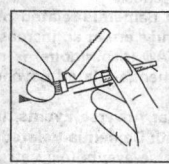

17. Tap the syringe gently to make any air bubbles rise to the top. Remove air in syringe by depressing the plunger rod while holding the needle in an upright position. Inject the entire contents of the syringe intramuscularly (IM) into the selected gluteal or deltoid muscle of the patient within 2 minutes to avoid settling. Gluteal injection should be made into the upper-outer quadrant of the gluteal area. **DO NOT ADMINISTER INTRAVENOUSLY.**

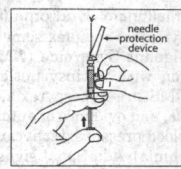

needle protection device

WARNING: To avoid a needle stick injury with a contaminated needle:
• Do not use free hand to press the Needle-Pro® safety device over the needle.
• Do not intentionally disengage the Needle-Pro® safety device.
• Do not attempt to straighten the needle or engage Needle-Pro® safety device if the needle is bent or damaged.
• Do not mishandle the Needle-Pro® safety device, as it may cause the needle to protrude from the Needle-Pro® safety device.

18. After injection is complete, press the needle into the orange Needle-Pro® safety device using a one-handed technique. Perform a one-handed technique by GENTLY pressing the orange Needle-Pro® safety device against a table top or other hard, flat surface. AS THE ORANGE NEEDLE-PRO® SAFETY DEVICE IS PRESSED, THE NEEDLE WILL FIRMLY ENGAGE INTO THE ORANGE NEEDLE-PRO® SAFETY DEVICE. Visually confirm that the needle is fully engaged into the orange Needle-Pro® safety device before discarding. Discard needle appropriately. Also discard the other (unused) needle provided in the dose pack.

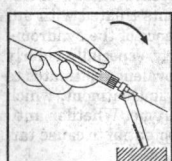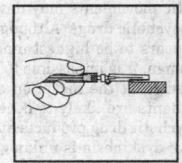

Upon suspension of the microspheres in the diluent, it is recommended to use RISPERDAL® CONSTA® immediately. If RISPERDAL® CONSTA® is not administered within 2 minutes of reconstitution, settling of the microspheres will occur and resuspension by shaking is necessary prior to administration. Keeping the vial upright, shake vigorously back and forth for as long as it takes to resuspend the microspheres. Once in suspension, the product may remain at room temperature (do not expose to temperatures above 77°F (25°C)). RISPERDAL® CONSTA® must be used within 6 hours of suspension.

Parenteral drug products should be inspected visually for particulate matter and discoloration prior to administration, whenever solution and container permit.

3   DOSAGE FORMS AND STRENGTHS

RISPERDAL® CONSTA® is available in dosage strengths of 12.5 mg, 25 mg, 37.5 mg, and 50 mg risperidone. It is provided as a dose pack, consisting of a vial containing the risperidone microspheres, a pre-filled syringe containing 2 mL of diluent for RISPERDAL® CONSTA®, a SmartSite® Needle-Free Vial Access Device, and two Needle-Pro® safety needles for intramuscular injection (a 21 G UTW 1-inch needle with needle protection device for deltoid administration and a 20 G TW 2-inch needle with needle protection device for gluteal administration).

4   CONTRAINDICATIONS

RISPERDAL® CONSTA® (risperidone) is contraindicated in patients with a known hypersensitivity to the product.

5   WARNINGS AND PRECAUTIONS

5.1   Increased Mortality in Elderly Patients with Dementia-Related Psychosis

Elderly patients with dementia-related psychosis treated with antipsychotic drugs are at an increased risk of death. RISPERDAL® CONSTA® (risperidone) is not approved for the treatment of dementia-related psychosis (see Boxed Warning).

5.2   Cerebrovascular Adverse Events, Including Stroke, in Elderly Patients with Dementia-Related Psychosis

Cerebrovascular adverse events (e.g., stroke, transient ischemic attack), including fatalities, were reported in patients (mean age 85 years; range 73–97) in trials of oral risperidone in elderly patients with dementia-related psychosis. In placebo-controlled trials, there was a significantly higher incidence of cerebrovascular adverse events in patients treated with oral risperidone compared to patients treated with placebo. RISPERDAL® CONSTA® is not approved for the treatment of patients with dementia-related psychosis [See also Boxed Warning and Warnings and Precautions (5.1)]

5.3   Neuroleptic Malignant Syndrome (NMS)

A potentially fatal symptom complex sometimes referred to as Neuroleptic Malignant Syndrome (NMS) has been reported in association with antipsychotic drugs. Clinical manifestations of NMS are hyperpyrexia, muscle rigidity, altered mental status, and evidence of autonomic instability (irregular pulse or blood pressure, tachycardia, diaphoresis, and cardiac dysrhythmia). Additional signs may include elevated creatine phosphokinase, myoglobinuria (rhabdomyolysis), and acute renal failure.

The diagnostic evaluation of patients with this syndrome is complicated. In arriving at a diagnosis, it is important to identify cases in which the clinical presentation includes both serious medical illness (e.g., pneumonia, systemic infection, etc.) and untreated or inadequately treated extrapyramidal signs and symptoms (EPS). Other important considerations in the differential diagnosis include central anticholinergic toxicity, heat stroke, drug fever, and primary central nervous system pathology.

The management of NMS should include: (1) immediate discontinuation of antipsychotic drugs and other drugs not essential to concurrent therapy; (2) intensive symptomatic treatment and medical monitoring; and (3) treatment of any concomitant serious medical problems for which specific treatments are available. There is no general agreement about specific pharmacological treatment regimens for uncomplicated NMS.

If a patient requires antipsychotic drug treatment after recovery from NMS, the potential reintroduction of drug therapy should be carefully considered. The patient should be carefully monitored, since recurrences of NMS have been reported.

5.4   Tardive Dyskinesia

A syndrome of potentially irreversible, involuntary, dyskinetic movements may develop in patients treated with antipsychotic drugs. Although the prevalence of the syndrome appears to be highest among the elderly, especially elderly women, it is impossible to rely upon prevalence estimates to predict, at the inception of antipsychotic treatment, which patients are likely to develop the syndrome. Whether antipsychotic drug products differ in their potential to cause tardive dyskinesia is unknown.

The risk of developing tardive dyskinesia and the likelihood that it will become irreversible are believed to increase as the duration of treatment and the total cumulative dose of antipsychotic drugs administered to the patient increase. However, the syndrome can develop, although much less commonly, after relatively brief treatment periods at low doses.

There is no known treatment for established cases of tardive dyskinesia, although the syndrome may remit, partially or completely, if antipsychotic treatment is withdrawn. Antipsychotic treatment, itself, however, may suppress (or partially suppress) the signs and symptoms of the syndrome and thereby may possibly mask the underlying process. The effect that symptomatic suppression has upon the long-term course of the syndrome is unknown.

Given these considerations, RISPERDAL® CONSTA® should be prescribed in a manner that is most likely to minimize the occurrence of tardive dyskinesia. Chronic antipsychotic treatment should generally be reserved for patients who suffer from a chronic illness that: (1) is known to respond to antipsychotic drugs, and (2) for whom alternative, equally effective, but potentially less harmful treatments are not available or appropriate. In patients who do require chronic treatment, the smallest dose and the shortest duration of treatment producing a satisfactory clinical response should be sought. The need for continued treatment should be reassessed periodically.

If signs and symptoms of tardive dyskinesia appear in a patient treated with RISPERDAL® CONSTA®, drug discontinuation should be considered. However, some patients may require treatment with RISPERDAL® CONSTA® despite the presence of the syndrome.

5.5   Hyperglycemia and Diabetes Mellitus

Hyperglycemia, in some cases extreme and associated with ketoacidosis or hyperosmolar coma or death, has been reported in patients treated with atypical antipsychotics including RISPERDAL®. Assessment of the relationship between atypical antipsychotic use and glucose abnormalities is complicated by the possibility of an increased background risk of diabetes mellitus in patients with schizophrenia and the increasing incidence of diabetes mellitus in the general population. Given these confounders, the relationship between atypical antipsychotic use and hyperglycemia-related adverse events is not completely understood. However, epidemiological studies suggest an increased risk of treatment-emergent hyperglycemia-related adverse events in patients treated with the atypical antipsychotics. Precise risk estimates for hyperglycemia-related adverse events in patients treated with atypical antipsychotics are not available.

Patients with an established diagnosis of diabetes mellitus who are started on atypical antipsychotics should be monitored regularly for worsening of glucose control. Patients with risk factors for diabetes mellitus (e.g., obesity, family history of diabetes) who are starting treatment with atypical antipsychotics should undergo fasting blood glucose testing at the beginning of treatment and periodically during treatment. Any patient treated with atypical antipsychotics should be monitored for symptoms of hyperglycemia including polydipsia, polyuria, polyphagia, and weakness. Patients who develop symptoms of hyperglycemia during treatment with atypical antipsychotics should undergo fasting blood glucose testing. In some cases, hyperglycemia has resolved when the atypical antipsychotic was discontinued; however, some patients required continuation of anti-diabetic treatment despite discontinuation of the suspect drug.

5.6   Hyperprolactinemia

As with other drugs that antagonize dopamine D_2 receptors, risperidone elevates prolactin levels and the elevation persists during chronic administration. Risperidone is associated with higher levels of prolactin elevation than other antipsychotic agents.

Hyperprolactinemia may suppress hypothalamic GnRH, resulting in reduced pituitary gonadotropin secretion. This, in turn, may inhibit reproductive function by impairing gonadal steroidogenesis in both female and male patients. Galactorrhea, amenorrhea, gynecomastia, and impotence have been reported in patients receiving prolactin-elevating compounds. Long-standing hyperprolactinemia when associated with hypogonadism may lead to decreased bone density in both female and male subjects.

Tissue culture experiments indicate that approximately one-third of human breast cancers are prolactin dependent in vitro, a factor of potential importance if the prescription of these drugs is contemplated in a patient with previously detected breast cancer. An increase in pituitary gland, mammary gland, and pancreatic islet cell neoplasia (mammary adenocarcinomas, pituitary and pancreatic adenomas) was observed in the risperidone carcinogenicity studies conducted in mice and rats [see Nonclinical Toxicology (13.1)]. Neither clinical studies nor epidemiologic studies conducted to date have shown an association between chronic administration of this class of drugs and tumorigenesis in humans; the available evidence is considered too limited to be conclusive at this time.

5.7   Orthostatic Hypotension

RISPERDAL® CONSTA® may induce orthostatic hypotension associated with dizziness, tachycardia, and in some patients, syncope, especially during the initial dose-titration period with oral risperidone, probably reflecting its alpha-adrenergic antagonistic properties. Syncope was reported in 0.8% (12/1499 patients) of patients treated with RISPERDAL® CONSTA® in multiple-dose studies. Patients should be instructed in nonpharmacologic interventions that help to reduce the occurrence of orthostatic hypotension (e.g., sitting on the edge of the bed for several minutes before attempting to stand in the morning and slowly rising from a seated position).

RISPERDAL® CONSTA® should be used with particular caution in (1) patients with known cardiovascular disease (history of myocardial infarction or ischemia, heart failure, or conduction abnormalities), cerebrovascular disease, and conditions which would predispose patients to hypotension, e.g., dehydration and hypovolemia, and (2) in the elderly and patients with renal or hepatic impairment. Monitoring of orthostatic vital signs should be considered in all such patients, and a dose reduction should be considered if hypotension occurs. Clinically significant hypotension has been observed with concomitant use of oral RISPERDAL® and antihypertensive medication.

5.8   Leukopenia, Neutropenia, and Agranulocytosis

Class Effect: In clinical trial and/or postmarketing experience, events of leukopenia/neutropenia have been reported temporally related to antipsychotic agents, including RISPERDAL® CONSTA®. Agranulocytosis has also been reported.

Possible risk factors for leukopenia/neutropenia include pre-existing low white blood cell count (WBC) and a history of drug-induced leukopenia/neutropenia. Patients with a history of a clinically significant low WBC or a drug-induced leukopenia/neutropenia should have their complete blood count (CBC) monitored frequently during the first few months of therapy and discontinuation of RISPERDAL® CONSTA® should be considered at the first sign of a clinically significant decline in WBC in the absence of other causative factors.

Patients with clinically significant neutropenia should be carefully monitored for fever or other symptoms or signs of infection and treated promptly if such symptoms or signs occur. Patients with severe neutropenia (absolute neutrophil count <1000/mm^3) should discontinue RISPERDAL® CONSTA® and have their WBC followed until recovery.

5.9   Potential for Cognitive and Motor Impairment

Somnolence was reported by 5% of patients treated with RISPERDAL® CONSTA® in multiple-dose trials. Since risperidone has the potential to impair judgment, thinking, or motor skills, patients should be cautioned about operating hazardous machinery, including automobiles, until they are reasonably certain that treatment with RISPERDAL® CONSTA® does not affect them adversely.

5.10   Seizures

During premarketing testing, seizures occurred in 0.3% (5/1499 patients) of patients treated with RISPERDAL® CONSTA®. Therefore, RISPERDAL® CONSTA® should be used cautiously in patients with a history of seizures.

5.11   Dysphagia

Esophageal dysmotility and aspiration have been associated with antipsychotic drug use. Aspiration pneumonia is a common cause of morbidity and mortality in patients with advanced Alzheimer's dementia. RISPERDAL® CONSTA® and other antipsychotic drugs should be used cautiously in patients at risk for aspiration pneumonia. [See also Boxed Warning and Warnings and Precautions (5.1)]

5.12   Priapism

Priapism has been reported during postmarketing surveillance [see Adverse Reactions (6.9)]. Severe priapism may require surgical intervention.

5.13   Thrombotic Thrombocytopenic Purpura (TTP)

A single case of TTP was reported in a 28 year-old female patient receiving oral RISPERDAL® in a large, open premarketing experience (approximately 1300 patients). She experienced jaundice, fever, and bruising, but eventually recovered after receiving plasmapheresis. The relationship to RISPERDAL® therapy is unknown.

5.14   Body Temperature Regulation

Disruption of body temperature regulation has been attributed to antipsychotic agents. Both hyperthermia and hypothermia have been reported in association with oral RISPERDAL® or RISPERDAL® CONSTA® use. Caution is advised when prescribing RISPERDAL® CONSTA® for patients who will be exposed to temperature extremes.

5.15   Administration

RISPERDAL® CONSTA® should be injected into the deltoid or gluteal muscle, and care must be taken to avoid inadvertent injection into a blood vessel. [See Dosage and Administration (2) and Adverse Reactions (6.8)]

5.16   Antiemetic Effect

Risperidone has an antiemetic effect in animals; this effect may also occur in humans, and may mask signs and symptoms of overdosage with certain drugs or of conditions such as intestinal obstruction, Reye's syndrome, and brain tumor.

5.17   Suicide

There is an increased risk of suicide attempt in patients with schizophrenia or bipolar disorder, and close supervision of high-risk patients should accompany drug therapy. RISPERDAL® CONSTA® is to be administered by a health care professional [see Dosage and Administration (2)]; therefore, suicide due to an overdose is unlikely.

5.18   Use in Patients with Concomitant Illness

Clinical experience with RISPERDAL® CONSTA® in patients with certain concomitant systemic illnesses is limited. Patients with Parkinson's Disease or Dementia with Lewy Bodies who receive antipsychotics, including RISPERDAL® CONSTA®, are reported to have an increased sensitivity to antipsychotic medications. Manifestations of this increased sensitivity have been reported to include confusion, obtundation, postural instability with frequent falls, extrapyramidal symptoms, and clinical features consistent with the neuroleptic malignant syndrome. Caution is advisable when using RISPERDAL® CONSTA® in patients with diseases or conditions that could affect metabolism or hemodynamic responses. RISPERDAL® CONSTA® has not been evaluated or used to any appreciable extent in patients with a recent history of myocardial infarction or unstable heart disease. Patients with these diagnoses were excluded from clinical studies during the product's premarket testing.

Increased plasma concentrations of risperidone and 9-hydroxyrisperidone occur in patients with severe renal impairment (creatinine clearance <30 mL/min/1.73 m²) treated with oral RISPERDAL®; an increase in the free fraction of risperidone is also seen in patients with severe hepatic impairment. Patients with renal or hepatic impairment should be carefully titrated on oral RISPERDAL® before treatment with RISPERDAL® CONSTA® is initiated at a dose of 25 mg. A lower initial dose of 12.5 mg may be appropriate when clinical factors warrant dose adjustment, such as in patients with renal or hepatic impairment [see Dosage and Administration (2.4)].

5.19 Osteodystrophy and Tumors in Animals

RISPERDAL® CONSTA® produced osteodystrophy in male and female rats in a 1-year toxicity study and a 2-year carcinogenicity study at a dose of 40 mg/kg administered IM every 2 weeks.

RISPERDAL® CONSTA® produced renal tubular tumors (adenoma, adenocarcinoma) and adrenomedullary pheochromocytomas in male rats in the 2-year carcinogenicity study at 40 mg/kg administered IM every 2 weeks. In addition, RISPERDAL® CONSTA® produced an increase in a marker of cellular proliferation in renal tissue in males in the 1-year toxicity study and in renal tumor-bearing males in the 2-year carcinogenicity study at 40 mg/kg administered IM every 2 weeks. (Cellular proliferation was not measured at the low dose or in females in either study.)

The effect dose for osteodystrophy and the tumor findings is 8 times the IM maximum recommended human dose (MRHD) (50 mg) on a mg/m² basis and is associated with a plasma exposure (AUC) 2 times the expected plasma exposure (AUC) at the IM MRHD. The no-effect dose for these findings was 5 mg/kg (equal to the IM MRHD on a mg/m² basis). Plasma exposure (AUC) at the no-effect dose was one third the expected plasma exposure (AUC) at the IM MRHD.

Neither the renal or adrenal tumors, nor osteodystrophy, were seen in studies of orally administered risperidone. Osteodystrophy was not observed in dogs at doses up to 14 times (based on AUC) the IM MRHD in a 1-year toxicity study.

The renal tubular and adrenomedullary tumors in male rats and other tumor findings are described in more detail in Section 13.1 (Carcinogenicity, Mutagenesis, Impairment of Fertility).

The relevance of these findings to human risk is unknown.

5.20 Monitoring: Laboratory Tests

No specific laboratory tests are recommended.

6 ADVERSE REACTIONS

The following are discussed in more detail in other sections of the labeling:

- Increased mortality in elderly patients with dementia-related psychosis [see Boxed Warning and Warnings and Precautions (5.1)]
- Cerebrovascular adverse events, including stroke, in elderly patients with dementia-related psychosis [see Warnings and Precautions (5.2)]
- Neuroleptic malignant syndrome [see Warnings and Precautions (5.3)]
- Tardive dyskinesia [see Warnings and Precautions (5.4)]
- Hyperglycemia and diabetes mellitus [see Warnings and Precautions (5.5)]
- Hyperprolactinemia [see Warnings and Precautions (5.6)]
- Orthostatic hypotension [see Warnings and Precautions (5.7)]
- Leukopenia/Neutropenia and Agranulocytosis [see Warnings and Precautions (5.8)]
- Potential for cognitive and motor impairment [see Warnings and Precautions (5.9)]
- Seizures [see Warnings and Precautions (5.10)]
- Dysphagia [see Warnings and Precautions (5.11)]
- Priapism [see Warnings and Precautions (5.12)]
- Thrombotic Thrombocytopenic Purpura (TTP) [see Warnings and Precautions (5.13)]
- Disruption of body temperature regulation [see Warnings and Precautions (5.14)]

- Avoidance of inadvertent injection into a blood vessel [see Warnings and Precautions (5.15)]
- Antiemetic effect [see Warnings and Precautions (5.16)]
- Suicide [see Warnings and Precautions (5.17)]
- Increased sensitivity in patients with Parkinson's disease or those with dementia with Lewy bodies [see Warnings and Precautions (5.18)]
- Diseases or conditions that could affect metabolism or hemodynamic responses [see Warnings and Precautions (5.18)]
- Osteodystrophy and tumors in animals [see Warnings and Precautions (5.19)]

The most common adverse reactions in clinical trials in patients with schizophrenia (≥ 5%) were headache, parkinsonism, dizziness, akathisia, fatigue, constipation, dyspepsia, sedation, weight increased, pain in extremity, and dry mouth. The most common adverse reactions in the double-blind, placebo-controlled periods of the bipolar disorder trials were weight increased (5% in the monotherapy trial) and tremor and parkinsonism (≥ 10% in the adjunctive treatment trial).

The most common adverse reactions that were associated with discontinuation from the 12-week double-blind, placebo-controlled trial in patients with schizophrenia (causing discontinuation in ≥ 1% of patients) were agitation, depression, anxiety, and akathisia. Adverse reactions that were associated with discontinuation from the double-blind, placebo-controlled periods of the bipolar disorder trials were hyperglycemia (one patient in the monotherapy trial) and hypokinesia and tardive dyskinesia (one patient each in the adjunctive treatment trial).

The data described in this section are derived from a clinical trial database consisting of 2392 patients exposed to one or more doses of RISPERDAL® CONSTA® for the treatment of schizophrenia. Of these 2392 patients, 332 were patients who received RISPERDAL® CONSTA® while participating in a 12-week double-blind, placebo-controlled trial. Two hundred two (202) of the 332 were schizophrenia patients who received 25 mg or 50 mg RISPERDAL® CONSTA®. The conditions and duration of treatment with RISPERDAL® CONSTA® in the other clinical trials varied greatly and included (in overlapping categories) double-blind, fixed- and flexible-dose, placebo- or active-controlled studies and open-label phases of studies, inpatients and outpatients, and short-term (up to 12 weeks) and longer-

term (up to 4 years) exposures. Safety was assessed by collecting adverse events and performing physical examinations, vital signs, body weights, laboratory analyses, and ECGs.

In addition to the studies in patients with schizophrenia, safety data are presented from a trial assessing the efficacy and safety of RISPERDAL® CONSTA® when administered as monotherapy for maintenance treatment in patients with bipolar I disorder. The subjects in this multi-center, double-blind, placebo-controlled study were adult patients who met DSM-IV criteria for Bipolar Disorder Type I and who were stable on risperidone (oral or long-acting injection), were stable on other antipsychotics or mood stabilizers, or were experiencing an acute episode. After a 3-week period of treatment with open-label oral risperidone (n=440), subjects who demonstrated an initial response to oral risperidone in this period and those who were stable on risperidone (oral or long-acting injection) at study entry entered into a 26-week stabilization period of open-label RISPERDAL® CONSTA® (n=501). Subjects who demonstrated a maintained response during this period were then randomized into a 24-month double-blind, placebo-controlled period in which they received RISPERDAL® CONSTA® (n=154) or placebo (n=149) as monotherapy. Subjects who relapsed or who completed the double-blind period could choose to enter an 8-week open-label RISPERDAL® CONSTA® extension period (n=160).

Safety data are also presented from a trial assessing the efficacy and safety of RISPERDAL® CONSTA® when administered as adjunctive maintenance treatment in patients with bipolar disorder. The subjects in this multi-center, double-blind, placebo-controlled study were adult patients who met DSM-IV criteria for Bipolar Disorder Type I or Type II and who experienced at least 4 episodes of mood disorder requiring psychiatric/clinical intervention in the previous 12 months, including at least 2 episodes in the 6 months prior to the start of the study. At the start of this study, all patients (n = 275) entered into a 16-week open-label treatment phase in which they received RISPERDAL® CONSTA® in addition to continuing their treatment as usual, which consisted of various mood stabilizers (primarily lithium and valproate), antidepressants, and/or anxiolytics. Patients who reached remission at the end of this 16-week open-label treatment phase (n = 139) were then

Table 1. Adverse Reactions in ≥ 2% of RISPERDAL® CONSTA®-Treated Patients with Schizophrenia in a 12-Week Double-Blind, Placebo-Controlled Trial

System/Organ Class Adverse Reaction	Percentage of Patients Reporting Event		
	RISPERDAL® CONSTA®		Placebo
	25 mg (N=99)	50 mg (N=103)	(N=98)
Eye disorders			
Vision blurred	2	3	0
Gastrointestinal disorders			
Constipation	5	7	1
Dry mouth	0	7	1
Dyspepsia	6	6	0
Nausea	3	4	5
Toothache	1	3	0
Salivary hypersecretion	4	1	0
General disorders and administration site conditions			
Fatigue*	3	9	0
Edema peripheral	2	3	1
Pain	4	1	0
Pyrexia	2	1	0
Infections and infestations			
Upper respiratory tract infection	2	0	1
Investigations			
Weight increased	5	4	2
Weight decreased	4	1	1
Musculoskeletal and connective tissue disorders			
Pain in extremity	6	2	1
Nervous system disorders			
Headache	15	21	12
Parkinsonism *	8	15	9
Dizziness	7	11	6
Akathisia *	4	11	6
Sedation *	5	6	3
Tremor	0	3	0
Syncope	2	1	0
Hypoesthesia	2	0	0
Respiratory, thoracic and mediastinal disorders			
Cough	4	2	3
Sinus congestion	2	0	0
Skin and subcutaneous tissue disorders			
Acne	2	2	0
Dry skin	2	0	0

*Fatigue includes fatigue and asthenia. Parkinsonism includes extrapyramidal disorder, musculoskeletal stiffness, muscle rigidity, and bradykinesia. Akathisia includes akathisia and restlessness. Sedation includes sedation and somnolence.

randomized into a 52-week double-blind, placebo-controlled phase in which they received RISPERDAL® CONSTA® (n = 72) or placebo (n = 67) as adjunctive treatment in addition to continuing their treatment as usual. Patients who did not reach remission at the end of the 16-week open-label treatment phase could choose to continue to receive RISPERDAL® CONSTA® as adjunctive therapy in an open-label manner, in addition to continuing their treatment as usual, for up to an additional 36 weeks as clinically indicated for a total period of up to 52 weeks; these patients (n = 70) were also included in the evaluation of safety.

Adverse events during exposure to study treatment were obtained by general inquiry and recorded by clinical investigators using their own terminology. Consequently, to provide a meaningful estimate of the proportion of individuals experiencing adverse events, events were grouped in standardized categories using MedDRA terminology.

Throughout this section, adverse reactions are reported. Adverse reactions are adverse events that were considered to be reasonably associated with the use of RISPERDAL® CONSTA® (adverse drug reactions) based on the comprehensive assessment of the available adverse event information. A causal association for RISPERDAL® CONSTA® often cannot be reliably established in individual cases. Further, because clinical trials are conducted under widely varying conditions, adverse reaction rates observed in the clinical trials of a drug cannot be directly compared to rates in the clinical trials of another drug and may not reflect the rates observed in clinical practice.

The majority of all adverse reactions were mild to moderate in severity.

6.1 Commonly-Observed Adverse Reactions in Double-Blind, Placebo-Controlled Clinical Trials - Schizophrenia

Table 1 lists the adverse reactions reported in 2% or more of RISPERDAL® CONSTA®-treated patients with schizophrenia in one 12-week double-blind, placebo-controlled trial.

[See table 1 at top of previous page]

6.2 Commonly-Observed Adverse Reactions in Double-Blind, Placebo-Controlled Clinical Trials – Bipolar Disorder

Table 2 lists the treatment-emergent adverse reactions reported in 2% or more of RISPERDAL® CONSTA®-treated patients in the 24-month double-blind, placebo-controlled treatment period of the trial assessing the efficacy and safety of RISPERDAL® CONSTA® when administered as monotherapy for maintenance treatment in patients with Bipolar I Disorder.

Table 2. Adverse Reactions in ≥2% of Patients with Bipolar I Disorder Treated with RISPERDAL® CONSTA® as Monotherapy in a 24-Month Double-Blind, Placebo-Controlled Trial

	Percentage of Patients Reporting Event	
System/Organ Class Adverse Reaction	**RISPERDAL® CONSTA® (N=154)**	**Placebo (N=149)**
Investigations		
Weight increased	5	1
Nervous system disorders		
Dizziness	3	1
Vascular disorders		
Hypertension	3	1

Table 3 lists the treatment-emergent adverse reactions reported in 4% or more of patients in the 52-week double-blind, placebo-controlled treatment phase of a trial assessing the efficacy and safety of RISPERDAL® CONSTA® when administered as adjunctive maintenance treatment in patients with bipolar disorder.

Table 3. Adverse Reactions in ≥4% of Patients with Bipolar Disorder Treated with RISPERDAL® CONSTA® as Adjunctive Therapy in a 52-Week Double-Blind, Placebo-Controlled Trial

	Percentage of Patients Reporting Event	
System/Organ Class Adverse Reaction	**RISPERDAL® CONSTA® + Treatment as Usual* (N=72)**	**Placebo + Treatment as Usual* (N=67)**
General disorders and administration site conditions		
Gait abnormal	4	0
Infections and infestations		
Upper respiratory tract infection	6	3
Investigations		
Weight increased	7	1
Metabolism and nutrition disorders		
Decreased appetite	6	1
Increased appetite	4	0
Musculoskeletal and connective tissue disorders		
Arthralgia	4	3
Nervous system disorders		
Tremor	24	16
Parkinsonism†	15	6
Dyskinesia†	6	3
Sedation‡	7	1
Disturbance in attention	4	0
Reproductive system and breast disorders		
Amenorrhea	4	1
Respiratory, thoracic and mediastinal disorders		
Cough	4	1

*Patients received double-blind RISPERDAL® CONSTA® or placebo in addition to continuing their treatment as usual, which included mood stabilizers, antidepressants, and/or anxiolytics.

†Parkinsonism includes muscle rigidity, hypokinesia, cogwheel rigidity, and bradykinesia. Dyskinesia includes muscle twitching and dyskinesia.

‡Sedation includes sedation and somnolence.

6.3 Other Adverse Reactions Observed During the Premarketing Evaluation of RISPERDAL® CONSTA®

The following additional adverse reactions occurred in < 2% of the RISPERDAL® CONSTA®-treated patients in the above schizophrenia double-blind, placebo-controlled trial dataset, in < 2% of the RISPERDAL® CONSTA®-treated patients in the above double-blind, placebo-controlled period of the monotherapy bipolar disorder trial dataset, or in < 4% of the RISPERDAL® CONSTA®-treated patients in the above double-blind, placebo-controlled period of the adjunctive treatment bipolar disorder trial dataset. The following also includes additional adverse reactions reported at any frequency in RISPERDAL® CONSTA®-treated patients who participated in the open-label phases of the above bipolar disorder studies and in other studies, including double-blind, active-controlled and open-label studies in schizophrenia and bipolar disorder.

Blood and lymphatic system disorders: anemia, neutropenia

Cardiac disorders: tachycardia, atrioventricular block first degree, palpitations, sinus bradycardia, bundle branch block left, bradycardia, sinus tachycardia, bundle branch block right

Ear and labyrinth disorders: ear pain, vertigo

Endocrine disorders: hyperprolactinemia

Eye disorders: conjunctivitis, visual acuity reduced

Gastrointestinal disorders: diarrhea, vomiting, abdominal pain upper, abdominal pain, stomach discomfort, gastritis

General disorders and administration site conditions: injection site pain, chest discomfort, chest pain, influenza like illness, sluggishness, malaise, induration, injection site induration, injection site swelling, injection site reaction, face edema

Immune system disorders: hypersensitivity

Infections and infestations: nasopharyngitis, influenza, bronchitis, urinary tract infection, rhinitis, respiratory tract infection, ear infection, pneumonia, lower respiratory tract infection, pharyngitis, sinusitis, viral infection, infection, localized infection, cystitis, gastroenteritis, subcutaneous abscess

Injury and poisoning: fall, procedural pain

Investigations: blood prolactin increased, alanine aminotransferase increased, electrocardiogram abnormal, gamma-glutamyl transferase increased, blood glucose increased, hepatic enzyme increased, aspartate aminotransferase increased, electrocardiogram QT prolonged, glucose urine present

Metabolism and nutritional disorders: anorexia, hyperglycemia

Musculoskeletal, connective tissue and bone disorders: posture abnormal, myalgia, back pain, buttock pain, muscular weakness, neck pain, musculoskeletal chest pain

Nervous system disorders: coordination abnormal, dystonia, tardive dyskinesia, drooling, paresthesia, dizziness postural, convulsion, akinesia, hypokinesia, dysarthria

Psychiatric disorders: insomnia, agitation, anxiety, sleep disorder, depression, initial insomnia, libido decreased, nervousness

Renal and urinary disorders: urinary incontinence

Reproductive system and breast disorders: galactorrhea, oligomenorrhea, erectile dysfunction, sexual dysfunction, ejaculation disorder, gynecomastia, breast discomfort, menstruation irregular, menstruation delayed, menstrual disorder, ejaculation delayed

Respiratory, thoracic and mediastinal disorders: nasal congestion, pharyngolaryngeal pain, dyspnea, rhinorrhea

Skin and subcutaneous tissue disorders: rash, eczema, pruritus generalized, pruritus

Vascular disorders: hypotension, orthostatic hypotension

6.4 Discontinuations Due to Adverse Reactions

Schizophrenia

Approximately 11% (22/202) of RISPERDAL® CONSTA®-treated patients in the 12-week double-blind, placebo-controlled schizophrenia trial discontinued treatment due to an adverse event, compared with 13% (13/98) who received placebo. The adverse reactions associated with discontinuation in two or more RISPERDAL® CONSTA®-treated patients were: agitation (3%), depression (2%), anxiety (1%), and akathisia (1%).

Bipolar Disorder

In the 24-month double-blind, placebo-controlled treatment period of the trial assessing the efficacy and safety of RISPERDAL® CONSTA® when administered as monotherapy for maintenance treatment in patients with bipolar I disorder, 1 (0.6%) of 154 RISPERDAL® CONSTA®-treated patients discontinued due to an adverse reaction (hyperglycemia).

In the 52-week double-blind phase of the placebo-controlled trial in which RISPERDAL® CONSTA® was administered as adjunctive therapy to patients with bipolar disorder in addition to continuing with their treatment as usual, approximately 4% (3/72) of RISPERDAL® CONSTA®-treated patients discontinued treatment due to an adverse event, compared with 1.5% (1/67) of placebo-treated patients. Adverse reactions associated with discontinuation in RISPERDAL® CONSTA®-treated patients were: hypokinesia (one patient) and tardive dyskinesia (one patient).

6.5 Dose Dependency of Adverse Reactions in Clinical Trials

Extrapyramidal Symptoms:

Two methods were used to measure extrapyramidal symptoms (EPS) in the 12-week double-blind, placebo-controlled trial comparing three doses of RISPERDAL® CONSTA® (25 mg, 50 mg, and 75 mg) with placebo in patients with schizophrenia, including: (1) the incidence of spontaneous reports of EPS symptoms; and (2) the change from baseline to endpoint on the total score (sum of the subscale scores for parkinsonism, dystonia, and dyskinesia) of the Extrapyramidal Symptom Rating Scale (ESRS).

As shown in Table 1, the overall incidence of EPS-related adverse reactions (akathisia, dystonia, parkinsonism, and tremor) in patients treated with 25 mg RISPERDAL® CONSTA® was comparable to that of patients treated with placebo; the incidence of EPS-related adverse reactions was higher in patients treated with 50 mg RISPERDAL® CONSTA®.

The median change from baseline to endpoint in total ESRS score showed no worsening in patients treated with RISPERDAL® CONSTA® compared with patients treated with placebo: 0 (placebo group); -1 (25-mg group, significantly less than the placebo group); and 0 (50-mg group).

Dystonia

Class Effect: Symptoms of dystonia, prolonged abnormal contractions of muscle groups, may occur in susceptible individuals during the first few days of treatment. Dystonic symptoms include: spasm of the neck muscles, sometimes progressing to tightness of the throat, swallowing difficulty, difficulty breathing, and/or protrusion of the tongue. While these symptoms can occur at low doses, they occur more frequently and with greater severity with high potency and at higher doses of first generation antipsychotic drugs. An elevated risk of acute dystonia is observed in males and younger age groups.

6.6 Changes in Body Weight

In the 12-week double-blind, placebo-controlled trial in patients with schizophrenia, 9% of patients treated with RISPERDAL® CONSTA®, compared with 6% of patients treated with placebo, experienced a weight gain of >7% of body weight at endpoint.

In the 24-month double-blind, placebo-controlled treatment period of a trial assessing the efficacy and safety of RISPERDAL® CONSTA® when administered as monotherapy for maintenance treatment in patients with bipolar I disorder, 11.6% of patients treated with RISPERDAL® CONSTA® compared with 2.8% of patients treated with placebo experienced a weight gain of >7% of body weight at endpoint.

In the 52-week double-blind, placebo-controlled trial in patients with bipolar disorder, 26.8% of patients treated with RISPERDAL® CONSTA® as adjunctive treatment in addition to continuing their treatment as usual, compared with 27.3% of patients treated with placebo in addition to continuing their treatment as usual, experienced a weight gain of >7% of body weight at endpoint.

6.7 Changes in ECG

The electrocardiograms of 202 schizophrenic patients treated with 25 mg or 50 mg RISPERDAL® CONSTA® and 98 schizophrenic patients treated with placebo in the 12-

week double-blind, placebo-controlled trial were evaluated. Compared with placebo, there were no statistically significant differences in QTc intervals (using Fridericia's and linear correction factors) during treatment with RISPERDAL® CONSTA®.

The electrocardiograms of 227 patients with Bipolar I Disorder were evaluated in the 24-month double-blind, placebo-controlled period. There were no clinically relevant differences in QTc intervals (using Fridericia's and linear correction factors) during treatment with RISPERDAL® CONSTA® compared to placebo.

The electrocardiograms of 85 patients with bipolar disorder were evaluated in the 52-week double-blind, placebo-controlled trial. There were no statistically significant differences in QTc intervals (using Fridericia's and linear correction factors) during treatment with RISPERDAL® CONSTA® 25 mg, 37.5 mg, or 50 mg when administered as adjunctive treatment in addition to continuing treatment as usual compared to placebo.

6.8   Pain Assessment and Local Injection Site Reactions
The mean intensity of injection pain reported by patients with schizophrenia using a visual analog scale (0 = no pain to 100 = unbearably painful) decreased in all treatment groups from the first to the last injection (placebo: 16.7 to 12.6; 25 mg: 12.0 to 9.0; 50 mg: 18.2 to 11.8). After the sixth injection (Week 10), investigator ratings indicated that 1% of patients treated with 25 mg or 50 mg RISPERDAL® CONSTA® experienced redness, swelling, or induration at the injection site.

In a separate study to observe local-site tolerability in which RISPERDAL® CONSTA® was administered into the deltoid muscle every 2 weeks over a period of 8 weeks, no patient discontinued treatment due to local injection site pain or reaction. Clinician ratings indicated that only mild redness, swelling, or induration at the injection site was observed in subjects treated with 37.5 mg or 50 mg RISPERDAL® CONSTA® at 2 hours after deltoid injection. All ratings returned to baseline at the predose assessment of the next injection 2 weeks later. No moderate or severe reactions were observed in any subject.

6.9   Postmarketing Experience
The following adverse reactions have been identified during postapproval use of risperidone; because these reactions are reported voluntarily from a population of uncertain size, it is not possible to reliably estimate their frequency: agranulocytosis, alopecia, anaphylactic reaction, angioedema, atrial fibrillation, diabetes mellitus, diabetic ketoacidosis in patients with impaired glucose metabolism, hypoglycemia, hypothermia, inappropriate antidiuretic hormone secretion, intestinal obstruction, jaundice, mania, pancreatitis, priapism, QT prolongation, sleep apnea syndrome, thrombocytopenia, urinary retention, and water intoxication. In addition, the following adverse reactions have been observed during postapproval use of RISPERDAL® CONSTA®: cerebrovascular disorders, including cerebrovascular accidents, and diabetes mellitus aggravated.

Retinal artery occlusion after injection of RISPERDAL® CONSTA® has been reported during postmarketing surveillance. This has been reported in the presence of abnormal arteriovenous anastomosis.

Serious injection site reactions including abscess, cellulitis, cyst, hematoma, necrosis, nodule, and ulcer have been reported with RISPERDAL® CONSTA® during postmarketing surveillance. Isolated cases required surgical intervention.

7   DRUG INTERACTIONS

The interactions of RISPERDAL® CONSTA® with coadministration of other drugs have not been systematically evaluated. The drug interaction data provided in this section is based on studies with oral RISPERDAL®.

7.1   Centrally-Acting Drugs and Alcohol
Given the primary CNS effects of risperidone, caution should be used when RISPERDAL® CONSTA® is administered in combination with other centrally-acting drugs or alcohol.

7.2   Drugs with Hypotensive Effects
Because of its potential for inducing hypotension, RISPERDAL® CONSTA® may enhance the hypotensive effects of other therapeutic agents with this potential.

7.3   Levodopa and Dopamine Agonists
RISPERDAL® CONSTA® may antagonize the effects of levodopa and dopamine agonists.

7.4   Amitriptyline
Amitriptyline did not affect the pharmacokinetics of risperidone or of risperidone and 9-hydroxyrisperidone combined following concomitant administration with oral RISPERDAL®.

7.5   Cimetidine and Ranitidine
Cimetidine and ranitidine increased the bioavailability of oral risperidone by 64% and 26%, respectively. However, cimetidine did not affect the AUC of risperidone and 9-hydroxyrisperidone combined, whereas ranitidine increased the AUC of risperidone and 9-hydroxyrisperidone combined by 20%.

7.6   Clozapine
Chronic administration of clozapine with risperidone may decrease the clearance of risperidone.

7.7   Lithium
Repeated doses of oral RISPERDAL® (3 mg twice daily) did not affect the exposure (AUC) or peak plasma concentrations (C_{max}) of lithium (n=13).

7.8   Valproate
Repeated doses of oral RISPERDAL® (4 mg once daily) did not affect the pre-dose or average plasma concentrations and exposure (AUC) of valproate (1000 mg/day in three divided doses) compared to placebo (n=21). However, there was a 20% increase in valproate peak plasma concentration (C_{max}) after concomitant administration of oral RISPERDAL®.

7.9   Digoxin
Oral RISPERDAL® (0.25 mg twice daily) did not show a clinically relevant effect on the pharmacokinetics of digoxin.

7.10   Topiramate
Oral RISPERDAL® administered at doses from 1–6 mg/day concomitantly with topiramate 400 mg/day resulted in a 23% decrease in risperidone C_{max} and a 33% decrease in risperidone $AUC_{0-12\ hour}$ at steady state. Minimal reductions in the exposure to risperidone and 9-hydroxyrisperidone combined, and no change for 9-hydroxyrisperidone were observed. This interaction is unlikely to be of clinical significance. There was no clinically relevant effect of oral RISPERDAL® on the pharmacokinetics of topiramate.

7.11   Drugs That Inhibit CYP 2D6 and Other CYP Isozymes
Risperidone is metabolized to 9-hydroxyrisperidone by CYP 2D6, an enzyme that is polymorphic in the population and that can be inhibited by a variety of psychotropic and other drugs [see Clinical Pharmacology (12.3)]. Drug interactions that reduce the metabolism of risperidone to 9-hydroxyrisperidone would increase the plasma concentrations of risperidone and lower the concentrations of 9-hydroxyrisperidone. Analysis of clinical studies involving a modest number of poor metabolizers (n=70 patients) does not suggest that poor and extensive metabolizers have different rates of adverse effects. No comparison of effectiveness in the two groups has been made.

In vitro studies showed that drugs metabolized by other CYP isozymes, including 1A1, 1A2, 2C9, 2C19, and 3A4, are only weak inhibitors of risperidone metabolism.

Fluoxetine and Paroxetine
Fluoxetine (20 mg once daily) and paroxetine (20 mg once daily), CYP 2D6 inhibitors, have been shown to increase the plasma concentration of risperidone 2.5–2.8 fold and 3–9 fold respectively. Fluoxetine did not affect the plasma concentration of 9-hydroxyrisperidone. Paroxetine lowered the concentration of 9-hydroxyrisperidone by about 10%. When either concomitant fluoxetine or paroxetine is initiated or discontinued, the physician should re-evaluate the dose of RISPERDAL® CONSTA®. When initiation of fluoxetine or paroxetine is considered, patients may be placed on a lower dose of RISPERDAL® CONSTA® between 2 to 4 weeks before the planned start of fluoxetine or paroxetine therapy to adjust for the expected increase in plasma concentrations of risperidone. When fluoxetine or paroxetine is initiated in patients receiving the recommended dose of 25 mg RISPERDAL® CONSTA®, it is recommended to continue treatment with the 25-mg dose unless clinical judgment necessitates lowering the RISPERDAL® CONSTA® dose to 12.5 mg or necessitates interruption of RISPERDAL® CONSTA® treatment. When RISPERDAL® CONSTA® is initiated in patients already receiving fluoxetine or paroxetine, a starting dose of 12.5 mg can be considered. The efficacy of the 12.5 mg dose has not been investigated in clinical trials. [See also Dosage and Administration (2.5)]. The effects of discontinuation of concomitant fluoxetine or paroxetine therapy on the pharmacokinetics of risperidone and 9-hydroxyrisperidone have not been studied.

Erythromycin
There were no significant interactions between oral RISPERDAL® and erythromycin.

7.12   Carbamazepine and Other CYP 3A4 Enzyme Inducers
Carbamazepine co-administration with oral RISPERDAL® decreased the steady-state plasma concentrations of risperidone and 9-hydroxyrisperidone by about 50%. Plasma concentrations of carbamazepine did not appear to be affected. Co-administration of other known CYP 3A4 enzyme inducers (e.g., phenytoin, rifampin, and phenobarbital) with risperidone may cause similar decreases in the combined plasma concentrations of risperidone and 9-hydroxyrisperidone, which could lead to decreased efficacy of RISPERDAL® CONSTA® treatment. At the initiation of therapy with carbamazepine or other known hepatic enzyme inducers, patients should be closely monitored during the first 4–8 weeks, since the dose of RISPERDAL® CONSTA® may need to be adjusted. A dose increase, or additional oral RISPERDAL®, may need to be considered. On discontinuation of carbamazepine or other CYP 3A4 hepatic enzyme inducers, the dosage of RISPERDAL® CONSTA® should be re-evaluated and, if necessary, decreased. Patients may be placed on a lower dose of RISPERDAL® CONSTA® between 2 to 4 weeks before the planned discontinuation of carbamazepine or other CYP 3A4 enzyme inducers to adjust for the expected increase in plasma concentrations of risperidone plus 9-hydroxyrisperidone. For patients treated with the recommended dose of 25 mg RISPERDAL® CONSTA® and discontinuing from carbamazepine or other CYP 3A4 enzyme inducers, it is recommended to continue treatment with the 25-mg dose unless clinical judgment necessitates lowering the RISPERDAL® CONSTA® dose to 12.5 mg or necessitates interruption of RISPERDAL® CONSTA® treatment. The efficacy of the 12.5 mg dose has not been investigated in clinical trials. [See also Dosage and Administration (2.5)]

7.13   Drugs Metabolized by CYP 2D6
In vitro studies indicate that risperidone is a relatively weak inhibitor of CYP 2D6. Therefore, RISPERDAL® CONSTA® is not expected to substantially inhibit the clearance of drugs that are metabolized by this enzymatic pathway. In drug interaction studies, oral RISPERDAL® did not significantly affect the pharmacokinetics of donepezil and galantamine, which are metabolized by CYP 2D6.

8   USE IN SPECIFIC POPULATIONS

8.1   Pregnancy
Pregnancy Category C.
The teratogenic potential of oral risperidone was studied in three embryofetal development studies in Sprague-Dawley and Wistar rats (0.63–10 mg/kg or 0.4 to 6 times the oral maximum recommended human dose [MRHD] on a mg/m^2 basis) and in one embryofetal development study in New Zealand rabbits (0.31–5 mg/kg or 0.4 to 6 times the oral MRHD on a mg/m^2 basis). The incidence of malformations was not increased compared to control in offspring of rats or rabbits given 0.4 to 6 times the oral MRHD on a mg/m^2 basis. In three reproductive studies in rats (two peri/postnatal development studies and a multigenerational study), there was an increase in pup deaths during the first 4 days of lactation at doses of 0.16–5 mg/kg or 0.1 to 3 times the oral MRHD on a mg/m^2 basis. It is not known whether these deaths were due to a direct effect on the fetuses or pups or to effects on the dams.

There was no no-effect dose for increased rat pup mortality. In one peri/post-natal development study, there was an increase in stillborn rat pups at a dose of 2.5 mg/kg or 1.5 times the oral MRHD on a mg/m^2 basis. In a cross-fostering study in Wistar rats, toxic effects on the fetus or pups, as evidenced by a decrease in the number of live pups and an increase in the number of dead pups at birth (Day 0), and a decrease in birth weight in pups of drug-treated dams were observed. In addition, there was an increase in deaths by Day 1 among pups of drug-treated dams, regardless of whether or not the pups were cross-fostered. Risperidone also appeared to impair maternal behavior in that pup body weight gain and survival (from Days 1 to 4 of lactation) were reduced in pups born to control but reared by drug-treated dams. These effects were all noted at the one dose of risperidone tested, i.e., 5 mg/kg or 3 times the oral MRHD on a mg/m^2 basis.

No studies were conducted with RISPERDAL® CONSTA®. Placental transfer of risperidone occurs in rat pups. There are no adequate and well-controlled studies in pregnant women. However, there was one report of a case of agenesis of the corpus callosum in an infant exposed to risperidone in utero. The causal relationship to oral RISPERDAL® therapy is unknown. Reversible extrapyramidal symptoms in the neonate were observed following postmarketing use of risperidone during the last trimester of pregnancy.
RISPERDAL® CONSTA® should be used during pregnancy only if the potential benefit justifies the potential risk to the fetus.

8.2   Labor and Delivery
The effect of RISPERDAL® CONSTA® on labor and delivery in humans is unknown.

8.3   Nursing Mothers
Risperidone and 9-hydroxyrisperidone are also excreted in human breast milk. Therefore, women should not breastfeed during treatment with RISPERDAL® CONSTA® and for at least 12 weeks after the last injection.

8.4   Pediatric Use
RISPERDAL® CONSTA® has not been studied in children younger than 18 years old.

8.5   Geriatric Use
In an open-label study, 57 clinically stable, elderly patients (≥65 years old) with schizophrenia or schizoaffective disorder received RISPERDAL® CONSTA® every 2 weeks for up to 12 months. In general, no differences in the tolerability of RISPERDAL® CONSTA® were observed between otherwise healthy elderly and nonelderly patients. Therefore,

dosing recommendations for otherwise healthy elderly patients are the same as for nonelderly patients. Because elderly patients exhibit a greater tendency to orthostatic hypotension than nonelderly patients, elderly patients should be instructed in nonpharmacologic interventions that help to reduce the occurrence of orthostatic hypotension (e.g., sitting on the edge of the bed for several minutes before attempting to stand in the morning and slowly rising from a seated position). In addition, monitoring of orthostatic vital signs should be considered in elderly patients for whom orthostatic hypotension is of concern *[see Warnings and Precautions (5.7)]*.

Concomitant use with Furosemide in Elderly Patients with Dementia-Related Psychosis

In two of four placebo-controlled trials in elderly patients with dementia-related psychosis, a higher incidence of mortality was observed in patients treated with furosemide plus oral risperidone when compared to patients treated with oral risperidone alone or with oral placebo plus furosemide. No pathological mechanism has been identified to explain this finding, and no consistent pattern for cause of death was observed. An increase of mortality in elderly patients with dementia-related psychosis was seen with the use of oral risperidone regardless of concomitant use with furosemide. RISPERDAL® CONSTA® is not approved for the treatment of patients with dementia-related psychosis. *[See Boxed Warning and Warnings and Precautions (5.1)]*

9 DRUG ABUSE AND DEPENDENCE

9.1 Controlled Substance

RISPERDAL® CONSTA® (risperidone) is not a controlled substance.

9.2 Abuse

RISPERDAL® CONSTA® has not been systematically studied in animals or humans for its potential for abuse. Because RISPERDAL® CONSTA® is to be administered by health care professionals, the potential for misuse or abuse by patients is low.

9.3 Dependence

RISPERDAL® CONSTA® has not been systematically studied in animals or humans for its potential for tolerance or physical dependence.

10 OVERDOSAGE

10.1 Human Experience

No cases of overdose were reported in premarketing studies with RISPERDAL® CONSTA®. Because RISPERDAL® CONSTA® is to be administered by health care professionals, the potential for overdosage by patients is low.

In premarketing experience with oral RISPERDAL®, there were eight reports of acute RISPERDAL® overdosage, with estimated doses ranging from 20 to 300 mg and no fatalities. In general, reported signs and symptoms were those resulting from an exaggeration of the drug's known pharmacological effects, i.e., drowsiness and sedation, tachycardia and hypotension, and extrapyramidal symptoms. One case, involving an estimated overdose of 240 mg, was associated with hyponatremia, hypokalemia, prolonged QT, and widened QRS. Another case, involving an estimated overdose of 36 mg, was associated with a seizure.

Postmarketing experience with oral RISPERDAL® includes reports of acute overdose, with estimated doses of up to 360 mg. In general, the most frequently reported signs and symptoms are those resulting from an exaggeration of the drug's known pharmacological effects, i.e., drowsiness, sedation, tachycardia, hypotension, and extrapyramidal symptoms. Other adverse reactions reported since market introduction related to oral RISPERDAL® overdose include prolonged QT interval and convulsions. Torsade de pointes has been reported in association with combined overdose of oral RISPERDAL® and paroxetine.

10.2 Management of Overdosage

In case of acute overdosage, establish and maintain an airway and ensure adequate oxygenation and ventilation. Cardiovascular monitoring should commence immediately and should include continuous electrocardiographic monitoring to detect possible arrhythmias. If antiarrhythmic therapy is administered, disopyramide, procainamide, and quinidine carry a theoretical hazard of QT prolonging effects that might be additive to those of risperidone. Similarly, it is reasonable to expect that the alpha-blocking properties of bretylium might be additive to those of risperidone, resulting in problematic hypotension.

There is no specific antidote to risperidone. Therefore, appropriate supportive measures should be instituted. The possibility of multiple drug involvement should be considered. Hypotension and circulatory collapse should be treated with appropriate measures, such as intravenous fluids and/or sympathomimetic agents (epinephrine and dopamine should not be used, since beta stimulation may worsen hypotension in the setting of risperidone-induced alpha blockade). In cases of severe extrapyramidal symptoms, anticholinergic medication should be administered. Close medical supervision and monitoring should continue until the patient recovers.

11 DESCRIPTION

Risperidone is a psychotropic agent belonging to the chemical class of benzisoxazole derivatives. The chemical designation is 3-[2-[4-(6-fluoro-1,2-benzisoxazol-3-yl)-1-piperidinyl]ethyl]-6,7,8,9-tetrahydro-2-methyl-4H-pyrido[1,2-a]pyrimidin-4-one. Its molecular formula is $C_{23}H_{27}FN_4O_2$ and its molecular weight is 410.49. The structural formula is:

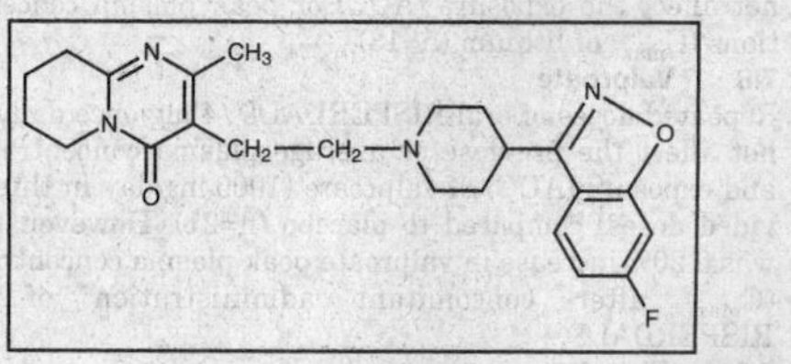

Risperidone is practically insoluble in water, freely soluble in methylene chloride, and soluble in methanol and 0.1 N HCl.

RISPERDAL® CONSTA® (risperidone) Long-Acting Injection is a combination of extended-release microspheres for injection and diluent for parenteral use.

The extended-release microspheres formulation is a white to off-white, free-flowing powder that is available in dosage strengths of 12.5 mg, 25 mg, 37.5 mg, or 50 mg risperidone per vial. Risperidone is micro-encapsulated in 7525 polylactide-co-glycolide (PLG) at a concentration of 381 mg risperidone per gram of microspheres.

The diluent for parenteral use is a clear, colorless solution. Composition of the diluent includes polysorbate 20, sodium carboxymethyl cellulose, disodium hydrogen phosphate dihydrate, citric acid anhydrous, sodium chloride, sodium hydroxide, and water for injection. The microspheres are suspended in the diluent prior to injection.

RISPERDAL® CONSTA® is provided as a dose pack, consisting of a vial containing the microspheres, a pre-filled syringe containing the diluent, a SmartSite® Needle-Free Vial Access Device, and two Needle-Pro® safety needles (a 21 G UTW 1-inch needle with needle protection device for deltoid administration and a 20 G TW 2-inch needle with needle protection device for gluteal administration).

12 CLINICAL PHARMACOLOGY

12.1 Mechanism of Action

The mechanism of action of RISPERDAL® CONSTA®, as with other drugs used to treat schizophrenia, is unknown. However, it has been proposed that the drug's therapeutic activity in schizophrenia is mediated through a combination of dopamine Type 2 (D_2) and serotonin Type 2 ($5HT_2$) receptor antagonism.

RISPERDAL® is a selective monoaminergic antagonist with high affinity (Ki of 0.12 to 7.3 nM) for the serotonin Type 2 ($5HT_2$), dopamine Type 2 (D_2), $\alpha 1$ and $\alpha 2$ adrenergic, and H_1 histaminergic receptors. RISPERDAL® acts as an antagonist at other receptors, but with lower potency. RISPERDAL® has low to moderate affinity (Ki of 47 to 253 nM) for the serotonin $5HT_{1C}$, $5HT_{1D}$, and $5HT_{1A}$ receptors, weak affinity (Ki of 620 to 800 nM) for the dopamine D_1 and haloperidol-sensitive sigma site, and no affinity (when tested at concentrations $>10^{-5}$ M) for cholinergic muscarinic or $\beta 1$ and $\beta 2$ adrenergic receptors.

12.2 Pharmacodynamics

The clinical effect from RISPERDAL® CONSTA® results from the combined concentrations of risperidone and its major metabolite, 9-hydroxyrisperidone *[see Clinical Pharmacology (12.3)]*. Antagonism at receptors other than D_2 and $5HT_2$ *[see Clinical Pharmacology (12.1)]* may explain some of the other effects of RISPERDAL® CONSTA®.

12.3 Pharmacokinetics

Absorption

After a single intramuscular (gluteal) injection of RISPERDAL® CONSTA®, there is a small initial release of the drug (< 1% of the dose), followed by a lag time of 3 weeks. The main release of the drug starts from 3 weeks onward, is maintained from 4 to 6 weeks, and subsides by 7 weeks following the intramuscular (IM) injection. Therefore, oral antipsychotic supplementation should be given during the first 3 weeks of treatment with RISPERDAL® CONSTA® to maintain therapeutic levels until the main release of risperidone from the injection site has begun *[see Dosage and Administration (2)]*. Following single doses of RISPERDAL® CONSTA®, the pharmacokinetics of risperidone, 9-hydroxyrisperidone (the major metabolite), and risperidone plus 9-hydroxyrisperidone were linear in the dosing range of 12.5 mg to 50 mg.

The combination of the release profile and the dosage regimen (IM injections every 2 weeks) of RISPERDAL® CONSTA® results in sustained therapeutic concentrations. Steady-state plasma concentrations are reached after 4 injections and are maintained for 4 to 6 weeks after the last injection. Following multiple doses of 25 mg and 50 mg RISPERDAL® CONSTA®, plasma concentrations of risperidone, 9-hydroxyrisperidone, and risperidone plus 9-hydroxyrisperidone were linear.

Deltoid and gluteal intramuscular injections at the same doses are bioequivalent and, therefore, interchangeable.

Distribution

Once absorbed, risperidone is rapidly distributed. The volume of distribution is 1–2 L/kg. In plasma, risperidone is bound to albumin and $\alpha 1$-acid glycoprotein. The plasma protein binding of risperidone is approximately 90%, and that of its major metabolite, 9-hydroxyrisperidone, is 77%. Neither risperidone nor 9-hydroxyrisperidone displaces each other from plasma binding sites. High therapeutic concentrations of sulfamethazine (100 mcg/mL), warfarin (10 mcg/mL), and carbamazepine (10 mcg/mL) caused only a slight increase in the free fraction of risperidone at 10 ng/mL and of 9-hydroxyrisperidone at 50 ng/mL, changes of unknown clinical significance.

Metabolism and Drug Interactions

Risperidone is extensively metabolized in the liver. The main metabolic pathway is through hydroxylation of risperidone to 9-hydroxyrisperidone by the enzyme, CYP 2D6. A minor metabolic pathway is through N-dealkylation. The main metabolite, 9-hydroxyrisperidone, has similar pharmacological activity as risperidone. Consequently, the clinical effect of the drug results from the combined concentrations of risperidone plus 9-hydroxyrisperidone.

CYP 2D6, also called debrisoquin hydroxylase, is the enzyme responsible for metabolism of many neuroleptics, antidepressants, antiarrhythmics, and other drugs. CYP 2D6 is subject to genetic polymorphism (about 6%–8% of Caucasians, and a very low percentage of Asians, have little or no activity and are "poor metabolizers") and to inhibition by a variety of substrates and some non-substrates, notably quinidine. Extensive CYP 2D6 metabolizers convert risperidone rapidly into 9-hydroxyrisperidone, whereas poor CYP 2D6 metabolizers convert it much more slowly. Although extensive metabolizers have lower risperidone and higher 9-hydroxyrisperidone concentrations than poor metabolizers, the pharmacokinetics of risperidone and 9-hydroxyrisperidone combined, after single and multiple doses, are similar in extensive and poor metabolizers.

The interactions of RISPERDAL® CONSTA® with coadministration of other drugs have not been systematically evaluated in human subjects. Drug interactions are based primarily on experience with oral RISPERDAL®. Risperidone could be subject to two kinds of drug-drug interactions. First, inhibitors of CYP 2D6 interfere with conversion of risperidone to 9-hydroxyrisperidone *[see Drug Interactions (7.11)]*. This occurs with quinidine, giving essentially all recipients a risperidone pharmacokinetic profile typical of poor metabolizers. The therapeutic benefits and adverse effects of RISPERDAL® in patients receiving quinidine have not been evaluated, but observations in a modest number (n#70) of poor metabolizers given oral RISPERDAL® do not suggest important differences between poor and extensive metabolizers. Second, co-administration of carbamazepine and other known enzyme inducers (e.g., phenytoin, rifampin, and phenobarbital) with oral RISPERDAL® cause a decrease in the combined plasma concentrations of risperidone and 9-hydroxyrisperidone *[see Drug Interactions (7.12)]*. It would also be possible for risperidone to interfere with metabolism of other drugs metabolized by CYP 2D6. Relatively weak binding of risperidone to the enzyme suggests this is unlikely *[see Drug Interactions (7.11)]*.

Excretion

Risperidone and its metabolites are eliminated via the urine and, to a much lesser extent, via the feces. As illustrated by a mass balance study of a single 1 mg oral dose of ^{14}C-risperidone administered as solution to three healthy male volunteers, total recovery of radioactivity at 1 week was 84%, including 70% in the urine and 14% in the feces. The apparent half-life of risperidone plus 9-hydroxyrisperidone following RISPERDAL® CONSTA® administration is 3 to 6 days, and is associated with a monoexponential decline in plasma concentrations. This half-life of 3–6 days is related to the erosion of the microspheres and subsequent absorption of risperidone. The clearance of risperidone and risperidone plus 9-hydroxyrisperidone was 13.7 L/h and 5.0 L/h in extensive CYP 2D6 metabolizers, and 3.3 L/h and 3.2 L/h in poor CYP 2D6 metabolizers, respectively. No accumulation of risperidone was observed during long-term use (up to 12 months) in patients treated every 2 weeks with 25 mg or 50 mg RISPERDAL® CONSTA®. The elimination phase is complete approximately 7 to 8 weeks after the last injection.

Renal Impairment

In patients with moderate to severe renal disease treated with oral RISPERDAL®, clearance of the sum of risperidone and its active metabolite decreased by 60% compared with young healthy subjects. Although patients with renal impairment were not studied with RISPERDAL® CONSTA®, it is recommended that patients with renal impairment be carefully titrated on oral RISPERDAL® before treatment with RISPERDAL® CONSTA® is initiated at a dose of 25 mg. A lower initial dose of 12.5 mg may be appropriate when clinical factors warrant dose adjustment, such as in patients with renal impairment *[see Dosage and Administration (2.4)]*.

Hepatic Impairment

While the pharmacokinetics of oral RISPERDAL® in subjects with liver disease were comparable to those in young healthy subjects, the mean free fraction of risperidone in plasma was increased by about 35% because of the diminished concentration of both albumin and α1-acid glycoprotein. Although patients with hepatic impairment were not studied with RISPERDAL® CONSTA®, it is recommended that patients with hepatic impairment be carefully titrated on oral RISPERDAL® before treatment with RISPERDAL® CONSTA® is initiated at a dose of 25 mg. A lower initial dose of 12.5 mg may be appropriate when clinical factors warrant dose adjustment, such as in patients with hepatic impairment *[see Dosage and Administration (2.4)]*.

Elderly

In an open-label trial, steady-state concentrations of risperidone plus 9-hydroxyrisperidone in otherwise healthy elderly patients (≥65 years old) treated with RISPERDAL® CONSTA® for up to 12 months fell within the range of values observed in otherwise healthy nonelderly patients. Dosing recommendations are the same for otherwise healthy elderly patients and nonelderly patients *[see Dosage and Administration (2)]*.

Race and Gender Effects

No specific pharmacokinetic study was conducted to investigate race and gender effects, but a population pharmacokinetic analysis did not identify important differences in the disposition of risperidone due to gender (whether or not corrected for body weight) or race.

13 NONCLINICAL TOXICOLOGY

13.1 Carcinogenesis, Mutagenesis, Impairment of Fertility

Carcinogenesis - Oral

Carcinogenicity studies were conducted in Swiss albino mice and Wistar rats. Risperidone was administered in the diet at doses of 0.63, 2.5, and 10 mg/kg for 18 months to mice and for 25 months to rats. These doses are equivalent to 2.4, 9.4, and 37.5 times the oral maximum recommended human dose (MRHD) for schizophrenia (16 mg/day) on a mg/kg basis, or 0.2, 0.75, and 3 times the oral MRHD (mice) or 0.4, 1.5, and 6 times the oral MRHD (rats) on a mg/m^2 basis. A maximum tolerated dose was not achieved in male mice. There was a significant increase in pituitary gland adenomas in female mice at doses 0.75 and 3 times the oral MRHD on a mg/m^2 basis. There was a significant increase in endocrine pancreatic adenomas in male rats at doses 1.5 and 6 times the oral MRHD on a mg/m^2 basis. Mammary gland adenocarcinomas were significantly increased in female mice at all doses tested (0.2, 0.75, and 3 times the oral MRHD on a mg/m^2 basis), in female rats at all doses tested (0.4, 1.5, and 6 times the oral MRHD on a mg/m^2 basis), and in male rats at a dose 6 times the oral MRHD on a mg/m^2 basis.

Carcinogenesis - Intramuscular

RISPERDAL® CONSTA® was evaluated in a 24-month carcinogenicity study in which SPF Wistar rats were treated every 2 weeks with intramuscular (IM) injections of either 5 mg/kg or 40 mg/kg of risperidone. These doses are 1 and 8 times the MRHD (50 mg) on a mg/m^2 basis. A control group received injections of 0.9% NaCl, and a vehicle control group was injected with placebo microspheres. There was a significant increase in pituitary gland adenomas, endocrine pancreas adenomas, and adrenomedullary pheochromocytomas at 8 times the IM MRHD on a mg/m^2 basis. The incidence of mammary gland adenocarcinomas was significantly increased in female rats at both doses (1 and 8 times the IM MRHD on a mg/m^2 basis). A significant increase in renal tubular tumors (adenoma, adenocarcinomas) was observed in male rats at 8 times the IM MRHD on a mg/m^2 basis. Plasma exposures (AUC) in rats were 0.3 and 2 times (at 5 and 40 mg/kg, respectively) the expected plasma exposure (AUC) at the IM MRHD.

Dopamine D_2 receptor antagonists have been shown to chronically elevate prolactin levels in rodents. Serum prolactin levels were not measured during the carcinogenicity studies of oral risperidone; however, measurements taken during subchronic toxicity studies showed that oral risperidone elevated serum prolactin levels 5- to 6-fold in mice and rats at the same doses used in the oral carcinogenicity studies. Serum prolactin levels increased in a dose-dependent manner up to 6- and 1.5-fold in male and female rats, respectively, at the end of the 24-month treatment with RISPERDAL® CONSTA® every 2 weeks. Increases in the incidence of pituitary gland, endocrine pancreas, and mammary gland neoplasms have been found in rodents after chronic administration of other antipsychotic drugs and may be prolactin-mediated.

The relevance for human risk of the findings of prolactin-mediated endocrine tumors in rodents is unknown *[see Warnings and Precautions (5.6)]*.

Mutagenesis

No evidence of mutagenic potential for oral risperidone was found in the *in vitro* Ames reverse mutation test, *in vitro* mouse lymphoma assay, *in vitro* rat hepatocyte DNA-repair assay, *in vivo* oral micronucleus test in mice, the sex-linked recessive lethal test in *Drosophila*, or the *in vitro* chromosomal aberration test in human lymphocytes or in Chinese hamster cells.

In addition, no evidence of mutagenic potential was found in the *in vitro* Ames reverse mutation test for RISPERDAL® CONSTA®.

Impairment of Fertility

Oral risperidone (0.16 to 5 mg/kg) was shown to impair mating, but not fertility, in Wistar rats in three reproductive studies (two mating and fertility studies and a multigenerational study) at doses 0.1 to 3 times the oral maximum recommended human dose (MRHD) (16 mg/day) on a mg/m^2 basis. The effect appeared to be in females, since impaired mating behavior was not noted in the mating and fertility study in which males only were treated. In a subchronic study in Beagle dogs in which oral risperidone was administered at doses of 0.31 to 5 mg/kg, sperm motility and concentration were decreased at doses 0.6 to 10 times the oral MRHD on a mg/m^2 basis. Dose-related decreases were also noted in serum testosterone at the same doses. Serum testosterone and sperm values partially recovered, but remained decreased after treatment was discontinued. No no-effect doses were noted in either rat or dog.

No mating and fertility studies were conducted with RISPERDAL® CONSTA®.

14 CLINICAL STUDIES

14.1 Schizophrenia

The effectiveness of RISPERDAL® CONSTA® in the treatment of schizophrenia was established, in part, on the basis of extrapolation from the established effectiveness of the oral formulation of risperidone. In addition, the effectiveness of RISPERDAL® CONSTA® in the treatment of schizophrenia was established in a 12-week, placebo-controlled trial in adult psychotic inpatients and outpatients who met the DSM-IV criteria for schizophrenia.

Efficacy data were obtained from 400 patients with schizophrenia who were randomized to receive injections of 25 mg, 50 mg, or 75 mg RISPERDAL® CONSTA® or placebo every 2 weeks. During a 1-week run-in period, patients were discontinued from other antipsychotics and were titrated to a dose of 4 mg oral RISPERDAL®. Patients who received RISPERDAL® CONSTA® were given doses of oral RISPERDAL® (2 mg for patients in the 25-mg group, 4 mg for patients in the 50-mg group, and 6 mg for patients in the 75-mg group) for the 3 weeks after the first injection to provide therapeutic plasma concentrations until the main release phase of risperidone from the injection site had begun. Patients who received placebo injections were given placebo tablets.

Efficacy was evaluated using the Positive and Negative Syndrome Scale (PANSS), a validated, multi-item inventory, composed of five subscales to evaluate positive symptoms, negative symptoms, disorganized thoughts, uncontrolled hostility/excitement, and anxiety/depression.

The primary efficacy variable in this trial was change from baseline to endpoint in the total PANSS score. The mean total PANSS score at baseline for schizophrenic patients in this study was 81.5.

Total PANSS scores showed significant improvement in the change from baseline to endpoint in schizophrenic patients treated with each dose of RISPERDAL® CONSTA® (25 mg, 50 mg, or 75 mg) compared with patients treated with placebo. While there were no statistically significant differences between the treatment effects for the three dose groups, the effect size for the 75 mg dose group was actually numerically less than that observed for the 50 mg dose group.

Subgroup analyses did not indicate any differences in treatment outcome as a function of age, race, or gender.

14.2 Bipolar Disorder - Monotherapy

The effectiveness of RISPERDAL® CONSTA® for the maintenance treatment of Bipolar I Disorder was established in a multicenter, double-blind, placebo-controlled study of adult patients who met DSM-IV criteria for Bipolar Disorder Type I, who were stable on medications or experiencing an acute manic or mixed episode.

A total of 501 patients were treated during a 26-week open-label period with RISPERDAL® CONSTA® (starting dose of 25 mg, and titrated, if deemed clinically desirable, to 37.5 mg or 50 mg; in patients not tolerating the 25 mg dose, the dose could be reduced to 12.5 mg). In the open-label phase, 303 (60%) patients were judged to be stable and were randomized to double-blind treatment with either the same dose of RISPERDAL® CONSTA® or placebo and monitored for relapse. The primary endpoint was time to relapse to any mood episode (depression, mania, hypomania, or mixed).

Time to relapse was delayed in patients receiving RISPERDAL® CONSTA® monotherapy as compared to placebo. The majority of relapses were due to manic rather than depressive symptoms. Based on their bipolar disorder history, subjects entering this study had had, on average, more manic episodes than depressive episodes.

14.3 Bipolar Disorder - Adjunctive Therapy

The effectiveness of RISPERDAL® CONSTA® as an adjunct to treatment with lithium or valproate for the maintenance treatment of Bipolar Disorder was established in a multicenter, randomized, double-blind, placebo-controlled study of adult patients who met DSM-IV criteria for Bipolar Disorder Type I and who experienced at least 4 episodes of mood disorder requiring psychiatric/clinical intervention in the previous 12 months, including at least 2 episodes in the 6 months prior to the start of the study.

A total of 240 patients were treated during a 16-week open-label period with RISPERDAL® CONSTA® (starting dose of 25 mg, and titrated, if deemed clinically desirable, to 37.5 mg or 50 mg), as adjunctive therapy in addition to continuing their treatment as usual for their bipolar disorder, which consisted of mood stabilizers (primarily lithium and valproate), antidepressants, and/or anxiolytics. All oral antipsychotics were discontinued after the first three weeks of the initial RISPERDAL® CONSTA® injection. In the open-label phase, 124 (51.7%) were judged to be stable for at least the last 4 weeks and were randomized to double-blind treatment with either the same dose of RISPERDAL® CONSTA® or placebo in addition to continuing their treatment as usual and monitored for relapse during a 52-week period. The primary endpoint was time to relapse to any new mood episode (depression, mania, hypomania, or mixed).

Time to relapse was delayed in patients receiving adjunctive therapy with RISPERDAL® CONSTA® as compared to placebo. The relapse types were about half depressive and half manic or mixed episodes.

16 HOW SUPPLIED/STORAGE AND HANDLING

RISPERDAL® CONSTA® (risperidone) is available in dosage strengths of 12.5 mg, 25 mg, 37.5 mg, or 50 mg risperidone. It is provided as a dose pack, consisting of a vial containing the risperidone microspheres, a pre-filled syringe containing 2 mL of diluent for RISPERDAL® CONSTA®, a SmartSite® Needle-Free Vial Access Device, and two Needle-Pro® safety needles for intramuscular injection (a 21 G UTW 1-inch needle with needle protection device for deltoid administration and a 20 G TW 2-inch needle with needle protection device for gluteal administration).

12.5-mg vial/kit (NDC 50458-309-11): 41 mg (equivalent to 12.5 mg of risperidone) of a white to off-white powder provided in a vial with a violet flip-off cap (NDC 50458-309-01).

25-mg vial/kit (NDC 50458-306-11): 78 mg (equivalent to 25 mg of risperidone) of a white to off-white powder provided in a vial with a pink flip-off cap (NDC 50458-306-01).

37.5-mg vial/kit (NDC 50458-307-11): 116 mg (equivalent to 37.5 mg of risperidone) of a white to off-white powder provided in a vial with a green flip-off cap (NDC 50458-307-01).

50-mg vial/kit (NDC 50458-308-11): 152 mg (equivalent to 50 mg of risperidone) of a white to off-white powder provided in a vial with a blue flip-off cap (NDC 50458-308-01).

Storage and Handling

The entire dose pack should be stored in the refrigerator (36°–46°F; 2°–8°C) and protected from light.

If refrigeration is unavailable, RISPERDAL® CONSTA® can be stored at temperatures not exceeding 77°F (25°C) for no more than 7 days prior to administration. Do not expose unrefrigerated product to temperatures above 77°F (25°C).

Keep out of reach of children.

17 PATIENT COUNSELING INFORMATION

Physicians are advised to discuss the following issues with patients for whom they prescribe RISPERDAL® CONSTA®.

17.1 Orthostatic Hypotension

Patients should be advised of the risk of orthostatic hypotension and instructed in nonpharmacologic interventions that help to reduce the occurrence of orthostatic hypotension (e.g., sitting on the edge of the bed for several minutes before attempting to stand in the morning and slowly rising from a seated position) *[see Warnings and Precautions (5.7)]*.

17.2 Interference with Cognitive and Motor Performance

Because RISPERDAL® CONSTA® has the potential to impair judgment, thinking, or motor skills, patients should be cautioned about operating hazardous machinery, including automobiles, until they are reasonably certain that treatment with RISPERDAL® CONSTA® does not affect them adversely *[see Warnings and Precautions (5.9)]*.

17.3 Pregnancy

Patients should be advised to notify their physician if they become pregnant or intend to become pregnant during therapy and for at least 12 weeks after the last injection of RISPERDAL® CONSTA® [see Use in Specific Populations (8.1)].

17.4 Nursing

Patients should be advised not to breast-feed an infant during treatment and for at least 12 weeks after the last injection of RISPERDAL® CONSTA® [see Use in Specific Populations (8.3)].

17.5 Concomitant Medication

Patients should be advised to inform their physicians if they are taking, or plan to take, any prescription or over-the-counter drugs, since there is a potential for interactions [see Drug Interactions (7)].

17.6 Alcohol

Patients should be advised to avoid alcohol during treatment with RISPERDAL® CONSTA® [see Drug Interactions (7.1)].

10130505
Revised April 2010
©Ortho-McNeil-Janssen Pharmaceuticals, Inc. 2007
Risperidone is manufactured by:
Janssen Pharmaceutical Ltd.
Wallingstown, Little Island, County Cork, Ireland
Microspheres are manufactured by:
Alkermes, Inc.
Wilmington, Ohio
Diluent is manufactured by:
Vetter Pharma Fertigung GmbH & Co. KG
Ravensburg or Langenargen, Germany
or
Cilag AG
Schaffhausen, Switzerland
or
Ortho Biotech Products, L.P.
Raritan, NJ
RISPERDAL® CONSTA® is manufactured for:
Janssen, Division of Ortho-McNeil-Janssen Pharmaceuticals, Inc.
Titusville, NJ 08560
Shown in Product Identification Guide, page 317

TYLENOL® WITH CODEINE   ℂⅢ ℞

[ti 'len-awl co' dĕn]
(acetaminophen and codeine phosphate)
Tablets

DESCRIPTION

TYLENOL® with Codeine is supplied in tablet form for oral administration.
Acetaminophen, 4'-hydroxyacetanilide, a slightly bitter, white, odorless, crystalline powder, is a non-opiate, non-salicylate analgesic and antipyretic. It has the following structural formula:

$C_8H_9NO_2$ M.W. 151.16

Codeine phosphate, 7,8-didehydro-4, 5α-epoxy-3-methoxy-17-methylmorphinan-6α-ol phosphate (1:1) (salt) hemihydrate, a white crystalline powder, is a narcotic analgesic and antitussive. It has the following structural formula:

$C_{18}H_{21}NO_3 \cdot H_3PO_4 \cdot \frac{1}{2}H_2O$ M.W. 406.37

Each tablet contains:
Acetaminophen .... 300 mg
No. 3 Codeine Phosphate .... 30 mg
(Warning: May be habit forming)
Acetaminophen .... 300 mg
No. 4 Codeine Phosphate .... 60 mg
(Warning: May be habit forming)
In addition, each tablet contains the following inactive ingredients:
TYLENOL® with Codeine No. 3 contains powdered cellulose, magnesium stearate, sodium metabisulfite†, pregelatinized starch (corn), and modified starch (corn).

TYLENOL® with Codeine No. 4 contains powdered cellulose, magnesium stearate, sodium metabisulfite†, pregelatinized starch (corn), and corn starch.
†See WARNINGS

CLINICAL PHARMACOLOGY

This product combines the analgesic effects of a centrally acting analgesic, codeine, with a peripherally acting analgesic, acetaminophen.

Pharmacokinetics

The behavior of the individual components is described below.
Codeine
Codeine is rapidly absorbed from the gastrointestinal tract. It is rapidly distributed from the intravascular spaces to the various body tissues, with preferential uptake by parenchymatous organs such as the liver, spleen and kidney. Codeine crosses the blood-brain barrier and is found in fetal tissue and breast milk. The plasma concentration does not correlate with brain concentration or relief of pain; however, codeine is not bound to plasma proteins and does not accumulate in body tissues.
The plasma half-life is about 2.9 hours. The elimination of codeine is primarily via the kidneys, and about 90% of an oral dose is excreted by the kidneys within 24 hours of dosing. The urinary secretion products consist of free and glucuronide conjugated codeine (about 70%), free and conjugated norcodeine (about 10%), free and conjugated morphine (about 10%) normorphine (4%), and hydrocodone (1%). The remainder of the dose is excreted in the feces.
At therapeutic doses, the analgesic effect reaches a peak within 2 hours and persists between 4 and 6 hours.
See OVERDOSAGE for toxicity information.
Acetaminophen
Acetaminophen is rapidly absorbed from the gastrointestinal tract and is distributed throughout most body tissues. The plasma half-life is 1.25 to 3 hours, but may be increased by liver damage and following overdosage. Elimination of acetaminophen is principally by liver metabolism (conjugation) and subsequent renal excretion of metabolites. Approximately 85% of an oral dose appears in the urine within 24 hours of administration, most as the glucuronide conjugate, with small amounts of other conjugates and unchanged drug.
See OVERDOSAGE for toxicity information.

INDICATIONS AND USAGE

TYLENOL® with Codeine (acetaminophen and codeine phosphate) tablets are indicated for the relief of mild to moderately severe pain.

CONTRAINDICATIONS

This product should not be administered to patients who have previously exhibited hypersensitivity to codeine or acetaminophen.

WARNINGS

In the presence of head injury or other intracranial lesions, the respiratory depressant effects of codeine and other narcotics may be markedly enhanced, as well as their capacity for elevating cerebrospinal fluid pressure. Narcotics also produce other CNS depressant effects, such as drowsiness, that may further obscure the clinical course of the patients with head injuries.
Codeine or other narcotics may obscure signs on which to judge the diagnosis or clinical course of patients with acute abdominal conditions.
Codeine is habit forming and potentially abusable. Consequently, the extended use of this product is not recommended.
TYLENOL® with Codeine (acetaminophen and codeine phosphate) tablets contain sodium metabisulfite, a sulfite that may cause allergic-type reactions including anaphylactic symptoms and life-threatening or less severe asthmatic episodes in certain susceptible people. The overall prevalence of sulfite sensitivity in the general population is unknown and probably low. Sulfite sensitivity is seen more frequently in asthmatic than in nonasthmatic people.

PRECAUTIONS

General

TYLENOL® with Codeine (acetaminophen and codeine phosphate) tablets should be prescribed with caution in certain special-risk patients, such as the elderly or debilitated, and those with severe impairment of renal or hepatic function, head injuries, elevated intracranial pressure, acute abdominal conditions, hypothyroidism, urethral stricture, Addison's disease, or prostatic hypertrophy.

Ultra-Rapid Metabolizers of Codeine

Some individuals may be ultra-rapid metabolizers due to a specific CYP2D6*2×2 genotype. These individuals convert codeine into its active metabolite, morphine, more rapidly and completely than other people. This rapid conversion results in higher than expected serum morphine levels. Even

at labeled dosage regimens, individuals who are ultra-rapid metabolizers may experience overdose symptoms such as extreme sleepiness, confusion, or shallow breathing.
The prevalence of this CYP2D6 phenotype varies widely and has been estimated at 0.5 to 1% in Chinese and Japanese, 0.5 to 1% in Hispanics, 1 to 10% in Caucasians, 3% in African Americans, and 16 to 28% in North Africans, Ethiopians, and Arabs. Data is not available for other ethnic groups.
When physicians prescribe codeine-containing drugs, they should choose the lowest effective dose for the shortest period of time and inform their patients about these risks and the signs of morphine overdose (see PRECAUTIONS – Nursing Mothers).

Information for Patients

Codeine may impair the mental and/or physical abilities required for the performance of potentially hazardous tasks such as driving a car or operating machinery. Such tasks should be avoided while taking this product.
Alcohol and other CNS depressants may produce an additive CNS depression, when taken with this combination product, and should be avoided.
Codeine may be habit forming. Patients should take the drug only for as long as it is prescribed, in the amounts prescribed, and no more frequently than prescribed.
Caution patients that some people have a variation in a liver enzyme and change codeine into morphine more rapidly and completely than other people. These people are ultra-rapid metabolizers and are more likely to have higher-than-normal levels of morphine in their blood after taking codeine, which can result in overdose symptoms such as extreme sleepiness, confusion, or shallow breathing. In most cases, it is unknown if someone is an ultra-rapid codeine metabolizer.
Nursing mothers taking codeine can also have higher morphine levels in their breast milk if they are ultra-rapid metabolizers. These higher levels of morphine in breast milk may lead to life-threatening or fatal side effects in nursing babies. Instruct nursing mothers to watch for signs of morphine toxicity in their infants including increased sleepiness (more than usual), difficulty breastfeeding, breathing difficulties, or limpness. Instruct nursing mothers to talk to the baby's doctor immediately if they notice these signs and, if they cannot reach the doctor right away, to take the baby to an emergency room or call 911 (or local emergency services).

Laboratory Tests

In patients with severe hepatic or renal disease, effects of therapy should be monitored with serial liver and/or renal function tests.

Drug Interactions

This drug may enhance the effects of other narcotic analgesics, alcohol, general anesthetics, tranquilizers such as chlordiazepoxide, sedative-hypnotics, or other CNS depressants, causing increased CNS depression.

Drug/Laboratory Test Interactions

Codeine may increase serum amylase levels.
Acetaminophen may produce false-positive test results for urinary 5-hydroxyindoleacetic acid.

Carcinogenesis, Mutagenesis, Impairment of Fertility

No adequate studies have been conducted in animals to determine whether acetaminophen and codeine have a potential for carcinogenesis or mutagenesis. No adequate studies have been conducted in animals to determine whether acetaminophen has a potential for impairment of fertility.
Acetaminophen and codeine have been found to have no mutagenic potential using the Ames Salmonella-Microsomal Activation test, the Basc test on Drosophila germ cells, and the Micronucleus test on mouse bone marrow.

Pregnancy

Teratogenic Effects: Pregnancy Category C.
Codeine:
A study in rats and rabbits reported no teratogenic effect of codeine administered during the period of organogenesis in doses ranging from 5 to 120 mg/kg. In the rat, doses at the 120 mg/kg level, in the toxic range for the adult animal, were associated with an increase in embryo resorption at the time of implantation. In another study a single 100 mg/kg dose of codeine administered to pregnant mice reportedly resulted in delayed ossification in the offspring.
There are no adequate and well-controlled studies in pregnant women. TYLENOL® with Codeine (acetaminophen and codeine phosphate) tablets should be used during pregnancy only if the potential benefit justifies the potential risk to the fetus.
Nonteratogenic Effects:
Dependence has been reported in newborns whose mothers took opiates regularly during pregnancy. Withdrawal signs include irritability, excessive crying, tremors, hyperreflexia, fever, vomiting, and diarrhea. These signs usually appear during the first few days of life.

Labor and Delivery

Narcotic analgesics cross the placental barrier. The closer to delivery and the larger the dose used, the greater the possibility of respiratory depression in the newborn. Narcotic analgesics should be avoided during labor if delivery of a premature infant is anticipated. If the mother has received narcotic analgesics during labor, newborn infants should be observed closely for signs of respiratory depression. Resuscitation may be required (see OVERDOSAGE). The effect of codeine, if any, on the later growth, development, and functional maturation of the child is unknown.

Nursing Mothers

Acetaminophen is excreted in breast milk in small amounts, but the significance of its effect on nursing infants is not known. Because of the potential for serious adverse reactions in nursing infants from acetaminophen, a decision should be made whether to discontinue the drug, taking into account the importance of the drug to the mother.

Codeine is secreted into human milk. In women with normal codeine metabolism (normal CYP2D6 activity), the amount of codeine secreted into human milk is low and dose-dependent. Despite the common use of codeine products to manage postpartum pain, reports of adverse events in infants are rare. However, some women are ultra-rapid metabolizers of codeine. These women achieve higher-than-expected serum levels of codeine's active metabolite, morphine, leading to higher-than-expected levels of morphine in breast milk and potentially dangerously high serum morphine levels in their breastfed infants. Therefore, maternal use of codeine can potentially lead to serious adverse reactions, including death, in nursing infants.

The prevalence of this CYP2D6 phenotype varies widely and has been estimated at 0.5 to 1% in Chinese and Japanese, 0.5 to 1% in Hispanics, 1 to 10% in Caucasians, 3% in African Americans, and 16 to 28% in North Africans, Ethiopians, and Arabs. Data is not available for other ethnic groups.

The risk of infant exposure to codeine and morphine through breast milk should be weighed against the benefits of breastfeeding for both the mother and baby. Caution should be exercised when codeine is administered to a nursing woman. If a codeine containing product is selected, the lowest dose should be prescribed for the shortest period of time to achieve the desired clinical effect. Mothers using codeine should be informed about when to seek immediate medical care and how to identify the signs and symptoms of neonatal toxicity, such as drowsiness or sedation, difficulty breastfeeding, breathing difficulties, and decreased tone, in their baby. Nursing mothers who are ultra-rapid metabolizers may also experience overdose symptoms such as extreme sleepiness, confusion, or shallow breathing. Prescribers should closely monitor mother-infant pairs and notify treating pediatricians about the use of codeine during breastfeeding (see PRECAUTIONS – General, Ultra-Rapid Metabolizers of Codeine).

ADVERSE REACTIONS

The most frequently observed adverse reactions include drowsiness, lightheadedness, dizziness, sedation, shortness of breath, nausea and vomiting. These effects seem to be more prominent in ambulatory than in non-ambulatory patients, and some of these adverse reactions may be alleviated if the patient lies down.

Other adverse reactions include allergic reactions, euphoria, dysphoria, constipation, abdominal pain, pruritus, rash, thrombocytopenia, and agranulocytosis.

At higher doses, codeine has most of the disadvantages of morphine including respiratory depression.

DRUG ABUSE AND DEPENDENCE

Controlled Substance

TYLENOL® with Codeine (acetaminophen and codeine phosphate) tablets are classified as a Schedule III controlled substance.

Abuse and Dependence

Codeine can produce drug dependence of the morphine type and, therefore, has the potential for being abused. Psychological dependence, physical dependence, and tolerance may develop upon repeated administration and it should be prescribed and administered with the same degree of caution appropriate to the use of other oral narcotic medications.

OVERDOSAGE

Following an acute overdosage, toxicity may result from codeine or acetaminophen.

Signs and Symptoms

Codeine

Toxicity from codeine poisoning includes the opioid triad of: pinpoint pupils, depression of respiration, and loss of consciousness. Convulsions may occur.

Acetaminophen

In acetaminophen overdosage, dose-dependent, potentially fatal hepatic necrosis is the most serious adverse effect. Renal tubular necrosis, hypoglycemic coma and thrombocytopenia may also occur.

Early symptoms following a potentially hepatotoxic overdose may include: nausea, vomiting, diaphoresis and general malaise. Clinical and laboratory evidence of hepatic toxicity may not be apparent until 48 to 72 hours post-ingestion.

In adults, hepatic toxicity has rarely been reported with acute overdoses of less than 10 grams or fatalities with less than 15 grams.

Treatment

A single or multiple overdose with acetaminophen and codeine is a potentially lethal polydrug overdose and consultation with a regional poison control center is recommended.

Immediate treatment includes support of cardiorespiratory function and measures to reduce drug absorption. Vomiting should be induced mechanically, or with syrup of ipecac, if the patient is alert (adequate pharyngeal and laryngeal reflexes). Oral activated charcoal (1 g/kg) should follow gastric emptying. The first dose should be accompanied by an appropriate cathartic. If repeated doses are used, the cathartic might be included with alternate doses as required. Hypotension is usually hypovolemic and should respond to fluids. Vasopressors and other supportive measures should be employed as indicated. A cuffed endo-tracheal tube should be inserted before gastric lavage of the unconscious patient and, when necessary, to provide assisted respiration.

Meticulous attention should be given to maintaining adequate pulmonary ventilation. In severe cases of intoxication, peritoneal dialysis, or preferably hemodialysis, may be considered. If hypoprothrombinemia occurs due to acetaminophen overdose, vitamin K should be administered intravenously.

Naloxone, a narcotic antagonist, can reverse respiratory depression and coma associated with opioid overdose. Naloxone hydrochloride 0.4 mg to 2 mg is given parenterally. Since the duration of action of codeine may exceed that of the naloxone, the patient should be kept under continuous surveillance and repeated doses of the antagonist should be administered as needed to maintain adequate respiration. A narcotic antagonist should not be administered in the absence of clinically significant respiratory or cardiovascular depression.

If the dose of acetaminophen may have exceeded 140 mg/kg, acetylcysteine should be administered as early as possible. Serum acetaminophen levels should be obtained, since levels four or more hours following ingestion help predict acetaminophen toxicity. Do not await acetaminophen assay results before initiating treatment. Hepatic enzymes should be obtained initially, and repeated at 24-hour intervals. Methemoglobinemia over 30% should be treated with methylene blue by slow intravenous administration.

Toxic Doses (for adults)

Acetaminophen: toxic dose 10 g
Codeine: toxic dose 240 mg

DOSAGE AND ADMINISTRATION

Dosage should be adjusted according to severity of pain and response of the patient.

The usual adult dosage is:

	Single Doses (Range)	Maximum 24-Hour Dose
Codeine phosphate	15 mg to 60 mg	360 mg
Acetaminophen	300 mg to 1000 mg	4000 mg

Doses may be repeated up to every 4 hours.

The prescriber must determine the number of tablets per dose, and the maximum number of tablets per 24 hours, based upon the above dosage guidance. This information should be conveyed in the prescription.

It should be kept in mind, however, that tolerance to codeine can develop with continued use and that the incidence of untoward effects is dose related. Adult doses of codeine higher than 60 mg fail to give commensurate relief of pain but merely prolong analgesia and are associated with an appreciably increased incidence of undesirable side effects. Equivalently high doses in children would have similar effects.

HOW SUPPLIED

TYLENOL® with Codeine (acetaminophen and codeine phosphate) tablets are white, round, flat-faced, beveled edged tablet imprinted "McNEIL" on one side and "TYLENOL CODEINE" and either "3" or "4" on the other side and are supplied as follows:

TYLENOL® with Codeine No. 3 bottle of 100 tablets – NDC 50458-513-60

TYLENOL® with Codeine No. 3 bottle of 1000 tablets – NDC 50458-513-80

TYLENOL® with Codeine No. 4 bottle of 100 tablets – NDC 50458-515-60

TYLENOL® with Codeine No. 4 bottle of 500 tablets – NDC 50458-515-70

Store TYLENOL® with Codeine tablets at 20° to 25°C (68° to 77°F). (See USP Controlled Room Temperature.)

Dispense in tight, light-resistant container as defined in the official compendium.

Manufactured by:
Janssen Ortho, LLC
Gurabo, Puerto Rico 00778

Manufactured for:
PriCara®,
Division of Ortho-McNeil-Janssen Pharmaceuticals, Inc.
Raritan, New Jersey 08869

Revised April 2009   10186600

© Ortho-McNeil-Janssen Pharmaceuticals, Inc. 2000

Shown in Product Identification Guide, page 317

Otsuka America Pharmaceutical, Inc.

**2440 RESEARCH BOULEVARD
ROCKVILLE, MD 20850**

Direct Inquiries to:
Medical Affairs
Otsuka America Pharmaceutical, Inc.
(800) 441-6763
FAX: (301) 721-7044
To Request Routine or Emergency Medical Information, or to Report an Adverse Experience:
(800) 438-9927

SAMSCA™   ℞
(tolvaptan)
tablets for oral use

HIGHLIGHTS OF PRESCRIBING INFORMATION
These highlights do not include all the information needed to use SAMSCA safely and effectively. See full prescribing information for SAMSCA.
SAMSCA™ (tolvaptan) tablets for oral use
Initial U.S. Approval: 05/2009

> **WARNING: INITIATE AND RE-INITIATE IN A HOSPITAL AND MONITOR SERUM SODIUM**
> *See full prescribing information for complete boxed warning.*
> - **SAMSCA should be initiated and re-initiated in patients only in a hospital where serum sodium can be monitored closely.**
> - **Too rapid correction of hyponatremia (e.g., >12 mEq/L/24 hours) can cause osmotic demyelination resulting in dysarthria, mutism, dysphagia, lethargy, affective changes, spastic quadriparesis, seizures, coma and death. In susceptible patients, including those with severe malnutrition, alcoholism or advanced liver disease, slower rates of correction may be advisable.**

——INDICATIONS AND USAGE——

SAMSCA is a selective vasopressin V_2-receptor antagonist indicated for the treatment of clinically significant hypervolemic and euvolemic hyponatremia [serum sodium <125 mEq/L or less marked hyponatremia that is symptomatic and has resisted correction with fluid restriction], including patients with heart failure, cirrhosis, and Syndrome of Inappropriate Antidiuretic Hormone (SIADH) (1).

Important Limitations:
- Patients requiring intervention to raise serum sodium urgently to prevent or to treat serious neurological symptoms should not be treated with SAMSCA (1).
- It has not been established that SAMSCA provides a symptomatic benefit to patients (1).

——DOSAGE AND ADMINISTRATION——

- SAMSCA should be initiated and re-initiated in a hospital (2.1).
- The recommended starting dose is 15 mg once daily. Dosage may be increased at intervals ≥24 hr to 30 mg once daily, and to a maximum of 60 mg once daily as needed to raise serum sodium. Monitor serum sodium and volume status (2.1)

——DOSAGE FORMS AND STRENGTHS——

- Tablets: 15 mg and 30 mg (3)

——CONTRAINDICATIONS——

- Do not administer to patients requiring urgent intervention to raise serum sodium acutely (4.1).
- Do not use in patients who are unable to sense or to respond appropriately to thirst (4.2).
- Do not use in patients with hypovolemic hyponatremia (4.3).
- Do not use with strong CYP 3A inhibitors (4.4).

- Do not administer to patients who are anuric as no benefit is expected (4.5)

————————WARNINGS/PRECAUTIONS————————

- Monitor serum sodium and neurologic status as serious neurologic sequelae can result from over rapid correction of sodium (5.1).
- Because of the potential increased risk of gastrointestinal bleeding in patients with cirrhosis, use in patients with cirrhosis only when the need to treat outweighs this risk (5.2).
- Dehydration and hypovolemia may require intervention (5.3).
- Avoid use with hypertonic saline (5.4).
- Avoid use with CYP 3A inducers and moderate CYP 3A inhibitors (5.5).
- Consider dose reduction if co-administered with P-gp inhibitors (5.5).
- Monitor serum potassium in patients with potassium >5 mEq/L or on drugs known to increase potassium (5.6).

————————ADVERSE REACTIONS————————

Most common adverse reactions (≥5% placebo) are thirst, dry mouth, asthenia, constipation, pollakiuria or polyuria, and hyperglycemia (6.1).

To report SUSPECTED ADVERSE REACTIONS, contact Otsuka at 1-877-726-7220 or FDA at 1-800-FDA-1088 (*www.fda.gov/medwatch*).

————————USE IN SPECIFIC POPULATIONS————————

- Pregnancy: Based on animal data, may cause fetal harm (8.1).
- Nursing mothers: Discontinue drug or nursing taking into consideration importance of drug to mother (8.3).
- Pediatric Use: There are no studies (8.4).

See 17 for PATIENT COUNSELING INFORMATION and Medication Guide.

Revised: 05/2009

FULL PRESCRIBING INFORMATION: CONTENTS*
WARNING: INITIATE AND RE-INITIATE IN A HOSPITAL AND MONITOR SERUM SODIUM

FULL PRESCRIBING INFORMATION

> **WARNING: INITIATE AND RE-INITIATE IN A HOSPITAL AND MONITOR SERUM SODIUM**
> **SAMSCA (tolvaptan) should be initiated and re-initiated in patients only in a hospital where serum sodium can be monitored closely.**
> **Too rapid correction of hyponatremia (e.g., >12 mEq/L/24 hours) can cause osmotic demyelination resulting in dysarthria, mutism, dysphagia, lethargy, affective changes, spastic quadriparesis, seizures, coma and death. In susceptible patients, including those with severe malnutrition, alcoholism or advanced liver disease, slower rates of correction may be advisable.**

1 INDICATIONS AND USAGE

SAMSCA™ is indicated for the treatment of clinically significant hypervolemic and euvolemic hyponatremia (serum sodium <125 mEq/L or less marked hyponatremia that is symptomatic and has resisted correction with fluid restriction), including patients with heart failure, cirrhosis, and Syndrome of Inappropriate Antidiuretic Hormone (SIADH).

Important Limitations

Patients requiring intervention to raise serum sodium urgently to prevent or to treat serious neurological symptoms should not be treated with SAMSCA.

It has not been established that raising serum sodium with SAMSCA provides a symptomatic benefit to patients.

2 DOSAGE AND ADMINISTRATION

2.1 Usual Dosage in Adults

Patients should be in a hospital for initiation and re-initiation of therapy to evaluate the therapeutic response and because too rapid correction of hyponatremia can cause osmotic demyelination resulting in dysarthria, mutism, dysphagia, lethargy, affective changes, spastic quadriparesis, seizures, coma and death.

The usual starting dose for SAMSCA is 15 mg administered once daily without regard to meals. Increase the dose to 30 mg once daily, after at least 24 hours, to a maximum of 60 mg once daily, as needed to achieve the desired level of serum sodium. During initiation and titration, frequently monitor for changes in serum electrolytes and volume. Avoid fluid restriction during the first 24 hours of therapy. Patients receiving SAMSCA should be advised that they can continue ingestion of fluid in response to thirst [see Warnings and Precautions (5.1)].

2.2 Drug Withdrawal

Following discontinuation from SAMSCA, patients should be advised to resume fluid restriction and should be monitored for changes in serum sodium and volume status.

2.3 Special Populations

There is no need to adjust dose based on age, gender, race, cardiac or hepatic function [see Use In Specific Populations (8) and Clinical Pharmacology (12.3)].

Renal Impairment

There is no need to adjust the dose in patients with mild to severe renal impairment (creatinine clearance 10-79 mL/min) as there is no increase in exposure to tolvaptan; tolvaptan has not been evaluated in patients with creatinine clearance <10 mL/min or in patients undergoing dialysis. No benefit can be expected in patients who are anuric [see Contraindications (4.5) and Clinical Pharmacology (12.3)].

2.4 Co-Administration with CYP 3A Inhibitors, CYP 3A Inducers and P-gp Inhibitors

CYP 3A Inhibitors

Tolvaptan is metabolized by CYP 3A, and use with strong CYP 3A inhibitors causes a marked (5-fold) increase in exposure [see Contraindications (4.4)]. The effect of moderate CYP 3A inhibitors on tolvaptan exposure has not been assessed. Avoid co-administration of SAMSCA and moderate CYP 3A inhibitors [see Warnings and Precautions (5.5), Drug Interactions (7.1)].

CYP 3A Inducers

Co-administration of SAMSCA with potent CYP 3A inducers (e.g., rifampin) reduces tolvaptan plasma concentrations by 85%. Therefore, the expected clinical effects of SAMSCA may not be observed at the recommended dose. Patient response should be monitored and the dose adjusted accordingly [see Warnings and Precautions (5.5), Drug Interactions (7.1)].

P-gp Inhibitors

Tolvaptan is a substrate of P-gp. Co-administration of SAMSCA with inhibitors of P-gp (e.g., cyclosporine) may necessitate a decrease in SAMSCA dose [see Warnings and Precautions (5.5), Drug Interactions (7.1)].

3 DOSAGE FORMS AND STRENGTHS

SAMSCA (tolvaptan) is available in 15 mg and 30 mg tablets [see How Supplied/Storage and Handling (16)].

4 CONTRAINDICATIONS

SAMSCA is contraindicated in the following conditions:

4.1 Urgent need to raise serum sodium acutely

SAMSCA has not been studied in a setting of urgent need to raise serum sodium acutely.

4.2 Inability of the patient to sense or appropriately respond to thirst

Patients who are unable to auto-regulate fluid balance are at substantially increased risk of incurring an overly rapid correction of serum sodium, hypernatremia and hypovolemia.

4.3 Hypovolemic hyponatremia

Risks associated with worsening hypovolemia, including complications such as hypotension and renal failure, outweigh possible benefits.

4.4 Concomitant use of strong CYP 3A inhibitors

Ketoconazole 200 mg administered with tolvaptan increased tolvaptan exposure by 5-fold. Larger doses would be expected to produce larger increases in tolvaptan exposure. There is not adequate experience to define the dose adjustment that would be needed to allow safe use of tolvaptan with strong CYP 3A inhibitors such as clarithromycin, ketoconazole, itraconazole, ritonavir, indinavir, nelfinavir, saquinavir, nefazodone, and telithromycin.

4.5 Anuric patients

In patients unable to make urine, no clinical benefit can be expected.

5 WARNINGS AND PRECAUTIONS

5.1 Too Rapid Correction of Serum Sodium Can Cause Serious Neurologic Sequelae (see BOXED WARNING)

Osmotic demyelination syndrome is a risk associated with too rapid correction of hyponatremia (e.g., >12 mEq/L/24 hours). Osmotic demyelination results in dysarthria, mutism, dysphagia, lethargy, affective changes, spastic quadriparesis, seizures, coma or death. In susceptible patients, including those with severe malnutrition, alcoholism or advanced liver disease, slower rates of correction may be advisable. In controlled clinical trials in which tolvaptan was administered in titrated doses starting at 15 mg once daily, 7% of tolvaptan-treated subjects with a serum sodium <130 mEq/L had an increase in serum sodium greater than 8 mEq/L at approximately 8 hours and 2% had an increase greater than 12 mEq/L at 24 hours. Approximately 1% of placebo-treated subjects with a serum sodium <130 mEq/L had a rise greater than 8 mEq/L at 8 hours and no patient had a rise greater than 12 mEq/L/24 hours. None of the patients in these studies had evidence of osmotic demyelination syndrome or related neurological sequelae, but such complications have been reported following too-rapid correction of serum sodium. Patients treated with SAMSCA should be monitored to assess serum sodium concentrations and neurologic status, especially during initiation and after titration. Subjects with SIADH or very low baseline serum sodium concentrations may be at greater risk for too-rapid correction of serum sodium. In patients receiving SAMSCA who develop too rapid a rise in serum sodium, discontinue or interrupt treatment with SAMSCA and consider administration of hypotonic fluid. Fluid restriction during the first 24 hours of therapy with SAMSCA may increase the likelihood of overly-rapid correction of serum sodium, and should generally be avoided.

5.2 Gastrointestinal Bleeding in Patients with Cirrhosis

In patients with cirrhosis treated with tolvaptan in hyponatremia trials, gastrointestinal bleeding was reported in 6 out of 63 (10%) tolvaptan-treated patients and 1 out of 57 (2%) placebo-treated patients. SAMSCA should be used in cirrhotic patients only when the need to treat outweighs this risk.

5.3 Dehydration and Hypovolemia

SAMSCA therapy induces copious aquaresis, which is normally partially offset by fluid intake. Dehydration and hypovolemia can occur, especially in potentially volume-depleted patients receiving diuretics or those who are fluid restricted. In multiple-dose, placebo-controlled trials in which 607 hyponatremic patients were treated with tolvaptan, the incidence of dehydration was 3.3% for tolvaptan and 1.5% for placebo-treated patients. In patients receiving SAMSCA who develop medically significant signs or symptoms of hypovolemia, interrupt or discontinue SAMSCA therapy and provide supportive care with careful management of vital signs, fluid balance and electrolytes. Fluid restriction during therapy with SAMSCA may increase the risk of dehydration and hypovolemia. Patients receiving SAMSCA should continue ingestion of fluid in response to thirst.

5.4 Co-administration with Hypertonic Saline

There is no experience with concomitant use of SAMSCA and hypertonic saline. Concomitant use with hypertonic saline is not recommended.

IMPORTANT NOTICE: Updated drug information is sent bi-monthly via the PDR® Update Insert. For *monthly* email updates, register at PDR.net.

5.5 Drug Interactions

Other Drugs Affecting Exposure to Tolvaptan

CYP 3A Inhibitors

Tolvaptan is a substrate of CYP 3A. CYP 3A inhibitors can lead to a marked increase in tolvaptan concentrations *[see Dosage and Administration (2.4), Drug Interactions (7.1)]*. Do not use SAMSCA (tolvaptan) with strong inhibitors of CYP 3A *[see Contraindications (4.4)]* and avoid concomitant use with moderate CYP 3A inhibitors.

CYP 3A Inducers

Avoid co-administration of CYP 3A inducers (e.g., rifampin, rifabutin, rifapentin, barbiturates, phenytoin, carbamazepine, St. John's Wort) with SAMSCA, as this can lead to a reduction in the plasma concentration of tolvaptan and decreased effectiveness of SAMSCA treatment. If co-administered with CYP 3A inducers, the dose of SAMSCA may need to be increased *[see Dosage and Administration (2.4), Drug Interactions (7.1)]*.

P-gp Inhibitors

The dose of SAMSCA may have to be reduced when SAMSCA is co-administered with P-gp inhibitors, e.g., cyclosporine *[see Dosage and Administration (2.4), Drug Interactions (7.1)]*.

5.6 Hyperkalemia or Drugs that Increase Serum Potassium

Treatment with tolvaptan is associated with an acute reduction of the extracellular fluid volume which could result in increased serum potassium. Serum potassium levels should be monitored after initiation of tolvaptan treatment in patients with a serum potassium >5 mEq/L as well as those who are receiving drugs known to increase serum potassium levels.

6 ADVERSE REACTIONS

6.1 Clinical Trials Experience

Because clinical trials are conducted under widely varying conditions, adverse reactions rates observed in the clinical trials of a drug cannot be directly compared to rates in the clinical trials of another drug and may not reflect the rates observed in practice. The adverse event information from clinical trials does, however, provide a basis for identifying the adverse events that appear to be related to drug use and for approximating rates.

In multiple-dose, placebo-controlled trials, 607 hyponatremic patients (serum sodium <135 mEq/L) were treated with SAMSCA. The mean age of these patients was 62 years; 70% of patients were male and 82% were Caucasian. One hundred eighty nine (189) tolvaptan-treated patients had a serum sodium <130 mEq/L, and 52 patients had a serum sodium <125 mEq/L. Hyponatremia was attributed to cirrhosis in 17% of patients, heart failure in 68% and SIADH/other in 16%. Of these patients, 223 were treated with the recommended dose titration (15 mg titrated to 60 mg as needed to raise serum sodium).

Overall, over 4,000 patients have been treated with oral doses of tolvaptan in open-label or placebo-controlled clinical trials. Approximately 650 of these patients had hyponatremia; approximately 219 of these hyponatremic patients were treated with tolvaptan for 6 months or more.

The most common adverse reactions (incidence ≥5% more than placebo) seen in two 30-day, double-blind, placebo-controlled hyponatremia trials in which tolvaptan was administered in titrated doses (15 mg to 60 mg once daily) were thirst, dry mouth, asthenia, constipation, pollakiuria or polyuria and hyperglycemia. In these trials, 10% (23/223) of tolvaptan-treated patients discontinued treatment because of an adverse event, compared to 12% (26/220) of placebo-treated patients; no adverse reaction resulting in discontinuation of trial medication occurred at an incidence of >1% in tolvaptan-treated patients.

Table 1 lists the adverse reactions reported in tolvaptan-treated patients with hyponatremia (serum sodium <135 mEq/L) and at a rate at least 2% greater than placebo-treated patients in two 30-day, double-blind, placebo-controlled trials. In these studies, 223 patients were exposed to tolvaptan (starting dose 15 mg, titrated to 30 and 60 mg as needed to raise serum sodium). Adverse events resulting in death in these trials were 6% in tolvaptan-treated-patients and 6% in placebo-treated patients.

Table 1. Adverse Reactions (>2% more than placebo) in Tolvaptan-Treated Patients in Double-Blind, Placebo-Controlled Hyponatremia Trials

System Organ Class MedDRA Preferred Term	Tolvaptan 15 mg/ day-60 mg/ day (N = 223) n (%)	Placebo (N = 220) n (%)
Gastrointestinal Disorders		
Dry mouth	28 (13)	9 (4)
Constipation	16 (7)	4 (2)
General Disorders and Administration Site Conditions		
Thirst[a]	35 (16)	11 (5)
Asthenia	19 (9)	9 (4)
Pyrexia	9 (4)	2 (1)
Metabolism and Nutrition Disorders		
Hyperglycemia[b]	14 (6)	2 (1)
Anorexia[c]	8 (4)	2 (1)
Renal and Urinary Disorders		
Pollakiuria or polyuria[d]	25 (11)	7 (3)

The following terms are subsumed under the referenced ADR in Table 1:
[a] polydipsia;
[b] diabetes mellitus;
[c] decreased appetite;
[d] urine output increased, micturition urgency, nocturia

In a subgroup of patients with hyponatremia (N = 475, serum sodium <135 mEq/L) enrolled in a double-blind, placebo-controlled trial (mean duration of treatment was 9 months) of patients with worsening heart failure, the following adverse reactions occurred in tolvaptan-treated patients at a rate at least 2% greater than placebo: mortality (42% tolvaptan, 38% placebo), nausea (21% tolvaptan, 16% placebo), thirst (12% tolvaptan, 2% placebo), dry mouth (7% tolvaptan, 2% placebo) and polyuria or pollakiuria (4% tolvaptan, 1% placebo).

The following adverse reactions occurred in <2% of hyponatremic patients treated with SAMSCA (tolvaptan) and at a rate greater than placebo in double-blind placebo-controlled trials (N = 607 tolvaptan; N = 518 placebo) or in <2% of patients in an uncontrolled trial of patients with hyponatremia (N = 111) and are not mentioned elsewhere in the label.

Blood and Lymphatic System Disorders: Disseminated intravascular coagulation

Cardiac Disorders: Intracardiac thrombus, ventricular fibrillation

Investigations: Prothrombin time prolonged

Gastrointestinal Disorders: Ischemic colitis

Metabolism and Nutrition Disorders: Diabetic ketoacidosis

Musculoskeletal and Connective Tissue Disorders: Rhabdomyolysis

Nervous System: Cerebrovascular accident

Renal and Urinary Disorders: Urethral hemorrhage

Reproductive System and Breast Disorders (female): Vaginal hemorrhage

Respiratory, Thoracic, and Mediastinal Disorders: Pulmonary embolism, respiratory failure

Vascular disorder: Deep vein thrombosis

7 DRUG INTERACTIONS

7.1 Effects of Drugs on Tolvaptan

Ketoconazole and Other Strong CYP 3A Inhibitors

SAMSCA is metabolized primarily by CYP 3A. Ketoconazole is a strong inhibitor of CYP 3A and also an inhibitor of P-gp. Co-administration of SAMSCA and ketoconazole 200 mg daily results in a 5-fold increase in exposure to tolvaptan. Co-administration of SAMSCA with 400 mg ketoconazole daily or with other strong CYP 3A inhibitors (e.g., clarithromycin, itraconazole, telithromycin, saquinavir, nelfinavir, ritonavir and nefazodone) at the highest labeled dose would be expected to cause an even greater increase in tolvaptan exposure. Thus, SAMSCA and strong CYP 3A inhibitors should not be co-administered *[see Dosage and Administration (2.4) and Contraindications (4.4)]*.

Moderate CYP 3A Inhibitors

The impact of moderate CYP 3A inhibitors (e.g., erythromycin, fluconazole, aprepitant, diltiazem and verapamil) on the exposure to co-administered tolvaptan has not been assessed. A substantial increase in the exposure to tolvaptan would be expected when SAMSCA is co-administered with moderate CYP 3A inhibitors. Co-administration of SAMSCA with moderate CYP 3A inhibitors should therefore generally be avoided *[see Dosage and Administration (2.4) and Warnings and Precautions (5.5)]*.

Grapefruit Juice

Co-administration of grapefruit juice and SAMSCA results in a 1.8-fold increase in exposure to tolvaptan *[see Dose and Administration (2.4) and Warnings and Precautions (5.5)]*.

P-gp Inhibitors

Reduction in the dose of SAMSCA may be required in patients concomitantly treated with P-gp inhibitors, such as e.g., cyclosporine, based on clinical response *[see Dose and Administration (2.4) and Warnings and Precautions (5.5)]*.

Rifampin and Other CYP 3A Inducers

Rifampin is an inducer of CYP 3A and P-gp. Co-administration of rifampin and SAMSCA reduces exposure to tolvaptan by 85%. Therefore, the expected clinical effects of SAMSCA (tolvaptan) in the presence of rifampin and other inducers (e.g., rifabutin, rifapentin, barbiturates, phenytoin, carbamazepine and St. John's Wort) may not be observed at the usual dose levels of SAMSCA. The dose of SAMSCA may have to be increased *[Dosage and Administration (2.4) and Warnings and Precautions (5.5)]*.

Lovastatin, Digoxin, Furosemide, and Hydrochlorothiazide

Co-administration of lovastatin, digoxin, furosemide, and hydrochlorothiazide with SAMSCA has no clinically relevant impact on the exposure to tolvaptan.

7.2 Effects of Tolvaptan on Other Drugs

Digoxin

Digoxin is a P-gp substrate and SAMSCA is a P-gp inhibitor. Co-administration of SAMSCA and digoxin results in a 1.3-fold increase in the exposure to digoxin.

Warfarin, Amiodarone, Furosemide, and Hydrochlorothiazide

Co-administration of tolvaptan does not appear to alter the pharmacokinetics of warfarin, furosemide, hydrochlorothiazide, or amiodarone (or its active metabolite, desethylamiodarone) to a clinically significant degree.

Lovastatin

SAMSCA is a weak inhibitor of CYP 3A. Co-administration of lovastatin and SAMSCA increases the exposure to lovastatin and its active metabolite lovastatin-β hydroxyacid by factors of 1.4 and 1.3, respectively. This is not a clinically relevant change.

Pharmacodynamic Interactions

Tolvaptan produces a greater 24 hour urine volume/excretion rate than does furosemide or hydrochlorothiazide. Concomitant administration of tolvaptan with furosemide or hydrochlorothiazide results in a 24 hour urine volume/excretion rate that is similar to the rate after tolvaptan administration alone.

Although specific interaction studies were not performed, in clinical studies tolvaptan was used concomitantly with beta-blockers, angiotensin receptor blockers, angiotensin converting enzyme inhibitors and potassium sparing diuretics. Adverse reactions of hyperkalemia were approximately 1-2% higher when tolvaptan was administered with angiotensin receptor blockers, angiotensin converting enzyme inhibitors and potassium sparing diuretics compared to administration of these medications with placebo. Serum potassium levels should be monitored during concomitant drug therapy.

8 USE IN SPECIFIC POPULATIONS

8.1 Pregnancy

Pregnancy Category C.

There are no adequate and well controlled studies of SAMSCA use in pregnant women. In animal studies, cleft palate, brachymelia, microphthalmia, skeletal malformations, decreased fetal weight, delayed fetal ossification, and embryo-fetal death occurred. SAMSCA should be used during pregnancy only if the potential benefit justifies the potential risk to the fetus.

In embryo-fetal development studies, pregnant rats and rabbits received oral tolvaptan during organogenesis. Rats received 2 to 162 times the maximum recommended human dose (MRHD) of tolvaptan (on a body surface area basis). Reduced fetal weights and delayed fetal ossification occurred at 162 times the MRHD. Signs of maternal toxicity (reduction in body weight gain and food consumption) occurred at 16 and 162 times the MRHD. When pregnant rabbits received oral tolvaptan at 32 to 324 times the MRHD (on a body surface area basis), there were reductions in maternal body weight gain and food consumption at all doses, and increased abortions at the mid and high doses (about 97 and 324 times the MRHD). At 324 times the MRHD, there were increased rates of embryo-fetal death, fetal microphthalmia, open eyelids, cleft palate, brachymelia and skeletal malformations *[see Nonclinical Toxicology (13.3)]*.

8.2 Labor and Delivery

The effect of SAMSCA on labor and delivery in humans is unknown.

8.3 Nursing Mothers

It is not known whether SAMSCA is excreted into human milk. Tolvaptan is excreted into the milk of lactating rats. Because many drugs are excreted into human milk and because of the potential for serious adverse reactions in nursing infants from SAMSCA, a decision should be made to discontinue nursing or SAMSCA, taking into consideration the importance of SAMSCA to the mother.

8.4 Pediatric Use

Safety and effectiveness of SAMSCA in pediatric patients have not been established.

8.5 Geriatric Use

Of the total number of hyponatremic subjects treated with SAMSCA (tolvaptan) in clinical studies, 42% were 65 and over, while 19% were 75 and over. No overall differences in safety or effectiveness were observed between these subjects and younger subjects, and other reported clinical experience has not identified differences in responses between the elderly and younger patients, but greater sensitivity of some older individuals cannot be ruled out. Increasing age has no effect on tolvaptan plasma concentrations.

8.6 Use in Patients with Hepatic Impairment

Moderate and severe hepatic impairment do not affect exposure to tolvaptan to a clinically relevant extent. No dose adjustment of tolvaptan is necessary.

8.7 Use in Patients with Renal Impairment

Exposure and response to tolvaptan are similar in patients with a creatinine clearance 10-79 mL/min and in patients without renal impairment. No dose adjustment is necessary. Exposure and response to tolvaptan in patients with a creatinine clearance <10 mL/min or in patients on chronic dialysis have not been studied. No benefit can be expected in patients who are anuric [see Contraindications (4.5)].

8.8 Use in Patients with Congestive Heart Failure

The exposure to tolvaptan in patients with congestive heart failure is not clinically relevantly increased. No dose adjustment is necessary.

10 OVERDOSAGE

Single oral doses up to 480 mg and multiple doses up to 300 mg once daily for 5 days have been well tolerated in studies in healthy subjects. There is no specific antidote for tolvaptan intoxication. The signs and symptoms of an acute overdose can be anticipated to be those of excessive pharmacologic effect: a rise in serum sodium concentration, polyuria, thirst, and dehydration/hypovolemia.

The oral LD_{50} of tolvaptan in rats and dogs is >2000 mg/kg. No mortality was observed in rats or dogs following single oral doses of 2000 mg/kg (maximum feasible dose). A single oral dose of 2000 mg/kg was lethal in mice, and symptoms of toxicity in affected mice included decreased locomotor activity, staggering gait, tremor and hypothermia.

If overdose occurs, estimation of the severity of poisoning is an important first step. A thorough history and details of overdose should be obtained, and a physical examination should be performed. The possibility of multiple drug involvement should be considered.

Treatment should involve symptomatic and supportive care, with respiratory, ECG and blood pressure monitoring and water/electrolyte supplements as needed. A profuse and prolonged aquaresis should be anticipated, which, if not matched by oral fluid ingestion, should be replaced with intravenous hypotonic fluids, while closely monitoring electrolytes and fluid balance.

ECG monitoring should begin immediately and continue until ECG parameters are within normal ranges. Dialysis may not be effective in removing tolvaptan because of its high binding affinity for human plasma protein (>99%). Close medical supervision and monitoring should continue until the patient recovers.

11 DESCRIPTION

Tolvaptan is (±)-4'-[(7-chloro-2,3,4,5-tetrahydro-5-hydroxy-1H-1-benzazepin-1-yl) carbonyl]-o-tolu-m-toluidide. The empirical formula is $C_{26}H_{25}ClN_2O_3$. Molecular weight is 448.94. The chemical structure is:

SAMSCA tablets for oral use contain 15 mg or 30 mg of tolvaptan. Inactive ingredients include corn starch, hydroxypropyl cellulose, lactose monohydrate, low-substituted hydroxypropyl cellulose, magnesium stearate and microcrystalline cellulose and FD&C Blue No. 2 Aluminum Lake as colorant.

12 CLINICAL PHARMACOLOGY

12.1 Mechanism of Action

Tolvaptan is a selective vasopressin V_2-receptor antagonist with an affinity for the V_2-receptor that is 1.8 times that of native arginine vasopressin (AVP). Tolvaptan affinity for the V_2-receptor is 29 times greater than for the V_{1a}-receptor. When taken orally, 15 to 60 mg doses of tolvaptan antagonize the effect of vasopressin and cause an increase in urine water excretion that results in an increase in free water clearance (aquaresis), a decrease in urine osmolality, and a resulting increase in serum sodium concentrations. Urinary excretion of sodium and potassium and plasma potassium concentrations are not significantly changed. Tolvaptan metabolites have no or weak antagonist activity for human V_2-receptors compared with tolvaptan.

Plasma concentrations of native AVP may increase (avg. 2-9 pg/mL) with tolvaptan administration.

Table 2. Effects of Treatment with Tolvaptan 15 mg/day to 60 mg/day

	Tolvaptan 15 mg/day-60 mg/day	Placebo	Estimated Effect (95% CI)
Subjects with Serum Sodium <135 mEq/L (ITT population)			
Change in average daily serum [Na+] AUC baseline to Day 4 (mEq/L) Mean (SD) N	4.0 (2.8) 213	0.4 (2.4) 203	3.7 (3.3-4.2) p <0.0001
Change in average daily serum [Na+] AUC baseline to Day 30 (mEq/L) Mean (SD) N	6.2 (4.0) 213	1.8 (3.7) 203	4.6 (3.9-5.2) p <0.0001
Percent of Patients Needing Fluid Restriction*	14% 30/215	25% 51/206	p <0.01
Subgroup with Serum Sodium <130 mEq/L			
Change in average daily serum [Na+] AUC baseline to Day 4 (mEq/L) Mean (SD) N	4.8 (3.0) 110	0.7 (2.5) 105	4.2 (3.5-5.0) p <0.0001
Change in average daily serum [Na+] AUC baseline to Day 30 (mEq/L) Mean (SD) N	7.9 (4.1) 110	2.6 (4.2) 105	5.5 (4.4-6.5) p <0.0001
Percent of Patients Needing Fluid Restriction*	19% 21/110	36% 38/106	p <0.01
Subgroup with Serum Sodium <125 mEq/L			
Change in average daily serum [Na+] AUC baseline to Day 4 (mEq/L) Mean (SD) N	5.7 (3.8) 26	1.0 (1.8) 30	5.3 (3.8-6.9) p <0.0001
Change in average daily serum [Na+] AUC baseline to Day 30 (mEq/L) Mean (SD) N	10.0 (4.8) 26	4.1 (4.5) 30	5.7 (3.1-8.3) p <0.0001
Percent of Patients Needing Fluid Restriction*	35% 9/26	50% 15/30	p = 0.14

*Fluid Restriction defined as <1L/day at any time during treatment period.

12.2 Pharmacodynamics

In healthy subjects receiving a single dose of SAMSCA (tolvaptan) 60 mg, the onset of the aquaretic and sodium increasing effects occurs within 2 to 4 hours post-dose. A peak effect of about a 6 mEq increase in serum sodium and about 9 mL/min increase in urine excretion rate is observed between 4 and 8 hours post-dose; thus, the pharmacological activity lags behind the plasma concentrations of tolvaptan. About 60% of the peak effect on serum sodium is sustained at 24 hours post-dose, but the urinary excretion rate is no longer elevated by this time. Doses above 60 mg tolvaptan do not increase aquaresis or serum sodium further. The effects of tolvaptan in the recommended dose range of 15 to 60 mg once daily appear to be limited to aquaresis and the resulting increase in sodium concentration.

In a parallel-arm, double-blind (for tolvaptan and placebo), placebo- and positive-controlled, multiple dose study of the effect of tolvaptan on the QTc interval, 172 healthy subjects were randomized to tolvaptan 30 mg, tolvaptan 300 mg, placebo, or moxifloxacin 400 mg once daily. At both the 30 mg and 300 mg doses, no significant effect of administering tolvaptan on the QTc interval was detected on Day 1 and Day 5. At the 300 mg dose, peak tolvaptan plasma concentrations were approximately 4-fold higher than the peak concentrations following a 30 mg dose. Moxifloxacin increased the QT interval by 12 ms at 2 hours after dosing on Day 1 and 17 ms at 1 hour after dosing on Day 5, indicating that the study was adequately designed and conducted to detect tolvaptan's effect on the QT interval, had an effect been present.

12.3 Pharmacokinetics

In healthy subjects the pharmacokinetics of tolvaptan after single doses of up to 480 mg and multiple doses up to 300 mg once daily have been examined. Area under the curve (AUC) increases proportionally with dose. After administration of doses ≥60 mg, however, Cmax increases less than proportionally with dose. The pharmacokinetic properties of tolvaptan are stereospecific, with a steady-state ratio of the S-(-) to the R-(+) enantiomer of about 3. The absolute bioavailability of tolvaptan is unknown. At least 40% of the dose is absorbed as tolvaptan or metabolites. Peak concentrations of tolvaptan are observed between 2 and 4 hours post-dose. Food does not impact the bioavailability of tolvaptan. In vitro data indicate that tolvaptan is a substrate and inhibitor of P-gp. Tolvaptan is highly plasma protein bound (99%) and distributed into an apparent volume of distribution of about 3 L/kg. Tolvaptan is eliminated entirely by non-renal routes and mainly, if not exclusively, metabolized by CYP 3A. After oral dosing, clearance is about 4 mL/min/kg and the terminal phase half-life is about 12 hours. The accumulation factor of tolvaptan with the once-daily regimen is 1.3 and the trough concentrations amount to ≤16% of the peak concentrations, suggesting a dominant half-life somewhat shorter than 12 hours. There is marked inter- subject variation in peak and average exposure to tolvaptan with a percent coefficient of variation ranging between 30 and 60%.

In patients with hyponatremia of any origin the clearance of tolvaptan is reduced to about 2 mL/min/kg. Moderate or severe hepatic impairment or congestive heart failure decrease the clearance and increase the volume of distribution of tolvaptan, but the respective changes are not clinically relevant. Exposure and response to tolvaptan in subjects with creatinine clearance ranging between 79 and 10 mL/min and patients with normal renal function are not different.

13 NONCLINICAL TOXICOLOGY

13.1 Carcinogenesis, Mutagenesis, Impairment of Fertility

Up to two years of oral administration of tolvaptan to male and female rats at doses up to 1000 mg/kg/day (162 times the maximum recommended human dose [MRHD] on a body surface area basis), to male mice at doses up to 60 mg/kg/day (5 times the MRHD) and to female mice at doses up to 100 mg/kg/day (8 times the MRHD) did not increase the incidence of tumors.

Tolvaptan tested negative for genotoxicity in in vitro (bacterial reverse mutation assay and chromosomal aberration test in Chinese hamster lung fibroblast cells) and in vivo (rat micronucleus assay) test systems.

In a fertility study in which male and female rats were orally administered tolvaptan at 100, 300 or 1000 mg/kg/day, the highest dose level was associated with significantly fewer corpora lutea and implants than control.

13.3 Reproductive and Developmental Toxicology

In pregnant rats, oral administration of tolvaptan at 10, 100 and 1000 mg/kg/day during organogenesis was associated with a reduction in maternal body weight gain and food consumption at 100 and 1000 mg/kg/day, and reduced fetal weight and delayed ossification of fetuses at 1000 mg/kg/day (162 times the MRHD on a body surface area basis). Oral administration of tolvaptan at 100, 300 and 1000 mg/kg/day to pregnant rabbits during organogenesis was associated with reductions in maternal body weight gain and food consumption at all doses, and abortions at mid- and high-doses. At 1000 mg/kg/day (324 times the MRHD), increased incidences of embryo-fetal death, fetal microphthalmia, open eyelids, cleft palate, brachymelia and skeletal malformations were observed. There are no adequate and well-controlled studies of SAMSCA (tolvaptan) in pregnant women. SAMSCA should be used in pregnancy only if the potential benefit justifies the risk to the fetus.

14 CLINICAL STUDIES

14.1 Hyponatremia

In two double-blind, placebo-controlled, multi-center studies (SALT-1 and SALT-2), a total of 424 patients with euvolemic or hypervolemic hyponatremia (serum sodium <135 mEq/L) resulting from a variety of underlying causes (heart failure, liver cirrhosis, syndrome of inappropriate antidiuretic hormone [SIADH] and others) were treated for 30 days with tolvaptan or placebo, then followed for an additional 7 days after withdrawal. Symptomatic patients, patients likely to require saline therapy during the course of therapy, patients with acute and transient hyponatremia associated with head trauma or postoperative state and patients with hyponatremia due to primary polydipsia, uncontrolled adrenal insufficiency or uncontrolled hypothyroidism were excluded. Patients were randomized to receive either placebo (N = 220) or tolvaptan (N = 223) at an initial oral dose of 15 mg once daily. The mean serum sodium concentration at study entry was 129 mEq/L. Fluid restriction was to be avoided if possible during the first 24 hours of therapy to avoid overly rapid correction of serum sodium, and during the first 24 hours of therapy 87% of patients had no fluid restriction. Thereafter, patients could resume or initiate fluid restriction (defined as daily fluid intake of ≤1.0 liter/day) as clinically indicated.

The dose of tolvaptan could be increased at 24 hour intervals to 30 mg once daily, then to 60 mg once daily, until either the maximum dose of 60 mg or normonatremia (serum sodium >135 mEq/L) was reached. Serum sodium concentrations were determined at 8 hours after study drug initiation and daily up to 72 hours, within which time titration was typically completed. Treatment was maintained for 30 days with additional serum sodium assessments on Days 11, 18, 25 and 30. On the day of study discontinuation, all patients resumed previous therapies for hyponatremia and were reevaluated 7 days later. The primary endpoint for these studies was the average daily AUC for change in serum sodium from baseline to Day 4 and baseline to Day 30 in patients with a serum sodium less than 135 mEq/L. Compared to placebo, tolvaptan caused a statistically greater increase in serum sodium (p <0.0001) during both periods in both studies (see Table 2). For patients with a serum sodium of <130 mEq/L or <125 mEq/L, the effects at Day 4 and Day 30 remained significant (see Table 2). This effect was also seen across all disease etiology subsets (e.g., CHF, cirrhosis, SIADH/other).

[See table 2 at top of previous page]

In patients with hyponatremia (defined as <135 mEq/L), serum sodium concentration increased to a significantly greater degree in tolvaptan-treated patients compared to placebo-treated patients as early as 8 hours after the first dose, and the change was maintained for 30 days. The percentage of patients requiring fluid restriction (defined as ≤1 L/day at any time during the treatment period) was also significantly less (p <0.0017) in the tolvaptan-treated group (30/215, 14%) as compared with the placebo-treated group (51/206, 25%).

Figure 1 shows the change from baseline in serum sodium by visit in patients with serum sodium <135 mEq/L. Within 7 days of tolvaptan discontinuation, serum sodium concentrations in tolvaptan-treated patients declined to levels similar to those of placebo-treated patients.

[See figure 1 at top of next column]

[See figure 2 in next column]

In the open-label study SALTWATER, 111 patients, 94 of them hyponatremic (serum sodium <135 mEq/L), previously on tolvaptan or placebo therapy were given tolvaptan as a titrated regimen (15 to 60 mg once daily) after having returned to standard care for at least 7 days. By this time, their baseline mean serum sodium concentration had fallen to between their original baseline and post-placebo therapy level. Upon initiation of therapy, average serum sodium concentrations increased to approximately the same levels as observed for those previously treated with tolvaptan, and were sustained for at least a year. Figure 3 shows results from 111 patients enrolled in the SALTWATER Study.

[See figure 3 in next column]

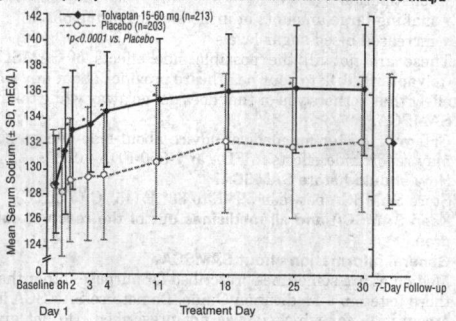

Figure 1: Pooled SALT Studies: Analysis of Mean Serum Sodium (± SD, mEq/L) by Visit - Patients with Baseline Serum Sodium <135 mEq/L

*p-value <0.0001 for all visits during tolvaptan treatment compared to placebo

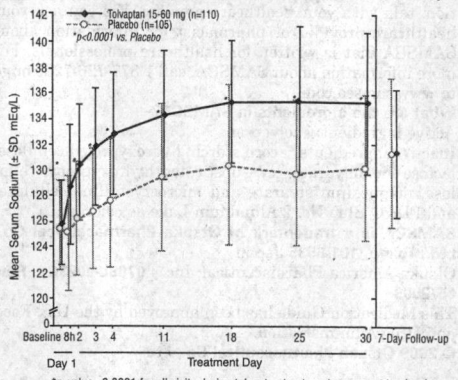

Figure 2: Pooled SALT Studies: Analysis of Mean Serum Sodium (± SD, mEq/L) by Visit - Patients with Baseline Serum Sodium <130 mEq/L

*p-value <0.0001 for all visits during tolvaptan treatment compared to placebo

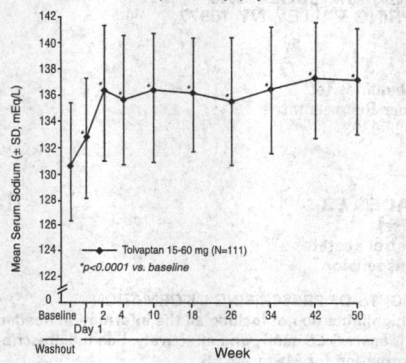

Figure 3: SALTWATER: Analysis of Mean Serum Sodium (± SD, mEq/L) by Visit

*p-value <0.0001 for all visits during tolvaptan treatment compared to baseline

14.2 Heart Failure

In a phase 3 double-blind, placebo-controlled study (EVEREST), 4133 patients with worsening heart failure were randomized to tolvaptan or placebo as an adjunct to standard of care. Long-term tolvaptan treatment (mean duration of treatment of 0.75 years) had no demonstrated effect, either favorable or unfavorable, on all-cause mortality [HR (95% CI): 0.98 (0.9, 1.1)] or the combined endpoint of CV mortality or subsequent hospitalization for worsening HF [HR (95% CI): 1.0 (0.9, 1.1)].

16 HOW SUPPLIED/STORAGE AND HANDLING

How Supplied

SAMSCA™ (tolvaptan) tablets are available in the following strengths and packages.

SAMSCA 15 mg tablets are non-scored, blue, triangular, shallow-convex, debossed with "OTSUKA" and "15" on one side.

Blister of 10   NDC 59148-020-50

SAMSCA 30 mg tablets are non-scored, blue, round, shallow-convex, debossed with "OTSUKA" and "30" on one side.

Blister of 10   NDC 59148-021-50

Storage and Handling

Store at 25 °C (77 °F), excursions permitted between 15 °C and 30 °C (59 °F to 86 °F) [see USP controlled Room Temperature].

Keep out of reach of children.

17 PATIENT COUNSELING INFORMATION

As a part of patient counseling, healthcare providers must review the SAMSCA (tolvaptan) Medication Guide with every patient [see FDA-Approved Medication Guide (17.3)].

17.1 Concomitant Medication

Advise patients to inform their physician if they are taking or plan to take any prescription or over-the-counter drugs since there is a potential for interactions.

Strong and Moderate CYP 3A inhibitors and Pg-p inhibitors

Advise patients to inform their physician if they use strong (e.g., ketoconazole, itraconazole, clarithromycin, telithromycin, nelfinavir, saquinavir, indinavir, ritonavir) or moderate CYP 3A inhibitors (e.g., aprepitant, erythromycin, diltiazem, verapamil, fluconazol) or P-gp inhibitors (e.g., cyclosporine) [see Dosage and Administration (2.4), Contraindications (4.4), Warnings and Precautions (5.5) and Drug Interactions (7.1)].

17.2 Nursing

Advise patients not to breastfeed an infant if they are taking SAMSCA [see Use In Specific Populations (8.3)].

17.3 FDA-Approved Medication Guide

MEDICATION GUIDE

SAMSCA™ (sam-sca)

tolvaptan

Tablets

Read the Medication Guide that comes with SAMSCA before you take it and each time you get a new prescription. There may be new information. This Medication Guide does not take the place of talking to your healthcare provider about your medical condition or your treatment. Share this important information with members of your household.

What is the most important information I should know about SAMSCA?

SAMSCA may make the salt (sodium) level in your blood rise too fast. This can increase your risk of a serious condition called osmotic demyelination syndrome (ODS). ODS can lead to coma or death. ODS can also cause new symptoms such as:

- trouble speaking
- swallowing trouble or feeling like food or liquid gets stuck while swallowing
- drowsiness
- confusion
- mood changes
- trouble controlling body movement (involuntary movement) and weakness in muscles of the arms and legs
- seizures

You or a family member should tell your healthcare provider right away if you have any of these symptoms even if they begin later in treatment. Also tell you healthcare provider about any other new symptoms while taking SAMSCA.

You may be more at risk for ODS if you have:

- liver disease
- not eaten for a long period of time (malnourished)
- very low sodium level in your blood
- been drinking large amounts of alcohol for a long period of time (chronic alcoholism)

To lessen your risk of ODS while taking SAMSCA:

- **Treatment with SAMSCA should be started and re-started only in a hospital, where the sodium levels in your blood can be checked closely.**
- Do not take SAMSCA if you can not tell if you are thirsty.
- To prevent losing too much body water (dehydration), have water available to drink at all times while taking SAMSCA. Unless your healthcare provider tells you otherwise, drink when you are thirsty.
- If your healthcare provider tells you to keep taking SAMSCA after you leave a hospital, it is important that you do not stop and re-start SAMSCA on your own. You may need to go back to a hospital to re-start SAMSCA. Talk to your healthcare provider right away if you stop taking SAMSCA for any reason.
- It is important to stay under the care of your healthcare provider while taking SAMSCA and follow their instructions.

What is SAMSCA?

SAMSCA is a prescription medicine used to help increase low sodium levels in the blood, in adults with conditions such as heart failure, liver disease, and certain hormone imbalances. SAMSCA helps raise salt levels in your blood by removing extra body water as urine.

It is not known if SAMSCA is safe or works in children.

Who should not take SAMSCA (tolvaptan)?

Do not take SAMSCA if:
- the sodium level in your blood must be increased right away.
- you can not replace fluids by drinking or you can not feel if you are thirsty.
- you are dizzy, faint, or your kidneys are not working normally because you have lost too much body fluid.
- you take certain medicines. These medicines could cause you to have too much SAMSCA in your blood:
  - the antibiotic medicines, clarithromycin (Biaxin, Biaxin XL) or telithromycin (Ketek)
  - the antifungal medicines, ketoconazole (Nizoral) or itraconazole (Sporonox)
  - the anti-HIV medicines, ritonavir (Kaletra, Norvir), indinavir (Crixivan), nelfinavir (Viracept), and saquinavir (Invirase)
  - the antidepressant medicine, nefazodone hydrochloride
- your body is not able to make urine. SAMSCA will not help your condition.

What should I tell my healthcare provider before taking SAMSCA?

Tell your healthcare provider about all your medical conditions, including if you:
- have kidney problems and your body can not make urine.
- can not feel if you are thirsty. See "What is the most important information I should know about SAMSCA?"
- have any allergies. See the end of this Medication Guide for a list of the ingredients in SAMSCA.
- are pregnant or plan to become pregnant. It is not known if SAMSCA will harm your unborn baby.
- are breast-feeding. It is not known if SAMSCA passes into your breast milk. You and your healthcare provider should decide if you will take SAMSCA or breast-feed. You should not do both.

Tell your healthcare provider about all the medicines you take, including prescription and non-prescription medicines, vitamins, and herbal supplements.

Using SAMSCA with certain medicines could cause you to have too much SAMSCA in your blood. See "Who should not take SAMSCA?"

SAMSCA may affect the way other medicines work, and other medicines may affect how SAMSCA works.

Know the medicines you take. Keep a list of them and show it to your healthcare provider and pharmacist when you get a new medicine.

How should I take SAMSCA?

- See "What is the most important information I should know about SAMSCA?"
- Take SAMSCA exactly as prescribed by your healthcare provider.
- Take SAMSCA one time each day.
- You can take SAMSCA with or without food.
- Do not drink grapefruit juice during treatment with SAMSCA. This could cause you to have too much SAMSCA in your blood.
- Certain medicines or illnesses may keep you from drinking fluids or may cause you to lose too much body fluid, such as vomiting or diarrhea. If you have these problems, call your healthcare provider right away.
- Do not miss or skip doses of SAMSCA. If you miss a dose, take it as soon as you remember. If it is near the time of the next dose, skip the missed dose. Just take the next dose at your regular time. Do not take 2 doses at the same time.
- **If you take too much SAMSCA, call your healthcare provider right away.** If you take an overdose of SAMSCA, you may need to go to a hospital.
- If your healthcare provider tells you to stop taking SAMSCA, follow their instructions about limiting the amount of fluid you should drink.

What are the possible side effects of SAMSCA?

SAMSCA can cause serious side effects including:
- See "What is the most important information I should know about SAMSCA?"
- **Loss of too much body fluid (dehydration). Tell your healthcare provider if you:**
  - have vomiting or diarrhea, and cannot drink normally.
  - feel dizzy or faint. These may be symptoms that you have lost too much body fluid.
- **Bleeding from the gastrointestinal tract in people with liver disease.** Tell your healthcare provider right away if you have any of these bleeding symptoms:
  - you vomit bright red blood
  - you vomit dark blood clots, or material that looks like coffee-grounds
  - your stools are black or look like tar
  - you pass blood or stool mixed with blood
  - your stool is bright red or has maroon colored blood in it

Call your healthcare provider right away, if you have any of these symptoms.

The most common side effects of SAMSCA are:
- thirst
- dry mouth

- weakness
- constipation
- making large amounts of urine and urinating often
- increased blood sugar levels

These are not all the possible side effects of SAMSCA (tolvaptan). Talk to your healthcare provider about any side effect that bothers you or that does not go away while taking SAMSCA.

Call your doctor for medical advice about side effects. You may report side effects to FDA at 1-800-FDA-1088.

How should I store SAMSCA?

Store SAMSCA between 59° F to 86° F (15° C to 30° C).

Keep SAMSCA and all medicines out of the reach of children.

General Information about SAMSCA

Medicines are sometimes prescribed for purposes other than those listed in a Medication Guide. Do not use SAMSCA for a condition for which it was not prescribed. Do not give SAMSCA to other people, even if they have the same symptoms you have. It may harm them.

This Medication Guide summarizes the most important information about SAMSCA. If you would like more information, talk with your healthcare provider. You can ask your healthcare provider or pharmacist for information about SAMSCA that is written for healthcare professionals. For more information about SAMSCA, call 1-877-726-7220 or go to www.samsca.com.

What are the ingredients in SAMSCA?

Active ingredient: tolvaptan.

Inactive ingredients: corn starch, hydroxypropyl cellulose, lactose monohydrate, low-substituted hydroxypropyl cellulose, magnesium stearate and microcrystalline cellulose, and FD&C Blue No. 2 Aluminum Lake as colorant.

SAMSCA is a trademark of Otsuka Pharmaceutical Co., Ltd., Tokyo, 101-8535 Japan

Otsuka America Pharmaceutical, Inc.   0708L-0023C   Rev. 05/2009

This Medication Guide has been approved by the U.S. Food and Drug Administration.

© 2009 Otsuka Pharmaceutical Co., Ltd.

Par Pharmaceutical, Inc.
**ONE RAM RIDGE ROAD
SPRING VALLEY, NY 10977**

Direct Inquiries to:
Customer Representative
(800) 828-9393

MEGACE® ES   ℞
[me-gāse]
**(megestrol acetate)
Oral Suspension**

HIGHLIGHTS OF PRESCRIBING INFORMATION

These highlights do not include all the information needed to use Megace® ES safely and effectively. See full prescribing information for Megace® ES.

Megace ES (megestrol acetate) Oral Suspension
Initial U.S. Approval: 1993

————————INDICATIONS AND USAGE————————

Megace® ES oral suspension is a progestin indicated for the treatment of anorexia, cachexia, or an unexplained significant weight loss in patients with a diagnosis of acquired immunodeficiency syndrome (AIDS) (1.0).

————DOSAGE AND ADMINISTRATION————

The recommended adult initial dosage of Megace® ES oral suspension is 625 mg/day (5 mL/day or one teaspoon daily). Shake container well before using (2.0).

————DOSAGE FORMS AND STRENGTHS————

Oral suspension containing 125 mg of megestrol acetate per mL (3.0).

————————CONTRAINDICATIONS————————

- History of hypersensitivity to megestrol acetate or any component of the formulation (4.1).
- Known or suspected pregnancy (4.2)(8.1).

————WARNINGS AND PRECAUTIONS————

- Women of childbearing potential should be advised to avoid becoming pregnant (5.2).
- Use with caution in patients with a history of thromboembolic disease (5.1).
- Clinical cases of overt Cushing's Syndrome have been reported in association with the *chronic use of megestrol acetate*. In addition, clinical cases of adrenal insufficiency have been observed in patients receiving or being withdrawn from chronic megestrol acetate therapy in the stressed and non-stressed state (5.3).
- New onset and exacerbation of pre-existing diabetes have been reported (5.4).

————————ADVERSE REACTIONS————————

To report SUSPECTED ADVERSE REACTIONS, contact Par Pharmaceutical, Inc. at 1-800-828-9393, option 3 or FDA at 1-800-FDA-1088 or www.fda.gov/medwatch.

The most common adverse events occurring in > 5% of all patients receiving 800mg/20mL of megestrol acetate oral suspension and enrolled in the two clinical efficacy trials were nausea, diarrhea, impotence, rash, flatulence, hypertension, and asthenia (6.2).

————————DRUG INTERACTIONS————————

Due to a significant decrease in Indinavir exposure, administration of a higher dose of indinavir should be considered when coadministering with megestrol acetate (7.1, 12.3).

————USE IN SPECIFIC POPULATIONS————

- **Geriatrics:** In general, dose selection for an elderly patient should be cautious, usually starting at the low end of the dosing range, reflecting the greater frequency of decreased hepatic, renal or cardiac function, and of concomitant disease or other therapy (8.5).
- **Nursing Mothers:** Because of the potential for adverse effects on the newborn, nursing should be discontinued if Megace® ES oral suspension is required (8.3).

See 17 for PATIENT COUNSELING INFORMATION

Revised: 08/2010

FULL PRESCRIBING INFORMATION

1   INDICATIONS AND USAGE

Megace® ES oral suspension is indicated for the treatment of anorexia, cachexia, or an unexplained, significant weight loss in patients with a diagnosis of acquired immunodeficiency syndrome (AIDS).

1.1   Limitations of Use

Other Treatable Causes

Therapy with megestrol acetate for weight loss should only be instituted after treatable causes of weight loss are sought and addressed. These treatable causes include possible malignancies, systemic infections, gastrointestinal disorders affecting absorption, endocrine disease, renal disease or psychiatric diseases.

Prophylactic Use

Megestrol acetate is not intended for prophylactic use to avoid weight loss.

2   DOSAGE AND ADMINISTRATION

The recommended adult initial dosage of Megace® ES oral suspension is 625 mg/day (5 mL/day or one teaspoon daily). **Please refer to the table below for correct dosing and administration.** Shake container well before using.

Table 1: Differences in Dosing between Megace® ES and Megace® oral suspension

	Megace® ES Oral Suspension	Megace® and other megestrol acetate oral suspensions
mg/mL	125 mg/mL	40 mg/mL
Recommended Daily Dose	625 mg	800 mg
Daily Volume Intake	5 mL (teaspoon)	20 mL (dosing cup)

3 DOSAGE FORMS AND STRENGTHS

Megace® ES is a milky white, lemon-lime flavored oral suspension containing 125 mg of megestrol acetate per mL. Megace® ES does not contain the same amount of megestrol acetate as Megace® oral suspension or any of the other megestrol acetate oral suspensions (2.0).

4 CONTRAINDICATIONS
4.1 Hypersensitivity Reaction
History of hypersensitivity to megestrol acetate or any component of the formulation.
4.2 Pregnancy
Known or suspected pregnancy.

5 WARNINGS AND PRECAUTIONS
5.1 General
• Effects on HIV viral replication have not been determined.
• Use with caution in patients with a history of thromboembolic disease.
5.2 Fetal Effects
Megestrol acetate may cause fetal harm when administered to a pregnant woman. For animal data on fetal effects, *see NONCLINICAL TOXICOLOGY: Impairment of Fertility (13.1)*. There are no adequate and well-controlled studies in pregnant women. If this drug is used during pregnancy, or if the patient becomes pregnant while taking (receiving) this drug, the patient should be apprised of the potential hazard to the fetus. Women of childbearing potential should be advised to avoid becoming pregnant.
5.3 Adrenal Insufficiency
The glucocorticoid activity of megestrol acetate oral suspension has not been fully evaluated. Clinical cases of overt Cushing's Syndrome have been reported in association with the chronic use of megestrol acetate. In addition, clinical cases of adrenal insufficiency have been observed in patients receiving or being withdrawn from chronic megestrol acetate therapy in the stressed and non-stressed state. Furthermore, adrenocorticotropin (ACTH) stimulation testing has revealed the frequent occurrence of asymptomatic pituitary-adrenal suppression in patients treated with chronic megestrol acetate therapy. Therefore, the possibility of adrenal insufficiency should be considered in any patient receiving or being withdrawn from chronic Megace® ES therapy who presents with symptoms and/or signs suggestive of hypoadrenalism (e.g., hypotension, nausea, vomiting, dizziness, or weakness) in either the stressed or non-stressed state. Laboratory evaluation for adrenal insufficiency and consideration of replacement or stress doses of a rapidly acting glucocorticoid are strongly recommended in such patients. Failure to recognize inhibition of the hypothalamic-pituitary adrenal axis may result in death. Finally, in patients who are receiving or being withdrawn from chronic Megace® ES therapy, consideration should be given to the use of empiric therapy with stress doses of a rapidly acting glucocorticoid during stress or serious intercurrent illness (e.g., surgery, infection).
5.4 Diabetes
Clinical cases of new onset diabetes mellitus and exacerbation of pre-existing diabetes mellitus have been reported in association with the chronic use of megestrol acetate.

6 ADVERSE REACTIONS
6.1 Serious and Otherwise Important Adverse Reactions
The following serious reactions and otherwise important adverse drug reactions are discussed in greater detail in other sections of the labeling:
• Hypersensitivity [*see Contraindications(4.1)*]
• Pregnancy [*see Contraindications (4.2)*]
• Fetal Effects [*see Warnings and Precautions (5.2)*]
• Thromboembolic Disease [*see Warnings and Precautions (5.1)*]
• Adrenal Insufficiency [*see Warnings and Precaution (5.3)*]
6.2 Clinical Trial Experience
Because clinical trials are conducted under widely varying conditions, adverse reactions observed in the clinical trials

Table 2: Adverse Events

Percent of Patients Reporting Adverse Events

	Trial 1 (N=236)				Trial 2 (N=87)		Open Label Trial
	Placebo				Placebo		
Megestrol Acetate, mg/day	0	100	400	800	0	800	1200
No. of Patients	N=34	N=68	N=69	N=65	N=38	N=49	N=176
Diarrhea	15	13	8	15	8	6	10
Impotence	3	4	6	14	0	4	7
Rash	9	9	4	12	3	2	6
Flatulence	9	0	1	9	3	10	6
Hypertension	0	0	0	8	0	0	4
Asthenia	3	2	3	6	8	4	5
Insomnia	0	3	4	6	0	0	1
Nausea	9	4	0	5	3	4	5
Anemia	6	3	3	5	0	0	0
Fever	3	6	4	5	3	2	1
Libido Decreased	3	4	0	5	0	2	1
Dyspepsia	0	0	3	3	5	4	2
Hyperglycemia	3	0	0	3	0	0	3
Headache	6	10	1	3	3	0	3
Pain	6	0	0	2	5	6	4
Vomiting	9	3	0	2	3	6	4
Pneumonia	6	2	0	2	3	0	1
Urinary Frequency	0	0	1	2	5	2	1

of a drug cannot be directly compared to rates in the clinical trials of another drug and may not reflect the rates observed in practice.

Adverse events which occurred in at least 5% of patients in any arm of the two clinical efficacy trials and the open trial for megestrol acetate oral suspension are listed below by treatment group. All patients listed had at least one post baseline visit during the 12 study weeks.
[See table 2 above]
Adverse events which occurred in 1% to 3% of all patients enrolled in the two clinical efficacy trials with at least one follow-up visit during the first 12 weeks of the study are listed below by body system. Adverse events occurring less than 1% are not included. There were no significant differences between incidence of these events in patients treated with megestrol acetate and patients treated with placebo.
Body as a Whole—abdominal pain, chest pain, infection, moniliasis and sarcoma
Cardiovascular System—cardiomyopathy and palpitation
Digestive System—constipation, dry mouth, hepatomegaly, increased salivation and oral moniliasis
Hemic and Lymphatic System—leukopenia
Metabolic and Nutritional—LDH increased, edema and peripheral edema
Nervous System—paresthesia, confusion, convulsion, depression, neuropathy, hypesthesia and abnormal thinking
Respiratory System—dyspnea, cough, pharyngitis and lung disorder
Skin and Appendages—alopecia, herpes, pruritus, vesiculobullous rash, sweating and skin disorder
Special Senses—amblyopia
Urogenital System—albuminuria, urinary incontinence, urinary tract infection and gynecomastia
6.3 Postmarketing Experience
Postmarketing reports associated with megestrol acetate oral suspension include thromboembolic phenomena including thrombophlebitis, deep vein thrombosis, and pulmonary embolism; and glucose intolerance [see *WARNINGS and PRECAUTIONS (5.1, 5.4)*].

7 DRUG INTERACTIONS
7.1 Indinavir
Due to the significant decrease in the exposure of indinavir by megestrol acetate, administration of a higher dose of indinavir should be considered when coadministering with megestrol acetate [See Clinical Pharmacology (12.3)].

7.2 Zidovudine and Rifabutin
No dosage adjustment for zidovudine and rifabutin is needed when megestrol acetate is coadministered with these drugs [See Clinical pharmacology (12.3)].

8 USE IN SPECIFIC POPULATIONS
8.1 Pregnancy
Pregnancy Category X [*see WARNINGS and PRECAUTIONS: (5.2)*]. No adequate animal teratology information is available at clinically relevant doses. Pregnant rats treated with low doses of megestrol acetate (0.02-fold the recommended clinical dose resulted in a reduction in fetal weight and number of live births, and feminization of male fetuses.
8.3 Nursing Mothers
Because of the potential for adverse effects on the newborn, nursing should be discontinued if Megace® ES oral suspension is required.
8.4 Pediatric Use
Safety and effectiveness in pediatric patients have not been established.
8.5 Geriatric Use
Clinical studies of megestrol acetate oral suspension in the treatment of anorexia, cachexia, or an unexplained significant weight loss in patients with AIDS did not include sufficient numbers of patients aged 65 years and older to determine whether they respond differently than younger patients. Other reported clinical experience has not identified differences in responses between elderly and younger patients. In general, dose selection for an elderly patient should be cautious, usually starting at the low end of the dosing range, reflecting the greater frequency of decreased hepatic, renal, or cardiac function, and of concomitant disease or other drug therapy.

Megestrol acetate is known to be substantially excreted by the kidney, and the risk of toxic reactions to this drug may be greater in patients with impaired renal function. Because elderly patients are more likely to have decreased renal function, care should be taken in dose selection, and it may be useful to monitor renal function.
8.6 Use in HIV Infected Women
Megestrol acetate has had limited use in HIV infected women.

All 10 women in the clinical trials reported breakthrough bleeding.

Table 3: Megestrol Acetate Oral Suspension Clinical Efficacy Trials

	Trial 1 Study Accrual Dates 11/88 to 12/90				Trial 2 Study Accrual Dates 5/89 to 4/91	
Megestrol Acetate, mg/day	0	100	400	800	0	800
Entered Patients	38	82	75	75	48	52
Evaluable Patients	28	61	53	53	29	36
Mean Change in Weight (lb.)						
Baseline to 12 Weeks	0.0	2.9	9.3	10.7	-2.1	11.2
% Patients ≥5 Pound Gain						
at Last Evaluation in 12 Weeks	21	44	57	64	28	47
Mean Changes in Body Composition*:						
Fat Body Mass (lb.)	0.0	2.2	2.9	5.5	1.5	5.7
Lean Body Mass (lb.)	-1.7	-0.3	1.5	2.5	-1.6	-0.6
Water (liters)	-1.3	-0.3	0.0	0.0	-0.1	-0.1
% Patients with Improved Appetite:						
At Time of Maximum Weight Change	50	72	72	93	48	69
At Last Evaluation in 12 Weeks	50	72	68	89	38	67
Mean Change in Daily Caloric Intake:						
Baseline to Time of Maximum Weight Change	-107	326	308	646	30	464

*Based on bioelectrical impedance analysis determinations at last evaluation in 12 weeks.

10 OVERDOSAGE

No serious unexpected side effects have resulted from studies involving megestrol acetate oral suspension administered in dosages as high as 1200 mg/day. Megestrol acetate has not been tested for dialyzability; however, due to its low solubility it is postulated that dialysis would not be an effective means of treating overdose.

11 DESCRIPTION

Megace® ES oral suspension contains megestrol acetate, a synthetic derivative of the naturally occurring steroid hormone, progesterone. Megestrol acetate is a white, crystalline solid chemically designated as 17-Hydroxy-6-methyl pregna-4,6-diene-3,20-dione acetate. Solubility at 37° C in water is 2 mcg per mL, solubility in plasma is 24 mcg per mL. Its molecular weight is 384.52.

The chemical formula is $C_{24}H_{32}O_4$ and the structural formula is represented as follows:

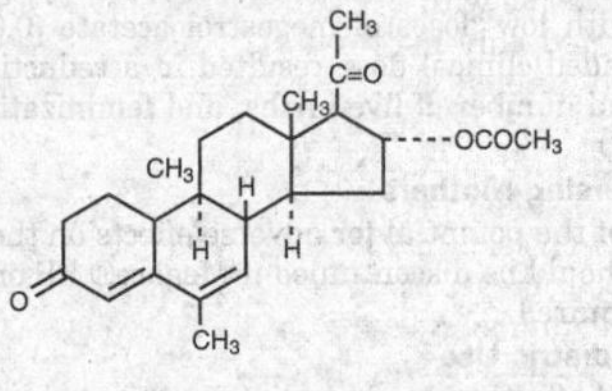

Figure 1. Megestrol Acetate Chemical Structure

Megace® ES is an oral suspension containing 125 mg of megestrol acetate per mL.

Megace® ES oral suspension contains the following inactive ingredients: alcohol (max 0.06% v/v from flavor), artificial lime flavor, citric acid monohydrate, docusate sodium, hydroxypropyl methylcellulose (hypromellose), natural and artificial lemon flavor, purified water, sodium benzoate, sodium citrate dihydrate, and sucrose.

12 CLINICAL PHARMACOLOGY

12.1 Mechanism of Action

Several investigators have reported on the appetite enhancing property of megestrol acetate and its possible use in cachexia. The precise mechanism by which megestrol acetate produces effects in anorexia and cachexia is unknown at the present time.

12.3 Pharmacokinetics

Absorption and Distribution

Mean plasma concentrations of megestrol acetate after administration of 625 mg (125 mg/mL) of Megace® ES oral suspension are equivalent under fed conditions to 800 mg (40 mg/mL) of megestrol acetate oral suspension in healthy volunteers.

In order to characterize the dose proportionality of Megace® ES, pharmacokinetic studies across a range of doses were conducted when administered under fasting and fed conditions. Pharmacokinetics of megestrol acetate was linear in the dosing range between 150 mg and 675 mg after Megace® ES administration regardless of meal condition. The mean peak plasma concentration (Cmax) and the mean area under the concentration time-curve (AUC) after a high fat meal were increased by 48% and 36%, respectively, compared to those under fasting condition after 625 mg Megace® ES administration. This food effect is less than that seen for the original formulation, megestrol acetate 800mg/20mL, where a high fat meal significantly increased AUC and Cmax of megestrol acetate to 2-fold and 7-fold, respectively, compared to those under the fasting condition. There was no difference in safety following administration in the fed state, therefore Megace® ES could be taken without regard to meals.

Plasma steady state pharmacokinetics of megestrol acetate were evaluated in 10 adult, cachectic male adult patients with acquired immunodeficiency syndrome (AIDS) and an involuntary weight loss greater than 10% of baseline who received single oral doses of 800 mg/day of megestrol acetate oral suspension for 21 days. The mean (±1SD) Cmax of megestrol acetate was 753 (±539) ng/mL. The mean AUC was 10476 (±7788) ng × hr/mL. Median Tmax value was five hours.

In another study, 24 asymptomatic HIV seropositive male adult subjects were dosed once daily with 750 mg of megestrol acetate oral suspension for 14 days. Mean Cmax and AUC values were 490 (±238) ng/mL and 6779 (±3048) hr × ng/mL, respectively. The Median Tmax value was three hours. The mean Cmin value was 202 (±101) ng/mL. The mean % of fluctuation value was 107 (±40).

Metabolism and Excretion

The major route of drug elimination in humans is urine. When radio-labeled megestrol acetate was administered to humans in doses of 4 to 90 mg, the urinary excretion within 10 days ranged from 56.5% to 78.4% (mean 66.4%) and fecal excretion ranged from 7.7% to 30.3% (mean 19.8%). The total recovered radioactivity varied between 83.1% and 94.7% (mean 86.2%).

Megestrol acetate metabolites which were identified in urine constituted 5% to 8% of the dose administered. Respiratory excretion as labeled carbon dioxide and fat storage may have accounted for at least part of the radioactivity not found in urine and feces.

The mean elimination half-life of megestrol ranged from 20 to 50 hours in healthy subjects.

Specific Populations

The pharmacokinetics of megestrol acetate has not been studied in specific population, for example, pediatric, renal impairment, and hepatic impairment.

Drug Interactions

The effects of indinavir, zidovudine or rifabutin on the pharmacokinetics of megestrol acetate were not studied.

Zidovudine

Pharmacokinetic studies show that there are no significant alterations in exposure of zidovudine when megestrol acetate is administered with this drug.

Rifabutin

Pharmacokinetic studies show that there are no significant alterations in exposure of rifabutin when megestrol acetate is administered with this drug.

Indinavir

A pharmacokinetic study in healthy male subjects demonstrated that coadministration of megestrol acetate (675 mg for 14 days) and indinavir (single dose 800 mg) results in a significant decrease in the pharmacokinetic parameters (~32% for Cmax and ~21% for AUC) of indinavir.

13 NONCLINICAL TOXICOLOGY

13.1 Carcinogenesis and Mutagenesis and Impairment of Fertility

Data on carcinogenesis were obtained from studies conducted in dogs, monkeys and rats treated with megestrol acetate at doses up to 0.01 to 0.1–fold the recommended clinical dose (13.3 mg/kg/day) based on body mass. No males were used in the dog and monkey studies. In female beagles, megestrol acetate (0.01, 0.1 or 0.25 mg/kg/day) administered for up to 7 years induced both benign and malignant tumors of the breast. In female monkeys, no tumors were found following 10 years of treatment with 0.01, 0.1 or 0.5 mg/kg/day megestrol acetate. Pituitary tumors were observed in female rats treated with 3.9 or 10 mg/kg/day of megestrol acetate for 2 years. The relationship of these tumors in rats and dogs to humans is unknown but should be considered in assessing the risk-to-benefit ratio when prescribing Megace® ES oral suspension and in surveillance of patients on therapy.

Megestrol acetate induced unscheduled DNA synthesis in primary cultures of human hepatocytes, but not in rat hepatocytes. Megetrol administered to mice increased the frequency of sister chromatid exchange and chromosomal aberrations in bone marrow cells after single intraperiotonial doses of 16.25 and 32.50 mg/kg. Perinatal/postnatal (segment III) toxicity studies were performed in rats at doses up to 0.02–fold the recommended clinical dose (13.3 mg/kg/day) based on body mass. In these low dose studies, the reproductive capability of male offspring of megestrol acetate-treated females was impaired. Similar results were obtained in dogs. No toxicity data are currently available on male reproduction (spermatogenesis)[see WARNINGS and PRECAUTIONS (5.2)].

13.2 Animal Pharmacology and/or Toxicology

Long-term treatment with Megace® ES may increase the risk of respiratory infections. A trend toward increased frequency of respiratory infections, decreased lymphocyte counts and increased neutrophil counts was observed in a two-year chronic toxicity/carcinogenicity study of megestrol acetate conducted in rats.

14 CLINICAL STUDIES

Megestrol acetate oral suspension at a dose of 800 mg/20 mL is equivalent to 625 mg/5 mL of Megace® ES under the fed condition. The clinical efficacy of megestrol acetate oral suspension was assessed in two clinical trials as described below.

Trial 1

One was a multicenter, randomized, double-blind, placebo-controlled study comparing megestrol acetate (MA) at doses of 100 mg, 400 mg, and 800 mg per day versus placebo in AIDS patients with anorexia/cachexia and significant weight loss. Of the 270 patients entered on study, 195 met all inclusion/exclusion criteria, had at least two additional post baseline weight measurements over a 12 week period or had one post baseline weight measurement but dropped out for therapeutic failure. The percent of patients gaining five or more pounds at maximum weight gain in 12 study weeks was statistically significantly greater for the 800 mg (64%) and 400 mg (57%) MA-treated groups than for the placebo group (24%). Mean weight increased from baseline to last evaluation in 12 study weeks in the 800 mg MA-treated group by 7.8 pounds, the 400 mg MA group by 4.2 pounds, the 100 mg MA group by 1.9 pounds and decreased in the placebo group by 1.6 pounds. Mean weight changes at 4, 8 and 12 weeks for patients evaluable for efficacy in the two clinical trials is shown graphically. Changes in body composition during the 12 study weeks as measured by bioelectrical impedance analysis showed increases in non-water body weight in the MA-treated groups. In addition, edema developed or worsened in only 3 patients.

Greater percentages of MA-treated patients in the 800 mg group (89%), the 400 mg group (68%) and the 100 mg group (72%), than in the placebo group (50%), showed an improvement in appetite at last evaluation during the 12 study weeks. A statistically significant difference was observed between the 800 mg MA-treated group and the placebo group in the change in caloric intake from baseline to time of maximum weight change. Patients were asked to assess weight change, appetite, appearance, and overall perception of well-being in a 9 question survey. At maximum weight change only the 800 mg MA-treated group gave responses that were statistically significantly more favorable to all questions when compared to the placebo-treated group. A dose response was noted in the survey with positive responses correlating with higher dose for all questions.

Trial 2

The second trial was a multicenter, randomized, double-blind, placebo-controlled study comparing megestrol acetate 800 mg/day versus placebo in AIDS patients with anorexia/cachexia and significant weight loss. Of the 100 patients entered on study, 65 met all inclusion/exclusion criteria, had at least two additional post baseline weight measurements over a 12 week period or had one post baseline weight measurement but dropped out for therapeutic failure. Patients in the 800 mg MA-treated group had a statistically significantly larger increase in mean maximum weight change than patients in the placebo group. From baseline to study week 12, mean weight increased by 11.2 pounds in the MA-treated group and decreased 2.1 pounds in the placebo group. Changes in body composition as measured by bioelectrical impedance analysis showed increases in non-water weight in the MA-treated group (see clinical studies table). No edema was reported in the MA-treated group. A greater percentage of MA-treated patients (67%) than placebo-treated patients (38%) showed an improvement in appetite at last evaluation during the 12 study weeks; this difference was statistically significant. There were no statistically significant differences between treatment groups in mean caloric change or in daily caloric intake at time to maximum weight change. In the same 9 question survey referenced in the first trial, patients' assessments of weight change, appetite, appearance, and overall perception of well-being showed increases in mean scores in MA-treated patients as compared to the placebo group.

In both trials, patients tolerated the drug well and no statistically significant differences were seen between the treatment groups with regard to laboratory abnormalities, new opportunistic infections, lymphocyte counts, T4 counts, T8 counts, or skin reactivity tests [see ADVERSE REACTIONS (6.0)].

[See table 3 at top of previous page]

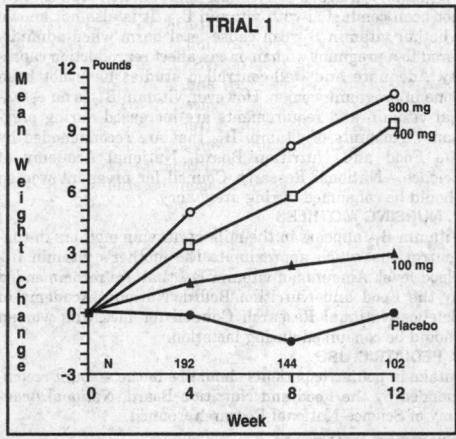

Figure 2: Mean Weight Change for Patients Evaluable for Efficacy in Trial 1

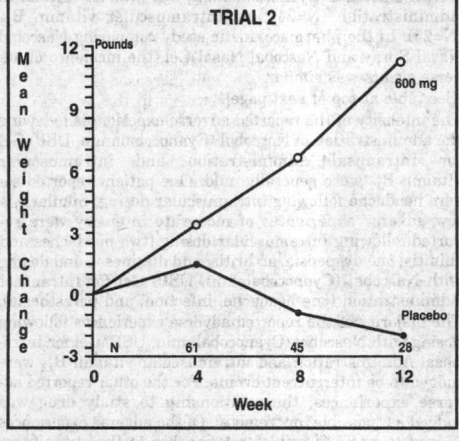

Figure 3: Mean Weight Change for Patients Evaluable for Efficacy in Trial 2

16 HOW SUPPLIED/STORAGE AND HANDLING

16.1 How Supplied

Megace® ES oral suspension is a milky white, lemon-lime flavored oral suspension containing 125 mg of megestrol acetate per mL. Available in bottles of 150 mL (5 fl oz) NDC 49884-949-69.

16.2 Storage

Store Megace® ES oral suspension between 15°-25° C (59°-77° F) and dispense in a tight container. Protect from heat.

16.3 Safe Handling

Health Hazard Data

There is no threshold limit value established by OSHA, NIOSH, or ACGIH. Exposure or overdose at levels approaching recommended dosing levels could result in side effects described above [see WARNINGS and PRECAUTIONS (5.0)andADVERSE REACTIONS (6.0)]. Women at risk of pregnancy should avoid such exposure.

17 PATIENT COUNSELING INFORMATION

The prescriber should inform the patient about the product differences to avoid overdosing or underdosing of megestrol acetate. The recommended adult dosage of Megace® ES is one teaspoon (5 mL) once a day [see table in DOSAGE and ADMINISTRATION (2.0)]

Patients using Megace® ES should receive the following instructions:

• This medication is to be used as directed by the physician.

• Megace® ES (625 mg/5 mL) does not contain the same amount of megestrol acetate as Megace® oral suspension or any of the other megestrol acetate oral suspensions. Megace® ES contains 625 mg of megestrol acetate per 5 mL (125mg/mL) whereas Megace® oral suspension and other megestrol acetate oral suspensions contain 800 mg per 20 mL (40 mg/mL).

• Report any adverse reaction experiences while taking this medication.

• Use contraception while taking this medication if you are a woman capable of becoming pregnant.

• Notify your physician if you become pregnant while taking this medication.

Manufactured by:

PAR PHARMACEUTICAL, INC.
Spring Valley, New York 10977
Revised: 07/10
OS949-52-1-04
Megace® is a registered trademark of Bristol-Myers Squibb Company licensed to Par Pharmaceutical, Inc.

NASCOBAL®   ℞

[naz-ko-bahl]
(Cyanocobalamin, USP)
Nasal Spray
A prescription B₁₂ nasal spray that is a simple alternative to monthly shots
One Spray, One Nostril, Once a Week
Pain-free, Convenient, Safe, Effective

Prescribing Information for Nascobal (Cyanocobalamin, USP) Nasal Spray

DESCRIPTION

Cyanocobalamin is a synthetic form of vitamin B_{12} with equivalent vitamin B_{12} activity. The chemical name is 5,6-dimethyl-benzimidazolyl cyanocobamide. The cobalt content is 4.35%. The molecular formula is $C_{63}H_{88}CoN_{14}O_{14}P$, which corresponds to a molecular weight of 1355.38 and the following structural formula:

Cyanocobalamin occurs as dark red crystals or orthorhombic needles or crystalline red powder. It is very hygroscopic in the anhydrous form, and sparingly to moderately soluble in water (1:80). Its pharmacologic activity is destroyed by heavy metals (iron) and strong oxidizing or reducing agents (vitamin C), but not by autoclaving for short periods of time (15-20 minutes) at 121°C. The vitamin B_{12} coenzymes are very unstable in light.

Nascobal® Nasal Spray is a solution of Cyanocobalamin, USP (vitamin B_{12}) for administration as a spray to the nasal mucosa. Each bottle of Nascobal Nasal Spray contains 2.3 mL of a 500 mcg/0.1 mL solution of cyanocobalamin with sodium citrate, citric acid, glycerin and benzalkonium chloride in purified water. The spray solution has a pH between 4.5 and 5.5. The spray pump unit must be fully primed (see Dosage and Administration) prior to initial use. After initial priming, each spray delivers an average of 500 mcg of cyanocobalamin and the 2.3 mL of spray solution contained in the bottle will deliver 8 doses of Nascobal Nasal Spray. The unit must be re-primed before each dose. (see Dosage and Administration).

CLINICAL PHARMACOLOGY

GENERAL PHARMACOLOGY AND MECHANISM OF ACTION

Vitamin B_{12} is essential to growth, cell reproduction, hematopoiesis, and nucleoprotein and myelin synthesis. Cells characterized by rapid division (e.g., epithelial cells, bone marrow, myeloid cells) appear to have the greatest requirement for vitamin B_{12}. Vitamin B_{12} can be converted to coenzyme B_{12} in tissues, and as such is essential for conversion of methylmalonate to succinate and synthesis of methionine from homocysteine, a reaction which also requires folate. In the absence of coenzyme B_{12}, tetrahydrofolate cannot be regenerated from its inactive storage form, 5-methyl tetrahydrofolate, and a functional folate deficiency occurs. Vitamin B_{12} also may be involved in maintaining sulfhydryl (SH) groups in the reduced form required by many SH-activated enzyme systems. Through these reactions, vitamin B_{12} is associated with fat and carbohydrate metabolism and protein synthesis. Vitamin B_{12} deficiency results in megaloblastic anemia, GI lesions, and neurologic damage that begins with an inability to produce myelin and is followed by gradual degeneration of the axon and nerve head. Cyanocobalamin is the most stable and widely used form of vitamin B_{12}, and has hematopoietic activity apparently identical to that of the antianemia factor in purified liver extract. The information below, describing the clinical pharmacology of cyanocobalamin, has been derived from studies with injectable vitamin B_{12}.

Vitamin B_{12} is quantitatively and rapidly absorbed from intramuscular and subcutaneous sites of injection. It is bound to plasma proteins and stored in the liver. Vitamin B_{12} is excreted in the bile and undergoes some enterohepatic recycling. Absorbed vitamin B_{12} is transported via specific B_{12} binding proteins, transcobalamin I and II, to the various tissues. The liver is the main organ for vitamin B_{12} storage. Parenteral (intramuscular) administration of vitamin B_{12} completely reverses the megaloblastic anemia and GI symptoms of vitamin B_{12} deficiency; the degree of improvement in neurologic symptoms depends on the duration and severity of the lesions, although progression of the lesions is immediately arrested.

Gastrointestinal absorption of vitamin B_{12} depends on the presence of sufficient intrinsic factor and calcium ions. Intrinsic factor deficiency causes pernicious anemia, which may be associated with subacute combined degeneration of the spinal cord. Prompt parenteral administration of vitamin B_{12} prevents progression of neurologic damage.

The average diet supplies about 4 to 15 mcg/day of vitamin B_{12} in a protein-bound form that is available for absorption after normal digestion. Vitamin B_{12} is not present in foods of plant origin, but is abundant in foods of animal origin. In people with normal absorption, deficiencies have been reported only in strict vegetarians who consume no products of animal origin (including no milk products or eggs).

Vitamin B_{12} is bound to intrinsic factor during transit through the stomach; separation occurs in the terminal ileum in the presence of calcium, and vitamin B_{12} enters the mucosal cell for absorption. It is then transported by the transcobalamin binding proteins. A small amount (approximately 1% of the total amount ingested) is absorbed by simple diffusion, but this mechanism is adequate only with very large doses. Oral absorption is considered too undependable to rely on in patients with pernicious anemia or other conditions resulting in malabsorption of vitamin B_{12}. Colchicine, para-aminosalicylic acid, and heavy alcohol intake for longer than 2 weeks may produce malabsorption of vitamin B_{12}.

PHARMACOKINETICS

Absorption

A three way crossover study in 25 fasting healthy subjects was conducted to compare the bioavailability of the B_{12} nasal spray to the B_{12} nasal gel and to evaluate the relative bioavailability of the nasal formulations as compared to the intramuscular injection. The peak concentrations after administration of intranasal spray were reached in 1.25 +/- 1.9 hours. The average peak concentration of B_{12} obtained after baseline correction following administration of intranasal spray was 757.96 +/- 532.17 pg/mL. The bioavailability of the nasal spray relative to the intramuscular injection was found to be 6.1%. The bioavailability of the B_{12} nasal spray was found to be 10% less than the B_{12} nasal gel. The 90% confidence intervals for the log$_e$ - transformed $AUC_{(0-t)}$ and C_{max} was 71.71%-114.19% and 71.6%-118.66% respectively.

In pernicious anemia patients, once weekly intranasal dosing with 500 mcg B_{12} gel resulted in a consistent increase in pre-dose serum B_{12} levels during one month of treatment ($p < 0.003$) above that seen one month after 100 mcg intramuscular dose (Figure).

Distribution

In the blood, B_{12} is bound to transcobalamin II, a specific B-globulin carrier protein, and is distributed and stored primarily in the liver and bone marrow.

Elimination

About 3-8 mcg of B_{12} is secreted into the GI tract daily via the bile; in normal subjects with sufficient intrinsic factor, all but about 1 mcg is re-absorbed. When B_{12} is administered in doses which saturate the binding capacity of plasma proteins and the liver, the unbound B_{12} is rapidly eliminated in the urine. Retention of B_{12} in the body is dose-dependent. About 80-90% of an intramuscular dose up to 50 mcg is retained in the body; this percentage drops to 55% for a 100 mcg dose, and decreases to 15% when a 1000 mcg dose is given.

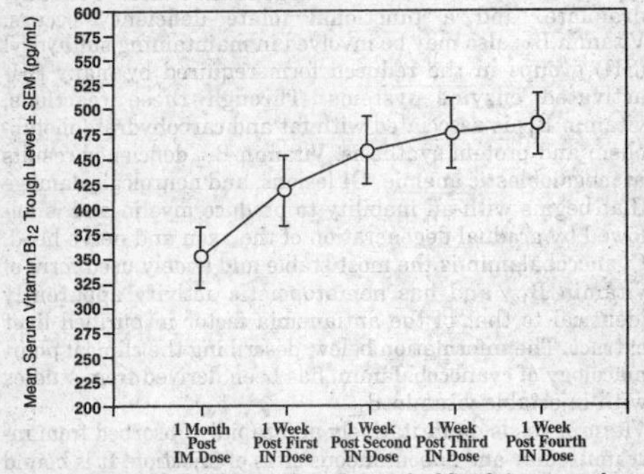

Figure. Vitamin B12 Serum Trough Levels After Intramuscular Solution (IM) of 100 mcg and Nasal Gel (IN) Administration of 500 mcg Cyanocobalamin After Weekly Doses.

INDICATIONS AND USAGE

Nascobal Nasal Spray is indicated for the maintenance of normal hematologic status in pernicious anemia patients who are in remission following intramuscular vitamin B_{12} therapy and who have no nervous system involvement.

Nascobal Nasal Spray is also indicated as a supplement for other vitamin B_{12} deficiencies, including:

I. Dietary deficiency of vitamin B_{12} occurring in strict vegetarians (Isolated vitamin B_{12} deficiency is very rare).

II. Malabsorption of vitamin B_{12} resulting from structural or functional damage to the stomach, where intrinsic factor is secreted, or to the ileum, where intrinsic factor facilitates vitamin B_{12} absorption. These conditions include HIV infection, AIDS, Crohn's disease, tropical sprue, and nontropical sprue (idiopathic steatorrhea, gluten-induced enteropathy). Folate deficiency in these patients is usually more severe than vitamin B_{12} deficiency.

III. Inadequate secretion of intrinsic factor, resulting from lesions that destroy the gastric mucosa (ingestion of corrosives, extensive neoplasia), and a number of conditions associated with a variable degree of gastric atrophy (such as multiple sclerosis, HIV infection, AIDS, certain endocrine disorders, iron deficiency, and subtotal gastrectomy). Total gastrectomy always produces vitamin B_{12} deficiency. Structural lesions leading to vitamin B_{12} deficiency include regional ileitis, ileal resections, malignancies, etc.

IV. Competition for vitamin B_{12} by intestinal parasites or bacteria. The fish tapeworm (Diphyllobothrium latum) absorbs huge quantities of vitamin B_{12} and infested patients often have associated gastric atrophy. The blind loop syndrome may produce deficiency of vitamin B_{12} or folate.

V. Inadequate utilization of vitamin B_{12}. This may occur if antimetabolites for the vitamin are employed in the treatment of neoplasia.

It may be possible to treat the underlying disease by surgical correction of anatomic lesions leading to small bowel bacterial overgrowth, expulsion of fish tapeworm, discontinuation of drugs leading to vitamin malabsorption (see "Drug/Laboratory Test Interactions"), use of a gluten free diet in nontropical sprue, or administration of antibiotics in tropical sprue. Such measures remove the need for long-term administration of vitamin B_{12}.

Requirements of vitamin B_{12} in excess of normal (due to pregnancy, thyrotoxicosis, hemolytic anemia, hemorrhage, malignancy, hepatic and renal disease) can usually be met with intranasal or oral supplementation.

Nascobal Nasal Spray is not suitable for vitamin B_{12} absorption test (Schilling Test).

CONTRAINDICATION

Sensitivity to cobalt and/or vitamin B_{12} or any component of the medication is a contraindication.

WARNINGS

Patients with early Leber's disease (hereditary optic nerve atrophy) who were treated with vitamin B_{12} suffered severe and swift optic atrophy.

Hypokalemia and sudden death may occur in severe megaloblastic anemia which is treated intensely with vitamin B_{12}. Folic acid is not a substitute for vitamin B_{12} although it may improve vitamin B_{12}-deficient megaloblastic anemia. Exclusive use of folic acid in treating vitamin B_{12}-deficient megaloblastic anemia could result in progressive and irreversible neurologic damage.

Anaphylactic shock and death have been reported after parenteral vitamin B_{12} administration. No such reactions have been reported in clinical trials with Nascobal Nasal Spray or Nascobal Nasal Gel.

Blunted or impeded therapeutic response to vitamin B_{12} may be due to such conditions as infection, uremia, drugs having bone marrow suppressant properties such as chloramphenicol, and concurrent iron or folic acid deficiency.

PRECAUTIONS

1. GENERAL

An intradermal test dose of parenteral vitamin B_{12} is recommended before Nascobal Nasal Spray is administered to patients suspected of cyanocobalamin sensitivity. Vitamin B_{12} deficiency that is allowed to progress for longer than three months may produce permanent degenerative lesions of the spinal cord. Doses of folic acid greater than 0.1 mg per day may result in hematologic remission in patients with vitamin B_{12} deficiency. Neurologic manifestations will not be prevented with folic acid, and if not treated with vitamin B_{12}, irreversible damage will result.

Doses of vitamin B_{12} exceeding 10 mcg daily may produce hematologic response in patients with folate deficiency. Indiscriminate administration may mask the true diagnosis. The validity of diagnostic vitamin B_{12} or folic acid blood assays could be compromised by medications, and this should be considered before relying on such tests for therapy.

Vitamin B_{12} is not a substitute for folic acid and since it might improve folic acid deficient megaloblastic anemia, indiscriminate use of vitamin B_{12} could mask the true diagnosis.

Hypokalemia and thrombocytosis could occur upon conversion of severe megaloblastic to normal erythropoiesis with vitamin B_{12} therapy. Therefore, serum potassium levels and the platelet count should be monitored carefully during therapy.

Vitamin B_{12} deficiency may suppress the signs of polycythemia vera. Treatment with vitamin B_{12} may unmask this condition.

If a patient is not properly maintained with Nascobal® Nasal Spray, intramuscular vitamin B_{12} is necessary for adequate treatment of the patient. No single regimen fits all cases, and the status of the patient observed in follow-up is the final criterion for adequacy of therapy.

The effectiveness of Nascobal Nasal Spray in patients with nasal congestion, allergic rhinitis and upper respiratory infections has not been determined. Therefore, treatment with Nascobal Nasal Spray should be deferred until symptoms have subsided.

2. INFORMATION FOR PATIENTS

Patients with pernicious anemia should be instructed that they will require weekly intranasal administration of Nascobal Nasal Spray for the remainder of their lives. Failure to do so will result in return of the anemia and in development of incapacitating and irreversible damage to the nerves of the spinal cord. Also, patients should be warned about the danger of taking folic acid in place of vitamin B_{12}, because the former may prevent anemia but allow progression of subacute combined degeneration of the spinal cord. (Hot foods may cause nasal secretions and a resulting loss of medication; therefore, patients should be told to administer Nascobal Nasal Spray at least one hour before or one hour after ingestion of hot foods or liquids).

A vegetarian diet which contains no animal products (including milk products or eggs) does not supply any vitamin B_{12}. Therefore, patients following such a diet should be advised to take Nascobal Nasal Spray weekly. The need for vitamin B_{12} is increased by pregnancy and lactation. Deficiency has been recognized in infants of vegetarian mothers who were breast fed, even though the mothers had no symptoms of deficiency at the time.

Because the nasal dosage forms of Vitamin B_{12} have a lower absorption than intramuscular dosage, nasal dosage forms are administered weekly, rather than the monthly intramuscular dosage. As shown in the Figure above, at the end of a month, weekly nasal administration results in significantly higher serum Vitamin B_{12} levels than after intramuscular administration. The patient should also understand the importance of returning for follow-up blood tests every 3 to 6 months to confirm adequacy of the therapy.

Careful instructions on the actuator assembly, removal of the safety clip, priming of the actuator and nasal administration of Nascobal Nasal Spray should be given to the patient. Although instructions for patients are supplied with individual bottles, procedures for use should be demonstrated to each patient.

3. LABORATORY TESTS

Hematocrit, reticulocyte count, vitamin B_{12} folate and iron levels should be obtained prior to treatment. If folate levels are low, folic acid should also be administered. All hematologic parameters should be normal when beginning treatment with Nascobal® Nasal Spray.

Vitamin B_{12} blood levels and peripheral blood counts must be monitored initially at one month after the start of treatment with Nascobal® Nasal Spray, and then at intervals of 3 to 6 months.

A decline in the serum levels of B_{12} after one month of treatment with B_{12} nasal spray may indicate that the dose may need to be adjusted upward. Patients should be seen one month after each dose adjustment; continued low levels of serum B_{12} may indicate that the patient is not a candidate for this mode of administration.

Patients with pernicious anemia have about 3 times the incidence of carcinoma of the stomach as in the general population, so appropriate tests for this condition should be carried out when indicated.

4. DRUG/LABORATORY TEST INTERACTIONS

Persons taking most antibiotics, methotrexate or pyrimethamine invalidate folic acid and vitamin B_{12} diagnostic blood assays.

Colchicine, para-aminosalicylic acid and heavy alcohol intake for longer than 2 weeks may produce malabsorption of vitamin B_{12}.

5. CARCINOGENESIS, MUTAGENESIS, IMPAIRMENT OF FERTILITY

Long-term studies in animals to evaluate carcinogenic potential have not been done. There is no evidence from long-term use in patients with pernicious anemia that vitamin B_{12} is carcinogenic. Pernicious anemia is associated with an increased incidence of carcinoma of the stomach, but this is believed to be related to the underlying pathology and not to treatment with vitamin B_{12}.

6. PREGNANCY

Pregnancy Category C: Animal reproduction studies have not been conducted with vitamin B_{12}. It is also not known whether vitamin B_{12} can cause fetal harm when administered to a pregnant woman or can affect reproduction capacity. Adequate and well-controlled studies have not been done in pregnant women. However, vitamin B_{12} is an essential vitamin and requirements are increased during pregnancy. Amounts of vitamin B_{12} that are recommended by the Food and Nutrition Board, National Academy of Science - National Research Council for pregnant women should be consumed during pregnancy.

7. NURSING MOTHERS

Vitamin B_{12} appears in the milk of nursing mothers in concentrations which approximate the mother's vitamin B_{12} blood level. Amounts of vitamin B_{12} that are recommended by the Food and Nutrition Board, National Academy of Science-National Research Council for lactating women should be consumed during lactation.

8. PEDIATRIC USE

Intake in pediatric patients should be in the amount recommended by the Food and Nutrition Board, National Academy of Science-National Research Council.

ADVERSE REACTIONS

The incidence of adverse experiences described in the Table below are based on data from a short-term clinical trial in vitamin B_{12} deficient patients in hematologic remission receiving Nascobal (Cyanocobalamin, USP) Gel for Intranasal Administration (N=24) and intramuscular vitamin B_{12} (N=25). In the pharmacokinetic study comparing Nascobal Nasal Spray and Nascobal Nasal Gel, the incidence of adverse events was similar.

[See table at top of next page]

The intensity of the reported adverse experiences following the administration of Nascobal (Cyanocobalamin, USP) Gel for Intranasal Administration and intramuscular vitamin B_{12} were generally mild. One patient reported severe headache following intramuscular dosing. Similarly, a few adverse experiences of moderate intensity were reported following intramuscular dosing (two headaches and rhinitis; one dyspepsia, arthritis, and dizziness), and dosing with Nascobal (Cyanocobalamin, USP) Gel for Intranasal Administration (one headache, infection, and paresthesia). The majority of the reported adverse experiences following dosing with Nascobal (Cyanocobalamin, USP) Gel for Intranasal Administration and intramuscular vitamin B_{12} were judged to be intercurrent events. For the other reported adverse experiences, the relationship to study drug was judged as "possible" or "remote". Of the adverse experiences judged to be of "possible" relationship to the study drug, anxiety, incoordination, and nervousness were reported following intramuscular vitamin B_{12} and headache, nausea, and rhinitis were reported following dosing with Nascobal (Cyanocobalamin, USP) Gel for Intranasal Administration. The following adverse reactions have been reported with parenteral vitamin B_{12}:

Generalized: Anaphylactic shock and death (See Warnings and Precautions).

Cardiovascular: Pulmonary edema and congestive heart failure early in treatment; peripheral vascular thrombosis.

Hematological: Polycythemia vera.

Gastrointestinal: Mild transient diarrhea.

Dermatological: Itching; transitory exanthema.

Miscellaneous: Feeling of swelling of the entire body.

OVERDOSAGE

No overdosage has been reported with Nascobal Nasal Spray, Nascobal (Cyanocobalamin, USP) Gel for Intranasal Administration or parenteral vitamin B_{12}.

DOSAGE AND ADMINISTRATION

The recommended initial dose of Nascobal Nasal Spray is one spray (500 mcg) administered in ONE nostril once weekly. Nascobal Nasal Spray should be administered at least one hour before or one hour after ingestion of hot foods or liquids. Periodic monitoring of serum B_{12} levels should be obtained to establish adequacy of therapy.

Priming (Activation) of Pump

Before the first dose and administration, the pump must be primed. Remove the clear plastic cover and the plastic safety clip from the pump. To prime the pump, place nozzle between the first and second finger with the thumb on the bottom of the bottle. Pump the unit firmly and quickly until the first appearance of spray. Then prime the pump an additional 2 times. Now the nasal spray is ready for use. The unit must be re-primed before each dose. Prime the pump **once** immediately before each administration of doses 2 through 8.

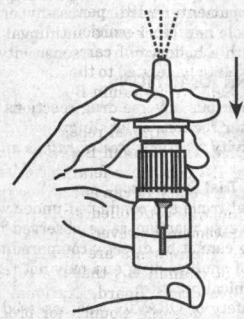

See LABORATORY TESTS for monitoring B_{12} levels and adjustment of dosage.

HOW SUPPLIED

Nascobal Nasal Spray is available as a spray in 3 mL glass bottles containing 2.3 mL of solution. It is available in a dosage strength of 500 mcg per actuation (0.1 mL/actuation). A screw-on actuator is provided. This actuator, following priming, will deliver 0.1 mL of the spray. Nascobal Nasal Spray is provided in a carton containing a nasal spray actuator with dust cover, a bottle of nasal spray solution, and a package insert. One bottle will deliver 8 doses (NDC 49884-270-14).

PHARMACIST ASSEMBLY INSTRUCTIONS FOR NASCOBAL NASAL SPRAY

The pharmacist should assemble the Nascobal Nasal Spray unit prior to dispensing to the patient, according to the following instructions:

1. Open the carton and remove the spray actuator and spray solution bottle.
2. Assemble Nascobal Nasal Spray by first unscrewing the white cap from the spray solution bottle and screwing the actuator unit tightly onto the bottle. Make sure the clear dust cover is on the pump unit.
3. Return the Nascobal Nasal Spray bottle to the carton for dispensing to the patient.

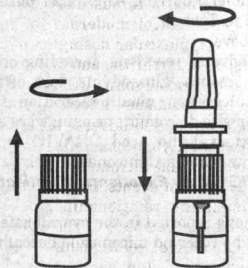

Table Adverse Experiences by Body System, Number of Patients and Number of Occurrences by Treatment Following Intramuscular and Intranasal Administration of Cyanocobalamin.

Body System	Adverse Experience	Number of Patients (Occurrences)	
		Vitamin B_{12} Nasal Gel, 500 mcg N=24	Intramuscular Vitamin B_{12}, 100 mcg N=25
Body as a Whole	Asthenia	1 (1)	4 (4)
	Back Pain	0 (0)	1 (1)
	Generalized Pain	0 (0)	2 (3)
	Headache	1 (2) *	5 (11)
	Infection[a]	3 (4)	3 (3)
Cardiovascular System	Peripheral Vascular Disorder	0 (0)	1 (1)
Digestive System	Dyspepsia	0 (0)	1 (2)
	Glossitis	1 (1)	0 (0)
	Nausea	1 (1) *	1 (1)
	Nausea & Vomiting	0 (0)	1 (1)
	Vomiting	0 (0)	1 (1)
Musculoskeletal System	Arthritis	0 (0)	2 (2)
	Myalgia	0 (0)	1 (1)
Nervous System	Abnormal Gait	0 (0)	1 (1)
	Anxiety	0 (0)	1 (1) *
	Dizziness	0 (0)	3 (3)
	Hypoesthesia	0 (0)	1 (1)
	Incoordination	0 (0)	1 (2) *
	Nervousness	0 (0)	1 (3) *
	Paresthesia	1 (1)	1 (1)
Respiratory System	Dyspnea	0 (0)	1 (1)
	Rhinitis	1 (1) *	2 (2)

[a] Sore throat, common cold

*There may be a possible relationship between these adverse experiences and the study drugs. These adverse experiences could have also been produced by the patient's clinical state or other concomitant therapy.

INFORMATION FOR PATIENTS

Patients with pernicious anemia should be instructed that they will require weekly intranasal administration of Nascobal Nasal Spray for the remainder of their lives. Failure to do so will result in return of the anemia and in development of incapacitating and irreversible damage to the nerves of the spinal cord. Also, patients should be warned about the danger of taking folic acid in place of vitamin B_{12}, because the former may prevent anemia but allow progression of subacute combined degeneration of the spinal cord. (Hot foods may cause nasal secretions and a resulting loss of medication; therefore, patients should be told to administer Nascobal Nasal Spray at least one hour before or one hour after ingestion of hot foods or liquids).

A vegetarian diet which contains no animal products (including milk products or eggs) does not supply any vitamin B_{12}. Therefore, patients following such a diet should be advised to take Nascobal Nasal Spray weekly. The need for vitamin B_{12} is increased by pregnancy and lactation. Deficiency has been recognized in infants of vegetarian mothers who were breast fed, even though the mothers had no symptoms of deficiency at the time.

Because the nasal dosage forms of Vitamin B_{12} have a lower absorption than intramuscular dosage, nasal dosage forms are administered weekly, rather than the monthly intramuscular dosage. As shown in the Figure above, at the end of a month, weekly nasal administration results in significantly higher serum Vitamin B_{12} levels than after intramuscular administration. The patient should also understand the importance of returning for follow-up blood tests every 3 to 6 months to confirm adequacy of the therapy.

Careful instructions on the actuator assembly, removal of safety clip, priming of the actuator and nasal administration of Nascobal Nasal Spray should be given to the patient.

Although instructions for patients are supplied with individual bottles, procedures for use should be demonstrated to each patient.

STORAGE CONDITIONS

Protect from light. Keep covered in carton until ready to use. Store upright at controlled room temperature 15°C to 30°C (59°F to 86°F). Protect from freezing.

To report suspected adverse reactions, contact Par Pharmaceutical Companies, Inc. at 1-800-828-9393.

Distributed by:

Par Pharmaceutical Companies, Inc.
Spring Valley, NY, 10977
Rev. 03/09

ORAVIG
[OR-a-vig]
(miconazole)
buccal tablets

℞

HIGHLIGHTS OF PRESCRIBING INFORMATION

These highlights do not include all the information needed to use ORAVIG safely and effectively. See full prescribing information for ORAVIG.

ORAVIG (miconazole) buccal tablets
Initial U.S. Approval: 1974

——————INDICATIONS AND USAGE——————

ORAVIG is an azole antifungal indicated for the local treatment of oropharyngeal candidiasis in adults (1).

————DOSAGE AND ADMINISTRATION————

- Application of one ORAVIG 50 mg buccal tablet to the gum region once daily for 14 consecutive days (2.1).
- Instruct patients not to crush, chew, or swallow tablets (2.2).

Table 1 Adverse Reactions (Treatment-Emergent) Occurring in ≥ 2% of HIV-Infected Patients in the Controlled Clinical Trial

Adverse Reaction (MedDRA v 9.1 System Organ Class and Preferred Term)	ORAVIG N = 290 (%)	Clotrimazole troches N = 287 (%)
Patients with any adverse reaction during the study	158 (54.5)	146 (50.9)
Gastrointestinal disorders	25.9	23.7
Diarrhea	9.0	8.0
Nausea	6.6	7.7
Vomiting	3.8	3.1
Dry mouth	2.8	1.7
Abdominal pain upper	1.7	2.8
Infections and infestations	15.9	17.1
Upper respiratory infection	2.1	2.4
Gastroenteritis	1.4	2.8
Nervous system disorders	13.1	8.4
Headache	7.6	6.6
Ageusia	2.4	0.3
Blood and lymphatic disorders	6.9	8.4
Anemia	2.8	1.7
Lymphopenia	1.7	2.1
Neutropenia	0.7	2.1
General disorders and administration site conditions	6.6	8.0
Fatigue	2.8	2.1
Pain	1.0	2.8
Respiratory/thoracic	5.2	7.7
Cough	2.8	1.7
Pharyngeal pain	0.7	2.4
Investigations	5.5	6.3
Increased GGT	1.0	2.8

Table 2: Adverse Reactions (Treatment-Emergent) Occurring in ≥ 2% of Patients with Head and Neck Cancer who had Received Radiation Therapy (Controlled Clinical Trial)

Adverse Reaction (MedDRA v 9.1 System Organ Class and Preferred Term)	ORAVIG N = 147 (%)	Miconazole gel N = 147 (%)
Patients with at least one adverse reaction	30 (20.4)	32 (21.8)
Gastrointestinal disorders	8.8	13.6
Abdominal pain, upper	1.4	2.0
Oral discomfort	2.7	2.7
Nausea	0.7	2.7
Vomiting	0.7	2.0
Glossodynia	0	2.0
Nervous system disorders	5.4	1.4
Dysgeusia	4.1	0
Skin and subcutaneous	3.4	0.7
Pruritus	2.0	0.7

───────DOSAGE FORMS AND STRENGTHS───────
50 mg buccal tablets (3).

───────CONTRAINDICATIONS───────
Known hypersensitivity to miconazole, milk protein concentrate, or any other component of the product (4).

───────WARNINGS AND PRECAUTIONS───────
Hypersensitivity reactions: Anaphylactic reactions have been reported in patients receiving miconazole. Discontinue ORAVIG immediately at the first sign of hypersensitivity (5.1).

───────ADVERSE REACTIONS───────
Most common adverse reactions (≥2%) are diarrhea, headache, nausea, dysgeusia, upper abdominal pain, and vomiting (6.1).

To report SUSPECTED ADVERSE REACTIONS, contact Par Pharmaceutical, Inc. at 1-800-828-9393 or FDA at 1-800-FDA-1088 or www.fda.gov/medwatch.

───────DRUG INTERACTIONS───────
Warfarin: Miconazole may enhance anticoagulant effect. Monitor prothrombin time, INR, and watch for bleeding (7.1).

───────USE IN SPECIFIC POPULATIONS───────
• Pregnancy: Based on animal data, may cause fetal harm (8.1).
• Nursing Mothers: Caution should be exercised when administered to a nursing woman (8.3).
• Pediatric Use: Safety and efficacy not established in patients less than 16 years of age (8.4).

See 17 for PATIENT COUNSELING INFORMATION and FDA-approved patient labeling

Revised: 05/2010

FULL PRESCRIBING INFORMATION: CONTENTS*

FULL PRESCRIBING INFORMATION

1 INDICATIONS AND USAGE

ORAVIG is indicated for the local treatment of oropharyngeal candidiasis (OPC) in adults.

2 DOSAGE AND ADMINISTRATION

2.1 Basic Dosing Information
The recommended dosing schedule for ORAVIG is the application of one 50 mg buccal tablet to the upper gum region (canine fossa) once daily for 14 consecutive days.

2.2 Administration Instructions
ORAVIG should be applied in the morning, after brushing the teeth. The tablet should be applied with dry hands. The rounded side surface of the tablet should be placed against the upper gum just above the incisor tooth (canine fossa) and held in place with slight pressure over the upper lip for 30 seconds to ensure adhesion. The tablet is round on one side for comfort, but either side of the tablet can be applied to the gum.
Once applied, ORAVIG stays in position and gradually dissolves. [See Clinical Pharmacology (12.3)] Subsequent applications of ORAVIG should be made to alternate sides of the mouth. Before applying the next tablet, the patient should clear away any remaining tablet material. In addition,

• ORAVIG should not be crushed, chewed or swallowed.
• Food and drink can be taken normally when ORAVIG is in place but chewing gum should be avoided.
• If ORAVIG does not adhere or falls off within the first 6 hours, the same tablet should be repositioned immediately. If the tablet still does not adhere, a new tablet should be placed.
• If ORAVIG is swallowed within the first 6 hours, the patient should drink a glass of water and a new tablet should be applied only once.
• If ORAVIG falls off or is swallowed after it was in place for 6 hours or more, a new tablet should not be applied until the next regularly scheduled dose. [See Patient Counseling Information (17)].

3 DOSAGE FORMS AND STRENGTHS

ORAVIG is a buccal tablet containing 50 mg of miconazole. ORAVIG tablets are round, off-white tablets, with a rounded side and a flat side. The tablets are marked with an "L" on the flat side.

4 CONTRAINDICATIONS

ORAVIG is contraindicated in patients with known hypersensitivity (e.g., anaphylaxis) to miconazole, milk protein concentrate, or any other component of the product.

5 WARNINGS AND PRECAUTIONS
5.1 Hypersensitivity
Allergic reactions, including anaphylactic reactions and hypersensitivity, have been reported with the administration of miconazole products, including ORAVIG. Discontinue ORAVIG immediately at the first sign of hypersensitivity. There is no information regarding cross-hypersensitivity between miconazole and other azole antifungal agents. Monitor patients with a history of hypersensitivity to azoles.

6 ADVERSE REACTIONS
The following serious adverse drug reactions are discussed in detail in other sections of labeling:
• Hypersensitivity reactions [see Warnings and Precautions (5.1)]

6.1 Clinical Trial Experience
Because clinical trials are conducted under widely varying conditions, adverse reaction rates observed in the clinical trials of a drug cannot be directly compared to rates in the clinical trials of another drug and may not reflect the rates observed in clinical practice.
The overall safety of ORAVIG was assessed in 480 adult subjects: 315 HIV-infected subjects, 147 subjects with head and neck cancer, and 18 healthy subjects.

HIV Infected Patients
Two trials were conducted in immunocompromised HIV infected patients: one randomized, double-blind, double-dummy, active-controlled design (N = 290 ORAVIG, 287 control) and one non-comparative trial (N = 25).
In the randomized, double blind trial (Study 1), 290 HIV infected subjects used ORAVIG once daily for 14 days, and 287 subjects used 10 mg clotrimazole troches five times daily for 14 days. Adverse reactions occurring in ≥ 2% of patients in either treatment are presented in Table 1.
[See table 1 above]
Overall local adverse reactions, including oral discomfort, oral burning, oral pain, gingival pain, gingival swelling, gingival pruritus, tongue ulceration, mouth ulceration, glossodynia, dry mouth, application site pain or discomfort, toothache, loss of taste, and altered taste, were reported by 35 (12.1%) patients who received miconazole buccal tablet compared to 27 (9.4%) patients who received clotrimazole troches.

Head and Neck Cancer Patients
In the randomized, open-label comparative trial of oropharyngeal candidiasis in patients with head and neck cancer who had received radiation therapy (Study 2), 147 patients used ORAVIG once daily for 14 days and 147 patients used 125 mg of miconazole oral gel four times daily for 14 days. Adverse reactions occurring in ≥2% of patients in either arm are listed in Table 2.
[See table 2 above]
Overall local adverse reactions, including oral discomfort, oral pain, dry mouth, glossodynia, loss of taste, altered taste, tongue ulceration, mouth ulceration, tooth disorder, and application site discomfort or pain, were experienced by 14 (9.5%) patients who used ORAVIG compared to 16 (10.9%) patients who used miconazole gel.

Overall ORAVIG Safety Experience In Patients and Healthy Subjects
Adverse reactions reported in the overall safety database of 480 subjects who received miconazole buccal tablet is listed in Table 3.

Table 3 Adverse Reactions Reported in ≥ 2% of Patients and Healthy Subjects who Received ORAVIG in Clinical Trials

Adverse reaction (MedDRA v 9.1 System Organ Class and Preferred Term)	ORAVIG N = 480 (%)
Patients with at least one AE	209 (43.5)
Gastrointestinal disorders	**20.6**
Diarrhea	6.0
Nausea	4.6
Abdominal pain upper	2.5
Vomiting	2.5
Infections and infestations	**11.9**
Nervous system disorders	**10.6**
Headache	5.0
Dysgeusia	2.9

Discontinuation of ORAVIG due to adverse drug reactions occurred in 0.6% overall.

7 DRUG INTERACTIONS

7.1 Warfarin
Concomitant administration of miconazole and warfarin has resulted in enhancement of anticoagulant effect. Cases of bleeding and bruising following the concomitant use of warfarin and topical, intravaginal, or oral miconazole were reported. Closely monitor prothrombin time, International Normalized Ratio (INR), or other suitable anticoagulation tests if ORAVIG is administered concomitantly with warfarin. Also monitor for evidence of bleeding.

7.2 Drugs Metabolized Through CYP2C9 and 3A4
No formal drug interaction studies have been performed with ORAVIG. Miconazole is a known inhibitor of CYP2C9 and CYP3A4. Although the systemic absorption of miconazole following ORAVIG administration is minimal and plasma concentrations of miconazole are substantially lower than when given intravenously, the potential for interaction with drugs metabolized through CYP2C9 and CYP3A4 such as oral hypoglycemics, phenytoin, or ergot alkaloids cannot be ruled out.

8 USE IN SPECIFIC POPULATIONS

8.1 Pregnancy
Pregnancy Category C
There are no adequate and well-controlled clinical trials of ORAVIG in pregnant women. ORAVIG should not be used during pregnancy unless the potential benefit to the mother outweighs the potential risk to the fetus.
Miconazole nitrate administered orally at doses of 80 mg/kg/day or higher to pregnant rats or rabbits crossed the placenta and resulted in embryo- and fetotoxicity, including increased fetal resorptions. These doses also resulted in prolonged gestation and dystocia in rats, but not in rabbits. Embryofetotoxicity was not observed in intravenous studies with miconazole at lower doses of 40 mg/kg/day in rats and 20 mg/kg/day in rabbits, which are approximately 8 times higher than the dose a patient would receive if she swallowed an ORAVIG buccal tablet, based on body surface area comparisons. Teratogenicity was not reported in any animal study with miconazole.

8.3 Nursing Mothers
It is not known whether this drug is excreted in human milk. Because many drugs are excreted in human milk, caution should be exercised when ORAVIG is administered to a nursing woman.

8.4 Pediatric Use
Safety and effectiveness of ORAVIG in pediatric patients below the age of 16 years have not been established. The ability of pediatric patients to comply with the application instructions has not been evaluated. Use in younger children is not recommended due to potential risk of choking.

8.5 Geriatric Use
Clinical studies of ORAVIG did not include sufficient numbers of subjects aged 65 and over to determine whether they respond differently from younger subjects.

8.6 Hepatic Impairment
Miconazole is metabolized by the liver. While miconazole systemic exposure is minimal following the application of ORAVIG, ORAVIG should be administered with caution in patients with hepatic impairment.

8.7 Renal Impairment
Less than 1% of miconazole is excreted as unchanged drug in the urine; therefore, no adjustment to therapy is necessary in patients with renal impairment.

10 OVERDOSAGE
Overdose with miconazole in humans has not been reported in the literature.
Miconazole absorption and systemic exposure following application of ORAVIG are minimal [see Clinical Pharmacology (12.3)]. Symptomatic and supportive care is the basis for management.

11 DESCRIPTION
ORAVIG (miconazole) buccal tablets are applied topically to the gum once daily and release miconazole as the buccal tablet gradually dissolves [see Clinical Pharmacology (12.3)].
Miconazole is an imidazole antifungal agent and is described chemically as 1-[(2RS)-2-[(2,4-dichlorobenzyl)oxy]-2-(2,4-dichlorophenyl)ethyl]-1H-imidazole with an empirical formula of $C_{18}H_{14}C_{14}N_2O$ and a molecular weight of 416.13. The structural formula is shown in Figure 1.

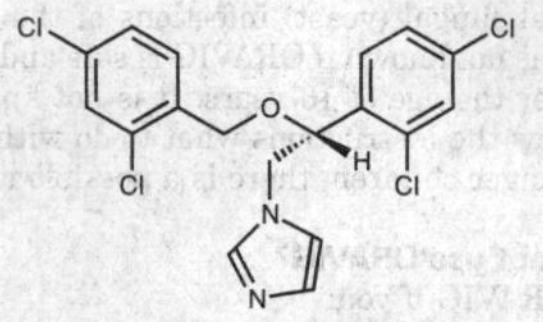

Figure 1: Structural Formula of Miconazole

Miconazole drug substance is a white to almost white powder.
ORAVIG contains 50 mg of miconazole base, USP and the following inactive ingredients: hypromellose, USP; milk protein concentrate; corn starch, NF; lactose monohydrate, NF; sodium lauryl sulfate, NF; magnesium stearate, NF; and talc, USP.

12 CLINICAL PHARMACOLOGY

12.1 Mechanism of Action
Miconazole is an antifungal [see Clinical Pharmacology (12.4)].

12.3 Pharmacokinetics
Absorption and Distribution
Salivary
Single dose application of ORAVIG containing 50 mg of miconazole to the buccal mucosa of 18 healthy volunteers provided mean maximum salivary concentrations of 15 mcg/mL at 7 hours after application of the tablet. This provided an average saliva exposure to miconazole estimated from the AUC (0-24h) of 55.23 mcg•h/mL. The pharmacokinetic parameters of miconazole in the saliva of healthy volunteers are provided in Table 4.

Table 4: Pharmacokinetic (PK) Parameters of Miconazole in Saliva Following Application of a Single ORAVIG 50 mg Tablet in Healthy Volunteers (N = 18)

Salivary PK Parameters (N = 18)	Mean ± SD (Min-Max)
AUC_{0-24h} (mcg·h/mL)	55.2 ± 35.1 (0.5–128.3)
C_{max} (mcg/mL)	15.1 ± 16.2 (0.5–64.8)
T_{max} (hour)	7* (2.0–24.1)

*Median

In healthy volunteers, the duration of buccal adhesion was on average 15 hours following a single dose application of ORAVIG 50 mg.
Plasma
Plasma concentrations of miconazole were below the lower limit of quantification (0.4 mcg/mL) in 157/162 (97%) samples from healthy volunteers following single-dose application of ORAVIG 50 mg. Measurable plasma concentrations ranged from 0.5 to 0.83 mcg/mL.
Plasma concentrations of miconazole evaluated after 7 days of treatment in 40 HIV positive patients were all below the limit of quantification (0.1 mcg/mL).
Metabolism and Excretion
Most of the absorbed miconazole is metabolized by the liver with less than 1% of the administered dose found unchanged in urine. In healthy volunteers, the terminal half-life is 24 hours following systemic administration. There are no active metabolites of miconazole.
Food Effect
There was no formal food effect study conducted with ORAVIG; however, in clinical studies patients were allowed to eat and drink while taking ORAVIG.

12.4 Microbiology
Mechanism of Action
Miconazole inhibits the enzyme cytochrome P450 14α-demethylase which leads to inhibition of ergosterol synthesis, an essential component of the fungal cell membrane. Miconazole also affects the synthesis of triglycerides and fatty acids and inhibits oxidative and peroxidative enzymes, increasing the amount of reactive oxygen species within the cell.

Activity in vitro and in vivo
Miconazole is active against Candida albicans, C. parapsilosis, and C. tropicalis. Correlation between minimum inhibitory concentration (MIC) results in vitro and clinical outcome has yet to be established.
Drug Resistance
In vitro studies have shown that some Candida strains that demonstrate reduced susceptibility to one antifungal azole may also exhibit reduced susceptibility to other azoles suggesting cross-resistance.
Clinically relevant resistance to systemically utilized triazoles may occur in Candida species. Resistance may occur by multiple mechanisms such as changes in amino acids and/or in the regulation of the target enzyme and of a variety of efflux pump proteins. Multiple mechanisms may coexist in the same isolate. Resistance breakpoints, correlating in vitro activity with clinical efficacy, have not been established for miconazole.

13 NONCLINICAL TOXICOLOGY

13.1 Carcinogenesis, Mutagenesis, Impairment of Fertility
Carcinogenicity studies with miconazole have not been conducted.
Miconazole nitrate was not genotoxic when tested in vitro in a bacterial reverse mutation (Ames) assay or in an in vivo mouse bone marrow micronucleus test. Intraperitoneal injections of miconazole to mice induced chromosomal aberrations in spermatocytes and bone marrow cells, and morphologic abnormalities in sperm at doses similar to or below clinical doses. However, no impairment of fertility was observed in intravenous studies with miconazole at 40 mg/kg/day in rats or 20 mg/kg/day in rabbits, which are approximately 8 times higher than the dose a patient would receive if she swallowed an ORAVIG buccal tablet, based on body surface area comparisons.

13.2 Animal Toxicology and/or Pharmacology
Local tolerance studies (LLNA sensitization test and tolerance study on the jugal mucosa of hamster) did not reveal any toxicity.

14 CLINICAL STUDIES
Study in HIV Infected Patients
The efficacy and safety of ORAVIG in the treatment of OPC was evaluated in a randomized, double-blind, double-dummy, multicenter trial comparing ORAVIG 50 mg once daily for 14 consecutive days (n = 290) with clotrimazole troches 10 mg 5 times per day for 14 days (n = 287) in HIV-positive patients with OPC. Seventy-five percent of patients were not receiving highly active antiretroviral treatment, 5% had CD4+ cell count < 50 cells/mm³, and 17% had a history of previous OPC. The mean viral load was 117,000 copies/mL. Patients were required to have symptoms and microbiological documentation of OPC for study entry. Most of the infections were caused by C. albicans (85%), followed by C. tropicalis (9%), and C. parapsilosis (3%). About 2% of the subjects were infected with more than one Candida species.
Clinical cure [defined as a complete resolution of both signs and symptoms of OPC at the test of cure (TOC) visit (days 17-22)], and clinical relapse by days 35-38 (21-24 days after end of therapy) are presented in Table 5. Mycological cure [defined as eradication (i.e., no yeast isolates) of Candida species] at the TOC visit (days 17-22) is also reported in the table.

Table 5: Clinical Cure and Mycological Cure at the TOC Visit and Relapse at Days 35-38 in HIV Infected Patients

	ORAVIG 50 mg N=290ᵃ (%)	Clotrimazole troches N=287ᵃ (%)
Clinical cure†	176 (60.7%)	187 (65.2%)
Clinical relapse‡		
Yesᵇ	48 (27.3%)	52 (27.8%)
No	124 (70.5%)	133 (71.1%)
Missing	4 (2.3%)	2 (1.1%)
Mycological cure	79 (27.2%)	71 (24.7%)

ᵃ Analysis population includes all randomized patients who took at least 1 dose of study medication. One randomized subject excluded from the ORAVIG arm.
ᵇ In those subjects who relapsed, the mean time to relapse was 15.3 days (SD 4.6) and 15.7 days (SD 6.6), in the ORAVIG and Clotrimazole treatment arms, respectively.
† Difference in clinical cure rates (ORAVIG-miconazole) was -4.5%, with a 95% CI: (-12.4%, 3.4%).
‡ Percentage based on those who had clinical cure.

Study in Head and Neck Cancer Patients
The efficacy and safety of ORAVIG 50 mg was evaluated in an open-label, randomized, multicenter trial comparing ORAVIG 50 mg once daily for 14 days to miconazole oral gel 125 mg four times daily for 14 days in head and neck cancer patients who had received radiation therapy. Most of the

infections were caused by *C. albicans* (71%), and *C. tropicalis* (8%). About 7% of the subjects were infected with more than one *Candida* species. Success rates of treatment at day 14 [defined as a complete (complete disappearance of candidiasis lesions) or partial response (improvement by at least 2 points of the score for extent of oral lesion compared with the score at day 1) based on a blind assessment] are shown in Table 6. Also reported in Table 6 are relapse rate at day 30, and mycologic cure assessed at day 14.

Table 6: Clinical Success and Mycological Cure at Day 14, in Patients with Head and Neck Cancer who had Received Radiation Therapy

	ORAVIG 50 mg N=148[a] (%)	Miconazole oral gel N=146[a] (%)
Success rate (CR+PR)[b]	79 (53.4%)	69 (46.6%)
CR†	74 (50.0%)	64 (43.8%)
Clinical relapse‡		
Yes[c]	14 (18.9%)	8 (12.5%)
No	59 (79.7%)	56 (87.5%)
Missing	1 (1.4%)	0
Mycological cure	66 (44.6%)	78 (53.4%)

[a] Analysis population includes all subjects who received at least one dose of study medication. Reasons for not receiving treatment included negative mycological culture, informed consent withdrawn, or lost during screening. Six patients excluded per arm.
[b] CR: complete response; PR: partial response
[c] In those subjects who relapsed, the mean time to relapse was 18.8 days (SD 16.3) and 20.6 days (SD 13.5), in the ORAVIG and Miconazole oral gel group, respectively.
† Difference in clinical complete response rates (ORAVIG-Miconazole oral gel) was 6.2%, with a 95% CI: (-5.2%, 17.6%).
‡ Percentage based on those who had complete response.

16   HOW SUPPLIED/STORAGE AND HANDLING
ORAVIG 50 mg buccal tablets are supplied as off-white tablets containing 50 mg of miconazole. ORAVIG tablets have a rounded side and a flat side. ORAVIG tablets are packaged in bottles of 14 tablets (NDC 49884-082-26).
ORAVIG should be stored at 20 to 25°C (68 to 77 °F) [see USP controlled room temperature] excursions between 15 and 30°C are permitted at room temperature. Protect from moisture, and keep out of reach of children.

17   PATIENT COUNSELING INFORMATION
See FDA-approved patient labeling.
17.1   Instructions for Use
The tablet should be used immediately after removal from the bottle.
• Instruct patients not to crush, chew, or swallow the tablet.
• The rounded side of the tablet should be applied to the upper gum above the incisor tooth in the morning, after brushing the teeth.
• The tablet should be held in place for 30 seconds with a slight pressure of the finger over the upper lip to make the tablet stick to the gum.
• The tablet may be used if it sticks to the cheek, inside of the lip or the gum.
• If the tablet does not adhere, it should be repositioned.
• As the ORAVIG tablet absorbs moisture from the mouth, it will slowly dissolve over time and should be left in place—there is no need to remove the tablet.
• Subsequent applications of ORAVIG should be made to alternate sides of the gum.
• If ORAVIG does not stick or falls off within the first 6 hours, the same tablet should be repositioned immediately. If the tablet does not adhere, a new tablet should be placed.
• If ORAVIG is swallowed within the first 6 hours, the patient should drink a glass of water and a new tablet should be applied only once.
• If ORAVIG falls off or is swallowed after it was in place for 6 hours or more, a new tablet should not be applied until the next, regularly scheduled dose.
Patients should avoid situations that could interfere with the sticking of the tablet including:
• touching or pressing the tablet after placement
• wearing upper denture
• chewing gum
• hitting tablet when brushing teeth
• rinsing mouth too vigorously
17.2   Hypersensitivity and Other Adverse Reactions
Patients who develop hives, skin rash, or other symptoms of an allergic reaction, and patients who develop swelling or pain, at the tablet application site should stop ORAVIG and contact a healthcare provider. Patients may experience other adverse reactions including diarrhea, headache, nausea, and change in taste.

FDA-APPROVED PATIENT LABELING
Oravig (OR-a-vig)
(miconazole)
Buccal Tablets
Read the Patient Information that comes with ORAVIG before you start taking it and each time you get a refill. There may be new information. This leaflet does not take the place of talking with your doctor or about your medical condition or your treatment.
What is ORAVIG?
ORAVIG is a prescription antifungal medicine used in adults to treat fungal (yeast) infections of the mouth and the throat. It is not known if ORAVIG is safe and effective in children under the age of 16 years. It is not known if children can follow the instructions what to do with the buccal tablet. In younger children, there is a possible risk of choking.
Who should not use ORAVIG?
Do not use ORAVIG if you:
• are allergic to miconazole (M-Zole, Monistat, Vusion)
• are allergic to milk protein concentrate
• are allergic to any of the ingredients in ORAVIG. See the end of this Patient Information leaflet for a complete list of ingredients in ORAVIG
What should I tell my doctor before using ORAVIG?
Before taking ORAVIG, tell your doctor if you:
• have liver problems
• have any other medical conditions
• are pregnant or plan to become pregnant. It is not known if ORAVIG will harm your unborn baby. Talk to your doctor if you are pregnant or plan to become pregnant.
• are breast-feeding or plan to breast-feed. It is not known if ORAVIG passes into your breast milk. Talk to your doctor about the best way to feed your baby if you use ORAVIG.
Tell your doctor about all the medicines you take, including prescription and nonprescription medicines, vitamins, and herbal supplements.
ORAVIG may affect the way other medicines work, and other medicines may affect how ORAVIG works. Especially tell your doctor if you take:
• a diabetes medicine
• phenytoin (Dilantin, Phenytek)
• an ergot medicine. Ask your doctor or pharmacist if you are not sure if your medicine is an ergot medicine.
• the blood thinner medicine warfarin sodium (Coumadin, Jantoven)
Know the medicines you take. Keep a list of them to show your doctor and pharmacist when you get a new medicine.
How should I use ORAVIG?
• Always use ORAVIG exactly as your doctor tells you. ORAVIG is usually applied in the morning after you brush your teeth.
• ORAVIG is placed 1 time each day to your upper gum for 14 days.
• You may eat and drink while using ORAVIG.
• Do not crush, chew or swallow ORAVIG.
• You should change where you place ORAVIG, between the left and right side of your upper gum with each use.
• It is okay if ORAVIG sticks to your cheek, the inside of your lip or your gum. If ORAVIG does not stick or falls off of your gum within the first 6 hours, re-apply it. If it still does not stick, replace it with a new tablet.
• If you swallow ORAVIG within the first 6 hours of placing, drink a glass of water and place a new ORAVIG to your gum.
• If ORAVIG falls off or is swallowed after it was in place for 6 hours or more, do not apply a new ORAVIG. Just place your next dose at your regular time.
• Check to see if ORAVIG is still in place after you brush your teeth, rinse your mouth, eat, or drink.
How to use ORAVIG?
• Before applying the tablet,
1. Locate the area on the upper gum, just above either the left or the right incisor. The incisor tooth is the tooth just to the right or left of your two front teeth (See Figure A)

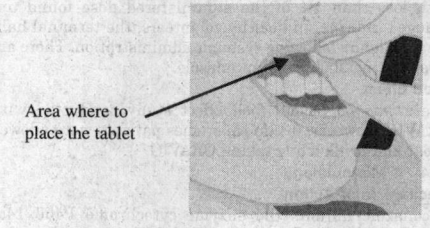

Area where to place the tablet

Figure A

2. Take one ORAVIG tablet out of the bottle. ORAVIG is round on one side and flat on the other side (Figure B). The tablet is marked with an "L" on the flat side.

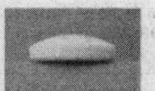
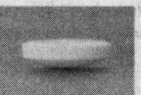
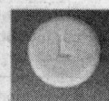

Figure B

Applying the ORAVIG tablet,
3. Place the flat side of the ORAVIG tablet on your dry fingertip. Gently push the rounded side of the tablet against your upper gum in the area shown in Figure C. Push the ORAVIG tablet up as high as it will go on your gum. The flat side will be facing the inside of your lip.

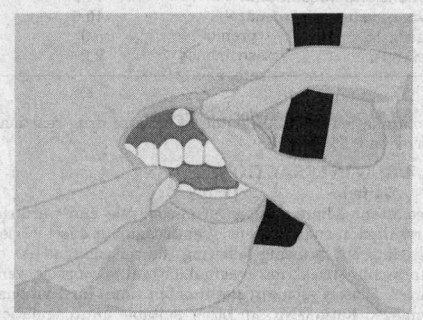

Figure C

4. Hold the ORAVIG tablet in place by applying a slight pressure with your finger on the outside of your upper lip for 30 seconds. This will make the tablet stick to your gum (See Figure D).

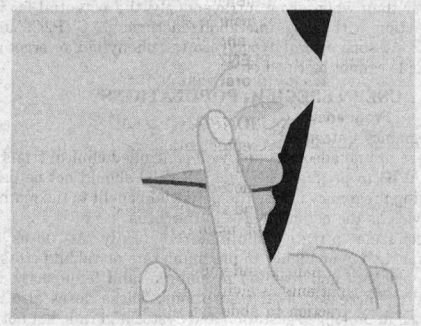

Figure D

5. Leave the tablet in place until it dissolves.
6. Before applying your next dose, be sure to clear away any remaining ORAVIG tablet material.
What should I avoid while using ORAVIG?
You should avoid activities that may prevent ORAVIG from sticking to your gum, including:
• touching or pressing ORAVIG after placement
• wearing upper denture that interfere with placement of the tablet
• chewing-gum.
• hitting tablet when brushing your teeth
• rinsing your mouth too vigorously
What are the possible side effects of ORAVIG?
ORAVIG may cause serious side effects including:
Allergic reactions. Tell your doctor or get emergency medical help right away if you have any of the symptoms below:
• skin rash or hives
• swelling of your face, eyes, lips, tongue or throat
• trouble swallowing or breathing
The most common side effects of ORAVIG include:
• diarrhea
• change in taste
• headache
• upper stomach (abdominal) pain
• nausea
• vomiting
Tell your doctor if you have any side effect that bothers you or that does not go away. These are not all the possible side effects of ORAVIG. For more information, ask your doctor or pharmacist.
Call your doctor for medical advice about side effects. You may report side effects to FDA at 1-800-FDA-1088.
How should I store ORAVIG?
• Store ORAVIG between 68 to 77 °F (20 to 25°C)
• Keep ORAVIG dry
Keep ORAVIG and all medicine out of the reach of children.

General information about the safe and effective use of ORAVIG

Medicines are sometimes prescribed for purposes other than those listed in a Patient Information Leaflet. Do not use ORAVIG for a condition for which it was not prescribed. Do not give ORAVIG to other people, even if they have the same symptoms that you have. It may harm them. This Patient Information Leaflet summarizes the most important information about ORAVIG. If you would like more information, talk with your doctor. You can ask your pharmacist or doctor for information about ORAVIG that is written for health professionals. You can also visit www.oravig.com for more information.

What are the ingredients in ORAVIG?

Active ingredient: miconazole

Inactive ingredients: hypromellose, milk protein concentrate, corn starch, lactose monohydrate, sodium lauryl sulfate, magnesium stearate, and talc.

Manufactured By:
Catalent Germany Shorndorf GmbH
Steinbeisstraße 2
73614 Schorndorf
Germany
Distributed By:
Strativa Pharmaceuticals, a Division of Par Pharmaceutical, Inc.
Woodcliff Lake, NJ 07677
Revised 05/2010
US patent numbers: 6,916,485
©2010 Par Pharmaceutical, Inc.

ZUPLENZ®
[ZOO-plenz]
(ondansetron)
Oral Soluble Film

℞

HIGHLIGHTS OF PRESCRIBING INFORMATION
These highlights do not include all the information needed to use ZUPLENZ® safely and effectively. See full prescribing information for ZUPLENZ.
ZUPLENZ (ondansetron) oral soluble film
Initial U.S. Approval: 1991

──────INDICATIONS AND USAGE──────
ZUPLENZ is a 5-HT₃ receptor antagonist indicated for:
- Prevention of nausea and vomiting associated with highly emetogenic cancer chemotherapy. (1.1).
- Prevention of nausea and vomiting associated with initial and repeat courses of moderately emetogenic cancer chemotherapy (1.2).
- Prevention of nausea and vomiting associated with radiotherapy in patients receiving total body irradiation, single high-dose fraction to abdomen, or daily fractions to the abdomen (1.3).
- Prevention of postoperative nausea and/or vomiting. (1.4).

──────DOSAGE AND ADMINISTRATION──────
- **Prevention of nausea and vomiting associated with highly emetogenic cancer chemotherapy:** The adult oral dosage is 24 mg given successively as three 8 mg films administered 30 minutes before the start of chemotherapy. (2.1)
- **Prevention of nausea and vomiting associated with moderately emetogenic cancer chemotherapy:**
  - Adult and pediatric patients 12 years of age and older: One 8mg film 30 minutes before chemotherapy followed by an 8 mg dose 8 hours later. Administer one 8mg film twice a day (every 12 hours) for 1 to 2 days after completion of chemotherapy. (2.2)
  - Pediatric patients 4 through 11 years of age: One 4 mg film three times a day. Administer the first dose 30 minutes before chemotherapy, with subsequent doses 4 and 8 hours later. Administer one 4 mg film three times a day (every 8 hours) for 1 to 2 days after completion of chemotherapy. (2.2)
- **Prevention of nausea and vomiting associated with radiotherapy:** The adult dosage is one 8 mg film three times a day. (2.3)
- **Postoperative nausea and vomiting:** The adult dose is 16 mg given successively as two 8 mg films 1 hour before anesthesia. (2.4)
- See dosage adjustment for patients with impaired hepatic function. (2.5)

──────DOSAGE FORMS AND STRENGTHS──────
- 4 mg and 8 mg oral soluble film (3)

──────CONTRAINDICATIONS──────
- Concomitant use of apomorphine. (4)
- Hypersensitivity to ondansetron. (4)

──────WARNINGS AND PRECAUTIONS──────
- Hypersensitivity reactions, including anaphylaxis and brochospasm, have been reported in patients who have exhibited hypersensitivity to other selective 5-HT₃ receptor antagonists (5.1).

- Rarely and predominantly with intravenous ondansetron, transient electrocardiographic changes, including QT interval prolongation, have been reported (5.2).
- The use of ondansetron in patients following abdominal surgery or in patients with chemotherapy-induced nausea and vomiting may mask a progressive ileus and/or gastric distension (5.3).

──────ADVERSE REACTIONS──────
To report suspected adverse reactions, contact Par Pharmaceutical, Inc. at 1-800-828-9393 or FDA at 1-800-FDA-1088 or www.fda.gov/medwatch.
- The most common adverse drug events (≥5%) in chemotherapy–induced nausea and vomiting and radiotherapy-induced nausea and vomiting trials were: headache, malaise/fatigue, constipation, and diarrhea. (6.1).
- The most common adverse event (≥5%) reported in postoperative nausea and vomiting trials was headache. (6.1).

──────DRUG INTERACTIONS──────
- Apomorphine - profound hypotension and loss of consciousness. (7.1)

──────USE IN SPECIFIC POPULATIONS──────
- **Pediatrics:** The safety and effectiveness in pediatric patients have only been established for the prevention of nausea and vomiting associated with moderately emetogenic cancer chemotherapy for patients four years of age and older (8.4). For dosage recommendations see (2.2).
- **Impaired Hepatic Function:** In severe hepatic impairment (Child-Pugh score of 10 or greater)², a total daily dose of 8 mg should not be exceeded (8.7).

See 17 for PATIENT COUNSELING INFORMATION
Revised: 07/2010

FULL PRESCRIBING INFORMATION: CONTENTS*

* Sections or subsections omitted from the full prescribing information are not listed

---

FULL PRESCRIBING INFORMATION

1 INDICATIONS AND USAGE

1.1 Prevention of Nausea and Vomiting Associated With Highly Emetogenic Cancer Chemotherapy
ZUPLENZ (ondansetron) oral soluble film is indicated for the prevention of nausea and vomiting associated with highly emetogenic cancer chemotherapy, including cisplatin ≥50 mg/m² [see Clinical Studies (14.1)]

1.2 Prevention of Nausea and Vomiting Associated With Moderately Emetogenic Cancer Chemotherapy
ZUPLENZ is indicated for the prevention of nausea and vomiting associated with initial and repeat courses of moderately emetogenic cancer chemotherapy [see Clinical Studies (14.1)].

1.3 Prevention of Nausea and Vomiting Associated With Radiotherapy
ZUPLENZ is indicated for the prevention of nausea and vomiting associated with radiotherapy in patients receiving either total body irradiation, single high-dose fraction to the abdomen, or daily fractions to the abdomen [see Clinical Studies (14.2)].

1.4 Prevention of Postoperative Nausea and/or Vomiting
ZUPLENZ is indicated for the prevention of postoperative nausea and/or vomiting. As with other antiemetics, routine prophylaxis is not recommended for patients in whom there is little expectation that nausea and/or vomiting will occur postoperatively. In patients where nausea and/or vomiting must be avoided postoperatively, ZUPLENZ is recommended even where the incidence of postoperative nausea and/or vomiting is low [see Clinical Studies (14.3)].

2 DOSAGE AND ADMINISTRATION

2.1 Prevention of Nausea and Vomiting Associated With Highly Emetogenic Cancer Chemotherapy
Adults
The recommended adult oral dosage of ZUPLENZ (ondansetron) oral soluble film is 24 mg given successively as three 8 mg films administered 30 minutes before the start of single-day highly emetogenic chemotherapy, including cisplatin ≥50 mg/m². Each ZUPLENZ oral soluble film should be allowed to dissolve completely before administering the next film. [see Dosage and Administration (2.6)]. Multiday, single-dose administration of a 24 mg dosage has not been studied.

Pediatrics
Safety and effectiveness of ZUPLENZ in pediatric patients have not been established for this indication.

2.2 Prevention of Nausea and Vomiting Associated With Moderately Emetogenic Cancer Chemotherapy
Adults
The recommended adult oral dosage is one 8 mg ZUPLENZ oral soluble film given twice a day. The first dose should be administered 30 minutes before the start of emetogenic chemotherapy, with a subsequent dose 8 hours after the first dose. One 8 mg ZUPLENZ oral soluble film should be administered twice a day (every 12 hours) for 1 to 2 days after completion of chemotherapy [see Dosage and Administration (2.6)].

Pediatrics
For pediatric patients 12 years of age and older, the dosage is the same as for adults. For pediatric patients 4 through 11 years of age, the dosage is one 4 mg ZUPLENZ oral soluble film given three times a day. The first dose should be administered 30 minutes before the start of emetogenic chemotherapy, with subsequent doses 4 and 8 hours after the first dose. One 4 mg ZUPLENZ oral soluble film should be administered three times a day (every 8 hours) for 1 to 2 days after completion of chemotherapy [see Dosage and Administration (2.6)].

Table 1: Adverse Events Reported in ≥5% of Adult Patients After Single Day Therapy Ondansetron HCl Tablets [Highly Emetogenic Chemotherapy (cisplatin dose ≥50 mg/m²)]

Adverse Event	Ondansetron 24 mg once daily N=300	Ondansetron 8 mg twice a day N=124	Ondansetron 32 mg once daily N=117
Headache	33 (11%)	16 (13%)	17 (15%)
Diarrhea	13 (4%)	9 (7%)	3 (3%)

Table 2: Adverse Events Reported in ≥5% of Adult Patients After Three Days of Therapy With Ondansetron HCl Tablets [Moderately Emetogenic Chemotherapy (primarily cyclophosphamide-based regimens)]

Adverse Event	Ondansetron 8 mg twice daily N=242	Ondansetron 8 mg three times day. N=415	Placebo N=262
Headache	58 (24%)	113 (27%)	34 (13%)
Malaise/fatigue	32 (13%)	37 (9%)	6 (2%)
Constipation	22 (9%)	26 (6%)	1 (<1%)
Diarrhea	15 (6%)	16 (4%)	10 (4%)

2.3 Prevention of Nausea and Vomiting Associated With Radiotherapy

Adults

The recommended adult oral dosage of ZUPLENZ oral soluble film is one 8 mg film given three times a day *[see Dosage and Administration (2.6)]*.

For total body irradiation, one 8 mg ZUPLENZ oral soluble film should be administered 1 to 2 hours before each fraction of radiotherapy administered each day.

For single high-dose fraction radiotherapy to the abdomen, one 8 mg ZUPLENZ oral soluble film should be administered 1 to 2 hours before radiotherapy, with subsequent doses every 8 hours after the first dose for 1 to 2 days after completion of radiotherapy.

For daily fractionated radiotherapy to the abdomen, one 8 mg ZUPLENZ oral soluble film should be administered 1 to 2 hours before radiotherapy, with subsequent doses every 8 hours after the first dose for each day radiotherapy is given.

Pediatrics

Safety and effectiveness of ZUPLENZ in pediatric patients have not been established for this indication.

2.4 Prevention of Postoperative Nausea and/or Vomiting

Adults

The recommended adult oral dosage of ZUPLENZ oral soluble film is 16 mg given successively as two 8 mg films 1 hour before induction of anesthesia. Each ZUPLENZ oral soluble film should be allowed to dissolve completely before administering the next film *[see Dosage and Administration (2.6)]*.

Pediatrics

Safety and effectiveness of ZUPLENZ in pediatric patients have not been established for this indication.

2.5 Dosage Adjustment for Patients with Impaired Hepatic Function

In patients with severe hepatic impairment (Child-Pugh score of 10 or greater)², clearance is reduced and apparent volume of distribution is increased with a resultant increase in plasma half-life *[see Clinical Pharmacology (12.3)]*. In such patients, a total daily dose of 8 mg should not be exceeded.

2.6 Important Administration Instructions

With dry hands, fold the pouch along the dotted line to expose the tear notch. While still folded, tear the pouch carefully along the edge and remove the ZUPLENZ oral soluble film from the pouch. Immediately place the film on top of the tongue where it dissolves in 4 to 20 seconds. Once the ZUPLENZ oral soluble film is dissolved, swallow with or without liquid *[see Clinical Pharmacology (12.3)]*. Wash hands after taking ZUPLENZ.

3 DOSAGE FORMS AND STRENGTHS

ZUPLENZ (ondansetron) oral soluble film is available in 4 mg and 8mg strengths. The thin white opaque films are rectangularly shaped strips with a printed identifier in black ink of "4 mg" for ZUPLENZ 4 mg or "8 mg" for ZUPLENZ 8mg.

4 CONTRAINDICATIONS

The concomitant use of apomorphine with ondansetron is contraindicated based on reports of profound hypotension and loss of consciousness when apomorphine was administered with ondansetron.

ZUPLENZ (ondansetron) oral soluble film is contraindicated for patients known to have hypersensitivity to the drug. Anaphylactic reactions have been reported in patients taking ondansetron.

5 WARNINGS AND PRECAUTIONS

5.1 Hypersensitivity

Hypersensitivity reactions, including anaphylaxis and bronchospasm, have been reported in patients who have exhibited hypersensitivity to other selective 5-HT₃ receptor antagonists.

5.2 Electrocardiographic Changes

Rarely and predominantly with intravenous ondansetron, transient electrocardiographic changes, including QT interval prolongation, have been reported.

5.3 Masking of Progressive Ileus and/or Gastric Distension

The use of ZUPLENZ in patients following abdominal surgery or in patients with chemotherapy-induced nausea and vomiting may mask a progressive ileus and/or gastric distension.

5.4 Effect on Peristalsis

ZUPLENZ is not a drug that stimulates gastric or intestinal peristalsis. It should not be used instead of nasogastric suction.

6 ADVERSE REACTIONS

6.1 Clinical Trial Experience

Because clinical trials are conducted under widely varying conditions, adverse reaction rates observed in the clinical trials of a drug cannot be directly compared to rates in the clinical trials of another drug and may not reflect the rates observed in clinical practice.

The following adverse events have been reported in clinical trials of patients treated with ondansetron, the active ingredient of ZUPLENZ. A causal relationship to therapy with ondansetron was unclear in many cases.

Chemotherapy-Induced Nausea and Vomiting

[See table 1 above]

[See table 2 above]

Central Nervous System: There have been rare reports consistent with, but not diagnostic of, extrapyramidal reactions in patients receiving ondansetron.

Hepatic: In 723 patients receiving cyclophosphamide-based chemotherapy in US clinical trials, AST and/or ALT values have been reported to exceed twice the upper limit of normal in approximately 1% to 2% of patients receiving ondansetron HCl tablets. The increases were transient and did not appear to be related to dose or duration of therapy. On repeat exposure, similar transient elevations in transaminase values occurred in some courses, but symptomatic hepatic disease did not occur. The role of cancer chemotherapy in these biochemical changes cannot be clearly determined. There have been reports of liver failure and death in patients with cancer receiving concurrent medications including potentially hepatotoxic cytotoxic chemotherapy and antibiotics. The etiology of the liver failure is unclear.

Integumentary: Rash has occurred in approximately 1% of patients receiving ondansetron.

Other: Rare cases of anaphylaxis, bronchospasm, tachycardia, angina (chest pain), hypokalemia, electrocardiographic alterations, vascular occlusive events, and grand mal seizures have been reported. Except for bronchospasm and anaphylaxis, the relationship to ondansetron was unclear.

Radiation-Induced Nausea and Vomiting

The adverse events reported in patients receiving ondansetron HCl tablets and concurrent radiotherapy were similar to those reported in patients receiving ondansetron HCl tablets and concurrent chemotherapy. The most frequently reported adverse events were headache, constipation, and diarrhea.

Postoperative Nausea and Vomiting

Table 3: Adverse Events Reported in ≥5% of Adult Patients After Single Dose Therapy With Ondansetron HCl Tablets

Adverse Event [a,b]	Ondansetron 16 mg N=550	Placebo N=531
Headache	49 (9%)	27 (5%)
Hypoxia	49 (9%)	35 (7%)
Pyrexia	45 (8%)	34 (6%)
Dizziness	36 (7%)	34 (6%)
Gynecological disorder	36 (7%)	33 (6%)
Anxiety/agitation	33 (6%)	29 (5%)
Urinary retention	28 (5%)	18 (3%)
Pruritus	27 (5%)	20 (4%)

[a] Adverse Events: With the exception of headache, rates of these events were not significantly different in the ondansetron and placebo groups.
[b] Patients were receiving multiple concomitant perioperative and postoperative medications.

6.2 Postmarketing Experience

The following events have been identified during post-approval use of ondansetron. Because these events are reported voluntarily from a population of uncertain size, it is not always possible to reliably estimate their frequency or establish a causal relationship to drug exposure. The events have been chosen for inclusion due to a combination of their seriousness, frequency of reporting, or potential causal connection to ondansetron.

Cardiovascular: Rarely and predominantly with intravenous ondansetron, transient ECG changes including QT interval prolongation have been reported.

General: Flushing. Rare cases of hypersensitivity reactions, sometimes severe (e.g., anaphylaxis reactions, angioedema, bronchospasm, shortness of breath, hypotension, laryngeal edema, stridor) have also been reported. Laryngospasm, shock, and cardiopulmonary arrest have occurred during allergic reactions in patients receiving injectable ondansetron.

Hepatobiliary: Liver enzyme abnormalities

Lower Respiratory: Hiccups

Neurology: Oculogyric crisis, appearing alone, as well as with other dystonic reactions

Skin: Urticaria

Eye Disorders: Cases of transient blindness, predominantly during intravenous administration, have been reported. These cases of transient blindness were reported to resolve within a few minutes up to 48 hours.

7 DRUG INTERACTIONS

Ondansetron does not itself appear to induce or inhibit the cytochrome P-450 drug-metabolizing enzyme system of the liver *[see Clinical Pharmacology (12.3)]*. Because ondansetron is metabolized by hepatic cytochrome P-450 drug-metabolizing enzymes (CYP3A4, CYP2D6, CYP1A2), inducers or inhibitors of these enzymes may change the clearance and, hence, the half-life of ondansetron. On the basis of available data, no dosage adjustment is recommended for patients on these drugs.

7.1 Apomorphine

Based on reports of profound hypotension and loss of consciousness when apomorphine was administered with ondansetron, the concomitant use of apomorphine with ondansetron is contraindicated *[see Contraindications (4)]*.

7.2 Phenytoin, Carbamazepine, Rifampicin

In patients treated with potent inducers of CYP3A4 (i.e., phenytoin, carbamazepine, and rifampicin), the clearance of ondansetron was significantly increased and ondansetron blood concentrations were decreased. In a pharmacokinetic study of 16 epileptic patients maintained chronically on CYP3A4 inducers, carbamazepine, or phenytoin, reduction in AUC, Cmax, and T½ of ondansetron was observed.[1] However, on the basis of available data, no dosage adjustment for ondansetron is recommended for patients on these drugs.[1,3]

7.3 Tramadol

Although there are no data on pharmacokinetic drug interactions between ondansetron and tramadol, data from two small studies indicate that concomitant use of ondansetron may result in reduced analgesic activity of tramadol. Patients in the studies self administered tramadol more frequently, leading to an increased cumulative dose in patient controlled administration (PCA) of tramadol.[4,5]

7.4 Chemotherapy

In humans, carmustine, etoposide, and cisplatin do not affect the pharmacokinetics of ondansetron.

In a crossover study in 76 pediatric patients, intravenous ondansetron did not increase blood levels of high-dose methotrexate.

7.5 Temazepam

The coadministration of ondansetron had no effect on the pharmacokinetics and pharmacodynamics of temazepam.

7.6 Antacids

Bioavailability of ondansetron is unaffected by antacids.

7.7 Alfentanil and Atracurium

Ondansetron does not alter respiratory depressant effects produced by alfentanil or the degree of neuromuscular blockade produced by atracurium. Interactions with general or local anesthetics have not been studied.

8 USE IN SPECIFIC POPULATIONS

8.1 Pregnancy

Pregnancy Category B. Reproduction studies have been performed in pregnant rats and rabbits at daily oral doses up to 15 and 30 mg/kg/day, respectively, (approximately 8 and 30 times the human dose of 16mg/day, based on body surface area), and have revealed no evidence of impaired fertility or harm to the fetus due to ondansetron. There are, however, no adequate and well-controlled studies in pregnant women. Because animal reproduction studies are not always predictive of human response, ZUPLENZ (ondansetron) oral soluble film should be used during pregnancy only if clearly needed.

8.3 Nursing Mothers

Ondansetron is excreted in the milk of rats. It is not known whether ondansetron is excreted in human milk. Because many drugs are excreted in human milk, caution should be exercised when ZUPLENZ oral soluble film is administered to a nursing woman.

8.4 Pediatric Use

Little information is available about dosage in pediatric patients less than 4 years of age. For dosage recommendations in the prevention of nausea and vomiting associated with moderately emetogenic cancer chemotherapy for patients 4 years of age and older *[see Dosage and Administration (2.2)]*. The safety and effectiveness in pediatric patients have not been established for the following indications: prevention of nausea and vomiting associated with highly emetogenic cancer chemotherapy, prevention of nausea and vomiting associated with radiotherapy, and prevention of postoperative nausea and/or vomiting.

8.5 Geriatric Use

Of the total number of subjects enrolled in cancer chemotherapy-induced and postoperative nausea and vomiting in US- and foreign-controlled clinical trials, for which there were subgroup analyses, 938 were 65 years of age and over. No overall differences in safety or effectiveness were observed between these subjects and younger subjects, and other reported clinical experience has not identified differences in responses between the elderly and younger patients, but greater sensitivity of some older individuals cannot be ruled out. Dosage adjustment is not needed in patients over the age of 65 *[see Clinical Pharmacology (12.3)]*.

8.6 Renal Impairment

The dosage recommendation is the same as for the general population. There is no experience beyond first-day administration of ondansetron.

8.7 Hepatic Impairment

In patients with severe hepatic impairment (Child-Pugh score of 10 or greater)[2], clearance is reduced and apparent volume of distribution is increased with a resultant increase in plasma half-life *[see Clinical Pharmacology (12.3)]*. In such patients, a total daily dose of 8 mg should not be exceeded.

9 DRUG ABUSE AND DEPENDENCE

Animal studies have shown that ondansetron is not discriminated as a benzodiazepine nor does it substitute for benzodiazepines in direct addiction studies.

10 OVERDOSAGE

There is no specific antidote for ondansetron overdose. Patients should be managed with appropriate supportive therapy. Individual intravenous doses as large as 150 mg and total daily intravenous doses as large as 252 mg have been inadvertently administered without significant adverse events. These doses are more than 10 times the recommended daily dose.

In addition to the adverse events listed above, the following events have been described in the setting of ondansetron overdose: "Sudden blindness" (amaurosis) of 2 to 3 minutes' duration plus severe constipation occurred in 1 patient that was administered 72 mg of ondansetron intravenously as a single dose. Hypotension (and faintness) occurred in a patient that took 48 mg of ondansetron HCl tablets. Following infusion of 32 mg over only a 4-minute period, a vasovagal episode with transient second-degree heart block was observed. In all instances, the events resolved completely.

Table 4: Mean Pharmacokinetic Parameters by Gender in Healthy Volunteers After A Single 8 mg ZUPLENZ Oral Soluble Film Dose

Gender	Mean Weight (kg)	n	C_{max} (ng/mL)	T_{max} (h)	$T_{1/2}$ (h)	AUC (h•ng/mL)
M F	62 56.7	39 7	35.2 49.1	1.67 1.7	4.54 5.39	207 323

11 DESCRIPTION

ZUPLENZ (ondansetron) oral soluble film is a white opaque orally dissolving film designed to be applied on top of the tongue where it will dissolve in 4 to 20 seconds and then is swallowed with saliva.

ZUPLENZ does not require water to aid dissolution or swallowing.

The active ingredient in ZUPLENZ is ondansetron base, the racemic form of ondansetron, and a selective blocking agent of the serotonin 5-HT_3 receptor type. Chemically it is (±) 1, 2, 3, 9-tetrahydro-9-methyl-3-[(2-methyl-1H-imidazol-1-yl)methyl]-4H-carbazol-4-one.

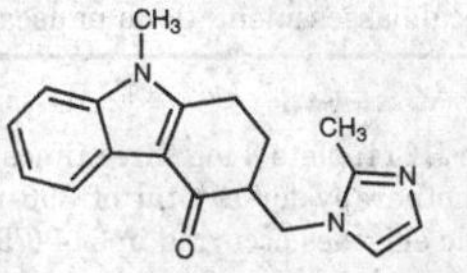

Figure 1: Structural formula of ondansetron

The empirical formula is $C_{18}H_{19}N_3O$ representing a molecular weight of 293.3. Each 4 mg ZUPLENZ oral soluble film for oral administration contains 4 mg ondansetron base. Each 8 mg ZUPLENZ oral soluble film for oral administration contains 8 mg ondansetron base. Each ZUPLENZ oral soluble film also contains the inactive ingredients butylated hydroxyltoluene, calcium carbonate, colloidal silicon dioxide, erythritol, hydroxypropyl methylcellulose, monoammonium glycyrrhizinate, peppermint flavor, polyethylene oxide, sodium bicarbonate, sucralose, titanium dioxide and xanthan gum.

12 CLINICAL PHARMACOLOGY

12.1 Mechanism of Action Section

Ondansetron is a selective 5-HT_3 receptor antagonist. While its mechanism of action has not been fully characterized, ondansetron is not a dopamine-receptor antagonist. Serotonin receptors of the 5-HT_3 type are present both peripherally on vagal nerve terminals and centrally in the chemoreceptor trigger zone of the area postrema. It is not certain whether ondansetron's antiemetic action is mediated centrally, peripherally, or in both sites. However, cytotoxic chemotherapy appears to be associated with release of serotonin from the enterochromaffin cells of the small intestine. In humans, urinary 5-HIAA (5-hydroxyindoleacetic acid) excretion increases after cisplatin administration in parallel with the onset of emesis. The released serotonin may stimulate the vagal afferents through the 5-HT_3 receptors and initiate the vomiting reflex.

12.2 Pharmacodynamics

In normal volunteers, single intravenous doses of 0.15 mg/kg of ondansetron had no effect on esophageal motility, gastric motility, lower esophageal sphincter pressure, or small intestinal transit time. Multiday administration of ondansetron has been shown to slow colonic transit in normal volunteers. Ondansetron has no effect on plasma prolactin concentrations.

12.3 Pharmacokinetics

Absorption

Ondansetron is well absorbed from the gastrointestinal tract and undergoes some first-pass metabolism. After a single dose of ZUPLENZ (ondansetron) oral soluble film 8 mg under fasting conditions (n=46), the peak plasma concentrations were achieved in 1.3 hours and the mean elimination half-life was 4.6 hours in healthy subjects. The mean (±S.D.) C_{max} and AUC were 37.28 (±14.9) ng/mL and 225 (±88.1) ng•h/mL, respectively. In the same study, mean ondansetron C_{max} and AUC following administration of 8 mg ZUPLENZ oral soluble film were comparable to those after 8 mg ondansetron ODT (orally disintegrating tablet). The systemic exposure after administration of ZUPLENZ oral soluble film 8 mg with or without water was found to be comparable.

In a study using ondansetron tablets, ondansetron systemic exposure did not increase proportionately to dose. AUC from a 16 mg tablet was 24% greater than predicted from an 8 mg tablet dose. This may reflect some reduction of first-pass metabolism at higher oral doses.

Food Effect

When ZUPLENZ 8 mg was administered with a high fat meal, the mean time to peak plasma concentration (T_{max}) was delayed by approximately 1 hour while AUC was similar to that under fasting conditions. Under the same fed conditions, both C_{max} and AUC were comparable between ZUPLENZ 8 mg and ondansetron ODT 8 mg.

Distribution

Plasma protein binding of ondansetron as measured in vitro was 70% to 76% over the concentration range of 10 to 500 ng/mL. Circulating drug also distributes into erythrocytes.

Metabolism and Excretion

Ondansetron is extensively metabolized in humans, with approximately 5% of a radiolabeled dose recovered as the parent compound from the urine. The primary metabolic pathway is hydroxylation on the indole ring followed by subsequent glucuronide or sulfate conjugation. Although some nonconjugated metabolites have pharmacologic activity, these are not found in plasma at concentrations likely to significantly contribute to the biological activity of ondansetron. The metabolites are observed in the urine.

In vitro metabolism studies have shown that ondansetron is a substrate for human hepatic cytochrome P-450 enzymes, including CYP1A2, CYP2D6, and CYP3A4. In terms of overall ondansetron turnover, CYP3A4 played the predominant role. Because of the multiplicity of metabolic enzymes capable of metabolizing ondansetron, it is likely that inhibition or loss of one enzyme (e.g., CYP2D6 genetic deficiency) will be compensated by others and may result in little change in overall rates of ondansetron elimination. Ondansetron elimination may be affected by cytochrome P-450 inducers.

Gender Effects

Gender differences were shown in the disposition of ondansetron given as a single dose. The extent and rate of ondansetron's absorption is greater in women than men. It is not known whether these gender-related differences were clinically important.

[See table 4 above]

Elderly

A reduction in clearance and increase in elimination half-life are seen in patients over 75 years of age. In clinical trials with cancer patients, safety and efficacy was similar in patients over 65 years of age and those under 65 years of age; there was an insufficient number of patients over 75 years of age to permit conclusions in that age-group. No dosage adjustment is recommended in the elderly.

Hepatic Impairment

In patients with mild-to-moderate hepatic impairment, clearance is reduced 2-fold and mean half-life is increased to 11.6 hours compared to 5.7 hours in healthy subjects. In patients with severe hepatic impairment (Child-Pugh score of 10 or greater)[2], clearance is reduced 2-fold to 3-fold and apparent volume of distribution is increased with a resultant increase in half-life to 20 hours. In patients with severe hepatic impairment, a total daily dose of 8 mg should not be exceeded.

Renal Impairment

Due to the very small contribution (5%) of renal clearance to the overall clearance, renal impairment was not expected to significantly influence the total clearance of ondansetron. However, ondansetron oral mean plasma clearance was reduced by about 50% in patients with severe renal impairment (creatinine clearance <30 mL/min). This reduction in clearance is variable and was not consistent with an increase in half-life. No reduction in dose or dosing frequency in these patients is warranted.

13 NONCLINICAL TOXICOLOGY

13.1 Carcinogenesis, Mutagenesis, Impairment of Fertility

Carcinogenic effects were not seen in 2-year studies in rats and mice with oral ondansetron doses up to 10 mg/kg/day and 30 mg/kg/day, respectively (approximately 5 and 8 times the human dose of 16 mg/day, based on body surface area). Ondansetron was not mutagenic in standard tests for mutagenicity. Oral administration of ondansetron up to 15 mg/kg/day (approximately 8 times the human dose of 16 mg/day, based on body surface area) did not affect fertility or general reproductive performance of male and female rats.

14 CLINICAL STUDIES

The clinical efficacy of ondansetron, the active ingredient of ZUPLENZ, was assessed in clinical trials as described below.

14.1 Chemotherapy-Induced Nausea and Vomiting
Highly Emetogenic Chemotherapy

In 2 randomized, double-blind, monotherapy trials, a single 24 mg ondansetron HCl tablet was superior to a relevant historical placebo control in the prevention of nausea and vomiting associated with highly emetogenic cancer chemotherapy, including cisplatin $\geq$50 mg/m². Steroid administration was excluded from these clinical trials. More than 90% of patients receiving a cisplatin dose $\geq$50 mg/m² in the historical placebo comparator experienced vomiting in the absence of antiemetic therapy.

The first trial compared oral doses of ondansetron 24 mg once a day, 8 mg twice a day, and 32 mg once a day in 357 adult cancer patients receiving chemotherapy regimens containing cisplatin $\geq$50 mg/m². A total of 66% of patients in the ondansetron 24 mg once-a-day group, 55% in the ondansetron 8 mg twice-a-day group, and 55% in the ondansetron 32 mg once-a-day group completed the 24-hour study period with no emetic episodes and no rescue antiemetic medications, the primary endpoint of efficacy. Each of the 3 treatment groups was shown to be statistically significantly superior to a historical placebo control.

In the same trial, 56% of patients receiving oral ondansetron 24 mg once a day experienced no nausea during the 24-hour study period, compared with 36% of patients in the oral ondansetron 8-mg twice-a-day group (p = 0.001) and 50% in the oral ondansetron 32-mg once-a-day group.

In a second trial, efficacy of the oral ondansetron 24-mg once-a-day regimen in the prevention of nausea and vomiting associated with highly emetogenic cancer chemotherapy, including cisplatin $\geq$50 mg/m², was confirmed.

Moderately Emetogenic Chemotherapy

In 1 double-blind US study in 67 patients, ondansetron HCl tablets 8 mg administered twice a day were significantly more effective than placebo in preventing vomiting induced by cyclophosphamide-based chemotherapy containing doxorubicin. Treatment response is based on the total number of emetic episodes over the 3-day study period. The results of this study are summarized in Table 5.

Table 5: Emetic Episodes: Treatment Response After Ondansetron HCl Tablets 8 mg Twice A Day

	Ondansetron Tablet 8 mg twice Daily[a]	Placebo	p Value
Number of patients	33	34	
Treatment response			
0 emetic episodes	20 (61%)	2 (6%)	<0.001
1-2 emetic episodes	6 (18%)	8 (24%)	
>2 emetic episodes/withdrawn	7 (21%)	24 (71%)	<0.001
Median number of emetic episodes	0.0	Undefined[b]	
Median time to first emetic episode (h)	Undefined[c]	6.5	

[a] The first dose was administered 30 minutes before the start of emetogenic chemotherapy, with a subsequent dose 8 hours after the first dose. An 8 mg ondansetron HCl tablet was administered twice a day for 2 days after completion of chemotherapy.
[b] Median undefined since at least 50% of the patients were withdrawn or had more than 2 emetic episodes.
[c] Median undefined since at least 50% of patients did not have any emetic episodes.

In 1 double-blind US study in 336 patients, ondansetron HCl tablets 8 mg administered twice a day were as effective as ondansetron HCl tablets 8 mg administered 3 times a day in preventing nausea and vomiting induced by cyclophosphamide-based chemotherapy containing either methotrexate or doxorubicin.

Treatment response is based on the total number of emetic episodes over the 3-day study period. The results of this study are summarized in Table 6.

[See table 6 above]

Retreatment

In uncontrolled trials, 148 patients receiving cyclophosphamide-based chemotherapy were re-treated

Table 6: Emetic Episodes: Treatment Response After Ondansetron HCl Tablets 8 mg Twice A Day and Three Times A Day

	Ondansetron 8 mg twice Daily[a]	Ondansetron 8 mg three times Daily[b]
Number of patients	165	171
Treatment response		
0 emetic episodes	101 (61%)	99 (58%)
1-2 emetic episodes	16 (10%)	17 (10%)
>2 emetic episodes/withdrawn	48 (29%)	55 (32%)
Median number of emetic episodes	0.0	0.0
Median time to first emetic episode (h)	Undefined[c]	Undefined[c]
Median nausea scores (0-100)[d]	6	6

[a] The first dose was administered 30 minutes before the start of emetogenic chemotherapy, with a subsequent dose 8 hours after the first dose. An 8 mg ondansetron HCl tablet was administered twice a day for 2 days after completion of chemotherapy.
[b] The first dose was administered 30 minutes before the start of emetogenic chemotherapy, with subsequent doses 4 and 8 hours after the first dose. An 8 mg ondansetron HCl tablet was administered 3 times daily for 2 days after completion of chemotherapy.
[c] Median undefined since at least 50% of patients did not have any emetic episodes.
[d] Visual analog scale assessment: 0=no nausea, 100=nausea as bad as it can be.

with ondansetron HCl tablets 8 mg three times daily during subsequent chemotherapy for a total of 396 re-treatment courses. No emetic episodes occurred in 314 (79%) of the re-treatment courses, and only 1 to 2 emetic episodes occurred in 43 (11%) of the re-treatment courses.

Pediatrics

Three open-label, uncontrolled, foreign trials have been performed with 182 pediatric patients 4 to 18 years old with cancer who were given a variety of cisplatin or non-cisplatin regimens. In these foreign trials, the initial dose of ondansetron HCl injection ranged from 0.04 to 0.87 mg/kg for a total dose of 2.16mg to 12 mg. This was followed by the administration of ondansetron HCl tablets ranging from 4mg to 24 mg daily for 3 days. In these studies, 58% of the 170 evaluable patients had a complete response (no emetic episodes) on day 1. Two studies showed the response rates for patients less than 12 years of age who received ondansetron HCl tablets 4 mg three times a daily to be similar to those in patients 12 to 18 years of age who received ondansetron HCl tablets 8 mg three times daily. Thus, prevention of emesis in these pediatric patients was essentially the same as for patients older than 18 years of age. Overall, ondansetron HCl tablets were well tolerated in these pediatric patients.

14.2 Radiation-Induced Nausea and Vomiting
Total Body Irradiation

In a randomized, double-blind study in 20 patients, ondansetron HCl tablets (8 mg given 1.5 hours before each fraction of radiotherapy for 4 days) were significantly more effective than placebo in preventing vomiting induced by total body irradiation. Total body irradiation consisted of 11 fractions (120 cGy per fraction) over 4 days for a total of 1,320 cGy. Patients received 3 fractions for 3 days, then 2 fractions on day 4.

Single High-Dose Fraction Radiotherapy

Ondansetron was significantly more effective than metoclopramide with respect to complete control of emesis (0 emetic episodes) in a double-blind trial in 105 patients receiving single high-dose radiotherapy (800 to 1,000 cGy) over an anterior or posterior field size of $\geq$80 cm² to the abdomen. Patients received the first dose of ondansetron HCl tablets (8 mg) or metoclopramide (10 mg) 1 to 2 hours before radiotherapy. If radiotherapy was given in the morning, 2 additional doses of study treatment were given (1 tablet late afternoon and 1 tablet before bedtime). If radiotherapy was given in the afternoon, patients took only 1 further tablet that day before bedtime. Patients continued the oral medication on a three times daily basis for 3 days.

Daily Fractionated Radiotherapy

Ondansetron was significantly more effective than prochlorperazine with respect to complete control of emesis (0 emetic episodes) in a double-blind trial in 135 patients receiving a 1- to 4-week course of fractionated radiotherapy (180 cGy doses) over a field size of >100 cm² to the abdomen. Patients received the first dose of ondansetron HCl tablets (8 mg) or prochlorperazine (10 mg) 1 to 2 hours before the patient received the first daily radiotherapy fraction, with 2 subsequent doses on a three times a day basis. Patients continued the oral medication on a three times daily basis on each day of radiotherapy.

14.3 Postoperative Nausea and Vomiting

Surgical patients who received ondansetron 1 hour before the induction of general balanced anesthesia (barbiturate: thiopental, methohexital, or thiamylal; opioid: alfentanil, sufentanil, morphine, or fentanyl; nitrous oxide; neuromuscular blockade: succinylcholine/curare or gallamine and/or vecuronium, pancuronium, or atracurium; and supplemental isoflurane or enflurane) were evaluated in 2 double-blind studies (1 US study, 1 foreign) involving 865 patients. Ondansetron HCl tablets (16 mg) were significantly more effective than placebo in preventing postoperative nausea and vomiting.

The study populations in all trials thus far consisted of women undergoing inpatient surgical procedures. No studies have been performed in males. No controlled clinical study comparing ondansetron HCl tablets to ondansetron injection has been performed.

15 REFERENCES

1. Britto MR, Hussey EK, Mydlow P, et al. Effect of enzyme inducers on ondansetron (OND) metabolism in humans. Clin Pharmacol Ther. 1997;61:228.
2. Pugh RNH, Murray-Lyon IM, Dawson JL, Pietroni MC, Williams R. Transection of the oesophagus for bleeding oesophageal varices. Brit J Surg. 1973;60:646-649.
3. Villikka K, Kivisto KT, Neuvonen PJ. The effect of rifampin on the pharmacokinetics of oral and intravenous ondansetron. Clin Pharmacol Ther. 1999;65:377-381.
4. De Witte JL, Schoenmaekers B, Sessler DI, et al. Anesth Analg. 2001;92:1319-1321.
5. Arcioni R, della Rocca M, Romanò R, et al. Anesth Analg. 2002;94:1553-1557.

16 HOW SUPPLIED/STORAGE AND HANDLING

ZUPLENZ (ondansetron) oral soluble film 4 mg and ZUPLENZ (ondansetron) oral soluble film 8 mg, are supplied as thin rectangular white opaque films in individual foil-foil sealed child resistant pouches. Individual films are identified by "4 mg" or "8 mg", according to the respective strengths, which is printed using pharmaceutical grade edible ink.

Individual pouches of ZUPLENZ 4 mg oral soluble film (NDC 49884-324-52) are packaged in boxes of 10 (NDC 49884-324-62).

Individual pouches of ZUPLENZ 8 mg oral soluble film (NDC 49884-325-52) are packaged in boxes of 10 (NDC 49884-325-62).

Store at controlled room temperature 20° to 25°C (68° to 77°F). Store pouches in cartons. Keep product in pouch until ready to use.

17 PATIENT COUNSELING INFORMATION

See FDA-Approved Patient Labeling

17.1 Instructions for use

Advise patients to carefully read the "Patient Information" and "Instructions for Use" accompanying each package of ZUPLENZ (ondansetron) oral soluble film.

Inform patients that ZUPLENZ film may cause headache, malaise/fatigue, constipation, and diarrhea. The patient should report the use of all medications, especially apomorphine, to their health care provider. Concomitant use of apomorphine and ondansetron may cause a significant drop in blood pressure and loss of consciousness.

Inform patients that ZUPLENZ may cause hypersensitivity reactions, some as severe as anaphylaxis and bronchospasm. The patient should report any hypersensitivity reactions to this and other 5-HT₃ receptor antagonists to their health care provider.

Instruct patients on how to use ZUPLENZ films:

The patient should keep the film in the pouch until ready to use and not chew or swallow the film. With dry hands, the patient should fold the pouch along the dotted line to expose the tear notch. While still folded, the patient should tear the pouch carefully along the edge and remove the ZUPLENZ oral soluble film from the pouch. The patient should immediately place the film on top of the tongue where it dissolves in 4 to 20 seconds, and then swallow with saliva. Once the film dissolves, the patient may swallow liquid but it is not required. The patient should wash his hands after taking ZUPLENZ.

PATIENT INFORMATION

ZUPLENZ (ZOO-plenz)
(ondansetron)
Oral Soluble Film

Read the Patient Information that comes with ZUPLENZ before you start taking it and each time you get a refill. There may be new information. This leaflet does not take the place of talking with your doctor about your medical condition or treatment.

What is ZUPLENZ?

ZUPLENZ is a prescription medicine that is used in adults to prevent nausea and vomiting:

- Caused by certain cancer chemotherapy medicines, radiation therapy to your stomach-area (abdomen), or radiation therapy to your entire body.
- that may happen after surgery

In children aged 4 years and older, ZUPLENZ is only used to prevent nausea and vomiting due to certain cancer chemotherapy medicines.

It is not known if ZUPLENZ is safe and works in children to prevent nausea and vomiting with radiation therapy, or nausea and vomiting that may happen after surgery in children.

Who should not take ZUPLENZ?

Do not take ZUPLENZ if you take apomorphine hydrochloride (Apokyn).

Do not take ZUPLENZ if you have had an allergic reaction to ZUPLENZ or are allergic to any of its ingredients. See the end of this leaflet for a complete list of ingredients in ZUPLENZ.

Ask your doctor if you are not sure.

What should I tell my doctor before taking ZUPLENZ?

Before you take ZUPLENZ oral soluble film, tell your doctor if you:

- have liver problems
- have any other medical conditions
- are pregnant or plan to become pregnant. It is not known if ZUPLENZ will harm your unborn baby.
- are breastfeeding or plan to breastfeed. It is not known if ZUPLENZ passes into your breast milk.
- have had an allergic reaction to another medicine for nausea and vomiting.

Tell your doctor about all the medicines you take, including prescription and non-prescription, vitamins, and herbal supplements.

Some medicines may affect how ZUPLENZ works, and ZUPLENZ may affect how other medicines work. Using ZUPLENZ with certain other medicines may cause serious side effects. Especially tell your doctor if you take:

- apomorphine hydrochloride (Apokyn)
- tramadol hydrochloride (Ultram, Ultram ER, Ryzolt)
- another medicine for nausea and vomiting

Ask your doctor or pharmacist if you are not sure if your medicine is listed above.

Know the medicines you take. Keep a list of them to show to your doctor or pharmacist each time you start a new medicine.

How should I take ZUPLENZ?

Take ZUPLENZ exactly as your doctor tells you to take it.

- An adult should help a young child use this medicine.
- See the "Instructions for Use" at the end of this leaflet.

What are the possible side effects of ZUPLENZ?

ZUPLENZ may cause serious side effects, including:

- **severe allergic reactions. Stop taking ZUPLENZ and tell your doctor right away if you have any of these signs or symptoms of an allergic reaction with ZUPLENZ:**
- **rash**
- **hives**
- **itching**
- **trouble breathing**
- **chest tightness or chest pain**
- **swelling of your mouth, face, lips, or tongue**
- **heart rhythm changes**

The most common side effects of ZUPLENZ are:

- headache
- tiredness and body discomfort
- constipation
- diarrhea

These are not all the possible side effects of ZUPLENZ. For more information, ask your doctor or your pharmacist.

Call your doctor for medical advice about side effects. You may report side effects to FDA at 1-800-FDA-1088.

How should I store ZUPLENZ?

- Store ZUPLENZ at room temperature, 68°F to 77°F (20°C to 25°C).
- Keep the film in the foil pouch until ready to use. Keep foil pouches in the carton.
- Use the film strip right away, after you take it from the pouch.

Keep ZUPLENZ and all medicines out of the reach of children.

General information about ZUPLENZ

Medicines are sometimes used for purposes other than those listed in Patient Information leaflets. Do not use ZUPLENZ for a condition for which it was not prescribed. Do not give ZUPLENZ to other people, even if they have the same condition that you have. It may harm them.

This Patient Information leaflet summarizes the most important information about ZUPLENZ. If you would like more information, talk with your doctor. You can ask your doctor or pharmacist for information about ZUPLENZ that is written for healthcare professionals. You can also visit www.ZUPLENZ.com or call 1-800-828-9393.

What are the ingredients in ZUPLENZ?

Active ingredient: ondansetron

Inactive ingredients: butylated hydroxytoluene, calcium carbonate, colloidal silicon dioxide, erythritol, hydroxypropyl methylcellulose, monoammonium glycyrrhizinate, peppermint flavor, polyethylene oxide, sodium bicarbonate, sucralose, titanium oxide and xanthan gum.

Manufactured By:
Monosol Rx, LLC
Portage, IN 46368
Distributed By:
Strativa Pharmaceuticals, a division of Par Pharmaceutical, Inc.
Issued: July 2010
©2010 Par Pharmaceutical, Inc.

INSTRUCTIONS FOR USE

ZUPLENZ (ZOO-plenz)
(ondansetron)
Oral Soluble Film

1. Keep the film in the foil pouch until ready to use. Use the film right away, after you take it from the pouch.

2. Make sure your hands are dry.

3. Fold the pouch along the dotted line to expose the tear notch. See Figure A.

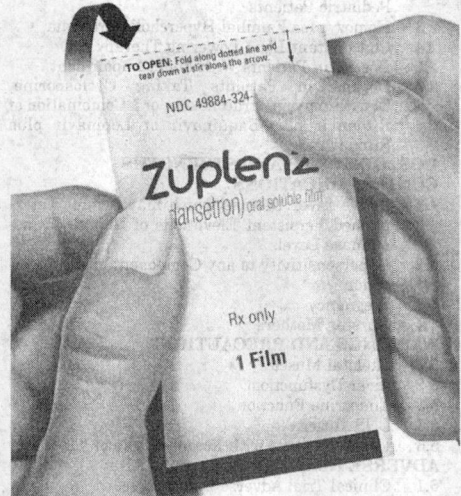

Figure A

4. While still folded, tear the pouch carefully along the edge. See Figure B.
[See figure B at top of next column]

5. Take the ZUPLENZ film strip from the pouch. See Figure C.
[See figure C in next column]

6. Put the ZUPLENZ film on top of your tongue, where it will dissolve in 4 to 20 seconds. See Figure D.
[See figure D in next column]

7. Do not chew or swallow the film whole.

8. Swallow after the film dissolves. You may swallow the dissolved film with or without liquid.

9. Wash your hands after taking ZUPLENZ.

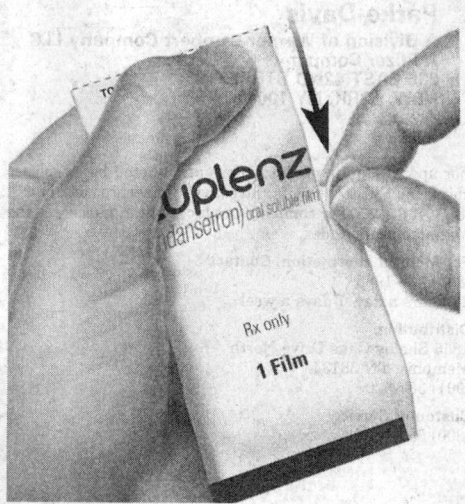

Figure B

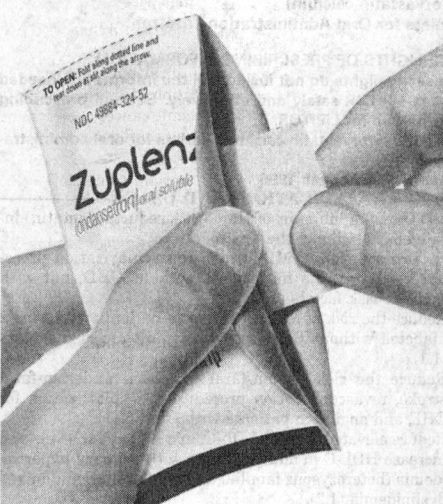

Figure C

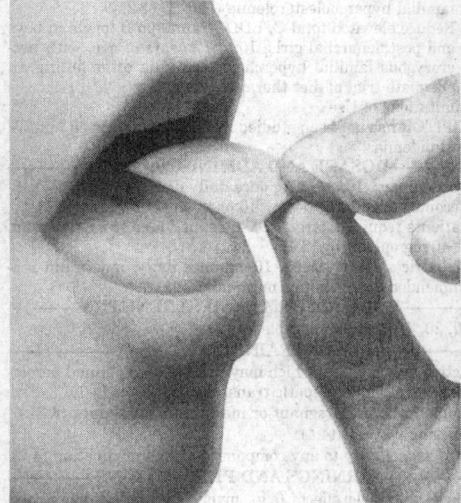

Figure D

Manufactured By:
Monosol Rx, LLC
Portage, IN 46368
Distributed By:
Strativa Pharmaceuticals, a division of Par Pharmaceutical, Inc.
Woodcliff Lake, NJ 07677
Issued July 2010
©2010 Par Pharmaceutical, Inc.

Parke-Davis
A Division of Warner-Lambert Company LLC
A Pfizer Company
235 EAST 42ND STREET
NEW YORK, NY 10017-5755

For updates to the product information listed below, please check the Pfizer Web site, http://www.pfizerpro.com, or call (800) 438-1985. For complete product listing, please see the Manufacturers' Index.

For Medical Information, Contact:
(800) 438-1985
24 hours a day, 7 days a week

Distribution:
1855 Shelby Oaks Drive North
Memphis, TN 38134
(901) 387-5200

Customer Service:
(800) 533-4535

LIPITOR®
[lĭ′pĭ-tōr]
(atorvastatin calcium)
Tablets for Oral Administration

℞

HIGHLIGHTS OF PRESCRIBING INFORMATION
These highlights do not include all the information needed to use LIPITOR safely and effectively. See full prescribing information for LIPITOR.
LIPITOR® (atorvastatin calcium) Tablets for oral administration
Initial U.S. Approval: 1996

——————INDICATIONS AND USAGE——————
LIPITOR is an inhibitor of HMG-CoA reductase (statin) indicated as an adjunct therapy to diet to:
• Reduce the risk of MI, stroke, revascularization procedures, and angina in patients without CHD, but with multiple risk factors (1.1).
• Reduce the risk of MI and stroke in patients with type 2 diabetes without CHD, but with multiple risk factors (1.1).
• Reduce the risk of non-fatal MI, fatal and non-fatal stroke, revascularization procedures, hospitalization for CHF, and angina in patients with CHD (1.1).
• Reduce elevated total-C, LDL-C, apo B, and TG levels and increase HDL-C in adult patients with primary hyperlipidemia (heterozygous familial and nonfamilial) and mixed dyslipidemia (1.2).
• Reduce elevated TG in patients with hypertriglyceridemia and primary dysbetalipoproteinemia (1.2).
• Reduce total-C and LDL-C in patients with homozygous familial hypercholesterolemia (HoFH) (1.2).
• Reduce elevated total-C, LDL-C, and apo B levels in boys and postmenarchal girls, 10 to 17 years of age, with heterozygous familial hypercholesterolemia after failing an adequate trial of diet therapy (1.2).
Limitations of Use
LIPITOR has not been studied in *Fredrickson* Types I and V dyslipidemias.

——————DOSAGE AND ADMINISTRATION——————
Dose range: 10 to 80 mg once daily (2.1).
Recommended start dose: 10 or 20 mg once daily (2.1).
Patients requiring large LDL-C reduction (>45%) may start at 40 mg once daily (2.1).
Pediatric starting dose: 10 mg once daily; maximum recommended dose: 20 mg once daily (2.2).

——————DOSAGE FORMS AND STRENGTHS——————
10, 20, 40, and 80 mg tablets (3).

——————CONTRAINDICATIONS——————
Active liver disease, which may include unexplained persistent elevations in hepatic transaminase levels (4.1).
Women who are pregnant or may become pregnant (4.3).
Nursing mothers (4.4).
Hypersensitivity to any component of this medication (4.2).

——————WARNINGS AND PRECAUTIONS——————
Skeletal muscle effects (e.g., myopathy and rhabdomyolysis): Risks increase when higher doses are used concomitantly with cyclosporine, fibrates, and strong CYP3A4 inhibitors (e.g., clarithromycin, itraconazole, HIV protease inhibitors). Predisposing factors include advanced age (> 65), uncontrolled hypothyroidism, and renal impairment. Rare cases of rhabdomyolysis with acute renal failure secondary to myoglobinuria have been reported. In cases of myopathy or rhabdomyolysis, therapy should be temporarily withheld or discontinued (5.1).
Liver enzyme abnormalities and monitoring: Persistent elevations in hepatic transaminases can occur. Monitor liver enzymes before and during treatment (5.2).

A higher incidence of hemorrhagic stroke was seen in patients without CHD but with stroke or TIA within the previous 6 months in the LIPITOR 80 mg group vs. placebo (5.5).

——————ADVERSE REACTIONS——————
The most commonly reported adverse reactions (incidence ≥ 2%) in patients treated with LIPITOR in placebo-controlled trials regardless of causality were: nasopharyngitis, arthralgia, diarrhea, pain in extremity, and urinary tract infection (6.1).
To report SUSPECTED ADVERSE REACTIONS, contact Pfizer at (1-800-438-1985 and www.pfizer.com) or FDA at 1-800-FDA-1088 or www.fda.gov/medwatch.

——————DRUG INTERACTIONS——————
Drug Interactions Associated with Increased Risk of Myopathy/Rhabdomyolysis (2.6, 5.1, 7, 12.3)

Interacting Agents	Prescribing Recommendations
Cyclosporine	Do not exceed 10 mg atorvastatin daily
Clarithromycin, itraconazole, HIV protease inhibitors (ritonavir plus saquinavir or lopinavir plus ritonavir)	Caution when exceeding doses > 20 mg atorvastatin daily. The lowest dose necessary should be used.

• Digoxin: Patients should be monitored appropriately (7.5).
• Oral Contraceptives: Values for norethindrone and ethinyl estradiol may be increased (7.6).
• Rifampin should be simultaneously co-administered with LIPITOR (7.4).

——————USE IN SPECIFIC POPULATIONS——————
• Hepatic impairment: Plasma concentrations markedly increased in patients with chronic alcoholic liver disease (12.3).
See 17 for PATIENT COUNSELING INFORMATION
Revised: [6/2009]

FULL PRESCRIBING INFORMATION: CONTENTS*
1 INDICATIONS AND USAGE
 1.1 Prevention of Cardiovascular Disease
 1.2 Hyperlipidemia
 1.3 Limitations of Use
2 DOSAGE AND ADMINISTRATION
 2.1 Hyperlipidemia
 2.2 Heterozygous Familial Hypercholesterolemia in Pediatric Patients
 2.3 Homozygous Familial Hypercholesterolemia
 2.4 Concomitant Lipid-Lowering Therapy
 2.5 Dosage in Patients With Renal Impairment
 2.6 Dosage in Patients Taking Cyclosporine, Clarithromycin, Itraconazole, or a Combination of Ritonavir plus Saquinavir or Lopinavir plus Ritonavir
3 DOSAGE FORMS AND STRENGTHS
4 CONTRAINDICATIONS
 4.1 Active Liver Disease which may include Unexplained Persistent Elevations of Hepatic Transaminase Levels
 4.2 Hypersensitivity to any Component of this Medication
 4.3 Pregnancy
 4.4 Nursing Mothers
5 WARNINGS AND PRECAUTIONS
 5.1 Skeletal Muscle
 5.2 Liver Dysfunction
 5.3 Endocrine Function
 5.4 CNS Toxicity
 5.5 Use in Patients with Recent Stroke or TIA
6 ADVERSE REACTIONS
 6.1 Clinical Trial Adverse Experiences
 6.2 Postintroduction Reports
 6.3 Pediatric Patients (ages 10-17 years)
7 DRUG INTERACTIONS
 7.1 Strong Inhibitors of Cytochrome P450 3A4: Clarithromycin Combination of Protease Inhibitors Itraconazole
 7.2 Grapefruit Juice
 7.3 Cyclosporine
 7.4 Rifampin or other Inducers of Cytochrome P450 3A4
 7.5 Digoxin
 7.6 Oral Contraceptives
 7.7 Warfarin
8 USE IN SPECIFIC POPULATIONS
 8.1 Pregnancy
 8.3 Nursing Mothers
 8.4 Pediatric Use
 8.5 Geriatric Use
 8.6 Hepatic Impairment
10 OVERDOSAGE
11 DESCRIPTION
12 CLINICAL PHARMACOLOGY
 12.1 Mechanism of Action
 12.2 Pharmacodynamics
 12.3 Pharmacokinetics
13 NONCLINICAL TOXICOLOGY
 13.1 Carcinogenesis, Mutagenesis, Impairment of Fertility
14 CLINICAL STUDIES
 14.1 Prevention of Cardiovascular Disease
 14.2 Hyperlipidemia and Mixed Dyslipidemia
 14.3 Hypertriglyceridemia
 14.4 Dysbetalipoproteinemia
 14.5 Homozygous Familial Hypercholesterolemia
 14.6 Heterozygous Familial Hypercholesterolemia in Pediatric Patients
15 REFERENCES
16 HOW SUPPLIED/STORAGE AND HANDLING
17 PATIENT COUNSELING INFORMATION
 17.1 Muscle Pain
 17.2 Liver Enzymes
 17.3 Pregnancy
 17.4 Breastfeeding
*Sections or subsections omitted from the full prescribing information are not listed.

FULL PRESCRIBING INFORMATION

1 INDICATIONS AND USAGE
Therapy with lipid-altering agents should be only one component of multiple risk factor intervention in individuals at significantly increased risk for atherosclerotic vascular disease due to hypercholesterolemia. Drug therapy is recommended as an adjunct to diet when the response to a diet restricted in saturated fat and cholesterol and other nonpharmacologic measures alone has been inadequate. In patients with CHD or multiple risk factors for CHD, LIPITOR can be started simultaneously with diet.

1.1 Prevention of Cardiovascular Disease
In adult patients without clinically evident coronary heart disease, but with multiple risk factors for coronary heart disease such as age, smoking, hypertension, low HDL-C, or a family history of early coronary heart disease, LIPITOR is indicated to:
• Reduce the risk of myocardial infarction
• Reduce the risk of stroke
• Reduce the risk for revascularization procedures and angina
In patients with type 2 diabetes, and without clinically evident coronary heart disease, but with multiple risk factors for coronary heart disease such as retinopathy, albuminuria, smoking, or hypertension, LIPITOR is indicated to:
• Reduce the risk of myocardial infarction
• Reduce the risk of stroke
In patients with clinically evident coronary heart disease, LIPITOR is indicated to:
• Reduce the risk of non-fatal myocardial infarction
• Reduce the risk of fatal and non-fatal stroke
• Reduce the risk for revascularization procedures
• Reduce the risk of hospitalization for CHF
• Reduce the risk of angina

1.2 Hyperlipidemia
LIPITOR is indicated:
• As an adjunct to diet to reduce elevated total-C, LDL-C, apo B, and TG levels and to increase HDL-C in patients with primary hypercholesterolemia (heterozygous familial and nonfamilial) and mixed dyslipidemia (*Fredrickson* Types IIa and IIb);
• As an adjunct to diet for the treatment of patients with elevated serum TG levels (*Fredrickson* Type IV);
• For the treatment of patients with primary dysbetalipoproteinemia (*Fredrickson* Type III) who do not respond adequately to diet;
• To reduce total-C and LDL-C in patients with homozygous familial hypercholesterolemia as an adjunct to other lipid-lowering treatments (e.g., LDL apheresis) or if such treatments are unavailable;
• As an adjunct to diet to reduce total-C, LDL-C, and apo B levels in boys and postmenarchal girls, 10 to 17 years of age, with heterozygous familial hypercholesterolemia if after an adequate trial of diet therapy the following findings are present:
 a. LDL-C remains ≥ 190 mg/dL or
 b. LDL-C remains ≥ 160 mg/dL and:
  • there is a positive family history of premature cardiovascular disease or
  • two or more other CVD risk factors are present in the pediatric patient

1.3 Limitations of Use
LIPITOR has not been studied in conditions where the major lipoprotein abnormality is elevation of chylomicrons (*Fredrickson* Types I and V).

2 DOSAGE AND ADMINISTRATION

2.1 Hyperlipidemia (Heterozygous Familial and Nonfamilial) and Mixed Dyslipidemia (*Fredrickson* Types IIa and IIb)
The recommended starting dose of LIPITOR is 10 or 20 mg once daily. Patients who require a large reduction in LDL-C (more than 45%) may be started at 40 mg once daily. The dosage range of LIPITOR is 10 to 80 mg once daily. LIPITOR can be administered as a single dose at any time of the day, with or without food. The starting dose and maintenance doses of LIPITOR should be individualized according to patient characteristics such as goal of therapy and response (see current *NCEP Guidelines*). After initiation and/or upon titration of LIPITOR, lipid levels should be analyzed within 2 to 4 weeks and dosage adjusted accordingly.

2.2 Heterozygous Familial Hypercholesterolemia in Pediatric Patients (10-17 years of age)
The recommended starting dose of LIPITOR is 10 mg/day; the maximum recommended dose is 20 mg/day (doses greater than 20 mg have not been studied in this patient population). Doses should be individualized according to the recommended goal of therapy (see current *NCEP Pediatric Panel Guidelines, Clinical Pharmacology (12),* and *Indications and Usage (1.2)*]. Adjustments should be made at intervals of 4 weeks or more.

2.3 Homozygous Familial Hypercholesterolemia
The dosage of LIPITOR in patients with homozygous FH is 10 to 80 mg daily. LIPITOR should be used as an adjunct to other lipid-lowering treatments (e.g., LDL apheresis) in these patients or if such treatments are unavailable.

2.4 Concomitant Lipid-Lowering Therapy
LIPITOR may be used with bile acid resins. The combination of HMG-CoA reductase inhibitors (statins) and fibrates should generally be used with caution [see *Warnings and Precautions, Skeletal Muscle (5.1), Drug Interactions (7)*].

2.5 Dosage in Patients With Renal Impairment
Renal disease does not affect the plasma concentrations nor LDL-C reduction of LIPITOR; thus, dosage adjustment in patients with renal dysfunction is not necessary [see *Warnings and Precautions, Skeletal Muscle (5.1), Clinical Pharmacology, Pharmacokinetics (12.3)*].

2.6 Dosage in Patients Taking Cyclosporine, Clarithromycin, Itraconazole, or a Combination of Ritonavir plus Saquinavir or Lopinavir plus Ritonavir
In patients taking cyclosporine, therapy should be limited to LIPITOR 10 mg once daily. In patients taking clarithromycin, itraconazole, or in patients with HIV taking a combination of ritonavir plus saquinavir or lopinavir plus ritonavir, for doses of LIPITOR exceeding 20 mg, appropriate clinical assessment is recommended to ensure that the lowest dose necessary of LIPITOR is employed [see *Warnings and Precautions, Skeletal Muscle (5.1), Drug Interactions (7)*].

3 DOSAGE FORMS AND STRENGTHS
White, elliptical, film-coated tablets containing 10, 20, 40, and 80 mg atorvastatin calcium.

4 CONTRAINDICATIONS

4.1 Active liver disease, which may include unexplained persistent elevations in hepatic transaminase levels
4.2 Hypersensitivity to any component of this medication
4.3 Pregnancy
Women who are pregnant or may become pregnant. LIPITOR may cause fetal harm when administered to a pregnant woman. Serum cholesterol and triglycerides increase during normal pregnancy, and cholesterol or cholesterol derivatives are essential for fetal development. Atherosclerosis is a chronic process and discontinuation of lipid-lowering drugs during pregnancy should have little impact on the outcome of long-term therapy of primary hypercholesterolemia. There are no adequate and well-controlled studies of LIPITOR use during pregnancy; however in rare reports, congenital anomalies were observed following intrauterine exposure to statins. In rat and rabbit animal reproduction studies, atorvastatin revealed no evidence of teratogenicity. LIPITOR SHOULD BE ADMINISTERED TO WOMEN OF CHILDBEARING AGE ONLY WHEN SUCH PATIENTS ARE HIGHLY UNLIKELY TO CONCEIVE AND HAVE BEEN INFORMED OF THE POTENTIAL HAZARDS. If the patient becomes pregnant while taking this drug, LIPITOR should be discontinued immediately and the patient apprised of the potential hazard to the fetus [see *Use in Specific Populations (8.1)*].

4.4 Nursing mothers
It is not known whether atorvastatin is excreted into human milk; however a small amount of another drug in this class does pass into breast milk. Because statins have the potential for serious adverse reactions in nursing infants, women who require LIPITOR treatment should not breast-feed their infants [see *Use in Specific Populations (8.3)*].

5 WARNINGS AND PRECAUTIONS

5.1 Skeletal Muscle
Rare cases of rhabdomyolysis with acute renal failure secondary to myoglobinuria have been reported with LIPITOR and with other drugs in this class. A history of renal impairment may be a risk factor for the development of rhabdomyolysis. Such patients merit closer monitoring for skeletal muscle effects.

Atorvastatin, like other statins, occasionally causes myopathy, defined as muscle aches or muscle weakness in conjunction with increases in creatine phosphokinase (CPK) values >10 times ULN. The concomitant use of higher doses of atorvastatin with certain drugs such as cyclosporine and strong CYP3A4 inhibitors (e.g., clarithromycin, itraconazole, and HIV protease inhibitors) increases the risk of myopathy/rhabdomyolysis.

Myopathy should be considered in any patient with diffuse myalgias, muscle tenderness or weakness, and/or marked elevation of CPK. Patients should be advised to report promptly unexplained muscle pain, tenderness, or weakness, particularly if accompanied by malaise or fever. LIPITOR therapy should be discontinued if markedly elevated CPK levels occur or myopathy is diagnosed or suspected.

The risk of myopathy during treatment with drugs in this class is increased with concurrent administration of cyclosporine, fibric acid derivatives, erythromycin, clarithromycin, combination of ritonavir plus saquinavir or lopinavir plus ritonavir, niacin, or azole antifungals. Physicians considering combined therapy with LIPITOR and fibric acid derivatives, erythromycin, clarithromycin, a combination of ritonavir plus saquinavir or lopinavir plus ritonavir, immunosuppressive drugs, azole antifungals, or lipid-modifying doses of niacin should carefully weigh the potential benefits and risks and should carefully monitor patients for any signs or symptoms of muscle pain, tenderness, or weakness, particularly during the initial months of therapy and during any periods of upward dosage titration of either drug. Lower starting and maintenance doses of atorvastatin should be considered when taken concomitantly with the aforementioned drugs (see *Drug Interactions (7)*). Periodic creatine phosphokinase (CPK) determinations may be considered in such situations, but there is no assurance that such monitoring will prevent the occurrence of severe myopathy. Prescribing recommendations for interacting agents are summarized in Table 1 [see also *Dosage and Administration (2.6), Drug Interactions (7), Clinical Pharmacology (12.3)*].

Table 1. Drug Interactions Associated with Increased Risk of Myopathy/Rhabdomyolysis

Interacting Agents	Prescribing Recommendations
Cyclosporine	Do not exceed 10 mg atorvastatin daily
Clarithromycin, itraconazole, HIV protease inhibitors (ritonavir plus saquinavir or lopinavir plus ritonavir)	Caution when exceeding doses > 20mg atorvastatin daily. The lowest dose necessary should be used.

LIPITOR therapy should be temporarily withheld or discontinued in any patient with an acute, serious condition suggestive of a myopathy or having a risk factor predisposing to the development of renal failure secondary to rhabdomyolysis (e.g., severe acute infection, hypotension, major surgery, trauma, severe metabolic, endocrine and electrolyte disorders, and uncontrolled seizures).

5.2 Liver Dysfunction
Statins, like some other lipid-lowering therapies, have been associated with biochemical abnormalities of liver function. **Persistent elevations (>3 times the upper limit of normal [ULN] occurring on 2 or more occasions) in serum transaminases occurred in 0.7% of patients who received LIPITOR in clinical trials. The incidence of these abnormalities was 0.2%, 0.2%, 0.6%, and 2.3% for 10, 20, 40, and 80 mg, respectively.**

One patient in clinical trials developed jaundice. Increases in liver function tests (LFT) in other patients were not associated with jaundice or other clinical signs or symptoms. Upon dose reduction, drug interruption, or discontinuation, transaminase levels returned to or near pretreatment levels without sequelae. Eighteen of 30 patients with persistent LFT elevations continued treatment with a reduced dose of LIPITOR.

It is recommended that liver function tests be performed prior to and at 12 weeks following both the initiation of therapy and any elevation of dose, and periodically (e.g., semiannually) thereafter. Liver enzyme changes generally occur in the first 3 months of treatment with LIPITOR. Patients who develop increased transaminase levels should be monitored until the abnormalities resolve. Should an increase in ALT or AST of >3 times ULN persist, reduction of dose or withdrawal of LIPITOR is recommended.

LIPITOR should be used with caution in patients who consume substantial quantities of alcohol and/or have a history of liver disease. Active liver disease or unexplained persistent transaminase elevations are contraindications to the use of LIPITOR [see *Contraindications (4.1)*].

5.3 Endocrine Function
Statins interfere with cholesterol synthesis and theoretically might blunt adrenal and/or gonadal steroid production. Clinical studies have shown that LIPITOR does not reduce basal plasma cortisol concentration or impair adrenal reserve. The effects of statins on male fertility have not been studied in adequate numbers of patients. The effects, if any, on the pituitary-gonadal axis in premenopausal women are unknown. Caution should be exercised if a statin is administered concomitantly with drugs that may decrease the levels or activity of endogenous steroid hormones, such as ketoconazole, spironolactone, and cimetidine.

5.4 CNS Toxicity
Brain hemorrhage was seen in a female dog treated for 3 months at 120 mg/kg/day. Brain hemorrhage and optic nerve vacuolation were seen in another female dog that was sacrificed in moribund condition after 11 weeks of escalating doses up to 280 mg/kg/day. The 120 mg/kg dose resulted in a systemic exposure approximately 16 times the human plasma area-under-the-curve (AUC, 0-24 hours) based on the maximum human dose of 80 mg/day. A single tonic convulsion was seen in each of 2 male dogs (one treated at 10 mg/kg/day and one at 120 mg/kg/day) in a 2-year study. No CNS lesions have been observed in mice after chronic treatment for up to 2 years at doses up to 400 mg/kg/day or in rats at doses up to 100 mg/kg/day. These doses were 6 to 11 times (mouse) and 8 to 16 times (rat) the human AUC (0-24) based on the maximum recommended human dose of 80 mg/day.

CNS vascular lesions, characterized by perivascular hemorrhages, edema, and mononuclear cell infiltration of perivascular spaces, have been observed in dogs treated with other members of this class. A chemically similar drug in this class produced optic nerve degeneration (Wallerian degeneration of retinogeniculate fibers) in clinically normal dogs in a dose-dependent fashion at a dose that produced plasma drug levels about 30 times higher than the mean drug level in humans taking the highest recommended dose.

5.5 Use in Patients with Recent Stroke or TIA
In a post-hoc analysis of the Stroke Prevention by Aggressive Reduction in Cholesterol Levels (SPARCL) study where LIPITOR 80 mg vs. placebo was administered in 4,731 subjects without CHD who had a stroke or TIA within the preceding 6 months, a higher incidence of hemorrhagic stroke was seen in the LIPITOR 80 mg group compared to placebo (55, 2.3% atorvastatin vs. 33, 1.4% placebo; HR: 1.68, 95% CI: 1.09, 2.59; p=0.0168). The incidence of fatal hemorrhagic stroke was similar across treatment groups (17 vs. 18 for the atorvastatin and placebo groups, respectively). The incidence of nonfatal hemorrhagic stroke was significantly higher in the atorvastatin group (38, 1.6%) as compared to the placebo group (16, 0.7%). Some baseline characteristics, including hemorrhagic and lacunar stroke on study entry, were associated with a higher incidence of hemorrhagic stroke in the atorvastatin group [see *Adverse Reactions (6.1)*].

6 ADVERSE REACTIONS
The following serious adverse reactions are discussed in greater detail in other sections of the label:
Rhabdomyolysis and myopathy [see *Warnings and Precautions (5.1)*]
Liver enzyme abnormalities [see *Warnings and Precautions (5.2)*]

6.1 Clinical Trial Adverse Experiences
Because clinical trials are conducted under widely varying conditions, the adverse reaction rates observed in the clinical studies of a drug cannot be directly compared to rates in the clinical trials of another drug and may not reflect the rates observed in clinical practice.

In the LIPITOR placebo-controlled clinical trial database of 16,066 patients (8755 LIPITOR vs. 7311 placebo; age range 10–93 years, 39% women, 91% Caucasians, 3% Blacks, 2% Asians, 4% other) with a median treatment duration of 53 weeks, 9.7% of patients on LIPITOR and 9.5% of the patients on placebo discontinued due to adverse reactions regardless of causality. The five most common adverse reactions in patients treated with LIPITOR that led to treatment discontinuation and occurred at a rate greater than placebo were: myalgia (0.7%), diarrhea (0.5%), nausea (0.4%), alanine aminotransferase increase (0.4%), and hepatic enzyme increase (0.4%).

The most commonly reported adverse reactions (incidence ≥ 2% and greater than placebo) regardless of causality, in

Table 2. Clinical adverse reactions occurring in ≥ 2% in patients treated with any dose of LIPITOR and at an incidence greater than placebo regardless of causality (% of patients).

Adverse Reaction*	Any dose N=8755	10 mg N=3908	20 mg N=188	40 mg N=604	80 mg N=4055	Placebo N=7311
Nasopharyngitis	8.3	12.9	5.3	7.0	4.2	8.2
Arthralgia	6.9	8.9	11.7	10.6	4.3	6.5
Diarrhea	6.8	7.3	6.4	14.1	5.2	6.3
Pain in extremity	6.0	8.5	3.7	9.3	3.1	5.9
Urinary tract infection	5.7	6.9	6.4	8.0	4.1	5.6
Dyspepsia	4.7	5.9	3.2	6.0	3.3	4.3
Nausea	4.0	3.7	3.7	7.1	3.8	3.5
Musculoskeletal pain	3.8	5.2	3.2	5.1	2.3	3.6
Muscle Spasms	3.6	4.6	4.8	5.1	2.4	3.0
Myalgia	3.5	3.6	5.9	8.4	2.7	3.1
Insomnia	3.0	2.8	1.1	5.3	2.8	2.9
Pharyngolaryngeal pain	2.3	3.9	1.6	2.8	0.7	2.1

* Adverse Reaction ≥ 2% in any dose greater than placebo

patients treated with LIPITOR in placebo controlled trials (n=8755) were: nasopharyngitis (8.3%), arthralgia (6.9%), diarrhea (6.8%), pain in extremity (6.0%), and urinary tract infection (5.7%).

Table 2 summarizes the frequency of clinical adverse reactions, regardless of causality, reported in ≥ 2% and at a rate greater than placebo in patients treated with LIPITOR (n=8755), from seventeen placebo-controlled trials.

[See table 2 above]

Other adverse reactions reported in placebo-controlled studies include:

Body as a whole: malaise, pyrexia; *Digestive system:* abdominal discomfort, eructation, flatulence, hepatitis, cholestasis;

Musculoskeletal system: musculoskeletal pain, muscle fatigue, neck pain, joint swelling; *Metabolic and nutritional system:* transaminases increase, liver function test abnormal, blood alkaline phosphatase increase, creatine phosphokinase increase, hyperglycemia; *Nervous system:* nightmare; *Respiratory system:* epistaxis; *Skin and appendages:* urticaria; *Special senses:* vision blurred, tinnitus; *Urogenital system:* white blood cells urine positive.

Anglo-Scandinavian Cardiac Outcomes Trial (ASCOT)

In ASCOT [see *Clinical Studies (14.1)*] involving 10,305 participants (age range 40–80 years, 19% women; 94.6% Caucasians, 2.6% Africans, 1.5% South Asians, 1.3% mixed/other) treated with LIPITOR 10 mg daily (n=5,168) or placebo (n=5,137), the safety and tolerability profile of the group treated with LIPITOR was comparable to that of the group treated with placebo during a median of 3.3 years of follow-up.

Collaborative Atorvastatin Diabetes Study (CARDS)

In CARDS [see *Clinical Studies (14.1)*] involving 2,838 subjects (age range 39–77 years, 32% women; 94.3% Caucasians, 2.4% South Asians, 2.3% Afro-Caribbean, 1.0% other) with type 2 diabetes treated with LIPITOR 10 mg daily (n=1,428) or placebo (n=1,410), there was no difference in the overall frequency of adverse reactions or serious adverse reactions between the treatment groups during a median follow-up of 3.9 years. No cases of rhabdomyolysis were reported.

Treating to New Targets Study (TNT)

In TNT [see *Clinical Studies (14.1)*] involving 10,001 subjects (age range 29–78 years, 19% women; 94.1% Caucasians, 2.9% Blacks, 1.0% Asians, 2.0% other) with clinically evident CHD treated with LIPITOR 10 mg daily (n=5006) or LIPITOR 80 mg daily (n=4995), there were more serious adverse reactions and discontinuations due to adverse reactions in the high-dose atorvastatin group (92, 1.8%; 497, 9.9%, respectively) as compared to the low-dose group (69, 1.4%; 404, 8.1%, respectively) during a median follow-up of 4.9 years. Persistent transaminase elevations (≥3 × ULN twice within 4–10 days) occurred in 62 (1.3%) individuals with atorvastatin 80 mg and in nine (0.2%) individuals with atorvastatin 10 mg. Elevations of CK (≥ 10 × ULN) were low overall, but were higher in the high-dose atorvastatin treatment group (13, 0.3%) compared to the low-dose atorvastatin group (6, 0.1%).

Incremental Decrease in Endpoints through Aggressive Lipid Lowering Study (IDEAL)

In IDEAL [see *Clinical Studies (14.1)*] involving 8,888 subjects (age range 26–80 years, 19% women; 99.3% Caucasians, 0.4% Asians, 0.3% Blacks, 0.04% other) treated with LIPITOR 80 mg/day (n=4439) or simvastatin 20–40 mg daily (n=4449), there was no difference in the overall frequency of adverse reactions or serious adverse reactions between the treatment groups during a median follow-up of 4.8 years.

Stroke Prevention by Aggressive Reduction in Cholesterol Levels (SPARCL)

In SPARCL involving 4731 subjects (age range 21–92 years, 40% women; 93.3% Caucasians, 3.0% Blacks, 0.6% Asians, 3.1% other) without clinically evident CHD but with a stroke or transient ischemic attack (TIA) within the previous 6 months treated with LIPITOR 80 mg (n=2365) or placebo (n=2366) for a median follow-up of 4.9 years, there was a higher incidence of persistent hepatic transaminase elevations (≥ 3 × ULN twice within 4–10 days) in the atorvastatin group (0.9%) compared to placebo (0.1%). Elevations of CK (>10 × ULN) were rare, but were higher in the atorvastatin group (0.1%) compared to placebo (0.0%). Diabetes was reported as an adverse reaction in 144 subjects (6.1%) in the atorvastatin group and 89 subjects (3.8%) in the placebo group [see *Warnings and Precautions (5.5)*].

In a post-hoc analysis, LIPITOR 80 mg reduced the incidence of ischemic stroke (218/2365, 9.2% vs. 274/2366, 11.6%) and increased the incidence of hemorrhagic stroke (55/2365, 2.3% vs. 33/2366, 1.4%) compared to placebo. The incidence of fatal hemorrhagic stroke was similar between groups (17 LIPITOR vs. 18 placebo). The incidence of non-fatal hemorrhagic strokes was significantly greater in the atorvastatin group (38 non-fatal hemorrhagic strokes) as compared to the placebo group (16 non-fatal hemorrhagic strokes). Subjects who entered the study with a hemorrhagic stroke appeared to be at increased risk for hemorrhagic stroke [7 (16%) LIPITOR vs. 2 (4%) placebo].

There were no significant differences between the treatment groups for all-cause mortality: 216 (9.1%) in the LIPITOR 80 mg/day group vs. 211 (8.9%) in the placebo group. The proportions of subjects who experienced cardiovascular death were numerically smaller in the LIPITOR 80 mg group (3.3%) than in the placebo group (4.1%). The proportions of subjects who experienced non-cardiovascular death were numerically larger in the LIPITOR 80 mg group (5.0%) than in the placebo group (4.0%).

6.2 Postmarketing Experience

The following adverse reactions have been identified during postapproval use of LIPITOR. Because these reactions are reported voluntarily from a population of uncertain size, it is not always possible to reliably estimate their frequency or establish a causal relationship to drug exposure.

Adverse reactions associated with LIPITOR therapy reported since market introduction, that are not listed above, regardless of causality assessment, include the following: anaphylaxis, angioneurotic edema, bullous rashes (including erythema multiforme, Stevens-Johnson syndrome, and toxic epidermal necrolysis), rhabdomyolysis, fatigue, tendon rupture, hepatic failure, dizziness, memory impairment, depression, and peripheral neuropathy.

6.3 Pediatric Patients (ages 10-17 years)

In a 26-week controlled study in boys and postmenarchal girls (n=140, 31% female; 92% Caucasians, 1.6% Blacks, 1.6% Asians, 4.8% other), the safety and tolerability profile of LIPITOR 10 to 20 mg daily was generally similar to that of placebo [see *Clinical Studies (14.6)* and *Use in Special Populations, Pediatric Use (8.4)*].

7 DRUG INTERACTIONS

The risk of myopathy during treatment with statins is increased with concurrent administration of fibric acid derivatives, lipid-modifying doses of niacin, cyclosporine, or strong CYP 3A4 inhibitors (e.g., clarithromycin, HIV protease inhibitors, and itraconazole) [see *Warnings and Precautions, Skeletal Muscle (5.1)* and *Clinical Pharmacology (12.3)*].

7.1 Strong Inhibitors of CYP 3A4: LIPITOR is metabolized by cytochrome P450 3A4. Concomitant administration of LIPITOR with strong inhibitors of CYP 3A4 can lead to increases in plasma concentrations of atorvastatin. The extent of interaction and potentiation of effects depend on the variability of effect on CYP 3A4.

Clarithromycin: Atorvastatin AUC was significantly increased with concomitant administration of LIPITOR 80 mg with clarithromycin (500 mg twice daily) compared to that of LIPITOR alone [see *Clinical Pharmacology (12.3)*]. Therefore, in patients taking clarithromycin, caution should be used when the LIPITOR dose exceeds 20 mg [see *Warnings and Precautions, Skeletal Muscle (5.1)* and *Dosage and Administration (2.6)*].

Combination of Protease Inhibitors: Atorvastatin AUC was significantly increased with concomitant administration of LIPITOR 40 mg with ritonavir plus saquinavir (400 mg twice daily) or LIPITOR 20 mg with lopinavir plus ritonavir (400 mg + 100 mg twice daily) compared to that of LIPITOR alone [see *Clinical Pharmacology (12.3)*]. Therefore, in patients taking HIV protease inhibitors, caution should be used when the LIPITOR dose exceeds 20 mg [see *Warnings and Precautions, Skeletal Muscle (5.1)* and *Dosage and Administration (2.6)*].

Itraconazole: Atorvastatin AUC was significantly increased with concomitant administration of LIPITOR 40 mg and itraconazole 200 mg [see *Clinical Pharmacology (12.3)*]. Therefore, in patients taking itraconazole, caution should be used when the LIPITOR dose exceeds 20 mg [see *Warnings and Precautions, Skeletal Muscle (5.1)* and *Dosage and Administration (2.6)*].

7.2 Grapefruit Juice: Contains one or more components that inhibit CYP 3A4 and can increase plasma concentrations of atorvastatin, especially with excessive grapefruit juice consumption (>1.2 liters per day).

7.3 Cyclosporine: Atorvastatin and atorvastatin-metabolites are substrates of the OATP1B1 transporter. Inhibitors of the OATP1B1 (e.g., cyclosporine) can increase the bioavailability of atorvastatin. Atorvastatin AUC was significantly increased with concomitant administration of LIPITOR 10 mg and cyclosporine 5.2 mg/kg/day compared to that of LIPITOR alone [see *Clinical Pharmacology (12.3)*]. In cases where co-administration of LIPITOR with cyclosporine is necessary, the dose of LIPITOR should not exceed 10 mg [see *Warnings and Precautions, Skeletal Muscle (5.1)*].

7.4 Rifampin or other Inducers of Cytochrome P450 3A4: Concomitant administration of LIPITOR with inducers of cytochrome P450 3A4 (e.g., efavirenz, rifampin) can lead to variable reductions in plasma concentrations of atorvastatin. Due to the dual interaction mechanism of rifampin, simultaneous co-administration of LIPITOR with rifampin is recommended, as delayed administration of LIPITOR after administration of rifampin has been associated with a significant reduction in atorvastatin plasma concentrations.

7.5 Digoxin: When multiple doses of LIPITOR and digoxin were coadministered, steady state plasma digoxin concentrations increased by approximately 20%. Patients taking digoxin should be monitored appropriately.

7.6 Oral Contraceptives: Co-administration of LIPITOR and an oral contraceptive increased AUC values for norethindrone and ethinyl estradiol [see *Clinical Pharmacology (12.3)*]. These increases should be considered when selecting an oral contraceptive for a woman taking LIPITOR.

7.7 Warfarin: LIPITOR had no clinically significant effect on prothrombin time when administered to patients receiving chronic warfarin treatment.

8 USE IN SPECIFIC POPULATIONS

8.1 Pregnancy

Pregnancy Category X

LIPITOR is contraindicated in women who are or may become pregnant. Serum cholesterol and triglycerides increase during normal pregnancy. Lipid lowering drugs offer no benefit during pregnancy because cholesterol and cholesterol derivatives are needed for normal fetal development. Atherosclerosis is a chronic process, and discontinuation of lipid-lowering drugs during pregnancy should have little impact on long-term outcomes of primary hypercholesterolemia therapy.

There are no adequate and well-controlled studies of atorvastatin use during pregnancy. There have been rare reports of congenital anomalies following intrauterine exposure to statins. In a review of about 100 prospectively followed pregnancies in women exposed to other statins, the incidences of congenital anomalies, spontaneous abortions, and fetal deaths/stillbirths did not exceed the rate expected in the general population. However, this study was only able to exclude a three-to-four-fold increased risk of congenital anomalies over background incidence. In 89% of these cases, drug treatment started before pregnancy and stopped during the first trimester when pregnancy was identified.

Atorvastatin crosses the rat placenta and reaches a level in fetal liver equivalent to that of maternal plasma. Atorvastatin was not teratogenic in rats at doses up to 300 mg/kg/day or in rabbits at doses up to 100 mg/kg/day. These doses resulted in multiples of about 30 times (rat) or 20 times (rabbit) the human exposure based on surface area (mg/m^2) [see *Contraindications, Pregnancy (4.3)*].

In a study in rats given 20, 100, or 225 mg/kg/day, from gestation day 7 through to lactation day 21 (weaning), there was decreased pup survival at birth, neonate, weaning, and maturity in pups of mothers dosed with 225 mg/kg/day. Body weight was decreased on days 4 and 21 in pups of mothers dosed at 100 mg/kg/day; pup body weight was decreased at birth and at days 4, 21, and 91 at 225 mg/kg/day. Pup development was delayed (rotorod performance at 100 mg/kg/day and acoustic startle at 225 mg/kg/day; pinnae detachment and eye-opening at 225 mg/kg/day). These doses correspond to 6 times (100 mg/kg) and 22 times (225 mg/kg) the human AUC at 80 mg/day.

Statins may cause fetal harm when administered to a pregnant woman. LIPITOR should be administered to women of childbearing potential only when such patients are highly unlikely to conceive and have been informed of the potential hazards. If the woman becomes pregnant while taking LIPITOR, it should be discontinued immediately and the patient advised again as to the potential hazards to the fetus and the lack of known clinical benefit with continued use during pregnancy.

8.3 Nursing Mothers

It is not known whether atorvastatin is excreted in human milk, but a small amount of another drug in this class does pass into breast milk. Nursing rat pups had plasma and liver drug levels of 50% and 40%, respectively, of that in their mother's milk. Animal breast milk drug levels may not accurately reflect human breast milk levels. Because another drug in this class passes into human milk and because statins have a potential to cause serious adverse reactions in nursing infants, women requiring LIPITOR treatment should be advised not to nurse their infants [see *Contraindications (4)*].

8.4 Pediatric Use

Safety and effectiveness in patients 10-17 years of age with heterozygous familial hypercholesterolemia have been evaluated in a controlled clinical trial of 6 months' duration in adolescent boys and postmenarchal girls. Patients treated with LIPITOR had an adverse experience profile generally similar to that of patients treated with placebo. The most common adverse experiences observed in both groups, regardless of causality assessment, were infections. **Doses greater than 20 mg have not been studied in this patient population.** In this limited controlled study, there was no significant effect on growth or sexual maturation in boys or on menstrual cycle length in girls [see *Clinical Studies (14.6); Adverse Reactions, Pediatric Patients (ages 10-17 years) (6.3); and Dosage and Administration, Heterozygous Familial Hypercholesterolemia in Pediatric Patients (10-17 years of age) (2.2)*]. Adolescent females should be counseled on appropriate contraceptive methods while on LIPITOR therapy [see *Contraindications, Pregnancy (4.3) and Use in Specific Populations, Pregnancy (8.1)*]. **LIPITOR has not been studied in controlled clinical trials involving prepubertal patients or patients younger than 10 years of age.** Clinical efficacy with doses up to 80 mg/day for 1 year have been evaluated in an uncontrolled study of patients with homozygous FH including 8 pediatric patients [see *Clinical Studies, Homozygous Familial Hypercholesterolemia (14.5)*].

8.5 Geriatric Use

Of the 39,828 patients who received LIPITOR in clinical studies, 15,813 (40%) were ≥65 years old and 2,800 (7%) were ≥75 years old. No overall differences in safety or effectiveness were observed between these subjects and younger subjects, and other reported clinical experience has not identified differences in responses between the elderly and younger patients, but greater sensitivity of some older adults cannot be ruled out. Since advanced age (≥65 years) is a predisposing factor for myopathy, LIPITOR should be prescribed with caution in the elderly.

8.6 Hepatic Impairment

Lipitor is contraindicated in patients with active liver disease which may include unexplained persistent elevations in hepatic transaminase levels [see *Contraindications (4) and Pharmacokinetics (12.3)*].

10 OVERDOSAGE

There is no specific treatment for LIPITOR overdosage. In the event of an overdose, the patient should be treated symptomatically, and supportive measures instituted as required. Due to extensive drug binding to plasma proteins, hemodialysis is not expected to significantly enhance LIPITOR clearance.

11 DESCRIPTION

LIPITOR is a synthetic lipid-lowering agent. Atorvastatin is an inhibitor of 3-hydroxy-3-methylglutaryl-coenzyme A (HMG-CoA) reductase. This enzyme catalyzes the conversion of HMG-CoA to mevalonate, an early and rate-limiting step in cholesterol biosynthesis.

Atorvastatin calcium is [R-(R*, R*)]-2-(4-fluorophenyl)-β, δ-dihydroxy-5-(1-methylethyl)-3-phenyl-4-[(phenylamino)-carbonyl]-1H-pyrrole-1-heptanoic acid, calcium salt (2:1) trihydrate. The empirical formula of atorvastatin calcium is $(C_{33}H_{34}FN_2O_5)_2Ca\cdot 3H_2O$ and its molecular weight is 1209.42. Its structural formula is:

TABLE 3. Effect of Co-administered Drugs on the Pharmacokinetics of Atorvastatin

Co-administered drug and dosing regimen	Atorvastatin		
	Dose (mg)	Change in AUC[&]	Change in Cmax[&]
#Cyclosporine 5.2 mg/kg/day, stable dose	10 mg QD for 28 days	↑ 8.7 fold	↑ 10.7 fold
#Lopinavir 400 mg BID/ritonavir 100 mg BID, 14 days	20 mg QD for 4 days	↑ 5.9 fold	↑ 4.7 fold
#Ritonavir 400 mg BID/saquinavir 400mg BID, 15 days	40 mg QD for 4 days	↑ 3.9 fold	↑ 4.3 fold
#Clarithromycin 500 mg BID, 9 days	80 mg QD for 8 days	↑ 4.4 fold	↑ 5.4 fold
#Itraconazole 200 mg QD, 4 days	40 mg SD	↑ 3.3 fold	↑ 20%
#Grapefruit Juice, 240 mL QD*	40 mg, SD	↑ 37%	↑ 16%
Diltiazem 240 mg QD, 28 days	40 mg, SD	↑ 51%	No change
Erythromycin 500 mg QID, 7 days	10 mg, SD	↑ 33%	↑ 38%
Amlodipine 10 mg, single dose	80 mg, SD	↑ 15%	↓ 12%
Cimetidine 300 mg QD, 4 weeks	10 mg QD for 2 weeks	↓ Less than 1%	↓ 11%
Colestipol 10 mg BID, 28 weeks	40 mg QD for 28 weeks	Not determined	↓ 26%**
Maalox TC® 30 mL QD, 17 days	10 mg QD for 15 days	↓ 33%	↓ 34%
Efavirenz 600 mg QD, 14 days	10 mg for 3 days	↓ 41%	↓ 1%
#Rifampin 600 mg QD, 7 days (co-administered)[†]	40 mg SD	↑ 30%	↑ 2.7 fold
#Rifampin 600 mg QD, 5 days (doses separated)[†]	40 mg SD	↓ 80%	↓ 40%
#Gemfibrozil 600mg BID, 7 days	40mg SD	↑ 35%	↓ Less than 1%
#Fenofibrate 160mg QD, 7 days	40mg SD	↑ 3%	↑ 2%

& Data given as x-fold change represent a simple ratio between co-administration and atorvastatin alone (i.e., 1-fold = no change). Data given as % change represent % difference relative to atorvastatin alone (i.e., 0% = no change).

See Sections 5.1 and 7 for clinical significance.

* Greater increases in AUC (up to 2.5 fold) and/or Cmax (up to 71%) have been reported with excessive grapefruit consumption (≥ 750 mL - 1.2 liters per day).

** Single sample taken 8-16 h post dose.

† Due to the dual interaction mechanism of rifampin, simultaneous co-administration of atorvastatin with rifampin is recommended, as delayed administration of atorvastatin after administration of rifampin has been associated with a significant reduction in atorvastatin plasma concentrations.

Atorvastatin calcium is a white to off-white crystalline powder that is insoluble in aqueous solutions of pH 4 and below. Atorvastatin calcium is very slightly soluble in distilled water, pH 7.4 phosphate buffer, and acetonitrile; slightly soluble in ethanol; and freely soluble in methanol.

LIPITOR Tablets for oral administration contain 10, 20, 40, or 80 mg atorvastatin and the following inactive ingredients: calcium carbonate, USP; candelilla wax, FCC; croscarmellose sodium, NF; hydroxypropyl cellulose, NF; lactose monohydrate, NF; magnesium stearate, NF; microcrystalline cellulose, NF; Opadry White YS-1-7040 (hypromellose, polyethylene glycol, talc, titanium dioxide); polysorbate 80, NF; simethicone emulsion.

12 CLINICAL PHARMACOLOGY

12.1 Mechanism of Action

LIPITOR is a selective, competitive inhibitor of HMG-CoA reductase, the rate-limiting enzyme that converts 3-hydroxy-3-methylglutaryl-coenzyme A to mevalonate, a precursor of sterols, including cholesterol. Cholesterol and triglycerides circulate in the bloodstream as part of lipoprotein complexes. With ultracentrifugation, these complexes separate into HDL (high-density lipoprotein), IDL (intermediate-density lipoprotein), LDL (low-density lipoprotein), and VLDL (very-low-density lipoprotein) fractions. Triglycerides (TG) and cholesterol in the liver are incorporated into VLDL and released into the plasma for delivery to peripheral tissues. LDL is formed from VLDL and is catabolized primarily through the high-affinity LDL receptor. Clinical and pathologic studies show that elevated plasma levels of total cholesterol (total-C), LDL-cholesterol (LDL-C), and apolipoprotein B (apo B) promote human atherosclerosis and are risk factors for developing cardiovascular disease, while increased levels of HDL-C are associated with a decreased cardiovascular risk.

In animal models, LIPITOR lowers plasma cholesterol and lipoprotein levels by inhibiting HMG-CoA reductase and cholesterol synthesis in the liver and by increasing the number of hepatic LDL receptors on the cell surface to enhance uptake and catabolism of LDL; LIPITOR also reduces LDL production and the number of LDL particles. LIPITOR reduces LDL-C in some patients with homozygous familial hypercholesterolemia (FH), a population that rarely responds to other lipid-lowering medication(s).

A variety of clinical studies have demonstrated that elevated levels of total-C, LDL-C, and apo B (a membrane complex for LDL-C) promote human atherosclerosis. Similarly, decreased levels of HDL-C (and its transport complex, apo A) are associated with the development of atherosclerosis. Epidemiologic investigations have established that cardiovascular morbidity and mortality vary directly with the level of total-C and LDL-C, and inversely with the level of HDL-C.

LIPITOR reduces total-C, LDL-C, and apo B in patients with homozygous and heterozygous FH, nonfamilial forms of hypercholesterolemia, and mixed dyslipidemia. LIPITOR also reduces VLDL-C and TG and produces variable increases in HDL-C and apolipoprotein A-1. LIPITOR reduces total-C, LDL-C, VLDL-C, apo B, TG, and non-HDL-C, and increases HDL-C in patients with isolated hypertriglyceridemia. LIPITOR reduces intermediate density lipoprotein cholesterol (IDL-C) in patients with dysbetalipoproteinemia.

Like LDL, cholesterol-enriched triglyceride-rich lipoproteins, including VLDL, intermediate density lipoprotein (IDL), and remnants, can also promote atherosclerosis. Elevated plasma triglycerides are frequently found in a triad with low HDL-C levels and small LDL particles, as well as in association with non-lipid metabolic risk factors for

TABLE 4. Effect of Atorvastatin on the Pharmacokinetics of Co-administered Drugs

Atorvastatin	Co-administered drug and dosing regimen		
	Drug/Dose (mg)	Change in AUC	Change in Cmax
80 mg QD for 15 days	Antipyrine, 600 mg SD	↑ 3%	↓ 11%
80 mg QD for 14 days	# Digoxin 0.25 mg QD, 20 days	↑ 15%	↑ 20%
40 mg QD for 22 days	Oral contraceptive QD, 2 months - norethindrone 1mg - ethinyl estradiol 35µg	↑ 28% ↑ 19%	↑ 23% ↑ 30%

See Section 7 for clinical significance.

TABLE 5. Overview of Efficacy Results in TNT

Endpoint	Atorvastatin 10 mg (N=5006)		Atorvastatin 80 mg (N=4995)		HRa (95%CI)
PRIMARY ENDPOINT	n	(%)	n	(%)	
First major cardiovascular endpoint	548	(10.9)	434	(8.7)	0.78 (0.69, 0.89)
Components of the Primary Endpoint					
CHD death	127	(2.5)	101	(2.0)	0.80 (0.61, 1.03)
Non-fatal, non-procedure related MI	308	(6.2)	243	(4.9)	0.78 (0.66, 0.93)
Resuscitated cardiac arrest	26	(0.5)	25	(0.5)	0.96 (0.56, 1.67)
Stroke (fatal and non-fatal)	155	(3.1)	117	(2.3)	0.75 (0.59, 0.96)
SECONDARY ENDPOINTS*					
First CHF with hospitalization	164	(3.3)	122	(2.4)	0.74 (0.59, 0.94)
First PVD endpoint	282	(5.6)	275	(5.5)	0.97 (0.83, 1.15)
First CABG or other coronary revascularization procedureb	904	(18.1)	667	(13.4)	0.72 (0.65, 0.80)
First documented angina endpointb	615	(12.3)	545	(10.9)	0.88 (0.79, 0.99)
All-cause mortality	282	(5.6)	284	(5.7)	1.01 (0.85, 1.19)
Components of All-Cause Mortality					
Cardiovascular death	155	(3.1)	126	(2.5)	0.81 (0.64, 1.03)
Noncardiovascular death	127	(2.5)	158	(3.2)	1.25 (0.99, 1.57)
Cancer death	75	(1.5)	85	(1.7)	1.13 (0.83, 1.55)
Other non-CV death	43	(0.9)	58	(1.2)	1.35 (0.91, 2.00)
Suicide, homicide and other traumatic non-CV death	9	(0.2)	15	(0.3)	1.67 (0.73, 3.82)

a Atorvastatin 80 mg: atorvastatin 10 mg
b Component of other secondary endpoints
* Secondary endpoints not included in primary endpoint
HR=hazard ratio; CHD=coronary heart disease; CI=confidence interval; MI=myocardial infarction; CHF=congestive heart failure; CV=cardiovascular; PVD=peripheral vascular disease; CABG=coronary artery bypass graft
Confidence intervals for the Secondary Endpoints were not adjusted for multiple comparisons

coronary heart disease. As such, total plasma TG has not consistently been shown to be an independent risk factor for CHD. Furthermore, the independent effect of raising HDL or lowering TG on the risk of coronary and cardiovascular morbidity and mortality has not been determined.

12.2 Pharmacodynamics

LIPITOR, as well as some of its metabolites, are pharmacologically active in humans. The liver is the primary site of action and the principal site of cholesterol synthesis and LDL clearance. Drug dosage, rather than systemic drug concentration, correlates better with LDL-C reduction. Individualization of drug dosage should be based on therapeutic response [see *Dosage and Administration (2)*].

12.3 Pharmacokinetics

Absorption: LIPITOR is rapidly absorbed after oral administration; maximum plasma concentrations occur within 1 to 2 hours. Extent of absorption increases in proportion to LIPITOR dose. The absolute bioavailability of atorvastatin (parent drug) is approximately 14% and the systemic availability of HMG-CoA reductase inhibitory activity is approximately 30%. The low systemic availability is attributed to presystemic clearance in gastrointestinal mucosa and/or hepatic first-pass metabolism. Although food decreases the rate and extent of drug absorption by approximately 25%

and 9%, respectively, as assessed by Cmax and AUC, LDL-C reduction is similar whether LIPITOR is given with or without food. Plasma LIPITOR concentrations are lower (approximately 30% for Cmax and AUC) following evening drug administration compared with morning. However, LDL-C reduction is the same regardless of the time of day of drug administration [see *Dosage and Administration (2)*].

Distribution: Mean volume of distribution of LIPITOR is approximately 381 liters. LIPITOR is ≥98% bound to plasma proteins. A blood/plasma ratio of approximately 0.25 indicates poor drug penetration into red blood cells. Based on observations in rats, LIPITOR is likely to be secreted in human milk [see *Contraindications, Nursing Mothers (4.4)* and *Use in Specific Populations, Nursing Mothers (8.3)*].

Metabolism: LIPITOR is extensively metabolized to ortho- and parahydroxylated derivatives and various beta-oxidation products. *In vitro* inhibition of HMG-CoA reductase by ortho- and parahydroxylated metabolites is equivalent to that of LIPITOR. Approximately 70% of circulating inhibitory activity for HMG-CoA reductase is attributed to active metabolites. *In vitro* studies suggest the importance of LIPITOR metabolism by cytochrome P450 3A4, consistent with increased plasma concentrations of LIPITOR in humans following co-administration with erythromycin, a known inhibitor of this isozyme [see *Drug*

Interactions (7.1)]. In animals, the ortho-hydroxy metabolite undergoes further glucuronidation.

Excretion: LIPITOR and its metabolites are eliminated primarily in bile following hepatic and/or extra-hepatic metabolism; however, the drug does not appear to undergo enterohepatic recirculation. Mean plasma elimination half-life of LIPITOR in humans is approximately 14 hours, but the half-life of inhibitory activity for HMG-CoA reductase is 20 to 30 hours due to the contribution of active metabolites. Less than 2% of a dose of LIPITOR is recovered in urine following oral administration.

Specific Populations

Geriatric: Plasma concentrations of LIPITOR are higher (approximately 40% for Cmax and 30% for AUC) in healthy elderly subjects (age ≥65 years) than in young adults. Clinical data suggest a greater degree of LDL-lowering at any dose of drug in the elderly patient population compared to younger adults [see *Use in Specific Populations, Geriatric Use (8.5)*].

Pediatric: Pharmacokinetic data in the pediatric population are not available.

Gender: Plasma concentrations of LIPITOR in women differ from those in men (approximately 20% higher for Cmax and 10% lower for AUC); however, there is no clinically significant difference in LDL-C reduction with LIPITOR between men and women.

Renal Impairment: Renal disease has no influence on the plasma concentrations or LDL-C reduction of LIPITOR; thus, dose adjustment in patients with renal dysfunction is not necessary [see *Dosage and Administration, Dosage in Patients with Renal Impairment (2.5), Warnings and Precautions, Skeletal Muscle (5.1)*].

Hemodialysis: While studies have not been conducted in patients with end-stage renal disease, hemodialysis is not expected to significantly enhance clearance of LIPITOR since the drug is extensively bound to plasma proteins.

Hepatic Impairment: In patients with chronic alcoholic liver disease, plasma concentrations of LIPITOR are markedly increased. Cmax and AUC are each 4-fold greater in patients with Childs-Pugh A disease. Cmax and AUC are approximately 16-fold and 11-fold increased, respectively, in patients with Childs-Pugh B disease [see *Contraindications (4.1)*].

[See table 3 at top of previous page]
[See table 4 above]

13 NONCLINICAL TOXICOLOGY

13.1 Carcinogenesis, Mutagenesis, Impairment of Fertility

In a 2-year carcinogenicity study in rats at dose levels of 10, 30, and 100 mg/kg/day, 2 rare tumors were found in muscle in high-dose females: in one, there was a rhabdomyosarcoma and, in another, there was a fibrosarcoma. This dose represents a plasma AUC (0-24) value of approximately 16 times the mean human plasma drug exposure after an 80 mg oral dose.

A 2-year carcinogenicity study in mice given 100, 200, or 400 mg/kg/day resulted in a significant increase in liver adenomas in high-dose males and liver carcinomas in high-dose females. These findings occurred at plasma AUC (0–24) values of approximately 6 times the mean human plasma drug exposure after an 80 mg oral dose.

In vitro, atorvastatin was not mutagenic or clastogenic in the following tests with and without metabolic activation: the Ames test with *Salmonella typhimurium* and *Escherichia coli*, the HGPRT forward mutation assay in Chinese hamster lung cells, and the chromosomal aberration assay in Chinese hamster lung cells. Atorvastatin was negative in the *in vivo* mouse micronucleus test.

Studies in rats performed at doses up to 175 mg/kg (15 times the human exposure) produced no changes in fertility. There was aplasia and aspermia in the epididymis of 2 of 10 rats treated with 100 mg/kg/day of atorvastatin for 3 months (16 times the human AUC at the 80 mg dose); testis weights were significantly lower at 30 and 100 mg/kg and epididymal weight was lower at 100 mg/kg. Male rats given 100 mg/kg/day for 11 weeks prior to mating had decreased sperm motility, spermatid head concentration, and increased abnormal sperm. Atorvastatin caused no adverse effects on semen parameters, or reproductive organ histopathology in dogs given doses of 10, 40, or 120 mg/kg for two years.

14 CLINICAL STUDIES

14.1 Prevention of Cardiovascular Disease

In the Anglo-Scandinavian Cardiac Outcomes Trial (ASCOT), the effect of LIPITOR on fatal and non-fatal coronary heart disease was assessed in 10,305 hypertensive patients 40–80 years of age (mean of 63 years), without a previous myocardial infarction and with TC levels ≤251 mg/dL (6.5 mmol/L). Additionally, all patients had at least 3 of the following cardiovascular risk factors: male gender (81.1%), age >55 years (84.5%), smoking (33.2%), diabetes (24.3%), history of CHD in a first-degree relative (26%), TC:HDL >6 (14.3%), peripheral vascular disease

(5.1%), left ventricular hypertrophy (14.4%), prior cerebrovascular event (9.8%), specific ECG abnormality (14.3%), proteinuria/albuminuria (62.4%). In this double-blind, placebo-controlled study, patients were treated with antihypertensive therapy (Goal BP <140/90 mm Hg for nondiabetic patients; <130/80 mm Hg for diabetic patients) and allocated to either LIPITOR 10 mg daily (n=5168) or placebo (n=5137), using a covariate adaptive method which took into account the distribution of nine baseline characteristics of patients already enrolled and minimized the imbalance of those characteristics across the groups. Patients were followed for a median duration of 3.3 years.

The effect of 10 mg/day of LIPITOR on lipid levels was similar to that seen in previous clinical trials.

LIPITOR significantly reduced the rate of coronary events [either fatal coronary heart disease (46 events in the placebo group vs. 40 events in the LIPITOR group) or non-fatal MI (108 events in the placebo group vs. 60 events in the LIPITOR group)] with a relative risk reduction of 36% [(based on incidences of 1.9% for LIPITOR vs. 3.0% for placebo), p=0.0005 (see Figure 1)]. The risk reduction was consistent regardless of age, smoking status, obesity, or presence of renal dysfunction. The effect of LIPITOR was seen regardless of baseline LDL levels. Due to the small number of events, results for women were inconclusive.

Figure 1: Effect of LIPITOR 10 mg/day on Cumulative Incidence of Non-Fatal Myocardial Infarction or Coronary Heart Disease Death (in ASCOT-LLA)

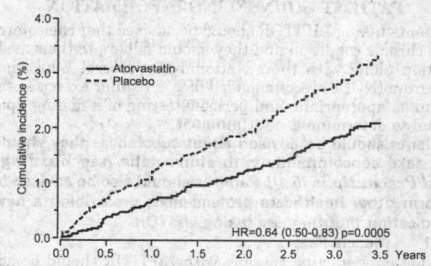

LIPITOR also significantly decreased the relative risk for revascularization procedures by 42%. Although the reduction of fatal and non-fatal strokes did not reach a predefined significance level (p=0.01), a favorable trend was observed with a 26% relative risk reduction (incidences of 1.7% for LIPITOR and 2.3% for placebo). There was no significant difference between the treatment groups for death due to cardiovascular causes (p=0.51) or noncardiovascular causes (p=0.17).

In the Collaborative Atorvastatin Diabetes Study (CARDS), the effect of LIPITOR on cardiovascular disease (CVD) endpoints was assessed in 2838 subjects (94% white, 68% male), ages 40–75 with type 2 diabetes based on WHO criteria, without prior history of cardiovascular disease and with LDL ≤ 160 mg/dL and TG ≤ 600 mg/dL. In addition to diabetes, subjects had 1 or more of the following risk factors: current smoking (23%), hypertension (80%), retinopathy (30%), or microalbuminuria (9%) or macroalbuminuria (3%). No subjects on hemodialysis were enrolled in the study. In this multicenter, placebo-controlled, double-blind clinical trial, subjects were randomly allocated to either LIPITOR 10 mg daily (1429) or placebo (1411) in a 1:1 ratio and were followed for a median duration of 3.9 years. The primary endpoint was the occurrence of any of the major cardiovascular events: myocardial infarction, acute CHD death, unstable angina, coronary revascularization, or stroke. The primary analysis was the time to first occurrence of the primary endpoint.

Baseline characteristics of subjects were: mean age of 62 years, mean HbA$_{1c}$ 7.7%; median LDL-C 120 mg/dL; median TC 207 mg/dL; median TG 151 mg/dL; median HDL-C 52 mg/dL.

The effect of LIPITOR 10 mg/day on lipid levels was similar to that seen in previous clinical trials.

LIPITOR significantly reduced the rate of major cardiovascular events (primary endpoint events) (83 events in the LIPITOR group vs. 127 events in the placebo group) with a relative risk reduction of 37%, HR 0.63, 95% CI (0.48, 0.83) (p=0.001) (see Figure 2). An effect of LIPITOR was seen regardless of age, sex, or baseline lipid levels.

LIPITOR significantly reduced the risk of stroke by 48% (21 events in the LIPITOR group vs. 39 events in the placebo group), HR 0.52, 95% CI (0.31, 0.89) (p=0.016) and reduced the risk of MI by 42% (38 events in the LIPITOR group vs. 64 events in the placebo group), HR 0.58, 95.1% CI (0.39, 0.86) (p=0.007). There was no significant difference between the treatment groups for angina, revascularization procedures, and acute CHD death.

TABLE 6. Dose Response in Patients With Primary Hyperlipidemia (Adjusted Mean % Change From Baseline)[a]

Dose	N	TC	LDL-C	Apo B	TG	HDL-C	Non-HDL-C/HDL-C
Placebo	21	4	4	3	10	-3	7
10	22	-29	-39	-32	-19	6	-34
20	20	-33	-43	-35	-26	9	-41
40	21	-37	-50	-42	-29	6	-45
80	23	-45	-60	-50	-37	5	-53

[a] Results are pooled from 2 dose-response studies.

TABLE 7. Mean Percentage Change From Baseline at Endpoint (Double-Blind, Randomized, Active-Controlled Trials)

Treatment (Daily Dose)	N	Total-C	LDL-C	Apo B	TG	HDL-C	Non-HDL-C/HDL-C
Study 1							
LIPITOR 10 mg	707	-27[a]	-36[a]	-28[a]	-17[a]	+7	-37[a]
Lovastatin 20 mg	191	-19	-27	-20	-6	+7	-28
95% CI for Diff[1]		-9.2, -6.5	-10.7, -7.1	-10.0, -6.5	-15.2, -7.1	-1.7, 2.0	-11.1, -7.1
Study 2							
LIPITOR 10 mg	222	-25[b]	-35[b]	-27[b]	-17[b]	+6	-36[b]
Pravastatin 20 mg	77	-17	-23	-17	-9	+8	-28
95% CI for Diff[1]		-10.8, -6.1	-14.5, -8.2	-13.4, -7.4	-14.1, -0.7	-4.9, 1.6	-11.5, -4.1
Study 3							
LIPITOR 10 mg	132	-29[c]	-37[c]	-34[c]	-23[c]	+7	-39[c]
Simvastatin 10 mg	45	-24	-30	-30	-15	+7	-33
95% CI for Diff[1]		-8.7, -2.7	-10.1, -2.6	-8.0, -1.1	-15.1, -0.7	-4.3, 3.9	-9.6, -1.9

[1] A negative value for the 95% CI for the difference between treatments favors LIPITOR for all except HDL-C, for which a positive value favors LIPITOR. If the range does not include 0, this indicates a statistically significant difference.
[a] Significantly different from lovastatin, ANCOVA, p ≤0.05
[b] Significantly different from pravastatin, ANCOVA, p ≤0.05
[c] Significantly different from simvastatin, ANCOVA, p ≤0.05

There were 61 deaths in the LIPITOR group vs. 82 deaths in the placebo group (HR 0.73, p=0.059).

Figure 2: Effect of LIPITOR 10 mg/day on Time to Occurrence of Major Cardiovascular Event (myocardial infarction, acute CHD death, unstable angina, coronary revascularization, or stroke) in CARDS

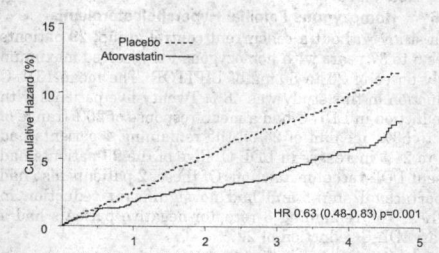

In the Treating to New Targets Study (TNT), the effect of LIPITOR 80 mg/day vs. LIPITOR 10 mg/day on the reduction in cardiovascular events was assessed in 10,001 subjects (94% white, 81% male, 38% ≥65 years) with clinically evident coronary heart disease who had achieved a target LDL-C level <130 mg/dL after completing an 8-week, open-label, run-in period with LIPITOR 10 mg/day. Subjects were randomly assigned to either 10 mg/day or 80 mg/day of LIPITOR and followed for a median duration of 4.9 years. The primary endpoint was the time-to-first occurrence of any of the following major cardiovascular events (MCVE): death due to CHD, non-fatal myocardial infarction, resuscitated cardiac arrest, and fatal and non-fatal stroke. The mean LDL-C, TC, TG, non-HDL, and HDL cholesterol levels at 12 weeks were 73, 145, 128, 98, and 47 mg/dL during treatment with 80 mg of LIPITOR and 99, 177, 152, 129, and 48 mg/dL during treatment with 10 mg of LIPITOR.

Treatment with LIPITOR 80 mg/day significantly reduced the rate of MCVE (434 events in the 80 mg/day group vs. 548 events in the 10 mg/day group) with a relative risk reduction of 22%, HR 0.78, 95% CI (0.69, 0.89), p=0.0002 (see Figure 3 and Table 5). The overall risk reduction was consistent regardless of age (<65, ≥65) or gender.

[See figure 3 at top of next column]
[See table 5 on previous page]
Of the events that comprised the primary efficacy endpoint, treatment with LIPITOR 80 mg/day significantly reduced the rate of non-fatal, non-procedure related MI and fatal and non-fatal stroke, but not CHD death or resuscitated cardiac arrest (Table 5). Of the predefined secondary endpoints, treatment with LIPITOR 80 mg/day significantly re-

Figure 3: Effect of LIPITOR 80 mg/day vs. 10 mg/day on Time to Occurrence of Major Cardiovascular Events (TNT)

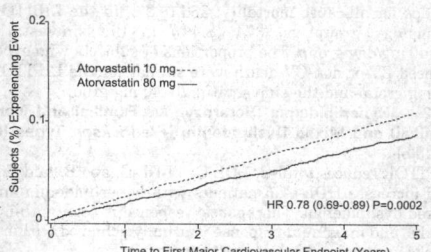

duced the rate of coronary revascularization, angina, and hospitalization for heart failure, but not peripheral vascular disease. The reduction in the rate of CHF with hospitalization was only observed in the 8% of patients with a prior history of CHF.

There was no significant difference between the treatment groups for all-cause mortality (Table 5). The proportions of subjects who experienced cardiovascular death, including the components of CHD death and fatal stroke, were numerically smaller in the LIPITOR 80 mg group than in the LIPITOR 10 mg treatment group. The proportions of subjects who experienced noncardiovascular death were numerically larger in the LIPITOR 80 mg group than in the LIPITOR 10 mg treatment group.

In the Incremental Decrease in Endpoints Through Aggressive Lipid Lowering Study (IDEAL), treatment with LIPITOR 80 mg/day was compared to treatment with simvastatin 20–40 mg/day in 8,888 subjects up to 80 years of age with a history of CHD to assess whether reduction in CV risk could be achieved. Patients were mainly male (81%), white (99%) with an average age of 61.7 years, and an average LDL-C of 121.5 mg/dL at randomization; 76% were on statin therapy. In this prospective, randomized, open-label, blinded endpoint (PROBE) trial with no run-in period, subjects were followed for a median duration of 4.8 years. The mean LDL-C, TC, TG, HDL, and non-HDL cholesterol levels at Week 12 were 78, 145, 115, 45, and 100 mg/dL during treatment with 80 mg of LIPITOR and 105, 179, 142, 47, and 132 mg/dL during treatment with 20–40 mg of simvastatin.

There was no significant difference between the treatment groups for the primary endpoint, the rate of first major coronary event (fatal CHD, non-fatal MI, and resuscitated cardiac arrest): 411 (9.3%) in the LIPITOR 80 mg/day group vs. 463 (10.4%) in the simvastatin 20–40 mg/day group, HR 0.89, 95% CI (0.78, 1.01), p=0.07.

TABLE 8. Combined Patients With Isolated Elevated TG: Median (min, max) Percentage Change From Baseline

	Placebo (N=12)	LIPITOR 10 mg (N=37)	LIPITOR 20 mg (N=13)	LIPITOR 80 mg (N=14)
Triglycerides	-12.4 (-36.6, 82.7)	-41.0 (-76.2, 49.4)	-38.7 (-62.7, 29.5)	-51.8 (-82.8, 41.3)
Total-C	-2.3 (-15.5, 24.4)	-28.2 (-44.9, -6.8)	-34.9 (-49.6, -15.2)	-44.4 (-63.5, -3.8)
LDL-C	3.6 (-31.3, 31.6)	-26.5 (-57.7, 9.8)	-30.4 (-53.9, 0.3)	-40.5 (-60.6, -13.8)
HDL-C	3.8 (-18.6, 13.4)	13.8 (-9.7, 61.5)	11.0 (-3.2, 25.2)	7.5 (-10.8, 37.2)
VLDL-C	-1.0 (-31.9, 53.2)	-48.8 (-85.8, 57.3)	-44.6 (-62.2, -10.8)	-62.0 (-88.2, 37.6)
non-HDL-C	-2.8 (-17.6, 30.0)	-33.0 (-52.1, -13.3)	-42.7 (-53.7, -17.4)	-51.5 (-72.9, -4.3)

TABLE 9. Open-Label Crossover Study of 16 Patients With Dysbetalipoproteinemia (Fredrickson Type III)

	Median (min, max) at Baseline (mg/dL)	Median % Change (min, max)	
		LIPITOR 10 mg	LIPITOR 80 mg
Total-C	442 (225, 1320)	-37 (-85, 17)	-58 (-90, -31)
Triglycerides	678 (273, 5990)	-39 (-92, -8)	-53 (-95, -30)
IDL-C + VLDL-C	215 (111, 613)	-32 (-76, 9)	-63 (-90, -8)
non-HDL-C	411 (218, 1272)	-43 (-87, -19)	-64 (-92, -36)

TABLE 10. Lipid-altering Effects of LIPITOR in Adolescent Boys and Girls with Heterozygous Familial Hypercholesterolemia or Severe Hypercholesterolemia (Mean Percentage Change From Baseline at Endpoint in Intention-to-Treat Population)

DOSAGE	N	Total-C	LDL-C	HDL-C	TG	Apolipoprotein B
Placebo	47	-1.5	-0.4	-1.9	1.0	0.7
LIPITOR	140	-31.4	-39.6	2.8	-12.0	-34.0

There were no significant differences between the treatment groups for all-cause mortality: 366 (8.2%) in the LIPITOR 80 mg/day group vs. 374 (8.4%) in the simvastatin 20–40 mg/day group. The proportions of subjects who experienced CV or non-CV death were similar for the LIPITOR 80 mg group and the simvastatin 20–40 mg group.

14.2 Hyperlipidemia (Heterozygous Familial and Nonfamilial) and Mixed Dyslipidemia (Fredrickson Types IIa and IIb)

LIPITOR reduces total-C, LDL-C, VLDL-C, apo B, and TG, and increases HDL-C in patients with hyperlipidemia and mixed dyslipidemia. Therapeutic response is seen within 2 weeks, and maximum response is usually achieved within 4 weeks and maintained during chronic therapy.

LIPITOR is effective in a wide variety of patient populations with hyperlipidemia, with and without hypertriglyceridemia, in men and women, and in the elderly.

In two multicenter, placebo-controlled, dose-response studies in patients with hyperlipidemia, LIPITOR given as a single dose over 6 weeks, significantly reduced total-C, LDL-C, apo B, and TG. (Pooled results are provided in Table 6.)

[See table 6 at top of previous page]

In patients with Fredrickson Types IIa and IIb hyperlipoproteinemia pooled from 24 controlled trials, the median (25th and 75th percentile) percent changes from baseline in HDL-C for LIPITOR 10, 20, 40, and 80 mg were 6.4 (-1.4, 14), 8.7 (0, 17), 7.8 (0, 16), and 5.1 (-2.7, 15), respectively. Additionally, analysis of the pooled data demonstrated consistent and significant decreases in total-C, LDL-C, TG, total-C/HDL-C, and LDL-C/HDL-C.

In three multicenter, double-blind studies in patients with hyperlipidemia, LIPITOR was compared to other statins. After randomization, patients were treated for 16 weeks with either LIPITOR 10 mg per day or a fixed dose of the comparative agent (Table 7).

[See table 7 on previous page]

The impact on clinical outcomes of the differences in lipid-altering effects between treatments shown in Table 7 is not known. Table 7 does not contain data comparing the effects of LIPITOR 10 mg and higher doses of lovastatin, pravastatin, and simvastatin. The drugs compared in the studies summarized in the table are not necessarily interchangeable.

14.3 Hypertriglyceridemia (Fredrickson Type IV)

The response to LIPITOR in 64 patients with isolated hypertriglyceridemia treated across several clinical trials is shown in the table below (Table 8). For the LIPITOR-treated patients, median (min, max) baseline TG level was 565 (267–1502).

[See table 8 above]

14.4 Dysbetalipoproteinemia (Fredrickson Type III)

The results of an open-label crossover study of 16 patients (genotypes: 14 apo E2/E2 and 2 apo E3/E2) with dysbetalipoproteinemia (Fredrickson Type III) are shown in the table below (Table 9).

[See table 9 above]

14.5 Homozygous Familial Hypercholesterolemia

In a study without a concurrent control group, 29 patients ages 6 to 37 years with homozygous FH received maximum daily doses of 20 to 80 mg of LIPITOR. The mean LDL-C reduction in this study was 18%. Twenty-five patients with a reduction in LDL-C had a mean response of 20% (range of 7% to 53%, median of 24%); the remaining 4 patients had 7% to 24% increases in LDL-C. Five of the 29 patients had absent LDL-receptor function. Of these, 2 patients also had a portacaval shunt and had no significant reduction in LDL-C. The remaining 3 receptor-negative patients had a mean LDL-C reduction of 22%.

14.6 Heterozygous Familial Hypercholesterolemia in Pediatric Patients

In a double-blind, placebo-controlled study followed by an open-label phase, 187 boys and postmenarchal girls 10-17 years of age (mean age 14.1 years) with heterozygous familial hypercholesterolemia (FH) or severe hypercholesterolemia, were randomized to LIPITOR (n=140) or placebo (n=47) for 26 weeks and then all received LIPITOR for 26 weeks. Inclusion in the study required 1) a baseline LDL-C level ≥ 190 mg/dL or 2) a baseline LDL-C level ≥ 160 mg/dL and positive family history of FH or documented premature cardiovascular disease in a first or second-degree relative. The mean baseline LDL-C value was 218.6 mg/dL (range: 138.5–385.0 mg/dL) in the LIPITOR group compared to 230.0 mg/dL (range: 160.0–324.5 mg/dL) in the placebo group. The dosage of LIPITOR (once daily) was 10 mg for the first 4 weeks and uptitrated to 20 mg if the LDL-C level was > 130 mg/dL. The number of LIPITOR-treated patients who required uptitration to 20 mg after Week 4 during the double-blind phase was 80 (57.1%).

LIPITOR significantly decreased plasma levels of total-C, LDL-C, triglycerides, and apolipoprotein B during the 26-week double-blind phase (see Table 10).

[See table 10 above]

The mean achieved LDL-C value was 130.7 mg/dL (range: 70.0–242.0 mg/dL) in the LIPITOR group compared to 228.5 mg/dL (range: 152.0–385.0 mg/dL) in the placebo group during the 26-week double-blind phase.

The safety and efficacy of doses above 20 mg have not been studied in controlled trials in children. The long-term efficacy of LIPITOR therapy in childhood to reduce morbidity and mortality in adulthood has not been established.

15 REFERENCES

[1] National Cholesterol Education Program (NCEP): Highlights of the Report of the Expert Panel on Blood Cholesterol Levels in Children and Adolescents, *Pediatrics*. 89(3): 495-501. 1992.

16 HOW SUPPLIED/STORAGE AND HANDLING

10 mg tablets: coded "PD 155" on one side and "10" on the other.
NDC 0071-0155-23 bottles of 90
NDC 0071-0155-34 bottles of 5000
NDC 0071-0155-40 10 × 10 unit dose blisters
20 mg tablets: coded "PD 156" on one side and "20" on the other.
NDC 0071-0156-23 bottles of 90
NDC 0071-0156-40 10 × 10 unit dose blisters
NDC 0071-0156-94 bottles of 5000
40 mg tablets: coded "PD 157" on one side and "40" on the other.
NDC 0071-0157-23 bottles of 90
NDC 0071-0157-73 bottles of 500
NDC 0071-0157-88 bottles of 2500
NDC 0071-0157-40 10 × 10 unit dose blisters
80 mg tablets: coded "PD 158" on one side and "80" on the other.
NDC 0071-0158-23 bottles of 90
NDC 0071-0158-73 bottles of 500
NDC 0071-0158-88 bottles of 2500
NDC 0071-0158-92 8 × 8 unit dose blisters
Storage
Store at controlled room temperature 20 - 25°C (68 - 77°F) [see USP].

17 PATIENT COUNSELING INFORMATION

Patients taking LIPITOR should be advised that cholesterol is a chronic condition and they should adhere to their medication along with their National Cholesterol Education Program (NCEP)-recommended diet, a regular exercise program as appropriate, and periodic testing of a fasting lipid panel to determine goal attainment.

Patients should be advised about substances they should not take concomitantly with atorvastatin [see Warnings and Precautions (5.1)]. Patients should also be advised to inform other healthcare professionals prescribing a new medication that they are taking LIPITOR.

17.1 Muscle Pain

All patients starting therapy with LIPITOR should be advised of the risk of myopathy and told to report promptly any unexplained muscle pain, tenderness, or weakness. The risk of this occurring is increased when taking certain types of medication or consuming larger quantities (>1 liter) of grapefruit juice. They should discuss all medication, both prescription and over the counter, with their healthcare professional.

17.2 Liver Enzymes

It is recommended that liver function tests be performed prior to and at 12 weeks following both the initiation of therapy and any elevation of dose, and periodically (e.g., semiannually) thereafter.

17.3 Pregnancy

Women of childbearing age should be advised to use an effective method of birth control to prevent pregnancy while using LIPITOR. Discuss future pregnancy plans with your patients, and discuss when to stop LIPITOR if they are trying to conceive. Patients should be advised that if they become pregnant, they should stop taking LIPITOR and call their healthcare professional.

17.4 Breastfeeding

Women who are breastfeeding should be advised to not use LIPITOR. Patients who have a lipid disorder and are breastfeeding, should be advised to discuss the options with their healthcare professional.

Rx Only
LAB-0021-24.0
Revised June 2009
PATIENT INFORMATION
LIPITOR®
atorvastatin calcium
tablets
(LIP-ih-tore)®
Read the Patient Information that comes with LIPITOR before you start taking it and each time you get a refill. There may be new information. This leaflet does not take the place of talking with your doctor about your condition or treatment.
If you have any questions about LIPITOR, ask your doctor or pharmacist.
What is LIPITOR?
LIPITOR is a prescription medicine that lowers cholesterol in your blood. It lowers the LDL-C ("bad" cholesterol) and triglycerides in your blood. It can raise your HDL-C ("good" cholesterol) as well. LIPITOR is for adults and children over 10 whose cholesterol does not come down enough with exercise and a low-fat diet alone.
LIPITOR can lower the risk for heart attack, stroke, certain types of heart surgery, and chest pain in patients who have heart disease or risk factors for heart disease such as:

- age, smoking, high blood pressure, low HDL-C, heart disease in the family.

LIPITOR can lower the risk for heart attack or stroke in patients with diabetes and risk factors such as:

- eye problems, kidney problems, smoking, or high blood pressure.

LIPITOR starts to work in about 2 weeks.

What is Cholesterol?

Cholesterol and triglycerides are fats that are made in your body. They are also found in foods. You need some cholesterol for good health, but too much is not good for you. Cholesterol and triglycerides can clog your blood vessels. It is especially important to lower your cholesterol if you have heart disease, smoke, have diabetes or high blood pressure, are older, or if heart disease starts early in your family.

Who Should Not Take LIPITOR?

Do not take LIPITOR if you:

- are pregnant or think you may be pregnant, or are planning to become pregnant. Lipitor may harm your unborn baby. If you get pregnant, stop taking LIPITOR and call your doctor right away.
- are breast feeding. LIPITOR can pass into your breast milk and may harm your baby.
- have liver problems.
- are allergic to LIPITOR or any of its ingredients. The active ingredient is atorvastatin. See the end of this leaflet for a complete list of ingredients in LIPITOR.

LIPITOR has not been studied in children under 10 years of age.

Before You Start LIPITOR

Tell your doctor if you:

- have muscle aches or weakness
- drink more than 2 glasses of alcohol daily
- have diabetes
- have a thyroid problem
- have kidney problems

Some medicines should not be taken with LIPITOR. Tell your doctor about all the medicines you take, including prescription and non-prescription medicines, vitamins, and herbal supplements. LIPITOR and certain other medicines can interact causing serious side effects. Especially tell your doctor if you take medicines for:

- your immune system
- cholesterol
- infections
- birth control
- heart failure
- HIV or AIDS

Know all the medicines you take. Keep a list of them with you to show your doctor and pharmacist.

How Should I Take LIPITOR?

- Take LIPITOR exactly as prescribed by your doctor. Do not change your dose or stop LIPITOR without talking to your doctor. Your doctor may do blood tests to check your cholesterol levels during your treatment with LIPITOR. Your dose of LIPITOR may be changed based on these blood test results.
- Take LIPITOR each day at any time of day at about the same time each day. LIPITOR can be taken with or without food.
  Don't break LIPITOR tablets before taking.
- Your doctor should start you on a low-fat diet before giving you LIPITOR. Stay on this low-fat diet when you take LIPITOR.
- If you miss a dose of LIPITOR, take it as soon as you remember. Do not take LIPITOR if it has been more than 12 hours since you missed your last dose. Wait and take the next dose at your regular time. Do not take 2 doses of LIPITOR at the same time.
- If you take too much LIPITOR or overdose, call your doctor or Poison Control Center right away. Or go to the nearest emergency room.

What Should I Avoid While Taking LIPITOR?

- Talk to your doctor before you start any new medicines. This includes prescription and non-prescription medicines, vitamins, and herbal supplements. LIPITOR and certain other medicines can interact causing serious side effects.
- Do not get pregnant. If you get pregnant, stop taking LIPITOR right away and call your doctor.

What are the Possible Side Effects of LIPITOR?

LIPITOR can cause serious side effects. These side effects have happened only to a small number of people. Your doctor can monitor you for them. These side effects usually go away if your dose is lowered or LIPITOR is stopped. These serious side effects include:

- **Muscle problems.** LIPITOR can cause serious muscle problems that can lead to kidney problems, including kidney failure. You have a higher chance for muscle problems if you are taking certain other medicines with LIPITOR.
- **Liver problems.** LIPITOR can cause liver problems. Your doctor may do blood tests to check your liver before you start taking LIPITOR, and while you take it.

Call your doctor right away if you have:

- muscle problems like weakness, tenderness, or pain that happen without a good reason, especially if you also have a fever or feel more tired than usual.
- allergic reactions including swelling of the face, lips, tongue, and/or throat that may cause difficulty in breathing or swallowing which may require treatment right away.
- nausea and vomiting.
- passing brown or dark-colored urine.
- you feel more tired than usual
- your skin and whites of your eyes get yellow.
- stomach pain.
- allergic skin reactions.

In clinical studies, patients reported the following common side effects while taking LIPITOR: diarrhea, upset stomach, muscle and joint pain, and alterations in some laboratory blood tests.

The following additional side effects have been reported with LIPITOR: tiredness, and tendon problems.

Talk to your doctor or pharmacist if you have side effects that bother you or that will not go away.

These are not all the side effects of LIPITOR. Ask your doctor or pharmacist for a complete list.

How do I store LIPITOR

- Store LIPITOR at room temperature, 68 to 77°F (20 to 25°C).
- Do not keep medicine that is out of date or that you no longer need.
- **Keep LIPITOR and all medicines out of the reach of children.** Be sure that if you throw medicine away, it is out of the reach of children.

General Information About LIPITOR

Medicines are sometimes prescribed for conditions that are not mentioned in patient information leaflets. Do not use LIPITOR for a condition for which it was not prescribed. Do not give LIPITOR to other people, even if they have the same problem you have. It may harm them.

This leaflet summarizes the most important information about LIPITOR. If you would like more information, talk with your doctor. You can ask your doctor or pharmacist for information about LIPITOR that is written for health professionals. Or you can go to the LIPITOR website at www.lipitor.com.

What are the Ingredients in LIPITOR?

Active Ingredient: atorvastatin calcium

Inactive Ingredients: calcium carbonate, USP; candelilla wax, FCC; croscarmellose sodium, NF; hydroxypropyl cellulose, NF; lactose monohydrate, NF; magnesium stearate, NF; microcrystalline cellulose, NF; Opadry White YS-1-7040 (hypromellose, polyethylene glycol, talc, titanium dioxide); polysorbate 80, NF; simethicone emulsion.

Rx Only

Distributed by:
Parke-Davis
Division of Pfizer Inc, NY, NY 10017
**Manufactured by Pfizer Ireland
Pharmaceuticals
Dublin, Ireland**
LAB-0348-4.0   June 2009

PBM Pharmaceuticals, Inc.
**204 NORTH MAIN STREET
GORDONSVILLE, VA 22942**

Direct Inquiries to:
Customer Service
866-366-6282
Fax 866-435-1487

ANIMI-3®

[ă-nĭ-mĭ̄ 3]

Each Capsule contains:

Folic Acid	1 mg
Vitamin B$_6$	12.5 mg
Vitamin B$_{12}$	500 mcg
Omega-3 Acids	500 mg
-Docosahexaenoic Acid (DHA)	350 mg
-Eicosapentaenoic Acid (EPA)	35 mg
Phytosterols	200 mg

Patent Pending
Rx Only

DESCRIPTION

Animi-3® Capsules are intended for oral administration. Each Capsule Contains: 1 mg Folic Acid USP, 12.5 mg Vitamin B-6 (Pyridoxine Hydrochloride, USP), 500 mcg Vitamin B-12 (Cyanocobalamin, USP), 200 mg Phytosterols and

Pharmaceutical Grade Omega-3 Fish Oil providing 500 mg Omega-3 Acids; including 350 mg Docosahexaenoic Acid (DHA) and 35 mg Eicosapentaenoic Acid (EPA). Also Contains: Bleached Lecithin NF, Ascorbic Acid USP, Mixed Tocopherols NF, Ascorbyl Palmitate NF and a soft shell capsule (which contains; Gelatin USP, Glycerin NF, Titanium Dioxide USP, FD&C Red 40 and USP Purified Water).

INDICATION

Animi-3® Capsules are indicated for improving nutritional status in conditions requiring Essential Fatty Acid, Vitamin B12, B6 and Folic Acid supplementation as well as for patients where cholesterol levels are a concern.

CONTRAINDICATIONS

This product is contraindicated in patients with a known hypersensitivity to any of the ingredients.

PRECAUTIONS

Folic Acid in doses above 0.1 mg daily may obscure pernicious anemia in that hematological remission can occur while neurological manifestations remain progressive.

Pediatric Use
Safety and effectiveness in pediatric patients have not been established.

Pregnancy and Lactation
The safety of phytosterols has not been studied in pregnant or breastfeeding women. There is no evidence that dietary intakes of naturally occurring phytosterols, such as those consumed by vegetarian women, adversely affects pregnancy or lactation.

ADVERSE REACTIONS

Allergic sensitization has been reported following oral, enteral and parenteral administration of folic acid.

DOSAGE AND ADMINISTRATION

Adults – One to Four capsules daily or as directed by a physician.

HOW SUPPLIED

Animi-3® supplied as red opaque oblong Capsules. Each Capsule is imprinted with "Animi-3" in black opacode.
Animi-3® Capsules are available in bottles of 60 capsules (NDC 66213-541-60).
Keep out of reach of children.
Dispense in a well-closed, tight light-resistant container as defined in the USP using a child-resistant closure.
Storage Conditions: Store at 20-25°C (68-77°F). See USP Controlled Room Temperature. Protect from light and moisture.
PBM Pharmaceuticals, Inc.
Gordonsville, VA 22942
Rev. 0507
© 2004 All Rights Reserved.
PHM 08240 SST
PBM Pharmaceuticals
800-485-9828
www.animi-3.com

Shown in Product Identification Guide, page 317

DONNATAL EXTENTABS®   ℞
Rev. 06/07
℞ Only

DESCRIPTION

Each Donnatal Extentabs® tablet contains:

Phenobarbital, USP (¾ gr.)	48.6 mg
Hyoscyamine Sulfate, USP	0.3111 mg
Atropine Sulfate, USP	0.0582 mg
Scopolamine Hydrobromide, USP	0.0195 mg

Each Donnatal Extentabs® tablet contains the equivalent of three Donnatal® tablets. Extentabs are designed to release the ingredients gradually to provide effects for up to twelve (12) hours.

In addition, each tablet contains the following inactive ingredients: Anhydrous Lactose, Calcium Sulfate Granular, Colloidal Silicon Dioxide, Dibasic Calcium Phosphate, Lactose Monohydrate, Magnesium Stearate, and Stearic Acid. Film Coating and Polishing Solution contains: D&C Yellow #10 Aluminum Lake, FD&C Blue #1 Aluminum Lake, Hydroxypropyl Methylcellulose, Polydextrose, Polyethylene Glycol, Titanium Dioxide, and Triacetin. The printing ink contains Titanium Dioxide.

ACTIONS

This drug combination provides natural belladonna alkaloids in a specific, fixed ratio combined with phenobarbital to provide peripheral anticholinergic/antispasmodic action and mild sedation.

INDICATIONS

Based on a review of this drug by the National Academy of Sciences - National Research Council and/or other information, FDA has classified the following indications as "possibly" effective:

For use as adjunctive therapy in the treatment of irritable bowel syndrome (irritable colon, spastic colon, mucous colitis) and acute enterocolitis.

May also be useful as adjunctive therapy in the treatment of duodenal ulcer. IT HAS NOT BEEN SHOWN CONCLUSIVELY WHETHER ANTICHOLINERGIC/ANTISPASMODIC DRUGS AID IN THE HEALING OF A DUODENAL ULCER, DECREASE THE RATE OF RECURRENCES OR PREVENT COMPLICATIONS.

CONTRAINDICATIONS

Glaucoma, obstructive uropathy (for example, bladder neck obstruction due to prostatic hypertrophy); obstructive disease of the gastrointestinal tract (as in achalasia, pyloroduodenal stenosis, etc.); paralytic ileus, intestinal atony of the elderly or debilitated patient; unstable cardiovascular status in acute hemorrhage; severe ulcerative colitis especially if complicated by toxic megacolon; myasthenia gravis; hiatal hernia associated with reflux esophagitis.

Donnatal Extentabs® is contraindicated in patients with known hypersensitivity to any of the ingredients. Phenobarbital is contraindicated in acute intermittent porphyria and in those patients in whom phenobarbital produces restlessness and/or excitement.

WARNINGS

In the presence of a high environmental temperature, heat prostration can occur with belladonna alkaloids (fever and heatstroke due to decreased sweating).

Diarrhea may be an early symptom of incomplete intestinal obstruction, especially in patients with ileostomy or colostomy. In this instance treatment with this drug would be inappropriate and possibly harmful.

Donnatal Extentabs® may produce drowsiness or blurred vision. The patient should be warned, should these occur, not to engage in activities requiring mental alertness, such as operating a motor vehicle or other machinery, and not to perform hazardous work.

Phenobarbital may decrease the effect of anticoagulants and necessitate larger doses of the anticoagulant for optimal effect. When phenobarbital is discontinued, the dose of the anticoagulant may have to be decreased.

Phenobarbital may be habit forming and should not be administered to individuals known to be addiction prone or to those with a history of physical and/or psychological dependence upon drugs.

Since barbiturates are metabolized in the liver, they should be used with caution and initial doses should be small in patients with hepatic dysfunction.

PRECAUTIONS

Use with caution in patients with: autonomic neuropathy, hepatic or renal disease, hyperthyroidism, coronary heart disease, congestive heart failure, cardiac arrhythmias, tachycardia, and hypertension.

Belladonna alkaloids may produce a delay in gastric emptying (antral stasis) which would complicate the management of gastric ulcer.

Theoretically, with overdosage, a curare-like action may occur.

Carcinogenesis, mutagenesis: Long-term studies in animals have not been performed to evaluate carcinogenic potential.

Pregnancy Category C: Animal reproduction studies have not been conducted with Donnatal Extentabs®. It is not known whether Donnatal Extentabs® can cause fetal harm when administered to a pregnant woman or can affect reproduction capacity. Donnatal Extentabs® should be given to a pregnant woman only if clearly needed.

Nursing mothers: It is not known whether this drug is excreted in human milk. Because many drugs are excreted in human milk, caution should be exercised when Donnatal Extentabs® is administered to a nursing mother.

ADVERSE REACTIONS

Adverse reactions may include xerostomia; urinary hesitancy and retention; blurred vision; tachycardia; palpitation; mydriasis; cycloplegia; increased ocular tension; loss of taste sense; headache; nervousness; drowsiness; weakness; dizziness; insomnia; nausea; vomiting; impotence; suppression of lactation; constipation; bloated feeling; musculoskeletal pain; severe allergic reaction or drug idiosyncrasies, including anaphylaxis, urticaria and other dermal manifestations; and decreased sweating. Acquired hypersensitivity to barbituates consists chiefly in allergic reactions that occur especially in persons who tend to have asthma, urticaria, angioedema and similar conditions. Hypersensitivity reactions in this category include localized swelling, particularly of the eyelids, cheeks, or lips, and erythematous dermatitis. Rarely, exfoliative dermatitis (e.g. Stevens-Johnson syndrome and toxic epidermal necrolysis) may be caused by phenobarbital and can prove fatal. The skin eruption may be associated with fever, delirium, and marked degenerative changes in the liver and other parenchymatous organs. In a few cases, megaloblastic anemia has been associated with the chronic use of phenobarbital. Elderly patients may react with symptoms of excitement, agitation, drowsiness, and other untoward manifestations to even small doses of the drug.

Phenobarbital may produce excitement in some patients, rather than a sedative effect. In patients habituated to barbiturates, abrupt withdrawal may produce delirium or convulsions.

DOSAGE AND ADMINISTRATION

The dosage of Donnatal Extentabs® should be adjusted to the needs of the individual patient to assure symptomatic control with a minimum of adverse reactions. The usual dose is one tablet every twelve (12) hours. If indicated, one tablet every eight (8) hours may be given.

OVERDOSAGE

The signs and symptoms of overdose are headache, nausea, vomiting, blurred vision, dilated pupils, hot and dry skin, dizziness, dryness of the mouth, difficulty in swallowing, and CNS stimulation. Treatment should consist of gastric lavage, emetics, and activated charcoal. If indicated, parenteral cholinergic agents such as physostigmine or bethanechol chloride should be added.

HOW SUPPLIED

Donnatal Extentabs® Tablets are supplied as: film coated green, round, compressed tablets printed "P421" in black ink.

Bottles of 100 tablets

Bottles of 500 tablets

Store at 20-25°C (68-77°F) [See USP Controlled Room Temperature]. Protect from light and moisture.

Dispense in a well-closed, light-resistant container as defined in the USP using a child-resistant closure.

Also available: Donnatal® Tablets in bottles of 100 and 1000 tablets and Donnatal® Elixir in 4 fl oz bottles and 1 pint bottles.

Manufactured For:

PBM Pharmaceuticals, Inc.

Gordonsville, VA 22942

Manufactured By:

West-ward Pharmaceutical Corp.

Eatontown, NJ 07724

Revised June 2007

Shown in Product Identification Guide, page 317

Pfizer Inc.

235 EAST 42ND STREET
NEW YORK, NY 10017–5755

For updates to the product information listed below, please check the Pfizer Web site, http://www.pfizerpro.com, or call (800) 438-1985. For complete product listing, please see the Manufacturers' Index.

For Medical Information, Contact:

(800) 438-1985

24 hours a day, 7 days a week

Distribution:

1855 Shelby Oaks Drive North

Memphis, TN 38134

(901) 387-5200

Customer Service:

(800) 533-4535

Pfizer companies include:

Agouron Pharmaceuticals

Parke-Davis – see Parke-Davis

Pharmacia & Upjohn – see Pharmacia & Upjohn

G.D. Searle & Co. – see G.D. Searle & Co.

CADUET®

[*CAD-oo-et*]

(amlodipine besylate/atorvastatin calcium)

Tablets

Rx

DESCRIPTION

CADUET® (amlodipine besylate and atorvastatin calcium) tablets combine the calcium channel blocker amlodipine besylate with the lipid-lowering agent atorvastatin calcium. The amlodipine besylate component of CADUET is chemically described as 3-ethyl-5-methyl ($\pm$)-2-[(2-amino-ethoxy)methyl]-4-(o-chlorophenyl)-1,4-dihydro-6-methyl-3,5-pyridinedicarboxylate, monobenzenesulphonate. Its empirical formula is $C_{20}H_{25}ClN_2O_5 \cdot C_6H_6O_3S$.

The atorvastatin calcium component of CADUET is chemically described as [R-(R*, R*)]-2-(4-fluorophenyl)-β,δ-dihydroxy-5-(1-methylethyl)-3-phenyl-4-[(phenylamino) carbonyl]-1H-pyrrole-1-heptanoic acid, calcium salt (2:1) trihydrate. Its empirical formula is $(C_{33}H_{34}FN_2O_5)_2Ca \cdot 3H_2O$. The structural formulae for amlodipine besylate and atorvastatin calcium are shown below.

Amlodipine besylate

Atorvastatin calcium

CADUET contains amlodipine besylate, a white to off-white crystalline powder, and atorvastatin calcium, also a white to off-white crystalline powder. Amlodipine besylate has a molecular weight of 567.1 and atorvastatin calcium has a molecular weight of 1209.42. Amlodipine besylate is slightly soluble in water and sparingly soluble in ethanol. Atorvastatin calcium is insoluble in aqueous solutions of pH 4 and below. Atorvastatin calcium is very slightly soluble in distilled water, pH 7.4 phosphate buffer, and acetonitrile; slightly soluble in ethanol, and freely soluble in methanol. CADUET tablets are formulated for oral administration in the following strength combinations:

[See table 1 at top of next page]

Each tablet also contains calcium carbonate, croscarmellose sodium, microcrystalline cellulose, pregelatinized starch, polysorbate 80, hydroxypropyl cellulose, purified water, colloidal silicon dioxide (anhydrous), magnesium stearate, Opadry® II White 85F28751 (polyvinyl alcohol, titanium dioxide, PEG 3000 and talc) or Opadry® II Blue 85F10919 (polyvinyl alcohol, titanium dioxide, PEG 3000, talc and FD&C blue #2). Combinations of atorvastatin with 2.5 mg and 5 mg amlodipine are film coated white, and combinations of atorvastatin with 10 mg amlodipine are film coated blue.

CLINICAL PHARMACOLOGY

Mechanism of Action

CADUET

CADUET is a combination of two drugs, a dihydropyridine calcium channel blocker amlodipine and an HMG-CoA reductase inhibitor atorvastatin. The amlodipine component of CADUET inhibits the transmembrane influx of calcium ions into vascular smooth muscle and cardiac muscle. The atorvastatin component of CADUET is a selective, competitive inhibitor of HMG-CoA reductase (statin), the rate-limiting enzyme that converts 3-hydroxy-3-methylglutaryl-coenzyme A to mevalonate, a precursor of sterols, including cholesterol.

Amlodipine

Experimental data suggest that amlodipine binds to both dihydropyridine and nondihydropyridine binding sites. The contractile processes of cardiac muscle and vascular smooth muscle are dependent upon the movement of extracellular calcium ions into these cells through specific ion channels. Amlodipine inhibits calcium ion influx across cell membranes selectively, with a greater effect on vascular smooth muscle cells than on cardiac muscle cells. Negative inotropic effects can be detected *in vitro* but such effects have not been seen in intact animals at therapeutic doses. Serum calcium concentration is not affected by amlodipine. Amlodipine is a peripheral arterial vasodilator that acts directly on vascular smooth muscle to cause a reduction in peripheral vascular resistance and reduction in blood pressure.

The precise mechanisms by which amlodipine relieves angina have not been fully delineated, but are thought to include the following:

Exertional Angina: In patients with exertional angina, amlodipine reduces the total peripheral resistance (afterload) against which the heart works and reduces the rate pressure product, and thus myocardial oxygen demand, at any given level of exercise.

Vasospastic Angina: Amlodipine has been demonstrated to block constriction and restore blood flow in coronary arteries and arterioles in response to calcium, potassium epinephrine, serotonin, and thromboxane A_2 analog in experimental animal models and in human coronary vessels *in vitro*. This inhibition of coronary spasm is responsible for the effectiveness of amlodipine in vasospastic (Prinzmetal's or variant) angina.

Atorvastatin

Cholesterol and triglycerides circulate in the bloodstream as part of lipoprotein complexes. With ultracentrifugation, these complexes separate into HDL (high-density lipoprotein), IDL (intermediate-density lipoprotein), LDL (low-density lipoprotein), and VLDL (very-low-density lipoprotein) fractions. Triglycerides (TG) and cholesterol in the liver are incorporated into VLDL and released into the plasma for delivery to peripheral tissues. LDL is formed from VLDL and is catabolized primarily through the high-affinity LDL receptor.

Clinical and pathologic studies show that elevated plasma levels of total cholesterol (total-C), LDL-cholesterol (LDL-C), and apolipoprotein B (apo B) promote human atherosclerosis and are risk factors for developing cardiovascular disease, while increased levels of HDL-C are associated with a decreased cardiovascular risk.

Epidemiologic investigations have established that cardiovascular morbidity and mortality vary directly with the level of total-C and LDL-C, and inversely with the level of HDL-C.

In animal models, atorvastatin lowers plasma cholesterol and lipoprotein levels by inhibiting HMG-CoA reductase and cholesterol synthesis in the liver and by increasing the number of hepatic LDL receptors on the cell-surface to enhance uptake and catabolism of LDL; atorvastatin also reduces LDL production and the number of LDL particles.

Atorvastatin reduces total-C, LDL-C, and apo B in patients with homozygous and heterozygous familial hypercholesterolemia (FH), nonfamilial forms of hypercholesterolemia, and mixed dyslipidemia. Atorvastatin also reduces VLDL-C and TG and produces variable increases in HDL-C and apolipoprotein A-1. Atorvastatin reduces total-C, LDL-C, VLDL-C, apo B, TG, and non-HDL-C, and increases HDL-C in patients with isolated hypertriglyceridemia. Atorvastatin reduces intermediate density lipoprotein cholesterol (IDL-C) in patients with dysbetalipoproteinemia.

Like LDL, cholesterol-enriched triglyceride-rich lipoproteins, including VLDL, intermediate density lipoprotein (IDL), and remnants, can also promote atherosclerosis. Elevated plasma triglycerides are frequently found in a triad with low HDL-C levels and small LDL particles, as well as in association with non-lipid metabolic risk factors for coronary heart disease. As such, total plasma TG has not consistently been shown to be an independent risk factor for CHD. Furthermore, the independent effect of raising HDL or lowering TG on the risk of coronary and cardiovascular morbidity and mortality has not been determined.

Pharmacokinetics and Metabolism

Absorption

Studies with amlodipine: After oral administration of therapeutic doses of amlodipine alone, absorption produces peak plasma concentrations between 6 and 12 hours. Absolute bioavailability has been estimated to be between 64% and 90%.

Studies with atorvastatin: After oral administration alone, atorvastatin is rapidly absorbed; maximum plasma concentrations occur within 1 to 2 hours. Extent of absorption increases in proportion to atorvastatin dose. The absolute bioavailability of atorvastatin (parent drug) is approximately 14% and the systemic availability of HMG-CoA reductase inhibitory activity is approximately 30%. The low systemic availability is attributed to presystemic clearance in gastrointestinal mucosa and/or hepatic first-pass metabolism. Plasma atorvastatin concentrations are lower (approximately 30% for Cmax and AUC) following evening drug administration compared with morning. However, LDL-C reduction is the same regardless of the time of day of drug administration (see **DOSAGE AND ADMINISTRATION**).

Studies with CADUET: Following oral administration of CADUET peak plasma concentrations of amlodipine and atorvastatin are seen at 6 to 12 hours and 1 to 2 hours post dosing, respectively. The rate and extent of absorption (bioavailability) of amlodipine and atorvastatin from CADUET are not significantly different from the bioavailability of amlodipine and atorvastatin administered separately (see above).

Table 1. CADUET Tablet Strengths

	2.5 mg/10mg	2.5 mg/20mg	2.5 mg/40mg	5 mg/10 mg	5 mg/20 mg	5 mg/40 mg	5 mg/80 mg	10 mg/10 mg	10 mg/20 mg	10 mg/40 mg	10 mg/80 mg
amlodipine equivalent (mg)	2.5	2.5	2.5	5	5	5	5	10	10	10	10
atorvastatin equivalent (mg)	10	20	40	10	20	40	80	10	20	40	80

TABLE 2. Effect of Co-administered Drugs on the Pharmacokinetics of Atorvastatin

Co-administered drug and dosing regimen	Atorvastatin		
	Dose (mg)	Change in AUC[&]	Change in Cmax[&]
#Cyclosporine 5.2 mg/kg/day, stable dose	10 mg QD for 28 days	↑ 8.7-fold	↑ 10.7-fold
#Lopinavir 400 mg BID/ritonavir 100 mg BID, 14 days	20 mg QD for 4 days	↑ 5.9-fold	↑ 4.7-fold
#Ritonavir 400 mg BID/saquinavir 400mg BID, 15 days	40 mg QD for 4 days	↑ 3.9-fold	↑ 4.3-fold
#Clarithromycin 500 mg BID, 9 days	80 mg QD for 8 days	↑ 4.4-fold	↑ 5.4-fold
#Itraconazole 200 mg QD, 4 days	40 mg SD	↑ 3.3-fold	↑ 20%
#Grapefruit Juice, 240 mL QD*	40 mg, SD	↑ 37%	↑ 16%
Diltiazem 240 mg QD, 28 days	40 mg, SD	↑ 51%	No change
Erythromycin 500 mg QID, 7 days	10 mg, SD	↑ 33%	↑ 38%
Amlodipine 10 mg, single dose	80 mg, SD	↑ 15%	↓ 12%
Cimetidine 300 mg QD, 4 weeks	10 mg QD for 2 weeks	↓ Less than 1%	↓ 11%
Colestipol 10 mg BID, 28 weeks	40 mg QD for 28 weeks	Not determined	↓ 26%**
Maalox TC® 30 mL QD, 17 days	10 mg QD for 15 days	↓ 33%	↓ 34%
Efavirenz 600 mg QD, 14 days	10 mg for 3 days	↓ 41%	↓ 1%
#Rifampin 600 mg QD, 7 days (co-administered)[†]	40 mg SD	↑ 30%	↑ 2.7-fold
#Rifampin 600 mg QD, 5 days (doses separated)[†]	40 mg SD	↓ 80%	↓ 40%
#Gemfibrozil 600mg BID, 7 days	40mg SD	↑ 35%	↓ Less than 1%
#Fenofibrate 160mg QD, 7 days	40mg SD	↑ 3%	↑ 2%

& Data given as x-fold change represent a simple ratio between co-administration and atorvastatin alone (i.e., 1-fold = no change). Data given as % change represent % difference relative to atorvastatin alone (i.e., 0% = no change).
# See WARNINGS, Skeletal Muscle and PRECAUTIONS, Drug Interactions for clinical significance.
* Greater increases in AUC (up to 2.5-fold) and/or Cmax (up to 71%) have been reported with excessive grapefruit consumption (≥ 750 mL-1.2 liters per day).
**Single sample taken 8-16 h post dose.
† Due to the dual interaction mechanism of rifampin, simultaneous co-administration of atorvastatin with rifampin is recommended, as delayed administration of atorvastatin after administration of rifampin has been associated with a significant reduction in atorvastatin plasma concentrations.

The bioavailability of amlodipine from CADUET was not affected by food. Food decreases the rate and extent of absorption of atorvastatin from CADUET by approximately 32% and 11%, respectively, as it does with atorvastatin when given alone. LDL-C reduction is similar whether atorvastatin is given with or without food.

Distribution

Studies with amlodipine: *Ex vivo* studies have shown that approximately 93% of the circulating amlodipine drug is bound to plasma proteins in hypertensive patients. Steady-state plasma levels of amlodipine are reached after 7 to 8 days of consecutive daily dosing.

Studies with atorvastatin: Mean volume of distribution of atorvastatin is approximately 381 liters. Atorvastatin is ≥98% bound to plasma proteins. A blood/plasma ratio of approximately 0.25 indicates poor drug penetration into red blood cells. Based on observations in rats, atorvastatin calcium is likely to be secreted in human milk (see **CONTRAINDICATIONS, Pregnancy and Lactation**, and **PRECAUTIONS, Nursing Mothers**).

Metabolism

Studies with amlodipine: Amlodipine is extensively (about 90%) converted to inactive metabolites via hepatic metabolism.

Studies with atorvastatin: Atorvastatin is extensively metabolized to ortho- and parahydroxylated derivatives and various beta-oxidation products. *In vitro* inhibition of HMG-CoA reductase by ortho- and parahydroxylated metabolites is equivalent to that of atorvastatin. Approximately 70% of circulating inhibitory activity for HMG-CoA reductase is attributed to active metabolites. *In vitro* studies suggest the importance of atorvastatin metabolism by cytochrome P450 3A4, consistent with increased plasma concentrations of atorvastatin in humans following coadministration with erythromycin, a known inhibitor of this isozyme (see **PRECAUTIONS, Drug Interactions**). In animals, the ortho-hydroxy metabolite undergoes further glucuronidation.

Excretion

Studies with amlodipine: Elimination from the plasma is biphasic with a terminal elimination half-life of about 30-50 hours. Ten percent of the parent amlodipine compound and 60% of the metabolites of amlodipine are excreted in the urine.

Studies with atorvastatin: Atorvastatin and its metabolites are eliminated primarily in bile following hepatic and/or extra-hepatic metabolism; however, the drug does not appear to undergo enterohepatic recirculation. Mean plasma elimination half-life of atorvastatin in humans is approximately 14 hours, but the half-life of inhibitory activity for HMG-CoA reductase is 20 to 30 hours due to the contribution of active metabolites. Less than 2% of a dose of atorvastatin is recovered in urine following oral administration.

Specific Populations

Geriatric

Studies with amlodipine: Elderly patients have decreased clearance of amlodipine with a resulting increase in AUC of approximately 40-60%, and a lower initial dose of amlodipine may be required.

Studies with atorvastatin: Plasma concentrations of atorvastatin are higher (approximately 40% for Cmax and 30% for AUC) in healthy elderly subjects (age ≥65 years)

TABLE 3. Effect of Atorvastatin on the Pharmacokinetics of Co-administered Drugs

Atorvastatin	Co-administered drug and dosing regimen		
	Drug/Dose (mg)	Change in AUC	Change in Cmax
80 mg QD for 15 days	Antipyrine, 600 mg SD	↑ 3%	↓ 11%
80 mg QD for 14 days	#Digoxin 0.25 mg QD, 20 days	↑ 15%	↑ 20%
40 mg QD for 22 days	Oral contraceptive QD, 2 months - norethindrone 1mg - ethinyl estradiol 35µg	 ↑ 28% ↑ 19%	 ↑ 23% ↑ 30%

See PRECAUTIONS, Drug Interactions for clinical significance.

than in young adults. Clinical data suggest a greater degree of LDL-lowering at any dose of atorvastatin in the elderly population compared to younger adults (see **PRECAUTIONS, Geriatric Use**).

Pediatric

Studies with amlodipine: Sixty-two hypertensive patients aged 6 to 17 years received doses of amlodipine between 1.25 mg and 20 mg. Weight-adjusted clearance and volume of distribution were similar to values in adults.

Studies with atorvastatin: Pharmacokinetic data in the pediatric population are not available.

Gender

Studies with atorvastatin: Plasma concentrations of atorvastatin in women differ from those in men (approximately 20% higher for Cmax and 10% lower for AUC); however, there is no clinically significant difference in LDL-C reduction with atorvastatin between men and women.

Renal Impairment

Studies with amlodipine: The pharmacokinetics of amlodipine are not significantly influenced by renal impairment. Patients with renal failure may therefore receive the usual initial amlodipine dose.

Studies with atorvastatin: Renal disease has no influence on the plasma concentrations or LDL-C reduction of atorvastatin; thus, dose adjustment of atorvastatin in patients with renal dysfunction is not necessary (see **DOSAGE AND ADMINISTRATION** and **WARNINGS, Skeletal Muscle**).

Hemodialysis

While studies have not been conducted in patients with end-stage renal disease, hemodialysis is not expected to clear atorvastatin or amlodipine since both drugs are extensively bound to plasma proteins.

Hepatic Impairment

Atorvastatin is contraindicated in patients with active liver disease.

Studies with amlodipine: Elderly patients and patients with hepatic insufficiency have decreased clearance of amlodipine with a resulting increase in AUC of approximately 40-60%.

Studies with atorvastatin: In patients with chronic alcoholic liver disease, plasma concentrations of atorvastatin are markedly increased. Cmax and AUC are each 4-fold greater in patients with Childs-Pugh A disease. Cmax and AUC of atorvastatin are approximately 16-fold and 11-fold increased, respectively, in patients with Childs-Pugh B disease (see **CONTRAINDICATIONS**).

Heart Failure

Studies with amlodipine: In patients with moderate to severe heart failure, the increase in AUC for amlodipine was similar to that seen in the elderly and in patients with hepatic insufficiency.

Pharmacokinetic Studies of Atorvastatin and Co-Administered Drugs

[See table 2 on previous page]

[See table 3 above]

Pharmacodynamics

Hemodynamic Effects of Amlodipine: Following administration of therapeutic doses to patients with hypertension, amlodipine produces vasodilation resulting in a reduction of supine and standing blood pressures. These decreases in blood pressure are not accompanied by a significant change in heart rate or plasma catecholamine levels with chronic dosing. Although the acute intravenous administration of amlodipine decreases arterial blood pressure and increases heart rate in hemodynamic studies of patients with chronic stable angina, chronic administration of oral amlodipine in clinical trials did not lead to clinically significant changes in heart rate or blood pressures in normotensive patients with angina.

With chronic once daily oral administration of amlodipine, antihypertensive effectiveness is maintained for at least 24 hours. Plasma concentrations correlate with effect in both young and elderly patients. The magnitude of reduction in blood pressure with amlodipine is also correlated with the height of pretreatment elevation; thus, individuals with moderate hypertension (diastolic pressure 105-114 mmHg) had about a 50% greater response than patients with mild hypertension (diastolic pressure 90-104 mmHg). Normotensive subjects experienced no clinically significant change in blood pressures (+1/–2 mmHg).

In hypertensive patients with normal renal function, therapeutic doses of amlodipine resulted in a decrease in renal vascular resistance and an increase in glomerular filtration rate and effective renal plasma flow without change in filtration fraction or proteinuria.

As with other calcium channel blockers, hemodynamic measurements of cardiac function at rest and during exercise (or pacing) in patients with normal ventricular function treated with amlodipine have generally demonstrated a small increase in cardiac index without significant influence on dP/dt or on left ventricular end diastolic pressure or volume. In hemodynamic studies, amlodipine has not been associated with a negative inotropic effect when administered in the therapeutic dose range to intact animals and man, even when co-administered with beta-blockers to man. Similar findings, however, have been observed in normals or well-compensated patients with heart failure with agents possessing significant negative inotropic effects.

Electrophysiologic Effects of Amlodipine: Amlodipine does not change sinoatrial nodal function or atrioventricular conduction in intact animals or man. In patients with chronic stable angina, intravenous administration of 10 mg did not significantly alter A-H and H-V conduction and sinus node recovery time after pacing. Similar results were obtained in patients receiving amlodipine and concomitant beta blockers. In clinical studies in which amlodipine was administered in combination with beta-blockers to patients with either hypertension or angina, no adverse effects on electrocardiographic parameters were observed. In clinical trials with angina patients alone, amlodipine therapy did not alter electrocardiographic intervals or produce higher degrees of AV blocks.

LDL-C Reduction with Atorvastatin: Atorvastatin as well as some of its metabolites are pharmacologically active in humans. The liver is the primary site of action and the principal site of cholesterol synthesis and LDL clearance. Drug dosage, rather than systemic drug concentration, correlates better with LDL-C reduction. Individualization of drug dosage should be based on therapeutic response (see **DOSAGE AND ADMINISTRATION**).

Clinical Studies

Clinical Studies with Amlodipine

Amlodipine Effects in Hypertension

Adult Patients: The antihypertensive efficacy of amlodipine has been demonstrated in a total of 15 double-blind, placebo-controlled, randomized studies involving 800 patients on amlodipine and 538 on placebo. Once daily administration produced statistically significant placebo-corrected reductions in supine and standing blood pressures at 24 hours postdose, averaging about 12/6 mmHg in the standing position and 13/7 mmHg in the supine position in patients with mild to moderate hypertension. Maintenance of the blood pressure effect over the 24-hour dosing interval was observed, with little difference in peak and trough effect. Tolerance was not demonstrated in patients studied for up to 1 year. The 3 parallel, fixed doses, dose response studies showed that the reduction in supine and standing blood pressures was dose-related within the recommended dosing range. Effects on diastolic pressure were similar in young and older patients. The effect on systolic pressure was greater in older patients, perhaps because of greater baseline systolic pressure. Effects were similar in black patients and in white patients.

Pediatric Patients: Two-hundred sixty-eight hypertensive patients aged 6 to 17 years were randomized first to amlodipine 2.5 or 5 mg once daily for 4 weeks and then randomized again to the same dose or to placebo for another 4 weeks. Patients receiving 5 mg amlodipine at the end of 8 weeks had lower blood pressure than those secondarily randomized to placebo. The magnitude of the treatment effect is difficult to interpret, but it is probably less than 5 mmHg systolic on the 5 mg dose. Adverse events were similar to those seen in adults.

Amlodipine Effects in Chronic Stable Angina: The effectiveness of 5-10 mg/day of amlodipine in exercise-induced angina has been evaluated in 8 placebo-controlled, double-blind clinical trials of up to 6 weeks duration involving 1038 patients (684 amlodipine, 354 placebo) with chronic stable angina. In 5 of the 8 studies, significant increases in exercise time (bicycle or treadmill) were seen with the 10 mg dose. Increases in symptom-limited exercise time averaged 12.8% (63 sec) for amlodipine 10 mg, and averaged 7.9% (38 sec) for amlodipine 5 mg. Amlodipine 10 mg also increased time to 1 mm ST segment deviation in several studies and decreased angina attack rate. The sustained efficacy of amlodipine in angina patients has been demonstrated over long-term dosing. In patients with angina, there were no clinically significant reductions in blood pressures (4/1 mmHg) or changes in heart rate (+0.3 bpm).

Amlodipine Effects in Vasospastic Angina: In a double-blind, placebo-controlled clinical trial of 4 weeks duration in 50 patients, amlodipine therapy decreased attacks by approximately 4/week compared with a placebo decrease of approximately 1/week (p<0.01). Two of 23 amlodipine and 7 of 27 placebo patients discontinued from the study due to lack of clinical improvement.

Amlodipine Effects in Documented Coronary Artery Disease: In PREVENT, 825 patients with angiographically documented coronary artery disease were randomized to amlodipine (5-10 mg once daily) or placebo and followed for 3 years. Although the study did not show significance on the primary objective of change in coronary luminal diameter as assessed by quantitative coronary angiography, the data suggested a favorable outcome with respect to fewer hospitalizations for angina and revascularization procedures in patients with CAD.

CAMELOT enrolled 1318 patients with CAD recently documented by angiography, without left main coronary disease and without heart failure or an ejection fraction <40%. Patients (76% males, 89% Caucasian, 93% enrolled at US sites, 89% with a history of angina, 52% without PCI, 4% with PCI and no stent, and 44% with a stent) were randomized to double-blind treatment with either amlodipine (5–10 mg once daily) or placebo in addition to standard care that included aspirin (89%), statins (83%), beta-blockers (74%), nitroglycerin (50%), anti-coagulants (40%), and diuretics (32%), but excluded other calcium channel blockers. The mean duration of follow-up was 19 months. The primary endpoint was the time to first occurrence of one of the following events: hospitalization for angina pectoris, coronary revascularization, myocardial infarction, cardiovascular death, resuscitated cardiac arrest, hospitalization for heart failure, stroke/TIA, or peripheral vascular disease. A total of 110 (16.6%) and 151 (23.1%) first events occurred in the amlodipine and placebo groups respectively for a hazard ratio of 0.691 (95% CI: 0.540-0.884, p= 0.003). The primary endpoint is summarized in Figure 1 below. The outcome of this study was largely derived from the prevention of hospitalizations for angina and the prevention of revascularization procedures (see Table 4). Effects in various subgroups are shown in Figure 2.

In a angiographic substudy (n=274) conducted within CAMELOT, there was no significant difference between amlodipine and placebo on the change of atheroma volume in the coronary artery as assessed by intravascular ultrasound.

Figure 1: Kaplan-Meier analysis of composite clinical outcomes for amlodipine versus placebo

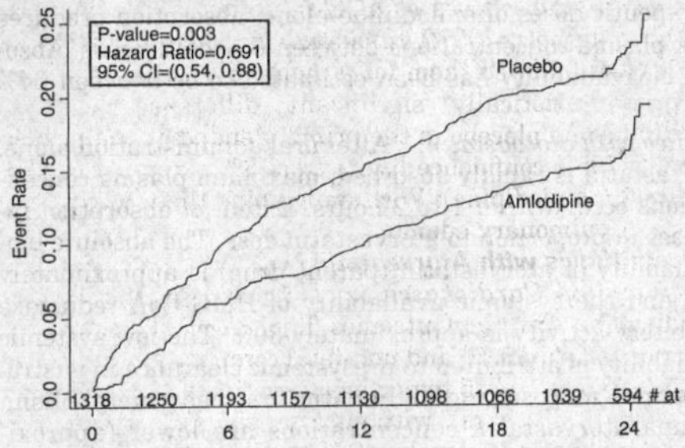

[See figure 2 at top of next page]

Table 4 below summarizes the significant composite endpoint and clinical outcomes from the composites of the primary endpoint. The other components of the primary endpoint including cardiovascular death, resuscitated cardiac arrest, myocardial infarction, hospitalization for heart failure, stroke/TIA, or peripheral vascular disease did not demonstrate a significant difference between amlodipine and placebo.

Figure 2 – Effects on primary endpoint of amlodipine versus placebo across subgroups

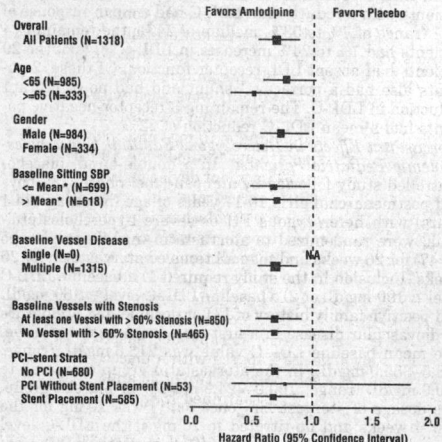

*The mean sitting baseline SBP is 129 mmHg

Table 4. Incidence of Significant Clinical Outcomes for CAMELOT

Clinical Outcomes N (%)	Amlodipine (N=663)	Placebo (N=655)	Risk Reduction (p-value)
Composite CV Endpoint	110 (16.6)	151 (23.1)	31% (0.003)
Hospitalization for Angina*	51 (7.7)	84 (12.8)	42% (0.002)
Coronary Revascularization*	78 (11.8)	103 (15.7)	27% (0.033)

*Total patients with these events

Amlodipine Effects in Patients with Congestive Heart Failure: Amlodipine has been compared to placebo in four 8-12 week studies of patients with NYHA class II/III heart failure, involving a total of 697 patients. In these studies, there was no evidence of worsened heart failure based on measures of exercise tolerance, NYHA classification, symptoms, or LVEF. In a long-term (follow-up at least 6 months, mean 13.8 months) placebo-controlled mortality/morbidity study of amlodipine 5-10 mg in 1153 patients with NYHA classes III (n=931) or IV (n=222) heart failure on stable doses of diuretics, digoxin, and ACE inhibitors, amlodipine had no effect on the primary endpoint of the study which was the combined endpoint of all-cause mortality and cardiac morbidity (as defined by life-threatening arrhythmia, acute myocardial infarction, or hospitalization for worsened heart failure), or on NYHA classification, or symptoms of heart failure. Total combined all-cause mortality and cardiac morbidity events were 222/571 (39%) for patients on amlodipine and 246/583 (42%) for patients on placebo; the cardiac morbid events represented about 25% of the endpoints in the study.

Another study (PRAISE-2) randomized patients with NYHA class III (80%) or IV (20%) heart failure without clinical symptoms or objective evidence of underlying ischemic disease, on stable doses of ACE inhibitor (99%), digitalis (99%) and diuretics (99%), to placebo (n=827) or amlodipine (n=827) and followed them for a mean of 33 months. There was no statistically significant difference between amlodipine and placebo in the primary endpoint of all cause mortality (95% confidence limits from 8% reduction to 29% increase on amlodipine). With amlodipine there were more reports of pulmonary edema.

Clinical Studies with Atorvastatin

Prevention of Cardiovascular Disease: In the Anglo-Scandinavian Cardiac Outcomes Trial (ASCOT), the effect of atorvastatin on fatal and non-fatal coronary heart disease was assessed in 10,305 hypertensive patients 40-80 years of age (mean of 63 years), without a previous myocardial infarction and with TC levels ≤251 mg/dl (6.5 mmol/l). Additionally all patients had at least 3 of the following cardiovascular risk factors: male gender (81.1%), age >55 years (84.5%), smoking (33.2%), diabetes (24.3%), history of CHD in a first-degree relative (26%), TC:HDL >6 (14.3%), peripheral vascular disease (5.1%), left ventricular hypertrophy (14.4%), prior cerebrovascular event (9.8%), specific ECG abnormality (14.3%), proteinuria/albuminuria (62.4%)]. In this double-blind, placebo-controlled study, patients were treated with anti-hypertensive therapy (Goal BP <140/90 mm Hg for non-diabetic patients; <130/80 mm Hg for diabetic patients) and allocated to either atorvastatin

10 mg daily (n=5168) or placebo (n=5137), using a covariate adaptive method which took into account the distribution of nine baseline characteristics of patients already enrolled and minimized the imbalance of those characteristics across the groups. Patients were followed for a median duration of 3.3 years.

The effect of 10 mg/day of atorvastatin on lipid levels was similar to that seen in previous clinical trials.

Atorvastatin significantly reduced the rate of coronary events [either fatal coronary heart disease (46 events in the placebo group vs. 40 events in the atorvastatin group) or nonfatal MI (108 events in the placebo group vs. 60 events in the atorvastatin group)] with a relative risk reduction of 36% [(based on incidences of 1.9% for atorvastatin vs. 3.0% for placebo), p=0.0005 (see Figure 3)]. The risk reduction was consistent regardless of age, smoking status, obesity or presence of renal dysfunction. The effect of atorvastatin was seen regardless of baseline LDL levels. Due to the small number of events, results for women were inconclusive.

Figure 3: Effect of Atorvastatin 10 mg/day on Cumulative Incidence of Nonfatal Myocardial Infarction or Coronary Heart Disease Death (in ASCOT-LLA)

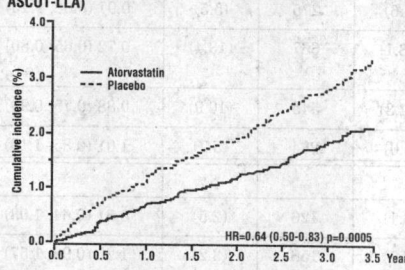

Atorvastatin also significantly decreased the relative risk for revascularization procedures by 42%. Although the reduction of fatal and non-fatal strokes did not reach a pre-defined significance level (p 0.01), a favorable trend was observed with a 26% relative risk reduction (incidences of 1.7% for atorvastatin and 2.3% for placebo). There was no significant difference between the treatment groups for death due to cardiovascular causes (p=0.51) or noncardiovascular causes (p=0.17).

In the Collaborative Atorvastatin Diabetes Study (CARDS), the effect of atorvastatin on cardiovascular disease (CVD) endpoints was assessed in 2838 subjects (94% White, 68% male), ages 40-75 with type 2 diabetes based on WHO criteria, without prior history of cardiovascular disease and with LDL ≤ 160 mg/dL and TG ≤ 600 mg/dL. In addition to diabetes, subjects had 1 or more of the following risk factors: current smoking (23%), hypertension (80%), retinopathy (30%), or microalbuminuria (9%) or macroalbuminuria (3%). No subjects on hemodialysis were enrolled in the study. In this multicenter, placebo-controlled, double-blind clinical trial, subjects were randomly allocated to either atorvastatin 10 mg daily (1429) or placebo (1411) in a 1:1 ratio and were followed for a median duration of 3.9 years. The primary endpoint was the occurrence of any of the major cardiovascular events: myocardial infarction, acute CHD death, unstable angina, coronary revascularization, or stroke. The primary analysis was the time to first occurrence of the primary endpoint.

Baseline characteristics of subjects were: mean age of 62 years, mean HbA₁c 7.7%; median LDL-C 120 mg/dL; median TC 207 mg/dL; median TG 151 mg/dL; median HDL-C 52 mg/dL.

The effect of atorvastatin 10 mg/day on lipid levels was similar to that seen in previous clinical trials.

Atorvastatin significantly reduced the rate of major cardiovascular events (primary endpoint events) (83 events in the atorvastatin group vs 127 events in the placebo group) with a relative risk reduction of 37%, HR 0.63, 95% CI (0.48,0.83) (p=0.001) (see Figure 4). An effect of atorvastatin was seen regardless of age, sex, or baseline lipid levels.

Figure 4. Effect of Atorvastatin 10 mg/day on Time to Occurrence of Major Cardiovascular Events (myocardial infarction, acute CHD death, unstable angina, coronary revascularization, or stroke) in CARDS.

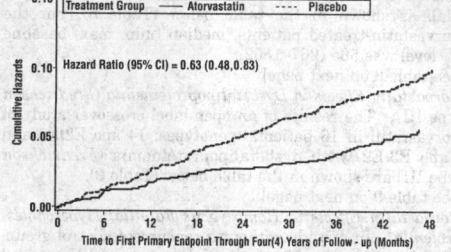

Atorvastatin significantly reduced the risk of stroke by 48% (21 events in the atorvastatin group vs. 39 events in the placebo group), HR 0.52, 95% CI (0.31, 0.89) (p=0.016) and reduced the risk of MI by 42% (38 events in the atorvastatin group vs. 64 events in the placebo group), HR 0.58, 95.1% CI (0.39, 0.86) (p=0.007). There was no significant difference between the treatment groups for angina, revascularization procedures, and acute CHD death.

There were 61 deaths in the atorvastatin group vs. 82 deaths in the placebo group, (HR 0.73, p=0.059).

In the Treating to New Targets Study (TNT), the effect of LIPITOR 80 mg/day vs. LIPITOR 10 mg/day on the reduction in cardiovascular events was assessed in 10,001 subjects (94% white, 81% male, 38% ≥65 years) with clinically evident coronary heart disease who had achieved a target LDL-C level <130 mg/dL after completing an 8-week, open-label, run-in period with LIPITOR 10 mg/day. Subjects were randomly assigned to either 10 mg/day or 80 mg/day of LIPITOR and followed for a median duration of 4.9 years. The primary endpoint was the time-to-first occurrence of any of the following major cardiovascular events (MCVE): death due to CHD, non-fatal myocardial infarction, resuscitated cardiac arrest, and fatal and non-fatal stroke. The mean LDL-C, TC, TG, non-HDL, and HDL cholesterol levels at 12 weeks were 73, 145, 128, 98, and 47 mg/dL during treatment with 80 mg of LIPITOR and 99, 177, 152, 129, and 48 mg/dL during treatment with 10 mg of LIPITOR.

Treatment with LIPITOR 80 mg/day significantly reduced the rate of MCVE (434 events in the 80mg/day group vs. 548 events in the 10 mg/day group) with a relative risk reduction of 22%, HR 0.78, 95% CI (0.69,0.89), p=0.0002 (see Figure 5 and Table 5). The overall risk reduction was consistent regardless of age (<65, ≥65) or gender.

Figure 5. Effect of LIPITOR 80 mg/day vs. 10 mg/day on Time to Occurrence of Major Cardiovascular Events (TNT)

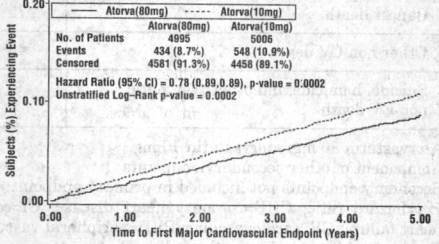

[See table 5 at top of next page]

Of the events that comprised the primary efficacy endpoint, treatment with LIPITOR 80 mg/day significantly reduced the rate of non-fatal, non-procedure related MI and fatal and non-fatal stroke, but not CHD death or resuscitated cardiac arrest (Table 5). Of the predefined secondary endpoints, treatment with LIPITOR 80 mg/day significantly reduced the rate of coronary revascularization, angina, and hospitalization for heart failure, but not peripheral vascular disease. The reduction in the rate of CHF with hospitalization was only observed in the 8% of patients with a prior history of CHF.

There was no significant difference between the treatment groups for all-cause mortality (Table 5). The proportions of subjects who experienced cardiovascular death, including the components of CHD death and fatal stroke, were numerically smaller in the LIPITOR 80 mg group than in the LIPITOR 10 mg treatment group. The proportions of subjects who experienced noncardiovascular death were numerically larger in the LIPITOR 80 mg group than in the LIPITOR 10 mg treatment group.

In the Incremental Decrease in Endpoints Through Aggressive Lipid Lowering Study (IDEAL), treatment with LIPITOR 80 mg/day was compared to treatment with simvastatin 20–40 mg/day in 8,888 subjects up to 80 years of age with a history of CHD to assess whether reduction in CV risk could be achieved. Patients were mainly male (81%), white (99%) with an average age of 61.7 years, and an average LDL-C of 121.5 mg/dL at randomization; 76% were on statin therapy. In this prospective, randomized, open-label, blinded endpoint (PROBE) trial with no run-in period, subjects were followed for a median duration of 4.8 years. The mean LDL-C, TC, TG, HDL, and non-HDL cholesterol levels at Week 12 were 78, 145, 115, 45, and 100 mg/dL during treatment with 80 mg of LIPITOR and 105, 179, 142, 47, and 132 mg/dL during treatment with 20–40 mg of simvastatin.

There was no significant difference between the treatment groups for the primary endpoint, the rate of first major coronary event (fatal CHD, nonfatal MI and resuscitated cardiac arrest): 411 (9.3%) in the LIPITOR 80 mg/day group vs. 463 (10.4%) in the simvastatin 20–40 mg/day group, HR 0.89, 95% CI (0.78, 1.01), p=0.07.

There were no significant differences between the treatment groups for all-cause mortality: 366 (8.2%) in the LIPITOR

TABLE 5. Overview of Efficacy Results in TNT

Endpoint	Atorvastatin 10 mg (N=5006)		Atorvastatin 80 mg (N=4995)		HR[a] (95%CI)
PRIMARY ENDPOINT	n	(%)	n	(%)	
First major cardiovascular endpoint	548	(10.9)	434	(8.7)	0.78 (0.69, 0.89)
Components of the Primary Endpoint					
CHD death	127	(2.5)	101	(2.0)	0.80 (0.61, 1.03)
Non-fatal, non-procedure related MI	308	(6.2)	243	(4.9)	0.78 (0.66, 0.93)
Resuscitated cardiac arrest	26	(0.5)	25	(0.5)	0.96 (0.56, 1.67)
Stroke (fatal and non-fatal)	155	(3.1)	117	(2.3)	0.75 (0.59, 0.96)
SECONDARY ENDPOINTS*					
First CHF with hospitalization	164	(3.3)	122	(2.4)	0.74 (0.59, 0.94)
First PVD endpoint	282	(5.6)	275	(5.5)	0.97 (0.83, 1.15)
First CABG or other coronary revascularization procedure[b]	904	(18.1)	667	(13.4)	0.72 (0.65, 0.80)
First documented angina endpoint[b]	615	(12.3)	545	(10.9)	0.88 (0.79, 0.99)
All cause mortality	282	(5.6)	284	(5.7)	1.01 (0.85, 1.19)
Components of all cause mortality					
Cardiovascular death	155	(3.1)	126	(2.5)	0.81 (0.64, 1.03)
Noncardiovascular death	127	(2.5)	158	(3.2)	1.25 (0.99, 1.57)
Cancer death	75	(1.5)	85	(1.7)	1.13 (0.83, 1.55)
Other non-CV death	43	(0.9)	58	(1.2)	1.35 (0.91, 2.00)
Suicide, homicide and other traumatic non-CV death	9	(0.2)	15	(0.3)	1.67 (0.73, 3.82)

a Atorvastatin 80 mg: atorvastatin 10 mg
b Component of other secondary endpoints
* Secondary endpoints not included in primary endpoint
    HR=hazard ratio; CHD=coronary heart disease; CI=confidence interval; MI=myocardial infarction; CHF=congestive heart failure; CV=cardiovascular; PVD=peripheral vascular disease; CABG=coronary artery bypass graft
    Confidence intervals for the Secondary Endpoints were not adjusted for multiple comparisons.

Table 6. Dose-Response in Patients With Primary Hyperlipidemia (Adjusted Mean Percent Change From Baseline)[a]

Dose	N	TC	LDL-C	Apo B	TG	HDL-C	Non-HDL-C/HDL-C
Placebo	21	4	4	3	10	-3	7
10	22	-29	-39	-32	-19	6	-34
20	20	-33	-43	-35	-26	9	-41
40	21	-37	-50	-42	-29	6	-45
80	23	-45	-60	-50	-37	5	-53

a Results are pooled from 2 dose-response studies.

80 mg/day group vs. 374 (8.4%) in the simvastatin 20–40 mg/day group. The proportions of subjects who experienced CV or non-CV death were similar for the LIPITOR 80 mg group and the simvastatin 20–40 mg group.
Atorvastatin Studies in Hyperlipidemia (Heterozygous Familial and Nonfamilial) and Mixed Dyslipidemia (Fredrickson Types IIa and IIb): Atorvastatin reduces total-C, LDL-C, VLDL-C, apo B, and TG, and increases HDL-C in patients with hyperlipidemia and mixed dyslipidemia. Therapeutic response is seen within 2 weeks, and maximum response is usually achieved within 4 weeks and maintained during chronic therapy.
Atorvastatin is effective in a wide variety of patient populations with hyperlipidemia, with and without hypertriglyceridemia, in men and women, and in the elderly.
In two multicenter, placebo-controlled, dose-response studies in patients with hyperlipidemia, atorvastatin given as a single dose over 6 weeks, significantly reduced total-C, LDL-C, apo B, and TG (pooled results are provided in Table 6).
[See table 6 above]
In patients with *Fredrickson* Types IIa and IIb hyperlipoproteinemia pooled from 24 controlled trials, the median (25th and 75th percentile) percent changes from baseline in HDL-C for atorvastatin 10, 20, 40, and 80 mg were 6.4 (-1.4, 14), 8.7 (0, 17), 7.8 (0, 16), and 5.1 (-2.7, 15), respectively. Additionally, analysis of the pooled data demonstrated consistent and significant decreases in total-C, LDL-C, TG, total-C/HDL-C, and LDL-C/HDL-C.

In three multicenter, double-blind studies in patients with hyperlipidemia, atorvastatin was compared to other statins. After randomization, patients were treated for 16 weeks with either atorvastatin 10 mg per day or a fixed dose of the comparative agent (Table 7).
[See table 7 on next page]
The impact on clinical outcomes of the differences in lipid-altering effects between treatments shown in Table 7 is not known. Table 7 does not contain data comparing the effects of atorvastatin 10 mg and higher doses of lovastatin, pravastatin, and simvastatin. The drugs compared in the studies summarized in the table are not necessarily interchangeable.
Atorvastatin Effects in Hypertriglyceridemia (Fredrickson Type IV): The response to atorvastatin in 64 patients with isolated hypertriglyceridemia treated across several clinical trials is shown in the table below (Table 8). For the atorvastatin-treated patients, median (min, max) baseline TG level was 565 (267–1502).
[See table 8 on next page]
Atorvastatin Effects in Dysbetalipoproteinemia (Fredrickson Type III): The results of an open-label crossover study of atorvastatin in 16 patients (genotypes: 14 apo E2/E2 and 2 apo E3/E2) with dysbetalipoproteinemia (*Fredrickson Type III*) are shown in the table below (Table 9).
[See table 9 on next page]
Atorvastatin Effects in Homozygous Familial Hypercholesterolemia: In a study without a concurrent control group, 29 patients ages 6 to 37 years with homozygous FH received

maximum daily doses of 20 to 80 mg of atorvastatin. The mean LDL-C reduction in this study was 18%. Twenty-five patients with a reduction in LDL-C had a mean response of 20% (range of 7% to 53%, median of 24%); the remaining 4 patients had 7% to 24% increases in LDL-C. Five of the 29 patients had absent LDL-receptor function. Of these, 2 patients also had a portacaval shunt and had no significant reduction in LDL-C. The remaining 3 receptor-negative patients had a mean LDL-C reduction of 22%.
Atorvastatin Effects in Heterozygous Familial Hypercholesterolemic Pediatric Patients: In a double-blind, placebo-controlled study followed by an open-label phase, 187 boys and postmenarchal girls 10-17 years of age (mean age 14.1 years) with heterozygous FH or severe hypercholesterolemia, were randomized to atorvastatin (n=140) or placebo (n=47) for 26 weeks and then all received atorvastatin for 26 weeks. Inclusion in the study required 1) a baseline LDL-C level ≥ 190 mg/dL or 2) a baseline LDL-C level ≥ 160 mg/dL and positive family history of FH or documented premature cardiovascular disease in a first- or second-degree relative. The mean baseline LDL-C value was 218.6 mg/dL (range: 138.5–385.0 mg/dL) in the atorvastatin group compared to 230.0 mg/dL (range: 160.0–324.5 mg/dL) in placebo group. The dosage of atorvastatin (once daily) was 10 mg for the first 4 weeks and up-titrated to 20 mg if the LDL-C level was > 130 mg/dL. The number of atorvastatin-treated patients who required up-titration to 20 mg after Week 4 during the double-blind phase was 80 (57.1%).
Atorvastatin significantly decreased plasma levels of total-C, LDL-C, triglycerides, and apolipoprotein B during the 26 week double-blind phase (see Table 10).
[See table 10 on next page]
The mean achieved LDL-C value was 130.7 mg/dL (range: 70.0-242.0 mg/dL) in the atorvastatin group compared to 228.5 mg/dL (range: 152.0–385.0 mg/dL) in the placebo group during the 26 week double-blind phase.
The safety and efficacy of atorvastatin doses above 20 mg have not been studied in controlled trials in children. The long-term efficacy of atorvastatin therapy in childhood to reduce morbidity and mortality in adulthood has not been established.
Clinical Study of Combined Amlodipine and Atorvastatin in Patients with Hypertension and Dyslipidemia
In a double-blind, placebo-controlled study, a total of 1660 patients with co-morbid hypertension and dyslipidemia received once daily treatment with eight dose combinations of amlodipine and atorvastatin (5/10, 10/10, 5/20, 10/20, 5/40, 10/40, 5/80, or 10/80 mg), amlodipine alone (5 mg or 10 mg), atorvastatin alone (10 mg, 20 mg, 40 mg, or 80 mg) or placebo. In addition to concomitant hypertension and dyslipidemia, 15% of the patients had diabetes mellitus, 22% were smokers and 14% had a positive family history of cardiovascular disease. At eight weeks, all eight combination-treatment groups of amlodipine and atorvastatin demonstrated statistically significant dose-related reductions in systolic blood pressure (SBP), diastolic blood pressure (DBP) and LDL-C compared to placebo, with no overall modification of effect of either component on SBP, DBP and LDL-C (Table 11).
[See table 11 at top of page 2784]

INDICATIONS AND USAGE

CADUET (amlodipine and atorvastatin) is indicated in patients for whom treatment with both amlodipine and atorvastatin is appropriate.
Amlodipine
1. *Hypertension:* Amlodipine is indicated for the treatment of hypertension. It may be used alone or in combination with other antihypertensive agents;
2. *Coronary Artery Disease (CAD)*
   Chronic Stable Angina: Amlodipine is indicated for the treatment of chronic stable angina. Amlodipine may be used alone or in combination with other antianginal or antihypertensive agents;
   Vasospastic Angina (Prinzmetal's or Variant Angina): Amlodipine is indicated for the treatment of confirmed or suspected vasospastic angina. Amlodipine may be used as monotherapy or in combination with other antianginal drugs.
   Angiographically Documented CAD: In patients with recently documented CAD by angiography and without heart failure or an ejection fraction <40%, amlodipine is indicated to reduce the risk of hospitalization due to angina and to reduce the risk of a coronary revascularization procedure.
AND
Atorvastatin
Therapy with lipid-altering agents should be only one component of multiple risk factor intervention in individuals at significantly increased risk for atherosclerotic vascular disease due to hypercholesterolemia. Drug therapy is recommended as an adjunct to diet when the response to a diet restricted in saturated fat and cholesterol and other non-pharmacologic measures alone has been inadequate. In patients with CHD or multiple risk factors for CHD, the atorvastatin component of CADUET can be started simultaneously with diet restriction.
1. *Prevention of Cardiovascular Disease:*
   In adult patients without clinically evident coronary heart disease, but with multiple risk factors for coronary

heart disease such as age, smoking, hypertension, low HDL-C, or a family history of early coronary heart disease, atorvastatin is indicated to:
- Reduce the risk of myocardial infarction
- Reduce the risk of stroke
- Reduce the risk for revascularization procedures and angina

In patients with type 2 diabetes, and without clinically evident coronary heart disease, but with multiple risk factors for coronary heart disease such as retinopathy, albuminuria, smoking, or hypertension, LIPITOR is indicated to:
- Reduce the risk of myocardial infarction
- Reduce the risk of stroke;

In patients with clinically evident coronary heart disease, LIPITOR is indicated to:
- Reduce the risk of non-fatal myocardial infarction
- Reduce the risk of fatal and non-fatal stroke
- Reduce the risk for revascularization procedures
- Reduce the risk of hospitalization for CHF
- Reduce the risk of angina

2. *Heterozygous Familial and Nonfamilial Hyperlipidemia:* Atorvastatin is indicated as an adjunct to diet to reduce elevated total-C, LDL-C, apo B, and TG levels and to increase HDL-C in patients with primary hypercholesterolemia (heterozygous familial and nonfamilial) and mixed dyslipidemia (*Fredrickson* Types IIa and IIb);
3. *Elevated Serum TG Levels:* Atorvastatin is indicated as an adjunct to diet for the treatment of patients with elevated serum TG levels (*Fredrickson* Type IV);
4. *Primary Dysbetalipoproteinemia:* Atorvastatin is indicated for the treatment of patients with primary dysbetalipoproteinemia (*Fredrickson* Type III) who do not respond adequately to diet;
5. *Homozygous Familial Hypercholesterolemia:* Atorvastatin is indicated to reduce total-C and LDL-C in patients with homozygous familial hypercholesterolemia as an adjunct to other lipid-lowering treatments (e.g., LDL apheresis) or if such treatments are unavailable;
6. *Pediatric Patients:* Atorvastatin is indicated as an adjunct to diet to reduce total-C, LDL-C, and apo B levels in boys and post-menarchal girls, 10 to 17 years of age, with heterozygous familial hypercholesterolemia if after

an adequate trial of diet therapy the following findings are present:
a. LDL-C remains ≥ 190 mg/dL or
b. LDL-C remains ≥ 160 mg/dL and:
  - there is a positive family history of premature cardiovascular disease or
  - two or more other CVD risk factors are present in the pediatric patients.

The antidyslipidemic component of CADUET has not been studied in conditions where the major lipoprotein abnormality is elevation of chylomicrons (*Fredrickson* Types I and V).

CONTRAINDICATIONS

CADUET contains atorvastatin and is therefore contraindicated in patients with active liver disease, which may include unexplained persistent elevations in hepatic transaminase levels.

CADUET is contraindicated in patients with known hypersensitivity to any component of this medication.

Pregnancy and Lactation

CADUET contains atorvastatin and is therefore contraindicated in women who are pregnant or may become pregnant. The atorvastatin component of CADUET may cause fetal harm when administered to a pregnant woman. Serum cholesterol and triglycerides increase during normal pregnancy, and cholesterol or cholesterol derivatives are essential for fetal development. Atherosclerosis is a chronic process and discontinuation of lipid-lowering drugs during pregnancy should have little impact on the outcome of long-term therapy of primary hypercholesterolemia.

There are no adequate and well-controlled studies of atorvastatin use during pregnancy; however in rare reports congenital anomalies were observed following intrauterine exposure to statins. In rat and rabbit animal reproduction studies, atorvastatin revealed no evidence of teratogenicity. CADUET, WHICH INCLUDES ATORVASTATIN, SHOULD BE ADMINISTERED TO WOMEN OF CHILDBEARING AGE ONLY WHEN SUCH PATIENTS ARE HIGHLY UNLIKELY TO CONCEIVE AND HAVE BEEN INFORMED OF THE POTENTIAL HAZARDS. If the patient becomes pregnant while taking this drug, therapy should be discontinued immediately and the patient apprised of the potential hazard to the fetus (see **PRECAUTIONS, Pregnancy**).

It is not known whether atorvastatin or amlodipine are excreted into human milk; however a small amount of another statin does pass into breast milk. Because statins have the potential for serious adverse reactions in nursing infants, women taking CADUET should not breastfeed their infants (see **PRECAUTIONS, Nursing Mothers**).

WARNINGS

Skeletal Muscle

Rare cases of rhabdomyolysis with acute renal failure secondary to myoglobinuria have been reported with the atorvastatin component of CADUET and with other statins. A history of renal impairment may be a risk factor for the development of rhabdomyolysis. Such patients merit closer monitoring for skeletal muscle effects.

The atorvastatin component of CADUET, like other statins, occasionally causes myopathy, defined as muscle aches or muscle weakness in conjunction with increases in creatine phosphokinase (CPK) values >10 times ULN. The concomitant use of higher doses of atorvastatin with certain drugs such as cyclosporine and strong CYP3A4 inhibitors (e.g., clarithromycin, itraconazole and HIV protease inhibitors) increases the risk of myopathy/rhabdomyolysis.

Myopathy should be considered in any patient with diffuse myalgias, muscle tenderness or weakness, or marked elevation of CPK. Patients should be advised to report promptly unexplained muscle pain, tenderness or weakness, particularly if accompanied by malaise or fever. CADUET therapy should be discontinued if markedly elevated CPK levels occur or myopathy is diagnosed or suspected.

The risk of myopathy during treatment with statins is increased with concurrent administration of cyclosporine, fibric acid derivatives, erythromycin, clarithromycin, combination of ritonavir plus saquinavir or lopinavir plus ritonavir, niacin, or azole antifungals. Physicians considering combined therapy with CADUET and fibric acid derivatives, erythromycin, clarithromycin, a combination of ritonavir plus saquinavir or lopinavir plus ritonavir, immunosuppressive drugs, azole antifungals, or lipid-modifying doses of niacin should carefully weigh the potential benefits and risks and should carefully monitor patients for any signs or symptoms of muscle pain, tenderness, or weakness, particularly during the initial months of therapy and during any periods of upward dosage titration of either drug. Lower starting and maintenance doses of atorvastatin should be considered when taken concomitantly with the aforementioned drugs (see **PRECAUTIONS, Drug Interactions**). Periodic creatine phosphokinase (CPK) determinations may be considered in such situations, but there is no assurance that such monitoring will prevent the occurrence of severe myopathy.

Table 7. Mean Percent Change From Baseline at Endpoint (Double-Blind, Randomized, Active-Controlled Trials)

Treatment (Daily Dose)	N	Total-C	LDL-C	Apo B	TG	HDL-C	Non-HDL-C/ HDL-C
Study 1							
Atorvastatin 10 mg	707	-27[a]	-36[a]	-28[a]	-17[a]	+7	-37[a]
Lovastatin 20 mg	191	-19	-27	-20	-6	+7	-28
95% CI for Diff[1]		-9.2, -6.5	-10.7, -7.1	-10.0, -6.5	-15.2, -7.1	-1.7, 2.0	-11.1, -7.1
Study 2							
Atorvastatin 10 mg	222	-25[b]	-35[b]	-27[b]	-17[b]	+6	-36[b]
Pravastatin 20 mg	77	-17	-23	-17	-9	+8	-28
95% CI for Diff[1]		-10.8, -6.1	-14.5, -8.2	-13.4, -7.4	-14.1, -0.7	-4.9, 1.6	-11.5, -4.1
Study 3							
Atorvastatin 10 mg	132	-29[c]	-37[c]	-34[c]	-23[c]	+7	-39[c]
Simvastatin 10 mg	45	-24	-30	-30	-15	+7	-33
95% CI for Diff[1]		-8.7, -2.7	-10.1, -2.6	-8.0, -1.1	-15.1, -0.7	-4.3, 3.9	-9.6, -1.9

[1] A negative value for the 95% CI for the difference between treatments favors atorvastatin for all except HDL-C, for which a positive value favors atorvastatin. If the range does not include 0, this indicates a statistically significant difference.
[a] Significantly different from lovastatin, ANCOVA, p ≤0.05
[b] Significantly different from pravastatin, ANCOVA, p ≤0.05
[c] Significantly different from simvastatin, ANCOVA, p ≤0.05

Table 8. Combined Patients With Isolated Elevated TG: Median (min, max) Percent Changes From Baseline

	Placebo (N=12)	Atorvastatin 10 mg (N=37)	Atorvastatin 20 mg (N=13)	Atorvastatin 80 mg (N=14)
Triglycerides	-12.4 (-36.6, 82.7)	-41.0 (-76.2, 49.4)	-38.7 (-62.7, 29.5)	-51.8 (-82.8, 41.3)
Total-C	-2.3 (-15.5, 24.4)	-28.2 (-44.9, -6.8)	-34.9 (-49.6, -15.2)	-44.4 (-63.5, -3.8)
LDL-C	3.6 (-31.3, 31.6)	-26.5 (-57.7, 9.8)	-30.4 (-53.9, 0.3)	-40.5 (-60.6, -13.8)
HDL-C	3.8 (-18.6, 13.4)	13.8 (-9.7, 61.5)	11.0 (-3.2, 25.2)	7.5 (-10.8, 37.2)
VLDL-C	-1.0 (-31.9, 53.2)	-48.8 (-85.8, 57.3)	-44.6 (-62.2, -10.8)	-62.0 (-88.2, 37.6)
non-HDL-C	-2.8 (-17.6, 30.0)	-33.0 (-52.1, -13.3)	-42.7 (-53.7, -17.4)	-51.5 (-72.9, -4.3)

Table 9. Open-Label Crossover Study of 16 Patients With Dysbetalipoproteinemia (*Fredrickson* Type III)

	Median (min, max) at Baseline (mg/dL)	Median % Change (min, max)	
		Atorvastatin 10 mg	Atorvastatin 80 mg
Total-C	442 (225, 1320)	-37 (-85, 17)	-58 (-90, -31)
Triglycerides	678 (273, 5990)	-39 (-92, -8)	-53 (-95, -30)
IDL-C + VLDL-C	215 (111, 613)	-32 (-76, 9)	-63 (-90, -8)
non-HDL-C	411 (218, 1272)	-43 (-87, -19)	-64 (-92, -36)

Table 10. Lipid-altering Effects of Atorvastatin in Adolescent Boys and Girls with Heterozygous Familial Hypercholesterolemia or Severe Hypercholesterolemia (Mean Percent Change From Baseline at Endpoint in Intention-to-Treat Population)

DOSAGE	N	Total-C	LDL-C	HDL-C	TG	Apolipoprotein B
Placebo	47	-1.5	-0.4	-1.9	1.0	0.7
Atorvastatin	140	-31.4	-39.6	2.8	-12.0	-34.0

Table 11. Efficacy in Terms of Reduction in Blood Pressure and LDL-C

Efficacy of the Combined Treatments in Reducing Systolic BP

Parameter/Analysis		ATO 0 mg	ATO 10 mg	ATO 20 mg	ATO 40 mg	ATO 80 mg
AML 0 mg	Mean change (mmHg)	-3.0	-4.5	-6.2	-6.2	-6.4
	Difference versus placebo (mmHg)	–	-1.5	-3.2	-3.2	-3.4
AML 5 mg	Mean change (mmHg)	-12.8	-13.7	-15.3	-12.7	-12.2
	Difference versus placebo (mmHg)	-9.8	-10.7	-12.3	-9.7	-9.2
AML 10 mg	Mean change (mmHg)	-16.2	-15.9	-16.1	-16.3	-17.6
	Difference versus placebo (mmHg)	-13.2	-12.9	-13.1	-13.3	-14.6

Efficacy of the Combined Treatments in Reducing Diastolic BP

Parameter/Analysis		ATO 0 mg	ATO 10 mg	ATO 20 mg	ATO 40 mg	ATO 80 mg
AML 0 mg	Mean change (mmHg)	-3.3	-4.1	-3.9	-5.1	-4.1
	Difference versus placebo (mmHg)	–	-0.8	-0.6	-1.8	-0.8
AML 5 mg	Mean change (mmHg)	-7.6	-8.2	-9.4	-7.3	-8.4
	Difference versus placebo (mmHg)	-4.3	-4.9	-6.1	-4.0	-5.1
AML 10 mg	Mean change (mmHg)	-10.4	-9.1	-10.6	-9.8	-11.1
	Difference versus placebo (mmHg)	-7.1	-5.8	-7.3	-6.5	-7.8

Efficacy of the Combined Treatments in Reducing LDL-C (% change)

Parameter/Analysis		ATO 0 mg	ATO 10 mg	ATO 20 mg	ATO 40 mg	ATO 80 mg
AML 0 mg	Mean % change	-1.1	-33.4	-39.5	-43.1	-47.2
AML 5 mg	Mean % change	-0.1	-38.7	-42.3	-44.9	-48.4
AML 10 mg	Mean % change	-2.5	-36.6	-38.6	-43.2	-49.1

Prescribing recommendations for atorvastatin, a component of CADUET, and interacting agents are summarized in Table 12 (see **DOSAGE AND ADMINISTRATION, PRECAUTIONS, Drug Interactions,** and **CLINICAL PHARMACOLOGY**).

TABLE 12
Atorvastatin Drug Interactions Associated with Increased Risk of Myopathy/Rhabdomyolysis

Interacting Agents	Prescribing Recommendations
Cyclosporine	Do not exceed 10 mg atorvastatin daily
Clarithromycin, Itraconazole, HIV protease inhibitors (ritonavir plus saquinavir or lopinavir plus ritonavir,)	Caution when exceeding doses > 20mg atorvastatin daily. The lowest dose necessary should be used.

In patients taking CADUET, therapy should be temporarily withheld or discontinued in any patient with an acute, serious condition suggestive of a myopathy or having a risk factor predisposing to the development of renal failure secondary to rhabdomyolysis (e.g., severe acute infection, hypotension, major surgery, trauma, severe metabolic, endocrine and electrolyte disorders, and uncontrolled seizures).

Liver Dysfunction
Statins, like the atorvastatin component of CADUET and like some other lipid-lowering therapies, have been associated with biochemical abnormalities of liver function. **Persistent elevations (>3 times the upper limit of normal [ULN] occurring on 2 or more occasions) in serum transaminases occurred in 0.7% of patients who received atorvastatin in clinical trials. The incidence of these abnormalities was 0.2%, 0.2%, 0.6%, and 2.3% for 10, 20, 40, and 80 mg, respectively.**
In clinical trials in patients taking the atorvastatin component of CADUET, the following has been observed. One patient in clinical trials developed jaundice. Increases in liver function tests (LFT) in other patients were not associated with jaundice or other clinical signs or symptoms. Upon dose reduction, drug interruption, or discontinuation, transaminase levels returned to or near pre-treatment levels without sequelae. Eighteen of 30 patients, with persistent LFT elevations continued treatment with a reduced dose of atorvastatin.
It is recommended that liver function tests be performed prior to and at 12 weeks following both the initiation of therapy and any elevation of dose, and periodically (e.g.,

semiannually) thereafter. Liver enzyme changes generally occur in the first 3 months of treatment with the atorvastatin component of CADUET. Patients who develop increased transaminase levels should be monitored until the abnormalities resolve. Should an increase in ALT or AST of >3 times ULN persist, reduction of dose or withdrawal of CADUET is recommended.
Active liver disease or unexplained persistent transaminase elevations are contraindications to the use of CADUET (see **CONTRAINDICATIONS**).

Increased Angina and/or Myocardial Infarction
Worsening angina and acute myocardial infarction can develop after starting or increasing the dose of amlodipine, particularly in patients with severe obstructive coronary artery disease.

PRECAUTIONS
Hypotension
Symptomatic hypotension is possible, particularly in patients with severe aortic stenosis. Because of the gradual onset of action, acute hypotension is unlikely.

Beta-Blocker Withdrawal
The amlodipine component of CADUET is not a beta-blocker and therefore gives no protection against the dangers of abrupt beta-blocker withdrawal; any such withdrawal should be by gradual reduction of the dose of beta-blocker.

Endocrine Function
Statins, such as the atorvastatin component of CADUET interfere with cholesterol synthesis and theoretically might blunt adrenal and/or gonadal steroid production. Clinical studies have shown that atorvastatin does not reduce basal plasma cortisol concentration or impair adrenal reserve. The effects of statins on male fertility have not been studied in adequate numbers of patients. The effects, if any, on the pituitary-gonadal axis in premenopausal women are unknown. Use caution when administering a statin with drugs that may decrease the levels or activity of endogenous steroid hormones, such as ketoconazole, spironolactone, and cimetidine.

CNS Toxicity
Studies with atorvastatin: Brain hemorrhage was seen in a female dog treated with atorvastatin calcium for 3 months at a dose equivalent to 120 mg atorvastatin/kg/day. Brain hemorrhage and optic nerve vacuolation were seen in another female dog that was sacrificed in moribund condition after 11 weeks of escalating doses of atorvastatin calcium equivalent to up to 280 mg atorvastatin/kg/day. The 120 mg/kg dose of atorvastatin resulted in a systemic exposure approximately 16 times the human plasma area-under-the-curve (AUC, 0-24 hours) based on the maximum human dose of 80 mg/day. A single tonic convulsion was seen in each of 2 male dogs (one treated with atorvastatin calcium at a dose equivalent to 10 mg atorvastatin/kg/day

and one at a dose equivalent to 120 mg atorvastatin/kg/day) in a 2-year study. No CNS lesions have been observed in mice after chronic treatment for up to 2 years at doses of atorvastatin calcium equivalent to up to 400 mg atorvastatin/kg/day or in rats at doses equivalent to up to 100 mg atorvastatin/kg/day. These doses were 6 to 11 times (mouse) and 8 to 16 times (rat) the human AUC (0-24) based on the maximum recommended human dose of 80 mg atorvastatin/day.
CNS vascular lesions, characterized by perivascular hemorrhages, edema, and mononuclear cell infiltration of perivascular spaces, have been observed in dogs treated with other statins. A chemically similar drug in this class produced optic nerve degeneration (Wallerian degeneration of retinogeniculate fibers) in clinically normal dogs in a dose-dependent fashion at a dose that produced plasma drug levels about 30 times higher than the mean drug level in humans taking the highest recommended dose.
Use in Patients with Recent Stroke or TIA
Studies with atorvastatin: In a post-hoc analysis of the Stroke Prevention by Aggressive Reduction in Cholesterol Levels (SPARCL) study where atorvastatin 80 mg vs. placebo was administered in 4,731 subjects without CHD who had a stroke or TIA within the preceding 6 months, a higher incidence of hemorrhagic stroke was seen in the atorvastatin 80 mg group compared to placebo (55, 2.3% atorvastatin vs. 33, 1.4% placebo; HR: 1.68, 95% CI: 1.09, 2.59; p=0.0168). The incidence of fatal hemorrhagic stroke was similar across treatment groups (17 vs. 18 for the atorvastatin and placebo groups, respectively). The incidence of nonfatal hemorrhagic stroke was significantly higher in the atorvastatin group (38, 1.6%) as compared to the placebo group (16, 0.7%). Some baseline characteristics, including hemorrhagic and lacunar stroke on study entry, were associated with a higher incidence of hemorrhagic stroke in the atorvastatin group (see **ADVERSE REACTIONS, The Atorvastatin Component of CADUET**).
Information for Patients
Because of the risk of myopathy with statins, the drug class to which the atorvastatin component of CADUET belongs, advise patients to promptly report unexplained muscle pain, tenderness, or weakness, particularly if accompanied by malaise or fever.
Drug Interactions
Data from a drug-drug interaction study involving 10 mg of amlodipine and 80 mg of atorvastatin in healthy subjects indicate that the pharmacokinetics of amlodipine are not altered when the drugs are coadministered. The effect of amlodipine on the pharmacokinetics of atorvastatin showed no effect on the Cmax: 91% (90% confidence interval: 80 to 103%), but the AUC of atorvastatin increased by 18% (90% confidence interval: 109 to 127%) in the presence of amlodipine, which was not clinically meaningful.
No drug interaction studies have been conducted with CADUET and other drugs, although studies have been conducted in the individual amlodipine and atorvastatin components, as described below:
Studies with Amlodipine:
In vitro data in human plasma indicate that amlodipine has no effect on the protein binding of drugs tested (digoxin, phenytoin, warfarin, and indomethacin).
Cimetidine: Co-administration of amlodipine with cimetidine did not alter the pharmacokinetics of amlodipine.
Maalox® (antacid): Co-administration of the antacid Maalox with a single dose of amlodipine had no significant effect on the pharmacokinetics of amlodipine.
Sildenafil: A single 100 mg dose of sildenafil (Viagra®) in subjects with essential hypertension had no effect on the pharmacokinetic parameters of amlodipine. When amlodipine and sildenafil were used in combination, each agent independently exerted its own blood pressure lowering effect.
Digoxin: Co-administration of amlodipine with digoxin did not change serum digoxin levels or digoxin renal clearance in normal volunteers.
Ethanol (alcohol): Single and multiple 10 mg doses of amlodipine had no significant effect on the pharmacokinetics of ethanol.
Warfarin: Co-administration of amlodipine with warfarin did not change the warfarin prothrombin response time.
In clinical trials, amlodipine has been safely administered with thiazide diuretics, beta-blockers, angiotensin-converting enzyme inhibitors, long-acting nitrates, sublingual nitroglycerin, digoxin, warfarin, non-steroidal anti-inflammatory drugs, antibiotics, and oral hypoglycemic drugs.
Studies with Atorvastatin:
The risk of myopathy during treatment with statins is increased with concurrent administration of fibric acid derivatives, lipid-modifying doses of niacin, cyclosporine, or strong CYP 3A4 inhibitors (e.g., clarithromycin, HIV protease inhibitors, and itraconazole) (see **WARNINGS, Skeletal Muscle,** and **CLINICAL PHARMACOLOGY**).
Strong Inhibitors of CYP 3A4: Atorvastatin is metabolized by cytochrome P450 3A4. Concomitant administration of atorvastatin with strong inhibitors of CYP 3A4 can lead to increases in plasma concentrations of atorvastatin. The extent of interaction and potentiation of effects depends on the variability of effect on CYP 3A4.

Clarithromycin: Atorvastatin AUC was significantly increased with concomitant administration of atorvastatin 80 mg with clarithromycin (500 mg twice daily) compared to that of atorvastatin alone (see **CLINICAL PHARMACOLOGY**). Therefore, in patients taking clarithromycin, use caution when administering atorvastatin doses >20 mg (see **WARNINGS, Skeletal Muscle,** and **DOSAGE AND ADMINISTRATION**).

Combination of Protease Inhibitors: Atorvastatin AUC was significantly increased with concomitant administration of atorvastatin 40 mg with ritonavir plus saquinavir (400 mg twice daily) or atorvastatin 20 mg with lopinavir plus ritonavir (400 mg + 100 mg twice daily) compared to that of atorvastatin alone (see **CLINICAL PHARMACOLOGY**). Therefore, in patients taking HIV protease inhibitors, use caution when administering atorvastatin doses >20 mg (see **WARNINGS, Skeletal Muscle,** and **DOSAGE AND ADMINISTRATION**).

Itraconazole: Atorvastatin AUC was significantly increased with concomitant administration of atorvastatin 40 mg and itraconazole 200 mg (see **CLINICAL PHARMACOLOGY**). Therefore, in patients taking itraconazole, use caution when administering atorvastatin doses >20 mg (see **WARNINGS, Skeletal Muscle,** and **DOSAGE AND ADMINISTRATION**).

Grapefruit juice: Contains one or more components that inhibit CYP 3A4 and can increase plasma concentrations of atorvastatin, especially with excessive grapefruit juice consumption (>1.2 liters per day).

Cyclosporine: Atorvastatin and atorvastatin-metabolites are substrates of the OATP1B1 transporter. Inhibitors of the OATP1B1 (e.g., cyclosporine) can increase the bioavailability of atorvastatin. Atorvastatin AUC was significantly increased with concomitant administration of atorvastatin 10 mg and cyclosporine 5.2 mg/kg/day compared to that of atorvastatin alone (see **CLINICAL PHARMACOLOGY**). In cases where coadministration of atorvastatin with cyclosporine is necessary, the dose of atorvastatin should not exceed 10 mg (see **WARNINGS, Skeletal Muscle**).

Rifampin or other Inducers of Cytochrome P450 3A4: Concomitant administration of atorvastatin with inducers of cytochrome P450 3A4 (e.g., efavirenz, rifampin) can lead to variable reductions in plasma concentrations of atorvastatin. Due to the dual interaction mechanism of rifampin, simultaneous co-administration of atorvastatin with rifampin is recommended, as delayed administration of atorvastatin after administration of rifampin has been associated with a significant reduction in atorvastatin plasma concentrations.

Digoxin: When multiple doses of atorvastatin and digoxin were coadministered, steady-state plasma digoxin concentrations increased by approximately 20%. Patients taking digoxin should be monitored appropriately.

Oral Contraceptives: Coadministration of atorvastatin and an oral contraceptive increased AUC values for norethindrone and ethinyl estradiol (see **CLINICAL PHARMACOLOGY**). These increases should be considered when selecting an oral contraceptive for a woman taking CADUET.

Warfarin: Atorvastatin had no clinically significant effect on prothrombin time when administered to patients receiving chronic warfarin treatment.

Drug/Laboratory Test Interactions
None known.

Carcinogenesis, Mutagenesis, Impairment of Fertility
Studies with amlodipine: Rats and mice treated with amlodipine maleate in the diet for up to two years, at concentrations calculated to provide daily dosage levels of 0.5, 1.25, and 2.5 mg amlodipine/kg/day, showed no evidence of a carcinogenic effect of the drug. For the mouse, the highest dose was, on a mg/m² basis, similar to the maximum recommended human dose of 10 mg amlodipine/day*. For the rat, the highest dose level was, on a mg/m² basis, about twice the maximum recommended human dose*.

Mutagenicity studies conducted with amlodipine maleate revealed no drug related effects at either the gene or chromosome levels.

There was no effect on the fertility of rats treated orally with amlodipine maleate (males for 64 days and females for 14 days prior to mating) at doses up to 10 mg amlodipine/kg/day (8 times* the maximum recommended human dose of 10 mg/day on a mg/m² basis).
*Based on patent weight of 50 kg.

Studies with atorvastatin: In a 2-year carcinogenicity study with atorvastatin calcium in rats at dose levels equivalent to 10, 30, and 100 mg atorvastatin/kg/day, 2 rare tumors were found in muscle in high-dose females: in one, there was a rhabdomyosarcoma and, in another, there was a fibrosarcoma. This dose represents a plasma AUC (0-24) value of approximately 16 times the mean human plasma drug exposure after an 80 mg oral dose.

A 2-year carcinogenicity study in mice given atorvastatin calcium at dose levels equivalent to 100, 200, and 400 mg atorvastatin/kg/day resulted in a significant increase in liver adenomas in high-dose males and liver carcinomas in

high-dose females. These findings occurred at plasma AUC (0-24) values of approximately 6 times the mean human plasma drug exposure after an 80 mg oral dose.

In vitro, atorvastatin was not mutagenic or clastogenic in the following tests with and without metabolic activation: the Ames test with *Salmonella typhimurium* and *Escherichia coli,* the HGPRT forward mutation assay in Chinese hamster lung cells, and the chromosomal aberration assay in Chinese hamster lung cells. Atorvastatin was negative in the *in vivo* mouse micronucleus test.

There were no effects on fertility when rats were given atorvastatin calcium at doses equivalent to up to 175 mg atorvastatin/kg/day (15 times the human exposure). There was aplasia and aspermia in the epididymides of 2 of 10 rats treated with atorvastatin calcium at a dose equivalent to 100 mg atorvastatin/kg/day for 3 months (16 times the human AUC at the 80 mg dose); testis weights were significantly lower at 30 and 100 mg/kg/day and epididymal weight was lower at 100 mg/kg/day. Male rats given the equivalent of 100 mg atorvastatin/kg/day for 11 weeks prior to mating had decreased sperm motility, spermatid head concentration, and increased abnormal sperm. Atorvastatin caused no adverse effects on semen parameters, or reproductive organ histopathology in dogs given doses of atorvastatin calcium equivalent to 10, 40, or 120 mg atorvastatin/kg/day for two years.

Pregnancy

Pregnancy Category X (see CONTRAINDICATIONS)
CADUET contains atorvastatin and is therefore contraindicated in women who are pregnant or may become pregnant. The atorvastatin component of CADUET may cause fetal harm when administered to a pregnant woman. CADUET should be administered to women of child-bearing potential only when such patients are highly unlikely to conceive and have been informed of the potential hazards. If the woman becomes pregnant while taking CADUET, it should be discontinued immediately and the patient advised again as to the potential hazards to the fetus, and the lack of known clinical benefit with continued use during pregnancy.

Serum cholesterol and triglycerides increase during normal pregnancy, and cholesterol products are essential for fetal development. Atherosclerosis is a chronic process, and discontinuation of lipid-lowering drugs during pregnancy should have little impact on long-term outcomes of primary hypercholesterolemia therapy.

Studies with amlodipine: No evidence of teratogenicity or other embryo/fetal toxicity was found when pregnant rats and rabbits were treated orally with amlodipine maleate at doses up to 10 mg amlodipine/kg/day (respectively 8 times* and 23 times* the maximum recommended human dose of 10 mg/day on a mg/m² basis) during their respective periods of major organogenesis. However, litter size was significantly decreased (by about 50%) and the number of intrauterine deaths was significantly increased (about 5-fold) in rats receiving amlodipine maleate at 10 mg amlodipine/kg/day for 14 days before mating and throughout mating and gestation. Amlodipine maleate has been shown to prolong both the gestation period and the duration of labor in rats at this dose. There are no adequate and well-controlled studies in pregnant women.
*Based on patient weight of 50 kg.

Studies with atorvastatin: There are no adequate and well-controlled studies of atorvastatin use during pregnancy. There have been rare reports of congenital anomalies following intrauterine exposure to statins. In a review of about 100 prospectively followed pregnancies in women exposed to other statins, the incidences of congenital anomalies, spontaneous abortions, and fetal deaths/stillbirths did not exceed the rate expected in the general population. However, this study was only able to exclude a three-to-four-fold increased risk of congenital anomalies over background incidence. In 89% of these cases, drug treatment started before pregnancy and stopped during the first trimester when pregnancy was identified.

Atorvastatin crosses the rat placenta and reaches a level in fetal liver equivalent to that of maternal plasma. Atorvastatin was not teratogenic in rats at doses of atorvastatin calcium equivalent to up to 300 mg atorvastatin/kg/day or in rabbits at doses of atorvastatin calcium equivalent to up to 100 mg atorvastatin/kg/day. These doses resulted in multiples of about 30 times (rat) or 20 times (rabbit) the human exposure based on surface area (mg/m²).

In a study in rats given atorvastatin calcium at doses equivalent to 20, 100, or 225 mg atorvastatin/kg/day, from gestation day 7 through to lactation day 21 (weaning), there was decreased pup survival at birth, neonate, weaning, and maturity for pups of mothers dosed with 225 mg/kg/day. Body weight was decreased on days 4 and 21 for pups of mothers dosed at 100 mg/kg/day; pup body weight was decreased at birth and at days 4, 21, and 91 at 225 mg/kg/day. Pup development was delayed (rotorod performance at 100 mg/kg/day and acoustic startle at 225 mg/kg/day; pin-

nae detachment and eye opening at 225 mg/kg/day). These doses of atorvastatin correspond to 6 times (100 mg/kg) and 22 times (225 mg/kg) the human AUC at 80 mg/day.

Labor and Delivery
No studies have been conducted in pregnant women on the effect of CADUET, amlodipine or atorvastatin on the mother or the fetus during labor or delivery, or on the duration of labor or delivery. Amlodipine has been shown to prolong the duration of labor in rats.

Nursing Mothers
Studies with amlodipine: It is not known whether the amlodipine component of CADUET is excreted in human milk.

Studies with atorvastatin: It is not known whether the atorvastatin component of CADUET is excreted in human milk, but a small amount of another drug in this class does pass into breast milk. Nursing rat pups taking atorvastatin had plasma and liver drug levels of 50% and 40%, respectively, of that in their mother's milk. Animal breast milk drug levels may not accurately reflect human breast milk levels. Because another drug in this class passes into human milk and because statins have a potential to cause serious adverse reactions in nursing infants, women taking CADUET, which includes atorvastatin, should be advised not to nurse their infants (see **CONTRAINDICATIONS**).

Pediatric Use
There have been no studies conducted to determine the safety or effectiveness of CADUET in pediatric populations.
Studies with amlodipine: The effect of amlodipine on blood pressure in patients less than 6 years of age is not known.
Studies with atorvastatin: Safety and effectiveness in patients 10-17 years of age with heterozygous familial hypercholesterolemia have been evaluated in controlled clinical trials of 6 months duration in adolescent boys and postmenarchal girls. Patients treated with atorvastatin had an adverse experience profile generally similar to that of patients treated with placebo, the most common adverse experiences observed in both groups, regardless of causality assessment, were infections. **Doses greater than 20 mg have not been studied in this patient population.** In this limited controlled study, there was no significant effect on growth or sexual maturation in boys or on menstrual cycle length in girls. See **CLINICAL PHARMACOLOGY, Clinical Studies** section; **ADVERSE REACTIONS,** *Pediatric Patients;* and **DOSAGE AND ADMINISTRATION,** *Pediatric Patients (10-17 years of age) with Heterozygous Familial Hypercholesterolemia.* Adolescent females should be counseled on appropriate contraceptive methods while on atorvastatin therapy (see **CONTRAINDICATIONS** and **PRECAUTIONS, Pregnancy**). **Atorvastatin has not been studied in controlled clinical trials involving pre-pubertal patients or patients younger than 10 years of age.**

Clinical efficacy with doses of atorvastatin up to 80 mg/day for 1 year have been evaluated in an uncontrolled study of patients with homozygous FH including 8 pediatric patients. See **CLINICAL PHARMACOLOGY, Clinical Studies,** *Atorvastatin Effects in Homozygous Familial Hypercholesterolemia.*

Geriatric Use
There have been no studies conducted to determine the safety or effectiveness of CADUET in geriatric populations.
In studies with amlodipine: Clinical studies of amlodipine did not include sufficient numbers of subjects aged 65 and over to determine whether they respond differently from younger subjects. Other reported clinical experience has not identified differences in responses between the elderly and younger patients. In general, dose selection of the amlodipine component of CADUET for an elderly patient should be cautious, usually starting at the low end of the dosing range, reflecting the greater frequency of decreased hepatic, renal, or cardiac function, and of concomitant disease or other drug therapy. Elderly patients have decreased clearance of amlodipine with a resulting increase of AUC of approximately 40-60%, and a lower initial dose may be required (see **DOSAGE AND ADMINISTRATION**).

In studies with atorvastatin: Of the 39,828 patients who received LIPITOR in clinical studies, 15,813 (40%) were ≥65 years old and 2,800 (7%) were ≥75 years old. No overall differences in safety or effectiveness were observed between these subjects and younger subjects, and other reported clinical experience has not identified differences in responses between the elderly and younger patients, but greater sensitivity of some older adults cannot be ruled out. Advanced age (≥65 years) is a predisposing factor for myopathy.

ADVERSE REACTIONS
CADUET
CADUET (amlodipine besylate/atorvastatin calcium) has been evaluated for safety in 1092 patients in double-blind placebo controlled studies treated for co-morbid hypertension and dyslipidemia. In general, treatment with CADUET was well tolerated. For the most part, adverse experiences have been mild or moderate in severity. In clinical trials

Table 13. Clinical adverse reactions occurring in ≥ 2% in patents treated with any dose of LIPITOR and at an incidence greater than placebo regardless of causality (% of patients).

Adverse Reaction*	Any dose N=8755	10 mg N=3908	20 mg N=188	40 mg N=604	80 mg N=4055	Placebo N=7311
Nasopharyngitis	8.3	12.9	5.3	7.0	4.2	8.2
Arthralgia	6.9	8.9	11.7	10.6	4.3	6.5
Diarrhea	6.8	7.3	6.4	14.1	5.2	6.3
Pain in extremity	6.0	8.5	3.7	9.3	3.1	5.9
Urinary tract infection	5.7	6.9	6.4	8.0	4.1	5.6
Dyspepsia	4.7	5.9	3.2	6.0	3.3	4.3
Nausea	4.0	3.7	3.7	7.1	3.8	3.5
Musculoskeletal pain	3.8	5.2	3.2	5.1	2.3	3.6
Muscle Spasms	3.6	4.6	4.8	5.1	2.4	3.0
Myalgia	3.5	3.6	5.9	8.4	2.7	3.1
Insomnia	3.0	2.8	1.1	5.3	2.8	2.9
Pharyngolaryngeal pain	2.3	3.9	1.6	2.8	0.7	2.1

*Adverse Reaction ≥2% in any dose greater than placebo

with CADUET, no adverse experiences peculiar to this combination have been observed. Adverse experiences are similar in terms of nature, severity, and frequency to those reported previously with amlodipine and atorvastatin.

The following information is based on the clinical experience with amlodipine and atorvastatin.

The Amlodipine Component of CADUET

Amlodipine has been evaluated for safety in more than 11,000 patients in U.S. and foreign clinical trials. In general, treatment with amlodipine was well tolerated at doses up to 10 mg daily. Most adverse reactions reported during therapy with amlodipine were of mild or moderate severity. In controlled clinical trials directly comparing amlodipine (N=1730) in doses up to 10 mg to placebo (N=1250), discontinuation of amlodipine due to adverse reactions was required in only about 1.5% of patients and was not significantly different from placebo (about 1%). The most common side effects are headache and edema. The incidence (%) of side effects which occurred in a dose related manner are as follows:

Adverse Event	amlodipine 2.5 mg N=275	5.0 mg N=296	10.0 mg N=268	Placebo N=520
Edema	1.8	3.0	10.8	0.6
Dizziness	1.1	3.4	3.4	1.5
Flushing	0.7	1.4	2.6	0.0
Palpitations	0.7	1.4	4.5	0.6

Other adverse experiences which were not clearly dose related but which were reported with an incidence greater than 1.0% in placebo-controlled clinical trials include the following:

Placebo-Controlled Studies

Adverse Event	amlodipine (%) (N=1730)	Placebo (%) (N=1250)
Headache	7.3	7.8
Fatigue	4.5	2.8
Nausea	2.9	1.9
Abdominal Pain	1.6	0.3
Somnolence	1.4	0.6

For several adverse experiences that appear to be drug and dose related, there was a greater incidence in women than men associated with amlodipine treatment as shown in the following table:

Adverse Event	amlodipine M=% (N=1218)	F=% (N=512)	Placebo M=% (N=914)	F=% (N=336)
Edema	5.6	14.6	1.4	5.1
Flushing	1.5	4.5	0.3	0.9
Palpitations	1.4	3.3	0.9	0.9
Somnolence	1.3	1.6	0.8	0.3

The following events occurred in ≤1% but >0.1% of patients treated with amlodipine in controlled clinical trials or under conditions of open trials or marketing experience where a causal relationship is uncertain; they are listed to alert the physician to a possible relationship:

Cardiovascular: arrhythmia (including ventricular tachycardia and atrial fibrillation), bradycardia, chest pain, hypotension, peripheral ischemia, syncope, tachycardia, postural dizziness, postural hypotension, vasculitis.

Central and Peripheral Nervous System: hypoesthesia, neuropathy peripheral, paresthesia, tremor, vertigo.

Gastrointestinal: anorexia, constipation, dyspepsia,** dysphagia, diarrhea, flatulence, pancreatitis, vomiting, gingival hyperplasia.

General: allergic reaction, asthenia,** back pain, hot flushes, malaise, pain, rigors, weight gain, weight decrease.

Musculoskeletal System: arthralgia, arthrosis, muscle cramps,** myalgia.

Psychiatric: sexual dysfunction (male** and female), insomnia, nervousness, depression, abnormal dreams, anxiety, depersonalization.

Respiratory System: dyspnea,** epistaxis.

Skin and Appendages: angioedema, erythema multiforme, pruritus,** rash,** rash erythematous, rash maculopapular.

**These events occurred in less than 1% in placebo-controlled trials, but the incidence of these side effects was between 1% and 2% in all multiple dose studies.

Special Senses: abnormal vision, conjunctivitis, diplopia, eye pain, tinnitus.

Urinary System: micturition frequency, micturition disorder, nocturia.

Autonomic Nervous System: dry mouth, sweating increased.

Metabolic and Nutritional: hyperglycemia, thirst.

Hemopoietic: leukopenia, purpura, thrombocytopenia.

The following events occurred in ≤0.1% of patients treated with amlodipine in controlled clinical trials or under conditions of open trials or marketing experience: cardiac failure, pulse irregularity, extrasystoles, skin discoloration, urticaria, skin dryness, alopecia, dermatitis, muscle weakness, twitching, ataxia, hypertonia, migraine, cold and clammy skin, apathy, agitation, amnesia, gastritis, increased appetite, loose stools, coughing, rhinitis, dysuria, polyuria, parosmia, taste perversion, abnormal visual accommodation, and xerophthalmia.

Other reactions occurred sporadically and cannot be distinguished from medications or concurrent disease states such as myocardial infarction and angina.

Amlodipine therapy has not been associated with clinically significant changes in routine laboratory tests. No clinically relevant changes were noted in serum potassium, serum glucose, total triglycerides, total cholesterol, HDL cholesterol, uric acid, blood urea nitrogen, or creatinine.

In the CAMELOT and PREVENT studies (see **CLINICAL PHARMACOLOGY Clinical Studies, *Clinical Studies with Amlodipine***) the adverse event profile was similar to that reported previously (see above), with the most common adverse event being peripheral edema.

The following postmarketing event has been reported infrequently with amlodipine treatment where a causal relationship is uncertain: gynecomastia. In postmarketing experience, jaundice and hepatic enzyme elevations (mostly consistent with cholestasis or hepatitis) in some cases severe enough to require hospitalization have been reported in association with use of amlodipine.

Amlodipine has been used safely in patients with chronic obstructive pulmonary disease, well-compensated congestive heart failure, peripheral vascular disease, diabetes mellitus, and abnormal lipid profiles.

The Atorvastatin Component of CADUET

The following serious adverse reactions are discussed in greater detail in other sections of the label:

Rhabdomyolysis and myopathy (see **WARNINGS, Skeletal Muscle**)

Liver enzyme abnormalities (see **WARNINGS, Liver Dysfunction**)

Clinical Adverse Experiences

Because clinical trials are conducted under widely varying conditions, the adverse reaction rates observed in the clinical studies of a drug cannot be directly compared to rates in the clinical trials of another drug and may not reflect the rates observed in clinical practice.

In the LIPITOR placebo-controlled clinical trial database of 16,066 patients (8755 LIPITOR vs. 7311 placebo; age range 10–93 years, 39% women, 91% Caucasians, 3% Blacks, 2% Asians, 4% other) with a median treatment duration of 53 weeks, 9.7% of patients on LIPITOR and 9.5% of the patients on placebo discontinued due to adverse reactions regardless of causality. The five most common adverse reactions in patients treated with LIPITOR that led to treatment discontinuation and occurred at a rate greater than placebo were: myalgia (0.7%), diarrhea (0.5%), nausea (0.4%), alanine aminotransferase increase (0.4%), and hepatic enzyme increase (0.4%).

The most commonly reported adverse reactions (incidence ≥ 2% and greater than placebo) regardless of causality, in patients treated with LIPITOR in placebo controlled trials (n=8755) were: nasopharyngitis (8.3%), arthralgia (6.9%), diarrhea (6.8%), pain in extremity (6.0%), and urinary tract infection (5.7%).

Table 13 summarizes the frequency of clinical adverse reactions, regardless of causality, reported in ≥ 2% and at a rate greater than placebo in patients treated with LIPITOR (n=8755), from seventeen placebo-controlled trials.

[See table 13 at left]

Other adverse reactions reported in placebo-controlled studies include:

Body as a whole: malaise, pyrexia; *Digestive system:* abdominal discomfort, eructation, flatulence, hepatitis, cholestasis; *Musculoskeletal system:* musculoskeletal pain, muscle fatigue, neck pain, joint swelling; *Metabolic and nutritional system:* transaminases increase, liver function test abnormal, blood alkaline phosphatase increase, creatine phosphokinase increase, hyperglycemia; *Nervous system:* nightmare; *Respiratory system:* epistaxis; *Skin and appendages:* urticaria; *Special senses:* vision blurred, tinnitus; *Urogenital system:* white blood cells urine positive.

Anglo-Scandinavian Cardiac Outcomes Trial (ASCOT)

In ASCOT (see **CLINICAL PHARMACOLOGY, Clinical Studies, *Clinical Studies with Atorvastatin***) involving 10,305 participants (age range 40–80 years, 19% women; 94.6% Caucasians, 2.6% Africans, 1.5% South Asians, 1.3% mixed/other) treated with atorvastatin 10 mg daily (n=5,168) or placebo (n=5,137), the safety and tolerability profile of the group treated with atorvastatin was comparable to that of the group treated with placebo during a median of 3.3 years of follow-up.

Collaborative Atorvastatin Diabetes Study (CARDS)

In CARDS (see **CLINICAL PHARMACOLOGY, Clinical Studies, *Clinical Studies with Atorvastatin***) involving 2838 subjects (age range 39–77 years, 32% women; 94.3% Caucasians, 2.4% South Asians, 2.3% Afro-Caribbean, 1.0% other) with type 2 diabetes treated with LIPITOR 10 mg daily (n=1428) or placebo (n=1410), there was no difference in the overall frequency of adverse reactions or serious adverse reactions between the treatment groups during a median follow-up of 3.9 years. No cases of rhabdomyolysis were reported.

Treating to New Targets Study (TNT)

In TNT (see **CLINICAL PHARMACOLOGY, Clinical Studies**) involving 10,001 subjects (age range 29–78 years, 19% women; 94.1% Caucasians, 2.9% Blacks, 1.0% Asians, 2.0% other) with clinically evident CHD treated with LIPITOR 10 mg daily (n=5006) or LIPITOR 80 mg daily (n=4995), there were more serious adverse reactions and discontinuations due to adverse reactions in the high-dose atorvastatin group (92, 1.8%; 497, 9.9%, respectively) as compared to the low-dose group (69, 1.4%; 404, 8.1%, respectively) during a median follow-up of 4.9 years. Persistent transaminase elevations (≥3 × ULN twice within 4-10 days) occurred in 62 (1.3%) individuals with atorvastatin 80 mg and in nine (0.2%) individuals with atorvastatin 10 mg. Elevations of CK (≥ 10 × ULN) were low overall, but were higher in the high-dose atorvastatin treatment group (13, 0.3%) compared to the low-dose atorvastatin group (6, 0.1%).

Incremental Decrease in Endpoints Through Aggressive Lipid Lowering Study (IDEAL)

In IDEAL (see **CLINICAL PHARMACOLOGY, Clinical Studies**) involving 8,888 subjects (age range 26–80 years, 19% women; 99.3% Caucasians, 0.4% Asians, 0.3% Blacks, 0.04% other) treated with LIPITOR 80 mg/day (n=4439) or simvastatin 20-40 mg daily (n=4449), there was no difference in the overall frequency of adverse reactions or serious adverse reactions between the treatment groups during a median follow-up of 4.8 years.

Stroke Prevention by Aggressive Reduction in Cholesterol Levels (SPARCL)

In SPARCL involving 4731 subjects (age range 21–92 years, 40% women; 93.3% Caucasians, 3.0% Blacks, 0.6% Asians, 3.1% other) without clinically evident CHD but with a stroke or transient ischemic attack (TIA) within the previous 6 months treated with LIPITOR 80 mg (n=2365) or placebo (n=2366) for a median follow-up of 4.9 years, there was a higher incidence of persistent hepatic transaminase elevations (≥ 3 × ULN twice within 4–10 days) in the atorvastatin group (0.9%) compared to placebo (0.1%). Elevations of CK (>10 × ULN) were rare, but were higher in the atorvastatin group (0.1%) compared to placebo (0.0%).

Diabetes was reported as an adverse reaction in 144 subjects (6.1%) in the atorvastatin group and 89 subjects (3.8%) in the placebo group (see **PRECAUTIONS**).

In a post-hoc analysis, LIPITOR 80 mg reduced the incidence of ischemic stroke (218/2365, 9.2% vs. 274/2366, 11.6%) and increased the incidence of hemorrhagic stroke (55/2365, 2.3% vs. 33/2366, 1.4%) compared to placebo. The incidence of fatal hemorrhagic stroke was similar between groups (17 LIPITOR vs. 18 placebo). The incidence of non-fatal hemorrhagic strokes was significantly greater in the atorvastatin group (38 non-fatal hemorrhagic strokes) as compared to the placebo group (16 non-fatal hemorrhagic strokes). Subjects who entered the study with a hemorrhagic stroke appeared to be at increased risk for hemorrhagic stroke [7 (16%) LIPITOR vs. 2 (4%) placebo].

There were no significant differences between the treatment groups for all-cause mortality: 216 (9.1%) in the LIPITOR 80 mg/day group vs. 211 (8.9%) in the placebo group. The proportions of subjects who experienced cardiovascular death were numerically smaller in the LIPITOR 80 mg group (3.3%) than in the placebo group (4.1%). The proportions of subjects who experienced non-cardiovascular death were numerically larger in the LIPITOR 80 mg group (5.0%) than in the placebo group (4.0%).

Postintroduction Reports with Atorvastatin

The following adverse reactions have been identified during postapproval use of the atorvastatin component of CADUET. Because these reactions are reported voluntarily from a population of uncertain size, it is not always possible to reliably estimate their frequency or establish a causal relationship to drug exposure.

Adverse reactions associated with atorvastatin therapy reported since market introduction, that are not listed above, regardless of causality assessment, include the following: anaphylaxis, angioneurotic edema, bullous rashes (including erythema multiforme, Stevens-Johnson syndrome, and toxic epidermal necrolysis), rhabdomyolysis, fatigue, tendon rupture, hepatic failure, dizziness, memory impairment, depression, and peripheral neuropathy.

Pediatric Patients (ages 10-17 years)

In a 26-week controlled study in boys and postmenarchal girls (n=140, 31% female; 92% Caucasians, 1.6% Blacks, 1.6% Asians, 4.8% other), the safety and tolerability profile of atorvastatin 10 to 20 mg daily was generally similar to that of placebo (see **CLINICAL PHARMACOLOGY, Clinical Studies** section and **PRECAUTIONS, Pediatric Use**).

OVERDOSAGE

There is no information on overdosage with CADUET in humans.

Information on Amlodipine

Single oral doses of amlodipine maleate equivalent to 40 mg amlodipine/kg and 100 mg amlodipine/kg in mice and rats, respectively, caused deaths. Single oral amlodipine maleate doses equivalent to 4 or more mg amlodipine/kg in dogs (11 or more times the maximum recommended clinical dose on a mg/m^2 basis) caused a marked peripheral vasodilation and hypotension.

Overdosage might be expected to cause excessive peripheral vasodilation with marked hypotension and possibly a reflex tachycardia. In humans, experience with intentional overdosage of amlodipine is limited. Reports of intentional overdosage include a patient who ingested 250 mg and was asymptomatic and was not hospitalized; another (120 mg) was hospitalized, underwent gastric lavage and remained normotensive; the third (105 mg) was hospitalized and had hypotension (90/50 mmHg) which normalized following plasma expansion. A patient who took 70 mg amlodipine and an unknown quantity of benzodiazepine in a suicide attempt developed shock which was refractory to treatment and died the following day with abnormally high benzodiazepine plasma concentration. A case of accidental drug overdose has been documented in a 19-month-old male who ingested 30 mg amlodipine (about 2 mg/kg). During the emergency room presentation, vital signs were stable with no evidence of hypotension, but a heart rate of 180 bpm. Ipecac was administered 3.5 hours after ingestion and on subsequent observation (overnight) no sequelae were noted.

If overdose should occur, begin active cardiac and respiratory monitoring. Perform frequent blood pressure measurements. Should hypotension occur, initiate cardiovascular support including elevation of the extremities and administration of fluids. If hypotension remains unresponsive to these conservative measures, consider administration of vasopressors (such as phenylephrine) with specific attention to circulating volume and urine output. As amlodipine is highly protein bound, hemodialysis is not likely to be of benefit.

Information on Atorvastatin

There is no specific treatment for atorvastatin overdosage. In the event of an overdose, the patient should be treated symptomatically, and supportive measures instituted as required. Due to extensive drug binding to plasma proteins, hemodialysis is not expected to significantly enhance atorvastatin clearance.

Table 14. CADUET Packaging Configurations

	CADUET			
Package Configuration	Tablet Strength (amlodipine besylate/atorvastatin calcium) mg	NDC #	Engraving	Tablet Color
Bottle of 30	2.5/10	0069-2960-30	CDT 251	White
Bottle of 30	2.5/20	0069-2970-30	CDT 252	White
Bottle of 30	2.5/40	0069-2980-30	CDT 254	White
Bottle of 30	5/10	0069-2150-30	CDT 051	White
Bottle of 30	5/20	0069-2170-30	CDT 052	White
Bottle of 30	5/40	0069-2190-30	CDT 054	White
Bottle of 30	5/80	0069-2260-30	CDT 058	White
Bottle of 30	10/10	0069-2160-30	CDT 101	Blue
Bottle of 30	10/20	0069-2180-30	CDT 102	Blue
Bottle of 30	10/40	0069-2250-30	CDT 104	Blue
Bottle of 30	10/80	0069-2270-30	CDT 108	Blue

DOSAGE AND ADMINISTRATION

Dosage of CADUET must be individualized on the basis of both effectiveness and tolerance for each individual component in the treatment of hypertension/angina and hyperlipidemia.

Amlodipine (Hypertension or angina)

Adults: The usual initial antihypertensive oral dose of amlodipine is 5 mg once daily with a maximum dose of 10 mg once daily. Small, fragile, or elderly individuals, or patients with hepatic insufficiency may be started on 2.5 mg once daily and this dose may be used when adding amlodipine to other antihypertensive therapy.

Dosage should be adjusted according to each patient's need. In general, titration should proceed over 7 to 14 days so that the physician can fully assess the patient's response to each dose level. Titration may proceed more rapidly, however, if clinically warranted, provided the patient is assessed frequently.

The recommended dose of amlodipine for chronic stable or vasospastic angina is 5-10 mg, with the lower dose suggested in the elderly and in patients with hepatic insufficiency. Most patients will require 10 mg for adequate effect. See **ADVERSE REACTIONS** section for information related to dosage and side effects.

The recommended dose range of amlodipine for patients with coronary artery disease is 5-10 mg once daily. In clinical studies the majority of patients required 10 mg (see **CLINICAL PHARMACOLOGY, Clinical studies**).

Children: The effective antihypertensive oral dose of amlodipine in pediatric patients ages 6-17 years is 2.5 mg to 5 mg once daily. Doses in excess of 5 mg daily have not been studied in pediatric patients (see **CLINICAL PHARMACOLOGY**).

Atorvastatin (Hyperlipidemia)

Hyperlipidemia (Heterozygous Familial and Nonfamilial) and Mixed Dyslipidemia (Fredrickson Types IIa and IIb)

The recommended starting dose of atorvastatin is 10 or 20 mg once daily. Patients who require a large reduction in LDL-C (more than 45%) may be started at 40 mg once daily. The dosage range of atorvastatin is 10 to 80 mg once daily. Atorvastatin can be administered as a single dose at any time of the day, with or without food. The starting dose and maintenance doses of atorvastatin should be individualized according to patient characteristics such as goal of therapy and response (see current *NCEP Guidelines*). After initiation and/or upon titration of atorvastatin, lipid levels should be analyzed within 2 to 4 weeks and dosage adjusted accordingly.

Heterozygous Familial Hypercholesterolemia in Pediatric Patients (10-17 years of age)

The recommended starting dose of atorvastatin is 10 mg/day; the maximum recommended dose is 20 mg/day (doses greater than 20 mg have not been studied in this patient population). Doses should be individualized according to the recommended goal of therapy (see current NCEP Pediatric Panel Guidelines[1], **CLINICAL PHARMACOLOGY**, and **INDICATIONS AND USAGE**). Adjustments should be made at intervals of 4 weeks or more.

[1]National Cholesterol Education Program (NCEP): Highlights of the Report of the Expert Panel on Blood Cholesterol Levels in Children Adolescents. *Pediatrics*. 89(3):495-501. 1992.

Homozygous Familial Hypercholesterolemia

The dosage of atorvastatin in patients with homozygous FH is 10 to 80 mg daily. Atorvastatin should be used as an adjunct to other lipid-lowering treatments (e.g., LDL apheresis) in these patients or if such treatments are unavailable. Note: a 2.5/80 mg CADUET tablet is not available. Management of patients needing a 2.5/80 mg combination requires individual assessments of dyslipidemia and therapy with the individual components as a 2.5/80 mg CADUET tablet is not available.

Concomitant Lipid Lowering Therapy

Atorvastatin may be used with bile acid resins. Monitor for signs of myopathy in patients receiving the combination of statins and fibrates (see **WARNINGS, Skeletal Muscle**, and **PRECAUTIONS, Drug Interactions**).

Dosage in Patients With Renal Impairment

Renal disease does not affect the plasma concentrations nor LDL-C reduction of atorvastatin; thus, dosage adjustment in patients with renal dysfunction is not necessary (see **WARNINGS, Skeletal Muscle**, and **CLINICAL PHARMACOLOGY, Specific Populations**).

Dosage in Patients Taking Cyclosporine, Clarithromycin, Itraconazole, or a Combination of Ritonavir plus Saquinavir or Lopinavir plus Ritonavir

In patients taking cyclosporine, therapy should be limited to LIPITOR 10 mg once daily. In patients taking clarithromycin, itraconazole or in patients with HIV taking a combination of ritonavir plus saquinavir or lopinavir plus ritonavir, for doses of atorvastatin exceeding 20 mg, appropriate clinical assessment is recommended to ensure that the lowest dose necessary of atorvastatin is employed (see **WARNINGS, Skeletal Muscle**, and **PRECAUTIONS, Drug Interactions**).

CADUET

CADUET may be substituted for its individually titrated components. Patients may be given the equivalent dose of CADUET or a dose of CADUET with increased amounts of amlodipine, atorvastatin or both for additional antianginal effects, blood pressure lowering, or lipid lowering effect.

CADUET may be used to provide additional therapy for patients already on one of its components. As initial therapy for one indication and continuation of treatment of the other, the recommended starting dose of CADUET should be selected based on the continuation of the component being used and the recommended starting dose for the added monotherapy.

CADUET may be used to initiate treatment in patients with hyperlipidemia and either hypertension or angina. The recommended starting dose of CADUET should be based on the appropriate combination of recommendations for the monotherapies. The maximum dose of the amlodipine component of CADUET is 10 mg once daily. The maximum dose of the atorvastatin component of CADUET is 80 mg once daily.

See above for detailed information related to the dosing and administration of amlodipine and atorvastatin.

HOW SUPPLIED

CADUET® tablets contain amlodipine besylate and atorvastatin calcium equivalent to amlodipine and atorvastatin in the dose strengths described below.

CADUET tablets are differentiated by tablet color/size and are engraved with "Pfizer" on one side and a unique number

on the other side. CADUET tablets are supplied for oral administration in the following strengths and package configurations:
[See table 14 at top of previous page]
Store at 25°C (77°F); excursions permitted to 15-30°C (59-86°F) [see USP Controlled Room Temperature].
Rx only
Manufactured by:
Pfizer Ireland Pharmaceuticals
Dublin, Ireland
Distributed by
Pfizer Labs
Division of Pfizer Inc, NY, NY 10017
LAB-0276-15.0
Revised January 2010

PATIENT INFORMATION

Caduet®
amlodipine besylate/atorvastatin calcium
from 5mg/10mg to 10mg/80mg tablets
(CAD-oo-et)

Read the patient information that comes with CADUET before you start taking it, and each time you get a refill. There may be new information. This information does not replace talking with your doctor about your condition or treatment. If you have any questions about CADUET, ask your doctor or pharmacist.

What is CADUET?
CADUET is a prescription drug that combines Norvasc® (amlodipine besylate) and Lipitor® (atorvastatin calcium) in one pill.

CADUET is used in adults who need both Norvasc and Lipitor.
Norvasc is used to treat:
- High blood pressure (hypertension) and
- Chest pain (angina) and
- Blocked arteries of the heart (coronary artery disease)

Lipitor is used to lower the levels of "bad" cholesterol and triglycerides in your blood. It can also raise the levels of "good" cholesterol.
Lipitor is also used to lower the risk for heart attack, stroke, certain types of heart surgery, and chest pain in patients who have heart disease or risk factors for heart disease such as:
- age, smoking, high blood pressure, low HDL-C, heart disease in the family

Lipitor can lower the risk for heart attack or stroke in patients with diabetes and risk factors such as:
- diabetic eye or kidney problems, smoking, or high blood pressure.

CADUET has not been studied in children.

Who should not use CADUET?
Do not use CADUET if you:
- Are pregnant or think you may be pregnant, or are planning to become pregnant. CADUET may harm your unborn baby. If you get pregnant, stop taking CADUET and call your doctor right away.
- Are breastfeeding. CADUET can pass into your breast milk and may harm your baby. Do not breastfeed if you take CADUET.
- Have liver problems.
- Are allergic to anything in CADUET. The active ingredients are atorvastatin calcium and amlodipine besylate. See the end of this leaflet for a complete list of ingredients.

What should I tell my doctor before taking CADUET?
Tell your doctor about all of your health conditions, including, if you have:
- heart disease
- muscle aches or weakness
- diabetes
- thyroid problems
- kidney problems
- or drink more than 2 glasses of alcohol daily

Tell your doctor about all the medicines you take including prescription and nonprescription medicines, vitamins and herbal supplements. CADUET and some other medicines can interact, causing serious side effects. Especially tell your doctor if you take medicines for:
- your immune system
- infections
- cholesterol
- birth control
- heart failure
- HIV (AIDS)

You can use nitroglycerin and CADUET together. If you take nitroglycerin for chest pain (angina), do not stop taking it while taking CADUET.
Know all the medicines you take. Keep a list of them with you to show your doctor and pharmacist.

How should I take CADUET?
- Take CADUET once a day, exactly as your doctor tells you. Do not change your dose or stop CADUET without talking to your doctor.
- Take CADUET each day at any time of day, at about the same time each day. CADUET can be taken with or without food.
- Do not break the tablets before taking them. Talk to your doctor if you have a problem swallowing pills.
- Your doctor should start you on a low-fat diet before giving you CADUET. Stay on this low-fat diet when you take CADUET.
- CADUET comes in many different strengths. Your doctor will test your cholesterol and blood pressure to find the right dose for you.
- If you miss a dose, take it as soon as you remember. Do not take CADUET if it has been more than 12 hours since your missed dose. Just take the next dose at your regular time. Do not take 2 doses of CADUET at the same time.
- If too much CADUET is taken by accident, call your doctor or poison control center, or go to the nearest emergency room.

What should I avoid while taking CADUET?
- Avoid getting pregnant. If you get pregnant, stop taking CADUET right away and call your doctor.
- Do not breastfeed. CADUET can pass into your breast milk and may harm your baby.

What are possible side effects of CADUET?
CADUET can cause serious side effects. These side effects happen only to a small number of people. Your doctor can monitor you for them. These side effects usually go away if your dose is lowered or CADUET is stopped. These serious side effects include:
- **Muscle problems.** CADUET can cause serious muscle problems that can lead to kidney problems, including kidney failure. You have a higher chance for muscle problems if you are taking certain other medicines with CADUET.
- **Liver problems.** CADUET can cause liver problems. Your doctor may do blood tests to check your liver before you start taking CADUET and while you take it.

Call your doctor right away if:
- you have muscle problems like weakness, tenderness, or pain that happen without a good reason, especially if you also have a fever or feel more tired than usual
- allergic reactions including swelling of the face, lips, tongue, and/or throat that may cause difficulty in breathing or swallowing which may require treatment right away.
- you have nausea and vomiting, stomach pain
- you are passing brown or dark-colored urine
- you feel more tired than usual
- your skin and white of your eyes get yellow
- allergic skin reactions.
- **Chest pain that does not go away or gets worse.** Sometimes, when you start CADUET or increase your dose, chest pain can get worse or a heart attack can happen. If this happens, call your doctor or go to the emergency room right away.

Common side effects of CADUET include:
- headache
- tiredness
- stomach pain
- upset stomach
- dizziness
- extreme sleepiness
- nausea
- diarrhea
- swelling of your legs or ankles (edema)
- hot or warm feeling in your face (flushing)
- irregular heartbeat (arrhythmia)
- very fast heartbeat (heart palpitations)
- muscle and joint pain
- alterations in some laboratory blood tests

Additional side effects have been reported: tendon problems.
Talk to your doctor or pharmacist about side effects that bother you or do not go away.
There are other side effects of CADUET. Ask your doctor or pharmacist for a complete list.

How do I store CADUET?
- Store CADUET at room temperature, 68 to 77°F (20 to 25°C).
- Do not keep medicine that is out-of-date or that you no longer need.
- **Keep CADUET and all medicines out of the reach of children.** Keep medicines in places where children cannot get it.

General information about CADUET
Medicines are sometimes prescribed for conditions that are not mentioned in patient information leaflets. Do not use CADUET for a condition for which it was not prescribed. Do not give CADUET to other people, even if they have the same problem you have. It may harm them.
This leaflet summarizes the most important information about CADUET. If you want more information, talk with your doctor. Ask your doctor or pharmacist for information about CADUET written for health professionals. You can also go to the CADUET website at www.CADUET.com, or call 866-514-0900.

What is high blood pressure (hypertension)?
You have high blood pressure when the force of blood against the walls of your arteries stays high. This can damage your heart and other parts of your body. Drugs that lower blood pressure lower your risk of having a stroke or heart attack.

What is angina (chest pain)?
Angina is a pain that keeps coming back when part of your heart does not get enough blood. It feels like something is pressing or squeezing your chest under the breastbone. Sometimes you can feel it in your shoulders, arms, neck, jaw, or back.

What is cholesterol?
Cholesterol is a fat-like substance made in your body. It is also found in foods. You need some cholesterol for good health, but too much is not good for you. Cholesterol can clog your blood vessels.

What is a heart attack?
A heart attack occurs when heart muscle does not get enough blood. Symptoms include chest pain, trouble breathing, nausea, and weakness. Heart muscle cells may be damaged or die. The heart cannot pump well or may stop beating.

What is a stroke?
A stroke occurs when nerve cells in the brain do not get enough blood. The cells may be damaged or die. The damaged cells may cause weakness or problems speaking or thinking.

WHAT ARE THE INGREDIENTS IN CADUET?
Active ingredients: amlodipine besylate, atorvastatin calcium
Inactive ingredients: calcium carbonate, croscarmellose sodium, microcrystalline cellulose, pregelatinized starch, polysorbate 80, hydroxypropyl cellulose, purified water, colloidal silicon dioxide (anhydrous), magnesium stearate
Film coating: Opadry® II White 85F28751 (polyvinyl alcohol, titanium dioxide, PEG 3000 and talc) or Opadry® II Blue 85F10919 (polyvinyl alcohol, titanium dioxide, PEG 3000, talc, and FD&C blue #2)
Rx only
Manufactured by Pfizer Ireland Pharmaceuticals
Dublin, Ireland
Distributed by
Pfizer Labs
Division of Pfizer Inc, NY, NY 10017
LAB-0347- 3.0
Issued July 2009

CHANTIX® ℞

[chan-tiks]
(varenicline)
Tablets

HIGHLIGHTS OF PRESCRIBING INFORMATION
These highlights do not include all the information needed to use CHANTIX safely and effectively. See full prescribing information for CHANTIX.
CHANTIX® (varenicline) Tablets
Initial U.S. Approval: 2006

WARNING: SERIOUS NEUROPSYCHIATRIC EVENTS
See full prescribing information for complete boxed warning.
- **Serious neuropsychiatric events have been reported in patients taking CHANTIX. (5.1 and 6.2)**
- **Advise patients and caregivers that the patient should stop taking CHANTIX and contact a healthcare provider immediately if agitation, hostility, depressed mood, or changes in behavior or thinking that are not typical for the patient are observed, or if the patient develops suicidal ideation or suicidal behavior while taking CHANTIX or shortly after discontinuing CHANTIX. (5.1 and 6.2)**
- **Weigh the risks of CHANTIX against benefits of its use. CHANTIX has been demonstrated to increase the likelihood of abstinence from smoking for as long as one year compared to treatment with placebo. The health benefits of quitting smoking are immediate and substantial. (5.1 and 6.2)**

RECENT MAJOR CHANGES

Boxed Warning	7/2009
Contraindications	4/2010
Known Hypersensitivity (4)	
Warnings and Precautions	7/2009
Neuropsychiatric Symptoms and Suicidality (5.1), Angioedema and Hypersensitivity Reactions (5.2), Serious Skin Reactions (5.3), Accidental Injury (5.4)	

INDICATIONS AND USAGE
CHANTIX is a nicotinic receptor partial agonist indicated for use as an aid to smoking cessation treatment. (1 and 2.1)

DOSAGE AND ADMINISTRATION
- Begin CHANTIX dosing one week before the date set by the patient to stop smoking. (2.1)
- Starting week: 0.5 mg once daily on days 1-3 and 0.5 mg twice daily on days 4-7. (2.1)
- Continuing weeks: 1 mg twice daily for a total of 12 weeks. (2.1)
- An additional 12 weeks of treatment is recommended for successful quitters to increase likelihood of long-term abstinence. (2.1)
- Renal impairment: Reduce the dose in patients with severe renal impairment (estimated creatinine clearance <30 mL/min). (2.2)

- Consider dose reduction for patients who cannot tolerate adverse effects. (2.1)
- Another attempt at treatment is recommended for those who fail to stop smoking or relapse when factors contributing to the failed attempt have been addressed. (2.1)
- Provide patients with appropriate educational materials and counseling to support the quit attempt. (2.1)

————————DOSAGE FORMS AND STRENGTHS————————

Tablets: 0.5 mg and 1 mg (3)

————————CONTRAINDICATIONS————————

History of serious hypersensitivity or skin reactions to CHANTIX (4)

————————WARNINGS AND PRECAUTIONS————————

- **Angioedema and hypersensitivity reactions:** Such reactions, including angioedema, infrequently life threatening, have been reported. Instruct patients to discontinue CHANTIX and immediately seek medical care if symptoms occur. (5.2 and 6.2)
- **Serious skin reactions:** Rare, potentially life-threatening skin reactions have been reported. Instruct patients to discontinue CHANTIX and contact a healthcare provider immediately at first appearance of skin rash with mucosal lesions. (5.3 and 6.2)
- **Accidental injury:** Accidental injuries (e.g., traffic accidents) have been reported. Instruct patients to use caution driving or operating machinery until they know how CHANTIX may affect them. (5.4)
- **Nausea:** Nausea is the most common adverse reaction (up to 30% incidence rate). Dose reduction may be helpful. (5.5)

————————ADVERSE REACTIONS————————

Most common adverse reactions (>5% and twice the rate seen in placebo-treated patients) were nausea, abnormal (e.g., vivid, unusual, or strange) dreams, constipation, flatulence, and vomiting. (6.1)

To report SUSPECTED ADVERSE REACTIONS, contact Pfizer Inc at 1-800-438-1985 or FDA at 1-800-FDA-1088 or www.fda.gov/medwatch.

————————DRUG INTERACTIONS————————

- Other smoking cessation therapies: Safety and efficacy in combination with other smoking cessation therapies has not been established. Coadministration of varenicline and transdermal nicotine resulted in a high rate of discontinuation due to adverse events. (7.1)
- Effect of smoking cessation: Pharmacokinetics or pharmacodynamics of certain drugs may be altered due to smoking cessation with CHANTIX, necessitating dose adjustment. (7.2)

————————USE IN SPECIFIC POPULATIONS————————

- Pregnancy: CHANTIX should be used during pregnancy only if the potential benefit justifies the potential risk to the fetus (8.1)
- Nursing Mothers: Discontinue drug or nursing taking into consideration importance of drug to mother (8.3)
- Pediatric Use: Safety and effectiveness not established (8.4)
- Renal Impairment: Dosage adjustment is required for severe renal impairment (2.2, 8.6)

See 17 for PATIENT COUNSELING INFORMATION and Medication Guide

Revised: 04/2010

FULL PRESCRIBING INFORMATION

> **WARNING: SERIOUS NEUROPSYCHIATRIC EVENTS**
> Serious neuropsychiatric events including, but not limited to, depression, suicidal ideation, suicide attempt and completed suicide have been reported in patients taking CHANTIX. Some reported cases may have been complicated by the symptoms of nicotine withdrawal in patients who stopped smoking. Depressed mood may be a symptom of nicotine withdrawal. Depression, rarely including suicidal ideation, has been reported in smokers undergoing a smoking cessation attempt without medication. However, some of these symptoms have occurred in patients taking CHANTIX who continued to smoke.
> All patients being treated with CHANTIX should be observed for neuropsychiatric symptoms including changes in behavior, hostility, agitation, depressed mood, and suicide-related events, including ideation, behavior, and attempted suicide. These symptoms, as well as worsening of pre-existing psychiatric illness and completed suicide, have been reported in some patients attempting to quit smoking while taking CHANTIX in the postmarketing experience. When symptoms were reported, most were during CHANTIX treatment, but some were following discontinuation of CHANTIX therapy.
> These events have occurred in patients with and without preexisting psychiatric disease. Patients with serious psychiatric illness such as schizophrenia, bipolar disorder, and major depressive disorder did not participate in the premarketing studies of CHANTIX, and the safety and efficacy of CHANTIX in such patients has not been established.
> Advise patients and caregivers that the patient should stop taking CHANTIX and contact a healthcare provider immediately if agitation, hostility, depressed mood, or changes in behavior or thinking that are not typical for the patient are observed, or if the patient develops suicidal ideation or suicidal behavior. In many postmarketing cases, resolution of symptoms after discontinuation of CHANTIX was reported, although in some cases the symptoms persisted; therefore, ongoing monitoring and supportive care should be provided until symptoms resolve.
> The risks of CHANTIX should be weighed against the benefits of its use. CHANTIX has been demonstrated to increase the likelihood of abstinence from smoking for as long as one year compared to treatment with placebo. The health benefits of quitting smoking are immediate and substantial. *[see Warnings and Precautions (5.1) and Adverse Reactions 6.2)]*

1   INDICATIONS AND USAGE

CHANTIX is indicated for use as an aid to smoking cessation treatment.

2   DOSAGE AND ADMINISTRATION

2.1   Usual Dosage for Adults

Smoking cessation therapies are more likely to succeed for patients who are motivated to stop smoking and who are provided additional advice and support. Provide patients with appropriate educational materials and counseling to support the quit attempt.

The patient should set a date to stop smoking. Begin CHANTIX dosing one week before this date.

CHANTIX should be taken after eating and with a full glass of water.

The recommended dose of CHANTIX is 1 mg twice daily following a 1-week titration as follows:

Days 1–3:	0.5 mg once daily
Days 4–7:	0.5 mg twice daily
Day 8–end of treatment:	1 mg twice daily

Patients should be treated with CHANTIX for 12 weeks. For patients who have successfully stopped smoking at the end of 12 weeks, an additional course of 12 weeks' treatment with CHANTIX is recommended to further increase the likelihood of long-term abstinence.

Patients who do not succeed in stopping smoking during 12 weeks of initial therapy, or who relapse after treatment, should be encouraged to make another attempt once factors contributing to the failed attempt have been identified and addressed.

Consider a temporary or permanent dose reduction in patients who cannot tolerate the adverse effects of CHANTIX.

2.2   Dosage in Special Populations

Patients with Impaired Renal Function: No dosage adjustment is necessary for patients with mild to moderate renal impairment. For patients with severe renal impairment (estimated creatinine clearance <30 mL/min), the recommended starting dose of CHANTIX is 0.5 mg once daily. The dose may then be titrated as needed to a maximum dose of 0.5 mg twice a day. For patients with end-stage renal disease undergoing hemodialysis, a maximum dose of 0.5 mg once daily may be administered if tolerated *[see Use in Specific Populations (8.6) and Clinical Pharmacology (12.3)].*

Elderly and Patients with Impaired Hepatic Function: No dosage adjustment is necessary for patients with hepatic impairment. Because elderly patients are more likely to have decreased renal function, care should be taken in dose selection, and it may be useful to monitor renal function *[see Use in Specific Populations (8.5)].*

3   DOSAGE FORMS AND STRENGTHS

Capsular, biconvex tablets: 0.5 mg (white to off-white, debossed with "*Pfizer*" on one side and "CHX 0.5" on the other side) and 1 mg (light blue, debossed with "*Pfizer*" on one side and "CHX 1.0" on the other side)

4   CONTRAINDICATIONS

CHANTIX is contraindicated in patients with a known history of serious hypersensitivity reactions or skin reactions to CHANTIX

5   WARNINGS AND PRECAUTIONS

5.1   Neuropsychiatric Symptoms and Suicidality

Serious neuropsychiatric symptoms have been reported in patients being treated with CHANTIX *[see Boxed Warning and Adverse Reactions (6.2)].* These postmarketing reports have included changes in mood (including depression and mania), psychosis, hallucinations, paranoia, delusions, homicidal ideation, hostility, agitation, anxiety, and panic, as well as suicidal ideation, suicide attempt, and completed suicide. Some reported cases may have been complicated by the symptoms of nicotine withdrawal in patients who stopped smoking. Depressed mood may be a symptom of nicotine withdrawal. Depression, rarely including suicidal ideation, has been reported in smokers undergoing a smoking cessation attempt without medication. However, some of these symptoms have occurred in patients taking CHANTIX who continued to smoke. When symptoms were reported, most were during CHANTIX treatment, but some were following discontinuation of CHANTIX therapy.

These events have occurred in patients with and without pre-existing psychiatric disease; some patients have experienced worsening of their psychiatric illnesses. All patients being treated with CHANTIX should be observed for neuropsychiatric symptoms or worsening of pre-existing psychiatric illness. Patients with serious psychiatric illness such as schizophrenia, bipolar disorder, and major depressive disorder did not participate in the premarketing studies of CHANTIX, and the safety and efficacy of CHANTIX in such patients has not been established.

Advise patients and caregivers that the patient should stop taking CHANTIX and contact a healthcare provider immediately if agitation, depressed mood, changes in behavior or thinking that are not typical for the patient are observed, or if the patient develops suicidal ideation or suicidal behavior. In many postmarketing cases, resolution of symptoms after discontinuation of CHANTIX was reported, although in some cases the symptoms persisted, therefore, ongoing monitoring and supportive care should be provided until symptoms resolve.

The risks of CHANTIX should be weighed against the benefits of its use. CHANTIX has been demonstrated to increase the likelihood of abstinence from smoking for as long as one year compared to treatment with placebo. The health benefits of quitting smoking are immediate and substantial.

5.2 Angioedema and Hypersensitivity Reactions

There have been postmarketing reports of hypersensitivity reactions including angioedema in patients treated with CHANTIX *[see Adverse Reactions (6.2), and Patient Counseling Information (17.10)]*. Clinical signs included swelling of the face, mouth (tongue, lips, and gums), extremities, and neck (throat and larynx). There were infrequent reports of life-threatening angioedema requiring emergent medical attention due to respiratory compromise. Instruct patients to discontinue CHANTIX and immediately seek medical care if they experience these symptoms.

5.3 Serious Skin Reactions

There have been postmarketing reports of rare but serious skin reactions, including Stevens-Johnson Syndrome and erythema multiforme, in patients using CHANTIX *[see Adverse Reactions (6.2)]*. As these skin reactions can be life-threatening, instruct patients to stop taking CHANTIX and contact a healthcare provider immediately at the first appearance of a skin rash with mucosal lesions or any other signs of hypersensitivity.

5.4 Accidental Injury

There have been postmarketing reports of traffic accidents, near-miss incidents in traffic, or other accidental injuries in patients taking CHANTIX. In some cases, the patients reported somnolence, dizziness, loss of consciousness or difficulty concentrating that resulted in impairment, or concern about potential impairment, in driving or operating machinery. Advise patients to use caution driving or operating machinery or engaging in other potentially hazardous activities until they know how CHANTIX may affect them.

5.5 Nausea

Nausea was the most common adverse reaction reported with CHANTIX treatment. Nausea was generally described as mild or moderate and often transient; however, for some patients, it was persistent over several months. The incidence of nausea was dose-dependent. Initial dose-titration was beneficial in reducing the occurrence of nausea. For patients treated to the maximum recommended dose of 1 mg twice daily following initial dosage titration, the incidence of nausea was 30% compared with 10% in patients taking a comparable placebo regimen. In patients taking CHANTIX 0.5 mg twice daily following initial titration, the incidence was 16% compared with 11% for placebo. Approximately 3% of patients treated with CHANTIX 1 mg twice daily in studies involving 12 weeks of treatment discontinued treatment prematurely because of nausea. For patients with intolerable nausea, a dose reduction should be considered.

6 ADVERSE REACTIONS

The following serious adverse reactions were reported in postmarketing experience and are discussed in greater detail in other sections of the labeling:

- Neuropsychiatric symptoms and suicidality *[see Boxed Warning and Warnings and Precautions (5.1)]*
- Angioedema and hypersensitivity reactions *[see Warnings and Precautions (5.2)]*
- Serious skin reactions *[see Warnings and Precautions (5.3)]*
- Accidental injury *[see Warnings and Precautions (5.4)]*

In the placebo-controlled studies, the most common adverse events associated with CHANTIX (>5% and twice the rate seen in placebo-treated patients) were nausea, abnormal (vivid, unusual, or strange) dreams, constipation, flatulence, and vomiting.

The treatment discontinuation rate due to adverse events in patients dosed with 1 mg twice daily was 12% for CHANTIX, compared to 10% for placebo in studies of three months' treatment. In this group, the discontinuation rates that are higher than placebo for the most common adverse events in CHANTIX-treated patients were as follows: nausea (3% vs. 0.5% for placebo), insomnia (1.2% vs. 1.1% for placebo), and abnormal dreams (0.3% vs. 0.2% for placebo). Smoking cessation, with or without treatment, is associated with nicotine withdrawal symptoms and has also been associated with the exacerbation of underlying psychiatric illness.

6.1 Clinical Trials Experience

Because clinical trials are conducted under widely varying conditions, the adverse reactions rates observed in the clinical studies of a drug cannot be directly compared to rates in the clinical trials of another drug and may not reflect the rates observed in clinical practice.

During the premarketing development of CHANTIX, over 4500 subjects were exposed to CHANTIX, with over 450 treated for at least 24 weeks and approximately 100 for a year. Most study participants were treated for 12 weeks or less.

The most common adverse event associated with CHANTIX treatment is nausea, occurring in 30% of patients treated at the recommended dose, compared with 10% in patients taking a comparable placebo regimen *[see Warnings and Precautions (5.5)]*.

Table 1 shows the adverse events for CHANTIX and placebo in the 12-week fixed dose studies with titration in the first week [Studies 2 (titrated arm only), 4, and 5]. Adverse events were categorized using the Medical Dictionary for Regulatory Activities (MedDRA, Version 7.1).

MedDRA High Level Group Terms (HLGT) reported in ≥ 5% of patients in the CHANTIX 1 mg twice daily dose group, and more commonly than in the placebo group, are listed, along with subordinate Preferred Terms (PT) reported in ≥ 1% of CHANTIX patients (and at least 0.5% more frequent than placebo). Closely related Preferred Terms such as 'Insomnia', 'Initial insomnia', 'Middle insomnia', 'Early morning awakening' were grouped, but individual patients reporting two or more grouped events are only counted once.

[See table 1 at left]

The overall pattern and frequency of adverse events during the longer-term trials was similar to those described in Table 1, though several of the most common events were reported by a greater proportion of patients with long-term use (e.g., nausea was reported in 40% of patients treated with CHANTIX 1 mg twice daily in a one-year study, compared to 8% of placebo-treated patients).

Following is a list of treatment-emergent adverse events reported by patients treated with CHANTIX during all clinical trials. The listing does not include those events already listed in the previous tables or elsewhere in labeling, those events for which a drug cause was remote, those events which were so general as to be uninformative, and those events reported only once which did not have a substantial probability of being acutely life-threatening.

Blood and Lymphatic System Disorders. *Infrequent:* anemia, lymphadenopathy. *Rare:* leukocytosis, splenomegaly, thrombocytopenia.

Cardiac Disorders. *Infrequent:* angina pectoris, arrhythmia, bradycardia, myocardial infarction, palpitations, tachycardia, ventricular extrasystoles. *Rare:* acute coronary syndrome, atrial fibrillation, cardiac flutter, cor pulmonale, coronary artery disease.

Ear and Labyrinth Disorders. *Infrequent:* tinnitus, vertigo. *Rare:* deafness, Meniere's disease.

Endocrine Disorders. *Infrequent:* thyroid gland disorders.

Eye Disorders. *Infrequent:* conjunctivitis, dry eye, eye irritation, eye pain, vision blurred, visual disturbance. *Rare:* acquired night blindness, blindness transient, cataract subcapsular, ocular vascular disorder, photophobia, vitreous floaters

Gastrointestinal Disorders. *Frequent:* diarrhea. *Infrequent:* dysphagia, enterocolitis, eructation, esophagitis, gastritis, gastrointestinal hemorrhage, mouth ulceration. *Rare:* gastric ulcer, intestinal obstruction, pancreatitis acute.

General Disorders and Administration Site Conditions. *Frequent:* chest pain, edema, influenza-like illness. *Infrequent:* chest discomfort, chills, pyrexia.

Hepatobiliary Disorders. *Infrequent:* gall bladder disorder

Investigations. *Frequent:* liver function test abnormal, weight increased. *Infrequent:* electrocardiogram abnormal, muscle enzyme increased, urine analysis abnormal.

Metabolism and Nutrition Disorders. *Infrequent:* diabetes mellitus, hyperlipidemia, hypokalemia. *Rare:* hypoglycemia.

Musculoskeletal and Connective Tissue Disorders. *Frequent:* arthralgia, back pain, muscle cramp, musculoskeletal pain, myalgia. *Infrequent:* arthritis, osteoporosis. *Rare:* myositis.

Table 1: Common Treatment Emergent AEs (%) in the Fixed-Dose, Placebo-Controlled Studies (≥ 1% in the 1 mg BID CHANTIX Group, and 1 mg BID CHANTIX at least 0.5% more than Placebo)

SYSTEM ORGAN CLASS High Level Group Term Preferred Term	CHANTIX 0.5 mg BID N=129	CHANTIX 1 mg BID N=821	Placebo N=805
GASTROINTESTINAL (GI)			
GI Signs and Symptoms			
Nausea	16	30	10
Abdominal Pain *	5	7	5
Flatulence	9	6	3
Dyspepsia	5	5	3
Vomiting	1	5	2
GI Motility/Defecation Conditions			
Constipation	5	8	3
Gastroesophageal reflux disease	1	1	0
Salivary Gland Conditions			
Dry mouth	4	6	4
PSYCHIATRIC DISORDERS			
Sleep Disorder/Disturbances			
Insomnia **	19	18	13
Abnormal dreams	9	13	5
Sleep disorder	2	5	3
Nightmare	2	1	0
NERVOUS SYSTEM			
Headaches			
Headache	19	15	13
Neurological Disorders NEC			
Dysgeusia	8	5	4
Somnolence	3	3	2
Lethargy	2	1	0
GENERAL DISORDERS			
General Disorders NEC			
Fatigue/Malaise/Asthenia	4	7	6
RESPIR/THORACIC/MEDIAST			
Respiratory Disorders NEC			
Rhinorrhea	0	1	0
Dyspnea	2	1	1
Upper Respiratory Tract Disorder	7	5	4
SKIN/SUBCUTANEOUS TISSUE			
Epidermal and Dermal Conditions			
Rash	1	3	2
Pruritus	0	1	1
METABOLISM & NUTRITION			
Appetite/General Nutrit. Disorders			
Increased appetite	4	3	2
Decreased appetite/Anorexia	1	2	1

* Includes PTs Abdominal (pain, pain upper, pain lower, discomfort, tenderness, distension) and Stomach discomfort
** Includes PTs Insomnia/Initial insomnia/Middle insomnia/Early morning awakening

Nervous System Disorders. *Frequent:* disturbance in attention, dizziness, sensory disturbance. *Infrequent:* amnesia, migraine, parosmia, psychomotor hyperactivity, restless legs syndrome, syncope, tremor. *Rare:* balance disorder, cerebrovascular accident, convulsion, dysarthria, facial palsy, mental impairment, multiple sclerosis, nystagmus, psychomotor skills impaired, transient ischemic attack, visual field defect.

Psychiatric Disorders. *Infrequent:* disorientation, dissociation, libido decreased, mood swings, thinking abnormal. *Rare:* bradyphrenia, euphoric mood.

Renal and Urinary Disorders. *Frequent:* polyuria. *Infrequent:* nephrolithiasis, nocturia, urethral syndrome, urine abnormality. *Rare:* renal failure acute, urinary retention.

Reproductive System and Breast Disorders. *Rare:* sexual dysfunction. *Frequent:* menstrual disorder. *Infrequent:* erectile dysfunction.

Respiratory, Thoracic and Mediastinal Disorders. *Frequent:* epistaxis, respiratory disorders. *Infrequent:* asthma. *Rare:* pleurisy, pulmonary embolism.

Skin and Subcutaneous Tissue Disorders. *Frequent:* hyperhidrosis. *Infrequent:* acne, dry skin, eczema, erythema, psoriasis, urticaria. *Rare:* photosensitivity reaction.

Vascular Disorders. *Frequent:* hot flush. *Infrequent:* thrombosis.

6.2 Postmarketing Experience

The following adverse events have been reported during post-approval use of CHANTIX. Because these events are reported voluntarily from a population of uncertain size, it is not possible to reliably estimate their frequency or establish a causal relationship to drug exposure.

There have been reports of depression, mania, psychosis, hallucinations, paranoia, delusions, homicidal ideation, aggression, hostility, anxiety, and panic, as well as suicidal ideation, suicide attempt, and completed suicide in patients attempting to quit smoking while taking CHANTIX *[see Boxed Warning, Warnings and Precautions (5.1)]*. Smoking cessation with or without treatment is associated with nicotine withdrawal symptoms and the exacerbation of underlying psychiatric illness. Not all patients had known pre-existing psychiatric illness and not all had discontinued smoking.

There have been reports of hypersensitivity reactions, including angioedema *[see Warnings and Precautions (5.2)]*.

There have also been reports of serious skin reactions, including Stevens-Johnson Syndrome and erythema multiforme, in patients taking CHANTIX *[see Warnings and Precautions (5.3)]*.

7 DRUG INTERACTIONS

Based on varenicline characteristics and clinical experience to date, CHANTIX has no clinically meaningful pharmacokinetic drug interactions *[see Clinical Pharmacology (12.3)]*.

7.1 Use With Other Drugs for Smoking Cessation

Safety and efficacy of CHANTIX in combination with other smoking cessation therapies have not been studied.

Bupropion: Varenicline (1 mg twice daily) did not alter the steady-state pharmacokinetics of bupropion (150 mg twice daily) in 46 smokers. The safety of the combination of bupropion and varenicline has not been established.

Nicotine replacement therapy (NRT): Although co-administration of varenicline (1 mg twice daily) and transdermal nicotine (21 mg/day) for up to 12 days did not affect nicotine pharmacokinetics, the incidence of nausea, headache, vomiting, dizziness, dyspepsia, and fatigue was greater for the combination than for NRT alone. In this study, eight of twenty-two (36%) patients treated with the combination of varenicline and NRT prematurely discontinued treatment due to adverse events, compared to 1 of 17 (6%) of patients treated with NRT and placebo.

7.2 Effect of Smoking Cessation on Other Drugs

Physiological changes resulting from smoking cessation, with or without treatment with CHANTIX, may alter the pharmacokinetics or pharmacodynamics of certain drugs (e.g., theophylline, warfarin, insulin) for which dosage adjustment may be necessary.

8 USE IN SPECIFIC POPULATIONS

8.1 Pregnancy

Pregnancy Category C.

There are no adequate and well-controlled studies of CHANTIX use in pregnant women. In animal studies, CHANTIX caused decreased fetal weights, increased auditory startle response, and decreased fertility in offspring. CHANTIX should be used during pregnancy only if the potential benefit justifies the potential risk to the fetus.

In reproductive and developmental toxicity studies, pregnant rats and rabbits received varenicline succinate during organogenesis at oral doses up to 15 and 30 mg/kg/day, respectively. These exposures were 36 (rats) and 50 (rabbits) times the human exposure (based on AUC) at the maximum recommended human dose (MRHD) of 1 mg BID. While no fetal structural abnormalities occurred in either species, reduced fetal weights occurred in rabbits at the highest dose (exposures 50 times the human exposure at the MRHD based on AUC). Fetal weight reduction did not occur at animal exposures 23 times the human exposure at the MRHD based on AUC.

In a pre- and postnatal development study, pregnant rats received up to 15 mg/kg/day of oral varenicline succinate from organogenesis through lactation. These resulted in exposures up to 36 times the human exposure (based on AUC) at the MRHD of 1 mg BID. Decreased fertility and increased auditory startle response occurred in offspring.

8.3 Nursing Mothers

It is not known whether CHANTIX is excreted in human milk. In animal studies varenicline was excreted in milk of lactating animals. Because many drugs are excreted in human milk and because of the potential for serious adverse reactions in nursing infants from CHANTIX, a decision should be made whether to discontinue nursing or to discontinue the drug, taking into account the importance of the drug to the mother.

8.4 Pediatric Use

Safety and effectiveness of CHANTIX in pediatric patients have not been established.

8.5 Geriatric Use

A combined single- and multiple-dose pharmacokinetic study demonstrated that the pharmacokinetics of 1 mg varenicline given once daily or twice daily to 16 healthy elderly male and female smokers (aged 65-75 yrs) for 7 consecutive days was similar to that of younger subjects. No overall differences in safety or effectiveness were observed between these subjects and younger subjects, and other reported clinical experience has not identified differences in responses between the elderly and younger patients, but greater sensitivity of some older individuals cannot be ruled out.

Varenicline is known to be substantially excreted by the kidney, and the risk of toxic reactions to this drug may be greater in patients with impaired renal function. Because elderly patients are more likely to have decreased renal function, care should be taken in dose selection, and it may be useful to monitor renal function *[see Dosage and Administration (2.2)]*.

No dosage adjustment is recommended for elderly patients.

8.6 Renal Impairment

Varenicline is substantially eliminated by renal glomerular filtration along with active tubular secretion. Dose reduction is not required in patients with mild to moderate renal impairment. For patients with severe renal impairment (estimated creatinine clearance <30 mL/min), and for patients with end-stage renal disease undergoing hemodialysis, dosage adjustment is needed. *[see Dosage and Administration (2.2) and Clinical Pharmacology (12.3)]*.

9 DRUG ABUSE AND DEPENDENCE

9.1 Controlled Substance

Varenicline is not a controlled substance.

9.3 Dependence

Humans: Fewer than 1 out of 1000 patients reported euphoria in clinical trials with CHANTIX. At higher doses (greater than 2 mg), CHANTIX produced more frequent reports of gastrointestinal disturbances such as nausea and vomiting. There is no evidence of dose-escalation to maintain therapeutic effects in clinical studies, which suggests that tolerance does not develop. Abrupt discontinuation of CHANTIX was associated with an increase in irritability and sleep disturbances in up to 3% of patients. This suggests that, in some patients, varenicline may produce mild physical dependence which is not associated with addiction.

In a human laboratory abuse liability study, a single oral dose of 1 mg varenicline did not produce any significant positive or negative subjective responses in smokers. In non-smokers, 1 mg varenicline produced an increase in some positive subjective effects, but this was accompanied by an increase in negative adverse effects, especially nausea. A single oral dose of 3 mg varenicline uniformly produced unpleasant subjective responses in both smokers and non-smokers.

Animals: Studies in rodents have shown that varenicline produces behavioral responses similar to those produced by nicotine. In rats trained to discriminate nicotine from saline, varenicline produced full generalization to the nicotine cue. In self-administration studies, the degree to which varenicline substitutes for nicotine is dependent upon the requirement of the task. Rats trained to self-administer nicotine under easy conditions continued to self-administer varenicline to a degree comparable to that of nicotine; however in a more demanding task, rats self-administered varenicline to a lesser extent than nicotine. Varenicline pretreatment also reduced nicotine self-administration.

10 OVERDOSAGE

In case of overdose, standard supportive measures should be instituted as required.

Varenicline has been shown to be dialyzed in patients with end stage renal disease *[see Clinical Pharmacology (12.3)]*, however, there is no experience in dialysis following overdose.

11 DESCRIPTION

CHANTIX tablets contain varenicline (as the tartrate salt), which is a partial agonist selective for $\alpha_4\beta_2$ nicotinic acetylcholine receptor subtypes.

Varenicline, as the tartrate salt, is a powder which is a white to off-white to slightly yellow solid with the following chemical name: 7,8,9,10-tetrahydro-6,10-methano-6*H*-pyrazino[2,3- h][3] benzazepine, (2*R*,3*R*)-2,3-dihydroxybutanedioate (1:1). It is highly soluble in water. Varenicline tartrate has a molecular weight of 361.35 Daltons, and a molecular formula of $C_{13}H_{13}N_3 \bullet C_4H_6O_6$. The chemical structure is:

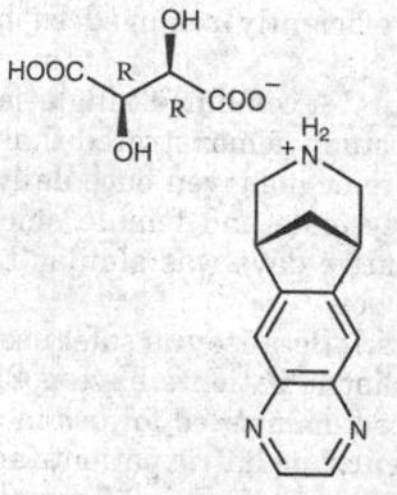

CHANTIX is supplied for oral administration in two strengths: a 0.5 mg capsular biconvex, white to off-white, film-coated tablet debossed with *"Pfizer"* on one side and "CHX 0.5" on the other side and a 1 mg capsular biconvex, light blue film-coated tablet debossed with *"Pfizer"* on one side and "CHX 1.0" on the other side. Each 0.5 mg CHANTIX tablet contains 0.85 mg of varenicline tartrate equivalent to 0.5 mg of varenicline free base; each 1mg CHANTIX tablet contains 1.71 mg of varenicline tartrate equivalent to 1 mg of varenicline free base. The following inactive ingredients are included in the tablets: microcrystalline cellulose, anhydrous dibasic calcium phosphate, croscarmellose sodium, colloidal silicon dioxide, magnesium stearate, Opadry® White (for 0.5 mg), Opadry® Blue (for 1 mg), and Opadry® Clear.

12 CLINICAL PHARMACOLOGY

12.1 Mechanism of Action

Varenicline binds with high affinity and selectivity at α4β2 neuronal nicotinic acetylcholine receptors. The efficacy of CHANTIX in smoking cessation is believed to be the result of varenicline's activity at α4β2 sub-type of the nicotinic receptor where its binding produces agonist activity, while simultaneously preventing nicotine binding to these receptors.

Electrophysiology studies *in vitro* and neurochemical studies *in vivo* have shown that varenicline binds to α4β2 neuronal nicotinic acetylcholine receptors and stimulates receptor-mediated activity, but at a significantly lower level than nicotine. Varenicline blocks the ability of nicotine to activate α4β2 receptors and thus to stimulate the central nervous mesolimbic dopamine system, believed to be the neuronal mechanism underlying reinforcement and reward experienced upon smoking. Varenicline is highly selective and binds more potently to α4β2 receptors than to other common nicotinic receptors (>500-fold α3β4, >3500- fold α7, >20,000-fold α1βγδ), or to non-nicotinic receptors and transporters (>2000-fold). Varenicline also binds with moderate affinity (Ki = 350 nM) to the 5-HT3 receptor.

12.3 Pharmacokinetics

Absorption/Distribution: Maximum plasma concentrations of varenicline occur typically within 3-4 hours after oral administration. Following administration of multiple oral doses of varenicline, steady-state conditions were reached within 4 days. Over the recommended dosing range, varenicline exhibits linear pharmacokinetics after single or repeated doses. In a mass balance study, absorption of varenicline was virtually complete after oral administration and systemic availability was ~90%. Oral bioavailability of varenicline is unaffected by food or time-of-day dosing. Plasma protein binding of varenicline is low (≤20%) and independent of both age and renal function.

Metabolism/Elimination: The elimination half-life of varenicline is approximately 24 hours. Varenicline undergoes minimal metabolism, with 92% excreted unchanged in the urine. Renal elimination of varenicline is primarily through glomerular filtration along with active tubular secretion possibly via the organic cation transporter, OCT2.

Pharmacokinetics in Special Patient Populations: There are no clinically meaningful differences in varenicline pharmacokinetics due to age, race, gender, smoking status, or use of concomitant medications, as demonstrated in specific pharmacokinetic studies and in population pharmacokinetic analyses.

Renal Impairment: Varenicline pharmacokinetics were unchanged in subjects with mild renal impairment (estimated creatinine clearance >50 mL/min and ≤80 mL/min). In subjects with moderate renal impairment (estimated creatinine clearance ≥30 mL/min and ≤50 mL/min), varenicline exposure increased 1.5-fold compared with subjects with normal renal function (estimated creatinine clearance >80 mL/min). In subjects with severe renal impairment (estimated creatinine clearance <30 mL/min), varenicline exposure was increased 2.1-fold. In subjects with end-stage-renal disease (ESRD) undergoing a three-hour session of hemodialysis for three days a week, varenicline exposure was increased 2.7-fold following 0.5 mg once daily administration for 12 days. The plasma Cmax and AUC of varenicline noted in this setting were similar to those of healthy subjects receiving 1 mg twice daily. *[see Dosage and Administration (2.2), and Use in Specific Populations (8.6)]*. Additionally, in subjects with ESRD, varenicline was efficiently removed by hemodialysis *[see Overdosage (10)]*.

Geriatric Patients: A combined single- and multiple-dose pharmacokinetic study demonstrated that the pharmacokinetics of 1 mg varenicline given once daily or twice daily to 16 healthy elderly male and female smokers (aged 65-75 yrs) for 7 consecutive days was similar to that of younger subjects.

Pediatric Patients: Because the safety and effectiveness of CHANTIX in pediatric patients have not been established, CHANTIX is not recommended for use in patients under 18 years of age. When 22 pediatric patients aged 12 to 17 years (inclusive) received a single 0.5 mg or 1 mg dose of varenicline, the pharmacokinetics of varenicline were approximately dose-proportional between the 0.5 mg and 1 mg doses. Systemic exposure, as assessed by AUC (0-∞), and renal clearance of varenicline were comparable to those of an adult population.

Hepatic Impairment: Due to the absence of significant hepatic metabolism, varenicline pharmacokinetics should be unaffected in patients with hepatic impairment.

Drug-Drug Interactions: Drug interaction studies were performed with varenicline and digoxin, warfarin, transdermal nicotine, bupropion, cimetidine, and metformin. No clinically meaningful pharmacokinetic drug-drug interactions have been identified.

In vitro studies demonstrated that varenicline does not inhibit the following cytochrome P450 enzymes (IC50 >6400 ng/mL): 1A2, 2A6, 2B6, 2C8, 2C9, 2C19, 2D6, 2E1, and 3A4/5. Also, in human hepatocytes *in vitro*, varenicline does not induce the cytochrome P450 enzymes 1A2 and 3A4.

In vitro studies demonstrated that varenicline does not inhibit human renal transport proteins at therapeutic concentrations. Therefore, drugs that are cleared by renal secretion (e.g., metformin [see below]) are unlikely to be affected by varenicline.

In vitro studies demonstrated the active renal secretion of varenicline is mediated by the human organic cation transporter OCT2. Co-administration with inhibitors of OCT2 (e.g., cimeditine [see below]) may not necessitate a dose adjustment of CHANTIX as the increase in systemic exposure to CHANTIX is not expected to be clinically meaningful. Furthermore, since metabolism of varenicline represents less than 10% of its clearance, drugs known to affect the cytochrome P450 system are unlikely to alter the pharmacokinetics of CHANTIX *[see Clinical Pharmacology (12.3)]*; therefore, a dose adjustment of CHANTIX would not be required.

Metformin: When co-administered to 30 smokers, varenicline (1 mg twice daily) did not alter the steady-state pharmacokinetics of metformin (500 mg twice daily), which is a substrate of OCT2. Metformin had no effect on varenicline steady-state pharmacokinetics.

Cimetidine: Co-administration of an OCT2 inhibitor, cimetidine (300 mg four times daily), with varenicline (2 mg single dose) to 12 smokers increased the systemic exposure of varenicline by 29% (90% CI: 21.5%, 36.9%) due to a reduction in varenicline renal clearance.

Digoxin: Varenicline (1 mg twice daily) did not alter the steady-state pharmacokinetics of digoxin administered as a 0.25 mg daily dose in 18 smokers.

Warfarin: Varenicline (1 mg twice daily) did not alter the pharmacokinetics of a single 25 mg dose of (R, S)-warfarin in 24 smokers. Prothrombin time (INR) was not affected by varenicline. Smoking cessation itself may result in changes to warfarin pharmacokinetics *[see Drug Interactions (7.2)]*.

Use with Other Drugs for Smoking Cessation:

Bupropion: Varenicline (1 mg twice daily) did not alter the steady-state pharmacokinetics of bupropion (150 mg twice daily) in 46 smokers *[see Drug Interactions (7.1)]*.

Nicotine replacement therapy (NRT): Although co-administration of varenicline (1 mg twice daily) and transdermal nicotine (21 mg/day) for up to 12 days did not affect nicotine pharmacokinetics, the incidence of adverse reactions was greater for the combination than for NRT alone *[see Drug Interactions (7.1)]*.

13 NONCLINICAL TOXICOLOGY

13.1 Carcinogenesis, Mutagenesis, Impairment of Fertility

Carcinogenesis: Lifetime carcinogenicity studies were performed in CD-1 mice and Sprague-Dawley rats. There was no evidence of a carcinogenic effect in mice administered varenicline by oral gavage for 2 years at doses up to 20 mg/kg/day (47 times the maximum recommended human daily exposure based on AUC). Rats were administered varenicline (1, 5, and 15 mg/kg/day) by oral gavage for 2 years. In male rats (n = 65 per sex per dose group), incidences of hibernoma (tumor of the brown fat) were increased at the mid dose (1 tumor, 5 mg/kg/day, 23 times the maximum recommended human daily exposure based on AUC) and maximum dose (2 tumors, 15 mg/kg/day, 67 times the maximum recommended human daily exposure based on AUC). The clinical relevance of this finding to humans has not been established. There was no evidence of carcinogenicity in female rats.

Mutagenesis: Varenicline was not genotoxic, with or without metabolic activation, in the following assays: Ames bacterial mutation assay; mammalian CHO/HGPRT assay; and tests for cytogenetic aberrations *in vivo* in rat bone marrow and *in vitro* in human lymphocytes.

Impairment of Fertility: There was no evidence of impairment of fertility in either male or female Sprague-Dawley rats administered varenicline succinate up to 15 mg/kg/day (67 and 36 times, respectively, the maximum recommended human daily exposure based on AUC at 1 mg twice daily). However, a decrease in fertility was noted in the offspring of pregnant rats who were administered varenicline succinate at an oral dose of 15 mg/kg/day (36 times the maximum recommended human daily exposure based on AUC at 1 mg BID). This decrease in fertility in the offspring of treated female rats was not evident at an oral dose of 3 mg/kg/day (9 times the maximum recommended human daily exposure based on AUC at 1 mg twice daily).

14 CLINICAL STUDIES

The efficacy of CHANTIX in smoking cessation was demonstrated in six clinical trials in which a total of 3659 chronic cigarette smokers (≥10 cigarettes per day) were treated with CHANTIX. In all clinical studies, abstinence from smoking was determined by patient self-report and verified by measurement of exhaled carbon monoxide (CO≤10 ppm) at weekly visits. Among the CHANTIX-treated patients enrolled in these studies, the completion rate was 65%. Except for the dose-ranging study (Study 1) and the maintenance of abstinence study (Study 6), patients were treated for 12 weeks and then were followed for 40 weeks post-treatment. Most patients enrolled in these trials were white (79-96%). All studies enrolled almost equal numbers of men and women. The average age of patients in these studies was 43 years. Patients on average had smoked about 21 cigarettes per day for an average of approximately 25 years.

In all studies, patients were provided with an educational booklet on smoking cessation and received up to 10 minutes of smoking cessation counseling at each weekly treatment visit according to Agency for Healthcare Research and Quality guidelines. Patients set a date to stop smoking (target quit date [TQD]) with dosing starting 1 week before this date.

14.1 Initiation of Abstinence

Study 1: This was a six-week dose-ranging study comparing CHANTIX to placebo. This study provided initial evidence that CHANTIX at a total dose of 1 mg per day or 2 mg per day was effective as an aid to smoking cessation.

Table 2: Continuous Abstinence, Weeks 9 through 12 (95% confidence interval)

	CHANTIX 0.5 mg BID	CHANTIX 1 mg BID	CHANTIX Flexible	Bupropion SR	Placebo
Study 2	45% (39%, 51%)	51% (44%, 57%)			12% (6%, 18%)
Study 3			40% (32%, 48%)		12% (7%, 17%)
Study 4		44% (38%, 49%)		30% (25%, 35%)	17% (13%, 22%)
Study 5		44% (38%, 49%)		30% (25%, 35%)	18% (14%, 22%)

BID = twice daily

Study 2: This study of 627 patients compared CHANTIX 1 mg per day and 2 mg per day with placebo. Patients were treated for 12 weeks (including one week titration) and then were followed for 40 weeks post-treatment. CHANTIX was given in two divided doses daily. Each dose of CHANTIX was given in two different regimens, with and without initial dose titration, to explore the effect of different dosing regimens on tolerability. For the titrated groups, dosage was titrated up over the course of one week, with full dosage achieved starting with the second week of dosing. The titrated and nontitrated groups were pooled for efficacy analysis.

Forty-five percent of patients receiving CHANTIX 1 mg per day (0.5 mg twice daily) and 51% of patients receiving 2 mg per day (1 mg twice daily) had CO-confirmed continuous abstinence during weeks 9 through 12 compared to 12% of patients in the placebo group (Figure 1). In addition, 31% of the 1 mg per day group and 31% of the 2 mg per day group were continuously abstinent from one week after TQD through the end of treatment as compared to 8% of the placebo group.

Study 3: This flexible-dosing study of 312 patients examined the effect of a patient-directed dosing strategy of CHANTIX or placebo. After an initial one-week titration to a dose of 0.5 mg twice daily, patients could adjust their dosage as often as they wished between 0.5 mg once daily to 1 mg twice daily per day. Sixty-nine percent of patients titrated to the maximum allowable dose at any time during the study. For 44% of patients, the modal dose selected was 1 mg twice daily; for slightly over half of the study participants, the modal dose selected was 1 mg/day or less.

Of the patients treated with CHANTIX, 40% had CO-confirmed continuous abstinence during weeks 9 through 12 compared to 12% in the placebo group. In addition, 29% of the CHANTIX group were continuously abstinent from one week after TQD through the end of treatment as compared to 9% of the placebo group.

Study 4 and Study 5: These identical double-blind studies compared CHANTIX 2 mg per day, bupropion sustained-release (SR) 150 mg twice daily, and placebo. Patients were treated for 12 weeks and then were followed for 40 weeks post-treatment. The CHANTIX dosage of 1 mg twice daily was achieved using a titration of 0.5 mg once daily for the initial 3 days followed by 0.5 mg twice daily for the next 4 days. The bupropion SR dosage of 150 mg twice daily was achieved using a 3-day titration of 150 mg once daily. Study 4 enrolled 1022 patients and Study 5 enrolled 1023 patients. Patients inappropriate for bupropion treatment or patients who had previously used bupropion were excluded.

In Study 4, patients treated with CHANTIX had a superior rate of CO-confirmed abstinence during weeks 9 through 12 (44%) compared to patients treated with bupropion SR (30%) or placebo (17%). The bupropion SR quit rate was also superior to placebo. In addition, 29% of the CHANTIX group were continuously abstinent from one week after TQD through the end of treatment as compared to 12% of the placebo group and 23% of the bupropion SR group.

Similarly in Study 5, patients treated with CHANTIX had a superior rate of CO-confirmed abstinence during weeks 9 through 12 (44%) compared to patients treated with bupropion SR (30%) or placebo (18%). The bupropion SR quit rate was also superior to placebo. In addition, 29% of the CHANTIX group were continuously abstinent from one week after TQD through the end of treatment as compared to 11% of the placebo group and 21% of the bupropion SR group.

Figure 1: Continuous Abstinence, Weeks 9 through 12

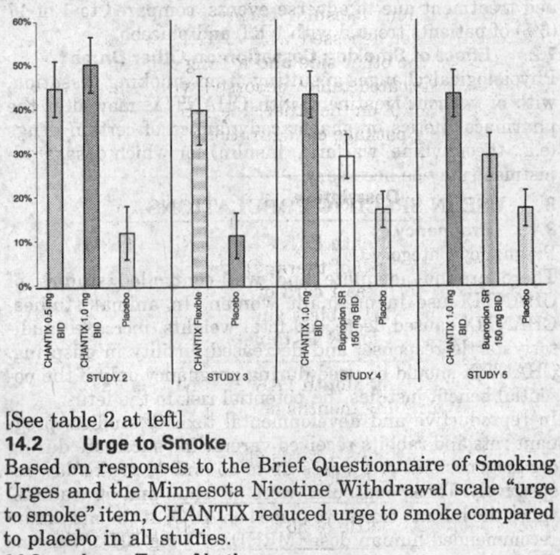

[See table 2 at left]

14.2 Urge to Smoke

Based on responses to the Brief Questionnaire of Smoking Urges and the Minnesota Nicotine Withdrawal scale "urge to smoke" item, CHANTIX reduced urge to smoke compared to placebo in all studies.

14.3 Long-Term Abstinence

Studies 1 through 5 included 40 weeks of post-treatment follow-up. In each study, CHANTIX-treated patients were more likely to maintain abstinence throughout the follow-up period than were patients treated with placebo (Figure 2, Table 3).

Figure 2: Continuous Abstinence, Weeks 9 through 52

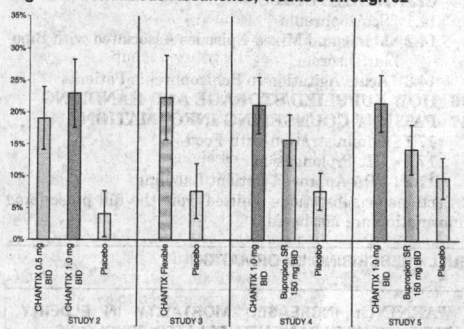

[See table 3 above]

Study 6: This study assessed the effect of an additional 12 weeks of CHANTIX therapy on the likelihood of long-term abstinence. Patients in this study (n=1927) were treated with open-label CHANTIX 1 mg twice daily for 12 weeks. Patients who had stopped smoking for at least a week by Week 12 (n= 1210) were then randomized to double-blind treatment with CHANTIX (1 mg twice daily) or placebo for an additional 12 weeks and then followed for 28 weeks post-treatment.

The continuous abstinence rate from Week 13 through Week 24 was higher for patients continuing treatment with CHANTIX (70%) than for patients switching to placebo (50%). Superiority to placebo was also maintained during 28 weeks post-treatment follow-up (CHANTIX 54% versus placebo 39%).

In Figure 3 below, the x-axis represents the study week for each observation, allowing a comparison of groups at similar times after discontinuation of CHANTIX; post-CHANTIX follow-up begins at Week 13 for the placebo group and Week 25 for the CHANTIX group. The y-axis represents the percentage of patients who had been abstinent for the last week of CHANTIX treatment and remained abstinent at the given timepoint.

Figure 3: Continuous Abstinence Rate during Nontreatment Follow-Up

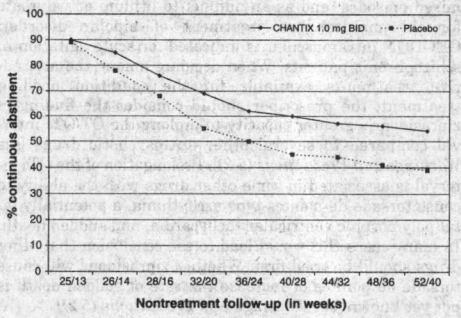

16 HOW SUPPLIED/STORAGE AND HANDLING

CHANTIX is supplied for oral administration in two strengths: a 0.5 mg capsular biconvex, white to off-white, film-coated tablet debossed with "*Pfizer*" on one side and "CHX 0.5" on the other side and a 1 mg capsular biconvex, light blue film-coated tablet debossed with "*Pfizer*" on one side and "CHX 1.0" on the other side. CHANTIX is supplied in the following package configurations:

	Description	NDC
Packs	Starting Month PAK (First month of therapy): Pack includes 1 card of 0.5 mg × 11 tablets and 3 cards of 1 mg × 14 tablets	NDC 0069-0471-97
	Continuing Month PAK (Continuing months of therapy): Pack includes 4 cards of 1 mg × 14 tablets	NDC 0069-0469-97
Bottles	0.5 mg - bottle of 56	NDC 0069-0468-56
	1 mg - bottle of 56	NDC 0069-0469-56

Table 3: Continuous Abstinence, Weeks 9 through 52 (95% confidence interval) across different studies

	CHANTIX 0.5 mg BID	CHANTIX 1 mg BID	CHANTIX Flexible	Bupropion SR	Placebo
Study 2	19% (14%, 24%)	23% (18%, 28%)			4% (1%, 8%)
Study 3			22% (16%, 29%)		8% (3%, 12%)
Study 4		21% (17%, 26%)		16% (12%, 20%)	8% (5%, 11%)
Study 5		22% (17%, 26%)		14% (11%, 18%)	10% (7%, 13%)

BID = twice daily

Store at 25°C (77°F); excursions permitted to 15–30°C (59–86°F) (see USP Controlled Room Temperature).

17 PATIENT COUNSELING INFORMATION

See Medication Guide

17.1 Set Quit Date and Continue to Attempt to Quit if Lapse
Instruct patients to set a date to quit smoking and to initiate CHANTIX treatment one week before the quit date. Encourage patients to continue to attempt to quit if they have early lapses after quit day [see Dosage and Administration (2.1)].

17.2 How To Take
Advise patients that CHANTIX should be taken after eating, and with a full glass of water [see Dosage and Administration (2.1)].

17.3 Starting Week Dosage
Instruct patients on how to titrate CHANTIX, beginning at a dose of 0.5 mg/day. Explain that one 0.5 mg tablet should be taken daily for the first three days, and that for the next four days, one 0.5 mg tablet should be taken in the morning and one 0.5 mg tablet should be taken in the evening [see Dosage and Administration (2.1)].

17.4 Continuing Weeks Dosage
Advise patients that, after the first seven days, the dose should be increased to one 1 mg tablet in the morning and one 1 mg tablet in the evening [see Dosage and Administration (2.1)].

17.5 Dosage Adjustment for CHANTIX or Other Drugs
Inform patients that nausea and insomnia are side effects of CHANTIX and are usually transient; however, advise patients that if they are persistently troubled by these symptoms, they should notify the prescribing physician so that a dose reduction can be considered.
Inform patients that some drugs may require dose adjustment after quitting smoking [see Dosage and Administration (2.1)].

17.6 Counseling and Support
Provide patients with educational materials and necessary counseling to support an attempt at quitting smoking [see Dosage and Administration (2.1)].

17.7 Neuropsychiatric Symptoms
Inform patients that some patients have experienced changes in mood (including depression and mania), psychosis, hallucinations, paranoia, delusions, homicidal ideation, aggression, anxiety, and panic, as well as suicidal ideation and suicide when attempting to quit smoking while taking CHANTIX. If patients develop agitation, hostility, depressed mood, or changes in behavior or thinking that are not typical for them, or if patients develop suicidal ideation or behavior, they should be urged to discontinue CHANTIX and report these symptoms to their healthcare provider immediately [see Boxed Warning, Warnings and Precautions (5.1), Adverse Reactions (6.2)].

17.8 History of Psychiatric Illness
Encourage patients to reveal any history of psychiatric illness prior to initiating treatment.

17.9 Nicotine Withdrawal
Inform patients that quitting smoking, with or without CHANTIX, may be associated with nicotine withdrawal symptoms (including depression or agitation) or exacerbation of pre-existing psychiatric illness.

17.10 Angioedema
Inform patients that there have been reports of angioedema, with swelling of the face, mouth (lip, gum, tongue) and neck (larynx and pharynx) that can lead to life-threatening respiratory compromise. Instruct patients to discontinue CHANTIX and immediately seek medical care if they experience these symptoms [see Warnings and Precautions (5.2), and Adverse Reactions (6.2)].

17.11 Serious Skin Reactions
Inform patients that serious skin reactions, such as Stevens-Johnson Syndrome and erythema multiforme, were reported by some patients taking CHANTIX. Advise patients to stop taking CHANTIX at the first sign of rash with mucosal lesions or skin reaction and contact a healthcare provider immediately [see Warnings and Precautions (5.3), and Adverse Reactions (6.2)].

17.12 Driving or Operating Machinery
Advise patients to use caution driving or operating machinery until they know how quitting smoking and/or varenicline may affect them [see Warnings and Precautions (5.5)].

17.13 Vivid, Unusual, or Strange Dreams
Inform patients that they may experience vivid, unusual or strange dreams during treatment with CHANTIX.

17.14 Pregnancy and Lactation
Patients who are pregnant or breastfeeding or planning to become pregnant should be advised of: the risks of smoking to a pregnant mother and her developing baby, the potential risks of CHANTIX use during pregnancy and breastfeeding, and the benefits of smoking cessation with and without CHANTIX [see Use in Specific Populations (8.1 and 8.3)].
Distributed by
Pfizer Labs
Division of Pfizer Inc, NY, NY 10017
LAB-0327-12.0

GEODON®   ℞

[gē-ō-dŏn]
**(ziprasidone HCl)
capsules**

GEODON

**(ziprasidone mesylate)
injection for intramuscular use**

HIGHLIGHTS OF PRESCRIBING INFORMATION
These highlights do not include all the information needed to use GEODON safely and effectively. See full prescribing information for GEODON.
GEODON (ziprasidone HCl) capsules
GEODON (ziprasidone mesylate) injection for intramuscular use
Initial U.S. Approval: 2001

> **WARNING: INCREASED MORTALITY IN ELDERLY PATIENTS WITH DEMENTIA-RELATED PSYCHOSIS**
> *See full prescribing information for complete boxed warning*
> • Elderly patients with dementia-related psychosis treated with antipsychotic drugs are at an increased risk of death compared to placebo treatment (5.1)
> • GEODON is not approved for elderly patients with dementia-related psychosis (5.1)

———RECENT MAJOR CHANGES———
Warnings and Precautions:
Leukopenia, Neutropenia, and Agranulocytosis   8/2009
Indications and Usage: Bipolar Disorder Maintenance treatment (as an adjunct to lithium or valproate) [1.2]
Dosage and Administration: Bipolar Disorder Maintenance treatment (as an adjunct to lithium or valproate) [2.2]

———INDICATIONS AND USAGE———
GEODON is an atypical antipsychotic. In choosing among treatments, prescribers should be aware of the capacity of GEODON to prolong the QT interval and may consider the use of other drugs first (5.2)
GEODON is indicated as an oral formulation for the:
Treatment of schizophrenia. (1.1)
• Adults: Efficacy was established in four 4-6 week trials and one maintenance trial in adult patients with schizophrenia (14.1)
Acute treatment as monotherapy of manic or mixed episodes associated with bipolar I disorder (1.2)
• Adults: Efficacy was established in two 3-week trials in adult patients with manic or mixed episodes. (14.2)
Maintenance treatment of bipolar I disorder as an adjunct to lithium or valproate. (1.2)
• Adults: Efficacy was established in one maintenance trial in adult patients. (14.2)

GEODON as an intramuscular injection is indicated for the: Acute treatment of agitation in schizophrenic patients. (1.3)
- Adults: Efficacy was established in two short-term trials in agitated patients with schizophrenia. (1.3)

DOSAGE AND ADMINISTRATION

Give oral doses with food.
- Schizophrenia: Initiate at 20 mg twice daily. Daily dosage may be adjusted up to 80 mg twice daily. Dose adjustments should occur at intervals of not less than 2 days. Safety and efficacy has been demonstrated in doses up to 100 mg twice daily. The lowest effective dose should be used. (2.1)
- Acute treatment of manic/mixed episodes of bipolar I disorder: Initiate at 40 mg twice daily. Increase to 60 mg or 80 mg twice daily on day 2 of treatment. Subsequent dose adjustments should be based on tolerability and efficacy within the range of 40-80 mg twice daily. (2.2)
- Maintenance treatment of bipolar I disorder as an adjunct to lithium or valproate: Continue treatment at the same dose on which the patient was initially stabilized, within the range of 40-80 mg twice daily. (2.2)
- Acute treatment of agitation associated with schizophrenia (intramuscular administration): 10 mg-20 mg up to a maximum dose of 40 mg per day. Doses of 10 mg may be administered every 2 hours. Doses of 10 mg may be administered every 2 hours. Doses of 20 mg may be administered every 4 hours (2.3)

DOSAGE FORMS AND STRENGTHS
- Capsules: 20 mg, 40 mg, 60 mg, and 80 mg (3)
- Intramuscular injection: 20 mg/mL single-use vials (3)

CONTRAINDICATIONS
- Do not use in patients with a known history of QT prolongation (4.1)
- Do not use in patients with recent acute myocardial infarction (4.1)
- Do not use in patients with uncompensated heart failure (4.1)
- Do not use in combination with other drugs that have demonstrated QT prolongation (4.1)
- Do not use in patients with known hypersensitivity to ziprasidone (4.2)

WARNINGS AND PRECAUTIONS
- *QT Interval Prolongation*: GEODON use should be avoided in patients with bradycardia, hypokalemia or hypomagnesemia, congenital prolongation of the QT interval, or in combination with other drugs that have demonstrated QT prolongation (5.2)
- *Neuroleptic Malignant Syndrome* (NMS): Potentially fatal symptom complex has been reported with antipsychotic drugs. Manage with immediate discontinuation of drug and close monitoring. (5.3)
- *Tardive Dyskinesia*: May develop acutely or chronically (5.4)
- *Hyperglycemia and Diabetes Mellitus* (DM): Any patient treated with atypical antipsychotics should be monitored for symptoms of hyperglycemia including polydipsia, polyuria, polyphagia, and weakness. When starting treatment, patients with DM risk factors should undergo blood glucose testing before and during treatment (5.5)
- *Rash*: Discontinue in patients who develop a rash without an identified cause (5.6)
- *Orthostatic Hypotension*: Use with caution in patients with known cardiovascular or cerebrovascular disease (5.7)
- *Leukopenia, Neutropenia, and Agranulocytosis* has been reported with antipsychotics. Patients with a pre-existing low white blood cell count (WBC) or a history of leukopenia/neutropenia should have their complete blood count (CBC) monitored frequently during the first few months of therapy and should discontinue Geodon at the first sign of a decline in WBC in the absence of other causative factors.
- *Seizures*: Use cautiously in patients with a history of seizures or with conditions that lower seizure threshold (5.8)
- *Potential for Cognitive and Motor impairment*: Patients should use caution when operating machinery (5.11)
- *Suicide*: Closely supervise high-risk patients (5.14)

ADVERSE REACTIONS
Commonly observed adverse reactions (incidence ≥5% and at least twice the incidence for placebo) were:
- *Schizophrenia*: Somnolence, respiratory tract infection (6.1)
- *Manic and Mixed Episodes Associated with Bipolar Disorder*: Somnolence, extrapyramidal symptoms, dizziness, akathisia, abnormal vision, asthenia, vomiting (6.1)
- *Intramuscular administration* (≥5% and at least twice the lowest intramuscular ziprasidone group): Headache, nausea, somnolence (6.1)

To report SUSPECTED ADVERSE REACTIONS, contact Pfizer Inc at 1-800-438-1985 or FDA at 1-800-FDA-1088 or **www.fda.gov/medwatch**.

DRUG INTERACTIONS
- Ziprasidone should not be used in combination with other drugs that have demonstrated QT prolongation (4.1, 7.3)
- The absorption of ziprasidone is increased up to two-fold in the presence of food (7.9)
- The full prescribing information contains additional drug interactions (7).

USE IN SPECIFIC POPULATIONS
- *Pregnancy*: Ziprasidone should be used during pregnancy only if the potential benefit justifies the potential risk (8.1).
- *Nursing Mothers*: Breast feeding is not recommended (8.3)
- *Pediatric Use*: Safety and effectiveness for pediatric patients has not been established (8.4)
- *Renal Impairment*: Intramuscular ziprasidone should be administered with caution to patients with impaired renal function as the cyclodextrin excipient is cleared by renal filtration (8.10)

See 17 for PATIENT COUNSELING INFORMATION and FDA-approved patient labeling.

Revised: [11/2009]

FULL PRESCRIBING INFORMATION

> **WARNING: INCREASED MORTALITY IN ELDERLY PATIENTS WITH DEMENTIA-RELATED PSYCHOSIS**
> Elderly patients with dementia-related psychosis treated with antipsychotic drugs are at an increased risk of death. Analyses of seventeen placebo-controlled trials (modal duration of 10 weeks), largely in patients taking atypical antipsychotic drugs, revealed a risk of death in drug-treated patients of between 1.6 to 1.7 times the risk of death in placebo-treated patients. Over the course of a typical 10-week controlled trial, the rate of death in drug-treated patients was about 4.5%, compared to a rate of about 2.6% in the placebo group. Although the causes of death were varied, most of the deaths appeared to be either cardiovascular (e.g., heart failure, sudden death) or infectious (e.g., pneumonia) in nature. Observational studies suggest that, similar to atypical antipsychotic drugs, treatment with conventional antipsychotic drugs may increase mortality. The extent to which the findings of increased mortality in observational studies may be attributed to the antipsychotic drug as opposed to some characteristic(s) of the patients is not clear. GEODON (ziprasidone) is not approved for the treatment of patients with Dementia-Related Psychosis [see Warnings and Precautions (5.1)]).

1 INDICATIONS AND USAGE

GEODON is indicated for the treatment of schizophrenia, as monotherapy for the acute treatment of bipolar manic or mixed episodes, and as an adjunct to lithium or valproate for the maintenance treatment of bipolar disorder. GEODON intramuscular is indicated for acute agitation in schizophrenic patients. When deciding among the alternative treatments available for the condition needing treatment, the prescriber should consider the finding of ziprasidone's greater capacity to prolong the QT/QTc interval compared to several other antipsychotic drugs [see Warnings and Precautions (5.2)]. Prolongation of the QTc interval is associated in some other drugs with the ability to cause torsade de pointes-type arrhythmia, a potentially fatal polymorphic ventricular tachycardia, and sudden death. In many cases this would lead to the conclusion that other drugs should be tried first. Whether ziprasidone will cause torsade de pointes or increase the rate of sudden death is not yet known [see Warnings and Precautions (5.2)]

Schizophrenia
Geodon is indicated for the treatment of schizophrenia. The efficacy of oral ziprasidone was established in four short-term (4- and 6-week) controlled trials of adult schizophrenic inpatients and in one maintenance trial of stable adult schizophrenic inpatients [see Clinical Studies (14.1)].

1.2 Bipolar I Disorder
Geodon is indicated as monotherapy for the acute treatment of manic or mixed episodes associated with bipolar I disorder. Efficacy was established in two 3-week monotherapy studies in adult patients. [see Clinical Studies (14.2)].
Geodon is indicated as an adjunct to lithium or valproate for the maintenance treatment of bipolar I disorder. Efficacy was established in a maintenance trial in adult patients. The efficacy of Geodon as monotherapy for the maintenance treatment of bipolar I disorder has not been systematically evaluated in controlled clinical trials. [see Clinical Studies (14.2)].

1.3 Acute Agitation in Schizophrenic Patients
GEODON intramuscular is indicated for the treatment of acute agitation in schizophrenic patients for whom treatment with ziprasidone is appropriate and who need intramuscular antipsychotic medication for rapid control of agitation. The efficacy of intramuscular ziprasidone for acute agitation in schizophrenia was established in single day controlled trials of agitated schizophrenic inpatients. [see Clinical Trials (14.1)]
"Psychomotor agitation" is defined in DSM-IV as "excessive motor activity associated with a feeling of inner tension."

Schizophrenic patients experiencing agitation often manifest behaviors that interfere with their diagnosis and care, e.g., threatening behaviors, escalating or urgently distressing behavior, or self-exhausting behavior, leading clinicians to the use of intramuscular antipsychotic medications to achieve immediate control of the agitation.

Since there is no experience regarding the safety of administering ziprasidone intramuscular to schizophrenic patients already taking oral ziprasidone, the practice of co-administration is not recommended.

Ziprasidone intramuscular is intended for intramuscular use only and should not be administered intravenously.

2 DOSAGE AND ADMINISTRATION

2.1 Schizophrenia

Dose Selection

GEODON Capsules should be administered at an initial daily dose of 20 mg twice daily with food. In some patients, daily dosage may subsequently be adjusted on the basis of individual clinical status up to 80 mg twice daily. Dosage adjustments, if indicated, should generally occur at intervals of not less than 2 days, as steady-state is achieved within 1 to 3 days. In order to ensure use of the lowest effective dose, patients should ordinarily be observed for improvement for several weeks before upward dosage adjustment.

Efficacy in schizophrenia was demonstrated in a dose range of 20 mg to 100 mg twice daily in short-term, placebo-controlled clinical trials. There were trends toward dose response within the range of 20 mg to 80 mg twice daily, but results were not consistent. An increase to a dose greater than 80 mg twice daily is not generally recommended. The safety of doses above 100 mg twice daily has not been systematically evaluated in clinical trials [see Clinical Studies (14.1)].

Maintenance Treatment

While there is no body of evidence available to answer the question of how long a patient treated with ziprasidone should remain on it, a maintenance study in patients who had been symptomatically stable and then randomized to continue ziprasidone or switch to placebo demonstrated a delay in time to relapse for patients receiving Geodon. [see Clinical Studies (14.1)]. No additional benefit was demonstrated for doses above 20 mg twice daily. Patients should be periodically reassessed to determine the need for maintenance treatment.

2.2 Bipolar I Disorder

Acute Treatment of Manic or Mixed Episodes

Dose Selection--Oral ziprasidone should be administered at an initial daily dose of 40 mg twice daily with food. The dose may then be increased to 60 mg or 80 mg twice daily on the second day of treatment and subsequently adjusted on the basis of tolerance and efficacy within the range 40 mg-80 mg twice daily. In the flexible-dose clinical trials, the mean daily dose administered was approximately 120 mg [see Clinical Studies (14.2)].

Maintenance Treatment (as an adjunct to lithium or valproate)

Continue treatment at the same dose on which the patient was initially stabilized, within the range of 40 mg-80 mg twice daily with food. Patients should be periodically reassessed to determine the need for maintenance treatment. [see Clinical Studies (14.2)]

2.3 Acute Treatment of Agitation in Schizophrenia

Intramuscular Dosing

The recommended dose is 10 mg to 20 mg administered as required up to a maximum dose of 40 mg per day. Doses of 10 mg may be administered every two hours; doses of 20 mg may be administered every four hours up to a maximum of 40 mg/day. Intramuscular administration of ziprasidone for more than three consecutive days has not been studied.

If long-term therapy is indicated, oral ziprasidone hydrochloride capsules should replace the intramuscular administration as soon as possible.

Since there is no experience regarding the safety of administering ziprasidone intramuscular to schizophrenic patients already taking oral ziprasidone, the practice of co-administration is not recommended.

Ziprasidone intramuscular is intended for intramuscular use only and should not be administered intravenously.

Intramuscular Preparation for Administration

GEODON for Injection (ziprasidone mesylate) should only be administered by intramuscular injection and should not be administered intravenously. Single-dose vials require reconstitution prior to administration.

Add 1.2 mL of Sterile Water for Injection to the vial and shake vigorously until all the drug is dissolved. Each mL of reconstituted solution contains 20 mg ziprasidone. To administer a 10 mg dose, draw up 0.5 mL of the reconstituted solution. To administer a 20 mg dose, draw up 1.0 mL of the reconstituted solution. Any unused portion should be discarded. Since no preservative or bacteriostatic agent is present in this product, aseptic technique must be used in preparation of the final solution. This medicinal product must not be mixed with other medicinal products or solvents other than Sterile Water for Injection. Parenteral drug products should be inspected visually for particulate matter and discoloration prior to administration, whenever solution and container permit.

2.4 Dosing in Special Populations

Oral: Dosage adjustments are generally not required on the basis of age, gender, race, or renal or hepatic impairment. Geodon is not approved for use in children or adolescents.

Intramuscular: Ziprasidone intramuscular has not been systematically evaluated in elderly patients or in patients with hepatic or renal impairment. As the cyclodextrin excipient is cleared by renal filtration, ziprasidone intramuscular should be administered with caution to patients with impaired renal function. Dosing adjustments are not required on the basis of gender or race [see Use in Specific Populations (8)].

3 DOSAGE FORMS AND STRENGTHS

GEODON Capsules are differentiated by capsule color/size and are imprinted in black ink with "Pfizer" and a unique number. GEODON Capsules are supplied for oral administration in 20 mg (blue/white), 40 mg (blue/blue), 60 mg (white/white), and 80 mg (blue/white) capsules. They are supplied in the following strengths and package configurations:

GEODON Capsules	
Capsule Strength (mg)	Imprint
20	396
40	397
60	398
80	399

GEODON for Injection is available in a single-dose vial as ziprasidone mesylate (20 mg ziprasidone/mL when reconstituted according to label instructions) [see Dosage and Administration (2.3)]. Each mL of ziprasidone mesylate for injection (when reconstituted) affords a colorless to pale pink solution that contains 20 mg of ziprasidone and 4.7 mg of methanesulfonic acid solubilized by 294 mg of sulfobutylether β-cyclodextrin sodium (SBECD).

4 CONTRAINDICATIONS

4.1 QT Prolongation

Because of ziprasidone's dose-related prolongation of the QT interval and the known association of fatal arrhythmias with QT prolongation by some other drugs, ziprasidone is contraindicated:

- in patients with a known history of QT prolongation (including congenital long QT syndrome)
- in patients with recent acute myocardial infarction
- in patients with uncompensated heart failure

Pharmacokinetic/pharmacodynamic studies between ziprasidone and other drugs that prolong the QT interval have not been performed. An additive effect of ziprasidone and other drugs that prolong the QT interval cannot be excluded. Therefore, ziprasidone should not be given with:

- dofetilide, sotalol, quinidine, other Class Ia and III antiarrhythmics, mesoridazine, thioridazine, chlorpromazine, droperidol, pimozide, sparfloxacin, gatifloxacin, moxifloxacin, halofantrine, mefloquine, pentamidine, arsenic trioxide, levomethadyl acetate, dolasetron mesylate, probucol or tacrolimus.
- other drugs that have demonstrated QT prolongation as one of their pharmacodynamic effects and have this effect described in the full prescribing information as a contraindication or a boxed or bolded warning [see Warnings and Precautions (5.2)].

4.2 Hypersensitivity

Ziprasidone is contraindicated in individuals with a known hypersensitivity to the product.

5 WARNINGS AND PRECAUTIONS

5.1 Increased Mortality in Elderly Patients with Dementia-Related Psychosis

Elderly patients with dementia-related psychosis treated with antipsychotic drugs are at an increased risk of death. GEODON is not approved for the treatment of dementia-related psychosis. [see Boxed Warning]

5.2 QT Prolongation and Risk of Sudden Death

Ziprasidone use should be avoided in combination with other drugs that are known to prolong the QTc interval [see Contraindications (4.1), Drug Interactions (7.4)]. Additionally, clinicians should be alert to the identification of other drugs that have been consistently observed to prolong the QTc interval. Such drugs should not be prescribed with ziprasidone. Ziprasidone should also be avoided in patients with congenital long QT syndrome and in patients with a history of cardiac arrhythmias [see Contraindications (4)].

A study directly comparing the QT/QTc prolonging effect of oral ziprasidone with several other drugs effective in the treatment of schizophrenia was conducted in patient volunteers. In the first phase of the trial, ECGs were obtained at the time of maximum plasma concentration when the drug was administered alone. In the second phase of the trial, ECGs were obtained at the time of maximum plasma concentration while the drug was co-administered with an inhibitor of the CYP4503A4 metabolism of the drug.

In the first phase of the study, the mean change in QTc from baseline was calculated for each drug, using a sample-based correction that removes the effect of heart rate on the QT interval. The mean increase in QTc from baseline for ziprasidone ranged from approximately 9 to 14 msec greater than for four of the comparator drugs (risperidone, olanzapine, quetiapine, and haloperidol), but was approximately 14 msec less than the prolongation observed for thioridazine.

In the second phase of the study, the effect of ziprasidone on QTc length was not augmented by the presence of a metabolic inhibitor (ketoconazole 200 mg twice daily).

In placebo-controlled trials, oral ziprasidone increased the QTc interval compared to placebo by approximately 10 msec at the highest recommended daily dose of 160 mg. In clinical trials with oral ziprasidone, the electrocardiograms of 2/2988 (0.06%) patients who received GEODON and 1/440 (0.23%) patients who received placebo revealed QTc intervals exceeding the potentially clinically relevant threshold of 500 msec. In the ziprasidone-treated patients, neither case suggested a role of ziprasidone. One patient had a history of prolonged QTc and a screening measurement of 489 msec; QTc was 503 msec during ziprasidone treatment. The other patient had a QTc of 391 msec at the end of treatment with ziprasidone and upon switching to thioridazine experienced QTc measurements of 518 and 593 msec.

Some drugs that prolong the QT/QTc interval have been associated with the occurrence of torsade de pointes and with sudden unexplained death. The relationship of QT prolongation to torsade de pointes is clearest for larger increases (20 msec and greater) but it is possible that smaller QT/QTc prolongations may also increase risk, or increase it in susceptible individuals. Although torsade de pointes has not been observed in association with the use of ziprasidone in premarketing studies and experience is too limited to rule out an increased risk, there have been rare postmarketing reports (in the presence of multiple confounding factors) [see Adverse Reactions (6.2)].

A study evaluating the QT/QTc prolonging effect of intramuscular ziprasidone, with intramuscular haloperidol as a control, was conducted in patient volunteers. In the trial, ECGs were obtained at the time of maximum plasma concentration following two injections of ziprasidone (20 mg then 30 mg) or haloperidol (7.5 mg then 10 mg) given four hours apart. Note that a 30 mg dose of intramuscular ziprasidone is 50% higher than the recommended therapeutic dose. The mean change in QTc from baseline was calculated for each drug, using a sample-based correction that removes the effect of heart rate on the QT interval. The mean increase in QTc from baseline for ziprasidone was 4.6 msec following the first injection and 12.8 msec following the second injection. The mean increase in QTc from baseline for haloperidol was 6.0 msec following the first injection and 14.7 msec following the second injection. In this study, no patients had a QTc interval exceeding 500 msec. As with other antipsychotic drugs and placebo, sudden unexplained deaths have been reported in patients taking ziprasidone at recommended doses. The premarketing experience for ziprasidone did not reveal an excess risk of mortality for ziprasidone compared to other antipsychotic drugs or placebo, but the extent of exposure was limited, especially for the drugs used as active controls and placebo. Nevertheless, ziprasidone's larger prolongation of QTc length compared to several other antipsychotic drugs raises the possibility that the risk of sudden death may be greater for ziprasidone than for other available drugs for treating schizophrenia. This possibility needs to be considered in deciding among alternative drug products [see Indications and Usage (1)].

Certain circumstances may increase the risk of the occurrence of torsade de pointes and/or sudden death in association with the use of drugs that prolong the QTc interval, including (1) bradycardia; (2) hypokalemia or hypomagnesemia; (3) concomitant use of other drugs that prolong the QTc interval; and (4) presence of congenital prolongation of the QT interval.

It is recommended that patients being considered for ziprasidone treatment who are at risk for significant electrolyte disturbances, hypokalemia in particular, have baseline serum potassium and magnesium measurements. Hypokalemia (and/or hypomagnesemia) may increase the risk of QT prolongation and arrhythmia. Hypokalemia may result from diuretic therapy, diarrhea, and other causes. Patients with low serum potassium and/or magnesium should be repleted with those electrolytes before proceeding with treatment. It is essential to periodically monitor serum electrolytes in patients for whom diuretic therapy is introduced during ziprasidone treatment. Persistently prolonged QTc intervals may also increase the risk of further prolongation and arrhythmia, but it is not clear that routine screening ECG measures are effective in detecting such patients. Rather, ziprasidone should be avoided in patients with histories of significant cardiovascular illness, e.g., QT prolongation, recent acute myocardial infarction, uncompensated heart failure, or cardiac arrhythmia. Ziprasidone should be discontinued in patients who are found to have persistent QTc measurements >500 msec.

For patients taking ziprasidone who experience symptoms that could indicate the occurrence of torsade de pointes, e.g., dizziness, palpitations, or syncope, the prescriber should initiate further evaluation, e.g., Holter monitoring may be useful.

5.3 Neuroleptic Malignant Syndrome (NMS)

A potentially fatal symptom complex sometimes referred to as Neuroleptic Malignant Syndrome (NMS) has been reported in association with administration of antipsychotic drugs. Clinical manifestations of NMS are hyperpyrexia, muscle rigidity, altered mental status, and evidence of autonomic instability (irregular pulse or blood pressure, tachycardia, diaphoresis, and cardiac dysrhythmia). Additional signs may include elevated creatinine phosphokinase, myoglobinuria (rhabdomyolysis), and acute renal failure.

The diagnostic evaluation of patients with this syndrome is complicated. In arriving at a diagnosis, it is important to exclude cases where the clinical presentation includes both serious medical illness (e.g., pneumonia, systemic infection, etc.) and untreated or inadequately treated extrapyramidal signs and symptoms (EPS). Other important considerations in the differential diagnosis include central anticholinergic toxicity, heat stroke, drug fever, and primary central nervous system (CNS) pathology.

The management of NMS should include: (1) immediate discontinuation of antipsychotic drugs and other drugs not essential to concurrent therapy; (2) intensive symptomatic treatment and medical monitoring; and (3) treatment of any concomitant serious medical problems for which specific treatments are available. There is no general agreement about specific pharmacological treatment regimens for NMS.

If a patient requires antipsychotic drug treatment after recovery from NMS, the potential reintroduction of drug therapy should be carefully considered. The patient should be carefully monitored, since recurrences of NMS have been reported.

5.4 Tardive Dyskinesia

A syndrome of potentially irreversible, involuntary, dyskinetic movements may develop in patients undergoing treatment with antipsychotic drugs. Although the prevalence of the syndrome appears to be highest among the elderly, especially elderly women, it is impossible to rely upon prevalence estimates to predict, at the inception of antipsychotic treatment, which patients are likely to develop the syndrome. Whether antipsychotic drug products differ in their potential to cause tardive dyskinesia is unknown.

The risk of developing tardive dyskinesia and the likelihood that it will become irreversible are believed to increase as the duration of treatment and the total cumulative dose of antipsychotic drugs administered to the patient increase. However, the syndrome can develop, although much less commonly, after relatively brief treatment periods at low doses.

There is no known treatment for established cases of tardive dyskinesia, although the syndrome may remit, partially or completely, if antipsychotic treatment is withdrawn. Antipsychotic treatment itself, however, may suppress (or partially suppress) the signs and symptoms of the syndrome, and thereby may possibly mask the underlying process. The effect that symptomatic suppression has upon the long-term course of the syndrome is unknown.

Given these considerations, ziprasidone should be prescribed in a manner that is most likely to minimize the occurrence of tardive dyskinesia. Chronic antipsychotic treatment should generally be reserved for patients who suffer from a chronic illness that (1) is known to respond to antipsychotic drugs, and (2) for whom alternative, equally effective, but potentially less harmful treatments are not available or appropriate. In patients who do require chronic treatment, the smallest dose and the shortest duration of treatment producing a satisfactory clinical response should be sought. The need for continued treatment should be reassessed periodically.

If signs and symptoms of tardive dyskinesia appear in a patient on ziprasidone, drug discontinuation should be considered. However, some patients may require treatment with ziprasidone despite the presence of the syndrome.

5.5 Hyperglycemia and Diabetes Mellitus

Hyperglycemia, in some cases extreme and associated with ketoacidosis or hyperosmolar coma or death, has been reported in patients treated with atypical antipsychotics. There have been few reports of hyperglycemia or diabetes in patients treated with GEODON. Although fewer patients have been treated with GEODON, it is not known if this more limited experience is the sole reason for the paucity of such reports. Assessment of the relationship between atypical antipsychotic use and glucose abnormalities is complicated by the possibility of an increased background risk of diabetes mellitus in patients with schizophrenia and the increasing incidence of diabetes mellitus in the general population. Given these confounders, the relationship between atypical antipsychotic use and hyperglycemia-related adverse reactions is not completely understood. However, epidemiological studies, which did not include GEODON, suggest an increased risk of treatment-emergent hyperglycemia-related adverse reactions in patients treated with the atypical antipsychotics included in these studies. Because GEODON was not marketed at the time these studies were performed, it is not known if GEODON is associated with this increased risk. Precise risk estimates for hyperglycemia-related adverse reactions in patients treated with atypical antipsychotics are not available.

Patients with an established diagnosis of diabetes mellitus who are started on atypical antipsychotics should be monitored regularly for worsening of glucose control. Patients with risk factors for diabetes mellitus (e.g., obesity, family history of diabetes) who are starting treatment with atypical antipsychotics should undergo fasting blood glucose testing at the beginning of treatment and periodically during treatment. Any patient treated with atypical antipsychotics should be monitored for symptoms of hyperglycemia including polydipsia, polyuria, polyphagia, and weakness. Patients who develop symptoms of hyperglycemia during treatment with atypical antipsychotics should undergo fasting blood glucose testing. In some cases, hyperglycemia has resolved when the atypical antipsychotic was discontinued; however, some patients required continuation of antidiabetic treatment despite discontinuation of the suspect drug.

5.6 Rash

In premarketing trials with ziprasidone, about 5% of patients developed rash and/or urticaria, with discontinuation of treatment in about one-sixth of these cases. The occurrence of rash was related to dose of ziprasidone, although the finding might also be explained by the longer exposure time in the higher dose patients. Several patients with rash had signs and symptoms of associated systemic illness, e.g., elevated WBCs. Most patients improved promptly with adjunctive treatment with antihistamines or steroids and/or upon discontinuation of ziprasidone, and all patients experiencing these reactions were reported to recover completely. Upon appearance of rash for which an alternative etiology cannot be identified, ziprasidone should be discontinued.

5.7 Orthostatic Hypotension

Ziprasidone may induce orthostatic hypotension associated with dizziness, tachycardia, and, in some patients, syncope, especially during the initial dose-titration period, probably reflecting its α_1-adrenergic antagonist properties. Syncope was reported in 0.6% of the patients treated with ziprasidone.

Ziprasidone should be used with particular caution in patients with known cardiovascular disease (history of myocardial infarction or ischemic heart disease, heart failure or conduction abnormalities), cerebrovascular disease, or conditions which would predispose patients to hypotension (dehydration, hypovolemia, and treatment with antihypertensive medications).

5.8 Leukopenia, Neutropenia, and Agranulocytosis

In clinical trial and postmarketing experience, events of leukopenia/neutropenia have been reported temporally related to antipsychotic agents. Agranulocytosis (including fatal cases) has also been reported.

Possible risk factors for leukopenia/neutropenia include pre-existing low white blood cell count (WBC) and history of drug induced leukopenia/neutropenia. Patients with a pre-existing low WBC or a history of drug induced leukopenia/neutropenia should have their complete blood count (CBC) monitored frequently during the first few months of therapy and should discontinue Geodon at the first sign of decline in WBC in the absence of other causative factors.

Patients with neutropenia should be carefully monitored for fever or other symptoms or signs of infection and treated promptly if such symptoms or signs occur. Patients with severe neutropenia (absolute neutrophil count <1000/mm3) should discontinue Geodon and have their WBC followed until recovery.

5.9 Seizures

During clinical trials, seizures occurred in 0.4% of patients treated with ziprasidone. There were confounding factors that may have contributed to the occurrence of seizures in many of these cases. As with other antipsychotic drugs, ziprasidone should be used cautiously in patients with a history of seizures or with conditions that potentially lower the seizure threshold, e.g., Alzheimer's dementia. Conditions that lower the seizure threshold may be more prevalent in a population of 65 years or older.

5.10 Dysphagia

Esophageal dysmotility and aspiration have been associated with antipsychotic drug use. Aspiration pneumonia is a common cause of morbidity and mortality in elderly patients, in particular those with advanced Alzheimer's dementia. Ziprasidone and other antipsychotic drugs should be used cautiously in patients at risk for aspiration pneumonia [see Boxed Warning].

5.11 Hyperprolactinemia

As with other drugs that antagonize dopamine D_2 receptors, ziprasidone elevates prolactin levels in humans. Increased prolactin levels were also observed in animal studies with this compound, and were associated with an increase in mammary gland neoplasia in mice; a similar effect was not observed in rats [see Nonclinical Toxicology (13.1)]. Tissue culture experiments indicate that approximately one-third of human breast cancers are prolactin-dependent in vitro, a factor of potential importance if the prescription of these drugs is contemplated in a patient with previously detected breast cancer. Although disturbances such as galactorrhea, amenorrhea, gynecomastia, and impotence have been reported with prolactin-elevating compounds, the clinical significance of elevated serum prolactin levels is unknown for most patients. Neither clinical studies nor epidemiologic studies conducted to date have shown an association between chronic administration of this class of drugs and tumorigenesis in humans; the available evidence is considered too limited to be conclusive at this time.

5.12 Potential for Cognitive and Motor Impairment

Somnolence was a commonly reported adverse reaction in patients treated with ziprasidone. In the 4- and 6-week placebo-controlled trials, somnolence was reported in 14% of patients on ziprasidone compared to 7% of placebo patients. Somnolence led to discontinuation in 0.3% of patients in short-term clinical trials. Since ziprasidone has the potential to impair judgment, thinking, or motor skills, patients should be cautioned about performing activities requiring mental alertness, such as operating a motor vehicle (including automobiles) or operating hazardous machinery until they are reasonably certain that ziprasidone therapy does not affect them adversely.

5.13 Priapism

One case of priapism was reported in the premarketing database. While the relationship of the reaction to ziprasidone use has not been established, other drugs with alpha-adrenergic blocking effects have been reported to induce priapism, and it is possible that ziprasidone may share this capacity. Severe priapism may require surgical intervention.

5.14 Body Temperature Regulation

Although not reported with ziprasidone in premarketing trials, disruption of the body's ability to reduce core body temperature has been attributed to antipsychotic agents. Appropriate care is advised when prescribing ziprasidone for patients who will be experiencing conditions which may contribute to an elevation in core body temperature, e.g., exercising strenuously, exposure to extreme heat, receiving concomitant medication with anticholinergic activity, or being subject to dehydration.

5.15 Suicide

The possibility of a suicide attempt is inherent in psychotic illness or bipolar disorder, and close supervision of high-risk patients should accompany drug therapy. Prescriptions for ziprasidone should be written for the smallest quantity of capsules consistent with good patient management in order to reduce the risk of overdose.

5.16 Patients with concomitant illnesses

Clinical experience with ziprasidone in patients with certain concomitant systemic illnesses is limited [see Use in Specific Populations (8.6), (8.7)]

Ziprasidone has not been evaluated or used to any appreciable extent in patients with a recent history of myocardial infarction or unstable heart disease. Patients with these diagnoses were excluded from premarketing clinical studies. Because of the risk of QTc prolongation and orthostatic hypotension with ziprasidone, caution should be observed in cardiac patients [see Warnings and Precautions (5.2), (5.7)]

5.17 Laboratory Tests

Patients being considered for ziprasidone treatment that are at risk of significant electrolyte disturbances should have baseline serum potassium and magnesium measurements. Low serum potassium and magnesium should be replaced before proceeding with treatment. Patients who are started on diuretics during Ziprasidone therapy need periodic monitoring of serum potassium and magnesium. Ziprasidone should be discontinued in patients who are found to have persistent QTc measurements >500 msec. [see Warnings and Precautions (5.2)]

6 ADVERSE REACTIONS

6.1 Clinical Trials Experience

Because clinical trials are conducted under widely varying conditions, adverse reaction rates observed in the clinical trials of a drug cannot be directly compared to rates in the clinical trials of another drug and may not reflect the rates observed in practice.

Clinical trials for oral ziprasidone included approximately 5700 patients and/or normal subjects exposed to one or more doses of ziprasidone. Of these 5700, over 4800 were patients who participated in multiple-dose effectiveness trials, and their experience corresponded to approximately 1831 patient-years. These patients include: (1) 4331 patients who participated in multiple-dose trials, predominantly in schizophrenia, representing approximately 1698 patient-years of exposure as of February 5, 2000; and (2) 472 patients who participated in bipolar mania trials representing approximately 133 patient-years of exposure. An additional 127 patients with bipolar disorder participated in a long-term maintenance treatment study representing approximately 74.7 patient-years of exposure to ziprasidone. The conditions and duration of treatment with ziprasidone included open-label and double-blind studies, inpatient and outpatient studies, and short-term and longer-term exposure.

Clinical trials for intramuscular ziprasidone included 570 patients and/or normal subjects who received one or more injections of ziprasidone. Over 325 of these subjects participated in trials involving the administration of multiple doses.

Adverse reactions during exposure were obtained by collecting voluntarily reported adverse experiences, as well as results of physical examinations, vital signs, weights, laboratory analyses, ECGs, and results of ophthalmologic examinations.

The stated frequencies of adverse reactions represent the proportion of individuals who experienced, at least once, a treatment-emergent adverse reaction of the type listed. A reaction was considered treatment emergent if it occurred for the first time or worsened while receiving therapy following baseline evaluation.

Adverse Findings Observed in Short-Term, Placebo-Controlled Trials with Oral Ziprasidone

The following findings are based on the short-term placebo-controlled premarketing trials for schizophrenia (a pool of two 6-week, and two 4-week fixed-dose trials) and bipolar mania (a pool of two 3-week flexible-dose trials) in which ziprasidone was administered in doses ranging from 10 to 200 mg/day.

Commonly Observed Adverse Reactions in Short Term Placebo-Controlled Trials

The following adverse reactions were the most commonly observed adverse reactions associated with the use of ziprasidone (incidence of 5% or greater) and not observed at an equivalent incidence among placebo-treated patients (ziprasidone incidence at least twice that for placebo):

Schizophrenia trials (see Table 1)
• Somnolence
• Respiratory Tract Infection
Bipolar trials (see Table 2)
• Somnolence
• Extrapyramidal Symptoms which includes the following adverse reaction terms: extrapyramidal syndrome, hypertonia, dystonia, dyskinesia, hypokinesia, tremor, paralysis and twitching. None of these adverse reactions occurred individually at an incidence greater than 10% in bipolar mania trials.
• Dizziness which includes the adverse reaction terms dizziness and lightheadedness.
• Akathisia
• Abnormal Vision
• Asthenia
• Vomiting

SCHIZOPHRENIA

Adverse Reactions Associated with Discontinuation of Treatment in Short-Term, Placebo-Controlled Trials of Oral Ziprasidone

Approximately 4.1% (29/702) of ziprasidone-treated patients in short-term, placebo-controlled studies discontinued treatment due to an adverse reaction, compared with about 2.2% (6/273) on placebo. The most common reaction associated with dropout was rash, including 7 dropouts for rash among ziprasidone patients (1%) compared to no placebo patients [See Warnings and Precautions (5.6)].

Adverse Reactions Occurring at an Incidence of 2% or More Among Ziprasidone-Treated Patients in Short-Term, Oral, Placebo-Controlled Trials

Table 1 enumerates the incidence, rounded to the nearest percent, of treatment-emergent adverse reactions that occurred during acute therapy (up to 6 weeks) in predominantly patients with schizophrenia, including only those reactions that occurred in 2% or more of patients treated with ziprasidone and for which the incidence in patients treated with ziprasidone was greater than the incidence in placebo-treated patients.

Table 1: Treatment-Emergent Adverse Reaction Incidence In Short-Term Oral Placebo-Controlled Trials – Schizophrenia

Body System/Adverse Reaction	Percentage of Patients Reporting Reaction	
	Ziprasidone (N=702)	Placebo (N=273)
Body as a Whole		
Asthenia	5	3
Accidental Injury	4	2
Chest Pain	3	2
Cardiovascular		
Tachycardia	2	1
Digestive		
Nausea	10	7
Constipation	9	8
Dyspepsia	8	7
Diarrhea	5	4
Dry Mouth	4	2
Anorexia	2	1
Nervous		
Extrapyramidal Symptoms*	14	8
Somnolence	14	7
Akathisia	8	7
Dizziness**	8	6
Respiratory		
Respiratory Tract Infection	8	3
Rhinitis	4	2
Cough Increased	3	1
Skin and Appendages		
Rash	4	3
Fungal Dermatitis	2	1
Special Senses		
Abnormal Vision	3	2

* Extrapyramidal Symptoms includes the following adverse reaction terms: extrapyramidal syndrome, hypertonia, dystonia, dyskinesia, hypokinesia, tremor, paralysis and twitching. None of these adverse reactions occurred individually at an incidence greater than 5% in schizophrenia trials.

** Dizziness includes the adverse reaction terms dizziness and lightheadedness.

Dose Dependency of Adverse Reactions in Short-Term, Fixed-Dose, Placebo-Controlled Trials

An analysis for dose response in the schizophrenia 4-study pool revealed an apparent relation of adverse reaction to dose for the following reactions: asthenia, postural hypotension, anorexia, dry mouth, increased salivation, arthralgia, anxiety, dizziness, dystonia, hypertonia, somnolence, tremor, rhinitis, rash, and abnormal vision.

Extrapyramidal Symptoms (EPS)—The incidence of reported EPS (which included the adverse reaction terms extrapyramidal syndrome, hypertonia, dystonia, dyskinesia, hypokinesia, tremor, paralysis and twitching) for ziprasidone-treated patients in the short-term, placebo-controlled schizophrenia trials was 14% vs. 8% for placebo. Objectively collected data from those trials on the Simpson-Angus Rating Scale (for EPS) and the Barnes Akathisia Scale (for akathisia) did not generally show a difference between ziprasidone and placebo.

Dystonia—*Class Effect:* Symptoms of dystonia, prolonged abnormal contractions of muscle groups, may occur in susceptible individuals during the first few days of treatment. Dystonic symptoms include: spasm of the neck muscles, sometimes progressing to tightness of the throat, swallowing difficulty, difficulty breathing, and/or protrusion of the tongue. While these symptoms can occur at low doses, they occur more frequently and with greater severity with high potency and at higher doses of first generation antipsychotic drugs. An elevated risk of acute dystonia is observed in males and younger age groups.

Vital Sign Changes—Ziprasidone is associated with orthostatic hypotension [see Warnings and Precautions (5.7)]

Weight Gain—The proportions of patients meeting a weight gain criterion of ≥7% of body weight were compared in a pool of four 4- and 6-week placebo-controlled schizophrenia clinical trials, revealing a statistically significantly greater incidence of weight gain for ziprasidone (10%) compared to placebo (4%). A median weight gain of 0.5 kg was observed in ziprasidone patients compared to no median weight change in placebo patients. In this set of clinical trials, weight gain was reported as an adverse reaction in 0.4% and 0.4% of ziprasidone and placebo patients, respectively. During long-term therapy with ziprasidone, a categorization of patients at baseline on the basis of body mass index (BMI) revealed the greatest mean weight gain and highest incidence of clinically significant weight gain (>7% of body weight) in patients with low BMI (<23) compared to normal (23-27) or overweight patients (>27). There was a mean weight gain of 1.4 kg for those patients with a "low" baseline BMI, no mean change for patients with a "normal" BMI, and a 1.3 kg mean weight loss for patients who entered the program with a "high" BMI.

ECG Changes—Ziprasidone is associated with an increase in the QTc interval [see Warnings and Precautions (5.2)]. In the schizophrenia trials, ziprasidone was associated with a mean increase in heart rate of 1.4 beats per minute compared to a 0.2 beats per minute decrease among placebo patients.

Other Adverse Reactions Observed During the Premarketing Evaluation of Oral Ziprasidone

Following is a list of COSTART terms that reflect treatment-emergent adverse reactions as defined in the introduction to the **ADVERSE REACTIONS** section reported by patients treated with ziprasidone in schizophrenia trials at multiple doses >4 mg/day within the database of 3834 patients. All reported reactions are included except those already listed in Table 1 or elsewhere in labeling, those reaction terms that were so general as to be uninformative, reactions reported only once and that did not have a substantial probability of being acutely life-threatening, reactions that are part of the illness being treated or are otherwise common as background reactions, and reactions considered unlikely to be drug-related. It is important to emphasize that, although the reactions reported occurred during treatment with ziprasidone, they were not necessarily caused by it.

Adverse reactions are further categorized by body system and listed in order of decreasing frequency according to the following definitions:

Frequent—adverse reactions occurring in at least 1/100 patients (≥1.0% of patients) (only those not already listed in the tabulated results from placebo-controlled trials appear in this listing);

Infrequent—adverse reactions occurring in 1/100 to 1/1000 patients (in 0.1-1.0% of patients)

Rare—adverse reactions occurring in fewer than 1/1000 patients (<0.1% of patients).

Body as a Whole
Frequent   abdominal pain, flu syndrome, fever, accidental fall, face edema, chills, photosensitivity reaction, flank pain, hypothermia, motor vehicle accident

Cardiovascular System
Frequent   tachycardia, hypertension, postural hypotension
Infrequent   bradycardia, angina pectoris, atrial fibrillation
Rare   first degree AV block, bundle branch block, phlebitis, pulmonary embolus, cardiomegaly, cerebral infarct, cerebrovascular accident, deep thrombophlebitis, myocarditis, thrombophlebitis

Digestive System
Frequent   anorexia, vomiting
Infrequent   rectal hemorrhage, dysphagia, tongue edema

Rare	gum hemorrhage, jaundice, fecal impaction, gamma glutamyl transpeptidase increased, hematemesis, cholestatic jaundice, hepatitis, hepatomegaly, leukoplakia of mouth, fatty liver deposit, melena

Endocrine

Rare	hypothyroidism, hyperthyroidism, thyroiditis

Hemic and Lymphatic System

Infrequent	anemia, ecchymosis, leukocytosis, leukopenia, eosinophilia, lymphadenopathy
Rare	thrombocytopenia, hypochromic anemia, lymphocytosis, monocytosis, basophilia, lymphedema, polycythemia, thrombocythemia

Metabolic and Nutritional Disorders

Infrequent	thirst, transaminase increased, peripheral edema, hyperglycemia, creatine phosphokinase increased, alkaline phosphatase increased, hypercholesteremia, dehydration, lactic dehydrogenase increased, albuminuria, hypokalemia
Rare	BUN increased, creatinine increased, hyperlipemia, hypocholesteremia, hyperkalemia, hypochloremia, hypoglycemia, hyponatremia, hypoproteinemia, glucose tolerance decreased, gout, hyperchloremia, hyperuricemia, hypocalcemia, hypoglycemic reaction, hypomagnesemia, ketosis, respiratory alkalosis

Musculoskeletal System

Frequent	myalgia
Infrequent	tenosynovitis
Rare	myopathy

Nervous System

Frequent	agitation, extrapyramidal syndrome, tremor, dystonia, hypertonia, dyskinesia, hostility, twitching, paresthesia, confusion, vertigo, hypokinesia, hyperkinesia, abnormal gait, oculogyric crisis, hypesthesia, ataxia, amnesia, cogwheel rigidity, delirium, hypotonia, akinesia, dysarthria, withdrawal syndrome, buccoglossal syndrome, choreoathetosis, diplopia, incoordination, neuropathy
Infrequent	paralysis
Rare	myoclonus, nystagmus, torticollis, circumoral paresthesia, opisthotonos, reflexes increased, trismus

Respiratory System

Frequent	dyspnea
Infrequent	pneumonia, epistaxis
Rare	hemoptysis, laryngismus

Skin and Appendages

Infrequent	maculopapular rash, urticaria, alopecia, eczema, exfoliative dermatitis, contact dermatitis, vesiculobullous rash

Special Senses

Frequent	fungal dermatitis
Infrequent	conjunctivitis, dry eyes, tinnitus, blepharitis, cataract, photophobia
Rare	eye hemorrhage, visual field defect, keratitis, keratoconjunctivitis

Urogenital System

Infrequent	impotence, abnormal ejaculation, amenorrhea, hematuria, menorrhagia, female lactation, polyuria, urinary retention, metrorrhagia, male sexual dysfunction, anorgasmia, glycosuria
Rare	gynecomastia, vaginal hemorrhage, nocturia, oliguria, female sexual dysfunction, uterine hemorrhage

BIPOLAR DISORDER
Acute Treatment of Manic or Mixed Episodes
Adverse Reactions Associated with Discontinuation of Treatment in Short Term, Placebo-Controlled Trials
Approximately 6.5% (18/279) of ziprasidone-treated patients in short-term, placebo-controlled studies discontinued treatment due to an adverse reaction, compared with about 3.7% (5/136) on placebo. The most common reactions associated with dropout in the ziprasidone-treated patients were akathisia, anxiety, depression, dizziness, dystonia, rash and vomiting, with 2 dropouts for each of these reactions among ziprasidone patients (1%) compared to one placebo patient each for dystonia and rash (1%) and no placebo patients for the remaining adverse reactions.
Adverse Reactions Occurring at an Incidence of 2% or More Among Ziprasidone-Treated Patients in Short-Term, Oral, Placebo-Controlled Trials
Table 2 enumerates the incidence, rounded to the nearest percent, of treatment-emergent adverse reactions that occurred during acute therapy (up to 3 weeks) in patients with bipolar mania, including only those reactions that

occurred in 2% or more of patients treated with ziprasidone and for which the incidence in patients treated with ziprasidone was greater than the incidence in placebo-treated patients.

Table 2: Treatment-Emergent Adverse Reactions Incidence In Short-Term Oral Placebo-Controlled Trials – Manic and Mixed Episodes Associated with Bipolar Disorder

	Percentage of Patients Reporting Reaction	
Body System/Adverse Reaction	Ziprasidone (N=279)	Placebo (N=136)
Body as a Whole		
Headache	18	17
Asthenia	6	2
Accidental Injury	4	1
Cardiovascular		
Hypertension	3	2
Digestive		
Nausea	10	7
Diarrhea	5	4
Dry Mouth	5	4
Vomiting	5	2
Increased Salivation	4	0
Tongue Edema	3	1
Dysphagia	2	0
Musculoskeletal		
Myalgia	2	0
Nervous		
Somnolence	31	12
Extrapyramidal Symptoms*	31	12
Dizziness**	16	7
Akathisia	10	5
Anxiety	5	4
Hypesthesia	2	1
Speech Disorder	2	0
Respiratory		
Pharyngitis	3	1
Dyspnea	2	1
Skin and Appendages		
Fungal Dermatitis	2	1
Special Senses		
Abnormal Vision	6	3

* Extrapyramidal Symptoms includes the following adverse reaction terms: extrapyramidal syndrome, hypertonia, dystonia, dyskinesia, hypokinesia, tremor, paralysis and twitching. None of these adverse reactions occurred individually at an incidence greater than 10% in bipolar mania trials.
** Dizziness includes the adverse reaction terms dizziness and lightheadedness.

Explorations for interactions on the basis of gender did not reveal any clinically meaningful differences in the adverse reaction occurrence on the basis of this demographic factor.
Weight Gain—During a 6-month placebo-controlled bipolar maintenance study in adults with ziprasidone as an adjunct to lithium or valproate, the incidence of clinically significant weight gain (≥7% of body weight) during the double-blind period was 5.6% for both ziprasidone and placebo treatment groups who completed the 6 months of observation for relapse. Interpretation of these findings should take into con-

sideration that only patients who adequately tolerated ziprasidone entered the maintenance phase of this study, and there were substantial dropouts by the 6 month endpoint.
INTRAMUSCULAR ZIPRASIDONE
Adverse Reactions Occurring at an Incidence of 1% or More Among Ziprasidone-Treated Patients in Short-Term Trials of Intramuscular Ziprasidone
Table 4 enumerates the incidence, rounded to the nearest percent, of treatment-emergent adverse reactions that occurred during acute therapy with intramuscular ziprasidone in 1% or more of patients.
In these studies, the most commonly observed adverse reactions associated with the use of intramuscular ziprasidone (incidence of 5% or greater) and observed at a rate on intramuscular ziprasidone (in the higher dose groups) at least twice that of the lowest intramuscular ziprasidone group were headache (13%), nausea (12%), and somnolence (20%).
[See table at top of next page]
6.2   Postmarketing Experience
The following adverse reactions have been identified during post approval use of GEODON. Because these reactions are reported voluntarily from a population of uncertain size, it is not always possible to reliably estimate their frequency or establish a causal relationship to drug exposure.
Adverse reaction reports not listed above that have been received since market introduction include rare occurrences of the following: *Cardiac Disorders:* Tachycardia, torsade de pointes (in the presence of multiple confounding factors), *[See Warnings and Precautions (5.2)]; Digestive System Disorders:* Swollen Tongue; *Reproductive System and Breast Disorders:* Galactorrhea, priapism; *Nervous System Disorders:* Facial Droop, neuroleptic malignant syndrome, serotonin syndrome (alone or in combination with serotonergic medicinal products), tardive dyskinesia; *Psychiatric Disorders:* Insomnia, mania/hypomania; *Skin and subcutaneous Tissue Disorders:* Allergic reaction (such as allergic dermatitis, angioedema, orofacial edema, urticaria), rash; *Urogenital System Disorders:* Enuresis, urinary incontinence; *Vascular Disorders:* Postural hypotension, syncope.

7   DRUG INTERACTIONS
Drug-drug interactions can be pharmacodynamic (combined pharmacologic effects) or pharmacokinetic (alteration of plasma levels). The risks of using ziprasidone in combination with other drugs have been evaluated as described below. All interactions studies have been conducted with oral ziprasidone. Based upon the pharmacodynamic and pharmacokinetic profile of ziprasidone, possible interactions could be anticipated:
7.1   Metabolic Pathway
Approximately two-thirds of ziprasidone is metabolized via reduction by aldehyde oxidase. There are no known clinically relevant inhibitors or inducers of aldehyde oxidase. Less than one-third of ziprasidone metabolic clearance is mediated by cytochrome P450 catalyzed oxidation.
7.2   In Vitro Studies
An *in vitro* enzyme inhibition study utilizing human liver microsomes showed that ziprasidone had little inhibitory effect on CYP1A2, CYP2C9, CYP2C19, CYP2D6 and CYP3A4, and thus would not likely interfere with the metabolism of drugs primarily metabolized by these enzymes. There is little potential for drug interactions with ziprasidone due to displacement *[See Clinical Pharmacology (12.3)].*
7.3   Pharmacodynamic Interactions
Ziprasidone should not be used with any drug that prolongs the QT interval *[See Contraindications (4.1)].*
Given the primary CNS effects of ziprasidone, caution should be used when it is taken in combination with other centrally acting drugs.
Because of its potential for inducing hypotension, ziprasidone may enhance the effects of certain antihypertensive agents.
Ziprasidone may antagonize the effects of levodopa and dopamine agonists.
7.4   Pharmacokinetic Interactions
Carbamazepine
Carbamazepine is an inducer of CYP3A4; administration of 200 mg twice daily for 21 days resulted in a decrease of approximately 35% in the AUC of ziprasidone.
This effect may be greater when higher doses of carbamazepine are administered.
Ketoconazole
Ketoconazole, a potent inhibitor of CYP3A4, at a dose of 400 mg QD for 5 days, increased the AUC and Cmax of ziprasidone by about 35-40%. Other inhibitors of CYP3A4 would be expected to have similar effects.
Cimetidine
Cimetidine at a dose of 800 mg QD for 2 days did not affect ziprasidone pharmacokinetics.

Antacid

The co-administration of 30 mL of Maalox® with ziprasidone did not affect the pharmacokinetics of ziprasidone.

7.5   Lithium

Ziprasidone at a dose of 40 mg twice daily administered concomitantly with lithium at a dose of 450 mg twice daily for 7 days did not affect the steady-state level or renal clearance of lithium. Ziprasidone dosed adjunctively to lithium in a maintenance trial of bipolar patients did not affect mean therapeutic lithium levels.

7.6   Oral Contraceptives

In vivo studies have revealed no effect of ziprasidone on the pharmacokinetics of estrogen or progesterone components. Ziprasidone at a dose of 20 mg twice daily did not affect the pharmacokinetics of concomitantly administered oral contraceptives, ethinyl estradiol (0.03 mg) and levonorgestrel (0.15 mg).

7.7   Dextromethorphan

Consistent with *in vitro* results, a study in normal healthy volunteers showed that ziprasidone did not alter the metabolism of dextromethorphan, a CYP2D6 model substrate, to its major metabolite, dextrorphan. There was no statistically significant change in the urinary dextromethorphan/dextrorphan ratio.

7.8   Valproate

A pharmacokinetic interaction of ziprasidone with valproate is unlikely due to the lack of common metabolic pathways for the two drugs. Ziprasidone dosed adjunctively to valproate in a maintenance trial of bipolar patients did not affect mean therapeutic valproate levels.

7.9   Other Concomitant Drug Therapy

Population pharmacokinetic analysis of schizophrenic patients enrolled in controlled clinical trials has not revealed evidence of any clinically significant pharmacokinetic interactions with benztropine, propranolol, or lorazepam.

7.10   Food Interaction

The absolute bioavailability of a 20 mg dose under fed conditions is approximately 60%. The absorption of ziprasidone is increased up to two-fold in the presence of food *[see Clinical Pharmacology (12.3)]*.

8   USE IN SPECIFIC POPULATIONS

8.1   Pregnancy

Pregnancy Category C—In animal studies ziprasidone demonstrated developmental toxicity, including possible teratogenic effects at doses similar to human therapeutic doses. When ziprasidone was administered to pregnant rabbits during the period of organogenesis, an increased incidence of fetal structural abnormalities (ventricular septal defects and other cardiovascular malformations and kidney alterations) was observed at a dose of 30 mg/kg/day (3 times the MRHD of 200 mg/day on a mg/m² basis). There was no evidence to suggest that these developmental effects were secondary to maternal toxicity. The developmental no-effect dose was 10 mg/kg/day (equivalent to the MRHD on a mg/m² basis). In rats, embryofetal toxicity (decreased fetal weights, delayed skeletal ossification) was observed following administration of 10 to 160 mg/kg/day (0.5 to 8 times the MRHD on a mg/m² basis) during organogenesis or throughout gestation, but there was no evidence of teratogenicity. Doses of 40 and 160 mg/kg/day (2 and 8 times the MRHD on a mg/m² basis) were associated with maternal toxicity. The developmental no-effect dose was 5 mg/kg/day (0.2 times the MRHD on a mg/m² basis).

There was an increase in the number of pups born dead and a decrease in postnatal survival through the first 4 days of lactation among the offspring of female rats treated during gestation and lactation with doses of 10 mg/kg/day (0.5 times the MRHD on a mg/m² basis) or greater. Offspring developmental delays and neurobehavioral functional impairment were observed at doses of 5 mg/kg/day (0.2 times the MRHD on a mg/m² basis) or greater. A no-effect level was not established for these effects.

There are no adequate and well-controlled studies in pregnant women. Ziprasidone should be used during pregnancy only if the potential benefit justifies the potential risk to the fetus.

8.2   Labor and Delivery

The effect of ziprasidone on labor and delivery in humans is unknown.

8.3   Nursing Mothers

It is not known whether ziprasidone or its metabolites are excreted in human milk. It is recommended that women receiving ziprasidone should not breastfeed.

8.4   Pediatric Use

The safety and effectiveness of ziprasidone in pediatric patients have not been established.

8.5   Geriatric Use

Of the total number of subjects in clinical studies of ziprasidone, 2.4 percent were 65 and over. No overall differences in safety or effectiveness were observed between these subjects and younger subjects, and other reported clinical experience has not identified differences in responses

Table 4: Treatment-Emergent Adverse Reaction Incidence In Short-Term Fixed-Dose Intramuscular Trials

Body System/Adverse Reaction	Percentage of Patients Reporting Reaction		
	Ziprasidone 2 mg (N=92)	Ziprasidone 10 mg (N=63)	Ziprasidone 20 mg (N=41)
Body as a Whole			
Headache	3	13	5
Injection Site Pain	9	8	7
Asthenia	2	0	0
Abdominal Pain	0	2	0
Flu Syndrome	1	0	0
Back Pain	1	0	0
Cardiovascular			
Postural Hypotension	0	0	5
Hypertension	2	0	0
Bradycardia	0	0	2
Vasodilation	1	0	0
Digestive			
Nausea	4	8	12
Rectal Hemorrhage	0	0	2
Diarrhea	3	3	0
Vomiting	0	3	0
Dyspepsia	1	3	2
Anorexia	0	2	0
Constipation	0	0	2
Tooth Disorder	1	0	0
Dry Mouth	1	0	0
Nervous			
Dizziness	3	3	10
Anxiety	2	0	0
Insomnia	3	0	0
Somnolence	8	8	20
Akathisia	0	2	0
Agitation	2	2	0
Extrapyramidal Syndrome	2	0	0
Hypertonia	1	0	0
Cogwheel Rigidity	1	0	0
Paresthesia	0	2	0
Personality Disorder	0	2	0
Psychosis	1	0	0
Speech Disorder	0	2	0
Respiratory			
Rhinitis	1	0	0
Skin and Appendages			
Furunculosis	0	2	0
Sweating	0	0	2
Urogenital			
Dysmenorrhea	0	2	0
Priapism	1	0	0

between the elderly and younger patients, but greater sensitivity of some older individuals cannot be ruled out. Nevertheless, the presence of multiple factors that might increase the pharmacodynamic response to ziprasidone, or cause poorer tolerance or orthostasis, should lead to consideration of a lower starting dose, slower titration, and careful monitoring during the initial dosing period for some elderly patients.
Ziprasidone intramuscular has not been systematically evaluated in elderly patients (65 years and over).

8.6 Renal Impairment

Because ziprasidone is highly metabolized, with less than 1% of the drug excreted unchanged, renal impairment alone is unlikely to have a major impact on the pharmacokinetics of ziprasidone. The pharmacokinetics of ziprasidone following 8 days of 20 mg twice daily dosing were similar among subjects with varying degrees of renal impairment (n=27), and subjects with normal renal function, indicating that dosage adjustment based upon the degree of renal impairment is not required. Ziprasidone is not removed by hemodialysis.
Intramuscular ziprasidone has not been systematically evaluated in elderly patients or in patients with hepatic or renal impairment. As the cyclodextrin excipient is cleared by renal filtration, ziprasidone intramuscular should be administered with caution to patients with impaired renal function *[see Clinical Pharmacology (12)]*.

8.7 Hepatic Impairment

As ziprasidone is cleared substantially by the liver, the presence of hepatic impairment would be expected to increase the AUC of ziprasidone; a multiple-dose study at 20 mg twice daily for 5 days in subjects (n=13) with clinically significant (Childs-Pugh Class A and B) cirrhosis revealed an increase in AUC_{0-12} of 13% and 34% in Childs-Pugh Class A and B, respectively, compared to a matched control group (n=14). A half-life of 7.1 hours was observed in subjects with cirrhosis compared to 4.8 hours in the control group.

8.8 Age and Gender Effects

In a multiple-dose (8 days of treatment) study involving 32 subjects, there was no difference in the pharmacokinetics of ziprasidone between men and women or between elderly (>65 years) and young (18 to 45 years) subjects. Additionally, population pharmacokinetic evaluation of patients in controlled trials has revealed no evidence of clinically significant age or gender-related differences in the pharmacokinetics of ziprasidone. Dosage modifications for age or gender are, therefore, not recommended.

8.9 Smoking

Based on *in vitro* studies utilizing human liver enzymes, ziprasidone is not a substrate for CYP1A2; smoking should therefore not have an effect on the pharmacokinetics of ziprasidone. Consistent with these *in vitro* results, population pharmacokinetic evaluation has not revealed any significant pharmacokinetic differences between smokers and nonsmokers.

9 DRUG ABUSE AND DEPENDENCE

9.3 Dependence

Ziprasidone has not been systematically studied, in animals or humans, for its potential for abuse, tolerance, or physical dependence. While the clinical trials did not reveal any tendency for drug-seeking behavior, these observations were not systematic and it is not possible to predict on the basis of this limited experience the extent to which ziprasidone will be misused, diverted, and/or abused once marketed. Consequently, patients should be evaluated carefully for a history of drug abuse, and such patients should be observed closely for signs of ziprasidone misuse or abuse (e.g., development of tolerance, increases in dose, drug-seeking behavior).

10 OVERDOSAGE

10.1 Human Experience

In premarketing trials involving more than 5400 patients and/or normal subjects, accidental or intentional overdosage of oral ziprasidone was documented in 10 patients. All of these patients survived without sequelae. In the patient taking the largest confirmed amount, 3,240 mg, the only symptoms reported were minimal sedation, slurring of speech, and transitory hypertension (200/95).
Adverse reactions reported with ziprasidone overdose included extrapyramidal symptoms, somnolence, tremor, and anxiety. *[see Adverse Reactions (6.2)]*

10.2 Management of Overdosage

In case of acute overdosage, establish and maintain an airway and ensure adequate oxygenation and ventilation. Intravenous access should be established, and gastric lavage (after intubation, if patient is unconscious) and administration of activated charcoal together with a laxative should be considered. The possibility of obtundation, seizure, or dystonic reaction of the head and neck following overdose may create a risk of aspiration with induced emesis.
Cardiovascular monitoring should commence immediately and should include continuous electrocardiographic monitoring to detect possible arrhythmias. If antiarrhythmic therapy is administered, disopyramide, procainamide, and quinidine carry a theoretical hazard of additive QT-prolonging effects that might be additive to those of ziprasidone.
Hypotension and circulatory collapse should be treated with appropriate measures such as intravenous fluids. If sympathomimetic agents are used for vascular support, epinephrine and dopamine should not be used, since beta stimulation combined with α_1 antagonism associated with ziprasidone may worsen hypotension. Similarly, it is reasonable to expect that the alpha-adrenergic-blocking properties of bretylium might be additive to those of ziprasidone, resulting in problematic hypotension.
In cases of severe extrapyramidal symptoms, anticholinergic medication should be administered. There is no specific antidote to ziprasidone, and it is not dialyzable. The possibility of multiple drug involvement should be considered. Close medical supervision and monitoring should continue until the patient recovers.

11 DESCRIPTION

GEODON is available as capsules (ziprasidone hydrochloride) for oral administration and as an injection (ziprasidone mesylate) for intramuscular use only. Ziprasidone is a psychotropic agent that is chemically unrelated to phenothiazine or butyrophenone antipsychotic agents. It has a molecular weight of 412.94 (free base), with the following chemical name: 5-[2-[4-(1,2-benzisothiazol-3-yl)-1-piperazinyl]ethyl]-6-chloro-1,3-dihydro-2*H*-indol-2-one. The empirical formula of $C_{21}H_{21}ClN_4OS$ (free base of ziprasidone) represents the following structural formula:

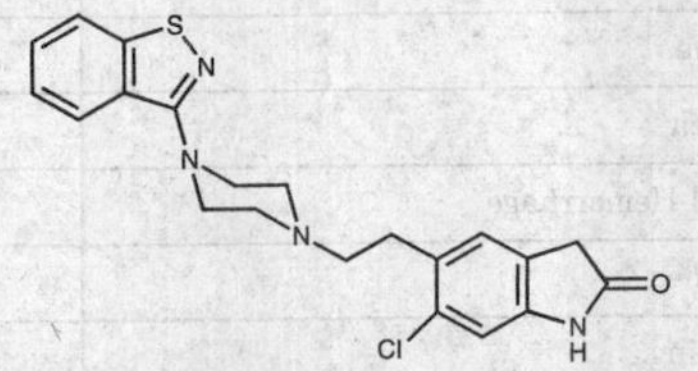

GEODON Capsules contain a monohydrochloride, monohydrate salt of ziprasidone. Chemically, ziprasidone hydrochloride monohydrate is 5-[2-[4-(1,2-benzisothiazol-3-yl)-1-piperazinyl]ethyl]-6-chloro-1,3-dihydro-2*H*-indol-2-one, monohydrochloride, monohydrate. The empirical formula is $C_{21}H_{21}ClN_4OS \bullet HCl \bullet H_2O$ and its molecular weight is 467.42. Ziprasidone hydrochloride monohydrate is a white to slightly pink powder.
GEODON Capsules are supplied for oral administration in 20 mg (blue/white), 40 mg (blue/blue), 60 mg (white/white), and 80 mg (blue/white) capsules. GEODON Capsules contain ziprasidone hydrochloride monohydrate, lactose, pregelatinized starch, and magnesium stearate.
GEODON for Injection contains a lyophilized form of ziprasidone mesylate trihydrate. Chemically, ziprasidone mesylate trihydrate is 5-[2-[4-(1,2-benzisothiazol-3-yl)-1-piperazinyl]ethyl]-6-chloro-1,3-dihydro-2*H*-indol-2-one, methanesulfonate, trihydrate. The empirical formula is $C_{21}H_{21}ClN_4OS \bullet CH_3SO_3H \bullet 3H_2O$ and its molecular weight is 563.09.
GEODON for Injection is available in a single-dose vial as ziprasidone mesylate (20 mg ziprasidone/mL when reconstituted according to label instructions) *[See Dosage and Administration (2.3)]*. Each mL of ziprasidone mesylate for injection (when reconstituted) contains 20 mg of ziprasidone and 4.7 mg of methanesulfonic acid solubilized by 294 mg of sulfobutylether ß-cyclodextrin sodium (SBECD).

12 CLINICAL PHARMACOLOGY

12.1 Mechanism of Action

The mechanism of action of ziprasidone, as with other drugs having efficacy in schizophrenia, is unknown. However, it has been proposed that this drug's efficacy in schizophrenia is mediated through a combination of dopamine type 2 (D_2) and serotonin type 2 ($5HT_2$) antagonism. As with other drugs having efficacy in bipolar disorder, the mechanism of action of ziprasidone in bipolar disorder is unknown.

12.2 Pharmacodynamics

Ziprasidone exhibited high *in vitro* binding affinity for the dopamine D_2 and D_3, the serotonin $5HT_{2A}$, $5HT_{2C}$, $5HT_{1A}$, $5HT_{1D}$, and α_1-adrenergic receptors (K_i s of 4.8, 7.2, 0.4, 1.3, 3.4, 2, and 10 nM, respectively), and moderate affinity for the histamine H_1 receptor (K_i=47 nM). Ziprasidone functioned as an antagonist at the D_2, $5HT_{2A}$, and $5HT_{1D}$ receptors, and as an agonist at the $5HT_{1A}$ receptor. Ziprasidone inhibited synaptic reuptake of serotonin and norepinephrine. No appreciable affinity was exhibited for other receptor/binding sites tested, including the cholinergic muscarinic receptor (IC_{50} >1 µM). Antagonism at receptors other than dopamine and $5HT_2$ with similar receptor affinities may explain some of the other therapeutic and side effects of ziprasidone. Ziprasidone's antagonism of histamine H_1 receptors may explain the somnolence observed with this drug. Ziprasidone's antagonism of α_1-adrenergic receptors may explain the orthostatic hypotension observed with this drug.

12.3 Pharmacokinetics

Oral Pharmacokinetics

Ziprasidone's activity is primarily due to the parent drug. The multiple-dose pharmacokinetics of ziprasidone are dose-proportional within the proposed clinical dose range, and ziprasidone accumulation is predictable with multiple dosing. Elimination of ziprasidone is mainly via hepatic metabolism with a mean terminal half-life of about 7 hours within the proposed clinical dose range. Steady-state concentrations are achieved within one to three days of dosing. The mean apparent systemic clearance is 7.5 mL/min/kg. Ziprasidone is unlikely to interfere with the metabolism of drugs metabolized by cytochrome P450 enzymes.
Absorption: Ziprasidone is well absorbed after oral administration, reaching peak plasma concentrations in 6 to 8 hours. The absolute bioavailability of a 20 mg dose under fed conditions is approximately 60%. The absorption of ziprasidone is increased up to two-fold in the presence of food.
Distribution: Ziprasidone has a mean apparent volume of distribution of 1.5 L/kg. It is greater than 99% bound to plasma proteins, binding primarily to albumin and α_1-acid glycoprotein. The *in vitro* plasma protein binding of ziprasidone was not altered by warfarin or propranolol, two highly protein-bound drugs, nor did ziprasidone alter the binding of these drugs in human plasma. Thus, the potential for drug interactions with ziprasidone due to displacement is minimal.
Metabolism and Elimination: Ziprasidone is extensively metabolized after oral administration with only a small amount excreted in the urine (<1%) or feces (<4%) as unchanged drug. Ziprasidone is primarily cleared via three metabolic routes to yield four major circulating metabolites, benzisothiazole (BITP) sulphoxide, BITP-sulphone, ziprasidone sulphoxide, and S-methyl-dihydroziprasidone. Approximately 20% of the dose is excreted in the urine, with approximately 66% being eliminated in the feces. Unchanged ziprasidone represents about 44% of total drug-related material in serum. *In vitro* studies using human liver subcellular fractions indicate that S-methyl-dihydroziprasidone is generated in two steps. The data indicate that the reduction reaction is mediated by aldehyde oxidase and the subsequent methylation is mediated by thiol methyltransferase. *In vitro* studies using human liver microsomes and recombinant enzymes indicate that CYP3A4 is the major CYP contributing to the oxidative metabolism of ziprasidone. CYP1A2 may contribute to a much lesser extent. Based on *in vivo* abundance of excretory metabolites, less than one-third of ziprasidone metabolic clearance is mediated by cytochrome P450 catalyzed oxidation and approximately two-thirds via reduction by aldehyde oxidase. There are no known clinically relevant inhibitors or inducers of aldehyde oxidase.

Intramuscular Pharmacokinetics

Systemic Bioavailability: The bioavailability of ziprasidone administered intramuscularly is 100%. After intramuscular administration of single doses, peak serum concentrations typically occur at approximately 60 minutes post-dose or earlier and the mean half-life ($T_{1/2}$) ranges from two to five hours. Exposure increases in a dose-related manner and following three days of intramuscular dosing, little accumulation is observed.
Metabolism and Elimination: Although the metabolism and elimination of IM ziprasidone have not been systematically evaluated, the intramuscular route of administration would not be expected to alter the metabolic pathways.

13 NONCLINICAL TOXICOLOGY

13.1 Carcinogenesis, Mutagenesis, Impairment of Fertility

Carcinogenesis

Lifetime carcinogenicity studies were conducted with ziprasidone in Long Evans rats and CD-1 mice. Ziprasidone was administered for 24 months in the diet at doses of 2, 6, or 12 mg/kg/day to rats, and 50, 100, or 200 mg/kg/day to mice (0.1 to 0.6 and 1 to 5 times the maximum recommended human dose [MRHD] of 200 mg/day on a mg/m^2 basis, respectively). In the rat study, there was no evidence of an increased incidence of tumors compared to controls. In male mice, there was no increase in incidence of tumors relative to controls. In female mice, there were dose-related increases in the incidences of pituitary gland adenoma and carcinoma, and mammary gland adenocarcinoma at all doses tested (50 to 200 mg/kg/day or 1 to 5 times the MRHD on a mg/m^2 basis). Proliferative changes in the pituitary and mammary glands of rodents have been observed following chronic administration of other antipsychotic agents and are considered to be prolactin-mediated. Increases in serum prolactin were observed in a 1-month dietary study in female, but not male, mice at 100 and 200 mg/kg/day (or 2.5 and 5 times the MRHD on a mg/m^2 basis). Ziprasidone had no effect on serum prolactin in rats in a 5-week dietary study at the doses that were used in the carcinogenicity study. The relevance for human risk of the findings of prolactin-mediated endocrine tumors in rodents is unknown *[see Warnings and Precautions (5.11)]*.

Mutagenesis

Ziprasidone was tested in the Ames bacterial mutation assay, the *in vitro* mammalian cell gene mutation mouse lymphoma assay, the *in vitro* chromosomal aberration assay in human lymphocytes, and the *in vivo* chromosomal aberration assay in mouse bone marrow. There was a reproducible mutagenic response in the Ames assay in one strain of *S. typhimurium* in the absence of metabolic activation. Positive results were obtained in both the *in vitro* mammalian cell gene mutation assay and the *in vitro* chromosomal aberration assay in human lymphocytes.

Impairment of Fertility

Ziprasidone was shown to increase time to copulation in Sprague-Dawley rats in two fertility and early embryonic development studies at doses of 10 to 160 mg/kg/day (0.5 to 8 times the MRHD of 200 mg/day on a mg/m^2 basis). Fertility rate was reduced at 160 mg/kg/day (8 times the MRHD on a mg/m^2 basis). There was no effect on fertility at 40 mg/kg/day (2 times the MRHD on a mg/m^2 basis). The effect on fertility appeared to be in the female since fertility was not impaired when males given 160 mg/kg/day (8 times the MRHD on a mg/m^2 basis) were mated with untreated females. In a 6-month study in male rats given 200 mg/kg/day (10 times the MRHD on a mg/m^2 basis) there were no treatment-related findings observed in the testes.

14 CLINICAL STUDIES

14.1 Schizophrenia

The efficacy of oral ziprasidone in the treatment of schizophrenia was evaluated in 5 placebo-controlled studies, 4 short-term (4- and 6-week) trials and one maintenance trial. All trials were in adult inpatients, most of whom met DSM III-R criteria for schizophrenia. Each study included 2 to 3 fixed doses of ziprasidone as well as placebo. Four of the 5 trials were able to distinguish ziprasidone from placebo; one short-term study did not. Although a single fixed-dose haloperidol arm was included as a comparative treatment in one of the three short-term trials, this single study was inadequate to provide a reliable and valid comparison of ziprasidone and haloperidol.

Several instruments were used for assessing psychiatric signs and symptoms in these studies. The Brief Psychiatric Rating Scale (BPRS) and the Positive and Negative Syndrome Scale (PANSS) are both multi-item inventories of general psychopathology usually used to evaluate the effects of drug treatment in schizophrenia. The BPRS psychosis cluster (conceptual disorganization, hallucinatory behavior, suspiciousness, and unusual thought content) is considered a particularly useful subset for assessing actively psychotic schizophrenic patients. A second widely used assessment, the Clinical Global Impression (CGI), reflects the impression of a skilled observer, fully familiar with the manifestations of schizophrenia, about the overall clinical state of the patient. In addition, the Scale for Assessing Negative Symptoms (SANS) was employed for assessing negative symptoms in one trial.

The results of the oral ziprasidone trials in schizophrenia follow:

In a 4-week, placebo-controlled trial (n=139) comparing 2 fixed doses of ziprasidone (20 and 60 mg twice daily) with placebo, only the 60 mg dose was superior to placebo on the BPRS total score and the CGI severity score. This higher dose group was not superior to placebo on the BPRS psychosis cluster or on the SANS.

In a 6-week, placebo-controlled trial (n=302) comparing 2 fixed doses of ziprasidone (40 and 80 mg twice daily) with placebo, both dose groups were superior to placebo on the BPRS total score, the BPRS psychosis cluster, the CGI severity score and the PANSS total and negative subscale scores. Although 80 mg twice daily had a numerically greater effect than 40 mg twice daily, the difference was not statistically significant.

In a 6-week, placebo-controlled trial (n=419) comparing 3 fixed doses of ziprasidone (20, 60, and 100 mg twice daily) with placebo, all three dose groups were superior to placebo on the PANSS total score, the BPRS total score, the BPRS psychosis cluster, and the CGI severity score. Only the 100 mg twice daily dose group was superior to placebo on the PANSS negative subscale score. There was no clear evidence for a dose-response relationship within the 20 mg twice daily to 100 mg twice daily dose range.

In a 4-week, placebo-controlled trial (n=200) comparing 3 fixed doses of ziprasidone (5, 20, and 40 mg twice daily), none of the dose groups was statistically superior to placebo on any outcome of interest.

A study was conducted in stable chronic or subchronic (CGI-S ≤5 at baseline) schizophrenic inpatients (n=294) who had been hospitalized for not less than two months. After a 3-day single-blind placebo run-in, subjects were randomized to one of 3 fixed doses of ziprasidone (20 mg, 40 mg, or 80 mg twice daily) or placebo and observed for relapse. Patients were observed for "impending psychotic relapse," defined as CGI-improvement score of ≥6 (much worse or very much worse) and/or scores ≥6 (moderately severe) on the hostility or uncooperativeness items of the PANSS on two consecutive days. Ziprasidone was significantly superior to placebo in time to relapse, with no significant difference between the different dose groups. There were insufficient data to examine population subsets based on age and race. Examination of population subsets based on gender did not reveal any differential responsiveness.

14.2 Bipolar I Disorder

Acute Manic and Mixed Episodes Associated with Bipolar I Disorder

The efficacy of ziprasidone was established in 2 placebo-controlled, double-blind, 3-week monotherapy studies in patients meeting DSM-IV criteria for bipolar I disorder, manic or mixed episode with or without psychotic features. Primary rating instruments used for assessing manic symptoms in these trials were: (1) the Mania Rating Scale (MRS), which is derived from the Schedule for Affective Disorders and Schizophrenia-Change Version (SADS-CB) with items grouped as the Manic Syndrome subscale (elevated mood, less need for sleep, excessive energy, excessive activity, grandiosity), the Behavior and Ideation subscale (irritability, motor hyperactivity, accelerated speech, racing thoughts, poor judgment) and impaired insight; and (2) the Clinical Global Impression-Severity of Illness Scale (CGI-S), which was used to assess the clinical significance of treatment response.

The results of the oral ziprasidone trials in adult bipolar I disorder, manic/mixed episode follow: in a 3-week placebo-controlled trial (n=210), the dose of ziprasidone was 40 mg twice daily on Day 1 and 80 mg twice daily on Day 2. Titration within the range of 40-80 mg twice daily (in 20 mg twice daily increments) was permitted for the duration of the study. Ziprasidone was significantly more effective than placebo in reduction of the MRS total score and the CGI-S score. The mean daily dose of ziprasidone in this study was 132 mg. In a second 3-week placebo-controlled trial (n=205), the dose of ziprasidone was 40 mg twice daily on Day 1. Titration within the range of 40-80 mg twice daily (in 20 mg twice daily increments) was permitted for the duration of study (beginning on Day 2). Ziprasidone was significantly more effective than placebo in reduction of the MRS total score and the CGI-S score. The mean daily dose of ziprasidone in this study was 112 mg.

Maintenance Therapy

The efficacy of ziprasidone as adjunctive therapy to lithium or valproate in the maintenance treatment of bipolar I disorder was established in a placebo-controlled trial in patients who met DSM-IV criteria for bipolar I disorder. The trial included patients whose most recent episode was manic or mixed, with or without psychotic features. In the open-label phase, patients were required to be stabilized on ziprasidone plus lithium or valproic acid for at least 8 weeks in order to be randomized. In the double-blind randomized phase, patients continued treatment with lithium or valproic acid and were randomized to receive either ziprasidone (administered twice daily totaling 80 mg to 160 mg per day) or placebo. Generally, in the maintenance phase, patients continued on the same dose on which they were stabilized during the stabilization phase. The primary endpoint in this study was time to recurrence of a mood episode (manic, mixed or depressed episode) requiring intervention, which was defined as any of the following: discontinuation due to a mood episode, clinical intervention for a mood episode (e.g., initiation of medication or hospitalization), or Mania Rating Scale score ≥18 or a MADRS score ≥18 (on 2 consecutive assessments no more than 10 days apart). A total of 584 subjects were treated in the open-label stabilization period. In the double-blind randomization period, 127 subjects were treated with ziprasidone, and 112 subjects were treated with placebo. Ziprasidone was superior to placebo in increasing the time to recurrence of a mood episode. The types of relapse events observed included depressive, manic, and mixed episodes. Depressive, manic, and mixed episodes accounted for 53%, 34%, and 13%, respectively, of the total number of relapse events in the study.

14.3 Acute Agitation in Schizophrenic Patients

The efficacy of intramuscular ziprasidone in the management of agitated schizophrenic patients was established in two short-term, double-blind trials of schizophrenic subjects who were considered by the investigators to be "acutely agitated" and in need of IM antipsychotic medication. In addition, patients were required to have a score of 3 or more on at least 3 of the following items of the PANSS: anxiety, tension, hostility and excitement. Efficacy was evaluated by analysis of the area under the curve (AUC) of the Behavioural Activity Rating Scale (BARS) and Clinical Global Impression (CGI) severity rating. The BARS is a seven point scale with scores ranging from 1 (difficult or unable to rouse) to 7 (violent, requires restraint). Patients' scores on the BARS at baseline were mostly 5 (signs of overt activity [physical or verbal], calms down with instructions) and as determined by investigators, exhibited a degree of agitation that warranted intramuscular therapy. There were few patients with a rating higher than 5 on the BARS, as the most severely agitated patients were generally unable to provide informed consent for participation in premarketing clinical trials.

Both studies compared higher doses of ziprasidone intramuscular with a 2 mg control dose. In one study, the higher dose was 20 mg, which could be given up to 4 times in the 24 hours of the study, at interdose intervals of no less than 4 hours. In the other study, the higher dose was 10 mg, which could be given up to 4 times in the 24 hours of the study, at interdose intervals of no less than 2 hours.

The results of the intramuscular ziprasidone trials follow:

(1) In a one-day, double-blind, randomized trial (n=79) involving doses of ziprasidone intramuscular of 20 mg or 2 mg, up to QID, ziprasidone intramuscular 20 mg was statistically superior to ziprasidone intramuscular 2 mg, as assessed by AUC of the BARS at 0 to 4 hours, and by CGI severity at 4 hours and study endpoint.

(2) In another one-day, double-blind, randomized trial (n=117) involving doses of ziprasidone intramuscular of 10 mg or 2 mg, up to QID, ziprasidone intramuscular 10 mg was statistically superior to ziprasidone intramuscular 2 mg, as assessed by AUC of the BARS at 0 to 2 hours, but not by CGI severity.

16 HOW SUPPLIED/STORAGE AND HANDLING

GEODON Capsules are differentiated by capsule color/size and are imprinted in black ink with "Pfizer" and a unique number. GEODON Capsules are supplied for oral administration in 20 mg (blue/white), 40 mg (blue/blue), 60 mg (white/white), and 80 mg (blue/white) capsules. They are supplied in the following strengths and package configurations:

GEODON Capsules

Package Configuration	Capsule Strength (mg)	NDC Code	Imprint
Bottles of 60	20	NDC-0049-3960-60	396
Bottles of 60	40	NDC-0049-3970-60	397
Bottles of 60	60	NDC-0049-3980-60	398
Bottles of 60	80	NDC-0049-3990-60	399
Unit dose/80	20	NDC-0049-3960-41	396
Unit dose/80	40	NDC-0049-3970-41	397
Unit dose/80	60	NDC-0049-3980-41	398
Unit dose/80	80	NDC-0049-3990-41	399

GEODON Capsules should be stored at 25°C (77°F); excursions permitted to 15-30°C (59-86°F) [See USP Controlled Room Temperature].

GEODON for Injection is available in a single-dose vial as ziprasidone mesylate (20 mg ziprasidone/mL when reconstituted according to label instructions) *[see Dosage and Administration (2.3)]*. Each mL of ziprasidone mesylate for injection (when reconstituted) affords a colorless to pale pink solution that contains 20 mg of ziprasidone and 4.7 mg of methanesulfonic acid solubilized by 294 mg of sulfobutylether ß-cyclodextrin sodium (SBECD).

GEODON for Injection

Package	Concentration	NDC Code
Single-use Vials	20 mg/mL	NDC-0049-3920-83

GEODON for Injection should be stored at 25°C (77°F); excursions permitted to 15-30°C (59-86°F) [See USP Controlled Room Temperature] in dry form. Protect from light. Following reconstitution, GEODON for Injection can be stored, when protected from light, for up to 24 hours at 15°-30°C (59°-86°F) or up to 7 days refrigerated, 2°-8°C (36°-46°F).

17 PATIENT COUNSELING INFORMATION

See *FDA-Approved Patient Labeling (17.3)*.

Please refer to the patient package insert. To assure safe and effective use of GEODON, the information and instructions provided in the patient information should be discussed with patients.

17.1 Administration with Food

Patients should be instructed to take GEODON Capsules with food for optimal absorption. The absorption of ziprasidone is increased up to two-fold in the presence of food [see Drug Interactions (7.8) and Clinical Pharmacology (12.3)].

17.2 QTc Prolongation

Patients should be advised to inform their health care providers of the following: History of QT prolongation; recent acute myocardial infarction; uncompensated heart failure; prescription of other drugs that have demonstrated QT prolongation; risk for significant electrolyte abnormalities; and history of cardiac arrhythmia [see Contraindications (4.1) and Warnings and Precautions (5.2)].

Patients should be instructed to report the onset of any conditions that put them at risk for significant electrolyte disturbances, hypokalemia in particular, including but not limited to the initiation of diuretic therapy or prolonged diarrhea. In addition, patients should be instructed to report symptoms such as dizziness, palpitations, or syncope to the prescriber [see Warnings and Precautions (5.2)].

17.3 FDA-Approved Patient Labeling

PATIENT SUMMARY OF INFORMATION ABOUT
GEODON® Capsules

(ziprasidone HCl)

Information for patients taking GEODON or their caregivers

This summary contains important information about GEODON. It is not meant to take the place of your doctor's instructions. Read this information carefully before you take GEODON. Ask your doctor or pharmacist if you do not understand any of this information or if you want to know more about GEODON.

What Is GEODON?

GEODON is a type of prescription medicine called a psychotropic, also known as an atypical antipsychotic. GEODON can be used to treat symptoms of schizophrenia and acute manic or mixed episodes associated with bipolar disorder. GEODON can also be used as maintenance treatment of bipolar disorder when added to lithium or valproate.

Who Should Take GEODON?

Only your doctor can know if GEODON is right for you. GEODON may be prescribed for you if you have schizophrenia or bipolar disorder.

Symptoms of schizophrenia may include:

- hearing voices, seeing things, or sensing things that are not there (hallucinations)
- beliefs that are not true (delusions)
- unusual suspiciousness (paranoia)
- becoming withdrawn from family and friends

Symptoms of manic or mixed episodes of bipolar disorder may include:

- extremely high or irritable mood
- increased energy, activity, and restlessness
- racing thoughts or talking very fast
- easily distracted
- little need for sleep

If you show a response to GEODON, your symptoms may improve. If you continue to take GEODON there is less chance of your symptoms returning. Do not stop taking the capsules even when you feel better without first discussing it with your doctor.

It is also important to remember that GEODON capsules should be taken with food.

What is the most important safety information I should know about GEODON?

GEODON is not approved for the treatment of patients with dementia-related psychosis. Elderly patients with a diagnosis of psychosis related to dementia treated with antipsychotics are at an increased risk of death when compared to patients who are treated with placebo (a sugar pill).

GEODON is an effective drug to treat the symptoms of schizophrenia and the manic or mixed episodes of bipolar disorder. However, one potential side effect is that it may change the way the electrical current in your heart works more than some other drugs. The change is small and it is not known whether this will be harmful, but some other drugs that cause this kind of change have in rare cases caused dangerous heart rhythm abnormalities. Because of this, GEODON should be used only after your doctor has considered this risk for GEODON against the risks and benefits of other medications available for treating schizophrenia or bipolar manic and mixed episodes.

Your risk of dangerous changes in heart rhythm can be increased if you are taking certain other medicines and if you already have certain abnormal heart conditions. Therefore, it is important to tell your doctor about any other medicines that you take, including nonprescription medicines, supplements, and herbal medicines. You must also tell your doctor about any heart problems you have or have had.

Who should NOT take GEODON?

Elderly patients with a diagnosis of psychosis related to dementia. GEODON is not approved for the treatment of these patients.

Anything that can increase the chance of a heart rhythm abnormality should be avoided. Therefore, do not take GEODON if:

- You have certain heart diseases, for example, long QT syndrome, a recent heart attack, severe heart failure, or certain irregularities of heart rhythm (discuss the specifics with your doctor)
- You are currently taking medications that should not be taken in combination with ziprasidone, for example, dofetilide, sotalol, quinidine, other Class Ia and III antiarrhythmics, mesoridazine, thioridazine, chlorpromazine, droperidol, pimozide, sparfloxacin, gatifloxacin, moxifloxacin, halofantrine, mefloquine, pentamidine, arsenic trioxide, levomethadyl acetate, dolasetron mesylate, probucol or tacrolimus.

What To Tell Your Doctor Before You Start GEODON

Only your doctor can decide if GEODON is right for you. Before you start GEODON, be sure to tell your doctor if you:

- have had any problem with the way your heart beats or any heart related illness or disease
- any family history of heart disease, including recent heart attack
- have had any problem with fainting or dizziness
- are taking or have recently taken any prescription medicines
- are taking any over-the-counter medicines you can buy without a prescription, including natural/herbal remedies
- have had any problems with your liver
- are pregnant, might be pregnant, or plan to get pregnant
- are breast feeding
- are allergic to any medicines
- have ever had an allergic reaction to ziprasidone or any of the other ingredients of GEODON capsules. Ask your doctor or pharmacist for a list of these ingredients
- have low levels of potassium or magnesium in your blood

Your doctor may want you to get additional laboratory tests to see if GEODON is an appropriate treatment for you.

GEODON And Other Medicines

There are some medications that may be unsafe to use when taking GEODON, and there are some medicines that can affect how well GEODON works. While you are on GEODON, check with your doctor before starting any new prescription or over-the-counter medications, including natural/herbal remedies.

How To Take GEODON

- Take GEODON only as directed by your doctor.
- Swallow the capsules whole.
- Take GEODON capsules with food.
- It is best to take GEODON at the same time each day.
- GEODON may take a few weeks to work. It is important to be patient.
- Do not change your dose or stop taking your medicine without your doctor's approval.
- Remember to keep taking your capsules, even when you feel better.

Possible Side Effects

Because these problems could mean you're having a heart rhythm abnormality, contact your doctor IMMEDIATELY if you:

- Faint or lose consciousness
- Feel a change in the way that your heart beats (palpitations)

Common side effects of GEODON include the following and should also be discussed with your doctor if they occur:

- Feeling unusually tired or sleepy
- Nausea or upset stomach
- Constipation
- Dizziness
- Restlessness
- Abnormal muscle movements, including tremor, shuffling, and uncontrolled involuntary movements
- Diarrhea
- Rash
- Increased cough/runny nose

If you develop any side effects that concern you, talk with your doctor. It is particularly important to tell your doctor if you have diarrhea, vomiting, or another illness that can cause you to lose fluids. Your doctor may want to check your blood to make sure that you have the right amount of important salts after such illnesses.

For a list of all side effects that have been reported, ask your doctor or pharmacist for the GEODON Professional Package Insert.

What To Do For An Overdose

In case of an overdose, call your doctor or poison control center right away or go to the nearest emergency room.

Other Important Safety Information

A serious condition called neuroleptic malignant syndrome (NMS) can occur with all antipsychotic medications including GEODON. Signs of NMS include very high fever, rigid muscles, shaking, confusion, sweating, or increased heart rate and blood pressure. NMS is a rare but serious side effect that could be fatal. Therefore, tell your doctor if you experience any of these signs.

Adverse reactions related to high blood sugar (hyperglycemia), sometimes serious, have been reported in patients treated with atypical antipsychotics. There have been few reports of hyperglycemia or diabetes in patients treated with GEODON, and it is not known if GEODON is associated with these reactions. Patients treated with an atypical antipsychotic should be monitored for symptoms of hyperglycemia.

Dizziness caused by a drop in your blood pressure may occur with GEODON, especially when you first start taking this medication or when the dose is increased. If this happens, be careful not to stand up too quickly, and talk to your doctor about the problem.

Before taking GEODON, tell your doctor if you are pregnant or plan on becoming pregnant. It is advised that you don't breast feed an infant if you are taking GEODON.

Because GEODON can cause sleepiness, be careful when operating machinery or driving a motor vehicle.

Since medications of the same drug class as GEODON may interfere with the ability of the body to adjust to heat, it is best to avoid situations involving high temperature or humidity.

It is best to avoid consuming alcoholic beverages while taking GEODON.

Call your doctor immediately if you take more than the amount of GEODON prescribed by your doctor.

GEODON has not been shown to be safe or effective in the treatment of children and teenagers under the age of 18 years old.

Keep GEODON and all medicines out of the reach of children.

How To Store GEODON

Store GEODON capsules at room temperature (59°-86°F or 15°-30°C).

For More Information About GEODON

This sheet is only a summary. GEODON is a prescription medicine and only your doctor can decide if it is right for you. If you have any questions or want more information about GEODON, talk with your doctor or pharmacist. You can also visit www.geodon.com.

Distributed by
Roerig
Division of Pfizer Inc, NY, NY 10017
LAB-0273-16.0   Revised November 2009

LYRICA®   Ⓒ ℞
[leer-ē-ka]
(pregabalin)
Capsules

LYRICA   Ⓒ ℞
(pregabalin)
Oral Solution

HIGHLIGHTS OF PRESCRIBING INFORMATION
These highlights do not include all the information needed to use LYRICA safely and effectively. See full prescribing information for LYRICA.

LYRICA (pregabalin) Capsules, Ⓒ
LYRICA (pregabalin) Oral Solution, Ⓒ
Initial U.S. Approval: 2004

————————RECENT MAJOR CHANGES————————

Dosage and Administration, Oral Solution Concentration and Dispensing (2.6)	12/2009
Warnings and Precautions, Suicidal Behavior and Ideation (5.4)	4/2009
Use in Specific Populations, Pregnancy (8.1)	4/2009
Patient Counseling Information, Medication Guide (17.1)	4/2009
Patient Counseling Information, Suicidal Thinking and Behavior (17.4)	4/2009
Patient Counseling Information, Use in Pregnancy (17.12)	4/2009

————————INDICATIONS AND USAGE————————

LYRICA is indicated for:

- Neuropathic pain associated with diabetic peripheral neuropathy (DPN) (1.1)
- Post herpetic neuralgia (PHN) (1.2)
- Adjunctive therapy for adult patients with partial onset seizures (1.3)
- Fibromyalgia (1.4)

————————DOSAGE AND ADMINISTRATION————————

DPN Pain (2.1):
- Administer in 3 divided doses per day
- Begin dosing at 150 mg/day
- May be increased to a maximum of 300 mg/day within 1 week.

PHN (2.2):
- Administer in 2 or 3 divided doses per day
- Begin dosing at 150 mg/day

- May be increased to 300 mg/day within 1 week
- Maximum dose of 600 mg/day.

Adjunctive Therapy for Adult Patients with Partial Onset Seizures (2.3):
- Administer in 2 or 3 divided doses per day
- Begin dosing at 150 mg/day
- Maximum dose of 600 mg/day.

Fibromyalgia (2.4):
- Administer in 2 divided doses per day
- Begin dosing at 150 mg/day
- May be increased to 300 mg/day within 1 week
- Maximum dose of 450 mg/day.

Dose should be adjusted in patients with reduced renal function. (2.5)
Oral Solution Concentration and Dispensing (2.6)

————DOSAGE FORMS AND STRENGTHS————

- Capsules: 25mg, 50 mg, 75 mg, 100 mg, 150 mg, 200 mg, 225 mg, and 300 mg. (3)
- Oral Solution: 20 mg/mL. (3)

————————CONTRAINDICATIONS————————

- Known hypersensitivity to pregabalin or any of its components. (4)

————WARNINGS AND PRECAUTIONS————

- Angioedema (e.g. swelling of the throat, head and neck) can occur, and may be associated with life-threatening respiratory compromise requiring emergency treatment. Discontinue LYRICA immediately in these cases. (5.1)
- Hypersensitivity reactions (e.g. hives, dyspnea, and wheezing) can occur. Discontinue LYRICA immediately in these patients. (5.2)
- Increased seizure frequency may occur in patients with seizure disorders if LYRICA is rapidly discontinued. Withdraw LYRICA gradually over a minimum of 1 week. (5.3)
- Antiepileptic drugs, including LYRICA, increase the risk of suicidal thoughts or behavior. (5.4)
- LYRICA may cause peripheral edema. Exercise caution when co-administering LYRICA and thiazolidinedione antidiabetic agents. (5.5)
- LYRICA may cause dizziness and somnolence and impair patients' ability to drive or operate machinery. (5.6)

————————ADVERSE REACTIONS————————

Most common adverse reactions (≥ 5% and twice placebo) are dizziness, somnolence, dry mouth, edema, blurred vision, weight gain and thinking abnormal (primarily difficulty with concentration/attention). (6.1)

To report SUSPECTED ADVERSE REACTIONS, contact Pfizer at (800) 438-1985 or FDA at 1-800-FDA-1088 or www.fda.gov/medwatch

————USE IN SPECIFIC POPULATIONS————

To enroll in the North American Antiepileptic Drug Pregnancy Registry call 1-888-233-2334 (toll free). (8.1)

See 17 for PATIENT COUNSELING INFORMATION and FDA-approved Medication Guide

Revised: 9/2010

FULL PRESCRIBING INFORMATION: CONTENTS*

*Sections or subsections omitted from the full prescribing information are not listed

FULL PRESCRIBING INFORMATION

1 INDICATIONS AND USAGE

LYRICA is indicated for:

1.1 Management of neuropathic pain associated with diabetic peripheral neuropathy

1.2 Management of postherpetic neuralgia

1.3 Adjunctive therapy for adult patients with partial onset seizures

1.4 Management of fibromyalgia

2 DOSAGE AND ADMINISTRATION

LYRICA is given orally with or without food.

When discontinuing LYRICA, taper gradually over a minimum of 1 week.

2.1 Neuropathic pain associated with diabetic peripheral neuropathy

The maximum recommended dose of LYRICA is 100 mg three times a day (300 mg/day) in patients with creatinine clearance of at least 60 mL/min. Begin dosing at 50 mg three times a day (150 mg/day). The dose may be increased to 300 mg/day within 1 week based on efficacy and tolerability. Because LYRICA is eliminated primarily by renal excretion, adjust the dose in patients with reduced renal function [see Dosage and Administration (2.5)].

Although LYRICA was also studied at 600 mg/day, there is no evidence that this dose confers additional significant benefit and this dose was less well tolerated. In view of the dose-dependent adverse reactions, treatment with doses above 300 mg/day is not recommended [see Adverse Reactions (6.1)].

2.2 Postherpetic neuralgia

The recommended dose of LYRICA is 75 to 150 mg two times a day, or 50 to 100 mg three times a day (150 to 300 mg/day) in patients with creatinine clearance of at least 60 mL/min. Begin dosing at 75 mg two times a day, or 50 mg three times a day (150 mg/day). The dose may be increased to 300 mg/day within 1 week based on efficacy and tolerability. Because LYRICA is eliminated primarily by renal excretion, adjust the dose in patients with reduced renal function [see Dosage and Administration (2.5)].

Patients who do not experience sufficient pain relief following 2 to 4 weeks of treatment with 300 mg/day, and who are able to tolerate LYRICA, may be treated with up to 300 mg two times a day, or 200 mg three times a day (600 mg/day). In view of the dose-dependent adverse reactions and the higher rate of treatment discontinuation due to adverse reactions, reserve dosing above 300 mg/day for those patients who have on-going pain and are tolerating 300 mg daily [see Adverse Reactions (6.1)].

2.3 Adjunctive therapy for adult patients with partial onset seizures

LYRICA at doses of 150 to 600 mg/day has been shown to be effective as adjunctive therapy in the treatment of partial onset seizures in adults. Both the efficacy and adverse event profiles of LYRICA have been shown to be dose-related. Administer the total daily dose in two or three divided doses. In general, it is recommended that patients be started on a total daily dose no greater than 150 mg/day (75 mg two times a day, or 50 mg three times a day). Based on individual patient response and tolerability, the dose may be increased to a maximum dose of 600 mg/day.

Because LYRICA is eliminated primarily by renal excretion, adjust the dose in patients with reduced renal function [see Dosage and Administration (2.5)].

The effect of dose escalation rate on the tolerability of LYRICA has not been formally studied.

The efficacy of add-on LYRICA in patients taking gabapentin has not been evaluated in controlled trials. Consequently, dosing recommendations for the use of LYRICA with gabapentin cannot be offered.

2.4 Management of Fibromyalgia

The recommended dose of LYRICA for fibromyalgia is 300 to 450 mg/day. Begin dosing at 75 mg two times a day (150 mg/day). The dose may be increased to 150 mg two times a day (300 mg/day) within 1 week based on efficacy and tolerability. Patients who do not experience sufficient benefit with 300 mg/day may be further increased to 225 mg two times a day (450 mg/day). Although LYRICA was also studied at 600 mg/day, there is no evidence that this dose confers additional benefit and this dose was less well tolerated. In view of the dose-dependent adverse reactions, treatment with doses above 450 mg/day is not recommended [see Adverse Reactions (6.1)]. Because LYRICA is eliminated primarily by renal excretion, adjust the dose in patients with reduced renal function [see Dosage and Administration (2.5)].

$$CLcr = \frac{[140 - age\ (years)] \times weight\ (kg)}{72 \times serum\ creatinine\ (mg/dL)} \quad (\times\ 0.85\ for\ female\ patients)$$

Table 1. Pregabalin Dosage Adjustment Based on Renal Function

Creatinine Clearance (CLcr) (mL/min)	Total Pregabalin Daily Dose (mg/day)*				Dose Regimen
≥60	150	300	450	600	BID or TID
30–60	75	150	225	300	BID or TID
15–30	25–50	75	100–150	150	QD or BID
<15	25	25–50	50–75	75	QD
Supplementary dosage following hemodialysis (mg)†					

Patients on the 25 mg QD regimen: take one supplemental dose of 25 mg or 50 mg
Patients on the 25–50 mg QD regimen: take one supplemental dose of 50 mg or 75 mg
Patients on the 50–75 mg QD regimen: take one supplemental dose of 75 mg or 100 mg
Patients on the 75 mg QD regimen: take one supplemental dose of 100 mg or 150 mg

TID = Three divided doses; BID = Two divided doses; QD = Single daily dose.
* Total daily dose (mg/day) should be divided as indicated by dose regimen to provide mg/dose.
† Supplementary dose is a single additional dose.

Table 2 Risk by indication for antiepileptic drugs in the pooled analysis

Indication	Placebo Patients with Events Per 1000 Patients	Drug Patients with Events Per 1000 Patients	Relative Risk: Incidence of Events in Drug Patients/Incidence in Placebo Patients	Risk Difference: Additional Drug Patients with Events Per 1000 Patients
Epilepsy	1.0	3.4	3.5	2.4
Psychiatric	5.7	8.5	1.5	2.9
Other	1.0	1.8	1.9	0.9
Total	2.4	4.3	1.8	1.9

2.5 Patients with Renal Impairment

In view of dose-dependent adverse reactions and since LYRICA is eliminated primarily by renal excretion, adjust the dose in patients with reduced renal function. Base the dose adjustment in patients with renal impairment on creatinine clearance (CLcr), as indicated in Table 1. To use this dosing table, an estimate of the patient's CLcr in mL/min is needed. CLcr in mL/min may be estimated from serum creatinine (mg/dL) determination using the Cockcroft and Gault equation:

[See first table at top of previous page]

Next, refer to the Dosage and Administration section to determine the recommended total daily dose based on indication, for a patient with normal renal function (CLcr ≥60 mL/min). Then refer to Table 1 to determine the corresponding renal adjusted dose.

(For example: A patient initiating LYRICA therapy for postherpetic neuralgia with normal renal function (CLcr ≥60 mL/min), receives a total daily dose of 150 mg/day pregabalin. Therefore, a renal impaired patient with a CLcr of 50 mL/min would receive a total daily dose of 75 mg/day pregabalin administered in two or three divided doses.)

For patients undergoing hemodialysis, adjust the pregabalin daily dose based on renal function. In addition to the daily dose adjustment, administer a supplemental dose immediately following every 4-hour hemodialysis treatment (see Table 1).

[See table 1 on previous page]

2.6 Oral Solution Concentration and Dispensing

The oral solution is 20 mg pregabalin per milliliter (mL) and prescriptions should be written in milligrams (mg). The pharmacist will calculate the applicable dose in mL for dispensing (e.g., 150 mg equals 7.5 mL oral solution).

3 DOSAGE FORMS AND STRENGTHS

Capsules: 25 mg, 50 mg, 75 mg, 100 mg, 150 mg, 200 mg, 225 mg, and 300 mg
Oral Solution: 20 mg/mL
[see Description (11) and How Supplied/Storage and Handling (16)].

4 CONTRAINDICATIONS

LYRICA is contraindicated in patients with known hypersensitivity to pregabalin or any of its components. Angioedema and hypersensitivity reactions have occurred in patients receiving pregabalin therapy.

5 WARNINGS AND PRECAUTIONS

5.1 Angioedema

There have been postmarketing reports of angioedema in patients during initial and chronic treatment with LYRICA. Specific symptoms included swelling of the face, mouth (tongue, lips, and gums), and neck (throat and larynx). There were reports of life-threatening angioedema with respiratory compromise requiring emergency treatment. Discontinue LYRICA immediately in patients with these symptoms.

Exercise caution when prescribing LYRICA to patients who have had a previous episode of angioedema. In addition, patients who are taking other drugs associated with angioedema (e.g., angiotensin converting enzyme inhibitors [ACE-inhibitors]) may be at increased risk of developing angioedema.

5.2 Hypersensitivity

There have been postmarketing reports of hypersensitivity in patients shortly after initiation of treatment with LYRICA. Adverse reactions included skin redness, blisters, hives, rash, dyspnea, and wheezing. Discontinue LYRICA immediately in patients with these symptoms.

5.3 Withdrawal of Antiepileptic Drugs (AEDs)

As with all AEDs, withdraw LYRICA gradually to minimize the potential of increased seizure frequency in patients with seizure disorders. If LYRICA is discontinued, taper the drug gradually over a minimum of 1 week.

5.4 Suicidal Behavior and Ideation

Antiepileptic drugs (AEDs), including LYRICA, increase the risk of suicidal thoughts or behavior in patients taking these drugs for any indication. Monitor patients treated with any AED for any indication for the emergence or worsening of depression, suicidal thoughts or behavior, and/or any unusual changes in mood or behavior.

Pooled analyses of 199 placebo-controlled clinical trials (mono- and adjunctive therapy) of 11 different AEDs showed that patients randomized to one of the AEDs had approximately twice the risk (adjusted Relative Risk 1.8, 95% CI: 1.2, 2.7) of suicidal thinking or behavior compared to patients randomized to placebo. In these trials, which had a median treatment duration of 12 weeks, the estimated incidence rate of suicidal behavior or ideation among 27,863 AED-treated patients was 0.43%, compared to 0.24% among 16,029 placebo-treated patients, representing an increase of approximately one case of suicidal thinking or behavior for every 530 patients treated. There were four suicides in drug-treated patients in the trials and none in placebo-treated patients, but the number is too small to allow any conclusion about drug effect on suicide.

The increased risk of suicidal thoughts or behavior with AEDs was observed as early as one week after starting drug treatment with AEDs and persisted for the duration of treatment assessed. Because most trials included in the analysis did not extend beyond 24 weeks, the risk of suicidal thoughts or behavior beyond 24 weeks could not be assessed.

The risk of suicidal thoughts or behavior was generally consistent among drugs in the data analyzed. The finding of increased risk with AEDs of varying mechanisms of action and across a range of indications suggests that the risk applies to all AEDs used for any indication. The risk did not vary substantially by age (5-100 years) in the clinical trials analyzed. Table 2 shows absolute and relative risk by indication for all evaluated AEDs.

[See table 2 above]

The relative risk for suicidal thoughts or behavior was higher in clinical trials for epilepsy than in clinical trials for psychiatric or other conditions, but the absolute risk differences were similar for the epilepsy and psychiatric indications.

Anyone considering prescribing LYRICA or any other AED must balance the risk of suicidal thoughts or behavior with the risk of untreated illness. Epilepsy and many other illnesses for which AEDs are prescribed are themselves associated with morbidity and mortality and an increased risk of suicidal thoughts and behavior. Should suicidal thoughts and behavior emerge during treatment, the prescriber needs to consider whether the emergence of these symptoms in any given patient may be related to the illness being treated.

Inform patients, their caregivers, and families that LYRICA and other AEDs increase the risk of suicidal thoughts and behavior and advise them of the need to be alert for the emergence or worsening of the signs and symptoms of depression, any unusual changes in mood or behavior, or the emergence of suicidal thoughts, behavior, or thoughts about self-harm. Report behaviors of concern immediately to healthcare providers.

5.5 Peripheral Edema

LYRICA treatment may cause peripheral edema. In short-term trials of patients without clinically significant heart or peripheral vascular disease, there was no apparent association between peripheral edema and cardiovascular complications such as hypertension or congestive heart failure. Peripheral edema was not associated with laboratory changes suggestive of deterioration in renal or hepatic function.

In controlled clinical trials the incidence of peripheral edema was 6% in the LYRICA group compared with 2% in the placebo group. In controlled clinical trials, 0.5% of LYRICA patients and 0.2% placebo patients withdrew due to peripheral edema.

Higher frequencies of weight gain and peripheral edema were observed in patients taking both LYRICA and a thiazolidinedione antidiabetic agent compared to patients taking either drug alone. The majority of patients using thiazolidinedione antidiabetic agents in the overall safety database were participants in studies of pain associated with diabetic peripheral neuropathy. In this population, peripheral edema was reported in 3% (2/60) of patients who were using thiazolidinedione antidiabetic agents only, 8% (69/859) of patients who were treated with LYRICA only, and 19% (23/120) of patients who were on both LYRICA and thiazolidinedione antidiabetic agents. Similarly, weight gain was reported in 0% (0/60) of patients on thiazolidinediones only; 4% (35/859) of patients on LYRICA only; and 7.5% (9/120) of patients on both drugs.

As the thiazolidinedione class of antidiabetic drugs can cause weight gain and/or fluid retention, possibly exacerbating or leading to heart failure, exercise caution when co-administering LYRICA and these agents.

Because there are limited data on congestive heart failure patients with New York Heart Association (NYHA) Class III or IV cardiac status, exercise caution when using LYRICA in these patients.

5.6 Dizziness and Somnolence

LYRICA may cause dizziness and somnolence. Inform patients that LYRICA-related dizziness and somnolence may impair their ability to perform tasks such as driving or operating machinery *[see Patient Counseling Information (17.5)].*

In the LYRICA controlled trials, dizziness was experienced by 31% of LYRICA-treated patients compared to 9% of placebo-treated patients; somnolence was experienced by 22% of LYRICA-treated patients compared to 7% of placebo-treated patients. Dizziness and somnolence generally began shortly after the initiation of LYRICA therapy and occurred more frequently at higher doses. Dizziness and somnolence were the adverse reactions most frequently leading to withdrawal (4% each) from controlled studies. In LYRICA-treated patients reporting these adverse reactions in short-term, controlled studies, dizziness persisted until the last dose in 30% and somnolence persisted until the last dose in 42% of patients.

5.7 Weight Gain

LYRICA treatment may cause weight gain. In LYRICA controlled clinical trials of up to 14 weeks, a gain of 7% or more over baseline weight was observed in 9% of LYRICA-treated patients and 2% of placebo-treated patients. Few patients treated with LYRICA (0.3%) withdrew from controlled trials due to weight gain. LYRICA associated weight gain was related to dose and duration of exposure, but did not appear to be associated with baseline BMI, gender, or age. Weight gain was not limited to patients with edema *[see Warnings and Precautions (5.5)].*

Although weight gain was not associated with clinically important changes in blood pressure in short-term controlled studies, the long-term cardiovascular effects of LYRICA-associated weight gain are unknown.

Among diabetic patients, LYRICA-treated patients gained an average of 1.6 kg (range: -16 to 16 kg), compared to an average 0.3 kg (range: -10 to 9 kg) weight gain in placebo patients. In a cohort of 333 diabetic patients who received LYRICA for at least 2 years, the average weight gain was 5.2 kg.

While the effects of LYRICA-associated weight gain on glycemic control have not been systematically assessed, in controlled and longer-term open label clinical trials with diabetic patients, LYRICA treatment did not appear to be associated with loss of glycemic control (as measured by HbA_{1C}).

5.8 Abrupt or Rapid Discontinuation

Following abrupt or rapid discontinuation of LYRICA, some patients reported symptoms including insomnia, nausea, headache, and diarrhea. Taper LYRICA gradually over a minimum of 1 week rather than discontinuing the drug abruptly.

5.9 Tumorigenic Potential

In standard preclinical *in vivo* lifetime carcinogenicity studies of LYRICA, an unexpectedly high incidence of hemangiosarcoma was identified in two different strains of mice *[see Nonclinical Toxicology (13.1)]*. The clinical significance of this finding is unknown. Clinical experience during LYRICA's premarketing development provides no direct means to assess its potential for inducing tumors in humans.

In clinical studies across various patient populations, comprising 6396 patient-years of exposure in patients >12 years of age, new or worsening-preexisting tumors were reported in 57 patients. Without knowledge of the background incidence and recurrence in similar populations not treated with LYRICA, it is impossible to know whether the incidence seen in these cohorts is or is not affected by treatment.

5.10 Ophthalmological Effects

In controlled studies, a higher proportion of patients treated with LYRICA reported blurred vision (7%) than did patients treated with placebo (2%), which resolved in a majority of cases with continued dosing. Less than 1% of patients discontinued LYRICA treatment due to vision-related events (primarily blurred vision).

Prospectively planned ophthalmologic testing, including visual acuity testing, formal visual field testing and dilated funduscopic examination, was performed in over 3600 patients. In these patients, visual acuity was reduced in 7% of patients treated with LYRICA, and 5% of placebo-treated patients. Visual field changes were detected in 13% of LYRICA-treated, and 12% of placebo-treated patients. Funduscopic changes were observed in 2% of LYRICA-treated and 2% of placebo-treated patients.

Although the clinical significance of the ophthalmologic findings is unknown, inform patients to notify their physician if changes in vision occur. If visual disturbance persists, consider further assessment. Consider more frequent assessment for patients who are already routinely monitored for ocular conditions [see Patient Counseling Information (17.8)].

5.11 Creatine Kinase Elevations
LYRICA treatment was associated with creatine kinase elevations. Mean changes in creatine kinase from baseline to the maximum value were 60 U/L for LYRICA-treated patients and 28 U/L for the placebo patients. In all controlled trials across multiple patient populations, 1.5% of patients on LYRICA and 0.7% of placebo patients had a value of creatine kinase at least three times the upper limit of normal. Three LYRICA treated subjects had events reported as rhabdomyolysis in premarketing clinical trials. The relationship between these myopathy events and LYRICA is not completely understood because the cases had documented factors that may have caused or contributed to these events. Instruct patients to promptly report unexplained muscle pain, tenderness, or weakness, particularly if these muscle symptoms are accompanied by malaise or fever. Discontinue treatment with LYRICA if myopathy is diagnosed or suspected or if markedly elevated creatine kinase levels occur.

5.12 Decreased Platelet Count
LYRICA treatment was associated with a decrease in platelet count. LYRICA-treated subjects experienced a mean maximal decrease in platelet count of $20 \times 10^3/\mu L$, compared to $11 \times 10^3/\mu L$ in placebo patients. In the overall database of controlled trials, 2% of placebo patients and 3% of LYRICA patients experienced a potentially clinically significant decrease in platelets, defined as 20% below baseline value and $<150 \times 10^3/\mu L$. A single LYRICA treated subject developed severe thrombocytopenia with a platelet count less than $20 \times 10^3/\mu L$. In randomized controlled trials, LYRICA was not associated with an increase in bleeding-related adverse reactions.

5.13 PR Interval Prolongation
LYRICA treatment was associated with PR interval prolongation. In analyses of clinical trial ECG data, the mean PR interval increase was 3–6 msec at LYRICA doses ≥300 mg/day. This mean change difference was not associated with an increased risk of PR increase ≥25% from baseline, an increased percentage of subjects with on-treatment PR >200 msec, or an increased risk of adverse reactions of second or third degree AV block.
Subgroup analyses did not identify an increased risk of PR prolongation in patients with baseline PR prolongation or in patients taking other PR prolonging medications. However, these analyses cannot be considered definitive because of the limited number of patients in these categories.

6 ADVERSE REACTIONS
6.1 Clinical Trials Experience
Because clinical trials are conducted under widely varying conditions, adverse reaction rates observed in the clinical trials of a drug cannot be directly compared to rates in the clinical trials of another drug and may not reflect the rates observed in practice.

In all controlled and uncontrolled trials across various patient populations during the premarketing development of LYRICA, more than 10,000 patients have received LYRICA. Approximately 5000 patients were treated for 6 months or more, over 3100 patients were treated for 1 year or longer, and over 1400 patients were treated for at least 2 years.

Adverse Reactions Most Commonly Leading to Discontinuation in All Premarketing Controlled Clinical Studies
In premarketing controlled trials of all populations combined, 14% of patients treated with LYRICA and 7% of patients treated with placebo discontinued prematurely due to adverse reactions. In the LYRICA treatment group, the adverse reactions most frequently leading to discontinuation were dizziness (4%) and somnolence (3%). In the placebo group, 1% of patients withdrew due to dizziness and <1% withdrew due to somnolence. Other adverse reactions that led to discontinuation from controlled trials more frequently in the LYRICA group compared to the placebo group were ataxia, confusion, asthenia, thinking abnormal, blurred vision, incoordination, and peripheral edema (1% each).

Most Common Adverse Reactions in All Premarketing Controlled Clinical Studies
In premarketing controlled trials of all patient populations combined, dizziness, somnolence, dry mouth, edema, blurred vision, weight gain, and "thinking abnormal" (primarily difficulty with concentration/attention) were more commonly reported by subjects treated with LYRICA than by subjects treated with placebo (≥5% and twice the rate of that seen in placebo).

Controlled Studies with Neuropathic Pain Associated with Diabetic Peripheral Neuropathy
Adverse Reactions Leading to Discontinuation
In clinical trials in patients with neuropathic pain associated with diabetic peripheral neuropathy, 9% of patients

Table 3 Treatment-emergent adverse reaction incidence in controlled trials in Neuropathic Pain Associated with Diabetic Peripheral Neuropathy (Events in at least 1% of all LYRICA-treated patients and at least numerically more in all LYRICA than in the placebo group)

Body system - Preferred term	75 mg/day [N=77] %	150 mg/day [N=212] %	300 mg/day [N=321] %	600 mg/day [N=369] %	All PGB* [N=979] %	Placebo [N=459] %
Body as a whole						
Asthenia	4	2	4	7	5	2
Accidental injury	5	2	2	6	4	3
Back pain	0	2	1	2	2	0
Chest pain	4	1	1	2	2	1
Face edema	0	1	1	2	1	0
Digestive system						
Dry mouth	3	2	5	7	5	1
Constipation	0	2	4	6	4	2
Flatulence	3	0	2	3	2	1
Metabolic and nutritional disorders						
Peripheral edema	4	6	9	12	9	2
Weight gain	0	4	4	6	4	0
Edema	0	2	4	2	2	0
Hypoglycemia	1	3	2	1	2	1
Nervous system						
Dizziness	8	9	23	29	21	5
Somnolence	4	6	13	16	12	3
Neuropathy	9	2	2	5	4	3
Ataxia	6	1	2	4	3	1
Vertigo	1	2	2	4	3	1
Confusion	0	1	2	3	2	1
Euphoria	0	0	3	2	2	0
Incoordination	1	0	2	2	2	0
Thinking abnormal†	1	0	1	3	2	0
Tremor	1	1	1	2	1	0
Abnormal gait	1	0	1	3	1	0
Amnesia	3	1	0	2	1	0
Nervousness	0	1	1	1	1	0
Respiratory system						
Dyspnea	3	0	2	2	2	1
Special senses						
Blurry vision‡	3	1	3	6	4	2
Abnormal vision	1	0	1	1	1	0

* PGB: pregabalin

† Thinking abnormal primarily consists of events related to difficulty with concentration/attention but also includes events related to cognition and language problems and slowed thinking.

‡ Investigator term; summary level term is amblyopia

treated with LYRICA and 4% of patients treated with placebo discontinued prematurely due to adverse reactions. In the LYRICA treatment group, the most common reasons for discontinuation due to adverse reactions were dizziness (3%) and somnolence (2%). In comparison, <1% of placebo patients withdrew due to dizziness and somnolence. Other reasons for discontinuation from the trials, occurring with greater frequency in the LYRICA group than in the placebo group, were asthenia, confusion, and peripheral edema. Each of these events led to withdrawal in approximately 1% of patients.

Most Common Adverse Reactions
Table 3 lists all adverse reactions, regardless of causality, occurring in ≥1% of patients with neuropathic pain associated with diabetic neuropathy in the combined LYRICA group for which the incidence was greater in this combined LYRICA group than in the placebo group. A majority of pregabalin-treated patients in clinical studies had adverse reactions with a maximum intensity of "mild" or "moderate".

[See table 3 above]
Controlled Studies in Postherpetic Neuralgia
Adverse Reactions Leading to Discontinuation
In clinical trials in patients with postherpetic neuralgia, 14% of patients treated with LYRICA and 7% of patients treated with placebo discontinued prematurely due to adverse reactions. In the LYRICA treatment group, the most common reasons for discontinuation due to adverse reactions were dizziness (4%) and somnolence (3%). In comparison, less than 1% of placebo patients withdrew due to dizziness and somnolence. Other reasons for discontinuation from the trials, occurring in greater frequency in the LYRICA group than in the placebo group, were confusion (2%), as well as peripheral edema, asthenia, ataxia, and abnormal gait (1% each).

Most Common Adverse Reactions
Table 4 lists all adverse reactions, regardless of causality, occurring in ≥ 1% of patients with neuropathic pain associated with postherpetic neuralgia in the combined LYRICA group for which the incidence was greater in this combined LYRICA group than in the placebo group. In addition, an event is included, even if the incidence in the all LYRICA group is not greater than in the placebo group, if the incidence of the event in the 600 mg/day group is more than twice that in the placebo group. A majority of pregabalin-

treated patients in clinical studies had adverse reactions with a maximum intensity of "mild" or "moderate". Overall, 12.4% of all pregabalin-treated patients and 9.0% of all placebo-treated patients had at least one severe event while 8% of pregabalin-treated patients and 4.3% of placebo-treated patients had at least one severe treatment-related adverse event.

[See table 4 at top of next page]
Controlled Add-On Studies in Adjunctive Therapy for Adult Patients with Partial Onset Seizures
Adverse Reactions Leading to Discontinuation
Approximately 15% of patients receiving LYRICA and 6% of patients receiving placebo in add-on epilepsy trials discontinued prematurely due to adverse reactions. In the LYRICA treatment group, the adverse reactions most frequently leading to discontinuation were dizziness (6%), ataxia (4%), and somnolence (3%). In comparison, <1% of patients in the placebo group withdrew due to each of these events. Other adverse reactions that led to discontinuation of at least 1% of patients in the LYRICA group and at least twice as frequently compared to the placebo group were asthenia, diplopia, blurred vision, thinking abnormal, nausea, tremor, vertigo, headache, and confusion (which each led to withdrawal in 2% or less of patients).

Most Common Adverse Reactions
Table 5 lists all dose-related adverse reactions occurring in at least 2% of all LYRICA-treated patients. Dose-relatedness was defined as the incidence of the adverse event in the 600 mg/day group was at least 2% greater than the rate in both the placebo and 150 mg/day groups. In these studies, 758 patients received LYRICA and 294 patients received placebo for up to 12 weeks. Because patients were also treated with 1 to 3 other AEDs, it is not possible to determine whether the following adverse reactions can be ascribed to LYRICA alone, or the combination of LYRICA and other AEDs. A majority of pregabalin-treated patients in clinical studies had adverse reactions with a maximum intensity of "mild" or "moderate".

[See table 5 at top of page 2807]
Controlled Studies with Fibromyalgia
Adverse Reactions Leading to Discontinuation
In clinical trials of patients with fibromyalgia, 19% of patients treated with pregabalin (150–600 mg/day) and 10% of patients treated with placebo discontinued prematurely due

Table 4 Treatment-emergent adverse reaction incidence in controlled trials in Neuropathic Pain Associated with Postherpetic Neuralgia (Events in at least 1% of all LYRICA-treated patients and at least numerically more in all LYRICA than in the placebo group)

Body system - Preferred term	75 mg/d [N=84] %	150 mg/d [N=302] %	300 mg/d [N=312] %	600 mg/d [N=154] %	All PGB* [N=852] %	Placebo [N=398] %
Body as a whole						
Infection	14	8	6	3	7	4
Headache	5	9	5	8	7	5
Pain	5	4	5	5	5	4
Accidental injury	4	3	3	5	3	2
Flu syndrome	1	2	2	1	2	1
Face edema	0	2	1	3	2	1
Digestive system						
Dry mouth	7	7	6	15	8	3
Constipation	4	5	5	5	5	2
Flatulence	2	1	2	3	2	1
Vomiting	1	1	3	3	2	1
Metabolic and nutritional disorders						
Peripheral edema	0	8	16	16	12	4
Weight gain	1	2	5	7	4	0
Edema	0	1	2	6	2	1
Musculoskeletal system						
Myasthenia	1	1	1	1	1	0
Nervous system						
Dizziness	11	18	31	37	26	9
Somnolence	8	12	18	25	16	5
Ataxia	1	2	5	9	5	1
Abnormal gait	0	2	4	8	4	1
Confusion	1	2	3	7	3	0
Thinking abnormal†	0	2	1	6	2	2
Incoordination	2	2	1	3	2	0
Amnesia	0	1	1	4	2	0
Speech disorder	0	0	1	3	1	0
Respiratory system						
Bronchitis	0	1	1	3	1	1
Special senses						
Blurry vision‡	1	5	5	9	5	3
Diplopia	0	2	2	4	2	0
Abnormal vision	0	1	2	5	2	0
Eye Disorder	0	1	1	2	1	0
Urogenital System						
Urinary Incontinence	0	1	1	2	1	0

* PGB: pregabalin
† Thinking abnormal primarily consists of events related to difficulty with concentration/attention but also includes events related to cognition and language problems and slowed thinking.
‡ Investigator term; summary level term is amblyopia

to adverse reactions. In the pregabalin treatment group, the most common reasons for discontinuation due to adverse reactions were dizziness (6%) and somnolence (3%). In comparison, <1% of placebo-treated patients withdrew due to dizziness and somnolence. Other reasons for discontinuation from the trials, occurring with greater frequency in the pregabalin treatment group than in the placebo treatment group, were fatigue, headache, balance disorder, and weight increased. Each of these adverse reactions led to withdrawal in approximately 1% of patients.

Most Common Adverse Reactions
Table 6 lists all adverse reactions, regardless of causality, occurring in ≥2% of patients with fibromyalgia in the 'all pregabalin' treatment group for which the incidence was greater than in the placebo treatment group. A majority of pregabalin-treated patients in clinical studies experienced adverse reactions with a maximum intensity of "mild" or "moderate".
[See table 6 at top of page 2808]

Other Adverse Reactions Observed During the Clinical Studies of LYRICA
Following is a list of treatment-emergent adverse reactions reported by patients treated with LYRICA during all clinical trials. The listing does not include those events already listed in the previous tables or elsewhere in labeling, those events for which a drug cause was remote, those events which were so general as to be uninformative, and those events reported only once which did not have a substantial probability of being acutely life-threatening.
Events are categorized by body system and listed in order of decreasing frequency according to the following definitions: *frequent* adverse reactions are those occurring on one or more occasions in at least 1/100 patients; *infrequent* adverse reactions are those occurring in 1/100 to 1/1000 patients; *rare* reactions are those occurring in fewer than 1/1000 patients. Events of major clinical importance are described in the *Warnings and Precautions* section (5).
Body as a Whole—*Frequent:* Abdominal pain, Allergic reaction, Fever, *Infrequent:* Abscess, Cellulitis, Chills, Malaise, Neck rigidity, Overdose, Pelvic pain, Photosensitivity reaction, *Rare:* Anaphylactoid reaction, Ascites, Granuloma,

Hangover effect, Intentional Injury, Retroperitoneal Fibrosis, Shock
Cardiovascular System—*Infrequent:* Deep thrombophlebitis, Heart failure, Hypotension, Postural hypotension, Retinal vascular disorder, Syncope; *Rare:* ST Depressed, Ventricular Fibrillation
Digestive System—*Frequent:* Gastroenteritis, Increased appetite; *Infrequent:* Cholecystitis, Cholelithiasis, Colitis, Dysphagia, Esophagitis, Gastritis, Gastrointestinal hemorrhage, Melena, Mouth ulceration, Pancreatitis, Rectal hemorrhage, Tongue edema; *Rare:* Aphthous stomatitis, Esophageal Ulcer, Periodontal abscess
Hemic and Lymphatic System—*Frequent:* Ecchymosis; *Infrequent:* Anemia, Eosinophilia, Hypochromic anemia, Leukocytosis, Leukopenia, Lymphadenopathy, Thrombocytopenia; *Rare:* Myelofibrosis, Polycythemia, Prothrombin decreased, Purpura, Thrombocythemia
Metabolic and Nutritional Disorders—*Rare:* Glucose Tolerance Decreased, Urate Crystalluria
Musculoskeletal System—*Frequent:* Arthralgia, Leg cramps, Myalgia, Myasthenia; *Infrequent:* Arthrosis; *Rare:* Chondrodystrophy, Generalized Spasm
Nervous System—*Frequent:* Anxiety, Depersonalization, Hypertonia, Hypesthesia, Libido decreased, Nystagmus, Paresthesia, Stupor, Twitching; *Infrequent:* Abnormal dreams, Agitation, Apathy, Aphasia, Circumoral paresthesia, Dysarthria, Hallucinations, Hostility, Hyperalgesia, Hyperesthesia, Hyperkinesia, Hypokinesia, Hypotonia, Libido increased, Myoclonus, Neuralgia, *Rare:* Addiction, Cerebellar syndrome, Cogwheel rigidity, Coma, Delirium, Delusions, Dysautonomia, Dyskinesia, Dystonia, Encephalopathy, Extrapyramidal syndrome, Guillain-Barré syndrome, Hypalgesia, Intracranial hypertension, Manic reaction, Paranoid reaction, Peripheral neuritis, Personality disorder, Psychotic depression, Schizophrenic reaction, Sleep disorder, Torticollis, Trismus
Respiratory System—*Rare:* Apnea, Atelectasis, Bronchiolitis, Hiccup, Laryngismus, Lung edema, Lung fibrosis, Yawn
Skin and Appendages—*Frequent:* Pruritus; *Infrequent:* Alopecia, Dry skin, Eczema, Hirsutism, Skin ulcer, Urticaria, Vesiculobullous rash; *Rare:* Angioedema, Exfoliative derma-

titis, Lichenoid dermatitis, Melanosis, Nail Disorder, Petechial rash, Purpuric rash, Pustular rash, Skin atrophy, Skin necrosis, Skin nodule, Stevens-Johnson syndrome, Subcutaneous nodule
Special senses—*Frequent:* Conjunctivitis, Diplopia, Otitis media, Tinnitus; *Infrequent:* Abnormality of accommodation, Blepharitis, Dry eyes, Eye hemorrhage, Hyperacusis, Photophobia, Retinal edema, Taste loss, Taste perversion; *Rare:* Anisocoria, Blindness, Corneal ulcer, Exophthalmos, Extraocular palsy, Iritis, Keratitis, Keratoconjunctivitis, Miosis, Mydriasis, Night blindness, Ophthalmoplegia, Optic atrophy, Papilledema, Parosmia, Ptosis, Uveitis
Urogenital System—*Frequent:* Anorgasmia, Impotence, Urinary frequency, Urinary incontinence; *Infrequent:* Abnormal ejaculation, Albuminuria, Amenorrhea, Dysmenorrhea, Dysuria, Hematuria, Kidney calculus, Leukorrhea, Menorrhagia, Metrorrhagia, Nephritis, Oliguria, Urinary retention, Urine abnormality; *Rare:* Acute kidney failure, Balanitis, Bladder Neoplasm, Cervicitis, Dyspareunia, Epididymitis, Female lactation, Glomerulitis, Ovarian disorder, Pyelonephritis
Comparison of Gender and Race
The overall adverse event profile of pregabalin was similar between women and men. There are insufficient data to support a statement regarding the distribution of adverse experience reports by race.

6.2 Post-marketing Experience
The following adverse reactions have been identified during postapproval use of LYRICA. Because these reactions are reported voluntarily from a population of uncertain size, it is not always possible to reliably estimate their frequency or establish a causal relationship to drug exposure.
Nervous System Disorders—Headache
Gastrointestinal Disorders—Nausea, Diarrhea

7 DRUG INTERACTIONS
Since LYRICA is predominantly excreted unchanged in the urine, undergoes negligible metabolism in humans (<2% of a dose recovered in urine as metabolites), and does not bind to plasma proteins, its pharmacokinetics are unlikely to be affected by other agents through metabolic interactions or protein binding displacement. *In vitro* and *in vivo* studies showed that LYRICA is unlikely to be involved in significant pharmacokinetic drug interactions. Specifically, there are no pharmacokinetic interactions between pregabalin and the following antiepileptic drugs: carbamazepine, valproic acid, lamotrigine, phenytoin, phenobarbital, and topiramate. Important pharmacokinetic interactions would also not be expected to occur between LYRICA and commonly used antiepileptic drugs [see Clinical Pharmacology (12)].
Pharmacodynamics
Multiple oral doses of LYRICA were co-administered with oxycodone, lorazepam, or ethanol. Although no pharmacokinetic interactions were seen, additive effects on cognitive and gross motor functioning were seen when LYRICA was co-administered with these drugs. No clinically important effects on respiration were seen.

8 USE IN SPECIFIC POPULATIONS
8.1 Pregnancy
Pregnancy Category C. Increased incidences of fetal structural abnormalities and other manifestations of developmental toxicity, including lethality, growth retardation, and nervous and reproductive system functional impairment, were observed in the offspring of rats and rabbits given pregabalin during pregnancy, at doses that produced plasma pregabalin exposures (AUC) ≥5 times human exposure at the maximum recommended dose (MRD) of 600 mg/day.
When pregnant rats were given pregabalin (500, 1250, or 2500 mg/kg) orally throughout the period of organogenesis, incidences of specific skull alterations attributed to abnormally advanced ossification (premature fusion of the jugal and nasal sutures) were increased at ≥1250 mg/kg, and incidences of skeletal variations and retarded ossification were increased at all doses. Fetal body weights were decreased at the highest dose. The low dose in this study was associated with a plasma exposure (AUC) approximately 17 times human exposure at the MRD of 600 mg/day. A no-effect dose for rat embryo-fetal developmental toxicity was not established.
When pregnant rabbits were given LYRICA (250, 500, or 1250 mg/kg) orally throughout the period of organogenesis, decreased fetal body weight and increased incidences of skeletal malformations, visceral variations, and retarded ossification were observed at the highest dose. The no-effect dose for developmental toxicity in rabbits (500 mg/kg) was associated with a plasma exposure approximately 16 times human exposure at the MRD.
In a study in which female rats were dosed with LYRICA (50, 100, 250, 1250, or 2500 mg/kg) throughout gestation and lactation, offspring growth was reduced at ≤ 100 mg/kg and offspring survival was decreased at ≥250 mg/kg. The effect on offspring survival was pronounced at doses ≥1250 mg/kg, with 100% mortality in high-dose litters.

When offspring were tested as adults, neurobehavioral abnormalities (decreased auditory startle responding) were observed at ≥250 mg/kg and reproductive impairment (decreased fertility and litter size) was seen at 1250 mg/kg. The no-effect dose for pre- and postnatal developmental toxicity in rats (50 mg/kg) produced a plasma exposure approximately 2 times human exposure at the MRD.

There are no adequate and well-controlled studies in pregnant women. Use LYRICA during pregnancy only if the potential benefit justifies the potential risk to the fetus.

To provide information regarding the effects of in utero exposure to LYRICA, physicians are advised to recommend that pregnant patients taking LYRICA enroll in the North American Antiepileptic Drug (NAAED) Pregnancy Registry. This can be done by calling the toll free number 1-888-233-2334, and must be done by patients themselves. Information on the registry can also be found at the website http://www.aedpregnancyregistry.org/.

8.2 Labor and Delivery
The effects of LYRICA on labor and delivery in pregnant women are unknown. In the prenatal-postnatal study in rats, pregabalin prolonged gestation and induced dystocia at exposures ≥50 times the mean human exposure ($AUC_{(0-24)}$ of 123 µg·hr/mL) at the maximum recommended clinical dose of 600 mg/day.

8.3 Nursing Mothers
It is not known if pregabalin is excreted in human milk; it is, however, present in the milk of rats. Because many drugs are excreted in human milk, and because of the potential for tumorigenicity shown for pregabalin in animal studies, decide whether to discontinue nursing or to discontinue the drug, taking into account the importance of the drug to the mother.

8.4 Pediatric Use
The safety and efficacy of pregabalin in pediatric patients have not been established.

In studies in which pregabalin (50 to 500 mg/kg) was orally administered to young rats from early in the postnatal period (Postnatal Day 7) through sexual maturity, neurobehavioral abnormalities (deficits in learning and memory, altered locomotor activity, decreased auditory startle responding and habituation) and reproductive impairment (delayed sexual maturation and decreased fertility in males and females) were observed at doses ≥50 mg/kg. The neurobehavioral changes of acoustic startle persisted at ≥250 mg/kg and locomotor activity and water maze performance at ≥500 mg/kg in animals tested after cessation of dosing and, thus, were considered to represent long-term effects. The low effect dose for developmental neurotoxicity and reproductive impairment in juvenile rats (50 mg/kg) was associated with a plasma pregabalin exposure (AUC) approximately equal to human exposure at the maximum recommended dose of 600 mg/day. A no-effect dose was not established.

8.5 Geriatric Use
In controlled clinical studies of LYRICA in neuropathic pain associated with diabetic peripheral neuropathy, 246 patients were 65 to 74 years of age, and 73 patients were 75 years of age or older.

In controlled clinical studies of LYRICA in neuropathic pain associated with postherpetic neuralgia, 282 patients were 65 to 74 years of age, and 379 patients were 75 years of age or older.

In controlled clinical studies of LYRICA in epilepsy, there were only 10 patients 65 to 74 years of age, and 2 patients who were 75 years of age or older.

No overall differences in safety and efficacy were observed between these patients and younger patients.

In controlled clinical studies of LYRICA in fibromyalgia, 106 patients were 65 years of age or older. Although the adverse reaction profile was similar between the two age groups, the following neurological adverse reactions were more frequent in patients 65 years of age or older: dizziness, vision blurred, balance disorder, tremor, confusional state, coordination abnormal, and lethargy.

LYRICA is known to be substantially excreted by the kidney, and the risk of toxic reactions to LYRICA may be greater in patients with impaired renal function. Because LYRICA is eliminated primarily by renal excretion, adjust the dose for elderly patients with renal impairment [see Dosage and Administration (2.5)].

9 DRUG ABUSE AND DEPENDENCE
9.1 Controlled Substance
LYRICA is a Schedule V controlled substance.

LYRICA is not known to be active at receptor sites associated with drugs of abuse. As with any CNS active drug, carefully evaluate patients for history of drug abuse and observe them for signs of LYRICA misuse or abuse (e.g., development of tolerance, dose escalation, drug-seeking behavior).

9.2 Abuse
In a study of recreational users (N=15) of sedative/hypnotic drugs, including alcohol, LYRICA (450mg, single dose) re-

Table 5. Dose-related treatment-emergent adverse reaction incidence in controlled trials in adjunctive therapy for adult patients with partial onset seizures (Events in at least 2% of all LYRICA-treated patients and the adverse reaction in the 600 mg/day group was ≥2% the rate in both the placebo and 150 mg/day groups)

Body System - Preferred Term	150 mg/d [N = 185] %	300 mg/d [N = 90] %	600 mg/d [N = 395] %	All PGB* [N = 670]† %	Placebo [N = 294] %
Body as a Whole					
Accidental Injury	7	11	10	9	5
Pain	3	2	5	4	3
Digestive System					
Increased Appetite	2	3	6	5	1
Dry Mouth	1	2	6	4	1
Constipation	1	1	7	4	2
Metabolic and Nutritional Disorders					
Weight Gain	5	7	16	12	1
Peripheral Edema	3	3	6	5	2
Nervous System					
Dizziness	18	31	38	32	11
Somnolence	11	18	28	22	11
Ataxia	6	10	20	15	4
Tremor	3	7	11	8	4
Thinking Abnormal‡	4	8	9	8	2
Amnesia	3	2	6	5	2
Speech Disorder	1	2	7	5	1
Incoordination	1	3	6	4	1
Abnormal Gait	1	3	5	4	0
Twitching	0	4	5	4	1
Confusion	1	2	5	4	2
Myoclonus	1	0	4	2	0
Special Senses					
Blurred Vision§	5	8	12	10	4
Diplopia	5	7	12	9	4
Abnormal Vision	3	1	5	4	1

* PGB: pregabalin
† Excludes patients who received the 50 mg dose in Study E1.
‡ Thinking abnormal primarily consists of events related to difficulty with concentration/attention but also includes events related to cognition and language problems and slowed thinking.
§ Investigator term; summary level term is amblyopia.

ceived subjective ratings of "good drug effect," "high" and "liking" to a degree that was similar to diazepam (30mg, single dose). In controlled clinical studies in over 5500 patients, 4 % of LYRICA-treated patients and 1 % of placebo-treated patients overall reported euphoria as an adverse reaction, though in some patient populations studied, this reporting rate was higher and ranged from 1 to 12%.

9.3 Dependence
In clinical studies, following abrupt or rapid discontinuation of LYRICA, some patients reported symptoms including insomnia, nausea, headache or diarrhea [see Warnings and Precautions (5.8)], suggestive of physical dependence.

10 OVERDOSAGE
Signs, Symptoms and Laboratory Findings of Acute Overdosage in Humans
There is limited experience with overdose of LYRICA. The highest reported accidental overdose of LYRICA during the clinical development program was 8000 mg, and there were no notable clinical consequences.

Treatment or Management of Overdose
There is no specific antidote for overdose with LYRICA. If indicated, elimination of unabsorbed drug may be attempted by emesis or gastric lavage; observe usual precautions to maintain the airway. General supportive care of the patient is indicated including monitoring of vital signs and observation of the clinical status of the patient. Contact a Certified Poison Control Center for up-to-date information on the management of overdose with LYRICA.

Although hemodialysis has not been performed in the few known cases of overdose, it may be indicated by the patient's clinical state or in patients with significant renal impairment. Standard hemodialysis procedures result in significant clearance of pregabalin (approximately 50% in 4 hours).

11 DESCRIPTION
Pregabalin is described chemically as (S)-3-(aminomethyl)-5-methylhexanoic acid. The molecular formula is $C_8H_{17}NO_2$ and the molecular weight is 159.23. The chemical structure of pregabalin is:

Pregabalin is a white to off-white, crystalline solid with a pK_{a1} of 4.2 and a pK_{a2} of 10.6. It is freely soluble in water and both basic and acidic aqueous solutions. The log of the partition coefficient (n-octanol/0.05M phosphate buffer) at pH 7.4 is −1.35.

LYRICA (pregabalin) Capsules are administered orally and are supplied as imprinted hard-shell capsules containing 25, 50, 75, 100, 150, 200, 225, and 300 mg of pregabalin, along with lactose monohydrate, cornstarch, and talc as inactive ingredients. The capsule shells contain gelatin and titanium dioxide. In addition, the orange capsule shells contain red iron oxide and the white capsule shells contain sodium lauryl sulfate and colloidal silicon dioxide. Colloidal silicon dioxide is a manufacturing aid that may or may not be present in the capsule shells. The imprinting ink contains shellac, black iron oxide, propylene glycol, and potassium hydroxide.

LYRICA (pregabalin) oral solution, 20 mg/mL, is administered orally and is supplied as a clear, colorless solution contained in a 16 fluid ounce white HDPE bottle with a polyethylene-lined closure. The oral solution contains 20 mg/mL of pregabalin, along with methylparaben, propylparaben, monobasic sodium phosphate anhydrous, dibasic sodium phosphate anhydrous, sucralose, artificial strawberry #11545 and purified water as inactive ingredients.

12 CLINICAL PHARMACOLOGY
12.1 Mechanism of Action
LYRICA (pregabalin) binds with high affinity to the alpha$_2$-delta site (an auxiliary subunit of voltage-gated calcium channels) in central nervous system tissues. Although the mechanism of action of pregabalin is unknown, results with genetically modified mice and with compounds structurally related to pregabalin (such as gabapentin) suggest that binding to the alpha$_2$-delta subunit may be involved in pregabalin's antinociceptive and antiseizure effects in animal models. In vitro, pregabalin reduces the calcium-dependent release of several neurotransmitters, possibly by modulation of calcium channel function.

While pregabalin is a structural derivative of the inhibitory neurotransmitter gamma-aminobutyric acid (GABA), it does not bind directly to GABA$_A$, GABA$_B$, or benzodiazepine receptors, does not augment GABA$_A$ responses in cultured neurons, does not alter rat brain GABA concentration or have acute effects on GABA uptake or degradation. However, in cultured neurons prolonged application of pregabalin increases the density of GABA transporter protein and increases the rate of functional GABA transport. Pregabalin does not block sodium channels, is not active at opiate receptors, and does not alter cyclooxygenase enzyme activity. It is inactive at serotonin and dopamine receptors and does not inhibit dopamine, serotonin, or noradrenaline reuptake.

12.3 Pharmacokinetics
Pregabalin is well absorbed after oral administration, is eliminated largely by renal excretion, and has an elimination half-life of about 6 hours.

Table 6 Treatment-emergent adverse reaction incidence in controlled trials in Fibromyalgia (Events in at least 2% of all LYRICA-treated patients and occurring more frequently in the all pregabalin-group than in the placebo treatment group)

System Organ Class - Preferred term	150 mg/d [N=132] %	300 mg/d [N=502] %	450 mg/d [N=505] %	600 mg/d [N=378] %	All PGB* [N=1517] %	Placebo [N=505] %
Ear and Labyrinth Disorders						
Vertigo	2	2	2	1	2	0
Eye Disorders						
Vision blurred	8	7	7	12	8	1
Gastrointestinal Disorders						
Dry mouth	7	6	9	9	8	2
Constipation	4	4	7	10	7	2
Vomiting	2	3	3	2	3	2
Flatulence	1	1	2	2	2	1
Abdominal distension	2	2	2	2	2	1
General Disorders and Administrative Site Conditions						
Fatigue	5	7	6	8	7	4
Edema peripheral	5	5	6	9	6	2
Chest pain	2	1	2	2	2	1
Feeling abnormal	1	3	2	2	2	0
Edema	1	2	1	2	2	1
Feeling drunk	1	2	1	2	2	0
Infections and Infestations						
Sinusitis	4	5	7	5	5	4
Investigations						
Weight increased	8	10	10	14	11	2
Metabolism and Nutrition Disorders						
Increased appetite	4	3	5	7	5	1
Fluid retention	2	3	3	2	2	1
Musculoskeletal and Connective Tissue Disorders						
Arthralgia	4	3	3	6	4	2
Muscle spasms	2	4	4	4	4	2
Back pain	2	3	4	3	3	3
Nervous System Disorders						
Dizziness	23	31	43	45	38	9
Somnolence	13	18	22	22	20	4
Headache	11	12	14	10	12	12
Disturbance in attention	4	4	6	6	5	1
Balance disorder	2	3	6	9	5	0
Memory impairment	1	3	4	4	3	0
Coordination abnormal	2	1	2	2	2	1
Hypoaesthesia	2	2	3	2	2	1
Lethargy	2	2	1	2	2	0
Tremor	0	1	3	2	2	0
Psychiatric Disorders						
Euphoric Mood	2	5	6	7	6	1
Confusional state	0	2	3	4	3	0
Anxiety	2	2	2	2	2	1
Disorientation	1	0	2	1	2	0
Depression	2	2	2	2	2	2
Respiratory, Thoracic and Mediastinal Disorders						
Pharyngolaryngeal pain	2	1	3	3	2	2

*PGB: pregabalin

Absorption and Distribution

Following oral administration of LYRICA capsules under fasting conditions, peak plasma concentrations occur within 1.5 hours. Pregabalin oral bioavailability is ≥90% and is independent of dose. Following single- (25 to 300 mg) and multiple-dose (75 to 900 mg/day) administration, maximum plasma concentrations (C_{max}) and area under the plasma concentration-time curve (AUC) values increase linearly. Following repeated administration, steady state is achieved within 24 to 48 hours. Multiple-dose pharmacokinetics can be predicted from single-dose data.

The rate of pregabalin absorption is decreased when given with food, resulting in a decrease in C_{max} of approximately 25% to 30% and an increase in T_{max} to approximately 3 hours. However, administration of pregabalin with food has no clinically relevant effect on the total absorption of pregabalin. Therefore, pregabalin can be taken with or without food.

Pregabalin does not bind to plasma proteins. The apparent volume of distribution of pregabalin following oral administration is approximately 0.5 L/kg. Pregabalin is a substrate for system L transporter which is responsible for the transport of large amino acids across the blood brain barrier. Although there are no data in humans, pregabalin has been shown to cross the blood brain barrier in mice, rats, and monkeys. In addition, pregabalin has been shown to cross the placenta in rats and is present in the milk of lactating rats.

Metabolism and Elimination

Pregabalin undergoes negligible metabolism in humans. Following a dose of radio-labeled pregabalin, approximately 90% of the administered dose was recovered in the urine as unchanged pregabalin. The N-methylated derivative of pregabalin, the major metabolite of pregabalin found in urine, accounted for 0.9% of the dose. In preclinical studies, pregabalin (S-enantiomer) did not undergo racemization to the R-enantiomer in mice, rats, rabbits, or monkeys.

Pregabalin is eliminated from the systemic circulation primarily by renal excretion as unchanged drug with a mean elimination half-life of 6.3 hours in subjects with normal renal function. Mean renal clearance was estimated to be 67.0 to 80.9 mL/min in young healthy subjects. Because pregabalin is not bound to plasma proteins this clearance rate indicates that renal tubular reabsorption is involved. Pregabalin elimination is nearly proportional to creatinine clearance (CLcr) [see Dosage and Administration, (2.5)].

12.4 Pharmacokinetics in Special Populations

Race

In population pharmacokinetic analyses of the clinical studies in various populations, the pharmacokinetics of LYRICA were not significantly affected by race (Caucasians, Blacks, and Hispanics).

Gender

Population pharmacokinetic analyses of the clinical studies showed that the relationship between daily dose and LYRICA drug exposure is similar between genders.

Renal Impairment and Hemodialysis

Pregabalin clearance is nearly proportional to creatinine clearance (CLcr). Dosage reduction in patients with renal dysfunction is necessary. Pregabalin is effectively removed from plasma by hemodialysis. Following a 4-hour hemodialysis treatment, plasma pregabalin concentrations are reduced by approximately 50%. For patients on hemodialysis, dosing must be modified [see Dosage and Administration (2.5)].

Elderly

Pregabalin oral clearance tended to decrease with increasing age. This decrease in pregabalin oral clearance is consistent with age-related decreases in CLcr. Reduction of pregabalin dose may be required in patients who have age-related compromised renal function [see Dosage and Administration, (2.5)].

Pediatric Pharmacokinetics

Pharmacokinetics of pregabalin have not been adequately studied in pediatric patients.

Drug Interactions

In Vitro Studies

Pregabalin, at concentrations that were, in general, 10-times those attained in clinical trials, does not inhibit human CYP1A2, CYP2A6, CYP2C9, CYP2C19, CYP2D6, CYP2E1, and CYP3A4 enzyme systems. In vitro drug interaction studies demonstrate that pregabalin does not induce CYP1A2 or CYP3A4 activity. Therefore, an increase in the metabolism of coadministered CYP1A2 substrates (e.g. theophylline, caffeine) or CYP 3A4 substrates (e.g. midazolam, testosterone) is not anticipated.

In Vivo Studies

The drug interaction studies described in this section were conducted in healthy adults, and across various patient populations.

Gabapentin

The pharmacokinetic interactions of pregabalin and gabapentin were investigated in 12 healthy subjects following concomitant single-dose administration of 100-mg pregabalin and 300-mg gabapentin and in 18 healthy subjects following concomitant multiple-dose administration of 200-mg pregabalin every 8 hours and 400-mg gabapentin every 8 hours. Gabapentin pharmacokinetics following single- and multiple-dose administration were unaltered by pregabalin coadministration. The extent of pregabalin absorption was unaffected by gabapentin coadministration, although there was a small reduction in rate of absorption.

Oral Contraceptive

Pregabalin coadministration (200 mg three times a day) had no effect on the steady-state pharmacokinetics of norethindrone and ethinyl estradiol (1 mg/35 μg, respectively) in healthy subjects.

Lorazepam

Multiple-dose administration of pregabalin (300 mg twice a day) in healthy subjects had no effect on the rate and extent of lorazepam single-dose pharmacokinetics and single-dose administration of lorazepam (1 mg) had no effect on the steady-state pharmacokinetics of pregabalin.

Oxycodone

Multiple-dose administration of pregabalin (300 mg twice a day) in healthy subjects had no effect on the rate and extent of oxycodone single-dose pharmacokinetics. Single-dose administration of oxycodone (10 mg) had no effect on the steady-state pharmacokinetics of pregabalin.

Ethanol

Multiple-dose administration of pregabalin (300 mg twice a day) in healthy subjects had no effect on the rate and extent of ethanol single-dose pharmacokinetics and single-dose administration of ethanol (0.7 g/kg) had no effect on the steady-state pharmacokinetics of pregabalin.

Phenytoin, carbamazepine, valproic acid, and lamotrigine

Steady-state trough plasma concentrations of phenytoin, carbamazepine and carbamazepine 10,11 epoxide, valproic acid, and lamotrigine were not affected by concomitant pregabalin (200 mg three times a day) administration.

Population pharmacokinetic analyses in patients treated with pregabalin and various concomitant medications suggest the following:

Therapeutic class	Specific concomitant drug studied
Concomitant drug has no effect on the pharmacokinetics of pregabalin	
Hypoglycemics Diuretics	Glyburide, insulin, metformin Furosemide
Antiepileptic Drugs	Tiagabine
Concomitant drug has no effect on the pharmacokinetics of pregabalin and pregabalin has no effect on the pharmacokinetics of concomitant drug	
Antiepileptic Drugs	Carbamazepine, lamotrigine, phenobarbital, phenytoin, topiramate, valproic acid

13 NONCLINICAL TOXICOLOGY

13.1 Carcinogenesis, Mutagenesis, Impairment of Fertility

Carcinogenesis

A dose-dependent increase in the incidence of malignant vascular tumors (hemangiosarcomas) was observed in two strains of mice (B6C3F1 and CD-1) given pregabalin (200, 1000, or 5000 mg/kg) in the diet for two years. Plasma pregabalin exposure (AUC) in mice receiving the lowest dose that increased hemangiosarcomas was approximately equal to the human exposure at the maximum recommended dose (MRD) of 600 mg/day. A no-effect dose for induction of hemangiosarcomas in mice was not established. No evidence of carcinogenicity was seen in two studies in Wistar rats following dietary administration of pregabalin for two years at doses (50, 150, or 450 mg/kg in males and 100, 300, or 900 mg/kg in females) that were associated with plasma exposures in males and females up to approximately 14 and 24 times, respectively, human exposure at the MRD.

Mutagenesis
Pregabalin was not mutagenic in bacteria or in mammalian cells *in vitro*, was not clastogenic in mammalian systems *in vitro* and *in vivo*, and did not induce unscheduled DNA synthesis in mouse or rat hepatocytes.

Impairment of Fertility
In fertility studies in which male rats were orally administered pregabalin (50 to 2500 mg/kg) prior to and during mating with untreated females, a number of adverse reproductive and developmental effects were observed. These included decreased sperm counts and sperm motility, increased sperm abnormalities, reduced fertility, increased preimplantation embryo loss, decreased litter size, decreased fetal body weights, and an increased incidence of fetal abnormalities. Effects on sperm and fertility parameters were reversible in studies of this duration (3–4 months). The no-effect dose for male reproductive toxicity in these studies (100 mg/kg) was associated with a plasma pregabalin exposure (AUC) approximately 3 times human exposure at the maximum recommended dose (MRD) of 600 mg/day.

In addition, adverse reactions on reproductive organ (testes, epididymides) histopathology were observed in male rats exposed to pregabalin (500 to 1250 mg/kg) in general toxicology studies of four weeks or greater duration. The no-effect dose for male reproductive organ histopathology in rats (250 mg/kg) was associated with a plasma exposure approximately 8 times human exposure at the MRD.

In a fertility study in which female rats were given pregabalin (500, 1250, or 2500 mg/kg) orally prior to and during mating and early gestation, disrupted estrous cyclicity and an increased number of days to mating were seen at all doses, and embryolethality occurred at the highest dose. The low dose in this study produced a plasma exposure approximately 9 times that in humans receiving the MRD. A no-effect dose for female reproductive toxicity in rats was not established.

Human Data
In a double-blind, placebo-controlled clinical trial to assess the effect of pregabalin on sperm motility, 30 healthy male subjects were exposed to pregabalin at a dose of 600 mg/day. After 3 months of treatment (one complete sperm cycle), the difference between placebo- and pregabalin-treated subjects in mean percent sperm with normal motility was <4% and neither group had a mean change from baseline of more than 2%. Effects on other male reproductive parameters in humans have not been adequately studied.

13.2 Animal Toxicology and/or Pharmacology

Dermatopathy
Skin lesions ranging from erythema to necrosis were seen in repeated-dose toxicology studies in both rats and monkeys. The etiology of these skin lesions is unknown. At the maximum recommended human dose (MRD) of 600 mg/day, there is a 2-fold safety margin for the dermatological lesions. The more severe dermatopathies involving necrosis were associated with pregabalin exposures (as expressed by plasma AUCs) of approximately 3 to 8 times those achieved in humans given the MRD. No increase in incidence of skin lesions was observed in clinical studies.

Ocular Lesions
Ocular lesions (characterized by retinal atrophy [including loss of photoreceptor cells] and/or corneal inflammation/mineralization) were observed in two lifetime carcinogenicity studies in Wistar rats. These findings were observed at plasma pregabalin exposures (AUC) ≥2 times those achieved in humans given the maximum recommended dose of 600 mg/day. A no-effect dose for ocular lesions was not established. Similar lesions were not observed in lifetime carcinogenicity studies in two strains of mice or in monkeys treated for 1 year.

14 CLINICAL STUDIES

14.1 Neuropathic pain associated with diabetic peripheral neuropathy
The efficacy of the maximum recommended dose of LYRICA for the management of neuropathic pain associated with diabetic peripheral neuropathy was established in three double-blind, placebo-controlled, multicenter studies with three times a day dosing, two of which studied the maximum recommended dose. Patients were enrolled with either Type 1 or Type 2 diabetes mellitus and a diagnosis of painful distal symmetrical sensorimotor polyneuropathy for 1 to 5 years. A total of 89% of patients completed Studies DPN 1 and DPN 2. The patients had a minimum mean baseline pain score of ≥4 on an 11-point numerical pain rating scale ranging from 0 (no pain) to 10 (worst possible pain). The

baseline mean pain scores across the two studies ranged from 6.1 to 6.7. Patients were permitted up to 4 grams of acetaminophen per day as needed for pain, in addition to pregabalin. Patients recorded their pain daily in a diary.

Study DPN 1: This 5-week study compared LYRICA 25, 100, or 200 mg three times a day with placebo. Treatment with LYRICA 100 and 200 mg three times a day statistically significantly improved the endpoint mean pain score and increased the proportion of patients with at least a 50% reduction in pain score from baseline. There was no evidence of a greater effect on pain scores of the 200 mg three times a day dose than the 100 mg three times a day dose, but there was evidence of dose dependent adverse reactions [see Adverse Reactions (6.1)]. For a range of degrees of improvement in pain from baseline to study endpoint, Figure 1 shows the fraction of patients achieving that degree of improvement. The figure is cumulative, so that patients whose change from baseline is, for example, 50%, are also included at every level of improvement below 50%. Patients who did not complete the study were assigned 0% improvement. Some patients experienced a decrease in pain as early as Week 1, which persisted throughout the study.

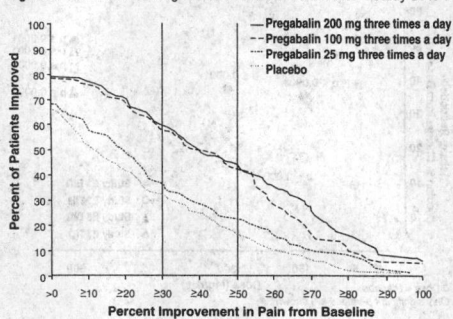

Figure 1: Patients Achieving Various Levels of Pain Relief – Study DPN 1

Study DPN 2: This 8-week study compared LYRICA 100 mg three times a day with placebo. Treatment with LYRICA 100 mg three times a day statistically significantly improved the endpoint mean pain score and increased the proportion of patients with at least a 50% reduction in pain score from baseline. For various degrees of improvement in pain from baseline to study endpoint, Figure 2 shows the fraction of patients achieving that degree of improvement. The figure is cumulative, so that patients whose change from baseline is, for example, 50%, are also included at every level of improvement below 50%. Patients who did not complete the study were assigned 0% improvement. Some patients experienced a decrease in pain as early as Week 1, which persisted throughout the study.

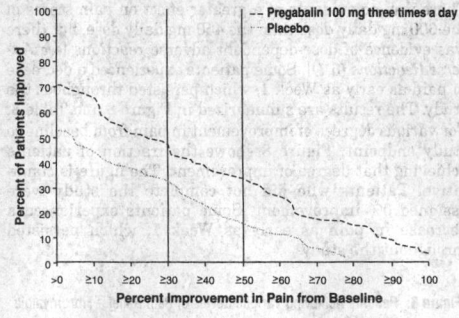

Figure 2: Patients Achieving Various Levels of Pain Relief – Study DPN 2

14.2 Postherpetic Neuralgia
The efficacy of LYRICA for the management of postherpetic neuralgia was established in three double-blind, placebo-controlled, multicenter studies. These studies enrolled patients with neuralgia persisting for at least 3 months following healing of herpes zoster rash and a minimum baseline score of ≥4 on an 11-point numerical pain rating scale ranging from 0 (no pain) to 10 (worst possible pain). Seventy-three percent of patients completed the studies. The baseline mean pain scores across the 3 studies ranged from 6 to 7. Patients were permitted up to 4 grams of acetaminophen per day as needed for pain, in addition to pregabalin. Patients recorded their pain daily in a diary.

Study PHN 1: This 13-week study compared LYRICA 75, 150, and 300 mg twice daily with placebo. Patients with creatinine clearance (CLcr) between 30 to 60 mL/min were randomized to 75 mg, 150 mg, or placebo twice daily. Patients

with creatinine clearance greater than 60 mL/min were randomized to 75 mg, 150 mg, 300 mg or placebo twice daily. In patients with creatinine clearance greater than 60 mL/min treatment with all doses of LYRICA statistically significantly improved the endpoint mean pain score and increased the proportion of patients with at least a 50% reduction in pain score from baseline. Despite differences in dosing based on renal function, patients with creatinine clearance between 30 to 60 mL/min tolerated LYRICA less well than patients with creatinine clearance greater than 60 mL/min as evidenced by higher rates of discontinuation due to adverse reactions. For various degrees of improvement in pain from baseline to study endpoint, Figure 3 shows the fraction of patients achieving that degree of improvement. The figure is cumulative, so that patients whose change from baseline is, for example, 50%, are also included at every level of improvement below 50%. Patients who did not complete the study were assigned 0% improvement. Some patients experienced a decrease in pain as early as Week 1, which persisted throughout the study.

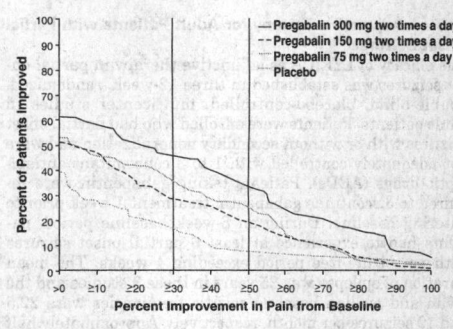

Figure 3: Patients Achieving Various Levels of Pain Relief – Study PHN 1

Study PHN 2: This 8-week study compared LYRICA 100 or 200 mg three times a day with placebo, with doses assigned based on creatinine clearance. Patients with creatinine clearance between 30 to 60 mL/min were treated with 100 mg three times a day, and patients with creatinine clearance greater than 60 mL/min were treated with 200 mg three times daily. Treatment with LYRICA statistically significantly improved the endpoint mean pain score and increased the proportion of patients with at least a 50% reduction in pain score from baseline. For various degrees of improvement in pain from baseline to study endpoint, Figure 4 shows the fraction of patients achieving that degree of improvement. The figure is cumulative, so that patients whose change from baseline is, for example, 50%, are also included at every level of improvement below 50%. Patients who did not complete the study were assigned 0% improvement. Some patients experienced a decrease in pain as early as Week 1, which persisted throughout the study.

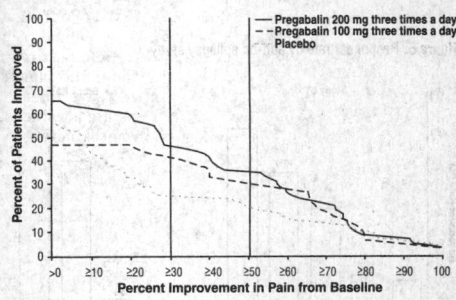

Figure 4: Patients Achieving Various Levels of Pain Relief – Study PHN 2

Study PHN 3: This 8-week study compared LYRICA 50 or 100 mg three times a day with placebo with doses assigned regardless of creatinine clearance. Treatment with LYRICA 50 and 100 mg three times a day statistically significantly improved the endpoint mean pain score and increased the proportion of patients with at least a 50% reduction in pain score from baseline. Patients with creatinine clearance between 30 to 60 mL/min tolerated LYRICA less well than patients with creatinine clearance greater than 60 mL/min as evidenced by markedly higher rates of discontinuation due to adverse reactions. For various degrees of improvement in pain from baseline to study endpoint, Figure 5 shows the fraction of patients achieving that degree of improvement. The figure is cumulative, so that patients whose change from baseline is, for example, 50%, are also included at every level of improvement below 50%. Patients who did not complete the study were assigned 0% improvement. Some patients experienced a decrease in pain as early as Week 1, which persisted throughout the study.

Figure 5: Patients Achieving Various Levels of Pain Relief – Study PHN 3

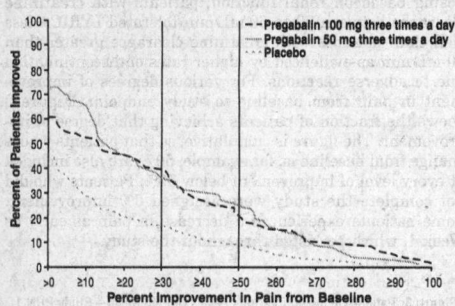

14.3 Adjunctive Therapy for Adult Patients with Partial Onset Seizures

The efficacy of LYRICA as adjunctive therapy in partial onset seizures was established in three 12-week, randomized, double-blind, placebo-controlled, multicenter studies in adult patients. Patients were enrolled who had partial onset seizures with or without secondary generalization and were not adequately controlled with 1 to 3 concomitant antiepileptic drugs (AEDs). Patients taking gabapentin were required to discontinue gabapentin treatment 1 week prior to entering baseline. During an 8-week baseline period, patients had to experience at least 6 partial onset seizures with no seizure-free period exceeding 4 weeks. The mean duration of epilepsy was 25 years in these 3 studies and the mean and median baseline seizure frequencies were 22.5 and 10 seizures per month, respectively. Approximately half of the patients were taking 2 concurrent AEDs at baseline. Among the LYRICA-treated patients, 80% completed the double-blind phase of the studies.

Table 7 shows median baseline seizure rates and median percent reduction in seizure frequency by dose.
[See table 7 above]

In the first study (E1), there was evidence of a dose-response relationship for total daily doses of Lyrica between 150 and 600 mg/day; a dose of 50 mg/day was not effective. In the first study (E1), each daily dose was divided into two equal doses (twice a day dosing). In the second study (E2), each daily dose was divided into three equal doses (three times a day dosing). In the third study (E3), the same total daily dose was divided into two equal doses for one group (twice a day dosing) and three equal doses for another group (three times a day dosing). While the three times a day dosing group in Study E3 performed numerically better than the twice a day dosing group, this difference was small and not statistically significant.

A secondary outcome measure included the responder rate (proportion of patients with ≥50% reduction from baseline in partial seizure frequency). The following figure displays responder rate by dose for two of the studies.

Figure 6. Responder rate by add-on epilepsy study

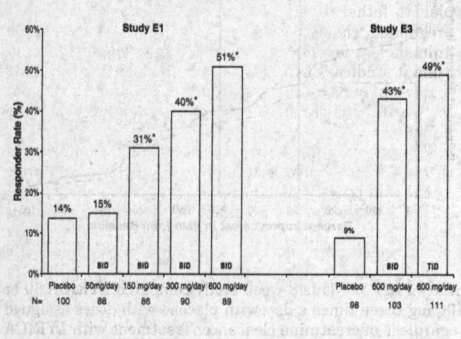

*statistically significant vs placebo

[See figure 7 at top of next column]
Subset evaluations of the antiseizure efficacy of LYRICA showed no clinically important differences as a function of age, gender, or race.

14.4 Management of Fibromyalgia

The efficacy of LYRICA for management of fibromyalgia was established in one 14-week, double-blind, placebo-controlled, multicenter study (F1) and one six-month, randomized withdrawal study (F2). Studies F1 and F2 enrolled

Table 7: Seizure Response in Controlled, Add-On Epilepsy Studies

Daily Dose of Pregabalin	Dosing Regimen	N	Baseline Seizure Frequency/mo	Median % Change from Baseline	p-value, vs. placebo
Study E1					
Placebo	BID	100	9.5	0	
50 mg/day	BID	88	10.3	-9	0.4230
150 mg/day	BID	86	8.8	-35	0.0001
300 mg/day	BID	90	9.8	-37	0.0001
600 mg/day	BID	89	9.0	-51	0.0001
Study E2					
Placebo	TID	96	9.3	1	
150 mg/day	TID	99	11.5	-17	0.0007
600 mg/day	TID	92	12.3	-43	0.0001
Study E3					
Placebo	BID/TID	98	11	-1	
600 mg/day	BID	103	9.5	-36	0.0001
600 mg/day	TID	111	10	-48	0.0001

Figure 7. Seizure Reduction by Dose (All Partial Onset Seizures) for Studies E1, E2, and E3

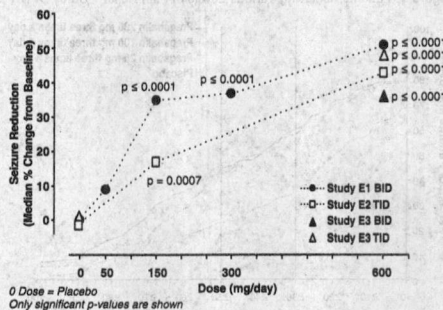

0 Dose = Placebo
Only significant p-values are shown

patients with a diagnosis of fibromyalgia using the American College of Rheumatology (ACR) criteria (history of widespread pain for 3 months, and pain present at 11 or more of the 18 specific tender point sites). The studies showed a reduction in pain by visual analog scale. In addition, improvement was demonstrated based on a patient global assessment (PGIC), and on the Fibromyalgia Impact Questionnaire (FIQ).

Study F1: This 14-week study compared LYRICA total daily doses of 300 mg, 450 mg and 600 mg with placebo. Patients were enrolled with a minimum mean baseline pain score of greater than or equal to 4 on an 11-point numeric pain rating scale and a score of greater than or equal to 40 mm on the 100 mm pain visual analog scale (VAS). The baseline mean pain score in this trial was 6.7. Responders to placebo in an initial one-week run-in phase were not randomized into subsequent phases of the study. A total of 64% of patients randomized to LYRICA completed the study. There was no evidence of a greater effect on pain scores of the 600 mg daily dose than the 450 mg daily dose, but there was evidence of dose-dependent adverse reactions [see Adverse Reactions (6.1)]. Some patients experienced a decrease in pain as early as Week 1, which persisted throughout the study. The results are summarized in Figure 8 and Table 8. For various degrees of improvement in pain from baseline to study endpoint, Figure 8 shows the fraction of patients achieving that degree of improvement. The figure is cumulative. Patients who did not complete the study were assigned 0% improvement. Some patients experienced a decrease in pain as early as Week 1, which persisted throughout the study.

Figure 8: Patients Achieving Various Levels of Pain Relief – Fibromyalgia Study F1

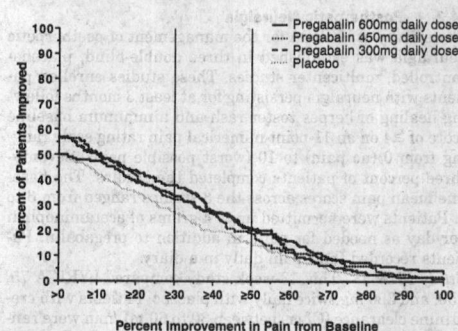

Table 8: Patient Global Response in Fibromyalgia Study F1

Patient Global Impression of Change		
Treatment Group (mg/day)	% Any Improvement	95% CI
Placebo	47.6	(40.0, 55.2)
PGB 300	68.1	(60.9, 75.3)
PGB 450	77.8	(71.5, 84.0)
PGB 600	66.1	(59.1, 73.1)

PGB = Pregabalin

Study F2: This randomized withdrawal study compared LYRICA with placebo. Patients were titrated during a 6-week open-label dose optimization phase to a total daily dose of 300 mg, 450 mg, or 600 mg. Patients were considered to be responders if they had both: 1) at least a 50% reduction in pain (VAS) and, 2) rated their overall improvement on the PGIC as "much improved" or "very much improved." Those who responded to treatment were then randomized in the double-blind treatment phase to either the dose achieved in the open-label phase or to placebo. Patients were treated for up to 6 months following randomization. Efficacy was assessed by time to loss of therapeutic response, defined as 1) less than 30% reduction in pain (VAS) from open-label baseline during two consecutive visits of the double-blind phase, or 2) worsening of FM symptoms necessitating an alternative treatment. Fifty-four percent of patients were able to titrate to an effective and tolerable dose of LYRICA during the 6-week open-label phase. Of the patients entering the randomized treatment phase assigned to remain on LYRICA, 38% of patients completed 26 weeks of treatment versus 19% of placebo-treated patients.

When considering return of pain or withdrawal due to adverse events as loss of response (LTR), treatment with LYRICA resulted in a longer time to loss of therapeutic response than treatment with placebo. Fifty-three percent of the pregabalin-treated subjects compared to 33% of placebo patients remained on study drug and maintained a therapeutic response to Week 26 of the study. Treatment with LYRICA also resulted in a longer time to loss of response based on the FIQ[1], and longer time to loss of overall assessment of patient status, as measured by the PGIC[2].

[1] Time to worsening of the FIQ was defined as the time to a 1-point increase from double-blind baseline in each of the subscales, and a 5-point increase from double-blind baseline evaluation for the FIQ total score.
[2] Time to PGIC lack of improvement was defined as time to PGIC assessments indicating less improvement than "much improvement."

[See figure 9 at top of next page]

16 HOW SUPPLIED/STORAGE AND HANDLING

25 mg capsules:
White, hard-gelatin capsule printed with black ink "Pfizer" on the cap, "PGN 25" on the body; available in:
Bottles of 90: NDC 0071-1012-68
50 mg capsules:
White, hard-gelatin capsule printed with black ink "Pfizer" on the cap, "PGN 50" and an ink band on the body, available in:
Bottles of 90: NDC 0071-1013-68
Unit-Dose Blister Packages of 100: NDC 0071-1013-41
75 mg capsules:
White/orange hard gelatin capsule printed with black ink "Pfizer" on the cap, "PGN 75" on the body; available in:

Figure 9: Time to Loss of Therapeutic Response, Fibromyalgia Study F2 (Kaplan-Meier Analysis)

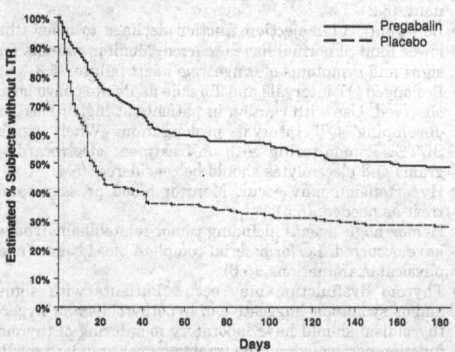

Bottles of 90: NDC 0071-1014-68
Unit-Dose Blister Packages of 100: NDC 0071-1014-41
100 mg capsules:
Orange, hard-gelatin capsule printed with black ink "Pfizer" on the cap, "PGN 100" on the body, available in:
Bottles of 90: NDC 0071-1015-68
Unit-Dose Blister Packages of 100: NDC 0071-1015-41
150 mg capsules:
White hard gelatin capsule printed with black ink "Pfizer" on the cap, "PGN 150" on the body, available in:
Bottles of 90: NDC 0071-1016-68
Unit-Dose Blister Packages of 100: NDC 0071-1016-41
200 mg capsules:
Light orange hard gelatin capsule printed with black ink "Pfizer" on the cap, "PGN 200" on the body, available in:
Bottles of 90: NDC 0071-1017-68
225 mg capsules:
White/light orange hard gelatin capsule printed with black ink "Pfizer" on the cap, "PGN 225" on the body; available in:
Bottles of 90: NDC 0071-1019-68
300 mg capsules:
White/orange hard gelatin capsule printed with black ink "Pfizer" on the cap, "PGN 300" on the body, available in:
Bottles of 90: NDC 0071-1018-68
20 mg/mL oral solution:
16 fluid ounce white high density polyethylene (HDPE) bottle with a polyethylene-lined closure:
16 fluid ounce bottle NDC 0071-1020-01
Storage and Handling
Store at 25°C (77°F); excursions permitted to 15°C to 30°C (59°F to 86°F) (see USP Controlled Room Temperature). For the oral solution, use within 45 days of first opening the bottle.

See FDA-Approved Medication Guide

17 PATIENT COUNSELING INFORMATION

17.1 Medication Guide
Inform patients of the availability of a Medication Guide, and instruct them to read the Medication Guide prior to taking LYRICA. Instruct patients to take LYRICA only as prescribed.

17.2 Angioedema
Advise patients that LYRICA may cause angioedema, with swelling of the face, mouth (lip, gum, tongue) and neck (larynx and pharynx) that can lead to life-threatening respiratory compromise. Instruct patients to discontinue LYRICA and immediately seek medical care if they experience these symptoms [see Warnings and Precautions (5.1)].

17.3 Hypersensitivity
Advise patients that LYRICA has been associated with hypersensitivity reactions such as wheezing, dyspnea, rash, hives, and blisters. Instruct patients to discontinue LYRICA and immediately seek medical care if they experience these symptoms [see Warnings and Precautions (5.2)].

17.4 Suicidal Thinking and Behavior
Patients, their caregivers, and families should be counseled that AEDs, including LYRICA, may increase the risk of suicidal thoughts and behavior and should be advised of the need to be alert for the emergence or worsening of symptoms of depression, any unusual changes in mood or behavior, or the emergence of suicidal thoughts, behavior, or thoughts about self-harm. Report behaviors of concern immediately to healthcare providers [see Warnings and Precautions (5.4)].

17.5 Dizziness and Somnolence
Counsel patients that LYRICA may cause dizziness, somnolence, blurred vision and other CNS signs and symptoms. Accordingly, advise patients not to drive, operate complex machinery, or engage in other hazardous activities until they have gained sufficient experience on LYRICA to gauge whether or not it affects their mental, visual, and/or motor performance adversely [see Warnings and Precautions (5.6)].

17.6 Weight Gain and Edema
Counsel patients that LYRICA may cause edema and weight gain. Advise patients that concomitant treatment with LYRICA and a thiazolidinedione antidiabetic agent may lead to an additive effect on edema and weight gain. For patients with preexisting cardiac conditions, this may increase the risk of heart failure. [see Warnings and Precautions (5.5 and 5.7)].

17.7 Abrupt or Rapid Discontinuation
Advise patients to take LYRICA as prescribed. Abrupt or rapid discontinuation may result in insomnia, nausea, headache, or diarrhea. [see Warnings and Precautions (5.8)].

17.8 Ophthalmological Effects
Counsel patients that LYRICA may cause visual disturbances. Inform patients that if changes in vision occur, they should notify their physician [see Warnings and Precautions (5.10)].

17.9 Creatine Kinase Elevations
Instruct patients to promptly report unexplained muscle pain, tenderness, or weakness, particularly if accompanied by malaise or fever. [see Warnings and Precautions (5.11)].

17.10 CNS Depressants
Inform patients who require concomitant treatment with central nervous system depressants such as opiates or benzodiazepines that they may experience additive CNS side effects, such as somnolence.

17.11 Alcohol
Tell patients to avoid consuming alcohol while taking LYRICA, as LYRICA may potentiate the impairment of motor skills and sedating effects of alcohol.

17.12 Use in Pregnancy
Instruct patients to notify their physician if they become pregnant or intend to become pregnant during therapy, and to notify their physician if they are breast feeding or intend to breast feed during therapy [see Use In Specific Populations (8.1) and (8.3)].
Encourage patients to enroll in the NAAED Pregnancy Registry if they become pregnant. This registry is collecting information about the safety of antiepileptic drugs during pregnancy. To enroll, patients can call the toll free number 1-888-233-2334 [see Use In Specific Populations (8.1)].

17.13 Male Fertility
Inform men being treated with LYRICA who plan to father a child of the potential risk of male-mediated teratogenicity. In preclinical studies in rats, pregabalin was associated with an increased risk of male-mediated teratogenicity. The clinical significance of this finding is uncertain [see Nonclinical Toxicology (13.1)].

17.14 Dermatopathy
Instruct diabetic patients to pay particular attention to skin integrity while being treated with LYRICA. Some animals treated with pregabalin developed skin ulcerations, although no increased incidence of skin lesions associated with LYRICA was observed in clinical trials [see Nonclinical Toxicology (13.2)].

Capsules manufactured by:
Pfizer Pharmaceuticals LLC
Vega Baja, PR 00694
Oral Solution manufactured by:
Pfizer Inc
Kalamazoo, MI 49001
Distributed by
Parke-Davis
Division of Pfizer Inc, NY, NY 10017
LAB-0294-17.0

MEDICATION GUIDE
LYRICA (LEER-i-kah)
(pregabalin)
Capsules and Oral Solution, Ⓥ
Read this Medication Guide before you start taking LYRICA and each time you get a refill. There may be new information. This information does not take the place of talking to your healthcare provider about your medical condition or treatment. If you have any questions about LYRICA, ask your healthcare provider or pharmacist.
What is the most important information I should know about LYRICA?
1. LYRICA may cause serious, even life-threatening, allergic reactions.
Stop taking LYRICA and call your healthcare provider right away if you have any of these signs of a serious allergic reaction:
• swelling of your face, mouth, lips, gums, tongue, throat or neck
• trouble breathing
• rash, hives (raised bumps) or blisters
2. Like other antiepileptic drugs, LYRICA may cause suicidal thoughts or actions in a very small number of people, about 1 in 500.
Call a healthcare provider right away if you have any of these symptoms, especially if they are new, worse, or worry you:
• thoughts about suicide or dying

• attempts to commit suicide
• new or worse depression
• new or worse anxiety
• feeling agitated or restless
• panic attacks
• trouble sleeping (insomnia)
• new or worse irritability
• acting aggressive, being angry, or violent
• acting on dangerous impulses
• an extreme increase in activity and talking (mania)
• other unusual changes in behavior or mood
If you have suicidal thoughts or actions, do not stop LYRICA without first talking to a healthcare provider.
• Stopping LYRICA suddenly can cause serious problems.
• Suicidal thoughts or actions can be caused by things other than medicines. If you have suicidal thoughts or actions, your healthcare provider may check for other causes.
How can I watch for early symptoms of suicidal thoughts and actions?
• Pay attention to any changes, especially sudden changes, in mood, behaviors, thoughts, or feelings.
• Keep all follow-up visits with your healthcare provider as scheduled.
• Call your healthcare provider between visits as needed, especially if you are worried about symptoms.
3. LYRICA may cause swelling of your hands, legs and feet. This swelling can be a serious problem for people with heart problems.
4. LYRICA may cause dizziness and sleepiness.
Do not drive a car, work with machines, or do other dangerous activities until you know how LYRICA affects you. Ask your healthcare provider about when it will be okay to do these activities.
What is LYRICA?
LYRICA is a prescription medicine used in adults, 18 years and older, to treat:
• pain from damaged nerves (neuropathic pain) that happens with diabetes
• pain from damaged nerves (neuropathic pain) that follows healing of shingles
• partial seizures when taken together with other seizure medicines
• fibromyalgia (pain all over your body)
LYRICA has not been studied in children under 18 years of age.
Who Should Not Take LYRICA?
Do not take LYRICA if you are allergic to pregabalin or any of the ingredients in LYRICA. See "What is the most important information I should know about LYRICA?" for the signs of an allergic reaction. See the end of this leaflet for a complete list of ingredients in LYRICA.
What should I tell my healthcare provider before taking LYRICA?
Before taking LYRICA, tell your healthcare provider about all your medical conditions, including if you:
• have or have had depression, mood problems or suicidal thoughts or behavior
• have kidney problems or get kidney dialysis
• have heart problems including heart failure
• have a bleeding problem or a low blood platelet count
• have abused prescription medicines, street drugs, or alcohol in the past
• have ever had swelling of your face, mouth, tongue, lips, gums, neck, or throat (angioedema)
• plan to father a child. Animal studies have shown that pregabalin, the active ingredient in LYRICA, made male animals less fertile and caused sperm to change. Also, in animal studies, birth defects were seen in the offspring (babies) of male animals treated with pregabalin. It is not known if these problems can happen in people who take LYRICA.
• **are pregnant or plan to become pregnant. It is not known if LYRICA will harm your unborn baby.** You and your healthcare provider will have to decide if you should take LYRICA while you are pregnant. If you become pregnant while taking LYRICA, talk to your healthcare provider about registering with the North American Antiepileptic Drug Pregnancy Registry. You can enroll in this registry by calling 1-888-233-2334. The purpose of this registry is to collect information about the safety of antiepileptic drugs during pregnancy.
• **are breastfeeding. It is not known if LYRICA passes into breast milk and if it can harm your baby.** You and your healthcare provider should discuss whether you should take LYRICA or breast-feed, but you should not do both
Tell your healthcare provider about all the medicines you take including prescription and non-prescription medicines, vitamins or herbal supplements. LYRICA and other medicines may affect each other causing side effects. Especially tell your healthcare provider if you take:
• angiotensin converting enzyme (ACE) inhibitors, which are used to treat many conditions, including high blood

pressure. You may have a higher chance for swelling and hives if these medicines are taken with LYRICA. See "What is the most important information I should know about LYRICA?"

- Avandia (rosiglitazone), Avandamet (contains rosiglitazone and metformin), or Actos (pioglitazone) for diabetes. You may have a higher chance of weight gain or swelling of your hands or feet if these medicines are taken with LYRICA. See "What are the possible side effects of LYRICA."
- any narcotic pain medicine (such as oxycodone), tranquilizers or medicines for anxiety (such as lorazepam). You may have a higher chance for dizziness and sleepiness if these medicines are taken with LYRICA.
- any medicines that make you sleepy

Know the medicines you take. Keep a list of them with you to show your healthcare provider and pharmacist each time you get a new medicine. Do not start a new medicine without talking with your healthcare provider.

How should I take LYRICA?
- Take LYRICA exactly as prescribed. Your healthcare provider will tell you how much LYRICA to take and when to take it. Take LYRICA at the same times each day.
- LYRICA may be taken with or without food.
- Your healthcare provider may change your dose. Do not change your dose without talking to your healthcare provider.
- Do not stop taking LYRICA without talking to your healthcare provider. If you stop taking LYRICA suddenly you may have headaches, nausea, diarrhea or trouble sleeping. If you have epilepsy and you stop taking LYRICA suddenly, you may have seizures more often. Talk with your healthcare provider about how to stop LYRICA slowly.
- If you miss a dose, take it as soon as you remember. If it is almost time for your next dose, just skip the missed dose. Take the next dose at your regular time. **Do not take two doses at the same time.**
- If you take too much LYRICA, call your healthcare provider or poison control center, or go to the nearest emergency room right away.

What should I avoid while taking LYRICA?
- **Do not drive a car, work with machines, or do other dangerous activities until you know how LYRICA affects you.**
- **Do not drink alcohol while taking LYRICA.** LYRICA and alcohol can affect each other and increase side effects such as sleepiness and dizziness.

What are the possible side effects of LYRICA?
LYRICA may cause serious side effects, including:
- See "What is the most important information I should know about LYRICA?"
- **muscle problems, muscle pain, soreness, or weakness.** If you have these symptoms, especially if you feel sick and have a fever, tell your healthcare provider right away.
- **problems with your eyesight, including blurry vision.** Call your healthcare provider if you have any changes in your eyesight.
- **weight gain.** If you have diabetes, weight gain may affect the management of your diabetes. Weight gain can also be a serious problem for people with heart problems.
- **feeling "high"**
The most common side effects of LYRICA are:
- dizziness
- blurry vision
- weight gain
- sleepiness
- trouble concentrating
- swelling of hands and feet
- dry mouth

LYRICA caused skin sores in animal studies. Skin sores did not happen in studies in people. If you have diabetes, you should pay attention to your skin while taking LYRICA and tell your healthcare provider about any sores or skin problems.
Tell your healthcare provider about any side effect that bothers you or that does not go away.
These are not all the possible side effects of LYRICA. For more information, ask your healthcare provider or pharmacist.
Call your doctor for medical advice about side effects. You may report side effects to FDA at 1-800-FDA-1088.

How should I store LYRICA?
- Store LYRICA capsules and oral solution at room temperature, 59°F to 86°F (15°C to 30°C) in its original package.
- LYRICA Oral Solution **must be used** within 45 days of first opening the bottle.
- Safely throw away any LYRICA that is out of date or no longer needed.
- **Keep LYRICA and all medicines out of the reach of children.**

General information about LYRICA
Medicines are sometimes prescribed for purposes other than those listed in a Medication Guide. Do not use LYRICA for a condition for which it was not prescribed. Do not give LYRICA to other people, even if they have the same symptoms you have. It may harm them.
This Medication Guide summarizes the most important information about LYRICA. If you would like more information, talk with your healthcare provider. You can ask your healthcare provider or pharmacist for information about LYRICA that is written for health professionals.
You can also visit the LYRICA website at www.LYRICA.com or call 1-866-459-7422 (1-866-4LYRICA).

What are the ingredients In LYRICA?
Active ingredient: pregabalin
Inactive ingredients:
LYRICA capsules: lactose monohydrate, cornstarch, talc
Capsule shell: gelatin and titanium dioxide; Orange capsule shell: red iron oxide; White capsule shell: sodium lauryl sulfate, colloidal silicon dioxide. Colloidal silicon dioxide is a manufacturing aid that may or may not be present in the capsule shells.
Imprinting ink: shellac, black iron oxide, propylene glycol, potassium hydroxide.
LYRICA oral solution: methylparaben, propylparaben, monobasic sodium phosphate anhydrous, dibasic sodium phosphate anhydrous, sucralose, artificial strawberry #11545 and purified water.
This Medication Guide has been approved by the U.S. Food and Drug Administration.
Capsules manufactured by:
Pfizer Pharmaceuticals LLC
Vega Baja, PR 00694
Oral Solution manufactured by:
Pfizer Inc.
Kalamazoo, MI 49001
Distributed by
Parke-Davis
Division of Pfizer Inc, NY, NY 10017
LAB-0299-7.0
December 2009

SUTENT® ℞
[*su TENT*]
(sunitinib malate)
capsules, oral

HIGHLIGHTS OF PRESCRIBING INFORMATION
These highlights do not include all the information needed to use SUTENT safely and effectively. See full prescribing information for SUTENT.
SUTENT® (sunitinib malate) capsules, oral
Initial U.S. Approval: 2006

WARNING: HEPATOTOXICITY
See full prescribing information for complete boxed warning.
Hepatotoxicity has been observed in clinical trials and post-marketing experience. This hepatotoxicity may be severe, and deaths have been reported. *[See Warnings and Precautions (5.1)]*

————**RECENT MAJOR CHANGES**————

Boxed Warning	7/2010
Warnings and Precautions, Hepatotoxicity (5.1)	7/2010
Warnings and Precautions, Left Ventricular Dysfunction (5.3)	2/2010
Warnings and Precautions, Hemorrhagic Events (5.6)	2/2010

————**INDICATIONS AND USAGE**————
SUTENT is a kinase inhibitor indicated for the treatment of:
- Gastrointestinal stromal tumor after disease progression on or intolerance to imatinib mesylate. (1.1)
- Advanced renal cell carcinoma. (1.2)

————**DOSAGE AND ADMINISTRATION**————
- 50 mg orally once daily, with or without food, 4 weeks on treatment followed by 2 weeks off. (2.1)
- Dose interruptions and/or dose adjustments of 12.5 mg recommended based on individual safety and tolerability. (2.2)

————**DOSAGE FORMS AND STRENGTHS**————
- Capsules: 12.5 mg, 25 mg, 50 mg (3)

————**CONTRAINDICATIONS**————
- None (4)

————**WARNINGS AND PRECAUTIONS**————
- Hepatotoxicity, including liver failure, has been observed. Monitor liver function tests before initiation of treatment, during each cycle of treatment, and as clinically indicated. SUTENT should be interrupted for Grade 3 or 4 drug-related hepatic adverse events and discontinued if there is no resolution. Do not restart SUTENT if patients subsequently experience severe changes in liver function tests or have other signs and symptoms of liver failure. (5.1)

- Women of childbearing potential should be advised of the potential hazard to the fetus and to avoid becoming pregnant. (5.2)
- Left ventricular ejection fraction declines to below the lower limit of normal have occurred. Monitor patients for signs and symptoms of congestive heart failure. (5.3)
- Prolonged QT intervals and Torsade de Pointes have been observed. Use with caution in patients at higher risk for developing QT interval prolongation. When using SUTENT, monitoring with on-treatment electrocardiograms and electrolytes should be considered. (5.4)
- Hypertension may occur. Monitor blood pressure and treat as needed. (5.5)
- Hemorrhagic events including tumor-related hemorrhage have occurred. Perform serial complete blood counts and physical examinations. (5.6)
- Thyroid dysfunction may occur. Patients with signs and/or symptoms suggestive of hypothyroidism or hyperthyroidism should have laboratory monitoring of thyroid function performed and be treated as per standard medical practice. (5.7)
- Adrenal hemorrhage was observed in animal studies. Monitor adrenal function in case of stress such as surgery, trauma or severe infection. (5.8)

————**ADVERSE REACTIONS**————
- The most common adverse reactions (≥20%) are fatigue, asthenia, fever, diarrhea, nausea, mucositis/stomatitis, vomiting, dyspepsia, abdominal pain, constipation, hypertension, peripheral edema, rash, hand-foot syndrome, skin discoloration, dry skin, hair color changes, altered taste, headache, back pain, arthralgia, extremity pain, cough, dyspnea, anorexia, and bleeding. (6)

To report SUSPECTED ADVERSE REACTIONS, contact Pfizer, Inc. at 1-800-438-1985 or FDA at 1-800-FDA-1088 or *www.fda.gov/medwatch.*

————**DRUG INTERACTIONS**————
- CYP3A4 Inhibitors: Consider dose reduction of SUTENT when administered with strong CYP3A4 inhibitors. (7.1)
- CYP3A4 Inducers: Consider dose increase of SUTENT when administered with CYP3A4 inducers. (7.2)

See 17 for PATIENT COUNSELING INFORMATION and FDA-approved patient labeling.

Revised: 7/2010

FULL PRESCRIBING INFORMATION: CONTENTS*
WARNING: HEPATOTOXICITY
1 INDICATIONS AND USAGE
  1.1 Gastrointestinal stromal tumor
  1.2 Advanced renal cell carcinoma
2 DOSAGE AND ADMINISTRATION
  2.1 Recommended Dose
  2.2 Dose Modification
3 DOSAGE FORMS AND STRENGTHS
4 CONTRAINDICATIONS
5 WARNINGS AND PRECAUTIONS
  5.1 Hepatotoxicity
  5.2 Pregnancy
  5.3 Left Ventricular Dysfunction
  5.4 QT Interval Prolongation and Torsade de Pointes
  5.5 Hypertension
  5.6 Hemorrhagic Events
  5.7 Thyroid Dysfunction
  5.8 Adrenal Function
  5.9 Laboratory Tests
6 ADVERSE REACTIONS
  6.1 Adverse Reactions in GIST Study A
  6.2 Adverse Reactions in the Treatment-Naïve RCC Study
  6.3 Venous Thromboembolic Events
  6.4 Reversible Posterior Leukoencephalopathy Syndrome
  6.5 Pancreatic and Hepatic Function
  6.6 Post-marketing Experience
7 DRUG INTERACTIONS
  7.1 CYP3A4 Inhibitors
  7.2 CYP3A4 Inducers
  7.3 In Vitro Studies of CYP Inhibition and Induction
8 USE IN SPECIFIC POPULATIONS
  8.1 Pregnancy
  8.3 Nursing Mothers
  8.4 Pediatric Use
  8.5 Geriatric Use
  8.6 Hepatic Impairment
10 OVERDOSAGE
11 DESCRIPTION
12 CLINICAL PHARMACOLOGY
  12.1 Mechanism of Action
  12.3 Pharmacokinetics
  12.4 Cardiac Electrophysiology
13 NONCLINICAL TOXICOLOGY
  13.1 Carcinogenesis, Mutagenesis, Impairment of Fertility

* Sections or subsections omitted from the full prescribing information are not listed.

FULL PRESCRIBING INFORMATION:

WARNING: HEPATOTOXICITY
Hepatotoxicity has been observed in clinical trials and post-marketing experience. This hepatotoxicity may be severe, and deaths have been reported. *[See Warnings and Precautions (5.1)]*

1 INDICATIONS AND USAGE

1.1 Gastrointestinal Stromal Tumor (GIST)

SUTENT is indicated for the treatment of gastrointestinal stromal tumor after disease progression on or intolerance to imatinib mesylate.

1.2 Advanced Renal Cell Carcinoma (RCC)

SUTENT is indicated for the treatment of advanced renal cell carcinoma.

2 DOSAGE AND ADMINISTRATION

2.1 Recommended Dose

The recommended dose of SUTENT for gastrointestinal stromal tumor (GIST) and advanced renal cell carcinoma (RCC) is one 50 mg oral dose taken once daily, on a schedule of 4 weeks on treatment followed by 2 weeks off (Schedule 4/2). SUTENT may be taken with or without food.

2.2 Dose Modification

Dose interruption and/or dose modification in 12.5 mg increments or decrements is recommended based on individual safety and tolerability.

Strong CYP3A4 inhibitors such as ketoconazole may **increase** sunitinib plasma concentrations. Selection of an alternate concomitant medication with no or minimal enzyme inhibition potential is recommended. A dose reduction for SUTENT to a minimum of 37.5 mg daily should be considered if SUTENT must be co-administered with a strong CYP3A4 inhibitor *[see Drug Interactions (7.1) and Clinical Pharmacology (12.3)]*.

CYP3A4 inducers such as rifampin may **decrease** sunitinib plasma concentrations. Selection of an alternate concomitant medication with no or minimal enzyme induction potential is recommended. A dose increase for SUTENT to a maximum of 87.5 mg daily should be considered if SUTENT must be co-administered with a CYP3A4 inducer. If dose is increased, the patient should be monitored carefully for toxicity *[see Drug Interactions (7.2) and Clinical Pharmacology (12.3)]*.

3 DOSAGE FORMS AND STRENGTHS

12.5 mg capsules
Hard gelatin capsule with orange cap and orange body, printed with white ink "Pfizer" on the cap and "STN 12.5 mg" on the body.
25 mg capsules
Hard gelatin capsule with caramel cap and orange body, printed with white ink "Pfizer" on the cap and "STN 25 mg" on the body.
50 mg capsules
Hard gelatin capsule with caramel top and caramel body, printed with white ink "Pfizer" on the cap and "STN 50 mg" on the body.

4 CONTRAINDICATIONS

None

5 WARNINGS AND PRECAUTIONS

5.1 Hepatotoxicity

SUTENT has been associated with hepatotoxicity, which may result in liver failure or death. Liver failure has been observed in clinical trials (7/2281 [0.3%]) and post-marketing experience. Liver failure signs include jaundice, elevated transaminases and/or hyperbilirubinemia in conjunction with encephalopathy, coagulopathy, and/or renal failure. Monitor liver function tests (ALT, AST, bilirubin) before initiation of treatment, during each cycle of treatment, and as clinically indicated. SUTENT should be interrupted for Grade 3 or 4 drug-related hepatic adverse events and discontinued if there is no resolution. Do not restart SUTENT if patients subsequently experience severe changes in liver function tests or have other signs and symptoms of liver failure.

Safety in patients with ALT or AST >2.5 × ULN or, if due to liver metastases, >5.0 × ULN has not been established.

5.2 Pregnancy

Pregnancy Category D

As angiogenesis is a critical component of embryonic and fetal development, inhibition of angiogenesis following administration of SUTENT should be expected to result in adverse effects on pregnancy. There are no adequate and well-controlled studies of SUTENT in pregnant women. If the drug is used during pregnancy, or if the patient becomes pregnant while receiving this drug, the patient should be apprised of the potential hazard to the fetus. Women of childbearing potential should be advised to avoid becoming pregnant while receiving treatment with SUTENT.

Sunitinib was evaluated in pregnant rats (0.3, 1.5, 3.0, 5.0 mg/kg/day) and rabbits (0.5, 1, 5, 20 mg/kg/day) for effects on the embryo. Significant increases in the incidence of embryolethality and structural abnormalities were observed in rats at the dose of 5 mg/kg/day (approximately 5.5 times the systemic exposure [combined AUC of sunitinib + primary active metabolite] in patients administered the recommended daily doses [RDD]). Significantly increased embryolethality was observed in rabbits at 5 mg/kg/day while developmental effects were observed at ≥1 mg/kg/day (approximately 0.3 times the AUC in patients administered the RDD of 50 mg/day). Developmental effects consisted of fetal skeletal malformations of the ribs and vertebrae in rats. In rabbits, cleft lip was observed at 1 mg/kg/day and cleft lip and cleft palate were observed at 5 mg/kg/day (approximately 2.7 times the AUC in patients administered the RDD). Neither fetal loss nor malformations were observed in rats dosed at ≤3 mg/kg/day (approximately 2.3 times the AUC in patients administered the RDD).

5.3 Left Ventricular Dysfunction

In the presence of clinical manifestations of congestive heart failure (CHF), discontinuation of SUTENT is recommended. The dose of SUTENT should be interrupted and/or reduced in patients without clinical evidence of CHF but with an ejection fraction <50% and >20% below baseline.

Cardiovascular events, including heart failure, myocardial disorders and cardiomyopathy, some of which were fatal, have been reported through post-marketing experience. More patients treated with SUTENT experienced decline in left ventricular ejection fraction (LVEF) than patients receiving either placebo or interferon-α (IFN-α). In the double-blind treatment phase of GIST Study A, 22/209 patients (11%) on SUTENT and 3/102 patients (3%) on placebo had treatment-emergent LVEF values below the lower limit of normal (LLN). Nine of 22 GIST patients on SUTENT with LVEF changes recovered without intervention. Five patients had documented LVEF recovery following intervention (dose reduction: one patient; addition of antihypertensive or diuretic medications: four patients). Six patients went off study without documented recovery. Additionally, three patients on SUTENT had Grade 3 reductions in left ventricular systolic function to LVEF <40%; two of these patients died without receiving further study drug. No GIST patients on placebo had Grade 3 decreased LVEF. In the double-blind treatment phase of GIST Study A, 1 patient on SUTENT and 1 patient on placebo died of diagnosed heart failure; 2 patients on SUTENT and 2 patients on placebo died of treatment-emergent cardiac arrest.

In the treatment-naïve RCC study, 103/375 (27%) and 54/360 (15%) patients on SUTENT and IFN-α, respectively, had an LVEF value below the LLN. Twenty-six patients on SUTENT (7%) and seven on IFN-α (2%) experienced declines in LVEF to >20% below baseline and to below 50%. Left ventricular dysfunction was reported in four patients (1%) and CHF in two patients (<1%) who received SUTENT.

Patients who presented with cardiac events within 12 months prior to SUTENT administration, such as myocardial infarction (including severe/unstable angina), coronary/peripheral artery bypass graft, symptomatic CHF, cerebrovascular accident or transient ischemic attack, or pulmonary embolism were excluded from SUTENT clinical studies. It is unknown whether patients with these concomitant conditions may be at a higher risk of developing drug-related left ventricular dysfunction. Physicians are advised to weigh this risk against the potential benefits of the drug. **These patients should be carefully monitored for clinical signs and symptoms of CHF while receiving SUTENT. Baseline and periodic evaluations of LVEF should also be considered while these patients are receiving SUTENT. In patients without cardiac risk factors, a baseline evaluation of ejection fraction should be considered.**

5.4 QT Interval Prolongation and Torsade de Pointes

SUTENT has been shown to prolong the QT interval in a dose dependent manner, which may lead to an increased risk for ventricular arrhythmias including Torsade de Pointes. Torsade de Pointes has been observed in <0.1% of SUTENT-exposed patients.

SUTENT should be used with caution in patients with a history of QT interval prolongation, patients who are taking antiarrhythmics, or patients with relevant pre-existing cardiac disease, bradycardia, or electrolyte disturbances. When using SUTENT, periodic monitoring with on-treatment electrocardiograms and electrolytes (magnesium, potassium) should be considered. Concomitant treatment with strong CYP3A4 inhibitors, which may increase sunitinib plasma concentrations, should be used with caution and dose reduction of SUTENT should be considered *[see Dosage and Administration (2.2)]*.

5.5 Hypertension

Patients should be monitored for hypertension and treated as needed with standard anti-hypertensive therapy. In cases of severe hypertension, temporary suspension of SUTENT is recommended until hypertension is controlled. Of patients receiving SUTENT for treatment-naïve RCC, 127/375 patients (34%) receiving SUTENT compared with 13/360 patients (4%) on IFN-α experienced hypertension. Grade 3 hypertension was observed in 50/375 treatment-naïve RCC patients (13%) on SUTENT compared to 1/360 patients (<1%) on IFN-α. While all-grade hypertension was similar in GIST patients on SUTENT compared to placebo, Grade 3 hypertension was reported in 9/202 GIST patients on SUTENT (4%), and none of the GIST patients on placebo. No Grade 4 hypertension was reported. SUTENT dosing was reduced or temporarily delayed for hypertension in 21/375 patients (6%) on the treatment-naive RCC study. Four treatment-naïve RCC patients, including one with malignant hypertension, and no GIST patients discontinued treatment due to hypertension. Severe hypertension (>200 mmHg systolic or 110 mmHg diastolic) occurred in 8/202 GIST patients on SUTENT (4%), 1/102 GIST patients on placebo (1%), and in 32/375 treatment-naïve RCC patients (9%) on SUTENT and 3/360 patients (1%) on IFN-α.

5.6 Hemorrhagic Events

Hemorrhagic events reported through post-marketing experience, some of which were fatal, have included GI, respiratory, tumor, urinary tract and brain hemorrhages. In patients receiving SUTENT in a clinical trial for treatment-naïve RCC, 140/375 patients (37%) had bleeding events compared with 35/360 patients (10%) receiving IFN-α. Bleeding events occurred in 37/202 patients (18%) receiving SUTENT in the double-blind treatment phase of GIST Study A, compared to 17/102 patients (17%) receiving placebo. Epistaxis was the most common hemorrhagic adverse event reported. Less common bleeding events in GIST or RCC patients included rectal, gingival, upper gastrointestinal, genital, and wound bleeding. In the double-blind treatment phase of GIST Study A, 14/202 patients (7%) receiving SUTENT and 9/102 patients (9%) on placebo had Grade 3 or 4 bleeding events. In addition, one patient in GIST Study A taking placebo had a fatal gastrointestinal bleeding event during Cycle 2. Most events in RCC patients were Grade 1 or 2; there was one Grade 5 event of gastric bleed in a treatment-naïve patient.

Tumor-related hemorrhage has been observed in patients treated with SUTENT. These events may occur suddenly, and in the case of pulmonary tumors may present as severe and life-threatening hemoptysis or pulmonary hemorrhage. Fatal pulmonary hemorrhage occurred in 2 patients receiving SUTENT on a clinical trial of patients with metastatic non-small cell lung cancer (NSCLC). Both patients had squamous cell histology. SUTENT is not approved for use in patients with NSCLC. Treatment-emergent Grade 3 and 4 tumor hemorrhage occurred in 5/202 patients (3%) with GIST receiving SUTENT on Study A. Tumor hemorrhages were observed as early as Cycle 1 and as late as Cycle 6. One of these five patients received no further drug following tumor hemorrhage. None of the other four patients discontinued treatment or experienced dose delay due to tumor hemorrhage. No patients with GIST in the Study A placebo arm were observed to undergo intratumoral hemorrhage. Clinical assessment of these events should include serial complete blood counts (CBCs) and physical examinations.

Serious, sometimes fatal gastrointestinal complications including gastrointestinal perforation, have occurred rarely in patients with intra-abdominal malignancies treated with SUTENT.

5.7 Thyroid Dysfunction

Baseline laboratory measurement of thyroid function is recommended and patients with hypothyroidism or hyperthyroidism should be treated as per standard medical practice prior to the start of SUTENT treatment. All patients should be observed closely for signs and symptoms of thyroid dysfunction on SUTENT treatment. Patients with signs and/or symptoms suggestive of thyroid dysfunction should have laboratory monitoring of thyroid function performed and be treated as per standard medical practice.

Treatment-emergent acquired hypothyroidism was noted in eight GIST patients (4%) on SUTENT versus one (1%) on placebo. Hypothyroidism was reported as an adverse reaction in sixty-one patients (16%) on SUTENT in the treatment-naïve RCC study and in three patients (<1%) in the IFN-α arm.

Cases of hyperthyroidism, some followed by hypothyroidism, have been reported in clinical trials and through post-marketing experience.

Table 1. Adverse Reactions Reported in Study A in at Least 10% of GIST Patients who Received SUTENT in the Double-Blind Treatment Phase and More Commonly Than in Patients Given Placebo*

Adverse Reaction, n (%)	GIST			
	SUTENT (n=202)		Placebo (n=102)	
	All Grades	Grade 3/4	All Grades	Grade 3/4
Any		114 (56)		52 (51)
Gastrointestinal				
Diarrhea	81 (40)	9 (4)	27 (27)	0 (0)
Mucositis/stomatitis	58 (29)	2 (1)	18 (18)	2 (2)
Constipation	41 (20)	0 (0)	14 (14)	2 (2)
Cardiac				
Hypertension	31 (15)	9 (4)	11 (11)	0 (0)
Dermatology				
Skin discoloration	61 (30)	0 (0)	23 (23)	0 (0)
Rash	28 (14)	2 (1)	9 (9)	0 (0)
Hand-foot syndrome	28 (14)	9 (4)	10 (10)	3 (3)
Neurology				
Altered taste	42 (21)	0 (0)	12 (12)	0 (0)
Musculoskeletal				
Myalgia/limb pain	28 (14)	1 (1)	9 (9)	1 (1)
Metabolism/Nutrition				
Anorexia[a]	67 (33)	1 (1)	30 (29)	5 (5)
Asthenia	45 (22)	10 (5)	11 (11)	3 (3)

* Common Terminology Criteria for Adverse Events (CTCAE), Version 3.0
[a] Includes decreased appetite

Table 2. Laboratory Abnormalities Reported in Study A in at Least 10% of GIST Patients Who Received SUTENT or Placebo in the Double-Blind Treatment Phase*

Laboratory Parameter, n (%)	GIST			
	SUTENT (n=202)		Placebo (n=102)	
	All Grades*	Grade 3/4*[a]	All Grades*	Grade 3/4*[b]
Any		68 (34)		22 (22)
Gastrointestinal				
AST/ALT	78 (39)	3 (2)	23 (23)	1 (1)
Lipase	50 (25)	20 (10)	17 (17)	7 (7)
Alkaline phosphatase	48 (24)	7 (4)	21 (21)	4 (4)
Amylase	35 (17)	10 (5)	12 (12)	3 (3)
Total bilirubin	32 (16)	2 (1)	8 (8)	0 (0)
Indirect bilirubin	20 (10)	0 (0)	4 (4)	0 (0)
Cardiac				
Decreased LVEF	22 (11)	2 (1)	3 (3)	0 (0)
Renal/Metabolic				
Creatinine	25 (12)	1 (1)	7 (7)	0 (0)
Potassium decreased	24 (12)	1 (1)	4 (4)	0 (0)
Sodium increased	20 (10)	0 (0)	4 (4)	1 (1)
Hematology				
Neutrophils	107 (53)	20 (10)	4 (4)	0 (0)
Lymphocytes	76 (38)	0 (0)	16 (16)	0 (0)
Platelets	76 (38)	10 (5)	4 (4)	0 (0)
Hemoglobin	52 (26)	6 (3)	22 (22)	2 (2)

LVEF=Left ventricular ejection fraction
* Common Terminology Criteria for Adverse Events (CTCAE), Version 3.0
[a] Grade 4 laboratory abnormalities in patients on SUTENT included alkaline phosphatase (1%), lipase (2%), creatinine (1%), potassium decreased (1%), neutrophils (2%), hemoglobin (2%), and platelets (1%).
[b] Grade 4 laboratory abnormalities in patients on placebo included amylase (1%), lipase (1%) and hemoglobin (2%).

5.8 Adrenal Function
Physicians prescribing SUTENT are advised to monitor for adrenal insufficiency in patients who experience stress such as surgery, trauma or severe infection.

Adrenal toxicity was noted in non-clinical repeat dose studies of 14 days to 9 months in rats and monkeys at plasma exposures as low as 0.7 times the AUC observed in clinical studies. Histological changes of the adrenal gland were characterized as hemorrhage, necrosis, congestion, hypertrophy and inflammation. In clinical studies, CT/MRI obtained in 336 patients after exposure to one or more cycles of SUTENT demonstrated no evidence of adrenal hemorrhage or necrosis. ACTH stimulation testing was performed in approximately 400 patients across multiple clinical trials of SUTENT. Among patients with normal baseline ACTH stimulation testing, one patient developed consistently abnormal test results during treatment that are unexplained and may be related to treatment with SUTENT. Eleven additional patients with normal baseline testing had abnormalities in the final test performed, with peak cortisol levels of 12-16.4 mcg/dL (normal >18 mcg/dL) following stimulation. None of these patients were reported to have clinical evidence of adrenal insufficiency.

5.9 Laboratory Tests
CBCs with platelet count and serum chemistries including phosphate should be performed at the beginning of each treatment cycle for patients receiving treatment with SUTENT.

6 ADVERSE REACTIONS
The data described below reflect exposure to SUTENT in 577 patients who participated in the double-blind treatment phase of a placebo-controlled trial (n=202) for the treatment of GIST [see Clinical Studies (14.1)] or an active-controlled trial (n=375) for the treatment of RCC [see Clinical Studies (14.2)]. The patients received a starting oral dose of 50 mg daily on Schedule 4/2 in repeated cycles.

The most common adverse reactions (≥20%) in patients with GIST or RCC are fatigue, asthenia, fever, diarrhea, nausea, mucositis/stomatitis, vomiting, dyspepsia, abdominal pain, constipation, hypertension, peripheral edema, rash, hand-foot syndrome, skin discoloration, dry skin, hair color changes, altered taste, headache, back pain, arthralgia, extremity pain, cough, dyspnea, anorexia, and bleeding. The potentially serious adverse reactions of hepatotoxicity, left ventricular dysfunction, QT interval prolongation, hemorrhage, hypertension, thyroid dysfunction, and adrenal function are discussed in Warnings and Precautions (5). Other adverse reactions occurring in GIST and RCC studies are described below.

Because clinical trials are conducted under widely varying conditions, adverse reaction rates observed in the clinical trials of a drug cannot be directly compared to rates in the clinical trials of another drug and may not reflect the rates observed in practice.

6.1 Adverse Reactions in GIST Study A
Median duration of blinded study treatment was two cycles for patients on SUTENT (mean 3.0, range 1-9) and one cycle (mean 1.8, range 1-6) for patients on placebo at the time of the interim analysis. Dose reductions occurred in 23 patients (11%) on SUTENT and none on placebo. Dose interruptions occurred in 59 patients (29%) on SUTENT and 31 patients (30%) on placebo. The rates of treatment-emergent, non-fatal adverse reactions resulting in permanent discontinuation were 7% and 6% in the SUTENT and placebo groups, respectively.

Most treatment-emergent adverse reactions in both study arms were Grade 1 or 2 in severity. Grade 3 or 4 treatment-emergent adverse reactions were reported in 56% versus 51% of patients on SUTENT versus placebo, respectively, in the double-blind treatment phase of the trial. Table 1 compares the incidence of common (≥10%) treatment-emergent adverse reactions for patients receiving SUTENT and reported more commonly in patients receiving SUTENT than in patients receiving placebo.

[See table 1 above]

In the double-blind treatment phase of GIST Study A, oral pain other than mucositis/stomatitis occurred in 12 patients (6%) on SUTENT versus 3 (3%) on placebo. Hair color changes occurred in 15 patients (7%) on SUTENT versus 4 (4%) on placebo. Alopecia was observed in 10 patients (5%) on SUTENT versus 2 (2%) on placebo.

Table 2 provides common (≥10%) treatment-emergent laboratory abnormalities.

[See table 2 at left]

After an interim analysis, the study was unblinded, and patients on the placebo arm were given the opportunity to receive open-label SUTENT treatment [see Clinical Studies (14.1)]. For 241 patients randomized to the SUTENT arm, including 139 who received SUTENT in both the double-blind and open-label treatment phases, the median duration of SUTENT treatment was 6 cycles (mean 8.5, range 1–44). For the 255 patients who ultimately received open-label SUTENT treatment, median duration of study treatment was 6 cycles (mean 7.8, range 1–37) from the time of the unblinding. A total of 118 patients (46%) required dosing interruptions, and a total of 72 patients (28%) required dose reductions. The incidence of treatment-emergent adverse reactions resulting in permanent discontinuation was 20%. The most common Grade 3 or 4 treatment-related adverse reactions experienced by patients receiving SUTENT in the open-label treatment phase were fatigue (10%), hypertension (8%), asthenia (5%), diarrhea (5%), hand-foot syndrome (5%), nausea (4%), abdominal pain (3%), anorexia (3%), mucositis (2%), vomiting (2%), and hypothyroidism (2%).

6.2 Adverse Reactions in the Treatment-Naïve RCC Study
The as-treated patient population for the treatment-naïve RCC study included 735 patients, 375 randomized to SUTENT and 360 randomized to IFN-α. The median duration of treatment was 11.1 months (range: 0.4–46.1) for SUTENT treatment and 4.1 months (range: 0.1–45.6) for IFN-α treatment. Dose interruptions occurred in 202 patients (54%) on SUTENT and 141 patients (39%) on IFN-α. Dose reductions occurred in 194 patients (52%) on SUTENT and 98 patients (27%) on IFN-α. Discontinuation rates due to adverse reactions were 20% for SUTENT and 24% for IFN-α. Most treatment-emergent adverse reactions in both study arms were Grade 1 or 2 in severity. Grade 3 or 4 treatment-emergent adverse reactions were reported in 77% versus 55% of patients on SUTENT versus IFN-α, respectively.

Table 3 compares the incidence of common (≥10%) treatment-emergent adverse reactions for patients receiving SUTENT versus IFN-α.

[See table 3 at right and on next page]
Treatment-emergent Grade 3/4 laboratory abnormalities are presented in Table 4.
[See table 4 at top of page 2817]

6.3 Venous Thromboembolic Events

Seven patients (3%) on SUTENT and none on placebo in the double-blind treatment phase of GIST Study A experienced venous thromboembolic events; five of the seven were Grade 3 deep venous thrombosis (DVT), and two were Grade 1 or 2. Four of these seven GIST patients discontinued treatment following first observation of DVT.

Thirteen (3%) patients receiving SUTENT for treatment-naïve RCC had venous thromboembolic events reported. Seven (2%) of these patients had pulmonary embolism, one was Grade 2 and six were Grade 4, and six (2%) patients had DVT, including three Grade 3. One patient was permanently withdrawn from SUTENT due to pulmonary embolism; dose interruption occurred in two patients with pulmonary embolism and one with DVT. In treatment-naïve RCC patients receiving IFN-α, six (2%) venous thromboembolic events occurred; one patient (<1%) experienced a Grade 3 DVT and five patients (1%) had pulmonary embolism, all Grade 4.

6.4 Reversible Posterior Leukoencephalopathy Syndrome

There have been rare (<1%) reports of subjects presenting with seizures and radiological evidence of reversible posterior leukoencephalopathy syndrome (RPLS). None of these subjects had a fatal outcome to the event. Patients with seizures and signs/symptoms consistent with RPLS, such as hypertension, headache, decreased alertness, altered mental functioning, and visual loss, including cortical blindness should be controlled with medical management including control of hypertension. Temporary suspension of SUTENT is recommended; following resolution, treatment may be resumed at the discretion of the treating physician.

6.5 Pancreatic and Hepatic Function

If symptoms of pancreatitis or hepatic failure are present, patients should have SUTENT discontinued. Pancreatitis was observed in 5 (1%) patients receiving SUTENT for treatment-naïve RCC compared to 1 (<1%) patient receiving IFN-α. Hepatotoxicity was observed in patients receiving SUTENT [See Boxed Warning and Warnings and Precautions (5.1)].

6.6 Post-marketing Experience

The following adverse reactions have been identified during post-approval use of SUTENT. Because these reactions are reported voluntarily from a population of uncertain size, it is not always possible to reliably estimate their frequency or establish a causal relationship to drug exposure.

Cases of serious infection (with or without neutropenia), in some cases with fatal outcome, have been reported.

Cases of myopathy and/or rhabdomyolysis with or without acute renal failure, in some cases with fatal outcome, have been reported. Patients with signs or symptoms of muscle toxicity should be managed as per standard medical practice.

Thrombotic microangiopathy has been reported in patients on SUTENT. Suspension of SUTENT is recommended; following resolution, treatment may be resumed at the discretion of the treating physician.

Cases of fatal hemorrhage associated with thrombocytopenia have been reported.

Pulmonary embolism, in some cases with fatal outcome, has been reported.

Cases of renal impairment and/or failure, in some cases with fatal outcome, have been reported.

Cases of proteinuria and rare cases of nephrotic syndrome have been reported. Baseline urinalysis is recommended, and patients should be monitored for the development or worsening of proteinuria. The safety of continued SUTENT treatment in patients with moderate to severe proteinuria has not been systematically evaluated. Discontinue SUTENT in patients with nephrotic syndrome.

Hypersensitivity reactions, including angioedema, have been reported.

Cases of fistula formation, sometimes associated with tumor necrosis and/or regression, in some cases with fatal outcome, have been reported.

7 DRUG INTERACTIONS

7.1 CYP3A4 Inhibitors

Strong CYP3A4 inhibitors such as ketoconazole may increase sunitinib plasma concentrations. Selection of an alternate concomitant medication with no or minimal enzyme inhibition potential is recommended. Concurrent administration of SUTENT with the strong CYP3A4 inhibitor, ketoconazole, resulted in 49% and 51% increases in the combined (sunitinib + primary active metabolite) C_{max} and $AUC_{0-\infty}$ values, respectively, after a single dose of SUTENT in healthy volunteers. Co-administration of SUTENT with strong inhibitors of the CYP3A4 family (e.g., ketoconazole, itraconazole, clarithromycin, atazanavir, indinavir, nefazodone, nelfinavir, ritonavir, saquinavir, telithromycin, vori-

conazole) may increase sunitinib concentrations. Grapefruit may also increase plasma concentrations of sunitinib. A dose reduction for SUTENT should be considered when it must be co-administered with strong CYP3A4 inhibitors [see Dosage and Administration (2.2)].

7.2 CYP3A4 Inducers

CYP3A4 inducers such as rifampin may decrease sunitinib plasma concentrations. Selection of an alternate concomitant medication with no or minimal enzyme induction potential is recommended. Concurrent administration of SUTENT with the strong CYP3A4 inducer, rifampin, resulted in a 23% and 46% reduction in the combined (sunitinib + primary active metabolite) C_{max} and $AUC_{0-\infty}$ values, respectively, after a single dose of SUTENT in healthy volunteers. Co-administration of SUTENT with inducers of the CYP3A4 family (e.g., dexamethasone, phenytoin, carbamazepine, rifampin, rifabutin, rifapentin, phenobarbital, St. John's Wort) may decrease sunitinib concentrations. St. John's Wort may decrease sunitinib plasma concentrations unpredictably. Patients receiving SUTENT should not take St. John's Wort concomitantly. A dose increase for SUTENT should be considered when it must be co-administered with CYP3A4 inducers [see Dosage and Administration (2.2)].

7.3 In Vitro Studies of CYP Inhibition and Induction

In vitro studies indicated that sunitinib does not induce or inhibit major CYP enzymes. The in vitro studies in human liver microsomes and hepatocytes of the activity of CYP isoforms CYP1A2, CYP2A6, CYP2B6, CYP2C8, CYP2C9, CYP2C19, CYP2D6, CYP2E1, CYP3A4/5, and CYP4A9/11 indicated that sunitinib and its primary active metabolite are unlikely to have any clinically relevant drug-drug interactions with drugs that may be metabolized by these enzymes.

8 USE IN SPECIFIC POPULATIONS

8.1 Pregnancy

Pregnancy Category D [see Warnings and Precautions (5.2)].

8.3 Nursing Mothers

Sunitinib and its metabolites are excreted in rat milk. In lactating female rats administered 15 mg/kg, sunitinib and its metabolites were extensively excreted in milk at concentrations up to 12-fold higher than in plasma. It is not known whether sunitinib or its primary active metabolite are excreted in human milk. Because drugs are commonly excreted in human milk and because of the potential for serious adverse reactions in nursing infants, a decision should be made whether to discontinue nursing or to discontinue the drug taking into account the importance of the drug to the mother [see Nonclinical Toxicology (13.1)].

8.4 Pediatric Use

The safety and efficacy of SUTENT in pediatric patients have not been established.

Physeal dysplasia was observed in cynomolgus monkeys with open growth plates treated for ≥ 3 months (3 month dosing 2, 6, 12 mg/kg/day; 8 cycles of dosing 0.3, 1.5, 6.0 mg/kg/day) with sunitinib at doses that were > 0.4 times the RDD based on systemic exposure (AUC). In developing

Table 3. Adverse Reactions Reported in at Least 10% of Patients with RCC Who Received SUTENT or IFN-α*

Adverse Reaction, n (%)	Treatment-Naïve RCC			
	SUTENT (n=375)		IFN-α (n=360)	
	All Grades	Grade 3/4[a]	All Grades	Grade 3/4[b]
Any	372 (99)	290 (77)	355 (99)	197 (55)
Constitutional				
Fatigue	233 (62)	55 (15)	202 (56)	54 (15)
Asthenia	96 (26)	42 (11)	81 (22)	21 (6)
Fever	84 (22)	3 (1)	134 (37)	1 (<1)
Weight decreased	60 (16)	1 (<1)	60 (17)	3 (1)
Chills	53 (14)	3 (1)	111 (31)	0 (0)
Chest Pain	50 (13)	7 (2)	24 (7)	3 (1)
Influenza like illness	18 (5)	0 (0)	54 (15)	1 (<1)
Gastrointestinal				
Diarrhea	246 (66)	37 (10)	76 (21)	1 (<1)
Nausea	216 (58)	21 (6)	147 (41)	6 (2)
Mucositis/stomatitis	178 (47)	13 (3)	19 (5)	2 (<1)
Vomiting	148 (39)	19 (5)	62 (17)	4 (1)
Dyspepsia	128 (34)	8 (2)	16 (4)	0 (0)
Abdominal pain[c]	113 (30)	20 (5)	42 (12)	5 (1)
Constipation	85 (23)	4 (1)	49 (14)	1 (<1)
Dry mouth	50 (13)	0 (0)	27 (7)	1 (<1)
GERD/reflux esophagitis	47 (12)	1 (<1)	3 (1)	0 (0)
Flatulence	52 (14)	0 (0)	8 (2)	0 (0)
Oral pain	54 (14)	2 (<1)	2 (1)	0 (0)
Glossodynia	40 (11)	0 (0)	2 (1)	0 (0)
Hemorrhoids	38 (10)	0 (0)	6 (2)	0 (0)
Cardiac				
Hypertension	127 (34)	50 (13)	13 (4)	1 (<1)
Edema, peripheral	91 (24)	7 (2)	17 (5)	2 (1)
Ejection fraction decreased	61 (16)	10 (3)	19 (5)	6 (2)
Dermatology				
Rash	109 (29)	6 (2)	39 (11)	1 (<1)
Hand-foot syndrome	108 (29)	32 (8)	3 (1)	0 (0)
Skin discoloration/ yellow skin	94 (25)	1 (<1)	0 (0)	0 (0)
Dry skin	85 (23)	1 (<1)	26 (7)	0 (0)
Hair color changes	75 (20)	0 (0)	1 (<1)	0 (0)
Alopecia	51 (14)	0 (0)	34 (9)	0 (0)
Erythema	46 (12)	2 (<1)	5 (1)	0 (0)
Pruritus	44 (12)	1 (<1)	24 (7)	1 (<1)
Neurology				
Altered taste[d]	178 (47)	1 (<1)	54 (15)	0 (0)
Headache	86 (23)	4 (1)	69 (19)	0 (0)
Dizziness	43 (11)	2 (<1)	50 (14)	2 (1)
Musculoskeletal				
Back pain	105 (28)	19 (5)	52 (14)	7 (2)
Arthralgia	111 (30)	10 (3)	69 (19)	4 (1)
Pain in extremity/ limb discomfort	150 (40)	19 (5)	107 (30)	7 (2)

(Table continued on next page)

Table 3 *(cont.)*. Adverse Reactions Reported in at Least 10% of Patients with RCC Who Received SUTENT or IFN-α*

Adverse Reaction, n (%)	Treatment-Naïve RCC			
	SUTENT (n=375)		IFN-α (n=360)	
	All Grades	Grade 3/4[a]	All Grades	Grade 3/4[b]
Endocrine				
Hypothyroidism	61 (16)	6 (2)	3 (1)	0 (0)
Respiratory				
Cough	100 (27)	3 (1)	51 (14)	1 (<1)
Dyspnea	99 (26)	24 (6)	71 (20)	15 (4)
Nasopharyngitis	54 (11)	0 (0)	8 (2)	0 (0)
Oropharyngeal Pain	51 (14)	2 (<1)	9 (2)	0 (0)
Upper respiratory tract infection	43 (11)	2 (<1)	9 (2)	0 (0)
Metabolism/Nutrition				
Anorexia[e]	182 (48)	11 (3)	153 (42)	7 (2)
Hemorrhage/Bleeding				
Bleeding, all sites	140 (37)	16 (4)[f]	35 (10)	3 (1)
Psychiatric				
Insomnia	57 (15)	3 (<1)	37 (10)	0 (0)
Depression[g]	40 (11)	0 (0)	51 (14)	5 (1)

* Common Terminology Criteria for Adverse Events (CTCAE), Version 3.0
[a] Grade 4 ARs in patients on SUTENT included back pain (1%), arthralgia (<1%), dyspnea (<1%), asthenia (<1%), fatigue (<1%), limb pain (<1%) and rash (<1%).
[b] Grade 4 ARs in patients on IFN-α included dyspnea (1%), fatigue (1%), abdominal pain (<1%) and depression (<1%).
[c] Includes flank pain
[d] Includes ageusia, hypogeusia and dysgeusia
[e] Includes decreased appetite
[f] Includes one patient with Grade 5 gastric hemorrhage
[g] Includes depressed mood

rats treated continuously for 3 months (1.5, 5.0 and 15.0 mg/kg) or 5 cycles (0.3, 1.5, and 6.0 mg/kg/day), bone abnormalities consisted of thickening of the epiphyseal cartilage of the femur and an increase of fracture of the tibia at doses ≥ 5 mg/kg (approximately 10 times the RDD based on AUC). Additionally, caries of the teeth were observed in rats at >5 mg/kg. The incidence and severity of physeal dysplasia were dose-related and were reversible upon cessation of treatment; however findings in the teeth were not. A no effect level was not observed in monkeys treated continuously for 3 months, but was 1.5 mg/kg/day when treated intermittently for 8 cycles. In rats the no effect level in bones was ≤ 2 mg/kg/day.

8.5 Geriatric Use
Of 825 GIST and RCC patients who received SUTENT on clinical studies, 277 (34%) were 65 and over. No overall differences in safety or effectiveness were observed between younger and older patients.

8.6 Hepatic Impairment
No dose adjustment is required when administering SUTENT to patients with Child-Pugh Class A or B hepatic impairment. Sunitinib and its primary metabolite are primarily metabolized by the liver. Systemic exposures after a single dose of SUTENT were similar in subjects with mild or moderate (Child-Pugh Class A and B) hepatic impairment compared to subjects with normal hepatic function. SUTENT was not studied in subjects with severe (Child-Pugh Class C) hepatic impairment. Studies in cancer patients have excluded patients with ALT or AST >2.5 × ULN or, if due to liver metastases, >5.0 × ULN.

10 OVERDOSAGE
Treatment of overdose with SUTENT should consist of general supportive measures. There is no specific antidote for overdosage with SUTENT. If indicated, elimination of unabsorbed drug should be achieved by emesis or gastric lavage. A few cases of accidental overdose have been reported; these cases were associated with adverse reactions consistent with the known safety profile of SUTENT, or without adverse reactions. A case of intentional overdose involving the ingestion of 1,500 mg of SUTENT in an attempted suicide was reported without adverse reaction. In non-clinical studies mortality was observed following as few as 5 daily doses of 500 mg/kg (3000 mg/m²) in rats. At this dose, signs of toxicity included impaired muscle coordination, head shakes, hypoactivity, ocular discharge, piloerection and gastrointestinal distress. Mortality and similar signs of toxicity were observed at lower doses when administered for longer durations.

11 DESCRIPTION
SUTENT, an oral multi-kinase inhibitor, is the malate salt of sunitinib. Sunitinib malate is described chemically as

Butanedioic acid, hydroxy-, (2S)-, compound with *N*-[2-(diethylamino)ethyl]-5-[(*Z*)-(5-fluoro-1,2-dihydro-2-oxo-3*H*-indol-3-ylidine)methyl]-2,4-dimethyl-1*H*-pyrrole-3-carboxamide (1:1). The molecular formula is $C_{22}H_{27}FN_4O_2 \cdot C_4H_6O_5$ and the molecular weight is 532.6 Daltons. The chemical structure of sunitinib malate is:

Sunitinib malate is a yellow to orange powder with a pKa of 8.95. The solubility of sunitinib malate in aqueous media over the range pH 1.2 to pH 6.8 is in excess of 25 mg/mL. The log of the distribution coefficient (octanol/water) at pH 7 is 5.2.
SUTENT (sunitinib malate) capsules are supplied as printed hard shell capsules containing sunitinib malate equivalent to 12.5 mg, 25 mg or 50 mg of sunitinib together with mannitol, croscarmellose sodium, povidone (K-25) and magnesium stearate as inactive ingredients.
The orange gelatin capsule shells contain titanium dioxide, and red iron oxide. The caramel gelatin capsule shells contain titanium dioxide, red iron oxide, yellow iron oxide and black iron oxide. The white printing ink contains shellac, propylene glycol, sodium hydroxide, povidone and titanium dioxide.

12 CLINICAL PHARMACOLOGY
12.1 Mechanism of Action
Sunitinib is a small molecule that inhibits multiple receptor tyrosine kinases (RTKs), some of which are implicated in tumor growth, pathologic angiogenesis, and metastatic progression of cancer. Sunitinib was evaluated for its inhibitory activity against a variety of kinases (>80 kinases) and was identified as an inhibitor of platelet-derived growth factor receptors (PDGFRα and PDGFRβ), vascular endothelial growth factor receptors (VEGFR1, VEGFR2 and VEGFR3), stem cell factor receptor (KIT), Fms-like tyrosine kinase-3 (FLT3), colony stimulating factor receptor Type 1 (CSF-1R), and the glial cell-line derived neurotrophic factor receptor (RET). Sunitinib inhibition of the activity of these RTKs has been demonstrated in biochemical and cellular assays, and inhibition of function has been demonstrated in cell proliferation assays. The primary metabolite exhibits similar potency compared to sunitinib in biochemical and cellular assays.

Sunitinib inhibited the phosphorylation of multiple RTKs (PDGFRβ, VEGFR2, KIT) in tumor xenografts expressing RTK targets *in vivo* and demonstrated inhibition of tumor growth or tumor regression and/or inhibited metastases in some experimental models of cancer. Sunitinib demonstrated the ability to inhibit growth of tumor cells expressing dysregulated target RTKs (PDGFR, RET, or KIT) *in vitro* and to inhibit PDGFRβ- and VEGFR2-dependent tumor angiogenesis *in vivo*.

12.3 Pharmacokinetics
The pharmacokinetics of sunitinib and sunitinib malate have been evaluated in 135 healthy volunteers and in 266 patients with solid tumors.
Maximum plasma concentrations (C_{max}) of sunitinib are generally observed between 6 and 12 hours (T_{max}) following oral administration. Food has no effect on the bioavailability of sunitinib. SUTENT may be taken with or without food.
Binding of sunitinib and its primary active metabolite to human plasma protein *in vitro* was 95% and 90%, respectively, with no concentration dependence in the range of 100–4000 ng/mL. The apparent volume of distribution (Vd/F) for sunitinib was 2230 L. In the dosing range of 25-100 mg, the area under the plasma concentration-time curve (AUC) and C_{max} increase proportionally with dose.
Sunitinib is metabolized primarily by the cytochrome P450 enzyme, CYP3A4, to produce its primary active metabolite, which is further metabolized by CYP3A4. The primary active metabolite comprises 23 to 37% of the total exposure. Elimination is via feces. In a human mass balance study of [^{14}C]sunitinib, 61% of the dose was eliminated in feces, with renal elimination accounting for 16% of the administered dose. Sunitinib and its primary active metabolite were the major drug-related compounds identified in plasma, urine, and feces, representing 91.5%, 86.4% and 73.8% of radioactivity in pooled samples, respectively. Minor metabolites were identified in urine and feces but generally not found in plasma. Total oral clearance (CL/F) ranged from 34 to 62 L/hr with an inter-patient variability of 40%. Following administration of a single oral dose in healthy volunteers, the terminal half-lives of sunitinib and its primary active metabolite are approximately 40 to 60 hours and 80 to 110 hours, respectively. With repeated daily administration, sunitinib accumulates 3- to 4-fold while the primary metabolite accumulates 7- to 10-fold. Steady-state concentrations of sunitinib and its primary active metabolite are achieved within 10 to 14 days. By Day 14, combined plasma concentrations of sunitinib and its active metabolite ranged from 62.9–101 ng/mL. No significant changes in the pharmacokinetics of sunitinib or the primary active metabolite were observed with repeated daily administration or with repeated cycles in the dosing regimens tested.
The pharmacokinetics were similar in healthy volunteers and in the solid tumor patient populations tested, including patients with GIST and RCC.
Pharmacokinetics in Special Populations
Population pharmacokinetic analyses of demographic data indicate that there are no clinically relevant effects of age, body weight, creatinine clearance, race, gender, or ECOG score on the pharmacokinetics of SUTENT or the primary active metabolite.
Pediatric Use: The pharmacokinetics of SUTENT have not been evaluated in pediatric patients.
Renal Insufficiency: No clinical studies of SUTENT were conducted in patients with impaired renal function. Studies that were conducted excluded patients with serum creatinine > 2.0 × ULN. Population pharmacokinetic analyses have shown that sunitinib pharmacokinetics were unaltered in patients with calculated creatinine clearances in the range of 42–347 mL/min.
Hepatic Insufficiency: Systemic exposures after a single dose of SUTENT were similar in subjects with mild (Child-Pugh Class A) or moderate (Child-Pugh Class B) hepatic impairment compared to subjects with normal hepatic function.

12.4 Cardiac Electrophysiology
See Warnings and Precautions (5.4).

13 NONCLINICAL TOXICOLOGY
13.1 Carcinogenesis, Mutagenesis, Impairment of Fertility
Although definitive carcinogenicity studies with sunitinib have not been completed, carcinoma and hyperplasia of the Brunner's gland of the duodenum have been observed at the highest dose tested in H2ras transgenic mice administered doses of 0, 10, 25, 75, or 200 mg/kg/day for 28 days. Sunitinib did not cause genetic damage when tested in *in vitro* assays (bacterial mutation [AMES Assay], human lymphocyte chromosome aberration) and an *in vivo* rat bone marrow micronucleus test.
Effects on the female reproductive system were identified in a 3-month repeat dose monkey study (2, 6, 12 mg/kg/day), where ovarian changes (decreased follicular development) were noted at 12 mg/kg/day (approximately 5.1 times the

Table 4. Laboratory Abnormalities Reported in at Least 10% of Treatment-Naïve RCC Patients Who Received SUTENT or IFN-α

Laboratory Parameter, n (%)	Treatment-Naïve RCC			
	SUTENT (n=375)		IFN-α (n=360)	
	All Grades*	Grade 3/4*[a]	All Grades*	Grade 3/4*[b]
Gastrointestinal				
AST	211 (56)	6 (2)	136 (38)	8 (2)
ALT	192 (51)	10 (3)	144 (40)	9 (2)
Lipase	211 (56)	69 (18)	165 (46)	29 (8)
Alkaline phosphatase	171 (46)	7 (2)	132 (37)	6 (2)
Amylase	130 (35)	22 (6)	114 (32)	12 (3)
Total bilirubin	75 (20)	3 (1)	8 (2)	0 (0)
Indirect bilirubin	49 (13)	4 (1)	3 (1)	0 (0)
Renal/Metabolic				
Creatinine	262 (70)	2 (<1)	183 (51)	1 (<1)
Creatine kinase	183 (49)	9 (2)	40 (11)	4 (1)
Uric acid	173 (46)	54 (14)	119 (33)	29 (8)
Calcium decreased	156 (42)	4 (1)	145 (40)	4 (1)
Phosphorus	116 (31)	22 (6)	87 (24)	23 (6)
Albumin	106 (28)	4 (1)	72 (20)	0 (0)
Glucose increased	86 (23)	21 (6)	55 (15)	22 (6)
Sodium decreased	75 (20)	31 (8)	55 (15)	13 (4)
Glucose decreased	65 (17)	0 (0)	43 (12)	1 (<1)
Potassium increased	61 (16)	13 (3)	61 (17)	15 (4)
Calcium increased	50 (13)	2 (<1)	35 (10)	5 (1)
Potassium decreased	49 (13)	3 (1)	7 (2)	1 (<1)
Sodium increased	48 (13)	0 (0)	38 (10)	0 (0)
Hematology				
Neutrophils	289 (77)	65 (17)	178 (49)	31 (9)
Hemoglobin	298 (79)	29 (8)	250 (69)	18 (5)
Platelets	255 (68)	35 (9)	85 (24)	2 (1)
Lymphocytes	256 (68)	66 (18)	245 (68)	93 (26)
Leukocytes	293 (78)	29 (8)	202 (56)	8 (2)

* Common Terminology Criteria for Adverse Events (CTCAE), Version 3.0
[a] Grade 4 laboratory abnormalities in patients on SUTENT included uric acid (14%), lipase (3%), neutrophils (2%), lymphocytes (2%), hemoglobin (2%), platelets (1%), amylase (1%), ALT (<1%), creatine kinase (<1%), creatinine (<1%), glucose increased (<1%), calcium decreased (<1%), phosphorous (<1%), potassium increased (<1%), and sodium decreased (<1%).
[b] Grade 4 laboratory abnormalities in patients on IFN-α included uric acid (8%), lymphocytes (2%), lipase (1%), neutrophils (1%), amylase (<1%), calcium increased (<1%), glucose decreased (<1%), potassium increased (<1%), and hemoglobin (<1%).

Table 5. GIST Efficacy Results from Study A (Double-Blind Treatment Phase)

Efficacy Parameter	SUTENT (n=207)	Placebo (n=105)	P-value (log-rank test)	HR (95% CI)
Time to Tumor Progression[a] [median, weeks (95% CI)]	27.3 (16.0, 32.1)	6.4 (4.4, 10.0)	<0.0001*	0.33 (0.23, 0.47)
Progression-free Survival[b] [median, weeks (95% CI)]	24.1 (11.1, 28.3)	6.0 (4.4, 9.9)	<0.0001	0.33 (0.24, 0.47)
Objective Response Rate (PR) [%, (95% CI)]	6.8 (3.7, 11.1)	0	0.006[c]	

CI=Confidence interval, HR=Hazard ratio, PR=Partial response
*A comparison is considered statistically significant if the p-value is < 0.00417 (O'Brien Fleming stopping boundary)
[a] Time from randomization to progression; deaths prior to documented progression were censored at time of last radiographic evaluation
[b] Time from randomization to progression or death due to any cause
[c] Pearson chi-square test

portive care. Other objectives included Progression-Free Survival (PFS), Objective Response Rate (ORR), and Overall Survival (OS). Patients were randomized (2:1) to receive either 50 mg SUTENT or placebo orally, once daily, on Schedule 4/2 until disease progression or withdrawal from the study for another reason. Treatment was unblinded at the time of disease progression. Patients randomized to placebo were then offered crossover to open-label SUTENT, and patients randomized to SUTENT were permitted to continue treatment per investigator judgment.

At the time of a pre-specified interim analysis, the intent-to-treat (ITT) population included 312 patients. Two-hundred seven (207) patients were randomized to the SUTENT arm, and 105 patients were randomized to the placebo arm. Demographics were comparable between the SUTENT and placebo groups with regard to age (69% vs 72% <65 years for SUTENT vs. placebo, respectively), gender (Male: 64% vs. 61%), race (White: 88% both arms, Asian: 5% both arms, Black: 4% both arms, remainder not reported), and Performance Status (ECOG 0: 44% vs. 46%, ECOG 1: 55% vs. 52%, and ECOG 2: 1 vs. 2%). Prior treatment included surgery (94% vs. 93%) and radiotherapy (8% vs. 15%). Outcome of prior imatinib treatment was also comparable between arms with intolerance (4% vs. 4%), progression within 6 months of starting treatment (17% vs. 16%), or progression beyond 6 months (78% vs. 80%) balanced.

The planned interim efficacy and safety analysis was performed after 149 TTP events had occurred. There was a statistically significant advantage for SUTENT over placebo in TTP, meeting the primary endpoint. Efficacy results are summarized in Table 5 and the Kaplan-Meier curve for TTP is in Figure 1.
[See table 5 below]

Figure 1. Kaplan-Meier Curve of TTP in GIST Study A (Intent-to-Treat Population)

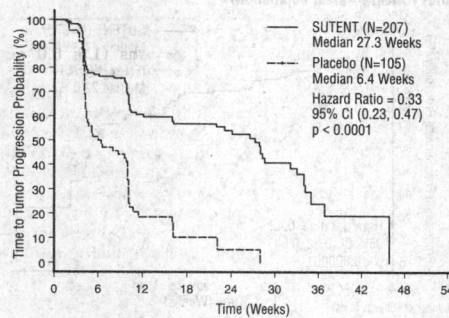

SUTENT (N=207) Median 27.3 Weeks
Placebo (N=105) Median 6.4 Weeks
Hazard Ratio = 0.33
95% CI (0.23, 0.47)
p < 0.0001

The final ITT population enrolled in the double-blind treatment phase of the study included 243 patients randomized to the SUTENT arm and 118 patients randomized to the placebo arm. After the primary endpoint was met at the interim analysis, the study was unblinded, and patients on the placebo arm were offered open-label SUTENT treatment. Ninety-nine of the patients initially randomized to placebo crossed over to receive SUTENT in the open-label treatment phase. At the protocol specified final analysis of OS, the median OS was 72.7 weeks for the SUTENT arm and 64.9 weeks for the placebo arm [HR= 0.876, 95% CI (0.679, 1.129)].

Study B
Study B was an open-label, multi-center, single-arm, dose-escalation study conducted in patients with GIST following progression on or intolerance to imatinib. Following identification of the recommended Phase 2 regimen (50 mg once daily on Schedule 4/2), 55 patients in this study received the 50 mg dose of SUTENT on treatment Schedule 4/2. Partial responses were observed in 5 of 55 patients [9.1% PR rate, 95% CI (3.0, 20.0)].

14.2   Renal Cell Carcinoma
Treatment-Naïve RCC
A multi-center, international randomized study comparing single-agent SUTENT with IFN-α was conducted in patients with treatment-naïve RCC. The objective was to compare Progression-Free Survival (PFS) in patients receiving SUTENT versus patients receiving IFN-α. Other endpoints included Objective Response Rate (ORR), Overall Survival (OS) and safety. Seven hundred fifty (750) patients were randomized (1:1) to receive either 50 mg SUTENT once daily on Schedule 4/2 or to receive IFN-α administered subcutaneously at 9 MIU three times a week. Patients were treated until disease progression or withdrawal from the study.

The ITT population included 750 patients, 375 randomized to SUTENT and 375 randomized to IFN-α. Demographics were comparable between the SUTENT and IFN-α groups with regard to age (59% vs. 67% <65 years for SUTENT vs. IFN-α, respectively), gender (Male: 71% vs. 72%), race

AUC in patients administered the RDD), while uterine changes (endometrial atrophy) were noted at ≥2 mg/kg/day (approximately 0.4 times the AUC in patients administered the RDD). With the addition of vaginal atrophy, the uterine and ovarian effects were reproduced at 6 mg/kg/day in the 9-month monkey study (0.3, 1.5 and 6 mg/kg/day administered daily for 28 days followed by a 14 day respite; the 6 mg/kg dose produced a mean AUC that was approximately 0.8 times the AUC in patients administered the RDD). A no effect level was not identified in the 3 month study; 1.5 mg/kg/day represents a no effect level in monkeys administered sunitinib for 9 months.
Although fertility was not affected in rats, SUTENT may impair fertility in humans. In female rats, no fertility effects were observed at doses of ≤5.0 mg/kg/day [(0.5, 1.5, 5.0 mg/kg/day) administered for 21 days up to gestational day 7; the 5.0 mg/kg dose produced an AUC that was approximately 5 times the AUC in patients administered the RDD], however significant embryolethality was observed at the 5.0 mg/kg dose. No reproductive effects were observed in male rats dosed (1, 3 or 10 mg/kg/day) for 58 days prior to

mating with untreated females. Fertility, copulation, conception indices, and sperm evaluation (morphology, concentration, and motility) were unaffected by sunitinib at doses ≤10 mg/kg/day (the 10 mg/kg/day dose produced a mean AUC that was approximately 25.8 times the AUC in patients administered the RDD).

14   CLINICAL STUDIES
The clinical safety and efficacy of SUTENT have been studied in patients with gastrointestinal stromal tumor (GIST) after progression on or intolerance to imatinib mesylate, and in patients with renal cell carcinoma (RCC).
14.1   Gastrointestinal Stromal Tumor
GIST Study A
Study A was a two-arm, international, randomized, double-blind, placebo-controlled trial of SUTENT in patients with GIST who had disease progression during prior imatinib mesylate (imatinib) treatment or who were intolerant of imatinib. The objective was to compare Time-to-Tumor Progression (TTP) in patients receiving SUTENT plus best supportive care versus patients receiving placebo plus best sup-

Table 6. Treatment-Naïve RCC Efficacy Results (interim analysis)

Efficacy Parameter	SUTENT (n=375)	IFN-α (n=375)	P-value (log-rank test)	HR (95% CI)
Progression-Free Survival[a] [median, weeks (95% CI)]	47.3 (42.6, 50.7)	22.0 (16.4, 24.0)	<0.000001[b]	0.415 (0.320, 0.539)
Objective Response Rate[a] [%, (95% CI)]	27.5 (23.0, 32.3)	5.3 (3.3, 8.1)	<0.001[c]	NA

CI=Confidence interval, NA=Not applicable
[a] Assessed by blinded core radiology laboratory; 90 patients' scans had not been read at time of analysis
[b] A comparison is considered statistically significant if the p-value is < 0.0042 (O'Brien Fleming stopping boundary)
[c] Pearson Chi-square test

(White: 94% vs. 91%, Asian: 2% vs. 3%, Black: 1% vs. 2%, remainder not reported), and Performance Status (ECOG 0: 62% vs. 61%, ECOG 1: 38% each arm, ECOG 2: 0 vs. 1%). Prior treatment included nephrectomy (91% vs. 89%) and radiotherapy (14% each arm). The most common site of metastases present at screening was the lung (78% vs. 80%, respectively), followed by the lymph nodes (58% vs. 53%, respectively) and bone (30% each arm); the majority of the patients had multiple (2 or more) metastatic sites at baseline (80% vs. 77%, respectively).

There was a statistically significant advantage for SUTENT over IFN-α in the endpoint of PFS (see Table 6 and Figure 2). In the pre-specified stratification factors of LDH (>1.5 ULN vs. ≤1.5 ULN), ECOG performance status (0 vs. 1), and prior nephrectomy (yes vs. no), the hazard ratio favored SUTENT over IFN-α. The ORR was higher in the SUTENT arm (see Table 6).

[See table 6 above]

Figure 2. Kaplan-Meier Curve of PFS in Treatment-Naïve RCC Study (Intent-to-Treat Population)

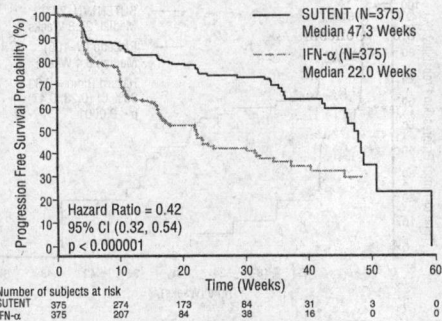

Number of subjects at risk						
SUTENT	375	274	173	84	31	3	0
IFN-α	375	207	84	38	16	0	0

At the protocol-specified final analysis of OS, the median OS was 114.6 weeks for the SUTENT arm and 94.9 weeks for the IFN-α arm [HR= 0.821, 95% CI (0.673, 1.001)]. The median OS for the IFN-α arm includes 25 patients who discontinued IFN-α treatment because of disease progression and crossed over to treatment with SUTENT as well as 121 patients (32%) on the IFN-α arm who received post-study cancer treatment with SUTENT.

Cytokine-Refractory RCC
The use of single agent SUTENT in the treatment of cytokine-refractory RCC was investigated in two single-arm, multi-center studies. All patients enrolled into these studies experienced failure of prior cytokine-based therapy. In Study 1, failure of prior cytokine therapy was based on radiographic evidence of disease progression defined by RECIST or World Health Organization (WHO) criteria during or within 9 months of completion of 1 cytokine therapy treatment (IFN-α, interleukin-2, or IFN-α plus interleukin-2; patients who were treated with IFN-α alone must have received treatment for at least 28 days). In Study 2, failure of prior cytokine therapy was defined as disease progression or unacceptable treatment-related toxicity. The endpoint for both studies was ORR. Duration of Response (DR) was also evaluated.

One hundred six patients (106) were enrolled into Study 1, and 63 patients were enrolled into Study 2. Patients received 50 mg SUTENT on Schedule 4/2. Therapy was continued until the patients met withdrawal criteria or had progressive disease. The baseline age, gender, race and ECOG performance statuses of the patients were comparable between Studies 1 and 2. Approximately 86-94% of patients in the two studies were White. Men comprised 65% of the pooled population. The median age was 57 years and ranged from 24 to 87 years in the studies. All patients had an ECOG performance status <2 at the screening visit. The baseline malignancy and prior treatment history of the patients were comparable between Studies 1 and 2. Across the two studies, 95% of the pooled population of patients had at least some component of clear-cell histology. All pa-

tients in Study 1 were required to have a histological clear-cell component. Most patients enrolled in the studies (97% of the pooled population) had undergone nephrectomy; prior nephrectomy was required for patients enrolled in Study 1. All patients had received one previous cytokine regimen. Metastatic disease present at the time of study entry included lung metastases in 81% of patients. Liver metastases were more common in Study 1 (27% vs. 16% in Study 2) and bone metastases were more common in Study 2 (51% vs. 25% in Study 1); 52% of patients in the pooled population had at least 3 metastatic sites. Patients with known brain metastases or leptomeningeal disease were excluded from both studies.

The ORR and DR data from Studies 1 and 2 are provided in Table 7. There were 36 PRs in Study 1 as assessed by a core radiology laboratory for an ORR of 34.0% (95% CI 25.0, 43.8). There were 23 PRs in Study 2 as assessed by the investigators for an ORR of 36.5% (95% CI 24.7, 49.6). The majority (>90%) of objective disease responses were observed during the first four cycles; the latest reported response was observed in Cycle 10. DR data from Study 1 is premature as only 9 of 36 patients (25%) responding to treatment had experienced disease progression or died at the time of the data cutoff.

Table 7. Cytokine-Refractory RCC Efficacy Results

Efficacy Parameter	Study 1 (N=106)	Study 2 (N=63)
Objective Response Rate [%, (95% CI)]	34.0[a] (25.0, 43.8)	36.5[b] (24.7, 49.6)
Duration of Response (DR) [median, weeks (95% CI)]	* (42.0, **)	54[b] (34.3, 70.1)

CI=Confidence interval
* Median DR has not yet been reached
** Data not mature enough to determine upper confidence limit
[a] Assessed by blinded core radiology laboratory
[b] Assessed by investigators

16   HOW SUPPLIED/STORAGE AND HANDLING

12.5 mg Capsules
Hard gelatin capsule with orange cap and orange body, printed with white ink "Pfizer" on the cap, "STN 12.5 mg" on the body; available in:
Bottles of 28:   NDC 0069-0550-38
25 mg Capsules
Hard gelatin capsule with caramel cap and orange body, printed with white ink "Pfizer" on the cap, "STN 25 mg" on the body; available in:
Bottles of 28:   NDC 0069-0770-38
50 mg Capsules
Hard gelatin capsule with caramel cap and caramel body, printed with white ink "Pfizer" on the cap, "STN 50 mg" on the body; available in:
Bottles of 28:   NDC 0069-0980-38
Store at 25°C (77°F); excursions permitted to 15-30°C (59-86°F) [see USP Controlled Room Temperature].

17   PATIENT COUNSELING INFORMATION

See 17.5 for FDA-Approved Patient Labeling.
17.1   Gastrointestinal Disorders
Gastrointestinal disorders such as diarrhea, nausea, stomatitis, dyspepsia, and vomiting were the most commonly reported gastrointestinal events occurring in patients who received SUTENT. Supportive care for gastrointestinal adverse events requiring treatment may include anti-emetic or anti-diarrheal medication.
17.2   Skin Effects
Skin discoloration possibly due to the drug color (yellow) occurred in approximately one third of patients. Patients should be advised that depigmentation of the hair or skin may occur during treatment with SUTENT. Other possible

dermatologic effects may include dryness, thickness or cracking of skin, blister or rash on the palms of the hands and soles of the feet.
17.3   Other Common Events
Other commonly reported adverse events included fatigue, high blood pressure, bleeding, swelling, mouth pain/irritation and taste disturbance.
17.4   Concomitant Medications
Patients should be advised to inform their health care providers of all concomitant medications, including over-the-counter medications and dietary supplements [see Drug Interactions (7)].
17.5   FDA-Approved Patient Labeling
LAB-0317-14.0
MEDICATION GUIDE
SUTENT (su TENT)
(sunitinib malate)
Read the Medication Guide that comes with SUTENT before you start taking it and each time you get a refill. There may be new information. This Medication Guide does not take the place of talking to your healthcare provider about your medical condition or treatment. If you have any questions about SUTENT, ask your healthcare provider or pharmacist.
What is the most important information I should know about SUTENT?
SUTENT can cause serious liver problems, including death.
• **Tell your healthcare provider right away if you develop any of the following signs and symptoms of liver problems during treatment with SUTENT:**
    • **itching**
    • **yellow eyes or skin,**
    • **dark urine, and**
    • **pain or discomfort in the right upper stomach area.**
• Your healthcare provider should do blood tests to check your liver function before you start taking SUTENT and during treatment.
What is SUTENT?
SUTENT is a prescription medicine used to treat:
1. GIST (gastrointestinal stromal tumor), a rare cancer of the stomach, bowel, or esophagus, when:
    • the medicine Gleevec® (imatinib mesylate) did not stop the cancer from growing, or
    • when you cannot take Gleevec®.
2. Advanced kidney cancer (advanced renal cell carcinoma or RCC).
It is not known if SUTENT is safe and effective in children.
What should I tell my healthcare provider before taking SUTENT?
Before taking SUTENT tell your healthcare provider if you:
• have any heart problems
• have high blood pressure
• have thyroid problems
• have kidney function problems (other than cancer)
• have liver problems
• have any bleeding problem
• have seizures
• have any other medical conditions
• are pregnant, could be pregnant or plan to become pregnant. SUTENT may harm an unborn baby. You should not become pregnant while taking SUTENT. Tell your healthcare provider right away if you become pregnant while taking SUTENT.
• are breastfeeding or plan to breastfeed. You and your healthcare provider should decide if you will take SUTENT or breastfeed. You should not do both.
Tell your healthcare provider about all the medicines you take, including prescription medicines and non-prescription medicines, vitamins, and herbal supplements. Using SUTENT with certain other medicines can cause serious side effects.
Know the medicines you take. Keep a list of them to show your healthcare provider and pharmacist when you get a new medicine. Talk with your healthcare provider before starting any new medicines.
How should I take SUTENT?
• Take SUTENT exactly the way your healthcare provider tells you.
• Take SUTENT 1 time each day with or without food.
• Do not open the SUTENT capsules.
• Do not drink grapefruit juice or eat grapefruit during your treatment with SUTENT. They may cause you to have too much SUTENT in your body.
SUTENT is usually taken for 4 weeks (28 days) and then stopped for 2 weeks (14 days). This is 1 cycle of treatment.
    • You will repeat this cycle of taking SUTENT for 4 weeks and then stopping it for 2 weeks, as long as your healthcare provider tells you to.
• Your healthcare provider may do blood tests before each cycle of treatment.
• If you miss a dose, take it as soon as you remember. Do not take it if it is close to your next dose. Just take the

next dose at your regular time. Do not take more than 1 dose of SUTENT at a time. Tell your healthcare provider about any missed dose.

- Call your healthcare provider right away, if you take too much SUTENT.

What are possible side effects of SUTENT?
SUTENT may cause serious side effects including:

- See "What is the most important information I should know about SUTENT?"
- **Heart problems.** Heart problems may include heart failure and heart muscle problems (cardiomyopathy). Tell your healthcare provider if you feel very tired, are short of breath, or have swollen feet and ankles.
- **Abnormal heart rhythm changes.** Your healthcare provider may do electrocardiograms and blood tests to watch for these problems during your treatment with SUTENT. Tell your healthcare provider if you feel dizzy, faint, or have abnormal heartbeats while taking SUTENT.
- **High blood pressure.** Your healthcare provider may check your blood pressure during treatment with SUTENT. Your healthcare provider may prescribe medicine for you to treat high blood pressure, if needed.
- **Bleeding sometimes leading to death.** Tell your healthcare provider right away if you have any of these symptoms or a serious bleeding problem during treatment with SUTENT.
  - painful, swollen stomach (abdomen)
  - vomiting blood
  - black, sticky stools
  - bloody urine
  - headache or change in your mental status

Your healthcare provider can tell you other symptoms to watch for.

- **Hormone problems, including thyroid and adrenal gland problems.** Your healthcare provider may do tests to check your thyroid and adrenal gland function during SUTENT treatment. Tell your doctor if you have any of the following signs and symptoms during treatment with SUTENT:
  - tiredness that worsens and does not go away
  - loss of appetite
  - heat intolerance
  - feeling nervous or agitated, tremors
  - sweating
  - nausea or vomiting
  - diarrhea
  - fast heart rate
  - weight gain or weight loss
  - feeling depressed
  - irregular menstrual periods or no menstrual periods
  - headache
  - hair loss

Common side effects of SUTENT include:

- The medicine in SUTENT is yellow, and it may make your skin look yellow. Your skin and hair may get lighter in color.
- tiredness
- weakness
- fever
- gastrointestinal symptoms, including diarrhea, nausea, vomiting, mouth sores, upset stomach, abdominal pain, and constipation. Talk with your healthcare provider about ways to handle these problems.
- rash or other skin changes, including drier, thicker, or cracking skin.
- blisters or a rash on the palms of your hands and soles of your feet.
- taste changes
- loss of appetite
- pain or swelling in your arms or legs
- cough
- shortness of breath
- bleeding, such as nosebleeds or bleeding from cuts.

Call your healthcare provider if you have any swelling or bleeding during treatment with SUTENT.

These are not all the possible side effects of SUTENT. For more information, ask your healthcare provider or pharmacist. Call your doctor for medical advice about side effects. You may report side effects to FDA at 1-800-FDA-1088.

How do I store SUTENT?

- Store SUTENT at room temperature, between 59°F and 86°F (15°C to 30°C).

Keep SUTENT and all medicines out of the reach of children.

General information about SUTENT
Medicines are sometimes prescribed for purposes other than those listed in a Medication Guide. Do not use SUTENT for a condition for which it was not prescribed. Do not give SUTENT to other people, even if they have the same symptoms you have. It may harm them.
This Medication Guide gives the most important information about SUTENT. For more information about SUTENT, talk with your healthcare provider or pharmacist. You can ask your healthcare provider or pharmacist for information about SUTENT that is written for health professionals.

For more information go to www.SUTENT.com or call 1-877-5-SUTENT.

What are the ingredients in SUTENT?
Active ingredient: sunitinib malate
Inactive ingredients: mannitol, croscarmellose sodium, povidone (K-25), magnesium stearate **Orange gelatin capsule shell:** titanium dioxide, red iron oxide **Caramel gelatin capsule shell:** titanium dioxide, red iron oxide, yellow iron oxide, black iron oxide **White printing ink:** shellac, propylene glycol, sodium hydroxide, povidone, titanium dioxide
Distributed by:
Pfizer Labs
Division of Pfizer Inc
New York, NY 10017
Issued July 2010
This Medication Guide has been approved by the U.S. Food and Drug Administration.
Gleevec® is a registered trademark of Novartis Pharmaceuticals Corp
LAB-0361-3.0

TOVIAZ® ℞
[TOH-vee-as]
(fesoterodine fumarate)
For oral administration

HIGHLIGHTS OF PRESCRIBING INFORMATION
These highlights do not include all the information needed to use Toviaz safely and effectively. See full prescribing information for Toviaz.
Toviaz® (fesoterodine fumarate)
For oral administration
Initial U.S. Approval: October 31, 2008

———INDICATIONS AND USAGE———
Toviaz is indicated for the treatment of overactive bladder with symptoms of urge urinary incontinence, urgency, and frequency. (1)

———DOSAGE AND ADMINISTRATION———
The recommended starting dose of Toviaz is 4 mg once daily. Based upon individual response and tolerability, the dose may be increased to 8 mg once daily. (2)
The daily dose of Toviaz should not exceed 4 mg in the following populations:
- Patients with severe renal impairment (CL$_{CR}$ <30 mL/min) (2)
- Patients taking potent CYP3A4 inhibitors, such as ketoconazole, itraconazole and clarithromycin. (2)
Toviaz is not recommended for use in patients with severe hepatic impairment (Child-Pugh C). (2)
Toviaz should be taken with liquid and swallowed whole. Toviaz can be administered with or without food, and should not be chewed, divided, or crushed. (2)

———DOSAGE FORMS AND STRENGTHS———
Toviaz 4 mg extended-release tablets are light blue, oval, biconvex, film-coated and engraved with "FS" on one side. (3)
Toviaz 8 mg extended-release tablets are blue, oval, biconvex, film-coated and engraved with "FT" on one side. (3)

———CONTRAINDICATIONS———
Toviaz is contraindicated in patients with urinary retention, gastric retention, or uncontrolled narrow-angle glaucoma. Toviaz is also contraindicated in patients with known hypersensitivity to the drug or its ingredients. (4)

———WARNINGS AND PRECAUTIONS———
- Toviaz should be administered with caution to patients with clinically significant bladder outlet obstruction because of the risk of urinary retention. (5.1)
- Toviaz, like other antimuscarinic drugs, should be used with caution in patients with decreased gastrointestinal motility, such as those with severe constipation. (5.2)
- Toviaz should be used with caution in patients being treated for narrow-angle glaucoma, and only where the potential benefits outweigh the risks (5.3)
- Doses of Toviaz greater than 4 mg are not recommended in patients taking a potent CYP3A4 inhibitor (e.g. ketoconazole, itraconazole, clarithromycin).In patients taking weak or moderate CYP3A4 inhibitors (e.g. erythromycin), careful assessment of tolerability at the 4 mg daily dose is advised prior to increasing the daily dose to 8 mg. (5.6)
- Toviaz should be used with caution in patients with myasthenia gravis, a disease characterized by decreased cholinergic activity at the neuromuscular junction. (5.7)

———ADVERSE REACTIONS———
The most frequently reported adverse events (≥4%) for Toviaz were: dry mouth (placebo, 7%; Toviaz 4 mg, 19%; Toviaz 8 mg, 35%) and constipation (placebo, 2%; Toviaz 4 mg, 4%; Toviaz 8 mg, 6%). (6)
To report SUSPECTED ADVERSE REACTIONS, contact Pfizer Inc. at 1-800-438-1985 or FDA at 1-800-FDA-1088 or www.fda.gov/medwatch.

———DRUG INTERACTIONS———
- Doses of Toviaz greater than 4mg are not recommended in patients taking potent CYP3A4 inhibitors. The effects of

weak or moderate CYP3A4 inhibitors were not examined. (7.2)
- No dosing adjustments are recommended in the presence of CYP3A4 inducers or CYP2D6 inhibitors. (7.3, 7.4)
- There were no changes in the plasma concentrations of combined oral contraceptives containing ethinyl estradiol and levonorgestrel. (7.6)

———USE IN SPECIFIC POPULATIONS———
- *Pregnancy and Nursing Mothers:* Toviaz should be used during pregnancy only if the potential benefit outweighs the potential risk to the fetus. (8.1)
Toviaz should not be administered during nursing unless the potential benefit outweighs the potential risk to the neonate. (8.3)
- *Pediatric Use:* The safety and effectiveness of Toviaz in pediatric patients have not been established. (8.4)
- *Geriatric Use:* No dose adjustment is recommended for the elderly. (8.5)
- *Renal impairment:* Doses of Toviaz greater than 4 mg are not recommended in patients with severe renal impairment. (8.6)
- *Hepatic impairment:* Subjects with severe hepatic impairment (Child-Pugh C) have not been studied; therefore Toviaz is not recommended for use in these patients. (8.7)

See 17 for PATIENT COUNSELING INFORMATION and FDA-approved patient labeling.

Revised: [3/2010]

FULL PRESCRIBING INFORMATION: CONTENTS*
*Sections or subsections omitted from the full prescribing information are not listed.

FULL PRESCRIBING INFORMATION

1 INDICATIONS AND USAGE
Toviaz® is indicated for the treatment of overactive bladder with symptoms of urge urinary incontinence, urgency, and frequency.

2 DOSAGE AND ADMINISTRATION
The recommended starting dose of Toviaz is 4 mg once daily. Based upon individual response and tolerability, the dose may be increased to 8 mg once daily.
The daily dose of Toviaz should not exceed 4 mg in the following populations:
- Patients with severe renal impairment (CL$_{CR}$ <30 mL/min).

Table 3 Adverse events with an incidence exceeding the placebo rate and reported by ≥1% of patients from double-blind, placebo-controlled Phase 3 trials of 12 weeks treatment duration

System organ class/Preferred term	Placebo N=554 %	Toviaz 4mg/day N=554 %	Toviaz 8mg/day N=566 %
Gastrointestinal disorders			
Dry mouth	7.0	18.8	34.6
Constipation	2.0	4.2	6.0
Dyspepsia	0.5	1.6	2.3
Nausea	1.3	0.7	1.9
Abdominal pain upper	0.5	1.1	0.5
Infections			
Urinary tract infection	3.1	3.2	4.2
Upper respiratory tract infection	2.2	2.5	1.8
Eye disorders			
Dry eyes	0	1.4	3.7
Renal and urinary disorders			
Dysuria	0.7	1.3	1.6
Urinary retention	0.2	1.1	1.4
Respiratory disorders			
Cough	0.5	1.6	0.9
Dry Throat	0.4	0.9	2.3
General disorders			
Edema peripheral	0.7	0.7	1.2
Musculoskeletal disorders			
Back pain	0.4	2.0	0.9
Psychiatric disorders			
Insomnia	0.5	1.3	0.4
Investigations			
ALT increased	0.9	0.5	1.2
GGT increased	0.4	0.4	1.2
Skin disorders			
Rash	0.5	0.7	1.1

ALT=alanine aminotransferase, GGT=gamma glutamyltransferase

- Patients taking potent CYP3A4 inhibitors, such as ketoconazole, itraconazole and clarithromycin.

Toviaz is not recommended for use in patients with severe hepatic impairment (Child-Pugh C) [see *WARNINGS AND PRECAUTIONS* (5.4, 5.6, 5.7), *USE IN SPECIFIC POPULATIONS* (8.6, 8.7), and *DRUG INTERACTIONS* (7.2)].

Toviaz should be taken with liquid and swallowed whole. Toviaz can be administered with or without food, and should not be chewed, divided, or crushed.

3 DOSAGE FORMS AND STRENGTHS

Toviaz (fesoterodine fumarate) extended-release tablets 4 mg are light blue, oval, biconvex, film-coated and engraved with "FS" on one side.

Toviaz (fesoterodine fumarate) extended-release tablets 8 mg are blue, oval, biconvex, film-coated and engraved with "FT" on one side.

4 CONTRAINDICATIONS

Toviaz is contraindicated in patients with urinary retention, gastric retention, or uncontrolled narrow-angle glaucoma. Toviaz is also contraindicated in patients with known hypersensitivity to the drug or its ingredients.

5 WARNINGS AND PRECAUTIONS

5.1   Bladder Outlet Obstruction: Toviaz should be administered with caution to patients with clinically significant bladder outlet obstruction because of the risk of urinary retention [see *CONTRAINDICATIONS* (4)].

5.2   Decreased Gastrointestinal Motility: Toviaz, like other antimuscarinic drugs, should be used with caution in patients with decreased gastrointestinal motility, such as those with severe constipation.

5.3   Controlled Narrow-Angle Glaucoma: Toviaz should be used with caution in patients being treated for narrow-angle glaucoma, and only where the potential benefits outweigh the risks [see *CONTRAINDICATIONS* (4)].

5.4   Hepatic Impairment: Toviaz has not been studied in patients with severe hepatic impairment and therefore is not recommended for use in this patient population [see *USE IN SPECIFIC POPULATIONS* (8.7) and *DOSAGE AND ADMINISTRATION* (2)].

5.5   Renal Impairment: Doses of Toviaz greater than 4 mg are not recommended in patients with severe renal impairment [see *USE IN SPECIFIC POPULATIONS* (8.6) and *DOSAGE AND ADMINISTRATION* (2)].

5.6   Concomitant Administration with CYP3A4 Inhibitors: Doses of Toviaz greater than 4 mg are not recommended in patients taking a potent CYP3A4 inhibitor (e.g. ketoconazole, itraconazole, clarithromycin).

In patients taking weak or moderate CYP3A4 inhibitors (e.g. erythromycin), careful assessment of tolerability at the 4 mg daily dose is advised prior to increasing the daily dose to 8 mg. While this specific interaction potential was not examined by clinical study, some pharmacokinetic interaction is expected, albeit less than that observed with potent CYP3A4 inhibitors [see *DRUG INTERACTIONS* (7.2) and *DOSAGE AND ADMINISTRATION* (2)].

5.7   Myasthenia Gravis: Toviaz should be used with caution in patients with myasthenia gravis, a disease characterized by decreased cholinergic activity at the neuromuscular junction.

6 ADVERSE REACTIONS

The safety of Toviaz was evaluated in Phase 2 and 3 controlled trials in a total of 2859 patients with overactive bladder of which 2288 were treated with fesoterodine. Of this total, 782 received Toviaz 4 mg/day, and 785 received Toviaz 8 mg/day in Phase 2 or 3 studies with treatment periods of 8 or 12 weeks. Approximately 80% of these patients had >10 weeks exposure to Toviaz in these trials.

A total of 1964 patients participated in two 12-week, Phase 3 efficacy and safety studies and subsequent open-label extension studies. In these 2 studies combined, 554 patients received Toviaz 4 mg/day and 566 patients received Toviaz 8 mg/day.

In Phase 2 and 3 placebo-controlled trials combined, the incidences of serious adverse events in patients receiving placebo, Toviaz 4 mg, and Toviaz 8 mg were 1.9%, 3.5%, and 2.9%, respectively. All serious adverse events were judged to be not related or unlikely to be related to study medication by the investigator, except for four patients receiving Toviaz who reported one serious adverse event each: angina, chest pain, gastroenteritis, and QT prolongation on ECG.

The most commonly reported adverse event in patients treated with Toviaz was dry mouth. The incidence of dry mouth was higher in those taking 8 mg/day (35%) and in those taking 4 mg/day (19%), as compared to placebo (7%). Dry mouth led to discontinuation in 0.4%, 0.4%, and 0.8% of patients receiving placebo, Toviaz 4 mg, and Toviaz 8 mg, respectively. For those patients who reported dry mouth, most had their first occurrence of the event within the first month of treatment.

The second most commonly reported adverse event was constipation. The incidence of constipation was 2% in those taking placebo, 4% in those taking 4 mg/day, and 6% in those taking 8 mg.

Table 3 lists adverse events, regardless of causality, that were reported in the combined Phase 3, randomized, placebo-controlled trials at an incidence greater than placebo and in 1% or more of patients treated with Toviaz 4 or 8 mg once daily for up to 12 weeks.
[See table 3 at left]

Patients also received Toviaz for up to three years in open-label extension phases of one Phase 2 and two Phase 3 controlled trials. In all open label trials combined, 857, 701, 529, and 105 patients received Toviaz for at least 6 months, 1 year, 2 years, and 3 years respectively. The adverse events observed during long-term, open-label studies were similar to those observed in the 12-week, placebo-controlled studies, and included dry mouth, constipation, dry eyes, dyspepsia and abdominal pain. Similar to the controlled studies, most adverse events of dry mouth and constipation were mild to moderate in intensity. Serious adverse events, judged to be at least possibly related to study medication by the investigator, and reported more than once during the open-label treatment period of up to 3 years included urinary retention (3 cases), diverticulitis (3 cases), constipation (2 cases), irritable bowel syndrome (2 cases), and electrocardiogram QT corrected interval prolongation (2 cases).

7 DRUG INTERACTIONS

7.1   Antimuscarinic Drugs: Coadministration of Toviaz with other antimuscarinic agents that produce dry mouth, constipation, urinary retention, and other anticholinergic pharmacological effects may increase the frequency and/or severity of such effects. Anticholinergic agents may potentially alter the absorption of some concomitantly administered drugs due to anticholinergic effects on gastrointestinal motility.

7.2   CYP3A4 Inhibitors: Doses of Toviaz greater than 4mg are not recommended in patients taking potent CYP3A4 inhibitors, such as ketoconazole, itraconazole and clarithromycin. Coadministration of the potent CYP3A4 inhibitor ketoconazole with fesoterodine led to approximately a doubling of the maximum concentration (C_{max}) and area under the concentration versus time curve (AUC) of 5-hydroxymethyl tolterodine (5-HMT), the active metabolite of fesoterodine. Compared with CYP2D6 extensive metabolizers not taking ketoconazole, further increases in the exposure to 5-HMT were observed in subjects who were CYP2D6 poor metabolizers taking ketoconazole [see *CLINICAL PHARMACOLOGY (12.3)*, *WARNINGS AND PRECAUTIONS (5.7)* and *DOSAGE AND ADMINISTRATION (2)*].

The effects of weak or moderate CYP3A4 inhibitors were not examined.

7.3   CYP3A4 Inducers: No dosing adjustments are recommended in the presence of CYP3A4 inducers, such as rifampin and carbamazepine. Following induction of CYP3A4 by coadministration of rifampin 600 mg once a day, C_{max} and AUC of the active metabolite of fesoterodine decreased by approximately 70% and 75%, respectively, after oral administration of Toviaz 8 mg. The terminal half-life of the active metabolite was not changed.

7.4   CYP2D6 Inhibitors: The interaction with CYP2D6 inhibitors was not tested clinically. In poor metabolizers for CYP2D6, representing a maximum CYP2D6 inhibition, C_{max} and AUC of the active metabolite are increased 1.7- and 2-fold, respectively.

No dosing adjustments are recommended in the presence of CYP2D6 inhibitors.

7.5   Drugs Metabolized by Cytochrome P450: In vitro data indicate that at therapeutic concentrations, the active metabolite of fesoterodine does not have the potential to inhibit or induce Cytochrome P450 enzyme systems [see CLINICAL PHARMACOLOGY (12.3)].

7.6   Oral Contraceptives: In the presence of fesoterodine, there are no clinically significant changes in the plasma concentrations of combined oral contraceptives containing ethinyl estradiol and levonorgestrel [see CLINICAL PHARMACOLOGY (12.3)].

7.7   Drug-Laboratory Test Interactions: Interactions between Toviaz and laboratory tests have not been studied.

8 USE IN SPECIFIC POPULATIONS

8.1   Pregnancy: Pregnancy Category C. There are no adequate and well-controlled studies using Toviaz in pregnant women.

No dose-related teratogenicity was observed in reproduction studies performed in mice and rabbits. In mice at 6 to 27 times the expected exposure at the maximum recommended human dose (MRHD) of 8 mg based on AUC (75 mg/kg/day, oral), increased resorptions and decreased live fetuses were observed. One fetus with cleft palate was observed at each dose (15, 45 and 75 mg/kg/day), at an incidence within the background historical range. In rabbits treated at 3 to 11 times the MRHD (27 mg/kg/day, oral), incompletely ossified sternebrae (retardation of bone development) were observed in fetuses. In rabbits at 9 to 11 times the MRHD (4.5 mg/kg/day, subcutaneous), maternal toxicity and incompletely ossified sternebrae were observed in fetuses (at an incidence within the background historical range). In rabbits at 3 times the MRHD (1.5 mg/kg/day, subcutaneous), decreased maternal food consumption in the absence of any fetal effects was observed. Oral administration of 30 mg/kg/day fesoterodine to mice in a pre- and post-natal development study resulted in decreased body weight of the dams and delayed ear opening of the pups. No effects were noted on mating and reproduction of the F_1 dams or on the F_2 offspring.

Toviaz should be used during pregnancy only if the potential benefit outweighs the potential risk to the fetus.

8.3 Nursing Mothers: It is not known whether fesoterodine is excreted in human milk. Toviaz should not be administered during nursing unless the potential benefit outweighs the potential risk to the neonate.

8.4 Pediatric Use: The pharmacokinetics of fesoterodine have not been evaluated in pediatric patients. The safety and effectiveness of Toviaz in pediatric patients have not been established.

8.5 Geriatric Use: No dose adjustment is recommended for the elderly. The pharmacokinetics of fesoterodine are not significantly influenced by age.

Of 1567 patients who received Toviaz 4mg/day or 8mg/day in the Phase 2 and 3, placebo-controlled, efficacy and safety studies, 515 (33%) were 65 years of age or older, and 140 (9%) were 75 years of age or older. No overall differences in safety or effectiveness were observed between patients younger than 65 years of age and those 65 years of age or older in these studies; however, the incidence of antimuscarinic adverse events, including dry mouth, constipation, dyspepsia, increase in residual urine, dizziness (at 8mg only) and urinary tract infection, was higher in patients 75 years of age and older as compared to younger patients. [*see* ***CLINICAL STUDIES*** *(14) and* ***ADVERSE REACTIONS*** *(6)*].

8.6 Renal Impairment: In patients with severe renal impairment (CL_{CR} < 30 mL/min), Cmax and AUC are increased 2.0- and 2.3-fold, respectively. Doses of Toviaz greater than 4 mg are not recommended in patients with severe renal impairment. In patients with mild or moderate renal impairment (CL_{CR} ranging from 30-80 mL/min), C_{max} and AUC of the active metabolite are increased up to 1.5- and 1.8-fold respectively, as compared to healthy subjects. No dose adjustment is recommended in patients with mild or moderate renal impairment [*see* ***WARNINGS AND PRECAUTIONS*** *(5.5) and* ***DOSAGE AND ADMINISTRATION*** *(2)*].

8.7 Hepatic Impairment: Patients with severe hepatic impairment (Child-Pugh C) have not been studied; therefore Toviaz is not recommended for use in these patients. In patients with moderate (Child-Pugh B) hepatic impairment, C_{max} and AUC of the active metabolite are increased 1.4- and 2.1-fold, respectively, as compared to healthy subjects. No dose adjustment is recommended in patients with mild or moderate hepatic impairment [*see* ***WARNINGS AND PRECAUTIONS*** *(5.4) and* ***DOSAGE AND ADMINISTRATION*** *(2)*].

8.8 Gender: No dose adjustment is recommended based on gender. The pharmacokinetics of fesoterodine are not significantly influenced by gender.

8.9 Race: Available data indicate that there are no differences in the pharmacokinetics of fesoterodine between Caucasian and Black healthy subjects following administration of Toviaz.

10 OVERDOSAGE

Overdosage with Toviaz can result in severe anticholinergic effects. Treatment should be symptomatic and supportive. In the event of overdosage, ECG monitoring is recommended.

11 DESCRIPTION

Toviaz contains fesoterodine fumarate and is an extended-release tablet. Fesoterodine is rapidly de-esterified to its active metabolite, (R)-2-(3-diisopropylamino-1-phenylpropyl)-4-hydroxymethyl-phenol, or 5-hydroxymethyl tolterodine, which is a muscarinic receptor antagonist.

Chemically, fesoterodine fumarate is designated as isobutyric acid 2-((R)-3-diisopropylammonium-1-phenylpropyl)-4-(hydroxymethyl) phenyl ester hydrogen fumarate. The empirical formula is $C_{30}H_{41}NO_7$ and its molecular weight is 527.66. The structural formula is:

Table 1 Summary of geometric mean [CV] pharmacokinetic parameters for the active metabolite after a single dose of Toviaz 4 mg and 8 mg in extensive and poor CYP2D6 metabolizers

Parameter	Toviaz 4 mg EM (n=16)	Toviaz 4 mg PM (n=8)	Toviaz 8 mg EM (n=16)	Toviaz 8 mg PM (n=8)
C_{max} (ng/mL)	1.89 [43%]	3.45 [54%]	3.98 [28%]	6.90 [39%]
AUC_{0-tz} (ng*h/mL)	21.2 [38%]	40.5 [31%]	45.3 [32%]	88.7 [36%]
t_{max} (h)[a]	5 [2-6]	5 [5-6]	5 [3-6]	5 [5-6]
$t_{1/2}$ (h)	7.31 [27%]	7.31 [30%]	8.59 [41%]	7.66 [21%]

EM = extensive CYP2D6 metabolizer, PM = poor CYP2D6 metabolizer, CV=coefficient of variation
C_{max} = maximum plasma concentration, AUC_{0-tz} = area under the concentration time curve from zero up to the last measurable plasma concentration, t_{max} = time to reach C_{max}, $t_{1/2}$= terminal half-life
[a] Data presented as median (range)

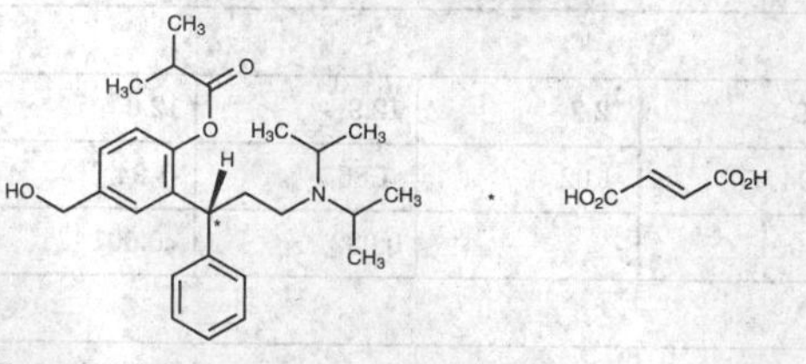

The asterisk (*) indicates the chiral carbon.

Fesoterodine fumarate is a white to off-white powder, which is freely soluble in water. Each Toviaz extended-release tablet contains either 4 mg or 8 mg of fesoterodine fumarate and the following inactive ingredients: glyceryl behenate, hypromellose, indigo carmine aluminum lake, lactose monohydrate, soya lecithin, microcrystalline cellulose, polyethylene glycol, polyvinyl alcohol, talc, titanium dioxide, and xylitol.

12 CLINICAL PHARMACOLOGY

12.1 Mechanism of Action:

Fesoterodine is a competitive muscarinic receptor antagonist. After oral administration, fesoterodine is rapidly and extensively hydrolyzed by nonspecific esterases to its active metabolite, 5-hydroxymethyl tolterodine, which is responsible for the antimuscarinic activity of fesoterodine.

Muscarinic receptors play a role in contractions of urinary bladder smooth muscle and stimulation of salivary secretion. Inhibition of these receptors in the bladder is presumed to be the mechanism by which fesoterodine produces its effects.

12.2 Pharmacodynamics:

In a urodynamic study involving patients with involuntary detrusor contractions, the effects after the administration of fesoterodine on the volume at first detrusor contraction and bladder capacity were assessed. Administration of fesoterodine increased the volume at first detrusor contraction and bladder capacity in a dose-dependent manner. These findings are consistent with an antimuscarinic effect on the bladder.

Cardiac Electrophysiology: The effect of fesoterodine 4 mg and 28 mg on the QT interval was evaluated in a double-blind, randomized, placebo- and positive-controlled (moxifloxacin 400 mg once a day) parallel trial with once-daily treatment over a period of 3 days in 261 male and female subjects aged 44 to 65 years. Electrocardiographic parameters were measured over a 24-hour period at pre-dose, after the first administration, and after the third administration of study medication. Fesoterodine 28 mg was chosen because this dose, when administered to CYP2D6 extensive metabolizers, results in an exposure to the active metabolite that is similar to the exposure in a CYP2D6 poor metabolizer receiving fesoterodine 8 mg together with CYP3A4 blockade. Corrected QT intervals (QTc) were calculated using Fridericia's correction and a linear individual correction method. Analyses of 24-hour average QTc, time-matched baseline-corrected QTc, and time-matched placebo-subtracted QTc intervals indicate that fesoterodine at doses of 4 and 28 mg/day did not prolong the QT interval. The sensitivity of the study was confirmed by positive QTc prolongation by moxifloxacin.

Toviaz is associated with an increase in heart rate that correlates with increasing dose. In the study described above, when compared to placebo, the mean increase in heart rate associated with a dose of 4 mg/day and 28 mg/day of fesoterodine was 3 beats/minute and 11 beats/minute respectively.

In the two, phase 3, placebo-controlled studies in patients with overactive bladder, the mean increase in heart rate compared to placebo was approximately 3-4 beats/minute in the 4 mg/day group and 3-5 beats/minute in the 8 mg/day group.

12.3 Pharmacokinetics:

Absorption: After oral administration, fesoterodine is well absorbed. Due to rapid and extensive hydrolysis by nonspecific esterases to its active metabolite 5-hydroxymethyl tolterodine, fesoterodine cannot be detected in plasma. Bioavailability of the active metabolite is 52%. After single or multiple-dose oral administration of fesoterodine in doses from 4 mg to 28 mg, plasma concentrations of the active metabolite are proportional to the dose. Maximum plasma levels are reached after approximately 5 hours. No accumulation occurs after multiple-dose administration.

A summary of pharmacokinetic parameters for the active metabolite after a single dose of Toviaz 4 mg and 8 mg in extensive and poor metabolizers of CYP2D6 is provided in Table 1.

[See table 1 above]

Effect of Food: There is no clinically relevant effect of food on the pharmacokinetics of fesoterodine. In a study of the effects of food on the pharmacokinetics of fesoterodine in 16 healthy male volunteers, concomitant food intake increased the active metabolite of fesoterodine AUC by approximately 19% and C_{max} by 18%. [*see* ***DOSAGE AND ADMINISTRATION*** *(2)*]

Distribution: Plasma protein binding of the active metabolite is low (approximately 50%) and is primarily bound to albumin and alpha-1-acid glycoprotein. The mean steady-state volume of distribution following intravenous infusion of the active metabolite is 169 L.

Metabolism: After oral administration, fesoterodine is rapidly and extensively hydrolyzed to its active metabolite. The active metabolite is further metabolized in the liver to its carboxy, carboxy-N-desisopropyl, and N-desisopropyl metabolites via two major pathways involving CYP2D6 and CYP3A4. None of these metabolites contribute significantly to the antimuscarinic activity of fesoterodine.

Variability in CYP2D6 Metabolism: A subset of individuals (approximately 7% of Caucasians and approximately 2% of African Americans) are poor metabolizers for CYP2D6. C_{max} and AUC of the active metabolite are increased 1.7- and 2-fold, respectively, in CYP2D6 poor metabolizers as compared to extensive metabolizers.

Excretion: Hepatic metabolism and renal excretion contribute significantly to the elimination of the active metabolite. After oral administration of fesoterodine, approximately 70% of the administered dose was recovered in urine as the active metabolite (16%), carboxy metabolite (34%), carboxy-N-desisopropyl metabolite (18%), or N-desisopropyl metabolite (1%), and a smaller amount (7%) was recovered in feces.

The terminal half-life of the active metabolite is approximately 4 hours following an intravenous administration. The apparent terminal half-life following oral administration is approximately 7 hours.

Pharmacokinetics in Specific Populations:

Geriatric Patients: Following a single 8 mg oral dose of fesoterodine, the mean (±SD) AUC and C_{max} for the active metabolite 5-hydroxymethyl tolterodine in 12 elderly men (mean age 67 years) were 51.8 ± 26.1 h*ng/mL and 3.8 ± 1.7 ng/mL respectively. In the same study, the mean (±SD) AUC and C_{max} in 12 young men (mean age 30 years) were 52.0 ± 31.5 h*ng/mL and 4.1 ± 2.1 ng/mL, respectively. The pharmacokinetics of fesoterodine were not significantly influenced by age [*see* ***USE IN SPECIFIC POPULATIONS*** *(8.5)*].

Pediatric Patients: The pharmacokinetics of fesoterodine have not been evaluated in pediatric patients [*see* ***USE IN SPECIFIC POPULATIONS*** *(8.4)*].

Gender: Following a single 8 mg oral dose of fesoterodine, the mean (±SD) AUC and Cmax for the active metabolite 5-hydroxymethyl tolterodine in 12 elderly men (mean age 67 years) were 51.8 ± 26.1 h*ng/mL and 3.8 ± 1.7 ng/mL respectively. In the same study, the mean (±SD) AUC and Cmax in 12 elderly women (mean age 68 years) were 56.0 ± 28.8 h*ng/mL and 4.6 ± 2.3 ng/mL, respectively. The pharmacokinetics of fesoterodine were not significantly influenced by gender [*see* ***USE IN SPECIFIC POPULATIONS*** *(8.8)*].

Race: The effects of Caucasian or Black race on the pharmacokinetics of fesoterodine were examined in a study of 12 Caucasian and 12 Black African young male volunteers. Each subject received a single oral dose of 8mg fesoterodine. The mean (±SD) AUC and Cmax for the active metabolite

Table 2 Mean baseline and change from baseline to Week 12 for urge urinary incontinence episodes, number of micturitions, and volume voided per micturition

Parameter	Study 1			Study 2		
	Placebo N=279	Toviaz 4mg/day N=265	Toviaz 8mg/day N=276	Placebo N=266	Toviaz 4mg/day N=267	Toviaz 8mg/day N=267
Number of urge incontinence episodes per 24 hours[a]						
Baseline	3.7	3.8	3.7	3.7	3.9	3.9
Change from baseline	-1.20	-2.06	-2.27	-1.00	-1.77	-2.42
p-value vs placebo	-	0.001	<0.001	-	<0.003	<0.001
Number of micturitions per 24 hours						
Baseline	12.0	11.6	11.9	12.2	12.9	12.0
Change from baseline	-1.02	-1.74	-1.94	-1.02	-1.86	-1.94
p-value vs placebo	-	<0.001	<0.001	-	0.032	<0.001
Voided volume per micturition (mL)						
Baseline	150	160	154	159	152	156
Change from baseline	10	27	33	8	17	33
p-value vs placebo	-	<0.001	<0.001	-	0.150	<0.001

vs=versus

a Only those patients who were urge incontinent at baseline were included for the analysis of number of urge incontinence episodes per 24 hours: In Study 1, the number of these patients was 211, 199, and 223 in the placebo, Toviaz 4 mg/day and Toviaz 8 mg/day groups, respectively. In Study 2, the number of these patients was 205, 228, and 218, respectively.

5-hydroxymethyl tolterodine in Caucasian males were 73.0 ± 27.8 h*ng/mL and 6.1 ± 2.7 ng/mL respectively. The mean (±SD) AUC and Cmax in Black males were 65.8 ± 23.2 h*ng/mL and 5.5 ± 1.9 ng/mL, respectively. The pharmacokinetics of fesoterodine were not significantly influenced by race [see **USE IN SPECIFIC POPULATIONS** (8.9)].

Renal Impairment: In patients with mild or moderate renal impairment (CL_{CR} ranging from 30-80 mL/min), C_{max} and AUC of the active metabolite are increased up to 1.5- and 1.8-fold respectively, as compared to healthy subjects. In patients with severe renal impairment (CL_{CR} < 30 mL/min), C_{max} and AUC are increased 2.0- and 2.3-fold, respectively.

In patients with mild or moderate renal impairment, no dose adjustment is recommended. Doses of Toviaz greater than 4 mg are not recommended in patients with severe renal impairment [see **USE IN SPECIFIC POPULATIONS** (8.6), **WARNINGS AND PRECAUTIONS** (5.5) and **DOSAGE AND ADMINISTRATION** (2)].

Hepatic Impairment: In patients with moderate (Child-Pugh B) hepatic impairment, C_{max} and AUC of the active metabolite are increased 1.4- and 2.1-fold, respectively, as compared to healthy subjects.

No dose adjustment is recommended in patients with mild or moderate hepatic impairment. Subjects with severe hepatic impairment (Child-Pugh C) have not been studied; therefore Toviaz is not recommended for use in these patients [see **USE IN SPECIFIC POPULATIONS** (8.7), **WARNINGS AND PRECAUTIONS** (5.4) and **DOSAGE AND ADMINISTRATION** (2)].

Drug-Drug Interactions:

Drugs Metabolized by Cytochrome P450: At therapeutic concentrations, the active metabolite of fesoterodine does not inhibit CYP1A2, 2B6, 2C8, 2C9, 2C19, 2D6, 2E1, or 3A4, or induce CYP1A2, 2B6, 2C9, 2C19, or 3A4 in vitro [see **DRUG INTERACTIONS** (7.5)].

CYP3A4 Inhibitors: Following blockade of CYP3A4 by co-administration of the potent CYP3A4 inhibitor ketoconazole 200 mg twice a day for 5 days, C_{max} and AUC of the active metabolite of fesoterodine increased 2.0- and 2.3-fold, respectively, after oral administration of Toviaz 8 mg to CYP2D6 extensive metabolizers. In CYP2D6 poor metabolizers, C_{max} and AUC of the active metabolite of fesoterodine increased 2.1- and 2.5-fold, respectively, during co-administration of ketoconazole 200 mg twice a day for 5 days. C_{max} and AUC were 4.5- and 5.7-fold higher, respectively, in subjects who were CYP2D6 poor metabolizers and taking ketoconazole compared to subjects who were CYP2D6 extensive metabolizers and not taking ketoconazole. In a separate study coadministering fesoterodine with ketoconazole 200 mg once a day for 5 days, the C_{max} and AUC values of the active metabolite of fesoterodine were increased 2.2-fold in CYP2D6 extensive metabolizers and 1.5- and 1.9-fold, respectively, in CYP2D6 poor metabolizers.

C_{max} and AUC were 3.4- and 4.2-fold higher, respectively, in subjects who were CYP2D6 poor metabolizers and taking ketoconazole compared to subjects who were CYP2D6 extensive metabolizers and not taking ketoconazole.

Therefore, doses of Toviaz greater than 4mg are not recommended in patients taking potent CYP3A4 inhibitors, such as ketoconazole, itraconazole and clarithromycin [see **DRUG INTERACTIONS** (7.2)], **WARNINGS AND PRECAUTIONS** (5.6) and **DOSAGE AND ADMINISTRATION** (2)].

The effects of weak or moderate CYP3A4 inhibitors were not examined.

CYP3A4 Inducers: Following induction of CYP3A4 by coadministration of rifampicin 600 mg once a day, C_{max} and AUC of the active metabolite of fesoterodine decreased by approximately 70% and 75%, respectively, after oral administration of Toviaz 8 mg. The terminal half-life of the active metabolite was not changed.

Induction of CYP3A4 may lead to reduced plasma levels. No dosing adjustments are recommended in the presence of CYP3A4 inducers [see **DRUG INTERACTIONS** (7.3)].

CYP2D6 Inhibitors: The interaction with CYP2D6 inhibitors was not studied. In poor metabolizers for CYP2D6, representing a maximum CYP2D6 inhibition, C_{max} and AUC of the active metabolite are increased 1.7- and 2-fold, respectively.

No dosing adjustments are recommended in the presence of CYP2D6 inhibitors [see **DRUG INTERACTIONS** (7.4)].

Oral Contraceptives: Thirty healthy female subjects taking an oral contraceptive containing 0.03 mg ethinyl estradiol and 0.15 mg levonorgestrel were evaluated in a 2-period crossover study. Each subject was randomized to receive concomitant administration of either placebo or fesoterodine 8 mg once daily on days 1–14 of hormone cycle for 2 consecutive cycles. Pharmacokinetics of ethinyl estradiol and levonorgestrel were assessed on day 13 of each cycle. Fesoterodine increased the AUC and C_{max} of ethinyl estradiol by 1–3% and decreased the AUC and C_{max} of levonorgestrel by 11–13% [see **DRUG INTERACTIONS** (7.6)].

13   NONCLINICAL TOXICOLOGY

13.1   Carcinogenesis, Mutagenesis, Impairment of Fertility: No evidence of drug-related carcinogenicity was found in 24-month studies with oral administration to mice and rats. The highest tolerated doses in mice (females 45 to 60 mg/kg/day, males 30 to 45 mg/kg/day) correspond to 11to19 times (females) and 4 to 9 times (males) the estimated human AUC values reached with fesoterodine 8 mg, which is the Maximum Recommended Human Dose (MRHD). In rats, the highest tolerated dose (45 to 60 mg/kg/day) corresponds to 3 to 8 times (females) and 3 to 14 times (males), the estimated human AUC at the MRHD.

Fesoterodine was not mutagenic or genotoxic in vitro (Ames tests, chromosome aberration tests) or in vivo (mouse micronucleus test).

Fesoterodine had no effect on reproductive function, fertility, or early embryonic development of the fetus at non-maternally toxic doses in mice. The maternal No-Observed-Effect Level (NOEL) and the NOEL for effects on reproduction and early embryonic development were both 15 mg/kg/day. Based on AUC, the systemic exposure was 0.6 to 1.5 times higher in mice than in humans at the MRHD, whereas based on peak plasma concentrations, the exposure in mice was 5 to 9 times higher. The Lowest-Observed-Effect Level (LOEL) for maternal toxicity was 45 mg/kg/day.

14   CLINICAL STUDIES

Toviaz extended-release tablets were evaluated in two, Phase 3, randomized, double-blind, placebo-controlled, 12-week studies for the treatment of overactive bladder with symptoms of urge urinary incontinence, urgency, and urinary frequency. Entry criteria required that patients have symptoms of overactive bladder for ≥ 6-months duration, at least 8 micturitions per day, and at least 6 urinary urgency episodes or 3 urge incontinence episodes per 3-day diary period. Patients were randomized to a fixed dose of Toviaz 4 or 8 mg/day or placebo. In one of these studies, 290 patients were randomized to an active control arm (an oral antimuscarinic agent). For the combined studies, a total of 554 patients received placebo, 554 patients received Toviaz 4 mg/day, and 566 patients received Toviaz 8 mg/day. The majority of patients were Caucasian (91%) and female (79%) with a mean age of 58 years (range 19-91 years).

The primary efficacy endpoints were the mean change in the number of urge urinary incontinence episodes per 24 hours and the mean change in the number of micturitions (frequency) per 24 hours. An important secondary endpoint was the mean change in the voided volume per micturition.

Results for the primary endpoints and for mean change in voided volume per micturition from the two 12-week clinical studies of Toviaz are reported in Table 2.

[See table 2 at left]

Figures 1-4: The following figures show change from baseline over time in number of micturitions and urge urinary incontinence episodes per 24 h in the two studies.

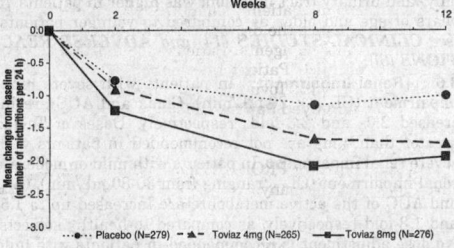

Figure 1: Change in Number of Micturitions per 24 h (Study 1)

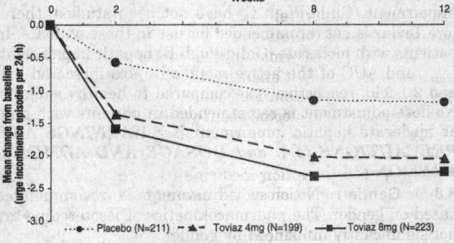

Figure 2: Change in Urge Incontinence Episodes per 24 h (Study 1)

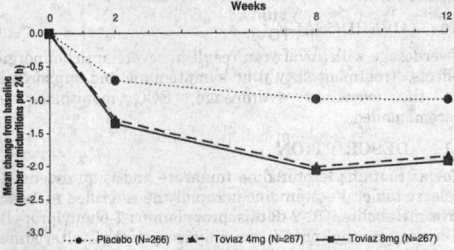

Figure 3: Change in Number of Micturitions per 24 h (Study 2)

[See figure 4 at top of next page]

A reduction in number of urge urinary incontinence episodes per 24 hours was observed for both doses as compared to placebo as early as two weeks after starting Toviaz therapy.

Figure 4: Change in Urge Incontinence Episodes per 24 h (Study 2)

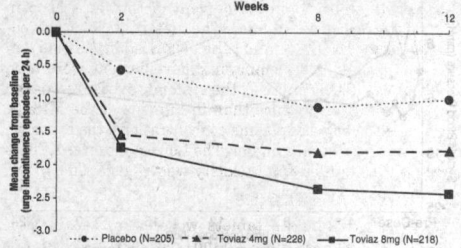

--- Placebo (N=205) --▲-- Toviaz 4mg (N=228) --■-- Toviaz 8mg (N=218)

16   HOW SUPPLIED/STORAGE AND HANDLING

Toviaz (fesoterodine fumarate) extended-release tablets 4 mg are light blue, oval, biconvex, film-coated and engraved with "FS" on one side. They are supplied as follows:

Bottles of 30	NDC 0069-0242-30
Bottles of 90	NDC 0069-0242-68
Unit Dose Package of 100	NDC 0069-0242-41

Toviaz (fesoterodine fumarate) extended-release tablets 8 mg are blue, oval, biconvex, film-coated and engraved with "FT" on one side. They are supplied as follows:

Bottles of 30	NDC 0069-0244-30
Bottles of 90	NDC 0069-0244-68
Unit Dose Package of 100	NDC 0069-0244-41

Store at 20° to 25°C (68° to 77°F); excursions permitted between 15° to 30°C (59° to 86°F) [see USP Controlled Room Temperature]. Protect from moisture.

17   PATIENT COUNSELING INFORMATION

See FDA-Approved Patient Labeling (17.2)

17.1   Information for Patients:

Patients should be informed that Toviaz, like other antimuscarinic agents, may produce clinically significant adverse effects related to antimuscarinic pharmacological activity including constipation and urinary retention. Toviaz, like other antimuscarinics, may be associated with blurred vision, therefore, patients should be advised to exercise caution until the drug's effects on the patient have been determined. Heat prostration (due to decreased sweating) can occur when Toviaz, like other antimuscarinic drugs, is used in a hot environment. Patients should also be informed that alcohol may enhance the drowsiness caused by Toviaz, like other anticholinergic agents. Patients should read the patient leaflet entitled "Patient Information TOVIAZ" before starting therapy with Toviaz.

17.2   FDA Approved Patient Labeling

Rx Only
Manufactured by:
SCHWARZ PHARMA PRODUKTIONS-GmbH
08056 Zwickau, Germany
Distributed by:
Pfizer Labs
Division of Pfizer Inc, NY, NY 10017
LAB-0381-4.0
Revised March 2010

Patient Information
TOVIAZ® (TOH-vee-as)
(fesoterodine fumarate)
extended-release tablets

Read the Patient Information that comes with TOVIAZ before you start taking it and each time you get a refill. There may be new information. This leaflet does not take the place of talking with your doctor about your medical condition or your treatment.

What is TOVIAZ?
TOVIAZ is a prescription medicine used in **adults** to treat symptoms of a condition called **overactive bladder**, including:
• Urge urinary incontinence—leaking or wetting accidents due to a strong need to urinate,
• Urinary urgency—having a strong need to urinate right away,
• Urinary frequency—having to urinate too often.
TOVIAZ has not been studied in children.

Who should not take TOVIAZ?
Do not take TOVIAZ if you:
• Are not able to empty your bladder (urinary retention)
• Have delayed or slow emptying of your stomach (gastric retention)
• Have an eye problem called "uncontrolled narrow-angle glaucoma"
• Are allergic to TOVIAZ or any of its ingredients. See the end of this leaflet for a complete list of ingredients.

What should I tell my doctor before starting TOVIAZ?
Before starting TOVIAZ, tell your doctor about all of your medical and other conditions that may affect the use of TOVIAZ, including:
• Stomach or intestinal problems or problems with constipation
• Problems emptying your bladder or if you have a weak urine stream

• Treatment for an eye problem called narrow-angle glaucoma
• Kidney problems
• Liver problems
• A condition called myasthenia gravis
• If you are pregnant or trying to become pregnant. It is not known if TOVIAZ can harm your unborn baby.
• If you are breastfeeding. It is not known if TOVIAZ passes into breast milk or if it can harm your baby. Talk to your doctor about the best way to feed your baby if you take TOVIAZ.

Before starting on TOVIAZ, tell your doctor about all the medicines you take, including prescription and nonprescription medicines, vitamins and herbal products. Toviaz may affect the way other medicines work, and other medicines may affect how TOVIAZ works. Especially tell your doctor if you are taking antibiotics or antifungal medicines.

Know all the medicines you take. Keep a list of them with you to show your doctor and pharmacist each time you get a new medicine.

How should I take TOVIAZ?
• Take TOVIAZ exactly as your doctor tells you to take it.
• Your doctor may give you the lower 4 mg dose of Toviaz if you have certain medical conditions, such as severe kidney problems.
• Take TOVIAZ with liquid and swallow the tablet whole. Do not chew, divide, or crush the tablet.
• You can take TOVIAZ with or without food.
• If you miss a dose of TOVIAZ, begin taking TOVIAZ again the next day. Do not take 2 doses of TOVIAZ in the same day.

If you take too much TOVIAZ, call your doctor or go to an emergency department right away.

What are the possible side effects of TOVIAZ?
The most common side effects of TOVIAZ are:
• Dry mouth
• Constipation
TOVIAZ may cause other less common side effects, including:
• Dry eyes
• Trouble emptying the bladder
Tell your doctor if you have any side effects that bother you or that do not go away.
Call your doctor for medical advice about side effects. You may report side effects to the FDA at 1-800-FDA-1088.
These are not all of the possible side effects of TOVIAZ. For a complete list, ask your doctor.

What else should I keep in mind while taking TOVIAZ?
• Use caution in driving, operating machinery, or doing other dangerous activities until you know how TOVIAZ affects you. Blurred vision and drowsiness are possible side effects of medicines such as TOVIAZ.
• Use caution in hot environments. Decreased sweating and severe heat illness can occur when medicines such as TOVIAZ are used in a hot environment.
• Drinking alcohol while taking medicines such as TOVIAZ may cause increased drowsiness.

How should I store TOVIAZ?
• Store TOVIAZ at room temperature, 68° to 77°F (20° to 25°C); brief periods permitted between 59° to 86°F (15° to 30°C)
• Protect the medicine from moisture by keeping the bottle closed tightly.
• Safely throw away TOVIAZ that is out of date or no longer needed.

Keep TOVIAZ and all medicines out of the reach of children.

General information about TOVIAZ
Medicines are sometimes prescribed for conditions that are not mentioned in patient information leaflets. Only use TOVIAZ the way your doctor tells you. Do not give TOVIAZ to other people, even if they have the same symptoms you have. It may harm them.
This leaflet summarizes the most important information about TOVIAZ. If you would like more information, talk with your doctor. You can ask your doctor for information about TOVIAZ that is written for healthcare professionals. You can also call 1-877-9-TOVIAZ (1-877-986-8429) or go to www.TOVIAZ.com.

What are the ingredients in TOVIAZ?
Active ingredient: fesoterodine fumarate
Inactive ingredients: glyceryl behenate, hypromellose, indigo carmine aluminum lake, lactose monohydrate, soya lecithin, microcrystalline cellulose, polyethylene glycol, polyvinyl alcohol, talc, titanium dioxide, and xylitol.
Manufactured by:
SCHWARZ PHARMA PRODUKTIONS-GmbH
08056 Zwickau, Germany
Distributed by:
Pfizer Labs
Division of Pfizer Inc, NY, NY 10017
LAB-0382-4.0
Revised March 2010

VIAGRA®
[vI-AG-ra]
(sildenafil citrate)
Tablets

Rx

DESCRIPTION

VIAGRA®, an oral therapy for erectile dysfunction, is the citrate salt of sildenafil, a selective inhibitor of cyclic guanosine monophosphate (cGMP)-specific phosphodiesterase type 5 (PDE5).

Sildenafil citrate is designated chemically as 1-[[3-(6,7-dihydro-1-methyl-7-oxo-3-propyl-1*H*-pyrazolo[4,3-*d*]pyrimidin-5-yl)-4-ethoxyphenyl]sulfonyl]-4-methylpiperazine citrate and has the following structural formula:

Sildenafil citrate is a white to off-white crystalline powder with a solubility of 3.5 mg/mL in water and a molecular weight of 666.7. VIAGRA (sildenafil citrate) is formulated as blue, film-coated rounded-diamond-shaped tablets equivalent to 25 mg, 50 mg and 100 mg of sildenafil for oral administration. In addition to the active ingredient, sildenafil citrate, each tablet contains the following inactive ingredients: microcrystalline cellulose, anhydrous dibasic calcium phosphate, croscarmellose sodium, magnesium stearate, hypromellose, titanium dioxide, lactose, triacetin, and FD & C Blue #2 aluminum lake.

CLINICAL PHARMACOLOGY

Mechanism of Action
The physiologic mechanism of erection of the penis involves release of nitric oxide (NO) in the corpus cavernosum during sexual stimulation. NO then activates the enzyme guanylate cyclase, which results in increased levels of cyclic guanosine monophosphate (cGMP), producing smooth muscle relaxation in the corpus cavernosum and allowing inflow of blood. Sildenafil has no direct relaxant effect on isolated human corpus cavernosum, but enhances the effect of nitric oxide (NO) by inhibiting phosphodiesterase type 5 (PDE5), which is responsible for degradation of cGMP in the corpus cavernosum. When sexual stimulation causes local release of NO, inhibition of PDE5 by sildenafil causes increased levels of cGMP in the corpus cavernosum, resulting in smooth muscle relaxation and inflow of blood to the corpus cavernosum. Sildenafil at recommended doses has no effect in the absence of sexual stimulation.

Studies *in vitro* have shown that sildenafil is selective for PDE5. Its effect is more potent on PDE5 than on other known phosphodiesterases (10-fold for PDE6, >80-fold for PDE1, >700-fold for PDE2, PDE3, PDE4, PDE7, PDE8, PDE9, PDE10, and PDE11). The approximately 4,000-fold selectivity for PDE5 versus PDE3 is important because PDE3 is involved in control of cardiac contractility. Sildenafil is only about 10-fold as potent for PDE5 compared to PDE6, an enzyme found in the retina which is involved in the phototransduction pathway of the retina. This lower selectivity is thought to be the basis for abnormalities related to color vision observed with higher doses or plasma levels (see **Pharmacodynamics**).

In addition to human corpus cavernosum smooth muscle, PDE5 is also found in lower concentrations in other tissues including platelets, vascular and visceral smooth muscle, and skeletal muscle. The inhibition of PDE5 in these tissues by sildenafil may be the basis for the enhanced platelet antiaggregatory activity of nitric oxide observed *in vitro*, an inhibition of platelet thrombus formation *in vivo* and peripheral arterial-venous dilatation *in vivo*.

Pharmacokinetics and Metabolism
VIAGRA is rapidly absorbed after oral administration, with a mean absolute bioavailability of 41% (range 25-63%). Its pharmacokinetics are dose-proportional over the recommended dose range. It is eliminated predominantly by hepatic metabolism (mainly cytochrome P450 3A4) and is converted to an active metabolite with properties similar to the parent, sildenafil. The concomitant use of potent cytochrome P450 3A4 inhibitors (e.g., erythromycin, ketoconazole, itraconazole) as well as the nonspecific CYP inhibitor, cimetidine, is associated with increased plasma levels of sildenafil (see **DOSAGE AND ADMINISTRATION**). Both sildenafil and the metabolite have terminal half lives of about 4 hours.

Mean sildenafil plasma concentrations measured after the administration of a single oral dose of 100 mg to healthy male volunteers is depicted below:

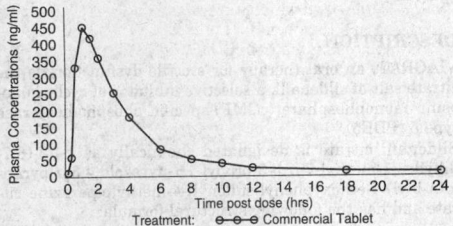

Figure 1: Mean Sildenafil Plasma Concentrations in Healthy Male Volunteers.

Absorption and Distribution: VIAGRA is rapidly absorbed. Maximum observed plasma concentrations are reached within 30 to 120 minutes (median 60 minutes) of oral dosing in the fasted state. When VIAGRA is taken with a high fat meal, the rate of absorption is reduced, with a mean delay in T_{max} of 60 minutes and a mean reduction in C_{max} of 29%. The mean steady state volume of distribution (Vss) for sildenafil is 105 L, indicating distribution into the tissues. Sildenafil and its major circulating N-desmethyl metabolite are both approximately 96% bound to plasma proteins. Protein binding is independent of total drug concentrations. Based upon measurements of sildenafil in semen of healthy volunteers 90 minutes after dosing, less than 0.001% of the administered dose may appear in the semen of patients.

Metabolism and Excretion: Sildenafil is cleared predominantly by the CYP3A4 (major route) and CYP2C9 (minor route) hepatic microsomal isoenzymes. The major circulating metabolite results from N-desmethylation of sildenafil, and is itself further metabolized. This metabolite has a PDE selectivity profile similar to sildenafil and an *in vitro* potency for PDE5 approximately 50% of the parent drug. Plasma concentrations of this metabolite are approximately 40% of those seen for sildenafil, so that the metabolite accounts for about 20% of sildenafil's pharmacologic effects.

After either oral or intravenous administration, sildenafil is excreted as metabolites predominantly in the feces (approximately 80% of administered oral dose) and to a lesser extent in the urine (approximately 13% of the administered oral dose). Similar values for pharmacokinetic parameters were seen in normal volunteers and in the patient population, using a population pharmacokinetic approach.

Pharmacokinetics in Special Populations

Geriatrics: Healthy elderly volunteers (65 years or over) had a reduced clearance of sildenafil, resulting in approximately 84% and 107% higher plasma AUC values of sildenafil and its active N-desmethyl metabolite, respectively, compared to those seen in healthy younger volunteers (18-45 years). Due to age-differences in plasma protein binding, the corresponding increase in the AUC of free (unbound) sildenafil and its active N-desmethyl metabolite were 45% and 57%, respectively.

Renal Insufficiency: In volunteers with mild (CLcr=50-80 mL/min) and moderate (CLcr=30-49 mL/min) renal impairment, the pharmacokinetics of a single oral dose of VIAGRA (50 mg) were not altered. In volunteers with severe (CLcr=<30 mL/min) renal impairment, sildenafil clearance was reduced, resulting in approximately doubling of AUC and C_{max} compared to age-matched volunteers with no renal impairment.

In addition, N-desmethyl metabolite AUC and C_{max} values significantly increased 200% and 79% respectively in subjects with severe renal impairment compared to subjects with normal renal function.

Hepatic Insufficiency: In volunteers with hepatic cirrhosis (Child-Pugh A and B), sildenafil clearance was reduced, resulting in increases in AUC (85%) and C_{max} (47%) compared to age-matched volunteers with no hepatic impairment. The pharmacokinetics of sildenafil in patients with severely impaired hepatic function (Child Pugh class C) have not been studied.

Therefore, age >65, hepatic impairment and severe renal impairment are associated with increased plasma levels of sildenafil. A starting oral dose of 25 mg should be considered in those patients (see **DOSAGE AND ADMINISTRATION**).

Pharmacodynamics

Effects of VIAGRA on Erectile Response: In eight double-blind, placebo-controlled crossover studies of patients with either organic or psychogenic erectile dysfunction, sexual stimulation resulted in improved erections, as assessed by an objective measurement of hardness and duration of erections (RigiScan®), after VIAGRA administration compared with placebo. Most studies assessed the efficacy of VIAGRA approximately 60 minutes post dose. The erectile response, as assessed by RigiScan®, generally increased with increasing sildenafil dose and plasma concentration. The time course of effect was examined in one study, showing an effect for up to 4 hours but the response was diminished compared to 2 hours.

Effects of VIAGRA on Blood Pressure: Single oral doses of sildenafil (100 mg) administered to healthy volunteers produced decreases in sitting blood pressure (mean maximum decrease in systolic/diastolic blood pressure of 8.3/5.3 mmHg). The decrease in sitting blood pressure was most notable approximately 1-2 hours after dosing, and was not different than placebo at 8 hours. Similar effects on blood pressure were noted with 25 mg, 50 mg and 100 mg of VIAGRA, therefore the effects are not related to dose or plasma levels within this dosage range. Larger effects were recorded among patients receiving concomitant nitrates (see **CONTRAINDICATIONS**).

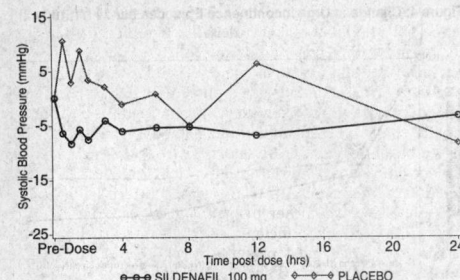

Figure 2: Mean Change from Baseline in Sitting Systolic Blood Pressure, Healthy Volunteers.

Effects of VIAGRA on Cardiac Parameters: Single oral doses of sildenafil up to 100 mg produced no clinically relevant changes in the ECGs of normal male volunteers. Studies have produced relevant data on the effects of VIAGRA on cardiac output. In one small, open-label, uncontrolled, pilot study, eight patients with stable ischemic heart disease underwent Swan-Ganz catheterization. A total dose of 40 mg sildenafil was administered by four intravenous infusions.

The results from this pilot study are shown in Table 1; the mean resting systolic and diastolic blood pressures decreased by 7% and 10% compared to baseline in these patients. Mean resting values for right atrial pressure, pulmonary artery pressure, pulmonary artery occluded pressure and cardiac output decreased by 28%, 28%, 20% and 7% respectively. Even though this total dosage produced plasma sildenafil concentrations which were approximately 2 to 5 times higher than the mean maximum plasma concentrations following a single oral dose of 100 mg in healthy male volunteers, the hemodynamic response to exercise was preserved in these patients.

[See table 1 below]

In a double-blind study, 144 patients with erectile dysfunction and chronic stable angina limited by exercise, not receiving chronic oral nitrates, were randomized to a single dose of placebo or VIAGRA 100 mg 1 hour prior to exercise testing. The primary endpoint was time to limiting angina in the evaluable cohort. The mean times (adjusted for baseline) to onset of limiting angina were 423.6 and 403.7 seconds for sildenafil (N=70) and placebo, respectively. These results demonstrated that the effect of VIAGRA on the primary endpoint was statistically non-inferior to placebo.

Effects of VIAGRA on Vision: At single oral doses of 100 mg and 200 mg, transient dose-related impairment of color discrimination (blue/green) was detected using the Farnsworth-Munsell 100-hue test, with peak effects near the time of peak plasma levels. This finding is consistent with the inhibition of PDE6, which is involved in phototransduction in the retina. An evaluation of visual function at doses up to twice the maximum recommended dose revealed no effects of VIAGRA on visual acuity, intraocular pressure, or pupillometry.

Clinical Studies

In clinical studies, VIAGRA was assessed for its effect on the ability of men with erectile dysfunction (ED) to engage in sexual activity and in many cases specifically on the ability to achieve and maintain an erection sufficient for satisfactory sexual activity. VIAGRA was evaluated primarily at doses of 25 mg, 50 mg and 100 mg in 21 randomized, double-blind, placebo-controlled trials of up to 6 months in duration, using a variety of study designs (fixed dose, titration, parallel, crossover). VIAGRA was administered to more than 3,000 patients aged 19 to 87 years, with ED of various etiologies (organic, psychogenic, mixed) with a mean duration of 5 years. VIAGRA demonstrated statistically significant improvement compared to placebo in all 21 studies. The studies that established benefit demonstrated improvements in success rates for sexual intercourse compared with placebo.

The effectiveness of VIAGRA was evaluated in most studies using several assessment instruments. The primary measure in the principal studies was a sexual function questionnaire (the International Index of Erectile Function - IIEF) administered during a 4-week treatment-free run-in period, at baseline, at follow-up visits, and at the end of double-blind, placebo-controlled, at-home treatment. Two of the questions from the IIEF served as primary study endpoints; categorical responses were elicited to questions about (1) the ability to achieve erections sufficient for sexual intercourse and (2) the maintenance of erections after penetration. The patient addressed both questions at the final visit for the last 4 weeks of the study. The possible categorical responses to these questions were (0) no attempted intercourse, (1) never or almost never, (2) a few times, (3) sometimes, (4) most times, and (5) almost always or always. Also collected as part of the IIEF was information about other aspects of sexual function, including information on erectile function, orgasm, desire, satisfaction with intercourse, and overall sexual satisfaction. Sexual function data were also

TABLE 1. HEMODYNAMIC DATA IN PATIENTS WITH STABLE ISCHEMIC HEART DISEASE AFTER IV ADMINISTRATION OF 40 MG SILDENAFIL

Means ± SD	At rest			
	n	Baseline (B2)	n	Sildenafil (D1)
PAOP (mmHg)	8	8.1 ± 5.1	8	6.5 ± 4.3
Mean PAP (mmHg)	8	16.7 ± 4	8	12.1 ± 3.9
Mean RAP (mmHg)	7	5.7 ± 3.7	8	4.1 ± 3.7
Systolic SAP (mmHg)	8	150.4 ± 12.4	8	140.6 ± 16.5
Diastolic SAP (mmHg)	8	73.6 ± 7.8	8	65.9 ± 10
Cardiac output (L/min)	8	5.6 ± 0.9	8	5.2 ± 1.1
Heart rate (bpm)	8	67 ± 11.1	8	66.9 ± 12

Means ± SD	After 4 minutes of exercise			
	n	Baseline	n	Sildenafil
PAOP (mmHg)	8	36.0 ± 13.7	8	27.8 ± 15.3
Mean PAP (mmHg)	8	39.4 ± 12.9	8	31.7 ± 13.2
Mean RAP (mmHg)	-	-	-	-
Systolic SAP (mmHg)	8	199.5 ± 37.4	8	187.8 ± 30.0
Diastolic SAP (mmHg)	8	84.6 ± 9.7	8	79.5 ± 9.4
Cardiac output (L/min)	8	11.5 ± 2.4	8	10.2 ± 3.5
Heart rate (bpm)	8	101.9 ± 11.6	8	99.0 ± 20.4

recorded by patients in a daily diary. In addition, patients were asked a global efficacy question and an optional partner questionnaire was administered.

The effect on one of the major end points, maintenance of erections after penetration, is shown in Figure 3, for the pooled results of 5 fixed-dose, dose-response studies of greater than one month duration, showing response according to baseline function. Results with all doses have been pooled, but scores showed greater improvement at the 50 and 100 mg doses than at 25 mg. The pattern of responses was similar for the other principal question, the ability to achieve an erection sufficient for intercourse. The titration studies, in which most patients received 100 mg, showed similar results. Figure 3 shows that regardless of the baseline levels of function, subsequent function in patients treated with VIAGRA was better than that seen in patients treated with placebo. At the same time, on-treatment function was better in treated patients who were less impaired at baseline.

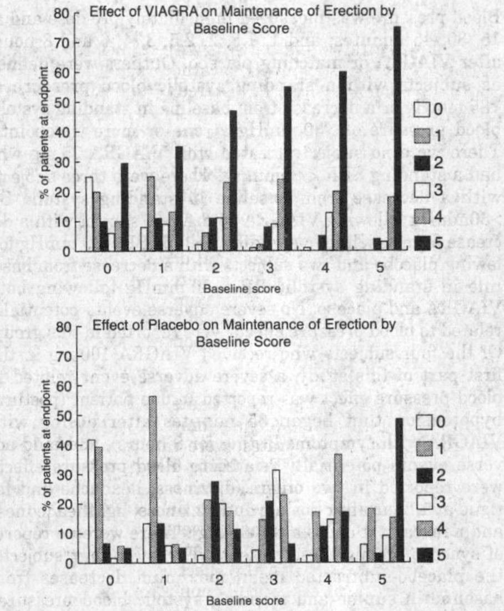

Figure 3. Effect of VIAGRA and Placebo on Maintenance of Erection by Baseline Score.

The frequency of patients reporting improvement of erections in response to a global question in four of the randomized, double-blind, parallel, placebo-controlled fixed dose studies (1797 patients) of 12 to 24 weeks duration is shown in Figure 4. These patients had erectile dysfunction at baseline that was characterized by median categorical scores of 2 (a few times) on principal IIEF questions. Erectile dysfunction was attributed to organic (58%; generally not characterized, but including diabetes and excluding spinal cord injury), psychogenic (17%), or mixed (24%) etiologies. Sixty-three percent, 74%, and 82% of the patients on 25 mg, 50 mg and 100 mg of VIAGRA, respectively, reported an improvement in their erections, compared to 24% on placebo. In the titration studies (n=644) (with most patients eventually receiving 100 mg), results were similar.

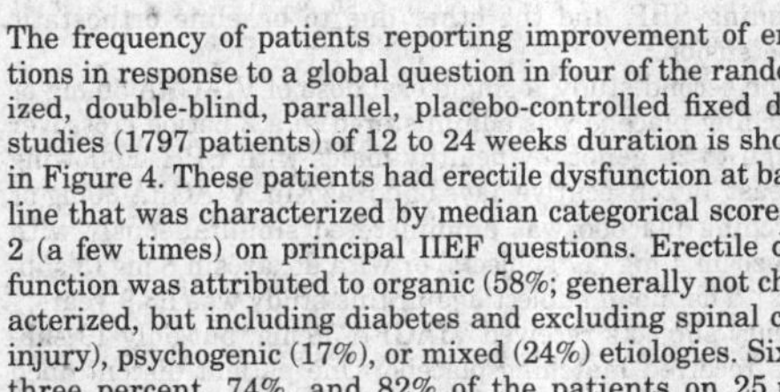

Overall treatment p<0.0001

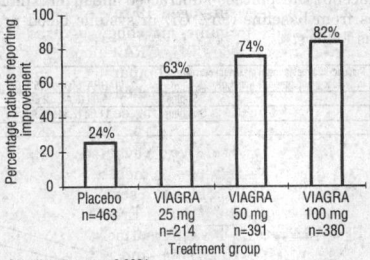

Figure 4. Percentage of Patients Reporting an Improvement in Erections.

The patients in studies had varying degrees of ED. One-third to one-half of the subjects in these studies reported successful intercourse *at least once* during a 4-week, treatment-free run-in period.

In many of the studies, of both fixed dose and titration designs, daily diaries were kept by patients. In these studies, involving about 1600 patients, analyses of patient diaries showed no effect of VIAGRA on rates of attempted intercourse (about 2 per week), but there was clear treatment-related improvement in sexual function: per patient weekly success rates averaged 1.3 on 50-100 mg of VIAGRA vs 0.4 on placebo; similarly, group mean success rates (total successes divided by total attempts) were about 66% on VIAGRA vs about 20% on placebo.

During 3 to 6 months of double-blind treatment or longer-term (1 year), open-label studies, few patients withdrew from active treatment for any reason, including lack of effectiveness. At the end of the long-term study, 88% of patients reported that VIAGRA improved their erections.

Men with untreated ED had relatively low baseline scores for all aspects of sexual function measured (again using a 5-point scale) in the IIEF. VIAGRA improved these aspects of sexual function: frequency, firmness and maintenance of erections; frequency of orgasm; frequency and level of desire; frequency, satisfaction and enjoyment of intercourse; and overall relationship satisfaction.

One randomized, double-blind, flexible-dose, placebo-controlled study included only patients with erectile dysfunction attributed to complications of diabetes mellitus (n=268). As in the other titration studies, patients were started on 50 mg and allowed to adjust the dose up to 100 mg or down to 25 mg of VIAGRA; all patients, however, were receiving 50 mg or 100 mg at the end of the study. There were highly statistically significant improvements on the two principal IIEF questions (frequency of successful penetration during sexual activity and maintenance of erections after penetration) on VIAGRA compared to placebo. On a global improvement question, 57% of VIAGRA patients reported improved erections versus 10% on placebo. Diary data indicated that on VIAGRA, 48% of intercourse attempts were successful versus 12% on placebo.

One randomized, double-blind, placebo-controlled, crossover, flexible-dose (up to 100 mg) study of patients with erectile dysfunction resulting from spinal cord injury (n=178) was conducted. The changes from baseline in scoring on the two end point questions (frequency of successful penetration during sexual activity and maintenance of erections after penetration) were highly statistically significantly in favor of VIAGRA. On a global improvement question, 83% of patients reported improved erections on VIAGRA versus 12% on placebo. Diary data indicated that on VIAGRA, 59% of attempts at sexual intercourse were successful compared to 13% on placebo.

Across all trials, VIAGRA improved the erections of 43% of radical prostatectomy patients compared to 15% on placebo.

Subgroup analyses of responses to a global improvement question in patients with psychogenic etiology in two fixed-dose studies (total n=179) and two titration studies (total n=149) showed 84% of VIAGRA patients reported improvement in erections compared with 26% of placebo. The changes from baseline in scoring on the two end point questions (frequency of successful penetration during sexual activity and maintenance of erections after penetration) were highly statistically significantly in favor of VIAGRA. Diary data in two of the studies (n=178) showed rates of successful intercourse per attempt of 70% for VIAGRA and 29% for placebo.

A review of population subgroups demonstrated efficacy regardless of baseline severity, etiology, race and age. VIAGRA was effective in a broad range of ED patients, including those with a history of coronary artery disease, hypertension, other cardiac disease, peripheral vascular disease, diabetes mellitus, depression, coronary artery bypass graft (CABG), radical prostatectomy, transurethral resection of the prostate (TURP) and spinal cord injury, and in patients taking antidepressants/antipsychotics and antihypertensives/diuretics.

Analysis of the safety database showed no apparent difference in the side effect profile in patients taking VIAGRA with and without antihypertensive medication. This analysis was performed retrospectively, and was not powered to detect any pre-specified difference in adverse reactions.

INDICATION AND USAGE

VIAGRA is indicated for the treatment of erectile dysfunction.

CONTRAINDICATIONS

Consistent with its known effects on the nitric oxide/cGMP pathway (see **CLINICAL PHARMACOLOGY**), VIAGRA was shown to potentiate the hypotensive effects of nitrates, and its administration to patients who are using organic nitrates, either regularly and/or intermittently, in any form is therefore contraindicated.

After patients have taken VIAGRA, it is unknown when nitrates, if necessary, can be safely administered. Based on the pharmacokinetic profile of a single 100 mg oral dose given to healthy normal volunteers, the plasma levels of sildenafil at 24 hours post dose are approximately 2 ng/mL (compared to peak plasma levels of approximately 440 ng/mL) (see **CLINICAL PHARMACOLOGY: Pharmacokinetics and Metabolism**). In the following patients: age >65, hepatic impairment (e.g., cirrhosis), severe renal impairment (e.g., creatinine clearance <30 mL/min), and concomitant use of potent cytochrome P450 3A4 inhibitors (erythromycin), plasma levels of sildenafil at 24 hours post dose have been found to be 3 to 8 times higher than those seen in healthy volunteers. Although plasma levels of sildenafil at 24 hours post dose are much lower than at peak concentration, it is unknown whether nitrates can be safely coadministered at this time point.

VIAGRA is contraindicated in patients with a known hypersensitivity to any component of the tablet.

WARNINGS

There is a potential for cardiac risk of sexual activity in patients with preexisting cardiovascular disease. Therefore, treatments for erectile dysfunction, including VIAGRA, should not be generally used in men for whom sexual activity is inadvisable because of their underlying cardiovascular status.

VIAGRA has systemic vasodilatory properties that resulted in transient decreases in supine blood pressure in healthy volunteers (mean maximum decrease of 8.4/5.5 mmHg), (see **CLINICAL PHARMACOLOGY: Pharmacodynamics**). While this normally would be expected to be of little consequence in most patients, prior to prescribing VIAGRA, physicians should carefully consider whether their patients with underlying cardiovascular disease could be affected adversely by such vasodilatory effects, especially in combination with sexual activity.

Patients with the following underlying conditions can be particularly sensitive to the actions of vasodilators including VIAGRA – those with left ventricular outflow obstruction (e.g. aortic stenosis, idiopathic hypertrophic subaortic stenosis) and those with severely impaired autonomic control of blood pressure.

There is no controlled clinical data on the safety or efficacy of VIAGRA in the following groups; if prescribed, this should be done with caution.

- Patients who have suffered a myocardial infarction, stroke, or life-threatening arrhythmia within the last 6 months;
- Patients with resting hypotension (BP <90/50) or hypertension (BP >170/110);
- Patients with cardiac failure or coronary artery disease causing unstable angina;
- Patients with retinitis pigmentosa (a minority of these patients have genetic disorders of retinal phosphodiesterases).

Prolonged erection greater than 4 hours and priapism (painful erections greater than 6 hours in duration) have been reported infrequently since market approval of VIAGRA. In the event of an erection that persists longer than 4 hours, the patient should seek immediate medical assistance. If priapism is not treated immediately, penile tissue damage and permanent loss of potency could result.

The concomitant administration of the protease inhibitor ritonavir substantially increases serum concentrations of sildenafil (**11-fold increase in AUC**). If VIAGRA is prescribed to patients taking ritonavir, caution should be used. Data from subjects exposed to high systemic levels of sildenafil are limited. Visual disturbances occurred more commonly at higher levels of sildenafil exposure. Decreased blood pressure, syncope, and prolonged erection were reported in some healthy volunteers exposed to high doses of sildenafil (200-800 mg). To decrease the chance of adverse events in patients taking ritonavir, a decrease in sildenafil dosage is recommended (see **Drug Interactions, ADVERSE REACTIONS** and **DOSAGE AND ADMINISTRATION**).

PRECAUTIONS

General

The evaluation of erectile dysfunction should include a determination of potential underlying causes and the identification of appropriate treatment following a complete medical assessment.

Before prescribing VIAGRA, it is important to note the following:

Caution is advised when Phosphodiesterase Type 5 (PDE5) inhibitors are co-administered with alpha-blockers. PDE5 inhibitors, including VIAGRA, and alpha-adrenergic blocking agents are both vasodilators with blood pressure lowering effects. When vasodilators are used in combination, an additive effect on blood pressure may be anticipated. In some patients, concomitant use of these two drug classes can lower blood pressure significantly (see Drug Interactions) leading to symptomatic hypotension (e.g. dizziness, lightheadedness, fainting).

Consideration should be given to the following:

- Patients should be stable on alpha-blocker therapy prior to initiating a PDE5 inhibitor. Patients who demonstrate hemodynamic instability on alpha-blocker therapy alone are at increased risk of symptomatic hypotension with concomitant use of PDE5 inhibitors.
- In those patients who are stable on alpha-blocker therapy, PDE5 inhibitors should be initiated at the lowest dose.
- In those patients already taking an optimized dose of a PDE5 inhibitor, alpha-blocker therapy should be initiated

at the lowest dose. Stepwise increase in alpha-blocker dose may be associated with further lowering of blood pressure when taking a PDE5 inhibitor.

- Safety of combined use of PDE5 inhibitors and alpha-blockers may be affected by other variables, including intravascular volume depletion and other anti-hypertensive drugs.

Viagra has systemic vasodilatory properties and may augment the blood pressure lowering effect of other anti-hypertensive medications.

Patients on multiple antihypertensive medications were included in the pivotal clinical trials for VIAGRA. In a separate drug interaction study, when amlodipine, 5 mg or 10 mg, and VIAGRA, 100 mg were orally administered concomitantly to hypertensive patients mean additional blood pressure reduction of 8 mmHg systolic and 7 mmHg diastolic were noted (see **Drug Interactions**).

The safety of VIAGRA is unknown in patients with bleeding disorders and patients with active peptic ulceration.

VIAGRA should be used with caution in patients with anatomical deformation of the penis (such as angulation, cavernosal fibrosis or Peyronie's disease), or in patients who have conditions which may predispose them to priapism (such as sickle cell anemia, multiple myeloma, or leukemia).

The safety and efficacy of combinations of VIAGRA with other treatments for erectile dysfunction have not been studied. Therefore, the use of such combinations is not recommended.

In humans, VIAGRA has no effect on bleeding time when taken alone or with aspirin. *In vitro* studies with human platelets indicate that sildenafil potentiates the antiaggregatory effect of sodium nitroprusside (a nitric oxide donor). The combination of heparin and VIAGRA had an additive effect on bleeding time in the anesthetized rabbit, but this interaction has not been studied in humans.

Information for Patients

Physicians should discuss with patients the contraindication of VIAGRA with regular and/or intermittent use of organic nitrates.

Physicians should advise patients of the potential for VIAGRA to augment the blood pressure lowering effect of alpha-blockers and anti-hypertensive medications. Concomitant administration of VIAGRA and an alpha-blocker may lead to symptomatic hypotension in some patients. Therefore, when VIAGRA is co-administered with alpha-blockers, patients should be stable on alpha-blocker therapy prior to initiating VIAGRA treatment and VIAGRA should be initiated at the lowest dose.

Physicians should discuss with patients the potential cardiac risk of sexual activity in patients with preexisting cardiovascular risk factors. Patients who experience symptoms (e.g., angina pectoris, dizziness, nausea) upon initiation of sexual activity should be advised to refrain from further activity and should discuss the episode with their physician.

Physicians should advise patients to stop use of all PDE5 inhibitors, including VIAGRA, and seek medical attention in the event of a sudden loss of vision in one or both eyes. Such an event may be a sign of non-arteritic anterior ischemic optic neuropathy (NAION), a cause of decreased vision including permanent loss of vision, that has been reported rarely post-marketing in temporal association with the use of all PDE5 inhibitors. It is not possible to determine whether these events are related directly to the use of PDE5 inhibitors or to other factors. Physicians should also discuss with patients the increased risk of NAION in individuals who have already experienced NAION in one eye, including whether such individuals could be adversely affected by use of vasodilators, such as PDE5 inhibitors (see **POST-MARKETING EXPERIENCE/Special Senses**).

Physicians should advise patients to stop taking PDE5 inhibitors, including VIAGRA, and seek prompt medical attention in the event of sudden decrease or loss of hearing. These events, which may be accompanied by tinnitus and dizziness, have been reported in temporal association to the intake of PDE5 inhibitors, including VIAGRA. It is not possible to determine whether these events are related directly to the use of PDE5 inhibitors or to other factors (see **ADVERSE REACTIONS, CLINICAL TRIALS and POST-MARKETING EXPERIENCE**).

Physicians should warn patients that prolonged erections greater than 4 hours and priapism (painful erections greater than 6 hours in duration) have been reported infrequently since market approval of VIAGRA. In the event of an erection that persists longer than 4 hours, the patient should seek immediate medical assistance. If priapism is not treated immediately, penile tissue damage and permanent loss of potency may result.

Physicians should inform patients not to take VIAGRA with other PDE5 inhibitors including REVATIO. Sildenafil is also marketed as REVATIO for the treatment of pulmonary arterial hypertension. The safety and efficacy of VIAGRA with other PDE5 inhibitors, including REVATIO, have not been studied.

The use of VIAGRA offers no protection against sexually transmitted diseases. Counseling of patients about the protective measures necessary to guard against sexually transmitted diseases, including the Human Immunodeficiency Virus (HIV), may be considered.

Drug Interactions

Effects of Other Drugs on VIAGRA

***In vitro* studies:** Sildenafil metabolism is principally mediated by the cytochrome P450 (CYP) isoforms 3A4 (major route) and 2C9 (minor route). Therefore, inhibitors of these isoenzymes may reduce sildenafil clearance and inducers of these isoenzymes may increase sildenafil clearance.

***In vivo* studies:** Cimetidine (800 mg), a nonspecific CYP inhibitor, caused a 56% increase in plasma sildenafil concentrations when coadministered with VIAGRA (50 mg) to healthy volunteers.

When a single 100 mg dose of VIAGRA was administered with erythromycin, a specific CYP3A4 inhibitor, at steady state (500 mg bid for 5 days), there was a 182% increase in sildenafil systemic exposure (AUC). In addition, in a study performed in healthy male volunteers, coadministration of the HIV protease inhibitor saquinavir, also a CYP3A4 inhibitor, at steady state (1200 mg tid) with VIAGRA (100 mg single dose) resulted in a 140% increase in sildenafil C_{max} and a 210% increase in sildenafil AUC. VIAGRA had no effect on saquinavir pharmacokinetics. Stronger CYP3A4 inhibitors such as ketoconazole or itraconazole would be expected to have still greater effects, and population data from patients in clinical trials did indicate a reduction in sildenafil clearance when it was coadministered with CYP3A4 inhibitors (such as ketoconazole, erythromycin, or cimetidine) (see **DOSAGE AND ADMINISTRATION**).

In another study in healthy male volunteers, coadministration with the HIV protease inhibitor ritonavir, which is a highly potent P450 inhibitor, at steady state (500 mg bid) with VIAGRA (100 mg single dose) resulted in a 300% (4-fold) increase in sildenafil C_{max} and a 1000% (11-fold) increase in sildenafil plasma AUC. At 24 hours the plasma levels of sildenafil were still approximately 200 ng/mL, compared to approximately 5 ng/mL when sildenafil was dosed alone. This is consistent with ritonavir's marked effects on a broad range of P450 substrates. VIAGRA had no effect on ritonavir pharmacokinetics (see **DOSAGE AND ADMINISTRATION**).

Although the interaction between other protease inhibitors and sildenafil has not been studied, their concomitant use is expected to increase sildenafil levels.

In a study of healthy male volunteers, co-administration of sildenafil at steady state (80 mg t.i.d.) with endothelin receptor antagonist bosentan (a moderate inducer of CYP3A4, CYP2C9 and possibly of cytochrome P450 2C19) at steady state (125 mg b.i.d.) resulted in a 63% decrease of sildenafil AUC and a 55% decrease in sildenafil C_{max}. Concomitant administration of strong CYP3A4 inducers, such as rifampin, is expected to cause greater decreases in plasma levels of sildenafil.

Single doses of antacid (magnesium hydroxide/aluminum hydroxide) did not affect the bioavailability of VIAGRA.

Pharmacokinetic data from patients in clinical trials showed no effect on sildenafil pharmacokinetics of CYP2C9 inhibitors (such as tolbutamide, warfarin), CYP2D6 inhibitors (such as selective serotonin reuptake inhibitors, tricyclic antidepressants), thiazide and related diuretics, ACE inhibitors, and calcium channel blockers. The AUC of the active metabolite, N-desmethyl sildenafil, was increased 62% by loop and potassium-sparing diuretics and 102% by nonspecific beta-blockers. These effects on the metabolite are not expected to be of clinical consequence.

Effects of VIAGRA on Other Drugs

***In vitro* studies:** Sildenafil is a weak inhibitor of the cytochrome P450 isoforms 1A2, 2C9, 2C19, 2D6, 2E1 and 3A4 (IC50 >150 µM). Given sildenafil peak plasma concentrations of approximately 1 µM after recommended doses, it is unlikely that VIAGRA will alter the clearance of substrates of these isoenzymes.

***In vivo* studies:** Three double-blind, placebo-controlled, randomized, two-way crossover studies were conducted to assess the interaction of VIAGRA with doxazosin, an alpha-adrenergic blocking agent.

In the first study, a single oral dose of VIAGRA 100 mg or matching placebo was administered in a 2-period crossover design to 4 generally healthy males with benign prostatic hyperplasia (BPH). Following at least 14 consecutive daily doses of doxazosin, VIAGRA 100 mg or matching placebo was administered simultaneously with doxazosin. Following a review of the data from these first 4 subjects (details provided below), the VIAGRA dose was reduced to 25 mg. Thereafter, 17 subjects were treated with VIAGRA 25 mg or matching placebo in combination with doxazosin 4 mg (15 subjects) or doxazosin 8mg (2 subjects). The mean subject age was 66.5 years.

For the 17 subjects who received VIAGRA 25 mg and matching placebo, the placebo-subtracted mean maximum decreases from baseline (95% CI) in systolic blood pressure were as follows:

Placebo-subtracted mean maximum decrease in systolic blood pressure (mm Hg)	VIAGRA 25 mg
Supine	7.4 (-0.9, 15.7)
Standing	6.0 (-0.8, 12.8)

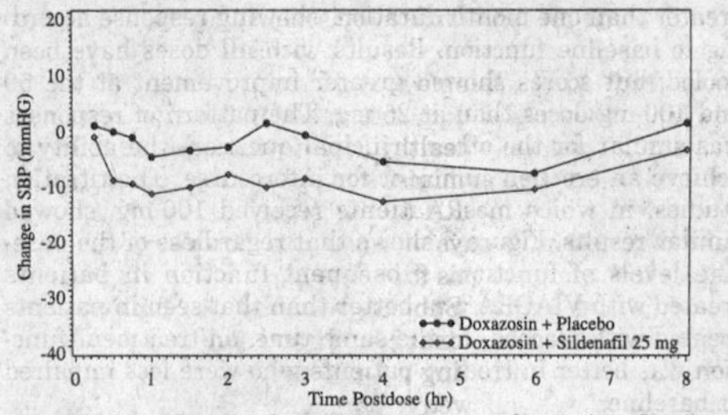

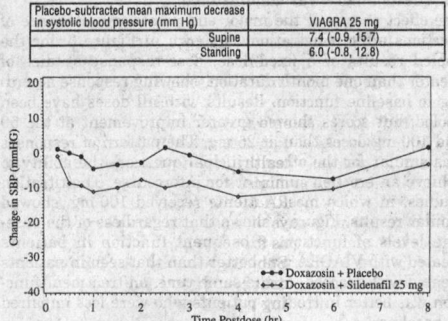

Figure 5: Mean Standing Systolic Blood Pressure Change from Baseline

Blood pressure was measured immediately pre-dose and at 15, 30, 45 minutes, and 1, 1.5, 2, 2.5, 3, 4, 6 and 8 hours after VIAGRA or matching placebo. Outliers were defined as subjects with a standing systolic blood pressure of <85 mmHg or a decrease from baseline in standing systolic blood pressure of >30 mmHg at one or more timepoints. There were no subjects treated with VIAGRA 25 mg who had a standing SBP < 85mmHg. There were three subjects with a decrease from baseline in standing systolic BP >30mmHg following VIAGRA 25 mg, one subject with a decrease from baseline in standing systolic BP > 30 mmHg following placebo and two subjects with a decrease from baseline in standing systolic BP > 30 mmHg following both VIAGRA and placebo. No severe adverse events potentially related to blood pressure effects were reported in this group.

Of the four subjects who received VIAGRA 100 mg in the first part of this study, a severe adverse event related to blood pressure effect was reported in one patient (postural hypotension that began 35 minutes after dosing with VIAGRA with symptoms lasting for 8 hours), and mild adverse events potentially related to blood pressure effects were reported in two others (dizziness, headache and fatigue at 1 hour after dosing; and dizziness, lightheadedness and nausea at 4 hours after dosing). There were no reports of syncope among these patients. For these four subjects, the placebo-subtracted mean maximum decreases from baseline in supine and standing systolic blood pressures were 14.8 mmHg and 21.5 mmHg, respectively. Two of these subjects had a standing SBP < 85mmHg. Both of these subjects were protocol violators, one due to a low baseline standing SBP, and the other due to baseline orthostatic hypotension.

In the second study, a single oral dose of VIAGRA 50 mg or matching placebo was administered in a 2-period crossover design to 20 generally healthy males with BPH. Following at least 14 consecutive days of doxazosin, VIAGRA 50mg or matching placebo was administered simultaneously with doxazosin 4 mg (17 subjects) or with doxazosin 8 mg (3 subjects). The mean subject age in this study was 63.9 years.

Twenty subjects received VIAGRA 50 mg, but only 19 subjects received matching placebo. One patient discontinued the study prematurely due to an adverse event of hypotension following dosing with VIAGRA 50 mg. This patient had been taking minoxidil, a potent vasodilator, during the study.

For the 19 subjects who received both VIAGRA and matching placebo, the placebo-subtracted mean maximum decreases from baseline (95% CI) in systolic blood pressure were as follows:

Placebo-subtracted mean maximum decrease in systolic blood pressure (mm Hg)	VIAGRA 50 mg (95% CI)
Supine	9.08 (5.48, 12.68)
Standing	11.62 (7.34, 15.90)

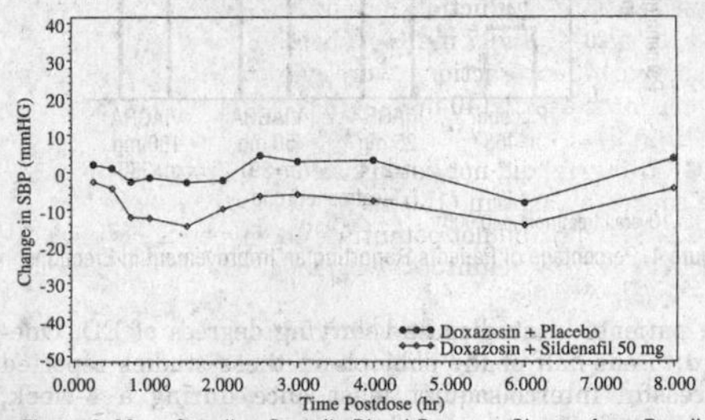

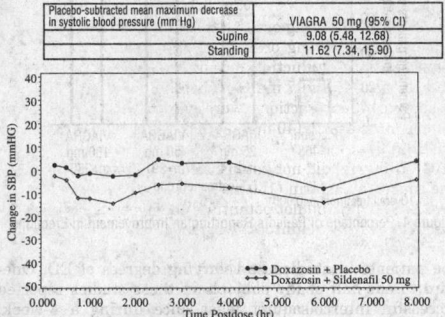

Figure 6: Mean Standing Systolic Blood Pressure Change from Baseline

Blood pressure was measured after administration of VIAGRA at the same times as those specified for the first doxazosin study. There were two subjects who had a standing SBP of < 85 mmHg. In these two subjects, hypotension was reported as a moderately severe adverse event, beginning at approximately 1 hour after administration of

VIAGRA 50 mg and resolving after approximately 7.5 hours. There was one subject with a decrease from baseline in standing systolic BP >30mmHg following VIAGRA 50 mg and one subject with a decrease from baseline in standing systolic BP > 30 mmHg following both VIAGRA 50 mg and placebo. There were no severe adverse events potentially related to blood pressure and no episodes of syncope reported in this study.

In the third study, a single oral dose of VIAGRA 100 mg or matching placebo was administered in a 3-period crossover design to 20 generally healthy males with BPH. In dose period 1, subjects were administered open-label doxazosin and a single dose of VIAGRA 50 mg simultaneously, after at least 14 consecutive days of doxazosin. If a subject did not successfully complete this first dosing period, he was discontinued from the study. Subjects who had successfully completed the previous doxazosin interaction study (using VIAGRA 50 mg), including no significant hemodynamic adverse events, were allowed to skip dose period 1. Treatment with doxazosin continued for at least 7 days after dose period 1. Thereafter, VIAGRA 100mg or matching placebo was administered simultaneously with doxazosin 4 mg (14 subjects) or doxazosin 8 mg (6 subjects) in standard crossover fashion. The mean subject age in this study was 66.4 years. Twenty-five subjects were screened. Two were discontinued after study period 1: one failed to meet pre-dose screening qualifications and the other experienced symptomatic hypotension as a moderately severe adverse event 30 minutes after dosing with open-label VIAGRA 50 mg. Of the twenty subjects who were ultimately assigned to treatment, a total of 13 subjects successfully completed dose period 1, and seven had successfully completed the previous doxazosin study (using VIAGRA 50 mg).

For the 20 subjects who received VIAGRA 100 mg and matching placebo, the placebo-subtracted mean maximum decreases from baseline (95% CI) in systolic blood pressure were as follows:

Placebo-subtracted mean maximum decrease in systolic blood pressure (mm Hg)	VIAGRA 100 mg
Supine	7.9 (4.6, 11.1)
Standing	4.3 (-1.8, 10.3)

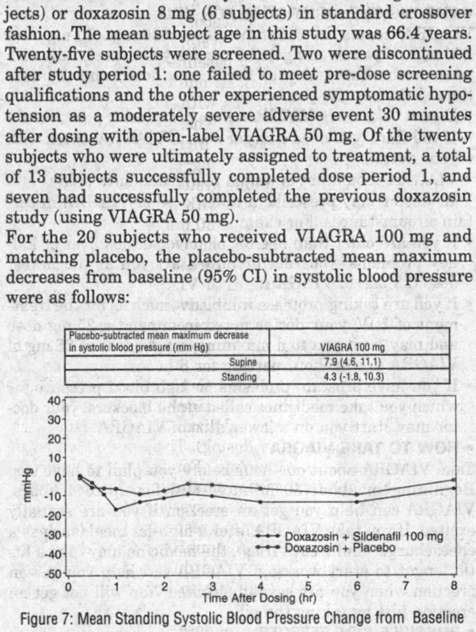

Figure 7: Mean Standing Systolic Blood Pressure Change from Baseline

Blood pressure was measured after administration of VIAGRA at the same times as those specified for the previous doxazosin studies. There were three subjects who had a standing SBP of < 85 mmHg. All three were taking VIAGRA 100 mg, and all three reported mild adverse events at the time of reductions in standing SBP, including vasodilation and lightheadedness. There were four subjects with a decrease from baseline in standing systolic BP >30mmHg following VIAGRA 100 mg, one subject with a decrease from baseline in standing systolic BP > 30 mmHg following placebo and one subject with a decrease from baseline in standing systolic BP > 30 mmHg following both VIAGRA and placebo. While there were no severe adverse events potentially related to blood pressure reported in this study, one subject reported moderate vasodilatation after both VIAGRA 50 mg and 100 mg. There were no episodes of syncope reported in this study.

When VIAGRA 100 mg oral was coadministered with amlodipine, 5 mg or 10 mg oral, to hypertensive patients, the mean additional reduction on supine blood pressure was 8 mmHg systolic and 7 mmHg diastolic.

No significant interactions were shown with tolbutamide (250 mg) or warfarin (40 mg), both of which are metabolized by CYP2C9.

VIAGRA (50 mg) did not potentiate the increase in bleeding time caused by aspirin (150 mg).

VIAGRA (50 mg) did not potentiate the hypotensive effect of alcohol in healthy volunteers with mean maximum blood alcohol levels of 0.08%.

In a study of healthy male volunteers, sildenafil (100 mg) did not affect the steady state pharmacokinetics of the HIV protease *inhibitors, saquinavir and ritonavir,* both of which are CYP3A4 substrates.

Sildenafil at steady state (80 mg t.i.d.) resulted in a 50% increase in AUC and a 42% increase in C_{max} of bosentan (125 mg b.i.d.).

Carcinogenesis, Mutagenesis, Impairment of Fertility

Sildenafil was not carcinogenic when administered to rats for 24 months at a dose resulting in total systemic drug exposure (AUCs) for unbound sildenafil and its major metabolite of 29- and 42-times, for male and female rats, respectively, the exposures observed in human males given the Maximum Recommended Human Dose (MRHD) of 100 mg. Sildenafil was not carcinogenic when administered to mice for 18-21 months at dosages up to the Maximum Tolerated Dose (MTD) of 10 mg/kg/day, approximately 0.6 times the MRHD on a mg/m^2 basis.

Sildenafil was negative in *in vitro* bacterial and Chinese hamster ovary cell assays to detect mutagenicity, and *in vitro* human lymphocytes and *in vivo* mouse micronucleus assays to detect clastogenicity.

There was no impairment of fertility in rats given sildenafil up to 60 mg/kg/day for 36 days to females and 102 days to males, a dose producing an AUC value of more than 25 times the human male AUC.

There was no effect on sperm motility or morphology after single 100 mg oral doses of VIAGRA in healthy volunteers.

Pregnancy, Nursing Mothers and Pediatric Use

VIAGRA is not indicated for use in newborns, children, or women.

Pregnancy Category B. No evidence of teratogenicity, embryotoxicity or fetotoxicity was observed in rats and rabbits which received up to 200 mg/kg/day during organogenesis. These doses represent, respectively, about 20 and 40 times the MRHD on a mg/m^2 basis in a 50 kg subject. In the rat pre- and postnatal development study, the no observed adverse effect dose was 30 mg/kg/day given for 36 days. In the nonpregnant rat the AUC at this dose was about 20 times human AUC. There are no adequate and well-controlled studies of sildenafil in pregnant women.

Geriatric Use: Healthy elderly volunteers (65 years or over) had a reduced clearance of sildenafil (see **CLINICAL PHARMACOLOGY: Pharmacokinetics in Special Populations**). Since higher plasma levels may increase both the efficacy and incidence of adverse events, a starting dose of 25 mg should be considered (see **DOSAGE AND ADMINISTRATION**).

ADVERSE REACTIONS

CLINICAL TRIALS:

VIAGRA was administered to over 3700 patients (aged 19-87 years) during pre-marketing clinical trials worldwide. Over 550 patients were treated for longer than one year.

In placebo-controlled clinical studies, the discontinuation rate due to adverse events for VIAGRA (2.5%) was not significantly different from placebo (2.3%). The adverse events were generally transient and mild to moderate in nature.

In trials of all designs, adverse events reported by patients receiving VIAGRA were generally similar. In fixed-dose studies, the incidence of some adverse events increased with dose. The nature of the adverse events in flexible-dose studies, which more closely reflect the recommended dosage regimen, was similar to that for fixed-dose studies.

When VIAGRA was taken as recommended (on an as-needed basis) in flexible-dose, placebo-controlled clinical trials, the following adverse events were reported:

TABLE 2. ADVERSE EVENTS REPORTED BY ≥2% OF PATIENTS TREATED WITH VIAGRA AND MORE FREQUENT ON DRUG THAN PLACEBO IN PRN FLEXIBLE-DOSE PHASE II/III STUDIES

Adverse Event	Percentage of Patients Reporting Event	
	VIAGRA N=734	PLACEBO N=725
Headache	16%	4%
Flushing	10%	1%
Dyspepsia	7%	2%
Nasal Congestion	4%	2%
Urinary Tract Infection	3%	2%
Abnormal Vision†	3%	0%
Diarrhea	3%	1%
Dizziness	2%	1%
Rash	2%	1%

† Abnormal Vision: Mild and transient, predominantly color tinge to vision, but also increased sensitivity to light or blurred vision. In these studies, only one patient discontinued due to abnormal vision.

Other adverse reactions occurred at a rate of >2%, but equally common on placebo: respiratory tract infection, back pain, flu syndrome, and arthralgia.

In fixed-dose studies, dyspepsia (17%) and abnormal vision (11%) were more common at 100 mg than at lower doses. At doses above the recommended dose range, adverse events were similar to those detailed above but generally were reported more frequently.

The following events occurred in <2% of patients in controlled clinical trials; a causal relationship to VIAGRA is uncertain. Reported events include those with a plausible relation to drug use; omitted are minor events and reports too imprecise to be meaningful:

Body as a whole: face edema, photosensitivity reaction, shock, asthenia, pain, chills, accidental fall, abdominal pain, allergic reaction, chest pain, accidental injury.

Cardiovascular: angina pectoris, AV block, migraine, syncope, tachycardia, palpitation, hypotension, postural hypotension, myocardial ischemia, cerebral thrombosis, cardiac arrest, heart failure, abnormal electrocardiogram, cardiomyopathy.

Digestive: vomiting, glossitis, colitis, dysphagia, gastritis, gastroenteritis, esophagitis, stomatitis, dry mouth, liver function tests abnormal, rectal hemorrhage, gingivitis.

Hemic and Lymphatic: anemia and leukopenia.

Metabolic and Nutritional: thirst, edema, gout, unstable diabetes, hyperglycemia, peripheral edema, hyperuricemia, hypoglycemic reaction, hypernatremia.

Musculoskeletal: arthritis, arthrosis, myalgia, tendon rupture, tenosynovitis, bone pain, myasthenia, synovitis.

Nervous: ataxia, hypertonia, neuralgia, neuropathy, paresthesia, tremor, vertigo, depression, insomnia, somnolence, abnormal dreams, reflexes decreased, hypesthesia.

Respiratory: asthma, dyspnea, laryngitis, pharyngitis, sinusitis, bronchitis, sputum increased, cough increased.

Skin and Appendages: urticaria, herpes simplex, pruritus, sweating, skin ulcer, contact dermatitis, exfoliative dermatitis.

Special Senses: sudden decrease or loss of hearing, mydriasis, conjunctivitis, photophobia, tinnitus, eye pain, ear pain, eye hemorrhage, cataract, dry eyes.

Urogenital: cystitis, nocturia, urinary frequency, breast enlargement, urinary incontinence, abnormal ejaculation, genital edema and anorgasmia.

POST-MARKETING EXPERIENCE:

Cardiovascular and cerebrovascular

Serious cardiovascular, cerebrovascular, and vascular events, including myocardial infarction, sudden cardiac death, ventricular arrhythmia, cerebrovascular hemorrhage, transient ischemic attack, hypertension, subarachnoid and intracerebral hemorrhages, and pulmonary hemorrhage have been reported post-marketing in temporal association with the use of VIAGRA. Most, but not all, of these patients had preexisting cardiovascular risk factors. Many of these events were reported to occur during or shortly after sexual activity, and a few were reported to occur shortly after the use of VIAGRA without sexual activity. Others were reported to have occurred hours to days after the use of VIAGRA and sexual activity. It is not possible to determine whether these events are related directly to VIAGRA, to sexual activity, to the patient's underlying cardiovascular disease, to a combination of these factors, or to other factors (see **WARNINGS** for further important cardiovascular information).

Special senses:

Cases of sudden decrease or loss of hearing have been reported postmarketing in temporal association with the use of PDE5 inhibitors, including VIAGRA. In some of the cases, medical conditions and other factors were reported that may have also played a role in the otologic adverse events. In many cases, medical follow-up information was limited. It is not possible to determine whether these reported events are related directly to the use of VIAGRA, to the patient's underlying risk factors for hearing loss, a combination of these factors, or to other factors (see **PRECAUTIONS, Information for Patients**).

Other events

Other events reported post-marketing to have been observed in temporal association with VIAGRA and not listed in the clinical trial adverse reactions section above include:

Nervous: seizure, seizure recurrence, anxiety, and transient global amnesia.

Urogenital: prolonged erection, priapism (see **WARNINGS**), and hematuria.

Special Senses: diplopia, temporary vision loss/decreased vision, ocular redness or bloodshot appearance, ocular burning, ocular swelling/pressure, increased intraocular pressure, retinal vascular disease or bleeding, vitreous detachment/traction, paramacular edema and epistaxis.

Non-arteritic anterior ischemic optic neuropathy (NAION), a cause of decreased vision including permanent loss of vision, has been reported rarely post-marketing in temporal association with the use of phosphodiesterase type 5 (PDE5) inhibitors, including VIAGRA. Most, but not all, of these patients had underlying anatomic or vascular risk factors for developing NAION, including but not necessarily limited to: low cup to disc ratio ("crowded disc"), age over 50, diabetes, hypertension, coronary artery disease, hyperlipidemia and smoking. It is not possible to determine whether these events are related directly to the use of PDE5 inhibitors, to the patient's underlying vascular risk factors or anatomical defects, to a combination of these factors, or to other factors (see **PRECAUTIONS/Information for Patients**).

OVERDOSAGE

In studies with healthy volunteers of single doses up to 800 mg, adverse events were similar to those seen at lower doses but incidence rates and severities were increased.

	25 mg	50 mg	100 mg
Obverse	VGR25	VGR50	VGR100
Reverse	PFIZER	PFIZER	PFIZER
Bottle of 30	NDC-0069-4200-30	NDC-0069-4210-30	NDC-0069-4220-30
Bottle of 100	N/A	NDC-0069-4210-66	NDC-0069-4220-66

In cases of overdose, standard supportive measures should be adopted as required. Renal dialysis is not expected to accelerate clearance as sildenafil is highly bound to plasma proteins and it is not eliminated in the urine.

DOSAGE AND ADMINISTRATION

For most patients, the recommended dose is 50 mg taken, as needed, approximately 1 hour before sexual activity. However, VIAGRA may be taken anywhere from 4 hours to 0.5 hour before sexual activity. Based on effectiveness and toleration, the dose may be increased to a maximum recommended dose of 100 mg or decreased to 25 mg. The maximum recommended dosing frequency is once per day.

The following factors are associated with increased plasma levels of sildenafil: age >65 (40% increase in AUC), hepatic impairment (e.g., cirrhosis, 80%), severe renal impairment (creatinine clearance <30 mL/min, 100%), and concomitant use of potent cytochrome P450 3A4 inhibitors [ketoconazole, itraconazole, erythromycin (182%), saquinavir (210%)]. Since higher plasma levels may increase both the efficacy and incidence of adverse events, a starting dose of 25 mg should be considered in these patients.

Ritonavir greatly increased the systemic level of sildenafil in a study of healthy, non-HIV infected volunteers (11-fold increase in AUC, see **Drug Interactions**.) Based on these pharmacokinetic data, it is recommended not to exceed a maximum single dose of 25 mg of VIAGRA in a 48 hour period.

VIAGRA was shown to potentiate the hypotensive effects of nitrates and its administration in patients who use nitric oxide donors or nitrates in any form is therefore contraindicated.

When VIAGRA is co-administered with an alpha-blocker, patients should be stable on alpha-blocker therapy prior to initiating VIAGRA treatment and VIAGRA should be initiated at the lowest dose (see **Drug Interactions**).

HOW SUPPLIED

VIAGRA® (sildenafil citrate) is supplied as blue, film-coated, rounded-diamond-shaped tablets containing sildenafil citrate equivalent to the nominally indicated amount of sildenafil as follows:
[See table above]

Recommended Storage: Store at 25°C (77°F); excursions permitted to 15-30°C (59-86°F) [see USP Controlled Room Temperature].

Rx only
Distributed by
Pfizer Labs
Division of Pfizer Inc, NY, NY 10017
LAB-0221-11.0   Revised January 2010

PATIENT SUMMARY OF INFORMATION ABOUT VIAGRA®

(sildenafil citrate) tablets

This summary contains important information about VIAGRA®. It is not meant to take the place of your doctor's instructions. Read this information carefully before you start taking VIAGRA. Ask your doctor or pharmacist if you do not understand any of this information or if you want to know more about VIAGRA.

This medicine can help many men when it is used as prescribed by their doctors. However, VIAGRA is not for everyone. It is intended for use only by men who have a condition called erectile dysfunction. **VIAGRA must never be used by men who are taking medicines that contain nitrates of any kind, at any time. This includes nitroglycerin. If you take VIAGRA with any nitrate medicine your blood pressure could suddenly drop to an unsafe or life threatening level.**

• WHAT IS VIAGRA?

VIAGRA is a pill used to treat erectile dysfunction (impotence) in men. It can help many men who have erectile dysfunction get and keep an erection when they become sexually excited (stimulated).

You will not get an erection just by taking this medicine. VIAGRA helps a man with erectile dysfunction get an erection only when he is sexually excited.

• HOW SEX AFFECTS THE BODY

When a man is sexually excited, the penis rapidly fills with more blood than usual. The penis then expands and hardens. This is called an erection. After the man is done having sex, this extra blood flows out of the penis back into the body. The erection goes away. If an erection lasts for a long

time (more than 6 hours), it can permanently damage your penis. You should call a doctor immediately if you ever have a prolonged erection that lasts more than 4 hours.

Some conditions and medicines interfere with this natural erection process. The penis cannot fill with enough blood. The man cannot have an erection. This is called erectile dysfunction if it becomes a frequent problem.

During sex, your heart works harder. Therefore sexual activity may not be advisable for people who have heart problems. Before you start any treatment for erectile dysfunction, ask your doctor if your heart is healthy enough to handle the extra strain of having sex. If you have chest pains, dizziness or nausea during sex, stop having sex and immediately tell your doctor you have had this problem.

• HOW VIAGRA WORKS

VIAGRA enables many men with erectile dysfunction to respond to sexual stimulation. When a man is sexually excited, VIAGRA helps the penis fill with enough blood to cause an erection. After sex is over, the erection goes away.

• VIAGRA IS NOT FOR EVERYONE

As noted above (*How Sex Affects the Body*), ask your doctor if your heart is healthy enough for sexual activity.

If you take any medicines that contain nitrates – either regularly or as needed – you should never take VIAGRA. If you take VIAGRA with any nitrate medicine or recreational drug containing nitrates, your blood pressure could suddenly drop to an unsafe level. You could get dizzy, faint, or even have a heart attack or stroke. Nitrates are found in many prescription medicines that are used to treat angina (chest pain due to heart disease) such as:

- nitroglycerin (sprays, ointments, skin patches or pastes, and tablets that are swallowed or dissolved in the mouth)
- isosorbide mononitrate and isosorbide dinitrate (tablets that are swallowed, chewed, or dissolved in the mouth)

Nitrates are also found in recreational drugs such as amyl nitrate or nitrite ("poppers"). If you are not sure if any of your medicines contain nitrates, or if you do not understand what nitrates are, ask your doctor or pharmacist.

VIAGRA is only for patients with erectile dysfunction. VIAGRA is not for newborns, children, or women. Do not let anyone else take your VIAGRA. VIAGRA must be used only under a doctor's supervision.

• WHAT VIAGRA DOES NOT DO

- VIAGRA does not cure erectile dysfunction. It is a treatment for erectile dysfunction.
- VIAGRA does not protect you or your partner from getting sexually transmitted diseases, including HIV—the virus that causes AIDS.
- VIAGRA is not a hormone or an aphrodisiac.

• WHAT TO TELL YOUR DOCTOR BEFORE YOU BEGIN VIAGRA

Only your doctor can decide if VIAGRA is right for you. VIAGRA can cause mild, temporary lowering of your blood pressure. You will need to have a thorough medical exam to diagnose your erectile dysfunction and to find out if you can safely take VIAGRA alone or with your other medicines. Your doctor should determine if your heart is healthy enough to handle the extra strain of having sex.

Be sure to tell your doctor if you:

- have ever had any heart problems (e.g., angina, chest pain, heart failure, irregular heart beats, heart attack or narrowing of the aortic valve)
- have ever had a stroke
- have low or high blood pressure
- have ever had severe vision loss
- have a rare inherited eye disease called retinitis pigmentosa
- have ever had any kidney problems
- have ever had any liver problems
- have ever had any blood problems, including sickle cell anemia or leukemia
- are allergic to sildenafil or any of the other ingredients of VIAGRA tablets
- have a deformed penis, Peyronie's disease, or ever had an erection that lasted more than 4 hours
- have stomach ulcers or any types of bleeding problems
- are taking any other medicines

• VIAGRA AND OTHER MEDICINES

Some medicines can change the way VIAGRA works. Tell your doctor about **any medicines** you are taking. Do not start or stop taking any medicines before checking with your doctor or pharmacist. This includes prescription and nonprescription medicines or remedies:

- Remember, VIAGRA should never be used with medicines that contain nitrates (see *VIAGRA Is Not for Everyone*).
- If you are taking medicines called alpha-blockers for the treatment of high blood pressure or prostate problems, your blood pressure could suddenly drop. You could get dizzy or faint.
- If you are taking a protease inhibitor, your dose may be adjusted (please see *Finding the Right Dose for You*).
- VIAGRA should not be used with any other medical treatments that cause erections. These treatments include pills, medicines that are injected or inserted into the penis, implants or vacuum pumps.
- VIAGRA contains sildenafil, which is the same medicine found in another drug called REVATIO. REVATIO is used to treat a rare disease called pulmonary arterial hypertension. VIAGRA should not be used with REVATIO.

• FINDING THE RIGHT DOSE FOR YOU

VIAGRA comes in different doses (25 mg, 50 mg and 100 mg). If you do not get the results you expect, talk with your doctor. You and your doctor can determine the dose that works best for you.

- Do not take more VIAGRA than your doctor prescribes.
- If you think you need a larger dose of VIAGRA, check with your doctor.
- VIAGRA should not be taken more than once a day.

Your doctor may prescribe a lower dose of VIAGRA in certain circumstances. For example:

- If you are older than age 65, or have serious liver or kidney problems, your doctor may start you at the lowest dose (25 mg) of VIAGRA.
- If you are taking protease inhibitors, such as for the treatment of HIV, your doctor may recommend a 25 mg dose and may limit you to a maximum single dose of 25 mg of VIAGRA in a 48 hour period.
- If you have prostate problems or high blood pressure for which you take medicines called alpha blockers, your doctor may start you on a lower dose of VIAGRA.

• HOW TO TAKE VIAGRA

Take VIAGRA about one hour before you plan to have sex. Beginning in about 30 minutes and for up to 4 hours, VIAGRA can help you get an erection if you are sexually excited. If you take VIAGRA after a high-fat meal (such as a cheeseburger and french fries), the medicine may take a little longer to start working. VIAGRA can help you get an erection when you are sexually excited. You will not get an erection just by taking the pill.

• POSSIBLE SIDE EFFECTS

Like all medicines, VIAGRA can cause some side effects. These effects are usually mild to moderate and usually don't last longer than a few hours. Some of these side effects are more likely to occur with higher doses. The most common side effects of VIAGRA are headache, flushing of the face, and upset stomach. Less common side effects that may occur are temporary changes in color vision (such as trouble telling the difference between blue and green objects or having a blue color tinge to them), eyes being more sensitive to light, or blurred vision.

In rare instances, men taking PDE5 inhibitors (oral erectile dysfunction medicines, including VIAGRA) reported a sudden decrease or loss of vision in one or both eyes. It is not possible to determine whether these events are related directly to these medicines, to other factors such as high blood pressure or diabetes, or to a combination of these. If you experience sudden decrease or loss of vision, stop taking PDE5 inhibitors, including VIAGRA, and call a doctor right away.

In rare instances, men have reported an erection that lasts many hours. You should call a doctor immediately if you ever have an erection that lasts more than 4 hours. If not treated right away, permanent damage to your penis could occur (see *How Sex Affects the Body*).

Sudden loss or decrease in hearing, sometimes with ringing in the ears and dizziness, has been rarely reported in people taking PDE5 inhibitors, including VIAGRA. It is not possible to determine whether these events are related directly to the PDE5 inhibitors, to other diseases or medications, to other factors, or to a combination of factors. If you experience these symptoms, stop taking VIAGRA and contact a doctor right away.

Heart attack, stroke, irregular heart beats, and death have been reported rarely in men taking VIAGRA. Most, but not all, of these men had heart problems before taking this medicine. It is not possible to determine whether these events were directly related to VIAGRA.

VIAGRA may cause other side effects besides those listed on this sheet. If you want more information or develop any side effects or symptoms you are concerned about, call your doctor.

IMPORTANT NOTICE: Updated drug information is sent bi-monthly via the PDR® Update Insert. For *monthly* email updates, register at PDR.net.

• ACCIDENTAL OVERDOSE
In case of accidental overdose, call your doctor right away.
• STORING VIAGRA
Keep VIAGRA out of the reach of children. Keep VIAGRA in its original container. Store at 25°C (77°F); excursions permitted to 15-30°C (59-86°F) [see USP Controlled Room Temperature].
• FOR MORE INFORMATION ON VIAGRA
VIAGRA is a prescription medicine used to treat erectile dysfunction. Only your doctor can decide if it is right for you. This sheet is only a summary. If you have any questions or want more information about VIAGRA, talk with your doctor or pharmacist, visit www.viagra.com, or call 1-888-4VIAGRA.
Distributed by
Pfizer Labs
Division of Pfizer Inc, NY, NY 10017
LAB-0220-7.0
January 2010

Pharmaceutical Associates, Inc.
A Subsidiary of Beach Products, Inc.
201 DELAWARE STREET
GREENVILLE, SC 29605

Direct Inquiries to:
Clete Harmon, Sr. Vice President.
PH: (800) 845-8210
(864) 277-7282
FAX: (864) 236-0116
www.paipharma.com

INSTITUTIONAL UNIT DOSE / TRADE PACKAGE

NDC Prefix: 00121-

_____

PRODUCT LISTING

ACETAMINOPHEN ORAL SOLUTION USP   OTC
(160 mg per 5 mL)
Unit Dose 5 mL, 10.15 mL, and 20.3 mL
ACETAMINOPHEN ORAL SUSPENSION USP   OTC
(160 mg/5 mL)
Unit dose 5 mL, 10.15 mL, 20.3 mL
ACETAMINOPHEN and CODEINE PHOSPHATE   © ℞
ORAL SOLUTION USP
(120 mg/12 mg per 5 mL)
Unit Dose 5 mL, 10 mL, 12.5 mL, and 15 mL
Bottles of 4 fl oz and 16 fl oz
ALUMINUM HYDROXIDE GEL USP   OTC
(320 mg per 5 mL)
Unit Dose 30 mL
Bottles of 12 fl oz and 16 fl oz
ALUMINUM HYDROXIDE GEL CONCENTRATE   OTC
(600 mg per 5 mL)
Bottles of 12 fl oz
AMANTADINE HYDROCHLORIDE   ℞
ORAL SOLUTION USP
(50 mg per 5 mL)
Unit Dose 10 mL
Bottles of 16 fl oz
CALCIUM CARBONATE ORAL SUSPENSION   OTC
(1250 mg / 5mL)
Unit Dose 5 mL
Bottle of 16 fl oz
CETIRIZINE HYDROCHLORIDE SYRUP   ℞
(5 mg / 5 mL)
Unit Dose 5 mL
CHLORAL HYDRATE ORAL SOLUTION USP   © ℞
(500 mg per 5 mL)
Unit Dose 5 mL
Bottles of 16 fl oz
CIMETIDINE HYDROCHLORIDE ORAL SOLUTION   ℞
(300 mg per 5 mL)
Bottles of 8 fl oz and 16 fl oz
DIPHENHYDRAMINE HYDROCHLORIDE   ℞
ORAL SOLUTION USP
(12.5 mg per 5 mL)
Unit Dose 5 mL, 10 mL, and 20 mL
DOCUSATE SODIUM LIQUID   OTC
(50 mg per 5 mL)
Unit Dose 10 mL and 25 mL
Bottles of 16 fl oz
DOCUSATE SODIUM SYRUP USP   OTC
(20 mg per 5 mL)
Unit Dose 25 mL
Bottles of 16 fl oz

ETHOSUXIMIDE SYRUP   ℞
(250 mg per 5 mL)
Bottles of 16 fl oz
FERROUS SULFATE ORAL SOLUTION USP   OTC
(300 mg per 5 mL)
Unit Dose 5 mL
FLUOXETINE ORAL SOLUTION USP   ℞
(20 mg per 5 mL)
Unit Dose 5 mL
Bottles of 4 fl oz
FLUPHENAZINE HYDROCHLORIDE ELIXIR USP   ℞
(2.5 mg per 5 mL)
Bottles of 60 mL and 16 fl oz
FLUPHENAZINE HYDROCHLORIDE ORAL SOLUTION ℞
USP Concentrate
(5 mg per 1 mL)
Bottles of 4 fl oz
GUAIFENESIN ORAL SOLUTION USP   OTC
(100 mg per 5 mL)
Unit Dose 5 mL, 10 mL, and 15 mL
Bottles of 4 fl oz, 8 fl oz and 16 fl oz
GUAIFENESIN AND CODEINE PHOSPHATE   OTC
ORAL SOLUTION USP (Alcohol free)
(100 mg/10 mg per 5 mL)
Unit Dose 5 mL and 10 mL
Bottles of 4 fl oz and 16 fl oz
GUAIFENESIN SYRUP and DEXTROMETHORPHAN   OTC
(100 mg/10 mg per 5 mL)
Unit Dose 5 mL and 10 mL
Bottles of 4 fl oz, 8 fl oz and 16 fl oz
GUAIFENESIN SYRUP and DEXTROMETHORPHAN
(Maximum Strength)
200 mg/10 mg per 5 mL
Unit Dose 5 mL, 10 mL
Bottles of 4 fl oz and 8 fl oz
HALOPERIDOL ORAL SOLUTION USP   ℞
(Concentrate)
(2 mg per 1 mL)
Unit Dose 5 mL
Bottles of 4 fl oz
HYDROCODONE BITARTRATE and   © ℞
ACETAMINOPHEN ORAL SOLUTION
(7.5 mg/500 mg per 15 mL)
Unit Dose 5 mL, 10 mL and 15 mL
Bottles of 4 fl oz and 16 fl oz
HYDROCODONE BITARTRATE and   © ℞
ACETAMINOPHEN ORAL SOLUTION
(10 mg / 325 mg per 15 mL)
Unit Dose 7.5 mL and 15 mL
HYDROCODONE BITARTRATE and   © ℞
HOMATROPINE METHYLBROMIDE SYRUP
(5 mg/1.5 mg per 5 mL)
Unit Dose 5 mL
IBUPROFEN ORAL SUSPENSION USP   ℞
(100 mg per 5 mL)
Unit Dose 5 mL
LACTULOSE SOLUTION USP   ℞
(10 g per 15 mL)
Unit Dose 15 mL and 30 mL
Bottles of 8 fl oz, 16 fl oz, and 32 fl oz
LEVETIRACETAM ORAL SOLUTION   ℞
(500 mg / 5 mL)
Unit Dose 5 mL
MAG-AL LIQUID   OTC
(Magnesium Hydroxide 1200 mg / 30 mL)
(Aluminum Hydroxide 1200 mg / 30 mL)
Unit Dose 30 mL
MAG-AL Plus   OTC
(Magnesium Hydroxide 1200 mg / 30 mL)
(Aluminum Hydroxide 1200 mg / 30 mL)
(Simethicone 120 mg / 30 mL)
Unit Dose 30 mL
MAG-AL Plus XS   OTC
(Magnesium Hydroxide 2400 mg / 30 mL)
(Aluminum Hydroxide 2400 mg / 30 mL)
(Simethicone 240 mg / 30 mL)
Unit Dose 30 mL
MAG-AL Ultimate Strength   OTC
(Magnesium Hydroxide 2000 mg / 20 mL)
(Aluminum Hydroxide 2000 mg/ 20 mL)
Unit Dose 20 mL
MEGESTROL ACETATE ORAL SUSPENSION   ℞
(400 mg per 10 mL)
Unit Dose 10 mL and 20 mL
METOCLOPRAMIDE ORAL SOLUTION USP   ℞
(5 mg per 5 mL)
Unit Dose 10 mL
Bottles of 16 fl oz
MILK OF MAGNESIA   OTC
(8% Suspension)
(400 mg per 5 mL)
Unit Dose 30 mL

MILK OF MAGNESIA CONCENTRATE   OTC
(24% Suspension)
(2400 mg per 10 mL)
Unit Dose 10 mL
MINERAL OIL   OTC
Unit Dose 30 mL
NORTRIPTYLINE HYDROCHLORIDE ORAL   ℞
SOLUTION USP
(10 mg per 5 mL)
Bottles of 16 fl oz
NYSTATIN ORAL SUSPENSION USP   ℞
500,000 units / 5 mL
Unit Dose 5 mL
OXYBUTYNIN CHLORIDE SYRUP USP   ℞
(5 mg per 5 mL)
Unit Dose 5 mL
Bottles of 16 fl oz
PHENOBARBITAL ORAL SOLUTION USP   © ℞
(20 mg per 5 mL)
Unit Dose 5 mL, 7.5 mL, and 15 mL
Bottle of 16 fl oz
PINK BISMUTH   OTC
(Bismuth Subsalicylate 524 mg / 30 mL)
Unit Dose 30 mL
POTASSIUM CHLORIDE ORAL SOLUTION USP 10% ℞
(20 mEq per 15 mL)
Unit Dose 15 mL and 30 mL
POTASSIUM CHLORIDE ORAL SOLUTION USP 20% ℞
(40 mEq per 15 mL)
Unit Dose 15 mL
Bottles of 16 fl oz
POTASSIUM CITRATE and CITRIC ACID   ℞
ORAL SOLUTION USP
(1100 mg/334 mg per 5 mL)
Bottles of 16 fl oz
PREDNISOLONE SODIUM PHOSPHATE   ℞
ORAL SOLUTION
(15 mg/5 mL)
Bottles of 8 fl oz
PROMETHAZINE HYDROCHLORIDE and CODEINE   © ℞
PHOSPHATE SYRUP
(6.25 mg/10 mg per 5 mL)
Unit Dose 5 mL
PSEUDOEPHEDRINE HYDROCHLORIDE ORAL
SOLUTION USP   OTC
(30 mg per 5 mL)
Bottles of 4 fl oz
RANITIDINE SYRUP (ORAL SOLUTION USP)   ℞
(150 mg/10 mL)
Unit Dose 10mL
Bottles of 16 fl. oz.
SENNA SYRUP - SENNA LEAF EXTRACT
(176 mg/5 mL)
Unit Dose 15 mL
Bottles of 8 fl oz
SODIUM CITRATE and CITRIC ACID ORAL   ℞
SOLUTION USP
(500 mg/334 mg per 5 mL)
Unit Dose 15 mL and 30 mL
Bottles of 16 fl oz
SORBITOL SOLUTION USP   OTC
(70% w/w)
Unit Dose 30 mL
Bottles of 16 fl oz
SORE THROAT SPRAY   OTC
(Phenol 1.4%) Cherry
Bottles of 6 fl oz
SUCRALFATE SUSPENSION   ℞
(1 g per 10 mL)
Unit Dose 10 mL
SULFAMETHOXAZOLE and TRIMETHOPRIM   ℞
ORAL SUSPENSION USP
(800 mg / 160 mg per 20 mL)
Unit Dose 20 mL
THEOPHYLLINE ORAL SOLUTION   ℞
(80 mg / 15 mL)
Unit Dose 15 mL
TRICITRATES ORAL SOLUTION   ℞
(550 mg/500 mg/334 mg per 5 mL)
Bottles of 16 fl oz
TRICITRATES SF ORAL SOLUTION   ℞
(550 mg/500 mg/334 mg per 5 mL)
Bottles of 16 fl oz
TRIHEXYPHENIDYL HYDROCHLORIDE   ℞
ELIXIR USP
(2 mg per 5 mL)
Bottles of 16 fl oz
VALPROIC ACID ORAL SOLUTION USP   ℞
(250 mg per 5 mL)
Unit Dose 5 mL
Bottles of 16 fl oz.

Pharmacia & Upjohn
A Division of Pfizer
235 EAST 42ND STREET
NEW YORK, NY 10017-5755

For updates to the product information listed below, please check the Pfizer Web site, http://www.pfizerpro.com, or call (800) 438-1985. For complete product listing, please see the Manufacturers' Index.

For Medical Information, Contact:
(800) 438-1985
24 hours a day, 7 days a week

Distribution:
1855 Shelby Oaks Drive North
Memphis, TN 38134
(901) 387-5200

Customer Service:
(800) 533-4535

AROMASIN®
[ă-rō-mă-sīn]
(exemestane) tablets

℞

DESCRIPTION
AROMASIN® Tablets for oral administration contain 25 mg of exemestane, an irreversible, steroidal aromatase inactivator. Exemestane is chemically described as 6-methylenandrosta-1,4-diene-3,17-dione. Its molecular formula is $C_{20}H_{24}O_2$ and its structural formula is as follows:

The active ingredient is a white to slightly yellow crystalline powder with a molecular weight of 296.41. Exemestane is freely soluble in N, N-dimethylformamide, soluble in methanol, and practically insoluble in water.
Each AROMASIN Tablet contains the following inactive ingredients: mannitol, crospovidone, polysorbate 80, hypromellose, colloidal silicon dioxide, microcrystalline cellulose, sodium starch glycolate, magnesium stearate, simethicone, polyethylene glycol 6000, sucrose, magnesium carbonate, titanium dioxide, methylparaben, and polyvinyl alcohol.

CLINICAL PHARMACOLOGY
Mechanism of Action
Breast cancer cell growth may be estrogen-dependent. Aromatase is the principal enzyme that converts androgens to estrogens both in pre- and postmenopausal women. While the main source of estrogen (primarily estradiol) is the ovary in premenopausal women, the principal source of circulating estrogens in postmenopausal women is from conversion of adrenal and ovarian androgens (androstenedione and testosterone) to estrogens (estrone and estradiol) by the aromatase enzyme in peripheral tissues. Estrogen deprivation through aromatase inhibition is an effective and selective treatment for some postmenopausal patients with hormone-dependent breast cancer.
Exemestane is an irreversible, steroidal aromatase inactivator, structurally related to the natural substrate androstenedione. It acts as a false substrate for the aromatase enzyme, and is processed to an intermediate that binds irreversibly to the active site of the enzyme causing its inactivation, an effect also known as "suicide inhibition." Exemestane significantly lowers circulating estrogen concentrations in postmenopausal women, but has no detectable effect on adrenal biosynthesis of corticosteroids or aldosterone. Exemestane has no effect on other enzymes involved in the steroidogenic pathway up to a concentration at least 600 times higher than that inhibiting the aromatase enzyme.
Pharmacokinetics
Following oral administration to healthy postmenopausal women, exemestane is rapidly absorbed. After maximum plasma concentration is reached, levels decline polyexponentially with a mean terminal half-life of about 24 hours. Exemestane is extensively distributed and is cleared from the systemic circulation primarily by metabolism. The pharmacokinetics of exemestane are dose proportional after single (10 to 200 mg) or repeated oral doses (0.5 to 50 mg). Following repeated daily doses of exemestane 25 mg, plasma concentrations of unchanged drug are similar to levels measured after a single dose.

Table 1. Demographic and Baseline Tumor Characteristics from the IES Study of Postmenopausal Women with Early Breast Cancer (ITT Population)

Parameter	Exemestane (N = 2352)		Tamoxifen (N = 2372)	
Age (years):				
Median age (range)	63.0 (38.0–96.0)		63.0 (31.0–90.0)	
Race, n (%):				
Caucasian	2315	(98.4)	2333	(98.4)
Hispanic	13	(0.6)	13	(0.5)
Asian	10	(0.4)	9	(0.4)
Black	7	(0.3)	10	(0.4)
Other/not reported	7	(0.3)	7	(0.3)
Nodal status, n (%):				
Negative	1217	(51.7)	1228	(51.8)
Positive	1051	(44.7)	1044	(44.0)
1–3 Positive nodes	721	(30.7)	708	(29.8)
4–9 Positive nodes	239	(10.2)	244	(10.3)
>9 Positive nodes	88	(3.7)	86	(3.6)
Not reported	3	(0.1)	6	(0.3)
Unknown or missing	84	(3.6)	100	(4.2)
Histologic type, n (%):				
Infiltrating ductal	1777	(75.6)	1830	(77.2)
Infiltrating lobular	341	(14.5)	321	(13.5)
Other	231	(9.8)	213	(9.0)
Unknown or missing	3	(0.1)	8	(0.3)
Receptor status*, n (%):				
ER and PgR Positive	1331	(56.6)	1319	(55.6)
ER Positive and PgR Negative/Unknown	677	(28.8)	692	(29.2)
ER Unknown and PgR Positive**/Unknown	288	(12.2)	291	(12.3)
ER Negative and PgR Positive	6	(0.3)	7	(0.3)
ER Negative and PgR Negative/Unknown (none positive)	48	(2.0)	58	(2.4)
Missing	2	(0.1)	5	(0.2)
Tumor Size, n (%):				
≤ 0.5 cm	58	(2.5)	46	(1.9)
> 0.5–1.0 cm	315	(13.4)	302	(12.7)
> 1.0–2 cm	1031	(43.8)	1033	(43.5)
> 2.0–5.0 cm	833	(35.4)	883	(37.2)
> 5.0 cm	62	(2.6)	59	(2.5)
Not reported	53	(2.3)	49	(2.1)
Tumor Grade, n (%):				
G1	397	(16.9)	393	(16.6)
G2	977	(41.5)	1007	(42.5)
G3	454	(19.3)	428	(18.0)
G4	23	(1.0)	19	(0.8)
Unknown/Not assessed/Not reported	501	(21.3)	525	(22.1)

* Results for receptor status include the results of the post-randomization testing of specimens from subjects for whom receptor status was unknown at randomization.
**Only one subject in the exemestane group had unknown ER status and positive PgR status.

Pharmacokinetic parameters in postmenopausal women with advanced breast cancer following single or repeated doses have been compared with those in healthy, postmenopausal women. Exemestane appeared to be more rapidly absorbed in the women with breast cancer than in the healthy women, with a mean t_{max} of 1.2 hours in the women with breast cancer and 2.9 hours in the healthy women. After repeated dosing, the average oral clearance in women with advanced breast cancer was 45% lower than the oral clearance in healthy postmenopausal women, with corresponding higher systemic exposure. Mean AUC values following repeated doses in women with breast cancer (75.4 ng•h/mL) were about twice those in healthy women (41.4 ng•h/mL).
Absorption: Following oral administration of radiolabeled exemestane, at least 42% of radioactivity was absorbed from the gastrointestinal tract. Exemestane plasma levels increased by approximately 40% after a high-fat breakfast.
Distribution: Exemestane is distributed extensively into tissues. Exemestane is 90% bound to plasma proteins and the fraction bound is independent of the total concentration. Albumin and α_1-acid glycoprotein both contribute to the binding. The distribution of exemestane and its metabolites into blood cells is negligible.
Metabolism and Excretion: Following administration of radiolabeled exemestane to healthy postmenopausal women, the cumulative amounts of radioactivity excreted in urine and feces were similar (42 ± 3% in urine and 42 ± 6% in feces over a 1-week collection period). The amount of drug excreted unchanged in urine was less than 1% of the dose. Exemestane is extensively metabolized, with levels of the unchanged drug in plasma accounting for less than 10% of the total radioactivity. The initial steps in the metabolism of exemestane are oxidation of the methylene group in position 6 and reduction of the 17-keto group with subsequent formation of many secondary metabolites. Each metabolite accounts only for a limited amount of drug-related material. The metabolites are inactive or inhibit aromatase with decreased potency compared with the parent drug. One metabolite may have androgenic activity (see Pharmacodynamics, Other Endocrine Effects). Studies using human liver preparations indicate that cytochrome P-450 3A4 (CYP 3A4) is the principal isoenzyme involved in the oxidation of exemestane.
Special Populations
Geriatric: Healthy postmenopausal women aged 43 to 68 years were studied in the pharmacokinetic trials. Age-related alterations in exemestane pharmacokinetics were not seen over this age range.
Gender: The pharmacokinetics of exemestane following administration of a single, 25-mg tablet to fasted healthy males (mean age 32 years) were similar to the pharmacokinetics of exemestane in fasted healthy postmenopausal women (mean age 55 years).
Race: The influence of race on exemestane pharmacokinetics has not been evaluated.
Hepatic Insufficiency: The pharmacokinetics of exemestane have been investigated in subjects with moderate or severe hepatic insufficiency (Childs-Pugh B or C). Following a single 25-mg oral dose, the AUC of exemestane was approximately 3 times higher than that observed in healthy volunteers (see PRECAUTIONS).
Renal Insufficiency: The AUC of exemestane after a single 25-mg dose was approximately 3 times higher in subjects with moderate or severe renal insufficiency (creatinine clearance <35 mL/min/1.73 m^2) compared with the AUC in healthy volunteers (see PRECAUTIONS).
Pediatric: The pharmacokinetics of exemestane have not been studied in pediatric patients.
Drug-Drug Interactions
Exemestane is metabolized by cytochrome P-450 3A4 (CYP 3A4) and aldoketoreductases. It does not inhibit any

of the major CYP isoenzymes, including CYP 1A2, 2C9, 2D6, 2E1, and 3A4. In a clinical pharmacokinetic study, ketoconazole showed no significant influence on the pharmacokinetics of exemestane. Although no other formal drug-drug interaction studies have been conducted, significant effects on exemestane clearance by CYP isoenzymes inhibitors appear unlikely. In a pharmacokinetic interaction study of 10 healthy postmenopausal volunteers pretreated with potent CYP 3A4 inducer rifampicin 600 mg daily for 14 days followed by a single dose of exemestane 25 mg, the mean plasma C_{max} and $AUC_{0-\infty}$ of exemestane were decreased by 41% and 54%, respectively (see PRECAUTIONS and DOSAGE AND ADMINISTRATION).

Pharmacodynamics

Effect on Estrogens: Multiple doses of exemestane ranging from 0.5 to 600 mg/day were administered to postmenopausal women with advanced breast cancer. Plasma estrogen (estradiol, estrone, and estrone sulfate) suppression was seen starting at a 5-mg daily dose of exemestane, with a maximum suppression of at least 85% to 95% achieved at a 25-mg dose. Exemestane 25 mg daily reduced whole body aromatization (as measured by injecting radiolabeled androstenedione) by 98% in postmenopausal women with breast cancer. After a single dose of exemestane 25 mg, the maximal suppression of circulating estrogens occurred 2 to 3 days after dosing and persisted for 4 to 5 days.

Effect on Corticosteroids: In multiple-dose trials of doses up to 200 mg daily, exemestane selectivity was assessed by examining its effect on adrenal steroids. Exemestane did not affect cortisol or aldosterone secretion at baseline or in response to ACTH at any dose. Thus, no glucocorticoid or mineralocorticoid replacement therapy is necessary with exemestane treatment.

Other Endocrine Effects: Exemestane does not bind significantly to steroidal receptors, except for a slight affinity for the androgen receptor (0.28% relative to dihydrotestosterone). The binding affinity of its 17-dihydrometabolite for the androgen receptor, however, is 100-times that of the parent compound. Daily doses of exemestane up to 25 mg had no significant effect on circulating levels of androstenedione, dehydroepiandrosterone sulfate, or 17-hydroxyprogesterone, and were associated with small decreases in circulating levels of testosterone. Increases in testosterone and androstenedione levels have been observed at daily doses of 200 mg or more. A dose-dependent decrease in sex hormone binding globulin (SHBG) has been observed with daily exemestane doses of 2.5 mg or higher. Slight, nondose-dependent increases in serum luteinizing hormone (LH) and follicle-stimulating hormone (FSH) levels have been observed even at low doses as a consequence of feedback at the pituitary level. Exemestane 25 mg daily had no significant effect on thyroid function [free triiodothyronine (FT3), free thyroxine (FT4) and thyroid stimulating hormone (TSH)].

Coagulation and Lipid Effects: In study 027 of postmenopausal women with early breast cancer treated with exemestane (N=73) or placebo (N=73), there was no change in the coagulation parameters activated partial thromboplastin time [APTT], prothrombin time [PT] and fibrinogen. Plasma HDL cholesterol was decreased 6–9% in exemestane treated patients; total cholesterol, LDL cholesterol, triglycerides, apolipoprotein-A1, apolipoprotein-B, and lipoprotein-a were unchanged. An 18% increase in homocysteine levels was also observed in exemestane treated patients compared with a 12% increase seen with placebo.

CLINICAL STUDIES

Adjuvant Treatment in Early Breast Cancer

The Intergroup Exemestane Study 031 (IES) was a randomized, double-blind, multicenter, multinational study comparing exemestane (25 mg/day) versus tamoxifen (20 or 30 mg/day) in postmenopausal women with early breast cancer. Patients who remained disease-free after receiving adjuvant tamoxifen therapy for 2 to 3 years were randomized to receive 3 to 2 years of AROMASIN or tamoxifen to complete a total of 5 years of hormonal therapy.

The primary objective of the study was to determine whether, in terms of disease-free survival, it was more effective to switch to AROMASIN rather than continuing tamoxifen therapy for the remainder of five years. Disease-free survival was defined as the time from randomization to time of local or distant recurrence of breast cancer, contralateral invasive breast cancer, or death from any cause.

The secondary objectives were to compare the two regimens in terms of overall survival and long-term tolerability. Time to contralateral invasive breast cancer and distant recurrence-free survival were also evaluated.

A total of 4724 patients in the intent-to-treat (ITT) analysis were randomized to AROMASIN (exemestane tablets) 25 mg once daily (N = 2352) or to continue to receive tamoxifen once daily at the same dose received before randomization (N = 2372). Demographics and baseline tumor characteristics are presented in Table 1. Prior breast cancer therapy is summarized in Table 2.

Table 2. Prior Breast Cancer Therapy of Patients in the IES Study of Postmenopausal Women with Early Breast Cancer (ITT Population)

Parameter	Exemestane (N = 2352)		Tamoxifen (N = 2372)	
Type of surgery, n (%):				
Mastectomy	1232	(52.4)	1242	(52.4)
Breast-conserving	1116	(47.4)	1123	(47.3)
Unknown or missing	4	(0.2)	7	(0.3)
Radiotherapy to the breast, n (%):				
Yes	1524	(64.8)	1523	(64.2)
No	824	(35.5)	843	(35.5)
Not reported	4	(0.2)	6	(0.3)
Prior therapy, n (%):				
Chemotherapy	774	(32.9)	769	(32.4)
Hormone replacement therapy	567	(24.1)	561	(23.7)
Bisphosphonates	43	(1.8)	34	(1.4)
Duration of tamoxifen therapy at randomization (months):				
Median (range)	28.5 (15.8–52.2)		28.4 (15.6–63.0)	
Tamoxifen dose, n (%):				
20 mg	2270	(96.5)	2287	(96.4)
30 mg*	78	(3.3)	75	(3.2)
Not reported	4	(0.2)	10	(0.4)

The 30 mg dose was used only in Denmark, where this dose was the standard of care.

Table 3. Primary Endpoint Events (ITT Population)

Event	First Events N (%)	
	Exemestane (N = 2352)	Tamoxifen (N = 2372)
Loco-regional recurrence	34 (1.45)	45 (1.90)
Distant recurrence	126 (5.36)	183 (7.72)
Second primary – contralateral breast cancer	7 (0.30)	25 (1.05)
Death – breast cancer	1 (0.04)	6 (0.25)
Death – other reason	41 (1.74)	43 (1.81)
Death – missing/unknown	3 (0.13)	5 (0.21)
Ipsilateral breast cancer	1 (0.04)	0
Total number of events	**213 (9.06)**	**307 (12.94)**

[See table 1 at top of previous page]
[See table 2 above]

After a median duration of therapy of 27 months and with a median follow-up of 34.5 months, 520 events were reported, 213 in the AROMASIN group and 307 in the tamoxifen group (Table 3).

[See table above]

Disease-free survival in the intent-to-treat population was statistically significantly improved [Hazard Ratio (HR) = 0.69, 95% CI: 0.58, 0.82, P = 0.00003, Table 4, Figure 1] in the AROMASIN arm compared to the tamoxifen arm. In the hormone receptor-positive subpopulation representing about 85% of the trial patients, disease-free survival was also statistically significantly improved (HR = 0.65, 95% CI: 0.53, 0.79, P = 0.00001) in the AROMASIN arm compared to the tamoxifen arm. Consistent results were observed in the subgroups of patients with node negative or positive disease, and patients who had or had not received prior chemotherapy. Overall survival was not significantly different in the two groups, with 116 deaths occurring in the AROMASIN group and 137 in the tamoxifen group.

[See table 4 at top of next page]

[See figure 1 at top of next column]

Treatment of Advanced Breast Cancer

Exemestane 25 mg administered once daily was evaluated in a randomized double-blind, multicenter, multinational comparative study and in two multicenter single-arm studies of postmenopausal women with advanced breast cancer who had disease progression after treatment with tamoxifen for metastatic disease or as adjuvant therapy. Some patients also have received prior cytotoxic therapy, either as adjuvant treatment or for metastatic disease.

The primary purpose of the three studies was evaluation of objective response rate (complete response [CR] and partial response [PR]). Time to tumor progression and overall survival were also assessed in the comparative trial. Response

Figure 1. Disease Free Survival in the IES Study of Postmenopausal Women with Early Breast Cancer (ITT Population)

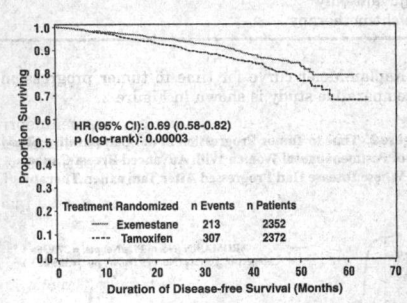

HR (95% CI): 0.69 (0.58-0.82)
p (log-rank): 0.00003

Treatment Randomized	n Events	n Patients
Exemestane	213	2352
Tamoxifen	307	2372

rates were assessed based on World Health Organization (WHO) criteria, and in the comparative study, were submitted to an external review committee that was blinded to patient treatment. In the comparative study, 769 patients were randomized to receive AROMASIN (exemestane tablets) 25 mg once daily (N = 366) or megestrol acetate 40 mg four times daily (N = 403). Demographics and baseline characteristics are presented in Table 5.

[See table 5 on next page]

The efficacy results from the comparative study are shown in Table 6. The objective response rates observed in the two treatment arms showed that AROMASIN was not different from megestrol acetate. Response rates for AROMASIN from the two single-arm trials were 23.4% and 28.1%.

[See table 6 at top of page 2833]

There were too few deaths occurring across treatment groups to draw conclusions on overall survival differences.

Table 4. Efficacy Results from the IES Study in Postmenopausal Women with Early Breast Cancer

ITT Population	Hazard Ratio (95% CI)	p-value (log-rank test)
Disease free survival	0.69 (0.58–0.82)	0.00003
Time to contralateral breast cancer	0.32 (0.15–0.72)	0.00340
Distant recurrence free survival	0.74 (0.62–0.90)	0.00207
Overall survival	0.86 (0.67–1.10)	0.22962
ER and/or PgR positive		
Disease free survival	0.65 (0.53–0.79)	0.00001
Time to contralateral breast cancer	0.22 (0.08–0.57)	0.00069
Distant recurrence free survival	0.73 (0.59–0.90)	0.00367
Overall survival	0.88 (0.67–1.17)	0.37460

Table 5. Demographics and Baseline Characteristics from the Comparative Study of Postmenopausal Women with Advanced Breast Cancer Whose Disease Had Progressed after Tamoxifen Therapy

Parameter	AROMASIN (N=366)	Megestrol Acetate (N=403)
Median Age (range)	65 (35–89)	65 (30–91)
ECOG Performance Status		
0	167 (46%)	187 (46%)
1	162 (44%)	172 (43%)
2	34 (9%)	42 (10%)
Receptor Status		
ER and/or PgR +	246 (67%)	274 (68%)
ER and PgR unknown	116 (32%)	128 (32%)
Responders to prior tamoxifen	68 (19%)	85 (21%)
NE for response to prior tamoxifen	46 (13%)	41 (10%)
Site of Metastasis		
Visceral ± other sites	207 (57%)	239 (59%)
Bone only	61 (17%)	73 (18%)
Soft tissue only	54 (15%)	51 (13%)
Bone & soft tissue	43 (12%)	38 (9%)
Measurable Disease	287 (78%)	314 (78%)
Prior Tamoxifen Therapy		
Adjuvant or Neoadjuvant	145 (40%)	152 (38%)
Advanced Disease, Outcome		
CR, PR or SD≥ 6 months	179 (49%)	210 (52%)
SD< 6 months, PD or NE	42 (12%)	41 (10%)
Prior Chemotherapy		
For advanced disease ± adjuvant	58 (16%)	67 (17%)
Adjuvant only	104 (28%)	108 (27%)
No chemotherapy	203 (56%)	226 (56%)

The Kaplan-Meier curve for time to tumor progression in the comparative study is shown in Figure 2.

Figure 2. Time to Tumor Progression in the Comparative Study of Postmenopausal Women With Advanced Breast Cancer Whose Disease Had Progressed After Tamoxifen Therapy

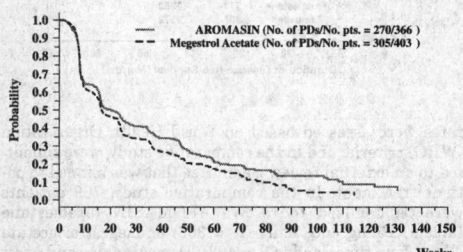

AROMASIN (No. of PDs/No. pts. = 270/366)
Megestrol Acetate (No. of PDs/No. pts. = 305/403)

INDICATIONS AND USAGE

AROMASIN is indicated for adjuvant treatment of postmenopausal women with estrogen-receptor positive early breast cancer who have received two to three years of tamoxifen and are switched to AROMASIN for completion of a total of five consecutive years of adjuvant hormonal therapy.

AROMASIN is indicated for the treatment of advanced breast cancer in postmenopausal women whose disease has progressed following tamoxifen therapy.

CONTRAINDICATIONS

AROMASIN Tablets are contraindicated in patients with a known hypersensitivity to the drug or to any of the excipients.

WARNINGS

AROMASIN Tablets may cause fetal harm when administered to a pregnant woman. Radioactivity related to ^{14}C-exemestane crossed the placenta of rats following oral administration of 1 mg/kg exemestane. The concentration of exemestane and its metabolites was approximately equivalent in maternal and fetal blood. When rats were administered exemestane from 14 days prior to mating until either days 15 or 20 of gestation, and resuming for the 21 days of lactation, an increase in placental weight was seen at 4 mg/kg/day (approximately 1.5 times the recommended human daily dose on a mg/m^2 basis). Prolonged gestation and abnormal or difficult labor was observed at doses equal to or greater than 20 mg/kg/day. Increased resorption, reduced number of live fetuses, decreased fetal weight, and retarded ossification were also observed at these doses. No malformations were noted when exemestane was administered to pregnant rats during the organogenesis period at doses up to 810 mg/kg/day (approximately 320 times the recommended human dose on a mg/m^2 basis). Daily doses of exemestane, given to rabbits during organogenesis caused a decrease in placental weight at 90 mg/kg/day (approximately 70 times the recommended human daily dose on a mg/m^2 basis). Abortions, an increase in resorptions, and a reduction in fetal body weight were seen at 270 mg/kg/day. There was no increase in the incidence of malformations in rabbits at doses up to 270 mg/kg/day (approximately 210 times the recommended human dose on a mg/m^2 basis). There are no studies in pregnant women using AROMASIN. AROMASIN is indicated for postmenopausal women. If there is exposure to AROMASIN during pregnancy, the patient should be apprised of the potential hazard to the fetus and potential risk for loss of the pregnancy.

PRECAUTIONS

General. AROMASIN Tablets should not be administered to premenopausal women. AROMASIN should not be coadministered with estrogen-containing agents as these could interfere with its pharmacologic action.

Hepatic Insufficiency. The pharmacokinetics of exemestane have been investigated in subjects with moderate or severe hepatic insufficiency (Childs-Pugh B or C). Following a single 25-mg oral dose, the AUC of exemestane was approximately 3 times higher than that observed in healthy volunteers. The safety of chronic dosing in patients with moderate or severe hepatic impairment has not been studied. Based on experience with exemestane at repeated doses up to 200 mg daily that demonstrated a moderate increase in non-life threatening adverse events, dosage adjustment does not appear to be necessary.

Renal Insufficiency. The AUC of exemestane after a single 25-mg dose was approximately 3 times higher in subjects with moderate or severe renal insufficiency (creatinine clearance <35 mL/min/1.73 m^2) compared with the AUC in healthy volunteers. The safety of chronic dosing in patients with moderate or severe renal impairment has not been studied. Based on experience with exemestane at repeated doses up to 200 mg daily that demonstrated a moderate increase in non-life threatening adverse events, dosage adjustment does not appear to be necessary.

Laboratory Tests. In patients with early breast cancer the incidence of hematological abnormalities of Common Toxicity Criteria (CTC) grade ≥1 were lower in the exemestane treatment group, compared with tamoxifen. Incidence of CTC grade 3 or 4 abnormalities was low (approximately 0.1%) in both treatment groups. Approximately 20% of patients receiving exemestane in clinical studies in advanced breast cancer, experienced CTC grade 3 or 4 lymphocytopenia. Of these patients, 89% had a pre-existing lower grade lymphopenia. Forty percent of patients either recovered or improved to a lesser severity while on treatment. Patients did not have a significant increase in viral infections, and no opportunistic infections were observed. Elevations of serum levels of AST, ALT, alkaline phosphatase and gamma glutamyl transferase > 5 times the upper value of the normal range (i.e., ≥ CTC grade 3) have been rarely reported in patients treated for advanced breast cancer but appear mostly attributable to the underlying presence of liver and/or bone metastases. In the comparative study in advanced breast cancer patients, CTC grade 3 or 4 elevation of gamma glutamyl transferase without documented evidence of liver metastasis was reported in 2.7% of patients treated with AROMASIN and in 1.8% of patients treated with megestrol acetate.

In patients with early breast cancer, elevations in bilirubin, alkaline phosphatase, and creatinine were more common in those receiving exemestane than either tamoxifen or placebo. Treatment emergent bilirubin elevations (any CTC grade) occurred in 5.3% of exemestane patients and 0.8% of tamoxifen patients on the IES, and in 6.9% of exemestane treated patients vs. 0% of placebo treated patients on the 027 study. CTC grade 3–4 increases in bilirubin occurred in 0.9% of exemestane treated patients compared to 0.1% of tamoxifen treated patients. Alkaline phosphatase elevations of any CTC grade occurred in 15.0% of exemestane treated patients on the IES compared to 2.6% of tamoxifen treated patients, and in 13.7% of exemestane treated patients compared to 6.9% of placebo treated patients on study 027. Creatinine elevations occurred in 5.8% of exemestane treated patients and 4.3% of tamoxifen treated patients on the IES and in 5.5% of exemestane treated patients and 0% of placebo treated patients on study 027.

Reductions in bone mineral density (BMD) over time are seen with exemestane use. Table 7 describes changes in BMD from baseline to 24 months in patients receiving exemestane compared to patients receiving tamoxifen (IES) or placebo (027). Concomitant use of bisphosponates, Vitamin D supplementation and Calcium was not allowed. [See table 7 on next page]

Drug Interactions. Exemestane is extensively metabolized by CYP 3A4, but coadministration of ketoconazole, a potent inhibitor of CYP 3A4, has no significant effect on exemestane pharmacokinetics. Significant pharmacokinetic interactions mediated by inhibition of CYP isoenzymes therefore appear unlikely. Co-medications that induce CYP 3A4 (e.g., rifampicin, phenytoin, carbamazepine, phenobarbital, or St. John's wort) may significantly decrease exposure to exemestane. Dose modification is recommended for patients who are also receiving a potent CYP 3A4

Table 6. Efficacy Results from the Comparative Study of Postmenopausal Women with Advanced Breast Cancer Whose Disease Had Progressed after Tamoxifen Therapy

Response Characteristics	AROMASIN (N=366)		Megestrol Acetate (N=403)
Objective Response Rate = CR + PR (%)	15.0		12.4
Difference in Response Rate (AR-MA)		2.6	
95% C.I.		7.5, -2.3	
CR (%)	2.2		1.2
PR (%)	12.8		11.2
SD ≥ 24 Weeks (%)	21.3		21.1
Median Duration of Response (weeks)	76.1		71.0
Median TTP (weeks)	20.3		16.6
Hazard Ratio (AR-MA)		0.84	

Abbreviations: CR = complete response, PR = partial response, SD = stable disease (no change), TTP = time to tumor progression, C.I. = confidence interval, MA = megestrol acetate, AR = AROMASIN

Table 7: Percent Change in BMD from Baseline to 24 months, Exemestane vs. Control[1]

BMD	IES		027	
	Exemestane N=29	Tamoxifen N=38	Exemestane N=59	Placebo N=65
Lumbar spine (%)	-3.14	-0.18	-3.51	-2.35
Femoral neck (%)	-4.15	-0.33	-4.57	-2.59

[1] For patients who had 24-month data.

inducer (see DOSAGE AND ADMINISTRATION and CLINICAL PHARMACOLOGY).

Drug/Laboratory Tests Interactions. No clinically relevant changes in the results of clinical laboratory tests have been observed.

Carcinogenesis, Mutagenesis, Impairment of Fertility. A 2-year carcinogenicity study in mice at doses of 50, 150 and 450 mg/kg/day exemestane (gavage), resulted in an increased incidence of hepatocellular adenomas and/or carcinomas in both genders at the high dose level. Plasma $AUC_{(0-24hr)}$ at the high dose were 2575 ± 386 and 5667 ± 1833 ng.hr/mL in males and females (approx. 34 and 75 fold the AUC in postmenopausal patients at the recommended clinical dose). An increased incidence of renal tubular adenomas was observed in male mice at the high dose of 450 mg/kg/day. Since the doses tested in mice did not achieve an MTD, neoplastic findings in organs other than liver and kidneys remain unknown.

A separate carcinogenicity study was conducted in rats at the doses of 30, 100 and 315 mg/kg/day exemestane (gavage) for 92 weeks in males and 2 years in females. No evidence of carcinogenic activity up to the highest dose tested of 315 mg/kg/day was observed in females. The male rat study was inconclusive since it was terminated prematurely at Week 92. At the highest dose, plasma $AUC_{(0-24hr)}$ levels in male (1418 ± 287 ng.hr/mL) and female (2318 ± 1067 ng.hr/mL) rats were 19 and 31 fold higher than those measured in postmenopausal cancer patients, receiving the recommended clinical dose.

Exemestane was not mutagenic in vitro in bacteria (Ames test) or mammalian cells (V79 Chinese hamster lung cells). Exemestane was clastogenic in human lymphocytes in vitro without metabolic activation but was not clastogenic in vivo (micronucleus assay in mouse bone marrow). Exemestane did not increase unscheduled DNA synthesis in rat hepatocytes when tested in vitro.

In a pilot reproductive study in rats, male rats were treated with doses of 125–1000 mg/kg/day exemestane, beginning 63 days prior to and during cohabitation. Untreated female rats showed reduced fertility when mated to males treated with ≥500 mg/kg/day exemestane (≥200 times the recommended human dose on a mg/m² basis). In a separate study, exemestane was given to female rats at 4–100 mg/kg/day beginning 14 days prior to mating and through day 15 or 20 of gestation. Exemestane increased the placental weights at ≥4 mg/kg/day (≥1.5 times the human dose on a mg/m² basis). Exemestane showed no effects on ovarian function, mating behavior, and conception rate in rats given doses up to 20 mg/kg/day (approximately 8 times the recommended human dose on a mg/m² basis), however, decreases in mean litter size and fetal body weight, along with delayed ossification were evidenced at ≥20 mg/kg/day. In general toxicology studies, changes in the ovary, including hyperplasia, an increase in the incidence of ovarian cysts and a decrease in corpora lutea were observed with variable frequency in mice, rats and dogs at doses that ranged from 3–20 times the human dose on a mg/m² basis.

Pregnancy. Pregnancy Category D. See WARNINGS.

Nursing Mothers. AROMASIN is only indicated in postmenopausal women. However, radioactivity related to exemestane appeared in rat milk within 15 minutes of oral administration of radiolabeled exemestane. Concentrations of exemestane and its metabolites were approximately equivalent in the milk and plasma of rats for 24 hours after a single oral dose of 1 mg/kg ^{14}C-exemestane. It is not known whether exemestane is excreted in human milk. Because many drugs are excreted in human milk, caution should be exercised if a nursing woman is inadvertently exposed to AROMASIN (see WARNINGS).

Pediatric Use. The safety and effectiveness of AROMASIN in pediatric patients have not been evaluated.

Geriatric Use. The use of AROMASIN in geriatric patients does not require special precautions.

ADVERSE REACTIONS

Adjuvant Treatment of Early Breast Cancer

AROMASIN tolerability in postmenopausal women with early breast cancer was evaluated in two well-controlled trials: the IES study (see CLINICAL STUDIES) and the 027 study (a randomized, placebo-controlled, double-blind, parallel group study specifically designed to assess the effects of exemestane on bone metabolism, hormones, lipids and coagulation factors over 2 years of treatment).

Certain adverse events, expected based on the known pharmacological properties and side effect profiles of test drugs, were actively sought through a positive checklist. Signs and symptoms were graded for severity using CTC in both studies. Within the IES study, the presence of some illnesses/conditions was monitored through a positive checklist without assessment of severity. These included myocardial infarction, other cardiovascular disorders, gynecological disorders, osteoporosis, osteoporotic fractures, other primary cancer, and hospitalizations.

The median duration of adjuvant treatment was 27.4 months and 27.3 months for patients receiving AROMASIN or tamoxifen, respectively, within the IES study and 23.9 months for patients receiving AROMASIN or placebo within the 027 study. Median duration of observation after randomization for AROMASIN was 34.5 months and for tamoxifen was 34.6 months. Median duration of observation was 30 months for both groups in the 027 study.

AROMASIN was generally well tolerated and adverse events were usually mild to moderate. Within the IES study discontinuations due to adverse events occurred in 6.3% and 5.1% of patients receiving AROMASIN and tamoxifen, respectively, and in 12.3% and 4.1% of patients receiving exemestane or placebo within study 027. Deaths due to any cause were reported for 1.3% of the exemestane-treated patients and 1.4% of the tamoxifen-treated patients within the IES study. There were 6 deaths due to stroke on the exemestane arm compared to 2 on tamoxifen. There were 5 deaths due to cardiac failure on the exemestane arm compared to 2 on tamoxifen.

The incidence of cardiac ischemic events (myocardial infarction, angina and myocardial ischemia) was 1.6% in exemestane treated patients and 0.6% in tamoxifen treated patients in the IES study. Cardiac failure was observed in 0.4% of exemestane treated patients and 0.3% of tamoxifen treated patients.

Treatment-emergent adverse events and illnesses including all causalities and occurring with an incidence of ≥5% in either treatment group of the IES study during or within one month of the end of treatment are shown in Table 8.

Table 8. Incidence (%) of Adverse Events of all Grades[1] and Illnesses Occurring in (≥5%) of Patients in Any Treatment Group in Study IES in Postmenopausal Women with Early Breast Cancer

Body system and Adverse Event by MedDRA dictionary	% of patients	
	AROMASIN 25 mg daily (N=2252)	Tamoxifen 20 mg daily[2] (N=2280)
Eye		
Visual disturbances[3]	5.0	3.8
Gastrointestinal		
Nausea[3]	8.5	8.7
General Disorders		
Fatigue[3]	16.1	14.7
Musculoskeletal		
Arthralgia	14.6	8.6
Pain in limb	9.0	6.4
Back pain	8.6	7.2
Osteoarthritis	5.9	4.5
Nervous System		
Headache[3]	13.1	10.8
Dizziness[3]	9.7	8.4
Psychiatric		
Insomnia[3]	12.4	8.9
Depression	6.2	5.6
Skin & Subcutaneous Tissue		
Increased sweating[3]	11.8	10.4
Vascular		
Hot flushes[3]	21.2	19.9
Hypertension	9.8	8.4

[1] Graded according to Common Toxicity Criteria; [2] 75 patients received tamoxifen 30 mg daily; [3] Event actively sought.

In the IES study, as compared to tamoxifen, AROMASIN was associated with a higher incidence of events in the musculoskeletal disorders and in the nervous system disorders, including the following events occurring with frequency lower than 5%: osteoporosis [4.6% vs. 2.8%], osteochondrosis and trigger finger [0.3% vs 0 for both events], paresthesia [2.6% vs. 0.9%], carpal tunnel syndrome [2.4% vs. 0.2%], and neuropathy [0.6% vs. 0.1%]. Diarrhea was also more frequent in the exemestane group (4.2% vs. 2.2%). Clinical fractures were reported in 94 patients receiving exemestane (4.2%) and 71 patients receiving tamoxifen (3.1%). After a median duration of therapy of about 30 months and a median follow-up of about 52 months, gastric ulcer was observed at a slightly higher frequency in the AROMASIN group compared to tamoxifen (0.7% versus <0.1%). The majority of patients on AROMASIN with gastric ulcer received concomitant treatment with non-steroidal anti-inflammatory agents and/or had a prior history.

Tamoxifen was associated with a higher incidence of muscle cramps [3.1% vs. 1.5%], thromboembolism [2.0% vs. 0.9%], endometrial hyperplasia [1.7% vs. 0.6%], and uterine polyps [2.4% vs. 0.4%].

Common adverse events occurring on study 027 are described in Table 9.

Table 9: Incidence of Selected Treatment-Emergent Adverse Events of all CTC Grades* Occurring in ≥ 5% of Patients in Either Arm on Study 027

Adverse Event	Exemestane N=73 (% incidence)	Placebo N=73 (% incidence)
Hot flushes	32.9	24.7
Arthralgia	28.8	28.8
Increased Sweating	17.8	20.6
Alopecia	15.1	4.1
Hypertension	15.1	6.9
Insomnia	13.7	15.1
Nausea	12.3	16.4

Fatigue	11.0	19.2
Abdominal pain	11.0	13.7
Depression	9.6	6.9
Diarrhea	9.6	1.4
Dizziness	9.6	9.6
Dermatitis	8.2	1.4
Headache	6.9	4.1
Myalgia	5.5	4.1
Edema	5.5	6.9
Anxiety	4.1	5.5

* Most events were CTC grade 1–2

Treatment of Advanced Breast Cancer

A total of 1058 patients were treated with exemestane 25 mg once daily in the clinical trials program. Exemestane was generally well tolerated, and adverse events were usually mild to moderate. Only one death was considered possibly related to treatment with exemestane; an 80-year-old woman with known coronary artery disease had a myocardial infarction with multiple organ failure after 9 weeks on study treatment. In the clinical trials program, only 3% of the patients discontinued treatment with exemestane because of adverse events, mainly within the first 10 weeks of treatment; late discontinuations because of adverse events were uncommon (0.3%).

In the comparative study, adverse reactions were assessed for 358 patients treated with AROMASIN and 400 patients treated with megestrol acetate. Fewer patients receiving AROMASIN discontinued treatment because of adverse events than those treated with megestrol acetate (2% vs. 5%). Adverse events that were considered drug related or of indeterminate cause included hot flashes (13% vs. 5%), nausea (9% vs. 5%), fatigue (8% vs. 10%), increased sweating (4% vs. 8%), and increased appetite (3% vs. 6%). The proportion of patients experiencing an excessive weight gain (>10% of their baseline weight) was significantly higher with megestrol acetate than with AROMASIN (17% vs. 8%). Table 10 shows the adverse events of all CTC grades, regardless of causality, reported in 5% or greater of patients in the study treated either with AROMASIN or megestrol acetate.

Table 10. Incidence (%) of Adverse Events of all Grades* and Causes Occurring in ≥5% of Advanced Breast Cancer Patients In Each Treatment Arm in the Comparative Study

Body system and Adverse Event by WHO ART dictionary	AROMASIN 25 mg once daily (N=358)	Megestrol Acetate 40 mg QID (N=400)
Autonomic Nervous		
Increased sweating	6	9
Body as a Whole		
Fatigue	22	29
Hot flashes	13	5
Pain	13	13
Influenza-like symptoms	6	5
Edema (includes edema, peripheral edema, leg edema)	7	6
Cardiovascular		
Hypertension	5	6
Nervous		
Depression	13	9
Insomnia	11	9
Anxiety	10	11
Dizziness	8	6
Headache	8	7
Gastrointestinal		
Nausea	18	12
Vomiting	7	4
Abdominal pain	6	11
Anorexia	6	5
Constipation	5	8
Diarrhea	4	5
Increased appetite	3	6

Respiratory		
Dyspnea	10	15
Coughing	6	7

* Graded according to Common Toxicity Criteria

Less frequent adverse events of any cause (from 2% to 5%) reported in the comparative study for patients receiving AROMASIN 25 mg once daily were fever, generalized weakness, paresthesia, pathological fracture, bronchitis, sinusitis, rash, itching, urinary tract infection, and lymphedema. Additional adverse events of any cause observed in the overall clinical trials program (N = 1058) in 5% or greater of patients treated with exemestane 25 mg once daily but not in the comparative study included pain at tumor sites (8%), asthenia (6%) and fever (5%). Adverse events of any cause reported in 2% to 5% of all patients treated with exemestane 25 mg in the overall clinical trials program but not in the comparative study included chest pain, hypoesthesia, confusion, dyspepsia, arthralgia, back pain, skeletal pain, infection, upper respiratory tract infection, pharyngitis, rhinitis, and alopecia.

Post-marketing Experience

The following adverse reactions have been identified during post approval use of Aromasin. Because reactions are reported voluntarily from a population of uncertain size, it is not always possible to reliably estimate their frequency or establish a causal relationship to drug exposure.

Cases of hepatitis including cholestatic hepatitis have been observed in clinical trials and reported through post-marketing surveillance.

OVERDOSAGE

Clinical trials have been conducted with exemestane given as a single dose to healthy female volunteers at doses as high as 800 mg and daily for 12 weeks to postmenopausal women with advanced breast cancer at doses as high as 600 mg. These dosages were well tolerated. There is no specific antidote to overdosage and treatment must be symptomatic. General supportive care, including frequent monitoring of vital signs and close observation of the patient, is indicated.

A male child (age unknown) accidentally ingested a 25-mg tablet of exemestane. The initial physical examination was normal, but blood tests performed 1 hour after ingestion indicated leucocytosis (WBC 25000/mm^3 with 90% neutrophils). Blood tests were repeated 4 days after the incident and were normal. No treatment was given.

In mice, mortality was observed after a single oral dose of exemestane of 3200 mg/kg, the lowest dose tested (about 640 times the recommended human dose on a mg/m^2 basis). In rats and dogs, mortality was observed after single oral doses of exemestane of 5000 mg/kg (about 2000 times the recommended human dose on a mg/m^2 basis) and of 3000 mg/kg (about 4000 times the recommended human dose on a mg/m^2 basis), respectively.

Convulsions were observed after single doses of exemestane of 400 mg/kg and 3000 mg/kg in mice and dogs (approximately 80 and 4000 times the recommended human dose on a mg/m^2 basis), respectively.

DOSAGE AND ADMINISTRATION

The recommended dose of AROMASIN in early and advanced breast cancer is one 25 mg tablet once daily after a meal.

In postmenopausal women with early breast cancer who have been treated with 2–3 years of tamoxifen, treatment with AROMASIN should continue in the absence of recurrence or contralateral breast cancer until completion of five years of adjuvant endocrine therapy.

For patients with advanced breast cancer, treatment with AROMASIN should continue until tumor progression is evident.

For patients receiving AROMASIN with a potent CYP 3A4 inducer such as rifampicin or phenytoin, the recommended dose of AROMASIN is 50 mg once daily after a meal.

The safety of chronic dosing in patients with moderate or severe hepatic or renal impairment has not been studied. Based on experience with exemestane at repeated doses up to 200 mg daily that demonstrated a moderate increase in non-life threatening adverse events, dosage adjustment does not appear to be necessary (see CLINICAL PHARMACOLOGY, Special Populations and PRECAUTIONS).

HOW SUPPLIED

AROMASIN Tablets are round, biconvex, and off-white to slightly gray. Each tablet contains 25 mg of exemestane. The tablets are printed on one side with the number "7663" in black. AROMASIN is packaged in HDPE bottles with a child-resistant screw cap, supplied in packs of 30 tablets.

30-tablet HDPE bottle   NDC 0009-7663-04

Store at 25°C (77°F); excursions permitted to 15°–30°C (59°–86°F) [see USP Controlled Room Temperature].

Rx only

Distributed by
Pharmacia & Upjohn Company
Division of Pfizer Inc, NY, NY 10017
LAB-0098-11.0
Revised October 2008

PATIENT INFORMATION

AROMASIN® (ah ROME ah sin)
(exemestane tablets)

Read the patient information leaflet that comes with AROMASIN before you start taking it. Read the leaflet each time you get a refill. There may be new information. This leaflet does not replace talking with your doctor about your condition or treatment. If you have any questions about AROMASIN, ask your nurse, doctor, or pharmacist.

What is AROMASIN?

AROMASIN is used in women who are past menopause. It is used in:
* **Early breast cancer** (cancer that has *not* spread outside the breast). AROMASIN lowers the risk the cancer will come back. It is for women who:
  * Have cancer that needs the female hormone estrogen to grow *and*
  * Had surgery for breast cancer, and possibly other treatments for breast cancer including radiation or chemotherapy *and*
  * Have taken tamoxifen for 2 to 3 years *and*
  * Are switching to AROMASIN to finish 5 years in a row of hormonal therapy.
* **Advanced breast cancer** (cancer that has spread), to treat cancer that came back after treatment with tamoxifen.

Certain breast cancers need the female hormone estrogen to grow (estrogen receptor-positive cancer).

While you are taking AROMASIN, your body stops making estrogen. AROMASIN may slow or stop the growth of the cancer.

AROMASIN is hormone therapy. It is not chemotherapy. It is not hormone replacement therapy (HRT).

Who should not take AROMASIN?

Do not take AROMASIN if:
* You are allergic to AROMASIN or anything in it. The active ingredient is exemestane. There is a list of what is in AROMASIN at the end of this leaflet.

What should I tell my doctor before taking AROMASIN?

Tell your doctor about all your medical conditions. Be sure to tell your doctor if you:
* Are still having menstrual periods (are not past menopause). AROMASIN is only for women who are past menopause.
* Are pregnant or could be pregnant. Taking AROMASIN during pregnancy may cause birth defects or miscarriage.
* Are breast-feeding. Do not breast-feed while you are being treated with AROMASIN.
* Have liver or kidney problems.

Tell your doctor about all the medicines you take. Include prescription and nonprescription medicines, herbal remedies, and vitamins.

AROMASIN and other medicines may affect how each other work.

Be sure to tell your doctor if you take:
* Medicines with estrogen, such as Premarin®, other hormone replacement therapy, or birth control pills or patches. AROMASIN should not be taken with these medicine as they could affect how well AROMASIN works.
* Rifadin® (rifampin)
* Dilantin® (phenytoin), Tegretol® (carbamazepine), or Luminal® (phenobarbital)
* St. John's wort

Know what medicines you take. Keep a list of them with you. Show it to your doctor or pharmacist each time you get a new prescription.

What are possible side effects of AROMASIN?

Serious Side Effects
* Bone loss. AROMASIN may reduce your bone density (BMD) over time. This may raise your risk for bone fractures.
* Chest pain, heart failure or stroke. A small number of women had chest pain, heart failure or a stroke while taking AROMASIN.

Common Side Effects
* hot flashes
* headache
* depression
* difficultly in breathing
* feeling tired
* trouble sleeping
* feeling anxious
* joint pain
* increased sweating
* upset stomach

Your doctor may do blood tests to check your liver and kidney function during treatment.

These are not all the side effects with AROMASIN. Ask your cancer nurse or doctor for a more complete list.

How should I take AROMASIN?

- Take your dose of AROMASIN once a day, every day, after a meal. AROMASIN comes in 25mg tablets you take by mouth. Your doctor will tell you how many AROMASIN tablets to take for your dose.
- Try to take your treatment at the same time each day.
- Take your medicine for as long as your doctor tells you.
- Tell your doctor if you do not feel well after starting AROMASIN.
- If you miss a dose of AROMASIN, take it as soon as you remember. If it is close to your next dose, just take your next dose at your regular time.
- Don't take more than one dose of AROMASIN at a time.
- Make a note of when your prescription will run out. That way, you can get it refilled on time.

How do I store AROMASIN?

- Keep AROMASIN and all medicines out of the reach of children.
- Store AROMASIN at room temperature, 77°F (25°C), in its original container.

General information about AROMASIN

Doctors can prescribe medicines for conditions that are not in the patient information leaflet. Use AROMASIN only for what your doctor prescribed. Do not give it to other people, even if they have the same conditions you have. It may harm them.

This leaflet gives the most important information about AROMASIN. For more information about AROMASIN, talk with your doctor, nurse, or pharmacist. You can visit our Web site at www.AROMASIN.com, or call 1-888-AROMASIN (1-888-276-6274).

What is in AROMASIN?

Active ingredient: exemestane

Inactive ingredients: mannitol, crospovidone, polysorbate 80, hypromellose, colloidal silicon dioxide, microcrystalline cellulose, sodium starch glycolate, magnesium stearate, simethicone, polyethylene glycol 6000, sucrose, magnesium carbonate, titanium dioxide, methylparaben, and polyvinyl alcohol

MADE IN ITALY

Rx only

Distributed by Pharmacia & Upjohn Company LLC
Division of Pfizer Inc New York, NY 10017

Printed in the USA.

Created: January 2009
LAB-0399-1.0

DETROL® ℞

[DE-trol]
tolterodine tartrate tablets

DESCRIPTION

DETROL Tablets contain tolterodine tartrate. The active moiety, tolterodine, is a muscarinic receptor antagonist. The chemical name of tolterodine tartrate is (R)-2-[3-[bis(1-methylethyl)-amino]1-phenylpropyl]-4-methylphenol [R-(R*,R*)]-2,3dihydroxybutanedioate (1:1) (salt). The empirical formula of tolterodine tartrate is $C_{26}H_{37}NO_7$, and its molecular weight is 475.6. The structural formula of tolterodine tartrate is represented below:

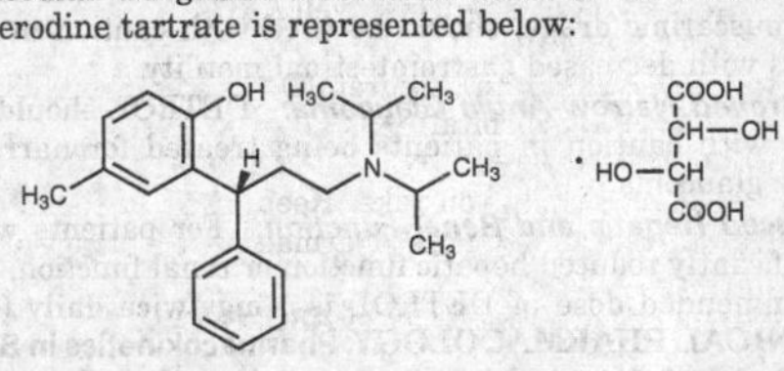

Tolterodine tartrate is a white, crystalline powder. The pKa value is 9.87 and the solubility in water is 12 mg/mL. It is soluble in methanol, slightly soluble in ethanol, and practically insoluble in toluene. The partition coefficient (Log D) between n-octanol and water is 1.83 at pH 7.3.

DETROL Tablets for oral administration contain 1 or 2 mg of tolterodine tartrate. The inactive ingredients are colloidal anhydrous silica, calcium hydrogen phosphate dihydrate, cellulose microcrystalline, hypromellose, magnesium stearate, sodium starch glycolate (pH 3.0 to 5.0), stearic acid, and titanium dioxide.

CLINICAL PHARMACOLOGY

Tolterodine is a competitive muscarinic receptor antagonist. Both urinary bladder contraction and salivation are mediated via cholinergic muscarinic receptors.

After oral administration, tolterodine is metabolized in the liver, resulting in the formation of the 5-hydroxymethyl derivative, a major pharmacologically active metabolite. The 5-hydroxymethyl metabolite, which exhibits an antimuscarinic activity similar to that of tolterodine, contributes significantly to the therapeutic effect. Both tolterodine and the 5-hydroxymethyl metabolite exhibit a high specificity for muscarinic receptors, since both show negligible activity or affinity for other neurotransmitter receptors and other potential cellular targets, such as calcium channels.

Table 1. Summary of Mean (±SD) Pharmacokinetic Parameters of Tolterodine and its Active Metabolite (5-hydroxymethyl metabolite) in Healthy Volunteers

	Tolterodine					5-Hydroxymethyl Metabolite			
Phenotype (CYP2D6)	t_{max} (h)	C_{max}* (μg/L)	C_{avg}* (μg/L)	$t_{1/2}$ (h)	CL/F (L/h)	t_{max} (h)	C_{max}* (μg/L)	C_{avg}* (μg/L)	$t_{1/2}$ (h)
Single-dose									
EM	1.6±1.5	1.6±1.2	0.50±0.35	2.0±0.7	534±697	1.8±1.4	1.8±0.7	0.62±0.26	3.1±0.7
PM	1.4±0.5	10±4.9	8.3±4.3	6.5±1.6	17±7.3	-†	-	-	-
Multiple-dose									
EM	1.2±0.5	2.6±2.8	0.58±0.54	2.2±0.4	415±377	1.2±0.5	2.4±1.3	0.92±0.46	2.9±0.4
PM	1.9±1.0	19±7.5	12±5.1	9.6±1.5	11±4.2	-	-	-	-

* Parameter was dose-normalized from 4 mg to 2 mg.
C_{max} = Maximum plasma concentration; t_{max} = Time of occurrence of C_{max};
C_{avg} = Average plasma concentration; $t_{1/2}$ = Terminal elimination half-life; CL/F = Apparent oral clearance.
EM = Extensive metabolizers; PM = Poor metabolizers.
† - = not applicable.

Tolterodine has a pronounced effect on bladder function. Effects on urodynamic parameters before and 1 and 5 hours after a single 6.4 mg dose of tolterodine immediate release were determined in healthy volunteers. The main effects of tolterodine at 1 and 5 hours were an increase in residual urine, reflecting an incomplete emptying of the bladder, and a decrease in detrusor pressure. These findings are consistent with an antimuscarinic action on the lower urinary tract.

Pharmacokinetics

Absorption: In a study with ^{14}C-tolterodine solution in healthy volunteers who received a 5-mg oral dose, at least 77% of the radiolabeled dose was absorbed. Tolterodine immediate release is rapidly absorbed, and maximum serum concentrations (C_{max}) typically occur within 1 to 2 hours after dose administration. C_{max} and area under the concentration-time curve (AUC) determined after dosage of tolterodine immediate release are dose-proportional over the range of 1 to 4 mg.

Effect of Food: Food intake increases the bioavailability of tolterodine (average increase 53%), but does not affect the levels of the 5-hydroxymethyl metabolite in extensive metabolizers. This change is not expected to be a safety concern and adjustment of dose is not needed.

Distribution: Tolterodine is highly bound to plasma proteins, primarily α_1-acid glycoprotein. Unbound concentrations of tolterodine average 3.7% ± 0.13% over the concentration range achieved in clinical studies. The 5-hydroxymethyl metabolite is not extensively protein bound, with unbound fraction concentrations averaging 36% ± 4.0%. The blood to serum ratio of tolterodine and the 5-hydroxymethyl metabolite averages 0.6 and 0.8, respectively, indicating that these compounds do not distribute extensively into erythrocytes. The volume of distribution of tolterodine following administration of a 1.28-mg intravenous dose is 113 ± 26.7 L.

Metabolism: Tolterodine is extensively metabolized by the liver following oral dosing. The primary metabolic route involves the oxidation of the 5-methyl group and is mediated by the cytochrome P450 2D6 (CYP2D6) and leads to the formation of a pharmacologically active 5-hydroxymethyl metabolite. Further metabolism leads to formation of the 5-carboxylic acid and *N*-dealkylated 5-carboxylic acid metabolites, which account for 51% ± 14% and 29% ± 6.3% of the metabolites recovered in the urine, respectively.

Variability in Metabolism: A subset (about 7%) of the population is devoid of CYP2D6, the enzyme responsible for the formation of the 5-hydroxymethyl metabolite of tolterodine. The identified pathway of metabolism for these individuals ("poor metabolizers") is dealkylation via cytochrome P450 3A4 (CYP3A4) to *N*-dealkylated tolterodine. The remainder of the population is referred to as "extensive metabolizers." Pharmacokinetic studies revealed that tolterodine is metabolized at a slower rate in poor metabolizers than in extensive metabolizers; this results in significantly higher serum concentrations of tolterodine and in negligible concentrations of the 5-hydroxymethyl metabolite.

Excretion: Following administration of a 5-mg oral dose of ^{14}C-tolterodine solution to healthy volunteers, 77% of radioactivity was recovered in urine and 17% was recovered in feces in 7 days. Less than 1% (<2.5% in poor metabolizers) of the dose was recovered as intact tolterodine, and 5% to 14% (<1% in poor metabolizers) was recovered as the active 5-hydroxymethyl metabolite.

A summary of mean (± standard deviation) pharmacokinetic parameters of tolterodine immediate release and the 5-hydroxymethyl metabolite in extensive (EM) and poor (PM) metabolizers is provided in Table 1. These data were obtained following single and multiple doses of tolterodine 4 mg administered twice daily to 16 healthy male volunteers (8 EM, 8 PM).

[See table 1 above]

Pharmacokinetics in Special Populations

Age: In Phase 1, multiple-dose studies in which tolterodine immediate release 4 mg (2 mg bid) was administered, serum concentrations of tolterodine and of the 5-hydroxymethyl metabolite were similar in healthy elderly volunteers (aged 64 through 80 years) and healthy young volunteers (aged less than 40 years). In another Phase 1 study, elderly volunteers (aged 71 through 81 years) were given tolterodine immediate release 2 or 4 mg (1 or 2 mg bid). Mean serum concentrations of tolterodine and the 5-hydroxymethyl metabolite in these elderly volunteers were approximately 20% and 50% higher, respectively, than reported in young healthy volunteers. However, no overall differences were observed in safety between older and younger patients on tolterodine in Phase 3, 12-week, controlled clinical studies; therefore, no tolterodine dosage adjustment for elderly patients is recommended (see **PRECAUTIONS, Geriatric Use**).

Pediatric: The pharmacokinetics of tolterodine have not been established in pediatric patients.

Gender: The pharmacokinetics of tolterodine immediate release and the 5-hydroxymethyl metabolite are not influenced by gender. Mean C_{max} of tolterodine (1.6 μg/L in males versus 2.2 μg/L in females) and the active 5-hydroxymethyl metabolite (2.2 μg/L in males versus 2.5 μg/L in females) are similar in males and females who were administered tolterodine immediate release 2 mg. Mean AUC values of tolterodine (6.7 μg•h/L in males versus 7.8 μg•h/L in females) and the 5-hydroxymethyl metabolite (10 μg•h/L in males versus 11 μg•h/L in females) are also similar. The elimination half-life of tolterodine for both males and females is 2.4 hours, and the half-life of the 5-hydroxymethyl metabolite is 3.0 hours in females and 3.3 hours in males.

Race: Pharmacokinetic differences due to race have not been established.

Renal Insufficiency: Renal impairment can significantly alter the disposition of tolterodine immediate release and its metabolites. In a study conducted in patients with creatinine clearance between 10 and 30 mL/min, tolterodine immediate release and the 5-hydroxymethyl metabolite levels were approximately 2–3 fold higher in patients with renal impairment than in healthy volunteers. Exposure levels of other metabolites of tolterodine (e.g., tolterodine acid, *N*-dealkylated tolterodine acid, *N*-dealkylated tolterodine, and *N*-dealkylated hydroxylated tolterodine) were significantly higher (10–30 fold) in renally impaired patients as compared to the healthy volunteers. The recommended dosage for patients with significantly reduced renal function is DETROL 1 mg twice daily (see **PRECAUTIONS, General** and **DOSAGE AND ADMINISTRATION**).

Hepatic Insufficiency: Liver impairment can significantly alter the disposition of tolterodine immediate release. In a study conducted in cirrhotic patients, the elimination half-life of tolterodine immediate release was longer in cirrhotic patients (mean, 7.8 hours) than in healthy, young, and elderly volunteers (mean, 2 to 4 hours). The clearance of orally administered tolterodine was substantially lower in cirrhotic patients (1.0 ± 1.7 L/h/kg) than in the healthy volunteers (5.7 ± 3.8 L/h/kg). The recommended dose for patients with significantly reduced hepatic function is DETROL 1 mg twice daily (see **PRECAUTIONS, General** and **DOSAGE AND ADMINISTRATION**).

Drug-Drug Interactions

Fluoxetine: Fluoxetine is a selective serotonin reuptake inhibitor and a potent inhibitor of CYP2D6 activity. In a study

Table 2. Mean (CI) change in QTc from baseline to steady state (Day 4 of dosing) at T_{max} (relative to placebo)

Drug/Dose	N	QTcF (msec) (manual)	QTcF (msec) (machine)	QTcP (msec) (manual)	QTcP (msec) (machine)
Tolterodine 2 mg BID[1]	48	5.01 (0.28, 9.74)	1.16 (-2.99, 5.30)	4.45 (-0.37, 9.26)	2.00 (-1.81, 5.81)
Tolterodine 4 mg BID[1]	48	11.84 (7.11, 16.58)	5.63 (1.48, 9.77)	10.31 (5.49, 15.12)	8.34 (4.53, 12.15)
Moxifloxacin 400 mg QD[2]	45	19.26[3] (15.49, 23.03)	8.90 (4.77, 13.03)	19.10[3] (15.32, 22.89)	9.29 (5.34, 13.24)

[1] At T_{max} of 1 hr; 95% Confidence Interval
[2] At T_{max} of 2 hr; 90% Confidence Interval
[3] The effect on QT interval with 4 days of moxifloxacin dosing in this QT trial may be greater than typically observed in QT trials of other drugs.

Table 3. 95% Confidence Intervals (CI) for the Difference between DETROL (2 mg bid) and Placebo for the Mean Change at Week 12 from Baseline in Study 007

	DETROL (SD) N=514	Placebo (SD) N=508	Difference (95% CI)
Number of Incontinence Episodes per Week			
Mean baseline	23.2	23.3	
Mean change from baseline	-10.6 (17)	-6.9 (15)	-3.7 (-5.7, -1.6)
Number of Micturitions per 24 Hours			
Mean baseline	11.1	11.3	
Mean change from baseline	-1.7 (3.3)	-1.2 (2.9)	-0.5* (-0.9, -0.1)
Volume Voided per Micturition (mL)			
Mean baseline	137	136	
Mean change from baseline	29 (47)	14 (41)	15* (9, 21)

SD = Standard Deviation.
* The difference between DETROL and placebo was statistically significant.

to assess the effect of fluoxetine on the pharmacokinetics of tolterodine immediate release and its metabolites, it was observed that fluoxetine significantly inhibited the metabolism of tolterodine immediate release in extensive metabolizers, resulting in a 4.8-fold increase in tolterodine AUC. There was a 52% decrease in C_{max} and a 20% decrease in AUC of the 5-hydroxymethyl metabolite. Fluoxetine thus alters the pharmacokinetics in patients who would otherwise be extensive metabolizers of tolterodine immediate release to resemble the pharmacokinetic profile in poor metabolizers. The sums of unbound serum concentrations of tolterodine immediate release and the 5-hydroxymethyl metabolite are only 25% higher during the interaction. No dose adjustment is required when DETROL and fluoxetine are coadministered.

Other Drugs Metabolized by Cytochrome P450 Isoenzymes: Tolterodine immediate release does not cause clinically significant interactions with other drugs metabolized by the major drug metabolizing CYP enzymes. In vivo drug-interaction data show that tolterodine immediate release does not result in clinically relevant inhibition of CYP1A2, 2D6, 2C9, 2C19, or 3A4 as evidenced by lack of influence on the marker drugs caffeine, debrisoquine, S-warfarin, and omeprazole. In vitro data show that tolterodine immediate release is a competitive inhibitor of CYP2D6 at high concentrations (Ki 1.05 μM), while tolterodine immediate release as well as the 5-hydroxymethyl metabolite are devoid of any significant inhibitory potential regarding the other isoenzymes.

CYP3A4 Inhibitors: The effect of 200 mg daily dose of ketoconazole on the pharmacokinetics of tolterodine immediate release was studied in 8 healthy volunteers, all of whom were poor metabolizers (see **Pharmacokinetics**, Variability in Metabolism for discussion of poor metabolizers). In the presence of ketoconazole, the mean C_{max} and AUC of tolterodine increased by 2 and 2.5 fold, respectively. Based on these findings, other potent CYP3A inhibitors such as other azole antifungals (eg, itraconazole, miconazole) or macrolide antibiotics (eg, erythromycin, clarithromycin) or cyclosporine or vinblastine may also lead to increases of tolterodine plasma concentrations (see **PRECAUTIONS** and **DOSAGE AND ADMINISTRATION**).

Warfarin: In healthy volunteers, coadministration of tolterodine immediate release 4 mg (2 mg bid) for 7 days and a single dose of warfarin 25 mg on day 4 had no effect on prothrombin time, Factor VII suppression, or on the pharmacokinetics of warfarin.

Oral Contraceptives: Tolterodine immediate release 4 mg (2 mg bid) had no effect on the pharmacokinetics of an oral contraceptive (ethinyl estradiol 30 μg/levonorgestrel 150 μg) as evidenced by the monitoring of ethinyl estradiol and levonorgestrel over a 2-month cycle in healthy female volunteers.

Diuretics: Coadministration of tolterodine immediate release up to 8 mg (4 mg bid) for up to 12 weeks with diuretic agents, such as indapamide, hydrochlorothiazide, triamterene, bendroflumethiazide, chlorothiazide, methylchlorothiazide, or furosemide, did not cause any adverse electrocardiographic (ECG) effects.

Cardiac Electrophysiology
The effect of 2 mg BID and 4 mg BID of tolterodine immediate release (IR) on the QT interval was evaluated in a 4-way crossover, double-blind, placebo- and active-controlled (moxifloxacin 400 mg QD) study in healthy male (N=25) and female (N=23) volunteers aged 18–55 years. Study subjects [approximately equal representation of CYP2D6 extensive metabolizers (EMs) and poor metabolizers (PMs)] completed sequential 4-day periods of dosing with moxifloxacin 400 mg QD, tolterodine 2 mg BID, tolterodine 4 mg BID, and placebo. The 4 mg BID dose of tolterodine IR (two times the highest recommended dose) was chosen because this dose results in tolterodine exposure similar to that observed upon coadministration of tolterodine 2 mg BID with potent CYP3A4 inhibitors in patients who are CYP2D6 poor metabolizers (see **PRECAUTIONS, Drug Interactions**). QT interval was measured over a 12-hour period following dosing, including the time of peak plasma concentration (T_{max}) of tolterodine and at steady state (Day 4 of dosing).

Table 2 summarizes the mean change from baseline to steady state in corrected QT interval (QTc) relative to placebo at the time of peak tolterodine (1 hour) and moxifloxacin (2 hour) concentrations. Both Fridericia's (QTcF) and a population-specific (QTcP) method were used to correct QT interval for heart rate. No single QT correction method is known to be more valid than others. QT interval was measured manually and by machine, and data from both are presented. The mean increase of heart rate associated with a 4 mg/day dose of tolterodine in this study was 2.0 beats/minute and 6.3 beats/minute with 8 mg/day tolterodine. The change in heart rate with moxifloxacin was 0.5 beats/minute.

[See table 2 above]
The reason for the difference between machine and manual read of QT interval is unclear.
The QT effect of tolterodine immediate release tablets appeared greater for 8 mg/day (two times the therapeutic dose) compared to 4 mg/day. The effect of tolterodine

8 mg/day was not as large as that observed after four days of therapeutic dosing with the active control moxifloxacin. However, the confidence intervals overlapped.
Tolterodine's effect on QT interval was found to correlate with plasma concentration of tolterodine. There appeared to be a greater QTc interval increase in CYP2D6 poor metabolizers than in CYP2D6 extensive metabolizers after tolterodine treatment in this study.
This study was not designed to make direct statistical comparisons between drugs or dose levels. There has been no association of Torsade de Pointes in the international post-marketing experience with DETROL or DETROL LA (see **PRECAUTIONS, Patients with Congenital or Acquired QT Prolongation**).

CLINICAL STUDIES

DETROL Tablets were evaluated for the treatment of overactive bladder with symptoms of urge urinary incontinence, urgency, and frequency in four randomized, double-blind, placebo-controlled, 12-week studies. A total of 853 patients received DETROL 2 mg twice daily and 685 patients received placebo. The majority of patients were Caucasian (95%) and female (78%), with a mean age of 60 years (range, 19 to 93 years). At study entry, nearly all patients perceived they had urgency and most patients had increased frequency of micturitions and urge incontinence. These characteristics were well balanced across treatment groups for the studies.
The efficacy endpoints for study 007 (see Table 3) included the change from baseline for:
• Number of incontinence episodes per week
• Number of micturitions per 24 hours (averaged over 7 days)
• Volume of urine voided per micturition (averaged over 2 days)
The efficacy endpoints for studies 008, 009, and 010 (see Table 4) were identical to the above endpoints with the exception that the number of incontinence episodes was per 24 hours (averaged over 7 days).
[See table 3 at left]
[See table 4 at top of next page]

INDICATIONS AND USAGE

DETROL Tablets are indicated for the treatment of overactive bladder with symptoms of urge urinary incontinence, urgency, and frequency.

CONTRAINDICATIONS

DETROL Tablets are contraindicated in patients with urinary retention, gastric retention, or uncontrolled narrow-angle glaucoma. DETROL is also contraindicated in patients who have demonstrated hypersensitivity to the drug or its ingredients.

PRECAUTIONS
General
Risk of Urinary Retention and Gastric Retention: DETROL Tablets should be administered with caution to patients with clinically significant bladder outflow obstruction because of the risk of urinary retention and to patients with gastrointestinal obstructive disorders, such as pyloric stenosis, because of the risk of gastric retention (see **CONTRAINDICATIONS**).
Decreased Gastrointestinal Motility: DETROL, like other antimuscarinic drugs, should be used with caution in patients with decreased gastrointestinal motility.
Controlled Narrow-Angle Glaucoma: DETROL should be used with caution in patients being treated for narrow-angle glaucoma.
Reduced Hepatic and Renal Function: For patients with significantly reduced hepatic function or renal function, the recommended dose of DETROL is 1 mg twice daily (see **CLINICAL PHARMACOLOGY, Pharmacokinetics in Special Populations**).
Myasthenia Gravis: DETROL should be used with caution in patients with myasthenia gravis, a disease characterized by decreased cholinergic activity at the neuromuscular junction.

Patients with Congenital or Acquired QT Prolongation
In a study of the effect of tolterodine immediate release tablets on the QT interval (See **CLINICAL PHARMACOLOGY, Cardiac Electrophysiology**), the effect on the QT interval appeared greater for 8 mg/day (two times the therapeutic dose) compared to 4 mg/day and was more pronounced in CYP2D6 poor metabolizers (PM) than extensive metabolizers (EMs). The effect of tolterodine 8 mg/day was not as large as that observed after four days of therapeutic dosing with the active control moxifloxacin. However, the confidence intervals overlapped. These observations should be considered in clinical decisions to prescribe DETROL for patients with a known history of QT prolongation or patients who are taking Class IA (e.g., quinidine, procainamide) or Class III (e.g., amiodarone, sotalol) antiarrhythmic medications (see **PRECAUTIONS, Drug**

Interactions). There has been no association of Torsade de Pointes in the international post-marketing experience with DETROL or DETROL LA.

Information for Patients

Patients should be informed that antimuscarinic agents such as DETROL may produce the following effects: blurred vision, dizziness, or drowsiness. Patients should be advised to exercise caution in decisions to engage in potentially dangerous activities until the drug's effects have been determined.

Drug Interactions

CYP3A4 Inhibitors: Ketoconazole, an inhibitor of the drug metabolizing enzyme CYP3A4, significantly increased plasma concentrations of tolterodine when coadministered to subjects who were poor metabolizers (see **CLINICAL PHARMACOLOGY**, Variability in Metabolism and **Drug-Drug Interactions**). For patients receiving ketoconazole or other potent CYP3A4 inhibitors such as other azole antifungals (e.g., itraconazole, miconazole) or macrolide antibiotics (e.g., erythromycin, clarithromycin) or cyclosporine or vinblastine, the recommended dose of DETROL is 1 mg twice daily (see **DOSAGE AND ADMINISTRATION**).

Drug-Laboratory-Test Interactions

Interactions between tolterodine and laboratory tests have not been studied.

Carcinogenesis, Mutagenesis, Impairment of Fertility

Carcinogenicity studies with tolterodine were conducted in mice and rats. At the maximum tolerated dose in mice (30 mg/kg/day), female rats (20 mg/kg/day), and male rats (30 mg/kg/day), AUC values obtained for tolterodine were 355, 291, and 462 µg•h/L, respectively. In comparison, the human AUC value for a 2-mg dose administered twice daily is estimated at 34 µg•h/L. Thus, tolterodine exposure in the carcinogenicity studies was 9- to 14-fold than expected in humans. No increase in tumors was found in either mice or rats.

No mutagenic effects of tolterodine were detected in a battery of *in vitro* tests, including bacterial mutation assays (Ames test) in 4 strains of *Salmonella typhimurium* and in 2 strains of *Escherichia coli*, a gene mutation assay in L5178Y mouse lymphoma cells, and chromosomal aberration tests in human lymphocytes. Tolterodine was also negative *in vivo* in the bone marrow micronucleus test in the mouse.

In female mice treated for 2 weeks before mating and during gestation with 20 mg/kg/day (corresponding to AUC value of about 500 µg•h/L), neither effects on reproductive performance or fertility were seen. Based on AUC values, the systemic exposure was about 15-fold higher in animals than in humans. In male mice, a dose of 30 mg/kg/day did not induce any adverse effects on fertility.

Pregnancy

Pregnancy Category C. At oral doses of 20 mg/kg/day (approximately 14 times the human exposure), no anomalies or malformations were observed in mice. When given at doses of 30 to 40 mg/kg/day, tolterodine has been shown to be embryolethal, reduce fetal weight, and increase the incidence of fetal abnormalities (cleft palate, digital abnormalities, intra-abdominal hemorrhage, and various skeletal abnormalities, primarily reduced ossification) in mice. At these doses, the AUC values were about 20- to 25-fold higher than in humans. Rabbits treated subcutaneously at a dose of 0.8 mg/kg/day achieved an AUC of 100 µg•h/L, which is about 3-fold higher than that resulting from the human dose. This dose did not result in any embryotoxicity or teratogenicity. There are no studies of tolterodine in pregnant women. Therefore, DETROL should be used during pregnancy only if the potential benefit for the mother justifies the potential risk to the fetus.

Nursing Mothers

Tolterodine is excreted into the milk in mice. Offspring of female mice treated with tolterodine 20 mg/kg/day during the lactation period had slightly reduced body weight gain. The offspring regained the weight during the maturation phase. It is not known whether tolterodine is excreted in human milk; therefore, DETROL should not be administered during nursing. A decision should be made whether to discontinue nursing or to discontinue DETROL in nursing mothers.

Pediatric Use

Efficacy in the pediatric population has not been demonstrated.

Two pediatric phase 3 randomized, placebo-controlled, double-blind, 12-week studies were conducted using tolterodine extended release (DETROL LA) capsules. A total of 710 pediatric patients (486 on DETROL LA and 224 on placebo) aged 5–10 years with urinary frequency and urge urinary incontinence were studied. The percentage of patients with urinary tract infections was higher in patients treated with DETROL LA (6.6%) compared to patients who received placebo (4.5%). Aggressive, abnormal and hyperactive behavior and attention disorders occurred in 2.9% of children treated with DETROL LA compared to 0.9% of children treated with placebo.

Table 4. 95% Confidence Intervals (CI) for the Difference between DETROL (2 mg bid) and Placebo for the Mean Change at Week 12 from Baseline in Studies 008, 009, 010

Study		DETROL (SD)	Placebo (SD)	Difference (95% CI)
Number of Incontinence Episodes per 24 Hours				
008	Number of patients	93	40	
	Mean baseline	2.9	3.3	
	Mean change from baseline	-1.3 (3.2)	-0.9 (1.5)	0.5 (-1.3,0.3)
009	Number of patients	116	55	
	Mean baseline	3.6	3.5	
	Mean change from baseline	-1.7 (2.5)	-1.3 (2.5)	-0.4 (-1.0,0.2)
010	Number of patients	90	50	
	Mean baseline	3.7	3.5	
	Mean change from baseline	-1.6 (2.4)	-1.1 (2.1)	-0.5 (-1.1,0.1)
Number of Micturitions per 24 Hours				
008	Number of patients	118	56	
	Mean baseline	11.5	11.7	
	Mean change from baseline	-2.7 (3.8)	-1.6 (3.6)	-1.2* (-2.0,-0.4)
009	Number of patients	128	64	
	Mean baseline	11.2	11.3	
	Mean change from baseline	-2.3 (2.1)	-1.4 (2.8)	-0.9* (-1.5,-0.3)
010	Number of patients	108	56	
	Mean baseline	11.6	11.6	
	Mean change from baseline	-1.7 (2.3)	-1.4 (2.8)	-0.38 (-1.1,0.3)
Volume Voided per Micturition (mL)				
008	Number of patients	118	56	
	Mean baseline	166	157	
	Mean change from baseline	38 (54)	6 (42)	32* (18,46)
009	Number of patients	129	64	
	Mean baseline	155	158	
	Mean change from baseline	36 (50)	10 (47)	26* (14,38)
010	Number of patients	108	56	
	Mean baseline	155	160	
	Mean change from baseline	31 (45)	13 (52)	18* (4,32)

SD = Standard Deviation.
* The difference between DETROL and placebo was statistically significant.

Table 5. Incidence* (%) of Adverse Events Exceeding Placebo Rate and Reported in >1% of Patients Treated with DETROL Tablets (2 mg bid) in 12-week, Phase 3 Clinical Studies

Body System	Adverse Event	% DETROL N=986	% Placebo N=683
Autonomic Nervous	accommodation abnormal	2	1
	dry mouth	35	10
General	chest pain	2	1
	fatigue	4	3
	headache	7	5
	influenza-like symptoms	3	2
Central/Peripheral Nervous	vertigo/dizziness	5	3
Gastrointestinal	abdominal pain	5	3
	constipation	7	4
	diarrhea	4	3
	dyspepsia	4	1
Urinary	dysuria	2	1
Skin/Appendages	dry skin	1	0
Musculoskeletal	arthralgia	2	1
Vision	xerophthalmia	3	2
Psychiatric	somnolence	3	2
Metabolic/Nutritional	weight gain	1	0
Resistance Mechanism	infection	1	0

*in nearest integer.

Geriatric Use

Of the 1120 patients who were treated in the four Phase 3, 12-week clinical studies of DETROL, 474 (42%) were 65 to 91 years of age. No overall differences in safety were observed between the older and younger patients (see **CLINICAL PHARMACOLOGY, Pharmacokinetics in Special Populations**).

ADVERSE REACTIONS

The Phase 2 and 3 clinical trial program for DETROL Tablets included 3071 patients who were treated with DETROL (N=2133) or placebo (N=938). The patients were treated with 1, 2, 4, or 8 mg/day for up to 12 months. No differences in the safety profile of tolterodine were identified based on age, gender, race, or metabolism.

The data described below reflect exposure to DETROL 2 mg bid in 986 patients and to placebo in 683 patients exposed for 12 weeks in five Phase 3, controlled clinical studies. Because clinical trials are conducted under widely varying conditions, adverse reaction rates observed in the clinical trials of a drug cannot be directly compared to rates in the clinical trials of another drug and may not reflect the rates observed in practice. The adverse reaction information from clinical trials does, however, provide a basis for identifying the adverse events that appear to be related to drug use and approximating rates.

Sixty-six percent of patients receiving DETROL 2 mg bid reported adverse events versus 56% of placebo patients. The most common adverse events reported by patients receiving DETROL were dry mouth, headache, constipation, vertigo/dizziness, and abdominal pain. Dry mouth, constipation, abnormal vision (accommodation abnormalities), urinary retention, and xerophthalmia are expected side effects of antimuscarinic agents.

Dry mouth was the most frequently reported adverse event for patients treated with DETROL 2 mg bid in the Phase 3 clinical studies, occurring in 34.8% of patients treated with DETROL and 9.8% of placebo-treated patients. One percent of patients treated with DETROL discontinued treatment due to dry mouth.

The frequency of discontinuation due to adverse events was highest during the first 4 weeks of treatment. Seven percent of patients treated with DETROL 2 mg bid discontinued treatment due to adverse events versus 6% of placebo patients. The most common adverse events leading to discontinuation of DETROL were dizziness and headache.

Three percent of patients treated with DETROL 2 mg bid reported a serious adverse event versus 4% of placebo patients. Significant ECG changes in QT and QTc have not been demonstrated in clinical-study patients treated with DETROL 2 mg bid. Table 5 lists the adverse events reported in 1% or more of the patients treated with DETROL 2 mg bid in the 12-week studies. The adverse events are reported regardless of causality.

[See table 5 on previous page]

Post-marketing Surveillance

The following events have been reported in association with tolterodine use in worldwide post-marketing experience: *General:* anaphylactoid reactions, including angioedema; *Cardiovascular:* tachycardia, palpitations, peripheral edema; *Central/Peripheral Nervous:* confusion, disorientation, memory impairment, hallucinations.

Reports of aggravation of symptoms of dementia (e.g. confusion, disorientation, delusion) have been reported after tolterodine therapy was initiated in patients taking cholinesterase inhibitors for the treatment of dementia.

Because these spontaneously reported events are from the worldwide post-marketing experience, the frequency of events and the role of tolterodine in their causation cannot be reliably determined.

OVERDOSAGE

A 27-month-old child who ingested 5 to 7 DETROL Tablets 2 mg was treated with a suspension of activated charcoal and was hospitalized overnight with symptoms of dry mouth. The child fully recovered.

Management of Overdosage

Overdosage with DETROL can potentially result in severe central anticholinergic effects and should be treated accordingly.

ECG monitoring is recommended in the event of overdosage. In dogs, changes in the QT interval (slight prolongation of 10% to 20%) were observed at a suprapharmacologic dose of 4.5 mg/kg, which is about 68 times higher than the recommended human dose. In clinical trials of normal volunteers and patients, QT interval prolongation was observed with tolterodine immediate release at doses up to 8 mg (4 mg bid) and higher doses were not evaluated (see **PRECAUTIONS, Patients with Congenital or Acquired QT Prolongation**).

DOSAGE AND ADMINISTRATION

The initial recommended dose of DETROL Tablets is 2 mg twice daily. The dose may be lowered to 1 mg twice daily based on individual response and tolerability. For patients with significantly reduced hepatic or renal function or who are currently taking drugs that are potent inhibitors of CYP3A4, the recommended dose of DETROL is 1 mg twice daily (see **PRECAUTIONS, General** and **PRECAUTIONS, Drug Interactions**).

HOW SUPPLIED

DETROL Tablets 1 mg (white, round, biconvex, film-coated tablets engraved with arcs above and below the letters "TO") and **DETROL Tablets 2 mg** (white, round, biconvex, film-coated tablets engraved with arcs above and below the letters "DT") are supplied as follows:

Bottles of 60
1 mg   NDC 0009-4541-02
2 mg   NDC 0009-4544-02
Bottles of 500
1 mg   NDC 0009-4541-03
2 mg   NDC 0009-4544-03
Unit Dose Pack of 140
1 mg   NDC 0009-4541-01
2 mg   NDC 0009-4544-01

Store at 25°C (77°F); excursions permitted to 15–30°C (59–86°F) [see USP Controlled Room Temperature] (DTL).

Rx only
Distributed by
Pharmacia & Upjohn Company
Division of Pfizer Inc, NY, NY 10017
LAB-0257-8.0
Revised March 2008

DETROL® LA   ℞
[*DE-trol el-ay*]
(tolterodine tartrate extended release capsules)
For oral administration

HIGHLIGHTS OF PRESCRIBING INFORMATION
These highlights do not include all the information needed to use Detrol® LA safely and effectively. See full prescribing information for Detrol LA.
Detrol® LA (tolterodine tartrate extended release capsules)
For oral administration
Initial U.S. Approval: December 2000

——————INDICATIONS AND USAGE——————
Detrol LA is an antimuscarinic indicated for the treatment of overactive bladder with symptoms of urge urinary incontinence, urgency, and frequency. (1)

————DOSAGE AND ADMINISTRATION————
• 4 mg capsules taken orally once daily with water and swallowed whole. (2.1)
• 2 mg capsules taken orally once daily with water and swallowed whole in the presence of:
  • mild to moderate hepatic impairment (Child-Pugh class A or B) (2.2)
  • severe renal impairment [Creatinine Clearance (CCr) 10-30 mL/min] (2.2)
  • drugs that are potent CYP3A4 inhibitors. (2.2)
• DETROL LA is not recommended for use in patients with CCr <10 mL/min. (2.2)
• Detrol LA is not recommended for use in patients with severe hepatic impairment (Child-Pugh Class C) (2.2)

——————DOSAGE FORMS AND STRENGTHS——————
• Capsules: 2 mg and 4 mg (3)

——————CONTRAINDICATIONS——————
• Urinary retention (4)
• Gastric retention (4)
• Uncontrolled narrow-angle glaucoma (4)

——————WARNINGS AND PRECAUTIONS——————
• Urinary Retention: use caution in patients with clinically significant bladder outflow obstruction because of the risk of urinary retention. (5.1)
• Gastrointestinal Disorders: use caution in patients with gastrointestinal obstructive disorders or decreased gastrointestinal motility because of the risk of gastric retention. (5.2)
• Controlled Narrow-Angle Glaucoma: use caution in patients being treated for narrow-angle glaucoma. (5.3)
• Myasthenia Gravis: use caution in patients with myasthenia gravis. (5.6)
• QT Prolongation: Consider observations from the thorough QT study in clinical decisions to prescribe DETROL LA to patients with a known history of QT prolongation or to patients who are taking Class IA (e.g., quinidine, procainamide) or Class III (e.g., amiodarone, sotalol) antiarrhythmic medications. (5.7)

——————ADVERSE REACTIONS——————
The most common adverse reactions (incidence ≥4% and >placebo) were dry mouth, headache, constipation and abdominal pain. (6.1)
To report SUSPECTED ADVERSE REACTIONS, contact Pfizer Inc. at 1-800-438-1985 or FDA at 1-800-FDA-1088 or *www.fda.gov/medwatch*

——————DRUG INTERACTIONS——————
• Potent CYP3A4 inhibitors: Co-administration may increase systemic exposure to DETROL LA. Reduce DETROL LA dose to 2 mg once daily. (7.2)
• Other Anticholinergics (antimuscarinics): Concomitant use with other anticholinergic agents may increase the frequency and/or severity of dry mouth, constipation, blurred vision and other anticholinergic pharmacological effects. (7.6)

——————USE IN SPECIFIC POPULATIONS——————
• Pregnancy and Lactation: DETROL LA should be used during pregnancy only if the potential benefit for the mother justifies the potential risk to the fetus. DETROL LA should not be administered during nursing. (8.1, 8.3)
• Pediatric Use: Efficacy in the pediatric population has not been demonstrated. Safety information from a study of a total of 710 pediatric patients (486 on DETROL LA, 224 on placebo) is available. (8.4)
• Renal Impairment: DETROL LA is not recommended for use in patients with CCr <10 mL/min. Dose adjustment in severe renal impairment (CCr: 10-30 mL/min). (8.6)

• *Hepatic Impairment:* Not recommended for use in severe hepatic impairment (Child Pugh Class C). Dose adjustment in mild to moderate hepatic impairment (Child Pugh Class A, B). (8.7)
See 17 for PATIENT COUNSELING INFORMATION and FDA-approved patient labeling.
                                                    Revised: [12/2009]

FULL PRESCRIBING INFORMATION: CONTENTS*
1   INDICATIONS AND USAGE
2   DOSAGE AND ADMINISTRATION
    2.1   Dosing Information
    2.2   Dosage Adjustment in Specific Populations
    2.3   Dosage Adjustment in Presence of Concomitant Drugs
3   DOSAGE FORMS AND STRENGTHS
4   CONTRAINDICATIONS
5   WARNINGS AND PRECAUTIONS
    5.1   Urinary Retention
    5.2   Gastrointestinal Disorders
    5.3   Controlled Narrow-Angle Glaucoma
    5.4   Hepatic Impairment
    5.5   Renal Impairment
    5.6   Myasthenia Gravis
    5.7   Use in Patients with Congenital or Acquired QT Prolongation
6   ADVERSE REACTIONS
    6.1   Clinical Trials Experience
    6.2   Post-marketing Experience
7   DRUG INTERACTIONS
    7.1   Potent CYP2D6 Inhibitors
    7.2   Potent CYP3A4 Inhibitors
    7.3   Other interactions
    7.4   Other drugs metabolized by cytochrome p450 isoenzymes
    7.5   Drug-Laboratory-Test Interactions
    7.6   Other Anticholinergics
8   USE IN SPECIFIC POPULATIONS
    8.1   Pregnancy
    8.3   Nursing Mothers
    8.4   Pediatric Use
    8.5   Geriatric Use
    8.6   Renal Impairment
    8.7   Hepatic Impairment
    8.8   Gender
    8.9   Race
10   OVERDOSAGE
11   DESCRIPTION
12   CLINICAL PHARMACOLOGY
    12.1   Mechanism of Action
    12.2   Pharmacodynamics
    12.3   Pharmacokinetics
13   NONCLINICAL TOXICOLOGY
    13.1   Carcinogenesis, Mutagenesis, Impairment of Fertility
14   CLINICAL STUDIES
16   HOW SUPPLIED/STORAGE AND HANDLING
17   PATIENT COUNSELING INFORMATION
    17.1   Information for Patients
    17.2   FDA Approved Patient Labeling
*Sections or subsections omitted from the full prescribing information are not listed.

FULL PRESCRIBING INFORMATION

1   INDICATIONS AND USAGE

DETROL LA Capsules is indicated for the treatment of overactive bladder with symptoms of urge urinary incontinence, urgency, and frequency [see *CLINICAL STUDIES* (14)].

2   DOSAGE AND ADMINISTRATION
2.1   Dosing Information
The recommended dose of DETROL LA Capsules is 4 mg once daily with water and swallowed whole.. The dose may be lowered to 2 mg daily based on individual response and tolerability; however, limited efficacy data are available for DETROL LA 2 mg [see *CLINICAL STUDIES* (14)].
2.2   Dosage Adjustment in Specific Populations
For patients with mild to moderate hepatic impairment (Child-Pugh Class A or B) or severe renal impairment (CCr 10-30 mL/min), the recommended dose of DETROL LA is 2 mg once daily. DETROL LA is not recommended for use in patients with severe hepatic impairment (Child-Pugh Class C). Patients with CCr<10 mL/min have not been studied and use of DETROL LA in this population is not recommended [see *WARNINGS AND PRECAUTIONS (5.4), USE IN SPECIFIC POPULATIONS (8.6, 8.7)*].
2.3   Dosage Adjustment in Presence of Concomitant Drugs
For patients who are taking drugs that are potent inhibitors of CYP3A4 [e.g. ketoconazole, clarithromycin, ritonavir], the recommended dose of DETROL LA is 2 mg once daily [see *DRUG INTERACTIONS (7.2)*].

3   DOSAGE FORMS AND STRENGTHS

The 2 mg capsules are blue-green with symbol and 2 printed in white ink.
The 4 mg capsules are blue with symbol and 4 printed in white ink.

4 CONTRAINDICATIONS

- urinary retention
- gastric retention
- uncontrolled narrow-angle glaucoma

[see *WARNINGS AND PRECAUTIONS (5.1), (5.3)*].

5 WARNINGS AND PRECAUTIONS

5.1 Urinary Retention

Administer DETROL LA Capsules with caution to patients with clinically significant bladder outflow obstruction because of the risk of urinary retention. [see *CONTRAINDICATIONS (4)*].

5.2 Gastrointestinal Disorders

Administer DETROL LA with caution in patients with gastrointestinal obstructive disorders because of the risk of gastric retention.

DETROL LA, like other antimuscarinic drugs, may decrease gastrointestinal motility and should be used with caution in patients with conditions associated with decreased gastrointestinal motility (e.g. intestinal atony) [see *CONTRAINDICATIONS (4)*].

5.3 Controlled Narrow-Angle Glaucoma

Administer DETROL LA with caution in patients being treated for narrow-angle glaucoma [see *CONTRAINDICATIONS (4)*].

5.4 Hepatic Impairment

The clearance of orally administered tolterodine immediate release was substantially lower in cirrhotic patients than in the healthy volunteers. For patients with mild to moderate hepatic impairment (Child-Pugh Class A or B), the recommended dose for DETROL LA is 2 mg once daily. DETROL LA is not recommended for use in patients with severe hepatic impairment (Child-Pugh Class C) [see *DOSAGE AND ADMINISTRATION (2.2) and USE IN SPECIFIC POPULATIONS (8.6)*].

5.5 Renal Impairment

Renal impairment can significantly alter the disposition of tolterodine and its metabolites. The dose of DETROL LA should be reduced to 2 mg once daily in patients with severe renal impairment (CCr: 10-30 mL/min). Patients with CCr<10 mL/min have not been studied and use of DETROL LA in this population is not recommended [see *DOSAGE AND ADMINISTRATION (2.2), and USE IN SPECIFIC POPULATIONS (8.7)*].

5.6 Myasthenia Gravis

Administer DETROL LA with caution in patients with myasthenia gravis, a disease characterized by decreased cholinergic activity at the neuromuscular junction.

5.7 Use in Patients with Congenital or Acquired QT Prolongation

In a study of the effect of tolterodine immediate release tablets on the QT interval [see *CLINICAL PHARMACOLOGY (12.2)*] the effect on the QT interval appeared greater for 8 mg/day (two times the therapeutic dose) compared to 4 mg/day and was more pronounced in CYP2D6 poor metabolizers (PM) than extensive metabolizers (EMs). The effect of tolterodine 8 mg/day was not as large as that observed after four days of therapeutic dosing with the active control moxifloxacin. However, the confidence intervals overlapped.

These observations should be considered in clinical decisions to prescribe DETROL LA to patients with a known history of QT prolongation or to patients who are taking Class IA (e.g., quinidine, procainamide) or Class III (e.g., amiodarone, sotalol) antiarrhythmic medications. There has been no association of Torsade de Pointes in the international post-marketing experience with DETROL or DETROL LA.

6 ADVERSE REACTIONS

Because clinical trials are conducted under widely varying conditions, adverse reaction rates observed in the clinical trials of a drug cannot be directly compared to rates in the clinical trials of another drug and may not reflect the rates observed in practice.

6.1 Clinical Trials Experience

The efficacy and safety of DETROL LA Capsules was evaluated in 1073 patients (537 assigned to DETROL LA; 536 assigned to placebo) who were treated with 2, 4, 6, or 8 mg/day for up to 15 months. These include a total of 1012 patients (505 randomized to DETROL LA 4 mg once daily and 507 randomized to placebo) enrolled in a randomized, placebo-controlled, double-blind, 12-week clinical efficacy and safety study.

Adverse events were reported in 52% (n=263) of patients receiving DETROL LA and in 49% (n=247) of patients receiving placebo. The most common adverse events reported by patients receiving DETROL LA were dry mouth, headache, constipation, and abdominal pain. Dry mouth was the most frequently reported adverse event for patients treated with DETROL LA occurring in 23.4% of patients treated with DETROL LA and 7.7% of placebo-treated patients. Dry mouth, constipation, abnormal vision (accommodation abnormalities), urinary retention, and dry eyes are expected side effects of antimuscarinic agents. A serious adverse event was reported by 1.4% (n=7) of patients receiving DETROL LA and by 3.6% (n=18) of patients receiving placebo.

Table 1 lists the adverse events, regardless of causality, that were reported in the randomized, double-blind, placebo-controlled 12-week study at an incidence greater than placebo and in greater than or equal to 1% of patients treated with DETROL LA 4 mg once daily.

[See table 1 above]

The frequency of discontinuation due to adverse events was highest during the first 4 weeks of treatment. Similar percentages of patients treated with DETROL LA or placebo discontinued treatment due to adverse events. Dry mouth was the most common adverse event leading to treatment discontinuation among patients receiving DETROL LA [n=12 (2.4%) vs. placebo n=6 (1.2%)].

6.2 Post-marketing Experience

The following events have been reported in association with tolterodine use in worldwide post-marketing experience: *General:* anaphylactoid reactions, including angioedema; *Cardiovascular:* tachycardia, palpitations, peripheral edema; *Gastrointestinal:* diarrhea; *Central/Peripheral Nervous:* confusion, disorientation, memory impairment, hallucinations.

Reports of aggravation of symptoms of dementia (e.g., confusion, disorientation, delusion) have been reported after tolterodine therapy was initiated in patients taking cholinesterase inhibitors for the treatment of dementia.

Because these spontaneously reported events are from the worldwide post-marketing experience, the frequency of events and the role of tolterodine in their causation cannot be reliably determined.

7 DRUG INTERACTIONS

7.1 Potent CYP2D6 Inhibitors

Fluoxetine, a potent inhibitor of CYP2D6 activity, significantly inhibited the metabolism of tolterodine immediate release in CYP2D6 extensive metabolizers, resulting in a 4.8-fold increase in tolterodine AUC. There was a 52% decrease in C_{max} and a 20% decrease in AUC of 5-hydroxymethyl tolterodine (5-HMT), the pharmacologically active metabolite of tolterodine [see *CLINICAL PHARMACOLOGY (12.1)*]. The sums of unbound serum concentrations of tolterodine and 5-HMT are only 25% higher during the interaction. No dose adjustment is required when tolterodine and fluoxetine are co-administered [see *CLINICAL PHARMACOLOGY (12.3)*].

7.2 Potent CYP3A4 Inhibitors

Ketoconazole (200 mg daily), a potent CYP3A4 inhibitor, increased the mean C_{max} and AUC of tolterodine by 2- and 2.5-fold, respectively in CYP2D6 poor metabolizers.

For patients receiving ketoconazole or other potent CYP3A4 inhibitors such as itraconazole, clarithromycin or ritonavir, the recommended dose of DETROL LA is 2 mg once daily [see *DOSAGE AND ADMINISTRATION (2.2), CLINICAL PHARMACOLOGY (12.3)*].

7.3 Other interactions

No clinically relevant interactions have been observed when tolterodine was co-administered with warfarin, with a combined oral contraceptive drug containing ethinyl estradiol and levonorgestrel, or with diuretics [see *CLINICAL PHARMACOLOGY (12.3)*].

7.4 Other drugs metabolized by Cytochrome P450 Isoenzymes

In vivo drug-interaction data show that tolterodine immediate release does not result in clinically relevant inhibition of CYP1A2, 2D6, 2C9, 2C19, or 3A4 as evidenced by lack of influence on the marker drugs caffeine, debrisoquine, S-warfarin, and omeprazole [see *CLINICAL PHARMACOLOGY (12.3)*].

7.5 Drug-Laboratory-Test Interactions

Interactions between tolterodine and laboratory tests have not been studied.

7.6 Other Anticholinergics

The concomitant use of DETROL LA with other anticholinergic (antimuscarinic) agents may increase the frequency and/or severity of dry mouth, constipation, blurred vision, somnolence and other anticholinergic pharmacological effects.

8 USE IN SPECIFIC POPULATIONS

8.1 Pregnancy

Pregnancy Category C.

At approximately 9-12 times the clinical exposure to the pharmacologically active components of DETROL® LA, no anomalies or malformations were observed in mice (based on the AUC of tolterodine and its 5-HMT metabolite at a dose of 20 mg/kg/day). At 14-18 times the exposure (doses of 30 to 40 mg/kg/day) in mice, tolterodine has been shown to be embryolethal and reduce fetal weight, and increase the incidence of fetal abnormalities (cleft palate, digital abnormalities, intra-abdominal hemorrhage, and various skeletal abnormalities, primarily reduced ossification). Pregnant rabbits treated subcutaneously at about 0.3-2.5 times the clinical exposure (dose of 0.8 mg/kg/day) did not show any embryotoxicity or teratogenicity. There are no studies of tolterodine in pregnant women. Therefore, DETROL LA should be used during pregnancy only if the potential benefit for the mother justifies the potential risk to the fetus.

8.3 Nursing Mothers

Tolterodine is excreted into the milk in mice. Offspring of female mice treated with tolterodine 20 mg/kg/day during the lactation period had slightly reduced body weight gain. The offspring regained the weight during the maturation phase.

It is not known whether tolterodine is excreted in human milk; therefore, DETROL LA should not be administered during nursing. A decision should be made whether to discontinue nursing or to discontinue DETROL LA in nursing mothers.

8.4 Pediatric Use

Efficacy in the pediatric population has not been demonstrated.

The pharmacokinetics of tolterodine extended release capsules have been evaluated in pediatric patients ranging in age from 11–15 years. The dose-plasma concentration relationship was linear over the range of doses assessed. Parent/metabolite ratios differed according to CYP2D6

Table 1. Incidence* (%) of Adverse Events Exceeding Placebo Rate and Reported in ≥1% of Patients Treated with DETROL LA (4 mg daily) in a 12-week, Phase 3 Clinical Trial

Body System	Adverse Event	% DETROL LA n=505	% Placebo n=507
Autonomic Nervous	dry mouth	23	8
General	headache	6	5
	fatigue	2	1
Central/Peripheral Nervous	dizziness	2	1
Gastrointestinal	constipation	6	4
	abdominal pain	4	2
	dyspepsia	3	1
Vision	xerophthalmia	3	2
	vision abnormal	1	0
Psychiatric	somnolence	3	2
	anxiety	1	0
Respiratory	sinusitis	2	1
Urinary	dysuria	1	0

*in nearest integer.

Table 2. Mean (CI) change in QT_c from baseline to steady state (Day 4 of dosing) at T_{max} (relative to placebo)

Drug/Dose	N	QT_cF (msec) (manual)	QT_cF (msec) (machine)	QT_cP (msec) (manual)	QT_cP (msec) (machine)
Tolterodine 2 mg BID*	48	5.01 (0.28, 9.74)	1.16 (-2.99, 5.30)	4.45 (-0.37, 9.26)	2.00 (-1.81, 5.81)
Tolterodine 4 mg BID*	48	11.84 (7.11, 16.58)	5.63 (1.48, 9.77)	10.31 (5.49, 15.12)	8.34 (4.53, 12.15)
Moxifloxacin 400 mg QD†	45	19.26‡ (15.49, 23.03)	8.90 (4.77, 13.03)	19.10‡ (15.32, 22.89)	9.29 (5.34, 13.24)

* At T_{max} of 1 hr; 95% Confidence Interval.
† At T_{max} of 2 hr; 90% Confidence Interval.
‡ The effect on QT interval with 4 days of moxifloxacin dosing in this QT trial may be greater than typically observed in QT trials of other drugs.

metabolizer status [*see* ***CLINICAL PHARMACOLOGY*** *(12.3)*]. CYP2D6 extensive metabolizers had low serum concentrations of tolterodine and high concentrations of the active metabolite 5-HMT, while poor metabolizers had high concentrations of tolterodine and negligible active metabolite concentrations.

A total of 710 pediatric patients (486 on DETROL LA, 224 on placebo) aged 5–10 with urinary frequency and urge incontinence were studied in two randomized, placebo-controlled, double-blind, 12-week studies. The percentage of patients with urinary tract infections was higher in patients treated with DETROL LA (6.6%) compared to patients who received placebo (4.5%). Aggressive, abnormal and hyperactive behavior and attention disorders occurred in 2.9% of children treated with DETROL LA compared to 0.9% of children treated with placebo.

8.5 Geriatric Use

No overall differences in safety were observed between the older and younger patients treated with tolterodine.

In multiple-dose studies in which tolterodine immediate release 4 mg (2 mg bid) was administered, serum concentrations of tolterodine and of 5-HMT were similar in healthy elderly volunteers (aged 64 through 80 years) and healthy young volunteers (aged less than 40 years). In another clinical study, elderly volunteers (aged 71 through 81 years) were given tolterodine immediate release 2 or 4 mg (1 or 2 mg bid). Mean serum concentrations of tolterodine and 5-HMT in these elderly volunteers were approximately 20% and 50% higher, respectively, than concentrations reported in young healthy volunteers. However, no overall differences were observed in safety between older and younger patients on tolterodine in the Phase 3, 12-week, controlled clinical studies; therefore, no tolterodine dosage adjustment for elderly patients is recommended.

8.6 Renal Impairment

Renal impairment can significantly alter the disposition of tolterodine immediate release and its metabolites. In a study conducted in patients with creatinine clearance between 10 and 30 mL/min, tolterodine and 5-HMT levels were approximately 2–3 fold higher in patients with renal impairment than in healthy volunteers. Exposure levels of other metabolites of tolterodine (e.g., tolterodine acid, *N*-dealkylated tolterodine acid, *N*-dealkylated tolterodine and *N*-dealkylated hydroxy tolterodine) were significantly higher (10–30 fold) in renally impaired patients as compared to the healthy volunteers. The recommended dose for patients with severe renal impairment (CCr: 10-30 mL/min) is DETROL LA 2 mg daily. Patients with CCr<10 mL/min have not been studied and use of DETROL LA in this population is not recommended [*see* ***DOSAGE AND ADMINISTRATION*** *(2.2) and* ***WARNINGS and PRECAUTIONS*** *(5.5)*]. DETROL LA has not been studied in patients with mild to moderate renal impairment [CCr 30-80 mL/min].

8.7 Hepatic Impairment

Liver impairment can significantly alter the disposition of tolterodine immediate release. In a study of tolterodine immediate release conducted in cirrhotic patients (Child-Pugh Class A and B), the elimination halflife of tolterodine immediate release was longer in cirrhotic patients (mean, 7.8 hours) than in healthy, young, and elderly volunteers (mean, 2 to 4 hours). The clearance of orally administered tolterodine immediate release was substantially lower in cirrhotic patients (1.0 ± 1.7 L/h/kg) than in the healthy volunteers (5.7 ± 3.8 L/h/kg). The recommended dose for patients with mild to moderate hepatic impairment (Child-Pugh Class A or B) is DETROL LA 2 mg once daily. DETROL LA is not recommended for use in patients with severe hepatic impairment (Child-Pugh Class C) [*see* ***DOSAGE AND ADMINISTRATION*** *(2.2) and* ***WARNINGS AND PRECAUTIONS*** *(5.4)*].

8.8 Gender

The pharmacokinetics of tolterodine immediate release and 5-HMT are not influenced by gender. Mean C_{max} of tolterodine immediate release (1.6 μg/L in males versus 2.2 μg/L in females) and the active 5-HMT (2.2 μg/L in males versus 2.5 μg/L in females) are similar in males and females who were administered tolterodine immediate release 2 mg. Mean AUC values of tolterodine (6.7 μg•h/L in males versus 7.8 μg•h/L in females) and 5-HMT (10 μg•h/L in males versus 11 μg•h/L in females) are also similar. The elimination half-life of tolterodine immediate release for both males and females is 2.4 hours, and the half-life of 5-HMT is 3.0 hours in females and 3.3 hours in males.

8.9 Race

Pharmacokinetic differences due to race have not been established.

10 OVERDOSAGE

Overdosage with DETROL LA Capsules can potentially result in severe central anticholinergic effects and should be treated accordingly.

ECG monitoring is recommended in the event of overdosage. In dogs, changes in the QT interval (slight prolongation of 10% to 20%) were observed at a suprapharmacologic dose of 4.5 mg/kg, which is about 68 times higher than the recommended human dose. In clinical trials of normal volunteers and patients, QT interval prolongation was observed with tolterodine immediate release at doses up to 8 mg (4 mg bid) and higher doses were not evaluated [*see* ***WARNINGS AND PRECAUTIONS*** *(5.6) and* ***CLINICAL PHARMACOLOGY*** *(12.2)*].

A 27-month-old child who ingested 5 to 7 tolterodine immediate release 2 mg tablets was treated with a suspension of activated charcoal and was hospitalized overnight with symptoms of dry mouth. The child fully recovered.

11 DESCRIPTION

DETROL LA Capsules contain tolterodine tartrate. The active moiety, tolterodine, is a muscarinic receptor antagonist. The chemical name of tolterodine tartrate is (R)-N, N-diisopropyl-3-(2-hydroxy-5- methylphenyl)-3-phenylpropanamine L-hydrogen tartrate. The empirical formula of tolterodine tartrate is $C_{26}H_{37}NO_7$. Its structure is:

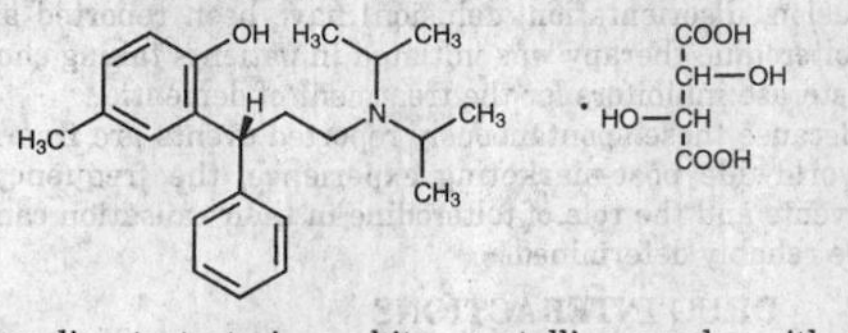

Tolterodine tartrate is a white, crystalline powder with a molecular weight of 475.6.. The pK_a value is 9.87 and the solubility in water is 12 mg/mL. It is soluble in methanol, slightly soluble in ethanol, and practically insoluble in toluene. The partition coefficient (Log D) between n-octanol and water is 1.83 at pH 7.3.

DETROL LA 4 mg capsule for oral administration contains 4 mg of tolterodine tartrate. Inactive ingredients are sucrose, starch, hypromellose, ethylcellulose, medium chain triglycerides, oleic acid, gelatin, and FD&C Blue #2.

DETROL LA 2 mg capsule for oral administration contains 2 mg of tolterodine tartrate, and the following inactive ingredients: sucrose, starch, hypromellose, ethylcellulose, medium chain triglycerides, oleic acid, gelatin, yellow iron oxide, and FD&C Blue #2.

Both the 2 mg and 4 mg capsule strengths are imprinted with a pharmaceutical grade printing ink that contains shellac glaze, titanium dioxide, propylene glycol, and simethicone.

12 CLINICAL PHARMACOLOGY

12.1 Mechanism of Action

Tolterodine acts as a competitive antagonist of acetylcholine at postganglionic muscarinic receptors. Both urinary bladder contraction and salivation are mediated via cholinergic muscarinic receptors.

After oral administration, tolterodine is metabolized in the liver, resulting in the formation of 5-hydroxymethyl tolterodine (5-HMT), the major pharmacologically active metabolite. 5-HMT, which exhibits an antimuscarinic activity similar to that of tolterodine, contributes significantly to the therapeutic effect. Both tolterodine and 5-HMT exhibit a high specificity for muscarinic receptors, since both show negligible activity or affinity for other neurotransmitter receptors and other potential cellular targets, such as calcium channels.

12.2 Pharmacodynamics

Tolterodine has a pronounced effect on bladder function. Effects on urodynamic parameters before and 1 and 5 hours after a single 6.4-mg dose of tolterodine immediate release were determined in healthy volunteers. The main effects of tolterodine at 1 and 5 hours were an increase in residual urine, reflecting an incomplete emptying of the bladder, and a decrease in detrusor pressure. These findings are consistent with an antimuscarinic action on the lower urinary tract.

Cardiac Electrophysiology

The effect of 2 mg BID and 4 mg BID of DETROL immediate release (tolterodine IR) tablets on the QT interval was evaluated in a 4-way crossover, double-blind, placebo- and active-controlled (moxifloxacin 400 mg QD) study in healthy male (N=25) and female (N=23) volunteers aged 18–55 years. Study subjects [approximately equal representation of CYP2D6 extensive metabolizers (EMs) and poor metabolizers (PMs)] completed sequential 4-day periods of dosing with moxifloxacin 400 mg QD, tolterodine 2 mg BID, tolterodine 4 mg BID, and placebo. The 4 mg BID dose of tolterodine IR (two times the highest recommended dose) was chosen because this dose results in tolterodine exposure similar to that observed upon coadministration of tolterodine 2 mg BID with potent CYP3A4 inhibitors in patients who are CYP2D6 poor metabolizers [*see* ***DRUG INTERACTIONS*** *(7.2)*]. QT interval was measured over a 12-hour period following dosing, including the time of peak plasma concentration (T_{max}) of tolterodine and at steady state (Day 4 of dosing).

Table 2 summarizes the mean change from baseline to steady state in corrected QT interval (QT_c) relative to placebo at the time of peak tolterodine (1 hour) and moxifloxacin (2 hour) concentrations. Both Fridericia's (QT_cF) and a population-specific (QT_cP) method were used to correct QT interval for heart rate. No single QT correction method is known to be more valid than others. QT interval was measured manually and by machine, and data from both are presented. The mean increase of heart rate associated with a 4 mg/day dose of tolterodine in this study was 2.0 beats/minute and 6.3 beats/minute with 8 mg/day tolterodine. The change in heart rate with moxifloxacin was 0.5 beats/minute.

[See table 2 above]

The reason for the difference between machine and manual read of QT interval is unclear.

The QT effect of tolterodine immediate release tablets appeared greater for 8 mg/day (two times the therapeutic dose) compared to 4 mg/day. The effect of tolterodine 8 mg/day was not as large as that observed after four days of therapeutic dosing with the active control moxifloxacin. However, the confidence intervals overlapped.

Tolterodine's effect on QT interval was found to correlate with plasma concentration of tolterodine. There appeared to be a greater QT_c interval increase in CYP2D6 poor metabolizers than in CYP2D6 extensive metabolizers after tolterodine treatment in this study.

This study was not designed to make direct statistical comparisons between drugs or dose levels. There has been no association of Torsade de Pointes in the international post-marketing experience with DETROL or DETROL LA [*see* ***WARNINGS and PRECAUTIONS*** *(5.6)*].

12.3 Pharmacokinetics

Absorption: In a study with ^{14}C-tolterodine solution in healthy volunteers who received a 5-mg oral dose, at least 77% of the radiolabeled dose was absorbed. C_{max} and area under the concentration-time curve (AUC) determined after dosage of tolterodine immediate release are dose-proportional over the range of 1 to 4 mg. Based on the sum of unbound serum concentrations of tolterodine and 5-HMT ("active moiety"), the AUC of tolterodine extended release 4 mg daily is equivalent to tolterodine immediate release 4 mg (2 mg bid). C_{max} and C_{min} levels of tolterodine extended release are about 75% and 150% of tolterodine immediate release, respectively. Maximum serum concentrations of tolterodine extended release are observed 2 to 6 hours after dose administration.

Effect of Food: There is no effect of food on the pharmacokinetics of tolterodine extended release.

Distribution: Tolterodine is highly bound to plasma proteins, primarily α_1-acid glycoprotein. Unbound concentrations of tolterodine average 3.7% ± 0.13% over the concentration range achieved in clinical studies. 5-HMT is not extensively protein bound, with unbound fraction concentrations averaging 36% ± 4.0%. The blood to serum ratio of tolterodine and 5-HMT averages 0.6 and 0.8, respectively, indicating that these compounds do not distribute extensively into erythrocytes. The volume of distribution of tolterodine following administration of a 1.28-mg intravenous dose is 113 ± 26.7 L.

Metabolism: Tolterodine is extensively metabolized by the liver following oral dosing. The primary metabolic route involves the oxidation of the 5-methyl group and is mediated by the cytochrome P450 2D6 (CYP2D6) and leads to the formation of a pharmacologically active metabolite, 5-HMT. Further metabolism leads to formation of the 5-carboxylic acid and N-dealkylated 5-carboxylic acid metabolites, which account for 51% ± 14% and 29% ± 6.3% of the metabolites recovered in the urine, respectively.

Variability in Metabolism: A subset of individuals (approximately 7% of Caucasians and approximately 2% of African Americans) are poor metabolizers for CYP2D6, the enzyme responsible for the formation of 5-HMT from tolterodine. The identified pathway of metabolism for these individuals ("poor metabolizers") is dealkylation via cytochrome P450 3A4 (CYP3A4) to N-dealkylated tolterodine. The remainder of the population is referred to as "extensive metabolizers." Pharmacokinetic studies revealed that tolterodine is metabolized at a slower rate in poor metabolizers than in extensive metabolizers; this results in significantly higher serum concentrations of tolterodine and in negligible concentrations of 5-HMT.

Excretion: Following administration of a 5-mg oral dose of ^{14}C-tolterodine solution to healthy volunteers, 77% of radioactivity was recovered in urine and 17% was recovered in feces in 7 days. Less than 1% (<2.5% in poor metabolizers) of the dose was recovered as intact tolterodine, and 5% to 14% (<1% in poor metabolizers) was recovered as 5-HMT.

A summary of mean (± standard deviation) pharmacokinetic parameters of tolterodine extended release and 5-HMT in extensive (EM) and poor (PM) metabolizers is provided in Table 3. These data were obtained following single and multiple doses of tolterodine extended release administered daily to 17 healthy male volunteers (13 EM, 4 PM).

[See table 3 above]

Drug Interactions:

Potent CYP2D6 inhibitors: Fluoxetine is a selective serotonin reuptake inhibitor and a potent inhibitor of CYP2D6 activity. In a study to assess the effect of fluoxetine on the pharmacokinetics of tolterodine immediate release and its metabolites, it was observed that fluoxetine significantly inhibited the metabolism of tolterodine immediate release in extensive metabolizers, resulting in a 4.8-fold increase in tolterodine AUC. There was a 52% decrease in C_{max} and a 20% decrease in AUC of 5-hydroxymethyl tolterodine (5-HMT, the pharmacologically active metabolite of tolterodine). Fluoxetine thus alters the pharmacokinetics in patients who would otherwise be CYP2D6 extensive metabolizers of tolterodine immediate release to resemble the pharmacokinetic profile in poor metabolizers. The sums of unbound serum concentrations of tolterodine immediate release and 5-HMT are only 25% higher during the interaction. No dose adjustment is required when tolterodine and fluoxetine are co-administered.

Potent CYP3A4 inhibitors: The effect of a 200-mg daily dose of ketoconazole on the pharmacokinetics of tolterodine immediate release was studied in 8 healthy volunteers, all of whom were CYP2D6 poor metabolizers. In the presence of ketoconazole, the mean C_{max} and AUC of tolterodine increased by 2- and 2.5-fold, respectively. Based on these findings, other potent CYP3A4 inhibitors may also lead to increases of tolterodine plasma concentrations.

For patients receiving ketoconazole or other potent CYP3A4 inhibitors such as itraconazole, miconazole, clarithromycin, ritonavir, the recommended dose of DETROL LA is 2 mg daily [see *DOSAGE AND ADMINISTRATION* (2.3)].

Warfarin: In healthy volunteers, coadministration of tolterodine immediate release 4 mg (2 mg bid) for 7 days and a single dose of warfarin 25 mg on day 4 had no effect on prothrombin time, Factor VII suppression, or on the pharmacokinetics of warfarin.

Oral Contraceptives: Tolterodine immediate release 4 mg (2 mg bid) had no effect on the pharmacokinetics of an oral contraceptive (ethinyl estradiol 30 μg/levo-norgestrel 150 μg) as evidenced by the monitoring of ethinyl estradiol and levo-norgestrel over a 2-month period in healthy female volunteers.

Diuretics: Coadministration of tolterodine immediate release up to 8 mg (4 mg bid) for up to 12 weeks with diuretic agents, such as indapamide, hydrochlorothiazide, triamterene, bendroflumethiazide, chlorothiazide, methylchlorothiazide, or furosemide, did not cause any adverse electrocardiographic (ECG) effects.

Effect of tolterodine on other drugs metabolized by Cytochrome P450 enzymes: Tolterodine immediate release does not cause clinically significant interactions with other drugs metabolized by the major drug-metabolizing CYP enzymes. *In vivo* drug-interaction data show that tolterodine immediate release does not result in clinically relevant in-

Table 3 Summary of Mean (±SD) Pharmacokinetic Parameters of Tolterodine Extended Release and its Active Metabolite (5-Hydroxymethyl Tolterodine) in Healthy Volunteers

	Tolterodine				5-Hydroxymethyl Tolterodine			
	t_{max}* (h)	C_{max} (μg/L)	C_{avg} (μg/L)	$t_{1/2}$ (h)	t_{max}* (h)	C_{max} (μg/L)	C_{avg} (μg/L)	$t_{1/2}$ (h)
Single dose 4 mg[†] EM	4(2–6)	1.3(0.8)	0.8(0.57)	8.4(3.2)	4(3–6)	1.6(0.5)	1.0(0.32)	8.8(5.9)
Multiple dose 4 mg EM	4(2–6)	3.4(4.9)	1.7(2.8)	6.9(3.5)	4(2–6)	2.7(0.90)	1.4(0.6)	9.9(4.0)
PM	4(3–6)	19(16)	13(11)	18(16)	—‡	—	—	—

C_{max} = Maximum serum concentration; t_{max} = Time of occurrence of C_{max};
C_{avg} = Average serum concentration; $t_{1/2}$ = Terminal elimination half-life.
* Data presented as median (range).
† Parameter dose-normalized from 8 to 4 mg for the single-dose data.
‡ = not applicable.

Table 4. 95% Confidence Intervals (CI) for the Difference between DETROL LA (4 mg daily) and Placebo for Mean Change at Week 12 from Baseline*

	DETROL LA (n=507)	Placebo (n=508)[†]	Treatment Difference, vs. Placebo (95% CI)
Number of incontinence episodes/week			
Mean Baseline	22.1	23.3	-4.8 ‡
Mean Change from Baseline	−11.8 (SD 17.8)	−6.9 (SD 15.4)	(−6.9, −2.8)
Number of micturitions/day			
Mean Baseline	10.9	11.3	-0.6 ‡
Mean Change from Baseline	−1.8 (SD 3.4)	−1.2 (SD 2.9)	(−1.0, −0.2)
Volume voided per micturition (mL)			
Mean Baseline	141	136	20 ‡
Mean Change from Baseline	34 (SD 51)	14 (SD 41)	(14, 26)

SD = Standard Deviation.
* Intent-to-treat analysis.
† 1 to 2 patients missing in placebo group for each efficacy parameter.
‡ The difference between DETROL LA and placebo was statistically significant.

hibition of CYP1A2, 2D6, 2C9, 2C19, or 3A4 as evidenced by lack of influence on the marker drugs caffeine, debrisoquine, S-warfarin, and omeprazole. *In vitro* data show that tolterodine immediate release is a competitive inhibitor of CYP2D6 at high concentrations (K_i 1.05 μM), while tolterodine immediate release as well as the 5-HMT are devoid of any significant inhibitory potential regarding other isoenzymes.

13 NONCLINICAL TOXICOLOGY

13.1 Carcinogenesis, Mutagenesis, Impairment of Fertility

Carcinogenicity studies with tolterodine were conducted in mice and rats. At the maximum tolerated dose in mice (30 mg/kg/day), female rats (20 mg/kg/day), and male rats (30 mg/kg/day), exposure margins were approximately 6-9 times, 7 times, and 11 times the clinical exposure to the pharmacologically active components of DETROL® LA (based on AUC of tolterodine and its 5-HMT metabolite). At these exposure margins, no increase in tumors was found in either mice or rats.

No mutagenic or genotoxic effects of tolterodine were detected in a battery of *in vitro* tests, including bacterial mutation assays (Ames test) in 4 strains of *Salmonella typhimurium* and in 2 strains of *Escherichia coli*, a gene mutation assay in L5178Y mouse lymphoma cells, and chromosomal aberration tests in human lymphocytes. Tolterodine was also negative *in vivo* in the bone marrow micronucleus test in the mouse.

In female mice treated for 2 weeks before mating and during gestation with 20 mg/kg/day (about 9-12 times the clinical exposure via AUC), neither effects on reproductive performance or fertility were seen. In male mice, a dose of 30 mg/kg/day did not induce any adverse effects on fertility.

14 CLINICAL STUDIES

DETROL LA Capsules 2 mg were evaluated in 29 patients in a Phase 2 dose-effect study. DETROL LA 4 mg was evaluated for the treatment of overactive bladder with symptoms of urge urinary incontinence and frequency in a randomized, placebo-controlled, multicenter, double-blind,

Phase 3, 12-week study. A total of 507 patients received DETROL LA 4 mg once daily in the morning and 508 received placebo. The majority of patients were Caucasian (95%) and female (81%), with a mean age of 61 years (range, 20 to 93 years). In the study, 642 patients (42%) were 65 to 93 years of age. The study included patients known to be responsive to tolterodine immediate release and other anticholinergic medications, however, 47% of patients never received prior pharmacotherapy for overactive bladder. At study entry, 97% of patients had at least 5 urge incontinence episodes per week and 91% of patients had 8 or more micturitions per day.

The primary efficacy assessment was change in mean number of incontinence episodes per week at week 12 from baseline. Secondary efficacy measures included change in mean number of micturitions per day and mean volume voided per micturition at week 12 from baseline.

Patients treated with DETROL LA experienced a statistically significant decrease in number of urinary incontinence per week from baseline to last assessment (week 12) compared with placebo as well as a decrease in the average daily urinary frequency and an increase in the average urine volume per void.

Mean change from baseline in weekly incontinence episodes, urinary frequency, and volume voided between placebo and DETROL LA are summarized in Table 4.

[See table 4 above]

16 HOW SUPPLIED/STORAGE AND HANDLING

DETROL LA Capsules are supplied as follows:
[See table above]
Store at 20°–25°C (68°–77°F); excursions permitted to 15–30°C (59–86°F) [see USP Controlled Room Temperature].
Protect from light.

17 PATIENT COUNSELING INFORMATION

See *FDA-Approved Patient Labeling (17.2)*.

17.1 Information for Patients

Patients should be informed that antimuscarinic agents such as DETROL LA may produce the following effects: blurred vision, dizziness, or drowsiness. Patients should be advised to exercise caution in decisions to engage in potentially dangerous activities until the drug's effects have been determined.

17.2   FDA Approved Patient Labeling

Rx only

Distributed by

Pharmacia & Upjohn Company

Division of Pfizer Inc, NY, NY 10017

LAB-0256-7.0

Revised December 2009

PATIENT INFORMATION

DETROL® LA (DE-trol el-ay)

(tolterodine tartrate extended release capsules)

Read the Patient Information that comes with DETROL LA before you start using it and each time you get a refill. There may be new information. This leaflet does not take the place of talking with your doctor about your condition or your treatment. Only your doctor can determine if treatment with DETROL LA is right for you.

What is DETROL LA?

DETROL LA is a prescription medicine for **adults** used to treat the following symptoms due to a condition called **overactive bladder**:

- having a strong need to urinate with leaking or wetting accidents (urge urinary incontinence)
- having a strong need to urinate right away (urgency)
- having to urinate often (frequency)

DETROL LA did not help the symptoms of overactive bladder when studied in children.

What is overactive bladder?

Overactive bladder happens when you cannot control your bladder muscle. When the muscle contracts too often or cannot be controlled, you get symptoms of overactive bladder, which are leakage of urine (urge urinary incontinence), needing to urinate right away (urgency), and needing to urinate often (frequency).

Who should not take DETROL LA?

Do not take DETROL LA if:

- you have trouble emptying your bladder (also called "urinary retention")
- your stomach empties slowly (also called "gastric retention")
- you have an eye problem called "uncontrolled narrow-angle glaucoma"
- you are allergic to DETROL LA or to any of its ingredients. See the end of this leaflet for a complete list of ingredients

What should I tell my doctor before starting DETROL LA?

Before starting DETROL LA, tell your doctor about all of your medical conditions, including if you:

- have any stomach or intestinal problems
- have trouble emptying your bladder or you have a weak urine stream
- have an eye problem called narrow-angle glaucoma
- have liver problems
- have kidney problems
- have a condition called myasthenia gravis
- or any family members have a rare heart condition called QT prolongation (long QT syndrome)
- are pregnant or trying to become pregnant. It is not known if DETROL LA could harm your unborn baby
- are breastfeeding. It is not known if DETROL LA passes into your milk and if it can harm your child

Tell your doctor about all the medicines you take, including prescription and non-prescription medicines, vitamins and herbal supplements. Other drugs can affect how your body handles DETROL LA. Your doctor may use a lower dose of DETROL LA if you are taking:

- Certain medicines for fungus or yeast infections such as Nizoral® (ketoconazole), Sporanox® (itraconazole), or Monistat® (miconazole)
- Certain medicines for bacteria infections such as Biaxin® (clarithromycin)
- Certain medicines for treatment of HIV infection such as Norvir® (ritonavir), Invirase® (saquinavir), Reyataz® (atazanavir)
- Sandimmune® (cyclosporine) or Velban® (vinblastine)

Know the medicines you take. Keep a list of them with you to show your doctor or pharmacist each time you get a new medicine.

How should I take DETROL LA?

- Take DETROL LA exactly as prescribed. Your doctor will prescribe the dose that is right for you. Do not change your dose unless told to do so by your doctor.
- Take DETROL LA capsules once a day with liquid. Swallow the whole capsule. Tell your doctor if you cannot swallow a capsule.
- DETROL LA can be taken with or without food.
- Take DETROL LA the same time each day.
- If you miss a dose of DETROL LA, begin taking DETROL LA again the next day. Do not take 2 doses of DETROL LA in the same day.

- If you took more than your prescribed dose of DETROL LA, call your doctor, or poison control center, or go to the hospital emergency room.

What are possible side effects of DETROL LA?

The most common side effects with DETROL LA are:

- dry mouth
- headache
- constipation
- stomach pain

Medicines like DETROL LA can cause blurred vision, dizziness, or drowsiness.

Use caution while driving or doing other dangerous activities until you know how DETROL LA affects you.

Call your doctor for medical advice about side effects. You may report side effects to the FDA at 1-800-FDA-1088.

These are not all the side effects with DETROL LA. For a complete list, ask your doctor or pharmacist.

How do I store DETROL LA?

- Store DETROL LA at room temperature, 68°-77°F (20°-25°C); brief periods permitted between 59°-86°F (15°-30°C). Protect from light. Keep in a dry place.
- **Keep DETROL LA and all medicines out of the reach of children.**

General Information about DETROL LA

Medicines are sometimes prescribed for conditions that are not in the patient information leaflet. Only use DETROL LA the way your doctor tells you. Do not share it with other people even if they have the same symptoms you have. It may harm them.

This leaflet summarizes the most important information about DETROL LA. If you would like more information, talk with your doctor. You can ask your doctor or pharmacist for information about DETROL LA that is written for health professionals. You can also visit www.DETROLLA.com on the Internet, or call 1-888-4-DETROL (1-888-433-8765).

What are the ingredients in DETROL LA?

Active ingredients: tolterodine tartrate

Inactive ingredients: sucrose, starch, hypromellose, ethylcellulose, medium chain triglycerides, oleic acid, gelatin, and FD&C Blue #2. 2 mg capsule also contains yellow iron oxide. Capsules have pharmaceutical grade printing ink that contains shellac glaze, titanium dioxide, propylene glycol, and simethicone.

Distributed by:

Pharmacia & Upjohn

Division of Pfizer Inc, NY, NY 10017

December 2009   LAB-0312-4.0

Registered trademarks are the property of their respective owners.

GENOTROPIN®   ℞

[gen-ō'' trō-pĭn]

(somatropin [rDNA origin] for injection)

HIGHLIGHTS OF PRESCRIBING INFORMATION

These highlights do not include all the information needed to use Genotropin safely and effectively. See full prescribing information for Genotropin.

GENOTROPIN® (somatropin [rDNA origin] for injection)

Initial U.S. Approval: 1995

————————**RECENT MAJOR CHANGES**————————

Indications and Usage (1.1)

  Idiopathic Short Stature   5/2008

Dosage and Administration (2.1)

  Idiopathic Short Stature   5/2008

————————**INDICATIONS AND USAGE**————————

GENOTROPIN is a recombinant human growth hormone indicated for:

- **Pediatric:** Treatment of children with growth failure due to growth hormone deficiency (GHD), Prader-Willi syndrome, Small for Gestational Age, Turner syndrome, and Idiopathic Short Stature (1.1)
- **Adult:** Treatment of adults with either adult onset or childhood onset GHD (1.2)

————————**DOSAGE AND ADMINISTRATION**————————

GENOTROPIN should be administered subcutaneously (2)

- **Pediatric GHD:** 0.16 to 0.24 mg/kg/week (2.1)
- **Prader-Willi Syndrome:** 0.24 mg/kg/week (2.1)
- **Small for Gestational Age:** Up to 0.48 mg/kg/week (2.1)
- **Turner Syndrome:** 0.33 mg/kg/week (2.1)
- **Idiopathic Short Stature:** up to 0.47 mg/kg/week (2.1)
- **Adult GHD:** Either a non-weight based or a weight based dosing regimen may be followed, with doses adjusted based on treatment response and IGF-I concentrations (2.2)
- **Non-weight based dosing:** A starting dose of approximately **0.2mg/day (range, 0.15-0.30 mg/day) may be used** without consideration of body weight, and increased gradually every 1-2 months by increments of approximately 0.1-0.2 mg/day. (2.2)

- **Weight based dosing:** The recommended initial dose is **not more than** 0.04 mg/kg/week; the dose may be increased as tolerated to not more than 0.08 mg/kg/week at 4–8 week intervals. (2.2)
- GENOTROPIN cartridges are color-coded to correspond to a specific GENOTROPIN PEN delivery device (2.3)
- Injection sites should always be rotated to avoid lipoatrophy (2.3)

————————**DOSAGE FORMS AND STRENGTHS**————————

GENOTROPIN lyophilized powder in a two-chamber color-coded cartridge (3):

- 5 mg (green tip) and 12 mg (purple tip) (with preservative)

GENOTROPIN MINIQUICK Growth Hormone Delivery Device containing a two-chamber cartridge (without preservative):

- 0.2 mg, 0.4 mg, 0.6 mg, 0.8 mg, 1.0 mg, 1.2 mg, 1.4 mg, 1.6 mg, 1.8 mg, and 2.0 mg

————————**CONTRAINDICATIONS**————————

- Acute Critical Illness (4.1, 5.1)
- Children with Prader-Willi syndrome who are severely obese or have severe respiratory impairment – reports of sudden death (4.2, 5.2)
- Active Malignancy (4.3)
- Active Proliferative or Severe Non-Proliferative Diabetic Retinopathy (4.4)
- Children with closed epiphyses (4.5)
- Known hypersensitivity to somatropin or m-cresol (4.6)

————————**WARNINGS AND PRECAUTIONS**————————

Acute Critical Illness: Potential benefit of treatment continuation should be weighed against the potential risk (5.1).

- Prader-Willi syndrome in Children: Evaluate for signs of upper airway obstruction and sleep apnea before initiation of treatment.

Discontinue treatment if these signs occur (5.2).

- Neoplasm: Monitor patients with preexisting tumors for progression or recurrence. Increased risk of a second neoplasm in childhood cancer survivors treated with somatropin—in particular meningiomas in patients treated with radiation to the head for their first neoplasm (5.3).
- Impaired Glucose Tolerance and Diabetes Mellitus: May be unmasked. Periodically monitor glucose levels in all patients. Doses of concurrent antihyperglycemic drugs in diabetics may require adjustment (5.4).
- Intracranial Hypertension: Exclude preexisting papilledema. May develop and is usually reversible after discontinuation or dose reduction (5.5).
- Fluid Retention: (i.e., edema, arthralgia, carpal tunnel syndrome – especially in adults): May occur frequently. Reduce dose as necessary (5.6).
- Hypopituitarism: Closely monitor other hormone replacement therapies (5.7)
- Hypothyroidism: May first become evident or worsen (5.8).
- Slipped Capital Femoral Epiphysis: May develop. Evaluate children with the onset of a limp or hip/knee pain (5.9).
- Progression of Preexisting Scoliosis: May develop (5.10).

————————**ADVERSE REACTIONS**————————

Other common somatropin-related adverse reactions include injection site reactions/rashes and lipoatrophy (6.1) and headaches (6.3).

To report SUSPECTED ADVERSE REACTIONS, contact Pfizer Inc. at 1-800-438-1985 or FDA at 1-800-FDA-1088 or *www.fda.gov/medwatch*.

————————**DRUG INTERACTIONS**————————

Inhibition of 11β-Hydroxysteroid Dehydrogenase Type 1: May require the initiation of glucocorticoid replacement therapy. Patients treated with glucocorticoid replacement for previously diagnosed hypoadrenalism may require an increase in their maintenance doses (7.1, 7.2).

- Glucocorticoid Replacement: Should be carefully adjusted (7.2)
- Cytochrome P450-Metabolized Drugs: Monitor carefully if used with somatropin (7.3)
- Oral Estrogen: Larger doses of somatropin may be required in women (7.4)
- Insulin and/or Oral Hypoglycemic Agents: May require adjustment (7.5)

See 17 for PATIENT COUNSELING INFORMATION

Revised: 8/2009

————————————————————————

FULL PRESCRIBING INFORMATION: CONTENTS*

1 INDICATIONS AND USAGE

  1.1   Pediatric Patients

  1.2   Adult Patients

2 DOSAGE AND ADMINISTRATION

  2.1   Dosing of Pediatric Patients

  2.2   Dosing of Adult Patients

  2.3   Preparation and Administration

3 DOSAGE FORMS AND STRENGTHS

4 CONTRAINDICATIONS

  4.1   Acute Critical Illness

  4.2   Prader-Willi Syndrome in Children

  4.3   Active Malignancy

  4.4   Diabetic Retinopathy

  4.5   Closed Epiphyses

*Sections or subsections omitted from the full prescribing information are not listed.

FULL PRESCRIBING INFORMATION

1 INDICATIONS AND USAGE
1.1 Pediatric Patients
GENOTROPIN (somatropin [rDNA origin] for injection) is indicated for the treatment of pediatric patients who have growth failure due to an inadequate secretion of endogenous growth hormone.

GENOTROPIN (somatropin [rDNA origin] for injection) is indicated for the treatment of pediatric patients who have growth failure due to Prader-Willi syndrome (PWS). The diagnosis of PWS should be confirmed by appropriate genetic testing (see CONTRAINDICATIONS).

GENOTROPIN (somatropin [rDNA origin] for injection) is indicated for the treatment of growth failure in children born small for gestational age (SGA) who fail to manifest catch-up growth by age 2 years.

GENOTROPIN (somatropin [rDNA origin] for injection) is indicated for the treatment of growth failure associated with Turner syndrome.

GENOTROPIN (somatropin [rDNA origin] for injection) is indicated for the treatment of idiopathic short stature (ISS), also called non-growth hormone-deficient short stature, defined by height standard deviation score (SDS) ≤-2.25, and associated with growth rates unlikely to permit attainment of adult height in the normal range, in pediatric patients whose epiphyses are not closed and for whom diagnostic evaluation excludes other causes associated with short stature that should be observed or treated by other means.

1.2 Adult Patients
GENOTROPIN (somatropin [rDNA origin] for injection) is indicated for replacement of endogenous growth hormone in adults with growth hormone deficiency who meet either of the following two criteria:

Adult Onset (AO): Patients who have growth hormone deficiency, either alone or associated with multiple hormone deficiencies (hypopituitarism), as a result of pituitary disease, hypothalamic disease, surgery, radiation therapy, or trauma; or

Childhood Onset (CO): Patients who were growth hormone deficient during childhood as a result of congenital, genetic, acquired, or idiopathic causes.

Patients who were treated with somatropin for growth hormone deficiency in childhood and whose epiphyses are closed should be reevaluated before continuation of somatropin therapy at the reduced dose level recommended for growth hormone deficient adults. According to current standards, confirmation of the diagnosis of adult growth hormone deficiency in both groups involves an appropriate growth hormone provocative test with two exceptions: (1) patients with multiple other pituitary hormone deficiencies due to organic disease; and (2) patients with congenital/genetic growth hormone deficiency.

2 DOSAGE AND ADMINISTRATION
The weekly dose should be divided into 6 or 7 subcutaneous injections. GENOTROPIN must not be injected intravenously.

Therapy with GENOTROPIN should be supervised by a physician who is experienced in the diagnosis and management of pediatric patients with growth failure associated with growth hormone deficiency (GHD), Prader-Willi syndrome (PWS), Turner syndrome (TS), those who were born small for gestational age (SGA) or Idiopathic Short Stature (ISS), and adult patients with either childhood onset or adult onset GHD.

2.1 Dosing of Pediatric Patients
General Pediatric Dosing Information
The GENOTROPIN dosage and administration schedule should be individualized based on the growth response of each patient.

Response to somatropin therapy in pediatric patients tends to decrease with time. However, in pediatric patients, the failure to increase growth rate, particularly during the first year of therapy, indicates the need for close assessment of compliance and evaluation for other causes of growth failure, such as hypothyroidism, undernutrition, advanced bone age and antibodies to recombinant human GH (rhGH). Treatment with GENOTROPIN for short stature should be discontinued when the epiphyses are fused.

Pediatric Growth Hormone Deficiency (GHD)
Generally, a dose of 0.16 to 0.24 mg/kg body weight/week is recommended.

Prader-Willi Syndrome
Generally, a dose of 0.24 mg/kg body weight/week is recommended.

Turner Syndrome
Generally, a dose of 0.33 mg/kg body weight/week is recommended.

Idiopathic Short Stature
Generally, a dose up to 0.47 mg/kg of body weight/week is recommended.

Small for Gestational Age[a]
Generally, a dose of 0.48 mg/kg body weight/week is recommended.

[a] Recent literature has recommended initial treatment with larger doses of somatropin (e.g., 0.48 mg/kg/week), especially in very short children (i.e., height SDS <-3), and/or older/pubertal children, and that a reduction in dosage (e.g., gradually towards 0.24 mg/kg/week) should be considered if substantial catch-up growth is observed during the first few years of therapy. On the other hand, in younger SGA children (e.g., approximately <4 years) (who respond the best in general) with less severe short stature (i.e., baseline height SDS values between -2 and -3), consideration should be given to initiating treatment at a lower dose (e.g., 0.24 mg/kg/week), and titrating the dose as needed over time. In all children, clinicians should carefully monitor the growth response, and adjust the somatropin dose as necessary.

2.2 Dosing of Adult Patients
Adult Growth Hormone Deficiency (GHD)
Either of two approaches to GENOTROPIN dosing may be followed: a non-weight based regimen or a weight based regimen.

Non-weight based—based on published consensus guidelines, a starting dose of approximately 0.2 mg/day (range, 0.15-0.30 mg/day) may be used without consideration of body weight. This dose can be increased gradually every 1-2 months by increments of approximately 0.1-0.2 mg/day, according to individual patient requirements based on the clinical response and serum insulin-like growth factor I (IGF-I) concentrations. The dose should be decreased as necessary on the basis of adverse events and/or serum IGF-I concentrations above the age- and gender-specific normal range. Maintenance dosages vary considerably from person to person, and between male and female patients.

Weight based—based on the dosing regimen used in the original adult GHD registration trials, the recommended dosage at the start of treatment is not more than 0.04 mg/kg/week. The dose may be increased according to individual patient requirements to not more than 0.08 mg/kg/week at 4–8 week intervals. Clinical response, side effects, and de-

termination of age- and gender-adjusted serum IGF-I concentrations should be used as guidance in dose titration. A lower starting dose and smaller dose increments should be considered for older patients, who are more prone to the adverse effects of somatropin than younger individuals. In addition, obese individuals are more likely to manifest adverse effects when treated with a weight-based regimen. In order to reach the defined treatment goal, estrogen-replete women may need higher doses than men. Oral estrogen administration may increase the dose requirements in women.

2.3 Preparation and Administration
The GENOTROPIN 5 and 12 mg cartridges are color-coded to help ensure proper use with the GENOTROPIN Pen delivery device. The 5 mg cartridge has a green tip to match the green pen window on the Pen 5, while the 12 mg cartridge has a purple tip to match the purple pen window on the Pen 12.

Parenteral drug products should always be inspected visually for particulate matter and discoloration prior to administration, whenever solution and container permit. GENOTROPIN MUST NOT BE INJECTED if the solution is cloudy or contains particulate matter. Use it only if it is clear and colorless.

GENOTROPIN may be given in the thigh, buttocks, or abdomen; the site of SC injections should be rotated daily to help prevent lipoatrophy.

3 DOSAGE FORMS AND STRENGTHS
GENOTROPIN lyophilized powder:
• **5 mg two-chamber cartridge (green tip, with preservative)** concentration of 5 mg/mL (approximately 15 IU/mL)
• **12 mg two-chamber cartridge (purple tip, with preservative)** concentration of 12 mg/mL (approximately 36 IU/mL)
GENOTROPIN MINIQUICK Growth Hormone Delivery Device containing a two-chamber cartridge of GENOTROPIN (without preservative)
• **0.2 mg, 0.4 mg, 0.6 mg, 0.8 mg, 1.0 mg, 1.2 mg, 1.4 mg, 1.6 mg, 1.8 mg, and 2.0 mg**

4 CONTRAINDICATIONS
4.1 Acute Critical Illness
Treatment with pharmacologic amounts of somatropin is contraindicated in patients with acute critical illness due to complications following open heart surgery, abdominal surgery or multiple accidental trauma, or those with acute respiratory failure. Two placebo-controlled clinical trials in non-growth hormone deficient adult patients (n=522) with these conditions in intensive care units revealed a significant increase in mortality (41.9% vs. 19.3%) among somatropin-treated patients (doses 5.3–8 mg/day) compared to those receiving placebo [see Warnings and Precautions (5.1)].

4.2 Prader-Willi Syndrome in Children
Somatropin is contraindicated in patients with Prader-Willi syndrome who are severely obese, have a history of upper airway obstruction or sleep apnea, or have severe respiratory impairment. There have been reports of sudden death when somatropin was used in such patients [see Warnings and Precautions (5.2)].

4.3 Active Malignancy
In general, somatropin is contraindicated in the presence of active malignancy. Any preexisting malignancy should be inactive and its treatment complete prior to instituting therapy with somatropin. Somatropin should be discontinued if there is evidence of recurrent activity. Since growth hormone deficiency may be an early sign of the presence of a pituitary tumor (or, rarely, other brain tumors), the presence of such tumors should be ruled out prior to initiation of treatment. Somatropin should not be used in patients with any evidence of progression or recurrence of an underlying intracranial tumor.

4.4 Diabetic Retinopathy
Somatropin is contraindicated in patients with active proliferative or severe non-proliferative diabetic retinopathy.

4.5 Closed Epiphyses
Somatropin should not be used for growth promotion in pediatric patients with closed epiphyses.

4.6 Hypersensitivity
GENOTROPIN is contraindicated in patients with a known hypersensitivity to somatropin or any of its excipients. The 5 mg and 12 mg presentations of GENOTROPIN lyophilized powder contain m-cresol as a preservative. These products should not be used by patients with a known sensitivity to this preservative. The GENOTROPIN MINIQUICK presentations are preservative-free (see HOW SUPPLIED). Localized reactions are the most common hypersensitivity reactions.

5 WARNINGS AND PRECAUTIONS
5.1 Acute Critical Illness
Increased mortality in patients with acute critical illness due to complications following open heart surgery, abdominal surgery or multiple accidental trauma, or those with acute respiratory failure has been reported after treatment with pharmacologic amounts of somatropin [see Contraindi-

cations (4.1)]. The safety of continuing somatropin treatment in patients receiving replacement doses for approved indications who concurrently develop these illnesses has not been established. Therefore, the potential benefit of treatment continuation with somatropin in patients having acute critical illnesses should be weighed against the potential risk.

5.2 Prader-Willi Syndrome in Children
There have been reports of fatalities after initiating therapy with somatropin in pediatric patients with Prader-Willi syndrome who had one or more of the following risk factors: severe obesity, history of upper airway obstruction or sleep apnea, or unidentified respiratory infection. Male patients with one or more of these factors may be at greater risk than females. Patients with Prader-Willi syndrome should be evaluated for signs of upper airway obstruction and sleep apnea before initiation of treatment with somatropin. If during treatment with somatropin, patients show signs of upper airway obstruction (including onset of or increased snoring) and/or new onset sleep apnea, treatment should be interrupted. All patients with Prader-Willi syndrome treated with somatropin should also have effective weight control and be monitored for signs of respiratory infection, which should be diagnosed as early as possible and treated aggressively [see Contraindications (4.2)].

5.3 Neoplasms
Patients with preexisting tumors or growth hormone deficiency secondary to an intracranial lesion should be examined routinely for progression or recurrence of the underlying disease process. In pediatric patients, clinical literature has revealed no relationship between somatropin replacement therapy and central nervous system (CNS) tumor recurrence or new extracranial tumors. However, in childhood cancer survivors, an increased risk of a second neoplasm has been reported in patients treated with somatropin after their first neoplasm. Intracranial tumors, in particular meningiomas, in patients treated with radiation to the head for their first neoplasm, were the most common of these second neoplasms. In adults, it is unknown whether there is any relationship between somatropin replacement therapy and CNS tumor recurrence.
Patients should be monitored carefully for any malignant transformation of skin lesions.

5.4 Glucose Intolerance
Treatment with somatropin may decrease insulin sensitivity, particularly at higher doses in susceptible patients. As a result, previously undiagnosed impaired glucose tolerance and overt diabetes mellitus may be unmasked during somatropin treatment. Therefore, glucose levels should be monitored periodically in all patients treated with somatropin, especially in those with risk factors for diabetes mellitus, such as obesity, Turner syndrome, or a family history of diabetes mellitus. Patients with preexisting type 1 or type 2 diabetes mellitus or impaired glucose tolerance should be monitored closely during somatropin therapy. The doses of antihyperglycemic drugs (i.e., insulin or oral agents) may require adjustment when somatropin therapy is instituted in these patients.

5.5 Intracranial Hypertension
Intracranial hypertension (IH) with papilledema, visual changes, headache, nausea and/or vomiting has been reported in a small number of patients treated with somatropin products. Symptoms usually occurred within the first eight (8) weeks after the initiation of somatropin therapy. In all reported cases, IH-associated signs and symptoms rapidly resolved after cessation of therapy or a reduction of the somatropin dose. Funduscopic examination should be performed routinely before initiating treatment with somatropin to exclude preexisting papilledema, and periodically during the course of somatropin therapy. If papilledema is observed by funduscopy during somatropin treatment, treatment should be stopped. If somatropin-induced IH is diagnosed, treatment with somatropin can be restarted at a lower dose after IH-associated signs and symptoms have resolved. Patients with Turner syndrome and Prader-Willi syndrome may be at increased risk for the development of IH.

5.6 Fluid Retention
Fluid retention during somatropin replacement therapy in adults may occur. Clinical manifestations of fluid retention are usually transient and dose dependent.

5.7 Hypopituitarism
Patients with hypopituitarism (multiple pituitary hormone deficiencies) should have their other hormonal replacement treatments closely monitored during somatropin treatment.

5.8 Hypothyroidism
Undiagnosed/untreated hypothyroidism may prevent an optimal response to somatropin, in particular, the growth response in children. Patients with Turner syndrome have an inherently increased risk of developing autoimmune thyroid disease and primary hypothyroidism. In patients with growth hormone deficiency, central (secondary) hypothyroidism may first become evident or worsen during somatropin treatment. Therefore, patients treated with

somatropin should have periodic thyroid function tests and thyroid hormone replacement therapy should be initiated or appropriately adjusted when indicated.

5.9 Slipped Capital Femoral Epiphyses in Pediatric Patients
Slipped capital femoral epiphyses may occur more frequently in patients with endocrine disorders (including GHD and Turner syndrome) or in patients undergoing rapid growth. Any pediatric patient with the onset of a limp or complaints of hip or knee pain during somatropin therapy should be carefully evaluated.

5.10 Progression of Preexisting Scoliosis in Pediatric Patients
Progression of scoliosis can occur in patients who experience rapid growth. Because somatropin increases growth rate, patients with a history of scoliosis who are treated with somatropin should be monitored for progression of scoliosis. However, somatropin has not been shown to increase the occurrence of scoliosis. Skeletal abnormalities including scoliosis are commonly seen in untreated Turner syndrome patients. Scoliosis is also commonly seen in untreated patients with Prader-Willi syndrome. Physicians should be alert to these abnormalities, which may manifest during somatropin therapy.

5.11 Otitis Media and Cardiovascular Disorders in Turner Syndrome
Patients with Turner syndrome should be evaluated carefully for otitis media and other ear disorders since these patients have an increased risk of ear and hearing disorders. Somatropin treatment may increase the occurrence of otitis media in patients with Turner syndrome. In addition, patients with Turner syndrome should be monitored closely for cardiovascular disorders (e.g., stroke, aortic aneurysm/dissection, hypertension) as these patients are also at risk for these conditions.

5.12 Local and Systemic Reactions
When somatropin is administered subcutaneously at the same site over a long period of time, tissue atrophy may result. This can be avoided by rotating the injection site [see Dosage and Administration. (2.3)].
As with any protein, local or systemic allergic reactions may occur. Parents/Patients should be informed that such reactions are possible and that prompt medical attention should be sought if allergic reactions occur.

5.13 Laboratory Tests
Serum levels of inorganic phosphorus, alkaline phosphatase, parathyroid hormone (PTH) and IGF-I may increase during somatropin therapy.

6 ADVERSE REACTIONS
6.1 Most Serious and/or Most Frequently Observed Adverse Reactions
This list presents the most serious[b] and/or most frequently observed[a] adverse reactions during treatment with somatropin:
- [b] Sudden death in pediatric patients with Prader-Willi syndrome with risk factors including severe obesity, history of upper airway obstruction or sleep apnea and unidentified respiratory infection [see Contraindications (4.2) and Warnings and Precautions (5.2)]
- [b] Intracranial tumors, in particular meningiomas, in teenagers/young adults treated with radiation to the head as children for a first neoplasm and somatropin [see Contraindications (4.3) and Warnings and Precautions (5.3)]
- [a], [b] Glucose intolerance including impaired glucose tolerance/impaired fasting glucose as well as overt diabetes mellitus [see Warnings and Precautions (5.4)]
- [b] Intracranial hypertension [see Warnings and Precautions (5.5)]
- [b] Significant diabetic retinopathy [see Contraindications (4.4)]
- [b] Slipped capital femoral epiphysis in pediatric patients [see Warnings and Precautions (5.8)]
- [b] Progression of preexisting scoliosis in pediatric patients [see Warnings and Precautions (5.9)]
- [a] Fluid retention manifested by edema, arthralgia, myalgia, nerve compression syndromes including carpal tunnel syndrome/paraesthesias [see Warnings and Precautions (5.6)]
- [a] Unmasking of latent central hypothyroidism [see Warnings and Precautions (5.7)]
- [a] Injection site reactions/rashes and lipoatrophy (as well as rare generalized hypersensitivity reactions) [see Warnings and Precautions (5.11)]

6.2 Clinical Trials Experience
Because clinical trials are conducted under varying conditions, adverse reaction rates observed during the clinical trials performed with one somatropin formulation cannot always be directly compared to the rates observed during the clinical trials performed with a second somatropin formulation, and may not reflect the adverse reaction rates observed in practice.

Clinical Trials in children with GHD
In clinical studies with GENOTROPIN in pediatric GHD patients, the following events were reported infrequently: injection site reactions, including pain or burning associated with the injection, fibrosis, nodules, rash, inflammation, pigmentation, or bleeding; lipoatrophy; headache; hematuria; hypothyroidism; and mild hyperglycemia.

Clinical Trials in PWS
In two clinical studies with GENOTROPIN in pediatric patients with Prader-Willi syndrome, the following drug-related events were reported: edema, aggressiveness, arthralgia, benign intracranial hypertension, hair loss, headache, and myalgia.

Clinical Trials in children with SGA
In clinical studies of 273 pediatric patients born small for gestational age treated with GENOTROPIN, the following clinically significant events were reported: mild transient hyperglycemia, one patient with benign intracranial hypertension, two patients with central precocious puberty, two patients with jaw prominence, and several patients with aggravation of preexisting scoliosis, injection site reactions, and self-limited progression of pigmented nevi. Anti-hGH antibodies were not detected in any of the patients treated with GENOTROPIN.

Clinical Trials in children with Turner Syndrome
In two clinical studies with GENOTROPIN in pediatric patients with Turner syndrome, the most frequently reported adverse events were respiratory illnesses (influenza, tonsillitis, otitis, sinusitis), joint pain, and urinary tract infection. The only treatment-related adverse event that occurred in more than 1 patient was joint pain.

Clinical Trials in children with Idiopathic Short Stature
In two open-label clinical studies with GENOTROPIN in pediatric patients with ISS, the most commonly encountered adverse events include upper respiratory tract infections, influenza, tonsillitis, nasopharyngitis, gastroenteritis, headaches, increased appetite, pyrexia, fracture, altered mood, and arthralgia. In one of the two studies, during Genotropin treatment, the mean IGF-1 standard deviation (SD) scores were maintained in the normal range. IGF-1 SD scores above +2 SD were observed as follows: 1 subject (3%), 10 subjects (30%) and 16 subjects (38%) in the untreated control, 0. 23 and the 0.47 mg/kg/week groups, respectively, had at least one measurement; while 0 subjects (0%), 2 subjects (7%) and 6 subjects (14%) had two or more consecutive IGF-1 measurements above +2 SD.

Clinical Trials in adults with GHD
In clinical trials with GENOTROPIN in 1,145 GHD adults, the majority of the adverse events consisted of mild to moderate symptoms of fluid retention, including peripheral swelling, arthralgia, pain and stiffness of the extremities, peripheral edema, myalgia, paresthesia, and hypoesthesia. These events were reported early during therapy, and tended to be transient and/or responsive to dosage reduction.
Table 1 displays the adverse events reported by 5% or more of adult GHD patients in clinical trials after various durations of treatment with GENOTROPIN. Also presented are the corresponding incidence rates of these adverse events in placebo patients during the 6-month double-blind portion of the clinical trials.
[See table 1 at top of next page]

Post-Trial Extension Studies in Adults
In expanded post-trial extension studies, diabetes mellitus developed in 12 of 3,031 patients (0.4%) during treatment with GENOTROPIN. All 12 patients had predisposing factors, e.g., elevated glycated hemoglobin levels and/or marked obesity, prior to receiving GENOTROPIN. Of the 3,031 patients receiving GENOTROPIN, 61 (2%) developed symptoms of carpal tunnel syndrome, which lessened after dosage reduction or treatment interruption (52) or surgery (9). Other adverse events that have been reported include generalized edema and hypoesthesia.

Anti-hGH Antibodies
As with all protein drugs, a small percentage of patients may develop antibodies to the protein. GH antibodies with binding capacities lower than 2 mg/L have not been associated with growth attenuation. In a very small number of patients, when binding capacity was greater than 2 mg/L, interference with the growth response was observed.
In 419 pediatric patients evaluated in clinical studies with GENOTROPIN lyophilized powder, 244 had been treated previously with GENOTROPIN or other growth hormone preparations and 175 had received no previous growth hormone therapy. Antibodies to growth hormone (anti-hGH antibodies) were present in six previously treated patients at baseline. Three of the six became negative for anti-hGH antibodies during 6 to 12 months of treatment with GENOTROPIN. Of the remaining 413 patients, eight (1.9%) developed detectable anti-hGH antibodies during treatment with GENOTROPIN; none had an antibody binding capacity > 2 mg/L. There was no evidence that the growth response to GENOTROPIN was affected in these antibody-positive patients.

Periplasmic Escherichia coli Peptides

Preparations of GENOTROPIN contain a small amount of periplasmic *Escherichia coli* peptides (PECP). Anti-PECP antibodies are found in a small number of patients treated with GENOTROPIN, but these appear to be of no clinical significance.

6.3 Post-Marketing Surveillance

Because these adverse events are reported voluntarily from a population of uncertain size, it is not always possible to reliably estimate their frequency or establish a causal relationship to drug exposure. The adverse events reported during post-marketing surveillance do not differ from those listed/discussed above in Sections 6.1 and 6.2 in children and adults.

Leukemia has been reported in a small number of GHD children treated with somatropin, somatrem (methionylated rhGH) and GH of pituitary origin. It is uncertain whether these cases of leukemia are related to GH therapy, the pathology of GHD itself, or other associated treatments such as radiation therapy. On the basis of current evidence, experts have not been able to conclude that GH therapy *per se* was responsible for these cases of leukemia. The risk for children with GHD, if any, remains to be established *[see Contraindications (4.3) and Warnings and Precautions (5.3)]*.

The following additional adverse reactions have been observed during the appropriate use of somatropin: headaches (children and adults), gynecomastia (children), and pancreatitis (children).

7 DRUG INTERACTIONS

7.1 11β-Hydroxysteroid Dehydrogenase Type 1

The microsomal enzyme 11β-hydroxysteroid dehydrogenase type 1 (11βHSD-1) is required for conversion of cortisone to its active metabolite, cortisol, in hepatic and adipose tissue. GH and somatropin inhibit 11βHSD-1. Consequently, individuals with untreated GH deficiency have relative increases in 11βHSD-1 and serum cortisol. Introduction of somatropin treatment may result in inhibition of 11βHSD-1 and reduced serum cortisol concentrations. As a consequence, previously undiagnosed central (secondary) hypoadrenalism may be unmasked and glucocorticoid replacement may be required in patients treated with somatropin. In addition, patients treated with glucocorticoid replacement for previously diagnosed hypoadrenalism may require an increase in their maintenance or stress doses following initiation of somatropin treatment; this may be especially true for patients treated with cortisone acetate and prednisone since conversion of these drugs to their biologically active metabolites is dependent on the activity of 11βHSD-1.

7.2 Pharmacologic Glucocorticoid Therapy and Supraphysiologic Glucocortioid Treatment

Pharmacologic glucocorticoid therapy and supraphysiologic glucocorticoid treatment may attenuate the growth promoting effects of somatropin in children. Therefore, glucocorticoid replacement dosing should be carefully adjusted in children receiving concomitant somatropin and glucocorticoid treatments to avoid both hypoadrenalism and an inhibitory effect on growth.

7.3 Cytochrome P450-Metabolized Drugs

Limited published data indicate that somatropin treatment increases cytochrome P450 (CYP450)-mediated antipyrine clearance in man. These data suggest that somatropin administration may alter the clearance of compounds known to be metabolized by CYP450 liver enzymes (e.g., corticosteroids, sex steroids, anticonvulsants, cyclosporine). Careful monitoring is advisable when somatropin is administered in combination with other drugs known to be metabolized by CYP450 liver enzymes. However, formal drug interaction studies have not been conducted.

7.4 Oral Estrogen

In patients on oral estrogen replacement, a larger dose of somatropin may be required to achieve the defined treatment goal *[see Dosage and Administration (2.2)]*.

7.5 Insulin and/or Oral Hypoglycemic Agents

In patients with diabetes mellitus requiring drug therapy, the dose of insulin and/or oral agent may require adjustment when somatropin therapy is initiated *[see Warnings and Precautions (5.4)]*.

8 USE IN SPECIFIC POPULATIONS

8.1 Pregnancy

Pregnancy Category B. Reproduction studies carried out with GENOTROPIN at doses of 0.3, 1, and 3.3 mg/kg/day administered SC in the rat and 0.08, 0.3, and 1.3 mg/kg/day administered intramuscularly in the rabbit (highest doses approximately 24 times and 19 times the recommended human therapeutic levels, respectively, based on body surface area) resulted in decreased maternal body weight gains but were not teratogenic. In rats receiving SC doses during gametogenesis and up to 7 days of pregnancy, 3.3 mg/kg/day (approximately 24 times human dose) produced anestrus or extended estrus cycles in females and fewer and less motile sperm in males. When given to pregnant female rats (days 1 to 7 of gestation) at 3.3 mg/kg/day a very slight increase in fetal deaths was observed. At 1 mg/kg/day (approximately seven times human dose) rats showed slightly extended estrus cycles, whereas at 0.3 mg/kg/day no effects were noted.

Table 1

Adverse Events Reported by ≥ 5% of 1,145 Adult GHD Patients During Clinical Trials of GENOTROPIN and Placebo, Grouped by Duration of Treatment

Adverse Event	Double Blind Phase		Open Label Phase GENOTROPIN		
	Placebo 0–6 mo. n = 572 % Patients	GENOTROPIN 0–6 mo. n = 573 % Patients	6–12 mo. n = 504 % Patients	12–18 mo. n = 63 % Patients	18–24 mo. n = 60 % Patients
Swelling, peripheral	5.1	17.5*	5.6	0	1.7
Arthralgia	4.2	17.3*	6.9	6.3	3.3
Upper respiratory infection	14.5	15.5	13.1	15.9	13.3
Pain, extremities	5.9	14.7*	6.7	1.6	3.3
Edema, peripheral	2.6	10.8*	3.0	0	0
Paresthesia	1.9	9.6*	2.2	3.2	0
Headache	7.7	9.9	6.2	0	0
Stiffness of extremities	1.6	7.9*	2.4	1.6	0
Fatigue	3.8	5.8	4.6	6.3	1.7
Myalgia	1.6	4.9*	2.0	4.8	6.7
Back pain	4.4	2.8	3.4	4.8	5.0

* Increased significantly when compared to placebo, $P \leq .025$: Fisher's Exact Test (one-sided)

n = number of patients receiving treatment during the indicated period.

% = percentage of patients who reported the event during the indicated period.

In perinatal and postnatal studies in rats, GENOTROPIN doses of 0.3, 1, and 3.3 mg/kg/day produced growth-promoting effects in the dams but not in the fetuses. Young rats at the highest dose showed increased weight gain during suckling but the effect was not apparent by 10 weeks of age. No adverse effects were observed on gestation, morphogenesis, parturition, lactation, postnatal development, or reproductive capacity of the offsprings due to GENOTROPIN. There are, however, no adequate and well-controlled studies in pregnant women. Because animal reproduction studies are not always predictive of human response, this drug should be used during pregnancy only if clearly needed.

8.3 Nursing Mothers

There have been no studies conducted with GENOTROPIN in nursing mothers. It is not known whether this drug is excreted in human milk. Because many drugs are excreted in human milk, caution should be exercised when GENOTROPIN is administered to a nursing woman.

8.5 Geriatric Use

The safety and effectiveness of GENOTROPIN in patients aged 65 and over have not been evaluated in clinical studies. Elderly patients may be more sensitive to the action of GENOTROPIN, and therefore may be more prone to develop adverse reactions. A lower starting dose and smaller dose increments should be considered for older patients *[see Dosage and Administration (2.2)]*.

10 OVERDOSAGE

Short-Term

Short-term overdosage could lead initially to hypoglycemia and subsequently to hyperglycemia. Furthermore, overdose with somatropin is likely to cause fluid retention.

Long-Term

Long-term overdosage could result in signs and symptoms of gigantism and/or acromegaly consistent with the known effects of excess growth hormone *[see Dosage and Administration (2)]*.

11 DESCRIPTION

GENOTROPIN lyophilized powder contains somatropin [rDNA origin], which is a polypeptide hormone of recombinant DNA origin. It has 191 amino acid residues and a molecular weight of 22,124 daltons. The amino acid sequence of the product is identical to that of human growth hormone of pituitary origin (somatropin). GENOTROPIN is synthesized in a strain of *Escherichia coli* that has been modified by the addition of the gene for human growth hormone. GENOTROPIN is a sterile white lyophilized powder intended for subcutaneous injection.

GENOTROPIN 5 mg is dispensed in a two-chamber cartridge. The front chamber contains recombinant somatropin 5.8 mg (approximately 17.4 IU), glycine 2.2 mg, mannitol 1.8 mg, sodium dihydrogen phosphate anhydrous 0.32 mg, and disodium phosphate anhydrous 0.31 mg; the rear chamber contains 0.3% m-Cresol (as a preservative) and mannitol 45 mg in 1.14 mL water for injection. The GENOTROPIN 5 mg two-chambered cartridge contains 5.8 mg of somatropin. The reconstituted concentration is 5mg/ml. The cartridge contains overfill to allow for delivery of 1ml containing the stated amount of GENOTROPIN – 5 mg.

GENOTROPIN 12mg is dispensed in a two-chamber cartridge. The front chamber contains recombinant somatropin 13.8 mg (approximately 41.4 IU), glycine 2.3 mg, mannitol 14.0 mg, sodium dihydrogen phosphate anhydrous 0.47 mg, and disodium phosphate anhydrous 0.46 mg; the rear chamber contains 0.3% m-Cresol (as a preservative) and mannitol 32 mg in 1.13 mL water for injection. The GENOTROPIN 12 mg two-chambered cartridge contains 13.8 mg of somatropin. The reconstituted concentration is 12 mg/ml. The cartridge contains overfill to allow for delivery of 1ml containing the stated amount of GENOTROPIN – 12 mg.

GENOTROPIN MINIQUICK® is dispensed as a single-use syringe device containing a two-chamber cartridge. GENOTROPIN MINIQUICK is available as individual doses of 0.2 mg to 2.0 mg in 0.2 mg increments. The front chamber contains recombinant somatropin 0.22 to 2.2 mg (approximately 0.66 to 6.6 IU), glycine 0.23 mg, mannitol 1.14 mg, sodium dihydrogen phosphate 0.05 mg, and disodium phosphate anhydrous 0.027 mg; the rear chamber contains mannitol 12.6 mg in water for injection 0.275 mL. The reconstituted GENOTROPIN MINIQUICK two-chamber cartridge contains overfill to allow for delivery of 0.25 ml containing the stated amount of GENOTROPIN.

GENOTROPIN is a highly purified preparation. The reconstituted recombinant somatropin solution has an osmolality of approximately 300 mOsm/kg, and a pH of approximately 6.7. The concentration of the reconstituted solution varies by strength and presentation (see HOW SUPPLIED).

12 CLINICAL PHARMACOLOGY

12.1 Mechanism of Action

In vitro, preclinical, and clinical tests have demonstrated that GENOTROPIN lyophilized powder is therapeutically equivalent to human growth hormone of pituitary origin and achieves similar pharmacokinetic profiles in normal adults. In pediatric patients who have growth hormone deficiency (GHD), have Prader-Willi syndrome (PWS), were born small for gestational age (SGA), have Turner syndrome (TS), or have Idiopathic short stature (ISS), treatment with GENOTROPIN stimulates linear growth. In patients with GHD or PWS, treatment with GENOTROPIN also normalizes concentrations of IGF-I (Insulin-like Growth Factor-I/Somatomedin C). In adults with GHD, treatment with GENOTROPIN results in reduced fat mass, increased lean body mass, metabolic alterations that include beneficial changes in lipid metabolism, and normalization of IGF-I concentrations.

In addition, the following actions have been demonstrated for GENOTROPIN and/or somatropin.

12.2 Pharmacodynamics

Tissue Growth

A. *Skeletal Growth:* GENOTROPIN stimulates skeletal growth in pediatric patients with GHD, PWS, SGA, TS, or ISS. The measurable increase in body length after administration of GENOTROPIN results from an effect on the epiphyseal plates of long bones. Concentrations of IGF-I, which may play a role in skeletal growth, are generally low in the serum of pediatric patients with GHD, PWS, or SGA, but tend to increase during treatment with GENOTROPIN. Elevations in mean serum alkaline phosphatase concentration are also seen.

B. *Cell Growth:* It has been shown that there are fewer skeletal muscle cells in short-statured pediatric patients who lack endogenous growth hormone as compared with the normal pediatric population. Treatment with somatropin results in an increase in both the number and size of muscle cells.

Protein Metabolism

Linear growth is facilitated in part by increased cellular protein synthesis. Nitrogen retention, as demonstrated by

Table 2
Mean SC Pharmacokinetic Parameters in Adult GHD Patients

	Bioavailability (%) (N=15)	T_{max} (hours) (N=16)	CL/F (L/hr × kg) (N=16)	Vss/F (L/kg) (N=16)	$T_{1/2}$ (hours) (N=16)
Mean (± SD)	80.5 *	5.9 (± 1.65)	0.3 (± 0.11)	1.3 (± 0.80)	3.0 (± 1.44)
95% CI	70.5–92.1	5.0–6.7	0.2–0.4	0.9–1.8	2.2–3.7

T_{max} = time of maximum plasma concentration
CL/F = plasma clearance
Vss/F = volume of distribution
$T_{1/2}$ = terminal half-life
SD = standard deviation
CI = confidence interval
* The absolute bioavailability was estimated under the assumption that the log-transformed data follow a normal distribution. The mean and standard deviation of the log-transformed data were mean = 0.22 (± 0.241).

Table 3
Efficacy of GENOTROPIN in Pediatric Patients with Prader-Willi Syndrome (Mean ± SD)

	Study 1		Study 2	
	GENOTROPIN (0.24 mg/kg/week) n=15	Untreated Control n=12	GENOTROPIN (0.36 mg/kg/week) n=7	Untreated Control n=9
Linear growth (cm)				
Baseline height	112.7 ± 14.9	109.5 ± 12.0	120.3 ± 17.5	120.5 ± 11.2
Growth from months 0 to 12	11.6* ± 2.3	5.0 ± 1.2	10.7* ± 2.3	4.3 ± 1.5
Height Standard Deviation Score (SDS) for age				
Baseline SDS	-1.6 ± 1.3	-1.8 ± 1.5	-2.6 ± 1.7	-2.1 ± 1.4
SDS at 12 months	-0.5[†] ± 1.3	-1.9 ± 1.4	-1.4[†] ± 1.5	-2.2 ± 1.4

* p ≤ 0.001
[†] p ≤ 0.002 (when comparing SDS change at 12 months)

Table 4
Effect of GENOTROPIN on Body Composition in Pediatric Patients with Prader-Willi Syndrome (Mean ± SD)

	GENOTROPIN n=14	Untreated Control n=10
Fat mass (kg)		
Baseline	12.3 ± 6.8	9.4 ± 4.9
Change from months 0 to 12	-0.9* ± 2.2	2.3 ± 2.4
Lean body mass (kg)		
Baseline	15.6 ± 5.7	14.3 ± 4.0
Change from months 0 to 12	4.7* ± 1.9	0.7 ± 2.4
Lean body mass/Fat mass		
Baseline	1.4 ± 0.4	1.8 ± 0.8
Change from months 0 to 12	1.0* ± 1.4	-0.1 ± 0.6
Body weight (kg)[†]		
Baseline	27.2 ± 12.0	23.2 ± 7.0
Change from months 0 to 12	3.7[‡] ± 2.0	3.5 ± 1.9

* p < 0.005
[†] n=15 for the group receiving GENOTROPIN; n=12 for the Control group
[‡] n.s.

decreased urinary nitrogen excretion and serum urea nitrogen, follows the initiation of therapy with GENOTROPIN.

Carbohydrate Metabolism
Pediatric patients with hypopituitarism sometimes experience fasting hypoglycemia that is improved by treatment with GENOTROPIN. Large doses of growth hormone may impair glucose tolerance.

Lipid Metabolism
In GHD patients, administration of somatropin has resulted in lipid mobilization, reduction in body fat stores, and increased plasma fatty acids.

Mineral Metabolism
Somatropin induces retention of sodium, potassium, and phosphorus. Serum concentrations of inorganic phosphate are increased in patients with GHD after therapy with GENOTROPIN. Serum calcium is not significantly altered by GENOTROPIN. Growth hormone could increase calciuria.

Body Composition
Adult GHD patients treated with GENOTROPIN at the recommended adult dose (see DOSAGE AND ADMINISTRATION) demonstrate a decrease in fat mass and an increase in lean body mass. When these alterations are coupled with the increase in total body water, the overall effect of GENOTROPIN is to modify body composition, an effect that is maintained with continued treatment.

12.3   Pharmacokinetics
Absorption
Following a 0.03 mg/kg subcutaneous (SC) injection in the thigh of 1.3 mg/mL GENOTROPIN to adult GHD patients, approximately 80% of the dose was systemically available as compared with that available following intravenous dosing. Results were comparable in both male and female patients. Similar bioavailability has been observed in healthy adult male subjects.

In healthy adult males, following an SC injection in the thigh of 0.03 mg/kg, the extent of absorption (AUC) of a concentration of 5.3 mg/mL GENOTROPIN was 35% greater than that for 1.3 mg/mL GENOTROPIN. The mean (± standard deviation) peak (C_{max}) serum levels were 23.0 (± 9.4) ng/mL and 17.4 (± 9.2) ng/mL, respectively.

In a similar study involving pediatric GHD patients, 5.3 mg/mL GENOTROPIN yielded a mean AUC that was 17% greater than that for 1.3 mg/mL GENOTROPIN. The mean C_{max} levels were 21.0 ng/mL and 16.3 ng/mL, respectively.

Adult GHD patients received two single SC doses of 0.03 mg/kg of GENOTROPIN at a concentration of 1.3 mg/mL, with a one- to four-week washout period between injections. Mean C_{max} levels were 12.4 ng/mL (first injection) and 12.2 ng/mL (second injection), achieved at approximately six hours after dosing.

There are no data on the bioequivalence between the 12 mg/mL formulation and either the 1.3 mg/mL or the 5.3 mg/mL formulations.

Distribution
The mean volume of distribution of GENOTROPIN following administration to GHD adults was estimated to be 1.3 (± 0.8) L/kg.

Metabolism
The metabolic fate of GENOTROPIN involves classical protein catabolism in both the liver and kidneys. In renal cells, at least a portion of the breakdown products are returned to the systemic circulation. The mean terminal half-life of intravenous GENOTROPIN in normal adults is 0.4 hours, whereas subcutaneously administered GENOTROPIN has a half-life of 3.0 hours in GHD adults. The observed difference is due to slow absorption from the subcutaneous injection site.

Excretion
The mean clearance of subcutaneously administered GENOTROPIN in 16 GHD adult patients was 0.3 (± 0.11) L/hrs/kg.

Special Populations
Pediatric: The pharmacokinetics of GENOTROPIN are similar in GHD pediatric and adult patients.
Gender: No gender studies have been performed in pediatric patients; however, in GHD adults, the absolute bioavailability of GENOTROPIN was similar in males and females.
Race: No studies have been conducted with GENOTROPIN to assess pharmacokinetic differences among races.
Renal or hepatic insufficiency: No studies have been conducted with GENOTROPIN in these patient populations.
[See table 2 above]

13   NONCLINICAL TOXICOLOGY
13.1   Carcinogenesis, Mutagenesis, Impairment of Fertility
Carcinogenicity studies have not been conducted with GENOTROPIN. No potential mutagenicity of GENOTROPIN was revealed in a battery of tests including induction of gene mutations in bacteria (the Ames test), gene mutations in mammalian cells grown in vitro (mouse L5178Y cells), and chromosomal damage in intact animals (bone marrow cells in rats). See PREGNANCY section for effect on fertility.

14   CLINICAL STUDIES
14.1   Adult Growth Hormone Deficiency (GHD)
GENOTROPIN lyophilized powder was compared with placebo in six randomized clinical trials involving a total of 172 adult GHD patients. These trials included a 6-month double-blind treatment period, during which 85 patients received GENOTROPIN and 87 patients received placebo, followed by an open-label treatment period in which participating patients received GENOTROPIN for up to a total of 24 months. GENOTROPIN was administered as a daily SC injection at a dose of 0.04 mg/kg/week for the first month of treatment and 0.08 mg/kg/week for subsequent months.

Beneficial changes in body composition were observed at the end of the 6-month treatment period for the patients receiving GENOTROPIN as compared with the placebo patients. Lean body mass, total body water, and lean/fat ratio increased while total body fat mass and waist circumference decreased. These effects on body composition were maintained when treatment was continued beyond 6 months. Bone mineral density declined after 6 months of treatment but returned to baseline values after 12 months of treatment.

14.2   Prader-Willi Syndrome (PWS)
The safety and efficacy of GENOTROPIN in the treatment of pediatric patients with Prader-Willi syndrome (PWS) were evaluated in two randomized, open-label, controlled

clinical trials. Patients received either GENOTROPIN or no treatment for the first year of the studies, while all patients received GENOTROPIN during the second year. GENOTROPIN was administered as a daily SC injection, and the dose was calculated for each patient every 3 months. In Study 1, the treatment group received GENOTROPIN at a dose of 0.24 mg/kg/week during the entire study. During the second year, the control group received GENOTROPIN at a dose of 0.48 mg/kg/week. In Study 2, the treatment group received GENOTROPIN at a dose of 0.36 mg/kg/week during the entire study. During the second year, the control group received GENOTROPIN at a dose of 0.36 mg/kg/week.

Patients who received GENOTROPIN showed significant increases in linear growth during the first year of study, compared with patients who received no treatment (see Table 3). Linear growth continued to increase in the second year, when both groups received treatment with GENOTROPIN.

[See table 3 on previous page]

Changes in body composition were also observed in the patients receiving GENOTROPIN (see Table 4). These changes included a decrease in the amount of fat mass, and increases in the amount of lean body mass and the ratio of lean-to-fat tissue, while changes in body weight were similar to those seen in patients who received no treatment. Treatment with GENOTROPIN did not accelerate bone age, compared with patients who received no treatment.

[See table 4 on previous page]

14.3 SGA

Pediatric Patients Born Small for Gestational Age (SGA) Who Fail to Manifest Catch-up Growth by Age 2

The safety and efficacy of GENOTROPIN in the treatment of children born small for gestational age (SGA) were evaluated in 4 randomized, open-label, controlled clinical trials. Patients (age range of 2 to 8 years) were observed for 12 months before being randomized to receive either GENOTROPIN (two doses per study, most often 0.24 and 0.48 mg/kg/week) as a daily SC injection or no treatment for the first 24 months of the studies. After 24 months in the studies, all patients received GENOTROPIN.

Patients who received any dose of GENOTROPIN showed significant increases in growth during the first 24 months of study, compared with patients who received no treatment (see Table 5). Children receiving 0.48 mg/kg/week demonstrated a significant improvement in height standard deviation score (SDS) compared with children treated with 0.24 mg/kg/week. Both of these doses resulted in a slower but constant increase in growth between months 24 to 72 (data not shown).

[See table 5 above]

14.4 Turner Syndrome

Two randomized, open-label, clinical trials were conducted that evaluated the efficacy and safety of GENOTROPIN in Turner syndrome patients with short stature. Turner syndrome patients were treated with GENOTROPIN alone or GENOTROPIN plus adjunctive hormonal therapy (ethinylestradiol or oxandrolone). A total of 38 patients were treated with GENOTROPIN alone in the two studies. In Study 055, 22 patients were treated for 12 months, and in Study 092, 16 patients were treated for 12 months. Patients received GENOTROPIN at a dose between 0.13 to 0.33 mg/kg/week.

SDS for height velocity and height are expressed using either the Tanner (Study 055) or Sempé (Study 092) standards for age-matched normal children as well as the Ranke standard (both studies) for age-matched, untreated Turner syndrome patients. As seen in Table 5, height velocity SDS and height SDS values were smaller at baseline and after treatment with GENOTROPIN when the normative standards were utilized as opposed to the Turner syndrome standard.

Both studies demonstrated statistically significant increases from baseline in all of the linear growth variables (i.e., mean height velocity, height velocity SDS, and height SDS) after treatment with GENOTROPIN (see Table 6). The linear growth response was greater in Study 055 wherein patients were treated with a larger dose of GENOTROPIN.

[See table 6 above]

14.5 Idiopathic Short Stature

The long-term efficacy and safety of GENOTROPIN in patients with idiopathic short stature (ISS) were evaluated in one randomized, open-label, clinical trial that enrolled 177 children. Patients were enrolled on the basis of short stature, stimulated GH secretion > 10 ng/mL, and prepubertal status (criteria for idiopathic short stature were retrospectively applied and included 126 patients). All patients were observed for height progression for 12 months and were subsequently randomized to Genotropin or observation only and followed to final height. Two Genotropin doses were evaluated in this trial: 0.23 mg/kg/week (0.033 mg/kg/day) and 0.47 mg/kg/week (0.067 mg/kg/day). Baseline patient characteristics for the ISS patients who remained prepubertal

Table 5
Efficacy of GENOTROPIN in Children Born Small for Gestational Age (Mean ± SD)

	GENOTROPIN (0.24 mg/kg/week) n=76	GENOTROPIN (0.48 mg/kg/week) n=93	Untreated Control n=40
Height Standard Deviation Score (SDS) Baseline SDS	-3.2 ± 0.8	-3.4 ± 1.0	-3.1 ± 0.9
SDS at 24 months	-2.0 ± 0.8	-1.7 ± 1.0	-2.9 ± 0.9
Change in SDS from baseline to month 24	1.2* ± 0.5	1.7*† ± 0.6	0.1 ± 0.3

* p = 0.0001 vs Untreated Control group
† p = 0.0001 vs group treated with GENOTROPIN 0.24 mg/kg/week

Table 6
Growth Parameters (mean ± SD) after 12 Months of Treatment with GENOTROPIN in Pediatric Patients with Turner Syndrome in Two Open Label Studies

	GENOTROPIN 0.33 mg/kg/week Study 055^ n=22	GENOTROPIN 0.13-0.23 mg/kg/week Study 092# n=16
Height Velocity (cm/yr)		
Baseline	4.1 ± 1.5	3.9 ± 1.0
Month 12	7.8 ± 1.6	6.1 ± 0.9
Change from baseline (95% CI)	3.7 (3.0, 4.3)	2.2 (1.5, 2.9)
Height Velocity SDS (Tanner^/Sempé# Standards)	(n=20)	
Baseline	-2.3 ± 1.4	-1.6 ± 0.6
Month 12	2.2 ± 2.3	0.7 ± 1.3
Change from baseline (95% CI)	4.6 (3.5, 5.6)	2.2 (1.4, 3.0)
Height Velocity SDS (Ranke Standard)		
Baseline	-0.1 ± 1.2	-0.4 ± 0.6
Month 12	4.2 ± 1.2	2.3 ± 1.2
Change from baseline (95% CI)	4.3 (3.5, 5.0)	2.7 (1.8, 3.5)
Height SDS (Tanner^/Sempé# Standards)		
Baseline	-3.1 ± 1.0	-3.2 ± 1.0
Month 12	-2.7 ± 1.1	-2.9 ± 1.0
Change from baseline (95% CI)	0.4 (0.3, 0.6)	0.3 (0.1, 0.4)
Height SDS (Ranke Standard)		
Baseline	-0.2 ± 0.8	-0.3 ± 0.8
Month 12	0.6 ± 0.9	0.1 ± 0.8
Change from baseline (95% CI)	0.8 (0.7, 0.9)	0.5 (0.4, 0.5)

SDS = Standard Deviation Score
Ranke standard based on age-matched, untreated Turner syndrome patients
Tanner^/Sempé# standards based on age-matched normal children
p<0.05, for all changes from baseline

tal at randomization (n= 105) were: mean (± SD): chronological age 11.4 (1.3) years, height SDS -2.4 (0.4), height velocity SDS -1.1 (0.8), and height velocity 4.4 (0.9) cm/yr, IGF-1 SDS -0.8 (1.4). Patients were treated for a median duration of 5.7 years. Results for final height SDS are displayed by treatment arm in Table 7. GENOTROPIN therapy improved final height in ISS children relative to untreated controls. The observed mean gain in final height was 9.8 cm for females and 5.0 cm for males for both doses combined compared to untreated control subjects. A height gain of 1 SDS was observed in 10% of untreated subjects, 50% of subjects receiving 0.23 mg/kg/week and 69% of subjects receiving 0.47 mg/kg/week.

[See table 7 at top of next page]

16 HOW SUPPLIED/STORAGE AND HANDLING

GENOTROPIN lyophilized powder is available in the following packages:

5 mg two-chamber cartridge (with preservative)
concentration of 5 mg/mL (approximately 15 IU/mL)
For use with the GENOTROPIN PEN® 5 Growth Hormone Delivery Device and/or the GENOTROPIN MIXER™ Growth Hormone Reconstitution Device.
Package of 1   NDC 0013-2626-81
12 mg two-chamber cartridge (with preservative)
concentration of 12 mg/mL (approximately 36 IU/mL)
For use with the GENOTROPIN PEN 12 Growth Hormone Delivery Device and/or the GENOTROPIN MIXER Growth Hormone Reconstitution Device.
Package of 1   NDC 0013-2646-81
GENOTROPIN MINIQUICK Growth Hormone Delivery Device containing a two-chamber cartridge of GENOTROPIN (without preservative)

After reconstitution, each GENOTROPIN MINIQUICK delivers 0.25 mL, regardless of strength. Available in the following strengths, each in a package of 7:

0.2 mg	NDC 0013-2649-02
0.4 mg	NDC 0013-2650-02
0.6 mg	NDC 0013-2651-02
0.8 mg	NDC 0013-2652-02
1.0 mg	NDC 0013-2653-02
1.2 mg	NDC 0013-2654-02
1.4 mg	NDC 0013-2655-02
1.6 mg	NDC 0013-2656-02
1.8 mg	NDC 0013-2657-02
2.0 mg	NDC 0013-2658-02

Storage and Handling
Except as noted below, store GENOTROPIN lyophilized powder under refrigeration at 2° to 8°C (36° to 46°F). Do not freeze. Protect from light.

The 5 mg and 12 mg cartridges of GENOTROPIN contain a diluent with a preservative. Thus, after reconstitution, they may be stored under refrigeration for up to 28 days.

The GENOTROPIN MINIQUICK Growth Hormone Delivery Device should be refrigerated prior to dispensing, but may be stored at or below 25°C (77°F) for up to three months after dispensing. The diluent has no preservative. After reconstitution, the GENOTROPIN MINIQUICK may be stored under refrigeration for up to 24 hours before use. The GENOTROPIN MINIQUICK should be used only once and then discarded.

17 PATIENT COUNSELING INFORMATION

Patients being treated with GENOTROPIN (and/or their parents) should be informed about the potential benefits and risks associated with GENOTROPIN treatment [in

Table 7. Final height SDS results for pre-pubertal patients with ISS*

	Untreated (n=30)	GEN 0.033 (n=30)	GEN 0.067 (n=42)	GEN 0.033 vs. Untreated (95% CI)	GEN 0.067 vs. Untreated (95% CI)
Baseline height SDS					
Final height SDS minus baseline	0.41 (0.58)	0.95 (0.75)	1.36 (0.64)	+0.53 (0.20, 0.87) p=0.0022	+0.94 (0.63, 1.26) p<0.0001
Baseline predicted ht					
Final height SDS minus baseline predicted final height SDS	0.23 (0.66)	0.73 (0.63)	1.05 (0.83)	+0.60 (0.09, 1.11) p=0.0217	+0.90 (0.42, 1.39) p=0.0004

* Mean (SD) are observed values.
** Least square means based on ANCOVA (final height SDS and final height SDS minus baseline predicted height SDS were adjusted for baseline height SDS).

particular, see Adverse Reactions (6.1) for a listing of the most serious and/or most frequently observed adverse reactions associated with somatropin treatment in children and adults]. This information is intended to better educate patients (and caregivers); it is not a disclosure of all possible adverse or intended effects.

Patients and caregivers who will administer GENOTROPIN should receive appropriate training and instruction on the proper use of GENOTROPIN from the physician or other suitably qualified health care professional. A puncture-resistant container for the disposal of used syringes and needles should be strongly recommended. Patients and/or parents should be thoroughly instructed in the importance of proper disposal, and cautioned against any reuse of needles and syringes. This information is intended to aid in the safe and effective administration of the medication.

GENOTROPIN is supplied in a two-chamber cartridge, with the lyophilized powder in the front chamber and a diluent in the rear chamber. A reconstitution device is used to mix the diluent and powder. The two-chamber cartridge contains overfill in order to deliver the stated amount of GENOTROPIN

The GENOTROPIN 5 mg and 12 mg cartridges are color-coded to help ensure proper use with the GENOTROPIN Pen delivery device. The 5 mg cartridge has a green tip to match the green pen window on the Pen 5, while the 12 mg cartridge has a purple tip to match the purple pen window on the Pen 12.

Follow the directions for reconstitution provided with each device. **Do not shake**; shaking may cause denaturation of the active ingredient.

Please see accompanying directions for use of the reconstitution and/or delivery device.

Manufactured by:
Vetter Pharma-Fertigung GmbH & Co. KG
Ravensburg, Germany
Or
Vetter Pharma-Fertigung GmbH & Co. KG
Langenargen, Germany
Rx only
Distributed by
Pharmacia & Upjohn Company
Division of Pfizer Inc, NY, NY 10017
LAB-0222-16.0
Revised August 2009

ZYVOX® ℞

[zī-vŏks]
(linezolid) injection
(linezolid) tablets
(linezolid) for oral suspension

To reduce the development of drug-resistant bacteria and maintain the effectiveness of ZYVOX formulations and other antibacterial drugs, ZYVOX should be used only to treat or prevent infections that are proven or strongly suspected to be caused by bacteria.

DESCRIPTION

ZYVOX I.V. Injection, ZYVOX Tablets, and ZYVOX for Oral Suspension contain linezolid, which is a synthetic antibacterial agent of the oxazolidinone class. The chemical name for linezolid is (S)-N-[[3-[3-Fluoro-4-(4-morpholinyl)phenyl]-2-oxo-5-oxazolidinyl] methyl]-acetamide.

The empirical formula is $C_{16}H_{20}FN_3O_4$. Its molecular weight is 337.35, and its chemical structure is represented below:

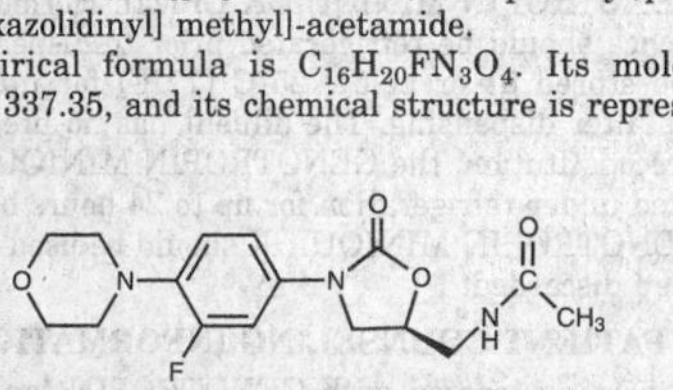

ZYVOX I.V. Injection is supplied as a ready-to-use sterile isotonic solution for intravenous infusion. Each mL contains 2 mg of linezolid. Inactive ingredients are sodium citrate, citric acid, and dextrose in an aqueous vehicle for intravenous administration. The sodium (Na^+) content is 0.38 mg/mL (5 mEq per 300-mL bag; 3.3 mEq per 200-mL bag; and 1.7 mEq per 100-mL bag).

ZYVOX Tablets for oral administration contain 400 mg or 600 mg linezolid as film-coated compressed tablets. Inactive ingredients are corn starch, microcrystalline cellulose, hydroxypropylcellulose, sodium starch glycolate, magnesium stearate, hypromellose, polyethylene glycol, titanium dioxide, and carnauba wax. The sodium (Na^+) content is 1.95 mg per 400-mg tablet and 2.92 mg per 600-mg tablet (0.1 mEq per tablet, regardless of strength).

ZYVOX for Oral Suspension is supplied as an orange-flavored granule/powder for constitution into a suspension for oral administration. Following constitution, each 5 mL contains 100 mg of linezolid. Inactive ingredients are sucrose, citric acid, sodium citrate, microcrystalline cellulose and carboxymethylcellulose sodium, aspartame, xanthan gum, mannitol, sodium benzoate, colloidal silicon dioxide, sodium chloride, and flavors (see **PRECAUTIONS, Information for Patients**). The sodium (Na^+) content is 8.52 mg per 5 mL (0.4 mEq per 5 mL).

CLINICAL PHARMACOLOGY

Pharmacodynamics

In a randomized, positive- and placebo-controlled crossover thorough QT study, 40 healthy subjects were administered a single ZYVOX 600 mg dose via a 1 hour IV infusion, a single ZYVOX 1200 mg dose via a 1 hour IV infusion, placebo, and a single oral dose of positive control. At both the 600 mg and 1200 mg ZYVOX doses, no significant effect on QTc interval was detected at peak plasma concentration or at any other time.

Pharmacokinetics

The mean pharmacokinetic parameters of linezolid in adults after single and multiple oral and intravenous (IV) doses are summarized in Table 1. Plasma concentrations of linezolid at steady-state after oral doses of 600 mg given every 12 hours (q12h) are shown in Figure 1.

[See table 1 at top of next page]

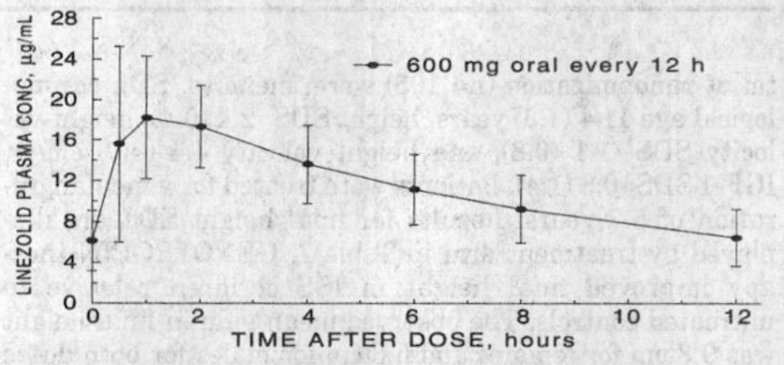

Figure 1. Plasma Concentrations of Linezolid in Adults at Steady-State Following Oral Dosing Every 12 Hours (Mean ± Standard Deviation, n=16)

Absorption: Linezolid is rapidly and extensively absorbed after oral dosing. Maximum plasma concentrations are reached approximately 1 to 2 hours after dosing, and the absolute bioavailability is approximately 100%. Therefore, linezolid may be given orally or intravenously without dose adjustment.

Linezolid may be administered without regard to the timing of meals. The time to reach the maximum concentration is delayed from 1.5 hours to 2.2 hours and C_{max} is decreased by about 17% when high fat food is given with linezolid. However, the total exposure measured as $AUC_{0-\infty}$ values is similar under both conditions.

Distribution: Animal and human pharmacokinetic studies have demonstrated that linezolid readily distributes to well-perfused tissues. The plasma protein binding of linezolid is approximately 31% and is concentration-independent. The volume of distribution of linezolid at steady-state averaged 40 to 50 liters in healthy adult volunteers.

Linezolid concentrations have been determined in various fluids from a limited number of subjects in Phase 1 volunteer studies following multiple dosing of linezolid. The ratio of linezolid in saliva relative to plasma was 1.2 to 1 and for sweat relative to plasma was 0.55 to 1.

Metabolism: Linezolid is primarily metabolized by oxidation of the morpholine ring, which results in two inactive ring-opened carboxylic acid metabolites: the aminoethoxyacetic acid metabolite (A), and the hydroxyethyl glycine metabolite (B). Formation of metabolite A is presumed to be formed via an enzymatic pathway whereas metabolite B is mediated by a non-enzymatic chemical oxidation mechanism in vitro. In vitro studies have demonstrated that linezolid is minimally metabolized and may be mediated by human cytochrome P450. However, the metabolic pathway of linezolid is not fully understood.

Excretion: Nonrenal clearance accounts for approximately 65% of the total clearance of linezolid. Under steady-state conditions, approximately 30% of the dose appears in the urine as linezolid, 40% as metabolite B, and 10% as metabolite A. The renal clearance of linezolid is low (average 40 mL/min) and suggests net tubular reabsorption. Virtually no linezolid appears in the feces, while approximately 6% of the dose appears in the feces as metabolite B, and 3% as metabolite A.

A small degree of nonlinearity in clearance was observed with increasing doses of linezolid, which appears to be due to lower renal and nonrenal clearance of linezolid at higher concentrations. However, the difference in clearance was small and was not reflected in the apparent elimination half-life.

Special Populations

Geriatric: The pharmacokinetics of linezolid are not significantly altered in elderly patients (65 years or older). Therefore, dose adjustment for geriatric patients is not necessary.

Pediatric: The pharmacokinetics of linezolid following a single IV dose were investigated in pediatric patients ranging in age from birth through 17 years (including premature and full-term neonates), in healthy adolescent subjects ranging in age from 12 through 17 years, and in pediatric patients ranging in age from 1 week through 12 years. The pharmacokinetic parameters of linezolid are summarized in Table 2 for the pediatric populations studied and healthy adult subjects after administration of single IV doses.

The C_{max} and the volume of distribution (V_{ss}) of linezolid are similar regardless of age in pediatric patients. However, clearance of linezolid varies as a function of age. With the exclusion of pre-term neonates less than one week of age, clearance is most rapid in the youngest age groups ranging from >1 week old to 11 years, resulting in lower single-dose systemic exposure (AUC) and shorter half-life as compared with adults. As age of pediatric patients increases, the clearance of linezolid gradually decreases, and by adolescence mean clearance values approach those observed for the adult population. There is wider inter-subject variability in linezolid clearance and systemic drug exposure (AUC) across all pediatric age groups as compared with adults.

Similar mean daily AUC values were observed in pediatric patients from birth to 11 years of age dosed every 8 hours (q8h) relative to adolescents or adults dosed every 12 hours (q12h). Therefore, the dosage for pediatric patients up to 11 years of age should be 10 mg/kg q8h. Pediatric patients 12 years and older should receive 600 mg q12h (see **DOSAGE AND ADMINISTRATION**).

[See table 2 on next page]

Gender: Females have a slightly lower volume of distribution of linezolid than males. Plasma concentrations are higher in females than in males, which is partly due to body weight differences. After a 600-mg dose, mean oral clearance is approximately 38% lower in females than in males. However, there are no significant gender differences in mean apparent elimination-rate constant or half-life. Thus, drug exposure in females is not expected to substantially increase beyond levels known to be well tolerated. Therefore, dose adjustment by gender does not appear to be necessary.

Renal Insufficiency: The pharmacokinetics of the parent drug, linezolid, are not altered in patients with any degree of renal insufficiency; however, the two primary metabolites of linezolid may accumulate in patients with renal insufficiency, with the amount of accumulation increasing with the severity of renal dysfunction (see Table 3). The clinical significance of accumulation of these two metabolites has not been determined in patients with severe renal insufficiency. Because similar plasma concentrations of linezolid are achieved regardless of renal function, no dose adjustment is recommended for patients with renal insufficiency. However, given the absence of information on the clinical significance of accumulation of the primary metabolites, use of linezolid in patients with renal insufficiency should be weighed against the potential risks of accumulation of these metabolites. Both linezolid and the two metabolites are eliminated by dialysis. No information is available on the effect of peritoneal dialysis on the pharmacokinetics of linezolid. Approximately 30% of a dose was eliminated in a 3-hour dialysis session beginning 3 hours after the dose of

linezolid was administered; therefore, linezolid should be given after hemodialysis.
[See table 3 at top of next page]

Hepatic Insufficiency: The pharmacokinetics of linezolid are not altered in patients (n=7) with mild-to-moderate hepatic insufficiency (Child-Pugh class A or B). On the basis of the available information, no dose adjustment is recommended for patients with mild-to-moderate hepatic insufficiency. The pharmacokinetics of linezolid in patients with severe hepatic insufficiency have not been evaluated.

Drug-Drug Interactions

Drugs Metabolized by Cytochrome P450: Linezolid is not an inducer of cytochrome P450 (CYP450) in rats. In addition, linezolid does not inhibit the activities of clinically significant human CYP isoforms (e.g., 1A2, 2C9, 2C19, 2D6, 2E1, 3A4). Therefore, linezolid is not expected to affect the pharmacokinetics of other drugs metabolized by these major enzymes. Concurrent administration of linezolid does not substantially alter the pharmacokinetic characteristics of (S)-warfarin, which is extensively metabolized by CYP2C9. Drugs such as warfarin and phenytoin, which are CYP2C9 substrates, may be given with linezolid without changes in dosage regimen.

Antibiotics:

Aztreonam: The pharmacokinetics of linezolid or aztreonam are not altered when administered together.

Gentamicin: The pharmacokinetics of linezolid or gentamicin are not altered when administered together.

Rifampin: The effect of rifampin on the pharmacokinetics of linezolid was evaluated in a study of 16 healthy adult males. Volunteers were administered oral linezolid 600 mg twice daily for 5 doses with and without rifampin 600 mg once daily for 8 days. Coadministration of rifampin with linezolid resulted in a 21% decrease in linezolid C_{max} [90% CI, 15% - 27%] and a 32% decrease in linezolid AUC_{0-12} [90% CI, 27% - 37%]. The mechanism of this interaction is not fully understood and may be related to the induction of hepatic enzymes (see **PRECAUTIONS, Drug Interactions**).

Monoamine Oxidase Inhibition: Linezolid is a reversible, nonselective inhibitor of monoamine oxidase. Therefore, linezolid has the potential for interaction with adrenergic and serotonergic agents.

Adrenergic Agents: A significant pressor response has been observed in normal adult subjects receiving linezolid and tyramine doses of more than 100 mg. Therefore, patients receiving linezolid need to avoid consuming large amounts of foods or beverages with high tyramine content (see **PRECAUTIONS, Information for Patients**).

A reversible enhancement of the pressor response of either pseudoephedrine HCl (PSE) or phenylpropanolamine HCl (PPA) is observed when linezolid is administered to healthy normotensive subjects (see **PRECAUTIONS, Drug Interactions**). A similar study has not been conducted in hypertensive patients. The interaction studies conducted in normotensive subjects evaluated the blood pressure and heart rate effects of placebo, PPA or PSE alone, linezolid alone, and the combination of steady-state linezolid (600 mg q12h for 3 days) with two doses of PPA (25 mg) or PSE (60 mg) given 4 hours apart. Heart rate was not affected by any of the treatments. Blood pressure was increased with both combination treatments. Maximum blood pressure levels were seen 2 to 3 hours after the second dose of PPA or PSE, and returned to baseline 2 to 3 hours after peak. The results of the PPA study follow, showing the mean (and range) maximum systolic blood pressure in mm Hg: placebo = 121 (103 to 158); linezolid = 120 (107 to 135); PPA alone = 125 (106 to 139); PPA with linezolid = 147 (129 to 176). The results from the PSE study were similar to those in the PPA study. The mean maximum increase in systolic blood pressure over baseline was 32 mm Hg (range: 20-52 mm Hg) and 38 mm Hg (range: 18-79 mm Hg) during co-administration of linezolid with pseudoephedrine or phenylpropanolamine, respectively.

Serotonergic Agents: The potential drug-drug interaction with dextromethorphan was studied in healthy volunteers. Subjects were administered dextromethorphan (two 20-mg doses given 4 hours apart) with or without linezolid. No serotonin syndrome effects (confusion, delirium, restlessness, tremors, blushing, diaphoresis, hyperpyrexia) have been observed in normal subjects receiving linezolid and dextromethorphan.

MICROBIOLOGY

Linezolid is a synthetic antibacterial agent of a new class of antibiotics, the oxazolidinones, which has clinical utility in the treatment of infections caused by aerobic Gram-positive bacteria. The in vitro spectrum of activity of linezolid also includes certain Gram-negative bacteria and anaerobic bacteria. Linezolid inhibits bacterial protein synthesis through a mechanism of action different from that of other antibacterial agents; therefore, cross-resistance between linezolid and other classes of antibiotics is unlikely. Linezolid binds to a site on the bacterial 23S ribosomal RNA of the 50S subunit and prevents the formation of a functional 70S initiation complex, which is an essential component of the bacterial translation process. The results of time-kill studies have shown linezolid to be bacteriostatic against enterococci and staphylococci. For streptococci, linezolid was found to be bactericidal for the majority of strains.

In clinical trials, resistance to linezolid developed in 6 patients infected with *Enterococcus faecium* (4 patients received 200 mg q12h, lower than the recommended dose, and 2 patients received 600 mg q12h). In a compassionate use program, resistance to linezolid developed in 8 patients with *E. faecium* and in 1 patient with *Enterococcus faecalis*. All patients had either unremoved prosthetic devices or undrained abscesses. Resistance to linezolid occurs in vitro at a frequency of 1×10^{-9} to 1×10^{-11}. In vitro studies have shown that point mutations in the 23S rRNA are associated with linezolid resistance. Reports of vancomycin-resistant *E. faecium* becoming resistant to linezolid during its clinical use have been published.[1] In one report nosocomial spread of vancomycin- and linezolid-resistant *E. faecium* occurred[2]. There has been a report of *Staphylococcus aureus* (methicillin-resistant) developing resistance to linezolid during its clinical use.[3] The linezolid resistance in these organisms was associated with a point mutation in the 23S rRNA (substitution of thymine for guanine at position 2576) of the organism. When antibiotic-resistant organisms are encountered in the hospital, it is important to emphasize infection control policies.[4, 5] Resistance to linezolid has not been reported in *Streptococcus* spp., including *Streptococcus pneumoniae*.

In vitro studies have demonstrated additivity or indifference between linezolid and vancomycin, gentamicin, rifampin, imipenem-cilastatin, aztreonam, ampicillin, or streptomycin.

Table 1. Mean (Standard Deviation) Pharmacokinetic Parameters of Linezolid in Adults

Dose of Linezolid	C_{max} µg/mL	C_{min} µg/mL	T_{max} hrs	AUC * µg·h/mL	$t_{1/2}$ hrs	CL mL/min
400 mg tablet						
single dose†	8.10 (1.83)	—	1.52 (1.01)	55.10 (25.00)	5.20 (1.50)	146 (67)
every 12 hours	11.00 (4.37)	3.08 (2.25)	1.12 (0.47)	73.40 (33.50)	4.69) (1.70)	110 (49)
600 mg tablet						
single dose	12.70 (3.96)	—	1.28 (0.66)	91.40 (39.30)	4.26 (1.65)	127 (48)
every 12 hours	21.20 (5.78)	6.15 (2.94)	1.03 (0.62)	138.00 (42.10)	5.40 (2.06)	80 (29)
600 mg IV injection‡						
single dose	12.90 (1.60)	—	0.50 (0.10)	80.20 (33.30)	4.40 (2.40)	138 (39)
every 12 hours	15.10 (2.52)	3.68 (2.36)	0.51 (0.03)	89.70 (31.00)	4.80 (1.70)	123 (40)
600 mg oral suspension						
single dose	11.00 (2.76)	—	0.97 (0.88)	80.80 (35.10)	4.60 (1.71)	141 (45)

* AUC for single dose = $AUC_{0-\infty}$; for multiple-dose = $AUC_{0-\tau}$
† Data dose-normalized from 375 mg
‡ Data dose-normalized from 625 mg, IV dose was given as 0.5-hour infusion.
C_{max} = Maximum plasma concentration; C_{min} = Minimum plasma concentration; T_{max} = Time to C_{max}; AUC = Area under concentration-time curve; $t_{1/2}$ = Elimination half-life; CL = Systemic clearance

Table 2. Pharmacokinetic Parameters of Linezolid in Pediatrics and Adults Following a Single Intravenous Infusion of 10 mg/kg or 600 mg Linezolid (Mean: (%CV); [Min, Max Values])

Age Group	C_{max} µg/mL	V_{ss} L/kg	AUC* µg·h/mL	$t_{1/2}$ hrs	CL mL/min/kg
Neonatal Patients					
Pre-term** < 1 week (N=9)†	12.7 (30%) [9.6, 22.2]	0.81 (24%) [0.43, 1.05]	108 (47%) [41, 191]	5.6 (46%) [2.4, 9.8]	2.0 (52%) [0.9, 4.0]
Full-term*** < 1 week (N=10)†	11.5 (24%) [8.0, 18.3]	0.78 (20%) [0.45, 0.96]	55 (47%) [19, 103]	3.0 (55%) [1.3, 6.1]	3.8 (55%) [1.5, 8.8]
Full-term*** ≥ 1 week to ≤ 28 days (N=10)†	12.9 (28%) [7.7, 21.6]	0.66 (29%) [0.35, 1.06]	34 (21%) [23, 50]	1.5 (17%) [1.2, 1.9]	5.1 (22%) [3.3, 7.2]
Infant Patients					
> 28 days to < 3 Months (N=12)†	11.0 (27%) [7.2, 18.0]	0.79 (26%) [0.42, 1.08]	33 (26%) [17, 48]	1.8 (28%) [1.2, 2.8]	5.4 (32%) [3.5, 9.9]
Pediatric Patients					
3 months through 11 years† (N=59)	15.1 (30%) [6.8, 36.7]	0.69 (28%) [0.31, 1.50]	58 (54%) [19, 153]	2.9 (53%) [0.9, 8.0]	3.8 (53%) [1.0, 8.5]
Adolescent Subjects and Patients					
12 through 17 years‡ (N=36)	16.7 (24%) [9.9, 28.9]	0.61 (15%) [9.9, 28.9]	95 (44%) [32, 178]	4.1 (46%) [1.3, 8.1]	2.1 (53%) [.09, 5.2]
Adult Subjects§ (N=29)	12.5 (21%) [8.2, 19.3]	0.65 (16%) [0.45, 0.84]	91 (33%) [53, 155]	4.9 (35%) [1.8, 8.3]	1.7 (34%) [0.9, 3.3]

* AUC = Single dose $AUC_{0-\infty}$
** In this data set, "pre-term" is defined as <34 weeks gestational age (Note: Only 1 patient enrolled was pre-term with a postnatal age between 1 week and 28 days)
*** In this data set, "full-term" is defined as ≥34 weeks gestational age
† Dose of 10 mg/kg
‡ Dose of 600 mg or 10 mg/kg up to a maximum of 600 mg
§ Dose normalized to 600 mg
C_{max} = Maximum plasma concentration; V_{ss}= Volume of distribution; AUC = Area under concentration-time curve; $t_{1/2}$ = Apparent elimination half-life; CL = Systemic clearance normalized for body weight

Table 3. Mean (Standard Deviation) AUCs and Elimination Half-lives of Linezolid and Metabolites A and B in Patients with Varying Degrees of Renal Insufficiency After a Single 600-mg Oral Dose of Linezolid

Parameter	Healthy Subjects CL_{CR} > 80 mL/min	Moderate Renal Impairment 30 < CL_{CR} < 80 mL/min	Severe Renal Impairment 10 < CL_{CR} < 30 mL/min	Hemodialysis-Dependent	
				Off Dialysis*	On Dialysis
Linezolid					
$AUC_{0-\infty}$, µg h/mL	110 (22)	128 (53)	127 (66)	141 (45)	83 (23)
$t_{1/2}$, hours	6.4 (2.2)	6.1 (1.7)	7.1 (3.7)	8.4 (2.7)	7.0 (1.8)
Metabolite A					
AUC_{0-48}, µg h/mL	7.6 (1.9)	11.7 (4.3)	56.5 (30.6)	185 (124)	68.8 (23.9)
$t_{1/2}$, hours	6.3 (2.1)	6.6 (2.3)	9.0 (4.6)	NA	NA
Metabolite B					
AUC_{0-48}, µg h/mL	30.5 (6.2)	51.1 (38.5)	203 (92)	467 (102)	239 (44)
$t_{1/2}$, hours	6.6 (2.7)	9.9 (7.4)	11.0 (3.9)	NA	NA

* between hemodialysis sessions
NA = Not applicable

Table 4. Susceptibility Interpretive Criteria for Linezolid

Pathogen	Susceptibility Interpretive Criteria					
	Minimal Inhibitory Concentrations (MIC in µg/mL)			Disk Diffusion (Zone Diameters in mm)		
	S	I	R	S	I	R
Enterococcus spp	≤2	4	≥8	≥23	21-22	≤20
Staphylococcus spp[a]	≤4	—	—	≥21	—	—
Streptococcus pneumoniae[a]	≤2[b]	—	—	≥21[c]	—	—
Streptococcus spp other than *S pneumoniae*[a]	≤2[b]	—	—	≥21[c]	—	—

[a] The current absence of data on resistant strains precludes defining any categories other than "Susceptible." Strains yielding test results suggestive of a "nonsusceptible" category should be retested, and if the result is confirmed, the isolate should be submitted to a reference laboratory for further testing.
[b] These interpretive standards for *S. pneumoniae* and *Streptococcus* spp. other than *S. pneumoniae* are applicable only to tests performed by broth microdilution using cation-adjusted Mueller-Hinton broth with 2 to 5% lysed horse blood inoculated with a direct colony suspension and incubated in ambient air at 35°C for 20 to 24 hours.
[c] These zone diameter interpretive standards are applicable only to tests performed using Mueller-Hinton agar supplemented with 5% defibrinated sheep blood inoculated with a direct colony suspension and incubated in 5% CO_2 at 35°C for 20 to 24 hours.

Linezolid has been shown to be active against most isolates of the following microorganisms, both in vitro and in clinical infections, as described in the **INDICATIONS AND USAGE** section.
Aerobic and facultative Gram-positive microorganisms
Enterococcus faecium (vancomycin-resistant strains only)
Staphylococcus aureus (including methicillin-resistant strains)
Streptococcus agalactiae
Streptococcus pneumoniae (including multi-drug resistant isolates [MDRSP]*)
Streptococcus pyogenes
The following in vitro data are available, but their clinical significance is unknown. At least 90% of the following microorganisms exhibit an in vitro minimum inhibitory concentration (MIC) less than or equal to the susceptible breakpoint for linezolid. However, the safety and effectiveness of linezolid in treating clinical infections due to these microorganisms have not been established in adequate and well-controlled clinical trials.
*MDRSP refers to isolates resistant to two or more of the following antibiotics: penicillin, second-generation cephalosporins, macrolides, tetracycline, and trimethoprim/sulfamethoxazole.
Aerobic and facultative Gram-positive microorganisms
Enterococcus faecalis (including vancomycin-resistant strains)
Enterococcus faecium (vancomycin-susceptible strains)
Staphylococcus epidermidis (including methicillin-resistant strains)
Staphylococcus haemolyticus
Viridans group streptococci

Aerobic and facultative Gram-negative microorganisms
Pasteurella multocida
Susceptibility Testing Methods
NOTE: Susceptibility testing by dilution methods requires the use of linezolid susceptibility powder.
When available, the results of in vitro susceptibility tests should be provided to the physician as periodic reports which describe the susceptibility profile of nosocomial and community-acquired pathogens. These reports should aid the physician in selecting the most effective antimicrobial.
Dilution Techniques: Quantitative methods are used to determine antimicrobial minimum inhibitory concentrations (MICs). These MICs provide estimates of the susceptibility of bacteria to antimicrobial compounds. The MICs should be determined using a standardized procedure. Standardized procedures are based on a dilution method[6,7] (broth or agar) or equivalent with standardized inoculum concentrations and standardized concentrations of linezolid powder. The MIC values should be interpreted according to criteria provided in Table 4.
Diffusion Techniques: Quantitative methods that require measurement of zone diameters also provide reproducible estimates of the susceptibility of bacteria to antimicrobial compounds. One such standardized procedure[7,8] requires the use of standardized inoculum concentrations. This procedure uses paper disks impregnated with 30 µg of linezolid to test the susceptibility of microorganisms to linezolid. The disk diffusion interpretive criteria are provided in Table 4.
[See table 4 above]
A report of "Susceptible" indicates that the pathogen is likely to be inhibited if the antimicrobial compound in the

blood reaches the concentrations usually achievable. A report of "Intermediate" indicates that the result should be considered equivocal, and, if the microorganism is not fully susceptible to alternative, clinically feasible drugs, the test should be repeated. This category implies possible clinical applicability in body sites where the drug is physiologically concentrated or in situations where high dosage of drug can be used. This category also provides a buffer zone which prevents small uncontrolled technical factors from causing major discrepancies in interpretation. A report of "Resistant" indicates that the pathogen is not likely to be inhibited if the antimicrobial compound in the blood reaches the concentrations usually achievable; other therapy should be selected.
Quality Control
Standardized susceptibility test procedures require the use of quality control microorganisms to control the technical aspects of the test procedures. Standard linezolid powder should provide the following range of values noted in Table 5.
NOTE: Quality control microorganisms are specific strains of organisms with intrinsic biological properties relating to resistance mechanisms and their genetic expression within bacteria; the specific strains used for microbiological quality control are not clinically significant.

Table 5. Acceptable Quality Control Ranges for Linezolid to be Used in Validation of Susceptibility Test Results

QC Strain	Acceptable Quality Control Ranges	
	Minimum Inhibitory Concentration (MIC in µg/mL)	Disk Diffusion (Zone Diameters in mm)
Enterococcus faecalis ATCC 29212	1 - 4	Not applicable
Staphylococcus aureus ATCC 29213	1 - 4	Not applicable
Staphylococcus aureus ATCC 25923	Not applicable	25 - 32
Streptococcus pneumoniae ATCC 49619[d]	0.50 - 2[e]	25 - 34[f]

[d] This organism may be used for validation of susceptibility test results when testing *Streptococcus* spp. other than *S. pneumoniae*.
[e] This quality control range for *S. pneumoniae* is applicable only to tests performed by broth microdilution using cation-adjusted Mueller-Hinton broth with 2 to 5% lysed horse blood inoculated with a direct colony suspension and incubated in ambient air at 35°C for 20 to 24 hours.
[f] This quality control zone diameter range is applicable only to tests performed using Mueller-Hinton agar supplemented with 5% defibrinated sheep blood inoculated with a direct colony suspension and incubated in 5% CO_2 at 35°C for 20 to 24 hours.

INDICATIONS AND USAGE

ZYVOX formulations are indicated in the treatment of the following infections caused by susceptible strains of the designated microorganisms (see **PRECAUTIONS, Pediatric Use** and **DOSAGE AND ADMINISTRATION** and **CLINICAL STUDIES**). Linezolid is not indicated for the treatment of Gram-negative infections. It is critical that specific Gram-negative therapy be initiated immediately if a concomitant Gram-negative pathogen is documented or suspected (see **WARNINGS**).
Vancomycin-Resistant *Enterococcus faecium* infections, including cases with concurrent bacteremia (see **CLINICAL STUDIES**).
Nosocomial pneumonia caused by *Staphylococcus aureus* (methicillin-susceptible and -resistant strains), or *Streptococcus pneumoniae* (including multi-drug resistant strains [MDRSP]).
Complicated skin and skin structure infections, including diabetic foot infections, without concomitant osteomyelitis, caused by *Staphylococcus aureus* (methicillin-susceptible and -resistant strains), *Streptococcus pyogenes,* or *Streptococcus agalactiae*. ZYVOX has not been studied in the treatment of decubitus ulcers.

Uncomplicated skin and skin structure infections caused by *Staphylococcus aureus* (methicillin-susceptible only) or *Streptococcus pyogenes*.

Community-acquired pneumonia caused by *Streptococcus pneumoniae* (including multi-drug resistant strains [MDRSP]*), including cases with concurrent bacteremia, or *Staphylococcus aureus* (methicillin-susceptible strains only).

To reduce the development of drug-resistant bacteria and maintain the effectiveness of ZYVOX and other antibacterial drugs, ZYVOX should be used only to treat or prevent infections that are proven or strongly suspected to be caused by susceptible bacteria. When culture and susceptibility information are available, they should be considered in selecting or modifying antibacterial therapy. In the absence of such data, local epidemiology and susceptibility patterns may contribute to the empiric selection of therapy.

*MDRSP refers to isolates resistant to two or more of the following antibiotics: penicillin, second-generation cephalosporins, macrolides, tetracycline, and trimethoprim/sulfamethoxazole.

CONTRAINDICATIONS

ZYVOX formulations are contraindicated for use in patients who have known hypersensitivity to linezolid or any of the other product components.

Monoamine Oxidase Inhibitors

Linezolid should not be used in patients taking any medicinal product which inhibits monoamine oxidases A or B (e.g., phenelzine, isocarboxazid) or within two weeks of taking any such medicinal product.

Potential Interactions Producing Elevation of Blood Pressure

Unless patients are monitored for potential increases in blood pressure, linezolid should not be administered to patients with uncontrolled hypertension, pheochromocytoma, thyrotoxicosis and/or patients taking any of the following types of medications: directly and indirectly acting sympathomimetic agents (e.g., pseudoephedrine), vasopressive agents (e.g., epinephrine, norepinephrine), dopaminergic agents (e.g., dopamine, dobutamine) (see **PRECAUTIONS, Drug Interactions**).

Potential Serotonergic Interactions

Unless patients are carefully observed for signs and/or symptoms of serotonin syndrome, linezolid should not be administered to patients with carcinoid syndrome and/or patients taking any of the following medications: serotonin re-uptake inhibitors, tricyclic antidepressants, serotonin 5-HT1 receptor agonists (triptans), meperidine or buspirone (see **PRECAUTIONS, General** and **Drug Interactions**).

WARNINGS

Myelosuppression (including anemia, leukopenia, pancytopenia, and thrombocytopenia) has been reported in patients receiving linezolid. In cases where the outcome is known, when linezolid was discontinued, the affected hematologic parameters have risen toward pretreatment levels. Complete blood counts should be monitored weekly in patients who receive linezolid, particularly in those who receive linezolid for longer than two weeks, those with preexisting myelosuppression, those receiving concomitant drugs that produce bone marrow suppression, or those with a chronic infection who have received previous or concomitant antibiotic therapy. Discontinuation of therapy with linezolid should be considered in patients who develop or have worsening myelosuppression.

In adult and juvenile dogs and rats, myelosuppression, reduced extramedullary hematopoiesis in spleen and liver, and lymphoid depletion of thymus, lymph nodes, and spleen were observed (see **ANIMAL PHARMACOLOGY**).

Mortality Imbalance in an Investigational Study in Patients with Catheter-Related Bloodstream Infections, including those with catheter-site infections

An imbalance in mortality was seen in patients treated with linezolid relative to vancomycin/dicloxacillin/oxacillin in an open-label study in seriously ill patients with intravascular catheter-related infections [78/363 (21.5%) vs. 58/363 (16.0%); odds ratio 1.426, 95% CI 0.970, 2.098]. While causality has not been established, this observed imbalance occurred primarily in linezolid-treated patients in whom either Gram-negative pathogens, mixed Gram-negative and Gram-positive pathogens, or no pathogen were identified at baseline, but was not seen in patients with Gram-positive infections only.

Linezolid is not approved and should not be used for the treatment of patients with catheter-related bloodstream infections or catheter-site infections.

Linezolid has no clinical activity against Gram-negative pathogens and is not indicated for the treatment of Gram-negative infections. It is critical that specific Gram-negative therapy be initiated immediately if a concomitant Gram-negative pathogen is documented or suspected (see **INDICATIONS AND USAGE**).

Clostridium difficile associated diarrhea (CDAD) has been reported with use of nearly all antibacterial agents, including ZYVOX, and may range in severity from mild diarrhea to fatal colitis. Treatment with antibacterial agents alters the normal flora of the colon leading to overgrowth of *C. difficile*.

C. difficile produces toxins A and B which contribute to the development of CDAD. Hypertoxin producing strains of *C. difficile* cause increased morbidity and mortality, as these infections can be refractory to antimicrobial therapy and may require colectomy. CDAD must be considered in all patients who present with diarrhea following antibiotic use. Careful medical history is necessary since CDAD has been reported to occur over two months after the administration of antibacterial agents.

If CDAD is suspected or confirmed, ongoing antibiotic use not directed against *C. difficile* may need to be discontinued. Appropriate fluid and electrolyte management, protein supplementation, antibiotic treatment of *C. difficile*, and surgical evaluation should be instituted as clinically indicated.

PRECAUTIONS

General

Lactic Acidosis

Lactic acidosis has been reported with the use of ZYVOX. In reported cases, patients experienced repeated episodes of nausea and vomiting. Patients who develop recurrent nausea or vomiting, unexplained acidosis, or a low bicarbonate level while receiving ZYVOX should receive immediate medical evaluation.

Serotonin Syndrome

Spontaneous reports of serotonin syndrome associated with the co-administration of ZYVOX and serotonergic agents, including antidepressants such as selective serotonin reuptake inhibitors (SSRIs), have been reported (see PRECAUTIONS, Drug Interactions).

Where administration of ZYVOX and concomitant serotonergic agents is clinically appropriate, patients should be closely observed for signs and symptoms of serotonin syndrome such as cognitive dysfunction, hyperpyrexia, hyperreflexia and incoordination. If signs or symptoms occur physicians should consider discontinuation of either one or both agents. If the concomitant serotonergic agent is withdrawn, discontinuation symptoms can be observed (see package insert of the specified agent(s) for a description of the associated discontinuation symptoms).

Peripheral and Optic Neuropathy

Peripheral and optic neuropathy have been reported in patients treated with ZYVOX, primarily those patients treated for longer than the maximum recommended duration of 28 days. In cases of optic neuropathy that progressed to loss of vision, patients were treated for extended periods beyond the maximum recommended duration. Visual blurring has been reported in some patients treated with ZYVOX for less than 28 days.

If patients experience symptoms of visual impairment, such as changes in visual acuity, changes in color vision, blurred vision, or visual field defect, prompt ophthalmic evaluation is recommended. **Visual function should be monitored in all patients taking ZYVOX for extended periods (≥ 3 months) and in all patients reporting new visual symptoms regardless of length of therapy with ZYVOX.** If peripheral or optic neuropathy occurs, the continued use of ZYVOX in these patients should be weighed against the potential risks.

Convulsions

Convulsions have been reported in patients when treated with linezolid. In some of these cases, a history of seizures or risk factors for seizures was reported.

The use of antibiotics may promote the overgrowth of non-susceptible organisms. Should superinfection occur during therapy, appropriate measures should be taken.

ZYVOX has not been studied in patients with uncontrolled hypertension, pheochromocytoma, carcinoid syndrome, or untreated hyperthyroidism.

The safety and efficacy of ZYVOX formulations given for longer than 28 days have not been evaluated in controlled clinical trials.

Prescribing ZYVOX in the absence of a proven or strongly suspected bacterial infection or a prophylactic indication is unlikely to provide benefit to the patient and increases the risk of the development of drug-resistant bacteria.

Information for Patients

Patients should be advised that:

- ZYVOX may be taken with or without food.
- They should inform their physician if they have a history of hypertension.
- Large quantities of foods or beverages with high tyramine content should be avoided while taking ZYVOX. Quantities of tyramine consumed should be less than 100 mg per meal. Foods high in tyramine content include those that may have undergone protein changes by aging, fermentation, pickling, or smoking to improve flavor, such as aged cheeses (0 to 15 mg tyramine per ounce); fermented or air-dried meats (0.1 to 8 mg tyramine per ounce); sauerkraut (8 mg tyramine per 8 ounces); soy sauce (5 mg tyramine per 1 teaspoon); tap beers (4 mg tyramine per 12 ounces); red wines (0 to 6 mg tyramine per 8 ounces). The tyramine content of any protein-rich food may be increased if stored for long periods or improperly refrigerated.[9,10]

- They should inform their physician if taking medications containing pseudoephedrine HCl or phenylpropanolamine HCl, such as cold remedies and decongestants.
- They should inform their physician if taking serotonin reuptake inhibitors or other antidepressants.
- *Phenylketonurics:* Each 5 mL of the 100 mg/5 mL ZYVOX for Oral Suspension contains 20 mg phenylalanine. The other ZYVOX formulations do not contain phenylalanine. Contact your physician or pharmacist.
- They should inform their physician if they experience changes in vision.
- They should inform their physician if they have a history of seizures.
- Diarrhea is a common problem caused by antibiotics, which usually ends when the antibiotic is discontinued. Sometimes after starting treatment with antibiotics, patients can develop watery and bloody stools (with or without stomach cramps and fever) even as late as two or more months after having taken the last dose of the antibiotic. If this occurs, patients should contact their physician as soon as possible.

Patients should be counseled that antibacterial drugs including ZYVOX should only be used to treat bacterial infections. They do not treat viral infections (e.g., the common cold). When ZYVOX is prescribed to treat a bacterial infection, patients should be told that although it is common to feel better early in the course of therapy, the medication should be taken exactly as directed. Skipping doses or not completing the full course of therapy may (1) decrease the effectiveness of the immediate treatment and (2) increase the likelihood that bacteria will develop resistance and will not be treatable by ZYVOX or other antibacterial drugs in the future.

Drug Interactions (see also CLINICAL PHARMACOLOGY, Drug-Drug Interactions)

Monoamine Oxidase Inhibition: Linezolid is a reversible, nonselective inhibitor of monoamine oxidase. Therefore, linezolid has the potential for interaction with adrenergic and serotonergic agents.

Adrenergic Agents: Some individuals receiving ZYVOX may experience a reversible enhancement of the pressor response to indirect-acting sympathomimetic agents, vasopressor or dopaminergic agents. Commonly used drugs such as phenylpropanolamine and pseudoephedrine have been specifically studied. Initial doses of adrenergic agents, such as dopamine or epinephrine, should be reduced and titrated to achieve the desired response.

Serotonergic Agents: Co-administration of linezolid and serotonergic agents was not associated with serotonin syndrome in Phase 1, 2 or 3 studies. Spontaneous reports of serotonin syndrome associated with co-administration of ZYVOX and serotonergic agents, including antidepressants such as selective serotonin reuptake inhibitors (SSRIs), have been reported. Patients who are treated with ZYVOX and concomitant serotonergic agents should be closely observed as described in the PRECAUTIONS, General Section.

Strong CYP450 Inducers: In a study in healthy volunteers, co-administration of rifampin with oral linezolid resulted in a 21% decrease in linezolid C_{max} and a 32% decrease in linezolid AUC_{0-12}. The clinical significance of this interaction is unknown. Other strong inducers of hepatic enzymes (e.g. carbamazepine, phenytoin, phenobarbital) could cause a similar or smaller decrease in linezolid exposure (see **CLINICAL PHARMACOLOGY, Drug-Drug Interactions**).

Drug-Laboratory Test Interactions

There are no reported drug-laboratory test interactions.

Carcinogenesis, Mutagenesis, Impairment of Fertility

Lifetime studies in animals have not been conducted to evaluate the carcinogenic potential of linezolid. Neither mutagenic nor clastogenic potential was found in a battery of tests including: assays for mutagenicity (Ames bacterial reversion and CHO cell mutation), an in vitro unscheduled DNA synthesis (UDS) assay, an in vitro chromosome aberration assay in human lymphocytes, and an in vivo mouse micronucleus assay.

Linezolid did not affect the fertility or reproductive performance of adult female rats. It reversibly decreased fertility and reproductive performance in adult male rats when given at doses ≥ 50 mg/kg/day, with exposures approximately equal to or greater than the expected human exposure level (exposure comparisons are based on AUCs). The reversible fertility effects were mediated through altered spermatogenesis. Affected spermatids contained abnormally formed and oriented mitochondria and were non-viable.

Epithelial cell hypertrophy and hyperplasia in the epididymis was observed in conjunction with decreased fertility. Similar epididymal changes were not seen in dogs.

In sexually mature male rats exposed to drug as juveniles, mildly decreased fertility was observed following treatment with linezolid through most of their period of sexual development (50 mg/kg/day from days 7 to 36 of age, and 100 mg/kg/day from days 37 to 55 of age), with exposures up to 1.7-fold greater than mean AUCs observed in pediatric patients aged 3 months to 11 years. Decreased fertility was not observed with shorter treatment periods, corresponding to exposure in utero through the early neonatal period (gestation day 6 through postnatal day 5), neonatal exposure (postnatal days 5 to 21), or to juvenile exposure (postnatal days 22 to 35). Reversible reductions in sperm motility and altered sperm morphology were observed in rats treated from postnatal day 22 to 35.

Pregnancy

Teratogenic Effects. Pregnancy Category C: Linezolid was not teratogenic in mice, rats, or rabbits at exposure levels 6.5-fold (in mice), equivalent to (in rats), or 0.06-fold (in rabbits) the expected human exposure level, based on AUCs. However, embryo and fetal toxicities were seen (see **Non-teratogenic Effects**). There are no adequate and well-controlled studies in pregnant women. ZYVOX should be used during pregnancy only if the potential benefit justifies the potential risk to the fetus.

Non-teratogenic Effects

In mice, embryo and fetal toxicities were seen only at doses that caused maternal toxicity (clinical signs and reduced body weight gain). A dose of 450 mg/kg/day (6.5-fold the estimated human exposure level based on AUCs) correlated with increased postimplantational embryo death, including total litter loss, decreased fetal body weights, and an increased incidence of costal cartilage fusion.

In rats, mild fetal toxicity was observed at 15 and 50 mg/kg/day (exposure levels 0.22-fold to approximately equivalent to the estimated human exposure, respectively based on AUCs). The effects consisted of decreased fetal body weights and reduced ossification of sternebrae, a finding often seen in association with decreased fetal body weights. Slight maternal toxicity, in the form of reduced body weight gain, was seen at 50 mg/kg/day.

In rabbits, reduced fetal body weight occurred only in the presence of maternal toxicity (clinical signs, reduced body weight gain and food consumption) when administered at a dose of 15 mg/kg/day (0.06-fold the estimated human exposure based on AUCs).

When female rats were treated with 50 mg/kg/day (approximately equivalent to the estimated human exposure based on AUCs) of linezolid during pregnancy and lactation, survival of pups was decreased on postnatal days 1 to 4. Male and female pups permitted to mature to reproductive age, when mated, showed an increase in preimplantation loss.

Nursing Mothers

Linezolid and its metabolites are excreted in the milk of lactating rats. Concentrations in milk were similar to those in maternal plasma. It is not known whether linezolid is excreted in human milk. Because many drugs are excreted in human milk, caution should be exercised when ZYVOX is administered to a nursing woman.

Pediatric Use

The safety and effectiveness of ZYVOX for the treatment of pediatric patients with the following infections are supported by evidence from adequate and well-controlled studies in adults, pharmacokinetic data in pediatric patients, and additional data from a comparator-controlled study of Gram-positive infections in pediatric patients ranging in age from birth through 11 years (see **INDICATIONS AND USAGE** and **CLINICAL STUDIES**):

• nosocomial pneumonia
• complicated skin and skin structure infections
• community-acquired pneumonia (also supported by evidence from an uncontrolled study in patients ranging in age from 8 months through 12 years)
• vancomycin-resistant *Enterococcus faecium* infections

The safety and effectiveness of ZYVOX for the treatment of pediatric patients with the following infection have been established in a comparator-controlled study in pediatric patients ranging in age from 5 through 17 years (see **CLINICAL STUDIES**):

• uncomplicated skin and skin structure infections caused by *Staphylococcus aureus* (methicillin-susceptible strains only) or *Streptococcus pyogenes*

Pharmacokinetic information generated in pediatric patients with ventriculoperitoneal shunts showed variable cerebrospinal fluid (CSF) linezolid concentrations following single and multiple dosing of linezolid; therapeutic concentrations were not consistently achieved or maintained in the CSF. Therefore, the use of linezolid for the empiric treatment of pediatric patients with central nervous system infections is not recommended.

The C_{max} and the volume of distribution (V_{ss}) of linezolid are similar regardless of age in pediatric patients. However, linezolid clearance is a function of age. Excluding neonates less than a week of age, clearance is most rapid in the youngest age groups ranging from >1 week old to 11 years, resulting in lower single-dose systemic exposure (AUC) and shorter half-life as compared with adults. As age of pediatric patients increases, the clearance of linezolid gradually decreases, and by adolescence, mean clearance values approach those observed for the adult population. There is wider inter-subject variability in linezolid clearance and in systemic drug exposure (AUC) across all pediatric age groups as compared with adults.

Similar mean daily AUC values were observed in pediatric patients from birth to 11 years of age dosed q8h relative to adolescents or adults dosed q12h. Therefore, the dosage for pediatric patients up to 11 years of age should be 10 mg/kg q8h. Pediatric patients 12 years and older should receive 600 mg q12h.

Recommendations for the dosage regimen for pre-term neonates less than 7 days of age (gestational age less than 34 weeks) are based on pharmacokinetic data from 9 pre-term neonates. Most of these pre-term neonates have lower systemic linezolid clearance values and larger AUC values than many full-term neonates and older infants. Therefore, these pre-term neonates should be initiated with a dosing regimen of 10 mg/kg q12h. Consideration may be given to the use of a 10 mg/kg q8h regimen in neonates with a suboptimal clinical response. All neonatal patients should receive 10 mg/kg q8h by 7 days of life (see **CLINICAL PHARMACOLOGY, Special Populations, Pediatric** and **DOSAGE AND ADMINISTRATION**).

In limited clinical experience, 5 out of 6 (83%) pediatric patients with infections due to Gram-positive pathogens with MICs of 4 μg/mL treated with ZYVOX had clinical cures. However, pediatric patients exhibit wider variability in linezolid clearance and systemic exposure (AUC) compared with adults. In pediatric patients with a sub-optimal clinical response, particularly those with pathogens with MIC of 4 μg/mL, lower systemic exposure, site and severity of infection, and the underlying medical condition should be considered when assessing clinical response (see **CLINICAL PHARMACOLOGY, Special Populations, Pediatric** and **DOSAGE AND ADMINISTRATION**).

Geriatric Use

Of the 2046 patients treated with ZYVOX in Phase 3 comparator-controlled clinical trials, 589 (29%) were 65 years or older and 253 (12%) were 75 years or older. No overall differences in safety or effectiveness were observed between these patients and younger patients.

ANIMAL PHARMACOLOGY

Target organs of linezolid toxicity were similar in juvenile and adult rats and dogs. Dose- and time-dependent myelosuppression, as evidenced by bone marrow hypocellularity/decreased hematopoiesis, decreased extramedullary hematopoiesis in spleen and liver, and decreased levels of circulating erythrocytes, leukocytes, and platelets have been seen in animal studies. Lymphoid depletion occurred in thymus, lymph nodes, and spleen. Generally, the lymphoid findings were associated with anorexia, weight loss, and suppression of body weight gain, which may have contributed to the observed effects.

In rats administered linezolid orally for 6 months, nonreversible, minimal to mild axonal degeneration of sciatic nerves was observed at 80 mg/kg/day; minimal degeneration of the sciatic nerve was also observed in 1 male at this dose level at a 3-month interim necropsy. Sensitive morphologic evaluation of perfusion-fixed tissues was conducted to investigate evidence of optic nerve degeneration. Minimal to moderate optic nerve degeneration was evident in 2 male rats after 6 months of dosing, but the direct relationship to drug was equivocal because of the acute nature of the finding and its asymmetrical distribution. The nerve degeneration observed was microscopically comparable to spontaneous unilateral optic nerve degeneration reported in aging rats and may be an exacerbation of common background change.

These effects were observed at exposure levels that are comparable to those observed in some human subjects. The hematopoietic and lymphoid effects were reversible, although in some studies, reversal was incomplete within the duration of the recovery period.

ADVERSE REACTIONS

Adult Patients

The safety of ZYVOX formulations was evaluated in 2046 adult patients enrolled in seven Phase 3 comparator-controlled clinical trials, who were treated for up to 28 days. In these studies, 85% of the adverse events reported with ZYVOX were described as mild to moderate in intensity. Table 6 shows the incidence of adverse events reported in at least 2% of patients in these trials. The most common adverse events in patients treated with ZYVOX were diarrhea (incidence across studies: 2.8% to 11.0%), headache (inci-

Table 7. Incidence (%) of Drug-Related Adverse Events Occurring in >1% of Adult Patients Treated with ZYVOX in Comparator-Controlled Clinical Trials

Adverse Event	Uncomplicated Skin and Skin Structure Infections		All Other Indications	
	ZYVOX 400 mg PO q12h (n=548)	Clarithromycin 250 mg PO q12h (n=537)	ZYVOX 600 mg q12h (n=1498)	All Other Comparators* (n=1464)
% of patients with 1 drug-related adverse event	25.4	19.6	20.4	14.3
% of patients discontinuing due to drug-related adverse events†	3.5	2.4	2.1	1.7
Diarrhea	5.3	4.8	4.0	2.7
Nausea	3.5	3.5	3.3	1.8
Headache	2.7	2.2	1.9	1.0
Taste alteration	1.8	2.0	0.9	0.2
Vaginal moniliasis	1.6	1.3	1.0	0.4
Fungal infection	1.5	0.2	0.1	<0.1
Abnormal liver function tests	0.4	0	1.3	0.5
Vomiting	0.9	0.4	1.2	0.4
Tongue discoloration	1.1	0	0.2	0
Dizziness	1.1	1.5	0.4	0.3
Oral moniliasis	0.4	0	1.1	0.4

* Comparators included cefpodoxime proxetil 200 mg PO q12h; ceftriaxone 1 g IV q12h; dicloxacillin 500 mg PO q6h; oxacillin 2 g IV q6h; vancomycin 1 g IV q12h.
† The most commonly reported drug-related adverse events leading to discontinuation in patients treated with ZYVOX were nausea, headache, diarrhea, and vomiting.

dence across studies: 0.5% to 11.3%), and nausea (incidence across studies: 3.4% to 9.6%).

Table 6. Incidence (%) of Adverse Events Reported in ≥2% of Adult Patients in Comparator-Controlled Clinical Trials with ZYVOX

Event	ZYVOX (n=2046)	All Comparators* (n=2001)
Diarrhea	8.3	6.3
Headache	6.5	5.5
Nausea	6.2	4.6
Vomiting	3.7	2.0
Insomnia	2.5	1.7
Constipation	2.2	2.1
Rash	2.0	2.2
Dizziness	2.0	1.9
Fever	1.6	2.1

*Comparators included cefpodoxime proxetil 200 mg PO q12h; ceftriaxone 1 g IV q12h; clarithromycin 250 mg PO q12h; dicloxacillin 500 mg PO q6h; oxacillin 2 g IV q6h; vancomycin 1 g IV q12h.

Other adverse events reported in Phase 2 and Phase 3 studies included oral moniliasis, vaginal moniliasis, hypertension, dyspepsia, localized abdominal pain, pruritus, and tongue discoloration.

Table 7 shows the incidence of drug-related adverse events reported in at least 1% of adult patients in these trials by dose of ZYVOX.

[See table 7 at top of previous page]

Pediatric Patients

The safety of ZYVOX formulations was evaluated in 215 pediatric patients ranging in age from birth through 11 years, and in 248 pediatric patients aged 5 through 17 years (146 of these 248 were age 5 through 11 and 102 were age 12 to 17). These patients were enrolled in two Phase 3 comparator-controlled clinical trials and were treated for up to 28 days. In these studies, 83% and 99%, respectively, of the adverse events reported with ZYVOX were described as mild to moderate in intensity. In the study of hospitalized pediatric patients (birth through 11 years) with Gram-positive infections, who were randomized 2 to 1 (linezolid:vancomycin), mortality was 6.0% (13/215) in the linezolid arm and 3.0% (3/101) in the vancomycin arm. However, given the severe underlying illness in the patient population, no causality could be established. Table 8 shows the incidence of adverse events reported in at least 2% of pediatric patients treated with ZYVOX in these trials.

[See table 8 at right]

Table 9 shows the incidence of drug-related adverse events reported in more than 1% of pediatric patients (and more than 1 patient) in either treatment group in the comparator-controlled Phase 3 trials.

[See table 9 at top of next page]

Laboratory Changes

ZYVOX has been associated with thrombocytopenia when used in doses up to and including 600 mg every 12 hours for up to 28 days. In Phase 3 comparator-controlled trials, the percentage of adult patients who developed a substantially low platelet count (defined as less than 75% of lower limit of normal and/or baseline) was 2.4% (range among studies: 0.3 to 10.0%) with ZYVOX and 1.5% (range among studies: 0.4 to 7.0%) with a comparator. In a study of hospitalized pediatric patients ranging in age from birth through 11 years, the percentage of patients who developed a substantially low platelet count (defined as less than 75% of lower limit of normal and/or baseline) was 12.9% with ZYVOX and 13.4% with vancomycin. In an outpatient study of pediatric patients aged from 5 through 17 years, the percentage of patients who developed a substantially low platelet count was 0% with ZYVOX and 0.4% with cefadroxil. Thrombocytopenia associated with the use of ZYVOX appears to be dependent on duration of therapy, (generally greater than 2 weeks of treatment). The platelet counts for most patients returned to the normal range/baseline during the follow-up period. No related clinical adverse events were identified in Phase 3 clinical trials in patients developing thrombocytopenia. Bleeding events were identified in thrombocytopenic patients in a compassionate use program for ZYVOX; the role of linezolid in these events cannot be determined (see **WARNINGS**).

Table 8. Incidence (%) of Adverse Events Reported in ≥2% of Pediatric Patients Treated with ZYVOX in Comparator-Controlled Clinical Trials

Event	Uncomplicated Skin and Skin Structure Infections*		All Other Indications†	
	ZYVOX (n=248)	Cefadroxil (n=251)	ZYVOX (n=215)	Vancomycin (n=101)
Fever	2.9	3.6	14.1	14.1
Diarrhea	7.8	8.0	10.8	12.1
Vomiting	2.9	6.4	9.4	9.1
Sepsis	0	0	8.0	7.1
Rash	1.6	1.2	7.0	15.2
Headache	6.5	4.0	0.9	0
Anemia	0	0	5.6	7.1
Thrombocytopenia	0	0	4.7	2.0
Upper respiratory infection	3.7	5.2	4.2	1.0
Nausea	3.7	3.2	1.9	0
Dyspnea	0	0	3.3	1.0
Reaction at site of injection or of vascular catheter	0	0	3.3	5.1
Trauma	3.3	4.8	2.8	2.0
Pharyngitis	2.9	1.6	0.5	1.0
Convulsion	0	0	2.8	2.0
Hypokalemia	0	0	2.8	3.0
Pneumonia	0	0	2.8	2.0
Thrombocythemia	0	0	2.8	2.0
Cough	2.4	4.0	0.9	1.0
Generalized abdominal pain	2.4	2.8	0.9	2.0
Localized abdominal pain	2.4	2.8	0.5	1.0
Apnea	0	0	2.3	2.0
Gastrointestinal bleeding	0	0	2.3	1.0
Generalized edema	0	0	2.3	1.0
Loose stools	1.6	0.8	2.3	3.0
Localized pain	2.0	1.6	0.9	0
Skin disorder	2.0	0	0.9	1.0

* Patients 5 through 11 years of age received ZYVOX 10 mg/kg PO q12h or cefadroxil 15 mg/kg PO q12h. Patients 12 years or older received ZYVOX 600 mg PO q12h or cefadroxil 500 mg PO q12h.
† Patients from birth through 11 years of age received ZYVOX 10 mg/kg IV/PO q8h or vancomycin 10 to 15 mg/kg IV q6-24h, depending on age and renal clearance.

Changes seen in other laboratory parameters, without regard to drug relationship, revealed no substantial differences between ZYVOX and the comparators. These changes were generally not clinically significant, did not lead to discontinuation of therapy, and were reversible. The incidence of adult and pediatric patients with at least one substantially abnormal hematologic or serum chemistry value is presented in Tables 10, 11, 12, and 13.

[See table 10 on next page]
[See table 11 at top of page 2855]
[See table 12 on page 2855]
[See table 13 on page 2855]

Postmarketing Experience

Myelosuppression (including anemia, leukopenia, pancytopenia, and thrombocytopenia) has been reported during postmarketing use of ZYVOX (see **WARNINGS**). Peripheral neuropathy, and optic neuropathy sometimes progressing to loss of vision, have been reported in patients treated with ZYVOX. Lactic acidosis has been reported with the use of ZYVOX (see **PRECAUTIONS**). Although these reports have primarily been in patients treated for longer than the maximum recommended duration of 28 days, these events have also been reported in patients receiving shorter courses of therapy. Serotonin syndrome has been reported in patients receiving concomitant serotonergic agents, including antidepressants such as selective serotonin reuptake inhibitors (SSRIs) and ZYVOX (see **PRECAUTIONS**). Convulsions have been reported with the use of ZYVOX (see **PRECAUTIONS**). Anaphylaxis, angioedema, and bullous skin disorders such as those described as Stevens Johnson syndrome have been reported. Superficial tooth discoloration and tongue discoloration have been reported with the use of linezolid. The tooth discoloration was removable with professional dental cleaning (manual descaling) in cases with known outcome. These events have been chosen for inclusion due to either their seriousness, frequency of reporting, possible causal connection to ZYVOX, or a combination of these factors. Because they are reported voluntarily from a population of unknown size, estimates of frequency cannot be made and causal relationship cannot be precisely established.

OVERDOSAGE

In the event of overdosage, supportive care is advised, with maintenance of glomerular filtration. Hemodialysis may facilitate more rapid elimination of linezolid. In a Phase 1 clinical trial, approximately 30% of a dose of linezolid was

Table 9. Incidence (%) of Drug-related Adverse Events Occurring in >1% of Pediatric Patients (and >1 Patient) in Either Treatment Group in Comparator-Controlled Clinical Trials

Event	Uncomplicated Skin and Skin Structure Infections*		All Other Indications†	
	ZYVOX (n=248)	Cefadroxil (n=251)	ZYVOX (n=215)	Vancomycin (n=101)
% of patients with ≥1 drug-related adverse event	19.2	14.1	18.8	34.3
% of patients discontinuing due to a drug-related adverse event	1.6	2.4	0.9	6.1
Diarrhea	5.7	5.2	3.8	6.1
Nausea	3.3	2.0	1.4	0
Headache	2.4	0.8	0	0
Loose stools	1.2	0.8	1.9	0
Thrombocytopenia	0	0	1.9	0
Vomiting	1.2	2.4	1.9	1.0
Generalized abdominal pain	1.6	1.2	0	0
Localized abdominal pain	1.6	1.2	0	0
Anemia	0	0	1.4	1.0
Eosinophilia	0.4	0.4	1.4	0
Rash	0.4	1.2	1.4	7.1
Vertigo	1.2	0.4	0	0
Oral moniliasis	0	0	0.9	4.0
Fever	0	0	0.5	3.0
Pruritus at non-application site	0.4	0	0	2.0
Anaphylaxis	0	0	0	10.1‡

* Patients 5 through 11 years of age received ZYVOX 10 mg/kg PO q12h or cefadroxil 15 mg/kg PO q12h. Patients 12 years or older received ZYVOX 600 mg PO q12h or cefadroxil 500 mg PO q12h.
† Patients from birth through 11 years of age received ZYVOX 10 mg/kg IV/PO q8h or vancomycin 10 to 15 mg/kg IV q6-24h, depending on age and renal clearance.
‡ These reports were of 'red-man syndrome', which were coded as anaphylaxis.

Table 10. Percent of Adult Patients who Experienced at Least One Substantially Abnormal* Hematology Laboratory Value in Comparator-Controlled Clinical Trials with ZYVOX

Laboratory Assay	Uncomplicated Skin and Skin Structure Infections		All Other Indications	
	ZYVOX 400 mg q12h	Clarithromycin 250 mg q12h	ZYVOX 600 mg q12h	All Other Comparators†
Hemoglobin (g/dL)	0.9	0.0	7.1	6.6
Platelet count (× 10³/mm³)	0.7	0.8	3.0	1.8
WBC (× 10³/mm³)	0.2	0.6	2.2	1.3
Neutrophils (× 10³/mm³)	0.0	0.2	1.1	1.2

* <75% (<50% for neutrophils) of Lower Limit of Normal (LLN) for values normal at baseline; <75% (<50% for neutrophils) of LLN and of baseline for values abnormal at baseline.
† Comparators included cefpodoxime proxetil 200 mg PO q12h; ceftriaxone 1 g IV q12h; dicloxacillin 500 mg PO q6h; oxacillin 2 g IV q6h; vancomycin 1 g IV q12h.

removed during a 3-hour hemodialysis session beginning 3 hours after the dose of linezolid was administered. Data are not available for removal of linezolid with peritoneal dialysis or hemoperfusion. Clinical signs of acute toxicity in animals were decreased activity and ataxia in rats and vomiting and tremors in dogs treated with 3000 mg/kg/day and 2000 mg/kg/day, respectively.

DOSAGE AND ADMINISTRATION
The recommended dosage for ZYVOX formulations for the treatment of infections is described in Table 14.
[See table 14 at top of page 2856]
Adult patients with infection due to MRSA should be treated with ZYVOX 600 mg q12h.
In limited clinical experience, 5 out of 6 (83%) pediatric patients with infections due to Gram-positive pathogens with MICs of 4 µg/mL treated with ZYVOX had clinical cures. However, pediatric patients exhibit wider variability in linezolid clearance and systemic exposure (AUC) compared with adults. In pediatric patients with a sub-optimal clinical response, particularly those with pathogens with MIC of 4 µg/mL, lower systemic exposure, site and severity of infection, and the underlying medical condition should be considered when assessing clinical response (see CLINICAL PHARMACOLOGY, Special Populations, Pediatric and PRECAUTIONS, Pediatric Use).
In controlled clinical trials, the protocol-defined duration of treatment for all infections ranged from 7 to 28 days. Total treatment duration was determined by the treating physician based on site and severity of the infection, and on the patient's clinical response.

No dose adjustment is necessary when switching from intravenous to oral administration. Patients whose therapy is started with ZYVOX I.V. Injection may be switched to either ZYVOX Tablets or Oral Suspension at the discretion of the physician, when clinically indicated.
Intravenous Administration
ZYVOX I.V. Injection is supplied in single-use, ready-to-use infusion bags (see HOW SUPPLIED for container sizes). Parenteral drug products should be inspected visually for particulate matter prior to administration. Check for minute leaks by firmly squeezing the bag. If leaks are detected, discard the solution, as sterility may be impaired.
ZYVOX I.V. Injection should be administered by intravenous infusion over a period of 30 to 120 minutes. **Do not use this intravenous infusion bag in series connections.** Additives should not be introduced into this solution. If ZYVOX I.V. Injection is to be given concomitantly with another drug, each drug should be given separately in accordance with the recommended dosage and route of administration for each product. In particular, physical incompatibilities resulted when ZYVOX I.V. Injection was combined with the following drugs during simulated Y-site administration: amphotericin B, chlorpromazine HCl, diazepam, pentamidine isothionate, erythromycin lactobionate, phenytoin sodium, and trimethoprim-sulfamethoxazole. Additionally, chemical incompatibility resulted when ZYVOX I.V. Injection was combined with ceftriaxone sodium.
If the same intravenous line is used for sequential infusion of several drugs, the line should be flushed before and after infusion of ZYVOX I.V. Injection with an infusion solution compatible with ZYVOX I.V. Injection and with any other drug(s) administered via this common line (see **Compatible Intravenous Solutions**).
Compatible Intravenous Solutions
5% Dextrose Injection, USP
0.9% Sodium Chloride Injection, USP
Lactated Ringer's Injection, USP
Keep the infusion bags in the overwrap until ready to use. Store at room temperature. Protect from freezing. ZYVOX I.V. Injection may exhibit a yellow color that can intensify over time without adversely affecting potency.
Constitution of Oral Suspension
ZYVOX for Oral Suspension is supplied as a powder/granule for constitution. Gently tap bottle to loosen powder. Add a total of 123 mL distilled water in two portions. After adding the first half, shake vigorously to wet all of the powder. Then add the second half of the water and shake vigorously to obtain a uniform suspension. After constitution, each 5 mL of the suspension contains 100 mg of linezolid. Before using, gently mix by inverting the bottle 3 to 5 times. **DO NOT SHAKE**. Store constituted suspension at room temperature. Use within 21 days after constitution.

HOW SUPPLIED
Injection
ZYVOX I.V. Injection is available in single-use, ready-to-use flexible plastic infusion bags in a foil laminate overwrap. The infusion bags and ports are latex-free. The infusion bags are available in the following package sizes:
100 mL bag (200 mg linezolid)   NDC 0009-5137-01
200 mL bag (400 mg linezolid)   NDC 0009-5139-01
300 mL bag (600 mg linezolid)   NDC 0009-5140-01
Tablets
ZYVOX Tablets are available as follows:
400 mg (white, oblong, film-coated tablets printed with "ZYVOX 400mg")
100 tablets in HDPE bottle   NDC 0009-5134-01
20 tablets in HDPE bottle   NDC 0009-5134-02
Unit dose packages of 30 tablets   NDC 0009-5134-03
600 mg (white, capsule-shaped, film-coated tablets printed with "ZYVOX 600 mg")
100 tablets in HDPE bottle   NDC 0009-5135-01
20 tablets in HDPE bottle   NDC 0009-5135-02
Unit dose packages of 30 tablets   NDC 0009-5135-03
Oral Suspension
ZYVOX for Oral Suspension is available as a dry, white to off-white, orange-flavored granule/powder. When constituted as directed, each bottle will contain 150 mL of a suspension providing the equivalent of 100 mg of linezolid per each 5 mL. ZYVOX for Oral Suspension is supplied as follows:
100 mg/5 mL in 240-mL glass bottles   NDC 0009-5136-01
Storage of ZYVOX Formulations
Store at 25°C (77°F); excursions permitted to 15-30°C (59-86°F) [see USP Controlled Room Temperature]. Protect from light. Keep bottles tightly closed to protect from moisture. It is recommended that the infusion bags be kept in the overwrap until ready to use. Protect infusion bags from freezing.

Table 11. Percent of Adult Patients who Experienced at Least One Substantially Abnormal* Serum Chemistry Laboratory Value in Comparator-Controlled Clinical Trials with ZYVOX

Laboratory Assay	Uncomplicated Skin and Skin Structure Infections		All Other Indications	
	ZYVOX 400 mg q12h	Clarithromycin 250 mg q12h	ZYVOX 600 mg q12h	All Other Comparators[†]
AST (U/L)	1.7	1.3	5.0	6.8
ALT (U/L)	1.7	1.7	9.6	9.3
LDH (U/L)	0.2	0.2	1.8	1.5
Alkaline phosphatase (U/L)	0.2	0.2	3.5	3.1
Lipase (U/L)	2.8	2.6	4.3	4.2
Amylase (U/L)	0.2	0.2	2.4	2.0
Total bilirubin (mg/dL)	0.2	0.0	0.9	1.1
BUN (mg/dL)	0.2	0.0	2.1	1.5
Creatinine (mg/dL)	0.2	0.0	0.2	0.6

* >2 × Upper Limit of Normal (ULN) for values normal at baseline;
  >2 × ULN and >2 × baseline for values abnormal at baseline.
[†] Comparators included cefpodoxime proxetil 200 mg PO q12h; ceftriaxone 1 g IV q12h; dicloxacillin 500 mg PO q6h; oxacillin 2 g IV q6h; vancomycin 1 g IV q12h.

Table 12. Percent of Pediatric Patients who Experienced at Least One Substantially Abnormal* Hematology Laboratory Value in Comparator-Controlled Clinical Trials with ZYVOX

Laboratory Assay	Uncomplicated Skin and Skin Structure Infections[†]		All Other Indications[‡]	
	ZYVOX	Cefadroxil	ZYVOX	Vancomycin
Hemoglobin (g/dL)	0.0	0.0	15.7	12.4
Platelet count (× 10^3/mm^3)	0.0	0.4	12.9	13.4
WBC (× 10^3/mm^3)	0.8	0.8	12.4	10.3
Neutrophils (× 10^3/mm^3)	1.2	0.8	5.9	4.3

* <75% (<50% for neutrophils) of Lower Limit of Normal (LLN) for values normal at baseline;
  <75% (<50% for neutrophils) of LLN and <75% (<50% for neutrophils, <90% for hemoglobin if baseline <LLN) of baseline for values abnormal at baseline.
[†] Patients 5 through 11 years of age received ZYVOX 10 mg/kg PO q12h or cefadroxil 15 mg/kg PO q12h. Patients 12 years or older received ZYVOX 600 mg PO q12h or cefadroxil 500 mg PO q12h.
[‡] Patients from birth through 11 years of age received ZYVOX 10 mg/kg IV/PO q8h or vancomycin 10 to 15 mg/kg IV q6-24h, depending on age and renal clearance.

Table 13. Percent of Pediatric Patients who Experienced at Least One Substantially Abnormal* Serum Chemistry Laboratory Value in Comparator-Controlled Clinical Trials with ZYVOX

Laboratory Assay	Uncomplicated Skin and Skin Structure Infections[†]		All Other Indications[‡]	
	ZYVOX	Cefadroxil	ZYVOX	Vancomycin
ALT (U/L)	0.0	0.0	10.1	12.5
Lipase (U/L)	0.4	1.2	—	—
Amylase (U/L)	—	—	0.6	1.3
Total bilirubin (mg/dL)	—	—	6.3	5.2
Creatinine (mg/dL)	0.4	—	2.4	1.0

* >2 × Upper Limit of Normal (ULN) for values normal at baseline; >2 × ULN and >2 (>1.5 for total bilirubin) × baseline for values abnormal at baseline.
[†] Patients 5 through 11 years of age received ZYVOX 10 mg/kg PO q12h or cefadroxil 15 mg/kg PO q12h. Patients 12 years or older received ZYVOX 600 mg PO q12h or cefadroxil 500 mg PO q12h.
[‡] Patients from birth through 11 years of age received ZYVOX 10 mg/kg IV/PO q8h or vancomycin 10 to 15 mg/kg IV q6-24h, depending on age and renal clearance.

CLINICAL STUDIES
Adults
Vancomycin-Resistant Enterococcal Infections
Adult patients with documented or suspected vancomycin-resistant enterococcal infection were enrolled in a randomized, multi-center, double-blind trial comparing a high dose of ZYVOX (600 mg) with a low dose of ZYVOX (200 mg) given every 12 hours (q12h) either intravenously (IV) or orally for 7 to 28 days. Patients could receive concomitant aztreonam or aminoglycosides. There were 79 patients randomized to high-dose linezolid and 66 to low-dose linezolid. The intent-to-treat (ITT) population with documented vancomycin-resistant enterococcal infection at baseline consisted of 65 patients in the high-dose arm and 52 in the low-dose arm.

The cure rates for the ITT population with documented vancomycin-resistant enterococcal infection at baseline are presented in Table 15 by source of infection. These cure rates do not include patients with missing or indeterm[...] outcomes. The cure rate was higher in the high-dose a[...] than in the low-dose arm, although the difference was n[...] statistically significant at the 0.05 level.

Table 15. Cure Rates at the Test-of-Cure Visit for ITT Adult Patients with Documented Vancomycin-Resistant Enterococcal Infections at Baseline

Source of Infection	Cured	
	ZYVOX 600 mg q12h n/N (%)	ZYVOX 200 mg q12h n/N (%)
Any site	39/58 (67)	24/46 (52)
Any site with associated bacteremia	10/17 (59)	4/14 (29)
Bacteremia of unknown origin	5/10 (50)	2/7 (29)
Skin and skin structure	9/13 (69)	5/5 (100)
Urinary tract	12/19 (63)	12/20 (60)
Pneumonia	2/3 (67)	0/1 (0)
Other*	11/13 (85)	5/13 (39)

*Includes sources of infection such as hepatic abscess, biliary sepsis, necrotic gall bladder, pericolonic abscess, pancreatitis, and catheter-related infection.

Nosocomial Pneumonia
Adult patients with clinically and radiologically documented nosocomial pneumonia were enrolled in a randomized, multi-center, double-blind trial. Patients were treated for 7 to 21 days. One group received ZYVOX I.V. Injection 600 mg q12h, and the other group received vancomycin 1 g q12h IV. Both groups received concomitant aztreonam (1 to 2 g every 8 hours IV), which could be continued if clinically indicated. There were 203 linezolid-treated and 193 vancomycin-treated patients enrolled in the study. One hundred twenty-two (60%) linezolid-treated patients and 103 (53%) vancomycin-treated patients were clinically evaluable. The cure rates in clinically evaluable patients were 57% for linezolid-treated patients and 60% for vancomycin-treated patients. The cure rates in clinically evaluable patients with ventilator-associated pneumonia were 47% for linezolid-treated patients and 40% for vancomycin-treated patients. A modified intent-to-treat (MITT) analysis of 94 linezolid-treated patients and 83 vancomycin-treated patients included subjects who had a pathogen isolated before treatment. The cure rates in the MITT analysis were 57% in linezolid-treated patients and 46% in vancomycin-treated patients. The cure rates by pathogen for microbiologically evaluable patients are presented in Table 16.

Table 16. Cure Rates at the Test-of-Cure Visit for Microbiologically Evaluable Adult Patients with Nosocomial Pneumonia

Pathogen	Cured	
	ZYVOX n/N (%)	Vancomycin n/N (%)
Staphylococcus aureus	23/38 (61)	14/23 (61)
Methicillin-resistant *S. aureus*	13/22 (59)	7/10 (70)
Streptococcus pneumoniae	9/9 (100)	9/10 (90)

Pneumonia caused by multi-drug resistant *S. pneumoniae* (MDRSP*)
ZYVOX was studied for the treatment of community-acquired (CAP) and hospital-acquired (HAP) pneumonia due to MDRSP by pooling clinical data from seven comparative and non-comparative Phase 2 and Phase 3 studies involving adult and pediatric patients. The pooled MITT population consisted of all patients with *S. pneumoniae* isolated at baseline; the pooled ME population consisted of patients satisfying criteria for microbiologic evaluability. The pooled MITT population with CAP included 15 patients (41%) with severe illness (risk classes IV and V) as assessed by a prediction rule[11]. The pooled clinical cure rates for patients with CAP due to MDRSP were 35/48 (73%) in the MITT and 33/36 (92%) in the ME populations respectively. The pooled clinical cure rates for patients with HAP due to MDRSP were 12/18 (67%) in the MITT and 10/12 (83%) in the ME populations respectively.

...al cure rates for
...ly-evaluable patients with
... who were treated with ZYVOX
...d by antibiotic susceptibility)

Screening	Clinical Cure	
	n/N[a]	(%)
Penicillin-resistant	14/16	88
2nd generation cephalosporin-resistant[b]	19/22	86
Macrolide-resistant[c]	29/30	97
Tetracycline-resistant	22/24	92
Trimethoprim/sulfamethoxazole-resistant	18/21	86

a) n= pooled number of patients treated successfully; N= pooled number of patients having MDRSP isolates that exhibited resistance to the listed antibiotic
b) 2nd-generation cephalosporin tested was cefuroxime
c) macrolide tested was erythromycin

* MDRSP refers to isolates resistant to two or more of the following antibiotics: penicillin, second-generation cephalosporins, macrolides, tetracycline, and trimethoprim/sulfamethoxazole.

Complicated Skin and Skin Structure Infections

Adult patients with clinically documented complicated skin and skin structure infections were enrolled in a randomized, multi-center, double-blind, double-dummy trial comparing study medications administered IV followed by medications given orally for a total of 10 to 21 days of treatment. One group of patients received ZYVOX I.V. Injection 600 mg q12h followed by ZYVOX Tablets 600 mg q12h; the other group received oxacillin 2 g every 6 hours (q6h) IV followed by dicloxacillin 500 mg q6h orally. Patients could receive concomitant aztreonam if clinically indicated. There were 400 linezolid-treated and 419 oxacillin-treated patients enrolled in the study. Two hundred forty-five (61%) linezolid-treated patients and 242 (58%) oxacillin-treated patients were clinically evaluable. The cure rates in clinically evaluable patients were 90% in linezolid-treated patients and 85% in oxacillin-treated patients. A modified intent-to-treat (MITT) analysis of 316 linezolid-treated patients and 313 oxacillin-treated patients included subjects who met all criteria for study entry. The cure rates in the MITT analysis were 86% in linezolid-treated patients and 82% in oxacillin-treated patients. The cure rates by pathogen for microbiologically evaluable patients are presented in Table 18.

Table 18. Cure Rates at the Test-of-Cure Visit for Microbiologically Evaluable Adult Patients with Complicated Skin and Skin Structure Infections

Pathogen	Cured	
	ZYVOX n/N (%)	Oxacillin/ Dicloxacillin n/N (%)
Staphylococcus aureus	73/83 (88)	72/84 (86)
Methicillin-resistant *S. aureus*	2/3 (67)	0/0 (–)
Streptococcus agalactiae	6/6 (100)	3/6 (50)
Streptococcus pyogenes	18/26 (69)	21/28 (75)

A separate study provided additional experience on the use of ZYVOX in the treatment of methicillin-resistant *Staphylococcus aureus* (MRSA) infections. This was a randomized, open-label trial in hospitalized adult patients with documented or suspected MRSA infection.
One group of patients received ZYVOX I.V. Injection 600 mg q12h followed by ZYVOX Tablets 600 mg q12h. The other group of patients received vancomycin 1 g q12h IV. Both groups were treated for 7 to 28 days, and could receive concomitant aztreonam or gentamicin if clinically indicated. The cure rates in microbiologically evaluable patients with MRSA skin and skin structure infection were 26/33 (79%) for linezolid-treated patients and 24/33 (73%) for vancomycin-treated patients.

Diabetic Foot Infections

Adult diabetic patients with clinically documented complicated skin and skin structure infections ("diabetic foot infections") were enrolled in a randomized (2:1 ratio), multi-center, open-label trial comparing study medications administered IV or orally for a total of 14 to 28 days of treatment. One group of patients received ZYVOX 600 mg q12h IV or orally; the other group received ampicillin/sulbactam 1.5 to 3 g IV or amoxicillin/clavulanate 500 to 875 mg every 8 to 12 hours (q8-12h) orally. In countries where ampicillin/sulbactam is not marketed, amoxicillin/clavulanate 500 mg to 2 g every 6 hours (q6h) was used for the intravenous regimen. Patients in the comparator group could also be treated with vancomycin 1 g q12h IV if MRSA was isolated from the foot infection. Patients in either treatment group who had Gram-negative bacilli isolated from the infection site could also receive aztreonam 1 to 2 g q8-12h IV. All patients were eligible to receive appropriate adjunctive treatment methods, such as debridement and off-loading, as typically required in the treatment of diabetic foot infections, and most patients received these treatments. There were 241 linezolid-treated and 120 comparator-treated patients in the intent-to-treat (ITT) study population. Two hundred twelve (86%) linezolid-treated patients and 105 (85%) comparator-treated patients were clinically evaluable. In the ITT population, the cure rates were 68.5% (165/241) in linezolid-treated patients and 64% (77/120) in comparator-treated patients, where those with indeterminate and missing outcomes were considered failures. The cure rates in the clinically evaluable patients (excluding those with indeterminate and missing outcomes) were 83% (159/192) and 73% (74/101) in the linezolid- and comparator-treated patients, respectively. A critical post-hoc analysis focused on 121 linezolid-treated and 60 comparator-treated patients who had a Gram-positive pathogen isolated from the site of infection or from blood, who had less evidence of underlying osteomyelitis than the overall study population, and who did not receive prohibited antimicrobials. Based upon that analysis, the cure rates were 71% (86/121) in the linezolid-treated patients and 63% (38/60) in the comparator-treated patients. None of the above analyses were adjusted for the use of adjunctive therapies. The cure rates by pathogen for microbiologically evaluable patients are presented in Table 19.

Table 19. Cure Rates at the Test-of-Cure Visit for Microbiologically Evaluable Adult Patients with Diabetic Foot Infections

Pathogen	Cured	
	ZYVOX n/N (%)	Comparator n/N (%)
Staphylococcus aureus	49/63 (78)	20/29 (69)
Methicillin-resistant *S. aureus*	12/17 (71)	2/3 (67)
Streptococcus agalactiae	25/29 (86)	9/16 (56)

Pediatric Patients
Infections Due to Gram-positive Organisms
A safety and efficacy study provided experience on the use of ZYVOX in pediatric patients for the treatment of nosocomial pneumonia, complicated skin and skin structure infections, catheter-related bacteremia, bacteremia of unidentified source, and other infections due to Gram-positive

Table 14. Dosage Guidelines for ZYVOX

Infection*	Dosage and Route of Administration		Recommended Duration of Treatment (consecutive days)
	Pediatric Patients[†] (Birth through 11 Years of Age)	Adults and Adolescents (12 Years and Older)	
Complicated skin and skin structure infections	10 mg/kg IV or oral[‡] q8h	600 mg IV or oral[‡] q12h	10 to 14
Community-acquired pneumonia, including concurrent bacteremia			
Nosocomial pneumonia			
Vancomycin-resistant *Enterococcus faecium* infections, including concurrent bacteremia	10 mg/kg IV or oral[‡] q8h	600 mg IV or oral[‡] q12h	14 to 28
Uncomplicated skin and skin structure infections	<5 yrs: 10 mg/kg oral[‡] q8h 5-11 yrs: 10 mg/kg oral[‡] q12h	Adults: 400 mg oral[‡] q12h Adolescents: 600 mg oral[‡] q12h	10 to 14

* Due to the designated pathogens (see **INDICATIONS AND USAGE**)
† **Neonates <7 days:** Most pre-term neonates < 7 days of age (gestational age < 34 weeks) have lower systemic linezolid clearance values and larger AUC values than many full-term neonates and older infants. These neonates should be initiated with a dosing regimen of 10 mg/kg q12h. Consideration may be given to the use of 10 mg/kg q8h regimen in neonates with a sub-optimal clinical response. All neonatal patients should receive 10 mg/kg q8h by 7 days of life (see **CLINICAL PHARMACOLOGY, Special Populations, Pediatric**).
‡ Oral dosing using either ZYVOX Tablets or ZYVOX for Oral Suspension

Table 20. Cure Rates at the Test-of-Cure Visit for Intent to Treat, Modified Intent to Treat, and Clinically Evaluable Pediatric Patients by Baseline Diagnosis

Population	ITT		MITT*		Clinically Evaluable	
	ZYVOX n/N (%)	Vancomycin n/N (%)	ZYVOX n/N (%)	Vancomycin n/N (%)	ZYVOX n/N (%)	Vancomycin n/N (%)
Any diagnosis	150/186 (81)	69/83 (83)	86/108 (80)	44/49 (90)	106/117 (91)	49/54 (91)
Bacteremia of unidentified source	22/29 (76)	11/16 (69)	8/12 (67)	7/8 (88)	14/17 (82)	7/9 (78)
Catheter-related bacteremia	30/41 (73)	8/12 (67)	25/35 (71)	7/10 (70)	21/25 (84)	7/9 (78)
Complicated skin and skin structure infections	61/72 (85)	31/34 (91)	37/43 (86)	22/23 (96)	46/49 (94)	26/27 (96)
Nosocomial pneumonia	13/18 (72)	11/12 (92)	5/6 (83)	4/4 (100)	7/7 (100)	5/5 (100)
Other infections	24/26 (92)	8/9 (89)	11/12 (92)	4/4 (100)	18/19 (95)	4/4 (100)

* MITT = ITT patients with an isolated Gram-positive pathogen at baseline

bacterial pathogens, including methicillin-resistant -susceptible *Staphylococcus aureus* and vancomycin-resistant *Enterococcus faecium*. Pediatric patients ranging in age from birth through 11 years with infections caused by the documented or suspected Gram-positive organisms were enrolled in a randomized, open-label, comparator-controlled trial. One group of patients received ZYVOX I.V. Injection 10 mg/kg every 8 hours (q8h) followed by ZYVOX for Oral Suspension 10 mg/kg q8h. A second group received vancomycin 10 to 15 mg/kg IV every 6 to 24 hours, depending on age and renal clearance. Patients who had confirmed VRE infections were placed in a third arm of the study and received ZYVOX 10 mg/kg q8h IV and/or orally. All patients were treated for a total of 10 to 28 days and could receive concomitant Gram-negative antibiotics if clinically indicated. In the intent-to-treat (ITT) population, there were 206 patients randomized to linezolid and 102 patients randomized to vancomycin. One hundred seventeen (57 %) linezolid-treated patients and 55 (54%) vancomycin-treated patients were clinically evaluable. The cure rates in ITT patients were 81% in patients randomized to linezolid and 83% in patients randomized to vancomycin (95% Confidence Interval of the treatment difference; -13%, 8%). The cure rates in clinically evaluable patients were 91% in linezolid-treated patients and 91% in vancomycin-treated patients (95% CI; -11%, 11%). Modified intent-to-treat (MITT) patients included ITT patients who, at baseline, had a Gram-positive pathogen isolated from the site of infection or from blood. The cure rates in MITT patients were 80% in patients randomized to linezolid and 90% in patients randomized to vancomycin (95% CI; -23%, 3%). The cure rates for ITT, MITT, and clinically evaluable patients are presented in Table 20. After the study was completed, 13 additional patients ranging from 4 days through 16 years of age were enrolled in an open-label extension of the VRE arm of the study. Table 21 provides clinical cure rates by pathogen for microbiologically evaluable patients including microbiologically evaluable patients with vancomycin-resistant *Enterococcus faecium* from the extension of this study. [See table 20 on previous page]

Table 21. Cure Rates at the Test-of-Cure Visit for Microbiologically Evaluable Pediatric Patients with Infections due to Gram-positive Pathogens

	Microbiologically Evaluable	
Pathogen	**ZYVOX** n/N (%)	**Vancomycin** n/N (%)
Vancomycin-resistant *Enterococcus faecium*	6/8 (75)*	0/0 (-)
Staphylococcus aureus	36/38 (95)	23/24 (96)
Methicillin-resistant *S. aureus*	16/17 (94)	9/9 (100)
Streptococcus pyogenes	2/2 (100)	1/2 (50)

* Includes data from 7 patients enrolled in the open-label extension of this study.

REFERENCES
1. Gonzales RD, PC Schreckenberger, MB Graham, et al. Infections due to vancomycin-resistant *Enterococcus faecium* resistant to linezolid. The Lancet 2001;357: 1179.
2. Herrero IA, NC Issa, R Patel. Nosocomial spread of linezolid-resistant, vancomycin-resistant *Enterococcus faecium*. The New England Journal of Medicine 2002; 346:867-869.
3. Tsiodras S, HS Gold, G Sakoulas, et al. Linezolid resistance in a clinical isolate of *Staphylococcus aureus*. The Lancet 2001;358:207-208.
4. Goldman DA, RA Weinstein, RP Wenzel, et al. Strategies to prevent and control the emergence and spread of antimicrobial-resistant microorganisms in hospitals. A challenge to hospital leadership. The Journal of the American Medical Association 1996;275:234-240.
5. Centers for Disease Control and Prevention. Guideline for hand hygiene in health-care settings: Recommendations of the Healthcare Infection Control Practices Advisory Committee and the HIPAC/SHEA/APIC/IDSA Hand Hygiene Task Force. Morbidity and Mortality Weekly Report 2002;51 (RR-16).
6. National Committee for Clinical Laboratory Standards. Methods for Dilution Antimicrobial Susceptibility Tests for Bacteria that Grow Aerobically. Fifth Edition. Approved Standard NCCLS Document M7-A5, Vol. 20, No. 2, NCCLS, Wayne, PA, January 2000.
7. National Committee for Clinical Laboratory Standards. Twelfth Informational Supplement. Approved NCCLS Document M100-S12, Vol. 21, No. 1, NCCLS, Wayne, PA, January 2002.
8. National Committee for Clinical Laboratory Standards. Performance Standards for Antimicrobial Disk Susceptibility Tests. Seventh Edition. Approved Standard NCCLS Document M2-A7, Vol. 20, No. 1, NCCLS, Wayne, PA, January 2000.
9. Walker SE et al. Tyramine content of previously restricted foods in monoamine oxidase inhibitor diets. Journal of Clinical Psychopharmacology 1996;16(5): 383-388.
10. DaPrada M et al. On tyramine, food, beverages and the reversible MAO inhibitor moclobemide. Journal of Neural Transmission 1988; [Supplement] 26:31-56.
11. Fine MJ, Auble TE, Yealy DM, et al. A Prediction Rule to Identify Low-Risk Patients with Community-Acquired Pneumonia. The New England Journal of Medicine. 1997;336 (4):243-250.

Rx only
Distributed by
Pharmacia & Upjohn Company
Division of Pfizer Inc, NY, NY 10017
LAB-0139-20.0
Revised June 2010

Progenics Pharmaceuticals, Inc.
777 OLD SAW MILL RIVER ROAD
TARRYTOWN, NY 10591

For Product Information Contact:
800-934-5556
For All Other Inquiries:
Tel: 914-789-2800
Fax: 914-789-2817
Email: info@progenics.com

RELISTOR® ℞
[rel'-i-store]
(methylnaltrexone bromide)
Subcutaneous Injection

HIGHLIGHTS OF PRESCRIBING INFORMATION
These highlights do not include all the information needed to use RELISTOR safely and effectively. See full prescribing information for RELISTOR.
RELISTOR (methylnaltrexone bromide) Subcutaneous Injection
Initial U.S. Approval: 2008

——————**RECENT MAJOR CHANGES**——————
Warnings and Precautions, Intestinal
Perforation (5.2)   [05/2010]
Dosage & Administration, Dosing (2.2)   [07/2010]

——————**INDICATIONS AND USAGE**——————
RELISTOR is indicated for the treatment of opioid-induced constipation in patients with advanced illness who are receiving palliative care, when response to laxative therapy has not been sufficient. Use of RELISTOR beyond four months has not been studied. (1)

——————**DOSAGE AND ADMINISTRATION**——————
RELISTOR is administered as a subcutaneous injection. The usual schedule is one dose every other day, as needed, but no more frequently than one dose in a 24-hour period. (2.2)
The recommended dose of RELISTOR is 8 mg for patients weighing 38 to less than 62 kg (84 to less than 136 lb) or 12 mg for patients weighing 62 to 114 kg (136 to 251 lb). Patients whose weights fall outside of these ranges should be dosed at 0.15 mg/kg. See the table below to determine the correct injection volume. (2.2)

Patient Weight		Injection Volume	Dose
Pounds	**Kilograms**		
Less than 84	Less than 38	**See below***	0.15 mg/kg
84 to less than 136	38 to less than 62	**0.4 mL**	8 mg
136 to 251	62 to 114	**0.6 mL**	12 mg
More than 251	More than 114	**See below***	0.15 mg/kg

* The injection volume for these patients should be calculated using one of the following (2.2):
• Multiply the patient weight in pounds by 0.0034 and round up the volume to the nearest 0.1 mL.
• Multiply the patient weight in kilograms by 0.0075 and round up the volume to the nearest 0.1 mL.

Only patients requiring an 8 mg or 12 mg dose shoul prescribed pre-filled syringes (2.2, 3).
In patients with severe renal impairment (creatinine cle ance less than 30 mL/min), dose reductions of RELISTOR by one half is recommended. (8.6)

——————**DOSAGE FORMS AND STRENGTHS**——————
RELISTOR is available in the following dosage forms:
• Single-use vial containing 12 mg/0.6 mL solution for subcutaneous injection.
• Single-use pre-filled syringe containing 8 mg/0.4 mL solution for subcutaneous injection.
• Single-use pre-filled syringe containing 12 mg/0.6 mL solution for subcutaneous injection.

——————**CONTRAINDICATIONS**——————
• RELISTOR is contraindicated in patients with known or suspected mechanical gastrointestinal obstruction. (4)

——————**WARNINGS AND PRECAUTIONS**——————
If severe or persistent diarrhea occurs during treatment, advise patients to discontinue therapy with RELISTOR and consult their physician. (5.1)
Rare cases of gastrointestinal (GI) perforation have been reported in advanced illness patients. Use RELISTOR with caution in patients with known or suspected lesions of the GI tract. (5.2)

——————**ADVERSE REACTIONS**——————
The most common (> 5%) adverse reactions reported with RELISTOR are abdominal pain, flatulence, nausea, dizziness, diarrhea and hyperhidrosis. (6.1)
To report SUSPECTED ADVERSE REACTIONS, contact Wyeth Pharmaceuticals Inc. at 1-800-934-5556 or FDA at 1-800-FDA-1088 or www.fda.gov/medwatch

——————**DRUG INTERACTIONS**——————
In an *in vitro* study, methylnaltrexone bromide was a weak inhibitor of cytochrome P450 (CYP) isozyme CYP2D6 activity, but in an *in vivo* study it did not significantly affect the metabolism of the CYP2D6 substrate, dextromethorphan (7.1)

——————**USE IN SPECIFIC POPULATIONS**——————
Pediatric Use: Safety and efficacy of RELISTOR have not been established in pediatric patients. (8.4)
See 17 for PATIENT COUNSELING INFORMATION and FDA-approved patient labeling

Revised: 09/2010

FULL PRESCRIBING INFORMATION: CONTENTS*
1 **INDICATIONS AND USAGE**
2 **DOSAGE AND ADMINISTRATION**
  2.1 General Dosing Information
  2.2 Dosing
  2.3 Preparation for Injection
3 **DOSAGE FORMS AND STRENGTHS**
4 **CONTRAINDICATIONS**
5 **WARNINGS AND PRECAUTIONS**
  5.1 Severe or Persistent Diarrhea
  5.2 Intestinal Perforation
  5.3 Peritoneal Catheters
6 **ADVERSE REACTIONS**
  6.1 Clinical Trial Experience
  6.2 Postmarketing Experience
7 **DRUG INTERACTIONS**
  7.1 Drugs Metabolized by Cytochrome P450 Isozymes
  7.2 Drugs Renally Excreted
8 **USE IN SPECIFIC POPULATIONS**
  8.1 Pregnancy
  8.2 Labor and Delivery
  8.3 Nursing Mothers
  8.4 Pediatric Use
  8.5 Geriatric Use
  8.6 Renal Impairment
  8.7 Hepatic Impairment
9 **DRUG ABUSE AND DEPENDENCE**
  9.1 Controlled Substance
  9.2 Abuse
  9.3 Dependence
10 **OVERDOSAGE**
  10.1 Human Experience
  10.2 Management of Overdosage
11 **DESCRIPTION**
12 **CLINICAL PHARMACOLOGY**
  12.1 Mechanism of Action
  12.2 Pharmacodynamics
  12.3 Pharmacokinetics
  12.4 Effect on Cardiac Repolarization
13 **NONCLINICAL TOXICOLOGY**
  13.1 Carcinogenesis, Mutagenesis, Impairment of Fertility
  13.2 Animal Toxicology and/or Pharmacology
14 **CLINICAL STUDIES**
16 **HOW SUPPLIED/STORAGE AND HANDLING**
  16.1 Storage
17 **PATIENT COUNSELING INFORMATION**
* Sections or subsections omitted from the full prescribing information are not listed

ON

D USAGE

...ted for the treatment of opioid-induced ...patients with advanced illness who are re- ...ative care, when response to laxative therapy ...been sufficient. Use of RELISTOR beyond four ...ths has not been studied.

2 DOSAGE AND ADMINISTRATION

2.1 General Dosing Information

FOR SUBCUTANEOUS INJECTION ONLY

RELISTOR should be injected in the upper arm, abdomen or thigh.

2.2 Dosing

RELISTOR is administered as a subcutaneous injection. The usual schedule is one dose every other day, as needed, but no more frequently than one dose in a 24-hour period [*see Clinical Studies (14)*].

The recommended dose of RELISTOR is 8 mg for patients weighing 38 to less than 62 kg (84 to less than 136 lb) or 12 mg for patients weighing 62 to 114 kg (136 to 251 lb). Patients whose weight falls outside of these ranges should be dosed at 0.15 mg/kg. See the table below to determine the correct injection volume. The pre-filled syringe is designed to deliver a fixed dose; therefore, patients requiring dosing calculated on a mg/kg basis should not be prescribed pre-filled syringes.

Patient Weight		Injection Volume	Dose
Pounds	Kilograms		
Less than 84	Less than 38	**See below***	0.15 mg/kg
84 to less than 136	38 to less than 62	**0.4 mL**	8 mg
136 to 251	62 to 114	**0.6 mL**	12 mg
More than 251	More than 114	**See below***	0.15 mg/kg

* The injection volume for these patients should be calculated using one of the following:

- Multiply the patient weight in pounds by 0.0034 and round up the volume to the nearest 0.1 mL.
- Multiply the patient weight in kilograms by 0.0075 and round up the volume to the nearest 0.1 mL.

Use in Patients with Severe Renal Impairment

In patients with severe renal impairment (creatinine clearance less than 30 mL/min), dose reduction of RELISTOR by one-half is recommended [*see Use in Specific Populations (8.6)*].

The pre-filled syringe is designed to deliver a fixed dose; therefore, patients with severe renal impairment should not be prescribed pre-filled syringes unless their body weight calculated dose is 8 mg or 12 mg.

2.3 Preparation for Injection

RELISTOR is a sterile, clear, and colorless to pale yellow aqueous solution. Parenteral drug products should be inspected visually for particulate matter and discoloration prior to administration, whenever solution and container permit. If any of these are present, the vial should not be used.

Preparation of RELISTOR Using the Single-use Vial

Once drawn into the syringe, if immediate administration is not possible, store at ambient room temperature and administer within 24 hours [*see Patient Counseling Information (17)*].

Preparation of RELISTOR Using the Single-use Pre-filled Syringe

Do not remove the pre-filled syringe from the tray until ready to administer.

3 DOSAGE FORMS AND STRENGTHS

RELISTOR is available in the following dosage forms and strengths. Only patients requiring an 8 mg or 12 mg dose should be prescribed pre-filled syringes.

- Single-use vial containing 12 mg/0.6 mL solution for subcutaneous injection [*see Dosage and Administration (2.2)*].
- Single-use pre-filled syringe containing 8 mg/0.4 mL solution for subcutaneous injection, with a 29-gauge × ½-inch fixed needle and a needle guard [*see Dosage and Administration (2.2)*].
- Single-use pre-filled syringe containing 12 mg/0.6 mL solution for subcutaneous injection, with a 29-gauge × ½-inch fixed needle and a needle guard [*see Dosage and Administration (2.2)*].

4 CONTRAINDICATIONS

RELISTOR is contraindicated in patients with known or suspected mechanical gastrointestinal obstruction.

5 WARNINGS AND PRECAUTIONS

5.1 Severe or Persistent Diarrhea

If severe or persistent diarrhea occurs during treatment, advise patients to discontinue therapy with RELISTOR and consult their physician.

5.2 Intestinal Perforation

Rare cases of gastrointestinal (GI) perforation have been reported in advanced illness patients with conditions that may be associated with localized or diffuse reduction of structural integrity in the wall of the GI tract (i.e., cancer, peptic ulcer, Ogilvie's syndrome). Perforations have involved varying regions of the GI tract: (e.g., stomach, duodenum, colon).

Use RELISTOR with caution in patients with known or suspected lesions of the GI tract. Advise patients to discontinue therapy with RELISTOR and promptly notify their physician if they develop severe, persistent, and/or worsening abdominal symptoms.

5.3 Peritoneal Catheters

Use of RELISTOR has not been studied in patients with peritoneal catheters.

6 ADVERSE REACTIONS

6.1 Clinical Trial Experience

Because clinical trials are conducted under varying conditions, adverse reaction rates observed in the clinical trials of a drug may not reflect the rates observed in practice.

The safety of RELISTOR was evaluated in two, double-blind, placebo-controlled trials in patients with advanced illness receiving palliative care: Study 1 included a single-dose, double-blind, placebo-controlled period, whereas Study 2 included a 14-day multiple dose, double-blind, placebo-controlled period [see *Clinical Studies (14)*]. In both studies, patients had advanced illness with a life expectancy of less than 6 months and received care to control their symptoms. The majority of patients had a primary diagnosis of incurable cancer; other primary diagnoses included end-stage COPD/emphysema, cardiovascular disease/heart failure, Alzheimer's disease/dementia, HIV/AIDS, or other advanced illnesses. Patients were receiving opioid therapy (median daily baseline oral morphine equivalent dose = 172 mg), and had opioid-induced constipation (either <3 bowel movements in the preceding week or no bowel movement for 2 days). Both the methylnaltrexone bromide and placebo patients were on a stable laxative regimen for at least 3 days prior to study entry and continued on their regimen throughout the study.

The adverse reactions in patients receiving RELISTOR are shown in table below.

Adverse Reactions from all Doses in Double-Blind, Placebo-Controlled Clinical Studies of RELISTOR*

Adverse Reaction	RELISTOR N = 165	Placebo N = 123
Abdominal Pain	47 (28.5%)	12 (9.8%)
Flatulence	22 (13.3%)	7 (5.7%)
Nausea	19 (11.5%)	6 (4.9%)
Dizziness	12 (7.3%)	3 (2.4%)
Diarrhea	9 (5.5%)	3 (2.4%)
Hyperhidrosis	11 (6.7%)	8 (6.5%)

*Doses: 0.075, 0.15, and 0.30 mg/kg/dose

6.2 Postmarketing Experience

Rare cases of gastrointestinal (GI) perforation have been reported in advanced illness patients with conditions that may be associated with localized or diffuse reduction of structural integrity in the wall of the GI tract (i.e., cancer, peptic ulcer, Ogilvie's syndrome). Perforations have involved varying regions of the GI tract: (e.g., stomach, duodenum, colon). Because these reactions are reported voluntarily from a population of uncertain size, it is not always possible to reliably estimate their frequency or establish a causal relationship to drug exposure.

7 DRUG INTERACTIONS

7.1 Drugs Metabolized by Cytochrome P450 Isozymes

In *in vitro* drug metabolism studies methylnaltrexone bromide did not significantly inhibit the activity of cytochrome P450 (CYP) isozymes CYP1A2, CYP2A6, CYP2C9, CYP2C19 or CYP3A4, while it is a weak inhibitor of CYP2D6. In a clinical drug interaction study in healthy adult male subjects, a subcutaneous dose of 0.30 mg/kg of methylnaltrexone bromide did not significantly affect the metabolism of dextromethorphan, a CYP2D6 substrate.

7.2 Drugs Renally Excreted

The potential for drug interactions between methylnaltrexone bromide and drugs that are actively secreted by the kidney has not been investigated in humans.

8 USE IN SPECIFIC POPULATIONS

8.1 Pregnancy

Pregnancy Category B

Reproduction studies have been performed in pregnant rats at intravenous doses up to about 14 times the recommended maximum human subcutaneous dose of 0.3 mg/kg based on the body surface area and in pregnant rabbits at intravenous doses up to about 17 times the recommended maximum human subcutaneous dose based on the body surface area and have revealed no evidence of impaired fertility or harm to the fetus due to methylnaltrexone bromide. There are no adequate and well-controlled studies in pregnant women. Because animal reproduction studies are not always predictive of human response, methylnaltrexone bromide should be used during pregnancy only if clearly needed.

8.2 Labor and Delivery

Effects of RELISTOR on mother, fetus, duration of labor, and delivery are unknown. There were no effects on the mother, labor, delivery, or on offspring survival and growth in rats following subcutaneous injection of methylnaltrexone bromide at dosages up to 25 mg/kg/day.

8.3 Nursing Mothers

Results from an animal study using [^{3}H]-labeled methylnaltrexone bromide indicate that methylnaltrexone bromide is excreted via the milk of lactating rats. It is not known whether this drug is excreted in human milk. Because many drugs are excreted in human milk, caution should be exercised when RELISTOR is administered to a nursing woman.

8.4 Pediatric Use

Safety and efficacy of RELISTOR have not been established in pediatric patients.

8.5 Geriatric Use

In the phase 2 and 3 double-blind studies, a total of 77 (24%) patients aged 65-74 years (54 methylnaltrexone bromide, 23 placebo) and a total of 100 (31.2%) patients aged 75 years or older (61 methylnaltrexone bromide, 39 placebo) were enrolled. There was no difference in the efficacy or safety profile of these elderly patients when compared to younger patients. Therefore, no dose adjustment is recommended based on age.

8.6 Renal Impairment

No dose adjustment is required in patients with mild or moderate renal impairment. Dose-reduction by one half is recommended in patients with severe renal impairment (creatinine clearance less than 30 mL/min).

In a study of volunteers with varying degrees of renal impairment receiving a single dose of 0.30 mg/kg methylnaltrexone bromide, renal impairment had a marked effect on the renal excretion of methylnaltrexone bromide. Severe renal impairment decreased the renal clearance of methylnaltrexone bromide by 8- to 9-fold and resulted in a 2-fold increase in total methylnaltrexone bromide exposure (AUC). C_{max} was not significantly changed. No studies were performed in patients with end-stage renal impairment requiring dialysis.

8.7 Hepatic Impairment

No dose adjustment is required for patients with mild or moderate hepatic impairment. The effect of mild and moderate hepatic impairment on the systemic exposure to methylnaltrexone bromide has been studied in 8 subjects each, with Child-Pugh Class A and B, compared to healthy subjects. Results showed no meaningful effect of hepatic impairment on the AUC or C_{max} of methylnaltrexone bromide. The effect of severe hepatic impairment on the pharmacokinetics of methylnaltrexone bromide has not been studied.

9 DRUG ABUSE AND DEPENDENCE

9.1 Controlled Substance

Methylnaltrexone bromide is not a controlled substance.

9.2 Abuse

RELISTOR is a peripherally-acting mu-opioid receptor antagonist with no known risk of abuse.

9.3 Dependence

RELISTOR is a peripherally-acting mu-opioid receptor antagonist with no known risk of dependency.

10 OVERDOSAGE

10.1 Human Experience

During clinical trials of RELISTOR administered subcutaneously, no cases of methylnaltrexone bromide overdose were reported. In a study of healthy volunteers (n = 41), a single dose of 0.50 mg/kg administered as a subcutaneous injection was well-tolerated. A study of healthy volunteers noted orthostatic hypotension associated with a dose of 0.64 mg/kg administered as an IV bolus.

10.2 Management of Overdosage

No specific information is available on the treatment of overdose with RELISTOR. In the event of overdose, employ the usual supportive measures, e.g., clinical monitoring and supportive therapy as dictated by the patient's clinical status. Signs or symptoms of orthostatic hypotension should be monitored, and treatment should be initiated, as appropriate.

11 DESCRIPTION

RELISTOR (methylnaltrexone bromide) Subcutaneous Injection, a peripherally-acting mu-opioid receptor antagonist, is a sterile, clear and colorless to pale yellow aqueous solution. The chemical name for methylnaltrexone bromide is (*R*)-*N*-(cyclopropylmethyl) noroxymorphone methobromide. The molecular formula is $C_{21}H_{26}NO_4Br$, and the molecular weight is 436.36.

Each 3 mL vial contains 12 mg of methylnaltrexone bromide in 0.6 mL of water. The excipients are 3.9 mg sodium chloride USP, 0.24 mg edetate calcium disodium USP, and 0.18 mg glycine hydrochloride. During manufacture, the pH may have been adjusted with hydrochloric acid and/or sodium hydroxide.

Each 8 mg/0.4 mL pre-filled syringe (1 mL syringe) contains 8 mg of methylnaltrexone bromide in 0.4 mL of water. The excipients are 2.6 mg sodium chloride USP, 0.16 mg edetate calcium disodium USP, and 0.12 mg glycine hydrochloride.

Each 12 mg/0.6 mL pre-filled syringe (1 mL syringe) contains 12 mg of methylnaltrexone bromide in 0.6 mL of water. The excipients are 3.9 mg sodium chloride USP, 0.24 mg edetate calcium disodium USP, and 0.18 mg glycine hydrochloride.

The structural formula is:

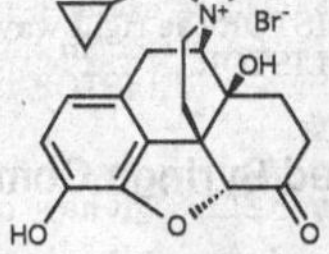

12 CLINICAL PHARMACOLOGY

12.1 Mechanism of Action

Methylnaltrexone bromide is a selective antagonist of opioid binding at the mu-opioid receptor. As a quaternary amine, the ability of methylnaltrexone bromide to cross the blood-brain barrier is restricted. This allows methylnaltrexone bromide to function as a peripherally-acting mu-opioid receptor antagonist in tissues such as the gastrointestinal tract, thereby decreasing the constipating effects of opioids without impacting opioid-mediated analgesic effects on the central nervous system.

12.2 Pharmacodynamics

Use of opioids induces slowing of gastrointestinal motility and transit. Antagonism of gastrointestinal mu-opioid receptors by methylnaltrexone bromide inhibits opioid-induced delay of gastrointestinal transit time in a dose-dependent manner in rats. The effects of methylnaltrexone bromide on central mu-opioid receptors were evaluated in a pharmacodynamic study in which subjects received a dose of remifentanil, sufficient to produce pupiliary constriction, followed by placebo, naloxone, or methylnaltrexone. Following remifentanil administration, the methylnaltrexone and placebo groups showed no change in pupiliary constriction while the naloxone group showed a marked change over the time interval tested.

12.3 Pharmacokinetics

Absorption

Following subcutaneous administration, methylnaltrexone bromide is absorbed rapidly, with peak concentrations (C_{max}) achieved at approximately 0.5 hours. Across the range of doses evaluated peak plasma concentration and area under the plasma concentration-time curve (AUC) increase in a dose-proportional manner, as shown in the table below.

PHARMACOKINETIC PARAMETERS OF METHYLNALTREXONE BROMIDE FOLLOWING SINGLE SUBCUTANEOUS DOSES

Parameter	0.15 mg/kg	0.30 mg/kg	0.50 mg/kg
C_{max} (ng/mL)[a]	117 (32.7)	239 (62.2)	392 (147.9)
t_{max} (hr)[b]	0.5 (0.25-0.75)	0.5 (0.25-0.75)	0.5 (0.25-0.75)
AUC_{24} (ng•hr/mL)[a]	175 (36.6)	362 (63.8)	582 (111.2)

[a] Expressed as mean (SD).
[b] Expressed as median (range).

Distribution

Methylnaltrexone bromide undergoes moderate tissue distribution. The steady-state volume of distribution (Vss) is approximately 1.1 L/kg. The fraction of methylnaltrexone bromide bound to human plasma proteins is 11.0% to 15.3%, as determined by equilibrium dialysis.

Metabolism

In a mass balance study, approximately 60% of the administered radioactivity recovered with 5 distinct metabolites and none of the detected metabolites was in amounts over 6% of administered radioactivity. Conversion to methyl-6-naltrexol isomers (5% of total) and methylnaltrexone sulfate (1.3% of total) appear to be the primary pathways of metabolism. N-demethylation of methylnaltrexone to produce naltrexone is not significant.

Excretion

Methylnaltrexone bromide is eliminated primarily as the unchanged drug (85% of administered radioactivity). Approximately half of the dose is excreted in the urine and somewhat less in feces. The terminal half-life ($t_{1/2}$) is approximately 8 hours.

12.4 Effect on Cardiac Repolarization

In a randomized, double blind placebo- and (open-label) moxifloxacin-controlled 4-period crossover study, 56 healthy subjects were administered methylnaltrexone bromide 0.3 mg/kg and methylnaltrexone bromide 0.64 mg/kg by IV infusion over 20 minutes, placebo, and a single oral dose of moxifloxacin. At both the 0.3 mg/kg and 0.64 mg/kg methylnaltrexone bromide doses, no significant effect on the QTc interval was detected.

13 NONCLINICAL TOXICOLOGY

13.1 Carcinogenesis, Mutagenesis, Impairment of Fertility

Carcinogenesis, Mutagenesis, Impairment of Fertility

Carcinogenesis

Long-term studies in animals have not been performed to evaluate the carcinogenic potential of methylnaltrexone bromide.

Mutagenesis

Methylnaltrexone bromide was negative in the Ames test, chromosome aberration tests in Chinese hamster ovary cells and human lymphocytes, in the mouse lymphoma cell forward mutation tests and in the *in vivo* mouse micronucleus test.

Impairment of Fertility

Methylnaltrexone bromide at subcutaneous doses up to 150 mg/kg/day (about 81 times the recommended maximum human subcutaneous dose based on the body surface area) was found to have no adverse effect on fertility and reproductive performance of male and female rats.

13.2 Animal Toxicology and/or Pharmacology

A single subcutaneous dose of 500 mg/kg of methylnaltrexone bromide was not lethal to rats.

Reproduction studies have been performed in pregnant rats at intravenous doses up to 25 mg/kg/day (about 14 times the recommended maximum human subcutaneous dose of 0.3 mg/kg based on the body surface area) and in pregnant rabbits at intravenous doses up to 16 mg/kg/day (about 17 times the recommended maximum human subcutaneous dose based on the body surface area) and have revealed no evidence of impaired fertility or harm to the fetus due to methylnaltrexone bromide.

In an *in vitro* human cardiac potassium ion channel (hERG) assay, methylnaltrexone bromide caused concentration-dependent inhibition of hERG current (1%, 12%, 13% and 40% inhibition at 30, 100, 300 and 1000 µM concentrations, respectively). Methylnaltrexone bromide had a hERG IC_{50} of > 1000 µM. In isolated dog Purkinje fibers, methylnaltrexone bromide caused prolongations in action potential duration (APD). The highest tested concentration (10 µM) in the dog Purkinje fiber study was about 18 and 37 times the C_{max} at human subcutaneous (SC) doses of 0.3 and 0.15 mg/kg, respectively. In isolated rabbit Purkinje fibers, methylnaltrexone bromide (up to 100 µM) did not have an effect on APD, compared to vehicle control. The highest methylnaltrexone bromide concentration (100 µM) tested was about 186 and 373 times the human C_{max} at SC doses of 0.3 and 0.15 mg/kg, respectively. In anesthetized dogs, methylnaltrexone bromide caused decreases in blood pressure, heart rate, cardiac output, left ventricular pressure, left ventricular end diastolic pressure, and +dP/dt at ≥ 1 mg/kg. In conscious dogs, methylnaltrexone bromide caused a dose-related increase in QTc interval. After a single IV dosage of 20 mg/kg to beagle dogs, predicted C_{max} and AUC values were approximately 482 and 144 times, respectively, the exposure at human SC dose of 0.15 mg/kg and 241 times and 66 times, respectively, the exposure at a human SC dose of 0.3 mg/kg. In conscious guinea pigs, methylnaltrexone caused mild prolongation of QTc (4% over baseline) at 20 mg/kg, IV. A thorough QTc assessment was conducted in humans [*see Pharmacokinetics (12.4)*].

In juvenile rats administered intravenous methylnaltrexone bromide for 13 weeks, adverse clinical signs such as convulsions, tremors and labored breathing occurred at dosages of 3 and 10 mg/kg/day (about 3.2 and 11 times, respectively, the recommended human dose of 0.15 mg/kg based on the body surface area). Similar a clinical signs were seen in adult rats at 20 mg/kg/day (22 times the recommended human dose of 0.15 mg/kg b on the body surface area). Juvenile rats were found to more sensitive to the toxicity of RELISTOR when compare to adults. The no observed adverse effect levels (NOAELs) in juvenile and adult rats were 1 and 5 mg/kg/day, respectively (about 1.1 and 5.4 times respectively, the recommended human dose of 0.15 mg/kg based on the body surface area).

In juvenile dogs administered intravenous methylnaltrexone bromide for 13 weeks, juvenile dogs had a toxicity profile similar to adult dogs. Following IV administration of methylnaltrexone bromide for 13 weeks, decreased heart rate (13.2 % reduction compared to pre-dose) in juvenile dogs and prolonged QTc interval in juvenile (9.6% compared to control) and adult (up to 15% compared to control) dogs occurred at 20 mg/kg/day (about 72 times the recommended human subcutaneous doses of 0.15 mg/kg based on the body surface area). Clinical signs consistent with effects on the CNS (including tremors and decreased activity) occurred in both juvenile and adult dogs. The NOAELs in juvenile and adult dogs were 5 mg/kg/day (about 18 times the recommended human subcutaneous doses of 0.15 mg/kg based on the body surface area).

14 CLINICAL STUDIES

The efficacy and safety of RELISTOR in the treatment of opioid-induced constipation in advanced illness patients receiving palliative care was demonstrated in two randomized, double-blind, placebo-controlled studies. In these studies, the median age was 68 years (range 21-100); 51% were females. In both studies, patients had advanced illness with a life expectancy of less than 6 months and received care to control their symptoms. The majority of patients had a primary diagnosis of incurable cancer; other primary diagnoses included end-stage COPD/emphysema, cardiovascular disease/heart failure, Alzheimer's disease/dementia, HIV/AIDS, or other advanced illnesses. Prior to screening, patients had been receiving palliative opioid therapy (median daily baseline oral morphine equivalent dose = 172 mg), and had opioid-induced constipation (either <3 bowel movements in the preceding week or no bowel movement for >2 days). Patients were on a stable opioid regimen ≥ 3 days prior to randomization (not including PRN or rescue pain medication) and received their opioid medication during the study as clinically needed. Patients maintained their regular laxative regimen for at least 3 days prior to study entry, and throughout the study. Rescue laxatives were prohibited from 4 hours before to 4 hours after taking an injection of study medication.

Study 1 compared a single, double-blind, subcutaneous dose of RELISTOR 0.15 mg/kg, or RELISTOR 0.3 mg/kg versus placebo. The double-blind dose was followed by an open-label 4-week dosing period, where RELISTOR could be used as needed, no more frequently than 1 dose in a 24 hour period. Throughout both study periods, patients maintained their regular laxative regimen. A total of 154 patients (47 RELISTOR 0.15 mg/kg, 55 RELISTOR 0.3 mg/kg, 52 placebo) were enrolled and treated in the double-blind period. The primary endpoint was the proportion of patients with a rescue-free laxation within 4 hours of the double-blind dose of study medication. RELISTOR-treated patients had a significantly higher rate of laxation within 4 hours of the double-blind dose (62% for 0.15 mg/kg and 58% for 0.3 mg/kg) than did placebo-treated patients (14%); $p < 0.0001$ for each dose versus placebo (Figure 1).

Study 2 compared double-blind, subcutaneous doses of RELISTOR given every other day for 2 weeks versus placebo. Patients received opioid medication ≥ 2 weeks prior to receiving study medication. During the first week (days 1, 3, 5, 7) patients received either 0.15 mg/kg RELISTOR or placebo. In the second week the patient's assigned dose could be increased to 0.30 mg/kg if the patient had 2 or fewer rescue-free laxations up to day 8. At any time, the patient's assigned dose could be reduced based on tolerability. Data from 133 (62 RELISTOR, 71 placebo) patients were analyzed. There were 2 primary endpoints: proportion of patients with a rescue-free laxation within 4 hours of the first dose of study medication and proportion of patients with a rescue-free laxation within 4 hours after at least 2 of the first 4 doses of study medication. RELISTOR-treated patients had a higher rate of laxation within 4 hours of the first dose (48%) than placebo-treated patients (16%); $p < 0.0001$ (Figure 1). RELISTOR-treated patients also had significantly higher rates of laxation within 4 hours after at least 2 of the first 4 doses (52%) than did placebo-treated patients (9%); $p < 0.0001$. In both studies, in approximately 30% of patients, laxation was reported within 30 minutes of a dose of RELISTOR.

[See figure 1 at top of next page]

In both studies, there was no evidence of differential effects of age or gender on safety or efficacy. No meaningful subgroup analysis could be conducted on race because the study

□ Placebo
■ RELISTOR 0.15 mg/kg
□ RELISTOR 0.30 mg/kg

58%

48%

20%
10%
0%

14%

16%

(n=52) (n=47) (n=55)   (n=71) (n=62)
Study 1   Study 2

*p < 0.0001 vs. Placebo

Figure 1. Laxation Response Within 4 Hours of the First Dose

population was predominantly Caucasian (88%). The rates of discontinuation due to adverse events during the double blind placebo controlled clinical trials (Study 1 and Study 2) were comparable between RELISTOR (1.2%) and placebo (2.4%).

Durability of Response
Durability of response was demonstrated in Study 2, in which the laxation response rate was consistent from dose 1 through dose 7 over the course of the 2-week, double-blind period.
The efficacy and safety of methylnaltrexone bromide was also demonstrated in open-label treatment administered from Day 2 through Week 4 in Study 1, and in two open-label extension studies (Study 1EXT and Study 2EXT) in which RELISTOR was given as needed for up to 4 months. During open-label treatment, patients maintained their regular laxative regimen. A total of 136, 21, and 82 patients received at least 1 open-label dose in studies 1, 1EXT, and 2EXT, respectively. Laxation response rates observed during double-blind treatment with RELISTOR were maintained over the course of 3 to 4 months of open-label treatment.

Opioid Use and Pain Scores
There was no relationship between baseline opioid dose and laxation response in methylnaltrexone bromide-treated patients in these studies. In addition, median daily opioid dose did not vary meaningfully from baseline in either RELISTOR-treated patients or in placebo-treated patients. There were no clinically relevant changes in pain scores from baseline in either the methylnaltrexone bromide or placebo-treated patients.

16   HOW SUPPLIED/STORAGE AND HANDLING

NDC NUMBER	PACK SIZE	CONTENTS
0008-1218-01	1 vial per carton	one 12 mg/0.6 mL single-use vial
0008-2513-02	7 trays per kit	Each tray contains: one 12 mg/0.6 mL single use vial, one 1 cc (mL) syringe with retractable (27-gauge × ½-inch) needle (VanishPoint®), two alcohol swabs
0008-1225-10	7 pre-filled syringes per carton	seven 8 mg/0.4 mL single-use pre-filled syringes with needle guard system
0008-1218-10	7 pre-filled syringes per carton	seven 12 mg/0.6 mL single-use pre-filled syringes with needle guard system

16.1   Storage
RELISTOR® should be stored at 20-25°C (68-77°F); excursions permitted to 15-30°C (59-86°F) [see USP Controlled Room Temperature]. Do not freeze. **Protect from light.**

17   PATIENT COUNSELING INFORMATION
[See FDA-Approved Patient Labeling] Instruct patients that the usual schedule is one dose every other day, as needed, but no more frequently than one dose in a 24-hour period. In approximately 30% of patients in clinical trials, laxation was reported within 30 minutes of a dose of RELISTOR; therefore, advise patients to be within close proximity to toilet facilities once the drug is administered.
Instruct patients not to continue taking RELISTOR if they experience severe or persistent diarrhea. Instruct patients that common side effects of RELISTOR include transient abdominal pain, nausea and vomiting.
Instruct patients not to continue taking RELISTOR and to promptly notify their physician if they experience severe,

persistent, and/or worsening abdominal symptoms because these could be symptoms of intestinal perforation [*see Warnings and Precautions (5.2)*].
Instruct patients to discontinue RELISTOR if they stop taking their opioid pain medication.

PATIENT INFORMATION
RELISTOR® [rel´- i- store]
(methylnaltrexone bromide)
Subcutaneous Injection
Read the Patient Information that comes with RELISTOR before you start using it and each time you get a refill. There may be new information. This leaflet does not take the place of talking with your healthcare provider about your medical condition or your treatment.

What is RELISTOR?
RELISTOR is a prescription medicine used to treat constipation that is caused by prescription pain medicines, called opioids, in patients receiving supportive care for their advanced illness, when other medicines for constipation, called laxatives, have not worked well enough.

Who should not take RELISTOR?
Do not take RELISTOR if you have or may have a blockage in your intestines called a mechanical bowel obstruction. Symptoms of this blockage are vomiting, stomach pain, and swelling of your abdomen. Talk to your healthcare provider if you have any of these symptoms before taking RELISTOR.

What should I tell my healthcare provider before taking RELISTOR?
Tell your healthcare provider about all of your medical conditions, including if you:
- are pregnant or plan to become pregnant. It is not known if RELISTOR can harm your unborn baby. If you become pregnant while using RELISTOR, tell your healthcare provider right away.
- are breast-feeding or plan to breast-feed. It is not known if RELISTOR passes into your breast milk.
- have kidney problems.

Tell your healthcare provider about all medicines you take. Continue taking your other medicines for constipation unless your healthcare provider tells you to stop taking them.

How should I take RELISTOR?
- Take RELISTOR exactly as your healthcare provider tells you.
- Take RELISTOR by an injection under the skin (subcutaneous injection) of the upper arm, abdomen, or thigh.
- Do not take more than one dose in a 24-hour period.
- Most patients have a bowel movement within a few minutes to a few hours after taking a dose of RELISTOR.
- If you stop taking your prescription pain medicine, check with your healthcare provider before continuing to take RELISTOR.
- If you take more RELISTOR than prescribed, talk to your healthcare provider right away.

See the detailed Patient Instructions for Use at the end of this Patient Information leaflet for information about how to prepare and inject RELISTOR.

What are the possible side effects of RELISTOR?
Common side effects of RELISTOR include:
- **abdominal (stomach) pain**
- **gas**
- **nausea**
- **dizziness**
- **diarrhea**
- **sweating**
- If you get diarrhea that is severe or does not stop while taking RELISTOR, stop taking RELISTOR and call your healthcare provider.
- If you get abdominal pain that is severe or will not go away, or nausea or vomiting that is new or worse, stop taking RELISTOR and call your healthcare provider.

These are not all of the possible side effects of RELISTOR. Tell your healthcare provider if you have any side effect that bothers you or that does not go away.
Call your doctor for medical advice about side effects. You may report side effects to FDA at 1-800-FDA-1088.

How should I store RELISTOR?
- Store RELISTOR vials or pre-filled syringes at 68 to 77°F (20 to 25°C).
- Do not freeze RELISTOR.
- Keep RELISTOR away from light until you are ready to use it.
- If RELISTOR has been drawn into a syringe and you are unable to use the medicine right away, keep the syringe at room temperature for up to 24 hours. The syringe does not need to be kept away from light during the 24-hour period.

Keep RELISTOR and all medicines, needles and syringes out of the reach of children.

General information about RELISTOR
Medicines are sometimes prescribed for conditions that are not mentioned in patient information leaflets. Do not use RELISTOR for a condition for which it was not prescribed. Do not give RELISTOR to other people, even if they have the same symptoms that you have. It may harm them.
This leaflet summarizes the most important information about RELISTOR. If you would like more information, talk with your doctor. You can ask your pharmacist or doctor for information about RELISTOR that is written for healthcare providers. For more information, go to WWW.RELISTOR.COM or call 1-800-934-5556.

What are the ingredients in RELISTOR?
Active ingredient: methylnaltrexone bromide
Inactive ingredients: sodium chloride, edetate calcium disodium USP, glycine hydrochloride.
During manufacture, the pH may have been adjusted with hydrochloric acid and/or sodium hydroxide.
Wyeth®
Marketed by:
Wyeth Pharmaceuticals Inc.
Philadelphia, PA 19101
Progenics®
Pharmaceuticals
Under license from:
Progenics Pharmaceuticals, Inc.
Tarrytown, NY 10591
Patient Instructions for Use of RELISTOR PRE-FILLED SYRINGE
Introduction
The following instructions explain how to prepare and give an injection of RELISTOR the right way, when using a pre-filled syringe of RELISTOR.

Pre-filled Syringe Components

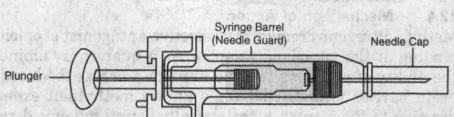

Syringe Barrel (Needle Guard)   Needle Cap
Plunger

The Patient Instructions for Use includes the following steps:
Step 1:   Choosing and preparing an injection site
Step 2:   Preparing the injection for pre-filled syringe
Step 3:   Injecting RELISTOR
Step 4:   Disposing of supplies
Before starting, read and make sure that you understand the Patient Instructions for Use. If you have any questions, talk to your healthcare provider.
Gather the supplies you will need for your injection. These include:
1. RELISTOR pre-filled syringe
2. Alcohol swab
3. Cotton ball or gauze
4. Adhesive bandage
Important Notes:
- Do not use a RELISTOR pre-filled syringe more than one time, even if there is medicine left in the syringe.
- Store RELISTOR pre-filled syringes at 68°F to 77°F (20°C to 25°C). Do not freeze RELISTOR. Keep RELISTOR away from light until you are ready to use it. For more information about how to store RELISTOR, see the section called "How should I store RELISTOR?" in the FDA-Approved Patient Labeling.
- Safely throw away RELISTOR pre-filled syringes after use (see Step 4 below).
- To avoid needle-stick injuries, do not recap used needles.
- Avoid touching the trigger fingers of the RELISTOR pre-filled syringe to keep from activating the safety device too soon. The safety device (needle guard) is activated by pressure from the plunger on the trigger fingers (Figure 1).

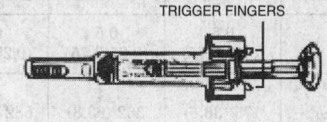

TRIGGER FINGERS

Figure 1

Step 1:   Choosing and preparing an injection site
1. Choose an injection site - abdomen, thighs, or upper arms. See shaded areas in Figures 2 and 3 below. Do not inject at the exact same spot each time (rotate injection

sites). Do not inject into areas where the skin is tender, bruised, red or hard. Avoid areas with scars or stretch marks.

Figure 2. Abdomen or thigh – use these sites when injecting yourself or another person.

Figure 3. Upper arm – use this site only when injecting another person.

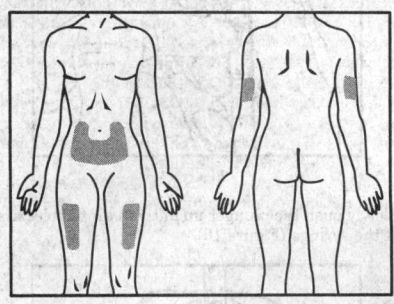

Figure 2   Figure 3

2. Clean the injection site with an alcohol swab and let it air-dry. Do not touch this area again before giving the injection (Figure 4).

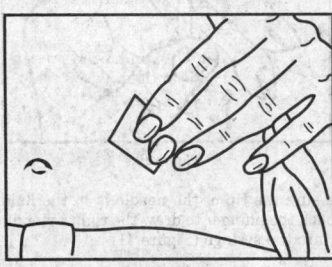

Figure 4

Step 2:   Preparing the injection for pre-filled syringe

1. Find a quiet place. Choose a flat, clean, well-lit working surface.
2. Wash your hands with soap and warm water before preparing for the injection.
3. Look at the pre-filled syringe of RELISTOR (Figure 5). Make sure that the dose prescribed by your healthcare provider matches the dose on the pre-filled syringe label. Look at the plunger rod of the syringe. If the dose prescribed by your healthcare provider is 8 mg, the plunger rod will be yellow; if the prescribed dose is 12 mg, the plunger rod of the syringe will be purple (Figure 5).

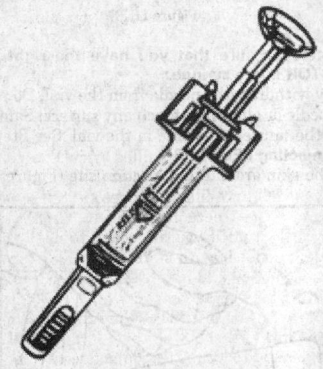

Figure 5

4. The liquid in the pre-filled syringe should be clear and colorless to pale yellow, and should not have any particles in it. If not, do not use the pre-filled syringe, and call your healthcare provider.
5. Firmly hold the barrel of the pre-filled syringe and pull the needle cap straight off (Figure 6). Do not touch the needle or allow it to touch any surface.

[See figure 6 at top of next column]

Step 3:   Injecting RELISTOR

1. Pinch the skin around the injection site (Figure 7).

[See figure 7 in next column]

2. Insert the full length of the needle into the skin at a 45-degree angle with a quick "dart-like" motion (Figure 8).

[See figure 8 in next column]

Let go of skin and slowly push down on the plunger with your thumb until the pre-filled syringe is empty (Figure 9). This will release the needle safety device.

[See figure 9 in next column]

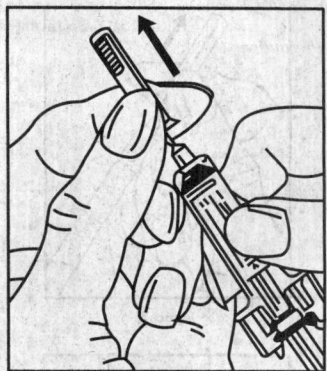

Figure 6

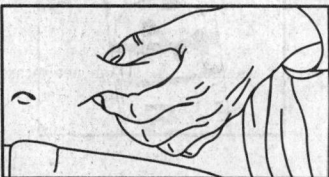

Figure 7

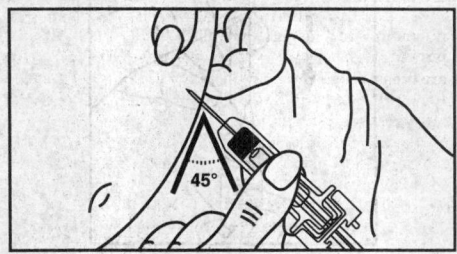

Figure 8

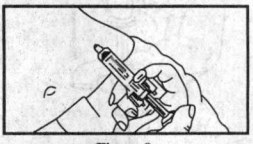

Figure 9

3. Continue to hold pressure on the plunger with your thumb and quickly pull the needle out of the skin. Be careful to keep the needle at the same angle as it was inserted. Then remove your thumb from the plunger to allow the protective sleeve to cover the needle (Figure 10). There may be a little bleeding at the injection site.

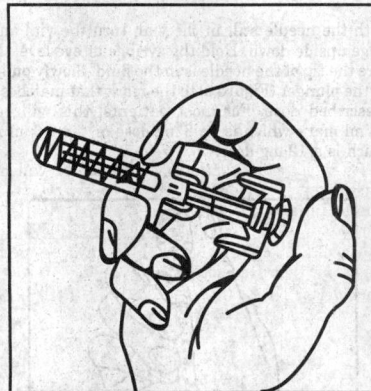

Figure 10

4. Hold a cotton ball or gauze over the injection site (Figure 11). Do not rub the injection site. Apply an adhesive bandage to the injection site if needed.

[See figure 11 in next column]

Step 4:   Disposing of supplies

• **Do not re-use the pre-filled syringe or recap the needle. Place used pre-filled syringe in a closeable, puncture-resistant container.** You may use a sharps container (such

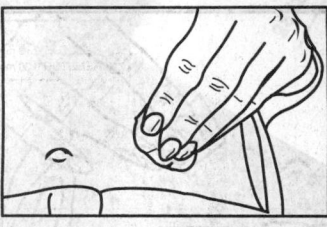

Figure 11

as a red biohazard container), a hard plastic container (such as a detergent bottle), or metal container (such as an empty coffee can). Ask your healthcare provider for instructions on the right way to throw away (dispose of) the container. There may be state and local laws about how you should throw away used needles and syringes.

• If you have any questions, talk to your healthcare provider or pharmacist.

Patient Instructions for Use of RELISTOR® VIAL AND STANDARD SYRINGE AND NEEDLE

Introduction

The following instructions explain how to prepare and give an injection of RELISTOR the right way, when using a vial of RELISTOR, and a standard syringe.

The Patient Instructions for Use includes the following steps:

Step 1:   Choosing and preparing an injection site
Step 2:   Preparing the injection
Step 3:   Preparing the syringe
Step 4:   Injecting RELISTOR
Step 5:   Disposing of supplies

Before starting, read and make sure that you understand the Patient Instructions for Use. If you have any questions, talk to your healthcare provider.

Gather the supplies you will need for your injection. These include:

1. RELISTOR vial
2. 1 mL syringe with a 27-gauge needle for subcutaneous use
3. 2 alcohol swabs
4. Cotton ball or gauze
5. Adhesive bandage

Important Notes:

• **Use the syringes and needles prescribed by your healthcare provider.**
• **Do not use a RELISTOR vial more than one time, even if there is medicine left in the vial.**
• **If RELISTOR has been drawn into a syringe and you are unable to use the medicine right away, keep the syringe at room temperature for up to 24 hours. The syringe does not need to be kept away from light during the 24-hour period. For more information about how to store RELISTOR, see the section called "How should I store RELISTOR?" in the FDA-Approved Patient Labeling.**
• **Safely throw away RELISTOR vials after use.**
• **Do not re-use syringes or needles.**
• **To avoid needle stick injuries, do not recap used needles.**

Step 1:   Choosing and preparing an injection site

1. Choose an injection site—abdomen, thighs, or upper arms. See shaded areas in Figures 1 and 2 below. Do not inject at the exact same spot each time (rotate injection sites). Do not inject into areas where the skin is tender, bruised, red or hard. Avoid areas with scars or stretch marks.

Figure 1. Abdomen or thigh – use these sites when injecting yourself or another person.

Figure 2. Upper arm – use this site only when injecting another person.

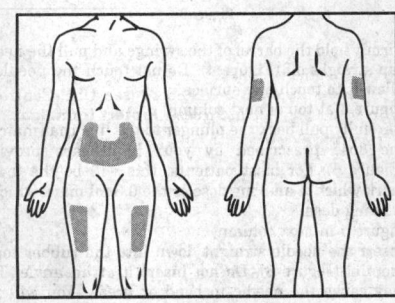

Figure 1   Figure 2

2. Clean the injection site with an alcohol swab and let it air dry. Do not touch this area again before giving the injection (Figure 3).

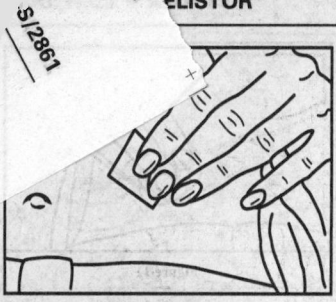

Figure 3

Step 2: Preparing the injection

1. Find a quiet place. Choose a flat, clean, well-lit working surface.
2. Wash your hands with soap and warm water before preparing for the injection.
3. Look at the vial of RELISTOR (Figure 1). The liquid in the vial should be clear and colorless to pale yellow, and should not have any particles in it. If not, do not use the vial, and call your healthcare provider.

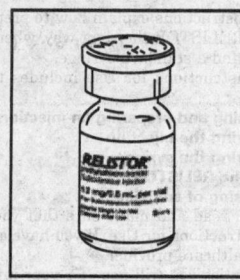

Figure 1

Step 3: Preparing the syringe

1. Remove the cap from the RELISTOR vial (Figure 2).

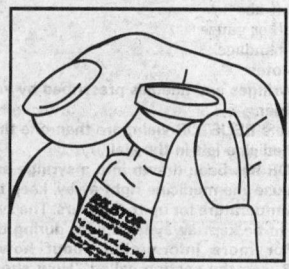

Figure 2

2. Wipe the rubber stopper with an alcohol swab (Figure 3).

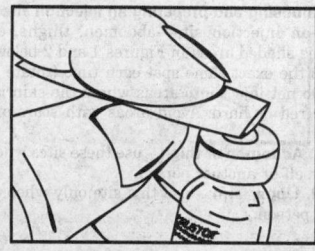

Figure 3

3. Firmly hold the barrel of the syringe and pull the needle cap straight off (Figure 4). Do not touch the needle or allow it to touch any surface.
[See figure 4 at top of next column]
4. Carefully pull back the plunger to the line that matches the dose prescribed by your healthcare provider (Figure 5). For most patients, this will be the 0.4 ml mark which is an 8 mg dose or the 0.6 ml mark which is a 12 mg dose.
[See figure 5 in next column]
5. Insert the needle straight down into the rubber top of the vial (Figure 6). Do not insert it at an angle. This may cause the needle to bend or break. You will feel some resistance as the needle passes through the rubber top.
[See figure 6 in next column]
6. Gently push down the plunger until all of the air is out of the syringe and has gone into the vial (Figure 7).
[See figure 7 in next column]

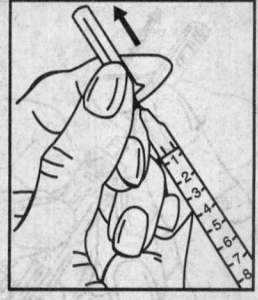

Figure 4

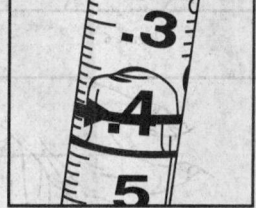

Figure 5

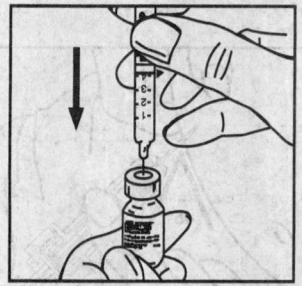

Figure 6

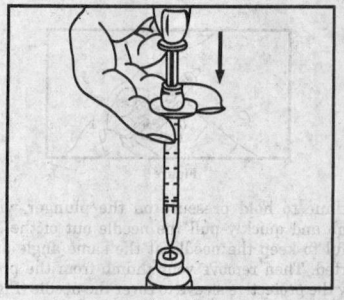

Figure 7

7. With the needle still in the vial, turn the vial and syringe upside down. Hold the syringe at eye level. Make sure the tip of the needle is in the fluid. Slowly pull back on the plunger (Figure 8) to the mark that matches your prescribed dose. For most patients, this will be the 0.4 ml mark which is an 8 mg dose or the 0.6 ml mark which is a 12 mg dose.

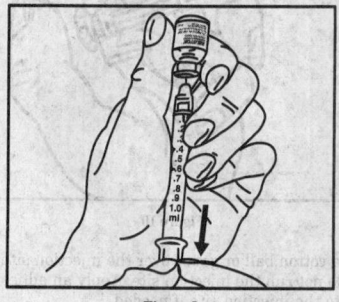

Figure 8

8. With the needle still in the vial, gently tap the side of the syringe to make any air bubbles rise to the top (Figure 9).

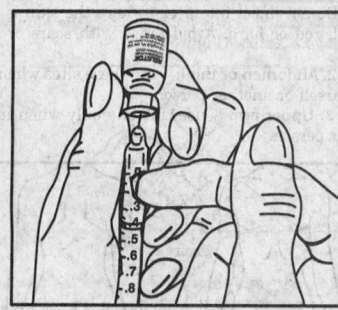

Figure 9

9. Slowly push the plunger up until all air bubbles are out of the syringe (Figure 10).

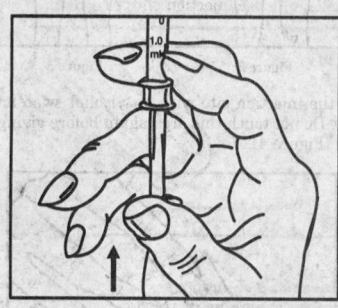

Figure 10

10. Make sure the tip of the needle is in the fluid. Slowly pull back the plunger to draw the right amount of liquid back into the syringe (Figure 11).

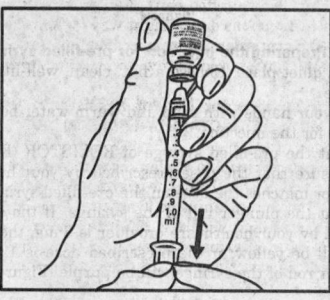

Figure 11

Check to be sure that you have the right dose of RELISTOR in the syringe.

11. Slowly withdraw the needle from the vial. Do not touch the needle or allow it to touch any surface. Safely throw away the unused medicine in the vial. See Step 5.

Step 4: Injecting RELISTOR

1. Pinch the skin around the injection site (Figure 12).

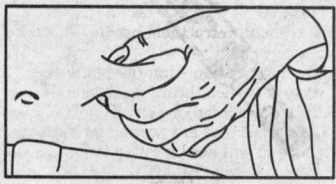

Figure 12

2. Insert the full length of the needle into the skin at a 45-degree angle with a quick "dart-like" motion (Figure 13).

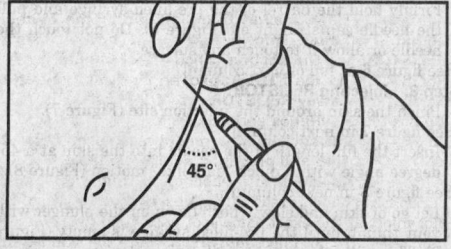

Figure 13

3. Let go of skin and slowly push down on the plunger until the syringe is empty (Figure 14).

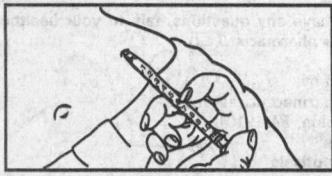

Figure 14

4. When the syringe is empty, quickly pull the needle out of the skin, being careful to keep it at the same angle as it was inserted. There may be a little bleeding at the injection site.
5. Hold a cotton ball or gauze over the injection site (Figure 15). Do not rub the injection site. Apply an adhesive bandage to the injection site if needed.

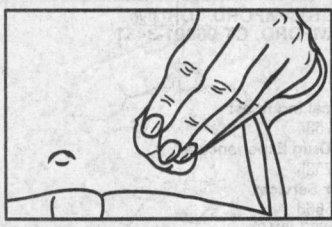

Figure 15

Step 5: Disposing of supplies
• Do not re-use a syringe or needle.
• Do not recap a used needle.
• Place used needle, syringes, and vials in a closeable, puncture-resistant container. You may use a sharps container (such as a red biohazard container), a hard plastic container (such as a detergent bottle), or metal container (such as an empty coffee can). Ask your healthcare provider for instructions on the right way to throw away (dispose of) the container. There may be state and local laws about how you should throw away used needles and syringes.

Patient Instructions for Use of RELISTOR® VIAL AND SYRINGE WITH RETRACTABLE NEEDLE IN TRAY
Introduction:
The following instructions explain how to prepare and give an injection of RELISTOR the right way, when using a RELISTOR tray containing a syringe with a retractable needle. A retractable needle is one that is pulled back so that it is covered after use, to prevent needle stick injury.
The Patient Instructions for Use includes the following steps:
Step 1: Choosing and preparing an injection site
Step 2: Preparing the injection
Step 3: Preparing the syringe
Step 4: Injecting RELISTOR
Step 5: Disposing of supplies
Before starting, read and make sure that you understand the Patient Instructions for Use. Familiarize yourself with the RELISTOR tray, which contains the supplies you need for an injection. If you have any questions, talk to your healthcare provider. Your tray should include the following:
1. RELISTOR vial
2. 1 mL syringe with retractable needle (VanishPoint®)
3. 2 alcohol swabs
4. Prescribing Information - information about RELISTOR that is written for healthcare professionals
5. Patient Instructions for Use of RELISTOR - instructions about RELISTOR that are written for patients
In addition, you will need a cotton ball or gauze, and you may need an adhesive bandage.
Important Notes:
• Do not use a RELISTOR vial more than one time, even if there is medicine left in the vial.
• If RELISTOR has been drawn into a syringe and you are unable to use the medicine right away, keep the syringe at room temperature for up to 24 hours. The syringe does not need to be kept away from light during the 24-hour period. For more information about how to store RELISTOR, see the section called "How should I store RELISTOR?" in the FDA-Approved Patient Labeling.
• Safely throw away RELISTOR vials after use.
• Do not reuse syringes and needles.
• To avoid needle stick injuries, do not recap used needles.
Step 1: Choosing and preparing an injection site
1. Choose an injection site—abdomen, thighs, or upper arms. See shaded areas in Figures 12 and 13 below. Do not inject at the exact same spot each time (rotate injection sites). Do not inject into areas where the skin is tender, bruised, red, or hard. Avoid areas with scars or stretch marks.

Figure 1. Abdomen or thigh – use these sites when injecting yourself or another person.
Figure 2. Upper arm – use this site only when injecting another person.

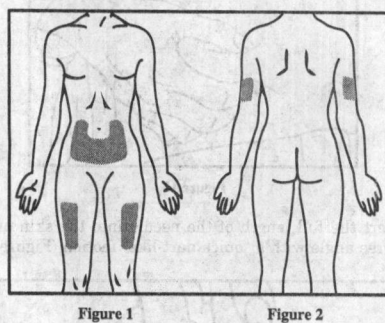

Figure 1   Figure 2

2. Clean the injection site with an alcohol swab and let it air dry. Do not touch this area again before giving the injection (Figure 3).

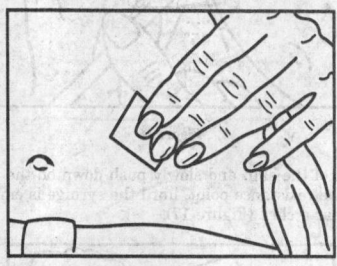

Figure 3

Step 2: Preparing the injection
1. Find a quiet place. Choose a flat, clean, well-lit working surface.
2. Wash your hands with soap and warm water before preparing for the injection.
3. Look at the vial of RELISTOR (Figure 4). The liquid in the vial should be clear and colorless to pale yellow, and should not have any particles in it. If not, do not use the vial and call your healthcare provider.

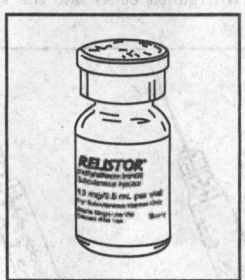

Figure 4

Step 3: Preparing the syringe
1. Remove the cap from the vial containing RELISTOR (Figure 5).

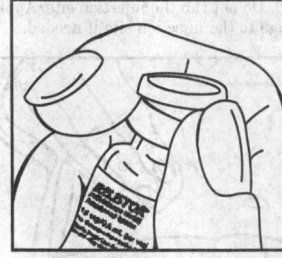

Figure 5

2. Wipe the rubber stopper with an alcohol swab (Figure 6).
[See figure 6 at top of next column]
3. Firmly hold the barrel of the syringe and remove the needle cap straight off (Figure 7. Do not touch the needle or allow it to touch any surface.
[See figure 7 in next column]
4. Carefully pull back on the plunger to the line that matches the dose prescribed by your healthcare provider (Figure 8). For most patients, this will be the

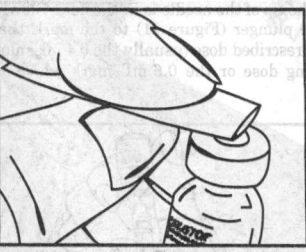

Figure 6

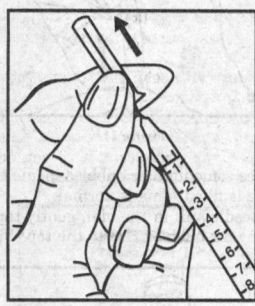

Figure 7

0.4 mL mark which is an 8 mg dose or the 0.6 mL mark which is a 12 mg dose.

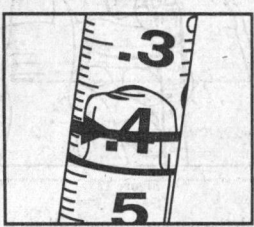

Figure 8

5. Insert the needle straight down into the rubber top of the RELISTOR vial (Figure 9). Do not insert it at an angle. This may cause the needle to bend or break. You will feel some resistance as the needle passes through the rubber top.

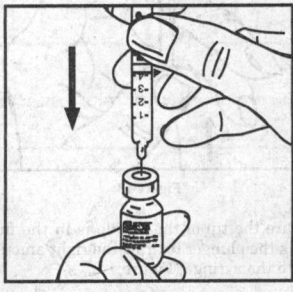

Figure 9

6. Gently push down the plunger until you feel resistance, and most of the air has gone out of the syringe and into the vial (Figure 10). **Do not push past the resistance point.** Doing this will make the needle retract (pull back) into the syringe barrel.

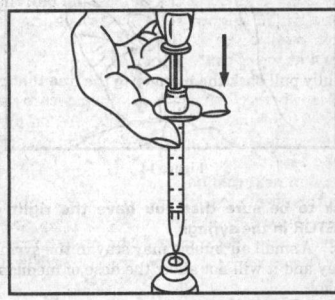

Figure 10

7. With the needle still in the vial, turn the vial and syringe upside down. Hold the syringe at eye level. Make

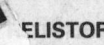
...n the fluid. Slowly pull back ...the mark that matches ...the 0.4 mL mark which is ...mL mark which is a 12 mg

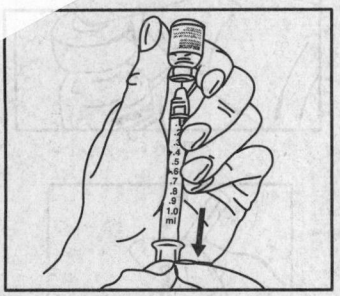

Figure 11

You may see some fluid or bubbles inside the vial when the syringe is filled. This is normal.

8. With the needle still in the vial, gently tap the syringe to make any air bubbles rise to the top (Figure 12).

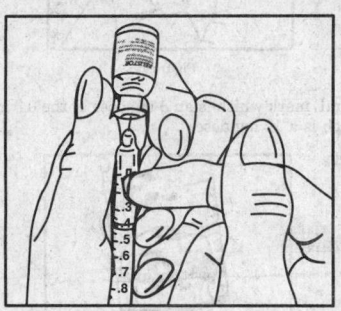

Figure 12

9. Slowly push the plunger up until all air bubbles are out of the syringe (Figure 13).

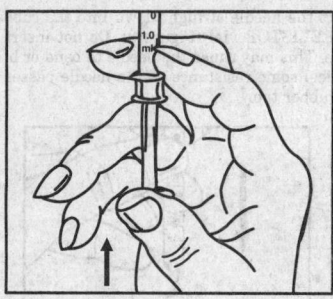

Figure 13

10. Make sure the tip of the needle is in the fluid. Slowly pull back the plunger to draw the right amount of liquid back into the syringe (Figure 14).

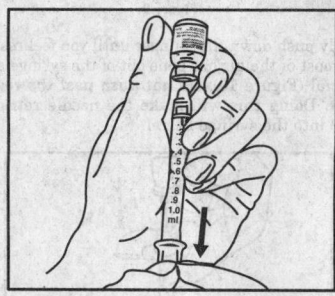

Figure 14

Check to be sure that you have the right dose of RELISTOR in the syringe.

Note: A small air bubble may stay in the syringe. This is okay and it will not affect the dose of medicine in the syringe.

11. Slowly withdraw the needle from the vial (do not touch the needle or allow the needle to touch any surface). Safely throw away the unused medicine in the vial. See Step 5.

Step 4: Injecting RELISTOR

1. Pinch the skin around the injection site as you were instructed (Figure 15).

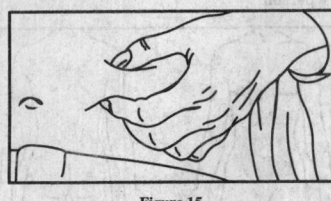

Figure 15

2. Insert the full length of the needle into the skin at 45-degree angle with a "quick dart-like" motion (Figure 16).

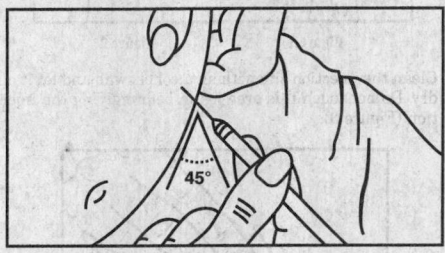

Figure 16

3. Let go of the skin and slowly push down on the plunger past the resistance point, until the syringe is empty and you hear a click (Figure 17).

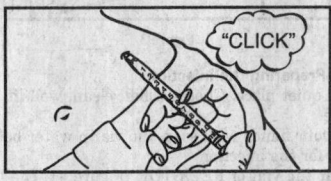

Figure 17

4. The click sound means that the needle (Figure 18) has been retracted (pulled back) into the syringe barrel (Figure 19).

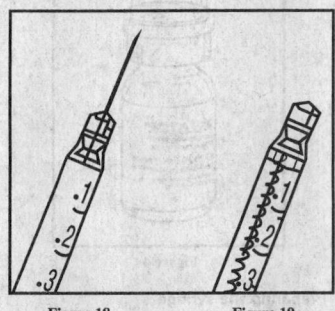

Figure 18   **Figure 19**

5. Hold a cotton ball or gauze over the injection site (Figure 20). Do not rub the injection site. Apply an adhesive bandage to the injection site if needed.

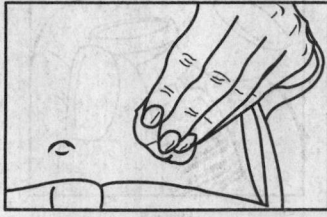

Figure 20

Step 5: Disposing of supplies
- **Do not** re-use a syringe or needle.
- **Do not** recap a used needle.
- Place used needles, syringes and vials in a closeable, puncture-resistant container. You may use a sharps container (such as a red biohazard container), a hard plastic container (such as a detergent bottle), or a metal container (such as an empty coffee can). Ask your healthcare provider for instructions on the right way to throw away

(dispose of) the container. There may be state and local laws about how you should throw away used needles and syringes.
- **If you have any questions, talk to your healthcare provider or pharmacist.**

Wyeth®
Marketed by:
Wyeth Pharmaceuticals Inc.
Philadelphia, PA 19101
Progenics®
Pharmaceuticals
Under license from:
Progenics Pharmaceuticals, Inc.
Tarrytown, NY 10591
W10531C005
ET01
(09-2010)

Purdue Pharma L.P.
ONE STAMFORD FORUM
STAMFORD, CT 06901-3431

For Medical Inquiries:
888-726-7535
Adverse Drug Experiences:
888-726-7535
Customer Service:
800-877-5666
FAX 800-877-3210

BUTRANS™   Ⓒ ℞
[BYOO-trans]
(buprenorphine)
Transdermal System for Transdermal Administration

HIGHLIGHTS OF PRESCRIBING INFORMATION
These highlights do not include all the information needed to use Butrans™ safely and effectively. See full prescribing information for Butrans.
Butrans (buprenorphine) Transdermal System for transdermal administration CIII
Initial U.S. Approval: 1981

WARNING: POTENTIAL FOR ABUSE and IMPORTANCE OF PROPER PATIENT SELECTION
See full prescribing information for complete boxed warning.
- **Butrans is indicated for the management of moderate to severe chronic pain in patients requiring a continuous, around-the-clock opioid analgesic for an extended period of time. (1)**
- **Butrans contains buprenorphine which is a mu opioid partial agonist and a Schedule III controlled substance. (9.1)**
- **Assess patients for their clinical risks for opioid abuse or addiction prior to prescribing opioids. (2.2)**
- **Do not exceed a dose of one 20 mcg/hour Butrans system due to the risk of QTc interval prolongation. (2.3)**
- **Avoid exposing the Butrans application site and surrounding area to direct external heat sources. Temperature-dependent increases in buprenorphine release from the system may result in overdose and death. (5.11)**

————INDICATIONS AND USAGE————
Butrans is indicated for the management of moderate to severe chronic pain in patients requiring a continuous, around-the-clock opioid analgesic for an extended period of time. (1)

————DOSAGE AND ADMINISTRATION————
- Each Butrans is intended to be worn for 7 days. (2.1)
- In opioid-naïve patients, the initial dose of Butrans should always be 5 mcg/hour. (2.2)
- For patients already receiving opioids, consult conversion instructions. (2.2)
- Do not increase the Butrans dose until the patient has been exposed continually to the previous dose for 72 hours. (2.3)
- After removal, wait a minimum of 3 weeks before applying to the same site (2.1)
- When Butrans is no longer required by the patient, taper the dose as part of a comprehensive treatment plan. (2.5)

————DOSAGE FORMS AND STRENGTHS————
- Transdermal system, 5 mcg/hour, 10 mcg/hour, and 20 mcg/hour. (3)

————CONTRAINDICATIONS————
- Patients who have significant respiratory depression (4, 5.1, 5.2)

- Patients who have severe bronchial asthma (4)
- Patients who have or are suspected of having paralytic ileus (4, 5.16)
- Patients who have known hypersensitivity to any of its components or the active ingredient, buprenorphine (4)
- The management of acute pain or in patients who require opioid analgesia for a short period of time (4)
- The management of post-operative pain, including use after out-patient or day surgeries (4)
- The management of mild pain (4)
- The management of intermittent pain (e.g., use on an as-needed basis [prn]) (4)

————WARNINGS AND PRECAUTIONS————

- Use with extreme caution in patients at risk of respiratory depression. (5.1, 7.2)
- Use with caution in patients who are receiving other central nervous system (CNS) depressants. (5.2, 7.2, 12.2)
- Additive CNS effects are expected when used with alcohol, benzodiazepines, other opioids, or illicit drugs. (5.3, 7.2)
- Avoid in patients with Long QT Syndrome, family history of Long QT Syndrome, or those taking Class IA or Class III antiarrhythmic medications. (5.4, 12.2)
- Butrans may worsen increased intracranial pressure and obscure its signs, such as level of consciousness or pupillary signs. (5.5)
- Use with caution in patients at increased risk of hypotension and in patients in circulatory shock. (5.6, 12.2)
- Ileus may occur. Monitor for decreased bowel motility in postoperative patients. (5.16)
- Use with caution in patients with biliary tract disease, including acute pancreatitis. (5.16)

————ADVERSE REACTIONS————

Most common adverse reactions (≥5%) include: nausea, headache, application site pruritus, dizziness, constipation, somnolence, vomiting, application site erythema, dry mouth, and application site rash.

To report SUSPECTED ADVERSE REACTIONS, contact Purdue Pharma L.P. at 1-888-726-7535 or FDA at 1-800-FDA-1088 or www.fda.gov/medwatch.

————DRUG INTERACTIONS————

- Agents that induce CYP3A4 enzymatic activity may alter the metabolism of buprenorphine but the clinical significance of these interactions is not known. (7.1)
- CNS depressants may interact with Butrans resulting in respiratory and CNS depression - use caution in prescribing Butrans for patients receiving benzodiazepines or other depressants and warn patients against concomitant self-administration/misuse. (7.2)
- Muscle relaxants may enhance the action of Butrans and produce an increased degree of respiratory depression. (7.2)

————USE IN SPECIFIC POPULATIONS————

- Pregnancy: Butrans is not recommended for use during pregnancy. (8.1)
- Nursing Mothers: Breast-feeding is not advised in mothers treated with Butrans. (8.3)
- Pediatric Use: Safety and effectiveness of Butrans have not been established in patients below 18 years. (8.4)
- Geriatric Use: While no dose adjustment is recommended on the basis of age, administer Butrans with caution in elderly patients. (8.5)
- Hepatic Impairment: Butrans has not been evaluated in patients with severe hepatic impairment and should be administered with caution. (8.6)

See 17 for PATIENT COUNSELING INFORMATION and Medication Guide.

Revised: August 2010

FULL PRESCRIBING INFORMATION: CONTENTS*
BOXED WARNING
*Sections or subsections omitted from the full prescribing information are not listed.

FULL PRESCRIBING INFORMATION

WARNING: IMPORTANCE OF PROPER PATIENT SELECTION, POTENTIAL FOR ABUSE, AND LIMITATIONS OF USE
Proper Patient Selection
Butrans is a transdermal formulation of buprenorphine indicated for the management of moderate to severe chronic pain in patients requiring a continuous, around-the-clock opioid analgesic for an extended period of time. (1)
Potential for Abuse
Butrans contains buprenorphine which is a mu opioid partial agonist and a Schedule III controlled substance. Butrans can be abused in a manner similar to other opioid agonists, legal or illicit. Consider the abuse potential when prescribing or dispensing Butrans in situations where the physician or pharmacist is concerned about an increased risk of misuse, abuse, or diversion. (9)

Persons at increased risk for opioid abuse include those with a personal or family history of substance abuse (including drug or alcohol abuse or addiction) or mental illness (e.g., major depression). Assess patients for their clinical risks for opioid abuse or addiction prior to being prescribed opioids. Routinely monitor all patients receiving opioids for signs of misuse, abuse and addiction. (2.2)
Limitations of Use
Do not exceed a dose of one 20 mcg/hour Butrans system due to the risk of QTc interval prolongation. (2.3)
Avoid exposing the Butrans application site and surrounding area to direct external heat sources. Temperature-dependent increases in buprenorphine release from the system may result in overdose and death. (5.11)

---

1   INDICATIONS AND USAGE
Butrans is indicated for the management of moderate to severe chronic pain in patients requiring a continuous, around-the-clock opioid analgesic for an extended period of time.

2   DOSAGE AND ADMINISTRATION

2.1   General Principles
Selection of patients for treatment with Butrans is governed by the same principles that apply to the use of similar opioid analgesics. Physicians should individualize treatment in every case, using non-opioid analgesics, opioids on an as-needed basis and/or combination products, and chronic opioid therapy in a progressive plan of pain management such as outlined by the World Health Organization, the American Pain Society, and Federation of State Medical Boards Model Policy.

Butrans is for transdermal use (on intact skin) only.

Do not use Butrans if the pouch seal is broken or the patch is cut, damaged, or changed in any way. Do not cut Butrans. Each Butrans is intended to be worn for 7 days.

Apply Butrans to the upper outer arm, upper chest, upper back or the side of the chest. These four sites (each present on both sides of the body) provide 8 possible application sites. Rotate Butrans among the 8 described skin sites. After Butrans removal, wait a minimum of 21 days before reapplying to the same skin site [see Clinical Pharmacology (12.3)].

Apply Butrans to a hairless or nearly hairless skin site. If none are available, the hair at the site should be clipped, not shaven. Do not apply Butrans to irritated skin. If the application site must be cleaned, clean the site with water only. Do not use soaps, alcohol, oils, lotions, or abrasive devices. Allow the skin to dry before applying Butrans.

If problems with adhesion of Butrans occur, the edges may be taped with first aid tape.

If Butrans falls off during the 7 days dosing interval, dispose of the transdermal system properly and place a new Butrans on at a different skin site [see How Supplied/Storage and Handling (16)].

2.2   Initiation of Therapy
It is critical to initiate the dosing regimen individually for each patient. Overestimating the Butrans dose when converting patients from another opioid medication can result in fatal overdose with the first dose [see Overdosage (10)]. Consider the following when selecting the initial dose of Butrans:
1. The total daily dose, potency, and specific characteristics of the opioid the patient has been taking previously;
2. The reliability of the relative potency estimate used to calculate the equivalent buprenorphine dose needed (when converting from other opioids or opioid-combination products);
3. The patient's degree of tolerance to the respiratory-depressant and sedating effects of opioids;
4. The age, general condition, and medical status of the patient;
5. Concurrent non-opioid analgesic and other medications;
6. The type and severity of the patient's pain;
7. The balance between pain control and adverse drug experiences;
8. Risk factors for abuse, addiction, or diversion, including a prior history of abuse, addiction, or diversion.

The following dosing recommendations, therefore, can only be considered as suggested approaches to what is actually a series of clinical decisions over time in the management of the pain of each individual patient.

Opioid-Naïve Patients
For opioid-naïve patients, initiate treatment with Butrans 5 mcg/hour. Thereafter, individually titrate the dose as described in Section 2.3 Dose Titration to a level that provides adequate analgesia and minimizes side effects. Dose may be titrated to the next higher level after a minimum of 72 hours.

Conversion from Other Opioids to Butrans
There is a potential for buprenorphine to precipitate withdrawal in patients who are already on opioids. For conversion from other opioids to Butrans (see Table 1), taper the patient's current around-the-clock opioids for up to 7 days to no more than 30 mg of morphine or equivalent per day before beginning treatment with Butrans. Patients may use short-acting analgesics as needed until analgesic efficacy with Butrans is attained.

For patients whose daily dose was less than 30 mg of oral morphine or equivalent, initiate treatment with Butrans 5 mcg/hour. For patients whose daily dose was between 30 and 80 mg morphine equivalents, initiate treatment with Butrans 10 mcg/hour (see Table 1). Thereafter, individually titrate the dose as described in Section 2.3 Dose Titration.

Table 1: Dose Estimation for Conversion of Oral Morphine Equivalents to Butrans

Current Opioid Analgesic	Current Daily Dose	
Oral Morphine Equivalent	<30 mg	30-80 mg
	↓	↓
Recommended Butrans Starting Dose	5 mcg/hour	10 mcg/hour

Use caution when prescribing Butrans to opioid-experienced patients requiring high doses of opioids (more than 80 mg/day of oral morphine equivalents). Butrans 20 mcg/hour may not provide adequate analgesia for patients requiring greater than 80 mg/day oral morphine equivalents.

2.3 Dose Titration

Based on the patient's requirement for supplemental short-acting analgesics, upward titration may be instituted with a minimum Butrans titration interval of 72 hours, based on the pharmacokinetic profile and time to reach steady state levels [see Clinical Pharmacology (12.3)]. Individually titrate the dose, under close supervision, to a level that provides adequate analgesia with tolerable side effects.

The maximum Butrans dose is 20 mcg/hour. **Do not exceed a dose of one 20 mcg/hour Butrans system due to the risk of QTc interval prolongation.** In a clinical trial, Butrans 40 mcg/hour (given as two Butrans 20 mcg/hour systems) resulted in prolongation of the QTc interval [see Warnings and Precautions (5.4) and Clinical Pharmacology (12.2)]. During periods of changing analgesic requirements, including initial titration, frequent contact is recommended between the prescriber, other members of the healthcare team, the patient, and the caregiver/family. Advise patients and caregivers/family members of the potential side effects.

2.4 Maintenance of Therapy and Supplemental Analgesia

The intent of the titration period is to establish a patient-specific weekly Butrans dose that will maintain adequate analgesia with tolerable side effects for as long as pain management is necessary. Immediate-release opioid and non-opioid medications can be used as supplemental analgesia during Butrans therapy.

During chronic opioid analgesic therapy with Butrans, reassess the continued need for around-the-clock opioid analgesic therapy periodically.

2.5 Cessation of Therapy

When the patient no longer requires therapy with Butrans, taper the dose gradually to prevent signs and symptoms of withdrawal in the physically-dependent patient; consider introduction of an appropriate immediate-release opioid medication. Undertake discontinuation of therapy as part of a comprehensive treatment plan.

2.6 Patients with Hepatic Impairment

Start patients with mild to moderate hepatic impairment with the Butrans 5 mcg/hour dose. Thereafter, individually titrate the dose to a level that provides adequate analgesia and tolerable side effects, under the close supervision of the prescriber. Butrans has not been evaluated in patients with severe hepatic impairment. As Butrans is only intended for 7-day application, consider use of an alternate analgesic that may permit more flexibility with the dosing in patients with severe hepatic impairment [see Warnings and Precautions (5.1), Use In Specific Populations (8.6), and Clinical Pharmacology (12.3)].

3 DOSAGE FORMS AND STRENGTHS

Butrans is available as:
- Butrans 5 mcg/hour Transdermal System (dimensions: 45 mm by 45 mm)
- Butrans 10 mcg/hour Transdermal System (dimensions: 45 mm by 68 mm)
- Butrans 20 mcg/hour Transdermal System (dimensions: 72 mm by 72 mm)

4 CONTRAINDICATIONS

Butrans is contraindicated in:
- patients who have significant respiratory depression
- patients who have severe bronchial asthma
- patients who have or are suspected of having paralytic ileus
- patients who have known hypersensitivity to any of its components or the active ingredient, buprenorphine
- the management of acute pain or in patients who require opioid analgesia for a short period of time
- the management of post-operative pain, including use after out-patient or day surgeries
- the management of mild pain
- the management of intermittent pain (e.g., use on an as needed basis [prn])

5 WARNINGS AND PRECAUTIONS

5.1 Respiratory Depression

Respiratory depression is the chief hazard of Butrans. Respiratory depression occurs more frequently in elderly or debilitated patients as well as those suffering from conditions accompanied by hypoxia or hypercapnia when even moderate therapeutic doses may dangerously decrease pulmonary ventilation, and when opioids, including Butrans, are given in conjunction with other agents that depress respiration. Profound sedation, unresponsiveness, infrequent deep ("sighing") breaths or atypical snoring frequently accompany opioid-induced respiratory depression.

Use Butrans with extreme caution in patients with any of the following:
- significant chronic obstructive pulmonary disease or cor pulmonale

- other risk of substantially decreased respiratory reserve such as asthma, severe obesity, sleep apnea, myxedema, clinically significant kyphoscoliosis, and central nervous system (CNS) depression
- hypoxia
- hypercapnia
- pre-existing respiratory depression

5.2 CNS Depression

Butrans may cause somnolence, dizziness, alterations in judgment and alterations in levels of consciousness, including coma.

5.3 Interactions with Alcohol, Central Nervous System Depressants, and Illicit Drugs

Hypotension, profound sedation, coma or respiratory depression may result if Butrans is added to a regimen that includes other CNS depressants (e.g., sedatives, anxiolytics, hypnotics, neuroleptics, muscle relaxants, other opioids). Therefore, use caution when deciding to initiate therapy with Butrans in patients who are taking other CNS depressants. Take into account the types of other medications being taken, the duration of therapy with them, and the patient's response to those medicines, including the degree of tolerance that has developed to CNS depression. Consider the patient's use, if any, of alcohol and/or illicit drugs that cause CNS depression. If the decision to begin Butrans is made, start with a lower Butrans dose than usual.

Consider using a lower initial dose of a CNS depressant when given to a patient currently taking Butrans due to the potential of additive CNS depressant effects.

5.4 QTc Prolongation

A positive-controlled study of the effects of Butrans on the QTc interval in healthy subjects demonstrated no clinically meaningful effect at a Butrans dose of 10 mcg/hour; however, a Butrans dose of 40 mcg/hour (given as two Butrans 20 mcg/hour Transdermal Systems) was observed to prolong the QTc interval [see Clinical Pharmacology (12.2)].

Consider these observations in clinical decisions when prescribing Butrans to patients with hypokalemia or clinically unstable cardiac disease, including: unstable atrial fibrillation, symptomatic bradycardia, unstable congestive heart failure, or active myocardial ischemia. Avoid the use of Butrans in patients with a history of Long QT Syndrome or an immediate family member with this condition, or those taking Class IA antiarrhythmic medications (e.g., quinidine, procainamide, disopyramide) or Class III antiarrhythmic medications (e.g., sotalol, amiodarone, dofetilide).

5.5 Head Injury

The respiratory depressant effects of opioids, including Butrans, include carbon dioxide retention, which can lead to an elevation of cerebrospinal fluid pressure. This effect may be exaggerated in the presence of head injury, intracranial lesions, or other sources of pre-existing increased intracranial pressure. Butrans may produce miosis that is independent of ambient light, and altered consciousness, either of which may obscure neurologic signs associated with increased intracranial pressure in persons with head injuries.

5.6 Hypotensive Effects

Butrans may cause severe hypotension. There is an added risk to individuals whose ability to maintain blood pressure has been compromised by a depleted blood volume, or after concurrent administration with drugs such as phenothiazines or other agents which compromise vasomotor tone. Buprenorphine may produce orthostatic hypotension in ambulatory patients. Administer Butrans with caution to patients in circulatory shock, since vasodilation produced by the drug may further reduce cardiac output and blood pressure.

5.7 Misuse, Abuse, and Diversion of Opioids

Butrans contains buprenorphine, a partial agonist at the mu opioid receptor and a Schedule III controlled substance. Opioid agonists have potential for being abused, are sought by drug abusers and people with addiction disorders, and are subject to criminal diversion.

Butrans can be abused in a manner similar to other opioid agonists, legal or illicit. Consider this potential for abuse when prescribing or dispensing Butrans in situations where the prescriber or pharmacist is concerned about an increased risk of misuse, abuse, or diversion. Monitor all patients receiving opioids for signs of abuse, misuse, and addiction. Furthermore, assess patients for their potential for opioid abuse prior to being prescribed opioid therapy. Persons at increased risk for opioid abuse include those with a personal or family history of substance abuse (including drug or alcohol abuse) or mental illness (e.g., depression). Opioids may still be appropriate for use in these patients; however, they will require intensive monitoring for signs of abuse.

Notwithstanding concerns about abuse, addiction, and diversion, provide proper management of pain. However, all patients treated with opioid agonists require careful monitoring for signs of abuse and addiction, since use of opioid agonist analgesic products carries the risk of addiction even under appropriate medical use [see Drug Abuse and Depen-

dence (9.2)]. Data are not available to establish the true incidence of addiction in patients with chronic pain treated with opioids.

Abuse of Butrans poses a significant risk to the abuser that could potentially result in overdose or death [see Drug Abuse and Dependence (9)].

Contact your state professional licensing board or state controlled substances authority for information on how to prevent and detect abuse or diversion of this product.

5.8 Hepatotoxicity

Although not observed in Butrans chronic pain clinical trials, cases of cytolytic hepatitis and hepatitis with jaundice have been observed in individuals receiving sublingual buprenorphine for the treatment of opioid dependence, both in clinical trials and through post-marketing adverse event reports. The spectrum of abnormalities ranges from transient asymptomatic elevations in hepatic transaminases to case reports of hepatic failure, hepatic necrosis, hepatorenal syndrome, and hepatic encephalopathy. In many cases, the presence of pre-existing liver enzyme abnormalities, infection with hepatitis B or hepatitis C virus, concomitant usage of other potentially hepatotoxic drugs, and ongoing injection drug abuse may have played a causative or contributory role. In other cases, insufficient data were available to determine the etiology of the abnormality. The possibility exists that buprenorphine had a causative or contributory role in the development of the hepatic abnormality in some cases. For patients at increased risk of hepatotoxicity (e.g., patients with a history of excessive alcohol intake, intravenous drug abuse or liver disease), baseline and periodic monitoring of liver function during treatment with Butrans is recommended. A biological and etiological evaluation is recommended when a hepatic event is suspected.

5.9 Application Site Skin Reactions

In rare cases, severe application site skin reactions with signs of marked inflammation including "burn," "discharge," and "vesicles" have occurred. Time of onset varies, ranging from days to months following the initiation of Butrans treatment. Instruct patients to promptly report the development of severe application site reactions and discontinue therapy.

5.10 Anaphylactic/Allergic Reactions

Cases of acute and chronic hypersensitivity to buprenorphine have been reported both in clinical trials and in the post-marketing experience. The most common signs and symptoms include rashes, hives, and pruritus. Cases of bronchospasm, angioneurotic edema, and anaphylactic shock have been reported. A history of hypersensitivity to buprenorphine is a contraindication to the use of Butrans.

5.11 Application of External Heat

Advise patients and their caregivers to avoid exposing the Butrans application site and surrounding area to direct external heat sources, such as heating pads or electric blankets, heat or tanning lamps, saunas, hot tubs, and heated water beds, etc., while wearing the system because an increase in absorption of buprenorphine may occur [see Clinical Pharmacology (12.3)]. Advise patients against exposure of the Butrans application site and surrounding area to hot water or prolonged exposure to direct sunlight. There is a potential for temperature-dependent increases in buprenorphine released from the system resulting in possible overdose and death.

5.12 Patients with Fever

Patients wearing Butrans systems who develop fever or increased core body temperature due to strenuous exertion should be monitored for opioid side effects and the Butrans dose should be adjusted if necessary [see Dosage and Administration (2.4)].

5.13 Driving and Operating Machinery

Butrans may impair the mental and physical abilities needed to perform potentially hazardous activities such as driving a car or operating machinery. Caution patients accordingly.

5.14 Seizures

Butrans, as with other opioids, may aggravate seizure disorders, may lower seizure threshold, and therefore, may induce seizures in some clinical settings. Use Butrans with caution in patients with a history of seizure disorders.

5.15 Special Risk Groups

Use Butrans with caution in the following conditions, due to increased risk of adverse reactions: alcoholism; delirium tremens; adrenocortical insufficiency; CNS depression; debilitation; kyphoscoliosis associated with respiratory compromise; myxedema or hypothyroidism; prostatic hypertrophy or urethral stricture; severe impairment of hepatic, pulmonary or renal function; and toxic psychosis.

5.16 Use in Pancreatic/Biliary Tract Disease and Other Gastrointestinal Conditions

Butrans may cause spasm of the sphincter of Oddi. Use with caution in patients with biliary tract disease, including acute pancreatitis. Opioids, including Butrans, may cause increased serum amylase.

The administration of Butrans may obscure the diagnosis or clinical course in patients with acute abdominal conditions. Use Butrans with caution in patients who are at risk of developing ileus.

5.17 Use in Addiction Treatment

Butrans has not been studied and is not approved for use in the management of addictive disorders.

5.18 MAO Inhibitors

Butrans is not recommended for use in patients who have received MAO inhibitors within 14 days, because severe and unpredictable potentiation by MAO inhibitors has been reported with opioid analgesics.

6 ADVERSE REACTIONS

The following adverse reactions described elsewhere in the labeling include:

- Respiratory Depression [see Warnings and Precautions (5.1)]
- CNS Depression [see Warnings and Precautions (5.2)]
- QTc Prolongation [see Warnings and Precautions (5.4)]
- Hypotensive Effects [see Warnings and Precautions (5.6)]
- Application Site Skin Reactions [see Warnings and Precautions (5.9)]
- Anaphylactic/Allergic Reactions [see Warnings and Precautions (5.10)]
- Seizures [see Warnings and Precautions (5.14)]

6.1 Clinical Trial Experience

Because clinical trials are conducted under widely varying conditions, adverse reaction rates observed in the clinical trials of a drug cannot be directly compared to rates in the clinical trials of another drug and may not reflect the rates observed in practice.

A total of 5415 patients were treated with Butrans in controlled and open-label chronic pain clinical trials. Nine hundred twenty-four subjects were treated for approximately six months and 183 subjects were treated for approximately one year. The clinical trial population consisted of patients with persistent moderate to severe pain.

The most common adverse reactions (≥5%) reported by patients in clinical trials comparing Butrans 10 or 20 mcg/hour to placebo are shown in Tables 2, and comparing Butrans 20 mcg/hour to Butrans 5 mcg/hour are shown in Table 3 below:

Table 2: Adverse Events Reported in ≥ 5% of Patients during the Open-Label Titration Period and Double-Blind Treatment Period: Opioid-Naïve Patients

MedDRA Preferred Term	Open-Label Titration Period Butrans	Double-Blind Treatment Period Butrans	Double-Blind Treatment Period Placebo
	(N = 1024)	(N = 256)	(N = 283)
Nausea	23%	13%	11%
Dizziness	10%	4%	1%
Headache	10%	5%	5%
Application site pruritus	8%	4%	7%
Somnolence	8%	2%	2%
Vomiting	8%	4%	2%
Constipation	7%	4%	1%

Table 3: Adverse Events Reported in ≥ 5% of Patients during the Open-Label Titration Period and Double-Blind Treatment Period: Opioid-Experienced Patients

MedDRA Preferred Term	Open-Label Titration Period Butrans	Double-Blind Treatment Period Butrans 20	Double-Blind Treatment Period Butrans 5
	(N = 1160)	(N = 219)	(N = 221)
Nausea	15%	12%	8%
Headache	11%	11%	5%
Application site pruritus	9%	13%	5%
Somnolence	6%	5%	2%
Vomiting	5%	5%	2%
Dizziness	5%	5%	2%
Constipation	4%	6%	3%
Application site erythema	3%	10%	5%
Application site rash	3%	9%	6%
Application site irritation	2%	5%	3%

The following table lists adverse events that were reported in at least 2.0% of patients in four placebo/active-controlled titration-to-effect trials.

Table 4: Adverse Events Reported in Titration-to-Effect Placebo/Active-Controlled Clinical Trials with Incidence ≥2%

MedDRA Preferred Term	Butrans (N = 392)	Placebo (N = 261)
Nausea	23%	8%
Dizziness	16%	8%
Headache	16%	11%
Application site pruritus	15%	12%
Constipation	14%	5%
Somnolence	14%	5%
Vomiting	11%	2%
Peripheral edema	7%	3%
Dry mouth	7%	2%
Application site erythema	7%	2%
Application site rash	6%	6%
Fatigue	5%	1%
Hyperhidrosis	4%	1%
Pruritus	4%	1%
Fall	4%	2%
Diarrhea	3%	2%
Pain in extremity	3%	2%
Insomnia	3%	2%
Dyspnea	3%	1%
Dyspepsia	3%	3%
Urinary tract infection	3%	2%
Back pain	3%	2%
Joint swelling	3%	1%
Hypoesthesia	2%	1%
Arthralgia	2%	2%
Stomach discomfort	2%	1%
Rash	2%	1%
Anorexia	2%	1%
Paraesthesia	2%	1%
Tremor	2%	<1%
Confusional State	2%	3%

The adverse events seen in controlled and open-label studies are presented below in the following manner: most common (≥5%), common (≥1%-<5%), and less common (<1%). The most common adverse events (≥5%) reported by patients treated with Butrans in the clinical trials were nausea, headache, application site pruritus, dizziness, constipation, somnolence, vomiting, application site erythema, dry mouth, and application site rash.

The common (≥1% to <5%) adverse events reported by patients treated with Butrans in the clinical trials organized by MedDRA (Medical Dictionary for Regulatory Activities) System Organ Class were:

Gastrointestinal disorders: diarrhea, dyspepsia, and upper abdominal pain

General disorders and administration site conditions: fatigue, peripheral edema, application site irritation, pain, pyrexia, chest pain, and asthenia

Infections and infestations: urinary tract infection, upper respiratory tract infection, nasopharyngitis, influenza, sinusitis, and bronchitis

Injury, poisoning and procedural complications: fall

Metabolism and nutrition disorders: anorexia

Musculoskeletal and connective tissue disorders: back pain, arthralgia, pain in extremity, muscle spasms, musculoskeletal pain, joint swelling, neck pain, and myalgia

Nervous system disorders: hypoesthesia, tremor, migraine, and paresthesia

Psychiatric disorders: insomnia, anxiety, and depression

Respiratory, thoracic and mediastinal disorders: dyspnea, pharyngolaryngeal pain, and cough

Skin and subcutaneous tissue disorders: pruritus, hyperhidrosis, rash, and generalized pruritus

Vascular disorders: hypertension

Other less common adverse events, including those known to occur with opioid treatment, that were seen in <1% of the patients in the Butrans trials include the following in alphabetical order:

Abdominal distention, abdominal pain, accidental injury, affect lability, agitation, alanine aminotransferase increased, angina pectoris, angioedema, apathy, application site dermatitis, asthma aggravated, bradycardia, chills, confusional state, contact dermatitis, coordination abnormal, dehydration, depressed level of consciousness, depressed mood, depersonalization, disorientation, disturbance in attention, diverticulitis, drug hypersensitivity, drug withdrawal syndrome, dry eye, dry skin, dysarthria, dysgeusia, dysmenorrhea, dysphagia, euphoric mood, face edema, flatulence, flushing, gait disturbance, hallucination, hiccups, hot flush, hyperventilation, hypotension, hypoventilation, ileus, insomnia, libido decreased, loss of consciousness, malaise, memory impairment, mental impairment, mental status changes, miosis, muscle weakness, nervousness, nightmare, orthostatic hypotension, palpitations, psychotic disorder, respiration abnormal, respiratory depression, respiratory distress, respiratory failure, restlessness, rhinitis, sedation, sexual dysfunction, syncope, tachycardia, tinnitus, urinary hesitation, urinary incontinence, urinary retention, urticaria, vasodilatation, vertigo, vision blurred, visual disturbance, weight decreased, and wheezing.

7 DRUG INTERACTIONS

7.1 Metabolic Drug Interactions

CYP3A4 Inhibitors

Co-administration of ketoconazole, a strong CYP3A4 inhibitor, with Butrans, did not have any effect on Cmax and AUC of buprenorphine. Based on this observation, pharmacokinetics of Butrans is not expected to be affected by co-administration of CYP3A4 inhibitors.

However, certain protease inhibitors (PIs) with CYP3A4 inhibitory activity such as atazanavir and atazanavir/ritonavir resulted in elevated levels of buprenorphine and norbuprenorphine following sublingual administration of buprenorphine and naloxone. Patients in this study reported increased sedation, and symptoms of opiate excess have been found in post-marketing reports of patients receiving sublingual buprenorphine and atazanavir with and without ritonavir concomitantly. It should be noted that atazanavir is both a CYP3A4 and UGT1A1 inhibitor. As such, the drug-drug interaction potential for buprenorphine with CYP3A4 inhibitors is likely to be dependent on the route of administration as well as the specificity of enzyme inhibition [see Clinical Pharmacology (12.3)].

CYP3A4 Inducers

The interaction between buprenorphine and CYP3A4 enzyme inducers has not been studied; therefore it is recommended that patients receiving Butrans be closely monitored for reduced efficacy if inducers of CYP3A4 (e.g. phenobarbital, carbamazepine, phenytoin, rifampin) are co-administered [see Clinical Pharmacology (12.3)].

7.2 Non-Metabolic Drug Interactions

Benzodiazepines

There have been a number of reports regarding coma and death associated with the misuse and abuse of the combination of buprenorphine and benzodiazepines. In many, but not all of these cases, buprenorphine was misused by self-injection of crushed buprenorphine tablets. Preclinical studies have shown that the combination of benzodiazepines and buprenorphine altered the usual ceiling effect on buprenorphine-induced respiratory depression, making the respiratory effects of buprenorphine appear similar to those of full opioid agonists. Prescribe Butrans with caution to patients taking benzodiazepines or other drugs that act on the central nervous system regardless of whether these drugs are taken on the advice of a physician or are being abused/misused. Warn patients that it is extremely dangerous to self-administer benzodiazepines while taking Butrans, and caution patients to use benzodiazepines concurrently with Butrans only as directed by their physician.

Skeletal Muscle Relaxants

Butrans, like other opioids, may interact with skeletal muscle relaxants to enhance neuromuscular blocking action and increase respiratory depression.

8 USE IN SPECIFIC POPULATIONS

8.1 Pregnancy

Pregnancy Category C

There are no adequate and well-controlled studies with Butrans in pregnant women. Butrans should be used during pregnancy only if the potential benefit justifies the potential risk to the mother and the fetus. In animal studies, buprenorphine caused an increase in the number of stillborn offspring, reduced litter size, and reduced offspring growth in rats at maternal exposure levels that were approximately 10 times that of human subjects who received one Butrans 20 mcg/hour, the maximum recommended human dose (MRHD).

Teratogenic Effects

Studies in rats and rabbits demonstrated no evidence of teratogenicity following Butrans or subcutaneous (SC) administration of buprenorphine during the period of major organogenesis. Rats were administered up to one Butrans 20 mcg/hour every 3 days (gestation days 6, 9, 12, & 15) or received daily SC buprenorphine up to 5 mg/kg (gestation days 6-17). Rabbits were administered four Butrans 20 mcg/hour every 3 days (gestation days 6, 9, 12, 15, 18, & 19) or received daily SC buprenorphine up to 5 mg/kg (gestation days 6-19). No teratogenicity was observed at any dose. Area under the curve (AUC) values for buprenorphine with Butrans application and SC injection were approximately 140 and 110 times that of human subjects who received the MRHD of one Butrans 20 mcg/hour.

Non-Teratogenic Effects

In a peri- and post-natal study conducted in pregnant and lactating rats, administration of buprenorphine either as Butrans or SC buprenorphine was associated with toxicity to offspring. Buprenorphine was present in maternal milk. Pregnant rats were administered 1/4 of one Butrans 5 mcg/hour every 3 days or received daily SC buprenorphine at doses of 0.05, 0.5, or 5 mg/kg from gestation day 6 to lactation day 21 (weaning). Administration of Butrans or SC buprenorphine at 0.5 or 5 mg/kg caused maternal toxicity and an increase in the number of stillborns, reduced litter size, and reduced offspring growth at maternal exposure levels that were approximately 10 times that of human subjects who received the MRHD of one Butrans 20 mcg/hour. Maternal toxicity was also observed at the no observed adverse effect level (NOAEL) for offspring.

8.2 Labor and Delivery

The safety of Butrans given during labor and delivery has not been established.

Opioids cross the placenta and may produce respiratory depression and psychophysiologic effects in neonates. Butrans is not recommended for use in women immediately prior to and during labor, when use of shorter-acting analgesics or other analgesic techniques are more appropriate. Occasionally, opioid analgesics may prolong labor through actions which temporarily reduce the strength, duration and frequency of uterine contractions. However this effect is not consistent and may be offset by an increased rate of cervical dilatation, which tends to shorten labor.

Closely observe neonates whose mothers received opioid analgesics during labor for signs of respiratory depression. Have a specific opioid antagonist, such as naloxone or nalmefene, available for reversal of opioid-induced respiratory depression in the neonate.

Neonates whose mothers have been taking opioids chronically may also exhibit withdrawal signs, either at birth and/or in the nursery, because they have developed physical dependence. This is not, however, synonymous with addiction. Neonatal opioid withdrawal syndrome, unlike opioid withdrawal syndrome in adults, may be life-threatening and should be treated according to protocols developed by neonatology experts.

8.3 Nursing Mothers

Buprenorphine has been detected in low concentrations in human milk. Breast-feeding is not advised in mothers treated with Butrans.

8.4 Pediatric Use

The safety and efficacy of Butrans in patients under 18 years of age has not been established. Butrans is not recommended for use in pediatric patients.

8.5 Geriatric Use

Of the total number of subjects in the clinical trials (5,415), Butrans was administered to 1,377 patients aged 65 years and older. Of those, 457 patients were 75 years of age and older. In the clinical program, the incidences of selected Butrans-related AEs were higher in older subjects. The incidences of application site AEs were slightly higher among subjects <65 years of age than those ≥ 65 years of age for both Butrans and placebo treatment groups.

In a single-dose study of healthy elderly and healthy young subjects treated with Butrans 10 mcg/hour, the pharmacokinetics and safety outcomes were similar. In a separate dose-escalation safety study, the pharmacokinetics in the healthy elderly and hypertensive elderly subjects taking thiazide diuretics were similar to those in the healthy young adults. In the elderly groups evaluated, adverse event rates were similar to or lower than rates in healthy young adult subjects, except for constipation and urinary retention, which were more common in the elderly. Although specific dose adjustments on the basis of advanced age are not re-

quired for pharmacokinetic reasons, use caution in the elderly population to ensure safe use [see Dosage and Administration (2.4) and Clinical Pharmacology (12.3)].

8.6 Hepatic Impairment

In a study utilizing intravenous buprenorphine, peak plasma levels (C_{max}) and exposure (AUC) of buprenorphine in patients with mild and moderate hepatic impairment did not increase as compared to those observed in subjects with normal hepatic function. Butrans has not been evaluated in patients with severe hepatic impairment and should be administered with caution [see Dosage and Administration (2.4), and Clinical Pharmacology (12.3)].

8.7 Renal Impairment

The pharmacokinetics of buprenorphine is not altered during the course of renal failure [see Clinical Pharmacology (12.3)].

8.8 Gender Differences

There was no significant gender effect observed for Butrans with respect to either the incidence of adverse events or pharmacokinetics [see Clinical Pharmacology (12.3)].

9 DRUG ABUSE AND DEPENDENCE

9.1 Controlled Substance

Butrans contains buprenorphine, a mu opioid partial agonist and Schedule III controlled substance. Butrans can be abused and is subject to misuse, abuse, addiction and criminal diversion.

9.2 Abuse

Abuse of Butrans poses a hazard of overdose and death. This risk is increased with compromise of the Butrans Transdermal System and with concurrent abuse of alcohol or other substances. Butrans has been diverted for nonmedical use.

All patients treated with opioids, including Butrans, require careful monitoring for signs of abuse and addiction, because use of opioid analgesic products carries the risk of addiction even under appropriate medical use.

Addiction is a primary, chronic, neurobiologic disease, with genetic, psychosocial, and environmental factors influencing its development and manifestations. It is characterized by behaviors that include one or more of the following: impaired control over drug use, compulsive use, continued use despite harm, and craving. Opioid drugs are sought by people with substance use disorders (abuse or addiction, the latter of which is also called "substance dependence") and criminals who supply them by diverting medicines out of legitimate distribution channels. Butrans is a target for theft and diversion.

"Drug-seeking" behavior is very common in persons with substance use disorders. Drug-seeking tactics include, but are not limited to, emergency calls or visits near the end of office hours, refusal to undergo appropriate examination, testing or referral, repeated "loss" of prescriptions, altering or forging of prescriptions and reluctance to provide prior medical records or contact information for other treating physician(s). "Doctor shopping" to obtain additional prescriptions is common among people with untreated substance use disorders, and criminals who divert controlled substances.

Abuse and addiction are separate and distinct from physical dependence and tolerance. Physicians should be aware that addiction may not be accompanied by concurrent tolerance and symptoms of physical dependence in all addicts. In addition, abuse of opioids can occur in the absence of true addiction and is characterized by misuse for nonmedical purposes, often in combination with other psychoactive substances. Since Butrans may be diverted for non-medical use, careful record-keeping of prescribing information, including quantity, frequency, and renewal requests is strongly advised.

The risks of misuse and abuse should be considered when prescribing or dispensing Butrans. Concerns about abuse and addiction, should not prevent the proper management of pain, however. Treatment of pain should be individualized, balancing the potential benefits and risks for each patient.

Butrans is intended for transdermal use only. Compromising the transdermal delivery system will result in the uncontrolled delivery of buprenorphine and pose a significant risk to the abuser that could result in overdose and death [see Warnings and Precautions (5.1)]. The risk of fatal overdose is further increased when buprenorphine is abused concurrently with alcohol or other CNS depressants, including other opioids and benzodiazepines [see Warnings and Precautions (5.3)]. Abuse may occur by applying the transdermal system in the absence of legitimate purpose, or by swallowing, snorting or injecting buprenorphine extracted from the transdermal system.

Proper assessment of the patient, proper prescribing practices, periodic re-evaluation of therapy, proper dispensing and correct storage and handling are appropriate measures that help to limit misuse and abuse of opioid drugs. Careful record-keeping of prescribing information, including quantity, frequency, and renewal requests is strongly advised.

Healthcare professionals should contact their State Professional Licensing Board or State Controlled Substances Authority for information on how to prevent and detect abuse or diversion of this product.

9.3 Physical Dependence and Tolerance

Tolerance is a state of adaptation in which exposure to a drug induces changes that result in a diminution of one or more of the drug's effects over time. Tolerance could occur to both the desired and undesired effects of drugs, and may develop at different rates for different effects.

Physical dependence to an opioid is manifested by characteristic withdrawal signs and symptoms after abrupt discontinuation of a drug, significant dose reduction, or upon administration of an antagonist. Physical dependence and tolerance are not unusual during chronic opioid analgesic therapy.

The opioid abstinence or withdrawal syndrome in adults is characterized by some or all of the following: restlessness, lacrimation, rhinorrhea, yawning, perspiration, chills, piloerection, myalgia, mydriasis, irritability, anxiety, backache, joint pain, weakness, abdominal cramps, insomnia, nausea, anorexia, vomiting, diarrhea, or increased blood pressure, respiratory rate, or heart rate [see Use In Specific Populations (8.2)]

Infants born to mothers physically dependent on opioids will also be physically dependent and may exhibit respiratory difficulties and withdrawal symptoms.

In general, opioids should not be abruptly discontinued [see Dosage and Administration (2.5)].

10 OVERDOSAGE

10.1 Symptoms

Acute overdosage with Butrans can be manifested by respiratory depression, somnolence progressing to stupor or coma, skeletal muscle flaccidity, cold and clammy skin, constricted pupils, bradycardia, hypotension, partial or complete airway obstruction, atypical snoring and death.

Deaths due to overdose have been reported with abuse and misuse of buprenorphine. Review of case reports has indicated that the risk of fatal overdose is further increased when Butrans is abused concurrently with alcohol or other CNS depressants, including other opioids.

10.2 Treatment

In cases of overdose, remove Butrans immediately. It is important to take the pharmacokinetic profile of Butrans into account when treating overdose. Even in the face of improvement, continued medical monitoring is required because of the possibility of extended effects as opioid continues to be absorbed from the skin. After removal of Butrans, the mean buprenorphine concentrations decrease approximately 50% in 12 hours (range 10-24 hours) with an apparent terminal half-life of approximately 26 hours. Due to this long apparent terminal half-life, patients may require monitoring and treatment for at least 24 hours.

In the treatment of Butrans overdosage, primary attention should be given to the maintenance of a patent airway, and of effective ventilation (clearance of CO_2) and oxygenation, whether by spontaneous, assisted or controlled respiration. Supportive measures (including oxygen and vasopressors) should be employed in the management of circulatory shock and pulmonary edema accompanying overdose as indicated. Cardiac arrest or arrhythmias may require cardiac massage or defibrillation.

Naloxone may not be effective in reversing any respiratory depression produced by buprenorphine. High doses of naloxone, 10-35 mg/70 kg, may be of limited value in the management of buprenorphine overdose. The onset of naloxone effect may be delayed by 30 minutes or more. Doxapram hydrochloride (a respiratory stimulant) has also been used. Since the duration of action of Butrans may exceed that of the antagonist, keep the patient under continued surveillance and administer repeated doses of the antagonist according to the antagonist labeling as needed to maintain adequate respiration. Maintenance of adequate ventilation is essential when managing Butrans overdose and more important than specific antidote treatment with an opioid antagonist such as naloxone.

Do not administer opioid antagonists in the absence of clinically significant respiratory or circulatory depression secondary to buprenorphine overdose. In patients who are physically dependent on any opioid agonist including Butrans, an abrupt partial or complete reversal of opioid effects may precipitate an acute abstinence or withdrawal syndrome. The severity of the withdrawal syndrome produced will depend on the degree of physical dependence and the dose of the antagonist administered. See the prescribing information for the specific opioid antagonist for details of its proper use.

11 DESCRIPTION

Butrans is a transdermal system providing systemic delivery of buprenorphine, a mu opioid partial agonist analgesic, continuously for 7 days. The chemical name of buprenorphine is 6,14-ethenomorphinan-7-methanol, 17-(cyclopropylmethyl)- α-(1,1-dimethylethyl)-4, 5-epoxy-18,

19-dihydro-3-hydroxy-6-methoxy-α-methyl-, [5α, 7α, (S)]. The structural formula is:

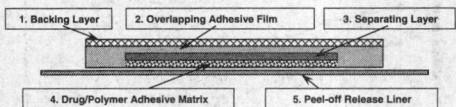

The molecular weight of buprenorphine is 467.6; the empirical formula is $C_{29}H_{41}NO_4$. Buprenorphine occurs as a white or almost white powder and is very slightly soluble in water, freely soluble in acetone, soluble in methanol and ether, and slightly soluble in cyclohexane. The pKa is 8.5 and the melting point is about 217°C.

System Components and Structure

Three different strengths of Butrans are available: 5, 10, and 20 mcg/hour (Table 5). The active component of the system is buprenorphine. The remaining components are pharmacologically inactive. The proportion of buprenorphine mixed in the adhesive matrix is the same in each of the 3 strengths. The amount of buprenorphine released from each system per hour is proportional to the active surface area of the system. The skin is the limiting barrier to diffusion from the system into the bloodstream.

Table 5: Butrans Product Specifications

Buprenorphine Delivery Rate (mcg/hour)	Active Surface Area (cm²)	Total Buprenorphine Content (mg)
Butrans 5	6.25	5
Butrans 10	12.5	10
Butrans 20	25	20

Butrans is a rectangular or square, beige-colored system consisting of a protective liner and functional layers. Proceeding from the outer surface toward the surface adhering to the skin, the layers are (1) a beige-colored web backing layer; (2) an adhesive rim without buprenorphine; (3) a separating layer over the buprenorphine-containing adhesive matrix; (4) the buprenorphine-containing adhesive matrix; and (5) a peel-off release liner. Before use, the release liner covering the adhesive layer is removed and discarded.

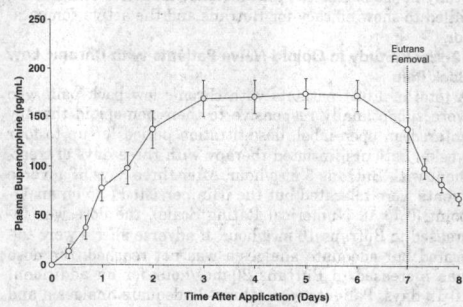

Figure 1 Cross-Section Diagram of Butrans (not to scale).

The active ingredient in Butrans is buprenorphine. The inactive ingredients in each system are: levulinic acid, oleyl oleate, povidone, and polyacrylate cross-linked with aluminum.

12 CLINICAL PHARMACOLOGY

12.1 Mechanism of Action

Buprenorphine is a partial agonist at mu opioid receptors. Buprenorphine is also an antagonist at kappa opioid receptors, an agonist at delta opioid receptors, and a partial agonist at ORL-1 (nociceptin) receptors. Its clinical actions result from binding to the opioid receptors.

12.2 Pharmacodynamics

Central Nervous System Effects

Buprenorphine binds to and dissociates from the mu opioid receptor slowly.

Cardiovascular Effects

Buprenorphine may cause a reduction in blood pressure

Electrophysiology

The effect of Butrans 10 mcg/hour and 2 × Butrans 20 mcg/hour on QTc interval was evaluated in a double-blind (Butrans vs. placebo), randomized, placebo and active-controlled (moxifloxacin 400 mg, open label), parallel-group, dose-escalating, single-dose study in 132 healthy male and female subjects aged 18 to 55 years. The dose escalation sequence for Butrans during the titration period was: Butrans 5 mcg/hour for 3 days, then Butrans 10 mcg/hour for 3 days, then Butrans 20 mcg/hour for 3 days, then 2 × Butrans 20 mcg/hour for 4 days. The QTc evaluation was performed during the third day of Butrans 10 mcg/hour and the fourth day of 2 × Butrans 20 mcg/hour when the plasma levels of buprenorphine were at steady state for the corresponding doses [see Warnings and Precautions (5.4)].

There was no clinically meaningful effect on mean QTc with a Butrans dose of 10 mcg/hour. A Butrans dose of 40 mcg/hour (given as two 20 mcg/hour Butrans Transdermal Systems) prolonged mean QTc by a maximum of 9.2 (90% CI: 5.2-13.3) msec across the 13 assessment time points.

Endocrine Effects

Opioids may influence the hypothalamic-pituitary-adrenal or -gonadal axes. Some changes that can be seen include an increase in serum prolactin, and decreases in plasma cortisol and testosterone. Clinical symptoms may be manifest from these hormonal changes.

Other Effects

Buprenorphine causes dose-related miosis and produces urinary retention in some patients.

In-vitro and animal studies indicate various effects of naturally-occurring opioids, such as morphine, on components of the immune system. The clinical significance of these findings is unknown. Whether buprenorphine, a semi-synthetic opioid, has immunological effects similar to morphine is unknown.

12.3 Pharmacokinetics

Each Butrans system provides delivery of buprenorphine for 7 days (see Figure 2). Steady state was achieved during the first application by Day 3.

Figure 2
Buprenorphine Plasma Concentrations (pg/mL)
Mean (±SE), Butrans 10 mcg/hour Application for 7 Days
(N = 23 Healthy Subjects)

Butrans 5, 10, and 20 mcg/hour provide dose-proportional total buprenorphine exposures (AUC) following 7-day applications (see Table 6). Plasma buprenorphine concentrations after titration showed no further change over the 60-day period studied. After removal of Butrans, mean buprenorphine concentrations decrease approximately 50% within 10-24 h, followed by decline with an apparent terminal half-life of approximately 26 hours.

Table 6: Pharmacokinetic Parameters of Butrans in Healthy Subjects (Single 7-day Application) Mean (%CV)

Dose (mcg/hour)	AUCinf (pg·h/mL)	Cmax (pg/mL)
Butrans 5	12087 (37)	176 (67)
Butrans 10	27035 (29)	191 (34)
Butrans 20	54294 (36)	471 (49)

Absorption

Transdermal delivery studies showed that intact human skin is permeable to buprenorphine. In clinical pharmacology studies, the median time for Butrans 10 mcg/hour to deliver quantifiable buprenorphine concentrations (≥25 pg/mL) was approximately 17 hours. The absolute bioavailability of Butrans relative to IV administration, following a 7-day application, is approximately 15% for all doses (Butrans 5, 10, and 20 mcg/hour).

Distribution

Buprenorphine is approximately 96% bound to plasma proteins, mainly to alpha- and beta-globulin.

Studies of IV buprenorphine have shown a large volume of distribution (approximately 430 L), implying extensive distribution of buprenorphine.

Following IV administration, buprenorphine and its metabolites are secreted into bile and excreted in urine. CSF buprenorphine concentrations appear to be approximately 15-25% of concurrent plasma concentrations.

Metabolism

Buprenorphine metabolism in the skin following Butrans application is negligible. Following transdermal application, buprenorphine is eliminated via hepatic metabolism, with subsequent biliary excretion and renal excretion of soluble metabolites.

Buprenorphine primarily undergoes N-dealkylation by CYP3A4 to norbuprenorphine and glucuronidation by UGT-isoenzymes (mainly UGT1A1 and 2B7) to buprenorphine

3-O-glucuronide. Norbuprenorphine, the major metabolite, is also glucuronidated (mainly UGT1A3) prior to excretion. Norbuprenorphine is the only known active metabolite of buprenorphine. It has been shown to be a respiratory depressant in rats, but only at concentrations at least 50-fold greater than those observed following application to humans of Butrans 20 mcg/hour.

Since metabolism and excretion of buprenorphine occur mainly via hepatic elimination, reductions in hepatic blood flow induced by some general anesthetics (e.g., halothane) and other drugs may result in a decreased rate of hepatic elimination of the drug, resulting in increased plasma concentrations.

Excretion

Following intramuscular administration of 2 mcg/kg dose of buprenorphine, approximately 70% of the dose was excreted in feces within 7 days. Approximately 27% was excreted in urine. The total clearance of buprenorphine is approximately 55 L/hour in postoperative patients.

Drug Interactions

Effect of CYP3A4 inhibitors

In a drug-drug interaction study, Butrans 10 mcg/hour (single dose × 7 days) was co-administered with 200 mg ketoconazole, a strong CYP3A4 inhibitor or ketoconazole placebo twice daily for 11 days and the pharmacokinetics of buprenorphine and its metabolites were evaluated. Plasma buprenorphine concentrations did not accumulate during co-medication with ketoconazole 200 mg twice daily. Based on the results from this study, metabolism during therapy with Butrans is not expected to be affected by co-administration of CYP3A4 inhibitors [see Drug Interactions (7.1)].

Antiretroviral agents have been evaluated for CYP3A4 mediated interactions with sublingual buprenorphine. Nucleoside reverse transcriptase inhibitors (NRTIs) and non-nucleoside reverse transcriptase inhibitors (NNRTIs) do not appear to have clinically significant interactions with buprenorphine. However, certain protease inhibitors (PIs) with CYP3A4 inhibitory activity such as atazanavir and atazanavir/ritonavir resulted in elevated levels of buprenorphine and norbuprenorphine when buprenorphine and naloxone were administered sublingually. C_{max} and AUC for buprenorphine increased by up to 1.6 and 1.9 fold, and C_{max} and AUC for norbuprenorphine increased by up to 1.6 and 2.0 fold respectively, when sublingual buprenorphine was administered with these PIs. Patients in this study reported increased sedation, and symptoms of opiate excess have been found in post-marketing reports of patients receiving buprenorphine and atazanavir with and without ritonavir concomitantly. It should be noted that atazanavir is both a CYP3A4 and UGT1A1 inhibitor. As such, the drug-drug interaction potential for buprenorphine with CYP3A4 inhibitors is likely to be dependent on the route of administration as well as the specificity of enzyme inhibition [see Drug Interactions (7.1)].

Effect of CYP3A4 inducers on buprenorphine

The interaction between buprenorphine and CYP3A4 inducers has not been studied.

Application Site

A study in healthy subjects demonstrated that the pharmacokinetic profile of buprenorphine delivered by Butrans 10 mcg/hour is similar when applied to the upper outer arm, upper chest, upper back, or the side of the chest [see Dosage and Administration (2.3)].

The reapplication of Butrans 10 mcg/hour after various rest periods to the same application site in healthy subjects showed that the minimum rest period needed to avoid variability in drug absorption is 3 weeks (21 days) [see Dosage and Administration (2.3)].

External Heat

In a study of healthy subjects, application of a heating pad directly on the Butrans 10 mcg/hour system caused a 26-55% increase in blood concentrations of buprenorphine. Concentrations returned to normal within 5 hours after the heat was removed. For this reason, applying heating pads directly to the Butrans system during system wear should be avoided [see Warnings and Precautions (5.11)].

Endotoxin Challenge

Fever may increase the permeability of the skin, leading to increased buprenorphine concentrations during Butrans treatment. As a result, febrile patients are at increased risk for the possibility of Butrans-related reactions during treatment with Butrans. Monitor patients with febrile illness for adverse effects and consider dose adjustment [see Warnings and Precautions (5.10)]. In a crossover study of healthy subjects receiving endotoxin or placebo challenge during Butrans 10 mcg/hour wear, the AUC and C_{max} were similar despite a physiologic response of mild fever to endotoxin.

Flux Determination

Buprenorphine flux for the 7-day application period was established to be 5, 10, and 20 mcg/hour, for Butrans containing 5, 10, and 20 mg of buprenorphine, respectively.

Specific Populations

Gender

In a pooled data analysis utilizing data from several studies that administered Butrans 10 mcg/hour to healthy subjects, no differences in buprenorphine C_{max} and AUC or body-weight normalized C_{max} and AUC were observed between males and females treated with Butrans *[see Use In Specific Populations (8.8)]*.

Geriatric

Following a single application of Butrans 10 mcg/hour to 12 healthy young adults (mean age 32 years) and 12 healthy elderly subjects (mean age 72 years), the pharmacokinetic profile of Butrans was similar in healthy elderly and healthy young adult subjects, though the elderly subjects showed a trend toward higher plasma concentrations immediately after Butrans removal. Both groups eliminated buprenorphine at similar rates after system removal *[see Dosage and Administration (2.4) and Use In Specific Populations (8.5)]*.

In a study of healthy young subjects, healthy elderly subjects, and elderly subjects treated with thiazide diuretics, Butrans at a fixed dose-escalation schedule (Butrans 5 mcg/hour for 3 days, followed by Butrans 10 mcg/hour for 3 days and Butrans 20 mcg/hour for 7 days) produced similar mean plasma concentration vs. time profiles for each of the three subject groups. There were no significant differences between groups in buprenorphine C_{max} or AUC *[see Dosage and Administration (2.4) and Use In Specific Populations (8.5)]*.

Pediatrics

Butrans has not been studied in children and is not recommended for pediatric use.

Renal Impairment

No studies in patients with renal impairment have been performed with Butrans.

In an independent study, the effect of impaired renal function on buprenorphine pharmacokinetics after IV bolus and after continuous IV infusion administrations was evaluated. It was found that plasma buprenorphine concentrations were similar in patients with normal renal function and in patients with impaired renal function or renal failure. In a separate investigation of the effect of intermittent hemodialysis on buprenorphine plasma concentrations in chronic pain patients with end-stage renal disease who were treated with a transdermal buprenorphine product (marketed outside the US) up to 70 mcg/hour, no significant differences in buprenorphine plasma concentrations before or after hemodialysis were observed *[see Dosage and Administration (2.4) and Use In Specific Populations (8.7)]*.

No notable relationship was observed between estimated creatinine clearance rates and steady-state buprenorphine concentrations among patients during Butrans therapy *[see Use In Specific Populations (8.7)]*.

Hepatic Impairment

The pharmacokinetics of buprenorphine following an IV infusion of 0.3 mg of buprenorphine was compared in 8 patients with mild impairment (Child-Pugh A), 4 patients with moderate impairment (Child-Pugh B) and 12 subjects with normal hepatic function. Buprenorphine and norbuprenorphine exposure did not increase in the mild and moderate hepatic impairment patients.

Butrans has not been evaluated in patients with severe (Child-Pugh C) hepatic impairment *[See Dosage and Administration (2.4), Warnings and Precautions (5.1) and Use In Specific Populations (8.6)]*.

13 NONCLINICAL TOXICOLOGY

13.1 Carcinogenesis, Mutagenesis, Impairment of Fertility

Carcinogenesis

Buprenorphine administered daily by skin painting to Sprague Dawley rats for 100 weeks at dosages (20, 60, or 200 mg/kg) produced systemic exposures (based on area under the curve, AUC) that ranged from approximately 130 to 350 times that of human subjects administered the maximum recommended human dose (MRHD) of Butrans 20 mcg/hour. An increased incidence of benign testicular interstitial cell tumors, considered buprenorphine treatment-related, was observed in male rats compared with concurrent controls. The tumor incidence was also above the highest incidence in the historical control database of the testing facility. These tumors were noted at 60 mg/kg/day and higher at approximately 220 times the proposed MRHD based on AUC). The no observed effect level (NOEL) was 20 mg/kg/day (approximately 140 times the proposed MRHD based on AUC). The mechanism leading to the tumor findings and relevance to humans is unknown.

Buprenorphine was administered by skin painting to hemizygous Tg.AC mice over a 6-month study period. At the dosages administered daily (18.75, 37.5, 150, or 600 mg/kg/day), buprenorphine was not carcinogenic or tumorigenic at systemic exposure to buprenorphine, based on AUC, of up to approximately 1000 times that of human subjects administered Butrans 20 mcg/hour, the MRHD.

Mutagenesis

Buprenorphine was not genotoxic in 3 in-vitro genetic toxicology studies (bacterial mutagenicity test, mouse lymphoma assay, chromosomal aberration assay in human peripheral blood lymphocytes), and in one in vivo mouse micronucleus test).

Impairment of fertility

Butrans (1/4 of a Butrans 5 mcg/hour, one Butrans 5 mcg/hour, or one Butrans 20 mcg/hour) every 3 days in males for 4 weeks prior to mating for a total of 10 weeks and in females for 2 weeks prior to mating through gestation day 7) had no effect on fertility or general reproductive performance of rats at AUC-based exposure levels as high as approximately 65 times (females) and 100 times (males) that for human subjects who received Butrans 20 mcg/hour, the MRHD.

14 CLINICAL STUDIES

The efficacy of Butrans has been evaluated in four 12-week double-blind, controlled clinical trials in opioid-naïve and opioid-experienced patients with moderate to severe chronic low back pain or osteoarthritis using pain scores as the primary efficacy variable. Two of these studies, described below, demonstrated efficacy in patients with low back pain. One study in low back pain failed to show efficacy. One study in osteoarthritis, that included an active comparator, failed to show efficacy for Butrans and the active comparator.

12-Week Study in Opioid-Naïve Patients with Chronic Low Back Pain

A total of 1,024 patients with chronic low back pain who were suboptimally responsive to their non-opioid therapy entered an open-label, dose-titration period for up to four weeks. Patients initiated therapy with three days of treatment with Butrans 5 mcg/hour. After three days, if adverse events were tolerated but the pain persisted (≥5 on an 11-point, 0 to 10 Numerical Rating Scale), the dose was increased to Butrans 10 mcg/hour. If adverse effects were tolerated but adequate analgesia was not reached, the dose was increased to Butrans 20 mcg/hour for an additional 10-12 days. Patients who achieved adequate analgesia and tolerable adverse effects on Butrans were then randomized to remain on their titrated dose of Butrans or matching placebo. Fifty-three percent of the patients who entered the open-label titration period were able to titrate to a tolerable and effective dose and were randomized into a 12-week, double-blind treatment period. Twenty three percent of patients discontinued due to an adverse event from the open-label titration period and 14% discontinued due to lack of a therapeutic effect. The remaining ten percent of patients were dropped due to various administrative reasons.

During the first seven days of double-blind treatment patients were allowed up to two tablets per day of immediate-release oxycodone 5 mg as supplemental analgesia to minimize opioid withdrawal symptoms in patients randomized to placebo. Thereafter, the supplemental analgesia was limited to either acetaminophen 500 mg or ibuprofen 200 mg at a maximum of four tablets per day. Sixty-six percent of the patients treated with Butrans completed the 12-week treatment compared to 70% of the patients treated with placebo. Of the 256 patients randomized to Butrans, 9% discontinued due to lack of efficacy and 16% due to adverse events. Of the 283 patients randomized to placebo, 13% discontinued due to lack of efficacy and 7% due to adverse events.

Of the patients who were randomized, the mean pain (SE) NRS scores were 7.2 (0.08) and 7.2 (0.07) at screening and 2.6 (0.08) and 2.6 (0.07) at pre-randomization (beginning of double-blind phase) for the Butrans and placebo groups, respectively.

The score for average pain over the last 24 hours at the end of the study (Week 12/Early Termination) was statistically significantly lower for patients treated with Butrans compared with patients treated with placebo. The proportion of patients with various degrees of improvement, from screening to study endpoint, is shown Figure 3 below.

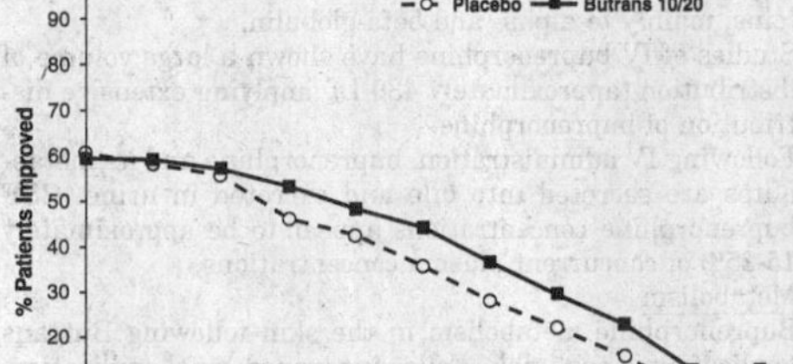

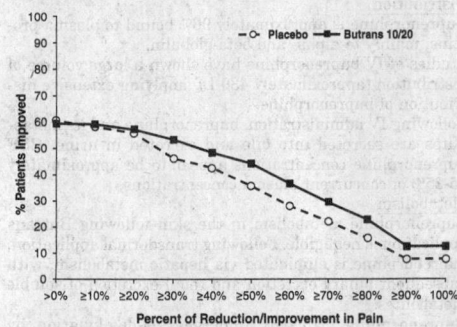

Figure 3 Percent Reduction in Pain Intensity

12-Week Study in Opioid-Experienced Patients with Chronic Low Back Pain

One thousand one hundred and sixty (1,160) patients on chronic opioid therapy (total daily dose 30-80 mg morphine equivalent) entered an open-label, dose-titration period with Butrans for up to 3 weeks, following taper of prior opioids. Patients initiated therapy with Butrans 10 mcg/hour for three days. After three days, if the patient tolerated the adverse effects, the dose was increased to Butrans 20 mcg/hour for up to 18 days. Patients with adequate analgesia and tolerable adverse effects on Butrans 20 mcg/hour were randomized to remain on Butrans 20 mcg/hour or were switched to a low-dose control (Butrans 5 mcg/hour) or an active control. Fifty-seven percent of the patients who entered the open-label titration period were able to titrate to and tolerate the adverse effects of Butrans 20 mcg/hour and were randomized into a 12-week double-blind treatment phase. Twelve percent of patients discontinued due to an adverse event and 21% discontinued due to lack of a therapeutic effect during the open-label titration period. During the double-blind period, patients were permitted to take ibuprofen (200 mg tablets) or acetaminophen (500 mg tablets) every 4 hours as needed for supplemental analgesia (up to 3200 mg of ibuprofen and 4 grams of acetaminophen daily). Sixty seven percent of patients treated with Butrans 20 mcg/hour and 58% of patients treated with Butrans 5 mcg/hour completed the 12-week treatment. Of the patients discontinuing the double-blind treatment early from the Butrans 20 mcg/hour group, 11% were for lack of efficacy and 13% were for adverse events. In the Butrans 5 mcg/hour group, 24% discontinued early due to lack of efficacy and 6% due to adverse events. Of the patients who were able to be randomized in the double-blind period, the mean pain (SE) NRS scores were 6.4 (0.08) and 6.5 (0.08) at screening and were 2.8 (0.08) and 2.9 (0.08) at pre-randomization (beginning of Double-Blind Period) for the Butrans 5 mcg/hour and Butrans 20 mcg/hour, respectively.

The score for average pain over the last 24 hours at Week 12 was statistically significantly lower for subjects treated with Butrans 20 mcg/hour compared to subjects treated with Butrans 5 mcg/hour. A higher proportion of Butrans 20 mcg/hour patients (49%) had at least a 30% reduction in pain score from screening to study endpoint when compared to Butrans 5 mcg/hour patients (33%). The proportion of patients with various degrees of improvement from screening to study endpoint is shown in Figure 4 below.

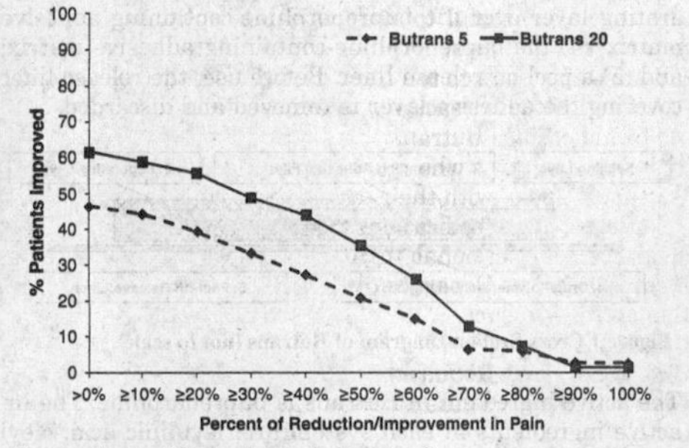

Figure 4 Percent Reduction in Pain Intensity

16 HOW SUPPLIED/STORAGE AND HANDLING

Butrans (buprenorphine) Transdermal System is supplied in cartons containing 4 individually-packaged systems and a pouch containing 4 Patch-Disposal Units.

Butrans 5 mcg/hour Transdermal System, 4-count carton **NDC 59011-750-04**

Butrans 10 mcg/hour Transdermal System, 4-count carton **NDC 59011-751-04**

Butrans 20 mcg/hour Transdermal System, 4-count carton **NDC 59011-752-04**

Store at 25°C (77°F); excursions permitted between 15°C-30°C (59°F-86°F).

Special Handling Instructions

If the buprenorphine-containing adhesive matrix accidentally contacts the skin, wash the area with water. Do not use soap, alcohol, or other solvents to remove the adhesive because they may enhance the absorption of the drug.

When changing the system, remove Butrans, fold it over on itself, and flush it down the toilet. Alternatively, Butrans can be sealed in the Patch-Disposal Unit provided and then disposed of in the trash. Never throw Butrans away in the trash without sealing it in the Patch-Disposal Unit.

Apply immediately after removal from the individually sealed pouch. Do not use Butrans if the pouch seal is broken or the patch is cut, damaged, or changed in any way. Butrans is for transdermal use only.

Keep Butrans out of the reach of children and pets.

17 PATIENT COUNSELING INFORMATION

See MEDICATION GUIDE (including Instructions for Use) as appended at the end of the full prescribing information.

17.1 Information for Patients and Caregivers

Provide the following information to patients receiving Butrans or their caregivers:

1. Advise patients to carefully follow instructions for the application, removal, and disposal of Butrans. Each week, apply Butrans to a different site based on the 8 described skin sites, with a minimum of 3 weeks between applications to a previously used site.
2. Advise patients to apply Butrans to a hairless or nearly hairless skin site. If none are available, instruct patients to clip the hair at the site and not to shave the area. Instruct patients not to apply to irritated skin. If the application site must be cleaned, use clear water only. Soaps, alcohol, oils, lotions, or abrasive devices should not be used. Allow the skin to dry before applying Butrans.
3. Advise the patient to wear Butrans continuously for 7 days.
4. Advise patients to talk to their doctor if they have any pain or bothersome side effects while they are using Butrans. The dose may have to be changed.
5. Advise patients not to increase or decrease the Butrans dose they are using without first speaking to their doctor.
6. Advise patients that Butrans may impair mental and/or physical ability required for the performance of potentially hazardous tasks (e.g., driving, operating heavy machinery).
7. Advise patients who are taking Butrans not to drink alcohol. They should also avoid taking sleep aids and CNS depressants, unless a doctor prescribes them.
8. Advise patients that while wearing Butrans, they should avoid exposing the Butrans site to external heat sources, such as heating pads, electric blankets, heat lamps, saunas, hot tubs, heated water beds, etc, because an increase in absorption of buprenorphine may occur that could lead to an overdose or death.
9. Advise women who become pregnant, or who plan to become pregnant, to ask their doctor about the effects that Butrans may have on themselves and their pregnancy.
10. Advise patients that buprenorphine is a drug that some people may abuse. They should use Butrans only as directed, and not give it to anyone other than the individual for whom it was prescribed. Protect it from theft. Be especially careful to keep this medication away from children and pets.
11. Advise patients to tell their doctor if they have a history of serious skin reactions to adhesives, as they may not be able to use Butrans.
12. Advise patients who must stop using Butrans that they should speak with their doctor to manage the transition to other pain medications.

Healthcare professionals can telephone Purdue Pharma's Medical Services Department (1-888-726-7535) for information on this product.

CAUTION

DEA Order Form Required.

Distributed by: Purdue Pharma L.P., Stamford, CT 06901-3431

Manufactured by: LTS Lohmann Therapie-Systeme AG, Andernach, Germany

U.S. Patent Numbers 5,681,413; 5,804,215; 6,264,980; 6,315,854; 6,344,211; RE41408; RE41489; RE41571.

302546-0A

Revised: August 2010

© 2010, Purdue Pharma L.P.

MEDICATION GUIDE

Butrans™ (BYOO-trans) CIII

(buprenorphine)

Transdermal System

Keep Butrans in a safe place away from children. Accidental use by a child is a medical emergency and can result in death. If a child accidentally uses Butrans, get emergency help right away.

Read the Medication Guide that comes with Butrans before you start using it and each time you get a refill. There may be new information. This Medication Guide does not take the place of talking to your doctor about your medical condition or your treatment. Make sure you read and understand all the instructions for using Butrans. Talk to your doctor if you have questions.

What is the most important information I should know about Butrans?

- Butrans overdose can cause serious and life-threatening breathing problems.
- Butrans is a skin patch that contains the strong opioid pain medicine (narcotic) buprenorphine.

- Butrans is used to treat moderate to severe chronic pain that continues around-the-clock and is expected to last for a long period of time.
- Butrans is not for pain that:
  ○ you only have once in while ("as needed")
  ○ is expected to last for only a short time or pain due to surgery
- **Serious and life-threatening breathing problems can happen with Butrans, especially during the first 24 to 72 hours after you apply a new patch.** This can happen because of an overdose or if the dose you are using is too high for you.
- **Call your doctor right away or get emergency medical help if you:**
  ○ have trouble breathing
  ○ have changes in breathing
    ■ unusual deep "sighing" breathing
    ■ slow or shallow breathing
    ■ new or unusual snoring
  ○ have a slow heartbeat
  ○ have severe sleepiness
  ○ have cold, clammy skin
  ○ feel faint, dizzy, confused, or cannot think, walk, or talk normally
- **Do not place direct heat on Butrans.** Exposure of Butrans to direct heat may cause too much of the medicine in Butrans to pass into your body. This can lead to overdose and death. Keep the Butrans system away from:
  • heating pads
  • electric blankets
  • heaters
  • tanning lamps
  • saunas
  • hot tubs
  • heated waterbeds
  • hot baths
  • sunbathing
- **Place the Butrans patch only on clean skin. Do not use Butrans on broken, irritated and cracked skin.**
- **Do not use Butrans if the seal on the protective pouch is broken or if the patch is cut, damaged or changed.** Do not cut the patch.

What is Butrans?

Butrans is a prescription medicine used to treat moderate to severe chronic pain that continues around-the-clock and is expected to last for a long period of time.

Butrans is a controlled substance (CIII) because it contains buprenorphine that can be a target for people who abuse prescription medicines or street drugs. Prevent theft, misuse and abuse. Keep Butrans in a safe place to protect from being stolen. Never give Butrans to anyone else, even if they have the same symptoms you have. It may harm them or even cause death. Selling or giving away this medicine is against the law.

It is not known if Butrans is safe and effective in children.

Who should not use Butrans?

Do not use Butrans if you:

- have trouble breathing, severe asthma or severe lung problems.
- have a bowel blockage called paralytic ileus.
- are allergic to any of the ingredients in Butrans. See the end of this Medication Guide for a list of the ingredients in Butrans. Ask your doctor if you are not sure.

Talk to your doctor before taking this medicine if you have any of these conditions listed above.

What should I tell my doctor before using Butrans?

Butrans may not be right for you. Before taking Butrans, tell your doctor if you:

- have trouble breathing or lung problems
- have or a family member has a history of a heart problem called Long QT syndrome
- have or have had head injury or brain problems
- have low blood pressure
- have liver or kidney problems
- have hepatitis B or hepatitis C
- have or have had convulsions or seizures
- have severe scoliosis
- have thyroid problems
- have prostate problems or trouble urinating
- have adrenal gland problems, such as Addison's disease
- have a past or present drinking problem or alcoholism, or a family history of this problem
- have mental problems including major depression or hallucinations (seeing or hearing things that are not there)
- have a past or present drug abuse or addiction problem, or a family history of this problem
- have any other medical conditions
- are pregnant or plan to become pregnant
- are breast-feeding or plan to breast-feed. Butrans passes into your breast milk. You and your doctor should decide if

you will take Butrans or breast-feed. You should not do both. Talk to your doctor about the best way to feed your baby if you take Butrans.

Tell your doctor about all the medicines you take, including prescription and non-prescription medicines, vitamins, and herbal supplements. Some medicines may cause serious or life-threatening medical problems when taken with Butrans. Sometimes, the doses of certain medicines and Butrans need to be changed if used together.

Especially tell your doctor if you take:

- other pain medicines
- antidepressant medicines
- sleeping pills
- antihistamines
- anti-anxiety medicines
- muscle relaxants
- anti-nausea medicines
- sedative or tranquilizer medicines (medicines that make you sleepy)
- a medicine for abnormal heartbeats

You should not take Butrans if you already take a monoamine oxidase inhibitor (MAOI) medicine or within 14 days after you stop taking an MAOI medicine.

Ask your doctor if you are not sure if your medicine is one listed above.

Know the medicines you take. Keep a list of your medicines to show your doctor and pharmacist. Your doctor will tell you if it is safe to take other medicines while you are using Butrans.

How should I use Butrans?

- **See the "What is the most important information I should know about Butrans?"**
- **Butrans patch comes in three strengths.** Each Butrans patch has the strength listed on the patch. Your doctor will prescribe the patch that is right for you.
  ○ 5 mcg/hour
  ○ 10 mcg/hour
  ○ 20 mcg/hour
- **Before you start using Butrans:** If you already use a continuous around-the-clock medicine for your pain, your doctor will tell you how to slowly stop using it. Your doctor should prescribe a short-acting opioid pain medicine for you to use while your dose of Butrans is being adjusted to treat your moderate to severe continuous around-the-clock pain.
- **Use Butrans exactly as prescribed by your doctor.** Do not change your dose unless your doctor tells you to change it.
- **Do not apply Butrans more often than prescribed.**
- **Do not use more than one patch at the same time unless your doctor tells you to do so.**
- **You should wear 1 Butrans patch continuously for 7 days.**
- **If the patch comes off and accidentally** sticks to the skin of another person, take the patch off of that person right away, wash the area with clear water, and get medical care for them right away.
- **Use only water to wash your skin where you apply Butrans.** Do not use soap, alcohol, or other solvents to wash the area or remove any leftover adhesive from the patch.
- **See the detailed Instructions for Use that comes with this Medication Guide to learn how to apply Butrans the right way.** Talk to your doctor if you have any questions. Your doctor should show you how to use Butrans before you start to use it.
- **If you use more Butrans than your doctor prescribed,** or overdose, call your local emergency number or your local Poison Control Center right away at 1-800-222-1222 or get emergency help right away.
- **Call your doctor right away if you have any swelling or blistering around a patch site.**
- Do not apply any medicine, cream, or lotion on the skin at the Butrans application site before applying the patch. This might affect how the patch sticks to the skin and how the medicine is absorbed from the patch.
- Do not stop using Butrans without first talking to your doctor. Your doctor will give you instructions on how to stop using this medicine slowly to avoid uncomfortable symptoms.
- After you stop using Butrans patches flush used or unused patches down the toilet or dispose of the patches in household trash using the Patch-Disposal Unit. See the Instructions for Use that comes with this Medication Guide for disposal instructions.

What should I avoid while using Butrans?

- **You should not drive, operate heavy machinery, or do other dangerous activities,** until you know how you react to this medicine. Butrans can make you sleepy and cause you to feel dizzy or lightheaded. This may affect your ability to think and react. Ask your doctor when it is okay to do these activities.
- **You should not drink alcohol or use prescription or non-prescription medicines that have alcohol in them while using Butrans.** Alcohol can increase your chances of having serious side effects including death.

What are the possible side effects of Butrans?

Butrans can cause serious side effects that can lead to death, including:

- See "What is the most important information that I should know about Butrans?"
- **Serious breathing problems that can be life threatening. Call your doctor or get emergency medical help right away if you:**
  - have trouble breathing,
  - have extreme drowsiness with slowed breathing
  - have slow shallow breathing (little chest movement with breathing)
  - feel faint, very dizzy, confused, or have any other unusual symptoms
- **Severe skin reactions. Butrans can cause skin reactions at the site where the patch is applied.**
- **Allergic reactions. Rash, itching, and hives are the most common symptoms of an allergic reaction. Call your doctor if you have these symptoms. Get medical help right away if you have any of these symptoms of an allergic reaction while taking Butrans:**
  - swelling of your lips or tongue
  - breathing problems
  - wheezing
  - chest pain
- **Butrans can cause a drop in your blood pressure.** Low blood pressure can make you feel dizzy if you get up too fast from sitting or lying down. Low blood pressure is also more likely to happen if you take other medicines that can also lower your blood pressure. Severe low blood pressure can happen if you lose blood or take certain other medicines.
- **Liver problems.** Your skin or the white part of your eyes can turn yellow (jaundice), urine can turn dark, stools can turn light in color, you may have less of an appetite, and nausea. Your doctor may do tests before you start and while you take Butrans.
- **Butrans can increase your chances of having a seizure if you have history of seizures.** Tell your doctor if you have a seizure or convulsion while taking Butrans.
- **Butrans can cause physical dependence.** Do not stop using Butrans or any other opioid without talking to your doctor. You could become sick with uncomfortable withdrawal symptoms because your body has become used to these medicines. Physical dependence is not the same as drug addiction.
- **There is a chance of abuse or addiction with Butrans.** The chance is higher if you are or have been addicted to or abused other medicines, street drugs or alcohol in the past. You may have a greater risk of developing abuse or addiction again while using Butrans.

The most common side effects of Butrans include:

- nausea
- headache
- dizziness
- constipation
- drowsiness
- vomiting
- dry mouth and
- itching, redness, or rash at the patch site

Constipation (incomplete or hard bowel movements) is a very common side effect of all opioid medicines. Talk to your doctor about the use of laxatives (medicines to treat constipation) and stool softeners to prevent or treat constipation while using Butrans.

Talk to your doctor about any side effects that bother you or do not go away.

These are not all the possible side effects of Butrans. For a complete list, ask your doctor or pharmacist.

Call your doctor for medical advice about side effects. You may report side effects to FDA at 1-800-FDA-1088.

How should I store Butrans?

- Store Butrans at room temperature, between 59°F to 86°F (15°C to 30°C).
- Keep the Butrans patch in its unopened protective pouch until you are ready to use it.
- **Keep Butrans in a safe place out of the reach of children.**

General information about Butrans

Medicines are sometimes prescribed for purposes other than those listed in a Medication Guide. Do not use Butrans for a condition for which it was not prescribed. Do not give Butrans to other people for any reason, even if they have the same symptoms you have. It may harm them and it is against the law.

This Medication Guide summarizes the most important information about Butrans. If you would like more information, talk with your doctor. You can ask your doctor or pharmacist for information about Butrans that is written for doctors.

For questions about Butrans, call Purdue Pharma at 1-888-726-7535 or visit www.butransrems.com or www.purdue pharma.com.

What are the ingredients in Butrans?

Active ingredient: buprenorphine
Inactive ingredients: levulinic acid, oleyl oleate, povidone, and polyacrylate cross-linked with aluminum.
Distributed by:
Purdue Pharma L.P.
Stamford, CT 06901-3431
Manufactured by:
LTS Lohmann Therapie-Systeme AG
Andernach, Germany
U.S. Patent Numbers: 5,681,413; 5,804,215; 6,264,980; 6,315,854; 6,344,211; RE41408; RE41489; RE41571.
Revised: August 2010
©2010, Purdue Pharma L.P.
This Medication Guide has been approved by the U.S. Food and Drug Administration.

INSTRUCTIONS FOR USE

Butrans™ (BYOO-trans) CIII
(buprenorphine)
Transdermal System

Be sure that you read, understand, and follow these Instructions for Use before you use Butrans. Talk to your doctor or pharmacist if you have any questions.

Before applying Butrans:

- Do not use soap, alcohol, lotions, oils, or other products to remove any leftover medicine gel from a patch because this may cause more Butrans to pass through the skin.
- Each patch is sealed in its own protective pouch. Do not remove a patch from the pouch until you are ready to use it.
- Do not use a patch if the seal on the protective pouch is broken or if the patch is cut, damaged or changed in any way.
- Butrans patches are available in 3 different strengths and patch sizes. Make sure you have the right strength patch that has been prescribed for you.

Where to apply Butrans:

- Butrans should be applied to the **upper outer arm, upper chest, upper back, or the side of the chest** (See Figure 1). These 4 sites (located on both sides of the body) provide 8 possible Butrans application sites. You should change the skin site where you apply Butrans each week, making sure that at least 3 weeks (21 days) pass before you re-use the same skin site.

Figure 1

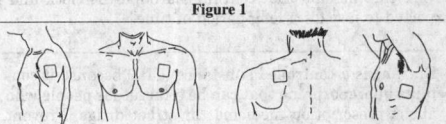

- Apply Butrans to **a hairless or nearly hairless skin site**. If needed, you can clip the hair at the skin site (See Figure 2). Do not shave the area. The skin site should not be irritated. **Use only water to clean** the application site. You should not use soaps, alcohol, oils, lotions, or abrasive devices. Allow the skin to dry before you apply the patch.

Figure 2

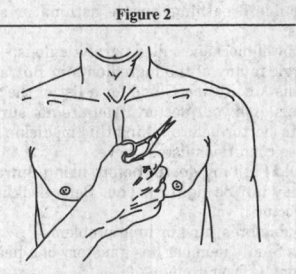

- The skin site should be free of cuts and irritation (rashes, swelling, redness, or other skin problems).

When to apply a new patch:

- When you apply a new patch, write down the date and time that the patch is applied. Use this to remember when the patch should be removed.
- Change the patch at the same time of day, one week (exactly 7 days) after you apply it.
- After removing and disposing of the patch, write down the time it was removed and how it was disposed.

How to apply Butrans:

- If you are wearing a patch, remember to remove it before applying a new one.
- Each patch is sealed in its own protective pouch.
- Use scissors to cut open the pouch along the dotted line (See Figure 3) and remove the patch. Do not remove the patch from the pouch until you are ready to use it. Do not use patches that have been cut or damaged in any way.

Figure 3

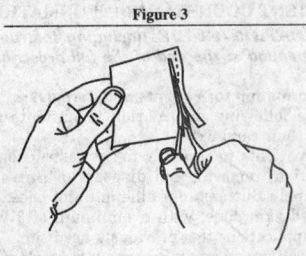

- Hold the patch with the protective liner facing you.
- Gently bend the patch (See Figures 4a and 4b) along the faint line and slowly peel the larger portion of the liner, which covers the sticky surface of the patch.

Figure 4a

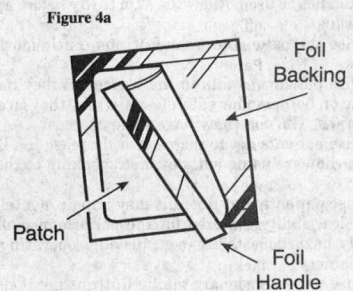

Foil Backing

Patch

Foil Handle

Figure 4b

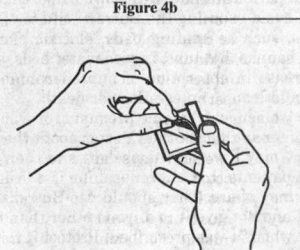

- Do not touch the sticky side of the patch with your fingers.
- Using the smaller portion of the protective liner as a handle (See Figure 5), apply the sticky side of the patch to one of the 8 body locations described above (see **Where to apply Butrans?**).

Figure 5

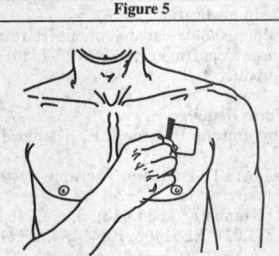

- While still holding the sticky side down, gently fold back the smaller portion of the patch. Grasp an edge of the remaining protective liner and slowly peel it off (See Figure 6).

Figure 6

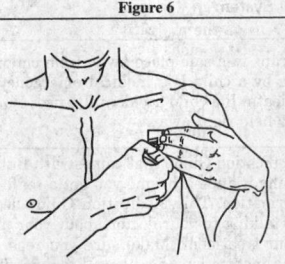

- Press the entire patch firmly into place with the palm (See Figure 7) of your hand over the patch, for about 15 seconds. Do not rub the patch.
[See figure 7 at top of next page]
- Make sure that the patch firmly sticks to the skin.
- Go over the edges with your fingers to assure good contact around the patch.

Figure 7

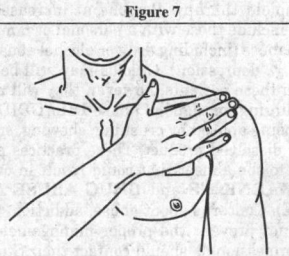

- Always wash your hands after applying or handling a patch.
- After the patch is applied, write down the date and time that the patch is applied. Use this to remember when the patch should be removed.

If the patch falls off right away after applying, throw it away and put a new one on at a different skin site **(see Disposing of Butrans Patch)**.

If a patch falls off, do not touch the sticky side of the patch with your fingers. A new patch should be applied to a different site. **Patches that fall off should not be re-applied. They must be thrown away correctly.**

If the edges of the Butrans patch start to loosen:
- Apply first aid tape only to the edges of the patch.
- If problems with the patch not sticking continue, cover the patch with special see-through adhesive dressings (for example Bioclusive or Tegaderm).
  ◦ Remove the backing from the transparent adhesive dressing and place it carefully and completely over the Butrans patch, smoothing it over the patch and your skin.
- **Never cover a Butrans patch with any other bandage or tape. It should only be covered with a special see-through adhesive dressing. Talk to your doctor or pharmacist about the kinds of dressing that should be used.**

If your patch falls off later, but before 1 week (7 days) of use, throw it away properly **(see Disposing of a Butrans Patch)** and apply a new patch at a different skin site. Be sure to let your doctor know that this has happened. Do not replace the new patch until 1 week (7 days) after you put it on (or as directed by your doctor).

Disposing of Butrans Patch:
Butrans patches must be disposed of by flushing them down the toilet or using the Patch-Disposal Unit.
To flush your Butrans patches down the toilet:
Remove your Butrans patch, fold the sticky sides of a used patch together (See Figure 8) and flush it down the toilet right away.

Figure 8

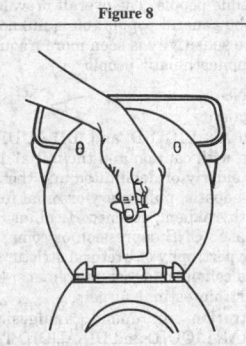

When disposing of unused Butrans patches you no longer need, remove the leftover patches from their protective pouch and remove the protective liner. Fold the patches in half with the sticky sides together, and flush the patches down the toilet.

Do not flush the pouch or the protective liner down the toilet. These items can be thrown away in the trash.

If you prefer not to flush the used patch down the toilet, you must use the Patch-Disposal Unit provided to you to discard the patch.

Never put used Butrans patches in the trash without first sealing them in the Patch-Disposal Unit.

To dispose of Butrans patches in household trash using the Patch-Disposal Unit:
Remove your patch and follow the directions printed on the Patch-Disposal Unit (See Figure 9) or see complete instructions below. **Use one Patch-Disposal Unit for each patch.**
[See figure 9 at top of next column]
1. Peel back the disposal unit liner to show the sticky surface (See Figure 10).
[See figure 10 in next column]

Figure 9

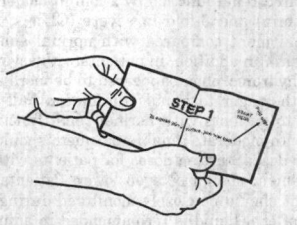

Figure 10

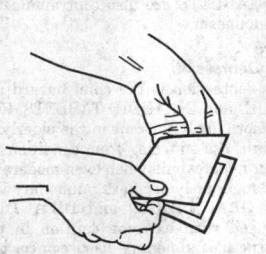

2. Place the sticky side of the used or unused patch to the indicated area on the disposal unit (See Figure 11).

Figure 11

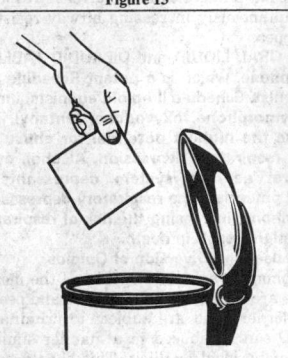

3. Close the disposal unit by folding the sticky sides together (See Figure 12). Press firmly and smoothly over the entire disposal unit so that the patch is sealed within.

Figure 12

4. The closed disposal unit, with the patch sealed inside may be thrown away in the trash (See Figure 13).

Figure 13

Do not put unused patches in household trash without first sealing them in the Patch-Disposal Unit.
Always remove the leftover patches from their protective pouch and remove the protective liner. The pouch and liner can be disposed of separately in the trash and should not be sealed in the Patch-Disposal Unit.

Distributed by:
Purdue Pharma L.P.
Stamford, CT 06901-3431
Manufactured by:
LTS Lohmann Therapie-Systeme AG
Andernach, Germany
Revised: August 2010
©2010, Purdue Pharma L.P.
Bioclusive is a trademark of Systagenix Wound Management (US), Inc.
Tegaderm is a trademark of 3M.
Shown in Product Identification Guide, page 317

DILAUDID®   ℂ ℞
(hydromorphone hydrochloride)
Oral Liquid
DILAUDID
(hydromorphone hydrochloride)
Tablets

> **WARNING: DILAUDID ORAL LIQUID AND DILAUDID TABLETS CONTAIN HYDROMORPHONE, WHICH IS A POTENT SCHEDULE II CONTROLLED OPIOID AGONIST. SCHEDULE II OPIOID AGONISTS, INCLUDING MORPHINE, OXYMORPHONE, OXYCODONE, FENTANYL, AND METHADONE, HAVE THE HIGHEST POTENTIAL FOR ABUSE AND RISK OF PRODUCING RESPIRATORY DEPRESSION. ALCOHOL, OTHER OPIOIDS AND CENTRAL NERVOUS SYSTEM DEPRESSANTS (SEDATIVE-HYPNOTICS) POTENTIATE THE RESPIRATORY DEPRESSANT EFFECTS OF HYDROMORPHONE, INCREASING THE RISK OF RESPIRATORY DEPRESSION THAT MIGHT RESULT IN DEATH.**

DESCRIPTION
DILAUDID (hydromorphone hydrochloride), a hydrogenated ketone of morphine, is an opioid analgesic.
The chemical name of DILAUDID (hydromorphone hydrochloride) is 4,5α-epoxy-3-hydroxy-17-methylmorphinan-6-one hydrochloride. The structural formula is:

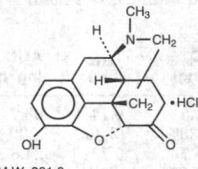

M.W. 321.8

Each 5 mL (1 teaspoon) of DILAUDID ORAL LIQUID contains 5 mg of hydromorphone hydrochloride. In addition, other ingredients include purified water, methylparaben, propylparaben, sucrose, and glycerin. DILAUDID ORAL LIQUID may contain traces of sodium metabisulfite.
Color Coded Tablets (for oral administration) contain:
2 mg hydromorphone hydrochloride (orange tablet) and D&C red #30 Lake dye, D&C yellow #10 Lake dye, lactose, and magnesium stearate. DILAUDID 2 mg TABLET may contain traces of sodium metabisulfite.
4 mg hydromorphone hydrochloride (yellow tablet) and D&C yellow #10 Lake dye, lactose, and magnesium stearate. DILAUDID 4 mg TABLET may contain traces of sodium metabisulfite.
8 mg hydromorphone hydrochloride (white tablet) and lactose anhydrous, and magnesium stearate. DILAUDID 8 mg TABLET may contain traces of sodium metabisulfite.

CLINICAL PHARMACOLOGY
Hydromorphone hydrochloride is a pure opioid agonist with the principal therapeutic activity of analgesia. A significant feature of the analgesia is that it can occur without loss of consciousness. Opioid analgesics also suppress the cough reflex and may cause respiratory depression, mood changes, mental clouding, euphoria, dysphoria, nausea, vomiting and electroencephalographic changes. Many of the effects described below are common to this class of mu-opioid agonist analgesics which includes morphine, oxycodone, hydrocodone, codeine and fentanyl. In some instances, data may not exist to distinguish the effects of DILAUDID ORAL LIQUID and DILAUDID TABLETS from those observed with other opioid analgesics. However, in the absence of data to the contrary, it is assumed that DILAUDID ORAL LIQUID and DILAUDID TABLETS would possess all the actions of mu-agonist opioids.

Central Nervous System
The precise mode of analgesic action of opioid analgesics is unknown. However, specific CNS opiate receptors have been identified. Opioids are believed to express their pharmacological effects by combining with these receptors.
Hydromorphone depresses the cough reflex by direct effect on the cough center in the medulla.
Hydromorphone depresses the respiratory reflex by a direct effect on brain stem respiratory centers. The mechanism of

respiratory depression also involves a reduction in the responsiveness of the brain stem respiratory centers to increases in carbon dioxide tension.

Hydromorphone causes miosis. Pinpoint pupils are a common sign of opioid overdose but are not pathognomonic (e.g., pontine lesions of hemorrhagic or ischemic origin may produce similar findings). Marked mydriasis rather than miosis may be seen with hypoxia in the setting of DILAUDID overdose.

Gastrointestinal Tract and Other Smooth Muscle
Gastric, biliary and pancreatic secretions are decreased by opioids such as hydromorphone. Hydromorphone causes a reduction in motility associated with an increase in tone in the gastric antrum and duodenum. Digestion of food in the small intestine is delayed and propulsive contractions are decreased. Propulsive peristaltic waves in the colon are decreased, and tone may be increased to the point of spasm. The end result is constipation. Hydromorphone can cause a marked increase in biliary tract pressure as a result of spasm of the sphincter of Oddi.

Cardiovascular System
Hydromorphone may produce hypotension as a result of either peripheral vasodilation or release of histamine, or both. Other manifestations of histamine release and/or peripheral vasodilation may include pruritus, flushing, and red eyes.

Pharmacokinetics and Metabolism
The analgesic activity of DILAUDID (hydromorphone hydrochloride) is due to the parent drug, hydromorphone. Hydromorphone is rapidly absorbed from the gastrointestinal tract after oral administration and undergoes extensive first-pass metabolism. Exposure of hydromorphone (C_{max} and AUC_{0-24}) is dose-proportional at a dose range of 2 and 8 mg. In vivo bioavailability following single-dose administration of the 8 mg tablet is approximately 24% (coefficient of variation 21%). Bioequivalence between the DILAUDID 8 mg TABLET and an equivalent dose of DILAUDID ORAL LIQUID has been demonstrated.

Absorption
After oral administration of DILAUDID 8 mg liquid or tablets, peak plasma hydromorphone concentrations are generally attained within ½ to 1-hour.

Mean (%cv) Dosage Form	C_{max} (ng)	T_{max} (hrs)	AUC (ng*hr/mL)	$T\frac{1}{2}$ (hrs)
8 mg Tablet	5.5 (33%)	0.74 (34%)	23.7 (28%)	2.6 (18%)
8 mg Oral Liquid	5.7 (31%)	0.73 (71%)	24.6 (29%)	2.8 (20%)

Food Effects
In a study conducted with a single 8 mg dose of hydromorphone (2 mg DILAUDID® IR tablets), food lowered C_{max} by 25%, prolonged T_{max} by 0.8 hour, and increased AUC by 35%. The effects may not be clinically relevant.

Distribution
At therapeutic plasma levels, hydromorphone is approximately 8-19% bound to plasma proteins. After an intravenous bolus dose, the steady state of volume distribution [mean (%cv)] is 302.9 (32%) liters.

Metabolism
Hydromorphone is extensively metabolized via glucuronidation in the liver, with greater than 95% of the dose metabolized to hydromorphone-3-glucuronide along with minor amounts of 6-hydroxy reduction metabolites.

Elimination
Only a small amount of the hydromorphone dose is excreted unchanged in the urine. Most of the dose is excreted as hydromorphone-3-glucuronide along with minor amounts of 6-hydroxy reduction metabolites. The systemic clearance is approximately 1.96 (20%) liters/minute. The terminal elimination half-life of hydromorphone after an intravenous dose is about 2.3 hours.

Special Populations
Hepatic Impairment
After oral administration of hydromorphone at a single 4 mg dose (2 mg Dilaudid IR Tablets), mean exposure to hydromorphone (C_{max} and AUC_∞) is increased 4-fold in patients with moderate (Child-Pugh Group B) hepatic impairment compared with subjects with normal hepatic function. Due to increased exposure of hydromorphone, patients with moderate hepatic impairment should be started at a lower dose and closely monitored during dose titration. Pharmacokinetics of hydromorphone in severe hepatic impairment patients has not been studied. Further increase in C_{max} and AUC of hydromorphone in this group is expected. As such, starting dose should be even more conservative. Use of oral liquid is recommended to adjust the dose (see **DOSAGE AND ADMINISTRATION**).

Renal Impairment
After oral administration of hydromorphone at a single 4 mg dose (2 mg Dilaudid IR Tablets), exposure to

hydromorphone (C_{max} and AUC_{0-48}) is increased in patients with impaired renal function by 2-fold in moderate (CLcr = 40-60 mL/min) and 3-fold in severe (CLcr < 30 mL/min) renal impairment compared with normal subjects (CLcr > 80 mL/min). In addition, in patients with severe renal impairment hydromorphone appeared to be more slowly eliminated with longer terminal elimination half-life (40 hr) compared to patients with normal renal function (15 hr). Patients with moderate renal impairment should be started on a lower dose. Starting doses for patients with severe renal impairment should be even lower. Patients with renal impairment should be closely monitored during dose titration. Use of oral liquid is recommended to adjust the dose (see **DOSAGE AND ADMINISTRATION**).

Pediatrics
Pharmacokinetics of hydromorphone have not been evaluated in children.

Geriatric
Age has no effect on the pharmacokinetics of hydromorphone.

Gender
Gender has little effect on the pharmacokinetics of hydromorphone. Females appear to have higher C_{max} (25%) than males with comparable AUC_{0-24} values. The difference observed in C_{max} may not be clinically relevant.

Pregnancy and Nursing Mothers
Hydromorphone crosses the placenta. Hydromorphone is also found in low levels in breast milk, and may cause respiratory compromise in newborns when administered during labor or delivery.

CLINICAL TRIALS
Analgesic effects of single doses of DILAUDID ORAL LIQUID administered to patients with post-surgical pain have been studied in double-blind controlled trials. In one study, both 5 mg and 10 mg of DILAUDID ORAL LIQUID provided significantly more analgesia than placebo. In another trial, 5 mg and 10 mg of DILAUDID ORAL LIQUID were compared to 30 mg and 60 mg of morphine sulfate oral liquid. The pain relief provided by 5 mg and 10 mg DILAUDID ORAL LIQUID was comparable to 30 mg and 60 mg oral morphine sulfate, respectively.

INDICATIONS AND USAGE
DILAUDID ORAL LIQUID and DILAUDID TABLETS are indicated for the management of pain in patients where an opioid analgesic is appropriate.

CONTRAINDICATIONS
DILAUDID ORAL LIQUID and DILAUDID TABLETS are contraindicated in: patients with known hypersensitivity to hydromorphone, patients with respiratory depression in the absence of resuscitative equipment, and in patients with status asthmaticus. DILAUDID ORAL LIQUID and DILAUDID TABLETS are also contraindicated for use in obstetrical analgesia.

WARNINGS
Respiratory Depression
Respiratory depression is the chief hazard of DILAUDID ORAL LIQUID and DILAUDID TABLETS. Respiratory depression is more likely to occur in the elderly, in the debilitated, and in those suffering from conditions accompanied by hypoxia or hypercapnia when even moderate therapeutic doses may dangerously decrease pulmonary ventilation.

DILAUDID ORAL LIQUID and DILAUDID TABLETS should be used with extreme caution in patients with chronic obstructive pulmonary disease or cor pulmonale, patients having a substantially decreased respiratory reserve, hypoxia, hypercapnia, or in patients with preexisting respiratory depression. In such patients even usual therapeutic doses of opioid analgesics may decrease respiratory drive while simultaneously increasing airway resistance to the point of apnea.

DILAUDID ORAL LIQUID and DILAUDID TABLETS contain hydromorphone, which is a potent Schedule II controlled opioid agonist. Schedule II opioid agonists, including morphine, oxymorphone, oxycodone, fentanyl, and methadone, have the highest potential for abuse and risk of producing respiratory depression. Alcohol, other opioids and central nervous system depressants (sedative-hypnotics) potentiate the respiratory depressant effects of hydromorphone, increasing the risk of respiratory depression that might result in death.

Misuse, Abuse, and Diversion of Opioids
Hydromorphone is an opioid agonist of the morphine-type. Such drugs are sought by drug abusers and people with addiction disorders and are subject to criminal diversion. DILAUDID can be abused in a manner similar to other opioid agonists, legal or illicit. This should be considered when prescribing or dispensing DILAUDID in situations where the physician or pharmacist is concerned about an increased risk of misuse, abuse, or diversion. Prescribers should monitor all patients receiving opioids for signs of abuse, misuse, and addiction. Furthermore, patients should be assessed for their potential for opioid abuse prior to being

prescribed opioid therapy. Persons at increased risk for opioid abuse include those with a personal or family history of substance abuse (including drug or alcohol abuse) or mental illness (e.g., depression). Opioids may still be appropriate for use in these patients, however, they will require intensive monitoring for signs of abuse DILAUDID has been reported as being abused by crushing, chewing, snorting, or injecting the dissolved product. These practices pose a significant risk to the abuser that could result in overdose or death (see **WARNINGS** and **DRUG ABUSE AND DEPENDENCE**). Concerns about abuse, addiction, and diversion should not prevent the proper management of pain. Healthcare professionals should contact their State Professional Licensing Board or State Controlled Substances Authority for information on how to prevent and detect abuse or diversion of this product.

Interactions with Alcohol and Drugs of Abuse
Hydromorphone may be expected to have additive effects when used in conjunction with alcohol, other opioids, or illicit drugs that cause central nervous system depression.

Neonatal Withdrawal Syndrome
Infants born to mothers physically dependent on DILAUDID will also be physically dependent and may exhibit respiratory difficulties and withdrawal symptoms (see **DRUG ABUSE AND DEPENDENCE**).

Head Injury and Increased Intracranial Pressure
The respiratory depressant effects of DILAUDID ORAL LIQUID and DILAUDID TABLETS with carbon dioxide retention and secondary elevation of cerebrospinal fluid pressure may be markedly exaggerated in the presence of head injury, other intracranial lesions, or preexisting increase in intracranial pressure. Opioid analgesics including DILAUDID ORAL LIQUID and DILAUDID TABLETS (hydromorphone hydrochloride) may produce effects on pupillary response and consciousness which can obscure the clinical course and neurologic signs of further increase in intracranial pressure in patients with head injuries.

Hypotensive Effect
Opioid analgesics, including DILAUDID ORAL LIQUID and DILAUDID TABLETS, may cause severe hypotension in an individual whose ability to maintain blood pressure has already been compromised by a depleted blood volume, or a concurrent administration of drugs such as phenothiazines or general anesthetics (see **PRECAUTIONS - Drug Interactions**). Therefore, DILAUDID ORAL LIQUID and DILAUDID TABLETS should be administered with caution to patients in circulatory shock, since vasodilation produced by the drug may further reduce cardiac output and blood pressure.

Sulfites
Contains sodium metabisulfite, a sulfite that may cause allergic-type reactions including anaphylactic symptoms and life-threatening or less severe asthmatic episodes in certain susceptible people. The overall prevalence of sulfite sensitivity in the general population is unknown and probably low. Sulfite sensitivity is seen more frequently in asthmatic than in nonasthmatic people.

PRECAUTIONS
Special Risk Patients
DILAUDID ORAL LIQUID and DILAUDID TABLETS should be given with caution and the initial dose should be reduced in the elderly or debilitated and those with severe impairment of hepatic, pulmonary or renal functions; myxedema or hypothyroidism; adrenocortical insufficiency (e.g., Addison's Disease); CNS depression or coma; toxic psychoses; prostatic hypertrophy or urethral stricture; gall bladder disease; acute alcoholism; delirium tremens; kyphoscoliosis or following gastrointestinal surgery.

The administration of opioid analgesics including DILAUDID ORAL LIQUID and DILAUDID TABLETS may obscure the diagnoses or clinical course in patients with acute abdominal conditions and may aggravate preexisting convulsions in patients with convulsive disorders.

Reports of mild to severe seizures and myoclonus have been reported in severely compromised patients, administered high doses of parenteral hydromorphone, for cancer and severe pain. Opioid administration at very high doses is associated with seizures and myoclonus in a variety of diseases where pain control is the primary focus.

Use in Drug and Alcohol Dependent Patients
DILAUDID should be used with caution in patients with alcoholism and other drug dependencies due to the increased frequency of opioid tolerance, dependence, and the risk of addiction observed in these patient populations. Abuse of DILAUDID in combination with other CNS depressant drugs can result in serious risk to the patient.

Hydromorphone is an opioid with no approved use in the management of addictive disorders.

Use in Ambulatory Patients
DILAUDID ORAL LIQUID and DILAUDID TABLETS may impair mental and/or physical ability required for the performance of potentially hazardous tasks (e.g. driving,

operating machinery). Patients should be cautioned accordingly. DILAUDID may produce orthostatic hypotension in ambulatory patients.

Use in Biliary Tract Disease

Opioid analgesics, including DILAUDID ORAL LIQUID and DILAUDID TABLETS, should also be used with caution in patients about to undergo surgery of the biliary tract since it may cause spasm of the sphincter of Oddi.

Tolerance and Physical Dependence

Tolerance is the need for increasing doses of opioids to maintain a defined effect such as analgesia (in the absence of disease progression or other external factors). Physical dependence is manifested by withdrawal symptoms after abrupt discontinuation of a drug or upon administration of an antagonist. Physical dependence and tolerance are not unusual during chronic opioid therapy.

The opioid abstinence or withdrawal syndrome is characterized by some or all of the following: restlessness, lacrimation, rhinorrhea, yawning, perspiration, chills, myalgia, mydriasis. Other symptoms also may develop, including: irritability, anxiety, backache, joint pain, weakness, abdominal cramps, insomnia, nausea, anorexia, vomiting, diarrhea, or increased blood pressure, respiratory rate, or heart rate.

In general, opioids used regularly should not be abruptly discontinued.

Information for Patients/Caregivers

Patients receiving DILAUDID (hydromorphone hydrochloride) ORAL LIQUID or DILAUDID TABLETS or their caregivers should be given the following information by the physician, nurse, or pharmacist:

1. Patients should be aware that DILAUDID tablets contain hydromorphone, which is a morphine-like substance and which could cause severe adverse effects including respiratory depression and even death if not taken according to the prescriber's directions.
2. Patients should be advised to report pain and adverse experiences occurring during therapy. Individualization of dosage is essential to make optimal use of this medication.
3. Patients should be advised not to adjust the dose of DILAUDID without consulting the prescribing professional.
4. Patients should be advised that DILAUDID may impair mental and/or physical ability required for the performance of potentially hazardous tasks (e.g., driving, operating heavy machinery).
5. Patients should not combine DILAUDID with alcohol or other central nervous system depressants (sleep aids, tranquilizers) except by the orders of the prescribing physician, because dangerous additive effects may occur, resulting in serious injury or death.
6. Women of childbearing potential who become, or are planning to become pregnant should be advised to consult their physician regarding the effects of analgesics and other drug use during pregnancy on themselves and their unborn child.
7. Patients should be advised that DILAUDID is a potential drug of abuse. They should protect it from theft, and it should never be given to anyone other than the individual for whom it was prescribed.
8. Patients should be advised that if they have been receiving treatment with DILAUDID for more than a few weeks and cessation of therapy is indicated, it may be appropriate to taper the DILAUDID dose, rather than abruptly discontinue it, due to the risk of precipitating withdrawal symptoms. Their physician can provide a dose schedule to accomplish a gradual discontinuation of the medication.
9. Patients should be instructed to keep DILAUDID in a secure place out of the reach of children. When DILAUDID is no longer needed, the unused tablets should be destroyed by flushing down the toilet.

Drug Interactions

Drug Interactions with Other CNS Depressants

The concomitant use of other central nervous system depressants including sedatives or hypnotics, general anesthetics, phenothiazines, tranquilizers and alcohol may produce additive depressant effects. Respiratory depression, hypotension and profound sedation or coma may occur. When such combined therapy is contemplated, the dose of one or both agents should be reduced. DILAUDID should not be taken with alcohol. Opioid analgesics, including DILAUDID ORAL LIQUID and DILAUDID TABLETS, may enhance the action of neuromuscular blocking agents and produce an excessive degree of respiratory depression. Interactions with Mixed Agonist/Antagonist Opioid Analgesics

Agonist/antagonist analgesics (i.e., pentazocine, nalbuphine, butorphanol, and buprenorphine) should be administered with caution to a patient who has received or is receiving a course of therapy with a pure opioid agonist analgesic such as hydromorphone. In this situation, mixed agonist/

antagonist analgesics may reduce the analgesic effect of hydromorphone and/or may precipitate withdrawal symptoms in these patients.

Carcinogenesis, Mutagenesis, Impairment of Fertility

No carcinogenicity studies have been conducted in animals. Hydromorphone was not mutagenic in the *in vitro* Ames reverse mutation assay or the human lymphocyte chromosome aberration assay. Hydromorphone was not clastogenic in the *in vivo* mouse micronucleus assay.

No effects on fertility, reproductive performance, or reproductive organ morphology were observed in male or female rats given oral doses up to 7 mg/kg/day, which is equivalent to the human dose of 2.5-10 mg every 3 to 6 hours for oral liquid, and 3-fold higher than the human dose of 2-4 mg every 4 to 6 hours for the tablet on a body surface area basis.

Pregnancy

Pregnancy Category C

No effects on teratogenicity or embryotoxicity were observed in female rats given oral doses up to 7 mg/kg/day, which is approximately equivalent to the human dose of 2.5-10 mg every 3 to 6 hours for oral liquid, and 3-fold higher than the human dose of 2-4 mg every 4 to 6 hours for the tablet on a body surface area basis. Hydromorphone produced skull malformations (exencephaly and cranioschisis) in Syrian hamsters given oral doses up to 20 mg/kg during the peak of organogenesis (gestation days 8-9). The skull malformations were observed at doses approximately 2-fold higher the human dose of 2.5-10 mg every 3 to 6 hours for oral liquid, and 7-fold higher than the human dose of 2-4 mg every 4 to 6 hours for the tablet on a body surface area basis. There are no adequate and well-controlled studies of DILAUDID in pregnant women.

Hydromorphone crosses the placenta, resulting in fetal exposure. DILAUDID ORAL LIQUID and DILAUDID TABLETS should be used in pregnant women only if the potential benefit justifies the potential risk to the fetus (see **Labor and Delivery** and **DRUG ABUSE AND DEPENDENCE**).

Nonteratogenic Effects

Babies born to mothers who have been taking opioids regularly prior to delivery will be physically dependent. The withdrawal signs include irritability and excessive crying, tremors, hyperactive reflexes, increased respiratory rate, increased stools, sneezing, yawning, vomiting, and fever. The intensity of the syndrome does not always correlate with the duration of maternal opioid use or dose. There is no consensus on the best method of managing withdrawal. Approaches to the treatment of this syndrome have included supportive care and, when indicated, drugs such as paregoric or phenobarbital.

Labor and Delivery

DILAUDID ORAL LIQUID and DILAUDID TABLETS are contraindicated in Labor and Delivery (see **CONTRAINDICATIONS**).

Nursing Mothers

Low levels of opioid analgesics have been detected in human milk. As a general rule, nursing should not be undertaken while a patient is receiving DILAUDID ORAL LIQUID and DILAUDID TABLETS since it, and other drugs in this class, may be excreted in the milk.

Pediatric Use

Safety and effectiveness in children have not been established.

Geriatric Use

Clinical studies of DILAUDID did not include sufficient numbers of subjects aged 65 and over to determine whether they respond differently from younger subjects. In general, dose selection for an elderly patient should be cautious, usually starting at the low end of the dosing range, reflecting the greater frequency of decreased hepatic, renal, or cardiac function, and of concomitant disease or other drug therapy (see **INDIVIDUALIZATION OF DOSAGE** and **PRECAUTIONS**).

ADVERSE REACTIONS

The major hazards of DILAUDID ORAL LIQUID and DILAUDID TABLETS include respiratory depression and apnea. To a lesser degree, circulatory depression, respiratory arrest, shock and cardiac arrest have occurred.

The most frequently observed adverse effects are lightheadedness, dizziness, sedation, nausea, vomiting, sweating, flushing, dysphoria, euphoria, dry mouth, and pruritus. These effects seem to be more prominent in ambulatory patients and in those not experiencing severe pain.

Less Frequently Observed Adverse Reactions

General and CNS

Weakness, headache, agitation, tremor, uncoordinated muscle movements, alterations of mood (nervousness, apprehension, depression, floating feelings, dreams), muscle rigidity, paresthesia, muscle tremor, blurred vision, nystagmus, diplopia and miosis, transient hallucinations and disorientation, visual disturbances, insomnia, increased intracranial pressure

Cardiovascular

Flushing of the face, chills, tachycardia, bradycardia, palpitation, faintness, syncope, hypotension, hypertension

Respiratory

Bronchospasm and laryngospasm

Gastrointestinal

Constipation, biliary tract spasm, ileus, anorexia, diarrhea, cramps, taste alteration

Genitourinary

Urinary retention or hesitancy, antidiuretic effects

Dermatologic

Urticaria, other skin rashes, diaphoresis

OVERDOSAGE

Serious overdosage with DILAUDID ORAL LIQUID and DILAUDID TABLETS is characterized by respiratory depression, somnolence progressing to stupor or coma, skeletal muscle flaccidity, cold and clammy skin, constricted pupils, and sometimes bradycardia and hypotension. In serious overdosage, particularly following intravenous injection, apnea, circulatory collapse, cardiac arrest and death may occur.

In the treatment of overdosage, primary attention should be given to the reestablishment of adequate respiratory exchange through provision of a patent airway and institution of assisted or controlled ventilation. A potentially serious oral ingestion, if recent, should be managed with gut decontamination. In unconscious patients with a secure airway, instill activated charcoal (30-100 g in adults, 1-2 g/kg in infants) via a nasogastric tube. A saline cathartic or sorbitol may be added to the first dose of activated charcoal.

Supportive measures (including oxygen, vasopressors) should be employed in the management of circulatory shock and pulmonary edema accompanying overdose as indicated. Cardiac arrest or arrhythmias may require cardiac massage or defibrillation.

The opioid antagonist, naloxone, is a specific antidote against respiratory depression which may result from overdosage, or unusual sensitivity to DILAUDID ORAL LIQUID and DILAUDID TABLETS. Therefore, an appropriate dose of this antagonist should be administered, preferably by the intravenous route, simultaneously with efforts at respiratory resuscitation. Naloxone should not be administered in the absence of clinically significant respiratory or circulatory depression. Naloxone should be administered cautiously to persons who are known, or suspected to be physically dependent on DILAUDID ORAL LIQUID and DILAUDID TABLETS. In such cases, an abrupt or complete reversal of narcotic effects may precipitate an acute withdrawal syndrome. Since the duration of action of DILAUDID ORAL LIQUID and DILAUDID TABLETS may exceed that of the antagonist, the patient should be kept under continued surveillance; repeated doses of the antagonist may be required to maintain adequate respiration. Apply other supportive measures when indicated.

DOSAGE AND ADMINISTRATION

Dilaudid Oral Liquid

The usual adult oral dosage of DILAUDID ORAL LIQUID is one-half (2.5 mL) to two teaspoonfuls (10 mL) (2.5 mg-10 mg) every 3 to 6 hours as directed by the clinical situation. Oral dosages higher than the usual dosages may be required in some patients.

Dilaudid Tablets

The usual starting dose for DILAUDID tablets is 2 mg to 4 mg, orally, every 4 to 6 hours. Appropriate use of the DILAUDID TABLETS must be decided by careful evaluation of each clinical situation.

A gradual increase in dose may be required if analgesia is inadequate, as tolerance develops, or if pain severity increases. The first sign of tolerance is usually a reduced duration of effect. Patients with hepatic and renal impairment should be started on a lower starting dose (See **CLINICAL PHARMACOLOGY - Pharmacokinetics and Metabolism**).

INDIVIDUALIZATION OF DOSAGE

The dosage of opioid analgesics like hydromorphone hydrochloride should be individualized for any given patient, since adverse events can occur at doses that may not provide complete freedom from pain.

Safe and effective administration of opioid analgesics to patients with acute or chronic pain depends upon a comprehensive assessment of the patient. The nature of the pain (severity, frequency, etiology, and pathophysiology) as well as the concurrent medical status of the patient will affect selection of the starting dosage.

In non-opioid-tolerant patients, therapy with hydromorphone is typically initiated at an oral dose of 2-4 mg every four hours, but elderly patients may require lower doses (see **PRECAUTIONS - Geriatric Use**).

In patients receiving opioids, both the dose and duration of analgesia will vary substantially depending on the patient's opioid tolerance. The dose should be selected and adjusted so that at least 3-4 hours of pain relief may be achieved. In patients taking opioid analgesics, the starting dose of DILAUDID should be based on prior opioid usage. This should be done by converting the total daily usage of the previous opioid to an equivalent total daily dosage of oral DILAUDID using an equianalgesic table (see below). For opioids not in the table, first estimate the equivalent total daily usage of oral morphine, then use the table to find the equivalent total daily dosage of DILAUDID.

Once the total daily dosage of DILAUDID has been estimated, it should be divided into the desired number of doses. Since there is individual variation in response to different opioid drugs, only 1/2 to 2/3 of the estimated dose of DILAUDID calculated from equivalence tables should be given for the first few doses, then increased as needed according to the patient's response.

Since the pharmacokinetics of hydromorphone are affected in hepatic and renal impairment with a consequent increase in exposure, patients with hepatic and renal impairment should be started on a lower starting dose (See **CLINICAL PHARMACOLOGY - Pharmacokinetics and Metabolism**).

In chronic pain, doses should be administered around-the-clock. A supplemental dose of 5-15% of the total daily usage may be administered every two hours on an "as-needed" basis.

Periodic reassessment after the initial dosing is always required. If pain management is not satisfactory and in the absence of significant opioid-induced adverse events, the hydromorphone dose may be increased gradually. If excessive opioid side effects are observed early in the dosing interval, the hydromorphone dose should be reduced. If this results in breakthrough pain at the end of the dosing interval, the dosing interval may need to be shortened. Dose titration should be guided more by the need for analgesia than the absolute dose of opioid employed.

OPIOID ANALGESIC EQUIVALENTS WITH APPROXIMATELY EQUIANALGESIC POTENCY*

Nonproprietary (Trade) Name	IM or SC Dose	ORAL Dose
Morphine sulfate	10 mg	40-60 mg
Hydromorphone HCl (DILAUDID)	1.3-2 mg	6.5-7.5 mg
Oxymorphone HCl (Numorphan)	1-1.1 mg	6.6 mg
Levorphanol tartrate (Levo-Dromoran)	2-2.3 mg	4 mg
Meperidine, pethidine HCl (Demerol)	75-100 mg	300-400 mg
Methadone HCl (Dolophine)	10 mg	10-20 mg

* Dosages, and ranges of dosages represented, are a compilation of estimated equipotent dosages from published references comparing opioid analgesics in cancer and severe pain.

DRUG ABUSE AND DEPENDENCE

DILAUDID ORAL LIQUID and DILAUDID TABLETS contain hydromorphone, a Schedule II controlled opioid agonist. Schedule II opioid substances which include morphine, oxycodone, oxymorphone, fentanyl, and methadone have the highest potential for abuse and risk of fatal overdose. Hydromorphone can be abused and is subject to criminal diversion.

Opioid analgesics may cause psychological and physical dependence. Physical dependence results in withdrawal symptoms in patients who abruptly discontinue the drug. Physical dependence usually does not occur to a clinically significant degree until after several weeks of continued opioid usage, but it may occur after as little as a week of opioid use. Physical dependence and tolerance are separate and distinct from abuse and addiction.

Addiction is a chronic, neurobiologic disease, with genetic, psychosocial, and environmental factors influencing its development and manifestations. It is characterized by behaviors that include one or more of the following: impaired control over drug use, compulsive use, continued use despite harm, and craving. Drug addiction is a treatable disease, utilizing a multidisciplinary approach, but relapse is common.

"Drug seeking" behavior is very common in addicts and drug abusers. Drug-seeking tactics include emergency calls or visits near the end of office hours, refusal to undergo appropriate examination, testing or referral, repeated "loss" of prescriptions, tampering with, forging or counterfeiting prescriptions and reluctance to provide prior medical records or contact information for other treating physician(s). "Doctor shopping" to obtain additional prescriptions is common among drug abusers, people suffering from untreated addiction and criminals seeking drugs to sell.

Physicians should be aware that addiction may not be accompanied by concurrent tolerance and symptoms of physical dependence in all addicts. In addition, abuse of opioids can occur in the absence of addiction and is characterized by misuse for non-medical purposes, often in combination with other psychoactive substances. Since DILAUDID ORAL LIQUID and DILAUDID TABLETS may be diverted for non-medical use, careful record keeping of prescribing information, including quantity, frequency, and renewal requests is strongly advised.

Proper assessment of the patient, proper prescribing practices, periodic re-evaluation of therapy, and proper dispensing and storage are appropriate measures that help to limit abuse of opioid drugs.

DILAUDID ORAL LIQUID and DILAUDID TABLETS are intended for oral use only. Misuse or abuse of DILAUDID ORAL LIQUID and DILAUDID TABLETS pose a risk of overdose and death. This risk is increased with concurrent abuse of alcohol and other CNS depressants. Parenteral drug abuse can potentially result in local tissue necrosis, infection, pulmonary granulomas, and increased risk of endocarditis and valvular heart injury. In addition, parenteral abuse is commonly associated with transmission of infectious diseases such as hepatitis and HIV.

SAFETY AND HANDLING INSTRUCTIONS

DILAUDID ORAL LIQUID and DILAUDID TABLETS pose little risk of direct exposure to health care personnel and should be handled and disposed of prudently in accordance with hospital or institutional policy. Significant absorption from dermal exposure is unlikely; accidental dermal exposure to DILAUDID ORAL LIQUID should be treated by removal of any contaminated clothing and rinsing the affected area with cool water. Patients and their families should be instructed to flush any DILAUDID ORAL LIQUID and DILAUDID TABLETS that are no longer needed.

Access to abuseable drugs such as DILAUDID ORAL LIQUID and DILAUDID TABLETS presents an occupational hazard for addiction in the health care industry. Routine procedures for handling controlled substances developed to protect the public may not be adequate to protect health care workers. Implementation of more effective accounting procedures and measures to restrict access to drugs of this class (appropriate to the practice setting) may minimize the risk of self-administration by health care providers.

HOW SUPPLIED

DILAUDID ORAL LIQUID is a clear, sweet, slightly viscous liquid. It is available in: Bottles of 1 pint (473 mL) - NDC# 59011-451-01

DILAUDID 2 mg TABLETS are orange, debossed with a P on one side and the number 2 on the opposite side. They are available in:

Bottles of 100 - NDC # 59011-452-10

Unit Dose Packages of 100 (4×25) - NDC # 59011-452-01

DILAUDID 4 mg TABLETS are yellow, debossed with a P on one side and the number 4 on the opposite side. They are available in:

Bottles of 100 - NDC # 59011-454-10

Unit Dose Packages of 100 (4×25) - NDC # 59011-454-01

Bottles of 500 - NDC # 59011-454-05

DILAUDID 8 mg TABLETS are white, triangular shaped tablets bisected and debossed with a "P" and an inverted "P" on one side and debossed with the number "8" on other side. They are available in:

Bottles of 100 - NDC# 59011-458-10

Healthcare professionals can telephone Purdue Pharma's Medical Services Department (1-888-726-7535) for information on this product.

STORAGE

Store at 25°C (77°F); excursions permitted to 15°-30°C (59°-86°F). [See USP Controlled Room Temperature]. Protect from light. A schedule **CS-II** Narcotic. DEA Order Form is Required.

Manufactured for Purdue Pharma L.P. Stamford CT 06901-3431

By Halo Pharmaceuticals, Inc.

Whippany, NJ 07981

Revised: October 21, 2009

302064-0C

Shown in Product Identification Guide, page 317

DILAUDID® and DILAUDID-HP® INJECTION

CII ℞

[Di-law-did]

1 mg/mL, 2 mg/mL, 4 mg/mL, and 10 mg/mL (hydromorphone hydrochloride)

C-II

WARNING: **DILAUDID-HP® (high potency, 10 mg/mL ampules and vials) is a more concentrated solution of hydromorphone than DILAUDID® INJECTION, and is intended for use only in opioid-tolerant patients. Do not confuse DILAUDID-HP with standard parenteral formulations of DILAUDID or other opioids, as overdose and death could result.**

DILAUDID INJECTION (1, 2, and 4 mg/mL ampules, sterile solution for parenteral administration) and DILAUDID-HP contain hydromorphone, a potent Schedule II opioid agonist.

Schedule II opioid agonists, including morphine, oxymorphone, hydromorphone, oxycodone, fentanyl and methadone, have the highest potential for abuse and risk of producing respiratory depression. Ethanol, other opioids, and other central nervous system depressants (e.g., sedative-hypnotics, skeletal muscle relaxants) can potentiate the respiratory-depressant effects of hydromorphone and increase the risk of adverse outcomes, including death.

DESCRIPTION

DILAUDID (hydromorphone hydrochloride), a hydrogenated ketone of morphine, is an opioid analgesic.

The chemical name of DILAUDID (hydromorphone hydrochloride) is 4,5α-epoxy-3-hydroxy-17-methylmorphinan-6-one hydrochloride. The structural formula is:

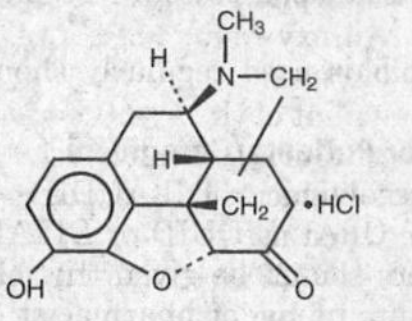

M.W. 321.8

DILAUDID INJECTION is available in ampules for parenteral administration. Each 1 mL of sterile aqueous solution contains 1 mg, 2 mg, or 4 mg hydromorphone hydrochloride with 0.2% sodium citrate and 0.2% citric acid solution.

DILAUDID INJECTION ampules are sterile. HIGH POTENCY DILAUDID (DILAUDID-HP) is available in AMBER ampules or single dose vials for intravenous (IV), subcutaneous (SC), or intramuscular (IM) administration. Each 1 mL of sterile aqueous solution contains 10 mg hydromorphone hydrochloride with 0.2% sodium citrate and 0.2% citric acid solution.

It is also available as lyophilized DILAUDID-HP for intravenous (IV), subcutaneous (SC), or intramuscular (IM) administration. Each single dose vial contains 250 mg sterile, lyophilized hydromorphone HCl to be reconstituted with 25 mL of Sterile Water for Injection USP to provide a solution containing 10 mg/mL. Hydrochloric acid or sodium hydroxide may be added to adjust pH.

CLINICAL PHARMACOLOGY

Hydromorphone hydrochloride is a pure opioid agonist with the principal therapeutic activity of analgesia. A significant feature of the analgesia is that it can occur without loss of consciousness. Opioid analgesics also suppress the cough reflex and may cause respiratory depression, mood changes, mental clouding, euphoria, dysphoria, nausea, vomiting and electroencephalographic changes. Many of the effects described below are common to the class of mu-opioid analgesics, which includes morphine, oxycodone, hydrocodone, codeine, and fentanyl. In some instances, data may not exist to demonstrate that DILAUDID INJECTION and DILAUDID-HP possess similar or different effects than those observed with other opioid analgesics. However, in the absence of data to the contrary, it is assumed that DILAUDID INJECTION and DILAUDID-HP would possess these effects.

Central Nervous System

The precise mode of analgesic action of opioid analgesics is unknown. However, specific CNS opiate receptors have been identified. Opioids are believed to express their pharmacological effects by combining with these receptors.

Hydromorphone depresses the cough reflex by direct effect on the cough center in the medulla.

Hydromorphone produces respiratory depression by direct effect on brain stem respiratory centers. The mechanism of respiratory depression also involves a reduction in the responsiveness of the brain stem respiratory centers to increases in carbon dioxide tension.

Hydromorphone causes miosis. Pinpoint pupils are a common sign of opioid overdose but are not pathognomonic (e.g., pontine lesions of hemorrhagic or ischemic origin may produce similar findings). Marked mydriasis rather than miosis may be seen with hypoxia in the setting of DILAUDID INJECTION or DILAUDID-HP overdose.

Gastrointestinal Tract and Other Smooth Muscle

Gastric, biliary and pancreatic secretions are decreased by opioids such as hydromorphone. Hydromorphone causes a reduction in motility associated with an increase in tone in the gastric antrum and duodenum. Digestion of food in the small intestine is delayed and propulsive contractions are decreased. Propulsive peristaltic waves in the colon are decreased, and tone may be increased to the point of spasm.

The end result is constipation. Hydromorphone can cause a marked increase in biliary tract pressure as a result of spasm of the sphincter of Oddi.

Cardiovascular System
Hydromorphone may produce hypotension as a result of either peripheral vasodilation, release of histamine, or both. Other manifestations of histamine release and/or peripheral vasodilation may include pruritus, flushing, and red eyes. Effects on the myocardium after intravenous administration of opioids are not significant in normal persons, vary with different opioid analgesic agents and vary with the hemodynamic state of the patient, state of hydration and sympathetic drive.

Pharmacokinetics and Metabolism
Distribution
At therapeutic plasma levels, hydromorphone is approximately 8-19% bound to plasma proteins. After an intravenous bolus dose, the steady state of volume of distribution [mean (%cv) is 302.9 (32%) liters.

Metabolism
Hydromorphone is extensively metabolized via glucuronidation in the liver, with greater than 95% of the dose metabolized to hydromorphone-3-glucuronide along with minor amounts of 6-hydroxy reduction metabolites.

Elimination
Only a small amount of the hydromorphone dose is excreted unchanged in the urine. Most of the dose is excreted as hydromorphone-3-glucuronide along with minor amounts of 6-hydroxy reduction metabolites. The systemic clearance is approximately 1.96 (20%) liters/minute. The terminal elimination half-life of hydromorphone after an intravenous dose is about 2.3 hours.

Special Populations
Hepatic Impairment
After oral administration of hydromorphone at a single 4 mg dose (2 mg Dilaudid IR Tablets), mean exposure to hydromorphone (C_{max} and AUC_∞) is increased 4 fold in patients with moderate (Child-Pugh Group B) hepatic impairment compared with subjects with normal hepatic function. Due to increased exposure of hydromorphone, patients with moderate hepatic impairment should be started at a lower dose and closely monitored during dose titration. The pharmacokinetics of hydromorphone in patients with severe hepatic impairment has not been studied. A further increase in Cmax and AUC of hydromorphone in this group is expected. As such, the starting dose should be even more conservative (see **DOSAGE AND ADMINISTRATION**).

Renal Impairment
After oral administration of hydromorphone at a single 4 mg dose (2 mg Dilaudid IR Tablets), mean exposure to hydromorphone (C_{max} and AUC_{0-48}) is increased in patients with impaired renal function by 2-fold, in moderate (CLcr = 40-60 mL/min) renal impairment and 3-fold in severe (CLcr < 30 mL/min) renal impairment compared with normal subjects (CLcr > 80 mL/min). In addition, in patients with severe renal impairment hydromorphone appeared to be more slowly eliminated with a longer terminal elimination half-life (40 hr) compared to patients with normal renal function (15 hr). Patients with moderate renal impairment should be started on a lower dose. Starting doses for patients with severe renal impairment should be even lower. Patients with renal impairment should be closely monitored during dose titration (see **DOSAGE AND ADMINISTRATION**).

Pediatrics
Pharmacokinetics of hydromorphone have not been evaluated in children.

Geriatric
The effect of age on the pharmacokinetics of hydromorphone has not been adequately evaluated.

Gender
Gender has little effect on the pharmacokinetics of hydromorphone. Females appear to have a higher C_{max} (25%) than males with comparable AUC_{0-24} values. The difference observed in C_{max} may not be clinically relevant.

Pregnancy and Nursing Mothers
Hydromorphone crosses the placenta. Hydromorphone is also found in low levels in breast milk, and may cause respiratory compromise in newborns when administered during labor or delivery.

CLINICAL TRIALS
Analgesic effects of single doses of DILAUDID ORAL LIQUID administered to patients with post-surgical pain have been studied in double-blind controlled trials. In one study, both 5 mg and 10 mg of DILAUDID ORAL LIQUID provided significantly more analgesia than placebo.

INDICATIONS AND USAGE
DILAUDID INJECTION is indicated for the management of pain in patients where an opioid analgesic is appropriate.
DILAUDID-HP is indicated for the relief of moderate-to-severe pain in opioid-tolerant patients who require larger than usual doses of opioids to provide adequate pain relief. Because DILAUDID-HP contains 10 mg of hydromorphone hydrochloride per mL, a smaller injection volume can be used than with other parenteral opioid formulations. Discomfort associated with the intramuscular or subcutaneous injection of an unusually large volume of solution can therefore be avoided.

CONTRAINDICATIONS
DILAUDID INJECTION and DILAUDID-HP are contraindicated in patients with known hypersensitivity to hydromorphone.
DILAUDID INJECTION and DILAUDID-HP are contraindicated in patients with respiratory depression in the absence of resuscitative equipment and in patients with status asthmaticus.
DILAUDID INJECTION and DILAUDID-HP are also contraindicated for use in obstetrical analgesia.
DILAUDID-HP is contraindicated in patients who are not already receiving large amounts of opioids.

WARNINGS
DILAUDID-HP (high potency, 10 mg/mL ampules and vials) is a more concentrated solution of hydromorphone than DILAUDID INJECTION, and is intended for use only in opioid-tolerant patients. Do not confuse DILAUDID-HP with standard parenteral formulations of DILAUDID or other opioids, as overdose and death could result.

Respiratory Depression
Respiratory depression is the chief hazard of DILAUDID INJECTION and DILAUDID-HP. Respiratory depression occurs most frequently in the elderly, in the debilitated, and in those suffering from conditions accompanied by hypoxia or hypercapnia, or upper airway obstruction, in whom even moderate therapeutic doses may dangerously decrease pulmonary ventilation.
DILAUDID INJECTION and DILAUDID-HP should be used with extreme caution in patients with chronic obstructive pulmonary disease or cor pulmonale, patients having a substantially decreased respiratory reserve, hypoxia, hypercapnia, or preexisting respiratory depression. In such patients even usual therapeutic doses of opioid analgesics may decrease respiratory drive while simultaneously increasing airway resistance to the point of apnea. Alternative nonopioid analgesics should be considered, and DILAUDID should be employed only under careful medical supervision at the lowest effective dose in such patients.

Misuse, Abuse, and Diversion of Opioids
DILAUDID INJECTION and DILAUDID-HP contain hydromorphone, an opioid agonist of the morphine-type, which is a potent Schedule II, controlled substance. Schedule II opioid agonists, including morphine, oxycodone, oxymorphone, fentanyl and methadone, have the highest potential for abuse and risk of fatal respiratory depression. Such drugs are sought by drug abusers and people with addiction disorders and are subject to criminal diversion.
DILAUDID INJECTION and DILAUDID-HP can be abused in a manner similar to other opioid agonists, legal or illicit. This should be considered when prescribing or dispensing DILAUDID INJECTION or DILAUDID-HP in situations where the physician or pharmacist is concerned about an increased risk of misuse, abuse, or diversion. Prescribers should monitor all patients receiving opioids for signs of abuse, misuse, and addiction. Furthermore, patients should be assessed for their potential for opioid abuse prior to being prescribed opioid therapy. Persons at increased risk for opioid abuse include those with a personal or family history of substance abuse (including drug or alcohol abuse) or mental illness (e.g., depression). Opioids may still be appropriate for use in these patients, however, they will require intensive monitoring for signs of abuse.
Concerns about abuse, addiction, and diversion should not prevent the proper management of pain.
Healthcare professionals should contact their State Professional Licensing Board or State Controlled Substances Authority for information on how to prevent and detect abuse or diversion of this product.

Interactions with Alcohol and Drugs of Abuse
Alcohol, other opioids and central nervous system depressants (sedative-hypnotics) potentiate the respiratory depressant effects of hydromorphone, increasing the risk of respiratory depression that might result in death.

Neonatal Withdrawal Syndrome
Infants born to mothers physically dependent on DILAUDID INJECTION or DILAUDID-HP will also be physically dependent and may exhibit respiratory difficulties and withdrawal symptoms. (see **DRUG ABUSE AND DEPENDENCE**).

Head Injury and Increased Intracranial Pressure
The respiratory depressant effects of DILAUDID INJECTION and DILAUDID-HP with carbon dioxide retention and secondary elevation of cerebrospinal fluid pressure may be markedly exaggerated in the presence of head injury, other intracranial lesions, or preexisting increase in intracranial pressure. Opioid analgesics including DILAUDID INJECTION and DILAUDID-HP may produce effects on pupillary response and consciousness which can obscure the clinical course and neurologic signs of further increase in pressure in patients with head injuries.

Hypotensive Effect
Opioid analgesics, including DILAUDID INJECTION and DILAUDID-HP, may cause severe hypotension in an individual whose ability to maintain his blood pressure has already been compromised by a depleted blood volume, or a concurrent administration of drugs such as phenothiazines or general anesthetics (see **PRECAUTIONS - Drug Interactions**). DILAUDID INJECTION and DILAUDID-HP may produce orthostatic hypotension in ambulatory patients. DILAUDID INJECTION and DILAUDID-HP should be administered with caution to patients in circulatory shock, since vasodilation produced by the drug may further reduce cardiac output and blood pressure.

Sulfites
DILAUDID INJECTION and DILAUDID-HP contain sodium metabisulfite, a sulfite that may cause allergic-type reactions including anaphylactic symptoms and life-threatening or less severe asthmatic episodes in certain susceptible people. The overall prevalence of sulfite sensitivity in the general population is unknown and probably low. Sulfite sensitivity is seen more frequently in asthmatic than in nonasthmatic people.

PRECAUTIONS
General
Because of its high concentration, the delivery of precise doses of DILAUDID-HP may be difficult if low doses of hydromorphone are required. Therefore, DILAUDID-HP should be used only if the amount of hydromorphone required can be delivered accurately with this formulation.

Gastrointestinal Effects
DILAUDID INJECTION and DILAUDID-HP should not be administered to patients with gastrointestinal obstruction, especially paralytic ileus, because hydromorphone diminishes the propulsive peristaltic wave in the gastrointestinal tract and may prolong the obstruction.
The administration of DILAUDID INJECTION or DILAUDID-HP may obscure the diagnosis or clinical course in patients with acute abdominal condition.

Use in Pancreatic/Biliary Tract Disease
DILAUDID INJECTION and DILAUDID-HP should be used with caution in patients with biliary tract disease, including acute pancreatitis, as hydromorphone may cause spasm of the sphincter of Oddi and diminish biliary and pancreatic secretions.

Special Risk Patients
DILAUDID INJECTION and DILAUDID-HP should be given with caution and the initial dose should be reduced in the elderly or debilitated and those with severe impairment of hepatic, pulmonary or renal function; myxedema or hypothyroidism; adrenocortical insufficiency (e.g., Addison's Disease); CNS depression or coma; toxic psychoses; prostatic hypertrophy or urethral stricture; acute alcoholism; delirium tremens; or kyphoscoliosis.
In the case of DILAUDID-HP, however, the patient is presumed to be receiving an opioid to which he or she exhibits tolerance and the initial dose of DILAUDID-HP selected should be estimated based on the relative potency of hydromorphone and the opioid previously used by the patient. (see **DOSAGE AND ADMINISTRATION**).
The administration of opioid analgesics including DILAUDID INJECTION and DILAUDID-HP may aggravate preexisting convulsions in patients with convulsive disorders.
Reports of mild to severe seizures and myoclonus have been reported in severely compromised patients, administered high doses of parenteral hydromorphone, for cancer and severe pain. Opioid administration at very high doses is associated with seizures and myoclonus in a variety of diseases where pain control is the primary focus.

Use in Drug and Alcohol Dependent Patients
DILAUDID INJECTION and DILAUDID-HP should be used with caution in patients with alcoholism and other drug dependencies due to the increased frequency of opioid tolerance, dependence, and the risk of addiction observed in these patient populations. Abuse of DILAUDID INJECTION or DILAUDID-HP in combination with other CNS depressant drugs can result in serious risk to the patient.
Hydromorphone is an opioid with no approved use in the management of addictive disorders.

Driving and Operating Machinery
DILAUDID INJECTION and DILAUDID-HP may impair mental and/or physical ability required for the performance of potentially hazardous tasks (e.g. driving, operating machinery). Patients should be cautioned accordingly. DILAUDID INJECTION and DILAUDID-HP may produce orthostatic hypotension in ambulatory patients.

Tolerance and Physical Dependence
Tolerance is the need for increasing doses of opioids to maintain a defined effect such as analgesia (in the absence of

disease progression or other external factors). Physical dependence is manifested by withdrawal symptoms after abrupt discontinuation of a drug or upon administration of an antagonist. Physical dependence and tolerance are not unusual during chronic opioid therapy.

The opioid abstinence or withdrawal syndrome is characterized by some or all of the following: restlessness, lacrimation, rhinorrhea, yawning, perspiration, chills, myalgia, mydriasis. Other symptoms also may develop, including: irritability, anxiety, backache, joint pain, weakness, abdominal cramps, insomnia, nausea, anorexia, vomiting, diarrhea, or increased blood pressure, respiratory rate, or heart rate.

In general, opioids used regularly should not be abruptly discontinued.

Information for Patients/Caregivers

Patients receiving DILAUDID (hydromorphone hydrochloride) or their caregivers should be given the following information by the physician, nurse, or pharmacist:

1. Patients should be aware that DILAUDID INJECTION and DILAUDID-HP contain hydromorphone, which is a morphine-like substance and which could cause severe adverse effects including respiratory depression and even death if not taken according to the prescriber's directions.
2. Patients should be advised to report pain and adverse experiences occurring during therapy. Individualization of dosage is essential to make optimal use of this medication.
3. Patients should be advised not to adjust the dose of DILAUDID INJECTION or DILAUDID-HP without consulting the prescribing professional.
4. Patients should be advised that DILAUDID INJECTION and DILAUDID-HP may impair mental and/or physical ability required for the performance of potentially hazardous tasks (e.g., driving, operating heavy machinery).
5. Patients should not combine DILAUDID INJECTION or DILAUDID-HP with alcohol or other central nervous system depressants (sleep aids, tranquilizers) except by the orders of the prescribing physician, because dangerous additive effects may occur, resulting in serious injury or death.
6. Women of childbearing potential who become, or are planning to become pregnant should be advised to consult their physician regarding the effects of analgesics and other drug use during pregnancy on themselves and their unborn child.
7. Patients should be advised that DILAUDID INJECTION and DILAUDID-HP are potential drugs of abuse. They should protect it from theft, and it should never be given to anyone other than the individual for whom it was prescribed.
8. Patients should be advised that if they have been receiving treatment with DILAUDID INJECTION or DILAUDID-HP for more than a few weeks and cessation of therapy is indicated, it may be appropriate to taper the DILAUDID INJECTION or DILAUDID-HP dose, rather than abruptly discontinue it, due to the risk of precipitating withdrawal symptoms. Their physician can provide a dose schedule to accomplish a gradual discontinuation of the medication.
9. Patients should be instructed to keep DILAUDID INJECTION and DILAUDID-HP in a secure place out of the reach of children.

Drug Interactions

Drug Interactions with other CNS Depressants

The concomitant use of other central nervous system depressants including sedatives or hypnotics, general anesthetics, phenothiazines, tranquilizers and alcohol may produce additive depressant effects. Respiratory depression, hypotension and profound sedation or coma may occur. When such combined therapy is contemplated, the dose of one or both agents should be reduced. Opioid analgesics, including DILAUDID INJECTION and DILAUDID-HP, may enhance the action of neuromuscular blocking agents and produce an increased degree of respiratory depression.

Interactions with Mixed Agonist/Antagonist Opioid Analgesics

Agonist/antagonist analgesics (i.e., pentazocine, nalbuphine, butorphanol, and buprenorphine) should be administered with caution to a patient who has received or is receiving a course of therapy with a pure opioid agonist analgesic such as hydromorphone. In this situation, mixed agonist/antagonist analgesics may reduce the analgesic effect of hydromorphone and/or may precipitate withdrawal symptoms in these patients.

Parenteral Administration

DILAUDID INJECTION may be given intravenously, but the injection should be given very slowly. Rapid intravenous injection of opioid analgesics increases the possibility of side effects such as hypotension and respiratory depression.

Reports of mild to severe seizures and myoclonus have been reported in severely compromised patients, administered high doses of parenteral hydromorphone, for cancer and severe pain. Opioid administration at very high doses is associated with seizures and myoclonus in a variety of diseases where pain control is the primary focus.

Experience with administration of DILAUDID-HP by the intravenous route is limited. Should intravenous administration be necessary, the injection should be given slowly, over at least 2 to 3 minutes.

Carcinogenesis, Mutagenesis, Impairment of Fertility

No carcinogenicity studies have been conducted in animals. Hydromorphone was not mutagenic in the *in vitro* Ames reverse mutation assay, or the human lymphocytes chromosome aberration assay. Hydromorphone was not clastogenic in the *in vivo* mouse micronucleus assay.

No effects on fertility, reproductive performance, or reproductive organ morphology were observed in male or female rats given oral doses up to 7 mg/kg/day which is equivalent to and 3-fold higher than the human dose of DILAUDID-HP when substituted for ORAL LIQUID or 8 mg TABLET, respectively, on a body surface area basis.

PREGNANCY

PREGNANCY CATEGORY C

No effects on teratogenicity or embryotoxicity were observed in female rats given oral doses up to 7 mg/kg/day which is equivalent to and 3-fold higher than the human dose of DILAUDID-HP, on a body surface area basis. Hydromorphone produced skull malformations (exencephaly and cranioschisis) in Syrian hamsters given oral doses up to 20 mg/kg during the peak of organogenesis (gestation days 8-9). The skull malformations were observed at doses approximately 2-fold and 7-fold higher than the human dose of DILAUDID-HP when substituted for ORAL LIQUID or 8 mg TABLET, respectively, on a body surface area basis. There are no adequate and well-controlled studies of DILAUDID INJECTION or DILAUDID-HP in pregnant women.

Hydromorphone crosses the placenta, resulting in fetal exposures. DILAUDID INJECTION or DILAUDID-HP should be used in pregnant women only if the potential benefit justifies the potential risk to the fetus (see **Labor and Delivery** and **DRUG ABUSE AND DEPENDENCE**).

Nonteratogenic Effects

Babies born to mothers who have been taking opioids regularly prior to delivery will be physically dependent. The withdrawal signs include irritability and excessive crying, tremors, hyperactive reflexes, increased respiratory rate, increased stools, sneezing, yawning, vomiting, and fever. The intensity of the syndrome does not always correlate with the duration of maternal opioid use or dose. There is no consensus on the best method of managing withdrawal. Approaches to the treatment of this syndrome have included supportive care and, when indicated, drugs such as paregoric or phenobarbital.

Labor and Delivery

DILAUDID INJECTION and DILAUDID-HP are contraindicated in Labor and Delivery (see **CONTRAINDICATIONS**).

Nursing Mothers

Low levels of opioid analgesics have been detected in human milk. As a general rule, nursing should not be undertaken while a patient is receiving DILAUDID INJECTION or DILAUDID-HP since it, and other drugs in this class, may be excreted in the milk.

Pediatric Use

Safety and effectiveness have not been established.

Geriatric Use

Clinical studies of DILAUDID INJECTION and DILAUDID-HP did not include sufficient numbers of subjects aged 65 and over to determine whether they respond differently from younger subjects. In general, dose selection for an elderly patient should be cautious, usually starting at the low end of the dosing range, reflecting the greater frequency of decreased hepatic, renal, or cardiac function, and of concomitant disease or other drug therapy. (see **DOSAGE AND ADMINISTRATION - Individualization Of Dosage** and **PRECAUTIONS**).

ADVERSE REACTIONS

The major hazards of DILAUDID INJECTION and DILAUDID-HP include respiratory depression and apnea. To a lesser degree, circulatory depression, respiratory arrest, shock and cardiac arrest have occurred.

The most frequently observed adverse effects are lightheadedness, dizziness, sedation, nausea, vomiting, sweating, flushing, dysphoria, euphoria, dry mouth, and pruritus. These effects seem to be more prominent in ambulatory patients and in those not experiencing severe pain.

Less Frequently Observed Adverse Reactions

General and CNS

Weakness, headache, agitation, tremor, uncoordinated muscle movements, alterations of mood (nervousness, apprehension, depression, floating feelings, dreams), muscle rigidity, paresthesia, muscle tremor, blurred vision, nystagmus, diplopia and miosis, transient hallucinations and disorientation, visual disturbances, insomnia, increased intracranial pressure

Cardiovascular

Flushing of the face, chills, tachycardia, bradycardia, palpitation, faintness, syncope, hypotension, hypertension

Respiratory

Bronchospasm and laryngospasm

Gastrointestinal

Constipation, biliary tract spasm, ileus, anorexia, diarrhea, cramps, taste alterations

Genitourinary

Urinary retention or hesitancy, antidiuretic effects

Dermatologic

Urticaria, other skin rashes, wheal and flare over the vein with intravenous injection, diaphoresis

Other

In clinical trials, neither local tissue irritation nor induration was observed at the site of subcutaneous injection of DILAUDID-HP; pain at the injection site was rarely observed.

OVERDOSAGE

Acute overdosage with DILAUDID INJECTION or DILAUDID-HP is characterized by respiratory depression, somnolence progressing to stupor or coma, skeletal muscle flaccidity, cold and clammy skin, constricted pupils, and sometimes bradycardia and hypotension. In serious overdosage, particularly following intravenous injection, apnea, circulatory collapse, cardiac arrest and death may occur.

Hydromorphone may cause miosis, even in total darkness. Pinpoint pupils are a sign of opioid overdose but are not pathognomonic (e.g., pontine lesions of hemorrhagic or ischemic origin may produce similar findings). Marked mydriasis rather than miosis may be seen with hypoxia in overdose situations.

In the treatment of overdosage, primary attention should be given to the reestablishment of a patent airway and institution of assisted or controlled ventilation. Supportive measures (including oxygen, vasopressors) should be employed in the management of circulatory shock and pulmonary edema accompanying overdose as indicated. Cardiac arrest or arrhythmias may require cardiac massage or defibrillation.

The opioid antagonist, naloxone, is a specific antidote against respiratory depression which may result from overdosage, or unusual sensitivity to DILAUDID INJECTION or DILAUDID-HP. Therefore, an appropriate dose of this antagonist should be administered, preferably by the intravenous route, simultaneously with efforts at respiratory resuscitation. Naloxone should not be administered in the absence of clinically significant respiratory or circulatory depression. Naloxone should be administered cautiously to persons who are known, or suspected to be physically dependent on DILAUDID INJECTION or DILAUDID-HP. In such cases, an abrupt or complete reversal of opioid effects may precipitate an acute withdrawal syndrome.

Since the duration of action of DILAUDID INJECTION and DILAUDID-HP may exceed that of the antagonist, the patient should be kept under continued surveillance; repeated doses of the antagonist may be required to maintain adequate respiration. Apply other supportive measures when indicated.

Opioid antagonists should not be administered in the absence of clinically significant respiratory or circulatory depression secondary to hydromorphone overdose. Such agents should be administered cautiously to persons who are known, or suspected to be physically dependent on hydromorphone. In such cases, an abrupt or complete reversal of opioid effects may precipitate an acute abstinence syndrome. In an individual physically dependant on opioids, administration of the usual dose antagonist will precipitate an acute withdrawal syndrome. The severity of the withdrawal symptoms experienced will depend on the degree of physical dependence and the dose of the antagonist administered. Use of an opioid antagonist should be reserved for cases where such treatment is clearly needed. If it is necessary to treat serious respiratory depression in the physically dependent patient, administration of the antagonist should be initiated with care and titrated with smaller than usual doses.

DOSAGE AND ADMINISTRATION

DILAUDID INJECTION

The usual starting dose is 1-2 mg *subcutaneously* or *intramuscularly* every 4 to 6 hours as necessary for pain control. The dose should be adjusted according to the severity of pain, as well as the patient's underlying disease, age, and size. Patients with terminal cancer may be tolerant to opioid analgesics and may, therefore, require higher doses for adequate pain relief. Intravenous or subcutaneous administration is usually not painful. Should intravenous administration be necessary, the injection should be given slowly, over at least 2 to 3 minutes, depending on the dose. A gradual increase in dose may be required if analgesia is inadequate, tolerance occurs, or if pain severity increases. The first sign of tolerance is usually a reduced duration of effect.

Patients with hepatic and renal impairment should be started on a lower starting dose (see **CLINICAL PHARMACOLOGY - Pharmacokinetics and Metabolism**).

If DILAUDID INJECTION is substituted for a different opioid analgesic, the equivalency tables below should be used as a guide to determine the appropriate dose of DILAUDID INJECTION.

DILAUDID-HP

DILAUDID-HP SHOULD BE GIVEN ONLY TO PATIENTS WHO ARE ALREADY RECEIVING LARGE DOSES OF OPIOIDS. DILAUDID-HP is indicated for relief of moderate-to-severe pain in opioid-tolerant patients. Thus, these patients will already have been treated with other opioid analgesics. If the patient is being changed from regular DILAUDID to DILAUDID-HP, similar doses should be used, depending on the patient's clinical response to the drug. If DILAUDID-HP is substituted for a different opioid analgesic, the following equivalency table should be used as a guide to determine the appropriate dose of DILAUDID-HP. Patients with hepatic and renal impairment should be started on a lower starting dose (see **CLINICAL PHARMACOLOGY - Pharmacokinetics and Metabolism**).

OPIOID ANALGESIC EQUIVALENTS WITH APPROXIMATELY EQUIANALGESIC POTENCY*		
Drug Substance	IM or SC** Dose	Oral Dose
Morphine Sulfate	10 mg	40–60 mg
Hydromorphone HCl	1.3–2 mg	6.5–7.5 mg
Oxymorphone HCl	1–1.1 mg	6.6 mg
Levorphanol tartrate	2–2.3 mg	4 mg
Meperidine HCl (pethidine HCl)	75–100 mg	300–400 mg
Methadone HCl	10 mg	10–20 mg
Nalbuphine HCl	12 mg	—
Butorphanol tartrate	1.5-2.5 mg	—

*Dosages, and ranges of dosages represented, are a compilation of estimated equipotent dosages from published references comparing opioid analgesics in cancer and severe pain.
**IM = intramuscular; SC = subcutaneous

Experience with administration of DILAUDID-HP by the intravenous route is limited. Should intravenous administration be necessary, the injection should be given slowly, over at least 2 to 3 minutes.

A gradual increase in dose may be required if analgesia is inadequate, tolerance occurs, or if pain severity increases. The first sign of tolerance is usually a reduced duration of effect.

NOTE: Parenteral drug products should be inspected visually for particulate matter and discoloration prior to administration, whenever solution and container permit. A slight yellowish discoloration may develop in DILAUDID INJECTION and DILAUDID-HP ampules. No loss of potency has been demonstrated. DILAUDID INJECTION and DILAUDID-HP injection are physically compatible and chemically stable for at least 24 hours at 25°C protected from light in most common large volume parenteral solutions.

500 mg/50 mL Vial*

To use this single dose presentation, do not penetrate the stopper with a syringe. Instead, remove both the aluminum flipseal and rubber stopper in a suitable work area such as under a laminar flow hood (or equivalent clean air compounding area). The contents may then be withdrawn for preparation of a single, large volume parenteral solution. Any unused portion should be discarded in an appropriate manner.

Reconstitution of Sterile Lyophilized DILAUDID-HP 250 mg*

Reconstitute immediately prior to use with 25 mL of Sterile Water for Injection USP to provide a sterile solution containing 10 mg/mL.

*The Packaging Of These Products Contain Dry Natural Rubber.

Individualization Of Dosage

The dosage of opioid analgesics like hydromorphone hydrochloride should be individualized for any given patient, since adverse events can occur at doses that may not provide complete freedom from pain.

Safe and effective administration of opioid analgesics to patients with acute or chronic pain depends upon a comprehensive assessment of the patient. The nature of the pain (severity, frequency, etiology, and pathophysiology), as well as the concurrent medical status of the patient, will affect selection of the starting dosage.

In patients receiving opioids, both the dose and duration of analgesia will vary substantially depending on the patient's opioid tolerance. The dose should be selected and adjusted so that at least 3-4 hours of pain relief may be achieved. In patients taking opioid analgesics, the starting dose of DILAUDID INJECTION or DILAUDID-HP should be based on prior opioid usage. This should be done by converting the total daily usage of the previous opioid to an equivalent total daily dosage of DILAUDID INJECTION or DILAUDID-HP using an equianalgesic table (see above). For opioids not in the table, first estimate the equivalent total daily usage of oral morphine, then use the table to find the equivalent total daily dosage of DILAUDID INJECTION or DILAUDID-HP.

Once the total daily dosage of DILAUDID INJECTION or DILAUDID-HP has been estimated, it should be divided into the desired number of doses. Since there is individual variation in response to different opioid drugs, only 1/2 to 2/3 of the estimated dose of DILAUDID INJECTION or DILAUDID-HP calculated from equivalence tables should be given for the first few doses, then increased as needed according to the patient's response.

Since the pharmacokinetics of hydromorphone are affected in hepatic and renal impairment with a consequent increase in exposure, patients with hepatic and renal impairment should be started on a lower starting dose (see **CLINICAL PHARMACOLOGY - Pharmacokinetics and Metabolism**).

In chronic pain, doses should be administered around-the-clock. A supplemental dose of 5-15% of the total daily usage may be administered every two hours on an "as-needed" basis.

Periodic reassessment after the initial dosing is always required. If pain management is not satisfactory, and in the absence of significant opioid-induced adverse events, the hydromorphone dose may be increased gradually. If excessive opioid side effects are observed early in the dosing interval, the hydromorphone hydrochloride dose should be reduced. If this results in breakthrough pain at the end of the dosing interval, the dosing interval may need to be shortened. Dose titration should be guided more by the need for analgesia than the absolute dose of opioid employed.

DRUG ABUSE AND DEPENDENCE

DILAUDID INJECTION and DILAUDID-HP contain hydromorphone, a Schedule II controlled opioid agonist. Schedule II opioid substances which include morphine, oxycodone, oxymorphone, fentanyl, and methadone have the highest potential for abuse and risk of fatal overdose. Hydromorphone can be abused and is subject to criminal diversion.

Opioid analgesics may cause psychological and physical dependence. Physical dependence results in withdrawal symptoms in patients who abruptly discontinue the drug. Physical dependence usually does not occur to a clinically significant degree until after several weeks of continued opioid usage, but it may occur after as little as a week of opioid use. Physical dependence and tolerance are separate and distinct from abuse and addiction.

Addiction is a chronic, neurobiologic disease, with genetic, psychosocial, and environmental factors influencing its development and manifestations. It is characterized by behaviors that include one or more of the following: impaired control over drug use, compulsive use, continued use despite harm, and craving. Drug addiction is a treatable disease, utilizing a multidisciplinary approach, but relapse is common.

"Drug seeking" behavior is very common in addicts and drug abusers. Drug-seeking tactics include emergency calls or visits near the end of office hours, refusal to undergo appropriate examination, testing or referral, repeated "loss" of prescriptions, tampering with, forging or counterfeiting prescriptions and reluctance to provide prior medical records or contact information for other treating physician(s). "Doctor shopping" to obtain additional prescriptions is common among drug abusers, people suffering from untreated addiction and criminals seeking drugs to sell.

Physicians should be aware that addiction may not be accompanied by concurrent tolerance and symptoms of physical dependence in all addicts. In addition, abuse of opioids can occur in the absence of addiction and is characterized by misuse for non-medical purposes, often in combination with other psychoactive substances. Since DILAUDID INJECTION and DILAUDID-HP may be diverted for non-medical use, careful record keeping of prescribing information, including quantity, frequency, and renewal requests is strongly advised.

Proper assessment of the patient, proper prescribing practices, periodic re-evaluation of therapy, and proper dispensing and storage are appropriate measures that help to limit abuse of opioid drugs.

DILAUDID INJECTION and DILAUDID-HP are intended for parenteral use only under the direct supervision of an appropriately licensed health care provider. Misuse or abuse of DILAUDID INJECTION or DILAUDID-HP poses a risk of overdose and death. This risk is increased with concurrent abuse of alcohol and other substances. Parenteral drug abuse is commonly associated with transmission of infectious diseases such as hepatitis and HIV.

SAFETY AND HANDLING INSTRUCTIONS

DILAUDID INJECTION and DILAUDID-HP pose little risk of direct exposure to health care personnel and should be handled and disposed of prudently in accordance with hospital or institutional policy. Patients and their families should be instructed to flush any DILAUDID INJECTION or DILAUDID-HP that is no longer needed.

Access to abusable drugs such as DILAUDID INJECTION and DILAUDID-HP presents an occupational hazard for addiction in the health care industry. Routine procedures for handling controlled substances developed to protect the public may not be adequate to protect health care workers. Implementation of more effective accounting procedures and measures to restrict access to drugs of this class (appropriate to the practice setting) may minimize the risk of self-administration by health care providers.

HOW SUPPLIED

DILAUDID INJECTION

DILAUDID INJECTION (hydromorphone hydrochloride) is available in CLEAR ampules. Each 1 mL of sterile aqueous solution contains 1 mg, 2 mg, or 4 mg hydromorphone hydrochloride with 0.2% sodium citrate and 0.2% citric acid solution. No added preservative. DILAUDID INJECTION ampules are sterile and are supplied as follows:

NDC 59011-441-10: Box of ten 1 mg/mL ampules
NDC 59011-442-10: Box of ten 2 mg/mL ampules
NDC 59011-442-25: Box of 25 2 mg/mL ampules
NDC 59011-444-10: Box of ten 4 mg/mL ampules

DILAUDID-HP

DILAUDID-HP (hydromorphone hydrochloride) is available in AMBER ampules and single dose vials. Each 1 mL of sterile aqueous solution contains 10 mg hydromorphone hydrochloride with 0.2% sodium citrate and 0.2% citric acid solution. No added preservative.

DILAUDID-HP Sterile Lyophilized Powder contains 250 mg of sterile, lyophilized hydromorphone HCl in a Single Dose Vial.

Hydrochloric acid or sodium hydroxide may be added to adjust pH.

DILAUDID-HP ampules and single dose vials are sterile and are supplied as follows:

NDC 59011-445-01: Box of ten 1mL (10 mg) ampules
NDC 59011-445-05: Box of ten 5mL (50 mg) ampules
NDC 59011-445-50: One 50 mL (500 mg) Single-Dose Vial*
NDC 59011-446-25: One 250 mg single dose vial*

*The Packaging of These Products Contain Dry Natural Rubber
Storage
PROTECT FROM LIGHT.
Keep covered in carton until time of use. Store at 20°-25°C (68°-77°F); excursions permitted to 15°-30°C (59°-86°F) [See USP Controlled Room Temperature].

A Schedule C-II Narcotic. DEA Order Form Required.
Revised December, 22 2009
302211-0B
Manufactured by
Hospira, Inc., Lake Forest, IL 60045, U.S.A.
for
Purdue Pharma L.P. Stamford, CT 06901-3431
U.S. Patent Number 6,589,960
Shown in Product Identification Guide, page 317

OXYCONTIN® Ⓒ ℞

[ŏks' ē-kŏn-tĭn]

(oxycodone hydrochloride controlled-release) Tablets

HIGHLIGHTS OF PRESCRIBING INFORMATION

These highlights do not include all the information needed to use OXYCONTIN® safely and effectively. See full prescribing information for OXYCONTIN.

OxyContin® (oxycodone hydrochloride controlled-release) Tablets CII
Initial U.S. Approval: 1982

WARNING: IMPORTANCE OF PROPER PATIENT SELECTION AND POTENTIAL FOR ABUSE
See full prescribing information for complete boxed warning.
• OxyContin contains oxycodone which is an opioid agonist and a Schedule II controlled substance with an abuse liability similar to morphine. (9)

- OxyContin is indicated for the management of moderate to severe pain when a continuous, around-the-clock opioid analgesic is needed for an extended period of time. (1)
- OxyContin is NOT intended for use on an as-needed basis. (1)
- OxyContin 60 mg and 80 mg Tablets, a single dose greater than 40 mg, or a total daily dose greater than 80 mg are only for use in opioid-tolerant patients to avoid fatal respiratory depression. (2.7)
- Patients should be assessed for their clinical risks for opioid abuse or addiction prior to being prescribed opioids. (2.2)
- OxyContin tablets must be swallowed whole and must not be cut, broken, chewed, crushed, or dissolved which can lead to rapid release and absorption of a potentially fatal dose of oxycodone. (2.1)
- The concomitant use with cytochrome P450 3A4 inhibitors such as macrolide antibiotics and protease inhibitors may result in an increase in oxycodone plasma concentrations and may cause potentially fatal respiratory depression. (7.2)

INDICATIONS AND USAGE

OxyContin is an opioid agonist indicated for:
- Management of moderate to severe pain when a continuous, around-the-clock opioid analgesic is needed for an extended period of time. (1)
- Not for use on an as-needed basis or in the immediate post-operative period. (1)

DOSAGE AND ADMINISTRATION

- Use low initial doses in patients who are not already opioid-tolerant, especially those who are receiving concurrent treatment with muscle relaxants, sedatives, or other central nervous system (CNS) active medications. (2.2)
- For patients already receiving opioids, use standard conversion ratio estimates. (2.2)
- Tablets must be swallowed whole and are not to be cut, broken, chewed, crushed, or dissolved (risk of potentially fatal dose). (2.1)

DOSAGE FORMS AND STRENGTHS

- Controlled-Release Tablets: 10 mg, 15 mg, 20 mg, 30 mg, 40 mg, 60 mg and 80 mg (3)

CONTRAINDICATIONS

- in patients who have significant respiratory depression (4)
- in patients who have or are suspected of having paralytic ileus (4)
- in patients who have acute or severe bronchial asthma (4)
- in patients with known hypersensitivity to oxycodone (4)

WARNINGS AND PRECAUTIONS

- Must be swallowed whole (5.1)
- May cause somnolence, dizziness, alterations in judgment and alterations in levels of consciousness, including coma. (5.2)
- Additive CNS effects are expected when used with alcohol, other opioids, or illicit drugs. (5.1, 5.3, 7.3)
- Use with caution in patients who are receiving other CNS depressants. (5.1, 5.3, 7.3)
- May cause respiratory depression, use with extreme caution in patients at risk of respiratory depression, elderly and debilitated patients (5.4)
- May aggravate convulsions in patients with convulsive disorders, and may induce or aggravate seizures in some clinical settings. (5.5)
- May worsen increased intracranial pressure and obscure its signs, such as level of consciousness or pupillary signs. (5.6)
- May cause hypotension, use with caution in patients at increased risk of hypotension and in patients in circulatory shock. (5.7)
- Concomitant use of CYP3A4 inhibitors may increase opioid effects (5.8)
- Mixed agonist/antagonist analgesics may precipitate withdrawal symptoms. (5.9)
- Use with caution in patients with biliary tract disease, including acute pancreatitis. (5.10)
- Use with caution in patients at risk for ileus. Monitor for decreased bowel motility in postoperative patients. (5.10)
- Tolerance may develop. (5.11)
- Use with caution in alcoholism; adrenocortical insufficiency; hypothyroidism; prostatic hypertrophy or urethral stricture; severe impairment of hepatic, pulmonary or renal function; and toxic psychosis. (5.12)
- May impair the mental and physical abilities needed to perform potentially hazardous activities such as driving a car or operating machinery. (5.13)
- No approved use in the treatment of addiction. (5.14)
- Not every urine drug test for "opioids" or "opiates" detects oxycodone reliably. (5.15)

ADVERSE REACTIONS

Most common adverse reactions (>5%) are constipation, nausea, somnolence, dizziness, vomiting, pruritus, headache, dry mouth, asthenia, and sweating.

To report Suspected Adverse Reactions, contact Purdue Pharma L.P. at 1-888-726-7535 or FDA at 1-800-FDA-1088 or www.fda.gov/medwatch.

DRUG INTERACTIONS

- OxyContin may enhance the neuromuscular blocking action of skeletal muscle relaxants and produce an increased degree of respiratory depression. (7.1)
- The CYP3A4 isoenzyme plays a major role in the metabolism of OxyContin, drugs that inhibit CYP3A4 activity may cause decreased clearance of oxycodone which could lead to an increase in oxycodone plasma concentrations. (7.2)
- Concurrent use of other CNS depressants may cause respiratory depression, hypotension, and profound sedation or coma. (7.3)
- Mixed agonist/antagonist analgesics may reduce the analgesic effect of oxycodone and may precipitate withdrawal symptoms in these patients. (7.4)

USE IN SPECIFIC POPULATIONS

- Labor and Delivery: Not recommended for use in women immediately prior to and during labor and delivery; (8.2)
- Nursing Mothers: Nursing should not be undertaken while a patient is receiving OxyContin. (8.3)
- Pediatrics: Safety and effectiveness in pediatric patients below the age of 18 have not been established. (8.4)
- Geriatrics: The initial dose may need to be reduced to 1/3 to ½ of the usual doses. (8.5)
- Hepatic impairment: Initiate therapy at 1/3 to 1/2 the usual doses and titrate carefully. (8.6)
- Renal impairment: Dose initiation should follow a conservative approach. (8.7)

See 17 for PATIENT COUNSELING INFORMATION and Medication Guide.
Revised: 08/2010

FULL PRESCRIBING INFORMATION

WARNING: IMPORTANCE OF PROPER PATIENT SELECTION AND POTENTIAL FOR ABUSE
OxyContin contains oxycodone which is an opioid agonist and a Schedule II controlled substance with an abuse liability similar to morphine. (9)
OxyContin can be abused in a manner similar to other opioid agonists, legal or illicit. This should be considered when prescribing or dispensing OxyContin in situations where the physician or pharmacist is concerned about an increased risk of misuse, abuse, or diversion. (9.2)
OxyContin is a controlled-release oral formulation of oxycodone hydrochloride indicated for the management of moderate to severe pain when a continuous, around-the-clock opioid analgesic is needed for an extended period of time. (1)
OxyContin is not intended for use on an as-needed basis. (1)
Patients considered opioid tolerant are those who are taking at least 60 mg oral morphine/day, 25 mcg transdermal fentanyl/hour, 30 mg oral oxycodone/day, 8 mg oral hydromorphone/day, 25 mg oral oxymorphone/day, or an equianalgesic dose of another opioid for one week or longer.
OxyContin 60 mg and 80 mg tablets, a single dose greater than 40 mg, or a total daily dose greater than 80 mg are only for use in opioid-tolerant patients, as they may cause fatal respiratory depression when administered to patients who are not tolerant to the respiratory-depressant or sedating effects of opioids. (2.7)
Persons at increased risk for opioid abuse include those with a personal or family history of substance abuse (including drug or alcohol abuse or addiction) or mental illness (e.g., major depression). Patients should be assessed for their clinical risks for opioid abuse or addiction prior to being prescribed opioids. All patients receiving opioids should be routinely monitored for signs of misuse, abuse and addiction. (2.2)
OxyContin must be swallowed whole and must not be cut, broken, chewed, crushed, or dissolved. Taking cut, broken, chewed, crushed or dissolved OxyContin tablets leads to rapid release and absorption of a potentially fatal dose of oxycodone. (2.1)
The concomitant use of OxyContin with all cytochrome P450 3A4 inhibitors such as macrolide antibiotics (e.g., erythromycin), azole-antifungal agents (e.g., ketoconazole), and protease inhibitors (e.g., ritonavir) may result in an increase in oxycodone plasma concentrations, which could increase or prolong adverse effects and may cause potentially fatal respiratory depression. Patients receiving OxyContin and a CYP3A4 inhibitor should be carefully monitored for an extended period of time and dosage adjustments should be made if warranted. (7.2)

1 INDICATIONS AND USAGE

OxyContin is a controlled-release oral formulation of oxycodone hydrochloride indicated for the management of moderate to severe pain when a continuous, around-the-clock opioid analgesic is needed for an extended period of time.

Limitations of Usage
OxyContin is not intended for use on an as-needed basis. OxyContin is not indicated for the management of pain in the immediate postoperative period (the first 12-24 hours following surgery), or if the pain is mild, or not expected to persist for an extended period of time. OxyContin is

indicated for postoperative use following the immediate post-operative period only if the patient is already receiving the drug prior to surgery or if the postoperative pain is expected to be moderate to severe and persist for an extended period of time. Physicians should individualize treatment, moving from parenteral to oral analgesics as appropriate. (See American Pain Society guidelines.)

OxyContin is not indicated for pre-emptive analgesia (pre-operative administration for the management of postoperative pain).

OxyContin is not indicated for rectal administration.

2 DOSAGE AND ADMINISTRATION

2.1 Safe Administration Instructions

OxyContin tablets must be swallowed whole and must not be cut, broken, chewed, crushed or dissolved. Taking cut, broken, chewed, crushed or dissolved OxyContin tablets leads to rapid release and absorption of a potentially fatal dose of oxycodone.

Selection of patients for treatment with OxyContin should be governed by the same principles that apply to the use of similar opioid analgesics. Physicians should individualize treatment using a progressive plan of pain management such as outlined by the World Health Organization, Federation of State Medical Boards Model Policy, and the American Pain Society. Healthcare professionals should follow appropriate pain management principles of careful assessment and ongoing monitoring.

2.2 Initiating Therapy with OxyContin

It is critical to initiate the dosing regimen for each patient individually. Attention should be given to:

- risk factors for abuse or addiction; including whether the patient has a previous or current substance abuse problem, a family history of substance abuse, or a history of mental illness or depression;
- the age, general condition and medical status of the patient;
- the patient's opioid exposure and opioid tolerance (if any);
- the daily dose, potency, and kind of the analgesic(s) the patient has been taking;
- the reliability of the conversion estimate used to calculate the dose of oxycodone;
- the special instructions for OxyContin 60 mg and 80 mg tablets, a single dose greater than 40 mg, **or total daily doses greater than 80 mg [see Dosage and Administration (2.7)];** and
- the balance between pain control and adverse reactions.

Use low initial doses of OxyContin in patients who are not already opioid-tolerant [see Dosage and Administration (2.7)], especially those who are receiving concurrent treatment with muscle relaxants, sedatives, or other CNS active medications [see Warnings and Precautions (5.1, 5.3) and Drug Interactions (7.1, 7.3)].

Experience indicates a reasonable starting dose of OxyContin for patients who are taking non-opioid analgesics and require continuous around-the-clock therapy for an extended period of time is 10 mg every 12 hours. Individually titrate OxyContin to a dose that provides adequate analgesia and minimizes adverse reactions while maintaining an every-twelve-hour dosing regimen.

For initiation of OxyContin therapy for patients previously taking opioids, the conversion ratios found in Table 1 are a reasonable starting point, although not verified in well-controlled, multiple-dose trials. No fixed conversion ratio is likely to be satisfactory in all patients, especially patients receiving large opioid doses. A reasonable approach for converting from existing opioid therapy to OxyContin is as follows:

- Discontinue all other around-the-clock opioid drugs when OxyContin therapy is initiated.
- Using standard conversion ratio estimates (see Table 1), multiply the mg/day of each of the current opioids to be converted by their appropriate multiplication factor to obtain the equivalent total daily dose of oral oxycodone.
- Divide the calculated 24-hour oxycodone dose in half to approximate the every 12-hour dose of OxyContin.
- Round down, if necessary, to the appropriate OxyContin tablet strengths available.
- Close observation and frequent titration are indicated until patients are stable on the new therapy.

TABLE 1
Multiplication Factors for Converting the Daily Dose of Current Opioids to the Daily Dose of Oral Oxycodone[1]*

(mg/Day Opioid × Factor = mg/Day Oral Oxycodone)	
Oral Opioid	Parenteral Opioid
Oxycodone	1	—
Codeine	0.15	—
Hydrocodone	0.9	—
Hydromorphone	4	20
Levorphanol	7.5	15
Meperidine	0.1	0.4
Methadone	1.5	3
Morphine	0.5	3

* To be used only for conversion to oral oxycodone. For patients receiving high-dose parenteral opioids, a more conservative conversion is warranted. For example, for high-dose parenteral morphine, use 1.5 instead of 3 as a multiplication factor.

2.3 Conversion from Transdermal Fentanyl to OxyContin

Eighteen hours following the removal of the transdermal fentanyl patch, OxyContin treatment can be initiated. Although there has been no systematic assessment of such conversion, a conservative oxycodone dose, approximately 10 mg every 12 hours of OxyContin, should be initially substituted for each 25 mcg/hr fentanyl transdermal patch. Follow the patient closely during conversion from transdermal fentanyl to OxyContin, as there is limited documented experience with this conversion.

2.4 Hepatic Impairment

For patients with hepatic impairment, start dosing patients at 1/3 to 1/2 the usual starting dose followed by careful dose titration [see Clinical Pharmacology (12.3)].

2.5 Managing Expected Opioid Adverse Reactions

Most patients receiving OxyContin, especially those who are opioid-naive, will experience adverse reactions. Patients do not usually become tolerant to the constipating effects of opioids, therefore, anticipate constipation and treat aggressively and prophylactically with a stimulant laxative with or without a stool softener. If nausea persists and is unacceptable to the patient, consider treatment with antiemetics or other modalities to relieve these symptoms.

2.6 Individualization of Dosage

Once therapy is initiated, assess pain relief and other opioid effects frequently. Titrate patients to adequate effect (generally mild or no pain with the regular use of no more than two doses of supplemental analgesia per 24 hours). Patients who experience breakthrough pain may require dosage adjustment or rescue medication. Because steady-state plasma concentrations are approximated within 24 to 36 hours, dosage adjustment may be carried out every 1 to 2 days.

There are no well-controlled clinical studies evaluating the safety and efficacy with dosing more frequently than every 12 hours. Increase the OxyContin dose by increasing the total daily dose, not by changing the 12-hour dosing interval. As a guideline, the total daily oxycodone dose usually can be increased by 25% to 50% of the current dose, each time an increase is clinically indicated.

If signs of excessive opioid-related adverse reactions are observed, the next dose may be reduced. If this adjustment leads to inadequate analgesia, a supplemental dose of immediate-release oxycodone may be given. Alternatively, non-opioid analgesic adjuvants may be employed. Adjust the dose to obtain an appropriate balance between pain relief and opioid-related adverse reactions.

During periods of changing analgesic requirements, including initial titration, maintain frequent contact between physician, other members of the healthcare team, the patient and, with proper consent, the caregiver/family.

2.7 Special Instructions for Patients who are not Opioid Tolerant

Do not begin treatment with OxyContin 60 mg and 80 mg Tablets, a single dose greater than 40 mg, or a total daily dose greater than 80 mg in patients who are not already tolerant to the respiratory-depressant and sedating effects of opioids. Use of these doses in patients who are not opioid tolerant may cause fatal respiratory depression. These doses are only for use in opioid-tolerant patients.

Patients considered opioid tolerant are those who are taking at least 60 mg oral morphine/day, 25 mcg transdermal fentanyl/hour, 30 mg oral oxycodone/day, 8 mg oral hydromorphone/day, 25 mg oral oxymorphone/day, or an equianalgesic dose of another opioid for one week or longer.

Instruct patients not to share or permit use by individuals other than the patient for whom OxyContin was prescribed, as such inappropriate use may have severe medical consequences, including death.

2.8 Continuation of Therapy

During chronic therapy, especially for non-cancer pain syndromes, reassess the continued need for around-the-clock opioid therapy regularly (e.g., every 6 to 12 months) as appropriate.

2.9 Cessation of Therapy

When the patient no longer requires therapy with OxyContin, taper the dose gradually to prevent signs and symptoms of withdrawal in the physically-dependent patient.

2.10 Conversion from OxyContin to Parenteral Opioids

To avoid overdose, follow conservative dose conversion ratios. When converting from OxyContin to parenteral opioids, it is advisable to calculate an equivalent parenteral dose and then initiate treatment at half of this calculated value.

3 DOSAGE FORMS AND STRENGTHS

- 10 mg film-coated tablets (round, white-colored, bi-convex tablets debossed with OP on one side and 10 on the other)
- 15 mg film-coated tablets (round, gray-colored, bi-convex tablets debossed with OP on one side and 15 on the other)
- 20 mg film-coated tablets (round, pink-colored, bi-convex tablets debossed with OP on one side and 20 on the other)
- 30 mg film-coated tablets (round, brown-colored, bi-convex tablets debossed with OP on one side and 30 on the other)
- 40 mg film-coated tablets (round, yellow-colored, bi-convex tablets debossed with OP on one side and 40 on the other)
- 60 mg film-coated tablets* (round, red-colored, bi-convex tablets debossed with OP on one side and 60 on the other)
- 80 mg film-coated tablets* (round, green-colored, bi-convex tablets debossed with OP on one side and 80 on the other)

* 60 mg and 80 mg tablets for use in opioid-tolerant patients only

4 CONTRAINDICATIONS

OxyContin is contraindicated in:

- patients who have significant respiratory depression
- patients who have or are suspected of having paralytic ileus
- patients who have acute or severe bronchial asthma
- patients who have known hypersensitivity to any of its components or the active ingredient, oxycodone.

5 WARNINGS AND PRECAUTIONS

5.1 Information Essential for Safe Administration

OxyContin tablets must be swallowed whole and must not be cut, broken, chewed, crushed, or dissolved. Taking cut, broken, chewed, crushed or dissolved OxyContin tablets leads to rapid release and absorption of a potentially fatal dose of oxycodone.

OxyContin 60 mg and 80 mg Tablets, a single dose greater than 40 mg, or a total daily dose greater than 80 mg are only for use in opioid-tolerant patients. Use of these doses in patients who are not opioid tolerant may cause fatal respiratory depression.

Instruct patients against use by individuals other than the patient for whom OxyContin was prescribed, as such inappropriate use may have severe medical consequences, including death.

Opioid analgesics have a narrow therapeutic index in certain patient populations, especially when combined with CNS depressant drugs, and should be reserved for cases where the benefits of opioid analgesia outweigh the known risks of respiratory depression, altered mental state, and postural hypotension.

5.2 CNS Depression

OxyContin may cause somnolence, dizziness, alterations in judgment and alterations in levels of consciousness, including coma.

5.3 Interactions with Alcohol, CNS Depressants and Illicit Drugs

Hypotension, profound sedation, coma or respiratory depression may result if OxyContin is added to a regimen that includes other CNS depressants (e.g., sedatives, anxiolytics, hypnotics, neuroleptics, other opioids). Therefore, use caution when deciding to initiate therapy with OxyContin in patients who are taking other CNS depressants. Take into account the types of other medications being taken, the duration of therapy with them, and the patient's response to those medicines, including the degree of tolerance that has developed to CNS depression. Consider the patient's use, if any, of alcohol and/or illicit drugs that cause CNS depression. If the decision to begin OxyContin is made, start with a lower OxyContin dose than usual. [see Drug Interactions (7.3)]

Consider using a lower initial dose of a CNS depressant when given to a patient currently taking OxyContin due to the potential of additive CNS depressant effects.

5.4 Respiratory Depression

Decreased respiratory drive resulting in respiratory depression is the chief hazard from the use or abuse of opioid agonists, including OxyContin. The risk of opioid-induced respiratory depression is increased, for example, in elderly [see Use In Specific Populations (8.5)] or debilitated patients; following large initial doses in any patient who is not tolerant to the respiratory-depressant or sedating effects of opioids; or when opioids are given in conjunction with other agents that either depress respiratory drive or consciousness.

Use OxyContin with extreme caution in patients with any of the following:

- significant chronic obstructive pulmonary disease or cor pulmonale
- other risk of substantially decreased respiratory reserve
- hypoxia
- hypercapnia
- pre-existing respiratory depression

Respiratory depression induced by opioids typically follows a pattern entailing first a shift in CO_2 responsiveness of the CNS respiratory drive center, which results in a decrease in the urge to breathe, despite the presence of hypercapnia. The increase in brain CO_2 can result in sedation that can accentuate the sedation from the opioid itself. Profound sedation, unresponsiveness, infrequent deep ("sighing") breaths or atypical snoring frequently accompany opioid-induced respiratory depression. Eventually, hypoxia ensues. In addition to further decreasing consciousness, hypoxia, along with hypercapnia, can predispose to life-threatening cardiac arrhythmias.

5.5 Seizures

Oxycodone, as with other opioids, may aggravate convulsions in patients with convulsive disorders, and may induce or aggravate seizures in some clinical settings. Use OxyContin with caution in patients with a history of seizure disorders.

5.6 Head Injury

The respiratory depressant effects of opioids include carbon dioxide retention, which can lead to an elevation of cerebrospinal fluid pressure. This effect may be exaggerated in the presence of head injury, intracranial lesions, or other sources of pre-existing increased intracranial pressure. Oxycodone may produce miosis that is independent of ambient light, and altered consciousness, either of which may obscure neurologic signs associated with increased intracranial pressure in persons with head injuries.

5.7 Hypotensive Effect

OxyContin may cause severe hypotension. There is an added risk to individuals whose ability to maintain blood pressure has been compromised by a depleted blood volume, or after concurrent administration with drugs such as phenothiazines or other agents which compromise vasomotor tone. Oxycodone may produce orthostatic hypotension in ambulatory patients. Administer OxyContin with caution to patients in circulatory shock, since vasodilation produced by the drug may further reduce cardiac output and blood pressure.

5.8 Cytochrome P450 3A4 Inhibitors and Inducers

Since the CYP3A4 isoenzyme plays a major role in the metabolism of OxyContin, drugs that alter CYP3A4 activity may cause changes in clearance of oxycodone which could lead to changes in oxycodone plasma concentrations.

The expected clinical results with CYP3A4 inhibitors would be an increase in oxycodone plasma concentrations and possibly increased or prolonged opioid effects. The expected clinical results with CYP3A4 inducers would be a decrease in oxycodone plasma concentrations, lack of efficacy or, possibly, development of an abstinence syndrome in a patient who had developed physical dependence to oxycodone.

If co-administration is necessary, caution is advised when initiating OxyContin treatment in patients currently taking, or discontinuing, CYP3A4 inhibitors or inducers. Evaluate these patients at frequent intervals and consider dose adjustments until stable drug effects are achieved. *[see Drug Interactions (7.2) and Clinical Pharmacology (12)]*

5.9 Interactions with Mixed Agonist/Antagonist Opioid Analgesics

It is generally not advisable to administer mixed agonist/antagonist analgesics (i.e., pentazocine, nalbuphine, and butorphanol) to a patient receiving OxyContin. In this situation, mixed agonist/antagonist analgesics may reduce the analgesic effect and may precipitate withdrawal symptoms in these patients.

5.10 Use in Pancreatic/Biliary Tract Disease and Other Gastrointestinal Conditions

Oxycodone may cause spasm of the sphincter of Oddi and should be used with caution in patients with biliary tract disease, including acute pancreatitis. Opioids may cause increases in the serum amylase.

The administration of OxyContin may obscure the diagnosis or clinical course in patients with acute abdominal conditions. Use OxyContin with caution in patients who are at risk of developing ileus.

5.11 Tolerance

Tolerance to opioids is demonstrated by the need for increasing doses to maintain adequate analgesic effect (in the absence of disease progression or other external factors). If tolerance develops, or if pain severity increases, a gradual increase in dose may be required. The first sign of tolerance is usually a reduced duration of effect. Tolerance to different effects of opioids may develop to varying degrees and at varying rates in a given individual. There is also interpatient variability in the rate and extent of tolerance that develops to various opioid effects, whether the effect is desirable (e.g., analgesia) or undesirable (e.g., nausea).

5.12 Special Risk Groups

Use OxyContin with caution in the following conditions, due to increased risk of adverse reactions: alcoholism; delirium tremens; adrenocortical insufficiency; CNS depression; debilitation; kyphoscoliosis associated with respiratory compromise; myxedema or hypothyroidism; prostatic hypertrophy or urethral stricture; severe impairment of hepatic, pulmonary or renal function; and toxic psychosis.

5.13 Driving and Operating Machinery

OxyContin may impair the mental and physical abilities needed to perform potentially hazardous activities such as driving a car or operating machinery. Caution patients accordingly.

5.14 Use in Addiction Treatment

OxyContin has no approved use in the treatment of addiction. Its proper usage in individuals with drug or alcohol addiction (substance dependence), either active or in remission, is for the management of pain requiring opioid analgesia.

5.15 Laboratory Monitoring

Not every urine drug test for "opioids" or "opiates" detects oxycodone reliably, especially those designed for in-office use. Further, many laboratories will report urine drug concentrations below a specified "cut-off" value as "negative". Therefore, if urine testing for oxycodone is considered in the clinical management of an individual patient, ensure that the sensitivity and specificity of the assay is appropriate, and use caution in interpreting results.

6 ADVERSE REACTIONS

The following adverse reactions described elsewhere in the labeling include:

- Respiratory depression *[see Boxed Warning, Warnings and Precautions (5.1, 5.4) and Overdosage (10)]*
- CNS depression *[see Warnings and Precautions (5.1, 5.2) and Overdosage (10)]*
- Hypotensive effects *[see Warning and Precautions (5.7) and Overdosage (10)]*
- Drug abuse, addiction, and dependence *[see Drug Abuse and Dependence (9.2, 9.3)]*
- Paralytic ileus *[see Warnings and Precautions (5.10)]*
- Seizures *[see Warnings and Precautions (5.5)]*

6.1 Clinical Trial Experience

Because clinical trials are conducted under widely varying conditions, adverse reaction rates observed in the clinical trials of a drug cannot be directly compared to rates in the clinical trials of another drug and may not reflect the rates observed in practice.

The safety of OxyContin was evaluated in double-blind clinical trials involving 713 patients with moderate to severe pain of various etiologies. In open-label studies of cancer pain, 187 patients received OxyContin in total daily doses ranging from 20 mg to 640 mg per day. The average total daily dose was approximately 105 mg per day. OxyContin may increase the risk of serious adverse reactions such as those observed with other opioid analgesics, including respiratory depression, apnea, respiratory arrest, circulatory depression, hypotension, or shock *[see Overdosage (10)]*.

The most common adverse reactions (>5%) reported by patients in clinical trials comparing OxyContin with placebo are shown in Table 2 below:

TABLE 2: Common Adverse Reactions (>5%)

Adverse Reaction	OxyContin (n=227)	Placebo (n=45)
	(%)	(%)
Constipation	(23)	(7)
Nausea	(23)	(11)
Somnolence	(23)	(4)
Dizziness	(13)	(9)
Pruritus	(13)	(2)
Vomiting	(12)	(7)
Headache	(7)	(7)
Dry Mouth	(6)	(2)
Asthenia	(6)	-
Sweating	(5)	(2)

In clinical trials, the following adverse reactions were reported in patients treated with OxyContin with an incidence between 1% and 5%:

Gastrointestinal disorders: abdominal pain, diarrhea, dyspepsia, gastritis, hiccups

General disorders and administration site conditions: chills, fever

Metabolism and nutrition disorders: anorexia

Musculoskeletal and connective tissue disorders: twitching

Psychiatric disorders: abnormal dreams, anxiety, confusion, dysphoria, euphoria, insomnia, nervousness, thought abnormalities

Respiratory, thoracic and mediastinal disorders: dyspnea, hiccups

Skin and subcutaneous tissue disorders: rash

Vascular disorders: postural hypotension

The following adverse reactions occurred **in less than 1% of patients** involved in clinical trials:

Blood and lymphatic system disorders: lymphadenopathy

Ear and labyrinth disorders: tinnitus

Eye disorders: abnormal vision

Gastrointestinal disorders: dysphagia, eructation, flatulence, gastrointestinal disorder, increased appetite, stomatitis

General disorders and administration site conditions: withdrawal syndrome (with and without seizures), edema, peripheral edema, thirst, malaise, chest pain, facial edema

Injury, poisoning and procedural complications: accidental injury

Investigations: ST depression

Metabolism and nutrition disorders: dehydration

Nervous system disorders: syncope, migraine, abnormal gait, amnesia, hyperkinesia, hypesthesia, hypotonia, paresthesia, speech disorder, stupor, tremor, vertigo, taste perversion

Psychiatric disorders: depression, agitation, depersonalization, emotional lability, hallucination

Renal and urinary disorders: dysuria, hematuria, polyuria, urinary retention

Reproductive system and breast disorders: impotence

Respiratory, thoracic and mediastinal disorders: cough increased, voice alteration

Skin and subcutaneous tissue disorders: dry skin, exfoliative dermatitis

6.2 Postmarketing Experience

The following adverse reactions have been identified during post-approval use of controlled-release oxycodone. Because these events are reported voluntarily from a population of uncertain size, it is not always possible to reliably estimate their frequency or establish a causal relationship to drug exposure: abuse, addiction, overdose, death, amenorrhea, symptoms associated with an anaphylactic or anaphylactoid reaction, cholestasis, dental caries, increased hepatic enzymes, muscular hypertonia, hyponatremia, ileus, palpitations (in the context of withdrawal), seizures, syndrome of inappropriate antidiuretic hormone secretion, and urticaria

7 DRUG INTERACTIONS

7.1 Neuromuscular Junction Blocking Agents

OxyContin may enhance the neuromuscular blocking action of true skeletal muscle relaxants (such as pancuronium) and produce an increased degree and/or duration of respiratory depression.

7.2 Agents Affecting Cytochrome P450 Isoenzymes

Inhibitors of CYP3A4:

Since the CYP3A4 isoenzyme plays a major role in the metabolism of OxyContin, drugs that inhibit CYP3A4 activity, such as macrolide antibiotics (e.g., erythromycin), azole-antifungal agents (e.g., ketoconazole), and protease inhibitors (e.g., ritonavir), may cause decreased clearance of oxycodone which could lead to an increase in oxycodone plasma concentrations. A published study showed that the co-administration of the antifungal drug, voriconazole, increased oxycodone AUC and C_{max} by 3.6 and 1.7 fold, respectively. Although clinical studies have not been conducted with other CYP3A4 inhibitors, the expected clinical results would be increased or prolonged opioid effects. If co-administration with OxyContin is necessary, caution is advised when initiating therapy with, currently taking, or discontinuing CYP450 inhibitors. Evaluate these patients at frequent intervals and consider dose adjustments until stable drug effects are achieved. *[see Clinical Pharmacology (12.3)]*

Inducers of CYP3A4:

CYP450 inducers, such as rifampin, carbamazepine, and phenytoin, may induce the metabolism of oxycodone and, therefore, may cause increased clearance of the drug which could lead to a decrease in oxycodone plasma concentrations, lack of efficacy or, possibly, development of an abstinence syndrome in a patient who had developed physical dependence to oxycodone. A published study showed that the co-administration of rifampin, a drug metabolizing enzyme inducer, decreased oxycodone (oral) AUC and Cmax by 86% and 63%, respectively. If co-administration with OxyContin is necessary, caution is advised when initiating therapy with, currently taking, or discontinuing CYP3A4 inducers. Evaluate these patients at frequent intervals and consider dose adjustments until stable drug effects are achieved.

Inhibitors of CYP2D6:

Oxycodone is metabolized in part to oxymorphone via cytochrome CYP2D6. While this pathway may be blocked by a variety of drugs (e.g., certain cardiovascular drugs including amiodarone and quinidine as well as polycyclic antidepressants), such blockade has not been shown to be of clinical significance during oxycodone treatment.

7.3 CNS Depressants

Start OxyContin at 1/3 to 1/2 of the usual dosage in patients who are concurrently receiving other CNS depressants including sedatives or hypnotics, general anesthetics, phenothiazines, centrally acting anti-emetics, tranquilizers, and alcohol because respiratory depression, hypotension, and profound sedation or coma may result. No specific interaction between oxycodone and monoamine oxidase inhibitors has been observed, but caution in the use of any opioid in patients taking this class of drugs is appropriate. *[see Warnings and Precautions (5.2)]*

7.4 Interactions with Mixed Agonist/Antagonist Opioid Analgesics

Mixed agonist/antagonist analgesics (i.e., pentazocine, nalbuphine, and butorphanol) should generally not be administered to a patient who has received or is receiving a course of therapy with a pure opioid agonist analgesic such as OxyContin. In this situation, mixed agonist/antagonist analgesics may reduce the analgesic effect of oxycodone and may precipitate withdrawal symptoms in these patients.

8 USE IN SPECIFIC POPULATIONS

8.1 Pregnancy

Category B:

There are no adequate and well-controlled studies of oxycodone use during pregnancy. Based on limited human data in the literature, oxycodone does not appear to increase the risk of congenital malformations. In animal reproduction and developmental toxicology studies, no evidence of fetal harm was observed. Because animal reproduction studies are not always predictive of human response, oxycodone should be used during pregnancy only if clearly needed.

Teratogenic Effects

The effect of oxycodone in human reproduction has not been adequately studied. Studies with oral doses of oxycodone hydrochloride in rats up to 8 mg/kg/day and rabbits up to 125 mg/kg/day, equivalent to 0.5 and 15 times an adult human dose of 160 mg/day, respectively on a mg/m^2 basis, did not reveal evidence of harm to the fetus due to oxycodone. In a pre- and postnatal toxicity study, female rats received oxycodone during gestation and lactation. There were no long-term developmental or reproductive effects in the pups. *[see Nonclinical Toxicology (13)]*

Non-Teratogenic Effects

Oxycodone hydrochloride was administered orally to female rats during gestation and lactation in a pre- and postnatal toxicity study. There were no drug-related effects on reproductive performance in these females or any long-term developmental or reproductive effects in pups born to these rats. Decreased body weight was found during lactation and the early post-weaning phase in pups nursed by mothers given the highest dose used (6 mg/kg/day, equivalent to approximately 0.4-times an adult human dose of 160 mg/day, on a mg/m^2 basis). However, body weight of these pups recovered.

8.2 Labor and Delivery

Opioids cross the placenta and may produce respiratory depression and psychophysiologic effects in neonates. OxyContin is not recommended for use in women immediately prior to and during labor, when use of shorter-acting analgesics or other analgesic techniques are more appropriate. Occasionally, opioid analgesics may prolong labor through actions which temporarily reduce the strength, duration and frequency of uterine contractions. However this effect is not consistent and may be offset by an increased rate of cervical dilatation, which tends to shorten labor.

Closely observe neonates whose mothers received opioid analgesics during labor for signs of respiratory depression. Have a specific opioid antagonist, such as naloxone or nalmefene, available for reversal of opioid-induced respiratory depression in the neonate.

Neonates whose mothers have been taking opioids chronically may also exhibit withdrawal signs, either at birth and/or in the nursery, because they have developed physical dependence. This is not, however, synonymous with addiction *[see Drug Abuse and Dependence (9.3)]*. Neonatal opioid withdrawal syndrome, unlike opioid withdrawal syndrome in adults, may be life-threatening and should be treated according to protocols developed by neonatology experts.

8.3 Nursing Mothers

Oxycodone has been detected in breast milk. Instruct patients not to undertake nursing while receiving OxyContin. Do not initiate OxyContin therapy while nursing because of the possibility of sedation or respiratory depression in the infant.

Withdrawal symptoms can occur in breast-fed infants when maternal administration of an opioid analgesic is stopped, or when breast-feeding is stopped.

8.4 Pediatric Use

Safety and effectiveness of OxyContin in pediatric patients below the age of 18 years have not been established.

8.5 Geriatric Use

In controlled pharmacokinetic studies in elderly subjects (greater than 65 years) the clearance of oxycodone was slightly reduced. Compared to young adults, the plasma concentrations of oxycodone were increased approximately 15% *[see Clinical Pharmacology (12.3)]*. Of the total number of subjects (445) in clinical studies of oxycodone hydrochloride controlled-release tablets, 148 (33.3%) were age 65 and older (including those age 75 and older) while 40 (9.0%) were age 75 and older. In clinical trials with appropriate initiation of therapy and dose titration, no untoward or unexpected adverse reactions were seen in the elderly patients who received oxycodone hydrochloride controlled-release tablets. Thus, the usual doses and dosing intervals may be appropriate for elderly patients. However, reduce the starting dose to 1/3 to ½ the usual dosage in debilitated, non-opioid-tolerant patients. Respiratory depression is the chief risk in elderly or debilitated patients, usually the result of large initial doses in patients who are not tolerant to opioids, or when opioids are given in conjunction with other agents that depress respiration. Titrate the dose of OxyContin cautiously in these patients.

8.6 Hepatic Impairment

A study of OxyContin in patients with hepatic impairment demonstrated greater plasma concentrations than those seen at equivalent doses in persons with normal hepatic function. Therefore, in the setting of hepatic impairment, start dosing patients at 1/3 to 1/2 the usual starting dose followed by careful dose titration *[see Clinical Pharmacology (12.3)]*.

8.7 Renal Impairment

In patients with renal impairment, as evidenced by decreased creatinine clearance (<60 mL/min), the concentrations of oxycodone in the plasma are approximately 50% higher than in subjects with normal renal function. Follow a conservative approach to dose initiation and adjust according to the clinical situation *[see Clinical Pharmacology (12.3)]*.

8.8 Gender Differences

In pharmacokinetic studies with OxyContin, opioid-naive females demonstrate up to 25% higher average plasma concentrations and greater frequency of typical opioid adverse events than males, even after adjustment for body weight. The clinical relevance of a difference of this magnitude is low for a drug intended for chronic usage at individualized dosages, and there was no male/female difference detected for efficacy or adverse events in clinical trials.

9 DRUG ABUSE AND DEPENDENCE

9.1 Controlled Substance

OxyContin contains oxycodone, which is a Schedule II controlled substance with an abuse liability similar to morphine. OxyContin, like morphine and other opioids used for analgesia, can be abused and is subject to criminal diversion.

9.2 Abuse

Abuse of OxyContin poses a hazard of overdose and death. This risk is increased with compromising the tablet and with concurrent abuse of alcohol or other substances.

With parenteral abuse, the tablet excipients can result in death, local tissue necrosis, infection, pulmonary granulomas, and increased risk of endocarditis and valvular heart injury. Parenteral drug abuse is commonly associated with transmission of infectious diseases, such as hepatitis and HIV.

Opioid drugs are sought by people with substance use disorders (abuse or addiction, the latter of which is also called "substance dependence") and criminals who supply them by diverting medicines out of legitimate distribution channels. OxyContin is a target for theft and diversion.

"Drug-seeking" behavior is very common in persons with substance use disorders. Drug-seeking tactics include, but are not limited to, emergency calls or visits near the end of office hours, refusal to undergo appropriate examination, testing or referral, repeated "loss" of prescriptions, altering or forging of prescriptions and reluctance to provide prior medical records or contact information for other treating physician(s). "Doctor shopping" to obtain additional prescriptions is common among people with untreated substance use disorders, and criminals who divert controlled substances.

The risks of misuse and abuse should be considered when prescribing or dispensing OxyContin. Concerns about abuse and addiction, should not prevent the proper management of pain, however. Treatment of pain should be individualized, balancing the potential benefits and risks for each patient.

Compromising an extended or controlled-release delivery system will result in the uncontrolled delivery of oxycodone and pose a significant risk to the abuser that could result in overdose and death *[see Warnings and Precautions (5.1)]*. The risk of fatal overdose is further increased when oxycodone is abused concurrently with alcohol or other CNS depressants, including other opioids *[see Warnings and Precautions (5.3)]*. Abuse may occur by taking intact tablets without legitimate purpose, by crushing and chewing or snorting the crushed formulation, or by injecting a solution made from the crushed formulation.

Drug addiction is characterized by compulsive abuse, repeated use for non-medical purposes, loss of control over intake, craving of psychic effects and continued abuse despite harm or risk of harm in medical, social, legal or occupational domains. There is a potential for drug addiction to develop following exposure to opioids, including oxycodone. Drug addiction is a treatable disease, but relapse is common.

Abuse and addiction are separate and distinct from physical dependence and tolerance. Physicians should be aware that addiction may not be accompanied by concurrent tolerance and physical dependence in all addicts. In addition, abuse of opioids can occur in the absence of addiction and is characterized by intentional misuse for non-medical purposes, often in combination with other psychoactive substances. OxyContin has been diverted for non-medical use.

Proper assessment of the patient, proper prescribing practices, periodic re-evaluation of therapy, proper dispensing and correct storage and handling are appropriate measures that help to limit misuse and abuse of opioid drugs. Careful record-keeping of prescribing information, including quantity, frequency, and renewal requests is strongly advised.

Healthcare professionals should contact their State Professional Licensing Board or State Controlled Substances Authority for information on how to prevent and detect abuse or diversion of this product.

9.3 Dependence

Physical dependence to an opioid is manifested by characteristic withdrawal signs and symptoms after abrupt discontinuation of a drug, significant dose reduction or upon administration of an antagonist. Physical dependence and tolerance are not unusual during chronic opioid therapy.

The opioid abstinence or withdrawal syndrome in adults is characterized by some or all of the following: restlessness, lacrimation, rhinorrhea, yawning, perspiration, chills, piloerection, myalgia, mydriasis, irritability, anxiety, backache, joint pain, weakness, abdominal cramps, insomnia, nausea, anorexia, vomiting, diarrhea, or increased blood pressure, respiratory rate, or heart rate. *[See Use In Specific Populations (8.2)]*

In general, opioids should not be abruptly discontinued *[see Dosage and Administration (2.9)]*.

10 OVERDOSAGE

Acute overdosage with OxyContin can be manifested by respiratory depression, somnolence progressing to stupor or coma, skeletal muscle flaccidity, cold and clammy skin, constricted pupils, bradycardia, hypotension, partial or complete airway obstruction, atypical snoring and death.

It is important to take the pharmacokinetic profile of OxyContin into account when treating overdose. Even in the face of improvement, continued medical monitoring is required because of the possibility of extended effects as opioid continues to be absorbed from ingested tablets.

Deaths due to overdose have been reported with abuse and misuse of whole OxyContin tablets, and with abuse and misuse by ingesting, inhaling, or injecting crushed tablets. Review of case reports has indicated that the risk of fatal overdose is further increased when OxyContin is abused concurrently with alcohol or other CNS depressants, including other opioids.

In the treatment of OxyContin overdosage, primary attention should be given to the maintenance of a patent airway, and of effective ventilation (clearance of CO_2) and oxygenation, whether by spontaneous, assisted or controlled respiration. Supportive measures (including oxygen and vasopressors) should be employed in the management of circulatory shock and pulmonary edema accompanying overdose as indicated. Cardiac arrest or arrhythmias may require cardiac massage or defibrillation.

The pure opioid antagonists such as naloxone or nalmefene are specific antidotes against respiratory depression from opioid overdose. Since the duration of action of OxyContin may exceed that of the antagonist, especially when the overdose involves intact tablets, keep the patient under continued surveillance and administer repeated doses of the antagonist according to the antagonist labeling as needed to maintain adequate respiration. Do not administer opioid antagonists in the absence of clinically significant respiratory or circulatory depression secondary to oxycodone overdose. In patients who are physically dependent on any opioid agonist including OxyContin, an abrupt partial or complete reversal of opioid effects may precipitate an acute abstinence (or withdrawal) syndrome. The severity of the withdrawal syndrome produced will depend on the degree of physical dependence and the dose of the antagonist administered. See the prescribing information for the specific opioid antagonist for details of its proper use.

11 DESCRIPTION

OxyContin (oxycodone hydrochloride controlled-release) is an opioid analgesic supplied in 10 mg, 15 mg, 20 mg, 30 mg, 40 mg, 60 mg and 80 mg tablets for oral administration. The tablet strengths describe the amount of oxycodone per tablet as the hydrochloride salt. The structural formula for oxycodone hydrochloride is as follows:

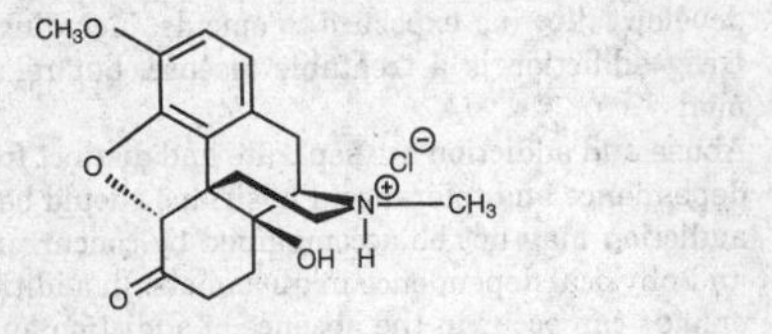

$C_{18}H_{21}NO_4 \cdot HCl$ MW 351.83

The chemical name is 4, 5α-epoxy-14-hydroxy-3-methoxy-17-methylmorphinan-6-one hydrochloride.

Oxycodone is a white, odorless crystalline powder derived from the opium alkaloid, thebaine. Oxycodone hydrochloride dissolves in water (1 g in 6 to 7 mL). It is slightly soluble in alcohol (octanol water partition coefficient 0.7).

The 10 mg, 15 mg, 20 mg, 30 mg, 40 mg, 60 mg and 80 mg tablets contain the following inactive ingredients: butylated hydroxytoluene (BHT), hypromellose, polyethylene glycol 400, polyethylene oxide, magnesium stearate, titanium dioxide.

The 10 mg tablets also contain: hydroxypropyl cellulose.

The 15 mg tablets also contain: black iron oxide, yellow iron oxide, and red iron oxide.

The 20 mg tablets also contain: polysorbate 80 and red iron oxide.

The 30 mg tablets also contain: polysorbate 80, red iron oxide, yellow iron oxide, and black iron oxide.

The 40 mg tablets also contain: polysorbate 80 and yellow iron oxide.

The 60 mg tablets also contain: polysorbate 80, red iron oxide and black iron oxide.

The 80 mg tablets also contain: hydroxypropyl cellulose, yellow iron oxide and FD&C Blue #2/Indigo Carmine Aluminum Lake.

12 CLINICAL PHARMACOLOGY

Oxycodone is a pure mu receptor opioid agonist whose principal therapeutic action is analgesia. Other members of the class known as opioid agonists include substances such as morphine, hydromorphone, fentanyl, codeine, hydrocodone and oxymorphone. Pharmacological effects of opioid agonists include anxiolysis, euphoria, feelings of relaxation, respiratory depression, constipation, miosis, and cough suppression, as well as analgesia. Increasing doses of pure mu receptor agonists are associated with increasing analgesia. There is no defined maximum dose; the ceiling to analgesic effectiveness is imposed only by adverse reactions, the more serious of which may include somnolence and respiratory depression.

12.1 Mechanism of Action

Central Nervous System

The precise mechanism of the analgesic action is unknown. However, specific CNS opioid receptors for endogenous compounds with opioid-like activity have been identified throughout the brain and spinal cord and are thought to play a role in the analgesic effects of this drug.

12.2 Pharmacodynamics

A single-dose, double-blind, placebo- and dose-controlled study was conducted using OxyContin (10, 20, and 30 mg) in an analgesic pain model involving 182 patients with moderate to severe pain. OxyContin doses of 20 mg and 30 mg produced statistically significant pain reduction compared to placebo.

Central Nervous System

Oxycodone produces respiratory depression by direct action on brain stem respiratory centers. The respiratory depression involves both a reduction in the responsiveness of the brain stem respiratory centers to increases in CO_2 tension and to electrical stimulation. Oxycodone depresses the cough reflex by direct effect on the cough center in the medulla. Antitussive effects may occur with doses lower than those usually required for analgesia.

Oxycodone causes miosis, even in total darkness. Pinpoint pupils are a sign of opioid overdose but are not pathognomonic (e.g., pontine lesions of hemorrhagic or ischemic origin may produce similar findings). Marked mydriasis rather than miosis may be seen with hypoxia in the setting of oxycodone overdose *[See Overdosage (10)]*.

Gastrointestinal Tract and Other Smooth Muscle

Oxycodone causes a reduction in motility associated with an increase in smooth muscle tone in the antrum of the stomach and duodenum. Digestion of food in the small intestine is delayed and propulsive contractions are decreased. Propulsive peristaltic waves in the colon are decreased, while tone may be increased to the point of spasm resulting in constipation. Other opioid-induced effects may include a reduction in gastric, biliary and pancreatic secretions, spasm of sphincter of Oddi, and transient elevations in serum amylase.

Cardiovascular System

Oxycodone may produce release of histamine with or without associated peripheral vasodilation. Manifestations of histamine release and/or peripheral vasodilation may include pruritus, flushing, red eyes, sweating, and/or orthostatic hypotension.

Endocrine System

Opioids may influence the hypothalamic-pituitary-adrenal or -gonadal axes. Some changes that can be seen include an increase in serum prolactin, and decreases in plasma cortisol and testosterone. Clinical signs and symptoms may be manifest from these hormonal changes.

Immune System

In vitro and animal studies indicate that opioids have a variety of effects on immune functions, depending on the context in which they are used. The clinical significance of these findings is unknown.

Concentration – Efficacy Relationships

Studies in normal volunteers and patients reveal predictable relationships between oxycodone dosage and plasma oxycodone concentrations, as well as between concentration and certain expected opioid effects, such as pupillary constriction, sedation, overall subjective "drug effect", analgesia and feelings of "relaxation".

The minimum effective analgesic concentration will vary widely among patients, especially among patients who have been previously treated with potent agonist opioids. As a result, patients must be treated with individualized titration of dosage to the desired effect. The minimum effective analgesic concentration of oxycodone for any individual patient may increase over time due to an increase in pain, the development of a new pain syndrome and/or the development of analgesic tolerance.

Concentration – Adverse Reaction Relationships

There is a relationship between increasing oxycodone plasma concentration and increasing frequency of dose-related opioid adverse reactions such as nausea, vomiting, CNS effects, and respiratory depression. In opioid-tolerant patients, the situation may be altered by the development of tolerance to opioid-related side effects.

The dose of OxyContin must be individualized *[see Dosage and Administration (2.6)]*, because the effective analgesic dose for some patients will be too high to be tolerated by other patients.

12.3 Pharmacokinetics

The activity of OxyContin is primarily due to the parent drug oxycodone. OxyContin is designed to provide delivery of oxycodone over 12 hours.

Cutting, breaking, chewing, crushing or dissolving OxyContin impairs the controlled-release delivery mechanism and results in the rapid release and absorption of a potentially fatal dose of oxycodone.

Oxycodone release from OxyContin is pH independent. The oral bioavailability of oxycodone is 60% to 87%. The relative oral bioavailability of oxycodone from OxyContin to that from immediate-release oral dosage forms is 100%. Upon repeated dosing with OxyContin in healthy subjects in pharmacokinetic studies, steady-state levels were achieved within 24-36 hours. Oxycodone is extensively metabolized and eliminated primarily in the urine as both conjugated and unconjugated metabolites. The apparent elimination half-life of oxycodone following the administration of OxyContin was 4.5 hours compared to 3.2 hours for immediate-release oxycodone.

Absorption

About 60% to 87% of an oral dose of oxycodone reaches the central compartment in comparison to a parenteral dose. This high oral bioavailability is due to low pre-systemic and/or first-pass metabolism.

Plasma Oxycodone Concentration Over Time

Dose proportionality has been established for OxyContin 10 mg, 15 mg, 20 mg, 30 mg, 40 mg, 60 mg, and 80 mg tablet strengths for both peak plasma concentrations (C_{max}) and extent of absorption (AUC) *(see Table 3)*. Given the short elimination half-life of oxycodone, steady-state plasma concentrations of oxycodone are achieved within 24-36 hours of initiation of dosing with OxyContin. In a study comparing 10 mg of OxyContin every 12 hours to 5 mg of immediate-release oxycodone every 6 hours, the two treatments were found to be equivalent for AUC and C_{max}, and similar for C_{min} (trough) concentrations.

TABLE 3
Mean [% coefficient of variation]

Regimen	Dosage Form	AUC (ng·hr/mL)*	C_{max} (ng/mL)	T_{max} (hr)
Single Dose†	10 mg	136 [27]	11.5 [27]	5.11 [21]
	15 mg	196 [28]	16.8 [29]	4.59 [19]
	20 mg	248 [25]	22.7 [25]	4.63 [22]
	30 mg	377 [24]	34.6 [21]	4.61 [19]
	40 mg	497 [27]	47.4 [30]	4.40 [22]
	60 mg	705 [22]	64.6 [24]	4.15 [26]
	80 mg	908 [21]	87.1 [29]	4.27 [26]

* for single-dose AUC = $AUC_{0\text{-}inf}$

† data obtained while subjects received naltrexone which can enhance absorption

Food Effects

Food has no significant effect on the extent of absorption of oxycodone from OxyContin.

Distribution

Following intravenous administration, the steady-state volume of distribution (Vss) for oxycodone was 2.6 L/kg. Oxycodone binding to plasma protein at 37°C and a pH of 7.4 was about 45%. Once absorbed, oxycodone is distributed to skeletal muscle, liver, intestinal tract, lungs, spleen, and brain. Oxycodone has been found in breast milk *[see Use In Specific Populations (8.3)]*.

Metabolism

Oxycodone is extensively metabolized by multiple metabolic pathways to produce noroxycodone, oxymorphone and noroxymorphone, which are subsequently glucuronidated. Noroxycodone and noroxymorphone are the major circulating metabolites. CYP3A mediated N-demethylation to noroxycodone is the primary metabolic pathway of oxycodone with a lower contribution from CYP2D6 mediated O-demethylation to oxymorphone. Therefore, the formation of these and related metabolites can, in theory, be affected by other drugs *(see Drug-Drug Interactions)*.

Noroxycodone exhibits very weak anti-nociceptive potency compared to oxycodone, however, it undergoes further oxidation to produce noroxymorphone, which is active at opioid receptors. Although noroxymorphone is an active metabolite and present at relatively high concentrations in circulation, it does not appear to cross the blood-brain barrier to a significant extent. Oxymorphone, is present in the plasma only at low concentrations and undergoes further metabolism to form its glucuronide and noroxymorphone. Oxymorphone has been shown to be active and possessing analgesic activity but its contribution to analgesia following oxycodone administration is thought to be clinically insignificant. Other metabolites (α- and β-oxycodol, noroxycodol and oxymorphol) may be present at very low concentrations and demonstrate limited penetration in to the brain as compared to oxycodone. The enzymes responsible for keto-reduction and glucuronidation pathways in oxycodone metabolism have not been established.

Excretion

Oxycodone and its metabolites are excreted primarily via the kidney. The amounts measured in the urine have been reported as follows: free and conjugated oxycodone 8.9%, free noroxycodone 23%, free oxymorphone less than 1%, conjugated oxymorphone 10%, free and conjugated noroxymorphone 14%, reduced free and conjugated metabolites up to 18%. The total plasma clearance was approximately 1.4 L/min in adults.

Special Populations

Elderly (≥65 years)

The plasma concentrations of oxycodone are only nominally affected by age, being 15% greater in elderly as compared to young subjects (age 21-45).

Gender

Across individual pharmacokinetic studies, average plasma oxycodone concentrations for female subjects were up to 25% higher than for male subjects on a body weight adjusted basis. The reason for this difference is unknown *[see Use In Specific Populations (8.8)]*.

Renal Impairment

Data from a pharmacokinetic study involving 13 patients with mild to severe renal dysfunction (creatinine clearance <60 mL/min) showed peak plasma oxycodone and noroxycodone concentrations 50% and 20% higher, respectively, and AUC values for oxycodone, noroxycodone, and oxymorphone 60%, 50%, and 40% higher than normal subjects, respectively. This was accompanied by an increase in sedation but not by differences in respiratory rate, pupillary constriction, or several other measures of drug effect. There was an increase in mean elimination t½ for oxycodone of 1 hour.

Hepatic Impairment

Data from a study involving 24 patients with mild to moderate hepatic dysfunction show peak plasma oxycodone and noroxycodone concentrations 50% and 20% higher, respectively, than healthy subjects. AUC values are 95% and 65% higher, respectively. Oxymorphone peak plasma concentrations and AUC values are lower by 30% and 40%. These differences are accompanied by increases in some, but not other, drug effects. The mean elimination t½ for oxycodone increased by 2.3 hours.

Drug-Drug Interactions

Oxycodone is extensively metabolized by multiple metabolic pathways. CYP3A4 is the major enzyme involved in noroxycodone formation followed by CYP2B6, CYP2C9/19 and CYP2D6. Drugs that inhibit CYP3A4 activity, such as macrolide antibiotics (e.g., erythromycin), azole-antifungal agents (e.g., ketoconazole), and protease inhibitors (e.g., ritonavir), may cause decreased clearance of oxycodone which could lead to an increase in oxycodone plasma concentrations. For example, a published study showed that the co-administration of the antifungal drug, voriconazole, increased oxycodone AUC and Cmax by 3.6 and 1.7 fold, respectively. Similarly, CYP450 inducers, such as rifampin, carbamazepine, and phenytoin, may induce the metabolism of oxycodone and, therefore, may cause increased clearance of the drug which could lead to a decrease in oxycodone plasma concentrations, lack of efficacy or, possibly, development of an abstinence syndrome in a patient who had developed physical dependence to oxycodone. A published study showed that the co-administration of rifampin, a drug metabolizing enzyme inducer, decreased oxycodone (oral) AUC and Cmax by 86% and 63%, respectively.

Oxymorphone is a minor metabolite, its formation is catalyzed primarily by CYP2D6 and to a small extent by CYP2C19. The formation of oxymorphone may be blocked by a variety of drugs (such as antipsychotics, beta blockers, antidepressants, etc.) that inhibit these enzymes. However, in a study involving ten subjects using quinidine, a known inhibitor of CYP2D6, the pharmacodynamic effects of oxycodone were unchanged. The genetic expression of CYP2D6 may have some influence in the pharmacokinetic properties of oxycodone.

The in vitro drug-drug interaction studies with noroxymorphone using human liver microsomes showed no significant inhibition of CYP2D6 and CYP3A4 activities which suggests that noroxymorphone may not alter the metabolism of other drugs that are metabolized by CYP2D6 and CYP3A4, and such blockade has not been shown to be of clinical significance with oxycodone. [see Drug Interactions (7.2)]

13   NONCLINICAL TOXICOLOGY

13.1   Carcinogenesis, Mutagenesis, Impairment of Fertility

Carcinogenesis

No animal studies to evaluate the carcinogenic potential of oxycodone have been conducted.

Mutagenesis

Oxycodone was genotoxic in the mouse lymphoma assay at concentrations of 50 mcg/mL or greater with metabolic activation and at 400 mcg/mL or greater without metabolic activation. Clastogenicity was observed with oxycodone in the presence of metabolic activation in one chromosomal aberration assay in human lymphocytes at concentrations greater than or equal to 1250 mcg/mL at 24 but not 48 hours of exposure. In a second chromosomal aberration assay with human lymphocytes, no structural clastogenicity was observed either with or without metabolic activation; however, in the absence of metabolic activation, oxycodone increased numerical chromosomal aberrations (polyploidy). Oxycodone was not genotoxic in the following assays: Ames S. typhimurium and E. coli test with and without metabolic activation at concentrations up to 5000 μg/plate, chromosomal aberration test in human lymphocytes (in the absence of metabolic activation) at concentrations up to 1500 μg/mL, and with activation after 48 hours of exposure at concentrations up to 5000 μg/mL, and in the in vivo bone marrow micronucleus assay in mice (at plasma levels up to 48 μg/mL).

Impairment of Fertility

In a study of reproductive performance, rats were administered a once daily gavage dose of the vehicle or oxycodone hydrochloride (0.5, 2, and 8 mg/kg). Male rats were dosed for 28 days before cohabitation with females, during the cohabitation and until necropsy (2-3 weeks post-cohabitation). Females were dosed for 14 days before cohabitation with males, during cohabitation and up to gestation day 6. Oxycodone hydrochloride did not affect reproductive function in male or female rats at any dose tested (≤8 mg/kg/day).

14   CLINICAL STUDIES

A double-blind, placebo-controlled, fixed-dose, parallel group, two-week study was conducted in 133 patients with persistent, moderate to severe pain, who were judged as having inadequate pain control with their current therapy. In this study, OxyContin 20 mg, but not 10 mg, was statistically significant in pain reduction compared with placebo.

15   REFERENCES

1. Adapted from Foley, KM. N Engl J Med, 1985; 313:84-95

16   HOW SUPPLIED/STORAGE AND HANDLING

OxyContin (oxycodone hydrochloride controlled-release) Tablets 10 mg are round, white-colored, bi-convex tablets debossed with OP on one side and 10 on the other and are supplied as child-resistant closure, opaque plastic bottles of 100 (NDC 59011-410-10) and unit dose packaging with 10 individually numbered tablets per card; two cards per glue end carton (NDC 59011-410-20)

OxyContin (oxycodone hydrochloride controlled-release) Tablets 15 mg are round, gray-colored, bi-convex tablets debossed with OP on one side and 15 on the other and are supplied as child-resistant closure, opaque plastic bottles of 100 (NDC 59011-415-10) and unit dose packaging with 10 individually numbered tablets per card; two cards per glue end carton (NDC 59011-415-20)

OxyContin (oxycodone hydrochloride controlled-release) Tablets 20 mg are round, pink-colored, bi-convex tablets debossed with OP on one side and 20 on the other and are supplied as child-resistant closure, opaque plastic bottles of 100 (NDC 59011-420-10) and unit dose packaging with 10 individually numbered tablets per card; two cards per glue end carton (NDC 59011-420-20)

OxyContin (oxycodone hydrochloride controlled-release) Tablets 30 mg are round, brown-colored, bi-convex tablets debossed with OP on one side and 30 on the other and are supplied as child-resistant closure, opaque plastic bottles of 100 (NDC 59011-430-10) and unit dose packaging with 10 individually numbered tablets per card; two cards per glue end carton (NDC 59011-430-20)

OxyContin (oxycodone hydrochloride controlled-release) Tablets 40 mg are round, yellow-colored, bi-convex tablets debossed with OP on one side and 40 on the other and are supplied as child-resistant closure, opaque plastic bottles of 100 (NDC 59011-440-10) and unit dose packaging with 10 individually numbered tablets per card; two cards per glue end carton (NDC 59011-440-20)

OxyContin (oxycodone hydrochloride controlled-release) Tablets 60 mg are round, red-colored, bi-convex tablets debossed with OP on one side and 60 on the other and are supplied as child-resistant closure, opaque plastic bottles of 100 (NDC 59011-460-10) and unit dose packaging with 10 individually numbered tablets per card; two cards per glue end carton (NDC 59011-460-20)

OxyContin (oxycodone hydrochloride controlled-release) Tablets 80 mg are round, green-colored, bi-convex tablets debossed with OP on one side and 80 on the other and are supplied as child-resistant closure, opaque plastic bottles of 100 (NDC 59011-480-10) and unit dose packaging with 10 individually numbered tablets per card; two cards per glue end carton (NDC 59011-480-20)

Store at 25°C (77°F); excursions permitted between 15°-30°C (59°-86°F).

Dispense in tight, light-resistant container.

17   PATIENT COUNSELING INFORMATION

See MEDICATION GUIDE as appended at the end of the full prescribing information

17.1   Information for Patients and Caregivers

Provide the following information to patients receiving OxyContin or their caregivers:

* Advise patients that OxyContin contains oxycodone, which is a morphine-like substance.
* Advise patients that OxyContin is designed to work properly only if swallowed whole. Taking cut, broken, chewed, crushed, or dissolved OxyContin Tablets can result in a fatal overdose.
* Advise patients to report adverse experiences, and episodes of increased or incident pain occurring during therapy. Individualization of dosage is essential to make optimal use of this medication.
* Advise patients not to adjust the dose of OxyContin without consulting the prescribing professional.
* Advise patients that OxyContin may impair mental and/or physical ability required for the performance of potentially hazardous tasks (e.g., driving, operating heavy machinery).
* Advise patients not to combine OxyContin with alcohol or other central nervous system depressants (e.g. sedatives, hypnotics) except by the orders of the prescribing physician, because dangerous additive effects may occur, resulting in serious injury or death.
* Advise women of childbearing potential who become, or are planning to become, pregnant to consult their physician regarding the effects of analgesics and other drug use during pregnancy on themselves and their unborn child.
* Advise patients that OxyContin is a drug with known abuse potential. They should protect it from theft, and it should never be given to anyone other than the individual for whom it was prescribed.
* Advise patients that if they have been receiving treatment with OxyContin for more than a few weeks and cessation of therapy is indicated, it may be appropriate to taper the OxyContin dose, rather than abruptly discontinue it, due to the risk of precipitating withdrawal symptoms. If tapering is appropriate, their prescriber can provide a dose schedule to gradually discontinue the medication.
* Advise patients to keep OxyContin in a secure place out of the reach of children. When OxyContin is no longer

needed, the unused tablets should be destroyed by flushing down the toilet.

Healthcare professionals can telephone Purdue Pharma's Medical Services Department (1-888-726-7535) for information on this product.

CAUTION

DEA Order Form Required.

©2010, Purdue Pharma L.P.

Purdue Pharma L.P.

Stamford, CT 06901-3431

U.S. Patent Numbers 5,508,042; 6,488,963; 7,129,248; 7,674,799; 7,674,800 and 7,683,072

301734-0C

May 10, 2010

MEDICATION GUIDE

OXYCONTIN® (ox-e-KON-tin) (CII)

(oxycodone hydrochloride controlled-release)

Tablets

Read this Medication Guide before you start taking OxyContin and each time you get a refill. There may be new information. This Medication Guide does not take the place of talking to your healthcare provider about your medical condition or your treatment.

What is the most important information I should know about OxyContin?

* **OxyContin can cause serious side effects, including addiction or death.**
* **Do not cut, break, chew, crush, or dissolve OxyContin before swallowing. If OxyContin is taken in this way, the medicine in the tablets will be released too fast. This is dangerous. It may cause you to stop breathing, and may lead to death.**
* OxyContin is not for use to treat pain that you only have once in a while ("as needed").
* **Do not take OxyContin 60 mg or 80 mg tablets unless you are "opioid tolerant."** Opioid tolerant means that you regularly use OxyContin or another opioid medicine for your constant (around-the-clock) pain and your body is used to it.
* **Do not take more than 40 mg of OxyContin in one dose or more than 80 mg of OxyContin in one day unless you are "opioid tolerant."** This may cause you to stop breathing and may lead to death.

---

* **OxyContin is a federally controlled substance** (CII) because it is a strong opioid pain medicine that can be abused by people who abuse prescription medicines or street drugs.
* **Prevent theft, misuse and abuse.** Keep OxyContin in a safe place, to keep it from being stolen. OxyContin can be a target for people who misuse or abuse prescription medicines or street drugs.
* **Never give OxyContin to anyone else, even if they have the same symptoms you have.** It may harm them and even cause death.
* Before taking OxyContin, tell your doctor if you or a family member have been addicted to or abused other medicines, street drugs, or alcohol, or if you have a history of mental illness.

---

* **Do not drink alcohol while using OxyContin. Using alcohol with OxyContin may increase your risk of dangerous side effects, including death.**
* **Certain medicines can interact with OxyContin and cause you to have high levels of oxycodone in your blood. This may cause you to stop breathing and lead to death. Before taking OxyContin, tell your healthcare provider if you take an antibiotic, an antifungal medicine, or an anti-HIV medicine.**

What is OxyContin?

* OxyContin is a prescription medicine used when an opioid medicine is needed to manage moderate to severe pain that continues around-the-clock and is expected to last for a long period of time.
* It is not known if OxyContin is safe and effective in children younger than 18 years.
* OxyContin is not for use:
  ○ to manage pain "as needed"
  ○ before surgery to manage any pain from your surgery
  ○ to manage pain after surgery if the pain is mild and is not expected to last for a long period of time
* If you already take OxyContin, it may be used to manage your pain after surgery if:
  ○ it has been at least 12 to 24 hours after your surgery, and
  ○ your pain from surgery is expected to be moderate to severe, and last for a long period of time.

Who should not take OxyContin?

Do not take OxyContin if you:

* are allergic to any of its ingredients. See the end of this Medication Guide for a list of the ingredients in OxyContin.
* have had a severe allergic reaction to a medicine that contains oxycodone. Ask your healthcare provider if you are not sure.
* are having an asthma attack or have severe asthma, trouble breathing, or lung problems
* have a bowel blockage called paralytic ileus

What should I tell my healthcare provider before taking OxyContin?

OxyContin may not be right for you. Before taking OxyContin, tell your doctor if you:
- have trouble breathing or lung problems
- have had a head injury
- have liver or kidney problems
- have adrenal gland problems, such as Addison's disease
- have severe scoliosis that affects your breathing
- have thyroid problems
- have enlargement of your prostate or a urethral stricture
- have or had convulsions or seizures
- have a past or present drinking problem or alcoholism
- have hallucinations or other severe mental problems
- have past or present substance abuse or drug addiction
- have any other medical conditions
- are pregnant or plan to become pregnant. If you take OxyContin regularly before your baby is born, your newborn baby may have signs of withdrawal because their body has become used to the medicine. Signs of withdrawal in a newborn baby can include:
  - irritability
  - crying more than usual
  - shaking (tremors)
  - jitteriness
  - breathing faster than normal
  - diarrhea or more stools than normal
  - sneezing
  - yawning
  - vomiting
  - fever

If you take OxyContin right before your baby is born, your baby could have breathing problems at birth.
- are breast-feeding. You should not take OxyContin if you are nursing. Some oxycodone from OxyContin passes into breast milk. A nursing baby could become very drowsy or have difficulty breathing or feeding well.

Tell your healthcare provider about all the medicines you take, including prescription and non-prescription medicines, vitamins, and herbal supplements. Sometimes the doses of medicines that you take with OxyContin may need to be changed if used together.
- See "What is the most important information I should know about OxyContin?"
- Be especially careful about taking other medicines that make you sleepy such as:
  - pain medicines
  - sleeping pills
  - anxiety medicines
  - antihistamines
  - anti-depressants
  - tranquilizers
  - anti-nausea medicine

Do not take other medicines without talking to your healthcare provider. Your healthcare provider will tell you if it is safe to take other medicines while you take OxyContin. Know the medicines you take. Keep a list of your medicines to show your healthcare provider and pharmacist.

How should I take OxyContin?
- See "What is the most important information I should know about OxyContin?"
- **Take OxyContin exactly as prescribed. Do not change your dose unless your healthcare provider tells you to.**
- **Swallow OxyContin tablets whole. Do not cut, break, chew, crush, or dissolve before swallowing.**
- Take OxyContin every 12 hours.
- You can take OxyContin with or without food.
- If you miss a dose, take it as soon as possible. Take your next dose 12 hours later. Do not take more than your prescribed dose of OxyContin. Call your healthcare provider if you are not sure about your dose of OxyContin or when to take it.
- **If you take more OxyContin than prescribed,** or overdose, call your local emergency number (such as 911) or your local Poison Control Center right away, or get emergency help.
- **Talk with your healthcare provider regularly about your pain** to see if you still need to take OxyContin.

What should I avoid while taking OxyContin?
- **Do not drink alcohol while using OxyContin. See "What is the most important information I should know about OxyContin?" Do not drive, operate heavy machinery, or do other dangerous activities, especially when you start taking OxyContin and when your dose is changed, until you know how you react to this medicine. OxyContin can make you sleepy, and also cause you to feel dizzy. Ask your healthcare provider to tell you when it is okay to do these activities.**

What are the possible side effects of OxyContin?
OxyContin can cause serious side effects, including:
- See "What is the most important information I should know about OxyContin?"
- **OxyContin can cause serious breathing problems that can become life-threatening, especially if OxyContin is** used the wrong way. Call your healthcare provider or get medical help right away if:
  - your breathing slows down
  - you have shallow breathing (little chest movement with breathing)
  - you feel faint, dizzy, confused, or
  - you have any other unusual symptoms

These can be signs or symptoms that you have taken too much OxyContin (overdose) or the dose is too high for you. **These symptoms may lead to serious problems or death if not treated right away.**
- **Central nervous system effects, including sleepiness, dizziness, passing out, becoming unconscious, or coma.**
- **OxyContin may cause a worsening of seizures in people who already have seizures.**
- **OxyContin can cause your blood pressure to drop.** This can make you feel dizzy and faint if you get up too fast from sitting or lying down. Low blood pressure is also more likely to happen if you take other medicines that can also lower your blood pressure. Severe low blood pressure can happen if you lost blood or take certain other medicines.
- **OxyContin can cause physical dependence.** Do not stop taking OxyContin or any other opioid without talking to your healthcare provider about how to slowly stop your medicine. You could become sick with uncomfortable withdrawal symptoms because your body has become used to these medicines. Physical dependence is not the same as drug addiction. Tell your healthcare provider if you have any of these signs or symptoms of withdrawal while slowly stopping OxyContin:
  - feel restless
  - tearing eyes
  - runny nose
  - yawning
  - sweating
  - chills or hair on your arms "standing up"
  - muscle aches, backache
  - dilated pupils of your eyes
  - feel irritable or anxious
  - nausea, loss of appetite, vomiting, diarrhea
  - increase in your blood pressure, breathing faster, or your heart beats faster
- **There is a chance of abuse or addiction with OxyContin.** The chance is higher if you are or have been addicted to or abused other medicines, street drugs, or alcohol, or if you have a history of mental problems.

The most common side effects of OxyContin include:
- constipation
- nausea
- drowsiness
- dizziness
- itching
- vomiting
- headache
- dry mouth
- weakness
- sweating

Some of these side effects may decrease with continued use. Talk with your healthcare provider if you continue to have these side effects. These are not all the possible side effects of OxyContin. For a complete list, ask your healthcare provider or pharmacist.

Constipation (not often enough or hard bowel movements) is a very common side effect of pain medicines (opioids) including OxyContin, and is unlikely to go away without treatment. Talk to your healthcare provider about dietary changes, and the use of laxatives (medicines to treat constipation) and stool softeners to prevent or treat constipation while taking OxyContin.

Call your doctor for medical advice about side effects. You may report side effects to FDA at 1–800–FDA–1088.

How should I store OxyContin?
- **Keep OxyContin out of the reach of children.** Accidental overdose by a child is dangerous and can lead to death.
- Store OxyContin at 59° F to 86° F (15° C to 30° C).
- Keep OxyContin in the container it comes in.
- Keep the container tightly closed and away from light.
- After you stop taking OxyContin, flush the unused tablets down the toilet.

General information about OxyContin
Medicines are sometimes prescribed for purposes other than those listed in a Medication Guide. Do not use OxyContin for a condition for which it was not prescribed. Never give your OxyContin to other people even if they have the same symptoms you have.

Selling or giving away OxyContin may harm others, even causing death, and is against the law.

This Medication Guide summarizes the most important information about OxyContin. If you would like more information, talk with your healthcare provider. You can ask your healthcare provider or pharmacist for infor- mation about OxyContin that is written for health professionals. For more information about OxyContin, go to www.purduepharma.com or call 1-888-726-7535.

What are the ingredients of OxyContin?
Active ingredient: oxycodone hydrochloride
Inactive ingredients in all strengths: butylated hydroxytoluene (BHT), hypromellose, polyethylene glycol 400, polyethylene oxide, magnesium stearate, titanium dioxide
- The 10 mg tablets also contain: hydroxypropyl cellulose.
- The 15 mg tablets also contain: black iron oxide, yellow iron oxide, and red iron oxide.
- The 20 mg tablets also contain: polysorbate 80 and red iron oxide.
- The 30 mg tablets also contain: polysorbate 80, red iron oxide, yellow iron oxide, and black iron oxide.
- The 40 mg tablets also contain: polysorbate 80 and yellow iron oxide.
- The 60 mg tablets also contain: polysorbate 80, red iron oxide and black iron oxide.
- The 80 mg tablets also contain: hydroxypropyl cellulose, yellow iron oxide and FD&C Blue #2/Indigo Carmine Aluminum Lake.

Always check to make sure that the medicine you are taking is the correct one. The dosage strength and appearance of each OxyContin tablet are as follows:
- 10 mg: white-colored with "OP" on one side and "10" on the other
- 15 mg: gray-colored with "OP" on one side and "15" on the other
- 20 mg: pink-colored with "OP" on one side and "20" on the other
- 30 mg: brown-colored with "OP" on one side and "30" on the other
- 40 mg: yellow-colored with "OP" on one side and "40" on the other
- 60 mg: red-colored with "OP" on one side and "60" on the other
- 80 mg: green-colored with "OP" on one side and "80" on the other

This Medication Guide has been approved by the U.S. Food and Drug Administration.
CAUTION
DEA Order Form Required.
©2010, Purdue Pharma L.P.
Purdue Pharma L.P.
Stamford, CT 06901-3431
U.S. Patent Numbers 5,508,042; 6,488,963; 7,129,248; 7,674,799; 7,674,800 and 7,683,072
301734-0C
May 10, 2010
Shown in Product Identification Guide, page 317

RYZOLT®   ℞
[RY-zolt]
(tramadol hydrochloride extended-release tablets)

DESCRIPTION
RYZOLT® (tramadol hydrochloride extended-release tablets) is a centrally acting analgesic composed of a dual-matrix delivery system with both immediate-release and extended-release characteristics. The chemical name for tramadol hydrochloride is (±)cis-2-[(dimethylamino) methyl]-1-(3-methoxyphenyl) cyclohexanol hydrochloride. Its structural formula is:

$C_{16}H_{25}NO_2 \cdot HCl$

The molecular weight of tramadol hydrochloride is 299.8. Tramadol hydrochloride is a white crystalline powder that is freely soluble in water and ethanol. RYZOLT® extended-release tablets are for oral administration and contain 100 mg, 200 mg or 300 mg of tramadol hydrochloride. The tablets are white to off-white in color. The inactive ingredients in the tablet are colloidal silicon dioxide, pregelatinized modified starch, hydrogenated vegetable oil, magnesium stearate, polyvinyl acetate, povidone, sodium lauryl sulfate and xanthan gum.

CLINICAL PHARMACOLOGY
Mechanism of Action
RYZOLT® is a centrally acting synthetic opioid analgesic. Although its mode of action is not completely understood, at least two complementary mechanisms that demonstrate three different types of activity appear applicable: binding of parent and M1 metabolite to μ-opioid receptors and weak inhibition of reuptake of norepinephrine and serotonin.
Opioid activity is due to both low affinity binding of the parent compound and higher affinity binding of the O-demethylated metabolite (M1) to mu-opioid receptors. In animal models, M1 is up to 6 times more potent than tramadol in producing analgesia and 200 times more potent

in mu-opioid binding. Tramadol-induced analgesia is only partially antagonized by the opiate antagonist naloxone in several animal tests. The relative contribution of both tramadol and M1 to human analgesia is dependent upon the plasma concentrations of each compound.

Tramadol has been shown to inhibit reuptake of norepinephrine and serotonin *in vitro*, as have some other opioid analgesics. These mechanisms may contribute independently to the overall analgesic profile of tramadol.

Apart from analgesia, tramadol hydrochloride administration may produce various symptoms (including dizziness, somnolence, nausea, constipation, sweating and pruritus) similar to that of other opioids. In contrast to morphine, tramadol has not been shown to cause histamine release. At therapeutic doses, tramadol has no effect on heart rate, left-ventricular function or cardiac index. Orthostatic hypotension has been observed.

Pharmacokinetics

The analgesic activity of tramadol hydrochloride is due to both parent drug and the M1 metabolite (see **CLINICAL PHARMACOLOGY, Mechanism of Action**).

RYZOLT® is formulated as a racemate and both tramadol and M1 are detected in the circulation.

The pharmacokinetics of tramadol and M1 are dose-proportional over a 100 to 300 mg dose range in healthy subjects.

Absorption

The median time to peak plasma concentrations of tramadol and M1 after multiple-dose administration of RYZOLT® 200 mg tablets to healthy subjects are attained at about 4 h and 5 h, respectively (Table 1 and Figure 1).

The pharmacokinetic parameter values for RYZOLT® 200 mg administered once daily and tramadol immediate-release 50 mg administered every six hours are provided in Table 1. The relative bioavailability of a 200 mg RYZOLT® tablet compared to a 50 mg immediate-release tablet dosed every six hours was approximately 95% in healthy subjects. [See table 1 above]

Steady-state plasma concentrations are reached within approximately 48 hours.

Figure 1. Mean Tramadol Plasma Concentrations at Steady State Following Five Days of Oral Administration of RYZOLT® 200 mg Once Daily and Immediate-Release Tramadol 50 mg Every 6 Hours.

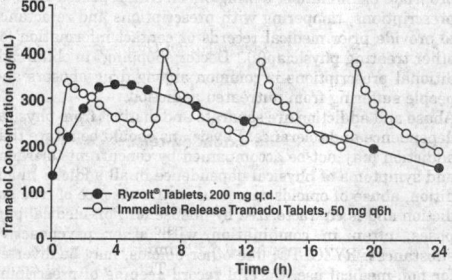

Figure 2. Mean M1 Plasma Concentrations at Steady State Following Five Days of Oral Administration of RYZOLT® 200 mg Once Daily and Immediate-Release Tramadol 50 mg Every 6 Hours

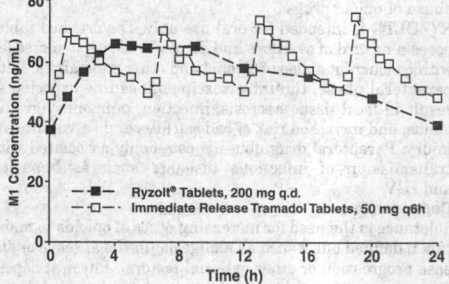

Food Effect

Co-administration with a high fat meal did not significantly affect AUC (overall exposure to tramadol); however, C_{max} (peak plasma concentration) increased 67% following a single 300 mg tablet administration and 54% following a single *200 mg tablet administration*. RYZOLT® was administered without regard to food in all clinical trials.

Distribution

The volume of distribution of tramadol is 2.6 and 2.9 L/kg in males and females, respectively, following a 100 mg intravenous dose. The binding of tramadol to human plasma proteins is approximately 20%. Protein binding also appears to be independent of concentration up to 10 µg/mL. Saturation of plasma protein binding occurs only at concentrations outside the clinically relevant range.

Metabolism

Tramadol is extensively metabolized after oral administration. The major metabolic pathways appear to be *N*- and *O*-demethylation and glucuronidation or sulfation in the liver. *N*-demethylation is mediated by CYP3A4 and CYP2B6. One metabolite (*O*-desmethyltramadol, denoted M1) is pharmacologically active in animal models. Formation of M1 is dependent on CYP2D6 and as such is subject to inhibition and polymorphism, which may affect the therapeutic response (see **PRECAUTIONS, Drug Interactions**).

Elimination

Tramadol is eliminated primarily through metabolism by the liver and the metabolites are eliminated primarily by the kidneys. Approximately 30% of the dose is excreted in the urine as unchanged drug, whereas 60% of the dose is excreted as metabolites. The remainder is excreted either as unidentified or as unextractable metabolites. After single administration of RYZOLT®, the mean terminal plasma elimination half-lives of racemic tramadol and racemic M1 are 6.5 ± 1.5 and 7.5 ± 1.4 hours, respectively.

Special Populations
Renal Impairment

Impaired renal function results in a decreased rate and extent of excretion of tramadol and its active metabolite, M1 in patients taking an immediate-release formulation of tramadol. RYZOLT® has not been studied in patients with renal impairment. The limited availability of dose strengths and once daily dosing of RYZOLT® do not permit the dosing flexibility required for safe use in patients with severe renal impairment. Therefore, RYZOLT® should not be used in patients with severe renal impairment (creatinine clearance less than 30 mL/min) (see **WARNINGS, Use in Renal and Hepatic Disease and DOSAGE AND ADMINISTRATION**). The total amount of tramadol and M1 removed during a 4-hour dialysis period is less than 7% of the administered dose.

Hepatic Impairment

The metabolism of tramadol and M1 is reduced in patients with advanced cirrhosis of the liver, resulting in both a larger area under the concentration time curve (AUC) for tramadol and longer mean tramadol and M1 elimination half-lives (13 hours for tramadol and 19 hours for M1) after the administration of tramadol immediate-release tablets. RYZOLT® has not been studied in patients with hepatic impairment. The limited availability of dose strengths and once daily dosing of RYZOLT® do not permit the dosing flexibility required for safe use in patients with hepatic impairment. Therefore, RYZOLT® should not be used in patients with hepatic impairment (see **WARNINGS, Use in Renal and Hepatic Disease and DOSAGE AND ADMINISTRATION**).

Geriatric Patients

Healthy elderly subjects aged 65 to 75 years administered an immediate-release formulation of tramadol, have plasma concentrations and elimination half-lives comparable to those observed in healthy subjects less than 65 years of age. In subjects over 75 years, mean maximum plasma concentrations are elevated (208 vs. 162 ng/mL) and the mean elimination half-life is prolonged (7 vs. 6 hours) compared to subjects 65 to 75 years of age. Adjustment of the daily dose is recommended for patients older than 75 years (see **DOSAGE AND ADMINISTRATION**).

Gender

Following a 100 mg IV dose of tramadol, plasma clearance was 6.4 mL/min/kg in males and 5.7 mL/min/kg in females. Following a single oral dose of immediate-release tramadol, and after adjusting for body weight, females had a 12% higher peak tramadol concentration and a 35% higher area under the concentration-time curve compared to males. The clinical significance of this difference is unknown.

Drug Interactions

The formation of the active metabolite of tramadol, M1, is mediated by CYP2D6, a polymorphic enzyme. Approxi-mately 7% of the population has reduced activity of CYP2D6. These individuals are "poor metabolizers" of debrisoquine, dextromethorphan and tricyclic antidepressants, among other drugs. In studies in healthy subjects administered immediate-release tramadol products, concentrations of tramadol were approximately 20% higher in "poor metabolizers" versus "extensive metabolizers", while M1 concentrations were 40% lower. *In vitro* drug interaction studies in human liver microsomes indicate that inhibitors of CYP2D6 (amitriptyline, quinidine and fluoxetine and its metabolite norfluoxetine,) inhibit the metabolism of tramadol to various degrees, suggesting that concomitant administration of these compounds could result in increases in tramadol concentrations and decreased concentrations of M1. The full pharmacological impact of these alterations in terms of either efficacy or safety is unknown.

Tramadol is also metabolized by CYP3A4. Administration of CYP3A4 inhibitors, such as ketoconazole and erythromycin, or inducers, such as rifampin and St. John's Wort, with RYZOLT® may affect the metabolism of tramadol leading to altered tramadol exposure (see **PRECAUTIONS**).

Quinidine

Quinidine is a selective inhibitor of CYP2D6, so that concomitant administration of quinidine and RYZOLT® may result in increased concentrations of tramadol and reduced concentrations of M1. The clinical consequences of these findings are unknown (see **PRECAUTIONS**). *In vitro* drug interaction studies in human liver microsomes indicate that tramadol has no effect on quinidine metabolism.

Carbamazepine

Carbamazepine, a CYP3A4 inducer, increases tramadol metabolism. Patients taking carbamazepine may have a significantly reduced analgesic effect of tramadol. Because of the seizure risk associated with tramadol, concomitant administration of RYZOLT® and carbamazepine is not recommended (see **PRECAUTIONS**).

Cimetidine

Concomitant administration of tramadol immediate-release tablets with cimetidine does not result in clinically significant changes in tramadol pharmacokinetics. No alteration of the RYZOLT® dosage regimen with cimetidine is recommended.

CLINICAL STUDIES

RYZOLT® was studied in four 12-week, randomized, double-blind, controlled studies in patients with moderate to severe pain due to osteoarthritis. Efficacy was demonstrated in one double-blind, placebo-controlled, randomized withdrawal design study. In this study, patients who experienced a reduction of pain and were able to tolerate RYZOLT® during an open-label titration period, were then randomized to RYZOLT® or to placebo for 12 weeks. Sixty-five percent of patients were able to successfully titrate onto RYZOLT®. After a washout, patients randomized to RYZOLT® were titrated to 200 mg or 300 mg of RYZOLT® based on tolerability and remained on that dose for the following 12-week period. Approximately 24% of patients discontinued during the randomized period of the study, with more patients discontinuing from the RYZOLT® arm due to adverse events (10% vs. 5%, respectively) and more patients discontinuing from the placebo arm than the RYZOLT® arm due to lack of efficacy (10% vs. 8%, respectively). Patients treated with RYZOLT® demonstrated a greater improvement in pain intensity, measured on an 11-point numerical rating scale, at the end of treatment compared to patients randomized to placebo. Figure 3 shows the fraction of patients achieving various degree of improvement in pain from baseline to the end of treatment (week 12). The figure is cumulative, so that patients whose change from baseline is, for example, 50%, are also included

Table 1. Mean (%CV) Steady-State Pharmacokinetic Parameter Values (n=26).

Pharmacokinetic Parameter	Tramadol		M1 Metabolite	
	RYZOLT® 200 mg Tablet Once-Daily	Immediate-release tramadol 50 mg Tablet Every 6 Hours	RYZOLT® 200 mg Tablet Once-Daily	Immediate-release tramadol 50 mg Tablet Every 6 Hours
AUC_{0-24} (ng•h/mL)	5991 (22)	6399 (28)	1361 (27)	1438 (23)
C_{max} (ng/mL)	345 (21)	423 (23)	71 (27)	79 (22)
C_{min} (ng/mL)	157 (31)	190 (34)	41 (30)	50 (29)
T_{max} (hr)*	4.0 (3.0–9.0)	1.0 (1.0–3.0)	5.0 (3.0–20)	1.5 (1.0–3.0)
Fluctuation (%)	77 (26)	91 (22)	53 (29)	49 (26)

* T_{max} is presented as Median (Range)

at every level of improvement below 50%. Patients who did not complete the study were assigned 0% improvement.

Figure 3. Proportion of Patients Achieving Various Levels of Pain Relief as Measured by 12-Week Pain Intensity.

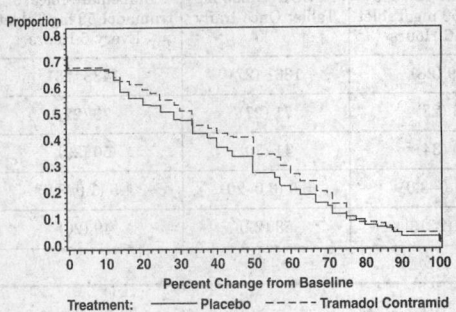

Treatment: —— Placebo ----- Tramadol Contramid

INDICATIONS AND USAGE

RYZOLT® is indicated for the management of moderate to moderately severe chronic pain in adults who require around-the-clock treatment of their pain for an extended period of time.

CONTRAINDICATIONS

RYZOLT® should not be administered to patients who have previously demonstrated hypersensitivity to tramadol, any other component of this product or opioids.

RYZOLT® is contraindicated in patients with significant respiratory depression in unmonitored settings or the absence of resuscitative equipment. RYZOLT® is also contraindicated in patients with acute or severe bronchial asthma or hypercapnia in unmonitored settings or the absence of resuscitative equipment.

WARNINGS

Seizure Risk

Seizures have been reported in patients receiving tramadol hydrochloride within the recommended dosage range. Spontaneous postmarketing reports indicate that seizure risk is increased with doses above the recommended range. Concomitant use of tramadol hydrochloride increases the seizure risk in patients taking:

- **Selective serotonin reuptake inhibitors (SSRI antidepressants or anorectics),**
- **Tricyclic antidepressants (TCAs), and other tricyclic compounds (e.g., cyclobenzaprine, promethazine, etc.), or**
- **Other opioids.**

Administration of RYZOLT® may enhance the seizure risk in patients taking:

- **Monoamine Oxidase (MAO) inhibitors (see WARNINGS, Use with MAO Inhibitors and Serotonin Re-uptake Inhibitors),**
- **Neuroleptics, or**
- **Other drugs that reduce the seizure threshold.**

Risk of convulsions may also be increased in patients with epilepsy, those with a history of seizures, or in patients with a recognized risk for seizure (such as head trauma, certain metabolic disorders, alcohol and drug withdrawal and CNS infections). In tramadol overdose, naloxone administration may increase the risk of seizures.

Suicide Risk

Do not prescribe RYZOLT® for patients who are suicidal or addiction-prone. Prescribe RYZOLT® with caution for patients taking tranquilizers or antidepressant drugs and for patients who use alcohol in excess. Serious potential consequences of overdosage with RYZOLT® are central nervous system depression, respiratory depression and death. In treating an overdose, primary attention should be given to maintaining adequate ventilation along with general supportive treatment (see **OVERDOSAGE**).

Serotonin Syndrome Risk

The development of a potentially life-threatening serotonin syndrome may occur with the use of tramadol products, including RYZOLT®, particularly with concomitant use of serotonergic drugs such as SSRIs, SNRIs, TCAs, MAOIs, and triptans, with drugs which impair metabolism of serotonin (including MAOIs), and with drugs which impair metabolism of tramadol (CYP2D6 and CYP3A4 inhibitors). This may occur within the recommended dose (see CLINICAL PHARMACOLOGY, Pharmacokinetics).

Serotonin syndrome may include mental-status changes (e.g., agitation, hallucinations, coma), autonomic instability (e.g., tachycardia, labile blood pressure, hyperthermia), neuromuscular aberrations (e.g., hyperreflexia, incoordination) and/or gastrointestinal symptoms (e.g., nausea, vomiting, diarrhea).

Tramadol products in excessive doses, either alone or in combination with other Central Nervous System (CNS) depressants, including alcohol, are a major cause of drug-related deaths. Fatalities within the first hour of overdosage

are not uncommon. Tramadol should not be taken in doses higher than those recommended by the physician. The judicious prescribing of tramadol is essential to the safe use of this drug. With patients who are depressed or suicidal, consideration should be given to the use of non-narcotic analgesics. Patients should be cautioned about the concomitant use of tramadol products and alcohol because of potentially serious CNS-additive effects of these agents. Because of its added depressant effects, tramadol should be prescribed with caution for those patients whose medical condition requires the concomitant administration of sedatives, tranquilizers, muscle relaxants, antidepressants, or other CNS-depressant drugs. Patients should be advised of the additive depressant effects of these combinations.

Many of the tramadol-related deaths have occurred in patients with previous histories of emotional disturbances or suicidal ideation or attempts as well as histories of misuse of tranquilizers, alcohol, and other CNS-active drugs. Some deaths have occurred as a consequence of the accidental ingestion of excessive quantities of tramadol alone or in combination with other drugs. Patients taking tramadol should be warned not to exceed the dose recommended by their physician.

Anaphylactoid Reactions

Serious and rarely fatal anaphylactoid reactions have been reported in patients receiving therapy with tramadol. When these events do occur, it is often following the first dose. Other reported allergic reactions include pruritus, hives, bronchospasm, angioedema, toxic epidermal necrolysis and Stevens-Johnson syndrome. Patients with a history of anaphylactoid reactions to other opioids may be at increased risk and therefore should not receive RYZOLT® (see **CONTRAINDICATIONS**).

Respiratory Depression

RYZOLT® should be administered cautiously in patients at risk for respiratory depression. In these patients, alternative non-opioid analgesics should be considered. When large doses of tramadol are administered with anesthetic medications or alcohol, respiratory depression may result. Respiratory depression should be treated as an overdose. If naloxone is to be administered, use cautiously because it may precipitate seizures (see **WARNINGS, Seizure Risk and OVERDOSAGE**).

Interaction with Central Nervous System (CNS) Depressants

RYZOLT® should be used with caution and in reduced dosages when administered to patients receiving CNS depressants such as alcohol, opioids, anesthetic agents, narcotics, phenothiazines, tranquilizers or sedative hypnotics. Tramadol increases the risk of CNS and respiratory depression in these patients.

Increased Intracranial Pressure or Head Trauma

RYZOLT® should be used with caution in patients with increased intracranial pressure or head injury. The respiratory depressant effects of opioids include carbon dioxide retention and secondary elevation of cerebrospinal fluid pressure, and may be markedly exaggerated in these patients. Additionally, pupillary changes (miosis) from tramadol may obscure the existence, extent, or course of intracranial pathology. Clinicians should also maintain a high index of suspicion for adverse drug reaction when evaluating altered mental status in these patients if they are receiving RYZOLT® (see **WARNINGS, Respiratory Depression**).

Use in Ambulatory Patients

RYZOLT® may impair the mental and physical abilities required for the performance of potentially hazardous tasks such as driving a car or operating machinery. Patients using this drug should be cautioned accordingly.

Use with MAO Inhibitors and Serotonin Re-uptake Inhibitors

RYZOLT® should be used with great caution in patients taking MAO inhibitors. Animal studies have shown increased deaths with combined administration of tramadol and MAO inhibitors. Concomitant use of tramadol products with MAO inhibitors or SSRIs increases the risk of adverse events, including seizure and serotonin syndrome.

Withdrawal

Withdrawal symptoms may occur if RYZOLT® is discontinued abruptly. These symptoms may include: anxiety, sweating, insomnia, rigors, pain, nausea, tremors, diarrhea, upper respiratory symptoms, piloerection, and rarely hallucinations.

In a 12 week study, 325 patients were followed for 3 and 7 days after discontinuation of treatment with RYZOLT®. The majority of reported post-treatment adverse events including withdrawal symptoms were mild to moderate in nature. Onset of the post-treatment adverse events occurred more frequently within the first three days after treatment was stopped. Less than 1% of patients taking RYZOLT® met the DSM-IV criteria for a diagnosis of opioid withdrawal.

Clinical experience suggests that signs and symptoms of withdrawal may be reduced by tapering medication when discontinuing tramadol therapy.

Misuse, Abuse and Diversion of Opioids

Tramadol is an opioid agonist of the morphine type. Such drugs are sought by drug abusers and people with addiction disorders and are subject to criminal diversion.

Like other opioid agonists, legal or illicit, tramadol can be abused. This should be considered when prescribing or dispensing RYZOLT® in situations where the healthcare professional is concerned about a risk of misuse, abuse, or diversion.

RYZOLT® could be abused by breaking, crushing, chewing, or dissolving the product which can result in the uncontrolled delivery of the opioid, and as a consequence poses a significant risk of overdose and death.

Concerns about abuse, addiction, and diversion should not prevent the proper management of pain.

Healthcare professionals should contact their State Professional Licensing Board or State Controlled Substances Authority for information on how to prevent and detect abuse or diversion of this product.

Interactions with Alcohol and Drugs of Abuse

Tramadol may be expected to have additive effects when used in conjunction with alcohol, other opioids or drugs, whether legal or illicit, which cause central nervous system depression.

DRUG ABUSE AND ADDICTION

Abuse

RYZOLT® is a mu-agonist opioid. Tramadol, like other opioids used in analgesia, can be abused and is subject to criminal diversion.

Addiction is a primary, chronic, neurobiologic disease, with genetic, psychosocial, and environmental factors influencing its development and manifestations. It is characterized by behaviors that include one or more of the following: impaired control over drug use, compulsive use, continued use despite harm, and craving. Drug addiction is a treatable disease, utilizing a multidisciplinary approach, but relapse is common.

Concerns about abuse and addiction should not prevent the proper management of pain. However all patients treated with opioids require careful monitoring for signs of abuse and addiction, because use of opioid analgesic products carries the risk of addiction even under appropriate medical use.

"Drug-seeking" behavior is very common in addicts and drug abusers. Drug-seeking tactics include emergency calls or visits near the end of office hours, refusal to undergo appropriate examination, testing or referral, repeated "loss" of prescriptions, tampering with prescriptions and reluctance to provide prior medical records or contact information for other treating physician(s). "Doctor shopping" to obtain additional prescriptions is common among drug abusers and people suffering from untreated addiction.

Abuse and addiction are separate and distinct from physical dependence and tolerance. Physicians should be aware that addiction may not be accompanied by concurrent tolerance and symptoms of physical dependence in all addicts. In addition, abuse of opioids can occur in the absence of true addiction and is characterized by misuse for non-medical purposes, often in combination with other psychoactive substances. RYZOLT®, like other opioids, may be diverted for non-medical use. Careful record-keeping of prescribing information, including quantity, frequency, and renewal requests is strongly advised.

Proper assessment of the patient, proper prescribing practices, periodic re-evaluation of therapy, and proper dispensing and storage are appropriate measures that help to limit abuse of opioid drugs.

RYZOLT® is intended for oral use only. The crushed tablet poses a hazard of overdose and death. This risk is increased with concurrent abuse of alcohol and other substances. With parenteral abuse, the tablet excipients can be expected to result in local tissue necrosis, infection, pulmonary granulomas, and increased risk of endocarditis and valvular heart injury. Parenteral drug abuse is commonly associated with transmission of infectious diseases such as hepatitis and HIV.

Dependence

Tolerance is the need for increasing doses of opioids to maintain a defined effect such as analgesia (in the absence of disease progression or other external factors). Physical dependence is manifested by withdrawal symptoms after abrupt discontinuation of a drug or upon administration of an antagonist.

The opioid abstinence or withdrawal syndrome is characterized by some or all of the following: restlessness, lacrimation, rhinorrhea, yawning, perspiration, chills, myalgia, and mydriasis. Other symptoms also may develop, including irritability, anxiety, backache, joint pain, weakness, abdominal cramps, insomnia, nausea, anorexia, vomiting, diarrhea, or increased blood pressure, respiratory rate, or heart rate. Generally, tolerance and/or withdrawal are more likely to occur the longer a patient is on continuous opioid therapy.

Risk of Overdosage

Serious potential consequences of overdosage with RYZOLT® are central nervous system depression, respiratory depression and death. In treating an overdose, primary attention should be given to maintaining adequate ventilation along with general supportive treatment (see **OVERDOSAGE**).

PRECAUTIONS

Acute Abdominal Conditions

The administration of RYZOLT® may complicate the clinical assessment of patients with acute abdominal conditions.

Use in Renal and Hepatic Disease

Impaired renal function results in a decreased rate and extent of excretion of tramadol and its active metabolite, M1 in patients taking an immediate-release formulation of tramadol. RYZOLT® has not been studied in patients with renal impairment. The limited availability of dose strengths and once daily dosing of RYZOLT® do not permit the dosing flexibility required for safe use in patients with severe renal impairment. Therefore, RYZOLT® should not be used in patients with severe renal impairment (see **CLINICAL PHARMACOLOGY and DOSAGE AND ADMINISTRATION**).

The metabolism of tramadol and M1 is reduced in patients with advanced cirrhosis of the liver. RYZOLT® has not been studied in patients with hepatic impairment. The limited availability of dose strengths and once daily dosing of RYZOLT® do not permit the dosing flexibility required for safe use in patients with hepatic impairment. Therefore, RYZOLT® should not be used in patients with hepatic impairment (see **CLINICAL PHARMACOLOGY and DOSAGE AND ADMINISTRATION**).

Information for Patients

Patients should be instructed that:

- RYZOLT® is for oral use only and should be swallowed whole with a sufficient quantity of liquid and not split, chewed, dissolved or crushed.
- RYZOLT® may cause seizures and/or serotonin syndrome with concomitant use of serotonergic agents (including SSRIs, SNRIs and triptans) or drugs that significantly reduce the metabolic clearance of tramadol.
- RYZOLT® should be taken once daily, at approximately the same time every day and that exceeding these instructions can result in respiratory depression, seizures or death.
- RYZOLT® should not be taken in doses exceeding the maximum recommended daily dose as exceeding these recommendations can result in respiratory depression, seizures or even death (see **DOSAGE AND ADMINISTRATION**).
- RYZOLT® may impair the mental and physical abilities required for the performance of potentially hazardous tasks such as driving a car or operating machinery. Patients using this drug should be cautioned accordingly.
- RYZOLT® should not be taken with alcohol-containing beverages.
- RYZOLT® should be used with caution when taking medications such as tranquilizers, hypnotics or other opiate containing analgesics.
- Female patients should be instructed to inform the physician if they are pregnant, think they might become pregnant, or are trying to become pregnant (see **PRECAUTIONS, Pregnancy, and Labor and Delivery**).
- Clinical experience suggests that signs and symptoms of withdrawal may be reduced by tapering medication when discontinuing tramadol therapy.
- Patients should be informed to keep RYZOLT® out of reach of children.

Use in Drug and Alcohol Addiction

RYZOLT® is an opioid with no approved use for the management of addictive disorders. Its proper usage in individuals with drug or alcohol dependence, either active or in remission is for the management of pain requiring opioid analgesia.

Drug Interactions

CYP2D6 and CYP3A4 Inhibitors: Concomitant administration of CYP2D6 and/or CYP3A4 inhibitors (see **CLINICAL PHARMACOLOGY, Pharmacokinetics**), such as quinidine, fluoxetine, paroxetine and amitriptyline (CYP2D6 inhibitors), and ketoconazole and erythromycin (CYP3A4 inhibitors), may reduce metabolic clearance of tramadol increasing the risk for serious adverse events including seizures and serotonin syndrome.

Serotonergic Drugs: There have been postmarketing reports of serotonin syndrome with use of tramadol and SSRIs/SNRIs or MAOIs and α2-adrenergic blockers. Caution is advised when RYZOLT® is coadministered with other drugs that may affect the serotonergic neurotransmitter systems, such as SSRIs, MAOIs, triptans, linezolid (an antibiotic which is a reversible non-selective MAOI), lithium, or St. John's Wort. If concomitant treatment of RYZOLT® with a drug affecting the serotonergic neurotransmitter system is clinically warranted, careful observation of the patient is advised, particularly during treatment initiation and dose increases (see **WARNINGS, Serotonin Syndrome**).

Triptans: Based on the mechanism of action of tramadol and the potential for serotonin syndrome, caution is advised when RYZOLT® is coadministered with a triptan. If concomitant treatment of RYZOLT® with a triptan is clinically warranted, careful observation of the patient is advised, particularly during treatment initiation and dose increases (see **WARNINGS, Serotonin Syndrome**).

Use with Carbamazepine

Patients taking carbamazepine, a CYP3A4 inducer, may have a significantly reduced analgesic effect. Because carbamazepine increases tramadol metabolism and because of the seizure risk associated with tramadol, concomitant administration of RYZOLT® and carbamazepine is not recommended.

Use with Quinidine

Tramadol is metabolized to M1 by CYP2D6. Quinidine is a selective inhibitor of that isoenzyme, so that concomitant administration of quinidine and tramadol products results in increased concentrations of tramadol and reduced concentrations of M1. The clinical consequences of these findings are unknown. *In vitro* drug interaction studies in human liver microsomes indicate that tramadol has no effect on quinidine metabolism.

Use with Digoxin and Warfarin

Post-marketing surveillance of tramadol has revealed rare reports of digoxin toxicity and alteration of warfarin effect, including elevation of prothrombin times.

Interaction With Central Nervous System (CNS) Depressants

RYZOLT® should be used with caution and in reduced dosages when administered to patients receiving CNS depressants such as alcohol, opioids, anesthetic agents, narcotics, phenothiazines, tranquilizers or sedative hypnotics. RYZOLT® increases the risk of CNS and respiratory depression in these patients.

Potential of Other Drugs to Affect Tramadol

In vitro drug interaction studies in human liver microsomes indicate that concomitant administration with inhibitors of CYP2D6 such as fluoxetine, paroxetine, and amitriptyline could result in some inhibition of the metabolism of tramadol.

Tramadol is partially metabolized by CYP3A4. Administration of CYP3A4 inhibitors, such as ketoconazole and erythromycin, or inducers, such as rifampin and St. John's Wort, with RYZOLT® may affect the metabolism of tramadol leading to altered tramadol exposure.

Potential for Tramadol to Affect Other Drugs

In vitro studies indicate that tramadol is unlikely to inhibit the CYP3A4-mediated metabolism of other drugs when administered concomitantly at therapeutic doses. Tramadol is a mild inducer of selected drug metabolism pathways measured in animals.

Carcinogenesis, Mutagenesis and Impairment of Fertility

A slight, but statistically significant increase in two common murine tumors, pulmonary and hepatic, was observed in a mouse carcinogenicity study, particularly in aged mice. Mice were dosed orally up to 30 mg/kg (90 mg/m^2 or 0.5 times the maximum daily human dosage of 185 mg/m^2) for approximately two years, although the study was not done with the Maximum Tolerated Dose. This finding is not believed to suggest risk in humans. No such finding occurred in a rat carcinogenicity study (dosing orally up to 30 mg/kg - 180 mg/m^2 equal to the maximum daily human dosage of tramadol).

Tramadol was not mutagenic in the following assays: Ames *Salmonella* microsomal activation test, CHO/HPRT mammalian cell assay, mouse lymphoma assay (in the absence of metabolic activation), dominant lethal mutation tests in mice, chromosome aberration test in Chinese hamsters, and bone marrow micronucleus tests in mice and Chinese hamsters. Positive mutagenic results occurred in the presence of metabolic activation in the mouse lymphoma assay and micronucleus test in rats. Relevance of the finding in humans is unknown.

No effects on fertility were observed for tramadol at oral dose levels up to 50 mg/kg (300 mg/m^2) in male rats and 75 mg/kg (450 mg/m^2) in female rats. These dosages are 1.6 and 2.4 times the maximum daily human dosage of 185 mg/m^2, respectively.

Pregnancy

Teratogenic Effects: Pregnancy Category C

Tramadol has been shown to be embryotoxic and fetotoxic in mice, (120 mg/kg or 360 mg/m^2), rats (≥25 mg/kg or 150 mg/m^2) and rabbits (≥75mg/kg or 900 mg/m^2) at maternally toxic dosages, but was not teratogenic at these dose levels. These dosages on an mg/m^2 basis are 1.9, 0.8 and 4.9 times the maximum daily human dosage (185 mg/m^2) for mouse, rat and rabbit, respectively.

No drug related teratogenic effects were observed in progeny of mice (up to 140 mg/kg or 420 mg/m^2), rats (up to 80 mg/kg or 480 mg/m^2) or rabbits (up to 300 mg/kg or 3600 mg/m^2) treated with tramadol by various routes. Embryo and fetal toxicity consisted primarily of decreased fetal weights, skeletal ossification and increased supernumerary ribs in maternally toxic dose levels. Transient delays in developmental or behavioral parameters were also seen in pups from rat dams allowed to deliver. Embryo and fetal lethality were reported only in one rabbit study at 300 mg/kg (3600 mg/m^2), a dose that would cause extreme maternal toxicity in the rabbit. The dosages listed for mouse, rat and rabbit are 2.2, 2.6 and 19.4 times the maximum daily human dosage (185 mg/m^2), respectively.

Non-teratogenic Effects

Tramadol was evaluated in peri- and post-natal studies in rats. Progeny of dams receiving oral (gavage) dose levels of 50 mg/kg (300 mg/m^2 or 1.6 times the maximum daily human RYZOLT® dosage) or greater had decreased weights, and pup survival was decreased early in lactation at 80 mg/kg (480 mg/m^2 or 2.6 times the maximum daily human dose).

There are no adequate and well-controlled studies in pregnant women. RYZOLT® should be used during pregnancy only if the potential benefit justifies the potential risk to the fetus. Neonatal seizures, neonatal withdrawal syndrome, fetal death and stillbirth have been reported during post-marketing surveillance of tramadol immediate-release products.

Labor and Delivery

RYZOLT® should not be used in pregnant women prior to or during labor unless the potential benefits outweigh the risks. Safe use in pregnancy has not been established. Chronic use during pregnancy may lead to physical dependence and post-partum withdrawal symptoms in the newborn (see **DRUG ABUSE AND ADDICTION**). Tramadol has been shown to cross the placenta. The mean ratio of serum tramadol in the umbilical veins compared to maternal veins was 0.83 for 40 women given tramadol during labor.

The effect of RYZOLT®, if any, on the later growth, development and functional maturation of the child is unknown.

Nursing Mother

RYZOLT® is not recommended for obstetrical preoperative medication or for post-delivery analgesia in nursing mothers because its safety in infants and newborns has not been studied. Following a single IV 100 mg dose of tramadol, the cumulative excretion in breast milk within 16 hours post-dose was 100 µg of tramadol (0.1% of the maternal dose) and 27 µg of M1.

Pediatric Use

The safety and efficacy of RYZOLT® in patients under 16 years of age has not been established. The use of RYZOLT® in the pediatric population is not recommended.

Geriatric Use

In general, caution should be used when selecting the dose for an elderly patient. Usually, dose administration should start at the low end of the dosing range, reflecting the greater frequency of decreased hepatic, renal or cardiac function and of concomitant disease or other drug therapy (see **CLINICAL PHARMACOLOGY and DOSAGE AND ADMINISTRATION**).

In 12-week clinical trials, RYZOLT® was administered to 534 patients aged 65 years and older. Of those, 68 patients were 75 years of age and older. Comparable incidence rates of patients experiencing adverse events were observed for patients older than 65 years of age compared with younger patients (< 65 years of age), except constipation for which the incidence was higher in older patients. RYZOLT® should be used with caution in patients older than 75 years of age (see **CLINICAL PHARMACOLOGY and DOSAGE AND ADMINISTRATION**).

ADVERSE REACTIONS

RYZOLT® was administered to a total of 2707 subjects (2406 patients and 301 healthy volunteers) during clinical studies, including four randomized double-blind studies (treatment ≥ 12 weeks) and two open-label long-term studies (treatment up to 12 months) in patients with moderate to severe pain due to osteoarthritis of the knee. A total of 844 patients were exposed to RYZOLT® for 12 weeks, 493 patients for 6 months and 243 patients for 12 months. Treatment emergent adverse events increased with dose from 100 mg to 300 mg in the three twelve-week, randomized, double-blind, placebo-controlled studies (Table 2).

[See table 2 at top of next page]

The majority of patients who experienced the most common adverse events (≥5%) reported mild to moderate symptoms. Less than 3% of adverse events were rated as severe. Overall, onset of these adverse events usually occurred within the first two weeks of treatment.

Adverse reactions with an incidence of 1.0% to <5.0%

Ear and labyrinth disorders: vertigo

Gastrointestinal disorders: abdominal pain, diarrhea, dry mouth, dyspepsia, upper abdominal pain

General disorders: fatigue, weakness

Investigations: weight decreased

Metabolism and nutrition disorders: anorexia

Musculoskeletal and connective tissue disorders: arthralgia

Table 2. Percentage of Patients with Incidence of Adverse Events ≥ 2% from Three 12-week Placebo-Controlled Studies (MDT3-002, MDT3-003 and MDT3-005).

ADVERSE EVENTS (MEDRA Preferred Terms)	RYZOLT®				Placebo
	100 mg	200 mg	300 mg	Total*	
	N=216	N=311	N=530	N=1095	N=668
Nausea	28 (13%)	42 (14%)	76 (14%)	179 (16%)	37 (6%)
Constipation	21 (10%)	36 (12%)	52 (10%)	140 (13%)	26 (4%)
Dizziness	16 (7%)	28 (9%)	52 (10%)	106 (10%)	18 (3%)
Somnolence	11 (5%)	22 (7%)	23 (4%)	77 (7%)	12 (2%)
Vomiting	7 (3%)	16 (5%)	31 (6%)	58 (5%)	4 (1%)
Pruritus	9 (4%)	15 (5%)	18 (3%)	51 (5%)	7 (1%)
Headache	10 (5%)	9 (3%)	15 (3%)	41 (4%)	21 (3%)
Sweating increased	1 (0%)	9 (3%)	14 (3%)	35 (3%)	5 (1%)
Dry mouth	7 (3%)	13 (4%)	6 (1%)	32 (3%)	8 (1%)
Fatigue	6 (3%)	7 (2%)	9 (2%)	26 (2%)	6 (1%)
Anorexia	4 (2%)	4 (1%)	10 (2%)	25 (2%)	2 (0%)
Vertigo	2 (1%)	3 (1%)	6 (1%)	21 (2%)	3 (0%)
Insomnia	2 (1%)	6 (2%)	9 (2%)	18 (2%)	8 (1%)

* Due to the difference in study design of MDT3-005, only the results of the double-blind phase of the study are presented and the dose specific results include maintenance period data only.

Nervous system disorders: headache, tremor
Psychiatric disorders: anxiety, insomnia
Skin and subcutaneous tissue disorders: pruritus, sweating increased
Vascular disorders: hot flushes
Adverse reactions with an incidence of <1.0%
Blood and lymphatic system disorders: anemia, thrombocytopenia
Cardiac disorders: bradycardia
Eye disorders: blurred vision, visual disturbance
Gastrointestinal disorders: abdominal discomfort, abdominal distension, abdominal tenderness, change in bowel habit, constipation aggravated, diverticulitis, diverticulum, dyspepsia aggravated, dysphagia, fecal impaction, gastric irritation, gastritis, gastrointestinal hemorrhage, gastrointestinal irritation, gastro-esophageal reflux disease, lower abdominal pain, pancreatitis aggravated, rectal hemorrhage, rectal prolapse, retching
General disorders: asthenia, malaise
Hepatobiliary disorders: biliary tract disorder, cholelithiasis
Immune system disorders: hypersensitivity
Investigations: alanine aminotransferase decreased, alanine aminotransferase increased, aspartate aminotransferase decreased, aspartate aminotransferase increased, blood amylase increased, blood creatinine increased, blood in stool, blood potassium abnormal, blood pressure increased gamma glutamyltransferase increased
Metabolism and nutrition disorders: appetite decreased, dehydration
Nervous system disorders: ataxia, disturbance in attention, dysarthria, gait abnormal, headache aggravated, mental impairment, sedation, seizure, sleep apnea syndrome, syncope, tremor
Psychiatric disorders: abnormal behavior, agitation, anxiety, confusion, depression, emotional disturbance, euphoric mood, indifference, irritability, libido decreased, nervousness, sleep disorder
Renal and urinary disorders: difficulty in micturition, urinary hesitation, urinary retention
Reproductive system and breast disorders: erectile dysfunction, sexual dysfunction
Respiratory, thoracic and mediastinal disorders: dyspnea
Skin and subcutaneous tissue disorders: allergic dermatitis, cold sweat, dermatitis, night sweats, pallor, generalized pruritus, urticaria
Vascular disorders: flushing, hypertension, hypotension, orthostatic hypotension

OVERDOSAGE

Acute overdosage with tramadol can be manifested by respiratory depression, somnolence progressing to stupor or coma, skeletal muscle flaccidity, cold and clammy skin, constricted pupils, bradycardia, hypotension and death.
Death due to overdose have been reported with abuse and misuse of tramadol, by ingesting, inhaling, or injecting the crushed tablets. The risk of fatal overdose is further increased when tramadol is abused concurrently with alcohol and other CNS depressants, including other opioids.
In the treatment of tramadol overdosage, primary attention should be given to the re-establishment of a patent airway and institution of assisted or controlled ventilation. Supportive measures (including oxygen and vasopressors) should be employed in the management of circulatory shock and pulmonary edema accompanying overdose as indicated. Cardiac arrest or arrhythmias may require cardiac massage or defibrillation.
While naloxone will reverse some (but not all) symptoms caused by overdosage with tramadol, the risk of seizures is also increased with naloxone administration. In animals, convulsions following the administration of toxic doses of tramadol could be suppressed with barbiturates or benzodiazepines but were increased with naloxone. Naloxone administration did not change the lethality of an overdose in mice. Hemodialysis is not expected to be helpful in an overdose because it removes less than 7% of the administered dose in a 4-hour dialysis period.

DOSAGE AND ADMINISTRATION

RYZOLT® extended-release tablets should be taken once a day. The tablets should be swallowed whole with liquid and not split, chewed, dissolved or crushed. RYZOLT® tablets produce a continuous release of active ingredient over 24 hours: a repeat dosage within 24 hours is not recommended.
Patients Not Currently on Tramadol Immediate-Release Products:
Treatment with RYZOLT® should be initiated at a dose of 100 mg/day. Daily doses should be titrated by 100 mg/day increments every 2-3 days (i.e., start 200 mg/day on day 3 or 4 of therapy) to achieve a balance between adequate pain control and tolerability for the individual patient. For patients requiring the 300 mg daily dose, titration should take at least 4 days (i.e. 300 mg/day on day 5). The usual daily dose is 200 or 300 mg. The daily dose and titration should be individualized for each patient. Therapy should be continued with the lowest effective dose. RYZOLT® should not be administered at a dose exceeding 300 mg per day.
Clinical experience suggests that signs and symptoms of withdrawal may be reduced by tapering medication when discontinuing tramadol therapy.
Patients Currently on Tramadol Immediate-Release Products:
For patients maintained on tramadol immediate release (IR) products, the 24-hour tramadol IR dose should be calculated and the patient should be initiated on a total daily dose of RYZOLT® rounded down to the next lowest 100 mg increment. The dose may subsequently be individualized according to patient need. Due to limitations in flexibility of dose selection with RYZOLT®, some patients maintained on tramadol IR products may not be able to convert to RYZOLT®. RYZOLT® should not be administered at a dose exceeding 300 mg per day. Do not use RYZOLT® with other tramadol products. (see **WARNINGS**).
Individualization of Dose
Good pain management practice dictates that analgesic dose be individualized according to patient need using the lowest beneficial dose. Studies with tramadol products in adults have shown that starting at the lowest possible dose and titrating upward will result in fewer discontinuations and increased tolerability.
Renal and Hepatic Disease
RYZOLT® should not be used in patients with:
• Creatinine clearance less than 30 mL/min,
• Hepatic impairment.
(see **WARNINGS, Use in Renal and Hepatic Disease**).
Geriatric patients (65 years of age and older)
In general, dose selection for patients over 65 years of age who may have decreased hepatic or renal function, or other concomitant diseases, should be initiated cautiously, usually starting at the low end of the dosing range. RYZOLT® should be administered with greater caution at the lowest effective dose in patients over 75 years, due to the potential for greater frequency of adverse events in this population.

HOW SUPPLIED

RYZOLT® (tramadol hydrochloride extended-release tablets) are supplied in a number of packages and dose strengths:

100-mg, white, beveled edge, round biconvex tablets, plain on one side and printed "PP 100" in black ink on the other side.
Bottle of 30 tablets – NDC 59011-334-30
Bottle of 90 tablets – NDC 59011-334-90
200-mg, white, beveled edge, round biconvex tablets, plain on one side and printed "PP 200" in black ink on the other side
Bottle of 30 tablets – NDC 59011-335-30
Bottle of 90 tablets – NDC 59011-335-90
300-mg, white, beveled edge, round biconvex tablets, plain on one side and printed "PP 300" in black ink on the other side
Bottle of 30 tablets – NDC 59011-336-30
Bottle of 90 tablets – NDC 59011-336-90
Store at 25°C (77°F); excursions permitted between 15-30°C (59–86°F). Dispense in a tight, light-resistant container.
Warning: keep out of reach of children.
Healthcare professionals can telephone Purdue Pharma's Medical Services Department (1-888-726-7535) for information on this product.
February 25, 2010
301397-0B
Manufactured by:
Confab Laboratories Inc
Saint-Hubert, Quebec, Canada J3Y 3X3
Distributed by:
Purdue Pharma L.P.
Stamford, CT 06901-3431
Licensed from Labopharm Europe Limited
U.S. Patent 6,607,748
RYZOLT® is a trademark of Purdue Pharma L.P.
Shown in Product Identification Guide, page 317

Regeneron Pharmaceuticals, Inc.
777 OLD SAW MILL RIVER ROAD
TARRYTOWN, NY 10591

For Medical Information Contact:
1-877-REGN-777 (1-877-734-6777)

ARCALYST®   ℞
[ARK-a-list]
(rilonacept)
Injection for Subcutaneous Use

HIGHLIGHTS OF PRESCRIBING INFORMATION
These highlights do not include all the information needed to use ARCALYST safely and effectively. See full prescribing information for ARCALYST.
ARCALYST® (rilonacept)
Injection for Subcutaneous Use
Initial U.S. Approval: 2008
————INDICATIONS AND USAGE————
ARCALYST (rilonacept) is an interleukin-1 blocker indicated for the treatment of Cryopyrin-Associated Periodic Syndromes (CAPS), including Familial Cold Auto-inflammatory Syndrome (FCAS) and Muckle-Wells Syndrome (MWS) in adults and children 12 and older. (1)
————DOSAGE AND ADMINISTRATION————
• Adult patients 18 yrs and older: Initiate treatment with a loading dose of 320 mg delivered as two, 2-mL, subcutaneous injections of 160 mg on the same day at two different sites. Continue dosing with a once-weekly injection of 160 mg administered as a single, 2-mL, subcutaneous injection. Do not administer ARCALYST more often than once weekly. (2)
• Pediatric patients aged 12 to 17 years: Initiate treatment with a loading dose of 4.4 mg/kg, up to a maximum of 320 mg, delivered as one or two subcutaneous injections with a maximum single-injection volume of 2 mL. Continue dosing with a once-weekly injection of 2.2 mg/kg, up to a maximum of 160 mg, administered as a single subcutaneous injection, up to 2 mL. If the initial dose is given as two injections, they should be given on the same day at two different sites. Do not administer ARCALYST more often than once weekly. (2)
————DOSAGE FORMS AND STRENGTHS————
Sterile, single-use 20-mL, glass vial containing 220 mg of rilonacept as a lyophilized powder for reconstitution. (3)
————CONTRAINDICATIONS————
None.
————WARNINGS AND PRECAUTIONS————
• Interleukin-1 blockade may interfere with immune response to infections. Serious, life-threatening infections have been reported in patients taking ARCALYST. Discontinue treatment with ARCALYST if a patient develops

a serious infection. Do not initiate treatment with ARCALYST in patients with active or chronic infections. (5.1)

- Hypersensitivity reactions associated with ARCALYST administration have been rare. If a hypersensitivity reaction occurs, discontinue administration of ARCALYST and initiate appropriate therapy. (5.5)
- Live vaccines should not be given concurrently with ARCALYST. Prior to initiation of therapy with ARCALYST, patients should receive all recommended vaccinations. (5.3)

————————ADVERSE REACTIONS————————

The most common adverse reactions reported by patients with CAPS treated with ARCALYST are injection-site reactions and upper respiratory tract infections. (6.2, 6.3)

To report SUSPECTED ADVERSE REACTIONS, contact Regeneron at 1-877-REGN-777 (1-877-734-6777) or FDA at 1-800-FDA-1088 or www.fda.gov/medwatch.

————————DRUG INTERACTIONS————————

No formal drug interaction studies have been conducted with ARCALYST. (7)

————————USE IN SPECIFIC POPULATIONS————————

Pregnancy–No human data. Based on animal data, may cause fetal harm. (8.1)

See 17 for PATIENT COUNSELING INFORMATION and FDA-approved patient labeling.

Revised: 04/2010

FULL PRESCRIBING INFORMATION: CONTENTS*

FULL PRESCRIBING INFORMATION

1 INDICATIONS AND USAGE

ARCALYST® (rilonacept) is an interleukin-1 blocker indicated for the treatment of Cryopyrin-Associated Periodic Syndromes (CAPS), including Familial Cold Autoinflammatory Syndrome (FCAS) and Muckle-Wells Syndrome (MWS) in adults and children 12 and older.

2 DOSAGE AND ADMINISTRATION

2.1 General Dosing Information

INJECTION FOR SUBCUTANEOUS USE ONLY.

2.2 Dosing

Adult patients 18 years and older: Treatment should be initiated with a loading dose of 320 mg delivered as two, 2 mL, subcutaneous injections of 160 mg each given on the same day at two different sites. Dosing should be continued with a once-weekly injection of 160 mg administered as a single, 2-mL, subcutaneous injection. ARCALYST should not be given more often than once weekly. Dosage modification is not required based on advanced age or gender.

Pediatric patients aged 12 to 17 years: Treatment should be initiated with a loading dose of 4.4 mg/kg, up to a maximum of 320 mg, delivered as one or two subcutaneous injections with a maximum single-injection volume of 2 mL. Dosing should be continued with a once-weekly injection of 2.2 mg/kg, up to a maximum of 160 mg, administered as a single subcutaneous injection, up to 2 mL. If the initial dose is given as two injections, they should be given on the same day at two different sites. ARCALYST should not be given more often than once weekly.

2.3 Preparation for Administration

Each single-use vial of ARCALYST contains a sterile, white to off-white, preservative-free, lyophilized powder. Reconstitution with 2.3 mL of preservative-free Sterile Water for Injection (supplied separately) is required prior to subcutaneous administration of the drug.

2.4 Administration

Using aseptic technique, withdraw 2.3 mL of preservative-free Sterile Water for Injection using a 27-gauge, ½-inch needle attached to a 3-mL syringe and inject the preservative-free Sterile Water for Injection into the drug product vial for reconstitution. The needle and syringe used for reconstitution with preservative-free Sterile Water for Injection should then be discarded and should not be used for subcutaneous injections. After the addition of preservative-free Sterile Water for Injection, the vial contents should be reconstituted by shaking the vial for approximately one minute and then allowing it to sit for one minute. The resulting 80-mg/mL solution is sufficient to allow a withdrawal volume of up to 2 mL for subcutaneous administration. The reconstituted solution is viscous, clear, colorless to pale yellow, and essentially free from particulates. Prior to injection, the reconstituted solution should be carefully inspected for any discoloration or particulate matter. If there is discoloration or particulate matter in the solution, the product in that vial should not be used.

Using aseptic technique, withdraw the recommended dose volume, up to 2 mL (160 mg), of the solution with a new 27-gauge, ½-inch needle attached to a new 3-mL syringe for subcutaneous injection. EACH VIAL SHOULD BE USED FOR A SINGLE DOSE ONLY. Discard the vial after withdrawal of drug.

Sites for subcutaneous injection, such as the abdomen, thigh, or upper arm, should be rotated. Injections should never be made at sites that are bruised, red, tender, or hard.

2.5 Stability and Storage

The lyophilized ARCALYST product is to be stored refrigerated at 2° to 8°C (36° to 46°F) inside the original carton to protect it from light. Do not use beyond the date stamped on the label. After reconstitution, ARCALYST may be kept at room temperature, should be protected from light, and should be used within three hours of reconstitution. ARCALYST does not contain preservatives; therefore, unused portions of ARCALYST should be discarded.

3 DOSAGE FORMS AND STRENGTHS

ARCALYST is supplied in sterile, single-use, 20-mL, glass vials. Each vial contains 220 mg of rilonacept as a white to off-white, preservative-free, lyophilized powder. Reconstitution with 2.3 mL of preservative-free Sterile Water for Injection is required prior to subcutaneous administration of the drug. The reconstituted ARCALYST is a viscous, clear, colorless to pale yellow, essentially free from particulates, 80-mg/mL solution.

4 CONTRAINDICATIONS

None.

5 WARNINGS AND PRECAUTIONS

5.1 Infections

Interleukin-1 (IL-1) blockade may interfere with the immune response to infections. Treatment with another medication that works through inhibition of IL-1 has been associated with an increased risk of serious infections, and serious infections have been reported in patients taking ARCALYST [see Clinical Studies (14)]. There was a greater incidence of infections in patients on ARCALYST compared with placebo. In the controlled portion of the study, one infection was reported as severe, which was bronchitis in a patient on ARCALYST.

In an open-label extension study, one patient developed bacterial meningitis and died [see Adverse Reactions (6.3)]. ARCALYST should be discontinued if a patient develops a serious infection. Treatment with ARCALYST should not be initiated in patients with an active or chronic infection.

In clinical studies, ARCALYST has not been administered concomitantly with tumor necrosis factor (TNF) inhibitors. An increased incidence of serious infections has been associated with administration of an IL-1 blocker in combination with TNF inhibitors. **Taking ARCALYST with TNF inhibitors is not recommended because this may increase the risk of serious infections.**

Drugs that affect the immune system by blocking TNF have been associated with an increased risk of reactivation of latent tuberculosis (TB). It is possible that taking drugs such as ARCALYST that block IL-1 increases the risk of TB or other atypical or opportunistic infections. Healthcare providers should follow current CDC guidelines both to evaluate for and to treat possible latent tuberculosis infections before initiating therapy with ARCALYST.

5.2 Immunosuppression

The impact of treatment with ARCALYST on active and/or chronic infections and the development of malignancies is not known [see Adverse Reactions (6.3)]. However, treatment with immunosuppressants, including ARCALYST, may result in an increase in the risk of malignancies.

5.3 Immunizations

Since no data are available on either the efficacy of live vaccines or on the risks of secondary transmission of infection by live vaccines in patients receiving ARCALYST, live vaccines should not be given concurrently with ARCALYST. In addition, because ARCALYST may interfere with normal immune response to new antigens, vaccinations may not be effective in patients receiving ARCALYST. No data are available on the effectiveness of vaccination with inactivated (killed) antigens in patients receiving ARCALYST. Because IL-1 blockade may interfere with immune response to infections, it is recommended that prior to initiation of therapy with ARCALYST adult and pediatric patients receive all recommended vaccinations, as appropriate, including pneumococcal vaccine and inactivated influenza vaccine. (See current Recommended Immunizations schedules at the website of the Centers for Disease Control. http://www.cdc.gov/vaccines/recs/schedules/).

5.4 Lipid Profile Changes

Patients should be monitored for changes in their lipid profiles and provided with medical treatment if warranted [see Adverse Reactions (6.7)].

5.5 Hypersensitivity

Hypersensitivity reactions associated with ARCALYST administration in the clinical studies were rare. If a hypersensitivity reaction occurs, administration of ARCALYST should be discontinued and appropriate therapy initiated.

6 ADVERSE REACTIONS

Six serious adverse reactions were reported by four patients during the clinical program. These serious adverse reactions were *Mycobacterium intracellulare* infection; gastrointestinal bleeding and colitis; sinusitis and bronchitis; and *Streptococcus pneumoniae* meningitis [see Adverse Reactions (6.3)].

The most commonly reported adverse reaction associated with ARCALYST was injection-site reaction (ISR) [see Adverse Reactions (6.2)]. The next most commonly reported adverse reaction was upper respiratory infection [see Adverse Reactions (6.3)].

Because clinical trials are conducted under widely varying conditions, adverse reaction rates observed in the clinical trials of a drug cannot be directly compared to rates in the clinical trials of another drug and may not reflect the rates observed in practice.

The data described herein reflect exposure to ARCALYST in 600 patients, including 85 exposed for at least 6 months and 65 exposed for at least one year. These included patients with CAPS, patients with other diseases, and healthy volunteers. Approximately 60 patients with CAPS have been treated weekly with 160 mg of ARCALYST. The pivotal trial population included 47 patients with CAPS. These patients were between the ages of 22 and 78 years (average 51 years). Thirty-one patients were female and 16 were male. All of the patients were White/Caucasian. Six pediatric patients (12-17 years) were enrolled directly into the open-label extension phase.

6.1 Clinical Trial Experience

Part A of the clinical trial was conducted in patients with CAPS who were naïve to treatment with ARCALYST. Part A of the study was a randomized, double-blind, placebo-controlled, six-week study comparing ARCALYST to placebo [see Clinical Studies (14)]. Table 1 reflects the frequency of adverse events reported by at least two patients during Part A.

Table 1: Most Frequent Adverse Reactions (Part A, Reported by at Least Two Patients)

Adverse Event	ARCALYST 160 mg (n = 23)	Placebo (n = 24)
Any AE	17 (74%)	13 (54%)
Injection-site reactions	11 (48%)	3 (13%)
Upper respiratory tract infection	6 (26%)	1 (4%)
Nausea	1 (4%)	3 (13%)

Diarrhea	1 (4%)	3 (13%)
Sinusitis	2 (9%)	1 (4%)
Abdominal pain upper	0	2 (8%)
Cough	2 (9%)	0
Hypoesthesia	2 (9%)	0
Stomach discomfort	1 (4%)	1 (4%)
Urinary tract infection	1 (4%)	1 (4%)

6.2 Injection-Site Reactions
In patients with CAPS, the most common and consistently reported adverse event associated with ARCALYST was injection-site reaction (ISR). The ISRs included erythema, swelling, pruritis, mass, bruising, inflammation, pain, edema, dermatitis, discomfort, urticaria, vesicles, warmth and hemorrhage. Most injection-site reactions lasted for one to two days. No ISRs were assessed as severe, and no patient discontinued study participation due to an ISR.

6.3 Infections
During Part A, the incidence of patients reporting infections was greater with ARCALYST (48%) than with placebo (17%). In Part B, randomized withdrawal, the incidence of infections were similar in the ARCALYST (18%) and the placebo patients (22%). Part A of the trial was initiated in the winter months, while Part B was predominantly performed in the summer months.
In placebo-controlled studies across a variety of patient populations encompassing 360 patients treated with rilonacept and 179 treated with placebo, the incidence of infections was 34% and 27% (2.15 per patient-exposure year and 1.81 per patient-exposure year), respectively, for rilonacept and placebo.
Serious Infections: One patient receiving ARCALYST for an unapproved indication in another study developed an infection in his olecranon bursa with *Mycobacterium intracellulare*. The patient was on chronic glucocorticoid treatment. The infection occurred after an intraarticular glucocorticoid injection into the bursa with subsequent local exposure to a suspected source of mycobacteria. The patient recovered after the administration of the appropriate antimicrobial therapy. One patient treated for another unapproved indication developed bronchitis/sinusitis, which resulted in hospitalization. One patient died in an open-label study of CAPS from *Streptococcus pneumoniae* meningitis.

6.4 Malignancies
[*see Warnings and Precautions (5.2)*].

6.5 Hematologic Events
One patient in a study in an unapproved indication developed transient neutropenia (ANC < 1 × 10^9/L) after receiving a large dose (2000 mg intravenously) of ARCALYST. The patient did not experience any infection associated with the neutropenia.

6.6 Immunogenicity
Antibodies directed against the receptor domains of rilonacept were detected by an ELISA assay in patients with CAPS after treatment with ARCALYST. Nineteen of 55 patients (35%) who had received ARCALYST for at least 6 weeks tested positive for treatment-emergent binding antibodies on at least one occasion. Of the 19, seven tested positive at the last assessment (Week 18 or 24 of the open-label extension period), and five patients tested positive for neutralizing antibodies on at least one occasion. There was no correlation of antibody activity and either clinical effectiveness or safety.
The data reflect the percentage of patients whose test results were positive for antibodies to the rilonacept receptor domains in specific assays, and are highly dependent on the sensitivity and specificity of the assays. The observed incidence of antibody (including neutralizing antibody) positivity in an assay is highly dependent on several factors including assay sensitivity and specificity, assay methodology, sample handling, timing of sample collection, concomitant medications, and underlying disease. For these reasons, comparison of the incidence of antibodies to rilonacept with the incidence of antibodies to other products may be misleading.

6.7 Lipid profiles
Cholesterol and lipid levels may be reduced in patients with chronic inflammation. Patients with CAPS treated with ARCALYST experienced increases in their mean total cholesterol, HDL cholesterol, LDL cholesterol, and triglycerides. The mean increases from baseline for total cholesterol, HDL cholesterol, LDL cholesterol, and triglycerides were 19 mg/dL, 2 mg/dL, 10 mg/dL, and 57 mg/dL respectively after 6 weeks of open-label therapy. Physicians should monitor the lipid profiles of their patients (for example after 2-3 months) and consider lipid-lowering therapies as needed based upon cardiovascular risk factors and current guidelines.

7 DRUG INTERACTIONS

7.1 TNF-blocking agent and IL-1 blocking agent
Specific drug interaction studies have not been conducted with ARCALYST. Concomitant administration of another drug that blocks IL-1 with a TNF-blocking agent in another patient population has been associated with an increased risk of serious infections and an increased risk of neutropenia. The concomitant administration of ARCALYST with TNF-blocking agents may also result in similar toxicities and is not recommended [*see Warnings and Precautions (5.1)*].
The concomitant administration of ARCALYST with other drugs that block IL-1 has not been studied. Based upon the potential for pharmacologic interactions between rilonacept and a recombinant IL-1ra, concomitant administration of ARCALYST and other agents that block IL-1 or its receptors is not recommended.

7.2 Cytochrome P450 Substrates
The formation of CYP450 enzymes is suppressed by increased levels of cytokines (e.g., IL-1) during chronic inflammation. Thus it is expected that for a molecule that binds to IL-1, such as rilonacept, the formation of CYP450 enzymes could be normalized. This is clinically relevant for CYP450 substrates with a narrow therapeutic index, where the dose is individually adjusted (e.g., warfarin). Upon initiation of ARCALYST, in patients being treated with these types of medicinal products, therapeutic monitoring of the effect or drug concentration should be performed and the individual dose of the medicinal product may need to be adjusted as needed.

8 USE IN SPECIFIC POPULATIONS

8.1 Pregnancy
Pregnancy Category C. There are no adequate and well-controlled studies of ARCALYST in pregnant women. Based on animal data, ARCALYST may cause fetal harm. An embryo-fetal developmental toxicity study was performed in cynomolgus monkeys treated with 0, 5, 15 or 30 mg/kg given twice a week (highest dose is approximately 3.7-fold higher than the human doses of 160 mg based on body surface area). The fetus of the only monkey with exposure to rilonacept during the later period of gestation showed multiple fusion and absence of the ribs and thoracic vertebral bodies and arches. Exposure to rilonacept during this time period was below that expected clinically. Likewise, in the cynomolgus monkey, all doses of rilonacept reduced serum levels of estradiol up to 64% compared to controls and increased the incidence of lumbar ribs compared to both control animals and historical control incidences. In perinatal and postnatal developmental toxicology studies in the mouse model using a murine analog of rilonacept (0, 20, 100 or 200 mg/kg), there was a 3-fold increase in the number of stillbirths in dams treated with 200 mg/kg three times per week (the highest dose is approximately 6-fold higher than the 160 mg maintenance dose based on body surface area). ARCALYST should be used during pregnancy only if the benefit justifies the potential risk to the fetus.
Nonteratogenic effects. A peri- and post-natal reproductive toxicology study was performed in which mice were subcutaneously administered a murine analogue of rilonacept at doses of 20, 100, 200 mg/kg three times per week (the highest dose is approximately 6-fold higher than the 160 mg maintenance dose based on body surface area). Results indicated an increased incidence in unscheduled deaths of the F_1 offspring during maturation at all doses tested.

8.3 Nursing Mothers
It is not known whether rilonacept is excreted in human milk. Because many drugs are excreted in human milk, caution should be exercised when ARCALYST is administered to a nursing woman.

8.4 Pediatric Use
Six pediatric patients with CAPS between the ages of 12 and 16 were treated with ARCALYST at a weekly, subcutaneous dose of 2.2 mg/kg (up to a maximum of 160 mg) for 24-weeks during the open-label extension phase. These patients showed improvement from baseline in their symptom scores and in objective markers of inflammation (e.g. Serum Amyloid A and C-Reactive Protein). The adverse events included injection site reactions and upper respiratory symptoms as were commonly seen in the adult patients. The trough drug levels for four pediatric patients measured at the end of the weekly dose interval (mean 20 mcg/mL, range 3.6 to 33 mcg/mL) were similar to those observed in adult patients with CAPS (mean 24 mcg/mL, range 7 to 56 mcg/mL).
Safety and effectiveness in pediatric patients below the age of 12 have not been established.
When administered to pregnant primates, rilonacept treatment may have contributed to alterations in bone ossification in the fetus. It is not known if ARCALYST will alter bone development in pediatric patients. Pediatric patients treated with ARCALYST should undergo appropriate monitoring for growth and development. [*see Use in Specific Populations (8.1)*]

8.5 Geriatric Use
In the placebo-controlled clinical studies in patients with CAPS and other indications, 70 patients randomized to treatment with ARCALYST were ≥ 65 years of age, and 6 were ≥ 75 years of age. In the CAPS clinical trial, efficacy, safety and tolerability were generally similar in elderly patients as compared to younger adults; however, only ten patients ≥ 65 years old participated in the trial. In an open-label extension study of CAPS, a 71 year old woman developed bacterial meningitis and died [*see Adverse Reactions (6.3)*]. Age did not appear to have a significant effect on steady-state trough concentrations in the clinical study.

8.6 Patients with Renal Impairment
No formal studies have been conducted to examine the pharmacokinetics of rilonacept administered subcutaneously in patients with renal impairment.

8.7 Patients with Hepatic Impairment
No formal studies have been conducted to examine the pharmacokinetics of rilonacept administered subcutaneously in patients with hepatic impairment.

10 OVERDOSAGE

There have been no reports of overdose with ARCALYST. Maximum weekly doses of up to 320 mg have been administered subcutaneously for up to approximately 18 months in a small number of patients with CAPS and up to 6 months in patients with an unapproved indication in clinical trials without evidence of dose-limiting toxicities. In addition, ARCALYST given intravenously at doses up to 2000 mg monthly in another patient population for up to six months were tolerated without dose-limiting toxicities. The maximum amount of ARCALYST that can be safely administered has not been determined.
In case of overdose, it is recommended that the patient be monitored for any signs or symptoms of adverse reactions or effects, and appropriate symptomatic treatment instituted immediately.

11 DESCRIPTION

Rilonacept is a dimeric fusion protein consisting of the ligand-binding domains of the extracellular portions of the human interleukin-1 receptor component (IL-1RI) and IL-1 receptor accessory protein (IL-1RAcP) linked in-line to the Fc portion of human IgG1. Rilonacept has a molecular weight of approximately 251 kDa. Rilonacept is expressed in recombinant Chinese hamster ovary (CHO) cells.
ARCALYST is supplied in single-use, 20-mL glass vials containing a sterile, white to off-white, lyophilized powder. Each vial of ARCALYST is to be reconstituted with 2.3 mL of Sterile Water for Injection. A volume of up to 2 mL can be withdrawn, which is designed to deliver 160 mg for subcutaneous administration only. The resulting solution is viscous, clear, colorless to pale yellow, and essentially free from particulates. Each vial contains 220 mg rilonacept. After reconstitution each vial contains 80 mg/mL rilonacept, 40 mM histidine, 50 mM arginine, 3.0% (w/v) polyethylene glycol 3350, 2.0% (w/v) sucrose, and 1.0% (w/v) glycine at a pH of 6.5 ± 0.3. No preservatives are present.

12 CLINICAL PHARMACOLOGY

12.1 Mechanism of Action
CAPS refer to rare genetic syndromes generally caused by mutations in the NLRP-3 [Nucleotide-binding domain, leucine rich family (NLR), pyrin domain containing 3] gene (also known as Cold-Induced Auto-inflammatory Syndrome-1 [*CIAS1*]). CAPS disorders are inherited in an autosomal dominant pattern with male and female offspring equally affected. Features common to all disorders include fever, urticaria-like rash, arthralgia, myalgia, fatigue, and conjunctivitis.
In most cases, inflammation in CAPS is associated with mutations in the NLRP-3 gene which encodes the protein cryopyrin, an important component of the inflammasome. Cryopyrin regulates the protease caspase-1 and controls the activation of interleukin-1 beta (IL-1β). Mutations in NLRP-3 result in an overactive inflammasome resulting in excessive release of activated IL-1β that drives inflammation.
Rilonacept blocks IL-1β signaling by acting as a soluble decoy receptor that binds IL-1β and prevents its interaction with cell surface receptors. Rilonacept also binds IL-1α and IL-1 receptor antagonist (IL-1ra) with reduced affinity. The equilibrium dissociation constants for rilonacept binding to IL-1β, IL-1α and IL-1ra were 0.5 pM, 1.4 pM and 6.1 pM, respectively.

12.2 Pharmacodynamics
C-Reactive Protein (CRP) and Serum Amyloid A (SAA) are indicators of inflammatory disease activity that are elevated in patients with CAPS. Elevated SAA has been associated with the development of systemic amyloidosis in patients with CAPS. Compared to placebo, treatment with ARCALYST resulted in sustained reductions from baseline in mean serum CRP and SAA to normal levels during the clinical trial. ARCALYST also normalized mean SAA from elevated levels.

12.3 Pharmacokinetics
The average trough levels of rilonacept were approximately 24 mcg/mL at steady-state following weekly subcutaneous doses of 160 mg for up to 48 weeks in patients with CAPS. The steady-state appeared to be reached by 6 weeks.

No pharmacokinetic data are available in patients with hepatic or renal impairment.

No study was conducted to evaluate the effect of age, gender, or body weight on rilonacept exposure. Based on limited data obtained from the clinical study, steady state trough concentrations were similar between male and female patients. Age (26-78 years old) and body weight (50-120 kg) did not appear to have a significant effect on trough rilonacept concentrations. The effect of race could not be assessed because only Caucasian patients participated in the clinical study, reflecting the epidemiology of the disease.

13 NONCLINICAL TOXICOLOGY

13.1 Carcinogenesis, Mutagenesis, Impairment of Fertility

Long-term animal studies have not been performed to evaluate the carcinogenic potential of rilonacept. The mutagenic potential of rilonacept was not evaluated.

Male and female fertility was evaluated in a mouse surrogate model using a murine analog of rilonacept. Male mice were treated beginning 8 weeks prior to mating and continuing through female gestation day 15. Female mice were treated for 2 weeks prior to mating and on gestation days 0, 3, and 6. The murine analog of rilonacept did not alter either male or female fertility parameters at doses up to 200 mg/kg (this dose is approximately 6-fold higher than the 160 mg maintenance dose based on body surface area).

14 CLINICAL STUDIES

The safety and efficacy of ARCALYST for the treatment of CAPS was demonstrated in a randomized, double-blind, placebo-controlled study with two parts (A and B) conducted sequentially in the same patients with FCAS and MWS.

Part A was a 6-week, randomized, double-blind, parallel-group period comparing ARCALYST at a dose of 160 mg weekly after an initial loading dose of 320 mg to placebo. Part B followed immediately after Part A and consisted of a 9-week, patient-blind period during which all patients received ARCALYST 160 mg weekly, followed by a 9-week, double-blind, randomized withdrawal period in which patients were randomly assigned to either remain on ARCALYST 160 mg weekly or to receive placebo. Patients were then given the option to enroll in a 24-week, open-label treatment extension phase in which all patients were treated with ARCALYST 160 mg weekly.

Using a daily diary questionnaire, patients rated the following five signs and symptoms of CAPS: joint pain, rash, feeling of fever/chills, eye redness/pain, and fatigue, each on a scale of 0 (none, no severity) to 10 (very severe). The study evaluated the mean symptom score using the change from baseline to the end of treatment.

The changes in mean symptom scores for the randomized parallel-group period (Part A) and the randomized withdrawal period (Part B) of the study are shown in Table 2. ARCALYST-treated patients had a larger reduction in the mean symptom score in Part A compared to placebo-treated patients. In Part B, mean symptom scores increased more in patients withdrawn to placebo compared to patients who remained on ARCALYST.

[See table 2 above]

Daily mean symptom scores over time for Part A are shown in Figure 1.

Figure 1: Group Mean Daily Symptom Scores by Treatment Group in Part A and Single-blind ARCALYST Treatment Phase from Week -3 to Week 15

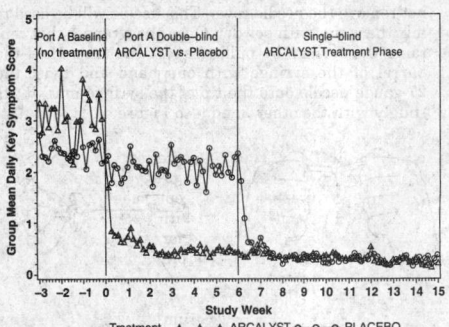

Improvement in symptom scores was noted within several days of initiation of ARCALYST therapy in most patients. In Part A, patients treated with ARCALYST experienced more improvement in each of the five components of the composite endpoint (joint pain, rash, feeling of fever/chills, eye redness/pain, and fatigue) than placebo-treated patients.

In Part A, a higher proportion of patients in the ARCALYST group experienced improvement from baseline in the composite score by at least 30% (96% vs. 29% of patients), by at least 50% (87% vs. 8%) and by at least 75% (70% vs. 0%) compared to the placebo group.

Table 2: Mean Symptom Scores

Part A	Placebo (n=24)	ARCALYST (n=23)	Part B	Placebo (n=23)	ARCALYST (n=22)
Pre-treatment Baseline Period (Weeks -3 to 0)	2.4	3.1	Active ARCALYST Baseline Period (Weeks 13 to 15)	0.2	0.3
Endpoint Period (Weeks 4 to 6)	2.1	0.5	Endpoint Period (Weeks 22 to 24)	1.2	0.4
LS* Mean Change from Baseline to Endpoint	-0.5	-2.4	LS* Mean Change from Baseline to Endpoint	0.9	0.1
95% confidence interval for difference between treatment groups	(-2.4, -1.3)**		95% confidence interval for difference between treatment groups	(-1.3, -0.4)**	

*Differences are adjusted using an analysis of covariance model with terms for treatment and Part A baseline.
** A confidence interval lying entirely below zero indicates a statistical difference favoring ARCALYST versus placebo.

Serum Amyloid A (SAA) and C-Reactive Protein (CRP) levels are acute phase reactants that are typically elevated in patients with CAPS with active disease. During Part A, mean levels of CRP decreased versus baseline for the ARCALYST treated patients, while there was no change for those on placebo (Table 3). ARCALYST also led to a decrease in SAA versus baseline to levels within the normal range.

Table 3. Mean Serum Amyloid A and C-Reactive Protein Levels Over Time in Part A

Part A	ARCALYST	Placebo
SAA (normal range: 0.7–6.4 mg/L)	(n=22)	(n=24)
Pre-treatment Baseline	60	110
Week 6	4	110
CRP (normal range: 0.0–8.4 mg/L)	(n= 21)	(n=24)
Pre-treatment Baseline	22	30
Week 6	2	28

During the open-label extension, reductions in mean symptom scores, serum CRP, and serum SAA levels were maintained for up to one year.

16 HOW SUPPLIED/STORAGE AND HANDLING

Each 20-mL glass vial of ARCALYST contains a sterile, white to off-white, preservative-free, lyophilized powder. ARCALYST is supplied in a carton containing four vials. (NDC 61755-001-01).

The lyophilized ARCALYST product is to be stored refrigerated at 2° to 8°C (36° to 46°F) inside the original carton to protect from light. Do not use beyond the date stamped on the label. After reconstitution, ARCALYST may be kept at room temperature, should be kept from light, and should be used within three hours of reconstitution. ARCALYST does not contain preservatives; therefore, unused portions of ARCALYST should be discarded. Discard the vial after a single withdrawal of drug.

17 PATIENT COUNSELING INFORMATION

See FDA-approved patient labeling.

The first injection of ARCALYST should be performed under the supervision of a qualified healthcare professional. If a patient or caregiver is to administer ARCALYST, he/she should be instructed on aseptic reconstitution of the lyophilized product and injection technique. The ability to inject subcutaneously should be assessed to ensure proper administration of ARCALYST, including rotation of injection sites. (*See Patient Information Leaflet for ARCALYST®*). ARCALYST should be reconstituted with preservative-free Sterile Water for Injection to be provided by the pharmacy. A puncture-resistant container for disposal of vials, needles and syringes should be used. Patients or caregivers should be instructed in proper vial, syringe, and needle disposal, and should be cautioned against reuse of these items.

Injection-site Reactions: Physicians should explain to patients that almost half of the patients in the clinical trials experienced a reaction at the injection site. Injection-site reactions may include pain, erythema, swelling, pruritis, bruising, mass, inflammation, dermatitis, edema, urticaria, vesicles, warmth, and hemorrhage. Patients should be cautioned to avoid injecting into an area that is already swollen or red. Any persistent reaction should be brought to the attention of the prescribing physician.

Infections: Patients should be cautioned that ARCALYST has been associated with serious, life-threatening infections, and not to initiate treatment with ARCALYST if they have a chronic or active infection. Patients should be counseled to contact their healthcare professional immediately if they develop an infection after starting ARCALYST. Treatment with ARCALYST should be discontinued if a patient develops a serious infection. Patients should be counseled not to take any IL-1 blocking drug, including ARCALYST, if they are also taking a drug that blocks TNF such as etanercept, infliximab, or adalimumab. Use of ARCALYST with other IL-1 blocking agents, such as anakinra, is not recommended.

Vaccinations: Prior to initiation of therapy with ARCALYST physicians should review with adult and pediatric patients their vaccination history relative to current medical guidelines for vaccine use, including taking into account the potential of increased risk of infection during treatment with ARCALYST.

REGENERON

Manufactured and distributed by:
Regeneron Pharmaceuticals, Inc.
777 Old Saw Mill River Road,
Tarrytown, NY 10591-6707, 1-877-REGN-777 (1-877-734-6777)
U.S. License Number 1760
NDC 61755-001-01

V3.0
Issue Date: 04/2010
Regeneron U.S. Patent 6,927,044 B2, 6,472,179 B2, 5,844,099 and other pending patents

PATIENT INFORMATION

ARCALYST® (ARK-a-list)
(rilonacept)
Injection for Subcutaneous Use

Read the patient information that comes with ARCALYST before you start taking it and each time you refill your prescription. There may be new information. The information in this leaflet does not take the place of talking with your healthcare provider about your medical condition and your treatment.

What is the most important information I should know about ARCALYST?

ARCALYST can affect your immune system. ARCALYST can lower the ability of your immune system to fight infections. Serious infections, including life-threatening infections and death have happened in patients taking ARCALYST. **Taking ARCALYST can make you more likely to get infections, including life-threatening serious infections, or may make any infection that you have worse.**

You should not begin treatment with ARCALYST if you have an infection or have infections that keep coming back (chronic infection).

After starting ARCALYST, if you get an infection, any sign of an infection including a fever, cough, flu-like symptoms, or have any open sores on your body, call your healthcare provider right away. **Treatment with ARCALYST should be stopped if you develop a serious infection.**

You should not take medicines that block Tumor Necrosis Factor (TNF), such as ENBREL® (etanercept), **Humira®** (adalimumab), **or Remicade®** (infliximab), **while you are taking ARCALYST. You should also not take other medicines that block Interleukin-1 (IL-1), such as Kineret®** (anakinra), **while taking ARCALYST. Taking ARCALYST with any of these medicines may increase your risk of getting a serious infection.**

Before starting treatment with ARCALYST, tell your healthcare provider if you:

- think you have an infection
- are being treated for an infection
- have signs of an infection, such as fever, cough, or flu-like symptoms
- have any open sores on your body
- have a history of infections that keep coming back
- have asthma. Patients with asthma may have an increased risk of infection.
- have diabetes or an immune system problem. People with these conditions have a higher chance for infections.
- have tuberculosis (TB), or if you have been in close contact with someone who has had tuberculosis.
- have or have had HIV, Hepatitis B, or Hepatitis C
- take other medicines that affect your immune system

Before you begin treatment with ARCALYST, talk with your healthcare provider about your vaccination history. Ask your healthcare provider whether you should receive any vaccinations, including pneumonia vaccine and flu vaccine, before you begin treatment with ARCALYST.

What is ARCALYST?

ARCALYST is a prescription medicine called an interleukin-1 (IL-1) blocker. ARCALYST is used to treat adults and children 12 years and older with Cryopyrin-Associated Periodic Syndromes (CAPS), including Familial Cold Auto-inflammatory Syndrome (FCAS) and Muckle Wells Syndrome (MWS). ARCALYST can help lessen the signs and symptoms of CAPS, such as rash, joint pain, fever, and tiredness, but it can also lead to serious side effects because of the effects on your immune system.

What should I tell my healthcare provider before taking ARCALYST?

ARCALYST may not be right for you. **Before taking ARCALYST, tell your healthcare provider about all of your medical conditions, including if you:**

- are scheduled to receive any vaccines. You should not receive live vaccines if you take ARCALYST.
- are pregnant or planning to become pregnant. It is not known if ARCALYST will harm your unborn child. Tell your healthcare provider right away if you become pregnant while taking ARCALYST.
- are breast-feeding or planning to breast-feed. It is not known if ARCALYST passes into your breast milk.

See "What is the most important information I should know about ARCALYST?"

Tell your healthcare provider about all the medicines you take, including prescription and non-prescription medicines, vitamins, and herbal supplements. Especially tell your healthcare provider if you take other medicines that affect your immune system, such as:

- other medicines that block IL-1, such as Kineret® (anakinra).
- medicines that block Tumor Necrosis Factor (TNF), such as ENBREL® (etanercept), Humira® (adalimumab), or Remicade® (infliximab).
- corticosteroids.

See "What is the most important information I should know about ARCALYST?"

Know the medicines you take. Keep a list of your medicines and show it to your healthcare provider and pharmacist every time you get a new prescription.

If you are not sure or have any questions about any of this information, ask your healthcare provider.

How should I take ARCALYST?

See the "Patient Instructions for Use" at the end of this leaflet.

- Take ARCALYST exactly as prescribed by your healthcare provider.
- ARCALYST is given by injection under the skin (subcutaneous injection) one time each week.
- Your healthcare provider will tell and show you or your caregiver:
  - how much ARCALYST to inject
  - how to prepare your dose
  - how to give the injection
- Do not try to give ARCALYST injections until you are sure that you or your caregiver understands how to prepare and inject your dose. Call your healthcare provider or pharmacist if you have any questions about preparing and injecting your dose, or if you or your caregiver would like more training.
- If you miss a dose of ARCALYST, inject it as soon as you remember, up to the day before your next scheduled dose. The next dose should be taken at the next regularly scheduled time. If you have any questions, contact your healthcare provider.
- If you accidentally take more ARCALYST than prescribed, call your healthcare provider.

What are the possible side effects of ARCALYST?

Serious side effects may occur while you are taking and after you finish taking ARCALYST including:

- **Serious Infections. See "What is the most important information I should know about taking ARCALYST?"** Treatment with ARCALYST should be discontinued if you develop a serious infection.

- **Allergic Reaction.** Call your healthcare provider or seek emergency care right away if you get any of the following symptoms of an allergic reaction while taking ARCALYST:
  - rash
  - swollen face
  - trouble breathing

Common side effects with ARCALYST include:

- **Injection-site reaction.** This includes: pain, redness, swelling, itching, bruising, lumps, inflammation, skin rash, blisters, warmth, and bleeding at the injection site.
- **Upper respiratory infection.**
- **Changes in your blood cholesterol and triglycerides (lipids).** Your healthcare provider will check you for this.

These are not all the possible side effects of ARCALYST. Tell your healthcare provider about any side effects that bother you or that do not go away. For more information ask your healthcare provider or pharmacist. Call your doctor for medical advice about side effects. You may report side effects to FDA at 1-800-FDA-1088.

How should I store ARCALYST?

- Keep ARCALYST in the carton it comes in.
- Store ARCALYST in a refrigerator between 36°F to 46°F (2°C to 8°C). Call your pharmacy if you have any questions.
- Always keep ARCALYST away from light.
- Refrigerated ARCALYST can be used until the expiration date printed on the vial and carton.
- ARCALYST may be kept at room temperature after mixing. ARCALYST should be used within **three hours** of mixing. Keep ARCALYST away from light.
- If you need to take ARCALYST with you when traveling, store the carton in a cool carrier with a cold pack and protect it from light.

Keep ARCALYST, injection supplies, and all other medicines out of reach of children.

What are the ingredients in ARCALYST?

Active ingredient: rilonacept.

Inactive ingredients: histidine, arginine, polyethylene glycol 3350, sucrose, and glycine.

General information about ARCALYST

Medicines are sometimes prescribed for conditions other than those listed in patient information leaflets. Do not use ARCALYST for a condition for which it was not prescribed. Do not give ARCALYST to other people even if they have the same condition. It may harm them.

This leaflet summarizes the most important information about ARCALYST. If you would like more information, speak with your healthcare provider. You can ask your healthcare provider or pharmacist for information about ARCALYST that was written for healthcare professionals. For more information about ARCALYST, call 1-877-REGN-777 (1-877-734-6777), or visit www.ARCALYST.com.

Patient instructions for use

It is important for you to read, understand and follow the instructions below exactly. Following the instructions correctly will help to make sure that you use, prepare, and inject the medicine the right way to prevent infection.

How do I prepare and give an injection of ARCALYST?

STEP 1: Setting up for an injection

1. Choose a table or other flat surface area to set up the supplies for your injection. Be sure that the area is clean or clean it with an antiseptic or soap and water first.
2. Wash your hands well with soap and water, and dry with a clean towel.
3. Put the following items on a table, or other flat surface, for each injection (see Figure 1):

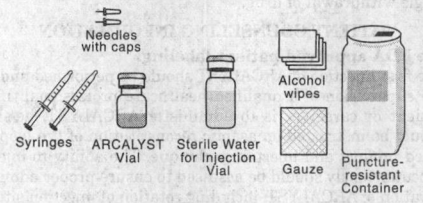

Figure 1

- 2 sterile, 3-milliliter (mL) disposable syringes with markings at each 0.1 mL (see Figure 2):
  - one needed for mixing (reconstitution) ARCALYST
  - one needed for injection

[See figure 2 at top of next column]

- 2 sterile disposable needles (27-gauge ½ inches):
  - one needed for mixing
  - one needed for injection
- 4 alcohol wipes
- 1 2×2 gauze pad
- 1 vial of ARCALYST (powder in vial)
- 1 vial of preservative-free Sterile Water for Injection
- 1 puncture-resistant container for disposal of used needles, syringes, and vials

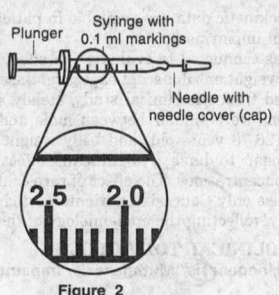

Figure 2

Note:

- Do not use Sterile Water for Injection, syringes or needles other than those provided by your pharmacy. Contact your pharmacy if you need replacement syringes or needles.
- Do not to touch the needles or the rubber stoppers on the vials with your hands. If you do touch a stopper, clean it with a fresh alcohol wipe.
- If you touch a needle or the needle touches any surface, throw away the entire syringe into the puncture-resistant container and start over with a new syringe.
- **Do not reuse needles or syringes.**
- To protect yourself and others from possible needle sticks, it is very important to throw away every syringe, with the needle attached, in the puncture-proof container right after use. *Do not try to recap the needle.*

STEP 2: Preparing vials

1. Check the expiration date on the carton of ARCALYST. Do not use the vial if the expiration date has passed. Contact your pharmacy for assistance.
2. Check the expiration date on the vial of Sterile Water for Injection. Do not use the vial if the expiration date has passed. Contact your pharmacy for assistance.
3. Remove the protective plastic cap from both vials.
4. Clean the top of each vial with an alcohol wipe. Use one wipe for each vial and wipe in one direction around the top of the vial (see Figure 3).

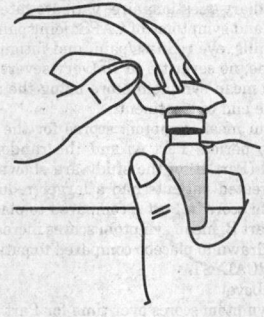

Figure 3

5. Open the wrapper that contains the 27-gauge needle by pulling apart the tabs and set it aside for later use. Do not remove the needle cover. This needle will be used to mix the water with powder. Open the wrapper that contains the syringe by pulling apart the tabs. Hold the barrel of the syringe with one hand and twist the 27-gauge needle onto the tip of the syringe until it fits snugly with the other hand (see Figure 4).

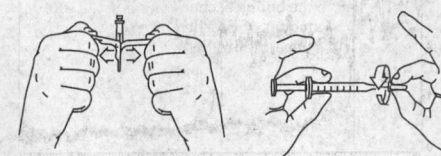

Figure 4

6. Hold the syringe at eye level. With the needle covered pull back the plunger to the 2.3 mL mark, filling the syringe with air (see Figure 5).

[See figure 5 at top of next page]

7. Hold the syringe in one hand, use the other hand to pull the needle cover straight off. Do not twist the needle as you pull off the cover. Place the needle cover aside. Hold the syringe in the hand that you will use to mix (reconstitute) your medicine. Hold the Sterile Water on a firm surface with your other hand. Slowly insert the needle straight through the rubber stopper. Do not bend

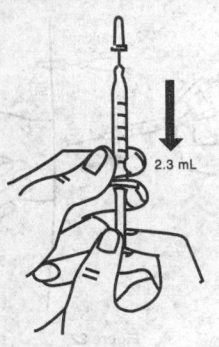

Figure 5

the needle. Push the plunger in all the way to push the air into the vial (see Figure 6).

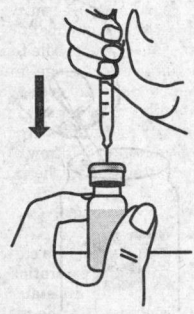

Figure 6

8. Hold the vial in one hand and the syringe in the other hand and carefully turn the vial upside down so that the needle is pointing straight up.
9. Make sure the tip of the needle is covered by the liquid and slowly pull back on the plunger to the 2.3 mL mark to withdraw the Sterile Water from the vial (see Figure 7).

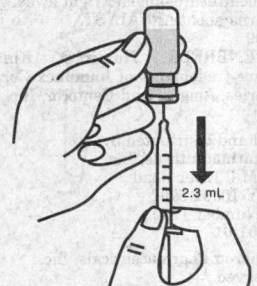

Figure 7

10. Keep the vial upside down and tap or flick the syringe with your fingers until any air bubbles rise to the top of the syringe.
11. To remove the air bubbles, gently push in the plunger so only the air is pushed out of the syringe and back into the bottle.
12. After removing the bubbles, check the syringe to be sure that the right amount of Sterile Water has been drawn into the syringe (see Figure 8).

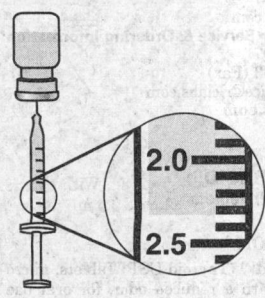

Figure 8

13. Carefully remove the syringe with needle from the Sterile Water vial. Do not touch the needle.

STEP 3: Mixing (reconstituting) ARCALYST

1. With one hand, hold the ARCALYST vial on a firm surface.
2. With the other hand, take the syringe with the Sterile Water and the same needle, and slowly insert the needle straight down through the rubber stopper of the ARCALYST vial. Push the plunger in all the way to inject the Sterile Water into the vial.
3. Direct the water stream to gently go down the side of the vial into the powder (see Figure 9).

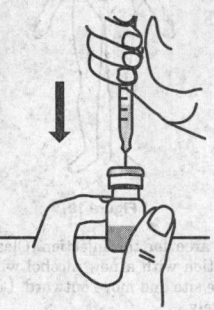

Figure 9

4. Remove the syringe and needle from the stopper and throw away the needle, syringe, and Sterile Water vial in the puncture-resistant container. Do not try to put the needle cover back on the needle.
5. Hold the vial containing the ARCALYST and sterile water for injection sideways (not upright) with your thumb and a finger at the top and bottom of the vial, and quickly shake the vial back and forth (side-to-side) for about 1 minute (see Figure 10).

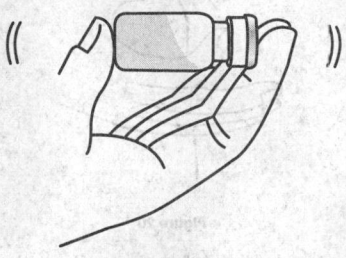

Figure 10

6. Put the vial back on the table and let the vial sit for about 1 minute.
7. Look at the vial for any particles or clumps of powder which have not dissolved.
8. If the powder has not completely dissolved, shake the vial quickly back and forth for 30 seconds more. Let the vial sit for about 1 minute.
9. Repeat Step 8 until the powder is completely dissolved and the solution is clear.
10. The mixed ARCALYST should be thick, clear, and colorless to pale yellow. Do not use the mixed liquid if it is discolored or cloudy, or if small particles are in it (see Figure 11).
    NOTE: Contact your pharmacy to report any mixed ARCALYST that is discolored or contains particles.

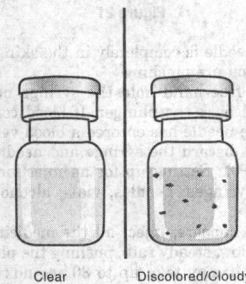

Clear   Discolored/Cloudy

Figure 11

11. ARCALYST may be kept at room temperature after mixing. ARCALYST should be used within **three hours** of mixing. Keep ARCALYST away from light.

STEP 4: Preparing the injection

1. Hold the ARCALYST vial on a firm surface and wipe the top of the ARCALYST vial with a new alcohol wipe (see Figure 12).

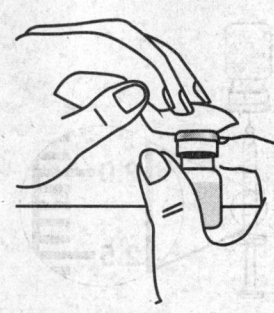

Figure 12

2. Take a new sterile, disposable needle and attach securely to a new syringe without removing the needle cover (see Figure 13).

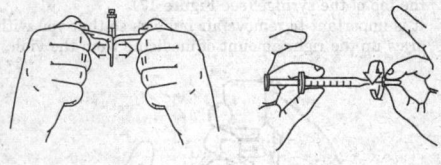

Figure 13

3. The amount of air you draw into the syringe should equal the amount of mixed ARCALYST that your healthcare provider has prescribed for you to inject.
4. To draw air into the syringe, hold the syringe at eye level. Do not remove the needle cover. Pull back the plunger on the syringe to the mark that is equal to the amount of mixed ARCALYST that your healthcare provider has prescribed for you to inject (see Figure 14).

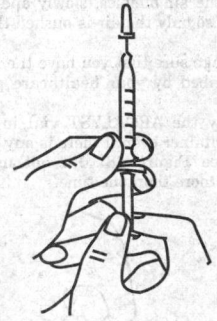

Figure 14

5. Remove the needle cover and be careful not to touch the needle. Keep the ARCALYST vial on a flat surface and slowly insert the needle straight down through the stopper. Push the plunger down and inject all the air into the vial (see Figure 15).

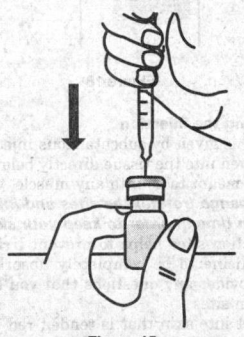

Figure 15

6. Hold the vial in one hand and the syringe in the other hand and carefully turn the vial upside down so that the needle is pointing straight up. Hold the vial at eye level.

7. Keep the tip of the needle in the liquid and slowly pull back on the plunger to the mark on the syringe that matches the amount of medicine prescribed by your healthcare provider (see Figure 16).

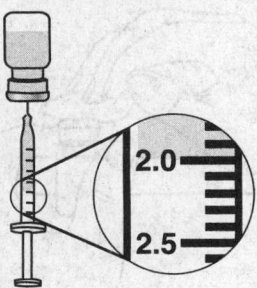

Figure 16

NOTE: The maximum adult dose of ARCALYST is 2 mL.

8. Keep the vial upside down with the needle straight up, and gently tap the syringe until any air bubbles rise to the top of the syringe (see Figure 17).
It is important to remove air bubbles so that you withdraw up the right amount of medicine from the vial.

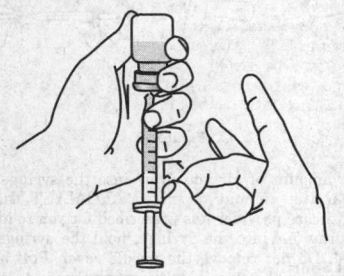

Figure 17

9. To remove the air bubbles, slowly and gently push in the plunger so only the air is pushed through the needle.
10. Check to make sure that you have the amount of medicine prescribed by your healthcare provider in the syringe.
11. Throw away the ARCALYST vial in the puncture-resistant container even if there is any medicine left in the vial (see Figure 18). Do not use any vial of ARCALYST more than one time.

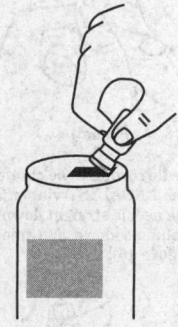

Figure 18

STEP 5: Giving the injection

1. ARCALYST is given by subcutaneous injection, an injection that is given into the tissue directly below the layers of skin. It is not meant to go into any muscle, vein, or artery. *You should change (rotate) the sites and inject in a different place each time in order to keep your skin healthy.* Rotating injection sites helps to prevent irritation and allows the medicine to be completely absorbed. Ask your healthcare provider any questions that you have about rotating injection sites.

• Do not inject into skin that is tender, red, or hard. If an area is tender or feels hardened, choose another site for injection until the tenderness or "hardening" goes away.
• Tell your healthcare provider about any skin reactions including redness, swelling, or hardening of the skin.
• Areas where you may inject ARCALYST include the left and right sides of the abdomen, and left and right thighs.

If someone else is giving the injection, the upper left and right arms may also be used for injection (see Figure 19): *(Do not inject within a 2-inch area around the navel)*

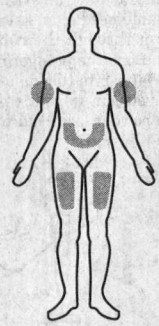

Figure 19

2. Choose the area for the injection. Clean the area in a circular motion with a new alcohol wipe. Begin at the center of the site and move outward. Let the alcohol air dry completely.
3. Take the cover off the needle and be careful not to touch the needle.
4. Hold the syringe in one hand like you would hold a pencil.
5. With the other hand gently pinch a fold of skin at the cleaned site for injection (see Figure 20).

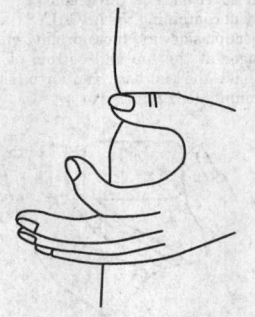

Figure 20

6. Use a quick "dartlike" motion to insert the needle straight into the skin (90 degree angle) (see Figure 21). Do not push down on the plunger while inserting the needle into the skin.
For small children or persons with little fat under the skin, you may need to hold the syringe and needle at a 45 degree angle (see Figure 21).

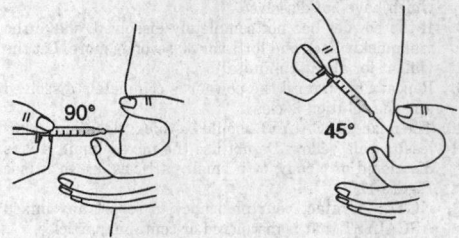

Figure 21

7. After the needle is completely in the skin, let go of the skin that you are pinching.
8. With your free hand hold the syringe near its base. Gently pull back the plunger. If blood comes into the syringe, the needle has entered a blood vessel. Remove the needle, discard the syringe and needle. Start over with "STEP 1: Setting up for an injection" using new supplies (syringes, needles, vials, alcohol swabs and gauze pad).
9. If no blood appears, inject all the medicine in the syringe at a slow, steady rate, pushing the plunger all the way down. It may take up to 30 seconds to inject the entire dose.
10. Pull the needle out of the skin, and hold a piece of sterile gauze over the injection site for several seconds (see Figure 22).
[See figure 22 at top of next column]
11. Do not replace the needle cover. Throw away the vials, used syringes and needles in the puncture-resistant

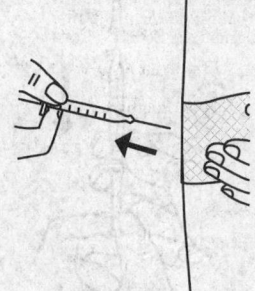

Figure 22

container (see Figure 23). Do not recycle the container. DO NOT throw away vials, needles, or syringes in the household trash or recycle.

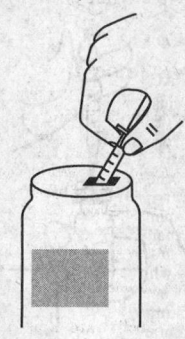

Figure 23

12. Keep the puncture-resistant container out of reach of children. When the container is about two-thirds full, dispose of it as instructed by your healthcare provider. Follow any special state or local laws about the right way to throw away needles and syringes.
13. Used alcohol wipes can be thrown away in the household trash.

Contact your healthcare provider right away with any questions or concerns about ARCALYST.

Issued 04/2009

Notes: 1. ENBREL®, Humira®, Kineret®, and Remicade®, are trademarks of Immunex Corporation, Abbott Laboratories, Amgen, and Centocor, Inc., respectively.

REGENERON

Manufactured and distributed by:
Regeneron Pharmaceuticals, Inc.
777 Old Saw Mill River Road
Tarrytown, NY 10591-6707
U.S. License Number 1760
NDC 61755-001-01

© 2008, Regeneron Pharmaceuticals, Inc.
All rights reserved.
V2.0
Issue Date: 04/24/2009
Regeneron U.S. Patents 6,927,044 B2, 6,472,179 B2, 5,844,099 and other pending patents
Shown in Product Identification Guide, page 317

RLC Labs, Inc.
CAVE CREEK, AZ 85331

For Product Information:
(877) 797-7997
sales@rlclabs.com
For Customer Service & Ordering Information:
(877) 797-7997
(623) 879-8683 (Fax)
customerservice@rlclabs.com
www.rlclabs.com

NATURE-THROID™   ℞
(Thyroid USP) Tablets

DESCRIPTION

Nature-Throid™ (Thyroid USP) Tablets, micro-coated, easy to swallow with a reduced odor, for oral use are natural preparations derived from porcine thyroid glands (T3 liothyronine is approximately four times as potent as T4 levothyroxine on a microgram for microgram basis). They provide 38 mcg levothyroxine (T4) and 9 mcg liothyronine (T3) for each 65 mg (1 Grain) of the labeled content of thyroid.

INACTIVE INGREDIENTS
Colloidal Silicon Dioxide, Dicalcium Phosphate, Lactose Monohydrate*, Magnesium Stearate, Microcrystalline Cellulose, Croscarmellose Sodium, Stearic Acid, Opadry II 85F19316 Clear.
*Present in traceable amount as part of Thyroid USP (diluent)
The structural formulas of liothyronine (T3) and levothyroxine (T4) are as follows:

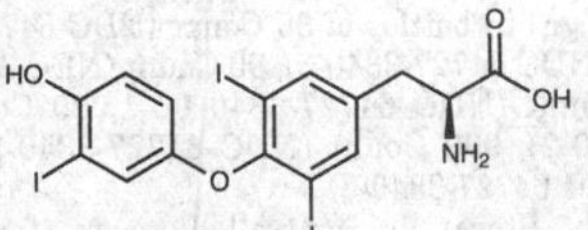

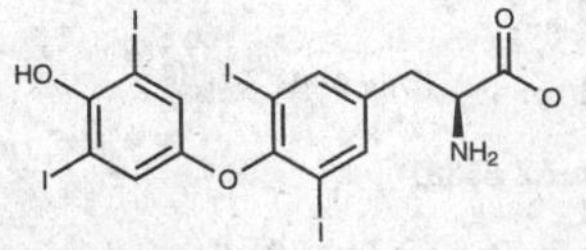

CLINICAL PHARMACOLOGY

The steps in the synthesis of the thyroid hormones are controlled by thyrotropin (Thyroid Stimulating Hormone, TSH) secreted by the anterior pituitary. This hormone's secretion is in turn controlled by a feedback mechanism affected by the thyroid hormones themselves and by thyrotropin releasing hormone (TRH), a tripeptide of hypothalamic origin. Endogenous thyroid hormone secretion is suppressed when exogenous thyroid hormones are administered to euthyroid individuals in excess of the normal gland's secretion.
The mechanisms by which thyroid hormones exert their physiologic action are not well understood. These hormones enhance oxygen consumption by most tissues of the body, increase the basal metabolic rate, and the metabolism of carbohydrates, lipids, and proteins. Thus, they exert a profound influence on every organ system in the body and are of particular importance in the development of the central nervous system.
The normal thyroid gland contains approximately 200 mcg of levothyroxine (T4) per gram of gland, and 15 mcg of liothyronine (T3) per gram. The ratio of these two hormones in the circulation does not represent the ratio in the thyroid gland, since about 80 percent of peripheral liothyronine (T3) comes from monodeiodination of levothyroxine (T4). Peripheral monodeiodination of levothyroxine (T4) at the 5 position (inner ring) also results in the formation of reverse liothyronine (T3), which is calorigenically inactive. Liothyronine (T3) levels are low in the fetus and newborn, in old age, in chronic caloric deprivation, hepatic cirrhosis, renal failure, surgical stress, and chronic illnesses representing what has been called the "T3 thyronine syndrome".

Pharmacokinetics
Animal studies have shown that levothyroxine (T4) is only partially absorbed from the gastrointestinal tract. The degree of absorption is dependent on the vehicle used for its administration and by the character of the intestinal contents, the intestinal flora, including plasma protein, and soluble dietary factors, all of which bind thyroid, thereby making it unavailable for diffusion. Only 41 percent is absorbed when given in a gelatin capsule, as opposed to 74 percent absorption when given with an albumin carrier.
Depending on other factors, absorption has varied from 48 to 79 percent of the administered dose. Fasting increases absorption. Malabsorption syndromes, as well as dietary factors, (children's soybean formula, concomitant use of anionic exchange resins such as cholestyramine) cause excessive fecal loss. Liothyronine (T3) is almost totally absorbed, 95 percent in 4 hours. The hormones contained in the natural preparations are absorbed in a manner similar to the synthetic hormones.
More than 99 percent of circulating hormones are bound to serum proteins, including thyroid-binding globulin (TBg), thyroid-binding pre-albumin (TBPA), and albumin (TBa), whose capacities and affinities vary for the hormones. The higher affinity of levothyroxine (T4) for both TBg and TBPA, as compared to liothyronine (T3), partially explains the higher serum levels and longer half-life of the former hormone. Both protein-bound hormones exist in reverse equilibrium with minute amounts of free hormone, the latter accounting for the metabolic activity. Deiodination of levothyroxine (T4) occurs at a number of sites, including liver, kidney, and other tissues. The conjugated hormone, in the form of glucuronide or sulfate, is found in the bile and gut where it may complete an enterohepatic circulation. Eighty-five percent of levothyroxine (T4) metabolized daily is deiodinated.

INDICATIONS AND USAGE

1. As replacement of supplemental therapy in patients with hypothyroidism of any etiology, except transient hypothyroidism during the recovery phase of subacute thyroiditis. This category includes cretinism, myxedema, and ordinary hypothyroidism in patients of any age (children, adults, the elderly), or state (including pregnancy); primary hypothyroidism resulting from functional deficiency, primary atrophy, partial or total absence of thyroid gland, or the effects of surgery, radiation, or drugs, with or without the presence of goiter; and secondary (pituitary), or tertiary (hypothalamic) hypothyroidism (See WARNINGS).
2. As pituitary TSH suppressants, in the treatment or prevention of various types of euthyroid goiters, including thyroid nodules, subacute, or chronic lymphocytic thyroiditis (Hashimoto's), multinodular goiter, and in the management of thyroid cancer.
3. As diagnostic agents in suppression tests to differentiate suspected mild hyperthyroidism or thyroid gland anatomy.

CONTRAINDICATIONS

Thyroid hormone preparations are generally contraindicated in patients with diagnosed, but as yet, uncorrected adrenal cortical insufficiency, untreated thyrotoxicosis, and apparent hypersensitivity to any of their active or extraneous constituents. There is no well documented evidence in the literature of true allergic or idiosyncratic reactions to thyroid hormone.

WARNINGS

Drugs with thyroid hormone activity, alone or together with other therapeutic agents, have been used for the treatment of obesity. In euthyroid patients, doses within the range of daily hormonal requirements are ineffective for weight reduction. Larger doses may produce serious or even life-threatening manifestations of toxicity, particularly when given in association with sympathomimetic amines such as those used for their anorectic effects.
The use of thyroid hormones in the therapy of obesity, alone or combined with other drugs, is unjustified and has been shown to be ineffective. Neither is their use justified for the treatment of male or female infertility unless this condition is accompanied by hypothyroidism.

PRECAUTIONS

General: Thyroid hormones should be used with great caution in a number of circumstances where the integrity of the cardiovascular system, particularly the coronary arteries, is suspected. These include patients with angina pectoris or the elderly, whom have a greater likelihood of occult cardiac disease. With these patients, therapy should be initiated with low doses, i.e. 16.25 - 32.5 mg. When, in such patients, a euthyroid state can only be reached at the expense of an aggravation of the cardiovascular disease, thyroid hormone dosage should be reduced.
Thyroid hormone therapy in patients with concomitant diabetes mellitus or diabetes insipidus or adrenal cortical insufficiency aggravates the intensity of their symptoms. Appropriate adjustments of the various therapeutic measures directed at these concomitant endocrine diseases are required. The therapy of myxedema coma requires simultaneous administration of glucorticoids (See DOSAGE AND ADMINISTRATION).
Hypothyroidism decreases and hyperthyroidism increases the sensitivity to oral anticoagulants. Prothrombin time should be closely monitored in thyroid treated patients on oral anticoagulants and dosage of the latter agents should be adjusted on the basis of frequent prothrombin time determinations. In infants, excessive doses of thyroid hormone preparations may produce craniosynostosis.
Information for the Patient: Patients on thyroid hormone preparations and parents of children on thyroid therapy should be informed that:
1. Replacement therapy is to be taken essentially for life, with the exception of cases of transient hypothyroidism, usually associated with thyroiditis, and in those patients receiving a therapeutic trial of the drug.
2. They should immediately report, during the course of therapy, any signs or symptoms of thyroid hormone toxicity, e.g., chest pain, increased pulse rate, palpitations, excessive sweating, heat intolerance, nervousness, or any other unusual event.
3. In case of concomitant diabetes mellitus, the daily dosage of antidiabetic medication may need readjustment as thyroid hormone replacement is achieved. If thyroid medication is stopped, a downward readjustment of the dosage of insulin or oral hypoglycemic agent may be necessary to avoid hypoglycemia. At all times, close monitoring of urinary glucose levels is mandatory in such patients.
4. In case of concomitant oral anticoagulant therapy, the prothrombin time should be measured frequently to determine if the dosage of oral anticoagulants is to be readjusted.
5. Partial loss of hair may be experienced by children in the first few months of thyroid therapy, but this is usually a transient phenomenon and later recovery is usually the rule.
Laboratory Tests: Treatment of patients with thyroid hormones requires the periodic assessment of thyroid status by means of appropriate laboratory tests, besides the full clinical evaluation. The TSH suppression test can be used to test the effectiveness of any thyroid preparation, bearing in mind the relative insensitivity of the infant pituitary to the negative feedback effect of thyroid hormones. SerumT4 levels can be used to test the effectiveness of all thyroid medications except T3. When the total serum T4 is low but TSH is normal, a test specific to assess unbound (free) T4 levels is warranted. Specific measurements of T4 and T3 by competitive protein binding or radioimmunoassay are not influenced by blood levels of organic or inorganic iodine.
Drug Interactions: Oral Anticoagulants—Thyroid hormones appear to increase catabolism of vitamin K-dependent clotting factors. If oral anticoagulants are also being given, compensatory increases in clotting factor synthesis are impaired. Patients stabilized on oral anticoagulants that are found to require thyroid replacement therapy should be watched very closely when thyroid is started. If a patient is truly hypothyroid, it is likely that a reduction in anticoagulant dosage will be required. No special precautions appear to be necessary when oral anticoagulant therapy is begun in a patient already stabilized on maintenance thyroid replacement therapy.
Insulin or Oral Hypoglycemic—Initiating thyroid replacement therapy may cause increases in insulin or oral hypoglycemic requirements. The effects seen are poorly understood and depend upon a variety of factors such as dose and type of thyroid preparations and endocrine status of the patient. Patients receiving insulin or oral hypoglycemic should be closely watched during initiation of thyroid replacement therapy.
Cholestyramine or Colestipol—Cholestyramine or Colestipol binds both levothyroxine (T4) and liothyronine (T3) in the intestine, thus impairing absorption of these thyroid hormones. In vitro studies indicate that the binding is not easily removed. Therefore, four to five hours should elapse between administration of Cholestyramine or Colestipol and thyroid hormones.
Estrogen, Oral Contraceptives—Estrogens tend to increase serum thyroxine-binding globulin (TBg). In a patient with a nonfunctioning thyroid gland who is receiving thyroid replacement therapy, free levothyroxine (T4) may be decreased when estrogens are started thus increasing thyroid requirements. However, if the patient's thyroid gland has sufficient function, the decreased free levothyroxine (T4) will result in a compensatory increase in levothyroxine (T4) output by the thyroid. Therefore, patients without a functioning thyroid gland who are on thyroid replacement therapy, may need to increase their thyroid dose if estrogens or estrogen-containing oral contraceptives are given.
Drug/Laboratory Test Interactions: The following drugs or moieties are known to interfere with laboratory tests performed in patients on thyroid hormone therapy: androgens, corticosteroids, estrogens, oral contraceptives containing estrogens, iodine-containing preparations, and the numerous preparations containing salicylates.
1. Changes in TBg concentration should be taken into consideration in the interpretation of levothyroxine (T4) and liothyronine (T3) values. In such cases, the unbound (free) hormone should be measured. Pregnancy, estrogens, and estrogen-containing oral contraceptives increase TBg concentrations. TBg may also be increased during infectious hepatitis. Decreases in TBg concentrations are observed in nephrosis, acromegaly, and after androgen or corticosteroid therapy. Familial hyper or hypothyroxine-binding-globulinemias have been described. The incidence of TBg deficiency approximates 1 in 9,000. The binding of levothyroxine by TBPA is inhibited by salicylates.
2. Medicinal or dietary iodine interferes with all in vivo tests of radio-iodine uptake, producing low uptakes which may not be relative of a true decrease in hormone synthesis.
3. The persistence of clinical and laboratory evidence of hypothyroidism in spite of adequate dosage replacement indicates; either poor patient compliance, poor absorption, excessive fecal loss, or inactivity of the preparation. Intracellular resistance to thyroid hormone is quite rare.
Carcinogenesis, Mutagenesis, and Impairment of Fertility: A reportedly apparent association between prolonged thyroid therapy and breast cancer has not been confirmed and patients on thyroid for established indications should not discontinue therapy. No confirmatory long-term studies in animals have been performed to evaluate carcinogenic potential, mutagenicity, or impairment of fertility in either males or females.
Pregnancy-Category A: Thyroid hormones do not readily cross the placental barrier. The clinical experience to date does not indicate any adverse effect on fetuses when thyroid hormones are administered to pregnant women. On the basis of current knowledge, thyroid replacement therapy to hypothyroid women should not be discontinued during pregnancy.
Nursing Mothers: Minimal amounts of thyroid hormones are excreted in human milk. Thyroid is not associated with serious adverse reactions and does not have a known

tumorigenic potential. However, caution should be exercised when thyroid is administered to a nursing woman.

Pediatric Use: Pregnant mothers provide little or no thyroid hormone to the fetus. The incidence of congenital hypothyroidism is relatively high (1:4,000) and the hypothyroid fetus would not derive any benefit from the small amounts of hormone crossing the placental barrier. Routine determination of serumT4 and/or TSH is strongly advised in neonates in view of the deleterious effects of thyroid deficiency on growth and development. Treatment should be initiated immediately upon diagnosis, and maintained for life, unless transient hypothyroidism is suspected; in which case, therapy may be interrupted for 2 to 8 weeks after the age of 3 years to reassess the condition. Cessation of therapy is justified in patients who have maintained a normal TSH during those 2 to 8 weeks.

Geriatric use: Clinical studies of Thyroid Tablets, USP did not include sufficient numbers of subjects aged 65 and over to determine whether they respond differently from younger subjects. Other reported clinical experience has not identified differences in responses between the elderly and younger patients. In general, dose selection for an elderly patient should be cautious, usually starting at the low end of the dosing range, reflecting the greater frequency of decreased hepatic, renal, or cardiac function, and of concomitant disease or other drug therapy.

ADVERSE REACTIONS

Adverse reactions other than those indicative of hyperthyroidism because of therapeutic overdosage, either initially or during the maintenance period, are rare (See OVERDOSAGE).

OVERDOSAGE

Signs and Symptoms: Excessive doses of thyroid result in a hypermetabolic state resembling in every respect the condition of endogenous origin. The condition may be self induced.

Treatment of Overdosage: Dosage should be reduced or therapy temporarily discontinued signs and symptoms of overdosage appear.

Treatment may be reinstituted at a lower dosage. In normal individuals, normal hypothalamic-pituitary-thyroid axis function is restored in 6 to 8 weeks after thyroid suppression.

Treatment of acute massive thyroid hormone overdosage is aimed at reducing gastrointestinal absorption of the drugs and counteracting central and peripheral effects, mainly those of increased sympathetic activity. Vomiting may be induced initially if further gastrointestinal absorption can reasonably be prevented and barring contraindications such as coma, convulsions, or loss of the gagging reflex. Treatment is symptomatic and supportive. Oxygen may be administered and ventilation maintained. Cardiac glycosides may be indicated if congestive heart failure develops. Measures to control fever, hypoglycemia, or fluid loss should be instituted if needed. Antiadrenergic agents, particularly propranolol, have been used advantageously in the treatment of increased sympathetic activity. Propranolol may be administered intravenously at a dosage of 1 to 3 mg, over a 10 minute period or orally, 80 to 160 mg/day, initially, especially when no contraindications exist for its use.

DOSAGE AND ADMINISTRATION

The dosage of thyroid hormones is determined by the indication and must in every case be individualized according to patient response and laboratory findings.

Thyroid hormones are given orally. In acute, emergency conditions, injectable levothyroxine sodium (T4) may be given intravenously when oral administration is not feasible or desirable (as in the treatment of myxedema coma, or during parenteral nutrition). Intramuscular administration is not advisable because of reported poor absorption.

Hypothyroidism: Therapy is usually instituted using low doses, with increments which depend on the cardiovascular status of the patient. The usual starting dose is 32.5 mg, with increment of 16.25 mg every 2 to 3 weeks. A lower starting dosage, 16.25 mg/day, is recommended in patients with longstanding myxedema, particularly if cardiovascular impairment is suspected, in which case extreme caution is recommended. The appearance of angina is an indication for reduction in dosage. Most patients require 65 - 130 mg/day. Failure to respond to doses of 195 mg suggests lack of compliance or malabsorption. Maintenance dosages 65 - 130 mg/day usually result in normal serum T4 and T3 levels. Adequate therapy usually results in normal TSH and T4 levels after 2 or 3 weeks of therapy.

Readjustment of thyroid hormone dosage should be made within the first four weeks of therapy, after proper clinical and laboratory evaluations, including serum levels of T4, bound and free, and TSH.

Liothyronine (T3) may be used in preference to levothyroxine (T4) during radio-isotope scanning procedures, since induction of hypothyroidism in those cases is more abrupt and can be of shorter duration. It may also be preferred when impairment of peripheral conversion of levothyroxine (T4) and liothyronine (T3) is suspected.

Myxedema Coma: Myxedema coma is usually precipitated in the hypothyroid patient of longstanding by intercurrent illness or drugs such as sedatives and anesthetics and should be considered a medical emergency. Therapy should be directed at the correction of electrolyte disturbances and possible infection, besides the administration of thyroid hormones. Corticosteroids should be administered routinely. Levothyroxine (T4) and Liothyronine (T3) may be administered via a nasogastric tube, but the preferred route of administration of both hormones is intravenous. Levothyroxine sodium (T4) is given at a starting dose of 400 mcg (100 mcg/mL) given rapidly, and is usually well tolerated, even in the elderly. This initial dose is followed by daily supplements of 100 to 200 mcg given IV. Normal T4 levels are achieved in 24 hours, followed in 3 days by threefold elevation of T3. Oral therapy with thyroid hormone would be resumed as soon as the clinical situation has been stabilized and the patient is able to take oral medication.

Thyroid Cancer: Exogenous thyroid hormone may produce regression of metastases from follicular and papillary carcinoma of the thyroid and is used as ancillary therapy of these conditions with radioactive iodine. TSH should be suppressed to low or undetectable levels. Therefore, larger amounts of thyroid hormone than those used for replacement therapy are required. Medullary carcinoma of the thyroid is usually unresponsive to this therapy.

Thyroid Suppression Therapy: Administration of thyroid hormone in doses higher than those produced physiologically by the gland results in suppression of the production of endogenous hormone. This is the basis for the thyroid suppression test and is used as an aid in the diagnosis of patients with signs of mild hyperthyroidism, in whom base line laboratory tests appear normal, or to demonstrate thyroid gland autonomy in patients with Grave's ophthalmopathy. 1 uptake is determined before and after the administration of the exogenous hormone. A fifty percent or greater suppression of uptake indicates a normal thyroid pituitary axis, and thus rules out thyroid gland autonomy.

For adults, the usual suppressive dose of levothyroxine (T4) is 1.56 mg/kg of body weight per day given for 7 to 10 days. These doses usually yield normal serum T4 and T3 levels and lack of response to TSH.

Thyroid hormones should be administered cautiously to patients in whom there is strong suspicion of thyroid gland autonomy, in view of the fact that the exogenous hormone effects will be additive to the endogenous source.

Pediatric Dosage: Pediatric dosage should follow the recommendations summarized in Table 1. In infants with congenital hypothyroidism, therapy with full doses should be instituted as soon as the diagnosis has been made.

TABLE 1. Recommended Pediatric Dosage for Congenital Hypothyroidism

Age	Dose per day	Daily dose per kg of body weight
0 - 6 months	16.25 - 32.5 mg	4.8-6.0 mg
6 - 12 months	32.5 - 48.75 mg	3.6-4.8 mg
1 - 5 years	48.75 - 65 mg	3.3-6.0 mg
6 - 12 years	65 - 97.5 mg	2.4-3.0 mg
Over 12 years	Over 97.5 mg	1.2-1.8 mg

HOW SUPPLIED

Nature-Throid™ (Thyroid USP) Tablets are supplied as follows:

16.25 mg. (1/4 gr.) in bottles of 30 Count (NDC 64727-3298-4), 60 Count (NDC 64727-3298-5), 90 Count (NDC 64727-3298-6), 100 Count (NDC 64727-3298-1), 1,000 Count (NDC 64727-3298-2), 990 Count (NDC 64727-3298-3) & 1,008 Count (NDC 64727-3298-8)

32.5 mg. (1/2 gr.) in bottles of 30 Count (NDC 64727-3299-4), 60 Count (NDC 64727-3299-5), 90 Count (NDC 64727-3299-6), 100 Count (NDC 64727-3299-1), 1,000 Count (NDC 64727-3299-2), 990 Count (NDC 64727-3299-3) & 1,008 Count (NDC 64727-3299-8)

65 mg. (1 gr.) in bottles of 30 Count (NDC 64727-3300-4), 60 Count (NDC 64727-3300-5), 90 Count (NDC 64727-3300-6), 100 Count (NDC 64727-3300-1), 1,000 Count (NDC 64727-3300-2), 990 Count (NDC 64727-3300-3) & 1,008 Count (NDC 64727-3300-8)

97.5 mg. (1 1/2 gr.) in bottles of 30 Count (NDC 64727-3305-4), 60 Count (NDC 64727-3305-5), 90 Count (NDC 64727-3305-6), 100 Count (NDC 64727-3305-1), 1,000 Count (NDC 64727-3305-2), 990 Count (NDC 64727-3305-3) & 1,008 Count (NDC 64727-3305-8)

130 mg. (2 gr.) in bottles of 30 Count (NDC 64727-3308-4), 60 Count (NDC 64727-3308-5), 90 Count (NDC 64727-3308-6), 100 Count (NDC 64727-3308-1), 1,000 Count (NDC 64727-3308-2), 990 Count (NDC 64727-3308-3) & 1,008 Count (NDC 64727-3308-8)

195 mg. (3 gr.) in bottles of 30 Count (NDC 64727-3312-4), 60 Count (NDC 64727-3312-5), 90 Count (NDC 64727-3312-6), 100 Count (NDC 64727-3312-1), 1,000 Count (NDC 64727-3312-2), 990 Count (NDC 64727-3312-3) & 1,008 Count (NDC 64727-3312-8)

260 mg. (4 gr.) in bottles of 30 Count (NDC 64727-3320-4), 60 Count (NDC 64727-33208-5), 90 Count (NDC 64727-3320-6), 100 Count (NDC 64727-3320-1), 1,000 Count (NDC 64727-3320-2), 990 Count (NDC 64727-3320-3) & 1,008 Count (NDC 64727-3320-8)

325 mg. (5 gr.) in bottles of 30 Count (NDC 64727-3340-4), 60 Count (NDC 64727-3340-5), 90 Count (NDC 64727-3340-6), 100 Count (NDC 64727-3340-1), 1,000 Count (NDC 64727-3340-2), 990 Count (NDC 64727-3340-3) & 1,008 Count (NDC 64727-3340-8)

STORAGE: Store at controlled room temperature; 15°-30°C (59°-86°F)

Dispense in tight, light-resistant containers as defined in the USP/NF

Rx Only.

Distributed by:
RLC LABS
Cave Creek, AZ 85331
R091007/01

Shown in Product Identification Guide, page 318

WESTHROID™ ℞

[*wĕs-throid*]
(Thyroid USP)
Tablets

DESCRIPTION

Westhroid™ (Thyroid USP) Tablets, micro-coated, easy to swallow with a reduced odor, for oral use are natural preparations derived from porcine thyroid glands (T3 liothyronine is approximately four times as potent asT4 levothyroxine on a microgram for microgram basis). They provide 38 mcg levothyroxine (T4) and 9 mcg liothyronine (T3) for each 65 mg (1 Grain) of the labeled content of thyroid.

INACTIVE INGREDIENTS

Colloidal Silicon Dioxide, Dicalcium Phosphate, Lactose Monohydrate*, Magnesium Stearate, Microcrystalline Cellulose, Croscarmellose Sodium, Stearic Acid, Opadry II 85F19316 Clear.

*Present in traceable amount as part of Thyroid USP (diluent)

The structural formulas of liothyronine (T3) and levothyroxine (T4) are as follows:

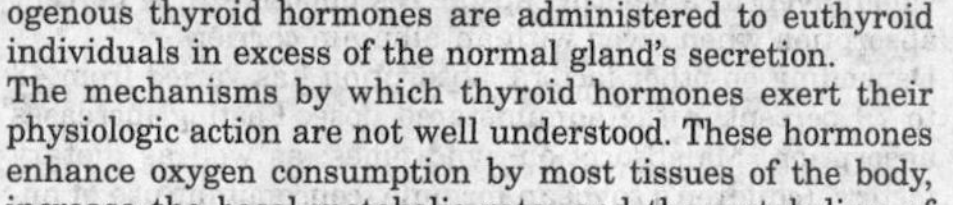

CLINICAL PHARMACOLOGY

The steps in the synthesis of the thyroid hormones are controlled by thyrotropin (Thyroid Stimulating Hormone, TSH) secreted by the anterior pituitary. This hormone's secretion is in turn controlled by a feedback mechanism affected by the thyroid hormones themselves and by thyrotropin releasing hormone (TRH), a tripeptide of hypothalamic origin. Endogenous thyroid hormone secretion is suppressed when exogenous thyroid hormones are administered to euthyroid individuals in excess of the normal gland's secretion.

The mechanisms by which thyroid hormones exert their physiologic action are not well understood. These hormones enhance oxygen consumption by most tissues of the body, increase the basal metabolic rate, and the metabolism of carbohydrates, lipids, and proteins. Thus, they exert a profound influence on every organ system in the body and are of particular importance in the development of the central nervous system.

The normal thyroid gland contains approximately 200 mcg of levothyroxine (T4) per gram of gland, and 15 mcg of liothyronine (T3) per gram. The ratio of these two hormones in the circulation does not represent the ratio in the thyroid gland, since about 80 percent of peripheral liothyronine (T3) comes from monodeiodination of levothyroxine (T4). Peripheral monodeiodination of levothyroxine (T4) at the 5 position (inner ring) also results in the formation of reverse liothyronine (T3), which is calorigenically inactive. Liothyronine (T3) levels are low in the fetus and newborn, in old age, in chronic caloric deprivation, hepatic cirrhosis, renal failure, surgical stress, and chronic illnesses representing what has been called the "T3 thyronine syndrome".

Pharmacokinetics

Animal studies have shown that levothyroxine (T4) is only partially absorbed from the gastrointestinal tract. The degree of absorption is dependent on the vehicle used for its administration and by the character of the intestinal contents, the intestinal flora, including plasma protein, and soluble dietary factors, all of which bind thyroid, thereby making it unavailable for diffusion. Only 41 percent is absorbed when given in a gelatin capsule, as opposed to 74 percent absorption when given with an albumin carrier. Depending on other factors, absorption has varied from 48 to 79 percent of the administered dose. Fasting increases absorption. Malabsorption syndromes, as well as dietary factors, (children's soybean formula, concomitant use of anionic exchange resins such as cholestyramine) cause excessive fecal loss. Liothyronine (T3) is almost totally absorbed, 95 percent in 4 hours. The hormones contained in the natural preparations are absorbed in a manner similar to the synthetic hormones.

More than 99 percent of circulating hormones are bound to serum proteins, including thyroid-binding globulin (TBg), thyroid-binding pre-albumin (TBPA), and albumin (TBa), whose capacities and affinities vary for the hormones. The higher affinity of levothyroxine (T4) for both TBg and TBPA, as compared to liothyronine (T3), partially explains the higher serum levels and longer half-life of the former hormone. Both protein-bound hormones exist in reverse equilibrium with minute amounts of free hormone, the latter accounting for the metabolic activity. Deiodination of levothyroxine (T4) occurs at a number of sites, including liver, kidney, and other tissues. The conjugated hormone, in the form of glucuronide or sulfate, is found in the bile and gut where it may complete an enterohepatic circulation. Eighty-five percent of levothyroxine (T4) metabolized daily is deiodinated.

INDICATIONS AND USAGE

1. As replacement of supplemental therapy in patients with hypothyroidism of any etiology, except transient hypothyroidism during the recovery phase of subacute thyroiditis. This category includes cretinism, myxedema, and ordinary hypothyroidism in patients of any age (children, adults, the elderly), or state (including pregnancy); primary hypothyroidism resulting from functional deficiency, primary atrophy, partial or total absence of thyroid gland, or the effects of surgery, radiation, or drugs, with or without the presence of goiter; and secondary (pituitary), or tertiary (hypothalamic) hypothyroidism (See WARNINGS).
2. As pituitary TSH suppressants, in the treatment or prevention of various types of euthyroid goiters, including thyroid nodules, subacute, or chronic lymphocytic thyroiditis (Hashimoto's), multinodular goiter, and in the management of thyroid cancer.
3. As diagnostic agents in suppression tests to differentiate suspected mild hyperthyroidism or thyroid gland anatomy.

CONTRAINDICATIONS

Thyroid hormone preparations are generally contraindicated in patients with diagnosed, but as yet, uncorrected adrenal cortical insufficiency, untreated thyrotoxicosis, and apparent hypersensitivity to any of their active or extraneous constituents. There is no well documented evidence in the literature of true allergic or idiosyncratic reactions to thyroid hormone.

WARNINGS

Drugs with thyroid hormone activity, alone or together with other therapeutic agents, have been used for the treatment of obesity. In euthyroid patients, doses within the range of daily hormonal requirements are ineffective for weight reduction. Larger doses may produce serious or even life-threatening manifestations of toxicity, particularly when given in association with sympathomimetic amines such as those used for their anorectic effects.

The use of thyroid hormones in the therapy of obesity, alone or combined with other drugs, is unjustified and has been shown to be ineffective. Neither is their use justified for the treatment of male or female infertility unless this condition is accompanied by hypothyroidism.

PRECAUTIONS

General: Thyroid hormones should be used with great caution in a number of circumstances where the integrity of the cardiovascular system, particularly the coronary arteries, is suspected. These include patients with angina pectoris or the elderly, whom have a greater likelihood of occult cardiac disease. With these patients, therapy should be initiated with low doses, i.e. 16.25 - 32.5 mg. When, in such patients, a euthyroid state can only be reached at the expense of an aggravation of the cardiovascular disease, thyroid hormone dosage should be reduced.

Thyroid hormone therapy in patients with concomitant diabetes mellitus or diabetes insipidus or adrenal cortical insufficiency aggravates the intensity of their symptoms. Appropriate adjustments of the various therapeutic measures directed at these concomitant endocrine diseases are required. The therapy of myxedema coma requires simultaneous administration of glucorticoids (See DOSAGE AND ADMINISTRATION).

Hypothyroidism decreases and hyperthyroidism increases the sensitivity to oral anticoagulants. Prothrombin time should be closely monitored in thyroid treated patients on oral anticoagulants and dosage of the latter agents should

be adjusted on the basis of frequent prothrombin time determinations. In infants, excessive doses of thyroid hormone preparations may produce craniosynostosis.

Information for the Patient: Patients on thyroid hormone preparations and parents of children on thyroid therapy should be informed that:

1. Replacement therapy is to be taken essentially for life, with the exception of cases of transient hypothyroidism, usually associated with thyroiditis, and in those patients receiving a therapeutic trial of the drug.
2. They should immediately report, during the course of therapy, any signs or symptoms of thyroid hormone toxicity, e.g., chest pain, increased pulse rate, palpitations, excessive sweating, heat intolerance, nervousness, or any other unusual event.
3. In case of concomitant diabetes mellitus, the daily dosage of antidiabetic medication may need readjustment as thyroid hormone replacement is achieved. If thyroid medication is stopped, a downward readjustment of the dosage of insulin or oral hypoglycemic agent may be necessary to avoid hypoglycemia. At all times, close monitoring of urinary glucose levels is mandatory in such patients.
4. In case of concomitant oral anticoagulant therapy, the prothrombin time should be measured frequently to determine if the dosage of oral anticoagulants is to be readjusted.
5. Partial loss of hair may be experienced by children in the first few months of thyroid therapy, but this is usually a transient phenomenon and later recovery is usually the rule.

Laboratory Tests: Treatment of patients with thyroid hormones requires the periodic assessment of thyroid status by means of appropriate laboratory tests, besides the full clinical evaluation. The TSH suppression test can be used to test the effectiveness of any thyroid preparation, bearing in mind the relative insensitivity of the infant pituitary to the negative feedback effect of thyroid hormones. Serum T4 levels can be used to test the effectiveness of all thyroid medications except T3. When the total serum T4 is low but TSH is normal, a test specific to assess unbound (free) T4 levels is warranted. Specific measurements of T4 and T3 by competitive protein binding or radioimmunoassay are not influenced by blood levels of organic or inorganic iodine.

Drug Interactions: Oral Anticoagulants-Thyroid hormones appear to increase catabolism of vitamin K- dependent clotting factors. If oral anticoagulants are also being given, compensatory increases in clotting factor synthesis are impaired. Patients stabilized on oral anticoagulants that are found to require thyroid replacement therapy should be watched very closely when thyroid is started. If a patient is truly hypothyroid, it is likely that a reduction in anticoagulant dosage will be required. No special precautions appear to be necessary when oral anticoagulant therapy is begun in a patient already stabilized on maintenance thyroid replacement therapy.

Insulin or Oral Hypoglycemic-Initiating thyroid replacement therapy may cause increases in insulin or oral hypoglycemic requirements. The effects seen are poorly understood and depend upon a variety of factors such as dose and type of thyroid preparations and endocrine status of the patient. Patients receiving insulin or oral hypoglycemic should be closely watched during initiation of thyroid replacement therapy.

Cholestyramine or Colestipol- Cholestyramine or Colestipol binds both levothyroxine (T4) and liothyronine (T3) in the intestine, thus impairing absorption of these thyroid hormones. In vitro studies indicate that the binding is not easily removed. Therefore, four to five hours should elapse between administration of Cholestyramine or Colestipol and thyroid hormones.

Estrogen, Oral Contraceptives- Estrogens tend to increase serum thyroxine-binding globulin (TBg). In a patient with a nonfunctioning thyroid gland who is receiving thyroid replacement therapy, free levothyroxine (T4) may be decreased when estrogens are started thus increasing thyroid requirements. However, if the patient's thyroid gland has sufficient function, the decreased free levothyroxine (T4) will result in a compensatory increase in levothyroxine (T4) output by the thyroid. Therefore, patients without a functioning thyroid gland who are on thyroid replacement therapy, may need to increase their thyroid dose if estrogens or estrogen-containing oral contraceptives are given.

Drug/Laboratory Test Interactions: The following drugs or moieties are known to interfere with laboratory tests performed in patients on thyroid hormone therapy: androgens, corticosteroids, estrogens, oral contraceptives containing estrogens, iodine-containing preparations, and the numerous preparations containing salicylates.

1. Changes in TBg concentration should be taken into consideration in the interpretation of levothyroxine (T4) and liothyronine (T3) values. In such cases, the unbound (free) hormone should be measured. Pregnancy, estrogens, and estrogen-containing oral contraceptives increase TBg concentrations. TBg may also be increased during infectious hepatitis. Decreases in TBg concentrations are observed in

nephrosis, acromegaly, and after androgen or corticosteroid therapy. Familial hyper or hypothyroxine-binding-globulinemias have been described. The incidence of TBg deficiency approximates 1 in 9,000. The binding of levothyroxine by TBPA is inhibited by salicylates.

2. Medicinal or dietary iodine interferes with all in vivo tests of radio-iodine uptake, producing low uptakes which may not be relative of a true decrease in hormone synthesis.
3. The persistence of clinical and laboratory evidence of hypothyroidism in spite of adequate dosage replacement indicates: either poor patient compliance, poor absorption, excessive fecal loss, or inactivity of the preparation. Intracellular resistance to thyroid hormone is quite rare.

Carcinogenesis, Mutagenesis, and Impairment of Fertility: A reportedly apparent association between prolonged thyroid therapy and breast cancer has not been confirmed and patients on thyroid for established indications should not discontinue therapy. No confirmatory long-term studies in animals have been performed to evaluate carcinogenic potential, mutagenicity, or impairment of fertility in either males or females.

Pregnancy-Category A: Thyroid hormones do not readily cross the placental barrier. The clinical experience to date does not indicate any adverse effect on fetuses when thyroid hormones are administered to pregnant women. On the basis of current knowledge, thyroid replacement therapy to hypothyroid women should not be discontinued during pregnancy.

Nursing Mothers: Minimal amounts of thyroid hormones are excreted in human milk. Thyroid is not associated with serious adverse reactions and does not have a known tumorigenic potential. However, caution should be exercised when thyroid is administered to a nursing woman.

Pediatric Use: Pregnant mothers provide little or no thyroid hormone to the fetus. The incidence of congenital hypothyroidism is relatively high (1:4,000) and the hypothyroid fetus would not derive any benefit from the small amounts of hormone crossing the placental barrier. Routine determination of serum T4 and/or TSH is strongly advised in neonates in view of the deleterious effects of thyroid deficiency on growth and development. Treatment should be initiated immediately upon diagnosis, and maintained for life, unless transient hypothyroidism is suspected; in which case, therapy may be interrupted for 2 to 8 weeks after the age of 3 years to reassess the condition. Cessation of therapy is justified in patients who have maintained a normal TSH during those 2 to 8 weeks.

Geriatric use: Clinical studies of Thyroid Tablets, USP did not include sufficient numbers of subjects aged 65 and over to determine whether they respond differently from younger subjects. Other reported clinical experience has not identified differences in responses between the elderly and younger patients. In general, dose selection for an elderly patient should be cautious, usually starting at the low end of the dosing range, reflecting the greater frequency of decreased hepatic, renal, or cardiac function, and of concomitant disease or other drug therapy.

ADVERSE REACTIONS

Adverse reactions other than those indicative of hyperthyroidism because of therapeutic overdosage, either initially or during the maintenance period, are rare (See OVERDOSAGE).

OVERDOSAGE

Signs and Symptoms: Excessive doses of thyroid result in a hypermetabolic state resembling in every respect the condition of endogenous origin. The condition may be self induced.

Treatment of Overdosage: Dosage should be reduced or therapy temporarily discontinued signs and symptoms of overdosage appear.

Treatment may be reinstituted at a lower dosage. In normal individuals, normal hypothalamic-pituitary-thyroid axis function is restored in 6 to 8 weeks after thyroid suppression.

Treatment of acute massive thyroid hormone overdosage is aimed at reducing gastrointestinal absorption of the drugs and counteracting central and peripheral effects, mainly those of increased sympathetic activity. Vomiting may be induced initially if further gastrointestinal absorption can reasonably be prevented and barring contraindications such as coma, convulsions, or loss of the gagging reflex. Treatment is symptomatic and supportive. Oxygen may be administered and ventilation maintained. Cardiac glycosides may be indicated if congestive heart failure develops. Measures to control fever, hypoglycemia, or fluid loss should be instituted if needed. Antiadrenergic agents, particularly propranolol, have been used advantageously in the treatment of increased sympathetic activity. Propranolol may be administered intravenously at a dosage of 1 to 3 mg, over a 10 minute period or orally, 80 to 160 mg/day, initially, especially when no contraindications exist for its use.

DOSAGE AND ADMINISTRATION

The dosage of thyroid hormones is determined by the indication and must in every case be individualized according to patient response and laboratory findings.

Thyroid hormones are given orally. In acute, emergency conditions, injectable levothyroxine sodium (T4) may be given intravenously when oral administration is not feasible or desirable (as in the treatment of myxedema coma, or during parenteral nutrition). Intramuscular administration is not advisable because of reported poor absorption.

Hypothyroidism: Therapy is usually instituted using low doses, with increments which depend on the cardiovascular status of the patient. The usual starting dose is 32.5 mg, with increment of 16.25 mg every 2 to 3 weeks. A lower starting dosage, 16.25 mg/day, is recommended in patients with longstanding myxedema, particularly if cardiovascular impairment is suspected, in which case extreme caution is recommended. The appearance of angina is an indication for reduction in dosage. Most patients require 65 - 130 mg/day. Failure to respond to doses of 195 mg suggests lack of compliance or malabsorption. Maintenance dosages 65 - 130 mg/day usually result in normal serum T4 and T3 levels. Adequate therapy usually results in normal TSH and T4 levels after 2 or 3 weeks of therapy.

Readjustment of thyroid hormone dosage should be made within the first four weeks of therapy, after proper clinical and laboratory evaluations, including serum levels of T4, bound and free, and TSH.

Liothyronine (T3) may be used in preference to levothyroxine (T4) during radio-isotope scanning procedures, since induction of hypothyroidism in those cases is more abrupt and can be of shorter duration. It may also be preferred when impairment of peripheral conversion of levothyroxine (T4) and liothyronine (T3) is suspected.

Myxedema Coma: Myxedema coma is usually precipitated in the hypothyroid patient of longstanding by intercurrent illness or drugs such as sedatives and anesthetics and should be considered a medical emergency. Therapy should be directed at the correction of electrolyte disturbances and possible infection, besides the administration of thyroid hormones. Corticosteroids should be administered routinely. Levothyroxine (T4) and Liothyronine (T3) may be administered via a nasogastric tube, but the preferred route of administration of both hormones is intravenous. Levothyroxine sodium (T4) is given at a starting dose of 400 mcg (100 mcg/mL) given rapidly, and is usually well tolerated, even in the elderly. This initial dose is followed by daily supplements of 100 to 200 mcg given IV. Normal T4 levels are achieved in 24 hours, followed in 3 days by threefold elevation of T3. Oral therapy with thyroid hormone would be resumed as soon as the clinical situation has been stabilized and the patient is able to take oral medication.

Thyroid Cancer: Exogenous thyroid hormone may produce regression of metastases from follicular and papillary carcinoma of the thyroid and is used as ancillary therapy of these conditions with radioactive iodine. TSH should be suppressed to low or undetectable levels. Therefore, larger amounts of thyroid hormone than those used for replacement therapy are required. Medullary carcinoma of the thyroid is usually unresponsive to this therapy.

Thyroid Suppression Therapy: Administration of thyroid hormone in doses higher than those produced physiologically by the gland results in suppression of the production of endogenous hormone. This is the basis for the thyroid suppression test and is used as an aid in the diagnosis of patients with signs of mild hyperthyroidism, in whom base line laboratory tests appear normal, or to demonstrate thyroid gland autonomy in patients with Grave's ophthalmopathy. 1 uptake is determined before and after administration of the exogenous hormone. A fifty percent or greater suppression of uptake indicates a normal thyroid pituitary axis, and thus rules out thyroid gland autonomy.

For adults, the usual suppressive dose of levothyroxine (T4) is 1.56 mg/kg of body weight per day given for 7 to 10 days. These doses usually yield normal serum T4 and T3 levels and lack of response to TSH.

Thyroid hormones should be administered cautiously to patients in whom there is strong suspicion of thyroid gland autonomy, in view of the fact that the exogenous hormone effects will be additive to the endogenous source.

Pediatric Dosage: Pediatric dosage should follow the recommendations summarized in Table 1. In infants with congenital hypothyroidism, therapy with full doses should be instituted as soon as the diagnosis has been made.

TABLE 1. Recommended Pediatric Dosage for Congenital Hypothyroidism

Age	Dose per day	Daily dose per kg of body weight
0 - 6 months	16.25 - 32.5 mg	4.8-6.0 mg
6 - 12 months	32.5 - 48.75 mg	3.6-4.8 mg
1 - 5 years	48.75 - 65 mg	3.3-6.0 mg
6 - 12 years	65 - 97.5 mg	2.4-3.0 mg
Over 12 years	Over 97.5 mg	1.2-1.8 mg

HOW SUPPLIED

Westhroid™ (Thyroid USP) Tablets are supplied as follows:
16.25 mg. (1/4 gr.) in bottles of 30 Count (NDC 64727-7065-4), 60 Count (NDC 64727-7065-5), 90 Count (NDC 64727-7065-6), 100 Count (NDC 64727-7065-1), 1,000 Count (NDC 64727-7065-2), 990 Count (NDC 64727-7065-3) & 1,008 Count (NDC 64727-7065-8)

32.5 mg. (1/2 gr.) in bottles of 30 Count (NDC 64727-7070-4), 60 Count (NDC 64727-7070-5), 90 Count (NDC 64727-7070-6), 100 Count (NDC 64727-7070-1), 1,000 Count (NDC 64727-7070-2), 990 Count (NDC 64727-7070-3) & 1,008 Count (NDC 64727-7070-8)

65 mg. (1 gr.) in bottles of 30 Count (NDC 64727-7073-4), 60 Count (NDC 64727-7073-5), 90 Count (NDC 64727-7073-6), 100 Count (NDC 64727-7073-1), 1,000 Count (NDC 64727-7073-2), 990 Count (NDC 64727-7073-3) & 1,008 Count (NDC 64727-7073-8)

97.5 mg. (1 1/2 gr.) in bottles of 30 Count (NDC 64727-7075-4), 60 Count (NDC 64727-7075-5), 90 Count (NDC 64727-7075-6), 100 Count (NDC 64727-7075-1), 1,000 Count (NDC 64727-7075-2), 990 Count (NDC 64727-7075-3) & 1,008 Count (NDC 64727-7075-8)

130 mg. (2 gr.) in bottles of 30 Count (NDC 64727-7080-4), 60 Count (NDC 64727-7080-5), 90 Count (NDC 64727-7080-6), 100 Count (NDC 64727-7080-1), 1,000 Count (NDC 64727-7080-2), 990 Count (NDC 64727-7080-3) & 1,008 Count (NDC 64727-7080-8)

195 mg. (3 gr.) in bottles of 30 Count (NDC 64727-7095-4), 60 Count (NDC 64727-7095-5), 90 Count (NDC 64727-7095-6), 100 Count (NDC 64727-7095-1), 1,000 Count (NDC 64727-7095-2), 990 Count (NDC 64727-7095-3) & 1,008 Count (NDC 64727-7095-8)

260 mg. (4 gr.) in bottles of 30 Count (NDC 64727-7100-4), 60 Count (NDC 64727-7100-5), 90 Count (NDC 64727-7100-6), 100 Count (NDC 64727-7100-1), 1,000 Count (NDC 64727-7100-2), 990 Count (NDC 64727-7100-3) & 1,008 Count (NDC 64727-7100-8)

325 mg. (5 gr.) in bottles of 30 Count (NDC 64727-7150-4), 60 Count (NDC 64727-7150-5), 90 Count (NDC 64727-7150-6), 100 Count (NDC 64727-7150-1), 1,000 Count (NDC 64727-7150-2), 990 Count (NDC 64727-7150-3) & 1,008 Count (NDC 64727-7150-8)

STORAGE: Store at controlled room temperature; 15°-30°C (59°-86°F)

Dispense in tight, light-resistant containers as defined in the USP/NF

Rx Only.

Distributed by:
RLC LABS
Cave Creek, AZ 85331
R091008/02

Shown in Product Identification Guide, page 318

Salix Pharmaceuticals, Inc.

1700 PERIMETER PARK DRIVE
MORRISVILLE, NC 27560

Direct Inquiries to:
(866) 669-7597 Phone
(919) 862-1817 Fax
www.salix.com
For adverse events, product quality complaints and patient information requests:
Product Information Center
(800) 508-0024 Phone
(510) 595-8183 Fax
E-mail: salix@medcomsol.com

APRISO™ ℞
[uh-pre-zoh]
(mesalamine)
Extended-Release Capsules

HIGHLIGHTS OF PRESCRIBING INFORMATION

These highlights do not include all the information needed to use APRISO safely and effectively. See full prescribing information for APRISO.

APRISO™ (mesalamine) extended-release capsules
Initial U.S. Approval: 1987

——————INDICATIONS AND USAGE——————

• APRISO is a locally-acting aminosalicylate indicated for the maintenance of remission of ulcerative colitis in adults (1)

——————DOSAGE AND ADMINISTRATION——————

• Four APRISO capsules once daily (1.5 g/day) in the morning with or without food. Do not co-administer with antacids (2)

——————DOSAGE FORMS AND STRENGTHS——————

• Extended-release capsules: 0.375 g (3)

——————CONTRAINDICATIONS——————

• Hypersensitivity to salicylates, aminosalicylates, or any component of APRISO capsules (4)

——————WARNINGS AND PRECAUTIONS——————

• Renal impairment may occur. Assess renal function at the beginning of treatment and periodically during therapy (5.1)
• Acute exacerbation of colitis symptoms can occur (5.2)
• Use caution with pre-existing liver disease (5.4)

——————ADVERSE REACTIONS——————

• The most common adverse reactions (incidence ≥3%) are headache, diarrhea, upper abdominal pain, nausea, nasopharyngitis, flu or flu-like illness, sinusitis (6.1)

To report SUSPECTED ADVERSE REACTIONS, contact Salix Pharmaceuticals, Inc. at 1-800-508-0024 or FDA at 1-800-FDA-1088 or www.fda.gov/medwatch.

——————DRUG INTERACTIONS——————

• Do not co-administer with antacids (7.1)

——————USE IN SPECIFIC POPULATIONS——————

• Use with caution in patients with renal disease (5.1)
• Monitor blood cell counts in geriatric patients (8.5)
• Advise patients with phenylketonuria that APRISO contains aspartame (17.1)

See 17 for PATIENT COUNSELING INFORMATION

Revised: 07/2009

FULL PRESCRIBING INFORMATION

1 INDICATIONS AND USAGE

APRISO capsules are indicated for the maintenance of remission of ulcerative colitis in patients 18 years of age and older.

2 DOSAGE AND ADMINISTRATION

The recommended dose for maintenance of remission of ulcerative colitis in adult patients is 1.5 g (four APRISO capsules) orally once daily in the morning. APRISO may be taken without regard to meals. APRISO should not be co-administered with antacids. An evaluation of renal function is recommended before initiating therapy with APRISO.

3 DOSAGE FORMS AND STRENGTHS

Extended-release capsules containing 0.375 g mesalamine.

4 CONTRAINDICATIONS

APRISO is contraindicated in patients with hypersensitivity to salicylates or aminosalicylates or to any of the components of APRISO capsules.

5 WARNINGS AND PRECAUTIONS

5.1 Renal Impairment

Renal impairment, including minimal change nephropathy, acute and chronic interstitial nephritis, and, rarely, renal failure, has been reported in patients given products such as APRISO that contain mesalamine or are converted to mesalamine.

It is recommended that patients have an evaluation of renal function prior to initiation of APRISO therapy and periodically while on therapy. Exercise caution when using APRISO in patients with known renal dysfunction or a history of renal disease.

In animal studies, the kidney was the principal organ for toxicity *[See Nonclinical Toxicology (13.2)]*

5.2 Mesalamine-Induced Acute Intolerance Syndrome

Mesalamine has been associated with an acute intolerance syndrome that may be difficult to distinguish from a flare of inflammatory bowel disease. Although the exact frequency of occurrence has not been determined, it has occurred in 3% of patients in controlled clinical trials of mesalamine or sulfasalazine. Symptoms include cramping, acute abdominal pain and bloody diarrhea, sometimes fever, headache, and rash. If acute intolerance syndrome is suspected, promptly discontinue treatment with APRISO.

5.3 Hypersensitivity

Some patients who have experienced a hypersensitivity reaction to sulfasalazine may have a similar reaction to APRISO capsules or to other compounds that contain or are converted to mesalamine.

5.4 Hepatic Impairment

There have been reports of hepatic failure in patients with pre-existing liver disease who have been administered mesalamine. Caution should be exercised when administering APRISO to patients with liver disease.

6 ADVERSE REACTIONS

6.1 Clinical Studies Experience

The data described below reflect exposure to APRISO in 557 patients, including 354 exposed for at least 6 months and 250 exposed for greater than one year. APRISO was studied in two placebo-controlled trials (n = 367 treated with APRISO) and in one open-label, long-term study (n = 190 additional patients). The population consisted of patients with ulcerative colitis; the mean age was 47 years, 54% were female, and 93% were white. Patients received doses of APRISO 1.5 g administered orally once per day for six months in the placebo-controlled trials and for up to 24 months in the open-label study.

Because clinical studies are conducted under widely varying conditions, adverse reaction rates observed in the clinical trials of a drug cannot be directly compared to rates in the clinical trials of another drug and may not reflect the rates observed in practice.

In the two placebo-controlled trials, 59% of APRISO-treated patients experienced an adverse reaction compared with 64% of placebo patients. Most adverse reactions with APRISO were mild or moderate in severity. Severe adverse reactions occurred in 6% of APRISO-treated patients and 5% of placebo-treated patients. Discontinuations due to adverse reactions occurred in 11% of APRISO-treated patients and 17% of placebo-treated patients; the most common adverse reaction resulting in study discontinuation was recurrence of ulcerative colitis (APRISO 6%, placebo 14%). The most common reactions reported with APRISO (≥3%) are shown in Table 1 below.

Table 1: Treatment-Emergent Adverse Reactions during Clinical Trials Occurring in at Least 3% of APRISO-Treated Patients and at a Greater Rate than with Placebo

MedDRA Preferred Term	APRISO 1.5g/day N=367	Placebo N=185
Headache	11%	8%
Diarrhea	8%	7%
Abdominal Pain Upper	5%	3%
Nausea	4%	3%
Nasopharyngitis	4%	3%
Influenza & Influenza-like illness	4%	4%
Sinusitis	3%	3%

The following adverse reactions, presented by body system, were reported at a frequency less than 3% in patients treated with APRISO for up to 24 months in controlled and open-label trials.

Ear and Labyrinth Disorders: tinnitus, vertigo
Dermatological Disorder: alopecia
Gastrointestinal: abdominal pain lower, rectal hemorrhage
Laboratory Abnormalities: increased triglycerides, decreased hematocrit and hemoglobin
General Disorders and Administration Site Disorders: fatigue
Hepatic: hepatitis cholestatic, transaminases increased
Renal Disorders: creatinine clearance decreased, hematuria
Musculoskeletal: pain, arthralgia
Respiratory: dyspnea

6.2 Adverse Reaction Information from Other Sources

The following adverse reactions have been identified during clinical trials of a product similar to APRISO and post approval use of other mesalamine-containing products such as APRISO. Because many of these reactions are reported voluntarily from a population of unknown size, it is not always possible to reliably estimate their frequency or establish a causal relationship to drug exposure.

Body as a Whole: lupus-like syndrome, drug fever
Cardiovascular: pericarditis, pericardial effusion, myocarditis
Gastrointestinal: pancreatitis, cholecystitis, gastritis, gastroenteritis, gastrointestinal bleeding, perforated peptic ulcer
Hepatic: jaundice, cholestatic jaundice, hepatitis, liver necrosis, liver failure, Kawasaki-like syndrome including changes in liver enzymes
Hematologic: agranulocytosis, aplastic anemia
Neurological/Psychiatric: peripheral neuropathy, Guillain-Barré syndrome, transverse myelitis
Respiratory/Pulmonary: eosinophilic pneumonia, interstitial pneumonitis
Skin: psoriasis, pyoderma gangrenosum, erythema nodosum
Renal/Urogenital: reversible oligospermia

7 DRUG INTERACTIONS

Based on in vitro studies, APRISO is not expected to inhibit the metabolism of drugs that are substrates of CYP1A2, CYP2C9, CYP2C19, CYP2D6, or CYP3A4.

7.1 Antacids

Because the dissolution of the coating of the granules in APRISO capsules depends on pH, APRISO capsules should not be co-administered with antacids.

8 USE IN SPECIFIC POPULATIONS

8.1 Pregnancy

Pregnancy Category B. Reproduction studies with mesalamine have been performed in rats at oral doses up to 320 mg/kg/day (about 1.7 times the recommended human dose based on a body surface area comparison) and rabbits at doses up to 495 mg/kg/day (about 5.4 times the recommended human dose based on a body surface area comparison) and have revealed no evidence of impaired fertility or harm to the fetus due to mesalamine. There are, however, no adequate and well-controlled studies in pregnant women. Because animal reproduction studies are not always predictive of human response, this drug should be used during pregnancy only if clearly needed.

Mesalamine is known to cross the placental barrier.

8.3 Nursing Mothers

Low concentrations of mesalamine and higher concentrations of its N-acetyl metabolite have been detected in human breast milk. The clinical significance of this has not been determined and there is limited experience of nursing women using mesalamine. Caution should be exercised when APRISO is administered to a nursing woman.

8.4 Pediatric Use

Safety and effectiveness of APRISO capsules in pediatric patients have not been established.

8.5 Geriatric Use

Clinical studies of APRISO did not include sufficient numbers of subjects aged 65 and over to determine whether they respond differently than younger subjects. Other reported clinical experience has not identified differences in responses between elderly and younger patients. In general, the greater frequency of decreased hepatic, renal, or cardiac function, and of concomitant disease or other drug therapy in elderly patients should be considered when prescribing APRISO.

Reports from uncontrolled clinical studies and postmarketing reporting systems suggested a higher incidence of blood dyscrasias, i.e., neutropenia, pancytopenia, in patients who were 65 years or older who were taking mesalamine-containing products such as APRISO. Caution should be taken to closely monitor blood cell counts during mesalamine therapy.

Mesalamine is known to be substantially excreted by the kidney, and the risk of adverse reactions to this drug may be greater in patients with impaired renal function. Because elderly patients are more likely to have decreased renal function, care should be taken when prescribing this drug therapy. *[see Warning and Precautions (5.1)]*.

10 OVERDOSAGE

APRISO is an aminosalicylate, and symptoms of salicylate toxicity include hematemesis, tachypnea, hyperpnea, tinnitus, deafness, lethargy, seizures, confusion, or dyspnea. Severe intoxication may lead to electrolyte and blood pH imbalance and potentially to other organ (e.g., renal and liver) involvement. There is no specific antidote for mesalamine overdose; however, conventional therapy for salicylate toxicity may be beneficial in the event of acute overdosage. This includes prevention of further gastrointestinal tract absorption by emesis and, if necessary, by gastric lavage. Fluid and electrolyte imbalance should be corrected by the administration of appropriate intravenous therapy. Adequate renal function should be maintained. APRISO is a pH-dependent delayed-release product and this factor should be considered when treating a suspected overdose.

11 DESCRIPTION

Each APRISO capsule is a delayed- and extended-release dosage form for oral administration. Each capsule contains 0.375 g of mesalamine USP (5-aminosalicylic acid, 5-ASA), an anti-inflammatory drug. The structural formula of mesalamine is:

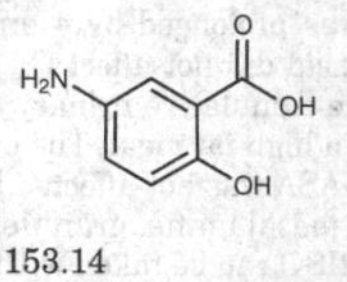

Molecular Weight: 153.14
Molecular Formula: $C_7H_7NO_3$

Each APRISO capsule contains granules composed of mesalamine in a polymer matrix with an enteric coating that dissolves at pH 6 and above.

The inactive ingredients of APRISO capsules are colloidal silicon dioxide, magnesium stearate, microcrystalline cellulose, simethicone emulsion ethylacrylate/methylmethacrylate copolymer nonoxynol 100 dispersion, hypromellose, methacrylic acid copolymer, talc, titanium dioxide, triethyl citrate, aspartame, anhydrous citric acid, povidone, vanilla flavor, and edible black ink.

12 CLINICAL PHARMACOLOGY

12.1 Mechanism of Action

The mechanism of action of mesalamine (5-ASA) is unknown, but appears to be local to the intestinal mucosa rather than systemic. Mucosal production of arachidonic acid metabolites, both through the cyclooxygenase pathways, i.e., prostanoids, and through the lipoxygenase pathways, i.e., leukotrienes and hydroxyeicosatetraenoic acids, is increased in patients with ulcerative colitis, and it is possible that 5-ASA diminishes inflammation by blocking production of arachidonic acid metabolites.

12.3 Pharmacokinetics

Absorption

The pharmacokinetics of 5-ASA and its metabolite, N-acetyl-5-aminosalicylic acid (N-Ac-5-ASA), were studied after a single and multiple oral doses of 1.5 g APRISO in a crossover study in healthy subjects under fasting conditions. In the multiple-dose period, each subject received APRISO 1.5 g (4×0.375 g capsules) every 24 hours (QD) for 7 consecutive days. Steady state was reached on Day 6 of QD dosing based on trough concentrations.

After single and multiple doses of APRISO, peak plasma concentrations were observed at about 4 hours post dose. At steady state, moderate increases (1.5-fold and 1.7-fold) in systemic exposure (AUC_{0-24}) to 5-ASA and N-Ac-5-ASA were observed when compared with a single-dose of APRISO.

Pharmacokinetic parameters after a single dose of 1.5 g APRISO and at steady state in healthy subjects under fasting condition are shown in Table 2.

Table 2: Single Dose and Multiple Dose Mean (±SD) Plasma Pharmacokinetic Parameters of Mesalamine (5-ASA) and N-Ac-5-ASA after 1.5 g APRISO Administration in Healthy Subjects

Mesalamine (5-ASA)	Single Dose (n=24)	Multiple Dose[c] (n=24)
AUC_{0-24} (μg*h/mL)	11 ± 5	17 ± 6
AUC_{0-inf} (μg*h/mL)	14 ± 5	-
C_{max} (μg/mL)	2.1 ± 1.1	2.7 ± 1.1
T_{max} (h)[a]	4 (2, 16)	4 (2, 8)
$t_{1/2}$ (h)[b]	9 ± 7	10 ± 8
N-Ac-5-ASA		
AUC_{0-24} (μg*h/mL)	26 ± 6	37 ± 9

AUC_{0-inf} (µg*h/mL)	51 ± 23	-
C_{max} (µg/mL)	2.8 ± 0.8	3.4 ± 0.9
T_{max} (h)[a]	4 (4, 12)	5 (2, 8)
$t_{1/2}$ (h)[b]	12 ± 11	14 ± 10

[a] Median (range);
[b] Harmonic mean (pseudo SD);
[c] after 7 days of treatment

In a separate study (n = 30), it was observed that under fasting conditions about 32% ± 11% (mean ± SD) of the administered dose was systemically absorbed based on the combined cumulative urinary excretion of 5-ASA and N-Ac-5-ASA over 96 hours post-dose.

The effect of a high fat meal intake on absorption of mesalamine granules (the same granules contained in APRISO capsules) was evaluated in 30 healthy subjects. Subjects received 1.6 g of mesalamine granules in sachet (2 × 0.8 g) following an overnight fast or a high fat meal in a crossover study. Under fed conditions, t_{max} for both 5-ASA and N-Ac-5-ASA was prolonged by 4 and 2 hours, respectively. A high fat meal did not affect C_{max} for 5-ASA, but a 27% increase in the cumulative urinary excretion of 5-ASA was observed with a high fat meal. The overall extent of absorption of N-Ac-5-ASA was not affected by a high fat meal. As APRISO and mesalamine granules in sachet were bioequivalent, APRISO can be taken without regard to food.

Distribution
In an *in vitro* study, at 2.5 µg/mL, mesalamine and N-Ac-5-ASA are 43 ± 6% and 78 ± 1% bound, respectively, to plasma proteins. Protein binding of N-Ac-5-ASA does not appear to be concentration dependent at concentrations ranging from 1 to 10 µg/mL.

Metabolism
The major metabolite of mesalamine is N-acetyl-5-aminosalicylic acid (N-Ac-5-ASA). It is formed by N-acetyltransferase activity in the liver and intestinal mucosa.

Elimination
Following single and multiple doses of APRISO, the mean half-lives were 9 to 10 hours for 5-ASA, and 12 to 14 hours for N-Ac-5-ASA. Of the approximately 32% of the dose absorbed, about 2% of the dose was excreted unchanged in the urine, compared with about 30% of the dose excreted as N-Ac-5-ASA.

In Vitro Drug-Drug Interaction Study
In an *in vitro* study using human liver microsomes, 5-ASA and its metabolite, N-Ac-5-ASA, were shown not to inhibit the major CYP enzymes evaluated (CYP1A2, CYP2C9, CYP2C19, CYP2D6, and CYP3A4). Therefore, mesalamine and its metabolite are not expected to inhibit the metabolism of other drugs that are substrates of CYP1A2, CYP2C9, CYP2C19, CYP2D6, or CYP3A4.

13 NONCLINICAL TOXICOLOGY
13.1 Carcinogenesis, Mutagenesis, Impairment of Fertility
Dietary mesalamine was not carcinogenic in rats at doses as high as 480 mg/kg/day, or in mice at 2000 mg/kg/day. These doses are about 2.6 and 5.4 times the recommended human dose of granulated mesalamine capsules of 1.5 g/day (30 mg/kg if 50 kg body weight assumed or 1110 mg/m²), respectively, based on body surface area. Mesalamine was negative in the Ames test, the mouse lymphoma cell (L5178Y/TK+/-) forward mutation test, the sister chromatid exchange assay in the Chinese hamster bone marrow test, and the mouse bone marrow micronucleus test. Mesalamine at oral doses up to 320 mg/kg (about 1.7 times the recommended human dose based on body surface area) was found to have no effect on fertility or reproductive performance in rats.

13.3 Animal Toxicology and/or Pharmacology
Renal Toxicity
Animal studies with mesalamine (13-week and 26-week oral toxicity studies in rats, and 26-week and 52-week oral toxicity studies in dogs) have shown the kidney to be the major target organ of mesalamine toxicity. Oral doses of 40 mg/kg/day (about 0.20 times the human dose, on the basis of body surface area) produced minimal to slight tubular injury, and doses of 160 mg/kg/day (about 0.90 times the human dose, on the basis of body surface area) or higher in rats produced renal lesions including tubular degeneration, tubular mineralization, and papillary necrosis. Oral doses of 60 mg/kg/day (about 1.1 times the human dose, on the basis of body surface area) or higher in dogs also produced renal lesions including tubular atrophy, interstitial cell infiltration, chronic nephritis, and papillary necrosis.

Overdosage
Single oral doses of 800 mg/kg (about 2.2 times the recommended human dose, on the basis of body surface area) and 1800 mg/kg (about 9.7 times the recommended human dose,

on the basis of body surface area) of mesalamine were lethal to mice and rats, respectively, and resulted in gastrointestinal and renal toxicity.

14 CLINICAL STUDIES
14.1 Ulcerative Colitis
Two similar, randomized, double-blind, placebo-controlled, multi-center studies were conducted in a total of 562 adult patients in remission from ulcerative colitis. The study populations had a mean age of 46 years (11% age 65 years or older), were 53% female, and were primarily white (92%). Ulcerative colitis disease activity was assessed using a modified Sutherland Disease Activity Index[1] (DAI), which is a sum of four subscores based on stool frequency, rectal bleeding, mucosal appearance on endoscopy, and physician's rating of disease activity. Each subscore can range from 0 to 3, for a total possible DAI score of 12.

At baseline, approximately 80% of patients had a total DAI score of 0 or 1.0. Patients were randomized 2:1 to receive either APRISO 1.5 g or placebo once daily in the morning for six months. Patients were assessed at baseline, 1 month, 3 months, and 6 months in the clinic, with endoscopy performed at baseline, at end of study, or if clinical symptoms developed. Relapse was defined as a rectal bleeding subscale score of 1 or more and a mucosal appearance subscale score of 2 or more using the DAI. The analysis of the intent-to-treat population was a comparison of the proportions of patients who remained relapse-free at the end of six months of treatment. For the table below (Table 3) all patients who prematurely withdrew from the study for any reason were counted as relapses.

In both studies, the proportion of patients who remained relapse-free at six months was greater for APRISO than for placebo.

Table 3: Percentage of Patients Relapse-Free* through 6 Months in APRISO Maintenance Studies

	APRISO 1.5 g/day % (# no relapse/N)	Placebo % (# no relapse/N)	Difference (95% C.I.)	P-value
Study 1	68% (143/209)	51% (49/96)	17% (5.5, 29.2)	<0.001
Study 2	71% (117/164)	59% (55/93)	12% (0, 24.5)	0.046

*Relapse counted as rectal bleeding score ≥ 1 and mucosal appearance score ≥ 2, or premature withdrawal from study.

Examination of gender subgroups did not identify difference in response to APRISO among these subgroups. There were too few elderly and too few African-American patients to adequately assess difference in effects in those populations. The use of APRISO for treating ulcerative colitis beyond six months has not been evaluated in controlled clinical trials.

15 REFERENCES
1. Sutherland LR, Martin F, Greer S, Robinson M, Greenberger N, Saibil F, *et al.* 5-Aminosalicylic acid enema in the treatment of distal ulcerative colitis, proctosigmoiditis, and proctitis. Gastroenterology 1987;92(6): 1894-1898.

16 HOW SUPPLIED/STORAGE AND HANDLING
APRISO is available as light blue opaque hard gelatin capsules containing 0.375 g mesalamine and with the letters "G" and "M" on either side of a black band imprinted on the capsule.
NDC 65649-103-02 Bottles of 120 capsules
NDC 65649-103-01 Bottles of 4 capsules
Storage:
Store at 20° to 25°C (68° to 77°F); excursions permitted between 15° and 30°C (59° and 86°F). See USP Controlled Room Temperature.

17 PATIENT COUNSELING INFORMATION
17.1 Patients with Phenylketonuria
• Inform patients with phenylketonuria (PKU) or their caregivers that each APRISO capsule contains aspartame equivalent to 0.56 mg of phenylalanine, so that the recommended adult dosing provides an equivalent of 2.24 mg of phenylalanine per day.
17.2 General Counseling Information
• Instruct patients not to take APRISO capsules with antacids, because it could affect the way APRISO dissolves.
• Instruct patients to contact a health care provider if they experience a worsening of ulcerative colitis symptoms, because it could be due to a reaction to APRISO.

Manufactured by Catalent Pharma Solutions for Salix Pharmaceuticals, Inc., Morrisville, NC 27560
* APRISO™ is a trademark of Salix Pharmaceuticals, Inc.
© 2008 Salix Pharmaceuticals, Inc.

Product protected by U.S. Patent No. 6,551,620 and U.S. Patent No. 7,547,451
VENART-113-1
Shown in Product Identification Guide, page 318

METOZOLV™ ODT
[MĔ-tō-zolv]
(metoclopramide hydrochloride)
Orally Disintegrating Tablets
℞

HIGHLIGHTS OF PRESCRIBING INFORMATION
These highlights do not include all the information needed to use METOZOLV ODT safely and effectively. See full prescribing information for METOZOLV ODT.
METOZOLV ODT (metoclopramide hydrochloride) orally disintegrating tablets
Initial U.S. Approval: 1976

> **WARNING: TARDIVE DYSKINESIA**
> *See full prescribing information for complete boxed warning.*
> Treatment with metoclopramide can cause tardive dyskinesia, a serious movement disorder that is often irreversible. The risk of developing tardive dyskinesia increases with the duration of treatment and the total cumulative dose.
> Metoclopramide therapy should be discontinued in patients who develop signs or symptoms of tardive dyskinesia. There is no known treatment for tardive dyskinesia. In some patients, symptoms may lessen or resolve after metoclopramide treatment is stopped.
> Treatment with metoclopramide for longer than 12 weeks should be avoided in all but rare cases where therapeutic benefit is thought to outweigh the risk of developing tardive dyskinesia. (5.1)

INDICATIONS AND USAGE
METOZOLV ODT is a dopamine receptor antagonist indicated for:
• **Relief of Symptomatic Gastroesophageal Reflux:** short-term (4 to 12 weeks) therapy for adults with symptomatic, documented gastroesophageal reflux who fail to respond to conventional therapy (1.1)
• **Diabetic Gastroparesis (Diabetic Gastric Stasis):** the relief of symptoms in adults associated with acute and recurrent diabetic gastroparesis (gastric stasis) (1.2)
Important Limitations:
• Therapy should not exceed 12 weeks in duration (1.3)
• METOZOLV ODT is recommended only for adults. The safety and effectiveness in pediatric patients have not been established (1.3)

DOSAGE AND ADMINISTRATION
• **Gastroesophageal Reflux Disease:** 10 mg to 15 mg dose up to four times daily at least 30 minutes before eating and at bedtime (2.2)
• **Diabetic Gastroparesis (Diabetic Gastric Stasis):** 10 mg dose four times daily at least 30 minutes before eating and at bedtime for two to eight weeks (2.3)

DOSAGE FORMS AND STRENGTHS
Orally Disintegrating Tablets: 5 mg and 10 mg (3)

CONTRAINDICATIONS
• Intestinal Obstruction, Hemorrhage, or Perforation (4.1)
• Pheochromocytoma (4.2)
• Known Sensitivity or Intolerance (4.3)
• Epilepsy (4.4)
• Concomitant Medications with Extrapyramidal Reactions (4.5)

WARNINGS AND PRECAUTIONS
• Tardive Dyskinesia (5.1)
• Acute Dystonic Reactions, Drug-induced Parkinsonism and Other Extrapyramidal Symptoms (5.2)
• Neuroleptic Malignant Syndrome (5.3)
• Depression (5.4)
• Hypertension (5.5)
• Congestive Heart Failure and Ventricular Arrhythmia (5.6)
• Withdrawal from Metoclopramide (5.7)

ADVERSE REACTIONS
The most common adverse reactions (> 2%) are headache, nausea, vomiting, fatigue, and somnolence (6.1).
To report suspected adverse reactions, contact Salix Pharmaceuticals, Inc. at 1-800-508-0024 or FDA at 1-800-FDA-1088 or www.fda.gov/medwatch.

DRUG INTERACTIONS
• Anticholinergic drugs: Antagonize effects of metoclopramide (7.1)
• Narcotic analgesic drugs: May increase sedation (7.1)
• Monoamine oxidase inhibitors: May cause hypertensive crisis (due to catecholamine release) (7.2)
• Altered drug absorption: May decrease absorption of drugs from the stomach and increase absorption of drugs from the small bowel (7.3)

- **Insulin:** Changes in food transit time may require adjustment of insulin dose or timing to avoid hypoglycemia (7.4)
- **Antidepressants, Antipsychotics, and Neuroleptics:** Concomitant use with metoclopramide is associated with increased risk of tardive dyskinesia and Neuroleptic Malignant Syndrome (7.5)

USE IN SPECIFIC POPULATIONS

- **Pediatric Use:** The safety and effectiveness of METOZOLV ODT in pediatric patients have not been established (8.4)
- **Geriatric Use:** Elderly patients may be more sensitive to adverse reactions such as sedation and drug-induced movement disorders. (8.5)
- **Impaired Renal Function:** Initial dosing may need to be reduced and titrated (8.6).

See 17 for PATIENT COUNSELING INFORMATION and Medication Guide

Revised: Sep 2009

FULL PRESCRIBING INFORMATION: CONTENTS*
WARNINGS: Tardive Dyskinesia

FULL PRESCRIBING INFORMATION

WARNING: TARDIVE DYSKINESIA
Treatment with metoclopramide can cause tardive dyskinesia, a serious movement disorder that is often irreversible. The risk of developing tardive dyskinesia increases with duration of treatment and total cumulative dose.
Metoclopramide therapy should be discontinued in patients who develop signs or symptoms of tardive dyskinesia. There is no known treatment for tardive dyski-

---

nesia. In some patients, symptoms may lessen or resolve after metoclopramide treatment is stopped. Treatment with metoclopramide for longer than 12 weeks should be avoided in all but rare cases where therapeutic benefit is thought to outweigh the risk of developing tardive dyskinesia.
[see Warnings and Precautions (5.1)]

1 INDICATIONS AND USAGE

1.1 Symptomatic Gastroesophageal Reflux Disease
METOZOLV ODT is indicated as short-term (4 to 12 weeks) therapy for adults with symptomatic, documented gastroesophageal reflux disease (GERD) who fail to respond to conventional therapy.

1.2 Diabetic Gastroparesis (Diabetic Gastric Stasis)
METOZOLV ODT is indicated for the relief of symptoms associated with acute and recurrent diabetic gastroparesis (gastric stasis) in adults.

1.3 Important Limitations
METOZOLV ODT is indicated for adults only. Therapy should not exceed 12 weeks in duration. The safety and effectiveness in pediatric patients have not been established.

2 DOSAGE AND ADMINISTRATION

2.1 Important Instructions for Use
Take on an empty stomach at least 30 minutes before eating since food can decrease the peak concentrations of drug in the bloodstream and/or the time it takes to achieve the maximum drug level in the bloodstream *[see Clinical Pharmacology (12.3)]*. Do not repeat dose if inadvertently taken with food.

Since the tablet absorbs moisture rapidly, only remove each dose from the packaging just prior to taking. Handle the tablet with dry hands and place on the tongue. If the tablet should break or crumble while handling, discard and remove a new tablet.

METOZOLV ODT disintegrates on the tongue in approximately one minute (with a range of 10 seconds to 14 minutes). METOZOLV ODT is designed to be taken without liquid; however, the effect on the pharmacokinetics of taking METOZOLV ODT with liquid is unknown.

2.2 Symptomatic Gastroesophageal Reflux Disease
For the relief of symptomatic, documented gastroesophageal reflux disease (GERD), therapy should not exceed 12 weeks in duration.

Take 10 mg to 15 mg dose of METOZOLV ODT up to four times daily (e.g., at least 30 minutes before each meal and at bedtime). Doses may vary depending upon the symptoms being treated and the clinical response. If symptoms only occur intermittently or at specific times of the day, metoclopramide may be used in single doses up to 20 mg prior to the symptoms rather than continuous treatment.

Since there is a poor correlation between symptomatic relief and healing of esophageal lesions, any therapy directed at esophageal lesions is best confirmed by endoscopic evaluation. Although experience with the effects of metoclopramide on esophageal erosions and ulcerations is limited, healing was documented in a controlled trial using four times daily therapy at 15 mg/dose. Prolonged treatment (>12 weeks) with metoclopramide should be avoided in all but rare cases where therapeutic benefit is thought to counterbalance the risks to the patient of developing tardive dyskinesia. *[see Warnings and Precautions (5.1)]*

2.3 Diabetic Gastroparesis (Diabetic Gastric Stasis)
For the relief of symptoms associated with diabetic gastroparesis (diabetic gastric stasis), therapy of two to eight weeks is recommended. Therapy should not exceed 12 weeks in duration.

Take a 10 mg dose of METOZOLV ODT up to four times a day (e.g., at least 30 minutes before each meal and at bedtime).

The initial route of administration should be determined by the severity of the presenting symptoms. If only the earliest manifestations of diabetic gastric stasis are present, oral administration of METOZOLV ODT may be initiated. However, if severe symptoms are present, therapy should begin with metoclopramide injection.

Administration of metoclopramide injection up to 10 days may be required before symptoms subside, at which time oral administration may be instituted. Since diabetic gastric stasis is frequently recurrent, METOZOLV ODT therapy should be reinstituted at the earliest manifestation.

2.4 Renal Impairment
Some patients, such as the elderly or those with impaired kidney function (creatinine clearance below 40 mL/min) may be more sensitive to the therapeutic dose or the adverse effects of metoclopramide. Therefore, these patients should start therapy at a lower dose (approximately half the recommended dosage) and the dose should be titrated according to their overall clinical response and/or adverse event profile. Dialysis is not likely to be an effective method of drug removal in overdose situations.

3 DOSAGE FORMS AND STRENGTHS
5 mg Tablets: Each white round 5 mg tablet is debossed with "5" on one side and plain on the other.
10 mg Tablets: Each white round 10 mg tablet is debossed with "10" on one side and plain on the other.

4 CONTRAINDICATIONS

4.1 Intestinal Obstruction, Hemorrhage, or Perforation
Do not use Metoclopramide whenever stimulation of gastrointestinal motility may be dangerous such as in the presence of gastrointestinal hemorrhage, mechanical obstruction, or perforation.

4.2 Pheochromocytoma
Metoclopramide is contraindicated in patients with pheochromocytoma because the drug may precipitate a hypertensive crisis, most likely due to release of catecholamines from the tumor. Such hypertensive crises may be controlled by phentolamine.

4.3 Known Sensitivity or Intolerance
Metoclopramide is contraindicated in patients with known sensitivity or intolerance to the drug.

4.4 Epilepsy
Do not use Metoclopramide in patients with epilepsy since the frequency and severity of seizures may be increased.

4.5 Concomitant Medications with Extrapyramidal Reactions
Do not use Metoclopramide in patients receiving other drugs which are likely to cause extrapyramidal reactions, since the frequency and severity of extrapyramidal reactions may be increased *[see Warnings and Precautions (5.2), Adverse Reactions (6.2) and Drug Interactions (7.5)]*.

5 WARNINGS AND PRECAUTIONS

5.1 Tardive Dyskinesia
Treatment with metoclopramide can cause tardive dyskinesia (TD) *[see Boxed Warning]*, a potentially irreversible and disfiguring disorder characterized by involuntary movements of the face, tongue, or extremities. Although the risk of TD with metoclopramide has not been extensively studied, one published study reported a TD prevalence of 20% among patients treated for at least 12 weeks. Treatment with metoclopramide for longer than 12 weeks should be avoided in all but rare cases where therapeutic benefit is thought to outweigh the risk of developing TD.

Although the risk of developing TD in the general population may be increased among the elderly, women, and diabetics, it is not possible to predict which patients will develop metoclopramide-induced TD. Both the risk of developing TD and the likelihood that TD will become irreversible increase with duration of treatment and total cumulative dose.

Metoclopramide should be discontinued in patients who develop signs or symptoms of TD. There is no known effective treatment for established cases of TD, although in some patients, TD may remit, partially or completely, within several weeks to months after metoclopramide is withdrawn.

Metoclopramide itself may suppress, or partially suppress, the signs of TD, thereby masking the underlying disease process. The effect of this symptomatic suppression upon the long-term course of TD is unknown. Therefore, metoclopramide should not be used for the symptomatic control of TD.

5.2 Acute Dystonic Reactions, Drug-induced Parkinsonism, and Other Extrapyramidal Symptoms
Extrapyramidal symptoms (EPS), manifested primarily as acute dystonic reactions, occur in approximately 1 in 500 patients treated with the usual adult dosages of 30 to 40 mg/day of metoclopramide. These usually are seen during the first 24 to 48 hours of treatment with metoclopramide, occur more frequently in pediatric patients and adult patients less than 30 years of age and are even more frequent at higher doses. These symptoms may include involuntary movements of limbs and facial grimacing, torticollis, oculogyric crisis, rhythmic protrusion of tongue, bulbar type of speech, trismus, or dystonic reactions resembling tetanus. Rarely, dystonic reactions may present as stridor and dyspnea, possibly due to laryngospasm. If these symptoms occur, inject 50 mg diphenhydramine hydrochloride intramuscularly. Benztropine mesylate, 1 to 2 mg intramuscularly, may also be used to reverse these reactions.

Drug-induced Parkinsonism can occur during metoclopramide therapy, more commonly within the first 6 months after beginning treatment, but also after longer periods. Parkinsonian symptoms generally subside within 2 to 3 months following discontinuation of metoclopramide. Patients with a history of Parkinson's disease should be given metoclopramide cautiously, if at all, since such patients can experience exacerbation of Parkinsonian symptoms when taking metoclopramide.

5.3 Neuroleptic Malignant Syndrome
There have been rare reports of an uncommon but potentially fatal symptom complex sometimes referred to as Neuroleptic Malignant Syndrome (NMS) associated with metoclopramide. Clinical manifestations of NMS include hyperthermia, muscle rigidity, altered consciousness, and

evidence of autonomic instability (irregular pulse or blood pressure, tachycardia, diaphoresis and cardiac arrhythmias). The diagnostic evaluation of patients with this syndrome is complicated. In arriving at a diagnosis, it is important to identify cases where the clinical presentation includes both serious medical illness (e.g., pneumonia, systemic infection) and untreated or inadequately treated extrapyramidal signs and symptoms (EPS). Other important considerations in the differential diagnosis include central anticholinergic toxicity, heat stroke, malignant hyperthermia, drug fever and primary central nervous system (CNS) pathology. The management of NMS should include immediate discontinuation of metoclopramide and other drugs not essential to concurrent therapy; intensive symptomatic treatment and medical monitoring; and, treatment of any concomitant serious medical problems for which specific treatments are available. Bromocriptine and dantrolene sodium have been used in treatment of NMS, but their effectiveness has not been established [see Adverse Reactions (6)].

5.4 Depression
Depression associated with metoclopramide use has occurred in patients with and without a history of depression. Symptoms ranged from mild to severe and included suicidal ideation and suicide. For those patients with a prior history of depression, metoclopramide should only be given if the expected benefits outweigh the potential risks.

5.5 Hypertension
In one study in hypertensive patients, intravenously administered metoclopramide was shown to release catecholamines; hence, caution should be exercised when metoclopramide is used in patients with hypertension. There are also clinical reports of hypertensive crises in some patients with undiagnosed pheochromocytoma, thus any rapid rise in blood pressure associated with METOZOLV ODT use should result in immediate cessation of metoclopramide use in those patients [see Contraindications (4.2)].

5.6 Congestive Heart Failure and Ventricular Arrhythmia
Since metoclopramide produces a transient increase in plasma aldosterone, patients with cirrhosis or congestive heart failure may be at risk of developing fluid retention and volume overload. If these side effects occur at any time in any patients during metoclopramide therapy, the drug should be discontinued.

5.7 Withdrawal from Metoclopramide
Adverse reactions, especially those involving the nervous system, may occur after stopping the use of METOZOLV ODT. A small number of patients may experience withdrawal symptoms after stopping that could include dizziness, nervousness, and/or headaches.

6 ADVERSE REACTIONS
6.1 Clinical Trials Experience
Because clinical trials are conducted under widely varying conditions, adverse reaction rates observed in the clinical trials of a drug cannot be directly compared to rates in the clinical studies of another drug and may not reflect the rates observed in clinical practice.

A total of 86 subjects entered three studies with METOZOLV ODT; 12 subjects entered a pilot bioavailability study (BA); 44 subjects entered a bioequivalence (BE) study, and 30 subjects entered a food-effect study. The adverse reactions from the BE and food-effect study are summarized in Table 1. The pilot BA study data are not included because it was performed with a formulation different from the METOZOLV ODT formulation.

The adverse experience profile seen with METOZOLV ODT was similar to metoclopramide tablets. Thirty-three (33) adverse reactions were reported after receiving METOZOLV ODT and 30 adverse reactions were reported after receiving metoclopramide tablets.

Table 1: Adverse Reactions in BE and Food-Effect Study in ≥ 2% of Subjects

Adverse Reaction	METOZOLV ODT $N^{1,3}$ (%)[2]	Metoclopramide tablets $N^{1,4}$ (%)[2]
Nausea	4 (4.2%)	4 (5.6%)
Vomiting	2 (2.1%)	1 (1.4%)
Fatigue	2 (2.1%)	2 (2.8%)
Headache	5 (5.2%)	3 (4.2%)
Somnolence	2 (2.1%)	2 (2.8%)
Dizziness	1 (1.0%)	3 (4.2%)

[1] N = number of subjects that reported adverse reactions

[2] Percent (%) occurrence = N divided by number of subjects dosed with respective study drug

[3] Number of subjects dosed with METOZOLV ODT: 68 under fasted conditions and 28 under fed conditions.

[4] Number of subjects dosed with metoclopramide tablets: 28 under fed conditions and 44 under fasted conditions.

The most frequently reported adverse reactions (greater than 2%) associated with METOZOLV ODT were: nausea, vomiting, fatigue, somnolence and headache. The most frequently reported adverse reactions (greater than 2%) associated with metoclopramide tablets were: nausea, headache, fatigue, somnolence, and dizziness. The combined data from the fasted BE study and the food-effect study did not demonstrate any significant differences in the adverse event profile for METOZOLV ODT compared to metoclopramide tablets.

6.2 Post-Marketing Experience
The following adverse reactions are from the cumulative post-marketing experience with metoclopramide tablets. Since the reactions are reported voluntarily from a population of uncertain size, it is not always possible to reliably estimate their frequency or establish a causal relationship to drug exposure.

CNS Effects: Restlessness, drowsiness, fatigue, and lassitude occur in approximately 10% of patients receiving the most commonly prescribed dosage of 10 mg four times a day. Insomnia, headache, confusion, dizziness, or depression with suicidal ideation occurs less frequently. The incidence of drowsiness is greater at higher doses. There are isolated reports of seizures without clear-cut relationship to metoclopramide. Rarely, hallucinations have been reported.

Extrapyramidal Syndromes (EPS):
Acute dystonic reactions, the most common type of EPS associated with metoclopramide, occur in approximately 0.2% of patients (1 in 500) treated with 30 to 40 mg of metoclopramide per day. Symptoms include involuntary movements of limbs, facial grimacing, torticollis, oculogyric crisis, rhythmic protrusion of tongue, bulbar type of speech, trismus, opisthotonus (tetanus-like reactions), and rarely, stridor and dyspnea possibly due to laryngospasm; ordinarily these symptoms are readily reversed by diphenhydramine [see Warnings and Precautions (5.1)].

Drug-induced Parkinsonian-like symptoms may include bradykinesia, tremor, cogwheel rigidity, mask-like facies [see Warnings and Precautions (5.2)].

Tardive dyskinesia is most frequently characterized by involuntary movements of the tongue, face, mouth, or jaw, and sometimes by involuntary movements of the trunk and/or extremities; movements may be choreoathetotic in appearance. Motor restlessness (akathisia) may include inability to sit still, pacing, and foot tapping. These symptoms may disappear spontaneously or respond to a reduction in dosage.

Neuroleptic Malignant Syndrome: Rare occurrences of Neuroleptic Malignant Syndrome (NMS) have been reported [see Warnings and Precautions (5.3)].

Endocrine Disturbances: Galactorrhea, amenorrhea, gynecomastia, and impotence secondary to hyperprolactinemia. Fluid retention secondary to transient elevation of aldosterone.

Cardiovascular: Hypotension, hypertension, supraventricular tachycardia, bradycardia, fluid retention, acute congestive heart failure, possible AV block.

Gastrointestinal: Nausea, bowel disturbances, primarily diarrhea.

Hepatic: Rarely, cases of hepatotoxicity characterized by such findings as jaundice and altered liver function tests, when metoclopramide was administered with other drugs with known hepatotoxic potential.

Renal: Urinary frequency and incontinence.

Hematologic: A few cases of neutropenia, leukopenia, or agranulocytosis, generally without clear-cut relationship to metoclopramide. Methemoglobinemia in adults and especially with overdosage in neonates. Sulfhemoglobinemia in adults.

Allergic Reactions: A few cases of rash, urticaria, or bronchospasm, especially in patients with a history of asthma. Rarely, angioneurotic edema, including glossal or laryngeal edema.

Miscellaneous: Visual disturbances. Porphyria.

7 DRUG INTERACTIONS
The effects of metoclopramide on gastrointestinal motility can impact the absorption of other drugs. The known drug-drug interactions are listed below.

7.1 Anticholinergic and Narcotic Analgesic Drugs
The effects of metoclopramide on gastrointestinal motility are antagonized by anticholinergic drugs and narcotic analgesics. Additive sedative effects can occur when metoclopramide is given with alcohol, sedatives, hypnotics, narcotics, or tranquilizers.

7.2 Monoamine Oxidase Inhibitors
Metoclopramide has been shown to release catecholamines in patients with essential hypertension suggests that it should be used cautiously, if at all, in patients taking monoamine oxidase (MAO) inhibitors.

7.3 Drug Absorption
Absorption of drugs from the stomach may be diminished by metoclopramide (e.g., digoxin), whereas the rate and/or extent of absorption of drugs from the small bowel may be increased (e.g., acetaminophen, tetracycline, levodopa, ethanol, cyclosporine).

7.4 Insulin
Because the action of metoclopramide will hasten the movement of food to the intestines and therefore the rate of absorption, insulin dosage or timing of dosage may require adjustment. Increasing movement of food to the intestines may lead to absorption of less glucose from a meal, hence less glucose in the circulation for a particular dose of administered insulin to act upon, resulting in hypoglycemia.

7.5 Antidepressants, Antipsychotics, and Neuroleptics
Concomitant use of metoclopramide should be avoided in patients taking antidepressants, antipsychotics, and/or neuroleptics that have been associated with extrapyramidal reactions such as tardive dyskinesia or Neuroleptic Malignant Syndrome (NMS) that have occurred in association with metoclopramide [see Warnings and Precautions (5.2), (5.3) and Adverse Reactions (6.2)].

8 USE IN SPECIFIC POPULATIONS
8.1 Pregnancy
Teratogenic Effects: Pregnancy Category B
Reproduction studies have been performed in rats at oral doses about 6 times the maximum recommended human dose calculated on the basis of surface area, and in rabbits at oral doses about 12 times the maximum recommended human dose calculated on the basis of surface area, and have revealed no evidence of impaired fertility or harm to the fetus due to metoclopramide. There are, however, no adequate and well-controlled studies in pregnant women. Because animal reproduction studies are not always predictive of human response, this drug should be used during pregnancy only if clearly needed.

8.2 Labor and Delivery
The use of metoclopramide in labor and delivery has not been studied.

8.3 Nursing Mothers
Metoclopramide is excreted in human milk. Caution should be exercised when metoclopramide is administered to a nursing mother. Because of the potential for serious adverse reactions from metoclopramide in nursing infants and because of the potential for tumorigenicity (including tumor promoting potential in rats), a decision should be made whether to discontinue nursing or to discontinue the drug, taking into account the importance of the drug to the mother.

8.4 Pediatric Use
The safety and effectiveness of METOZOLV ODT in pediatric patients have not been established.

The safety profile of METOZOLV ODT in adults cannot be extrapolated to pediatric patients. Dystonias and other extrapyramidal reactions associated with metoclopramide are more common in the pediatric population than in adults. In addition, neonates have reduced levels of NADH-cytochrome b5 reductase making them more susceptible to methemoglobinemia, a possible side effect of metoclopramide use in neonates.

Pediatric PK
The pharmacodynamics of metoclopramide following oral and intravenous administration in pediatric populations are highly variable and a concentration-effect relationship has not been established. Thus, there are insufficient data to conclude whether the pharmacokinetics of METOZOLV ODT in adults and the pediatric population are similar. Although there are insufficient data to support the efficacy of metoclopramide in pediatric patients with symptomatic gastroesophageal reflux disease (GERD) or cancer chemotherapy-related nausea and vomiting, the pharmacokinetics of metoclopramide have been studied in these patient populations and are summarized as follows.

In an open-label study, six pediatric patients (ranging in age from 3.5 weeks to 5.4 months) with GERD received metoclopramide 0.15 mg/kg oral solution every 6 hours for 10 doses. The mean peak plasma concentration of metoclopramide after the tenth dose was twice the level (56.8 mcg/L) compared to after the first dose (29 mcg/L) indicating drug accumulation with repeated dosing. However, the PK parameters after the tenth dose were comparable to those observed after the first dose for the mean time to reach peak concentrations (2.2 hr); half-life (4.1 hr); clearance (0.67 L/h/kg); and volume of distribution (4.4 L/kg). The youngest patient (3.5 weeks) showed a significantly longer half-life after the first dose (23.1 hr) compared to after the tenth dose (10.3 hr), suggesting the reduced clearance observed at birth may be a reflection of the immature hepatic and renal systems.

8.5 Geriatric Use

Clinical studies of metoclopramide did not include sufficient numbers of subjects aged 65 and over to determine whether elderly subjects respond differently from younger subjects. The risk of developing drug-induced Parkinsonism due to metoclopramide is dose-related. Geriatric patients should receive the lowest dose that is effective. If drug-induced Parkinsonism symptoms develop in a geriatric patient, METOZOLV ODT should be discontinued. The elderly may be at greater risk for tardive dyskinesia [see *Warnings and Precautions (5.1)*].

Sedation is a potential adverse event associated with metoclopramide use in the elderly.

Metoclopramide is known to be substantially excreted by the kidney, and the risk of toxic reactions to this drug may be greater in patients with impaired renal function. For these reasons, dose selection for an elderly patient should be cautious, starting at the low end of the dosing range, due to the greater frequency of decreased renal function, concomitant disease, or other drug therapy in the elderly. [see *Warnings and Precautions (5.4)*].

8.6 Other Special Populations

Patients with NADH-cytochrome b5 reductase deficiency are at an increased risk of developing methemoglobinemia and/or sulfhemoglobinemia when metoclopramide is administered. In patients with G6PD deficiency who experience metoclopramide-induced methemoglobinemia, methylene blue treatment is not recommended.

Since metoclopramide is excreted principally through the kidneys, therapy should be initiated at approximately one-half the recommended dose in those patients whose creatinine clearance is below 40 mL/min. Depending upon clinical efficacy and safety considerations, the dosage may be increased or decreased as appropriate. Metoclopramide has been safely used in patients with advanced liver disease whose renal function was normal.

10 OVERDOSAGE

Symptoms of overdosage may include drowsiness, disorientation, and extrapyramidal reactions. Anticholinergic or anti-Parkinson drugs or antihistamines with anticholinergic properties may be helpful in controlling the extrapyramidal reactions. Symptoms are self-limiting and may disappear within 24 hours.

Hemodialysis removes relatively little metoclopramide, probably because of the small amount of the drug in blood relative to tissues. Similarly, continuous ambulatory peritoneal dialysis does not remove significant amounts of drug. It is unlikely that dosage would need to be adjusted to compensate for losses through dialysis. Dialysis is not likely to be an effective method of drug removal in overdose situations.

Unintentional overdose has been reported in infants and children with the use of metoclopramide oral solution. While there was no consistent pattern to the reports associated with these overdoses, events included seizures, extrapyramidal reactions, and lethargy.

Methemoglobinemia has occurred in premature and full-term neonates who were given overdoses of metoclopramide (1 to 4 mg/kg/day orally, intramuscularly or intravenously for 1 to 3 or more days). Methemoglobinemia can be reversed by the intravenous administration of methylene blue. However, methylene blue may cause hemolytic anemia in patients with G6PD deficiency, which may be fatal.

11 DESCRIPTION

METOZOLV ODT is an orally disintegrating tablet formulation of metoclopramide hydrochloride. The 5 mg strength is a round white tablet debossed on one side with a "5" and plain on the other side; it is comprised of 5 mg metoclopramide (as 5.91 mg of metoclopramide hydrochloride) with gelatin, mannitol, mint flavoring, and Acesulfame K (artificial sweetener). The 10 mg strength is a round white tablet debossed on one side with a "10" and plain on the other side; it is comprised of 10 mg metoclopramide (as 11.82 mg of metoclopramide hydrochloride) with gelatin, mannitol, mint flavoring, and Acesulfame K.

The active ingredient, metoclopramide hydrochloride, is a white crystalline, odorless substance, freely soluble in water. Chemically, it is 4-amino-5-chloro-N-[2-(diethylamino)ethyl]-2-methoxy benzamide monohydrochloride monohydrate. Its molecular formula is $C_{14}H_{22}ClN_3O_2 \bullet HCl \bullet H_2O$. Its molecular weight is 354.3. The structural formula is shown in Figure 1.

Figure 1

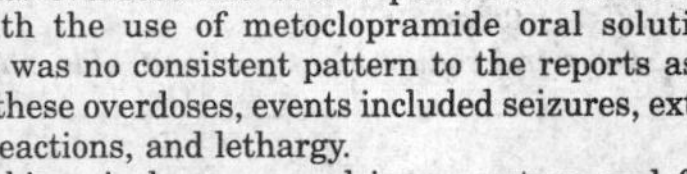

METOZOLV ODT includes the following inactive ingredients: gelatin, mannitol, mint flavoring, Acesulfame potassium (artificial sweetener), and trace amounts of sodium chloride and sodium hydroxide.

12 CLINICAL PHARMACOLOGY

12.1 Mechanism of Action

Metoclopramide stimulates motility of the upper gastrointestinal tract without stimulating gastric, biliary, or pancreatic secretions. While its mode of action is unclear, it appears to sensitize tissues to the action of acetylcholine. The effect on motility is not dependent on intact vagal innervation, but can be abolished by anticholinergic drugs. Metoclopramide increases the tone and amplitude of gastric (especially antral) contractions, relaxes the pyloric sphincter and the duodenal bulb, and increases peristalsis of the duodenum and jejunum resulting in accelerated gastric emptying and intestinal transit. It increases the resting tone of the lower esophageal sphincter. It has little, if any, effect on the motility of the colon or gallbladder.

The antiemetic properties of metoclopramide appear to be a result of its antagonism of central and peripheral dopamine receptors. Dopamine produces nausea and vomiting by stimulation of the medullary chemoreceptor trigger zone (CTZ), and metoclopramide blocks stimulation of the CTZ by agents like l-dopa or apomorphine, which are known to increase dopamine levels or to possess dopamine-like effects. Metoclopramide also abolishes the slowing of gastric emptying caused by apomorphine. Like the phenothiazines and related drugs, which are also dopamine antagonists, metoclopramide produces sedation and may produce extrapyramidal reactions [see *Warnings and Precautions (5.2), (5.3)*]. Metoclopramide inhibits the central and peripheral effects of apomorphine, induces release of prolactin, and causes a transient increase in circulating aldosterone levels, which may be associated with transient fluid retention.

12.2 Pharmacodynamics

The onset of pharmacological action of metoclopramide is 30 to 60 minutes following an oral dose; pharmacological effects persist for 1 to 2 hours. In patients with gastroesophageal reflux and low LESP (lower esophageal sphincter pressure), single oral doses of metoclopramide produce dose-related increases in LESP. Effects begin at about 5 mg and increase through 20 mg (the largest dose tested). The increase in LESP from a 5 mg dose lasts about 45 minutes and that of a 20 mg dose lasts between 2 and 3 hours. Increased rate of stomach emptying has been observed with single oral doses of 10 mg.

The principal effect of metoclopramide is on symptoms of post-prandial and daytime heartburn with less observed effect on nocturnal symptoms. If symptoms are confined to particular situations, such as following the evening meal, use of metoclopramide as single doses prior to the provocative situation should be considered, rather than using the drug throughout the day. Healing of esophageal ulcers and erosions has been endoscopically demonstrated at the end of a 12-week trial using doses of 15 mg taken four times a day. As there is no documented correlation between symptoms and healing of esophageal lesions, patients with documented lesions should be monitored endoscopically. For gastroparesis, the usual manifestations of delayed gastric emptying (e.g., nausea, vomiting, heartburn, persistent fullness after meals, and anorexia) appear to respond within different time intervals.

12.3 Pharmacokinetics

Adult PK of METOZOLV ODT

In a randomized, two-arm, two-way crossover study in 44 healthy adult (male and female) fasted subjects, METOZOLV ODT was bioequivalent to Reglan Tablets.

In a food-effect study with 28 subjects, METOZOLV ODT taken immediately after a high-fat meal had a 17% lower peak blood level than when taken after an overnight fast. The time to peak blood levels increased from about 1.75 hours under fasted conditions to 3 hours when taken immediately after a high-fat meal. The extent of metoclopramide absorbed (area under the curve) was comparable whether METOZOLV ODT was administered with or without food. The clinical effect of the decrease in peak plasma level if METOZOLV ODT is inadvertently taken with food is unknown.

Adult PK of Metoclopramide

Metoclopramide is rapidly and well absorbed. Relative to an intravenous dose of 20 mg, the absolute oral bioavailability of metoclopramide is 80% ± 15.5% as demonstrated in a crossover study of 18 subjects. Peak plasma concentrations occur at about 1 to 2 hr after a single oral dose. Similar time to peak is observed after individual doses at steady state. A single dose study of 12 subjects showed that the area under the drug concentration-time curve increases linearly with doses from 20 to 100 mg (results summarized in Table 2). Peak concentrations increase linearly with dose; time to peak concentrations remains the same; whole body clearance is unchanged; and the elimination rate remains the same. The average elimination half-life in individuals with normal renal function is 5 to 6 hr. Linear kinetic processes adequately describe the absorption and elimination of metoclopramide.

Table 2: Adult Pharmacokinetic Data

Parameter	Value
Vd (L/kg)	~ 3.5
Plasma Protein Binding	~ 30%
T ½	5 to 6 hours
Oral Bioavailability	80% ± 15.5%

Approximately 85% of the radioactivity of an orally administered dose appears in the urine within 72 hr. Of the 85% eliminated in the urine, about half is present as free or conjugated metoclopramide.

The drug is not extensively bound to plasma proteins (about 30%). The whole body volume of distribution is high (about 3.5 L/kg) which suggests extensive distribution of drug to the tissues.

The *in vivo* disintegration time (time reported between placing the tablet on the tongue and it completely disintegrated into fine particles) was approximately one minute (with a range of 10 seconds to 14 minutes). In the two clinical trials (N = 96) with a mean ± SD being 76.8 ± 110.6 seconds and a median of 53.5 seconds.

Renal impairment affects the clearance of metoclopramide. In a study with patients with varying degrees of renal impairment, a reduction in creatinine clearance was correlated with a reduction in plasma clearance, renal clearance, non-renal clearance, and increase in elimination half-life. The kinetics of metoclopramide in the presence of renal impairment remained linear. The reduction in clearance as a result of renal impairment suggests that reduction of maintenance dosage should be done to avoid drug accumulation.

13 NONCLINICAL TOXICOLOGY

13.1 Carcinogenesis, Mutagenesis, Impairment of Fertility

A 77-week study was conducted in rats with oral doses up to 40 mg/kg/day (about 5 times the maximum recommended human dose on surface area basis). Metoclopramide elevates prolactin levels and the elevation persists during chronic administration. Tissue culture experiments indicate that approximately one-third of human breast cancers are prolactin-dependent *in vitro*, a factor of potential importance if the prescription of metoclopramide is contemplated in a patient with previously detected breast cancer. Although disturbances such as galactorrhea, amenorrhea, gynecomastia, and impotence have been reported with prolactin-elevating drugs, the clinical significance of elevated serum prolactin levels is unknown for most patients. An increase in mammary neoplasms has been found in rodents after chronic administration of prolactin-stimulating neuroleptic drugs and metoclopramide. Neither clinical studies nor epidemiologic studies conducted to date, however, have shown an association between chronic administration of these drugs and mammary tumorigenesis; the available evidence is too limited to be conclusive at this time.

In a rat model for assessing the tumor promotion potential, a two-week oral treatment with metoclopramide at a dose of 260 mg/kg/day (about 35 times the maximum recommended human dose based on body surface area) enhanced the tumorigenic effect of N-nitrosodiethylamine.

Metoclopramide was positive in the *in vitro* Chinese hamster lung cell/HGPRT forward mutation assay for mutagenic effects and the *in vitro* human lymphocyte chromosome aberration assay for clastogenic effects. It was negative in the *in vitro* Ames mutation assay, the *in vitro* unscheduled DNA synthesis (UDS) assay with rat and human hepatocytes and the *in vivo* rat micronucleus assay.

Metoclopramide at intramuscular doses up to 20 mg/kg/day (about 3 times the maximum recommended human dose based on body surface area) was found to have no effect on fertility and reproductive performance of male and female rats.

16 HOW SUPPLIED/STORAGE AND HANDLING

5 mg Tablets: Available in blister pack with 10 tablets individually sealed in a foil-backed unit-dose container; a carton contains 10 cards (NDC 65649-431-02).

10 mg Tablets: Available in blister pack with 10 tablets individually sealed in a foil-backed unit-dose container; a carton contains 10 cards (NDC 65649-432-02).

Tablets should be stored at controlled room temperature, between 20°C and 25°C (68°F and 77°F).

17 PATIENT COUNSELING INFORMATION

- Instruct patients to take METOZOLV ODT at least 30 minutes before eating and at bedtime.

- A patient Medication Guide is available for METOZOLV ODT and printed at the end of the prescribing information. Instruct patients, families, and caregivers to read the Medication Guide and assist them in understanding its contents.
- Inform patients or their caregivers of serious potential issues associated with metoclopramide use such as tardive dyskinesia, extrapyramidal symptoms, and neuroleptic malignant syndrome. Advise patients to inform their physician if symptoms associated with these disorders occur during or after treatment with METOZOLV ODT.
- Inform patients that METOZOLV ODT may cause drowsiness, dizziness, or otherwise impair mental alertness or physical abilities required for the performance of hazardous tasks such as operating machinery or driving a motor vehicle. Sedation may be more pronounced in the elderly.
- Inform patients that the most common adverse reactions in patients treated with METOZOLV ODT or other metoclopramide-containing products are headache, nausea, vomiting, tiredness, sleepiness, dizziness, and restlessness.

Manufactured by:
Catalent UK Swindon Zydis Limited
Swindon, UK
Manufactured for:
Salix Pharmaceuticals, Inc.
Morrisville, North Carolina
VENART-144-0/Sep 2009

Medication Guide
METOZOLV™ (MĔ-tō-zolv) ODT
(metoclopramide hydrochloride)
Orally Disintegrating Tablets
Read the Medication Guide that comes with METOZOLV ODT before you take it and each time you get a refill. There may be new information. If you take another product that contains metoclopramide (such as REGLAN tablets, REGLAN ODT, REGLAN injection or metoclopramide oral solution), you should read the Medication Guide that comes with that product. Some of the information may be different. This Medication Guide does not take the place of talking with your doctor about your medical condition or your treatment.

What is the most important information I should know about METOZOLV ODT?
METOZOLV ODT can cause serious side effects, including:
Abnormal muscle movements called tardive dyskinesia (TD). These movements happen mostly in the face muscles. You cannot control these movements. They may not go away even after stopping METOZOLV ODT. There is no treatment for TD, but symptoms may lessen or go away over time after you stop taking METOZOLV ODT.
Your chances for getting TD go up:
- the longer you take METOZOLV ODT and the more METOZOLV ODT you take. You should not take METOZOLV ODT for more than 12 weeks.
- if you are older, especially if you are an older woman
- if you have diabetes
It is not possible for your doctor to know if **you** will get TD if you take METOZOLV ODT.
Call your doctor right away if you have movements you can not stop or control, such as:
- lip smacking, chewing, or puckering of your lips
- frowning or scowling
- sticking out your tongue
- blinking and moving your eyes
- shaking of your arms and legs
See the section "What are the possible side effects of METOZOLV ODT?" for more information about side effects.
What is METOZOLV ODT?
METOZOLV ODT is a prescription medicine used in adults:
- for 4 to 12 weeks to relieve heartburn symptoms of gastroesophageal reflux disease (GERD) when certain other treatments do not work.
- to relieve the symptoms of slow stomach emptying in people with diabetes.
It is not known if METOZOLV ODT is safe or works in children.
Who should not take METOZOLV ODT?
Do not take METOZOLV ODT if you:
- have stomach or intestine problems that could get worse with METOZOLV ODT, such as bleeding, blockage or a tear in your stomach or bowel wall
- have an adrenal tumor called pheochromocytoma
- are allergic to metoclopramide or any of the ingredients in METOZOLV ODT. See the end of this Medication Guide for a list of ingredients in METOZOLV ODT.
- take medicines that can cause uncontrolled movements, such as medicines for mental illness
- have seizures
What should I tell my doctor before taking METOZOLV ODT?
Before you take METOZOLV ODT, tell your doctor if you:
- have kidney or liver disease
- have depression or mental illness

- have high blood pressure
- have heart failure or heart rhythm problems
- have diabetes. Your dose of insulin may need to be changed.
- have Parkinson's disease
- have any other medical conditions
- drink alcohol
- are pregnant or plan to become pregnant. It is not known if METOZOLV ODT will harm your unborn baby.
- are breast-feeding or plan to breast-feed. METOZOLV ODT can pass into your milk and may harm your baby. You and your doctor should decide if you will take METOZOLV ODT or breast-feed. You should not do both.

Tell your doctor about all the medicines you take, including prescription and non-prescription medicines, vitamins, and herbal supplements. METOZOLV ODT and some medicines can affect each other and may not work as well, or cause possible side effects. Do not start any new medicine while taking METOZOLV ODT until you talk with your doctor.
Especially tell your doctor if you take:
- another medicine that contains metoclopramide, such as REGLAN tablets, REGLAN ODT, or metoclopramide oral syrup
- a blood pressure medicine
- a medicine for depression, especially a monoamine oxidase inhibitor (MAOI)
- an anti-psychotic medicine
- insulin
- medicines that can make you sleepy, such as anti-anxiety medicines, sleep medicines, and narcotics.
Ask your doctor or pharmacist if you are not sure if your medication is listed above.
Know the medicines you take. Keep a list of your medicines to show your doctor and pharmacist when you get new medicine.
How should I take METOZOLV ODT?
- METOZOLV ODT comes as a tablet that melts in your mouth.
- Take METOZOLV ODT exactly as prescribed by your doctor. Do not change your dose unless your doctor tells you to.
- You should not take METOZOLV ODT for more than 12 weeks.
- Take METOZOLV ODT at least 30 minutes before eating and at bedtime.
To take METOZOLV ODT:
1. Leave the tablet in the sealed blister METOZOLV ODT pack until you are ready to take it.
2. Use dry hands to open a blister and take out a tablet. If the tablet breaks or crumbles throw it away and take a new tablet out of the blister pack.
3. Put the tablet on your tongue right away. Let it melt and then swallow. You do not need water to take METOZOLV ODT.
If you take too much METOZOLV ODT, call your doctor or Poison Control Center.
What should I avoid while taking METOZOLV ODT?
- Do not drink alcohol while taking METOZOLV ODT. Alcohol may make some side effects of METOZOLV ODT worse, such as feeling sleepy.
- Do not drive, work with machines, or do dangerous tasks until you know how METOZOLV ODT affects you. METOZOLV ODT may cause sleepiness.
What are the possible side effects of METOZOLV ODT?
METOZOLV ODT can cause serious side effects, including:
- **Abnormal muscle movements.** See "What is the most important information I should know about METOZOLV ODT?"
- **Uncontrolled spasms of your face and neck muscles, or muscles of your body, arms, and legs (dystonia).** These muscle spasms can cause abnormal movements and body positions. These spasms usually start within the first 2 days of treatment. These spasms happen more often in children and adults younger than 30.
- **Depression, thoughts about suicide, and suicide.** Some people who take METOZOLV ODT may become depressed. You may have thoughts about hurting or killing yourself. Some people who have taken metoclopramide products have ended their own lives (suicide).
- **Neuroleptic Malignant Syndrome (NMS).** NMS is a rare but very serious condition that can happen with METOZOLV ODT. NMS can cause death and must be treated in a hospital. Symptoms of NMS include: high fever, stiff muscles, problems thinking, very fast or uneven heartbeat, and increased sweating.
- **Parkinsonism.** Symptoms include slight shaking, body stiffness, trouble moving or keeping your balance. If you have Parkinson's Disease, your symptoms may become worse while you are taking METOZOLV ODT.
- **High blood pressure.** METOZOLV ODT can cause your blood pressure to increase.
- **Too much body water.** People who have certain liver problems or heart failure and take METOZOLV ODT may

hold too much water in their body (fluid retention). Tell your doctor right away if you have sudden weight gain, or swelling of your hands, legs, or feet.
Call your doctor and get medical help right away if you:
- feel depressed or have thoughts about hurting or killing yourself
- have high fever, stiff muscles, problems thinking, very fast or uneven heartbeat, and increased sweating
- have muscle movements you cannot stop or control
- have muscle movements that are new or unusual
The most common side effects of METOZOLV ODT are:
- headache
- nausea
- vomiting
- tiredness
- sleepiness
You may have more side effects the longer you take METOZOLV ODT and the more METOZOLV ODT you take. You may still have side effects after you stop METOZOLV ODT. You may have symptoms from stopping (withdrawal) METOZOLV ODT such as headaches, and feeling dizzy or nervous.
Tell your doctor about any side effects that bother you or do not go away. These are not all the possible side effects of METOZOLV ODT.
Call your doctor for medical advice about side effects. You may report side effects to FDA at 1–800–FDA-1088.
How do I store METOZOLV ODT?
- Store METOZOLV ODT at room temperature, between 68°F to 77°F (20°C to 25°C).
- Keep METOZOLV ODT away from moisture.
- Throw away any METOZOLV ODT that is not used.
Keep METOZOLV ODT and all medicines away from children.
General information about METOZOLV ODT
Medicines are sometimes prescribed for purposes other than those listed in a Medication Guide. Do not use METOZOLV ODT for a condition for which it was not prescribed. Do not give METOZOLV ODT to other people, even if they have the same symptoms that you have. It may harm them.
This Medication Guide summarizes the most important information about METOZOLV ODT. If you would like more information about METOZOLV ODT, talk with your doctor. You can ask your doctor or pharmacist for information about METOZOLV ODT that is written for health professionals. For more information, call 1-866-669-7597.
What are the ingredients in METOZOLV ODT?
Active ingredients: metoclopramide hydrochloride
Inactive ingredients: gelatin, mannitol, mint flavoring, Acesulfame potassium (artificial sweetener), and trace amounts of sodium chloride and sodium hydroxide
Salix Pharmaceuticals, Inc.
Morrisville, NC 27560, USA
This Medication Guide has been approved by the U.S. Food and Drug Administration.
VENART-144-0/Sep 2009
Shown in Product Identification Guide, page 318

MOVIPREP®   ℞
[Movi-Prep]
(PEG-3350, Sodium Sulfate, Sodium Chloride, Potassium Chloride, Sodium Ascorbate and Ascorbic Acid for Oral Solution)

DESCRIPTION
MoviPrep® consists of 4 separate pouches (2 of pouch A and 2 of pouch B) containing white to yellow powder for reconstitution. Each pouch A contains 100 grams of polyethylene glycol (PEG) 3350, NF, 7.5 grams of sodium sulfate, USP, 2.691 grams of sodium chloride, USP, and 1.015 grams of potassium chloride, USP, plus the following excipients: aspartame, NF (sweetener), acesulfame potassium, NF (sweetener), and lemon flavoring. Each pouch B contains 4.7 grams of ascorbic acid, USP and 5.9 grams of sodium ascorbate, USP. When 1 pouch A and 1 pouch B are dissolved together in water to a volume of 1 liter, MoviPrep® (PEG-3350, sodium sulfate, sodium chloride, potassium chloride, sodium ascorbate, and ascorbic acid) is an oral solution having a lemon taste.
The entire, reconstituted, 2-liter MoviPrep® colon preparation contains 200 grams of PEG-3350, 15 grams of sodium sulfate, 5.38 grams of sodium chloride, 2.03 grams of potassium chloride, 9.4 grams of ascorbic acid, and 11.8 grams of sodium ascorbate plus the following excipients: aspartame (sweetener), acesulfame potassium (sweetener), and lemon flavoring.

CLINICAL PHARMACOLOGY
MoviPrep® produces a watery stool leading to cleansing of the colon. The osmotic activity of polyethylene glycol 3350, sodium sulfate, sodium chloride, potassium chloride,

sodium ascorbate, and ascorbic acid, when taken with 1 liter of additional clear fluid, usually results in no net absorption or excretion of ions or water.

The pharmacokinetics of MoviPrep® have not been studied in patients with renal or hepatic insufficiency.

CLINICAL STUDIES

The colon cleansing efficacy and safety of MoviPrep® was evaluated in two randomized, actively-controlled, multi-center, investigator-blinded, phase 3 trials in patients scheduled to have an elective colonoscopy.

In the first study, patients were randomized to one of the following two colon preparation treatments: 1) 2 liters of MoviPrep® with 1 additional liter of clear fluid split into two doses (during the evening before and the morning of the colonoscopy) and 2) 4 liters of polyethylene glycol plus electrolytes solution (4L PEG + E) split into two doses (during the evening before and the morning of the colonoscopy). Patients were allowed to have a morning breakfast, a light lunch, clear soup and/or plain yogurt for dinner. Dinner had to be completed at least one hour prior to initiation of the colon preparation administration.

The primary efficacy endpoint was the proportion of patients with effective colon cleansing as judged by blinded gastroenterologists on the basis of videotapes recorded during the colonoscopy. The blinded gastroenterologists graded the colon cleansing twice (during introduction and withdrawal of the colonoscope) and the poorer of the two assessments was used in the primary efficacy analysis.

The efficacy analysis included 308 adult patients who had an elective colonoscopy. Patients ranged in age from 18 to 88 years old (mean age about 59 years old) with 52% female and 48% male patients. Table 1 displays the results.

Table 1: Effectiveness of Overall Colon Cleansing in the Study of MoviPrep® vs 4 Liter Polyethylene Glycol plus Electrolytes Solution

	Responders A[2] or B[3] (%)	C[4] (%)	D[5] (%)
MoviPrep® (N=153)	88.9	9.8	1.3
4L PEG + E[1] (N=155)	94.8	4.5	0.6

[1] 4L PEG + E is 4 Liter Polyethylene Glycol plus Electrolytes Solution
[2] A: colon empty and clean or presence of clear liquid, but easily removed by suction
[3] B: brown liquid or semisolid remaining amounts of stool, fully removable by suction or displaceable, thus allowing a complete visualization of the gut mucosa
[4] C: semisolid amounts of stool, only partially removable with a risk of incomplete visualization of the gut mucosa
[5] D: semisolid or solid amounts of stool; consequently colonoscopy incomplete or needed to be terminated

4 L PEG+E's responder rate was not significantly higher than MoviPrep's responder rate.

In the second study, patients were randomized to one of the following two colon preparation treatments: 1) 2 liters of MoviPrep® with 1 additional liter of clear fluid in the evening prior to the colonoscopy and 2) 90 mL of oral sodium phosphate solution (90 mL OSPS) with at least 2 liters of additional clear fluid during the day and evening prior to the colonoscopy. Patients randomized to MoviPrep® therapy were allowed to have a morning breakfast; a light lunch; and clear soup and/or plain yogurt for dinner. Dinner had to be completed at least one hour prior to initiation of the colon preparation administration.

The primary efficacy endpoint was the proportion of patients with effective colon cleansing as judged by the colonoscopist and one blinded gastroenterologist (on the basis of videotapes recorded during the colonoscopy). In case of a discrepancy between the colonoscopist and the blinded gastroenterologist, a second blinded gastroenterologist made the final efficacy determination.

The efficacy analysis included 280 adult patients who had an elective colonoscopy. Patients ranged in age from 21 to 76 years old (mean age about 53 years old) with 47% female and 53% male patients. Table 2 displays the results.

Table 2: Effectiveness of Overall Colon Cleansing in the Study of MoviPrep® vs 90 mL Oral Sodium Phosphate Solution

	Responders A[2] or B[3] (%)	C[4] (%)	D[5] (%)
MoviPrep® (N=137)	73.0	23.4	3.6
90 mL OSPS[1] (N=143)	64.4	29.4	6.3

[1] OSPS is Oral Sodium Phosphate Solution
[2] A: empty and clean or clear liquid (transparent, yellow, or green)
[3] B: brown liquid or semisolid remaining small amounts of stool, fully removable by suction or displaceable allowing a complete visualization of the underlying mucosa
[4] C: semi solid only partially removable/displaceable stools; risk of incomplete examination of the underlying mucosa
[5] D: heavy and hard stool making the segment examination uninterpretable and, consequently, the colonoscopy needed to be terminated

MoviPrep's responder rate was not significantly higher than OSPS's responder rate.

INDICATIONS AND USAGE

MoviPrep® is indicated for cleansing of the colon as a preparation for colonoscopy in adults 18 years of age or older.

CONTRAINDICATIONS

MoviPrep® is contraindicated in patients who have had a severe hypersensitivity reaction to any of its components.

WARNINGS

There have been rare reports of generalized tonic-clonic seizures associated with use of polyethylene glycol colon preparation products in patients with no prior history of seizures. The seizure cases were associated with electrolyte abnormalities (e.g., hyponatremia, hypokalemia). The neurologic abnormalities resolved with correction of fluid and electrolyte abnormalities. Therefore, MoviPrep® should be used with caution in patients using concomitant medications that increase the risk of electrolyte abnormalities [such as diuretics or angiotensin converting enzyme (ACE)-inhibitors] or in patients with known or suspected hyponatremia. Consider performing baseline and post-colonoscopy laboratory tests (sodium, potassium, calcium, creatinine, and BUN) in these patients.

MoviPrep® should be used with caution in patients with severe ulcerative colitis, ileus, gastrointestinal obstruction or perforation, gastric retention, toxic colitis, or toxic megacolon.

PRECAUTIONS

General: Patients with impaired gag reflex and patients prone to regurgitation or aspiration should be observed during the administration of MoviPrep®. If a patient experiences severe bloating, abdominal distention, or abdominal pain, administration should be slowed or temporarily discontinued until the symptoms abate. If gastrointestinal obstruction or perforation is suspected, appropriate tests should be performed to rule out these conditions before administration of MoviPrep®.

Phenylketonurics: MoviPrep® contains phenylalanine – a maximum of 2.33 mg of phenylalanine per treatment.

No additional ingredients (e.g., flavorings) should be added to the MoviPrep® solution.

Since MoviPrep® contains sodium ascorbate and ascorbic acid, MoviPrep® should be used with caution in patients with glucose-6-phosphate dehydrogenase (G-6-PD) deficiency especially G-6-PD deficiency patients with an active infection, with a history of hemolysis, or taking concomitant medications known to precipitate hemolytic reactions.

Information for patients: MoviPrep® produces a watery stool which cleanses the colon before colonoscopy. It is recommended that patients receiving MoviPrep® be advised to adequately hydrate before, during, and after the use of MoviPrep®. Patients may have clear soup and/or plain yogurt for dinner, finishing the evening meal at least one hour prior to the start of MoviPrep® treatment. No solid food should be taken from the start of MoviPrep® treatment until after the colonoscopy.

The first bowel movement may occur approximately 1 hour after the start of MoviPrep® administration. Abdominal bloating and distention may occur before the first bowel movement. If severe abdominal discomfort or distention occurs, stop drinking temporarily or drink each portion at longer intervals until these symptoms disappear.

Drug Interactions: Oral medication administered within 1 hour of the start of administration of MoviPrep® may be flushed from the gastrointestinal tract and the medication may not be absorbed.

Carcinogenesis, Mutagenesis, Impairment of Fertility: Long-term studies in animals to evaluate the carcinogenic potential have not been performed with MoviPrep®. Studies to evaluate potential for impairment of fertility or mutagenic potential have not been performed with MoviPrep®.

Pregnancy: Teratogenic Effects: Pregnancy Category C. Animal reproduction studies have not been performed with MoviPrep®. It is also not known if MoviPrep® can cause fetal harm when administered to a pregnant woman or can affect reproductive capacity. MoviPrep® should be given to a pregnant woman only if clearly needed.

Nursing Mothers: Because many drugs are excreted in human milk, caution should be exercised when MoviPrep® is administered to a nursing woman.

Pediatric Use: The safety and effectiveness of MoviPrep® in pediatric patients has not been established.

Geriatric Use: Of the 413 patients in clinical studies receiving MoviPrep®, 91 (22%) patients were aged 65 or older, while 25 (6%) patients were over 75 years of age. No overall differences in safety or effectiveness were observed between geriatric patients and younger patients, and other reported clinical experience has not identified differences in responses between geriatric patients and younger patients, but greater sensitivity of some older individuals cannot be ruled out.

ADVERSE REACTIONS

In the MoviPrep® trials, abdominal distension, anal discomfort, thirst, nausea, and abdominal pain were some of the most common adverse reactions to MoviPrep® administration. Since diarrhea was considered as a part of the efficacy of MoviPrep®, diarrhea was not defined as an adverse reaction in the clinical studies. Tables 3 and 4 display the most common drug-related adverse reactions of MoviPrep® and its comparator in the controlled MoviPrep® trials.

Table 3: The Most Common Drug-Related Adverse Reactions[1] (≥ 2%) in the Study of MoviPrep® vs. 4 liter Polyethylene Glycol plus Electrolytes Solution

	MoviPrep® (split dose) N=180	4L PEG + E[2] N=179
	n (%=n/N)	n (%=n/N)
Malaise	35 (19.4)	32 (17.9)
Nausea	26 (14.4)	36 (20.1)
Abdominal pain	24 (13.3)	27 (15.1)
Vomiting	14 (7.8)	23 (12.8)
Upper abdominal pain	10 (5.6)	11 (6.1)
Dyspepsia	5 (2.8)	2 (1.1)

[1] Drug-related adverse reactions were adverse events that were possibly, probably, or definitely related to the study drug.

[2] 4L PEG + E is 4 liter Polyethylene Glycol plus Electrolytes Solution

Table 4: The Most Common Drug-Related Adverse Reactions[1] (≥ 5%) in the Study of MoviPrep® vs. 90 mL Oral Sodium Phosphate Solution

	MoviPrep® (evening-only) (full dose) N=169	90 mL OSPS[2] N=171
	n (%=n/N)	n (%=n/N)
Abdominal distension	101 (59.8)	70 (40.9)
Anal discomfort	87 (51.5)	89 (52.0)
Thirst	80 (47.3)	112 (65.5)
Nausea	80 (47.3)	80 (46.8)
Abdominal pain	66 (39.1)	55 (32.2)
Sleep disorder	59 (34.9)	49 (28.7)
Rigors	57 (33.7)	51 (29.8)
Hunger	51 (30.2)	121 (70.8)
Malaise	45 (26.6)	90 (52.6)
Vomiting	12 (7.1)	14 (8.2)
Dizziness	11 (6.5)	31 (18.1)
Headache	3 (1.8)	9 (5.3)

Hypokalemia	0 (0)	10 (5.8)
Hyperphosphatemia	0 (0)	10 (5.8)

[1] Drug-related adverse reactions were adverse events that were possibly, probably, or definitely related to the study drug. In addition to the recording of spontaneous adverse events, patients were also specifically asked about the occurrence of the following symptoms: shivering, anal irritations, abdominal bloating or fullness, sleep loss, nausea, vomiting, weakness, hunger sensation, abdominal cramps or pain, thirst sensation, and dizziness.
[2] OSPS is Oral Sodium Phosphate Solution

Isolated cases of urticaria, rhinorrhea, dermatitis, and anaphylactic reaction have been reported with PEG-based products and may represent allergic reactions.

Published literature contains isolated reports of serious adverse events following the administration of PEG-based products in patients over 60 years of age. These adverse events included upper gastrointestinal bleeding from a Mallory-Weiss tear, esophageal perforation, asystole, and acute pulmonary edema after aspirating the PEG-based preparation.

Postmarketing Experience

In addition to adverse events reported from clinical trials, the following adverse events have been identified during post-approval use of MoviPrep®. Because they are reported voluntarily from a population of unknown size, estimates of frequency cannot be made. These events have been chosen for inclusion due to either their seriousness, frequency of reporting or causal connection to MoviPrep®, or a combination of these factors.

General: Hypersensitivity reactions including anaphylaxis (some of which were severe, including shock), rash, urticaria, pruritus, lip, tongue and facial swelling, dyspnea, chest tightness and throat tightness. Fever, chills and dehydration.

OVERDOSAGE

There have been no reported cases of overdose with MoviPrep®. Purposeful or gross accidental ingestion of more than the recommended dose of MoviPrep® might be expected to lead to severe electrolyte disturbances, including hyponatremia and/or hypokalemia, as well as dehydration and hypovolemia, with signs and symptoms of these disturbances. The patient who has taken an overdose should be monitored carefully, and treated symptomatically for complications until stable.

DOSAGE AND ADMINISTRATION

The MoviPrep® dose for colon cleansing for adult patients is 2 liters (approximately 64 ounces) of MoviPrep® solution (with 1 additional liter of clear fluids) taken orally prior to the colonoscopy in one of the following ways:

1) Split-dose MoviPrep® regimen: The evening before the colonoscopy, take the first liter of MoviPrep® solution over one hour (one 8 ounce glass every 15 minutes) and then drink 0.5 liters (approximately 16 ounces) of clear fluid. Then, on the morning of the colonoscopy, take the second liter of MoviPrep® solution over one hour and then drink 0.5 liters of clear liquid at least one hour prior to the start of the colonoscopy; or

2) Evening-only (Full-dose) MoviPrep® regimen: Around 6 PM in the evening before the colonoscopy, take the first liter of MoviPrep® solution over one hour (one 8 ounce glass every 15 minutes) and then about 1.5 hours later take the second liter of MoviPrep® solution over one hour. In addition, take 1 liter (approximately 32 ounces) of additional clear liquid during the evening before the colonoscopy.

Preparation of the MoviPrep® solution: MoviPrep® solution is prepared by emptying the contents of 1 pouch A and 1 pouch B into a suitable glass container (or the container provided) and adding to the container 1 liter of lukewarm water. Mix the solution to ensure that the ingredients are completely dissolved. If the patient prefers, the MoviPrep® solution can be refrigerated prior to drinking. The reconstituted solution should be used within 24 hours. After consumption of the first liter of MoviPrep® solution, the above mixing procedure should be repeated with the second pouch A and pouch B to reconstitute the second liter of the MoviPrep® solution.

HOW SUPPLIED

MoviPrep® is supplied in powdered form. MoviPrep® is administered as an oral solution after reconstitution.
MoviPrep® is available in the following presentations:
Carton: The MoviPrep® carton contains a disposable container for reconstitution of MoviPrep® and an inner carton containing 4 pouches (2 of pouch A and 2 of pouch B). Pouch A contains polyethylene glycol (PEG) 3350 100 grams, sodium sulfate 7.5 grams, sodium chloride 2.69 grams, and potassium chloride 1.015 grams. Pouch B contains ascorbic acid 4.7 grams and sodium ascorbate 5.9 grams. 1 pouch A

and 1 pouch B should be dissolved together in 1 liter of lukewarm water. When reconstituted to 1 liter volume with water, the solution contains PEG-3350 29.6 mmol/L, sodium 181.6 mmol/L (of which not more than 56.2 mmol is absorbable), sulfate 52.8 mmol/L, chloride 59.8 mmol/L, potassium 14.2 mmol/L, and ascorbate 29.8 mmol/L.
NDC 65649-201-75
Rx only
STORAGE
Store carton/container at 25°C (77°F); excursions permitted to 15-30°C (59-86°F). When reconstituted, store upright and keep solution refrigerated. Use within 24 hours.
Manufactured by:
Norgine B.V.
Hogehilweg 7
1101 CA Amsterdam Zuidoost
Netherlands
For:
Salix Pharmaceuticals, Inc.
Morrisville, NC 27560
©2006 Salix Pharmaceuticals Inc.
VENART 53-4/JUN 10
Product protected by US Patent Nos. 7,169,381 and 7,658,914.
Shown in Product Identification Guide, page 318

OSMOPREP®　　　　　　　　　　　　　　　　Rx
[AhZ-MŌ-prĕp]
(sodium phosphate monobasic monohydrate and sodium phosphate dibasic anhydrous)
Tablet

WARNINGS

There have been rare, but serious reports of acute phosphate nephropathy in patients who received oral sodium phosphate products for colon cleansing prior to colonoscopy. Some cases have resulted in permanent impairment of renal function and some patients required long-term dialysis. While some cases have occurred in patients without identifiable risk factors, patients at increased risk of acute phosphate nephropathy may include those with increased age, hypovolemia, increased bowel transit time (such as bowel obstruction), active colitis, or baseline kidney disease, and those using medicines that affect renal perfusion or function (such as diuretics, angiotensin converting enzyme [ACE] inhibitors, angiotensin receptor blockers [ARBs], and possibly nonsteriodal anti-inflammatory drugs [NSAIDs]).
See **WARNINGS**.
It is important to use the dose and dosing regimen as recommended (pm/am split dose).
See **DOSAGE and ADMINISTRATION**.

DESCRIPTION

OsmoPrep® (sodium phosphate monobasic monohydrate, USP, and sodium phosphate dibasic anhydrous, USP) is a purgative used to clean the colon prior to colonoscopy. OsmoPrep is manufactured with a highly soluble tablet binder and does not contain microcrystalline cellulose (MCC). OsmoPrep Tablets are oval, white to off-white compressed tablets, debossed with "SLX" on one side of the bisect and "102" on the other side of the bisect. Each OsmoPrep tablet contains 1.102 grams of sodium phosphate monobasic monohydrate, USP and 0.398 grams of sodium phosphate dibasic anhydrous, USP for a total of 1.5 grams of sodium phosphate per tablet. Inert ingredients include polyethylene glycol 8000, NF; and magnesium stearate, NF. OsmoPrep is gluten-free.
The structural and molecular formulae and molecular weights of the active ingredients are shown below:
• Sodium phosphate monobasic monohydrate, USP
Molecular Formula: $NaH_2PO_4 \cdot H_2O$
Molecular Weight: 137.99

• Sodium phosphate dibasic anhydrous, USP
Molecular Formula: Na_2HPO_4
Molecular Weight: 141.96

OsmoPrep Tablets are for oral administration only.

CLINICAL PHARMACOLOGY

OsmoPrep Tablets, a dosing regimen containing 48 grams of sodium phosphate (32 tablets), induces diarrhea, which ef-

fectively cleanses the entire colon. Each administration has a purgative effect for approximately 1 to 3 hours. The primary mode of action is thought to be through the osmotic effect of sodium, causing large amounts of water to be drawn into the colon, promoting evacuation.

Pharmacokinetics

Pharmacokinetic studies with OsmoPrep have not been conducted. However, the following pharmacokinetic study was conducted with Visicol® tablets which contain the same active ingredients (sodium phosphate) as OsmoPrep. In addition, Visicol is administered at a dose that is 25% greater than the OsmoPrep dose.
An open-label pharmacokinetic study of Visicol in healthy volunteers was performed to determine the concentration-time profile of serum inorganic phosphorus levels after Visicol administration. All subjects received the approved Visicol dosing regimen (60 grams of sodium phosphate with a total liquid volume of 3.6 quarts) for colon cleansing. A 30 gram dose (20 tablets given as 3 tablets every 15 minutes with 8 ounces of clear liquids) was given beginning at 6 PM in the evening. The 30 gram dose (20 tablets given as 3 tablets every 15 minutes with 8 ounces of clear liquids) was repeated the following morning beginning at 6 AM. Twenty-three healthy subjects (mean age 57 years old; 57% male and 43% female; and 65% Hispanic, 30% Caucasian, and 4% African-American) participated in this pharmacokinetic study. The serum phosphorus level rose from a mean (± standard deviation) baseline of 4.0 (± 0.7) mg/dL to 7.7 (± 1.6 mg/dL), at a median of 3 hours after the administration of the first 30-gram dose of sodium phosphate tablets (see Figure 1). The serum phosphorus level rose to a mean of 8.4 (± 1.9) mg/dL, at a median of 4 hours after the administration of the second 30-gram dose of sodium phosphate tablets. The serum phosphorus level remained above baseline for a median of 24 hours after the administration of the initial dose of sodium phosphate tablets (range 16 to 48 hours).

Figure 1. Mean (± standard deviation) serum phosphorus concentrations

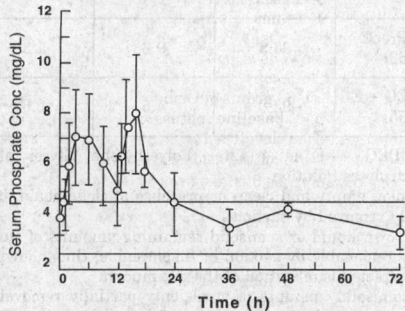

The upper (4.5 mg/dL) and lower (2.6 mg/dL) reference limits for serum phosphate are represented by solid bars.

Special Populations
Renal Insufficiency: The effect of renal dysfunction on the pharmacokinetics of OsmoPrep Tablets has not been studied. Since the inorganic form of phosphate in the circulating plasma is excreted almost entirely by the kidneys, patients with renal disease may have difficulty excreting a large phosphate load. Thus, OsmoPrep Tablets should be used with caution in patients with impaired renal function (see WARNINGS).
Hepatic Insufficiency: OsmoPrep Tablets have not been investigated in patients with hepatic failure.
Geriatric: In a single pharmacokinetic study of sodium phosphate tablets, which included 6 elderly volunteers, plasma half-life increased two-fold in subjects > 70 years of age compared to subjects < 50 years of age (3 subjects and 5 subjects, respectively).
Gender: No difference in serum phosphate AUC values were observed in the single pharmacokinetic study conducted with sodium phosphate tablets in 13 male and 10 female healthy volunteers.

CLINICAL STUDIES

The colon cleansing efficacy and safety of OsmoPrep was evaluated in 2 randomized, investigator-blinded, actively controlled, multicenter, U.S. trials in patients scheduled to have an elective colonoscopy. The trials consisted of a dose ranging and a confirmatory phase 3 study.
In the phase 3 trial, patients were randomized into one of the following three sodium phosphate treatment groups: 1) Visicol containing 60 grams of sodium phosphate given in split doses (30 grams in the evening before the colonoscopy and 30 grams on the next day) with at least 3.6 quarts of clear liquids; 2) OsmoPrep containing 60 grams of sodium phosphate given in split doses (30 grams in the evening before the colonoscopy and 30 grams on the next day) with 2.5 quarts of clear liquids; and 3) OsmoPrep containing 48 grams of sodium phosphate (30 grams in the evening

before the colonoscopy and 18 grams on the next day) with 2 quarts of clear liquids. Patients were instructed to eat a light breakfast before noon on the day prior to the colonoscopy and then were told to drink only clear liquids after noon on the day prior to the colonoscopy.

The primary efficacy endpoint was the overall colon cleansing response rate in the 4-point Colonic Contents Scale. Response was defined as a rating of "excellent" or "good" on the 4-point scale as determined by the blinded colonoscopist. This phase 3 study was planned to assess the non-inferiority of the two OsmoPrep groups compared to the Visicol group.

The efficacy analysis included 704 adult patients who had an elective colonoscopy. Patients ranged in age from 21 to 89 years old (mean age 56 years old) with 55% female and 45% male patients. Race was distributed as follows: 87% Caucasian, 10% African American, and 3% other race. The OsmoPrep 60 gram and 48 gram treatment groups demonstrated non-inferiority compared to Visicol. See Table 1 for the results.

[See table 1 at right]

Electrolyte Changes

In the OsmoPrep clinical studies, expected serum electrolyte changes (including phosphate, calcium, potassium, and sodium levels) have been observed in patients taking OsmoPrep. In the overwhelming majority of patients, electrolyte abnormalities were not associated with any adverse events.

In the OsmoPrep phase 3 study, 96%, 96%, and 93% of patients who took 60 grams of Visicol, 60 grams of OsmoPrep, and 48 grams of OsmoPrep, respectively, developed hyperphosphatemia (defined as phosphate level > 5.1 mg/dL) on the day of the colonoscopy. In this study, patients who took 60 grams of Visicol, 60 grams of OsmoPrep, and 48 grams of OsmoPrep had baseline mean phosphate levels of 3.5, 3.5, and 3.6 mg/dL and subsequently developed mean phosphate levels of 7.6, 7.9, and 7.1 mg/dL, respectively, on the day of the colonoscopy.

In the OsmoPrep phase 3 study, 20%, 22%, and 18% of patients who took 60 grams of Visicol, 60 grams of OsmoPrep, and 48 grams of OsmoPrep, respectively, developed hypokalemia (defined as a potassium level < 3.4 mEq/L) on the day of the colonoscopy. In this study, patients who took 60 grams of Visicol, 60 grams of OsmoPrep, and 48 grams of OsmoPrep all had baseline potassium levels of about 4.3 mEq/L and then developed a mean potassium level of 3.7 mEq/L on the day of the colonoscopy.

In the OsmoPrep phase 3 trial, several patients on all three sodium phosphate regimens developed hypocalcemia and hypernatremia that did not require treatment.

INDICATIONS AND USAGE

OsmoPrep Tablets are indicated for cleansing of the colon as a preparation for colonoscopy in adults 18 years of age or older.

CONTRAINDICATIONS

OsmoPrep Tablets are contraindicated in patients with biopsy-proven acute phosphate nephropathy.

OsmoPrep Tablets are contraindicated in patients with a known allergy or hypersensitivity to sodium phosphate salts or any of its ingredients.

WARNINGS

Administration of sodium phosphate products prior to colonoscopy for colon cleansing has resulted in fatalities due to significant fluid shifts, severe electrolyte abnormalities, and cardiac arrhythmias. These fatalities have been observed in patients with renal insufficiency, in patients with bowel perforation, and in patients who misused or overdosed sodium phosphate products. It is recommended that patients receiving OsmoPrep be advised to adequately hydrate before, during, and after the use of OsmoPrep.

Considerable caution should be advised before OsmoPrep Tablets are used in patients with the following illnesses: severe renal insufficiency (creatinine clearance less than 30 mL/minute), congestive heart failure, ascites, unstable angina, gastric retention, ileus, acute bowel obstruction, pseudo-obstruction of the bowel, severe chronic constipation, bowel perforation, acute colitis, toxic megacolon, gastric bypass or stapling surgery, or hypomotility syndrome.

Consider performing baseline and post-colonoscopy labs (phosphate, calcium, potassium, sodium, creatinine, and BUN) in patients who may be at increased risk for serious adverse events, including those with history of renal insufficiency, history of - or at greater risk of - acute phosphate nephropathy, known or suspected electrolyte disorders, seizures, arrhythmias, cardiomyopathy, prolonged QT, recent history of a MI and those with known or suspected hyperphosphatemia, hypocalcemia, hypokalemia, and hypernatremia. Also if patients develop vomiting and/or signs of dehydration then measure post-colonoscopy labs (phosphate, calcium, potassium, sodium, creatinine, and BUN).

Table 1: Phase 3 Study – Overall Colon Content Cleansing Response Rates[1]

Treatment Arm (grams of sodium phosphate)	No. of tablets taken at 6 PM on the day prior to colonoscopy	No. of tablets taken the next day[2]	Excellent	Good	Fair	Inadequate	Overall Response Rate (Excellent or Good)
OsmoPrep 32 tabs (48 g) n=236	20	12	76%	19%	3%	2%	95%
OsmoPrep 40 tabs (60 g) n=233	20	20	73%	24%	2%	1%	97%
Visicol 40 tabs (60 g) n=235	20	20	51%	43%	6%	0%	94%

[1] Colon-cleansing efficacy was based on response rate to treatment. A patient was considered to be a responder if overall colon cleansing was rated as "excellent" or "good" on a 4-point scale based on the amount of retained "colonic contents." Excellent was defined as >90% of mucosa seen, mostly liquid stool, minimal suctioning needed for adequate visualization. Good was defined as >90% of mucosa seen, mostly liquid stool, significant suctioning needed for adequate visualization. Fair was defined as >90% of mucosa seen, mixture of liquid and semisolid stool, could be suctioned and/or washed. Inadequate was defined as <90% of mucosa seen, mixture of semisolid and solid stool which could not be suctioned or washed.

[2] On the day of the colonoscopy, study medication was taken 3 to 5 hours before the start of the colonoscopy.

Renal Disease, Acute Phosphate Nephropathy, and Electrolyte Disorders

There have been rare, but serious, reports of renal failure, acute phosphate nephropathy, and nephrocalcinosis in patients who received oral sodium phosphate products (including oral sodium phosphate solutions and tablets) for colon cleansing prior to colonoscopy. These cases often resulted in permanent impairment of renal function and several patients required long-term dialysis. The time to onset is typically within days; however, in some cases, the diagnosis of these events has been delayed up to several months after the ingestion of these products. Patients at increased risk of acute phosphate nephropathy may include patients with the following: hypovolemia, baseline kidney disease, increased age, and patients using medicines that affect renal perfusion or function [such as diuretics, angiotensin converting enzyme (ACE) inhibitors, angiotensin receptor blockers, and possibly nonsteroidal anti-inflammatory drugs (NSAIDs)].

Use OsmoPrep with caution in patients with impaired renal function, patients with a history of acute phosphate nephropathy, known or suspected electrolyte disturbances (such as dehydration), or people taking concomitant medications that may affect electrolyte levels (such as diuretics). Patients with electrolyte abnormalities such as hypernatremia, hyperphosphatemia, hypokalemia, or hypocalcemia should have their electrolytes corrected before treatment with OsmoPrep Tablets.

Seizures

There have been rare reports of generalized tonic-clonic seizures and/or loss of consciousness associated with use of sodium phosphate products in patients with no prior history of seizures. The seizure cases were associated with electrolyte abnormalities (e.g., hyponatremia, hypokalemia, hypocalcemia, and hypomagnesemia) and low serum osmolality. The neurologic abnormalities resolved with correction of fluid and electrolyte abnormalities. OsmoPrep should be used with caution in patients with a history of seizures and in patients at higher risk of seizure [patients using concomitant medications that lower the seizure threshold (such as tricyclic antidepressants), patients withdrawing from alcohol or benzodiazepines, or patients with known or suspected hyponatremia].

Cardiac Arrhythmias

There have been rare, but serious, reports of arrhythmias associated with the use of sodium phosphate products. OsmoPrep should be used with caution in patients with higher risk of arrhythmias (patients with a history of cardiomyopathy, patients with prolonged QT, patients with a history of uncontrolled arrhythmias, and patients with a recent history of a myocardial infarction). Pre-dose and post-colonoscopy ECGs should be considered in patients with high risk of serious, cardiac arrhythmias.

PRECAUTIONS

General

Patients should be instructed to drink 8 ounces of clear liquids with each 4-tablet dose of OsmoPrep Tablets. Patients should take a total of 2 quarts of clear liquids with OsmoPrep. Inadequate fluid intake, as with any effective purgative, may lead to excessive fluid loss, hypovolemia, and dehydration. Dehydration from purgation may be exacerbated by inadequate oral fluid intake, vomiting, and/or use of diuretics.

Patients should be instructed not to administer additional laxative or purgative agents, particularly additional sodium phosphate-based purgative or enema products.

Prolongation of the QT interval has been observed in some patients who were dosed with sodium phosphate colon preparations. QT prolongation with sodium phosphate tablets has been associated with electrolyte imbalances, such as hypokalemia and hypocalcemia. OsmoPrep Tablets should be used with caution in patients who are taking medications known to prolong the QT interval, since serious complications may occur. Pre-dose and post-colonoscopy ECGs should be considered in patients with known prolonged QT.

Administration of OsmoPrep Tablets may induce colonic mucosal aphthous ulcerations, since this endoscopic finding was observed with other sodium phosphate cathartic preparations. In the OsmoPrep clinical program, aphthous ulcers were observed in 3% of patients who took the 48 gram OsmoPrep dosing regimen. This colonoscopic finding should be considered in patients with known or suspected inflammatory bowel disease.

Because published data suggest that sodium phosphate absorption may be enhanced in patients experiencing an acute exacerbation of chronic inflammatory bowel disease, OsmoPrep Tablets should be used with caution in such patients.

Drug Interactions

Medications administered in close proximity to OsmoPrep Tablets may not be absorbed from the gastrointestinal tract due to the rapid intestinal peristalsis and watery diarrhea induced by the purgative agent.

Carcinogenesis, Mutagenesis, Impairment of Fertility

Long-term studies in animals have not been performed to evaluate the carcinogenic potential of OsmoPrep. Studies to evaluate the effect of OsmoPrep on fertility or its mutagenic potential have not been performed.

Pregnancy. Teratogenic Effects: Pregnancy Category C

Animal reproduction studies have not been conducted with OsmoPrep. It is not known whether OsmoPrep can cause fetal harm when administered to a pregnant woman, or can affect reproduction capacity. OsmoPrep Tablets should be given to a pregnant woman only if clearly needed.

Pediatric Use

The safety and efficacy of OsmoPrep Tablets have not been demonstrated in patients less than 18 years of age.

Geriatric Use

In controlled colon preparation trials of OsmoPrep, 228 (24%) of 931 patients were 65 years of age or older. In addition, 49 (5%) of the 931 patients were 75 years of age or older.

Of the 228 geriatric patients in the trials, 134 patients (59%) received at least 48 grams of OsmoPrep. Of the 49 patients 75 years old or older in the trials, 27 (55%) patients received at least 48 grams of OsmoPrep. No overall differences in safety or effectiveness were observed between geriatric patients and younger patients. However, the mean phosphate levels in geriatric patients were greater than the

phosphate levels in younger patients after OsmoPrep administration. The mean colonoscopy-day phosphate levels in patients 18-64, 65-74, and ≥ 75 years old who received 48 grams of OsmoPrep in the phase 3 study were 7.0, 7.3, and 8.0 mg/dL, respectively. In addition, in all three sodium phosphate treatment groups, the mean phosphate levels in patients 18-64, 65-74, and ≥ 75 years old in the phase 3 study were 7.4, 7.9, and 8.0 mg/dL, respectively, after sodium phosphate administration. Greater sensitivity of some older individuals cannot be ruled out; therefore, OsmoPrep Tablets should be used with caution in geriatric patients.
Sodium phosphate is known to be substantially excreted by the kidney, and the risk of adverse reactions with sodium phosphate may be greater in patients with impaired renal function. Since geriatric patients are more likely to have impaired renal function, consider performing baseline and post-colonoscopy labs (phosphate, calcium, potassium, sodium, creatinine, and BUN) in these patients (see WARNINGS). It is recommended that patients receiving OsmoPrep be advised to adequately hydrate before, during, and after the use of OsmoPrep.

ADVERSE REACTIONS

Abdominal bloating, abdominal pain, nausea, and vomiting were the most common adverse events reported with the use of OsmoPrep Tablets. Dizziness and headache were reported less frequently. Since diarrhea was considered as a part of the efficacy of OsmoPrep, diarrhea was not defined as an adverse event in the clinical studies. Table 2 shows the most common adverse events associated with the use of 48 grams of OsmoPrep, 60 grams of OsmoPrep, and 60 grams of Visicol in the colon preparation trials (n=931).

Table 2: Frequency of Adverse Events of Any Severity Occurring in Greater Than 3% of Patients in the OsmoPrep Trials

	OsmoPrep 32 tabs (48 g) N=272	OsmoPrep 40 tabs (60 g) N=265	Visicol 40 tabs (60 g) N=268
Bloating	31%	39%	41%
Nausea	26%	37%	30%
Abdominal Pain	23%	24%	25%
Vomiting	4%	10%	9%

Postmarketing Experience

In addition to adverse events reported from clinical trials, the following adverse events have been identified during post-approval use of OsmoPrep. Because they are reported voluntarily from a population of unknown size, estimates of frequency cannot be made. These events have been chosen for inclusion due to either their seriousness, frequency of reporting or causal connection to OsmoPrep, or a combination of these factors.
General: Hypersensitivity reactions including anaphylaxis, rash, pruritus, urticaria, throat tightness, bronchospasm, dyspnea, pharyngeal edema, dysphagia, paresthesia and swelling of the lips and tongue, and facial swelling.
Cardiovascular: Arrhythmias
Nervous system: Seizures
Renal: Renal impairment, increased blood urea nitrogen (BUN), increased creatinine, acute renal failure, acute phosphate nephropathy, nephrocalcinosis, and renal tubular necrosis.

DRUG ABUSE AND DEPENDENCE

Laxatives and purgatives (including OsmoPrep) have the potential for abuse by bulimia nervosa patients who frequently have binge eating and vomiting.

OVERDOSAGE

There have been no reported cases of overdosage with OsmoPrep Tablets. Purposeful or accidental ingestion of more than the recommended dosage of OsmoPrep Tablets might be expected to lead to severe electrolyte disturbances, including hyperphosphatemia, hypocalcemia, hypernatremia, or hypokalemia, as well as dehydration and hypovolemia, with attendant signs and symptoms of these disturbances. Certain severe electrolyte disturbances resulting from overdose may lead to cardiac arrhythmias, seizure, renal failure, and death. The patient who has taken an overdosage should be monitored carefully, and treated symptomatically for complications until stable.

DOSAGE AND ADMINISTRATION

The recommended dose of OsmoPrep Tablets for colon cleansing for adult patients is 32 tablets (48 grams of sodium phosphate) taken orally with a total of 2 quarts of clear liquids in the following manner:
The evening before the colonoscopy procedure: Take 4 OsmoPrep Tablets with 8 ounces of clear liquids every 15 minutes for a total of 20 tablets.
On the day of the colonoscopy procedure: Starting 3-5 hours before the procedure, take 4 OsmoPrep Tablets with 8 ounces of clear liquids every 15 minutes for a total of 12 tablets.
Patients should be advised of the importance of taking the recommended fluid regimen. It is recommended that patients receiving OsmoPrep be advised to adequately hydrate before, during, and after the use of OsmoPrep.
Patients should not use OsmoPrep for colon cleansing within seven days of previous administration. No additional enema or laxative is required, and patients should be advised NOT to take additional agents, particularly those containing sodium phosphate.

HOW SUPPLIED

OsmoPrep Tablets are supplied in child-resistant bottles containing 100 tablets. Each tablet contains 1.102 g sodium phosphate monobasic monohydrate, USP and 0.398 g sodium phosphate dibasic anhydrous, USP for a total of 1.5 g of sodium phosphate per tablet.
Each bottle contains two silica desiccant packets, which should not be ingested.
NDC 65649-701-41 (100 tablet bottle)
Rx only.
Store at 25°C (77°F); excursions permitted to 15-30°C (59-86°F) [See USP Controlled Room Temperature]. Discard any unused portion.
Manufactured by:
WellSpring Pharmaceutical Canada Corp.
Oakville, Ontario Canada L6H 1M5
for:
Salix Pharmaceuticals, Inc.
Morrisville, NC 27560
Made in Canada
VENART-30-4
Revised March 2009
Product protected by US Patent No. 5,616,346 and other pending applications.

MEDICATION GUIDE

OsmoPrep® (AhZ-MŌ-prĕp) (sodium phosphate monobasic monohydrate, USP and sodium phosphate dibasic anhydrous, USP) Tablets
Read the Medication Guide that comes with OsmoPrep before you take it and each time you take it. This Medication Guide does not take the place of talking with your doctor about your medical condition or your treatment. If you have any questions about OsmoPrep, ask your doctor or pharmacist.

What is the most important information I should know about OsmoPrep?
OsmoPrep can cause serious side effects, including:
Serious kidney problems. Rare, but serious kidney problems can happen in people who take medicines made with sodium phosphate, including OsmoPrep, to clean your colon before colonoscopy. These kidney problems can sometimes lead to kidney failure or the need for dialysis for a long time. These problems often happen within a few days, but sometimes may happen several months after taking OsmoPrep.
Conditions that can make you more at risk for having serious kidney problems with OsmoPrep include if you:
- lose too much body fluid (dehydration)
- have slow moving bowels
- have bowels blocked with stool (constipation)
- have severe stomach pain or bloating
- have any disease that causes bowel irritation (colitis)
- have kidney disease
- have heart failure
- take water pills or non-steroidal anti-inflammatory drugs (NSAIDS)

Your age may also affect your risk for having kidney problems with OsmoPrep.
Before you start taking OsmoPrep tell your doctor if you:
- have kidney problems.
- take any medicines for blood pressure, heart disease, or kidney disease.

Severe fluid loss. People who take medicines that contain sodium phosphate can have severe loss of body fluid, with severe changes in body salts in the blood, and abnormal heart rhythms. These problems can lead to death.
Tell your doctor if you have any of these symptoms of loss of too much body fluid (dehydration) while taking OsmoPrep:
- vomiting
- dizziness
- urinating less often than normal
- headache

See "What are the possible side effects of OsmoPrep?" for more information about side effects.

What is OsmoPrep?
OsmoPrep is a prescription medicine used in adults 18 years and older, to clean your colon before a colonoscopy. OsmoPrep cleans your colon by causing you to have diarrhea. Cleaning your colon helps your doctor see the inside of your colon more clearly during the colonoscopy.
It is not known if OsmoPrep is safe and works in children under age 18.

Who should not take OsmoPrep?
Do not take OsmoPrep if:
- you have had a kidney biopsy that shows you have kidney problems because of too much phosphate
- you are allergic to sodium phosphate salts or any of the ingredients in OsmoPrep. See the end of this Medication Guide for a list of ingredients in OsmoPrep.

What should I tell my doctor before taking OsmoPrep?
Before taking OsmoPrep, tell your doctor about all of your medical conditions, including if you have:
- any of the medical conditions listed in the section "What is the most important information I should know about OsmoPrep?"
- irritation of the bowel (colitis). OsmoPrep can cause symptoms of irritable bowel disease to flare-up.
- damage to your bowels
- problems with abnormal heart beat
- had a recent heart attack or have other heart problems
- symptoms of too much body fluid loss (dehydration) including vomiting, dizziness, urinating less often than normal, or headache
- had stomach surgery
- a history of seizures
- if you drink alcohol
- are on a low salt diet
- are pregnant. It is not known if OsmoPrep will harm your unborn baby.

Tell your doctor about all the medicines you take, including prescription and non-prescription medicines, vitamins, and herbal supplements. Any medicine that you take close to the time that you take OsmoPrep may not work as well. Especially tell your doctor if you take:
- water pills (diuretics)
- medicines for blood pressure or heart problems
- medicines for kidney damage
- medicines for pain, such as aspirin or a non-steroidal anti-inflammatory drug (NSAID)
- a medicine for seizures
- a laxative for constipation in the last 7 days. You should not take another medicine that contains sodium phosphate while you take OsmoPrep.

Ask your doctor if you are not sure if your medicine is listed above.
Know the medicines you take. Keep a list of your medicines to show your doctor or pharmacist when you get a new prescription.

How should I take OsmoPrep?
- Take OsmoPrep exactly as prescribed by your doctor.
- **It is important for you to drink clear liquids before, during, and after taking OsmoPrep. This may help prevent kidney damage.** Examples of **clear liquids** are water, flavored water, lemonade (no pulp), ginger ale or apple juice. Do not drink any liquids colored purple or red.

You must read, understand, and follow these instructions to take OsmoPrep the right way:
On the evening before your colonoscopy, you will take a total of 20 OsmoPrep tablets, as follows:
1. Take 4 OsmoPrep tablets with 8 ounces of **clear liquids.**
2. **Wait 15 minutes.**
3. Take 4 more OsmoPrep tablets with 8 ounces of **clear liquids.**
4. Repeat steps 2 and 3 above, three more times. Make sure you wait 15 minutes after each time.

On the day of your colonoscopy, you will take a total of 12 OsmoPrep tablets, starting about 3 to 5 hours before your colonoscopy, as follows:
1. Take 4 OsmoPrep tablets with 8 ounces of **clear liquids.**
2. **Wait 15 minutes.**
3. Take 4 more OsmoPrep tablets with 8 ounces of **clear liquids.**
4. Repeat steps 2 and 3 one more time.

Tell your doctor if you have any of these symptoms while taking OsmoPrep:
- vomiting, dizziness, or if you urinate less often than normal. These may be signs that you have lost too much fluid while taking OsmoPrep.
- trouble drinking clear fluids
- severe stomach cramping, bloating, nausea, or headache.

If you take too much OsmoPrep, call your doctor or get medical help right away.

What should I avoid while taking OsmoPrep?
- You should not take other laxatives or enemas made with sodium phosphate, while taking OsmoPrep.
- You should not use OsmoPrep if you have already used it in the last 7 days.

What are the possible side effects of OsmoPrep?
OsmoPrep can cause serious side effects, including:
- See "What is the most important information I should know about OsmoPrep?"

- Seizures or fainting (black-outs). People who take a medicine that contains sodium phosphate, such as OsmoPrep, can have seizures or faint (become unconscious) even if they have not had seizures before. Tell your doctor right away if you have a seizure or faint while taking OsmoPrep
- Abnormal heart beat (arrhythmias)
- changes in your blood levels of calcium, phosphate, potassium, sodium

The most common side effects of OsmoPrep are:
- bloating
- stomach area (abdominal) pain
- nausea
- vomiting

These are not all the possible side effects of OsmoPrep. For more information, ask your doctor or pharmacist.
Call your doctor for medical advice about side effects. You may report side effects to FDA at 1-800-FDA-1088.

How do I store OsmoPrep?
- Store OsmoPrep at room temperature, between 59° F to 86° F (15° C to 30° C).
- Throw away any OsmoPrep that is not needed.
- **Keep OsmoPrep and all medicines out of the reach of children.**

General information about OsmoPrep
Medicines are sometimes prescribed for purposes other than those listed in a Medication Guide. Do not use OsmoPrep for a condition for which it was not prescribed. Do not give OsmoPrep to other people, even if they have the same symptoms that you have. It may harm them.
This Medication Guide summarizes the most important information about OsmoPrep. If you would like more information about OsmoPrep, talk with your doctor or pharmacist. You can ask your doctor or pharmacist for information that is written for healthcare professionals. For more information, call 1-866-669-7597 (toll-free) or go to www.Salix.com.

What are the ingredients in OsmoPrep?
Active ingredients: sodium phosphate monobasic monohydrate and sodium phosphate dibasic anhydrous
Inactive ingredients: polyethylene glycol 8000 and magnesium stearate
This Medication Guide has been approved by the U.S. Food and Drug Administration.
Revised March 2009
Salix Pharmaceuticals, Inc.
Morrisville, NC 27560, USA
This Medication Guide has been approved by the U.S. Food and Drug Administration.
VENART-30-4
Revised March 2009
Shown in Product Identification Guide, page 318

XIFAXAN®   ℞
[zuh FAX in]
(rifaximin)
Tablets

HIGHLIGHTS OF PRESCRIBING INFORMATION
These highlights do not include all the information needed to use XIFAXAN safely and effectively. See full prescribing information for XIFAXAN.
XIFAXAN® (rifaximin) Tablets
Initial U.S. Approval: 2004
To reduce the development of drug-resistant bacteria and maintain the effectiveness of XIFAXAN and other antibacterial drugs, XIFAXAN should be used only to treat or prevent infections that are proven or strongly suspected to be caused by bacteria.

———RECENT MAJOR CHANGES———
Indications and Usage,
Hepatic Encephalopathy (1.2)   03/2010
Dosage and Administration,
Hepatic Encephalopathy (2.2)   03/2010

———INDICATIONS AND USAGE———
XIFAXAN is a rifamycin antibacterial indicated for:
- The treatment of patients (≥ 12 years of age) with travelers' diarrhea (TD) caused by noninvasive strains of *Escherichia coli* (1.1)
- Reduction in risk of overt hepatic encephalopathy (HE) recurrence in patients ≥ 18 years of age (1.2)
Limitations of Use
- TD: Do not use in patients with diarrhea complicated by fever or blood in the stool or diarrhea due to pathogens other than *Escherichia coli* (1.1)

———DOSAGE AND ADMINISTRATION———
- Travelers' diarrhea: One 200 mg tablet taken orally three times a day for 3 days, with or without food (2.1)
- Hepatic encephalopathy: One 550 mg tablet taken orally two times a day, with or without food (2.2)

———DOSAGE FORMS AND STRENGTHS———
- 200 mg and 550 mg tablets (3)

———CONTRAINDICATIONS———
History of hypersensitivity to rifaximin, rifamycin antimicrobial agents, or any of the components of XIFAXAN (4.1)

———WARNINGS AND PRECAUTIONS———
- Travelers' Diarrhea Not Caused by *E. coli*: XIFAXAN was not effective in diarrhea complicated by fever and/or blood in the stool or diarrhea due to pathogens other than *E. coli*. If diarrhea symptoms get worse or persist for more than 24-48 hours, discontinue XIFAXAN and consider alternative antibiotics (5.1)
- *Clostridium difficile*-Associated Diarrhea: Evaluate if diarrhea occurs after therapy or does not improve or worsens during therapy (5.2)
- Hepatic Impairment: Use with caution in patients with severe (Child-Pugh C) hepatic impairment (5.4, 8.7)

———ADVERSE REACTIONS———
- Most common adverse reactions in travelers' diarrhea (≥ 5%): Flatulence, headache, abdominal pain, rectal tenesmus, defecation urgency and nausea (6.1)
- Most common adverse reactions in HE (≥ 10%): Peripheral edema, nausea, dizziness, fatigue, ascites, flatulence, and headache (6.1)

To report suspected adverse reactions, contact Salix Pharmaceuticals at 1-866-669-7597 and www.Salix.com or FDA at 1-800-FDA-1088 or *www.fda.gov/medwatch*

———USE IN SPECIFIC POPULATIONS———
- Pregnancy: Based on animal data, may cause fetal harm (8.1)
- Nursing Mothers: Discontinue nursing or drug, taking into account the importance of the drug to the mother (8.3)

See 17 for PATIENT COUNSELING INFORMATION
                                          Revised: Mar/2010

FULL PRESCRIBING INFORMATION: CONTENTS*
* Sections or subsections omitted from the full prescribing information are not listed

FULL PRESCRIBING INFORMATION

1   INDICATIONS AND USAGE
To reduce the development of drug-resistant bacteria and maintain the effectiveness of XIFAXAN and other antibacterial drugs, XIFAXAN when used to treat infection should be used only to treat or prevent infections that are proven or strongly suspected to be caused by susceptible bacteria. When culture and susceptibility information are available,

they should be considered in selecting or modifying antibacterial therapy. In the absence of such data, local epidemiology and susceptibility patterns may contribute to the empiric selection of therapy.

1.1   Travelers' Diarrhea
XIFAXAN 200 mg is indicated for the treatment of patients (≥ 12 years of age) with travelers' diarrhea caused by noninvasive strains of *Escherichia coli* [see Warnings and Precautions (5), Clinical Pharmacology (12.4) and Clinical Studies (14.1)].
Limitations of Use
XIFAXAN should not be used in patients with diarrhea complicated by fever or blood in the stool or diarrhea due to pathogens other than *Escherichia coli*.

1.2   Hepatic Encephalopathy
XIFAXAN 550 mg is indicated for reduction in risk of overt hepatic encephalopathy (HE) recurrence in patients ≥ 18 years of age.
In the trials of XIFAXAN for HE, 91% of the patients were using lactulose concomitantly. Differences in the treatment effect of those patients not using lactulose concomitantly could not be assessed.
XIFAXAN has not been studied in patients with MELD (Model for End-Stage Liver Disease) scores > 25, and only 8.6% of patients in the controlled trial had MELD scores over 19. There is increased systemic exposure in patients with more severe hepatic dysfunction [see Warnings and Precautions (5.4), Use in Specific Populations (8.7), Clinical Pharmacology (12.3)].

2   DOSAGE AND ADMINISTRATION
2.1   Dosage for Travelers' Diarrhea
The recommended dose of XIFAXAN is one 200 mg tablet taken orally three times a day for 3 days. XIFAXAN can be administered orally, with or without food [see Clinical Pharmacology (12.3)].

2.2   Dosage for Hepatic Encephalopathy
The recommended dose of XIFAXAN is one 550 mg tablet taken orally two times a day, with or without food [see Clinical Pharmacology (12.3)].

3   DOSAGE FORMS AND STRENGTHS
XIFAXAN is a pink-colored biconvex tablet and is available in the following strengths:
- 200 mg – a round tablet debossed with "Sx" on one side.
- 550 mg – an oval tablet debossed with "rfx" on one side.

4   CONTRAINDICATIONS
4.1   Hypersensitivity
XIFAXAN is contraindicated in patients with a hypersensitivity to rifaximin, any of the rifamycin antimicrobial agents, or any of the components in XIFAXAN. Hypersensitivity reactions have included exfoliative dermatitis, angioneurotic edema, and anaphylaxis [see Adverse Reactions (6.2)].

5   WARNINGS AND PRECAUTIONS
5.1   Travelers' Diarrhea Not Caused by *Escherichia coli*
XIFAXAN was not found to be effective in patients with diarrhea complicated by fever and/or blood in the stool or diarrhea due to pathogens other than *Escherichia coli*.
Discontinue XIFAXAN if diarrhea symptoms get worse or persist more than 24-48 hours and alternative antibiotic therapy should be considered.
XIFAXAN is not effective in cases of travelers' diarrhea due to *Campylobacter jejuni*. The effectiveness of XIFAXAN in travelers' diarrhea caused by *Shigella* spp. and *Salmonella* spp. has not been proven. XIFAXAN should not be used in patients where *Campylobacter jejuni*, *Shigella* spp., or *Salmonella* spp. may be suspected as causative pathogens.

5.2   *Clostridium difficile*-Associated Diarrhea
Clostridium difficile-associated diarrhea (CDAD) has been reported with use of nearly all antibacterial agents, including XIFAXAN, and may range in severity from mild diarrhea to fatal colitis. Treatment with antibacterial agents alters the normal flora of the colon which may lead to overgrowth of *C. difficile*.
C. difficile produces toxins A and B which contribute to the development of CDAD. Hypertoxin producing strains of *C. difficile* cause increased morbidity and mortality, as these infections can be refractory to antimicrobial therapy and may require colectomy. CDAD must be considered in all patients who present with diarrhea following antibiotic use. Careful medical history is necessary since CDAD has been reported to occur over two months after the administration of antibacterial agents.
If CDAD is suspected or confirmed, ongoing antibiotic use not directed against *C. difficile* may need to be discontinued. Appropriate fluid and electrolyte management, protein supplementation, antibiotic treatment of *C. difficile*, and surgical evaluation should be instituted as clinically indicated.

5.3   Development of Drug Resistant Bacteria
Prescribing XIFAXAN for travelers' diarrhea in the absence of a proven or strongly suspected bacterial infection or a prophylactic indication is unlikely to provide benefit to the patient and increases the risk of the development of drug-resistant bacteria.

5.4 Severe (Child-Pugh C) Hepatic Impairment

There is increased systemic exposure in patients with severe hepatic impairment. Animal toxicity studies did not achieve systemic exposures that were seen in patients with severe hepatic impairment. The clinical trials were limited to patients with MELD scores <25. Therefore, caution should be exercised when administering XIFAXAN to patients with severe hepatic impairment (Child-Pugh C) *[see Use in Specific Populations (8.7), Nonclinical Toxicology (13.2) and Clinical Studies (14.2)].*

6 ADVERSE REACTIONS

6.1 Clinical Studies Experience

Because clinical trials are conducted under widely varying conditions, adverse reaction rates observed in the clinical trials of a drug cannot be directly compared to rates in the clinical trials of another drug and may not reflect the rates observed in practice.

Travelers' Diarrhea

The safety of XIFAXAN 200 mg taken three times a day was evaluated in patients with travelers' diarrhea consisting of 320 patients in two placebo-controlled clinical trials with 95% of patients receiving three or four days of treatment with XIFAXAN. The population studied had a mean age of 31.3 (18-79) years of which approximately 3% were ≥ 65 years old, 53% were male and 84% were White, 11% were Hispanic.

Discontinuations due to adverse reactions occurred in 0.4% of patients. The adverse reactions leading to discontinuation were taste loss, dysentery, weight decrease, anorexia, nausea and nasal passage irrigation.

All adverse reactions for XIFAXAN 200 mg three times daily that occurred at a frequency ≥ 2% in the two placebo-controlled trials combined are provided in Table 1. (These include adverse reactions that may be attributable to the underlying disease.)

Table 1. All Adverse Reactions With an Incidence ≥2% Among Patients Receiving XIFAXAN Tablets, 200 mg Three Times Daily, in Placebo-Controlled Studies

MedDRA Preferred Term	Number (%) of Patients	
	XIFAXAN Tablets, 600 mg/day N = 320	Placebo N = 228
Flatulence	36 (11%)	45 (20%)
Headache	31 (10%)	21 (9%)
Abdominal Pain NOS*	23 (7%)	23 (10%)
Rectal Tenesmus	23 (7%)	20 (9%)
Defecation Urgency	19 (6%)	21 (9%)
Nausea	17 (5%)	19 (8%)
Constipation	12 (4%)	8 (4%)
Pyrexia	10 (3%)	10 (4%)
Vomiting NOS	7 (2%)	4 (2%)

* NOS: Not otherwise specified

The following adverse reactions, presented by body system, have also been reported in <2% of patients taking XIFAXAN in the two placebo-controlled clinical trials where the 200 mg tablet was taken three times a day for travelers' diarrhea. The following includes adverse reactions regardless of causal relationship to drug exposure.

Blood and Lymphatic System Disorders: Lymphocytosis, monocytosis, neutropenia
Ear and Labyrinth Disorders: Ear pain, motion sickness, tinnitus
Gastrointestinal Disorders: Abdominal distension, diarrhea NOS, dry throat, fecal abnormality NOS, gingival disorder NOS, inguinal hernia NOS, dry lips, stomach discomfort
General Disorders and Administration Site Conditions: Chest pain, fatigue, malaise, pain NOS, weakness
Infections and Infestations: Dysentery NOS, respiratory tract infection NOS, upper respiratory tract infection NOS
Injury and Poisoning: Sunburn
Investigations: Aspartate aminotransferase increased, blood in stool, blood in urine, weight decreased
Metabolic and Nutritional Disorders: Anorexia, dehydration
Musculoskeletal, Connective Tissue, and Bone Disorders: Arthralgia, muscle spasms, myalgia, neck pain

Nervous System Disorders: Abnormal dreams, dizziness, migraine NOS, syncope, loss of taste
Psychiatric Disorders: Insomnia
Renal and Urinary Disorders: Choluria, dysuria, hematuria, polyuria, proteinuria, urinary frequency
Respiratory, Thoracic, and Mediastinal Disorders: Dyspnea NOS, nasal passage irritation, nasopharyngitis, pharyngitis, pharyngolaryngeal pain, rhinitis NOS, rhinorrhea
Skin and Subcutaneous Tissue Disorders: Clamminess, rash NOS, sweating increased
Vascular Disorders: Hot flashes NOS

Hepatic Encephalopathy

The data described below reflect exposure to XIFAXAN 550 mg in 348 patients, including 265 exposed for 6 months and 202 exposed for more than a year (mean exposure was 364 days). The safety of XIFAXAN 550 mg taken two times a day for reducing the risk of overt hepatic encephalopathy recurrence in adult patients was evaluated in a 6-month placebo-controlled clinical trial (n = 140) and in a long term follow-up study (n = 280). The population studied had a mean age of 56.26 (range: 21-82) years; approximately 20% of the patients were ≥ 65 years old, 61% were male, 86% were White, and 4% were Black. Ninety-one percent of patients in the trial were taking lactulose concomitantly. All adverse reactions that occurred at an incidence ≥ 5% and at a higher incidence in XIFAXAN 550 mg-treated subjects than in the placebo group in the 6-month trial are provided in Table 2. (These include adverse events that may be attributable to the underlying disease).

Table 2: Adverse Reactions Occurring in ≥ 5% of Patients Receiving XIFAXAN and at a Higher Incidence Than Placebo

MedDRA Preferred Term	Number (%) of Patients	
	XIFAXAN Tablets 550 mg TWICE DAILY N = 140	Placebo N = 159
Edema peripheral	21 (15%)	13 (8%)
Nausea	20 (14%)	21 (13%)
Dizziness	18 (13%)	13 (8%)
Fatigue	17 (12%)	18 (11%)
Ascites	16 (11%)	15 (9%)
Muscle spasms	13 (9%)	11 (7%)
Pruritus	13 (9%)	10 (6%)
Abdominal pain	12 (9%)	13 (8%)
Abdominal distension	11 (8%)	12 (8%)
Anemia	11 (8%)	6 (4%)
Cough	10 (7%)	11 (7%)
Depression	10 (7%)	8 (5%)
Insomnia	10 (7%)	11 (7%)
Nasopharyngitis	10 (7%)	10 (6%)
Abdominal pain upper	9 (6%)	8 (5%)
Arthralgia	9 (6%)	4 (3%)
Back pain	9 (6%)	10 (6%)
Constipation	9 (6%)	10 (6%)
Dyspnea	9 (6%)	7 (4%)
Pyrexia	9 (6%)	5 (3%)
Rash	7 (5%)	6 (4%)

The following adverse reactions, presented by body system, have also been reported in the placebo-controlled clinical trial in greater than 2% but less than 5% of patients taking XIFAXAN 550 mg taken orally two times a day for hepatic encephalopathy. The following includes adverse events occurring at a greater incidence than placebo, regardless of causal relationship to drug exposure.

Ear and Labyrinth Disorders: Vertigo
Gastrointestinal Disorders: Abdominal pain lower, abdominal tenderness, dry mouth, esophageal variceal bleed, stomach discomfort

General Disorders and Administration Site Conditions: Chest pain, generalized edema, influenza like illness, pain NOS
Infections and Infestations: Cellulitis, pneumonia, rhinitis, upper respiratory tract infection NOS
Injury, Poisoning and Procedural Complications: Contusion, fall, procedural pain
Investigations: Weight increased
Metabolic and Nutritional Disorders: Anorexia, dehydration, hyperglycemia, hyperkalemia, hypoglycemia, hyponatremia
Musculoskeletal, Connective Tissue, and Bone Disorders: Myalgia, pain in extremity
Nervous System Disorders: Amnesia, disturbance in attention, hypoesthesia, memory impairment, tremor
Psychiatric Disorders: Confusional state
Respiratory, Thoracic, and Mediastinal Disorders: Epistaxis
Vascular Disorders: Hypotension

6.2 Postmarketing Experience

The following adverse reactions have been identified during post approval use of XIFAXAN. Because these reactions are reported voluntarily from a population of unknown size, estimates of frequency cannot be made. These reactions have been chosen for inclusion due to either their seriousness, frequency of reporting or causal connection to XIFAXAN.

Infections and Infestations

Cases of *C. difficile*-associated colitis have been reported *[see Warnings and Precautions (5.2)].*

General

Hypersensitivity reactions, including exfoliative dermatitis, rash, angioneurotic edema (swelling of face and tongue and difficulty swallowing), urticaria, flushing, pruritus and anaphylaxis have been reported. These events occurred as early as within 15 minutes of drug administration.

7 DRUG INTERACTIONS

In vitro studies have shown that rifaximin did not inhibit cytochrome P450 isoenzymes 1A2, 2A6, 2B6, 2C9, 2C19, 2D6, 2E1 and CYP3A4 at concentrations ranging from 2 to 200 ng/mL *[see Clinical Pharmacology (12.3)].* Rifaximin is not expected to inhibit these enzymes in clinical use.

An *in vitro* study has suggested that rifaximin induces CYP3A4 *[see Clinical Pharmacology (12.3)].* However, in patients with normal liver function, rifaximin at the recommended dosing regimen is not expected to induce CYP3A4. It is unknown whether rifaximin can have a significant effect on the pharmacokinetics of concomitant CYP3A4 substrates in patients with reduced liver function who have elevated rifaximin concentrations.

An *in vitro* study suggested that rifaximin is a substrate of P-glycoprotein. It is unknown whether concomitant drugs that inhibit P-glycoprotein can increase the systemic exposure of rifaximin *[see Clinical Pharmacology (12.3)].*

8 USE IN SPECIFIC POPULATIONS

8.1 Pregnancy

Pregnancy Category C

There are no adequate and well controlled studies in pregnant women. XIFAXAN should be used during pregnancy only if the potential benefit outweighs the potential risk to the fetus.

Rifaximin was teratogenic in rats at doses of 150 to 300 mg/kg (approximately 2.5 to 5 times the clinical dose for travelers' diarrhea [600 mg/day], and approximately 1.3 to 2.6 times the clinical dose for hepatic encephalopathy [1100 mg/day], adjusted for body surface area). Rifaximin was teratogenic in rabbits at doses of 62.5 to 1000 mg/kg (approximately 2 to 33 times the clinical dose for travelers' diarrhea [600 mg/day], and approximately 1.1 to 18 times the clinical dose for hepatic encephalopathy [1100 mg/day], adjusted for body surface area). These effects include cleft palate, agnathia, jaw shortening, hemorrhage, eye partially open, small eyes, brachygnathia, incomplete ossification, and increased thoracolumbar vertebrae.

8.3 Nursing Mothers

It is not known whether rifaximin is excreted in human milk. Because many drugs are excreted in human milk and because of the potential for adverse reactions in nursing infants from XIFAXAN, a decision should be made whether to discontinue nursing or to discontinue the drug, taking into account the importance of the drug to the mother.

8.4 Pediatric Use

The safety and effectiveness of XIFAXAN 200 mg in pediatric patients with travelers' diarrhea less than 12 years of age have not been established.

The safety and effectiveness of XIFAXAN 550 mg for HE have not been established in patients < 18 years of age.

8.5 Geriatric Use

Clinical studies with rifaximin 200 mg for travelers' diarrhea did not include sufficient numbers of patients aged 65 and over to determine whether they respond differently than younger subjects.

In the controlled trial with XIFAXAN 550 mg for hepatic encephalopathy, 19.4% were 65 and over, while 2.3% were 75 and over. No overall differences in safety or effectiveness were observed between these subjects and younger subjects, and other reported clinical experience has not identified differences in responses between the elderly and younger patients, but greater sensitivity of some older individuals cannot be ruled out.

8.6   Renal Impairment
The pharmacokinetics of rifaximin in patients with impaired renal function has not been studied.

8.7   Hepatic Impairment
Following administration of XIFAXAN 550 mg twice daily to patients with a history of hepatic encephalopathy, the systemic exposure (i.e., AUC_τ) of rifaximin was about 10-, 13-, and 20-fold higher in those patients with mild (Child-Pugh A), moderate (Child-Pugh B) and severe (Child-Pugh C) hepatic impairment, respectively, compared to that in healthy volunteers. No dosage adjustment is recommended because rifaximin is presumably acting locally. Nonetheless, caution should be exercised when XIFAXAN is administered to patients with severe hepatic impairment [see *Warnings and Precautions (5.4), Clinical Pharmacology (12.3), Nonclinical Toxicology (13.2), and Clinical Studies (14.2)*].

10   OVERDOSAGE
No specific information is available on the treatment of overdosage with XIFAXAN. In clinical studies at doses higher than the recommended dose (> 600 mg/day for travelers' diarrhea or > 1100 mg/day for hepatic encephalopathy), adverse reactions were similar in subjects who received doses higher than the recommended dose and placebo. In the case of overdosage, discontinue XIFAXAN, treat symptomatically, and institute supportive measures as required.

11   DESCRIPTION
XIFAXAN tablets contain rifaximin, a non-aminoglycoside semi-synthetic, nonsystemic antibiotic derived from rifamycin SV. Rifaximin is a structural analog of rifampin. The chemical name for rifaximin is (2S,16Z,18E,20S,21S,22R,23R,24R,25S,26S,27S,28E)-5,6,21,23,25-pentahydroxy-27-methoxy-2,4,11,16,20,22,24,26-octamethyl-2,7-(epoxypentadeca-[1,11,13]trienimino)-benzofuro[4,5-e]pyrido[1,2-á]-benzimidazole-1,15(2H)-dione,25-acetate. The empirical formula is $C_{43}H_{51}N_3O_{11}$ and its molecular weight is 785.9. The chemical structure is represented below:

XIFAXAN Tablets for oral administration are film-coated and contain 200 mg or 550 mg of rifaximin.
Inactive ingredients: Each tablet contains colloidal silicon dioxide, disodium edetate, glycerol palmitostearate, hypromellose, microcrystalline cellulose, propylene glycol, red iron oxide, sodium starch glycolate, talc, and titanium dioxide.

12   CLINICAL PHARMACOLOGY
12.1   Mechanism of Action
Rifaximin is an antibacterial drug [see *Clinical Pharmacology (12.4)*].

12.3   Pharmacokinetics
Absorption
Travelers' Diarrhea
Systemic absorption of rifaximin (200 mg three times daily) was evaluated in 13 subjects challenged with shigellosis on Days 1 and 3 of a three-day course of treatment. Rifaximin plasma concentrations and exposures were low and variable. There was no evidence of accumulation of rifaximin following repeated administration for 3 days (9 doses). Peak plasma rifaximin concentrations after 3 and 9 consecutive doses ranged from 0.81 to 3.4 ng/mL on Day 1 and 0.68 to 2.26 ng/mL on Day 3. Similarly, AUC_{0-last} estimates were 6.95 ± 5.15 ng•h/mL on Day 1 and 7.83 ± 4.94 ng•h/mL on Day 3. XIFAXAN is not suitable for treating systemic bacterial infections because of limited systemic exposure after oral administration [see *Warnings and Precautions (5.1)*].
Hepatic Encephalopathy
After a single dose and multiple doses of rifaximin 550 mg in healthy subjects, the mean time to reach peak plasma concentrations was about an hour. The pharmacokinetic (PK) parameters were highly variable and the accumulation ratio based on AUC was 1.37.
The PK of rifaximin in patients with a history of HE was evaluated after administration of XIFAXAN, 550 mg two

Table 3. Mean (± SD) Pharmacokinetic Parameters of Rifaximin at Steady-State in Patients with a History of Hepatic Encephalopathy by Child-Pugh Class[1]

	Healthy Subjects (n = 14)	Child-Pugh Class		
		A (n = 18)	B (n = 7)	C (n = 4)
AUC_{tau} (ng•h/mL)	12.3 ± 4.8	118 ± 67.8	161 ± 101	246 ± 120
C_{max} (ng/mL)	3.4 ± 1.6	19.5 ± 11.4	25.1 ± 12.6	35.5 ± 12.5
$T_{max}{}^2$ (h)	0.8 (0.5, 4.0)	1 (0.9, 10)	1 (0.97, 1)	1 (0, 2)

[1] Cross-study comparison with PK parameters in healthy subjects
[2] Median (range)

times a day. The PK parameters were associated with a high variability and mean rifaximin exposure (AUC_τ) in patients with a history of HE (147 ng•h/mL) was approximately 12-fold higher than that observed in healthy subjects following the same dosing regimen (12.3 ng•h/mL). When PK parameters were analyzed based on Child-Pugh Class A, B, and C, the mean AUC_τ was 10-, 13-, and 20-fold higher, respectively, compared to that in healthy subjects (Table 3).
[See table 3 above]
Food Effect in Healthy Subjects
A high-fat meal consumed 30 minutes prior to XIFAXAN dosing in healthy subjects delayed the mean time to peak plasma concentration from 0.75 to 1.5 hours and increased the systemic exposure (AUC) of rifaximin by 2-fold (Table 4).

Table 4. Mean (± SD) Pharmacokinetic Parameters After Single-Dose Administration of XIFAXAN Tablets 550 mg in Healthy Subjects Under Fasting and Fed Conditions (N = 12)

Parameter	Fasting	Fed
C_{max} (ng/mL)	4.1 ± 1.5	4.8 ± 4.3
Tmax[1] (h)	0.8 (0.5, 2.1)	1.5 (0.5, 4.1)
Half-Life (h)	1.8 ± 1.4	4.8 ± 1.3
AUC (ng•h/mL)	11.1 ± 4.2	22.5 ± 12

[1] Median (range)

XIFAXAN can be administered with or without food [see *Dosage and Administration (2.1 and 2.2)*].
Distribution
Rifaximin is moderately bound to human plasma proteins. *In vivo*, the mean protein binding ratio was 67.5% in healthy subjects and 62% in patients with hepatic impairment when XIFAXAN 550 mg was administered.
Metabolism and Excretion
In a mass balance study, after administration of 400 mg ^{14}C-rifaximin orally to healthy volunteers, of the 96.94% total recovery, 96.62% of the administered radioactivity was recovered in feces almost exclusively as the unchanged drug and 0.32% was recovered in urine mostly as metabolites with 0.03% as the unchanged drug. Rifaximin accounted for 18% of radioactivity in plasma. This suggests that the absorbed rifaximin undergoes metabolism with minimal renal excretion of the unchanged drug. The enzymes responsible for metabolizing rifaximin are unknown.
In a separate study, rifaximin was detected in the bile after cholecystectomy in patients with intact gastrointestinal mucosa, suggesting biliary excretion of rifaximin.
Specific Populations
Hepatic Impairment
The systemic exposure of rifaximin was markedly elevated in patients with hepatic impairment compared to healthy subjects. The mean AUC in patients with Child-Pugh Class C hepatic impairment was 2-fold higher than in patients with Child-Pugh Class A hepatic impairment (see Table 3), [see *Warnings and Precautions (5.4) and Use in Specific Populations (8.7)*].
Renal Impairment
The pharmacokinetics of rifaximin in patients with impaired renal function has not been studied.
Drug Interactions
In vitro drug interaction studies have shown that rifaximin, at concentrations ranging from 2 to 200 ng/mL, did not inhibit human hepatic cytochrome P450 isoenzymes 1A2, 2A6, 2B6, 2C9, 2C19, 2D6, 2E1, and 3A4.
In an *in vitro* study, rifaximin was shown to induce CYP3A4 at the concentration of 0.2 μM.
An *in vitro* study suggests that rifaximin is a substrate of P-glycoprotein. In the presence of P-glycoprotein inhibitor verapamil, the efflux ratio of rifaximin was reduced greater than 50% *in vitro*. The effect of P-glycoprotein inhibition on rifaximin was not evaluated *in vivo*.

The inhibitory effect of rifaximin on P-gp transporter was observed in an *in vitro* study. The effect of rifaximin on P-gp transporter was not evaluated *in vivo*.
Midazolam
The effect of rifaximin 200 mg administered orally every 8 hours for 3 days and for 7 days on the pharmacokinetics of a single dose of either midazolam 2 mg intravenous or midazolam 6 mg orally was evaluated in healthy subjects. No significant difference was observed in the metrics of systemic exposure or elimination of intravenous or oral midazolam or its major metabolite, 1'-hydroxymidazolam, between midazolam alone or together with rifaximin. Therefore, rifaximin was not shown to significantly affect intestinal or hepatic CYP3A4 activity for the 200 mg three times a day dosing regimen.
After XIFAXAN 550 mg was administered three times a day for 7 days and 14 days to healthy subjects, the mean AUC of single midazolam 2 mg orally was 3.8% and 8.8% lower, respectively, than when midazolam was administered alone. The mean C_{max} of midazolam was also decreased by 4-5% when XIFAXAN was administered for 7-14 days prior to midazolam administration. This degree of interaction is not considered clinically meaningful.
The effect of rifaximin on CYP3A4 in patients with impaired liver function who have elevated systemic exposure is not known.
Oral Contraceptives Containing 0.07 mg Ethinyl Estradiol and 0.5 mg Norgestimate
The oral contraceptive study utilized an open-label, crossover design in 28 healthy female subjects to determine if rifaximin 200 mg orally administered three times a day for 3 days (the dosing regimen for travelers' diarrhea) altered the pharmacokinetics of a single dose of an oral contraceptive containing 0.07 mg ethinyl estradiol and 0.5 mg norgestimate. Results showed that the pharmacokinetics of single doses of ethinyl estradiol and norgestimate were not altered by rifaximin [see *Drug Interactions (7)*].
Effect of rifaximin on oral contraceptives was not studied for XIFAXAN 550 mg twice a day, the dosing regimen for hepatic encephalopathy.
12.4   Microbiology
Mechanism of Action
Rifaximin is a non-aminoglycoside semi-synthetic antibacterial derived from rifamycin SV. Rifaximin acts by binding to the beta-subunit of bacterial DNA-dependent RNA polymerase resulting in inhibition of bacterial RNA synthesis. *Escherichia coli* has been shown to develop resistance to rifaximin *in vitro*. However, the clinical significance of such an effect has not been studied.
Rifaximin is a structural analog of rifampin. Organisms with high rifaximin minimum inhibitory concentration (MIC) values also have elevated MIC values against rifampin. Cross-resistance between rifaximin and other classes of antimicrobials has not been studied.
Rifaximin has been shown to be active against the following pathogen in clinical studies of infectious diarrhea as described in the *Indications and Usage (1)* section: *Escherichia coli* (enterotoxigenic and enteroaggregative strains).
For HE, rifaximin is thought to have an effect on the gastrointestinal flora.
Susceptibility Tests
In vitro susceptibility testing was performed according to the National Committee for Clinical Laboratory Standards (NCCLS) agar dilution method M7-A6 [see *References (15)*]. However, the correlation between susceptibility testing and clinical outcome has not been determined.

13   NONCLINICAL TOXICOLOGY
13.1   Carcinogenesis, Mutagenesis, Impairment of Fertility
Malignant schwannomas in the heart were significantly increased in male Crl:CD® (SD) rats that received rifaximin by oral gavage for two years at 150 to 250 mg/kg/day (doses equivalent to 2.4 to 4 times the recommended dose of 200 mg three times daily for travelers' diarrhea, and equivalent to 1.3 to 2.2 times the recommended dose of 550 mg twice daily for hepatic encephalopathy, based on relative

body surface area comparisons). There was no increase in tumors in Tg.rasH2 mice dosed orally with rifaximin for 26 weeks at 150 to 2000 mg/kg/day (doses equivalent to 1.2 to 16 times the recommended daily dose for travelers' diarrhea and equivalent to 0.7 to 9 times the recommended daily dose for hepatic encephalopathy, based on relative body surface area comparisons).

Rifaximin was not genotoxic in the bacterial reverse mutation assay, chromosomal aberration assay, rat bone marrow micronucleus assay, rat hepatocyte unscheduled DNA synthesis assay, or the CHO/HGPRT mutation assay. There was no effect on fertility in male or female rats following the administration of rifaximin at doses up to 300 mg/kg (approximately 5 times the clinical dose of 600 mg/day, and approximately 2.6 times the clinical dose of 1100 mg/day, adjusted for body surface area).

13.2 Animal Toxicology and/or Pharmacology

Oral administration of rifaximin for 3-6 months produced hepatic proliferation of connective tissue in rats (50 mg/kg/day) and fatty degeneration of liver in dogs (100 mg/kg/day). However, plasma drug levels were not measured in these studies. Subsequently, rifaximin was studied at doses as high as 300 mg/kg/day in rats for 6 months and 1000 mg/kg/day in dogs for 9 months, and no signs of hepatotoxicity were observed. The maximum plasma AUC $_{0\text{-}8\ hr}$ values from the 6 month rat and 9 month dog toxicity studies (range: 42-127 ng•h/mL) was lower than the maximum plasma AUC $_{0\text{-}8\ hr}$ values in cirrhotic patients (range: 19-306 ng•h/mL).

14 CLINICAL STUDIES

14.1 Travelers' Diarrhea

The efficacy of XIFAXAN given as 200 mg orally taken three times a day for 3 days was evaluated in 2 randomized, multi–center, double-blind, placebo-controlled studies in adult subjects with travelers' diarrhea. One study was conducted at clinical sites in Mexico, Guatemala, and Kenya (Study 1). The other study was conducted in Mexico, Guatemala, Peru, and India (Study 2). Stool specimens were collected before treatment and 1 to 3 days following the end of treatment to identify enteric pathogens. The predominant pathogen in both studies was *Escherichia coli*.

The clinical efficacy of XIFAXAN was assessed by the time to return to normal, formed stools and resolution of symptoms. The primary efficacy endpoint was time to last unformed stool (TLUS) which was defined as the time to the last unformed stool passed, after which clinical cure was declared. Table 5 displays the median TLUS and the number of patients who achieved clinical cure for the intent to treat (ITT) population of Study 1. The duration of diarrhea was significantly shorter in patients treated with XIFAXAN than in the placebo group. More patients treated with XIFAXAN were classified as clinical cures than were those in the placebo group.

Table 5. Clinical Response in Study 1 (ITT population)

	XIFAXAN (n=125)	Placebo (n=129)	Estimate (97.5% CI)	P-Value
Median TLUS (hours)	32.5	58.6	1.78[a] (1.26, 2.50)	0.0002
Clinical cure, n (%)	99 (79.2)	78 (60.5)	18.7[b] (5.3, 32.1)	0.001

[a] Hazard Ratio
[b] Difference in rates

Microbiological eradication (defined as the absence of a baseline pathogen in culture of stool after 72 hours of therapy) rates for Study 1 are presented in Table 6 for patients with any pathogen at baseline and for the subset of patients with *Escherichia coli* at baseline. *Escherichia coli* was the only pathogen with sufficient numbers to allow comparisons between treatment groups.

Even though XIFAXAN had microbiologic activity similar to placebo, it demonstrated a clinically significant reduction in duration of diarrhea and a higher clinical cure rate than placebo. Therefore, patients should be managed based on clinical response to therapy rather than microbiologic response.

Table 6. Microbiologic Eradication Rates in Study 1 Subjects with a Baseline Pathogen

	XIFAXAN	Placebo
Overall	48/70 (68.6)	41/61 (67.2)
E. coli	38/53 (71.7)	40/54 (74.1)

The results of Study 2 supported the results presented for Study 1. In addition, this study provided evidence that subjects treated with XIFAXAN with fever and/or blood in the stool at baseline had prolonged TLUS. These subjects had lower clinical cure rates than those without fever or blood in the stool at baseline. Many of the patients with fever and/or blood in the stool (dysentery-like diarrheal syndromes) had invasive pathogens, primarily *Campylobacter jejuni*, isolated in the baseline stool.

Also in this study, the majority of the subjects treated with XIFAXAN who had *Campylobacter jejuni* isolated as a sole pathogen at baseline failed treatment and the resulting clinical cure rate for these patients was 23.5% (4/17). In addition to not being different from placebo, the microbiologic eradication rates for subjects with *Campylobacter jejuni* isolated at baseline were much lower than the eradication rates seen for *Escherichia coli*.

In an unrelated open-label, pharmacokinetic study of oral XIFAXAN 200 mg taken every 8 hours for 3 days, 15 adult subjects were challenged with *Shigella flexneri* 2a, of whom 13 developed diarrhea or dysentery and were treated with XIFAXAN. Although this open-label challenge trial was not adequate to assess the effectiveness of XIFAXAN in the treatment of shigellosis, the following observations were noted: eight subjects received rescue treatment with ciprofloxacin either because of lack of response to XIFAXAN treatment within 24 hours (2), or because they developed severe dysentery (5), or because of recurrence of *Shigella flexneri* in the stool (1); five of the 13 subjects received ciprofloxacin although they did not have evidence of severe disease or relapse.

14.2 Hepatic Encephalopathy

The efficacy of XIFAXAN 550 mg taken orally two times a day was evaluated in a randomized, placebo-controlled, double-blind, multi-center 6-month trial of adult subjects from the U.S., Canada and Russia who were defined as being in remission (Conn score of 0 or 1) from hepatic encephalopathy (HE). Eligible subjects had ≥ 2 episodes of HE associated with chronic liver disease in the previous 6 months.

A total of 299 subjects were randomized to receive either XIFAXAN (n=140) or placebo (n=159) in this study. Patients had a mean age of 56 years (range, 21-82 years), 81% < 65 years of age, 61% were male and 86% White. At baseline, 67% of patients had a Conn score of 0 and 68% had an asterixis grade of 0. Patients had MELD scores of either ≤ 10 (27%) or 11 to 18 (64%) at baseline. No patients were enrolled with a MELD score of > 25. Nine percent of the patients were Child-Pugh Class C. Lactulose was concomitantly used by 91% of the patients in each treatment arm of the study. Per the study protocol, patients were withdrawn from the study after experiencing a breakthrough HE episode. Other reasons for early study discontinuation included: adverse reactions (XIFAXAN 6%; placebo 4%), patient request to withdraw (XIFAXAN 4%; placebo 6%) and other (XIFAXAN 7%; placebo 5%).

The primary endpoint was the time to first breakthrough overt HE episode. A breakthrough overt HE episode was defined as a marked deterioration in neurological function and an increase of Conn score to Grade ≥ 2. In patients with a baseline Conn score of 0, a breakthrough overt HE episode was defined as an increase in Conn score of 1 and asterixis grade of 1.

Breakthrough overt HE episodes were experienced by 31 of 140 subjects (22%) in the XIFAXAN group and by 73 of 159 subjects (46%) in the placebo group during the 6-month treatment period. Comparison of Kaplan-Meier estimates of event-free curves showed XIFAXAN significantly reduced the risk of HE breakthrough by 58% during the 6-month treatment period. Presented below in Figure 1 is the Kaplan-Meier event-free curve for all subjects (n = 299) in the study.

Figure 1: Kaplan-Meier Event-Free Curves[1] in HE Study (Time to First Breakthrough-HE Episode up to 6 Months of Treatment, Day 170) (ITT Population)

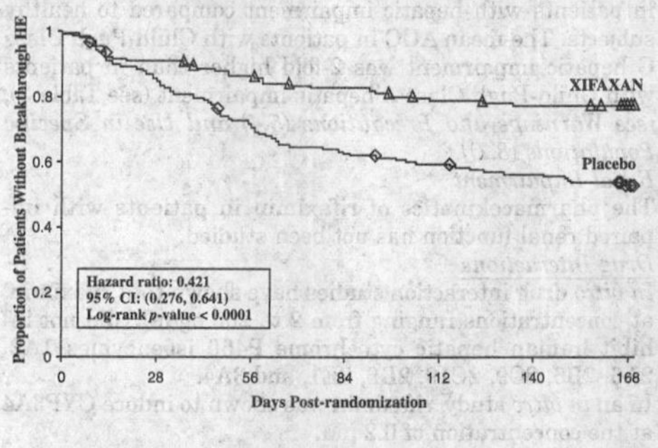

Note: Open diamonds and open triangles represent censored subjects.
[1]Event-free refers to non-occurrence of breakthrough HE.

When the results were evaluated by the following demographic and baseline characteristics, the treatment effect of XIFAXAN 550 mg in reducing the risk of breakthrough overt HE recurrence was consistent for: sex, baseline Conn score, duration of current remission and diabetes. The differences in treatment effect could not be assessed in the following subpopulations due to small sample size: non-White (n=42), baseline MELD > 19 (n=26), Child-Pugh C (n=31), and those without concomitant lactulose use (n=26).

HE-related hospitalizations (hospitalizations directly resulting from HE, or hospitalizations complicated by HE) were reported for 19 of 140 subjects (14%) and 36 of 159 subjects (23%) in the XIFAXAN and placebo groups respectively. Comparison of Kaplan-Meier estimates of event-free curves showed XIFAXAN significantly reduced the risk of HE-related hospitalizations by 50% during the 6-month treatment period. Comparison of Kaplan-Meier estimates of event-free curves is shown in Figure 2.

Figure 2: Kaplan-Meier Event-Free Curves[1] in Pivotal HE Study (Time to First HE-Related Hospitalization in HE Study up to 6 Months of Treatment, Day 170) (ITT Population)

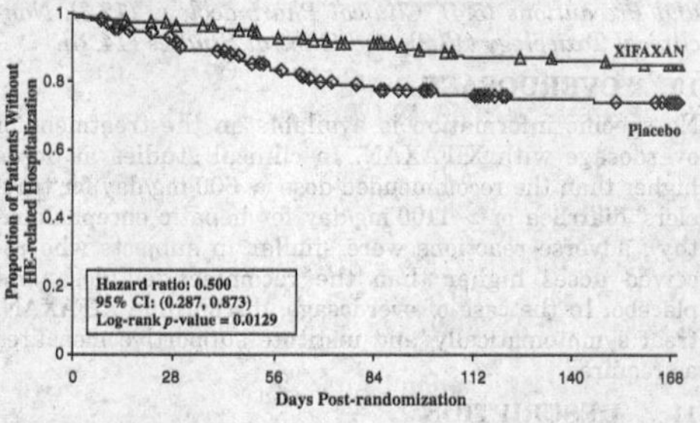

Note: Open diamonds and open triangles represent censored subjects.
[1]Event-free refers to non-occurrence of HE-related hospitalization.

15 REFERENCES

Methods for dilution antimicrobial susceptibility tests for bacteria that grow aerobically. National Committee for Clinical Laboratory Standards, Sixth Edition, Wayne PA. *Approved Standard NCCLS Document M7-A6* January 2003; 23 (2).

16 HOW SUPPLIED/STORAGE AND HANDLING

The 200 mg tablet is a pink-colored, round, biconvex tablet with "Sx" debossed on one side. It is available in the following presentations:

- NDC 65649-301-03, bottles of 30 tablets
- NDC 65649-301-41, bottles of 100 tablets
- NDC 65649-301-05, carton of 100 tablets, Unit Dose

The 550 mg tablet is a pink-colored, oval, biconvex tablet with "rfx" debossed on one side. It is available in the following presentations:

- NDC 65649-303-02, bottles of 60 tablets
- NDC 65649-303-03, carton of 60 tablets, Unit Dose

Storage

Store XIFAXAN Tablets at 20–25°C (68–77°F); excursions permitted to 15–30°C (59-86°F). See USP Controlled Room Temperature.

17 PATIENT COUNSELING INFORMATION

17.1 Persistent Diarrhea

For those patients being treated for travelers' diarrhea, discontinue XIFAXAN if diarrhea persists more than 24-48 hours or worsens. Advise the patient to seek medical care for fever and/or blood in the stool [see *Warnings and Precautions (5.1)*].

17.2 *Clostridium difficile*-Associated Diarrhea

Clostridium difficile-associated diarrhea (CDAD) has been reported with use of nearly all antibacterial agents, including XIFAXAN, and may range in severity from mild diarrhea to fatal colitis. Treatment with antibiotics alters the normal flora of the colon which may lead to *C. difficile*. Patients can develop watery and bloody stools (with or without stomach cramps and fever) even as late as two or more months after having taken the last dose of the antibiotic. If diarrhea occurs after therapy or does not improve or worsens during therapy, advise patients to contact a physician as soon as possible [see *Warnings and Precautions (5.4)*].

17.3 Administration with Food

Inform patients that XIFAXAN may be taken with or without food.

17.4 Antibacterial Resistance

Counsel patients that antibacterial drugs including XIFAXAN should only be used to treat bacterial infections. They do not treat viral infections (e.g., the common cold). When XIFAXAN is prescribed to treat a bacterial infection, patients should be told that although it is common to feel better early in the course of therapy, the medication should be taken exactly as directed. Skipping doses or not completing the full course of therapy may (1) decrease the effectiveness of the immediate treatment and (2) increase the likelihood that bacteria will develop resistance and will not be treatable by XIFAXAN or other antibacterial drugs in the future.

17.5   Severe Hepatic Impairment

Patients should be informed that in patients with severe hepatic impairment (Child-Pugh C) there is an increase in systemic exposure to XIFAXAN [see Warnings and Precautions (5.4)].

Manufactured for Salix Pharmaceuticals, Inc., Morrisville, NC 27560, under license from Alfa Wassermann S.p.A.

XIFAXAN® is a trademark of Salix Pharmaceuticals, Inc., under license from Alfa Wassermann S.p.A.

Copyright © Salix Pharmaceuticals, Inc.

VENART-156-0

Mar 2010

Product protected by US Patent Nos. 7,045,620 and 7,612,199 and other pending applications.

Web site: www.Salix.com

E-mail: customer.service@salix.com

1700 Perimeter Park Drive, Morrisville, NC 27560

Tel.866-669-SLXP (7597) Salix Pharmaceuticals, Inc.

All rights reserved.

Shown in Product Identification Guide, page 318

---

sanofi-aventis U.S.
**55 CORPORATE DRIVE
BRIDGEWATER, NJ 08807**

Direct Inquiries to:
Customer Service
55 Corporate Drive
PO Box 5925
Bridgewater, NJ 08807
(800) 207-8049

For Medical Information Contact:
Generally:
Medical Information Services
55 Corporate Drive
PO Box 5925
Bridgewater, NJ 08807
(800) 633-1610
For Oncology Medical Information
call (866) 662-6411

ALLEGRA®   Rx
[ə-'lĕgra]
**(fexofenadine hydrochloride)
tablets, ODT (orally disintegrating tablets) and oral suspension**

HIGHLIGHTS OF PRESCRIBING INFORMATION
These highlights do not include all the information needed to use ALLEGRA safely and effectively. See full prescribing information for ALLEGRA.

Initial U.S. Approval: 1996

RECENT MAJOR CHANGES
Dosage and Administration, ALLEGRA ODT (2.2)	[7/2007]
Dosage and Administration, ALLEGRA oral suspension (2.3)	[10/2006]

INDICATIONS AND USAGE
ALLEGRA is an H₁-receptor antagonist indicated for:
- Relief of symptoms associated with seasonal allergic rhinitis in patients ≥ 2 years of age (1.1)
- Treatment of uncomplicated skin manifestations of chronic idiopathic urticaria in patients ≥ 6 months of age (1.2)

DOSAGE AND ADMINISTRATION

Patient Population	ALLEGRA tablets (2.1)	ALLEGRA ODT (2.2)	ALLEGRA oral suspension (2.3)
Adults and children ≥ 12 years	60 mg twice daily[1], or 180 mg once daily[2]	N/A	N/A
Children 6 to 11 years	30 mg twice daily[1]	30 mg twice daily[1]	30 mg twice daily[1]
Children 2 to 5 years	N/A	N/A	30 mg twice daily[1]
Children 6 months to less than 2 years	N/A	N/A	15 mg twice daily[1,3]

[1] starting dose in patients with decreased renal function should be the recommended dose indicated above but administered once daily
[2] dose not for use in patients with decreased renal function
[3] indicated for chronic idiopathic urticaria only

- ALLEGRA tablets: take with water (2.1)
- ALLEGRA ODT: take on an empty stomach; allow to disintegrate on the tongue and swallow with or without water; do not remove from original blister package until time of administration; do not break or use partial tablets (2.2)

DOSAGE FORMS AND STRENGTHS
- ALLEGRA tablets: 30 mg, 60 mg, and 180 mg (3)
- ALLEGRA ODT: 30 mg (3)
- ALLEGRA oral suspension: 30 mg/5 mL (6 mg/mL) (3)

CONTRAINDICATIONS
Patients with known hypersensitivity to fexofenadine and any of the ingredients of ALLEGRA. (4)

WARNINGS AND PRECAUTIONS
ALLEGRA ODT contains phenylalanine, a component of aspartame. Other ALLEGRA products do not contain phenylalanine.

ADVERSE REACTIONS
The most common adverse reactions (≥ 2%) in subjects age 12 years and older were headache, back pain, dizziness, stomach discomfort, and pain in extremity. In subjects aged 6 to 11 years, cough, upper respiratory tract infection, pyrexia and otitis media were more frequently reported. In subjects aged 6 months to 5 years, vomiting, diarrhea, somnolence/fatigue and rhinorrhea were more frequently reported. (6.1)

Other adverse reactions have been reported. (6)

To report SUSPECTED ADVERSE REACTIONS, contact sanofi-aventis at 1-800-633-1610 or FDA at 1-800-FDA-1088 or www.fda.gov/medwatch.

DRUG INTERACTIONS
- Antacids: Do not take at the same time as aluminum and magnesium containing antacids (7.1)
- Fruit juice: Take with water; not fruit juice

USE IN SPECIFIC POPULATIONS
- Pregnancy: Use only if benefit justifies risk to fetus (8.1)
- Nursing Mothers: Use with caution (8.3)

See 17 for PATIENT COUNSELING INFORMATION

Revised: [7/2007]

FULL PRESCRIBING INFORMATION: CONTENTS*

FULL PRESCRIBING INFORMATION

1   INDICATIONS AND USAGE
1.1   Seasonal Allergic Rhinitis
ALLEGRA is indicated for the relief of symptoms associated with seasonal allergic rhinitis in adults and children 2 years of age and older.

1.2   Chronic Idiopathic Urticaria
ALLEGRA is indicated for treatment of uncomplicated skin manifestations of chronic idiopathic urticaria in adults and children 6 months of age and older.

2   DOSAGE AND ADMINISTRATION
2.1   ALLEGRA tablets
Seasonal Allergic Rhinitis and Chronic Idiopathic Urticaria
Adults and Children 12 Years and Older: The recommended dose of ALLEGRA tablets is 60 mg twice daily or 180 mg once daily with water. A dose of 60 mg once daily is recommended as the starting dose in patients with decreased renal function [see Clinical Pharmacology (12.3)].
Children 6 to 11 Years: The recommended dose of ALLEGRA tablets is 30 mg twice daily with water. A dose of 30 mg once daily is recommended as the starting dose in pediatric patients with decreased renal function [see Clinical Pharmacology (12.3)].

2.2   ALLEGRA ODT
Seasonal Allergic Rhinitis and Chronic Idiopathic Urticaria
Children 6 to 11 Years: ALLEGRA ODT is intended for use only in children 6 to 11 years of age. The recommended dose of ALLEGRA ODT is 30 mg twice daily. A dose of 30 mg once daily is recommended as the starting dose in pediatric patients with decreased renal function [see Clinical Pharmacology (12.3)].

ALLEGRA ODT is designed to disintegrate on the tongue, followed by swallowing with or without water. ALLEGRA ODT should be taken on an empty stomach. ALLEGRA ODT is not intended to be chewed.

ALLEGRA ODT should not be removed from the original blister package until the time of administration.

2.3   ALLEGRA oral suspension
Seasonal Allergic Rhinitis
Children 2 to 11 Years: The recommended dose of ALLEGRA oral suspension is 30 mg twice daily. A dose of 30 mg (5 mL) once daily is recommended as the starting dose in pediatric patients with decreased renal function [see Clinical Pharmacology (12.3)].
Shake bottle well, before each use.
Chronic Idiopathic Urticaria
Children 6 Months to 11 years: The recommended dose of ALLEGRA oral suspension is 30 mg (5 mL) twice daily for patients 2 to 11 years of age and 15 mg (2.5 mL) twice daily for patients 6 months to less than 2 years of age. For pediatric patients with decreased renal function, the recommended starting doses of ALLEGRA oral suspension are 30 mg (5 mL) once daily for patients 2 to 11 years of age and 15 mg (2.5 mL) once daily for patients 6 months to less than 2 years of age [see Clinical Pharmacology (12.3)].
Shake bottle well, before each use.

3   DOSAGE FORMS AND STRENGTHS
ALLEGRA tablets are available in 30 mg, 60 mg, and 180 mg strengths. ALLEGRA tablets are coated with a peach colored film coating. Tablets have the following unique shape and identifiers: 30 mg tablets are round, bi-convex and have 03 on one side and a scripted "e" on the other; 60 mg tablets are oval, bi-convex and have 06 on one side and a scripted "e" on the other; and 180 mg tablets are oblong, bi-convex and have 018 on one side and a scripted "e" on the other.

ALLEGRA ODT is available as a 30 mg orally disintegrating tablet and is white, flat-faced, ½-inch round shaped with beveled edges and debossed with a scripted "e" on one side and "311AV" on the other side.

ALLEGRA oral suspension is available as 30 mg/ 5 mL (6 mg/mL).

4   CONTRAINDICATIONS
ALLEGRA tablets, ALLEGRA ODT and ALLEGRA oral suspension are contraindicated in patients with known hypersensitivity to fexofenadine and any of the ingredients of ALLEGRA. Rare cases of hypersensitivity reactions with manifestations such as angioedema, chest tightness, dyspnea, flushing and systemic anaphylaxis have been reported.

5   WARNINGS AND PRECAUTIONS
5.1   Phenylketonurics
ALLEGRA ODT contains phenylalanine, a component of aspartame. Each 30 mg ALLEGRA ODT contains 5.3 mg phenylalanine. ALLEGRA products other than ALLEGRA ODT do not contain phenylalanine.

6 ADVERSE REACTIONS

6.1 Clinical Studies Experience

Because clinical trials are conducted under widely varying conditions, adverse reaction rates observed in the clinical trials of a drug cannot be directly compared to rates in the clinical trials of another drug and may not reflect the rates observed in practice.

The safety data described below reflect exposure to fexofenadine hydrochloride in 5083 patients in trials for allergic rhinitis and chronic idiopathic urticaria. In these trials, 3010 patients 12 years of age and older with seasonal allergic rhinitis received fexofenadine hydrochloride at doses of 20 to 240 mg twice daily or 120 to 180 mg once daily. A total of 646 patients 6 to 11 years of age with seasonal allergic rhinitis were exposed to fexofenadine hydrochloride at doses of 15 to 60 mg twice daily. The duration of treatment in these trials was 2 weeks. A total of 534 patients 6 months to 5 years of age with allergic rhinitis were exposed to fexofenadine hydrochloride at doses of 15 to 30 mg twice daily. The duration of treatment in these trials ranged from 1 day to 2 weeks. There were 893 patients 12 years of age and older with chronic idiopathic urticaria exposed to fexofenadine hydrochloride at doses of 20 to 240 mg twice daily or 180 mg once daily. The duration of treatment in these trials was 4 weeks.

Seasonal Allergic Rhinitis

Adults and Adolescents: In placebo-controlled seasonal allergic rhinitis clinical trials in subjects 12 years of age and older, 2439 subjects received fexofenadine hydrochloride capsules at doses of 20 mg to 240 mg twice daily. All adverse reactions that were reported by greater than 1% of subjects who received the recommended daily dose of fexofenadine hydrochloride (60 mg capsules twice daily) are listed in Table 1.

In another placebo-controlled clinical study in the United States, 571 subjects aged 12 years and older received fexofenadine hydrochloride tablets at doses of 120 or 180 mg once daily. Table 1 also lists adverse reactions that were reported by greater than 2% of subjects treated with fexofenadine hydrochloride tablets at doses of 180 mg once daily.

The incidence of adverse reactions, including somnolence/fatigue, was not dose-related and was similar across subgroups defined by age, gender, and race.

Table 1
Adverse reactions in subjects aged 12 years and older reported in placebo-controlled seasonal allergic rhinitis clinical trials in the United States
Twice-daily dosing with fexofenadine capsules at rates of greater than 1%

Adverse reaction	Fexofenadine 60 mg Twice Daily (n=680) Frequency	Placebo Twice Daily (n=674) Frequency
Dysmenorrhea	1.5%	0.3%

Once-daily dosing with fexofenadine hydrochloride tablets at rates of greater than 2%

Adverse reaction	Fexofenadine 180 mg Once Daily (n=283) Frequency	Placebo (n=293) Frequency
Headache	10.3%	7.2%
Back Pain	2.5%	1.4%

The frequency and magnitude of laboratory abnormalities were similar in fexofenadine hydrochloride- and placebo-treated subjects.

Pediatrics: Table 2 lists adverse reactions in subjects aged 6 years to 11 years of age which were reported by greater than 2% of subjects treated with fexofenadine hydrochloride tablets at a dose of 30 mg twice daily in placebo-controlled seasonal allergic rhinitis studies in the United States and Canada.

Table 2
Adverse reactions reported in placebo-controlled seasonal allergic rhinitis studies in pediatric subjects aged 6 years to 11 years in the United States and Canada at rates of greater than 2%

Adverse reaction	Fexofenadine 30 mg Twice Daily (n=209) Frequency	Placebo (n=229) Frequency
Cough	3.8%	1.3%
Upper Respiratory Tract Infection	2.9%	0.9%
Pyrexia	2.4%	0.9%
Otitis Media	2.4%	0.0%

Table 3 lists adverse reactions in subjects 6 months to 5 years of age which were reported by greater than 2% of subjects treated with fexofenadine hydrochloride in 3 open single- and multiple-dose pharmacokinetic studies and 3 placebo-controlled safety studies with fexofenadine hydrochloride capsule content (484 subjects) and suspension (50 subjects) at doses of 15 mg (108 subjects) and 30 mg (426 subjects) given twice a day.

[See table below]

Chronic Idiopathic Urticaria

Adverse reactions reported by subjects 12 years of age and older in placebo-controlled chronic idiopathic urticaria studies were similar to those reported in placebo-controlled seasonal allergic rhinitis studies.

In placebo-controlled chronic idiopathic urticaria clinical trials, 726 subjects 12 years of age and older received fexofenadine hydrochloride tablets at doses of 20 to 240 mg twice daily. Table 4 lists adverse reactions in subjects aged 12 years and older which were reported by greater than 2% of subjects treated with fexofenadine hydrochloride 60 mg tablets twice daily in controlled clinical studies in the United States and Canada.

In a placebo-controlled clinical study in the United States, 167 subjects aged 12 years and older received fexofenadine hydrochloride 180 mg tablets. Table 4 also lists adverse reactions that were reported by greater than 2% of subjects treated with fexofenadine hydrochloride tablets at doses of 180 mg once daily.

Table 4
Adverse reactions reported in subjects 12 years of age and older in placebo-controlled chronic idiopathic urticaria studies
Twice-daily dosing with fexofenadine hydrochloride in studies in the United States and Canada at rates of greater than 2%

Adverse reaction	Fexofenadine 60 mg Twice Daily (n=191) Frequency	Placebo (n=183) Frequency
Dizziness	2.1%	1.1%
Back Pain	2.1%	1.1%
Stomach discomfort	2.1%	0.6%
Pain in extremity	2.1%	0.0%

Once-daily dosing with fexofenadine hydrochloride in a study in the United States at rates of greater than 2%

Adverse reaction	Fexofenadine 180 mg Once Daily (n=167) Frequency	Placebo (n=92) Frequency
Headache	4.8%	3.3%

The safety of fexofenadine hydrochloride in the treatment of chronic idiopathic urticaria in pediatric patients 6 months to 11 years of age is based on the safety profile of fexofenadine hydrochloride in adults and pediatric patients at doses equal to or higher than the recommended dose [see *Use in Specific Populations (8.4)*].

6.2 Postmarketing Experience

In addition to the adverse reactions reported during clinical studies and listed above, the following adverse events have been identified during post-approval use of ALLEGRA. Because these events are reported voluntarily from a population of uncertain size, it is not always possible to reliably estimate their frequency or establish a causal relationship to drug exposure. Events that have been reported rarely during postmarketing experience include: insomnia, nervousness, sleep disorders or paroniria, and hypersensitivity reactions (including anaphylaxis, urticaria, angioedema, chest tightness, dyspnea, flushing, pruritus, and rash).

7 DRUG INTERACTIONS

7.1 Antacids

Fexofenadine hydrochloride should not be taken closely in time with aluminum and magnesium containing antacids. In healthy adult subjects, administration of 120 mg of fexofenadine hydrochloride (2×60 mg capsule) within 15 minutes of an aluminum and magnesium containing antacid (Maalox®) decreased fexofenadine AUC by 41% and C_{max} by 43%.

7.2 Erythromycin and Ketoconazole

Fexofenadine has been shown to exhibit minimal (ca. 5%) metabolism. However, co-administration of fexofenadine hydrochloride with either ketoconazole or erythromycin led to increased plasma concentrations of fexofenadine in healthy adult subjects. Fexofenadine had no effect on the pharmacokinetics of either erythromycin or ketoconazole. In 2 separate studies in healthy adult subjects, fexofenadine hydrochloride 120 mg twice daily (240 mg total daily dose) was co-administered with either erythromycin 500 mg every 8 hours or ketoconazole 400 mg once daily under steady-state conditions to healthy adult subjects (n=24, each study). No differences in adverse events or QT_c interval were observed when subjects were administered fexofenadine hydrochloride alone or in combination with either erythromycin or ketoconazole. The findings of these studies are summarized in the following table:

Table 5
Effects on steady-state fexofenadine pharmacokinetics after 7 days of co-administration with fexofenadine hydrochloride 120 mg every 12 hours in healthy adult subjects (n=24)

Concomitant Drug	C_{maxSS} (Peak plasma concentration)	$AUC_{ss(0-12h)}$ (Extent of systemic exposure)
Erythromycin (500 mg every 8 hrs)	+82%	+109%
Ketoconazole (400 mg once daily)	+135%	+164%

The changes in plasma levels were within the range of plasma levels achieved in adequate and well-controlled clinical trials.

The mechanism of these interactions has been evaluated in *in vitro*, *in situ*, and *in vivo* animal models. These studies indicate that ketoconazole or erythromycin co-administration enhances fexofenadine gastrointestinal absorption. This observed increase in the bioavailability of fexofenadine may be due to transport-related effects, such as p-glycoprotein. *In vivo* animal studies also suggest that in addition to enhancing absorption, ketoconazole decreases fexofenadine gastrointestinal secretion, while erythromycin may also decrease biliary excretion.

7.3 Fruit Juices

Fruit juices such as grapefruit, orange and apple may reduce the bioavailability and exposure of fexofenadine. This is based on the results from 3 clinical studies using histamine induced skin wheals and flares coupled with population pharmacokinetic analysis. The size of wheal and flare were significantly larger when fexofenadine hydrochloride was administered with either grapefruit or orange juices compared to water. Based on the literature reports, the same effects may be extrapolated to other fruit juices such as apple juice. The clinical significance of these observations is unknown. In addition, based on the population pharmacokinetics analysis of the combined data from grapefruit and orange juices studies with the data from a bioequivalence study, the bioavailability of fexofenadine was reduced by 36%. Therefore, to maximize the effects of fexofenadine, it is recommended that ALLEGRA tablets should be taken with water [see *Clinical Pharmacology (12.3) and Dosage and Administration (2.1)*].

ALLEGRA ODT can be taken with or without water [see *Clinical Pharmacology (12.3) and Dosage and Administration (2.2)*].

8 USE IN SPECIFIC POPULATIONS

8.1 Pregnancy

Teratogenic Effects: Pregnancy Category C. There was no evidence of teratogenicity in rats or rabbits at oral doses of terfenadine up to 300 mg/kg (which led to fexofenadine exposures that were approximately 4 and 30 times, respectively, the exposure at the maximum recommended human daily oral dose of 180 mg of fexofenadine hydrochloride based on comparison of AUCs).

Table 3
Adverse reactions reported in placebo-controlled studies in pediatric subjects with allergic rhinitis aged 6 months to 5 years of age at rates greater than 2%

Adverse reaction	Fexofenadine 15 mg Twice Daily (n=108) Frequency	Fexofenadine 30 mg Twice Daily (n=426) Frequency	Fexofenadine Total Twice Daily (n=534) Frequency	Placebo (n=430) Frequency
Vomiting	12.0%	4.2%	5.8%	8.6%
Diarrhea	3.7%	2.8%	3.0%	2.6%
Somnolence/Fatigue	2.8%	0.9%	1.3%	0.2%
Rhinorrhea	0.9%	2.1%	1.9%	0.9%

In mice, no adverse effects and no teratogenic effects during gestation were observed with fexofenadine hydrochloride at oral doses up to 3730 mg/kg (which led to fexofenadine exposures that were approximately 15 times the exposure at the maximum recommended human daily oral dose of 180 mg of fexofenadine hydrochloride based on comparison of AUCs).

There are no adequate and well controlled studies in pregnant women. Fexofenadine hydrochloride should be used during pregnancy only if the potential benefit justifies the potential risk to the fetus.

Nonteratogenic Effects: Dose-related decreases in pup weight gain and survival were observed in rats exposed to an oral dose of 150 mg/kg of terfenadine (which led to fexofenadine exposures that were approximately 3 times the exposure at the maximum recommended human daily oral dose of 180 mg of fexofenadine hydrochloride based on comparison of AUCs).

8.3 Nursing Mothers

It is not known if fexofenadine is excreted in human milk. There are no adequate and well-controlled studies in women during lactation. Because many drugs are excreted in human milk, caution should be exercised when fexofenadine hydrochloride is administered to a nursing woman.

8.4 Pediatric Use

The recommended doses of fexofenadine hydrochloride in pediatric patients 6 months to 11 years of age are based on cross-study comparison of the pharmacokinetics of fexofenadine in adults and pediatric subjects and on the safety profile of fexofenadine hydrochloride in both adult and pediatric subjects at doses equal to or higher than the recommended doses. The safety and effectiveness of fexofenadine hydrochloride in pediatric patients under 6 months of age have not been established.

The safety of fexofenadine hydrochloride is based on the administration of ALLEGRA tablets at a dose of 30 mg twice daily demonstrated in 438 pediatric subjects 6 years to 11 years of age in 2 placebo-controlled 2-week seasonal allergic rhinitis trials. The safety of fexofenadine hydrochloride at doses of 15 mg and 30 mg given once and twice a day has been demonstrated in 969 pediatric subjects (6 months to 5 years of age) with allergic rhinitis in 3 pharmacokinetic studies and 3 safety studies. The safety of fexofenadine hydrochloride for the treatment of chronic idiopathic urticaria in subjects 6 months to 11 years of age is based on cross-study comparison of the pharmacokinetics of ALLEGRA in adult and pediatric subjects and on the safety profile of fexofenadine in both adult and pediatric subjects at doses equal to or higher than the recommended dose.

The effectiveness of fexofenadine hydrochloride for the treatment of seasonal allergic rhinitis in subjects 6 to 11 years of age was demonstrated in 1 trial (n=411) in which ALLEGRA tablets 30 mg twice daily significantly reduced total symptom scores compared to placebo, along with extrapolation of demonstrated efficacy in subjects aged 12 years and above, and the pharmacokinetic comparisons in adults and children. The effectiveness of fexofenadine hydrochloride 30 mg twice daily for the treatment of seasonal allergic rhinitis in patients 2 to 5 years of age is based on the pharmacokinetic comparisons in adult and pediatric subjects and an extrapolation of the demonstrated efficacy of fexofenadine hydrochloride in adult subjects with this condition and the likelihood that the disease course, pathophysiology, and the drug's effect are substantially similar in pediatric patients to those in adult patients. The effectiveness of fexofenadine hydrochloride for the treatment of chronic idiopathic urticaria in patients 6 months to 11 years of age is based on the pharmacokinetic comparisons in adults and children and an extrapolation of the demonstrated efficacy of ALLEGRA in adults with this condition and the likelihood that the disease course, pathophysiology and the drug's effect are substantially similar in children to that of adult patients. Administration of a 15 mg dose of fexofenadine hydrochloride to pediatric subjects 6 months to less than 2 years of age and a 30 mg dose to pediatric subjects 2 to 11 years of age produced exposures comparable to those seen with a dose of 60 mg administered to adults.

8.5 Geriatric Use

Clinical studies of ALLEGRA tablets and capsules did not include sufficient numbers of subjects aged 65 years and over to determine whether this population responds differently from younger subjects. Other reported clinical experience has not identified differences in responses between the geriatric and younger subjects. This drug is known to be substantially excreted by the kidney, and the risk of toxic reactions to this drug may be greater in patients with impaired renal function. Because elderly patients are more likely to have decreased renal function, care should be taken in dose selection, and it may be useful to monitor renal function *[see Clinical Pharmacology (12.3)]*.

8.6 Renal Impairment

Based on increases in bioavailability and half-life, a dose of 60 mg once daily is recommended as the starting dose in adult patients with decreased renal function (mild, moderate or severe renal impairment). For pediatric patients with decreased renal function (mild, moderate or severe renal impairment), the recommended starting dose of fexofenadine is 30 mg once daily for patients 2 to 11 years of age and 15 mg once daily for patients 6 months to less than 2 years of age. *[See Dosage and Administration (2.2, 2.3) and Clinical Pharmacology (12.3)]*.

8.7 Hepatic Impairment

The pharmacokinetics of fexofenadine hydrochloride in subjects with hepatic impairment did not differ substantially from that observed in healthy subjects.

10 OVERDOSAGE

Dizziness, drowsiness, and dry mouth have been reported with fexofenadine hydrochloride overdose. Single doses of fexofenadine hydrochloride up to 800 mg (6 healthy subjects at this dose level), and doses up to 690 mg twice daily for 1 month (3 healthy subjects at this dose level) or 240 mg once daily for 1 year (234 healthy subjects at this dose level) were administered without the development of clinically significant adverse events as compared to placebo.

In the event of overdose, consider standard measures to remove any unabsorbed drug. Symptomatic and supportive treatment is recommended. Following administration of terfenadine, hemodialysis did not effectively remove fexofenadine, the major active metabolite of terfenadine, from blood (up to 1.7% removed).

No deaths occurred at oral doses of fexofenadine hydrochloride up to 5000 mg/kg in mice (110 times the maximum recommended daily oral dose in adults and children based on mg/m^2) and up to 5000 mg/kg in rats (230 times the maximum recommended daily oral dose in adults and 210 times the maximum recommended daily oral dose in children based on mg/m^2). Additionally, no clinical signs of toxicity or gross pathological findings were observed. In dogs, no evidence of toxicity was observed at oral doses up to 2000 mg/kg (300 times the maximum recommended daily oral dose in adults and 280 times the maximum recommended daily oral dose in children based on mg/m^2).

11 DESCRIPTION

Fexofenadine hydrochloride, the active ingredient of ALLEGRA tablets, ALLEGRA ODT and ALLEGRA oral suspension, is a histamine H_1-receptor antagonist with the chemical name (±)-4-[1 hydroxy-4-[4-(hydroxydiphenylmethyl)-1-piperidinyl]-butyl]-α, α-dimethyl benzeneacetic acid hydrochloride. It has the following chemical structure

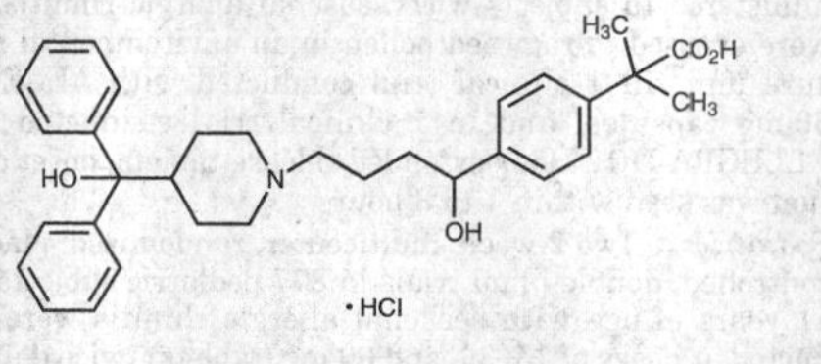

The molecular weight is 538.13 and the empirical formula is $C_{32}H_{39}NO_4$•HCl.

Fexofenadine hydrochloride is a white to off-white crystalline powder. It is freely soluble in methanol and ethanol, slightly soluble in chloroform and water, and insoluble in hexane. Fexofenadine hydrochloride is a racemate and exists as a zwitterion in aqueous media at physiological pH.

ALLEGRA is formulated as a tablet for oral administration. Each tablet contains 30, 60, or 180 mg fexofenadine hydrochloride (depending on the dosage strength) and the following excipients: croscarmellose sodium, magnesium stearate, microcrystalline cellulose, and pregelatinized starch. The aqueous tablet film coating is made from hypromellose, iron oxide blends, polyethylene glycol, povidone, silicone dioxide, and titanium dioxide.

ALLEGRA ODT is formulated for disintegration in the mouth immediately following administration. Each orally disintegrating tablet contains 30 mg fexofenadine hydrochloride and the following excipients: citric acid anhydrous, crospovidone, magnesium stearate, mannitol, methacrylate copolymer, microcrystalline cellulose, povidone K-30, sodium bicarbonate, sodium starch glycolate, aspartame, natural and artificial orange flavor, artificial cream flavor, and alcohol anhydrous; the alcohol is predominantly removed during the manufacturing process.

ALLEGRA oral suspension, a white uniform suspension, contains 6 mg fexofenadine hydrochloride per mL and the following excipients: propylene glycol, edetate disodium, propylparaben, butylparaben, xanthan gum, poloxamer 407, titanium dioxide, sodium phosphate monobasic monohydrate, sodium phosphate dibasic heptahydrate, artificial raspberry cream flavor, sucrose, xylitol and purified water.

12 CLINICAL PHARMACOLOGY

12.1 Mechanism of Action

Fexofenadine hydrochloride, the major active metabolite of terfenadine, is an antihistamine with selective H_1-receptor antagonist activity. Both enantiomers of fexofenadine hydrochloride displayed approximately equipotent antihistaminic effects. Fexofenadine hydrochloride inhibited antigen-induced bronchospasm in sensitized guinea pigs and histamine release from peritoneal mast cells in rats. The clinical significance of these findings is unknown. In laboratory animals, no anticholinergic or alpha$_1$-adrenergic blocking effects were observed. Moreover, no sedative or other central nervous system effects were observed. Radiolabeled tissue distribution studies in rats indicated that fexofenadine does not cross the blood-brain barrier.

12.2 Pharmacodynamics

Wheal and Flare: Human histamine skin wheal and flare studies in adults following single and twice daily doses of 20 and 40 mg fexofenadine hydrochloride demonstrated that the drug exhibits an antihistamine effect by 1 hour, achieves maximum effect at 2 to 3 hours, and an effect is still seen at 12 hours. There was no evidence of tolerance to these effects after 28 days of dosing. The clinical significance of these observations is unknown.

Histamine skin wheal and flare studies in 7 to 12 year old subjects showed that following a single dose of 30 or 60 mg, antihistamine effect was observed at 1 hour and reached a maximum by 3 hours. Greater than 49% inhibition of wheal area, and 74% inhibition of flare area were maintained for 8 hours following the 30 and 60 mg dose.

No statistically significant increase in mean QT_c interval compared to placebo was observed in 714 adult subjects with seasonal allergic rhinitis given fexofenadine hydrochloride capsules in doses of 60 to 240 mg twice daily for 2 weeks. Pediatric subjects from 2 placebo-controlled trials (n=855) treated with up to 60 mg fexofenadine hydrochloride twice daily demonstrated no significant treatment- or dose-related increases in QT_c. In addition, no statistically significant increase in mean QT_c interval compared to placebo was observed in 40 healthy adult subjects given fexofenadine hydrochloride as an oral solution at doses up to 400 mg twice daily for 6 days, or in 230 healthy adult subjects given fexofenadine hydrochloride 240 mg once daily for 1 year. In subjects with chronic idiopathic urticaria, there were no clinically relevant differences for any ECG intervals, including QT_c, between those treated with fexofenadine hydrochloride 180 mg once daily (n = 163) and those treated with placebo (n = 91) for 4 weeks.

12.3 Pharmacokinetics

The pharmacokinetics of fexofenadine hydrochloride in subjects with seasonal allergic rhinitis and subjects with chronic urticaria were similar to those in healthy subjects.

Absorption:

ALLEGRA tablets: Fexofenadine hydrochloride was absorbed following oral administration of a single dose of two 60 mg capsules to healthy male subjects with a mean time to maximum plasma concentration occurring at 2.6 hours post-dose. After administration of a single 60 mg capsule to healthy adult subjects, the mean maximum plasma concentration (Cmax) was 131 ng/mL. Following single dose oral administrations of either the 60 and 180 mg tablet to healthy adult male subjects, mean Cmax were 142 and 494 ng/mL, respectively. The tablet formulations are bioequivalent to the capsule when administered at equal doses. Fexofenadine hydrochloride pharmacokinetics are linear for oral doses up to a total daily dose of 240 mg (120 mg twice daily). The administration of the 60 mg capsule contents mixed with applesauce did not have a significant effect on the pharmacokinetics of fexofenadine in adults. Co-administration of 180 mg fexofenadine hydrochloride tablet with a high fat meal decreased the mean area under the curve (AUC) and (Cmax) of fexofenadine by 21 and 20% respectively.

ALLEGRA ODT: Fexofenadine hydrochloride was absorbed following single-dose oral administration of ALLEGRA ODT 30 mg to healthy adult subjects with a mean time to maximum plasma concentration occurring at approximately 2.0 hours post-dose. After single-dose administration of ALLEGRA 30 mg ODT to healthy adult subjects, the mean maximum plasma concentration (Cmax) was 88.0 ng/mL. ALLEGRA ODT 30 mg tablets are bioequivalent to the 30 mg ALLEGRA tablets. The administration of ALLEGRA ODT 30 mg with a high-fat meal decreased the AUC and Cmax by approximately 40% and 60% respectively and a 2-hour delay in the time to peak exposure (Tmax) was observed. ALLEGRA ODT should be taken on an empty stomach. The bioavailability of ALLEGRA ODT was comparable whether given with or without water *[see Dosage and Administration (2.2)]*.

ALLEGRA oral suspension: A dose of 5 mL of ALLEGRA oral suspension containing 30 mg of fexofenadine hydrochloride is bioequivalent to a 30 mg dose of ALLEGRA tablets. Following oral administration of a 30 mg dose of ALLEGRA oral suspension to healthy adult subjects, the mean Cmax was 118 ng/mL and occurred at approximately 1 hour. The administration of 30 mg ALLEGRA oral suspension with a high fat meal decreased the AUC and the mean

Cmax by approximately 30 and 47%, respectively in healthy adult subjects.

Distribution:

Fexofenadine hydrochloride is 60% to 70% bound to plasma proteins, primarily albumin and α_1-acid glycoprotein.

Metabolism:

Approximately 5% of the total dose of fexofenadine hydrochloride was eliminated by hepatic metabolism.

Elimination:

The mean elimination half-life of fexofenadine was 14.4 hours following administration of 60 mg twice daily in healthy adult subjects.

Human mass balance studies documented a recovery of approximately 80% and 11% of the [^{14}C] fexofenadine hydrochloride dose in the feces and urine, respectively. Because the absolute bioavailability of fexofenadine hydrochloride has not been established, it is unknown if the fecal component represents primarily unabsorbed drug or is the result of biliary excretion.

Special Populations:

Pharmacokinetics in renally and hepatically impaired subjects and geriatric subjects, obtained after a single dose of 80 mg fexofenadine hydrochloride, were compared to those from healthy subjects in a separate study of similar design.

Renally Impaired:

In subjects with mild to moderate (creatinine clearance 41-80 mL/min) and severe (creatinine clearance 11-40 mL/min) renal impairment, peak plasma concentrations of fexofenadine were 87% and 111% greater, respectively, and mean elimination half-lives were 59% and 72% longer, respectively, than observed in healthy subjects. Peak plasma concentrations in subjects on dialysis (creatinine clearance ≤10 mL/min) were 82% greater and half-life was 31% longer than observed in healthy subjects. Based on increases in bioavailability and half-life, a dose of 60 mg once daily is recommended as the starting dose in adult patients with decreased renal function. For pediatric patients with decreased renal function, the recommended starting dose of fexofenadine is 30 mg once daily for patients 2 to 11 years of age and 15 mg once daily for patients 6 months to less than 2 years of age [see Dosage and Administration (2.2, 2.3)].

Hepatically Impaired:

The pharmacokinetics of fexofenadine hydrochloride in subjects with hepatic impairment did not differ substantially from that observed in healthy subjects.

Geriatric Subjects:

In older subjects (≥65 years old), peak plasma levels of fexofenadine were 99% greater than those observed in younger subjects (<65 years old). Mean fexofenadine elimination half-lives were similar to those observed in younger subjects.

Pediatric Subjects:

A population pharmacokinetic analysis was performed with data from 77 pediatric subjects (6 months to 12 years of age) with allergic rhinitis and 136 adult subjects. The individual apparent oral clearance estimates of fexofenadine were on average 44% and 36% lower in pediatric subjects 6 to 12 years (n=14) and 2 to 5 years of age (n=21), respectively, compared to adult subjects.

Administration of a 15 mg dose of fexofenadine hydrochloride to pediatric subjects 6 months to less than 2 years of age and a 30 mg dose to pediatric subjects 2 to 11 years of age produced exposures comparable to those seen with a dose of 60 mg administered to adults.

Effect of Gender:

Across several trials, no clinically significant gender-related differences were observed in the pharmacokinetics of fexofenadine hydrochloride.

13   NONCLINICAL TOXICOLOGY

13. 1   Carcinogenesis, Mutagenesis, Impairment of Fertility

The carcinogenic potential of fexofenadine was assessed using terfenadine studies with adequate fexofenadine exposure (based on plasma area-under-the-concentration vs. time [AUC] values). No evidence of carcinogenicity was observed in an 18-month study in mice and in a 24-month study in rats at oral doses up to 150 mg/kg of terfenadine (which led to fexofenadine exposures that were approximately 3 and 5 times the exposure at the maximum recommended daily oral dose of fexofenadine hydrochloride in adults [180 mg] and children [60 mg] respectively).

In *in vitro* (Bacterial Reverse Mutation, CHO/HGPRT Forward Mutation, and Rat Lymphocyte Chromosomal Aberration assays) and *in vivo* (Mouse Bone Marrow Micronucleus assay) tests, fexofenadine hydrochloride revealed no evidence of mutagenicity.

In rat fertility studies, dose-related reductions in implants and increases in postimplantation losses were observed at an oral dose of 150 mg/kg of terfenadine (which led to fexofenadine exposures that were approximately 3 times the exposure at the maximum recommended human daily oral dose of 180 mg of fexofenadine hydrochloride based on comparison of AUCs). In mice, fexofenadine hydrochloride

produced no effect on male or female fertility at average oral doses up to 4438 mg/kg (which led to fexofenadine exposures that were approximately 13 times the exposure at the maximum recommended human daily oral dose of 180 mg of fexofenadine hydrochloride based on comparison of AUCs).

13. 2   Animal Toxicology and/or Pharmacology

In dogs (30 mg/kg/orally twice daily for 5 days) and rabbits (10 mg/kg, intravenously over 1 hour), fexofenadine hydrochloride did not prolong QT_c. In dogs, the plasma fexofenadine concentration was approximately 9 times the therapeutic plasma concentrations in adults receiving the maximum recommended human daily oral dose of 180 mg. In rabbits, the plasma fexofenadine concentration was approximately 20 times the therapeutic plasma concentration in adults receiving the maximum recommended human daily oral dose of 180 mg. No effect was observed on calcium channel current, delayed K^+ channel current, or action potential duration in guinea pig myocytes, or on the delayed rectifier K^+ channel cloned from human heart at concentrations up to 1×10^{-5} M of fexofenadine.

14   CLINICAL STUDIES

14.1   Seasonal Allergic Rhinitis

Adults: In three 2-week, multicenter, randomized, double-blind, placebo-controlled trials in subjects 12 to 68 years of age with seasonal allergic rhinitis (n=1634), fexofenadine hydrochloride 60 mg twice daily significantly reduced total symptom scores (the sum of the individual scores for sneezing, rhinorrhea, itchy nose/palate/throat, itchy/watery/red eyes) compared to placebo. Statistically significant reductions in symptom scores were observed following the first 60 mg dose, with the effect maintained throughout the 12-hour interval. In these studies, there was no additional reduction in total symptom scores with higher doses of fexofenadine hydrochloride up to 240 mg twice daily.

In one 2-week, multicenter, randomized, double-blind clinical trial in subjects 12 to 65 years of age with seasonal allergic rhinitis (n=863), fexofenadine hydrochloride 180 mg once daily significantly reduced total symptom scores (the sum of the individual scores for sneezing, rhinorrhea, itchy nose/palate/throat, itchy/watery/red eyes) compared to placebo. Although the number of subjects in some of the subgroups was small, there were no significant differences in the effect of fexofenadine hydrochloride across subgroups of subjects defined by gender, age, and race. Onset of action for reduction in total symptom scores, excluding nasal congestion, was observed at 60 minutes compared to placebo following a single 60 mg fexofenadine hydrochloride dose administered to subjects with seasonal allergic rhinitis who were exposed to ragweed pollen in an environmental exposure unit. In 1 clinical trial conducted with ALLEGRA 60 mg capsules, and in 1 clinical trial conducted with ALLEGRA-D 12 Hour extended release tablets, onset of action was seen within 1 to 3 hours.

Pediatrics: Two 2-week, multicenter, randomized, placebo-controlled, double-blind trials in 877 pediatric subjects 6 to 11 years of age with seasonal allergic rhinitis were conducted at doses of 15, 30, and 60 mg (tablets) twice daily. In 1 of these 2 studies, conducted in 411 pediatric subjects, all 3 doses of fexofenadine hydrochloride significantly reduced total symptom scores (the sum of the individual scores for sneezing, rhinorrhea, itchy nose/palate/throat, itchy/watery/red eyes) compared to placebo, however, a dose-response relationship was not seen. The 60 mg twice daily dose did not provide any additional benefit over the 30 mg twice daily dose in pediatric subjects 6 to 11 years of age.

Administration of a 30 mg dose to pediatric subjects 2 to 11 years of age produced exposures comparable to those seen with a dose of 60 mg administered to adults. [See Clinical Pharmacology (12.3)].

14.2   Chronic Idiopathic Urticaria

Two 4-week, multicenter, randomized, double-blind, placebo-controlled clinical trials compared four different doses of fexofenadine hydrochloride tablet (20, 60, 120, and 240 mg twice daily) to placebo in subjects aged 12 to 70 years with chronic idiopathic urticaria (n=726). Efficacy was demonstrated by a significant reduction in mean pruritus scores (MPS), mean number of wheals (MNW), and mean total symptom scores (MTSS, the sum of the MPS and MNW score). Although all 4 doses were significantly superior to placebo, symptom reduction was greater and efficacy was maintained over the entire 4-week treatment period with fexofenadine hydrochloride doses of ≥60 mg twice daily. However, no additional benefit of the 120 or 240 mg fexofenadine hydrochloride twice daily dose was seen over the 60 mg twice daily dose in reducing symptom scores. There were no significant differences in the effect of fexofenadine hydrochloride across subgroups of subjects defined by gender, age, weight, and race.

In one 4-week, multicenter, randomized, double-blind, placebo-controlled clinical trial in subjects 12 years of age and older with chronic idiopathic urticaria (n=259), fexofenadine hydrochloride 180 mg once daily significantly reduced the mean number of wheals (MNW), the mean pru-

ritus score (MPS), and the mean total symptom score (MTSS, the sum of the MPS and MNW scores). Similar reductions were observed for mean number of wheals and mean pruritus score at the end of the 24-hour dosing interval. Symptom reduction was greater with fexofenadine hydrochloride 180 mg than with placebo. Improvement was demonstrated within 1 day of treatment with fexofenadine hydrochloride 180 mg and was maintained over the entire 4-week treatment period. There were no significant differences in the effect of fexofenadine hydrochloride across subgroups of subjects defined by gender, age, and race.

16   HOW SUPPLIED/ STORAGE AND HANDLING

16.1   ALLEGRA tablets

ALLEGRA 30 mg tablets are available in: high-density polyethylene (HDPE) bottles of 100 (NDC 0088-1106-47) with a polypropylene screw cap containing a pulp/wax liner with heat-sealed foil inner seal and HDPE bottles of 500 (NDC 0088-1106-55) with a polypropylene screw cap containing a pulp/wax liner with heat-sealed foil inner seal.

ALLEGRA 60 mg tablets are available in: HDPE bottles of 100 (NDC 0088-1107-47) with a polypropylene screw cap containing a pulp/wax liner with heat-sealed foil inner seal; HDPE bottles of 500 (NDC 0088-1107-55) with a polypropylene screw cap containing a pulp/wax liner with heat-sealed foil inner seal; and aluminum foil-backed clear blister packs of 100 (NDC 0088-1107-49).

ALLEGRA 180 mg tablets are available in: HDPE bottles of 100 (NDC 0088-1109-47) with a polypropylene screw cap containing a pulp/wax liner with heat-sealed foil inner seal and HDPE bottles of 500 (NDC 0088-1109-55) with a polypropylene screw cap containing a pulp/wax liner with heat-sealed foil inner seal.

ALLEGRA tablets are coated with a peach colored film coating. Tablets have the following unique shape and identifiers: 30 mg tablets are round, bi-convex and have 03 on one side and a scripted "e" on the other; 60 mg tablets are oval, bi-convex and have 06 on one side and a scripted "e" on the other; and 180 mg tablets are oblong, bi-convex and have 018 on one side and a scripted "e" on the other.

Store ALLEGRA tablets at controlled room temperature 20-25°C (68-77°F). (See USP Controlled Room Temperature). Foil-backed blister packs containing ALLEGRA tablets should be protected from excessive moisture.

16.2   ALLEGRA ODT

ALLEGRA ODT 30 mg orally disintegrating tablets are available in aluminum-foil blister packs of 60 (NDC 0088-1113-30).

Each ALLEGRA ODT is white, flat-faced, 1/2-inch round shaped with beveled edges and debossed with a scripted "e" on one side and "311AV" on the other side.

Store ALLEGRA ODT at controlled room temperature 20-25°C (68-77°F). (See USP Controlled Room Temperature). Foil-backed blister packs containing ALLEGRA ODT should be protected from moisture. ALLEGRA ODT should not be removed from the original blister package until the time of administration.

16.3   ALLEGRA oral suspension

ALLEGRA oral suspension (fexofenadine hydrochloride, 30 mg/5 mL (6 mg/mL)) is available in an amber PET bottle containing 300 mL (NDC 0088-1097-20) of suspension.

Store ALLEGRA oral suspension at controlled room temperature 20-25°C (68-77°F). (See USP Controlled Room Temperature).

Shake bottle well, before each use.

17   PATIENT COUNSELING INFORMATION

Provide the following information to patients and parents/caregivers of pediatric patients taking ALLEGRA tablets, ALLEGRA ODT or ALLEGRA oral suspension:

• ALLEGRA tablets, ALLEGRA ODT or ALLEGRA oral suspension are prescribed for the relief of symptoms of seasonal allergic rhinitis or for the relief of symptoms of chronic idiopathic urticaria (hives). Instruct patients to take ALLEGRA only as prescribed. **Do not exceed the recommended dose.** If any untoward effects occur while taking ALLEGRA, discontinue use and consult a doctor.

• Patients who are hypersensitive to any of the ingredients should not use these products.

• Patients who are pregnant or nursing should use these products only if the potential benefit justifies the potential risk to the fetus or nursing infant.

• Advise patients and parents/caregivers of pediatric patients to store the medication in a tightly closed container in a cool, dry place, away from small children.

• Advise patients and parents/caregivers not to take ALLEGRA with fruit juices.

For ALLEGRA tablets: Advise patients to take the ALLEGRA tablets with water.

For ALLEGRA ODT: Advise patients to take their dose on an empty stomach. Allow ALLEGRA ODT to disintegrate on the tongue before swallowing, with or without water. ALLEGRA ODT is not intended to be chewed. Store ALLEGRA ODT in its original blister package. Do not remove ALLEGRA ODT from the original blister package until the time of administration.

Phenylketonurics: ALLEGRA ODT contains phenylalanine, a component of aspartame. Each 30-mg ALLEGRA ODT contains 5.3 mg phenylalanine. ALLEGRA products other than ALLEGRA ODT do not contain phenylalanine.

For ALLEGRA oral suspension: Advise patients and parents/caregivers of pediatric patients to shake the ALLEGRA oral suspension bottle well, before each use.

sanofi-aventis U.S. LLC
Bridgewater, NJ 08807
ALLEGRA ODT manufactured for:
sanofi-aventis U.S. LLC
Bridgewater, NJ 08807

Shown in Product Identification Guide, page 318

ALLEGRA-D® 12 HOUR ℞

[ə-'lĕgra-D]

(fexofenadine HCl 60 mg and pseudoephedrine HCl 120 mg) Extended-Release Tablets

DESCRIPTION

ALLEGRA-D® 12 HOUR (fexofenadine hydrochloride and pseudoephedrine hydrochloride) Extended-Release Tablets for oral administration contain 60 mg fexofenadine hydrochloride for immediate release and 120 mg pseudoephedrine hydrochloride for extended release. Tablets also contain as excipients: microcrystalline cellulose, pregelatinized starch, croscarmellose sodium, magnesium stearate, carnauba wax, stearic acid, silicon dioxide, hypromellose and polyethylene glycol.

Fexofenadine hydrochloride, one of the active ingredients of ALLEGRA-D 12 HOUR, is a histamine H_1-receptor antagonist with the chemical name (±)-4-[1-hydroxy-4-[4-(hydroxydiphenylmethyl)-1-piperidinyl]-butyl]-α,α-dimethyl benzeneacetic acid hydrochloride and the following chemical structure:

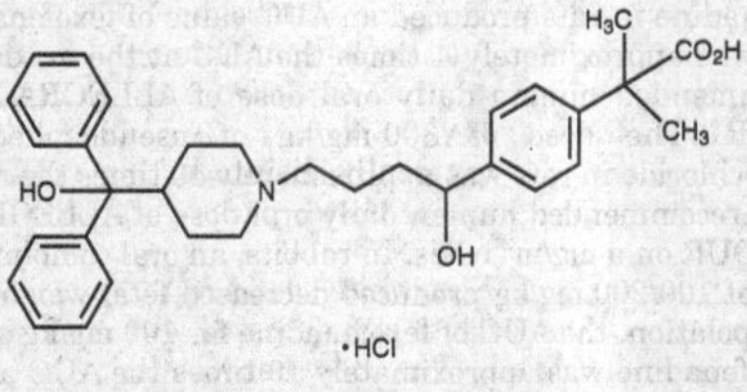

The molecular weight is 538.13 and the empirical formula is $C_{32}H_{39}NO_4$•HCl. Fexofenadine hydrochloride is a white to off-white crystalline powder. It is freely soluble in methanol and ethanol, slightly soluble in chloroform and water, and insoluble in hexane. Fexofenadine hydrochloride is a racemate and exists as a zwitterion in aqueous media at physiological pH.

Pseudoephedrine hydrochloride, the other active ingredient of ALLEGRA-D 12 HOUR, is an adrenergic (vasoconstrictor) agent with the chemical name [S-(R*,R*)]-α-[1-(methylamino)ethyl]-benzenemethanol hydrochloride and the following chemical structure:

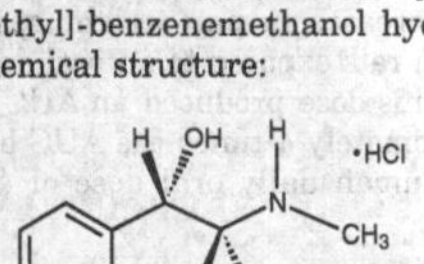

The molecular weight is 201.70. The molecular formula is $C_{10}H_{15}NO$•HCl. Pseudoephedrine hydrochloride occurs as fine, white to off-white crystals or powder, having a faint characteristic odor. It is very soluble in water, freely soluble in alcohol, and sparingly soluble in chloroform.

CLINICAL PHARMACOLOGY

Mechanism of Action

Fexofenadine hydrochloride, the major active metabolite of terfenadine, is an antihistamine with selective peripheral H_1-receptor antagonist activity. Fexofenadine hydrochloride inhibited antigen-induced bronchospasm in sensitized guinea pigs and histamine release from peritoneal mast cells in rats. In laboratory animals, no anticholinergic or alpha$_1$-adrenergic-receptor blocking effects were observed. Moreover, no sedative or other central nervous system effects were observed. Radiolabeled tissue distribution studies in rats indicated that fexofenadine does not cross the blood-brain barrier.

Pseudoephedrine hydrochloride is an orally active sympathomimetic amine and exerts a decongestant action on the nasal mucosa. Pseudoephedrine hydrochloride is recognized as an effective agent for the relief of nasal congestion due to allergic rhinitis. Pseudoephedrine produces peripheral effects similar to those of ephedrine and central effects similar to, but less intense than, amphetamines. It has the potential for excitatory side effects. At the recommended oral dose, it has little or no pressor effect in normotensive adults.

Pharmacokinetics

The pharmacokinetics of fexofenadine hydrochloride in subjects with seasonal allergic rhinitis were similar to those in healthy volunteers.

Absorption

The pharmacokinetics of fexofenadine hydrochloride and pseudoephedrine hydrochloride when administered separately have been well characterized. Fexofenadine pharmacokinetics were linear for oral doses of fexofenadine hydrochloride up to a total daily dose of 240 mg (120 mg twice daily). Peak fexofenadine plasma concentrations were similar between adolescent (12–16 years of age) and adult subjects.

The bioavailability of fexofenadine hydrochloride and pseudoephedrine hydrochloride from ALLEGRA-D 12 HOUR Extended-Release Tablets is similar to that achieved with separate administration of the components. Coadministration of fexofenadine and pseudoephedrine does not significantly affect the bioavailability of either component.

Fexofenadine hydrochloride was rapidly absorbed following single-dose administration of the 60 mg fexofenadine hydrochloride/120 mg pseudoephedrine hydrochloride tablet with median time to mean maximum fexofenadine plasma concentration of 191 ng/mL occurring 2 hours post-dose. Pseudoephedrine hydrochloride produced a mean single-dose pseudoephedrine peak plasma concentration of 206 ng/mL which occurred 6 hours post-dose. Following multiple dosing to steady-state, a fexofenadine peak concentration of 255 ng/mL was observed 2 hours post-dose. Following multiple dosing to steady-state, a pseudoephedrine peak concentration of 411 ng/mL was observed 5 hours post-dose. The administration of ALLEGRA-D 12 HOUR with a high fat meal decreased the bioavailability of fexofenadine by approximately 50% (AUC 42% and Cmax 46%). Time to maximum concentration (T_{max}) was delayed by 50%. The rate or extent of pseudoephedrine absorption was not affected by food. Therefore, ALLEGRA-D 12 HOUR should be taken on an empty stomach with water (see DOSAGE AND ADMINISTRATION).

Distribution

Fexofenadine is 60% to 70% bound to plasma proteins, primarily albumin and α_1-acid glycoprotein. The protein binding of pseudoephedrine in humans is not known. Pseudoephedrine hydrochloride is extensively distributed into extravascular sites (apparent volume of distribution between 2.6 and 3.5 L/kg).

Metabolism

Approximately 5% of the total dose of fexofenadine hydrochloride and less than 1% of the total oral dose of pseudoephedrine hydrochloride were eliminated by hepatic metabolism.

Elimination

The mean elimination half-life of fexofenadine was 14.4 hours following administration of 60 mg fexofenadine hydrochloride, twice daily, to steady-state in healthy volunteers. Human mass balance studies documented a recovery of approximately 80% and 11% of the [^{14}C] fexofenadine hydrochloride dose in the feces and urine, respectively. Because the absolute bioavailability of fexofenadine hydrochloride has not been established, it is unknown if the fecal component is primarily unabsorbed drug or the result of biliary excretion.

Pseudoephedrine has been shown to have a mean elimination half-life of 4–6 hours which is dependent on urine pH. The elimination half-life is decreased at urine pH lower than 6 and may be increased at urine pH higher than 8.

Special Populations

Pharmacokinetics in special populations (for renal, hepatic impairment, and age), obtained after a single dose of 80 mg fexofenadine hydrochloride, were compared to those from healthy subjects in a separate study of similar design.

Effect of Age

In older subjects (≥65 years old), peak plasma levels of fexofenadine were 99% greater than those observed in younger subjects (<65 years old). Mean fexofenadine elimination half-lives were similar to those observed in younger subjects.

Renally Impaired

In subjects with mild (creatinine clearance 41–80 mL/min) to severe (creatinine clearance 11–40 mL/min) renal impairment, peak plasma levels of fexofenadine were 87% and 111% greater, respectively, and mean elimination half-lives were 59% and 72% longer, respectively, than observed in healthy volunteers. Peak plasma levels in subjects on dialysis (creatinine clearance ≤10 mL/min) were 82% greater and half-life was 31% longer than observed in healthy volunteers.

No data are available on the pharmacokinetics of pseudoephedrine in renally-impaired subjects. However, most of the oral dose of pseudoephedrine hydrochloride (43–96%) is excreted unchanged in the urine. A decrease in renal function is, therefore, likely to decrease the clearance of pseudoephedrine significantly, thus prolonging the half-life and resulting in accumulation.

Based on increases in bioavailability and half-life of fexofenadine hydrochloride and pseudoephedrine hydrochloride, a dose of one tablet once daily is recommended as the starting dose in patients with decreased renal function (see DOSAGE AND ADMINISTRATION).

Hepatically Impaired

The pharmacokinetics of fexofenadine hydrochloride in subjects with hepatic disease did not differ substantially from that observed in healthy volunteers. The effect on pseudoephedrine pharmacokinetics is unknown.

Effect of Gender

Across several trials, no clinically significant gender-related differences were observed in the pharmacokinetics of fexofenadine hydrochloride.

Pharmacodynamics

Wheal and Flare

Human histamine skin wheal and flare studies following single and twice daily doses of 20 mg and 40 mg fexofenadine hydrochloride demonstrated that the drug exhibits an antihistamine effect by 1 hour, achieves maximum effect at 2–3 hours, and an effect is still seen at 12 hours. There was no evidence of tolerance to these effects after 28 days of dosing. The clinical significance of these observations is unknown.

Effects on QT_c

In dogs (30 mg/kg orally twice daily for 5 days) and rabbits (10 mg/kg intravenously over 1 hour), fexofenadine hydrochloride did not prolong QT_c at plasma concentrations that were at least 17 and 38 times, respectively, the therapeutic plasma concentrations in man (based on a 60 mg twice daily fexofenadine hydrochloride dose). No effect was observed on calcium channel current, delayed K^+ channel current, or action potential duration in guinea pig myocytes, Na^+ current in rat neonatal myocytes, or on the delayed rectifier K^+ channel cloned from human heart at concentrations up to 1×10^{-5} M of fexofenadine. This concentration was at least 21 times the therapeutic plasma concentration in man (based on a 60 mg twice daily fexofenadine hydrochloride dose).

No statistically significant increase in mean QT_c interval compared to placebo was observed in 714 subjects with seasonal allergic rhinitis given fexofenadine hydrochloride capsules in doses of 60 mg to 240 mg twice daily for 2 weeks or in 40 healthy volunteers given fexofenadine hydrochloride as an oral solution at doses up to 400 mg twice daily for 6 days.

A 1-year study designed to evaluate safety and tolerability of 240 mg of fexofenadine hydrochloride (n=240) compared to placebo (n=237) in healthy volunteers, did not reveal a statistically significant increase in the mean QT_c interval for the fexofenadine hydrochloride treated group when evaluated pretreatment and after 1, 2, 3, 6, 9, and 12 months of treatment.

Administration of the 60 mg fexofenadine hydrochloride/120 mg pseudoephedrine hydrochloride combination tablet for approximately 2 weeks to 213 subjects with seasonal allergic rhinitis demonstrated no statistically significant increase in the mean QT_c interval compared to fexofenadine hydrochloride administered alone (60 mg twice daily, n=215), or compared to pseudoephedrine hydrochloride (120 mg twice daily, n=215) administered alone.

Clinical Studies

In a 2-week, multicenter, randomized, double-blind, active-controlled trial in subjects 12–65 years of age with seasonal allergic rhinitis due to ragweed allergy (n=651), the 60 mg fexofenadine hydrochloride/120 mg pseudoephedrine hydrochloride combination tablet administered twice daily significantly reduced the intensity of sneezing, rhinorrhea, itchy nose/palate/throat, itchy/watery/red eyes, and nasal congestion.

In three, 2-week, multicenter, randomized, double-blind, placebo-controlled trials in subjects 12–68 years of age with seasonal allergic rhinitis (n=1634), fexofenadine hydrochloride 60 mg twice daily significantly reduced total symptom scores (the sum of the individual scores for sneezing, rhinorrhea, itchy nose/palate/throat, itchy/watery/red eyes) compared to placebo. Statistically significant reductions in symptom scores were observed following the first 60 mg dose, with the effect maintained throughout the 12-hour interval. In general, there was no additional reduction in total symptom scores with higher doses of fexofenadine hydrochloride up to 240 mg twice daily. Although the number of subjects in some of the subgroups was small, there were no significant differences in the effect of fexofenadine hydrochloride across subgroups of subjects defined by gender, age, and race. Onset of action for reduction in total symptom scores, excluding nasal congestion, was observed at 60 minutes compared to placebo following a single 60 mg fexofenadine hydrochloride dose administered to subjects with seasonal allergic rhinitis who were exposed to ragweed pollen in an environmental exposure unit.

INDICATIONS AND USAGE

ALLEGRA-D 12 HOUR Extended-Release Tablets are indicated for the relief of symptoms associated with seasonal allergic rhinitis in adults and children 12 years of age and older. Symptoms treated effectively include sneezing, rhinorrhea, itchy nose/palate/and/or throat, itchy/watery/red eyes, and nasal congestion.

ALLEGRA-D 12 HOUR should be administered when both the antihistaminic properties of fexofenadine hydrochloride and the nasal decongestant properties of pseudoephedrine hydrochloride are desired (see CLINICAL PHARMACOLOGY).

CONTRAINDICATIONS

ALLEGRA-D 12 HOUR is contraindicated in patients with known hypersensitivity to any of its ingredients.

Due to its pseudoephedrine component, ALLEGRA-D 12 HOUR is contraindicated in patients with narrow-angle glaucoma or urinary retention, and in patients receiving monoamine oxidase (MAO) inhibitor therapy or within fourteen (14) days of stopping such treatment (see Drug Interactions section). It is also contraindicated in patients with severe hypertension, or severe coronary artery disease, and in those who have shown idiosyncrasy to its components, to adrenergic agents, or to other drugs of similar chemical structures. Manifestations of patient idiosyncrasy to adrenergic agents include: insomnia, dizziness, weakness, tremor, or arrhythmias.

WARNINGS

Sympathomimetic amines should be used with caution in patients with hypertension, diabetes mellitus, ischemic heart disease, increased intraocular pressure, hyperthyroidism, renal impairment, or prostatic hypertrophy (see CONTRAINDICATIONS). Sympathomimetic amines may produce central nervous system stimulation with convulsions or cardiovascular collapse with accompanying hypotension.

PRECAUTIONS

General

Patients with decreased renal function should be given a lower initial dose (one tablet per day) because they have reduced elimination of fexofenadine and pseudoephedrine (see CLINICAL PHARMACOLOGY and DOSAGE AND ADMINISTRATION).

Information for Patients

Patients taking ALLEGRA-D 12 HOUR tablets should receive the following information: ALLEGRA-D 12 HOUR tablets are prescribed for the relief of symptoms of seasonal allergic rhinitis. Patients should be instructed to take ALLEGRA-D 12 HOUR tablets only as prescribed. **Do not exceed the recommended dose.** If nervousness, dizziness, or sleeplessness occur, discontinue use and consult the doctor. Patients should also be advised against the concurrent use of ALLEGRA-D 12 HOUR tablets with over-the-counter antihistamines and decongestants.

The product should not be used by patients who are hypersensitive to it or to any of its ingredients. Due to its pseudoephedrine component, this product should not be used by patients with narrow-angle glaucoma, urinary retention, or by patients receiving a monoamine oxidase (MAO) inhibitor or within 14 days of stopping use of MAO inhibitor. It also should not be used by patients with severe hypertension or severe coronary artery disease.

Patients should be told that this product should be used in pregnancy or lactation only if the potential benefit justifies the potential risk to the fetus or nursing infant. Patients should be advised to take the tablet on an empty stomach with water. Patients should be directed to swallow the tablet whole. Patients should be cautioned not to break or chew the tablet. Patients should also be instructed to store the medication in a tightly closed container in a cool, dry place, away from children.

Patients should be told that the inactive ingredients may occasionally be eliminated in the feces in a form that may resemble the original tablet (see DOSAGE AND ADMINISTRATION).

Drug Interactions

Fexofenadine hydrochloride and pseudoephedrine hydrochloride do not influence the pharmacokinetics of each other when administered concomitantly.

Fexofenadine has been shown to exhibit minimal (ca. 5%) metabolism. However, co-administration of fexofenadine hydrochloride with either ketoconazole or erythromycin led to increased plasma concentrations of fexofenadine. Fexofenadine had no effect on the pharmacokinetics of either erythromycin or ketoconazole. In 2 separate studies, fexofenadine hydrochloride 120 mg twice daily (twice the recommended dose) was co-administered with erythromycin 500 mg every 8 hours or ketoconazole 400 mg once daily under steady-state conditions to healthy volunteers (n=24, each study). No differences in adverse events or QT_c inter-

val were observed when subjects were administered fexofenadine hydrochloride alone or in combination with either erythromycin or ketoconazole. The findings of these studies are summarized in the following table.

Effects on Steady-State Fexofenadine Pharmacokinetics After 7 Days of Co-Administration with Fexofenadine Hydrochloride 120 mg Every 12 Hours (two times the recommended twice daily dose) in Healthy Volunteers (n=24)

Concomitant Drug	$C_{max\ SS}$ (Peak plasma concentration)	AUC_{SS} (0–12h) (Extent of systemic exposure)
Erythromycin (500 mg every 8 hrs)	+82%	+109%
Ketoconazole (400 mg once daily)	+135%	+164%

The changes in plasma levels were within the range of plasma levels achieved in adequate and well-controlled clinical trials.

The mechanism of these interactions has been evaluated in *in vitro*, *in situ*, and *in vivo* animal models. These studies indicate that ketoconazole or erythromycin co-administration enhances fexofenadine gastrointestinal absorption. This observed increase in the bioavailability of fexofenadine may be due to transport-related effects, such as p-glycoprotein. *In vivo* animal studies also suggest that in addition to enhancing absorption, ketoconazole decreases fexofenadine gastrointestinal secretion, while erythromycin may also decrease biliary excretion.

Due to the pseudoephedrine component, ALLEGRA-D 12 HOUR is contraindicated in patients taking monoamine oxidase inhibitors and for 14 days after stopping use of an MAO inhibitor. Concomitant use with antihypertensive drugs which interfere with sympathetic activity (e.g., methyldopa, mecamylamine, and reserpine) may reduce their antihypertensive effects. Increased ectopic pacemaker activity can occur when pseudoephedrine is used concomitantly with digitalis. Care should be taken in the administration of ALLEGRA-D 12 HOUR concomitantly with other sympathomimetic amines because combined effects on the cardiovascular system may be harmful to the patient (see WARNINGS).

Drug Interactions with Antacids

Administration of 120 mg of fexofenadine hydrochloride (2 × 60 mg capsule) within 15 minutes of an aluminum and magnesium containing antacid (Maalox®) decreased fexofenadine AUC by 41% and C_{max} by 43%. ALLEGRA-D 12 HOUR should not be taken closely in time with aluminum and magnesium containing antacids.

Interactions with Fruit Juices

Fruit juices such as grapefruit, orange and apple may reduce the bioavailability and exposure of fexofenadine. This is based on the results from 3 clinical studies using histamine induced skin wheals and flares coupled with population pharmacokinetic analysis. The size of wheal and flare were significantly larger when fexofenadine hydrochloride was administered with either grapefruit or orange juices compared to water. Based on the literature reports, the same effects may be extrapolated to other fruit juices such as apple juice. The clinical significance of these observations is unknown. In addition, based on the population pharmacokinetics analysis of the combined data from grapefruit and orange juices studies with the data from a bioequivalence study, the bioavailability of fexofenadine was reduced by 36%. Therefore, to maximize the effects of fexofenadine, it is recommended that ALLEGRA-D 12 HOUR should be taken with water (see DOSAGE AND ADMINISTRATION).

Carcinogenesis, Mutagenesis, Impairment of Fertility

There are no animal or *in vitro* studies on the combination product fexofenadine hydrochloride and pseudoephedrine hydrochloride to evaluate carcinogenesis, mutagenesis, or impairment of fertility.

The carcinogenic potential and reproductive toxicity of fexofenadine hydrochloride were assessed using terfenadine studies with adequate fexofenadine exposure (area-under-the plasma concentration versus time curve [AUC]). No evidence of carcinogenicity was observed when mice and rats were given daily oral doses up to 150 mg/kg of terfenadine for 18 and 24 months, respectively. In both species, 150 mg/kg of terfenadine produced AUC values of fexofenadine that were approximately 3 times the human AUC at the maximum recommended human daily oral dose of ALLEGRA-D 12 HOUR.

Two-year feeding studies in rats and mice conducted under the auspices of the National Toxicology Program (NTP) demonstrated no evidence of carcinogenic potential with ephedrine sulfate, a structurally related drug with pharma-

cological properties similar to pseudoephedrine, at doses up to 10 and 27 mg/kg, respectively (less than the maximum recommended human daily oral dose of pseudoephedrine hydrochloride on a mg/m² basis).

In *in vitro* (Bacterial Reverse Mutation, CHO/HGPRT Forward Mutation, and Rat Lymphocyte Chromosomal Aberration assays) and *in vivo* (Mouse Bone Marrow Micronucleus assay) tests, fexofenadine hydrochloride revealed no evidence of mutagenicity.

Reproduction and fertility studies with terfenadine in rats produced no effect on male or female fertility at oral doses up to 300 mg/kg/day. However, reduced implants and post implantation losses were reported at 300 mg/kg. A reduction in implants was also observed at an oral dose of 150 mg/kg/day. Oral doses of 150 and 300 mg/kg of terfenadine produced AUC values of fexofenadine that were approximately 4 times the AUC at the maximum recommended human daily oral dose of ALLEGRA-D 12 HOUR. In mice, fexofenadine produced no effect on male or female fertility at average dietary doses up to 4438 mg/kg (approximately 15 times the maximum recommended human daily oral dose of ALLEGRA-D 12 HOUR based on comparison of the AUCs).

Pregnancy

Teratogenic Effects

Category C. Terfenadine alone was not teratogenic in rats and rabbits at oral doses up to 300 mg/kg; 300 mg/kg of terfenadine produced fexofenadine AUC values that were approximately 4 and 30 times, respectively, the AUC at the maximum recommended human daily oral dose of ALLEGRA-D 12 HOUR.

In mice, no adverse effects and no teratogenic effects during gestation were observed with fexofenadine at dietary doses up to 3730 mg/kg (approximately 15 times the maximum recommended human daily oral dose of ALLEGRA-D 12 HOUR based on comparison of the AUCs).

The combination of terfenadine and pseudoephedrine hydrochloride in a ratio of 1:2 by weight was studied in rats and rabbits. In rats, an oral combination dose of 150/300 mg/kg produced reduced fetal weight and delayed ossification with a finding of wavy ribs. The dose of 150 mg/kg of terfenadine in rats produced an AUC value of fexofenadine that was approximately 4 times the AUC at the maximum recommended human daily oral dose of ALLEGRA-D 12 HOUR. The dose of 300 mg/kg of pseudoephedrine hydrochloride in rats was approximately 10 times the maximum recommended human daily oral dose of ALLEGRA-D 12 HOUR on a mg/m² basis. In rabbits, an oral combination dose of 100/200 mg/kg produced decreased fetal weight. By extrapolation, the AUC of fexofenadine for 100 mg/kg orally of terfenadine was approximately 10 times the AUC at the maximum recommended human daily oral dose of ALLEGRA-D 12 HOUR. The dose of 200 mg/kg of pseudoephedrine hydrochloride was approximately 15 times the maximum recommended human daily oral dose of ALLEGRA-D 12 HOUR on a mg/m² basis.

There are no adequate and well-controlled studies in pregnant women. ALLEGRA-D 12 HOUR should be used during pregnancy only if the potential benefit justifies the potential risk to the fetus.

Nonteratogenic Effects

Dose-related decreases in pup weight gain and survival were observed in rats exposed to an oral dose of 150 mg/kg of terfenadine; this dose produced an AUC of fexofenadine that was approximately 4 times the AUC at the maximum recommended human daily oral dose of ALLEGRA-D 12 HOUR.

Nursing Mothers

It is not known if fexofenadine is excreted in human milk. Because many drugs are excreted in human milk, caution should be used when fexofenadine hydrochloride is administered to a nursing woman. Pseudoephedrine hydrochloride administered alone distributes into breast milk of lactating human females. Pseudoephedrine concentrations in milk are consistently higher than those in plasma. The total amount of drug in milk as judged by AUC is 2 to 3 times greater than the plasma AUC. The fraction of a pseudoephedrine dose excreted in milk is estimated to be 0.4% to 0.7%. A decision should be made whether to discontinue nursing or to discontinue the drug, taking into account the importance of the drug to the mother. Caution should be exercised when ALLEGRA-D 12 HOUR is administered to nursing women.

Pediatric Use

Safety and effectiveness of ALLEGRA-D 12 HOUR in children below the age of 12 years have not been established. In addition, the doses of the individual components in ALLEGRA-D 12 HOUR exceed the recommended individual doses for pediatric patients under 12 years of age. ALLEGRA-D 12 HOUR is not recommended for pediatric patients under 12 years of age.

Geriatric Use

Clinical studies of ALLEGRA-D 12 HOUR did not include sufficient numbers of subjects aged 65 and older to determine whether they respond differently from younger subjects. Other reported clinical experience has not identified differences in responses between the elderly and younger subjects, although the elderly are more likely to have adverse reactions to sympathomimetic amines.

The pseudoephedrine component of ALLEGRA-D 12 HOUR is known to be substantially excreted by the kidney, and the risk of toxic reactions to this drug may be greater in patients with impaired renal function. Because elderly patients are more likely to have decreased renal function, care should be taken in dose selection, and it may be useful to monitor renal function.

ADVERSE REACTIONS
ALLEGRA-D 12 HOUR

In one clinical trial (n=651) in which 215 subjects with seasonal allergic rhinitis received the 60 mg fexofenadine hydrochloride/120 mg pseudoephedrine hydrochloride combination tablet twice daily for up to 2 weeks, adverse events were similar to those reported either in subjects receiving fexofenadine hydrochloride 60 mg alone (n=218 subjects) or in subjects receiving pseudoephedrine hydrochloride 120 mg alone (n=218). A placebo group was not included in this study.

The percent of subjects who withdrew prematurely because of adverse events was 3.7% for the fexofenadine hydrochloride/pseudoephedrine hydrochloride combination group, 0.5% for the fexofenadine hydrochloride group, and 4.1% for the pseudoephedrine hydrochloride group. All adverse events that were reported by greater than 1% of subjects who received the recommended daily dose of the fexofenadine hydrochloride/pseudoephedrine hydrochloride combination are listed in the following table.

[See table at right]

Many of the adverse events occurring in the fexofenadine hydrochloride/pseudoephedrine hydrochloride combination group were adverse events also reported predominately in the pseudoephedrine hydrochloride group, such as insomnia, headache, nausea, dry mouth, dizziness, agitation, nervousness, anxiety, and palpitation.

Fexofenadine Hydrochloride

In placebo-controlled clinical trials, which included 2461 subjects receiving fexofenadine hydrochloride at doses of 20 mg to 240 mg twice daily, adverse events were similar in fexofenadine hydrochloride and placebo-treated subjects. The incidence of adverse events, including drowsiness, was not dose related and was similar across subgroups defined by age, gender, and race. The percent of subjects who withdrew prematurely because of adverse events was 2.2% with fexofenadine hydrochloride vs 3.3% with placebo.

Events that have been reported during controlled clinical trials involving subjects with seasonal allergic rhinitis and chronic idiopathic urticaria at incidences less than 1% and similar to placebo and have been rarely reported during postmarketing surveillance include: insomnia, nervousness, and sleep disorders or paroniria. In rare cases, rash, urticaria, pruritus and hypersensitivity reactions with manifestations such as angioedema, chest tightness, dyspnea, flushing and systemic anaphylaxis have been reported.

Pseudoephedrine Hydrochloride

Pseudoephedrine hydrochloride may cause mild CNS stimulation in hypersensitive patients. Nervousness, excitability, restlessness, dizziness, weakness, or insomnia may occur. Headache, drowsiness, tachycardia, palpitation, pressor activity, cardiac arrhythmias and ischemic colitis have been reported. Sympathomimetic drugs have also been associated with other untoward effects such as fear, anxiety, tenseness, tremor, hallucinations, seizures, pallor, respiratory difficulty, dysuria, and cardiovascular collapse.

OVERDOSAGE

Most reports of fexofenadine hydrochloride overdose contain limited information. However, dizziness, drowsiness, and dry mouth have been reported. For the pseudoephedrine hydrochloride component of ALLEGRA-D 12 HOUR, information on acute overdose is limited to the marketing history of pseudoephedrine hydrochloride. Single doses of fexofenadine hydrochloride up to 800 mg (6 healthy volunteers at this dose level), and doses up to 690 mg twice daily for one month (3 healthy volunteers at this dose level), were administered without the development of clinically significant adverse events.

In large doses, sympathomimetics may give rise to giddiness, headache, nausea, vomiting, sweating, thirst, tachycardia, precordial pain, palpitations, difficulty in micturition, muscular weakness and tenseness, anxiety, restlessness, and insomnia. Many patients can present a toxic psychosis with delusions and hallucinations. Some may develop cardiac arrhythmias, circulatory collapse, convulsions, coma, and respiratory failure.

In the event of overdose, consider standard measures to remove any unabsorbed drug. Symptomatic and supportive treatment is recommended. Following administration of terfenadine, hemodialysis did not effectively remove

fexofenadine, the major active metabolite of terfenadine, from blood (up to 1.7% removed). The effect of hemodialysis on the removal of pseudoephedrine is unknown.

No deaths occurred in mature mice and rats at oral doses of fexofenadine hydrochloride up to 5000 mg/kg (approximately 170 and 340 times, respectively, the maximum recommended human daily oral dose of ALLEGRA-D 12 HOUR on a mg/m^2 basis.) The median oral lethal dose in newborn rats was 438 mg/kg (approximately 30 times the maximum recommended human daily oral dose of ALLEGRA-D 12 HOUR on a mg/m^2 basis). In dogs, no evidence of toxicity was observed at oral doses up to 2000 mg/kg (approximately 450 times the maximum recommended human daily oral dose on a mg/m^2 basis). The oral median lethal dose of pseudoephedrine hydrochloride in rats was 1674 mg/kg (approximately 55 times the maximum recommended human daily oral dose of ALLEGRA-D 12 HOUR on a mg/m^2 basis).

DOSAGE AND ADMINISTRATION

The recommended dose of ALLEGRA-D 12 HOUR Extended-Release Tablets is one tablet twice daily administered on an empty stomach with water for adults and children 12 years of age and older. It is recommended that the administration of ALLEGRA-D 12 HOUR with food should be avoided. A dose of one tablet once daily is recommended as the starting dose in patients with decreased renal function. (See CLINICAL PHARMACOLOGY and PRECAUTIONS.)

ALLEGRA-D 12 HOUR must be swallowed whole and never crushed or chewed. Occasionally, the inactive ingredients of ALLEGRA-D 12 HOUR may be eliminated in the feces in a form that may resemble the original tablet. (See PRECAUTIONS, Information for Patients.)

HOW SUPPLIED

ALLEGRA-D 12 HOUR Extended-Release Tablets contain 60 mg fexofenadine hydrochloride for immediate release and 120 mg pseudoephedrine hydrochloride for extended release. ALLEGRA-D 12 HOUR Extended-Release Tablets are available in high-density polyethylene (HDPE) bottles of 100 (NDC 0088-1090-47) with a polypropylene screw cap containing a pulp/wax liner with heat-sealed foil inner seal; HDPE bottles of 500 (NDC 0088-1090-55) with a polypropylene screw cap containing a pulp/wax liner with heat-sealed foil inner seal; and aluminum foil-backed clear blister packs of 100 (NDC 0088-1090-49).

ALLEGRA-D 12 HOUR is a two-layer tablet, one white layer and one tan layer with a clear film coating on the tablet. The tablets are engraved with "06/012D" on the white layer.

Store ALLEGRA-D 12 HOUR Extended-Release Tablets at 20–25°C (68–77°F). (See USP Controlled Room Temperature.)

Rev. December 2009

sanofi-aventis U.S. LLC
Bridgewater, NJ 08807
©2009 sanofi-aventis U.S. LLC
www.allegra.com

Shown in Product Identification Guide, page 318

ALLEGRA-D® 24 HOUR

[ə'lĕgra]
(fexofenadine HCl 180 mg and pseudoephedrine HCl 240 mg) Extended-Release Tablets

DESCRIPTION

ALLEGRA-D® 24 HOUR (fexofenadine hydrochloride and pseudoephedrine hydrochloride) Extended-Release Tablets for oral administration contain 180 mg fexofenadine hydrochloride for immediate release and 240 mg pseudoephedrine hydrochloride for extended release. Tablets also contain as excipients: microcrystalline cellulose, sodium chloride, cellulose acetate, polyethylene glycol, opadry white, povidone, talc, hypromellose, croscarmellose sodium, copovidone, titanium dioxide, magnesium stearate, colloidal silicon dioxide, brilliant blue aluminum lake, acetone, isopropyl alcohol, methyl alcohol, methylene chloride, water, and black ink.

Fexofenadine hydrochloride, one of the active ingredients of ALLEGRA-D 24 HOUR, is a histamine H$_1$-receptor antagonist with the chemical name (±)-4-[1-hydroxy-4-[4-(hydroxydiphenylmethyl)-1-piperidinyl]-butyl]-α, α-dimethyl benzeneacetic acid hydrochloride and the following chemical structure:

The molecular weight is 538.13 and the empirical formula is C$_{32}$H$_{39}$NO$_4$•HCl. Fexofenadine hydrochloride is a white to off-white crystalline powder. It is freely soluble in methanol and ethanol, slightly soluble in chloroform and water, and insoluble in hexane. Fexofenadine hydrochloride is a racemate and exists as a zwitterion in aqueous media at physiological pH.

Pseudoephedrine hydrochloride, the other active ingredient of ALLEGRA-D 24 HOUR, is an adrenergic (vasoconstrictor) agent with the chemical name [S-(R*,R*)]-α-[1-

Adverse Experiences Reported in One Active-Controlled Seasonal Allergic Rhinitis Clinical Trial at Rates of Greater than 1%

Adverse Experience	60 mg Fexofenadine Hydrochloride/120 mg Pseudoephedrine Hydrochloride Combination Tablet Twice Daily (n=215)	Fexofenadine Hydrochloride 60 mg Twice Daily (n=218)	Pseudoephedrine Hydrochloride 120 mg Twice Daily (n=218)
Headache	13.0%	11.5%	17.4%
Insomnia	12.6%	3.2%	13.3%
Nausea	7.4%	0.5%	5.0%
Dry Mouth	2.8%	0.5%	5.5%
Dyspepsia	2.8%	0.5%	0.9%
Throat Irritation	2.3%	1.8%	0.5%
Dizziness	1.9%	0.0%	3.2%
Agitation	1.9%	0.0%	1.4%
Back Pain	1.9%	0.5%	0.5%
Palpitation	1.9%	0.0%	0.9%
Nervousness	1.4%	0.5%	1.8%
Anxiety	1.4%	0.0%	1.4%
Upper Respiratory Infection	1.4%	0.9%	0.9%
Abdominal Pain	1.4%	0.5%	0.5%

(methylamino)ethyl]-benzenemethanol hydrochloride and the following chemical structure:

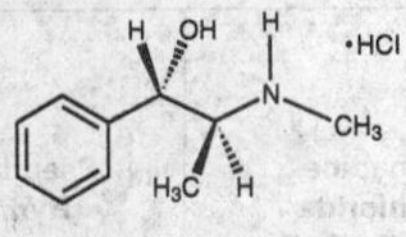

The molecular weight is 201.70 and the molecular formula is $C_{10}H_{15}NO \bullet HCl$. Pseudoephedrine hydrochloride occurs as fine, white to off-white crystals or powder, having a faint characteristic odor. It is very soluble in water, freely soluble in alcohol, and sparingly soluble in chloroform.

CLINICAL PHARMACOLOGY

Mechanism of Action

Fexofenadine hydrochloride, the major active metabolite of terfenadine, is an antihistamine with selective peripheral H_1-receptor antagonist activity. Fexofenadine hydrochloride inhibited antigen-induced bronchospasm in sensitized guinea pigs and histamine release from peritoneal mast cells in rats. In laboratory animals, no anticholinergic or alpha$_1$-adrenergic-receptor blocking effects were observed. Moreover, no sedative or other central nervous system effects were observed. Radiolabeled tissue distribution studies in rats indicated that fexofenadine does not cross the blood-brain barrier.

Pseudoephedrine hydrochloride is an orally active sympathomimetic amine and exerts a decongestant action on the nasal mucosa. Pseudoephedrine hydrochloride is recognized as an effective agent for the relief of nasal congestion due to allergic rhinitis. Pseudoephedrine produces peripheral effects similar to those of ephedrine and central effects similar to, but less intense than, amphetamines. It has the potential for excitatory side effects.

Pharmacokinetics

The pharmacokinetics of fexofenadine hydrochloride in subjects with seasonal allergic rhinitis were similar to those in healthy volunteers.

Absorption

Fexofenadine hydrochloride and pseudoephedrine hydrochloride administered as ALLEGRA-D 24 HOUR tablets are absorbed at a similar rate and are equally available under single-dose and steady-state conditions as the separate administration of the components. Coadministration of fexofenadine and pseudoephedrine does not significantly affect the bioavailability of either component. The administration of ALLEGRA-D 24 HOUR tablets 30 minutes or 1.5 hour after a high-fat meal decreased the bioavailability of fexofenadine by approximately 50% (AUC 42% and C_{max} 54%). Pseudoephedrine pharmacokinetics were unaffected when coadministered with a high-fat meal. Therefore, ALLEGRA-D 24 HOUR should be taken on an empty stomach with water (see DOSAGE AND ADMINISTRATION).

A pharmacokinetic study following single and multiple oral doses over 7 days of ALLEGRA-D 24 HOUR in 66 healthy volunteers showed that fexofenadine, the immediate release component of ALLEGRA-D 24 HOUR, was rapidly absorbed with mean maximum plasma concentrations of 634 ng/mL and 674 ng/mL after single and multiple doses, respectively. The median time to maximum concentration of fexofenadine was 1.8–2.0 hours post-dose. In the same study, the mean maximum plasma concentrations of pseudoephedrine, the extended-release component of ALLEGRA-D 24 HOUR, were 394 ng/mL and 495 ng/mL after single and multiple doses, respectively, with median time to maximum concentration of 12 hours post-dose. Pseudoephedrine concentrations at the end of the dosing interval (mean: 172 ng/mL) at steady state were equivalent to those observed from a comparator pseudoephedrine hydrochloride 240 mg tablet.

Distribution

Fexofenadine hydrochloride is 60% to 70% bound to plasma proteins, primarily albumin and α_1-acid glycoprotein. The protein binding of pseudoephedrine in humans is not known. Pseudoephedrine hydrochloride is extensively distributed into extravascular sites (apparent volume of distribution between 2.6 and 3.5 L/kg).

Metabolism

Approximately 5% of the total dose of fexofenadine hydrochloride and less than 1% of the total oral dose of pseudoephedrine hydrochloride were eliminated by hepatic metabolism.

Elimination

The mean terminal elimination half-life of fexofenadine was 14.6 hours following administration of ALLEGRA-D 24 HOUR tablets in healthy volunteers, which is consistent with observations from separate administration. Human mass balance studies documented a recovery of approximately 80% and 11% of the [^{14}C]-fexofenadine hydrochloride dose in the feces and urine, respectively. Because the absolute bioavailability of fexofenadine hydrochloride has not been established, it is unknown if the fecal component is primarily unabsorbed drug or the result of biliary excretion.

The mean terminal half-life of pseudoephedrine was 7 hours following single-dose administration of ALLEGRA-D 24 HOUR tablets.

Pseudoephedrine has been shown to have a mean elimination half-life of 4–6 hours which is dependent on urine pH. The elimination half-life is decreased at urine pH lower than 6 and may be increased at urine pH higher than 8.

Special Populations

Pharmacokinetics in special populations (for renal, hepatic impairment, and age), obtained after a single dose of 80 mg fexofenadine hydrochloride, were compared to those from healthy volunteers in a separate study of similar design.

Effect of Age

In older subjects (≥65 years old), peak plasma levels of fexofenadine were 99% greater than those observed in younger subjects (<65 years old). Mean fexofenadine elimination half-lives were similar to those observed in younger subjects.

Renally Impaired

In subjects with mild (creatinine clearance 41–80 mL/min) to severe (creatinine clearance 11–40 mL/min) renal impairment, peak plasma levels of fexofenadine were 87% and 111% greater, respectively, and mean elimination half-lives were 59% and 72% longer, respectively, than observed in healthy volunteers. Peak plasma levels in subjects on dialysis (creatinine clearance ≤10 mL/min) were 82% greater and half-life was 31% longer than observed in healthy volunteers. No data are available on the pharmacokinetics of pseudoephedrine in renally impaired subjects. However, most of the oral dose of pseudoephedrine hydrochloride (43–96%) is excreted unchanged in the urine. A decrease in renal function is, therefore, likely to decrease the clearance of pseudoephedrine significantly, thus prolonging the half-life and resulting in accumulation. (See PRECAUTIONS and DOSAGE AND ADMINISTRATION.)

Hepatically Impaired

The pharmacokinetics of fexofenadine hydrochloride in subjects with hepatic disease did not differ substantially from that observed in healthy volunteers. The effect on pseudoephedrine pharmacokinetics is unknown.

Effect of Gender

Across several trials, no clinically significant gender-related differences were observed in the pharmacokinetics of fexofenadine hydrochloride.

Pharmacodynamics

Wheal and Flare

Human histamine skin wheal and flare studies following single and twice daily doses of 20 mg and 40 mg fexofenadine hydrochloride demonstrated that the drug exhibits an antihistamine effect by 1 hour, achieves maximum effect at 2–3 hours, and an effect is still seen at 12 hours. There was no evidence of tolerance to these effects after 28 days of dosing. The clinical significance of these observations is unknown.

Effects on QT_c

In dogs (30 mg/kg orally twice daily for 5 days) and rabbits (10 mg/kg intravenously over 1 hour), fexofenadine hydrochloride did not prolong QT_c at plasma concentrations that were at least 7 and 15 times, respectively, the therapeutic plasma concentrations in man (based on a 180 mg once daily fexofenadine hydrochloride dose when administered as ALLEGRA-D 24 HOUR). No effect was observed on calcium channel current, delayed K^+ channel current, or action potential duration in guinea pig myocytes, Na^+ current in rat neonatal myocytes, or on the delayed rectifier K^+ channel cloned from human heart at concentrations up to 1×10^{-5} M of fexofenadine. This concentration was at least 8 times the therapeutic plasma concentration in man (based on a 180 mg once daily fexofenadine hydrochloride dose).

No statistically significant increase in mean QT_c interval compared to placebo was observed in 714 subjects with seasonal allergic rhinitis given fexofenadine hydrochloride capsules in doses of 60 mg to 240 mg twice daily for 2 weeks or in 40 healthy volunteers given fexofenadine hydrochloride as an oral solution at doses up to 400 mg twice daily for 6 days.

A 1-year study designed to evaluate safety and tolerability of 240 mg of fexofenadine hydrochloride (n=240) compared to placebo (n=237) in healthy volunteers, did not reveal a statistically significant increase in the mean QT_c interval for the fexofenadine hydrochloride treated group when evaluated pretreatment and after 1, 2, 3, 6, 9, and 12 months of treatment.

Administration of the 60 mg fexofenadine hydrochloride/120 mg pseudoephedrine hydrochloride combination tablet for approximately 2 weeks to 213 subjects with seasonal allergic rhinitis demonstrated no statistically significant increase in the mean QT_c interval compared to fexofenadine hydrochloride administered alone (60 mg twice daily, n=215), or compared to pseudoephedrine hydrochloride (120 mg twice daily, n=215) administered alone.

Clinical Studies

Clinical efficacy and safety studies were not conducted with ALLEGRA-D 24 HOUR Extended-Release Tablets. The effectiveness of ALLEGRA-D 24 HOUR for the treatment of seasonal allergic rhinitis is based on an extrapolation of the demonstrated efficacy of ALLEGRA 180 mg and the nasal decongestant properties of pseudoephedrine hydrochloride. In one 2-week, multicenter, randomized, double-blind clinical trial in subjects 12 to 65 years of age with seasonal allergic rhinitis (n=863), fexofenadine hydrochloride 180 mg once daily significantly reduced total symptom scores (the sum of the individual scores for sneezing, rhinorrhea, itchy nose/palate/throat, itchy/watery/red eyes) compared to placebo. Although the number of subjects in some of the subgroups was small, there were no significant differences in the effect of fexofenadine hydrochloride across subgroups of subjects defined by gender, age, and race.

INDICATIONS AND USAGE

ALLEGRA-D 24 HOUR Extended-Release Tablets are indicated for the relief of symptoms associated with seasonal allergic rhinitis in adults and children 12 years of age and older. Symptoms treated effectively include sneezing, rhinorrhea, itchy nose/palate/ and/or throat, itchy/watery/red eyes, and nasal congestion.

ALLEGRA-D 24 HOUR should be administered when both the antihistaminic properties of fexofenadine hydrochloride and the nasal decongestant properties of pseudoephedrine hydrochloride are desired (see CLINICAL PHARMACOLOGY).

CONTRAINDICATIONS

ALLEGRA-D 24 HOUR is contraindicated in patients with known hypersensitivity to any of its ingredients.

Due to its pseudoephedrine component, ALLEGRA-D 24 HOUR is contraindicated in patients with narrow-angle glaucoma or urinary retention, and in patients receiving monoamine oxidase (MAO) inhibitor therapy or within fourteen (14) days of stopping such treatment (see Drug Interactions section). It is also contraindicated in patients with severe hypertension, or severe coronary artery disease, and in those who have shown idiosyncrasy to its components, to adrenergic agents, or to other drugs of similar chemical structures. Manifestations of patient idiosyncrasy to adrenergic agents include: insomnia, dizziness, weakness, tremor, or arrhythmias.

WARNINGS

Sympathomimetic amines should be used with caution in patients with hypertension, diabetes mellitus, ischemic heart disease, increased intraocular pressure, hyperthyroidism, renal impairment, or prostatic hypertrophy (see CONTRAINDICATIONS). Sympathomimetic amines may produce central nervous system stimulation with convulsions or cardiovascular collapse with accompanying hypotension.

PRECAUTIONS

General

Because ALLEGRA-D 24 HOUR is a once-daily, fixed-dose combination that cannot be titrated and renal insufficiency increases the bioavailability and prolongs the half-life of fexofenadine hydrochloride and pseudoephedrine hydrochloride, ALLEGRA-D 24 HOUR tablets should generally be avoided in patients with renal insufficiency (see CLINICAL PHARMACOLOGY, and DOSAGE AND ADMINISTRATION).

Information for Patients

Patients taking ALLEGRA-D 24 HOUR tablets should receive the following information: ALLEGRA-D 24 HOUR tablets are prescribed for the relief of symptoms of seasonal allergic rhinitis. Patients should be instructed to take ALLEGRA-D 24 HOUR tablets only as prescribed. **Do not exceed the recommended dose.** If nervousness, dizziness, or sleeplessness occur, discontinue use and consult the doctor. Patients should also be advised against the concurrent use of ALLEGRA-D 24 HOUR tablets with over-the-counter antihistamines and decongestants.

The product should not be used by patients who are hypersensitive to it or to any of its ingredients. Due to its pseudoephedrine component, this product should not be used by patients with narrow-angle glaucoma, urinary retention, or by patients receiving a monoamine oxidase (MAO) inhibitor or within 14 days of stopping use of MAO inhibitor. It also should not be used by patients with severe hypertension or severe coronary artery disease.

Patients should be told that this product should be used in pregnancy or lactation only if the potential benefit justifies the potential risk to the fetus or nursing infant. Patients should be advised to take the tablet on an empty stomach with water. Patients should be directed to swallow the tablet whole. Patients should be cautioned not to break or chew the tablet. Patients should also be instructed to store the medication in a tightly closed container in a cool, dry place, away from children.

Drug Interactions

Fexofenadine hydrochloride and pseudoephedrine hydrochloride do not influence the pharmacokinetics of each other when administered concomitantly.

Fexofenadine has been shown to exhibit minimal (ca. 5%) metabolism. However, co-administration of fexofenadine hydrochloride with either ketoconazole or erythromycin led to increased plasma concentrations of fexofenadine. Fexofenadine had no effect on the pharmacokinetics of either erythromycin or ketoconazole. In 2 separate studies, fexofenadine hydrochloride 120 mg twice daily was co-administered with either erythromycin 500 mg every 8 hours or ketoconazole 400 mg once daily under steady-state conditions to healthy volunteers (n=24, each study). No differences in adverse events or QT_c interval were observed when subjects were administered fexofenadine hydrochloride alone or in combination with either erythromycin or ketoconazole. The findings of these studies are summarized in the following table:

Effects on steady-state fexofenadine pharmacokinetics after 7 days of co-administration with fexofenadine hydrochloride 120 mg every 12 hours (two times the recommended twice daily dose) in healthy volunteers (n=24)

Concomitant Drug	C_{maxSS} (Peak plasma concentration)	$AUC_{ss(0-12h)}$ (Extent of systemic exposure)
Erythromycin (500 mg every 8 hrs)	+82%	+109%
Ketoconazole (400 mg once daily)	+135%	+164%

The changes in plasma levels were within the range of plasma levels achieved in adequate and well-controlled clinical trials.

The mechanism of these interactions has been evaluated in *in vitro, in situ,* and *in vivo* animal models. These studies indicate that ketoconazole or erythromycin co-administration enhances fexofenadine gastrointestinal absorption. This observed increase in the bioavailability of fexofenadine may be due to transport-related effects, such as p-glycoprotein. *In vivo* animal studies also suggest that in addition to enhancing absorption, ketoconazole decreases fexofenadine gastrointestinal secretion, while erythromycin may also decrease biliary excretion.

Due to the pseudoephedrine component, ALLEGRA-D 24 HOUR is contraindicated in patients taking monoamine oxidase inhibitors and for 14 days after stopping use of an MAO inhibitor. Concomitant use with antihypertensive drugs which interfere with sympathetic activity (e.g., methyldopa, mecamylamine, and reserpine) may reduce their antihypertensive effects. Increased ectopic pacemaker activity can occur when pseudoephedrine is used concomitantly with digitalis. Care should be taken in the administration of ALLEGRA-D 24 HOUR concomitantly with other sympathomimetic amines because combined effects on the cardiovascular system may be harmful to the patient (see WARNINGS).

Drug Interactions with Antacids
Administration of 120 mg of fexofenadine hydrochloride (2 × 60 mg capsule) within 15 minutes of an aluminum and magnesium containing antacid (Maalox®) decreased fexofenadine AUC by 41% and C_{max} by 43%. ALLEGRA-D 24 HOUR should not be taken closely in time with aluminum and magnesium containing antacids.

Interactions with Fruit Juices
Fruit juices such as grapefruit, orange and apple may reduce the bioavailability and exposure of fexofenadine. This is based on the results from 3 clinical studies using histamine induced skin wheals and flares coupled with population pharmacokinetic analysis. The size of wheal and flare were significantly larger when fexofenadine hydrochloride was administered with either grapefruit or orange juices compared to water. Based on the literature reports, the same effects may be extrapolated to other fruit juices such as apple juice. The clinical significance of these observations is unknown. In addition, based on the population pharmacokinetics analysis of the combined data from grapefruit and orange juices studies with the bioequivalence study data, the bioavailability of fexofenadine was reduced by 36%. Therefore, to maximize the effects of fexofenadine, it is recommended that ALLEGRA-D 24 HOUR should be taken with water (see DOSAGE AND ADMINISTRATION).

Carcinogenesis, Mutagenesis, Impairment of Fertility
There are no animal or *in vitro* studies on the combination product fexofenadine hydrochloride and pseudoephedrine hydrochloride to evaluate carcinogenesis, mutagenesis, or impairment of fertility.

The carcinogenic potential and reproductive toxicity of fexofenadine hydrochloride were assessed using terfenadine studies with adequate fexofenadine exposure (area-under-the plasma concentration versus time curve [AUC]). No evidence of carcinogenicity was observed when mice and rats were given daily oral doses up to 150 mg/kg of terfenadine

for 18 and 24 months, respectively. In both species, 150 mg/kg of terfenadine produced AUC values of fexofenadine that were approximately 2 and 3 times, respectively, the exposure from the maximum recommended human daily oral dose of ALLEGRA-D 24 HOUR.

Two-year feeding studies in rats and mice conducted under the auspices of the National Toxicology Program (NTP) demonstrated no evidence of carcinogenic potential with ephedrine sulfate, a structurally related drug with pharmacological properties similar to pseudoephedrine, at doses up to 10 and 27 mg/kg, respectively (less than the maximum recommended human daily oral dose of pseudoephedrine hydrochloride on a mg/m² basis).

In *in vitro* (Bacterial Reverse Mutation, CHO/HGPRT Forward Mutation, and Rat Lymphocyte Chromosomal Aberration assays) and *in vivo* (Mouse Bone Marrow Micronucleus assay) tests, fexofenadine hydrochloride revealed no evidence of mutagenicity.

Reproduction and fertility studies with terfenadine in rats produced no effect on male or female fertility at oral doses up to 300 mg/kg/day (approximately 3 times the maximum recommended human daily oral dose of ALLEGRA-D 24 HOUR based on comparison of the AUCs of fexofenadine). However, reduced implants and post-implantation losses were reported at 300 mg/kg. A reduction in implants was also observed at an oral dose of 150 mg/kg/day (approximately 3 times the maximum recommended human daily oral dose of ALLEGRA-D 24 HOUR based on comparison of the AUCs). In mice, fexofenadine produced no effect on male or female fertility at average dietary doses up to 4438 mg/kg (approximately 10 times the maximum recommended human daily oral dose of ALLEGRA-D 24 HOUR based on comparison of the AUCs).

Pregnancy
Teratogenic Effects
Category C
Terfenadine alone was not teratogenic in rats at oral doses up to 300 mg/kg (approximately 3 times the maximum recommended human daily oral dose of ALLEGRA-D 24 HOUR based on comparison of the AUCs of fexofenadine) and in rabbits at oral doses up to 300 mg/kg (approximately 25 times the maximum recommended human daily oral dose of ALLEGRA-D 24 HOUR based on comparison of the AUCs of fexofenadine).

In mice, no adverse effects and no teratogenic effects during gestation were observed with fexofenadine at dietary doses up to 3730 mg/kg (approximately 10 times the maximum recommended human daily oral dose of ALLEGRA-D 24 HOUR based on comparison of the AUCs).

The combination of terfenadine and pseudoephedrine hydrochloride in a ratio of 1:2 by weight was studied in rats and rabbits. In rats, an oral combination dose of 150/300 mg/kg produced reduced fetal weight and delayed ossification with a finding of wavy ribs. The dose of 150 mg/kg of terfenadine in rats produced an AUC value of fexofenadine that was approximately 3 times the AUC of the maximum recommended human daily oral dose of ALLEGRA-D 24 HOUR. The dose of 300 mg/kg of pseudoephedrine hydrochloride in rats was approximately 10 times the maximum recommended human daily oral dose of ALLEGRA-D 24 HOUR on a mg/m² basis. In rabbits, an oral combination dose of 100/200 mg/kg produced decreased fetal weight. By extrapolation, the AUC of fexofenadine for 100 mg/kg orally of terfenadine was approximately 8 times the human AUC of the maximum recommended human daily oral dose of ALLEGRA-D 24 HOUR. The dose of 200 mg/kg of pseudoephedrine hydrochloride was approximately 15 times the maximum recommended human daily oral dose of ALLEGRA-D 24 HOUR on a mg/m² basis.

There are no adequate and well-controlled studies in pregnant women. ALLEGRA-D 24 HOUR should be used during pregnancy only if the potential benefit justifies the potential risk to the fetus.

Nonteratogenic Effects
Dose-related decreases in pup weight gain and survival were observed in rats exposed to an oral dose of 150 mg/kg of terfenadine; this dose produced an AUC of fexofenadine that was approximately 3 times the human AUC of the maximum recommended human daily oral dose of ALLEGRA-D 24 HOUR.

Nursing Mothers
It is not known if fexofenadine is excreted in human milk. Because many drugs are excreted in human milk, caution should be used when fexofenadine hydrochloride is administered to a nursing woman. Pseudoephedrine hydrochloride administered alone distributes into breast milk of lactating human females. Pseudoephedrine concentrations in milk are consistently higher than those in plasma. The total amount of drug in milk as judged by AUC is 2 to 3 times greater than the plasma AUC. The fraction of a pseudoephedrine dose excreted in milk is estimated to be 0.4% to 0.7%. A decision should be made whether to discontinue nursing or to discontinue the drug, taking into ac-

count the importance of the drug to the mother. Caution should be exercised when ALLEGRA-D 24 HOUR is administered to nursing women.

Pediatric Use
Safety and effectiveness of ALLEGRA-D 24 HOUR in children below the age of 12 years have not been established. In addition, the doses of the individual components in ALLEGRA-D 24 HOUR exceed the recommended individual doses for pediatric patients under 12 years of age. ALLEGRA-D 24 HOUR is not recommended for pediatric patients under 12 years of age.

Geriatric Use
Clinical studies of ALLEGRA-D 24 HOUR did not include sufficient numbers of subjects aged 65 and older to determine whether they respond differently from younger subjects. Other reported clinical experience has not identified differences in responses between the elderly and younger patients, although the elderly are more likely to have adverse reactions to sympathomimetic amines.

The pseudoephedrine component of ALLEGRA-D 24 HOUR is known to be substantially excreted by the kidney, and the risk of toxic reactions to this drug may be greater in patients with impaired renal function. Because elderly patients are more likely to have decreased renal function, it may be useful to monitor renal function.

ADVERSE REACTIONS
Fexofenadine Hydrochloride
In a placebo-controlled clinical study in the United States, which included 570 subjects with seasonal allergic rhinitis aged 12 years and older receiving fexofenadine hydrochloride tablets at doses of 120 or 180 mg once daily, adverse events were similar in fexofenadine hydrochloride and placebo-treated subjects. The following table lists adverse experiences that were reported by greater than 2% of subjects treated with fexofenadine hydrochloride tablets at doses of 180 mg once daily and that were more common with fexofenadine hydrochloride than placebo.

Once daily dosing with fexofenadine hydrochloride tablets at rates of greater than 2%

Adverse experience	Fexofenadine 180 mg once daily (n=283)	Placebo (n=293)
Headache	10.6%	7.5%
Upper Respiratory Tract Infection	3.2%	3.1%
Back Pain	2.8%	1.4%

Events that have been reported during controlled clinical trials involving subjects with seasonal allergic rhinitis at incidences less than 1% and similar to placebo and have been rarely reported during postmarketing surveillance include: insomnia, nervousness, and sleep disorders or paroniria. In rare cases, rash, urticaria, pruritus and hypersensitivity reactions with manifestations such as angioedema, chest tightness, dyspnea, flushing and systemic anaphylaxis have been reported.

Pseudoephedrine Hydrochloride
Pseudoephedrine hydrochloride may cause mild CNS stimulation in hypersensitive patients. Nervousness, excitability, restlessness, dizziness, weakness, or insomnia may occur. Headache, drowsiness, tachycardia, palpitation, pressor activity, cardiac arrhythmias and ischemic colitis have been reported. Sympathomimetic drugs have also been associated with other untoward effects such as fear, anxiety, tenseness, tremor, hallucinations, seizures, pallor, respiratory difficulty, dysuria, and cardiovascular collapse.

OVERDOSAGE
Most reports of fexofenadine hydrochloride overdose contain limited information. However, dizziness, drowsiness, and dry mouth have been reported. For the pseudoephedrine hydrochloride component of ALLEGRA-D 24 HOUR, information on acute overdose is limited to the marketing history of pseudoephedrine hydrochloride. Single doses of fexofenadine hydrochloride up to 800 mg (6 healthy volunteers at this dose level), and doses up to 690 mg twice daily for one month (3 healthy volunteers at this dose level), were administered without the development of clinically significant adverse events.

In large doses, sympathomimetics may give rise to giddiness, headache, nausea, vomiting, sweating, thirst, tachycardia, precordial pain, palpitations, difficulty in micturition, muscular weakness and tenseness, anxiety, restlessness, and insomnia. Many patients can present a toxic psychosis with delusions and hallucinations. Some may develop cardiac arrhythmias, circulatory collapse, convulsions, coma, and respiratory failure.

In the event of overdose, consider standard measures to remove any unabsorbed drug. Symptomatic and supportive treatment is recommended. Following administration of terfenadine, hemodialysis did not effectively remove fexofenadine, the major active metabolite of terfenadine, from blood (up to 1.7% removed). The effect of hemodialysis on the removal of pseudoephedrine is unknown.

No deaths occurred in mature mice and rats at oral doses of fexofenadine hydrochloride up to 5000 mg/kg (approximately 110 and 230 times, respectively, the maximum recommended human daily oral dose of ALLEGRA-D 24 HOUR on a mg/m^2 basis.) The median oral lethal dose in newborn rats was 438 mg/kg (approximately 20 times the maximum recommended human daily oral dose of ALLEGRA-D 24 HOUR on a mg/m^2 basis). In dogs, no evidence of toxicity was observed at oral doses up to 2000 mg/kg (approximately 300 times the maximum recommended human daily oral dose of ALLEGRA-D 24 HOUR on a mg/m^2 basis). The oral median lethal dose of pseudoephedrine hydrochloride in rats was 1674 mg/kg (approximately 55 times the maximum recommended human daily oral dose of ALLEGRA-D 24 HOUR on a mg/m^2 basis).

DOSAGE AND ADMINISTRATION

The recommended dose of ALLEGRA-D 24 HOUR Extended-Release Tablets is one tablet once daily administered on an empty stomach with water for adults and children 12 years of age and older. ALLEGRA-D 24 HOUR tablets should generally be avoided in patients with renal insufficiency. ALLEGRA-D 24 HOUR must be swallowed whole and never crushed or chewed.

HOW SUPPLIED

ALLEGRA-D 24 HOUR Extended-Release Tablets contain 180 mg fexofenadine hydrochloride for immediate release and 240 mg pseudoephedrine hydrochloride for extended release. ALLEGRA-D 24 HOUR Extended-Release Tablets are available in high-density polyethylene (HDPE) bottles of 100 (NDC 0088-1095-47), with an activated charcoal pouch. All bottles have a polypropylene screw cap containing a pulp/wax liner with heat-sealed foil inner seal.

ALLEGRA-D 24 HOUR Extended-Release Tablet is a white, round, film coated tablet. The tablet has 308AV printed on one side in black ink.

Store ALLEGRA-D 24 HOUR Extended-Release Tablets at 20–25°C (68–77°F). (See USP Controlled Room Temperature.)

Rev. December 2009
sanofi-aventis U.S. LLC
Bridgewater, NJ 08807
©2009 sanofi-aventis U.S. LLC
Shown in Product Identification Guide, page 318

AMBIEN®   © R
[ăm′bē-ən]
(zolpidem tartrate)
tablets

HIGHLIGHTS OF PRESCRIBING INFORMATION
These highlights do not include all the information needed to use AMBIEN safely and effectively. See full prescribing information for AMBIEN.
Ambien® (zolpidem tartrate) tablets CIV
Initial US Approval: 1992

————————INDICATIONS AND USAGE————————
Ambien is indicated for the short term treatment of insomnia characterized by difficulties with sleep initiation. Ambien has been shown to decrease sleep latency for up to 35 days in controlled clinical studies (1)

————————DOSAGE AND ADMINISTRATION————————
- Adult dose: 10 mg once daily immediately before bedtime (2.1)
- Elderly/debilitated patients/hepatically impaired: 5 mg once daily immediately before bedtime (2.2)
- Downward dosage adjustment may be necessary when used with CNS depressants (2.3)
- Should not be taken with or immediately after a meal (2.4)

————————DOSAGE FORMS AND STRENGTHS————————
5 mg and 10 mg tablets. Tablets not scored (3)

————————CONTRAINDICATIONS————————
Known hypersensitivity to zolpidem tartrate or to any of the inactive ingredients in the formulation (4)

————————WARNINGS AND PRECAUTIONS————————
- Need to evaluate for co-morbid diagnosis: Reevaluate if insomnia persists after 7 to 10 days of use (5.1)
- Severe anaphylactic/anaphylactoid reactions: Angioedema and anaphylaxis have been reported. Do not rechallenge if such reactions occur (5.2)
- Abnormal thinking, behavioral changes and complex behaviors: May include "sleep-driving" and hallucinations. Immediately evaluate any new onset behavioral changes (5.3)
- Depression: Worsening of depression or, suicidal thinking may occur. Prescribe the least amount feasible to avoid intentional overdose (5.3, 5.6)

- Withdrawal effects: Symptoms may occur with rapid dose reduction or discontinuation (5.4, 9.3)
- CNS depressant effects: Use can impair alertness and motor coordination. If used in combination with other CNS depressants, dose reductions may be needed due to additive effects. Do not use with alcohol (2.3, 5.5)
- Elderly/debilitated patients: Use lower dose due to impaired motor, cognitive performance and increased sensitivity (2.2, 5.6)
- Patients with hepatic impairment, mild to moderate COPD, impaired drug metabolism or hemodynamic responses, mild to moderate sleep apnea: Use with caution and monitor closely (5.6)

————————ADVERSE REACTIONS————————
- Most commonly observed adverse reactions were:
  Short-term (< 10 nights): Drowsiness, dizziness, and diarrhea
  Long-term (28 < 35 nights): Dizziness and drugged feelings (6.1)

To report SUSPECTED ADVERSE REACTIONS, contact sanofi-aventis U.S. LLC at 1-800-633-1610 or FDA at 1-800-FDA-1088, or http://www.fda.gov/medwatch

————————DRUG INTERACTIONS————————
- CNS depressants: Enhanced CNS-depressant effects with combination use. Use with alcohol causes additive psychomotor impairment (7.1)
- Imipramine: Decreased alertness observed with combination use (7.1)
- Chlorpromazine: Impaired alertness and psychomotor performance observed with combination use (7.1)
- Rifampin: Combination use decreases exposure to and effects of zolpidem (7.2)
- Ketoconazole: Combination use increases exposure to and effect of zolpidem (7.2)

————————USE IN SPECIFIC POPULATIONS————————
- Pregnancy: Crosses the placenta. No studies in pregnant women (8.1)
- Nursing mothers: Infant exposure via breast milk (8.3)
- Pediatric use: Safety and effectiveness not established. Hallucinations (incidence rate 7.4%) and other psychiatric and/or nervous system adverse reactions were observed frequently in a study of pediatric patients with Attention-Deficit/Hyperactivity Disorder (5.6, 8.4)

See 17 for PATIENT COUNSELING INFORMATION and Medication Guide

Revised: 09/2009

FULL PRESCRIBING INFORMATION

1   INDICATIONS AND USAGE

Ambien (zolpidem tartrate) is indicated for the short-term treatment of insomnia characterized by difficulties with sleep initiation. Ambien has been shown to decrease sleep latency for up to 35 days in controlled clinical studies *[see Clinical Studies (14)]*.

The clinical trials performed in support of efficacy were 4–5 weeks in duration with the final formal assessments of sleep latency performed at the end of treatment.

2   DOSAGE AND ADMINISTRATION

The dose of Ambien should be individualized.

2.1   Dosage in adults
The recommended dose for adults is 10 mg once daily immediately before bedtime. The total Ambien dose should not exceed 10 mg per day.

2.2   Special populations
Elderly or debilitated patients may be especially sensitive to the effects of zolpidem tartrate. Patients with hepatic insufficiency do not clear the drug as rapidly as normal subjects. The recommended dose of Ambien in both of these patient populations is 5 mg once daily immediately before bedtime *[see Warnings and Precautions (5.6)]*.

2.3   Use with CNS depressants
Dosage adjustment may be necessary when Ambien is combined with other CNS depressant drugs because of the potentially additive effects *[see Warnings and Precautions (5.5)]*.

2.4   Administration
The effect of Ambien may be slowed by ingestion with or immediately after a meal.

3   DOSAGE FORMS AND STRENGTHS

Ambien is available in 5 mg and 10 mg strength tablets for oral administration. Tablets are not scored.

Ambien 5 mg tablets are capsule-shaped, pink, film coated, with AMB 5 debossed on one side and 5401 on the other.

Ambien 10 mg tablets are capsule-shaped, white, film coated, with AMB 10 debossed on one side and 5421 on the other.

4   CONTRAINDICATIONS

Ambien is contraindicated in patients with known hypersensitivity to zolpidem tartrate or to any of the inactive ingredients in the formulation. Observed reactions include anaphylaxis and angioedema *[see Warnings and Precautions (5.2)]*.

5   WARNINGS AND PRECAUTIONS

5.1   Need to evaluate for co-morbid diagnoses
Because sleep disturbances may be the presenting manifestation of a physical and/or psychiatric disorder, symptomatic treatment of insomnia should be initiated only after a careful evaluation of the patient. **The failure of insomnia to remit after 7 to 10 days of treatment may indicate the presence of a primary psychiatric and/or medical illness that should be evaluated.** Worsening of insomnia or the emergence of new thinking or behavior abnormalities may be the consequence of an unrecognized psychiatric or physical disorder. Such findings have emerged during the course of treatment with sedative/hypnotic drugs, including zolpidem.

5.2   Severe anaphylactic and anaphylactoid reactions
Rare cases of angioedema involving the tongue, glottis or larynx have been reported in patients after taking the first or subsequent doses of sedative-hypnotics, including zolpidem. Some patients have had additional symptoms such as dyspnea, throat closing or nausea and vomiting that suggest anaphylaxis. Some patients have required medical therapy in the emergency department. If angioedema involves the throat, glottis or larynx, airway obstruction may occur and be fatal. Patients who develop angioedema after treatment with zolpidem should not be rechallenged with the drug.

5.3   Abnormal thinking and behavioral changes
A variety of abnormal thinking and behavior changes have been reported to occur in association with the use of sedative/hypnotics. Some of these changes may be characterized by decreased inhibition (e.g., aggressiveness and extroversion that seemed out of character), similar to effects produced by alcohol and other CNS depressants. Visual and auditory hallucinations have been reported as well as behavioral changes such as bizarre behavior, agitation and

depersonalization. In controlled trials, < 1% of adults with insomnia who received zolpidem reported hallucinations. In a clinical trial, 7.4% of pediatric patients with insomnia associated with attention-deficit/hyperactivity disorder (ADHD), who received zolpidem reported hallucinations *[see Use in Specific Populations (8.4)]*.

Complex behaviors such as "sleep-driving" (i.e., driving while not fully awake after ingestion of a sedative-hypnotic, with amnesia for the event) have been reported with sedative-hypnotics, including zolpidem. These events can occur in sedative-hypnotic-naive as well as in sedative-hypnotic-experienced persons. Although behaviors such as "sleep-driving" may occur with Ambien alone at therapeutic doses, the use of alcohol and other CNS depressants with Ambien appears to increase the risk of such behaviors, as does the use of Ambien at doses exceeding the maximum recommended dose. Due to the risk to the patient and the community, discontinuation of Ambien should be strongly considered for patients who report a "sleep-driving" episode. Other complex behaviors (e.g., preparing and eating food, making phone calls, or having sex) have been reported in patients who are not fully awake after taking a sedative-hypnotic. As with "sleep-driving", patients usually do not remember these events. Amnesia, anxiety and other neuro-psychiatric symptoms may occur unpredictably.

In primarily depressed patients, worsening of depression, including suicidal thoughts and actions (including completed suicides), has been reported in association with the use of sedative/hypnotics.

It can rarely be determined with certainty whether a particular instance of the abnormal behaviors listed above is drug induced, spontaneous in origin, or a result of an underlying psychiatric or physical disorder. Nonetheless, the emergence of any new behavioral sign or symptom of concern requires careful and immediate evaluation.

5.4 Withdrawal effects

Following the rapid dose decrease or abrupt discontinuation of sedative/hypnotics, there have been reports of signs and symptoms similar to those associated with withdrawal from other CNS-depressant drugs *[see Drug Abuse and Dependence (9)]*.

5.5 CNS depressant effects

Ambien, like other sedative/hypnotic drugs, has CNS-depressant effects. Due to the rapid onset of action, Ambien should only be taken immediately prior to going to bed. Patients should be cautioned against engaging in hazardous occupations requiring complete mental alertness or motor coordination such as operating machinery or driving a motor vehicle after ingesting the drug, including potential impairment of the performance of such activities that may occur the day following ingestion of Ambien. Ambien showed additive effects when combined with alcohol and should not be taken with alcohol. Patients should also be cautioned about possible combined effects with other CNS-depressant drugs. Dosage adjustments may be necessary when Ambien is administered with such agents because of the potentially additive effects.

5.6 Special populations

Use in the elderly and/or debilitated patients:

Impaired motor and/or cognitive performance after repeated exposure or unusual sensitivity to sedative/hypnotic drugs is a concern in the treatment of elderly and/or debilitated patients. Therefore, the recommended Ambien dosage is 5 mg in such patients to decrease the possibility of side effects *[see Dosage and Administration (2.2)]*. These patients should be closely monitored.

Use in patients with concomitant illness:

Clinical experience with Ambien (zolpidem tartrate) in patients with concomitant systemic illness is limited. Caution is advisable in using Ambien in patients with diseases or conditions that could affect metabolism or hemodynamic responses.

Although studies did not reveal respiratory depressant effects at hypnotic doses of zolpidem in normal subjects or in patients with mild to moderate chronic obstructive pulmonary disease (COPD), a reduction in the Total Arousal Index together with a reduction in lowest oxygen saturation and increase in the times of oxygen desaturation below 80% and 90% was observed in patients with mild-to-moderate sleep apnea when treated with Ambien (10 mg) when compared to placebo. Since sedative/hypnotics have the capacity to depress respiratory drive, precautions should be taken if Ambien is prescribed to patients with compromised respiratory function. Post-marketing reports of respiratory insufficiency, most of which involved patients with pre-existing respiratory impairment, have been received. Ambien should be used with caution in patients with sleep apnea syndrome or myasthenia gravis.

Data in end-stage renal failure patients repeatedly treated with Ambien did not demonstrate drug accumulation or alterations in pharmacokinetic parameters. No dosage adjustment in renally impaired patients is required; however, these patients should be closely monitored *[see Clinical Pharmacology (12.3)]*.

Incidence of Treatment-Emergent Adverse Experiences in Placebo-Controlled Clinical Trials Lasting up to 10 Nights (Percentage of patients reporting)

Body System/ Adverse Event*	Zolpidem (≤10mg) (N=685)	Placebo (N=473)
Central and Peripheral Nervous System		
Headache	7	6
Drowsiness	2	–
Dizziness	1	–
Gastrointestinal System		
Diarrhea	1	-

*Reactions reported by at least 1% of patients treated with Ambien and at a greater frequency than placebo.

A study in subjects with hepatic impairment did reveal prolonged elimination in this group; therefore, treatment should be initiated with 5 mg in patients with hepatic compromise, and they should be closely monitored *[see Dosage and Administration (2.2) and Clinical Pharmacology (12.3)]*.

Use in patients with depression:

As with other sedative/hypnotic drugs, Ambien should be administered with caution to patients exhibiting signs or symptoms of depression. Suicidal tendencies may be present in such patients and protective measures may be required. Intentional over-dosage is more common in this group of patients; therefore, the least amount of drug that is feasible should be prescribed for the patient at any one time.

Use in pediatric patients:

Safety and effectiveness of zolpidem have not been established in pediatric patients. In an 8-week study in pediatric patients (aged 6–17 years) with insomnia associated with ADHD, zolpidem did not decrease sleep latency compared to placebo. Hallucinations were reported in 7.4% of the pediatric patients who received zolpidem; none of the pediatric patients who received placebo reported hallucinations *[see Use in Specific Populations (8.4)]*.

6 ADVERSE REACTIONS

The following serious adverse reactions are discussed in greater detail in other sections of the labeling:

- Serious anaphylactic and anaphylactoid reactions *[see Warnings and Precautions (5.2)]*
- Abnormal thinking, behavior changes, and complex behaviors *[see Warnings and Precautions (5.3)]*
- Withdrawal effects *[see Warnings and Precautions (5.4)]*
- CNS-depressant effects *[see Warnings and Precautions (5.5)]*

6.1 Clinical trials experience

Associated with discontinuation of treatment:

Approximately 4% of 1,701 patients who received zolpidem at all doses (1.25 to 90 mg) in U.S. premarketing clinical trials discontinued treatment because of an adverse reaction. Reactions most commonly associated with discontinuation from U.S. trials were daytime drowsiness (0.5%), dizziness (0.4%), headache (0.5%), nausea (0.6%), and vomiting (0.5%).

Approximately 4% of 1,959 patients who received zolpidem at all doses (1 to 50 mg) in similar foreign trials discontinued treatment because of an adverse reaction. Reactions most commonly associated with discontinuation from these trials were daytime drowsiness (1.1%), dizziness/vertigo (0.8%), amnesia (0.5%), nausea (0.5%), headache (0.4%), and falls (0.4%).

Data from a clinical study in which selective serotonin reuptake inhibitor (SSRI)-treated patients were given zolpidem revealed that four of the seven discontinuations during double-blind treatment with zolpidem (n=95) were associated with impaired concentration, continuing or aggravated depression, and manic reaction; one patient treated with placebo (n=97) was discontinued after an attempted suicide.

Most commonly observed adverse reactions in controlled trials:

During short-term treatment (up to 10 nights) with Ambien at doses up to 10 mg, the most commonly observed adverse reactions associated with the use of zolpidem and seen at statistically significant differences from placebo treated patients were drowsiness (reported by 2% of zolpidem patients), dizziness (1%), and diarrhea (1%). During longer-term treatment (28 to 35 nights) with zolpidem at doses up to 10 mg, the most commonly observed adverse reactions associated with the use of zolpidem and seen at statistically significant differences from placebo treated patients were dizziness (5%) and drugged feelings (3%).

Adverse reactions observed at an incidence of ≥ 1% in controlled trials:

The following tables enumerate treatment-emergent adverse reactions frequencies that were observed at an incidence equal to 1% or greater among patients with insomnia who received zolpidem tartrate and at a greater incidence than placebo in U.S. placebo-controlled trials. Events reported by investigators were classified utilizing a modified World Health Organization (WHO) dictionary of preferred terms for the purpose of establishing event frequencies. The prescriber should be aware that these figures cannot be used to predict the incidence of side effects in the course of usual medical practice, in which patient characteristics and other factors differ from those that prevailed in these clinical trials. Similarly, the cited frequencies cannot be compared with figures obtained from other clinical investigators involving related drug products and uses, since each group of drug trials is conducted under a different set of conditions. However, the cited figures provide the physician with a basis for estimating the relative contribution of drug and nondrug factors to the incidence of side effects in the population studied.

The following table was derived from results of 11 placebo-controlled short-term U.S. efficacy trials involving zolpidem in doses ranging from 1.25 to 20 mg. The table is limited to data from doses up to and including 10 mg, the highest dose recommended for use.

[See table above]

The following table was derived from results of three placebo-controlled long-term efficacy trials involving Ambien (zolpidem tartrate). These trials involved patients with chronic insomnia who were treated for 28 to 35 nights with zolpidem at doses of 5, 10, or 15 mg. The table is limited to data from doses up to and including 10 mg, the highest dose recommended for use. The table includes only adverse events occurring at an incidence of at least 1% for zolpidem patients.

Incidence of Treatment-Emergent Adverse Experiences in Placebo-Controlled Clinical Trials Lasting up to 35 Nights (Percentage of patients reporting)

Body System/ Adverse Event*	Zolpidem (≤10mg) (N=152)	Placebo (N=161)
Autonomic Nervous System		
Dry mouth	3	1
Body as a Whole		
Allergy	4	1
Back Pain	3	2
Influenza-like symptoms	2	-
Chest pain	1	-
Cardiovascular System		
Palpitation	2	-
Central and Peripheral Nervous System		
Drowsiness	8	5
Dizziness	5	1
Lethargy	3	1
Drugged feeling	3	-
Lightheadedness	2	1
Depression	2	1
Abnormal dreams	1	-
Amnesia	1	-
Sleep disorder	1	-
Gastrointestinal System		
Diarrhea	3	2
Abdominal pain	2	2
Constipation	2	1
Respiratory System		
Sinusitis	4	2
Pharyngitis	3	1
Skin and Appendages		
Rash	2	1

*Reactions reported by at least 1% of patients treated with Ambien and at a greater frequency than placebo.

Dose relationship for adverse reactions:

There is evidence from dose comparison trials suggesting a dose relationship for many of the adverse reactions associated with zolpidem use, particularly for certain CNS and gastrointestinal adverse events.

Adverse event incidence across the entire preapproval database:

Ambien was administered to 3,660 subjects in clinical trials throughout the U.S., Canada, and Europe. Treatment-emergent adverse events associated with clinical trial participation were recorded by clinical investigators using terminology of their own choosing. To provide a meaningful estimate of the proportion of individuals experiencing treatment-emergent adverse events, similar types of untoward events were grouped into a smaller number of standardized event categories and classified utilizing a modified World Health Organization (WHO) dictionary of preferred terms.

The frequencies presented, therefore, represent the proportions of the 3,660 individuals exposed to zolpidem, at all doses, who experienced an event of the type cited on at least one occasion while receiving zolpidem. All reported treatment-emergent adverse events are included, except those already listed in the table above of adverse events in placebo-controlled studies, those coding terms that are so general as to be uninformative, and those events where a drug cause was remote. It is important to emphasize that, although the events reported did occur during treatment with Ambien, they were not necessarily caused by it.

Adverse events are further classified within body system categories and enumerated in order of decreasing frequency using the following definitions: frequent adverse events are defined as those occurring in greater than 1/100 subjects; infrequent adverse events are those occurring in 1/100 to 1/1,000 patients; rare events are those occurring in less than 1/1,000 patients.

Autonomic nervous system: Infrequent: increased sweating, pallor, postural hypotension, syncope. Rare: abnormal accommodation, altered saliva, flushing, glaucoma, hypotension, impotence, increased saliva, tenesmus.

Body as a whole: Frequent: asthenia. Infrequent: edema, falling, fatigue, fever, malaise, trauma. Rare: allergic reaction, allergy aggravated, anaphylactic shock, face edema, hot flashes, increased ESR, pain, restless legs, rigors, tolerance increased, weight decrease.

Cardiovascular system: Infrequent: cerebrovascular disorder, hypertension, tachycardia. Rare: angina pectoris, arrhythmia, arteritis, circulatory failure, extrasystoles, hypertension aggravated, myocardial infarction, phlebitis, pulmonary embolism, pulmonary edema, varicose veins, ventricular tachycardia.

Central and peripheral nervous system: Frequent: ataxia, confusion, euphoria, headache, insomnia, vertigo. Infrequent: agitation, anxiety, decreased cognition, detached, difficulty concentrating, dysarthria, emotional lability, hallucination, hypoesthesia, illusion, leg cramps, migraine, nervousness, paresthesia, sleeping (after daytime dosing), speech disorder, stupor, tremor. Rare: abnormal gait, abnormal thinking, aggressive reaction, apathy, appetite increased, decreased libido, delusion, dementia, depersonalization, dysphasia, feeling strange, hypokinesia, hypotonia, hysteria, intoxicated feeling, manic reaction, neuralgia, neuritis, neuropathy, neurosis, panic attacks, paresis, personality disorder, somnambulism, suicide attempts, tetany, yawning.

Gastrointestinal system: Frequent: dyspepsia, hiccup, nausea. Infrequent: anorexia, constipation, dysphagia, flatulence, gastroenteritis, vomiting. Rare: enteritis, eructation, esophagospasm, gastritis, hemorrhoids, intestinal obstruction, rectal hemorrhage, tooth caries.

Hematologic and lymphatic system: Rare: anemia, hyperhemoglobinemia, leukopenia, lymphadenopathy, macrocytic anemia, purpura, thrombosis.

Immunologic system: Infrequent: infection. Rare: abscess herpes simplex herpes zoster, otitis externa, otitis media.

Liver and biliary system: Infrequent: abnormal hepatic function, increased SGPT. Rare: bilirubinemia, increased SGOT.

Metabolic and nutritional: Infrequent: hyperglycemia, thirst. Rare: gout, hypercholesteremia, hyperlipidemia, increased alkaline phosphatase, increased BUN, periorbital edema.

Musculoskeletal system: Frequent: arthralgia, myalgia. Infrequent: arthritis. Rare: arthrosis, muscle weakness, sciatica, tendinitis.

Reproductive system: Infrequent: menstrual disorder, vaginitis. Rare: breast fibroadenosis, breast neoplasm, breast pain.

Respiratory system: Frequent: upper respiratory infection. Infrequent: bronchitis, coughing, dyspnea, rhinitis. Rare: bronchospasm, epistaxis, hypoxia, laryngitis, pneumonia.

Skin and appendages: Infrequent: pruritus. Rare: acne, bullous eruption, dermatitis, furunculosis, injection-site inflammation, photosensitivity reaction, urticaria.

Special senses: Frequent: diplopia, vision abnormal. Infrequent: eye irritation, eye pain, scleritis, taste perversion, tinnitus. Rare: conjunctivitis, corneal ulceration, lacrimation abnormal, parosmia, photopsia.

Urogenital system: Frequent: urinary tract infection. Infrequent: cystitis, urinary incontinence. Rare: acute renal failure, dysuria, micturition frequency, nocturia, polyuria, pyelonephritis, renal pain, urinary retention.

7 DRUG INTERACTIONS

7.1 CNS-active drugs

Since the systematic evaluations of zolpidem in combination with other CNS-active drugs have been limited, careful consideration should be given to the pharmacology of any CNS-active drug to be used with zolpidem. Any drug with CNS-depressant effects could potentially enhance the CNS-depressant effects of zolpidem.

Ambien was evaluated in healthy subjects in single-dose interaction studies for several CNS drugs. Imipramine in combination with zolpidem produced no pharmacokinetic interaction other than a 20% decrease in peak levels of imipramine, but there was an additive effect of decreased alertness. Similarly, chlorpromazine in combination with zolpidem produced no pharmacokinetic interaction, but there was an additive effect of decreased alertness and psychomotor performance. A study involving haloperidol and zolpidem revealed no effect of haloperidol on the pharmacokinetics or pharmacodynamics of zolpidem. The lack of a drug interaction following single-dose administration does not predict a lack following chronic administration.

An additive effect on psychomotor performance between alcohol and zolpidem was demonstrated [see Warnings and Precautions (5.5)].

A single-dose interaction study with zolpidem 10 mg and fluoxetine 20 mg at steady-state levels in male volunteers did not demonstrate any clinically significant pharmacokinetic or pharmacodynamic interactions. When multiple doses of zolpidem and fluoxetine at steady-state concentrations were evaluated in healthy females, the only significant change was a 17% increase in the zolpidem half-life. There was no evidence of an additive effect in psychomotor performance.

Following five consecutive nightly doses of zolpidem 10 mg in the presence of sertraline 50 mg (17 consecutive daily doses, at 7:00 am, in healthy female volunteers), zolpidem C_{max} was significantly higher (43%) and T_{max} was significantly decreased (53%). Pharmacokinetics of sertraline and N-desmethylsertraline were unaffected by zolpidem.

7.2 Drugs that affect drug metabolism via cytochrome P450

Some compounds known to inhibit CYP3A may increase exposure to zolpidem. The effect of inhibitors of other P450 enzymes has not been carefully evaluated.

A randomized, double-blind, crossover interaction study in ten healthy volunteers between itraconazole (200 mg once daily for 4 days) and a single dose of zolpidem (10 mg) given 5 hours after the last dose of itraconazole resulted in a 34% increase in $AUC_{0-\infty}$ of zolpidem. There were no significant pharmacodynamic effects of zolpidem on subjective drowsiness, postural sway, or psychomotor performance.

A randomized, placebo-controlled, crossover interaction study in eight healthy female subjects between five consecutive daily doses of rifampin (600 mg) and a single dose of zolpidem (20 mg) given 17 hours after the last dose of rifampin showed significant reductions of the AUC (–73%), C_{max} (–58%), and $T_{1/2}$ (–36%) of zolpidem together with significant reductions in the pharmacodynamic effects of zolpidem.

A randomized double-blind crossover interaction study in twelve healthy subjects showed that co-administration of a single 5 mg dose of zolpidem tartrate with ketoconazole, a potent CYP3A4 inhibitor, given as 200 mg twice daily for 2 days increased C_{max} of zolpidem by a factor of 1.3 and increased the total AUC of zolpidem by a factor of 1.7 compared to zolpidem alone and prolonged the elimination half-life by approximately 30% along with an increase in the pharmacodynamic effects of zolpidem. Caution should be used when ketoconazole is given with zolpidem and consideration should be given to using a lower dose of zolpidem when ketoconazole and zolpidem are given together. Patients should be advised that use of Ambien with ketoconazole may enhance the sedative effects.

7.3 Other drugs with no interaction with zolpidem

A study involving cimetidine/zolpidem and ranitidine/zolpidem combinations revealed no effect of either drug on the pharmacokinetics or pharmacodynamics of zolpidem. Zolpidem had no effect on digoxin pharmacokinetics and did not affect prothrombin time when given with warfarin in normal subjects.

7.4 Drug-laboratory test interactions

Zolpidem is not known to interfere with commonly employed clinical laboratory tests. In addition, clinical data indicate that zolpidem does not cross-react with benzodiazepines, opiates, barbiturates, cocaine, cannabinoids, or amphetamines in two standard urine drug screens.

8 USE IN SPECIFIC POPULATIONS

8.1 Pregnancy

Pregnancy Category C

There are no adequate and well-controlled studies in pregnant women. Ambien should be used during pregnancy only if the potential benefit outweighs the potential risk to the fetus.

Oral studies of zolpidem in pregnant rats and rabbits showed adverse effects on the development of offspring only at doses greater than the maximum recommended human dose (MRHD of 10 mg/day). These doses were also maternally toxic in animals. A teratogenic effect was not observed in these studies. Administration to pregnant rats during the period of organogenesis produced dose-related maternal toxicity and decreases in fetal skull ossification at doses 25 to 125 times the MRHD. The no-effect dose for embryo-fetal toxicity was between 4 and 5 times the MRHD. Treatment of pregnant rabbits during organogenesis resulted in maternal toxicity at all doses studied and increased post-implantation embryo-fetal loss and under-ossification of fetal sternebrae at the highest dose (over 35 times the MRHD). The no-effect level for embryo-fetal toxicity was between 9 and 10 times the MRHD. Administration to rats during the latter part of pregnancy and throughout lactation produced maternal toxicity and decreased pup growth and survival at doses approximately 25 to 125 times the MRHD. The no-effect dose for offspring toxicity was between 4 and 5 times the MRHD.

Studies to assess the effects on children whose mothers took zolpidem during pregnancy have not been conducted. There is a published case report documenting the presence of zolpidem in human umbilical cord blood. Children born of mothers taking sedative/hypnotic drugs may be at some risk for withdrawal symptoms from the drug during the postnatal period. In addition, neonatal flaccidity has been reported in infants born of mothers who received sedative/hypnotic drugs during pregnancy. Cases of severe neonatal respiratory depression have been reported when zolpidem was used with other CNS depressants at the end of pregnancy.

8.2 Labor and delivery

Ambien has no established use in labor and delivery [see Pregnancy (8.1)].

8.3 Nursing mothers

Studies in lactating mothers indicate that the half-life of zolpidem is similar to that in young normal subjects (2.6 ± 0.3 hr). Between 0.004% and 0.019% of the total administered dose is excreted into milk. The effect of zolpidem on the nursing infant is not known. Caution should be exercised when Ambien is administered to a nursing mother.

8.4 Pediatric use

Safety and effectiveness of zolpidem have not been established in pediatric patients.

In an 8-week controlled study, 201 pediatric patients (aged 6-17 years) with insomnia associated with attention-deficit/hyperactivity disorder (90% of the patients were using psychoanaleptics) were treated with an oral solution of zolpidem (n=136), or placebo (n=65). Zolpidem did not significantly decrease latency to persistent sleep, compared to placebo, as measured by polysomnography after 4 weeks of treatment. Psychiatric and nervous system disorders comprised the most frequent (> 5%) treatment emergent adverse reactions observed with zolpidem versus placebo and included dizziness (23.5% vs. 1.5%), headache (12.5% vs. 9.2%), and hallucinations (7.4% vs. 0%) [see Warnings and Precautions (5.6)]. Ten patients on zolpidem (7.4%) discontinued treatment due to an adverse reaction.

8.5 Geriatric use

A total of 154 patients in U.S. controlled clinical trials and 897 patients in non-U.S. clinical trials who received zolpidem were ≥ 60 years of age. For a pool of U.S. patients receiving zolpidem at doses of ≤ 10 mg or placebo, there were three adverse reactions occurring at an incidence of at least 3% for zolpidem and for which the zolpidem incidence was at least twice the placebo incidence (i.e., they could be considered drug related).

Adverse Event	Zolpidem	Placebo
Dizziness	3%	0%
Drowsiness	5%	2%
Diarrhea	3%	1%

A total of 30/1,959 (1.5%) non-U.S. patients receiving zolpidem reported falls, including 28/30 (93%) who were ≥ 70 years of age. Of these 28 patients, 23 (82%) were receiving zolpidem doses > 10 mg. A total of 24/1,959 (1.2%) non-U.S. patients receiving zolpidem reported confusion, including 18/24 (75%) who were ≥ 70 years of age. Of these 18 patients, 14 (78%) were receiving zolpidem doses > 10 mg.

The dose of Ambien in elderly patients is 5 mg to minimize adverse effects related to impaired motor and/or cognitive performance and unusual sensitivity to sedative/hypnotic drugs *[see Warnings and Precautions (5.6)]*.

9 DRUG ABUSE AND DEPENDENCE

9.1 Controlled substance

Zolpidem tartrate is classified as a Schedule IV controlled substance by federal regulation.

9.2 Abuse

Abuse and addiction are separate and distinct from physical dependence and tolerance. Abuse is characterized by misuse of the drug for non-medical purposes, often in combination with other psychoactive substances. Tolerance is a state of adaptation in which exposure to a drug induces changes that result in a diminution of one or more of the drug effects over time. Tolerance may occur to both desired and undesired effects of drugs and may develop at different rates for different effects.

Addiction is a primary, chronic, neurobiological disease with genetic, psychosocial, and environmental factors influencing its development and manifestations. It is characterized by behaviors that include one or more of the following: impaired control over drug use, compulsive use, continued use despite harm, and craving. Drug addiction is a treatable disease, using a multidisciplinary approach, but relapse is common.

Studies of abuse potential in former drug abusers found that the effects of single doses of zolpidem tartrate 40 mg were similar, but not identical, to diazepam 20 mg, while zolpidem tartrate 10 mg was difficult to distinguish from placebo.

Because persons with a history of addiction to, or abuse of, drugs or alcohol are at increased risk for misuse, abuse and addiction of zolpidem, they should be monitored carefully when receiving zolpidem or any other hypnotic.

9.3 Dependence

Physical dependence is a state of adaptation that is manifested by a specific withdrawal syndrome that can be produced by abrupt cessation, rapid dose reduction, decreasing blood level of the drug, and/or administration of an antagonist.

Sedative/hypnotics have produced withdrawal signs and symptoms following abrupt discontinuation. These reported symptoms range from mild dysphoria and insomnia to a withdrawal syndrome that may include abdominal and muscle cramps, vomiting, sweating, tremors, and convulsions. The following adverse events which are considered to meet the DSM-III-R criteria for uncomplicated sedative/hypnotic withdrawal were reported during U.S. clinical trials following placebo substitution occurring within 48 hours following last zolpidem treatment: fatigue, nausea, flushing, lightheadedness, uncontrolled crying, emesis, stomach cramps, panic attack, nervousness, and abdominal discomfort. These reported adverse events occurred at an incidence of 1% or less. However, available data cannot provide a reliable estimate of the incidence, if any, of dependence during treatment at recommended doses. Post-marketing reports of abuse, dependence and withdrawal have been received.

10 OVERDOSAGE

10.1 Signs and symptoms

In postmarketing experience of overdose with zolpidem tartrate alone, or in combination with CNS-depressant agents, impairment of consciousness ranging from somnolence to coma, cardiovascular and/or respiratory compromise, and fatal outcomes have been reported.

10.2 Recommended treatment

General symptomatic and supportive measures should be used along with immediate gastric lavage where appropriate. Intravenous fluids should be administered as needed. Zolpidem's sedative hypnotic effect was shown to be reduced by flumazenil and therefore may be useful; however, flumazenil administration may contribute to the appearance of neurological symptoms (convulsions). As in all cases of drug overdose, respiration, pulse, blood pressure, and other appropriate signs should be monitored and general supportive measures employed. Hypotension and CNS depression should be monitored and treated by appropriate medical intervention.

Sedating drugs should be withheld following zolpidem overdosage, even if excitation occurs. The value of dialysis in the treatment of overdosage has not been determined, although hemodialysis studies in patients with renal failure receiving therapeutic doses have demonstrated that zolpidem is not dialyzable.

As with the management of all overdosage, the possibility of multiple drug ingestion should be considered. The physician may wish to consider contacting a poison control center for up-to-date information on the management of hypnotic drug product overdosage.

11 DESCRIPTION

Ambien (zolpidem tartrate) is a non-benzodiazepine hypnotic of the imidazopyridine class and is available in 5 mg and 10 mg strength tablets for oral administration.

Chemically, zolpidem is N,N,6-trimethyl-2-p-tolylimidazo [1,2-a] pyridine-3-acetamide L-(+)-tartrate (2:1). It has the following structure:

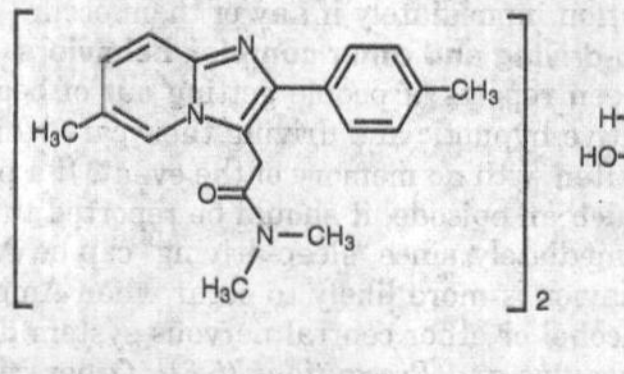

Zolpidem tartrate is a white to off-white crystalline powder that is sparingly soluble in water, alcohol, and propylene glycol. It has a molecular weight of 764.88.

Each Ambien tablet includes the following inactive ingredients: hydroxypropyl methylcellulose, lactose, magnesium stearate, mico-crystalline cellulose, polyethylene glycol, sodium starch glycolate, and titanium dioxide. The 5 mg tablet also contains FD&C Red No. 40, iron oxide colorant, and polysorbate 80.

12 CLINICAL PHARMACOLOGY

12.1 Mechanism of action

Subunit modulation of the $GABA_A$ receptor chloride channel macromolecular complex is hypothesized to be responsible for sedative, anticonvulsant, anxiolytic, and myorelaxant drug properties. The major modulatory site of the $GABA_A$ receptor complex is located on its alpha (α) subunit and is referred to as the benzodiazepine (BZ) or omega (ω) receptor. At least three subtypes of the (ω) receptor have been identified.

Zolpidem, the active moiety of zolpidem tartrate, is a hypnotic agent with a chemical structure unrelated to benzodiazepines, barbiturates, pyrrolopyrazines, pyrazolopyrimidines or other drugs with known hypnotic properties, it interacts with a GABA-BZ receptor complex and shares some of the pharmacological properties of the benzodiazepines. In contrast to the benzodiazepines, which nonselectively bind to and activate all BZ receptor subtypes, zolpidem *in vitro* binds the (BZ_1) receptor preferentially with a high affinity ratio of the $alpha_1/alpha_5$ subunits. The (BZ_1) receptor is found primarily on the Lamina IV of the sensorimotor cortical regions, substantia nigra (pars reticulata), cerebellum molecular layer, olfactory bulb, ventral thalamic complex, pons, inferior colliculus, and globus pallidus. This selective binding of zolpidem on the (BZ_1) receptor is not absolute, but it may explain the relative absence of myorelaxant and anticonvulsant effects in animal studies as well as the preservation of deep sleep (stages 3 and 4) in human studies of zolpidem at hypnotic doses.

12.3 Pharmacokinetics

The pharmacokinetic profile of Ambien is characterized by rapid absorption from the gastrointestinal tract and a short elimination half-life ($T_{1/2}$) in healthy subjects.

In a single-dose crossover study in 45 healthy subjects administered 5 and 10 mg zolpidem tartrate tablets, the mean peak concentrations (C_{max}) were 59 (range: 29 to 113) and 121 (range: 58 to 272) ng/mL, respectively, occurring at a mean time (T_{max}) of 1.6 hours for both. The mean Ambien elimination half-life was 2.6 (range: 1.4 to 4.5) and 2.5 (range: 1.4 to 3.8) hours, for the 5 and 10 mg tablets, respectively. Ambien is converted to inactive metabolites that are eliminated primarily by renal excretion. Ambien demonstrated linear kinetics in the dose range of 5 to 20 mg. Total protein binding was found to be 92.5 ± 0.1% and remained constant, independent of concentration between 40 and 790 ng/mL. Zolpidem did not accumulate in young adults following nightly dosing with 20 mg zolpidem tartrate tablets for 2 weeks.

A food-effect study in 30 healthy male subjects compared the pharmacokinetics of Ambien 10 mg when administered while fasting or 20 minutes after a meal. Results demonstrated that with food, mean AUC and C_{max} were decreased by 15% and 25%, respectively, while mean T_{max} was prolonged by 60% (from 1.4 to 2.2 hr). The half-life remained unchanged. These results suggest that, for faster sleep onset, Ambien should not be administered with or immediately after a meal.

Special Populations

Elderly

In the elderly, the dose for Ambien should be 5 mg *[see Warnings and Precautions (5) and Dosage and Administration (2)]*. This recommendation is based on several studies in which the mean C_{max}, $T_{1/2}$, and AUC were significantly increased when compared to results in young adults. In one study of eight elderly subjects (> 70 years), the means for C_{max}, $T_{1/2}$, and AUC significantly increased by 50% (255 vs. 384 ng/mL), 32% (2.2 vs. 2.9 hr), and 64% (955 vs. 1,562 ng•hr/mL), respectively, as compared to younger adults (20 to 40 years) following a single 20 mg oral dose. Ambien did not accumulate in elderly subjects following nightly oral dosing of 10 mg for 1 week.

Hepatic Impairment

The pharmacokinetics of Ambien in eight patients with chronic hepatic insufficiency were compared to results in healthy subjects. Following a single 20 mg oral zolpidem tartrate dose, mean C_{max} and AUC were found to be two times (250 vs. 499 ng/mL) and five times (788 vs. 4,203 ng•hr/mL) higher, respectively, in hepatically-compromised patients. T_{max} did not change. The mean half-life in cirrhotic patients of 9.9 hr (range: 4.1 to 25.8 hr) was greater than that observed in normal subjects of 2.2 hr (range: 1.6 to 2.4 hr). Dosing should be modified accordingly in patients with hepatic insufficiency *[see Dosage and Administration (2.2) and Warnings and Precautions (5.6)]*.

Renal Impairment

The pharmacokinetics of zolpidem tartrate were studied in 11 patients with end-stage renal failure (mean Cl_{Cr} = 6.5 ± 1.5 mL/min) undergoing hemodialysis three times a week, who were dosed with zolpidem tartrate 10 mg orally each day for 14 or 21 days. No statistically significant differences were observed for C_{max}, T_{max}, half-life, and AUC between the first and last day of drug administration when baseline concentration adjustments were made. On day 1, C_{max} was 172 ± 29 ng/mL (range: 46 to 344 ng/mL). After repeated dosing for 14 or 21 days, C_{max} was 203 ± 32 ng/mL (range: 28 to 316 ng/mL). On day 1, T_{max} was 1.7 ± 0.3 hr (range: 0.5 to 3.0 hr); after repeated dosing T_{max} was 0.8 ± 0.2 hr (range: 0.5 to 2.0 hr). This variation is accounted for by noting that last-day serum sampling began 10 hours after the previous dose, rather than after 24 hours. This resulted in residual drug concentration and a shorter period to reach maximal serum concentration. On day 1, $T_{1/2}$ was 2.4 ± 0.4 hr (range: 0.4 to 5.1 hr). After repeated dosing, $T_{1/2}$ was 2.5 ± 0.4 hr (range: 0.7 to 4.2 hr). AUC was 796 ± 159 ng•hr/mL after the first dose and 818 ± 170 ng•hr/mL after repeated dosing. Zolpidem was not hemodialyzable. No accumulation of unchanged drug appeared after 14 or 21 days. Zolpidem pharmacokinetics were not significantly different in renally impaired patients. No dosage adjustment is necessary in patients with compromised renal function. However, as a general precaution, these patients should be closely monitored.

13 NONCLINICAL TOXICOLOGY

13.1 Carcinogenesis, mutagenesis, impairment of fertility

Carcinogenesis:

Zolpidem was administered to rats and mice for 2 years at dietary dosages of 4, 18, and 80 mg/kg/day. In mice, these doses are 26 to 520 times or 2 to 35 times the maximum 10 mg human dose on a mg/kg or mg/m^2 basis, respectively. In rats these doses are 43 to 876 times or 6 to 115 times the maximum 10 mg human dose on a mg/kg or mg/m^2 basis, respectively. No evidence of carcinogenic potential was observed in mice. Renal liposarcomas were seen in 4/100 rats (3 males, 1 female) receiving 80 mg/kg/day and a renal lipoma was observed in one male rat at the 18 mg/kg/day dose. Incidence rates of lipoma and liposarcoma for zolpidem were comparable to those seen in historical controls and the tumor findings are thought to be a spontaneous occurrence.

Mutagenesis:

Zolpidem did not have mutagenic activity in several tests including the Ames test, genotoxicity in mouse lymphoma cells in vitro, chromosomal aberrations in cultured human lymphocytes, unscheduled DNA synthesis in rat hepatocytes in vitro, and the micronucleus test in mice.

Impairment of fertility:

In a rat reproduction study, the high dose (100 mg base/kg) of zolpidem resulted in irregular estrus cycles and prolonged precoital intervals, but there was no effect on male or female fertility after daily oral doses of 4 to 100 mg base/kg or 5 to 130 times the recommended human dose in mg/m^2. No effects on any other fertility parameters were noted.

14 CLINICAL STUDIES

14.1 Transient insomnia

Normal adults experiencing transient insomnia (n = 462) during the first night in a sleep laboratory were evaluated in a double-blind, parallel group, single-night trial comparing two doses of zolpidem (7.5 and 10 mg) and placebo. Both zolpidem doses were superior to placebo on objective (polysomnographic) measures of sleep latency, sleep duration, and number of awakenings.

Normal elderly adults (mean age 68) experiencing transient insomnia (n = 35) during the first two nights in a sleep laboratory were evaluated in a double-blind, crossover, 2-night trial comparing four doses of zolpidem (5, 10, 15 and 20 mg) and placebo. All zolpidem doses were superior to placebo on the two primary PSG parameters (sleep latency and efficiency) and all four subjective outcome measures (sleep duration, sleep latency, number of awakenings, and sleep quality).

14.2 Chronic insomnia

Zolpidem was evaluated in two controlled studies for the treatment of patients with chronic insomnia (most closely resembling primary insomnia, as defined in the APA

Diagnostic and Statistical Manual of Mental Disorders, DSM-IV™). Adult outpatients with chronic insomnia (n = 75) were evaluated in a double-blind, parallel group, 5-week trial comparing two doses of zolpidem tartrate and placebo. On objective (polysomnographic) measures of sleep latency and sleep efficiency, zolpidem 10 mg was superior to placebo on sleep latency for the first 4 weeks and on sleep efficiency for weeks 2 and 4. Zolpidem was comparable to placebo on number of awakenings at both doses studied.

Adult outpatients (n=141) with chronic insomnia were also evaluated, in a double-blind, parallel group, 4-week trial comparing two doses of zolpidem and placebo. Zolpidem 10 mg was superior to placebo on a subjective measure of sleep latency for all 4 weeks, and on subjective measures of total sleep time, number of awakenings, and sleep quality for the first treatment week.

Increased wakefulness during the last third of the night as measured by polysomnography has not been observed in clinical trials with Ambien.

14.3 Studies pertinent to safety concerns for sedative/hypnotic drugs

Next-day residual effects:

Next-day residual effects of Ambien were evaluated in seven studies involving normal subjects. In three studies in adults (including one study in a phase advance model of transient insomnia) and in one study in elderly subjects, a small but statistically significant decrease in performance was observed in the Digit Symbol Substitution Test (DSST) when compared to placebo. Studies of Ambien in non-elderly patients with insomnia did not detect evidence of next-day residual effects using the DSST, the Multiple Sleep Latency Test (MSLT), and patient ratings of alertness.

Rebound effects:

There was no objective (polysomnographic) evidence of rebound insomnia at recommended doses seen in studies evaluating sleep on the nights following discontinuation of Ambien (zolpidem tartrate). There was subjective evidence of impaired sleep in the elderly on the first post-treatment night at doses above the recommended elderly dose of 5 mg.

Memory impairment:

Controlled studies in adults utilizing objective measures of memory yielded no consistent evidence of next-day memory impairment following the administration of Ambien. However, in one study involving zolpidem doses of 10 and 20 mg, there was a significant decrease in next-morning recall of information presented to subjects during peak drug effect (90 minutes post-dose), i.e., these subjects experienced anterograde amnesia. There was also subjective evidence from adverse event data for anterograde amnesia occurring in association with the administration of Ambien, predominantly at doses above 10 mg.

Effects on sleep stages:

In studies that measured the percentage of sleep time spent in each sleep stage, Ambien has generally been shown to preserve sleep stages. Sleep time spent in stages 3 and 4 (deep sleep) was found comparable to placebo with only inconsistent, minor changes in REM (paradoxical) sleep at the recommended dose.

16 HOW SUPPLIED/STORAGE AND HANDLING

Ambien 5 mg tablets are capsule-shaped, pink, film coated, with AMB 5 debossed on one side and 5401 on the other and supplied as:

NDC Number	Size
0024-5401-31	bottle of 100
0024-5401-34	carton of 100 unit dose
0024-5401-50	bottle of 500

Ambien 10 mg tablets are capsule-shaped, white, film coated, with AMB 10 debossed on one side and 5421 on the other and supplied as:

NDC Number	Size
0024-5421-31	bottle of 100
0024-5421-34	carton of 100 unit dose
0024-5421-50	bottle of 500

Store at controlled room temperature 20°–25°C (68°–77°F).

17 PATIENT COUNSELING INFORMATION

Prescribers or other healthcare professionals should inform patients, their families, and their caregivers about the benefits and risks associated with treatment with sedative-hypnotics, should counsel them in its appropriate use, and should instruct them to read the accompanying Medication Guide *[see Medication Guide (17.4)]*.

17.1 Severe anaphylactic and anaphylactoid reactions

Inform patients that severe anaphylactic and anaphylactoid reactions have occurred with zolpidem. Describe the signs/symptoms of these reactions and advise patients to seek medical attention immediately if any of them occur.

17.2 Sleep-driving and other complex behaviors

There have been reports of people getting out of bed after taking a sedative-hypnotic and driving their cars while not fully awake, often with no memory of the event. If a patient experiences such an episode, it should be reported to his or her doctor immediately, since "sleep-driving" can be dangerous. This behavior is more likely to occur when Ambien is taken with alcohol or other central nervous system depressants *[see Warnings and Precautions (5.3)]*. Other complex behaviors (e.g., preparing and eating food, making phone calls, or having sex) have been reported in patients who are not fully awake after taking a sedative-hypnotic. As with "sleep-driving", patients usually do not remember these events.

In addition, patients should be advised to report all concomitant medications to the prescriber. Patients should be instructed to report events such as "sleep-driving" and other complex behaviors immediately to the prescriber.

17.3 Administration instructions

Patients should be counseled to take Ambien right before they get into bed and only when they are able to stay in bed a full night (7-8 hours) before being active again. Ambien tablets should not be taken with or immediately after a meal. Advise patients NOT to take Ambien when drinking alcohol.

17.4 Medication Guide

MEDICATION GUIDE

AMBIEN® (ām'bē-ən) Tablets C-IV

(zolpidem tartrate)

Read the Medication Guide that comes with AMBIEN before you start taking it and each time you get a refill. There may be new information. This Medication Guide does not take the place of talking to your doctor about your medical condition or treatment.

What is the most important information I should know about AMBIEN?

After taking AMBIEN, you may get up out of bed while not being fully awake and do an activity that you do not know you are doing. The next morning, you may not remember that you did anything during the night. You have a higher chance for doing these activities if you drink alcohol or take other medicines that make you sleepy with AMBIEN. Reported activities include:

- driving a car ("sleep-driving")
- making and eating food
- talking on the phone
- having sex
- sleep-walking

Call your doctor right away if you find out that you have done any of the above activities after taking AMBIEN.

Important:

1. Take AMBIEN exactly as prescribed

- Do not take more AMBIEN than prescribed.
- Take AMBIEN right before you get in bed, not sooner.

2. Do not take AMBIEN if you:

- drink alcohol
- take other medicines that can make you sleepy. Talk to your doctor about all of your medicines. Your doctor will tell you if you can take AMBIEN with your other medicines.
- cannot get a full night's sleep

What is AMBIEN?

AMBIEN is a sedative-hypnotic (sleep) medicine. AMBIEN is used in adults for the short-term treatment of a sleep problem called insomnia. Symptoms of insomnia include:

- trouble falling asleep

AMBIEN is not for children.

AMBIEN is a federally controlled substance (C-IV) because it can be abused or lead to dependence. Keep AMBIEN in a safe place to prevent misuse and abuse. Selling or giving away AMBIEN may harm others, and is against the law. Tell your doctor if you have ever abused or have been dependent on alcohol, prescription medicines or street drugs.

Who should not take AMBIEN?

Do not take AMBIEN if you are allergic to anything in it. See the end of this Medication Guide for a complete list of ingredients in AMBIEN.

AMBIEN may not be right for you. Before starting AMBIEN, tell your doctor about all of your health conditions, including if you:

- have a history of depression, mental illness, or suicidal thoughts
- have a history of drug or alcohol abuse or addiction
- have kidney or liver disease
- have a lung disease or breathing problems
- are pregnant, planning to become pregnant, or breast-feeding

Tell your doctor about all of the medicines you take including prescription and nonprescription medicines, vitamins and herbal supplements. Medicines can interact with each other, sometimes causing serious side effects. **Do not take AMBIEN with other medicines that can make you sleepy.**

Know the medicines you take. Keep a list of your medicines with you to show your doctor and pharmacist each time you get a new medicine.

How should I take AMBIEN?

- Take AMBIEN exactly as prescribed. Do not take more AMBIEN than prescribed for you.
- **Take AMBIEN right before you get into bed.**
- **Do not take AMBIEN unless you are able to stay in bed a full night (7-8 hours) before you must be active again.**
- For faster sleep onset, AMBIEN should NOT be taken with or immediately after a meal.
- Call your doctor if your insomnia worsens or is not better within 7 to 10 days. This may mean that there is another condition causing your sleep problem.
- If you take too much AMBIEN or overdose, call your doctor or poison control center right away, or get emergency treatment.

What are the possible side effects of AMBIEN?

Serious side effects of AMBIEN include:

- **getting out of bed while not being fully awake and do an activity that you do not know you are doing.** (See "What is the most important information I should know about AMBIEN?)
- **abnormal thoughts and behavior.** Symptoms include more outgoing or aggressive behavior than normal, confusion, agitation, hallucinations, worsening of depression, and suicidal thoughts or actions.
- **memory loss**
- **anxiety**
- **severe allergic reactions.** Symptoms include swelling of the tongue or throat, trouble breathing, and nausea and vomiting. Get emergency medical help if you get these symptoms after taking AMBIEN.

Call your doctor right away if you have any of the above side effects or any other side effects that worry you while using AMBIEN.

The most common side effects of AMBIEN are:

- drowsiness
- dizziness
- diarrhea
- "drugged feelings"
- You may still feel drowsy the next day after taking AMBIEN. **Do not drive or do other dangerous activities after taking AMBIEN until you feel fully awake.**

After you stop taking a sleep medicine, you may have symptoms for 1 to 2 days such as: trouble sleeping, nausea, flushing, lightheadedness, uncontrolled crying, vomiting, stomach cramps, panic attack, nervousness, and stomach area pain.

These are not all the side effects of AMBIEN. Ask your doctor or pharmacist for more information.

Call your doctor for medical advice about side effects. You may report side effects to FDA at 1–800–FDA–1088.

How should I store AMBIEN?

- Store AMBIEN at room temperature, 68° to 77°F (20° to 25°C).
- **Keep AMBIEN and all medicines out of reach of children.**

General Information about AMBIEN

- Medicines are sometimes prescribed for purposes other than those listed in a Medication Guide.
- Do not use AMBIEN for a condition for which it was not prescribed.
- Do not share AMBIEN with other people, even if you think they have the same symptoms that you have. It may harm them and it is against the law.

This Medication Guide summarizes the most important information about AMBIEN. If you would like more information, talk with your doctor. You can ask your doctor or pharmacist for information about AMBIEN that is written for healthcare professionals. For more information about AMBIEN, call 1-800-633-1610.

What are the ingredients in AMBIEN?

Active Ingredient: Zolpidem tartrate

Inactive Ingredients: hydroxypropyl methylcellulose, lactose, magnesium stearate, micro-crystalline cellulose, polyethylene glycol, sodium starch glycolate, and titanium dioxide. In addition, the 5 mg tablet contains FD&C Red No. 40, iron oxide colorant, and polysorbate 80.

Rx Only

This Medication Guide has been approved by the U.S. Food and Drug Administration.

sanofi-aventis U.S. LLC
Bridgewater, NJ 08807
September 2009

Shown in Product Identification Guide, page 318

AMBIEN CR®   ℂⱽ ℞
[a -m'be-ə n see ahr]
(zolpidem tartrate extended-release)
tablets

HIGHLIGHTS OF PRESCRIBING INFORMATION
These highlights do not include all the information needed to use Ambien CR safely and effectively. See full prescribing information for Ambien CR.
Ambien CR® (zolpidem tartrate extended-release) tablets - CIV
Initial U.S. Approval: 1992

INDICATIONS AND USAGE
Ambien CR is indicated for the treatment of insomnia characterized by difficulties with sleep onset and/or sleep maintenance. (1)

DOSAGE AND ADMINISTRATION
- Adult dose: 12.5 mg once daily immediately before bedtime (2.1)
- Elderly/debilitated/hepatically impaired patients: 6.25 mg once daily immediately before bedtime (2.2)
- Tablets to be swallowed whole, not to be crushed, divided or chewed. Should not be taken with or immediately after a meal (2.4)

DOSAGE FORMS AND STRENGTHS
6.25 mg and 12.5 mg extended-release tablets. Tablets not scored (3)

CONTRAINDICATIONS
Known hypersensitivity to zolpidem tartrate or to any of the inactive ingredients in the formulation (4)

WARNINGS AND PRECAUTIONS
- Need to evaluate for co-morbid diagnoses: Revaluate if insomnia persists after 7 to 10 days of use (5.1)
- Severe anaphylactic/anaphylactoid reactions: Angioedema and anaphylaxis have been reported. Do not rechallenge if such reactions occur (5.2)
- Abnormal thinking, behavioral changes, complex behaviors: May include "sleep-driving" and hallucinations. Immediately evaluate any new onset behavioral changes (5.3)
- Depression: Worsening of depression or, suicidal thinking may occur. Prescribe the least amount feasible to avoid intentional overdose (5.3, 5.6)
- Withdrawal effects: Symptoms may occur with rapid dose reduction or discontinuation (5.4, 9.2)
- CNS depressant effects: Use can impair alertness and motor coordination. If used in combination with other CNS depressants, dose reductions may be needed due to additive effects. Do not use with alcohol (2.3, 5.5)
- Elderly/debilitated patients: Use lower dose due to impaired motor, cognitive performance and increased sensitivity (2.2, 5.6)
- Patients with hepatic impairment, mild to moderate COPD, impaired drug metabolism or hemodynamic responses, mild to moderate sleep apnea: Use with caution and monitor closely (5.6)

ADVERSE REACTIONS
Most commonly observed adverse reactions (> 10% in either elderly or adult patients) are: headache, next-day somnolence and dizziness (6.1)

To report SUSPECTED ADVERSE REACTIONS, contact sanofi-aventis U.S. LLC at 1-800-633-1610 or FDA at 1-800-FDA-1088 or http://www.fda.gov/medwatch.

DRUG INTERACTIONS
- CNS depressants: Enhanced CNS-depressant effects with combination use. Use with alcohol causes additive psychomotor impairment (7.1)
- Imipramine: Decreased alertness observed with combination use. (7.1)
- Chlorpromazine: Impaired alertness and psychomotor performance observed with combination use (7.1)
- Rifampin: Combination use decreases exposure to and effects of zolpidem (7.2)
- Ketoconazole: Combination use increases exposure to and effect of zolpidem (7.2)

USE IN SPECIFIC POPULATIONS
- Pregnancy: Crosses the placenta. No studies in pregnant women. (8.1)
- Nursing mothers: Infant exposure via breast milk (8.3)
- Pediatric use: Safety and effectiveness not established. Hallucinations (incidence rate 7.4%) and other psychiatric and/or nervous system adverse reactions were observed frequently in a study of pediatric patients with Attention-Deficit/Hyperactivity Disorder (5.6, 8.4)

See 17 for PATIENT COUNSELING INFORMATION and Medication Guide

Revised: 09/2009

FULL PRESCRIBING INFORMATION: CONTENTS *

FULL PRESCRIBING INFORMATION

1   INDICATIONS AND USAGE
Ambien CR (zolpidem tartrate extended-release tablets) is indicated for the treatment of insomnia characterized by difficulties with sleep onset and/or sleep maintenance (as measured by wake time after sleep onset).
The clinical trials performed in support of efficacy were up to 3 weeks (using polysomnography measurement up to 2 weeks in both adult and elderly patients) and 24 weeks (using patient-reported assessment in adult patients only) in duration [see Clinical Studies (14)].

2   DOSAGE AND ADMINISTRATION
The dose of Ambien CR should be individualized.

2.1   Dosage in adults
The recommended dose of Ambien CR for adults is 12.5 mg once daily immediately before bedtime. The total Ambien CR dose should not exceed 12.5 mg per day.

2.2   Special populations
Elderly or debilitated patients may be especially sensitive to the effects of zolpidem tartrate. Patients with hepatic insufficiency do not clear the drug as rapidly as normals. The recommended dose of Ambien CR in both of these patient populations is 6.25 mg once daily immediately before bedtime [see Warnings and Precautions (5.6)].

2.3   Use with CNS depressants
Dosage adjustments may be necessary when Ambien CR is combined with other CNS depressant drugs because of the potentially additive effects [see Warnings and Precautions (5.5)].

2.4   Administration
Ambien CR extended-release tablets should be swallowed whole, and not be divided, crushed, or chewed. The effect of Ambien CR may be slowed by ingestion with or immediately after a meal.

3   DOSAGE FORMS AND STRENGTHS
Ambien CR is available as extended-release tablets containing 6.25 mg or 12.5 mg of zolpidem tartrate for oral administration. Tablets are not scored.

Ambien CR 6.25 mg tablets are pink, round, bi-convex, and debossed with A~ on one side.

Ambien CR 12.5 mg tablets are blue, round, bi-convex, and debossed with A~ on one side.

4   CONTRAINDICATIONS
Ambien CR is contraindicated in patients with known hypersensitivity to zolpidem tartrate or to any of the inactive ingredients in the formulation. Observed reactions include anaphylaxis and angioedema [see Warnings and Precautions (5.2)].

5   WARNINGS AND PRECAUTIONS
5.1   Need to evaluate for co-morbid diagnoses
Because sleep disturbances may be the presenting manifestation of a physical and/or psychiatric disorder, symptomatic treatment of insomnia should be initiated only after a careful evaluation of the patient. The failure of insomnia to remit after 7 to 10 days of treatment may indicate the presence of a primary psychiatric and/or medical illness that should be evaluated. Worsening of insomnia or the emergence of new thinking or behavior abnormalities may be the consequence of an unrecognized psychiatric or physical disorder. Such findings have emerged during the course of treatment with sedative/hypnotic drugs, including zolpidem.

5.2   Severe anaphylactic and anaphylactoid reactions
Rare cases of angioedema involving the tongue, glottis or larynx have been reported in patients after taking the first or subsequent doses of sedative-hypnotics, including zolpidem. Some patients have had additional symptoms such as dyspnea, throat closing or nausea and vomiting that suggest anaphylaxis. Some patients have required medical therapy in the emergency department. If angioedema involves the throat, glottis or larynx, airway obstruction may occur and be fatal. Patients who develop angioedema after treatment with zolpidem should not be rechallenged with the drug.

5.3   Abnormal thinking and behavioral changes
A variety of abnormal thinking and behavior changes have been reported to occur in association with the use of sedative/hypnotics. Some of these changes may be characterized by decreased inhibition (e.g. aggressiveness and extroversion that seemed out of character), similar to effects produced by alcohol and other CNS depressants. Visual and auditory hallucinations have been reported as well as behavioral changes such as bizarre behavior, agitation and depersonalization. In controlled trials, <1% of adults with insomnia who received zolpidem reported hallucinations. In a clinical trial, 7.4% of pediatric patients with insomnia associated with attention-deficit/hyperactivity disorder (ADHD), who received zolpidem reported hallucinations [see Use in Specific Populations (8.4)].

Complex behaviors such as "sleep-driving" (i.e., driving while not fully awake after ingestion of a sedative-hypnotic, with amnesia for the event) have been reported with sedative-hypnotics, including zolpidem. These events can occur in sedative-hypnotic-naive as well as in sedative-hypnotic-experienced persons. Although behaviors such as "sleep-driving" may occur with Ambien CR alone at therapeutic doses, the use of alcohol and other CNS depressants with Ambien CR appears to increase the risk of such behaviors, as does the use of Ambien CR at doses exceeding the maximum recommended dose. Due to the risk to the patient and the community, discontinuation of Ambien CR should be strongly considered for patients who report a "sleep-driving" episode. Other complex behaviors (e.g., preparing and eating food, making phone calls, or having sex) have been reported in patients who are not fully awake after taking a sedative-hypnotic. As with "sleep-driving", patients usually do not remember these events. Amnesia, anxiety and other neuro-psychiatric symptoms may occur unpredictably.

In primarily depressed patients, worsening of depression, including suicidal thoughts and actions (including completed suicides), have been reported in association with the use of sedative/hypnotics.

It can rarely be determined with certainty whether a particular instance of the abnormal behaviors listed above is drug induced, spontaneous in origin, or a result of an underlying psychiatric or physical disorder. Nonetheless, the emergence of any new behavioral sign or symptom of concern requires careful and immediate evaluation.

5.4   Withdrawal effects
Following the rapid dose decrease or abrupt discontinuation of sedative/hypnotics, there have been reports of signs and symptoms similar to those associated with withdrawal from other CNS-depressant drugs [see Drug Abuse and Dependence (9)].

5.5   CNS depressant effects
Ambien CR, like other sedative/hypnotic drugs, has CNS-depressant effects. Due to the rapid onset of action, Ambien CR should only be taken immediately prior to going to bed. Patients should be cautioned against engaging in hazardous occupations requiring complete mental alertness or motor

coordination such as operating machinery or driving a motor vehicle after ingesting the drug, including potential impairment of the performance of such activities that may occur the day following ingestion of Ambien CR. Ambien CR showed additive effects when combined with alcohol and should not be taken with alcohol. Patients should also be cautioned about possible combined effects with other CNS-depressant drugs. Dosage adjustments may be necessary when Ambien CR is administered with such agents because of the potentially additive effects.

5.6   Special populations
Use in the elderly and/or debilitated patients: Impaired motor and/or cognitive performance after repeated exposure or unusual sensitivity to sedative/hypnotic drugs is a concern in the treatment of elderly and/or debilitated patients. Therefore, the recommended Ambien CR dosage is 6.25 mg in such patients to decrease the possibility of side effects *[see Dosage and Administration (2.2)]*. These patients should be closely monitored.

Use in patients with concomitant illness: Clinical experience with Ambien CR (zolpidem tartrate) in patients with concomitant systemic illness is limited. Caution is advisable in using Ambien CR in patients with diseases or conditions that could affect metabolism or hemodynamic responses.

Although studies did not reveal respiratory depressant effects at hypnotic doses of zolpidem in normals or in patients with mild to moderate chronic obstructive pulmonary disease (COPD), a reduction in the Total Arousal Index together with a reduction in lowest oxygen saturation and increase in the times of oxygen desaturation below 80% and 90% was observed in patients with mild-to-moderate sleep apnea when treated with an immediate-release formulation of zolpidem tartrate (10 mg) when compared to placebo. Since sedative/hypnotics have the capacity to depress respiratory drive, precautions should be taken if Ambien CR is prescribed to patients with compromised respiratory function. Post-marketing reports of respiratory insufficiency, most of which involved patients with pre-existing respiratory impairment, have been received. Ambien CR should be used with caution in patients with sleep apnea syndrome or myasthenia gravis.

Data in end-stage renal failure patients repeatedly treated with an immediate-release formulation of zolpidem tartrate (10 mg) did not demonstrate drug accumulation or alterations in pharmacokinetic parameters. No dosage adjustment in renally impaired patients is required; however, these patients should be closely monitored *[see Clinical Pharmacology (12.3)]*.

A study in subjects with hepatic impairment did reveal prolonged elimination in this group; therefore, treatment should be initiated with Ambien CR 6.25 mg in patients with hepatic compromise, and they should be closely monitored *[see Dosage and Administration (2.2) and Clinical Pharmacology (12.3)]*.

Use in patients with depression: As with other sedative/hypnotic drugs, Ambien CR should be administered with caution to patients exhibiting signs or symptoms of depression. Suicidal tendencies may be present in such patients and protective measures may be required. Intentional overdosage is more common in this group of patients; therefore, the least amount of drug that is feasible should be prescribed for the patient at any one time.

Use in pediatric patients: Safety and effectiveness of zolpidem has not been established in pediatric patients. In an 8-week study in pediatric patients (aged 6–17 years) with insomnia associated with ADHD given an immediate-release oral solution of zolpidem tartrate, zolpidem did not decrease sleep latency compared to placebo. Hallucinations were reported in 7.4% of the pediatric patients who received zolpidem; none of the pediatric patients who received placebo reported hallucinations *[see Use in Specific Populations (8.4)]*.

6   ADVERSE REACTIONS
The following serious adverse reactions are discussed in greater detail in other sections of the labeling:
• Serious anaphylactic and anaphylactoid reactions *[see Warnings and Precautions (5.2)]*
• Abnormal thinking, behavior changes, and complex behaviors *[see Warnings and Precautions (5.3)]*
• Withdrawal effects *[see Warnings and Precautions (5.4)]*
• CNS-depressant effects *[see Warnings and Precautions (5.5)]*

6.1   Clinical trials experience
Associated with discontinuation of treatment: In 3-week clinical trials in adults and elderly patients (> 65 years), 3.5% (7/201) patients receiving Ambien CR 6.25 or 12.5 mg discontinued treatment due to an adverse reaction as compared to 0.9% (2/216) of patients on placebo. The reaction most commonly associated with discontinuation in patients treated with Ambien CR was somnolence (1%).

In a 6-month study in adult patients (18–64 years of age), 8.5% (57/669) of patients receiving Ambien CR 12.5 mg as compared to 4.6% on placebo (16/349) discontinued

treatment due to an adverse reaction. Reactions most commonly associated with discontinuation of Ambien CR included anxiety (anxiety, restlessness or agitation) reported in 1.5% (10/669) of patients as compared to 0.3% (1/349) of patients on placebo, and depression (depression, major depression or depressed mood) reported in 1.5% (10/669) of patients as compared to 0.3% (1/349) of patients on placebo. Data from a clinical study in which selective serotonin reuptake inhibitor- (SSRI-) treated patients were given zolpidem revealed that four of the seven discontinuations during double-blind treatment with zolpidem (n=95) were associated with impaired concentration, continuing or aggravated depression, and manic reaction; one patient treated with placebo (n =97) was discontinued after an attempted suicide.

Most commonly observed adverse reactions in controlled trials: During treatment with Ambien CR in adults and elderly at daily doses of 12.5 mg and 6.25 mg, respectively, each for three weeks, the most commonly observed adverse reactions associated with the use of Ambien CR were headache, next-day somnolence, and dizziness.

In the 6-month trial evaluating Ambien CR 12.5 mg, the adverse reaction profile was consistent with that reported in short-term trials, except for a higher incidence of anxiety (6.3% for Ambien CR versus 2.6% for placebo).

Adverse reactions observed at an incidence of ≥1% in controlled trials: The following tables enumerate treatment-emergent adverse reaction frequencies that were observed at an incidence equal to 1% or greater among patients with insomnia who received Ambien CR in placebo-controlled trials. Events reported by investigators were classified utilizing the MedDRA dictionary for the purpose of establishing event frequencies. The prescriber should be aware that these figures cannot be used to predict the incidence of side effects in the course of usual medical practice, in which patient characteristics and other factors differ from those that prevailed in these clinical trials. Similarly, the cited frequencies cannot be compared with figures obtained from other clinical investigators involving related drug products and uses, since each group of drug trials is conducted under a different set of conditions. However, the cited figures provide the physician with a basis for estimating the relative contribution of drug and nondrug factors to the incidence of side effects in the population studied.

The following tables were derived from results of two placebo-controlled efficacy trials involving Ambien CR. These trials involved patients with primary insomnia who were treated for 3 weeks with Ambien CR at doses of 12.5 mg (Table 1) or 6.25 mg (Table 2), respectively. The tables include only adverse reactions occurring at an incidence of at least 1% for Ambien CR patients and with an incidence greater than that seen in the placebo patients.

Table 1. Incidences of Treatment-Emergent Adverse Reactions in a 3-Week Placebo-Controlled Clinical Trial in Adults (percentage of patients reporting)

Body System/Adverse Reaction *	Ambien CR 12.5 mg (N = 102)	Placebo (N = 110)
Infections and infestations		
Influenza	3	0
Gastroenteritis	1	0
Labyrinthitis	1	0
Metabolism and nutrition disorders		
Appetite disorder	1	0
Psychiatric disorders		
Hallucinations [†]	4	0
Disorientation	3	2
Anxiety	2	0
Depression	2	0
Psychomotor retardation	2	0
Binge eating	1	0
Depersonalization	1	0
Disinhibition	1	0
Euphoric mood	1	0
Mood swings	1	0
Stress symptoms	1	0
Nervous system disorders		
Headache	19	16
Somnolence	15	2
Dizziness	12	5
Memory disorders [‡]	3	0
Balance disorder	2	0
Disturbance in attention	2	0
Hypoesthesia	2	1
Ataxia	1	0
Paresthesia	1	0
Eye disorders		
Visual disturbance	3	0
Eye redness	2	0
Vision blurred	2	1
Altered visual depth perception	1	0
Asthenopia	1	0
Ear and labyrinth disorders		
Vertigo	2	0
Tinnitus	1	0
Respiratory, thoracic and mediastinal disorders		
Throat irritation	1	0
Gastrointestinal disorders		
Nausea	7	4
Constipation	2	0
Abdominal discomfort	1	0
Abdominal tenderness	1	0
Frequent bowel movements	1	0
Gastroesophageal reflux disease	1	0
Vomiting	1	0
Skin and subcutaneous tissue disorders		
Rash	1	0
Skin wrinkling	1	0
Urticaria	1	0
Musculoskeletal and connective tissue disorders		
Back pain	4	3
Myalgia	4	0
Neck pain	1	0
Reproductive system and breast disorders		
Menorrhagia	1	0
General disorders and administration site conditions		
Fatigue	3	2
Asthenia	1	0
Chest discomfort	1	0

Investigations		
Blood pressure increased	1	0
Body temperature increased	1	0
Injury, poisoning and procedural complications		
Contusion	1	0
Social circumstances		
Exposure to poisonous plant	1	0

* Reactions reported by at least 1% of patients treated with Ambien CR and at greater frequency than in the placebo group.

† Hallucinations included hallucinations NOS as well as visual and hypnogogic hallucinations.

‡ Memory disorders include: memory impairment, amnesia, anterograde amnesia.

Table 2. Incidences of Treatment-Emergent Adverse Reactions in a 3-Week Placebo-Controlled Clinical Trial in Elderly (percentage of patients reporting)

Body System/Adverse Reaction *	Ambien CR 6.25 mg (N=99)	Placebo (N=106)
Infections and infestations		
Nasopharyngitis	6	4
Lower respiratory tract infection	1	0
Otitis externa	1	0
Upper respiratory tract infection	1	0
Psychiatric disorders		
Anxiety	3	2
Psychomotor retardation	2	0
Apathy	1	0
Depressed mood	1	0
Nervous system disorders		
Headache	14	11
Dizziness	8	3
Somnolence	6	5
Burning sensation	1	0
Dizziness postural	1	0
Memory disorders †	1	0
Muscle contractions involuntary	1	0
Paresthesia	1	0
Tremor	1	0
Cardiac disorders		
Palpitations	2	0
Respiratory, thoracic and mediastinal disorders		
Dry throat	1	0
Gastrointestinal disorders		
Flatulence	1	0
Vomiting	1	0
Skin and subcutaneous tissue disorders		
Rash	1	0
Urticaria	1	0

Musculoskeletal and connective tissue disorders		
Arthralgia	2	0
Muscle cramp	2	1
Neck pain	2	0
Renal and urinary disorders		
Dysuria	1	0
Reproductive system and breast disorders		
Vulvovaginal dryness	1	0
General disorders and administration site conditions		
Influenza like illness	1	0
Pyrexia	1	0
Injury, poisoning and procedural complications		
Neck injury	1	0

* Reactions reported by at least 1% of patients treated with Ambien CR and at greater frequency than in the placebo group.

† Memory disorders include: memory impairment, amnesia, anterograde amnesia.

Dose relationship for adverse reactions: There is evidence from dose comparison trials suggesting a dose relationship for many of the adverse reactions associated with zolpidem use, particularly for certain CNS and gastrointestinal adverse events.

Other adverse reactions observed during the premarketing evaluation of Ambien CR: Other treatment-emergent adverse reactions associated with participation in Ambien CR studies (those reported at frequencies of <1%) were not different in nature or frequency to those seen in studies with immediate-release zolpidem tartrate, which are listed below.

Adverse Events Observed During the Premarketing Evaluation of Immediate-Release Zolpidem Tartrate:

Immediate-release zolpidem tartrate was administered to 3,660 subjects in clinical trials throughout the U.S., Canada, and Europe. Treatment-emergent adverse events associated with clinical trial participation were recorded by clinical investigators using terminology of their own choosing. To provide a meaningful estimate of the proportion of individuals experiencing treatment-emergent adverse events, similar types of untoward events were grouped into a smaller number of standardized event categories and classified utilizing a modified World Health Organization (WHO) dictionary of preferred terms.

The frequencies presented, therefore, represent the proportions of the 3,660 individuals exposed to zolpidem, at all doses, who experienced an event of the type cited on at least one occasion while receiving zolpidem. All reported treatment-emergent adverse events are included, except those already listed in the table above of adverse events in placebo-controlled studies, those coding terms that are so general as to be uninformative, and those events where a drug cause was remote. It is important to emphasize that, although the events reported did occur during treatment with Ambien, they were not necessarily caused by it.

Adverse events are further classified within body system categories and enumerated in order of decreasing frequency using the following definitions: frequent adverse events are defined as those occurring in greater than 1/100 subjects; infrequent adverse events are those occurring in 1/100 to 1/1,000 patients; rare events are those occurring in less than 1/1,000 patients.

Autonomic nervous system: Frequent: dry mouth. Infrequent: increased sweating, pallor, postural hypotension, syncope. Rare: abnormal accommocation, altered saliva, flushing, glaucoma, hypotension, impotence, increased saliva, tenesmus.

Body as a whole: Frequent: asthenia. Infrequent: chest pain, edema, falling, fever, malaise, trauma. Rare: allergic reaction, allergy aggravated, anaphylactic shock, face edema, hot flashes, increased ESR, pain, restless legs, rigors, tolerance increased, weight decrease.

Cardiovascular system: Infrequent: cerebrovascular disorder, hypertension, tachycardia. Rare: angina pectoris, arrhythmia, arteritis, circulatory failure, extrasystoles, hypertension aggravated, myocardial infarction, phlebitis,

pulmonary embolism, pulmonary edema, varicose veins, ventricular tachycardia.

Central and peripheral nervous system: Frequent: ataxia, confusion, drowsiness, drugged feeling, euphoria, insomnia, lethargy, lightheadedness, vertigo. Infrequent: agitation, decreased cognition, detached, difficulty concentrating, dysarthria, emotional lability, hallucination, hypoesthesia, illusion, leg cramps, migraine, nervousness, paresthesia, sleeping (after daytime dosing), speech disorder, stupor, tremor. Rare: abnormal gait, abnormal thinking, aggressive reaction, apathy, appetite increased, decreased libido, delusion, dementia, depersonalization, dysphasia, feeling strange, hypokinesia, hypotonia, hysteria, intoxicated feeling, manic reaction, neuralgia, neuritis, neuropathy, neurosis, panic attacks, paresis, personality disorder, somnambulism, suicide attempts, tetany, yawning.

Gastrointestinal system: Frequent: diarrhea, dyspepsia, hiccup. Infrequent: anorexia, constipation, dysphagia, flatulence, gastroenteritis. Rare: enteritis, eructation, esophagospasm, gastritis, hemorrhoids, intestinal obstruction, rectal hemorrhage, tooth caries.

Hematologic and lymphatic system: Rare: anemia, hyperhemoglobinemia, leukopenia, lymphadenopathy, macrocytic anemia, purpura, thrombosis.

Immunologic system: Infrequent: infection. Rare: abscess herpes simplex herpes zoster, otitis externa, otitis media.

Liver and biliary system: Infrequent: abnormal hepatic function, increased SGPT. Rare: bilirubinemia, increased SGOT.

Metabolic and nutritional: Infrequent: hyperglycemia, thirst. Rare: gout, hypercholesteremia, hyperlipidemia, increased alkaline phosphatase, increased BUN, periorbital edema.

Musculoskeletal system: Infrequent: arthritis. Rare: arthrosis, muscle weakness, sciatica, tendinitis.

Reproductive system: Infrequent: menstrual disorder, vaginitis. Rare: breast fibroadenosis, breast neoplasm, breast pain.

Respiratory system: Frequent: sinusitis. Infrequent: bronchitis, coughing, dyspnea. Rare: bronchospasm, epistaxis, hypoxia, laryngitis, pneumonia.

Skin and appendages: Infrequent: pruritus. Rare: acne, bullous eruption, dermatitis, furunculosis, injection-site inflammation, photosensitivity reaction, urticaria.

Special senses: Frequent: diplopia, vision abnormal. Infrequent: eye irritation, eye pain, scleritis, taste perversion, tinnitus. Rare: conjunctivitis, corneal ulceration, lacrimation abnormal, parosmia, photopsia.

Urogenital system: Frequent: urinary tract infection. Infrequent: cystitis, urinary incontinence. Rare: acute renal failure, dysuria, micturition frequency, nocturia, polyuria, pyelonephritis, renal pain, urinary retention.

7 DRUG INTERACTIONS

7.1 CNS-active drugs

Since the systematic evaluations of zolpidem in combination with other CNS-active drugs have been limited, careful consideration should be given to the pharmacology of any CNS-active drug to be used with zolpidem. Any drug with CNS-depressant effects could potentially enhance the CNS-depressant effects of zolpidem.

An immediate-release formulation of zolpidem tartrate was evaluated in healthy subjects in single-dose interaction studies for several CNS drugs. Imipramine in combination with zolpidem produced no pharmacokinetic interaction other than a 20% decrease in peak levels of imipramine, but there was an additive effect of decreased alertness. Similarly, chlorpromazine in combination with zolpidem produced no pharmacokinetic interaction, but there was an additive effect of decreased alertness and psychomotor performance. A study involving haloperidol and zolpidem revealed no effect of haloperidol on the pharmacokinetics or pharmacodynamics of zolpidem. The lack of a drug interaction following single-dose administration does not predict a lack following chronic administration.

An additive effect on psychomotor performance between alcohol and zolpidem was demonstrated *[see Warnings and Precautions (5.5)]*.

A single-dose interaction study with zolpidem 10 mg and fluoxetine 20 mg at steady-state levels in male volunteers did not demonstrate any clinically significant pharmacokinetic or pharmacodynamic interactions. When multiple doses of zolpidem and fluoxetine at steady-state concentrations were evaluated in healthy females, the only significant change was a 17% increase in the zolpidem half-life. There was no evidence of an additive effect in psychomotor performance.

Following five consecutive nightly doses of zolpidem 10 mg in the presence of sertraline 50 mg (17 consecutive daily doses, at 7:00 am, in healthy female volunteers), zolpidem C_{max} was significantly higher (43%) and T_{max} was significantly decreased (53%). Pharmacokinetics of sertraline and N-desmethylsertraline were unaffected by zolpidem.

7.2 Drugs that affect drug metabolism via cytochrome P450

Some compounds known to inhibit CYP3A may increase exposure to zolpidem. The effect of inhibitors of other P450 enzymes has not been carefully evaluated.

A randomized, double-blind, crossover interaction study in ten healthy volunteers between itraconazole (200 mg once daily for 4 days) and a single dose of zolpidem (10 mg) given 5 hours after the last dose of itraconazole resulted in a 34% increase in $AUC_{0-\infty}$ of zolpidem. There were no significant pharmacodynamic effects of zolpidem on subjective drowsiness, postural sway, or psychomotor performance.

A randomized, placebo-controlled, crossover interaction study in eight healthy female subjects between five consecutive daily doses of rifampin (600 mg) and a single dose of an immediate-release formulation of zolpidem tartrate (20 mg) given 17 hours after the last dose of rifampin showed significant reductions of the AUC (–73%), C_{max} (–58%), and $T_{1/2}$ (–36%) of zolpidem together with significant reductions in the pharmacodynamic effects of zolpidem.

A randomized double-blind crossover interaction study in twelve healthy subjects showed that co-administration of a single 5 mg dose of immediate-release zolpidem tartrate with ketoconazole, a potent CYP3A4 inhibitor, given as 200 mg twice daily for 2 days increased C_{max} of zolpidem by a factor of 1.3 and increased the total AUC of zolpidem by a factor of 1.7 compared to zolpidem alone and prolonged the elimination half-life by approximately 30% along with an increase in the pharmacodynamic effects of zolpidem. Caution should be used when ketoconazole is given with zolpidem and consideration should be given to using a lower dose of zolpidem when ketoconazole and zolpidem are given together. Patients should be advised that use of Ambien CR with ketoconazole may enhance the sedative effects.

7.3 Other drugs with no interaction with zolpidem

A study involving cimetidine/zolpidem and ranitidine/zolpidem combinations revealed no effect of either drug on the pharmacokinetics or pharmacodynamics of zolpidem.

Zolpidem had no effect on digoxin pharmacokinetics and did not affect prothrombin time when given with warfarin in normal subjects.

7.4 Drug-laboratory test interactions

Zolpidem is not known to interfere with commonly employed clinical laboratory tests. In addition, clinical data indicate that zolpidem does not cross-react with benzodiazepines, opiates, barbiturates, cocaine, cannabinoids, or amphetamines in two standard urine drug screens.

8 USE IN SPECIFIC POPULATIONS

8.1 Pregnancy

Pregnancy Category C

There are no adequate and well-controlled studies of Ambien CR in pregnant women. Ambien CR should be used during pregnancy only if the potential benefit outweighs the potential risk to the fetus.

Oral studies of zolpidem in pregnant rats and rabbits showed adverse effects on the development of offspring only at doses greater than the maximum recommended human dose (MRHD of 12.5 mg/day). These doses were also maternally toxic in animals. A teratogenic effect was not observed in these studies. Administration to pregnant rats during the period of organogenesis produced dose-related maternal toxicity and decreases in fetal skull ossification at doses 20 to 100 times the MRHD. The no-effect dose for embryo-fetal toxicity was 4 times the MRHD. Treatment of pregnant rabbits during organogenesis resulted in maternal toxicity at all doses studied and increased post-implantation embryo-fetal loss and under-ossification of fetal sternebrae at the highest dose (30 times the MRHD). The no-effect level for embryo-fetal toxicity was approximately 8 times the MRHD. Administration to rats during the latter part of pregnancy and throughout lactation produced maternal toxicity and decreased pup growth and survival at doses approximately 20 to 100 times the MRHD. The no-effect dose for offspring toxicity was approximately 4 times the MRHD.

Studies to assess the effects on children whose mothers took zolpidem during pregnancy have not been conducted. There is a published case report documenting the presence of zolpidem in human umbilical cord blood. Children born of mothers taking sedative/hypnotic drugs may be at some risk for withdrawal symptoms from the drug during the postnatal period. In addition, neonatal flaccidity has been reported in infants born of mothers who received sedative/hypnotic drugs during pregnancy. Cases of severe neonatal respiratory depression have been reported when zolpidem was used with other CNS depressants at the end of pregnancy.

8.2 Labor and delivery

Ambien CR has no established use in labor and delivery *[see Pregnancy (8.1)]*.

8.3 Nursing mothers

Studies in lactating mothers indicate that the half-life of zolpidem is similar to that in young normal subjects (2.6 ± 0.3 hr). Between 0.004% and 0.019% of the total administered dose is excreted into milk. The effect of zolpidem on the nursing infant is not known. Caution should be exercised when Ambien CR is administered to a nursing mother.

8.4 Pediatric use

Safety and effectiveness of zolpidem have not been established in pediatric patients.

In an 8-week controlled study, 201 pediatric patients (aged 6–17 years) with insomnia associated with attention-deficit/hyperactivity disorder (90% of the patients were using psychoanaleptics), were treated with an oral solution of zolpidem (n=136), or placebo (n = 65). Zolpidem did not significantly decrease latency to persistent sleep, compared to placebo, as measured by polysomnography after 4 weeks of treatment. Psychiatric and nervous system disorders comprised the most frequent (> 5%) treatment emergent adverse reactions observed with zolpidem versus placebo and included dizziness (23.5% vs. 1.5%), headache (12.5% vs. 9.2%), and hallucinations (7.4% vs. 0%) *[see Warnings and Precautions (5.6)]*. Ten patients on zolpidem (7.4%) discontinued treatment due to an adverse reaction.

FDA has not required pediatric studies of Ambien CR in the pediatric population based on these efficacy and safety findings.

8.5 Geriatric use

A total of 99 elderly (≥ 65 years of age) received daily doses of 6.25 mg Ambien CR in a 3-week placebo-controlled study. The adverse reaction profile of Ambien CR 6.25 mg in this population was similar to that of Ambien CR 12.5 mg in younger adults (≤ 64 years of age). Dizziness was reported in 8% of Ambien CR-treated patients compared with 3% of those treated with placebo.

The dose of Ambien CR in elderly patients is 6.25 mg to minimize adverse effects related to impaired motor and/or cognitive performance and unusual sensitivity to sedative/hypnotic drugs *[see Warnings and Precautions (5.6)]*.

9 DRUG ABUSE AND DEPENDENCE

9.1 Controlled substance

Zolpidem tartrate is classified as a Schedule IV controlled substance by federal regulation.

9.2 Abuse

Abuse and addiction are separate and distinct from physical dependence and tolerance. Abuse is characterized by misuse of the drug for non-medical purposes, often in combination with other psychoactive substances. Tolerance is a state of adaptation in which exposure to a drug induces changes that result in a diminution of one or more of the drug effects over time. Tolerance may occur to both desired and undesired effects of drugs and may develop at different rates for different effects.

Addiction is a primary, chronic, neurobiological disease with genetic, psychosocial, and environmental factors influencing its development and manifestations. It is characterized by behaviors that include one or more of the following: impaired control over drug use, compulsive use, continued use despite harm, and craving. Drug addiction is a treatable disease, using a multidisciplinary approach, but relapse is common.

Studies of abuse potential in former drug abusers found that the effects of single doses of zolpidem tartrate 40 mg were similar, but not identical, to diazepam 20 mg, while zolpidem tartrate 10 mg effects were difficult to distinguish from placebo.

Because persons with a history of addiction to, or abuse of, drugs or alcohol are at increased risk for misuse, abuse and addiction of zolpidem, they should be monitored carefully when receiving zolpidem or any other hypnotic.

9.3 Dependence

Physical dependence is a state of adaptation that is manifested by a specific withdrawal syndrome that can be produced by abrupt cessation, rapid dose reduction, decreasing blood level of the drug, and/or administration of an antagonist.

Sedative/hypnotics have produced withdrawal signs and symptoms following abrupt discontinuation. These reported symptoms range from mild dysphoria and insomnia to a withdrawal syndrome that may include abdominal and muscle cramps, vomiting, sweating, tremors, and convulsions. The following adverse events, which are considered to meet the DSM-III-R criteria for uncomplicated sedative/hypnotic withdrawal, were reported during U.S. clinical trials following placebo substitution occurring within 48 hours following last zolpidem treatment: fatigue, nausea, flushing, lightheadedness, uncontrolled crying, emesis, stomach cramps, panic attack, nervousness, and abdominal discomfort. These reported adverse events occurred at an incidence of 1% or less. However, available data cannot provide a reliable estimate of the incidence, if any, of dependence during treatment at recommended doses. Postmarketing reports of abuse, dependence and withdrawal have been received.

10 OVERDOSAGE

10.1 Signs and symptoms

In postmarketing experience of overdose with zolpidem tartrate alone, or in combination with CNS-depressant agents, impairment of consciousness ranging from somnolence to coma, cardiovascular and/or respiratory compromise and fatal outcomes have been reported.

10.2 Recommended treatment

General symptomatic and supportive measures should be used along with immediate gastric lavage where appropriate. Intravenous fluids should be administered as needed. Zolpidem's sedative hypnotic effect was shown to be reduced by flumazenil and therefore may be useful; however, flumazenil administration may contribute to the appearance of neurological symptoms (convulsions). As in all cases of drug overdose, respiration, pulse, blood pressure, and other appropriate signs should be monitored and general supportive measures employed. Hypotension and CNS depression should be monitored and treated by appropriate medical intervention. Sedating drugs should be withheld following zolpidem overdosage, even if excitation occurs. The value of dialysis in the treatment of overdosage has not been determined, although hemodialysis studies in patients with renal failure receiving therapeutic doses have demonstrated that zolpidem is not dialyzable.

As with the management of all overdosage, the possibility of multiple drug ingestion should be considered. The physician may wish to consider contacting a poison control center for up-to-date information on the management of hypnotic drug product overdosage.

11 DESCRIPTION

Ambien CR contains zolpidem tartrate, a non-benzodiazepine hypnotic of the imidazopyridine class. Ambien CR (zolpidem tartrate extended-release tablets) is available in 6.25 mg and 12.5 mg strength tablets for oral administration.

Chemically, zolpidem is N,N,6-trimethyl-2-p-tolylimidazo [1,2-a] pyridine-3-acetamide L-(+)-tartrate (2:1). It has the following structure:

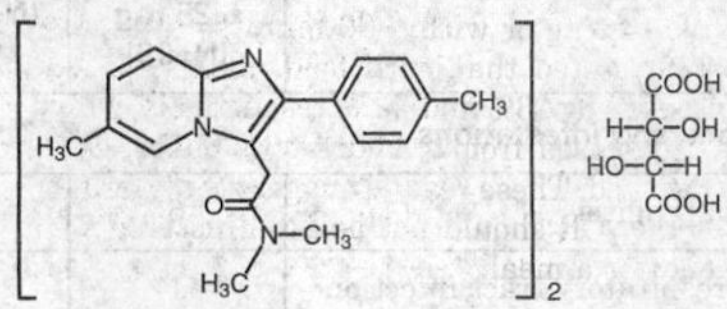

Zolpidem tartrate is a white to off-white crystalline powder that is sparingly soluble in water, alcohol, and propylene glycol. It has a molecular weight of 764.88.

Ambien CR consists of a coated two-layer tablet: one layer that releases its drug content immediately and another layer that allows a slower release of additional drug content. The 6.25 mg Ambien CR tablet contains the following inactive ingredients: colloidal silicon dioxide, hypromellose, lactose monohydrate, magnesium stearate, microcrystalline cellulose, polyethylene glycol, potassium bitartrate, red ferric oxide, sodium starch glycolate, and titanium dioxide. The 12.5 mg Ambien CR tablet contains the following inactive ingredients: colloidal silicon dioxide, FD&C Blue #2, hypromellose, lactose monohydrate, magnesium stearate, microcrystalline cellulose, polyethylene glycol, potassium bitartrate, sodium starch glycolate, titanium dioxide, and yellow ferric oxide.

12 CLINICAL PHARMACOLOGY

12.1 Mechanism of action

Subunit modulation of the $GABA_A$ receptor chloride channel macromolecular complex is hypothesized to be responsible for sedative, anticonvulsant, anxiolytic, and myorelaxant drug properties. The major modulatory site of the $GABA_A$ receptor complex is located on its alpha (α) subunit and is referred to as the benzodiazepine (BZ) receptor.

Zolpidem, the active moiety of zolpidem tartrate, is a hypnotic agent with a chemical structure unrelated to benzodiazepines, barbiturates, pyrrolopyrazines, pyrazolopyrimidines, or other drugs with known hypnotic properties. In contrast to the benzodiazepines, which nonselectively bind to and activate all BZ receptor subtypes, zolpidem *in vitro* binds the BZ_1 receptor preferentially with a high affinity ratio of the $alpha_1/alpha_5$ subunits. The BZ_1 receptor is found primarily on the Lamina IV of the sensorimotor cortical regions, substantia nigra (pars reticulata), cerebellum molecular layer, olfactory bulb, ventral thalamic complex, pons, inferior colliculus, and globus pallidus. This selective binding of zolpidem on the BZ_1 receptor is not absolute, but it may explain the relative absence of myorelaxant and anticonvulsant effects in animal studies as well as the preservation of deep sleep (stages 3 and 4) in human studies of zolpidem at hypnotic doses.

12.3 Pharmacokinetics

Ambien CR exhibits biphasic absorption characteristics, which results in rapid initial absorption from the gastrointestinal tract similar to zolpidem tartrate immediate-release, then provides extended plasma concentrations beyond three hours after administration. A study in 24 healthy male subjects was conducted to compare mean zolpidem plasma concentration-time profiles obtained after single oral administration of Ambien CR 12.5 mg and of an immediate-release formulation of zolpidem tartrate (10 mg). The terminal elimination half-life observed with Ambien CR (12.5 mg) was similar to that obtained with immediate-release zolpidem tartrate (10 mg). The mean plasma concentration-time profiles are shown in Figure 1.

Figure 1: Mean plasma concentration-time profiles for Ambien CR (12.5 mg) and immediate-release zolpidem tartrate (10 mg)

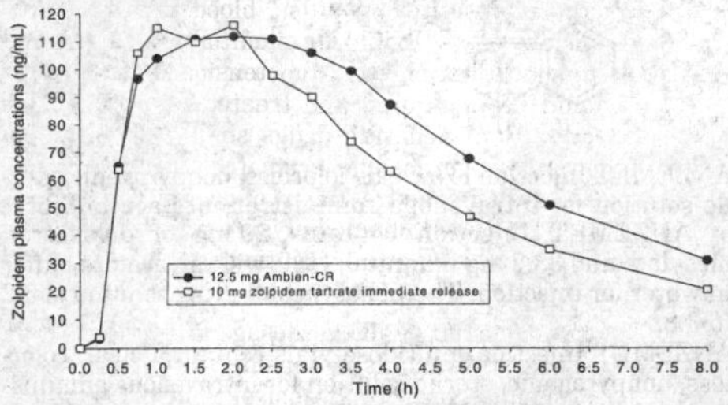

In adult and elderly patients treated with Ambien CR, there was no evidence of accumulation after repeated once-daily dosing for up to two weeks.

Absorption:

Following administration of Ambien CR, administered as a single 12.5 mg dose in healthy male adult subjects, the mean peak concentration (C_{max}) of zolpidem was 134 ng/mL (range: 68.9 to 197 ng/ml) occurring at a median time (T_{max}) of 1.5 hours. The mean AUC of zolpidem was 740 ng•hr/mL (range: 295 to 1359 ng•hr/mL).

A food-effect study in 45 healthy subjects compared the pharmacokinetics of Ambien CR 12.5 mg when administered while fasting or within 30 minutes after a meal. Results demonstrated that with food, mean AUC and C_{max} were decreased by 23% and 30%, respectively, while median T_{max} was increased from 2 hours to 4 hours. The half-life was not changed. These results suggest that, for faster sleep onset, Ambien CR should not be administered with or immediately after a meal.

Distribution:

Total protein binding was found to be 92.5 ± 0.1% and remained constant, independent of concentration between 40 and 790 ng/mL.

Metabolism:

Zolpidem is converted to inactive metabolites that are eliminated primarily by renal excretion.

Elimination:

When Ambien CR was administered as a single 12.5 mg dose in healthy male adult subjects, the mean zolpidem elimination half-life was 2.8 hours (range: 1.62 to 4.05 hr).

Special Populations

Elderly:

In 24 elderly (≥ 65 years) healthy subjects administered a single 6.25 mg dose of Ambien CR, the mean peak concentration (C_{max}) of zolpidem was 70.6 (range: 35.0 to 161) ng/mL occurring at a median time (T_{max}) of 2.0 hours. The mean AUC of zolpidem was 413 ng•hr/mL (range: 124 to 1190 ng•hr/mL) and the mean elimination half-life was 2.9 hours (range: 1.59 to 5.50 hours).

Hepatic Impairment:

Ambien CR was not studied in patients with hepatic impairment. The pharmacokinetics of an immediate-release formulation of zolpidem tartrate in eight patients with chronic hepatic insufficiency were compared to results in healthy subjects. Following a single 20-mg oral zolpidem tartrate dose, mean C_{max} and AUC were found to be two times (250 vs. 499 ng/mL) and five times (788 vs. 4,203 ng•hr/mL) higher, respectively, in hepatically compromised patients. T_{max} did not change. The mean half-life in cirrhotic patients of 9.9 hr (range: 4.1 to 25.8 hr) was greater than that observed in normal subjects of 2.2 hr (range: 1.6 to 2.4 hr). Dosing should be modified accordingly in patients with hepatic insufficiency *[see Dosage and Administration (2.2) and Warnings and Precautions (5.6)]*.

Renal Impairment:

Ambien CR was not studied in patients with renal impairment. The pharmacokinetics of an immediate-release formulation of zolpidem tartrate were studied in 11 patients with end-stage renal failure (mean Cl_{Cr} = 6.5 ± 1.5 mL/min) undergoing hemodialysis three times a week, who were dosed with zolpidem tartrate 10 mg orally each day for 14 or 21 days. No statistically significant differences were observed for C_{max}, T_{max}, half-life, and AUC between the first and last day of drug administration when baseline concentration adjustments were made. On day 1, C_{max} was 172 ± *29 ng/mL (range: 46 to 344 ng/mL)*. After repeated dosing for 14 or 21 days, C_{max} was 203 ± 32 ng/mL (range: 28 to 316 ng/mL). On day 1, T_{max} was 1.7 ± 0.3 hr (range: 0.5 to 3.0 hr); after repeated dosing T_{max} was 0.8 ± 0.2 hr (range: 0.5 to 2.0 hr). This variation is accounted for by noting that last-day serum sampling began 10 hours after the previous dose, rather than after 24 hours. This resulted in residual drug concentration and a shorter period to reach maximal serum concentration. On day 1, $T_{1/2}$ was 2.4 ± 0.4 hr (range: 0.4 to 5.1 hr). After repeated dosing, $T_{1/2}$ was 2.5 ± 0.4 hr (range: 0.7 to 4.2 hr). AUC was 796 ± 159 ng•hr/mL after the first dose and 818 ± 170 ng•hr/mL after repeated dosing. Zolpidem was not hemodialyzable. No accumulation of unchanged drug appeared after 14 or 21 days. Zolpidem pharmacokinetics were not significantly different in renally-impaired patients. No dosage adjustment is necessary in patients with compromised renal function. However, as a general precaution, these patients should be closely monitored.

13 NONCLINICAL TOXICOLOGY

13.1 Carcinogenesis, mutagenesis, impairment of fertility

Carcinogenesis:

Zolpidem tartrate was administered to CD-1 mice and Sprague-Dawley rats for two years at dietary dosages of 4, 18, and 80 mg/kg/day. No evidence of carcinogenic potential was observed in either mice or rats at doses up to 80 mg base/kg/day (40 and 80 times the maximum recommended human dose [MRHD] of Ambien CR 12.5 mg [10 mg zolpidem base], respectively, on a mg/m^2 basis).

Mutagenesis:

Zolpidem did not have mutagenic activity in several tests including an *in vitro* bacterial reverse mutation (Ames) assay, an *in vitro* mammalian gene forward mutation assay in mouse lymphoma cells, and an *in vitro* unscheduled DNA synthesis in rat hepatocytes. Zolpidem was not clastogenic in an *in vitro* chromosomal aberration assay in human lymphocytes or in an *in vivo* micronucleus test in mice.

Impairment of fertility:

Zolpidem tartrate was administered by oral gavage to Sprague-Dawley rats at doses of 4, 20, or 100 mg base/kg/day. Treatment of males began 71 days prior to mating and continued through mating while treatment of females began 14 days prior to mating and continued through mating, gestation, and weaning which occurred on post partum Day 25. Zolpidem administered at 100 mg base/kg was associated with irregular estrus cycles and prolonged pre-coital intervals, but did not produce a decline in fertility. The no-effect dose was 20 mg base/kg/day (20 times the MRHD of Ambien CR on a mg/m^2 basis).

14 CLINICAL STUDIES

14.1 Controlled clinical trials

Ambien CR was evaluated in three placebo-controlled studies for the treatment of patients with chronic primary insomnia (as defined in the APA Diagnostic and Statistical Manual of Mental Disorders, DSM IV).

Adult outpatients (18–64 years) with primary insomnia (N=212) were evaluated in a double-blind, randomized, parallel-group, 3-week trial comparing Ambien CR 12.5 mg and placebo. Ambien CR 12.5 mg decreased wake time after sleep onset (WASO) for the first 7 hours during the first 2 nights and for the first 5 hours after 2 weeks of treatment. Ambien CR 12.5 mg was superior to placebo on objective measures (polysomnography recordings) of sleep induction (by decreasing latency to persistent sleep [LPS]) during the first 2 nights of treatment and after 2 weeks of treatment. Ambien CR 12.5 mg was also superior to placebo on the patient reported global impression regarding the aid to sleep after the first 2 nights and after 3 weeks of treatment.

Elderly outpatients (≥ 65 years) with primary insomnia (N=205) were evaluated in a double-blind, randomized, parallel-group, 3-week trial comparing Ambien CR 6.25 mg and placebo. Ambien CR 6.25 mg decreased wake time after sleep onset (WASO) for the first 6 hours during the first 2 nights and the first 4 hours after 2 weeks of treatment. Ambien CR 6.25 mg was superior to placebo on objective measures (polysomnography recordings) of sleep induction (by decreasing LPS) during the first 2 nights of treatment and after 2 weeks on treatment. Ambien CR 6.25 mg was superior to placebo on the patient reported global impression regarding the aid to sleep after the first 2 nights and after 3 weeks of treatment.

In both studies, in patients treated with Ambien CR, polysomnography showed increased wakefulness at the end of the night compared to placebo-treated patients.

In a 24-week double-blind, placebo controlled, randomized study in adult outpatients (18–64 years) with primary insomnia (N=1025), Ambien CR 12.5 mg administered as needed (3 to 7 nights per week) was superior to placebo over 24 weeks, on patient global impression regarding aid to sleep, and on patient-reported specific sleep parameters for sleep induction and sleep maintenance with no significant increased frequency of drug intake observed over time.

14.2 Studies pertinent to safety concerns for sedative/hypnotic drugs

Next-day residual effects: In five clinical studies [three controlled studies in adults (18–64 years of age) administered Ambien CR 12.5 mg and two controlled studies in the elderly (≥ 65 years of age) administered Ambien CR 6.25 mg or 12.5 mg], the effect of Ambien CR on vigilance, memory, or motor function were assessed using neurocognitive tests. In these studies, no significant decrease in performance was observed eight hours after a nighttime dose. In addition, no evidence of next-day residual effects was detected with Ambien CR 12.5 mg and 6.25 mg using self-ratings of sedation.

During the 3-week studies, next-day somnolence was reported by 15% of the adult patients who received 12.5 mg Ambien CR versus 2% of the placebo group; next-day somnolence was reported by 6% of the elderly patients who received 6.25 mg Ambien CR versus 5% of the placebo group *[see Adverse Reactions (6)]*. In a 6-month study, the overall incidence of next-day somnolence was 5.7% in the Ambien CR group as compared to 2% in the placebo group.

Rebound effects: Rebound insomnia, defined as a dose-dependent worsening in sleep parameters (latency, sleep efficiency, and number of awakenings) compared with baseline following discontinuation of treatment, is observed with short- and intermediate-acting hypnotics. In the two 3-week placebo-controlled studies in patients with primary insomnia, a rebound effect was only observed on the first night after abrupt discontinuation of Ambien CR. On the second night, there was no worsening compared to baseline in the Ambien CR group.

In a 6-month placebo-controlled study in which Ambien CR was taken as needed (3 to 7 nights per week), within the first month a rebound effect was observed for Total Sleep Time (not for WASO) during the first night off medication. After this first month period, no further rebound insomnia was observed. After final treatment discontinuation no rebound was observed.

16 HOW SUPPLIED/STORAGE AND HANDLING

Ambien CR 6.25 mg tablets are composed of two layers[1] and are coated, pink, round, bi-convex, debossed with A~ on one side and supplied as:

NDC Number	Size
0024-5501-31	bottle of 100
0024-5501-50	bottle of 500
0024-5501-10	carton of 30 unit dose
0024-5501-34	carton of 100 unit dose

Ambien CR 12.5 mg tablets are composed of two layers[1] and are coated, blue, round, bi-convex, debossed with A~ on one side and supplied as:

NDC Number	Size
0024-5521-31	bottle of 100
0024-5521-50	bottle of 500
0024-5521-10	carton of 30 unit dose
0024-5521-34	carton of 100 unit dose

1Layers are covered by the coating and are indistinguishable.

Store between 15°–25° C (59°–77°F). Limited excursions permissible up to 30° C (86°F)

17 PATIENT COUNSELING INFORMATION

Prescribers or other healthcare professionals should inform patients, their families, and their caregivers about the benefits and risks associated with treatment with sedative-hypnotics, should counsel them in its appropriate use, and should instruct them to read the accompanying Medication Guide *[see Medication Guide (17.4)]*.

17.1 Severe anaphylactic and anaphylactoid reactions

Inform patients that severe anaphylactic and anaphylactoid reactions have occurred with zolpidem. Describe the signs/symptoms of these reactions and advise patients to seek medical attention immediately if any of them occur.

17.2 Sleep-driving and other complex behaviors

There have been reports of people getting out of bed after taking a sedative-hypnotic and driving their cars while not fully awake, often with no memory of the event. If a patient experiences such an episode, it should be reported to his or her doctor immediately, since "sleep-driving" can be dangerous. This behavior is more likely to occur when Ambien CR is taken with alcohol or other central nervous system depressants *[see Warnings and Precautions (5.3)]*. Other complex behaviors (e.g., preparing and eating food, making phone calls, or having sex) have been reported in patients who are not fully awake after taking a sedative-hypnotic. As with "sleep-driving", patients usually do not remember these events.

In addition, patients should be advised to report all concomitant medications to the prescriber. Patients should be instructed to report events such as "sleep-driving" and other complex behaviors immediately to the prescriber.

17.3 Administration instructions

Patients should be counseled to take Ambien right before they get into bed and only when they are able to stay in bed a full night (7– 8 hours) before being active again. Ambien CR tablets should not be crushed, divided, or chewed, and should not be taken with or immediately after a meal. Advise patients NOT to take Ambien CR when drinking alcohol.

17.4 Medication Guide

MEDICATION GUIDE

AMBIEN CR® (ām′bē-ən see ahr) **C-IV**

(zolpidem tartrate extended-release tablets)

Read the Medication Guide that comes with AMBIEN CR before you start taking it and each time you get a refill. There may be new information. This Medication Guide does not take the place of talking to your doctor about your medical condition or treatment.

What is the most important information I should know about AMBIEN CR?

After taking AMBIEN CR, you may get up out of bed while not being fully awake and do an activity that you do not know you are doing. The next morning, you may not remember that you did anything during the night. You have a higher chance for doing these activities if you drink alcohol or take other medicines that make you sleepy with AMBIEN CR. Reported activities include:

- driving a car ("sleep-driving")
- making and eating food
- talking on the phone
- having sex
- sleep-walking

Call your doctor right away if you find out that you have done any of the above activities after taking AMBIEN CR.

Important:

1. Take AMBIEN CR exactly as prescribed

- Do not take more AMBIEN CR than prescribed.
- Take AMBIEN CR right before you get in bed, not sooner.

2. Do not take AMBIEN CR if you:

- drink alcohol
- take other medicines that can make you sleepy. Talk to your doctor about all of your medicines. Your doctor will tell you if you can take AMBIEN CR with your other medicines.
- cannot get a full night's sleep

What is AMBIEN CR?

AMBIEN CR is a sedative-hypnotic (sleep) medicine. AMBIEN CR is used in adults for the treatment of a sleep problem called insomnia. Symptoms of insomnia include:

- trouble falling asleep
- waking up often during the night

AMBIEN CR is not for children.

> AMBIEN CR is a federally controlled substance (C-IV) because it can be abused or lead to dependence. Keep AMBIEN CR in a safe place to prevent misuse and abuse. Selling or giving away AMBIEN CR may harm others, and is against the law. Tell your doctor if you have ever abused or have been dependent on alcohol, prescription medicines or street drugs.

Who should not take AMBIEN CR?

Do not take AMBIEN CR if you are allergic to anything in it. See the end of this Medication Guide for a complete list of ingredients in AMBIEN CR.

AMBIEN CR may not be right for you. Before starting AMBIEN CR, tell your doctor about all of your health conditions, including if you:

- have a history of depression, mental illness, or suicidal thoughts
- have a history of drug or alcohol abuse or addiction
- have kidney or liver disease
- have a lung disease or breathing problems
- are pregnant, planning to become pregnant, or breast-feeding

Tell your doctor about all of the medicines you take including prescription and nonprescription medicines, vitamins and herbal supplements. Medicines can interact with each other, sometimes causing serious side effects. **Do not take AMBIEN CR with other medicines that can make you sleepy.**

Know the medicines you take. Keep a list of your medicines with you to show your doctor and pharmacist each time you get a new medicine.

How should I take AMBIEN CR?

- Take AMBIEN CR exactly as prescribed. Do not take more AMBIEN CR than prescribed for you.
- **Take AMBIEN CR right before you get into bed.**
- **Do not take AMBIEN CR unless you are able to stay in bed a full night (7–8 hours) before you must be active again.**
- Swallow AMBIEN CR Tablets whole. Do not chew or break the tablets. Tell your doctor if you cannot swallow tablets whole.
- For faster sleep onset, AMBIEN CR should NOT be taken with or immediately after a meal.
- Call your doctor if your insomnia worsens or is not better within 7 to 10 days. This may mean that there is another condition causing your sleep problems.
- If you take too much AMBIEN CR or overdose, call your doctor or poison control center right away, or get emergency treatment.

What are the possible side effects of AMBIEN CR?

Serious side effects of AMBIEN CR include:

- **getting out of bed while not being fully awake and do an activity that you do not know you are doing.** (See "What is the most important information I should know about AMBIEN CR?)
- **abnormal thoughts and behavior.** Symptoms include more outgoing or aggressive behavior than normal, confusion, agitation, hallucinations, worsening of depression, and suicidal thoughts or actions.
- **memory loss**
- **anxiety**
- **severe allergic reactions.** Symptoms include swelling of the tongue or throat, trouble breathing, and nausea and vomiting. Get emergency medical help if you get these symptoms after taking AMBIEN CR.

Call your doctor right away if you have any of the above side effects or any other side effects that worry you while using AMBIEN CR.

The most common side effects of AMBIEN CR are:

- headache
- sleepiness
- dizziness
- You may still feel drowsy the next day after taking AMBIEN CR. **Do not drive or do other dangerous activities after taking AMBIEN CR until you feel fully awake.**

After you stop taking a sleep medicine, you may have symptoms for 1 to 2 days such as: trouble sleeping, nausea, flushing, lightheadedness, uncontrolled crying, vomiting, stomach cramps, panic attack, nervousness, and stomach area pain.

These are not all the side effects of AMBIEN CR. Ask your doctor or pharmacist for more information.

Call your doctor for medical advice about side effects. You may report side effects to FDA at 1–800–FDA–1088.

How should I store AMBIEN CR?

- Store AMBIEN CR at room temperature, 59° to 77°F (15° to 25° C).
- **Keep AMBIEN CR and all medicines out of reach of children.**

General Information about AMBIEN CR

- Medicines are sometimes prescribed for purposes other than those listed in a Medication Guide.
- Do not use AMBIEN CR for a condition for which it was not prescribed.
- Do not share AMBIEN CR with other people, even if you think they have the same symptoms that you have. It may harm them and it is against the law.

This Medication Guide summarizes the most important information about AMBIEN CR. If you would like more information, talk with your doctor. You can ask your doctor or pharmacist for information about AMBIEN CR that is written for healthcare professionals. For more information about AMBIEN CR, call 1-800-633-1610 or visit www.ambiencr.com.

What are the ingredients in AMBIEN CR?

Active Ingredient: Zolpidem tartrate

Inactive Ingredients: The 6.25 mg tablets contain: colloidal silicon dioxide, hypromellose, lactose monohydrate, magnesium stearate, microcrystalline cellulose, polyethylene glycol, potassium bitartrate, red ferric oxide, sodium starch glycolate, and titanium dioxide. The 12.5 mg tablets contain: colloidal silicon dioxide, FD&C Blue #2, hypromellose, lactose monohydrate, magnesium stearate, microcrystalline cellulose, polyethylene glycol, potassium bitartrate, sodium starch glycolate, titanium dioxide, and yellow ferric oxide.

This Medication Guide has been approved by the U.S. Food and Drug Administration.

sanofi-aventis U.S. LLC
Bridgewater, NJ 08807
September 2009

Shown in Product Identification Guide, page 318

ANZEMET® INJECTION ℞

[*an-zĕmĕt*]

(dolasetron mesylate injection)

DESCRIPTION

ANZEMET (dolasetron mesylate) is an antinauseant and antiemetic agent. Chemically, dolasetron mesylate is (2α,6α,8α,9aβ)-octahydro-3-oxo-2,6-methano-2*H*-quinolizin-8-yl-1*H*-indole-3-carboxylate monomethanesulfonate, monohydrate. It is a highly specific and selective serotonin subtype 3 ($5\text{-}HT_3$) receptor antagonist both in vitro and in vivo. Dolasetron mesylate has the following structural formula:

[See chemical structure at top of next column]

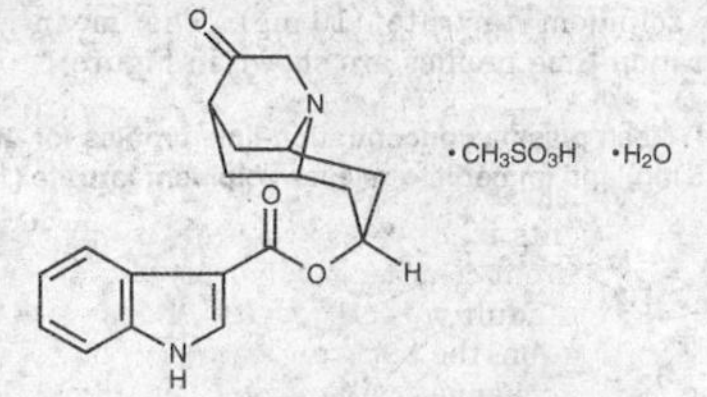

The empirical formula is $C_{19}H_{20}N_2O_3 \cdot CH_3SO_3H \cdot H_2O$, with a molecular weight of 438.50. Approximately 74% of dolasetron mesylate monohydrate is dolasetron base.

Dolasetron mesylate monohydrate is a white to off-white powder that is freely soluble in water and propylene glycol, slightly soluble in ethanol, and slightly soluble in normal saline.

ANZEMET Injection is a clear, colorless, nonpyrogenic, sterile solution for intravenous administration. Each milliliter of ANZEMET Injection contains 20 mg of dolasetron mesylate and 38.2 mg mannitol, USP, with an acetate buffer in water for injection. The pH of the resulting solution is 3.2 to 3.8.

ANZEMET Injection multidose vials contain a clear, colorless, nonpyrogenic, sterile solution for intravenous administration. Each ANZEMET multidose vial contains 25 mL (500 mg) dolasetron mesylate. Each milliliter contains 20 mg dolasetron mesylate, 29 mg mannitol, USP, and 5 mg phenol, USP, with an acetate buffer in water for injection. The pH of the resulting solution is 3.2 to 3.7.

CLINICAL PHARMACOLOGY

Dolasetron and its active metabolite, hydrodolasetron (MDL 74,156), are selective serotonin $5\text{-}HT_3$ receptor antagonists not shown to have activity at other known serotonin receptors and with low affinity for dopamine receptors. The serotonin $5\text{-}HT_3$ receptors are located on the nerve terminals of the vagus in the periphery and centrally in the chemoreceptor trigger zone of the area postrema. It is thought that chemotherapeutic agents produce nausea and vomiting by releasing serotonin from the enterochromaffin cells of the small intestine, and that the released serotonin then activates $5\text{-}HT_3$ receptors located on vagal efferents to initiate the vomiting reflex.

Acute, usually reversible, ECG changes (PR and QT_c prolongation; QRS widening), caused by dolasetron mesylate, have been observed in healthy volunteers and in controlled clinical trials. The active metabolites of dolasetron may block sodium channels, a property unrelated to its ability to block $5\text{-}HT_3$ receptors. QT_c prolongation is primarily due to QRS widening. Dolasetron appears to prolong both depolarization and, to a lesser extent, repolarization time. The magnitude and frequency of the ECG changes increased with dose (related to peak plasma concentrations of hydrodolasetron but not the parent compound). These ECG interval prolongations usually returned to baseline within 6 to 8 hours, but in some patients were present at 24 hour follow up. Dolasetron mesylate administration has little or no effect on blood pressure.

In healthy volunteers (N=64), dolasetron mesylate in single intravenous doses up to 5 mg/kg produced no effect on pupil size or meaningful changes in EEG tracings. Results from neuropsychiatric tests revealed that dolasetron mesylate did not alter mood or concentration. Multiple daily doses of dolasetron have had no effect on colonic transit in humans. Dolasetron mesylate has no effect on plasma prolactin concentrations.

Pharmacokinetics in Humans

Intravenous dolasetron mesylate is rapidly eliminated ($t_{1/2}$<10 min) and completely metabolized to the most clinically relevant species, hydrodolasetron.

The reduction of dolasetron to hydrodolasetron is mediated by a ubiquitous enzyme, carbonyl reductase. Cytochrome P-450 (CYP)2D6 is primarily responsible for the subsequent hydroxylation of hydrodolasetron and both CYP3A and flavin monooxygenase are responsible for the N-oxidation of hydrodolasetron.

Hydrodolasetron is excreted in the urine unchanged (53.0% of administered intravenous dose). Other urinary metabolites include hydroxylated glucuronides and N-oxide.

Hydrodolasetron appeared rapidly in plasma, with a maximum concentration occurring approximately 0.6 hour after the end of intravenous treatment, and was eliminated with a mean half-life of 7.3 hours (%CV=24) and an apparent clearance of 9.4 mL/min/kg (%CV=28) in 24 adults. Hydrodolasetron is eliminated by multiple routes, including renal excretion and, after metabolism, mainly glucuronidation, and hydroxylation. Hydrodolasetron exhibits linear pharmacokinetics over the intravenous dose range of 50 to 200 mg and they are independent of infusion rate. Doses lower than 50 mg have not been studied. Two thirds of the administered dose is recovered in the urine and one third in the feces. Hydrodolasetron is widely distributed in the body with a mean apparent volume of distribution of 5.8 L/kg (%CV=25, N=24) in adults.

Sixty-nine to 77% of hydrodolasetron is bound to plasma protein. In a study with ^{14}C labeled dolasetron, the distribution of radioactivity to blood cells was not extensive. The binding of hydrodolasetron to α_1-acid glycoprotein is approximately 50%. The pharmacokinetics of hydrodolasetron are linear and similar in men and women.

The pharmacokinetics of hydrodolasetron, in special and targeted patient populations following intravenous administration of ANZEMET Injection, are summarized in Table 1. The pharmacokinetics of hydrodolasetron are similar in adult (young and elderly) healthy volunteers and in adult cancer patients receiving chemotherapeutic agents. The apparent clearance of hydrodolasetron in pediatric and adolescent patients is 1.4 times to twofold higher than in adults. The apparent clearance of hydrodolasetron is not affected by age in adult cancer patients. Following intravenous administration, the apparent clearance of hydrodolasetron remains unchanged with severe hepatic impairment and decreases 47% with severe renal impairment. No dose adjustment is necessary for elderly patients (see PRECAUTIONS, Geriatric Use) or for patients with hepatic or renal impairment.

In a pharmacokinetic study in pediatric cancer patients (ages 3 to 11, N=25; ages 12 to 17, N=21) given a single 0.6, 1.2, 1.8, or 2.4 mg/kg dose of ANZEMET Injection intravenously, apparent clearance values were highest and half-lives were lowest in the youngest age group. For the 3 to 11 and the 12 to 17 year age groups, all receiving doses between 0.6 to 2.4 mg/kg, mean apparent clearances are 2 and 1.3 times greater, respectively, than for healthy adults receiving the same range of doses.

Thirty-two pediatric cancer patients ages 3 to 11 years (N=19) and 12 to 17 years (N=13), received 0.6, 1.2, or 1.8 mg/kg ANZEMET Injection diluted with either apple or apple-grape juice and administered orally. In this study, the mean apparent clearances were 3 times greater in the younger pediatric group and 1.8 times greater in the older pediatric group than those observed in healthy adult volunteers. Across this spectrum of pediatric patients, maximum plasma concentrations were 0.6 to 0.7 times those observed in healthy adults receiving similar doses.

In a pharmacokinetic study in 18 pediatric patients (2 to 11 years of age) undergoing surgery with general anesthesia and administered a single 1.2 mg/kg intravenous dose of ANZEMET Injection, mean apparent clearance was greater (40%) and terminal half-life shorter (36%) for hydrodolasetron than in healthy adults receiving the same dose.

For 12 pediatric patients, ages 2 to 12 years receiving 1.2 mg/kg ANZEMET Injection diluted in apple or apple-grape juice and administered orally, the mean apparent clearance was 34% greater and half-life was 21% shorter than in healthy adults receiving the same dose.

[See table 1 above]

Clinical Studies

Prevention of Cancer Chemotherapy-Induced Nausea and Vomiting

ANZEMET Injection administered intravenously at a dose of 1.8 mg/kg gave similar results in preventing nausea and vomiting as the other selective serotonin 5-HT$_3$ receptor antagonists studied as active comparators. It was more effective than metoclopramide. Efficacy was based on complete response rates (0 emetic episodes and no rescue medication).

Cisplatin Based Chemotherapy

A randomized, double-blind trial compared single intravenous doses of ANZEMET Injection with metoclopramide in 226 (160 men and 66 women) adult cancer patients receiving ≥80 mg/m² cisplatin. ANZEMET Injection at a dose of 1.8 mg/kg was significantly more effective than metoclopramide in the prevention of chemotherapy-induced nausea and vomiting in this study (Table 2).

[See table 2 above]

A second randomized, double-blind trial compared single intravenous doses of ANZEMET Injection with intravenous ondansetron in 609 (377 men and 232 women) adult cancer patients receiving ≥70 mg/m² cisplatin. A single intravenous 1.8 mg/kg dose of ANZEMET Injection was shown to be equivalent to a single intravenous 32 mg dose of ondansetron (Table 3).

[See table 3 at right]

Another randomized, double-blind trial compared single IV doses of ANZEMET with a single 3-mg IV dose of granisetron in 474 (315 men and 159 women) patients receiving ≥80 mg/m² cisplatin chemotherapy.

A single intravenous 1.8-mg/kg dose of ANZEMET gave similar results as those from granisetron.

Cyclophosphamide Based Chemotherapy

In a study of ANZEMET Injection in 309 patients (96 men and 213 women) receiving moderately emetogenic chemotherapy such as cyclophosphamide based regimens, a single *intravenous 1.8 mg/kg* dose of ANZEMET Injection was equivalent to metoclopramide administered as a 2 mg/kg intravenous bolus followed by 3 mg/kg intravenously over 8 hours. Complete response rates were 63% and 52%, respectively, p=0.12.

Prevention of Postoperative Nausea and Vomiting

ANZEMET Injection administered intravenously at a dose of 12.5 mg approximately 15 minutes before the cessation of general balanced anesthesia (short-acting barbiturate, nitrous oxide, narcotic and analgesic, and skeletal muscle re-

laxant) was significantly more effective than placebo in preventing postoperative nausea and vomiting. No increased efficacy was seen with higher doses.

One trial compared single intravenous ANZEMET Injection doses of 12.5, 25, 50, and 100 mg with placebo in 635 women surgical patients undergoing laparoscopic procedures. ANZEMET Injection at a dose of 12.5 mg was statistically superior to placebo for complete response (no vomiting, no rescue medication) (p=.0003). Complete response rates were 50% and 31%, respectively.

Another trial compared single intravenous ANZEMET Injection doses of 12.5, 25, 50, and 100 mg with placebo in 1030 (722 women and 308 men) surgical patients. In women, the 12.5 mg dose was statistically superior to placebo for complete response. The complete response rates were 50% and 40%, respectively. However, in men, there was no statistically significant difference in complete response between any ANZEMET dose and placebo.

Treatment of Postoperative Nausea and/or Vomiting

Two randomized, double-blinded trials compared single intravenous ANZEMET Injection doses of 12.5, 25, 50, and 100 mg with placebo in 124 male and 833 female patients who had undergone surgery with general balanced anesthesia and presented with early postoperative nausea or vomiting requiring antiemetic treatment.

In both studies, the 12.5 mg intravenous dose of ANZEMET was statistically superior to placebo for complete response (no vomiting, no escape medication). No significant increased efficacy was seen with higher doses.

INDICATIONS AND USAGE

ANZEMET Injection is indicated for the following:

- **(1) the prevention of nausea and vomiting associated with initial and repeat courses of emetogenic cancer chemotherapy, including high dose cisplatin;**

Table 1. Pharmacokinetic Values for Plasma Hydrodolasetron Following Intravenous Administration of ANZEMET Injection*

	Age (years)	Dose	CL$_{app}$ (mL/min/kg)	t$_{1/2}$ (h)	C$_{max}$ (ng/mL)
Young Healthy Volunteers (N=24)	19–40	100 mg	9.4 (28%)	7.3 (24%)	320 (25%)
Elderly Healthy Volunteers (N=15)	65–75	2.4 mg/kg	8.3 (30%)	6.9 (22%)	620 (31%)
Cancer Patients					
Adults (N=273)	19–87	0.6–3.0 mg/kg	10.2 (34%)[†]	7.5 (43%)[†]	505 (26%)[‡]
Adolescents (N=21)	12–17	0.6–3.0 mg/kg	12.5 (37%)	5.5 (31%)	562 (45%)[§]
Children (N=25)	3–11	0.6–2.4 mg/kg	19.2 (30%)	4.4 (24%)	505 (100%)[¶]
Pediatric Surgery Patients (N=18)	2–11	1.2 mg/kg	13.1 (47%)	4.8 (23%)	255 (22%)
Patients with Severe Renal Impairment (N=12) (Creatinine clearance ≤10 mL/min)	28–74	200 mg	5.0 (33%)	10.9 (30%)	867 (31%)
Patients with Severe Hepatic Impairment (N=3)	42–52	150 mg	9.6 (19%)	11.7 (22%)	396 (45%)

CL$_{app}$: apparent clearance t$_{1/2}$: terminal elimination half-life ( ): coefficient of variation in %
* mean values
† results from population kinetic study
‡ results from adult cancer study (dose=1.8 mg/kg, N=8)
§ results from adolescents (dose=1.8 mg/kg, N=7)
¶ results from children (dose=1.8 mg/kg, N=5)

Table 2. Prevention of Chemotherapy-Induced Nausea and Emesis from Cisplatin Chemotherapy*

	ANZEMET Injection 1.8 mg/kg[†]	Metoclopramide[‡]	*p*-value
Number of Patients	72	69	
Response Over 24 Hours			
Complete Response[§]	41 (57%)	24 (35%)	0.0009
Nausea Score[¶]	4	30	0.0400

* Dose ≥80 mg/m²
† Administered intravenously
‡ 3 mg/kg intravenous bolus and 0.5 mg/kg/h intravenously over 8 h.
§ No emetic episodes and no rescue medication.
¶ Median 24-h change from baseline nausea score using visual analog scale (VAS): Score range 0="none" to 100="nausea as bad as it could be."

Table 3. Prevention of Chemotherapy-Induced Nausea and Emesis from Cisplatin Chemotherapy*

	ANZEMET Injection 1.8 mg/kg[†]	Ondansetron 32 mg[‡]	*p*-value
Number of Patients	198	206	
Response Over 24 Hours			
Complete Response[§]	88 (44%)	88 (43%)	NS
Nausea Score[¶]	10	16	NS

* Dose ≥70 mg/m²
† Administered intravenously
‡ Includes 12 patients who received 3 doses 0.15 mg/kg of ondansetron intravenously.
§ No emetic episodes and no rescue medication.
¶ Median 24-h change from baseline nausea score using visual analog scale (VAS): Score range 0="none" to 100="nausea as bad as it could be."

- **(2) the prevention of postoperative nausea and vomiting.** As with other antiemetics, routine prophylaxis is not recommended for patients in whom there is little expectation that nausea and/or vomiting will occur postoperatively. In patients where nausea and/or vomiting must be avoided postoperatively, ANZEMET Injection is recommended even where the incidence of postoperative nausea and/or vomiting is low;
- **(3) the treatment of postoperative nausea and/or vomiting.**

CONTRAINDICATIONS

ANZEMET Injection is contraindicated in patients known to have hypersensitivity to the drug.

WARNINGS

ANZEMET can cause ECG interval changes (PR, QT_c, JT prolongation and QRS widening). These changes are related in magnitude and frequency to blood levels of the active metabolite. These changes are self-limiting with declining blood levels. Some patients have interval prolongations for 24 hours or longer. Interval prolongation could lead to cardiovascular consequences, including heart block or cardiac arrhythmias. These have rarely been reported.

A cardiac conduction abnormality observed on an intraoperative cardiac rhythm monitor (interpreted as complete heart block) was reported in a 61-year-old woman who received 200 mg ANZEMET for the prevention of postoperative nausea and vomiting. This patient was also taking verapamil. A similar event also interpreted as complete heart block was reported in one patient receiving placebo.

A 66-year-old man with Stage IV non-Hodgkins lymphoma died suddenly 6 hours after receiving 1.8 mg/kg (119 mg) intravenous ANZEMET Injection. This patient had other potential risk factors including substantial exposure to doxorubicin and concomitant cyclophosphamide.

Pediatric Use

Dolasetron should be administered with caution in pediatric patients who have or may develop prolongation of cardiac conduction intervals, particularly QT_c. Rare cases of sustained supraventricular and ventricular arrhythmias, cardiac arrest leading to death, and myocardial infarction have been reported in children and adolescents (See Precautions, General, and Adverse Reactions – Postmarketing Experience).

PRECAUTIONS

General

Dolasetron should be administered with caution in patients who have or may develop prolongation of cardiac conduction intervals, particularly QT_c. These include patients with hypokalemia or hypomagnesemia, patients taking diuretics with potential for inducing electrolyte abnormalities, patients with congenital QT syndrome, patients taking anti-arrhythmic drugs or other drugs which lead to QT prolongation, and cumulative high dose anthracycline therapy.

Cross hypersensitivity reactions have been reported in patients who received other selective 5-HT_3 receptor antagonists. These reactions have not been seen with dolasetron mesylate.

Drug Interactions

The potential for clinically significant drug-drug interactions posed by dolasetron and hydrodolasetron appears to be low for drugs commonly used in chemotherapy or surgery, because hydrodolasetron is eliminated by multiple routes. See PRECAUTIONS, General for information about potential interaction with other drugs that prolong the QT_c interval.

When oral dolasetron (200 mg once daily) was coadministered with cimetidine (300 mg four times daily) for 7 days, the systemic exposure (i.e., AUC) of hydrodolasetron increased by 24% and the maximum plasma concentration of hydrodolasetron increased by 15%. When oral dolasetron (200 mg once daily) was coadministered with rifampin (600 mg once daily) for 7 days, the systemic exposure of hydrodolasetron decreased by 28% and the maximum plasma concentration of hydrodolasetron decreased by 17%.

ANZEMET Injection has been safely coadministered with drugs used in chemotherapy and surgery. As with other agents which prolong ECG intervals, caution should be exercised in patients taking drugs which prolong ECG intervals, particularly QT_c.

In patients taking furosemide, nifedipine, diltiazem, ACE inhibitors, verapamil, glyburide, propranolol, and various chemotherapy agents, no effect was shown on the clearance of hydrodolasetron. Clearance of hydrodolasetron decreased by about 27% when dolasetron mesylate was administered intravenously concomitantly with atenolol. ANZEMET did not influence anesthesia recovery time in patients. Dolasetron mesylate did not inhibit the antitumor activity of four chemotherapeutic agents (cisplatin, 5-fluorouracil, doxorubicin, cyclophosphamide) in four murine models.

Carcinogenesis, Mutagenesis, Impairment of Fertility

In a 24-month carcinogenicity study, there was a statistically significant (P<0.001) increase in the incidence of combined hepatocellular adenomas and carcinomas in male mice treated with 150 mg/kg/day and above. In this study, mice (CD-1) were treated orally with dolasetron mesylate 75, 150 or 300 mg/kg/day (225, 450 or 900 mg/m^2/day). For a 50 kg person of average height (1.46 m^2 body surface area), these doses represent 3.4, 6.8 and 13.5 times the recommended clinical dose (66.6 mg/m^2, intravenous) on a body surface area basis. No increase in liver tumors was observed at a dose of 75 mg/kg/day in male mice and at doses up to 300 mg/kg/day in female mice.

In a 24-month rat (Sprague-Dawley) carcinogenicity study, oral dolasetron mesylate was not tumorigenic at doses up to 150 mg/kg/day (900 mg/m^2/day, 13.5 times the recommended human dose based on body surface area) in male rats and 300 mg/kg/day (1800 mg/m^2/day, 27 times the recommended human dose based on body surface area) in female rats.

Dolasetron mesylate was not genotoxic in the Ames test, the rat lymphocyte chromosomal aberration test, the Chinese hamster ovary (CHO) cell (HGPRT) forward mutation test, the rat hepatocyte unscheduled DNA synthesis (UDS) test or the mouse micronucleus test.

Dolasetron mesylate was found to have no effect on fertility and reproductive performance at oral doses up to 100 mg/kg/day (600 mg/m^2/day, 9 times the recommended human dose based on body surface area) in female rats and up to 400 mg/kg/day (2400 mg/m^2/day, 36 times the recommended human dose based on body surface area) in male rats.

Pregnancy

Teratogenic Effects

Pregnancy Category B

Teratology studies have not revealed evidence of impaired fertility or harm to the fetus due to dolasetron mesylate. These studies have been performed in pregnant rats at intravenous doses up to 60 mg/kg/day (5.4 times the recommended human dose based on body surface area) and pregnant rabbits at intravenous doses up to 20 mg/kg/day (3.2 times the recommended human dose based on body surface area). There are, however, no adequate and well-controlled studies in pregnant women. Because animal reproduction studies are not always predictive of human response, this drug should be used during pregnancy only if clearly needed.

Nursing Mothers

It is not known whether dolasetron mesylate is excreted in human milk. Because many drugs are excreted in human milk, caution should be exercised when ANZEMET Injection is administered to a nursing woman.

Pediatric Use

Dolasetron should be administered with caution in pediatric patients who have or may develop prolongation of cardiac conduction intervals, particularly QT_c. Rare cases of sustained supraventricular and ventricular arrhythmias, cardiac arrest leading to death, and myocardial infarction have been reported in children and adolescents (See Warnings and Adverse Reactions – Postmarketing Experience).

Four open-label, noncomparative pharmacokinetic studies have been performed in a total of 108 pediatric patients receiving emetogenic chemotherapy or undergoing surgery with general anesthesia. These patients received ANZEMET Injection either intravenously or orally in juice. Pediatric patients from 2 to 17 years of age participated in these trials, which included intravenous ANZEMET Injection doses of 0.6, 1.2, 1.8, or 2.4 mg/kg, and oral doses of 0.6, 1.2, or 1.8 mg/kg. There is no experience in pediatric patients under 2 years of age. Overall, ANZEMET Injection was well tolerated in these pediatric patients. Efficacy information collected in pediatric patients receiving cancer chemotherapy are consistent with those obtained in adults. No efficacy information was collected in the pediatric postoperative nausea and vomiting studies.

Geriatric Use

Prevention of cancer chemotherapy-induced nausea and vomiting (CINV)

In controlled clinical trials in the prevention of chemotherapy-induced nausea and vomiting, 723 (32%) of 2264 patients were 65 years of age or older. Of the 723 geriatric patients in the trial, 563 received intravenous ANZEMET Injection. No overall differences in safety or effectiveness were observed between geriatric and younger patients, and other reported clinical experience has not identified differences in responses between geriatric and younger patients, but greater sensitivity of some older individuals cannot be ruled out.

Prevention and treatment of post-operative nausea and vomiting (PONV)

Controlled clinical studies in the prevention and treatment of post-operative nausea and vomiting did not include sufficient numbers of patients aged 65 years or older – only 57 (2%) geriatric patients (43 received intravenous ANZEMET Injection) out of 3289 total patients participated in the controlled PONV trials – to determine whether they respond differently from younger patients. Other reported clinical experiences have not identified differences in responses between geriatric and younger patients. In general, dose selection for an elderly patient should be cautious, usually starting at the low end of the dosing range, reflecting the greater frequency of decreased hepatic, renal, or cardiac function, and of concomitant disease or other drug therapy.

The pharmacokinetics, including clearance of intravenous ANZEMET Injection, in elderly and younger patients are similar (see **CLINICAL PHARMACOLOGY, Pharmacokinetics in Humans**). Dosage adjustment is not needed in patients over the age of 65.

ADVERSE REACTIONS

Chemotherapy Patients

In controlled clinical trials, 2265 adult patients received ANZEMET Injection. The overall adverse event rates were similar with 1.8 mg/kg ANZEMET Injection and ondansetron or granisetron. Patients were receiving concurrent chemotherapy, predominantly high-dose (≥50 mg/m^2) cisplatin. Following is a combined listing of all adverse events reported in ≥2% of patients in these controlled trials (Table 4).

TABLE 4. ADVERSE EVENTS ≥2% FROM CHEMOTHERAPY-INDUCED NAUSEA AND VOMITING STUDIES

Event	ANZEMET Injection 1.8 mg/kg (n=695)		Ondansetron/ Granisetron* (n=356)	
Headache	169	(24.3%)	73	(20.5%)
Diarrhea	86	(12.4%)	25	(7.0%)
Fever	30	(4.3%)	18	(5.1%)
Fatigue	25	(3.6%)	12	(3.4%)
Hepatic Function Abnormal†	25	(3.6%)	12	(3.4%)
Abdominal Pain	22	(3.2%)	7	(2.0%)
Hypertension	20	(2.9%)	9	(2.5%)
Pain	17	(2.4%)	7	(2.0%)
Dizziness	15	(2.2%)	7	(2.0%)
Chills/Shivering	14	(2.0%)	6	(1.7%)

* Ondansetron 32 mg intravenous, granisetron 3 mg intravenous.

† Includes events coded as SGOT- and/or SGPT-increased (see also Liver and Biliary System below)

Postoperative Patients

In controlled clinical trials with 2550 adult patients, headache and dizziness were reported more frequently with 12.5 mg ANZEMET Injection than with placebo. Rates of other adverse events were similar. Following is a listing of all adverse events reported in ≥2% of patients receiving either placebo or 12.5 mg ANZEMET Injection for the prevention or treatment of postoperative nausea and vomiting in controlled clinical trials (Table 5).

Table 5. Adverse Events ≥2% from Placebo-Controlled Postoperative Nausea and Vomiting Studies

Event	ANZEMET Injection 12.5 mg (n=615)	Placebo (n=739)
Headache	58 (9.4%)	51 (6.9%)
Dizziness	34 (5.5%)	23 (3.1%)
Drowsiness	15 (2.4%)	18 (2.4%)
Pain	15 (2.4%)	21 (2.8%)
Urinary Retention	12 (2.0%)	16 (2.2%)

In clinical trials, the following infrequently reported adverse events, assessed by investigators as treatment-related or causality unknown, occurred following oral or intravenous administration of ANZEMET to adult patients receiving concomitant cancer chemotherapy or surgery:

Cardiovascular: Hypotension; rarely–edema, peripheral edema. The following events also occurred rarely and with a similar frequency as placebo and/or active comparator: Mobitz I AV block, chest pain, orthostatic hypotension, myocardial ischemia, syncope, severe bradycardia, and palpitations. See PRECAUTIONS section for information on potential effects on ECG.

In addition, the following asymptomatic treatment-emergent ECG changes were seen at rates less than or equal to those for active or placebo controls: bradycardia,

tachycardia, T wave change, ST-T wave change, sinus arrhythmia, extrasystole (APCs or VPCs), poor R-wave progression, bundle branch block (left and right), nodal arrhythmia, U wave change, atrial flutter/fibrillation.
Furthermore, severe hypotension, bradycardia and syncope have been reported immediately or closely following IV administration.
Dermatologic: Rash, increased sweating.
Gastrointestinal System: Constipation, dyspepsia, abdominal pain, anorexia; rarely–pancreatitis.
Hearing, Taste and Vision: Taste perversion, abnormal vision; rarely–tinnitus, photophobia.
Hematologic: Rarely–hematuria, epistaxis, prothrombin time prolonged, PTT increased, anemia, purpura/hematoma, thrombocytopenia.
Hypersensitivity: Rarely–anaphylactic reaction, facial edema, urticaria.
Liver and Biliary System: Transient increases in AST (SGOT) and/or ALT (SGPT) values have been reported as adverse events in less than 1% of adult patients receiving ANZEMET in clinical trials. The increases did not appear to be related to dose or duration of therapy and were not associated with symptomatic hepatic disease. Similar increases were seen with patients receiving active comparator. Rarely–hyperbilirubinemia, increased GGT.
Metabolic and Nutritional: Rarely–alkaline phosphatase increased.
Musculoskeletal: Rarely–myalgia, arthralgia.
Nervous System: Flushing, vertigo, paraesthesia, tremor; rarely–ataxia, twitching.
Psychiatric: Agitation, sleep disorder, depersonalization; rarely–confusion, anxiety, abnormal dreaming.
Respiratory System: Rarely–dyspnea, bronchospasm.
Urinary System: Rarely–dysuria, polyuria, acute renal failure.
Vascular (Extracardiac): Local pain or burning on IV administration; rarely–peripheral ischemia, thrombophlebitis/phlebitis.

Postmarketing Experience

There are rare reports of wide complex tachycardia or ventricular tachycardia and of ventricular fibrillation cardiac arrest following intravenous administration.

OVERDOSAGE

A 59-year-old man with metastatic melanoma and no known pre-existing cardiac conditions developed severe hypotension and dizziness 40 minutes after receiving a 15 minute intravenous infusion of 1000 mg (13 mg/kg) of dolasetron mesylate. Treatment for the overdose consisted of infusion of 500 mL of a plasma expander, dopamine, and atropine. The patient had normal sinus rhythm and prolongation of PR, QRS and QT_c intervals on an ECG recorded 2 hours after the infusion. The patient's blood pressure was normal 3 hours after the event and the ECG intervals returned to baseline on follow-up. The patient was released from the hospital 6 hours after the event.
Following a suspected overdose of ANZEMET Injection, a patient found to have second-degree or higher AV conduction block with ECG should undergo cardiac telemetry monitoring.
There is no known specific antidote for dolasetron mesylate, and patients with suspected overdose should be managed with supportive therapy. Individual doses as large as 5 mg/kg intravenously or 400 mg orally have been safely given to healthy volunteers or cancer patients.
It is not known if dolasetron mesylate is removed by hemodialysis or peritoneal dialysis.
A 7-year-old boy received 6 mg/kg dolasetron mesylate orally before surgery. No symptoms occurred and no treatment was required.
Single intravenous doses of dolasetron mesylate at 160 mg/kg in male mice and 140 mg/kg in female mice and rats of both sexes (6.3 to 12.6 times the recommended human dose based on body surface area) were lethal. Symptoms of acute toxicity were tremors, depression and convulsions.

DOSAGE AND ADMINISTRATION

The recommended dose of ANZEMET Injection should not be exceeded.

Prevention of Cancer Chemotherapy-Induced Nausea and Vomiting

Adults
The recommended intravenous dosage of ANZEMET Injection from clinical trial results is 1.8 mg/kg given as a single dose approximately 30 minutes before chemotherapy (see Administration). Alternatively, for most patients, a fixed dose of 100 mg can be administered over 30 seconds.
Pediatric Patients
The recommended intravenous dosage in pediatric patients 2 to 16 years of age is 1.8 mg/kg given as a single dose approximately 30 minutes before chemotherapy, up to a maximum of 100 mg (see Administration). Safety and effectiveness in pediatric patients under 2 years of age have not been established.
ANZEMET Injection mixed in apple or apple-grape juice may be used for oral dosing of pediatric patients. When ANZEMET Injection is administered orally, the recommended dosage in pediatric patients 2 to 16 years of age is 1.8 mg/kg up to a maximum 100 mg dose given within 1 hour before chemotherapy.
The diluted product may be kept up to 2 hours at room temperature before use.
Use in the Elderly, in Renal Failure Patients, or in Hepatically Impaired Patients
No dosage adjustment is recommended.

Prevention or Treatment of Postoperative Nausea and/or Vomiting

Adults
The recommended intravenous dosage of ANZEMET Injection is 12.5 mg given as a single dose approximately 15 minutes before the cessation of anesthesia (prevention) or as soon as nausea or vomiting presents (treatment).
Pediatric Patients
The recommended intravenous dosage in pediatric patients 2 to 16 years of age is 0.35 mg/kg, with a maximum dose of 12.5 mg, given as a single dose approximately 15 minutes before the cessation of anesthesia or as soon as nausea or vomiting presents. Safety and effectiveness in pediatric patients under 2 years of age have not been established.
ANZEMET Injection mixed in apple or apple-grape juice may be used for oral dosing of pediatric patients. When ANZEMET Injection is administered orally, the recommended oral dosage in pediatric patients 2 to 16 years of age is 1.2 mg/kg up to a maximum 100-mg dose given within 2 hours before surgery. The diluted product may be kept up to 2 hours at room temperature before use.
Use in the Elderly, in Renal Failure Patients, or in Hepatically Impaired Patients
No dosage adjustment is recommended.

ADMINISTRATION

ANZEMET Injection can be safely infused intravenously as rapidly as 100 mg/30 seconds or diluted in a compatible intravenous solution (see below) to 50 mL and infused over a period of up to 15 minutes. ANZEMET Injection should not be mixed with other drugs. Flush the infusion line before and after administration of ANZEMET Injection.

STABILITY

After dilution, ANZEMET Injection is stable under normal lighting conditions at room temperature for 24 hours or under refrigeration for 48 hours with the following compatible intravenous fluids: 0.9% sodium chloride injection, 5% dextrose injection, 5% dextrose and 0.45% sodium chloride injection, 5% dextrose and Lactated Ringer's injection, Lactated Ringer's injection, and 10% mannitol injection. Although ANZEMET Injection is chemically and physically stable when diluted as recommended, sterile precautions should be observed because diluents generally do not contain preservative. After dilution, do not use beyond 24 hours, or 48 hours if refrigerated.
Parenteral drug products should be inspected visually for particulate matter and discoloration before administration whenever solution and container permit.

HOW SUPPLIED

ANZEMET Injection (dolasetron mesylate injection) is supplied as a clear, colorless solution in single and multidose vials, and Carpuject® sterile cartridges with Luer Lock.

ANZEMET® Injection
(dolasetron mesylate injection)
20 mg/mL

Strength	Description	NDC Number
12.5 mg	0.625mL single-use vial* (Box of 6)	0088-1208-06
12.5 mg	0.625mL fill in single-use 2mL Carpuject with Luer Lock† (Box of 10)	0088-1208-76
100 mg/5 mL	5mL single-use vial*	0088-1206-32
500 mg/25 mL	25mL multi-dose vial*	0088-1209-26

* sanofi-aventis U.S. LLC
Bridgewater, NJ 08807
Origin Italy
† Mfd by Hospira, Inc.
McPherson, KS 67460 USA

Store at 20–25°C (68–77°F) with excursions permitted to 15–30°C (59–86°F) [See USP Controlled Room Temperature]. Protect from light.
Prescribing information as of October 2009

Mfd. for: sanofi-aventis U.S. LLC
Bridgewater, NJ 08807
Carpuject is a registered trademark of Hospira Inc.

Shown in Product Identification Guide, page 318

ANZEMET® TABLETS ℞

[*an-zĕmĕt*]
(dolasetron mesylate)

DESCRIPTION

ANZEMET (dolasetron mesylate) is an antinauseant and antiemetic agent. Chemically, dolasetron mesylate is (2α,6α,8α,9aβ)-octahydro-3-oxo-2,6-methano-2*H*-quinolizin-8-yl-1*H*-indole-3-carboxylate monomethanesulfonate, monohydrate. It is a highly specific and selective serotonin subtype 3 (5-HT_3) receptor antagonist both in vitro and in vivo.
Dolasetron mesylate has the following structural formula:

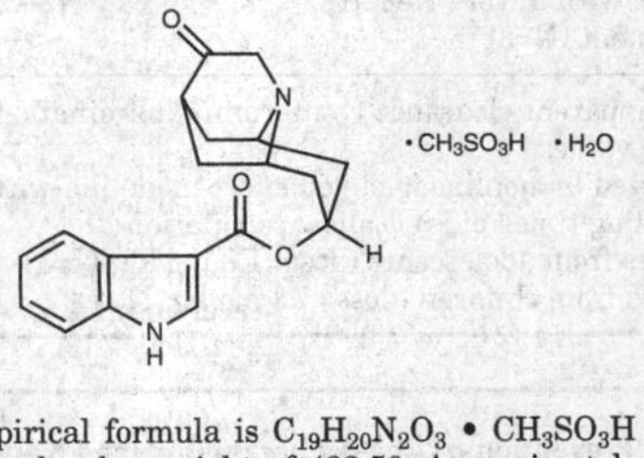

The empirical formula is $C_{19}H_{20}N_2O_3 \bullet CH_3SO_3H \bullet H_2O$, with a molecular weight of 438.50. Approximately 74% of dolasetron mesylate monohydrate is dolasetron base.
Dolasetron mesylate monohydrate is a white to off-white powder that is freely soluble in water and propylene glycol, slightly soluble in ethanol, and slightly soluble in normal saline.
Each ANZEMET Tablet for oral administration contains dolasetron mesylate (as the monohydrate) and also contains the inactive ingredients: carnauba wax, croscarmellose sodium, hypromellose, lactose, magnesium stearate, polyethylene glycol, polysorbate 80, pregelatinized starch, synthetic red iron oxide, titanium dioxide, and white wax. The tablets are printed with black ink, which contains lecithin, pharmaceutical glaze, propylene glycol, and synthetic black iron oxide.

CLINICAL PHARMACOLOGY

Dolasetron mesylate and its active metabolite, hydrodolasetron (MDL 74,156), are selective serotonin 5-HT_3 receptor antagonists not shown to have activity at other known serotonin receptors and with low affinity for dopamine receptors. The serotonin 5-HT_3 receptors are located on the nerve terminals of the vagus in the periphery and centrally in the chemoreceptor trigger zone of the area postrema. It is thought that chemotherapeutic agents produce nausea and vomiting by releasing serotonin from the enterochromaffin cells of the small intestine, and that the released serotonin then activates 5-HT_3 receptors located on vagal efferents to initiate the vomiting reflex.
Acute, usually reversible, ECG changes (PR and QT_c prolongation; QRS widening), caused by dolasetron mesylate, have been observed in healthy volunteers and in controlled clinical trials. The active metabolites of dolasetron may block sodium channels, a property unrelated to its ability to block 5-HT_3 receptors. QT_c prolongation is primarily due to QRS widening. Dolasetron appears to prolong both depolarization and, to a lesser extent, repolarization time. The magnitude and frequency of the ECG changes increased with dose (related to peak plasma concentrations of hydrodolasetron but not the parent compound). These ECG interval prolongations usually returned to baseline within 6 to 8 hours, but in some patients were present at 24 hour follow up. Dolasetron mesylate administration has little or no effect on blood pressure.
In healthy volunteers (N=64), dolasetron mesylate in single intravenous doses up to 5 mg/kg produced no effect on pupil size or meaningful changes in EEG tracings. Results from neuropsychiatric tests revealed that dolasetron mesylate did not alter mood or concentration. Multiple daily doses of dolasetron have had no effect on colonic transit in humans. Dolasetron has no effect on plasma prolactin concentrations.

Pharmacokinetics in Humans

Oral dolasetron is well absorbed, although parent drug is rarely detected in plasma due to rapid and complete metabolism to the most clinically relevant species, hydrodolasetron.
The reduction of dolasetron to hydrodolasetron is mediated by a ubiquitous enzyme, carbonyl reductase. Cytochrome P-450 (CYP)2D6 is primarily responsible for the subsequent hydroxylation of hydrodolasetron and both CYP3A and flavin monooxygenase are responsible for the N-oxidation of hydrodolasetron.

Table 1. Pharmacokinetic Values for Plasma Hydrodolasetron Following Oral Administration of ANZEMET*

	Age (years)	Dose	CL_{app} (mL/min/kg)	$t_{1/2}$ (h)	C_{max} (ng/mL)
Young Healthy Volunteers (N=30)	19–45	200 mg	13.4 (29%)	8.1 (18%)	556 (28%)
Elderly Healthy Volunteers (N=15)	65–75	2.4 mg/kg	9.5 (36%)	7.2 (32%)	662 (28%)
Cancer Patients					
Adults (N=61)[†]	24–84	25–200 mg	12.9 (49%)	7.9 (43%)	- -[‡]
Adolescents (N=13)	12–17	0.6–1.8 mg/kg	26.5 (67%)	6.4 (30%)	374[§] (32%)
Children (N=19)	3–11	0.6–1.8 mg/kg	44.2 (49%)	5.5 (39%)	217[¶] (67%)
Pediatric Surgery Patients (N=11)	2–12	1.2 mg/kg	20.8 (49%)	5.9 (24%)	159 (32%)
Patients with Severe Renal Impairment (N=12 (Creatinine clearance ≤10 mL/min)	28–74	200 mg	7.2 (48%)	10.7 (29%)	701 (21%)
Patients with Severe Hepatic Impairment (N=3)	42–52	150 mg	8.8 (57%)	11.0 (36%)	410 (12%)

CL_{app}: apparent clearance $t_{1/2}$: terminal elimination half-life ( ): coefficient of variation in %
* mean values
† analyzed by nonlinear mixed effect modeling with data pooled across dose strengths
‡ sampling times did not allow calculation
§ results from adolescents (dose=1.8 mg/kg, N=3)
¶ results from children (dose=1.8 mg/kg, N=7)

Table 2. Prevention of Chemotherapy-Induced Nausea and Vomiting from Moderately Emetogenic Chemotherapy

	ANZEMET Tablets				
Response Over 24 Hours	25 mg (N=78)	50 mg (N=83)	100 mg* (N=80)	200 mg (N=78)	*p*-value for Linear Trend
Complete Response[†]	24 (31%)	34 (41%)	49 (61%)	46 (59%)	P<.0001
Nausea Score[‡]	49	10	11	7	P=.0006

* The recommended dose
† No emetic episodes and no rescue medication.
‡ Median 24-h change from baseline nausea score using visual analog scale (VAS): Score range 0="none" to 100="nausea as bad as it could be."

Table 3. Prevention of Postoperative Nausea and Vomiting

	ANZEMET Tablets				
Response Over 24 Hours	25 mg (N=159)	50 mg (N=166)	100 mg* (N=154)	200 mg (N=154)	Placebo (N=156)
Complete Response[†]	71 (45%)	95 (57%)[‡]	78 (51%)[‡]	73 (47%)[‡]	55 (35%)
Nausea Score[§]	5[‡]	4[‡]	5[‡]	6[‡]	15

* The recommended dose
† No emetic episodes and no rescue medication.
‡ *p*<.05 vs placebo
§ Median 24-h change from baseline nausea score using visual analog scale (VAS): Score range 0="none" to 100="nausea as bad as it could be."

Hydrodolasetron is excreted in the urine unchanged (61.0% of administered oral dose). Other urinary metabolites include hydroxylated glucuronides and N-oxide.

Hydrodolasetron appears rapidly in plasma, with a maximum concentration occurring approximately 1 hour after dosing, and is eliminated with a mean half-life of 8.1 hours (%CV=18%) and an apparent clearance of 13.4 mL/min/kg (%CV=29%) in 30 adults. The apparent absolute bioavailability of oral dolasetron, determined by the major active metabolite hydrodolasetron, is approximately 75%. Orally administered dolasetron intravenous solution and tablets are bioequivalent. Food does not affect the bioavailability of dolasetron taken by mouth.

Hydrodolasetron is eliminated by multiple routes, including renal excretion and, after metabolism, mainly, glucuronidation and hydroxylation. Two thirds of the administered dose is recovered in the urine and one third in the feces. Hydrodolasetron is widely distributed in the body with a mean apparent volume of distribution of 5.8 L/kg (%CV=25%, N=24) in adults.

Sixty-nine to 77% of hydrodolasetron is bound to plasma protein. In a study with ^{14}C labeled dolasetron, the distribution of radioactivity to blood cells was not extensive. Approximately 50% of hydrodolasetron is bound to α_1-acid glycoprotein. The pharmacokinetics of hydrodolasetron are linear and similar in men and women.

The pharmacokinetics of hydrodolasetron, in special and targeted patient populations following oral administration of dolasetron, are summarized in Table 1. The pharmacokinetics of hydrodolasetron are similar in adult (young and elderly) healthy volunteers and in adult cancer patients receiving chemotherapeutic agents. The apparent clearance following oral administration of hydrodolasetron is approximately 1.6- to 3.4-fold higher in children and adolescents than in adults. The clearance following oral administration of hydrodolasetron is not affected by age in adult cancer patients. The apparent oral clearance of hydrodolasetron decreases 42% with severe hepatic impairment and 44% with severe renal impairment. No dose adjustment is necessary for elderly patients (see PRECAUTIONS, Geriatric Use) or for patients with hepatic or renal impairment.

The pharmacokinetics of ANZEMET Tablets have not been studied in the pediatric population. However, the following pharmacokinetic data are available on intravenous ANZEMET Injection administered orally to children. Thirty-two pediatric cancer patients ages 3 to 11 years (N=19) and 12 to 17 years (N=13), received 0.6, 1.2, or 1.8 mg/kg ANZEMET Injection diluted with either apple or apple-grape juice and administered orally. In this study, the mean apparent clearances of hydrodolasetron were 3 times greater in the younger pediatric group and 1.8 times greater in the older pediatric group than those observed in healthy adult volunteers. Across this spectrum of pediatric patients, maximum plasma concentrations were 0.6 to 0.7 times those observed in healthy adults receiving similar doses. For 12 pediatric patients, ages 2 to 12 years receiving 1.2 mg/kg ANZEMET Injection diluted in apple or apple-grape juice and administered orally, the mean apparent clearance was 34% greater and half-life was 21% shorter than in healthy adults receiving the same dose.
[See table 1 at left]

Clinical Studies

Prevention of Cancer Chemotherapy-Induced Nausea and Vomiting

Oral ANZEMET at a dose of 100 mg prevents nausea and vomiting associated with moderately emetogenic cancer therapy as shown by 24 hour efficacy data from two double-blind studies. Efficacy was based on complete response (ie, no vomiting, no rescue medication).

The first randomized, double-blind trial compared single oral ANZEMET doses of 25, 50, 100 and 200 mg in 60 men and 259 women cancer patients receiving cyclophosphamide and/or doxorubicin. There was no statistically significant difference in complete response between the 100 mg and 200 mg dose. Results are summarized in Table 2.
[See table 2 at left]

Another trial also compared single oral ANZEMET doses of 25, 50, 100, and 200 mg in 307 patients receiving moderately emetogenic chemotherapy. In this study, the 100 mg ANZEMET dose gave a 73% complete response rate.

Prevention of Postoperative Nausea and Vomiting

ANZEMET Tablets at a dose of 100 mg administered orally 1-2 hours before surgery and before general balanced anesthesia (short-acting barbiturate, nitrous oxide, narcotic analgesic, and skeletal muscle relaxant) was significantly more effective than placebo in preventing postoperative nausea and vomiting. Efficacy was based on complete response rates (0 emetic episodes and no rescue medication over 24 hours). No increased efficacy was seen with higher doses.

One trial compared single ANZEMET Tablet doses of 25, 50, 100, and 200 mg with placebo in 789 women undergoing gynecological surgery. In this study the 100 mg dose produced a complete response rate statistically superior to placebo. The study results are summarized in Table 3.
[See table 3 at left]

Another trial also compared single oral ANZEMET doses of 25, 50, 100, and 200 mg with placebo in 373 women undergoing gynecological surgery. In this study, the 100 mg ANZEMET dose gave a 54% complete response rate as compared to the 29% rate of placebo.

INDICATIONS AND USAGE

ANZEMET Tablets are indicated for:
- **1)the prevention of nausea and vomiting associated with moderately emetogenic cancer chemotherapy, including initial and repeat courses;**
- **2)the prevention of postoperative nausea and vomiting.**

CONTRAINDICATIONS

ANZEMET Tablets are contraindicated in patients known to have hypersensitivity to the drug.

WARNINGS

ANZEMET can cause ECG interval changes (PR, QT_c, JT prolongation and QRS widening). These changes are related in magnitude and frequency to blood levels of the active metabolite. These changes are self-limiting with declining blood levels. Some patients have interval prolongations for 24 hours or longer. Interval prolongation could lead to cardiovascular consequences, including heart block or cardiac arrhythmias. These have rarely been reported.

A cardiac conduction abnormality observed on an intraoperative cardiac rhythm monitor (interpreted as complete heart block) was reported in a 61-year-old woman who received 200 mg ANZEMET for the prevention of postoperative nausea and vomiting. This patient was also taking verapamil. A similar event also interpreted as complete heart block was reported in one patient receiving placebo.

A 66-year-old man with Stage IV non-Hodgkins lymphoma died suddenly 6 hours after receiving 1.8 mg/kg (119 mg) intravenous ANZEMET Injection. This patient had other potential risk factors including substantial exposure to doxorubicin and concomitant cyclophosphamide.

Pediatric Use

Dolasetron should be administered with caution in pediatric patients who have or may develop prolongation of cardiac conduction intervals, particularly QT_c. Rare cases of sustained supraventricular and ventricular arrhythmias, cardiac arrest leading to death, and myocardial infarction have been reported in children and adolescents (See Precautions, General, and Adverse Reactions – Postmarketing Experience).

PRECAUTIONS

General

Dolasetron should be administered with caution in patients who have or may develop prolongation of cardiac

conduction intervals, particularly QT_c. These include patients with hypokalemia or hypomagnesemia, patients taking diuretics with potential for inducing electrolyte abnormalities, patients with congenital QT syndrome, patients taking anti-arrhythmic drugs or other drugs which lead to QT prolongation, and cumulative high dose anthracycline therapy.

Cross hypersensitivity reactions have been reported in patients who received other selective $5\text{-}HT_3$ receptor antagonists. These reactions have not been seen with dolasetron mesylate.

Drug Interactions

The potential for clinically significant drug-drug interactions posed by dolasetron and hydrodolasetron appears to be low for drugs commonly used in chemotherapy or surgery, because hydrodolasetron is eliminated by multiple routes. See PRECAUTIONS, General for information about potential interaction with other drugs that prolong the QT_c interval.

When oral dolasetron (200 mg once daily) was coadministered with cimetidine (300 mg four times daily) for 7 days, the systemic exposure (i.e., AUC) of hydrodolasetron increased by 24% and the maximum plasma concentration of hydrodolasetron increased by 15%. When oral dolasetron (200 mg once daily) was coadministered with rifampin (600 mg once daily) for 7 days, the systemic exposure of hydrodolasetron decreased by 28% and the maximum plasma concentration of hydrodolasetron decreased by 17%.

ANZEMET has been safely coadministered with drugs used in chemotherapy and surgery. As with other agents which prolong ECG intervals, caution should be exercised in patients taking drugs which prolong ECG intervals, particularly QT_c.

In patients taking furosemide, nifedipine, diltiazem, ACE inhibitors, verapamil, glyburide, propranolol, and various chemotherapy agents, no effect was shown on the clearance of hydrodolasetron. Clearance of hydrodolasetron decreased by about 27% when dolasetron mesylate was administered intravenously concomitantly with atenolol. ANZEMET did not influence anesthesia recovery time in patients. Dolasetron mesylate did not inhibit the antitumor activity of four chemotherapeutic agents (cisplatin, 5-fluorouracil, doxorubicin, cyclophosphamide) in four murine models.

Carcinogenesis, Mutagenesis, Impairment of Fertility

In a 24-month carcinogenicity study, there was a statistically significant (P<0.001) increase in the incidence of combined hepatocellular adenomas and carcinomas in male mice treated with 150 mg/kg/day and above. In this study, mice (CD-1) were treated orally with dolasetron mesylate 75, 150, or 300 mg/kg/day (225, 450 or 900 mg/m^2/day). For a 50 kg person of average height (1.46 m^2 body surface area), these doses represent 3, 6, and 12 times the recommended clinical dose (74 mg/m^2) on a body surface area basis. No increase in liver tumors was observed at a dose of 75 mg/kg/day in male mice and at doses up to 300 mg/kg/day in female mice.

In a 24-month rat (Sprague-Dawley) carcinogenicity study, oral dolasetron mesylate was not tumorigenic at doses up to 150 mg/kg/day (900 mg/m^2/day, 12 times the recommended human dose based on body surface area) in male rats and 300 mg/kg/day (1800 mg/m^2/day, 24 times the recommended human dose based on body surface area) in female rats.

Dolasetron mesylate was not genotoxic in the Ames test, the rat lymphocyte chromosomal aberration test, the Chinese hamster ovary (CHO) cell (HGPRT) forward mutation test, the rat hepatocyte unscheduled DNA synthesis (UDS) test or the mouse micronucleus test.

Dolasetron mesylate was found to have no effect on fertility and reproductive performance at oral doses up to 100 mg/kg/day (600 mg/m^2/day, 8 times the recommended human dose based on body surface area) in female rats and up to 400 mg/kg/day (2400 mg/m^2/day, 32 times the recommended human dose based on body surface area) in male rats.

Pregnancy

Teratogenic Effects

Pregnancy Category B

Teratology studies have not revealed evidence of impaired fertility or harm to the fetus due to dolasetron mesylate. These studies have been performed in pregnant rats at oral doses up to 100 mg/kg/day (8 times the recommended human dose based on body surface area) and pregnant rabbits at oral doses up to 100 mg/kg/day (16 times the recommended human dose based on body surface area). There are, however, no adequate and well-controlled studies in pregnant women. Because animal reproduction studies are not always predictive of human response, this drug should be used during pregnancy only if clearly needed.

Nursing Mothers

It is not known whether dolasetron mesylate is excreted in human milk. Because many drugs are excreted in human milk, caution should be exercised when ANZEMET Tablets are administered to a nursing woman.

Pediatric Use

Dolasetron should be administered with caution in pediatric patients who have or may develop prolongation of cardiac conduction intervals, particularly QT_c. Rare cases of sustained supraventricular and ventricular arrhythmias, cardiac arrest leading to death, and myocardial infarction have been reported in children and adolescents (See Warnings and Adverse Reactions – Postmarketing Experience).

ANZEMET Tablets are expected to be as safe and effective as when ANZEMET Injection is given orally to pediatric patients. ANZEMET Tablets are recommended for children old enough to swallow tablets (see CLINICAL PHARMACOLOGY, Pharmacokinetics in Humans).

Geriatric Use

Prevention of cancer chemotherapy-induced nausea and vomiting (CINV)

In controlled clinical trials in the prevention of chemotherapy-induced nausea and vomiting, 301 (29%) of 1026 patients were 65 years of age or older. Of the 301 geriatric patients in the trial, 282 received oral ANZEMET Tablets. No overall differences in safety or effectiveness were observed between geriatric and younger patients, and other reported clinical experience has not identified differences in responses between geriatric and younger patients, but greater sensitivity of some older individuals cannot be ruled out.

Prevention and treatment of post-operative nausea and vomiting (PONV)

Controlled clinical studies in the prevention and treatment of post-operative nausea and vomiting did not include sufficient numbers of patients aged 65 years or older – only 5 (0.4%) geriatric patients (all 5 received intravenous ANZEMET Injection) out of 1167 total patients participated in the controlled PONV trials – to determine whether they respond differently from the younger patients. Other reported clinical experiences have not identified differences in responses between geriatric and younger patients. In general, dose selection for an elderly patient should be cautious, usually starting at the low end of the dosing range, reflecting the greater frequency of decreased hepatic, renal, or cardiac function, and of concomitant disease or other drug therapy.

The pharmacokinetics, including clearance of oral ANZEMET Tablets, in elderly and younger patients are similar (see CLINICAL PHARMACOLOGY, Pharmacokinetics in Humans). Dosage adjustment is not needed in patients over the age of 65.

ADVERSE REACTIONS

Chemotherapy Patients

In controlled clinical trials, 943 adult cancer patients received ANZEMET Tablets. These patients were receiving concurrent chemotherapy, predominantly cyclophosphamide and doxorubicin regimens. The following adverse events were reported in ≥2% of patients receiving either ANZEMET 25 mg or ANZEMET 100 mg tablets for prevention of cancer chemotherapy induced nausea and vomiting in controlled clinical trials (Table 4).

Table 4. Adverse Events ≥2% from Chemotherapy-Induced Nausea and Vomiting Studies

	ANZEMET	
Event	25 mg (N=235)	100 mg (N=227)
Headache	42 (17.9%)	52 (22.9%)
Fatigue	6 (2.6%)	13 (5.7%)
Diarrhea	5 (2.1%)	12 (5.3%)
Bradycardia	12 (5.1%)	9 (4.0%)
Dizziness	3 (1.3%)	7 (3.1%)
Pain	0	7 (3.1%)
Tachycardia	7 (3.0%)	6 (2.6%)
Dyspepsia	7 (3.0%)	5 (2.2%)
Chills/Shivering	3 (1.3%)	5 (2.2%)

Postoperative Patients

In controlled clinical trials, 936 adult female patients have received oral ANZEMET for the prevention of postoperative nausea and vomiting. Following is a listing of all adverse events reported in ≥ 2% of patients receiving either placebo or ANZEMET for prevention of postoperative nausea and vomiting in controlled clinical trials (Table 5).

Table 5. Adverse Events ≥2% from Placebo-Controlled Postoperative Nausea and Vomiting Studies

Event	ANZEMET 100 mg (N=228)	Placebo (N=231)
Headache	16 (7.0%)	11 (4.8%)
Hypotension	12 (5.3%)	15 (6.5%)
Dizziness	10 (4.4%)	0 (0.0%)
Fever	8 (3.5%)	7 (3.0%)
Pruritus	7 (3.1%)	8 (3.5%)
Oliguria	6 (2.6%)	3 (1.3%)
Hypertension	5 (2.2%)	7 (3.0%)
Tachycardia	5 (2.2%)	2 (0.9%)

In clinical trials, the following infrequently reported adverse events, assessed by investigators as treatment-related or causality unknown, occurred following oral or intravenous administration of ANZEMET to adult patients receiving concomitant cancer chemotherapy or surgery:

Cardiovascular: Hypotension; rarely–edema, peripheral edema. The following events also occurred rarely and with a similar frequency as placebo and/or active comparator: Mobitz I AV block, chest pain, orthostatic hypotension, myocardial ischemia, syncope, severe bradycardia, and palpitations. See PRECAUTIONS section for information on potential effects on ECG.

In addition, the following asymptomatic treatment-emergent ECG changes were seen at rates less than or equal to those for active or placebo controls: bradycardia, T wave change, ST-T wave change, sinus arrhythmia, extrasystole (APCs or VPCs), poor R-wave progression, bundle branch block (left and right), nodal arrhythmia, U wave change, atrial flutter/fibrillation.

Furthermore, severe hypotension, bradycardia and syncope have been reported immediately or closely following IV administration.

Dermatologic: Rash, increased sweating.

Gastrointestinal System: Constipation, dyspepsia, abdominal pain, anorexia; rarely–pancreatitis.

Hearing, Taste and Vision: Taste perversion, abnormal vision; rarely–tinnitus, photophobia.

Hematologic: Rarely–hematuria, epistaxis, prothrombin time prolonged, PTT increased, anemia, purpura/hematoma, thrombocytopenia.

Hypersensitivity: Rarely–anaphylactic reaction, facial edema, urticaria.

Liver and Biliary System: Transient increases in AST (SGOT) and/or ALT (SGPT) values have been reported as adverse events in less than 1% of adult patients receiving ANZEMET in clinical trials. The increases did not appear to be related to dose or duration of therapy and were not associated with symptomatic hepatic disease. Similar increases were seen with patients receiving active comparator. Rarely–hyperbilirubinemia, increased GGT.

Metabolic and Nutritional: Rarely–alkaline phosphatase increased.

Musculoskeletal: Rarely–myalgia, arthralgia.

Nervous System: Flushing, vertigo, paresthesia, tremor; rarely–ataxia, twitching.

Psychiatric: Agitation, sleep disorder, depersonalization; rarely–confusion, anxiety, abnormal dreaming.

Respiratory System: Rarely–dyspnea, bronchospasm.

Urinary System: Rarely–dysuria, polyuria, acute renal failure.

Vascular (Extracardiac): Local pain or burning on IV administration; rarely–peripheral ischemia, thrombophlebitis/phlebitis.

Postmarketing Experience

There are rare reports of wide complex tachycardia or ventricular tachycardia and of ventricular fibrillation cardiac arrest following intravenous administration.

OVERDOSAGE

A 59-year-old man with metastatic melanoma and no known pre-existing cardiac conditions developed severe hypotension and dizziness 40 minutes after receiving a 15 minute intravenous infusion of 1000 mg (13 mg/kg) of dolasetron mesylate. Treatment for the overdose consisted of infusion of 500 mL of a plasma expander, dopamine, and atropine. The patient had normal sinus rhythm and prolongation of PR, QRS and QT_c intervals on an ECG recorded 2 hours after the infusion. The patient's blood pressure was normal 3 hours after the event and the ECG intervals returned to baseline on follow-up. The patient was released from the hospital 6 hours after the event.

ANZEMET®
Tablets (dolasetron mesylate)

Strength	Quantity	NDC Number	Description
50 mg	5 ct Bottle 10 ct Unit Dose Pack	0088-1202-05 0088-1202-43	Light pink, film coated, round tablet imprinted with "A" on one side and "50" on the other.
100 mg	5 ct Bottle 10 ct Unit Dose 5 ct Blister Pack	0088-1203-05 0088-1203-43 0088-1203-29	Pink, film coated, elongated oval tablet imprinted with "100" on one side and "ANZAMET" on the other.

Following a suspected overdose of ANZEMET Injection, a patient found to have second-degree or higher AV conduction block with ECG should undergo cardiac telemetry monitoring.

There is no known specific antidote for dolasetron mesylate, and patients with suspected overdose should be managed with supportive therapy. Individual doses as large as 5 mg/kg intravenously or 400 mg orally have been safely given to healthy volunteers or cancer patients.

It is not known if dolasetron mesylate is removed by hemodialysis or peritoneal dialysis.

A 7-year-old boy received 6 mg/kg of dolasetron mesylate orally before surgery. No symptoms occurred and no treatment was required.

Single intravenous doses of dolasetron mesylate at 160 mg/kg in male mice and 140 mg/kg in female mice and rats of both sexes (6.3 to 12.6 times the recommended human dose based on body surface area) were lethal. Symptoms of acute toxicity were tremors, depression and convulsions.

DOSAGE AND ADMINISTRATION
The recommended doses of ANZEMET Tablets should not be exceeded.

Prevention of Cancer Chemotherapy-Induced Nausea and Vomiting
Adults
The recommended oral dosage of ANZEMET (dolasetron mesylate) is 100 mg given within one hour before chemotherapy.
Pediatric Patients
The recommended oral dosage in pediatric patients 2 to 16 years of age is 1.8 mg/kg given within one hour before chemotherapy, up to a maximum of 100 mg. Safety and effectiveness in pediatric patients under 2 years of age have not been established.
Use in the Elderly, Renal Failure Patients, or Hepatically Impaired Patients
No dosage adjustment is recommended. (See Pharmacokinetics in Humans.)

Prevention of Postoperative Nausea and Vomiting
Adults
The recommended oral dosage of ANZEMET (dolasetron mesylate) is 100 mg within two hours before surgery.
Pediatric Patients
The recommended oral dosage in pediatric patients 2 to 16 years of age is 1.2 mg/kg given within two hours before surgery, up to a maximum of 100 mg. Safety and effectiveness in pediatric patients under 2 years of age have not been established.
Use in the Elderly, Renal Failure Patients, or Hepatically Impaired Patients
No dosage adjustment is recommended. (See Pharmacokinetics in Humans.)

HOW SUPPLIED
[See table above]
Store at controlled room temperature 20–25°C (68–77°F). Protect from light.
Prescribing Information as of October 2009
Manufactured by: Patheon Pharmaceuticals Inc.
Cincinnati, OH 45237
Manufactured for: sanofi-aventis U.S. LLC
Bridgewater, NJ 08807
©2009 sanofi-aventis U.S. LLC
Shown in Product Identification Guide, page 318

APIDRA®   ℞
[a'pĭ-dră]
insulin glulisine [rDNA origin]injection
solution for injection
APIDRA SOLOSTAR
(insulin glulisine)
injection, solution for subcutaneous use

HIGHLIGHTS OF PRESCRIBING INFORMATION
These highlights do not include all the information needed to use APIDRA safely and effectively. See full prescribing information for APIDRA.
APIDRA (insulin glulisine [rDNA origin] injection) solution for injection

APIDRA SOLOSTAR (insulin glulisine) injection, solution for subcutaneous use
Initial U.S. Approval: 2004

───────RECENT MAJOR CHANGES───────

Indications and Usage (1)	10/2008

───────INDICATIONS AND USAGE───────
APIDRA is a rapid acting human insulin analog indicated to improve glycemic control in adults and children with diabetes mellitus. (1)

───────DOSAGE AND ADMINISTRATION───────
The dosage of APIDRA must be individualized (2.1)

Subcutaneous Injection	Administer within 15 minutes before a meal or within 20 minutes after starting a meal. Use in a regimen with an intermediate or long-acting insulin. (2.1, 2.2)
Continuous Subcutaneous Infusion Pump	APIDRA must not be mixed or diluted when used in an external insulin infusion pump. (2.3)
Intravenous Infusion	Infuse intravenously (0.05 Units/mL to 1 Units/mL APIDRA in 0.9% sodium chloride using polyvinyl chloride infusion bags) only under strict medical supervision with close monitoring of blood glucose and potassium. (2.4)

───────DOSAGE FORMS AND STRENGTHS───────
APIDRA 100 units/mL (U-100) is available as: (3)
• 10 mL vials
• 3 mL cartridge system for use in OptiClik® (Insulin Delivery Device)
• 3 mL SoloStar® prefilled pen

───────CONTRAINDICATIONS───────
• Do not use during episodes of hypoglycemia (4)
• Do not use in patients with hypersensitivity to APIDRA or any of its excipients (4)

───────WARNINGS AND PRECAUTIONS───────
• Dose adjustment and monitoring: Closely monitor blood glucose in all patients treated with insulin. Change insulin regimens cautiously and only under medical supervision. (5.1)
• Hypoglycemia: Most common adverse reaction of insulin therapy and may be life-threatening (5.2)
• Allergic reactions: Severe, life-threatening, generalized allergy, including anaphylaxis, can occur with any insulin, including APIDRA (5.3)
• Hypokalemia: All insulins, including APIDRA can cause hypokalemia, which if untreated, may result in respiratory paralysis, ventricular arrhythmia, and death (5.4)
• Renal or hepatic impairment: Like all insulins, may require a reduction in the APIDRA dose (5.5)
• Mixing: APIDRA for subcutaneous injection should not be mixed with insulins other than NPH insulin. Do not mix APIDRA with any insulin for intravenous administration or for use in a continuous infusion pump (5.6)
• Pump use: Change the APIDRA in the pump reservoir every 48 hours (5.7)
• Intravenous use: Frequently monitor for hypoglycemia and hypokalemia. (5.8)

───────ADVERSE REACTIONS───────
Adverse reactions commonly associated with APIDRA include hypoglycemia, allergic reactions, injection site reactions, lipodystrophy, pruritus, and rash. (6.1)

To report SUSPECTED ADVERSE REACTIONS, contact sanofi-aventis at 1-800-633-1610 or FDA at 1-800-FDA-1088 or www.fda.gov/medwatch

───────DRUG INTERACTIONS───────
• Certain drugs affect glucose metabolism and may necessitate insulin dose adjustment (7)

• The signs of hypoglycemia may be reduced or absent in patients taking anti-adrenergic drugs (e.g., beta-blockers, clonidine, guanethidine, and reserpine). (7)

───────USE IN SPECIFIC POPULATIONS───────
• APIDRA has not been studied in children under 4 years of age (8.4)

See 17 for PATIENT COUNSELING INFORMATION and FDA-approved patient labeling

Revised: 02/2009

FULL PRESCRIBING INFORMATION: CONTENTS*

FULL PRESCRIBING INFORMATION

1 INDICATIONS AND USAGE
APIDRA is indicated to improve glycemic control in adults and children with diabetes mellitus.

2 DOSAGE AND ADMINISTRATION
2.1 Dosage considerations
APIDRA is a recombinant insulin analog that is equipotent to human insulin (i.e. one unit of APIDRA has the same glucose-lowering effect as one unit of regular human insulin) when given intravenously. When given subcutaneously, APIDRA has a more rapid onset of action and a shorter duration of action than regular human insulin.
The dosage of APIDRA must be individualized. Blood glucose monitoring is essential in all patients receiving insulin therapy.
The total daily insulin requirement may vary and is usually between 0.5 to 1 Unit/kg/day. Insulin requirements may be altered during stress, major illness, or with changes in exercise, meal patterns, or coadministered drugs.
2.2 Subcutaneous administration
APIDRA should be given within 15 minutes before a meal or within 20 minutes after starting a meal.
APIDRA given by subcutaneous injection should generally be used in regimens with an intermediate or long-acting insulin.

APIDRA should be administered by subcutaneous injection in the abdominal wall, thigh, or upper arm. Injection sites should be rotated within the same region (abdomen, thigh or upper arm) from one injection to the next to reduce the risk of lipodystrophy *[See Adverse Reactions (6.1)]*.

2.3 Continuous subcutaneous infusion (insulin pump)

APIDRA may be administered by continuous subcutaneous infusion in the abdominal wall. Do not use diluted or mixed insulins in external insulin pumps. Infusion sites should be rotated within the same region to reduce the risk of lipodystrophy *[See Adverse Reactions (6.1)]*. The initial programming of the external insulin infusion pump should be based on the total daily insulin dose of the previous regimen.

The following insulin pumps[1] have been used in APIDRA clinical trials conducted by sanofi-aventis, the manufacturer of APIDRA:

- Disetronic® H-Tron® plus V100 and D-Tron® with Disetronic catheters (Rapid™, Rapid C™, Rapid D™, and Tender™)
- MiniMed® Models 506, 507, 507c and 508 with MiniMed catheters (Sof-set Ultimate QR™, and Quick-set™).

Before using a different insulin pump with APIDRA, read the pump label to make sure the pump has been evaluated with APIDRA.

Physicians and patients should carefully evaluate information on pump use in the APIDRA prescribing information, Patient Information Leaflet, and the pump manufacturer's manual. APIDRA-specific information should be followed for in-use time, frequency of changing infusion sets, or other details specific to APIDRA usage, because APIDRA-specific information may differ from general pump manual instructions.

Based on *in vitro* studies which have shown loss of the preservative, metacresol and insulin degradation, APIDRA in the reservoir should be changed at least every 48 hours. APIDRA in clinical use should not be exposed to temperatures greater than 98.6°F (37°C). *[See Warnings and Precautions (5.7) and How Supplied/Storage and Handling (16.2)]*.

2.4 Intravenous administration

APIDRA can be administered intravenously under medical supervision for glycemic control with close monitoring of blood glucose and serum potassium to avoid hypoglycemia and hypokalemia. For intravenous use, APIDRA should be used at concentrations of 0.05 Units/mL to 1 Unit/mL insulin glulisine in infusion systems using polyvinyl chloride (PVC) bags. APIDRA has been shown to be stable only in normal saline solution (0.9% sodium chloride). Parenteral drug products should be inspected visually for particulate matter and discoloration prior to administration, whenever solution and container permit. Do not administer insulin mixtures intravenously.

3 DOSAGE FORMS AND STRENGTHS

APIDRA 100 units per mL (U-100) is available as:
- 10 mL vials
- 3 mL cartridges for use in the OptiClik® Insulin Delivery Device
- 3 mL SoloStar prefilled pen

4 CONTRAINDICATIONS

APIDRA is contraindicated:
- during episodes of hypoglycemia
- in patients who are hypersensitive to APIDRA or to any of its excipients
  When used in patients with known hypersensitivity to APIDRA or its excipients, patients may develop localized or generalized hypersensitivity reactions *[See Adverse Reactions (6.1)]*.

5 WARNINGS AND PRECAUTIONS

5.1 Dosage adjustment and monitoring

Glucose monitoring is essential for patients receiving insulin therapy. Changes to an insulin regimen should be made cautiously and only under medical supervision. Changes in insulin strength, manufacturer, type, or method of administration may result in the need for a change in insulin dose. Concomitant oral antidiabetic treatment may need to be adjusted.

As with all insulin preparations, the time course of action for APIDRA may vary in different individuals or at different times in the same individual and is dependent on many conditions, including the site of injection, local blood supply, or local temperature. Patients who change their level of physical activity or meal plan may require adjustment of insulin *dosages*.

5.2 Hypoglycemia

Hypoglycemia is the most common adverse reaction of insulin therapy, including APIDRA. The risk of hypoglycemia increases with tighter glycemic control. Patients must be educated to recognize and manage hypoglycemia. Severe hypoglycemia may lead to unconsciousness and/or convulsions and may result in temporary or permanent impairment of brain function or death. Severe hypoglycemia requiring the assistance of another person and/or parenteral

glucose infusion or glucagon administration has been observed in clinical trials with insulin, including trials with APIDRA.

The timing of hypoglycemia usually reflects the time-action profile of the administered insulin formulations. Other factors such as changes in food intake (e.g., amount of food or timing of meals), injection site, exercise, and concomitant medications may also alter the risk of hypoglycemia *[See Drug Interactions (7)]*.

As with all insulins, use caution in patients with hypoglycemia unawareness and in patients who may be predisposed to hypoglycemia (e.g., the pediatric population and patients who fast or have erratic food intake). The patient's ability to concentrate and react may be impaired as a result of hypoglycemia. This may present a risk in situations where these abilities are especially important, such as driving or operating other machinery.

Rapid changes in serum glucose levels may induce symptoms similar to hypoglycemia in persons with diabetes, regardless of the glucose value. Early warning symptoms of hypoglycemia may be different or less pronounced under certain conditions, such as longstanding diabetes, diabetic nerve disease, use of medications such as beta-blockers *[See Drug Interactions (7)]*, or intensified diabetes control. These situations may result in severe hypoglycemia (and, possibly, loss of consciousness) prior to the patient's awareness of hypoglycemia.

Intravenously administered insulin has a more rapid onset of action than subcutaneously administered insulin, requiring closer monitoring for hypoglycemia.

5.3 Hypersensitivity and allergic reactions

Severe, life-threatening, generalized allergy, including anaphylaxis, can occur with insulin products, including APIDRA *[See Adverse reactions (6.1)]*.

5.4 Hypokalemia

All insulin products, including APIDRA, cause a shift in potassium from the extracellular to intracellular space, possibly leading to hypokalemia. Untreated hypokalemia may cause respiratory paralysis, ventricular arrhythmia, and death. Use caution in patients who may be at risk for hypokalemia (e.g., patients using potassium-lowering medications, patients taking medications sensitive to serum potassium concentrations). Monitor glucose and potassium frequently when APIDRA is administered intravenously.

5.5 Renal or hepatic impairment

Frequent glucose monitoring and insulin dose reduction may be required in patients with renal or hepatic impairment *[See Clinical Pharmacology (12.4)]*.

5.6 Mixing of insulins

APIDRA for subcutaneous injection should not be mixed with insulin preparations other than NPH insulin. If APIDRA is mixed with NPH insulin, APIDRA should be drawn into the syringe first. Injection should occur immediately after mixing.

Do not mix APIDRA with other insulins for intravenous administration or for use in a continuous subcutaneous infusion pump.

APIDRA for intravenous administration should not be diluted with solutions other than 0.9% sodium chloride (normal saline). The efficacy and safety of mixing APIDRA with diluents or other insulins for use in external subcutaneous infusion pumps have not been established.

5.7 Subcutaneous insulin infusion pumps

When used in an external insulin pump for subcutaneous infusion, APIDRA should not be diluted or mixed with any other insulin. APIDRA in the reservoir should be changed at least every 48 hours. APIDRA should not be exposed to temperatures greater than 98.6°F (37°C).

Malfunction of the insulin pump or infusion set or insulin degradation can rapidly lead to hyperglycemia and ketosis. Prompt identification and correction of the cause of hyperglycemia or ketosis is necessary. Interim subcutaneous injections with APIDRA may be required. Patients using continuous subcutaneous insulin infusion pump therapy must be trained to administer insulin by injection and have alternate insulin therapy available in case of pump failure. *[See Dosage and Administration (2.3), How Supplied/ Storage and Handling (16), and Patient Counseling Information (17.2)]*.

5.8 Intravenous administration

When APIDRA is administered intravenously, glucose and potassium levels must be closely monitored to avoid potentially fatal hypoglycemia and hypokalemia.

Do not mix APIDRA with other insulins for intravenous administration. APIDRA may be diluted only in normal saline solution.

5.9 Drug interactions

Some medications may alter insulin requirements and the risk for hypoglycemia or hyperglycemia *[See Drug Interactions (7)]*.

6 ADVERSE REACTIONS

The following adverse reactions are discussed elsewhere:
- Hypoglycemia *[See Warnings and Precautions (5.2)]*
- Hypokalemia *[See Warnings and Precautions (5.4)]*

6.1 Clinical trial experience

Because clinical trials are conducted under widely varying designs, the adverse reaction rates reported in one clinical trial may not be easily compared to those rates reported in another clinical trial, and may not reflect the rates actually observed in clinical practice.

The frequencies of adverse drug reactions during APIDRA clinical trials in patients with type 1 diabetes mellitus and type 2 diabetes mellitus are listed in the tables below.

Table 1: Treatment –emergent adverse events in pooled studies of adults with type 1 diabetes (adverse events with frequency ≥ 5%)

	APIDRA, % (n=950)	All comparators*, % (n=641)
Nasopharyngitis	10.6	12.9
Hypoglycemia†	6.8	6.7
Upper respiratory tract infection	6.6	5.6
Influenza	4.0	5.0

* Insulin lispro, regular human insulin, insulin aspart
† Only severe symptomatic hypoglycemia

Table 2: Treatment –emergent adverse events in pooled studies of adults with type 2 diabetes (adverse events with frequency ≥ 5%)

	APIDRA, % (n=883)	Regular human insulin, % (n=883)
Upper respiratory tract infection	10.5	7.7
Nasopharyngitis	7.6	8.2
Edema peripheral	7.5	7.8
Influenza	6.2	4.2
Arthralgia	5.9	6.3
Hypertension	3.9	5.3

- *Pediatrics*

Table 3 summarizes the adverse reactions occurring with frequency higher than 5% in a clinical study in children and adolescents with type 1 diabetes treated with APIDRA (n=277) or insulin lispro (n=295).

Table 3: Treatment –emergent adverse events in children and adolescents with type 1 diabetes (adverse reactions with frequency ≥ 5%)

	APIDRA, % (n=277)	Lispro, % (n=295)
Nasopharyngitis	9.0	9.5
Upper respiratory tract infection	8.3	10.8
Headache	6.9	11.2
Hypoglycemic seizure	6.1	4.7

- *Severe symptomatic hypoglycemia*

Hypoglycemia is the most commonly observed adverse reaction in patients using insulin, including APIDRA *[See Warnings and Precautions (5.2)]*. The rates and incidence of severe symptomatic hypoglycemia, defined as hypoglycemia requiring intervention from a third party, were comparable for all treatment regimens (see Table 4). In the phase 3 clinical trial, children and adolescents with type 1 diabetes had a higher incidence of severe symptomatic hypoglycemia in the two treatment groups compared to adults with type 1 diabetes. (see Table 4) *[See Clinical Studies (14)]*.

[See table 4 at top of next page]

- *Insulin initiation and intensification of glucose control*

Intensification or rapid improvement in glucose control has been associated with a transitory, reversible ophthalmologic refraction disorder, worsening of diabetic retinopathy, and acute painful peripheral neuropathy. However, long-term glycemic control decreases the risk of diabetic retinopathy and neuropathy.

Table 4: Severe Symptomatic Hypoglycemia*

	Type 1 Diabetes Adults 12 weeks with insulin glargine			Type 1 Diabetes Adults 26 weeks with insulin glargine		Type 2 Diabetes Adults 26 weeks with NPH human insulin		Type 1 Diabetes Pediatrics 26 weeks	
	APIDRA Pre-meal	APIDRA Post-meal	Regular Human Insulin	APIDRA	Insulin Lispro	APIDRA	Regular Human Insulin	APIDRA	Insulin Lispro
Events per month per patient	0.05	0.05	0.13	0.02	0.02	0.00	0.00	0.09	0.08
Percent of patients (n/total N)	8.4% (24/286)	8.4% (25/296)	10.1% (28/278)	4.8% (16/339)	4.0% (13/333)	1.4% (6/416)	1.2% (5/420)	16.2% (45/277)	19.3% (57/295)

* Severe symptomatic hypoglycemia defined as a hypoglycemic event requiring the assistance of another person that met one of the following criteria:
the event was associated with a whole blood referenced blood glucose <36mg/dL or the event was associated with prompt recovery after oral carbohydrate, intravenous glucose or glucagon administration.

• *Lipodystrophy*
Long-term use of insulin, including APIDRA, can cause lipodystrophy at the site of repeated insulin injections or infusion. Lipodystrophy includes lipohypertrophy (thickening of adipose tissue) and lipoatrophy (thinning of adipose tissue), and may affect insulin absorption. Rotate insulin injection or infusion sites within the same region to reduce the risk of lipodystrophy. *[See Dosage and Administration (2.2, 2.3)].*

• *Weight gain*
Weight gain can occur with insulin therapy, including APIDRA, and has been attributed to the anabolic effects of insulin and the decrease in glucosuria.

• *Peripheral Edema*
Insulin, including APIDRA, may cause sodium retention and edema, particularly if previously poor metabolic control is improved by intensified insulin therapy.

• *Adverse Reactions with Continuous Subcutaneous Insulin Infusion (CSII)*
In a 12-week randomized study in patients with type 1 diabetes (n=59), the rates of catheter occlusions and infusion site reactions were similar for APIDRA and insulin aspart treated patients (Table 5).

Table 5: Catheter Occlusions and Infusion Site Reactions.

	APIDRA (n=29)	insulin aspart (n=30)
Catheter occlusions/month	0.08	0.15
Infusion site reactions	10.3% (3/29)	13.3% (4/30)

• *Allergic Reactions*
Local Allergy
As with any insulin therapy, patients taking APIDRA may experience redness, swelling, or itching at the site of injection. These minor reactions usually resolve in a few days to a few weeks, but in some occasions may require discontinuation of APIDRA. In some instances, these reactions may be related to factors other than insulin, such as irritants in a skin cleansing agent or poor injection technique.
Systemic Allergy
Severe, life-threatening, generalized allergy, including anaphylaxis, may occur with any insulin, including APIDRA. Generalized allergy to insulin may cause whole body rash (including pruritus), dyspnea, wheezing, hypotension, tachycardia, or diaphoresis.
In controlled clinical trials up to 12 months duration, potential systemic allergic reactions were reported in 79 of 1833 patients (4.3%) who received APIDRA and 58 of 1524 patients (3.8%) who received the comparator short-acting insulins. During these trials treatment with APIDRA was permanently discontinued in 1 of 1833 patients due to a potential systemic allergic reaction.
Localized reactions and generalized myalgias have been reported with the use of metacresol, which is an excipient of APIDRA.
Antibody Production
In a study in patients with type 1 diabetes (n=333), the concentrations of insulin antibodies that react with both human insulin and insulin glulisine (cross-reactive insulin antibodies) remained near baseline during the first 6 months of the study in the patients treated with APIDRA. A decrease in antibody concentration was observed during the following 6 months of the study. In a study in patients with type 2 diabetes (n=411), a similar increase in cross-reactive insulin antibody concentration was observed in the patients

treated with APIDRA and in the patients treated with human insulin during the first 9 months of the study. Thereafter the concentration of antibodies decreased in the APIDRA patients and remained stable in the human insulin patients. There was no correlation between cross-reactive insulin antibody concentration and changes in HbA1c, insulin doses, or incidence of hypoglycemia. The clinical significance of these antibodies is not known.
APIDRA did not elicit a significant antibody response in a study of children and adolescents with type 1 diabetes.

6.2   Postmarketing experience
The following adverse reactions have been identified during post-approval use of APIDRA.
Because these reactions are reported voluntarily from a population of uncertain size, it is not always possible to estimate reliably their frequency or establish a causal relationship to drug exposure.
Medication errors have been reported in which other insulins, particularly long-acting insulins, have been accidentally administered instead of APIDRA *[See Patient Counseling Information (17)].*

7   DRUG INTERACTIONS
A number of drugs affect glucose metabolism and may necessitate insulin dose adjustment and particularly close monitoring.
Drugs that may increase the blood glucose-lowering effect of insulins including APIDRA, and therefore increase the risk of hypoglycemia, include oral antidiabetic products, pramlintide, ACE inhibitors, disopyramide, fibrates, fluoxetine, monoamine oxidase inhibitors, propoxyphene, pentoxifylline, salicylates, somatostatin analogs, and sulfonamide antibiotics.
Drugs that may reduce the blood-glucose-lowering effect of APIDRA include corticosteroids, niacin, danazol, diuretics, sympathomimetic agents (e.g., epinephrine, albuterol, terbutaline), glucagon, isoniazid, phenothiazine derivatives, somatropin, thyroid hormones, estrogens, progestogens (e.g., in oral contraceptives), protease inhibitors, and atypical antipsychotics.
Beta-blockers, clonidine, lithium salts, and alcohol may either increase or decrease the blood-glucose-lowering effect of insulin.
Pentamidine may cause hypoglycemia, which may sometimes be followed by hyperglycemia.
The signs of hypoglycemia may be reduced or absent in patients taking anti-adrenergic drugs such as beta-blockers, clonidine, guanethidine, and reserpine.

8   USE IN SPECIFIC POPULATIONS
8.1   Pregnancy
Pregnancy Category C: Reproduction and teratology studies have been performed with insulin glulisine in rats and rabbits using regular human insulin as a comparator. Insulin glulisine was given to female rats throughout pregnancy at subcutaneous doses up to 10 Units/kg once daily (dose resulting in an exposure 2 times the average human dose, based on body surface area comparison) and did not have any remarkable toxic effects on embryo-fetal development.
Insulin glulisine was given to female rabbits throughout pregnancy at subcutaneous doses up to 1.5 Units/kg/day (dose resulting in an exposure 0.5 times the average human dose, based on body surface area comparison). Adverse effects on embryo-fetal development were only seen at maternal toxic dose levels inducing hypoglycemia. Increased incidence of post-implantation losses and skeletal defects were observed at a dose level of 1.5 Units/kg once daily (dose resulting in an exposure 0.5 times the average human dose, based on body surface area comparison) that also caused

mortality in dams. A slight increased incidence of post-implantation losses was seen at the next lower dose level of 0.5 Units/kg once daily (dose resulting in an exposure 0.2 times the average human dose, based on body surface area comparison) which was also associated with severe hypoglycemia but there were no defects at that dose. No effects were observed in rabbits at a dose of 0.25 Units/kg once daily (dose resulting in an exposure 0.1 times the average human dose, based on body surface area comparison). The effects of insulin glulisine did not differ from those observed with subcutaneous regular human insulin at the same doses and were attributed to secondary effects of maternal hypoglycemia.
There are no well-controlled clinical studies of the use of APIDRA in pregnant women. Because animal reproduction studies are not always predictive of human response, this drug should be used during pregnancy only if the potential benefit justifies the potential risk to the fetus. It is essential for patients with diabetes or a history of gestational diabetes to maintain good metabolic control before conception and throughout pregnancy. Insulin requirements may decrease during the first trimester, generally increase during the second and third trimesters, and rapidly decline after delivery. Careful monitoring of glucose control is essential in these patients.

8.3   Nursing mothers
It is unknown whether insulin glulisine is excreted in human milk. Because many drugs are excreted in human milk, caution should be exercised when APIDRA is administered to a nursing woman. Use of APIDRA is compatible with breastfeeding, but women with diabetes who are lactating may require adjustments of their insulin doses.

8.4   Pediatric use
The safety and effectiveness of subcutaneous injections of APIDRA have been established in pediatric patients (age 4 to 17 years) with type 1 diabetes *[See Clinical Studies (14.4)].* APIDRA has not been studied in pediatric patients with type 1 diabetes younger than 4 years of age and in pediatric patients with type 2 diabetes.
As in adults, the dosage of APIDRA must be individualized in pediatric patients based on metabolic needs and frequent monitoring of blood glucose.

8.5   Geriatric use
In clinical trials (n=2408), APIDRA was administered to 147 patients ≥65 years of age and 27 patients ≥75 years of age. The majority of this small subset of elderly patients had type 2 diabetes. The change in HbA1c values and hypoglycemia frequencies did not differ by age. Nevertheless, caution should be exercised when APIDRA is administered to geriatric patients.

10   OVERDOSAGE
Excess insulin may cause hypoglycemia and, particularly when given intravenously, hypokalemia. Mild episodes of hypoglycemia usually can be treated with oral glucose. Adjustments in drug dosage, meal patterns, or exercise may be needed. More severe episodes of hypoglycemia with coma, seizure, or neurologic impairment may be treated with intramuscular/subcutaneous glucagon or concentrated intravenous glucose. Sustained carbohydrate intake and observation may be necessary because hypoglycemia may recur after apparent clinical recovery. Hypokalemia must be corrected appropriately.

11   DESCRIPTION
APIDRA® (insulin glulisine [rDNA origin] injection) is a rapid-acting human insulin analog used to lower blood glucose. Insulin glulisine is produced by recombinant DNA technology utilizing a non-pathogenic laboratory strain of *Escherichia coli* (K12). Insulin glulisine differs from human insulin in that the amino acid asparagine at position B3 is replaced by lysine and the lysine in position B29 is replaced by glutamic acid. Chemically, insulin glulisine is 3^B-lysine-29^B-glutamic acid-human insulin, has the empirical formula $C_{258}H_{384}N_{64}O_{78}S_6$ and a molecular weight of 5823 and has the following structural formula:

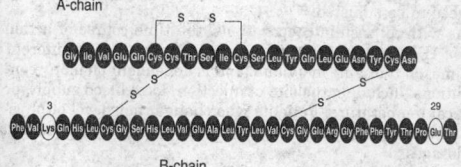

APIDRA is a sterile, aqueous, clear, and colorless solution. Each milliliter of APIDRA contains 100 units (3.49 mg) insulin glulisine, 3.15 mg metacresol, 6 mg tromethamine, 5 mg sodium chloride, 0.01 mg polysorbate 20, and water for injection. APIDRA has a pH of approximately 7.3. The pH is adjusted by addition of aqueous solutions of hydrochloric acid and/or sodium hydroxide.

12   CLINICAL PHARMACOLOGY

12.1   Mechanism of action

Regulation of glucose metabolism is the primary activity of insulins and insulin analogs, including insulin glulisine. Insulins lower blood glucose by stimulating peripheral glucose uptake by skeletal muscle and fat, and by inhibiting hepatic glucose production. Insulins inhibit lipolysis and proteolysis, and enhance protein synthesis.

The glucose lowering activities of APIDRA and of regular human insulin are equipotent when administered by the intravenous route. After subcutaneous administration, the effect of APIDRA is more rapid in onset and of shorter duration compared to regular human insulin. *[See Pharmacodynamics (12.2)].*

12.2   Pharmacodynamics

Studies in healthy volunteers and patients with diabetes demonstrated that APIDRA has a more rapid onset of action and a shorter duration of activity than regular human insulin when given subcutaneously.

In a study in patients with type 1 diabetes (n= 20), the glucose-lowering profiles of APIDRA and regular human insulin were assessed at various times in relation to a standard meal at a dose of 0.15 Units/kg. (Figure 1.)

The maximum blood glucose excursion (ΔGLU_{max}; baseline subtracted glucose concentration) for APIDRA injected 2 minutes before a meal was 65 mg/dL compared to 64 mg/dL for regular human insulin injected 30 minutes before a meal (see Figure 1A), and 84 mg/dL for regular human insulin injected 2 minutes before a meal (see Figure 1B). The maximum blood glucose excursion for APIDRA injected 15 minutes after the start of a meal was 85 mg/dL compared to 84 mg/dL for regular human insulin injected 2 minutes before a meal (see Figure 1C).

Figure 1. Serial mean blood glucose collected up to 6 hours following a single dose of APIDRA and regular human insulin. APIDRA given 2 minutes (APIDRA - pre) before the start of a meal compared to regular human insulin given 30 minutes (Regular - 30 min) before start of the meal (Figure 1A) and compared to regular human insulin (Regular - pre) given 2 minutes before a meal (Figure 1B). APIDRA given 15 minutes (APIDRA - post) after start of a meal compared to regular human insulin (Regular - pre) given 2 minutes before a meal (Figure 1C). On the x-axis zero (0) is the start of a 15-minute meal.

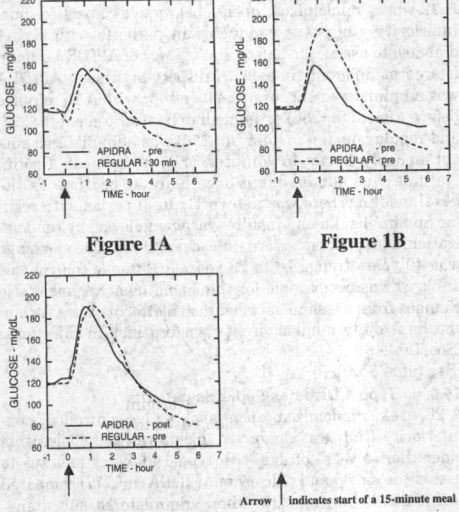

Figure 1A   **Figure 1B**

Figure 1C

Arrow ↑ indicates start of a 15-minute meal

In a randomized, open-label, two-way crossover study, 16 healthy male subjects received an intravenous infusion of APIDRA or regular human insulin with saline diluent at a rate of 0.8 milliUnits/kg/min for two hours. Infusion of the same dose of APIDRA or regular human insulin produced equivalent glucose disposal at steady state.

12.3   Pharmacokinetics

Absorption and bioavailability

Pharmacokinetic profiles in healthy volunteers and patients with diabetes (type 1 or type 2) demonstrated that absorption of insulin glulisine was faster than that of regular human insulin.

In a study in patients with type 1 *diabetes (n=20) after subcutaneous administration of 0.15 Units/kg, the median time to maximum concentration (T_{max}) was 60 minutes (range 40 to 120 minutes) and the peak concentration (C_{max}) was 83 microUnits/mL (range 40 to 131 microUnits/mL) for insulin glulisine compared to a median T_{max} of 120 minutes (range 60 to 239 minutes) and a C_{max} of 50 microUnits/mL (range 35 to 71 microUnits/mL) for regular human insulin. (Figure 2)

Figure 2. Pharmacokinetic profiles of insulin glulisine and regular human insulin in patients with type 1 diabetes after a dose of 0.15 Units/kg.

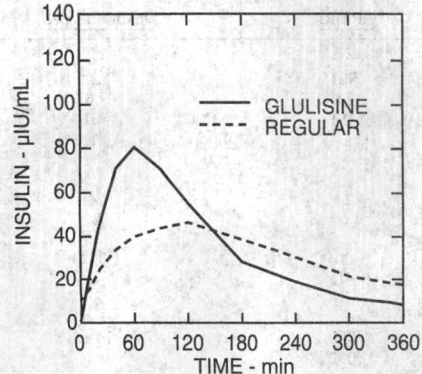

Insulin glulisine and regular human insulin were administered subcutaneously at a dose of 0.2 Units/kg in an euglycemic clamp study in patients with type 2 diabetes (n=24) and a body mass index (BMI) between 20 and 36 kg/m². The median time to maximum concentration (T_{max}) was 100 minutes (range 40 to 120 minutes) and the median peak concentration (C_{max}) was 84 microUnits/mL (range 53 to 165 microUnits/mL) for insulin glulisine compared to a median T_{max} of 240 minutes (range 80 to 360 minutes) and a median C_{max} of 41 microUnits/mL (range 33 to 61 microUnits/mL) for regular human insulin. (Figure 3.)

Figure 3. Pharmacokinetic profiles of insulin glulisine and regular human insulin in patients with type 2 diabetes after a subcutaneous dose of 0.2 Units/kg.

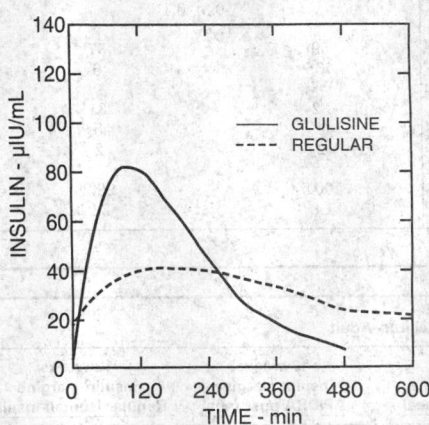

When APIDRA was injected subcutaneously into different areas of the body, the time-concentration profiles were similar. The absolute bioavailability of insulin glulisine after subcutaneous administration is approximately 70%, regardless of injection area (abdomen 73%, deltoid 71%, thigh 68%).

In a clinical study in healthy volunteers (n=32) the total insulin glulisine bioavailability was similar after subcutaneous injection of insulin glulisine and NPH insulin (premixed in the syringe) and following separate simultaneous subcutaneous injections. There was 27% attenuation of the maximum concentration (C_{max}) of APIDRA after premixing; however, the time to maximum concentration (T_{max}) was not affected. No data are available on mixing APIDRA with insulin preparations other than NPH insulin. *[See Clinical Studies (14)].*

Distribution and elimination

The distribution and elimination of insulin glulisine and regular human insulin after intravenous administration are similar with volumes of distribution of 13 and 21 L and half-lives of 13 and 17 minutes, respectively. After subcutaneous administration, insulin glulisine is eliminated more rapidly than regular human insulin with an apparent half-life of 42 minutes compared to 86 minutes.

12.4   Clinical pharmacology in specific populations

Pediatric patients

The pharmacokinetic and pharmacodynamic properties of APIDRA and regular human insulin were assessed in a study conducted in children 7 to 11 years old (n=10) and adolescents 12 to 16 years old (n=10) with type 1 diabetes. The relative differences in pharmacokinetics and pharmacodynamics between APIDRA and regular human insulin in these patients with type 1 diabetes were similar to those in healthy adult subjects and adults with type 1 diabetes.

Race

A study in 24 healthy Caucasians and Japanese subjects compared the pharmacokinetics and pharmacodynamics after subcutaneous injection of insulin glulisine, insulin lispro, and regular human insulin. With subcutaneous injection of insulin glulisine, Japanese subjects had a greater initial exposure (33%) for the ratio of $AUC_{(0-1h)}$ to $AUC_{(0-clamp\ end)}$ than Caucasians (21%) although the total exposures were similar. There were similar findings with insulin lispro and regular human insulin.

Obesity

Insulin glulisine and regular human insulin were administered subcutaneously at a dose of 0.3 Units/kg in a euglycemic clamp study in obese, non-diabetic subjects (n=18) with a body mass index (BMI) between 30 and 40 kg/m². The median time to maximum concentration (T_{max}) was 85 minutes (range 49 to 150 minutes) and the median peak concentration (C_{max}) was 192 microUnits/mL (range 98 to 380 microUnits/mL) for insulin glulisine compared to a median T_{max} of 150 minutes (range 90 to 240 minutes) and a median C_{max} of 86 microUnits/mL (range 43 to 175 microUnits/mL) for regular human insulin.

The more rapid onset of action and shorter duration of activity of APIDRA and insulin lispro compared to regular human insulin were maintained in an obese non-diabetic population (n= 18). (Figure 4.)

Figure 4. Glucose infusion rates (GIR) in a euglycemic clamp study after subcutaneous injection of 0.3 Units/kg of APIDRA, insulin lispro or regular human insulin in an obese population.

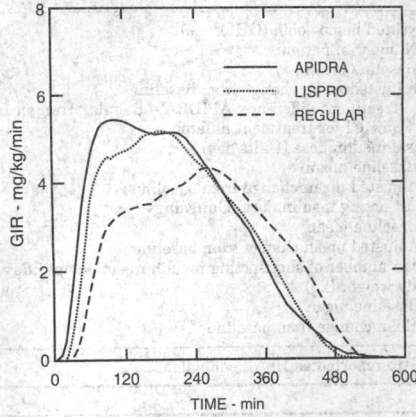

Renal impairment

Studies with human insulin have shown increased circulating levels of insulin in patients with renal failure. In a study performed in 24 non-diabetic subjects with normal renal function (Cl_{Cr} >80 mL/min), moderate renal impairment (30–50 mL/min) and severe renal impairment (<30 mL/min), the subjects with moderate and severe renal impairment had increased exposure to insulin glulisine by 29% to 40% and reduced clearance of insulin glulisine by 20% to 25% compared to subjects with normal renal function. *[See Warnings and Precautions (5.4)].*

Hepatic impairment

The effect of hepatic impairment on the pharmacokinetics and pharmacodynamics of APIDRA has not been studied. Some studies with human insulin have shown increased circulating levels of insulin in patients with liver failure. *[See Warnings and Precautions (5.4)].*

Gender

The effect of gender on the pharmacokinetics and pharmacodynamics of APIDRA has not been studied.

Pregnancy

The effect of pregnancy on the pharmacokinetics and pharmacodynamics of APIDRA has not been studied.

Smoking

The effect of smoking on the pharmacokinetics and pharmacodynamics of APIDRA has not been studied.

13   NONCLINICAL TOXICOLOGY

13.1   Carcinogenesis, mutagenesis, impairment of fertility

Standard 2-year carcinogenicity studies in animals have not been performed. In Sprague Dawley rats, a 12-month repeat dose toxicity study was conducted with insulin glulisine at subcutaneous doses of 2.5, 5, 20 or 50 Units/kg twice daily (dose resulting in an exposure 1, 2, 8, and 20 times the average human dose, based on body surface area comparison). There was a non-dose dependent higher incidence of mammary gland tumors in female rats administered insulin glulisine compared to untreated controls. The incidence of

Table 6: Type 1 Diabetes Mellitus–Adult

Treatment duration Treatment in combination with:	26 weeks Insulin glargine	
	APIDRA	Insulin Lispro
Glycated hemoglobin (GHb)* (%)		
Number of patients	331	322
Baseline mean	7.6	7.6
Adjusted mean change from baseline	-0.1	-0.1
Treatment difference: APIDRA – Insulin Lispro	0.0	
95% CI for treatment difference	(-0.1; 0.1)	
Basal insulin dose (Units/day)		
Baseline mean	24	24
Adjusted mean change from baseline	0	2
Short-acting insulin dose (Units/day)		
Baseline mean	30	31
Adjusted mean change from baseline	-1	-1
Mean number of short-acting insulin injections per day	3	3
Body weight (kg)		
Baseline mean	73.9	74.1
Mean change from baseline	0.6	0.3

* GHb reported as HbA_{1c} equivalent

Table 7: Type 2 Diabetes Mellitus–Adult

Treatment duration Treatment in combination with:	26 weeks NPH human insulin	
	APIDRA	Regular Human Insulin
Glycated hemoglobin (GHb)* (%)		
Number of patients	404	403
Baseline mean	7.6	7.5
Adjusted mean change from baseline	-0.5	-0.3
Treatment difference: APIDRA – Regular Human Insulin	-0.2	
95% CI for treatment difference	(-0.3; -0.1)	
Basal insulin dose (Units/day)		
Baseline mean	59	57
Adjusted mean change from baseline	6	6
Short-acting insulin dose (Units/day)		
Baseline mean	32	31
Adjusted mean change from baseline	4	5
Mean number of short-acting insulin injections per day	2	2
Body weight (kg)		
Baseline mean	100.5	99.2
Mean change from baseline	1.8	2.0

* GHb reported as HbA_{1c} equivalent

Table 8: Pre- and Post-Meal Administration in Type 1 Diabetes Mellitus–Adult

Treatment duration Treatment in combination with:	12 weeks insulin glargine APIDRA pre meal	12 weeks insulin glargine APIDRA post meal	12 weeks insulin glargine Regular Human Insulin
Glycated hemoglobin (GHb)* (%)			
Number of patients	268	276	257
Baseline mean	7.7	7.7	7.6
Adjusted mean change from baseline†	-0.3	-0.1	-0.1
Basal insulin dose (Units/day)			
Baseline mean	29	29	28
Adjusted mean change from baseline	1	0	1
Short-acting insulin dose (Units/day)			
Baseline mean	29	29	27
Adjusted mean change from baseline	-1	-1	2
Mean number of short-acting insulin injections per day	3	3	3
Body weight (kg)			
Baseline mean	79.2	80.3	78.9
Mean change from baseline	0.3	-0.3	0.3

* GHb reported as HbA_{1c} equivalent
† Adjusted mean change from baseline treatment difference (98.33% CI for treatment difference):
  APIDRA pre meal vs. Regular Human Insulin - 0.1 (-0.3; 0.0)
  APIDRA post meal vs. Regular Human Insulin 0.0 (-0.1; 0.2)
  APIDRA post meal vs. pre meal 0.2 (0.0; 0.3)

14.1 Type 1 Diabetes-Adults

A 26-week, randomized, open-label, active-controlled, non-inferiority study was conducted in patients with type 1 diabetes to assess the safety and efficacy of APIDRA (n= 339) compared to insulin lispro (n= 333) when administered subcutaneously within 15 minutes before a meal. Insulin glargine was administered once daily in the evening as the basal insulin. There was a 4-week run-in period with insulin lispro and insulin glargine prior to randomization. Most patients were Caucasian (97%). Fifty eight percent of the patients were men. The mean age was 39 years (range 18 to 74 years). Glycemic control, the number of daily short-acting insulin injections and the total daily doses of APIDRA and insulin lispro were similar in the two treatment groups (Table 6).
[See table 6 at left]

14.2 Type 2 Diabetes-Adults

A 26-week, randomized, open-label, active-controlled, non-inferiority study was conducted in insulin-treated patients with type 2 diabetes to assess the safety and efficacy of APIDRA (n= 435) given within 15 minutes before a meal compared to regular human insulin (n=441) administered 30 to 45 minutes prior to a meal. NPH human insulin was given twice a day as the basal insulin. All patients participated in a 4-week run-in period with regular human insulin and NPH human insulin. Eighty-five percent of patients were Caucasian and 11% were Black. The mean age was 58 years (range 26 to 84 years). The average body mass index (BMI) was 34.6 kg/m². At randomization, 58% of the patients were taking an oral antidiabetic agent. These patients were instructed to continue use of their oral antidiabetic agent at the same dose throughout the trial. The majority of patients (79%) mixed their short-acting insulin with NPH human insulin immediately prior to injection. The reductions from baseline in GHb were similar between the 2 treatment groups (see Table 7). No differences between APIDRA and regular human insulin groups were seen in the number of daily short-acting insulin injections or basal or short-acting insulin doses. (See Table 7.)
[See table 7 at left]

14.3 Type 1 Diabetes-Adults: Pre- and post-meal administration

A 12-week, randomized, open-label, active-controlled, non-inferiority study was conducted in patients with type 1 diabetes to assess the safety and efficacy of APIDRA administered at different times with respect to a meal. APIDRA was administered subcutaneously either within 15 minutes before a meal (n=286) or immediately after a meal (n=296) and regular human insulin (n= 278) was administered subcutaneously 30 to 45 minutes prior to a meal. Insulin glargine was administered once daily at bedtime as the basal insulin. There was a 4-week run-in period with regular human insulin and insulin glargine followed by randomization. Most patients were Caucasian (94%). The mean age was 40 years (range 18 to 73 years). Glycemic control (see Table 8) was comparable for the 3 treatment regimens. No changes from baseline between the treatments were seen in the total daily number of short-acting insulin injections. (See Table 8.)
[See table 8 at left]

14.4 Type 1 Diabetes-Pediatric patients

A 26-week, randomized, open-label, active-controlled, non-inferiority study was conducted in children and adolescents older than 4 years of age with type 1 diabetes mellitus to assess the safety and efficacy of APIDRA (n= 277) compared to insulin lispro (n= 295) when administered subcutaneously within 15 minutes before a meal. Patients also received insulin glargine (administered once daily in the evening) or NPH insulin (administered once in the morning and once in the evening). There was a 4-week run-in period with insulin lispro and insulin glargine or NPH prior to randomization. Most patients were Caucasian (91%). Fifty percent of the patients were male. The mean age was 12.5 years (range 4 to 17 years). Mean BMI was 20.6 kg/m². Glycemic control (see Table 9) was comparable for the two treatment regimens.
[See table 9 at top of next page]

14.5 Type 1 Diabetes-Adults: Continuous subcutaneous insulin infusion

A 12-week randomized, active control study (APIDRA versus insulin aspart) conducted in adults with type 1 diabetes (APIDRA n= 29, insulin aspart n=30) evaluated the use of APIDRA in an external continuous subcutaneous insulin pump. All patients were Caucasian. The mean age was 46 years (range 21 to 73 years). The mean GHb increased from baseline to endpoint in both treatment groups (from 6.8% to 7.0% for APIDRA; from 7.1% to 7.2% for insulin aspart).

mammary tumors for insulin glulisine and regular human insulin was similar. The relevance of these findings to humans is not known. Insulin glulisine was not mutagenic in the following tests: Ames test, *in vitro* mammalian chromosome aberration test in V79 Chinese hamster cells, and *in vivo* mammalian erythrocyte micronucleus test in rats.
In fertility studies in male and female rats at subcutaneous doses up to 10 Units/kg once daily (dose resulting in an exposure 2 times the average human dose, based on body surface area comparison), no clear adverse effects on male and female fertility, or general reproductive performance of animals were observed.

14 CLINICAL STUDIES

The safety and efficacy of APIDRA was studied in adult patients with type 1 and type 2 diabetes (n =1833) and in children and adolescent patients (4 to 17 years) with type 1 diabetes (n=572). The primary efficacy parameter in these trials was glycemic control, assessed using glycated hemoglobin (GHb reported as HbA_{1c} equivalent).

16 HOW SUPPLIED/STORAGE AND HANDLING

16.1 How supplied

APIDRA 100 units per mL (U-100) is available as:

10 mL vials	NDC 0088-2500-33
3 mL cartridge system*, package of 5	NDC 0088-2500-52
3 mL SoloStar prefilled pen, package of 5	NDC 0088-2502-05

* Cartridge systems are for use only in OptiClik® (Insulin Delivery Device)

Pen needles are not included in the packs.
BD Ultra-Fine™ pen needles[1] to be used in conjunction with OptiClik are sold separately and are manufactured by Becton Dickinson and Company.
Solostar is compatible with all pen needles from Becton Dickinson and Company, Ypsomed and Owen Mumford.

16.2 Storage

Do not use after the expiration date (see carton and container).

Unopened Vial/Cartridge System/SoloStar
Unopened APIDRA vials, cartridge systems and SoloStar should be stored in a refrigerator, 36°F–46°F (2°C–8°C). Protect from light. APIDRA should not be stored in the freezer and it should not be allowed to freeze. Discard it if it has been frozen.
Unopened vials/cartridge systems/SoloStar not stored in a refrigerator must be used within 28 days.

Open (In-Use) Vial:
Opened vials, whether or not refrigerated, must be used within 28 days. If refrigeration is not possible, the open vial in use can be kept unrefrigerated for up to 28 days away from direct heat and light, as long as the temperature is not greater than 77°F (25°C).

Open (In-Use) Cartridge System:
The opened (in-use) cartridge system inserted in OptiClik® should NOT be refrigerated but should be kept below 77°F (25°C) away from direct heat and light. The opened (in-use) cartridge system must be discarded after 28 days. Do not store OptiClik®, with or without cartridge system, in a refrigerator at any time.

Open (In-Use) SoloStar prefilled pen:
The opened (in-use) SoloStar should **NOT** be refrigerated but should be kept below 77°F (25°C) away from direct heat and light. The opened (in-use) SoloStar kept at room temperature must be discarded after 28 days.

Infusion sets:
Infusion sets (reservoirs, tubing, and catheters) and the APIDRA in the reservoir should be discarded after 48 hours of use or after exposure to temperatures that exceed 98.6°F (37°C).

Intravenous use:
Infusion bags prepared as indicated under DOSAGE AND ADMINISTRATION (2.4) are stable at room temperature for 48 hours.

16.3 Preparation and handling

After dilution for intravenous use, the solution should be inspected visually for particulate matter and discoloration prior to administration. Do not use the solution if it has become cloudy or contains particles; use only if it is clear and colorless. APIDRA is not compatible with Dextrose solution and Ringers solution and, therefore, cannot be used with these solution fluids. The use of APIDRA with other solutions has not been studied and is, therefore, not recommended.
Cartridge system: If OptiClik® (the Insulin Delivery Device for APIDRA) malfunctions, APIDRA may be drawn from the cartridge system into a U-100 syringe and injected.

17 PATIENT COUNSELING INFORMATION

See FDA-approved patient labeling.

17.1 Instructions for all patients

Patients should be instructed on self-management procedures including glucose monitoring, proper injection technique, and management of hypoglycemia and hyperglycemia.
Patients must be instructed on handling of special situations such as intercurrent conditions (illness, stress, or emotional disturbances), an inadequate or skipped insulin dose, inadvertent administration of an increased insulin *dose*, inadequate food intake, and skipped meals.
Refer patients to the APIDRA Patient Information Leaflet for additional information.
Women with diabetes should be advised to inform their doctor if they are pregnant or are contemplating pregnancy.
Accidental mix-ups between APIDRA and other insulins, particularly long-acting insulins, have been reported. To avoid medication errors between APIDRA and other insulins, patients should be instructed to always check the insulin label before each injection.

Table 9: Results from a 26-week study in pediatric patients with type 1 diabetes mellitus

Number of patients Basal Insulin	APIDRA 271 NPH or insulin glargine	Lispro 291 NPH or insulin glargine
Glycated hemoglobin (GHb)* (%)		
Baseline mean	8.2	8.2
Adjusted mean change from baseline	0.1	0.2
Treatment Difference: Mean (95% confidence interval)	-0.1 (-0.2, 0.1)	
Basal insulin dose (Units/kg/day)		
Baseline mean	0.5	0.5
Mean change from baseline	0.0	0.0
Short-acting insulin dose (Units/kg/day)		
Baseline mean	0.5	0.5
Mean change from baseline	0.0	0.0
Mean number of short-acting insulin injections per day	3	3
Baseline mean body weight (kg)	51.5	50.8
Mean weight change from baseline (kg)	2.2	2.2

* GHb reported as HbA_{1c} equivalent

17.2 For patients using continuous subcutaneous insulin pumps

Patients using external pump infusion therapy should be trained appropriately.
The following insulin pumps[1] have been used in APIDRA clinical trials conducted by sanofi-aventis, the manufacturer of APIDRA:
• Disetronic® H-Tron® plus V100 and D-Tron® with Disetronic catheters (Rapid™, Rapid C™, Rapid D™, and Tender™)
• MiniMed® Models 506, 507, 507c and 508 with MiniMed catheters (Sof-set Ultimate QR™, and Quick-set™).
Before using a different insulin pump with APIDRA, read the pump label to make sure the pump has been evaluated with APIDRA.
To minimize insulin degradation, infusion set occlusion, and loss of the preservative (metacresol), the infusion sets (reservoir, tubing, and catheter) and the APIDRA in the reservoir should be replaced every 48 hours and a new infusion site should be selected. The temperature of the insulin may exceed ambient temperature when the pump housing, cover, tubing or sport case is exposed to sunlight or radiant heat. Insulin exposed to temperatures higher than 98.6°F (37°C) should be discarded. Infusion sites that are erythematous, pruritic, or thickened should be reported to the healthcare professional, and a new site selected because continued infusion may increase the skin reaction or alter the absorption of APIDRA.
Pump or infusion set malfunctions or insulin degradation can lead to rapid hyperglycemia and ketosis. This is especially pertinent for rapid-acting insulin analogs that are more rapidly absorbed through skin and have a shorter duration of action. Prompt identification and correction of the cause of hyperglycemia or ketosis is necessary. Problems include pump malfunction, infusion set occlusion, leakage, disconnection or kinking, and degraded insulin. Less commonly, hypoglycemia from pump malfunction may occur. If these problems cannot be promptly corrected, patients should resume therapy with subcutaneous insulin injection and contact their healthcare professional. *[See Dosage and Administration (2.3), Warnings and Precautions (5.7), and How Supplied/Storage and Handling (16)].*

---

[1]The brands listed are the registered trademarks of their respective owners and are not trademarks of sanofi-aventis U.S. LLC

sanofi-aventis U.S. LLC
Bridgewater, NJ 08807
©2009 sanofi-aventis U.S. LLC

PATIENT INFORMATION
APIDRA (uh PEE druh)
(insulin glulisine [recombinant DNA origin] injection) solution for injection
Read the Patient Information that comes with APIDRA before you start taking it and each time you get a refill. There may be new information. This leaflet does not take the place of talking with your healthcare provider about your diabetes or treatment. If you have questions about APIDRA or about diabetes, talk with your healthcare provider.

What is APIDRA?
APIDRA is a man-made insulin used to control high blood sugar in adults and children with diabetes mellitus.
It is not known if APIDRA is safe or effective in:
• children under age 4 with type 1 diabetes
• children with type 2 diabetes

Who should NOT take APIDRA?
Do not take APIDRA:
• when your blood sugar is too low (hypoglycemia). See the section, "What are the possible side effects of APIDRA?"

• if you are allergic to any of the ingredients in APIDRA. See the end of this leaflet for a complete list of ingredients. Ask your healthcare provider if you are not sure.

What should I tell my healthcare provider before taking APIDRA?
Medical conditions can affect your insulin needs. Tell your healthcare provider about all of your medical conditions, including if you:
• **have liver or kidney problems.**
• **are pregnant, plan to become pregnant, or are breast-feeding.** It is not known if APIDRA will harm your unborn baby or nursing child. You and your healthcare provider should talk about the best way to manage your diabetes while you are pregnant or breast-feeding. It is especially important to keep good control of your blood sugar during pregnancy.
Tell your healthcare provider about all the medicines you take, including prescription and non-prescription medicines, vitamins, and herbal supplements.
Know the medicines you take. Keep a list of your medicines with you and show it to your healthcare provider and pharmacist when you get a new medicine.

How should I take APIDRA?
• Take APIDRA exactly as prescribed.
• Do not make any changes to your dose or type of insulin unless told to do so by your healthcare provider.
• Know your insulin. Make sure you know:
  • the type and strength of insulin prescribed for you
  • the amount of insulin you take
  • the best time for you to take your insulin. This may change if you take a different type of insulin or if the way you give your insulin changes for example, using an insulin pump instead of giving injections under the skin (subcutaneous injections).
• APIDRA starts working faster than regular insulin, but does not work as long.
• APIDRA is usually used with a longer-acting insulin when given by injection under the skin (subcutaneous), or by itself when using an insulin pump.
• **Read the instructions for use that come with your APIDRA.** Talk to your healthcare provider if you have any questions. Your healthcare provider should show you how to inject APIDRA before you start taking it.
• Your healthcare provider will prescribe the best type of APIDRA for you. APIDRA is available in:
  • 3 mL cartridge system for use in OptiClik® Insulin Delivery Device
  • 3 mL SoloStar® prefilled pen
  • 10 mL vials
• You need a prescription to get APIDRA. Always be sure you receive the right insulin from the pharmacy.
• Check your blood sugar level before each use of APIDRA. Ask your healthcare provider what your blood sugars should be and when you should check your blood sugar levels.
• Check the label to make sure you have the correct insulin type. This is especially important if you also take long-acting insulin.
• APIDRA should look clear and colorless. Do not use APIDRA if it looks cloudy, colored, or has particles in it. Talk with your pharmacist or healthcare provider if you have any questions.
• If you take too much APIDRA, your blood sugar may fall low (hypoglycemia). You can treat mild low blood sugar (hypoglycemia) by drinking or eating something sugary right away.
• **Do not share needles, insulin pens or syringes with others.**

Your dose of APIDRA may need to be changed because of:

- illness
- stress
- other medicines you take
- change in diet
- change in physical activity or exercise
- travel

Check your blood sugar and stay on the diet and exercise plan as prescribed by your healthcare provider.

What should I consider while taking APIDRA?

- Alcohol may affect your blood sugar when you take APIDRA
- **Driving and operating machinery.** You may have trouble paying attention or reacting if you have low blood sugar (hypoglycemia). Be careful when you drive a car or operate machinery. Ask your healthcare provider if it is alright for you to drive if you have:
  - low blood sugar (hypoglycemia)
  - decreased or no warning signs of low blood sugar

What are the possible side effects of APIDRA?
APIDRA can cause serious side effects, including:

- **Low blood sugar (hypoglycemia).** Symptoms of low blood sugar may include:
  - feeling anxious, or irritable, mood changes
  - trouble concentrating or feeling confused
  - tingling in your hands, feet, lips, or tongue
  - feeling dizzy, light-headed, or drowsy
  - nightmares or trouble sleeping
  - headache
  - blurred vision
  - slurred speech
  - a fast heart beat
  - sweating
  - shakiness
  - walking unsteady

Very low blood sugar (hypoglycemia) can cause unconsciousness (passing out), seizures, and death. Talk to your healthcare provider about how to tell if you have low blood sugar and what to do if this happens while taking APIDRA. Know your symptoms of low blood sugar. Follow your healthcare provider's instructions for treating your low blood sugar.

Talk to your healthcare provider if low blood sugar is a problem for you. Your dose of APIDRA may need to be changed.

- **Serious allergic reactions.**

Get medical help right away if you have any of these symptoms of a severe allergic reaction:
  - a rash all over your body
  - shortness of breath
  - trouble breathing (wheezing)
  - fast pulse
  - sweating
  - feel faint (due to low blood pressure)
- **Low potassium** in your blood. Your doctor will check you for this.

Common side effects include:

- **Reactions at the injection site** (local allergic reaction). You may get redness, swelling and itching at the injection site. If you keep having skin reactions or they are serious talk to your healthcare provider.
- **Skin thickening or pits at the injection site.** Do not inject insulin into skin where this has happened. Choose an injection area (upper arm, thigh, or stomach area). Change injection sites within the area you choose with each dose. **Do not inject into the exact same spot for each injection.**
- Weight gain

Tell your healthcare provider about any side effect that bothers you or that does not go away. These are not all of the possible side effects of APIDRA.

Call your doctor for medical advice about side effects. You may report side effects to FDA at 1-800-332-1088.

How should I store APIDRA?

- See the Patient Instructions for Use that come with your APIDRA for specific storage instructions.

Unopened APIDRA:

- Do not use APIDRA after the expiration date stamped on the label.
- Keep all unopened APIDRA in the refrigerator between 36°F to 46°F (2°C to 8°C).
- Do not freeze. Do not use APIDRA if it has been frozen.
- Keep APIDRA away from direct heat and light.
- Unopened vials, cartridge systems and SoloStar that were not kept in a refrigerator must be used within 28 days after opening.

General Information about APIDRA

Medicines are sometimes prescribed for conditions that are not mentioned in patient information leaflets. Do not use APIDRA for a condition for which it was not prescribed. Do not give APIDRA to other people, even if they have the same symptoms you have. It may harm them.

This leaflet summarizes the most important information about APIDRA. If you would like more information, talk with your healthcare provider. You can ask your healthcare provider for information about APIDRA that is written for healthcare providers. For more information about APIDRA call 1-800-633-1610 or go to www.apidra.com.

What are the ingredients in APIDRA?

Active ingredient: insulin glulisine
Inactive ingredients: metacresol, tromethamine, sodium chloride, polysorbate 20, water for injection, hydrochloric acid or sodium hydroxide

ADDITIONAL INFORMATION

DIABETES FORECAST is a national magazine designed especially for patients with diabetes and their families and is available by subscription from the American Diabetes Association, (ADA), P.O. Box 363, Mt. Morris, IL 61054-0363, 1-800-DIABETES (1-800-342-2383). You may also visit the ADA website at www.diabetes.org.

Another publication, **COUNTDOWN**, is available from the Juvenile Diabetes Research Foundation International (JDRF), 120 Wall Street, 19th Floor, New York, New York 10005, 1-800-JDF-CURE (1-800-533-2873). You may also visit the JDRF website at www.jdf.org.

To get more information about diabetes, check with your healthcare provider or diabetes educator or visit www.DiabetesWatch.com.

For more information about APIDRA or OptiClik® call 1-800-633-1610 or visit www.apidra.com or www.opticlik.com.
Rev. February 2009
sanofi-aventis U.S. LLC
Bridgewater NJ 08807
©2009 sanofi-aventis U.S. LLC

PATIENT INSTRUCTIONS FOR USE
APIDRA 10 mL vial (100 Units/mL)
This Instructions for Use has two parts:
Part 1 Use with a syringe
Part 2 Use with an external insulin infusion pump
Be sure to read, understand and follow these instructions before taking APIDRA.

Part 1 Use with a syringe
If you will give yourself subcutaneous injections of APIDRA:

- You should take APIDRA within 15 minutes before a meal or within 20 minutes after starting a meal.
- Do not inject APIDRA if you are not going to eat within 15 minutes.
- Inject APIDRA into the skin of your upper arm, thigh, or stomach area. Do not inject APIDRA into a vein or into a muscle.
- Choose an injection area (upper arm, thigh, or stomach area). Change injection sites within the area you choose with each dose. **Do not inject into the exact same spot for each injection.**
- Do not mix APIDRA with insulins other than NPH, for subcutaneous injections. If mixing APIDRA with NPH insulin, draw up APIDRA into the syringe first. Inject the mixture right away.
- Use the needles and syringes prescribed by your healthcare provider.

Before every injection make sure you have the following items:

- Alcohol swabs
- Needle and syringe
- Insulin vial
- Puncture resistant container. See "How do I dispose of used needles and syringes?".

Drawing the insulin into a syringe

- 1. Use a new syringe each time you give an injection of APIDRA.

Preparing for an injection

- 2. Wash your hands with soap and water. Before you start to prepare your injection, check the label to make sure that you are taking the right type of insulin.
- 3. Look at the APIDRA in the vial. It should look clear. Do not use this vial of APIDRA if the solution is colored, or cloudy, or if you see particles in it.
- 4. If you are using a new vial, remove the protective cap. **Do not** remove the stopper.

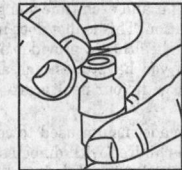

- 5. Wipe the rubber stopper with an alcohol swab. You do not have to shake the APIDRA before use.
[See figure at top of next column]
- 6. Use the needles and syringes prescribed by your healthcare provider. APIDRA 10 mL vials come with 100 units of insulin in 1 mL of APIDRA.

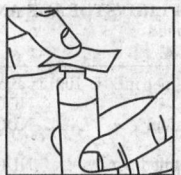

- 7. Use a new needle and syringe for each injection. Use disposable syringes and needles only one time.
- 8. Draw air into the syringe equal to the insulin dose prescribed by your healthcare provider.

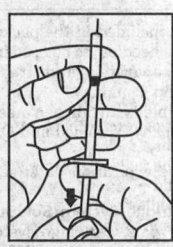

- 9. Put the needle through the rubber stopper of the vial and push the plunger to inject the air into the vial.

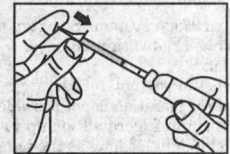

- 10. Leave the syringe in the vial and turn both upside down. Hold the syringe and vial firmly in one hand.
- 11. Make sure the tip of the needle is in the insulin solution. With your free hand, pull back on the plunger to draw the correct dose of insulin into the syringe.

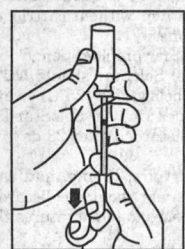

- 12 Before you take the needle out of the vial, check the syringe for air bubbles. If you see bubbles in the syringe, hold the syringe straight up and tap the side of the syringe with your finger a few times to make any air bubbles float to the top. Gently push the air bubbles out with the plunger and draw insulin back into the syringe until you have the correct dose. If you are mixing APIDRA with NPH insulin, check with your healthcare provider on how to mix it the right way.

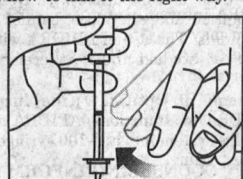

- 13. Remove the needle from the vial. Do not let the needle touch anything. You are now ready to inject.

Giving the injection
Do the injection exactly as shown to you by your healthcare provider. Inject APIDRA under your skin.

- 14. Choose an injection area (for example upper arm, thigh or stomach area). Change injection sites within the area you choose. **Do not inject in the same spot.**
- 15. Clean the area with an alcohol swab. Let the injection site dry before you inject.

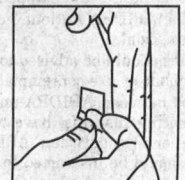

- 16. Pinch the skin. Insert the needle into the skin. Release the skin.
- 17. Inject the dose by slowly pushing in the plunger of the syringe all the way, making sure you have injected all the insulin. Keep the needle in the skin for at least 10 seconds.

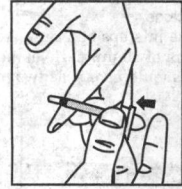

Pull the needle out of your skin, gently press the injection site with a finger for several seconds. **Do not rub the area.**
- 18. Do not recap the needle. Recapping can lead to a needle stick injury and passing of infection. See "How do I dispose of used needles and syringes?".

If your injection is given by another person, this person must also be careful to prevent accidental needle stick injury and passing infections.

How do I dispose of used needles and syringes?
- 19. Check with your healthcare provider's office for instructions about the right way to dispose of used needles and syringes. There may be local or state laws about how to dispose of used needles and syringes. Do not dispose of used needles or syringes in household trash and do not recycle them.
- 20. Put used needles and syringes in a container specially made for throwing away syringes and needles (called a "sharps" container) or a hard plastic container with a screw-on cap or a metal container with a plastic lid labeled "Used Syringes". These containers should be sealed and dispose of the right way.

See "How should I store APIDRA?" in the Patient Information leaflet that comes With APIDRA for complete instructions on how to store APIDRA vials.

Part 2 Use with an external insulin pump:
Be sure to read, understand, and follow these instructions before using APIDRA with an external insulin infusion pump. Always read the instruction manual for your pump. If you will be using an insulin pump:
- APIDRA should be given into the stomach area.
- Change injection sites in the stomach area.
- **Do not mix APIDRA with other insulins and do not dilute APIDRA.**
- Use only insulin pumps that have been specially tested with APIDRA.
Follow your healthcare provider or pharmacist instructions for which insulin pumps may be used.
- Change the infusion set (reservoir, tubing, and catheter), and the APIDRA in the reservoir every 2 days (48 hours). Change all of these parts sooner if they have been exposed to temperatures higher than 98.6°F (37°C).

Important information about using APIDRA with an external insulin infusion pump
- **Do not mix APIDRA with any other insulin or liquid when used in a pump.**
- If your APIDRA infusion pump set is not working the right way, you may not get the right amount of insulin that can cause:
  - low blood sugar (hypoglycemia)
  - high blood sugar (hyperglycemia)
  - high amounts of sugar and ketones in your blood or urine
- When you start using APIDRA by infusion pump, your insulin dose may need to be adjusted. Check with your healthcare provider before making any changes to your insulin dose.

How to use APIDRA with an external insulin infusion pump?
- Check with your healthcare provider or pharmacist to see if your pump and infusion set can be used with APIDRA. See the instruction manual of your specific pump on proper use of insulin in a pump. Call your healthcare provider if you have questions about using the pump.
- Change the infusion set, reservoir with insulin, and injection site:
  - at least every 48 hours, change more often than every 48 hours if you have high blood sugar (hyperglycemia), or the pump alarm sounds.
  - if the insulin has been in temperatures over 98.6°F (37°C). Dark colored pump cases or sport covers can increase this type of heat. The location where the pump is worn may affect the temperature.
If you get reactions at the injections infusion site you may need to change infusion sites more often.

If your APIDRA infusion pump is not working the right way, follow these steps:
- Use insulin from a new vial of APIDRA if infusion pump alarms do not respond to all of the following:
  - a repeat injection or bolus of APIDRA
  - a change in the infusion set and the reservoir
  - a change in the infusion injection site
- If the same problems happen again, do not use your infusion pump with APIDRA. You may need to restart insulin injections with syringes and needles.
  - Contact your healthcare provider right away.
  - See section I of the Instructions for Use ("Use with a syringe") for the steps for giving injections of APIDRA using syringes and needles.
  - Continue to check your blood sugar often.

How should I store APIDRA 10 mL vial?
- Keep in the refrigerator or below 77°F (25°C).
- Keep vials away from direct heat and light.
- Dispose of any opened vial after 28 days after the first use, even if there is insulin left in the vial.

Rev. February 2009
sanofi-aventis U.S. LLC
Bridgewater NJ 08807
©2009 sanofi-aventis U.S. LLC

PATIENT INSTRUCTIONS FOR USE
APIDRA 3 mL cartridge system (100 Units/mL)
Be sure to read, understand, and follow these instructions before using your APIDRA 3 mL cartridge system. **Also read and follow the step-by-step instructions in the "OptiClik® Instructions for Use Leaflet" that comes with OptiClik. If you do not follow the instructions, you may take too much or too little insulin.** Your healthcare provider should show you how to use the APIDRA 3 mL cartridge system and OptiClik to inject APIDRA before you use it for the first time. Ask your healthcare provider if you have any questions.

Important Information
If you will give yourself subcutaneous injections of APIDRA:
- You should take APIDRA within 15 minutes before a meal or within 20 minutes after starting a meal.
- Do not inject APIDRA if you are not going to eat within 15 minutes.
- Inject APIDRA into the skin of your upper arm, stomach area, or thigh. Do not inject APIDRA into a vein or into a muscle.
- Choose an injection area (upper arm, thigh, or stomach area). Change injection sites within the area you choose with each dose. Do not inject into the exact same spot for each injection.
- Only use your APIDRA 3 mL cartridge system with OptiClik, a reusable insulin delivery device.
- Use a new needle each time you give an APIDRA injection.
- Use BD Ultra-Fine pen needles with the OptiClik. The needles do not come with the APIDRA 3 mL cartridge system or OptiClik. You will need to buy these from a pharmacy. Talk to your healthcare provider if you have questions.
- **Needles, OptiClik and cartridge systems must not be shared.**

Getting ready
Make sure you have the following items:
- OptiClik insulin delivery device
- Pen needles
- Alcohol swab
- APIDRA cartridge system
- Puncture resistant container. See "How do I dispose of used needles and cartridge systems?

Preparing for an injection
- Wash your hands with soap and water before you start to touch the cartridge system or the OptiClik.
- Use a new needle for each injection.
- Always perform the safety test before use (see the OptiClik Instruction Leaflet).
- Do not use APIDRA if the solution is colored, cloudy, or if you see particles in it.
- Choose an injection area (for example upper arm, thigh, or stomach area). Change injection sites within the area you choose. **Do not inject into the exact same spot for each injection.**
- After injecting APIDRA, leave the needle in the skin for at least 10 seconds. Then pull the needle straight out. Gently press the injection site for a few seconds. **Do not rub the area.**
- Handle OptiClik® with care
- Do not use OptiClik if it is damaged or if you are not sure that it is working correctly.

How do I dispose of used needles and cartridge systems?
- Check with your healthcare provider for instructions about the right way to dispose of used needles and pens. There may be local or state laws about how to dispose of used needles and pens. Do not dispose of used needles or pens in household trash and do not recycle.
- Put used needles and used empty cartridge systems in a container made specially for disposing of used syringes and needles (called a "sharps" container) or a hard plastic container (such as detergent bottles), with a screw-on cap, or metal container with a plastic lid labeled "Used Syringes". These containers should be sealed and disposed of the right way.

How should I store APIDRA cartridge system?
- Store the opened cartridge system in the OptiClik (Insulin Delivery Device) below 77°F (25°C). Do not refrigerate.
- Keep away from direct heat and light.
- Dispose of any used APIDRA cartridge system 28 days after the first use even if there is insulin left in the cartridge.

If your blood glucose reading is high or low, tell your healthcare provider so the dose can be changed.
If you have lost your OptiClik Instruction Leaflet or have a question, go to www.opticlik.com or call 1-800-633-1610.
Rev. February 2009
sanofi-aventis U.S. LLC
Bridgewater NJ 08807
©2009 sanofi-aventis U.S. LLC

OptiClik®
INSTRUCTION LEAFLET
Your healthcare professional has decided that OptiClik® is right for you. Before using OptiClik®, your healthcare provider should provide training for the use of the pen and injection technique, or direct you to the appropriate person to get training.

Read these instructions carefully before using your OptiClik. Read both sides of the leaflet. If you are not able to follow all the instructions completely on your own, use OptiClik only if you have help from a person who is able to follow the instructions.

Hold the pen as shown in this leaflet. The word "OptiClik" must be readable to the left of the digital dose display to ensure the correct reading of the dose. **If you do not follow these instructions completely, you may get too much or too little insulin.**

OptiClik is a reusable pen for the injection of insulin. You can set doses from 1 to 80 units in steps of 1 unit. OptiClik can only be used with 3 mL (300 units) Lantus or Apidra® cartridge (U-100) systems.

OptiClik is available in different colors. If you use two different types of insulin with OptiClik, you should use a different color pen for each insulin.

Keep this leaflet for future reference for each time you use OptiClik.

If you have any questions about OptiClik or about diabetes, ask your health care professional, go to **www.opticlik.com** or call sanofi-aventis at 1-800-633-1610.

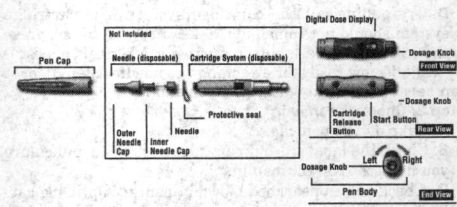

Important information for use of OptiClik:
- Always attach a new needle before each use. BD Ultra-Fine needles are available from BD Consumer Healthcare. Contact your healthcare professional for further information.
- Always perform the safety test before each injection (see Step 4).
- If you use two different types of insulin with OptiClik, you should use a different color pen for each insulin. Always check the label of your insulin before use.
- Accidental pressing of the start button or the cartridge release button may interfere with normal operation. Avoid accidentally pressing these buttons.
- This pen is only for your use. Do not share it with anyone else.
- If your injection is given by another person, special caution must be taken by this person to avoid accidental needle penetration and transmission of infection.
- OptiClik should not be used near electrical and electronic equipment.
- Never use OptiClik if it is damaged or if you are not sure that it is working properly.
- Always have a back-up method for delivering your insulin.
- **Do not store your OptiClik in a refrigerator**

Step 1: Insert a new Cartridge System
[See figure at top of next page]
- **A.** Make sure the dosage knob is pushed in.
- **B.** Check the label on your cartridge system to make sure you have the correct insulin. Using the wrong insulin

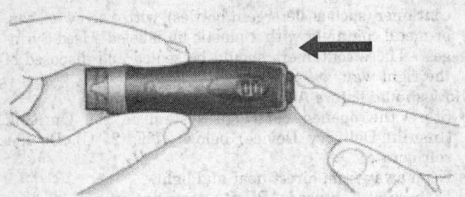

may result in unwanted changes in blood sugar that could be harmful to your health.

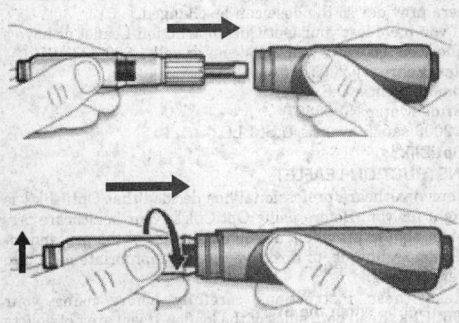

- **C.** Insert the cartridge system straight into the pen body. Make sure that it clicks in.
  - If you meet resistance, wiggle the cartridge system while inserting it.
  If the cartridge system does not click into the pen body properly, do not use force:
  - Check that the dosage knob is pressed in before you start
  - Take the cartridge system out and try again, aligning it carefully.
  - Try pressing the release button as you insert the cartridge.

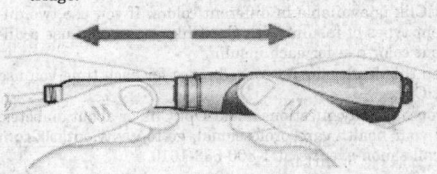

- **D.** Try pulling out the cartridge system. The cartridge system should not come out. Make sure you do not press the cartridge release button during or after this check.
OptiClik is now ready for attaching the needle (Step 3), or it can be stored with the attached pen cap.

Step 2: Check the insulin
- **A.** Take off the pen cap.
- **B.** Check the label on your cartridge system to make sure you have the correct insulin.
- **C.** Check the appearance of your insulin. OptiClik cartridge systems, Lantus or Apidra, only contain clear insulin. Do not use this cartridge system if the insulin is cloudy, colored or has particles.

Step 3: Attach the needle
Always use a new sterile needle for each injection. This helps prevent contamination, and potential needle blocks.
- **A.** Wipe the rubber seal on the end of the cartridge system with alcohol.

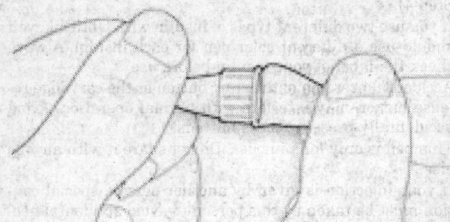

- **B** Remove the protective seal from a new needle.

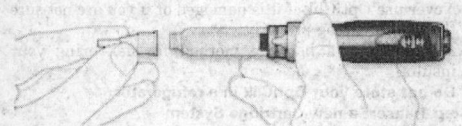

- **C.** Line up the needle with the pen, and keep it straight as you attach it (screw or push on, depending on the needle type.).

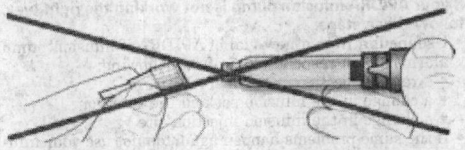

- If the needle is not kept straight while you attach it, it can damage the rubber seal and cause leakage, or the needle can be bend.

Step 4: Perform a Safety Test
Always perform the safety test before each injection. This ensures that you get an accurate dose by:
- ensuring that pen and needle work properly
- removing air bubbles
Do not press the cartridge release button during these steps.

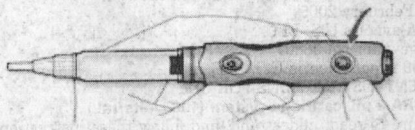

- **A.** Press the start button. The dosage knob comes out.

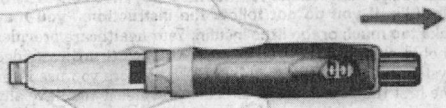

- **B.** "00" appears in the digital dose display.

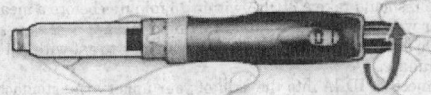

- **C.** Select a dose of 1 unit by turning the dosage knob forward (clockwise) until it clicks.

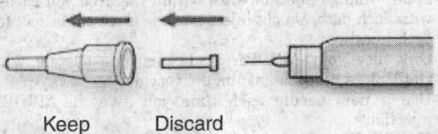

Keep   Discard

- **D.** Take off the outer needle cap and keep it to remove the used needle after injection. Take off the inner needle cap and discard it.

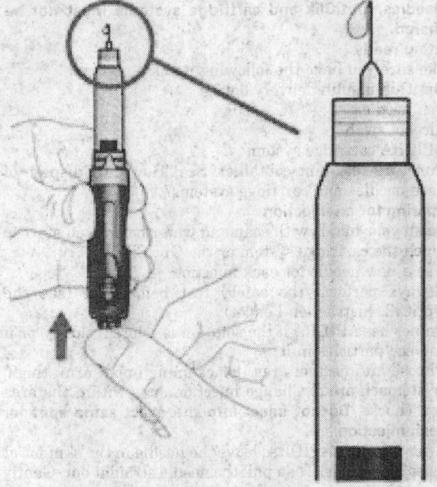

- **E.** Hold the pen with the needle pointing up.
- **F.** Tap the insulin reservoir so that any air bubbles rise up towards the needle.
- **G.** Press the dosage knob fully until it stays in. **Check that insulin comes out of the needle tip.** If it does not you must repeat the test until it does.
With a new cartridge system, or if there are air bubbles in the cartridge system, you may have to perform the safety test several times before insulin is seen.
If no insulin comes out, first check:
- that '01' was visible on the dose display
- that the cartridge system is properly inserted (see Step 1) and then repeat the safety test.

If still no insulin comes out, then:
- Check for air bubbles and repeat the safety test two more times using a dose of **2 units** instead of 1 unit.
- If still no insulin comes out, the needle may be blocked. Change the needle and try again.
- If no insulin comes out after changing the needle, your cartridge system may be damaged. Do not use this cartridge system. Insert a new one.

Step 5: Select the dose
You can set the dose in steps of 1 unit, from a minimum of 1 unit to a maximum of 80 units. If you need a dose greater than 80 units, you should give it as two or more injections.

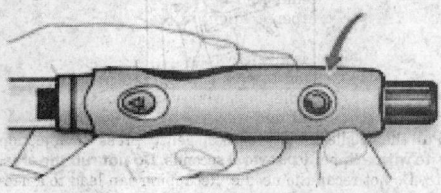

- **A.** Press the start button.

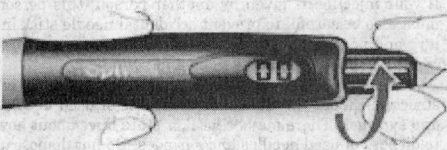

- **B.** Select your required dose by turning the dosage knob forward to the right. Make sure that the dosage knob is not in between two dose steps. You must feel and hear a click.
  - If you have selected a dose that is too high, simply turn the dosage knob backwards to the left.
  - Do not dial past 80. If you do dial past 80, follow the instructions in B. "Questions and answers" section I, to reset the pen.
  - You cannot turn the dosage knob past the number of units left in the cartridge system. Do not force the dosage knob to turn. In this case, either you can inject what is remaining in this cartridge system and complete your dose with a new cartridge system, or use a new cartridge system for your full dose.

Step 6: Inject the dose

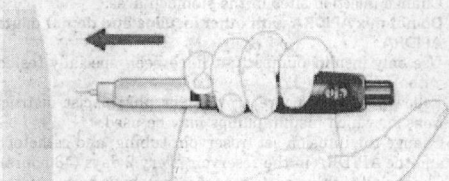

- **A.** Clean the area of skin to be injected with rubbing alcohol.
- **B.** Use the injection method as instructed by your healthcare professional
- **C.** Insert the needle into the skin.

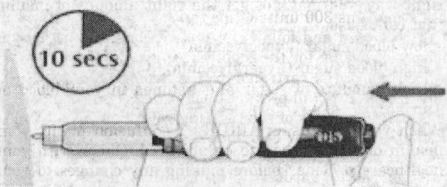

10 secs

- **D.** Deliver the dose by pressing the dosage knob all the way in. Do not press the cartridge release button or the start button while injecting.
  - If the dosage knob cannot be pressed down, you may have turned the dosage knob so that it is between two dose steps. The pen prevents you from pressing down the dosage knob if you are between two dose steps. Turn the dosage knob to the left or right to the correct dose.
- **E.** Keep the dosage knob pressed all the way in. Slowly count to 10, then make sure that the dosage knob stays in before you withdraw the needle from the skin. This ensures that the full dosage is delivered.
After injecting your dose, the digital dose display will not go back to "0" but will show the delivered dose for 2 minutes. Do not re-inject your dose as this may result in an overdose.

Step 7: Remove and discard the needle
Always remove the needle after each injection and store OptiClik without a needle attached. This prevents entry of

---

air into the insulin reservoir and leakage of insulin, which can cause inaccurate dosing.

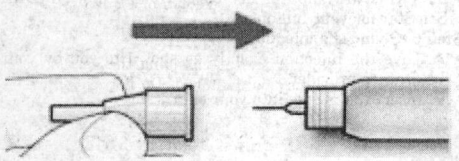

- **A.** Put the outer needle cap back on the needle, and use it to unscrew the needle from the pen. To reduce the risk of accidental needle penetration, never replace the inner needle cap.
  - If your injection is given by another person, special caution must be taken by this person when removing and disposing the needle. Follow recommended safety measures for removal and disposal of needles (e.g. a one handed capping technique) in order to reduce the risk of accidental needle penetration and transmission of infectious diseases.

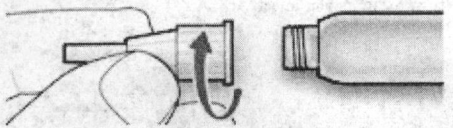

- **B.** Dispose of the needle safely, as instructed by your healthcare professional. For safe disposal of needles see (A.) GENERAL NOTES, Needles for OptiClik.
- **C.** Always put the pen cap back on the pen body, then store the pen until your next injection.

Step 8: Replacing an empty cartridge system

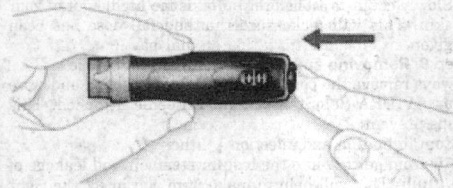

- **A.** Make sure the dosage knob is pushed in.

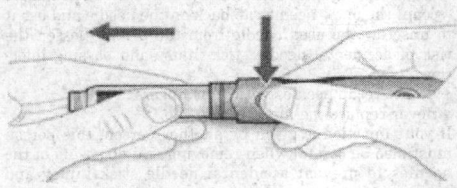

- **B.** Press the cartridge release button, and remove the entire cartridge system. Dispose of the cartridge system.

Start again at Step 1.

A. GENERAL NOTES

Cartridge system

The cartridge system is available separately. Each cartridge system contains 300 units of insulin.

Be sure to read and follow the instructions in the patient information leaflet for the insulin.

Do not remove the cartridge system from packaging until ready to use. This will prevent dust or dirt from getting into the mechanical parts of the cartridge system.

When you need a new cartridge system, take it out of the refrigerator 1–2 hours before you inject to allow it to warm up to room temperature. Cold insulin is more painful to inject.

Do not open or manipulate the cartridge system in any way.

Needles for OptiClik

BD Ultra-Fine needles are available from BD Consumer Healthcare.

Needles may vary from country to country and may not be interchangeable. If you intend to travel abroad, make sure that you have sufficient needles and insulin with you.

Needle disposal

Used needles should be placed in sharps containers (such as red biohazard containers), hard plastic containers (such as detergent bottles), or metal containers (such as an empty coffee can). Such containers should be sealed and disposed of properly.

B. QUESTIONS AND ANSWERS

I. Dose-setting

You hear no clicking sound during dose-setting:

The cartridge system may have been inserted incorrectly. Check by trying to pull the cartridge system gently out. If

the cartridge system comes out, reinsert it completely following the instructions in Step 1. Perform a safety test before dialing your dose.

If you still hear no clicking sound, try a new cartridge system and listen for clicking sound. In case there is still no clicking sound, obtain a new OptiClik.

If insulin drips from the needle tip during dose-setting Or, if you have dialed to 80 and then continued to dial:

The maximum dose of OptiClik is 80 units. If you continue to dial after reaching 80 units, insulin will drip from the needle and the display will continue to show "80".

- DO NOT dial back to your required dose, instead dial back to "00".
- Then press the dosage knob to eject excess insulin and to reset OptiClik. OptiClik is now again ready for dose setting.

If you need a dose greater than 80 units, you should give it as two or more injections.

If you cannot turn the dosage knob to set your dose:

Do not force the dosage knob to turn any further.

- a) You are turning to the left and trying to dial down below zero. Turn the dosage knob forward to the right to dial your dose.
- b) The cartridge system is almost empty and no longer contains a sufficient amount of insulin for the dose you need.
  - 1) EITHER, inject the partial dose that is in this cartridge system, then change the cartridge system and complete your dose from the new cartridge system.
  - 2) OR, change the cartridge system and give your complete dose from the new cartridge system. Dial back (to the left) to "00" before releasing the old cartridge system.
- c) You have dialed past the maximum dose of 80 units and either have no needle attached or the needle is blocked.
  - Dial completely backward to "00"
  - Attach a new needle and then perform a safety test before dialing your dose.

The dosage knob does not stop at "00":

When turned back completely, the dosage knob should stop with the dose display at "00", however, sometimes it may stop at "02" or "01". Make sure that a needle is attached, then press the dosage knob down (insulin will appear at the tip of the needle). OptiClik is now ready for use.

The dosage knob no longer turns after a new cartridge system has been inserted:

Check that the cartridge system is firmly clicked in. Reseat the cartridge system and try again. If it still does not work, try again with a new cartridge system. Otherwise, get a new OptiClik.

The dosage knob does not come out after you pressed the start button:

Do not pull out the dosage knob. Check that the cartridge system is firmly clicked in (see Step 1C and D).

II. Insulin injection

The dosage knob cannot be pressed down for the insulin injection:

- a) You have dialed between two dose steps (see Step 5B).
- b) The needle may be blocked or defective. Use a new needle.

The dosage knob does not stay down at the end of injection:

Make sure you are not accidentally pressing the start button at the same time.

After withdrawing the needle from your skin, more than one drop of insulin drips from the needle:

It is possible that you may not have injected your full insulin dose. DO NOT try to make up for the shortfall in your insulin dose by giving a second injection (otherwise you will be at risk for low blood sugar).

Please check your blood sugar and consult with your healthcare professional. You can avoid the problem next time by taking the following steps:

- a) Remove any air bubbles that may be present in the cartridge system (see step 4).
- b) After delivering the insulin dose, slowly count to 10 before withdrawing the needle from your skin.

III. Digital dose display functions

Reading the dose display

To read the dose correctly, hold OptiClik as shown in Step 5B, Select the dose. The printed "OptiClik" must be readable left of the dose display. Do not hold the pen upside down when reading the dose display; otherwise you may misread the dose on the digital dose display.

Dose display energy save function

The dose display switches off after two minutes of no activity, to conserve battery power.

The dose display goes blank during dose setting

The device has been inactive for 2 minutes (e.g. if you were interrupted in the middle of your injection preparations) and the display has turned off to conserve battery power. Turn the dosage knob one click forward. OptiClik should now be ready to use again; check the digital dose display and adjust for the right dose if needed.

No numbers appear on the Digital Dose Display when the start button is pressed or when the dosage knob is released:

Press the dosage knob. Start with a Safety Test (Step 4). If there are still no numbers on the digital dose display, you should obtain a new OptiClik.

⊡ is displayed:

The dosage knob has been forced into the negative range with excessive force. The cartridge system might be damaged and needs to be replaced. Remove this cartridge system (step 8) and start again at Step 1 with a new cartridge system.

⊡ and ⊡ flash alternately:

- a) The dosage knob has been forced into the negative range and was pushed in. The cartridge system might be damaged and needs to be replaced. Remove this cartridge system (step 8) and start again at Step 1 with a new cartridge system.
- b) The dosage knob has been turned too quickly.
  - EITHER, dispose of the unknown pre-set dose by pressing the dosage knob. Set your dose (Step 5) and inject your dose (Step 6).

OR, turn the dosage knob slowly backward until it stops, and then push the dosage knob in. Restart OptiClik and dial your dose.

IV. Lifetime of OptiClik and the battery information.

Lifetime of OptiClik:

OptiClik has a lifetime of 3 years after first use.

⊡ flashes when the Start Button is pressed:

OptiClik is reaching the end of its lifetime (3 years). The digital dose display will continue to operate for about 4 more weeks. Please obtain a new OptiClik.

⊡ stays when the Start Button is pressed:

OptiClik has reached the end of its lifetime. When you continue to turn the dosage knob, the display still shows ⊡. Please obtain a new OptiClik.

Battery information:

⊡ flashes when the Start Button is pressed:

Your battery is running out. Please obtain a new OptiClik as soon as possible.

⊡ is displayed when the Start Button is pressed:

Your battery has run out. Please obtain a new OptiClik.

C. STORAGE INSTRUCTIONS

Never store OptiClik in a refrigerator. Protect OptiClik from moisture and direct heat.

Always store OptiClik without the needle attached.

When OptiClik is stored, push the dosage knob in. This conserves the battery and ensures that the pen functions throughout its scheduled lifetime.

To avoid dust or dirt from getting into the pen body, always replace the pen cap.

Once the cartridge system is in use, it can be used for up to 28 days under normal carrying conditions (for Lantus, below 86°F [30°C]; for Apidra, below 77°F [25°C]). For specific insulin storage information, see "Patient Information" for Lantus or Apidra 3 mL Cartridge System for cartridge system storage information.

D. CARING FOR YOUR OPTICLIK

Care, cleaning, and maintenance instructions

Handle OptiClik carefully. Regularly clean your OptiClik, by using a clean damp cloth. Dirt can impede the operation. DO NOT use cleaning agents. Use an alcohol swab only for cleaning the cartridge system's rubber seal.

Damage to OptiClik

OptiClik may become damaged by rough handling, dropping, or turning of the dosage knob by force. Make sure that no dirt comes in contact with the mechanical parts. You should always make sure that:

- 1) The cartridge system is not damaged.
- 2) The start Button, dosage knob, and digital dose display still operate properly.

Do not use tools on OptiClik. If you are not sure whether or not your OptiClik is damaged, contact your health care professional or call 1-800-633-1610. If damaged, it is no longer safe to use it. In an emergency, you can draw up the insulin from the cartridge system using a U-100 insulin syringe.

APIDRA® SoloStar®

(insulin glulisine [rDNA origin] injection)

3 mL prefilled pen

Patient Instructions for Use

Be sure that you read, understand and follow these instructions before you use your APIDRA SoloStar®. Talk with your healthcare provider about the right way to use your APIDRA SoloStar before you use it for the first time. Keep this leaflet in case you need to look at it again later.

APIDRA SoloStar should not be used by people who are blind or have severe vision problems, without the help of a person who has good eyesight and who is trained to use the APIDRA SoloStar the right way.

APIDRA SoloStar is a disposable prefilled pen used to inject APIDRA. Each APIDRA SoloStar has 300 units of insulin which can be used for many doses. You can select a dose from 1 to 80 units. The pen plunger moves with each dose.

The plunger will only move to the end of the cartridge when 300 units of insulin have been given.

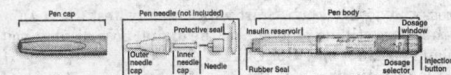

If you will give yourself subcutaneous injections of APIDRA:
• You should take APIDRA within 15 minutes before a meal or within 20 minutes after starting a meal.
• Do not inject APIDRA if you are not going to eat within 15 minutes.
• Inject APIDRA into the skin of your upper arm, thigh, or stomach area. Do not inject APIDRA into a vein or into a muscle.
• Choose an injection area (upper arm, thigh, or stomach area). Change injection sites within the area you choose with each dose. **Do not inject into the exact same spot for each injection.**

Important information for use of APIDRA SoloStar:
• Use a new needle for each injection. APIDRA Solostar may be used with pen needles from Becton Dickinson and Company, Ypsomed and Owen Mumford. Contact your healthcare provider for further information.
• Do a safety test before each injection. (See step 3.)
• Do not share your APIDRA SoloStar with others even if they have diabetes.
• If your injection is given by another person, this person must be careful to avoid accidental needle stick injury and prevent passing (transmission of) infection.
• Do not use APIDRA SoloStar if it is damaged or if you are not sure that it is working correctly.
• Always carry an extra APIDRA SoloStar prefilled pen in case your APIDRA SoloStar is lost or damaged.

Step 1. Preparing for an injection
Make sure you have the following items:
• Apidra SoloStar
• Pen needles
• Alcohol swab
• Puncture resistant container. See "How do I dispose of used needles and APIDRA SoloStar?".
• **A.** Check the label on your APIDRA SoloStar to make sure you have the right insulin. The APIDRA Solostar is blue. It has a dark blue injection button with a raised ring on the top.
• **B.** Check the expiration date, located on the carton or the label of your APIDRA SoloStar to make sure the date has not passed. Do not use an APIDRA SoloStar if the date has passed.
• **C.** Take off the pen cap.
• **D.** Look at the insulin in your APIDRA SoloStar. Check to make sure that the insulin looks clear. Do not use this APIDRA SoloStar if the insulin is cloudy, colored, or has particles in it.

Step 2. Attaching the needle
Always use a new sterile needle for each injection to help prevent contamination, and potential needle blocks.
Read the pen needle "Instructions for Use" before you use them.
Please note: Pen needles may look different. The pen needles shown are for illustrative purposes only.
• **A.** Wipe the Rubber Seal with alcohol.
• **B.** Remove the protective seal from the new pen needle.
• **C.** Line up the needle with the pen, and keep it straight as you attach it (screw or push on, depending on the needle type).

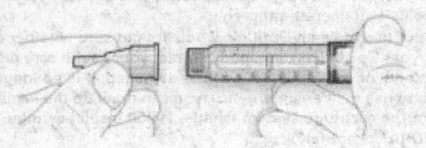

• If you do not keep the needle straight while you attach it this can damage the rubber seal, and cause leakage of insulin, or break the needle.

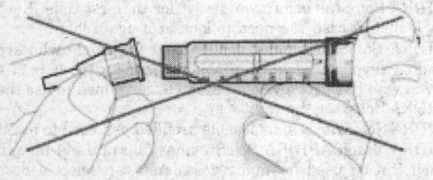

Step 3. Doing a Safety test
Do a safety test before each injection to make sure that you get the correct dose of APIDRA. The safety test:
• makes sure that the pen and needle work properly
• removes air bubbles
• **A.** Select a dose of 2 units by turning the dosage selector.

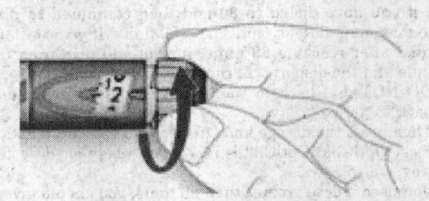

• **B.** Take off the outer needle cap and keep it to remove the used needle after injection. Take off the inner needle cap and dispose of it.

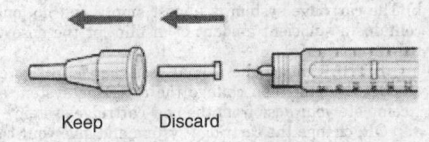

Keep   Discard

• **C.** Hold the pen with the needle pointing upwards.
• **D.** Tap the insulin reservoir so that any air bubbles rise up towards the needle.
• **E.** Press the injection button all the way in. Check if insulin comes out of the needle tip.

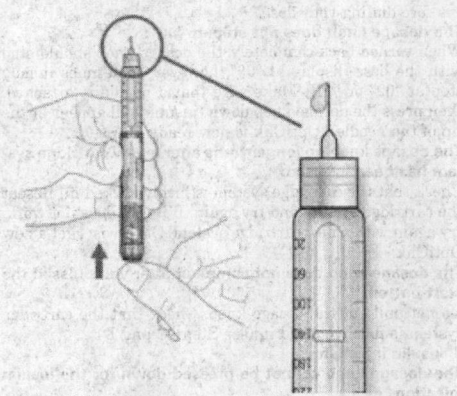

You may have to do the safety test more than once before you see the insulin.
• If no insulin comes out, check for air bubbles and repeat the safety test two more times to remove them.
• If still no insulin comes out, the needle may be blocked. Change the needle and try again.
• If no insulin comes out after changing the needle, your APIDRA SoloStar may be damaged. Do not use this APIDRA SoloStar.

Step 4. Selecting your dose
Select the APIDRA dose prescribed by your healthcare provider. You can select the insulin dose in steps of 1 unit, from a minimum of 1 unit to a maximum of 80 units. If you need a dose larger than 80 units, you should give it as two or more injections.
• **A.** Check that the dose window shows "0" after the safety test.
• **B.** Select your needed dose (in the example below, the selected dose is 30 units). If you turn past your dose, you can turn back down.

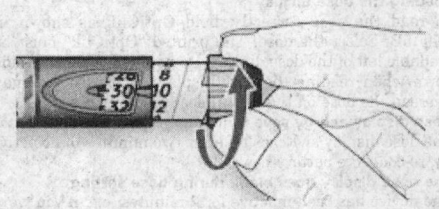

• Do not push the injection button while turning, insulin will come out.
• You cannot turn the dosage selector passed the number of units left in the pen. Do not force the dosage selector to

turn. In this case, either you can inject the amount of insulin that is still in the pen and finish your dose with a new APIDRA SoloStar or you can use a new APIDRA SoloStar for your full dose.

Step 5. Giving the injection
• **A.** Give the injection exactly as shown to you by your healthcare provider.
• **B.** Insert the needle into your skin.

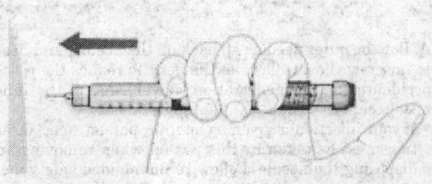

• **C.** Inject the dose by pressing the injection button in all the way. Only push the injection button when you are ready to inject. The number in the dose window will return to "0" as you inject.

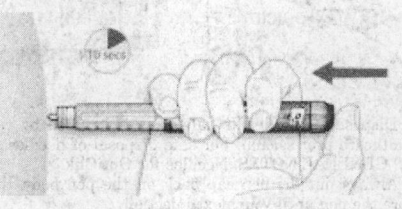

• **D.** Keep the injection button pressed all the way in. Slowly count to 10 before you take the needle out of your skin. This will make sure that the full dose has been given.

Step 6. Removing and disposing of the pen needle
Always remove the pen needle after each injection and store your APIDRA SoloStar without a needle attached. This helps prevent:
• Contamination and infection
• Air from getting into the insulin reservoir and leakage of insulin. This will help to make sure you inject the right dose of insulin.
• **A.** Follow the instructions from your healthcare provider when removing and disposing of the needle. For example "scoop" the outer needle cap back on the needle and use it to unscrew the used needle from the pen. To lessen the risk of accidental needle stick injury and passing infection:
  • do not recap needles with your fingers
  • never replace the inner needle cap.
  If your injection is given by another person, this person must also be careful when removing and disposing of the needles to prevent accidental needle stick injury and passing infection.
• **B.** Dispose of the needle the right way into your special puncture resistant container (See "How Do I Dispose of used needles and APIDRA SoloStar?")
• **C.** Always put the pen cap back on the pen, then store the APIDRA SoloStar until your next injection.

How do I dispose of used needles and APIDRA SoloStar?
• Check with your healthcare provider for instructions about the right way to dispose of used needles and APIDRA SoloStars. There may be local or state laws about how to throw away used needles and APIDRA SoloStar. Do not dispose of used needles or APIDRA SoloStar in household trash and do not recycle them.
• Put used needles and used empty APIDRA SoloStar in a container made specially for disposing of used syringes and needles (called a "sharps" container) or a hard plastic container (such as empty detergent bottles), with a screw-on cap, or metal container with a plastic lid labeled "Used Syringes". These containers should be sealed and disposed of the right way.

How should I Store APIDRA SoloStar?
• Do not refrigerate APIDRA SoloStar after first use.
• Keep at room temperature below 77°F (25°C).
• Dispose of any opened APIDRA SoloStar 28 days after first use.

Maintenance
• Protect your APIDRA SoloStar from dust and dirt.
• You can clean the outside of your APIDRA SoloStar by wiping it with a damp cloth.
• Do not soak, wash or lubricate the pen as this may damage it.
• Handle your APIDRA SoloStar with care. Avoid situations where your APIDRA SoloStar might be damaged. If you are concerned that your APIDRA SoloStar may be damaged, use a new one.

If you have any questions about APIDRA SoloStar or about diabetes, ask your healthcare provider, go to www.apidra.com or call sanofi-aventis U.S. at 1-800-633-1610.
sanofi-aventis U.S. LLC
Bridgewater, NJ 08807
Date of revision:
February 2009
©2009 sanofi-aventis U.S. LLC
Revised: 02/2009   Distributed by: sanofi-aventis S.A.

APLENZIN™   ℞
(bupropion hydrobromide)
Tablet, Film Coated, Extended Release for Oral use

HIGHLIGHTS OF PRESCRIBING INFORMATION
These highlights do not include all the information needed to use Aplenzin™ safely and effectively. See full prescribing information for Aplenzin.
Aplenzin (bupropion hydrobromide) Tablet, Film Coated, Extended Release for Oral use
Initial U.S. Approval: 1985

WARNING: SUICIDALITY AND ANTIDEPRESSANT DRUGS
See full prescribing information for complete boxed warning.
- **Antidepressants increased the risk compared to placebo of suicidal thinking and behavior (suicidality) in children, adolescents, and young adults in short-term studies of major depressive disorder (MDD) and other psychiatric disorders (5.1) (8.4)**
- **Anyone considering the use of Aplenzin or any other antidepressant in a child, adolescent, or young adult must balance this risk with the clinical need. (8.4)**
- **Short-term studies did not show an increase in the risk of suicidality with antidepressants compared to placebo in adults beyond age 24; there was a reduction in risk with antidepressants compared to placebo in adults aged 65 and older. (5.1)**
- **Depression and certain other psychiatric disorders are themselves associated with increases in the risk of suicide. (5.1)**
- **Patients of all ages who are started on antidepressant therapy should be monitored appropriately and observed closely for clinical worsening, suicidality, or unusual changes in behavior. (5.1)**
- **Families and caregivers should be advised of the need for close observation and communication with the prescriber. (17)**
- **Aplenzin is not approved for use in pediatric patients. [See WARNINGS and PRECAUTIONS: Clinical Worsening and Suicide Risk (5.1) and USE IN SPECIFIC POPULATIONS: Pediatric Use (8.4)]**

INDICATIONS AND USAGE
Aplenzin is an aminoketone antidepressant indicated for the treatment of: Major depressive disorder (1)
Periodically reevaluate long-term usefulness for the individual patient. (1)

DOSAGE AND ADMINISTRATION
General: Increase dose gradually to reduce seizure risk and other effects (2.1)
Recommendations for Adults:
- Start: 174 mg/day. Usual target: 348 mg/day. (2.2)
  Periodically reassess dose and need for maintenance treatment (2.3)
- Switching from Wellbutrin®, Wellbutrin SR®, Wellbutrin XL® (2.4)
  Patients should be given equivalent daily doses, if possible
- Impaired Hepatic Function, Impaired Renal Function (2.5, 2.6) Reduce dose and/or frequency. Severe cirrhosis: max. 174 mg/48 hours

DOSAGE FORMS AND STRENGTHS
- 174 mg Aplenzin extended-release tablets (3)
- 348 mg Aplenzin extended-release tablets (3)
- 522 mg Aplenzin extended-release tablets (3)

CONTRAINDICATIONS
- Patients with seizure disorder (4)
- Patients using other bupropion products, including Zyban® (4)
- Current or prior diagnosis of bulimia or anorexia nervosa (4)
- Abrupt discontinuation of alcohol, sedatives (incl. benzodiazepines) (4)
- Use of MAO inhibitor; stop at least 2 weeks prior to bupropion use (4)
- Patients allergic to any of the ingredients of Aplenzin (4)

WARNINGS AND PRECAUTIONS
- Suicide risk: Closely monitor high risk patients and all other patients (BOXED WARNING, 5.1, 8.4)

- Risk of activation of psychosis and/or mixed/manic episodes (5.2)
  Screen patients for bipolar disorder. Aplenzin is not approved for bipolar depression (5.3)
- Seizure risk: Can be minimized by limiting daily dose to 522 mg and slow dose increase. Extreme caution with high risk patients (5.4, 4, 7.4)
- Hepatic impairment: Use with caution; reduce dose and/or frequency. Severe hepatic cirrhosis: Extreme caution; max. 174 mg/48 hours (5.5)
- Potential for hepatotoxicity (5.6)
- Risk of restlessness, agitation, anxiety, insomnia (5.7); risk of neuropsychiatric events, incl. delusions, hallucinations, psychosis, concentration disturbance, paranoia, confusion (5.8)
- Loss of appetite should be considered if weight loss is a concern (5.9)
- Risk of anaphylactic/oid reactions; erythema multiforme, Stevens-Johnson syndrome; risk of arthralgia, myalgia, and fever with rash and other symptoms suggestive of delayed hypersensitivity (5.10)
- Risk of severe hypertension; may require acute treatment. Caution in patients with recent history of MI or unstable heart disease (5.11)

ADVERSE REACTIONS
Most common adverse reactions are (incidence ≥ 5%; ≥ 2× placebo rate):   Dry mouth, nausea, insomnia, dizziness, pharyngitis, abdominal pain, agitation, anxiety, tremor, palpitation, sweating, tinnitus, myalgia, anorexia, urinary frequency, rash (6.1)
To report SUSPECTED ADVERSE REACTIONS, contact BTA Pharmaceuticals at (866-246-8245 (opt. 3) or FDA at 1-800-FDA-1088 or *www.fda.gov/medwatch*.

DRUG INTERACTIONS
- CYP2B6 substrates or inhibitors (e.g. cyclophosphamide, orphenadrine, thiotepa), efavirenz, fluvoxamine, norfluoxetine, nelfinavir, paroxetine, ritonavir, sertraline: May increase bupropion activity (7)
- Carbamazepine, phenobarbital, phenytoin: May induce bupropion metabolism (7)
- Bupropion may be an inducer of drug metabolizing enzymes (7)
- Drugs metabolized by CYP2D6, e.g. certain antidepressants (e.g., nortriptyline, imipramine, desipramine, paroxetine, fluoxetine, sertraline), antipsychotics (e.g., haloperidol, risperidone, thioridazine), beta-blockers (e.g., metoprolol), and Type 1C antiarrhythmics (e.g., propafenone, flecainide):   Consider dose reduction when using with bupropion. Bupropion & hydroxybupropion inhibit CYP2D6 (7.1)
- MAO inhibitors: Increase bupropion toxicity. Contraindicated (4, 7.2)
- Levodopa, amantadine: Cautious bupropion dosing (7.3)
- Drugs that lower seizure threshold: Cautious bupropion dosing (5.4, 7.4)
- Nicotine transdermal system: Monitor for severe hypertension (5.11)
- Alcohol: Minimize consumption or avoid (7.6)

USE IN SPECIFIC POPULATIONS
- Pregnancy: Use only if benefit outweighs potential risk to the fetus (8.1)
- Nursing: Breast feeding or drug should be discontinued (8.3)
- Children: Safety & effectiveness not established. Balance risk/need (8.4)
- Renal Impairment: Reduce dose and/or frequency (8.6)
- Hepatic impairment: Use with caution; reduce dose and/or frequency. Severe cirrhosis: Extreme caution; max. 174 mg/48 hours (8.7)
See 17 for PATIENT COUNSELING INFORMATION and FDA-approved patient labeling.

Revised: [10/2008]

FULL PRESCRIBING INFORMATION: CONTENTS*
WARNING: SUICIDALITY AND ANTIDEPRESSANT DRUGS

*Sections or subsections omitted from the full prescribing information are not listed.

FULL PRESCRIBING INFORMATION

WARNING: SUICIDALITY AND ANTIDEPRESSANT DRUGS
Antidepressants increased the risk compared to placebo of suicidal thinking and behavior (suicidality) in children, adolescents, and young adults in short-term studies of major depressive disorder (MDD) and other psychiatric disorders. Anyone considering the use of Aplenzin™ or any other antidepressant in a child, adolescent, or young adult must balance this risk with the clinical need. Short-term studies did not show an increase in the risk of suicidality with antidepressants compared to placebo in adults beyond age 24; there was a reduction in risk with antidepressants compared to placebo in adults aged 65 and older. Depression and certain other psychiatric disorders are themselves associated with increases in the risk of suicide. Patients of all ages who are started on antidepressant therapy should be monitored appropriately and observed closely for clinical worsening, suicidality, or unusual changes in behavior. **Families and caregivers should be advised of the need for close observation and communication with the prescriber. Aplenzin is not approved for use in pediatric patients. [See *WARNINGS AND PRECAUTIONS: Clinical Worsening and Suicide Risk (5.1) and USE IN SPECIFIC POPULATIONS: Pediatric Use (8.4)]***

---

1   INDICATIONS AND USAGE

Aplenzin™ (bupropion hydrobromide extended-release tablets) is indicated for the treatment of major depressive disorder.

The efficacy of bupropion in the treatment of a major depressive episode was established in two 4-week controlled trials of inpatients and in one 6-week controlled trial of outpatients whose diagnoses corresponded most closely to the Major Depression category of the APA Diagnostic and Statistical Manual (DSM) [see *CLINICAL STUDIES (14)*].

A major depressive episode (DSM-IV) implies the presence of 1) depressed mood or 2) loss of interest or pleasure; in addition, at least 5 of the following symptoms have been present during the same 2-week period and represent a change from previous functioning: depressed mood, markedly diminished interest or pleasure in usual activities, significant change in weight and/or appetite, insomnia or hypersomnia, psychomotor agitation or retardation, increased fatigue, feelings of guilt or worthlessness, slowed thinking or impaired concentration, a suicide attempt, or suicidal ideation.

The efficacy of bupropion in maintaining an antidepressant response for up to 44 weeks following 8 weeks of acute treatment was demonstrated in a placebo-controlled trial with the sustained-release formulation of bupropion [see *CLINICAL STUDIES (14)*]. Nevertheless, the physician who elects to use Aplenzin for extended periods should periodically reevaluate the long-term usefulness of the drug for the individual patient.

2 DOSAGE AND ADMINISTRATION

2.1 General Dosing Considerations

It is particularly important to administer Aplenzin Tablets in a manner most likely to minimize the risk of seizure [see *WARNINGS AND PRECAUTIONS: Seizures (5.4)*]. Gradual escalation in dosage is also important if agitation, motor restlessness, and insomnia, often seen during the initial days of treatment, are to be minimized. If necessary, these effects may be managed by temporary reduction of dose or the short-term administration of an intermediate to long-acting sedative hypnotic. A sedative hypnotic usually is not required beyond the first week of treatment. Insomnia may also be minimized by avoiding bedtime doses. If distressing, untoward effects supervene, dose escalation should be stopped. Aplenzin should be swallowed whole and not crushed, divided, or chewed. Aplenzin may be taken without regard to meals.

2.2 Initial Treatment

The usual adult target dose for Aplenzin Tablets is 348 mg/day (equivalent to 300 mg/day bupropion HCl), given once daily in the morning. Dosing with Aplenzin Tablets should begin at 174-mg/day (equivalent to 150 mg/day bupropion HCl) given as a single daily dose in the morning. If the 174 mg initial dose is adequately tolerated, an increase to the 348-mg/day target dose, given as once daily, may be made as early as day 4 of dosing. There should be an interval of at least 24 hours between successive doses.

Increasing the Dosage Above 348 mg/day: As with other antidepressants, the full antidepressant effect of Aplenzin Tablets may not be evident until 4 weeks of treatment or longer. An increase in dosage to the maximum of 522 mg/day, given as a single dose, may be considered for patients in whom no clinical improvement is noted after several weeks of treatment at 348 mg/day.

2.3 Maintenance Treatment

It is generally agreed that acute episodes of depression require several months or longer of sustained pharmacological therapy beyond response to the acute episode. It is unknown whether or not the dose of Aplenzin needed for maintenance treatment is identical to the dose needed to achieve an initial response. Patients should be periodically reassessed to determine the need for maintenance treatment and the appropriate dose for such treatment.

2.4 Switching Patients from WELLBUTRIN®, WELLBUTRIN SR® or WELLBUTRIN XL®

When switching patients from WELLBUTRIN®, WELLBUTRIN SR® or WELLBUTRIN XL® Tablets to Aplenzin, give the equivalent total daily dose when possible (522 mg bupropion HBr are equivalent to 450 mg bupropion HCl; 348 mg bupropion HBr are equivalent to 300 mg bupropion HCl; 174 mg bupropion HBr are equivalent to 150 mg bupropion HCl). Patients who are currently being treated with WELLBUTRIN® Tablets at 300 mg/day (for example, 100 mg 3 times a day) may be switched to Aplenzin 348 mg once daily. Patients who are currently being treated with WELLBUTRIN SR® Sustained-Release Tablets at 300 mg/day (for example, 150 mg twice daily) may be switched to Aplenzin 348 mg once daily.

2.5 Dosage Adjustment for Patients With Impaired Hepatic Function

Aplenzin should be used with extreme caution in patients with severe hepatic cirrhosis. The dose should not exceed 174 mg every other day in these patients. Aplenzin should be used with caution in patients with hepatic impairment (including mild to moderate hepatic cirrhosis) and a reduced frequency and/or dose should be considered in patients with mild to moderate hepatic cirrhosis [see *WARNINGS AND PRECAUTIONS: Hepatic Impairment (5.5), USE IN SPE-*

CIFIC POPULATIONS: Hepatic Impairment (8.7) and *CLINICAL PHARMACOLOGY: Pharmacokinetics (12.3)*].

2.6 Dosage Adjustment for Patients With Impaired Renal Function

Aplenzin should be used with caution in patients with renal impairment and a reduced frequency and/or dose should be considered [see *USE IN SPECIFIC POPULATIONS: Renal Impairment (8.6)* and *CLINICAL PHARMACOLOGY: Pharmacokinetics (12.3)*].

3 DOSAGE FORMS AND STRENGTHS

Aplenzin Extended-Release Tablets, 174 mg of bupropion hydrobromide, are white to off white, round tablets printed with "BR" over "174" in bottles of 30 tablets.

Aplenzin Extended-Release Tablets, 348 mg of bupropion hydrobromide, are white to off white, round tablets printed with "BR" over "348" in bottles of 30 tablets.

Aplenzin Extended-Release Tablets, 522 mg of bupropion hydrobromide, are white to off white, round tablets printed with "BR" over "522" in bottles of 30 tablets.

4 CONTRAINDICATIONS

Aplenzin is contraindicated in patients with a seizure disorder.

Aplenzin is contraindicated in patients treated with ZYBAN® (bupropion hydrochloride) Sustained-Release Tablets; WELLBUTRIN® (bupropion hydrochloride immediate-release formulation); WELLBUTRIN SR® (bupropion hydrochloride sustained-release formulation); WELLBUTRIN XL® (bupropion hydrochloride extended-release formulation); or any other medications that contain bupropion because the incidence of seizure is dose dependent.

Aplenzin is contraindicated in patients with a current or prior diagnosis of bulimia or anorexia nervosa because of a higher incidence of seizures noted in patients treated for bulimia with the immediate-release formulation of bupropion.

Aplenzin is contraindicated in patients undergoing abrupt discontinuation of alcohol or sedatives (including benzodiazepines).

The concurrent administration of Aplenzin Tablets and a monoamine oxidase (MAO) inhibitor is contraindicated. At least 14 days should elapse between discontinuation of an MAO inhibitor and initiation of treatment with Aplenzin Tablets.

Aplenzin is contraindicated in patients who have shown an allergic response to bupropion or the other ingredients that make up Aplenzin Tablets.

5 WARNINGS AND PRECAUTIONS

5.1 Clinical Worsening and Suicide Risk

Patients with major depressive disorder (MDD), both adult and pediatric, may experience worsening of their depression and/or the emergence of suicidal ideation and behavior (suicidality) or unusual changes in behavior, whether or not they are taking antidepressant medications, and this risk may persist until significant remission occurs. Suicide is a known risk of depression and certain other psychiatric disorders, and these disorders themselves are the strongest predictors of suicide. There has been a long-standing concern that antidepressants may have a role in inducing worsening of depression and the emergence of suicidality in certain patients during the early phases of treatment. Pooled analyses of short-term placebo-controlled trials of antidepressant drugs (SSRIs and others) show that these drugs increase the risk of suicidal thinking and behavior (suicidality) in children, adolescents, and young adults (ages 18-24) with major depressive disorder (MDD) and other psychiatric disorders. Short-term studies did not show an increase in the risk of suicidality with anti-depressants compared to placebo in adults beyond age 24; there was a reduction with antidepressants compared to placebo in adults aged 65 and older.

The pooled analyses of placebo-controlled trials in children and adolescents with MDD, obsessive compulsive disorder (OCD), or other psychiatric disorders included a total of 24 short-term trials of 9 antidepressant drugs in over 4,400 patients. The pooled analyses of placebo-controlled trials in adults with MDD or other psychiatric disorders included a total of 295 short-term trials (median duration of 2 months) of 11 antidepressant drugs in over 77,000 patients. There was considerable variation in risk of suicidality among drugs, but a tendency toward an increase in the younger patients for almost all drugs studied. There were differences in absolute risk of suicidality across the different indications, with the highest incidence in MDD. The risk differences (drug vs placebo), however, were relatively stable within age strata and across indications. These risk differences (drug-placebo difference in the number of cases of suicidality per 1,000 patients treated) are provided in Table 1.

Table 1

Age Range	Drug-Placebo Difference in Number of Cases of Suicidality per 1,000 Patients Treated
	Increases Compared to Placebo
<18	14 additional cases
18-24	5 additional cases
	Decreases Compared to Placebo
25-64	1 fewer case
≥65	6 fewer cases

No suicides occurred in any of the pediatric trials. There were suicides in the adult trials, but the number was not sufficient to reach any conclusion about drug effect on suicide.

It is unknown whether the suicidality risk extends to longer-term use, i.e., beyond several months. However, there is substantial evidence from placebo-controlled maintenance trials in adults with depression that the use of antidepressants can delay the recurrence of depression.

All patients being treated with antidepressants for any indication should be monitored appropriately and observed closely for clinical worsening, suicidality, and unusual changes in behavior, especially during the initial few months of a course of drug therapy, or at times of dose changes, either increases or decreases. [See *BOXED WARNING* and *USE IN SPECIFIC POPULATIONS: Pediatric Use (8.4)*]

The following symptoms, anxiety, agitation, panic attacks, insomnia, irritability, hostility, aggressiveness, impulsivity, akathisia (psychomotor restlessness), hypomania, and mania, have been reported in adult and pediatric patients being treated with antidepressants for major depressive disorder as well as for other indications, both psychiatric and nonpsychiatric. Although a causal link between the emergence of such symptoms and either the worsening of depression and/or the emergence of suicidal impulses has not been established, there is concern that such symptoms may represent precursors to emerging suicidality.

Consideration should be given to changing the therapeutic regimen, including possibly discontinuing the medication, in patients whose depression is persistently worse, or who are experiencing emergent suicidality or symptoms that might be precursors to worsening depression or suicidality, especially if these symptoms are severe, abrupt in onset, or were not part of the patient's presenting symptoms.

Families and caregivers of patients being treated with antidepressants for major depressive disorder or other indications, both psychiatric and nonpsychiatric, should be alerted about the need to monitor patients for the emergence of agitation, irritability, unusual changes in behavior, and the other symptoms described above, as well as the emergence of suicidality, and to report such symptoms immediately to health care providers. Such monitoring should include daily observation by families and caregivers. [See also *PATIENT COUNSELING INFORMATION (17)*] Prescriptions for Aplenzin should be written for the smallest quantity of tablets consistent with good patient management, in order to reduce the risk of overdose. Families and caregivers of adults being treated for depression should be similarly advised.

5.2 Activation of Psychosis and/or Mania

Antidepressants can precipitate manic episodes in bipolar disorder patients during the depressed phase of their illness and may activate latent psychosis in other susceptible patients. Aplenzin is expected to pose similar risks.

5.3 Screening Patients for Bipolar Disorder

A major depressive episode may be the initial presentation of bipolar disorder. It is generally believed (though not established in controlled trials) that treating such an episode with an antidepressant alone may increase the likelihood of precipitation of a mixed/manic episode in patients at risk for bipolar disorder. Whether any of the symptoms described above represent such a conversion is unknown. However, prior to initiating treatment with an antidepressant, patients with depressive symptoms should be adequately screened to determine if they are at risk for bipolar disorder; such screening should include a detailed psychiatric history, including a family history of suicide, bipolar disorder, and depression. It should be noted that Aplenzin is not approved for use in treating bipolar depression.

Patients should be made aware that Aplenzin contains bupropion, the same active ingredient found in ZYBAN®, used as an aid to smoking cessation treatment, and that Aplenzin should not be used in combination with ZYBAN®, or any other medications that contain bupropion, such as WELLBUTRIN XL® (bupropion hydrochloride extended-release formulation), WELLBUTRIN SR® (bupropion hydrochloride sustained-release formulation), or WELLBUTRIN® (bupropion hydrochloride immediate-release formulation). [See also *PATIENT COUNSELING INFORMATION (17)*]

5.4 Seizures

Bupropion is associated with a dose-related risk of seizures. The risk of seizures is also related to patient factors, clinical situations, and concomitant medications, which must be considered in selection of patients for therapy with Aplenzin. Aplenzin should be discontinued and not restarted in patients who experience a seizure while on treatment.

The seizure incidence with Aplenzin has not been formally evaluated in clinical trials. Studies in mice suggest the potential for a significant reduction in the risk of seizure with bupropion HBr as compared to bupropion HCl. The seizure incidence is not expected to be worse than presented below for comparable doses of the immediate-release and sustained release formulations of bupropion HCl.

• Dose

At doses up to 300 mg/day (equivalent to 348 mg/day of bupropion HBr) of the sustained-release formulation of bupropion hydrochloride (WELLBUTRIN SR®), the incidence of seizure is approximately 0.1% (1/1,000).

Data for the immediate-release formulation of bupropion hydrochloride revealed a seizure incidence of approximately 0.4% (i.e., 13 of 3,200 patients followed prospectively) in patients treated at doses in a range of 300 to 450 mg/day (equivalent to a range of 348 to 522 mg/day of bupropion HBr). This seizure incidence (0.4%) may exceed that of some other marketed antidepressants.

Additional data accumulated for the immediate-release formulation of bupropion hydrochloride suggested that the estimated seizure incidence increases almost tenfold between 450 and 600 mg/day (equivalent to 522 and 696 mg/day bupropion HBr). The 600 mg dose is twice the usual adult dose and one and one-third the maximum recommended daily dose (450 mg) of WELLBUTRIN XL® (equivalent to 522 mg Aplenzin) Tablets. This disproportionate increase in seizure incidence with dose incrementation calls for caution in dosing.

• Patient Factors

Predisposing factors that may increase the risk of seizure with bupropion use include history of head trauma or prior seizure, central nervous system (CNS) tumor, the presence of severe hepatic cirrhosis, and concomitant medications that lower seizure threshold.

• Clinical Situations

Circumstances associated with an increased seizure risk include, among others, excessive use of alcohol or sedatives (including benzodiazepines); addiction to opiates, cocaine, or stimulants; use of over-the-counter stimulants and anorectics; and diabetes treated with oral hypoglycemics or insulin.

• Concomitant Medications

Many medications (e.g., antipsychotics, antidepressants, theophylline, systemic steroids) are known to lower seizure threshold.

Recommendations for Reducing the Risk of Seizure; Retrospective analysis of clinical experience gained during the development of bupropion suggests that the risk of seizure may be minimized if

- the total daily dose of Aplenzin Tablets does *not* exceed 522 mg,
- the rate of incrementation of dose is gradual.

Aplenzin should be administered with extreme caution to patients with a history of seizure, cranial trauma, or other predisposition(s) toward seizure, or patients treated with other agents (e.g., antipsychotics, other antidepressants, theophylline, systemic steroids, etc.) that lower seizure threshold.

5.5 Hepatic Impairment

Aplenzin should be used with extreme caution in patients with severe hepatic cirrhosis. In these patients a reduced frequency and/or dose is required, as peak bupropion, as well as AUC, levels are substantially increased and accumulation is likely to occur in such patients to a greater extent than usual. The dose should not exceed 174 mg every other day in these patients.

Aplenzin should be used with caution in patients with hepatic impairment (including mild to moderate hepatic cirrhosis) and reduced frequency and/or dose should be considered in patients with mild to moderate hepatic cirrhosis. All patients with hepatic impairment should be closely monitored for possible adverse effects that could indicate high drug and metabolite levels.

See DOSAGE AND ADMINISTRATION: Dosage Adjustment for Patients With Impaired Hepatic Function (2.5), USE IN SPECIFIC POPULATIONS: Hepatic Impairment (8.7) and CLINICAL PHARMACOLOGY: Pharmacokinetics (12.3)

5.6 Potential for Hepatotoxicity

In rats receiving large doses of bupropion chronically, there was an increase in incidence of hepatic hyperplastic nodules and hepatocellular hypertrophy. In dogs receiving large doses of bupropion chronically, various histologic changes were seen in the liver, and laboratory tests suggesting mild hepatocellular injury were noted.

Table 2. Incidence of Agitation, Anxiety, and Insomnia in Placebo-Controlled Trials of WELLBUTRIN SR® (Bupropion HCl Sustained-release Tablets) for Major Depressive Disorder

Adverse Reaction Term	WELLBUTRIN SR® (Bupropion HCl) 300 mg/day* (n = 376)	WELLBUTRIN SR® (Bupropion HCl) 400 mg/day** (n = 114)	Placebo (n = 385)
Agitation	3%	9%	2%
Anxiety	5%	6%	3%
Insomnia	11%	16%	6%

* Equivalent to 348 mg/day bupropion HBr
**Equivalent to 464 mg/day bupropion HBr

Table 3. Incidence of Weight Gain and Weight Loss in Placebo-Controlled Trials of WELLBUTRIN SR® (Bupropion Hydrochloride Sustained-Release Tablets) for Major Depressive Disorder

Weight Change	WELLBUTRIN SR® (Bupropion HCl) 300 mg/day* (n = 339)	WELLBUTRIN SR® (Bupropion HCl) 400 mg/day** (n = 112)	Placebo (n = 347)
Gained >5 lbs	3%	2%	4%
Lost >5 lbs	14%	19%	6%

* Equivalent to 348 mg/day bupropion HBr
**Equivalent to 464 mg/day bupropion HBr

5.7 Agitation and Insomnia

Increased restlessness, agitation, anxiety, and insomnia, especially shortly after initiation of treatment, have been associated with treatment with bupropion.

Patients in placebo-controlled trials of major depressive disorder with WELLBUTRIN SR®, the sustained-release formulation of bupropion hydrochloride, experienced agitation, anxiety, and insomnia as shown in Table 2.

[See table 2 above]

In clinical studies of major depressive disorder, these symptoms were sometimes of sufficient magnitude to require treatment with sedative/hypnotic drugs.

Symptoms in these studies were sufficiently severe to require discontinuation of treatment in 1% and 2.6% of patients treated with 300 and 400 mg/day, respectively, of bupropion hydrochloride sustained-release tablets and 0.8% of patients treated with placebo.

5.8 Psychosis, Confusion, and Other Neuropsychiatric Phenomena

Depressed patients treated with bupropion have been reported to show a variety of neuropsychiatric signs and symptoms, including delusions, hallucinations, psychosis, concentration disturbance, paranoia, and confusion. In some cases, these symptoms abated upon dose reduction and/or withdrawal of treatment.

5.9 Altered Appetite and Weight

In placebo-controlled studies of major depressive disorder using WELLBUTRIN SR®, the sustained-release formulation of bupropion hydrochloride, patients experienced weight gain or weight loss as shown in Table 3.

[See table 3 above]

In studies conducted with the immediate-release formulation of bupropion hydrochloride, 35% of patients receiving tricyclic antidepressants gained weight, compared to 9% of patients treated with the immediate-release formulation of bupropion hydrochloride. If weight loss is a major presenting sign of a patient's depressive illness, the anorectic and/or weight-reducing potential of Aplenzin Tablets should be considered.

5.10 Allergic Reactions

Anaphylactoid/anaphylactic reactions characterized by symptoms such as pruritus, urticaria, angioedema, and dyspnea requiring medical treatment have been reported in clinical trials with bupropion. In addition, there have been rare spontaneous postmarketing reports of erythema multiforme, Stevens-Johnson syndrome, and anaphylactic shock associated with bupropion. A patient should stop taking Aplenzin and consult a doctor if experiencing allergic or anaphylactoid/anaphylactic reactions (e.g., skin rash, pruritus, hives, chest pain, edema, and shortness of breath) during treatment.

Arthralgia, myalgia, and fever with rash and other symptoms suggestive of delayed hypersensitivity have been reported in association with bupropion. These symptoms may resemble serum sickness.

5.11 Cardiovascular Effects

In clinical practice, hypertension, in some cases severe, requiring acute treatment, has been reported in patients receiving bupropion alone and in combination with nicotine replacement therapy. These reactions have been observed in both patients with and without evidence of preexisting hypertension.

Data from a comparative study of the sustained-release formulation of bupropion hydrochloride (ZYBAN® Sustained-Release Tablets), nicotine transdermal system (NTS), the combination of sustained-release bupropion hydrochloride plus NTS, and placebo as an aid to smoking cessation suggest a higher incidence of treatment-emergent hypertension in patients treated with the combination of sustained-release bupropion hydrochloride and NTS. In this study, 6.1% of patients treated with the combination of sustained-release bupropion hydrochloride and NTS had treatment-emergent hypertension compared to 2.5%, 1.6%, and 3.1% of patients treated with sustained-release bupropion hydrochloride, NTS, and placebo, respectively. The majority of these patients had evidence of preexisting hypertension. Three patients (1.2%) treated with the combination of ZYBAN® and NTS and 1 patient (0.4%) treated with NTS had study medication discontinued due to hypertension compared to none of the patients treated with ZYBAN® or placebo. Monitoring of blood pressure is recommended in patients who receive the combination of bupropion and nicotine replacement.

There is no clinical experience establishing the safety of Aplenzin Tablets in patients with a recent history of myocardial infarction or unstable heart disease. Therefore, care should be exercised if it is used in these groups. Bupropion was well tolerated in depressed patients who had previously developed orthostatic hypotension while receiving tricyclic antidepressants, and was also generally well tolerated in a group of 36 depressed inpatients with stable congestive heart failure (CHF). However, bupropion was associated with a rise in supine blood pressure in the study of patients with CHF, resulting in discontinuation of treatment in 2 patients for exacerbation of baseline hypertension.

5.12 Laboratory Tests

There are no specific laboratory tests recommended.

6 ADVERSE REACTIONS

The following risks are discussed in greater detail in other sections of the labeling:

- Clinical worsening and suicide risk [see WARNINGS AND PRECAUTIONS: Clinical Worsening and Suicide Risk (5.1)]
- Activation of Psychosis and/or Mania [see WARNINGS AND PRECAUTIONS: Activation of Psychosis and/or Mania (5.2) and WARNINGS AND PRECAUTIONS: Screening Patients for Bipolar Disorder (5.3)]
- Hepatotoxicity [see WARNINGS AND PRECAUTIONS: Potential for Hepatotoxicity (5.6)]
- Agitation and Insomnia [see WARNINGS AND PRECAUTIONS: Agitation and Insomnia (5.7)]
- Psychosis, confusion and other neuropsychiatric phenomena [see WARNINGS AND PRECAUTIONS: Psychosis, Confusion, and Other Neuropsychiatric Phenomena (5.8)]
- Altered appetite [see WARNINGS AND PRECAUTIONS: Altered Appetite and Weight (5.9)]

Table 4. Treatment Discontinuations Due to Adverse Reactions in Placebo-Controlled Trials for Major Depressive Disorder

Adverse Reaction Term	WELLBUTRIN SR® (Bupropion HCl) 300 mg/day* (n = 376)	WELLBUTRIN SR® (Bupropion HCl) 400 mg/day** (n = 114)	Placebo (n = 385)
Rash	2.4%	0.9%	0.0%
Nausea	0.8%	1.8%	0.3%
Agitation	0.3%	1.8%	0.3%
Migraine	0.0%	1.8%	0.3%

* Equivalent to 348 mg/day bupropion HBr
**Equivalent to 464 mg/day bupropion HBr

- Allergic reactions, including anaphylactoid/anaphylactic reactions, erythema multiforme, Stevens-Johnson syndrome and other symptoms suggestive of delayed hypersensitivity [see *WARNINGS AND PRECAUTIONS: Allergic Reactions (5.10)*]
- Hypertension [see *WARNINGS AND PRECAUTIONS: Cardiovascular Effects (5.11)*]

6.1 Commonly Observed Adverse Reactions in Controlled Clinical Trials

Adverse reactions from Table 5 occurring in at least 5% of patients treated with the sustained-release formulation of bupropion hydrochloride and at a rate at least twice the placebo rate are listed below for the 300- and 400-mg/day dose groups.

300 mg/day of WELLBUTRIN SR® (equivalent to 348 mg/day bupropion HBr): Anorexia, dry mouth, rash, sweating, tinnitus, and tremor.

400 mg/day of WELLBUTRIN SR® (equivalent to 464 mg/day bupropion HBr): Abdominal pain, agitation, anxiety, dizziness, dry mouth, insomnia, myalgia, nausea, palpitation, pharyngitis, sweating, tinnitus, and urinary frequency. Aplenzin is bioequivalent to WELLBUTRIN XL®, which has been demonstrated to have similar bioavailability both to the immediate-release formulation of bupropion and to the sustained-release formulation of bupropion. The information included under this subsection and under subsections 6.2 and 6.3 is based primarily on data from controlled clinical trials with WELLBUTRIN SR® Tablets, the sustained-release formulation of bupropion hydrochloride.

6.2 Adverse Reactions Leading to Discontinuation of Treatment With WELLBUTRIN® or WELLBUTRIN SR®

In placebo-controlled clinical trials, 9% and 11% of patients treated with 300 and 400 mg/day, respectively, of the sustained-release formulation of bupropion hydrochloride and 4% of patients treated with placebo discontinued treatment due to adverse reactions. The specific adverse reactions in these trials that led to discontinuation in at least 1% of patients treated with either 300 mg/day or 400 mg/day of WELLBUTRIN SR®, the sustained-release formulation of bupropion hydrochloride, and at a rate at least twice the placebo rate are listed in Table 4.

[See table 4 above]

In clinical trials with the immediate-release formulation of bupropion, 10% of patients and volunteers discontinued due to an adverse reaction. Reactions resulting in discontinuation, in addition to those listed above for the sustained-release formulation of bupropion hydrochloride, include vomiting, seizures, and sleep disturbances.

6.3 Adverse Reactions Occurring at an Incidence of 1% or More Among Patients Treated With WELLBUTRIN® or WELLBUTRIN SR®

Table 5 enumerates treatment-emergent adverse reactions that occurred among patients treated with 300 and 400 mg/day of the sustained-release formulation of bupropion hydrochloride and with placebo in controlled trials. Reactions that occurred in either the 300- or 400-mg/day group at an incidence of 1% or more and were more frequent than in the placebo group are included. Reported adverse reactions were classified using a COSTART-based Dictionary. Accurate estimates of the incidence of adverse reactions associated with the use of any drug are difficult to obtain. Estimates are influenced by drug dose, detection technique, setting, physician judgments, etc. The figures cited cannot be used to predict precisely the incidence of untoward reactions in the course of usual medical practice where patient characteristics and other factors differ from those that prevailed in the clinical trials. These incidence figures also cannot be compared with those obtained from other clinical studies involving related drug products as each group of drug trials is conducted under a different set of conditions. Finally, it is important to emphasize that the tabulation does not reflect the relative severity and/or clinical importance of the reactions. A better perspective on the serious adverse reactions associated with the use of bupropion is provided in the WARNINGS AND PRECAUTIONS section (5).

[See table 5 at top of next page]

Additional reactions to those listed in Table 5 that occurred at an incidence of at least 1% in controlled clinical trials of the immediate-release formulation of bupropion hydrochloride (300 to 600 mg/day) and that were numerically more frequent than placebo were: cardiac arrhythmias (5% vs 4%), hypertension (4% vs 2%), hypotension (3% vs 2%), tachycardia (11% vs 9%), appetite increase (4% vs 2%), dyspepsia (3% vs 2%), menstrual complaints (5% vs 1%), akathisia (2% vs 1%), impaired sleep quality (4% vs 2%), sensory disturbance (4% vs 3%), confusion (8% vs 5%), decreased libido (3% vs 2%), hostility (6% vs 4%), auditory disturbance (5% vs 3%), and gustatory disturbance (3% vs 1%).

6.4 Other Events Observed During the Clinical Development and Postmarketing Experience of Bupropion

In addition to the adverse events noted above, the following events have been reported in clinical trials and postmarketing experience with the sustained-release formulation of bupropion hydrochloride in depressed patients and in nondepressed smokers, as well as in clinical trials and postmarketing clinical experience with the immediate-release formulation of bupropion hydrochloride.

Adverse events for which frequencies are provided below occurred in clinical trials with the sustained-release formulation of bupropion hydrochloride. The frequencies represent the proportion of patients who experienced a treatment-emergent adverse event on at least one occasion in placebo-controlled studies for depression (n = 987) or smoking cessation (n = 1,013), or patients who experienced an adverse event requiring discontinuation of treatment in an open-label surveillance study with the sustained-release formulation of bupropion hydrochloride (n = 3,100). All treatment-emergent adverse events are included except those listed in Tables 2 through 5, those events listed in other safety-related sections, those adverse events subsumed under COSTART terms that are either overly general or excessively specific so as to be uninformative, those events not reasonably associated with the use of the drug, and those events that were not serious and occurred in fewer than 2 patients. Events of major clinical importance are described in the WARNINGS AND PRECAUTIONS section (5).

Events are further categorized by body system and listed in order of decreasing frequency according to the following definitions of frequency: Frequent adverse events are defined as those occurring in at least 1/100 patients. Infrequent adverse events are those occurring in 1/100 to 1/1,000 patients, while rare events are those occurring in less than 1/1,000 patients.

Adverse events for which frequencies are not provided occurred in clinical trials or postmarketing experience with bupropion. Only those adverse events not previously listed for sustained-release bupropion are included. The extent to which these events may be associated with Aplenzin is unknown.

Body (General)
Infrequent were chills, facial edema, musculoskeletal chest pain, and photosensitivity. Rare was malaise. Also observed were arthralgia, myalgia, and fever with rash and other symptoms suggestive of delayed hypersensitivity. These symptoms may resemble serum sickness [see *WARNINGS AND PRECAUTIONS: Allergic Reactions (5.10)*].

Cardiovascular
Infrequent were postural hypotension, stroke, tachycardia, and vasodilation. Rare was syncope. Also observed were complete atrioventricular block, extrasystoles, hypotension, hypertension (in some cases severe; [see *WARNINGS AND PRECAUTIONS: Cardiovascular Effects (5.11)*], myocardial infarction, phlebitis, and pulmonary embolism.

Digestive
Infrequent were abnormal liver function, bruxism, gastric reflux, gingivitis, glossitis, increased salivation, jaundice, mouth ulcers, stomatitis, and thirst. Rare was edema of tongue. Also observed were colitis, esophagitis, gastrointestinal hemorrhage, gum hemorrhage, hepatitis, intestinal perforation, liver damage, pancreatitis, and stomach ulcer.

Endocrine
Also observed were hyperglycemia, hypoglycemia, and syndrome of inappropriate antidiuretic hormone.

Hemic and Lymphatic
Infrequent was ecchymosis. Also observed were anemia, leukocytosis, leukopenia, lymphadenopathy, pancytopenia, and thrombocytopenia. Altered PT and/or INR, infrequently associated with hemorrhagic or thrombotic complications, were observed when bupropion was coadministered with warfarin.

Metabolic and Nutritional
Infrequent were edema and peripheral edema. Also observed was glycosuria.

Musculoskeletal
Infrequent were leg cramps. Also observed were muscle rigidity/fever/rhabdomyolysis and muscle weakness.

Nervous System
Infrequent were abnormal coordination, decreased libido, depersonalization, dysphoria, emotional lability, hostility, hyperkinesia, hypertonia, hypesthesia, suicidal ideation, and vertigo. Rare were amnesia, ataxia, derealization, and hypomania. Also observed were abnormal electroencephalogram (EEG), aggression, akinesia, aphasia, coma, delirium, delusions, dysarthria, dyskinesia, dystonia, euphoria, extrapyramidal syndrome, hallucinations, hypokinesia, increased libido, manic reaction, neuralgia, neuropathy, paranoid ideation, restlessness, and unmasking tardive dyskinesia.

Respiratory
Rare was bronchospasm. Also observed was pneumonia.

Skin
Rare was maculopapular rash. Also observed were alopecia, angioedema, exfoliative dermatitis, and hirsutism.

Special Senses
Infrequent were accommodation abnormality and dry eye. Also observed were deafness, diplopia, increased intraocular pressure, and mydriasis.

Urogenital
Infrequent were impotence, polyuria, and prostate disorder. Also observed were abnormal ejaculation, cystitis, dyspareunia, dysuria, gynecomastia, menopause, painful erection, salpingitis, urinary incontinence, urinary retention, and vaginitis.

7 DRUG INTERACTIONS

Few systemic data have been collected on the metabolism of bupropion following concomitant administration with other drugs or, alternatively, the effect of concomitant administration of bupropion on the metabolism of other drugs.

Because bupropion is extensively metabolized, the coadministration of other drugs may affect its clinical activity. In vitro studies indicate that bupropion is primarily metabolized to hydroxybupropion by the CYP2B6 isoenzyme. Therefore, the potential exists for a drug interaction between Aplenzin and drugs that are substrates or inhibitors of the CYP2B6 isoenzyme (e.g., orphenadrine, thiotepa, and cyclophosphamide). In addition, *in vitro* studies suggest that paroxetine, sertraline, norfluoxetine, and fluvoxamine as well as nelfinavir, ritonavir, and efavirenz inhibit the hydroxylation of bupropion. No clinical studies have been performed to evaluate this finding. The threohydrobupropion metabolite of bupropion does not appear to be produced by the cytochrome P450 isoenzymes. The effects of concomitant administration of cimetidine on the pharmacokinetics of bupropion and its active metabolites were studied in 24 healthy young male volunteers. Following oral administration of two 150-mg tablets of the sustained-release formulation of bupropion hydrochloride with and without 800 mg of cimetidine, the pharmacokinetics of bupropion and hydroxybupropion were unaffected. However, there were 16% and 32% increases in the AUC and C_{max}, respectively, of the combined moieties of threohydrobupropion and erythrohydrobupropion.

While not systematically studied, certain drugs may induce the metabolism of bupropion (e.g., carbamazepine, phenobarbital, phenytoin).

Multiple oral doses of bupropion had no statistically significant effects on the single dose pharmacokinetics of lamotrigine in 12 healthy volunteers.

Animal data indicated that bupropion may be an inducer of drug-metabolizing enzymes in humans. In one study, following chronic administration of bupropion hydrochloride, 100 mg 3 times daily to 8 healthy male volunteers for 14 days, there was no evidence of induction of its own metabolism. Nevertheless, there may be the potential for clinically important alterations of blood levels of coadministered drugs.

7.1 Drugs Metabolized By Cytochrome P450IID6 (CYP2D6)

Many drugs, including most antidepressants (SSRIs, many tricyclics), beta-blockers, antiarrhythmics, and antipsychotics are metabolized by the CYP2D6 isoenzyme. Although bupropion is not metabolized by this isoenzyme, bupropion and hydroxybupropion are inhibitors of CYP2D6 isoenzyme *in vitro*. In a study of 15 male subjects (ages 19 to 35 years) who were extensive metabolizers of the CYP2D6 isoenzyme, daily doses of bupropion hydrochloride given as 150 mg twice daily followed by a single dose of 50 mg desipramine increased the C_{max}, AUC, and $t_{1/2}$ of desipramine by an average of approximately 2-, 5-, and 2-fold, respectively. The effect was present for at least 7 days after the last dose of bupropion. Concomitant use of bupropion with other drugs metabolized by CYP2D6 has not been formally studied. Therefore, co-administration of bupropion with drugs that are metabolized by CYP2D6 isoenzyme including certain antidepressants (e.g., nortriptyline, imipramine, desipramine, paroxetine, fluoxetine, sertraline), antipsychotics (e.g., haloperidol, risperidone, thioridazine), beta-blockers (e.g., metoprolol), and Type 1C antiarrhythmics (e.g., propafenone, flecainide), should be approached with caution and should be initiated at the lower end of the dose range of the concomitant medication. If bupropion is added to the treatment regimen of a patient already receiving a drug metabolized by CYP2D6, the need to decrease the dose of the original medication should be considered, particularly for those concomitant medications with a narrow therapeutic index.

7.2 MAO Inhibitors
Studies in animals demonstrate that the acute toxicity of bupropion is enhanced by the MAO inhibitor phenelzine [see *CONTRAINDICATIONS (4)*].

7.3 Levodopa and Amantadine
Limited clinical data suggest a higher incidence of adverse experiences in patients receiving bupropion concurrently with either levodopa or amantadine. Administration of Aplenzin Tablets to patients receiving either levodopa or amantadine concurrently should be undertaken with caution, using small initial doses and gradual dose increases.

7.4 Drugs That Lower Seizure Threshold
Concurrent administration of Aplenzin Tablets and agents (e.g., antipsychotics, other antidepressants, theophylline, systemic steroids, etc.) that lower seizure threshold should be undertaken only with extreme caution [see *WARNINGS AND PRECAUTIONS: Seizures (5.4)*]. Low initial dosing and gradual dose increases should be employed.

7.5 Nicotine Transdermal System
See *WARNINGS AND PRECAUTIONS: Cardiovascular Effects (5.11)*.

7.6 Alcohol
In postmarketing experience, there have been rare reports of adverse neuropsychiatric events or reduced alcohol tolerance in patients who were drinking alcohol during treatment with bupropion. The consumption of alcohol during treatment with Aplenzin should be minimized or avoided [also see *CONTRAINDICATIONS (4)*].

8 USE IN SPECIFIC POPULATIONS
8.1 Pregnancy
Teratogenic Effects
Pregnancy Category C. In studies conducted in rats and rabbits, bupropion hydrochloride was administered orally at doses up to 450 and 150 mg/kg/day, respectively (approximately 11 and 7 times the maximum recommended human dose [MRHD], respectively, on a mg/m² basis), during the period of organogenesis. No clear evidence of teratogenic activity was found in either species; however, in rabbits, slightly increased incidences of fetal malformations and skeletal variations were observed at the lowest dose tested (25 mg/kg/day, approximately equal to the MRHD on a mg/m² basis) and greater. Decreased fetal weights were seen at 50 mg/kg and greater.
When rats were administered bupropion hydrochloride at oral doses of up to 300 mg/kg/day (approximately 7 times the MRHD on a mg/m² basis) prior to mating and throughout pregnancy and lactation, there were no apparent adverse effects on offspring development.
One study has been conducted in pregnant women. This retrospective, managed-care database study assessed the risk of congenital malformations overall, and cardiovascular malformations specifically, following exposure to bupropion in the first trimester compared to the risk of these malformations following exposure to other antidepressants in the first trimester and bupropion outside of the first trimester. This study included 7,005 infants with antidepressant exposure during pregnancy, 1,213 of whom were exposed to bupropion in the first trimester. The study showed no greater risk for congenital malformations overall, or cardiovascular malformations specifically, following first trimester bupropion exposure compared to exposure to all other antidepressants in the first trimester, or bupropion outside of the first trimester. The results of this study have not been corroborated. Aplenzin should be used during pregnancy only if the potential benefit justifies the potential risk to the fetus.

8.2 Labor and Delivery
The effect of Aplenzin Tablets on labor and delivery in humans is unknown.

8.3 Nursing Mothers
Like many other drugs, bupropion and its metabolites are secreted in human milk. Because of the potential for serious adverse reactions in nursing infants from Aplenzin Tablets, a decision should be made whether to discontinue nursing or to discontinue the drug, taking into account the importance of the drug to the mother.

8.4 Pediatric Use
Safety and effectiveness in the pediatric population have not been established [see *BOXED WARNING and WARNINGS AND PRECAUTIONS: Clinical Worsening and Suicide Risk (5.1)*]. Anyone considering the use of Aplenzin in a child or adolescent must balance the potential risks with the clinical need.

8.5 Geriatric Use
Of the approximately 6,000 patients who participated in clinical trials with bupropion hydrochloride sustained-release tablets (depression and smoking cessation studies), 275 were ≥65 years old and 47 were ≥75 years old. In addition, several hundred patients 65 and over participated in clinical trials using the immediate-release formulation of bupropion hydrochloride (depression studies). No overall differences in safety or effectiveness were observed between these subjects and younger subjects. Reported clinical experience has not identified differences in responses between

Table 5. Treatment-Emergent Adverse Reactions in Placebo-Controlled Trials* for Major Depressive Disorder

Body System/Adverse Reaction	WELLBUTRIN SR® (Bupropion HCl) 300 mg/day** (n = 376)	WELLBUTRIN SR® (Bupropion HCl) 400 mg/day*** (n = 114)	Placebo (n = 385)
Body (General)			
Headache	26%	25%	23%
Infection	8%	9%	6%
Abdominal pain	3%	9%	2%
Asthenia	2%	4%	2%
Chest pain	3%	4%	1%
Pain	2%	3%	2%
Fever	1%	2%	—
Cardiovascular			
Palpitation	2%	6%	2%
Flushing	1%	4%	—
Migraine	1%	4%	1%
Hot flashes	1%	3%	1%
Digestive			
Dry mouth	17%	24%	7%
Nausea	13%	18%	8%
Constipation	10%	5%	7%
Diarrhea	5%	7%	6%
Anorexia	5%	3%	2%
Vomiting	4%	2%	2%
Dysphagia	0%	2%	0%
Musculoskeletal			
Myalgia	2%	6%	3%
Arthralgia	1%	4%	1%
Arthritis	0%	2%	0%
Twitch	1%	2%	—
Nervous system			
Insomnia	11%	16%	6%
Dizziness	7%	11%	5%
Agitation	3%	9%	2%
Anxiety	5%	6%	3%
Tremor	6%	3%	1%
Nervousness	5%	3%	3%
Somnolence	2%	3%	2%
Irritability	3%	2%	2%
Memory decreased	—	3%	1%
Paresthesia	1%	2%	1%
Central nervous system stimulation	2%	1%	1%
Respiratory			
Pharyngitis	3%	11%	2%
Sinusitis	3%	1%	2%
Increased cough	1%	2%	1%
Skin			
Sweating	6%	5%	2%
Rash	5%	4%	1%
Pruritus	2%	4%	2%
Urticaria	2%	1%	0%
Special senses			
Tinnitus	6%	6%	2%
Taste perversion	2%	4%	—
Blurred vision or diplopia	3%	2%	2%
Urogenital			
Urinary frequency	2%	5%	2%
Urinary urgency	—	2%	0%
Vaginal hemorrhage†	0%	2%	—
Urinary tract infection	1%	0%	—

* Adverse reactions that occurred in at least 1% of patients treated with either 300 or 400 mg/day of the sustained-release formulation of bupropion hydrochloride, but equally or more frequently in the placebo group, were: abnormal dreams, accidental injury, acne, appetite increased, back pain, bronchitis, dysmenorrhea, dyspepsia, flatulence, flu syndrome, hypertension, neck pain, respiratory disorder, rhinitis, and tooth disorder.
** Equivalent to 348 mg/day bupropion HBr
*** Equivalent to 464 mg/day bupropion HBr
† Incidence based on the number of female patients.
— Hyphen denotes adverse reactions occurring in greater than 0 but less than 0.5% of patients.

the elderly and younger patients, but greater sensitivity of some older individuals cannot be ruled out.

A single-dose pharmacokinetic study demonstrated that the disposition of bupropion and its metabolites in elderly subjects was similar to that of younger subjects; however, another pharmacokinetic study, single and multiple dose, has suggested that the elderly are at increased risk for accumulation of bupropion and its metabolites **[see *CLINICAL PHARMACOLOGY: Pharmacokinetics (12.3)*]**.

Bupropion is extensively metabolized in the liver to active metabolites, which are further metabolized and excreted by the kidneys. The risk of toxic reaction to this drug may be greater in patients with impaired renal function. Because elderly patients are more likely to have decreased renal function, care should be taken in dose selection, and it may be useful to monitor renal function **[see *DOSAGE AND ADMINISTRATION: Dosage Adjustment in Patients With Impaired Renal Function (2.6)* and *USE IN SPECIFIC POPULATIONS: Renal Impairment (8.6)*]**.

8.6 Renal Impairment

There is limited information on the pharmacokinetics of bupropion in patients with renal impairment. An inter-study comparison between normal subjects and patients with end-stage renal failure demonstrated that the parent drug C_{max} and AUC values were comparable in the 2 groups, whereas the hydroxybupropion and threohydrobupropion metabolites had a 2.3- and 2.8-fold increase, respectively, in AUC for patients with end-stage renal failure. Bupropion is extensively metabolized in the liver to active metabolites, which are further metabolized and subsequently excreted by the kidneys. Aplenzin should be used with caution in patients with renal impairment and a reduced frequency and/or dose should be considered as bupropion and the metabolites of bupropion may accumulate in such patients to a greater extent than usual. The patient should be closely monitored for possible adverse effects that could indicate high drug or metabolite levels **[see *DOSAGE AND ADMINISTRATION: Dosage Adjustment for Patients With Impaired Renal Function (2.6)* and *CLINICAL PHARMACOLOGY: Pharmacokinetics (12.3)*]**.

8.7 Hepatic Impairment

Aplenzin should be used with extreme caution in patients with severe hepatic cirrhosis. In these patients a reduced frequency and/or dose is required, as peak bupropion, as well as AUC, levels are substantially increased and accumulation is likely to occur in such patients to a greater extent than usual. The dose should not exceed 174 mg every other day in these patients.

Aplenzin should be used with caution in patients with hepatic impairment (including mild to moderate hepatic cirrhosis) and reduced frequency and/or dose should be considered in patients with mild to moderate hepatic cirrhosis.

All patients with hepatic impairment should be closely monitored for possible adverse effects that could indicate high drug and metabolite levels.

See *DOSAGE AND ADMINISTRATION: Dosage Adjustment for Patients With Impaired Hepatic Function (2.5)* and *CLINICAL PHARMACOLOGY: Pharmacokinetics (12.3)*.

9 DRUG ABUSE AND DEPENDENCE

9.1 Controlled Substance

Bupropion is not a controlled substance.

9.2 Abuse

Humans

Controlled clinical studies of bupropion hydrochloride (immediate-release formulation) conducted in normal volunteers, in subjects with a history of multiple drug abuse, and in depressed patients showed some increase in motor activity and agitation/excitement.

In a population of individuals experienced with drugs of abuse, a single dose of 400 mg of bupropion hydrochloride produced mild amphetamine-like activity as compared to placebo on the Morphine-Benzedrine Subscale of the Addiction Research Center Inventories (ARCI), and a score intermediate between placebo and amphetamine on the Liking Scale of the ARCI. These scales measure general feelings of euphoria and drug desirability.

Findings in clinical trials, however, are not known to reliably predict the abuse potential of drugs. Nonetheless, evidence from single-dose studies does suggest that the recommended daily dosage of bupropion when administered in divided doses is not likely to be especially reinforcing to amphetamine or stimulant abusers. However, higher doses that could not be tested because of the risk of seizure might be modestly attractive to those who abuse stimulant drugs.

Animals

Studies in rodents and primates have shown that bupropion exhibits some pharmacologic actions common to psychostimulants. In rodents, it has been shown to increase locomotor activity, elicit a mild stereotyped behavioral response, and increase rates of responding in several schedule-controlled behavior paradigms. In primate models to assess the positive reinforcing effects of psychoactive drugs, bupropion was self-administered intravenously. In rats, bupropion produced amphetamine-like and cocaine-like discriminative stimulus effects in drug discrimination paradigms used to characterize the subjective effects of psychoactive drugs.

10 OVERDOSAGE

10.1 Human Overdose Experience

Overdoses of up to 30 g or more of bupropion have been reported. Seizure was reported in approximately one third of all cases. Other serious reactions reported with overdoses of bupropion alone included hallucinations, loss of consciousness, sinus tachycardia, and ECG changes such as conduction disturbances or arrhythmias. Fever, muscle rigidity, rhabdomyolysis, hypotension, stupor, coma, and respiratory failure have been reported mainly when bupropion was part of multiple drug overdoses.

Although most patients recovered without sequelae, deaths associated with overdoses of bupropion alone have been reported in patients ingesting large doses of the drug. Multiple uncontrolled seizures, bradycardia, cardiac failure, and cardiac arrest prior to death were reported in these patients.

10.2 Overdosage Management

Ensure an adequate airway, oxygenation, and ventilation. Monitor cardiac rhythm and vital signs. EEG monitoring is also recommended for the first 48 hours post-ingestion. General supportive and symptomatic measures are also recommended. Induction of emesis is not recommended. Gastric lavage with a large-bore orogastric tube with appropriate airway protection, if needed, may be indicated if performed soon after ingestion or in symptomatic patients. Activated charcoal should be administered. There is no experience with the use of forced diuresis, dialysis, hemoperfusion, or exchange transfusion in the management of bupropion overdoses. No specific antidotes for bupropion are known.

Due to the dose-related risk of seizures with Aplenzin, hospitalization following suspected overdose should be considered. Based on studies in animals, it is recommended that seizures be treated with intravenous benzodiazepine administration and other supportive measures, as appropriate.

In managing overdosage, consider the possibility of multiple drug involvement. The physician should consider contacting a poison control center for additional information on the treatment of any overdose. Telephone numbers for certified poison control centers are listed in the *Physicians' Desk Reference* (PDR).

11 DESCRIPTION

Aplenzin (bupropion hydrobromide), an antidepressant of the aminoketone class, is chemically unrelated to tricyclic, tetracyclic, selective serotonin re-uptake inhibitor, or other known antidepressant agents. Its structure closely resembles that of diethylpropion; it is related to phenylethylamines. It is designated as (±)-2-(tert-butylamino)-3′-chloropropiophenone hydrobromide. The molecular weight is 320.6. The molecular formula is $C_{13}H_{18}ClNO \bullet HBr$. Bupropion hydrobromide powder is white or almost white, crystalline, and soluble in water. It has a bitter taste and produces the sensation of local anesthesia on the oral mucosa. The structural formula is:

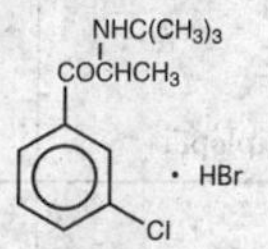
NHC(CH3)3
COCHCH3
• HBr
Cl

Aplenzin Tablets are supplied for oral administration as 174 mg, 348 mg, and 522 mg white to off white extended-release tablets. Each tablet contains the labeled amount of bupropion hydrobromide and the inactive ingredients: ethylcellulose aqueous dispersion, glyceryl behenate, polyvinyl alcohol, polyethylene glycol, povidone, and dibutyl sebacate. Carnauba wax is included in the 174 mg and 348 mg strengths. The tablets are printed with edible black ink.

The insoluble shell of the extended-release tablet may remain intact during gastrointestinal transit and is eliminated in the feces.

12 CLINICAL PHARMACOLOGY

12.1 Mechanism of Action

The mechanism of action of bupropion is unknown, as is the case with other antidepressants. However, it is presumed that this action is mediated by noradrenergic and/or dopaminergic mechanisms.

12.2 Pharmacodynamics

Bupropion is a relatively weak inhibitor of the neuronal uptake of norepinephrine and dopamine, and does not inhibit monoamine oxidase or the re-uptake of serotonin.

12.3 Pharmacokinetics

Bupropion is a racemic mixture. The pharmacologic activity and pharmacokinetics of the individual enantiomers have not been studied.

Following chronic dosing of Aplenzin 348 mg Tablets, the mean peak steady-state plasma concentration and area under the curve of bupropion were 134.3 (± 38.2) ng/mL and 1409 (± 346) ng•hr/mL, respectively. Steady-state plasma concentrations of bupropion were reached within 8 days. The elimination half-life (±SD) of bupropion after a single dose is 21.3 (± 6.7) hours.

In a study comparing 10-day dosing with Aplenzin Tablets 348 mg once daily and WELLBUTRIN XL® Tablets 300 mg once daily, following a 3-day titration with once daily WELLBUTRIN XL® Tablets 150 mg, Aplenzin peak plasma concentration and area under the curve for bupropion and the 3 metabolites (hydroxybupropion, threohydrobupropion, and erythrohydrobupropion) were equivalent to WELLBUTRIN XL® Tablets 300 mg, with the average being 8-14% lower.

In a single dose study, two Aplenzin Tablets 174 mg once daily and one Aplenzin Tablet 348 mg once daily were evaluated. Equivalence was demonstrated for peak plasma concentration and area under the curve for bupropion and the 3 metabolites.

Additionally, a multiple dose study compared 14-day dosing with Aplenzin Tablets 522 mg once daily to dosing with three Aplenzin Tablets 174 mg once daily, following a 3-day titration with one Aplenzin Tablet 174 mg once daily, and a succeeding 5-day titration with two Aplenzin tablets 174 mg once daily. Equivalence was demonstrated for peak plasma concentration and area under the curve for bupropion and the 3 metabolites.

These findings demonstrate that Aplenzin Tablets 174 mg, 348 mg and 522 mg are dose proportional. A 348 mg dose can be achieved by administering either one Aplenzin Tablet 348 mg or two Aplenzin Tablets 174 mg. A 522 mg dose can be achieved by administering either one Aplenzin Tablet 522 mg, three Aplenzin Tablets 174 mg, or one Aplenzin Tablet 174 mg plus one Aplenzin Tablet 348 mg.

Absorption

Following single oral administration of Aplenzin Tablets to healthy volunteers, the median time to peak plasma concentrations for bupropion was approximately 5 hours. The presence of food did not affect the peak concentration and time to peak plasma concentration of bupropion; area under the curve was increased by 19%.

Distribution

In vitro tests show that bupropion is 84% bound to human plasma proteins at concentrations up to 200 mcg/mL. The extent of protein binding of the hydroxybupropion metabolite is similar to that for bupropion, whereas the extent of protein binding of the threohydrobupropion metabolite is about half that seen with bupropion.

Metabolism

Bupropion is extensively metabolized in humans. Three metabolites have been shown to be active: hydroxybupropion, which is formed via hydroxylation of the *tert*-butyl group of bupropion, and the amino-alcohol isomers threohydrobupropion and erythrohydrobupropion, which are formed via reduction of the carbonyl group. *In vitro* findings suggest that cytochrome P450IIB6 (CYP2B6) is the principal isoenzyme involved in the formation of hydroxybupropion, while cytochrome P450 isoenzymes are not involved in the formation of threohydrobupropion. Oxidation of the bupropion side chain results in the formation of a glycine conjugate of meta-chlorobenzoic acid, which is then excreted as the major urinary metabolite. The potency and toxicity of the metabolites relative to bupropion have not been fully characterized. However, it has been demonstrated in an antidepressant screening test in mice that hydroxybupropion is one half as potent as bupropion, while threohydrobupropion and erythrohydrobupropion are 5-fold less potent than bupropion. This may be of clinical importance because the plasma concentrations of the metabolites are as high or higher than those of bupropion.

Because bupropion is extensively metabolized, there is the potential for drug-drug interactions, particularly with those agents that are metabolized by the cytochrome P450IIB6 (CYP2B6) isoenzyme. Although bupropion is not metabolized by cytochrome P450IID6 (CYP2D6), there is the potential for drug-drug interactions when bupropion is co-administered with drugs metabolized by this isoenzyme **[see *DRUG INTERACTIONS: Drugs Metabolized by Cytochrome P450IID6 (CYP2D6) (7.1)*]**.

Following chronic administration in healthy volunteers, peak plasma concentration of hydroxybupropion occurred approximately 6 hours after administration of Aplenzin tablets. The peak plasma concentrations of hydroxybupropion were approximately 9 times the peak level of the parent drug at steady state. The elimination half-life of hydroxybupropion is approximately 24.3 (± 4.9) hours, and its AUC at steady state is about 15.6 times that of bupropion. The times to peak concentrations for the erythrohydrobupropion and threohydrobupropion metabolites are similar to that of hydroxybupropion. However, the elimination half-lives of erythrohydrobupropion and threohydrobupropion are longer, approximately 31.1 (± 7.8) and 50.8 (± 8.5) hours, respectively, and steady-state AUCs were 1.5 and 6.8 times that of bupropion, respectively.

Bupropion and its metabolites exhibit linear kinetics following chronic administration of 300 to 450 mg/day of bupropion hydrochloride (equivalent to 348 mg and 522 mg of bupropion hydrobromide, respectively).

Elimination

Following oral administration of 200 mg of ^{14}C-bupropion in humans, 87% and 10% of the radioactive dose were recovered in the urine and feces, respectively. However, the fraction of the oral dose of bupropion excreted unchanged was only 0.5%, a finding consistent with the extensive metabolism of bupropion.

Population Subgroups

Factors or conditions altering metabolic capacity (e.g., liver disease, congestive heart failure [CHF], age, concomitant medications, etc.) or elimination may be expected to influence the degree and extent of accumulation of the active metabolites of bupropion. The elimination of the major metabolites of bupropion may be affected by reduced renal or hepatic function because they are moderately polar compounds and are likely to undergo further metabolism or conjugation in the liver prior to urinary excretion.

Hepatic

The effect of hepatic impairment on the pharmacokinetics of bupropion was characterized in 2 single-dose studies, one in patients with alcoholic liver disease and one in patients with mild to severe cirrhosis. The first study showed that the half-life of hydroxybupropion was significantly longer in 8 patients with alcoholic liver disease than in 8 healthy volunteers (32±14 hours versus 21±5 hours, respectively). Although not statistically significant, the AUCs for bupropion and hydroxybupropion were more variable and tended to be greater (by 53% to 57%) in patients with alcoholic liver disease. The differences in half-life for bupropion and the other metabolites in the 2 patient groups were minimal.

The second study showed no statistically significant differences in the pharmacokinetics of bupropion and its active metabolites in 9 patients with mild to moderate hepatic cirrhosis compared to 8 healthy volunteers. However, more variability was observed in some of the pharmacokinetic parameters for bupropion (AUC, C_{max}, and T_{max}) and its active metabolites ($t_{1/2}$) in patients with mild to moderate hepatic cirrhosis. In addition, in patients with severe hepatic cirrhosis, the bupropion C_{max} and AUC were substantially increased (mean difference: by approximately 70% and 3-fold, respectively) and more variable when compared to values in healthy volunteers; the mean bupropion half-life was also longer (29 hours in patients with severe hepatic cirrhosis vs 19 hours in healthy subjects). For the metabolite hydroxybupropion, the mean C_{max} was approximately 69% lower. For the combined amino-alcohol isomers threohydrobupropion and erythrohydrobupropion, the mean C_{max} was approximately 31% lower. The mean AUC increased by about 1½-fold for hydroxybupropion and about 2½-fold for threo/erythrohydrobupropion. The median T_{max} was observed 19 hours later for hydroxybupropion and 31 hours later for threo/erythrohydrobupropion. The mean half-lives for hydroxybupropion and threo/erythrohydrobupropion were increased 5- and 2-fold, respectively, in patients with severe hepatic cirrhosis compared to healthy volunteers [see DOSAGE AND ADMINISTRATION: Dosage Adjustment for Patients With Impaired Hepatic Function (2.5), WARNINGS AND PRECAUTIONS: Hepatic Impairment (5.5) and USE IN SPECIFIC POPULATIONS: Hepatic Impairment (8.7)].

Renal

There is limited information on the pharmacokinetics of bupropion in patients with renal impairment. An interstudy comparison between normal subjects and patients with endstage renal failure demonstrated that the parent drug C_{max} and AUC values were comparable in the 2 groups, whereas the hydroxybupropion and threohydrobupropion metabolites had a 2.3- and 2.8-fold increase, respectively, in AUC for patients with end-stage renal failure. The elimination of the major metabolites of bupropion may be reduced by impaired renal function [see DOSAGE AND ADMINISTRATION: Dosage Adjustment for Patients With Impaired Renal Function (2.6) and USE IN SPECIFIC POPULATIONS: Renal Impairment (8.6)].

Left Ventricular Dysfunction

During a chronic dosing study with bupropion in 14 depressed patients with left ventricular dysfunction (history of CHF or an enlarged heart on x-ray), no apparent effect on the pharmacokinetics of bupropion or its metabolites was revealed, compared to healthy volunteers.

Age

The effects of age on the pharmacokinetics of bupropion and its metabolites have not been fully characterized, but an exploration of steady-state bupropion concentrations from several depression efficacy studies involving patients dosed in a range of 300 to 750 mg/day, on a 3 times daily schedule, revealed no relationship between age (18 to 83 years) and

plasma concentration of bupropion. A single-dose pharmacokinetic study demonstrated that the disposition of bupropion and its metabolites in elderly subjects was similar to that of younger subjects. These data suggest there is no prominent effect of age on bupropion concentration; however, another pharmacokinetic study, single and multiple dose, has suggested that the elderly are at increased risk for accumulation of bupropion and its metabolites [see USE IN SPECIFIC POPULATIONS: Geriatric Use (8.5)].

Gender

Pooled analysis of bupropion pharmacokinetic data from 90 healthy male and 90 healthy female volunteers revealed no sex-related differences in the peak plasma concentrations of bupropion. The mean systemic exposure (AUC) was approximately 13% higher in male volunteers compared to female volunteers. The clinical significance of this finding is unknown.

Smokers

The effects of cigarette smoking on the pharmacokinetics of bupropion hydrochloride were studied in 34 healthy male and female volunteers; 17 were chronic cigarette smokers and 17 were nonsmokers. Following oral administration of a single 150-mg dose of bupropion, there was no statistically significant difference in C_{max}, half-life, T_{max}, AUC, or clearance of bupropion or its active metabolites between smokers and nonsmokers.

13   NONCLINICAL TOXICOLOGY

13.1   Carcinogenesis, Mutagenesis, Impairment of Fertility

Lifetime carcinogenicity studies were performed in rats and mice at doses up to 300 and 150 mg/kg/day bupropion hydrochloride, respectively. These doses are approximately 7 and 2 times the maximum recommended human dose (MRHD), respectively, on a mg/m^2 basis. In the rat study there was an increase in nodular proliferative lesions of the liver at doses of 100 to 300 mg/kg/day of bupropion hydrochloride (approximately 2 to 7 times the MRHD on a mg/m^2 basis); lower doses were not tested. The question of whether or not such lesions may be precursors of neoplasms of the liver is currently unresolved. Similar liver lesions were not seen in the mouse study, and no increase in malignant tumors of the liver and other organs was seen in either study. Bupropion produced a positive response (2 to 3 times control mutation rate) in 2 of 5 strains in one Ames bacterial mutagenicity assay, but was negative in another. Bupropion produced an increase in chromosomal aberrations in 1 of 3 in vivo rat bone marrow cytogenetic studies.

A fertility study in rats at doses up to 300 mg/kg/day revealed no evidence of impaired fertility.

14   CLINICAL STUDIES

The efficacy of bupropion as a treatment for major depressive disorder was established with the immediate-release formulation of bupropion hydrochloride in two 4-week, placebo-controlled trials in adult inpatients and in one 6-week, placebo-controlled trial in adult outpatients. In the first study, patients were titrated in a bupropion hydrochloride dose range of 300 to 600 mg/day of the immediate-release formulation on a 3 times daily schedule; 78% of patients received maximum doses of 450 mg/day or less. This trial demonstrated the effectiveness of bupropion on the Hamilton Depression Rating Scale (HDRS) total score, the depressed mood item (item 1) from that scale, and the Clinical Global Impressions (CGI) severity score. A second study included 2 fixed doses of the immediate-release formulation of bupropion hydrochloride (300 and 450 mg/day) and placebo. This trial demonstrated the effectiveness of bupropion, but only at the 450-mg/day dose of the immediate-release formulation; the results were positive for the HDRS total score and the CGI severity score, but not for HDRS item 1. In the third study, outpatients received 300 mg/day of the immediate-release formulation of bupropion hydrochloride. This study demonstrated the effectiveness of bupropion on the HDRS total score, HDRS item 1, the Montgomery-Asberg Depression Rating Scale, the CGI severity score, and the CGI improvement score.

In a longer-term study, outpatients meeting DSM-IV criteria for major depressive disorder, recurrent type, who had responded during an 8-week open trial on bupropion hydrochloride (150 mg twice daily of the sustained-release formulation) were randomized to continuation of their same dose of bupropion or placebo, for up to 44 weeks of observation for relapse. Response during the open phase was defined as CGI Improvement score of 1 (very much improved) or 2 (much improved) for each of the final 3 weeks. Relapse during the double-blind phase was defined as the investigator's judgment that drug treatment was needed for worsening depressive symptoms. Patients receiving continued bupropion treatment experienced significantly lower relapse rates over the subsequent 44 weeks compared to those receiving placebo.

Although there are no independent trials demonstrating the antidepressant effectiveness of Aplenzin or WELLBUTRIN XL®, studies have demonstrated similar bioavailability of

WELLBUTRIN XL® to both the immediate-release formulation and to the sustained-release formulation of bupropion under steady-state conditions, i.e., WELLBUTRIN XL® 300 mg once daily was shown to have bioavailability that was similar to that of 100 mg 3 times daily of the immediate-release formulation of bupropion and to that of 150 mg 2 times daily of the sustained-release formulation of bupropion, with regard to both peak plasma concentration and extent of absorption, for parent drug and metabolites. Further, it has been demonstrated that Aplenzin is bioequivalent to WELLBUTRIN XL®.

16   HOW SUPPLIED/STORAGE AND HANDLING

Aplenzin Extended-Release Tablets, 174 mg of bupropion hydrobromide, are white to off white, round tablets printed with "BR" over "174" in bottles of 30 tablets (NDC 0024-5810-30).

Aplenzin Extended-Release Tablets, 348 mg of bupropion hydrobromide, are white to off white, round tablets printed with "BR" over "348" in bottles of 30 tablets (NDC 0024-5811-30).

Aplenzin Extended-Release Tablets, 522 mg of bupropion hydrobromide, are white to off white, round tablets printed with "BR" over "522" in bottles of 30 tablets (NDC 0024-5812-30).

Store at 25°C (77°F); excursions permitted to 15-30°C (59-86°F) [see USP Controlled Room Temperature].

17   PATIENT COUNSELING INFORMATION

See FDA-approved patient labeling (Medication Guide) below.

17.1   Counseling Information

Prescribers or other health professionals should inform patients, their families, and their caregivers about the benefits and risks associated with treatment with Aplenzin and should counsel them in its appropriate use. A patient Medication Guide [see below: PATIENT COUNSELING INFORMATION: FDA-Approved Patient Labeling (17.2)] about "Antidepressant Medicines, Depression and Other Serious Mental Illnesses, and Suicidal Thoughts or Actions" and other important information about using Aplenzin is available for Aplenzin. The prescriber or health professional should instruct patients, their families, and their caregivers to read the Medication Guide and should assist them in understanding its contents. Patients should be given the opportunity to discuss the contents of the Medication Guide and to obtain answers to any questions they may have. The complete text of the Medication Guide is reprinted at the end of this document.

Patients should be advised of the following issues and asked to alert their prescriber if these occur while taking Aplenzin.

Clinical Worsening and Suicide Risk: Patients, their families, and their caregivers should be encouraged to be alert to the emergence of anxiety, agitation, panic attacks, insomnia, irritability, hostility, aggressiveness, impulsivity, akathisia (psychomotor restlessness), hypomania, mania, other unusual changes in behavior, worsening of depression, and suicidal ideation, especially early during antidepressant treatment and when the dose is adjusted up or down. Families and caregivers of patients should be advised to observe for the emergence of such symptoms on a day-to-day basis, since changes may be abrupt. Such symptoms should be reported to the patient's prescriber or health professional, especially if they are severe, abrupt in onset, or were not part of the patient's presenting symptoms. Symptoms such as these may be associated with an increased risk for suicidal thinking and behavior and indicate a need for very close monitoring and possibly changes in the medication.

Patients should be made aware that Aplenzin contains the same active ingredient (bupropion) found in ZYBAN®, which is used as an aid to smoking cessation treatment, and that Aplenzin should not be used in combination with ZYBAN® or any other medications that contain bupropion hydrochloride (such as WELLBUTRIN XL®, the extended-release formulation, WELLBUTRIN SR®, the sustained-release formulation, and WELLBUTRIN®, the immediate-release formulation).

Patients should be told that Aplenzin should be discontinued and not restarted if they experience a seizure while on treatment.

Patients should be told that any CNS-active drug like Aplenzin Tablets may impair their ability to perform tasks requiring judgment or motor and cognitive skills. Consequently, until they are reasonably certain that Aplenzin Tablets do not adversely affect their performance, they should refrain from driving an automobile or operating complex, hazardous machinery.

Patients should be told that the excessive use or abrupt discontinuation of alcohol or sedatives (including benzodiazepines) may alter the seizure threshold. Some patients have reported lower alcohol tolerance during treatment with bupropion. Patients should be advised that the consumption of alcohol should be minimized or avoided.

Patients should be advised to notify their physicians if they are taking or plan to take any prescription or over-the-counter drugs. Concern is warranted because Aplenzin Tablets and other drugs may affect each other's metabolism.
Patients should be advised to notify their physicians if they become pregnant or intend to become pregnant during therapy.
Patients should be advised to swallow Aplenzin Tablets whole so that the release rate is not altered. Do not chew, divide, or crush tablets.
Patients should be advised that they may notice in their stool something that looks like a tablet. This is normal. The medication in Aplenzin is contained in a non-absorbable shell that has been specially designed to slowly release drug in the body. When this process is completed, the empty shell is eliminated from the body.

17.2 FDA-Approved Patient Labeling (Medication Guide)

MEDICATION GUIDE

Aplenzin (*uh-PLEN-zin*)

(bupropion hydrobromide extended-release tablets)

Read this Medication Guide carefully before you start using Aplenzin and each time you get a refill. There may be new information. This information does not take the place of talking with your doctor about your medical condition or your treatment. If you have any questions about Aplenzin, ask your doctor or pharmacist.

IMPORTANT: Be sure to read both sections of this Medication Guide. The first section is about the risk of suicidal thoughts and actions with antidepressant medicines; the second section is entitled "What other important information should I know about Aplenzin?"

ANTIDEPRESSANT MEDICINES, DEPRESSION AND OTHER SERIOUS MENTAL ILLNESSES, AND SUICIDAL THOUGHTS OR ACTIONS

This section of the Medication Guide is only about the risk of suicidal thoughts and actions with antidepressant medicines. **Talk to your, or your family member's, healthcare provider about:**

- all risks and benefits of treatment with antidepressant medicines
- all treatment choices for depression or other serious mental illness

What is the most important information I should know about antidepressant medicines, depression and other serious mental illnesses, and suicidal thoughts or actions?

1. **Antidepressant medicines may increase suicidal thoughts or actions in some children, teenagers, and young adults within the first few months of treatment.**
2. **Depression and other serious mental illnesses are the most important causes of suicidal thoughts and actions. Some people may have a particularly high risk of having suicidal thoughts or actions.** These include people who have (or have a family history of) bipolar illness (also called manic-depressive illness) or suicidal thoughts or actions.
3. **How can I watch for and try to prevent suicidal thoughts and actions in myself or a family member?**
   - Pay close attention to any changes, especially sudden changes in mood, behaviors, thoughts, or feelings. This is very important when an antidepressant medicine is started or when the dose is changed.
   - Call the healthcare provider right away to report new or sudden changes in mood, behavior, thoughts, or feelings.
   - Keep all follow-up visits with the healthcare provider as scheduled. Call the healthcare provider between visits as needed, especially if you have concerns about symptoms.

Call a healthcare provider *right away* if you or your family member has any of the following symptoms, especially if they are new, worse, or worry you:

- thoughts about suicide or dying
- attempts to commit suicide
- new or worse depression
- new or worse anxiety
- feeling very agitated or restless
- panic attacks
- trouble sleeping (insomnia)
- new or worse irritability
- acting aggressive, being angry, or violent
- acting on dangerous impulses
- an extreme increase in activity and talking (mania)
- other unusual changes in behavior or mood

What else do I need to know about antidepressant medicines?

- **Never stop an antidepressant medicine without first talking to a healthcare provider.** Stopping an antidepressant medicine suddenly can cause other symptoms.
- **Antidepressants are medicines used to treat depression and other illnesses.** It is important to discuss all the risks of treating depression and also the risks of not treating it. Patients and their families or other caregivers should discuss all treatment choices with the healthcare provider, not just the use of antidepressants.
- **Antidepressant medicines have other side effects.** Talk to the healthcare provider about the side effects of the medicine prescribed for you or your family member.
- **Antidepressant medicines can interact with other medicines.** Know all of the medicines that you or your family member takes. Keep a list of all medicines to show the healthcare provider. Do not start new medicines without first checking with your healthcare provider.
- **Not all antidepressant medicines prescribed for children are FDA approved for use in children.** Talk to your child's healthcare provider for more information.

Aplenzin has not been studied in children under the age of 18 and is not approved for use in children and teenagers.

WHAT OTHER IMPORTANT INFORMATION SHOULD I KNOW ABOUT APLENZIN?

There is a chance of having a seizure (convulsion, fit) with Aplenzin, especially in people:

- with certain medical problems.
- who take certain medicines.

The chance of having seizures increases with higher doses of Aplenzin. For more information, see the sections "Who should not take Aplenzin?" and "What should I tell my doctor before using Aplenzin?" Tell your doctor about all of your medical conditions and all the medicines you take. **Do not take any other medicines while you are using Aplenzin unless your doctor has said it is okay to take them.**

If you have a seizure while taking Aplenzin, stop taking the tablets and call your doctor right away. Do not take Aplenzin again if you have a seizure.

What is Aplenzin?

Aplenzin is a prescription medicine used to treat adults with a certain type of depression called major depressive disorder.

Who should not take Aplenzin?

Do not take Aplenzin if you:

- have or had a seizure disorder or epilepsy.
- **are taking ZYBAN® (used to help people stop smoking) or any other medicines that contain bupropion, such as WELLBUTRIN® Tablets, or WELLBUTRIN SR® Sustained-Release Tablets, or WELLBUTRIN XL® Extended-Release Tablets.** Bupropion is the same active ingredient that is in Aplenzin.
- drink a lot of alcohol and abruptly stop drinking, or use medicines called sedatives (these make you sleepy) or benzodiazepines and you stop using them all of a sudden.
- have taken within the last 14 days medicine for depression called a monoamine oxidase inhibitor (MAOI), such as NARDIL® (phenelzine sulfate), PARNATE® (tranylcypromine sulfate), or MARPLAN® (isocarboxazid).
- have or had an eating disorder such as anorexia nervosa or bulimia.
- are allergic to the active ingredient in Aplenzin, bupropion, or to any of the inactive ingredients. See the end of this leaflet for a complete list of ingredients in Aplenzin.

What should I tell my doctor before using Aplenzin?

- **Tell your doctor about your medical conditions.** Tell your doctor if you:
  - **are pregnant or plan to become pregnant.** It is not known if Aplenzin can harm your unborn baby.
  - **are breastfeeding.** Aplenzin passes through your milk. It is not known if Aplenzin can harm your baby.
  - **have liver problems**, especially cirrhosis of the liver.
  - have kidney problems.
  - have an eating disorder such as anorexia nervosa or bulimia.
  - have had a head injury.
  - have had a seizure (convulsion, fit).
  - have a tumor in your nervous system (brain or spine).
  - have had a heart attack, heart problems, or high blood pressure.
  - are a diabetic taking insulin or other medicines to control your blood sugar.
  - drink a lot of alcohol.
  - abuse prescription medicines or street drugs.
- **Tell your doctor about all the medicines you take**, including prescription and non-prescription medicines, vitamins and herbal supplements. Many medicines increase your chances of having seizures or other serious side effects if you take them while you are using Aplenzin.

How should I take Aplenzin?

- Take Aplenzin exactly as prescribed by your doctor.
- **Do not chew, cut, or crush Aplenzin tablets.** You must swallow the tablets whole. **Tell your doctor if you cannot swallow medicine tablets.**
- Take Aplenzin at the same time each day.
- Take your doses of Aplenzin at least 24 hours apart.
- You may take Aplenzin with or without food.
- If you miss a dose, do not take an extra tablet to make up for the dose you forgot. Wait and take your next tablet at the regular time. **This is very important.** Too much Aplenzin can increase your chance of having a seizure.
- If you take too much Aplenzin, or overdose, call your local emergency room or poison control center right away.
- The Aplenzin tablet is covered by a shell that slowly releases the medicine inside your body. You may notice something in your stool that looks like a tablet. This is normal. This is the empty shell passing from your body.
- **Do not take any other medicines while using Aplenzin unless your doctor has told you it is okay.**
- If you are taking Aplenzin for the treatment of major depressive disorder, it may take several weeks for you to feel that Aplenzin is working. Once you feel better, it is important to keep taking Aplenzin exactly as directed by your doctor. Call your doctor if you do not feel Aplenzin is working for you.
- Do not change your dose or stop taking Aplenzin without talking with your doctor first.

What should I avoid while taking Aplenzin?

- Do not drink a lot of alcohol while taking Aplenzin. If you usually drink a lot of alcohol, talk with your doctor before suddenly stopping. If you suddenly stop drinking alcohol, you may increase your chance of having seizures.
- Do not drive a car or use heavy machinery until you know how Aplenzin affects you. Aplenzin can impair your ability to perform these tasks.

What are possible side effects of Aplenzin?

- **Seizures.** Some patients may get seizures while taking Aplenzin. **If you have a seizure while taking Aplenzin, stop taking the tablets and call your doctor right away.** Do not take Aplenzin again if you have a seizure.
- **Hypertension (high blood pressure).** Some patients may get high blood pressure, sometimes severe, while taking Aplenzin. The chance of high blood pressure may be increased if you also use nicotine replacement therapy (for example, a nicotine patch) to help you stop smoking.
- **Severe allergic reactions. Stop taking Aplenzin and call your doctor right away** if you get a rash, itching, hives, fever, swollen lymph glands, painful sores in the mouth or around the eyes, swelling of the lips or tongue, chest pain, or have trouble breathing. These could be signs of a serious allergic reaction.
- **Unusual thoughts or behaviors.** Some patients may have unusual thoughts or behaviors while taking Aplenzin, including delusions (believe you are someone else), hallucinations (seeing or hearing things that are not there), paranoia (feeling that people are against you), or feeling confused. If this happens to you, call your doctor.

Common side effects reported in studies of major depressive disorder include weight loss, loss of appetite, dry mouth, skin rash, sweating, ringing in the ears, shakiness, stomach pain, agitation, anxiety, dizziness, trouble sleeping, muscle pain, nausea, fast heartbeat, sore throat, and urinating more often.

If you have nausea, take your medicine with food. If you have trouble sleeping, do not take your medicine too close to bedtime.

Tell your doctor right away about any side effects that bother you.

These are not all the side effects of Aplenzin. For a complete list, ask your doctor or pharmacist.

Call your doctor for medical advice about side effects. You may report side effects to FDA at 1-800-FDA-1088 or contact BTA Pharmaceuticals at (866-246-8245 (opt. 3).

How should I store Aplenzin?

- Store Aplenzin at room temperature. Store out of direct sunlight. Keep Aplenzin in its tightly closed bottle.
- Aplenzin tablets may have an odor.

General Information about Aplenzin.

- Medicines are sometimes prescribed for purposes other than those listed in a Medication Guide. Do not use Aplenzin for a condition for which it was not prescribed. Do not give Aplenzin to other people, even if they have the same symptoms you have. It may harm them. Keep Aplenzin out of the reach of children.

This Medication Guide summarizes important information about Aplenzin. For more information, talk with your doctor. You can ask your doctor or pharmacist for information about Aplenzin that is written for health professionals or you can call toll-free [800-633-1610].

What are the ingredients in Aplenzin?

Active ingredient: bupropion hydrobromide.

Inactive ingredients: ethylcellulose aqueous dispersion, glyceryl behenate, polyvinyl alcohol, polyethylene glycol, povidone, and dibutyl sebacate. Carnauba wax is included in the 174 mg and 348 mg strengths. The tablets are printed with edible black ink.

The following are registered trademarks of their respective manufacturers: WELLBUTRIN®/GlaxoSmithKline, WELLBUTRIN SR®/GlaxoSmithKline, WELLBUTRIN XL®/GlaxoSmithKline, ZYBAN®/GlaxoSmithKline; PROZAC®/Eli Lilly and Company; ZOLOFT®/Pfizer Pharmaceuticals; LUVOX®/Solvay Pharmaceuticals, Inc.;

ANAFRANIL®/Mallinckrodt Inc.; NARDIL®/Warner Lambert Company; MARPLAN®/Oxford Pharmaceutical Services, Inc.

This Medication Guide has been approved by the U.S. Food and Drug Administration.

Rx only
Manufactured by:
Biovail Corporation
7150 Mississauga Rd
Mississauga, Ontario L5N 8M5
Manufactured for:
sanofi-aventis U.S. LLC
Bridgewater, NJ 08807
LB0060-00   Rev. 10/08   50090346
APZ-OCT08-F-Aa

AVALIDE®   Rx

[avă-līde]
**(irbesartan and hydrochlorothiazide)
tablet for oral use**

AVALIDE®

**(irbesartan and hydrochlorothiazide)
tablet, film coated for oral use**

HIGHLIGHTS OF PRESCRIBING INFORMATION

These highlights do not include all the information needed to use AVALIDE and effectively. See full prescribing information for AVALIDE.

AVALIDE (irbesartan and hydrochlorothiazide)
tablet for oral use
AVALIDE (irbesartan and hydrochlorothiazide)
tablet, film coated for oral use
Initial U.S. Approval: 1997

WARNING: USE IN PREGNANCY
See full prescribing information for complete boxed warning.
When pregnancy is detected, discontinue AVALIDE as soon as possible. When used in pregnancy during the second and third trimesters, drugs that act directly on the renin-angiotensin system can cause injury and even death to the developing fetus. (5.1)

INDICATIONS AND USAGE

AVALIDE is a combination of irbesartan, an angiotensin II receptor antagonist, and hydrochlorothiazide, a thiazide diuretic, indicated for hypertension:
• In patients not adequately controlled with monotherapy (1).
• As initial therapy in patients likely to need multiple drugs to achieve their blood pressure goals (1).

DOSAGE AND ADMINISTRATION

General Considerations
• Maximum effects within 2 to 4 weeks after dose change (2.1).
• Renal impairment: Not recommended for patients with severe renal impairment (creatinine clearance <30 mL/min) (2.1, 5.8).
Hypertension
• Not controlled on monotherapy: Initiate with 150/12.5 mg. Titrate to 300/12.5 mg then 300/25 mg if needed. One tablet daily (2.2).
• Replacement therapy: May be substituted for titrated components (2.3).
• Initial therapy: Initiate with 150/12.5 mg once daily for 1 to 2 weeks and titrate as needed up to maximum of 300/25 mg once daily (2.4).

DOSAGE FORMS AND STRENGTHS

• 150 mg irbesartan/12.5 mg hydrochlorothiazide tablets (3)
• 300 mg irbesartan/12.5 mg hydrochlorothiazide tablets (3)
• 300 mg irbesartan/25 mg hydrochlorothiazide tablets (3)

CONTRAINDICATIONS

• Hypersensitivity to any component of this product (4)
• Anuria (4)
• Hypersensitivity to sulfonamide-derived drugs (4)

WARNINGS AND PRECAUTIONS

• Symptomatic hypotension with intravascular volume- or sodium-depletion. Correct volume-depletion prior to administration. Not recommended as initial therapy in *volume-depleted* patients (2.4, 5.2).
• Impaired hepatic function: Thiazides should be used with caution as minor fluid and electrolyte imbalances may precipitate hepatic coma (5.7).
• Impaired renal function: Use with caution. Oliguria or azotemia with acute renal failure and/or death has been reported in medications affecting the renin-angiotensin-aldosterone system (5.8).
• Thiazide diuretics may cause an exacerbation or activation of systemic lupus erythematosus (5.4).

ADVERSE REACTIONS

Most common adverse events (≥5% on AVALIDE and more often than on placebo) are dizziness, fatigue, and musculoskeletal pain (6.1).

To report SUSPECTED ADVERSE REACTIONS, contact Bristol-Myers Squibb at 1-800-721-5072 or FDA at 1-800-FDA-1088 or www.fda.gov/medwatch

DRUG INTERACTIONS

Hydrochlorothiazide (7):
• Alcohol, Barbiturates, Narcotics: Potentiation of orthostatic hypotension
• Antidiabetic Drugs: Dosage adjustment of antidiabetic may be required
• Cholestyramine and colestipol: Reduced absorption of thiazides
• Corticosteroids, ACTH: Hypokalemia, electrolyte depletion
• Lithium: Reduced renal clearance and high risk of lithium toxicity when used with diuretics. Should not be given with diuretics.
• NSAIDs: Can reduce diuretic, natriuretic, and antihypertensive effects of diuretics. Observe patient closely.

USE IN SPECIFIC POPULATIONS

• Nursing Mothers: Potential for adverse effects in infant (8.3).

See 17 for PATIENT COUNSELING INFORMATION
                                        Revised: 11/2008

FULL PRESCRIBING INFORMATION: CONTENTS*

WARNING: USE IN PREGNANCY
1 INDICATIONS AND USAGE
2 DOSAGE AND ADMINISTRATION
    2.1 General Considerations
    2.2 Add-On Therapy
    2.3 Replacement Therapy
    2.4 Initial Therapy
3 DOSAGE FORMS AND STRENGTHS
4 CONTRAINDICATIONS
5 WARNINGS AND PRECAUTIONS
    5.1 Fetal/Neonatal Morbidity and Mortality
    5.2 Hypotension in Volume- or Salt-Depleted Patients
    5.3 Hypersensitivity Reaction
    5.4 Systemic Lupus Erythematosus
    5.5 Lithium Interaction
    5.6 Electrolyte and Metabolic Imbalances
    5.7 Hepatic Impairment
    5.8 Impaired Renal Function
6 ADVERSE REACTIONS
    6.1 Clinical Trials Experience
    6.2 Post-Marketing Experience
    6.3 Laboratory Abnormalities
7 DRUG INTERACTIONS
8 USE IN SPECIFIC POPULATIONS
    8.1 Pregnancy
    8.3 Nursing Mothers
    8.4 Pediatric Use
    8.5 Geriatric Use
10 OVERDOSAGE
11 DESCRIPTION
12 CLINICAL PHARMACOLOGY
    12.1 Mechanism of Action
    12.2 Pharmacodynamics
    12.3 Pharmacokinetics
13 NONCLINICAL TOXICOLOGY
    13.1 Carcinogenesis, Mutagenesis, Impairment of Fertility
    13.2 Animal Toxicology and/or Pharmacology
14 CLINICAL STUDIES
    14.1 Irbesartan Monotherapy
    14.2 Irbesartan-Hydrochlorothiazide
16 HOW SUPPLIED/STORAGE AND HANDLING
    16.1 How Supplied
    16.2 Storage
17 PATIENT COUNSELING INFORMATION
    17.1 Pregnancy
    17.2 Symptomatic Hypotension
* Sections or subsections omitted from the full prescribing information are not listed.

FULL PRESCRIBING INFORMATION

WARNING: USE IN PREGNANCY
When pregnancy is detected, discontinue AVALIDE as soon as possible. When used in pregnancy during the second and third trimesters, drugs that act directly on the renin-angiotensin system can cause injury and even death to the developing fetus. [See *Warnings and Precautions (5.1).*]

---

1   INDICATIONS AND USAGE

AVALIDE® (irbesartan-hydrochlorothiazide) Tablets is indicated for the treatment of hypertension.

AVALIDE may be used in patients whose blood pressure is not adequately controlled on monotherapy.

AVALIDE may also be used as initial therapy in patients who are likely to need multiple drugs to achieve their blood pressure goals.

The choice of AVALIDE as initial therapy for hypertension should be based on an assessment of potential benefits and risks.

Patients with stage 2 (moderate or severe) hypertension are at relatively high risk for cardiovascular events (such as strokes, heart attacks, and heart failure), kidney failure, and vision problems, so prompt treatment is clinically relevant. The decision to use a combination as initial therapy should be individualized and may be shaped by considerations such as the baseline blood pressure, the target goal, and the incremental likelihood of achieving goal with a combination compared with monotherapy.

Data from Studies V and VI [see *Clinical Trials (14.2)*] provide estimates of the probability of reaching a blood pressure goal with AVALIDE compared to irbesartan or HCTZ monotherapy. The relationship between baseline blood pressure and achievement of a SeSBP <140 or <130 mmHg or SeDBP <90 or <80 mmHg in patients treated with AVALIDE compared to patients treated with irbesartan or HCTZ monotherapy are shown in Figures 1a through 2b.

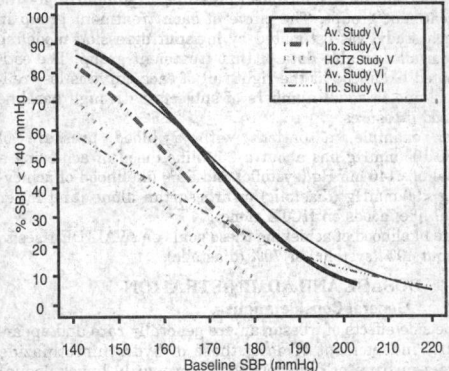

Figure 1a: Probability of Achieving SBP <140 mmHg in Patients from Initial Therapy Studies V (Week 8) and VI (Week 7)*

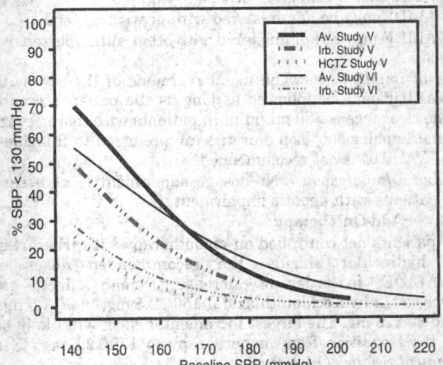

Figure 1b: Probability of Achieving SBP <130 mmHg in Patients from Initial Therapy Studies V (Week 8) and VI (Week 7)*

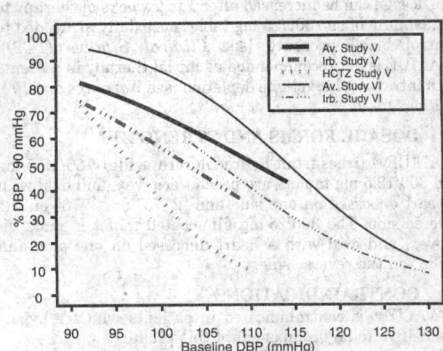

Figure 2a: Probability of Achieving DBP <90 mmHg in Patients from Initial Therapy Studies V (Week 8) and VI (Week 7)*

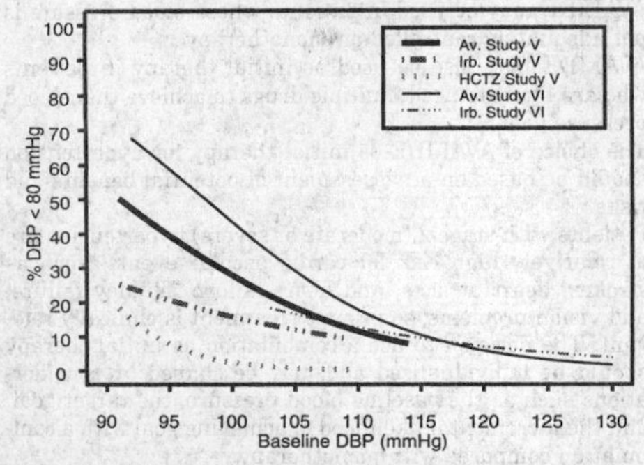

Figure 2b: Probability of Achieving DBP <80 mmHg in Patients from Initial Therapy Studies V (Week 8) and VI (Week 7)*

*For all probability curves, patients without blood pressure measurements at Week 7 (Study VI) and Week 8 (Study V) were counted as not reaching goal (intent-to-treat analysis).

The above graphs provide a rough approximation of the likelihood of reaching a targeted blood pressure goal (eg, Week 8 sitting systolic blood pressure ≤140 mmHg) for the treatment groups. The curve of each treatment group in each study was estimated by logistic regression modeling from all available data of that treatment group. The estimated likelihood at the right tail of each curve is less reliable due to small numbers of subjects with high baseline blood pressures.

For example, a patient with a blood pressure of 180/105 mmHg has about a 25% likelihood of achieving a goal of <140 mmHg (systolic) and 50% likelihood of achieving <90 mmHg (diastolic) on irbesartan alone (and lower still likelihoods on HCTZ alone).

The likelihood of achieving these goals on AVALIDE rises to about 40% (systolic) or 70% (diastolic).

2 DOSAGE AND ADMINISTRATION

2.1 General Considerations

The side effects of irbesartan are generally rare and apparently independent of dose; those of hydrochlorothiazide are a mixture of dose-dependent (primarily hypokalemia) and dose-independent phenomena (eg, pancreatitis), the former much more common than the latter. [See *Adverse Reactions (6)*.]

Maximum antihypertensive effects are attained within 2 to 4 weeks after a change in dose.

AVALIDE may be administered with or without food.

AVALIDE may be administered with other antihypertensive agents.

Renal impairment. The usual regimens of therapy with AVALIDE may be followed as long as the patient's creatinine clearance is >30 mL/min. In patients with more severe renal impairment, loop diuretics are preferred to thiazides, so AVALIDE is not recommended.

Hepatic impairment. No dosage adjustment is necessary in patients with hepatic impairment.

2.2 Add-On Therapy

In patients not controlled on monotherapy with irbesartan or hydrochlorothiazide, the recommended doses of AVALIDE, in order of increasing mean effect, are (irbesartan-hydrochlorothiazide) 150/12.5 mg, 300/12.5 mg, and 300/25 mg. The largest incremental effect will likely be in the transition from monotherapy to 150/12.5 mg. [See *Clinical Studies (14.2)*.]

2.3 Replacement Therapy

AVALIDE may be substituted for the titrated components.

2.4 Initial Therapy

The usual starting dose is AVALIDE 150/12.5 mg once daily. The dosage can be increased after 1 to 2 weeks of therapy to a maximum of one 300/25 mg tablet once daily as needed to control blood pressure [see *Clinical Studies (14.2)*]. AVALIDE is not recommended as initial therapy in patients with intravascular volume depletion [see *Warnings and Precautions (5.2)*].

3 DOSAGE FORMS AND STRENGTHS

AVALIDE® (irbesartan-hydrochlorothiazide) 150/12.5 mg and 300/12.5 mg tablets are peach, biconvex, and oval with a heart debossed on one side and "2775" or "2776" on the reverse side. The 300/25 mg film-coated tablet is pink, biconvex, and oval with a heart debossed on one side and "2788" on the reverse side.

4 CONTRAINDICATIONS

- AVALIDE is contraindicated in patients who are hypersensitive to any component of this product.
- Because of the hydrochlorothiazide component, this product is contraindicated in patients with anuria or hypersensitivity to other sulfonamide-derived drugs.

5 WARNINGS AND PRECAUTIONS

5.1 Fetal/Neonatal Morbidity and Mortality

AVALIDE can cause fetal harm when administered to a pregnant woman. If this drug is used during pregnancy, or if the patient becomes pregnant while taking this drug, the patient should be apprised of the potential hazard to the fetus [see *Use in Specific Populations (8.1)*]. In several dozen published cases, angiotensin converting enzyme (ACE) inhibitor use during the second and third trimesters of pregnancy was associated with fetal and neonatal injury, including hypotension, neonatal skull hypoplasia, anuria, reversible or irreversible renal failure, and death. Similar renal findings occur in reproductive toxicology studies in rats. Thiazides cross the placenta, and use of thiazides during pregnancy is associated with a risk of fetal or neonatal jaundice, thrombocytopenia, and possibly other adverse reactions that have occurred in adults.

5.2 Hypotension in Volume- or Salt-Depleted Patients

Excessive reduction of blood pressure was rarely seen in patients with uncomplicated hypertension treated with irbesartan alone (<0.1%) or with irbesartan-hydrochlorothiazide (approximately 1%). Initiation of antihypertensive therapy may cause symptomatic hypotension in patients with intravascular volume- or sodium-depletion, eg, in patients treated vigorously with diuretics or in patients on dialysis. Such volume depletion should be corrected prior to administration of antihypertensive therapy.

If hypotension occurs, the patient should be placed in the supine position and, if necessary, given an intravenous infusion of normal saline. A transient hypotensive response is not a contraindication to further treatment, which usually can be continued without difficulty once the blood pressure has stabilized.

5.3 Hypersensitivity Reaction

Hydrochlorothiazide

Hypersensitivity reactions to hydrochlorothiazide may occur in patients with or without a history of allergy or bronchial asthma, but are more likely in patients with such a history.

5.4 Systemic Lupus Erythematosus

Hydrochlorothiazide

Thiazide diuretics have been reported to cause exacerbation or activation of systemic lupus erythematosus.

5.5 Lithium Interaction

Hydrochlorothiazide

Lithium generally should not be given with thiazides. [See *Drug Interactions (7)*.]

5.6 Electrolyte and Metabolic Imbalances

Irbesartan-Hydrochlorothiazide

In double-blind clinical trials of various doses of irbesartan and hydrochlorothiazide, the incidence of hypertensive patients who developed hypokalemia (serum potassium <3.5 mEq/L) was 7.5% versus 6.0% for placebo; the incidence of hyperkalemia (serum potassium >5.7 mEq/L) was <1.0% versus 1.7% for placebo. No patient discontinued due to increases or decreases in serum potassium. On average, the combination of irbesartan and hydrochlorothiazide had no effect on serum potassium. Higher doses of irbesartan ameliorated the hypokalemic response to hydrochlorothiazide.

Hydrochlorothiazide

Periodic determination of serum electrolytes to detect possible electrolyte imbalance should be performed at appropriate intervals. All patients receiving thiazide therapy should be observed for clinical signs of fluid or electrolyte imbalance: hyponatremia, hypochloremic alkalosis, and hypokalemia. Serum and urine electrolyte determinations are particularly important when the patient is vomiting excessively or receiving parenteral fluids. Warning signs or symptoms of fluid and electrolyte imbalance, irrespective of cause, include dryness of mouth, thirst, weakness, lethargy, drowsiness, restlessness, confusion, seizures, muscle pains or cramps, muscular fatigue, hypotension, oliguria, tachycardia, and gastrointestinal disturbances such as nausea and vomiting.

Hypokalemia may develop, especially with brisk diuresis, when severe cirrhosis is present, or after prolonged therapy. Interference with adequate oral electrolyte intake will also contribute to hypokalemia. Hypokalemia may cause cardiac arrhythmia and may also sensitize or exaggerate the response of the heart to the toxic effects of digitalis (eg, increased ventricular irritability).

Although any chloride deficit is generally mild and usually does not require specific treatment except under extraordinary circumstances (as in liver disease or renal disease), chloride replacement may be required in the treatment of metabolic alkalosis.

Dilutional hyponatremia may occur in edematous patients in hot weather; appropriate therapy is water restriction, rather than administration of salt except in rare instances when the hyponatremia is life-threatening. In actual salt depletion, appropriate replacement is the therapy of choice.

Hyperuricemia may occur or frank gout may be precipitated in certain patients receiving thiazide therapy.

In diabetic patients, dosage adjustments of insulin or oral hypoglycemic agents may be required. Hyperglycemia may occur with thiazide diuretics. Thus, latent diabetes mellitus may become manifest during thiazide therapy.

The antihypertensive effects of the drug may be enhanced in the post-sympathectomy patient.

If progressive renal impairment becomes evident, consider withholding or discontinuing diuretic therapy.

Thiazides have been shown to increase the urinary excretion of magnesium; this may result in hypomagnesemia.

Thiazides may decrease urinary calcium excretion. Thiazides may cause intermittent and slight elevation of serum calcium in the absence of known disorders of calcium metabolism. Marked hypercalcemia may be evidence of hidden hyperparathyroidism. Thiazides should be discontinued before carrying out tests for parathyroid function.

Increases in cholesterol and triglyceride levels may be associated with thiazide diuretic therapy.

5.7 Hepatic Impairment

Hydrochlorothiazide

Thiazides should be used with caution in patients with impaired hepatic function or progressive liver disease, since minor alterations of fluid and electrolyte balance may precipitate hepatic coma.

5.8 Impaired Renal Function

As a consequence of inhibiting the renin-angiotensin-aldosterone system, changes in renal function may be anticipated in susceptible individuals. In patients whose renal function may depend on the activity of the renin-angiotensin-aldosterone system (eg, patients with severe congestive heart failure), treatment with ACE inhibitors has been associated with oliguria and/or progressive azotemia and (rarely) with acute renal failure and/or death. Irbesartan would be expected to behave similarly. In studies of ACE inhibitors in patients with unilateral or bilateral renal artery stenosis, increases in serum creatinine or BUN have been reported. There has been no known use of irbesartan in patients with unilateral or bilateral renal artery stenosis, but a similar effect should be anticipated.

Thiazides should be used with caution in severe renal disease. In patients with renal disease, thiazides may precipitate azotemia. Cumulative effects of the drug may develop in patients with impaired renal function.

6 ADVERSE REACTIONS

6.1 Clinical Trials Experience

Because clinical trials are conducted under widely varying conditions, adverse reaction rates observed in the clinical trials of a drug cannot be directly compared to rates in the clinical trials of another drug and may not reflect the rates observed in practice. The adverse reaction information from clinical trials does, however, provide a basis for identifying the adverse events that appear to be related to drug use and for approximating rates.

Irbesartan-Hydrochlorothiazide

AVALIDE (irbesartan-hydrochlorothiazide) Tablets has been evaluated for safety in 1694 patients treated for essential hypertension in 6 clinical trials. In Studies I through IV with AVALIDE, no adverse events peculiar to this combination drug product have been observed. Adverse events have been limited to those that were reported previously with irbesartan or hydrochlorothiazide (HCTZ). The overall incidence of adverse events was similar with the combination and placebo. In general, treatment with AVALIDE was well tolerated. For the most part, adverse events have been mild and transient in nature and have not required discontinuation of therapy. In controlled clinical trials, discontinuation of AVALIDE therapy due to clinical adverse events was required in only 3.6%. This incidence was significantly less (p=0.023) than the 6.8% of patients treated with placebo who discontinued therapy.

In these double-blind controlled clinical trials, the following adverse events reported with AVALIDE occurred in ≥1% of patients, and more often on the irbesartan-hydrochlorothiazide combination than on placebo, regardless of drug relationship:

[See table at top of next page]

The following adverse events were also reported at a rate of 1% or greater, but were as, or more, common in the placebo group: headache, sinus abnormality, cough, URI, pharyngitis, diarrhea, rhinitis, urinary tract infection, rash, anxiety/nervousness, and muscle cramp.

Adverse events occurred at about the same rates in men and women, older and younger patients, and black and non-black patients.

Adverse events in Studies V and VI were similar to those described above in Studies I through IV.

Irbesartan

Other adverse events that have been reported with irbesartan, without regard to causality, are listed below:

Body as a Whole: fever, chills, orthostatic effects, facial edema, upper extremity edema

Cardiovascular: flushing, hypertension, cardiac murmur, myocardial infarction, angina pectoris, hypotension, syncope, arrhythmic/conduction disorder, cardiorespiratory arrest, heart failure, hypertensive crisis
Dermatologic: pruritus, dermatitis, ecchymosis, erythema face, urticaria
Endocrine/Metabolic/Electrolyte Imbalances: sexual dysfunction, libido change, gout
Gastrointestinal: diarrhea, constipation, gastroenteritis, flatulence, abdominal distention
Musculoskeletal/Connective Tissue: musculoskeletal trauma, extremity swelling, muscle cramp, arthritis, muscle ache, musculoskeletal chest pain, joint stiffness, bursitis, muscle weakness
Nervous System: anxiety/nervousness, sleep disturbance, numbness, somnolence, vertigo, emotional disturbance, depression, paresthesia, tremor, transient ischemic attack, cerebrovascular accident
Renal/Genitourinary: prostate disorder
Respiratory: cough, upper respiratory infection, epistaxis, tracheobronchitis, congestion, pulmonary congestion, dyspnea, wheezing
Special Senses: vision disturbance, hearing abnormality, ear infection, ear pain, conjunctivitis
Hydrochlorothiazide
Other adverse events that have been reported with hydrochlorothiazide, without regard to causality, are listed below:
Body as a Whole: weakness
Digestive: pancreatitis, jaundice (intrahepatic cholestatic jaundice), sialadenitis, cramping, gastric irritation
Hematologic: aplastic anemia, agranulocytosis, leukopenia, hemolytic anemia, thrombocytopenia
Hypersensitivity: purpura, photosensitivity, urticaria, necrotizing angiitis (vasculitis and cutaneous vasculitis), fever, respiratory distress including pneumonitis and pulmonary edema, anaphylactic reactions
Metabolic: hyperglycemia, glycosuria, hyperuricemia
Musculoskeletal: muscle spasm
Nervous System/Psychiatric: restlessness
Renal: renal failure, renal dysfunction, interstitial nephritis
Skin: erythema multiforme including Stevens-Johnson syndrome, exfoliative dermatitis including toxic epidermal necrolysis
Special Senses: transient blurred vision, xanthopsia
Initial Therapy
In the moderate hypertension Study V (mean SeDBP between 90 and 110 mmHg), the types and incidences of adverse events reported for patients treated with AVALIDE were similar to the adverse event profile in patients on initial irbesartan or HCTZ monotherapy. There were no reported events of syncope in the AVALIDE treatment group and there was one reported event in the HCTZ treatment group. The incidences of pre-specified adverse events on AVALIDE, irbesartan, and HCTZ, respectively, were: 0.9%, 0%, and 0% for hypotension; 3.0%, 3.8%, and 1.0% for dizziness; 5.5%, 3.8%, and 4.8% for headache; 1.2%, 0%, and 1.0% for hyperkalemia; and 0.9%, 0%, and 0% for hypokalemia. The rates of discontinuation due to adverse events on AVALIDE, irbesartan alone, and HCTZ alone were 6.7%, 3.8%, and 4.8%.
In the severe hypertension (SeDBP ≥110 mmHg) Study VI, the overall pattern of adverse events reported through 7 weeks of follow-up was similar in patients treated with AVALIDE as initial therapy and in patients treated with irbesartan as initial therapy. The incidences of the pre-specified adverse events on AVALIDE and irbesartan, respectively, were: 0% and 0% for syncope; 0.6% and 0% for hypotension; 3.6% and 4.0% for dizziness; 4.3% and 6.6% for headache; 0.2% and 0% for hyperkalemia; and 0.6% and 0.4% for hypokalemia. The rates of discontinuation due to adverse events were 2.1% and 2.2%. [See *Clinical Studies (14.2)*.]

6.2   Post-Marketing Experience
The following adverse reactions have been identified during post-approval use of AVALIDE. Because these reactions are reported voluntarily from a population of uncertain size, it is not always possible to reliably estimate their frequency or establish a causal relationship to drug exposure. Decisions to include these reactions in labeling are typically based on one or more of the following factors: (1) seriousness of the reaction, (2) frequency of reporting, or (3) strength of causal connection to AVALIDE.
The following have been very rarely reported: urticaria; angioedema (involving swelling of the face, lips, pharynx, and/or tongue); and hepatitis. Hyperkalemia has been rarely reported.
Very rare cases of jaundice have been reported with irbesartan.
Rare cases of rhabdomyolysis have been reported in patients receiving angiotensin II receptor blockers.

6.3   Laboratory Abnormalities
In controlled clinical trials, clinically important changes in standard laboratory parameters were rarely associated with administration of AVALIDE.
Creatinine, Blood Urea Nitrogen: Minor increases in blood urea nitrogen (BUN) or serum creatinine were observed in

	Irbesartan/HCTZ (n=898) (%)	Placebo (n=236) (%)	Irbesartan (n=400) (%)	HCTZ (n=380) (%)
Body as a Whole				
Chest Pain	2	1	2	2
Fatigue	7	3	4	3
Influenza	3	1	2	2
Cardiovascular				
Edema	3	3	2	2
Tachycardia	1	0	1	1
Gastrointestinal				
Abdominal Pain	2	1	2	2
Dyspepsia/heartburn	2	1	0	2
Nausea/vomiting	3	0	2	0
Immunology				
Allergy	1	0	1	1
Musculoskeletal				
Musculoskeletal Pain	7	5	6	10
Nervous System				
Dizziness	8	4	6	5
Dizziness Orthostatic	1	0	1	1
Renal/Genitourinary				
Abnormality Urination	2	1	1	2

2.3% and 1.1%, respectively, of patients with essential hypertension treated with AVALIDE alone. No patient discontinued taking AVALIDE due to increased BUN. One patient discontinued taking AVALIDE due to a minor increase in serum creatinine.
Liver Function Tests: Occasional elevations of liver enzymes and/or serum bilirubin have occurred. In patients with essential hypertension treated with AVALIDE alone, one patient was discontinued due to elevated liver enzymes.
Serum Electrolytes: [See *Warnings and Precautions (5.2, 5.6)*.]

7   DRUG INTERACTIONS
Irbesartan
No significant drug-drug interactions have been reported with irbesartan. [See *Clinical Pharmacology (12.3)*.]
Hydrochlorothiazide
When administered concurrently the following drugs may interact with thiazide diuretics:
Alcohol, Barbiturates, or Narcotics: potentiation of orthostatic hypotension may occur.
Antidiabetic Drugs (oral agents and insulin): dosage adjustment of the antidiabetic drug may be required.
Other Antihypertensive Drugs: additive effect or potentiation.
Cholestyramine and Colestipol Resins: absorption of hydrochlorothiazide is impaired in the presence of anionic exchange resins. Single doses of either cholestyramine or colestipol resins bind the hydrochlorothiazide and reduce its absorption from the gastrointestinal tract by up to 85% and 43%, respectively.
Corticosteroids, ACTH: intensified electrolyte depletion, particularly hypokalemia.
Pressor Amines (eg, Norepinephrine): possible decreased response to pressor amines but not sufficient to preclude their use.
Skeletal Muscle Relaxants, Nondepolarizing (eg, Tubocurarine): possible increased responsiveness to the muscle relaxant.
Lithium: should not generally be given with diuretics. Diuretic agents reduce the renal clearance of lithium and add a high risk of lithium toxicity. Refer to the package insert for lithium preparations before use of such preparations with AVALIDE. [See *Warnings and Precautions (5.5)*.]
Non-steroidal Anti-inflammatory Drugs: in some patients, the administration of a non-steroidal anti-inflammatory agent can reduce the diuretic, natriuretic, and antihypertensive effects of loop, potassium-sparing and thiazide diuretics. Therefore, when AVALIDE (irbesartan-

hydrochlorothiazide) Tablets and non-steroidal anti-inflammatory agents are used concomitantly, the patient should be observed closely to determine if the desired effect of the diuretic is obtained.

8   USE IN SPECIFIC POPULATIONS
8.1   Pregnancy
Pregnancy Category D
See *Warnings and Precautions (5.1)*.
AVALIDE contains both irbesartan (an angiotensin II receptor antagonist) and hydrochlorothiazide (a thiazide diuretic). When administered during the second or third trimester of pregnancy, drugs that act directly on the renin-angiotensin system (RAS) can cause fetal and neonatal morbidity and death. Thiazides cross the placenta, and use of thiazides during pregnancy is associated with a risk of fetal or neonatal jaundice, thrombocytopenia, and possibly other adverse reactions that have occurred in adults. AVALIDE can cause fetal harm when administered to a pregnant woman. If this drug is used during pregnancy, or if the patient becomes pregnant while taking this drug, the patient should be apprised of the potential hazard to the fetus.
Angiotensin II receptor antagonists, like irbesartan, and ACE inhibitors exert similar effects on the RAS. In several dozen published cases, ACE inhibitor use during the second and third trimesters of pregnancy was associated with fetal and neonatal injury, including hypotension, neonatal skull hypoplasia, anuria, reversible or irreversible renal failure, and death. Oligohydramnios was also reported, presumably from decreased fetal renal function. In this setting, oligohydramnios was associated with fetal limb contractures, craniofacial deformation, and hypoplastic lung development. Prematurity, intrauterine growth retardation, and patent ductus arteriosus were also reported, although it is not clear whether these occurrences were due to exposure to the drug. These adverse effects do not appear to have resulted from intrauterine drug exposure that has been limited to the first trimester.
When pregnancy occurs in a patient using AVALIDE, the physician should discontinue AVALIDE treatment as soon as possible. The physician should inform the patient about potential risks to the fetus based on the time of gestational exposure to AVALIDE (first trimester only or later). If exposure occurs beyond the first trimester, an ultrasound examination should be done.
In rare cases when another antihypertensive agent cannot be used to treat the pregnant patient, serial ultrasound examinations should be performed to assess the intraamniotic environment. Routine fetal testing with non-stress tests, biophysical profiles, and/or contraction stress tests may be

appropriate based on gestational age and standards of care in the community. If oligohydramnios occurs in these situations, individualized decisions about continuing or discontinuing AVALIDE treatment and about pregnancy management should be made by the patient, her physician, and experts in the management of high risk pregnancy. Patients and physicians should be aware that oligohydramnios may not appear until after the fetus has sustained irreversible injury.

Infants with histories of *in utero* exposure to AVALIDE should be closely observed for hypotension, oliguria, and hyperkalemia. If oliguria occurs, these infants may require blood pressure and renal perfusion support. Exchange transfusion or dialysis may be required to reverse hypotension and/or support decreased renal function.

Irbesartan crosses the placenta in rats and rabbits. In pregnant rats given irbesartan at doses greater than the maximum recommended human dose (MRHD), fetuses showed increased incidences of renal pelvic cavitation, hydroureter and/or absence of renal papilla. Subcutaneous edema also occurred in fetuses at doses about 4 times the MRHD (based on body surface area). These anomalies occurred when pregnant rats received irbesartan through Day 20 of gestation but not when drug was stopped on gestation Day 15. The observed effects are believed to be late gestational effects of the drug. Pregnant rabbits given oral doses of irbesartan equivalent to 1.5 times the MRHD experienced a high rate of maternal mortality and abortion. Surviving females had a slight increase in early resorptions and a corresponding decrease in live fetuses [see *Nonclinical Toxicology (13.2)*]. Radioactivity was present in the rat and rabbit fetus during late gestation and in rat milk following oral doses of radiolabeled irbesartan.

When pregnant mice and rats were given hydrochlorothiazide at doses up to 3000 and 1000 mg/kg/day, respectively (about 600 and 400 times the MRHD) during their respective periods of major organogenesis, there was no evidence of fetal harm.

A development toxicity study was performed in rats with doses of 50/50 mg/kg/day and 150/150 mg/kg/day irbesartan-hydrochlorothiazide. Although the high dose combination appeared to be more toxic to the dams than either drug alone, there did not appear to be an increase in toxicity to the developing embryos.

8.3 Nursing Mothers

It is not known whether irbesartan is excreted in human milk, but irbesartan or some metabolite of irbesartan is secreted at low concentration in the milk of lactating rats. Thiazides appear in human milk. Because of the potential for adverse effects on the nursing infant, a decision should be made whether to discontinue nursing or discontinue the drug, taking into account the importance of the drug to the mother.

8.4 Pediatric Use

Safety and effectiveness in pediatric patients have not been established.

8.5 Geriatric Use

Of 1694 patients receiving AVALIDE in controlled clinical studies of hypertension, 264 (15.6%) were 65 years and over, while 45 (2.7%) were 75 years and over. No overall differences in safety or effectiveness were observed between these patients and younger patients, but greater sensitivity of some older individuals cannot be ruled out. [See *Clinical Pharmacology (12.3)* and *Clinical Studies (14)*.]

10 OVERDOSAGE

Irbesartan

No data are available in regard to overdosage in humans. However, daily doses of 900 mg for 8 weeks were well tolerated. The most likely manifestations of overdosage are expected to be hypotension and tachycardia; bradycardia might also occur from overdose. Irbesartan is not removed by hemodialysis.

To obtain up-to-date information about the treatment of overdosage, a good resource is a certified regional Poison Control Center. Telephone numbers of certified Poison Control Centers are listed in the *Physicians' Desk Reference* (PDR). In managing overdose, consider the possibilities of multiple-drug interactions, drug-drug interactions, and unusual drug kinetics in the patient.

Laboratory determinations of serum levels of irbesartan are not widely available, and such determinations have, in any event, no established role in the management of irbesartan overdose.

Acute oral toxicity studies with irbesartan in mice and rats indicated acute lethal doses were in excess of 2000 mg/kg, about 25- and 50-fold the MRHD (300 mg) on a mg/m^2 basis, respectively.

Hydrochlorothiazide

The most common signs and symptoms of overdose observed in humans are those caused by electrolyte depletion (hypokalemia, hypochloremia, hyponatremia) and dehydration resulting from excessive diuresis. If digitalis has also been administered, hypokalemia may accentuate cardiac arrhythmias. The degree to which hydrochlorothiazide is removed by hemodialysis has not been established. The oral LD_{50} of hydrochlorothiazide is greater than 10 g/kg in both mice and rats.

11 DESCRIPTION

AVALIDE (irbesartan-hydrochlorothiazide) Tablets is a combination of an angiotensin II receptor antagonist (AT_1 subtype), irbesartan, and a thiazide diuretic, hydrochlorothiazide (HCTZ).

Irbesartan is a non-peptide compound, chemically described as a 2-butyl-3-[*p*-(*o*-1*H*-tetrazol-5-ylphenyl)benzyl]-1,3-diazaspiro[4.4]non-1-en-4-one. Its empirical formula is $C_{25}H_{28}N_6O$, and its structural formula is:

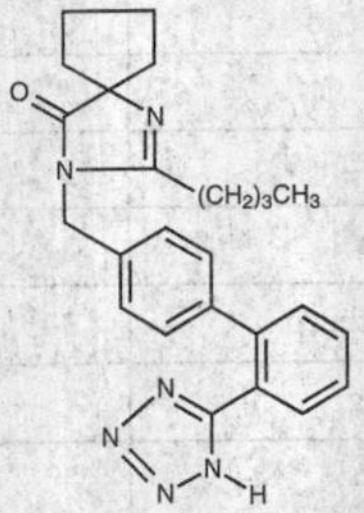

Irbesartan is a white to off-white crystalline powder with a molecular weight of 428.5. It is a nonpolar compound with a partition coefficient (octanol/water) of 10.1 at pH of 7.4. Irbesartan is slightly soluble in alcohol and methylene chloride and practically insoluble in water.

Hydrochlorothiazide is 6-chloro-3,4-dihydro-2*H*-1,2,4-benzothiadiazine-7-sulfonamide 1,1-dioxide. Its empirical formula is $C_7H_8ClN_3O_4S_2$ and its structural formula is:

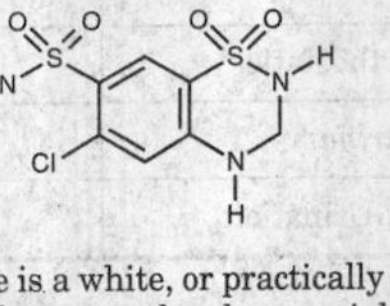

Hydrochlorothiazide is a white, or practically white, crystalline powder with a molecular weight of 297.7. Hydrochlorothiazide is slightly soluble in water and freely soluble in sodium hydroxide solution.

AVALIDE is available for oral administration in tablets containing either 150 mg or 300 mg of irbesartan combined with 12.5 mg of hydrochlorothiazide or 300 mg of irbesartan combined with 25 mg hydrochlorothiazide. Inactive ingredients include: lactose monohydrate, microcrystalline cellulose, pregelatinized starch, croscarmellose sodium, ferric oxide red, ferric oxide yellow, silicon dioxide, and magnesium stearate. In addition, the 300/25 mg pink film-coated tablet contains ferric oxide black, hypromellose-2910, PEG-3350, titanium dioxide, and carnauba wax.

12 CLINICAL PHARMACOLOGY

12.1 Mechanism of Action

Irbesartan

Angiotensin II is a potent vasoconstrictor formed from angiotensin I in a reaction catalyzed by angiotensin-converting enzyme (ACE, kininase II). Angiotensin II is the principal pressor agent of the RAS and also stimulates aldosterone synthesis and secretion by adrenal cortex, cardiac contraction, renal resorption of sodium, activity of the sympathetic nervous system, and smooth muscle cell growth. Irbesartan blocks the vasoconstrictor and aldosterone-secreting effects of angiotensin II by selectively binding to the AT_1 angiotensin II receptor. There is also an AT_2 receptor in many tissues, but it is not involved in cardiovascular homeostasis.

Irbesartan is a specific competitive antagonist of AT_1 receptors with a much greater affinity (more than 8500-fold) for the AT_1 receptor than for the AT_2 receptor, and no agonist activity.

Blockade of the AT_1 receptor removes the negative feedback of angiotensin II on renin secretion, but the resulting increased plasma renin activity and circulating angiotensin II do not overcome the effects of irbesartan on blood pressure.

Irbesartan does not inhibit ACE or renin or affect other hormone receptors or ion channels known to be involved in the cardiovascular regulation of blood pressure and sodium homeostasis. Because irbesartan does not inhibit ACE, it does not affect the response to bradykinin; whether this has clinical relevance is not known.

Hydrochlorothiazide

Hydrochlorothiazide is a thiazide diuretic. Thiazides affect the renal tubular mechanisms of electrolyte reabsorption, directly increasing excretion of sodium and chloride in approximately equivalent amounts. Indirectly, the diuretic action of hydrochlorothiazide reduces plasma volume, with consequent increases in plasma renin activity, increases in aldosterone secretion, increases in urinary potassium loss, and decreases in serum potassium. The renin-aldosterone link is mediated by angiotensin II, so coadministration of an angiotensin II receptor antagonist tends to reverse the potassium loss associated with these diuretics.

The mechanism of the antihypertensive effect of thiazides is not fully understood.

12.2 Pharmacodynamics

Irbesartan

In healthy subjects, single oral irbesartan doses of up to 300 mg produced dose-dependent inhibition of the pressor effect of angiotensin II infusions. Inhibition was complete (100%) 4 hours following oral doses of 150 mg or 300 mg and partial inhibition was sustained for 24 hours (60% and 40% at 300 mg and 150 mg, respectively).

In hypertensive patients, angiotensin II receptor inhibition following chronic administration of irbesartan causes a 1.5- to 2-fold rise in angiotensin II plasma concentration and a 2- to 3-fold increase in plasma renin levels. Aldosterone plasma concentrations generally decline following irbesartan administration, but serum potassium levels are not significantly affected at recommended doses.

In hypertensive patients, chronic oral doses of irbesartan (up to 300 mg) had no effect on glomerular filtration rate, renal plasma flow or filtration fraction. In multiple dose studies in hypertensive patients, there were no clinically important effects on fasting triglycerides, total cholesterol, HDL-cholesterol, or fasting glucose concentrations. There was no effect on serum uric acid during chronic oral administration and no uricosuric effect.

Hydrochlorothiazide

After oral administration of hydrochlorothiazide, diuresis begins within 2 hours, peaks in about 4 hours and lasts about 6 to 12 hours.

12.3 Pharmacokinetics

Irbesartan

Irbesartan is an orally active agent that does not require biotransformation into an active form. The oral absorption of irbesartan is rapid and complete with an average absolute bioavailability of 60% to 80%. Following oral administration of irbesartan, peak plasma concentrations of irbesartan are attained at 1.5 to 2 hours after dosing. Food does not affect the bioavailability of irbesartan.

Irbesartan exhibits linear pharmacokinetics over the therapeutic dose range.

The terminal elimination half-life of irbesartan averaged 11 to 15 hours. Steady-state concentrations are achieved within 3 days. Limited accumulation of irbesartan (<20%) is observed in plasma upon repeated once-daily dosing.

Hydrochlorothiazide

When plasma levels have been followed for at least 24 hours, the plasma half-life has been observed to vary between 5.6 and 14.8 hours.

Metabolism and Elimination

Irbesartan

Irbesartan is metabolized via glucuronide conjugation and oxidation. Following oral or intravenous administration of ^{14}C-labeled irbesartan, more than 80% of the circulating plasma radioactivity is attributable to unchanged irbesartan. The primary circulating metabolite is the inactive irbesartan glucuronide conjugate (approximately 6%). The remaining oxidative metabolites do not add appreciably to irbesartan's pharmacologic activity.

Irbesartan and its metabolites are excreted by both biliary and renal routes. Following either oral or intravenous administration of ^{14}C-labeled irbesartan, about 20% of radioactivity is recovered in the urine and the remainder in the feces, as irbesartan or irbesartan glucuronide.

In vitro studies of irbesartan oxidation by cytochrome P450 isoenzymes indicated irbesartan was oxidized primarily by 2C9; metabolism by 3A4 was negligible. Irbesartan was neither metabolized by, nor did it substantially induce or inhibit, isoenzymes commonly associated with drug metabolism (1A1, 1A2, 2A6, 2B6, 2D6, 2E1). There was no induction or inhibition of 3A4.

Hydrochlorothiazide

Hydrochlorothiazide is not metabolized but is eliminated rapidly by the kidney. At least 61% of the oral dose is eliminated unchanged within 24 hours.

Distribution

Irbesartan

Irbesartan is 90% bound to serum proteins (primarily albumin and α_1-acid glycoprotein) with negligible binding to cellular components of blood. The average volume of distribution is 53 to 93 liters. Total plasma and renal clearances are in the range of 157 to 176 mL/min and 3.0 to 3.5 mL/min, respectively. With repetitive dosing, irbesartan accumulates to no clinically relevant extent.

Studies in animals indicate that radiolabeled irbesartan weakly crosses the blood-brain barrier and placenta. Irbesartan is excreted in the milk of lactating rats.

Hydrochlorothiazide

Hydrochlorothiazide crosses the placental but not the blood-brain barrier and is excreted in breast milk.

Pediatric
Irbesartan-hydrochlorothiazide pharmacokinetics have not been investigated in patients <18 years of age.
Gender
No gender-related differences in pharmacokinetics were observed in healthy elderly (age 65 to 80 years) or in healthy young (age 18 to 40 years) subjects. In studies of hypertensive patients, there was no gender difference in half-life or accumulation, but somewhat higher plasma concentrations of irbesartan were observed in females (11% to 44%). No gender-related dosage adjustment is necessary.
Geriatric
In elderly subjects (age 65 to 80 years), irbesartan elimination half-life was not significantly altered, but AUC and C_{max} values were about 20% to 50% greater than those of young subjects (age 18 to 40 years). No dosage adjustment is necessary in the elderly.
Race
In healthy black subjects, irbesartan AUC values were approximately 25% greater than whites; there were no differences in C_{max} values.
Renal Insufficiency
The pharmacokinetics of irbesartan were not altered in patients with renal impairment or in patients on hemodialysis. Irbesartan is not removed by hemodialysis. No dosage adjustment is necessary in patients with mild to severe renal impairment unless a patient with renal impairment is also volume depleted. [See *Warnings and Precautions (5.2)*.]
Hepatic Insufficiency
The pharmacokinetics of irbesartan following repeated oral administration were not significantly affected in patients with mild to moderate cirrhosis of the liver. No dosage adjustment is necessary in patients with hepatic insufficiency.
Drug-Drug Interactions
No significant drug-drug pharmacokinetic (or pharmacodynamic) interactions have been found in interaction studies with hydrochlorothiazide, digoxin, warfarin, and nifedipine. *In vitro* studies show significant inhibition of the formation of oxidized irbesartan metabolites with the known cytochrome CYP 2C9 substrates/inhibitors sulphenazole, tolbutamide and nifedipine. However, in clinical studies the consequences of concomitant irbesartan on the pharmacodynamics of warfarin were negligible. Concomitant nifedipine or hydrochlorothiazide had no effect on irbesartan pharmacokinetics. Based on *in vitro* data, no interaction would be expected with drugs whose metabolism is dependent upon cytochrome P450 isoenzymes 1A1, 1A2, 2A6, 2B6, 2D6, 2E1, or 3A4.
In separate studies of patients receiving maintenance doses of warfarin, hydrochlorothiazide, or digoxin, irbesartan administration for 7 days had no effect on the pharmacodynamics of warfarin (prothrombin time) or the pharmacokinetics of digoxin. The pharmacokinetics of irbesartan were not affected by coadministration of nifedipine or hydrochlorothiazide.

13 NONCLINICAL TOXICOLOGY

13.1 Carcinogenesis, Mutagenesis, Impairment of Fertility

Irbesartan-Hydrochlorothiazide
No carcinogenicity studies have been conducted with the irbesartan-hydrochlorothiazide combination.
Irbesartan-hydrochlorothiazide was not mutagenic in standard *in vitro* tests (Ames microbial test and Chinese hamster mammalian-cell forward gene-mutation assay). Irbesartan-hydrochlorothiazide was negative in tests for induction of chromosomal aberrations (*in vitro*—human lymphocyte assay; *in vivo*—mouse micronucleus study).
The combination of irbesartan and hydrochlorothiazide has not been evaluated in definitive studies of fertility.
Irbesartan
No evidence of carcinogenicity was observed when irbesartan was administered at doses of up to 500/1000 mg/kg/day (males/females, respectively) in rats and 1000 mg/kg/day in mice for up to 2 years. For male and female rats, 500 mg/kg/day provided an average systemic exposure to irbesartan ($AUC_{0-24\ hours}$, bound plus unbound) about 3 and 11 times, respectively, the average systemic exposure in humans receiving the maximum recommended dose (MRD) of 300 mg irbesartan/day, whereas 1000 mg/kg/day (administered to females only) provided an average systemic exposure about 21 times that reported for humans at the MRD. For male and female mice, 1000 mg/kg/day provided an exposure to irbesartan about 3 and 5 times, respectively, the human exposure at 300 mg/day.
Irbesartan was not mutagenic in a battery of *in vitro* tests (Ames microbial test, rat hepatocyte DNA repair test, V79 mammalian-cell forward gene-mutation assay). Irbesartan was negative in several tests for induction of chromosomal aberrations (*in vitro*—human lymphocyte assay; *in vivo*—mouse micronucleus study).
Irbesartan had no adverse effects on fertility or mating of male or female rats at oral doses ≤650 mg/kg/day, the highest dose providing a systemic exposure to irbesartan ($AUC_{0-24\ hours}$, bound plus unbound) about 5 times that found in humans receiving the MRD of 300 mg/day.
Hydrochlorothiazide
Two-year feeding studies in mice and rats conducted under the auspices of the National Toxicology Program (NTP) uncovered no evidence of a carcinogenic potential of hydrochlorothiazide in female mice (at doses of up to approximately 600 mg/kg/day) or in male and female rats (at doses of up to approximately 100 mg/kg/day). The NTP, however, found equivocal evidence for hepatocarcinogenicity in male mice.
Hydrochlorothiazide was not genotoxic *in vitro* in the Ames mutagenicity assay of *Salmonella typhimurium* strains TA 98, TA 100, TA 1535, TA 1537, and TA 1538 and in the Chinese Hamster Ovary (CHO) test for chromosomal aberrations, or *in vivo* in assays using mouse germinal cell chromosomes, Chinese hamster bone marrow chromosomes, and the *Drosophila* sex-linked recessive lethal trait gene. Positive test results were obtained only in the *in vitro* CHO Sister Chromatid Exchange (clastogenicity) and in the Mouse Lymphoma Cell (mutagenicity) assays, using concentrations of hydrochlorothiazide from 43 to 1300 µg/mL, and in the *Aspergillus nidulans* non-disjunction assay at an unspecified concentration.
Hydrochlorothiazide had no adverse effects on the fertility of mice and rats of either sex in studies wherein these species were exposed, via their diet, to doses of up to 100 and 4 mg/kg, respectively, prior to mating and throughout gestation.

13.2 Animal Toxicology and/or Pharmacology

Reproductive Toxicology Studies
When pregnant rats were treated with irbesartan from day 0 to day 20 of gestation (oral doses of 50, 180, and 650 mg/kg/day), increased incidences of renal pelvic cavitation, hydroureter and/or absence of renal papilla were observed in fetuses at doses ≥50 mg/kg/day (approximately equivalent to the MRHD, 300 mg/day, on a body surface area basis). Subcutaneous edema was observed in fetuses at doses ≥180 mg/kg/day (about 4 times the MRHD on a body surface area basis). As these anomalies were not observed in rats in which irbesartan exposure (oral doses of 50, 150, and 450 mg/kg/day) was limited to gestation days 6 to 15, they appear to reflect late gestational effects of the drug. In pregnant rabbits, oral doses of 30 mg irbesartan/kg/day were associated with maternal mortality and abortion. Surviving females receiving this dose (about 1.5 times the MRHD on a body surface area basis) had a slight increase in early resorptions and a corresponding decrease in live fetuses. Irbesartan was found to cross the placental barrier in rats and rabbits.

14 CLINICAL STUDIES

14.1 Irbesartan Monotherapy

The antihypertensive effects of irbesartan were examined in 7 major placebo-controlled, 8- to 12-week trials in patients with baseline diastolic blood pressures of 95 to 110 mmHg. Doses of 1 to 900 mg were included in these trials in order to fully explore the dose-range of irbesartan. These studies allowed a comparison of once- or twice-daily regimens at 150 mg/day, comparisons of peak and trough effects, and comparisons of response by gender, age, and race. Two of the 7 placebo-controlled trials identified above and 2 additional placebo-controlled studies examined the antihypertensive effects of irbesartan and hydrochlorothiazide in combination.
The 7 studies of irbesartan monotherapy included a total of 1915 patients randomized to irbesartan (1 to 900 mg) and 611 patients randomized to placebo. Once-daily doses of 150 to 300 mg provided statistically and clinically significant decreases in systolic and diastolic blood pressure with trough (24-hour post-dose) effects after 6 to 12 weeks of treatment compared to placebo, of about 8 to 10/5 to 6 mmHg and 8 to 12/5 to 8 mmHg, respectively. No further increase in effect was seen at dosages greater than 300 mg. The dose-response relationships for effects on systolic and diastolic pressure are shown in Figures 3 and 4.
[See figure 3 at top of next column]
[See figure 4 in next column]
Once-daily administration of therapeutic doses of irbesartan gave peak effects at around 3 to 6 hours and, in one continuous ambulatory blood pressure monitoring study, again around 14 hours. This was seen with both once-daily and twice-daily dosing. Trough-to-peak ratios for systolic and diastolic response were generally between 60% to 70%. In a continuous ambulatory blood pressure monitoring study, once-daily dosing with 150 mg gave trough and mean 24-hour responses similar to those observed in patients receiving twice-daily dosing at the same total daily dose.
Analysis of age, gender, and race subgroups of patients showed that men and women, and patients over and under 65 years of age, had generally similar responses. Irbesartan was effective in reducing blood pressure regardless of race, although the effect was somewhat less in blacks (usually a low-renin population). Black patients typically show an improved response with the addition of a low dose diuretic (eg, 12.5 mg hydrochlorothiazide).

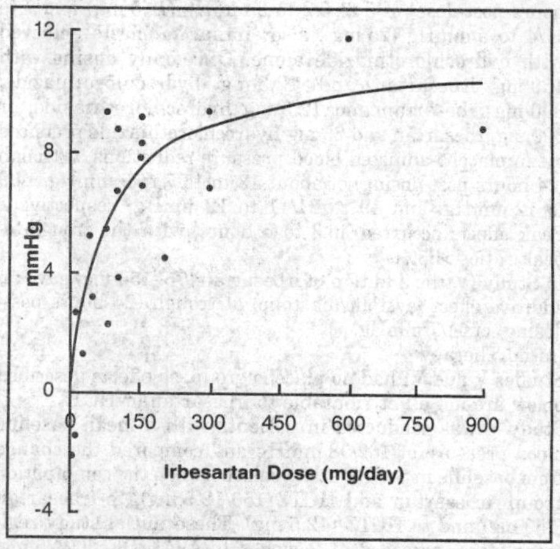

Figure 3. Placebo-subtracted reduction in trough SeSBP; integrated analysis

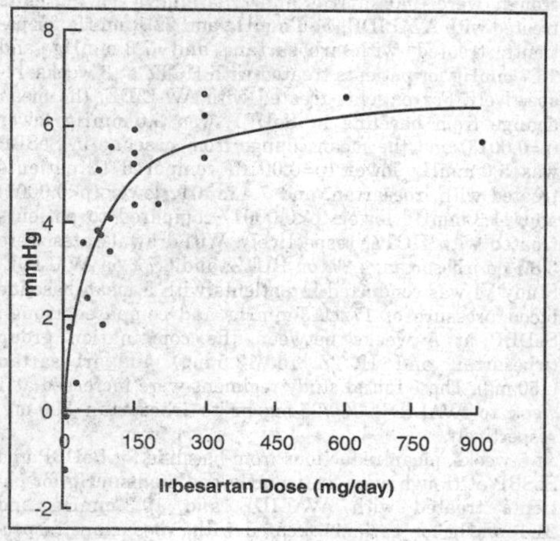

Figure 4. Placebo-subtracted reduction in trough SeDBP; integrated analysis

The effect of irbesartan is apparent after the first dose and is close to the full observed effect at 2 weeks. At the end of the 8-week exposure, about 2/3 of the antihypertensive effect was still present 1 week after the last dose. Rebound hypertension was not observed. There was essentially no change in average heart rate in irbesartan-treated patients in controlled trials.

14.2 Irbesartan-Hydrochlorothiazide

The antihypertensive effects of AVALIDE (irbesartan-hydrochlorothiazide) Tablets were examined in 4 placebo-controlled studies in patients with mild-moderate hypertension (mean seated diastolic blood pressure [SeDBP] between 90 and 110 mmHg), one study in patients with moderate hypertension (mean seated systolic blood pressure [SeSBP] 160 to 179 mmHg or SeDBP 100 to 109 mmHg), and one study in patients with severe hypertension (mean SeDBP ≥110 mmHg) of 8 to 12 weeks. These trials included 3149 patients randomized to fixed doses of irbesartan (37.5 to 300 mg) and concomitant hydrochlorothiazide (6.25 to 25 mg).
Study I was a factorial study that compared all combinations of irbesartan (37.5 mg, 100 mg, and 300 mg or placebo) and hydrochlorothiazide (6.25 mg, 12.5 mg, and 25 mg or placebo).
Study II compared the irbesartan-hydrochlorothiazide combinations of 75/12.5 mg and 150/12.5 mg to their individual components and placebo.
Study III investigated the ambulatory blood pressure responses to irbesartan-hydrochlorothiazide (75/12.5 mg and 150/12.5 mg) and placebo after 8 weeks of dosing.
Study IV investigated the effects of the addition of irbesartan (75 or 150 mg) in patients not controlled (SeDBP 93-120 mmHg) on hydrochlorothiazide (25 mg) alone. In Studies I–III, the addition of irbesartan 150 to 300 mg to hydrochlorothiazide doses of 6.25, 12.5, or 25 mg produced further dose-related reductions in blood pressure at trough of 8 to 10 mmHg/3 to 6 mmHg, similar to those achieved with the same monotherapy dose of irbesartan. The addition of hydrochlorothiazide to irbesartan produced further dose-related reductions in blood pressure at trough (24

hours post-dose) of 5 to 6/2 to 3 mmHg (12.5 mg) and 7 to 11/4 to 5 mmHg (25 mg), also similar to effects achieved with hydrochlorothiazide alone. Once-daily dosing with 150 mg irbesartan and 12.5 mg hydrochlorothiazide, 300 mg irbesartan and 12.5 mg hydrochlorothiazide, or 300 mg irbesartan and 25 mg hydrochlorothiazide produced mean placebo-adjusted blood pressure reductions at trough (24 hours post-dosing) of about 13 to 15/7 to 9 mmHg, 14/9 to 12 mmHg, and 19 to 21/11 to 12 mmHg, respectively. Peak effects occurred at 3 to 6 hours, with the trough-to-peak ratios >65%.

In Study IV, the addition of irbesartan (75–150 mg) gave an additive effect (systolic/diastolic) at trough (24 hours post-dosing) of 11/7 mmHg.

Initial Therapy

Studies V and VI had no placebo group, so effects described below are not all attributable to irbesartan or HCTZ.

Study V was conducted in patients with a mean baseline blood pressure of 162/98 mmHg and compared the change from baseline in SeSBP at 8 weeks between the combination group (irbesartan and HCTZ 150/12.5 mg), to irbesartan (150 mg) and to HCTZ (12.5 mg). These initial study regimens were increased at 2 weeks to AVALIDE 300/25 mg, irbesartan 300 mg, or to HCTZ 25 mg, respectively.

Mean reductions from baseline for SeDBP and SeSBP at trough were 14.6 mmHg and 27.1 mmHg for patients treated with AVALIDE, 11.6 mmHg and 22.1 mmHg for patients treated with irbesartan, and 7.3 mmHg and 15.7 mmHg for patients treated with HCTZ at 8 weeks, respectively. For patients treated with AVALIDE, the mean change from baseline in SeDBP was 3.0 mmHg lower (p=0.0013) and the mean change from baseline in SeSBP was 5.0 mmHg lower (p=0.0016) compared to patients treated with irbesartan, and 7.4 mmHg lower (p<0.0001) and 11.3 mmHg lower (p<0.0001) compared to patients treated with HCTZ, respectively. Withdrawal rates were 3.8% on irbesartan, 4.8% on HCTZ, and 6.7% on AVALIDE.

Study VI was conducted in patients with a mean baseline blood pressure of 172/113 mmHg and compared trough SeDBP at 5 weeks between the combination group (irbesartan and HCTZ 150/12.5 mg) and irbesartan (150 mg). These initial study regimens were increased at 1 week to AVALIDE 300/25 mg or to irbesartan 300 mg, respectively.

At 5 weeks, mean reductions from baseline for SeDBP and SeSBP at trough were 24.0 mmHg and 30.8 mmHg for patients treated with AVALIDE and 19.3 mmHg and 21.1 mmHg for patients treated with irbesartan, respectively. The mean SeDBP was 4.7 mmHg lower (p<0.0001) and the mean SeSBP was 9.7 mmHg lower (p<0.0001) in the group treated with AVALIDE than in the group treated with irbesartan. Patients treated with AVALIDE achieved more rapid blood pressure control with significantly lower SeDBP and SeSBP and greater blood pressure control at every assessment (Week 1, Week 3, Week 5, and Week 7). Maximum effects were seen at Week 7.

Withdrawal rates were 2.2% on irbesartan and 2.1% on AVALIDE.

In Studies I–VI, there was no difference in response for men and women or in patients over or under 65 years of age. Black patients had a larger response to hydrochlorothiazide than non-black patients and a smaller response to irbesartan. The overall response to the combination was similar for black and non-black patients.

16 HOW SUPPLIED/STORAGE AND HANDLING

16.1 How Supplied

AVALIDE® (irbesartan-hydrochlorothiazide) 150/12.5 mg and 300/12.5 mg tablets are peach, biconvex, and oval with a heart debossed on one side and "2775" or "2776" on the reverse side. The 300/25 mg film-coated tablet is pink, biconvex, and oval with a heart debossed on one side and "2788" on the reverse side. AVALIDE® Tablets are supplied as follows:

Irbesartan (mg)	HCTZ (mg)	NDC 0087-xxxx-xx for unit of use	
		Bottle of 30	Bottle of 90
150	12.5	2775-31	2775-32
300	12.5	2776-31	2776-32
300	25	2788-31	2788-32

16.2 Storage

Store at 25°C (77°F); excursions permitted to 15°C-30°C (59°F-86°F) [see USP Controlled Room Temperature].

17 PATIENT COUNSELING INFORMATION

17.1 Pregnancy

Female patients of childbearing age should be told that use of drugs like AVALIDE during the second or third trimesters of pregnancy can cause serious problems in the fetus and infant including: low blood pressure, poor development of skull bones, kidney failure, and death. These effects have not occurred with drug exposure limited to the first trimester. Women using AVALIDE who become pregnant should notify their physician as soon as possible.

17.2 Symptomatic Hypotension

Patients using AVALIDE should be told that they may feel lightheaded, especially during the first days of use. Patients should inform their physician if they feel lightheaded or faint. If fainting occurs, the patient should stop using AVALIDE and contact the prescribing doctor.

Patients using AVALIDE should be told that getting dehydrated can lower their blood pressure too much and lead to lightheadedness and possible fainting. Dehydration may occur with excessive sweating, diarrhea, or vomiting and with not drinking enough liquids.

Manufactured by:
Bristol-Myers Squibb Company
Princeton, New Jersey 08543 USA
Distributed by:
Bristol-Myers Squibb Sanofi-Synthelabo Partnership
New York, New York 10016
1243926A1
Rev November 2008

Shown in Product Identification Guide, page 318

AVAPRO® ℞

[ă-vă-prō]
(irbesartan) Tablets
Rx only

USE IN PREGNANCY
When used in pregnancy during the second and third trimesters, drugs that act directly on the renin-angiotensin system can cause injury and even death to the developing fetus. When pregnancy is detected, AVAPRO should be discontinued as soon as possible. See **WARNINGS: Fetal/Neonatal Morbidity and Mortality.**

DESCRIPTION

AVAPRO®* (irbesartan) is an angiotensin II receptor (AT_1 subtype) antagonist.

Irbesartan is a non-peptide compound, chemically described as a 2-butyl-3-[*p*-(*o*-1*H*-tetrazol-5-ylphenyl)benzyl]-1,3-diazaspiro[4.4]non-1-en-4-one.

Its empirical formula is $C_{25}H_{28}N_6O$, and the structural formula:

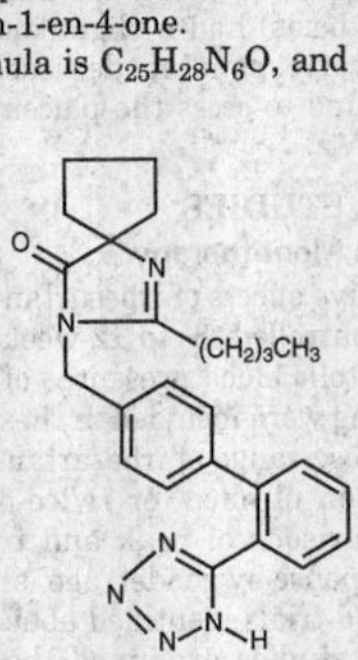

Irbesartan is a white to off-white crystalline powder with a molecular weight of 428.5. It is a nonpolar compound with a partition coefficient (octanol/water) of 10.1 at pH of 7.4. Irbesartan is slightly soluble in alcohol and methylene chloride and practically insoluble in water.

AVAPRO is available for oral administration in unscored tablets containing 75 mg, 150 mg, or 300 mg of irbesartan. Inactive ingredients include: lactose, microcrystalline cellulose, pregelatinized starch, croscarmellose sodium, poloxamer 188, silicon dioxide and magnesium stearate.

*Registered trademark of Sanofi-Synthelabo

CLINICAL PHARMACOLOGY

Mechanism of Action

Angiotensin II is a potent vasoconstrictor formed from angiotensin I in a reaction catalyzed by angiotensin-converting enzyme (ACE, kininase II). Angiotensin II is the principal pressor agent of the renin-angiotensin system (RAS) and also stimulates aldosterone synthesis and secretion by adrenal cortex, cardiac contraction, renal resorption of sodium, activity of the sympathetic nervous system, and smooth muscle cell growth. Irbesartan blocks the vasoconstrictor and aldosterone-secreting effects of angiotensin II by selectively binding to the AT_1 angiotensin II receptor. There is also an AT_2 receptor in many tissues, but it is not involved in cardiovascular homeostasis.

Irbesartan is a specific competitive antagonist of AT_1 receptors with a much greater affinity (more than 8500-fold) for the AT_1 receptor than for the AT_2 receptor and no agonist activity.

Blockade of the AT_1 receptor removes the negative feedback of angiotensin II on renin secretion, but the resulting increased plasma renin activity and circulating angiotensin II do not overcome the effects of irbesartan on blood pressure.

Irbesartan does not inhibit ACE or renin or affect other hormone receptors or ion channels known to be involved in the cardiovascular regulation of blood pressure and sodium homeostasis. Because irbesartan does not inhibit ACE, it does not affect the response to bradykinin; whether this has clinical relevance is not known.

Pharmacokinetics

Irbesartan is an orally active agent that does not require biotransformation into an active form. The oral absorption of irbesartan is rapid and complete with an average absolute bioavailability of 60-80%. Following oral administration of AVAPRO, peak plasma concentrations of irbesartan are attained at 1.5-2 hours after dosing. Food does not affect the bioavailability of AVAPRO.

Irbesartan exhibits linear pharmacokinetics over the therapeutic dose range.

The terminal elimination half-life of irbesartan averaged 11-15 hours. Steady-state concentrations are achieved within 3 days. Limited accumulation of irbesartan (<20%) is observed in plasma upon repeated once-daily dosing.

Metabolism and Elimination

Irbesartan is metabolized via glucuronide conjugation and oxidation. Following oral or intravenous administration of ^{14}C-labeled irbesartan, more than 80% of the circulating plasma radioactivity is attributable to unchanged irbesartan. The primary circulating metabolite is the inactive irbesartan glucuronide conjugate (approximately 6%). The remaining oxidative metabolites do not add appreciably to irbesartan's pharmacologic activity.

Irbesartan and its metabolites are excreted by both biliary and renal routes. Following either oral or intravenous administration of ^{14}C-labeled irbesartan, about 20% of radioactivity is recovered in the urine and the remainder in the feces, as irbesartan or irbesartan glucuronide.

In vitro studies of irbesartan oxidation by cytochrome P450 isoenzymes indicated irbesartan was oxidized primarily by 2C9; metabolism by 3A4 was negligible. Irbesartan was neither metabolized by, nor did it substantially induce or inhibit, isoenzymes commonly associated with drug metabolism (1A1, 1A2, 2A6, 2B6, 2D6, 2E1). There was no induction or inhibition of 3A4.

Distribution

Irbesartan is 90% bound to serum proteins (primarily albumin and α_1-acid glycoprotein) with negligible binding to cellular components of blood. The average volume of distribution is 53-93 liters. Total plasma and renal clearances are in the range of 157-176 and 3.0-3.5 mL/min, respectively. With repetitive dosing, irbesartan accumulates to no clinically relevant extent.

Studies in animals indicate that radiolabeled irbesartan weakly crosses the blood brain barrier and placenta. Irbesartan is excreted in the milk of lactating rats.

Special Populations

Gender

No gender-related differences in pharmacokinetics were observed in healthy elderly (age 65-80 years) or in healthy young (age 18-40 years) subjects. In studies of hypertensive patients, there was no gender difference in half-life or accumulation, but somewhat higher plasma concentrations of irbesartan were observed in females (11-44%). No gender-related dosage adjustment is necessary.

Geriatric

In elderly subjects (age 65-80 years), irbesartan elimination half-life was not significantly altered, but AUC and C_{max} values were about 20-50% greater than those of young subjects (age 18-40 years). No dosage adjustment is necessary in the elderly.

Race

In healthy black subjects, irbesartan AUC values were approximately 25% greater than whites; there were no differences in C_{max} values.

Renal Insufficiency

The pharmacokinetics of irbesartan were not altered in patients with renal impairment or in patients on hemodialysis. Irbesartan is not removed by hemodialysis. No dosage adjustment is necessary in patients with mild to severe renal impairment unless a patient with renal impairment is also volume depleted. (See **WARNINGS: Hypotension in Volume- or Salt-depleted Patients** and **DOSAGE AND ADMINISTRATION.**)

Hepatic Insufficiency

The pharmacokinetics of irbesartan following repeated oral administration were not significantly affected in patients with mild to moderate cirrhosis of the liver. No dosage adjustment is necessary in patients with hepatic insufficiency.

Drug Interactions

(See **PRECAUTIONS: Drug Interactions.**)

Pharmacodynamics

In healthy subjects, single oral irbesartan doses of up to 300 mg produced dose-dependent inhibition of the pressor effect of angiotensin II infusions. Inhibition was complete (100%) 4 hours following oral doses of 150 mg or 300 mg and partial inhibition was sustained for 24 hours (60% and 40% at 300 mg and 150 mg, respectively).

In hypertensive patients, angiotensin II receptor inhibition following chronic administration of irbesartan causes a 1.5- to 2-fold rise in angiotensin II plasma concentration and a 2- to 3-fold increase in plasma renin levels. Aldosterone plasma concentrations generally decline following irbesartan administration, but serum potassium levels are not significantly affected at recommended doses.

In hypertensive patients, chronic oral doses of irbesartan (up to 300 mg) had no effect on glomerular filtration rate, renal plasma flow or filtration fraction. In multiple dose studies in hypertensive patients, there were no clinically important effects on fasting triglycerides, total cholesterol, HDL-cholesterol, or fasting glucose concentrations. There was no effect on serum uric acid during chronic oral administration, and no uricosuric effect.

Clinical Studies

Hypertension

The antihypertensive effects of AVAPRO (irbesartan) were examined in seven (7) major placebo-controlled 8-12 week trials in patients with baseline diastolic blood pressures of 95-110 mmHg. Doses of 1-900 mg were included in these trials in order to fully explore the dose-range of irbesartan. These studies allowed comparison of once- or twice-daily regimens at 150 mg/day, comparisons of peak and trough effects, and comparisons of response by gender, age, and race. Two of the seven placebo-controlled trials identified above examined the antihypertensive effects of irbesartan and hydrochlorothiazide in combination.

The seven (7) studies of irbesartan monotherapy included a total of 1915 patients randomized to irbesartan (1-900 mg) and 611 patients randomized to placebo. Once-daily doses of 150 and 300 mg provided statistically and clinically significant decreases in systolic and diastolic blood pressure with trough (24 hours post-dose) effects after 6-12 weeks of treatment compared to placebo, of about 8-10/5-6 and 8-12/5-8 mmHg, respectively. No further increase in effect was seen at dosages greater than 300 mg. The dose-response relationships for effects on systolic and diastolic pressure are shown in Figures 1 and 2.

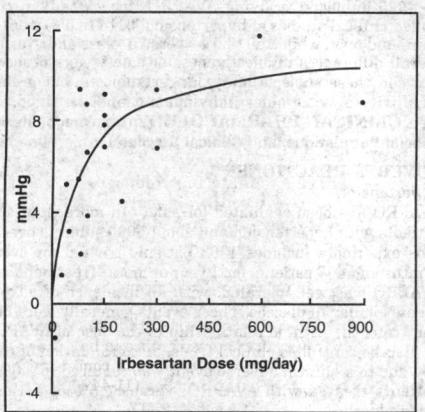

Figure 1.
Placebo-subtracted reduction in trough SeSBP; integrated analysis

[See figure 2 at top of next column]

Once-daily administration of therapeutic doses of irbesartan gave peak effects at around 3-6 hours and, in one ambulatory blood pressure monitoring study, again around 14 hours. This was seen with both once-daily and twice-daily dosing. Trough-to-peak ratios for systolic and diastolic response were generally between 60-70%. In a continuous ambulatory blood pressure monitoring study, once-daily dosing with 150 mg gave trough and mean 24-hour responses similar to those observed in patients receiving twice-daily dosing at the same total daily dose.

In controlled trials, the addition of irbesartan to hydrochlorothiazide doses of 6.25, 12.5, or 25 mg produced further dose-related reductions in blood pressure similar to those achieved with the same monotherapy dose of irbesartan. HCTZ also had an approximately additive effect.

Analysis of age, gender, and race subgroups of patients showed that men and women, and patients over and under 65 years of age, had generally similar responses. Irbesartan was effective in reducing blood pressure regardless of race, although the effect was somewhat less in blacks (usually a low-renin population).

Table 1: IDNT: Components of Primary Composite Endpoint

	AVAPRO N=579 (%)	Comparison With Placebo			Comparison With Amlodipine		
		Placebo N=569 (%)	Hazard Ratio	95% CI	Amlodipine N=567 (%)	Hazard Ratio	95% CI
Primary Composite Endpoint	32.6	39.0	0.80	0.66-0.97 (p=0.0234)	41.1	0.77	0.63-0.93
Breakdown of first occurring event contributing to primary endpoint							
2× creatinine	14.2	19.5	—	—	22.8	—	—
ESRD	7.4	8.3	—	—	8.8	—	—
Death	11.1	11.2	—	—	9.5	—	—
Incidence of total events over entire period of follow-up							
2× creatinine	16.9	23.7	0.67	0.52-0.87	25.4	0.63	0.49-0.81
ESRD	14.2	17.8	0.77	0.57-1.03	18.3	0.77	0.57-1.03
Death	15.0	16.3	0.92	0.69-1.23	14.6	1.04	0.77-1.40

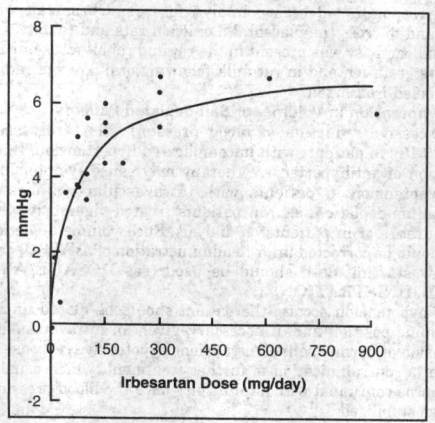

Figure 2.
Placebo-subtracted reduction in trough SeDBP; integrated analysis

The effect of irbesartan is apparent after the first dose, and it is close to its full observed effect at 2 weeks. At the end of an 8-week exposure, about 2/3 of the antihypertensive effect was still present one week after the last dose. Rebound hypertension was not observed. There was essentially no change in average heart rate in irbesartan-treated patients in controlled trials.

Nephropathy in Type 2 Diabetic Patients

The Irbesartan Diabetic Nephropathy Trial (IDNT) was a randomized, placebo- and active-controlled, double-blind multicenter study, conducted worldwide in 1715 patients with type 2 diabetes, hypertension (SeSBP >135 mmHg or SeDBP >85 mmHg), and nephropathy (serum creatinine 1.0 to 3.0 mg/dL in females or 1.2 to 3.0 mg/dL in males and proteinuria ≥900 mg/day). Patients were randomized to receive AVAPRO 75 mg, amlodipine 2.5 mg, or matching placebo once-daily. Patients were titrated to a maintenance dose of AVAPRO 300 mg, or amlodipine 10 mg, as tolerated. Additional antihypertensive agents (excluding ACE inhibitors, angiotensin II receptor antagonists and calcium channel blockers) were added as needed to achieve blood pressure goal (≤135/85 or 10 mmHg reduction in systolic blood pressure if higher than 160 mmHg) for patients in all groups.

The study population was 66.5% male, 72.9% below 65 years of age and 72% White, (Asian/Pacific Islander 5.0%, Black 13.3%, Hispanic 4.8%). The mean baseline seated systolic and diastolic blood pressures were 159 mmHg and 87 mmHg, respectively. The patients entered the trial with a mean serum creatinine of 1.7 mg/dL and mean proteinuria of 4144 mg/day.

The mean blood pressure achieved was 142/77 mmHg for AVAPRO, 142/76 mmHg for amlodipine, and 145/79 mmHg for placebo. Overall, 83.0% of patients received the target dose of irbesartan more than 50% of the time. Patients were followed for a mean duration of 2.6 years.

The primary composite endpoint was the time to occurrence of any one of the following events: doubling of baseline serum creatinine, end-stage renal disease (ESRD; defined by serum creatinine ≥6 mg/dL, dialysis, or renal transplan-

tation) or death. Treatment with AVAPRO resulted in a 20% risk reduction versus placebo (p=0.0234) (see Figure 3 and Table 1). Treatment with AVAPRO also reduced the occurrence of sustained doubling of serum creatinine as a separate endpoint (33%), but had no significant effect on ESRD alone and no effect on overall mortality (see Table 1).

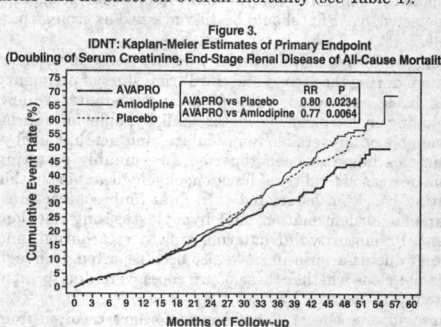

Figure 3.
IDNT: Kaplan-Meier Estimates of Primary Endpoint (Doubling of Serum Creatinine, End-Stage Renal Disease of All-Cause Mortality)

The percentages of patients experiencing an event during the course of the study can be seen in Table 1 below:
[See table 1 above]

The secondary endpoint of the study was a composite of cardiovascular mortality and morbidity (myocardial infarction, hospitalization for heart failure, stroke with permanent neurological deficit, amputation). There were no statistically significant differences among treatment groups in these endpoints. Compared with placebo, AVAPRO significantly reduced proteinuria by about 27%, an effect that was evident within 3 months of starting therapy. AVAPRO significantly reduced the rate of loss of renal function (glomerular filtration rate), as measured by the reciprocal of the serum creatinine concentration, by 18.2%. Table 2 presents results for demographic subgroups. Subgroup analyses are difficult to interpret and it is not known whether these observations represent true differences or chance effects. For the primary endpoint, AVAPRO's favorable effects were seen in patients also taking other antihypertensive medications (angiotensin II receptor antagonists, angiotensin-converting-enzyme inhibitors and calcium channel blockers were not allowed), oral hypoglycemic agents, and lipid-lowering agents.
[See table 2 at top of next page]

INDICATIONS AND USAGE

Hypertension

AVAPRO (irbesartan) is indicated for the treatment of hypertension. It may be used alone or in combination with other antihypertensive agents.

Nephropathy in Type 2 Diabetic Patients

AVAPRO is indicated for the treatment of diabetic nephropathy with an elevated serum creatinine and proteinuria (>300 mg/day) in patients with type 2 diabetes and hypertension. In this population, AVAPRO reduces the rate of progression of nephropathy as measured by the occurrence of doubling of serum creatinine or end-stage renal disease (need for dialysis or renal transplantation) (see **CLINICAL PHARMACOLOGY: Clinical Studies**).

CONTRAINDICATIONS

AVAPRO is contraindicated in patients who are hypersensitive to any component of this product.

Table 2: IDNT: Primary Efficacy Outcome Within Subgroups

Baseline Factors	AVAPRO N=579 (%)	Comparison With Placebo		
		Placebo N=569 (%)	Hazard Ratio	95% CI
Gender				
Male	27.5	36.7	0.68	0.53-0.88
Female	42.3	44.6	0.98	0.72-1.34
Race				
White	29.5	37.3	0.75	0.60-0.95
Non-White	42.6	43.5	0.95	0.67-1.34
Age (years)				
<65	31.8	39.9	0.77	0.62-0.97
≥65	35.1	36.8	0.88	0.61-1.29

WARNINGS

Fetal/Neonatal Morbidity and Mortality

Drugs that act directly on the renin-angiotensin system can cause fetal and neonatal morbidity and death when administered to pregnant women. Several dozen cases have been reported in the world literature in patients who were taking angiotensin-converting-enzyme inhibitors. When pregnancy is detected, AVAPRO should be discontinued as soon as possible.

The use of drugs that act directly on the renin-angiotensin system during the second and third trimesters of pregnancy has been associated with fetal and neonatal injury, including hypotension, neonatal skull hypoplasia, anuria, reversible or irreversible renal failure, and death. Oligohydramnios has also been reported, presumably resulting from decreased fetal renal function; oligohydramnios in this setting has been associated with fetal limb contractures, craniofacial deformation, and hypoplastic lung development. Prematurity, intrauterine growth retardation, and patent ductus arteriosus have also been reported, although it is not clear whether these occurrences were due to exposure to the drug.

These adverse effects do not appear to have resulted from intrauterine drug exposure that has been limited to the first trimester.

Mothers whose embryos and fetuses are exposed to an angiotensin II receptor antagonist only during the first trimester should be so informed. Nonetheless, when patients become pregnant, physicians should have the patient discontinue the use of AVAPRO as soon as possible.

Rarely (probably less often than once in every thousand pregnancies), no alternative to a drug acting on the renin-angiotensin system will be found. In these rare cases, the mothers should be apprised of the potential hazards to their fetuses, and serial ultrasound examinations should be performed to assess the intraamniotic environment.

If oligohydramnios is observed, AVAPRO should be discontinued unless it is considered life-saving for the mother. Contraction stress testing (CST), a non-stress test (NST), or biophysical profiling (BPP) may be appropriate depending upon the week of pregnancy. Patients and physicians should be aware, however, that oligohydramnios may not appear until after the fetus has sustained irreversible injury.

Infants with histories of in utero exposure to an angiotensin II receptor antagonist should be closely observed for hypotension, oliguria, and hyperkalemia. If oliguria occurs, attention should be directed toward support of blood pressure and renal perfusion. Exchange transfusion or dialysis may be required as means of reversing hypotension and/or substituting for disordered renal function.

When pregnant rats were treated with irbesartan from day 0 to day 20 of gestation (oral doses of 50, 180, and 650 mg/kg/day), increased incidences of renal pelvic cavitation, hydroureter and/or absence of renal papilla were observed in fetuses at doses ≥50 mg/kg/day (approximately equivalent to the maximum recommended human dose [MRHD], 300 mg/day, on a body surface area basis). Subcutaneous edema was observed in fetuses at doses ≥180 mg/kg/day (about 4 times the MRHD on a body surface area basis). As these anomalies were not observed in rats in which irbesartan exposure (oral doses of 50, 150, and 450 mg/kg/day) was limited to gestation days 6-15, they appear to reflect late gestational effects of the drug. In pregnant rabbits, oral doses of 30 mg irbesartan/kg/day were associated with maternal mortality and abortion. Surviving females receiving this dose (about 1.5 times the MRHD on a body surface area basis) had a slight increase in early resorptions and a corresponding decrease in live fetuses. Irbesartan was found to cross the placental barrier in rats and rabbits. Radioactivity was present in the rat and rabbit fetus during late gestation and in rat milk following oral doses of radiolabeled irbesartan.

Hypotension in Volume- or Salt-depleted Patients

Excessive reduction of blood pressure was rarely seen (<0.1%) in patients with uncomplicated hypertension. Initiation of antihypertensive therapy may cause symptomatic hypotension in patients with intravascular volume- or sodium-depletion, e.g., in patients treated vigorously with diuretics or in patients on dialysis. Such volume depletion should be corrected prior to administration of AVAPRO, or a low starting dose should be used (see DOSAGE AND ADMINISTRATION).

If hypotension occurs, the patient should be placed in the supine position and, if necessary, given an intravenous infusion of normal saline. A transient hypotensive response is not a contraindication to further treatment, which usually can be continued without difficulty once the blood pressure has stabilized.

PRECAUTIONS

Impaired Renal Function

As a consequence of inhibiting the renin-angiotensin-aldosterone system, changes in renal function may be anticipated in susceptible individuals. In patients whose renal function may depend on the activity of the renin-angiotensin-aldosterone system (e.g., patients with severe congestive heart failure), treatment with angiotensin-converting-enzyme inhibitors has been associated with oliguria and/or progressive azotemia and (rarely) with acute renal failure and/or death. AVAPRO would be expected to behave similarly.

In studies of ACE inhibitors in patients with unilateral or bilateral renal artery stenosis, increases in serum creatinine or BUN have been reported. There has been no known use of AVAPRO in patients with unilateral or bilateral renal artery stenosis, but a similar effect should be anticipated.

Information for Patients

Pregnancy

Female patients of childbearing age should be told about the consequences of second- and third-trimester exposure to drugs that act on the renin-angiotensin system, and they should also be told that these consequences do not appear to have resulted from intrauterine drug exposure that has been limited to the first trimester. These patients should be asked to report pregnancies to their physicians as soon as possible.

Drug Interactions

No significant drug-drug pharmacokinetic (or pharmacodynamic) interactions have been found in interaction studies with hydrochlorothiazide, digoxin, warfarin, and nifedipine. In vitro studies show significant inhibition of the formation of oxidized irbesartan metabolites with the known cytochrome CYP 2C9 substrates/inhibitors sulphenazole, tolbutamide and nifedipine. However, in clinical studies the consequences of concomitant irbesartan on the pharmacodynamics of warfarin were negligible. Based on in vitro data, no interaction would be expected with drugs whose metabolism is dependent upon cytochrome P450 isoenzymes 1A1, 1A2, 2A6, 2B6, 2D6, 2E1, or 3A4.

In separate studies of patients receiving maintenance doses of warfarin, hydrochlorothiazide, or digoxin, irbesartan administration for 7 days had no effect on the pharmacodynamics of warfarin (prothrombin time) or pharmacokinetics of digoxin. The pharmacokinetics of irbesartan were not affected by coadministration of nifedipine or hydrochlorothiazide.

Carcinogenesis, Mutagenesis, Impairment of Fertility

No evidence of carcinogenicity was observed when irbesartan was administered at doses of up to 500/1000 mg/kg/day (males/females, respectively) in rats and 1000 mg/kg/day in mice for up to two years. For male and female rats, 500 mg/kg/day provided an average systemic exposure to irbesartan (AUC_{0-24h}, bound plus unbound) about 3 and 11 times, respectively, the average systemic exposure in humans receiving the maximum recommended dose (MRD) of 300 mg irbesartan/day, whereas 1000 mg/kg/day (administered to females only) provided an average systemic exposure about 21 times that reported for humans at the MRD. For male and female mice, 1000 mg/kg/day provided an exposure to irbesartan about 3 and 5 times, respectively, the human exposure at 300 mg/day.

Irbesartan was not mutagenic in a battery of in vitro tests (Ames microbial test, rat hepatocyte DNA repair test, V79 mammalian-cell forward gene-mutation assay). Irbesartan was negative in several tests for induction of chromosomal aberrations (in vitro-human lymphocyte assay; in vivo-mouse micronucleus study).

Irbesartan had no adverse effects on fertility or mating of male or female rats at oral doses ≤650 mg/kg/day, the highest dose providing a systemic exposure to irbesartan (AUC_{0-24h}, bound plus unbound) about 5 times that found in humans receiving the maximum recommended dose of 300 mg/day.

Pregnancy

Pregnancy Categories C (first trimester) and D (second and third trimester)

See WARNINGS: Fetal/Neonatal Morbidity and Mortality.

Nursing Mothers

It is not known whether irbesartan is excreted in human milk, but irbesartan or some metabolite of irbesartan is secreted at low concentration in the milk of lactating rats. Because of the potential for adverse effects on the nursing infant, a decision should be made whether to discontinue nursing or discontinue the drug, taking into account the importance of the drug to the mother.

Pediatric Use

Irbesartan, in a study at a dose of up to 4.5 mg/kg/day, once daily, did not appear to lower blood pressure effectively in pediatric patients ages 6 to 16 years.

AVAPRO has not been studied in pediatric patients less than 6 years old.

Geriatric Use

Of 4925 subjects receiving AVAPRO (irbesartan) in controlled clinical studies of hypertension, 911 (18.5%) were 65 years and over, while 150 (3.0%) were 75 years and over. No overall differences in effectiveness or safety were observed between these subjects and younger subjects, but greater sensitivity of some older individuals cannot be ruled out. (See CLINICAL PHARMACOLOGY: Pharmacokinetics, Special Populations, and Clinical Studies.)

ADVERSE REACTIONS

Hypertension

AVAPRO has been evaluated for safety in more than 4300 patients with hypertension and about 5000 subjects overall. This experience includes 1303 patients treated for over 6 months and 407 patients for 1 year or more. Treatment with AVAPRO was well-tolerated, with an incidence of adverse events similar to placebo. These events generally were mild and transient with no relationship to the dose of AVAPRO. In placebo-controlled clinical trials, discontinuation of therapy due to a clinical adverse event was required in 3.3% of patients treated with AVAPRO, versus 4.5% of patients given placebo.

In placebo-controlled clinical trials, the following adverse event experiences reported in at least 1% of patients treated with AVAPRO (n=1965) and at a higher incidence versus placebo (n=641), excluding those too general to be informative and those not reasonably associated with the use of drug because they were associated with the condition being treated or are very common in the treated population, include: diarrhea (3% vs. 2%), dyspepsia/heartburn (2% vs. 1%), and fatigue (4% vs. 3%).

The following adverse events occurred at an incidence of 1% or greater in patients treated with irbesartan, but were at least as frequent or more frequent in patients receiving placebo: abdominal pain, anxiety/nervousness, chest pain, dizziness, edema, headache, influenza, musculoskeletal pain, pharyngitis, nausea/vomiting, rash, rhinitis, sinus abnormality, tachycardia and urinary tract infection.

Irbesartan use was not associated with an increased incidence of dry cough, as is typically associated with ACE inhibitor use. In placebo-controlled studies, the incidence of cough in irbesartan-treated patients was 2.8% versus 2.7% in patients receiving placebo.

The incidence of hypotension or orthostatic hypotension was low in irbesartan-treated patients (0.4%), unrelated to dosage, and similar to the incidence among placebo-treated patients (0.2%). Dizziness, syncope, and vertigo were reported with equal or less frequency in patients receiving irbesartan compared with placebo.

	75 mg	150 mg	300 mg
Debossing	2771	2772	2773
Bottle of 30	0087-2771-31	0087-2772-31	0087-2773-31
Bottle of 90	0087-2771-32	0087-2772-32	0087-2773-32
Bottle of 500		0087-2772-15	0087-2773-15
Blister of 100		0087-2772-35	

In addition, the following potentially important events occurred in less than 1% of the 1965 patients and at least 5 patients (0.3%) receiving irbesartan in clinical studies, and those less frequent, clinically significant events (listed by body system). It cannot be determined whether these events were causally related to irbesartan:

Body as a Whole: fever, chills, facial edema, upper extremity edema

Cardiovascular: flushing, hypertension, cardiac murmur, myocardial infarction, angina pectoris, arrhythmic/conduction disorder, cardio-respiratory arrest, heart failure, hypertensive crisis

Dermatologic: pruritus, dermatitis, ecchymosis, erythema face, urticaria

Endocrine/Metabolic/Electrolyte Imbalances: sexual dysfunction, libido change, gout

Gastrointestinal: constipation, oral lesion, gastroenteritis, flatulence, abdominal distention

Musculoskeletal/Connective Tissue: extremity swelling, muscle cramp, arthritis, muscle ache, musculoskeletal chest pain, joint stiffness, bursitis, muscle weakness

Nervous System: sleep disturbance, numbness, somnolence, emotional disturbance, depression, paresthesia, tremor, transient ischemic attack, cerebrovascular accident

Renal/Genitourinary: abnormal urination, prostate disorder

Respiratory: epistaxis, tracheobronchitis, congestion, pulmonary congestion, dyspnea, wheezing

Special Senses: vision disturbance, hearing abnormality, ear infection, ear pain, conjunctivitis, other eye disturbance, eyelid abnormality, ear abnormality

Nephropathy in Type 2 Diabetic Patients

In clinical studies in patients with hypertension and type 2 diabetic renal disease, the adverse drug experiences were similar to those seen in patients with hypertension with the exception of an increased incidence of orthostatic symptoms (dizziness, orthostatic dizziness, and orthostatic hypotension) observed in IDNT (proteinuria ≥900 mg/day, and serum creatinine ranging from 1.0-3.0 mg/dL). In this trial, orthostatic symptoms occurred more frequently in the AVAPRO group (dizziness 10.2%, orthostatic dizziness 5.4%, orthostatic hypotension 5.4%) than in the placebo group (dizziness 6.0%, orthostatic dizziness 2.7%, orthostatic hypotension 3.2%).

Post-Marketing Experience

The following have been very rarely reported in post-marketing experience: urticaria; angioedema (involving swelling of the face, lips, pharynx, and/or tongue); increased liver function tests; jaundice; and hepatitis. Hyperkalemia has been rarely reported.

Rare cases of rhabdomyolysis have been reported in patients receiving angiotensin II receptor blockers.

Laboratory Test Findings

Hypertension

In controlled clinical trials, clinically important differences in laboratory tests were rarely associated with administration of AVAPRO.

Creatinine, Blood Urea Nitrogen: Minor increases in blood urea nitrogen (BUN) or serum creatinine were observed in less than 0.7% of patients with essential hypertension treated with AVAPRO alone versus 0.9% on placebo. (See **PRECAUTIONS: Impaired Renal Function.**)

Hematologic: Mean decreases in hemoglobin of 0.2 g/dL were observed in 0.2% of patients receiving AVAPRO compared to 0.3% of placebo-treated patients. Neutropenia (<1000 cells/mm³) occurred at similar frequencies among patients receiving AVAPRO (0.3%) and placebo-treated patients (0.5%).

Nephropathy in Type 2 Diabetic Patients

Hyperkalemia: In IDNT (proteinuria ≥900 mg/day, and serum creatinine ranging from 1.0-3.0 mg/dL), the percent of patients with hyperkalemia (>6 mEq/L) was 18.6% in the AVAPRO group vs. 6.0% in the placebo group. Discontinuations due to hyperkalemia in the AVAPRO group were 2.1% vs. 0.4% in the placebo group.

OVERDOSAGE

No data are available in regard to overdosage in humans. However, daily doses of 900 mg for 8 weeks were well-tolerated. The most likely manifestations of overdosage are expected to be hypotension and tachycardia; bradycardia might also occur from overdose. Irbesartan is not removed by hemodialysis.

To obtain up-to-date information about the treatment of overdosage, a good resource is a certified regional Poison Control Center. Telephone numbers of certified Poison Control Centers are listed in the *Physicians' Desk Reference* (PDR). In managing overdose, consider the possibilities of multiple-drug interactions, drug-drug interactions, and unusual drug kinetics in the patient.

Laboratory determinations of serum levels of irbesartan are not widely available, and such determinations have, in any event, no known established role in the management of irbesartan overdose.

Acute oral toxicity studies with irbesartan in mice and rats indicated acute lethal doses were in excess of 2000 mg/kg, about 25- and 50-fold the maximum recommended human dose (300 mg) on a mg/m² basis, respectively.

DOSAGE AND ADMINISTRATION

AVAPRO may be administered with other antihypertensive agents and with or without food.

Hypertension

The recommended initial dose of AVAPRO (irbesartan) is 150 mg once daily. Patients requiring further reduction in blood pressure should be titrated to 300 mg once daily.

A low dose of a diuretic may be added, if blood pressure is not controlled by AVAPRO alone. Hydrochlorothiazide has been shown to have an additive effect (see **CLINICAL PHARMACOLOGY: Clinical Studies**). Patients not adequately treated by the maximum dose of 300 mg once daily are unlikely to derive additional benefit from a higher dose or twice-daily dosing.

No dosage adjustment is necessary in elderly patients, or in patients with hepatic impairment or mild to severe renal impairment.

Nephropathy in Type 2 Diabetic Patients

The recommended target maintenance dose is 300 mg once daily. There are no data on the clinical effects of lower doses of AVAPRO on diabetic nephropathy (see **CLINICAL PHARMACOLOGY: Clinical Studies**).

Volume- and Salt-depleted Patients

A lower initial dose of AVAPRO (75 mg) is recommended in patients with depletion of intravascular volume or salt (e.g., patients treated vigorously with diuretics or on hemodialysis) (see **WARNINGS: Hypotension in Volume- or Salt-depleted Patients**).

HOW SUPPLIED

AVAPRO® (irbesartan) is available as white to off-white biconvex oval tablets, debossed with a heart shape on one side and a portion of the NDC code on the other. Unit-of-use bottles contain 30, 90, or 500 tablets and blister packs contain 100 tablets, as follows:

[See table above]

Storage

Store at 25° C (77° F); excursions permitted to 15° C-30° C (59° F-86° F) [see USP Controlled Room Temperature].

Distributed by:

Bristol-Myers Squibb Sanofi-Synthelabo Partnership
New York, NY 10016

Bristol-Myers Squibb Company   sanofi aventis
1192328A2   Revised April 2007
1192327A2

Shown in Product Identification Guide, page 318

BENZACLIN® TOPICAL GEL   ℞

[ben-zA-clin]

(clindamycin - benzoyl peroxide gel)
Topical Gel: Clindamycin (1%) As Clindamycin Phosphate, Benzoyl Peroxide (5%)
For Dermatological Use Only - Not for Ophthalmic Use
Reconstitute Before Dispensing

DESCRIPTION

BenzaClin® Topical Gel contains clindamycin phosphate, (7(S)-chloro-7-deoxylincomycin-2-phosphate). Clindamycin phosphate is a water soluble ester of the semi-synthetic antibiotic produced by a 7(S)-chloro-substitution of the 7(R)-hydroxyl group of the parent antibiotic lincomycin.

Chemically, clindamycin phosphate is ($C_{18}H_{34}ClN_2O_8PS$). The structural formula for clindamycin is represented below:

Clindamycin phosphate has molecular weight of 504.97 and its chemical name is Methyl 7-chloro-6,7,8-trideoxy-6-(1-methyl-trans-4-propyl-L-2-pyrrolidinecarboxamido)-1-thio-L-threo-alpha-D-galacto-octopyranoside 2-(dihydrogen phosphate).

BenzaClin Topical Gel also contains benzoyl peroxide, for topical use.

Chemically, benzoyl peroxide is ($C_{14}H_{10}O_4$). It has the following structural formula:

Benzoyl peroxide has a molecular weight of 242.23.

Each gram of BenzaClin Topical Gel contains, as dispensed, 10 mg (1%) clindamycin as phosphate and 50 mg (5%) benzoyl peroxide in a base of carbomer, sodium hydroxide, dioctyl sodium sulfosuccinate, and purified water.

CLINICAL PHARMACOLOGY

An *in vitro* percutaneous penetration study comparing BenzaClin Topical Gel and topical 1% clindamycin gel alone, demonstrated there was no statistical difference in penetration between the two drugs. Mean systemic bioavailability of topical clindamycin in BenzaClin Topical Gel is suggested to be less than 1%.

Benzoyl peroxide has been shown to be absorbed by the skin where it is converted to benzoic acid. Less than 2% of the dose enters systemic circulation as benzoic acid. It is suggested that the lipophilic nature of benzoyl peroxide acts to concentrate the compound into the lipid-rich sebaceous follicle.

Pharmacokinetics

The pharmacokinetics (plasma and urine) of clindamycin from BenzaClin Topical Gel was studied in male and female patients (n=13) with acne vulgaris. BenzaClin Topical Gel (~2g) was applied topically to the face and back twice daily for four and a half (4.5) days. Quantifiable (>LOQ=1ng/mL) clindamycin plasma concentrations were obtained in six of thirteen subjects (46.2%) on Day 1 and twelve of thirteen subjects (92.3%) on Day 5. Peak plasma concentrations (C_{max}) of clindamycin ranged from 1.47 ng/mL to 2.77 ng/mL on Day 1 and 1.43 ng/mL to 7.18 ng/mL on Day 5. The AUC (0-12h) ranged from 2.74 ng.h/mL to 12.86 ng.h/mL on Day 1 and 11.4 ng.h/mL to 69.7 ng.h/mL on Day 5.

The amount of clindamycin excreted in the urine during the 12 hour dosing interval increased from a mean (SD) of 5745 (3130) ng on Day 1 to 12069 (7660) ng on Day 5. The mean % (SD) of the administered dose that was excreted in the urine ranged from 0.03% (0.02) to 0.08% (0.04).

A comparison of the single (Day 1) and multiple (Day 5) dose plasma and urinary concentrations of clindamycin indicates that there is accumulation of clindamycin following multiple dosing of BenzaClin Topical Gel. The degree of accumulation calculated from the plasma and urinary excretion data was ~2-fold.

Microbiology

The clindamycin and benzoyl peroxide components individually have been shown to have *in vitro* activity against *Propionibacterium acnes* an organism which has been associated with acne vulgaris; however, the clinical significance of this activity against *P. acnes* was not examined in clinical trials with this product.

CLINICAL STUDIES

In two adequate and well controlled clinical studies of 758 patients, 214 used BenzaClin, 210 used benzoyl peroxide, 168 used clindamycin, and 166 used vehicle. BenzaClin applied twice daily for 10 weeks was significantly more effective than vehicle in the treatment of moderate to moderately severe facial acne vulgaris. Patients were evaluated and acne lesions counted at each clinical visit; weeks 2, 4, 6, 8 and 10. The primary efficacy measures were the lesion counts and the investigator's global assessment evaluated at week 10. Patients were instructed to wash the face with a mild soap, using only the hands. Fifteen minutes after the face was thoroughly dry, application was made to the entire face. Non-medicated make-up could be applied one hour after the BenzaClin application. If a moisturizer was required, the patients were provided a moisturizer to be used as needed. Patients were instructed to avoid sun exposure. Percent reductions in lesion counts after treatment for 10 weeks in these two studies are shown below:

Study 1

BenzaClin n=120	Benzoyl peroxide n=120	Clindamycin n=120	Vehicle N=120
Mean percent reduction in inflammatory lesion counts			
46%	32%	16%	+ 3%
Mean percent reduction in non-inflammatory lesion counts			
22%	22%	9%	+1%
Mean percent reduction in total lesion counts			
36%	28%	15%	0.2%

Study 2

BenzaClin n=95	Benzoyl peroxide n=95	Clindamycin n=49	Vehicle N=48
Mean percent reduction in inflammatory lesion counts			
63%	53%	45%	42%
Mean percent reduction in non-inflammatory lesion counts			
54%	50%	39%	36%
Mean percent reduction in total lesion counts			
58%	52%	42%	39%

The BenzaClin group showed greater overall improvement than the benzoyl peroxide, clindamycin and vehicle groups as rated by the investigator.

INDICATIONS AND USAGE

BenzaClin Topical Gel is indicated for the topical treatment of acne vulgaris.

CONTRAINDICATIONS

BenzaClin Topical Gel is contraindicated in those individuals who have shown hypersensitivity to any of its components or to lincomycin. It is also contraindicated in those having a history of regional enteritis, ulcerative colitis, or antibiotic-associated colitis.

WARNINGS

ORALLY AND PARENTERALLY ADMINISTERED CLINDAMYCIN HAS BEEN ASSOCIATED WITH SEVERE COLITIS WHICH MAY RESULT IN PATIENT DEATH. USE OF THE TOPICAL FORMULATION OF CLINDAMYCIN RESULTS IN ABSORPTION OF THE ANTIBIOTIC FROM THE SKIN SURFACE. DIARRHEA, BLOODY DIARRHEA, AND COLITIS (INCLUDING PSEUDOMEMBRANOUS COLITIS) HAVE BEEN REPORTED WITH THE USE OF TOPICAL AND SYSTEMIC CLINDAMYCIN. STUDIES INDICATE A TOXIN(S) PRODUCED BY CLOSTRIDIA IS ONE PRIMARY CAUSE OF ANTIBIOTIC-ASSOCIATED COLITIS. THE COLITIS IS USUALLY CHARACTERIZED BY SEVERE PERSISTENT DIARRHEA AND SEVERE ABDOMINAL CRAMPS AND MAY BE ASSOCIATED WITH THE PASSAGE OF BLOOD AND MUCUS. ENDOSCOPIC EXAMINATION MAY REVEAL PSEUDOMEMBRANOUS COLITIS. STOOL CULTURE FOR *Clostridium Difficile* AND STOOL ASSAY FOR *C. difficile* TOXIN MAY BE HELPFUL DIAGNOSTICALLY. WHEN SIGNIFICANT DIARRHEA OCCURS, THE DRUG SHOULD BE DISCONTINUED. LARGE BOWEL ENDOSCOPY SHOULD BE CONSIDERED TO ESTABLISH A DEFINITIVE DIAGNOSIS IN CASES OF SEVERE DIARRHEA. ANTIPERISTALTIC AGENTS SUCH AS OPIATES AND DIPHENOXYLATE WITH ATROPINE MAY PROLONG AND/OR WORSEN THE CONDITION. DIARRHEA, COLITIS, AND PSEUDOMEMBRANOUS COLITIS HAVE BEEN OBSERVED TO BEGIN UP TO SEVERAL WEEKS FOLLOWING CESSATION OF ORAL AND PARENTERAL THERAPY WITH CLINDAMYCIN.

Mild cases of pseudomembranous colitis usually respond to drug discontinuation alone. In moderate to severe cases, consideration should be given to management with fluids and electrolytes, protein supplementation and treatment with an antibacterial drug clinically effective against *C. difficile* colitis.

PRECAUTIONS

General

For dermatological use only; not for ophthalmic use. Concomitant topical acne therapy should be used with caution

Size (Net Weight)	NDC 0066-	Benzoyl Peroxide Gel	Active Clindamycin Powder (In plastic vial)	Purified Water To Be Added to each vial
25 grams	0494-25	19.7g	0.3g	5 mL
35 grams (pump)	0494-35	27.6g	0.4g	7 mL
50 grams	0494-50	39.4g	0.6g	10 mL
50 grams (pump)	0494-55	39.4g	0.6g	10 mL
BenzaClin Care Kit: 50 grams BenzaClin (pump) with 20 ampoules Viscontour Serum	0495-55	39.4g	0.6g	10 mL

because a possible cumulative irritancy effect may occur, especially with the use of peeling, desquamating, or abrasive agents.

The use of antibiotic agents may be associated with the overgrowth of nonsusceptible organisms including fungi. If this occurs, discontinue use of this medication and take appropriate measures.

Avoid contact with eyes and mucous membranes.

Clindamycin and erythromycin containing products should not be used in combination. *In vitro* studies have shown antagonism between these two antimicrobials. The clinical significance of this *in vitro* antagonism is not known.

Information for Patients

Patients using BenzaClin Topical Gel should receive the following information and instructions:

1. BenzaClin Topical Gel is to be used as directed by the physician. It is for external use only. Avoid contact with eyes, and inside the nose, mouth, and all mucous membranes, as this product may be irritating.
2. This medication should not be used for any disorder other than that for which it was prescribed.
3. Patients should not use any other topical acne preparation unless otherwise directed by physician.
4. Patients should minimize or avoid exposure to natural or artificial sunlight (tanning beds or UVA/B treatment) while using BenzaClin Topical Gel. To minimize exposure to sunlight, a wide-brimmed hat or other protective clothing should be worn, and a sunscreen with SPF 15 rating or higher should be used.
5. Patients who develop allergic symptoms such as severe swelling or shortness of breath should discontinue BenzaClin Topical Gel and contact their physician immediately.
6. BenzaClin Topical Gel may bleach hair or colored fabric.
7. BenzaClin Topical Gel can be stored at room temperature up to 25°C (77°F) for 3 months. Do not freeze. Discard any unused product after 3 months.
8. Before applying BenzaClin Topical Gel to affected areas wash the skin gently, then rinse with warm water and pat dry.

Carcinogenesis, Mutagenesis, Impairment of Fertility

Benzoyl peroxide has been shown to be a tumor promoter and progression agent in a number of animal studies. The clinical significance of this is unknown.

Benzoyl peroxide in acetone at doses of 5 and 10 mg administered twice per week induced skin tumors in transgenic Tg.AC mice in a study using 20 weeks of topical treatment. In a 52 week dermal photocarcinogenicity study in hairless mice, the median time to onset of skin tumor formation was decreased and the number of tumors per mouse increased following chronic concurrent topical administration of BenzaClin Topical Gel with exposure to ultraviolet radiation (40 weeks of treatment followed by 12 weeks of observation).

In a 2-year dermal carcinogenicity study in rats, treatment with BenzaClin Topical Gel at doses of 100, 500 and 2000 mg/kg/day caused a dose-dependent increase in the incidence of keratoacanthoma at the treated skin site of male rats. The incidence of keratoacanthoma at the treated site of males treated with 2000 mg/kg/day (8 times the highest recommended adult human dose of 2.5 g BenzaClin Topical Gel, based on mg/m^2) was statistically significantly higher than that in the sham- and vehicle-controls.

Genotoxicity studies were not conducted with BenzaClin Topical Gel. Clindamycin phosphate was not genotoxic in *Salmonella typhimurium* or in a rat micronucleus test. Clindamycin phosphate sulfoxide, an oxidative degradation product of clindamycin phosphate and benzoyl peroxide, was not clastogenic in a mouse micronucleus test. Benzoyl peroxide has been found to cause DNA strand breaks in a variety of mammalian cell types, to be mutagenic in *S. typhimurium* tests by some but not all investigators, and to cause sister chromatid exchanges in Chinese hamster ovary cells. Studies have not been performed with BenzaClin

Topical Gel or benzoyl peroxide to evaluate the effect on fertility. Fertility studies in rats treated orally with up to 300 mg/kg/day of clindamycin (approximately 120 times the amount of clindamycin in the highest recommended adult human dose of 2.5 g BenzaClin Topical Gel, based on mg/m^2) revealed no effects on fertility or mating ability.

Pregnancy
Teratogenic Effects
Pregnancy Category C

Animal reproductive/developmental toxicity studies have not been conducted with BenzaClin Topical Gel or benzoyl peroxide. Developmental toxicity studies performed in rats and mice using oral doses of clindamycin up to 600 mg/kg/day (240 and 120 times amount of clindamycin in the highest recommended adult human dose based on mg/m^2, respectively) or subcutaneous doses of clindamycin up to 250 mg/kg/day (100 and 50 times the amount of clindamycin in the highest recommended adult human dose based on mg/m^2, respectively) revealed no evidence of teratogenicity.

There are no well-controlled trials in pregnant women treated with BenzaClin Topical Gel. It also is not known whether BenzaClin Topical Gel can cause fetal harm when administered to a pregnant woman.

Nursing Women

It is not known whether BenzaClin Topical Gel is excreted in human milk after topical application. However, orally and parenterally administered clindamycin has been reported to appear in breast milk. Because of the potential for serious adverse reactions in nursing infants, a decision should be made whether to discontinue nursing or to discontinue the drug, taking into account the importance of the drug to the mother.

Pediatric Use

Safety and effectiveness of this product in pediatric patients below the age of 12 have not been established.

ADVERSE REACTIONS

During clinical trials, the most frequently reported adverse event in the BenzaClin treatment group was dry skin (12%). The Table below lists local adverse events reported by at least 1% of patients in the BenzaClin and vehicle groups.

Local Adverse Events - all causalities in >/= 1% of patients		
	BenzaClin n = 420	Vehicle n = 168
Application site reaction	13 (3%)	1 (<1%)
Dry skin	50 (12%)	10 (6%)
Pruritus	8 (2%)	1 (<1%)
Peeling	9 (2%)	-
Erythema	6 (1%)	1 (<1%)
Sunburn	5 (1%)	

The actual incidence of dry skin might have been greater were it not for the use of a moisturizer in these studies. Anaphylaxis, as well as allergic reactions leading to hospitalization, have been reported during post-marketing use of clindamycin/benzoyl peroxide products. Because these reactions are reported voluntarily from a population of uncertain size, it is not always possible to reliably estimate their frequency or establish a causal relationship to drug exposure.

DOSAGE AND ADMINISTRATION

BenzaClin Topical Gel should be applied twice daily, morning and evening, or as directed by a physician, to affected areas after the skin is gently washed, rinsed with warm water and patted dry.

HOW SUPPLIED AND COMPOUNDING INSTRUCTIONS

[See table at top of previous page]

Prior to dispensing, tap the vial until powder flows freely. Add indicated amount of purified water to the vial (to the mark) and immediately shake to completely dissolve clindamycin. If needed, add additional purified water to bring level up to the mark. Add the solution in the vial to the gel and stir until homogenous in appearance (1 to 1½ minutes). For the 35 and 50 gram pumps only, reassemble jar with pump dispenser. **BenzaClin Topical Gel** (as reconstituted) can be stored at room temperature up to 25°C (77°F) for 3 months. Place a 3 month expiration date on the label immediately following mixing.

Store at room temperature up to 25°C (77°F) (See USP).

Do not freeze. Keep tightly closed. Keep out of the reach of children.

Prescribing Information as of June 2010.

Dermik Laboratories
a business of sanofi-aventis U.S. LLC
Bridgewater, NJ 08807
©2010 sanofi-aventis U.S. LLC

CARAC® CREAM, 0.5%

[ca-rack]

(fluorouracil cream)

FOR TOPICAL DERMATOLOGICAL USE ONLY (NOT FOR OPHTHALMIC, ORAL, OR INTRAVAGINAL USE)

Rx

DESCRIPTION

Carac® (fluorouracil cream) Cream, 0.5%, contains fluorouracil for topical dermatologic use. Chemically, fluorouracil is 5-fluoro-2,4(1H, 3H)-pyrimidinedione. The molecular formula is $C_4H_3FN_2O_2$. Fluorouracil has a molecular weight of 130.08.

Carac Cream contains 0.5% fluorouracil, with 0.35% being incorporated into a patented porous microsphere (Microsponge®)[1] composed of methyl methacrylate/glycol dimethacrylate crosspolymer and dimethicone. The cream formulation contains the following other inactive ingredients: Carbomer Homopolymer Type C, dimethicone, glycerin, methyl gluceth-20, methyl methacrylate/glycol dimethacrylate crosspolymer, methylparaben, octyl hydroxy stearate, polyethylene glycol 400, polysorbate 80, propylene glycol, propylparaben, purified water, sorbitan monooleate, stearic acid, and trolamine.

1Microsponge is a registered trademark of Cardinal Health, Inc. or one of its subsidiaries.

CLINICAL PHARMACOLOGY

There is evidence that the metabolism of fluorouracil in the anabolic pathway blocks the methylation reaction of deoxyuridylic acid to thymidylic acid. In this manner, fluorouracil interferes with the synthesis of deoxyribonucleic acid (DNA) and to a lesser extent inhibits the formation of ribonucleic acid (RNA). Since DNA and RNA are essential for cell division and growth, the effect of fluorouracil may be to create a thymine deficiency that provokes unbalanced growth and death of the cell. The effects of DNA and RNA deprivation are most marked on those cells that grow more rapidly and take up fluorouracil at a more rapid rate. The contribution to efficacy or safety of individual components of the vehicle has not been established.

Pharmacokinetics

A multiple-dose, randomized, open-label, parallel study was performed in 21 patients with actinic keratoses. Twenty patients had pharmacokinetic samples collected: 10 patients treated with Carac and 10 treated with Efudex®[2] 5% Cream. Patients were treated for a maximum of 28 days with *Carac*, 1 g once daily in the morning; or Efudex® 5% Cream, 1 g twice daily, in the morning and evening. Steady-state plasma concentrations and the amounts of fluorouracil in urine resulting from the topical application of either product were measured.

Three patients who received Carac and nine patients who received Efudex® 5% Cream had measurable plasma fluorouracil levels; however, only one patient receiving Carac and six patients receiving Efudex® 5% Cream had a

---

sufficient number of data points to calculate mean pharmacokinetic parameters.

Plasma Pharmacokinetic Summary

PK Parameter	Carac n=1	Efudex (Mean ± SD) n=6
C_{max}	0.77 ng/mL	11.49 ± 8.24 ng/mL
T_{max}	1.00 hr	1.03 ± 0.028 hr
AUC (0–24)	2.80 ng•hr/mL	22.39 ± 7.89 ng•hr/mL

Five of 10 patients receiving Carac and nine of 10 patients receiving Efudex® 5% Cream had measurable urine fluorouracil levels.

Urine Pharmacokinetic Summary

PK Parameter	Carac (Mean ± SD) (Range) n=10	Efudex (Mean ± SD) (Range) n=10
Cum Ae* (min-max)	2.74± 5.22 mcg (0–15.02)	119.8± 94.80 mcg (0–329.87)
Max excretion rate (min-max)	0.19 ± 0.52 mcg/hr (0–1.67)	40.27 ±47.14 mcg/hr (0–164.5)

* Cumulative urinary excretion

Both Carac and Efudex® 5% Cream demonstrated low measurable plasma concentrations for fluorouracil when administered under steady-state conditions. Cumulative urinary excretion of fluorouracil was low for Carac and for Efudex®, corresponding to 0.055% and 0.24% of the applied doses, respectively.

2Efudex is a registered trademark of ICN Pharmaceuticals, Inc.

Clinical Trials

Under the experimental conditions of the topical safety studies, Carac was not observed to cause contact sensitization. However, approximately 95% of subjects in the active arms of the Phase 3 clinical studies experienced facial irritation. Irritation is likely and sensitization is unlikely based on the results of the topical safety and Phase 3 studies.

Two Phase 3 identically designed, multi-center, vehicle-controlled, double-blind studies were conducted to evaluate the clinical safety and efficacy of Carac. Patients with 5 or more actinic keratoses (AKs) on the face or anterior bald scalp were randomly allocated to active or vehicle treatment in a 2:1 ratio. Patients were randomly allocated to treatment durations of 1, 2, or 4 weeks in a 1:1:1 ratio. They applied the study cream once daily to the entire face/anterior bald scalp. Each patient's clinical response was evaluated 4 weeks after the patient's last scheduled application of study cream. No additional post-treatment follow-up efficacy or safety assessments were performed beyond 4 weeks after the last scheduled application. The following graphs show the percentage of patients in whom 100% of treated lesions cleared, and the percentage of patients in whom 75% or more of treated lesions cleared. Treatment with Carac cream for 1, 2, or 4 weeks is compared to treatment with vehicle cream. Outcomes from 1, 2, and 4 weeks of treatment with vehicle cream are pooled because duration of treatment with vehicle had no substantive effect on clearance. Results from the two Phase 3 studies are shown separately. Although all treatment regimens of Carac studied demonstrated efficacy over vehicle for the treatment of actinic keratosis, continuing treatment up to 4 weeks as tolerated results in further lesion reduction and clearing.

Percentage of Subjects with 100% Clearance

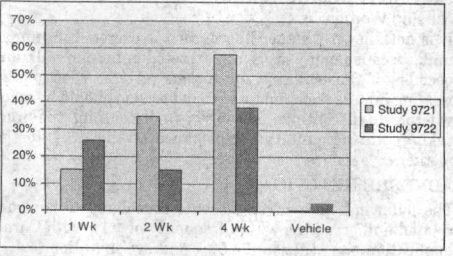

[See figure at top of next column]
Clinical efficacy and safety in the treatment of AKs on the ears and other sun-exposed areas were not evaluated in the studies.

Percentage of Subjects with at Least 75% Clearance

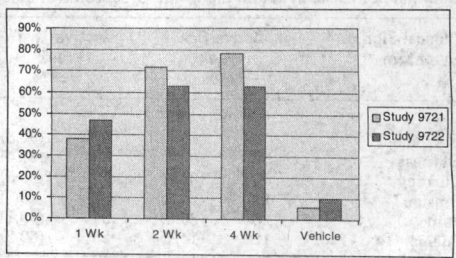

INDICATIONS AND USAGE

Carac is indicated for the topical treatment of multiple actinic or solar keratoses of the face and anterior scalp.

CONTRAINDICATIONS

Fluorouracil may cause fetal harm when administered to a pregnant woman. Fluorouracil is contraindicated in women who are or may become pregnant. If this drug is used during pregnancy, or if the patient becomes pregnant while taking this drug, the patient should be apprised of the potential hazard to the fetus.

No adequate and well-controlled studies have been conducted in pregnant women with either topical or parenteral forms of fluorouracil. One birth defect (ventricular septal defect) and cases of miscarriage have been reported when fluorouracil was applied to mucous membrane areas. Multiple birth defects have been reported in the fetus of a patient treated with intravenous fluorouracil.

Animal reproduction studies have not been conducted with Carac. Fluorouracil, the active ingredient, has been shown to be teratogenic in mice, rats, and hamsters when administered parenterally at doses greater than or equal to 10, 15 and 33 mg/kg/day, respectively, [4X, 11X and 20X, respectively, the Maximum Recommended Human Dose (MRHD) based on body surface area (BSA)]. Fluorouracil was administered during the period of organogenesis for each species. Embryolethal effects occurred in monkeys at parenteral doses greater than 40 mg/kg/day (65X the MRHD based on BSA) administered during the period of organogenesis.

Carac should not be used in patients with dihydropyrimidine dehydrogenase (DPD) enzyme deficiency. A large percentage of fluorouracil is catabolized by the enzyme dihydropyrimidine dehydrogenase (DPD). DPD enzyme deficiency can result in shunting of fluorouracil to the anabolic pathway, leading to cytotoxic activity and potential toxicities.

Carac is contraindicated in patients with known hypersensitivity to any of its components.

WARNINGS

The potential for a delayed hypersensitivity reaction to fluorouracil exists. Patch testing to prove hypersensitivity may be inconclusive.

Patients should discontinue therapy with Carac if symptoms of DPD enzyme deficiency develop.

Rarely, unexpected, systemic toxicity (e.g. stomatitis, diarrhea, neutropenia, and neurotoxicity) associated with parenteral administration of fluorouracil has been attributed to deficiency of dihydropyrimidine dehydrogenase "DPD" activity. One case of life threatening systemic toxicity has been reported with the topical use of 5% fluorouracil in a patient with a complete absence of DPD enzyme activity. Symptoms included severe abdominal pain, bloody diarrhea, vomiting, fever, and chills. Physical examination revealed stomatitis, erythematous skin rash, neutropenia, thrombocytopenia, inflammation of the esophagus, stomach, and small bowel. Although this case was observed with 5% fluorouracil cream, it is unknown whether patients with profound DPD enzyme deficiency would develop systemic toxicity with lower concentrations of topically applied fluorouracil.

Applications to mucous membranes should be avoided due to the possibility of local inflammation and ulceration.

PRECAUTIONS

General

There is a possibility of increased absorption through ulcerated or inflamed skin.

Information for the Patient

Patients using Carac should receive the following information and instructions:

1. This medication is to be used as directed.
2. This medication should not be used for any disorder other than that for which it was prescribed.
3. It is for external use only.
4. Avoid contact with the eyes, eyelids, nostrils, and mouth.

Summary of Facial Irritation Signs and Symptoms - Pooled Phase 3 Studies

Clinical Sign or Symptom	Active One Week N=85		Active Two Week N=87		Active Four Week N=85		ALL Active Treatments N=257		Vehicle Treatments N=127	
	n	%	n	%	n	%	n	%	n	%
Erythema	76	(89.4)	82	(94.3)	82	(96.5)	240	(93.4)	76	(59.8)
Dryness	59	(69.4)	76	(87.4)	79	(92.9)	214	(83.3)	60	(47.2)
Burning	51	(60.0)	70	(80.5)	71	(83.5)	192	(74.7)	28	(22.0)
Erosion	21	(24.7)	38	(43.7)	54	(63.5)	113	(44.0)	17	(13.4)
Pain	26	(30.6)	34	(39.1)	52	(61.2)	112	(43.6)	7	(5.5)
Edema	12	(14.1)	28	(32.2)	51	(60.0)	91	(35.4)	6	(4.7)

Summary of All Adverse Events Reported in ≥ 1% of Patients in the Combined Active Treatment and Vehicle Groups — Pooled Phase 3 Studies

Adverse Event	9721 and 9722 Combined				
	Active One Week N= 85	Active Two Week N= 87	Active Four Week N= 85	ALL Active Treatments N=257	Vehicle Treatments N=127
	n (%)	n (%)	n (%)	n (%)	n (%)
BODY AS A WHOLE	7 (8.2)	6 (6.9)	12 (14.1)	25 (9.7)	15 (11.8)
Headache	3 (3.5)	2 (2.3)	3 (3.5)	8 (3.1)	3 (2.4)
Common Cold	4 (4.7)	0	2 (2.4)	6 (2.3)	3 (2.4)
Allergy	0	2 (2.3)	1 (1.2)	3 (1.2)	2 (1.6)
Infection Upper Respiratory	0	0	0	0	2 (1.6)
MUSCULOSKELETAL	1 (1.2)	1 (1.1)	1 (1.2)	3 (1.2)	5 (3.9)
Muscle Soreness	0	0	0	0	2 (1.6)
RESPIRATORY	5 (5.9)	0	1 (1.2)	6 (2.3)	6 (4.7)
Sinusitis	4 (4.7)	0	0	4 (1.6)	2 (1.6)
SKIN & APPENDAGES	78 (91.8)	83 (95.4)	82 (96.5)	243 (94.6)	85 (66.9)
Application Site Reaction	78 (91.8)	83 (95.4)	82 (96.5)	243 (94.6)	83 (65.4)
Irritation Skin	1 (1.2)	0	2 (2.4)	3 (1.2)	0
SPECIAL SENSES	6 (7.1)	4 (4.6)	6 (7.1)	16 (6.2)	6 (4.7)
Eye Irritation	5 (5.9)	3 (3.4)	6 (7.1)	14 (5.4)	3 (2.4)

5. Cleanse affected area and wait 10 minutes before applying Carac.

6. Wash hands immediately after applying Carac.

7. Avoid prolonged exposure to sunlight or other forms of ultraviolet irradiation during treatment, as the intensity of the reaction may be increased.

8. Most patients using Carac get skin reactions where the medicine is used. These reactions include redness, dryness, burning, pain, erosion (loss of the upper layer of skin), and swelling. Irritation at the application site may persist for two or more weeks after therapy is discontinued. Treated areas may be unsightly during and after therapy.

9. If you develop abdominal pain, bloody diarrhea, vomiting, fever, or chills while on Carac therapy, stop the medication and contact your physician and/or pharmacist.

10. Report any side effects to the physician and/or pharmacist.

Laboratory Tests

To rule out the presence of a frank neoplasm, a biopsy may be considered for those areas failing to respond to treatment or recurring after treatment.

Carcinogenesis, Mutagenesis and Impairment of Fertility

Adequate long-term studies in animals to evaluate carcinogenic potential have not been conducted with fluorouracil. Studies with the active ingredient of Carac, fluorouracil, have shown positive effects in *in vitro* and *in vivo* tests for mutagenicity and on impairment of fertility in *in vivo* animal studies.

Fluorouracil produced morphological transformation of cells in *in vitro* cell transformation assays. Morphological transformation was also produced in an *in vitro* assay by a metabolite of fluorouracil, and the transformed cells produced malignant tumors when injected into immunosuppressed syngeneic mice. Fluorouracil has been shown to exert mutagenic activity in yeast cells, *Bacillus subtilis*, and *Drosophila* assays. In addition, fluorouracil has produced chromosome damage at concentrations of 1.0 and 2.0 mcg/mL in an *in vitro* hamster fibroblast assay, was positive in a microwell mouse lymphoma assay, and was positive in *in vivo* micronucleus assays in rats and mice following intraperitoneal administration. Some patients receiving cumulative doses of 0.24 to 1.0 g of fluorouracil parenterally have shown an increase in numerical and structural chromosome aberrations in peripheral blood lymphocytes.

Fluorouracil has been shown to impair fertility after parenteral administration in rats. Fluorouracil administered at intraperitoneal doses of 125 and 250 mg/kg has been shown to induce chromosomal aberrations and changes in chromosome organization of spermatogonia in rats. In mice, single-dose intravenous and intraperitoneal injections of fluorouracil have been reported to kill differentiated spermatogonia and spermatocytes at a dose of 500 mg/kg and produce abnormalities in spermatids at 50 mg/kg.

Pediatric Use

Actinic keratosis is not a condition seen within the pediatric population, except in association with rare genetic diseases. Carac should not be used in children. The safety and effectiveness of Carac have not been established in patients less than 18 years old.

Geriatric Use

No significant differences in safety and efficacy measures were demonstrated in patients age 65 and older compared to all other patients.

Pregnancy

Teratogenic Effects: Pregnancy Category X

See **CONTRAINDICATIONS**

Nursing Women

It is not known whether fluorouracil is excreted in human milk. Because many drugs are excreted in human milk and because of the potential for serious adverse reactions in nursing infants from fluorouracil, a decision should be made whether to discontinue nursing or to discontinue the drug, taking into account the importance of the drug to the mother.

ADVERSE REACTIONS

The following were adverse events considered to be drug-related and occurring with a frequency of ≥1% with Carac: application site reaction (94.6%), and eye irritation (5.4%). The signs and symptoms of facial irritation (application site reaction) are presented below.

[See first table above]

During clinical trials, irritation generally began on day 4 and persisted for the remainder of treatment. Severity of facial irritation at the last treatment visit was slightly be-

low baseline for the vehicle group, mild to moderate for the 1 week active treatment group, and moderate for the 2 and 4 week active treatment groups. Mean severity declined rapidly for each active group after completion of treatment and was below baseline for each group at the week 2 post-treatment follow-up visit.

Thirty-one patients (12% of those treated with Carac in the Phase 3 clinical studies) discontinued study treatment early due to facial irritation. Except for three patients, discontinuation of treatment occurred on or after day 11 of treatment.

Eye irritation adverse events, described as mild to moderate in intensity, were characterized as burning, watering, sensitivity, stinging and itching. These adverse events occurred across all treatment arms in one of the two Phase 3 studies. [See second table at left]

Adverse Experiences Reported by Body System

In the Phase 3 studies, no serious adverse event was considered related to study drug. A total of five patients, three in the active treatment groups and two in the vehicle group, experienced at least one serious adverse event. Three patients died as a result of adverse event(s) considered unrelated to study drug (stomach cancer, myocardial infarction and cardiac failure).

Post-treatment clinical laboratory tests other than pregnancy tests were not performed during the Phase 3 clinical studies. Clinical laboratory tests were performed during conduct of a Phase 2 study of 104 patients and 21 patients in a Phase 1 study. No abnormal serum chemistry, hematology, or urinalysis results in these studies were considered clinically significant.

DOSAGE AND ADMINISTRATION

Carac cream should be applied once a day to the skin where actinic keratosis lesions appear, using enough to cover the entire area with a thin film. Carac cream should not be applied near the eyes, nostrils or mouth. Carac cream should be applied ten minutes after thoroughly washing, rinsing, and drying the entire area. Carac cream may be applied using the fingertips. Immediately after application, the hands should be thoroughly washed. Carac should be applied up to 4 weeks as tolerated. Continued treatment up to 4 weeks results in greater lesion reduction. Local irritation is not markedly increased by extending treatment from 2 to 4 weeks, and is generally resolved within 2 weeks of cessation of treatment.

OVERDOSE

Ordinarily, topical overdosage will not cause acute problems. If Carac is accidentally ingested, induce emesis and gastric lavage. Administer symptomatic and supportive care as needed. If contact is made with the eye, flush with copious amounts of water.

HOW SUPPLIED

Cream - 30 gram tube NDC 0066-7150-30

Store at Controlled Room Temperature 20 to 25° C (68 to 77° F) [see USP].

Prescribing Information as of 2009.

Keep out of the reach of children.

Dermik Laboratories

a business of sanofi-aventis U.S. LLC

Bridgewater, NJ 08807

© 2009 sanofi-aventis U.S. LLC

PATIENT INFORMATION

Carac® Cream, 0.5%

(fluorouracil cream)

Read this leaflet carefully before you start to use your medicine. Read the information you get every time you get more medicine. There may be new information about the drug. This leaflet does not take the place of talks with your doctor. If you have any questions or are not sure about something, ask your doctor or pharmacist.

What is Carac?

Carac (Care ack) is a cream used by adults to treat skin conditions on the face and front part of the scalp called solar keratosis or actinic keratosis.

Who should not use Carac?

Do not use Carac

• if you are pregnant or might become pregnant. Carac may harm your unborn child.

• if you are nursing a baby. We do not know if Carac can pass to the baby through the milk.

• if you have dihydropyrimidine dehydrogenase (DPD) enzyme deficiency. The active ingredient in Carac, fluorouracil, can cause serious side effects in patients who are DPD enzyme deficient. If you have DPD enzyme deficiency and use medications containing fluorouracil, you may develop serious side effects such as stomach pain, bloody diarrhea, vomiting, fever, or chills.

• if you are allergic to the ingredients in Carac. Ask your doctor or pharmacist about the inactive ingredients.

• if under 18 years of age. Carac should not be used in children

Tell your doctor if you are able to become pregnant. Your doctor may advise you about birth control to avoid pregnancy.

How should I use Carac?

Use Carac once a day as instructed by your doctor. Use it only on your skin. You should use Carac for up to 4 weeks.

1. Clean the area where you will apply Carac. Rinse well and dry the area with a towel and wait 10 minutes before applying Carac.
2. Put Carac on your face as directed by your physician, using your fingertips. Use enough to cover the affected skin.
3. Avoid contact with your eyes, nostrils, and mouth.
4. Wash your hands as soon as you finish putting the Carac on your skin.
5. A moisturizer/sunscreen may be applied 2 hours after Carac has been applied. Do not use any other skin products including creams, lotions, medications or cosmetics -unless instructed by your doctor.

What should I avoid while using Carac?
Avoid sunlight or other ultraviolet light (such as tanning booths) as much as possible while using Carac. Sunlight may increase your side effects. When exposed to sunlight, wear a hat and use sunscreen.
Do not cover the treated skin with a dressing.
Do not breast feed or become pregnant while using Carac. If you do become pregnant, stop using Carac and tell your doctor right away.

What are the possible side effects of Carac?
Most patients using Carac get skin reactions where the medicine is used. These reactions include redness, dryness, burning, pain, erosion (loss of the upper layer of skin), and swelling. Irritation may continue for two or more weeks after treatment is over. The treated area may become unsightly during therapy.
Some patients get eye irritation. Eye irritation might consist of burning, sensitivity, itching, stinging, and watering. If you are concerned about side effects, talk to your doctor. A few patients have reported side effects such as stomach pain, diarrhea, vomiting, fever, or chills, possibly due to the lack of a specific enzyme, DPD, in their body. If you experience any of these symptoms, discontinue therapy immediately, and contact your doctor.

Storage information
Keep this medicine at room temperature (68–77° F/20–25° C). Throw away unused medicine.
Keep this medicine out of the reach of children.

General advice about prescription medicines
Medicines are sometimes prescribed for conditions that are not described in patient information leaflets. Do not use it for a condition for which it was not prescribed. This medicine is for your use only. Never give it to other people. It may harm them even if their skin problem appears to be the same as yours. Do not use **Carac** after the expiration date on the tube
Prescribing Information as of August 2009.
Dermik Laboratories
a business of sanofi-aventis U.S. LLC
Bridgewater, NJ 08807
© 2009 sanofi-aventis U.S. LLC
Revised: 10/2009   Distributed by: Dermik Laboratories

ELIGARD®
[ĕl'-ə gärd]
(leuprolide acetate for injectable suspension)
7.5 mg, 22.5 mg, 30 mg, 45 mg

℞

DESCRIPTION
ELIGARD® is a sterile polymeric matrix formulation of leuprolide acetate for subcutaneous injection. It is designed to deliver leuprolide acetate at a controlled rate over a one-, three-, four- or six-month therapeutic period.
Leuprolide acetate is a synthetic nonapeptide analog of naturally occurring gonadotropin releasing hormone (GnRH or LH-RH) that, when given continuously, inhibits pituitary gonadotropin secretion and suppresses testicular and ovarian steroidogenesis. The analog possesses greater potency than the natural hormone. The chemical name is 5-oxo-L-prolyl-L-histidyl-L-tryptophyl-L-seryl-L-tyrosyl-D-leucyl-L-leucyl-L-arginyl-N-ethyl-L-prolinamide acetate (salt) with the following structural formula:

ELIGARD® is prefilled and supplied in two separate, sterile syringes whose contents are mixed immediately prior to administration. The two syringes are joined and the single dose product is mixed until it is homogenous. ELIGARD® is administered subcutaneously, where it forms a solid drug delivery depot.
One syringe contains the ATRIGEL® Delivery System and the other contains leuprolide acetate. ATRIGEL® is a poly-

Table 1. ELIGARD® Delivery System Composition and Constituted Product Formulation

		ELIGARD® 7.5 mg	ELIGARD® 22.5 mg	ELIGARD® 30 mg	ELIGARD® 45 mg
ATRIGEL® Delivery System Syringe	Polymer	PLGH	PLG	PLG	PLG
	Polymer description	Copolymer containing carboxyl endgroups	Copolymer with hexanediol	Copolymer with hexanediol	Copolymer with hexanediol
	Polymer DL-lactide to Glycolide Molar Ratio	50:50	75:25	75:25	85:15
Constituted Product	Polymer delivered	82.5 mg	158.6 mg	211.5 mg	165 mg
	NMP delivered	160.0 mg	193.9 mg	258.5 mg	165 mg
	Leuprolide acetate delivered	7.5 mg	22.5 mg	30 mg	45 mg
	Approximate Leuprolide free base equivalent	7.0 mg	21 mg	28 mg	42 mg
	Approximate administered formulation weight	250 mg	375 mg	500 mg	375 mg
	Approximate injection volume	0.25 mL	0.375 mL	0.5 mL	0.375 mL

meric (non-gelatin containing) delivery system consisting of a biodegradable poly (DL-lactide-co-glycolide) (PLGH or PLG) polymer formulation dissolved in a biocompatible solvent, *N*-methyl-2-pyrrolidone (NMP).
Refer to Table 1 for the delivery system composition and constituted product formulation for each ELIGARD® product.
[See table 1 above]

CLINICAL PHARMACOLOGY
Leuprolide acetate, an LH-RH agonist, acts as a potent inhibitor of gonadotropin secretion when given continuously in therapeutic doses. Animal and human studies indicate that after an initial stimulation, chronic administration of leuprolide acetate results in suppression of testicular and ovarian steroidogenesis. This effect is reversible upon discontinuation of drug therapy.
In humans, administration of leuprolide acetate results in an initial increase in circulating levels of luteinizing hormone (LH) and follicle stimulating hormone (FSH), leading to a transient increase in levels of the gonadal steroids (testosterone and dihydrotestosterone in males, and estrone and estradiol in premenopausal females). However, continuous administration of leuprolide acetate results in decreased levels of LH and FSH. In males, testosterone is reduced to below castrate threshold (≤ 50 ng/dL). These decreases occur within two to four weeks after initiation of treatment. Long-term studies have shown that continuation of therapy with leuprolide acetate maintains testosterone below the castrate level for up to seven years.

PHARMACODYNAMICS
Following the first dose of ELIGARD®, mean serum testosterone concentrations transiently increased, then fell to below castrate threshold (≤ 50 ng/dL) within three weeks for all ELIGARD® concentrations.
Continued monthly treatment with ELIGARD® 7.5 mg maintained castrate testosterone suppression throughout the study. No breakthrough of testosterone concentrations above castrate threshold (> 50 ng/dL) occurred at any time during the study once castrate suppression was achieved (Figure 1).
One patient received less than a full dose of ELIGARD® 22.5 mg at baseline, never suppressed and withdrew from the study at Day 73. Of the 116 patients remaining in the study, 115 (99%) had serum testosterone levels below the castrate threshold by Month 1 (Day 28). By Day 35, 116 (100%) had serum testosterone levels below the castrate threshold. Once testosterone suppression was achieved, one patient (< 1%) demonstrated breakthrough (concentrations > 50 ng/dL after achieving castrate levels) following the initial injection; that patient remained below the castrate threshold following the second injection (Figure 2).
One patient withdrew from the ELIGARD® 30 mg study at Day 14. Of the 89 patients remaining in the study, 85 (96%) had serum testosterone levels below the castrate threshold by Month 1 (Day 28). By Day 42, 89 (100%) of patients attained castrate testosterone suppression. Once castrate testosterone suppression was achieved, three patients (3%) demonstrated breakthrough (concentrations > 50 ng/dL after achieving castrate levels) (Figure 3).
One patient at Day 1 and another patient at Day 29 were withdrawn from the ELIGARD® 45 mg study. Of the 109 patients remaining in the study, 108 (99.1%) had serum testosterone levels below the castrate threshold by Month 1 (Day 28). One patient did not achieve castrate suppression and was withdrawn from the study at Day 85. Once castrate

testosterone suppression was achieved, one patient (< 1%) demonstrated breakthrough (concentrations > 50 ng/dL after achieving castrate levels) (Figure 4).
Leuprolide acetate is not active when given orally.

PHARMACOKINETICS
Absorption
ELIGARD® 7.5 mg
The pharmacokinetics/pharmacodynamics observed during three once-monthly injections in 20 patients with advanced prostate cancer is shown in Figure 1. Mean serum leuprolide concentrations following the initial injection rose to 25.3 ng/mL (C_{max}) at approximately 5 hours after injection. After the initial increase following each injection, serum concentrations remained relatively constant (0.28–2.00 ng/mL).

Figure 1 Pharmacokinetic/Pharmacodynamic Response (N=20) to ELIGARD® 7.5 mg – Patients Dosed Initially and at Months 1 and 2

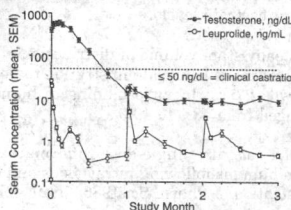

A reduced number of sampling timepoints resulted in the apparent decrease in C_{max} values with the second and third doses of ELIGARD® 7.5 mg (Figure 1).
ELIGARD® 22.5 mg
The pharmacokinetics/pharmacodynamics observed during two injections every three months (ELIGARD® 22.5 mg) in 22 patients with advanced prostate cancer is shown in Figure 2. Mean serum leuprolide concentrations rose to 127 ng/mL and 107 ng/mL at approximately 5 hours following the initial and second injections, respectively. After the initial increase following each injection, serum concentrations remained relatively constant (0.2–2.0 ng/mL).

Figure 2 Pharmacokinetic/Pharmacodynamic Response (N=22) to ELIGARD® 22.5 mg – Patients Dosed Initially and at Month 3

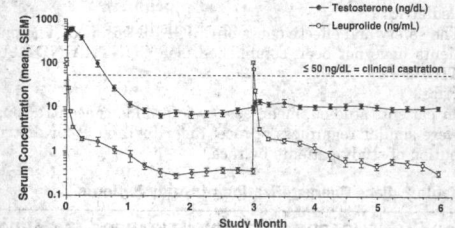

ELIGARD® 30 mg
The pharmacokinetics/pharmacodynamics observed during injections administered initially and at four months (ELIGARD® 30 mg) in 24 patients with advanced prostate cancer is shown in Figure 3. Mean serum leuprolide concentrations following the initial injection rose rapidly to 150 ng/mL (C_{max}) at approximately 3.3 hours after injection. After the initial increase following each injection, mean

serum concentrations remained relatively constant (0.1–1.0 ng/mL).

Figure 3 Pharmacokinetic/Pharmacodynamic Response (N=24) to ELIGARD® 30 mg – Patients Dosed Initially and at Month 4

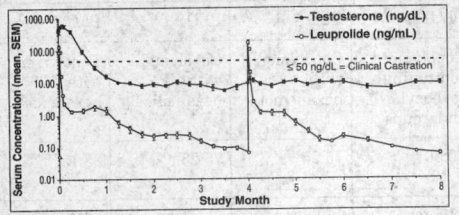

ELIGARD® 45 mg

The pharmacokinetics/pharmacodynamics observed during injections administered initially and at six months (ELIGARD® 45 mg) in 27 patients with advanced prostate cancer is shown in Figure 4. Mean serum leuprolide concentrations rose to 82.0 ng/mL and 102 ng/mL (C_{max}) at approximately 4.5 hours following the initial and second injections, respectively. After the initial increase following each injection, mean serum concentrations remained relatively constant (0.2–2.0 ng/mL).

Figure 4 Pharmacokinetic/Pharmacodynamic Response (N=27) to ELIGARD® 45 mg - Patients Dosed Initially and at Month 6

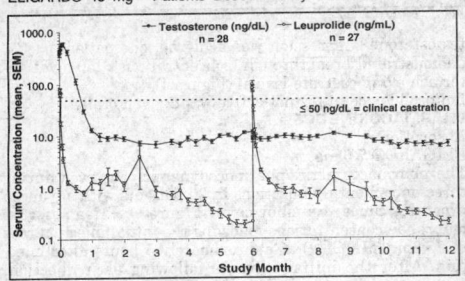

There was no evidence of significant accumulation during repeated dosing. Nondetectable leuprolide plasma concentrations have been occasionally observed during ELIGARD® administration, but testosterone levels were maintained at castrate levels.

Distribution

The mean steady-state volume of distribution of leuprolide following intravenous bolus administration to healthy male volunteers was 27 L.[1] In vitro binding to human plasma proteins ranged from 43% to 49%.

[1]Sennello LT et al. Single-dose pharmacokinetics of leuprolide in humans following intravenous and subcutaneous administration. J Pharm Sci 1986; 75(2): 158–160.

Metabolism

In healthy male volunteers, a 1-mg bolus of leuprolide administered intravenously revealed that the mean systemic clearance was 8.34 L/h, with a terminal elimination half-life of approximately 3 hours based on a two compartment model.[1]

No drug metabolism study was conducted with ELIGARD®. Upon administration with different leuprolide acetate formulations, the major metabolite of leuprolide acetate is a pentapeptide (M-1) metabolite.

Excretion

No drug excretion study was conducted with ELIGARD®.

Special Populations

Geriatrics

The majority of the patients (approximately 70%) studied in the clinical trials were age 70 and older.

Pediatrics

The safety and effectiveness of ELIGARD® in pediatric patients have not been established (see **CONTRAINDICATIONS**).

Race

In patients studied, mean serum leuprolide concentrations were similar regardless of race. Refer to Table 2 for distribution of study patients by race.

Table 2. Race Characterization of Study Patients

Race	ELIGARD® 7.5 mg	ELIGARD® 22.5 mg	ELIGARD® 30 mg	ELIGARD® 45 mg
White	26	19	18	17
Black	-	4	4	7
Hispanic	2	2	2	3

Table 3. Summary of ELIGARD® Clinical Studies

		7.5 mg	22.5 mg	30 mg	45 mg
Study number		AGL9904	AGL9909	AGL0001	AGL0205
Total Number of patients		120 (117 completed)	117* (111 completed[†])	90 (82 completed[‡])	111 (103 completed[§])
Jewett Stages	Stage A	-	2	2	5
	Stage B	-	19	38	43
	Stage C	89	60	16	19
	Stage D	31	36	34	44
Treatment		6 monthly injections	1 injection (4 patients)	1 injection (5 patients)	1 injection (5 patients)
			2 injections, one every three months (113 patients)	2 injections, one every four months (85 patients)	2 injections, one every six months (106 patients)
Duration of therapy		6 months	6 months	8 months	12 months
Mean testosterone concentration (ng/dL)	Baseline	361.3	367.1	385.5	367.7
	Day 2	574.6 (Day 3)	588.0	610.0	588.6
	Day 14	Below Baseline (Day 10)	Below Baseline	Below Baseline	Below Baseline
	Day 28	21.8	27.7 (Day 21)	17.2	16.7
	Conclusion	6.1	10.1	12.4	12.6
Number of patients below castrate threshold (≤ 50 ng/dL)	Day 28	112 of 119 (94.1%)	115 of 116 (99%)	85 of 89 (96%)	108 of 109 (99.1%)
	Day 35	-	116 (100%)	-	-
	Day 42	119 (100%)	-	89 (100%)	-
	Conclusion	117[¶] (100%)	111 (100%)	81 (99%)	102 (99%)

* One patient received less than a full dose at Baseline, never suppressed, and was withdrawn at Day 73 and given an alternate treatment.
† All non-evaluable patients who had attained castration by Day 28 maintained castration at each timepoint up to and including the time of withdrawal.
‡ One patient withdrew on Day 14. All 7 non-evaluable patients who had achieved castration by Day 28 maintained castration at each timepoint, up to and including the time of withdrawal.
§ Two patients were withdrawn prior to the Month 1 blood draw. One patient did not achieve castration and was withdrawn on Day 85. All 5 non-evaluable patients who attained castration by Day 28, maintained castration at each timepoint up to and including the time of withdrawal.
¶ Two patients withdrew for reasons unrelated to drug.

Renal and Hepatic Insufficiency

The pharmacokinetics of ELIGARD® in hepatically and renally impaired patients have not been determined

Drug-Drug Interactions

No pharmacokinetic drug-drug interaction studies were conducted with ELIGARD®.

CLINICAL STUDIES

One open-label, multicenter study was conducted with each ELIGARD® formulation (7.5 mg, 22.5 mg, 30 mg, and 45 mg) in patients with Jewett stage A though D prostate cancer who were treated with at least a single injection of study drug (Table 3). These studies evaluated the achievement and maintenance of castrate serum testosterone suppression over the duration of therapy (Figures 5–8).

During the AGL9904 study using ELIGARD® 7.5 mg, once testosterone suppression was achieved, no patients (0%) demonstrated breakthrough (concentration >50 ng/dL) at any time in the study.

During the AGL9909 study using ELIGARD® 22.5 mg, once testosterone suppression was achieved, only one patient (< 1%) demonstrated breakthrough following the initial injection; that patient remained below the castrate threshold following the second injection.

During the AGL0001 study using ELIGARD® 30 mg, once testosterone suppression was achieved, three patients (3%) demonstrated breakthrough. In the first of these patients, a single serum testosterone concentration of 53 ng/dL was reported on the day after the second injection. In this patient, castrate suppression was reported for all other timepoints. In the second patient, a serum testosterone concentration of 66 ng/dL was reported immediately prior to the second injection. This rose to a maximum concentration of 147 ng/dL

on the second day after the second injection. In this patient, castrate suppression was again reached on the seventh day after the second injection and was maintained thereafter. In the final patient, serum testosterone concentrations > 50 ng/dL were reported at 2 and at 8 hours after the second injection. Serum testosterone concentration rose to a maximum of 110 ng/dL on the third day after the second injection. In this patient, castrate suppression was again reached eighteen days after the second injection and was maintained until the final day of the study, when a single serum testosterone concentration of 55 ng/dL was reported. During the AGL0205 study using ELIGARD® 45 mg, once testosterone suppression was achieved, one patient (<1%) demonstrated breakthrough. This patient reached castrate suppression at Day 21 and remained suppressed until Day 308 when his testosterone level rose to 112 ng/dL. At Month 12 (Day 336), his testosterone was 210 ng/dL.

[See table 3 above]

Figure 5 ELIGARD® 7.5 mg Mean Serum Testosterone Concentrations (n=117)

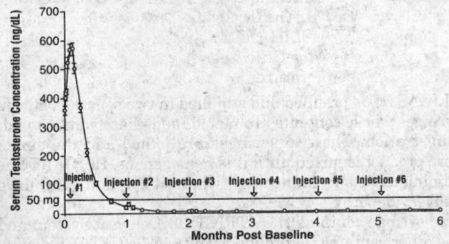

Figure 6 ELIGARD® 22.5 mg Mean Serum Testosterone Concentrations (n=111)

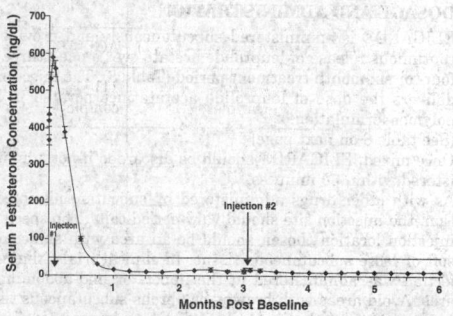

Figure 7 ELIGARD® 30 mg Mean Serum Testosterone Concentrations (n=90)

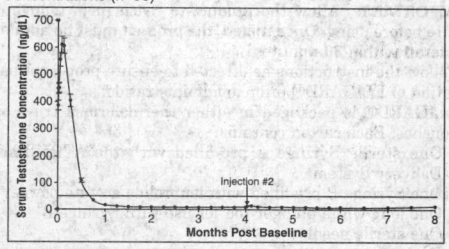

Figure 8 ELIGARD® 45 mg Mean Serum Testosterone Concentrations (n=103)

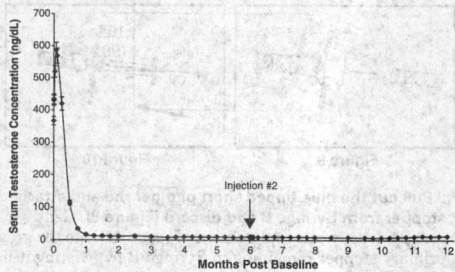

Serum PSA decreased in all patients in all studies whose Baseline values were elevated above the normal limit. Refer to Table 4 for a summary of the effectiveness of ELIGARD® in reducing serum PSA values.

Table 4 Effect of ELIGARD® on Patient Serum PSA Values

ELIGARD®	7.5 mg	22.5 mg	30 mg	45 mg
Mean PSA Reduction at Study Conclusion	94%	98%	86%	97%
Patients with Normal PSA at Study Conclusion*	94%	91%	93%	95%

*Among patients who presented with elevated levels at Baseline

Other secondary efficacy endpoints evaluated included WHO performance status, bone pain, urinary pain and urinary signs and symptoms. Refer to Table 5 for a summary of these endpoints.
[See table 5 above]

INDICATIONS AND USAGE

ELIGARD® is indicated for the palliative treatment of advanced prostate cancer.

CONTRAINDICATIONS

1. ELIGARD® is contraindicated in patients with hypersensitivity to GnRH, GnRH agonist analogs or any of the components of ELIGARD®. Anaphylactic reactions to synthetic GnRH or GnRH agonist analogs have been reported in the literature.[2]
2. ELIGARD® is contraindicated in women and in pediatric patients and was not studied in women or children. Moreover, leuprolide acetate can cause fetal harm when administered to a pregnant woman. Major fetal abnormalities were observed in rabbits but not in rats after administration of leuprolide acetate throughout gestation. There were increased fetal mortality and decreased fetal weights in rats and rabbits. The effects on fetal mor-

Table 5 Secondary Efficacy Endpoints

		ELIGARD® 7.5 mg	ELIGARD® 22.5 mg	ELIGARD® 30 mg	ELIGARD® 45 mg
Baseline	WHO Status = 0*	88%	94%	90%	90%
	WHO Status = 1[†]	11%	6%	10%	7%
	WHO Status = 2[‡]				3%
	Mean Bone Pain[§] (range)	1.22 (1–9)	1.20 (1–9)	1.20 (1–7)	1.38 (1–7)
	Mean Urinary Pain (range)	1.12 (1–5)	1.02 (1–2)	1.01 (1–2)	1.22 (1–8)
	Mean Urinary Signs and Symptoms (range)	Low	1.09 (1–4)	Low	Low
	Number of Patients with Prostate Abnormalities	102 (85%)	96 (82%)	66 (73%)	89 (80%)
Follow-up		Month 6	Month 6	Month 8	Month 12
	WHO Status = 0	Unchanged	96%	87%	94%
	WHO Status = 1	Unchanged	4%	12%	5%
	WHO Status = 2			1%	1%
	Mean Bone Pain (range)	1.26 (1–7)	1.22 (1–5)	1.19 (1–8)	1.31 (1–8)
	Mean Urinary Pain (range)	1.07 (1–8)	1.10 (1–8)	1.00 (1–1)	1.07 (1–5)
	Mean Urinary Signs and Symptoms (range)	Modestly Decreased	1.18 (1–7)	Modestly Decreased	Modestly Decreased
	Number of Patients with Prostate Abnormalities	77 (64%)	76 (65%)	54 (60%)	60 (58%)

* WHO Status = 0 classified as "fully active."
† WHO Status = 1 classified as "restricted in strenuous activity but ambulatory and able to carry out work of a light or sedentary nature."
‡ WHO Status = 2 classified as "ambulatory but unable to carry out work activities."
§ Pain score scale: 1 (no pain) to 10 (worst pain possible).

tality are expected consequences of the alterations in hormonal levels brought about by this drug. The possibility exists that spontaneous abortion may occur.

2MacLeod TL et al. Anaphylactic reaction to synthetic luteinizing hormone releasing hormone. Fertil Steril 1987 Sept; 48(3): 500–502.

WARNINGS

ELIGARD® 7.5 mg 22.5 mg 30 mg, like other LH-RH agonists, causes a transient increase in serum concentrations of testosterone during the first week of treatment. ELIGARD® 45 mg causes a transient increase in serum concentrations of testosterone during the first two weeks of treatment. Patients may experience worsening of symptoms or onset of new signs and symptoms during the first few weeks of treatment, including bone pain, neuropathy, hematuria, or bladder outlet obstruction. Isolated cases of ureteral obstruction and/or spinal cord compression, which may contribute to paralysis with or without fatal complications, have been observed in the palliative treatment of advanced prostate cancer using LH-RH agonists (see **PRECAUTIONS**).
If spinal cord compression or ureteral obstruction develops, standard treatment of these complications should be instituted.

PRECAUTIONS
General
Patients with metastatic vertebral lesions and/or with urinary tract obstruction should be closely observed during the first few weeks of therapy (see **WARNINGS** section).
Laboratory Tests
Response to ELIGARD® should be monitored by measuring serum concentrations of testosterone and prostate specific antigen periodically.
In the majority of patients, testosterone levels increased above Baseline during the first week, declining thereafter to Baseline levels or below by the end of the second or third week. Castrate levels were generally reached within two to four weeks.
Castrate testosterone levels were maintained for the duration of the treatment with ELIGARD® 7.5 mg. No increases to above the castrate level occurred in any of the patients. Castrate levels were generally maintained for the duration of treatment with ELIGARD® 22.5 mg.
Once castrate levels were achieved with ELIGARD® 30 mg, most (86/89) patients remained suppressed throughout the study.

Once castrate levels were achieved with ELIGARD® 45 mg, only one patient (< 1%) experienced a breakthrough, with testosterone levels > 50 ng/dL.
Results of testosterone determinations are dependent on assay methodology. It is advisable to be aware of the type and precision of the assay methodology to make appropriate clinical and therapeutic decisions.
Drug Interactions
See **PHARMACOKINETICS**.
Drug/Laboratory Test Interactions
Therapy with leuprolide acetate results in suppression of the pituitary-gonadal system. Results of diagnostic tests of pituitary gonadotropic and gonadal functions conducted during and after leuprolide therapy may be affected.
Carcinogenesis, Mutagenesis, Impairment of Fertility
Two-year carcinogenicity studies were conducted with leuprolide acetate in rats and mice. In rats, a dose-related increase of benign pituitary hyperplasia and benign pituitary adenomas was noted at 24 months when the drug was administered subcutaneously at high daily doses (0.6 to 4 mg/kg). There was a significant but not dose-related increase of pancreatic islet-cell adenomas in females and of testicular interstitial cell adenomas in males (highest incidence in the low dose group). In mice, no leuprolide acetate-induced tumors or pituitary abnormalities were observed at a dose as high as 60 mg/kg for two years. Patients have been treated with leuprolide acetate for up to three years with doses as high as 10 mg/day and for two years with doses as high as 20 mg/day without demonstrable pituitary abnormalities. No carcinogenicity studies have been conducted with ELIGARD®.
Mutagenicity studies have been performed with leuprolide acetate using bacterial and mammalian systems and with ELIGARD® 7.5 mg in bacterial systems. These studies provided no evidence of a mutagenic potential.
Pregnancy
Teratogenic Effects
Pregnancy category X
(see **CONTRAINDICATIONS**).
Pediatric Use
ELIGARD® is contraindicated in pediatric patients and was not studied in children (see **CONTRAINDICATIONS**).

ADVERSE REACTIONS
The safety of all ELIGARD® formulations was evaluated in clinical trials involving patients with advanced prostate cancer. In addition, the safety of ELIGARD® 7.5 mg was evaluated in 8 surgically castrated males (Table 7).

Table 6 Reported Injection Site Adverse Events

	7.5 mg	22.5 mg	30 mg	45 mg
Study Number	AGL9904	AGL9909	AGL0001	AGL0205
Number of patients	120	117	90	111
Treatment	1 injection every month up to 6 months	1 injection every 3 months up to 6 months	1 injection every 4 months up to 8 months	1 injection every 6 months up to 12 months
Number of injections	716	230	175	217
Transient burning/ stinging	248 (34.6%) injections; 84% reported as mild	50 (21.7%) injections; 86% reported as mild	35 (20%) injections; 100% reported as mild	35 (16%) injections; 91.4% reported as mild*
Pain (generally brief and mild)	4.3% of injections (18.3% of patients)	3.5% of injections (6.0% of patients)	2.3% of injections† (3.3% of patients)	4.6% of injections‡
Erythema (generally brief and mild)	2.6% of injections (12.5% of patients)	0.9% of injections§ (1.7% of patients)	1.1% of injections (2.2% of patients)	
Bruising (Mild)	2.5% of injections (11.7% of patients)	1.7% of injections (3.4% of patients)		2.3% of injections¶
Pruritis	1.4% of injections (9.2% of patients)	0.4% of injections (0.9% of patients)		
Induration	0.4% of injections (2.5% of patients)			
Ulceration	0.1% of injections (> 0.8% of patients)			

* Following injection of ELIGARD® 30 mg, three of the 35 burning/stinging events were reported as moderate.
† A single event reported as moderate pain resolved within two minutes and all 3 mild pain events resolved within several days following injection of ELIGARD® 30 mg.
‡ Transient pain was reported as mild in intensity in nine of ten (90%) events and moderate in intensity in one of ten (10%) events following injection of ELIGARD® 45 mg.
§ Erythema reported following 2 injections of ELIGARD® 22.5 mg. One report characterized the erythema as mild and it resolved within 7 days. The other report characterized the erythema as moderate and it resolved within 15 days. Neither patient experienced erythema at multiple injections.
¶ Mild bruising was reported following 5 (2.3%) study injections and moderate bruising was reported following 2 (<1%) study injections of ELIGARD® 45 mg.

ELIGARD®, like other LH-RH analogs, caused a transient increase in serum testosterone concentrations during the first one to two weeks of treatment. Therefore, potential exacerbations of signs and symptoms of the disease during the first weeks of treatment are of concern in patients with vertebral metastases and/or urinary obstruction or hematuria. If these conditions are aggravated, it may lead to neurological problems such as weakness and/or paresthesia of the lower limbs or worsening of urinary symptoms (see **WARNINGS** and **PRECAUTIONS**).
During the clinical trials, injection sites were closely monitored. Refer to Table 6 for a summary of reported injection site events.
[See table 6 above]
These localized adverse events were non-recurrent over time. No patient discontinued therapy due to an injection site adverse event.
The following possibly or probably related systemic adverse events occurred during clinical trials with ELIGARD®, and were reported in > 2% of patients (Table 7). Often, causality is difficult to assess in patients with metastatic prostate cancer. Reactions considered not drug-related are excluded.
[See table 7 at top of next page]
In addition, the following possibly or probably related systemic adverse events were reported by < 2% of the patients treated with ELIGARD® in these clinical studies.

Body System	Adverse Event
General	Sweating, insomnia, syncope, rigors, weakness, lethargy
Gastrointestinal	Flatulence, constipation, dyspepsia
Hematologic	Decreased red blood cell count, hematocrit and hemoglobin
Metabolic	Weight gain
Musculoskeletal	Tremor, backache, joint pain, muscle atrophy, limb pain
Nervous	Disturbance of smell and taste, depression, vertigo
Psychiatric	Insomnia, depression, loss of libido*
Renal/Urinary	Difficulties with urination, pain on urination, scanty urination, bladder spasm, blood in urine, urinary retention, urinary urgency, incontinence, nocturia, nocturia aggravated
Reproductive/ Urogenital:	Testicular soreness/pain, impotence*, decreased libido*, gynecomastia*, breast soreness/ tenderness*, testicular atrophy*, erectile dysfunction, penile disorder*, reduced penis size
Skin	Alopecia, clamminess, night sweats*, sweating increased*
Vascular	Hypertension, hypotension

*Expected pharmacological consequences of testosterone suppression.

Changes in Bone Density
Decreased bone density has been reported in the medical literature in men who have had orchiectomy or who have been treated with an LH-RH agonist analog.[3] It can be anticipated that long periods of medical castration in men will have effects on bone density.

[3]Hatano T et al. Incidence of bone fracture in patients receiving luteinizing hormone-releasing hormone agonists for prostate cancer. BJU International 2000 86: 449–452.

Post-Marketing
Pituitary apoplexy
During post-marketing surveillance, rare cases of pituitary apoplexy (a clinical syndrome secondary to infarction of the pituitary gland) have been reported after the administration of gonadotropin-releasing hormone agonists. In a majority of these cases, a pituitary adenoma was diagnosed with a majority of pituitary apoplexy cases occurring within 2 weeks of the first dose, and some within the first hour. In these cases, pituitary apoplexy has presented as sudden headache, vomiting, visual changes, ophthalmoplegia, altered mental status, and sometimes cardiovascular collapse. Immediate medical attention has been required.

OVERDOSAGE
In clinical trials using daily subcutaneous injections of leuprolide acetate in patients with prostate cancer, doses as high as 20 mg/day for up to two years caused no adverse effects differing from those observed with the 1 mg/day dose.

DOSAGE AND ADMINISTRATION
ELIGARD® is administered subcutaneously and provides continuous release of leuprolide acetate over a one-, three-, four- or six-month treatment period (Table 8). The injection delivers the dose of leuprolide acetate incorporated in a polymer formulation.
[See table 8 on next page]
Once mixed, ELIGARD® should be discarded if not administered within 30 minutes.
As with other drugs administered by subcutaneous injection, the injection site should vary periodically. The specific injection location chosen should be an area with sufficient soft or loose subcutaneous tissue. In clinical trials, the injection was administered in the upper- or mid-abdominal area. Avoid areas with brawny or fibrous subcutaneous tissue or locations that could be rubbed or compressed (i.e., with a belt or clothing waistband).
Mixing Procedure
IMPORTANT: Allow the product to reach room temperature before using. **Once mixed, the product must be administered within 30 minutes.**
Follow the instructions as directed to ensure proper preparation of ELIGARD® prior to administration:
ELIGARD® is packaged in either thermoformed trays or pouches. Each carton contains:
• One sterile Syringe A pre-filled with the ATRIGEL® Delivery System
• One Syringe B pre-filled with leuprolide acetate powder
• One long white plunger rod for use with Syringe B
• One sterile needle
• Desiccant pack(s)
• 1.On a clean field, open all of the packages and remove the contents. Discard the desiccant pack(s).

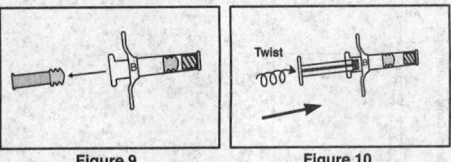

Figure 9   **Figure 10**

• 2.Pull out the blue-tipped short plunger rod and attached stopper from Syringe B and discard (Figure 9). Gently insert the long, white replacement plunger rod into the gray primary stopper remaining in Syringe B by twisting it in place (Figure 10).

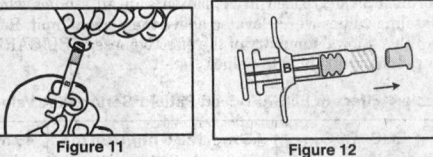

Figure 11   **Figure 12**

• 3.Unscrew the clear cap from Syringe A (Figure 11). Remove the gray rubber cap from Syringe B (Figure 12).

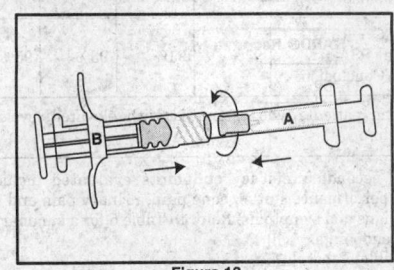

Figure 13

• 4.Join the two syringes together by pushing in and twisting until secure (Figure 13).

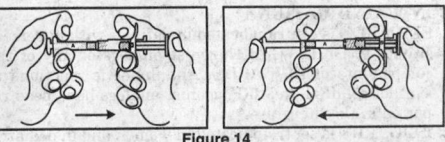

Figure 14

• 5.Inject the liquid contents of Syringe A into Syringe B containing the leuprolide acetate. Thoroughly mix the product by pushing the contents of both syringes back and forth between syringes (approximately 45 seconds) to obtain a uniform suspension (Figure 14). (7.5 mg PI, 22.5 mg PI, 30 mg PI, 45 mg PI) When thoroughly mixed,

Table 7 Summary of Possible or Probably Related Systemic Adverse Events Reported by > 2% of Patients treated with ELIGARD®

		7.5 mg	7.5 mg	22.5 mg	30 mg	45 mg
Study Number		AGL9904	AGL9802	AGL9909	AGL0001	AGL0205
Number of patients		120	8	117	90	111
Treatment		1 injection every month up to 6 months	1 injection (surgically castrated patients)	1 injection every 3 months up to 6 months	1 injection every 4 months up to 8 months	1 injection every 6 months up to 12 months
Body System	**Adverse Event**	Number (Percent)				
Body as a Whole	Malaise and Fatigue	21 (17.5 %)		7 (6.0%)	12 (13.3%)	13 (11.7%)
	Weakness					4 (3.6%)
Nervous System	Dizziness	4 (3.3%)			4 (4.4%)	
Vascular	Hot flashes/sweats	68 (56.7%)*	2 (25.0%)*	66 (56.4%)*	66 (73.3%)*	64 (57.7%)*
Renal/Urinary	Urinary frequency			3 (2.6%)	2 (2.2%)	
	Nocturia				2 (2.2%)	
Gastrointestinal	Nausea			4 (3.4%)	2 (2.2%)	
	Gastroenteritis/colitis	3 (2.5%)				
Skin	Pruritis			3 (2.6%)		
	Clamminess				4 (4.4%)*	
	Night sweats				3 (3.3%)*	3 (2.7%)*
	Alopecia				2 (2.2%)	
Musculoskeletal	Arthralgia			4 (3.4%)		
	Myalgia				2 (2.2%)	5 (4.5%)
	Pain in limb					3 (2.7%)
Reproductive	Testicular atrophy	6 (5.0%)			4 (4.4%)*	8 (7.2%)*
	Gynecomastia				2 (2.2%)*	4 (3.6%)*
	Testicular pain				2 (2.2%)	
Psychiatric	Decreased libido				3 (3.3%)*	

In the patient populations studied with ELIGARD® 7.5 mg, a total of 85 hot flashes/sweats adverse events were reported in 70 patients. Of these, 71 events (83%) were mild; 14 (16%) were moderate; 1 (1%) was severe.

In the patient population studied with ELIGARD® 22.5 mg, a total of 84 hot flashes/sweats adverse events were reported in 66 patients. Of these, 73 events (87%) were mild; 11 (13%) were moderate; none were severe.

In the patient population studied with ELIGARD® 30 mg, a total of 75 hot flash adverse events were reported in 66 patients. Of these, 57 events (76%) were mild; 16 (21%) were moderate; 2 (3%) were severe.

In the patient population studied with ELIGARD® 45 mg, a total of 89 hot flash adverse events were reported in 64 patients. Of these, 62 events (70%) were mild; 27 (30%) were moderate; none were severe.

* Expected pharmacological consequences of testosterone suppression.

Table 8 ELIGARD® Recommended Dosing

Dosage	7.5 mg	22.5 mg	30 mg	45 mg
Recommended dose	1 injection every month	1 injection every 3 months	1 injection every 4 months	1 injection every 6 months

the suspension will appear light tan to tan (ELIGARD® 7.5 mg) or colorless to pale yellow (ELIGARD®, 22.5 mg, 30 mg and 45 mg) in color. **Please Note: Product must be mixed as described; shaking will not provide adequate mixing of the product.**
[See figure 15 at top of third column]

- 6. Hold the syringes vertically with Syringe B on the bottom. The syringes should remain securely coupled. Draw the entire mixed product into Syringe B (short, wide syringe) by depressing the Syringe A plunger and slightly withdrawing the Syringe B plunger. Uncouple Syringe A while continuing to push down on the Syringe A plunger (Figure 15). **Note: Small air bubbles will remain in the formulation – this is acceptable.**
[See figures 16-18 next column]

- 7. Hold Syringe B upright. Remove the cap on the bottom of the sterile needle cartridge by twisting it (Figure 16). Attach the needle cartridge to the end of Syringe B (Figure 17) by pushing in and turning the needle until it is firmly seated. Do not twist the needle onto the syringe un-

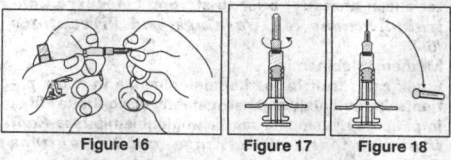

| Figure 16 | Figure 17 | Figure 18 |

til it is stripped. Pull off the clear needle cartridge cover prior to administration (Figure 18).

Administration Procedure

IMPORTANT: Allow the product to reach room temperature before using. **Once mixed, the product must be administered within 30 minutes.**

1. Choose an injection site on the abdomen, upper buttocks, or anywhere with adequate amounts of subcutaneous tissue that does not have excessive pigment, nodules, lesions, or hair. Since you can vary the injection site with a subcutaneous injection, choose an area that hasn't recently been used.

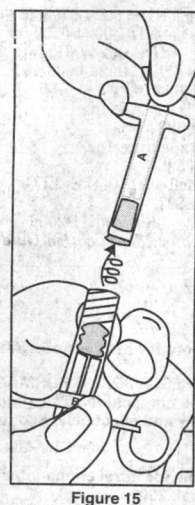

Figure 15

2. Cleanse the injection-site area with an alcohol swab.
3. Using the thumb and forefinger of your nondominant hand, grab and bunch the area of skin around the injection site.

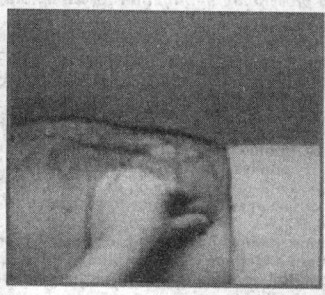

4. Using your dominant hand, insert the needle quickly at a 90° angle. The approximate angle you use will depend on the amount and fullness of the subcutaneous tissue and the length of the needle. After the needle is inserted, release the skin with your nondominant hand.

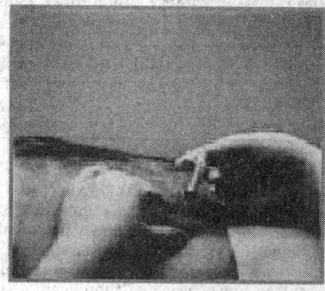

5. Inject the drug using a slow, steady push. Press down on the plunger until the syringe is empty.
6. Withdraw the needle quickly at the same angle used for insertion.
7. Discard all components safely in an appropriate biohazard container.

HOW SUPPLIED

ELIGARD® is available in a single use kit. The kit consists of a two-syringe mixing system, a sterile needle (Table 9), a silicone desiccant pouch to control moisture uptake, and a package insert for constitution and administration procedures. Each syringe is individually packaged. One contains the ATRIGEL® Delivery System and the other contains leuprolide acetate. When constituted, ELIGARD® is administered as a single dose.

Table 9. ELIGARD® Needle specifications

ELIGARD® formulation	Gauge	Length
7.5 mg	20-gauge	½-inch
22.5 mg	20-gauge	½-inch
30 mg	20-gauge	5/8-inch
45 mg	18-gauge	5/8-inch

ELIGARD® 7.5 mg – NDC 0024-0793-75
ELIGARD® 22.5 mg – NDC 0024-0222-05
ELIGARD® 30 mg – NDC 0024-0610-30
ELIGARD® 45 mg – NDC 0024-0605-45
Store at 2–8 °C (35.6–46.4 °F)
Manufactured by: TOLMAR, Inc.
Fort Collins, CO 80526
for: TOLMAR Therapeutics, Inc.
Fort Collins, CO 80526
Distributed by: sanofi-aventis U.S. LLC
Bridgewater, NJ 08807
44380, Rev 1 11/09   Revised 11/2009
Shown in Product Identification Guide, page 318

ELITEK®   Rx
[el-i-tek]
(rasburicase)
Powder for solution, for intravenous infusion

HIGHLIGHTS OF PRESCRIBING INFORMATION
These highlights do not include all the information needed to use ELITEK safely and effectively. See full prescribing information for ELITEK.
ELITEK (rasburicase)
Powder for solution, for intravenous infusion
Initial U.S. Approval: 2002

WARNING: ANAPHYLAXIS, HEMOLYSIS, METHE-MOGLOBINEMIA, AND INTERFERENCE WITH URIC ACID MEASUREMENTS
See full prescribing information for complete boxed warning.
- **Anaphylaxis:** Elitek can cause severe hypersensitivity reactions including anaphylaxis. Immediately and permanently discontinue Elitek if a serious hypersensitivity reaction occurs (4, 5.1, 6.2).
- **Hemolysis:** Do not administer Elitek to patients with glucose-6-phosphate dehydrogenase (G6PD) deficiency. Immediately and permanently discontinue Elitek if hemolysis occurs. Screen patients at higher risk for G6PD deficiency (e.g., patients of African or Mediterranean ancestry) prior to starting Elitek therapy (4, 5.2).
- **Methemoglobinemia:** Elitek can result in methemoglobinemia in some patients. Immediately and permanently discontinue Elitek if methemoglobinemia occurs (4, 5.3).
- **Interference with uric acid measurements:** Elitek enzymatically degrades uric acid in blood samples left at room temperature. Collect blood samples in pre-chilled tubes containing heparin and immediately immerse and maintain sample in an ice water bath. Assay plasma samples within 4 hours of collection (5.4).

---RECENT MAJOR CHANGES---

Indication and Usage (1)	10/2009
Dosage and Administration/Dosage (2.1)	10/2009

---INDICATIONS AND USAGE---
Elitek is a recombinant urate-oxidase indicated for initial management of plasma uric acid levels in pediatric and adult patients with leukemia, lymphoma, and solid tumor malignancies who are receiving anti-cancer therapy expected to result in tumor lysis and subsequent elevation of plasma uric acid (1).
Limitation of use: Elitek is indicated only for a single course of treatment (1).
---DOSAGE AND ADMINISTRATION---
- Administer at 0.2 mg/kg as an intravenous infusion over 30 minutes daily for up to 5 days (2.1).
- Do not administer as an intravenous bolus (2.3).
---DOSAGE FORMS AND STRENGTHS---
- 1.5 mg powder per single-use vial (3)
- 7.5 mg powder per single-use vial (3)
---CONTRAINDICATIONS---
- History of the following reactions to rasburicase: anaphylaxis, severe hypersensitivity, hemolysis, methemoglobinemia (4).
- Glucose-6-phosphate dehydrogenase (G6PD) deficiency (4).
---WARNINGS AND PRECAUTIONS---
- Anaphylaxis: See Boxed Warning, (5.1)
- Hemolysis: See Boxed Warning, (5.2)
- Methemoglobinemia: See Boxed Warning, (5.3)
- Laboratory Sample Handling Procedure: See Boxed Warning, (5.4)
---ADVERSE REACTIONS---
Most common adverse reactions (incidence ≥20%), occurring in patients with hematological malignancy and treated by chemotherapy are vomiting, nausea, pyrexia, peripheral edema, anxiety, headache, abdominal pain, constipation, and diarrhea (6.1).

To report SUSPECTED ADVERSE REACTIONS, contact sanofi-aventis U.S. LLC at 1-800-633-1610 or FDA at 1-800-FDA-1088 or *www.fda.gov/medwatch*
---USE IN SPECIFIC POPULATIONS---
- Pregnancy: May cause fetal harm. Use only if the potential benefit to the mother justifies the potential risk to the fetus (8.1).
- Nursing Mothers: Discontinue nursing or Elitek taking into account the importance of the drug to the mother (8.3).
See 17 for PATIENT COUNSELING INFORMATION
Revised: 02/2010

FULL PRESCRIBING INFORMATION: CONTENTS*
WARNING: ANAPHYLAXIS, HEMOLYSIS, METHEMOGLO-BINEMIA, AND INTERFERENCE WITH URIC ACID MEASUREMENTS
1 INDICATIONS AND USAGE
2 DOSAGE AND ADMINISTRATION
  2.1 Dosage
  2.2 Reconstitution Procedure
  2.3 Further Dilution and Administration
3 DOSAGE FORMS AND STRENGTHS
4 CONTRAINDICATIONS
5 WARNINGS AND PRECAUTIONS
  5.1 Anaphylaxis
  5.2 Hemolysis
  5.3 Methemoglobinemia
  5.4 Laboratory Sample Handling Procedure
6 ADVERSE REACTIONS
  6.1 Clinical Trials
  6.2 Immunogenicity
7 DRUG INTERACTIONS
8 USE IN SPECIFIC POPULATIONS
  8.1 Pregnancy
  8.3 Nursing Mothers
  8.4 Pediatric Use
  8.5 Geriatric Use
10 OVERDOSAGE
11 DESCRIPTION
12 CLINICAL PHARMACOLOGY
  12.1 Mechanism of Action
  12.2 Pharmacodynamics
  12.3 Pharmacokinetics
13 NONCLINICAL TOXICOLOGY
  13.1 Carcinogenesis, Mutagenesis, Impairment of Fertility
  13.3 Reproductive and Developmental Toxicology
14 CLINICAL STUDIES
  14.1 Pediatrics
  14.2 Studies in Adults
16 HOW SUPPLIED/STORAGE AND HANDLING
17 PATIENT COUNSELING INFORMATION
* Sections or subsections omitted from the full prescribing information are not listed

---

FULL PRESCRIBING INFORMATION

WARNING: ANAPHYLAXIS, HEMOLYSIS, METHEMO-GLOBINEMIA, AND INTERFERENCE WITH URIC ACID MEASUREMENTS
Anaphylaxis
Elitek® can cause severe hypersensitivity reactions including anaphylaxis. Immediately and permanently discontinue Elitek in patients who experience a serious hypersensitivity reaction [*see Contraindications (4), Warnings and Precautions (5.1), Adverse Reactions (6.2)*].
Hemolysis
Do not administer Elitek to patients with glucose-6-phosphate dehydrogenase (G6PD) deficiency. Immediately and permanently discontinue Elitek in patients developing hemolysis. Screen patients at higher risk for G6PD deficiency (e.g., patients of African or Mediterranean ancestry) prior to starting Elitek [*see Contraindications (4), Warnings and Precautions (5.2)*].
Methemoglobinemia
Elitek can result in methemoglobinemia in some patients. Immediately and permanently discontinue Elitek in patients developing methemoglobinemia [*see Contraindications (4), Warnings and Precautions (5.3)*].
Interference with Uric Acid Measurements
Elitek enzymatically degrades uric acid in blood samples left at room temperature. Collect blood samples in pre-chilled tubes containing heparin and immediately immerse and maintain sample in an ice water bath. Assay plasma samples within 4 hours of collection [*see Warnings and Precautions (5.4)*].

---

1 INDICATIONS AND USAGE
Elitek® is indicated for the initial management of plasma uric acid levels in pediatric and adult patients with leuke-

mia, lymphoma, and solid tumor malignancies who are receiving anti-cancer therapy expected to result in tumor lysis and subsequent elevation of plasma uric acid.
Limitation of use: Elitek is indicated only for a single course of treatment [*see Warnings and Precautions (5.1)*].

2 DOSAGE AND ADMINISTRATION
2.1 Dosage
The recommended dose of Elitek is 0.2 mg/kg as a 30 minute intravenous infusion daily for up to 5 days. Dosing beyond 5 days or administration of more than one course is not recommended.
2.2 Reconstitution Procedure
- Elitek must be reconstituted with the diluent provided in the carton.
- Reconstitute the 1.5 mg vial of Elitek with 1 mL of diluent. Reconstitute the 7.5 mg vial of Elitek with 5 mL of diluent. Mix by swirling gently. **Do not shake or vortex.**
- Inspect reconstituted Elitek visually for particulate matter and discoloration prior to administration. Discard solution if particulate matter is visible or product is discolored.
2.3 Further Dilution and Administration
- **Do not administer Elitek as a bolus injection.**
- Inject the calculated dose of reconstituted Elitek solution into an infusion bag containing the appropriate volume of 0.9% sterile sodium chloride, to achieve a final total volume of 50 mL.
- Infuse over 30 minutes through a separate line or flush line with at least 15 mL of normal saline prior to and after Elitek infusion.
- Do not use filters during reconstitution or infusion of Elitek.
- Store reconstituted or diluted solution at 2–8°C.
- Discard unused product solution 24 hours following reconstitution.

3 DOSAGE FORMS AND STRENGTHS
- 1.5 mg powder per single-use vial
- 7.5 mg powder per single-use vial

4 CONTRAINDICATIONS
Elitek is contraindicated in patients with a history of anaphylaxis or severe hypersensitivity to rasburicase or in patients with development of hemolytic reactions or methemoglobinemia with rasburicase [*see Boxed Warning, Warnings and Precautions (5)*].
Elitek is contraindicated in individuals deficient in glucose-6-phosphate dehydrogenase (G6PD) [*see Boxed Warning, Warnings and Precautions (5.2)*].

5 WARNINGS AND PRECAUTIONS
5.1 Anaphylaxis
The safety and efficacy of Elitek have been established only for a single course of treatment once daily for 5 days. Elitek can cause severe allergic reactions including anaphylaxis. In clinical studies, anaphylaxis was reported in <1% patients receiving Elitek. This can occur at any time during treatment including the first dose. Signs and symptoms of these reactions include bronchospasm, chest pain and tightness, dyspnea, hypoxia, hypotension, shock, and urticaria. Immediately and permanently discontinue Elitek administration in any patient developing clinical evidence of a serious hypersensitivity reaction [*see Boxed Warning, Contraindications (4), Adverse Reactions (6.2)*].
5.2 Hemolysis
Elitek is contraindicated in patients with G6PD deficiency because hydrogen peroxide is one of the major by-products of the conversion of uric acid to allantoin. In clinical studies, hemolysis occurs in <1% patients receiving Elitek; severe hemolytic reactions occurred within 2–4 days of the start of Elitek. Immediately and permanently discontinue Elitek administration in any patient developing hemolysis. Institute appropriate patient monitoring and support measures (e.g., transfusion support). Screen patients at higher risk for G6PD deficiency (e.g., patients of African or Mediterranean ancestry) prior to starting Elitek [*see Boxed Warning, Contraindications (4)*].
5.3 Methemoglobinemia
In clinical studies, methemoglobinemia occurred in <1% patients receiving Elitek. These included cases of serious hypoxemia requiring intervention with medical support measures. It is not known whether patients with deficiency of cytochrome b_5 reductase (formerly known as methemoglobin reductase) or of other enzymes with antioxidant activity are at increased risk for methemoglobinemia or hemolytic anemia. Immediately and permanently discontinue Elitek administration in any patient identified as having developed methemoglobinemia. Institute appropriate monitoring and support measures (e.g., transfusion support, methylene-blue administration) [*see Boxed Warning, Contraindications (4)*].
5.4 Laboratory Sample Handling Procedure
At room temperature, Elitek causes enzymatic degradation of the uric acid in blood/plasma/serum samples potentially

resulting in spuriously low plasma uric acid assay readings. The following special sample handling procedure must be followed to avoid *ex vivo* uric acid degradation.

Uric acid must be analyzed in plasma. Blood must be collected into pre-chilled tubes containing heparin anticoagulant. **Immediately immerse plasma samples for uric acid measurement in an ice water bath.** Plasma samples must be prepared by centrifugation in a pre-cooled centrifuge (4°C). Finally, the plasma must be maintained in an ice water bath and analyzed for uric acid within four hours of collection [*see Boxed Warning*].

6 ADVERSE REACTIONS

The following serious adverse reactions are discussed in greater detail in other sections of the prescribing information:

- Anaphylaxis [*see Boxed Warning, Contraindications (4), Warnings and Precautions (5.1)*]
- Hemolysis [*see Boxed Warning, Contraindications (4), Warnings and Precautions (5.2)*]
- Methemoglobinemia [*see Boxed Warning, Contraindications (4), Warnings and Precautions (5.3)*]

6.1 Clinical Trials

Because clinical trials are conducted under widely varying conditions, adverse reaction rates observed in the clinical trials of a drug cannot be directly compared to rates in the clinical trials of another drug and may not reflect the rates observed in practice.

The data below reflect exposure to Elitek in 265 pediatric and 82 adult patients enrolled in one active-controlled trial (Study 1), two uncontrolled trials (Studies 2 and 3), and an uncontrolled safety trial (n=82). Additional data were obtained from an expanded access program of 356 patients, for whom data collection was limited to serious adverse reactions. Among these 703 patients 63% were male, the median age was 10 years (range 10 days to 88 years), 73% were Caucasian, 9% African, 4% Asian, and 14% other/unknown. Among the 347 patients for whom all adverse reactions regardless of severity were assessed, the most frequently observed adverse reactions (incidence ≥10%) were vomiting (50%), fever (46%), nausea (27%), headache (26%), abdominal pain (20%), constipation (20%), diarrhea (20%), mucositis (15%), and rash (13%). In Study 1, an active control study, the following adverse reactions occurred more frequently in Elitek-treated subjects than allopurinol-treated subjects: vomiting, fever, nausea, diarrhea, and headache. Although the incidence of rash was similar in the two arms, severe rash was reported only in one Elitek-treated patient. Further studies, including one-active controlled study (Study 4) and four supportive studies, have been conducted in adult patients. In these studies, Elitek was administered to a total of 434 adult patients [58% male, 42% female; median age 56 years (range 18 years to 89 years); 52% Caucasian, 7% African, 14% Asian, 28% other/unknown].

Of these 434 patients, 275 adult patients with leukemia, lymphoma, or solid tumor malignancies at risk for hyperuricemia and tumor lysis syndrome (TLS) were randomized in an open label trial receiving either Elitek alone, Elitek in combination with allopurinol, or allopurinol alone (Study 4). A drug-related adverse reaction in Study 4 of any grade was experienced in 4.3% of Elitek-treated patients, 5.4% of Elitek/allopurinol-treated patients, and 1.1% of allopurinol-treated patients.

Table 1 presents the per patient incidence of adverse reactions by study arm in Study 4.

[See table 1 above]

Hypersensitivity reactions occurred in 4.3% of Elitek-treated patients and 1.1% of Elitek/allopurinol-treated patients in Study 4. Clinical manifestations of hypersensitivity included arthralgia, injection site irritation, peripheral edema, and rash.

The following serious adverse reactions occurred at a difference in incidence of ≥2% in patients receiving rasburicase compared to patients receiving allopurinol in randomized studies (Study 1 and Study 4): pulmonary hemorrhage, respiratory failure, supraventricular arrhythmias, ischemic coronary artery disorders, and abdominal and gastrointestinal infections.

The incidence of anaphylaxis, hemolysis, and methemoglobinemia was less than 1% of the 887 rasburicase-treated patients entered on these clinical trials.

6.2 Immunogenicity

As with all therapeutic proteins, there is potential for immunogenicity. Elitek can elicit anti-product antibodies that bind to rasburicase and in some instances inhibit the activity of rasburicase *in vitro* [*see Boxed Warning, Warnings and Precautions (5.1)*].

In clinical trials of pediatric patients with hematologic malignancies, 24/218 patients tested (11%) developed antibodies by day 28 following Elitek administration as assessed by qualitative ELISA.

Using quasi-quantitative immunoassays in rasburicase naïve adult patients with hematological malignancies, 47/260 (18%) patients were positive for anti-rasburicase immunoglobulin G (IgG), 21/260 (8%) patients were positive for anti-rasburicase neutralizing IgG, and 16/260 (6%) patients were positive for anti-rasburicase immunoglobulin E (IgE) from day 14 to 24 months after 5 daily doses of Elitek. The incidence of antibody responses detected is highly dependent on the sensitivity and specificity of the assay, which have not been fully evaluated. Additionally, the observed incidence of antibody positivity in an assay may be influenced by several factors, including serum sampling, timing and methodology, concomitant medications, and underlying disease. For these reasons, comparison of the incidence of antibodies to Elitek with the incidence of antibodies to other products may be misleading.

7 DRUG INTERACTIONS

No drug interaction studies have been conducted in humans.

Rasburicase does not metabolize allopurinol, cytarabine, methylprednisolone, methotrexate, 6-mercaptopurine, thioguanine, etoposide, daunorubicin, cyclophosphamide or vincristine *in vitro*. No metabolic-based drug interactions are therefore anticipated with these agents in patients.

In preclinical *in vivo* studies, rasburicase did not affect the activity of isoenzymes CYP1A, CYP2A, CYP2B, CYP2C, CYP2E, and CYP3A, suggesting no induction or inhibition potential. Clinically relevant P450-mediated drug-drug interactions are therefore not anticipated in patients treated with the recommended Elitek dose and dosing schedule.

8 USE IN SPECIFIC POPULATIONS

8.1 Pregnancy

Pregnancy Category C

There are no studies of rasburicase in pregnant women. Reproductive toxicity studies in rabbits treated during organogenesis with approximately 10 to 100 times the recommended human dose of rasburicase resulted in teratogenicity, including decreased fetal body weights and heart and great vessel malformations at all dose levels. Multiple heart and great vessel malformations were also observed in offspring of pregnant rats treated with approximately 250 times the recommended human dose of rasburicase. Other adverse effects were observed in rasburicase-treated pregnant rabbits at all dose levels tested and included pre- and post-implantation losses, abortions, and decreased uterine weights [*See Nonclinical Toxicology (13.3)*].

It is unknown whether rasburicase can cross the placental barrier in humans and result in fetal harm. Because of the observed teratogenic effects of rasburicase in animal reproductive studies, use rasburicase during pregnancy only if the potential benefit to the mother justifies the potential risk to the fetus.

8.3 Nursing Mothers

It is not known whether rasburicase is excreted in human milk. Because many drugs are excreted in human milk and because of the potential for serious adverse reactions in nursing infants from rasburicase, a decision should be made whether to discontinue nursing or to discontinue rasburicase, taking into account the importance of the drug to the mother.

8.4 Pediatric Use

The safety and efficacy of Elitek was studied in 246 pediatric patients ranging in age from 1 month to 17 years. There were insufficient numbers of patients between 0 and 6 months (n=7) to determine whether they respond differently from older children. Mean uric acid $AUC_{0-96\ hr}$ was higher in children <2 years of age (n=24; 150 ± s.e. 16 mg hr/dL) than those age 2 to 17 years (n=222; 108 ± s.e. 4 mg hr/dL). Children <2 years of age had a lower rate of achieving normal uric acid concentration by 48 hours [83% (95% CI: 62, 95)] than those 2 to 17 years [93% (95% CI: 89, 95)].

8.5 Geriatric Use

Of the total number of adults treated with Elitek (n=434) in clinical studies, 30% were aged 65 and over while 8% were aged 75 and over. No overall differences in pharmacokinetics, safety, and effectiveness were observed between the elderly and younger patients.

10 OVERDOSAGE

The maximum reported overdosage of Elitek is a single dose of 1.3 mg/kg. No adverse events occurred in reported cases of overdosage. Monitor patients who receive an overdose and initiate supportive measures if required.

11 DESCRIPTION

Elitek (rasburicase) is a recombinant urate-oxidase produced by a genetically modified *Saccharomyces cerevisiae* strain. The cDNA coding for rasburicase was cloned from a strain of *Aspergillus flavus*.

Rasburicase is a tetrameric protein with identical subunits. Each subunit is made up of a single 301 amino acid polypeptide chain with a molecular mass of about 34 kDa. The drug product is a sterile, white to off-white, lyophilized powder intended for intravenous administration following reconstitution with a diluent. Elitek is supplied in 3 mL and 10 mL colorless, glass vials containing rasburicase at a concentration of 1.5 mg/mL after reconstitution.

Elitek 1.5 mg presentation contains 1.5 mg rasburicase, 10.6 mg mannitol, 15.9 mg L-alanine, between 12.6 and 14.3 mg of dibasic sodium phosphate (lyophilized powder), and a diluent (1 mL Water for Injection, USP, and 1 mg Poloxamer 188).

Elitek 7.5 mg presentation contains 7.5 mg of rasburicase, 53 mg mannitol, 79.5 mg L-alanine, and between 63 and 71.5 mg dibasic sodium phosphate (lyophilized powder) and a diluent (5 mL Water for Injection, USP, and 5 mg Poloxamer 188).

12 CLINICAL PHARMACOLOGY

12.1 Mechanism of Action

In humans, uric acid is the final step in the catabolic pathway of purines. Rasburicase catalyzes enzymatic oxidation of poorly soluble uric acid into an inactive and more soluble metabolite (allantoin).

Table 1 – per patient incidence of selected adverse reactions by study arm in Study 4

Adverse Reaction*	Elitek (n=92)		Elitek/Allopurinol (n=92)		Allopurinol (n=91)	
	All Grades %	Grades 3,4 %	All Grades %	Grades 3,4 %	All Grades %	Grades 3,4 %
Nausea	57.6	1.1	60.9	1.1	54.9	2.2
Peripheral edema	50	2.2	43.5	3.3	42.9	6.6
Vomiting	38	1.1	37	0	30.8	1.1
Anxiety	23.9	3.3	17.4	0	17.6	0
Abdominal pain	21.7	3.3	33.7	4.3	25.3	2.2
Hypophosphatemia	17.4	4.3	22.8	6.5	16.5	6.6
Hyperbilirubinemia	16.3	3.3	14.1	2.2	7.7	4.4
Pharyngolaryngeal pain	14.1	1.1	20.7	0	9.9	0
Sepsis	12	5.4	7.6	6.5	4.4	4.4
Fluid overload	12	0	6.5	0	3.3	1.1
Increased alanine aminotransferase	10.9	3.3	27.2	4.3	17.6	2.2
Hyperphosphatemia	9.8	0	15.2	0	8.8	1.1

* Events were reported and graded according to NCI-CTC version 3.0 and presented as preferred terms MedDRA version 10.1.

* Overall incidence ≥10% in any Elitek arm and the difference between any Elitek arm versus the allopurinol arm ≥5%.

12.2 Pharmacodynamics

The measurement of plasma uric acid was used to evaluate the effectiveness of rasburicase in clinical studies. Following administration of either 0.15 or 0.20 mg/kg rasburicase daily for up to 5 days, plasma uric acid levels decreased within 4 hours and were maintained below 7.5 mg/dL in 98% of adult and 90% of pediatric patients for at least 7 days. There was no evidence of a dose response effect on uric acid control for doses between 0.15 and 0.20 mg/kg rasburicase.

12.3 Pharmacokinetics

The pharmacokinetics of rasburicase were evaluated in both pediatric and adult patients with leukemia, lymphoma or other hematological malignancies. Rasburicase exposure, as measured by $AUC_{0-24\ hr}$ and C_{max}, tended to increase with a dose range from 0.15 to 0.2 mg/kg. The mean terminal half-life was similar between pediatric and adult patients and ranged from 15.7 to 22.5 hours. The mean volume of distribution of rasburicase ranged from 110 to 127 mL/kg in pediatric patients and from 75.8 to 138 mL/kg in adult patients, respectively. Minimal accumulation of rasburicase (<1.3 fold) was observed between days 1 and 5 of dosing. In adults, age, gender, baseline liver enzymes and creatinine clearance did not impact the pharmacokinetics of rasburicase. A cross-study comparison revealed that after administration of rasburicase at 0.15 or 0.20 mg/kg, the geometric mean values of body-weight normalized clearance were approximately 40% lower in Japanese (n=20) than that in Caucasians (n=22).

13 NONCLINICAL TOXICOLOGY

13.1 Carcinogenesis, Mutagenesis, Impairment of Fertility

Carcinogenicity studies in animals to evaluate tumoriogenic potential of rasburicase have not been performed. Rasburicase was not mutagenic in the Ames, unscheduled DNA synthesis, chromosome analysis, mouse lymphoma, and micronucleus tests.

Rasburicase did not affect reproductive performance or fertility in male or female rats at a dose 50-fold higher (10 mg/kg) than the recommended human dose.

13.3 Reproductive and Developmental Toxicology

Pregnant rabbits dosed daily with 10 to 100 times the human dose of rasburicase during the period of organogenesis (gestation day 6–19) exhibited teratogenic effects, clinical signs of maternal toxicity including weight loss and mortality, decreases in uterine weights and viable fetuses, and increased fetal resorptions, post-implantation losses and abortions. Teratogenic effects included multiple heart and great vessel malformations at all dose levels. Multiple heart and great vessel malformations were also observed in offspring of pregnant rats treated with approximately 250 times the recommended human dose of rasburicase. There are no data available regarding the level of rasburicase exposure in the offspring.

14 CLINICAL STUDIES

14.1 Pediatrics

Elitek was administered in three studies to 265 patients with acute leukemia or non-Hodgkin's lymphoma. These clinical studies were largely limited to pediatric patients (246 of 265). Elitek was administered as a 30-minute infusion once (n=251) or twice (n=14) daily at a dose of 0.15 or 0.2 mg/kg/dose (total daily dose 0.2–0.4 mg/kg/day). Elitek was administered prior to and concurrent with anti-tumor therapy, which consisted of either systemic chemotherapy (n=196) or steroids (n=69).

Study 1

Study 1 was a randomized, open-label, controlled study conducted at six institutions, in which 52 pediatric patients were randomized to receive either Elitek (n=27) or allopurinol (n=25). The dose of allopurinol varied according to local institutional practice. Elitek was administered as an intravenous infusion over 30 minutes once (n=26) or twice (n=1) daily at a dose of 0.2 mg/kg/dose (total daily dose 0.2–0.4 mg/kg/day). Initiation of dosing was permitted at any time between 4 to 48 hours before the start of anti-tumor therapy and could be continued for 5 to 7 days after initiation of anti-tumor therapy. Patients were stratified at randomization on the basis of underlying malignant disease (leukemia or lymphoma) and baseline serum or plasma uric acid levels (<8 mg/dL and ≥8 mg/dL). The primary study objective was to demonstrate a greater reduction in uric acid concentration over 96 hours ($AUC_{0-96\ hr}$) in the Elitek group as compared to the allopurinol group. Uric acid $AUC_{0-96\ hr}$ was defined as the area under the curve for plasma uric acid levels (mg hr/dL), measured from the last value prior to the first dose of Elitek until 96 hours after that first dose. Plasma uric acid levels were used for all uric acid $AUC_{0-96\ hr}$ calculations [*see Warnings and Precautions (5.4)*].

The demographics of the two study arms (Elitek vs. allopurinol) were as follows: age <13 years (82% vs. 76%), males (59% vs. 72%), Caucasian (59% vs. 72%), ECOG performance status 0 (89% vs. 84%), and leukemia (74% vs. 76%).

Table 2 – Summary of Response Rates

	Arm A Elitek n=92	Arm B Elitek/Allopurinol n=92	Arm C Allopurinol n=91
Response Rate % (95% CI)	87% (80%, 94%)	78% (70%, 87%)	66% (56%, 76%)
Non-Response Rate %	13%	22%	34%
Failed to control uric acid	0	0	11%
Hyperuricemic treatment extended beyond 5 days	0	6.5%	4.4%
Missing uric acid samples	13%	15%	19%

The median interval, in hours, between initiation of Elitek and of anti-tumor treatment was 20 hours, with a range of 70 hours before to 10 hours after the initiation of anti-tumor treatment (n=24, data not reported for 3 patients).

The uric acid $AUC_{0-96\ hr}$ was significantly lower in the Elitek group (128 ± s.e. 14 mg hr/dL) as compared to the allopurinol group (328 ± s.e. 26 mg hr/dL). All but one patient in the Elitek arm had reduction and maintenance of uric acid levels to within or below the normal range during the treatment. The incidence of renal dysfunction was similar in the two study arms; one patient in the allopurinol arm developed acute renal failure.

Study 2

Study 2 was a multi-institutional, single-arm study conducted in 89 pediatric and 18 adult patients with hematologic malignancies. Patients received Elitek at a dose of 0.15 mg/kg/day. The primary efficacy objective was determination of the proportion of patients with maintained plasma uric acid concentration at 48 hours where maintenance of uric acid concentration was defined as: 1) achievement of uric acid concentration ≤6.5 mg/dL (patients <13 years) or ≤7.5 mg/dL (patients ≥13 years) within a designated time point (48 hours) from initiation of Elitek and maintained until 24 hours after the last administration of study drug; and 2) control of uric acid level without the need for allopurinol or other agents.

The study population demographics were: age <13 years (76%), males (61%), Caucasian (91%), ECOG performance status=0 (92%), and leukemia (89%).

The proportion of patients with maintenance of uric acid concentration at 48 hours in Study 2 was 99% (106/107).

Study 3

Study 3 was a multi-institutional, single-arm study conducted in 130 pediatric patients and 1 adult patient with hematologic malignancies. Patients received Elitek at either a dose of 0.15 mg/kg/day (n=12) or 0.2 mg/kg/day (n=119). The primary efficacy objective was determination of the proportion of patients with maintained plasma uric acid concentration at 48 hours as defined for Study 2 above. The study population demographics were: age <13 years (76%), Caucasian (83%), males (67%), ECOG=0 (67%), and leukemia (88%).

The proportion of patients with maintenance of uric acid concentration at 48 hours in Study 3 was 92% in the 0.15 mg/kg group (n=12) and 95% in the 0.2 mg/kg group (n=119).

Pooled Analyses of Studies 1, 2, and 3

Data from the 3 studies (n=265) were pooled and analyzed according to the plasma uric acid levels over time. The pre-treatment plasma uric acid concentration was ≥8 mg/dL in 61 patients and was <8 mg/dL in 200 patients. The median uric acid concentration at baseline, at 4 hours following the first dose of Elitek, and the per patient fall in plasma uric acid concentration from baseline to 4 hours were calculated in those patients with both pre-treatment and 4-hour post-treatment values. Among patients with pre-treatment uric acid ≥8 mg/dL [baseline median 10.6 mg/dL (range 8.1–36.4)], the median per-patient change in plasma uric acid concentration by 4 hours after the first dose was a decrease of 9.1 mg/dL (0.3–19.3 mg/dL). Among the patients with a pre-treatment plasma uric acid level <8 mg/dL [baseline median 4.6 mg/dL (range 0.2–7.9 mg/dL)], the median per-patient change in plasma uric acid concentration by 4 hours after the first dose was a decrease of 4.1 mg/dL (0.1–7.6 mg/dL).

[See figure at top of next column]

Figure 1 is a box and whisker plot of plasma uric acid levels inclusive of 261 of the 265 Elitek treated patients from Studies 1, 2, and 3. Of the 261 evaluable patients, plasma uric acid concentration was maintained [*see Study 2* for the definition of uric acid concentration maintenance], by 4 hours for 92% of patients (240/261), by 24 hours for 93% of patients (245/261), by 48 hours for 97% of patients (254/261), by 72 hours for 99% of patients (260/261), and by 96 hours for 100% of patients (261/261). Of the subset of 61 patients whose plasma uric acid level was elevated at baseline (≥8 mg/dL), plasma uric acid concentration was maintained by 4 hours for 72% of patients (44/61), by 24 hours for 80% of patients (49/61), by 48 hours for 92% of patients (56/61), by 72 hours for 98% of patients (60/61), and by 96 hours for 100% (61/61).

Figure 1. Box and Whisker Plot of Uric Acid Concentration at designated time blocks. ELITEK administration began immediately after baseline.

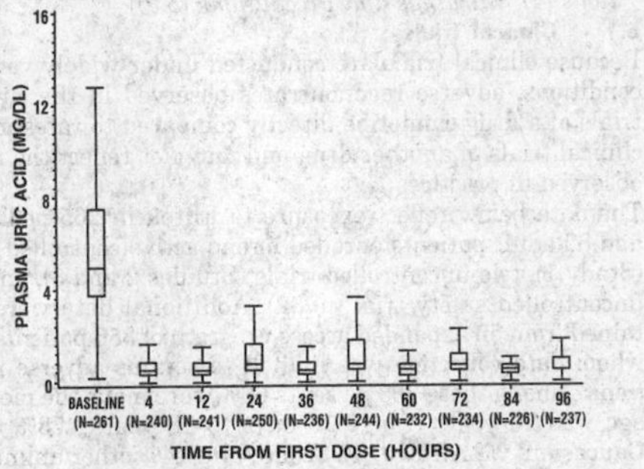

14.2 Studies in Adults

A total of 342 adults with either leukemia, lymphoma, or other hematologic malignancy received Elitek in five studies (one randomized study, Study 4, and four uncontrolled studies). Across the five studies, Elitek was administered at a dose of 0.15 mg/kg/day (n=38) or 0.2 mg/kg/day (n=304).

Study 4 was a randomized (1:1:1), multi-center, open-label study conducted in patients with leukemia, lymphoma, and solid tumor malignancies at risk for hyperuricemia and TLS. A total of 275 adult patients received at least one dose of study drug. The median age was 56 years, 62% were males, 80% were Caucasian, 66% had leukemia, 29% had lymphoma, 18% were hyperuricemic (uric acid ≥7.5mg/dL) at study entry. Patients in Arm A received Elitek for 5 days (n=92). Patients in Arm B received Elitek from day 1 through day 3 followed by oral allopurinol from day 3 through day 5 (overlap on day 3: Elitek and allopurinol administered approximately 12 hours apart) (n=92). Patients in Arm C received oral allopurinol for 5 days (n=91). Elitek was administered at the dose of 0.2 mg/kg/day as a 30-minute infusion once daily. Allopurinol was administered orally at the dose of 300 mg once a day. Patients were eligible for the study if they were either at high risk, or potential risk for TLS. The major endpoint of this study was the uric acid response rate defined as the proportion of patients with plasma uric acid levels ≤7.5 mg/dL from day 3 to day 7, after initiation of antihyperuricemic treatment.

Table 2 presents the response rates in the three treatment arms. The response rate in arm A was significantly greater than in arm C (p=0.0009). The response rate was higher for arm B compared to arm C; this difference was not statistically significant.

[See table 1 above]

There were no patients with documented failure to control uric acid in arms A or B. In arm C, 34% of patients did not have a uric acid response; 11% due to failure to control uric acid and 4.4% due to the need for extended antihyperuricemic treatment.

Box and whisker plots of uric acid over time for the patient population (Figure 2) show that in the two arms containing Elitek, uric acid levels were ≤2 mg/dL in 96% of patients at 4 hours of the day 1 dose.

[See figure 2 at top of next page]

Tumor lysis syndrome (TLS)

Clinical TLS was defined by changes in at least two or more laboratory parameters for hyperuricemia, hyperkalemia, hyperphosphatemia and hypocalcemia and at least one of the following events occurring within 7 days of treatment: renal failure/injury, need for renal dialysis, and/or serum creatinine increase >1.5 ULN, arrhythmia or seizure. Clin-

Figure 2 – Uric acid concentration over time – Patient population
Box and Whisker plot

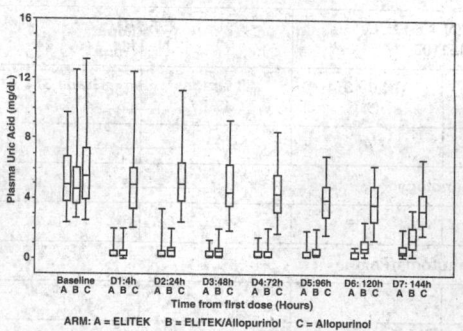

ARM: A = ELITEK   B = ELITEK/Allopurinol   C = Allopurinol

ical TLS occurred in 3% of Elitek-treated patients, 3% of Elitek/allopurinol-treated patients, and 4% of allopurinol-treated patients.

16   HOW SUPPLIED/STORAGE AND HANDLING

How Supplied
NDC 0024-5150-10:   One carton contains 3 single-use vials each containing 1.5 mg of rasburicase and 3 ampules each containing 1 mL diluent.
NDC 0024-5151-75:   One carton contains 1 single-use vial containing 7.5 mg of rasburicase and 1 ampule containing 5 mL diluent.
Storage and Handling
The lyophilized drug product and the diluent for reconstitution should be stored at 2–8°C (36–46°F). **Do not freeze.** Protect from light.

17   PATIENT COUNSELING INFORMATION

Instruct patients to notify their physician immediately if any of the following occur: allergic reaction, bronchospasm, chest pain or tightness, dyspnea, hypoxia, hypotension, shock or urticaria.

Manufactured by:
sanofi-aventis U.S. LLC
Bridgewater, NJ 08807
U.S. License No. 1752
Manufactured at:
GlaxoSmithKline
76960 Notre-Dame de Bondeville, France
Diluent manufactured at:
Hospira Inc.
Lake Forest, IL 60045
© 2010 sanofi-aventis U.S. LLC

ELOXATIN®
[eh-LOX-ah-tin]
(oxaliplatin)
powder, for solution for intravenous use
ELOXATIN®
(oxaliplatin)
injection, solution, concentrate for intravenous use   ℞

HIGHLIGHTS OF PRESCRIBING INFORMATION
These highlights do not include all the information needed to use ELOXATIN safely and effectively. See full prescribing information for ELOXATIN.
ELOXATIN (oxaliplatin) powder, for solution for intravenous use
ELOXATIN (oxaliplatin) injection, solution, concentrate for intravenous use
Initial U.S. Approval: 2002

WARNING: ANAPHYLACTIC REACTIONS
See full prescribing information for complete boxed warning.
Anaphylactic reactions to ELOXATIN have been reported, and may occur within minutes of ELOXATIN administration. Epinephrine, corticosteroids, and anti-histamines have been employed to alleviate symptoms. (5.1)

—————INDICATIONS AND USAGE—————
ELOXATIN is a platinum-based drug used in combination with infusional 5-fluorouracil/leucovorin, which is indicated for:
• adjuvant treatment of stage *III* colon cancer in patients who have undergone complete resection of the primary tumor.
• treatment of advanced colorectal cancer. (1)

—————DOSAGE AND ADMINISTRATION—————
• Administer ELOXATIN in combination with 5-fluorouracil/leucovorin every 2 weeks. (2.1):
  – Day 1:   ELOXATIN 85 mg/m² intravenous infusion in 250–500 mL 5% Dextrose Injection, USP and leucovo-

rin 200 mg/m² intravenous infusion in 5% Dextrose Injection, USP both given over 120 minutes at the same time in separate bags using a Y-line, followed by 5-fluorouracil 400 mg/m² intravenous bolus given over 2–4 minutes, followed by 5-fluorouracil 600 mg/m² intravenous infusion in 500 mL 5% Dextrose Injection, USP (recommended) as a 22-hour continuous infusion.
  – Day 2:   leucovorin 200 mg/m² intravenous infusion over 120 minutes, followed by 5-fluorouracil 400 mg/m² intravenous bolus given over 2–4 minutes, followed by 5-fluorouracil 600 mg/m² intravenous infusion in 500 mL 5% Dextrose Injection, USP (recommended) as a 22-hour continuous infusion.
• Reduce the dose of ELOXATIN to 75 mg/m² (adjuvant setting) or 65 mg/m² (advanced colorectal cancer) (2.2):
  – if there are persistent grade 2 neurosensory events that do not resolve.
  – after recovery from grade 3/4 gastrointestinal toxicities (despite prophylactic treatment) or grade 4 neutropenia or grade 3/4 thrombocytopenia. Delay next dose until neutrophils ≥1.5 × 10⁹/L and platelets ≥75 × 10⁹/L.
• Discontinue ELOXATIN if there are persistent Grade 3 neurosensory events. (2.2)
• Never reconstitute or prepare final dilution with a sodium chloride solution or other chloride-containing solutions. (2.3)

—————DOSAGE FORMS AND STRENGTHS—————
Single-use vials of 50 mg or 100 mg oxaliplatin as a sterile, preservative-free lyophilized powder for reconstitution. (3)
Single-use vials of 50 mg, 100 mg or 200 mg oxaliplatin as a sterile, preservative-free, aqueous solution at a concentration of 5 mg/ml. (3)

—————CONTRAINDICATIONS—————
• Known allergy to ELOXATIN or other platinum compounds. (4, 5.1)

—————WARNINGS AND PRECAUTIONS—————
• Allergic Reactions: Monitor for development of rash, urticaria, erythema, pruritis, bronchospasm, and hypotension. (5.1)
• Neuropathy: Reduce the dose or discontinue ELOXATIN if necessary. (5.2)
• Pulmonary Toxicity: May need to discontinue ELOXATIN until interstitial lung disease or pulmonary fibrosis are excluded. (5.3)
• Hepatotoxicity: Monitor liver function tests. (5.4)
• Pregnancy. Fetal harm can occur when administered to a pregnant woman. Women should be apprised of the potential harm to the fetus. (5.5, 8.1)

—————ADVERSE REACTIONS—————
• Most common adverse reactions (incidence ≥ 40%) were peripheral sensory neuropathy, neutropenia, thrombocytopenia, anemia, nausea, increase in transaminases and alkaline phosphatase, diarrhea, emesis, fatigue and stomatitis. Other adverse reactions, including serious adverse reactions, have been reported. (6.1)

To report SUSPECTED ADVERSE REACTIONS, contact sanofi-aventis U.S. LLC at 1-800-633-1610 or FDA at 1-800-FDA-1088 or www.fda.gov/medwatch
See 17 for PATIENT COUNSELING INFORMATION and FDA-approved patient labeling

Revised: 03/2009

FULL PRESCRIBING INFORMATION: CONTENTS*
WARNING: ANAPHYLACTIC REACTIONS

*Sections or subsections omitted from the full prescribing information are not listed

---

FULL PRESCRIBING INFORMATION

WARNING: ANAPHYLACTIC REACTIONS
Anaphylactic reactions to ELOXATIN have been reported, and may occur within minutes of ELOXATIN administration. Epinephrine, corticosteroids, and antihistamines have been employed to alleviate symptoms of anaphylaxis *[see Warnings and Precautions (5.1)]*.

---

1   INDICATIONS AND USAGE
ELOXATIN, used in combination with infusional 5-fluorouracil/leucovorin, is indicated for:
• adjuvant treatment of stage III colon cancer in patients who have undergone complete resection of the primary tumor.
• treatment of advanced colorectal cancer.

2   DOSAGE AND ADMINISTRATION
ELOXATIN (oxaliplatin injection) should be administered under the supervision of a qualified physician experienced in the use of cancer chemotherapeutic agents. Appropriate management of therapy and complications is possible only when adequate diagnostic and treatment facilities are readily available.

2.1   Dosage
Administer ELOXATIN in combination with 5-fluorouracil/leucovorin every 2 weeks. For advanced disease, treatment is recommended until disease progression or unacceptable toxicity. For adjuvant use, treatment is recommended for a total of 6 months (12 cycles):
Day 1:   ELOXATIN 85 mg/m² intravenous infusion in 250–500 mL 5% Dextrose injection, USP and leucovorin 200 mg/m² intravenous infusion in 5% Dextrose Injection, USP both given over 120 minutes at the same time in separate bags using a Y-line, followed by 5-fluorouracil 400 mg/m² intravenous bolus given over 2–4 minutes, followed by 5-fluorouracil 600 mg/m² intravenous infusion in 500 mL 5% Dextrose Injection, USP (recommended) as a 22-hour continuous infusion.
Day 2:   Leucovorin 200 mg/m² intravenous infusion over 120 minutes, followed by 5-fluorouracil 400 mg/m² intravenous bolus given over 2–4 minutes, followed by 5-fluorouracil 600 mg/m² intravenous infusion in 500 mL 5% Dextrose Injection, USP (recommended) as a 22-hour continuous infusion.

Figure 1

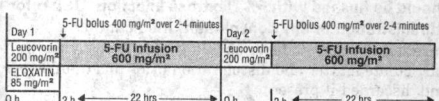

The administration of ELOXATIN does not require prehydration. Premedication with antiemetics, including 5-HT₃ blockers with or without dexamethasone, is recommended. For information on 5-fluorouracil and leucovorin, see the respective package inserts.

2.2   Dose Modification Recommendations
Prior to subsequent therapy cycles, patients should be evaluated for clinical toxicities and recommended laboratory tests *[see Warnings and Precautions (5.6)]*. Prolongation of infusion time for ELOXATIN from 2 hours to 6 hours may mitigate acute toxicities. The infusion times for 5-fluorouracil and leucovorin do not need to be changed.
Adjuvant Therapy in Patients with Stage III Colon Cancer
Neuropathy and other toxicities were graded using the NCI CTC scale version 1 *[see Warnings and Precautions (5.2)]*.

For patients who experience persistent Grade 2 neurosensory events that do not resolve, a dose reduction of ELOXATIN to 75 mg/m^2 should be considered. For patients with persistent Grade 3 neurosensory events, discontinuing therapy should be considered. The infusional 5-fluorouracil/leucovorin regimen need not be altered.

A dose reduction of ELOXATIN to 75 mg/m^2 and infusional 5-fluorouracil to 300 mg/m^2 bolus and 500 mg/m^2 22 hour infusion is recommended for patients after recovery from grade 3/4 gastrointestinal (despite prophylactic treatment) or grade 4 neutropenia or grade 3/4 thrombocytopenia. The next dose should be delayed until: neutrophils ≥1.5 × 10^9/L and platelets ≥75 × 10^9/L.

Dose Modifications in Therapy in Previously Untreated and Previously Treated Patients with Advanced Colorectal Cancer
Neuropathy was graded using a study-specific neurotoxicity scale *[see Warnings and Precautions (5.2)]*. Other toxicities were graded by the NCI CTC, Version 2.0.
For patients who experience persistent Grade 2 neurosensory events that do not resolve, a dose reduction of ELOXATIN to 65 mg/m^2 should be considered. For patients with persistent Grade 3 neurosensory events, discontinuing therapy should be considered. The 5-fluorouracil/leucovorin regimen need not be altered.
A dose reduction of ELOXATIN to 65 mg/m^2 and 5-fluorouracil by 20% (300 mg/m^2 bolus and 500 mg/m^2 22-hour infusion) is recommended for patients after recovery from grade 3/4 gastrointestinal (despite prophylactic treatment) or grade 4 neutropenia or grade 3/4 thrombocytopenia. The next dose should be delayed until: neutrophils ≥1.5 × 10^9/L and platelets ≥75 × 10^9/L.

2.3 Preparation of Infusion Solution
Powder for solution for infusion
Reconstitution or final dilution must never be performed with a sodium chloride solution or other chloride containing solutions.
The lyophilized powder is reconstituted by adding 10 mL (for the 50 mg vial) or 20 mL (for the 100 mg vial) of Water for Injection, USP or 5% Dextrose Injection, USP. **Do not administer the reconstituted solution without further dilution. The reconstituted solution must be further diluted in an infusion solution of 250–500 mL of 5% Dextrose Injection, USP.**
After reconstitution in the original vial, the solution may be stored up to 24 hours under refrigeration [2–8°C (36–46°F)]. After final dilution with 250–500 mL of 5% Dextrose Injection, USP, the shelf life is **6 hours at room temperature [20–25°C (68–77°F)] or up to 24 hours under refrigeration [2–8°C (36–46°F)].**
ELOXATIN is not light sensitive.
Concentrate for solution for infusion
Do not freeze and protect from light the concentrated solution.
A final dilution must never be performed with a sodium chloride solution or other chloride-containing solutions.
The solution must be further diluted in an infusion solution of 250–500 mL of 5% Dextrose Injection, USP.
After dilution with 250–500 mL of 5% Dextrose Injection, USP, the shelf life is **6 hours at room temperature [20–25°C (68–77°F)] or up to 24 hours under refrigeration [2–8°C (36–46°F)].** After final dilution, protection from light is not required.
ELOXATIN is incompatible in solution with alkaline medications or media (such as basic solutions of 5-fluorouracil) and must not be mixed with these or administered simultaneously through the same infusion line. **The infusion line should be flushed with 5% Dextrose Injection, USP prior to administration of any concomitant medication.**
Parenteral drug products should be inspected visually for particulate matter and discoloration prior to administration and discarded if present.
Needles or intravenous administration sets containing aluminum parts that may come in contact with ELOXATIN should not be used for the preparation or mixing of the drug. Aluminum has been reported to cause degradation of platinum compounds.

3 DOSAGE FORMS AND STRENGTHS
ELOXATIN is supplied in single-use vials containing 50 mg or 100 mg of oxaliplatin as a sterile, preservative-free lyophilized powder for reconstitution.
ELOXATIN is supplied in single-use vials containing 50 mg, 100 mg or 200 mg of oxaliplatin as a sterile, preservative-free, aqueous solution at a concentration of 5 mg/ml.

4 CONTRAINDICATIONS
ELOXATIN should not be administered to patients with a history of known allergy to ELOXATIN or other platinum compounds *[see Warnings and Precautions (5.1)]*.

Table 3 - Adverse Reactions Reported in Patients with Colon Cancer receiving Adjuvant Treatment (≥5% of all patients and with ≥1% NCI Grade 3/4 events)

Adverse reaction (WHO/Pref)	ELOXATIN + 5-FU/LV N=1108		5-FU/LV N=1111	
	All Grades (%)	Grade 3/4 (%)	All Grades (%)	Grade 3/4 (%)
Any Event	100	70	99	31
Allergy/Immunology				
Allergic Reaction	10	3	2	<1
Constitutional Symptoms/Pain				
Fatigue	44	4	38	1
Abdominal Pain	18	1	17	2
Dermatology/Skin				
Skin Disorder	32	2	36	2
Injection Site Reaction*	11	3	10	3
Gastrointestinal				
Nausea	74	5	61	2
Diarrhea	56	11	48	7
Vomiting	47	6	24	1
Stomatitis	42	3	40	2
Anorexia	13	1	8	<1
Fever/Infection				
Fever	27	1	12	1
Infection	25	4	25	3
Neurology				
Overall Peripheral Sensory Neuropathy	92	12	16	<1

*Includes thrombosis related to the catheter

5 WARNINGS AND PRECAUTIONS
5.1 Allergic Reactions
See boxed warning
Grade 3/4 hypersensitivity, including anaphylactic/anaphylactoid reactions, to ELOXATIN has been observed in 2–3% of colon cancer patients. These allergic reactions which can be fatal, can occur within minutes of administration and at any cycle, and were similar in nature and severity to those reported with other platinum-containing compounds, such as rash, urticaria, erythema, pruritus, and, rarely, bronchospasm and hypotension. The symptoms associated with hypersensitivity reactions reported in the previously untreated patients were urticaria, pruritus, flushing of the face, diarrhea associated with oxaliplatin infusion, shortness of breath, bronchospasm, diaphoresis, chest pains, hypotension, disorientation and syncope. These reactions are usually managed with standard epinephrine, corticosteroid, antihistamine therapy, and may require discontinuation of therapy. Drug-related deaths associated with platinum compounds from anaphylaxis have been reported.

5.2 Neuropathy
ELOXATIN is associated with two types of neuropathy:
An acute, reversible, primarily peripheral, sensory neuropathy that is of early onset, occurring within hours or one to two days of dosing, that resolves within 14 days, and that frequently recurs with further dosing. The symptoms may be precipitated or exacerbated by exposure to cold temperature or cold objects and they usually present as transient paresthesia, dysesthesia and hypoesthesia in the hands, feet, perioral area, or throat. Jaw spasm, abnormal tongue sensation, dysarthria, eye pain, and a feeling of chest pressure have also been observed. The acute, reversible pattern of sensory neuropathy was observed in about 56% of study patients who received ELOXATIN with 5-fluorouracil/leucovorin. In any individual cycle acute neurotoxicity was observed in approximately 30% of patients. In adjuvant patients the median cycle of onset for grade 3 peripheral sensory neuropathy was 9 in the previously treated patients the median number of cycles administered on the ELOXATIN with 5-fluorouracil/leucovorin combination arm was 6.
An acute syndrome of pharyngolaryngeal dysesthesia seen in 1–2% (grade 3/4) of patients previously untreated for advanced colorectal cancer, and the previously treated patients, is characterized by subjective sensations of dysphagia or dyspnea, without any laryngospasm or bronchospasm (no stridor or wheezing). Ice (mucositis prophylaxis) should be avoided during the infusion of ELOXATIN because cold temperature can exacerbate acute neurological symptoms. **A persistent (>14 days), primarily peripheral, sensory neuropathy that is usually characterized by paresthesias, dysesthesias, hypoesthesias, but may also include deficits in proprioception that can interfere with daily activities (e.g., writing, buttoning, swallowing, and difficulty walking from impaired proprioception).** These forms of neuropathy occurred in 48% of the study patients receiving ELOXATIN with 5-fluorouracil/leucovorin. Persistent neuropathy can occur without any prior acute neuropathy event. The majority of the patients (80%) who developed grade 3 persistent neuropathy progressed from prior Grade 1 or 2 events. These symptoms may improve in some patients upon discontinuation of ELOXATIN.
In the adjuvant colon cancer trial, neuropathy was graded using a prelisted module derived from the Neuro-Sensory section of the National Cancer Institute Common Toxicity Criteria (NCI CTC) scale, Version 1, as follows:

Table 1 - NCI CTC Grading for Neuropathy in Adjuvant Patients

Grade	Definition
Grade 0	No change or none
Grade 1	Mild paresthesias, loss of deep tendon reflexes
Grade 2	Mild or moderate objective sensory loss, moderate paresthesias
Grade 3	Severe objective sensory loss or paresthesias that interfere with function
Grade 4	Not applicable

Peripheral sensory neuropathy was reported in adjuvant patients treated with the ELOXATIN combination with a frequency of 92% (all grades) and 13% (grade 3). At the 28-day follow-up after the last treatment cycle, 60% of all patients had any grade (Grade 1=40%, Grade 2=16%, Grade 3=5%) peripheral sensory neuropathy decreasing to 39% at 6 months follow-up (Grade 1=31%, Grade 2=7%, Grade 3=1%) and 21% at 18 months of follow-up (Grade 1=17%, Grade 2=3%, Grade 3=1%).

In the advanced colorectal cancer studies, neuropathy was graded using a study-specific neurotoxicity scale, which was different from the NCI CTC scale, Version 2.0 (see below).

Table 2 - Grading Scale for Paresthesias/Dysesthesias in Advanced Colorectal Cancer Patients

Grade	Definition
Grade 1	Resolved and did not interfere with functioning
Grade 2	Interfered with function but not daily activities
Grade 3	Pain or functional impairment that interfered with daily activities
Grade 4	Persistent impairment that is disabling or life-threatening

Overall, neuropathy was reported in patients previously untreated for advanced colorectal cancer in 82% (all grades) and 19% (grade 3/4), and in the previously treated patients in 74% (all grades) and 7% (grade 3/4) events. Information regarding reversibility of neuropathy was not available from the trial for patients who had not been previously treated for colorectal cancer.

5.3   Pulmonary Toxicity
ELOXATIN has been associated with pulmonary fibrosis (<1% of study patients), which may be fatal. The combined incidence of cough and dyspnea was 7.4% (any grade) and <1% (grade 3) with no grade 4 events in the ELOXATIN plus infusional 5-fluorouracil/leucovorin arm compared to 4.5% (any grade) and no grade 3 and 0.1% grade 4 events in the infusional 5-fluorouracil/leucovorin alone arm in adjuvant colon cancer patients. In this study, one patient died from eosinophilic pneumonia in the ELOXATIN combination arm. The combined incidence of cough, dyspnea and hypoxia was 43% (any grade) and 7% (grade 3 and 4) in the ELOXATIN plus 5-fluorouracil/leucovorin arm compared to 32% (any grade) and 5% (grade 3 and 4) in the irinotecan plus 5-fluorouracil/leucovorin arm of unknown duration for patients with previously untreated colorectal cancer. In case of unexplained respiratory symptoms such as nonproductive cough, dyspnea, crackles, or radiological pulmonary infiltrates, ELOXATIN should be discontinued until further pulmonary investigation excludes interstitial lung disease or pulmonary fibrosis.

5.4   Hepatotoxicity
Hepatotoxicity as evidenced in the adjuvant study, by increase in transaminases (57% vs. 34%) and alkaline phosphatase (42% vs. 20%) was observed more commonly in the ELOXATIN combination arm than in the control arm. The incidence of increased bilirubin was similar on both arms. Changes noted on liver biopsies include: peliosis, nodular regenerative hyperplasia or sinusoidal alterations, perisinusoidal fibrosis, and veno-occlusive lesions. Hepatic vascular disorders should be considered, and if appropriate, should be investigated in case of abnormal liver function test results or portal hypertension, which cannot be explained by liver metastases *[see Clinical Trials Experience (6.1)]*.

5.5   Use in Pregnancy
Pregnancy Category D
ELOXATIN may cause fetal harm when administered to a pregnant woman. There are no adequate and well-controlled studies of ELOXATIN in pregnant women. Women of childbearing potential should be advised to avoid becoming pregnant while receiving treatment with ELOXATIN. *[see Use in Specific Populations (8.1)]*.

5.6   Recommended Laboratory Tests
Standard monitoring of the white blood cell count with differential, hemoglobin, platelet count, and blood chemistries (including ALT, AST, bilirubin and creatinine) is recommended before each ELOXATIN cycle *[see Dosage and Administration (2)]*.

There have been reports while on study and from postmarketing surveillance of prolonged prothrombin time and INR occasionally associated with hemorrhage in patients *who received* ELOXATIN plus 5-fluorouracil/leucovorin while on anticoagulants. Patients receiving ELOXATIN plus 5-fluorouracil/leucovorin and requiring oral anticoagulants may require closer monitoring.

6   ADVERSE REACTIONS
6.1   Clinical Trials Experience
Serious adverse reactions including anaphylaxis and allergic reactions, neuropathy, pulmonary toxicities and hepatotoxicities can occur *[See Warnings and Precautions (5.1)]*.

Table 5 – Adverse Reactions Reported in Patients Previously Untreated for Advanced Colorectal Cancer Clinical Trial (≥5% of all patients and with ≥1% NCI Grade 3/4 events)

Adverse reaction (WHO/Pref)	ELOXATIN + 5-FU/LV N=259		irinotecan + 5-FU/LV N=256		ELOXATIN + irinotecan N=258	
	All Grades (%)	Grade 3/4 (%)	All Grades (%)	Grade 3/4 (%)	All Grades (%)	Grade 3/4 (%)
Any Event	99	82	98	70	99	76
Allergy/Immunology						
Hypersensitivity	12	2	5	0	6	1
Cardiovascular						
Thrombosis	6	5	6	6	3	3
Hypotension	5	3	6	3	4	3
Constitutional Symptoms/Pain/Ocular/Visual						
Fatigue	70	7	58	11	66	16
Abdominal Pain	29	8	31	7	39	10
Myalgia	14	2	6	0	9	2
Pain	7	1	5	1	6	1
Vision abnormal	5	0	2	1	6	1
Neuralgia	5	0	0	0	2	1
Dermatology/Skin						
Skin reaction – hand/foot	7	1	2	1	1	0
Injection site reaction	6	0	1	0	4	1
Gastrointestinal						
Nausea	71	6	67	15	83	19
Diarrhea	56	12	65	29	76	25
Vomiting	41	4	43	13	64	23
Stomatitis	38	0	25	1	19	1
Anorexia	35	2	25	4	27	5
Constipation	32	4	27	2	21	2
Diarrhea-colostomy	13	2	16	7	16	3
Gastrointestinal NOS*	5	2	4	2	3	2
Hematology/Infection						
Infection normal ANC†	10	4	5	1	7	2
Infection low ANC†	8	8	12	11	9	8
Lymphopenia	6	2	4	1	5	2
Febrile neutropenia	4	4	15	14	12	11

(Table continued on next page)

Because clinical trials are conducted under widely varying conditions, adverse reaction rates observed in the clinical trials of a drug cannot be directly compared to rates in the clinical trials of another drug and may not reflect the rates observed in practice.

More than 1100 patients with stage II or III colon cancer and more than 4,000 patients with advanced colorectal cancer have been treated in clinical studies with ELOXATIN. The most common adverse reactions in patients with stage II or III colon cancer receiving adjuvant therapy were peripheral sensory neuropathy, neutropenia, thrombocytopenia, anemia, nausea, increase in transaminases and alkaline phosphatase, diarrhea, emesis, fatigue and stomatitis. The most common adverse reactions in previously untreated and treated patients were peripheral sensory neuropathies, fatigue, neutropenia, nausea, emesis, and diarrhea *[see Warnings and Precautions (5)]*.

Combination Adjuvant Therapy with ELOXATIN and Infusional 5-fluorouracil/leucovorin in Patients with Colon Cancer

One thousand one hundred and eight patients with stage II or III colon cancer, who had undergone complete resection of the primary tumor, have been treated in a clinical study with ELOXATIN in combination with infusional 5-fluorouracil/leucovorin *[see Clinical Studies (14)]*. The incidence of grade 3 or 4 adverse reactions was 70% on the ELOXATIN combination arm, and 31% on the infusional 5-fluorouracil/leucovorin arm. The adverse reactions in this trial are shown in the tables below. Discontinuation of treatment due to adverse reactions occurred in 15% of the patients receiving ELOXATIN and infusional 5-fluorouracil/leucovorin. Both 5-fluorouracil/leucovorin and ELOXATIN are associated with gastrointestinal or hematologic adverse reactions. When ELOXATIN is administered in combination with infusional 5-fluorouracil/leucovorin, the incidence of these events is increased.

The incidence of death within 28 days of last treatment, regardless of causality, was 0.5% (n=6) in both the ELOXATIN combination and infusional 5-fluorouracil/leucovorin, respectively. Deaths within 60 days from initiation of therapy were 0.3% (n=3) in both the ELOXATIN combination and infusional 5-fluorouracil/leucovorin arms, respectively. On the ELOXATIN combination arm, 3 deaths were due to sepsis/neutropenic sepsis, 2 from intracerebral bleeding and one from eosinophilic pneumonia. On the 5-fluorouracil/leucovorin arm, one death was due to suicide, 2 from Steven-Johnson Syndrome (1 patient also had sepsis), 1 unknown cause, 1 anoxic cerebral infarction and 1 probable abdominal aorta rupture.

The following table provides adverse reactions reported in the adjuvant therapy colon cancer clinical trial [see Clinical Studies (14)] by body system and decreasing order of frequency in the ELOXATIN and infusional 5-fluorouracil/leucovorin arm for events with overall incidences ≥ 5% and for NCI grade 3/4 events with incidences ≥ 1%.

[See table 3 at top of page 2980]

The following table provides adverse reactions reported in the adjuvant therapy colon cancer clinical trial [see Clinical Studies (14)] by body system and decreasing order of frequency in the ELOXATIN and infusional 5-fluorouracil/leucovorin arm for events with overall incidences ≥ 5% but with incidences <1% NCI grade 3/4 events.

Table 4 - Adverse Reactions Reported in Patients with Colon Cancer receiving Adjuvant Treatment (≥ 5% of all patients, but with <1% NCI Grade 3/4 events)

Adverse reaction (WHO/Pref)	Eloxatin + 5-FU/LV N=1108 All Grades (%)	5-FU/LV N=1111 All Grades (%)
Allergy/Immunology		
Rhinitis	6	8
Constitutional Symptoms/Pain/Ocular/Visual		
Epistaxis	16	12
Weight Increase	10	10
Conjunctivitis	9	15
Headache	7	5
Dyspnea	5	3
Pain	5	5
Lacrimation Abnormal	4	12
Dermatology/Skin		
Alopecia	30	28
Gastrointestinal		
Constipation	22	19
Taste Perversion	12	8
Dyspepsia	8	5
Metabolic		
Phosphate Alkaline increased	42	20
Neurology		
Sensory Disturbance	8	1

Although specific events can vary, the overall frequency of adverse reactions was similar in men and women and in patients <65 and ≥65 years. However, the following grade 3/4 events were more common in females: diarrhea, fatigue, granulocytopenia, nausea and vomiting. In patients ≥65 years old, the incidence of grade 3/4 diarrhea and granulocytopenia was higher than in younger patients. Insufficient subgroup sizes prevented analysis of safety by race. The following additional adverse reactions were reported in ≥2% and <5% of the patients in the ELOXATIN and infusional 5-fluorouracil/leucovorin combination arm (listed in decreasing order of frequency): pain, leukopenia, weight decrease, coughing.

The number of patients who developed secondary malignancies was similar; 62 in the ELOXATIN combination arm and 68 in the infusional 5-fluorouracil/leucovorin arm. An exploratory analysis showed that the number of deaths due to

Table 5 (cont.) – Adverse Reactions Reported in Patients Previously Untreated for Advanced Colorectal Cancer Clinical Trial (≥5% of all patients and with ≥1% NCI Grade 3/4 events)

Adverse reaction (WHO/Pref)	ELOXATIN + 5-FU/LV N=259 All Grades (%)	Grade 3/4 (%)	irinotecan + 5-FU/LV N=256 All Grades (%)	Grade 3/4 (%)	ELOXATIN + irinotecan N=258 All Grades (%)	Grade 3/4 (%)
Any Event	99	82	98	70	99	76
Hepatic/Metabolic/Laboratory/Renal						
Hyperglycemia	14	2	11	3	12	3
Hypokalemia	11	3	7	4	6	2
Dehydration	9	5	16	11	14	7
Hypoalbuminemia	8	0	5	2	9	1
Hyponatremia	8	2	7	4	4	1
Urinary frequency	5	1	2	1	3	1
Neurology						
Overall Neuropathy	82	19	18	2	69	7
Paresthesias	77	18	16	2	62	6
Pharyngo-laryngeal dysesthesias	38	2	1	0	28	1
Neuro-sensory	12	1	2	0	9	1
Neuro NOS*	1	0	1	0	1	0
Pulmonary						
Cough	35	1	25	1	17	1
Dyspnea	18	7	14	3	11	2
Hiccups	5	1	2	0	3	2

* Not otherwise specified
† Absolute neutrophil count

secondary malignancies was 1.96% in the ELOXATIN combination arm and 0.98% in infusional 5-fluorouracil/leucovorin arm.

In addition, the number of cardiovascular deaths was 1.4% in the ELOXATIN combination arm as compared to 0.7% in the infusional 5-fluorouracil/leucovorin arm. Clinical significance of these findings is unknown.

Patients Previously Untreated for Advanced Colorectal Cancer

Two hundred and fifty-nine patients were treated in the ELOXATIN and 5-fluorouracil/leucovorin combination arm of the randomized trial in patients previously untreated for advanced colorectal cancer [see Clinical Studies (14)]. The adverse reaction profile in this study was similar to that seen in other studies and the adverse reactions in this trial are shown in the tables below. Both 5-fluorouracil and ELOXATIN are associated with gastrointestinal and hematologic adverse reactions. When ELOXATIN is administered in combination with 5-fluorouracil, the incidence of these events is increased.

The incidence of death within 30 days of treatment in the previously untreated for advanced colorectal cancer study, regardless of causality, was 3% with the ELOXATIN and 5-fluorouracil/leucovorin combination, 5% with irinotecan plus 5-fluorouracil/leucovorin, and 3% with ELOXATIN plus irinotecan. Deaths within 60 days from initiation of therapy were 2.3% with the ELOXATIN and 5-fluorouracil/leucovorin combination, 5.1% with irinotecan plus 5-fluorouracil/leucovorin, and 3.1% with ELOXATIN plus irinotecan.

The following table provides adverse reactions reported in the previously untreated for advanced colorectal cancer study [see Clinical Studies (14)] by body system and decreasing order of frequency in the ELOXATIN and 5-fluorouracil/leucovorin combination arm for events with overall incidences ≥5% and for grade 3/4 events with incidences ≥1%.

[See table 5 on previous page and above]

The following table provides adverse reactions reported in the previously untreated for advanced colorectal cancer study [see Clinical Studies (14)] by body system and decreasing order of frequency in the ELOXATIN and 5-fluorouracil/leucovorin combination arm for events with overall incidences ≥5% but with incidences <1% NCI Grade 3/4 events.

Table 6 - Adverse Reactions Reported in Patients Previously Untreated for Advanced Colorectal Cancer Clinical Trial (≥5% of all patients but with < 1% NCI Grade 3/4 events)

Adverse reaction (WHO/Pref)	ELOXATIN + 5-FU/LV N=259 All Grades (%)	irinotecan + 5-FU/LV N=256 All Grades (%)	ELOXATIN + irinotecan N=258 All Grades (%)
Allergy/Immunology			
Rash	11	4	7
Rhinitis allergic	10	6	6
Cardiovascular			
Edema	15	13	10
Constitutional Symptoms/Pain/Ocular/Visual			
Headache	13	6	9
Weight loss	11	9	11
Epistaxis	10	2	2
Tearing	9	1	2
Rigors	8	2	7
Dysphasia	5	3	3
Sweating	5	6	12
Arthralgia	5	5	8
Dermatology/Skin			
Alopecia	38	44	67
Flushing	7	2	5

Table 7 – Adverse Reactions Reported In Previously Treated Colorectal Cancer Clinical Trial (≥5% of all patients and with ≥1% NCI Grade 3/4 events)

Adverse reaction (WHO/Pref)	5-FU/LV (N = 142)		ELOXATIN (N = 153)		ELOXATIN + 5-FU/LV (N = 150)	
	All Grades (%)	Grade 3/4 (%)	All Grades (%)	Grade 3/4 (%)	All Grades (%)	Grade 3/4 (%)
Any Event	98	41	100	46	99	73
Cardiovascular						
Dyspnea	11	2	13	7	20	4
Coughing	9	0	11	0	19	1
Edema	13	1	10	1	15	1
Thromboembolism	4	2	2	1	9	8
Chest Pain	4	1	5	1	8	1
Constitutional Symptoms/Pain						
Fatigue	52	6	61	9	68	7
Back Pain	16	4	11	0	19	3
Pain	9	3	14	3	15	2
Arthralgia	10		7		10	
Epistaxis	1		2		9	
Abnormal Lacrimation	6		1		7	
Rigors	6		9		7	
Dermatology/Skin						
Hand-Foot Syndrome	13		1		11	
Flushing	2		3		10	
Alopecia	3		3		7	
Gastrointestinal						
Constipation	23		31		32	
Dyspepsia	10		7		14	
Taste Perversion	1		5		13	
Mucositis	10		2		7	
Flatulence	6		3		5	
Hepatic/Metabolic/Laboratory/Renal						
Hematuria	4		0		6	
Dysuria	1		1		6	
Neurology						
Dizziness	8		7		13	
Insomnia	4		11		9	
Pulmonary						
Upper Resp Tract Infection	4		7		10	
Pharyngitis	10		2		9	
Hiccup	0		2		5	

(Table continued on next page)

Pruritis	6	4			2	
Dry Skin	6	2			5	
Gastrointestinal						
Taste perversion	14	6			8	
Dyspepsia	12	7			5	
Flatulence	9	6			5	
Mouth Dryness	5	2			3	
Hematology/Infection						
Fever normal ANC*	16	9			9	
Hepatic/Metabolic/Laboratory/Renal						
Hypocalcemia	7	5			4	
Elevated Creatinine	4	4			5	
Neurology						
Insomnia	13	9			11	
Depression	9	5			7	
Dizziness	8	6			10	
Anxiety	5	2			6	

*Absolute neutrophil count

Adverse reactions were similar in men and women and in patients <65 and ≥65 years, but older patients may have been more susceptible to diarrhea, dehydration, hypokalemia, leukopenia, fatigue and syncope. The following additional adverse reactions, at least possibly related to treatment and potentially important, were reported in ≥2% and <5% of the patients in the ELOXATIN and 5-fluorouracil/leucovorin combination arm (listed in decreasing order of frequency): metabolic, pneumonitis, catheter infection, vertigo, prothrombin time, pulmonary, rectal bleeding, dysuria, nail changes, chest pain, rectal pain, syncope, hypertension, hypoxia, unknown infection, bone pain, pigmentation changes, and urticaria.

Previously Treated Patients with Advanced Colorectal Cancer
Four hundred and fifty patients (about 150 receiving the combination of ELOXATIN and 5-fluorouracil/leucovorin) were studied in a randomized trial in patients with refractory and relapsed colorectal cancer *[see Clinical Studies (14)]*. The adverse reaction profile in this study was similar to that seen in other studies and the adverse reactions in this trial are shown in the tables below.
Thirteen percent of patients in the ELOXATIN and 5-fluorouracil/leucovorin combination arm and 18% in the 5-fluorouracil/leucovorin arm of the previously treated study had to discontinue treatment because of adverse effects related to gastrointestinal, or hematologic adverse reactions, or neuropathies. Both 5-fluorouracil and ELOXATIN are associated with gastrointestinal and hematologic adverse reactions. When ELOXATIN is administered in combination with 5-fluorouracil, the incidence of these events is increased.
The incidence of death within 30 days of treatment in the previously treated study, regardless of causality, was 5% with the ELOXATIN and 5-fluorouracil/leucovorin combination, 8% with ELOXATIN alone, and 7% with 5-fluorouracil/leucovorin. Of the 7 deaths that occurred on the ELOXATIN and 5-fluorouracil/leucovorin combination arm within 30 days of stopping treatment, 3 may have been treatment related, associated with gastrointestinal bleeding or dehydration.
The following table provides adverse reactions reported in the previously treated study *[see Clinical Studies (14)]* by body system and in decreasing order of frequency in the ELOXATIN and 5-fluorouracil/leucovorin combination arm for events with overall incidences ≥5% and for grade 3/4 events with incidences ≥1%. This table does not include hematologic and blood chemistry abnormalities; these are shown separately below.
[See table 7 above and on next page]
The following table provides adverse reactions reported in the previously treated study *[see Clinical Studies (14)]* by body system and in decreasing order of frequency in the ELOXATIN and 5-fluorouracil/leucovorin combination arm for events with overall incidences ≥5% but with incidences <1% NCI Grade 3/4 events.

Table 8 - Adverse Reactions Reported In Previously Treated Colorectal Cancer Clinical Trial (≥5% of all patients but with < 1% NCI Grade 3/4 events)

Adverse reaction (WHO/Pref)	5-FU/LV (N = 142) All Grades (%)	ELOXATIN (N = 153) All Grades (%)	ELOXATIN + 5-FU/LV (N = 150) All Grades (%)
Allergy/Immunology			
Rhinitis	4	6	15
Allergic Reaction	1	3	10
Rash	5	5	9
Cardiovascular			
Peripheral Edema	11	5	10
Constitutional Symptoms/Pain/Ocular/Visual			
Headache	8	13	17

Adverse reactions were similar in men and women and in patients <65 and ≥65 years, but older patients may have been more susceptible to dehydration, diarrhea, hypokalemia and fatigue. The following additional adverse reactions, at least possibly related to treatment and potentially important, were reported in ≥2% and <5% of the patients in the ELOXATIN and 5-fluorouracil/leucovorin combination arm (listed in decreasing order of frequency): anxiety, myalgia, erythematous rash, increased sweating, conjunctivitis, weight decrease, dry mouth, rectal hemorrhage, depression, ataxia, ascites, hemorrhoids, muscle weakness, nervousness, tachycardia, abnormal micturition frequency, dry skin, pruritus, hemoptysis, purpura, vaginal hemorrhage, melena, somnolence, pneumonia, proctitis, involuntary muscle contractions, intestinal obstruction, gingivitis, tenesmus, hot flashes, enlarged abdomen, urinary incontinence.

Hematologic Changes
The following tables list the hematologic changes occurring in ≥5% of patients, based on laboratory values and NCI grade, with the exception of those events occurring in adjuvant patients and anemia in the patients previously untreated for advanced colorectal cancer, respectively, which are based on AE reporting and NCI grade alone.
[See table 9 on next page]
[See table 10 at top of page 2985]
[See table 11 on page 2985]
Thrombocytopenia and Bleeding
Thrombocytopenia was frequently reported with the combination of ELOXATIN and infusional 5-fluorouracil/leucovorin. The incidence of all hemorrhagic events in the adjuvant and previously treated patients was higher on the ELOXATIN combination arm compared to the infusional 5-fluorouracil/leucovorin arm. These events included gastrointestinal bleeding, hematuria, and epistaxis. In the adjuvant trial, two patients died from intracerebral hemorrhages.
The incidence of Grade 3/4 thrombocytopenia was 2% in adjuvant patients with colon cancer. In patients treated for advanced colorectal cancer the incidence of Grade 3/4 thrombocytopenia was 3–5%, and the incidence of these events was greater for the combination of ELOXATIN and

5-fluorouracil/leucovorin over the irinotecan plus 5-fluorouracil/leucovorin or 5-fluorouracil/leucovorin control groups. Grade 3/4 gastrointestinal bleeding was reported in 0.2% of adjuvant patients receiving ELOXATIN and 5-fluorouracil/leucovorin. In the previously untreated patients, the incidence of epistaxis was 10% in the ELOXATIN and 5-fluorouracil/leucovorin arm, and 2% and 1%, respectively, in the irinotecan plus 5-fluorouracil/leucovorin or irinotecan plus ELOXATIN arms.

Neutropenia
Neutropenia was frequently observed with the combination of ELOXATIN and 5-fluorouracil/leucovorin, with Grade 3 and 4 events reported in 29% and 12% of adjuvant patients with colon cancer, respectively. In the adjuvant trial, 3 patients died from sepsis/neutropenic sepsis. Grade 3 and 4 events were reported in 35% and 18% of the patients previously untreated for advanced colorectal cancer, respectively. Grade 3 and 4 events were reported in 27% and 17% of previously treated patients, respectively. In adjuvant patients the incidence of either febrile neutropenia (0.7%) or documented infection with concomitant grade 3/4 neutropenia (1.1%) was 1.8% in the ELOXATIN and 5-fluorouracil/leucovorin arm. The incidence of febrile neutropenia in the patients previously untreated for advanced colorectal cancer was 15% (3% of cycles) in the irinotecan plus 5-fluorouracil/leucovorin arm and 4% (less than 1% of cycles) in the ELOXATIN and 5-fluorouracil/leucovorin combination arm. Additionally, in this same population, infection with grade 3 or 4 neutropenia was 12% in the irinotecan plus 5-fluorouracil/leucovorin, and 8% in the ELOXATIN and 5-fluorouracil/leucovorin combination. The incidence of febrile neutropenia in the previously treated patients was 1% in the 5-fluorouracil/leucovorin arm and 6% (less than 1% of cycles) in the ELOXATIN and 5-fluorouracil/leucovorin combination arm.

Gastrointestinal
In patients receiving the combination of ELOXATIN plus infusional 5-fluorouracil/leucovorin for adjuvant treatment for colon cancer the incidence of Grade 3/4 nausea and vomiting was greater than those receiving infusional 5-fluorouracil/leucovorin alone (see table). In patients previously untreated for advanced colorectal cancer receiving the combination of ELOXATIN and 5-fluorouracil/leucovorin, the incidence of Grade 3 and 4 vomiting and diarrhea was less compared to irinotecan plus 5-fluorouracil/leucovorin controls (see table). In previously treated patients receiving the combination of ELOXATIN and 5-fluorouracil/leucovorin, the incidence of Grade 3 and 4 nausea, vomiting, diarrhea, and mucositis/stomatitis increased compared to 5-fluorouracil/leucovorin controls (see table).
The incidence of gastrointestinal adverse reactions in the previously untreated and previously treated patients appears to be similar across cycles. Premedication with antiemetics, including 5-HT$_3$ blockers, is recommended. Diarrhea and mucositis may be exacerbated by the addition of ELOXATIN to 5-fluorouracil/leucovorin, and should be managed with appropriate supportive care. Since cold temperature can exacerbate acute neurological symptoms, ice (mucositis prophylaxis) should be avoided during the infusion of ELOXATIN.

Dermatologic
ELOXATIN did not increase the incidence of alopecia compared to 5-fluorouracil/leucovorin alone. No complete alopecia was reported. The incidence of Grade 3/4 skin disorders was 2% in both the ELOXATIN plus infusional 5-fluorouracil/leucovorin and the infusional 5-fluorouracil/leucovorin alone arms in the adjuvant colon cancer patients. The incidence of hand-foot syndrome in patients previously untreated for advanced colorectal cancer was 2% in the irinotecan plus 5-fluorouracil/leucovorin arm and 7% in the ELOXATIN and 5-fluorouracil/leucovorin combination arm. The incidence of hand-foot syndrome in previously treated patients was 13% in the 5-fluorouracil/leucovorin arm and 11% in the ELOXATIN and 5-fluorouracil/leucovorin combination arm.

Intravenous Site Reactions
Extravasation, in some cases including necrosis, has been reported. Injection site reaction, including redness, swelling, and pain, has been reported.

Anticoagulation and Hemorrhage
There have been reports while on study and from postmarketing surveillance of prolonged prothrombin time and INR occasionally associated with hemorrhage in patients who received ELOXATIN plus 5-fluorouracil/leucovorin while on anticoagulants. Patients receiving ELOXATIN plus 5-fluorouracil/leucovorin and requiring oral anticoagulants may require closer monitoring.

Renal
About 5-10% of patients in all groups had some degree of elevation of serum creatinine. The incidence of Grade 3/4 elevations in serum creatinine in the ELOXATIN and 5-fluorouracil/leucovorin combination arm was 1% in the previously treated patients. Serum creatinine measurements were not reported in the adjuvant trial.

Hepatic
Hepatotoxicity (defined as elevation of liver enzymes) appears to be related to ELOXATIN combination therapy [see *Warnings and Precautions (5.4)*]. The following tables list the clinical chemistry changes associated with hepatic tox-

Table 7 – Adverse Reactions Reported In Previously Treated Colorectal Cancer Clinical Trial (≥5% of all patients and with ≥1% NCI Grade 3/4 events)

Adverse reaction (WHO/Pref)	5-FU/LV (N = 142)		ELOXATIN (N = 153)		ELOXATIN + 5-FU/LV (N = 150)	
	All Grades (%)	Grade 3/4 (%)	All Grades (%)	Grade 3/4 (%)	All Grades (%)	Grade 3/4 (%)
Dermatology/Skin						
Injection Site Reaction	5	1	9	0	10	3
Gastrointestinal						
Diarrhea	44	3	46	4	67	11
Nausea	59	4	64	4	65	11
Vomiting	27	4	37	4	40	9
Stomatitis	32	3	14	0	37	3
Abdominal Pain	31	5	31	7	33	4
Anorexia	20	1	20	2	29	3
Gastroesophageal Reflux	3	0	1	0	5	2
Hematology/Infection						
Fever	23	1	25	1	29	1
Febrile Neutropenia	1	1	0	0	6	6
Hepatic/Metabolic/Laboratory/Renal						
Hypokalemia	3	1	3	2	9	4
Dehydration	6	4	5	3	8	3
Neurology						
Neuropathy	17	0	76	7	74	7
Acute	10	0	65	5	56	2
Persistent	9	0	43	3	48	6

Table 9 - Adverse Hematologic Reactions in Patients with Colon Cancer Receiving Adjuvant Therapy (≥5% of patients)

Hematology Parameter	ELOXATIN + 5-FU/LV (N=1108)		5-FU/LV (N=1111)	
	All Grades (%)	Grade 3/4 (%)	All Grades (%)	Grade 3/4 (%)
Anemia	76	1	67	<1
Neutropenia	79	41	40	5
Thrombocytopenia	77	2	19	<1

icity occurring in ≥5% of patients, based on adverse reactions reported and NCI CTC grade for adjuvant patients and patients previously untreated for advanced colorectal cancer, laboratory values and NCI CTC grade for previously treated patients.
[See table 12 on next page]
[See table 13 on next page]
[See table 14 on next page]

Thromboembolism
The incidence of thromboembolic events in adjuvant patients with colon cancer was 6% (1.8% grade 3/4) in the infusional 5-fluorouracil/leucovorin arm and 6% (1.2% grade 3/4) in the ELOXATIN and infusional 5-fluorouracil/leucovorin combined arm, respectively. The incidence was 6 and 9% of the patients previously untreated for advanced colorectal cancer and previously treated patients in the ELOXATIN and 5-fluorouracil/leucovorin combination arm, respectively.

6.2   Postmarketing Experience
The following adverse reactions have been identified during post-approval use of ELOXATIN. Because these reactions are reported voluntarily from a population of uncertain size, it is not always possible to reliably estimate their frequency or establish a causal relationship to drug exposure.
Body as a whole:
angioedema, anaphylactic shock
Central and peripheral nervous system disorders:
loss of deep tendon reflexes, dysarthria, Lhermitte's sign, cranial nerve palsies, fasciculations, convulsion
Liver and Gastrointestinal system disorders:
severe diarrhea/vomiting resulting in hypokalemia, colitis (including *Clostridium difficile* diarrhea), metabolic acido-

sis; ileus; intestinal obstruction, pancreatitis; veno-occlusive disease of liver also known as sinusoidal obstruction syndrome, and perisinusoidal fibrosis which rarely may progress.
Hearing and vestibular system disorders:
deafness
Platelet, bleeding, and clotting disorders:
immuno-allergic thrombocytopenia
prolongation of prothrombin time and of INR in patients receiving anticoagulants
Red Blood Cell disorders:
hemolytic uremic syndrome, immuno-allergic hemolytic anemia
Renal disorders:
Acute tubular necrosis, acute interstitial nephritis and acute renal failure.
Respiratory system disorders:
pulmonary fibrosis, and other interstitial lung diseases (sometimes fatal)
Vision disorders:
decrease of visual acuity, visual field disturbance, optic neuritis and transient vision loss (reversible following therapy discontinuation)

7   DRUG INTERACTIONS
No specific cytochrome P-450-based drug interaction studies have been conducted. No pharmacokinetic interaction between 85 mg/m² ELOXATIN and 5-fluorouracil/leucovorin has been observed in patients treated every 2 weeks. Increases of 5-fluorouracil plasma concentrations by approximately 20% have been observed with doses of 130 mg/m²

ELOXATIN dosed every 3 weeks. Because platinum-containing species are eliminated primarily through the kidney, clearance of these products may be decreased by co-administration of potentially nephrotoxic compounds; although, this has not been specifically studied [see Clinical Pharmacology (12.3)].

8 USE IN SPECIFIC POPULATIONS

8.1 Pregnancy

Pregnancy Category D

Based on direct interaction with DNA, ELOXATIN may cause fetal harm when administered to a pregnant woman. There are no adequate and well-controlled studies of ELOXATIN in pregnant women. Reproductive toxicity studies in rats demonstrated adverse effects on fertility and embryo-fetal development at maternal doses that were below the recommended human dose based on body surface area. If this drug is used during pregnancy or if the patient becomes pregnant while taking this drug, the patient should be apprised of the potential hazard to the fetus. Women of childbearing potential should be advised to avoid becoming pregnant and use effective contraception while receiving treatment with ELOXATIN.

Pregnant rats were administered oxaliplatin at less than one-tenth the recommended human dose based on body surface area during gestation days 1–5 (pre-implantation), 6–10, or 11–16 (during organogenesis). Oxaliplatin caused developmental mortality (increased early resorptions) when administered on days 6–10 and 11–16 and adversely affected fetal growth (decreased fetal weight, delayed ossification) when administered on days 6–10. Administration of oxaliplatin to male and female rats prior to mating resulted in 97% post-implantation loss in animals that received approximately one-seventh the recommended human dose based on the body surface area.

8.3 Nursing Mothers

It is not known whether ELOXATIN or its derivatives are excreted in human milk. Because many drugs are excreted in human milk and because of the potential for serious adverse reactions in nursing infants from ELOXATIN, a decision should be made whether to discontinue nursing or discontinue the drug, taking into account the importance of the drug to the mother.

8.4 Pediatric Use

The effectiveness of oxaliplatin in children has not been established. Oxaliplatin has been tested in 2 Phase I and 2 Phase II trials in 159 patients ages 7 months to 22 years with solid tumors (see below) and no significant activity observed.

In a Phase I/II study, oxaliplatin was administered as a 2-hour intravenous infusion on days 1, 8 and 15 every 4 weeks (1 cycle), for a maximum of 6 cycles, to 43 patients with refractory or relapsed malignant solid tumors, mainly neuroblastoma and osteosarcoma. Twenty eight pediatric patients in the Phase I study received oxaliplatin at 6 dose levels starting at 40 mg/m^2 with escalation to 110 mg/m^2. The dose limiting toxicity (DLT) was sensory neuropathy at the 110 mg/m^2 dose. Fifteen patients received oxaliplatin at a dose of 90 mg/m^2 intravenous in the Phase II portion of the study. At this dose, paresthesia (60%, G3/4: 7%), fever (40%, G3/4: 7%) and thrombocytopenia (40%, G3/4: 27%) were the main adverse reactions. No responses were observed.

In a second Phase I study, oxaliplatin was administered to 26 pediatric patients as a 2-hour intravenous infusion on day 1 every 3 weeks (1 cycle) at 5 dose levels starting at 100 mg/m^2 with escalation to 160 mg/m^2, for a maximum of 6 cycles. In a separate cohort, oxaliplatin 85 mg/m^2 was administered on day 1 every 2 weeks, for a maximum of 9 doses. Patients had metastatic or unresectable solid tumors mainly neuroblastoma and ganglioneuroblastoma. No responses were observed. The DLT was sensory neuropathy at the 160 mg/m^2 dose. Based on these studies, oxaliplatin 130 mg/m^2 as a 2-hour intravenous infusion on day 1 every 3 weeks (1 cycle) was used in subsequent Phase II studies. A dose of 85 mg/m^2 on day 1 every 2 weeks was also found to be tolerable.

In one Phase II study, 43 pediatric patients with recurrent or refractory embryonal CNS tumors received oxaliplatin 130 mg/m^2 every 3 weeks for a maximum of 12 months in absence of progressive disease or unacceptable toxicity. In patients < 10 kg the oxaliplatin dose used was 4.3 mg/kg. The most common adverse reactions reported were leukopenia (67%, G3/4: 12%), anemia (65%, G3/4: 5%), thrombocytopenia (65%, G3/4: 26%), vomiting (65%, G3/4: 7%), neutropenia (58%, G3/4: 16%) and sensory neuropathy (40%, G3/4: 5%). One partial response was observed.

In a second Phase II study, 47 pediatric patients with recurrent solid tumors, including Ewing sarcoma or peripheral PNET, osteosarcoma, rhabdomyosarcoma and neuroblastoma, received oxaliplatin 130 mg/m^2 every 3 weeks for a maximum of 12 months or 17 cycles. In patients ≤ 12 months old the oxaliplatin dose used was 4.3 mg/kg. The most common adverse reactions reported were sensory neuropathy (53%, G3/4: 15%), thrombocytopenia (40%, G3/4: 26%), anemia (40%, G3/4: 15%), vomiting (32%, G3/4: 0%), nausea (30%, G3/4: 2%) and AST increased (26%, G3/4: 4%). No responses were observed.

The pharmacokinetic parameters of ultrafiltrable platinum have been evaluated in 105 pediatric patients during the first cycle. The mean clearance in pediatric patients estimated by the population pharmacokinetic analysis was 4.7 L/h. The inter-patient variability of platinum clearance in pediatric cancer patients was 41%. Mean platinum pharmacokinetic parameters in ultrafiltrate were C_{max} of 0.75 ± 0.24 mcg/mL, AUC_{0-48} of 7.52 ± 5.07 mcg•h/mL and AUC_{inf} of 8.83 ± 1.57 mcg•h/mL at 85 mg/m^2 of oxaliplatin and C_{max} of 1.10 ± 0.43 mcg/mL, AUC_{0-48} of 9.74 ± 2.52 mcg•h/mL and AUC_{inf} of 17.3 ± 5.34 mcg•h/mL at 130 mg/m^2 of oxaliplatin.

8.5 Geriatric Use

No significant effect of age on the clearance of ultrafilterable platinum has been observed.

In the adjuvant therapy colon cancer randomized clinical trial, [see Clinical Studies (14)] 723 patients treated with ELOXATIN and infusional 5-fluorouracil/leucovorin were <65 years and 400 patients were ≥65 years.

A descriptive subgroup analysis demonstrated that the improvement in DFS for the ELOXATIN combination arm compared to the infusional 5-fluorouracil/leucovorin alone arm appeared to be maintained across genders. The effect of ELOXATIN in patients ≥65 years of age was not conclusive. Insufficient subgroup sizes prevented analysis by race.

Table 10 - Adverse Hematologic Reactions in Patients Previously Untreated for Advanced Colorectal Cancer (≥5% of patients)

Hematology Parameter	ELOXATIN + 5-FU/LV N=259		irinotecan + 5-FU/LV N=256		ELOXATIN + irinotecan N=258	
	All Grades (%)	Grade 3/4 (%)	All Grades (%)	Grade 3/4 (%)	All Grades (%)	Grade 3/4 (%)
Anemia	27	3	28	4	25	3
Leukopenia	85	20	84	23	76	24
Neutropenia	81	53	77	44	71	36
Thrombocytopenia	71	5	26	2	44	4

Table 11 - Adverse Hematologic Reactions in Previously Treated Patients (≥5% of patients)

Hematology Parameter	5-FU/LV (N=142)		ELOXATIN (N=153)		ELOXATIN + 5-FU/LV (N=150)	
	All Grades (%)	Grade 3/4 (%)	All Grades (%)	Grade 3/4 (%)	All Grades (%)	Grade 3/4 (%)
Anemia	68	2	64	1	81	2
Leukopenia	34	1	13	0	76	19
Neutropenia	25	5	7	0	73	44
Thrombocytopenia	20	0	30	3	64	4

Table 12 - Adverse Hepatic Reactions in Patients with Stage II or III Colon Cancer Receiving Adjuvant Therapy (≥5% of patients)

Hepatic Parameter	ELOXATIN + 5-FU/LV (N=1108)		5-FU/LV (N=1111)	
	All Grades (%)	Grade 3/4 (%)	All Grades (%)	Grade 3/4 (%)
Increase in transaminases	57	2	34	1
ALP increased	42	<1	20	<1
Bilirubinaemia	20	4	20	5

Table 13 – Adverse Hepatic – Clinical Chemistry Abnormalities in Patients Previously Untreated for Advanced Colorectal Cancer (≥5% of patients)

Clinical Chemistry	ELOXATIN + 5-FU/LV N=259		irinotecan + 5-FU/LV N=256		ELOXATIN + irinotecan N=258	
	All Grades (%)	Grade 3/4 (%)	All Grades (%)	Grade 3/4 (%)	All Grades (%)	Grade 3/4 (%)
ALT (SGPT-ALAT)	6	1	2	0	5	2
AST (SGOT-ASAT)	17	1	2	1	11	1
Alkaline Phosphatase	16	0	8	0	14	2
Total Bilirubin	6	1	3	1	3	2

Table 14 – Adverse Hepatic – Clinical Chemistry Abnormalities in Previously Treated Patients (≥5% of patients)

Clinical Chemistry	5-FU/LV (N=142)		ELOXATIN (N=153)		ELOXATIN + 5-FU/LV (N=150)	
	All Grades (%)	Grade 3/4 (%)	All Grades (%)	Grade 3/4 (%)	All Grades (%)	Grade 3/4 (%)
ALT (SGPT-ALAT)	28	3	36	1	31	0
AST (SGOT-ASAT)	39	2	54	4	47	0
Total Bilirubin	22	6	13	5	13	1

Patients ≥ 65 years of age receiving the ELOXATIN combination therapy experienced more grade 3–4 granulocytopenia than patients < 65 years of age (45% versus 39%).

In the previously untreated for advanced colorectal cancer randomized clinical trial *[see Clinical Studies (14)]* of ELOXATIN, 160 patients treated with ELOXATIN and 5-fluorouracil/leucovorin were < 65 years and 99 patients were ≥65 years. The same efficacy improvements in response rate, time to tumor progression, and overall survival were observed in the ≥65 year old patients as in the overall study population. In the previously treated for advanced colorectal cancer randomized clinical trial *[see Clinical Studies (14)]* of ELOXATIN, 95 patients treated with ELOXATIN and 5-fluorouracil/leucovorin were <65 years and 55 patients were ≥65 years. The rates of overall adverse reactions, including grade 3 and 4 events, were similar across and within arms in the different age groups in all studies. The incidence of diarrhea, dehydration, hypokalemia, leukopenia, fatigue and syncope were higher in patients ≥65 years old. No adjustment to starting dose was required in patients ≥65 years old.

8.6 Patients with Renal Impairment

The safety and effectiveness of the combination of ELOXATIN and 5-fluorouracil/leucovorin in patients with renal impairment have not been evaluated. The combination of ELOXATIN and 5-fluorouracil/leucovorin should be used with caution in patients with preexisting renal impairment since the primary route of platinum elimination is renal. Clearance of ultrafilterable platinum is decreased in patients with mild, moderate, and severe renal impairment. A pharmacodynamic relationship between platinum ultrafiltrate levels and clinical safety and effectiveness has not been established *[see Adverse Reactions (6.1) and Clinical Pharmacology (12.3)]*.

10 OVERDOSAGE

There is no known antidote for ELOXATIN overdose. In addition to thrombocytopenia, the anticipated complications of an ELOXATIN overdose include hypersensitivity reaction, myelosuppression, nausea, vomiting, diarrhea and neurotoxicity.

Several cases of overdoses have been reported with ELOXATIN. Adverse reactions observed were Grade 4 thrombocytopenia (<25,000/mm^3) without any bleeding, anemia, sensory neuropathy such as paresthesia, dysesthesia, laryngospasm and facial muscle spasms, gastrointestinal disorders such as nausea, vomiting, stomatitis, flatulence, abdomen enlarged and Grade 4 intestinal obstruction, Grade 4 dehydration, dyspnea, wheezing, chest pain, respiratory failure, severe bradycardia and death.

Patients suspected of receiving an overdose should be monitored, and supportive treatment should be administered. The maximum dose of oxaliplatin that has been administered in a single infusion is 825 mg.

11 DESCRIPTION

ELOXATIN® (oxaliplatin for injection and oxaliplatin injection) is an antineoplastic agent with the molecular formula $C_8H_{14}N_2O_4Pt$ and the chemical name of *cis*-[(1 *R*,2 *R*)-1,2-cyclohexanediamine-*N,N'*] [oxalato(2-)- *O,O'*] platinum. Oxaliplatin is an organoplatinum complex in which the platinum atom is complexed with 1,2-diaminocyclohexane(DACH) and with an oxalate ligand as a leaving group.

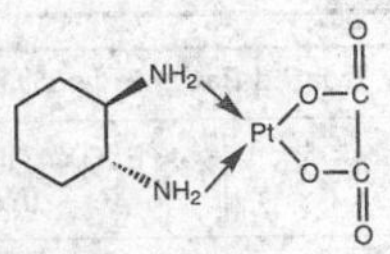

The molecular weight is 397.3. Oxaliplatin is slightly soluble in water at 6 mg/mL, very slightly soluble in methanol, and practically insoluble in ethanol and acetone.

Powder for solution for infusion:

ELOXATIN is supplied in vials containing 50 mg or 100 mg of oxaliplatin as a sterile, preservative-free lyophilized powder for reconstitution. Lactose monohydrate is present as an inactive ingredient at 450 mg and 900 mg in the 50 mg and 100 mg dosage strengths, respectively.

Concentrate for solution for infusion:

ELOXATIN is supplied in vials containing 50 mg, 100 mg or 200 mg of oxaliplatin as a sterile, preservative-free, aqueous solution at a concentration of 5 mg/ml. Water for Injection, USP is present as an inactive ingredient.

12 CLINICAL PHARMACOLOGY

12.1 Mechanism of Action

Oxaliplatin undergoes nonenzymatic conversion in physiologic solutions to active derivatives via displacement of the labile oxalate ligand. Several transient reactive species are formed, including monoaquo and diaquo DACH platinum, which covalently bind with macromolecules. Both inter- and intrastrand Pt-DNA crosslinks are formed. Crosslinks are formed between the *N*7 positions of two adjacent guanines (GG), adjacent adenine-guanines (AG), and guanines separated by an intervening nucleotide (GNG). These crosslinks inhibit DNA replication and transcription. Cytotoxicity is cell-cycle nonspecific.

In vivo studies have shown antitumor activity of oxaliplatin against colon carcinoma. In combination with 5-fluorouracil, oxaliplatin exhibits *in vitro* and *in vivo* antiproliferative activity greater than either compound alone in several tumor models [HT29 (colon), GR (mammary), and L1210 (leukemia)].

12.3 Pharmacokinetics

The reactive oxaliplatin derivatives are present as a fraction of the unbound platinum in plasma ultrafiltrate. The decline of ultrafilterable platinum levels following oxaliplatin administration is triphasic, characterized by two relatively short distribution phases ($t_{1/2\alpha}$; 0.43 hours and $t_{1/2\beta}$; 16.8 hours) and a long terminal elimination phase ($t_{1/2\gamma}$; 391 hours). Pharmacokinetic parameters obtained after a single 2-hour intravenous infusion of ELOXATIN at a dose of 85 mg/m^2 expressed as ultrafilterable platinum were C_{max} of 0.814 mcg/mL and volume of distribution of 440 L. Interpatient and intrapatient variability in ultrafilterable platinum exposure (AUC_{0-48hr}) assessed over 3 cycles was moderate to low (23% and 6%, respectively). A pharmacodynamic relationship between platinum ultrafiltrate levels and clinical safety and effectiveness has not been established.

Distribution

At the end of a 2-hour infusion of ELOXATIN, approximately 15% of the administered platinum is present in the systemic circulation. The remaining 85% is rapidly distributed into tissues or eliminated in the urine. In patients, plasma protein binding of platinum is irreversible and is greater than 90%. The main binding proteins are albumin and gamma-globulins. Platinum also binds irreversibly and accumulates (approximately 2-fold) in erythrocytes, where it appears to have no relevant activity. No platinum accumulation was observed in plasma ultrafiltrate following 85 mg/m^2 every two weeks.

Metabolism

Oxaliplatin undergoes rapid and extensive nonenzymatic biotransformation. There is no evidence of cytochrome P450-mediated metabolism *in vitro*.

Up to 17 platinum-containing derivatives have been observed in plasma ultrafiltrate samples from patients, including several cytotoxic species (monochloro DACH platinum, dichloro DACH platinum, and monoaquo and diaquo DACH platinum) and a number of noncytotoxic, conjugated species.

Elimination

The major route of platinum elimination is renal excretion. At five days after a single 2-hour infusion of ELOXATIN, urinary elimination accounted for about 54% of the platinum eliminated, with fecal excretion accounting for only about 2%. Platinum was cleared from plasma at a rate (10–17 L/h) that was similar to or exceeded the average human glomerular filtration rate (GFR; 7.5 L/h). There was no significant effect of gender on the clearance of ultrafilterable platinum. The renal clearance of ultrafilterable platinum is significantly correlated with GFR.

Pharmacokinetics in Special Populations

Pediatric

[See Use In Specific Patient Populations (8.4)].

Renal Impairment

The AUC_{0-48hr} of platinum in the plasma ultrafiltrate increases as renal function decreases. The AUC_{0-48hr} of platinum in patients with mild (creatinine clearance, CL_{cr} 50 to 80 mL/min), moderate (CL_{cr} 30 to <50 mL/min) and severe renal (CL_{cr} <30 mL/min) impairment is increased by about 60, 140 and 190%, respectively, compared to patients with normal renal function (CL_{cr} >80 mL/min) *[see Adverse Reactions (6), Drug Interactions (7) and Use In Specific Patient Populations (8.6)]*.

Drug - Drug Interactions

No pharmacokinetic interaction between 85 mg/m^2 of ELOXATIN and infusional 5-fluorouracil has been observed in patients treated every 2 weeks, but increases of 5-fluorouracil plasma concentrations by approximately 20% have been observed with doses of 130 mg/m^2 of ELOXATIN administered every 3 weeks. *In vitro*, platinum was not displaced from plasma proteins by the following medications: erythromycin, salicylate, sodium valproate, granisetron, and paclitaxel. *In vitro*, oxaliplatin is not metabolized by, nor does it inhibit, human cytochrome P450 isoenzymes. No P450-mediated drug-drug interactions are therefore anticipated in patients.

Since platinum-containing species are eliminated primarily through the kidney, clearance of these products may be decreased by co-administration of potentially nephrotoxic compounds, although this has not been specifically studied.

13 NONCLINICAL TOXICOLOGY

13.1 Carcinogenesis, Mutagenesis, Impairment of Fertility

Long-term animal studies have not been performed to evaluate the carcinogenic potential of oxaliplatin. Oxaliplatin was not mutagenic to bacteria (Ames test) but was mutagenic to mammalian cells *in vitro* (L5178Y mouse lymphoma assay). Oxaliplatin was clastogenic both *in vitro* (chromosome aberration in human lymphocytes) and *in vivo* (mouse bone marrow micronucleus assay).

In a fertility study, male rats were given oxaliplatin at 0, 0.5, 1, or 2 mg/kg/day for five days every 21 days for a total of three cycles prior to mating with females that received two cycles of oxaliplatin on the same schedule. A dose of 2 mg/kg/day (less than one-seventh the recommended human dose on a body surface area basis) did not affect pregnancy rate, but caused developmental mortality (increased early resorptions, decreased live fetuses, decreased live births) and delayed growth (decreased fetal weight).

Testicular damage, characterized by degeneration, hypoplasia, and atrophy, was observed in dogs administered oxaliplatin at 0.75 mg/kg/day × 5 days every 28 days for three cycles. A no effect level was not identified. This daily dose is approximately one-sixth of the recommended human dose on a body surface area basis.

14 CLINICAL STUDIES

14.1 Combination Adjuvant Therapy with ELOXATIN and Infusional 5-fluorouracil/leucovorin in Patients with Colon Cancer

An international, multicenter, randomized study compared the efficacy and evaluated the safety of ELOXATIN in combination with an infusional schedule of 5-fluorouracil/leucovorin to infusional 5-fluorouracil/leucovorin alone, in patients with stage II (Dukes' B2) or III (Dukes' C) colon cancer who had undergone complete resection of the primary tumor. The primary objective of the study was to compare the 3-year disease-free survival (DFS) in patients receiving ELOXATIN and infusional 5-fluorouracil/leucovorin to those receiving 5-fluorouracil/leucovorin alone. Patients were to be treated for a total of 6 months (i.e., 12 cycles). A total of 2246 patients were randomized; 1123 patients per study arm. Patients in the study had to be between 18 and 75 years of age, have histologically proven stage II (T_3-T_4 N0 M0; Dukes' B2) or III (any T N_{1-2} M0; Dukes' C) colon carcinoma (with the inferior pole of the tumor above the peritoneal reflection, i.e., ≥15 cm from the anal margin) and undergone (within 7 weeks prior to randomization) complete resection of the primary tumor without gross or microscopic evidence of residual disease. Patients had to have had no prior chemotherapy, immunotherapy or radiotherapy, and have an ECOG performance status of 0, 1, or 2 (KPS ≥ 60%), absolute neutrophil count (ANC) > 1.5×10^9/L, platelets ≥100×10^9/L, serum creatinine ≤ 1.25 × ULN total bilirubin < 2 × ULN, AST/ALT < 2 × ULN and carcinoembyrogenic antigen (CEA) < 10 ng/mL. Patients with preexisting peripheral neuropathy (NCI grade ≥ 1) were ineligible for this trial.

The following table shows the dosing regimens for the two arms of the study.

[See table 15 at left]

The following tables show the baseline characteristics and dosing of the patient population entered into this study. The baseline characteristics were well balanced between arms.

[See table 16 at top of next page]

[See table 17 on next page]

The following table and figures summarize the disease-free survival (DFS) results in the overall randomized population

Table 15 - Dosing Regimens in Adjuvant Therapy Study

Treatment Arm	Dose	Regimen
ELOXATIN + 5-FU/LV (FOLFOX4) (N=1123)	Day 1: ELOXATIN: 85 mg/m^2 (2-hour infusion) + LV: 200 mg/m^2 (2-hour infusion), followed by 5-FU: 400 mg/m^2 (bolus), 600 mg/m^2 (22-hour infusion) Day 2: LV: 200 mg/m^2 (2-hour infusion), followed by 5-FU: 400 mg/m^2 (bolus), 600 mg/m^2 (22-hour infusion)	every 2 weeks 12 cycles
5-FU/LV (N=1123)	Day 1: LV: 200 mg/m^2 (2-hour infusion), followed by 5-FU: 400 mg/m^2 (bolus), 600 mg/m^2 (22-hour infusion) Day 2: LV: 200 mg/m^2 (2-hour infusion), followed by 5-FU: 400 mg/m^2 (bolus), 600 mg/m^2 (22-hour infusion)	every 2 weeks 12 cycles

and in patients with stage II and III disease based on an ITT analysis. The median duration of follow-up was approximately 77 months.

[See table 18 at top of next page]

In the overall and stage III colon cancer populations DFS was statistically significantly improved in the ELOXATIN combination arm compared to infusional 5-fluorouracil/leucovorin alone. However, a statistically significant improvement in DFS was not noted in Stage II patients.

Figure 2 shows the DFS Kaplan-Meier curves for the comparison of ELOXATIN and infusional 5-fluorouracil/leucovorin combination and infusional 5-fluorouracil/leucovorin alone for the overall population (ITT analysis).

Figure 3 shows the DFS Kaplan-Meier curves for the comparison of ELOXATIN and infusional 5-fluorouracil/leucovorin combination and infusional 5-fluorouracil/leucovorin alone in Stage III patients.

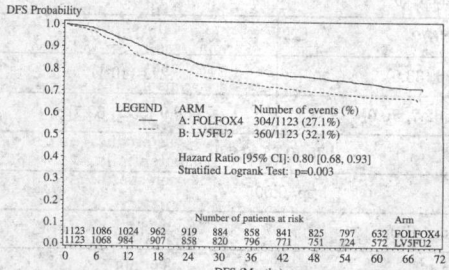

Figure 2 - DFS Kaplan-Meier curves by treatment arm (cutoff: 1 June 2006) – ITT population

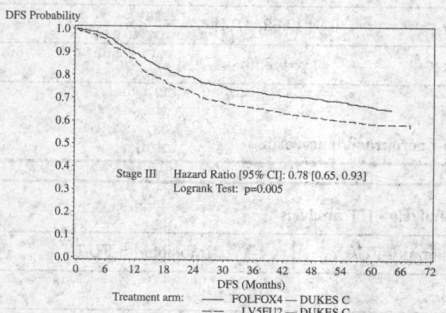

Figure 3 - DFS Kaplan-Meier curves by treatment arm in Stage III patients (cutoff: 1 June 2006) – ITT population

The following table summarizes the overall survival (OS) results in the overall randomized population and in patients with stage II and III disease, based on the ITT analysis.

[See table 19 on next page]

14.2   Combination Therapy with ELOXATIN and 5-fluorouracil/leucovorin in Patients Previously Untreated for Advanced Colorectal Cancer

A North American, multicenter, open-label, randomized controlled study was sponsored by the National Cancer Institute (NCI) as an intergroup study led by the North Central Cancer Treatment Group (NCCTG). The study had 7 arms at different times during its conduct, four of which were closed due to either changes in the standard of care, toxicity, or simplification. During the study, the control arm was changed to irinotecan plus 5-fluorouracil/leucovorin. The results reported below compared the efficacy and safety of two experimental regimens, ELOXATIN in combination with infusional 5-fluorouracil/leucovorin and a combination of ELOXATIN plus irinotecan, to an approved control regimen of irinotecan plus 5-fluorouracil/leucovorin in 795 concurrently randomized patients previously untreated for locally advanced or metastatic colorectal cancer. After completion of enrollment, the dose of irinotecan plus 5-fluorouracil/leucovorin was decreased due to toxicity. Patients had to be at least 18 years of age, have known locally advanced, locally recurrent, or metastatic colorectal adenocarcinoma not curable by surgery or amenable to radiation therapy with curative intent, histologically proven colorectal adenocarcinoma, measurable or evaluable disease, with an ECOG performance status 0, 1, or 2. Patients had to have granulocyte count $\geq 1.5 \times 10^9$/L, platelets $\geq 100 \times 10^9$/L, hemoglobin ≥ 9.0 gm/dL, creatinine $\leq 1.5 \times$ ULN, total bilirubin ≤ 1.5 mg/dL, AST $\leq 5 \times$ ULN, and alkaline phosphatase $\leq 5 \times$ ULN. Patients may have received adjuvant therapy for resected Stage II or III disease without recurrence within 12 months. The patients were stratified for ECOG performance status (0, 1 vs. 2), prior adjuvant chemotherapy (yes vs. no), prior immunotherapy (yes vs. no), and age (<65 vs. ≥65 years). Although no post study treatment was specified in the protocol, 65 to 72% of patients received additional post study chemotherapy after study treatment discontinuation on all arms. Fifty-eight percent of patients on the ELOXATIN plus 5-fluorouracil/leucovorin arm received an irinotecan-containing regimen and 23% of patients on the irinotecan plus 5-fluorouracil/leucovorin arm received oxaliplatin-containing regimens. Oxaliplatin was not commercially available during the trial.

Table 16 - Patient Characteristics in Adjuvant Therapy Study

	ELOXATIN + infusional 5-FU/LV N=1123	Infusional 5-FU/LV N=1123
Sex: Male (%)	56.1	52.4
Female (%)	43.9	47.6
Median age (years)	61.0	60.0
<65 years of age (%)	64.4	66.2
≥65 years of age (%)	35.6	33.8
Karnofsky Performance Status (KPS) (%)		
100	29.7	30.5
90	52.2	53.9
80	4.4	3.3
70	13.2	11.9
≤60	0.6	0.4
Primary site (%)		
Colon including cecum	54.6	54.4
Sigmoid	31.9	33.8
Recto sigmoid	12.9	10.9
Other including rectum	0.6	0.9
Bowel obstruction (%)		
Yes	17.9	19.3
Perforation (%)		
Yes	6.9	6.9
Stage at Randomization (%)		
II (T=3,4 N=0, M=0)	40.1	39.9
III (T=any, N=1,2, M=0)	59.6	59.3
IV (T=any, N=any, M=1)	0.4	0.8
Staging–T (%)		
T1	0.5	0.7
T2	4.5	4.8
T3	76.0	75.9
T4	19.0	18.5
Staging–N (%)		
N0	40.2	39.9
N1	39.4	39.4
N2	20.4	20.7
Staging–M (%)		
M1	0.4	0.8

Table 17 - Dosing in Adjuvant Therapy Study

	ELOXATIN + infusional 5-FU/LV N=1108	Infusional 5-FU/LV N=1111
Median Relative Dose Intensity (%)		
5-FU	84.4	97.7
ELOXATIN	80.5	N/A
Median Number of Cycles	12	12
Median Number of cycles with ELOXATIN	11	N/A

The following table presents the dosing regimens of the three arms of the study.
[See table 20 at top of next page]
The following table presents the demographics of the patient population entered into this study.
[See table 21 on next page]
The length of a treatment cycle was 2 weeks for the ELOXATIN and 5-fluorouracil/leucovorin regimen; 6 weeks for the irinotecan plus 5-fluorouracil/leucovorin regimen; and 3 weeks for the ELOXATIN plus irinotecan regimen. The median number of cycles administered per patient was 10 (23.9 weeks) for the ELOXATIN and 5-fluorouracil/leucovorin regimen, 4 (23.6 weeks) for the irinotecan plus 5-fluorouracil/leucovorin regimen, and 7 (21.0 weeks) for the ELOXATIN plus irinotecan regimen. Patients treated with the ELOXATIN and 5-fluorouracil/leucovorin combination had a significantly longer time to tumor progression based on investigator assessment, longer overall survival, and a significantly higher confirmed response rate based on investigator assessment compared to patients given irinotecan plus 5-fluorouracil/leucovorin. The following table summarizes the efficacy results.
[See table 22 at top of page 2990]
Figure 4 illustrates the Kaplan-Meier survival curves for the comparison of ELOXATIN and 5-fluorouracil/leucovorin combination and ELOXATIN plus irinotecan to irinotecan plus 5-fluorouracil/leucovorin.

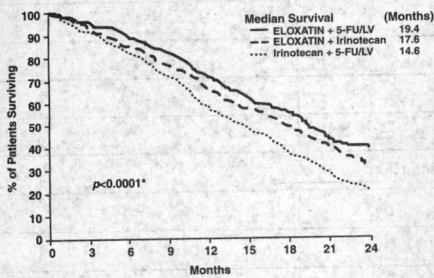

Figure 4 – Kaplan-Meier Overall Survival by treatment arm

A descriptive subgroup analysis demonstrated that the improvement in survival for ELOXATIN plus 5-fluorouracil/leucovorin compared to irinotecan plus 5-fluorouracil/leucovorin appeared to be maintained across age groups, prior adjuvant therapy, and number of organs involved. An estimated survival advantage in ELOXATIN plus 5-fluorouracil/leucovorin versus irinotecan plus 5-fluorouracil/leucovorin was seen in both genders; however it was greater among women than men. Insufficient subgroup sizes prevented analysis by race.

14.3 Combination Therapy with ELOXATIN and 5-fluorouracil/leucovorin in Previously Treated Patients with Advanced Colorectal Cancer

A multicenter, open-label, randomized, three-arm controlled study was conducted in the US and Canada comparing the efficacy and safety of ELOXATIN in combination with an infusional schedule of 5-fluorouracil/leucovorin to the same dose and schedule of 5-fluorouracil/leucovorin alone and to single agent oxaliplatin in patients with advanced colorectal cancer who had relapsed/progressed during or within 6 months of first-line therapy with bolus 5-fluorouracil/leucovorin and irinotecan. The study was intended to be analyzed for response rate after 450 patients were enrolled. Survival will be subsequently assessed in all patients enrolled in the completed study. Accrual to this study is complete, with 821 patients enrolled. Patients in the study had to be at least 18 years of age, have unresectable, measurable, histologically proven colorectal adenocarcinoma, with a Karnofsky performance status >50%. Patients had to have SGOT(AST) and SGPT(ALT) ≤2× the institution's upper limit of normal (ULN), unless liver metastases were present and documented at baseline by CT or MRI scan, in which case ≤5× ULN was permitted. Patients had to have alkaline phosphatase ≤2× the institution's ULN, unless liver metastases were present and documented at baseline by CT or MRI scan, in which cases ≤5× ULN was permitted. Prior radiotherapy was permitted if it had been completed at least 3 weeks before randomization.
The dosing regimens of the three arms of the study are presented in the table below.
[See table 23 on page 2990]
Patients entered into the study for evaluation of response must have had at least one unidimensional lesion measuring ≥20mm using conventional CT or MRI scans, or ≥10mm using a spiral CT scan. Tumor response and progression were assessed every 3 cycles (6 weeks) using the Response Evaluation Criteria in Solid Tumors (RECIST) until radiological documentation of progression or for 13

months following the first dose of study drug(s), whichever came first. Confirmed responses were based on two tumor assessments separated by at least 4 weeks.
The demographics of the patient population entered into this study are shown in the table below.
[See table 24 on page 2991]
The median number of cycles administered per patient was 6 for the ELOXATIN and 5-fluorouracil/leucovorin combination and 3 each for 5-fluorouracil/leucovorin alone and ELOXATIN alone.
Patients treated with the combination of ELOXATIN and 5-fluorouracil/leucovorin had an increased response rate compared to patients given 5-fluorouracil/leucovorin or oxaliplatin alone. The efficacy results are summarized in the tables below.
[See table 25 on page 2991]

[See table 26 on page 2991]
At the time of the interim analysis 49% of the radiographic progression events had occurred. In this interim analysis an estimated 2-month increase in median time to radiographic progression was observed compared to 5-fluorouracil/leucovorin alone.
Of the 13 patients who had tumor response to the combination of ELOXATIN and 5-fluorouracil/leucovorin, 5 were female and 8 were male, and responders included patients <65 years old and ≥65 years old. The small number of non-Caucasian participants made efficacy analyses in these populations uninterpretable.

15 REFERENCES
1. NIOSH Alert: Preventing occupational exposures to antineoplastic and other hazardous drugs in healthcare

Table 18 - Summary of DFS analysis – ITT analysis*

Parameter	ELOXATIN + Infusional 5-FU/LV	Infusional 5-FU/LV
Overall		
N	1123	1123
Number of events – relapse or death (%)	304 (27.1)	360 (32.1)
Disease-free survival % [95% CI][†]	73.3 [70.7, 76.0]	67.4 [64.6, 70.2]
Hazard ratio [95% CI][‡]	0.80 [0.68, 0.93]	
Stratified Logrank test	p=0.003	
Stage III (Dukes' C)		
N	672	675
Number of events–relapse or death (%)	226 (33.6)	271 (40.1)
Disease-free survival % [95% CI][†]	66.4 [62.7, 70.0]	58.9 [55.2, 62.7]
Hazard ratio [95% CI][‡]	0.78 [0.65, 0.93]	
Logrank test	p=0.005	
Stage II (Dukes' B2)		
N	451	448
Number of events–relapse or death (%)	78 (17.3)	89 (19.9)
Disease-free survival % [95% CI][†]	83.7 [80.2, 87.1]	79.9 [76.2, 83.7]
Hazard ratio [95% CI][‡]	0.84 [0.62, 1.14]	
Logrank test	p=0.258	

* Data cut off for disease free survival 1 June 2006
† Disease-free survival at 5 years
‡ A hazard ratio of less than 1.00 favors Eloxatin + Infusional 5-fluorouracil/leucovorin

Table 19 - Summary of OS analysis - ITT analysis*

Parameter	Eloxatin + Infusional 5-FU/LV	Infusional 5-FU/LV
Overall		
N	1123	1123
Number of death events (%)	245 (21.8)	283 (25.2)
Hazard ratio[†] [95% CI]	0.84 [0.71, 1.00]	
Stage III (Dukes' C)		
N	672	675
Number of death events (%)	182 (27.1)	220 (32.6)
Hazard ratio[†] [95% CI]	0.80 [0.65, 0.97]	
Stage II (Dukes' B2)		
N	451	448
Number of death events (%)	63 (14.0)	63 (14.1)
Hazard ratio[†] [95% CI]	1.00 [0.70, 1.41]	

* Data cut off for overall survival 16 January 2007
† A hazard ratio of less than 1.00 favors Eloxatin + Infusional 5-fluourouracil/leucovorin

settings. 2004. U.S. Department of Health and Human Services, Public Health Service, Centers for Disease Control and Prevention, National Institute for Occupational Safety and Health, DHHS (NIOSH) Publication No. 2004–165.
2. OSHA Technical Manual, TED 1-0.15A, Section VI: Chapter 2. Controlling Occupational Exposure to Hazardous Drugs. OSHA, 1999.
http://www.osha.gov/dts/osta/otm/otm_vi/otm_vi_2.html
3. American Society of Health-System Pharmacists. (2006) ASHP Guidelines on Handling Hazardous Drugs.
4. Polovich, M., White, J. M., & Kelleher, L.O. (eds.) 2005. Chemotherapy and biotherapy guidelines and recommendations for practice (2nd. ed.) Pittsburgh, PA: Oncology Nursing Society.

16 HOW SUPPLIED/STORAGE AND HANDLING

16.1 How Supplied

Powder for solution for infusion:
ELOXATIN is supplied in clear, glass, single-use vials with gray elastomeric stoppers and aluminum flip-off seals containing 50 mg or 100 mg of oxaliplatin as a sterile, preservative-free lyophilized powder for reconstitution. Lactose monohydrate is also present as an inactive ingredient.
NDC 0024-0596-02: 50 mg single-use vial with green flip-off seal individually packaged in a carton.
NDC 0024-0597-04: 100 mg single-use vial with dark blue flip-off seal individually packaged in a carton.
Concentrate for solution for infusion:
ELOXATIN is supplied in clear, glass, single-use vials with gray elastomeric stoppers and aluminum flip-off seals containing 50 mg, 100 mg or 200 mg of oxaliplatin as a sterile, preservative-free, aqueous solution at a concentration of 5 mg/ml. Water for Injection, USP is present as an inactive ingredient.
NDC 0024-0590-10: 50 mg single-use vial with green flip-off seal individually packaged in a carton.
NDC 0024-0591-20: 100 mg single-use vial with dark blue flip-off seal individually packaged in a carton.
NDC 0024-0592-40: 200 mg single-use vial with orange flip-off seal individually packaged in a carton.

16.2 Storage

Powder for solution for infusion:
Store under normal lighting conditions at 25°C (77°F); excursions permitted to 15–30°C (59–86°F) [see USP controlled room temperature].
Concentrate for solution for infusion:
Store at 25°C (77°F); excursions permitted to 15–30°C (59–86°F). Do not freeze and protect from light (keep in original outer carton).

16.3 Handling and Disposal

As with other potentially toxic anticancer agents, care should be exercised in the handling and preparation of infusion solutions prepared from ELOXATIN. The use of gloves is recommended. If a solution of ELOXATIN contacts the skin, wash the skin immediately and thoroughly with soap and water. If ELOXATIN contacts the mucous membranes, flush thoroughly with water.
Procedures for the handling and disposal of anticancer drugs should be considered. Several guidelines on the subject have been published [see References (15)]. There is no general agreement that all of the procedures recommended in the guidelines are necessary or appropriate.

17 PATIENT COUNSELING INFORMATION

17.1 Information for Patients

Patients and patients' caregivers should be informed of the expected side effects of ELOXATIN, particularly its neurologic effects, both the acute, reversible effects and the persistent neurosensory toxicity. Patients should be informed that the acute neurosensory toxicity may be precipitated or exacerbated by exposure to cold or cold objects. Patients should be instructed to avoid cold drinks, use of ice, and should cover exposed skin prior to exposure to cold temperature or cold objects.
Patients must be adequately informed of the risk of low blood cell counts and instructed to contact their physician immediately should fever, particularly if associated with persistent diarrhea, or evidence of infection develop.
Patients should be instructed to contact their physician if persistent vomiting, diarrhea, signs of dehydration, cough or breathing difficulties occur, or signs of allergic reaction appear.
No studies on the effects on the ability to drive and use machines have been performed. However oxaliplatin treatment resulting in an increase risk of dizziness, nausea and vomiting, and other neurologic symptoms that affect gait and balance may lead to a minor or moderate influence on the ability to drive and use machines.
Vision abnormalities, in particular transient vision loss (reversible following therapy discontinuation), may affect patients' ability to drive and use machines. Therefore, patients should be warned of the potential effect of these events on the ability to drive or use machines.

Table 20 – Dosing Regimens in Patients Previously Untreated for Advanced Colorectal Cancer Clinical Trial

Treatment Arm	Dose	Regimen
ELOXATIN + 5-FU/LV (FOLFOX4) (N=267)	Day 1: ELOXATIN: 85 mg/m^2 (2-hour infusion) + LV 200 mg/m^2 (2-hour infusion), followed by 5-FU: 400 mg/m^2 (bolus), 600 mg/m^2 (22-hour infusion) Day 2: LV 200 mg/m^2 (2-hour infusion), followed by 5-FU: 400 mg/m^2 (bolus), 600 mg/m^2 (22-hour infusion)	every 2 weeks
Irinotecan + 5-FU/LV (IFL) (N=264)	Day 1: irinotecan 125 mg/m^2 as a 90-min infusion + LV 20 mg/m^2 as a 15-min infusion or intravenous push, followed by 5-FU 500 mg/m^2 intravenous bolus weekly × 4	every 6 weeks
ELOXATIN + Irinotecan (IROX) (N=264)	Day 1: ELOXATIN: 85 mg/m^2 intravenous (2-hour infusion) + irinotecan 200 mg/m^2 intravenous over 30 minutes	every 3 weeks

Table 21 – Patient Demographics in Patients Previously Untreated for Advanced Colorectal Cancer Clinical Trial

	ELOXATIN + 5-FU/LV N=267	Irinotecan + 5-FU/LV N=264	ELOXATIN + irinotecan N=264
Sex: Male (%)	58.8	65.2	61.0
Female (%)	41.2	34.8	39.0
Median age (years)	61.0	61.0	61.0
<65 years of age (%)	61	62	63
≥65 years of age (%)	39	38	37
ECOG (%)			
0.1	94.4	95.5	94.7
2	5.6	4.5	5.3
Involved organs (%)			
Colon only	0.7	0.8	0.4
Liver only	39.3	44.3	39.0
Liver + other	41.2	38.6	40.9
Lung only	6.4	3.8	5.3
Other (including lymph nodes)	11.6	11.0	12.9
Not reported	0.7	1.5	1.5
Prior radiation (%)	3.0	1.5	3.0
Prior surgery (%)	74.5	79.2	81.8
Prior adjuvant (%)	15.7	14.8	15.2

17.2 FDA-Approved Patient Labeling

Patient Information
ELOXATIN® (eh-LOX-ah-tin) (OXALIplatin)
powder, for solution for intravenous use
and
ELOXATIN® (eh-LOX-ah-tin) (OXALIplatin)
concentrate, for solution for intravenous use
Read this information carefully before you start using ELOXATIN. It will help you learn more about ELOXATIN. This information does not take the place of talking to your doctor about your medical condition or your treatment. Ask your doctor about any questions you have.
What is the most important information I should know about ELOXATIN?
ELOXATIN can cause serious allergic reactions.
In people who get severe allergic reactions while taking platinum medicines, death can occur.
Get emergency help right away if you:
• **suddenly have trouble breathing.**
• **feel like your throat is closing up.**
Call your doctor right away if you have any signs of allergic reaction:
• rash
• flushed face
• hives
• itching
• swelling of your lips or tongue
• sudden cough
• dizziness or feel faint
• sweating
• chest pain

If you have vision problems while taking Eloxatin
• do not drive, operate heavy machines, or engage in dangerous activities.
See "What are the possible side effects of ELOXATIN" for information on other serious side effects.
What is ELOXATIN?
ELOXATIN is an anti-cancer (chemotherapy) medicine that is used with other anti-cancer medicines called 5-fluorouracil and leucovorin to treat adults with:
• stage III colon cancer after surgery to remove the tumor
• advanced colon or rectal cancer (colo-rectal cancer).
ELOXATIN with infusional 5-fluorouracil and leucovorin was shown to lower the chance of colon cancer returning when given to patients with stage III colon cancer after surgery to remove the tumor. ELOXATIN also increases survival in patients with stage III colon cancer. ELOXATIN with infusional 5-fluorouracil and leucovorin was also shown to increase survival, shrink tumors and delay growth of tumors in some patients with advanced colorectal cancer. It is not known if ELOXATIN works in children.
Who should not use ELOXATIN?
Do not use ELOXATIN if you are allergic to any of the ingredients in Eloxatin or other medicines that contain platinum. Cisplatin (Platinol®) and carboplatin (Paraplatin®) are other chemotherapy medicines that also contain platinum. See the end of this leaflet for a list of the ingredients ELOXATIN.
What should I tell my doctor before treatment with ELOXATIN?
Tell your doctor about all your medical conditions including, if you are:
• pregnant or planning to become pregnant. ELOXATIN may harm your unborn child. You should avoid becoming pregnant while taking ELOXATIN. Talk with your doctor about how to avoid pregnancy.

Table 22 – Summary of Efficacy*

	ELOXATIN + 5-FU/LV N=267	irinotecan + 5-FU/LV N=264	ELOXATIN + irinotecan N=264
Survival (ITT)			
Number of deaths N (%)	155 (58.1)	192 (72.7)	175 (66.3)
Median survival (months)	19.4	14.6	17.6
Hazard Ratio and (95% confidence interval)	0.65 (0.53–0.80)[†]		
P-value	<0.0001[†]	-	-
TTP (ITT, investigator assessment)			
Percentage of progressors	82.8	81.8	89.4
Median TTP (months)	8.7	6.9	6.5
Hazard Ratio and (95% confidence interval)[‡]	0.74 (0.61–0.89)[†]		
P-value	0.0014[†]		
Response Rate (investigator assessment)[§]			
Patients with measurable disease	210	212	215
Complete response N (%)	13 (6.2)	5 (2.4)	7 (3.3)
Partial response N (%)	82 (39.0)	64 (30.2)	67 (31.2)
Complete and partial response N (%)	95 (45.2)	69 (32.5)	74 (34.4)
95% confidence interval	(38.5–52.0)	(26.2–38.9)	(28.1–40.8)
P-value	0.0080[†]	-	-

* The numbers in the response rate and TTP analysis are based on unblinded investigator assessment.
[†] Compared to irinotecan plus 5-fluorouracil/leucovorin (IFL) arm
[‡] A hazard ratio of less than 1.00 favors Eloxatin + Infusional 5-fluorouracil/leucovorin
[§] Based on all patients with measurable disease at baseline

Table 23 – Dosing Regimens in Refractory and Relapsed Colorectal Cancer Clinical Trial

Treatment Arm	Dose	Regimen
ELOXATIN + 5-FU/LV (N=152)	Day 1: ELOXATIN: 85 mg/m^2 (2-hour infusion) + LV 200 mg/m^2 (2-hour infusion), followed by 5-FU: 400 mg/m^2 (bolus), 600 mg/m^2 (22-hour infusion) Day 2: LV 200 mg/m^2 (2-hour infusion), followed by 5-FU: 400 mg/m^2 (bolus), 600 mg/m^2 (22-hour infusion)	every 2 weeks
5-FU/LV (N=151)	Day 1: LV 200 mg/m^2 (2-hour infusion), followed by 5-FU: 400 mg/m^2 (bolus), 600 mg/m^2 (22-hour infusion) Day 2: LV 200 mg/m^2 (2-hour infusion), followed by 5-FU: 400 mg/m^2 (bolus), 600 mg/m^2 (22-hour infusion)	every 2 weeks
ELOXATIN (N=156)	Day 1: ELOXATIN 85 mg/m^2 (2-hour infusion)	every 2 weeks

- breast feeding or plan to breast feed. We do not know if ELOXATIN can pass through your milk and if it can harm your baby. You will need to decide whether to stop breast feeding or not to take ELOXATIN.

Tell your doctor about all the medicines you take, including prescription and non-prescription medicines, vitamins, and herbal supplements. ELOXATIN may affect how other medicines work in your body.

Know the medicines you take. Keep a list of them and show it to your doctor and pharmacist when you get a new medicine.

How is ELOXATIN given to me?
ELOXATIN is given to you through your veins (blood vessels).
- Your doctor will prescribe ELOXATIN in an amount that is right for you.
- Your doctor will treat you with several medicines for your cancer.
- It is very important that you do exactly what your doctor and nurse have taught you to do.
- Some medicines may be given to you before ELOXATIN to help prevent nausea and vomiting.
- ELOXATIN is given with 2 other chemotherapy medicines, leucovorin and 5-fluorouracil.
- Each treatment course is given to you over 2 days. You will receive ELOXATIN on the first day only.
- There are usually 14 days between each chemotherapy treatment course.

Treatment Day 1:
ELOXATIN and leucovorin are given through a thin plastic tube put into a vein (intravenous infusion or I.V.) and given for 2 hours. You will be watched by a healthcare provider during this time.
Right after the ELOXATIN and leucovorin are finished, 2 doses of 5-fluorouracil will be given. The first dose is given right away into your I.V. tube. The second dose will be given into your I.V. tube over the next 22 hours, using a pump device.

Treatment Day 2:
You will not get ELOXATIN on Day 2. Leucovorin and 5-fluorouracil will be given the same way as on Day 1.

During your treatment with ELOXATIN:
- It is important for you to keep all appointments. Call your doctor if you must miss an appointment. There may be special instructions for you.
- Your doctor may change how often you get ELOXATIN, how much you get, or how long the infusion will take.
- You and your doctor will discuss how many times you will get ELOXATIN.

The 5-fluorouracil will be given through your I.V. with a pump. If you have any problems with the pump or the tube, call your doctor, your nurse, or the person who is responsible for your pump. Do not let anyone other than a healthcare provider touch your infusion pump or tubing.

What activities should I avoid while on treatment with ELOXATIN?
- Avoid cold temperatures and cold objects. Cover your skin if you must go outside in cold temperatures.

- Do not drink cold drinks or use ice cubes in drinks.
- Do not put ice or ice packs on your body.

See the end of this leaflet ("How can I reduce the side effects caused by cold temperatures?") for more information.
Talk with your doctor and nurse about your level of activity during treatment with ELOXATIN. Follow their instructions.

What are the possible side effects of ELOXATIN?
ELOXATIN can cause serious side effects:
- **Serious allergic reactions.** See "What is the most important information I should know about ELOXATIN?"
- **Nerve problems (peripheral neuropathy).** ELOXATIN can affect how your nerves work and make you feel. Tell your doctor right away if you get any signs of nerve problems listed below:
  - Very sensitive to cold temperatures and cold objects
  - Trouble breathing, swallowing, or saying words, jaw tightness, odd feelings in your tongue, or chest pressure
  - Pain, tingling, burning (pins and needles, numb feeling) in your hands, feet, or around your mouth or throat, which may cause problems walking or performing activities of daily living.

  The first signs of nerve problems may happen with the first treatment. The nerve problems can also start up to 2 days after treatment. If you develop nerve problems, the amount of ELOXATIN in your next treatment may be changed or ELOXATIN treatment may be stopped.
  For information on ways to lessen or help with the nerve problems, see the end of this leaflet, "How can I reduce the side effects caused by cold temperatures?"
- **Lung problems (interstitial fibrosis).** Tell your doctor if you get a dry cough and have trouble breathing (shortness of breath) before your next treatment. These may be signs of a serious lung disease.
- **Liver problems (hepatotoxicity).** Your doctor will do blood tests to watch for this.
- **Harm to an unborn baby. ELOXATIN may cause harm to your unborn baby.** See "What should I tell my doctor before treatment with ELOXATIN?"

Common side effects with ELOXATIN include:
- decreased blood counts: Eloxatin can cause a decrease in neutrophils (a type of white blood cells important in fighting in bacterial infections), red blood cells (blood cells that carry oxygen to the tissues), and platelets (important for clotting and to control bleeding).

Call your doctor right away if you get any of the following signs of infection:
- Fever (temperature of 100.5 F or greater)
- Chills or shivering
- Cough that brings up mucus
- Burning or pain on urination
- Pain on swallowing
- Sore throat
- Redness or swelling at intravenous site
- Tell your doctor about any bleeding or bruising.
- nausea
- vomiting
- diarrhea
- constipation
- mouth sores
- stomach pain
- decreased appetite
- tiredness
- eyesight (visual) problems including reversible short-term loss of vision. Tell your doctor about any eyesight changes
- injection site reactions. Reactions may include redness, swelling, pain, tissue damage
- hair loss (alopecia)

Call your doctor if you get any of the following:
- Vomiting that does not go away
- Frequent, loose, watery bowel movements (Diarrhea)
- Signs of dehydration (too much water loss)
  ○ tiredness
  ○ thirst
  ○ dry mouth
  ○ lightheadedness (dizziness)
  ○ decreased urination

Tell your doctor if you have any side effect that bothers you or that does not go away. These are not all the possible side effects of ELOXATIN. For more information, ask your doctor or pharmacist.

Call your doctor for medical advice about side effects. You may report side effects to FDA at 1-800-FDA-1088.

How can I reduce the side effects caused by cold temperatures?
- Cover yourself with a blanket while you are getting your ELOXATIN infusion.
- Do not breathe deeply when exposed to cold air.
- Wear warm clothing in cold weather at all times. Cover your mouth and nose with a scarf or a pull-down cap (ski cap) to warm the air that goes to your lungs.
- Wear gloves when taking things from the freezer or refrigerator.
- Drink fluids warm or at room temperature.

- Always drink through a straw.
- **Do not** use ice chips if you have nausea or mouth sores. Ask your nurse about what you can use.
- Be aware that most metals are cold to touch, especially in the winter. These include your car door and mailbox. Wear gloves to touch cold objects.
- Do not run the air-conditioning at high levels in the house or in the car in hot weather.
- If your body gets cold, warm-up the affected part. If your hands get cold, wash them with warm water.
- Always let your nurse and doctor know **before** your next treatment how well you did since your last visit.

This list is not complete and your healthcare provider may have other useful tips for helping you with these side effects.

General information about the safe and effective use of ELOXATIN

Medicines are sometimes prescribed for conditions that are not mentioned in patient information leaflets.

This leaflet summarizes the most important information about ELOXATIN. If you would like more information, talk with your doctor. You can ask your doctor or pharmacist for information about ELOXATIN that is written for health professionals.

What are the ingredients in ELOXATIN?

Active ingredient: oxaliplatin

Powder for solution for infusion inactive ingredients: lactose monohydrate

Concentrate for solution for infusion inactive ingredients: water for injection

Paraplatin® and Platinol® are registered trademarks of Bristol-Myers Squibb Company.

Manufactured by:
sanofi-aventis U.S. LLC
Bridgewater, NJ 08807

Eloxatin is also manufactured by Ben Venue Laboratories Cleveland, OH 44146 0568 for sanofi-aventis U.S. LLC

©2009 sanofi-aventis U.S. LLC

Revised: 03/2009   sanofi-aventis U.S. LLC

Shown in Product Identification Guide, page 319

FERRLECIT®
(sodium ferric gluconate complex in sucrose injection)   ℞

DESCRIPTION

Ferrlecit® (sodium ferric gluconate complex in sucrose injection) is a stable macromolecular complex with an apparent molecular weight on gel chromatography of 289,000–440,000 daltons. The macromolecular complex is negatively charged at alkaline pH and is present in solution with sodium cations. The product has a deep red color indicative of ferric oxide linkages.

The structural formula is considered to be $[NaFe_2O_3(C_6H_{11}O_7)(C_{12}H_{22}O_{11}5]_{n\sim200}$.

Each sterile, single-use ampule of 5 mL of Ferrlecit for intravenous injection contains 62.5 mg (12.5 mg/mL) of elemental iron as the sodium salt of a ferric ion carbohydrate complex in an alkaline aqueous solution with approximately 20% sucrose w/v (195 mg/mL) in water for injection, pH 7.7–9.7.

Each mL contains 9 mg of benzyl alcohol as an inactive ingredient.

Therapeutic class: Hematinic

CLINICAL PHARMACOLOGY

Ferrlecit is used to replete the total body content of iron. Iron is critical for normal hemoglobin synthesis to maintain oxygen transport. Additionally, iron is necessary for metabolism and various enzymatic processes.

The total body iron content of an adult ranges from 2 to 4 grams. Approximately 2/3 is in hemoglobin and 1/3 is in reticuloendothelial (RE) storage (bone marrow, spleen, liver) bound to intracellular ferritin. The body highly conserves iron (daily loss of 0.03%) requiring supplementation of about 1 mg/day to replenish losses in healthy, nonmenstruating adults. The etiology of iron deficiency in hemodialysis patients is varied and can include blood loss and/or increased iron utilization (e.g., from epoetin therapy). The administration of exogenous epoetin increases red blood cell production and iron utilization. The increased iron utilization and blood losses in the hemodialysis patient may lead to absolute or functional iron deficiency. Iron deficiency is absolute when hematological indicators of iron stores are low. Patients with functional iron deficiency do not meet laboratory criteria for absolute iron deficiency but demonstrate an increase in hemoglobin/hematocrit or a decrease in epoetin dosage with stable hemoglobin/hematocrit when parenteral iron is administered.

Pharmacokinetics

Multiple sequential single dose intravenous pharmacokinetic studies were performed on 14 healthy iron-deficient volunteers. Entry criteria included hemoglobin ≥ 10.5 gm/dL and transferrin saturation $\leq 15\%$ (TSAT) or serum ferritin value ≤ 20 ng/mL. In the first stage, each subject was randomized 1:1 to undiluted Ferrlecit injection of either 125 mg/hr or 62.5 mg/0.5 hr (2.1 mg/min). Five days after the first stage, each subject was re-randomized 1:1 to undiluted Ferrlecit injection of either 125 mg/7 min or 62.5 mg/4 min (>15.5 mg/min).

Peak drug levels (C_{max}) varied significantly by dosage and by rate of administration with the highest C_{max} observed in the regimen in which 125 mg was administered in 7 minutes (19.0 mg/L). The initial volume of distribution (V_{Ferr}) of 6 L corresponds well to calculated blood volume. V_{Ferr} did not vary by dosage or rate of administration. The terminal elimination half-life (λ_z-HL) for drug bound iron was approximately 1 hour. λ_z-HL varied by dose but not by rate of administration. The shortest value (0.85 h) occurred in the 62.5 mg/4 min regimen; the longest value (1.45 h) occurred in the 125 mg/7 min regimen. Total clearance of Ferrlecit was 3.02 to 5.35 L/h. There was no significant variation by rate of administration. The AUC for Ferrlecit bound iron varied by dose from 17.5 mg-h/L (62.5 mg) to 35.6 mg-h/L (125 mg). There was no significant variation by rate of administration. Approximately 80% of drug bound iron was delivered to transferrin as a mononuclear ionic iron species

---

Table 24 – Patient Demographics in Refractory and Relapsed Colorectal Cancer Clinical Trial

	5-FU/LV (N = 151)	ELOXATIN (N = 156)	ELOXATIN + 5-FU/LV (N = 152)
Sex: Male (%)	54.3	60.9	57.2
Female (%)	45.7	39.1	42.8
Median age (years)	60.0	61.0	59.0
Range	21–80	27–79	22–88
Race (%)			
Caucasian	87.4	84.6	88.8
Black	7.9	7.1	5.9
Asian	1.3	2.6	2.6
Other	3.3	5.8	2.6
KPS (%)			
70–100	94.7	92.3	95.4
50–60	2.6	4.5	2.0
Not reported	2.6	3.2	2.6
Prior radiotherapy (%)	25.2	19.2	25.0
Prior pelvic radiation (%)	18.5	13.5	21.1
Number of metastatic sites (%)			
1	27.2	31.4	25.7
≥2	72.2	67.9	74.3
Liver involvement (%)			
Liver only	22.5	25.6	18.4
Liver + other	60.3	59.0	53.3

Table 25 - Response Rates (ITT Analysis)

Best Response	5-FU/LV (N=151)	ELOXATIN (N=156)	ELOXATIN + 5-FU/LV (N=152)
CR	0	0	0
PR	0	2 (1%)	13 (9%)
p-value	0.0002 for 5-FU/LV vs. ELOXATIN + 5-FU/LV		
95% CI	0–2.4%	0.2–4.6%	4.6–14.2%

Table 26 - Summary of Radiographic Time to Progression*

Arm	5-FU/LV (N=151)	ELOXATIN (N=156)	ELOXATIN + 5-FU/LV (N=152)
No. of Progressors	74	101	50
No. of patients with no radiological *evaluation beyond baseline*	22 (15%)	16 (10%)	17 (11%)
Median TTP (months)	2.7	1.6	4.6
95% CI	1.8–3.0	1.4–2.7	4.2–6.1

*This is not an ITT analysis. Events were limited to radiographic disease progression documented by independent review of radiographs. Clinical progression was not included in this analysis, and 18% of patients were excluded from the analysis based on unavailability of the radiographs for independent review.

within 24 hours of administration in each dosage regimen. Direct movement of iron from Ferrlecit to transferrin was not observed. Mean peak transferrin saturation did not exceed 100% and returned to near baseline by 40 hours after administration of each dosage regimen.

Pediatrics: Single dose intravenous pharmacokinetic analyses were performed on 48 iron-deficient pediatric hemodialysis patients. Twenty-two patients received 1.5 mg/kg Ferrlecit and 26 patients received 3.0 mg/kg Ferrlecit (maximum dose 125 mg). The mean Cmax, $AUC_{0-\infty}$, and terminal elimination half-life values for the 22 patients who received a 1.5 mg/kg dose were 12.9 mg/L, 95.0 mg•hr/L, and 2.0 hours, respectively. The mean Cmax, $AUC_{0-\infty}$, and terminal elimination half-life values for the 26 patients who received a 3.0 mg/kg dose were 22.8 mg/L, 170.9 mg•hr/L, and 2.5 hours, respectively.

In vitro experiments have shown that less than 1% of the iron species within Ferrlecit can be dialyzed through membranes with pore sizes corresponding to 12,000 to 14,000 daltons over a period of up to 270 minutes. Human studies in renally competent patients suggest the clinical insignificance of urinary excretion.

Drug-drug Interactions: Drug-drug interactions involving Ferrlecit have not been studied. However, like other parenteral iron preparations, Ferrlecit may be expected to reduce the absorption of concomitantly administered oral iron preparations.

CLINICAL STUDIES

Two clinical studies (Studies A and B) were conducted in adults and one clinical study was conducted in pediatric patients (Study C) to assess the efficacy and safety of Ferrlecit.

Study A

Study A was a three-center, randomized, open-label study of the safety and efficacy of two doses of Ferrlecit administered intravenously to iron-deficient hemodialysis patients. The study included both a dose-response concurrent control and an historical control. Enrolled patients received a test dose of Ferrlecit (25 mg of elemental iron) and were then randomly assigned to receive Ferrlecit at cumulative doses of either 500 mg (low dose) or 1000 mg (high dose) of elemental iron. Ferrlecit was given to both dose groups in eight divided doses during sequential dialysis sessions (a period of 16 to 17 days). At each dialysis session, patients in the low-dose group received Ferrlecit 62.5 mg of elemental iron over 30 minutes, and those in the high-dose group received Ferrlecit 125 mg of elemental iron over 60 minutes. The primary endpoint was the change in hemoglobin from baseline to the last available observation through Day 40.

Eligibility for this study included chronic hemodialysis patients with a hemoglobin below 10 g/dL (or hematocrit at or below 32%) and either serum ferritin below 100 ng/mL or transferrin saturation below 18%. Exclusion criteria included significant underlying disease or inflammatory conditions or an epoetin requirement of greater than 10,000 units three times per week. Parenteral iron and red cell transfusion were not allowed for two months before the study. Oral iron and red cell transfusion were not allowed during the study for Ferrlecit-treated patients.

The historical control population consisted of 25 chronic hemodialysis patients who received only oral iron supplementation for 14 months and did not receive red cell transfusion. All patients had stable epoetin doses and hematocrit values for at least two months before initiation of oral iron therapy.

The evaluated population consisted of 39 patients in the low-dose Ferrlecit (sodium ferric gluconate complex in sucrose injection) group (50% female, 50% male; 74% white, 18% black, 5% Hispanic, 3% Asian; mean age 54 years, range 22–83 years), 44 patients in the high-dose Ferrlecit group (50% female, 48% male, 2% unknown; 75% white, 11% black, 5% Hispanic, 7% other, 2% unknown; mean age 56 years, range 20–87 years), and 25 historical control patients (68% female, 32% male; 40% white, 32% black, 20% Hispanic, 4% Asian, 4% unknown; mean age 52 years, range 25–84 years).

The mean baseline hemoglobin and hematocrit were similar between treatment and historical control patients: 9.8 g/dL and 29% and 9.6 g/dL and 29% in low- and high-dose Ferrlecit-treated patients, respectively, and 9.4 g/dL and 29% in historical control patients. Baseline serum transferrin saturation was 20% in the low-dose group, 16% in the high-dose group, and 14% in the historical control. Baseline serum ferritin was 106 ng/mL in the low-dose group, 88 ng/mL in the high-dose group, and 606 ng/mL in the historical control.

Patients in the high-dose Ferrlecit group achieved significantly higher increases in hemoglobin and hematocrit than either patients in the low-dose Ferrlecit group or patients in the historical control group (oral iron). Patients in the low-dose Ferrlecit group did not achieve significantly higher increases in hemoglobin and hematocrit than patients receiving oral iron. See Table 1.

[See table 1 above]

Study B

Study B was a single-center, non-randomized, open-label, historically-controlled, study of the safety and efficacy of variable, cumulative doses of intravenous Ferrlecit in iron-deficient hemodialysis patients. Ferrlecit administration was identical to Study A. The primary efficacy variable was the change in hemoglobin from baseline to the last available observation through Day 50.

Inclusion and exclusion criteria were identical to those of Study A as was the historical control population. Sixty-three patients were evaluated in this study: 38 in the Ferrlecit-treated group (37% female, 63% male; 95% white, 5% Asian; mean age 56 years, range 22–84 years) and 25 in the historical control group (68% female, 32% male; 40% white, 32% black, 20% Hispanic, 4% Asian, 4% unknown; mean age 52 years, range 25–84 years).

Ferrlecit-treated patients were considered to have completed the study per protocol if they received at least eight Ferrlecit doses of either 62.5 mg or 125 mg of elemental iron. A total of 14 patients (37%) completed the study per protocol. Twelve (32%) Ferrlecit-treated patients received less than eight doses, and 12 (32%) patients had incomplete information on the sequence of dosing. Not all patients received Ferrlecit at consecutive dialysis sessions and many received oral iron during the study.

[See second table above]

Baseline hemoglobin and hematocrit values were similar between the treatment and control groups, and were 9.1 g/dL and 27.3%, respectively, for Ferrlecit-treated patients. Serum iron studies were also similar between treatment and control groups, with the exception of serum ferritin, which was 606 ng/mL for historical control patients, compared to 77 ng/mL for Ferrlecit-treated patients.

In this patient population, only the Ferrlecit-treated group achieved significant increase in hemoglobin and hematocrit from baseline. This increase was significantly greater than that seen in the historical oral iron treatment group. See Table 2.

Study C

Study C was a multicenter, randomized, open-label study of the safety and efficacy of two Ferrlecit dose regimens (1.5 mg/kg or 3.0 mg/kg of elemental iron) administered intravenously to 66 iron-deficient (transferrin saturation < 20% and/or serum ferritin < 100 ng/mL) pediatric hemodialysis patients, 6 to 15 years of age, inclusive who were receiving a stable erythropoietin dosing regimen.

Ferrlecit at a dose of 1.5 mg/kg or 3.0 mg/kg (up to a maximum dose of 125 mg of elemental iron) in 25 mL 0.9% sodium chloride was infused intravenously over 1 hour during each hemodialysis session for eight sequential dialysis sessions. Thirty-two patients received the 1.5 mg/kg dosing regimen (47% male, 53% female; 66% Caucasian, 25% Hispanic, and 3% Black, Asian, or Other; mean age 12.3 years). Thirty-four patients received the 3.0 mg/kg dosing regimen (56% male, 44% female; 77% Caucasian, 12% Hispanic, 9% Black, and 3% Other; mean age 12.0 years).

The primary endpoint was the change in hemoglobin concentration from baseline to 2 weeks after last Ferrlecit administration. Patients in both Ferrlecit dose groups had statistically significant changes from baseline in hemoglobin concentrations (Table 3). There was no significant difference between the treatment groups. Statistically significant improvements in hematocrit, transferrin saturation, serum ferritin, and reticulocyte hemoglobin concentrations compared to baseline values were observed 2 weeks after the last Ferrlecit infusion in both the 1.5 mg/kg and 3.0 mg/kg treatment groups (Table 3).

TABLE 1 Hemoglobin, Hematocrit, and Iron Studies

Study A	Mean Change from Baseline to Two Weeks After Cessation of Therapy		
	Ferrlecit 1000 mg IV (N=44)	Ferrlecit 500 mg IV (N=39)	Historical Control Oral Iron (N=25)
Hemoglobin (g/dL)	1.1*	0.3	0.4
Hematocrit (%)	3.6*	1.4	0.8
Transferrin Saturation (%)	8.5	2.8	6.1
Serum Ferritin (ng/mL)	199	132	NA

*$p<0.01$ versus both the 500 mg group and the historical control group.

Cumulative Ferrlecit Dose (mg of elemental iron)	62.5	250	375	562.5	625	750	1000	1125	1187.5
Patients (#)	1	1	2	1	10	4	12	6	1

TABLE 2 Hemoglobin, Hematocrit, and Iron Studies

Study B	Mean Change from Baseline to One Month After Treatment	
	Ferrlecit (N=38)	Oral Iron (N=25)
	change	change
Hemoglobin (g/dL)	1.3a,b	0.4
Hematocrit (%)	3.8a,b	0.2
Transferrin Saturation (%)	6.7b	1.7
Serum Ferritin (ng/dL)	73b	-145

a - $p<0.05$ on group comparison by the ANCOVA method.
b - $p<0.001$ from baseline by the paired t-test method.

TABLE 3 Hemoglobin, Hematocrit, and Iron Status

Study C	Mean Change From Baseline to Two Weeks After Cessation of Therapy in Patients Completing Treatment	
	1.5 mg/kg Ferrlecit* (N=25)	3.0 mg/kg Ferrlecit (N=32)
Hemoglobin (g/dL)	0.8*	0.9*
Hematocrit (%)	2.6*	3.0*
Transferrin Saturation (%)	5.5*	10.5*
Serum Ferritin (ng/mL)	192*	314*
Reticulocyte Hemoglobin Content (pg)	1.3*	1.2*

*$p < 0.03$ versus the baseline values

The increased hemoglobin concentrations were maintained at 4 weeks after the last Ferrlecit infusion in both the 1.5 mg/kg and the 3.0 mg/kg Ferrlecit dose treatment groups.

INDICATIONS AND USAGE

Ferrlecit (sodium ferric gluconate complex in sucrose injection) is indicated for treatment of iron deficiency anemia in adult patients and in pediatric patients age 6 years and older undergoing chronic hemodialysis who are receiving supplemental epoetin therapy.

CONTRAINDICATIONS

- All anemias not associated with iron deficiency.
- Hypersensitivity to Ferrlecit or any of its inactive components.
- Evidence of iron overload.

WARNINGS

Hypersensitivity reactions have been reported with injectable iron products. See PRECAUTIONS.

PRECAUTIONS

General: Iron is not easily eliminated from the body and accumulation can be toxic. Unnecessary therapy with parenteral iron will cause excess storage of iron with consequent possibility of iatrogenic hemosiderosis. Iron overload is particularly apt to occur in patients with hemoglobinopathies and other refractory anemias. Ferrlecit should not be administered to patients with iron overload. See OVERDOSAGE.

Hypersensitivity Reactions: One case of a life-threatening hypersensitivity reaction was observed in 1,097 patients who received a single dose of Ferrlecit in a postmarketing safety study. In the postmarketing spontaneous reporting system, life-threatening hypersensitivity reactions have been reported rarely in patients receiving Ferrlecit. See ADVERSE REACTIONS.

Hypotension: Hypotension associated with lightheadedness, malaise, fatigue, weakness or severe pain in the chest, back, flanks, or groin has been associated with administration of intravenous iron. These hypotensive reactions are not associated with signs of hypersensitivity and have usually resolved within one or two hours. Successful treatment may consist of observation or, if the hypotension causes symptoms, volume expansion. See ADVERSE REACTIONS.

Carcinogenesis, mutagenesis, impairment of fertility: Long term carcinogenicity studies in animals were not performed. Studies to assess the effects of Ferrlecit on fertility were not conducted. Ferrlecit was not mutagenic in the Ames test and the rat micronucleus test. It produced a clastogenic effect in an *in vitro* chromosomal aberration assay in Chinese hamster ovary cells.

Pregnancy Category B: Ferrlecit was not teratogenic at doses of elemental iron up to 100 mg/kg/day (300 mg/m^2/day) in mice and 20 mg/kg/day (120 mg/m^2/day) in rats. On a body surface area basis, these doses were 1.3 and 3.24 times the recommended human dose (125 mg/day or 92.5 mg/m^2/day) for a person of 50 kg body weight, average height and body surface area of 1.46 m^2. There were no adequate and well-controlled studies in pregnant women. Ferrlecit should be used during pregnancy only if the potential benefit justifies the potential risk to the fetus.

Nursing Mothers: It is not known whether this drug is excreted in human milk. Because many drugs are excreted in human milk, caution should be exercised when Ferrlecit is administered to a nursing woman.

Pediatric Use: Ferrlecit was shown to be safe and effective in pediatric patients ages 6 to 15 years (refer to CLINICAL STUDIES section). Safety and effectiveness in pediatric patients younger than 6 years of age have not been established.

Ferrlecit contains benzyl alcohol and therefore should not be used in neonates.

Geriatric Use: Clinical studies of Ferrlecit did not include sufficient numbers of subjects aged 65 and over to determine whether they respond differently from younger subjects. Other reported clinical experience has not identified differences in responses between the elderly and younger patients. In particular, 51/159 hemodialysis patients in North American clinical studies were aged 65 years or older. Among these patients, no differences in safety or efficacy as a result of age were identified. In general, dose selection for an elderly patient should be cautious, usually starting at the low end of the dosing range, reflecting the greater frequency of decreased hepatic, renal, or cardiac function, and of concomitant disease or other drug therapy.

ADVERSE REACTIONS

Exposure to Ferrlecit has been documented in over 1,400 patients on hemodialysis. This population included in 1,097 Ferrlecit-naïve patients who received a single-dose of Ferrlecit in a placebo-controlled, cross-over, post-marketing safety study. Undiluted Ferrlecit was administered over ten minutes (125 mg of Ferrlecit at 12.5 mg/min). No test dose was used. From a total of 1,498 Ferrlecit-treated patients in medical reports, North American trials, and post-marketing studies, twelve patients (0.8%) experienced serious reactions which precluded further therapy with Ferrlecit.

Hypersensitivity Reactions: See PRECAUTIONS. In the single-dose, post-marketing, safety study one patient experienced a life-threatening hypersensitivity reaction (diaphoresis, nausea, vomiting, severe lower back pain, dyspnea, and wheezing for 20 minutes) following Ferrlecit administration. Among 1,097 patients who received Ferrlecit in this study, there were 9 patients (0.8%) who had an adverse reaction that, in the view of the investigator, precluded further Ferrlecit administration (drug intolerance). These included one life-threatening reaction, six allergic reactions (pruritus ×2, facial flushing, chills, dyspnea/chest pain, and rash), and two other reactions (hypotension and nausea). Another 2 patients experienced (0.2%) allergic reactions not deemed to represent drug intolerance (nausea/malaise and nausea/dizziness) following Ferrlecit administration.

Seventy-two (7.0%) of the 1,034 patients who had prior iron dextran exposure had a sensitivity to at least one form of iron dextran (INFeD® or Dexferrum®). The patient who experienced a life-threatening adverse event following Ferrlecit administration during the study had a previous severe anaphylactic reaction to dextran in both forms (INFeD® and Dexferrum®). The incidences of both drug intolerance and suspected allergic events following first dose Ferrlecit administration were 2.8% in patients with prior iron dextran sensitivity compared to 0.8% in patients without prior iron dextran sensitivity.

In this study, 28% of the patients received concomitant angiotensin converting enzyme inhibitor (ACEi) therapy. The incidences of both drug intolerance or suspected allergic events following first dose Ferrlecit administration were 1.6% in patients with concomitant ACEi use compared to 0.7% in patients without concomitant ACEi use. The patient with a life-threatening event was not on ACEi therapy. One patient had facial flushing immediately on Ferrlecit exposure. No hypotension occurred and the event resolved rapidly and spontaneously without intervention other than drug withdrawal.

In multiple dose Studies A and B, no fatal hypersensitivity reactions occurred among the 126 patients who received Ferrlecit. Ferrlecit-associated hypersensitivity events in Study A resulting in premature study discontinuation occurred in three out of a total 88 (3.4%) Ferrlecit-treated patients. The first patient withdrew after the development of pruritus and chest pain following the test dose of Ferrlecit. The second patient, in the high-dose group, experienced nausea, abdominal and flank pain, fatigue and rash following the first dose of Ferrlecit. The third patient, in the low-dose group, experienced a "red blotchy rash" following the first dose of Ferrlecit. Of the 38 patients exposed to Ferrlecit in Study B, none reported hypersensitivity reactions.

Many chronic renal failure patients experience cramps, pain, nausea, rash, flushing, and pruritus.

In the postmarketing spontaneous reporting system, life-threatening hypersensitivity reactions have been reported rarely in patients receiving Ferrlecit.

Hypotension: See PRECAUTIONS. In the single dose safety study, post-administration hypotensive events were observed in 22/1,097 patients (2%) following Ferrlecit administration. Hypotension has also been reported following administration of Ferrlecit in European case reports. Of the 226 renal dialysis patients exposed to Ferrlecit and reported in the literature, 3 (1.3%) patients experienced hypotensive events, which were accompanied by flushing in two. All completely reversed after one hour without sequelae. Transient hypotension may occur during dialysis. Administration of Ferrlecit may augment hypotension caused by dialysis.

Among the 126 patients who received Ferrlecit in Studies A and B, one patient experienced a transient decreased level of consciousness without hypotension. Another patient discontinued treatment prematurely because of dizziness, lightheadedness, diplopia, malaise, and weakness without hypotension that resulted in a 3–4 hour hospitalization for observation following drug administration. The syndrome resolved spontaneously.

Adverse Laboratory Changes: No differences in laboratory findings associated with Ferrlecit (sodium ferric gluconate complex in sucrose injection) were reported in North American clinical trials when normalized against a National Institute of Health database on laboratory findings in 1,100 hemodialysis patients.

Most Frequent Adverse Reactions: In the single-dose, post-marketing safety study, 11% of patients who received Ferrlecit and 9.4% of patients who received placebo reported adverse reactions. The most frequent adverse reactions following Ferrlecit were: hypotension (2%), nausea, vomiting and/or diarrhea (2%), pain (0.7%), hypertension (0.6%), allergic reaction (0.5%), chest pain (0.5%), pruritus (0.5%), and back pain (0.4%). Similar adverse reactions were seen following placebo administration. However, because of the high baseline incidence of adverse events in the hemodialysis patient population, insufficient number of exposed patients, and limitations inherent to the cross-over, single dose study design, no comparison of event rates between Ferrlecit and placebo treatments can be made.

In multiple-dose Studies A and B, the most frequent adverse reactions following Ferrlecit were:

Body as a Whole: injection site reaction (33%), chest pain (10%), pain (10%), asthenia (7%), headache (7%), abdominal pain (6%), fatigue (6%), fever (5%), malaise, infection, abscess, back pain, chills, rigors, arm pain, carcinoma, flu-like syndrome, sepsis.

Nervous System: cramps (25%), dizziness (13%), paresthesias (6%), agitation, somnolence.

Respiratory System: dyspnea (11%), coughing (6%), upper respiratory infections (6%), rhinitis, pneumonia.

Cardiovascular System: hypotension (29%), hypertension (13%), syncope (6%), tachycardia (5%), bradycardia, vasodilatation, angina pectoris, myocardial infarction, pulmonary edema.

Gastrointestinal System: nausea, vomiting and/or diarrhea (35%), anorexia, rectal disorder, dyspepsia, eructation, flatulence, gastrointestinal disorder, melena.

Musculoskeletal System: leg cramps (10%), myalgia, arthralgia.

Skin and Appendages: pruritus (6%), rash, increased sweating.

Genitourinary System: urinary tract infection.

Special Senses: conjunctivitis, abnormal vision, ear disorder.

Metabolic and Nutritional Disorders: hyperkalemia (6%), generalized edema (5%), leg edema, peripheral edema, hypoglycemia, edema, hypervolemia, hypokalemia.

Hematologic System: abnormal erythrocytes (11%), anemia, leukocytosis, lymphadenopathy.

Other Adverse Reactions Observed During Clinical Trials: In the single-dose post-marketing safety study in 1,097 patients receiving Ferrlecit, the following additional events were reported in two or more patients: hypertonia, nervousness, dry mouth, and hemorrhage.

Pediatric Patients: In a clinical trial of 66 iron-deficient pediatric hemodialysis patients, 6 to 15 years of age, inclusive, who were receiving a stable erythropoietin dosing regimen, the most common adverse events, whether or not related to study drug, occurring in ≥5%, regardless of treatment group, were: hypotension (35%), headache (24%), hypertension (23%), tachycardia (17%), vomiting (11%), fever (9%), nausea (9%), abdominal pain (9%), pharyngitis (9%), diarrhea (8%), infection (8%), rhinitis (6%), and thrombosis (6%). More patients in the higher dose group (3.0 mg/kg) than in the lower dose group (1.5 mg/kg) experienced the following adverse events: hypotension (41% vs. 28%), tachycardia (21% vs. 13%), fever (15% vs. 3%), headache (29% vs. 19%), abdominal pain (15% vs. 3%), nausea (12% vs. 6%), vomiting (12% vs. 9%), pharyngitis (12% vs. 6%), and rhinitis (9% vs. 3%).

Postmarketing Surveillance: The following additional adverse reactions have been identified with the use of Ferrlecit from postmarketing spontaneous reports: dysgeusia, hypoesthesia, loss of consciousness, convulsion, skin discoloration, pallor, phlebitis, and shock. Because these reactions are reported voluntarily from a population of uncertain size, it is not always possible to reliably estimate their frequency or establish a causal relationship to drug exposure.

OVERDOSAGE

Dosages in excess of iron needs may lead to accumulation of iron in iron storage sites and hemosiderosis. Periodic monitoring of laboratory parameters of iron storage may assist in recognition of iron accumulation. Ferrlecit should not be administered in patients with iron overload.

Serum iron levels greater than 300 µg/dL may indicate iron poisoning which is characterized by abdominal pain, diarrhea, or vomiting which progresses to pallor or cyanosis, lassitude, drowsiness, hyperventilation due to acidosis, and cardiovascular collapse. Caution should be exercised in interpreting serum iron levels in the 24 hours following the administration of Ferrlecit since many laboratory assays will falsely overestimate serum or transferrin bound iron by measuring iron still bound to the Ferrlecit complex. Additionally, in the assessment of iron overload, caution should be exercised in interpreting serum ferritin levels in the week following Ferrlecit administration since, in clinical studies, serum ferritin exhibited a nonspecific rise which persisted for five days.

The Ferrlecit iron complex is not dialyzable.

Ferrlecit at elemental iron doses of 125 mg/kg, 78.8 mg/kg, 62.5 mg/kg and 250 mg/kg caused deaths to mice, rats, rabbits, and dogs respectively. The major symptoms of acute toxicity were decreased activity, staggering, ataxia, increases in the respiratory rate, tremor, and convulsions.

Individual doses exceeding 125 mg may be associated with a higher incidence and/or severity of adverse events based on information from postmarketing spontaneous reports. These adverse events included hypotension, nausea, vomiting, abdominal pain, diarrhea, dizziness, dyspnea, urticaria, chest pain, paresthesia, and peripheral swelling. Because these reactions are reported voluntarily from a population of uncertain size, it is not always possible to reliably estimate their frequency or establish a causal relationship to drug exposure.

DOSAGE AND ADMINISTRATION

The dosage of Ferrlecit is expressed in terms of mg of elemental iron. Each 5 mL sterile, single-use ampule contains 62.5 mg of elemental iron (12.5 mg/mL).

The recommended dosage of Ferrlecit for the repletion treatment of iron deficiency in hemodialysis patients is 10 mL of Ferrlecit (125 mg of elemental iron). Ferrlecit may be diluted in 100 mL of 0.9% sodium chloride administered by intravenous infusion over 1 hour. Ferrlecit may also be administered undiluted as a slow IV injection (at a rate of up to 12.5 mg/min). Most patients will require a minimum cumulative dose of 1.0 gram of elemental iron, administered over eight sessions at sequential dialysis treatments, to achieve a favorable hemoglobin or hematocrit response. Patients may continue to require therapy with intravenous iron at the lowest dose necessary to maintain target levels of hemoglobin, hematocrit, and laboratory parameters of iron storage within acceptable limits. Ferrlecit has been administered at sequential dialysis sessions by infusion or by slow IV injection during the dialysis session itself.

Data from Ferrlecit postmarketing spontaneous reports indicate that individual doses exceeding 125 mg may be associated with a higher incidence and/or severity of adverse events. See OVERDOSAGE.

Pediatric Dosage: The recommended pediatric dosage of Ferrlecit for the repletion treatment of iron deficiency in hemodialysis patients is 0.12 mL/kg Ferrlecit (1.5 mg/kg of elemental iron) diluted in 25 mL 0.9% sodium chloride and administered by intravenous infusion over 1 hour at eight sequential dialysis sessions. The maximum dosage should not exceed 125 mg per dose.

Note: Do not mix Ferrlecit with other medications, or add to parenteral nutrition solutions for intravenous infusion. The compatibility of Ferrlecit with intravenous infusion vehicles other than 0.9% sodium chloride has not been evaluated. Parenteral drug products should be inspected visually for particulate matter and discoloration before administration, whenever the solution and container permit.

If diluted in saline, use immediately after dilution.

HOW SUPPLIED

NDC 0024-2791-50

Ferrlecit is supplied in colorless glass ampules. Each sterile, single-use ampule contains 62.5 mg of elemental iron in 5 mL for intravenous use, packaged in cartons of 10 ampules.

Store at 20–25°C (68–77°F); excursions permitted to 15–30°C (59–86°F). Do not freeze. See USP Controlled Room Temperature.

Keep out of the reach of children.

Revised: January 2010
sanofi-aventis U.S. LLC
Bridgewater, NJ 08807
©2010 sanofi-aventis U.S. LLC

HYALGAN®
[*hi-al-gan*]
(Sodium Hyaluronate)

℞

CAUTION

Federal law restricts this device to sale by or on the order of a physician.

DESCRIPTION

Hyalgan® is a viscous solution consisting of a high molecular weight (500,000–730,000 daltons) fraction of purified natural sodium hyaluronate (Hyalectin®) in buffered physiological sodium chloride, having a pH of 6.8–7.5. The sodium hyaluronate is extracted from rooster combs. Hyaluronic acid is a natural complex sugar of the glycosaminoglycan family and is a long-chain polymer containing repeating disaccharide units of Na-glucuronate-N-acetylglucosamine.

INDICATIONS

Hyalgan® is indicated for the treatment of pain in osteoarthritis (OA) of the knee in patients who have failed to respond adequately to conservative nonpharmacologic therapy, and to simple analgesics, e.g., acetaminophen.

CONTRAINDICATIONS

- Do not administer to patients with known hypersensitivity to hyaluronate preparations.
- Intra-articular injections are contraindicated in cases of present infections or skin diseases in the area of the injection site to reduce the potential for developing septic arthritis.

WARNINGS

- Do not concomitantly use disinfectants containing quaternary ammonium salts for skin preparation because hyaluronic acid can precipitate in their presence.

- Anaphylactoid and allergic reactions have been reported with this product. See Adverse Events Section for more detail.
- Transient increases in inflammation in the injected knee following Hyalgan® injection in some patients with inflammatory arthritis such as rheumatoid arthritis or gouty arthritis have been reported.
- Patients should be carefully examined prior to administration to determine signs of acute inflammation, and the physician should evaluate whether Hyalgan® treatment should be initiated when objective signs of inflammation are present.

PRECAUTIONS

General

- The effectiveness of a single treatment cycle of less than 3 injections has not been established.
- The safety and effectiveness of the use of Hyalgan® in joints other than the knee have not been established.
- The safety and effectiveness of the use of Hyalgan® concomitantly with other intra-articular injectables have not been established.
- Use caution when injecting Hyalgan® into patients who are allergic to avian proteins, feathers, and egg products.
- Strict aseptic administration technique must be followed to avoid infections in the injection site.
- Remove joint effusion, if present, before injecting Hyalgan®.
- **STERILE CONTENTS.** The vial/syringe is intended for single use. The contents of the vial must be used immediately once the container has been opened. Discard any unused Hyalgan®.
- Do not use Hyalgan® if the package is opened or damaged. Store in the original packaging (protected from light) below 77° F (25° C). DO NOT FREEZE.

Information for Patients

- Provide patients with a copy of the Patient Information prior to use.
- Transient pain and/or swelling of the injected joint may occur after intra-articular injection of Hyalgan®.
- As with any invasive joint procedure, it is recommended that the patient avoid any strenuous activities or prolonged (i.e., more than 1 hour) weight-bearing activities such as jogging or tennis within 48 hours following the intra-articular injection.

Use in Specific Populations

- **Pregnancy:** *Teratogenic Effects*—Reproductive toxicity studies, including multigeneration studies, have been performed in rats and rabbits at doses up to 11 times the anticipated human dose (1.43 mg/kg per treatment cycle) and have revealed no evidence of impaired fertility or harm to the experimental animal fetus due to intra-articular injections of Hyalgan®. Animal reproduction studies are not always predictive of human response. The safety and effectiveness of Hyalgan® have not been established in pregnant women.
- **Nursing Mothers:** It is not known if Hyalgan® is excreted in human milk. The safety and effectiveness of Hyalgan® have not been established in lactating women.
- **Pediatrics:** The safety and effectiveness of Hyalgan® have not been demonstrated in children.

ADVERSE EVENTS

Hyalgan® was investigated in a pivotal clinical investigation conducted in the United States in which there were three arms (164 subjects treated with Hyalgan®; 168 with placebo; and 163 with naproxen) (refer to Table 1). Common adverse events reported for the Hyalgan®-treated subjects were gastrointestinal complaints, injection site pain, knee swelling/effusion, local skin reactions (rash, ecchymosis), pruritus, and headache. Swelling and effusion, local skin reactions (ecchymosis and rash), and headache occurred at equal frequency in the Hyalgan®- and placebo-treated groups. Hyalgan® treated subjects had 48/164 (29%) incidents of gastrointestinal complaints that were not statistically different from the placebo-treated group. A statistically significant difference in the occurrence of pain at the injection site was noted in the Hyalgan®-treated subjects:

38/164 (23%) in comparison to 22/168 (13%) in the placebo-treated subjects (p=0.022). There were 6/164 (4%) premature discontinuations in Hyalgan®-treated subjects due to injection site pain in comparison to 1/168 (<1%) in the placebo-treated subjects. These differences were not statistically significant. Two (2/164, 1.2%) Hyalgan®-treated subjects and 3/168 (1.8%) placebo-treated subjects were reported to have positive bacterial cultures of effusion aspirated from the treated knee. The two Hyalgan®-treated subjects and two of the placebo-treated subjects did not exhibit evidence of infection clinically or subsequently and were not treated with antibiotics. One of the placebo-treated subjects was hospitalized and received presumptive treatment for septic arthritis.

TABLE 1
Incidence[1] of Adverse Events Occurring in More Than 5% of All Subjects

Adverse Event	Hyalgan®	Placebo
	N = 164	N = 168
Gastrointestinal Complaints[2]	48 (29%)	59 (36%)
Injection site pain[3]	38 (23%)[4]	22 (13%)
Headache	30 (18%)	29 (17%)
Local skin[5]	23 (14%)	17 (10%)
Local joint pain and swelling[6]	21 (13%)	22 (13%)
Pruritus (local)	12 (7%)	7 (4%)

Notes: [1] Number and % of subjects
[2] Severe in 4 Hyalgan®-treated subjects and 4 placebo-treated subjects
[3] Severe in 5 Hyalgan®-treated subjects and 2 placebo-treated subjects
[4] Statistically significant (p=0.02)
[5] Includes ecchymosis and rash
[6] Severe in 2 Hyalgan®-treated subjects (1.2%) and 1 placebo-treated subject

Hyalgan® has been in clinical use in Europe since 1987. Analysis of the adverse events that have been reported with the use of Hyalgan® in Europe reveals that most of the events are related to local symptoms such as pain, swelling/effusion, and warmth or redness at the injection site. Usually such symptoms disappear within a few days by resting the affected joint and applying ice locally. Only sporadically have these events been more severe and longer lasting. Very rare cases of intra-articular infection have been reported. Strict aseptic technique must be followed in administering Hyalgan®. Systemic allergic reactions rarely have been recorded. Isolated cases of an anaphylactic or anaphylactic-like reaction have been reported in post-marketing experience and they all resolved. Allergic-type signs and symptoms such as rash, pruritus, and urticaria also are very rare. A few cases of fever were reported. In some instances, they were associated with local reactions, in other cases, no association other than temporal was found with the use of the product.

Adverse experience data from the literature contain no evidence of increased risk relating to retreatment with Hyalgan®. The frequency and severity of adverse events occurring during repeat treatment cycles did not increase over that reported for a single treatment cycle. (Carrabba et al., 1995; Carrabba et al., 1991; Kotz and Kolarz, 1999; Scali, 1995).

CLINICAL STUDY

The use of Hyalgan® as a treatment for pain in OA of the knee was investigated in a multicenter clinical trial conducted in the United States.

Study Design

This study was a double-masked, placebo and naproxen-controlled, multicenter prospective clinical trial with three treatment arms, as summarized in Table 2. A total of 495 subjects with moderate to severe pain was randomized (at baseline evaluation) into three treatment groups in a ratio of 1:1:1 Hyalgan®, placebo, or naproxen.

[See table 2 at left]

Patient Population and Demographics

The demographics of trial participants were comparable across treatment groups with regard to age, sex, race, height, weight, history of osteoarthritis, prior use of NSAIDs, prior physical therapy, and use of assistive devices (refer to Table 3).

TABLE 2 STUDY DESIGN

Routes of Administration	Hyalgan®	Placebo	Naproxen
s.c.	Lidocaine (1%)	Lidocaine (1%)	Lidocaine (1%)
i.a.*	Hyalgan® (20 mg/2 mL)	Phosphate-Buffered Saline (2 mL)	none
p.o./b.i.d.	Placebo for naproxen capsules	Placebo for naproxen capsules	Naproxen capsules (500 mg)
p.o./p.r.n. (not to exceed 4 grams/day)	Acetaminophen	Acetaminophen	Acetaminophen

Legend: s.c. = subcutaneous; i.a. = intra-articular; p.o. = by mouth; b.i.d. = twice a day; p.r.n. = as needed
*Synovial fluid was aspirated (when present) in the Hyalgan® and placebo groups.

TABLE 3
Demographic Characteristics of all Randomized Subjects

DEMOGRAPHIC VARIABLE	TREATMENT			
	Hyalgan® N = 164	Placebo N = 168	Naproxen N = 163	TOTAL N = 495
AGE (years):				
Mean	63.5	64.3	63.2	63.7
SD	10.1	10.0	9.2	9.8
Range	41-90	44-85	40-80	40-90
Gender [N (%)]:				
Female	99 (60.3)	91 (54.1)	99 (60.7)	289 (58.4)
Male	65 (39.6)	77 (45.8)	64 (39.3)	206 (41.6)
Race [N (%)]:				
Caucasian	137 (83.6)	135 (80.4)	133 (81.6)	405 (81.8)
Black	23 (14.0)	32 (19.0)	25 (15.3)	80 (16.2)
Other	4 (4.2)	1 (1.0)	5 (3.1)	10 (2.0)
Height (cm):				
Mean	167.8	168.6	167.6	168.0
SD	8.8	10.7	11.9	10.5
Range	145-190	142-193	102-198	102-198
Weight (kg):				
Mean	88.4	88.1	89.7	88.7
SD	18.0	18.2	18.4	18.2
Range	46-139	49-170	45-150	45-170
NSAIDs Use (N, %)	107 (65.2)	117 (69.6)	113 (69.3)	337 (68.1)
Use of Assistive Devices (N, %)	35 (21.3)	34 (20.2)	32 (19.6)	101 (20.4)
Physical Therapy (N, %)	20 (12.2)	17 (10.1)	25 (15.3)	62 (12.5)

Legend: cm = centimeters; kg = kilograms; SD = standard deviation

TABLE 4
Clinical Results

Evaluation	Success Criteria	Results
100 mm VAS for pain during 50 foot walk.	A statistically significant (alpha =0.05) reduction on mean VAS for Hyalgan® when compared to placebo at Week 26. This difference was also to exceed one fourth of the Standard Deviation of the mean change from baseline.	At Week 26, the difference between the Hyalgan®-treated group and the placebo-treated group adjusted means was 8.85 mm (p = 0.0043), which is a difference of approximately one-third of a standard deviation (Table 5).
Masked Evaluator Categorical Assessment of subject pain (0=none to 5=disabled) during the 48 hours preceding visits.	The number of Hyalgan®-treated subjects showing improvement at Week 26 was to be concordant with the VAS results; however, not required to be independently statistically significant.	At Week 26 the masked evaluator's categorical assessment of pain indicated that the Hyalgan®-treated subjects experienced less pain than the placebo-treated subjects (Table 6).
Subjects' Categorical Assessment of pain (0=none to 5=disabled) during the 48 hours preceding visits.	The number of Hyalgan®-treated subjects showing improvement at Week 26 was to be concordant with the VAS results; however, not required to be independently statistically significant.	At Week 26 the subjects' categorical assessment of pain indicated that the Hyalgan®-treated subjects experienced less pain than the placebo-treated subjects (Table 7).
Magnitude of the observed effect for Hyalgan® versus placebo on both the VAS and the categorical pain assessments.	At Week 26 the magnitude of the observed effect for Hyalgan® versus placebo on both the VAS and the categorical pain assessments were to be at least 50% of those observed for the naproxen group.	The improvement in pain on the VAS exhibited by the Hyalgan®-treated group relative to the placebo-treated group were at least 50% of the benefits exhibited by the naproxen-treated group relative to the placebo-treated group. The results of the categorical assessments by the masked evaluator and the subject indicated that improvement of the Hyalgan®-treated group relative to the placebo-treated group was at least 50% of the benefits exhibited by the naproxen-treated group relative to the placebo-treated group (Table 8).

[See table 3 above]

Evaluation Schedule

After meeting initial screening requirements NSAID therapy was discontinued. After 2 weeks, all subjects returned for baseline evaluations. The baseline evaluation included assessment of three primary effectiveness criteria; measurement of pain during a 50-foot walk test using a 100 mm Visual Analog Scale (VAS), a categorical assessment (0 = none to 5 = disabled) of pain, as assessed by a masked evaluator, during the 48 hours preceding the visit, and a categorical assessment (0 = none to 5 = disabled) of pain, as assessed by the subject, during the 48 hours preceding the visit.

All subjects who completed the NSAID washout period and met all entry requirements received their first injection after randomization. All subjects received subcutaneous lidocaine injections. Intra-articular injections (Hyalgan®, placebo) were administered weekly for a total of 5 injections (Weeks 0–4). The naproxen group received 500 mg of naproxen to be taken b.i.d. for 26 weeks. Subsequent visits and evaluations took place at Weeks 5, 9, 12, 16, 21, and 26.

Safety and effectiveness criteria were assessed and recorded at these time periods.

Clinical Results

For this trial, overall success for effectiveness was defined as meeting all four of the success criteria listed in Table 4 using scores from week 26. The criteria were met (refer to Tables 4 through 8).
[See table 4 below]
[See table 5 at top of next page]
[See table 6 on next page]
[See table 7 on next page]
[See table 8 on next page]

Additional Analyses

a. An analysis of study completers was performed as follows: Success was defined as 1) achieving a 20 mm decrease in the VAS for the 50-foot walk test by Week 5, and 2) maintaining this improvement through Week 26. In this analysis greater proportions of Hyalgan®-treated subjects (59/105, 56%) than either placebo (47/115, 41%) or naproxen-treated subjects (51/113, 45%) were successful under this definition. The Hyalgan®-placebo comparison was statistically significant (p=0.031, Fisher's Exact Test).

Since patients were not followed beyond Week 26, it is unknown how long pain relief continued. There are reports in the literature of some patients experiencing benefit beyond 26 weeks.

b. *Categorical Assessment of Pain - Subjects:* A longitudinal analysis of categorical assessment of pain by the subject, which analyzed the percentage of subjects who attained success revealed that a significantly higher percentage of Hyalgan®-treated subjects as compared to the placebo-treated subjects (55/105, 52% vs 43/115, 37%, p = 0.030, Fisher's Exact Test) achieved success (an improvement of greater than or equal to one point on the five-point scale) and maintained this success from Week 5 until Week 26.

Supplementary Clinical Information

Three randomized, controlled clinical investigations were performed that provide information about a three-injection treatment course of Hyalgan®. In all of the studies the patients were followed for 60 days.

Two studies provided a comparison to placebo. One of the placebo-controlled studies evaluated two treatment doses of Hyalgan®, 20 mg/2 mL and 40 mg/2 mL. The 20 mg/2 mL treatment arm included 19 knees, the 40 mg/2 ml included 20 knees, and the placebo arm included 18 knees. The other placebo study included 20 knees in the treatment group and 18 knees in the placebo-treatment group. The third study provided a comparison between patients treated with three weekly injections of Hyalgan® followed by 2 weekly treatments with arthrocentesis with patients treated with arthrocentesis for five weeks, and arthrocentesis and placebo injections for five weeks. Additional arms of this study assessed additional treatment regimens. Statistical evaluation of the data was performed at day 60. In this study only patients considered to be success were followed beyond day 60. These patients were followed for 180 days, however, due to the number of dropouts, statistical evaluation was not performed on data gathered at time points beyond day 60. The results of these investigations reported that the three-injection Hyalgan® treated patients experienced pain relief beginning at day 21 and continuing throughout the remaining 60-day observation period.

Safety

In order for the product to be considered safe, the incidence of severe swelling and pain consequent to intra-articular injection should be less than 5%. This criterion was met as indicated in Table 1. See the Adverse Events Section.

DETAILED DEVICE DESCRIPTION

Each vial or syringe contains:

Sodium Hyaluronate	20.0 mg
Sodium chloride	17.0 mg
Monobasic sodium phosphate • 2H2O	0.1 mg
Dibasic sodium phosphate • 12H2O	1.2 mg
Water for injection	q.s.* to 2.0 mL

* q.s. = up to

HOW SUPPLIED

Hyalgan® is supplied as a sterile, non-pyrogenic solution in 2 mL vials or 2 mL pre-filled syringes.

DIRECTIONS FOR USE

Hyalgan® is administered by intra-articular injection. A treatment cycle consists of five injections given at weekly intervals. Some patients may experience benefit with three injections given at weekly intervals. This has been noted in studies reported in the literature in which patients treated with three injections were followed for 60 days.

Precaution: Do not use Hyalgan® if the package is opened or damaged. Store in the original packaging (protected from light) below 77° F (25° C). DO NOT FREEZE.

Precaution: Strict aseptic administration technique must be followed.

Warning: Do not concomitantly use disinfectants containing quaternary ammonium salts for skin preparation because hyaluronic acid can precipitate in their presence.

TABLE 5
ANCOVA of 50-Foot Walk Test (mm) VAS by Week for All Completed Subjects

	Week							
	3	4	5	9	12	16	21	26
Adjusted Means Hyalgan®	27.23	21.54	19.29	20.04	20.26	20.83	18.44	17.88
Placebo	32.35	28.57	25.67	24.28	26.66	25.44	24.77	26.73
Hyalgan® versus Placebo	5.13	7.03	6.39	4.24	6.40	4.61	6.33	8.846
p-value	0.06	0.01	0.01	0.1	0.03	0.1	0.02	0.004

TABLE 6
Masked Evaluators' Categorical Assessments of Pain for Completed Subjects in Prior 48 Hours:
Level of Pain by Treatment Group at Baseline and Week 26

	NUMBER (%) OF SUBJECTS IN CATEGORY					
	Hyalgan®		Placebo		Naproxen	
	Baseline	Week 26	Baseline	Week 26	Baseline	Week 26
None (0)	0 (0.0)	27 (25.7)	0 (0.0)	15 (13.0)	0 (0.0)	17 (15.0)
Slight (1)	1 (1.0)	23 (21.9)	0 (0.0)	27 (23.5)	0 (0.0)	32 (28.3)
Mild (2)	2 (1.9)	24 (22.9)	2 (1.7)	29 (25.2)	2 (1.8)	27 (23.9)
Moderate (3)	69 (65.7)	26 (24.8)	85 (73.9)	34 (29.6)	79 (70.5)	28 (24.8)
Marked (4)	33 (31.4)	5 (4.8)	28 (24.3)	10 (8.7)	31 (27.7)	9 (8.0)
TOTAL	105 (100)	105 (100)	115 (100)	115 (100)	112* (100)	113 (100)

*One Naproxen treated subject was missing a Baseline assessment.

TABLE 7
Subjects' Categorical Assessments of Pain for Completed Subjects in Prior 48 Hours:
Level of Pain by Treatment Group at Baseline and Week 26

	NUMBER (%) OF SUBJECTS IN CATEGORY					
	Hyalgan®		Placebo		Naproxen	
	Baseline	Week 26	Baseline	Week 26	Baseline	Week 26
None (0)	1 (1.0)	23 (21.9)	0 (0.0)	14 (12.2)	0 (0.0)	13 (11.5)
Slight (1)	2 (1.9)	27 (25.7)	0 (0.0)	24 (20.9)	1 (0.9)	31 (27.4)
Mild (2)	6 (5.7)	19 (18.1)	8 (7.0)	24 (20.9)	7 (6.2)	26 (23.0)
Moderate (3)	62 (59.0)	26 (24.8)	78 (67.8)	40 (34.8)	72 (63.7)	31 (27.4)
Marked (4)	34 (32.4)	10 (9.5)	29 (25.2)	13 (11.3)	33 (29.2)	12 (10.6)
TOTAL	105 (100)	105 (100)	115 (100)	115 (100)	113 (100)	113 (100)

TABLE 8
Hyalgan® Effect as a Percentage of the Naproxen-Placebo Difference

Assessment	Hyalgan® (HYL)	Placebo (PLA)	Naproxen (NAP)	HYL-PLA	NAP-HYL	NAP-PLA	(HYL-PLA) % of (NAP-PLA)
VAS for 50 foot Walk Baseline Adjusted Mean Effect Sizes From ANCOVA				-8.85 mm on a 100 mm VAS	4.12 mm on a 100 mm VAS	-4.73* mm on a 100 mm VAS	187%
% of Subjects Improved by Masked Evaluators	78.1	69.6	73.2	8.5	-4.9	3.6	236%
% of Subjects Improved by Subjects	73.3	62.6	67.3	10.7	-6.0	4.7	228%

* Imputed as (NAP-HYL)+(HYL-PLA).
Note that Effectiveness Success Criterion D is satisfied since ((HYL-PLA) % of (NAP-PLA)) >50% for all three of the above pain assessments.

Inject subcutaneous lidocaine or similar local anesthetic prior to injection of Hyalgan®.
Precaution: Remove joint effusion, if present, before injection of Hyalgan®.
Do not use the same syringe for removing joint effusion and for injecting Hyalgan®.

Take care to remove the tip cap of the syringe and needle aseptically.
Inject Hyalgan® into the joint through a 20-gauge needle.
Precaution: The vial/syringe is intended for single use. The contents of the vial must be used immediately once the container has been opened. Discard any unused Hyalgan®.

Inject the full 2 mL in one knee only. If treatment is bilateral, a separate vial should be used for each knee.
MANUFACTURED BY
Fidia Farmaceutici S.p.A.
Via Ponte della Fabbrica 3/A - 35031 Abano Terme, Padua (PD), Italy
MANUFACTURED FOR
sanofi-aventis U.S. LLC
Bridgewater, NJ 08807
REFERENCES
1. M. Carrabba et al., 1991 Hyaluronic acid sodium salt (Hyalgan®) in the treatment of patients with osteoarthritis of the knee: a controlled trial versus Orgotein, Final Report, April 1991. Data on file.
2. M. Carrabba et al., 1995. Effectiveness and safety of 1, 3 and 5 injections of 20 mg/2 ml Hyalgan® in comparison with a placebo and with arthrocentesis only, in the treatment of knee osteoarthritis. European Journal of Rheumatology and Inflammation 15:25-31.
3. M. Dougados et al., 1993. High molecular weight sodium hyaluronate (hyalectin) in osteoarthritis of the knee: a one-year placebo-controlled trial. Osteoarthritis and Cartilage 1:97-103.
4. R. Kotz and G. Kolarz, 1997 published as R. Kotz and G. Kolarz, 1999. Intra-articular hyaluronic acid: duration of effect and results of repeated treatment cycles. The American Journal of Orthopedics, 28:5-7.
5. G. Leardini et al., 1987. Intra-articular sodium hyaluronate (Hyalgan®) in gonarthrosis. Clinical Trials Journal 24(4):341-350.
6. J.J. Scali, 1995. Intra-articular hyaluronic acid in the treatment of osteoarthritis of the knee: a long term study 15(1):57-62.
07241191
Revised January 2009　　　　　　684071/7
Shown in Product Identification Guide, page 319

JEVTANA®　　　　　　　　　　　R
[*JEV-TA-NA*]
(cabazitaxel)
Injection, 60 mg/1.5 mL, for intravenous infusion only

HIGHLIGHTS OF PRESCRIBING INFORMATION
These highlights do not include all the information needed to use JEVTANA safely and effectively. See full prescribing information for JEVTANA.
JEVTANA (cabazitaxel) Injection, 60 mg/1.5 mL, for intravenous infusion only
Initial U.S. Approval: 2010

> **WARNING**
> *See full prescribing information for complete boxed warning.*
> • Neutropenic deaths have been reported. Obtain frequent blood counts to monitor for neutropenia. Do not give JEVTANA if neutrophil counts are ≤1,500 cells/mm³. (2.2)(4)
> • Severe hypersensitivity can occur and may include generalized rash/ erythema, hypotension and bronchospasm. Discontinue JEVTANA immediately if severe reactions occur and administer appropriate therapy. (2.3)(5.2)
> • Contraindicated if history of severe hypersensitivity reactions to JEVTANA or to drugs formulated with polysorbate 80. (4)

——INDICATIONS AND USAGE——
JEVTANA is a microtubule inhibitor indicated in combination with prednisone for treatment of patients with hormone-refractory metastatic prostate cancer previously treated with a docetaxel-containing treatment regimen. (1)
——DOSAGE AND ADMINISTRATION——
Recommended dose: JEVTANA 25 mg/m² administered every three weeks as a one-hour intravenous infusion in combination with oral prednisone 10 mg administered daily throughout JEVTANA treatment. (2.1)
• JEVTANA requires two dilutions prior to administration (2.5)
• Use the **entire** contents of the accompanying diluent to achieve a concentration of 10 mg/mL JEVTANA. (2.5)
• PVC equipment should not be used (2.5)
• **Premedication Regimen:** Administer intravenously 30 minutes before each dose of JEVTANA:
• Antihistamine (dexchloropheniramine 5 mg or diphenhydramine 25 mg or equivalent antihistamine)
• Corticosteroid (dexamethasone 8 mg or equivalent steroid)
• H₂ antagonist (ranitidine 50 mg or equivalent H₂ antagonist) (2.3)

Antiemetic prophylaxis (oral or intravenous) is recommended as needed. (2.3)
- **Dosage Modifications:** See full prescribing information (2.2)

---------------------DOSAGE FORMS AND STRENGTHS---------------------
- Single use vial 60 mg/1.5 mL, supplied with diluent (5.7 mL) for JEVTANA (3)

-----------------------------CONTRAINDICATIONS-----------------------------
- Neutrophil counts of ≤1,500/mm^3 (2.2)(4)
- History of severe hypersensitivity to JEVTANA or polysorbate 80 (4)

------------------------WARNINGS AND PRECAUTIONS------------------------
- Neutropenia, febrile neutropenia: Neutropenic deaths have been reported. Monitor blood counts frequently to determine if initiation of G-CSF and/or dosage modification is needed. Primary prophylaxis with G-CSF should be considered in patients with high-risk clinical features. (2.2)(4)(5.1)
- Hypersensitivity: Severe hypersensitivity reactions can occur. Premedicate with corticosteroids and H2 antagonists. Discontinue infusion immediately if hypersensitivity is observed and treat as indicated. (4)(5.2)
- Gastrointestinal symptoms (nausea, vomiting, diarrhea): Mortality related to diarrhea has been reported. Rehydrate and treat with anti-emetics and anti-diarrheals as needed. If experiencing Grade ≥ 3 diarrhea, dosage should be modified. (2.2)(5.3)
- Renal failure, including cases with fatal outcomes, has been reported. Identify cause and manage aggressively. (5.4)
- Elderly patients: Patients ≥ 65 years of age were more likely to experience fatal outcomes not related to disease progression and certain adverse reactions, including neutropenia and febrile neutropenia. Monitor closely (5.5)(6)(8.5).
- Hepatic impairment: Patients with impaired hepatic function were excluded from the randomized clinical trial. Hepatic impairment is likely to increase the cabazitaxel concentrations. JEVTANA should not be given to patients with hepatic impairment. (5.6)(8.7)
- JEVTANA can cause fetal harm when administered to a pregnant woman. (5.7)(8.1)

-----------------------------ADVERSE REACTIONS-----------------------------
Most common all grades adverse reactions (≥10%) are neutropenia, anemia, leukopenia, thrombocytopenia, diarrhea, fatigue, nausea, vomiting, constipation, asthenia, abdominal pain, hematuria, back pain, anorexia, peripheral neuropathy, pyrexia, dyspnea, dysgeusia, cough, arthralgia, and alopecia. (6)

To report SUSPECTED ADVERSE REACTIONS, contact sanofi-aventis U.S. LLC at 1-800-633-1610 or FDA at 1-800-FDA-1088 or www.fda.gov/medwatch.

------------------------------DRUG INTERACTIONS------------------------------
- Use with caution in patients taking concomitant medicines that induce or inhibit CYP3A. (7)

See 17 for PATIENT COUNSELING INFORMATION and FDA-approved patient labeling

Revised: 07/2010

FULL PRESCRIBING INFORMATION: CONTENTS*
WARNING

* Sections or subsections omitted from the full prescribing information are not listed

FULL PRESCRIBING INFORMATION

> **WARNING**
>
> **Neutropenic deaths have been reported. In order to monitor the occurrence of neutropenia, frequent blood cell counts should be performed on all patients receiving JEVTANA. JEVTANA should not be given to patients with neutrophil counts of ≤1,500 cells/mm^3. Severe hypersensitivity reactions can occur and may include generalized rash/erythema, hypotension and bronchospasm. Severe hypersensitivity reactions require immediate discontinuation of the JEVTANA infusion and administration of appropriate therapy [see Warnings and Precautions (5.2)]. Patients should receive premedication [see Dosage and Administrations (2.3)]. JEVTANA must not be given to patients who have a history of severe hypersensitivity reactions to JEVTANA or to other drugs formulated with polysorbate 80 [see Contraindications (4)].**

---

1.   INDICATIONS AND USAGE

JEVTANA® is a microtubule inhibitor indicated in combination with prednisone for the treatment of patients with hormone-refractory metastatic prostate cancer previously treated with a docetaxel-containing treatment regimen.

2.   DOSAGE AND ADMINISTRATION

2.1   General Dosing Information
- The individual dosage of JEVTANA is based on calculation of the Body Surface Area (BSA) and is 25 mg/m^2 administered as a one-hour intravenous infusion every three weeks in combination with oral prednisone 10 mg administered daily throughout JEVTANA treatment.
- Premedication is recommended prior to treatment [see Dosage and Administration (2.3)].
- JEVTANA should be administered under the supervision of a qualified physician experienced in the use of antineoplastic medicinal products. Appropriate management of complications is possible only when the adequate diagnostic and treatment facilities are readily available.
- JEVTANA Injection single-use vial requires two dilutions prior to administration [see Dosage and Administration (2.5)].
- Do not use PVC infusion containers and polyurethane infusions sets for preparation and administration of JEVTANA infusion solution [see Dosage and Administration (2.5)].
- Both the JEVTANA Injection and the diluent vials contain an overfill to compensate for liquid loss during preparation.

2.2   Dose Modifications
The JEVTANA dose should be reduced to 20 mg/m^2 if patients experience the following adverse reactions.

Table 1: Recommended Dosage Modifications for Adverse Reactions in Patients Treated with JEVTANA

Toxicity	Dosage Modification
Prolonged grade ≥ 3 neutropenia (greater than 1 week) despite appropriate medication including G-CSF	Delay treatment until neutrophil count is > 1,500 cells/mm^3, then reduce dosage of JEVTANA to 20 mg/m^2. Use G-CSF for secondary prophylaxis.
Febrile neutropenia	Delay treatment until improvement or resolution, and until neutrophil count is > 1,500 cells/mm^3, then reduce dosage of JEVTANA to 20 mg/m^2. Use G-CSF for secondary prophylaxis.
Grade ≥ 3 diarrhea or persisting diarrhea despite appropriate medication, fluid and electrolytes replacement	Delay treatment until improvement or resolution, then reduce dosage of JEVTANA to 20 mg/m^2.

Discontinue JEVTANA treatment if a patient continues to experience any of these reactions at 20 mg/m^2.

2.3   Premedication
Premedicate at least 30 minutes prior to each dose of JEVTANA with the following intravenous medications to reduce the risk and/or severity of hypersensitivity:
- antihistamine (dexchlorpheniramine 5 mg, or diphenhydramine 25 mg or equivalent antihistamine),
- corticosteroid (dexamethasone 8 mg or equivalent steroid),
- H$_2$ antagonist (ranitidine 50 mg or equivalent H$_2$ antagonist).

Antiemetic prophylaxis is recommended and can be given orally or intravenously as needed.

2.4   Administration Precautions
JEVTANA is a cytotoxic anticancer drug and caution should be exercised when handling and preparing JEVTANA solutions, taking into account the use of containment devices, personal protective equipment (e.g., gloves), and preparation procedures. Please refer to *Handling and Disposal (16.3)*.

If JEVTANA Injection, first diluted solution, or second (final) dilution for intravenous infusion should come into contact with the skin, immediately and thoroughly wash with soap and water. If JEVTANA Injection, first diluted solution, or second (final) dilution for intravenous infusion should come into contact with mucosa, immediately and thoroughly wash with water.

2.5   Instructions for Preparation
Do not use PVC infusion containers or polyurethane infusions sets for preparation and administration of JEVTANA infusion solution.

Read this entire section carefully before mixing and diluting. JEVTANA requires two dilutions prior to administration. Please follow the preparation instructions provided below. **Note:** Both the JEVTANA Injection and the diluent vials contain an overfill to compensate for liquid loss during preparation. This overfill ensures that after dilution with the **entire** contents of the accompanying diluent, there is an initial diluted solution containing 10 mg/mL JEVTANA.

The following two-step dilution process must be carried out under aseptic conditions to prepare the second (final) infusion solution.

Set aside the JEVTANA Injection and supplied diluent vials. The JEVTANA Injection is a clear yellow to brownish-yellow viscous solution, if appropriately stored.

Step 1 – First Dilution

Each vial of JEVTANA (cabazitaxel) 60 mg/1.5 mL must first be mixed with the **entire contents** of supplied diluent. Once reconstituted, the resultant solution contains 10 mg/mL of JEVTANA.

When transferring the diluent, direct the needle onto the inside wall of JEVTANA vial and inject slowly to limit foaming. Remove the syringe and needle and gently mix the initial diluted solution by repeated inversions for at least 45 seconds to assure full mixing of the drug and diluent. Do not shake.

Let the solution stand for a few minutes to allow any foam to dissipate, and check that the solution is homogeneous and contains no visible particulate matter. It is not required that all foam dissipate prior to continuing the preparation process.

The resulting initial diluted JEVTANA solution (cabazitaxel 10 mg/mL) requires further dilution before administration. The second dilution should be done immediately (within 30 minutes) to obtain the final infusion as detailed in Step 2.

Step 2 – Second (Final) Dilution

Withdraw the recommended dose from the JEVTANA solution containing 10 mg/mL as prepared in Step 1 using a calibrated syringe and further dilute into a sterile 250 mL PVC-free container of either 0.9% sodium chloride solution or 5% dextrose solution for infusion. If a dose greater than 65 mg of JEVTANA is required, use a larger volume of the infusion vehicle so that a concentration of 0.26 mg/mL JEVTANA is not exceeded. The concentration of the JEVTANA final infusion solution should be between 0.10 mg/mL and 0.26 mg/mL.

JEVTANA should not be mixed with any other drugs. Remove the syringe and thoroughly mix the final infusion solution by gently inverting the bag or bottle.

JEVTANA final infusion solution (in either 0.9% sodium chloride solution or 5% dextrose solution) should be used within 8 hours at ambient temperature (including the one-hour infusion) or within a total of 24 hours if refrigerated (including the one-hour infusion).

As the final infusion solution is supersaturated, it may crystallize over time. Do not use if this occurs and discard. Inspect visually for particulate matter, any crystals and discoloration prior to administration. If the JEVTANA first diluted solution or second (final) infusion solution is not clear or appears to have precipitation, it should be discarded. Discard any unused portion.

2.6 Administration

The final JEVTANA infusion solution should be administered intravenously as a one-hour infusion at room temperature.

Use an in-line filter of 0.22 micrometer nominal pore size during administration.

The final JEVTANA infusion solution should be used immediately. However, in-use storage time can be longer under specific conditions, i.e. 8 hours under ambient conditions (including the one-hour infusion) or for a total of 24 hours if refrigerated (including the one-hour infusion) [see Dosage and Administration (2.5)].

3. DOSAGE FORMS AND STRENGTHS

JEVTANA (cabazitaxel) Injection 60 mg/1.5 mL is supplied as a kit consisting of the following:

- – JEVTANA Injection 60 mg/1.5 mL: contains 60 mg cabazitaxel in 1.5 mL polysorbate 80,
- – Diluent for JEVTANA Injection 60 mg/1.5 mL: contains approximately 5.7 mL of 13% (w/w) ethanol in water for injection.

4. CONTRAINDICATIONS

JEVTANA should not be used in patients with neutrophil counts of $\leq 1,500/mm^3$.

JEVTANA is contraindicated in patients who have a history of severe hypersensitivity reactions to cabazitaxel or to other drugs formulated with polysorbate 80.

5. WARNINGS AND PRECAUTIONS

5.1 Neutropenia

Five patients experienced fatal infectious adverse events (sepsis or septic shock). All had grade 4 neutropenia and one had febrile neutropenia. One additional patient's death was attributed to neutropenia without a documented infection. G-CSF may be administered to reduce the risks of neutropenia complications associated with JEVTANA use. Primary prophylaxis with G-CSF should be considered in patients with high-risk clinical features (age > 65 years, poor performance status, previous episodes of febrile neutropenia, extensive prior radiation ports, poor nutritional status, or other serious comorbidities) that predispose them to increased complications from prolonged neutropenia. Therapeutic use of G-CSF and secondary prophylaxis should be considered in all patients considered to be at increased risk for neutropenia complications.

Monitoring of complete blood counts is essential on a weekly basis during cycle 1 and before each treatment cycle thereafter so that the dose can be adjusted, if needed [see Dosage and Administration (2.2)].

JEVTANA should not be administered to patients with neutrophils $\leq 1,500/mm^3$ [see Contraindications (4)].

If a patient experiences febrile neutropenia or prolonged neutropenia (greater than one week) despite appropriate medication (e.g., G-CSF), the dose of JEVTANA should be reduced [see Dosage and Administration (2.2)]. Patients can restart treatment with JEVTANA only when neutrophil counts recover to a level > 1,500/mm³ [see Contraindications (4)].

5.2 Hypersensitivity Reactions

All patients should be premedicated prior to the initiation of the infusion of JEVTANA [see Dosage and Administration (2.3)]. Patients should be observed closely for hypersensitivity reactions, especially during the first and second infusions. Hypersensitivity reactions may occur within a few minutes following the initiation of the infusion of JEVTANA, thus facilities and equipment for the treatment of hypotension and bronchospasm should be available. Severe hypersensitivity reactions can occur and may include generalized rash/erythema, hypotension and bronchospasm. Severe hypersensitivity reactions require immediate discontinuation of the JEVTANA infusion and appropriate therapy. Patients with a history of severe hypersensitivity reactions should not be re-challenged with JEVTANA [see Contraindications (4)].

5.3 Gastrointestinal Symptoms

Nausea, vomiting and severe diarrhea, at times, may occur. Death related to diarrhea and electrolyte imbalance occurred in the randomized clinical trial. Intensive measures may be required for severe diarrhea and electrolyte imbalance. Patients should be treated with rehydration, anti-diarrheal or anti-emetic medications as needed. Treatment delay or dosage reduction may be necessary if patients experience Grade ≥ 3 diarrhea [see Dosage and Administration (2.2)].

5.4 Renal Failure

Renal failure, including four cases with fatal outcome, was reported in the randomized clinical trial. Most cases

Table 2 – Incidence of Reported Adverse Reactions* and Hematologic Abnormalities in $\geq 5\%$ of Patients Receiving JEVTANA in Combination with Prednisone or Mitoxantrone in Combination with Prednisone

	JEVTANA 25 mg/m² every 3 weeks with prednisone 10 mg daily n=371		Mitoxantrone 12 mg/m² every 3 weeks with prednisone 10 mg daily n=371	
	Grade 1–4 n (%)	Grade 3–4 n (%)	Grade 1–4 n (%)	Grade 3–4 n (%)
Any Adverse Reaction				
Blood and Lymphatic System Disorders				
Neutropenia[†]	347 (94%)	303 (82%)	325 (87%)	215 (58%)
Febrile Neutropenia	27 (7%)	27 (7%)	5 (1%)	5 (1%)
Anemia[†]	361 (98%)	39 (11%)	302 (82%)	18 (5%)
Leukopenia[†]	355 (96%)	253 (69%)	343 (93%)	157 (42%)
Thrombocytopenia[†]	176 (48%)	15 (4%)	160 (43%)	6 (2%)
Cardiac Disorders				
Arrhythmia[‡]	18 (5%)	4 (1%)	6 (2%)	1 (< 1%)
Gastrointestinal Disorders				
Diarrhea	173 (47%)	23 (6%)	39 (11%)	1 (< 1%)
Nausea	127 (34%)	7 (2%)	85 (23%)	1 (< 1%)
Vomiting	83 (22%)	6 (2%)	38 (10%)	0
Constipation	76 (20%)	4 (1%)	57 (15%)	2 (< 1%)
Abdominal Pain[§]	64 (17%)	7 (2%)	23 (6%)	0
Dyspepsia[¶]	36 (10%)	0	9 (2%)	0
General Disorders and Administration Site Conditions				
Fatigue	136 (37%)	18 (5%)	102 (27%)	11 (3%)
Asthenia	76 (20%)	17 (5%)	46 (12%)	9 (2%)
Pyrexia	45 (12%)	4 (1%)	23 (6%)	1 (< 1%)
Peripheral Edema	34 (9%)	2 (< 1%)	34 (9%)	2 (< 1%)
Mucosal Inflammation	22 (6%)	1 (< 1%)	10 (3%)	1 (< 1%)
Pain	20 (5%)	4 (1%)	18 (5%)	7 (2%)
Infections and Infestations				
Urinary Tract Infection[#]	29 (8%)	6 (2%)	12 (3%)	4 (1%)
Investigations				
Weight Decreased	32 (9%)	0	28 (8%)	1 (< 1%)
Metabolism and Nutrition Disorders				
Anorexia	59 (16%)	3 (< 1%)	39 (11%)	3 (< 1%)
Dehydration	18 (5%)	8 (2%)	10 (3%)	3 (< 1%)
Musculoskeletal and Connective Tissue Disorders				
Back Pain	60 (16%)	14 (4%)	45 (12%)	11 (3%)
Arthralgia	39 (11%)	4 (1%)	31 (8%)	4 (1%)
Muscle Spasms	27 (7%)	0	10 (3%)	0
Nervous System Disorders				
Peripheral Neuropathy[Þ]	50 (13%)	3 (< 1%)	12 (3.2%)	3 (< 1%)
Dysgeusia	41 (11%)	0	15 (4%)	0
Dizziness	30 (8%)	0	21 (6%)	2 (< 1%)
Headache	28 (8%)	0	19 (5%)	0
Renal and Urinary Tract Disorders				
Hematuria	62 (17%)	7 (2%)	13 (4%)	1 (< 1%)
Dysuria	25 (7%)	0	5 (1%)	0
Respiratory, Thoracic and Mediastinal Disorders				
Dyspnea	43 (12%)	4 (1%)	16 (4%)	2 (< 1%)
Cough	40 (11%)	0	22 (6%)	0
Skin and Subcutaneous Tissue Disorders				
Alopecia	37 (10%)	0	18 (5%)	0
Vascular Disorders				
Hypotension	20 (5%)	2 (<1 %)	9 (2%)	1 (< 1%)
Median Duration of Treatment	6 cycles		4 cycles	

* Graded using NCI CTCAE version 3
† Based on laboratory values, cabazitaxel: n =369, mitoxantrone: n = 370.
‡ Includes atrial fibrillation, atrial flutter, atrial tachycardia, atrioventricular block complete, bradycardia, palpitations, supraventricular tachycardia, tachyarrhythmia, and tachycardia.
§ Includes abdominal discomfort, abdominal pain lower, abdominal pain upper, abdominal tenderness, and GI pain.
¶ Includes gastroesophageal reflux disease and reflux gastritis.
# Includes urinary tract infection enterococcal and urinary tract infection fungal.
Þ Includes peripheral motor neuropathy and peripheral sensory neuropathy.

occurred in association with sepsis, dehydration, or obstructive uropathy [see Adverse Reactions (6.1)]. Some deaths due to renal failure did not have a clear etiology. Appropriate measures should be taken to identify causes of renal failure and treat aggressively.

5.5 Elderly Patients

In the randomized clinical trial, 3 of 131 (2%) patients < 65 years of age and 15 of 240 (6%) $\geq$ 65 years of age died of causes other than disease progression within 30 days of the last cabazitaxel dose. Patients $\geq$ 65 years of age are more likely to experience certain adverse reactions, including neutropenia and febrile neutropenia [see Adverse Reactions (6) and Use in Specific Populations (8.5)].

5.6 Hepatic Impairment

No dedicated hepatic impairment trial for JEVTANA has been conducted. Patients with impaired hepatic function (total bilirubin $\geq$ ULN, or AST and/or ALT $\geq 1.5 \times$ ULN) were excluded from the randomized clinical trial.

Cabazitaxel is extensively metabolized in the liver, and hepatic impairment is likely to increase cabazitaxel concentrations.

Hepatic impairment increases the risk of severe and life-threatening complications in patients receiving other drugs belonging to the same class as JEVTANA. JEVTANA should not be given to patients with hepatic impairment (total bilirubin $\geq$ ULN, or AST and/or ALT $\geq 1.5 \times$ ULN).

5.7 Pregnancy

Pregnancy category D.

JEVTANA can cause fetal harm when administered to a pregnant woman. In non-clinical studies in rats and rabbits, cabazitaxel was embryotoxic, fetotoxic, and abortifacient at exposures significantly lower than those expected at the recommended human dose level.

There are no adequate and well-controlled studies in pregnant women using JEVTANA. If this drug is used during pregnancy, or if the patient becomes pregnant while taking this drug, the patient should be apprised of the potential hazard to the fetus. Women of childbearing potential should be advised to avoid becoming pregnant during treatment with JEVTANA *[see Use in Specific Populations (8.1)]*.

6. ADVERSE REACTIONS

The following serious adverse reactions are discussed in greater detail in another section of the label:

- Neutropenia *[see Warnings and Precautions (5.1)]*.
- Hypersensitivity Reactions *[see Warnings and Precautions (5.2)]*.
- Gastrointestinal Symptoms *[see Warnings and Precautions (5.3)]*.
- Renal Failure *[see Warnings and Precautions (5.4)]*.

6.1 Clinical Trial Experience

Because clinical trials are conducted under widely varying conditions, the adverse reaction rates observed cannot be directly compared to rates in other trials and may not reflect the rates observed in clinical practice.

The safety of JEVTANA in combination with prednisone was evaluated in 371 patients with hormone-refractory metastatic prostate cancer treated in a single randomized trial, compared to mitoxantrone plus prednisone.

Deaths due to causes other than disease progression within 30 days of last study drug dose were reported in 18 (5%) JEVTANA-treated patients and 3 (< 1%) mitoxantrone-treated patients. The most common fatal adverse reactions in JEVTANA-treated patients were infections (n=5) and renal failure (n=4). The majority (4 of 5 patients) of fatal infection-related adverse reactions occurred after a single dose of JEVTANA. Other fatal adverse reactions in JEVTANA-treated patients included ventricular fibrillation, cerebral hemorrhage, and dyspnea.

The most common (≥ 10%) grade 1–4 adverse reactions were anemia, leukopenia, neutropenia, thrombocytopenia, diarrhea, fatigue, nausea, vomiting, constipation, asthenia, abdominal pain, hematuria, back pain, anorexia, peripheral neuropathy, pyrexia, dyspnea, dysguesia, cough, arthralgia, and alopecia.

The most common (≥ 5%) grade 3–4 adverse reactions in patients who received JEVTANA were neutropenia, leukopenia, anemia, febrile neutropenia, diarrhea, fatigue, and asthenia.

Treatment discontinuations due to adverse drug reactions occurred in 18% of patients who received JEVTANA and 8% of patients who received mitoxantrone. The most common adverse reactions leading to treatment discontinuation in the JEVTANA group were neutropenia and renal failure. Dose reductions were reported in 12% of JEVTANA-treated patients and 4% of mitoxantrone-treated patients. Dose delays were reported in 28% of JEVTANA-treated patients and 15% of mitoxantrone-treated patients.

[See table 2 at top of previous page]

Neutropenia and Associated Clinical Events:

Five patients experienced fatal infectious adverse events (sepsis or septic shock). All had grade 4 neutropenia and one had febrile neutropenia. One additional patient's death was attributed to neutropenia without a documented infection. Twenty-two (6%) patients discontinued JEVTANA treatment due to neutropenia, febrile neutropenia, infection, or sepsis. The most common adverse reaction leading to treatment discontinuation in the JEVTANA group was neutropenia (2%).

Hematuria:

Adverse events of hematuria, including those requiring medical intervention, were more common in JEVTANA-treated patients. The incidence of grade ≥ 2 hematuria was 6% in JEVTANA-treated patients and 2% in mitoxantrone-treated patients. Other factors associated with hematuria were well-balanced between arms and do not account for the increased rate of hematuria on the JEVTANA arm.

Hepatic Laboratory Abnormalities:

The incidences of grade 3–4 increased AST, increased ALT, and increased bilirubin were each ≤ 1%.

Elderly Population:

The following grade 1–4 adverse reactions were reported at rates ≥ 5% higher in patients 65 years of age or greater compared to younger patients: fatigue (40% vs. 30%), neutropenia (97% vs. 89%), asthenia (24% vs. 15%), pyrexia (15% vs. 8%), dizziness (10% vs. 5%), urinary tract infection (10% vs. 3%) and dehydration (7% vs. 2%), respectively.

The incidence of the following grade 3–4 adverse reactions were higher in patients ≥ 65 years of age compared to younger patients; neutropenia (87% vs. 74%), and febrile neutropenia (8% vs. 6%) *[see Use in Specific Populations (8.5)]*.

7. DRUG INTERACTIONS

No formal clinical drug-drug interaction trials have been conducted with JEVTANA.

Prednisone or prednisolone administered at 10 mg daily did not affect the pharmacokinetics of cabazitaxel.

7.1 Drugs That May Increase Cabazitaxel Plasma Concentrations

CYP3A4 Inhibitors: Cabazitaxel is primarily metabolized through CYP3A *[see Clinical Pharmacology (12.3)]*. Though no formal drug interaction trials have been conducted for JEVTANA, concomitant administration of strong CYP3A inhibitors (e.g., ketoconazole, itraconazole, clarithromycin, atazanavir, indinavir, nefazodone, nelfinavir, ritonavir, saquinavir, telithromycin, voriconazole) is expected to increase concentrations of cabazitaxel. Therefore, co-administration with strong CYP3A inhibitors should be avoided. Caution should be exercised with concomitant use of moderate CYP3A inhibitors.

7.2 Drugs That May Decrease Cabazitaxel Plasma Concentrations

CYP3A4 Inducers: Though no formal drug interaction trials have been conducted for JEVTANA, the concomitant administration of strong CYP3A inducers (e.g., phenytoin, carbamazepine, rifampin, rifabutin, rifapentin, phenobarbital) is expected to decrease cabazitaxel concentrations. Therefore, co-administration with strong CYP3A inducers should be avoided. In addition, patients should also refrain from taking St. John's Wort.

8. USE IN SPECIFIC POPULATIONS

8.1 Pregnancy

Pregnancy category D. See 'Warnings and Precautions' section.

JEVTANA can cause fetal harm when administered to a pregnant woman. There are no adequate and well-controlled studies of JEVTANA in pregnant women.

Non-clinical studies in rats and rabbits have shown that cabazitaxel is embryotoxic, fetotoxic, and abortifacient. Cabazitaxel was shown to cross the placenta barrier within 24 hours of a single intravenous administration of a 0.08 mg/kg dose (approximately 0.02 times the maximum recommended human dose-MRHD) to pregnant rats at gestational day 17.

Cabazitaxel administered once daily to female rats during organogenesis at a dose of 0.16 mg/kg/day (approximately 0.02–0.06 times the Cmax in patients with cancer at the recommended human dose) caused maternal and embryofetal toxicity consisting of increased post-implantation loss, embryolethality, and fetal deaths. Decreased mean fetal birth weight associated with delays in skeletal ossification were observed at doses ≥ 0.08 mg/kg (approximately 0.02 times the Cmax at the MRHD). *In utero* exposure to cabazitaxel did not result in fetal abnormalities in rats or rabbits at exposure levels significantly lower than the expected human exposures.

If this drug is used during pregnancy or if the patient becomes pregnant while taking this drug, the patient should be apprised of the potential hazard to the fetus. Women of childbearing potential should be advised to avoid becoming pregnant while taking JEVTANA.

8.3 Nursing Mothers

Cabazitaxel or cabazitaxel metabolites are excreted in maternal milk of lactating rats. It is not known whether this drug is excreted in human milk. Within 2 hours of a single intravenous administration of cabazitaxel to lactating rats at a dose of 0.08 mg/kg (approximately 0.02 times the maximum recommended human dose), radioactivity related to cabazitaxel was detected in the stomachs of nursing pups. This was detectable for up to 24 hours post-dose. Approximately 1.5% of the dose delivered to the mother was calculated to be delivered in the maternal milk. Because many drugs are excreted in human milk and because of the potential for serious adverse reactions in nursing infants from JEVTANA, a decision should be made whether to discontinue nursing or to discontinue the drug, taking into account the importance of the drug to the mother.

8.4 Pediatric Use

The safety and effectiveness of JEVTANA in pediatric patients have not been established.

8.5 Geriatric Use

Based on a population pharmacokinetic analysis, no significant difference was observed in the pharmacokinetics of cabazitaxel between patients < 65 years (n=100) and older (n=70).

Of the 371 patients with prostate cancer treated with JEVTANA every three weeks plus prednisone, 240 patients (64.7%) were 65 years of age and over, while 70 patients (18.9%) were 75 years of age and over. No overall differences in effectiveness were observed between patients ≥ 65 years of age and younger patients. Elderly patients (≥ 65 years of age) may be more likely to experience certain adverse reactions. The incidence of neutropenia, fatigue, asthenia, pyrexia, dizziness, urinary tract infection and dehydration occurred at rates ≥ 5% higher in patients who were 65 years of age or greater compared to younger patients *[see Adverse Reactions (6.1)]*.

8.6 Renal Impairment

No dedicated renal impairment trial for JEVTANA has been conducted. Based on the population pharmacokinetic analysis, no significant difference in clearance was observed in patients with mild (50 mL/min ≤ creatinine clearance (CLcr) < 80 mL/min) and moderate renal impairment (30 mL/min ≤ CLcr < 50 mL/min). No data are available for patients with severe renal impairment or end-stage renal disease *[see Clinical Pharmacology (12.3)]*. Caution should be used in patients with severe renal impairment (CLcr < 30 mL/min) and patients with end-stage renal diseases.

8.7 Hepatic Impairment

No dedicated hepatic impairment trial for JEVTANA has been conducted. The safety of JEVTANA has not been evaluated in patients with hepatic impairment *[see Warnings and Precautions (5.6)]*.

As cabazitaxel is extensively metabolized in the liver, hepatic impairment is likely to increase the cabazitaxel concentrations. Patients with impaired hepatic function (total bilirubin ≥ ULN, or AST and/or ALT ≥ 1.5 × ULN) were excluded from the randomized clinical trial.

10 OVERDOSAGE

There is no known antidote for JEVTANA overdose. Anticipated complications of overdose include exacerbation of adverse reactions such as bone marrow suppression and gastrointestinal disorders.

In case of overdose, the patient should be kept in a specialized unit where vital signs, chemistry and particular functions can be closely monitored. Patients should receive therapeutic G-CSF as soon as possible after discovery of overdose. Other appropriate symptomatic measures should be taken, as needed.

11 DESCRIPTION

JEVTANA (cabazitaxel) is an antineoplastic agent belonging to the taxane class. It is prepared by semi-synthesis with a precursor extracted from yew needles.

The chemical name of cabazitaxel is (2α,5β,7β,10β,13α)-4-acetoxy-13-({(2R,3S)-3-[(tertbutoxycarbonyl) amino]-2-hydroxy-3-phenylpropanoyl}oxy)-1-hydroxy-7,10-dimethoxy-9-oxo-5,20-epoxytax-11-en-2-yl benzoate – propan-2-one(1:1).

Cabazitaxel has the following structural formula:

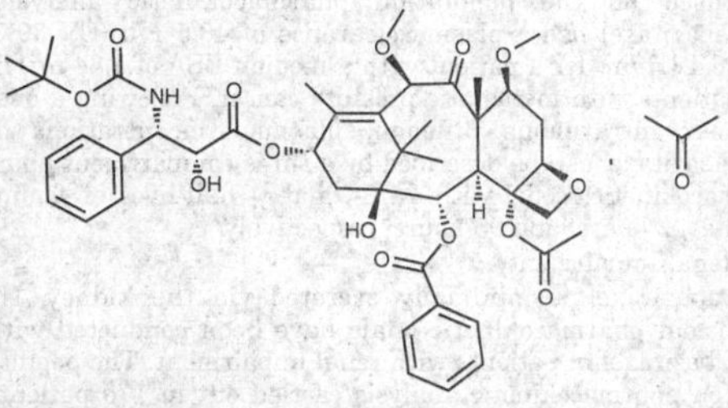

Cabazitaxel is a white to off-white powder with a molecular formula of $C_{45}H_{57}NO_{14}.C_3H_6O$ and a molecular weight of 894.01 (for the acetone solvate)/835.93 (for the solvent free). It is lipophilic, practically insoluble in water and soluble in alcohol.

JEVTANA (cabazitaxel) Injection 60 mg/1.5 mL is a sterile, non-pyrogenic, clear yellow to brownish-yellow viscous solution and is available in single-use vials containing 60 mg cabazitaxel (anhydrous and solvent free) and 1.56 g polysorbate 80.

Each mL contains 40 mg cabazitaxel (anhydrous) and 1.04 g polysorbate 80.

DILUENT for JEVTANA is a clear, colorless, sterile, and non-pyrogenic solution containing 13% (w/w) ethanol in water for injection, approximately 5.7 mL.

JEVTANA requires two dilutions prior to intravenous infusion. JEVTANA injection should be diluted only with the supplied DILUENT for JEVTANA, followed by dilution in either 0.9% sodium chloride solution or 5% dextrose solution.

12 CLINICAL PHARMACOLOGY

12.1 Mechanism of Action

Cabazitaxel is a microtubule inhibitor. Cabazitaxel binds to tubulin and promotes its assembly into microtubules while simultaneously inhibiting disassembly. This leads to the stabilization of microtubules, which results in the inhibition of mitotic and interphase cellular functions.

12.2 Pharmacodynamics

Cabazitaxel demonstrated antitumor activity against advanced human tumors xenografted in mice. Cabazitaxel is active in docetaxel-sensitive tumors. In addition, cabazitaxel demonstrated activity in tumor models insensitive to chemotherapy including docetaxel.

12.3 Pharmacokinetics

A population pharmacokinetic analysis was conducted in 170 patients with solid tumors at doses ranging from 10 to 30 mg/m^2 weekly or every three weeks.

Absorption

Based on the population pharmacokinetic analysis, after an intravenous dose of cabazitaxel 25 mg/m^2 every three weeks, the mean C_{max} in patients with metastatic prostate cancer was 226 ng/mL (CV 107%) and was reached at the end of the one-hour infusion (T_{max}). The mean AUC in patients with metastatic prostate cancer was 991 ng•h/mL (CV 34%).

No major deviation from the dose proportionality was observed from 10 to 30 mg/m^2 in patients with advanced solid tumors.

Distribution

The volume of distribution (V_{ss}) was 4,864 L (2,643 L/m^2 for a patient with a median BSA of 1.84 m^2) at steady state.

In vitro, the binding of cabazitaxel to human serum proteins was 89 to 92% and was not saturable up to 50,000 ng/mL, which covers the maximum concentration observed in clinical trials. Cabazitaxel is mainly bound to human serum albumin (82%) and lipoproteins (88% for HDL, 70% for LDL, and 56% for VLDL). The *in vitro* blood-to-plasma concentration ratio in human blood ranged from 0.90 to 0.99, indicating that cabazitaxel was equally distributed between blood and plasma.

Metabolism

Cabazitaxel is extensively metabolized in the liver (> 95%), mainly by the CYP3A4/5 isoenzyme (80% to 90%), and to a lesser extent by CYP2C8. Cabazitaxel is the main circulating moiety in human plasma. Seven metabolites were detected in plasma (including the 3 active metabolites issued from O-demethylation), with the main one accounting for 5% of cabazitaxel exposure. Around 20 metabolites of cabazitaxel are excreted into human urine and feces.

Based on *in vitro* studies, the potential for cabazitaxel to inhibit drugs that are substrates of other CYP isoenzymes (1A2,-2B6,-2C9, -2C8, -2C19, -2E1, -2D6, and 3A4/5) is low. In addition, cabazitaxel did not induce CYP isozymes *in vitro*.

Elimination

After a one-hour intravenous infusion [^{14}C]-cabazitaxel 25 mg/m^2, approximately 80% of the administered dose was eliminated within 2 weeks. Cabazitaxel is mainly excreted in the feces as numerous metabolites (76% of the dose); while renal excretion of cabazitaxel and metabolites account for 3.7% of the dose (2.3% as unchanged drug in urine).

Based on the population pharmacokinetic analysis, cabazitaxel has a plasma clearance of 48.5 L/h (CV 39%; 26.4 L/h/m^2 for a patient with a median BSA of 1.84 m^2) in patients with metastatic prostate cancer. Following a one-hour intravenous infusion, plasma concentrations of cabazitaxel can be described by a three-compartment pharmacokinetic model with α-, β-, and γ- half-lives of 4 minutes, 2 hours, and 95 hours, respectively.

Renal Impairment

Cabazitaxel is minimally excreted via the kidney. No formal pharmacokinetic trials have been conducted with cabazitaxel in patients with renal impairment. The population pharmacokinetic analysis carried out in 170 patients including 14 patients with moderate renal impairment (30 mL/min ≤ CLcr < 50 mL/min) and 59 patients with mild renal impairment (50 mL/min ≤ CLcr < 80 mL/min) showed that mild to moderate renal impairment did not have meaningful effects on the pharmacokinetics of cabazitaxel. No data are available for patients with severe renal impairment or end-stage renal disease *[see Use in Special Populations (8.6)]*.

Hepatic Impairment

No formal trials in patients with hepatic impairment have been conducted. As cabazitaxel is extensively metabolized in the liver, hepatic impairment is likely to increase the cabazitaxel concentrations *[see Warnings and Precautions (5.6), and Use in Special Populations (8.7)]*.

Drug interactions

As cabazitaxel is mainly metabolized by CYP3A *in vitro*, strong CYP3A inducers or inhibitors are expected to affect the pharmacokinetics of cabazitaxel.

Prednisone or prednisolone administered at 10 mg daily did not affect the pharmacokinetics of cabazitaxel.

In vitro, cabazitaxel did not inhibit the multidrug-resistance protein 1 (MRP1) or 2 (MRP2). *In vitro* cabazitaxel inhibited the transport of P-gp and BRCP, at concentrations at least 38 fold what is observed in clinical settings. Therefore, the *in vivo* risk of cabazitaxel to inhibit MRPs, P-gp, or BCRP is unlikely at the dose of 25 mg/m^2.

In vitro, cabazitaxel is a substrate of P-gp, but not a substrate of MRP1, MRP2, or BCRP.

13 NONCLINICAL TOXICOLOGY

13.1 Carcinogenesis, Mutagenesis, Impairment of Fertility

Long-term animal studies have not been performed to evaluate the carcinogenic potential of cabazitaxel.

Cabazitaxel was positive for clastogenesis in the *in vivo* micronucleus test, inducing an increase of micronuclei in rats at doses ≥ 0.5 mg/kg. Cabazitaxel increased numerical aberrations with or without metabolic activation in an *in vitro* test in human lymphocytes though no induction of structural aberrations was observed. Cabazitaxel did not induce mutations in the bacterial reverse mutation (Ames) test. The positive *in vivo* genotoxicity findings are consistent with the pharmacological activity of the compound (inhibition of tubulin depolymerization).

Cabazitaxel may impair fertility in humans. In a fertility study performed in female rats at cabazitaxel doses of 0.05, 0.1, or 0.2 mg/ kg/day there was no effect of administration of the drug on mating behavior or the ability to become pregnant. There was an increase in pre-implantation loss at the 0.2 mg/kg/day dose and an increase in early resorptions at doses ≥ 0.1 mg/kg/day (approximately 0.02–0.06 times the human clinical exposure based on Cmax). In multi-cycle studies following the clinically recommended dosing schedule, atrophy of the uterus was observed at the 5 mg/kg dose level (approximately the AUC in patients with cancer at the recommended human dose) along with necrosis of the corpora lutea at doses ≥ 1 mg/kg (approximately 0.2 times the AUC at the clinically recommended human dose).

Cabazitaxel did not affect mating performances or fertility of treated male rats at doses of 0.05, 0.1, or 0.2 mg/kg/day. In multiple-cycle studies following the clinically recommended dosing schedule, however, degeneration of seminal vesicle and seminiferous tubule atrophy in the testis were observed in rats treated intravenously with cabazitaxel at a dose of 1 mg/kg (approximately 0.2–0.35 times the AUC in patients with cancer at the recommended human dose), and minimal testicular degeneration (minimal epithelial single cell necrosis in epididymis) was observed in dogs treated with a dose of 0.5 mg/kg (approximately one-tenth of the AUC in patients with cancer at the recommended human dose).

14. CLINICAL STUDIES

The efficacy and safety of JEVTANA in combination with prednisone were evaluated in a randomized, open-label, international, multi-center study in patients with hormone-refractory metastatic prostate cancer previously treated with a docetaxel-containing treatment regimen.

A total of 755 patients were randomized to receive either JEVTANA 25 mg/m^2 intravenously every 3 weeks for a maximum of 10 cycles with prednisone 10 mg orally daily (n=378), or to receive mitoxantrone 12 mg/m^2 intravenously every 3 weeks for 10 cycles with prednisone 10 mg orally daily (n=377) for a maximum of 10 cycles.

This study included patients over 18 years of age with hormone-refractory metastatic prostate cancer either measurable by RECIST criteria or non-measurable disease with rising PSA levels or appearance of new lesions, and ECOG (Eastern Cooperative Oncology Group) performance status 0–2. Patients had to have neutrophils >1,500 cells/mm^3, platelets > 100,000 cells/mm^3, hemoglobin > 10 g/dL, creatinine < 1.5 × upper limit of normal (ULN), total bilirubin < 1×ULN, AST < 1.5 × ULN, and ALT < 1.5 × ULN. Patients with a history of congestive heart failure, or myocardial infarction within the last 6 months, or patients with uncontrolled cardiac arrhythmias, angina pectoris, and/or hypertension were not included in the study.

Demographics, including age, race, and ECOG performance status (0–2) were balanced between the treatment arms. The median age was 68 years (range 46–92) and the racial distribution for all groups was 83.9% Caucasian, 6.9% Asian, 5.3% Black, and 4% Others in the JEVTANA group. Efficacy results for the JEVTANA arm versus the control arm are summarized in Table 3 and Figure 1.

Table 3 - Efficacy of JEVTANA in the Treatment of Patients with Hormone Refractory Metastatic Prostate Cancer (Intent-to-Treat Analysis)

	JEVTANA + Prednisone n=378	Mitoxantrone + Prednisone n=377
Overall Survival		
Number of deaths (%)	234 (61.9 %)	279 (74%)
Median survival (month) (95% CI)	15.1 (14.1–16.3)	12.7 (11.6–13.7)
Hazard Ratio* (95% CI)	0.70 (0.59–0.83)	
p-value	<0.0001	

* Hazard ratio estimated using Cox model; a hazard ratio of less than 1 favors JEVTANA

[See figure 1 at top of next column]

Investigator-assessed tumor response of 14.4% (95%CI: 9.6–19.3) was higher for patients in the JEVTANA arm compared to 4.4% (95%CI: 1.6–7.2) for patients in the mitoxantrone arm, p=0.0005.

15. REFERENCES

1. NIOSH Alert: Preventing occupational exposures to antineoplastic and other hazardous drugs in healthcare settings. 2004. U.S. Department of Health and Human Services, Public Health Service, Centers for Disease Control and Prevention, National Institute for Occupational Safety and Health, DHHS (NIOSH) Publication No. 2004-165.

Figure 1 - Kaplan-Meier Overall Survival Curves

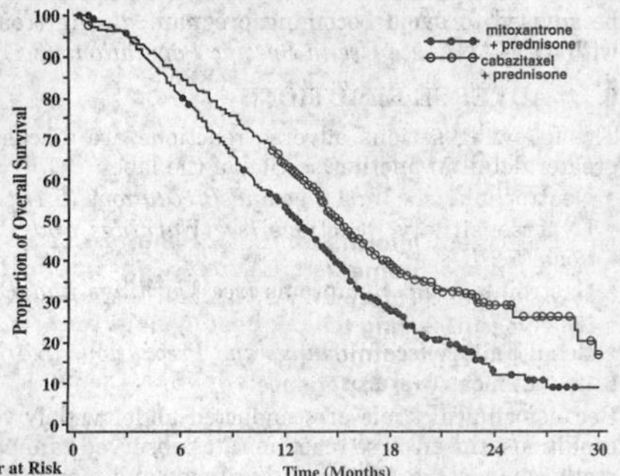

Number at Risk	0	6	12	18	24	30
mitoxantrone + prednisone	377	300	188	67	11	1
cabazitaxel + prednisone	378	321	231	90	28	4

2. OSHA Technical Manual, TED 1-0.15A, Section VI: Chapter 2. Controlling Occupational Exposure to Hazardous Drugs. OSHA, 1999. http://www.osha.gov/dts/osta/otm/otm_vi/otm_vi_2.html

3. American Society of Health-System Pharmacists. (2006) ASHP Guidelines on Handling Hazardous Drugs. *Am J Health-Syst Pharm 2006; 63:1172–1193.*

4. Polovich, M., White, J. M., & Kelleher, L.O. (eds.) 2005. Chemotherapy and biotherapy guidelines and recommendations for practice (2nd. ed.) Pittsburgh, PA: Oncology Nursing Society.

16. HOW SUPPLIED/STORAGE AND HANDLING

16.1 How Supplied

JEVTANA is supplied as a kit containing one single-use vial of JEVTANA (cabazitaxel) Injection (clear glass vial with a grey rubber closure, aluminum cap and light green plastic flip-off cap) and one vial of Diluent for JEVTANA (13% (w/w) ethanol in water for injection) in a clear glass vial with a grey rubber closure, gold-color aluminum cap and colorless plastic flip-off cap. Both items are in a blister pack in one carton.

NDC 0024-5824-11

16.2 Storage

JEVTANA Injection and Diluent for JEVTANA:

Store at 25°C (77°F); excursions permitted between 15°–30°C (59°–86°F).

Do not refrigerate.

Stability of the First Diluted Solution in the Vial:

First diluted solution of JEVTANA should be used immediately (within 30 minutes). Discard any unused portion *[see Dosage and Administration (2.5)]*.

Stability of the Second (Final) Dilution Solution in the Infusion Bag:

Fully prepared JEVTANA infusion solution (in either 0.9% sodium chloride solution or 5% dextrose solution) should be used within 8 hours at ambient temperature (including the one-hour infusion), or for a total of 24 hours (including the one-hour infusion) under the refrigerated conditions.

In addition, chemical and physical stability of the infusion solution has been demonstrated for 24 hours under refrigerated conditions. As both the first diluted solution and the second (final) infusion solution are supersaturated, the solutions may crystallize over time. If crystals and/or particulates appear, the solutions must not be used and should be discarded *[see Dosage and Administration (2.5)]*.

16.3 Handling and Disposal

Procedures for proper handling and disposal of antineoplastic drugs should be followed. Several guidelines on this subject have been published *[see References (15)]*. Any unused product or waste material should be disposed of in accordance with local requirements.

17. PATIENT COUNSELING INFORMATION

See FDA-Approved Patient Labeling

- Educate patients about the risk of potential hypersensitivity associated with JEVTANA. Confirm patients do not have a history of severe hypersensitivity reactions to cabazitaxel or to other drugs formulated with polysorbate 80. Instruct patients to immediately report signs of a hypersensitivity reaction.
- Explain the importance of routine blood cell counts. Instruct patients to monitor their temperature frequently and immediately report any occurrence of fever to the treating oncologist.
- Explain that it is important to take the oral prednisone as prescribed. Instruct patients to report if they were not compliant with oral corticosteroid regimen.
- Explain to patients that severe and fatal infections, dehydration, and renal failure have been associated with cabazitaxel exposure. Patients should immediately report fever, significant vomiting or diarrhea, decreased urinary output, and hematuria to the treating oncologist.

- Inform patients about the risk of drug interactions and the importance of providing a list of prescription and non-prescription drugs to the treating oncologist [see Drug Interactions (7)].
- Inform elderly patients that certain side effects may be more frequent or severe.

Patient Information
JEVTANA® (JEV-TA-NA)
(cabazitaxel)
Injection
Read this Patient Information before you start receiving JEVTANA and each time before you receive your infusion. There may be new information. This information does not take the place of talking to your doctor about your medical condition or your treatment.

What is the most important information I should know about JEVTANA?
JEVTANA may cause serious side effects including:
1. **Low white blood cells.** Low white blood cells can cause you to get serious infections, and may lead to death. People who are 65 years or older may be more likely to have these problems. Your doctor:
   - will do blood tests regularly to check your white blood cell counts during your treatment with JEVTANA.
   - may lower your dose of JEVTANA, change how often you receive it, or stop JEVTANA until your doctor decides that you have enough white blood cells.
   - may prescribe a medicine for you called G-CSF, to help prevent complications if your white blood cell count is too low.

   Tell your doctor right away if you have any of these symptoms of infection while receiving JEVTANA:
   - fever. Take your temperature often during treatment with JEVTANA.
   - cough
   - burning on urination
   - muscle aches

   Also, tell your doctor if you have any diarrhea during the time that your white blood cell count is low. Your doctor may prescribe treatment for you as needed.
2. **Severe allergic reactions.** Severe allergic reactions can happen within a few minutes after your infusion of JEVTANA starts, especially during the first and second infusions. Your doctor should prescribe medicines before each infusion to help prevent severe allergic reactions. Tell your doctor or nurse right away if you have any of these symptoms of a severe allergic reaction during or soon after an infusion of JEVTANA:
   - rash or itching
   - skin redness
   - feeling dizzy or faint
   - breathing problems
   - chest or throat tightness
   - swelling of face
3. **Gastrointestinal symptoms.** Vomiting and diarrhea can happen when you take JEVTANA. Severe vomiting and diarrhea with JEVTANA can lead to loss of too much body fluid (dehydration), or too much of your body salts (electrolytes). Death has happened from having severe diarrhea and losing too much body fluid or body salts with JEVTANA. Tell your doctor if you have vomiting or diarrhea. Your doctor will prescribe medicines to prevent or treat vomiting and diarrhea, as needed with JEVTANA. Tell your doctor if your symptoms get worse or do not get better. You may need to go to the hospital for treatment.
4. **Kidney failure.** Kidney failure may happen with JEVTANA, because of severe infection, loss of too much body fluid (dehydration), and other reasons, which may lead to death. Your doctor will check you for this problem and treat you if needed. Tell your doctor if you develop:
   - swelling of your face or body
   - decrease in the amount of urine that your body makes each day.

What is JEVTANA?
JEVTANA is a prescription anti-cancer medicine used with the steroid medicine prednisone. JEVTANA is used to treat people with prostate cancer that has worsened (progressed) after treatment with other anti-cancer medicines, including docetaxel. It is not known if JEVTANA is safe and works in children.

Who should not receive JEVTANA?
Do not receive JEVTANA if:
- your white blood cell (neutrophil count) is too low
- you have had a severe allergic reaction to cabazitaxel or other medicines that contain polysorbate 80. Ask your doctor if you are not sure.

What should I tell my doctor before receiving JEVTANA?
Before receiving JEVTANA, tell your doctor if you:
- had allergic reactions in the past
- have kidney or liver problems
- are over the age of 65
- have any other medical conditions
- if you are a female and:
   - are pregnant or plan to become pregnant. JEVTANA can harm your unborn baby. Talk to your doctor about

the best way for you to prevent pregnancy while you are receiving JEVTANA.
- are breastfeeding or plan to breastfeed. It is not known if JEVTANA passes into your breast milk. You and your doctor should decide if you will take JEVTANA or breastfeed. You should not do both.

Tell your doctor about all the medicines you take, including prescription and non-prescription medicines, vitamins, and herbal supplements. JEVTANA can interact with many other medicines. Do not take any new medicines without asking your doctor first. Your doctor will tell you if it is safe to take the new medicine with JEVTANA.

How will I receive JEVTANA?
- JEVTANA will be given to you by an intravenous (IV) infusion into your vein.
- Your treatment will take about 1 hour.
- JEVTANA is usually given every 3 weeks. Your doctor will decide how often you will receive JEVTANA.
- Your doctor will also prescribe another medicine called prednisone, for you to take by mouth every day during treatment with JEVTANA. Your doctor will tell you how and when to take your prednisone.

It is important that you take prednisone exactly as prescribed by your doctor. If you forget to take your prednisone, or do not take it on schedule, make sure to tell your doctor or nurse. Before each infusion of JEVTANA, you may receive other medicines to prevent or treat side effects.

What are the possible side effects of JEVTANA?
JEVTANA may cause serious side effects including:
- See "What is the most important information I should know about JEVTANA?"

Common side effects of JEVTANA include:
- **Low red blood cell count (anemia).** Your doctor will regularly check your red blood cell count. Symptoms of anemia include shortness of breath and tiredness.
- **Low blood platelet count.** Tell your doctor if you have any unusual bruising or bleeding.

• tiredness	• fever
• nausea	• shortness of breath
• constipation	• stomach (abdominal) pain
• weakness	• change in your sense of taste
• blood in the urine. Tell your doctor or nurse if you see blood in your urine.	• cough
	• joint pain
	• hair loss
• back pain	• numbness, tingling, burning or decreased sensation in your hands or feet
• decreased appetite	

Tell your doctor if you have any side effect that bothers you or that does not go away.
These are not all the possible side effects of JEVTANA. For more information, ask your doctor or pharmacist.
Call your doctor for medical advice about side effects. You may report side effects to FDA at 1-800-FDA-1088.

General information about JEVTANA
Medicines are sometimes prescribed for purposes other than those listed in a Patient Information leaflet.
This leaflet summarizes the most important information about JEVTANA. If you would like more information, talk with your doctor. You can ask your pharmacist or doctor for information about JEVTANA that is written for health professionals.
For more information, go to www.sanofi-aventis.us or call 1-800-633-1610.

What are the ingredients in JEVTANA?
Active ingredient: cabazitaxel
Inactive ingredient: polysorbate 80
sanofi-aventis U.S. LLC
Bridgewater, NJ 08807
Issued June 2010
JEVTANA® is a registered trademark of sanofi-aventis
©2010 sanofi-aventis U.S. LLC

KETEK®   Rx
[kē-tēk]
(telithromycin)
Tablets

> Ketek is contraindicated in patients with myasthenia gravis. There have been reports of fatal and life-threatening respiratory failure in patients with myasthenia gravis associated with the use of Ketek. (See **CONTRAINDICATIONS**.)

To reduce the development of drug-resistant bacteria and maintain the effectiveness of KETEK and other antibacte-

rial drugs, KETEK should be used only to treat infections that are proven or strongly suspected to be caused by bacteria.

DESCRIPTION
KETEK® tablets contain telithromycin, a semisynthetic antibacterial in the ketolide class for oral administration. Chemically, telithromycin is designated as Erythromycin, 3-de[(2,6-dideoxy-3-C-methyl-3-O-methyl-α-L-ribo-hexopyranosyl)oxy]-11,12-dideoxy-6-O-methyl-3-oxo-12,11-[oxycarbonyl[[4-[4-(3-pyridinyl)-1H-imidazol-1-yl]butyl]imino]]-. Telithromycin, a ketolide, differs chemically from the macrolide group of antibacterials by the lack of α-L-cladinose at position 3 of the erythronolide A ring, resulting in a 3-keto function. It is further characterized by a C11-12 carbamate substituted by an imidazolyl and pyridyl ring through a butyl chain. Its empirical formula is $C_{43}H_{65}N_5O_{10}$ and its molecular weight is 812.03. Telithromycin is a white to off-white crystalline powder. The following represents the chemical structure of telithromycin.

KETEK tablets are available as light-orange, oval, film-coated tablets, each containing 400 mg or 300 mg of telithromycin, and the following inactive ingredients: croscarmellose sodium, hypromellose, magnesium stearate, microcrystalline cellulose, polyethylene glycol, povidone, red ferric oxide, talc, titanium dioxide, and yellow ferric oxide.

CLINICAL PHARMACOLOGY

Pharmacokinetics
Absorption
Following oral administration, telithromycin reached maximal concentration at about 1 hour (0.5–4 hours).
It has an absolute bioavailability of 57% in both young and elderly subjects.
The rate and extent of absorption are unaffected by food intake, thus KETEK tablets can be given without regard to food.
In healthy adult subjects, peak plasma telithromycin concentrations of approximately 2 µg/mL are attained at a median of 1 hour after an 800-mg oral dose.
Steady-state plasma concentrations are reached within 2 to 3 days of once daily dosing with telithromycin 800 mg.
Following oral dosing, the mean terminal elimination half-life of telithromycin is 10 hours.
The pharmacokinetics of telithromycin after administration of single and multiple (7 days) once daily 800-mg doses to healthy adult subjects are shown in Table 1.

Table 1

Parameter	Mean (SD)	
	Single dose (n=18)	Multiple dose (n=18)
C_{max} (µg/mL)	1.9 (0.80)	2.27 (0.71)
T_{max} (h)*	1.0 (0.5–4.0)	1.0 (0.5–3.0)
$AUC_{(0-24)}$ (µg•h/mL)	8.25 (2.6)	12.5 (5.4)
Terminal $t_{1/2}$ (h)	7.16 (1.3)	9.81 (1.9)
C_{24h} (µg/mL)	0.03 (0.013)	0.07 (0.051)

SD=Standard deviation
C_{max}=Maximum plasma concentration
T_{max}=Time to C_{max}
AUC=Area under concentration vs. time curve
$t_{1/2}$=Terminal plasma half-life
C_{24h}=Plasma concentration at 24 hours post-dose
*Median (min–max) values

In a patient population, mean peak and trough plasma concentrations were 2.9 µg/mL (±1.55), (n=219) and 0.2 µg/mL (±0.22), (n=204), respectively, after 3 to 5 days of KETEK 800 mg once daily.
Distribution
Total in vitro protein binding is approximately 60% to 70% and is primarily due to human serum albumin.
Protein binding is not modified in elderly subjects and in patients with hepatic impairment.
The volume of distribution of telithromycin after intravenous infusion is 2.9 L/kg.

Telithromycin concentrations in bronchial mucosa, epithelial lining fluid, and alveolar macrophages after 800 mg once daily dosing for 5 days in patients are displayed in Table 2.

Table 2

	Hours post-dose	Mean concentration (µg/mL) Tissue or fluid	Plasma	Tissue/ Plasma Ratio
Bronchial mucosa	2	3.88*	1.86	2.11
	12	1.41*	0.23	6.33
	24	0.78*	0.08	12.11
Epithelial lining fluid	2	14.89	1.86	8.57
	12	3.27	0.23	13.8
	24	0.84	0.08	14.41
Alveolar macrophages	2	65	1.07	55
	8	100	0.605	180
	24	41	0.073	540

*Units in mg/kg

Telithromycin concentration in white blood cells exceeds the concentration in plasma and is eliminated more slowly from white blood cells than from plasma. Mean white blood cell concentrations of telithromycin peaked at 72.1 µg/mL at 6 hours, and remained at 14.1 µg/mL 24 hours after 5 days of repeated dosing of 600 mg once daily. After 10 days, repeated dosing of 600 mg once daily, white blood cell concentrations remained at 8.9 µg/mL 48 hours after the last dose.

Metabolism

In total, metabolism accounts for approximately 70% of the dose. In plasma, the main circulating compound after administration of an 800-mg radio-labeled dose was parent compound, representing 56.7% of the total radioactivity. The main metabolite represented 12.6% of the AUC of telithromycin. Three other plasma metabolites were quantified, each representing 3% or less of the AUC of telithromycin.

It is estimated that approximately 50% of its metabolism is mediated by CYP 450 3A4 and the remaining 50% is CYP 450-independent.

Elimination

The systemically available telithromycin is eliminated by multiple pathways as follows: 7% of the dose is excreted unchanged in feces by biliary and/or intestinal secretion; 13% of the dose is excreted unchanged in urine by renal excretion; and 37% of the dose is metabolized by the liver.

Special populations

Gender

There was no significant difference between males and females in mean AUC, C_{max}, and elimination half-life in two studies; one in 18 healthy young volunteers (18 to 40 years of age) and the other in 14 healthy elderly volunteers (65 to 92 years of age), given single and multiple once daily doses of 800 mg of KETEK.

Hepatic insufficiency

In a single-dose study (800 mg) in 12 patients and a multiple-dose study (800 mg) in 13 patients with mild to severe hepatic insufficiency (Child Pugh Class A, B and C), the C_{max}, AUC and $t_{1/2}$ of telithromycin were similar to those obtained in age- and sex-matched healthy subjects. In both studies, an increase in renal elimination was observed in hepatically impaired patients indicating that this pathway may compensate for some of the decrease in metabolic clearance. No dosage adjustment is recommended due to hepatic impairment.

(See **PRECAUTIONS, General** and **DOSAGE AND ADMINISTRATION**)

Renal insufficiency

In a multiple-dose study, 36 subjects with varying degrees of renal impairment received 400 mg, 600 mg, or 800 mg KETEK once daily for 5 days. There was a 1.4-fold increase in $C_{max,ss}$, and a 1.9-fold increase in AUC $(0–24)_{ss}$ at 800 mg multiple doses in the severely renally impaired group (CL_{CR} < 30 mL/min) compared to healthy volunteers. Renal excretion may serve as a compensatory elimination pathway for telithromycin in situations where metabolic clearance is impaired. Patients with severe renal impairment are prone to conditions that may impair their metabolic clearance. Therefore, in the presence of severe renal impairment (CL_{CR} < 30 mL/min), a reduced dosage of KETEK is recommended. (See **DOSAGE AND ADMINISTRATION**)

In a single-dose study in patients with end-stage renal failure on hemodialysis (n=10), the mean C_{max} and AUC values were similar to normal healthy subjects when KETEK was administered 2 hours post-dialysis. However, the effect of dialysis on removing telithromycin from the body has not been studied.

Multiple insufficiency

The effects of co-administration of ketoconazole in 12 subjects (age ≥ 60 years), with impaired renal function were studied (CL_{CR}=24 to 80 mL/min). In this study, when severe renal insufficiency (CL_{CR} < 30 mL/min, n=2) and concomitant impairment of CYP 3A4 metabolism pathway were present, telithromycin exposure (AUC (0–24)) was increased by approximately 4- to 5-fold compared with the exposure in healthy subjects with normal renal function receiving telithromycin alone. In the presence of severe renal impairment (CL_{CR} < 30 mL/min), with coexisting hepatic impairment, a reduced dosage of KETEK is recommended. (See **PRECAUTIONS, General** and **DOSAGE AND ADMINISTRATION**)

Geriatric

Pharmacokinetic data show that there is an increase of 1.4-fold in exposure (AUC) in 20 patients ≥ 65 years of age with community acquired pneumonia in a Phase III study, and a 2.0-fold increase in exposure (AUC) in 14 subjects ≥ 65 years of age as compared with subjects less than 65 years of age in a Phase I study. No dosage adjustment is required based on age alone.

Drug-drug interactions

Studies were performed to evaluate the effect of CYP 3A4 inhibitors on telithromycin and the effect of telithromycin on drugs that are substrates of CYP 3A4 and CYP 2D6. In addition, drug interaction studies were conducted with several other concomitantly prescribed drugs.

CYP 3A4 inhibitors

Itraconazole

A multiple-dose interaction study with itraconazole showed that C_{max} of telithromycin was increased by 22% and AUC by 54%.

Ketoconazole

A multiple-dose interaction study with ketoconazole showed that C_{max} of telithromycin was increased by 51% and AUC by 95%.

Grapefruit juice

When telithromycin was given with 240 mL of grapefruit juice after an overnight fast to healthy subjects, the pharmacokinetics of telithromycin were not affected.

CYP 3A4 substrates

Cisapride

Steady-state peak plasma concentrations of cisapride (an agent with the potential to increase QT interval) were increased by 95% when co-administered with repeated doses of telithromycin, resulting in significant increases in QTc. (See **CONTRAINDICATIONS**)

Simvastatin

When simvastatin was co-administered with telithromycin, there was a 5.3-fold increase in simvastatin C_{max}, an 8.9-fold increase in simvastatin AUC, a 15-fold increase in the simvastatin active metabolite C_{max}, and a 12-fold increase in the simvastatin active metabolite AUC. (See **PRECAUTIONS**)

In another study, when simvastatin and telithromycin were administered 12 hours apart, there was a 3.4-fold increase in simvastatin C_{max}, a 4.0-fold increase in simvastatin AUC, a 3.2-fold increase in the active metabolite C_{max}, and a 4.3-fold increase in the active metabolite AUC. (See **PRECAUTIONS**)

Midazolam

Concomitant administration of telithromycin with intravenous or oral midazolam resulted in 2- and 6-fold increases, respectively, in the AUC of midazolam due to inhibition of CYP 3A4-dependent metabolism of midazolam. (See **PRECAUTIONS**)

CYP 2D6 substrates

Paroxetine

There was no pharmacokinetic effect on paroxetine when telithromycin was co-administered.

Metoprolol

When metoprolol was co-administered with telithromycin, there was an increase of approximately 38% on the C_{max} and AUC of metoprolol, however, there was no effect on the elimination half-life of metoprolol. Telithromycin exposure is not modified with concomitant single-dose administration of metoprolol. (See **PRECAUTIONS, Drug interactions**)

Other drug interactions

Digoxin

The plasma peak and trough levels of digoxin were increased by 73% and 21%, respectively, in healthy volunteers when co-administered with telithromycin. However, trough plasma concentrations of digoxin (when equilibrium between plasma and tissue concentrations has been achieved) ranged from 0.74 to 2.17 ng/mL. There were no significant changes in ECG parameters and no signs of digoxin toxicity. (See **PRECAUTIONS**)

Theophylline

When theophylline was co-administered with repeated doses of telithromycin, there was an increase of approximately 16% and 17% on the steady-state C_{max} and AUC of theophylline. Co-administration of theophylline may worsen gastrointestinal side effects such as nausea and vomiting, especially in female patients. It is recommended that telithromycin should be taken with theophylline 1 hour apart to decrease the likelihood of gastrointestinal side effects.

Sotalol

Telithromycin has been shown to decrease the C_{max} and AUC of sotalol by 34% and 20%, respectively, due to decreased absorption.

Warfarin

When co-administered with telithromycin in healthy subjects, there were no pharmacodynamic or pharmacokinetic effects on racemic warfarin.

Oral contraceptives

When oral contraceptives containing ethinyl estradiol and levonorgestrel were co-administered with telithromycin, the steady-state AUC of ethinyl estradiol did not change and the steady-state AUC of levonorgestrel was increased by 50%. The pharmacokinetic/pharmacodynamic study showed that telithromycin did not interfere with the antiovulatory effect of oral contraceptives containing ethinyl estradiol and levonorgestrel.

Ranitidine, antacid

There was no clinically relevant pharmacokinetic interaction of ranitidine or antacids containing aluminum and magnesium hydroxide on telithromycin.

Rifampin

During concomitant administration of rifampin and KETEK in repeated doses, C_{max} and AUC of telithromycin were decreased by 79%, and 86%, respectively. (See **PRECAUTIONS, Drug Interactions**)

Microbiology

Telithromycin belongs to the ketolide class of antibacterials and is structurally related to the macrolide family of antibiotics. Telithromycin concentrates in phagocytes where it exhibits activity against intracellular respiratory pathogens. *In vitro,* telithromycin has been shown to demonstrate concentration-dependent bactericidal activity against isolates of *Streptococcus pneumoniae* (including multi-drug resistant isolates [MDRSP[1]]).

1MDRSP=Multi-drug resistant *Streptococcus pneumoniae* includes isolates known as PRSP (penicillin-resistant *Streptococcus pneumoniae*), and are isolates resistant to two or more of the following antimicrobials: penicillin, 2nd generation cephalosporins (e.g., cefuroxime), macrolides, tetracyclines, and trimethoprim/sulfamethoxazole.

Mechanism of action

Telithromycin blocks protein synthesis by binding to domains II and V of 23S rRNA of the 50S ribosomal subunit. By binding at domain II, telithromycin retains activity against gram-positive cocci (e.g., *Streptococcus pneumoniae*) in the presence of resistance mediated by methylases (*erm* genes) that alter the domain V binding site of telithromycin. Telithromycin may also inhibit the assembly of nascent ribosomal units.

Mechanism of resistance

Staphylococcus aureus and *Streptococcus pyogenes* with the constitutive macrolide-lincosamide-streptogramin B ($cMLS_B$) phenotype are resistant to telithromycin.

Mutants of *Streptococcus pneumoniae* derived in the laboratory by serial passage in subinhibitory concentrations of telithromycin have demonstrated resistance based on L22 riboprotein mutations (telithromycin MICs are elevated but still within the susceptible range), one of two reported mutations affecting the L4 riboprotein, and production of K-peptide. The clinical significance of these laboratory mutants is not known.

Cross resistance

Telithromycin does not induce resistance through methylase gene expression in erythromycin-inducibly resistant bacteria, a function of its 3-keto moiety. Telithromycin has not been shown to induce resistance to itself.

List of Microorganisms

Telithromycin has been shown to be active against most strains of the following microorganisms, both *in vitro* and in clinical settings as described in the **INDICATIONS AND USAGE** section.

Aerobic gram-positive microorganisms

Streptococcus pneumoniae (including multi-drug resistant isolates [MDRSP[2]])

Aerobic gram-negative microorganisms

Haemophilus influenzae

Moraxella catarrhalis

Other microorganisms

Chlamydophila (Chlamydia) pneumoniae

Mycoplasma pneumoniae

The following *in vitro* data are available, but their clinical significance is unknown.

At least 90% of the following microorganisms exhibit *in vitro* minimum inhibitory concentrations (MICs) less than or equal to the susceptible breakpoint for telithromycin. However, the safety and efficacy of telithromycin in treating clinical infections due to these microorganisms have not been established in adequate and well-controlled clinical trials.

Aerobic gram-positive microorganisms
Staphylococcus aureus (methicillin and erythromycin susceptible isolates only)
Streptococcus pyogenes (erythromycin susceptible isolates only)
Streptococci (Lancefield groups C and G)
Other microorganisms
Legionella pneumophila

2MDRSP=Multi-drug resistant *Streptococcus pneumoniae* includes isolates known as PRSP (penicillin-resistant *S. pneumoniae*), and are isolates resistant to two or more of the following antimicrobials: penicillin, 2nd generation cephalosporins (e.g., cefuroxime), macrolides, tetracyclines, and trimethoprim/sulfamethoxazole.

Susceptibility Test Methods

When available, the clinical microbiology laboratory should provide cumulative results of *in vitro* susceptibility test results for antimicrobial drugs used in local hospitals and practice areas to the physician as periodic reports that describe the susceptibility profile of nosocomial and community-acquired pathogens. These reports should aid the physician in selecting the most effective antimicrobial.

Dilution techniques

Quantitative methods are used to determine antimicrobial minimum inhibitory concentrations (MICs). These MICs provide estimates of the susceptibility of bacteria to antibacterial compounds. The MICs should be determined using a standardized procedure. Standardized procedures are based on dilution methods (broth or agar dilution)[1,3] or equivalent with standardized inoculum and concentrations of telithromycin powder. The MIC values should be interpreted according to criteria provided in Table 3.

Diffusion techniques

Quantitative methods that require measurement of zone diameters also provide reproducible estimates of the susceptibility of bacteria to antibiotics. One such standardized procedure[2,3] requires the use of standardized inoculum concentrations. This procedure uses paper disks impregnated with 15 µg telithromycin to test the susceptibility of microorganisms to telithromycin. Disc diffusion zone sizes should be interpreted according to criteria in Table 3.

Table 3. Susceptibility Test Result Interpretive Criteria for Telithromycin

Pathogen	Minimal Inhibitory Concentrations (µg/mL) S	I	R	Disk Diffusion (zone diameters in mm) S	I	R
Streptococcus pneumoniae	≤ 1	2	≥ 4	≥ 19	16–18	≤ 15
Haemophilus influenzae	≤ 4	8	≥ 16	≥ 15	12–14	≤ 11

A report of "Susceptible" indicates that the antimicrobial is likely to inhibit growth of the pathogen if the antibacterial compound in the blood reaches the concentrations usually achievable. A report of "Intermediate" indicates that the result should be considered equivocal, and, if the microorganism is not fully susceptible to alternative, clinically feasible drugs, the test should be repeated. This category implies possible clinical applicability in body sites where the drug is physiologically concentrated or in situations where high dosage of drug can be used. This category also provides a buffer zone that prevents small uncontrolled technical factors from causing major discrepancies in interpretation. A report of "Resistant" indicates that the antimicrobial is not likely to inhibit growth of the pathogen if the antimicrobial compound in the blood reaches the concentrations usually achievable; other therapy should be selected.

Quality control

Standardized susceptibility test procedures require the use of quality control microorganisms to determine the performance of the test procedures[1,2,3]. Standard telithromycin powder should provide the MIC ranges for the quality control organisms in Table 4. For the disk diffusion technique, the 15-µg telithromycin disk should provide the zone diameter ranges for the quality control organisms in Table 4.

Table 4. Acceptable Quality Control Ranges for Telithromycin

QC Strain	Minimum Inhibitory Concentrations (µg/mL)	Disk Diffusion (Zone diameter in mm)
Streptococcus pneumoniae ATCC 49619	0.004–0.03	27–33
Haemophilus influenzae ATCC 49247	1.0–4.0	17–23

ATCC = American Type Culture Collection

INDICATIONS AND USAGE

KETEK tablets are indicated for the treatment of community-acquired pneumonia (of mild to moderate severity) due to *Streptococcus pneumoniae*, (including multi-drug resistant isolates [MDRSP[3]]), *Haemophilus influenzae, Moraxella catarrhalis, Chlamydophila pneumoniae*, or *Mycoplasma pneumoniae*, for patients 18 years old and above.

To reduce the development of drug-resistant bacteria and maintain the effectiveness of KETEK and other antibacterial drugs, KETEK should be used only to treat infections that are proven or strongly suspected to be caused by susceptible bacteria. When culture and susceptibility information are available, they should be considered in selecting or modifying antibacterial therapy. In the absence of such data, local epidemiology and susceptibility patterns may contribute to the empiric selection of therapy.

3MDRSP, Multi-drug resistant *Streptococcus pneumoniae* includes isolates known as PRSP (penicillin-resistant *Streptococcus pneumoniae*), and are isolates resistant to two or more of the following antibiotics: penicillin, 2nd generation cephalosporins, e.g., cefuroxime, macrolides, tetracyclines and trimethoprim/sulfamethoxazole.

CONTRAINDICATIONS

KETEK is contraindicated in patients with myasthenia gravis. Exacerbations of myasthenia gravis have been reported in patients and sometimes occurred within a few hours of the first dose of telithromycin. Reports have included fatal and life-threatening acute respiratory failure with a rapid onset and progression.

KETEK is contraindicated in patients with previous history of hepatitis and/or jaundice associated with the use of KETEK tablets, or any macrolide antibiotic.

KETEK is contraindicated in patients with a history of hypersensitivity to telithromycin and/or any components of KETEK tablets, or any macrolide antibiotic.

Concomitant administration of KETEK with cisapride or pimozide is contraindicated. (See **CLINICAL PHARMACOLOGY, Drug-drug Interactions** and **PRECAUTIONS.**)

WARNINGS

Hepatotoxicity

Acute hepatic failure and severe liver injury, in some cases fatal, have been reported in patients treated with KETEK. These hepatic reactions included fulminant hepatitis and hepatic necrosis leading to liver transplant, and were observed during or immediately after treatment. In some of these cases, liver injury progressed rapidly and occurred after administration of a few doses of KETEK. (See **ADVERSE REACTIONS**)

Physicians and patients should monitor for the appearance of signs or symptoms of hepatitis, such as fatigue, malaise, anorexia, nausea, jaundice, bilirubinuria, acholic stools, liver tenderness or hepatomegaly. **Patients with signs or symptoms of hepatitis must be advised to discontinue KETEK and immediately seek medical evaluation, which should include liver function tests.** (See **ADVERSE REACTIONS, PRECAUTIONS, Information to Patients.**) If clinical hepatitis or transaminase elevations combined with other systemic symptoms occur, KETEK should be permanently discontinued.

Ketek must not be re-administered to patients with a previous history of hepatitis and/or jaundice associated with the use of KETEK tablets, or any macrolide antibiotic. (See **CONTRAINDICATIONS**)

In addition, less severe hepatic dysfunction associated with increased liver enzymes, hepatitis and in some cases jaundice was reported with the use of KETEK. These events associated with less severe forms of liver toxicity were reversible.

QTc prolongation

Telithromycin has the potential to prolong the QTc interval of the electrocardiogram in some patients. QTc prolongation may lead to an increased risk for ventricular arrhythmias, including torsades de pointes. Thus, telithromycin should be avoided in patients with congenital prolongation of the QTc interval, and in patients with ongoing proarrhythmic conditions such as uncorrected hypokalemia or hypomagnesemia, clinically significant bradycardia, and in patients receiving Class IA (e.g., quinidine and procainamide) or Class III (e.g., dofetilide) antiarrhythmic agents.

Cases of torsades de pointes have been reported post-marketing with KETEK. In clinical trials, no cardiovascular morbidity or mortality attributable to QTc prolongation occurred with telithromycin treatment in 4780 patients in clinical trials, including 204 patients having a prolonged QTc at baseline.

Visual disturbances*

KETEK may cause visual disturbances particularly in slowing the ability to accommodate and the ability to release accommodation. Visual disturbances included blurred vision, difficulty focusing, and diplopia. Most events were mild to moderate; however, severe cases have been reported.

Loss of Consciousness*

There have been post-marketing adverse event reports of transient loss of consciousness including some cases associated with vagal syndrome.

***Because of potential visual difficulties or loss of consciousness, patients should attempt to minimize activities such as driving a motor vehicle, operating heavy machinery or engaging in other hazardous activities during treatment with KETEK. If patients experience visual disorders or loss of consciousness while taking KETEK, patients should not drive a motor vehicle, operate heavy machinery or engage in other hazardous activities.** (See **PRECAUTIONS, Information for Patients**)

Pseudomembranous colitis

Clostridium difficile associated diarrhea (CDAD) has been reported with use of nearly all antibacterial agents, including KETEK, and may range in severity from mild diarrhea to fatal colitis. Treatment with antibacterial agents alters the normal flora of the colon leading to overgrowth of *C. difficile*.

C. difficile produces toxins A and B which contribute to the development of CDAD. Hypertoxin producing strains of *C. difficile* cause increased morbidity and mortality, as these infections can be refractory to antimicrobial therapy and may require colectomy. CDAD must be considered in all patients who present with diarrhea following antibiotic use. Careful medical history is necessary since CDAD has been reported to occur over two months after the administration of antibacterial agents.

If CDAD is suspected or confirmed, ongoing antibiotic use not directed against *C. difficile* may need to be discontinued. Appropriate fluid and electrolyte management, protein supplementation, antibiotic treatment of *C difficile*, and surgical evaluation should be instituted as clinically indicated.

PRECAUTIONS

General

Prescribing KETEK in the absence of a proven or strongly suspected bacterial infection or a prophylactic indication is unlikely to provide benefit to the patient and increases the risk of the development of drug-resistant bacteria.

Telithromycin is principally excreted via the liver and kidney. Telithromycin may be administered without dosage adjustment in the presence of hepatic impairment. In the presence of severe renal impairment (CL_{CR} < 30 mL/min), a reduced dosage of KETEK is recommended. (See **DOSAGE AND ADMINISTRATION**)

Information for patients

A Medication Guide is provided to patients when Ketek is dispensed. Patients should be instructed to read the MedGuide when Ketek is received. In addition, the complete text of the MedGuide is reprinted at the end of this document.

The following information and instructions should be communicated to the patient.

- KETEK may cause problems with vision particularly when looking quickly between objects close by and objects far away. These events include blurred vision, difficulty focusing, and objects looking doubled. Most events were mild to moderate; however, severe cases have been reported. Problems with vision were reported as having occurred after any dose during treatment, but most occurred following the first or second dose. These problems lasted several hours and in some patients came back with the next dose. (See **WARNINGS** and **ADVERSE REACTIONS.**)

Patients should be advised that avoiding quick changes in viewing between objects in the distance and objects nearby may help to decrease the effects of these visual difficulties.

- **Because of potential visual difficulties or loss of consciousness, patients should attempt to minimize activities such as driving a motor vehicle, operating heavy machinery or engaging in other hazardous activities during treatment with KETEK.**

If patients experience visual difficulties or loss of consciousness/fainting

- patients should seek advice from their physician before taking another dose
- patients should not drive a motor vehicle, operate heavy machinery, or engage in otherwise hazardous activities.

Patients should also be advised:

- **Ketek is contraindicated in patients with myasthenia gravis.** (See **CONTRAINDICATIONS**)
- of the possibility of liver injury, associated with KETEK, which in rare cases may be severe. **Patients developing signs or symptoms of liver injury should be instructed to discontinue KETEK and seek medical attention immediately.** Symptoms of liver injury may include nausea,

fatigue, anorexia, jaundice, dark urine, light-colored stools, pruritus, or tender abdomen. Ketek must not be taken by patients with a previous history of hepatitis/jaundice associated with the use of KETEK or macrolide antibiotics. (See **CONTRAINDICATIONS** and **WARNINGS**)

- antibacterial drugs including KETEK should only be used to treat bacterial infections. They do not treat viral infections (e.g., the common cold). When KETEK is prescribed to treat a bacterial infection, patients should be told that although it is common to feel better early in the course of therapy, the medication should be taken exactly as directed. Skipping doses or not completing the full course of therapy may (1) decrease the effectiveness of the immediate treatment and (2) increase the likelihood that bacteria will develop resistance and will not be treatable by KETEK or other antibacterial drugs in the future.
- KETEK has the potential to produce changes in the electrocardiogram (QTc interval prolongation) and that they should report any fainting occurring during drug treatment.
- KETEK should be avoided in patients receiving Class 1A (e.g., quinidine, procainamide) or Class III (e.g., dofetilide) antiarrhythmic agents.
- to inform their physician of any personal or family history of QTc prolongation or proarrhythmic conditions such as uncorrected hypokalemia, or clinically significant bradycardia.
- diarrhea is a common problem caused by antibiotics which usually ends when the antibiotic is discontinued. Sometimes after starting treatment with antibiotics, patients can develop watery and bloody stools (with or without stomach cramps and fever) even as late as two or more months after having taken the last dose of the antibiotic. If this occurs, patients should contact their physician as soon as possible.
- simvastatin, lovastatin, or atorvastatin should be avoided in patients receiving KETEK. If KETEK is prescribed, therapy with simvastatin, lovastatin, or atorvastatin should be stopped during the course of treatment. (See **CLINICAL PHARMACOLOGY, Drug-drug interactions**)
- KETEK tablets can be taken with or without food.
- to inform their physician of any other medications taken concurrently with KETEK, including over-the-counter medications and dietary supplements.

Drug interactions

Telithromycin is a strong inhibitor of the cytochrome P450 3A4 system. Co-administration of KETEK tablets and a drug primarily metabolized by the cytochrome P450 3A4 enzyme system may result in increased plasma concentration of the drug co-administered with telithromycin that could increase or prolong both the therapeutic and adverse effects. Therefore, appropriate dosage adjustments may be necessary for the drug co-administered with telithromycin.

The use of KETEK is contraindicated with cisapride. (See **CONTRAINDICATIONS** and **CLINICAL PHARMACOLOGY, Drug-drug interactions**)

The use of KETEK is contraindicated with pimozide. Although there are no studies looking at the interaction between KETEK and pimozide, there is a potential risk of increased pimozide plasma levels by inhibition of CYP 3A4 pathways by KETEK as with macrolides. (See **CONTRAINDICATIONS**)

In a pharmacokinetic study, simvastatin levels were increased due to CYP 3A4 inhibition by telithromycin. (See **CLINICAL PHARMACOLOGY, Drug-drug interactions**)

Similarly, an interaction may occur with lovastatin or atorvastatin. Although pravastatin is not metabolized by CYPs, hepatic cell OATP1 transporters play an important role in its elimination from the body. In vitro OATP1 transporter inhibition has been demonstrated for macrolides and telithromycin. Telithromycin slightly inhibits the in vitro transporter uptake of pravastatin. The in vivo relevance of this in vitro finding has not been established for telithromycin.

Fluvastatin is essentially metabolized via CYP2C9 and transporter inhibition was shown not to significantly increase fluvastatin exposure in patients. Consequently, no drug-drug interaction is expected when telithromycin is co-administered with fluvastatin.

Rosuvastatin is mainly excreted unchanged (only 10% is metabolized by CYP2C9). Although it is known to be a substrate of OATP1B1 *in vitro*, alternate transporting proteins are thought to be involved. Given the current available information, the relevance of these findings for drug-drug interaction with telithromycin has not been established.

High levels of HMG-CoA reductase inhibitors increase the risk of myopathy. Use of simvastatin, lovastatin, or atorvastatin concomitantly with KETEK should be avoided. If KETEK is prescribed, therapy with simvastatin, lovastatin, or atorvastatin should be suspended during the course of treatment. Patients concomitantly treated with statins should be carefully monitored for signs and symptoms of myopathy and rhabdomyolysis.

Monitoring of digoxin side effects or serum levels should be considered during concomitant administration of digoxin and KETEK. (See **CLINICAL PHARMACOLOGY, Drug-drug interactions.**)

Patients should be monitored with concomitant administration of midazolam and dosage adjustment of midazolam should be considered if necessary. Precaution should be used with other benzodiazepines, which are metabolized by CYP 3A4 and undergo a high first-pass effect (e.g., triazolam). (See **CLINICAL PHARMACOLOGY, Drug-drug interactions.**)

Concomitant treatment of KETEK with rifampin, a CYP 3A4 inducer, should be avoided. Concomitant administration of other CYP 3A4 inducers such as phenytoin, carbamazepine, or phenobarbital is likely to result in subtherapeutic levels of telithromycin and loss of effect. (See **CLINICAL PHARMACOLOGY, Other drug interactions.**)

In patients treated with metoprolol for heart failure, the increased exposure to metoprolol, a CYP 2D6 substrate, may be of clinical importance. Therefore, co-administration of KETEK and metoprolol in patients with heart failure should be considered with caution. (See **CLINICAL PHARMACOLOGY, Drug-drug interactions.**)

Spontaneous post-marketing reports suggest that administration of KETEK and oral anticoagulants concomitantly may potentiate the effects of the oral anticoagulants. Consideration should be given to monitoring prothrombin times/INR while patients are receiving KETEK and oral anticoagulants simultaneously.

No specific drug interaction studies have been performed to evaluate the following potential drug-drug interactions with KETEK. However, these drug interactions have been observed with macrolide products.

Drugs metabolized by the cytochrome P450 system such as carbamazepine, cyclosporine, tacrolimus, sirolimus, hexobarbital, and phenytoin: elevation of serum levels of these drugs may be observed when co-administered with telithromycin. As a result, increases or prolongation of the therapeutic and/or adverse effects of the concomitant drug may be observed.

Ergot alkaloid derivatives (such as ergotamine or dihydroergotamine): acute ergot toxicity characterized by severe peripheral vasospasm and dysesthesia has been reported when macrolide antibiotics were co-administered. Without further data, the co-administration of KETEK and these drugs is not recommended.

Laboratory test interactions

There are no reported laboratory test interactions.

Carcinogenesis, mutagenesis, impairment of fertility

Long-term studies in animals to determine the carcinogenic potential of KETEK have not been conducted.

Telithromycin showed no evidence of genotoxicity in four tests: gene mutation in bacterial cells, gene mutation in mammalian cells, chromosome aberration in human lymphocytes, and the micronucleus test in the mouse.

No evidence of impaired fertility in the rat was observed at doses estimated to be 0.61 times the human daily dose on a mg/m^2 basis. At doses of 1.8–3.6 times the human daily dose, at which signs of parental toxicity were observed, moderate reductions in fertility indices were noted in male and female animals treated with telithromycin.

Pregnancy

Teratogenic effects

Pregnancy Category C

Telithromycin was not teratogenic in the rat or rabbit. Reproduction studies have been performed in rats and rabbits, with effect on pre-post natal development studied in the rat. At doses estimated to be 1.8 times (900 mg/m^2) and 0.49 times (240 mg/m^2) the daily human dose of 800 mg (492 mg/m^2) in the rat and rabbit, respectively, no evidence of fetal terata was found. At doses higher than the 900 mg/m^2 and 240 mg/m^2 in rats and rabbits, respectively, maternal toxicity may have resulted in delayed fetal maturation. No adverse effects on prenatal and postnatal development of rat pups were observed at 1.5 times (750 mg/m^2/d) the daily human dose.

There are no adequate and well-controlled studies in pregnant women. Telithromycin should be used during pregnancy only if the potential benefit justifies the potential risk to the fetus.

Nursing mothers

Telithromycin is excreted in breast milk of rats. Telithromycin may also be excreted in human milk. Because many drugs are excreted in human milk, caution should be exercised when KETEK is administered to a nursing mother.

Pediatric use

The safety and effectiveness of KETEK in pediatric patients has not been established.

Geriatric use

In all Phase III clinical trials (n=4,780), KETEK was administered to 694 patients who were 65 years and older, including 231 patients who were 75 years and older. Efficacy and safety in elderly patients ≥ 65 years were generally similar to that observed in younger patients; however, greater sensitivity of some older individuals cannot be ruled out. No dosage adjustment is required based on age alone. (See **CLINICAL PHARMACOLOGY, Special populations, Geriatric** and **DOSAGE AND ADMINISTRATION.**)

ADVERSE REACTIONS

In Phase III clinical trials, 4,780 patients (n=2702 in controlled trials) received daily oral doses of KETEK 800 mg once daily for 5 days or 7 to 10 days. Most adverse events were mild to moderate in severity. In the combined Phase III studies, discontinuation due to treatment-emergent adverse events occurred in 4.4% of KETEK-treated patients and 4.3% of combined comparator-treated patients. Most discontinuations in the KETEK group were due to treatment-emergent adverse events in the gastrointestinal body system, primarily diarrhea (0.9% for KETEK vs. 0.7% for comparators), nausea (0.7% for KETEK vs. 0.5% for comparators).

All and possibly related treatment-emergent adverse events (TEAEs) occurring in controlled clinical studies in ≥ 2.0% of all patients are included below:

[See table 5 at left]

Table 5

All and Possibly Related Treatment-Emergent Adverse Events Reported in Controlled Phase III Clinical Studies (Percent Incidence)

Adverse Event*	All TEAEs		Possibly-Related TEAEs	
	KETEK n= 2702	Comparator† n= 2139	KETEK n= 2702	Comparator† n= 2139
Diarrhea	10.8%	8.6%	10.0%	8.0%
Nausea	7.9%	4.6%	7.0%	4.1%
Headache	5.5%	5.8%	2.0%	2.5%
Dizziness (excl. vertigo)	3.7%	2.7%	2.8%	1.5%
Vomiting	2.9%	2.2%	2.4%	1.4%
Loose Stools	2.3%	1.5%	2.1%	1.4%
Dysgeusia	1.6%	3.6%	1.5%	3.6%

* Based on a frequency of all and possibly related treatment-emergent adverse events of ≥ 2% in KETEK or comparator groups.

† Includes comparators from all controlled Phase III studies.

The following events judged by investigators to be at least possibly drug related were observed infrequently (≥ 0.2% and < 2%), in KETEK-treated patients in the controlled Phase III studies.

Gastrointestinal system: abdominal distension, dyspepsia, gastrointestinal upset, flatulence, constipation, gastroenteritis, gastritis, anorexia, oral candidiasis, glossitis, stomatitis, watery stools.

Liver and biliary system: abnormal liver function tests: increased transaminases, increased liver enzymes (e.g., ALT, AST) were usually asymptomatic and reversible. ALT elevations above 3 times the upper limit of normal were observed in 1.6%, and 1.7% of patients treated with KETEK and comparators, respectively. Hepatitis, with or without jaundice, occurred in 0.07% of patients treated with KETEK, and was reversible. (See **PRECAUTIONS, General**.)

Nervous system: dry mouth, somnolence, insomnia, vertigo, increased sweating

Body as a whole: abdominal pain, upper abdominal pain, fatigue

Special senses: Visual adverse events most often included blurred vision, diplopia, or difficulty focusing. Most events were mild to moderate; however, severe cases have been reported. Some patients discontinued therapy due to these adverse events. Visual adverse events were reported as having occurred after any dose during treatment, but most visual adverse events (65%) occurred following the first or second dose. Visual events lasted several hours and recurred upon subsequent dosing in some patients. For patients who continued treatment, some resolved on therapy while others continued to have symptoms until they completed the full course of treatment. (See **WARNINGS** and **PRECAUTIONS, Information for patients**.)

Females and patients under 40 years old experienced a higher incidence of telithromycin-associated visual adverse events. (See **CLINICAL STUDIES**.)

Urogenital system: vaginal candidiasis, vaginitis, vaginosis fungal

Skin: rash

Hematologic: increased platelet count

Other possibly related clinically-relevant events occurring in <0.2% of patients treated with KETEK from the controlled Phase III studies included: anxiety, bradycardia, eczema, elevated blood bilirubin, erythema multiforme, flushing, hypotension, increased blood alkaline phosphatase, increased eosinophil count, paresthesia, pruritus, urticaria.

Post-Marketing Adverse Event Reports

In addition to adverse events reported from clinical trials, the following events have been reported from worldwide post-marketing experience with KETEK.

Allergic: face edema, rare reports of severe allergic reactions, including angioedema and anaphylaxis.

Cardiovascular: atrial arrhythmias, palpitations

Gastrointestinal system: pancreatitis

Liver and biliary system: Hepatic dysfunction has been reported.

Severe and in some cases fatal hepatotoxicity, including fulminant hepatitis, hepatic necrosis and hepatic failure have been reported in patients treated with KETEK. These hepatic reactions were observed during or immediately after treatment. In some of these cases, liver injury progressed rapidly and occurred after administration of only a few doses of KETEK. (See **CONTRAINDICATIONS** and **WARNINGS**.) Severe reactions, in some but not all cases, have been associated with serious underlying diseases or concomitant medications.

Data from post-marketing reports and clinical trials show that most cases of hepatic dysfunction were mild to moderate. (See **PRECAUTIONS, General**.)

Musculoskeletal: muscle cramps, rare reports of exacerbation of myasthenia gravis. (See **CONTRAINDICATIONS**.)

Nervous system: loss of consciousness, in some cases associated with vagal syndrome.

OVERDOSAGE

In the event of acute overdosage, the stomach should be emptied by gastric lavage. The patient should be carefully monitored (e.g., ECG, electrolytes) and given symptomatic and supportive treatment. Adequate hydration should be maintained. The effectiveness of hemodialysis in an overdose situation with KETEK is unknown.

DOSAGE AND ADMINISTRATION

The dose of KETEK tablets is 800 mg (2 tablets of 400 mg) taken orally once every 24 hours, for 7–10 days. KETEK tablets can be administered with or without food.

KETEK may be administered without dosage adjustment in the presence of hepatic impairment.

In the presence of severe renal impairment (CL_{CR} < 30 mL/min), including patients who need dialysis, the dose should be reduced to KETEK 600 mg once daily. In patients undergoing hemodialysis, KETEK should be given after the dialysis session on dialysis days. (See **CLINICAL PHARMACOLOGY, Renal insufficiency**.)

In the presence of severe renal impairment (CL_{CR} < 30 mL/min), with coexisting hepatic impairment, the dose should be reduced to KETEK 400 mg once daily. (See **CLINICAL PHARMACOLOGY, Multiple insufficiency**.)

HOW SUPPLIED

KETEK® 400 mg tablets are supplied as light-orange, oval, film-coated tablets, imprinted "H3647" on one side and "400" on the other side. These are packaged in bottles and blister cards (Ketek Pak™ and unit dose) as follows:

Bottles of 60   (NDC 0088-2225-41)

Ketek Pak™, 10-tablet cards (2 tablets per blister cavity)   (NDC 0088-2225-07)

Unit dose package of 100

(blister pack)   (NDC 0088-2225-49)

KETEK® 300 mg tablets are supplied as light-orange, oval, film-coated tablets, imprinted "38AV" on one side and blank on the other side. These are packaged in bottles as follows:

Bottles of 20   (NDC 0088-2223-20)

Store at 25°C (77°F); excursions permitted to 15–30°C (59–86°F) [see USP Controlled Room Temperature].

CLINICAL STUDIES
Community-acquired pneumonia (CAP)

KETEK was studied in four randomized, double-blind, controlled studies and four open-label studies for the treatment of community-acquired pneumonia. Patients with mild to moderate CAP who were considered appropriate for oral outpatient treatment were enrolled in these trials. Patients with severe pneumonia were excluded based on any one of the following: ICU admission, need for parenteral antibiotics, respiratory rate > 30/minute, hypotension, altered mental status, < 90% oxygen saturation by pulse oximetry, or white blood cell count < 4000/mm³. Total number of clinically evaluable patients in the telithromycin group included 2016 patients.

[See table 6 above]

Clinical cure rates by pathogen from the four CAP controlled clinical trials in microbiologically evaluable patients given KETEK for 7–10 days or a comparator are displayed in Table 7.

Table 7. CAP: Clinical cure rate by pathogen at post-therapy follow-up (17–24 days)

Pathogen	KETEK	Comparator
Streptococcus pneumoniae	73/78 (93.6%)	63/70 (90.0%)
Haemophilus influenzae	39/47 (83.0%)	42/44 (95.5%)
Moraxella catarrhalis	12/14 (85.7%)	7/9 (77.8%)
Chlamydophila (Chlamydia) pneumoniae	23/25 (92.0%)	18/19 (94.7%)
Mycoplasma pneumoniae	22/23 (95.7%)	20/22 (90.9%)

Clinical cure rates for patients with CAP due to *Streptococcus pneumoniae* were determined from patients in controlled and uncontrolled trials. Of 333 evaluable patients with CAP due to *Streptococcus pneumoniae*, 312 (93.7%) achieved clinical success. Only patients considered appropriate for oral outpatient therapy were included in these trials. More severely ill patients were not enrolled. Blood cultures were obtained in all patients participating in the clinical trials of mild to moderate community-acquired pneumonia. In a limited number of outpatients with incidental pneumococcal bacteremia treated with KETEK, a clinical cure rate of 88% (67/76) has been observed. KETEK is not indicated for the treatment of severe community-acquired pneumonia or suspected pneumococcal bacteremia.

Clinical cure rates for patients with CAP due to multi-drug resistant *Streptococcus pneumoniae* (MDRSP*) were determined from patients in controlled and uncontrolled trials. Of 36 evaluable patients with CAP due to MDRSP, 33 (91.7%) achieved clinical success.

*MDRSP: Multi-drug resistant *Streptococcus pneumoniae* includes isolates known as PRSP (penicillin-resistant *Strep-*

Table 6. CAP: Clinical cure rate at post-therapy follow-up (17–24 days)

Controlled Studies	Patients (n)		Clinical cure rate	
	KETEK	Comparator	KETEK	Comparator
KETEK vs. clarithromycin 500 mg BID for 10 days	162	156	88.3%	88.5%
KETEK vs. trovafloxacin* 200 mg QD for 7 to 10 days	80	86	90.0%	94.2%
KETEK vs. amoxicillin 1000 mg TID for 10 days	149	152	94.6%	90.1%
KETEK for 7 days vs. clarithromycin 500 mg BID for 10 days	161	146	88.8%	91.8%

*This study was stopped prematurely after trovafloxacin was restricted for use in hospitalized patients with severe infection.

tococcus pneumoniae), and are isolates resistant to two or more of the following antibiotics: penicillin, 2nd generation cephalosporins, e.g., cefuroxime, macrolides, tetracyclines and trimethoprim/sulfamethoxazole.

Table 8. Clinical cure rate for 36 evaluable patients with MDRSP treated with KETEK in studies of community-acquired pneumonia

Screening Susceptibility	Clinical Success in Evaluable MDRSP Patients	
	n/N*	%
Penicillin-resistant	20/23	86.9
2nd generation cephalosporin-resistant	20/22	90.9
Macrolide-resistant	25/28	89.3
Trimethoprim/ sulfamethoxazole-resistant	24/27	88.9
Tetracycline-resistant†	11/13	84.6

* n = the number of patients successfully treated; N = the number with resistance to the listed drug of the 36 evaluable patients with CAP due to MDRSP.
† Includes isolates tested for resistance to either tetracycline or doxycycline.

Visual Adverse Events

Table 9 provides the incidence of all treatment-emergent visual adverse events in controlled Phase III studies by age and gender. The group with the highest incidence was females under the age of 40, while males over the age of 40 had rates of visual adverse events similar to comparator-treated patients.

Table 9. Incidence of All Treatment-Emergent Visual Adverse Events in Controlled Phase III Studies

Gender/Age	Telithromycin	Comparators*
Female ≤ 40	2.1% (14/682)	0.0% (0/534)
Female > 40	1.0% (7/703)	0.35% (2/574)
Male ≤ 40	1.2% (7/563)	0.48% (2/417)
Male > 40	0.27% (2/754)	0.33% (2/614)
Total	1.1% (30/2702)	0.28% (6/2139)

*Includes all comparators combined

ANIMAL PHARMACOLOGY

Repeated dose toxicity studies of 1, 3, and 6 months' duration with telithromycin conducted in rat, dog and monkey showed that the liver was the principal target for toxicity with elevations of liver enzymes and histological evidence of damage. There was evidence of reversibility after cessation of treatment. Plasma exposures based on free fraction of drug at the no observed adverse effect levels ranged from 1 to 10 times the expected clinical exposure.

Phospholipidosis (intracellular phospholipid accumulation) affecting a number of organs and tissues (e.g., liver, kidney, lung, thymus, spleen, gall bladder, mesenteric lymph nodes, GI-tract) has been observed with the administration of telithromycin in rats at repeated doses of 900 mg/m²/day (1.8× the human dose) or more for 1 month, and 300 mg/m²/day (0.61× the human dose) or more for 3–6 months. Similarly, phospholipidosis has been observed in dogs with telithromycin at repeated doses of 3000 mg/m²/day (6.1× the human dose) or more for 1 month and

1000 mg/m²/day (2.0× the human dose) or more for 3 months. The significance of these findings for humans is unknown.

Pharmacology/toxicology studies showed an effect both in prolonging QTc interval in dogs *in vivo* and *in vitro* action potential duration (APD) in rabbit Purkinje fibers. These effects were observed at concentrations of free drug at least 8.8 (in dogs) times those circulating in clinical use. *In vitro* electrophysiological studies (hERG assays) suggested an inhibition of the rapid activating component of the delayed rectifier potassium current (I_{Kr}) as an underlying mechanism.

Rev. February 2010
sanofi-aventis U.S. LLC
Bridgewater, NJ 08807
© 2010 sanofi-aventis U.S. LLC

REFERENCES

1. National Committee for Clinical Laboratory Standards. Methods for Dilution Antimicrobial Susceptibility Tests for Bacteria That Grow Aerobically – Sixth Edition; Approved Standard, NCCLS Document M7-A6, Vol. 23, No. 2, NCCLS, Wayne, PA, January, 2003.
2. National Committee for Clinical Laboratory Standards. Performance Standards for Antimicrobial Disk Susceptibility Tests - Eighth Edition; Approved Standard, NCCLS Document M2-A8, Vol. 23, No. 1, NCCLS, Wayne, PA, January, 2003.
3. National Committee for Clinical Laboratory Standards. Performance Standards for Antimicrobial Susceptibility Testing: Twelfth Informational Supplement; Approved Standard, NCCLS Document M2-A8 and M7-A6, Vol. 23, No. 1, NCCLS, Wayne, PA, January, 2004.

MEDICATION GUIDE

KETEK® (*KEE tek*) Tablets
(telithromycin)

Read the Medication Guide that comes with KETEK before you start taking it. Talk to your doctor if you have any questions about KETEK. This Medication Guide does not take the place of talking with your doctor about your medical condition or treatment.

What is the most important information I should know about KETEK?
* **1. Do not take KETEK if you have Myasthenia Gravis (a rare disease which causes muscle weakness). Worsening of myasthenia gravis symptoms including life-threatening breathing problems have happened in patients with myasthenia gravis after taking KETEK in some cases leading to death.**

KETEK can cause other serious side effects, including:
* **2. Severe liver damage (hepatoxicity).** Severe liver damage, in some cases leading to a liver transplant or death has happened in patients treated with KETEK. Severe liver damage has happened during treatment, even after a few doses, or right after treatment with KETEK has ended.

Stop KETEK and call your doctor right away if you have signs of liver problems. Do not take another dose of KETEK unless your doctor tells you to do so.

Signs of liver problems include:

• increased tiredness	• light-colored stools
• loss of appetite	• dark urine
• yellowing of the skin and/or eyes	• itchy skin
• right upper belly pain	

Do not take KETEK if you have ever had side effects of the liver while taking KETEK or macrolide antibiotics. Macrolide antibiotics include erythromycin, azithromycin (Zithromax®), clarithromycin (Biaxin®) or dirithromycin (Dynabac®).
* **3. Vision problems.** KETEK may cause blurred vision, trouble focusing, and double vision. You may notice vision problems if you look quickly from near objects to far objects.
* **4. Fainting.** You may faint especially if you are also having nausea, vomiting, and lightheadedness.

Be aware that vision problems and fainting while taking KETEK may affect your ability to drive or do dangerous activities. Limit driving and other dangerous activities.

If you have vision problems or faint while taking KETEK do not drive, operate heavy machines, or do dangerous activities.

Call your doctor before taking another dose of KETEK if you have vision problems or faint.

See "What are the possible side effects of KETEK?" for other side effects of KETEK.

What is KETEK?
KETEK is an antibiotic. KETEK is used to treat adults 18 years of age and older with a lung infection called "community acquired pneumonia" that is caused by certain bacteria germs.
* KETEK is not for other types of infections caused by bacteria
* KETEK, like other antibiotics, does not kill viruses.

Who should not take KETEK?
Do not take KETEK if you:
* have myasthenia gravis
* have had side effects on the liver while taking KETEK or macrolide antibiotics.
* have ever had an allergic reaction to KETEK or macrolide antibiotics.
* take cisapride (Propulsid®) or pimozide (Orap®).

KETEK may not be right for you. Before taking KETEK, tell your doctor about all of your medical conditions, including if you:
* have myasthenia gravis
* have liver problems
* have (or have a family history of) a heart problem called "QTc prolongation"
* have other heart problems
* are pregnant or breastfeeding
Tell your doctor about all of the medicines you take, including prescription and nonprescription medicines, vitamins, and herbal supplements. KETEK and other medicines may affect or interact with each other, sometimes causing serious side effects.

You should not take the following cholesterol lowering medicines while taking KETEK:
* simvastatin (Zocor®, Vytorin®)
* lovastatin (Mevacor®)
* atorvastatin (Lipitor®)
Know the medicines you take. Keep a list of your medicines with you to show your doctor or pharmacist.

Do not take other medicines with KETEK without first checking with your doctor. Your doctor will tell you if you can take other medicines with KETEK.

How should I take KETEK?
* Take KETEK exactly as your doctor tells you. Skipping doses or not taking all of an antibiotic may:
  * make the treatment not work as well
  * increase the chance that the bacteria will develop resistance to the antibiotic
* The usual dose is two 400 mg KETEK Tablets taken at the same time once a day for 7 to 10 days. If you have kidney disease, your doctor may prescribe a lower dose for you.
* Take KETEK with or without food.
* Swallow KETEK tablets whole.
* Call your doctor if you took too much KETEK.

What are the possible side effects of KETEK?
See "What is the most important information I should know about KETEK?" for worsening of myasthenia gravis symptoms, and serious liver, vision, and fainting side effects.

Other serious side effects include:
* **Pseudomembranous colitis** (an intestine infection). Pseudomembranous colitis can happen with most antibiotics, including KETEK. Call your doctor if you get watery diarrhea, diarrhea that does not go away, or bloody stools. You may also have stomach cramps and a fever. Pseudomembranous colitis can happen up to 2 months after you have finished your antibiotic.

The most common side effects of KETEK are nausea, headache, dizziness, vomiting, and diarrhea.

These are not all of the side effects of KETEK. Ask your doctor or pharmacist for more information.

Call your doctor for medical advice about side effects. You may report side effects to FDA at 1-800-FDA-1088.
You may also report side effects to sanofi-aventis U.S. at 1-800-633-1610.

How should I store KETEK?
* Store KETEK tablets at room temperature, 59° to 86°F (15° to 30°C).
* **Keep KETEK and all medicines out of the reach of children.**

General Information about KETEK
* Medicines are sometimes prescribed for purposes other than those listed in a Medication Guide.
* Do not use KETEK for a condition for which it was not prescribed.
* Do not share KETEK with other people, even if they have the same symptoms that you have. It may harm them.
This Medication Guide summarizes the most important information about KETEK. If you would like more informa-

tion, talk with your doctor. You can ask your doctor or pharmacist for information about KETEK that was written for healthcare professional. This information is also available on the KETEK website at www.KETEK.com.

What are the ingredients in KETEK?
Active Ingredient: telithromycin
Inactive Ingredients: croscarmellose sodium, hypromellose, magnesium stearate, microcrystalline cellulose, polyethylene glycol, povidone, red ferric oxide, talc, titanium dioxide, and yellow ferric oxide
Medication Guide as of June 2009
This Medication Guide has been approved by the U.S. Food and Drug Administration.
sanofi-aventis U.S. LLC
Bridgewater, NJ 08807
BIAXIN® (clarithromycin) is a registered trademark of Abbott Laboratories.
ZITHROMAX® (azithromycin) is a registered trademark of Pfizer Inc.
DYNABAC® (dirithromycin) is a registered trademark of Eli Lilly and Company.
PROPULSID® (cisapride) is a registered trademark of Johnson & Johnson.
ORAP® (pimozide) is a registered trademark of Teva Pharmaceuticals USA, Inc.
LIPITOR® (atorvastatin) is a registered trademark of Pfizer Inc.
ZOCOR® (simvastatin) is a registered trademark of Merck & Co Inc.
VYTORIN® (simvastatin and ezetimibe) is a registered trademark of Merck/Schering Plough Pharmaceuticals.
MEVACOR® (lovastatin) is a registered trademark of Merck & Co Inc..

Shown in Product Identification Guide, page 319

LANTUS® ℞
[lăn' tus]
(insulin glargine [rDNA origin] injection)
solution for subcutaneous injection

HIGHLIGHTS OF PRESCRIBING INFORMATION
These highlights do not include all the information needed to use LANTUS safely and effectively. See full prescribing information for LANTUS.
LANTUS (insulin glargine [rDNA origin] injection) solution for subcutaneous injection
Initial U.S. Approval: 2000

————INDICATIONS AND USAGE————
LANTUS is a long-acting human insulin analog indicated to improve glycemic control in adults and children with type 1 diabetes mellitus and in adults with type 2 diabetes mellitus. (1)
Important Limitations of Use:
* Not recommended for treating diabetic ketoacidosis. Use intravenous, short-acting insulin instead.

————DOSAGE AND ADMINISTRATION————
* The starting dose should be individualized based on the type of diabetes and whether the patient is insulin-naïve (2.1, 2.2, 2.3)
* Administer subcutaneously once daily at any time of day, but at the same time every day. (2.1)
* Rotate injection sites within an injection area (abdomen, thigh, or deltoid) to reduce the risk of lipodystrophy. (2.1)
* Converting from other insulin therapies may require adjustment of timing and dose of LANTUS. Closely monitor glucoses especially upon converting to LANTUS and during the initial weeks thereafter. (2.3)

————DOSAGE FORMS AND STRENGTHS————
Solution for injection 100 units/mL (U-100) in
* 10 mL vials
* 3 mL cartridge system for use in OptiClik (Insulin Delivery Device)
* 3 mL SoloStar disposable insulin device (3)

————CONTRAINDICATIONS————
Do not use in patients with hypersensitivity to LANTUS or one of its excipients (4)

————WARNINGS AND PRECAUTIONS————
* Dose adjustment and monitoring: Monitor blood glucose in all patients treated with insulin. Insulin regimens should be modified cautiously and only under medical supervision (5.1)
* Administration: Do not dilute or mix with any other insulin or solution. Do not administer subcutaneously via an insulin pump or intravenously because severe hypoglycemia can occur (5.2)
* Do not share reusable or disposable insulin devices or needles between patients (5.2)
* Hypoglycemia: Most common adverse reaction of insulin therapy and may be life-threatening (5.3, 6.1)
* Allergic reactions: Severe, life-threatening, generalized allergy, including anaphylaxis, can occur (5.4, 6.1)
* Renal or hepatic impairment: May require a reduction in the LANTUS dose (5.5, 5.6)

---ADVERSE REACTIONS---

Adverse reactions commonly associated with Lantus are:
• Hypoglycemia, allergic reactions, injection site reaction, lipodystrophy, pruritus, and rash. (6.1)

To report SUSPECTED ADVERSE REACTIONS, contact sanofi-aventis at 1-800-633-1610 or FDA at 1-800-FDA-1088 or www.fda.gov/medwatch.

---DRUG INTERACTIONS---

• Certain drugs may affect glucose metabolism, requiring insulin dose adjustment and close monitoring of blood glucose. (7)
• The signs of hypoglycemia may be reduced or absent in patients taking anti-adrenergic drugs (e.g., beta-blockers, clonidine, guanethidine, and reserpine). (7)

---USE IN SPECIFIC POPULATIONS---

• Pregnancy category C: Use during pregnancy only if the potential benefit justifies the potential risk to the fetus (8.1)
• Pediatric: Has not been studied in children with type 2 diabetes. Has not been studied in children with type 1 diabetes <6 years of age (8.4)

See 17 for PATIENT COUNSELING INFORMATION and FDA-approved patient labeling

                                    Revised: 09/2009

FULL PRESCRIBING INFORMATION: CONTENTS*

FULL PRESCRIBING INFORMATION

1. INDICATIONS AND USAGE

LANTUS is indicated to improve glycemic control in adults and children with type 1 diabetes mellitus and in adults with type 2 diabetes mellitus.
Important Limitations of Use:
• LANTUS is not recommended for the treatment of diabetic ketoacidosis. Intravenous short-acting insulin is the preferred treatment for this condition.

2. DOSAGE AND ADMINISTRATION
2.1 Dosing

LANTUS is a recombinant human insulin analog for once daily subcutaneous administration with potency that is approximately the same as the potency of human insulin. LANTUS exhibits a relatively constant glucose-lowering profile over 24 hours that permits once-daily dosing. LANTUS may be administered at any time during the day. LANTUS should be administered subcutaneously once a day at the same time every day. The dose of LANTUS must be individualized based on clinical response. Blood glucose monitoring is essential in all patients receiving insulin therapy.

Patients adjusting the amount or timing of dosing with LANTUS, should only do so under medical supervision with appropriate glucose monitoring [see Warnings and Precautions (5.1).]
In patients with type 1 diabetes, LANTUS must be used in regimens with short-acting insulin.
The intended duration of activity of LANTUS is dependent on injection into subcutaneous tissue [see Clinical pharmacology (12.2)]. LANTUS should not be administered intravenously or via an insulin pump. Intravenous administration of the usual subcutaneous dose could result in severe hypoglycemia [see Warnings and Precautions (5.3)].
As with all insulins, injection sites should be rotated within the same region (abdomen, thigh, or deltoid) from one injection to the next to reduce the risk of lipodystrophy [See Adverse Reactions (6.1)].
In clinical studies, there was no clinically relevant difference in insulin glargine absorption after abdominal, deltoid, or thigh subcutaneous administration. As for all insulins, the rate of absorption, and consequently the onset and duration of action, may be affected by exercise and other variables, such as stress, intercurrent illness, or changes in co-administered drugs or meal patterns.

2.2 Initiation of LANTUS therapy

The recommended starting dose of LANTUS in patients with type 1 diabetes should be approximately one-third of the total daily insulin requirements. Short-acting, premeal insulin should be used to satisfy the remainder of the daily insulin requirements.
The recommended starting dose of LANTUS in patients with type 2 diabetes who are not currently treated with insulin is 10 units (or 0.2 Units/kg) once daily, which should subsequently be adjusted to the patient's needs.
The dose of LANTUS should be adjusted according to blood glucose measurements. The dosage of LANTUS should be individualized under the supervision of a healthcare provider in accordance with the needs of the patient.

2.3 Converting to LANTUS from other insulin therapies

If changing from a treatment regimen with an intermediate- or long-acting insulin to a regimen with LANTUS, the amount and timing of shorter-acting insulins and doses of any oral anti-diabetic drugs may need to be adjusted.
• If transferring patients from once-daily NPH insulin to once-daily LANTUS, the recommended initial LANTUS dose is the same as the dose of NPH that is being discontinued.
• If transferring patients from twice-daily NPH insulin to once-daily LANTUS, the recommended initial LANTUS dose is 80% of the total NPH dose that is being discontinued. This dose reduction will lower the likelihood of hypoglycemia [see Warnings and Precautions (5.3)].

3. DOSAGE FORMS AND STRENGTHS

LANTUS solution for injection 100 Units per mL is available as:
• -10 mL Vial (1000 Units/10 mL)
• -3 mL Cartridge systems for use only in OptiClik® (300 Units/3 mL)
• -3 mL SoloStar® disposable insulin device (300 Units/3 mL)

4. CONTRAINDICATIONS

LANTUS is contraindicated in patients with hypersensitivity to LANTUS or one of its excipients.

5. WARNINGS AND PRECAUTIONS
5.1 Dosage adjustment and monitoring

Glucose monitoring is essential for all patients receiving insulin therapy. Changes to an insulin regimen should be made cautiously and only under medical supervision.
Changes in insulin strength, manufacturer, type, or method of administration may result in the need for a change in insulin dose or an adjustment in concomitant oral anti-diabetic treatment.
As with all insulin preparations, the time course of action for LANTUS may vary in different individuals or at different times in the same individual and is dependent on many conditions, including the local blood supply, local temperature, and physical activity.

5.2 Administration

Do not administer LANTUS intravenously or via an insulin pump. The intended duration of activity of LANTUS is dependent on injection into subcutaneous tissue
Intravenous administration of the usual subcutaneous dose could result in severe hypoglycemia [see Warnings and Precautions (5.3)].
Do not dilute or mix LANTUS with any other insulin or solution. If LANTUS is diluted or mixed, the solution may become cloudy, and the pharmacokinetic or pharmacodynamic profile (e.g., onset of action, time to peak effect) of LANTUS and the mixed insulin may be altered in an unpredictable manner. When LANTUS and regular human insulin were mixed immediately before injection in dogs, a delayed onset of action and a delayed time to maximum effect for regular

human insulin was observed. The total bioavailability of the mixture was also slightly decreased compared to separate injections of LANTUS and regular human insulin. The relevance of these observations in dogs to humans is unknown. Do not share disposable or reusable insulin devices or needles between patients, because doing so carries a risk for transmission of blood-borne pathogens.

5.3 Hypoglycemia

Hypoglycemia is the most common adverse reaction of insulin, including LANTUS. The risk of hypoglycemia increases with intensive glycemic control. Patients must be educated to recognize and manage hypoglycemia. Severe hypoglycemia can lead to unconsciousness or convulsions and may result in temporary or permanent impairment of brain function or death. Severe hypoglycemia requiring the assistance of another person or parenteral glucose infusion or glucagon administration has been observed in clinical trials with insulin, including trials with LANTUS.
The timing of hypoglycemia usually reflects the time-action profile of the administered insulin formulations. Other factors such as changes in food intake (e.g., amount of food or timing of meals), exercise, and concomitant medications may also alter the risk of hypoglycemia [See Drug Interactions (7)].
The prolonged effect of subcutaneous LANTUS may delay recovery from hypoglycemia. Patients being switched from twice daily NPH insulin to once-daily LANTUS should have their initial LANTUS dose reduced by 20% from the previous total daily NPH dose to reduce the risk of hypoglycemia [see Dosage and Administration (2.3)].
As with all insulins, use caution in patients with hypoglycemia unawareness and in patients who may be predisposed to hypoglycemia (e.g., the pediatric population and patients who fast or have erratic food intake). The patient's ability to concentrate and react may be impaired as a result of hypoglycemia. This may present a risk in situations where these abilities are especially important, such as driving or operating other machinery.
Early warning symptoms of hypoglycemia may be different or less pronounced under certain conditions, such as long-standing diabetes, diabetic neuropathy, use of medications such as beta-blockers, or intensified glycemic control. These situations may result in severe hypoglycemia (and, possibly, loss of consciousness) prior to the patient's awareness of hypoglycemia.

5.4 Hypersensitivity and allergic reactions

Severe, life-threatening, generalized allergy, including anaphylaxis, can occur with insulin products, including LANTUS.

5.5 Renal impairment

Due to its long duration of action, Lantus is not recommended during periods of rapidly declining renal function because of the risk for prolonged hypoglycemia.
Although studies have not been performed in patients with diabetes and renal impairment, a reduction in the LANTUS dose may be required in patients with renal impairment because of reduced insulin metabolism, similar to observations found with other insulins. [See Clinical Pharmacology (12.3)].

5.6 Hepatic impairment

Due to its long duration of action, Lantus is not recommended during periods of rapidly declining hepatic function because of the risk for prolonged hypoglycemia.
Although studies have not been performed in patients with diabetes and hepatic impairment, a reduction in the LANTUS dose may be required in patients with hepatic impairment because of reduced capacity for gluconeogenesis and reduced insulin metabolism, similar to observations found with other insulins. [See Clinical Pharmacology (12.3)].

5.7 Drug interactions

Some medications may alter insulin requirements and subsequently increase the risk for hypoglycemia or hyperglycemia [See Drug Interactions (7)].

6. ADVERSE REACTIONS

The following adverse reactions are discussed elsewhere:
• Hypoglycemia [See Warnings and Precautions (5.3)]
• Hypersensitivity and allergic reactions [See Warnings and Precautions (5.4)]

6.1 Clinical trial experience

Because clinical trials are conducted under widely varying designs, the adverse reaction rates reported in one clinical trial may not be easily compared to those rates reported in another clinical trial, and may not reflect the rates actually observed in clinical practice.
The frequencies of treatment-emergent adverse events during LANTUS clinical trials in patients with type 1 diabetes mellitus and type 2 diabetes mellitus are listed in the tables below.

Table 1: Treatment–emergent adverse events in pooled clinical trials up to 28 weeks duration in adults with type 1 diabetes (adverse events with frequency ≥ 5%)

	LANTUS, % (n=1257)	NPH, % (n=1070)
Upper respiratory tract infection	22.4	23.1
Infection*	9.4	10.3
Accidental injury	5.7	6.4
Headache	5.5	4.7

*Body System not Specified

Table 2: Treatment–emergent adverse events in pooled clinical trials up to 1 year duration in adults with type 2 diabetes (adverse events with frequency ≥ 5%)

	LANTUS, % (n=849)	NPH, % (n=714)
Upper respiratory tract infection	11.4	13.3
Infection*	10.4	11.6
Retinal vascular disorder	5.8	7.4

*Body System not Specified

Table 3: Treatment–emergent adverse events in a 5-year trial of adults with type 2 diabetes (adverse events with frequency ≥ 10%)

	LANTUS, % (n=514)	NPH, % (n=503)
Upper respiratory tract infection	29.0	33.6
Edema peripheral	20.0	22.7
Hypertension	19.6	18.9
Influenza	18.7	19.5
Sinusitis	18.5	17.9
Cataract	18.1	15.9
Bronchitis	15.2	14.1
Arthralgia	14.2	16.1
Pain in extremity	13.0	13.1
Back pain	12.8	12.3
Cough	12.1	7.4
Urinary tract infection	10.7	10.1
Diarrhea	10.7	10.3
Depression	10.5	9.7
Headache	10.3	9.3

Table 4: Treatment–emergent adverse events in a 28-week clinical trial of children and adolescents with type 1 diabetes (adverse events with frequency ≥ 5%)

	LANTUS, % (n=174)	NPH, % (n=175)
Infection*	13.8	17.7
Upper respiratory tract infection	13.8	16.0
Pharyngitis	7.5	8.6
Rhinitis	5.2	5.1

*Body System not Specified

• *Severe Hypoglycemia*
Hypoglycemia is the most commonly observed adverse reaction in patients using insulin, including LANTUS *[See Warnings and Precautions (5.3)]*. Tables 5 and 6 summarize

Table 5: Severe Symptomatic Hypoglycemia in Patients with Type 1 Diabetes

	Study A Type 1 Diabetes Adults 28 weeks In combination with regular insulin		Study B Type 1 Diabetes Adults 28 weeks In combination with regular insulin		Study C Type 1 Diabetes Adults 16 weeks In combination with insulin lispro		Study D Type 1 Diabetes Pediatrics 26 weeks In combination with regular insulin	
	LANTUS	NPH	LANTUS	NPH	LANTUS	NPH	LANTUS	NPH
Percent of patients (n/total N)	10.6 (31/292)	15.0 (44/293)	8.7 (23/264)	10.4 (28/270)	6.5 (20/310)	5.2 (16/309)	23.0 (40/174)	28.6 (50/175)

Table 6: Severe Symptomatic Hypoglycemia in Patients with Type 2 Diabetes

	Study E Type 2 Diabetes Adults 52 weeks In combination with oral agents		Study F Type 2 Diabetes Adults 28 weeks In combination with regular insulin		Study G Type 2 Diabetes Adults 5 years In combination with regular insulin	
	LANTUS	NPH	LANTUS	NPH	LANTUS	NPH
Percent of patients (n/total N)	1.7 (5/289)	1.1 (3/281)	0.4 (1/259)	2.3 (6/259)	7.8 (40/513)	11.9 (60/504)

Table 7. Number (%) of patients with 3 or more step progression on ETDRS scale at endpoint

	Lantus (%)	NPH (%)	Difference*,† (SE)	95% CI for difference
Per-protocol	53/374 (14.2%)	57/363 (15.7%)	-2.0% (2.6%)	-7.0% to +3.1%
Intent-to-Treat	63/502 (12.5%)	71/487 (14.6%)	-2.1% (2.1%)	-6.3% to +2.1%

* Difference = Lantus − NPH
† using a generalized linear model (SAS GENMOD) with treatment and baseline HbA1c strata (cutoff 9.0%) as the classified independent variables, and with binomial distribution and identity link function

the incidence of severe hypoglycemia in the LANTUS individual clinical trials. Severe symptomatic hypoglycemia was defined as an event with symptoms consistent with hypoglycemia requiring the assistance of another person and associated with either a blood glucose below 50 mg/dL (≤56 mg/dL in the 5-year trial) or prompt recovery after oral carbohydrate, intravenous glucose or glucagon administration.
The rates of severe symptomatic hypoglycemia in the LANTUS clinical trials (see Section 14 for a description of the study designs) were comparable for all treatment regimens (see Tables 5 and 6). In the pediatric phase 3 clinical trial, children and adolescents with type 1 diabetes had a higher incidence of severe symptomatic hypoglycemia in the two treatment groups compared to the adult trials with type 1 diabetes. (see Table 5) *[See Clinical Studies (14)]*.
[See table 5 above]
[See table 6 above]
• *Retinopathy*
Retinopathy was evaluated in the LANTUS clinical studies by analysis of reported retinal adverse events and fundus photography. The numbers of retinal adverse events reported for LANTUS and NPH insulin treatment groups were similar for patients with type 1 and type 2 diabetes. LANTUS was compared to NPH insulin in a 5-year randomized clinical trial that evaluated the progression of retinopathy as assessed with fundus photography using a grading protocol derived from the Early Treatment Diabetic Retinopathy Scale (ETDRS). Patients had type 2 diabetes (mean age 55 yrs) with no (86%) or mild (14%) retinopathy at baseline. Mean baseline HbA1c was 8.4%. The primary outcome was progression by 3 or more steps on the ETDRS scale at study endpoint. Patients with pre-specified post-baseline eye procedures (pan-retinal photocoagulation for proliferative or severe nonproliferative diabetic retinopathy, local photocoagulation for new vessels, and vitrectomy for diabetic retinopathy) were also considered as 3-step progressors regardless of actual change in ETDRS score from baseline. Retinopathy graders were blinded to treatment group assignment. The results for the primary endpoint are shown in Table 7 for both the per-protocol and Intent-to-Treat populations, and indicate similarity of Lantus to NPH in the progression of diabetic retinopathy as assessed by this outcome.
[See table 7 above]
• *Insulin initiation and intensification of glucose control*
Intensification or rapid improvement in glucose control has been associated with a transitory, reversible ophthalmologic refraction disorder, worsening of diabetic retinopathy, and acute painful peripheral neuropathy. However, long-term glycemic control decreases the risk of diabetic retinopathy and neuropathy.
• *Lipodystrophy*
Long-term use of insulin, including LANTUS, can cause lipodystrophy at the site of repeated insulin injections. Lipodystrophy includes lipohypertrophy (thickening of adipose tissue) and lipoatrophy (thinning of adipose tissue), and may affect insulin absorption. Rotate insulin injection or infusion sites within the same region to reduce the risk of lipodystrophy. *[See Dosage and Administration (2.1)]*.
• *Weight gain*
Weight gain can occur with insulin therapy, including LANTUS, and has been attributed to the anabolic effects of insulin and the decrease in glucosuria.
• *Peripheral Edema*
Insulin, including LANTUS, may cause sodium retention and edema, particularly if previously poor metabolic control is improved by intensified insulin therapy.
• *Allergic Reactions*
Local Allergy
As with any insulin therapy, patients taking LANTUS may experience injection site reactions, including redness, pain, itching, urticaria, edema, and inflammation. In clinical studies in adult patients, there was a higher incidence of treatment-emergent injection site pain in LANTUS-treated patients (2.7%) compared to NPH insulin-treated patients (0.7%). The reports of pain at the injection site did not result in discontinuation of therapy.
Rotation of the injection site within a given area from one injection to the next may help to reduce or prevent these reactions. In some instances, these reactions may be related to factors other than insulin, such as irritants in a skin cleansing agent or poor injection technique. Most minor reactions to insulin usually resolve in a few days to a few weeks.
Systemic Allergy
Severe, life-threatening, generalized allergy, including anaphylaxis, generalized skin reactions, angioedema, bronchospasm, hypotension, and shock may occur with any insulin, including LANTUS and may be life threatening.
• *Antibody production*
All insulin products can elicit the formation of insulin antibodies. The presence of such insulin antibodies may increase or decrease the efficacy of insulin and may require adjustment of the insulin dose. In phase 3 clinical trials of LANTUS, increases in titers of antibodies to insulin were observed in NPH insulin and insulin glargine treatment groups with similar incidences.
6.2   Postmarketing experience
The following adverse reactions have been identified during post-approval use of LANTUS.

Because these reactions are reported voluntarily from a population of uncertain size, it is not always possible to estimate reliably their frequency or establish a causal relationship to drug exposure.

Medication errors have been reported in which other insulins, particularly short-acting insulins, have been accidentally administered instead of LANTUS *[See Patient Counseling Information (17)]*. To avoid medication errors between LANTUS and other insulins, patients should be instructed to always verify the insulin label before each injection.

7. DRUG INTERACTIONS

A number of drugs affect glucose metabolism and may require insulin dose adjustment and particularly close monitoring.

The following are examples of drugs that may increase the blood-glucose-lowering effect of insulins including LANTUS and, therefore, increase the susceptibility to hypoglycemia: oral anti-diabetic products, pramlintide, angiotensin converting enzyme (ACE) inhibitors, disopyramide, fibrates, fluoxetine, monoamine oxidase inhibitors, propoxyphene, pentoxifylline, salicylates, somatostatin analogs, and sulfonamide antibiotics.

The following are examples of drugs that may reduce the blood-glucose-lowering effect of insulins including LANTUS: corticosteroids, niacin, danazol, diuretics, sympathomimetic agents (e.g., epinephrine, albuterol, terbutaline), glucagon, isoniazid, phenothiazine derivatives, somatropin, thyroid hormones, estrogens, progestogens (e.g., in oral contraceptives), protease inhibitors and atypical antipsychotic medications (e.g. olanzapine and clozapine).

Beta-blockers, clonidine, lithium salts, and alcohol may either potentiate or weaken the blood-glucose-lowering effect of insulin. Pentamidine may cause hypoglycemia, which may sometimes be followed by hyperglycemia.

The signs of hypoglycemia may be reduced or absent in patients taking sympatholytic drugs such as beta-blockers, clonidine, guanethidine, and reserpine.

8. USE IN SPECIFIC POPULATIONS

8.1 Pregnancy

Pregnancy Category C: Subcutaneous reproduction and teratology studies have been performed with insulin glargine and regular human insulin in rats and Himalayan rabbits. Insulin glargine was given to female rats before mating, during mating, and throughout pregnancy at doses up to 0.36 mg/kg/day, which is approximately 7 times the recommended human subcutaneous starting dose of 10 Units/day (0.008 mg/kg/day), based on mg/m^2. In rabbits, doses of 0.072 mg/kg/day, which is approximately 2 times the recommended human subcutaneous starting dose of 10 Units/day (0.008 mg/kg/day), based on mg/m^2, were administered during organogenesis. The effects of insulin glargine did not generally differ from those observed with regular human insulin in rats or rabbits. However, in rabbits, five fetuses from two litters of the high-dose group exhibited dilation of the cerebral ventricles. Fertility and early embryonic development appeared normal.

There are no well-controlled clinical studies of the use of LANTUS in pregnant women. Because animal reproduction studies are not always predictive of human response, this drug should be used during pregnancy only if the potential benefit justifies the potential risk to the fetus. It is essential for patients with diabetes or a history of gestational diabetes to maintain good metabolic control before conception and throughout pregnancy. Insulin requirements may decrease during the first trimester, generally increase during the second and third trimesters, and rapidly decline after delivery. Careful monitoring of glucose control is essential in these patients.

8.3 Nursing Mothers

It is unknown whether insulin glargine is excreted in human milk. Because many drugs, including human insulin, are excreted in human milk, caution should be exercised when LANTUS is administered to a nursing woman. Use of LANTUS is compatible with breastfeeding, but women with diabetes who are lactating may require adjustments of their insulin doses.

8.4 Pediatric Use

The safety and effectiveness of subcutaneous injections of LANTUS have been established in pediatric patients (age 6 to 15 years) with type 1 diabetes *[see Clinical Studies (14)]*. LANTUS has not been studied in pediatric patients younger than 6 years of age with type 1 diabetes. LANTUS has not been studied in pediatric patients with type 2 diabetes.

Based on the results of a study in pediatric patients, the dose recommendation when switching to LANTUS is the same as that described for adults *[see Dosage and Administration (2.3)* and *Clinical Studies (14)]*. As in adults, the dosage of LANTUS must be individualized in pediatric patients based on metabolic needs and frequent monitoring of blood glucose.

8.5 Geriatric Use

In controlled clinical studies comparing LANTUS to NPH insulin, 593 of 3890 patients (15%) with type 1 and type 2 diabetes were ≥65 years of age and 80 (2%) patients were ≥75 years of age. The only difference in safety or effectiveness in the subpopulation of patients ≥65 years of age compared to the entire study population was a higher incidence of cardiovascular events typically seen in an older population in both LANTUS and NPH insulin-treated patients. Nevertheless, caution should be exercised when LANTUS is administered to geriatric patients. In elderly patients with diabetes, the initial dosing, dose increments, and maintenance dosage should be conservative to avoid hypoglycemic reactions. Hypoglycemia may be difficult to recognize in the elderly *[See Warnings and Precautions (5.3)]*.

10. OVERDOSAGE

An excess of insulin relative to food intake, energy expenditure, or both may lead to severe and sometimes prolonged and life-threatening hypoglycemia. Mild episodes of hypoglycemia can usually be treated with oral carbohydrates. Adjustments in drug dosage, meal patterns, or exercise may be needed.

More severe episodes of hypoglycemia with coma, seizure, or neurologic impairment may be treated with intramuscular/subcutaneous glucagon or concentrated intravenous glucose. After apparent clinical recovery from hypoglycemia, continued observation and additional carbohydrate intake may be necessary to avoid recurrence of hypoglycemia.

11. DESCRIPTION

LANTUS (insulin glargine [rDNA origin] injection) is a sterile solution of insulin glargine for use as a subcutaneous injection. Insulin glargine is a recombinant human insulin analog that is a long-acting (up to 24-hour duration of action), parenteral blood-glucose-lowering agent *[See Clinical Pharmacology (12)]*. LANTUS is produced by recombinant DNA technology utilizing a non-pathogenic laboratory strain of *Escherichia coli* (K12) as the production organism. Insulin glargine differs from human insulin in that the amino acid asparagine at position A21 is replaced by glycine and two arginines are added to the C-terminus of the B-chain. Chemically, insulin glargine is 21^A-Gly-30^{B}a-L-Arg-30^{B}b-L-Arg-human insulin and has the empirical formula $C_{267}H_{404}N_{72}O_{78}S_6$ and a molecular weight of 6063. Insulin glargine has the following structural formula:

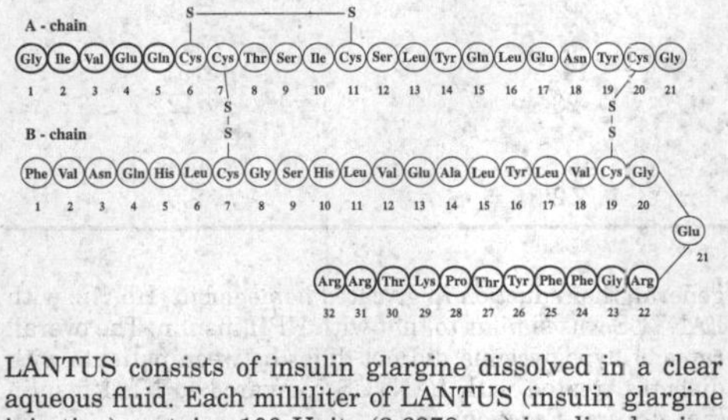

LANTUS consists of insulin glargine dissolved in a clear aqueous fluid. Each milliliter of LANTUS (insulin glargine injection) contains 100 Units (3.6378 mg) insulin glargine. The 10 mL vial presentation contains the following inactive ingredients per mL: 30 mcg zinc, 2.7 mg m-cresol, 20 mg glycerol 85%, 20 mcg polysorbate 20, and water for injection.

The 3 mL cartridge presentation contains the following inactive ingredients per mL: 30 mcg zinc, 2.7 mg m-cresol, 20 mg glycerol 85%, and water for injection.

The pH is adjusted by addition of aqueous solutions of hydrochloric acid and sodium hydroxide. LANTUS has a pH of approximately 4.

12. CLINICAL PHARMACOLOGY

12.1 Mechanism of Action

The primary activity of insulin, including insulin glargine, is regulation of glucose metabolism. Insulin and its analogs lower blood glucose by stimulating peripheral glucose uptake, especially by skeletal muscle and fat, and by inhibiting hepatic glucose production. Insulin inhibits lipolysis and proteolysis, and enhances protein synthesis.

12.2 Pharmacodynamics

Insulin glargine is a human insulin analog that has been designed to have low aqueous solubility at neutral pH. At pH 4, as in the LANTUS injection solution, insulin glargine is completely soluble. After injection into the subcutaneous tissue, the acidic solution is neutralized, leading to formation of microprecipitates from which small amounts of insulin glargine are slowly released, resulting in a relatively constant concentration/time profile over 24 hours with no pronounced peak. This profile allows once-daily dosing as a basal insulin.

In clinical studies, the glucose-lowering effect on a molar basis (i.e., when given at the same doses) of intravenous insulin glargine is approximately the same as that for human insulin. In euglycemic clamp studies in healthy subjects or in patients with type 1 diabetes, the onset of action of subcutaneous insulin glargine was slower than NPH insulin. The effect profile of insulin glargine was relatively constant with no pronounced peak and the duration of its effect was prolonged compared to NPH insulin. *Figure 1* shows results from a study in patients with type 1 diabetes conducted for a maximum of 24 hours after the injection. The median time between injection and the end of pharmacological effect was 14.5 hours (range: 9.5 to 19.3 hours) for NPH insulin, and 24 hours (range: 10.8 to >24.0 hours) (24 hours was the end of the observation period) for insulin glargine.

Figure 1. Activity Profile in Patients with Type 1 Diabetes

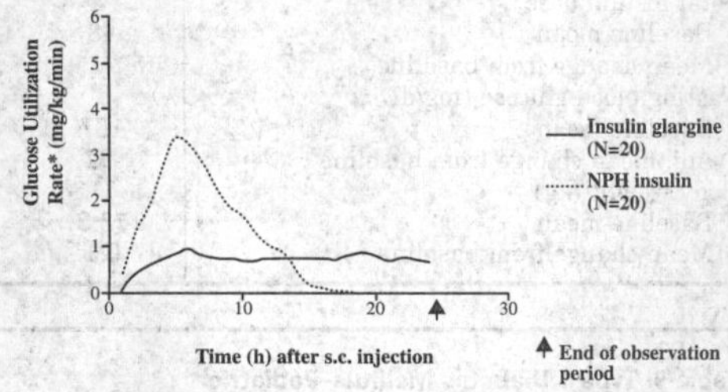

* Determined as amount of glucose infused to maintain constant plasma glucose levels (hourly mean values); indicative of insulin activity.

The longer duration of action (up to 24 hours) of LANTUS is directly related to its slower rate of absorption and supports once-daily subcutaneous administration. The time course of action of insulins, including LANTUS, may vary between individuals and within the same individual.

12.3 Pharmacokinetics

Absorption and Bioavailability. After subcutaneous injection of insulin glargine in healthy subjects and in patients with diabetes, the insulin serum concentrations indicated a slower, more prolonged absorption and a relatively constant concentration/time profile over 24 hours with no pronounced peak in comparison to NPH insulin. Serum insulin concentrations were thus consistent with the time profile of the pharmacodynamic activity of insulin glargine.

After subcutaneous injection of 0.3 Units/kg insulin glargine in patients with type 1 diabetes, a relatively constant concentration/time profile has been demonstrated. The duration of action after abdominal, deltoid, or thigh subcutaneous administration was similar.

Metabolism. A metabolism study in humans indicates that insulin glargine is partly metabolized at the carboxyl terminus of the B chain in the subcutaneous depot to form two active metabolites with in vitro activity similar to that of insulin, M1 (21^A-Gly-insulin) and M2 (21^A-Gly-des-30^B-Thr-insulin). Unchanged drug and these degradation products are also present in the circulation.

Special Populations

Age, Race, and Gender. Information on the effect of age, race, and gender on the pharmacokinetics of LANTUS is not available. However, in controlled clinical trials in adults (n=3890) and a controlled clinical trial in pediatric patients (n=349), subgroup analyses based on age, race, and gender did not show differences in safety and efficacy between insulin glargine and NPH insulin *[see Clinical Studies (14)]*.

Smoking. The effect of smoking on the pharmacokinetics/pharmacodynamics of LANTUS has not been studied.

Pregnancy. The effect of pregnancy on the pharmacokinetics and pharmacodynamics of LANTUS has not been studied *[see Use in Specific Populations (8.1)]*.

Obesity. In controlled clinical trials, which included patients with Body Mass Index (BMI) up to and including 49.6 kg/m^2, subgroup analyses based on BMI did not show differences in safety and efficacy between insulin glargine and NPH insulin *[see Clinical Studies (14)]*.

Renal Impairment. The effect of renal impairment on the pharmacokinetics of LANTUS has not been studied. However, some studies with human insulin have shown increased circulating levels of insulin in patients with renal failure. Careful glucose monitoring and dose adjustments of insulin, including LANTUS, may be necessary in patients with renal impairment *[See Warnings and Precautions (5.5)]*.

Hepatic Impairment. The effect of hepatic impairment on the pharmacokinetics of LANTUS has not been studied. However, some studies with human insulin have shown increased circulating levels of insulin in patients with liver failure. Careful glucose monitoring and dose adjustments of insulin, including LANTUS, may be necessary in patients with hepatic impairment *[See Warnings and Precautions (5.6)]*.

Table 8: Type 1 Diabetes Mellitus–Adult

Treatment duration Treatment in combination with	Study A 28 weeks Regular insulin		Study B 28 weeks Regular insulin		Study C 16 weeks Insulin lispro	
	LANTUS	NPH	LANTUS	NPH	LANTUS	NPH
Number of subjects treated	292	293	264	270	310	309
HbA1c						
Baseline HbA1c	8.0	8.0	7.7	7.7	7.6	7.7
Adj. mean change from baseline	+0.2	+0.1	-0.2	-0.2	-0.1	-0.1
LANTUS – NPH	+0.1		+0.1		0.0	
95% CI for Treatment difference	(0.0; +0.2)		(-0.1; +0.2)		(-0.1; +0.1)	
Basal insulin dose						
Baseline mean	21	23	29	29	28	28
Mean change from baseline	-2	0	-4	+2	-5	+1
Total insulin dose						
Baseline mean	48	52	50	51	50	50
Mean change from baseline	-1	0	0	+4	-3	0
Fasting blood glucose (mg/dL)						
Baseline mean	167	166	166	175	175	173
Adj. mean change from baseline	-21	-16	-20	-17	-29	-12
Body weight (kg)						
Baseline mean	73.2	74.8	75.5	75.0	74.8	75.6
Mean change from baseline	0.1	-00	0.7	1.0	0.1	0.5

Table 9: Type 1 Diabetes Mellitus–Pediatric

Treatment duration Treatment in combination with	Study D 28 weeks Regular insulin	
	LANTUS	NPH
Number of subjects treated	174	175
HbA1c		
Baseline mean	8.5	8.8
Adj. mean change from baseline	+0.3	+0.3
LANTUS – NPH	0.0	
95% CI for Treatment difference	(-0.2; +0.3)	
Basal insulin dose		
Baseline mean	19	19
Mean change from baseline	-1	+2
Total insulin dose		
Baseline mean	43	43
Mean change from baseline	+2	+3
Fasting blood glucose (mg/dL)		
Baseline mean	194	191
Adj. mean change from baseline	-23	-12
Body weight (kg)		
Baseline mean	45.5	44.6
Mean change from baseline	2.2	2.5

13. NONCLINICAL TOXICOLOGY

13.1 Carcinogenesis, Mutagenesis, Impairment of Fertility

In mice and rats, standard two-year carcinogenicity studies with insulin glargine were performed at doses up to 0.455 mg/kg, which was for the rat approximately 10 times and for the mouse approximately 5 times the recommended human subcutaneous starting dose of 10 Units/day (0.008 mg/kg/day), based on mg/m². The findings in female mice were not conclusive due to excessive mortality in all dose groups during the study. Histiocytomas were found at injection sites in male rats (statistically significant) and male mice (not statistically significant) in acid vehicle containing groups. These tumors were not found in female animals, in saline control, or insulin comparator groups using a different vehicle. The relevance of these findings to humans is unknown.

Insulin glargine was not mutagenic in tests for detection of gene mutations in bacteria and mammalian cells (Ames- and HGPRT-test) and in tests for detection of chromosomal aberrations (cytogenetics in vitro in V79 cells and in vivo in Chinese hamsters).

In a combined fertility and prenatal and postnatal study in male and female rats at subcutaneous doses up to 0.36 mg/kg/day, which was approximately 7 times the recommended human subcutaneous starting dose of 10 Units/day (0.008 mg/kg/day), based on mg/m², maternal toxicity due to dose-dependent hypoglycemia, including some deaths, was observed. Consequently, a reduction of the rearing rate occurred in the high-dose group only. Similar effects were observed with NPH insulin.

14. CLINICAL STUDIES

The safety and effectiveness of LANTUS given once-daily at bedtime was compared to that of once-daily and twice-daily NPH insulin in open-label, randomized, active-controlled, parallel studies of 2,327 adult patients and 349 pediatric patients with type 1 diabetes mellitus and 1,563 adult patients with type 2 diabetes mellitus (see Tables 8–11). In general, the reduction in glycated hemoglobin (HbA1c) with LANTUS was similar to that with NPH insulin. The overall rates of hypoglycemia did not differ between patients with diabetes treated with LANTUS compared to NPH insulin *[See Adverse Reactions (6.1)]*.

Type 1 Diabetes–Adult (see Table 8).

In two clinical studies (Studies A and B), patients with type 1 diabetes (Study A; n=585, Study B; n=534) were randomized to 28 weeks of basal-bolus treatment with LANTUS or NPH insulin. Regular human insulin was administered before each meal. LANTUS was administered at bedtime. NPH insulin was administered once daily at bedtime or in the morning and at bedtime when used twice daily.

In another clinical study (Study C), patients with type 1 diabetes (n=619) were randomized to 16 weeks of basal-bolus treatment with LANTUS or NPH insulin. Insulin lispro was used before each meal. LANTUS was administered once daily at bedtime and NPH insulin was administered once or twice daily.

In these 3 studies, LANTUS and NPH insulin had similar effects on HbA1c (Table 8) with a similar overall rate of hypoglycemia *[See Adverse Reactions (6.1)]*.

[See table 8 above]

Type 1 Diabetes–Pediatric (see Table 9).

In a randomized, controlled clinical study (Study D), pediatric patients (age range 6 to 15 years) with type 1 diabetes (n=349) were treated for 28 weeks with a basal-bolus insulin regimen where regular human insulin was used before each meal. LANTUS was administered once daily at bedtime and NPH insulin was administered once or twice daily. Similar effects on HbA1c (Table 9) and the incidence of hypoglycemia were observed in both treatment groups *[See Adverse Reactions (6.1)]*.

[See table 9 above]

Type 2 Diabetes–Adult (see Table 10).

In a randomized, controlled clinical study (Study E) (n=570), LANTUS was evaluated for 52 weeks in combination with oral anti-diabetic medications (a sulfonylurea, metformin, acarbose, or combinations of these drugs). LANTUS administered once daily at bedtime was as effective as NPH insulin administered once daily at bedtime in reducing HbA1c and fasting glucose (Table 10). The rate of hypoglycemia was similar in LANTUS and NPH insulin treated patients *[See Adverse Reactions (6.1)]*.

In a randomized, controlled clinical study (Study F), in patients with type 2 diabetes not using oral anti-diabetic medications (n=518), a basal-bolus regimen of LANTUS once daily at bedtime or NPH insulin administered once or twice daily was evaluated for 28 weeks. Regular human insulin was used before meals, as needed. LANTUS had similar effectiveness as either once- or twice-daily NPH insulin in reducing HbA1c and fasting glucose (Table 10) with a similar incidence of hypoglycemia *[See Adverse Reactions (6.1)]*.

In a randomized, controlled clinical study (Study G), patients with type 2 diabetes were randomized to 5 years of treatment with once-daily LANTUS or twice-daily NPH insulin. For patients not previously treated with insulin, the starting dose of LANTUS or NPH insulin was 10 units daily. Patients who were already treated with NPH insulin either continued on the same total daily NPH insulin dose or started LANTUS at a dose that was 80% of the total previous NPH insulin dose. The primary endpoint for this study was a comparison of the progression of diabetic retinopathy by 3 or more steps on the Early Treatment Diabetic Retinopathy Study (ETDRS) scale. HbA1c change from baseline was a secondary endpoint. Similar glycemic control in the 2 treatment groups was desired in order to not confound the interpretation of the retinal data. Patients or study personnel used an algorithm to adjust the LANTUS and NPH insulin doses to a target fasting plasma glucose ≤100 mg/dL. After the LANTUS or NPH insulin dose was adjusted, other anti-diabetic agents, including pre-meal insulin were to be adjusted or added. The LANTUS group had a smaller mean reduction from baseline in HbA1c compared to the NPH insulin group, which may be explained by the lower daily basal insulin doses in the LANTUS group (Table 10). Both treatment groups had a similar incidence of reported symptomatic hypoglycemia. The incidences of severe symptomatic hypoglycemia are given in Table 6 *[See Adverse Reactions (6.1)]*.

[See table 10 at top of next page]

LANTUS Timing of Daily Dosing (see Table 11).

The safety and efficacy of LANTUS administered pre-breakfast, pre-dinner, or at bedtime were evaluated in a randomized, controlled clinical study in patients with type 1 diabetes (study H, n=378). Patients were also treated with insulin lispro at mealtime. LANTUS administered at different times of the day resulted in similar reductions in HbA1c compared to that with bedtime administration (see Table 11). In these patients, data are available from 8-point home glucose monitoring. The maximum mean blood glucose was observed just prior to injection of LANTUS regardless of time of administration.

In this study, 5% of patients in the LANTUS-breakfast arm discontinued treatment because of lack of efficacy. No patients in the other two arms discontinued for this reason. The safety and efficacy of LANTUS administered pre-breakfast or at bedtime were also evaluated in a randomized, active-controlled clinical study (Study I, n=697) in patients with type 2 diabetes not adequately controlled on oral anti-diabetic therapy. All patients in this study also received glimepiride 3 mg daily. LANTUS given before breakfast was at least as effective in lowering HbA1c as LANTUS given at bedtime or NPH insulin given at bedtime (see Table 11).

[See table 11 on next page]

16. HOW SUPPLIED/STORAGE AND HANDLING

16.1 How supplied

LANTUS solution for injection 100 units per mL (U-100) is available as:

[See third table on next page]

Needles are not included in the packs.

BD Ultra-Fine™ needles[1] to be used in conjunction with SoloStar and OptiClik are sold separately and are manufactured by BD.

[1]The brands listed are the registered trademarks of their respective owners and are not trademarks of sanofi-aventis U.S. LLC

16.2 Storage

LANTUS should not be stored in the freezer and should not be allowed to freeze. Discard LANTUS if it has been frozen. Unopened Vial/Cartridge system/SoloStar disposable insulin device:

Unopened LANTUS vials, cartridge systems and SoloStar device should be stored in a refrigerator, 36°F–46°F (2°C–8°C). Discard after the expiration date.

Open (In-Use) Vial:

Vials must be discarded 28 days after being opened. If refrigeration is not possible, the open vial can be kept unrefrigerated for up to 28 days away from direct heat and light, as long as the temperature is not greater than 86°F (30°C).

Open (In-Use) Cartridge system:
The opened (in-use) cartridge system in OptiClik should NOT be refrigerated but should be kept at room temperature (below 86°F [30°C]) away from direct heat and light. The opened (in-use) cartridge system in OptiClik must be discarded 28 days after being opened. Do not store OptiClik, with or without cartridge system, in a refrigerator at any time.

Open (In-Use) SoloStar disposable insulin device:
The opened (in-use) SoloStar should NOT be refrigerated but should be kept at room temperature (below 86°F [30°C]) away from direct heat and light. The opened (in-use) SoloStar device must be discarded 28 days after being opened.

These storage conditions are summarized in the following table:
[See table at top of next page]

16.3 Preparation and handling

Parenteral drug products should be inspected visually prior to administration whenever the solution and the container permit. LANTUS must only be used if the solution is clear and colorless with no particles visible.

Mixing and diluting: LANTUS must NOT be diluted or mixed with any other insulin or solution [See Warnings and Precautions (5.2)].

Vial: The syringes must not contain any other medicinal product or residue.

Cartridge system/SoloStar: If OptiClik, the Insulin Delivery Device used with the LANTUS cartridge system, or SoloStar disposable insulin device, malfunctions, LANTUS may be drawn from the cartridge system or from SoloStar into a U-100 syringe and injected.

17. PATIENT COUNSELING INFORMATION

17.1 Instructions for patients

Patients should be informed that changes to insulin regimens must be made cautiously and only under medical supervision.

Patients should be informed about the potential side effects of insulin therapy, including lipodystrophy (and the need to rotate injection sites within the same body region), weight gain, allergic reactions, and hypoglycemia. Patients should be informed that the ability to concentrate and react may be impaired as a result of hypoglycemia. This may present a risk in situations where these abilities are especially important, such as driving or operating other machinery. Patients who have frequent hypoglycemia or reduced or absent warning signs of hypoglycemia should be advised to use caution when driving or operating machinery.

Accidental mix-ups between LANTUS and other insulins, particularly short-acting insulins, have been reported. To avoid medication errors between LANTUS and other insulins, patients should be instructed to always check the insulin label before each injection.

LANTUS must only be used if the solution is clear and colorless with no particles visible. Patients must be advised that LANTUS must NOT be diluted or mixed with any other insulin or solution.

Patients should be advised not to share disposable or reusable insulin devices or needles with other patients, because doing so carries a risk for transmission of blood-borne pathogens.

Patients should be instructed on self-management procedures including glucose monitoring, proper injection technique, and management of hypoglycemia and hyperglycemia. Patients must be instructed on handling of special situations such as intercurrent conditions (illness, stress, or emotional disturbances), an inadequate or skipped insulin dose, inadvertent administration of an increased insulin dose, inadequate food intake, and skipped meals.

Patients with diabetes should be advised to inform their health care professional if they are pregnant or are contemplating pregnancy. Refer patients to the LANTUS "Patient Information" for additional information.

17.2 FDA approved patient labeling

See attached document at end of Full Prescribing Information.

Rev. September 2009
sanofi-aventis U.S. LLC
Bridgewater, NJ 08807
©2009 sanofi-aventis U.S. LLC

Patient Information
LANTUS® 10 mL vial (1000 units per vial) 100 units per mL (U-100)
(insulin glargine [recombinant DNA origin] injection)

- What is the most important information I should know about LANTUS?
- What is LANTUS?
- Who should NOT take LANTUS?
- How should I use LANTUS?
- What kind of syringe should I use?
- Mixing with LANTUS

Table 10: Type 2 Diabetes Mellitus–Adult

Treatment duration Treatment in combination with	Study E 52 weeks Oral agents		Study F 28 weeks Regular insulin		Study G 5 years Regular insulin	
	LANTUS	NPH	LANTUS	NPH	LANTUS	NPH
Number of subjects treated	289	281	259	259	513	504
HbA1c						
Baseline mean	9.0	8.9	8.6	8.5	8.4	8.3
Adj. mean change from baseline	-0.5	-0.4	-0.4	-0.6	-0.6	-0.8
LANTUS – NPH	-C.1		+0.2		+0.2	
95% CI for Treatment difference	(-0.3; +0.1)		(0.0; +0.4)		(+0.1; +0.4)	
Basal insulin dose*						
Baseline mean	14	15	44.1	45.5	39	44
Mean change from baseline	+12	+9	-1	+7	+23	+30
Total insulin dose*						
Baseline mean	14	15	64	67	48	53
Mean change from baseline	+12	+9	+10	+13	+41	+40
Fasting blood glucose (mg/dL)						
Baseline mean	179	180	164	166	190	180
Adj. mean change from baseline	-49	-46	-24	-22	-45	-44
Body weight (kg)						
Baseline mean	83.5	82.1	89.6	90.7	100	99
Mean change from baseline	2.0	1.9	0.4	1.4	3.7	4.8

* In Study G, the baseline dose of basal or total insulin was the first available on-treatment dose prescribed during the study (on visit month 1.5).

Table 11: LANTUS Timing of Daily Dosing in Type 1 (Study H) and Type 2 (Study I) Diabetes Mellitus

Treatment duration Treatment in combination with:	Study H 24 weeks Insulin lispro			Study I 24 weeks Glimepiride		
	LANTUS Breakfast	LANTUS Dinner	LANTUS Bedtime	LANTUS Breakfast	LANTUS Bedtime	NPH Bedtime
Number of subjects treated*	112	124	128	234	226	227
HbA1c						
Baseline mean	7.6	7.5	7.6	9.1	9.1	9.1
Mean change from baseline	-0.2	-0.1	0.0	-1.3	-1.0	-0.8
Basal insulin dose (U)						
Baseline mean	22	23	21	19	20	19
Mean change from baseline	5	2	2	11	18	18
Total insulin dose (U)					NA	NA
Baseline mean	52	52	49	NA†		
Mean change from baseline	2	3	2			
Body weight (kg)						
Baseline mean	77.1	77.8	74.5	80.7	82	81
Mean change from baseline	0.7	0.1	0.4	3.9	3.7	2.9

** total number of patients evaluable for safety
* Intent to treat
† Not applicable

Dosage Unit/Strength	Package size	NDC # 0088
10 mL vials 100 Units/mL	Pack of 1	2220-33
3 mL cartridge system* 100 Units/mL	package of 5	2220-52
3 mL SoloStar® disposable insulin device 100 Units/mL	package of 5	2220-60

* Cartridge systems are for use only in OptiClik® (Insulin Delivery Device)

- Instructions for Use
  - How do I draw the insulin into the syringe?
  - How do I inject LANTUS?
- What can affect how much insulin I need?
- What are the possible side effects of LANTUS and other insulins?
- How should I store LANTUS?
- General Information about LANTUS

Read this "Patient Information" that comes with LANTUS (LAN-tus) before you start using it and each time you get a refill because there may be new information. This leaflet does not take the place of talking with your healthcare provider about your condition or treatment. If you have questions about LANTUS or about diabetes, talk with your healthcare provider.

What is the most important information I should know about LANTUS?

- **Do not change the insulin you are using without talking to your healthcare provider.** Any change of insulin should be made cautiously and only under medical supervision. Changes in insulin strength, manufacturer, type (for example: Regular, NPH, analogs), species (beef, pork, beef-pork, human) or method of manufacture (recombinant DNA versus animal source insulin) may need a change in the dose. This dose change may be needed right away or later on during the first several weeks or months on the new insulin. Doses of oral anti-diabetic medicines may also need to change, if your insulin is changed.
- **You must test your blood sugar levels while using an insulin, such as LANTUS.** Your healthcare provider will tell you how often you should test your blood sugar level, and what to do if it is high or low.
- **Do NOT dilute or mix LANTUS with any other insulin or solution.** It will not work and you may lose blood sugar control, which could be serious.
- **LANTUS** comes as U-100 insulin and contains 100 units of LANTUS per milliliter (mL). One milliliter of U-100 insulin contains 100 units of insulin. (1 mL = 1 cc).

What is Diabetes?

- Your body needs insulin to turn sugar (glucose) into energy. If your body does not make enough insulin, you need to take more insulin so you will not have too much sugar in your blood.

	Not in-use (unopened) Refrigerated	Not in-use (unopened) Room Temperature	In-use (opened) (See Temperature Below)
10 mL Vial	Until expiration date	28 days	28 days Refrigerated or room temperature
3 mL Cartridge system	Until expiration date	28 days	28 days Refrigerated or room temperature
3 mL Cartridge system inserted into OptiClik®			28 days Room temperature only (Do not refrigerate)
3 mL SoloStar® disposable insulin device	Until expiration date	28 days	28 days Room temperature only (Do not refrigerate)

- Insulin injections are important in keeping your diabetes under control. But the way you live, your diet, careful checking of your blood sugar levels, exercise, and planned physical activity, all work with your insulin to help you control your diabetes.

What is LANTUS?
- LANTUS (insulin glargine [recombinant DNA origin]) is a long-acting insulin. Because LANTUS is made by recombinant DNA technology (rDNA) and is chemically different from the insulin made by the human body, it is called an insulin analog. LANTUS is used to treat patients with diabetes for the control of high blood sugar. It is used once a day to lower blood sugar.
- LANTUS is a clear, colorless, sterile solution for injection under the skin (subcutaneously).
- The active ingredient in LANTUS is insulin glargine. The concentration of insulin glargine is 100 units per milliliter (mL), or U-100. LANTUS also contains zinc, metacresol, glycerol, polysorbate 20 and water for injection as inactive ingredients. Hydrochloric acid and/or sodium hydroxide may be added to adjust the pH.
- You need a prescription to get LANTUS. Always be sure you receive the right insulin from the pharmacy.

Who should NOT take LANTUS?
Do not take LANTUS if you are allergic to insulin glargine or any of the inactive ingredients in LANTUS. Check with your healthcare provider if you are not sure.
Before starting LANTUS, tell your healthcare provider about all your medical conditions including if you:
- **have liver or kidney problems.** Your dose may need to be adjusted.
- **are pregnant or plan to become pregnant.** It is not known if LANTUS may harm your unborn baby. It is very important to maintain control of your blood sugar levels during pregnancy. Your healthcare provider will decide which insulin is best for you during your pregnancy.
- **are breast-feeding or plan to breast-feed.** It is not known whether LANTUS passes into your milk. Many medicines, including insulin, pass into human milk, and could affect your baby. Talk to your healthcare provider about the best way to feed your baby.
- **about all the medicines you take including** prescription and non-prescription medicines, vitamins, and herbal supplements.

How should I use LANTUS?
See the "Instructions for Use" including the "How do I draw the insulin into the syringe?" section for additional information.
- Follow the instructions given by your healthcare provider about the type or types of insulin you are using. Do not make any changes with your insulin unless you have talked to your healthcare provider. Your insulin needs may change because of illness, stress, other medicines, or changes in diet or activity level. Talk to your healthcare provider about how to adjust your insulin dose.
- You may take LANTUS at any time during the day but you must take it at the same time every day.
- Only use LANTUS that is clear and colorless. If your LANTUS is cloudy or slightly colored, return it to your pharmacy for a replacement.
- Follow your healthcare provider's instructions for testing your blood sugar.
- Inject LANTUS under your skin (subcutaneously) in your upper arm, abdomen (stomach area), or thigh (upper leg). Never inject it into a vein or muscle.
- Change (rotate) injection sites within the same body area.

What kind of syringe should I use?
- Always use a syringe that is marked for U-100 insulin. If you use other than U-100 insulin syringe, you may get the wrong dose of insulin causing serious problems for you, such as a blood sugar level that is too low or too high. Always use a new needle and syringe each time you give LANTUS injection.
- **NEEDLES AND SYRINGES MUST NOT BE SHARED.**
- Disposable syringes and needles should be used only once. Used syringe and needle should be placed in sharps con-

tainers (such as red biohazard containers), hard plastic containers (such as detergent bottles), or metal containers (such as an empty coffee can). Such containers should be sealed and disposed of properly.

Mixing with LANTUS
- **Do NOT dilute or mix LANTUS with any other insulin or solution.** It will not work as intended and you may lose blood sugar control, which could be serious.

Instructions for Use
How do I draw the insulin into the syringe?
- **The syringe must be new and does not contain any other medicine.**
- **Do not mix LANTUS with any other type of insulin.**
Follow these steps:
1. Wash your hands with soap and water or with alcohol.
2. Check the insulin to make sure it is clear and colorless. Do not use the insulin after the expiration date stamped on the label, if it is colored or cloudy, or if you see particles in the solution.
3. If you are using a new vial, remove the protective cap. **Do not** remove the stopper.

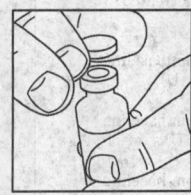

4. Wipe the top of the vial with an alcohol swab. You do not have to shake the vial of LANTUS before use.

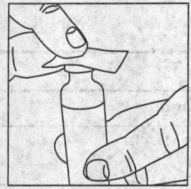

5. Use a new needle and syringe every time you give an injection. Use disposable syringes and needles only once. Throw them away properly. **Never** share needles and syringes.
6. Draw air into the syringe equal to your insulin dose. Put the needle through the rubber top of the vial and push the plunger to inject the air into the vial.

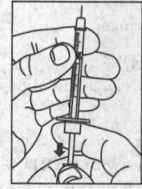 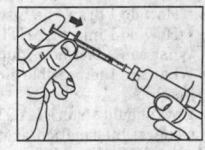

7. Leave the syringe in the vial and turn both upside down. Hold the syringe and vial firmly in one hand.
8. Make sure the tip of the needle is in the insulin. With your free hand, pull the plunger to withdraw the correct dose into the syringe.
[See figure at top of next column]
9. Before you take the needle out of the vial, check the syringe for air bubbles. If bubbles are in the syringe, hold the syringe straight up and tap the side of the syringe until the bubbles float to the top. Push the bubbles out

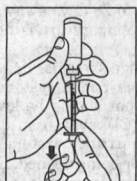

with the plunger and draw insulin back in until you have the correct dose.

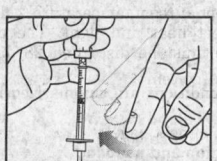

10. Remove the needle from the vial. Do not let the needle touch anything. You are now ready to inject.
How do I inject LANTUS?
Inject LANTUS under your skin. Take LANTUS as prescribed by your healthcare provider.
Follow these steps:
1. Decide on an injection area - either upper arm, thigh or abdomen. Injection sites within an injection area must be different from one injection to the next.
2. Use alcohol or soap and water to clean the injection site. The injection site should be dry before you inject.

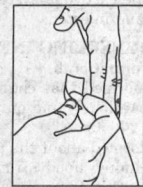

3. Pinch the skin. Stick the needle in the way your healthcare provider showed you. Release the skin.
4. Slowly push in the plunger of the syringe all the way, making sure you have injected all the insulin. Leave the needle in the skin for about 10 seconds.

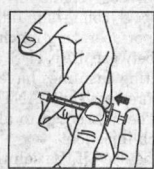

5. Pull the needle straight out and gently press on the spot where you injected yourself for several seconds. **Do not rub the area.**
6. Follow your healthcare providers instructions for throwing away the used needle and syringe. Do not recap the used needle. Used needle and syringe should be placed in sharps containers (such as red biohazard containers), hard plastic containers (such as detergent bottles), or metal containers (such as an empty coffee can). Such containers should be sealed and disposed of properly.

What can affect how much insulin I need?
Illness. Illness may change how much insulin you need. It is a good idea to think ahead and make a "sick day" plan with your healthcare provider in advance so you will be ready when this happens. Be sure to test your blood sugar more often and call your healthcare provider if you are sick.
Medicines. Many medicines can affect your insulin needs. Other medicines, including prescription and non-prescription medicines, vitamins, and herbal supplements, can change the way insulin works. You may need a different dose of insulin when you are taking certain other medicines. **Know all the medicines you take,** including prescription and non-prescription medicines, vitamins, and herbal supplements. You may want to keep a list of the medicines you take. You can show this list to your healthcare provider anytime you get a new medicine or refill. Your healthcare provider will tell you if your insulin dose needs to be changed.
Meals. The amount of food you eat can affect your insulin needs. If you eat less food, skip meals, or eat more food than usual, you may need a different dose of insulin. Talk to your healthcare provider if you change your diet so that you know how to adjust your LANTUS and other insulin doses.
Alcohol. Alcohol, including beer and wine, may affect the way LANTUS works and affect your blood sugar levels. Talk to your healthcare provider about drinking alcohol.

Exercise or Activity level. Exercise or activity level may change the way your body uses insulin. Check with your healthcare provider before you start an exercise program because your dose may need to be changed.

Travel. If you travel across time zones, talk with your healthcare provider about how to time your injections. When you travel, wear your medical alert identification. Take extra insulin and supplies with you.

Pregnancy or nursing. The effects of LANTUS on an unborn child or on a nursing baby are unknown. Therefore, tell your healthcare provider if you are planning to have a baby, are pregnant, or nursing a baby. Good control of diabetes is especially important during pregnancy and nursing.

What are the possible side effects of LANTUS and other insulins?

Insulins, including LANTUS, can cause hypoglycemia (low blood sugar), hyperglycemia (high blood sugar), allergy, and skin reactions.

Hypoglycemia (low blood sugar):

Hypoglycemia is often called an "insulin reaction" or "low blood sugar". It may happen when you do not have enough sugar in your blood. Common causes of hypoglycemia are illness, emotional or physical stress, too much insulin, too little food or missed meals, and too much exercise or activity.

Early warning signs of hypoglycemia may be different, less noticeable or not noticeable at all in some people. That is why it is important to check your blood sugar as you have been advised by your healthcare provider.

Hypoglycemia can happen with:

- **Taking too much insulin.** This can happen when too much insulin is injected.
- **Not enough carbohydrate (sugar or starch) intake.** This can happen if a meal or snack is missed or delayed.
- **Vomiting or diarrhea** that decreases the amount of sugar absorbed by your body.
- **Intake of alcohol.**
- **Medicines that affect insulin.** Be sure to discuss all your medicines with your healthcare provider. **Do not start any new medicines until you know how they may affect your insulin dose.**
- **Medical conditions that can affect your blood sugar levels or insulin.** These conditions include diseases of the adrenal glands, the pituitary, the thyroid gland, the liver, and the kidney.
- **Too much glucose use by the body.** This can happen if you exercise too much or have a fever.
- **Injecting insulin the wrong way or in the wrong injection area.**

Hypoglycemia can be mild to severe. Its onset may be rapid. Some patients have few or no warning symptoms, including:
- patients with diabetes for a long time
- patients with diabetic neuropathy (nerve problems)
- or patients using certain medicines for high blood pressure or heart problems.

Hypoglycemia may reduce your ability to drive a car or use mechanical equipment and you may risk injury to yourself or others.

Severe hypoglycemia can be dangerous and can cause temporary or permanent harm to your heart or brain. It may cause unconsciousness, seizures, or death.

Symptoms of hypoglycemia may include:
- anxiety, irritability, restlessness, trouble concentrating, personality changes, mood changes, or other abnormal behavior
- tingling in your hands, feet, lips, or tongue
- dizziness, light-headedness, or drowsiness
- nightmares or trouble sleeping
- headache
- blurred vision
- slurred speech
- palpitations (fast heart beat)
- sweating
- tremor (shaking)
- unsteady gait (walking).

If you have hypoglycemia often or it is hard for you to know if you have the symptoms of hypoglycemia, talk to your healthcare provider.

Mild to moderate hypoglycemia is treated by eating or drinking carbohydrates, such as fruit juice, raisins, sugar candies, milk or glucose tablets. Talk to your healthcare provider about the amount of carbohydrates you should eat to treat mild to moderate hypoglycemia.

Severe hypoglycemia may require the help of another person or emergency medical people. A person with hypoglycemia who is unable to take foods or liquids with sugar by mouth, or is unconscious needs medical help fast and will need treatment with a glucagon injection or glucose given intravenously (IV). Without medical help right away, serious reactions or even death could happen.

Hyperglycemia (high blood sugar):

Hyperglycemia happens when you have too much sugar in your blood. Usually, it means there is not enough insulin to break down the food you eat into energy your body can use.

Hyperglycemia can be caused by a fever, an infection, stress, eating more than you should, taking less insulin than prescribed, or it can mean your diabetes is getting worse.

Hyperglycemia can happen with:

- **Insufficient (too little) insulin.** This can happen from:
  - - injecting too little or no insulin
  - - incorrect storage (freezing, excessive heat)
  - - use after the expiration date.
- **Too much carbohydrate intake.** This can happen if you eat larger meals, eat more often, or increase the amount of carbohydrate in your meals.
- **Medicines that affect insulin.** Be sure to discuss all your medicines with your healthcare provider. **Do not start any new medicines until you know how they may affect your insulin dose.**
- **Medical conditions that affect insulin.** These medical conditions include fevers, infections, heart attacks, and stress.
- **Injecting insulin the wrong way or in the wrong injection area.**

Testing your blood or urine often will let you know if you have hyperglycemia. If your tests are often high, tell your healthcare provider so your dose of insulin can be changed. Hyperglycemia can be mild or severe. Hyperglycemia can **progress to diabetic ketoacidosis (DKA) or very high glucose levels (hyperosmolar coma) and result in unconsciousness and death.**

Although diabetic ketoacidosis occurs most often in patients with type 1 diabetes, it can also happen in patients with type 2 diabetes who become very sick. Because some patients get few symptoms of hyperglycemia, it is important to check your blood sugar/urine sugar and ketones regularly.

Symptoms of hyperglycemia include:
- confusion or drowsiness
- increased thirst
- decreased appetite, nausea, or vomiting
- rapid heart rate
- increased urination and dehydration (too little fluid in your body).

Symptoms of DKA also include:
- fruity smelling breath
- fast, deep breathing
- stomach area (abdominal) pain.

Severe or continuing hyperglycemia or DKA needs evaluation and treatment right away by your healthcare provider. Do not use LANTUS to treat diabetic ketoacidosis.

Other possible side effects of LANTUS include:

Serious allergic reactions:
Some times severe, life-threatening allergic reactions can happen with insulin. If you think you are having a severe allergic reaction, get medical help right away. Signs of insulin allergy include:
- rash all over your body
- shortness of breath
- wheezing (trouble breathing)
- fast pulse
- sweating
- low blood pressure.

Reactions at the injection site:
Injecting insulin can cause the following reactions on the skin at the injection site:
- little depression in the skin (lipoatrophy)
- skin thickening (lipohypertrophy)
- red, swelling, itchy skin (injection site reaction).

You can reduce the chance of getting an injection site reaction if you change (rotate) the injection site each time. An injection site reaction should clear up in a few days or a few weeks. If injection site reactions do not go away or keep happening, call your healthcare provider.

Tell your healthcare provider if you have any side effects that bother you.

These are not all the side effects of LANTUS. Ask your healthcare provider or pharmacist for more information.

How should I store LANTUS?

- **Unopened vial:**
Store new (unopened) LANTUS vials in a refrigerator (not the freezer) between 36°F to 46°F (2°C to 8°C). Do not freeze LANTUS. Keep LANTUS out of direct heat and light. If a vial has been frozen or overheated, throw it away.

- **Open (In-Use) vial:**
Once a vial is opened, you can keep it in a refrigerator or at room temperature (below 86°F [30°C]) but away from direct heat and light. Opened vial, either kept in a refrigerator or at room temperature, should be discarded 28

days after the first use even if it still contains LANTUS. Do not leave your insulin in a car on a summer day. These storage conditions are summarized in the following table:

[See table above]

- Do not use a vial of LANTUS after the expiration date stamped on the label.
- Do not use LANTUS if it is cloudy, colored, or if you see particles.

General Information about LANTUS

- Use LANTUS only to treat your diabetes. **Do not** give or share LANTUS with another person, even if they have diabetes also. It may harm them.
- This leaflet summarizes the most important information about LANTUS. If you would like more information, talk with your healthcare provider. You can ask your doctor or pharmacist for information about LANTUS that is written for healthcare professionals. For more information about LANTUS call 1-800-633-1610 or go to website www.lantus.com.

ADDITIONAL INFORMATION

DIABETES FORECAST is a national magazine designed especially for patients with diabetes and their families and is available by subscription from the American Diabetes Association (ADA), P.O.Box 363, Mt. Morris, IL 61054-0363, 1-800-DIABETES (1-800-342-2383). You may also visit the ADA website at www.diabetes.org.

Another publication, **COUNTDOWN**, is available from the Juvenile Diabetes Research Foundation International (JDRF), 120 Wall Street, 19th Floor, New York, New York 10005, 1-800-JDF-CURE (1-800-533-2873). You may also visit the JDRF website at www.jdf.org.

To get more information about diabetes, check with your healthcare professional or diabetes educator or visit www.DiabetesWatch.com.

Additional information about LANTUS can be obtained by calling 1-800-633-1610 or by visiting www.lantus.com.

Rev. March 2007
sanofi-aventis U.S. LLC
Bridgewater, NJ 08807
©2007 sanofi-aventis U.S. LLC

Patient Information
LANTUS® 3 mL cartridge system (300 units per cartridge system)
100 units per mL (U-100)
(insulin glargine [recombinant DNA origin] injection)
- What is the most important information I should know about LANTUS?
- What is LANTUS?
- Who should NOT take LANTUS?
- How should I use LANTUS?
- What kind of insulin Pen should I use?
- Mixing with LANTUS
- Instructions for Use
- What can affect how much insulin I need?
- What are the possible side effects of LANTUS and other insulins?
- How should I store LANTUS?
- General Information about LANTUS

Read this "Patient Information" that comes with LANTUS (LAN-tus) before you start using it and each time you get a refill because there may be new information. This leaflet does not take the place of talking with your healthcare provider about your condition or treatment. If you have questions about LANTUS or about diabetes, talk with your healthcare provider.

What is the most important information I should know about LANTUS?

- **Do not change the insulin you are using without talking to your healthcare provider.** Any change of insulin should be made cautiously and only under medical supervision. Changes in insulin strength, manufacturer, type (for example: Regular, NPH, analogs), species (beef, pork, beef-pork, human) or method of manufacture (recombinant DNA versus animal-source insulin) may need a change in the dose. This dose change may be needed right away or later on during the first several weeks or months on the new insulin. Doses of oral anti-diabetic medicines may also need to change, if your insulin is changed.
- **You must test your blood sugar levels while using an insulin, such as LANTUS.** Your healthcare provider will tell you how often you should test your blood sugar level, and what to do if it is high or low.

	Not in-use (unopened) Refrigerated	Not in-use (unopened) Room Temperature	In-use (opened) (See Temperature Below)
10 mL Vial	Until expiration date	28 days	28 days Refrigerated or room temperature

- **Do NOT dilute or mix LANTUS with any other insulin or solution.** It will not work and you may lose blood sugar control, which could be serious.
- **LANTUS** comes as U-100 insulin and contains 100 units of LANTUS per milliliter (mL). One milliliter of U-100 insulin contains 100 units of insulin. (1 mL = 1 cc).

What is Diabetes?

- Your body needs insulin to turn sugar (glucose) into energy. If your body does not make enough insulin, you need to take more insulin so you will not have too much sugar in your blood.
- Insulin injections are important in keeping your diabetes under control. But the way you live, your diet, careful checking of your blood sugar levels, exercise, and planned physical activity, all work with your insulin to help you control your diabetes.

What is LANTUS?

- LANTUS (insulin glargine [recombinant DNA origin]) is a long-acting insulin. Because LANTUS is made by recombinant DNA technology (rDNA) and is chemically different from the insulin made by the human body, it is called an insulin analog. LANTUS is used to treat patients with diabetes for the control of high blood sugar. It is used once a day to lower blood glucose.
- LANTUS is a clear, colorless, sterile solution for injection under the skin (subcutaneously).
- The active ingredient in LANTUS is insulin glargine. The concentration of insulin glargine is 100 units per milliliter (mL), or U-100. LANTUS also contains zinc, metacresol, glycerol, and water for injection as inactive ingredients. Hydrochloric acid and/ or sodium hydroxide may be added to adjust the pH.
- You need a prescription to get LANTUS. Always be sure you receive the right insulin from the pharmacy.

Who should NOT take LANTUS?

Do not take LANTUS if you are allergic to insulin glargine or any of the inactive ingredients in LANTUS. Check with your healthcare provider if you are not sure.

- **Before starting LANTUS, tell your healthcare provider about all your medical conditions including if you:**
  - **have liver or kidney problems.** Your dose may need to be adjusted.
  - **are pregnant or plan to become pregnant.** It is not known if LANTUS may harm your unborn baby. It is very important to maintain control of your blood sugar levels during pregnancy. Your healthcare provider will decide which insulin is best for you during your pregnancy.
  - **are breast-feeding or plan to breast-feed.** It is not known whether LANTUS passes into your milk. Many medicines, including insulin, pass into human milk, and could affect your baby. Talk to your healthcare provider about the best way to feed your baby.
  - **about all the medicines you take including** prescription and non-prescription medicines, vitamins and herbal supplements.

How should I use LANTUS?

See the "Instructions for OptiClik® Use" section for additional information.

- Follow the instructions given by your healthcare provider about the type or types of insulin you are using. Do not make any changes with your insulin unless you have talked to your healthcare provider. Your insulin needs may change because of illness, stress, other medicines, or changes in diet or activity level. Talk to your healthcare provider about how to adjust your insulin dose.
- You may take LANTUS at any time during the day but you must take it at the same time every day.
- Only use LANTUS that is clear and colorless. If your LANTUS is cloudy or slightly colored, return it to your pharmacy for a replacement.
- Follow your healthcare provider's instructions for testing your blood sugar.
- Inject LANTUS under your skin (subcutaneously) in your upper arm, abdomen (stomach area), or thigh (upper leg). Never inject it into a vein or muscle.
- Change (rotate) injection sites within the same body area.

What kind of insulin Pen should I use?

- Always use the OptiClik® device distributed by sanofi-aventis. If you use any other device than OptiClik® insulin Pen with this cartridge, you may get the wrong dose of insulin causing serious problems for you, such as a blood sugar level that is too low or too high. Always use a new needle each time you give LANTUS injection.
- **NEEDLES AND INSULIN PEN MUST NOT BE SHARED.**
- Disposable needle should be used only once. Used needle should be placed in sharps containers (such as red biohazard containers), hard plastic containers (such as detergent bottles), or metal containers (such as an empty coffee can). Such containers should be sealed and disposed of properly.

Mixing with LANTUS

- **Do NOT dilute or mix LANTUS with any other insulin or solution.** It will not work as intended and you may lose blood sugar control, which could be serious.

Instructions for OptiClik® Use

It is important to read, understand, and follow the step-by-step instructions in the "OptiClik® Instruction Leaflet" before using OptiClik® insulin Pen. Failure to follow the instructions may result in getting too much or too little insulin. If you have lost your leaflet or have a question, go to www.opticlik.com or call 1-800-633-1610.

The following general notes should be taken into consideration before injecting LANTUS:

- Always wash your hands before handling the cartridge system and/or the OptiClik® insulin Pen.
- Always attach a new needle before use. BD Ultra-Fine™ needles† are compatible with OptiClik. These are sold separately and are manufactured by BD.
- Always perform the safety test before use.
- Check the insulin solution in the cartridge system to make sure it is clear, colorless, and free of particles. If it is not, throw it away.
- Do NOT mix or dilute LANTUS with any other insulin or solution. LANTUS will not work if it is mixed or diluted and you may lose blood sugar control, which could be serious.
- Decide on an injection area - either upper arm, thigh, or abdomen. Do not use the same injection site as your last injection.
- After injecting LANTUS, leave the needle in the skin for an additional 10 seconds. Then pull the needle straight out. Gently press on the spot where you injected yourself for a few seconds. **Do not rub the area.**
- Do not drop the OptiClik® insulin Pen.

If your blood glucose reading is high or low, tell your healthcare provider so the dose can be adjusted.

What can affect how much insulin I need?

Illness. Illness may change how much insulin you need. It is a good idea to think ahead and make a "sick day" plan with your healthcare provider in advance so you will be ready when this happens. Be sure to test your blood sugar more often and call your healthcare provider if you are sick.

Medicines. Many medicines can affect your insulin needs. Other medicines, including prescription and non-prescription medicines, vitamins, and herbal supplements, can change the way insulin works. You may need a different dose of insulin when you are taking certain other medicines. **Know all the medicines you take,** including prescription and non-prescription medicines, vitamins and herbal supplements. You may want to keep a list of the medicines you take. You can show this list to your healthcare provider and pharmacists anytime you get a new medicine or refill. Your healthcare provider will tell you if your insulin dose needs to be changed.

Meals. The amount of food you eat can affect your insulin needs. If you eat less food, skip meals, or eat more food than usual, you may need a different dose of insulin. Talk to your healthcare provider if you change your diet so that you know how to adjust your LANTUS and other insulin doses.

Alcohol. Alcohol, including beer and wine, may affect the way LANTUS works and affect your blood sugar levels. Talk to your healthcare provider about drinking alcohol.

Exercise or Activity level. Exercise or activity level may change the way your body uses insulin. Check with your healthcare provider before you start an exercise program because your dose may need to be changed.

Travel. If you travel across time zones, talk with your healthcare provider about how to time your injections. When you travel, wear your medical alert identification. Take extra insulin and supplies with you.

Pregnancy or nursing. The effects of LANTUS on an unborn child or on a nursing baby are unknown. Therefore, tell your healthcare provider if you are planning to have a baby, are pregnant, or nursing a baby. Good control of diabetes is especially important during pregnancy and nursing.

What are the possible side effects of LANTUS and other insulins?

Insulins, including LANTUS, can cause hypoglycemia (low blood sugar), hyperglycemia (high blood sugar), allergy, and skin reactions.

Hypoglycemia (low blood sugar):

Hypoglycemia is often called an "insulin reaction" or "low blood sugar". It may happen when you do not have enough sugar in your blood. Common causes of hypoglycemia are illness, emotional or physical stress, too much insulin, too little food or missed meals, and too much exercise or activity.

Early warning signs of hypoglycemia may be different, less noticeable or not noticeable at all in some people. That is why it is important to check your blood sugar as you have been advised by your healthcare provider.

Hypoglycemia can happen with:

- **Taking too much insulin.** This can happen when too much insulin is injected.

- **Not enough carbohydrate (sugar or starch) intake.** This can happen if a meal or snack is missed or delayed.
- **Vomiting or diarrhea** that decreases the amount of sugar absorbed by your body.
- **Intake of alcohol.**
- **Medicines that affect insulin.** Be sure to discuss all your medicines with your healthcare provider. **Do not start any new medicines until you know how they may affect your insulin dose.**
- **Medical conditions that can affect your blood sugar levels or insulin.** These conditions include diseases of the adrenal glands, the pituitary, the thyroid gland, the liver, and the kidney.
- **Too much glucose use by the body.** This can happen if you exercise too much or have a fever.
- **Injecting insulin the wrong way or in the wrong injection area.**

Hypoglycemia can be mild to severe. Its onset may be rapid. Some patients have few or no warning symptoms, including:

- patients with diabetes for a long time
- patients with diabetic neuropathy (nerve problems)
- or patients using certain medicines for high blood pressure or heart problems.

Hypoglycemia may reduce your ability to drive a car or use mechanical equipment and you may risk injury to yourself or others. Severe hypoglycemia can be dangerous and can cause temporary or permanent harm to your heart or brain. **It may cause unconsciousness, seizures, or death.**

Symptoms of hypoglycemia may include:

- anxiety, irritability, restlessness, trouble concentrating, personality changes, mood changes, or other abnormal behavior
- tingling in your hands, feet, lips, or tongue
- dizziness, light-headedness, or drowsiness
- nightmares or trouble sleeping
- headache
- blurred vision
- slurred speech
- palpitations (fast heart beat)
- sweating
- tremor (shaking)
- unsteady gait (walking).

If you have hypoglycemia often or it is hard for you to know if you have the symptoms of hypoglycemia, talk to your healthcare provider.

Mild to moderate hypoglycemia is treated by eating or drinking carbohydrates such as fruit juice, raisins, sugar candies, milk or glucose tablets. Talk to your healthcare provider about the amount of carbohydrates you should eat to treat mild to moderate hypoglycemia.

Severe hypoglycemia may require the help of another person or emergency medical people. A person with hypoglycemia who is unable to take foods or liquids with sugar by mouth, or is unconscious needs medical help fast and will need treatment with a glucagon injection or glucose given intravenously (IV). Without medical help right away, serious reactions or even death could happen.

Hyperglycemia (high blood sugar):

Hyperglycemia happens when you have too much sugar in your blood. Usually, it means there is not enough insulin to break down the food you eat into energy your body can use. Hyperglycemia can be caused by a fever, an infection, stress, eating more than you should, taking less insulin than prescribed, or it can mean your diabetes is getting worse.

Hyperglycemia can happen with:

- **Insufficient (too little) insulin.** This can happen from:
  - -injecting too little or no insulin
  - -incorrect storage (freezing, excessive heat)
  - -use after the expiration date.
- **Too much carbohydrate intake.** This can happen if you eat larger meals, eat more often, or increase the amount of carbohydrate in your meals.
- **Medicines that affect insulin.** Be sure to discuss all your medicines with your healthcare provider. **Do not start any new medicines until you know how they may affect your insulin dose.**
- **Medical conditions that affect insulin.** These medical conditions include fevers, infections, heart attacks, and stress.
- **Injecting insulin the wrong way or in the wrong injection area.**

Testing your blood or urine often will let you know if you have hyperglycemia. If your tests are often high, tell your healthcare provider so your dose of insulin can be changed. Hyperglycemia can be mild or severe. It can **progress to diabetic ketoacidosis (DKA) or very high glucose levels (hyperosmolar coma) and result in unconsciousness and death.**

Although diabetic ketoacidosis occurs most often in patients with type 1 diabetes, it can also happen in patients with type 2 diabetes who become very sick. Because some patients get few symptoms of hyperglycemia, it is important to check your blood sugar/urine sugar and ketones regularly.

Symptoms of hyperglycemia include:
- confusion or drowsiness
- increased thirst
- decreased appetite, nausea, or vomiting
- rapid heart rate
- increased urination and dehydration (too little fluid in your body).

Symptoms of DKA also include:
- fruity smelling breath
- fast, deep breathing
- stomach area (abdominal) pain.

Severe or continuing hyperglycemia or DKA needs evaluation and treatment right away by your healthcare provider.
Do not use LANTUS to treat diabetic ketoacidosis.
Other possible side effects of LANTUS include:

Serious allergic reactions:
Some times severe, life-threatening allergic reactions can happen with insulin. If you think you are having a severe allergic reaction, get medical help right away. Signs of insulin allergy include:
- rash all over your body
- shortness of breath
- wheezing (trouble breathing)
- fast pulse
- sweating
- low blood pressure.

Reactions at the injection site:
Injecting insulin can cause the following reactions on the skin at the injection site:
- little depression in the skin (lipoatrophy)
- skin thickening (lipohypertrophy)
- red, swelling, itchy skin (injection site reaction).

You can reduce the chance of getting an injection site reaction if you change (rotate) the injection site each time. An injection site reaction should clear up in a few days or a few weeks. If injection site reactions do not go away or keep happening call your healthcare provider.
Tell your healthcare provider if you have any side effects that bother you.
These are not all the side effects of LANTUS. Ask your healthcare provider or pharmacist for more information.

How should I store LANTUS?
- **Unopened cartridge system:**
  Store new unopened LANTUS cartridge systems in a refrigerator (not the freezer) between 36 °F to 46 °F (2°C to 8°C). Do not freeze LANTUS. Keep LANTUS out of direct heat and light. If a cartridge system has been frozen or overheated, throw it away.
- **Open (In-Use) cartridge system:**
  Once a cartridge system is opened, you can keep it at room temperature (below 86°F [30°C]) but away from direct heat and light for 28 days. Cartridge system in OptiClik insulin Pen must be discarded 28 days after the first use even if it still contains LANTUS. The opened cartridge system in OptiClik® insulin Pen should be kept at room temperature (below 86°F [30°C]) and away from direct heat and light for up to 28 days. For example, do not leave it in a car on a summer day. Do not store OptiClik®, with or without cartridge system, in a refrigerator at any time.

These storage conditions are summarized in the following table:
[See table above]
- Do not use a cartridge system of LANTUS after the expiration date stamped on the label.
- Do not use LANTUS if it is cloudy, colored, or if you see particles.

General Information about LANTUS
- Use LANTUS only to treat your diabetes. **Do not** give or share LANTUS with another person, even if they have diabetes also. It may harm them.
- This leaflet summarizes the most important information about LANTUS. If you would like more information, talk with your healthcare provider. You can ask your healthcare provider or pharmacist for information about LANTUS that is written for healthcare professionals. For more information about LANTUS call 1-800-633-1610 or go to website www.lantus.com.

ADDITIONAL INFORMATION
DIABETES FORECAST is a national magazine designed especially for patients with diabetes and their families and is available by subscription from the American Diabetes Association (ADA), P.O. Box 363, Mt. Morris, IL 61054-0363, 1-800-DIABETES (1-800-342-2383). You may also visit the ADA website at www.diabetes.org.
Another publication, **COUNTDOWN**, is available from the Juvenile Diabetes Research Foundation International (JDRF), 120 Wall Street, 19th Floor, New York, New York 10005, 1-800-JDF-CURE (1-800-533-2873). You may also visit the JDRF website at www.jdf.org.
To get more information about diabetes, check with your healthcare professional or diabetes educator or visit www.DiabetesWatch.com.
Additional information about LANTUS can be obtained by calling 1-800-633-1610 or by visiting www.lantus.com.

	Not in-use (unopened) Refrigerated	Not in-use (unopened) Room Temperature	In-use (opened) (See Temperature Below)
3 mL Cartridge System	Until expiration date	28 days	28 days Refrigerated or room temperature
3 mL cartridge system inserted in OptiClik® insulin Pen			28 days Room temperature only (Do not refrigerate)

Rev. March 2007
sanofi-aventis U.S. LLC
Bridgewater, NJ 08807
©2007 sanofi-aventis U.S. LLC
OptiClik® is a registered trademark of sanofi-aventis U.S. LLC
†The brands listed are the trademarks of their respective owners and are not trademarks of sanofi-aventis U.S. LLC

OptiClik® INSTRUCTION LEAFLET
OptiClik® is a reusable insulin delivery device (insulin Pen) for use with 3 mL Lantus® or Apidra® cartridge (U-100) systems.
OptiClik® allows you to dial the dose in one-unit step increments between one unit and a maximum of 80 units per injection.
OptiClik® is available in different colors. For patients that use two different types of insulin, Lantus or Apidra, it is recommended to use a different color pen for each insulin. Read these instructions carefully before using your OptiClik®. Read both sides of the leaflet. If you are not able to follow all the instructions completely on your own, use OptiClik® only if you have help from a person who is able to follow the instructions. Hold the pen as shown in this leaflet. The word "OptiClik" must be readable to the left of the digital dose display to ensure the correct reading of the dose.
If you do not follow these instructions completely, you may get too much or too little insulin.
Keep this leaflet for future reference for each time you use OptiClik®.
You will find further useful information on the back side of this leaflet in the chapters:
- (A.) General Notes
- (B.) Troubleshooting
- (C.) Storage Instructions
- (D.) Other Information

Talk with your healthcare provider before using OptiClik® about proper injection technique. Before using OptiClik®, your healthcare provider should provide training for the use of the pen, or direct you to the appropriate person to get training.
If you have visual problems, use OptiClik® only if you have help from a trained person with good vision.
Additional items needed for use with OptiClik®
- Alcohol swabs
- BD Ultra-Fine needles
- 3 mL Lantus or Apidra Cartridge System, at room temperature

If you have any questions about OptiClik® or about diabetes, ask your healthcare professional, go to www.opticlik.com or call sanofi-aventis at 1-800-633-1610.

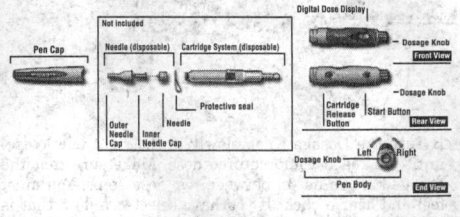

General Warnings and Precautions
This pen is only for your use. Do not share it with anyone else.
Insulin
Check the label on your Cartridge System to make sure you have the correct insulin before injecting. Using the wrong insulin may result in unwanted changes in blood sugar that could be harmful to your health.
Needles
You must use a new sterile needle (intact protective seal) for each injection. This prevents a blocked needle and air bubbles. In order to avoid injuries, replace Outer Needle Cap before removing and disposing of used needles.
Safety test
Before each injection, carry out the Safety Test (Step **3**). If you do not follow the instructions completely, you may get too much or too little insulin. Injecting too much or too little

insulin dose may lead to unwanted blood sugar changes (see the package leaflet for your insulin). Do not perform the safety test without the needle attached.
Damage to OptiClik®
OptiClik® may become damaged by rough handling, dropping, or turning of the Dosage Knob by force. Make sure that no dirt gets in contact with the mechanical parts. You should always make sure that:
- a)The Cartridge System is undamaged.
- b)The Start Button, Dosage Knob, and Digital Dose Display operate properly.

Do not use tools on OptiClik®. If you are not sure whether or not your OptiClik® is damaged, contact your healthcare professional or call 1-800-633-1610. If damaged, it is no longer safe to use. In an emergency, you can draw up the insulin from the Cartridge System using a U-100 insulin syringe.
OptiClik® should not be used near electrical and electronic equipment.

Step 1: Inserting the Cartridge System
Do not shake the Cartridge System before use. You should look at the solution in the Cartridge System before inserting it into OptiClik®. If the solution is cloudy, slightly colored, or has particles in it, do not use the Cartridge System.

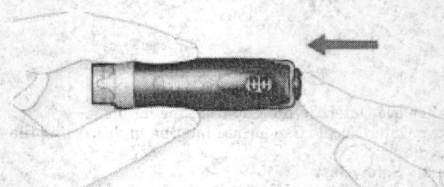

- **A** Make sure the Dosage Knob is pushed in.

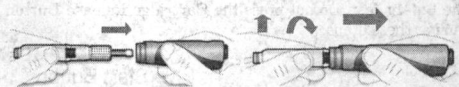

- **B** Hold the Pen Body with the release button facing up. Insert the Cartridge System straight into the Pen Body. If you meet resistance, slightly raise and rotate the Cartridge System while inserting it. Make sure that it clicks in. Do not use force.

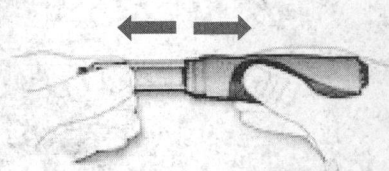

- **C** To make sure that the Cartridge System clicked in place properly, gently try pulling out the Cartridge System. The Cartridge System should not come out. Make sure you do not press the Cartridge Release button during or after this check.
OptiClik® is now ready for Step 2 (Attaching the needle), or it can be stored with the attached Pen Cap.
DO NOT STORE YOUR OPTICLIK® IN A REFRIGERATOR AFTER CARTRIDGE SYSTEM IS INSERTED IN OPTICLIK®
Step 2: Attaching the needle

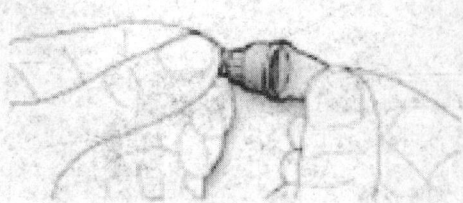

- **A** Peel off the Protective Seal on the needle.

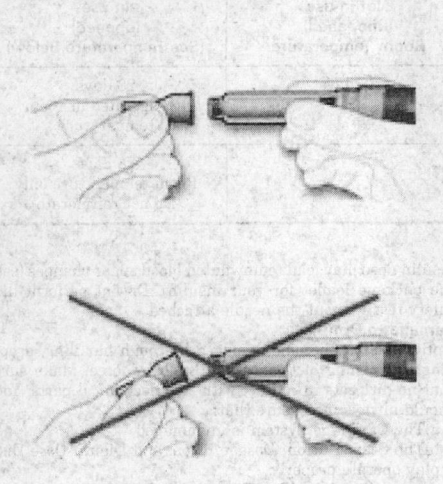

• **B** Use an alcohol swab to wipe the rubber seal on the end of the Cartridge System. Attach a new needle straight to the Cartridge System and screw into place without removing the Outer and Inner Needle Caps

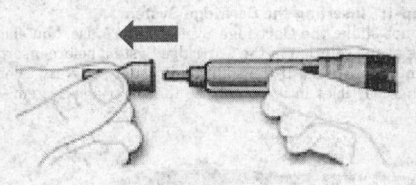

• **C** Remove Outer Needle Cap from the needle.
Save Outer Needle Cap for use later on in discarding the needle.

Step 3:   Safety Test
Before each injection, carry out the Safety Test or you may get too much or too little insulin.
Make sure a needle is attached to OptiClik® before you do the Safety Test. Do not press the Cartridge Release Button during these steps.

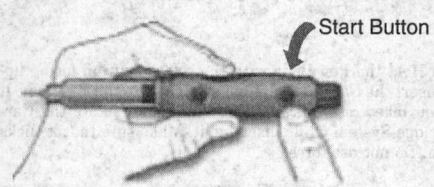

Start Button

• **A** Press the Start Button.

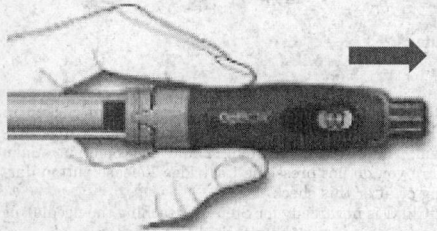

• **B** The Dosage Knob must come out. "00" appears in the Digital Dose Display.

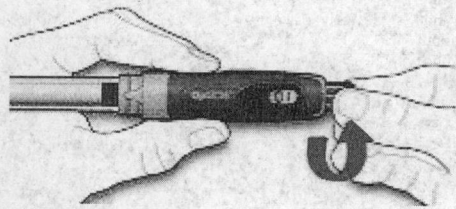

• **C** Turn the Dosage Knob to the right (clockwise) until it clicks. "01" appears in the Digital Dose Display.

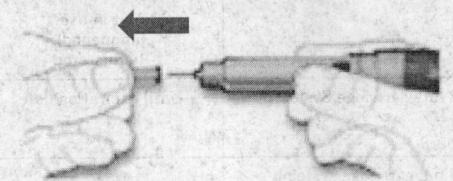

• **D** Remove and discard the Inner Needle Cap. Handle the exposed needle carefully.

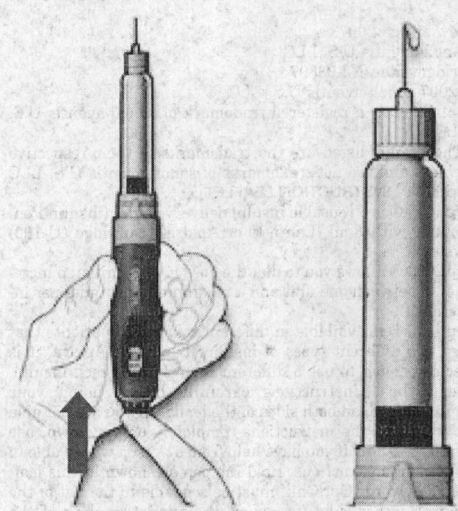

• **E** Hold OptiClik® with the needle pointing up.
Press the Dosage Knob fully until it stays in.
Insulin must appear at the tip of the needle. If not, repeat the Safety Test. When replacing an empty cartridge system with a new one, it might require repeating this procedure several times.
A Safety Test must be carried out before each injection.
Additional information about "Cartridge System" and "Removing air bubbles" is on the back side of this leaflet.

Step 4:   Setting the dose

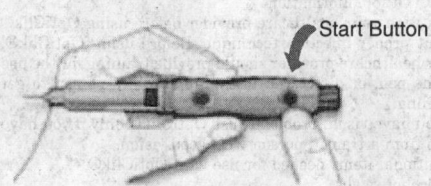

Start Button

• **A** Press the Start Button.

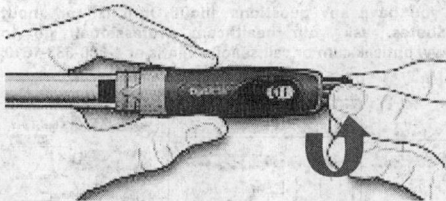

• **B** Turn the Dosage Knob slowly to the right (clockwise) until you reach your required dose. Make sure that the dosage knob is not in between two dose steps. You must feel and hear a click. If you have selected a dose that is too high, simply turn the Dosage Knob back (to the left). If you have dialed past 80 units, see (B.) TROUBLE-SHOOTING, Dose-setting on the back of this leaflet.

Step 5:   Injecting the dose

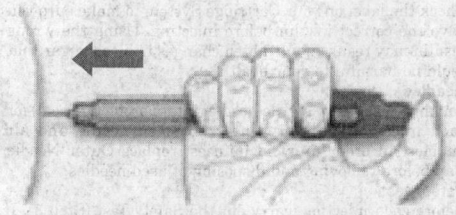

• **A** Check the label on your cartridge system to make sure you have the correct insulin before injecting. Clean the

---

injection area with alcohol. Insert the needle as recommended by your healthcare professional (e.g., lightly pinch a fold of skin on your upper arm, stomach, or thigh. Insert the needle straight into the pinched skin).

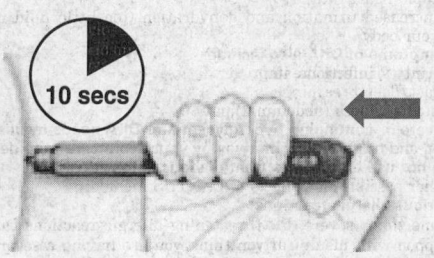

10 secs

• **B** Press the Dosage Knob slowly and completely. Slowly count to 10 while holding the Dosage Knob in before withdrawing the needle. The Dosage Knob must stay in. The Dosage Knob staying in after injection indicates the delivery of the full dose.
After injecting your dose, the Digital Dose Display will not go back to "0" but will show the delivered dose for 2 minutes. Do not re-inject your dose as this may result in an overdose.
Do not press the Cartridge Release Button or the Start Button while injecting.

Step 6:   Removing the needle

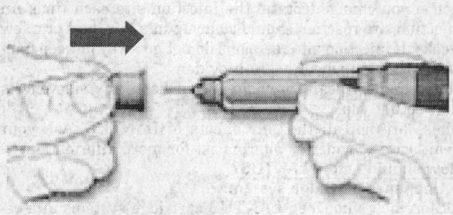

• **A** Replace Outer Needle Cap carefully.

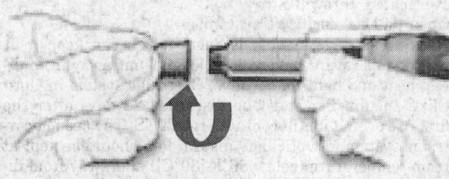

• **B** Remove the needle after the injection. For safe disposal of needles see (A.) GENERAL NOTES, Needles for Opti-Clik® on the back of this leaflet. Always replace Pen Cap on the Pen Body after use.
OptiClik® can be stored with the attached Cartridge System until your next injection. See (C.) STORAGE INSTRUCTIONS.

Step 7:   Replacing an empty Cartridge System

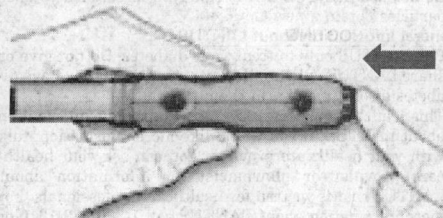

• **A** Make sure the Dosage Knob is pushed in.

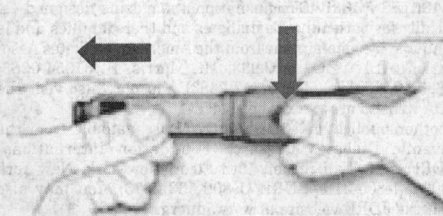

• **B** Press the Cartridge Release Button, and remove the entire Cartridge System. Dispose of the Cartridge System.
Start again at Step 1 (Inserting the Cartridge System).

IMPORTANT NOTICE: Updated drug information is sent bi-monthly via the PDR® Update Insert. For *monthly* email updates, register at PDR.net.

A. GENERAL NOTES
Cartridge System
The Cartridge System is sold separately. Before every injection, check the appearance of the solution in the Cartridge System and follow the instructions in the "Patient Information" leaflet for the insulin. It is important to follow the directions of this Instruction Leaflet closely to help avoid side effects (e.g., infections, improper dosing). Consult with your healthcare professional before using OptiClik®.

Before the use of an unopened, refrigerated Cartridge System, take it out of the refrigerator and leave it at room temperature for about 1 to 2 hours. Do not remove the Cartridge System from packaging until ready to use. This will prevent dust or dirt from getting into the mechanical parts of the Cartridge System. Use an alcohol swab to wipe the rubber seal on the end of the Cartridge System before inserting the needle. Do not open or manipulate the Cartridge System in any way.

Needles for OptiClik®
BD Ultra-Fine needles are available from BD Consumer Healthcare. Contact your healthcare professional for further information. Needles may vary from country to country and may not be interchangeable. If you intend to travel abroad, make sure that you have sufficient needles and insulin with you.

Never store OptiClik® with a needle attached. Storing OptiClik® with the needle attached may allow insulin to leak from OptiClik® and air bubbles to form in the Cartridge System. Used needles should be placed in sharps containers (such as red biohazard containers), hard plastic containers (such as detergent bottles), or metal containers (such as an empty coffee can). Such containers should be sealed and disposed of properly.

Removing air bubbles
Air bubbles must be removed before each injection during the Safety Test (Step 3 for Safety Test). If air bubbles still remain, repeat the Safety Test, turning the Dosage Knob to the right until "02" appears on the display. Gently tap the Cartridge System until the air rises to the top of the Cartridge System tip. Then press the Dosage Knob until it stays in. If necessary, keep repeating the Safety Test until insulin appears at the tip of the needle.

Setting the dose and Display feature
To read the dose correctly, hold OptiClik® as shown in Step 4B, Setting the dose. The printed "OptiClik" must be readable left of the dose display. Do not hold the pen upside down when reading the dose display; otherwise you may misread the dose on the Digital Dose Display.

The Digital Dose Display shows the delivered dose for 2 minutes after every injection and then turns off to conserve battery power. With the Dosage Knob released the display also switches off after 2 minutes.

How long will OptiClik® last
The expected lifetime of OptiClik® is 3 years.

▢ **flashes when the Start Button is pressed:**
OptiClik® is reaching the end of its expected lifetime (3 years). The Digital Dose Display will continue to operate for about 4 more weeks. Please obtain a new OptiClik®.

▢ **stays when the Start Button is pressed:**
OptiClik® has reached the end of its lifetime. When you continue to turn the Dosage Knob, the display still shows ▢ . Please obtain a new OptiClik®.

B. TROUBLESHOOTING
Safety test
No insulin appears at the needle tip during Step 3 (Safety Test):
Repeat Step 3 (Safety Test). If no insulin appears this time either, confirm that:
1. The needle is firmly in position. Replace a blocked or defective needle with a new one.
2. The Dosage Knob has been set correctly (always turn the Dosage Knob to the right/clockwise to preselect the dose). Turn the Dosage Knob one click to the right, equal to one unit.
3. The Cartridge System has been inserted correctly. Check by trying to pull the Cartridge System gently out. If the Cartridge System comes out, reinsert it completely, see Step 1 (Inserting the Cartridge System). Repeat Step 3 (Safety Test).
4. The Cartridge System is not empty. If it is empty, insert a new one. Repeat Step 3 (Safety Test).

You hear no clicking sound during dose-setting:
The Cartridge System may have been inserted incorrectly. Check by trying to pull the Cartridge System gently out. If the Cartridge System comes out, reinsert it completely, see Step 1 (Inserting the Cartridge System). Repeat Step 3 (Safety Test).
If you still hear no clicking sound, try a new Cartridge System and listen for clicking sound. If there is still no clicking sound, obtain a new OptiClik®.

Dose-setting
Insulin drips from the needle tip during dose-setting:
The maximum dose of OptiClik® is 80 units. If you continue to dial after reaching 80 units, insulin will drip from the needle and the display will continue to show "80". In such a case, DO NOT turn back to the required dose, instead dial back (to the left) to "00".
Press the Dosage Knob to expel excess insulin and to reset OptiClik®. OptiClik® is now again ready for dose setting. If you need a dose greater than 80 units, you should give it as two injection.

You feel resistance during dose-setting and the Dosage Knob will not turn further forward (to the right):
- a)You are turning to the left and trying to dial down below zero. Turn the Dosage Knob to the right to dial your dose.
- b)The Cartridge System is almost empty and no longer contains a sufficient amount of insulin for the dose you need. For example, if there are only 20 units left in the Cartridge System and you need 25 units, the dosage knob will stop at 20 units. You can choose to do one of the following:
  - 1)Do not force the Dosage Knob any further (to the right). Inject the partial dose (20 units in the example), and replace the empty Cartridge System with a new one. Perform the Safety Test as described in Step 3, then inject the remainder of the dose to equal your total prescribed dose. In the above example, the remaining dose is 5 units. OR
  - 2)Dial back (to the left) to "00". Follow Step 7 (Replacing an empty Cartridge System), Step 1 (Inserting the Cartridge System), Step 2 (Attaching the needle), and Step 3 (Safety Test).
- c)You have dialed (to the right) past the maximum dose of 80 units and have no needle (or a clogged needle) mounted. Dial completely back (to the left) to "00", and perform Step 2 (Attaching the needle) and Step 3 (Safety Test). Do not force the Dosage Knob to turn further.

The Dosage Knob does not stop at "00":
When turned back completely, the Dosage Knob should stop at "00", however, sometimes it may stop at "02" or "01". Make sure that a needle is attached; then press the Dosage Knob down (insulin will appear at the tip of the needle). OptiClik® is now ready for dose setting.

The Dosage Knob no longer turns after a new Cartridge System has been inserted:
Check that the Cartridge System is firmly clicked in. Reseat the Cartridge System and try again. If it still does not work, try again with a new Cartridge System, see Step 1 (Inserting the Cartridge System). Otherwise, get a new OptiClik®.

The Dosage Knob does not come out after you pressed the Start Button:
Do not pull out the Dosage Knob. Check that the Cartridge System is firmly clicked in, see Step 1B-Inserting the Cartridge System.

Insulin injection
The Dosage Knob cannot be pressed down for the insulin injection or it does not stay down:
1. In setting the dose, you have turned the Dosage Knob so that it is between two dose steps.
   Turn the Dosage Knob to the right or the left to the desired dose.
2. The needle may be blocked or defective. Use a new needle.
3. Avoid pushing the Start Button and Dosage Knob at the same time.

After withdrawing the needle from your skin, more than one drop of insulin drips from the needle:
It is possible that you may not have injected your full insulin dose. DO NOT try to make up for the shortfall in your insulin dose by giving a second injection (otherwise you will be at risk for low blood sugar).
Please check your blood sugar and consult with your healthcare professional.
You can avoid the problem next time by taking the following steps:
1. Remove any air bubbles that may be present in the Cartridge System
   (see "GENERAL NOTES: Removing air bubbles").
2. After delivering the insulin dose, slowly count to 10 before withdrawing the needle from your skin.

Cartridge System replacement
The Cartridge System and Pen Body do not click back together properly:
1. Check that the Dosage Knob is pushed in.
2. Check that you have put the Cartridge System correctly into the Pen Body. Take the Cartridge System out and insert it again (see under Step 7 for replacing an empty Cartridge System and Step 1 for inserting the Cartridge System). Repeat Step 2 for attaching the needle and Step 3 for Safety Test.

Digital Dose Display functions
▢ **is displayed:**
The Dosage Knob has been forced into the negative range with excessive force. The Cartridge System might be damaged and needs to be replaced. Follow the instructions under Step 7 to replace the Cartridge System and dispose of the damaged Cartridge System. Repeat Step 1 for inserting the Cartridge System, Step 2 for attaching the needle, and Step 3 for Safety Test.

▢ **and** ▢ **flash alternately:**
- a)The Dosage Knob has been forced into the negative range and was pushed in. The Cartridge System might be damaged and needs to be replaced. Repeat Step 7 for replacing an empty Cartridge System and dispose of the damaged Cartridge System. Repeat Step 1 for inserting the Cartridge System, Step 2 for attaching the needle, and Step 3 for Safety Test.
- b)The Dosage Knob has been turned too quickly. You can choose to do one of the following:
  - 1)Dispose of the unknown pre-set dose by pressing the Dosage Knob. Set your dose (Step 4) and inject your dose (Step 5). OR
  - 2)Turn the Dosage Knob slowly backward (to the left) until it stops, and then push the Dosage Knob in. Restart OptiClik® and dial your dose.

No numbers appear on the Digital Dose Display when the Start Button is pressed or when the Dosage Knob is released:
Press the Dosage Knob. Start with a Safety Test (Step 3). If there are still no numbers on Digital Dose Display, you should obtain a new OptiClik®.

The Digital Dose Display goes blank during dose setting (e.g., if you are interrupted in the middle of your injection preparations):
The energy save function has automatically come into operation. Turn the Dosage Knob one click further (to the right). OptiClik® should now be ready to use again; check the Digital Dose Display and adjust for the right dose if needed.

Battery Information
▢ **flashes when the Start Button is pressed:**
Your battery is running out. Please obtain a new OptiClik® as soon as possible.

▢ **is displayed when the Start Button is pressed:**
Your battery has run out. Please obtain a new OptiClik®.

C. STORAGE INSTRUCTIONS
Always store OptiClik® Pen Body at room temperature below 86°F (30°C). Do not store OptiClik®, (with or without the Cartridge System inserted), in a refrigerator at any time. Protect OptiClik® from moisture and direct heat. When OptiClik® is not in use, push the Dosage Knob in to conserve the battery and to ensure OptiClik® functions throughout its expected lifetime.

To avoid dust or dirt from getting into OptiClik®, always replace the Pen Cap.

Once the Cartridge System is used with OptiClik®, the Cartridge System can be used for up to 28 days under normal carrying conditions (for Lantus®, below 86°F [30°C]; for Apidra®, below 77°F [25°C]). For specific insulin storage information, see "Patient Information" for Lantus® or Apidra® 3 mL Cartridge System.

Do not store OptiClik® with the needle attached to the Cartridge System.

D. OTHER INFORMATION
Care, cleaning, and maintenance instructions
Handle OptiClik® carefully. To keep it clean, use a clean damp cloth. Clean it once a week. Dirt can impede the operation. DO NOT use cleaning agents. Use an alcohol swab only for cleaning the Cartridge System's rubber seal.

Lifetime
OptiClik® has a lifetime of 3 years. See "(A.) GENERAL NOTES, How long will OptiClik® last" for details.

Manufactured for and distributed by:
sanofi-aventis U.S. LLC
Bridgewater NJ 08807
OptiClik®, Lantus® and Apidra® are registered trademarks of sanofi-aventis U.S. LLC
For more information call toll free 1-800-633-1610 or visit www.opticlik.com
Date of revision:
December 2006
Patient Information
LANTUS® SOLOSTAR® 3 mL disposable insulin delivery device (300 units per device)
100 units per mL (U-100)
(insulin glargine [recombinant DNA origin] injection)
- What is the most important information I should know about LANTUS?
- What is LANTUS?
- Who should NOT take LANTUS?
- How should I use LANTUS?
- Mixing with LANTUS
- Instructions for Use
- What can affect how much insulin I need?
- What are the possible side effects of LANTUS and other insulins?
- How should I store LANTUS?
- General Information about LANTUS

Read this "Patient Information" that comes with LANTUS (LAN-tus) before you start using it and each time you get a refill because there may be new information. This leaflet does not take the place of talking with your healthcare provider about your condition or treatment. If you have questions about LANTUS or about diabetes, talk with your healthcare provider.

What is the most important information I should know about LANTUS?

- **Do not change the insulin you are using without talking to your healthcare provider.** Any change of insulin should be made cautiously and only under medical supervision. Changes in insulin strength, manufacturer, type (for example: Regular, NPH, analogs), species (beef, pork, beef-pork, human) or method of manufacture (recombinant DNA versus animal-source insulin) may need a change in the dose. This dose change may be needed right away or later on during the first several weeks or months on the new insulin. Doses of oral anti-diabetic medicines may also need to change, if your insulin is changed.
- **You must test your blood sugar levels while using an insulin, such as LANTUS.** Your healthcare provider will tell you how often you should test your blood sugar level, and what to do if it is high or low.
- **Do NOT dilute or mix LANTUS with any other insulin or solution.** It will not work and you may lose blood sugar control, which could be serious.
- **LANTUS** comes as U-100 insulin and contains 100 units of LANTUS per milliliter (mL). One milliliter of U-100 insulin contains 100 units of insulin. (1 mL = 1 cc).

What is Diabetes?

- Your body needs insulin to turn sugar (glucose) into energy. If your body does not make enough insulin, you need to take more insulin so you will not have too much sugar in your blood.
- Insulin injections are important in keeping your diabetes under control. But the way you live, your diet, careful checking of your blood sugar levels, exercise, and planned physical activity, all work with your insulin to help you control your diabetes.

What is LANTUS?

- LANTUS (insulin glargine [recombinant DNA origin]) is a long-acting insulin. . Because Lantus is made by recombinant DNA technology (rDNA) and is chemically different from the insulin made by the human body, it is called an insulin analog. LANTUS is used to treat patients with diabetes for the control of high blood sugar. It is used once a day to lower blood glucose.
- LANTUS is a clear, colorless, sterile solution for injection under the skin (subcutaneously).
- The active ingredient in LANTUS is insulin glargine. The concentration of insulin glargine is 100 units per milliliter (mL), or U-100. LANTUS also contains zinc, metacresol, glycerol, and water for injection as inactive ingredients. Hydrochloric acid and/ or sodium hydroxide may be added to adjust the pH.
- You need a prescription to get LANTUS. Always be sure you receive the right insulin from the pharmacy.

Who should NOT take LANTUS?

Do not take LANTUS if you are allergic to insulin glargine or any of the inactive ingredients in LANTUS. Check with your healthcare provider if you are not sure.

- **Before starting LANTUS, tell your healthcare provider about all your medical conditions including if you:**
  - **have liver or kidney problems.** Your dose may need to be adjusted.
  - **are pregnant or plan to become pregnant.** It is not known if LANTUS may harm your unborn baby. It is very important to maintain control of your blood sugar levels during pregnancy. Your healthcare provider will decide which insulin is best for you during your pregnancy.
  - **are breast-feeding or plan to breast-feed.** It is not known whether LANTUS passes into your milk. Many medicines, including insulin, pass into human milk, and could affect your baby. Talk to your healthcare provider about the best way to feed your baby.
  - **are taking any other medicines including** prescription and non-prescription medicines, vitamins and herbal supplements.

How should I use LANTUS?

See the "Instructions for SoloStar® Use" section for additional information.

- Follow the instructions given by your healthcare provider about the type or types of insulin you are using. Do not make any changes with your insulin unless you have talked to your healthcare provider. Your insulin needs may change because of illness, stress, other medicines, or changes in diet or activity level. Talk to your healthcare provider about how to adjust your insulin dose.
- You may take LANTUS at any time during the day but you must take it at the same time every day.

- Only use LANTUS that is clear and colorless. If your LANTUS is cloudy or slightly colored, return it to your pharmacy for a replacement.
- Follow your healthcare provider's instructions for testing your blood sugar.
- Inject LANTUS under your skin (subcutaneously) in your upper arm, abdomen (stomach area), or thigh (upper leg). Never inject it into a vein or muscle.
- Change (rotate) injection sites within the same body area.
- **NEEDLES AND SOLOSTAR® MUST NOT BE SHARED.**
- Disposable needles should be used only once. Used needle should be placed in sharps containers (such as red biohazard containers), hard plastic containers (such as detergent bottles), or metal containers (such as an empty coffee can). Such containers should be sealed and disposed of properly.

Mixing with LANTUS

- **Do NOT dilute or mix LANTUS with any other insulin or solution.** It will not work as intended and you may lose blood sugar control, which could be serious.

Instructions for SoloStar® Use

It is important to read, understand, and follow the step-by-step instructions in the "SoloStar® Instruction Leaflet" before using SoloStar® disposable insulin Pen. Failure to follow the instructions may result in getting too much or too little insulin. If you have lost your leaflet or have a question, go to www.lantus.com or call 1-800-633-1610.

The following general notes should be taken into consideration before injecting LANTUS:

- Always wash your hands before handling the SoloStar® disposable insulin Pen.
- Always attach a new needle before use. BD Ultra-Fine™ needles† are compatible with SoloStar. These are sold separately and are manufactured by BD.
- Always perform the safety test before use.
- Check the insulin solution in the pen to make sure it is clear, colorless, and free of particles. If it is not, throw it away.
- Do NOT mix or dilute LANTUS with any other insulin or solution. LANTUS will not work if it is mixed or diluted and you may lose blood sugar control, which could be serious.
- Decide on an injection area - either upper arm, thigh, or abdomen. Do not use the same injection site as your last injection.
- After injecting LANTUS, leave the needle in the skin for an additional 10 seconds. Then pull the needle straight out. Gently press on the spot where you injected yourself for a few seconds. **Do not rub the area.**
- Do not drop the SoloStar® disposable insulin Pen.

If your blood glucose reading is high or low, tell your healthcare provider so the dose can be adjusted.

What can affect how much insulin I need?

Illness. Illness may change how much insulin you need. It is a good idea to think ahead and make a "sick day" plan with your healthcare provider in advance so you will be ready when this happens. Be sure to test your blood sugar more often and call your healthcare provider if you are sick.

Medicines. Many medicines can affect your insulin needs. Other medicines, including prescription and non-prescription medicines, vitamins, and herbal supplements, can change the way insulin works. You may need a different dose of insulin when you are taking certain other medicines. **Know all the medicines you take,** including prescription and non-prescription medicines, vitamins and herbal supplements. You may want to keep a list of the medicines you take. You can show this list to your healthcare provider and pharmacists anytime you get a new medicine or refill. Your healthcare provider will tell you if your insulin dose needs to be changed.

Meals. The amount of food you eat can affect your insulin needs. If you eat less food, skip meals, or eat more food than usual, you may need a different dose of insulin. Talk to your healthcare provider if you change your diet so that you know how to adjust your LANTUS and other insulin doses.

Alcohol. Alcohol, including beer and wine, may affect the way LANTUS works and affect your blood sugar levels. Talk to your healthcare provider about drinking alcohol.

Exercise or Activity level. Exercise or activity level may change the way your body uses insulin. Check with your healthcare provider before you start an exercise program because your dose may need to be changed.

Travel. If you travel across time zones, talk with your healthcare provider about how to time your injections. When you travel, wear your medical alert identification. Take extra insulin and supplies with you.

Pregnancy or nursing. The effects of LANTUS on an unborn child or on a nursing baby are unknown. Therefore, tell your healthcare provider if you planning to have a baby, are pregnant, or nursing a baby. Good control of diabetes is especially important during pregnancy and nursing.

What are the possible side effects of LANTUS and other insulins?

Insulins, including LANTUS, can cause hypoglycemia (low blood sugar), hyperglycemia (high blood sugar), allergy, and skin reactions.

Hypoglycemia (low blood sugar):

Hypoglycemia is often called an "insulin reaction" or "low blood sugar". It may happen when you do not have enough sugar in your blood. Common causes of hypoglycemia are illness, emotional or physical stress, too much insulin, too little food or missed meals, and too much exercise or activity.

Early warning signs of hypoglycemia may be different, less noticeable or not noticeable at all in some people. That is why it is important to check your blood sugar as you have been advised by your healthcare provider.

Hypoglycemia can happen with:

- **Taking too much insulin.** This can happen when too much insulin is injected.
- **Not enough carbohydrate (sugar or starch) intake.** This can happen if a meal or snack is missed or delayed.
- **Vomiting or diarrhea** that decreases the amount of sugar absorbed by your body.
- **Intake of alcohol.**
- **Medicines that affect insulin.** Be sure to discuss all your medicines with your healthcare provider. **Do not start any new medicines until you know how they may affect your insulin dose.**
- **Medical conditions that can affect your blood sugar levels or insulin.** These conditions include diseases of the adrenal glands, the pituitary, the thyroid gland, the liver, and the kidney.
- **Too much glucose use by the body.** This can happen if you exercise too much or have a fever.
- **Injecting insulin the wrong way or in the wrong injection area.**

Hypoglycemia can be mild to severe. Its onset may be rapid. Some patients have few or no warning symptoms, including:

- patients with diabetes for a long time
- patients with diabetic neuropathy (nerve problems)
- or patients using certain medicines for high blood pressure or heart problems.

Hypoglycemia may reduce your ability to drive a car or use mechanical equipment and you may risk injury to yourself or others. Severe hypoglycemia can be dangerous and can cause temporary or permanent harm to your heart or brain. **It may cause unconsciousness, seizures, or death.**

Symptoms of hypoglycemia may include:

- anxiety, irritability, restlessness, trouble concentrating, personality changes, mood changes, or other abnormal behavior
- tingling in your hands, feet, lips, or tongue
- dizziness, light-headedness, or drowsiness
- nightmares or trouble sleeping
- headache
- blurred vision
- slurred speech
- palpitations (fast heart beat)
- sweating
- tremor (shaking)
- unsteady gait (walking).

If you have hypoglycemia often or it is hard for you to know if you have the symptoms of hypoglycemia, talk to your healthcare provider.

Mild to moderate hypoglycemia is treated by eating or drinking carbohydrates such as fruit juice, raisins, sugar candies, milk or glucose tablets. Talk to your healthcare provider about the amount of carbohydrates you should eat to treat mild to moderate hypoglycemia.

Severe hypoglycemia may require the help of another person or emergency medical people. A person with hypoglycemia who is unable to take foods or liquids with sugar by mouth, or is unconscious needs medical help fast and will need treatment with a glucagon injection or glucose given intravenously (IV). Without medical help right away, serious reactions or even death could happen.

Hyperglycemia (high blood sugar):

Hyperglycemia happens when you have too much sugar in your blood. Usually, it means there is not enough insulin to break down the food you eat into energy your body can use. Hyperglycemia can be caused by a fever, an infection, stress, eating more than you should, taking less insulin than prescribed, or it can mean your diabetes is getting worse.

Hyperglycemia can happen with:

- **Insufficient (too little) insulin.** This can happen from:
  - - injecting too little or no insulin
  - - incorrect storage (freezing, excessive heat)
  - - use after the expiration date.
- **Too much carbohydrate intake.** This can happen if you eat larger meals, eat more often, or increase the amount of carbohydrate in your meals.

	Not in-use (unopened) Refrigerated	Not in-use (unopened) Room Temperature	In-use (opened) Room Temperature (Do not refrigerate)
3 mL SoloStar® dispoable insulin device	Until expiration date	28 days	28 days

- Medicines that affect insulin. Be sure to discuss all your medicines with your healthcare provider. **Do not start any new medicines until you know how they may affect your insulin dose.**
- **Medical conditions that affect insulin.** These medical conditions include fevers, infections, heart attacks, and stress.
- **Injecting insulin the wrong way or in the wrong injection area.**

Testing your blood or urine often will let you know if you have hyperglycemia. If your tests are often high, tell your healthcare provider so your dose of insulin can be changed. Hyperglycemia can be mild or severe. It can **progress to diabetic ketoacidosis (DKA) or very high glucose levels (hyperosmolar coma) and result in unconsciousness and death.**

Although diabetic ketoacidosis occurs most often in patients with type 1 diabetes, it can also happen in patients with type 2 diabetes who become very sick. Because some patients get few symptoms of hyperglycemia, it is important to check your blood sugar/urine sugar and ketones regularly.

Symptoms of hyperglycemia include:
- confusion or drowsiness
- increased thirst
- decreased appetite, nausea, or vomiting
- rapid heart rate
- increased urination and dehydration (too little fluid in your body).

Symptoms of DKA also include:
- fruity smelling breath
- fast, deep breathing
- stomach area (abdominal) pain.

Severe or continuing hyperglycemia or DKA needs evaluation and treatment right away by your healthcare provider.
Do not use LANTUS to treat diabetic ketoacidosis.
Other possible side effects of LANTUS include:
Serious allergic reactions:
Some times severe, life-threatening allergic reactions can happen with insulin. If you think you are having a severe allergic reaction, get medical help right away. Signs of insulin allergy include:
- rash all over your body
- shortness of breath
- wheezing (trouble breathing)
- fast pulse
- sweating
- low blood pressure.

Reactions at the injection site:
Injecting insulin can cause the following reactions on the skin at the injection site:
- little depression in the skin (lipoatrophy)
- skin thickening (lipohypertrophy)
- red, swelling, itchy skin (injection site reaction)

You can reduce the chance of getting an injection site reaction if you change (rotate) the injection site each time. An injection site reaction should clear up in a few days or a few weeks. If injection site reactions do not go away or keep happening call your healthcare provider.
Tell your healthcare provider if you have any side effects that bother you.
These are not all the side effects of LANTUS. Ask your healthcare provider or pharmacist for more information.

How should I store LANTUS?
- **Unopened SoloStar®:**
Store new unopened SoloStar® disposable insulin pen in a refrigerator (not the freezer) between 36°F to 46°F (2°C to 8°C). Do not freeze LANTUS. Keep LANTUS out of direct heat and light. If a disposable insulin pen has been frozen or overheated, throw it away.

- **Open (In-Use) SoloStar®:**
Once SoloStar® is opened (in-use), SoloStar® should **NOT** be refrigerated but should be kept at room temperature (below 86°F [30°C]) away from direct heat and light. The opened (in-use) SoloStar® kept at room temperature must be discarded after 28 days.

These storage conditions are summarized in the following table:
[See table above]
- Do not use SoloStar® with LANTUS after the expiration date stamped on the label.
- Do not use LANTUS if it is cloudy, colored, or if you see particles.

General Information about LANTUS
- Use LANTUS only to treat your diabetes. **Do not** give or share LANTUS with another person, even if they have diabetes also. It may harm them.
- This leaflet summarizes the most important information about LANTUS. If you would like more information, talk with your healthcare provider. You can ask your healthcare provider or pharmacist for information about LANTUS that is written for healthcare professionals. For more information about LANTUS call 1-800-633-1610 or go to website www.lantus.com.

ADDITIONAL INFORMATION
DIABETES FORECAST is a national magazine designed especially for patients with diabetes and their families and is available by subscription from the American Diabetes Association (ADA), P.O. Box 363, Mt. Morris, IL 61054-0363, 1-800-DIABETES (1-800-342-2383). You may also visit the ADA website at www.diabetes.org.
Another publication, **COUNTDOWN**, is available from the Juvenile Diabetes Research Foundation International (JDRF), 120 Wall Street, 19th Floor, New York, New York 10005, 1-800-JDF-CURE (1-800-533-2873). You may also visit the JDRF website at www.jdf.org.
To get more information about diabetes, check with your healthcare professional or diabetes educator or visit www.DiabetesWatch.com.
Additional information about LANTUS can be obtained by calling 1-800-633-1610 or by visiting www.lantus.com.
Rev. March 2007
sanofi-aventis U.S. LLC
Bridgewater, NJ 08807
©2007 sanofi-aventis U.S. LLC
Lantus® and SoloStar® are a registered trademark of sanofi-aventis U.S. LLC
†The brands listed are the trademarks of their respective owners and are not trademarks of sanofi-aventis U.S. LLC

LANTUS® SOLOSTAR®
(insulin glargine [rDNA origin] injection)
Instruction Leaflet
Your healthcare professional has decided that SoloStar® is right for you. Talk with your healthcare professional about proper injection technique before using SoloStar®.
Read these instructions carefully before using your SoloStar®. If you are not able to follow all the instructions completely on your own, use SoloStar® only if you have help from a person who is able to follow the instructions.
Follow these instructions completely each time you use SoloStar® to ensure that you get an accurate dose. If you do not follow these instructions you may get too much or too little insulin, which may affect your blood glucose.
SoloStar® is a disposable pen for the injection of insulin. Each SoloStar® contains in total 300 units of insulin. You can set doses from 1 to 80 units in steps of 1 unit.
Keep this leaflet for future reference.
If you have any questions about SoloStar® or about diabetes, ask your healthcare professional, go to www.lantus.com or call sanofi aventis at 1-800-633-1610.

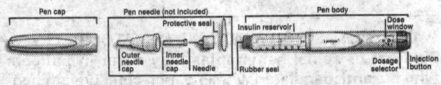

Important information for use of SoloStar®:
- Always attach a new needle before each use. BD Ultra-Fine needles are compatible with SoloStar®. These are sold separately and manufactured by BD. Contact your healthcare professional for further information.
- Always perform the safety test before each injection.
- This pen is only for your use. Do not share it with anyone else.
- If your injection is given by another person, special caution must be taken by this person to avoid accidental needle injury and transmission of infection.
- Never use SoloStar® if it is damaged or if you are not sure that it is working properly.
- Always have a spare SoloStar® in case your SoloStar® is lost or damaged.

Storage Instructions
Please check the leaflet for the insulin for complete instructions on how to store SoloStar®.
If your SoloStar® is in cool storage, take it out 1 to 2 hours before you inject to allow it to warm up. Cold insulin is more painful to inject.
Keep SoloStar® out of the reach and sight of children.
Keep SoloStar® in cool storage (36°F–46°F [2°C–8°C]) until first use. Do not allow it to freeze. Do not put it next to the freezer compartment of your refrigerator, or next to a freezer pack.
Once you take your SoloStar® out of cool storage, for use or as a spare, you can use it for up to 28 days. During this time it can be safely kept at room temperature up to 86°F (30°C). Do not use it after this time. SoloStar® in use must not be stored in a refrigerator.
Do not use SoloStar® after the expiration date printed on the label of the pen or on the carton.

Protect SoloStar® from light.
Discard your used SoloStar® as required by your local authorities.
Maintenance
Protect your SoloStar® from dust and dirt.
You can clean the outside of your SoloStar® by wiping it with a damp cloth.
Do not soak, wash or lubricate the pen as this may damage it.
Your SoloStar® is designed to work accurately and safely. It should be handled with care. Avoid situations where SoloStar® might be damaged. If you are concerned that your SoloStar® may be damaged, use a new one.
Step 1. Check the insulin
- A. Check the label on your SoloStar® to make sure you have the correct insulin. The Lantus® SoloStar® is grey with a purple injection button.
- B. Take off the pen cap.
- C. Check the appearance of your insulin. Lantus® is a clear insulin. Do not use this SoloStar® if the insulin is cloudy, colored or has particles.
Step 2. Attach the needle
Always use a new sterile needle for each injection. This helps prevent contamination, and potential needle blocks.
- A. Wipe the Rubber Seal with alcohol.
- B. Remove the protective seal from a new needle.
- C. Line up the needle with the pen, and keep it straight as you attach it (screw or push on, depending on the needle type).

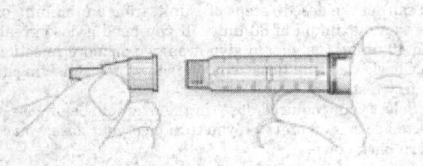

- If the needle is not kept straight while you attach it, it can damage the rubber seal and cause leakage, or break the needle.

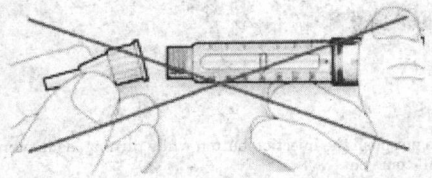

Step 3. Perform a Safety test
Always perform the Safety test before each injection. Performing the safety test ensures that you get an accurate dose by:
- ensuring that pen and needle work properly
- removing air bubbles
- A. Select a dose of 2 units by turning the dosage selector.

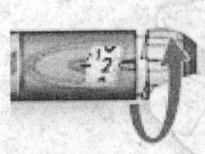

- B. Take off the outer needle cap and keep it to remove the used needle after injection. Take off the inner needle cap and discard it.
[See first figure at top of next page]
- C. Hold the pen with the needle pointing upwards.
- D. Tap the insulin reservoir so that any air bubbles rise up towards the needle.
- E. Press the injection button all the way in. Check if insulin comes out of the needle tip.
[See second figure on next page]

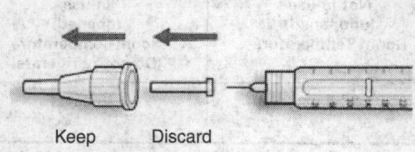

Keep   Discard

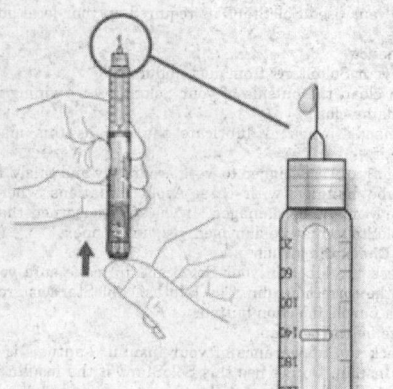

You may have to perform the safety test several times before insulin is seen.
- If no insulin comes out, check for air bubbles and repeat the safety test two more times to remove them.
- If still no insulin comes out, the needle may be blocked. Change the needle and try again.
- If no insulin comes out after changing the needle, your SoloStar® may be damaged. Do not use this SoloStar®.

Step 4. Select the dose
You can set the dose in steps of 1 unit, from a minimum of 1 unit to a maximum of 80 units. If you need a dose greater than 80 units, you should give it as two or more injections.
- **A.** Check that the dose window shows "0" following the safety test.
- **B.** Select your required dose (in the example below, the selected dose is 30 units). If you turn past your dose, you can turn back down.

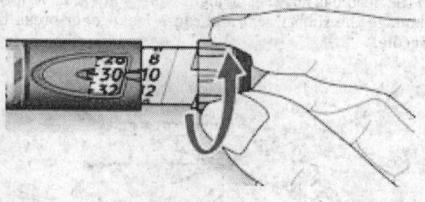

- Do not push the injection button while turning, as insulin will come out.
- You cannot turn the dosage selector past the number of units left in the pen. Do not force the dosage selector to turn. In this case, either you can inject what is remaining in the pen and complete your dose with a new SoloStar® or use a new SoloStar® for your full dose.

Step 5. Inject the dose
- **A.** Use the injection method as instructed by your healthcare professional.
- **B.** Insert the needle into the skin.

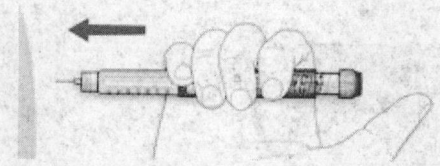

- **C.** Deliver the dose by pressing the injection button in all the way. The number in the dose window will return to "0" as you inject.
[See figure at top of next column]
- **D.** Keep the injection button pressed all the way in. **Slowly count to 10 before you withdraw the needle from the skin.** This ensures that the full dose will be delivered.

Step 6. Remove and discard the needle
Always remove the needle after each injection and store SoloStar® without a needle attached. This helps prevent:
- Contamination and/or infection

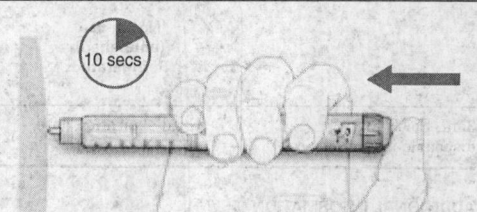

10 secs

- Entry of air into the insulin reservoir and leakage of insulin, which can cause inaccurate dosing.
- **A.** Put the outer needle cap back on the needle, and use it to unscrew the needle from the pen. To reduce the risk of accidental needle injury, never replace the inner needle cap.
  - If your injection is given by another person, special caution must be taken by this person when removing and disposing the needle. Follow recommended safety measures for removal and disposal of needles (e.g. a one handed capping technique) in order to reduce the risk of accidental needle injury and transmission of infectious diseases.
- **B.** Dispose of the needle safely. Used needles should be placed in sharps containers (such as red biohazard containers), hard plastic containers (such as detergent bottles), or metal containers (such as an empty coffee can). Such containers should be sealed and disposed of properly.
  If you are giving an injection to a third person, you should remove the needle in an approved manner to avoid needle-stick injuries.
- **C.** Always put the pen cap back on the pen, then store the pen until your next injection.

sanofi-aventis U.S. LLC
Bridgewater, NJ 08807
Country of Origin: Germany
Date of revision:
March 2007
©2007 sanofi-aventis U.S. LLC
Shown in Product Identification Guide, page 319

LOVENOX®
[lōōvə-nŏks]   ℞
(enoxaparin sodium injection)
for subcutaneous and intravenous use

HIGHLIGHTS OF PRESCRIBING INFORMATION
These highlights do not include all the information needed to use Lovenox safely and effectively. See full prescribing information for Lovenox.
Lovenox (enoxaparin sodium injection) for subcutaneous and intravenous use
Initial U.S. Approval: 1993

WARNING: SPINAL/EPIDURAL HEMATOMA
Epidural or spinal hematomas may occur in patients who are anticoagulated with low molecular weight heparins (LMWH) or heparinoids and are receiving neuraxial anesthesia or undergoing spinal puncture. These hematomas may result in long-term or permanent paralysis. Consider these risks when scheduling patients for spinal procedures. Factors that can increase the risk of developing epidural or spinal hematomas in these patients include:
• **Use of indwelling epidural catheters**
• **Concomitant use of other drugs that affect hemostasis, such as non-steroidal anti-inflammatory drugs (NSAIDs), platelet inhibitors, other anticoagulants**
• **A history of traumatic or repeated epidural or spinal punctures**
• **A history of spinal deformity or spinal surgery.**
Monitor patients frequently for signs and symptoms of neurological impairment. If neurological compromise is noted, urgent treatment is necessary.
Consider the benefits and risks before neuraxial intervention in patients anticoagulated or to be anticoagulated for thromboprophylaxis [see *Warnings and Precautions (5.1)* and *Drug Interactions (7)*].

RECENT MAJOR CHANGES

Boxed Warning, Warnings and Precautions (5.1)   (12/2009)

INDICATIONS AND USAGE
Lovenox is a low molecular weight heparin [LMWH] indicated for:
- Prophylaxis of deep vein thrombosis (DVT) in abdominal surgery, hip replacement surgery, knee replacement surgery, or medical patients with severely restricted mobility during acute illness (1.1)

- Inpatient treatment of acute DVT with or without pulmonary embolism (1.2)
- Outpatient treatment of acute DVT without pulmonary embolism. (1.2)
- Prophylaxis of ischemic complications of unstable angina and non-Q-wave myocardial infarction [MI] (1.3)
- Treatment of acute ST-segment elevation myocardial infarction [STEMI] managed medically or with subsequent percutaneous coronary intervention [PCI] (1.4)

DOSAGE AND ADMINISTRATION

Indication	Standard Regimen (2.1, 2.3)
DVT prophylaxis in abdominal surgery	40 mg SC once daily up to 12 days
DVT prophylaxis in knee replacement surgery	30 mg SC every 12 hours up to 14 days
DVT prophylaxis in hip replacement surgery	30 mg SC every 12 hours or 40 mg SC once daily up to 14 days
DVT prophylaxis in medical patients	40 mg SC once daily up to 14 days
Inpatient treatment of acute DVT with or without pulmonary embolism	1 mg/kg SC every 12 hours or 1.5 mg/kg SC once daily (with warfarin) up to 17 days
Outpatient treatment of acute DVT without pulmonary embolism	1 mg/kg SC every 12 hours (with warfarin) up to 17 days
Unstable angina and non-Q-wave MI	1 mg/kg SC every 12 hours (with aspirin) 2 to 8 days
Acute STEMI in patients <75 years of age [For dosing in subsequent PCI, see *Dosage and Administration (2.1)*]	30 mg single IV bolus plus a 1 mg/kg SC dose followed by 1 mg/kg SC every 12 hours at least 8 days (with aspirin)
Acute STEMI in patients ≥75 years of age	0.75 mg/kg SC every 12 hours (no bolus) at least 8 days (with aspirin)

- Adjust the dose for patients with severe renal impairment (2.2, 8.7)

DOSAGE FORMS AND STRENGTHS
100 mg/mL concentration (3.1):
- Prefilled syringes: 30 mg/0.3 mL, 40 mg/0.4 mL
- Graduated prefilled syringes: 60 mg/0.6 mL, 80 mg/0.8 mL, 100 mg/1 mL
- Multiple-dose vial: 300 mg/3 mL
150 mg/mL concentration (3.2):
- Graduated prefilled syringes: 120 mg/0.8 mL, 150 mg/1 mL

CONTRAINDICATIONS
- Active major bleeding (4)
- Thrombocytopenia with a positive *in vitro* test for antiplatelet antibody in the presence of enoxaparin sodium (4)
- Hypersensitivity to enoxaparin sodium (4)
- Hypersensitivity to heparin or pork products (4)
- Hypersensitivity to benzyl alcohol [for multi-dose formulation only] (4)

WARNINGS AND PRECAUTIONS
- Increased risk of hemorrhage: Use with caution in patients at risk (5.1)
- Percutaneous coronary revascularization: Obtain hemostasis at the puncture site before sheath removal (5.2)
- Concomitant medical conditions: Use with caution in patients with bleeding diathesis, uncontrolled arterial hypertension or history of recent gastrointestinal ulceration, diabetic retinopathy, renal dysfunction, or hemorrhage (5.3)
- History of heparin-induced thrombocytopenia: Use with caution (5.4)
- Thrombocytopenia: Monitor thrombocytopenia closely (5.5)
- Interchangeability with other heparins: Do not exchange with heparin or other LMWHs (5.6)
- Pregnant women with mechanical prosthetic heart valves and their fetuses, may be at increased risk and may need more frequent monitoring and dosage adjustment (5.7)

ADVERSE REACTIONS
Most common adverse reactions (>1%) were bleeding, anemia, thrombocytopenia, elevation of serum aminotransferase, diarrhea, and nausea (6.1).
To report SUSPECTED ADVERSE REACTIONS, contact sanofi-aventis at 1-800-633-1610 or FDA at 1-800-FDA-1088 or *www.fda.gov/medwatch*.

—DRUG INTERACTIONS—

Discontinue agents which may enhance hemorrhage risk prior to initiation of Lovenox or conduct close clinical and laboratory monitoring (5.9, 7)

—USE IN SPECIFIC POPULATIONS—

- Severe Renal Impairment: Adjust dose for patients with creatinine clearance <30mL/min (2.2, 8.7)
- Geriatric Patients: Monitor for increased risk of bleeding (8.5)
- Patients with mechanical heart valves: Not adequately studied (8.6)
- Hepatic Impairment: Use with caution. (8.8)
- Low-Weight Patients: Observe for signs of bleeding (8.9)

See 17 for PATIENT COUNSELING INFORMATION

Revised: 12/2009

FULL PRESCRIBING INFORMATION

WARNING: SPINAL/EPIDURAL HEMATOMAS

Epidural or spinal hematomas may occur in patients who are anticoagulated with low molecular weight heparins (LMWH) or heparinoids and are receiving neuraxial anesthesia or undergoing spinal puncture. These hematomas may result in long-term or permanent paralysis. Consider these risks when scheduling patients for spinal procedures. Factors that can increase the risk of developing epidural or spinal hematomas in these patients include:

- Use of indwelling epidural catheters
- Concomitant use of other drugs that affect hemostasis, such non-steroidal anti-inflammatory drugs (NSAIDs), platelet inhibitors, other anticoagulants.
- A history of traumatic or repeated epidural or spinal punctures
- A history of spinal deformity or spinal surgery

Monitor patients frequently for signs and symptoms of neurological impairment. If neurological compromise is noted, urgent treatment is necessary.

Consider the benefits and risks before neuraxial intervention in patients anticoagulated or to be anticoagulated for thromboprophylaxis [see *Warnings and Precautions (5.1)* and *Drug Interactions (7)*].

---

1 INDICATIONS AND USAGE

1.1 Prophylaxis of Deep Vein Thrombosis

Lovenox® is indicated for the prophylaxis of deep vein thrombosis (DVT), which may lead to pulmonary embolism (PE):

- in patients undergoing abdominal surgery who are at risk for thromboembolic complications [see *Clinical Studies (14.1)*].
- in patients undergoing hip replacement surgery, during and following hospitalization.
- in patients undergoing knee replacement surgery.
- in medical patients who are at risk for thromboembolic complications due to severely restricted mobility during acute illness.

1.2 Treatment of Acute Deep Vein Thrombosis

Lovenox is indicated for:

- the **inpatient treatment** of acute deep vein thrombosis **with or without pulmonary embolism**, when administered in conjunction with warfarin sodium.
- the **outpatient treatment** of acute deep vein thrombosis **without pulmonary embolism** when administered in conjunction with warfarin sodium.

1.3 Prophylaxis of Ischemic Complications of Unstable Angina and Non-Q-Wave Myocardial Infarction

Lovenox is indicated for the prophylaxis of ischemic complications of unstable angina and non-q-wave myocardial infarction, when concurrently administered with aspirin.

1.4 Treatment of Acute ST-Segment Elevation Myocardial Infarction

Lovenox, when administered concurrently with aspirin, has been shown to reduce the rate of the combined endpoint of recurrent myocardial infarction or death in patients with acute ST-segment elevation myocardial infarction (STEMI) receiving thrombolysis and being managed medically or with percutaneous coronary intervention (PCI).

2 DOSAGE AND ADMINISTRATION

All patients should be evaluated for a bleeding disorder before administration of Lovenox, unless the medication is needed urgently. Since coagulation parameters are unsuitable for monitoring Lovenox activity, routine monitoring of coagulation parameters is not required [see *Warnings and Precautions (5.9)*].

For subcutaneous use, Lovenox should not be mixed with other injections or infusions. For intravenous use (*i.e.*, for treatment of acute STEMI), Lovenox can be mixed with normal saline solution (0.9%) or 5% dextrose in water.

Lovenox is not intended for intramuscular administration.

2.1 Adult Dosage

Abdominal Surgery: In patients undergoing abdominal surgery who are at risk for thromboembolic complications, the recommended dose of Lovenox is **40 mg once a day** administered by SC injection with the initial dose given 2 hours prior to surgery. The usual duration of administration is 7 to 10 days; up to 12 days administration has been administered in clinical trials.

Hip or Knee Replacement Surgery: In patients undergoing hip or knee replacement surgery, the recommended dose of Lovenox is **30 mg every 12 hours** administered by SC injection. Provided that hemostasis has been established, the initial dose should be given 12 to 24 hours after surgery. For hip replacement surgery, a dose of **40 mg once a day** SC, given initially 12 (±3) hours prior to surgery, may be considered. Following the initial phase of thromboprophylaxis in hip replacement surgery patients, it is recommended that

continued prophylaxis with Lovenox 40 mg once a day be administered by SC injection for 3 weeks. The usual duration of administration is 7 to 10 days; up to 14 days administration has been administered in clinical trials.

Medical Patients During Acute Illness: In medical patients at risk for thromboembolic complications due to severely restricted mobility during acute illness, the recommended dose of Lovenox is **40 mg once a day** administered by SC injection. The usual duration of administration is 6 to 11 days; up to 14 days of Lovenox has been administered in the controlled clinical trial.

Treatment of Deep Vein Thrombosis with or without Pulmonary Embolism: In **outpatient treatment**, patients with acute deep vein thrombosis without pulmonary embolism who can be treated at home, the recommended dose of Lovenox is **1 mg/kg every 12 hours** administered SC. In **inpatient (hospital) treatment**, patients with acute deep vein thrombosis with pulmonary embolism or patients with acute deep vein thrombosis without pulmonary embolism (who are not candidates for outpatient treatment), the recommended dose of Lovenox is **1 mg/kg every 12 hours** administered SC **or 1.5 mg/kg once a day** administered SC at the same time every day. In both outpatient and inpatient (hospital) treatments, warfarin sodium therapy should be initiated when appropriate (usually within 72 hours of Lovenox). Lovenox should be continued for a minimum of 5 days and until a therapeutic oral anticoagulant effect has been achieved (International Normalization Ratio 2.0 to 3.0). The average duration of administration is 7 days; up to 17 days of Lovenox administration has been administered in controlled clinical trials.

Unstable Angina and Non-Q-Wave Myocardial Infarction: In patients with unstable angina or non-q-wave myocardial infarction, the recommended dose of Lovenox is **1 mg/kg** administered SC **every 12 hours** in conjunction with oral aspirin therapy (100 to 325 mg once daily). Treatment with Lovenox should be prescribed for a minimum of 2 days and continued until clinical stabilization. The usual duration of treatment is 2 to 8 days; up to 12.5 days of Lovenox has been administered in clinical trials [see *Warnings and Precautions (5.2)* and *Clinical Studies (14.5)*].

Treatment of Acute ST-Segment Elevation Myocardial Infarction: In patients with acute ST-segment elevation myocardial infarction, the recommended dose of Lovenox is **a single IV bolus of 30 mg** plus a 1 mg/kg SC dose followed by 1 mg/kg administered SC every 12 hours (maximum 100 mg for the first two doses only, followed by 1 mg/kg dosing for the remaining doses). Dosage adjustments are recommended in patients ≥75 years of age [see *Dosage and Administration (2.3)*]. All patients should receive aspirin as soon as they are identified as having STEMI and maintained with 75 to 325 mg once daily unless contraindicated.

When administered in conjunction with a thrombolytic (fibrin-specific or non-fibrin specific), Lovenox should be given between 15 minutes before and 30 minutes after the start of fibrinolytic therapy. In the pivotal clinical study, the Lovenox treatment duration was 8 days or until hospital discharge, whichever came first. An optimal duration of treatment is not known, but it is likely to be longer than 8 days.

For patients managed with percutaneous coronary intervention (PCI): If the last Lovenox SC administration was given less than 8 hours before balloon inflation, no additional dosing is needed. If the last Lovenox SC administration was given more than 8 hours before balloon inflation, an IV bolus of 0.3 mg/kg of Lovenox should be administered [see *Warnings and Precautions (5.2)*].

2.2 Renal Impairment

Although no dose adjustment is recommended in patients with moderate (creatinine clearance 30–50 mL/min) and mild (creatinine clearance 50–80 mL/min) renal impairment, all such patients should be observed carefully for signs and symptoms of bleeding.

The recommended prophylaxis and treatment dosage regimens for patients with severe renal impairment (creatinine clearance <30 mL/min) are described in Table 1 [see *Use in Specific Populations (8.6)* and *Clinical Pharmacology (12.3)*].

Table 1

Dosage Regimens for Patients with Severe Renal Impairment (creatinine clearance <30mL/minute)	
Indication	**Dosage Regimen**
Prophylaxis in abdominal surgery	30 mg administered SC once daily
Prophylaxis in hip or knee replacement surgery	30 mg administered SC once daily

Prophylaxis in medical patients during acute illness	30 mg administered SC once daily
Inpatient treatment of acute deep vein thrombosis with or without pulmonary embolism, when administered in conjunction with warfarin sodium	1 mg/kg administered SC once daily
Outpatient treatment of acute deep vein thrombosis without pulmonary embolism, when administered in conjunction with warfarin sodium	1 mg/kg administered SC once daily
Prophylaxis of ischemic complications of unstable angina and non-Q-wave myocardial infarction, when concurrently administered with aspirin	1 mg/kg administered SC once daily
Treatment of acute ST-segment elevation myocardial infarction in patients <75 years of age, when administered in conjunction with aspirin	30 mg single IV bolus plus a 1 mg/kg SC dose followed by 1 mg/kg administered SC once daily.
Treatment of acute ST-segment elevation myocardial infarction in geriatric patients ≥75 years of age, when administered in conjunction with aspirin	1 mg/kg administered SC once daily (**no** initial bolus)

2.3 Geriatric Patients with Acute ST-Segment Elevation Myocardial Infarction

For treatment of acute ST-segment elevation myocardial infarction in geriatric patients ≥75 years of age, **do not use an initial IV bolus**. Initiate dosing with **0.75 mg/kg SC every 12 hours (maximum 75 mg for the first two doses only, followed by 0.75 mg/kg dosing for the remaining doses)** [see *Use in Specific Populations (8.5)* and *Clinical Pharmacology (12.3)*].
No dose adjustment is necessary for other indications in geriatric patients unless kidney function is impaired [see *Dosage and Administration (2.2)*].

2.4 Administration

Lovenox is a clear, colorless to pale yellow sterile solution, and as with other parenteral drug products, should be inspected visually for particulate matter and discoloration prior to administration.
The use of a tuberculin syringe or equivalent is recommended when using Lovenox multiple-dose vials to assure withdrawal of the appropriate volume of drug.
Lovenox must not be administered by intramuscular injection. Lovenox is intended for use under the guidance of a physician.
For subcutaneous administration, patients may self-inject only if their physicians determine that it is appropriate and with medical follow-up, as necessary. Proper training in subcutaneous injection technique (with or without the assistance of an injection device) should be provided.
Subcutaneous Injection Technique: Patients should be lying down and Lovenox administered by deep SC injection. To avoid the loss of drug when using the 30 and 40 mg prefilled syringes, do not expel the air bubble from the syringe before the injection. Administration should be alternated between the left and right anterolateral and left and right posterolateral abdominal wall. The whole length of the needle should be introduced into a skin fold held between the thumb and forefinger; the skin fold should be held throughout the injection. To minimize bruising, do not rub the injection site after completion of the injection.
Lovenox prefilled syringes and graduated prefilled syringes are for single, one-time use only and are available with a system that shields the needle after injection.
1. Remove the needle shield by pulling it straight off the syringe (see Figure A). If adjusting the dose is required, the dose adjustment must be done prior to injecting the prescribed dose to the patient.
[See figure A at top of next column]
2. Inject using standard technique, pushing the plunger to the bottom of the syringe (see Figure B).
[See figure B in next column]
3. Remove the syringe from the injection site keeping your finger on the plunger rod (see Figure C).
[See figure C in next column]

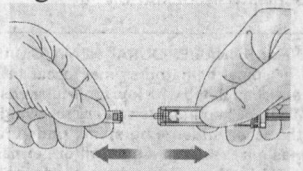

Figure A

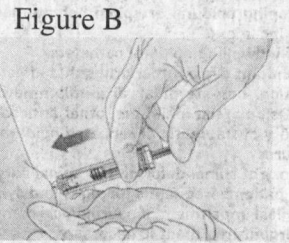

Figure B

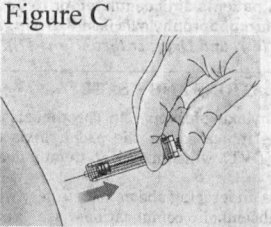

Figure C

4. Orient the needle away from you and others, and activate the safety system by firmly pushing the plunger rod. The protective sleeve will automatically cover the needle and an audible "click" will be heard to confirm shield activation (see Figure D).

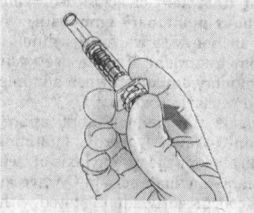

Figure D

5. Immediately dispose of the syringe in the nearest sharps container (see Figure E).

Figure E

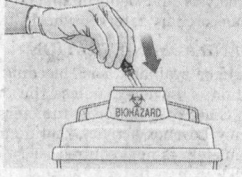

NOTE:
• The safety system can only be activated once the syringe has been emptied.
• Activation of the safety system must be done only after removing the needle from the patient's skin.
• Do not replace the needle shield after injection.
• The safety system should not be sterilized.
Activation of the safety system may cause minimal splatter of fluid. For optimal safety activate the system while orienting it downwards away from yourself and others.
Intravenous (Bolus) Injection Technique: For intravenous injection, the multiple-dose vial should be used. Lovenox should be administered through an intravenous line. Lovenox should not be mixed or co-administered with other medications. To avoid the possible mixture of Lovenox with other drugs, the intravenous access chosen should be flushed with a sufficient amount of saline or dextrose solution prior to and following the intravenous bolus administration of Lovenox to clear the port of drug. Lovenox may be safely administered with normal saline solution (0.9%) or 5% dextrose in water.

3 DOSAGE FORMS AND STRENGTHS
Lovenox is available in two concentrations:
3.1 100 mg/mL Concentration

-Prefilled Syringes	30 mg/0.3 mL, 40 mg/0.4 mL
-Graduated Prefilled Syringes	60 mg/0.6 mL, 80 mg/0.8 mL, 100 mg/1 mL
-Multiple-Dose Vials	300 mg/3 mL

3.2 150 mg/mL Concentration

-Graduated Prefilled Syringes	120 mg/0.8 mL, 150 mg/1 mL

4 CONTRAINDICATIONS
• Active major bleeding
• Thrombocytopenia associated with a positive *in vitro* test for anti-platelet antibody in the presence of enoxaparin sodium
• Known hypersensitivity to enoxaparin sodium (*e.g.*, pruritus, urticaria, anaphylactic/anaphylactoid reactions) [see *Adverse Reactions (6.2)*]
• Known hypersensitivity to heparin or pork products
• Known hypersensitivity to benzyl alcohol (which is in only the multi-dose formulation of Lovenox) [see *Warnings and Precautions (5.8)*]

5 WARNINGS AND PRECAUTIONS
5.1 Increased Risk of Hemorrhage
Cases of epidural or spinal hematomas have been reported with the associated use of Lovenox and spinal/epidural anesthesia or spinal puncture resulting in long-term or permanent paralysis. The risk of these events is higher with the use of post-operative indwelling epidural catheters, with the concomitant use of additional drugs affecting hemostasis such as NSAIDs, with traumatic or repeated epidural or spinal puncture, or in patients with a history of spinal surgery or spinal deformity [see *Boxed Warning, Adverse Reactions (6.2)* and *Drug Interactions (7)*].
Lovenox should be used with extreme caution in conditions with increased risk of hemorrhage, such as bacterial endocarditis, congenital or acquired bleeding disorders, active ulcerative and angiodysplastic gastrointestinal disease, hemorrhagic stroke, or shortly after brain, spinal, or ophthalmological surgery, or in patients treated concomitantly with platelet inhibitors.
Major hemorrhages including retroperitoneal and intracranial bleeding have been reported. Some of these cases have been fatal.
Bleeding can occur at any site during therapy with Lovenox. An unexplained fall in hematocrit or blood pressure should lead to a search for a bleeding site.
5.2 Percutaneous Coronary Revascularization Procedures
To minimize the risk of bleeding following the vascular instrumentation during the treatment of unstable angina, non-Q-wave myocardial infarction and acute ST-segment elevation myocardial infarction, adhere precisely to the intervals recommended between Lovenox doses. It is important to achieve hemostasis at the puncture site after PCI. In case a closure device is used, the sheath can be removed immediately. If a manual compression method is used, sheath should be removed 6 hours after the last IV/SC Lovenox. If the treatment with enoxaparin sodium is to be continued, the next scheduled dose should be given no sooner than 6 to 8 hours after sheath removal. The site of the procedure should be observed for signs of bleeding or hematoma formation [see *Dosage and Administration (2.1)*].
5.3 Use of Lovenox with Concomitant Medical Conditions
Lovenox should be used with care in patients with a bleeding diathesis, uncontrolled arterial hypertension or a history of recent gastrointestinal ulceration, diabetic retinopathy, renal dysfunction and hemorrhage.
5.4 History of Heparin-Induced Thrombocytopenia
Lovenox should be used with extreme caution in patients with a history of heparin-induced thrombocytopenia.
5.5 Thrombocytopenia
Thrombocytopenia can occur with the administration of Lovenox.
Moderate thrombocytopenia (platelet counts between 100,000/mm³ and 50,000/mm³) occurred at a rate of 1.3% in patients given Lovenox, 1.2% in patients given heparin, and 0.7% in patients given placebo in clinical trials.
Platelet counts less than 50,000/mm³ occurred at a rate of 0.1% in patients given Lovenox, in 0.2% of patients given heparin, and 0.4% of patients given placebo in the same trials.
Thrombocytopenia of any degree should be monitored closely. If the platelet count falls below 100,000/mm³,

Lovenox should be discontinued. Cases of heparin-induced thrombocytopenia with thrombosis have also been observed in clinical practice. Some of these cases were complicated by organ infarction, limb ischemia, or death [see *Warnings and Precautions (5.4)*].

5.6 Interchangeability with Other Heparins
Lovenox cannot be used interchangeably (unit for unit) with heparin or other low molecular weight heparins as they differ in manufacturing process, molecular weight distribution, anti-Xa and anti-IIa activities, units, and dosage. Each of these medicines has its own instructions for use.

5.7 Pregnant Women with Mechanical Prosthetic Heart Valves
The use of Lovenox for thromboprophylaxis in pregnant women with mechanical prosthetic heart valves has not been adequately studied. In a clinical study of pregnant women with mechanical prosthetic heart valves given enoxaparin (1 mg/kg twice daily) to reduce the risk of thromboembolism, 2 of 8 women developed clots resulting in blockage of the valve and leading to maternal and fetal death. Although a causal relationship has not been established these deaths may have been due to therapeutic failure or inadequate anticoagulation. No patients in the heparin/warfarin group (0 of 4 women) died. There also have been isolated postmarketing reports of valve thrombosis in pregnant women with mechanical prosthetic heart valves while receiving enoxaparin for thromboprophylaxis. Women with mechanical prosthetic heart valves may be at higher risk for thromboembolism during pregnancy, and, when pregnant, have a higher rate of fetal loss from stillbirth, spontaneous abortion and premature delivery. Therefore, frequent monitoring of peak and trough anti-Factor Xa levels, and adjusting of dosage may be needed [see *Use in Specific Populations (8.6)*].

5.8 Benzyl Alcohol
Lovenox multiple-dose vials contain benzyl alcohol as a preservative. The administration of medications containing benzyl alcohol as a preservative to premature neonates has been associated with a fatal "gasping syndrome". Because benzyl alcohol may cross the placenta, Lovenox multiple-dose vials, preserved with benzyl alcohol, should be used with caution in pregnant women and only if clearly needed [see *Use in Specific Populations (8.1)*].

5.9 Laboratory Tests
Periodic complete blood counts, including platelet count, and stool occult blood tests are recommended during the course of treatment with Lovenox. When administered at recommended prophylaxis doses, routine coagulation tests such as Prothrombin Time (PT) and Activated Partial Thromboplastin Time (aPTT) are relatively insensitive measures of Lovenox activity and, therefore, unsuitable for monitoring. Anti-Factor Xa may be used to monitor the anticoagulant effect of Lovenox in patients with significant renal impairment. If during Lovenox therapy abnormal coagulation parameters or bleeding should occur, anti-Factor Xa levels may be used to monitor the anticoagulant effects of Lovenox [see *Clinical Pharmacology (12.3)*].

6 ADVERSE REACTIONS
6.1 Clinical Trials Experience
The following serious adverse reactions are also discussed in other sections of the labeling:
- Spinal/epidural hematoma [see *Boxed Warning and Warnings and Precautions (5.1)*]
- Increased Risk of Hemorrhage [see *Warnings and Precautions (5.1)*]
- Thrombocytopenia [see *Warnings and Precautions (5.5)*]

Because clinical studies are conducted under widely varying conditions, adverse reaction rates observed in the clinical studies of a drug cannot be directly compared to rates in the clinical studies of another drug and may not reflect the rates observed in practice.

During clinical development for the approved indications, 15,918 patients were exposed to enoxaparin sodium. These included 1,228 for prophylaxis of deep vein thrombosis following abdominal surgery in patients at risk for thromboembolic complications, 1,368 for prophylaxis of deep vein thrombosis following hip or knee replacement surgery, 711 for prophylaxis of deep vein thrombosis in medical patients with severely restricted mobility during acute illness, 1,578 for prophylaxis of ischemic complications in unstable angina and non-Q-wave myocardial infarction, 10,176 for treatment of acute ST-elevation myocardial infarction, and 857 for treatment of deep vein thrombosis with or without pulmonary embolism. Enoxaparin sodium doses in the clinical trials for prophylaxis of deep vein thrombosis following abdominal or hip or knee replacement surgery or in medical patients with severely restricted mobility during acute illness ranged from 40 mg SC once daily to 30 mg SC twice daily. In the clinical studies for prophylaxis of ischemic complications of unstable angina and non-Q-wave myocardial infarction doses were 1 mg/kg every 12 hours and in the clinical studies for treatment of acute ST-segment elevation myocardial infarction enoxaparin sodium doses were a 30 mg IV bolus followed by 1 mg/kg every 12 hours SC.

Table 3 Major Bleeding Episodes Following Hip or Knee Replacement Surgery*

Indications	Dosing Regimen		
	Lovenox 40 mg q.d. SC	Lovenox 30 mg q12h SC	Heparin 15,000 U/24h SC
Hip Replacement Surgery without Extended Prophylaxis†		n = 786 31 (4%)	n = 541 32 (6%)
Hip Replacement Surgery with Extended Prophylaxis			
Peri-operative Period‡	n = 288 4 (2%)		
Extended Prophylaxis Period§	n = 221 0 (0%)		
Knee Replacement Surgery without Extended Prophylaxis†		n = 294 3 (1%)	n = 225 3 (1%)

* Bleeding complications were considered major: (1) if the hemorrhage caused a significant clinical event, or (2) if accompanied by a hemoglobin decrease ≥ 2 g/dL or transfusion of 2 or more units of blood products. Retroperitoneal and intracranial hemorrhages were always considered major. In the knee replacement surgery trials, intraocular hemorrhages were also considered major hemorrhages.
† Lovenox 30 mg every 12 hours SC initiated 12 to 24 hours after surgery and continued for up to 14 days after surgery
‡ Lovenox 40 mg SC once a day initiated up to 12 hours prior to surgery and continued for up to 7 days after surgery
§ Lovenox 40 mg SC once a day for up to 21 days after discharge

Hemorrhage
The incidence of major hemorrhagic complications during Lovenox treatment has been low.
The following rates of major bleeding events have been reported during clinical trials with Lovenox [see Tables 2 to 7].

Table 2 Major Bleeding Episodes Following Abdominal and Colorectal Surgery*

Indications	Dosing Regimen	
	Lovenox 40 mg q.d. SC	Heparin 5000 U q8h SC
Abdominal Surgery	n = 555 23 (4%)	n = 560 16 (3%)
Colorectal Surgery	n = 673 28 (4%)	n = 674 21 (3%)

* Bleeding complications were considered major: (1) if the hemorrhage caused a significant clinical event, or (2) if accompanied by a hemoglobin decrease ≥ 2 g/dL or transfusion of 2 or more units of blood products. Retroperitoneal, intraocular, and intracranial hemorrhages were always considered major.

[See table 3 above]
NOTE: At no time point were the 40 mg once a day pre-operative and the 30 mg every 12 hours post-operative hip replacement surgery prophylactic regimens compared in clinical trials.
Injection site hematomas during the extended prophylaxis period after hip replacement surgery occurred in 9% of the Lovenox patients versus 1.8% of the placebo patients.

Table 4 Major Bleeding Episodes in Medical Patients with Severely Restricted Mobility During Acute Illness*

Indications	Dosing Regimen		
	Lovenox† 20 mg q.d. SC	Lovenox† 40 mg q.d. SC	Placebo†
Medical Patients During Acute Illness	n = 351 1 (<1%)	n = 360 3 (<1%)	n = 362 2 (<1%)

* Bleeding complications were considered major: (1) if the hemorrhage caused a significant clinical event, (2) if the hemorrhage caused a decrease in hemoglobin ≥ 2 g/dL or transfusion of 2 or more units of blood products. Retroperitoneal and intracranial hemorrhages were always considered major although none were reported during the trial.
† The rates represent major bleeding on study medication up to 24 hours after last dose.

Table 5 Major Bleeding Episodes in Deep Vein Thrombosis with or without Pulmonary Embolism Treatment*

Indication	Dosing Regimen†		
	Lovenox 1.5 mg/kg q.d. SC	Lovenox 1 mg/kg q12h SC	Heparin aPTT Adjusted IV Therapy
Treatment of DVT and PE	n = 298 5 (2%)	n = 559 9 (2%)	n = 554 9 (2%)

* Bleeding complications were considered major: (1) if the hemorrhage caused a significant clinical event, or (2) if accompanied by a hemoglobin decrease ≥ 2 g/dL or transfusion of 2 or more units of blood products. Retroperitoneal, intraocular, and intracranial hemorrhages were always considered major.
† All patients also received warfarin sodium (dose-adjusted according to PT to achieve an INR of 2.0 to 3.0) commencing within 72 hours of Lovenox or standard heparin therapy and continuing for up to 90 days.

Table 6 Major Bleeding Episodes in Unstable Angina and Non-Q-Wave Myocardial Infarction

Indication	Dosing Regimen	
	Lovenox* 1 mg/kg q12h SC	Heparin* aPTT Adjusted IV Therapy
Unstable Angina and Non-Q-Wave MI†‡	n = 1578 17 (1%)	n = 1529 18 (1%)

* The rates represent major bleeding on study medication up to 12 hours after dose.
† Aspirin therapy was administered concurrently (100 to 325 mg per day).
‡ Bleeding complications were considered major: (1) if the hemorrhage caused a significant clinical event, or (2) if accompanied by a hemoglobin decrease by ≥ 3 g/dL or transfusion of 2 or more units of blood products. Intraocular, retroperitoneal, and intracranial hemorrhages were always considered major.

[See table 7 at top of next page]
Elevations of Serum Aminotransferases
Asymptomatic increases in aspartate (AST [SGOT]) and alanine (ALT [SGPT]) aminotransferase levels greater than three times the upper limit of normal of the laboratory reference range have been reported in up to 6.1% and 5.9% of patients, respectively, during treatment with Lovenox. Similar significant increases in aminotransferase levels have also been observed in patients and healthy volunteers treated with heparin and other low molecular weight heparins. Such elevations are fully reversible and are rarely associated with increases in bilirubin.
Since aminotransferase determinations are important in the differential diagnosis of myocardial infarction, liver dis-

ease, and pulmonary emboli, elevations that might be caused by drugs like Lovenox should be interpreted with caution.

Local Reactions
Mild local irritation, pain, hematoma, ecchymosis, and erythema may follow SC injection of Lovenox.

Adverse Reactions in Patients Receiving Lovenox for Prophylaxis or Treatment of DVT, PE:
Other adverse reactions that were thought to be possibly or probably related to treatment with Lovenox, heparin, or placebo in clinical trials with patients undergoing hip or knee replacement surgery, abdominal or colorectal surgery, or treatment for DVT and that occurred at a rate of at least 2% in the Lovenox group, are provided below [see Tables 8 to 11].

Table 8 Adverse Reactions Occurring at ≥2% Incidence in Lovenox-Treated Patients Undergoing Abdominal or Colorectal Surgery

	Dosing Regimen			
	Lovenox 40 mg q.d. SC n = 1228 %		Heparin 5000 U q8h SC n = 1234 %	
Adverse Reaction	Severe	Total	Severe	Total
Hemorrhage	<1	7	<1	6
Anemia	<1	3	<1	3
Ecchymosis	0	3	0	3

[See table 9 at right]

Table 10 Adverse Reactions Occurring at ≥2% Incidence in Lovenox-Treated Medical Patients with Severely Restricted Mobility During Acute Illness

	Dosing Regimen	
	Lovenox 40 mg q.d. SC n = 360 %	Placebo q.d. SC n = 362 %
Adverse Reaction		
Dyspnea	3.3	5.2
Thrombocytopenia	2.8	2.8
Confusion	2.2	1.1
Diarrhea	2.2	1.7
Nausea	2.5	1.7

[See table 11 at right]

Adverse Events in Lovenox-Treated Patients with Unstable Angina or Non-Q-Wave Myocardial Infarction:
Non-hemorrhagic clinical events reported to be related to Lovenox therapy occurred at an incidence of ≤1%.

Non-major hemorrhagic events, primarily injection site ecchymoses and hematomas, were more frequently reported in patients treated with SC Lovenox than in patients treated with IV heparin.

Serious adverse events with Lovenox or heparin in a clinical trial in patients with unstable angina or non-Q-wave myocardial infarction that occurred at a rate of at least 0.5% in the Lovenox group are provided below [see Table 12].

Table 12 Serious Adverse Events Occurring at ≥0.5% Incidence in Lovenox-Treated Patients with Unstable Angina or Non-Q-Wave Myocardial Infarction

	Dosing Regimen	
	Lovenox 1 mg/kg q12h SC n = 1578 n (%)	Heparin aPTT Adjusted IV Therapy n = 1529 n (%)
Adverse Event		
Atrial fibrillation	11 (0.70)	3 (0.20)
Heart failure	15 (0.95)	11 (0.72)
Lung edema	11 (0.70)	11 (0.72)
Pneumonia	13 (0.82)	9 (0.59)

Table 7 Major Bleeding Episodes in Acute ST-Segment Elevation Myocardial Infarction

		Dosing Regimen
Indication	Lovenox* Initial 30 mg IV bolus followed by 1 mg/kg q12h SC	Heparin* aPTT Adjusted IV Therapy
Acute ST-Segment Elevation Myocardial Infarction	n = 10176 n (%)	n = 10151 n (%)
- Major bleeding (including ICH)†	211 (2.1)	138 (1.4)
- Intracranial hemorrhages (ICH)	84 (0.8)	66 (0.7)

* The rates represent major bleeding (including ICH) up to 30 days
† Bleedings were considered major if the hemorrhage caused a significant clinical event associated with a hemoglobin decrease by ≥ 5 g/dL. ICH were always considered major.

Table 9 Adverse Reactions Occurring at ≥2% Incidence in Lovenox-Treated Patients Undergoing Hip or Knee Replacement Surgery

	Dosing Regimen									
	Lovenox 40 mg q.d. SC				Lovenox 30 mg q12h SC n = 1080 %		Heparin 15,000 U/24h SC n = 766 %		Placebo q12h SC n = 115 %	
	Peri-operative Period n = 288 * %		Extended Prophylaxis Period n = 131 † %							
Adverse Reaction	Severe	Total	Severe	Total	Severe	Total	Severe	Total	Severe	Total
Fever	0	8	0	0	<1	5	<1	4	0	3
Hemorrhage	<1	13	0	5	<1	4	1	4	0	3
Nausea					<1	3	<1	2	0	2
Anemia	0	16	0	<2	<1	2	2	5	<1	7
Edema					<1	2	<1	2	0	2
Peripheral edema	0	6	0	0	<1	3	<1	4	0	3

* Data represent Lovenox 40 mg SC once a day initiated up to 12 hours prior to surgery in 288 hip replacement surgery patients who received Lovenox peri-operatively in an unblinded fashion in one clinical trial.
† Data represent Lovenox 40 mg SC once a day given in a blinded fashion as extended prophylaxis at the end of the peri-operative period in 131 of the original 288 hip replacement surgery patients for up to 21 days in one clinical trial.

Table 11 Adverse Reactions Occurring at ≥2% Incidence in Lovenox-Treated Patients Undergoing Treatment of Deep Vein Thrombosis with or without Pulmonary Embolism

	Dosing Regimen					
	Lovenox 1.5 mg/kg q.d. SC n = 298 %		Lovenox 1 mg/kg q12h SC n = 559 %		Heparin aPTT Adjusted IV Therapy n = 544 %	
Adverse Reaction	Severe	Total	Severe	Total	Severe	Total
Injection Site Hemorrhage	0	5	0	3	<1	<1
Injection Site Pain	0	2	0	2	0	0
Hematuria	0	2	0	<1	<1	2

Adverse Reactions in Lovenox-Treated Patients with Acute ST-Segment Elevation Myocardial Infarction:
In a clinical trial in patients with acute ST-segment elevation myocardial infarction, the only adverse reaction that occurred at a rate of at least 0.5% in the Lovenox group was thrombocytopenia (1.5%).

6.2 Postmarketing Experience
There have been reports of epidural or spinal hematoma formation with concurrent use of Lovenox and spinal/epidural anesthesia or spinal puncture. The majority of patients had a post-operative indwelling epidural catheter placed for analgesia or received additional drugs affecting hemostasis such as NSAIDs. Many of the epidural or spinal hematomas caused neurologic injury, including long-term or permanent paralysis.

Local reactions at the injection site (e.g. nodules, inflammation, oozing), systemic allergic reactions (e.g. pruritus, urticaria, anaphylactic/anaphylactoid reactions), vesiculobullous rash, rare cases of hypersensitivity cutaneous vasculitis, purpura, skin necrosis (occurring at either the injection site or distant from the injection site), thrombocytosis, and thrombocytopenia with thrombosis [see Warnings and Precautions (5.5)] have been reported.

Cases of hyperkalemia have been reported. Most of these reports occurred in patients who also had conditions that tend toward the development of hyperkalemia (e.g., renal dysfunction, concomitant potassium-sparing drugs, administration of potassium, hematoma in body tissues). Very rare cases of hyperlipidemia have also been reported, with one case of hyperlipidemia, with marked hypertriglyceridemia, reported in a diabetic pregnant woman; causality has not been determined.

Because these reactions are reported voluntarily from a population of uncertain size, it is not possible to estimate reliably their frequency or to establish a causal relationship to drug exposure.

7 DRUG INTERACTIONS
Whenever possible, agents which may enhance the risk of hemorrhage should be discontinued prior to initiation of Lovenox therapy. These agents include medications such as: anticoagulants, platelet inhibitors including acetylsalicylic acid, salicylates, NSAIDs (including ketorolac tromethamine), dipyridamole, or sulfinpyrazone. If co-administration is essential, conduct close clinical and laboratory monitoring [see Warnings and Precautions (5.9)].

8 USE IN SPECIFIC POPULATIONS
8.1 Pregnancy
Pregnancy Category B
All pregnancies have a background risk of birth defect, loss, or other adverse outcome regardless of drug exposure. The

fetal risk summary below describes the potential of Lovenox to increase the risk of developmental abnormalities above the background risk.

Fetal Risk Summary

Lovenox does not cross the placenta, and is not expected to result in fetal exposure to the drug. Human data from a retrospective cohort study, which included 693 live births, suggest that Lovenox does not increase the risk of major developmental abnormalities. Based on animal data, enoxaparin is not predicted to increase the risk of major developmental abnormalities (see *Data*).

Clinical Considerations

Pregnancy alone confers an increased risk for thromboembolism that is even higher for women with thromboembolic disease and certain high risk pregnancy conditions. While not adequately studied, pregnant women with mechanical prosthetic heart valves may be at even higher risk for thrombosis [see *Warnings and Precautions (5.7)* and *Use in Specific Populations (8.6)*]. Pregnant women with thromboembolic disease, including those with mechanical prosthetic heart valves and those with inherited or acquired thrombophilias, have an increased risk of other maternal complications and fetal loss regardless of the type of anticoagulant used.

All patients receiving anticoagulants, including pregnant women, are at risk for bleeding. Pregnant women receiving enoxaparin should be carefully monitored for evidence of bleeding or excessive anticoagulation. Consideration for use of a shorter acting anticoagulant should be specifically addressed as delivery approaches [see *Boxed Warning*]. Hemorrhage can occur at any site and may lead to death of mother and/or fetus. Pregnant women should be apprised of the potential hazard to the fetus and the mother if enoxaparin is administered during pregnancy.

It is not known if monitoring of anti-Factor Xa activity and dose adjustment (by weight or anti-Factor Xa activity) of Lovenox affect the safety and the efficacy of the drug during pregnancy.

Cases of "gasping syndrome" have occurred in premature infants when large amounts of benzyl alcohol have been administered (99–405 mg/kg/day). The multiple-dose vial of Lovenox contains 15 mg benzyl alcohol per 1 mL as a preservative [see *Warnings and Precautions (5.8)*].

Data

- *Human Data* - There are no adequate and well-controlled studies in pregnant women.

  A retrospective study reviewed the records of 604 women who used enoxaparin during pregnancy. A total of 624 pregnancies resulted in 693 live births. There were 72 hemorrhagic events (11 serious) in 63 women. There were 14 cases of neonatal hemorrhage. Major congenital anomalies in live births occurred at rates (2.5%) similar to background rates.

  There have been postmarketing reports of fetal death when pregnant women received Lovenox. Causality for these cases has not been determined. Insufficient data, the underlying disease, and the possibility of inadequate anticoagulation complicate the evaluation of these cases.

  A clinical study using enoxaparin in pregnant women with mechanical prosthetic heart valves has been conducted [see *Warnings and Precautions (5.7)*].
- *Animal Data* - Teratology studies have been conducted in pregnant rats and rabbits at SC doses of enoxaparin up to 15 times the recommended human dose (by comparison with 2 mg/kg as the maximum recommended daily dose). There was no evidence of teratogenic effects or fetotoxicity due to enoxaparin. Because animal reproduction studies are not always predictive of human response, this drug should be used during pregnancy only if clearly needed.

8.3 Nursing Mothers

It is not known whether Lovenox is excreted in human milk. Because many drugs are excreted in human milk and because of the potential for serious adverse reactions in nursing infants from Lovenox, a decision should be made whether to discontinue nursing or discontinue Lovenox, taking into account the importance of Lovenox to the mother and the known benefits of nursing.

8.4 Pediatric Use

Safety and effectiveness of Lovenox in pediatric patients have not been established.

8.5 Geriatric Use

Prevention of Deep Vein Thrombosis in Hip, Knee and Abdominal Surgery; Treatment of Deep Vein Thrombosis, Prevention of Ischemic Complications of Unstable Angina and Non-Q-wave Myocardial Infarction

Over 2800 patients, 65 years and older, have received Lovenox in pivotal clinical trials. The efficacy of Lovenox in the geriatric (≥65 years) was similar to that seen in younger patients (<65 years). The incidence of bleeding complications was similar between geriatric and younger patients when 30 mg every 12 hours or 40 mg once a day doses of Lovenox were employed. The incidence of bleeding complications was higher in geriatric patients as compared to younger patients when Lovenox was administered at doses of 1.5 mg/kg once a day or 1 mg/kg every 12 hours. The risk of Lovenox-associated bleeding increased with age. Serious adverse events increased with age for patients receiving Lovenox. Other clinical experience (including postmarketing surveillance and literature reports) has not revealed additional differences in the safety of Lovenox between geriatric and younger patients. Careful attention to dosing intervals and concomitant medications (especially antiplatelet medications) is advised. Lovenox should be used with care in geriatric patients who may show delayed elimination of enoxaparin. Monitoring of geriatric patients with low body weight (<45 kg) and those predisposed to decreased renal function should be considered [see *Warnings and Precautions (5.9) and Clinical Pharmacology (12.3)*].

Treatment of Acute ST-Segment Elevation Myocardial Infarction

In the clinical study for treatment of acute ST-segment elevation myocardial infarction, there was no evidence of difference in efficacy between patients ≥75 years of age (n = 1241) and patients less than 75 years of age (n=9015). Patients ≥75 years of age did not receive a 30 mg IV bolus prior to the normal dosage regimen and had their SC dose adjusted to 0.75 mg/kg every 12 hours [see *Dosage and Administration (2.3)*]. The incidence of bleeding complications was higher in patients ≥65 years of age as compared to younger patients (<65 years).

8.6 Patients with Mechanical Prosthetic Heart Valves

The use of Lovenox has not been adequately studied for thromboprophylaxis in patients with mechanical prosthetic heart valves and has not been adequately studied for long-term use in this patient population. Isolated cases of prosthetic heart valve thrombosis have been reported in patients with mechanical prosthetic heart valves who have received enoxaparin for thromboprophylaxis. Some of these cases were pregnant women in whom thrombosis led to maternal and fetal deaths. Insufficient data, the underlying disease and the possibility of inadequate anticoagulation complicate the evaluation of these cases. Pregnant women with mechanical prosthetic heart valves may be at higher risk for thromboembolism [see *Warnings and Precautions (5.7)*].

8.7 Renal Impairment

In patients with renal impairment, there is an increase in exposure of enoxaparin sodium. All such patients should be observed carefully for signs and symptoms of bleeding. Because exposure of enoxaparin sodium is significantly increased in patients with severe renal impairment (creatinine clearance <30 mL/min), a dosage adjustment is recommended for therapeutic and prophylactic dosage ranges. No dosage adjustment is recommended in patients with moderate (creatinine clearance 30–50 mL/min) and mild (creatinine clearance 50–80 mL/min) renal impairment [see *Dosage and Administration (2.2)* and *Clinical Pharmacology (12.3)*]. In patients with renal failure, treatment with enoxaparin has been associated with the development of hyperkalemia [see *Adverse Reactions (6.2)*].

8.8 Hepatic Impairment

The impact of hepatic impairment on enoxaparin's exposure and antithrombotic effect has not been investigated. Caution should be exercised when administering enoxaparin to patients with hepatic impairment.

8.9 Low-Weight Patients

An increase in exposure of enoxaparin sodium with prophylactic dosages (non-weight adjusted) has been observed in low-weight women (<45 kg) and low-weight men (<57 kg). All such patients should be observed carefully for signs and symptoms of bleeding [see *Clinical Pharmacology (12.3)*].

10 OVERDOSAGE

Accidental overdosage following administration of Lovenox may lead to hemorrhagic complications. Injected Lovenox may be largely neutralized by the slow IV injection of protamine sulfate (1% solution). The dose of protamine sulfate should be equal to the dose of Lovenox injected: 1 mg protamine sulfate should be administered to neutralize 1 mg Lovenox, if enoxaparin sodium was administered in the previous 8 hours. An infusion of 0.5 mg protamine per 1 mg of enoxaparin sodium may be administered if enoxaparin sodium was administered greater than 8 hours previous to the protamine administration, or if it has been determined that a second dose of protamine is required. The second infusion of 0.5 mg protamine sulfate per 1 mg of Lovenox may be administered if the aPTT measured 2 to 4 hours after the first infusion remains prolonged.

If at least 12 hours have elapsed since the last enoxaparin sodium injection, protamine administration may not be required; however, even with higher doses of protamine, the aPTT may remain more prolonged than following administration of heparin. In all cases, the anti-Factor Xa activity is never completely neutralized (maximum about 60%). Particular care should be taken to avoid overdosage with protamine sulfate. Administration of protamine sulfate can cause severe hypotensive and anaphylactoid reactions. Because fatal reactions, often resembling anaphylaxis, have been reported with protamine sulfate, it should be given only when resuscitation techniques and treatment of anaphylactic shock are readily available. For additional information consult the labeling of protamine sulfate injection products.

11 DESCRIPTION

Lovenox is a sterile aqueous solution containing enoxaparin sodium, a low molecular weight heparin. The pH of the injection is 5.5 to 7.5.

Enoxaparin sodium is obtained by alkaline depolymerization of heparin benzyl ester derived from porcine intestinal mucosa. Its structure is characterized by a 2-O-sulfo-4-enepyranosuronic acid group at the non-reducing end and a 2-N,6-O-disulfo-D-glucosamine at the reducing end of the chain. About 20% (ranging between 15% and 25%) of the enoxaparin structure contains an 1,6 anhydro derivative on the reducing end of the polysaccharide chain. The drug substance is the sodium salt. The average molecular weight is about 4500 daltons. The molecular weight distribution is:

<2000 daltons	≤20%
2000 to 8000 daltons	≥68%
>8000 daltons	≤18%

STRUCTURAL FORMULA

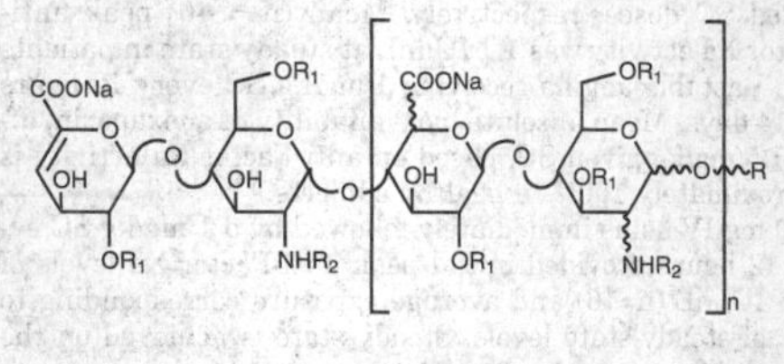
COONa
OR1
OH
O
OR1
NHR2
COONa
OR1
OH
OR1
NHR2
R
n

R_1 = H or SO_3Na and R_2 = SO_3Na or $COCH_3$

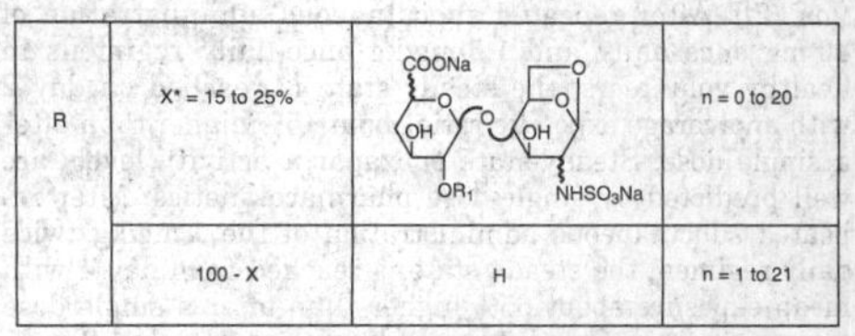
R
X* = 15 to 25%
COONa
OH
OH
OR1
NHSO3Na
n = 0 to 20
100 - X
H
n = 1 to 21

*X = Percent of polysaccharide chain containing 1,6 anhydro derivative on the reducing end.

Lovenox 100 mg/mL Concentration contains 10 mg enoxaparin sodium (approximate anti-Factor Xa activity of 1000 IU [with reference to the W.H.O. First International Low Molecular Weight Heparin Reference Standard]) per 0.1 mL Water for Injection.

Lovenox 150 mg/mL Concentration contains 15 mg enoxaparin sodium (approximate anti-Factor Xa activity of 1500 IU [with reference to the W.H.O. First International Low Molecular Weight Heparin Reference Standard]) per 0.1 mL Water for Injection.

The Lovenox prefilled syringes and graduated prefilled syringes are preservative-free and intended for use only as a single-dose injection. The multiple-dose vial contains 15 mg benzyl alcohol per 1 mL as a preservative [see *Dosage and Administration (2)* and *How Supplied (16)*].

12 CLINICAL PHARMACOLOGY

12.1 Mechanism of Action

Enoxaparin is a low molecular weight heparin which has antithrombotic properties.

12.2 Pharmacodynamics

In humans, enoxaparin given at a dose of 1.5 mg/kg subcutaneously (SC) is characterized by a higher ratio of anti-Factor Xa to anti-Factor IIa activity (mean ± SD, 14.0 ± 3.1) (based on areas under anti-Factor activity versus time curves) compared to the ratios observed for heparin (mean±SD, 1.22 ± 0.13). Increases of up to 1.8 times the control values were seen in the thrombin time (TT) and the activated partial thromboplastin time (aPTT). Enoxaparin at a 1 mg/kg dose (100 mg/mL concentration), administered SC every 12 hours to patients in a large clinical trial resulted in aPTT values of 45 seconds or less in the majority of patients (n = 1607). A 30 mg IV bolus immediately followed by a 1 mg/kg SC administration resulted in aPTT post-injection values of 50 seconds. The average aPTT prolongation value on Day 1 was about 16% higher than on Day 4.

12.3 Pharmacokinetics

Absorption: Pharmacokinetic trials were conducted using the 100 mg/mL formulation. Maximum anti-Factor Xa and anti-thrombin (anti-Factor IIa) activities occur 3 to 5 hours after SC injection of enoxaparin. Mean peak anti-Factor Xa activity was 0.16 IU/mL (1.58 mcg/mL) and 0.38 IU/mL (3.83 mcg/mL) after the 20 mg and the 40 mg clinically

Table 13 Pharmacokinetic Parameters* After 5 Days of 1.5 mg/kg SC Once Daily Doses of Enoxaparin Sodium Using 100 mg/mL or 200 mg/mL Concentrations

	Concentration	Anti-Xa	Anti-IIa	Heptest	aPTT
A_{max} (IU/mL or Δ sec)	100 mg/mL	1.37 ($\pm$0.23)	0.23 ($\pm$0.05)	105 ($\pm$17)	19 ($\pm$5)
	200 mg/mL	1.45 ($\pm$0.22)	0.26 ($\pm$0.05)	111 ($\pm$17)	22 ($\pm$7)
	90% CI	102–110%		102–111%	
t_{max}[†] (h)	100 mg/mL	3 (2–6)	4 (2–5)	2.5 (2–4.5)	3 (2–4.5)
	200 mg/mL	3.5 (2–6)	4.5 (2.5–6)	3.3 (2–5)	3 (2–5)
AUC (ss) (h*IU/mL or h* Δ sec)	100 mg/mL	14.26 ($\pm$2.93)	1.54 ($\pm$0.61)	1321 ($\pm$219)	
	200 mg/mL	15.43 ($\pm$2.96)	1.77 ($\pm$0.67)	1401 ($\pm$227)	
	90% CI	105–112%		103–109%	

* Means $\pm$ SD at Day 5 and 90% Confidence Interval (CI) of the ratio
† Median (range)

tested SC doses, respectively. Mean (n = 46) peak anti-Factor Xa activity was 1.1 IU/mL at steady state in patients with unstable angina receiving 1 mg/kg SC every 12 hours for 14 days. Mean absolute bioavailability of enoxaparin, after 1.5 mg/kg given SC, based on anti-Factor Xa activity is approximately 100% in healthy subjects.

A 30 mg IV bolus immediately followed by a 1 mg/kg SC every 12 hours provided initial peak anti-Factor Xa levels of 1.16 IU/mL (n=16) and average exposure corresponding to 84% of steady-state levels. Steady state is achieved on the second day of treatment.

Enoxaparin pharmacokinetics appear to be linear over the recommended dosage ranges [see *Dosage and Administration (2)*]. After repeated subcutaneous administration of 40 mg once daily and 1.5 mg/kg once-daily regimens in healthy volunteers, the steady state is reached on day 2 with an average exposure ratio about 15% higher than after a single dose. Steady-state enoxaparin activity levels are well predicted by single-dose pharmacokinetics. After repeated subcutaneous administration of the 1 mg/kg twice daily regimen, the steady state is reached from day 4 with mean exposure about 65% higher than after a single dose and mean peak and trough levels of about 1.2 and 0.52 IU/mL, respectively. Based on enoxaparin sodium pharmacokinetics, this difference in steady state is expected and within the therapeutic range.

Although not studied clinically, the 150 mg/mL concentration of enoxaparin sodium is projected to result in anticoagulant activities similar to those of 100 mg/mL and 200 mg/mL concentrations at the same enoxaparin dose. When a daily 1.5 mg/kg SC injection of enoxaparin sodium was given to 25 healthy male and female subjects using a 100 mg/mL or a 200 mg/mL concentration the following pharmacokinetic profiles were obtained [see Table 13]. [See table 13 above]

Distribution: The volume of distribution of anti-Factor Xa activity is about 4.3 L.
Elimination: Following intravenous (IV) dosing, the total body clearance of enoxaparin is 26 mL/min. After IV dosing of enoxaparin labeled with the gamma-emitter, ^{99m}Tc, 40% of radioactivity and 8 to 20% of anti-Factor Xa activity were recovered in urine in 24 hours. Elimination half-life based on anti-Factor Xa activity was 4.5 hours after a single SC dose to about 7 hours after repeated dosing. Significant anti-Factor Xa activity persists in plasma for about 12 hours following a 40 mg SC once a day dose. Following SC dosing, the apparent clearance (CL/F) of enoxaparin is approximately 15 mL/min.
Metabolism: Enoxaparin sodium is primarily metabolized in the liver by desulfation and/or depolymerization to lower molecular weight species with much reduced biological potency. Renal clearance of active fragments represents about 10% of the administered dose and total renal excretion of active and non-active fragments 40% of the dose.

Special Populations
Gender: Apparent clearance and A_{max} derived from anti-Factor Xa activity following single SC dosing (40 mg and 60 mg) were slightly higher in males than in females. The source of the gender difference in these parameters has not been conclusively identified; however, body weight may be a contributing factor.
Geriatric: Apparent clearance and A_{max} derived from anti-Factor Xa values following single and multiple SC dosing in geriatric subjects were close to those observed in young subjects. Following once a day SC dosing of 40 mg enoxaparin, the Day 10 mean area under anti-Factor Xa activity versus time curve (AUC) was approximately 15% greater than the mean Day 1 AUC value [see *Dosage and Administration (2.3)* and *Use in Specific Populations (8.5)*].
Renal Impairment: A linear relationship between anti-Factor Xa plasma clearance and creatinine clearance at steady state has been observed, which indicates decreased clearance of enoxaparin sodium in patients with reduced renal function. Anti-Factor Xa exposure represented by AUC, at steady state, is marginally increased in mild (creatinine clearance 50–80 mL/min) and moderate (creatinine clearance 30–50 mL/min) renal impairment after repeated subcutaneous 40 mg once-daily doses. In patients with severe renal impairment (creatinine clearance <30 mL/min), the AUC at steady state is significantly increased on average by 65% after repeated subcutaneous 40 mg once-daily doses [see *Dosage and Administration (2.2)* and *Use in Specific Populations (8.7)*].
Hemodialysis: In a single study, elimination rate appeared similar but AUC was two-fold higher than control population, after a single 0.25 or 0.5 mg/kg intravenous dose.
Hepatic Impairment: Studies with enoxaparin in patients with hepatic impairment have not been conducted and the impact of hepatic impairment on the exposure to enoxaparin is unknown [see *Use in Specific Populations (8.8)*].
Weight: After repeated subcutaneous 1.5 mg/kg once daily dosing, mean AUC of anti-Factor Xa activity is marginally higher at steady state in obese healthy volunteers (BMI 30–48 kg/m^2) compared to non-obese control subjects, while A_{max} is not increased.
When non-weight adjusted dosing was administered, it was found after a single-subcutaneous 40 mg dose, that anti-Factor Xa exposure is 52% higher in low-weight women (<45 kg) and 27% higher in low-weight men (<57 kg) when compared to normal weight control subjects [see *Use in Specific Populations (8.9)*].
Pharmacokinetic interaction: No pharmacokinetic interaction was observed between enoxaparin and thrombolytics when administered concomitantly.

13   NONCLINICAL TOXICOLOGY
13.1   Carcinogenesis, Mutagenesis, Impairment of Fertility
No long-term studies in animals have been performed to evaluate the carcinogenic potential of enoxaparin. Enoxaparin was not mutagenic in *in vitro* tests, including the Ames test, mouse lymphoma cell forward mutation test, and human lymphocyte chromosomal aberration test, and the *in vivo* rat bone marrow chromosomal aberration test. Enoxaparin was found to have no effect on fertility or reproductive performance of male and female rats at SC doses up to 20 mg/kg/day or 141 mg/m^2/day. The maximum human dose in clinical trials was 2.0 mg/kg/day or 78 mg/m^2/day (for an average body weight of 70 kg, height of 170 cm, and body surface area of 1.8 m^2).
13.2   Animal Toxicology and/or Pharmacology
A single SC dose of 46.4 mg/kg enoxaparin was lethal to rats. The symptoms of acute toxicity were ataxia, decreased motility, dyspnea, cyanosis, and coma.
13.3   Reproductive and Developmental Toxicology
Teratology studies have been conducted in pregnant rats and rabbits at SC doses of enoxaparin up to 30 mg/kg/day corresponding to 211 mg/m^2/day and 410 mg/m^2/day in rats and rabbits respectively. There was no evidence of teratogenic effects or fetotoxicity due to enoxaparin.

14   CLINICAL STUDIES
14.1   Prophylaxis of Deep Vein Thrombosis Following Abdominal Surgery in Patients at Risk for Thromboembolic Complications
Abdominal surgery patients at risk include those who are over 40 years of age, obese, undergoing surgery under general anesthesia lasting longer than 30 minutes or who have additional risk factors such as malignancy or a history of deep vein thrombosis (DVT) or pulmonary embolism (PE). In a double-blind, parallel group study of patients undergoing elective cancer surgery of the gastrointestinal, urological, or gynecological tract, a total of 1116 patients were enrolled in the study, and 1115 patients were treated. Patients ranged in age from 32 to 97 years (mean age 67 years) with 52.7% men and 47.3% women. Patients were 98% Caucasian, 1.1% Black, 0.4% Asian and 0.4% others. Lovenox 40 mg SC, administered once a day, beginning 2 hours prior to surgery and continuing for a maximum of 12 days after surgery, was comparable to heparin 5000 U every 8 hours SC in reducing the risk of DVT. The efficacy data are provided below [see Table 14].

Table 14 Efficacy of Lovenox in the Prophylaxis of Deep Vein Thrombosis Following Abdominal Surgery

	Dosing Regimen	
Indication	Lovenox 40 mg q.d. SC n (%)	Heparin 5000 U q8h SC n (%)
All Treated Abdominal Surgery Patients	555 (100)	560 (100)
Treatment Failures Total VTE* (%)	56 (10.1) (95% CI[†]: 8 to 13)	63 (11.3) (95% CI: 9 to 14)
DVT Only (%)	54 (9.7) (95% CI: 7 to 12)	61 (10.9) (95% CI: 8 to 13)

* VTE = Venous thromboembolic events which included DVT, PE, and death considered to be thromboembolic in origin.
† CI = Confidence Interval

In a second double-blind, parallel group study, Lovenox 40 mg SC once a day was compared to heparin 5000 U every 8 hours SC in patients undergoing colorectal surgery (one-third with cancer). A total of 1347 patients were randomized in the study and all patients were treated. Patients ranged in age from 18 to 92 years (mean age 50.1 years) with 54.2% men and 45.8% women. Treatment was initiated approximately 2 hours prior to surgery and continued for approximately 7 to 10 days after surgery. The efficacy data are provided below [see Table 15].

Table 15 Efficacy of Lovenox in the Prophylaxis of Deep Vein Thrombosis Following Colorectal Surgery

	Dosing Regimen	
Indication	Lovenox 40 mg q.d. SC n (%)	Heparin 5000 U q8h SC n (%)
All Treated Colorectal Surgery Patients	673 (100)	674 (100)
Treatment Failures Total VTE* (%)	48 (7.1) (95% CI[†]: 5 to 9)	45 (6.7) (95% CI: 5 to 9)
DVT Only (%)	47 (7.0) (95% CI: 5 to 9)	44 (6.5) (95% CI: 5 to 8)

* VTE = Venous thromboembolic events which included DVT, PE, and death considered to be thromboembolic in origin.
† CI = Confidence Interval

14.2   Prophylaxis of Deep Vein Thrombosis Following Hip or Knee Replacement Surgery
Lovenox has been shown to reduce the risk of post-operative deep vein thrombosis (DVT) following hip or knee replacement surgery.
In a double-blind study, Lovenox 30 mg every 12 hours SC was compared to placebo in patients with hip replacement. A total of 100 patients were randomized in the study and all patients were treated. Patients ranged in age from 41 to 84 years (mean age 67.1 years) with 45% men and 55% women. After hemostasis was established, treatment was initiated 12 to 24 hours after surgery and was continued for 10 to 14 days after surgery. The efficacy data are provided below [see Table 16].

Table 16 Efficacy of Lovenox in the Prophylaxis of Deep Vein Thrombosis Following Hip Replacement Surgery

Indication	Dosing Regimen	
	Lovenox 30 mg q12h SC n (%)	Placebo q12h SC n (%)
All Treated Hip Replacement Patients	50 (100)	50 (100)
Treatment Failures Total DVT (%)	5 (10)*	23 (46)
Proximal DVT (%)	1 (2)†	11 (22)

* p value versus placebo = 0.0002
† p value versus placebo = 0.0134

A double-blind, multicenter study compared three dosing regimens of Lovenox in patients with hip replacement. A total of 572 patients were randomized in the study and 568 patients were treated. Patients ranged in age from 31 to 88 years (mean age 64.7 years) with 63% men and 37% women. Patients were 93% Caucasian, 6% Black, <1% Asian, and 1% others. Treatment was initiated within two days after surgery and was continued for 7 to 11 days after surgery. The efficacy data are provided below [see Table 17].

Table 17 Efficacy of Lovenox in the Prophylaxis of Deep Vein Thrombosis Following Hip Replacement Surgery

Indication	Dosing Regimen		
	10 mg q.d. SC n (%)	30 mg q12h SC n (%)	40 mg q.d. SC n (%)
All Treated Hip Replacement Patients	161 (100)	208 (100)	199 (100)
Treatment Failures Total DVT (%)	40 (25)	22 (11)*	27 (14)
Proximal DVT (%)	17 (11)	8 (4)†	9 (5)

* p value versus Lovenox 10 mg once a day = 0.0008
† p value versus Lovenox 10 mg once a day = 0.0168

There was no significant difference between the 30 mg every 12 hours and 40 mg once a day regimens. In a double-blind study, Lovenox 30 mg every 12 hours SC was compared to placebo in patients undergoing knee replacement surgery. A total of 132 patients were randomized in the study and 131 patients were treated, of which 99 had total knee replacement and 32 had either unicompartmental knee replacement or tibial osteotomy. The 99 patients with total knee replacement ranged in age from 42 to 85 years (mean age 70.2 years) with 36.4% men and 63.6% women. After hemostasis was established, treatment was initiated 12 to 24 hours after surgery and was continued up to 15 days after surgery. The incidence of proximal and total DVT after surgery was significantly lower for Lovenox compared to placebo. The efficacy data are provided below [see Table 18].

Table 18 Efficacy of Lovenox in the Prophylaxis of Deep Vein Thrombosis Following Total Knee Replacement Surgery

Indication	Dosing Regimen	
	Lovenox 30 mg q12h SC n (%)	Placebo q12h SC n (%)
All Treated Total Knee Replacement Patients	47 (100)	52 (100)
Treatment Failures Total DVT (%)	5 (11)* (95% CI: 1 to 21)	32 (62) (95% CI: 47 to 76)
Proximal DVT (%)	0 (0)‡ (95% Upper CL§: 5)	7 (13) (95% CI: 3 to 24)

* p value versus placebo = 0.0001
† CI = Confidence Interval

Table 20 Efficacy of Lovenox in the Prophylaxis of Deep Vein Thrombosis in Medical Patients with Severely Restricted Mobility During Acute Illness

Indication	Dosing Regimen		
	Lovenox 20 mg q.d. SC n (%)	Lovenox 40 mg q.d. SC n (%)	Placebo n (%)
All Treated Medical Patients During Acute Illness	351 (100)	360 (100)	362 (100)
Treatment Failure* Total VTE† (%)	43 (12.3)	16 (4.4)	43 (11.9)
Total DVT (%)	43 (12.3) (95% CI‡ 8.8 to 15.7)	16 (4.4) (95% CI‡ 2.3 to 6.6)	41 (11.3) (95% CI‡ 8.1 to 14.6)
Proximal DVT (%)	13 (3.7)	5 (1.4)	14 (3.9)

* Treatment failures during therapy, between Days 1 and 14
† VTE = Venous thromboembolic events which included DVT, PE, and death considered to be thromboembolic in origin
‡ CI = Confidence Interval

‡ p value versus placebo = 0.013
§ CL = Confidence Limit

Additionally, in an open-label, parallel group, randomized clinical study, Lovenox 30 mg every 12 hours SC in patients undergoing elective knee replacement surgery was compared to heparin 5000 U every 8 hours SC. A total of 453 patients were randomized in the study and all were treated. Patients ranged in age from 38 to 90 years (mean age 68.5 years) with 43.7% men and 56.3% women. Patients were 92.5% Caucasian, 5.3% Black, and 0.6% others. Treatment was initiated after surgery and continued up to 14 days. The incidence of deep vein thrombosis was significantly lower for Lovenox compared to heparin.

Extended Prophylaxis of Deep Vein Thrombosis Following Hip Replacement Surgery: In a study of extended prophylaxis for patients undergoing hip replacement surgery, patients were treated, while hospitalized, with Lovenox 40 mg SC, initiated up to 12 hours prior to surgery for the prophylaxis of post-operative DVT. At the end of the peri-operative period, all patients underwent bilateral venography. In a double-blind design, those patients with no venous thromboembolic disease were randomized to a post-discharge regimen of either Lovenox 40 mg (n = 90) once a day SC or to placebo (n = 89) for 3 weeks. A total of 179 patients were randomized in the double-blind phase of the study and all patients were treated. Patients ranged in age from 47 to 87 years (mean age 69.4 years) with 57% men and 43% women. In this population of patients, the incidence of DVT during extended prophylaxis was significantly lower for Lovenox compared to placebo. The efficacy data are provided below [see Table 19].

Table 19 Efficacy of Lovenox in the Extended Prophylaxis of Deep Vein Thrombosis Following Hip Replacement Surgery

Indication (Post-Discharge)	Post-Discharge Dosing Regimen	
	Lovenox 40 mg q.d. SC n (%)	Placebo q.d. SC n (%)
All Treated Extended Prophylaxis Patients	90 (100)	89 (100)
Treatment Failures Total DVT (%)	6 (7)* (95% CI†: 3 to 14)	18 (20) (95% CI: 12 to 30)
Proximal DVT (%)	5 (6)‡ (95% CI: 2 to 13)	7 (8) (95% CI: 3 to 16)

* p value versus placebo = 0.008
† CI= Confidence Interval
‡ p value versus placebo = 0.537

In a second study, patients undergoing hip replacement surgery were treated, while hospitalized, with Lovenox 40 mg SC, initiated up to 12 hours prior to surgery. All patients were examined for clinical signs and symptoms of venous thromboembolism (VTE) disease. In a double-blind design, patients without clinical signs and symptoms of VTE disease were randomized to a post-discharge regimen of either Lovenox 40 mg (n = 131) once a day SC or to placebo (n = 131) for 3 weeks. A total of 262 patients were randomized in the study double-blind phase and all patients were

treated. Patients ranged in age from 44 to 87 years (mean age 68.5 years) with 43.1% men and 56.9% women. Similar to the first study the incidence of DVT during extended prophylaxis was significantly lower for Lovenox compared to placebo, with a statistically significant difference in both total DVT (Lovenox 21 [16%] versus placebo 45 [34%]; p = 0.001) and proximal DVT (Lovenox 8 [6%] versus placebo 28 [21%]; p = <0.001).

14.3   Prophylaxis of Deep Vein Thrombosis in Medical Patients with Severely Restricted Mobility During Acute Illness

In a double blind multicenter, parallel group study, Lovenox 20 mg or 40 mg once a day SC was compared to placebo in the prophylaxis of deep vein thrombosis (DVT) in medical patients with severely restricted mobility during acute illness (defined as walking distance of <10 meters for ≤3 days). This study included patients with heart failure (NYHA Class III or IV); acute respiratory failure or complicated chronic respiratory insufficiency (not requiring ventilatory support): acute infection (excluding septic shock); or acute rheumatic disorder [acute lumbar or sciatic pain, vertebral compression (due to osteoporosis or tumor), acute arthritic episodes of the lower extremities]. A total of 1102 patients were enrolled in the study, and 1073 patients were treated. Patients ranged in age from 40 to 97 years (mean age 73 years) with equal proportions of men and women. Treatment continued for a maximum of 14 days (median duration 7 days). When given at a dose of 40 mg once a day SC, Lovenox significantly reduced the incidence of DVT as compared to placebo. The efficacy data are provided below [see Table 20].

[See table 20 above]

At approximately 3 months following enrollment, the incidence of venous thromboembolism remained significantly lower in the Lovenox 40 mg treatment group versus the placebo treatment group.

14.4   Treatment of Deep Vein Thrombosis with or without Pulmonary Embolism

In a multicenter, parallel group study, 900 patients with acute lower extremity deep vein thrombosis (DVT) with or without pulmonary embolism (PE) were randomized to an inpatient (hospital) treatment of either (i) Lovenox 1.5 mg/kg once a day SC, (ii) Lovenox 1 mg/kg every 12 hours SC, or (iii) heparin IV bolus (5000 IU) followed by a continuous infusion (administered to achieve an aPTT of 55 to 85 seconds). A total of 900 patients were randomized in the study and all patients were treated. Patients ranged in age from 18 to 92 years (mean age 60.7 years) with 54.7% men and 45.3% women. All patients also received warfarin sodium (dose adjusted according to PT to achieve an International Normalization Ratio [INR] of 2.0 to 3.0), commencing within 72 hours of initiation of Lovenox or standard heparin therapy, and continuing for 90 days. Lovenox or standard heparin therapy was administered for a minimum of 5 days and until the targeted warfarin sodium INR was achieved. Both Lovenox regimens were equivalent to standard heparin therapy in reducing the risk of recurrent venous thromboembolism (DVT and/or PE). The efficacy data are provided below [see Table 21].

[See table 21 at top of next page]

Similarly, in a multicenter, open-label, parallel group study, patients with acute proximal DVT were randomized to Lovenox or heparin. Patients who could not receive outpatient therapy were excluded from entering the study. Outpatient exclusion criteria included the following: inability to receive outpatient heparin therapy because of associated comorbid conditions or potential for non-compliance and inability to attend follow-up visits as an outpatient because of geographic inaccessibility. Eligible patients could be treated in the hospital, but ONLY Lovenox patients were permitted to go home on therapy (72%). A total of 501 patients were randomized in the study and all patients were treated. Patients ranged in age from 19 to 96 years (mean age 57.8 years) with 60.5% men and 39.5% women. Patients were randomized to either Lovenox 1 mg/kg every 12 hours SC or heparin IV bolus (5000 IU) followed by a continuous infusion administered to achieve an aPTT of 60 to 85 seconds (in-patient treatment). All patients also received warfarin sodium as described in the previous study. Lovenox or standard heparin therapy was administered for a minimum of 5 days. Lovenox was equivalent to standard heparin therapy in reducing the risk of recurrent venous thromboembolism. The efficacy data are provided below [see Table 22].

Table 22 Efficacy of Lovenox in Treatment of Deep Vein Thrombosis

Indication	Dosing Regimen*	
	Lovenox 1 mg/kg q12h SC n (%)	Heparin aPTT Adjusted IV Therapy n (%)
All Treated DVT Patients	247 (100)	254 (100)
Patient Outcome Total VTE[†] (%)	13 (5.3)[‡]	17 (6.7)
DVT Only (%)	11 (4.5)	14 (5.5)
Proximal DVT (%)	10 (4.0)	12 (4.7)
PE (%)	2 (0.8)	3 (1.2)

* All patients were also treated with warfarin sodium commencing on the evening of the second day of Lovenox or standard heparin therapy.
† VTE = venous thromboembolic event (deep vein thrombosis [DVT] and/or pulmonary embolism [PE]).
‡ The 95% Confidence Intervals for the treatment difference for total VTE was: Lovenox versus heparin (-5.6 to 2.7).

14.5 Prophylaxis of Ischemic Complications in Unstable Angina and Non-Q-Wave Myocardial Infarction

In a multicenter, double-blind, parallel group study, patients who recently experienced unstable angina or non-Q-wave myocardial infarction were randomized to either Lovenox 1 mg/kg every 12 hours SC or heparin IV bolus (5000 U) followed by a continuous infusion (adjusted to achieve an aPTT of 55 to 85 seconds). A total of 3171 patients were enrolled in the study, and 3107 patients were treated. Patients ranged in age from 25–94 years (median age 64 years), with 33.4% of patients female and 66.6% male. Race was distributed as follows: 89.8% Caucasian, 4.8% Black, 2.0% Asian, and 3.5% other. **All** patients were also treated with aspirin 100 to 325 mg per day. Treatment was initiated within 24 hours of the event and continued until clinical stabilization, revascularization procedures, or hospital discharge, with a maximal duration of 8 days of therapy. The combined incidence of the triple endpoint of death, myocardial infarction, or recurrent angina was lower for Lovenox compared with heparin therapy at 14 days after initiation of treatment. The lower incidence of the triple endpoint was sustained up to 30 days after initiation of treatment. These results were observed in an analysis of both all-randomized and all-treated patients. The efficacy data are provided below [see Table 23].
[See table 23 above]
The combined incidence of death or myocardial infarction at all time points was lower for Lovenox compared to standard heparin therapy, but did not achieve statistical significance. The efficacy data are provided below [see Table 24].
[See table 24 at right]
In a survey one year following treatment, with information available for 92% of enrolled patients, the combined incidence of death, myocardial infarction, or recurrent angina remained lower for Lovenox versus heparin (32.0% vs 35.7%).
Urgent revascularization procedures were performed less frequently in the Lovenox group as compared to the heparin group, 6.3% compared to 8.2% (at 30 days (p = 0.047).

14.6 Treatment of Acute ST-Segment Elevation Myocardial Infarction

In a multicenter, double-blind, double-dummy, parallel group study, patients with acute ST-segment elevation myocardial infarction (STEMI) who were to be hospitalized within 6 hours of onset and were eligible to receive fibrinolytic therapy were randomized in a 1:1 ratio to receive either Lovenox or unfractionated heparin.

Table 21 Efficacy of Lovenox in Treatment of Deep Vein Thrombosis with or without Pulmonary Embolism

Indication	Dosing Regimen*		
	Lovenox 1.5 mg/kg q.d. SC n (%)	Lovenox 1 mg/kg q12h SC n (%)	Heparin aPTT Adjusted IV Therapy n (%)
All Treated DVT Patients with or without PE	298 (100)	312 (100)	290 (100)
Patient Outcome Total VTE[†] (%)	13 (4.4)[‡]	9 (2.9)[‡]	12 (4.1)
DVT Only (%)	11 (3.7)	7 (2.2)	8 (2.8)
Proximal DVT (%)	9 (3.0)	6 (1.9)	7 (2.4)
PE (%)	2 (0.7)	2 (0.6)	4 (1.4)

* All patients were also treated with warfarin sodium commencing within 72 hours of Lovenox or standard heparin therapy.
† VTE = venous thromboembolic event (DVT and/or PE)
‡ The 95% Confidence Intervals for the treatment differences for total VTE were:
Lovenox once a day versus heparin (-3.0 to 3.5)
Lovenox every 12 hours versus heparin (-4.2 to 1.7).

Table 23 Efficacy of Lovenox in the Prophylaxis of Ischemic Complications in Unstable Angina and Non-Q-Wave Myocardial Infarction (Combined Endpoint of Death, Myocardial Infarction, or Recurrent Angina)

Indication	Dosing Regimen*		Reduction (%)	p Value
	Lovenox 1 mg/kg q12h SC n (%)	Heparin aPTT Adjusted IV Therapy n (%)		
All Treated Unstable Angina and Non-Q-Wave MI Patients	1578 (100)	1529 (100)		
Timepoint[†] 48 Hours	96 (6.1)	112 (7.3)	1.2	0.120
14 Days	261 (16.5)	303 (19.8)	3.3	0.017
30 Days	313 (19.8)	358 (23.4)	3.6	0.014

* All patients were also treated with aspirin 100 to 325 mg per day.
† Evaluation timepoints are after initiation of treatment. Therapy continued for up to 8 days (median duration of 2.6 days).

Table 24 Efficacy of Lovenox in the Prophylaxis of Ischemic Complications in Unstable Angina and Non-Q-Wave Myocardial Infarction (Combined Endpoint of Death or Myocardial Infarction)

Indication	Dosing Regimen*		Reduction (%)	p Value
	Lovenox 1 mg/kg q12h SC n (%)	Heparin aPTT Adjusted IV Therapy n (%)		
All Treated Unstable Angina and Non-Q-Wave MI Patients	1578 (100)	1529 (100)		
Timepoint[†] 48 Hours	16 (1.0)	20 (1.3)	0.3	0.126
14 Days	76 (4.8)	93 (6.1)	1.3	0.115
30 Days	96 (6.1)	118 (7.7)	1.6	0.069

* All patients were also treated with aspirin 100 to 325 mg per day.
† Evaluation timepoints are after initiation of treatment. Therapy continued for up to 8 days (median duration of 2.6 days).

Study medication was initiated between 15 minutes before and 30 minutes after the initiation of fibrinolytic therapy. Unfractionated heparin was administered beginning with an IV bolus of 60 U/kg (maximum 4000 U) and followed with an infusion of 12 U/kg per hour (initial maximum 1000 U per hour) that was adjusted to maintain an aPTT of 1.5 to 2 times the control value. The IV infusion was to be given for at least 48 hours. The enoxaparin dosing strategy was adjusted according to the patient's age and renal function. For patients younger than 75 years of age, enoxaparin was given as a single 30 mg intravenous bolus plus a 1 mg/kg SC dose followed by an SC injection of 1 mg/kg every 12 hours. For patients at least 75 years of age, the IV bolus was not given and the SC dose was reduced to 0.75 mg/kg every 12 hours. For patients with severe renal insufficiency (estimated creatinine clearance of less than 30 mL per minute), the dose was to be modified to 1 mg/kg every 24 hours. The SC injections of enoxaparin were given until hospital discharge or for a maximum of eight days (whichever came first). The mean treatment duration for enoxaparin was 6.6 days. The mean treatment duration of unfractionated heparin was 54 hours.

When percutaneous coronary intervention was performed during study medication period, patients received antithrombotic support with blinded study drug. For patients on enoxaparin, the PCI was to be performed on enoxaparin (no switch) using the regimen established in previous studies, i.e. no additional dosing, if the last SC administration was less than 8 hours before balloon inflation, IV bolus of 0.3 mg/kg enoxaparin if the last SC administration was more than 8 hours before balloon inflation.

Table 25 Efficacy of Lovenox in the Treatment of Acute ST-Segment Elevation Myocardial Infarction

	Enoxaparin (N=10,256)	UFH (N=10,223)	Relative Risk (95% CI)	P Value
Outcome at 48 hours	n (%)	n (%)		
Death or Myocardial Re-infarction	478 (4.7)	531 (5.2)	0.90 (0.80 to 1.01)	0.08
Death	383 (3.7)	390 (3.8)	0.98 (0.85 to 1.12)	0.76
Myocardial Re-infarction	102 (1.0)	156 (1.5)	0.65 (0.51 to 0.84)	<0.001
Urgent Revascularization	74 (0.7)	96 (0.9)	0.77 (0.57 to 1.04)	0.09
Death or Myocardial Re-infarction or Urgent Revascularization	548 (5.3)	622 (6.1)	0.88 (0.79 to 0.98)	0.02
Outcome at 8 Days				
Death or Myocardial Re-infarction	740 (7.2)	954 (9.3)	0.77 (0.71 to 0.85)	<0.001
Death	559 (5.5)	605 (5.9)	0.92 (0.82 to 1.03)	0.15
Myocardial Re-infarction	204 (2.0)	378 (3.7)	0.54 (0.45 to 0.63)	<0.001
Urgent Revascularization	145 (1.4)	247 (2.4)	0.59 (0.48 to 0.72)	<0.001
Death or Myocardial Re-infarction or Urgent Revascularization	874 (8.5)	1181 (11.6)	0.74 (0.68 to 0.80)	<0.001
Outcome at 30 Days				
Primary efficacy endpoint (Death or Myocardial Re-infarction)	**1017 (9.9)**	**1223 (12.0)**	**0.83 (0.77 to 0.90)**	**0.000003**
Death	708 (6.9)	765 (7.5)	0.92 (0.84 to 1.02)	0.11
Myocardial Re-infarction	352 (3.4)	508 (5.0)	0.69 (0.60 to 0.79)	<0.001
Urgent Revascularization	213 (2.1)	286 (2.8)	0.74 (0.62 to 0.88)	<0.001
Death or Myocardial Re-infarction or Urgent Revascularization	1199 (11.7)	1479 (14.5)	0.81 (0.75 to 0.87)	<0.001

Note: Urgent revascularization denotes episodes of recurrent myocardial ischemia (without infarction) leading to the clinical decision to perform coronary revascularization during the same hospitalization. CI denotes confidence intervals.

Table 26 100 mg/mL Concentration

Dosage Unit/Strength*	Anti-Xa Activity†	Package Size (per carton)	Label Color	NDC # 0075-
Prefilled Syringes‡				
30 mg/0.3 mL	3000 IU	10 syringes	Medium Blue	0624-30
40 mg/0.4 mL	4000 IU	10 syringes	Yellow	0620-40
Graduated Prefilled Syringes‡				
60 mg/0.6 mL	6000 IU	10 syringes	Orange	0621-60
80 mg/0.8 mL	8000 IU	10 syringes	Brown	0622-80
100 mg/1 mL	10,000 IU	10 syringes	Black	0623-00
Multiple-Dose Vial§				
300 mg/3 mL	30,000 IU	1 vial	Red	0626-03

* Strength represents the number of milligrams of enoxaparin sodium in Water for Injection. Lovenox 30 and 40 mg prefilled syringes, and 60, 80, and 100 mg graduated prefilled syringes each contain **10 mg enoxaparin sodium per 0.1 mL Water for Injection.**
† Approximate anti-Factor Xa activity based on reference to the W.H.O. First International Low Molecular Weight Heparin Reference Standard.
‡ Each Lovenox prefilled syringe is for single, one-time use only and is affixed with a 27 gauge × 1/2 inch needle.
§ Each Lovenox multiple-dose vial contains 15 mg benzyl alcohol per 1 mL as a preservative.

Table 27 150 mg/mL Concentration

Dosage Unit / Strength*	Anti-Xa Activity†	Package Size (per carton)	Syringe Label Color	NDC # 0075-
Graduated Prefilled Syringes‡				
120 mg/0.8 mL	12,000 IU	10 syringes	Purple	2912-01
150 mg/1 mL	15,000 IU	10 syringes	Navy Blue	2915-01

* Strength represents the number of milligrams of enoxaparin sodium in Water for Injection. Lovenox 120 and 150 mg graduated prefilled syringes contain **15 mg enoxaparin sodium per 0.1 mL** Water for Injection.
† Approximate anti-Factor Xa activity based on reference to the W.H.O. First International Low Molecular Weight Heparin Reference Standard.
‡ Each Lovenox graduated prefilled syringe is for single, one-time use only and is affixed with a 27 gauge × 1/2 inch needle.

All patients were treated with aspirin for a minimum of 30 days. Eighty percent of patients received a fibrin-specific agent (19% tenecteplase, 5% reteplase and 55% alteplase) and 20% received streptokinase.
Among 20,479 patients in the ITT population, the mean age was 60 years, and 76% were male. Racial distribution was: 87% Caucasian, 9.8% Asian, 0.2% Black, and 2.8% other. Medical history included previous MI (13%), hypertension (44%), diabetes (15%) and angiographic evidence of CAD (5%). Concomitant medication included aspirin (95%), beta-blockers (86%), ACE inhibitors (78%), statins (70%) and clopidogrel (27%). The MI at entry was anterior in 43%, non-anterior in 56%, and both in 1%.

The primary efficacy end point was the composite of death from any cause or myocardial re-infarction in the first 30 days after randomization. Total follow-up was one year.
The rate of the primary efficacy end point (death or myocardial re-infarction) was 9.9% in the enoxaparin group, and 12.0% in the unfractionated heparin group, a 17% reduction in the relative risk, (P=0.000003) [see Table 25].
[See table 25 above]
The beneficial effect of enoxaparin on the primary end point was consistent across key subgroups including age, gender, infarct location, history of diabetes, history of prior myocardial infarction, fibrinolytic agent administered, and time to

treatment with study drug (see Figure 1); however, it is necessary to interpret such subgroup analyses with caution.

Figure 1. Relative Risks of and Absolute Event Rates for the Primary End Point at 30 Days in Various Subgroups *

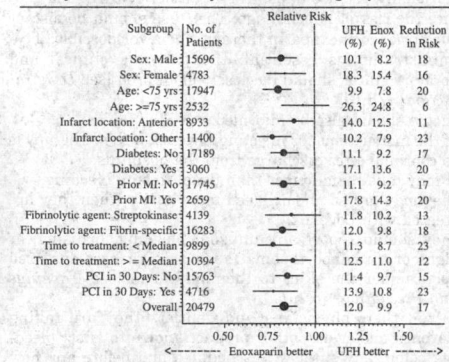

* The primary efficacy end point was the composite of death from any cause or myocardial re-infarction in the first 30 days. The overall treatment effect of enoxaparin as compared to the unfractionated heparin is shown at the bottom of the figure. For each subgroup, the circle is proportional to the number and represents the point estimate of the treatment effect and the horizontal lines represent the 95 percent confidence intervals. Fibrin-specific fibrinolytic agents included alteplase, tenecteplase and reteplase. Time to treatment indicates the time from the onset of symptoms to the administration of study drug (median, 3.2 hours).

The beneficial effect of enoxaparin on the primary end point observed during the first 30 days was maintained over a 12 month follow-up period (see Figure 2).

Figure 2 - Kaplan-Meier plot - death or myocardial re-infarction at 30 days - ITT population

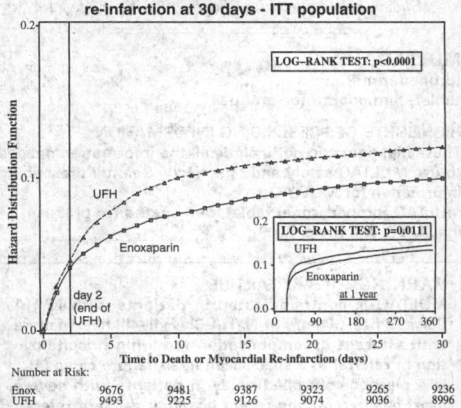

Number at Risk:						
Enox	9676	9481	9387	9323	9265	9236
UFH	9493	9225	9126	9074	9036	8996

There is a trend in favor of enoxaparin during the first 48 hours, but most of the treatment difference is attributed to a step increase in the event rate in the UFH group at 48 hours (seen in Figure 2), an effect that is more striking when comparing the event rates just prior to and just subsequent to actual times of discontinuation. These results provide evidence that UFH was effective and that it would be better if used longer than 48 hours. There is a similar increase in endpoint event rate when enoxaparin was discontinued, suggesting that it too was discontinued too soon in this study.
The rates of major hemorrhages (defined as requiring 5 or more units of blood for transfusion, or 15% drop in hematocrit or clinically overt bleeding, including intracranial hemorrhage) at 30 days were 2.1% in the enoxaparin group and 1.4% in the unfractionated heparin group. The rates of intracranial hemorrhage at 30 days were 0.8% in the enoxaparin group and 0.7% in the unfractionated heparin group. The 30-day rate of the composite endpoint of death, myocardial re-infarction or ICH (a measure of net clinical benefit) was significantly lower in the enoxaparin group (10.1%) as compared to the heparin group (12.2%).

16   HOW SUPPLIED/STORAGE AND HANDLING

Lovenox is available in two concentrations [see Tables 26 and 27]:
[See table 26 above]
[See table 27 above]
Store at 25°C (77°F); excursions permitted to 15–30°C (59–86°F) [see USP Controlled Room Temperature].
Do not store the multiple-dose vials for more than 28 days after the first use.
Keep out of the reach of children.

17   PATIENT COUNSELING INFORMATION

If patients have had neuraxial anesthesia or spinal puncture, and particularly, if they are taking concomitant NSAIDs, platelet inhibitors, or other anticoagulants, they should be informed to watch for signs and symptoms of spinal or epidural hematoma, such as tingling, numbness (especially in the lower limbs) and muscular weakness. If any of these symptoms occur the patient should contact his or her physician immediately.

Additionally, the use of aspirin and other NSAIDs may enhance the risk of hemorrhage. Their use should be discontinued prior to enoxaparin therapy whenever possible; if co-administration is essential, the patient's clinical and laboratory status should be closely monitored [see *Drug Interactions (7)*].

Patients should also be informed:

- of the instructions for injecting Lovenox if their therapy is to continue after discharge from the hospitals.
- it may take them longer than usual to stop bleeding.
- they may bruise and/or bleed more easily when they are treated with Lovenox.
- they should report any unusual bleeding, bruising, or signs of thrombocytopenia (such as a rash of dark red spots under the skin) to their physician [see *Warnings and Precautions (5.1, 5.5)*].
- to tell their physicians and dentists they are taking Lovenox and/or any other product known to affect bleeding before any surgery is scheduled and before any new drug is taken [see *Warnings and Precautions (5.3)*].
- to tell their physicians and dentists of all medications they are taking, including those obtained without a prescription, such as aspirin or other NSAIDs [see *Drug Interactions (7)*].

sanofi-aventis U.S. LLC
Bridgewater, NJ 08807
Multiple-dose vials are also manufactured by DSM Pharmaceuticals, Inc.
Greenville, NC 27835
© 2009 sanofi-aventis U.S. LLC
Shown in Product Identification Guide, page 319

MULTAQ ℞
(dronedarone)
tablet, film coated for oral use

HIGHLIGHTS OF PRESCRIBING INFORMATION
These highlights do not include all the information needed to use MULTAQ safely and effectively. See full prescribing information for MULTAQ.
MULTAQ (dronedarone) tablet, film coated for oral use
Initial U.S. Approval: 2009

> **WARNING: HEART FAILURE**
> MULTAQ is contraindicated in patients with NYHA Class IV heart failure or NYHA Class II – III heart failure with a recent decompensation requiring hospitalization or referral to a specialized heart failure clinic (4).
> In a placebo-controlled study in patients with severe heart failure requiring recent hospitalization or referral to a specialized heart failure clinic for worsening symptoms (the ANDROMEDA Study), patients given dronedarone had a greater than two-fold increase in mortality. Such patients should not be given dronedarone (14.3).

————INDICATIONS AND USAGE————
MULTAQ is an antiarrhythmic drug indicated to reduce the risk of cardiovascular hospitalization in patients with paroxysmal or persistent atrial fibrillation (AF) or atrial flutter (AFL), with a recent episode of AF/AFL and associated cardiovascular risk factors (i.e., age >70, hypertension, diabetes, prior cerebrovascular accident, left atrial diameter ≥50 mm or left ventricular ejection fraction [LVEF] <40%), who are in sinus rhythm or who will be cardioverted (1, 14).

————DOSAGE AND ADMINISTRATION————
One tablet of 400 mg twice a day with morning and evening meals (2)

————DOSAGE FORMS AND STRENGTHS————
400 mg film-coated tablets (3)

————CONTRAINDICATIONS————
- Class IV heart failure or symptomatic heart failure with a recent decompensation (Boxed Warning, 4)
- Second- or third-degree atrioventicular (AV) block or sick sinus syndrome (except when used in conjunction with a functioning pacemaker) (4)
- Bradycardia <50 bpm (4)
- Concomitant use of a strong CYP3A inhibitor (4)
- Concomitant use of drugs or herbal products that prolong the QT interval and may induce Torsade de Pointes (4)
- QTc Bazett interval ≥500 ms (4)
- Severe hepatic impairment (4)
- Pregnancy (4, 8.1)
- Nursing mothers (4, 8.3)

————WARNINGS AND PRECAUTIONS————
- Heart failure: If heart failure develops or worsens, consider the suspension or discontinuation of MULTAQ (5.1)
- Hypokalemia and hypomagnesemia: Maintain potassium and magnesium levels within the normal range (5.2)

- QT prolongation: Stop MULTAQ if QTc Bazett ≥500ms (5.3)
- Increase in creatinine: Within a week, MULTAQ causes a small increase in serum creatinine that does not reflect a change in underlying renal function (5.4)
- Teratogen: Women of childbearing potential should use effective contraception while using MULTAQ (5.5)

————ADVERSE REACTIONS————
Most common adverse reactions (≥2%) are diarrhea, nausea, abdominal pain, vomiting, and asthenia (6)

To report SUSPECTED ADVERSE REACTIONS, contact sanofi-aventis U.S. LLC at 1-800-633-1610 or FDA at 1-800-FDA-1088 or www.fda.gov/medwatch

————DRUG INTERACTIONS————
Dronedarone is metabolized by CYP 3A and is a moderate inhibitor of CYP 3A and CYP 2D6 and has potentially important pharmacodynamic interactions (7)
- Antiarrhythmics: Avoid concomitant use (4, 7.1)
- Digoxin: Consider discontinuation or halve dose of digoxin before treatment and monitor (7.1, 7.3)
- Calcium channel blockers (CCB): Initiate CCB with low dose and increase after ECG verification of tolerability (7.1, 7.2, 7.3)
- Beta-blockers: May provoke excessive bradycardia, Initiate with low dose and increase after ECG verification of tolerability (7.1, 7.3)
- CYP 3A inducers: Avoid concomitant use (7.2)
- Grapefruit juice: Avoid concomitant use (7.2)
- Statins: Follow label recommendations for concomitant use of certain statins with a CYP 3A and P-gP inhibitor like dronedarone (7.3)
- CYP 3A substrates with a narrow therapeutic index (e.g., sirolimus and tacrolimus): Monitor and adjust dosage of concomitant drug as needed when used with MULTAQ (7.3)

See 17 for PATIENT COUNSELING INFORMATION and Medication Guide

Revised: 07/2009

FULL PRESCRIBING INFORMATION: CONTENTS*
WARNING: HEART FAILURE
1 INDICATIONS AND USAGE
2 DOSAGE AND ADMINISTRATION
3 DOSAGE FORMS AND STRENGTHS
4 CONTRAINDICATIONS
5 WARNINGS AND PRECAUTIONS
  5.1 Patients with New or Worsening Heart Failure during Treatment
  5.2 Hypokalemia and Hypomagnesemia with Potassium-Depleting Diuretics
  5.3 QT Interval Prolongation
  5.4 Increase in Creatinine after Treatment Initiation
  5.5 Women of Childbearing Potential
6 ADVERSE REACTIONS
7 DRUG INTERACTIONS
  7.1 Pharmacodynamic Interactions
  7.2 Effects of Other Drugs on Dronedarone
  7.3 Effects of Dronedarone on Other Drugs
8 USE IN SPECIFIC POPULATIONS
  8.1 Pregnancy
  8.3 Nursing Mothers
  8.4 Pediatric Use
  8.5 Geriatric Use
  8.6 Renal Impairment
  8.7 Hepatic Impairment
10 OVERDOSAGE
11 DESCRIPTION
12 CLINICAL PHARMACOLOGY
  12.1 Mechanism of Action
  12.2 Pharmacodynamics
  12.3 Pharmacokinetics
13 NONCLINICAL TOXICOLOGY
  13.1 Carcinogenesis, Mutagenesis, Impairment of Fertility
  13.3 Developmental Toxicity
14 CLINICAL STUDIES
  14.1 ATHENA Study
  14.2 EURIDIS and ADONIS Studies
  14.3 ANDROMEDA Study (Increased Mortality in Patients with Severe Heart Failure)
16 HOW SUPPLIED/STORAGE AND HANDLING
17 PATIENT COUNSELING INFORMATION
  17.1 Information for Patients
  17.2 Medication Guide
* Sections or subsections omitted from the full prescribing information are not listed

FULL PRESCRIBING INFORMATION

> **WARNING: HEART FAILURE**
> MULTAQ is contraindicated in patients with NYHA Class IV heart failure, or NYHA Class II – III heart failure with a recent decompensation requiring hospitaliza-

---

tion or referral to a specialized heart failure clinic [see *Contraindications (4)*].
In a placebo-controlled study in patients with severe heart failure requiring recent hospitalization or referral to a specialized heart failure clinic for worsening symptoms (the ANDROMEDA Study), patients given dronedarone had a greater than two-fold increase in mortality. Such patients should not be given dronedarone [see *Clinical Studies (14.3)*].

1 INDICATIONS AND USAGE
MULTAQ® is indicated to reduce the risk of cardiovascular hospitalization in patients with paroxysmal or persistent atrial fibrillation (AF) or atrial flutter (AFL), with a recent episode of AF/AFL and associated cardiovascular risk factors (i.e., age >70, hypertension, diabetes, prior cerebrovascular accident, left atrial diameter ≥50 mm or left ventricular ejection fraction [LVEF] <40%), who are in sinus rhythm or who will be cardioverted [see *Clinical Studies (14)*].

2 DOSAGE AND ADMINISTRATION
The only recommended dosage of MULTAQ is 400 mg twice daily in adults. MULTAQ should be taken as one tablet with the morning meal and one tablet with the evening meal. Treatment with Class I or III antiarrhythmics (e.g., amiodarone, flecainide, propafenone, quinidine, disopyramide, dofetilide, sotalol) or drugs that are strong inhibitors of CYP3A (e.g., ketoconazole) must be stopped before starting MULTAQ [see *Contraindications (4)*].

3 DOSAGE FORMS AND STRENGTHS
MULTAQ 400 mg tablets are provided as white film-coated tablets for oral administration, oblong-shaped, engraved with a double wave marking on one side and "4142" code on the other side.

4 CONTRAINDICATIONS
MULTAQ is contraindicated in patients with:
- NYHA Class IV heart failure or NYHA Class II – III heart failure with a recent decompensation requiring hospitalization or referral to a specialized heart failure clinic [see *Boxed Warning and Clinical Studies (14.3)*]
- Second- or third-degree atrioventricular (AV) block or sick sinus syndrome (except when used in conjunction with a functioning pacemaker)
- Bradycardia <50 bpm
- Concomitant use of strong CYP 3A inhibitors, such as ketoconazole, itraconazole, voriconazole, cyclosporine, telithromycin, clarithromycin, nefazodone, and ritonavir [see *Drug Interactions (7.2)*]
- Concomitant use of drugs or herbal products that prolong the QT interval and might increase the risk of Torsade de Pointes, such as phenothiazine anti-psychotics, tricyclic antidepressants, certain oral macrolide antibiotics, and Class I and III antiarrhythmics
- QTc Bazett interval ≥500 ms or PR interval >280 ms
- Severe hepatic impairment
- Pregnancy (Category X): MULTAQ may cause fetal harm when administered to a pregnant woman. MULTAQ is contraindicated in women who are or may become pregnant. If this drug is used during pregnancy, or if the patient becomes pregnant while taking this drug, the patient should be apprised of the potential hazard to a fetus [see *Use in Specific Populations (8.1)*].
- Nursing mothers [see *Use in Specific Populations (8.3)*]

5 WARNINGS AND PRECAUTIONS

5.1 Patients with New or Worsening Heart Failure during Treatment
Advise patients to consult a physician if they develop signs or symptoms of heart failure, such as weight gain, dependent edema, or increasing shortness of breath. There are limited data available for AF/AFL patients who develop worsening heart failure during treatment with MULTAQ. If heart failure develops or worsens, consider the suspension or discontinuation of MULTAQ.

5.2 Hypokalemia and Hypomagnesemia with Potassium-Depleting Diuretics
Hypokalemia or hypomagnesemia may occur with concomitant administration of potassium-depleting diuretics. Potassium levels should be within the normal range prior to administration of MULTAQ and maintained in the normal range during administration of MULTAQ.

5.3 QT Interval Prolongation
Dronedarone induces a moderate (average of about 10 ms but much greater effects have been observed) QTc (Bazett) prolongation [see *Clinical Pharmacology (12.2) and Clinical Studies (14.1)*]. If the QTc Bazett interval is ≥500 ms, MULTAQ should be stopped [see *Contraindications (4)*].

5.4 Increase in Creatinine after Treatment Initiation
Serum creatinine levels increase by about 0.1 mg/dL following dronedarone treatment initiation.

The elevation has a rapid onset, reaches a plateau after 7 days and is reversible after discontinuation. If an increase in serum creatinine occurs and plateaus, this increased value should be used as the patient's new baseline. The change in creatinine levels has been shown to be the result of an inhibition of creatinine's tubular secretion, with no effect upon the glomerular filtration rate.

5.5 Women of Childbearing Potential

Premenopausal women who have not undergone a hysterectomy or oophorectomy must use effective contraception while using MULTAQ. Dronedarone caused fetal harm in animal studies at doses equivalent to recommended human doses. Women of childbearing potential should be counseled regarding appropriate contraceptive choices taking into consideration their underlying medical conditions and lifestyle preferences [see Use in Specific Populations (8.1)].

6 ADVERSE REACTIONS

The following safety concerns are described elsewhere in the label:

- New or worsening heart failure [see Warnings and Precautions (5.1)]
- Hypokalemia and hypomagnesemia with potassium-depleting diuretics [see Warnings and Precautions (5.2)]
- QT prolongation [see Warnings and Precautions (5.3)]

The safety evaluation of dronedarone 400 mg twice daily in patients with AF or AFL is based on 5 placebo controlled studies, ATHENA, EURIDIS, ADONIS, ERATO and DAFNE. In these studies, a total of 6285 patients were randomized and treated, 3282 patients with MULTAQ 400 mg twice daily, and 2875 with placebo. The mean exposure across studies was 12 months. In ATHENA, the maximum follow-up was 30 months.

In clinical trials, premature discontinuation because of adverse reactions occurred in 11.8% of the dronedarone-treated patients and in 7.7% of the placebo-treated group. The most common reasons for discontinuation of therapy with MULTAQ were gastrointestinal disorders (3.2% versus 1.8% in the placebo group) and QT prolongation (1.5% versus 0.5% in the placebo group).

The most frequent adverse reactions observed with MULTAQ 400 mg twice daily in the 5 studies were diarrhea, nausea, abdominal pain, vomiting, and asthenia.

Table 1 displays adverse reactions more common with dronedarone 400 mg twice daily than with placebo in AF or AFL patients, presented by system organ class and by decreasing order of frequency. Adverse laboratory and ECG effects are presented separately in Table 2.

Table 1: Adverse Drug Reactions that Occurred in at Least 1% of Patients and Were More Frequent than Placebo

	Placebo (N=2875)	Dronedarone 400 mg twice daily (N=3282)
Gastrointestinal		
Diarrhea	6%	9%
Nausea	3%	5%
Abdominal pain	3%	4%
Vomiting	1%	2%
Dyspeptic signs and symptoms	1%	2%
General		
Asthenic conditions	5%	7%
Cardiac		
Bradycardia	1%	3%
Skin and subcutaneous tissue		
Including rashes (generalized, macular, maculo-papular, erythematous), pruritus, eczema, dermatitis, dermatitis allergic	3%	5%

Photosensitivity reaction and dysgeusia have also been reported at an incidence less than 1% in patients treated with MULTAQ.

The following laboratory data/ECG parameters were reported with MULTAQ 400 mg twice daily.

Table 2: Laboratory data/ECG parameters not necessarily reported as adverse events

	Placebo	MULTAQ 400 mg twice daily
	(N=2875)	(N=3282)
Serum creatinine increased ≥10% five days after treatment initiation	21%	51%
	(N=2237)	(N=2701)
QTc Bazett prolonged (>450 ms in males >470 ms in females)	19%	28%

Assessment of demographic factors such as gender or age on the incidence of treatment-emergent adverse events did not suggest an excess of adverse events in any particular subgroup.

7 DRUG INTERACTIONS

Dronedarone is metabolized primarily by CYP 3A and is a moderate inhibitor of CYP 3A and CYP 2D6 [see Clinical Pharmacology (12.3)]. Dronedarone's blood levels can therefore be affected by inhibitors and inducers of CYP 3A, and dronedarone can interact with drugs that are substrates of CYP 3A and CYP 2D6.

Dronedarone has no significant potential to inhibit CYP 1A2, CYP 2C9, CYP 2C19, CYP 2C8 and CYP 2B6. It has the potential to inhibit P-glycoprotein (P-gP) transport. Pharmacodynamic interactions can be expected with beta-blockers; calcium antagonists and digoxin [see Drug Interactions (7.1)].

In clinical trials, patients treated with dronedarone received concomitant medications including beta-blockers, digoxin, calcium antagonists (including those with heart rate-lowering effects), statins and oral anticoagulants.

7.1 Pharmacodynamic Interactions

Drugs prolonging the QT interval (inducing Torsade de Pointes)

Co-administration of drugs prolonging the QT interval (such as certain phenothiazines, tricyclic antidepressants, certain macrolide antibiotics, and Class I and III antiarrhythmics) is contraindicated because of the potential risk of Torsade de Pointes-type ventricular tachycardia [see Contraindications (4)].

Digoxin

Digoxin can potentiate the electrophysiologic effects of dronedarone (such as decreased AV-node conduction). In clinical trials, increased levels of digoxin were observed when dronedarone was co-administered with digoxin. Gastrointestinal disorders were also increased.

Because of the pharmacokinetic interaction [see Drug Interaction (7.3)] and possible pharmacodynamic interaction, reconsider the need for digoxin therapy. If digoxin treatment is continued, halve the dose of digoxin, monitor serum levels closely, and observe for toxicity.

Calcium channel blockers

Calcium channel blockers with depressant effects on the sinus and AV nodes could potentiate dronedarone's effects on conduction.

Give low doses of calcium channel blockers initially and increase only after ECG verification of good tolerability [see Drug Interactions (7.3)].

Beta-blockers

In clinical trials, bradycardia was more frequently observed when dronedarone was given in combination with beta-blockers.

Give low dose of beta-blockers initially, and increase only after ECG verification of good tolerability [see Drug Interactions (7.3)].

7.2 Effects of Other Drugs on Dronedarone

Ketoconazole and other potent CYP 3A inhibitors

Repeated doses of ketoconazole, a strong CYP 3A inhibitor, resulted in a 17-fold increase in dronedarone exposure and a 9-fold increase in C_{max}. Concomitant use of ketoconazole as well as other potent CYP 3A inhibitors such as itraconazole, voriconazole, ritonavir, clarithromycin, and nefazodone is contraindicated [see Contraindications (4)].

Grapefruit juice

Grapefruit juice, a moderate inhibitor of CYP 3A, resulted in a 3-fold increase in dronedarone exposure and a 2.5-fold increase in C_{max}. Therefore, patients should avoid grapefruit juice beverages while taking MULTAQ.

Rifampin and other CYP 3A inducers

Rifampin decreased dronedarone exposure by 80%. Avoid rifampin or other CYP 3A inducers such as phenobarbital, carbamazepine, phenytoin, and St John's wort with dronedarone because they decrease its exposure significantly.

Calcium channel blockers

Verapamil and diltiazem are moderate CYP 3A inhibitors and increase dronedarone exposure by approximately 1.4- to 1.7-fold [see Drug Interactions (7.1, 7.3)].

Pantoprazole

Pantoprazole, a drug that increases gastric pH, did not have a significant effect on dronedarone pharmacokinetics.

7.3 Effects of Dronedarone on Other Drugs

Statins

Dronedarone increased simvastatin/simvastatin acid exposure by 4- and 2-fold, respectively.

Because of multiple mechanisms of interaction with statins (CYPs and transporters), follow statin label recommendations for use with CYP 3A and P-gP inhibitors such as dronedarone.

Calcium channel blockers

Dronedarone increases calcium channel blocker (verapamil, diltiazem or nifedipine) exposure by 1.4- to 1.5-fold [see Drug Interactions (7.1)].

Sirolimus, tacrolimus, and other CYP3A substrates with narrow therapeutic range

Dronedarone can increase plasma concentrations of tacrolimus, sirolimus, and other CYP 3A substrates with a narrow therapeutic range when given orally. Monitor plasma concentrations and adjust dosage appropriately.

Beta-blockers and other CYP 2D6 substrates

Dronedarone increased propranolol exposure by approximately 1.3-fold following single dose administration. Dronedarone increased metoprolol exposure by 1.6-fold following multiple dose administration [see Drug Interaction (7.1)]. Other CYP 2D6 substrates, including other beta-blockers, tricyclic antidepressants, and selective serotonin reuptake inhibitors (SSRIs) may have increased exposure upon co-administration with dronedarone.

Digoxin and P-glycoprotein substrates

Dronedarone increased digoxin exposure by 2.5-fold by inhibiting the P-gP transporter [see Drug Interactions (7.1)]. Other P-gP substrates are expected to have increased exposure when coadministered with dronedarone.

Warfarin and losartan (CYP 2C9 substrates)

In healthy subjects, dronedarone at a dose of 600 mg twice daily increased S-warfarin exposure by 1.2-fold with no change in R-warfarin and with no clinically significant increase in INR. In clinical trials in patients with AF/AFL, there was no observed excess risk of bleeding compared to placebo when dronedarone was co-administered with oral anticoagulants. Monitor INR per the warfarin label.

No interaction was observed between dronedarone and losartan.

Theophylline (CYP 1A2 substrate)

Dronedarone does not increase steady state theophylline exposure.

Oral contraceptives

No decreases in ethinylestradiol and levonorgestrel concentrations were observed in healthy subjects receiving dronedarone concomitantly with oral contraceptives.

8 USE IN SPECIFIC POPULATIONS

8.1 Pregnancy

Pregnancy Category X [see Contraindications (4)]

MULTAQ may cause fetal harm when administered to a pregnant woman. In animal studies, dronedarone is teratogenic in rats at the maximum recommended human dose (MRHD), and in rabbits at half the MRHD. If this drug is used during pregnancy or if the patient becomes pregnant while taking this drug, the patient should be apprised of the potential hazard to the fetus.

When pregnant rats received dronedarone at oral doses greater than or equal to the MRHD (on a mg/m^2 basis), fetuses had increased rates of external, visceral and skeletal malformations (cranioschisis, cleft palate, incomplete evagination of pineal body, brachygnathia, partially fused carotid arteries, truncus arteriosus, abnormal lobation of the liver, partially duplicated inferior vena cava, brachydactyly, ectrodactylia, syndactylia, and anterior and/or posterior club feet). When pregnant rabbits received dronedarone, at a dose approximately half the MRHD (on a mg/m^2 basis), fetuses had an increased rate of skeletal abnormalities (anomalous ribcage and vertebrae, pelvic asymmetry) at doses ≥20 mg/kg (the lowest dose tested and approximately half the MRHD on a mg/m^2 basis).

Actual animal doses: rat (≥80 mg/kg/day); rabbit (≥20 mg/kg)

8.3 Nursing Mothers

It is not known whether MULTAQ is excreted in human milk. Dronedarone and its metabolites are excreted in rat milk. During a pre- and post-natal study in rats, maternal dronedarone administration was associated with minor reduced body-weight gain in the offspring. Because many drugs are excreted in human milk and because of the potential for serious adverse reactions in nursing infants from MULTAQ, a decision should be made whether to discontinue nursing or to discontinue the drug, taking into account the importance of the drug to the mother *[see Contraindications (4)]*.

8.4 Pediatric Use

Safety and efficacy in children below the age of 18 years have not been established.

8.5 Geriatric Use

More than 4500 patients with AF or AFL aged 65 years or above were included in the MULTAQ clinical program (of whom more than 2000 patients were 75 years or older). Efficacy and safety were similar in elderly and younger patients.

8.6 Renal Impairment

Patients with renal impairment were included in clinical studies. Because renal excretion of dronedarone is minimal *[see Clinical Pharmacology (12.3)]*, no dosing alteration is needed.

8.7 Hepatic Impairment

Dronedarone is extensively metabolized by the liver. There is little clinical experience with moderate hepatic impairment and none with severe impairment. No dosage adjustment is recommended for moderate hepatic impairment *[see Contraindications (4) and Clinical Pharmacology (12.3)]*.

10 OVERDOSAGE

In the event of overdosage, monitor the patient's cardiac rhythm and blood pressure. Treatment should be supportive and based on symptoms.

It is not known whether dronedarone or its metabolites can be removed by dialysis (hemodialysis, peritoneal dialysis or hemofiltration).

There is no specific antidote available.

11 DESCRIPTION

Dronedarone HCl is a benzofuran derivative with the following chemical name:

N-{2-butyl-3-[4-(3-dibutylaminopropoxy)benzoyl]benzofuran-5-yl} methanesulfonamide, hydrochloride.

Dronedarone HCl is a white fine powder that is practically insoluble in water and freely soluble in methylene chloride and methanol.

Its empirical formula is $C_{31}H_{44}N_2O_5$ S, HCl with a relative molecular mass of 593.2. Its structural formula is:

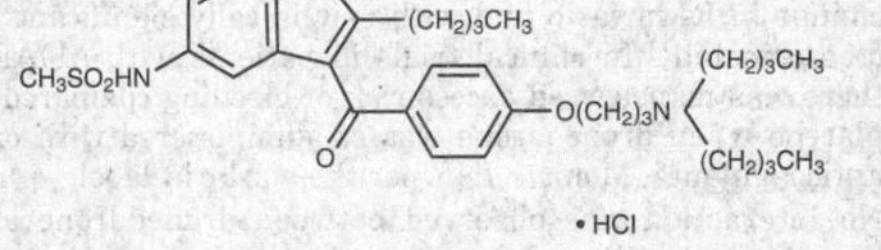

MULTAQ is provided as tablets for oral administration.

Each tablet of MULTAQ contains 400 mg of dronedarone (expressed as base).

The inactive ingredients are:

Core of the tablets—hypromellose, starch, crospovidone, poloxamer 407, lactose monohydrate, colloidal silicon dioxide, magnesium stearate.

Coating/polishing of the tablets—hypromellose, polyethylene glycol 6000, titanium dioxide, carnauba wax.

12 CLINICAL PHARMACOLOGY

12.1 Mechanism of Action

The mechanism of action of dronedarone is unknown. Dronedarone has antiarrhythmic properties belonging to all four Vaughan-Williams classes, but the contribution of each of these activities to the clinical effect is unknown.

12.2 Pharmacodynamics

Electrophysiological effects

Dronedarone exhibits properties of all four Vaughn-Williams antiarrhythmic classes, although it is unclear which of these are important in producing dronedarone's clinical effects. The effect of dronedarone on 12-lead ECG parameters (heart rate, PR, and QTc) was investigated in healthy subjects following repeated oral doses up to 1600 mg once daily or 800 mg twice daily for 14 days and 1600 mg twice daily for 10 days. In the dronedarone 400 mg twice daily group, there was no apparent effect on heart rate; a moderate heart rate lowering effect (about 4 bpm) was noted at 800 mg twice daily. There was a clear dose-dependent effect on PR-interval with an increase of +5 ms at 400 mg twice daily and up to +50 ms at 1600 mg twice daily. There was a moderate dose related effect on the QTc-interval with an increase of +10 ms at 400 mg twice daily and up to +25 ms with 1600 mg twice daily.

DAFNE study

DAFNE was a dose-response study in patients with recurrent AF, evaluating the effect of dronedarone in comparison with placebo in maintaining sinus rhythm. The doses of dronedarone in this study were 400, 600 and 800 mg twice a day. In this small study, doses above 400 mg were not more effective and were less well tolerated.

12.3 Pharmacokinetics

Dronedarone is extensively metabolized and has low systemic bioavailability; its bioavailability is increased by meals. Its elimination half life is 13–19 hours.

Absorption

Because of presystemic first pass metabolism the absolute bioavailability of dronedarone without food is low, about 4%. It increases to approximately 15% when dronedarone is administered with a high fat meal. After oral administration in fed conditions, peak plasma concentrations of dronedarone and the main circulating active metabolite (N-debutyl metabolite) are reached within 3 to 6 hours. After repeated administration of 400 mg twice daily, steady state is reached within 4 to 8 days of treatment and the mean accumulation ratio for dronedarone ranges from 2.6 to 4.5. The steady state C_{max} and exposure of the main N-debutyl metabolite is similar to that of the parent compound. The pharmacokinetics of dronedarone and its N-debutyl metabolite both deviate moderately from dose proportionality: a 2-fold increase in dose results in an approximate 2.5- to 3.0-fold increase with respect to C_{max} and AUC.

Distribution

The *in vitro* plasma protein binding of dronedarone and its N-debutyl metabolite is >98 % and not saturable. Both compounds bind mainly to albumin. After intravenous (IV) administration the volume of distribution at steady state is about 1400 L.

Metabolism

Dronedarone is extensively metabolized, mainly by CYP 3A. The initial metabolic pathway includes N-debutylation to form the active N-debutyl metabolite, oxidative deamination to form the inactive propanoic acid metabolite, and direct oxidation. The metabolites undergo further metabolism to yield over 30 uncharacterized metabolites. The N-debutyl metabolite exhibits pharmacodynamic activity but is 1/10 to 1/3 as potent as dronedarone

Excretion/Elimination

In a mass balance study with orally administered dronedarone (^{14}C-labeled) approximately 6% of the labeled dose was excreted in urine, mainly as metabolites (no unchanged compound excreted in urine), and 84% was excreted in feces, mainly as metabolites. Dronedarone and its N-debutyl active metabolite accounted for less than 15% of the resultant radioactivity in the plasma.

After IV administration the plasma clearance of dronedarone ranges from 130 to 150 L/h. The elimination half-life of dronedarone ranges from 13 to 19 hours.

Special populations

Gender

Dronedarone exposures are on average 30% higher in females than in males.

Race

Pharmacokinetic differences related to race were not formally assessed. However, based on a cross study comparison, following single dose administration (400 mg), Asian males (Japanese) have about a 2-fold higher exposure than Caucasian males. The pharmacokinetics of dronedarone in other races has not been assessed.

Elderly

Of the total number of subjects in clinical studies of dronedarone, 73% were 65 years of age and over and 34% were 75 and over. In patients aged 65 years old and above, dronedarone exposures are 23% higher than in patients less than 65 years old *[see Use in Specific Populations (8.5)]*.

Hepatic impairment

In subjects with moderate hepatic impairment, the mean dronedarone exposure increased by 1.3-fold relative to subjects with normal hepatic function and the mean exposure of the N-debutyl metabolite decreased by about 50%. Pharmacokinetic data were significantly more variable in subjects with moderate hepatic impairment.

The effect of severe hepatic impairment on the pharmacokinetics of dronedarone was not assessed *[see Contraindications (4)]*.

Renal impairment

Consistent with the low renal excretion of dronedarone, no pharmacokinetic difference was observed in subjects with mild or moderate renal impairment compared to subjects with normal renal function *[see Use in Specific Populations (8.6)]*. No pharmacokinetic difference was observed in patients with mild to severe renal impairment in comparison with patients with normal renal function.

13 NONCLINICAL TOXICOLOGY

13.1 Carcinogenesis, Mutagenesis, Impairment of Fertility

In studies in which dronedarone was administered to rats and mice for up to 2 years at doses of up to 70 mg/kg/day and 300 mg/kg/day, respectively, there was an increased incidence of histiocytic sarcomas in dronedarone-treated male mice (300 mg/kg/day or 5× the maximum recommended human dose based on AUC comparisons), mammary adenocarcinomas in dronedarone-treated female mice (300 mg/kg/day or 8× MRHD based on AUC comparisons) and hemangiomas in dronedarone-treated male rats (70 mg/kg/day or 5× MRHD based on AUC comparisons).

Dronedarone did not demonstrate genotoxic potential in the in vivo mouse micronucleus test, the Ames bacterial mutation assay, the unscheduled DNA synthesis assay, or an in vitro chromosomal aberration assay in human lymphocytes. S-9 processed dronedarone, however, was positive in a V79 transfected Chinese hamster V79 assay.

In fertility studies conducted with female rats, dronedarone given prior to breeding and implantation caused an increase in irregular estrus cycles and cessation of cycling at doses ≥10mg/kg (equivalent to 0.12× the MRHD on a mg/m^2 basis).

Corpora lutea, implantations and live fetuses were decreased at 100 mg/kg (equivalent to 1.2× the MRHD on a mg/m^2 basis). There were no reported effects on mating behavior or fertility of male rats at doses of up to 100 mg/kg/day.

13.3 Developmental Toxicity

Dronedarone was teratogenic in rats given oral doses ≥80 mg/kg/day (a dose equivalent to the maximum recommended human dose [MHRD] on a mg/m^2 basis), with fetuses showing external, visceral and skeletal malformations (cranioschisis, cleft palate, incomplete evagination of pineal body, brachygnathia, partially fused carotid arteries, truncus arteriosus, abnormal lobation of the liver, partially duplicated inferior vena cava, brachydactyly, ectrodactylia, syndactylia, and anterior and/or posterior club feet). In rabbits, dronedarone caused an increase in skeletal abnormalities (anomalous ribcage and vertebrae, pelvic asymmetry) at doses ≥20 mg/kg (the lowest dose tested and approximately half the MRHD on a mg/m^2 basis).

14 CLINICAL STUDIES

14.1 ATHENA Study

ATHENA was a multicenter, multinational, double blind, and randomized placebo-controlled study of dronedarone in 4628 patients with a recent history of AF/AFL who were in sinus rhythm or who were to be converted to sinus rhythm. The objective of the study was to determine whether dronedarone could delay death from any cause or hospitalization for cardiovascular reasons.

Initially patients were to be ≥70 years old, or <70 years old with at least one risk factor (including hypertension, diabetes, prior cerebrovascular accident, left atrial diameter ≥50 mm or LVEF<0.40). The inclusion criteria were later changed such that patients were to be ≥75 years old, or ≥70 years old with at least one risk factor. Patients had to have both AF/AFL and sinus rhythm documented within the previous 6 months. Patients could have been in AF/AFL or in sinus rhythm at the time of randomization, but patients not in sinus rhythm were expected to be either electrically or chemically converted to normal sinus rhythm after anticoagulation.

Subjects were randomized and treated for up to 30 months (median follow-up: 22 months) with either MULTAQ 400 mg twice daily (2301 patients) or placebo (2327 patients), in addition to conventional therapy for cardiovascular diseases that included beta-blockers (71%), ACE inhibitors or angiotensin II receptor blockers (ARBs) (69%), digoxin (14%), calcium antagonists (14%), statins (39%), oral anticoagulants (60%), aspirin (44%), other chronic antiplatelet therapy (6%) and diuretics (54%).

The primary endpoint of the study was the time to first hospitalization for cardiovascular reasons or death from any cause. Time to death from any cause, time to first hospitalization for cardiovascular reasons, and time to cardiovascular death and time to all causes of death were also explored.

Patients ranged in age from 23 to 97 years; 42% were 75 years old or older. Forty-seven percent (47%) of patients were female and a majority was Caucasian (89%). Approximately seventy percent (71%) of those enrolled had no history of heart failure. The median ejection fraction was 60%. Twenty-nine percent (29%) of patients had heart failure, mostly NYHA class II (17%). The majority had hypertension (86%) and structural heart disease (60%).

Results are shown in Table 3. MULTAQ reduced the combined endpoint of cardiovascular hospitalization or death from any cause by 24.2% when compared to placebo. This difference was entirely attributable to its effect on cardiovascular hospitalization, principally hospitalization related to AF.

Other endpoints, death from any cause and first hospitalization for cardiovascular reasons, are shown in Table 3. Secondary endpoints count all first events of a particular type, whether or not they were preceded by a different type of event.

[See table 3 at top of next page]

The Kaplan-Meier cumulative incidence curves showing the time to first event are displayed in Figure 1. The event curves separated early and continued to diverge over the 30 month follow-up period.

[See figure 1 at top of next page]

Reasons for hospitalization included major bleeding (1% in both groups), syncope (1% in both groups), and ventricular arrhythmia (<1% in both groups).

Figure 1: Kaplan-Meier Cumulative Incidence Curves from Randomization to First Cardiovascular Hospitalization or Death from any Cause

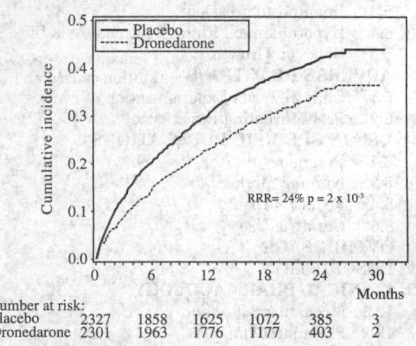

Number at risk:

Placebo	2327	1858	1625	1072	385	3
Dronedarone	2301	1963	1776	1177	403	2

The reduction in cardiovascular hospitalization or death from any cause was generally consistent in all subgroups based on baseline characteristics or medications (ACE inhibitors or ARBs; beta-blockers, digoxin, statins, calcium channel blockers, diuretics) (see Figure 2).

Figure 2: Relative Risk (MULTAQ versus placebo) Estimates with 95% Confidence Intervals According to Selected Baseline Characteristics: First Cardiovascular Hospitalization or Death from any Cause.

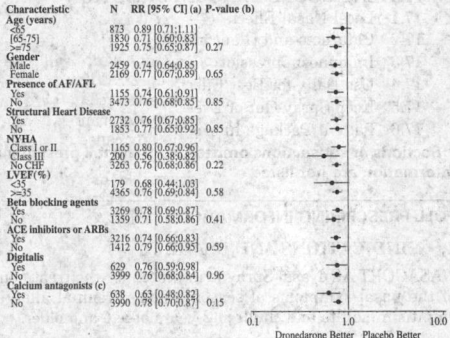

a Determined from Cox regression model
b P-value of interaction between baseline characteristics and treatment based on Cox regression model
c Calcium antagonists with heart rate lowering effects restricted to diltiazem, verapamil and bepridil

14.2 EURIDIS and ADONIS Studies

In EURIDIS and ADONIS, a total of 1237 patients in sinus rhythm with a prior episode of AF or AFL were randomized in an outpatient setting and treated with either MULTAQ 400 mg twice daily (n=828) or placebo (n=409) on top of conventional therapies (including oral anticoagulants, beta-blockers, ACE inhibitors or ARBs, chronic antiplatelet agents, diuretics, statins, digoxin, and calcium channel blockers). Patients had at least one ECG-documented AF/AFL episode during the 3 months prior to study entry but were in sinus rhythm for at least one hour. Patients ranged in age from 20 to 88 years, with the majority being Caucasian (97%), male (70%) patients. The most common comorbidities were hypertension (56.8%) and structural heart disease (41.5%), including coronary heart disease (21.8%). Patients were followed for 12 months.

In the pooled data from EURIDIS and ADONIS as well as in the individual trials, dronedarone delayed the time to first recurrence of AF/AFL (primary endpoint), lowering the risk of first AF/AFL recurrence during the 12-month study period by about 25%,with an absolute difference in recurrence rate of about 11% at 12 months.

14.3 ANDROMEDA Study (Increased Mortality in Patients with Severe Heart Failure)

Patients recently hospitalized with symptomatic heart failure and severe left ventricular systolic dysfunction (wall motion index ≤1.2) were randomized to either MULTAQ 400 mg twice daily or matching placebo, with a primary composite end point of all-cause mortality or hospitalization for heart failure. After enrollment of 627 of 1000 planned patients (310 and 317 in the dronedarone and placebo groups, respectively), and a median follow-up of 63 days, the trial was terminated because of excess mortality in the dronedarone group. Twenty-five (25) patients in the dronedarone group (8.1%) versus 12 patients in the placebo group (3.8%) had died, hazard ratio 2.13; 95% CI: 1.07 to 4.25; p=0.027. The main reason for death was worsening heart failure. There were also excess hospitalizations for cardiovascular reasons in the dronedarone group (71 versus 51 for placebo) *[see Boxed Warning and Contraindications (4)]*.

The populations enrolled in the ANDROMEDA and ATHENA studies were significantly different. The patients enrolled in ANDROMEDA had relatively severe heart failure and had been hospitalized, or referred to a specialty heart failure clinic, for worsening symptoms of heart failure, notably shortness of breath. Note that these patients may have been clinically improved at the time of enrollment and it is the history of decompensation that characterized them. Patients enrolled into ANDROMEDA were predominantly NYHA Class II (40%) and III (57%), and only 38% had a history of AF/AFL (25% had AF at randomization). In contrast, in ATHENA, 71% of patients had no heart failure, 25% were NYHA Class I or II, and only 4% were Class III. All patients had a history of AF/AFL.

16 HOW SUPPLIED/STORAGE AND HANDLING

MULTAQ 400-mg tablets are provided as white film-coated tablets for oral administration, oblong-shaped, engraved with a double wave marking on one side and "4142" code on the other side in:

Bottles of 60 tablets, NDC 0024-4142-60
Bottles of 180 tablets, NDC 0024-4142-18
Bottles of 500 tablets NDC 0024-4142-50
Box of 10 blisters (10 tablets per blister) NDC 0024-4142-10
Store at 25°C (77°F): excursions permitted to 15–30°C (59–86°F), [see USP controlled room temperature].

17 PATIENT COUNSELING INFORMATION

17.1 Information for Patients

[See Medication Guide (17.2)]

MULTAQ should be administered with a meal. Warn patients not to take MULTAQ with grapefruit juice.

If a dose is missed, patients should take the next dose at the regularly scheduled time and should not double the dose.

Advise patients to consult a physician if they develop signs or symptoms of worsening heart failure such as acute weight gain, dependent edema, or increasing shortness of breath.

Advise patients to inform their physician of any history of heart failure, rhythm disturbance other than atrial fibrillation or flutter or predisposing conditions such as uncorrected hypokalemia.

MULTAQ may interact with some drugs; therefore, advise patients to report to their doctor the use of any other prescription, non-prescription medication or herbal products, particularly St. John's wort.

17.2 Medication Guide

Medication Guide

MULTAQ (MUL-tak)

(dronedarone) Tablets

Read this Medication Guide before you start taking MULTAQ and each time you get a refill. There may be new information. This information does not take the place of talking with your doctor about your medical condition or your treatment.

What is the most important information I should know before taking MULTAQ?

MULTAQ is not for people with severe heart failure. People with severe heart failure who take MULTAQ have an increased chance of dying. Heart failure means your heart does not pump blood through your body as well as it should.

Do not take MULTAQ if you have severe heart failure:

• where any physical activity causes shortness of breath or you have shortness of breath while at rest or after a small amount of exercise.

• if you were hospitalized for heart failure within the last month even if you are better now.

Call your doctor right away if you have any signs and symptoms of worsening heart failure:

• shortness of breath or wheezing at rest

• wheezing, chest tightness or coughing up frothy sputum at rest, nighttime or after minor exercise

• trouble sleeping or waking up at night because of breathing problems

• using more pillows to prop yourself up at night so you can breathe more easily

• gaining more than 5 pounds quickly

• increasing swelling of feet or legs

What is MULTAQ?

MULTAQ is a prescription medicine used to lower the chance that you would need to go into the hospital for heart problems. It is meant for people who have had an abnormal heart rhythm called atrial fibrillation or atrial flutter in the last six months but who do not have that abnormal rhythm now or are about to be converted to a normal rhythm. It may be safely used for people who have had atrial fibrillation and atrial flutter who also have medical problems such as high blood pressure, stroke or diabetes.

It is not known if MULTAQ is safe and effective in children younger than age 18 years old.

Who should not take MULTAQ?

See "What is the most important information I should know about taking MULTAQ?"

Do not take MULTAQ if:

• You have severe heart failure or have recently been in the hospital for heart failure, even if you are better now.

• You have severe liver problems.

• You take certain medicines that can change the amount of MULTAQ that gets into your body. Do not use these medicines with MULTAQ:

  ◦ Nefazodone for depression

  ◦ Norvir® (ritonavir) for HIV infection

  ◦ Nizoral® (ketoconazole), and Sporanox® (itraconazole), and Vfend® (voriconazole) for fungal infections

  ◦ Ketek® (telithromycin), Biaxin® (clarithromycin) for bacterial infections

  ◦ Cyclosporine for organ transplant

• You take certain medicines that can lead to a dangerous abnormal heart rhythm:

  ◦ Some medicines for mental illness called phenothiazines

  ◦ Some medicines for depression called tricyclic antidepressants

  ◦ Some medicines for abnormal heart rhythm or fast heartbeat

  ◦ Some medicines for bacterial infection

  Ask your doctor if you are not sure if your medicine is one that is listed above.

• You are pregnant or plan to become pregnant. It is not known if MULTAQ will harm your unborn baby. Talk to your doctor if you are pregnant or plan to become pregnant.

• You are breast-feeding or plan to breastfeed. It is not known if MULTAQ passes into your breast milk. You and your doctor should decide if you will take MULTAQ or breastfeed. You should not do both.

Table 3: Incidence of Endpoint Events

	Placebo (N= 2327)	MULTAQ 400mg BID (N= 2301)	HR	95% CI	p-Value
Primary endpoint					
Cardiovascular hospitalization or death from any cause	913 (39.2%)	727 (31.6%)	0.76	[0.68–0.83]	<0.0001
Components of the endpoint (as first event)					
• Cardiovascular hospitalization	856 (36.8%)	669 (29.1%)			
• Death from any cause	57 (2.4%)	58 (2.5%)			
Secondary endpoints (any time in study)					
• Death from any cause	135 (5.8%)	115 (5.0%)	0.86	[0.67–1.11]	0.24
• Cardiovascular hospitalization	856 (36.8%)	669 (29.1%)	0.74	[0.67–0.82]	<0.0001
Components of the cardiovascular hospitalization endpoint (as first event)					
• AF and other supraventricular rhythm disorders	456 (19.6%)	292 (12.7%)	0.61	[0.53–0.71]	<0.0001
• Other	400 (17.2%)	377 (16.4%)	0.89	[0.77–1.03]	0.11

What should I tell my doctor before starting MULTAQ?
- If you have any other heart problems
- Tell your doctor about all the medicines you take, including any new medicines. Include all prescription and non-prescription medicines, vitamins and herbal remedies. MULTAQ and certain other medicines can react with each other, causing serious side effects. **Know the medicines you take.** Keep a list of them and show it to your doctor and pharmacist when you get a new medicine.

Be sure to tell your doctor and pharmacist if you take:
- medicine for high blood pressure, chest pain, or other heart conditions
- statin medicine to lower bad cholesterol
- medicine for TB (tuberculosis)
- medicine for seizures
- medicine for organ transplant
- herbal supplement called St. John's wort

Some of these medicines could keep MULTAQ from working well or make it more likely for you to have side effects.

How should I take MULTAQ?
- Take MULTAQ exactly as your doctor tells you.
- Take MULTAQ two times a day with food, once with your morning meal and once with your evening meal.
- Do not stop taking MULTAQ even if you are feeling well for a long time. The medicine may be working.
- If you miss a dose, wait and take your next dose at your regular time. Do not take 2 doses at the same time. Do not try to make up for a missed dose.

What should I avoid while taking MULTAQ?
- Do not drink grapefruit juice while you take MULTAQ. Grapefruit juice can increase the amount of MULTAQ in your blood and increase the likelihood that you will have a side effect of MULTAQ.

What are the possible side effects of MULTAQ?
- Slowed heartbeat (bradycardia)
- Stomach problems such as
  - diarrhea
  - nausea
  - vomiting
  - stomach area (abdominal) pain
  - indigestion
- feeling tired and weak
- skin problems such as redness, rash, and itching

Tell your doctor about any side effect that bothers you or that does not go away. These are not all the possible side effects of MULTAQ. For more information ask your doctor or pharmacist.

Call your doctor for medical advice about side effects. You may report side effects to FDA at 1-800-FDA-1088.

How should I store MULTAQ?
Store MULTAQ at room temperature (59–86°F, or 15–30°C).
Keep MULTAQ and all medicines out of the reach of children.

General information about MULTAQ
Medicines are sometimes used for purposes not mentioned in a Medication Guide. Do not use MULTAQ for a condition for which it was not prescribed. Do not give MULTAQ to other people, even if they have the same symptoms or condition. It may harm them.

This Medication Guide summarizes the most important information about MULTAQ. If you would like more information:
- Talk with your doctor
- Ask your doctor or pharmacist for information about MULTAQ that was written for health-care professionals
- For the latest information and Medication Guide, visit www.sanofi-aventis.us or call sanofi-aventis Medical Information Services at 1-800-633-1610 option 1. The Medication Guide may have changed since this copy was printed.

What are the ingredients in MULTAQ?
Active ingredient: dronedarone
Inactive ingredients: hypromellose, starch, crospovidone, poloxamer 407, lactose monohydrate, colloidal silicon dioxide, magnesium stearate polyethylene glycol 6000, titanium dioxide, carnauba wax
This Medication Guide has been approved by the U.S. Food and Drug Administration.

Issued July 2009
Manufactured by Sanofi Winthrop Industrie
1, rue de la Vierge
33440 Ambares, France
©sanofi-aventis, 2009
All rights reserved.
MULTAQ is a trademark of sanofi-aventis.
The brands listed are the registered trademarks of their respective owners and are not trademarks of sanofi-aventis U.S. LLC.
sanofi-aventis U.S. LLC
Bridgewater, NJ 08807
Revised: 07/2009   sanofi-aventis U.S. LLC
Shown in Product Identification Guide, page 319

NASACORT® AQ   ℞
[na' za-cort]
(triamcinolone acetonide)
Spray, Metered For Nasal Use

HIGHLIGHTS OF PRESCRIBING INFORMATION
These highlights do not include all the information needed to use NASACORT AQ safely and effectively. See full prescribing information for NASACORT AQ.
NASACORT AQ (triamcinolone acetonide) spray, metered for nasal use
Initial U.S. Approval: 1957

———————RECENT MAJOR CHANGES———————

Indications and Usage (1)	September 2008
Dosage and Administration (2.2)	September 2008

———————INDICATIONS AND USAGE———————
- NASACORT AQ Nasal Spray is a corticosteroid indicated for treatment of nasal symptoms of seasonal and perennial allergic rhinitis in adults and children 2 years of age and older. (1)

———————DOSAGE AND ADMINISTRATION———————
- *Adults and adolescents ≥ 12 years:* Starting and maximum dose is 220 mcg/day (two sprays in each nostril once daily). (2.1)
- *Children 6 to 12 years of age:* Starting dose is 110 mcg/day (one spray in each nostril once daily). Maximum dose is 220 mcg/day (two sprays per nostril once daily). (2.2)
- *Children 2 to 5 years of age:* Starting and maximum dose 110 mcg/day (one spray in each nostril once daily). (2.2)
- *Priming/Use:* Shake well before each use. Before using for the first time, release 5 sprays into the air away from the face. If the product is not used for more than 2 weeks, release 1 spray into the air before using. (2.3)

———————DOSAGE FORMS AND STRENGTHS———————
- Nasal Spray: 55 mcg triamcinolone acetonide in each spray. Supplied in 16.5 g bottle containing 120 actuations. Each 120 actuation bottle contains 9.075 mg triamcinolone acetonide. (3)

———————CONTRAINDICATIONS———————
- Do not administer to patients with history of hypersensitivity to triamcinolone acetonide or any ingredients of this product. (4)

———————WARNINGS AND PRECAUTIONS———————
- Epistaxis, nasal septal perforation, *Candida albicans* infection, impaired wound healing. Monitor patients periodically for signs of adverse effects on the nasal mucosa. Avoid use in patients with recent nasal septal ulcers, nasal surgery, or trauma. (5.1)
- Development of glaucoma or posterior subcapsular cataracts. Monitor patients closely with a change in vision or with a history of increased intraocular pressure, glaucoma, and/or cataracts. (5.2)
- Potential worsening of existing tuberculosis; fungal, bacterial, viral, or parasitic infections; or ocular herpes simplex. More serious or even fatal course of chickenpox or measles in susceptible patients. Use caution in patient with the above because of the potential for worsening of these infections. (5.3)
- Hypercorticism and adrenal suppression with very high dosages or at the regular dosage in susceptible individuals. If such changes occur, discontinue NASACORT AQ Nasal Spray slowly. (5.4)
- Potential reduction in growth velocity in children. Monitor growth routinely in pediatric patients receiving NASACORT AQ Nasal Spray. (5.5, 8.4)

———————ADVERSE REACTIONS———————
- Most common adverse reactions (>2% incidence) were pharyngitis, epistaxis, flu syndrome, cough increased, bronchitis, dyspepsia, tooth disorder, headache, pharyngolaryngeal pain, nasopharyngitis, abdominal upper pain, diarrhea, and excoriation. (6.1)
- Other adverse reactions, including serious adverse reactions, have been reported. (6.1)

To report SUSPECTED ADVERSE REACTIONS, contact sanofi-aventis U.S. LLC at 1-800-633-1610 or FDA at 1-800-FDA-1088 or www.fda.gov/medwatch

———————USE IN SPECIFIC POPULATIONS———————
NASACORT AQ should be used during pregnancy only if potential benefit justifies potential risk to fetus. (8.1)
See 17 for PATIENT COUNSELING INFORMATION and FDA-approved patient labeling

Revised: 10/2008

FULL PRESCRIBING INFORMATION: CONTENTS*

FULL PRESCRIBING INFORMATION

1.   INDICATIONS AND USAGE
NASACORT AQ Nasal Spray is indicated for the treatment of the nasal symptoms of seasonal and perennial allergic rhinitis in adults and children 2 years of age and older.

2.   DOSAGE AND ADMINISTRATION
Administer NASACORT AQ Nasal Spray by the intranasal route only. Shake NASACORT AQ Nasal Spray well before each use.

2.1   Adults and Adolescents 12 Years of Age and Older
The recommended starting and maximum dose is 220 mcg per day as two sprays in each nostril once daily. Titrate an individual patient to the minimum effective dose to reduce the possibility of side effects. When the maximum benefit has been achieved and symptoms have been controlled, reducing the dose to 110 mcg per day (one spray in each nostril once a day) has been shown to be effective in maintaining control of the allergic rhinitis symptoms.

2.2   Children 2 to 12 Years of Age
Children 6 to 12 years of age: The recommended starting dose is 110 mcg per day given as one spray in each nostril once daily. Children not responding adequately to 110 mcg per day may use 220 mcg (2 sprays in each nostril) once daily. Once symptoms have been controlled, the dosage may be decreased to 110 mcg once daily.

Children 2 to 5 years of age: The recommended and maximum dose is 110 mcg per day given as one spray in each nostril once daily.

NASACORT AQ Nasal Spray is not recommended for children under 2 years of age.

2.3   Administration Information
Priming: Prime NASACORT AQ Nasal Spray before using for the first time by shaking the contents well and releasing 5 sprays into the air away from the face. It will remain adequately primed for two weeks. If the product is not used for more than 2 weeks, then it can be adequately reprimed with one spray. Shake NASACORT AQ Nasal Spray well before each use.

If adequate relief of symptoms has not been obtained after 3 weeks of treatment, NASACORT AQ Nasal Spray should be discontinued. [*See Warnings and Precautions (5), Patient Counseling Information (17), and Adverse Reactions (6)*]

3.   DOSAGE FORMS AND STRENGTHS
NASACORT AQ Nasal Spray is a metered-dose pump spray containing the active ingredient triamcinolone acetonide. Each actuation delivers 55 mcg triamcinolone acetonide from the nasal actuator after an initial priming of 5 sprays. Each 16.5 gram bottle (120 actuations) contains 9.075 mg of triamcinolone acetonide. The bottle should be discarded

when the labeled-number of actuations have been reached even though the bottle is not completely empty.

4. CONTRAINDICATIONS

NASACORT AQ should not be administered to patients with a history of hypersensitivity to triamcinolone acetonide or to any of the other ingredients of this preparation.

5. WARNINGS AND PRECAUTIONS

5.1 Local Nasal Effects

Epistaxis: In clinical studies of 2 to 12 weeks duration, epistaxis was observed more frequently in patients treated with NASACORT AQ Nasal Spray than those who received placebo [see Adverse Reactions (6)].

Nasal Septal Perforation: In clinical trials, nasal septum perforation was reported in one adult patient treated with NASACORT AQ Nasal Spray.

Candida Infection: In clinical studies with NASACORT AQ Nasal Spray, the development of localized infections of the nose and pharynx with Candida albicans has rarely occurred. When such an infection develops it may require treatment with appropriate local or systemic therapy and discontinuation of NASACORT AQ Nasal Spray. Therefore, patients using NASACORT AQ Nasal Spray over several months or longer should be examined periodically for evidence of Candida infection or other signs of adverse effects on the nasal mucosa.

Impaired Wound Healing: Because of the inhibitory effect of corticosteroids on wound healing, patients who have experienced recent nasal ulcers, surgery, or trauma should not use NASACORT AQ Nasal Spray until healing has occurred.

5.2 Glaucoma and Cataracts

Nasal and inhaled corticosteroids may result in the development of glaucoma and/or cataracts. Therefore, close monitoring is warranted in patients with a change in vision or with a history of increased intraocular pressure, glaucoma and/or cataracts.

5.3 Immunosuppression

Persons who are using drugs that suppress the immune system are more susceptible to infections than healthy individuals. Chickenpox and measles, for example, can have a more serious or even fatal course in susceptible children or adults using corticosteroids. In children or adults who have not had these diseases or have not been properly immunized, particular care should be taken to avoid exposure. How the dose, route, and duration of corticosteroid administration affect the risk of developing a disseminated infection is not known. The contribution of the underlying disease and/or prior corticosteroid treatment to the risk is also not known. If exposed to chickenpox, prophylaxis with varicella zoster immune globulin (VZIG) may be indicated. If exposed to measles, prophylaxis with pooled intramuscular immunoglobulin (IG) may be indicated. (See the respective package inserts for complete VZIG and IG prescribing information.) If chickenpox develops, treatment with antiviral agents may be considered.

Corticosteroids should be used with caution, if at all, in patients with active or quiescent tuberculosis infections of the respiratory tract; untreated local or systemic fungal or bacterial infections; systemic viral or parasitic infections; or ocular herpes simplex because of the potential for worsening of these infections.

5.4 Hypothalamic-Pituitary-Adrenal Axis Effects

Hypercorticism and Adrenal Suppression: When intranasal steroids are used at higher than recommended dosages or in susceptible individuals at recommended dosages, systemic corticosteroid effects such as hypercoticism and adrenal suppression may appear. If such changes occur, the dosage of NASACORT AQ Nasal Spray should be discontinued slowly, consistent with accepted procedures for discontinuing oral corticosteroid therapy. The replacement of a systemic corticosteroid with a topical corticosteroid can be accompanied by signs of adrenal insufficiency. In addition, some patients may experience symptoms of corticosteroid withdrawal, e.g., joint and/or muscular pain, lassitude, and depression. Patients previously treated for prolonged periods with systemic corticosteroids and transferred to topical corticosteroids should be carefully monitored for acute adrenal insufficiency in response to stress. In those patients who have asthma or other clinical conditions requiring long-term systemic corticosteroid treatment, rapid decreases in systemic corticosteroid dosages may cause a severe exacerbation of their symptoms.

5.5 Effect on Growth

Corticosteroids may cause a reduction in growth velocity when administered to pediatric patients. Monitor the growth routinely of pediatric patients receiving NASACORT AQ Nasal Spray. To minimize the systemic effects of intranasal corticosteroids, including NASACORT AQ Nasal Spray, titrate each patient's dose to the lowest dosage that effectively controls his/her symptoms [see Use in Specific Populations (8.4)].

6. ADVERSE REACTIONS

Systemic and local corticosteroid use may result in the following:
* Epistaxis, Candida albicans infection, nasal septal perforation, impaired wound healing [see Warnings and Precautions (5.1)]
* Glaucoma and Cataracts [see Warnings and Precautions (5.2)]
* Immunosuppression [see Warnings and Precautions (5.3)]
* Hypothalamic-pituitary-adrenal (HPA) axis effects, including growth reduction [see Warnings and Precautions (5.4, 5.5), Use in Specific Populations (8.4)]

6.1 Clinical Trials Experience

In placebo-controlled, double-blind, and open-label clinical studies, 1483 adults and children 12 years and older received treatment with NASACORT AQ Nasal Spray. These patients were treated for an average duration of 51 days. In the controlled trials (2–5 weeks duration) from which the following adverse reaction data are derived, 1394 patients were treated with NASACORT AQ Nasal Spray for an average of 19 days. In a long-term, open-label study, 172 patients received treatment for an average duration of 286 days. Adverse reactions from 12 studies in adults and adolescent patients 12 to 17 years of age receiving NASACORT AQ Nasal Spray 27.5 mcg to 440 mcg once daily are summarized in Table 1.

In clinical trials, nasal septum perforation was reported in one adult patient who received NASACORT AQ Nasal Spray.

Table 1 - Adverse drug reactions > 2% and greater than placebo with NASACORT AQ Nasal Spray 220 mcg treatment in studies in adults and adolescents 12 years and older

Adverse reaction	Placebo (N=962) %	NASACORT AQ 220 mcg (N=857) %
Pharyngitis	3.6	5.1
Epistaxis	0.8	2.7
Cough increased	1.5	2.1

Coding dictionary for adverse events is Coding Symbols for Thesaurus of Adverse Reaction Terms (COSTART).

A total of 602 children 6 to 12 years of age were studied in 3 double-blind, placebo-controlled clinical trials. Of these, 172 received 110 mcg/day and 207 received 220 mcg/day of NASACORT AQ Nasal Spray for two, six, or twelve weeks. The longest average durations of treatment for patients receiving 110 mcg/day and 220 mcg/day were 76 days and 80 days, respectively. One percent of patients treated with NASACORT AQ were discontinued due to adverse experiences. No patient receiving 110 mcg/day and one patient receiving 220mcg/day discontinued due to a serious adverse event. A similar adverse reaction profile was observed in pediatric patients 6–12 years of age as compared to adolescents and adults with the exception of epistaxis which occurred in less than 2% of the children studied. Adverse reactions from 2 studies in children 4 to 12 years of age receiving NASACORT AQ Nasal Spray 110 mcg once daily are summarized in Table 2.

Table 2 - Adverse drug reactions > 2% and greater than placebo with NASACORT AQ Nasal Spray 110 mcg treatment in US studies in patients 4 to 12 years of age

Adverse reaction	Placebo (N=202) %	NASACORT AQ 110 mcg (N=179) %
Flu syndrome	7.4	8.9
Cough increased	6.4	8.4
Pharyngitis	6.4	7.8
Bronchitis	1.0	3.4
Dyspepsia	1.0	3.4
Tooth disorder	1.0	3.4

Coding dictionary for adverse events is Coding Symbols for Thesaurus of Adverse Reaction Terms (COSTART).

A total of 474 children 2 to 5 years of age were studied in a 4-week double-blind, placebo-controlled clinical trial. Of these, 236 received 110 mcg/day of NASACORT AQ Nasal Spray for a mean duration of 28 days. No patient discontinued due to a serious adverse event. Adverse reactions from

the single placebo-controlled study in children 2 to 5 years of age receiving NASACORT AQ Nasal Spray 110 mcg once daily are summarized in Table 3.

Table 3 - Adverse drug reactions > 2% and greater than placebo with NASACORT AQ Nasal Spray 110 mcg treatment in children 2 to 5 years of age

Adverse reactions	Placebo (N=238) %	NASACORT AQ 110 mcg (N=236) %
Headache	4.2	5.5
Pharyngolaryngeal pain	4.2	5.5
Epistaxis	5.0	5.1
Nasopharyngitis	3.8	5.1
Abdominal upper pain	0.8	4.7
Diarrhea	1.3	3.0
Asthma	2.1	2.5
Rash	1.7	2.5
Excoriation	0.0	2.5
Rhinorrhea	1.7	2.1

Coding dictionary for adverse events is Medical Dictionary for Regulatory Activities terminology (MedDRA) Version 8.1

In the event of accidental overdose, an increased potential for these adverse experiences may be expected, but acute systemic adverse experiences are unlikely. [See Overdosage (10)]

6.2 Post-Marketing Experience

In addition to the adverse drug reactions reported during clinical studies and listed above, the following adverse events have been identified during post-approval use of NASACORT AQ Nasal Spray. Because these events are reported voluntarily from a population of uncertain size, it is not always possible to reliably estimate their frequency or establish a causal relationship to drug exposure. Events that have been reported during post-marketing experience include: nasal discomfort and congestion, sneezing, alterations of taste and smell, nausea, insomnia, dizziness, fatigue, dyspnea, decreased blood cortisol, cataract, glaucoma, increased ocular pressure, pruritus, rash, and hypersensitivity.

8. USE IN SPECIFIC POPULATIONS

8.1 Pregnancy

Teratogenic Effects: Pregnancy Category C

There are no adequate and well-controlled studies of NASACORT AQ Nasal Spray in pregnant women. Triamcinolone acetonide was teratogenic in rats, rabbits, and monkeys. NASACORT AQ Nasal Spray, like other corticosteroids, should be used during pregnancy only if the potential benefit justifies the potential risk to the fetus. Since their introduction, experience with oral corticosteroids in pharmacologic as opposed to physiologic doses suggests that rodents are more prone to teratogenic effects from corticosteroids than humans. In addition, because there is a natural increase in glucocorticoid production during pregnancy, most women will require a lower exogenous corticosteroid dose and many will not need corticosteroid treatment during pregnancy.

In reproduction studies in rats and rabbits, triamcinolone acetonide administered by inhalation produced cleft palate and/or internal hydrocephaly and axial skeletal defects at exposures less than and 2 times, respectively, the maximum recommended daily intranasal dose in adults on a mcg/m^2 basis. In a monkey reproduction study, triamcinolone acetonide administered by inhalation produced cranial malformations at an exposure approximately 37 times the maximum recommended daily intranasal dose in adults on a mcg/m^2 basis.

8.3 Nursing Mothers

It is not known whether triamcinolone acetonide is excreted in human milk. Because other corticosteroids are excreted in human milk, caution should be exercised when NASACORT AQ Nasal Spray is administered to nursing women.

8.4 Pediatric Use

The safety and effectiveness of NASACORT AQ Nasal Spray has been evaluated in 464 children 2 to 5 years of age, 518 children 6 to 12 years of age, and 176 adolescents 12 to 17 years of age [see Clinical Studies (14)]. The safety and effectiveness of NASACORT AQ Nasal Spray in children below 2 years of age have not been established.

Controlled clinical studies have shown that intranasal corticosteroids may cause a reduction in growth velocity in pediatric patients. This effect has been observed in the absence of laboratory evidence of HPA axis suppression, suggesting that growth velocity is a more sensitive indicator of systemic corticosteroid exposure in pediatric patients than some commonly used tests of HPA axis function. The long-term effects of reduction in growth velocity associated with intranasal corticosteroids, including the impact of final adult height are unknown. The potential for "catch-up" growth following discontinuation of treatment with intranasal corticosteroids has not been adequately studied. The growth of pediatric patients receiving intranasal corticosteroids, including NASACORT AQ Nasal Spray, should be monitored routinely (e.g., via stadiometry). The potential growth effects of prolonged treatment should be weighed against the clinical benefits obtained and the risks/benefits of treatment alternatives. To minimize the systemic effects of intranasal corticosteroids, including NASACORT AQ Nasal Spray, each patient's dose should be titrated to the lowest dosage that effectively controls his/her symptoms.

The potential for NASACORT AQ Nasal Spray to cause growth suppression in susceptible patients and when given at higher than recommended dosages cannot be ruled out.

8.5 Geriatric Use

Clinical studies of NASACORT AQ did not include sufficient numbers of subjects aged 65 and over to determine whether they respond differently from younger subjects. Other reported clinical experience has not identified differences in responses between the elderly and younger patients. In general, dose selection for an elderly patient should be cautious, usually starting at the low end of the dosing range, reflecting the greater frequency of decreased hepatic, renal, or cardiac function, and of concomitant disease or other drug therapy.

10. OVERDOSAGE

Chronic overdosage may result in signs/symptoms of hypercorticism [*see Warnings and Precautions (5.4)*]. There are no data on the effects of acute or chronic overdosage with NASACORT AQ Nasal Spray. Because of low systemic bioavailability and an absence of acute drug-related systemic findings in clinical studies overdose is unlikely to require any therapy other than observation.

Acute overdosing with the intranasal dosage form is unlikely in view of the total amount of active ingredient present and low bioavailability of triamcinolone acetonide. In the event that the entire contents of the bottle were administered all at once, via either oral or nasal application, clinically significant systemic adverse events would most likely not result.

11. DESCRIPTION

Triamcinolone acetonide, USP, the active ingredient in NASACORT AQ Nasal Spray, is a corticosteroid with a molecular weight of 434.51 and with the chemical designation 9-Fluoro-11β,16α,17,21-tetrahydroxypregna-1,4-diene-3,20-dione cyclic 16,17-acetal with acetone ($C_{24}H_{31}FO_6$).

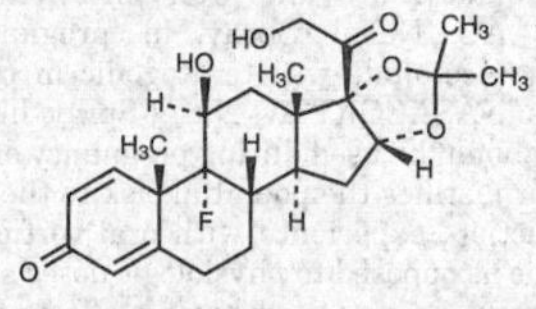

NASACORT AQ Nasal Spray is a thixotropic, water-based metered-dose pump spray formulation unit containing a microcrystalline suspension of triamcinolone acetonide in an aqueous medium. Microcrystalline cellulose, carboxymethylcellulose sodium, polysorbate 80, dextrose, benzalkonium chloride, and edetate disodium are contained in this aqueous medium; hydrochloric acid or sodium hydroxide may be added to adjust the pH to a target of 5.0 within a range of 4.5 and 6.0.

12. CLINICAL PHARMACOLOGY

12.1 Mechanism of Action

Triamcinolone acetonide is a synthetic fluorinated corticosteroid with approximately 8 times the potency of prednisone in animal models of inflammation.

Although the precise mechanism of corticosteroid antiallergic action is unknown, corticosteroids have been shown to have a wide range of actions on multiple cell types (e.g., mast cells, eosinophils, neutrophils, macrophages, lymphocytes) and mediators (e.g., histamine, eicosanoids, leukotrienes, cytokines) involved in inflammation.

12.2 Pharmacodynamics

In order to determine if systemic absorption plays a role in the effect of NASACORT AQ Nasal Spray on allergic rhinitis symptoms, a two week double-blind, placebo-controlled clinical study was conducted comparing NASACORT AQ, orally ingested triamcinolone acetonide, and placebo in 297 adult patients with seasonal allergic rhinitis. The study demonstrated that the therapeutic efficacy of NASACORT AQ Nasal Spray can be attributed to the topical effects of triamcinolone acetonide.

Adrenal Function: In order to evaluate the effects of systemic absorption on the Hypothalamic-Pituitary-Adrenal (HPA) axis, 3 clinical studies, one each in adults and in children 6–12 years of age and 2–5 years of age, were conducted.

The adult clinical study compared 220 mcg or 440 mcg NASACORT AQ per day, or 10 mg prednisone per day with placebo for 42 days. Adrenal response to a six-hour 250 mcg cosyntropin stimulation test showed that NASACORT AQ administered at doses of 220 mcg and 440 mcg had no statistically significant effect on HPA activity versus placebo. Conversely, oral prednisone at 10 mg/day significantly reduced the response to ACTH.

A study evaluating plasma cortisol response thirty and sixty minutes after 250 mcg cosyntropin stimulation in 80 pediatric patients 6 to 12 years of age who received 220 mcg or 440 mcg (twice the maximum recommended daily dose) daily for six weeks was conducted. No abnormal response to cosyntropin infusion (peak serum cortisol <18 mcg/dL) was observed in any pediatric patient after six weeks of dosing with NASACORT AQ at 440 mcg per day.

In pediatric patients 2 to 5 years of age, HPA axis assessment was performed; however, the results were inconclusive and an effect of NASACORT AQ Nasal Spray on adrenal function in children 2 to 5 years of age cannot be ruled out.

12.3 Pharmacokinetics

Based upon intravenous dosing of triamcinolone acetonide phosphate ester in adults, the half-life of triamcinolone acetonide was reported to be 88 minutes. The volume of distribution (Vd) reported was 99.5 L (SD ± 27.5) and clearance was 45.2 L/hour (SD ± 9.1) for triamcinolone acetonide. The plasma half-life of corticosteroids does not correlate well with the biologic half-life.

Pharmacokinetic characterization of the NASACORT AQ Nasal Spray formulation was determined in both normal adult subjects and patients with allergic rhinitis. Single dose intranasal administration of 220 mcg of NASACORT AQ Nasal Spray in normal adult subjects and patients demonstrated minimal absorption of triamcinolone acetonide. The mean peak plasma concentration was approximately 0.5 ng/mL (range: 0.1 to 1.0 ng/mL) and occurred at 1.5 hours post dose. The mean plasma drug concentration was less than 0.06 ng/mL at 12 hours, and below the assay detection limit (the minimum LOQ of the assay was 0.025 ng/ml) at 24 hours. The average terminal half-life was 3.1 hours. The range of mean $AUC_{0-\infty}$ values was 1.4 ng·hr/mL to 4.7 ng·hr/mL between doses of 110 mcg to 440 mcg in both patients and healthy volunteers. Dose proportionality was demonstrated in both normal adult subjects and in allergic rhinitis patients following single intranasal doses of 110 mcg or 220 mcg NASACORT AQ Nasal Spray. The C_{max} and $AUC_{0-\infty}$ of the 440 mcg dose increased less than proportionally when compared to 110 and 220 mcg doses.

Following multiple dose administration of NASACORT AQ 440 mcg once daily in pediatric patients 6 to 12 years of age, plasma drug concentrations, $AUC_{0-\infty}$, C_{max} and T_{max} were similar to those values observed in adult patients receiving the same dose. Intranasal administration of NASACORT AQ 110 mcg once daily in pediatric patients 2 to 5 years of age exhibited similar systemic exposure to that achieved in adult patients 20 to 49 years of age with intranasal administration of NASACORT AQ at a dose of 220 mcg once daily. Based on the population pharmacokinetic modeling, the apparent clearance and volume of distribution following intranasal administration of NASACORT AQ in pediatric patients 2 to 5 years of age were found to be approximately half of that in adults.

In animal studies using rats and dogs, three metabolites of triamcinolone acetonide have been identified. They are 6β-hydroxytriamcinolone acetonide, 21-carboxytriamcinolone acetonide and 21-carboxy-6β-hydroxytriamcinolone acetonide. All three metabolites are expected to be substantially less active than the parent compound due to (a) the dependence of anti-inflammatory activity on the presence of a 21-hydroxyl group, (b) the decreased activity observed upon 6-hydroxylation, and (c) the markedly increased water solubility favoring rapid elimination. There appeared to be some quantitative differences in the metabolites among species. No differences were detected in metabolic pattern as a function of route of administration.

13. NONCLINICAL TOXICOLOGY

13.1 Carcinogenesis, Mutagenesis, Impairment of Fertility

In a two-year study in rats, triamcinolone acetonide caused no treatment-related carcinogenicity at oral doses up to 1.0 mcg/kg (less than the maximum recommended daily intranasal dose in adults and children on a mcg/m^2 basis, respectively). In a two-year study in mice, triamcinolone acetonide caused no treatment-related carcinogenicity at oral doses up to 3.0 mcg/kg (less than the maximum recommended daily intranasal dose in adults and children on a mcg/m^2 basis, respectively).

No evidence of mutagenicity was detected from *in vitro* tests (a reverse mutation test in *Salmonella* bacteria and a forward mutation test in Chinese hamster ovary cells) conducted with triamcinolone acetonide.

In male and female rats, triamcinolone acetonide caused no change in pregnancy rate at oral doses up to 15.0 mcg/kg (less than the maximum recommended daily intranasal dose in adults on a mcg/m^2 basis). Triamcinolone acetonide caused increased fetal resorptions and stillbirths and decreases in pup weight and survival at doses of 5.0 mcg/kg and above (less than the maximum recommended daily intranasal dose in adults on a mcg/m^2 basis). At 1.0 mcg/kg (less than the maximum recommended daily intranasal dose in adults on a mcg/m^2 basis), it did not induce the above mentioned effects.

13.2 Animal Toxicology and/or Pharmacology

Triamcinolone acetonide was teratogenic in rats, rabbits, and monkeys. In rats, triamcinolone acetonide was teratogenic at an inhalation dose of 20 mcg/kg and above (approximately 7/10 of the maximum recommended daily intranasal dose in adults on a mcg/m^2 basis). In rabbits, triamcinolone acetonide was teratogenic at inhalation doses of 20 mcg/kg and above (approximately 2 times the maximum recommended daily intranasal dose in adults on a mcg/m^2 basis). In monkeys, triamcinolone acetonide was teratogenic at an inhalation dose of 500 mcg/kg (approximately 37 times the maximum recommended daily intranasal dose in adults on a mcg/m^2 basis). Dose-related teratogenic effects in rats and rabbits included cleft palate and/or internal hydrocephaly and axial skeletal defects, whereas the effects observed in the monkey were cranial malformations.

Hypoadrenalism may occur in infants born of mothers receiving corticosteroids during pregnancy. Such infants should be carefully observed.

14. CLINICAL STUDIES

The safety and efficacy of NASACORT AQ Nasal Spray have been evaluated in 10 double-blind, placebo-controlled clinical studies of two- to four-weeks duration in adults and children 12 years and older with seasonal or perennial allergic rhinitis. The number of patients treated with NASACORT AQ Nasal Spray in these studies was 1266; of these patients, 675 were males and 591 were females.

Overall, the results of these clinical studies in adults and children 12 years and older demonstrated that NASACORT AQ Nasal Spray 220 mcg once daily (2 sprays in each nostril), when compared to placebo, provides statistically significant relief of nasal symptoms of seasonal or perennial allergic rhinitis including sneezing, stuffiness, discharge, and itching.

The safety and efficacy of NASACORT AQ Nasal Spray, at doses of 110 mcg or 220 mcg once daily, have also been adequately studied in two double-blind, placebo-controlled studies of two- and twelve-weeks duration in children ages 6 through 12 years with seasonal and perennial allergic rhinitis. These studies included 341 males and 177 females. NASACORT AQ administered at either dose resulted in statistically significant reductions in the severity of nasal symptoms of allergic rhinitis.

The safety and efficacy of NASACORT AQ Nasal Spray in children 2 to 5 years of age with perennial allergic rhinitis with or without seasonal allergic rhinitis was studied in a single 4 week double blind, placebo controlled clinical study with a 24 week open label extension conducted in the United States. The study included 464 patients (266 males and 198 females) 2 to 5 years of age who received at least one dose of study medication (233 placebo, 231 NASACORT AQ 110 mcg once daily). Efficacy was determined over a four-week double-blind, placebo-controlled treatment period and was based on patient's parent or guardian recording of four nasal symptoms (total nasal symptom score, TNSS), congestion, itching, rhinorrhea, and sneezing on a 0–3 categorical severity scale (0=absent, 1=mild, 2=moderate, and 3=severe) once daily. Reflective scoring (rTNSS) required recording symptom severity over the previous 24 hours; the instantaneous scoring (iTNSS) required recording symptom severity at the time just prior to dosing. Baseline symptom severity was comparable between NASACORT AQ and placebo respectively, for iTNSS (7.52, 7.61) and rTNSS (7.96, 7.87). While the 24-hour iTNSS over the 4-week double-blind period was numerically improved with NASACORT AQ (-2.28) vs. placebo (-1.92), the difference was not statistically significant (difference from placebo -0.36; 95% CI [-0.77, 0.06]; p value = 0.095). For the 24-hour rTNSS over the 4 week double-blind treatment period, NASACORT AQ 110 mcg once daily provided statistically significantly greater improvement from baseline (-2.31) versus placebo (-1.87) (difference from placebo -0.44; 95% CI [-0.84, -0.04]; p value = 0.033).

16. HOW SUPPLIED/STORAGE AND HANDLING

16.1 How Supplied

NASACORT AQ Nasal Spray, 55 mcg per spray, is supplied in a white high-density polyethylene container with a metered-dose pump unit, white nasal adapter, and patient instructions (NDC 0075-1506-16).

The contents of one 16.5 gram bottle provide 120 actuations. After 120 actuations, the amount of triamcinolone acetonide delivered per actuation may not be consistent and the unit should be discarded. Each actuation delivers 55 mcg triamcinolone acetonide from the nasal actuator after an initial priming of 5 sprays [See *Administration Information (2.3)*].

In the Patient Package Information, patients are provided with a check-off form to track usage [See *Patient Counseling Information (17)*].

Keep out of reach of children.

16.2 Storage

Store at Controlled Room Temperature, 20 to 25°C (68 to 77°F).

17. PATIENT COUNSELING INFORMATION

See FDA-Approved Patient Labeling accompanying the product.

17.1 Local Nasal Effects

Patients should be informed that treatment with NASACORT AQ Nasal Spray may lead to adverse reactions, which include epistaxis and nasal ulceration. Candida infection may also occur with treatment with NASACORT AQ Nasal Spray. In addition, nasal corticosteroids are associated with nasal septal perforation and impaired wound healing. Patients who have experienced recent nasal ulcers, nasal surgery, or nasal trauma should not use NASACORT AQ Nasal Spray until healing has occurred [*see Warnings and Precautions (5.1)*].

17.2 Cataracts and Glaucoma

Patients should be informed that glaucoma and cataracts are associated with nasal and inhaled corticosteroid use. Patients should inform his/her heath care provider if a change in vision is noted while using NASACORT AQ Nasal Spray [*see Warnings and Precautions (5.2)*].

17.3 Immunosuppression

Patients who are on immunosuppressant doses of corticosteroids should be warned to avoid exposure to chickenpox or measles and, if exposed, to consult their physician without delay. Patients should be informed of potential worsening of existing tuberculosis, fungal, bacterial, viral or parasitic infections, or ocular herpes simplex [*see Warnings and Precautions (5.3)*].

17.4 Use Daily for Best Effect

Patients should use NASACORT AQ Nasal Spray on a regular once-daily basis for optimal effect. It is also important to shake the bottle well before each use. Do not blow your nose for 15 minutes after using the spray. NASACORT AQ Nasal Spray, like other corticosteroids, does not have an immediate effect on rhinitis symptoms. Although improvement in some patient symptoms may be seen within the first day of treatment, maximum benefit may not be reached for up to one week. The patient should not increase the prescribed dosage but should contact the physician if symptoms do not improve or if the condition worsens.

17.5 Keep Spray Out of Eyes

Patients should be informed to avoid spraying NASACORT AQ Nasal Spray in their eyes.

17.6 Patient Package Information

IMPORTANT: Please read these instructions carefully before using your NASACORT® AQ Nasal Spray

Nasacort® AQ (triamcinolone acetonide)

[na' za-cort]

Nasal Spray

Patient Information:

These instructions provide important information about Nasacort AQ. Ask your healthcare provider or pharmacist if you have any questions.

Important: For use as a nasal spray only.

What is Nasacort AQ?

Nasacort® AQ Nasal Spray is a prescription medicine called a corticosteroid used to treat nasal symptoms of seasonal and year around allergies in adults and children 2 years of age and older. When Nasacort AQ is sprayed in your nose, this medicine helps to lessen the symptoms of sneezing, runny nose, nasal itching and stuffy nose.

Nasacort AQ is not for children under the age of 2 years.

Who should use Nasacort AQ?

Do not use Nasacort AQ if you have had a reaction to triamcinolone acetonide or to any of the other ingredients in Nasacort AQ. See the end of this leaflet for a complete list of ingredients in Nasacort AQ.

What should I tell my healthcare provider before using Nasacort AQ?

Tell your healthcare provider if you are:

• pregnant or planning to become pregnant
• breastfeeding
• exposed to chickenpox or measles
• feeling unwell or have any symptoms that you do not understand

Tell your healthcare provider about all of the medicines you take, including prescription and non-prescription medicines, vitamins, and herbal supplements.

How do I use Nasacort AQ?

• Use Nasacort AQ exactly as your healthcare provider tells you.

• You will get the best results if you use Nasacort AQ regularly and without missing a dose. Do not take extra doses.

• Nasacort AQ should be used as a nasal spray only. Do not spray it in your eyes or mouth.

• Your healthcare provider will tell you how and when to use Nasacort AQ. Do not use more Nasacort AQ or take it more often than your healthcare provider tells you.

• The prescription label will usually tell you how many sprays to take and how often. If it does not or if you are unsure, ask your healthcare provider or pharmacist.

  • **For people aged 12 years and older**, the usual dose is **2 sprays in each nostril, one time each day.**

  • **For children aged 6 to 12 years**, the usual dose is **1 spray in each nostril, one time each day.** Your healthcare provider may tell you to take 2 sprays in each nostril **one time each** day.

  • **For children aged 2 to 5 years**, the usual dose is **1 spray in each nostril, one time each day.**

  • **An adult should help a young child use this medicine.** Do not stop taking Nasacort AQ without telling your healthcare provider. Before you throw away Nasacort AQ, talk to your healthcare provider to see if you need another prescription. If your healthcare provider tells you to continue using Nasacort AQ, throw away the empty or expired bottle and use a new bottle of Nasacort AQ.

• For detailed instructions, see the "Patient Instructions for Use" at the end of this leaflet.

• Some symptoms may get better on the first day of treatment. It generally takes one week of use to feel the most benefit.

• Protect your eyes from the spray. If you get the spray in your eyes, rinse your eyes well with water.

• If your symptoms do not improve, or if they become worse, contact your healthcare provider.

• Tell your healthcare provider if you have irritation, burning or stinging inside your nose that does not go away when using Nasacort AQ.

What are the possible side effects of Nasacort AQ?

Common side effects of Nasacort AQ include:

Sore throat, headache, and nosebleeds. If you have an increase in nosebleeds after using Nasacort AQ or the inside of your nose hurts, contact your healthcare provider.

Tell your healthcare provider if you have any side effect that bothers you or that does not go away. Call your doctor for medical advice about side effects. You may report side effects to the FDA at 1-800-FDA-1088.

Patient Instructions for Use

Read these instructions carefully before using your Nasacort AQ.

Before using the spray pump bottle:

• 1. Pull the blue cover and the clip off the spray pump unit. See figure A.

  If the top part of the spray pump comes off of the bottle when removing the cover, then re-insert the stem back into the pump.

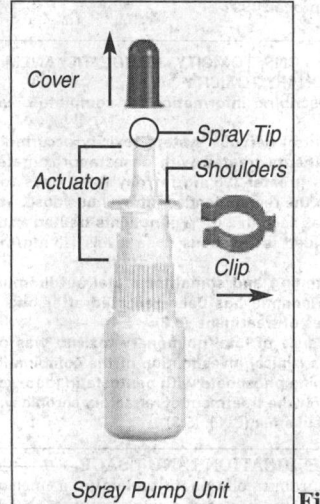

Cover

Spray Tip

Actuator

Shoulders

Clip

Spray Pump Unit

Figure A.

• 2. Shake the spray pump bottle before each use.

Priming the Spray Pump Bottle

• 3. Before using the spray pump bottle for the first time, it must be primed. To prime, put your thumb on the bottom of the bottle and your index and middle fingers on the "shoulders" of the bottle, and hold it upright. See figure B.

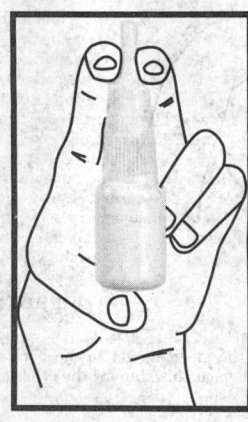

Figure B

• 4. Point the bottle away from your eyes. Push the bottle up with your thumb and against your two fingers **firmly** and **quickly** until a fine spray appears. Do this pumping action 5 times.

  Now your spray pump bottle is primed and ready for use. A fine mist can only be made by a rapid and firm pumping action.

• 5. Repeat priming the pump, if it has not been used for more than 2 weeks. To reprime, shake the spray pump bottle and pump it just one time. Now the spray pump bottle is reprimed.

Using the spray:

• 6. Gently blow your nose to clear it, if needed. For small children, be sure to help them gently blow their nose, as much as possible.

• 7. Pull off the blue cover and clip as shown in figure C. Shake the spray pump well.

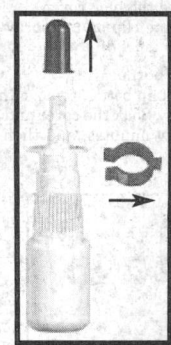

Figure C

• 8. Hold the spray pump firmly, with the index and middle finger on either side of the spray tip. Place your thumb on the bottom of the bottle. **Be careful** so that your fingers will not slip off the spray pump as you spray inside your nose. See figure D.

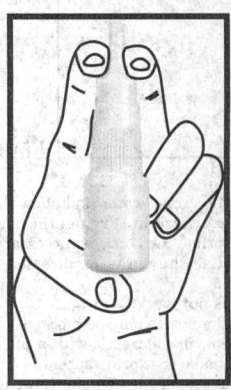

Figure D

• 9. Put the spray tip into one side of your nose. The tip should not reach far into the nose. Rest the side of your index finger against your upper lip. Tip your head back a little and aim the spray toward the back of your nose. See figure E.

[See figure E at top of next page]

• 10. Press against the other side of your nose with your finger so the nostril is closed. Pump the spray bottle by pushing on the bottom of the bottle with your thumb **firmly** and **quickly** for the full dose of medicine. Sniff gently at the

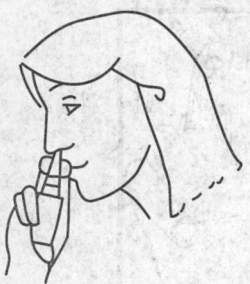

Figure E

same time to help the medicine get to the back of your nose. See figure F. Repeat this step for the other side.

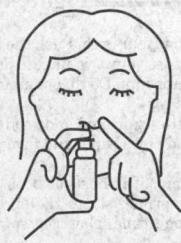

Figure F

- 11. Repeat steps 8, 9 and 10 if your healthcare provider tells you to use more than one spray in each nostril.
- 12. Do not blow your nose for 15 minutes after using the spray.
- 13. After use, wipe the nozzle on the spray bottle with a clean tissue, and replace the blue cover.
- 14. Keep the cover and the clip on the spray pump bottle when not in use.

Cleaning the spray pump bottle:
- 15. To clean the spray pump bottle, remove the blue cover and the spray nozzle only. Soak the cover and spray nozzle in warm water for a few minutes, and then rinse under cold water. See figure G.

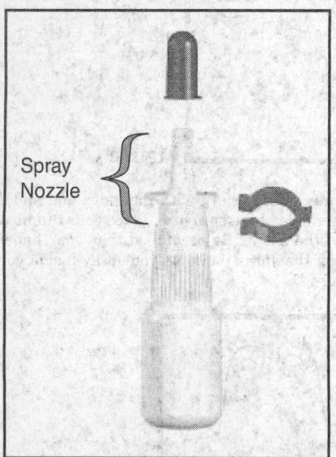

Spray Nozzle

Figure G

- 16. Shake or tap off the excess water and allow to air dry. Once the cap and spray nozzle are dry, put the nozzle back onto the bottle, and prime the bottle as necessary until a fine mist is made. Use the spray as directed by your healthcare provider.

If the spray bottle does not work:
The hole in the tip of the nozzle may be blocked. Never try to unblock the spray hole or enlarge it with a pin or other sharp object. This will make the spray mechanism not work correctly. Changing the size of the opening can change the amount of medicine you or your child will receive. This could cause an overdose of the medicine. To clean nasal spray pump bottle, refer to Step 15.

Important information
Repriming the spray pump is only necessary when it has not been used for more than 2 weeks. To reprime, shake the bottle and only pump the spray bottle one time. Do not reprime if you use the spray more often than every two weeks. Each Nasacort AQ bottle contains 120 doses of medicine plus a little extra for priming the pump. A check-off chart is included with your Nasacort AQ to help you keep track of

the number of sprays. This will help make sure that you receive 120 sprays of Nasacort AQ.

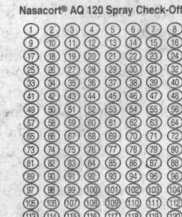

Nasacort® AQ 120 Spray Check-Off

- Keep this chart near your Nasacort AQ.
- Check off one circle each time you use this bottle of Nasacort AQ.
- When you reach 120 sprays, throw the bottle away.
- If you use more than 120 sprays, you will not get the right amount of medicine.

How should I store Nasacort AQ?
- Store Nasacort AQ between 68° to 77°F (20° to 25° C).
- After using 120 sprays, throw the medicine away, as directed by your healthcare provider, even if the bottle is not empty. You may not get enough medicine if you use the bottle after 120 sprays.

Keep Nasacort and all medicines out of the reach of children. General information about the safe and effective use of Nasacort AQ.
Medicines are sometimes prescribed for conditions that are not mentioned in patient information. Do not use Nasacort AQ for a condition for which it was not prescribed. Do not give Nasacort AQ to other people, even if they have the same symptoms that you have. It may harm them.
This leaflet summarizes the most important information about Nasacort AQ. If you would like more information, talk with your healthcare provider. You can ask your pharmacist or healthcare provider for information about Nasacort AQ that is written for health professionals.
For more information call 1-800-633-1610.

What are the ingredients in Nasacort AQ?
Active ingredient: triamcinolone acetonide
Inactive ingredients: Microcrystalline cellulose, carboxymethylcellulose sodium, polysorbate 80, dextrose, benzalkonium chloride, and edetate disodium are contained in this aqueous medium; hydrochloric acid or sodium hydroxide may be added to adjust the pH to a target of 5.0 within a range of 4.5 and 6.0.
sanofi-aventis U.S. LLC
Bridgewater, NJ 08807
© 2008 **sanofi-aventis U.S. LLC**
Revised: 10/2008   Distributed by: sanofi-aventis U.S. LLC
Shown in Product Identification Guide, page 319

OFORTA™   ℞
(fludarabine phosphate tablets)
for Oral Use

HIGHLIGHTS OF PRESCRIBING INFORMATION
These highlights do not include all the information needed to use Oforta™ safely and effectively. See full prescribing information for Oforta™.
Oforta™ (fludarabine phosphate tablets) for Oral Use.
Initial U.S. Approval: 1991

WARNING: CNS TOXICITY, HEMOLYTIC ANEMIA, AND PULMONARY TOXICITY
See full prescribing information for complete boxed warning.
- **Severe central nervous system toxicity occurred in 36% of patients treated with doses approximately four times greater (96 mg/m^2/day for 5 days to 7 days) than the recommended intravenous dose. This toxicity was seen in ≤0.2% of patients treated at the recommended intravenous dose levels (25 mg/m^2). (5.1)**
- **Life-threatening and sometimes fatal autoimmune hemolytic anemia has been reported after one or more cycles of treatment. (5.2)**
- **High incidence of fatal pulmonary toxicity was observed in a clinical investigation of the combination of fludarabine phosphate with pentostatin (deoxycoformycin) for the treatment of refractory chronic lymphocytic leukemia (CLL). (5.3)**

──INDICATIONS AND USAGE──
Oforta™ (fludarabine phosphate tablets) is a nucleotide metabolic inhibitor indicated as a single agent for the treatment of adult patients with B-cell chronic lymphocytic leukemia (CLL) whose disease has not responded to or has progressed during or after treatment with at least one standard alkylating-agent containing regimen. Studies demonstrating clinical benefit such as prolongation of survival or relief of symptoms have not been performed. A direct comparison of the clinical efficacy and safety of orally administered Oforta™ relative to intravenously administered fludarabine phosphate has not been studied. (1)

──DOSAGE AND ADMINISTRATION──
Note: The oral dose of Oforta™ is different than the intravenous fludarabine phosphate dose.
Chronic Lymphocytic Leukemia (CLL) (2.1):
- The recommended adult dose is 40 mg/m^2 administered daily for five consecutive days by the oral route.
- Begin each 5-day course of treatment every 28 days.
Renal Impairment (2.2):
- Reduce dose by 20% in patients with mild to moderate renal impairment (creatinine clearance 30 to 70 mL/min/ 1.73 m^2).
- Reduce dose by 50% in patients with severe renal impairment (creatinine clearance < 30 mL/min/1.73 m^2)

──DOSAGE FORMS AND STRENGTHS──
- 10 milligram tablets. (see 3)

──CONTRAINDICATIONS──
- None

──WARNINGS AND PRECAUTIONS──
- Severe bone marrow suppression, notably anemia, thrombocytopenia and neutropenia. Monitor blood counts before and during treatment. (5.2)
- Infections. Monitor for signs or symptoms of infection. (5.3)
- Tumor lysis syndrome. Take precautions for patients at high risk. (5.4)
- Transfusion-associated graft-versus-host disease. Use only irradiated blood products for transfusions. (5.6)
- Oforta™ dose should be adjusted in patients with mild to moderate (creatinine clearance 30 to 70 mL/ min/1.73 m^2) or severe (creatinine clearance < 30 mL/min/1.73 m^2) renal impairment. (5.7)
- Fetal harm may occur when administered to a pregnant woman. Women of childbearing potential and fertile males must take contraceptive measures during and at least for 6 months after the cessation of therapy. (5.9)

──ADVERSE REACTIONS──
Most common adverse reactions (incidence > 30%) include myelosuppression (neutropenia, thrombocytopenia and anemia). Fever, weakness, infection, pain, cough and anorexia were also reported as common adverse reactions. (6)
To report SUSPECTED ADVERSE REACTIONS, contact sanofi-aventis U.S. LLC at 1-800-633-1610 or FDA at 1-800-FDA-1088 or www.fda.gov/medwatch.

──DRUG INTERACTIONS──
- Oforta™ in combination with pentostatin is not recommended due to the risk of severe pulmonary toxicity. (5.3 and 7.1)

See 17 for PATIENT COUNSELING INFORMATION and FDA-approved patient labeling
                     Revised: 03/2009

FULL PRESCRIBING INFORMATION: CONTENTS*
WARNING: CNS TOXICITY, HEMOLYTIC ANEMIA, AND PULMONARY TOXICITY

17.3 Pregnancy
17.4 Handling and Disposal
* Sections or subsections omitted from the full prescribing information are not listed

FULL PRESCRIBING INFORMATION

> **WARNING: CNS TOXICITY, HEMOLYTIC ANEMIA, AND PULMONARY TOXICITY**
>
> Severe neurologic effects, including blindness, coma, and death were observed in dose-ranging studies in patients with acute leukemia when fludarabine phosphate was administered at high doses. This severe central nervous system toxicity occurred in 36% of patients treated with doses approximately four times greater (96 mg/m^2/day for 5 days to 7 days) than the recommended intravenous dose (25 mg/m^2/day). Similar severe central nervous system toxicity has been rarely ($\leq$0.2%) reported in patients treated at doses in the range of the dose recommended for chronic lymphocytic leukemia. [*See Warnings and Precautions (5.1)*] Periodic neurological assessments are recommended.
>
> Instances of life-threatening and sometimes fatal autoimmune hemolytic anemia have been reported after one or more cycles of treatment with fludarabine phosphate. Patients undergoing treatment with Oforta™ should be evaluated and closely monitored for hemolysis. [*See Warnings and Precautions (5.2)*]
>
> High incidence of fatal pulmonary toxicity was observed in a clinical investigation using fludarabine phosphate in combination with pentostatin (deoxycoformycin) for the treatment of refractory chronic lymphocytic leukemia (CLL). Therefore, the use of Oforta™ in combination with pentostatin is not recommended [*See Warnings and Precautions (5.3)*]

1 INDICATIONS AND USAGE

Oforta™ (fludarabine phosphate tablets) for oral use is indicated as a single agent for the treatment of adult patients with B-cell chronic lymphocytic leukemia (CLL) whose disease has not responded to or has progressed during or after treatment with at least one standard alkylating-agent containing regimen. Studies demonstrating clinical benefit such as prolongation of survival or relief of symptoms have not been performed. Studies providing a direct comparison of the clinical efficacy and safety of Oforta™ relative to intravenously administered fludarabine phosphate have not been performed.

2 DOSAGE AND ADMINISTRATION

2.1 Chronic Lymphocytic Leukemia (CLL)

The oral dose of Oforta™ is different than the intravenous fludarabine phosphate dose.

The recommended adult dose of Oforta™ is 40 mg/m^2 administered by mouth daily for five consecutive days. Each 5-day course of treatment should commence every 28 days. Dosage may be decreased or delayed based on evidence of hematologic or nonhematologic toxicity. Physicians should consider delaying or discontinuing the drug if neurotoxicity occurs. Oforta™ can be taken either on an empty stomach or with food. The tablets have to be swallowed whole with water; they should not be chewed or broken.

The following table provides guidance for determining the number of tablets of Oforta™ to be administered based on body surface area (BSA):

TABLE 1: SUGGESTED NUMBER OF TABLETS TO BE ADMINISTERED

Body Surface Area (BSA)	Calculated Total Dose Equivalent to 40 mg/m^2 BSA (rounded up or down to nearest 10 mg)	Total Number of Tablets
0.75–0.88	30 mg	3
0.89–1.13	40 mg	4
1.14–1.38	50 mg	5
1.39–1.63	60 mg	6
1.64–1.88	70 mg	7
1.89–2.13	80 mg	8
2.14–2.38	90 mg	9
2.39–2.50	100 mg	10

A number of clinical settings may predispose to increased toxicity from Oforta™. These include advanced age, renal insufficiency, and bone marrow impairment. Such patients should be monitored closely for excessive toxicity and the dose modified accordingly. The optimal duration of treatment has not been clearly established. It is recommended that three additional cycles of Oforta™ be administered following the achievement of a maximal response and then the drug should be discontinued.

2.2 Renal Impairment

• Reduce dose by 20% in patients with mild to moderate renal impairment (creatinine clearance 30 to 70 mL/min/1.73 m^2). [*See Warnings and Precautions (5.7)*]
• Reduce dose by 50% in patients with severe renal impairment (creatinine clearance < 30 mL/min/1.73 m^2). [*See Warnings and Precautions (5.7)*]

3 DOSAGE FORMS AND STRENGTHS

10 mg tablets that are capsule shaped and salmon pink in color, marked on one side with 'LN' in a regular hexagon.

4 CONTRAINDICATIONS

None

5 WARNINGS AND PRECAUTIONS

5.1 Neurotoxicity

Dose-dependent neurotoxicity has been observed with fludarabine phosphate. Dose levels approximately 4 times greater (96 mg/m^2/day for 5 days to 7 days) than the recommended intravenous dose (25 mg/m^2/day for 5 days) were associated with a syndrome characterized by delayed blindness, coma and death. Symptoms appeared from 21 days to 60 days following the last dose. Thirteen of 36 patients (36.1%) who received fludarabine phosphate intravenously at high doses ($\geq$ 96 mg/m^2/day for 5 days to 7 days per course) developed severe neurotoxicity, while only one of 443 patients (0.2%) who received the drug intravenously at low doses ($\leq$ 40 mg/m^2/day for 5 days per course) developed toxicity. In the pivotal clinical study conducted with Oforta™ administered at 40 mg/m^2, severe impairment of consciousness was reported in one patient. The effect of chronic administration of fludarabine phosphate on the central nervous system is unknown; however, patients have received the recommended dose for up to 15 courses of therapy. Physicians should consider delaying or discontinuing the drug if neurotoxicity occurs.

5.2 Bone Marrow Suppression

Severe bone marrow suppression, notably anemia, thrombocytopenia and neutropenia, has been reported in patients treated with fludarabine phosphate. In a study in adult solid tumor patients, the median time to nadir counts was 13 days (range, 3 days to 25 days) for granulocytes and 16 days (range, 2 days to 32 days) for platelets. Most patients had hematologic impairment at baseline either as a result of disease or as a result of prior myelosuppressive therapy. Cumulative myelosuppression may be seen. While chemotherapy-induced myelosuppression is often reversible, administration of Oforta™ requires careful hematologic monitoring.

Several instances of trilineage bone marrow hypoplasia or aplasia resulting in pancytopenia, sometimes resulting in death, have been reported in adult patients. The duration of clinically significant cytopenia in the reported cases has ranged from approximately 2 months to approximately 1 year. These episodes have occurred both in previously treated or untreated patients. One case of pancytopenia was reported in the pivotal clinical study conducted with Oforta™.

Instances of life-threatening and sometimes fatal autoimmune hemolytic anemia have been reported to occur after one or more cycles of treatment with fludarabine phosphate in patients with or without a previous history of autoimmune hemolytic anemia or a positive Coombs' test and who may or may not be in remission from their disease. Steroids may or may not be effective in controlling these hemolytic episodes. The majority of patients rechallenged with fludarabine phosphate developed a recurrence in the hemolytic process. The mechanism(s) which predispose patients to the development of this complication has not been identified. Patients undergoing treatment with Oforta™ should be evaluated and closely monitored for hemolysis.

5.3 Pulmonary Toxicity

A high incidence of fatal pulmonary toxicity was observed in a clinical investigation using fludarabine phosphate in combination with pentostatin (deoxycoformycin) for the treatment of refractory chronic lymphocytic leukemia (CLL) in adults. Therefore, the use of Oforta™ in combination with pentostatin is not recommended.

5.4 Infections

Of 133 adult patients with CLL who received intravenous fludarabine phosphate in two clinical trials, there were 29 fatalities during study. Approximately 50% of the fatalities were due to infection and 25% due to progressive disease. Of 183 adult patients with CLL that received Oforta™ in two clinical trials, there were 13 deaths. Approximately 50% of the deaths were due to progressive disease, while two patient deaths (15%) were attributed to infection. Monitor for signs and symptoms of infection.

5.5 Tumor Lysis Syndrome

Tumor lysis syndrome associated with fludarabine phosphate treatment has been reported in patients with CLL with large tumor burdens. Since Oforta™ can induce a response as early as the first week of treatment, precautions should be taken in those patients at risk of developing this complication.

5.6 Use of Transfusions

Transfusion-associated graft-versus-host disease has been observed rarely after transfusion of non-irradiated blood in fludarabine phosphate treated patients. Consideration should, therefore, be given to the use of irradiated blood products in those patients requiring transfusions while undergoing treatment with Oforta™.

5.7 Renal Impairment

Oforta™ must be administered cautiously in patients with renal impairment. Following dosing of the intravenous product, the total body clearance of 2-fluoro-ara-A has been shown to be directly correlated with creatinine clearance. Patients with mild to moderate impairment of renal function (creatinine clearance 30 to 70 mL/min/1.73 m^2) should have their Oforta™ dose reduced by 20% and be monitored closely. Patients with severe impairment of renal function (creatinine clearance < 30 mL/min/1.73 m^2) should have their Oforta™ dose reduced by 50% and be monitored closely.

5.8 Monitoring

• Hematologic and Nonhematologic Toxicity
Oforta™ is an antineoplastic agent with potentially significant toxic side effects. Patients undergoing therapy should be closely observed for signs of hematologic and nonhematologic toxicity. Periodic assessment of peripheral blood counts is recommended to detect the development of anemia, neutropenia and thrombocytopenia.
• Hematopoietic Suppression
During treatment, the patient's hematologic profile (particularly neutrophils and platelets) should be monitored regularly to determine the degree of hematopoietic suppression.
• Infections
Patients treated with Oforta™ appear to be at an increased risk of infection. Monitor for signs and symptoms of infection.

5.9 Pregnancy

Based on its mechanism of action, Oforta™ can cause fetal harm when administered to a pregnant woman. Fludarabine phosphate administered to rats and rabbits during organogenesis caused an increase in resorptions, skeletal and visceral malformation, and decreased fetal body weights. If Oforta™ is used during pregnancy, or if the patient becomes pregnant while taking this drug, the patient should be apprised of the potential hazard to the fetus. Women of childbearing potential should be advised to avoid becoming pregnant. Women of childbearing potential and fertile males must take contraceptive measures during and at least for 6 months after the cessation of therapy.
[*see Use in Specific Populations (8.1)*].

6 ADVERSE REACTIONS

6.1 Clinical Trials Experience

Because clinical trials are conducted under widely varying conditions, adverse reaction rates observed in the clinical trials of a drug cannot be directly compared to rates in the clinical trials of another drug and may not reflect the rates observed in practice.

The data described below reflect exposure to Oforta™ in 159 patients exposed to the drug. Oforta™ was studied primarily in Study 1 in 78 patients with CLL who received prior therapy and in Study 2 in 81 patients with CLL who had not received prior therapy.

Based on experience with the intravenous and oral use of fludarabine phosphate, the most common adverse reactions include myelosuppression (neutropenia, thrombocytopenia and anemia), fever and chills, infection, and nausea and vomiting. Other commonly reported events include malaise, fatigue, anorexia, and weakness. Serious opportunistic infections have occurred in patients with CLL treated with fludarabine phosphate. The most frequently reported adverse reactions and those reactions which are more clearly related to the drug, as reported in clinical studies conducted with intravenous and oral fludarabine phosphate, are arranged below according to body system.

Hematopoietic Systems
Hematologic events (neutropenia, thrombocytopenia, and/or anemia) were reported in the majority of patients with CLL treated with fludarabine phosphate. During intravenous fludarabine phosphate treatment of 133 patients with CLL, the absolute neutrophil count decreased to less than 500/mm^3 in 59% of patients, hemoglobin decreased from pretreatment values by at least 2 grams percent in 60%, and platelet count decreased from pretreatment values by at least 50% in 55%. Among 78 patients with B-CLL who were treated with Oforta™, the absolute neutrophil count decreased to less than 500/mm^3 in 37% of patients,

hemoglobin decreased from pretreatment values by at least 2 grams percent in 14%, and platelet count decreased from pretreatment values by at least 50% in 17% of patients. Myelosuppression may be severe, cumulative, and may affect multiple cell lines. Bone marrow fibrosis occurred in one CLL patient treated with fludarabine phosphate intravenously. In the pivotal oral fludarabine phosphate study (Study 1), there was one report of a non-fatal case of pancytopenia. Similarly, there was one case of non-fatal pancytopenia reported among the 133 patients with CLL treated with intravenous fludarabine phosphate.

Life-threatening and sometimes fatal autoimmune hemolytic anemias have been reported to occur in patients receiving fludarabine phosphate. [See Warnings and Precautions (5.2)] The majority of patients rechallenged with fludarabine phosphate developed a recurrence in the hemolytic process.

Metabolic
Tumor lysis syndrome has been reported in patients with CLL treated with fludarabine phosphate for injection. This complication may include hyperuricemia, hyperphosphatemia, hypocalcemia, metabolic acidosis, hyperkalemia, hematuria, urate crystalluria, and renal failure. The onset of this syndrome may be heralded by flank pain and hematuria.

Nervous System
Objective weakness, agitation, confusion, visual disturbances, and coma have occurred in patients with CLL treated with fludarabine phosphate at the recommended dose. Peripheral neuropathy and one case of wrist-drop have been observed with intravenous administration of fludarabine phosphate. In Study 1 for Oforta™, there was one report of severe impairment of consciousness that presented concurrent with hemolytic anemia. This patient had enrolled in the study with pre-existing peripheral neurotoxicity. [See Warnings and Precautions (5.1)]

Pulmonary System
Pneumonia, a frequent manifestation of infection in patients with CLL, was observed in two clinical trials conducted with intravenous fludarabine phosphate (16% and 22%) and in two clinical trials with Oforta™ (8% and 3%). Pulmonary hypersensitivity reactions to fludarabine phosphate characterized by dyspnea, cough and interstitial pulmonary infiltrate have been observed. In Study 1 conducted with Oforta™, severe pulmonary toxicity was reported in 5 of 78 patients, often in conjunction with respiratory or pulmonary infections and hence not regarded as isolated drug related pulmonary toxicity.

Gastrointestinal System
Gastrointestinal disturbances such as nausea and vomiting, anorexia, diarrhea, stomatitis and gastrointestinal bleeding have been reported in patients treated with fludarabine phosphate. Nausea and vomiting occurred in up to 38% of patients following treatment with Oforta™ in the clinical trials.

Cardiovascular
Edema has been frequently reported. One patient developed a pericardial effusion possibly related to treatment with Oforta™. No other severe cardiovascular events were considered to be drug related.

Genitourinary System
Hemorrhagic cystitis has been reported in patients treated intravenously with fludarabine phosphate.

Skin
Skin toxicity, consisting primarily of skin rashes, has been reported in patients treated with oral and intravenous fludarabine phosphate.

Data in Table 2 are derived from the 159 patients with CLL who received Oforta™ in Study 1 and Study 2.

TABLE 2: Incidence (≥5%) of Non-Hematologic Adverse Reactions in Patients with CLL Treated with Oforta™

ADVERSE REACTIONS	Study 1 (N=78) %	Study 2 (N=81) %
ANY ADVERSE REACTION	82	89
BODY AS A WHOLE	59	77
FEVER	26	11
INFECTION	12	17
PAIN	5	19
FLU SYNDROME	8	5
DIAPHORESIS	8	0
NEUROLOGICAL	19	41
WEAKNESS/FATIGUE (ASTHENIA)	13	31
SWEATING INCREASED	0	14
HEADACHE	9	9
PULMONARY	37	53
COUGH	21	0
COUGH INCREASED	0	6
PNEUMONIA	8	3
DYSPNEA	1	5
SINUSITIS	1	5
UPPER RESPIRATORY INFECTION	9	14
RHINITIS	3	11
BRONCHITIS	6	9
METABOLIC AND NUTRITIONAL	3	31
WEIGHT DECREASED	1	6
LACTIC DEHYDROGENASE INCREASED	0	6
PERIPHERAL EDEMA	0	7
GASTROINTESTINAL	41	28
NAUSEA	5	1
DIARRHEA	6	5
ANOREXIA	19	0
ABDOMINAL PAIN	8	10
CUTANEOUS	22	25
RASH	5	4
SKIN DISORDER	0	6
HERPES SIMPLEX	8	7
GENITOURINARY	8	14
URINARY TRACT INFECTION	4	5
CARDIOVASCULAR	14	17
CHEST PAIN	0	5
MUSCULOSKELETAL	10	19
BACK PAIN	4	9

6.2 Post Marketing Experience
The following adverse reactions have been identified during post approval use of Oforta™. Because these reactions are reported voluntarily from a population of uncertain size, it is not always possibly to reliably estimate their frequency or establish a causal relationship to drug exposure.

Hematopoietic Systems
Several instances of trilineage bone marrow hypoplasia or aplasia resulting in pancytopenia, sometimes resulting in death, have been reported in post-marketing surveillance. The duration of clinically significant cytopenia in the reported cases has ranged from approximately 2 months to approximately 1 year. These episodes have occurred both in previously treated or untreated patients.

Nervous System
In post-marketing experience, cases of progressive multifocal leukoencephalopathy have been reported. Most cases had a fatal outcome. Many of these cases were confounded by prior and/or concurrent chemotherapy. The median time to onset was approximately one year.

Pulmonary System
In post-marketing experience, cases of severe pulmonary toxicity have been observed with fludarabine phosphate use which resulted in acute respiratory distress syndrome, respiratory distress, pulmonary hemorrhage, pulmonary fibrosis, and respiratory failure. After exclusion of an infectious origin, some patients experienced symptom improvement with corticosteroids.

7 DRUG INTERACTIONS
7.1 Pentostatin
The use of Oforta™ in combination with pentostatin is not recommended due to the risk of severe pulmonary toxicity. [See Warnings and Precautions (5.6)]

8 USE IN SPECIFIC POPULATIONS
8.1 Pregnancy
"Pregnancy Category D. See 'Warnings and Precautions' section."
Based on its mechanism of action, Oforta™ can cause fetal harm when administered to a pregnant woman. There are no adequate and well-controlled studies of fludarabine phosphate in pregnant women. Fludarabine phosphate was embryolethal and teratogenic in both rats and rabbits. If Oforta™ is used during pregnancy, or if the patient becomes pregnant while taking this drug, the patient should be apprised of the potential hazard to the fetus. Women of childbearing potential should be advised to avoid becoming pregnant. Women of childbearing potential and fertile males must take contraceptive measures during and at least for 6 months after the cessation of therapy.
In rats, repeated intravenous doses of fludarabine phosphate at 1.5 times and 4.5 times the recommended human oral dose (40 mg/m²) administered during organogenesis caused an increase in resorptions, skeletal and visceral malformations (cleft palate, exencephaly, and fetal vertebrae deformities) and decreased fetal body weights. Maternal toxicity was not apparent at 1.5 times the human oral dose, and was limited to slight body weight decreases at 4.5 times the human oral dose. In rabbits, repeated intravenous doses of fludarabine phosphate at 2.4 times the human oral dose administered during organogenesis increased embryo and fetal lethality as indicated by increased resorptions and a decrease in live fetuses. A significant increase in malformations including cleft palate, hydrocephaly, adactyly,

brachydactyly, fusions of the digits, diaphragmatic hernia, heart/great vessel defects, and vertebrae/rib anomalies were seen in all dose levels (≥ 0.3 times the human oral dose).

8.3 Nursing Mothers
It is not known whether Oforta™ is excreted in human milk. Because many drugs are excreted in human milk and because of the potential for serious adverse reactions including tumorigenicity in nursing infants, a decision should be made to discontinue nursing or discontinue the drug, taking into account the importance of the drug to the mother.

8.4 Pediatric Use
Safety and effectiveness in pediatric patients have not been established.

8.5 Geriatric Use
Of 78 previously treated patients with B-CLL treated with Oforta™ 50% were ≥ age 65 and 3% were ≥ age 75. The response rate was generally lower among patients age 65 and older. Among previously treated patients (Study 1) age 65 and older, the overall objective response, according to standardized response criteria developed by the National Cancer Institute CLL Working Group (NCI criteria), was 41%. The safety profile among younger and older patients on study was similar. Other reported clinical experience has not identified differences in responses or safety between older and younger patients.

8.6 Patients with Renal Impairment
In patients receiving intravenous fludarabine phosphate, the total body clearance of the metabolite 2-fluoro-ara-adenine (2F-ara-A) correlated with the creatinine clearance, indicating the importance of the renal excretion pathway for the elimination of the drug. Renal clearance represented approximately 40% of the total body clearance. Patients with mild to moderate impairment (30 to 70 mL/min/1.73 m²) receiving 20% reduced fludarabine phosphate dose had a similar exposure compared to patients with normal renal function receiving the recommended dose (AUC; 21 nM•h/mL versus 20 nM•h/mL). Two patients with severe renal impairment (< 30 mL/min/1.73 m²) receiving 40% reduced fludarabine phosphate dose had a 40% increase in exposure compared to patients with normal renal function receiving the recommended dose. The mean total body clearance was 172 mL/min for patients with normal renal function, 124 mL/min for patients with mild to moderately impaired renal function, and 71 mL/min for the two patients with severe renal impairment.

10 OVERDOSAGE
High doses of fludarabine phosphate [See Indications and Usage (1.1) and Warnings and Precautions (5.1)] have been associated with an irreversible central nervous system toxicity characterized by delayed blindness, coma and death. High doses are also associated with severe thrombocytopenia and neutropenia due to bone marrow suppression. There is no known specific antidote for fludarabine phosphate overdosage. Treatment consists of drug discontinuation and supportive therapy. In Study 2, two patients ingested an overdose of 20% to 33% of Oforta™. No serious side effects were reported.

11 DESCRIPTION
The chemical name for fludarabine phosphate is 9H-Purin-6-amine,2-fluoro-9-(5-O-phosphono-β-D-arabinofuranosyl) (2-fluoro-ara-AMP). The molecular formula of fludarabine phosphate is $C_{10}H_{13}FN_5O_7P$ (MW 365.2) and the structure is provided in Figure 1

Figure 1: Chemical Structure of Fludarabine Phosphate

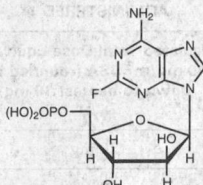

Oforta™ (fludarabine phosphate tablets) for oral administration contain fludarabine phosphate, a fluorinated nucleotide analog of the antiviral agent vidarabine, 9-beta -D-arabinofuranosyladenine (ara-A) that is relatively resistant to deamination by adenosine deaminase. Each tablet contains 10 mg of the active ingredient fludarabine phosphate. The tablet core consists of microcrystalline cellulose, lactose monohydrate, colloidal anhydrous silicon dioxide, croscarmellose sodium and magnesium stearate. The film-coat contains hypromellose, talc, titanium dioxide (E171) and ferric oxide pigment (red/E172, yellow/E172).

12 CLINICAL PHARMACOLOGY
12.1 Mechanism of Action
Fludarabine phosphate (2F-ara-AMP) is a synthetic purine nucleotide antimetabolite agent. Upon administration,

2F-ara-AMP is rapidly dephosphorylated in the plasma to 2F-ara-A, which then enters into the cell. Intracellularly, 2F-ara-A is converted to the 5'-triphosphate, 2-fluoro-ara-ATP (2F-ara-ATP). 2F-ara-ATP competes with deoxyadenosine triphosphate for incorporation into DNA. Once incorporated into DNA, 2F-ara-ATP functions as a DNA chain terminator, inhibits DNA polymerase alpha, gamma, and delta, and inhibits ribonucleoside diphosphate reductase. 2F-ara-A also inhibits DNA primase and DNA ligase I. The mechanism of action of this antimetabolite is not completely characterized and may be multi-faceted.

12.2 Pharmacodynamics
Cardiac Electrophysiology

In a randomized, uncontrolled, open-label, parallel study, patients with B-cell CLL were administered a single dose of Oforta™ 40 mg/m^2 (n = 42) or intravenous fludarabine phosphate 25 mg/m^2 (n=14). The maximum increase in the baseline-corrected mean change in QTcI (individual-corrected QT interval) following treatment with Oforta™ was less than 10 milliseconds.

12.3 Pharmacokinetics
Studies with the intravenous product have demonstrated that fludarabine phosphate is converted to the active metabolite, 2F-ara-A. Clinical pharmacology studies have focused on 2F-ara-A pharmacokinetics.

Following administration of the intravenous product, systemic plasma clearance of 2F-ara-A is approximately 117 mL/min to 145 mL/min. After five daily 30 minute intravenous infusions of 25 mg 2F-ara-AMP/m^2 to cancer patients, trough concentrations of 2F-ara-A increased by a factor of about 2. The terminal half-life of 2F-ara-A was approximately 20 hours. Plasma protein binding of 2F-ara-A was approximately 19% to 29%. A correlation was noted between the degree of absolute granulocyte count nadir and increased area under the concentration × time curve (AUC).

2F-ara-A exhibits dose proportional increases in AUC and Cmax after single oral doses of 50 mg, 70 mg or 90 mg of 2F-ara-AMP. Cmax of 2F-ara-A occurs 1 hour to 2 hours after single or multiple oral doses and is approximately 20 % to 30 % of the maximum plasma concentrations produced at the end of a 30 minute intravenous infusion of the same dose. The absolute oral bioavailability of 2F-ara-A is 50–65% following single and repeated doses of Oforta™. Similar systemic exposure (AUC) was observed after a single 40 mg/m^2 Oforta™ and a single 25 mg/m^2 fludarabine phosphate intravenous dose. The terminal half-life of 2F-ara-A was similar to that following intravenous administration; approximately 20 hours. The Cmax, AUC and terminal half-life of 2F-ara-A are unaffected when administered with a high fat meal, although Tmax is slightly delayed from 1.3 hours to 2.2 hours.

Following intravenous administration, renal clearance of 2F-ara-A represents approximately 40% of the total body clearance of fludarabine phosphate, and total body clearance is inversely correlated with serum creatinine and creatinine clearance. In two patients with median creatinine clearance of 22 mL/min/1.73 m^2, 2F-ara-A clearance was reduced by 56%. Dosage adjustment based on creatinine clearance is recommended as follows:

Reduce dose by 20% in patients with mild to moderate renal impairment (creatinine clearance 30 to 70 mL/min/1.73 m^2). [See Warnings and Precautions (5.7)]

Reduce dose by 50% in patients with severe renal impairment (creatinine clearance < 30 mL/min/1.73 m^2). [See Warnings and Precautions (5.7)]

13 NONCLINICAL TOXICOLOGY
13.1 Carcinogenesis, Mutagenesis, Impairment of Fertility
No animal carcinogenicity studies with Oforta™ have been conducted.

Oforta™ is a clastogen.

Fludarabine phosphate was clastogenic in vitro to Chinese hamster ovary cells (chromosome aberration assay) in the presence of metabolic activation and induced sister chromatid exchanges both in the presence and absence of metabolic activation. In addition, fludarabine phosphate was clastogenic in vivo (mouse micronucleus assay) but was not mutagenic to germ cells (dominant lethal test in male mice). Fludarabine phosphate was not mutagenic to bacteria (Ames test) or mammalian cells either in the presence or absence of metabolic activation.

Studies in mice, rats and dogs have demonstrated dose-related adverse effects on the male reproductive system. Observations consisted of a decrease in mean testicular weights in mice and rats with a trend toward decreased testicular weights in dogs and degeneration and necrosis of spermatogenic epithelium of the testes in mice, rats and dogs.

14 CLINICAL STUDIES
Study 1, a single-arm, open-label study of Oforta™ was conducted in 78 adult patients with CLL refractory to at least one prior standard alkylating-agent containing regimen. In this multicenter study patients were treated with Oforta™ at a dose of 40 mg/m^2 daily for 5 days every 28 days. The patient population median age was 64.5 years and consisted of 72% males and 28% females. Ninety-nine percent of the patients were Caucasian. The Rai stage for patients entering the study was: Stage 0 (3.9%), Stage I (20.5%), Stage II (32.1%), Stage III (11.5%), and Stage IV (32.1%). The mean number of treatment cycles was 5.1 with a mean daily dose of Oforta™ of 38 mg/m^2. The overall objective response, according to standardized response criteria developed by the National Cancer Institute CLL Working Group (NCI criteria), was 51%, including 18% complete responses and 33% partial responses. The overall response rate, according to standardized criteria developed by the International Workshop on CLL (IWCLL criteria), was 46%, including 21% complete responses and 26% partial responses. Data on duration of response was not collected.

In Study 2, a supportive single-arm, open-label study, Oforta™ was administered to 81 previously untreated patients with B-CLL. In this multicenter study each patient was treated with Oforta™ at a dose of 40 mg/m^2 daily for 5 days every 28 days. The patient population median age was 64.0 years and consisted of 63% males and 37% females. Ninety-nine percent of the patients were Caucasian. The Rai stage for patients entering the study was: Stage 0 (3.7%), Stage I (37.0%), Stage II (37.0%), Stage III (9.9%), and Stage IV (12.3%). The mean number of treatment cycles was 5.9 with a mean daily dose per patient of 71 mg to 74 mg. The overall responses rate, according to NCI criteria, was 80%, including 12% complete and 68% partial responses. The overall response rate, according to IWCLL criteria, was 72%, including 37% complete responses and 35% partial responses. The median duration of response was 22.9 months.

Study 3 was a supportive randomized controlled open label study in patients with previously untreated B-CLL that included fludarabine phosphate monotherapy and fludarabine phosphate combination therapy arms. In this study 107 evaluable patients received Oforta™ 40mg/m^2 orally daily for 5 days every 28 days. The overall response rate according to modified NCI criteria was 74% and the CR plus nodular PR rate was 41%.

15 REFERENCES
1. Preventing Occupational Exposures to Antineoplastic and Other Hazardous Drugs in Health Care Settings. NIOSH Alert 2004-165.
2. OSHA Technical Manual, TED 1-0.15A, Section VI: Chapter 2. Controlling Occupational Exposure to Hazardous Drugs. OSHA, 1999.
   http://www.osha.gov/dts/osta/otm/otm_vi/otm_vi_2.html
3. American Society of Health-System Pharmacists. ASHP guidelines on handling hazardous drugs. Am J Health-Syst Pharm. 2006;63:1172-1193.
4. Polovich, M., White, J. M., & Kelleher, L.O. (eds.) 2005. Chemotherapy and biotherapy guidelines and recommendations for practice (2nd. ed.) Pittsburgh, PA: Oncology Nursing Society.

16 HOW SUPPLIED/STORAGE AND HANDLING
HOW SUPPLIED
Oforta™ is supplied in 10 milligram tablets that are film-coated, capsule shaped, salmon pink in color, and marked on one side with 'LN' in a regular hexagon. Each film-coated tablet contains 10 mg fludarabine phosphate. The tablets are supplied in blisters, each blister strip containing 5 tablets. Packages of 15 and 20 tablets are available in child-resistant containers.

NDC 0024-5820-15: 15 – 10 milligram film-coated tablets per container. Each film-coated tablet is packaged in an individual blister package; 5 tablets per blister strip; 3 blister strips packaged in a plastic bottle with a child-resistant container closure; each bottle is packaged in an individual chipboard carton.

NDC0024-5820-20: 20 – 10 milligram film-coated tablets per container. Each film-coated tablet is packaged in an individual blister package; 5 tablets per blister strip; 4 blister strips packaged in a plastic bottle with a child-resistant container closure; each bottle is packaged in an individual chipboard carton.

STORAGE
Store under normal lighting conditions at 25°C (77°F); excursions permitted to 15–30°C (59–86°F) [see USP controlled room temperature].

HANDLING AND DISPOSAL
Procedures for proper handling and disposal should be considered. Consideration should be given to handling and disposal according to guidelines issued for cytotoxic drugs. Several guidelines on this subject have been published.[1-4] Caution should be exercised in the handling of Oforta™. **Push tablets through foil to open. Do not remove tablets from individual blisters until immediately prior to taking or administering each scheduled dose. Do not crush tablets.** Avoid exposure by direct contact of the skin or mucous membranes or by inhalation. If contact occurs, wash thoroughly with soap and water or wash the eyes immediately with gently flowing water for at least 15 minutes. Consult healthcare provider in case of a skin reaction or if the drug gets in the eyes.

17 PATIENT COUNSELING INFORMATION
17.1 Bone Marrow Suppression
Inform patients that Oforta™ decreases blood cell counts such as white blood cells, platelets, and red blood cells. Thus, it is important that periodic assessment of their blood count be performed to detect the development of neutropenia, thrombocytopenia and anemia. [See Warnings and Precautions (5.2)]

17.2 Infections
Instruct patients to notify their physician promptly if fever or other signs of infection such as chills, cough, or burning pain on urination occurs while on therapy. [See Warnings and Precautions (5.4)]

17.3 Pregnancy
Women of childbearing potential and fertile males must take contraceptive measures during and at least for 6 months after the cessation of therapy. Oforta™ may cause fetal harm when administered to a pregnant woman. [See Warnings and Precautions (5.9)]

17.4 Handling and Disposal
Instruct patients that caution should be exercised in the handling of Oforta™. Do not crush tablets. Avoid exposure by direct contact of the skin or mucous membranes or by inhalation. If contact occurs, wash thoroughly with soap and water or wash the eyes immediately with gently flowing water for at least 15 minutes. Consult healthcare provider in case of a skin reaction or if the drug gets in the eyes. Ask your healthcare provider or pharmacist for directions about how to safely dispose of Oforta™.

Manufactured for: sanofi-aventis U.S. LLC, Bridgewater, NJ 08807
©2009

OFORTA™ (oh-FORT-tuh)
(oral fludarabine phosphate tablets)

Read this Patient Information leaflet before you start taking OFORTA™ and each time you get a refill. There may be new information. This information does not take the place of talking with your healthcare provider about your medical condition or your treatment.

What Is OFORTA™?
OFORTA™ (oral fludarabine phosphate tablets) is a prescription anticancer medicine that slows or stops the growth of cancer cells in adults with chronic lymphocytic leukemia (CLL). OFORTA™ also stops or slows the growth of some healthy cells. This can cause side effects that you should know about and report to your healthcare provider.
OFORTA™ has not been studied in children.

What is the most important information I should know about OFORTA™?
On rare occasions people taking OFORTA™ can have life-threatening symptoms. If you:
• **have problems seeing**
• **feel very sleepy, tired, or confused**
• **have shortness of breath or have trouble breathing**
• **have yellow skin or dark urine**
Tell your healthcare provider right away.

What should I tell my healthcare provider before taking OFORTA™?
Before taking OFORTA™, tell your healthcare provider about all of your medical conditions, including if you:
• have kidney problems
• have bleeding problems
• are pregnant or plan to become pregnant. It is not known if OFORTA™ will harm your unborn baby. Talk to your doctor if you are pregnant or plan to become pregnant. Women should not get pregnant during treatment with OFORTA™ because the unborn baby may be harmed. Both men and women must take contraceptive measures during and for at least six months after cessation of therapy. Call your doctor right away if you become pregnant during or in the six months after treatment with OFORTA™.
• are breast-feeding or plan to breast-feed. It is not known if OFORTA™ passes into your breast milk. You and your healthcare provider should decide if you will take OFORTA™ or breast-feed. You should not do both.

Tell your healthcare provider about all the medicines you take including prescription and non-prescription medicines, vitamins, and herbal supplements. Using OFORTA™ with certain other medicines may affect each other. Using OFORTA™ with other medicines may cause serious side effects.
Know the medicines you take. Keep a list of them with you to show your healthcare provider.

How should I take OFORTA™?
• Take OFORTA™ exactly as your healthcare provider tells you to take it.
• Your healthcare provider will tell you how much and when to take OFORTA™.

- OFORTA™ can be taken with or without food.
- **Push tablets through foil to open. Do not remove tablets from individual blisters until immediately prior to taking or administering each scheduled dose.**
- OFORTA™ tablets have to be swallowed whole with water; they should never be chewed, crushed, or broken. If you cannot swallow OFORTA™ whole, ask your health-care provider if you can take another form of fludarabine.
- If you miss a dose call your healthcare provider.
- If you take too much call your healthcare provider.

What should I avoid while taking OFORTA™?
- Do not allow other people or pets to touch or take OFORTA™.
- Avoid letting the tablets (whole or broken) touch your skin
- Do not chew tablets or hold them in your mouth. Swallow tablets right away.
- Do not breathe in any powder or residue from a broken tablet.
- If you touch a broken tablet, wash the area thoroughly with soap and water.
- If any OFORTA™ gets in your eyes, wash your eyes right away with water for at least 15 minutes, and call your healthcare provider right away.
- Call your healthcare provider right away in case of a skin reaction.

What are the possible side effects of OFORTA™?
See "What is the most important information I should know about OFORTA™?"
OFORTA™ may cause serious side effects, including:
Low blood cell counts.
OFORTA™ lessens the number of blood cells that fight infection, help your blood to clot, and carry oxygen throughout your body. This can result in
- Infection
- Bleeding
- Tiredness.

Avoid activities that can raise your chances of these conditions. Your healthcare provider will check your blood counts so that you will know when you are most at risk for infection, bleeding, and tiredness.
Call your healthcare provider right away if you have a temperature of 100.5°F or above or do not feel well. Do not take a fever medicine until you check with your healthcare provider.
OFORTA™ may cause other side effects, including:
- nausea and vomiting
- loss of appetite
- skin rash
- swelling in your legs
- diarrhea
- redness and irritation inside your mouth (stomatitis)
- abdominal and muscle pain.

Tell your healthcare provider if you have any side effect that bothers you or that does not go away. These are not all the possible side effects of OFORTA™. For more information, ask your healthcare provider or pharmacist.
Call your doctor for medical advice about side effects. You may report side effects to the FDA at 1-800-FDA-1088.

How should I store and throw away OFORTA™?
- Store OFORTA™ at 59–86°F (15–30°C).
- Keep under normal light in a child-resistant container.
- Safely throw away medicine that is out of date or no longer needed.
- Do not put OFORTA™ in your regular household trash.
- Ask your healthcare provider or pharmacist for directions about how to safely throw away and handle OFORTA™.

Keep OFORTA™ and all medicines out of the reach of children.

General information about OFORTA™
Medicines are sometimes prescribed for conditions that are not mentioned in patient information. Do not use OFORTA™ for a condition for which it was not prescribed. Do not give OFORTA™ to other people, even if they have the same symptoms you have. It may harm them.
This patient information leaflet summarizes the most important information about OFORTA™. For more information about OFORTA™, talk with your healthcare provider. You can ask your healthcare provider or pharmacist for information about OFORTA™ that is written for health professionals. For more information call 1-800-633-1610.

What are the ingredients in OFORTA™?
Active ingredients: fludarabine phosphate
Inactive ingredients: microcrystalline cellulose, lactose monohydrate, colloidal anhydrous silicon dioxide, croscarmellose sodium and magnesium stearate. The film-coat contains hypromellose, talc, titanium dioxide (E171) and ferric oxide pigment (red/E172, yellow/E172).
Manufactured for: sanofi-aventis U.S. LLC, Bridgewater, NJ 08807
©2009
Revised: 03/2009   sanofi-aventis U.S. LLC

PLAVIX®
[plă-vĭcks]
(clopidogrel bisulfate)
tablets   ℞

HIGHLIGHTS OF PRESCRIBING INFORMATION
These highlights do not include all the information needed to use PLAVIX safely and effectively. See full prescribing information for PLAVIX.
PLAVIX (clopidogrel bisulfate) tablets
Initial U.S. Approval: 1997

WARNING: DIMINISHED EFFECTIVENESS IN POOR METABOLIZERS
See full prescribing information for complete boxed warning.
- **Effectiveness of Plavix depends on activation to an active metabolite by the cytochrome P450 (CYP) system, principally CYP2C19. (5.1)**
- **Poor metabolizers treated with Plavix at recommended doses exhibit higher cardiovascular event rates following acute coronary syndrome (ACS) or percutaneous coronary intervention (PCI) than patients with normal CYP2C19 function. (12.5)**
- **Tests are available to identify a patient's CYP2C19 genotype and can be used as an aid in determining therapeutic strategy. (12.5)**
- **Consider alternative treatment or treatment strategies in patients identified as CYP2C19 poor metabolizers. (2.3, 5.1)**

———RECENT MAJOR CHANGES———

Boxed Warning	03/2010
Dosage and Administration (2.3, 2.4)	08/2010
Warnings and Precautions (5.1, 5.2, 5.3)	08/2010

———INDICATIONS AND USAGE———
Plavix is a P2Y₁₂ platelet inhibitor indicated for:
- Acute coronary syndrome
  - For patients with non-ST-segment elevation ACS [unstable angina (UA)/non-ST-elevation myocardial infarction (NSTEMI)] including patients who are to be managed medically and those who are to be managed with coronary revascularization, Plavix has been shown to decrease the rate of a combined endpoint of cardiovascular death, myocardial infarction (MI), or stroke as well as the rate of a combined endpoint of cardiovascular death, MI, stroke, or refractory ischemia. (1.1)
  - For patients with ST-elevation myocardial infarction (STEMI), Plavix has been shown to reduce the rate of death from any cause and the rate of a combined endpoint of death, re-infarction, or stroke. The benefit for patients who undergo primary PCI is unknown. (1.1)
- Recent myocardial infarction (MI), recent stroke, or established peripheral arterial disease. Plavix has been shown to reduce the combined endpoint of new ischemic stroke (fatal or not), new MI (fatal or not), and other vascular death. (1.2)

———DOSAGE AND ADMINISTRATION———
- Acute coronary syndrome (2.1)
  - Non-ST-segment elevation ACS (UA/NSTEMI): 300 mg loading dose followed by 75 mg once daily, in combination with aspirin (75–325 mg once daily)
  - STEMI: 75 mg once daily, in combination with aspirin (75–325 mg once daily), with or without a loading dose and with or without thrombolytics
- Recent MI, recent stroke, or established peripheral arterial disease: 75 mg once daily (2.2)

———DOSAGE FORMS AND STRENGTHS———
Tablets: 75 mg, 300 mg (3)

———CONTRAINDICATIONS———
- Active pathological bleeding, such as peptic ulcer or intracranial hemorrhage (4.1)
- Hypersensitivity to clopidogrel or any component of the product (4.2)

———WARNINGS AND PRECAUTIONS———
- Reduced effectiveness in impaired CYP2C19 function: Avoid concomitant use with drugs that are strong or moderate CYP2C19 inhibitors (e.g., omeprazole). (5.1)
- Bleeding: Plavix increases risk of bleeding. Discontinue 5 days prior to elective surgery. (5.2)
- Discontinuation of Plavix: Premature discontinuation increases risk of cardiovascular events. (5.3)
- Recent transient ischemic attack or stroke: Combination use of Plavix and aspirin in these patients was not shown to be more effective than Plavix alone, but was shown to increase major bleeding. (5.4)
- Thrombotic thrombocytopenic purpura (TTP): TTP has been reported with Plavix, including fatal cases. (5.5)

———ADVERSE REACTIONS———
Bleeding, including life-threatening and fatal bleeding, is the most commonly reported adverse reaction. (6.1)
To report SUSPECTED ADVERSE REACTIONS, contact Bristol-Myers Squibb/Sanofi Pharmaceuticals Partnership at 1-800-633-1610 or FDA at 1-800-FDA-1088 or www.fda.gov/medwatch

———DRUG INTERACTIONS———
- Nonsteroidal anti-inflammatory drugs (NSAIDs): Combination use increases risk of gastrointestinal bleeding. (7.2)
- Warfarin: Combination use increases risk of bleeding. (7.3)

———USE IN SPECIFIC POPULATIONS———
Nursing mothers: Discontinue drug or nursing, taking into consideration importance of drug to mother. (8.3)
See 17 for PATIENT COUNSELING INFORMATION
Revised: 08/2010

FULL PRESCRIBING INFORMATION

WARNING: DIMINISHED EFFECTIVENESS IN POOR METABOLIZERS
The effectiveness of Plavix is dependent on its activation to an active metabolite by the cytochrome P450 (CYP) system, principally CYP2C19 *[see Warnings and Precautions (5.1)]*. **Plavix at recommended doses**

forms less of that metabolite and has a smaller effect on platelet function in patients who are CYP2C19 poor metabolizers. Poor metabolizers with acute coronary syndrome or undergoing percutaneous coronary intervention treated with Plavix at recommended doses exhibit higher cardiovascular event rates than do patients with normal CYP2C19 function. Tests are available to identify a patient's CYP2C19 genotype; these tests can be used as an aid in determining therapeutic strategy *[see Clinical Pharmacology (12.5)]*. Consider alternative treatment or treatment strategies in patients identified as CYP2C19 poor metabolizers *[see Dosage and Administration (2.3)]*.

1 INDICATIONS AND USAGE

1.1 Acute Coronary Syndrome (ACS)

- For patients with non-ST-segment elevation ACS [unstable angina (UA)/non-ST-elevation myocardial infarction (NSTEMI)], including patients who are to be managed medically and those who are to be managed with coronary revascularization, Plavix has been shown to decrease the rate of a combined endpoint of cardiovascular death, myocardial infarction (MI), or stroke as well as the rate of a combined endpoint of cardiovascular death, MI, stroke, or refractory ischemia.
- For patients with ST-elevation myocardial infarction (STEMI), Plavix has been shown to reduce the rate of death from any cause and the rate of a combined endpoint of death, re-infarction, or stroke. The benefit for patients who undergo primary percutaneous coronary intervention is unknown.

The optimal duration of Plavix therapy in ACS is unknown.

1.2 Recent MI, Recent Stroke, or Established Peripheral Arterial Disease

For patients with a history of recent myocardial infarction (MI), recent stroke, or established peripheral arterial disease, Plavix has been shown to reduce the rate of a combined endpoint of new ischemic stroke (fatal or not), new MI (fatal or not), and other vascular death.

2 DOSAGE AND ADMINISTRATION

2.1 Acute Coronary Syndrome

Plavix can be administered with or without food *[see Clinical Pharmacology (12.3)]*

- For patients with non-ST-elevation ACS (UA/NSTEMI), initiate Plavix with a single 300 mg oral loading dose and then continue at 75 mg once daily. Initiate aspirin (75–325 mg once daily) and continue in combination with Plavix *[see Clinical Studies (14.1)]*.
- For patients with STEMI, the recommended dose of Plavix is 75 mg once daily orally, administered in combination with aspirin (75–325 mg once daily), with or without thrombolytics. Plavix may be initiated with or without a loading dose *[see Clinical Studies (14.1)]*.

2.2 Recent MI, Recent Stroke, or Established Peripheral Arterial Disease

The recommended daily dose of Plavix is 75 mg once daily orally, with or without food *[see Clinical Pharmacology (12.3)]*.

2.3 CYP2C19 Poor Metabolizers

CYP2C19 poor metabolizer status is associated with diminished antiplatelet response to clopidogrel. Although a higher dose regimen in poor metabolizers increases antiplatelet response *[see Clinical Pharmacology (12.5)]*, an appropriate dose regimen for this patient population has not been established.

2.4 Use with Proton Pump Inhibitors (PPI)

Omeprazole, a moderate CYP2C19 inhibitor, reduces the pharmacological activity of Plavix if using omeprazole concomitantly or 12 hours apart with Plavix. Consider using another acid reducing agent with less CYP2C19 inhibitory activity. A higher dose regimen of clopidogrel concomitantly administered with omeprazole increases antiplatelet response; an appropriate dose regimen has not been established *[see Warnings and Precautions (5.1), Drug Interactions (7.1) and Clinical Pharmacology (12.5)]*.

3 DOSAGE FORMS AND STRENGTHS

- 75 mg tablets: Pink, round, biconvex, film-coated tablets debossed with "75" on one side and "1171" on the other
- 300 mg tablets: Pink, oblong, film-coated tablets debossed with "300" on one side and "1332" on the other

4 CONTRAINDICATIONS

4.1 Active Bleeding

Plavix is contraindicated in patients with active pathological bleeding such as peptic ulcer or intracranial hemorrhage.

4.2 Hypersensitivity

Plavix is contraindicated in patients with hypersensitivity (e.g., anaphylaxis) to clopidogrel or any component of the product *[see Adverse Reactions (6.2)]*.

Table 1: CURE Incidence of Bleeding Complications (% patients)

Event	Plavix (+ aspirin)* (n=6259)	Placebo (+ aspirin)* (n=6303)	p-value
Major bleeding[†]	3.7[‡]	2.7[§]	0.001
Life-threatening bleeding	2.2	1.8	0.13
Fatal	0.2	0.2	
5 g/dL hemoglobin drop	0.9	0.9	
Requiring surgical intervention	0.7	0.7	
Hemorrhagic strokes	0.1	0.1	
Requiring inotropes	0.5	0.5	
Requiring transfusion (≥4 units)	1.2	1.0	
Other major bleeding	1.6	1.0	0.005
Significantly disabling	0.4	0.3	
Intraocular bleeding with significant loss of vision	0.05	0.03	
Requiring 2–3 units of blood	1.3	0.9	
Minor bleeding ¶	5.1	2.4	< 0.001

* Other standard therapies were used as appropriate.

† Life-threatening and other major bleeding.

‡ Major bleeding event rate for Plavix + aspirin was dose-dependent on aspirin: <100 mg = 2.6%; 100–200 mg = 3.5%; >200 mg = 4.9%

Major bleeding event rates for Plavix + aspirin by age were: <65 years = 2.5%, ≥65 to <75 years = 4.1%, ≥75 years = 5.9%.

§ Major bleeding event rate for placebo + aspirin was dose-dependent on aspirin: <100 mg = 2.0%; 100–200 mg = 2.3%; >200 mg = 4.0%

Major bleeding event rates for placebo + aspirin by age were: <65 years = 2.1%, ≥65 to <75 years = 3.1%, ≥75 years = 3.6%

¶ Led to interruption of study medication.

---

5 WARNINGS AND PRECAUTIONS

5.1 Diminished Antiplatelet Activity Due to Impaired CYP2C19 Function

Clopidogrel is a prodrug. Inhibition of platelet aggregation by clopidogrel is due to an active metabolite. The metabolism of clopidogrel to its active metabolite can be impaired by genetic variations in CYP2C19 *[see Boxed Warning]* and by concomitant medications that interfere with CYP2C19. Avoid concomitant use of Plavix and strong or moderate CYP2C19 inhibitors.

Omeprazole, a moderate CYP2C19 inhibitor, has been shown to reduce the pharmacological activity of Plavix if given concomitantly or if given 12 hours apart. Consider using another acid reducing agent with less CYP2C19 inhibitory activity. Pantoprazole, a weak CYP2C19 inhibitor, had less effect on the pharmacological activity of Plavix than omeprazole *[see Drug Interactions (7.1) and Dosage and Administration (2.4)]*.

5.2 General Risk of Bleeding

Thienopyridines, including Plavix, increase the risk of bleeding. If a patient is to undergo surgery and an antiplatelet effect is not desired, discontinue Plavix five days prior to surgery. In patients who stopped therapy more than five days prior to CABG the rates of major bleeding were similar (event rate 4.4% Plavix + aspirin; 5.3% placebo + aspirin). In patients who remained on therapy within five days of CABG, the major bleeding rate was 9.6% for Plavix + aspirin, and 6.3% for placebo + aspirin.

Thienopyridines inhibit platelet aggregation for the lifetime of the platelet (7–10 days), so withholding a dose will not be useful in managing a bleeding event or the risk of bleeding associated with an invasive procedure. Because the half-life of clopidogrel's active metabolite is short, it may be possible to restore hemostasis by administering exogenous platelets; however, platelet transfusions within 4 hours of the loading dose or 2 hours of the maintenance dose may be less effective.

5.3 Discontinuation of Plavix

Avoid lapses in therapy, and if Plavix must be temporarily discontinued, restart as soon as possible. Premature discontinuation of Plavix may increase the risk of cardiovascular events.

5.4 Patients with Recent Transient Ischemic Attack (TIA) or Stroke

In patients with recent TIA or stroke who are at high risk for recurrent ischemic events, the combination of aspirin and Plavix has not been shown to be more effective than Plavix alone, but the combination has been shown to increase major bleeding.

5.5 Thrombotic Thrombocytopenic Purpura (TTP)

TTP, sometimes fatal, has been reported following use of Plavix, sometimes after a short exposure (<2 weeks). TTP is a serious condition that requires urgent treatment including plasmapheresis (plasma exchange). It is characterized by thrombocytopenia, microangiopathic hemolytic anemia (schistocytes [fragmented RBCs] seen on peripheral smear), neurological findings, renal dysfunction, and fever *[see Adverse Reactions (6.2)]*.

6 ADVERSE REACTIONS

The following serious adverse reactions are discussed below and elsewhere in the labeling:

- Bleeding *[see Warnings and Precautions (5.2)]*
- Thrombotic thrombocytopenic purpura *[see Warnings and Precautions (5.5)]*

6.1 Clinical Studies Experience

Because clinical trials are conducted under widely varying conditions and durations of follow up, adverse reaction rates observed in the clinical trials of a drug cannot be directly compared to rates in the clinical trials of another drug and may not reflect the rates observed in practice.

Plavix has been evaluated for safety in more than 54,000 patients, including over 21,000 patients treated for 1 year or more. The clinically important adverse reactions observed in trials comparing Plavix plus aspirin to placebo plus aspirin and trials comparing Plavix alone to aspirin alone are discussed below.

Bleeding

CURE

In CURE, Plavix use with aspirin was associated with an increase in major bleeding (primarily gastrointestinal and at puncture sites) compared to placebo with aspirin (see Table 1). The incidence of intracranial hemorrhage (0.1%) and fatal bleeding (0.2%) were the same in both groups. Other bleeding events that were reported more frequently in the clopidogrel group were epistaxis, hematuria, and bruise. The overall incidence of bleeding is described in Table 1.

[See table 1 above]

Ninety-two percent (92%) of the patients in the CURE study received heparin or low molecular weight heparin (LMWH), and the rate of bleeding in these patients was similar to the overall results.

COMMIT

In COMMIT, similar rates of major bleeding were observed in the Plavix and placebo groups, both of which also received aspirin (see Table 2).

[See table 2 at top of next page]

CAPRIE (Plavix vs. Aspirin)

In CAPRIE, gastrointestinal hemorrhage occurred at a rate of 2.0% in those taking Plavix vs. 2.7% in those taking aspirin; bleeding requiring hospitalization occurred in 0.7% and 1.1%, respectively. The incidence of intracranial hemorrhage was 0.4% for Plavix compared to 0.5% for aspirin. Other bleeding events that were reported more frequently in the Plavix group were epistaxis and hematoma.

Other Adverse Events

In CURE and CHARISMA, which compared Plavix plus aspirin to aspirin alone, there was no difference in the rate of adverse events (other than bleeding) between Plavix and placebo.

In CAPRIE, which compared Plavix to aspirin, pruritus was more frequently reported in those taking Plavix. No other difference in the rate of adverse events (other than bleeding) was reported.

6.2 Postmarketing Experience

The following adverse reactions have been identified during post-approval use of Plavix. Because these reactions are reported voluntarily from a population of an unknown size, it is not always possible to reliably estimate their frequency or establish a causal relationship to drug exposure.

- *Blood and lymphatic system disorders*: Agranulocytosis, aplastic anemia/pancytopenia, thrombotic thrombocytopenic purpura (TTP)

Table 2: Incidence of Bleeding Events in COMMIT (% patients)

Type of bleeding	Plavix (+ aspirin) (n=22961)	Placebo (+ aspirin) (n=22891)	p-value
Major* noncerebral or cerebral bleeding†	0.6	0.5	0.59
Major noncerebral	0.4	0.3	0.48
Fatal	0.2	0.2	0.90
Hemorrhagic stroke	0.2	0.2	0.91
Fatal	0.2	0.2	0.81
Other noncerebral bleeding (non-major)	3.6	3.1	0.005
Any noncerebral bleeding	3.9	3.4	0.004

* Major bleeds were cerebral bleeds or non-cerebral bleeds thought to have caused death or that required transfusion.
† The relative rate of major noncerebral or cerebral bleeding was independent of age. Event rates for Plavix + aspirin by age were: <60 years = 0.3%, ≥60 to <70 years = 0.7%, ≥70 years = 0.8%. Event rates for placebo + aspirin by age were: <60 years = 0.4%, ≥60 to <70 years = 0.6%, ≥70 years = 0.7%.

Table 3. Comparison of Clopidogrel Active Metabolite Exposure and Platelet Inhibition with and without Proton Pump Inhibitors, Omeprazole and Pantoprazole

Plavix plus	% Change from Plavix (300 mg/75 mg) alone					
	Cmax (ng/mL)		AUC		Platelet Inhibition* (%)	
	Day 1	Day 5	Day 1	Day 5†	Day 1	Day 5
Omeprazole‡ 80 mg	↓46%	↓42%	↓45%	↓40%	↓39%	↓21%
Pantoprazole 80 mg	↓24%	↓28%	↓20%	↓14%	↓15%	↓11%

* Inhibition of platelet aggregation with 5 mcM ADP
† AUC at Day 5 is AUC_{0-24}
‡ Similar results seen when Plavix and omeprazole were administered 12 hours apart.

- *Gastrointestinal disorders*: Gastrointestinal and retroperitoneal hemorrhage with fatal outcome, colitis (including ulcerative or lymphocytic colitis), pancreatitis, stomatitis
- *General disorders and administration site condition*: Fever, hemorrhage of operative wound
- *Hepato-biliary disorders*: Acute liver failure, hepatitis (non-infectious), abnormal liver function test
- *Immune system disorders*: Hypersensitivity reactions, anaphylactoid reactions, serum sickness
- *Musculoskeletal, connective tissue and bone disorders*: Musculoskeletal bleeding, myalgia, arthralgia, arthritis
- *Nervous system disorders*: Taste disorders, fatal intracranial bleeding
- *Eye disorders*: Eye (conjunctival, ocular, retinal) bleeding
- *Psychiatric disorders*: Confusion, hallucinations
- *Respiratory, thoracic and mediastinal disorders*: Bronchospasm, interstitial pneumonitis, respiratory tract bleeding
- *Renal and urinary disorders*: Glomerulopathy, increased creatinine levels
- *Skin and subcutaneous tissue disorders*: Maculopapular or erythematous rash, urticaria, bullous dermatitis, eczema, toxic epidermal necrolysis, Stevens-Johnson syndrome, angioedema, erythema multiforme, skin bleeding, lichen planus
- *Vascular disorders*: Vasculitis, hypotension

7 DRUG INTERACTIONS
7.1 CYP2C19 Inhibitors
Clopidogrel is metabolized to its active metabolite in part by CYP2C19. Concomitant use of drugs that inhibit the activity of this enzyme results in reduced plasma concentrations of the active metabolite of clopidogrel and a reduction in platelet inhibition [see Warnings and Precautions (5.1) and Dosage and Administration (2.4)].
Proton Pump Inhibitors (PPI)
A study was conducted with Plavix (300 mg loading dose followed by 75 mg/day) administered with a high dose (80 mg/day) of omeprazole. As shown in Table 3 below, with concomitant dosing of omeprazole, exposure (Cmax and AUC) to the clopidogrel active metabolite and platelet inhibition were substantially reduced. Similar reductions in exposure to the clopidogrel active metabolite and platelet inhibition were observed when Plavix and omeprazole were administered 12 hours apart (data not shown).
There are no adequate studies of a lower dose of omeprazole or a higher dose of Plavix in comparison with the approved dose of Plavix.
A study was conducted using Plavix (300 mg loading dose followed by 75 mg/day) and a high dose (80 mg/day) of pantoprazole, a PPI with less CYP2C19 inhibitory activity than omeprazole. The plasma concentrations of the clopidogrel active metabolite and the degree of platelet inhibition were less than observed with Plavix alone but were greater than observed when omeprazole 80 mg was co administered with 300 mg loading dose followed by 75 mg/day of Plavix (Table 3).
[See table 3 above]
7.2 Nonsteroidal Anti-Inflammatory Drugs (NSAIDs)
Coadministration of Plavix and NSAIDs increases the risk of gastrointestinal bleeding.
7.3 Warfarin (CYP2C9 Substrates)
Although the administration of clopidogrel 75 mg per day did not modify the pharmacokinetics of S-warfarin (a CYP2C9 substrate) or INR in patients receiving long-term warfarin therapy, coadministration of Plavix with warfarin increases the risk of bleeding because of independent effects on hemostasis.
However, at high concentrations *in vitro*, clopidogrel inhibits CYP2C9.

8 USE IN SPECIFIC POPULATIONS
8.1 Pregnancy
Pregnancy Category B
Reproduction studies performed in rats and rabbits at doses up to 500 and 300 mg/kg/day, respectively (65 and 78 times the recommended daily human dose, respectively, on a mg/m² basis), revealed no evidence of impaired fertility or fetotoxicity due to clopidogrel. There are, however, no adequate and well-controlled studies in pregnant women. Because animal reproduction studies are not always predictive of a human response, Plavix should be used during pregnancy only if clearly needed.
8.3 Nursing Mothers
Studies in rats have shown that clopidogrel and/or its metabolites are excreted in the milk. It is not known whether this drug is excreted in human milk. Because many drugs are excreted in human milk and because of the potential for serious adverse reactions in nursing infants from clopidogrel, a decision should be made whether to discontinue nursing or to discontinue the drug, taking into account the importance of the drug to the mother.
8.4 Pediatric Use
Safety and effectiveness in the pediatric population have not been established.
8.5 Geriatric Use
Of the total number of subjects in the CAPRIE and CURE controlled clinical studies, approximately 50% of patients treated with Plavix were 65 years of age and older, and 15% were 75 years and older. In COMMIT, approximately 58% of the patients treated with Plavix were 60 years and older, 26% of whom were 70 years and older.
The observed risk of thrombotic events with clopidogrel plus aspirin versus placebo plus aspirin by age category is provided in Figures 2 and 5 for the CURE and COMMIT trials, respectively [see Clinical Studies (14.1)]. The observed risk of bleeding events with clopidogrel plus aspirin versus placebo plus aspirin by age category is provided in Tables 1 and 2 for the CURE and COMMIT trials, respectively [see Adverse Reactions (6.1)]. No dosage adjustment is necessary in elderly patients.
8.6 Renal Impairment
Experience is limited in patients with severe and moderate renal impairment [see Clinical Pharmacology (12.2)].
8.7 Hepatic Impairment
No dosage adjustment is necessary in patients with hepatic impairment [see Clinical Pharmacology (12.2)].

10 OVERDOSAGE
Platelet inhibition by Plavix is irreversible and will last for the life of the platelet. Overdose following clopidogrel administration may result in bleeding complications. A single oral dose of clopidogrel at 1500 or 2000 mg/kg was lethal to mice and to rats and at 3000 mg/kg to baboons. Symptoms of acute toxicity were vomiting, prostration, difficult breathing, and gastrointestinal hemorrhage in animals.
Based on biological plausibility, platelet transfusion may restore clotting ability.

11 DESCRIPTION
Plavix (clopidogrel bisulfate) is a thienopyridine class inhibitor of $P2Y_{12}$ ADP platelet receptors. Chemically it is methyl (+)-(S)-α-(2-chlorophenyl)-6,7-dihydrothieno[3,2-c]pyridine-5(4H)-acetate sulfate (1:1). The empirical formula of clopidogrel bisulfate is $C_{16}H_{16}ClNO_2S \bullet H_2SO_4$ and its molecular weight is 419.9.
The structural formula is as follows:

Clopidogrel bisulfate is a white to off-white powder. It is practically insoluble in water at neutral pH but freely soluble at pH 1. It also dissolves freely in methanol, dissolves sparingly in methylene chloride, and is practically insoluble in ethyl ether. It has a specific optical rotation of about +56°.
Plavix for oral administration is provided as either pink, round, biconvex, debossed, film-coated tablets containing 97.875 mg of clopidogrel bisulfate which is the molar equivalent of 75 mg of clopidogrel base or pink, oblong, debossed film-coated tablets containing 391.5 mg of clopidogrel bisulfate which is the molar equivalent of 300 mg of clopidogrel base.
Each tablet contains hydrogenated castor oil, hydroxypropylcellulose, mannitol, microcrystalline cellulose and polyethylene glycol 6000 as inactive ingredients. The pink film coating contains ferric oxide, hypromellose 2910, lactose monohydrate, titanium dioxide and triacetin. The tablets are polished with Carnauba wax.

12 CLINICAL PHARMACOLOGY
12.1 Mechanism of Action
Clopidogrel is an inhibitor of platelet activation and aggregation through the irreversible binding of its active metabolite to the $P2Y_{12}$ class of ADP receptors on platelets.
12.2 Pharmacodynamics
Clopidogrel must be metabolized by CYP450 enzymes to produce the active metabolite that inhibits platelet aggregation. The active metabolite of clopidogrel selectively inhibits the binding of adenosine diphosphate (ADP) to its platelet $P2Y_{12}$ receptor and the subsequent ADP-mediated activation of the glycoprotein GPIIb/IIIa complex, thereby inhibiting platelet aggregation. This action is irreversible. Consequently, platelets exposed to clopidogrel's active metabolite are affected for the remainder of their lifespan (about 7 to 10 days). Platelet aggregation induced by agonists other than ADP is also inhibited by blocking the amplification of platelet activation by released ADP.
Dose-dependent inhibition of platelet aggregation can be seen 2 hours after single oral doses of Plavix. Repeated doses of 75 mg Plavix per day inhibit ADP-induced platelet aggregation on the first day, and inhibition reaches steady state between Day 3 and Day 7. At steady state, the average inhibition level observed with a dose of 75 mg Plavix per day was between 40% and 60%. Platelet aggregation and bleeding time gradually return to baseline values after treatment is discontinued, generally in about 5 days.
Geriatric Patients
Elderly (≥75 years) and young healthy subjects had similar effects on platelet aggregation.
Renally-Impaired Patients
After repeated doses of 75 mg Plavix per day, patients with severe renal impairment (creatinine clearance from 5 to 15 mL/min) and moderate renal impairment (creatinine clearance from 30 to 60 mL/min) showed low (25%) inhibition of ADP-induced platelet aggregation.
Hepatically-Impaired Patients
After repeated doses of 75 mg Plavix per day for 10 days in patients with severe hepatic impairment, inhibition of ADP-induced platelet aggregation was similar to that observed in healthy subjects.

Gender
In a small study comparing men and women, less inhibition of ADP-induced platelet aggregation was observed in women.

12.3 Pharmacokinetics
Clopidogrel is a prodrug and is metabolized to a pharmacologically active metabolite and inactive metabolites.

Absorption
After single and repeated oral doses of 75 mg per day, clopidogrel is rapidly absorbed. Absorption is at least 50%, based on urinary excretion of clopidogrel metabolites.

Effect of Food
Plavix can be administered with or without food. In a study in healthy male subjects when Plavix 75 mg per day was given with a standard breakfast, mean inhibition of ADP-induced platelet aggregation was reduced by less than 9%. The active metabolite AUC_{0-24} was unchanged in the presence of food, while there was a 57% decrease in active metabolite Cmax. Similar results were observed when a Plavix 300 mg loading dose was administered with a high-fat breakfast.

Metabolism
Clopidogrel is extensively metabolized by two main metabolic pathways: one mediated by esterases and leading to hydrolysis into an inactive carboxylic acid derivative (85% of circulating metabolites) and one mediated by multiple cytochrome P450 enzymes. Cytochromes first oxidize clopidogrel to a 2-oxo-clopidogrel intermediate metabolite. Subsequent metabolism of the 2-oxo-clopidogrel intermediate metabolite results in formation of the active metabolite, a thiol derivative of clopidogrel. This metabolic pathway is mediated by CYP2C19, CYP3A, CYP2B6 and CYP1A2. The active thiol metabolite binds rapidly and irreversibly to platelet receptors, thus inhibiting platelet aggregation for the lifespan of the platelet.

The Cmax of the active metabolite is twice as high following a single 300 mg clopidogrel loading dose as it is after four days of 75 mg maintenance dose. Cmax occurs approximately 30 to 60 minutes after dosing. In the 75 to 300 mg dose range, the pharmacokinetics of the active metabolite deviates from dose proportionality: increasing the dose by a factor of four results in 2.0- and 2.7-fold increases in Cmax and AUC, respectively.

Elimination
Following an oral dose of ^{14}C-labeled clopidogrel in humans, approximately 50% of total radioactivity was excreted in urine and approximately 46% in feces over the 5 days post-dosing. After a single, oral dose of 75 mg, clopidogrel has a half-life of approximately 6 hours. The half-life of the active metabolite is about 30 minutes.

12.5 Pharmacogenomics
CYP2C19 is involved in the formation of both the active metabolite and the 2-oxo-clopidogrel intermediate metabolite. Clopidogrel active metabolite pharmacokinetics and antiplatelet effects, as measured by *ex vivo* platelet aggregation assays, differ according to CYP2C19 genotype. Genetic variants of other CYP450 enzymes may also affect the formation of clopidogrel's active metabolite. The CYP2C19*1 allele corresponds to fully functional metabolism while the CYP2C19*2 and *3 alleles are nonfunctional. CYP2C19*2 and *3 account for the majority of reduced function alleles in white (85%) and Asian (99%) poor metabolizers. Other alleles associated with absent or reduced metabolism are less frequent, and include, but are not limited to, CYP2C19*4, *5, *6, *7, and *8. A patient with poor metabolizer status will possess two loss-of-function alleles as defined above. Published frequencies for poor CYP2C19 metabolizer genotypes are approximately 2% for whites, 4% for blacks and 14% for Chinese. Tests are available to determine a patient's CYP2C19 genotype.

A crossover study in 40 healthy subjects, 10 each in the four CYP2C19 metabolizer groups, evaluated pharmacokinetic and antiplatelet responses using 300 mg followed by 75 mg per day and 600 mg followed by 150 mg per day, each for a total of 5 days. Decreased active metabolite exposure and diminished inhibition of platelet aggregation were observed in the poor metabolizers as compared to the other groups. When poor metabolizers received the 600 mg/150 mg regimen, active metabolite exposure and antiplatelet response were greater than with the 300 mg/75 mg regimen (see Table 4). An appropriate dose regimen for this patient population has not been established in clinical outcome trials.
[See table above]

Some published studies suggest that intermediate metabolizers have decreased active metabolite exposure and diminished antiplatelet effects.

The relationship between CYP2C19 genotype and Plavix treatment outcome was evaluated in retrospective analyses of Plavix-treated subjects in CHARISMA (n=2428) and TRITON-TIMI 38 (n=1477), and in several published cohort studies. In TRITON-TIMI 38 and the majority of the cohort studies, the combined group of patients with either intermediate or poor metabolizer status had a higher rate of cardiovascular events (death, myocardial infarction, and stroke)

Table 4: Active Metabolite Pharmacokinetics and Antiplatelet Responses by CYP2C19 Metabolizer Status

	Dose	Ultrarapid (n=10)	Extensive (n=10)	Intermediate (n=10)	Poor (n=10)
Cmax (ng/mL)	300 mg (24 h)	24 (10)	32 (21)	23 (11)	11 (4)
	600 mg (24 h)	36 (13)	44 (27)	39 (23)	17 (6)
	75 mg (Day 5)	12 (6)	13 (7)	12 (5)	4 (1)
	150 mg (Day 5)	16 (9)	19 (5)	18 (7)	7 (2)
IPA (%)*	300 mg (24 h)	40 (21)	39 (28)	37 (21)	24 (26)
	600 mg (24 h)	51 (28)	49 (23)	56 (22)	32 (25)
	75 mg (Day 5)	56 (13)	58 (19)	60 (18)	37 (23)
	150 mg (Day 5)	68 (18)	73 (9)	74 (14)	61 (14)
VASP-PRI (%) †	300 mg (24 h)	73 (12)	68 (16)	78 (12)	91 (12)
	600 mg (24 h)	51 (20)	48 (20)	56 (26)	85 (14)
	75 mg (Day 5)	40 (9)	39 (14)	50 (16)	83 (13)
	150 mg (Day 5)	20 (10)	24 (10)	29 (11)	61 (18)

Values are mean (SD)
* Inhibition of platelet aggregation with 5mcM ADP; larger value indicates greater platelet inhibition
† Vasodilator-stimulated phosphoprotein – platelet reactivity index; smaller value indicates greater platelet inhibition

---

Table 5: Outcome Events in the CURE Primary Analysis

Outcome	Plavix (+ aspirin)* (n=6259)	Placebo (+ aspirin)* (n=6303)	Relative Risk Reduction (%) (95% CI)
Primary outcome (Cardiovascular death, MI, stroke)	582 (9.3%)	719 (11.4%)	20% (10.3, 27.9) p < 0.001
All Individual Outcome Events:†			
CV death	318 (5.1%)	345 (5.5%)	7% (-7.7, 20.6)
MI	324 (5.2%)	419 (6.6%)	23% (11.0, 33.4)
Stroke	75 (1.2%)	87 (1.4%)	14% (-17.7, 36.6)

* Other standard therapies were used as appropriate.
† The individual components do not represent a breakdown of the primary and co-primary outcomes, but rather the total number of subjects experiencing an event during the course of the study.

---

or stent thrombosis compared to extensive metabolizers. In CHARISMA and one cohort study, the increased event rate was observed only in poor metabolizers.

13 NONCLINICAL TOXICOLOGY
13.1 Carcinogenesis, Mutagenesis, Impairment of Fertility
There was no evidence of tumorigenicity when clopidogrel was administered for 78 weeks to mice and 104 weeks to rats at dosages up to 77 mg/kg per day, which afforded plasma exposures >25 times that in humans at the recommended daily dose of 75 mg.

Clopidogrel was not genotoxic in four *in vitro* tests (Ames test, DNA-repair test in rat hepatocytes, gene mutation assay in Chinese hamster fibroblasts, and metaphase chromosome analysis of human lymphocytes) and in one *in vivo* test (micronucleus test by oral route in mice).

Clopidogrel was found to have no effect on fertility of male and female rats at oral doses up to 400 mg/kg per day (52 times the recommended human dose on a mg/m^2 basis).

14 CLINICAL STUDIES
The clinical evidence of the efficacy of Plavix is derived from three double-blind trials involving 77,599 patients. The CAPRIE study (Clopidogrel vs. Aspirin in Patients at Risk of Ischemic Events) was a comparison of Plavix to aspirin. The CURE (Clopidogrel in Unstable Angina to Prevent Recurrent Ischemic Events) and the COMMIT/CCS-2 (Clopidogrel and Metoprolol in Myocardial Infarction Trial/ Second Chinese Cardiac Study) studies were comparisons of Plavix to placebo, given in combination with aspirin and other standard therapy. The CHARISMA (Clopidogrel for High Atherothrombotic Risk Ischemic Stabilization, Management, and Avoidance) study (n=15,603) also compared Plavix to placebo, given in combination with aspirin and other standard therapy.

14.1 Acute Coronary Syndrome
CURE
The CURE study included 12,562 patients with ACS without ST-elevation (UA or NSTEMI) and presenting within 24 hours of onset of the most recent episode of chest pain or symptoms consistent with ischemia. Patients were required to have either ECG changes compatible with new ischemia (without ST-elevation) or elevated cardiac enzymes or troponin I or T to at least twice the upper limit of normal. The patient population was largely Caucasian (82%) and included 38% women, and 52% patients ≥65 years of age. Patients were randomized to receive Plavix (300-mg loading dose followed by 75 mg once daily) or placebo, and were

treated for up to one year. Patients also received aspirin (75–325 mg once daily) and other standard therapies such as heparin. The use of GPIIb/IIIa inhibitors was not permitted for three days prior to randomization.

The number of patients experiencing the primary outcome (CV death, MI, or stroke) was 582 (9.3%) in the Plavix-treated group and 719 (11.4%) in the placebo-treated group, a 20% relative risk reduction (95% CI of 10%–28%; p < 0.001) for the Plavix-treated group (see Table 5).
[See table 5 above]

Most of the benefit of Plavix occurred in the first two months, but the difference from placebo was maintained throughout the course of the trial (up to 12 months) (see Figure 1).

Figure 1: Cardiovascular Death, Myocardial Infarction, and Stroke in the CURE Study

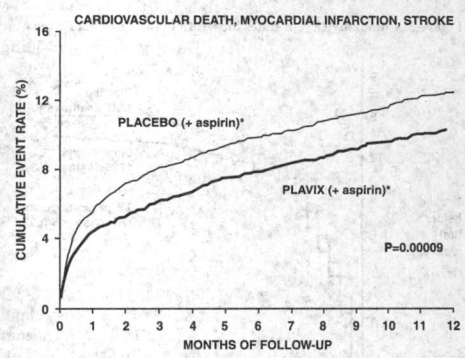

*Other standard therapies were used as appropriate

In CURE, the use of Plavix was associated with a lower incidence of CV death, MI or stroke in patient populations with different characteristics, as shown in Figure 2. The benefits associated with Plavix were independent of the use of other acute and long-term cardiovascular therapies, including heparin/LMWH, intravenous glycoprotein IIb/IIIa (GPIIb/IIIa) inhibitors, lipid-lowering drugs, beta-blockers, and ACE-inhibitors. The efficacy of Plavix was observed independently of the dose of aspirin (75–325 mg once daily).

The use of oral anticoagulants, non-study anti-platelet drugs, and chronic NSAIDs was not allowed in CURE.

Figure 2: Hazard Ratio for Patient Baseline Characteristics and On-Study Concomitant Medications/Interventions for the CURE Study

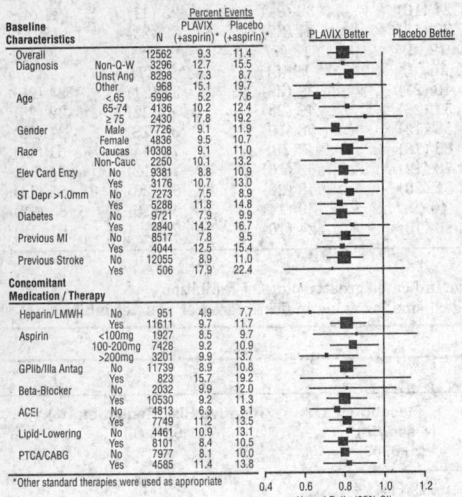

The use of Plavix in CURE was associated with a decrease in the use of thrombolytic therapy (71 patients [1.1%] in the Plavix group, 126 patients [2.0%] in the placebo group; relative risk reduction of 43%), and GPIIb/IIIa inhibitors (369 patients [5.9%] in the Plavix group, 454 patients [7.2%] in the placebo group, relative risk reduction of 18%). The use of Plavix in CURE did not affect the number of patients treated with CABG or PCI (with or without stenting), (2253 patients [36.0%] in the Plavix group, 2324 patients [36.9%] in the placebo group; relative risk reduction of 4.0%).

COMMIT
In patients with STEMI, the safety and efficacy of Plavix were evaluated in the randomized, placebo-controlled, double-blind study, COMMIT. COMMIT included 45,852 patients presenting within 24 hours of the onset of symptoms of myocardial infarction with supporting ECG abnormalities (*i.e.*, ST-elevation, ST-depression or left bundle-branch block). Patients were randomized to receive Plavix (75 mg once daily) or placebo, in combination with aspirin (162 mg per day), for 28 days or until hospital discharge, whichever came first.
The primary endpoints were death from any cause and the first occurrence of re-infarction, stroke or death.
The patient population included 28% women, 58% age ≥ 60 years (26% age ≥ 70 years), 55% patients who received thrombolytics, 68% who received ACE-inhibitors, and only 3% who underwent PCI.
As shown in Table 6 and Figures 3 and 4 below, Plavix significantly reduced the relative risk of death from any cause by 7% (p=0.029), and the relative risk of the combination of re-infarction, stroke or death by 9% (p=0.002).
[See table 6 above]

Figure 3: Cumulative Event Rates for Death in the COMMIT Study*

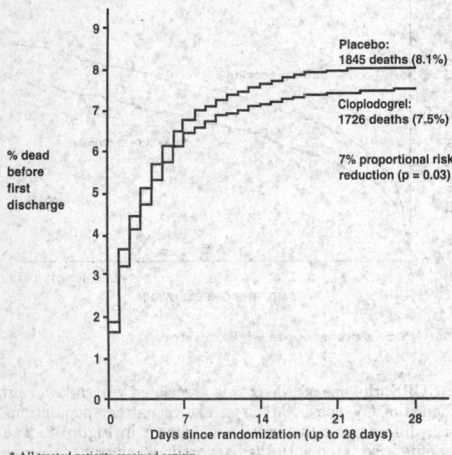

* All treated patients received aspirin.

[See figure 4 at top of next column]
The effect of Plavix did not differ significantly in various pre-specified subgroups as shown in Figure 5. The effect was also similar in non-prespecified subgroups including

Table 6: Outcome Events in the COMMIT Analysis

Event	Plavix (+ aspirin) (N=22961)	Placebo (+ aspirin) (N=22891)	Odds ratio (95% CI)	p-value
Composite endpoint: Death, MI, or Stroke*	2121 (9.2%)	2310 (10.1%)	0.91 (0.86, 0.97)	0.002
Death	1726 (7.5%)	1845 (8.1%)	0.93 (0.87, 0.99)	0.029
Non-fatal MI†	270 (1.2%)	330 (1.4%)	0.81 (0.69, 0.95)	0.011
Non-fatal Stroke†	127 (0.6%)	142 (0.6%)	0.89 (0.70, 1.13)	0.33

* The difference between the composite endpoint and the sum of death+non-fatal MI+non-fatal stroke indicates that 9 patients (2 clopidogrel and 7 placebo) suffered both a non-fatal stroke and a non-fatal MI.
† Non-fatal MI and non-fatal stroke exclude patients who died (of any cause).

Figure 4: Cumulative Event Rates for the Combined Endpoint Re-Infarction, Stroke or Death in the COMMIT Study*

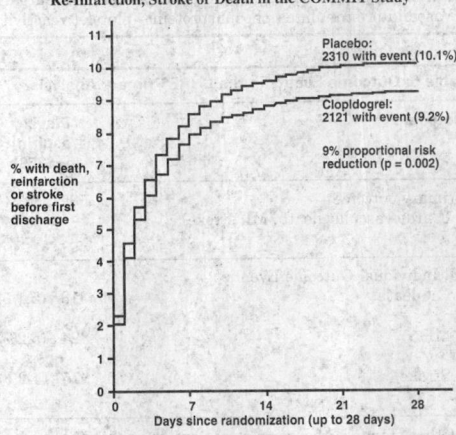

* All treated patients received aspirin.

those based on infarct location, Killip class or prior MI history (see Figure 6). Such subgroup analyses should be interpreted cautiously.

Figure 5: Effects of Adding Plavix to Aspirin on the Combined Primary Endpoint across Baseline and Concomitant Medication Subgroups for the COMMIT Study

Baseline Categorisation	Events (%) Clopidogrel (22 961)	Placebo (22 891)	Odds ratio & C.I. Clopidogrel better : Placebo better	Heterogeneity or trend test χ^2 (p-value)
Sex:				
Male	1274 (7.7%)	1416 (8.6%)		1.0 (0.3)
Female	847 (13.3%)	894 (14.0%)		
Age at entry (years):				
< 60	485 (5.0%)	512 (5.4%)		0.0 (0.9)
60-69	745 (10.1%)	835 (11.2%)		
70+	891 (14.9%)	963 (16.2%)		
Hours since onset:				
< 6	709 (9.2%)	830 (10.8%)		5.7 (0.02)
6 to <13	738 (9.8%)	808 (10.8%)		
13 to 24	674 (8.8%)	672 (8.8%)		
SBP (mmHg):				
< 120	797 (10.4%)	892 (11.5%)		1.0 (0.3)
120-139	693 (8.5%)	770 (9.5%)		
140-159	388 (8.5%)	399 (8.9%)		
160+	243 (9.2%)	249 (9.6%)		
Heart rate (bpm):				
< 70	268 (5.3%)	315 (6.2%)		0.0 (1.0)
70-89	698 (8.1%)	952 (8.5%)		
90-109	632 (12.3%)	683 (13.5%)		
110+	323 (19.9%)	350 (22.2%)		
Fibrinolytic agent given:				
Yes	1003 (8.8%)	1122 (9.9%)		0.7 (0.4)
No	1118 (9.7%)	1188 (10.3%)		
Prognostic index (3 equal groups):*				
Good	228 (3.7%)	282 (3.7%)		3.1 (0.08)
Average	574 (7.5%)	636 (8.3%)		
Poor	1319 (17.3%)	1392 (18.2%)		
Metoprolol allocation:				
Yes	1063 (9.3%)	1100 (9.7%)		2.4 (0.1)
No	1058 (9.2%)	1200 (10.5%)		
■ Total	2121 (9.2%)	2310 (10.1%)		Proportional reduction 9% SE 3 (p = 0.002)

Global Heterogeneity Test: $\chi^2_{15} = 16.4$; p = 0.4
◆■ 99% or ─ 95% confidence interval

* Three similar-sized prognostic index groups were based on absolute risk of primary composite outcome for each patient calculated from baseline prognostic variables (excluding allocated treatments) with a Cox regression model.

Figure 6: Effects of Adding Plavix to Aspirin in the Non-Prespecified Subgroups in the COMMIT Study

Categorisation	Events (%) Clopidogrel (22 961)	Placebo (22 891)	Odds ratio & C.I. Clopidogrel better : Placebo better	Heterogeneity or trend test χ^2 (p-value)
Killip class:				
I	1273 (7.3%)	1415 (8.2%)		0.6 (0.5)
II/III	848 (15.0%)	896 (16.0%)		
Previous MI				
Yes	177 (9.0%)	204 (11.1%)		1.6 (0.2)
No	1944 (9.3%)	2105 (100%)		
Infarct location:				
Anterior	1083 (9.6%)	1247 (10.8%)		1.9 (0.2)
Other	1038 (8.9%)	1063 (9.3%)		
■ Total	2121 (9.2%)	2310 (10.1%)		Proportional reduction 9% SE 3 (p=0.002)

Global Heterogeneity Test: $\chi^2_3 = 4.1$; p=0.3
■─■ 99% or ─ 95% confidence interval

14.2 Recent Myocardial Infarction, Recent Stroke, or Established Peripheral Arterial Disease
CAPRIE
The CAPRIE trial was a 19,185-patient, 304-center, international, randomized, double-blind, parallel-group study comparing Plavix (75 mg daily) to aspirin (325 mg daily). The patients randomized had: 1) recent histories of myocardial infarction (within 35 days); 2) recent histories of ischemic stroke (within 6 months) with at least a week of residual neurological signs; or 3) established peripheral arterial disease. Patients received randomized treatment for an average of 1.6 years (maximum of 3 years).
The trial's primary outcome was the time to first occurrence of new ischemic stroke (fatal or not), new myocardial infarction (fatal or not), or other vascular death. Deaths not easily attributable to nonvascular causes were all classified as vascular.

Table 7: Outcome Events in the CAPRIE Primary Analysis

Patients	Plavix n=9599	aspirin n=9586
Ischemic stroke (fatal or not)	438 (4.6%)	461 (4.8%)
MI (fatal or not)	275 (2.9%)	333 (3.5%)
Other vascular death	226 (2.4%)	226 (2.4%)
Total	939 (9.8%)	1020 (10.6%)

As shown in the table, Plavix was associated with a lower incidence of outcome events, primarily MI. The overall relative risk reduction (9.8% vs. 10.6%) was 8.7%, p=0.045. Similar results were obtained when all-cause mortality and all-cause strokes were counted instead of vascular mortality and ischemic strokes (risk reduction 6.9%). In patients who survived an on-study stroke or myocardial infarction, the incidence of subsequent events was lower in the Plavix group.
The curves showing the overall event rate are shown in Figure 7. The event curves separated early and continued to diverge over the 3-year follow-up period.

Figure 7: Fatal or Non-Fatal Vascular Events in the CAPRIE Study

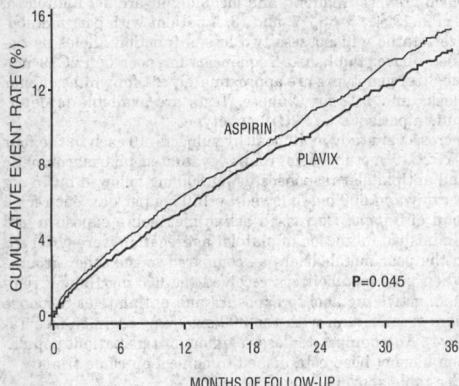

FATAL OR NON-FATAL VASCULAR EVENTS

The statistical significance favoring Plavix over aspirin was marginal (p=0.045). However, because aspirin is itself effective in reducing cardiovascular events in patients with recent myocardial infarction or stroke, the effect of Plavix is substantial.
The CAPRIE trial included a population that was randomized on the basis of 3 entry criteria. The efficacy of Plavix relative to aspirin was heterogeneous across these randomized subgroups (p=0.043). It is not clear whether this difference is real or a chance occurrence. Although the CAPRIE trial was not designed to evaluate the relative benefit of

Plavix over aspirin in the individual patient subgroups, the benefit appeared to be strongest in patients who were enrolled because of peripheral vascular disease (especially those who also had a history of myocardial infarction) and weaker in stroke patients. In patients who were enrolled in the trial on the sole basis of a recent myocardial infarction, Plavix was not numerically superior to aspirin.

14.3 Lack of Established Benefit of Plavix plus Aspirin in Patients with Multiple Risk Factors or Established Vascular Disease

CHARISMA

The CHARISMA trial was a 15,603 subject, randomized, double-blind, parallel group study comparing Plavix (75 mg daily) to placebo for prevention of ischemic events in patients with vascular disease or multiple risk factors for atherosclerosis. All subjects were treated with aspirin 75–162 mg daily. The mean duration of treatment was 23 months. The study failed to demonstrate a reduction in the occurrence of the primary endpoint, a composite of CV death, MI, or stroke. A total of 534 (6.9%) patients in the Plavix group versus 573 (7.4%) patients in the placebo group experienced a primary outcome event (p=0.22). Bleeding of all severities was more common in the subjects randomized to Plavix.

16 HOW SUPPLIED/STORAGE AND HANDLING

Plavix (clopidogrel bisulfate) 75 mg tablets are available as pink, round, biconvex, film-coated tablets debossed with "75" on one side and "1171" on the other. Tablets are provided as follows:

- NDC 63653-1171-6 Bottles of 30
- NDC 63653-1171-1 Bottles of 90
- NDC 63653-1171-5 Bottles of 500
- NDC 63653-1171-3 Blisters of 100

Plavix (clopidogrel bisulfate) 300 mg tablets are available as pink, oblong, film-coated tablets debossed with "300" on one side and "1332" on the other. Tablets are provided as follows:

- NDC 63653-1332-2 Unit-dose packages of 30
- NDC 63653-1332-3 Unit-dose packages of 100

Store at 25° C (77° F); excursions permitted to 15°–30° C (59°–86° F) [see USP Controlled Room Temperature].

17 PATIENT COUNSELING INFORMATION

17.1 Benefits and Risks

- Summarize the effectiveness features and potential side effects of Plavix.
- Tell patients to take Plavix exactly as prescribed.
- Remind patients not to discontinue Plavix without first discussing it with the physician who prescribed Plavix.

17.2 Bleeding

Inform patients that they:

- will bruise and bleed more easily.
- will take longer than usual to stop bleeding.
- should report any unanticipated, prolonged, or excessive bleeding, or blood in their stool or urine.

17.3 Other Signs and Symptoms Requiring Medical Attention

- Inform patients that TTP is a rare but serious condition that has been reported with Plavix and other drugs in this class of drugs.
- Instruct patients to get prompt medical attention if they experience any of the following symptoms that cannot otherwise be explained: fever, weakness, extreme skin paleness, purple skin patches, yellowing of the skin or eyes, or neurological changes.

17.4 Invasive Procedures

Instruct patients to:

- inform physicians and dentists that they are taking Plavix before any invasive procedure is scheduled.
- tell the doctor performing the invasive procedure to talk to the prescribing health care professional before stopping Plavix.

17.5 Concomitant Medications

Ask patients to list all prescription medications, over-the-counter medications, or dietary supplements they are taking or plan to take, including prescription or over-the-counter omeprazole, so the physician knows about other treatments that may affect how Plavix works (*e.g.*, warfarin and NSAIDs) *[see Warnings and Precautions (5)]*.

Distributed by:
Bristol-Myers Squibb/Sanofi Pharmaceuticals Partnership
Bridgewater, NJ 08807
Plavix® is a registered trademark.

Shown in Product Identification Guide, page 319

RILUTEK® ℞
[rĭl-ū-tĕk]
(riluzole)
tablet, film coated

DESCRIPTION

RILUTEK® (riluzole) is a member of the benzothiazole class. Chemically, riluzole is 2-amino-6-(trifluoromethoxy) benzothiazole. Its molecular formula is $C_8H_5F_3N_2OS$ and its molecular weight is 234.2. Its structural formula is as follows:

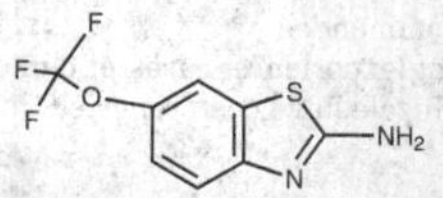

Riluzole is a white to slightly yellow powder that is very soluble in dimethylformamide, dimethylsulfoxide and methanol, freely soluble in dichloromethane, sparingly soluble in 0.1 N HCl and very slightly soluble in water and in 0.1 N NaOH. RILUTEK is available as a capsule-shaped, white, film-coated tablet for oral administration containing 50 mg of riluzole. Each tablet is engraved with "RPR 202" on one side.

Inactive Ingredients

Core: anhydrous dibasic calcium phosphate, USP; microcrystalline cellulose, NF; anhydrous colloidal silica, NF; magnesium stearate, NF; croscarmellose sodium, NF.
Film coating: hypromellose, USP; polyethylene glycol 6000; titanium dioxide, USP.

CLINICAL PHARMACOLOGY

Mechanism of Action

The etiology and pathogenesis of amyotrophic lateral sclerosis (ALS) are not known, although a number of hypotheses have been advanced. One hypothesis is that motor neurons, made vulnerable through either genetic predisposition or environmental factors, are injured by glutamate. In some cases of familial ALS the enzyme superoxide dismutase has been found to be defective.

The mode of action of RILUTEK is unknown. Its pharmacological properties include the following, some of which may be related to its effect: 1) an inhibitory effect on glutamate release, 2) inactivation of voltage-dependent sodium channels, and 3) ability to interfere with intracellular events that follow transmitter binding at excitatory amino acid receptors.

Riluzole has also been shown, in a single study, to delay median time to death in a transgenic mouse model of ALS. These mice express human superoxide dismutase bearing one of the mutations found in one of the familial forms of human ALS.

It is also neuroprotective in various *in vivo* experimental models of neuronal injury involving excitotoxic mechanisms. In *in vitro* tests, riluzole protected cultured rat motor neurons from the excitotoxic effects of glutamic acid and prevented the death of cortical neurons induced by anoxia. Due to its blockade of glutamatergic neurotransmission, riluzole also exhibits myorelaxant and sedative properties in animal models at doses of 30 mg/kg (about 20 times the recommended human daily dose) and anticonvulsant properties at a dose of 2.5 mg/kg (about 2 times the recommended human daily dose).

Pharmacokinetics

Riluzole is well-absorbed (approximately 90%), with average absolute oral bioavailability of about 60% (CV=30%). Pharmacokinetics are linear over a dose range of 25 to 100 mg given every 12 hours. A high fat meal decreases absorption, reducing AUC by about 20% and peak blood levels by about 45%. The mean elimination half-life of riluzole is 12 hours (CV=35%) after repeated doses. With multiple-dose administration, riluzole accumulates in plasma by about twofold and steady-state is reached in less than 5 days. Riluzole is 96% bound to plasma proteins, mainly to albumin and lipoproteins over the clinical concentration range.

The 50 mg market tablet was equivalent, with respect to AUC, to the tablet used in the dose ranging clinical trials, while the C_{max} was approximately 30% higher. Both tablets have been used in clinical trials. However, if doses greater than those recommended are given, it is likely that higher plasma levels will be achieved, the safety of which has not been established (see DOSAGE AND ADMINISTRATION).

Metabolism and Elimination

Riluzole is extensively metabolized to six major and a number of minor metabolites, not all of which have been identified. Some metabolites appear pharmacologically active in *in vitro* assays. The metabolism of riluzole is mostly hepatic and consists of cytochrome P450-dependent hydroxylation and glucuronidation.

There is marked interindividual variability in the clearance of riluzole, probably attributable to variability of CYP 1A2 activity, the principal isozyme involved in N-hydroxylation. *In vitro* studies using liver microsomes show that hydroxylation of the primary amine group producing N-hydroxyriluzole is the main metabolic pathway in human, monkey, dog and rabbit. In humans, cytochrome P450 1A2 is the principal isozyme involved in N-hydroxylation. *In vitro* studies predict that CYP 2D6, CYP 2C19, CYP 3A4 and CYP 2E1 are unlikely to contribute significantly to riluzole metabolism in humans. Whereas direct glucuroconjugation of riluzole (involving the glucurotransferase isoform UGT-HP4) is very slow in human liver microsomes, N-hydroxyriluzole is readily conjugated at the hydroxylamine group resulting in the formation of O- (>90%) and N-glucuronides.

Following a single 150 mg dose of ^{14}C-riluzole to 6 healthy males, 90% and 5% of the radioactivity was recovered in the urine and feces respectively over a period of 7 days. Glucuronides accounted for more than 85% of the metabolites in urine. Only 2% of a riluzole dose was recovered in the urine as unchanged drug.

Special Populations

Hepatic Impairment

The area-under-the-curve (AUC) of riluzole, after a single 50 mg oral dose, increases by about 1.7-fold in patients with mild chronic liver insufficiency (n=6; Child-Pugh's score A) and by about 3-fold in patients with moderate chronic liver insufficiency (n=6; Child-Pugh's score B) compared to healthy volunteers (n=12) (see WARNINGS and PRECAUTIONS). The pharmacokinetics of riluzole have not been studied in patients with severe hepatic impairment.

Renal Impairment

There is no significant difference in pharmacokinetic parameters between patients with moderate (n=5; creatinine clearance 30–50 $ml.min^{-1}$) and severe (n=7; creatinine clearance <30 $ml.min^{-1}$) renal insufficiency and healthy volunteers (n=12) after a single oral dose of 50 mg riluzole. The pharmacokinetics of riluzole have not been studied in patients undergoing hemodialysis.

Age

The pharmacokinetic parameters of riluzole after multiple dose administration (4.5 days of treatment at 50 mg riluzole b.i.d.) are not affected in the elderly (≥ 70 years).

Gender

No gender effect on riluzole pharmacokinetics has been found in young or elderly healthy subjects. However, in one placebo-controlled clinical trial with population pharmacokinetics, riluzole mean clearance was found to be 30% lower in female patients (corresponding to an approximate increase in AUC of 45%) as compared to male patients. No favorable or adverse effects of riluzole in relation to gender were seen in controlled trials, however.

Smoking

Patients who smoke cigarettes eliminate riluzole 20% faster than non-smoking patients, based on a population pharmacokinetic analysis on data from 128 ALS patients, of whom 19 were smokers. However, there is no need for dosage adjustment in these patients.

Race

A clinical study conducted to evaluate the pharmacokinetics of riluzole and its metabolite following repeated oral administration twice daily in healthy Japanese and Caucasian adult males showed that there were no significant racial differences in pharmacokinetic parameters between the Japanese and Caucasian subjects.

Clinical Trials

The efficacy of RILUTEK as a treatment of ALS was established in two adequate and well-controlled trials in which the time to tracheostomy or death was longer for patients randomized to RILUTEK than for those randomized to placebo.

These studies admitted patients with either familial or sporadic ALS, a disease duration of less than 5 years, and a baseline forced vital capacity greater than or equal to 60%.

In one study, performed in France and Belgium, 155 ALS patients were followed for at least 13 months (maximum duration 18 months) after being randomized to either 100 mg/day (given 50 mg BID) of RILUTEK or placebo.

Figure 1, which follows, displays the survival curves for time to death or tracheostomy. The vertical axis represents the proportion of individuals alive without tracheostomy at various times following treatment initiation (horizontal axis). Although these survival curves were not statistically significantly different when evaluated by the analysis specified in the study protocol (Logrank test p=0.12), the difference was found to be significant by another appropriate analysis (Wilcoxon test p=0.05). As seen, the study showed an early increase in survival in patients given riluzole. Among the patients in whom treatment failed during the study (tracheostomy or death) there was a difference between the treatment groups in median survival of approximately 90 days. There was no statistically significant difference in mortality at the end of the study.

[See figure 1 at top of next page]

In the second study, performed in both Europe and North America, 959 ALS patients were followed for at least 1 year (North American centers) and up to 18 months (European centers) after being randomized to either 50, 100, 200 mg/day of RILUTEK or placebo.

Figure 2, which follows, displays the survival curves for time to death or tracheostomy for patients randomized to either 100 mg/day of RILUTEK or placebo. Although these survival curves were not statistically significantly different when evaluated by the analysis specified in the study pro-

Figure 1: Kaplan-Meier Survival Curves

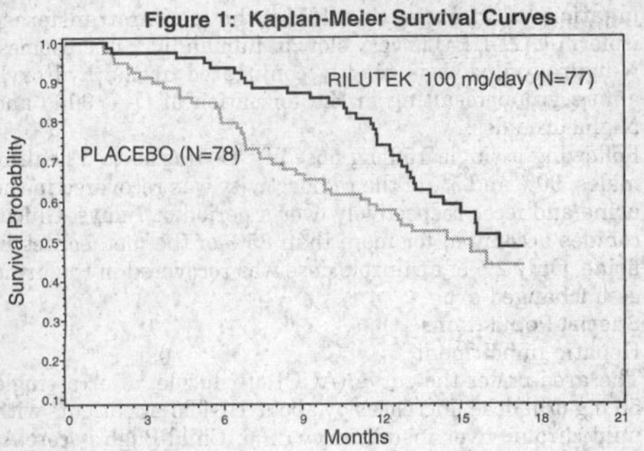

tocol (Logrank test p = 0.076), the difference was found to be significant by another appropriate analysis (Wilcoxon test p = 0.05). Not displayed in Figure 2 are the results of 50 mg/day of RILUTEK which could not be statistically distinguished from placebo and the results of 200 mg/day which are essentially identical to 100 mg/day. As seen, the study showed an early increase in survival in patients given riluzole. Among the patients in whom treatment failed during the study (tracheostomy or death) there was a difference between the treatment groups in median survival of approximately 60 days. There was no statistically significant difference in mortality at the end of the study.

Figure 2: Kaplan-Meier Survival Curves

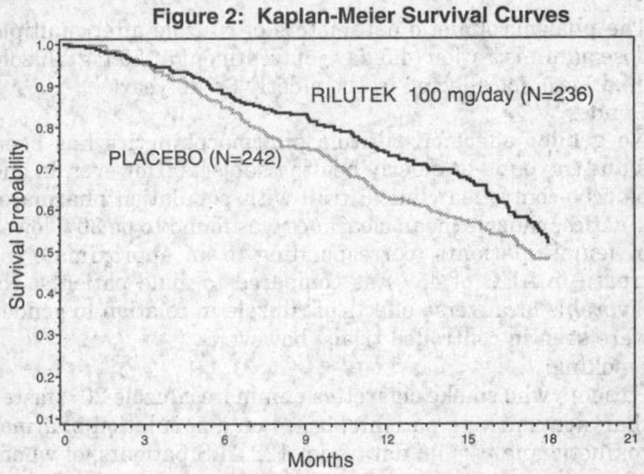

Although riluzole improved early survival in both studies, measures of muscle strength and neurological function did not show a benefit.

INDICATIONS AND USAGE

RILUTEK is indicated for the treatment of patients with amyotrophic lateral sclerosis (ALS). Riluzole extends survival and/or time to tracheostomy.

CONTRAINDICATIONS

RILUTEK is contraindicated in patients who have a history of severe hypersensitivity reactions to riluzole or any of the tablet components.

WARNINGS

Liver Injury / Monitoring Liver Chemistries

RILUTEK should be prescribed with care in patients with current evidence or history of abnormal liver function indicated by significant abnormalities in serum transaminase (ALT/SGPT; AST/SGOT), bilirubin, and/or gamma-glutamate transferase (GGT) levels (see PRECAUTIONS and DOSAGE AND ADMINISTRATION sections). Baseline elevations of several LFTs (especially elevated bilirubin) should preclude the use of RILUTEK.

RILUTEK, even in patients without a prior history of liver disease, causes serum aminotransferase elevations. Treatment should be discontinued if ALT levels are ≥ 5 × ULN or if clinical jaundice develops.

Experience in almost 800 ALS patients indicates that about 50% of riluzole-treated patients will experience at least one ALT/SGPT level above the upper limit of normal, about 8% will have elevations > 3 × ULN, and about 2% of patients will have elevations > 5 × ULN. A single non-ALS patient with epilepsy treated with concomitant carbamazepine and phenobarbital experienced marked, rapid elevations of liver enzymes with jaundice (ALT 26 × ULN, AST 17 × ULN, and bilirubin 11 × ULN) four months after starting RILUTEK; these returned to normal 7 weeks after treatment discontinuation.

Maximum increases in serum ALT usually occurred within 3 months after the start of riluzole therapy and were usually transient when < 5 times ULN. In trials, if ALT levels were < 5 times ULN, treatment continued and ALT levels usually returned to below 2 times ULN within 2 to 6 months. Treatment in studies was discontinued, however, if ALT levels exceeded 5 × ULN, so that there is no experience with continued treatment of ALS patients once ALT values exceed 5 times ULN. There were rare instances of jaundice. There is limited experience with rechallenge of patients who have had RILUTEK discontinued for ALT > 5 × ULN, but there is the possibility of increased ALT values reoccurring (see PRECAUTIONS: Laboratory Tests). Therefore, rechallenge is not recommended.

In postmarketing experience, cases of clinical hepatitis associated with riluzole have been reported, including with fatal outcome.

Neutropenia

Among approximately 4000 patients given riluzole for ALS, there were three cases of marked neutropenia (absolute neutrophil count less than 500/mm^3), all seen within the first 2 months of riluzole treatment. In one case, neutrophil counts rose on continued treatment. In a second case, counts rose after therapy was stopped. A third case was more complex, with marked anemia as well as neutropenia and the etiology of both is uncertain. Patients should be warned to report any febrile illness to their physicians. The report of a febrile illness should prompt treating physicians to check white blood cell counts.

Interstitial Lung Disease

Cases of interstitial lung disease (see ADVERSE REACTIONS) have been reported in patients treated with riluzole, some of them severe; upon further investigation, many of these cases were hypersensitivity pneumonitis. If respiratory symptoms develop such as dry cough and/or dyspnea, chest radiography should be performed, and in case of findings suggestive of interstitial lung disease or hypersensitivity pneumonitis (e.g., bilateral diffuse lung opacities), riluzole should be discontinued immediately. In the majority of the reported cases, symptoms resolved after drug discontinuation and symptomatic treatment.

PRECAUTIONS

Use in Patients with Concomitant Disease

RILUTEK should be used with caution in patients with concomitant liver insufficiency (see WARNINGS, CLINICAL PHARMACOLOGY). In particular, in cases of RILUTEK-induced hepatic injury manifested by elevated liver enzymes, the effect of the hepatic injury on RILUTEK metabolism is unknown.

Special Populations

Riluzole should be used with caution in elderly patients whose hepatic function may be compromised due to age. Also, female patients may possess a lower metabolic capacity to eliminate riluzole compared to males (see CLINICAL PHARMACOLOGY: Special Populations).

Information for the Patient

Patients should be advised to report any febrile illness to their physicians (see WARNINGS: Neutropenia).

Patients should be advised to report any cough or difficulties in breathing to their physicians (see WARNINGS: Interstitial Lung Disease).

Patients and caregivers should be advised that RILUTEK should be taken on a regular basis and at the same time of the day (*e.g.*, in the morning and evening) each day. If a dose is missed, take the next tablet as originally planned (see DOSAGE AND ADMINISTRATION).

Patients should be warned about the potential for dizziness, vertigo, or somnolence and advised not to drive or operate machinery until they have gained sufficient experience on RILUTEK to gauge whether or not it affects their mental and/or motor performance adversely.

Whether alcohol increases the risk of serious hepatotoxicity with RILUTEK is unknown; therefore, patients being treated with RILUTEK should be discouraged from drinking excessive amounts of alcohol.

Patients should also be made aware that RILUTEK should be stored at temperatures between 20°–25° C (68°–77°F) and protected from bright light.

RILUTEK must be kept out of the reach of children.

Laboratory Tests

Serum aminotransferases including ALT levels should be measured before and during riluzole therapy. Serum ALT levels should be evaluated every month during the first 3 months of treatment, every 3 months during the remainder of the first year, and periodically thereafter. Serum ALT levels should be evaluated more frequently in patients who develop elevations (see WARNINGS).

As noted in the WARNINGS Section, there is no experience with continued treatment of patients once ALT exceeds 5 × ULN. Treatment should be discontinued if ALT levels are ≥ 5 × ULN or if clinical jaundice develops. There is limited experience with rechallenge of patients who have had RILUTEK discontinued for ALT > 5 × ULN, but there is the possibility of increased ALT values reoccurring. Therefore, rechallenge is not recommended.

In the two controlled trials in patients with ALS, the frequency with which values for hemoglobin, hematocrit, and erythrocyte counts fell below the lower limit of normal was greater in RILUTEK-treated patients than in placebo-treated patients; however, these changes were mild and transient. The proportions of patients observed with abnormally low values for these parameters showed a dose-response relationship. Only one patient was discontinued from treatment because of severe anemia. The significance of this finding is unknown.

Drug Interactions

There have been no clinical studies designed to evaluate the interaction of riluzole with other drugs.

As with all drugs, the potential for interaction by a variety of mechanisms is a possibility.

Hepatotoxic Drugs

The clinical trials in ALS excluded patients on concomitant medications which were potentially hepatotoxic, (*e.g.*, allopurinol, methyldopa, sulfasalazine). Accordingly, there is no information about the safety of administering RILUTEK in conjunction with such medications. If the practitioner chooses to prescribe such a combination, caution should be exercised.

Drugs Highly Bound To Plasma Proteins

Riluzole is highly bound (96%) to plasma proteins, binding mainly to serum albumin and to lipoproteins. The effect of riluzole (up to 5 mcg/mL) on warfarin (5 mcg/mL) binding did not show any displacement of warfarin. Conversely, riluzole binding was unaffected by the addition of warfarin, digoxin, imipramine and quinine at high therapeutic concentrations.

Effect of Other Drugs On Riluzole Metabolism

In vitro studies using human liver microsomal preparations suggest that CYP 1A2 is the principal isozyme involved in the initial oxidative metabolism of riluzole and, therefore, potential interactions may occur when riluzole is given concurrently with agents that affect CYP 1A2 activity. Potential inhibitors of CYP 1A2 (*e.g.*, caffeine, phenacetin, theophylline, amitriptyline, and quinolones) could decrease the rate of riluzole elimination, while inducers of CYP 1A2 (*e.g.*, cigarette smoke, charcoal-broiled food, rifampicin, and omeprazole) could increase the rate of riluzole elimination.

Effect of Riluzole On the Metabolism of Other Drugs

CYP 1A2 is the principal isoenzyme involved in the initial oxidative metabolism of riluzole; potential interactions may occur when riluzole is given concurrently with other agents which are also metabolized primarily by CYP 1A2 (*e.g.*, theophylline, caffeine, and tacrine). Currently, it is not known whether riluzole has any potential for enzyme induction in humans.

Drug Laboratory Test Interactions

None known

Carcinogenesis, Mutagenesis, Impairment of Fertility

Riluzole was not carcinogenic in mice or rats when administered for 2 years at daily oral doses up to 20 mg/kg and 10 mg/kg, respectively, which are approximately equivalent to the maximum human dose on a mg/m^2 basis.

The genotoxic potential of riluzole was evaluated in the bacterial mutagenicity (Ames) test, the mouse lymphoma mutation assay in L5178Y cells, the *in vitro* chromosomal aberration assay in human lymphocytes and the *in vivo* rat cytogenetic assay and *in vivo* mouse micronucleus assay in bone marrow. There was no evidence of mutagenic or clastogenic potential in the Ames test, the mouse lymphoma assay, or the *in vivo* assays in the mouse and rat. There was an equivocal clastogenic response in the *in vitro* human lymphocyte chromosomal aberration assay, which was not reproduced in a second assay performed at equal or higher concentrations; riluzole was therefore considered non-clastogenic in the human lymphocyte assay.

N-hydroxyriluzole, the major active metabolite of riluzole, caused chromosomal damage in the *in vitro* mammalian mouse lymphoma assay and in the *in vitro* micronucleus assay that used the same mouse lymphoma cell line, L5178Y. N-hydroxyriluzole was not mutagenic in this cell line when tested in the HPRT gene mutation assay, and was negative in the Ames bacterial gene mutation assay (with and without rat or hamster S9), the *in vitro* UDS assay in rat hepatocytes, the chromosomal aberration test in human lymphocytes, and the *in vivo* mouse bone marrow micronucleus test.

Riluzole impaired fertility when administered to male and female rats prior to and during mating at an oral dose of 15 mg/kg or 1.5 times the maximum daily dose on a mg/m^2 basis (see PRECAUTIONS: "Pregnancy" for effects on fertility).

Pregnancy

Pregnancy category C

Oral administration of riluzole to pregnant animals during the period of organogenesis caused embryotoxicity in rats and rabbits at doses of 27 mg/kg and 60 mg/kg, respectively, or 2.6 and 11.5 times, respectively, the recommended maximum human daily dose on a mg/m^2 basis. Evidence of maternal toxicity was also observed at these doses.

When administered to rats prior to and during mating (males and females) and throughout gestation and lactation (females), riluzole produced adverse effects on pregnancy (decreased implantations, increased intrauterine death) and offspring viability and growth at an oral dose of 15 mg/kg or 1.5 times the maximum daily dose on a mg/m^2 basis.

There are no adequate and well-controlled studies in pregnant women. Riluzole should be used during pregnancy only if the potential benefit justifies the potential risk to the fetus.

Nursing Women

In rat studies, ^{14}C-riluzole was detected in maternal milk. It is not known whether riluzole is excreted in human breast milk. Because many drugs are excreted in human milk, and because the potential for serious adverse reactions in nursing infants from RILUTEK® is unknown, women should be advised not to breast-feed during treatment with RILUTEK.

Geriatric Use

Age-related compromised renal and hepatic function may cause a decrease in clearance of riluzole (see CLINICAL PHARMACOLOGY: Special Populations). In controlled clinical trials, about 30% of patients were over 65. There were no differences in adverse effects between younger and older patients.

Pediatric Use

The safety and the effectiveness of RILUTEK in pediatric patients have not been established.

ADVERSE REACTIONS

The most commonly observed AEs associated with the use of RILUTEK more frequently than placebo treated patients were: asthenia, nausea, dizziness, decreased lung function, diarrhea, abdominal pain, pneumonia, vomiting, vertigo, circumoral paresthesia, anorexia, and somnolence. Asthenia, nausea, dizziness, diarrhea, anorexia, vertigo, somnolence, and circumoral paresthesia were dose related.

Approximately 14% (n = 141) of the 982 individuals with ALS who received RILUTEK in pre-marketing clinical trials discontinued treatment because of an adverse experience. Of those patients who discontinued due to adverse events, the most commonly reported were: nausea, abdominal pain, constipation, and ALT elevations. In a dose response study in ALS patients, the rates of discontinuation of RILUTEK for asthenia, nausea, abdominal pain, and ALT elevation were dose related.

Incidence in Controlled ALS Clinical Studies

Table 1 lists treatment-emergent signs and symptoms that occurred in at least 2% of patients with ALS treated with RILUTEK (n=794) participating in placebo-controlled trials and were numerically greater in the patients treated with RILUTEK 100 mg/day than with placebo or for which a dose response relationship is suggested.

The prescriber should be aware that these figures cannot be used to predict the frequency of adverse experiences in the course of usual medical practice where patient characteristics and other factors may differ from those prevailing during clinical studies. Inspection of these frequencies, however, does provide the prescriber with one basis to estimate the relative contribution of drug and non-drug factors to the AE incidences in the population studied.

[See table 1 at right]

Other Adverse Events Observed

Other events which occurred in more than 2% of patients treated with RILUTEK 100 mg/day but equally or more frequently in the placebo group included: accidental injury, apnea, bronchitis, constipation, death, dysphagia, dyspnea, flu syndrome, heart arrest, increased sputum, pneumonia, and respiratory disorder.

The overall adverse event profile for RILUTEK was similar between females and males, and was independent of age. Because the largest non-white racial subgroup was only 2% of patients exposed to RILUTEK (18/794) in placebo-controlled trials, there are insufficient data to support a statement regarding the distribution of adverse experience reports by race. In ALS studies, dizziness did occur more commonly in females (11%) than in males (4%). There was not a difference between females and males in the rates of discontinuation of RILUTEK for individual adverse experiences.

Other Adverse Events Observed During All Clinical Trials

RILUTEK has been administered to 1713 individuals during all clinical trials, some of which were placebo-controlled. During these trials, all adverse events were recorded by the clinical investigators using terminology of their own choosing. To provide a meaningful estimate of the proportion of individuals having adverse events, similar types of events were grouped into a smaller number of standardized categories using modified COSTART dictionary terminology. The frequencies presented represent the proportion of the 1713 individuals exposed to RILUTEK who experienced an event of the type cited on at least one occasion while receiving RILUTEK. All reported events are included except those already listed in the previous table, those too general to be informative, and those not reasonably associated with the use of the drug.

Events are further classified within body system categories and enumerated in order of decreasing frequency using the following definitions: *frequent* adverse events are defined as those occurring in at least 1/100 patients; *infrequent* adverse events are those occurring in 1/100 to 1/1000 patients; *rare* adverse events are those occurring in fewer than 1/1000 patients.

Body as a Whole: *Frequent:* Hostility[1]. *Infrequent:* Abscess[1], sepsis[1], photosensitivity reaction[1], cellulitis, face edema[1], hernia, peritonitis, attempted suicide, injection site reaction, chills[1], flu syndrome, intentional injury, enlarged abdomen, neoplasm. *Rare:* Acrodynia, hypothermia, moniliasis[1], rheumatoid arthritis.

Digestive System: *Infrequent:* Increased appetite, intestinal obstruction[1], fecal impaction, gastrointestinal hemorrhage, gastrointestinal ulceration, gastritis[1], fecal incontinence, jaundice, hepatitis, glossitis, gum hemorrhage[1], pancreatitis, tenesmus, esophageal stenosis. *Rare:* Cheilitis[1], cholecystitis, hematemesis, melena[1], biliary pain, proctitis, pseudomembranous enterocolitis, enlarged salivary gland, tongue discoloration, tooth caries.

Immune System Disorders: *Infrequent:* Anaphylactoid reaction and anaphylaxis.

Nervous System: *Frequent:* Agitation[1], tremor. *Infrequent:* Hallucinations, personality disorder[1], abnormal thinking[1], coma, paranoid reaction[1], manic reaction, ataxia, extrapyramidal syndrome, hypokinesia, urinary retention, emotional lability, delusions, apathy, hypesthesia, incoordination, confusion[1], convulsion, leg cramps, amnesia, dysarthria, increased libido, stupor, subdural hematoma, abnormal gait, delirium, depersonalization, facial paralysis, hemiplegia, decreased libido, myoclonus. *Rare:* Abnormal dreams, acute brain syndrome, CNS depression, dementia, cerebral embolism, euphoria[1], hypotonia, ileus[1], peripheral neuritis, psychosis[1], psychotic depression, schizophrenic reaction, trismus, wristdrop.

Skin and Appendages: *Infrequent:* Skin ulceration, urticaria, psoriasis, seborrhea[1], skin disorder, fungal dermatitis[1]. *Rare:* Angioedema, contact dermatitis, erythema multiforme, furunculosis[1], skin moniliasis, skin granuloma, skin nodule.

Respiratory System: *Infrequent:* Hiccup, pleural disorder[1], asthma, epistaxis, hemoptysis, yawn, hyperventilation[1], lung edema[1], hypoventilation[1], lung carcinoma, hypoxia, laryngitis, pleural effusion, pneumothorax[1], respiratory moniliasis, stridor, interstitial lung disease, hypersensitivity pneumonitis.

Cardiovascular System: *Infrequent:* Syncope[1], hypotension, heart failure, migraine, peripheral vascular disease, angina pectoris[1], myocardial infarction[1], ventricular extrasystoles, cerebral hemorrhage, atrial fibrillation[1], bundle branch block, congestive heart failure, pericarditis, lower extremity embolus, myocardial ischemia[1], shock[1]. *Rare:* Bradycardia, cerebral ischemia, hemorrhage, mesenteric artery occlusion, subarachnoid hemorrhage, supraventricular tachycardia[1], thrombosis, ventricular fibrillation, ventricular tachycardia.

Metabolic and Nutritional Disorders: *Infrequent:* Gout[1], respiratory acidosis, edema, thirst[1], hypokalemia, hyponatremia, weight gain[1]. *Rare:* Generalized edema, hypercalcemia, hypercholesteremia.

Endocrine System: *Infrequent:* Diabetes mellitus, thyroid neoplasia. *Rare:* Diabetes insipidus, parathyroid disorder.

Hemic and Lymphatic System: *Infrequent:* Anemia[1], leukocytosis, leukopenia, ecchymosis. *Rare:* Neutropenia, aplastic anemia, cyanosis, hypochromic anemia, iron deficiency anemia, lymphadenopathy, petechiae[1], purpura.

Musculoskeletal System: *Infrequent:* Arthrosis, myasthenia[1], bone neoplasm. *Rare:* Bone necrosis, osteoporosis, tetany.

Special Senses: *Infrequent:* Amblyopia, ophthalmitis. *Rare:* Blepharitis, cataract, deafness, diplopia[1], ear pain,

Table 1 Adverse Events Occurring in Placebo-Controlled Clinical Trials

Body System/ Adverse Event*	Riluzole 50 mg/day (N=237)	Riluzole 100 mg/day (N=313)	Riluzole 200 mg/day (N=244)	Placebo (N=320)
Body as a Whole				
Asthenia	14.8	19.2	20.1	12.2
Headache	8.0	7.3	7.0	6.6
Abdominal pain	6.8	5.1	7.8	3.8
Back pain	1.7	3.2	4.1	2.5
Aggravation reaction	0.4	1.3	2.0	0.9
Malaise	0.4	0.6	1.2	0.0
Digestive				
Nausea	12.2	16.3	20.5	10.6
Vomiting	4.2	4.2	4.5	1.6
Dyspepsia	2.5	3.8	6.1	5.0
Anorexia	3.8	3.2	8.6	3.8
Diarrhea	5.5	2.9	9.0	3.1
Flatulence	2.5	2.6	2.0	1.9
Stomatitis	0.8	1.0	1.2	0.9
Tooth disorder	0.0	1.0	1.2	0.3
Oral Moniliasis	0.4	0.6	1.2	0.3
Nervous				
Hypertonia	5.9	6.1	5.3	5.9
Depression	4.2	4.5	6.1	5.0
Dizziness	5.1	3.8	12.7	2.5
Dry mouth	3.0	3.5	2.0	3.4
Insomnia	2.1	3.5	2.9	3.4
Somnolence	0.8	1.9	4.1	1.3
Vertigo	2.5	1.9	4.5	0.9
Circumoral paresthesia	1.3	1.6	3.3	0.0
Skin and Appendages				
Pruritus	3.8	3.8	2.5	3.1
Eczema	0.8	1.6	1.6	0.6
Alopecia	0.0	1.0	1.2	0.6
Exfoliative dermatitis	0.0	0.6	1.2	0.0
Respiratory				
Decreased lung function	13.1	10.2	16.0	9.4
Rhinitis	8.9	6.4	7.8	6.3
Increased cough	2.1	2.6	3.7	1.6
Sinusitis	0.4	1.0	1.6	0.9
Cardiovascular				
Hypertension	6.8	5.1	3.3	4.1
Tachycardia	1.3	2.6	2.0	1.3
Phlebitis	0.4	1.0	0.8	0.3
Palpitation	0.4	0.6	1.2	0.9
Postural hypotension	0.8	0.0	1.6	0.6
Metabolic and Nutritional Disorders				
Weight loss	4.6	4.8	3.7	4.7
Peripheral edema	4.2	2.9	3.3	2.2
Musculoskeletal System				
Arthralgia	5.1	3.5	1.6	3.4
Urogenital System				
Urinary tract infection	2.5	2.6	4.5	2.2
Dysuria	0.0	1.0	1.2	0.3

*Percentage of patients reporting events

glaucoma, hyperacusis, photophobia, taste loss, vestibular disorder.

Urogenital System: *Infrequent:* Urinary urgency, urine abnormality, urinary incontinence, kidney calculus, hematuria, impotence, prostate carcinoma, kidney pain, metrorrhagia, priapism. *Rare:* Amenorrhea, breast abscess, breast pain, nephritis[1], nocturia, pyelonephritis, enlarged uterine fibroids, uterine hemorrhage, vaginal moniliasis.

Laboratory Tests: *Infrequent:* Increased gamma glutamyl transferase, abnormal liver function/tests, increased alkaline phosphatase, positive direct Coombs test, increased gamma globulins. *Rare:* increased lactic dehydrogenase.

[1] = AE frequency ≤ to placebo

OVERDOSAGE

No specific antidote or information on treatment of overdosage with RILUTEK is available. In the event of overdose, RILUTEK therapy should be discontinued immediately. Experience with riluzole overdose in humans is limited. Neurological and psychiatric symptoms, acute toxic encephalopathy with stupor, coma, and methemoglobinemia have been observed in isolated cases. Treatment should be supportive and directed toward alleviating symptoms.

Severe methemoglobinemia may be rapidly reversible after treatment with methylene blue.

The estimated oral median lethal dose is 94 mg/kg and 39 mg/kg for male mice and rats, respectively.

DOSAGE AND ADMINISTRATION

The recommended dose for RILUTEK is 50 mg every 12 hours. No increased benefit can be expected from higher daily doses, but adverse events are increased.

RILUTEK tablets should be taken at least an hour before, or two hours after, a meal to avoid a food-related decrease in bioavailability.

Special Populations
Patients with Impaired Hepatic Function
see WARNINGS, PRECAUTIONS, CLINICAL PHARMACOLOGY.

HOW SUPPLIED

RILUTEK 50 mg tablets are white, film-coated, capsule-shaped and engraved with "RPR 202" on one side. RILUTEK is supplied in bottles of 60 tablets, NDC 0075-7700-60.

STORE AT CONTROLLED ROOM TEMPERATURE 20°–25°C (68°–77°F) AND PROTECT FROM BRIGHT LIGHT. KEEP OUT OF THE REACH OF CHILDREN.

Revised August 2009
sanofi-aventis U.S. LLC
Bridgewater, NJ 08807
© 2009 sanofi-aventis U.S. LLC
Revised: 08/2009   sanofi-aventis U.S. LLC
Shown in Product Identification Guide, page 319

TAXOTERE®   ℞
[tax-ō-tĕr]
(docetaxel)
Injection Concentrate, Intravenous Infusion (IV)

HIGHLIGHTS OF PRESCRIBING INFORMATION
These highlights do not include all the information needed to use TAXOTERE safely and effectively. See full prescribing information for TAXOTERE.
TAXOTERE (docetaxel) Injection Concentrate, Intravenous Infusion (IV). Initial U.S. Approval: 1996

WARNING: TOXIC DEATHS, HEPATOTOXICITY, NEUTROPENIA, HYPERSENSITIVITY REACTIONS, and FLUID RETENTION
See full prescribing information for complete boxed warning
- Treatment-related mortality increases with abnormal liver function, at higher doses, and in patients with NSCLC and prior platinum-based therapy receiving TAXOTERE at 100 mg/m² (5.1)
- Should not be given if bilirubin > ULN, or if AST and/or ALT > 1.5 × ULN concomitant with alkaline phosphatase > 2.5 × ULN. LFT elevations increase risk of severe or life-threatening complications. Obtain LFTs before each treatment cycle (8.6)
- Should not be given if neutrophil counts are < 1500 cells/mm³. Obtain frequent blood counts to monitor for neutropenia (4)
- Severe hypersensitivity, including very rare fatal anaphylaxis, has been reported in patients who received dexamethasone premedication. Severe reactions require immediate discontinuation of TAXOTERE and administration of appropriate therapy (5.4)
- Contraindicated if history of severe hypersensitivity reactions to TAXOTERE or to drugs formulated with polysorbate 80 (4)

- Severe fluid retention may occur despite dexamethasone (5.5)

---RECENT MAJOR CHANGES---
- -Dosage and administration (2.8, 2.9) 04/2010
- -Drug interactions (7) 04/2010

---INDICATIONS AND USAGE---
TAXOTERE is a microtubule inhibitor indicated for:
- **Breast Cancer (BC):** single agent for locally advanced or metastatic BC after chemotherapy failure; and with doxorubicin and cyclophosphamide as adjuvant treatment of operable node-positive BC (1.1)
- **Non-Small Cell Lung Cancer (NSCLC):** single agent for locally advanced or metastatic NSCLC after platinum therapy failure; and with cisplatin for unresectable, locally advanced or metastatic untreated NSCLC (1.2)
- **Hormone Refractory Prostate Cancer (HRPC):** with prednisone in androgen independent (hormone refractory) metastatic prostate cancer (1.3)
- **Gastric Adenocarcinoma (GC):** with cisplatin and fluorouracil for untreated, advanced GC, including the gastroesophageal junction (1.4)
- **Squamous Cell Carcinoma of the Head and Neck Cancer (SCCHN):** with cisplatin and fluorouracil for induction treatment of locally advanced SCCHN (1.5)

---DOSAGE AND ADMINISTRATION---
Administer in a facility equipped to manage possible complications (e.g., anaphylaxis). Administer intravenously (IV) over 1 hr every 3 weeks. PVC equipment is not recommended.
- BC locally advanced or metastatic: 60 mg/m² to 100 mg/m² single agent (2.1)
- BC adjuvant: 75 mg/m² administered 1 hour after doxorubicin 50 mg/m² and cyclophosphamide 500 mg/m² every 3 weeks for 6 cycles (2.1)
- NSCLC: after platinum therapy failure: 75 mg/m² single agent (2.2)
- NSCLC: chemotherapy-naive: 75 mg/m² followed by cisplatin 75 mg/m² (2.2)
- HRPC: 75 mg/m² with 5 mg prednisone twice a day continuously (2.3)
- GC: 75 mg/m² followed by cisplatin 75 mg/m² (both on day 1 only) followed by fluorouracil 750 mg/m² per day as a 24-hr IV (days 1–5), starting at end of cisplatin infusion (2.4)
- SCCHN: 75 mg/m² followed by cisplatin 75 mg/m² IV (day 1), followed by fluorouracil 750 mg/m² per day as a 24-hr IV (days 1–5), starting at end of cisplatin infusion; for 4 cycles (2.5)
- SCCHN: 75 mg/m² followed by cisplatin 100 mg/m² IV (day 1), followed by fluorouracil 1000 mg/m² per day as a 24-hr IV (days 1–4); for 3 cycles (2.5)

For all patients:
- Premedicate with oral corticosteroids (2.6)
- Adjust dose **as** needed (2.7)

---DOSAGE FORMS AND STRENGTHS---
Two vial TAXOTERE:
- 80 mg/2 mL and Diluent for Taxotere 80 mg,
- 20 mg/0.5 mL and Diluent for Taxotere 20 mg (3)

---CONTRAINDICATIONS---
- Hypersensitivity to docetaxel or polysorbate 80 (4)
- Neutrophil counts of <1500 cells/mm³ (4)

---WARNINGS AND PRECAUTIONS---
- Acute myeloid leukemia: In patients who received TAXOTERE, doxorubicin and cyclophosphamide, monitor for delayed myelodysplasia or myeloid leukemia (5.6)
- Cutaneous reactions: Reactions including erythema of the extremities with edema followed by desquamation may occur. Severe skin toxicity may require dose adjustment (5.7)
- Neurologic reactions: Reactions including. paresthesia, dysesthesia, and pain may occur. Severe neurosensory symptoms require dose adjustment or discontinuation if persistent. (5.8)
- Asthenia: Severe asthenia may occur and may require treatment discontinuation. (5.9)
- Pregnancy: Fetal harm can occur when administered to a pregnant woman. Women of childbearing potential should be advised not to become pregnant when receiving TAXOTERE (5.10, 8.1)

---ADVERSE REACTIONS---
Most common adverse reactions across all TAXOTERE indications are infections, neutropenia, anemia, febrile neutropenia, hypersensitivity, thrombocytopenia, neuropathy, dysgeusia, dyspnea, constipation, anorexia, nail disorders, fluid retention, asthenia, pain, nausea, diarrhea, vomiting, mucositis, alopecia, skin reactions, myalgia (6)

To report SUSPECTED ADVERSE REACTIONS, contact sanofi-aventis U.S. LLC at 1-800-633-1610 or FDA at 1-800-FDA-1088 or www.fda.gov/medwatch

---DRUG INTERACTIONS---
- Cytochrome P450 3A4 inducers, inhibitors, or substrates: May alter docetaxel metabolism. (7)

See 17 for PATIENT COUNSELING INFORMATION and FDA-approved patient labeling
Revised: 05/2010

FULL PRESCRIBING INFORMATION: CONTENTS*
WARNING: TOXIC DEATHS, HEPATOTOXICITY, NEUTROPENIA, HYPERSENSITIVITY REACTIONS, AND FLUID RETENTION

* Sections or subsections omitted from the full prescribing information are not listed

---

FULL PRESCRIBING INFORMATION

WARNING: TOXIC DEATHS, HEPATOTOXICITY, NEUTROPENIA, HYPERSENSITIVITY REACTIONS, AND FLUID RETENTION
The incidence of treatment-related mortality associated with TAXOTERE therapy is increased in patients with abnormal liver function, in patients receiving higher doses, and in patients with non-small cell lung carcinoma and a history of prior treatment with platinum-based chemotherapy who receive TAXOTERE as a single agent at a dose of 100 mg/m² *[see Warnings and Precautions (5.1)].*
TAXOTERE should not be given to patients with bilirubin > upper limit of normal (ULN), or to patients with AST and/or ALT >1.5 × ULN concomitant with alkaline phosphatase >2.5 × ULN. Patients with elevations of bilirubin or abnormalities of transaminase concurrent

with alkaline phosphatase are at increased risk for the development of grade 4 neutropenia, febrile neutropenia, infections, severe thrombocytopenia, severe stomatitis, severe skin toxicity, and toxic death. Patients with isolated elevations of transaminase >1.5 × ULN also had a higher rate of febrile neutropenia grade 4 but did not have an increased incidence of toxic death. Bilirubin, AST or ALT, and alkaline phosphatase values should be obtained prior to each cycle of TAXOTERE therapy [see Warnings and Precautions (5.2)].

TAXOTERE therapy should not be given to patients with neutrophil counts of <1500 cells/mm³. In order to monitor the occurrence of neutropenia, which may be severe and result in infection, frequent blood cell counts should be performed on all patients receiving TAXOTERE [see Warnings and Precautions (5.3)]. Severe hypersensitivity reactions characterized by generalized rash/erythema, hypotension and/or bronchospasm, or very rarely fatal anaphylaxis, have been reported in patients who received a 3-day dexamethasone premedication. Hypersensitivity reactions require immediate discontinuation of the TAXOTERE infusion and administration of appropriate therapy [see Warnings and Precautions (5.4)]. TAXOTERE must not be given to patients who have a history of severe hypersensitivity reactions to TAXOTERE or to other drugs formulated with polysorbate 80 [see Contraindications (4)].

Severe fluid retention occurred in 6.5% (6/92) of patients despite use of a 3-day dexamethasone premedication regimen. It was characterized by one or more of the following events: poorly tolerated peripheral edema, generalized edema, pleural effusion requiring urgent drainage, dyspnea at rest, cardiac tamponade, or pronounced abdominal distention (due to ascites) [see Warnings and Precautions (5.5)].

1. INDICATIONS AND USAGE

1.1 Breast Cancer
- TAXOTERE is indicated for the treatment of patients with locally advanced or metastatic breast cancer after failure of prior chemotherapy.
- TAXOTERE in combination with doxorubicin and cyclophosphamide is indicated for the adjuvant treatment of patients with operable node-positive breast cancer.

1.2 Non-Small Cell Lung Cancer
- TAXOTERE as a single agent is indicated for the treatment of patients with locally advanced or metastatic non-small cell lung cancer after failure of prior platinum-based chemotherapy.
- TAXOTERE in combination with cisplatin is indicated for the treatment of patients with unresectable, locally advanced or metastatic non-small cell lung cancer who have not previously received chemotherapy for this condition.

1.3 Prostate Cancer
- TAXOTERE in combination with prednisone is indicated for the treatment of patients with androgen independent (hormone refractory) metastatic prostate cancer.

1.4 Gastric Adenocarcinoma
- TAXOTERE in combination with cisplatin and fluorouracil is indicated for the treatment of patients with advanced gastric adenocarcinoma, including adenocarcinoma of the gastroesophageal junction, who have not received prior chemotherapy for advanced disease.

1.5 Head and Neck Cancer
- TAXOTERE in combination with cisplatin and fluorouracil is indicated for the induction treatment of patients with locally advanced squamous cell carcinoma of the head and neck (SCCHN).

2. DOSAGE AND ADMINISTRATION

For all indications, toxicities may warrant dosage adjustments [see Dosage and Administration (2.7)].

Administer in a facility equipped to manage possible complications (e.g. anaphylaxis).

2.1 Breast Cancer
- For locally advanced or metastatic breast cancer after failure of prior chemotherapy, the recommended dose of TAXOTERE is 60 mg/m² to 100 mg/m² administered intravenously over 1 hour every 3 weeks.
- For the adjuvant treatment of operable node-positive breast cancer, the recommended TAXOTERE dose is 75 mg/m² administered 1 hour after doxorubicin 50 mg/m² and cyclophosphamide 500 mg/m² every 3 weeks for 6 courses. Prophylactic G-CSF may be used to mitigate the risk of hematological toxicities [see Dosage and Administration (2.7)].

2.2 Non-Small Cell Lung Cancer
- For treatment after failure of prior platinum-based chemotherapy, TAXOTERE was evaluated as monotherapy, and the recommended dose is 75 mg/m² administered intravenously over 1 hour every 3 weeks. A dose of 100 mg/m² in patients previously treated with chemotherapy was associated with increased hematologic toxicity, infection, and treatment-related mortality in randomized, controlled trials [see Boxed Warning, Dosage and Administration (2.7), Warnings and Precautions (5), Clinical Studies (14)].
- For chemotherapy-naïve patients, TAXOTERE was evaluated in combination with cisplatin. The recommended dose of TAXOTERE is 75 mg/m² administered intravenously over 1 hour immediately followed by cisplatin 75 mg/m² over 30–60 minutes every 3 weeks [see Dosage and Administration (2.7)].

2.3 Prostate cancer
- For hormone-refractory metastatic prostate cancer, the recommended dose of TAXOTERE is 75 mg/m² every 3 weeks as a 1 hour intravenous infusion. Prednisone 5 mg orally twice daily is administered continuously [see Dosage and Administration (2.7)].

2.4 Gastric adenocarcinoma
- For gastric adenocarcinoma, the recommended dose of TAXOTERE is 75 mg/m² as a 1 hour intravenous infusion, followed by cisplatin 75 mg/m², as a 1 to 3 hour intravenous infusion (both on day 1 only), followed by fluorouracil 750 mg/m² per day given as a 24-hour continuous intravenous infusion for 5 days, starting at the end of the cisplatin infusion. Treatment is repeated every three weeks. Patients must receive premedication with antiemetics and appropriate hydration for cisplatin administration [see Dosage and Administration (2.7)].

2.5 Head and Neck Cancer
Patients must receive premedication with antiemetics, and appropriate hydration (prior to and after cisplatin administration). Prophylaxis for neutropenic infections should be administered. All patients treated on the TAXOTERE containing arms of the TAX323 and TAX324 studies received prophylactic antibiotics.
- Induction chemotherapy followed by radiotherapy (TAX323)
For the induction treatment of locally advanced inoperable SCCHN, the recommended dose of TAXOTERE is 75 mg/m² as a 1 hour intravenous infusion followed by cisplatin 75 mg/m² intravenously over 1 hour, on day one, followed by fluorouracil as a continuous intravenous infusion at 750 mg/m² per day for five days. This regimen is administered every 3 weeks for 4 cycles. Following chemotherapy, patients should receive radiotherapy [see Dosage and Administration (2.7)].
- Induction chemotherapy followed by chemoradiotherapy (TAX324)
For the induction treatment of patients with locally advanced (unresectable, low surgical cure, or organ preservation) SCCHN, the recommended dose of TAXOTERE is 75 mg/m² as a 1 hour intravenous infusion on day 1, followed by cisplatin 100 mg/m² administered as a 30-minute to 3 hour infusion, followed by fluorouracil 1000 mg/m²/day as a continuous infusion from day 1 to day 4. This regimen is administered every 3 weeks for 3 cycles. Following chemotherapy, patients should receive chemoradiotherapy [see Dosage and Administration (2.7)].

2.6 Premedication Regimen
- All patients should be premedicated with oral corticosteroids (see below for prostate cancer) such as dexamethasone 16 mg per day (e.g., 8 mg BID) for 3 days starting 1 day prior to TAXOTERE administration in order to reduce the incidence and severity of fluid retention as well as the severity of hypersensitivity reactions [see Boxed Warning, Warnings and Precautions (5.4)].
- For hormone-refractory metastatic prostate cancer, given the concurrent use of prednisone, the recommended premedication regimen is oral dexamethasone 8 mg, at 12 hours, 3 hours and 1 hour before the TAXOTERE infusion [see Warnings and Precautions (5.4)].

2.7 Dosage Adjustments During Treatment
Breast Cancer
Patients who are dosed initially at 100 mg/m² and who experience either febrile neutropenia, neutrophils <500 cells/mm³ for more than 1 week, or severe or cumulative cutaneous reactions during TAXOTERE therapy should have the dosage adjusted from 100 mg/m² to 75 mg/m². If the patient continues to experience these reactions, the dosage should either be decreased from 75 mg/m² to 55 mg/m² or the treatment should be discontinued. Conversely, patients who are dosed initially at 60 mg/m² and who do not experience febrile neutropenia, neutrophils <500 cells/mm³ for more than 1 week, severe or cumulative cutaneous reactions, or severe peripheral neuropathy during TAXOTERE therapy may tolerate higher doses. Patients who develop ≥grade 3 peripheral neuropathy should have TAXOTERE treatment discontinued entirely.
Combination Therapy with TAXOTERE in the Adjuvant Treatment of Breast Cancer
TAXOTERE in combination with doxorubicin and cyclophosphamide should be administered when the neutrophil count is ≥1,500 cells/mm³. Patients who experience febrile neutropenia should receive G-CSF in all subsequent cycles. Patients who continue to experience this reaction should remain on G-CSF and have their TAXOTERE dose reduced to 60 mg/m². Patients who experience grade 3 or 4 stomatitis should have their TAXOTERE dose decreased to 60 mg/m². Patients who experience severe or cumulative cutaneous reactions or moderate neurosensory signs and/or symptoms during TAXOTERE therapy should have their dosage of TAXOTERE reduced from 75 to 60 mg/m². If the patient continues to experience these reactions at 60 mg/m², treatment should be discontinued.
Non-Small Cell Lung Cancer
Monotherapy with TAXOTERE for NSCLC treatment after failure of prior platinum-based chemotherapy
Patients who are dosed initially at 75 mg/m² and who experience either febrile neutropenia, neutrophils <500 cells/mm³ for more than one week, severe or cumulative cutaneous reactions, or other grade 3/4 non-hematological toxicities during TAXOTERE treatment should have treatment withheld until resolution of the toxicity and then resumed at 55 mg/m². Patients who develop ≥grade 3 peripheral neuropathy should have TAXOTERE treatment discontinued entirely.
Combination therapy with TAXOTERE for chemotherapy-naïve NSCLC
For patients who are dosed initially at TAXOTERE 75 mg/m² in combination with cisplatin, and whose nadir of platelet count during the previous course of therapy is <25,000 cells/mm³, in patients who experience febrile neutropenia, and in patients with serious non-hematologic toxicities, the TAXOTERE dosage in subsequent cycles should be reduced to 65 mg/m². In patients who require a further dose reduction, a dose of 50 mg/m² is recommended. For cisplatin dosage adjustments, see manufacturers' prescribing information.
Prostate Cancer
Combination therapy with TAXOTERE for hormone-refractory metastatic prostate cancer
TAXOTERE should be administered when the neutrophil count is ≥1,500 cells/mm³. Patients who experience either febrile neutropenia, neutrophils <500 cells/mm³ for more than one week, severe or cumulative cutaneous reactions or moderate neurosensory signs and/or symptoms during TAXOTERE therapy should have the dosage of TAXOTERE reduced from 75 to 60 mg/m². If the patient continues to experience these reactions at 60 mg/m², the treatment should be discontinued.
Gastric or Head and Neck Cancer
TAXOTERE in combination with cisplatin and fluorouracil in gastric cancer or head and neck cancer
Patients treated with TAXOTERE in combination with cisplatin and fluorouracil must receive antiemetics and appropriate hydration according to current institutional guidelines. In both studies, G-CSF was recommended during the second and/or subsequent cycles in case of febrile neutropenia, or documented infection with neutropenia, or neutropenia lasting more than 7 days. If an episode of febrile neutropenia, prolonged neutropenia or neutropenic infection occurs despite G-CSF use, the TAXOTERE dose should be reduced from 75 to 60 mg/m². If subsequent episodes of complicated neutropenia occur the TAXOTERE dose should be reduced from 60 to 45 mg/m². In case of grade 4 thrombocytopenia the TAXOTERE dose should be reduced from 75 to 60 mg/m². Patients should not be retreated with subsequent cycles of TAXOTERE until neutrophils recover to a level >1,500 cells/mm³ and platelets recover to a level >100,000 cells/mm³. Discontinue treatment if these toxicities persist. [see Warnings and Precautions (5.3)].
Recommended dose modifications for toxicities in patients treated with TAXOTERE in combination with cisplatin and fluorouracil are shown in Table 1.

Table 1 - Recommended Dose Modifications for Toxicities in Patients Treated with TAXOTERE in Combination with Cisplatin and Fluorouracil

Toxicity	Dosage adjustment
Diarrhea grade 3	First episode: reduce fluorouracil dose by 20%. Second episode: then reduce TAXOTERE dose by 20%.
Diarrhea grade 4	First episode: reduce TAXOTERE and fluorouracil doses by 20%. Second episode: discontinue treatment.
Stomatitis/mucositis grade 3	First episode: reduce fluorouracil dose by 20%. Second episode: stop fluorouracil only, at all subsequent cycles.

	Third episode: reduce TAXOTERE dose by 20%.
Stomatitis/mucositis grade 4	First episode: stop fluorouracil only, at all subsequent cycles. Second episode: reduce TAXOTERE dose by 20%.

Liver dysfunction:
In case of AST/ALT >2.5 to ≤5 × ULN and AP ≤2.5 × ULN, or AST/ALT >1.5 to ≤5 × ULN and AP >2.5 to ≤5 × ULN, TAXOTERE should be reduced by 20%.
In case of AST/ALT >5 × ULN and/or AP >5 × ULN TAXOTERE should be stopped.
The dose modifications for cisplatin and fluorouracil in the gastric cancer study are provided below:
Cisplatin dose modifications and delays
Peripheral neuropathy: A neurological examination should be performed before entry into the study, and then at least every 2 cycles and at the end of treatment. In the case of neurological signs or symptoms, more frequent examinations should be performed and the following dose modifications can be made according to NCIC-CTC grade:
- Grade 2: Reduce cisplatin dose by 20%.
- Grade 3: Discontinue treatment.

Ototoxicity: In the case of grade 3 toxicity, discontinue treatment.
Nephrotoxicity: In the event of a rise in serum creatinine ≥grade 2 (>1.5 × normal value) despite adequate rehydration, CrCl should be determined before each subsequent cycle and the following dose reductions should be considered (see Table 2).
For other cisplatin dosage adjustments, also refer to the manufacturers' prescribing information.

Table 2 – Dose Reductions for Evaluation of Creatinine Clearance

Creatinine clearance result before next cycle	Cisplatin dose next cycle
CrCl ≥60 mL/min	Full dose of cisplatin was given. CrCl was to be repeated before each treatment cycle.
CrCl between 40 and 59 mL/min	Dose of cisplatin was reduced by 50% at subsequent cycle. If CrCl was >60 mL/min at end of cycle, full cisplatin dose was reinstituted at the next cycle. If no recovery was observed, then cisplatin was omitted from the next treatment cycle.
CrCl <40 mL/min	Dose of cisplatin was omitted in that treatment cycle only. If CrCl was still <40 mL/min at the end of cycle, cisplatin was discontinued. If CrCl was >40 and <60 mL/min at end of cycle, a 50% cisplatin dose was given at the next cycle. If CrCl was >60 mL/min at end of cycle, full cisplatin dose was given at next cycle.

CrCl = Creatinine clearance

Fluorouracil dose modifications and treatment delays
For diarrhea and stomatitis, see Table 1.
In the event of grade 2 or greater plantar-palmar toxicity, fluorouracil should be stopped until recovery. The fluorouracil dosage should be reduced by 20%.
For other greater than grade 3 toxicities, except alopecia and anemia, chemotherapy should be delayed (for a maximum of 2 weeks from the planned date of infusion) until resolution to grade ≤1 and then recommenced, if medically appropriate.
For other fluorouracil dosage adjustments, also refer to the manufacturers' prescribing information.
Combination Therapy with Strong CYP3A4 inhibitors:
Avoid using concomitant strong CYP3A4 inhibitors (e.g., ketoconazole, itraconazole, clarithromycin, atazanavir, indinavir, nefazodone, nelfinavir, ritonavir, saquinavir, telithromycin and voriconazole). There are no clinical data with a dose adjustment in patients receiving strong CYP3A4 inhibitors. Based on extrapolation from a pharmacokinetic study with ketoconazole in 7 patients, consider a 50% docetaxel dose reduction if patients require coadministration of a strong CYP3A4 inhibitor. *[see Drug Interactions (7), Clinical Pharmacology (12.3)]*.

2.8 Administration Precautions

TAXOTERE is a cytotoxic anticancer drug and, as with other potentially toxic compounds, caution should be exercised when handling and preparing TAXOTERE solutions. The use of gloves is recommended. Please refer to *[see How Supplied/ Storage and Handling (16.3)]*.
If TAXOTERE Injection Concentrate, initial diluted solution, or final dilution for infusion should come into contact with the skin, immediately and thoroughly wash with soap and water. If TAXOTERE Injection Concentrate, initial diluted solution, or final dilution for infusion should come into contact with mucosa, immediately and thoroughly wash with water.
Contact of the TAXOTERE concentrate with plasticized PVC equipment or devices used to prepare solutions for infusion is not recommended. In order to minimize patient exposure to the plasticizer DEHP (di-2-ethylhexyl phthalate), which may be leached from PVC infusion bags or sets, the final TAXOTERE dilution for infusion should be stored in bottles (glass, polypropylene) or plastic bags (polypropylene, polyolefin) and administered through polyethylene-lined administration sets.
Two-vial formulation (Injection Concentrate and Diluent)
TAXOTERE Injection Concentrate requires two dilutions prior to administration. Please follow the preparation instructions provided below. **Note:** Both the TAXOTERE Injection Concentrate and the diluent vials contain an overfill to compensate for liquid loss during preparation. This overfill ensures that after dilution with the **entire** contents of the accompanying diluent, there is an initial diluted solution containing 10 mg/mL docetaxel.
The table below provides the fill range of the Diluent, the approximate extractable volume of Diluent when the entire contents of the diluent vial are withdrawn, and the concentration of the initial diluted solution for TAXOTERE 20 mg and TAXOTERE 80 mg (see Table 3).
[See table 3 below]

2.9 Preparation and Administration

DO NOT use the two-vial formulation (Injection Concentrate and diluent) with the one-vial formulation.
Two-vial formulation (Injection Concentrate and Diluent)
A. Initial Diluted Solution
1. TAXOTERE vials should be stored between 2°C and 25°C (36°F and 77°F). If the vials are stored under refrigeration, allow the appropriate number of vials of TAXOTERE Injection Concentrate and diluent (13% ethanol in water for injection) vials to stand at room temperature for approximately 5 minutes.
2. Aseptically withdraw the entire contents of the appropriate diluent vial (approximately 1.8 mL for TAXOTERE 20 mg and approximately 7.1 mL for TAXOTERE 80 mg) into a syringe by partially inverting the vial, and transfer it to the appropriate vial of TAXOTERE Injection Concentrate. **If the procedure is followed as described, an initial diluted solution of 10 mg docetaxel/mL will result.**
3. Mix the initial diluted solution by repeated inversions for at least 45 seconds to assure full mixture of the concentrate and diluent. Do not shake.
4. The initial diluted TAXOTERE solution (10 mg docetaxel/mL) should be clear; however, there may be some foam on top of the solution due to the polysorbate 80. Allow the solution to stand for a few minutes to allow any foam to dissipate. It is not required that all foam dissipate prior to continuing the preparation process.
The initial diluted solution may be used immediately or stored either in the refrigerator or at room temperature for a maximum of 8 hours.

B. Final Dilution for Infusion
1. Aseptically withdraw the required amount of initial diluted TAXOTERE solution (10 mg docetaxel/mL) with a calibrated syringe and inject into a 250 mL infusion bag or bottle of either 0.9% Sodium Chloride solution or 5% Dextrose solution to produce a final concentration of 0.3 to 0.74 mg/mL.
If a dose greater than 200 mg of TAXOTERE is required, use a larger volume of the infusion vehicle so that a concentration of 0.74 mg/mL TAXOTERE is not exceeded.
2. Thoroughly mix the infusion by manual rotation.
3. As with all parenteral products, TAXOTERE should be inspected visually for particulate matter or discoloration prior to administration whenever the solution and container permit. If the TAXOTERE initial diluted solution or final dilution for intravenous infusion is not clear or appears to have precipitation, these should be discarded.

The final TAXOTERE dilution for infusion should be administered intravenously as a 1-hour infusion under ambient room temperature and lighting conditions.

2.10 Stability

TAXOTERE final dilution for infusion, if stored between 2°C and 25°C (36°F and 77°F) is stable for 4 hours. TAXOTERE final dilution for infusion (in either 0.9% Sodium Chloride solution or 5% Dextrose solution) should be used within 4 hours (including the 1 hour intravenous administration).

Table 3 – Initial Dilution of TAXOTERE Injection Concentrate

Product	Diluent 13% (w/w) ethanol in water for injection Fill Range (mL)	Approximate extractable volume of Diluent when entire contents are withdrawn (mL)	Concentration of the initial diluted solution (mg/mL docetaxel)
Taxotere® 20 mg/0.5 mL	1.88–2.08 mL	1.8 mL	10 mg/mL
Taxotere® 80 mg/2 mL	6.96–7.70 mL	7.1 mL	10 mg/mL

3. DOSAGE FORMS AND STRENGTHS

Two-vial formulation (Injection Concentrate and Diluent)
TAXOTERE 80 mg/2 mL
TAXOTERE (docetaxel) Injection Concentrate 80 mg/2 mL: 80 mg docetaxel in 2 mL polysorbate 80 and Diluent for TAXOTERE 80 mg (13% (w/w) ethanol in water for injection). Both items are in a blister pack in one carton.
TAXOTERE 20 mg/0.5 mL
TAXOTERE (docetaxel) Injection Concentrate 20 mg/0.5 mL: 20 mg docetaxel in 0.5 mL polysorbate 80 and Diluent for TAXOTERE 20 mg (13% (w/w) ethanol in water for injection). Both items are in a blister pack in one carton.

4. CONTRAINDICATIONS

- TAXOTERE is contraindicated in patients who have a history of severe hypersensitivity reactions to docetaxel or to other drugs formulated with polysorbate 80. Severe reactions, including anaphylaxis, have occurred *[see Warnings and Precautions (5.4)]*.
- TAXOTERE should not be used in patients with neutrophil counts of <1500 cells/mm^3.

5. WARNINGS AND PRECAUTIONS

5.1 Toxic Deaths

Breast Cancer
TAXOTERE administered at 100 mg/m^2 was associated with deaths considered possibly or probably related to treatment in 2.0% (19/965) of metastatic breast cancer patients, both previously treated and untreated, with normal baseline liver function and in 11.5% (7/61) of patients with various tumor types who had abnormal baseline liver function (AST and/or ALT >1.5 times ULN together with AP >2.5 times ULN). Among patients dosed at 60 mg/m^2, mortality related to treatment occurred in 0.6% (3/481) of patients with normal liver function, and in 3 of 7 patients with abnormal liver function. Approximately half of these deaths occurred during the first cycle. Sepsis accounted for the majority of the deaths.
Non-Small Cell Lung Cancer
TAXOTERE administered at a dose of 100 mg/m^2 in patients with locally advanced or metastatic non-small cell lung cancer who had a history of prior platinum-based chemotherapy was associated with increased treatment-related mortality (14% and 5% in two randomized, controlled studies). There were 2.8% treatment-related deaths among the 176 patients treated at the 75 mg/m^2 dose in the randomized trials. Among patients who experienced treatment-related mortality at the 75 mg/m^2 dose level, 3 of 5 patients had an ECOG PS of 2 at study entry *[see Dosage and Administration (2.2), Clinical Studies (14)]*.

5.2 Hepatic Impairment

Patients with combined abnormalities of transaminases and alkaline phosphatase should not be treated with TAXOTERE *[see Boxed Warning, Use in Specific Populations (8.6), Clinical studies (14)]*.

5.3 Hematologic Effects

Perform frequent peripheral blood cell counts on all patients receiving TAXOTERE. Patients should not be retreated with subsequent cycles of TAXOTERE until neutrophils recover to a level >1500 cells/mm^3 and platelets recover to a level > 100,000 cells/mm^3.
A 25% reduction in the dose of TAXOTERE is recommended during subsequent cycles following severe neutropenia (<500 cells/mm^3) lasting 7 days or more, febrile neutropenia, or a grade 4 infection in a TAXOTERE cycle *[see Dosage and Administration (2.7)]*.

Table 4 - Summary of Adverse Reactions in Patients Receiving TAXOTERE at 100 mg/m²

Adverse Reaction	All Tumor Types Normal LFTs* n=2045 %	All Tumor Types Elevated LFTs† n=61 %	Breast Cancer Normal LFTs* n=965 %
Hematologic			
Neutropenia			
<2000 cells/mm³	96	96	99
<500 cells/mm³	75	88	86
Leukopenia			
<4000 cells/mm³	96	98	99
<1000 cells/mm³	32	47	44
Thrombocytopenia			
<100,000 cells/mm³	8	25	9
Anemia			
<11 g/dL	90	92	94
<8 g/dL	9	31	8
Febrile Neutropenia‡	11	26	12
Septic Death	2	5	1
Non-Septic Death	1	7	1
Infections			
Any	22	33	22
Severe	6	16	6
Fever in Absence of Infection			
Any	31	41	35
Severe	2	8	2
Hypersensitivity Reactions			
Regardless of Premedication			
Any	21	20	18
Severe	4	10	3
With 3-day Premedication	n=92	n=3	n=92
Any	15	33	15
Severe	2	0	2
Fluid Retention			
Regardless of Premedication			
Any	47	39	60
Severe	7	8	9
With 3-day Premedication	n=92	n=3	n=92
Any	64	67	64
Severe	7	33	7
Neurosensory			
Any	49	34	58
Severe	4	0	6
Cutaneous			
Any	48	54	47
Severe	5	10	5
Nail Changes			
Any	31	23	41
Severe	3	5	4
Gastrointestinal			
Nausea	39	38	42
Vomiting	22	23	23
Diarrhea	39	33	43
Severe	5	5	6
Stomatitis			
Any	42	49	52
Severe	6	13	7
Alopecia	76	62	74
Asthenia			
Any	62	53	66
Severe	13	25	15
Myalgia			
Any	19	16	21
Severe	2	2	2
Arthralgia	9	7	8
Infusion Site Reactions	4	3	4

* Normal Baseline LFTs: Transaminases ≤1.5 times ULN or alkaline phosphatase ≤2.5 times ULN or isolated elevations of transaminases or alkaline phosphatase up to 5 times ULN
† Elevated Baseline LFTs: AST and/or ALT >1.5 times ULN concurrent with alkaline phosphatase >2.5 times ULN
‡ Febrile Neutropenia: ANC grade 4 with fever >38°C with intravenous antibiotics and/or hospitalization

Neutropenia (<2000 neutrophils/mm³) occurs in virtually all patients given 60 mg/m² to 100 mg/m² of TAXOTERE and grade 4 neutropenia (<500 cells/mm³) occurs in 85% of patients given 100 mg/m² and 75% of patients given 60 mg/m². Frequent monitoring of blood counts is, therefore, essential so that dose can be adjusted. TAXOTERE should not be administered to patients with neutrophils <1500 cells/mm³. Febrile neutropenia occurred in about 12% of patients given 100 mg/m² but was very uncommon in patients given 60 mg/m². Hematologic responses, febrile reactions and infections, and rates of septic death for different regimens are dose related [see Adverse Reactions (6.1), Clinical Studies (14)].

Three breast cancer patients with severe liver impairment (bilirubin >1.7 times ULN) developed fatal gastrointestinal bleeding associated with severe drug-induced thrombocytopenia. In gastric cancer patients treated with docetaxel in combination with cisplatin and fluorouracil (TCF), febrile neutropenia and/or neutropenic infection occurred in 12% of patients receiving G-CSF compared to 28% who did not. Patients receiving TCF should be closely monitored during the first and subsequent cycles for febrile neutropenia and neutropenic infection [see Dosage and Administration (2.7), Adverse Reactions (6)].

5.4   Hypersensitivity Reactions

Patients should be observed closely for hypersensitivity reactions, especially during the first and second infusions. Severe hypersensitivity reactions characterized by generalized rash/erythema, hypotension and/or bronchospasm, or very rarely fatal anaphylaxis, have been reported in patients premedicated with 3 days of corticosteroids. Severe hypersensitivity reactions require immediate discontinuation of the TAXOTERE infusion and aggressive therapy. Patients with a history of severe hypersensitivity reactions should not be rechallenged with TAXOTERE.

Hypersensitivity reactions may occur within a few minutes following initiation of a TAXOTERE infusion. If minor reactions such as flushing or localized skin reactions occur, interruption of therapy is not required. All patients should be premedicated with an oral corticosteroid prior to the initiation of the infusion of TAXOTERE [see Dosage and Administration (2.6)].

5.5   Fluid Retention

Severe fluid retention has been reported following TAXOTERE therapy. Patients should be premedicated with oral corticosteroids prior to each TAXOTERE administration to reduce the incidence and severity of fluid retention [see Dosage and Administration (2.6)]. Patients with pre-existing effusions should be closely monitored from the first dose for the possible exacerbation of the effusions.

When fluid retention occurs, peripheral edema usually starts in the lower extremities and may become generalized with a median weight gain of 2 kg.

Among 92 breast cancer patients premedicated with 3-day corticosteroids, moderate fluid retention occurred in 27.2% and severe fluid retention in 6.5%. The median cumulative dose to onset of moderate or severe fluid retention was 819 mg/m². Nine of 92 patients (9.8%) of patients discontinued treatment due to fluid retention: 4 patients discontinued with severe fluid retention; the remaining 5 had mild or moderate fluid retention. The median cumulative dose to treatment discontinuation due to fluid retention was 1021 mg/m². Fluid retention was completely, but sometimes slowly, reversible with a median of 16 weeks from the last infusion of TAXOTERE to resolution (range: 0 to 42+ weeks). Patients developing peripheral edema may be treated with standard measures, e.g., salt restriction, oral diuretic(s).

5.6   Acute Myeloid Leukemia

Treatment-related acute myeloid leukemia (AML) or myelodysplasia has occurred in patients given anthracyclines and/or cyclophosphamide, including use in adjuvant therapy for breast cancer. In the adjuvant breast cancer trial (TAX316) AML occurred in 3 of 744 patients who received TAXOTERE, doxorubicin and cyclophosphamide (TAC) and in 1 of 736 patients who received fluorouracil, doxorubicin and cyclophosphamide [see Clinical Studies (14.2)]. In TAC-treated patients, the risk of delayed myelodysplasia or myeloid leukemia requires hematological follow-up.

5.7   Cutaneous Reactions

Localized erythema of the extremities with edema followed by desquamation has been observed. In case of severe skin toxicity, an adjustment in dosage is recommended [see Dosage and Administration (2.7)]. The discontinuation rate due to skin toxicity was 1.6% (15/965) for metastatic breast cancer patients. Among 92 breast cancer patients premedicated with 3-day corticosteroids, there were no cases of severe skin toxicity reported and no patient discontinued TAXOTERE due to skin toxicity.

5.8   Neurologic Reactions

Severe neurosensory symptoms (e.g. paresthesia, dysesthesia, pain) were observed in 5.5% (53/965) of metastatic breast cancer patients, and resulted in treatment discontinuation in 6.1%. When these symptoms occur, dosage must be adjusted. If symptoms persist, treatment should be discontinued [see Dosage and Administration (2.7)]. Patients who experienced neurotoxicity in clinical trials and for whom follow-up information on the complete resolution of the event was available had spontaneous reversal of symptoms with a median of 9 weeks from onset (range: 0 to 106 weeks). Severe peripheral motor neuropathy mainly manifested as distal extremity weakness occurred in 4.4% (42/965).

5.9 Asthenia

Severe asthenia has been reported in 14.9% (144/965) of metastatic breast cancer patients but has led to treatment discontinuation in only 1.8%. Symptoms of fatigue and weakness may last a few days up to several weeks and may be associated with deterioration of performance status in patients with progressive disease.

5.10 Use in Pregnancy

TAXOTERE can cause fetal harm when administered to a pregnant woman. Docetaxel caused embryofetal toxicities including intrauterine mortality when administered to pregnant rats and rabbits during the period of organogenesis. Embryofetal effects in animals occurred at doses as low as 1/50 and 1/300 the recommended human dose on a body surface area basis.

There are no adequate and well-controlled studies in pregnant women using TAXOTERE. If TAXOTERE is used during pregnancy, or if the patient becomes pregnant while receiving this drug, the patient should be apprised of the potential hazard to the fetus. Women of childbearing potential should be advised to avoid becoming pregnant during therapy with TAXOTERE [see Use in Specific Populations (8.1)].

6. ADVERSE REACTIONS

The most serious adverse reactions from TAXOTERE are:
- Toxic Deaths [see Boxed Warning, Warning and Precautions (5.1)]
- Hepatotoxicity [see Boxed Warning, Warnings and Precautions (5.2)]
- Neutropenia [see Boxed Warning, Warnings and Precautions (5.3)]
- Hypersensitivity [see Boxed Warning, Warnings and Precautions (5.4)]
- Fluid Retention [see Boxed Warning, Warnings and Precautions (5.5)]

The most common adverse reactions across all TAXOTERE indications are infections, neutropenia, anemia, febrile neutropenia, hypersensitivity, thrombocytopenia, neuropathy, dysgeusia, dyspnea, constipation, anorexia, nail disorders, fluid retention, asthenia, pain, nausea, diarrhea, vomiting, mucositis, alopecia, skin reactions, and myalgia. Incidence varies depending on the indication.

Adverse reactions are described according to indication. Because clinical trials are conducted under widely varying conditions, adverse reaction rates observed in the clinical trials of a drug cannot be directly compared to rates in the clinical trials of another drug and may not reflect the rates observed in practice.

Responding patients may not experience an improvement in performance status on therapy and may experience worsening. The relationship between changes in performance status, response to therapy, and treatment-related side effects has not been established.

6.1 Clinical Trial Experience

Breast Cancer

Monotherapy with TAXOTERE for locally advanced or metastatic breast cancer after failure of prior chemotherapy

TAXOTERE 100 mg/m²: Adverse drug reactions occurring in at least 5% of patients are compared for three populations who received TAXOTERE administered at 100 mg/m² as a 1-hour infusion every 3 weeks: 2045 patients with various tumor types and normal baseline liver function tests; the subset of 965 patients with locally advanced or metastatic breast cancer, both previously treated and untreated with chemotherapy, who had normal baseline liver function tests; and an additional 61 patients with various tumor types who had abnormal liver function tests at baseline. These reactions were described using COSTART terms and were considered possibly or probably related to TAXOTERE. At least 95% of these patients did not receive hematopoietic support. The safety profile is generally similar in patients receiving TAXOTERE for the treatment of breast cancer and in patients with other tumor types (See Table 4).

[See table 4 at top of previous page]

Hematologic Reactions

Reversible marrow suppression was the major dose-limiting toxicity of TAXOTERE [see Warnings and Precautions (5.3)]. The median time to nadir was 7 days, while the median duration of severe neutropenia (<500 cells/mm³) was 7 days. Among 2045 patients with solid tumors and normal baseline LFTs, severe neutropenia occurred in 75.4% and lasted for more than 7 days in 2.9% of cycles.

Febrile neutropenia (<500 cells/mm³ with fever >38°C with intravenous antibiotics and/or hospitalization) occurred in 11% of patients with solid tumors, in 12.3% of patients with metastatic breast cancer, and in 9.8% of 92 breast cancer patients premedicated with 3-day corticosteroids.

Severe infectious episodes occurred in 6.1% of patients with solid tumors, in 6.4% of patients with metastatic breast cancer, and in 5.4% of 92 breast cancer patients premedicated with 3-day corticosteroids.

Table 5 - Hematologic Adverse Reactions in Breast Cancer Patients Previously Treated with Chemotherapy Treated at TAXOTERE 100 mg/m² with Normal or Elevated Liver Function Tests or 60 mg/m² with Normal Liver Function Tests

Adverse Reaction	TAXOTERE 100 mg/m²		TAXOTERE 60 mg/m²
	Normal LFTs* n=730 %	Elevated LFTs[†] n=18 %	Normal LFTs* n=174 %
Neutropenia			
Any <2000 cells/mm³	98	100	95
Grade 4 <500 cells/mm³	84	94	75
Thrombocytopenia			
Any <100,000 cells/mm³	11	44	14
Grade 4 <20,000 cells/mm³	1	17	1
Anemia <11 g/dL	95	94	65
Infection[‡]			
Any	23	39	1
Grade 3 and 4	7	33	0
Febrile Neutropenia[§]			
By Patient	12	33	0
By Course	2	9	0
Septic Death	2	6	1
Non-Septic Death	1	11	0

* Normal Baseline LFTs: Transaminases ≤1.5 times ULN or alkaline phosphatase ≤2.5 times ULN or isolated elevations of transaminases or alkaline phosphatase up to 5 times ULN
† Elevated Baseline LFTs: AST and/or ALT >1.5 times ULN concurrent with alkaline phosphatase >2.5 times ULN
‡ Incidence of infection requiring hospitalization and/or intravenous antibiotics was 8.5% (n=62) among the 730 patients with normal LFTs at baseline; 7 patients had concurrent grade 3 neutropenia, and 46 patients had grade 4 neutropenia.
§ Febrile Neutropenia: For 100 mg/m², ANC grade 4 and fever >38°C with intravenous antibiotics and/or hospitalization; for 60 mg/m², ANC grade 3/4 and fever >38.1°C

Table 6 - Non-Hematologic Adverse Reactions in Breast Cancer Patients Previously Treated with Chemotherapy Treated at TAXOTERE 100 mg/m² with Normal or Elevated Liver Function Tests or 60 mg/m² with Normal Liver Function Tests

Adverse Reaction	TAXOTERE 100 mg/m²		TAXOTERE 60 mg/m²
	Normal LFTs* n=730 %	Elevated LFTs[†] n=18 %	Normal LFTs* n=174 %
Acute Hypersensitivity Reaction Regardless of Premedication			
Any	13	6	1
Severe	1	0	0
Fluid Retention[‡] Regardless of Premedication			
Any	56	61	13
Severe	8	17	0
Neurosensory			
Any	57	50	20
Severe	6	0	0
Myalgia	23	33	3
Cutaneous			
Any	45	61	31
Severe	5	17	0
Asthenia			
Any	65	44	66
Severe	17	22	0
Diarrhea			
Any	42	28	NA
Severe	6	11	NA
Stomatitis			
Any	53	67	19
Severe	8	39	1

NA = not available
* Normal Baseline LFTs: Transaminases ≤1.5 times ULN or alkaline phosphatase ≤2.5 times ULN or isolated elevations of transaminases or alkaline phosphatase up to 5 times ULN
† Elevated Baseline Liver Function: AST and/or ALT >1.5 times ULN concurrent with alkaline phosphatase >2.5 times ULN
‡ Fluid Retention includes (by COSTART): edema (peripheral, localized, generalized, lymphedema, pulmonary edema, and edema otherwise not specified) and effusion (pleural, pericardial, and ascites); no premedication given with the 60 mg/m² dose

Thrombocytopenia (<100,000 cells/mm^3) associated with fatal gastrointestinal hemorrhage has been reported.

Hypersensitivity Reactions
Severe hypersensitivity reactions have been reported [see Boxed Warning, Warnings and Precautions (5.4)]. Minor events, including flushing, rash with or without pruritus, chest tightness, back pain, dyspnea, drug fever, or chills, have been reported and resolved after discontinuing the infusion and instituting appropriate therapy.

Fluid Retention.
Fluid retention can occur with the use of TAXOTERE [see Boxed Warning, Dosage and Administration (2.6), Warnings and Precautions (5.5)].

Cutaneous Reactions
Severe skin toxicity is discussed elsewhere in the label [see Warnings and Precautions (5.7)]. Reversible cutaneous reactions characterized by a rash including localized eruptions, mainly on the feet and/or hands, but also on the arms, face, or thorax, usually associated with pruritus, have been observed. Eruptions generally occurred within 1 week after TAXOTERE infusion, recovered before the next infusion, and were not disabling.
Severe nail disorders were characterized by hypo- or hyperpigmentation, and occasionally by onycholysis (in 0.8% of patients with solid tumors) and pain.

Neurologic Reactions
Neurologic reactions are discussed elsewhere in the label [see Warnings and Precautions (5.8)]

Gastrointestinal Reactions
Nausea, vomiting, and diarrhea were generally mild to moderate. Severe reactions occurred in 3–5% of patients with solid tumors and to a similar extent among metastatic breast cancer patients. The incidence of severe reactions was 1% or less for the 92 breast cancer patients premedicated with 3-day corticosteroids.
Severe stomatitis occurred in 5.5% of patients with solid tumors, in 7.4% of patients with metastatic breast cancer, and in 1.1% of the 92 breast cancer patients premedicated with 3-day corticosteroids.

Cardiovascular Reactions
Hypotension occurred in 2.8% of patients with solid tumors; 1.2% required treatment. Clinically meaningful events such as heart failure, sinus tachycardia, atrial flutter, dysrhythmia, unstable angina, pulmonary edema, and hypertension occurred rarely. Seven of 86 (8.1%) of metastatic breast cancer patients receiving TAXOTERE 100 mg/m^2 in a randomized trial and who had serial left ventricular ejection fractions assessed developed deterioration of LVEF by ≥10% associated with a drop below the institutional lower limit of normal.

Infusion Site Reactions
Infusion site reactions were generally mild and consisted of hyperpigmentation, inflammation, redness or dryness of the skin, phlebitis, extravasation, or swelling of the vein.

Hepatic Reactions
In patients with normal LFTs at baseline, bilirubin values greater than the ULN occurred in 8.9% of patients. Increases in AST or ALT >1.5 times the ULN, or alkaline phosphatase >2.5 times ULN, were observed in 18.9% and 7.3% of patients, respectively. While on TAXOTERE, increases in AST and/or ALT >1.5 times ULN concomitant with alkaline phosphatase >2.5 times ULN occurred in 4.3% of patients with normal LFTs at baseline. Whether these changes were related to the drug or underlying disease has not been established.

Hematologic and Other Toxicity: Relation to dose and baseline liver chemistry abnormalities
Hematologic and other toxicity is increased at higher doses and in patients with elevated baseline liver function tests (LFTs). In the following tables, adverse drug reactions are compared for three populations: 730 patients with normal LFTs given TAXOTERE at 100 mg/m^2 in the randomized and single arm studies of metastatic breast cancer after failure of previous chemotherapy; 18 patients in these studies who had abnormal baseline LFTs (defined as AST and/or ALT >1.5 times ULN concurrent with alkaline phosphatase >2.5 times ULN); and 174 patients in Japanese studies given TAXOTERE at 60 mg/m^2 who had normal LFTs (see Tables 5 and 6).
[See table 5 at top of previous page]
[See table 6 on previous page]
In the three-arm monotherapy trial, TAX313, which compared TAXOTERE 60 mg/m^2, 75 mg/m^2 and 100 mg/m^2 in advanced breast cancer, grade 3/4 or severe adverse reactions occurred in 49.0% of patients treated with TAXOTERE 60 mg/m^2 compared to 55.3% and 65.9% treated with 75 mg/m^2 and 100 mg/m^2 respectively. Discontinuation due to adverse reactions was reported in 5.3% of patients treated with 60 mg/m^2 vs. 6.9% and 16.5% for patients treated at 75 mg/m^2 and 100 mg/m^2 respectively. Deaths within 30 days of last treatment occurred in 4.0% of patients treated with 60 mg/m^2 compared to 5.3% and 1.6% for patients treated at 75 and 100 mg/m^2 respectively.
The following adverse reactions were associated with increasing docetaxel doses: fluid retention (26%, 38%, and 46% at 60 mg/m^2, 75 mg/m^2, and 100 mg/m^2 respectively), thrombocytopenia (7%, 11% and 12% respectively), neutropenia (92%, 94%, and 97% respectively), febrile neutropenia (5%, 7%, and 14% respectively), treatment-related grade 3/4 infection (2%, 3%, and 7% respectively) and anemia (87%, 94%, and 97% respectively).

Table 7 - Clinically Important Treatment Emergent Adverse Reactions Regardless of Causal Relationship in Patients Receiving TAXOTERE in Combination with Doxorubicin and Cyclophosphamide (TAX316).

Adverse Reaction	TAXOTERE 75 mg/m^2 + Doxorubicin 50 mg/m^2 + Cyclophosphamide 500 mg/m^2 (TAC) n=744 %		Fluorouracil 500 mg/m^2 + Doxorubicin 50 mg/m^2 + Cyclophosphamide 500 mg/m^2 (FAC) n=736 %	
	Any	Grade 3/4	Any	Grade 3/4
Anemia	92	4	72	2
Neutropenia	71	66	82	49
Fever in absence of infection	47	1	17	0
Infection	39	4	36	2
Thrombocytopenia	39	2	28	1
Febrile neutropenia	25	N/A	3	N/A
Neutropenic infection	12	N/A	6	N/A
Hypersensitivity reactions	13	1	4	0
Lymphedema	4	0	1	0
Fluid Retention*	35	1	15	0
Peripheral edema	27	0	7	0
Weight gain	13	0	9	0
Neuropathy sensory	26	0	10	0
Neuro-cortical	5	1	6	1
Neuropathy motor	4	0	2	0
Neuro-cerebellar	2	0	2	0
Syncope	2	1	1	0
Alopecia	98	N/A	97	N/A
Skin toxicity	27	1	18	0
Nail disorders	19	0	14	0
Nausea	81	5	88	10
Stomatitis	69	7	53	2
Vomiting	45	4	59	7
Diarrhea	35	4	28	2
Constipation	34	1	32	1
Taste perversion	28	1	15	0
Anorexia	22	2	18	1
Abdominal Pain	11	1	5	0
Amenorrhea	62	N/A	52	N/A
Cough	14	0	10	0
Cardiac dysrhythmias	8	0	6	0
Vasodilatation	27	1	21	1
Hypotension	2	0	1	0
Phlebitis	1	0	1	0
Asthenia	81	11	71	6
Myalgia	27	1	10	0
Arthralgia	19	1	9	0
Lacrimation disorder	11	0	7	0
Conjunctivitis	5	0	7	0

* COSTART term and grading system for events related to treatment.

Combination therapy with TAXOTERE in the adjuvant treatment of breast cancer
The following table presents treatment emergent adverse reactions observed in 744 patients, who were treated with TAXOTERE 75 mg/m^2 every 3 weeks in combination with doxorubicin and cyclophosphamide (see Table 7).

Table 8 - Treatment Emergent Adverse Reactions Regardless of Relationship to Treatment in Patients Receiving TAXOTERE as Monotherapy for Non-Small Cell Lung Cancer Previously Treated with Platinum-Based Chemotherapy*

Adverse Reaction	TAXOTERE 75 mg/m² n=176 %	Best Supportive Care n=49 %	Vinorelbine/Ifosfamide n=119 %
Neutropenia			
Any	84	14	83
Grade 3/4	65	12	57
Leukopenia			
Any	84	6	89
Grade 3/4	49	0	43
Thrombocytopenia			
Any	8	0	8
Grade 3/4	3	0	2
Anemia			
Any	91	55	91
Grade 3/4	9	12	14
Febrile Neutropenia†	6	NA‡	1
Infection			
Any	34	29	30
Grade 3/4	10	6	9
Treatment Related Mortality	3	NA‡	3
Hypersensitivity Reactions			
Any	6	0	1
Grade 3/4	3	0	0
Fluid Retention			
Any	34	ND§	23
Severe	3		3
Neurosensory			
Any	23	14	29
Grade 3/4	2	6	5
Neuromotor			
Any	16	8	10
Grade 3/4	5	6	3
Skin			
Any	20	6	17
Grade 3/4	1	2	1
Gastrointestinal			
Nausea			
Any	34	31	31
Grade 3/4	5	4	8
Vomiting			
Any	22	27	22
Grade 3/4	3	2	6
Diarrhea			
Any	23	6	12
Grade 3/4	3	0	4
Alopecia	56	35	50
Asthenia			
Any	53	57	54
Severe¶	18	39	23
Stomatitis			
Any	26	6	8
Grade 3/4	2	0	1

(Table continued on next page)

[See table 7 at top of previous page]
Of the 744 patients treated with TAC, 36.3% experienced severe treatment emergent adverse reactions compared to 26.6% of the 736 patients treated with FAC. Dose reductions due to hematologic toxicity occurred in 1% of cycles in the TAC arm versus 0.1% of cycles in the FAC arm. Six percent of patients treated with TAC discontinued treatment due to adverse reactions, compared to 1.1% treated with FAC; fever in the absence of infection and allergy being the most common reasons for withdrawal among TAC-treated patients. Two patients died in each arm within 30 days of their last study treatment; 1 death per arm was attributed to study drugs.

Fever and Infection
Fever in the absence of infection was seen in 46.5% of TAC-treated patients and in 17.1% of FAC-treated patients. Grade 3/4 fever in the absence of infection was seen in 1.3% and 0% of TAC- and FAC-treated patients respectively. Infection was seen in 39.4% of TAC-treated patients compared to 36.3% of FAC-treated patients. Grade 3/4 infection was seen in 3.9% and 2.2% of TAC-treated and FAC-treated patients respectively. There were no septic deaths in either treatment arm.

Gastrointestinal Reactions
In addition to gastrointestinal reactions reflected in the table above, 7 patients in the TAC arm were reported to have colitis/enteritis/large intestine perforation vs. one patient in the FAC arm. Five of the 7 TAC-treated patients required treatment discontinuation; no deaths due to these events occurred.

Cardiovascular Reactions
More cardiovascular reactions were reported in the TAC arm vs. the FAC arm; dysrhythmias, all grades (7.9% vs. 6.0%), hypotension, all grades (2.6% vs. 1.1%) and CHF (2.3% vs. 0.9%, at 70 months median follow-up). One patient in each arm died due to heart failure.

Acute Myeloid Leukemia (AML)
Treatment-related acute myeloid leukemia or myelodysplasia is known to occur in patients treated with anthracy-

clines and/or cyclophosphamide, including use in adjuvant therapy for breast cancer. AML occurs at a higher frequency when these agents are given in combination with radiation therapy. AML occurred in the adjuvant breast cancer trial (TAX316). The cumulative risk of developing treatment-related AML at 5 years in TAX316 was 0.4% for TAC-treated patients and 0.1% for FAC-treated patients. This risk of AML is comparable to the risk observed for other anthracyclines/cyclophosphamide containing adjuvant breast chemotherapy regimens.

Lung Cancer
Monotherapy with TAXOTERE for unresectable, locally advanced or metastatic NSCLC previously treated with platinum-based chemotherapy
TAXOTERE 75 mg/m²: Treatment emergent adverse drug reactions are shown in Table 8. Included in this table is safety data for a total of 176 patients with non-small cell lung carcinoma and a history of prior treatment with platinum-based chemotherapy who were treated in two randomized, controlled trials. These reactions were described using NCI Common Toxicity Criteria regardless of relationship to study treatment, except for the hematologic toxicities or where otherwise noted.
[See table 8 at left and on next page]
Combination therapy with TAXOTERE in chemotherapy-naïve advanced unresectable or metastatic NSCLC
Table 9 presents safety data from two arms of an open label, randomized controlled trial (TAX326) that enrolled patients with unresectable stage IIIB or IV non-small cell lung cancer and no history of prior chemotherapy. Adverse reactions were described using the NCI Common Toxicity Criteria except where otherwise noted.

Table 9 - Adverse Reactions Regardless of Relationship to Treatment in Chemotherapy-Naïve Advanced Non-Small Cell Lung Cancer Patients Receiving TAXOTERE in Combination with Cisplatin

Adverse Reaction	TAXOTERE 75 mg/m² + Cisplatin 75 mg/m² n=406 %	Vinorelbine 25 mg/m² + Cisplatin 100 mg/m² n=396 %
Neutropenia		
Any	91	90
Grade 3/4	74	78
Febrile Neutropenia	5	5
Thrombocytopenia		
Any	15	15
Grade 3/4	3	4
Anemia		
Any	89	94
Grade 3/4	7	25
Infection		
Any	35	37
Grade 3/4	8	8
Fever in absence of infection		
Any	33	29
Grade 3/4	< 1	1
Hypersensitivity Reaction*		
Any	12	4
Grade 3/4	3	<1
Fluid Retention†		
Any	54	42
All severe or life-threatening events	2	2
Pleural effusion		
Any	23	22
All severe or life-threatening events	2	2
Peripheral edema		
Any	34	18
All severe or life-threatening events	<1	<1
Weight gain		
Any	15	9
All severe or life-threatening events	<1	<1
Neurosensory		
Any	47	42
Grade 3/4	4	4

Adverse Reaction		
Neuromotor		
Any	19	17
Grade 3/4	3	6
Skin		
Any	16	14
Grade 3/4	<1	1
Nausea		
Any	72	76
Grade 3/4	10	17
Vomiting		
Any	55	61
Grade 3/4	8	16
Diarrhea		
Any	47	25
Grade 3/4	7	3
Anorexia†		
Any	42	40
All severe or life-threatening events	5	5
Stomatitis		
Any	24	21
Grade 3/4	2	1
Alopecia		
Any	75	42
Grade 3	<1	0
Asthenia†		
Any	74	75
All severe or life-threatening events	12	14
Nail Disorder†		
Any	14	<1
All severe events	<1	0
Myalgia†		
Any	18	12
All severe events	<1	<1

* Replaces NCI term "Allergy"
† COSTART term and grading system

Deaths within 30 days of last study treatment occurred in 31 patients (7.6%) in the docetaxel+cisplatin arm and 37 patients (9.3%) in the vinorelbine+cisplatin arm. Deaths within 30 days of last study treatment attributed to study drug occurred in 9 patients (2.2%) in the docetaxel+cisplatin arm and 8 patients (2.0%) in the vinorelbine+cisplatin arm. The second comparison in the study, vinorelbine+cisplatin versus TAXOTERE+carboplatin (which did not demonstrate a superior survival associated with TAXOTERE, *[see Clinical Studies (14.3)]*) demonstrated a higher incidence of thrombocytopenia, diarrhea, fluid retention, hypersensitivity reactions, skin toxicity, alopecia and nail changes on the TAXOTERE+carboplatin arm, while a higher incidence of anemia, neurosensory toxicity, nausea, vomiting, anorexia and asthenia was observed on the vinorelbine+cisplatin arm.

Prostate Cancer
Combination therapy with TAXOTERE in patients with prostate cancer
The following data are based on the experience of 332 patients, who were treated with TAXOTERE 75 mg/m^2 every 3 weeks in combination with prednisone 5 mg orally twice daily (see Table 10).

Table 10 - Clinically Important Treatment Emergent Adverse Reactions (Regardless of Relationship) in Patients with Prostate Cancer who Received TAXOTERE in Combination with Prednisone (TAX327)

Adverse Reaction	TAXOTERE 75 mg/m^2 every 3 weeks + prednisone 5 mg twice daily n=332 %		Mitoxantrone 12 mg/m^2 every 3 weeks + prednisone 5 mg twice daily n=335 %	
	Any	Grade 3/4	Any	Grade 3/4
Anemia	67	5	58	2
Neutropenia	41	32	48	22

Table 8 *(cont.)* - Treatment Emergent Adverse Reactions Regardless of Relationship to Treatment in Patients Receiving TAXOTERE as Monotherapy for Non-Small Cell Lung Cancer Previously Treated with Platinum-Based Chemotherapy*

Adverse Reaction	TAXOTERE 75 mg/m^2 n=176 %	Best Supportive Care n=49 %	Vinorelbine/Ifosfamide n=119 %
Pulmonary			
Any	41	49	45
Grade 3/4	21	29	19
Nail Disorder			
Any	11	0	2
Severe¶	1	0	0
Myalgia			
Any	6	0	3
Severe¶	0	0	0
Arthralgia			
Any	3	2	2
Severe¶	0	0	1
Taste Perversion			
Any	6	0	0
Severe¶	0	1	0

* Normal Baseline LFTs: Transaminases ≤1.5 times ULN or alkaline phosphatase ≤2.5 times ULN or isolated elevations of transaminases or alkaline phosphatase up to 5 times ULN
† Febrile Neutropenia: ANC grade 4 with fever >38°C with intravenous antibiotics and/or hospitalization
‡ Not Applicable;
§ Not Done
¶ COSTART term and grading system

Adverse Reaction				
Thrombocytopenia	3	1	8	1
Febrile neutropenia	3	N/A	2	N/A
Infection	32	6	20	4
Epistaxis	6	0	2	0
Allergic Reactions	8	1	1	0
Fluid Retention*	24	1	5	0
Weight Gain*	8	0	3	0
Peripheral Edema*	18	0	2	0
Neuropathy Sensory	30	2	7	0
Neuropathy Motor	7	2	3	1
Rash/ Desquamation	6	0	3	1
Alopecia	65	N/A	13	N/A
Nail Changes	30	0	8	0
Nausea	41	3	36	2
Diarrhea	32	2	10	1
Stomatitis/ Pharyngitis	20	1	8	0
Taste Disturbance	18	0	7	0
Vomiting	17	2	14	2
Anorexia	17	1	14	0
Cough	12	0	8	0
Dyspnea	15	3	9	1
Cardiac left ventricular function	10	0	22	1
Fatigue	53	5	35	5
Myalgia	15	0	13	1
Tearing	10	1	2	0
Arthralgia	8	1	5	1

* Related to treatment

Gastric Cancer
Combination therapy with TAXOTERE in gastric adenocarcinoma
Data in the following table are based on the experience of 221 patients with advanced gastric adenocarcinoma and no history of prior chemotherapy for advanced disease, who were treated with TAXOTERE 75 mg/m^2 in combination with cisplatin and fluorouracil (see Table 11).

Table 11 - Clinically Important Treatment Emergent Adverse Reactions Regardless of Relationship to Treatment in the Gastric Cancer Study

Adverse Reaction	TAXOTERE 75 mg/m^2 + cisplatin 75 mg/m^2 + fluorouracil 750 mg/m^2 n=221		Cisplatin 100 mg/m^2 + flourouracil 1000 mg/m^2 n=224	
	Any %	Grade 3/4 %	Any %	Grade 3/4 %
Anemia	97	18	93	26
Neutropenia	96	82	83	57
Fever in the absence of infection	36	2	23	1
Thrombocytopenia	26	8	39	14
Infection	29	16	23	10
Febrile neutropenia	16	N/A	5	N/A
Neutropenic infection	16	N/A	10	N/A
Allergic reactions	10	2	6	0
Fluid retention*	15	0	4	0
Edema*	13	0	3	0
Lethargy	63	21	58	18
Neurosensory	38	8	25	3
Neuromotor	9	3	8	3
Dizziness	16	5	8	2
Alopecia	67	5	41	1
Rash/itch	12	1	9	0

Table 12 – Clinically Important Treatment Emergent Adverse Reactions (Regardless of Relationship) in Patients with SCCHN Receiving Induction Chemotherapy with TAXOTERE in Combination with cisplatin and fluorouracil followed by radiotherapy (TAX323) or chemoradiotherapy (TAX324)

Adverse Reaction (by Body System)	TAX323 (n=355)				TAX324 (n=494)			
	TAXOTERE arm (n=174)		Comparator arm (n=181)		TAXOTERE arm (n=251)		Comparator arm (n=243)	
	Any %	Grade 3/4 %	Any %	Grade 3/4 %	Any %	Grade 3/4 %	Any %	Grade 3/4 %
Neutropenia	93	76	87	53	95	84	84	56
Anemia	89	9	88	14	90	12	86	10
Thrombocytopenia	24	5	47	18	28	4	31	11
Infection	27	9	26	8	23	6	28	5
Febrile neutropenia*	5	N/A	2	N/A	12	N/A	7	N/A
Neutropenic infection	14	N/A	8	N/A	12	N/A	8	N/A
Cancer pain	21	5	16	3	17	9	20	11
Lethargy	41	3	38	3	61	5	56	10
Fever in the absence of infection	32	1	37	0	30	4	28	3
Myalgia	10	1	7	0	7	0	7	2
Weight loss	21	1	27	1	14	2	14	2
Allergy	6	0	3	0	2	0	0	0
Fluid retention†	20	0	14	1	13	1	7	2
Edema only	13	0	7	0	12	1	6	1
Weight gain only	6	0	6	0	0	0	1	0
Dizziness	2	0	5	1	16	4	15	2
Neurosensory	18	1	11	1	14	1	14	0
Altered hearing	6	0	10	3	13	1	19	3
Neuromotor	2	1	4	1	9	0	10	2
Alopecia	81	11	43	0	68	4	44	1
Rash/itch	12	0	6	0	20	0	16	1
Dry skin	6	0	2	0	5	0	3	0
Desquamation	4	1	6	0	2	0	5	0
Nausea	47	1	51	7	77	14	80	14
Stomatitis	43	4	47	11	66	21	68	27
Vomiting	26	1	39	5	56	8	63	10
Diarrhea	33	3	24	4	48	7	40	3
Constipation	17	1	16	1	27	1	38	1
Anorexia	16	1	25	3	40	12	34	12
Esophagitis/dysphagia/Odynophagia	13	1	18	3	25	13	26	10
Taste, sense of smell altered	10	0	5	0	20	0	17	1
Gastrointestinal pain/cramping	8	1	9	1	15	2	10	2
Heartburn	6	0	6	0	13	2	13	1
Gastrointestinal bleeding	4	2	0	0	5	1	2	1
Cardiac dysrhythmia	2	2	2	1	6	3	5	3
Venous‡	3	2	6	2	4	2	5	4
Ischemia myocardial	2	2	1	0	2	1	1	1
Tearing	2	0	1	0	2	0	2	0
Conjunctivitis	1	0	1	0	1	0	0.4	0
Nail changes	8	0	0	0				
Skin desquamation	2	0	0	0				
Nausea	73	16	76	19				
Vomiting	67	15	73	19				
Anorexia	51	13	54	12				
Stomatitis	59	21	61	27				
Diarrhea	78	20	50	8				
Constipation	25	2	34	3				
Esophagitis/dysphagia/odynophagia	16	2	14	5				
Gastrointestinal pain/cramping	11	2	7	3				
Cardiac dysrhythmias	5	2	2	1				
Myocardial ischemia	1	0	3	2				
Tearing	8	0	2	0				
Altered hearing	6	0	13	2				

Clinically important treatment emergent adverse reactions based upon frequency, severity, and clinical impact.
* Febrile neutropenia: grade ≥2 fever concomitant with grade 4 neutropenia requiring intravenous antibiotics and/or hospitalization.
† Related to treatment.
‡ Includes superficial and deep vein thrombosis and pulmonary embolism

Clinically important treatment emergent adverse reactions were determined based upon frequency, severity, and clinical impact of the adverse reaction.
* Related to treatment

Head and Neck Cancer

Combination therapy with TAXOTERE in head and neck cancer

Table 12 summarizes the safety data obtained from patients that received induction chemotherapy with TAXOTERE 75 mg/m² in combination with cisplatin and fluorouracil followed by radiotherapy (TAX323; 174 patients) or chemoradiotherapy (TAX324; 251 patients). The treatment regimens are described in Section 14.6.
[See table 12 at left]

6.2 Post-marketing Experiences

The following adverse reactions have been identified from clinical trials and/or post-marketing surveillance. Because they are reported from a population of unknown size, precise estimates of frequency cannot be made.

Body as a whole: diffuse pain, chest pain, radiation recall phenomenon.

Cardiovascular: atrial fibrillation, deep vein thrombosis, ECG abnormalities, thrombophlebitis, pulmonary embolism, syncope, tachycardia, myocardial infarction.

Cutaneous: very rare cases of cutaneous lupus erythematosus and rare cases of bullous eruptions such as erythema multiforme, Stevens-Johnson syndrome, toxic epidermal necrolysis, and Scleroderma-like changes usually preceded by peripheral lymphedema. In some cases multiple factors may have contributed to the development of these effects. Severe hand and foot syndrome has been reported.

Gastrointestinal: abdominal pain, anorexia, constipation, duodenal ulcer, esophagitis, gastrointestinal hemorrhage, gastrointestinal perforation, ischemic colitis, colitis, intestinal obstruction, ileus, neutropenic enterocolitis and dehydration as a consequence to gastrointestinal events have been reported.

Hematologic: bleeding episodes. Disseminated intravascular coagulation (DIC), often in association with sepsis or multiorgan failure, has been reported. Cases of acute myeloid leukemia and myelodysplasic syndrome have been reported in association with TAXOTERE when used in combination with other chemotherapy agents and/or radiotherapy.

Hypersensitivity: rare cases of anaphylactic shock have been reported. Very rarely these cases resulted in a fatal outcome in patients who received premedication.

Hepatic: rare cases of hepatitis, sometimes fatal primarily in patients with pre-existing liver disorders, have been reported.

Neurologic: confusion, rare cases of seizures or transient loss of consciousness have been observed, sometimes appearing during the infusion of the drug.

Ophthalmologic: conjunctivitis, lacrimation or lacrimation with or without conjunctivitis. Excessive tearing which may be attributable to lacrimal duct obstruction has been reported. Rare cases of transient visual disturbances (flashes, flashing lights, scotomata) typically occurring during drug infusion and in association with hypersensitivity reactions have been reported. These were reversible upon discontinuation of the infusion.

Hearing: rare cases of ototoxicity, hearing disorders and/or hearing loss have been reported, including cases associated with other ototoxic drugs.

Respiratory: dyspnea, acute pulmonary edema, acute respiratory distress syndrome, interstitial pneumonia. Pulmonary fibrosis has been rarely reported. Rare cases of radiation pneumonitis have been reported in patients receiving concomitant radiotherapy.

Renal: renal insufficiency and renal failure have been reported, the majority of these cases were associated with concomitant nephrotoxic drugs.

7. DRUG INTERACTIONS

Docetaxel is a CYP3A4 substrate. *In vitro* studies have shown that the metabolism of docetaxel may be modified by the concomitant administration of compounds that induce, inhibit, or are metabolized by cytochrome P450 3A4.

In vivo studies showed that the exposure of docetaxel increased 2.2-fold when it was coadministered with ketoconazole, a potent inhibitor of CYP3A4. Protease inhibitors, particularly ritonavir, may increase the exposure of docetaxel. Concomitant use of TAXOTERE and drugs that inhibit CYP3A4 may increase exposure to docetaxel and should be avoided. In patients receiving treatment with TAXOTERE, close monitoring for toxicity and a TAXOTERE dose reduction could be considered if systemic administration of a potent CYP3A4 inhibitor cannot be avoided *[see Dosage and Administration (2.7) and Clinical Pharmacology (12.3)]*.

8. USE IN SPECIFIC POPULATIONS

8.1 Pregnancy

Pregnancy Category D *[see 'Warnings and Precautions' section]*

Based on its mechanism of action and findings in animals, TAXOTERE can cause fetal harm when administered to a pregnant woman. If TAXOTERE is used during pregnancy, or if the patient becomes pregnant while receiving this drug, the patient should be apprised of the potential hazard to the fetus. Women of childbearing potential should be advised to avoid becoming pregnant during therapy with TAXOTERE.

TAXOTERE can cause fetal harm when administered to a pregnant woman. Studies in both rats and rabbits at doses ≥0.3 and 0.03 mg/kg/day, respectively (about 1/50 and 1/300 the daily maximum recommended human dose on a mg/m^2 basis), administered during the period of organogenesis, have shown that TAXOTERE is embryotoxic and fetotoxic (characterized by intrauterine mortality, increased resorption, reduced fetal weight, and fetal ossification delay). The doses indicated above also caused maternal toxicity.

8.3 Nursing Mothers

It is not known whether docetaxel is excreted in human milk. Because many drugs are excreted in human milk, and because of the potential for serious adverse reactions in nursing infants from TAXOTERE, a decision should be made whether to discontinue nursing or to discontinue the drug, taking into account the importance of the drug to the mother.

8.4 Pediatric Use

The efficacy of TAXOTERE in pediatric patients as monotherapy or in combination has not been established. The overall safety profile of TAXOTERE in pediatric patients receiving monotherapy or TCF was consistent with the known safety profile in adults. TAXOTERE has been studied in a total of 289 pediatric patients: 239 in 2 trials with monotherapy and 50 in combination treatment with cisplatin and 5-fluoruracil (TCF).

TAXOTERE Monotherapy

TAXOTERE monotherapy was evaluated in a dose-finding phase 1 trial in 61 pediatric patients (median age 12.5 years, range 1–22 years) with a variety of refractory solid tumors. The recommended dose was 125 mg/m^2 as a 1-hour intravenous infusion every 21 days. The primary dose limiting toxicity was neutropenia.

The recommended dose for TAXOTERE monotherapy was evaluated in a phase 2 single-arm trial in 178 pediatric patients (median age 12 years, range 1–26 years) with a variety of recurrent/refractory solid tumors. Efficacy was not established with tumor response rates ranging from one complete response (CR) (0.6%) in a patient with undifferentiated sarcoma to four partial responses (2.2%) seen in one patient each with Ewing Sarcoma, neuroblastoma, osteosarcoma, and squamous cell carcinoma.

TAXOTERE in Combination

TAXOTERE was studied in combination with cisplatin and 5-fluorouracil (TCF) versus cisplatin and 5-fluorouracil (CF) for the induction treatment of nasopharyngeal carcinoma (NPC) in pediatric patients prior to chemoradiation consolidation. Seventy-five patients (median age 16 years, range 9 to 21 years) were randomized (2:1) to TAXOTERE (75 mg/m^2) in combination with cisplatin (75 mg/m^2) and 5-fluorouracil (750 mg/m^2) (TCF) or to cisplatin (80 mg/m^2) and 5-fluorouracil (1000 mg/m^2/day) (CF). The primary endpoint was the CR rate following induction treatment of NPC. One patient out of 50 in the TCF group (2%) had a complete response while none of the 25 patients in the CF group had a complete response.

Pharmacokinetics:

Pharmacokinetic parameters for docetaxel were determined in 2 pediatric solid tumor trials. Following docetaxel administration at 55 mg/m^2 to 235 mg/m^2 in a 1-hour intravenous infusion every 3 weeks in 25 patients aged 1 to 20 years (median 11 years), docetaxel clearance was 17.3± 10.9 L/h/m^2.

Docetaxel was administered in combination with cisplatin and 5-fluorouracil (TCF), at dose levels of 75 mg/m^2 in a 1-hour intravenous infusion day 1 in 28 patients aged 10 to 21 years (median 16 years, 17 patients were older than 16). Docetaxel clearance was 17.9±8.75 L/h/m^2, corresponding to an AUC of 4.20±2.57 µg•h/mL.

In summary, the body surface area adjusted clearance of docetaxel monotherapy and TCF combination in children were comparable to those in adults *[see Clinical Pharmacology (12.3)]*.

8.5 Geriatric Use

In general, dose selection for an elderly patient should be cautious, reflecting the greater frequency of decreased hepatic, renal, or cardiac function and of concomitant disease or other drug therapy in elderly patients.

Non-Small Cell Lung Cancer

In a study conducted in chemotherapy-naïve patients with NSCLC (TAX326), 148 patients (36%) in the TAXOTERE+cisplatin group were 65 years of age or greater. There were 128 patients (32%) in the vinorelbine+ cisplatin group 65 years of age or greater. In the TAXOTERE+cisplatin group, patients less than 65 years of age had a median survival of 10.3 months (95% CI: 9.1 months, 11.8 months) and patients 65 years or older had a median survival of 12.1 months (95% CI: 9.3 months, 14 months). In patients 65 years of age or greater treated with TAXOTERE+cisplatin, diarrhea (55%), peripheral edema (39%) and stomatitis (28%) were observed more frequently than in the vinorelbine+cisplatin group (diarrhea 24%, peripheral edema 20%, stomatitis 20%). Patients treated with TAXOTERE+cisplatin who were 65 years of age or greater were more likely to experience diarrhea (55%), infections (42%), peripheral edema (39%) and stomatitis (28%) compared to patients less than the age of 65 administered the same treatment (43%, 31%, 31% and 21%, respectively).

When TAXOTERE was combined with carboplatin for the treatment of chemotherapy-naïve, advanced non-small cell lung carcinoma, patients 65 years of age or greater (28%) experienced higher frequency of infection compared to similar patients treated with TAXOTERE+cisplatin, and a higher frequency of diarrhea, infection and peripheral edema than elderly patients treated with vinorelbine+cisplatin.

Prostate Cancer

Of the 333 patients treated with TAXOTERE every three weeks plus prednisone in the prostate cancer study (TAX327), 209 patients were 65 years of age or greater and 68 patients were older than 75 years. In patients treated with TAXOTERE every three weeks, the following treatment emergent adverse reactions occurred at rates ≥10% higher in patients 65 years of age or greater compared to younger patients: anemia (71% vs. 59%), infection (37% vs. 24%), nail changes (34% vs. 23%), anorexia (21% vs. 10%), weight loss (15% vs. 5%) respectively.

Breast Cancer

In the adjuvant breast cancer trial (TAX316), TAXOTERE in combination with doxorubicin and cyclophosphamide was administered to 744 patients of whom 48 (6%) were 65 years of age or greater. The number of elderly patients who received this regimen was not sufficient to determine whether there were differences in safety and efficacy between elderly and younger patients.

Gastric Cancer

Among the 221 patients treated with TAXOTERE in combination with cisplatin and fluorouracil in the gastric cancer study, 54 were 65 years of age or older and 2 patients were older than 75 years. In this study, the number of patients who were 65 years of age or older was insufficient to determine whether they respond differently from younger patients. However, the incidence of serious adverse reactions was higher in the elderly patients compared to younger patients. The incidence of the following adverse reactions (all grades, regardless of relationship): lethargy, stomatitis, diarrhea, dizziness, edema, febrile neutropenia/neutropenic infection occurred at rates ≥10% higher in patients who were 65 years of age or older compared to younger patients. Elderly patients treated with TCF should be closely monitored.

Head and Neck Cancer

Among the 174 and 251 patients who received the induction treatment with TAXOTERE in combination with cisplatin and fluorouracil (TPF) for SCCHN in the TAX323 and TAX324 studies, 18 (10%) and 32 (13%) of the patients were 65 years of age or older, respectively.

These clinical studies of TAXOTERE in combination with cisplatin and fluorouracil in patients with SCCHN did not include sufficient numbers of patients aged 65 and over to determine whether they respond differently from younger patients. Other reported clinical experience with this treatment regimen has not identified differences in responses between elderly and younger patients.

8.6 Hepatic Impairment

Patients with bilirubin >ULN should not receive TAXOTERE. Also, patients with AST and/or ALT >1.5 × ULN concomitant with alkaline phosphatase >2.5 × ULN should not receive TAXOTERE *[see Boxed Warning, Warnings and Precautions (5.2), Clinical Pharmacology (12.3)]*.

10. OVERDOSAGE

There is no known antidote for TAXOTERE overdosage. In case of overdosage, the patient should be kept in a specialized unit where vital functions can be closely monitored. Anticipated complications of overdosage include: bone marrow suppression, peripheral neurotoxicity, and mucositis. Patients should receive therapeutic G-CSF as soon as possible after discovery of overdose. Other appropriate symptomatic measures should be taken, as needed.

In two reports of overdose, one patient received 150 mg/m^2 and the other received 200 mg/m^2 as 1-hour infusions. Both patients experienced severe neutropenia, mild asthenia, cutaneous reactions, and mild paresthesia, and recovered without incident.

In mice, lethality was observed following single intravenous doses that were ≥154 mg/kg (about 4.5 times the human dose of 100 mg/m^2 on a mg/m^2 basis); neurotoxicity associated with paralysis, non-extension of hind limbs, and myelin degeneration was observed in mice at 48 mg/kg (about 1.5 times the human dose of 100 mg/m^2 basis). In male and female rats, lethality was observed at a dose of 20 mg/kg (comparable to the human dose of 100 mg/m^2 on a mg/m^2 basis) and was associated with abnormal mitosis and necrosis of multiple organs.

11. DESCRIPTION

Docetaxel is an antineoplastic agent belonging to the taxoid family. It is prepared by semisynthesis beginning with a precursor extracted from the renewable needle biomass of yew plants. The chemical name for docetaxel is (2R,3S)-N-carboxy-3-phenylisoserine,N-*tert*-butyl ester, 13-ester with 5β-20-epoxy-1,2α,4,7β,10β,13α-hexahydroxytax-11-en-9-one 4-acetate 2-benzoate, trihydrate. Docetaxel has the following structural formula:

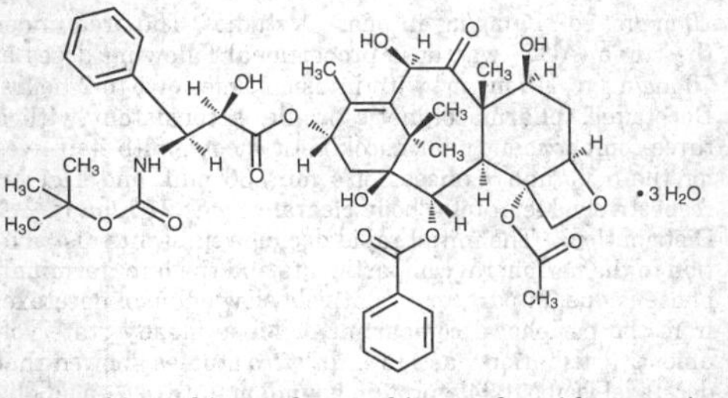

Docetaxel is a white to almost-white powder with an empirical formula of $C_{43}H_{53}NO_{14}$• $3H_2O$, and a molecular weight of 861.9. It is highly lipophilic and practically insoluble in water.

Two-vial formulation (Injection Concentrate and Diluent)

TAXOTERE (docetaxel) Injection Concentrate is a clear yellow to brownish-yellow viscous solution. TAXOTERE is sterile, non-pyrogenic, and is available in single-dose vials containing 20 mg (0.5 mL) or 80 mg (2 mL) docetaxel (anhydrous). Each mL contains 40 mg docetaxel (anhydrous) and 1040 mg polysorbate 80.

TAXOTERE Injection Concentrate requires dilution with Diluent prior to addition to the infusion bag. A sterile, non-pyrogenic, single-dose diluent is supplied for that purpose. The diluent for TAXOTERE contains 13% ethanol in water for injection, and is supplied in vials.

12. CLINICAL PHARMACOLOGY

12.1 Mechanism of Action

Docetaxel is an antineoplastic agent that acts by disrupting the microtubular network in cells that is essential for mitotic and interphase cellular functions. Docetaxel binds to free tubulin and promotes the assembly of tubulin into stable microtubules while simultaneously inhibiting their disassembly. This leads to the production of microtubule bundles without normal function and to the stabilization of microtubules, which results in the inhibition of mitosis in cells. Docetaxel's binding to microtubules does not alter the number of protofilaments in the bound microtubules, a feature which differs from most spindle poisons currently in clinical use.

12.3 Human Pharmacokinetics

Absorption: The pharmacokinetics of docetaxel have been evaluated in cancer patients after administration of

Table 13 - Efficacy of TAXOTERE in the Treatment of Breast Cancer Patients Previously Treated with an Anthracycline-Containing Regimen (Intent-to-Treat Analysis)

Efficacy Parameter	Docetaxel (n=203)	Mitomycin/Vinblastine (n=189)	p-value
Median Survival	11.4 months	8.7 months	
Risk Ratio*, Mortality (Docetaxel: Control) 95% CI (Risk Ratio)	0.73 0.58–0.93		p=0.01 Log Rank
Median Time to Progression	4.3 months	2.5 months	
Risk Ratio*, Progression (Docetaxel: Control) 95% CI (Risk Ratio)	0.75 0.61–0.94		p=0.01 Log Rank
Overall Response Rate Complete Response Rate	28.1% 3.4%	9.5% 1.6%	p<0.0001 Chi Square

* For the risk ratio, a value less than 1.00 favors docetaxel.

Table 14 - Efficacy of TAXOTERE in the Treatment of Breast Cancer Patients Previously Treated with an Alkylating-Containing Regimen (Intent-to-Treat Analysis)

Efficacy Parameter	Docetaxel (n=161)	Doxorubicin (n=165)	p-value
Median Survival	14.7 months	14.3 months	
Risk Ratio*, Mortality (Docetaxel: Control) 95% CI (Risk Ratio)	0.89 0.68–1.16		p=0.39 Log Rank
Median Time to Progression	6.5 months	5.3 months	
Risk Ratio*, Progression (Docetaxel: Control) 95% CI (Risk Ratio)	0.93 0.71–1.16		p=0.45 Log Rank
Overall Response Rate Complete Response Rate	45.3% 6.8%	29.7% 4.2%	p=0.004 Chi Square

* For the risk ratio, a value less than 1.00 favors docetaxel.

20 mg/m^2 to 115 mg/m^2 in phase 1 studies. The area under the curve (AUC) was dose proportional following doses of 70 mg/m^2 to 115 mg/m^2 with infusion times of 1 to 2 hours. Docetaxel's pharmacokinetic profile is consistent with a three-compartment pharmacokinetic model, with half-lives for the α, β, and γ phases of 4 min, 36 min, and 11.1 hr, respectively. Mean total body clearance was 21 L/h/m².
Distribution: The initial rapid decline represents distribution to the peripheral compartments and the late (terminal) phase is due, in part, to a relatively slow efflux of docetaxel from the peripheral compartment. Mean steady state volume of distribution was 113 L. In vitro studies showed that docetaxel is about 94% protein bound, mainly to α_1-acid glycoprotein, albumin, and lipoproteins. In three cancer patients, the in vitro binding to plasma proteins was found to be approximately 97%. Dexamethasone does not affect the protein binding of docetaxel.
Metabolism: In vitro drug interaction studies revealed that docetaxel is metabolized by the CYP3A4 isoenzyme, and its metabolism may be modified by the concomitant administration of compounds that induce, inhibit, or are metabolized by cytochrome P450 3A4 [see Drug Interactions (7)].
Elimination: A study of ¹⁴C-docetaxel was conducted in three cancer patients. Docetaxel was eliminated in both the urine and feces following oxidative metabolism of the tert-butyl ester group, but fecal excretion was the main elimination route. Within 7 days, urinary and fecal excretion accounted for approximately 6% and 75% of the administered radioactivity, respectively. About 80% of the radioactivity recovered in feces is excreted during the first 48 hours as 1 major and 3 minor metabolites with very small amounts (less than 8%) of unchanged drug.
Effect of Age: A population pharmacokinetic analysis was carried out after TAXOTERE treatment of 535 patients dosed at 100 mg/m^2. Pharmacokinetic parameters estimated by this analysis were very close to those estimated from phase 1 studies. The pharmacokinetics of docetaxel were not influenced by age.
Effect of Gender: The population pharmacokinetics analysis described above also indicated that gender did not influence the pharmacokinetics of docetaxel.
Hepatic Impairment: The population pharmacokinetic analysis described above indicated that in patients with clinical chemistry data suggestive of mild to moderate liver impairment (AST and/or ALT >1.5 times ULN concomitant with alkaline phosphatase >2.5 times ULN), total body clearance was lowered by an average of 27%, resulting in a 38% increase in systemic exposure (AUC). This average, however, includes a substantial range and there is, at present, no measurement that would allow recommendation for dose adjustment in such patients. Patients with combined abnormalities of transaminase and alkaline phosphatase should not be treated with TAXOTERE. Patients with severe hepatic impairment have not been studied. [see Warnings and Precautions (5.2) and Use in Specific Populations (8.6)]
Effect of Race: Mean total body clearance for Japanese patients dosed at the range of 10 mg/m^2 to 90 mg/m^2 was similar to that of European/American populations dosed at 100 mg/m^2, suggesting no significant difference in the elimination of docetaxel in the two populations.
Effect of Ketoconazole: The effect of ketoconazole (a strong CYP3A4 inhibitor) on the pharmacokinetics of docetaxel was investigated in 7 cancer patients. Patients were randomized to receive either docetaxel (100 mg/m^2 intravenous) alone or docetaxel (10 mg/m^2 intravenous) in combination with ketoconazole (200 mg orally once daily for 3 days) in a crossover design with a 3-week washout period. The results of this study indicated that the mean dose-normalized AUC of docetaxel was increased 2.2-fold and its clearance was reduced by 49% when docetaxel was co-administration with ketoconazole [see Dosage and Administration (2.7) and Drug-Drug Interactions (7)].
Effect of Combination Therapies:
• Dexamethasone: Docetaxel total body clearance was not modified by pretreatment with dexamethasone.
• Cisplatin: Clearance of docetaxel in combination therapy with cisplatin was similar to that previously observed following monotherapy with docetaxel. The pharmacokinetic profile of cisplatin in combination therapy with docetaxel was similar to that observed with cisplatin alone.
• Cisplatin and Fluorouracil: The combined administration of docetaxel, cisplatin and fluorouracil in 12 patients with solid tumors had no influence on the pharmacokinetics of each individual drug.
• Prednisone: A population pharmacokinetic analysis of plasma data from 40 patients with hormone-refractory metastatic prostate cancer indicated that docetaxel systemic clearance in combination with prednisone is similar to that observed following administration of docetaxel alone.

• Cyclophosphamide and Doxorubicin: A study was conducted in 30 patients with advanced breast cancer to determine the potential for drug-drug-interactions between docetaxel (75 mg/m^2), doxorubicin (50 mg/m^2), and cyclophosphamide (500 mg/m^2) when administered in combination. The coadministration of docetaxel had no effect on the pharmacokinetics of doxorubicin and cyclophosphamide when the three drugs were given in combination compared to coadministration of doxorubicin and cyclophosphamide only. In addition, doxorubicin and cyclophosphamide had no effect on docetaxel plasma clearance when the three drugs were given in combination compared to historical data for docetaxel monotherapy.

13. NONCLINICAL TOXICOLOGY
13.1 Carcinogenesis, Mutagenesis, Impairment of Fertility
Carcinogenicity studies with docetaxel have not been performed.
Docetaxel was clastogenic in the in vitro chromosome aberration test in CHO-K₁ cells and in the in vivo micronucleus test in mice administered doses of 0.39 to 1.56 mg/kg (about 1/60th to 1/15th the recommended human dose on a mg/m² basis). Docetaxel was not mutagenic in the Ames test or the CHO/HGPRT gene mutation assays.
Docetaxel did not reduce fertility in rats when administered in multiple intravenous doses of up to 0.3 mg/kg (about 1/50th the recommended human dose on a mg/m² basis), but decreased testicular weights were reported. This correlates with findings of a 10-cycle toxicity study (dosing once every 21 days for 6 months) in rats and dogs in which testicular atrophy or degeneration was observed at intravenous doses of 5 mg/kg in rats and 0.375 mg/kg in dogs (about 1/3rd and 1/15th the recommended human dose on a mg/m² basis, respectively). An increased frequency of dosing in rats produced similar effects at lower dose levels.

14. CLINICAL STUDIES
14.1 Locally Advanced or Metastatic Breast Cancer
The efficacy and safety of TAXOTERE have been evaluated in locally advanced or metastatic breast cancer after failure of previous chemotherapy (alkylating agent-containing regimens or anthracycline-containing regimens).
Randomized Trials
In one randomized trial, patients with a history of prior treatment with an anthracycline-containing regimen were assigned to treatment with TAXOTERE (100 mg/m^2 every 3 weeks) or the combination of mitomycin (12 mg/m^2 every 6 weeks) and vinblastine (6 mg/m^2 every 3 weeks). Two hundred three patients were randomized to TAXOTERE and 189 to the comparator arm. Most patients had received prior chemotherapy for metastatic disease; only 27 patients on the TAXOTERE arm and 33 patients on the comparator arm entered the study following relapse after adjuvant therapy. Three-quarters of patients had measurable, visceral metastases. The primary endpoint was time to progression. The following table summarizes the study results (See Table 13).
[See table 13 above]
In a second randomized trial, patients previously treated with an alkylating-containing regimen were assigned to treatment with TAXOTERE (100 mg/m^2) or doxorubicin (75 mg/m^2) every 3 weeks. One hundred sixty-one patients were randomized to TAXOTERE and 165 patients to doxorubicin. Approximately one-half of patients had received prior chemotherapy for metastatic disease, and one-half entered the study following relapse after adjuvant therapy. Three-quarters of patients had measurable, visceral metastases. The primary endpoint was time to progression. The study results are summarized below (See Table 14).
[See table 14 above]
In another multicenter open-label, randomized trial (TAX313), in the treatment of patients with advanced breast cancer who progressed or relapsed after one prior chemotherapy regimen, 527 patients were randomized to receive TAXOTERE monotherapy 60 mg/m^2 (n=151), 75 mg/m^2 (n=188) or 100 mg/m^2 (n=188). In this trial, 94% of patients had metastatic disease and 79% had received prior anthracycline therapy. Response rate was the primary endpoint. Response rates increased with TAXOTERE dose: 19.9% for the 60 mg/m^2 group compared to 22.3% for the 75 mg/m^2 and 29.8% for the 100 mg/m^2 group; pair-wise comparison between the 60 mg/m^2 and 100 mg/m^2 groups was statistically significant (p=0.037).
Single Arm Studies
TAXOTERE at a dose of 100 mg/m^2 was studied in six single arm studies involving a total of 309 patients with metastatic breast cancer in whom previous chemotherapy had failed. Among these, 190 patients had anthracycline-resistant breast cancer, defined as progression during an anthracycline-containing chemotherapy regimen for metastatic disease, or relapse during an anthracycline-containing adjuvant regimen. In anthracycline-resistant patients, the overall response rate was 37.9% (72/190; 95% C.I.: 31.0–44.8) and the complete response rate was 2.1%.

TAXOTERE was also studied in three single arm Japanese studies at a dose of 60 mg/m², in 174 patients who had received prior chemotherapy for locally advanced or metastatic breast cancer. Among 26 patients whose best response to an anthracycline had been progression, the response rate was 34.6% (95% C.I.: 17.2–55.7), similar to the response rate in single arm studies of 100 mg/m².

14.2   Adjuvant Treatment of Breast Cancer

A multicenter, open-label, randomized trial (TAX316) evaluated the efficacy and safety of TAXOTERE for the adjuvant treatment of patients with axillary-node-positive breast cancer and no evidence of distant metastatic disease. After stratification according to the number of positive lymph nodes (1–3, 4+), 1491 patients were randomized to receive either TAXOTERE 75 mg/m² administered 1-hour after doxorubicin 50 mg/m² and cyclophosphamide 500 mg/m² (TAC arm), or doxorubicin 50 mg/m² followed by fluorouracil 500 mg/m² and cyclophosphamide 500 mg/m² (FAC arm). Both regimens were administered every 3 weeks for 6 cycles. TAXOTERE was administered as a 1-hour infusion; all other drugs were given as intravenous bolus on day 1. In both arms, after the last cycle of chemotherapy, patients with positive estrogen and/or progesterone receptors received tamoxifen 20 mg daily for up to 5 years. Adjuvant radiation therapy was prescribed according to guidelines in place at participating institutions and was given to 69% of patients who received TAC and 72% of patients who received FAC.

Results from a second interim analysis (median follow-up 55 months) are as follows: In study TAX316, the docetaxel-containing combination regimen TAC showed significantly longer disease-free survival (DFS) than FAC (hazard ratio=0.74; 2-sided 95% CI=0.60, 0.92, stratified log rank p=0.0047). The primary endpoint, disease-free survival, included local and distant recurrences, contralateral breast cancer and deaths from any cause. The overall reduction in risk of relapse was 25.7% for TAC-treated patients. (See Figure 1).

At the time of this interim analysis, based on 219 deaths, overall survival was longer for TAC than FAC (hazard ratio=0.69, 2-sided 95% CI=0.53, 0.90). (See Figure 2). There will be further analysis at the time survival data mature.

Figure 1 - TAX316 Disease Free Survival K-M curve

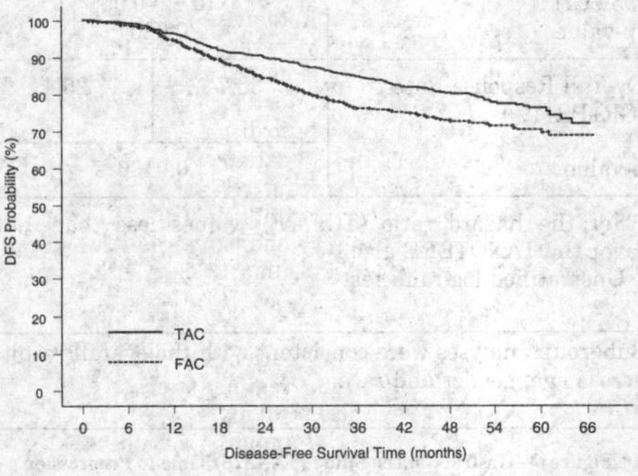

Figure 2 - TAX316 Overall Survival K-M Curve

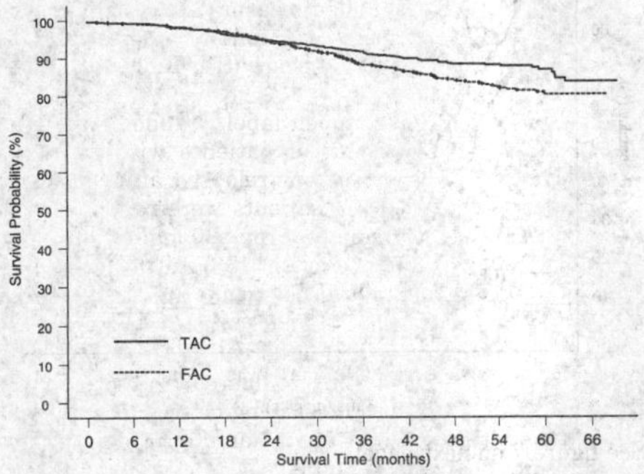

The following table describes the results of subgroup analyses for DFS and OS (See Table 15).
[See table 15 above]

14.3   Non-Small Cell Lung Cancer (NSCLC)

The efficacy and safety of TAXOTERE has been evaluated in patients with unresectable, locally advanced or metastatic non-small cell lung cancer whose disease has failed prior platinum-based chemotherapy or in patients who are chemotherapy-naïve.

Table 15 - Subset Analyses-Adjuvant Breast Cancer Study

Patient subset	Number of patients	Disease Free Survival		Overall Survival	
		Hazard ratio*	95% CI	Hazard ratio*	95% CI
No. of positive nodes					
Overall	744	0.74	(0.60, 0.92)	0.69	(0.53, 0.90)
1–3	467	0.64	(0.47, 0.87)	0.45	(0.29, 0.70)
4+	277	0.84	(0.63, 1.12)	0.93	(0.66, 1.32)
Receptor status					
Positive	566	0.76	(0.59, 0.98)	0.69	(0.48, 0.99)
Negative	178	0.68	(0.48, 0.97)	0.66	(0.44, 0.98)

* a hazard ratio of less than 1 indicates that TAC is associated with a longer disease free survival or overall survival compared to FAC.

Table 16 - Efficacy of TAXOTERE in the Treatment of Non-Small Cell Lung Cancer Patients Previously Treated with a Platinum-Based Chemotherapy Regimen (Intent-to-Treat Analysis)

	TAX317		TAX320	
	Docetaxel 75 mg/m² n=55	Best Supportive Care n=49	Docetaxel 75 mg/m² n=125	Control (V/I*) n=123
Overall Survival Log-rank Test	p=0.01		p=0.13	
Risk Ratio†, Mortality (Docetaxel: Control) 95% CI (Risk Ratio)	0.56 (0.35, 0.88)		0.82 (0.63, 1.06)	
Median Survival 95% CI	7.5 months‡ (5.5, 12.8)	4.6 months (3.7, 6.1)	5.7 months (5.1, 7.1)	5.6 months (4.4, 7.9)
% 1-year Survival 95% CI	37%‡§ (24, 50)	12% (2, 23)	30%‡§ (22, 39)	20% (13, 27)
Time to Progression 95% CI	12.3 weeks‡ (9.0, 18.3)	7.0 weeks (6.0, 9.3)	8.3 weeks (7.0, 11.7)	7.6 weeks (6.7, 10.1)
Response Rate 95% CI	5.5% (1.1, 15.1)	Not Applicable	5.7% (2.3, 11.3)	0.8% (0.0, 4.5)

* Vinorelbine/Ifosfamide
† a value less than 1.00 favors docetaxel.
‡ p≤0.05;
§ uncorrected for multiple comparisons;

Monotherapy with TAXOTERE for NSCLC Previously Treated with Platinum-Based Chemotherapy

Two randomized, controlled trials established that a TAXOTERE dose of 75 mg/m² was tolerable and yielded a favorable outcome in patients previously treated with platinum-based chemotherapy (see below). TAXOTERE at a dose of 100 mg/m², however, was associated with unacceptable hematologic toxicity, infections, and treatment-related mortality and this dose should not be used [see Boxed Warning, Dosage and Administration (2.7), Warnings and Precautions (5.3)].

One trial (TAX317), randomized patients with locally advanced or metastatic non-small cell lung cancer, a history of prior platinum-based chemotherapy, no history of taxane exposure, and an ECOG performance status ≤2 to TAXOTERE or best supportive care. The primary endpoint of the study was survival. Patients were initially randomized to TAXOTERE 100 mg/m² or best supportive care, but early toxic deaths at this dose led to a dose reduction to TAXOTERE 75 mg/m². A total of 104 patients were randomized in this amended study to either TAXOTERE 75 mg/m² or best supportive care.

In a second randomized trial (TAX320), 373 patients with locally advanced or metastatic non-small cell lung cancer, a history of prior platinum-based chemotherapy, and an ECOG performance status ≤2 were randomized to TAXOTERE 75 mg/m², TAXOTERE 100 mg/m² and a treatment in which the investigator chose either vinorelbine 30 mg/m² days 1, 8, and 15 repeated every 3 weeks or ifosfamide 2 g/m² days 1–3 repeated every 3 weeks. Forty percent of the patients in this study had a history of prior paclitaxel exposure. The primary endpoint was survival in both trials. The efficacy data for the TAXOTERE 75 mg/m² arm and the comparator arms are summarized in Table 16 and Figures 3 and 4 showing the survival curves for the two studies.

[See table 16 above]

Only one of the two trials (TAX317) showed a clear effect on survival, the primary endpoint; that trial also showed an increased rate of survival to one year. In the second study (TAX320) the rate of survival at one year favored TAXOTERE 75 mg/m².

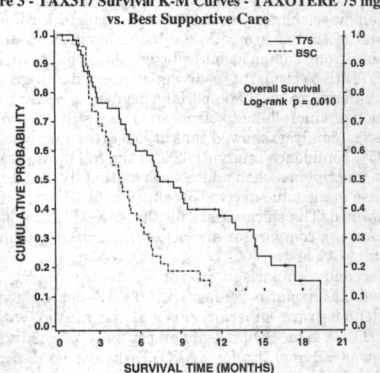

Figure 3 - TAX317 Survival K-M Curves - TAXOTERE 75 mg/m² vs. Best Supportive Care

[See figure 4 on next page]

Patients treated with TAXOTERE at a dose of 75 mg/m² experienced no deterioration in performance status and body weight relative to the comparator arms used in these trials.

Combination Therapy with TAXOTERE for Chemotherapy-Naïve NSCLC

In a randomized controlled trial (TAX326), 1218 patients with unresectable stage IIIB or IV NSCLC and no prior chemotherapy were randomized to receive one of three treatments: TAXOTERE 75 mg/m² as a 1 hour infusion immediately followed by cisplatin 75 mg/m² over 30 to 60 minutes every 3 weeks; vinorelbine 25 mg/m² administered over

Table 17 - Survival Analysis of TAXOTERE in Combination Therapy for Chemotherapy-Naïve NSCLC

Comparison †	Taxotere+Cisplatin n=408	Vinorelbine+Cisplatin n=405
Kaplan-Meier Estimate of Median Survival	10.9 months	10.0 months
p-value*	0.122	
Estimated Hazard Ratio†	0.88	
Adjusted 95% CI‡	(0.74, 1.06)	

* From the superiority test (stratified log rank) comparing TAXOTERE+cisplatin to vinorelbine+cisplatin
† Hazard ratio of TAXOTERE+cisplatin vs. vinorelbine+cisplatin. A hazard ratio of less than 1 indicates that TAXOTERE+cisplatin is associated with a longer survival.
‡ Adjusted for interim analysis and multiple comparisons.

Table 18 - Response and TTP Analysis of TAXOTERE in Combination Therapy for Chemotherapy-Naïve NSCLC

Endpoint	TAXOTERE+Cisplatin	Vinorelbine+Cisplatin	p-value
Objective Response Rate (95% CI)*	31.6% (26.5%, 36.8%)	24.4% (19.8%, 29.2%)	Not Significant
Median Time to Progression† (95% CI)*	21.4 weeks (19.3, 24.6)	22.1 weeks (18.1, 25.6)	Not Significant

* Adjusted for multiple comparisons.
† Kaplan-Meier estimates.

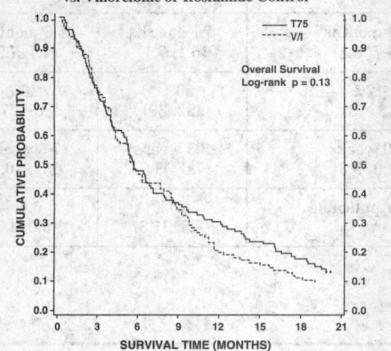

Figure 4 - TAX320 Survival K-M Curves - TAXOTERE 75 mg/m² vs. Vinorelbine or Ifosfamide Control

6–10 minutes on days 1, 8, 15, 22 followed by cisplatin 100 mg/m² administered on day 1 of cycles repeated every 4 weeks; or a combination of TAXOTERE and carboplatin. The primary efficacy endpoint was overall survival. Treatment with TAXOTERE+cisplatin did not result in a statistically significantly superior survival compared to vinorelbine+cisplatin (see table below). The 95% confidence interval of the hazard ratio (adjusted for interim analysis and multiple comparisons) shows that the addition of TAXOTERE to cisplatin results in an outcome ranging from a 6% inferior to a 26% superior survival compared to the addition of vinorelbine to cisplatin. The results of a further statistical analysis showed that at least (the lower bound of the 95% confidence interval) 62% of the known survival effect of vinorelbine when added to cisplatin (about a 2-month increase in median survival; Wozniak et al. JCO, 1998) was maintained. The efficacy data for the TAXOTERE+cisplatin arm and the comparator arm are summarized in Table 17. [See table 17 above]

The second comparison in the same three-arm study, vinorelbine+cisplatin versus TAXOTERE+carboplatin, did not demonstrate superior survival associated with the TAXOTERE arm (Kaplan-Meier estimate of median survival was 9.1 months for TAXOTERE +carboplatin compared to 10.0 months on the vinorelbine+cisplatin arm) and the TAXOTERE+carboplatin arm did not demonstrate preservation of at least 50% of the survival effect of vinorelbine added to cisplatin. Secondary endpoints evaluated in the trial included objective response and time to progression. There was no statistically significant difference between TAXOTERE+cisplatin and vinorelbine+cisplatin with respect to objective response and time to progression (see Table 18). [See table 18 above]

14.4   Hormone Refractory Prostate Cancer
The safety and efficacy of TAXOTERE in combination with prednisone in patients with androgen independent (hormone refractory) metastatic prostate cancer were evaluated in a randomized multicenter active control trial. A total of 1006 patients with Karnofsky Performance Status (KPS) ≥60 were randomized to the following treatment groups:
• TAXOTERE 75 mg/m² every 3 weeks for 10 cycles.
• TAXOTERE 30 mg/m² administered weekly for the first 5 weeks in a 6-week cycle for 5 cycles.
• Mitoxantrone 12 mg/m² every 3 weeks for 10 cycles.
All 3 regimens were administered in combination with prednisone 5 mg twice daily, continuously.
In the TAXOTERE every three week arm, a statistically significant overall survival advantage was demonstrated compared to mitoxantrone. In the TAXOTERE weekly arm, no overall survival advantage was demonstrated compared to the mitoxantrone control arm. Efficacy results for the TAXOTERE every 3 week arm versus the control arm are summarized in Table 19 and Figure 5.

Table 19 - Efficacy of TAXOTERE in the Treatment of Patients with Androgen Independent (Hormone Refractory) Metastatic Prostate Cancer (Intent-to-Treat Analysis)

	TAXOTERE + Prednisone every 3 weeks	Mitoxantrone + Prednisone every 3 weeks
Number of patients	335	337
Median survival (months)	18.9	16.5
95% CI	(17.0–21.2)	(14.4–18.6)
Hazard ratio	0.761	–
95% CI	(0.619–0.936)	–
p-value*	0.0094	–

* Stratified log rank test. Threshold for statistical significance = 0.0175 because of 3 arms.

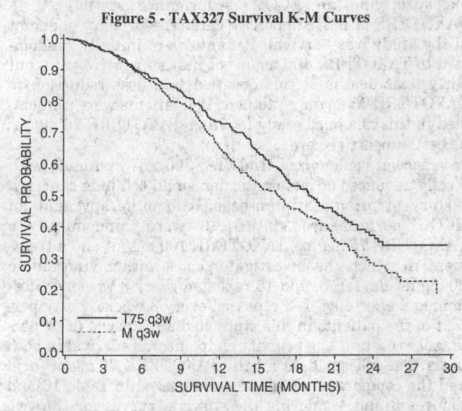

Figure 5 - TAX327 Survival K-M Curves

14.5   Gastric Adenocarcinoma
A multicenter, open-label, randomized trial was conducted to evaluate the safety and efficacy of TAXOTERE for the treatment of patients with advanced gastric adenocarcinoma, including adenocarcinoma of the gastroesophageal junction, who had not received prior chemotherapy for advanced disease. A total of 445 patients with KPS >70 were treated with either TAXOTERE (T) (75 mg/m² on day 1) in combination with cisplatin (C) (75 mg/m² on day 1) and fluorouracil (F) (750 mg/m² per day for 5 days) or cisplatin (100 mg/m² on day 1) and fluorouracil (1000 mg/m² per day for 5 days). The length of a treatment cycle was 3 weeks for the TCF arm and 4 weeks for the CF arm. The demographic characteristics were balanced between the two treatment arms. The median age was 55 years, 71% were male, 71% were Caucasian, 24% were 65 years of age or older, 19% had a prior curative surgery and 12% had palliative surgery. The median number of cycles administered per patient was 6 (with a range of 1–16) for the TCF arm compared to 4 (with a range of 1–12) for the CF arm. Time to progression (TTP) was the primary endpoint and was defined as time from randomization to disease progression or death from any cause within 12 weeks of the last evaluable tumor assessment or within 12 weeks of the first infusion of study drugs for patients with no evaluable tumor assessment after randomization. The hazard ratio (HR) for TTP was 1.47 (CF/TCF, 95% CI: 1.19–1.83) with a significantly longer TTP (p=0.0004) in the TCF arm. Approximately 75% of patients had died at the time of this analysis. Overall survival was significantly longer (p=0.0201) in the TCF arm with a HR of 1.29 (95% CI: 1.04–1.61). Efficacy results are summarized in Table 20 and Figures 6 and 7.

Table 20 - Efficacy of TAXOTERE in the treatment of patients with gastric adenocarcinoma

Endpoint	TCF n=221	CF n=224
Median TTP (months) (95%CI)	5.6 (4.86–5.91)	3.7 (3.45–4.47)
Hazard ratio* (95%CI)	0.68 (0.55–0.84)	
†p-value	0.0004	
Median survival (months) (95%CI)	9.2 (8.38–10.58)	8.6 (7.16–9.46)
Hazard ratio* (95%CI)	0.77 (0.62–0.96)	
†p-value	0.0201	
Overall Response Rate (CR+PR) (%)	36.7	25.4
p-value	0.0106	

* For the hazard ratio (TCF/CF), values less than 1.00 favor the TAXOTERE arm.
† Unstratified log-rank test

Subgroup analyses were consistent with the overall results across age, gender and race.

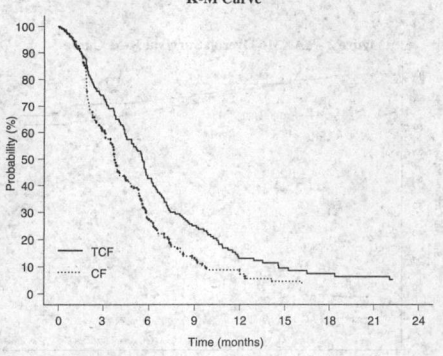

Figure 6 - Gastric Cancer Study (TAX325) Time to Progression K-M Curve

[See figure 7 on next page]

14.6   Head and Neck Cancer
Induction chemotherapy followed by radiotherapy (TAX323) The safety and efficacy of TAXOTERE in the induction treatment of patients with squamous cell carcinoma of the head and neck (SCCHN) was evaluated in a multicenter, open-label, randomized trial (TAX323). In this study, 358 patients with inoperable locally advanced SCCHN, and WHO performance status 0 or 1, were randomized to one of two treatment arms. Patients on the TAXOTERE arm received TAXOTERE (T) 75 mg/m² followed by cisplatin (P)

Figure 7 - Gastric Cancer Study (TAX325) Survival K-M Curve

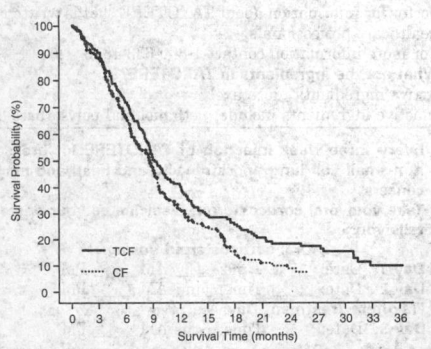

75 mg/m^2 on Day 1, followed by fluorouracil (F) 750 mg/m^2 per day as a continuous infusion on Days 1–5. The cycles were repeated every three weeks for 4 cycles. Patients whose disease did not progress received radiotherapy (RT) according to institutional guidelines (TPF/RT). Patients on the comparator arm received cisplatin (P) 100 mg/m^2 on Day 1, followed by fluorouracil (F) 1000 mg/m^2/day as a continuous infusion on Days 1–5. The cycles were repeated every three weeks for 4 cycles. Patients whose disease did not progress received RT according to institutional guidelines (PF/RT). At the end of chemotherapy, with a minimal interval of 4 weeks and a maximal interval of 7 weeks, patients whose disease did not progress received radiotherapy (RT) according to institutional guidelines. Locoregional therapy with radiation was delivered either with a conventional fraction regimen (1.8 Gy–2.0 Gy once a day, 5 days per week for a total dose of 66 to 70 Gy) or with an accelerated/hyperfractionated regimen (twice a day, with a minimum interfraction interval of 6 hours, 5 days per week, for a total dose of 70 to 74 Gy, respectively). Surgical resection was allowed following chemotherapy, before or after radiotherapy. The primary endpoint in this study, progression-free survival (PFS), was significantly longer in the TPF arm compared to the PF arm, p=0.0077 (median PFS: 11.4 vs. 8.3 months respectively) with an overall median follow up time of 33.7 months. Median overall survival with a median follow-up of 51.2 months was also significantly longer in favor of the TPF arm compared to the PF arm (median OS: 18.6 vs. 14.2 months respectively). Efficacy results are presented in Table 21 and Figures 8 and 9.
[See table 21 above]

Figure 8 - TAX323 Progression-Free Survival K-M Curve

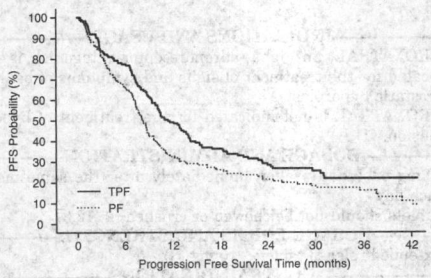

Figure 9 - TAX323 Overall Survival K-M Curve

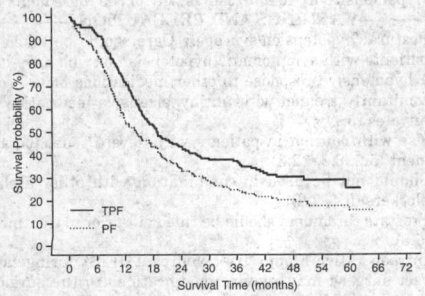

Induction chemotherapy followed by chemoradiotherapy (TAX324)
The safety and efficacy of TAXOTERE in the induction treatment of patients with locally advanced (unresectable,

---

Table 21 - Efficacy of TAXOTERE in the induction treatment of patients with inoperable locally advanced SCCHN (Intent-to-Treat Analysis)

ENDPOINT	TAXOTERE+Cisplatin+Fluorouracil n=177	Cisplatin+Fluorouracil n=181
Median progression free survival (months) (95%CI)	11.4 (10.1–14.0)	8.3 (7.4–9.1)
Adjusted Hazard ratio (95%CI) *p-value	0.71 (0.56–0.91) 0.0077	
Median survival (months) (95%CI)	18.6 (15.7–24.0)	14.2 (11.5–18.7)
Hazard ratio (95%CI) †p-value	0.71 (0.56–0.90) 0.0055	
Best overall response (CR + PR) to chemotherapy (%) (95%CI)	67.8 (60.4–74.6)	53.6 (46.0–61.0)
‡p-value	0.006	
Best overall response (CR + PR) to study treatment [chemotherapy +/– radiotherapy] (%) (95%CI)	72.3 (65.1–78.8)	58.6 (51.0–65.8)
‡p-value	0.006	

A Hazard ratio of less than 1 favors TAXOTERE+Cisplatin+Fluorouracil
* Stratified log-rank test based on primary tumor site
† Stratified log-rank test, not adjusted for multiple comparisons
‡ Chi square test, not adjusted for multiple comparisons

---

low surgical cure, or organ preservation) SCCHN was evaluated in a randomized, multicenter open-label trial (TAX324). In this study, 501 patients, with locally advanced SCCHN, and a WHO performance status of 0 or 1, were randomized to one of two treatment arms. Patients on the TAXOTERE arm received TAXOTERE (T) 75 mg/m^2 by intravenous infusion on day 1 followed by cisplatin (P) 100 mg/m^2 administered as a 30-minute to three-hour intravenous infusion, followed by the continuous intravenous infusion of fluorouracil (F) 1000 mg/m^2/day from day 1 to day 4. The cycles were repeated every 3 weeks for 3 cycles. Patients on the comparator arm received cisplatin (P) 100 mg/m^2 as a 30-minute to three-hour intravenous infusion on day 1 followed by the continuous intravenous infusion of fluorouracil (F) 1000 mg/m^2/day from day 1 to day 5. The cycles were repeated every 3 weeks for 3 cycles.
All patients in both treatment arms who did not have progressive disease were to receive 7 weeks of chemoradiotherapy (CRT) following induction chemotherapy 3 to 8 weeks after the start of the last cycle. During radiotherapy, carboplatin (AUC 1.5) was given weekly as a one-hour intravenous infusion for a maximum of 7 doses. Radiation was delivered with megavoltage equipment using once daily fractionation (2 Gy per day, 5 days per week for 7 weeks for a total dose of 70–72 Gy). Surgery on the primary site of disease and/or neck could be considered at anytime following completion of CRT.
The primary efficacy endpoint, overall survival (OS), was significantly longer (log-rank test, p=0.0058) with the TAXOTERE-containing regimen compared to PF [median OS: 70.6 versus 30.1 months respectively, hazard ratio (HR)=0.70, 95% confidence interval (CI)= 0.54–0.90]. Overall survival results are presented in Table 22 and Figure 10.

Table 22 - Efficacy of TAXOTERE in the induction treatment of patients with locally advanced SCCHN (Intent-to-Treat Analysis)

ENDPOINT	TAXOTERE+Cisplatin+Fluorouracil n=255	Cisplatin+Fluorouracil n=246
Median overall survival (months) (95% CI)	70.6 (49.0–NE)	30.1 (20.9–51.5)
Hazard ratio: (95% CI) *p-value	0.70 (0.54–0.90) 0.0058	

A Hazard ratio of less than 1 favors TAXOTERE+cisplatin+fluorouracil
NE - not estimable
* un-adjusted log-rank test

Figure 10 - TAX324 Overall Survival K-M Curve

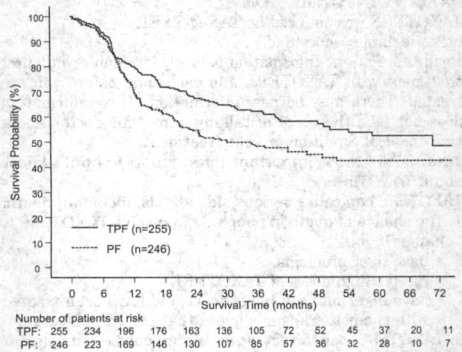

Number of patients at risk												
TPF:	255	234	196	176	163	136	105	72	52	45	37	20	11
PF:	246	223	169	146	130	107	85	57	36	32	28	10	7

15. REFERENCES

1. NIOSH Alert: Preventing occupational exposures to antineoplastic and other hazardous drugs in healthcare settings. 2004. U.S. Department of Health and Human Services, Public Health Service, Centers for Disease Control and Prevention, National Institute for Occupational Safety and Health, DHHS (NIOSH) Publication No. 2004-165.
2. OSHA Technical Manual, TED 1-0.15A, Section VI: Chapter 2. Controlling Occupational Exposure to Hazardous Drugs. OSHA, 1999. http://www.osha.gov/dts/osta/otm/otm_vi/otm_vi_2.html
3. American Society of Health-System Pharmacists. (2006) ASHP Guidelines on Handling Hazardous Drugs. *Am J Health-Syst Pharm.* 2006;63:1172–1193
4. Polovich, M., White, J. M., & Kelleher, L.O. (eds.) 2005. Chemotherapy and biotherapy guidelines and recommendations for practice (2nd. ed.) Pittsburgh, PA: Oncology Nursing Society.

16. HOW SUPPLIED/STORAGE AND HANDLING
16.1 How Supplied
Two vial formulation (Injection Concentrate and Diluent)
TAXOTERE Injection Concentrate is supplied in a single-dose vial as a sterile, pyrogen-free, non-aqueous, viscous solution with an accompanying sterile, non-pyrogenic, Diluent (13% ethanol in water for injection) vial.
TAXOTERE 80 mg/2 mL   (NDC 0075-8001-80)
TAXOTERE (docetaxel) Injection Concentrate 80 mg/2 mL: 80 mg docetaxel in 2 mL polysorbate 80 and Diluent for TAXOTERE 80 mg (13% (w/w) ethanol in water for injection). Both items are in a blister pack in one carton.

TAXOTERE 20 mg/0.5 mL   (NDC 0075-8001-20) TAXOTERE (docetaxel) Injection Concentrate 20 mg/0.5 mL: 20 mg docetaxel in 0.5 mL polysorbate 80 and Diluent for TAXOTERE 20 mg (13% (w/w) ethanol in water for injection). Both items are in a blister pack in one carton.

16.2   Storage
Store between 2°C and 25°C (36°F and 77°F). Retain in the original package to protect from bright light. Freezing does not adversely affect the product.

16.3   Handling and Disposal
Procedures for proper handling and disposal of anticancer drugs should be considered. Several guidelines on this subject have been published *[see References (15)].*

17.   PATIENT COUNSELING INFORMATION

See FDA-Approved Patient Labeling

- TAXOTERE may cause fetal harm. Advise patients to avoid becoming pregnant while receiving this drug. Women of childbearing potential should use effective contraceptives if receiving TAXOTERE *[see Warnings and Precautions (5.10) and Use in Specific Populations (8.1)].*
- Obtain detailed allergy and concomitant drug information from the patient prior to TAXOTERE administration.
- Explain the significance of oral corticosteroids such as dexamethasone administration to the patient to help facilitate compliance. Instruct patients to report if they were not compliant with oral corticosteroid regimen.
- Instruct patients to immediately report signs of a hypersensitivity reaction.
- Tell patients to watch for signs of fluid retention such as peripheral edema in the lower extremities, weight gain and dyspnea.
- Explain the significance of routine blood cell counts. Instruct patients to monitor their temperature frequently and immediately report any occurrence of fever.
- Instruct patients to report myalgia, cutaneous, or neurologic reactions.
- Explain to patients that side effects such as nausea, vomiting, diarrhea, constipation, fatigue, excessive tearing, infusion site reactions, and hair loss are associated with docetaxel administration.

PATIENT INFORMATION
TAXOTERE (pronounced as TAX-O-TEER)
(generic name = docetaxel)
Read this Patient Information before you receive your first treatment with TAXOTERE and each time before you are treated. There may be new information. This information does not take the place of talking with your doctor about your medical condition or your treatment.

What is the most important information I should know about TAXOTERE?
TAXOTERE can cause serious side effects, including death.
1. **The chance of death in people who receive TAXOTERE is higher if you:**
   - have liver problems
   - receive high doses of TAXOTERE
   - have non-small cell lung cancer and have been treated with chemotherapy medicines that contain platinum
2. **TAXOTERE can affect your blood cells.** Your doctor should do routine blood tests during treatment with TAXOTERE. This will include regular checks of your white blood cell counts. If your white blood cells are too low, your doctor may not treat you with TAXOTERE until you have enough white blood cells. People with low white blood counts can develop life-threatening infections. The earliest sign of infection may be fever. Follow your doctor's instructions for how often to take your temperature while taking TAXOTERE. Call your doctor right away if you have a fever.
3. **Serious allergic reactions** can happen in people who take TAXOTERE. Serious allergic reactions are medical emergencies that can lead to death and must be treated right away.
   Tell your doctor right away if you have any of these signs of a serious allergic reaction:
   - trouble breathing
   - sudden swelling of your face, lips, tongue, throat, or trouble swallowing
   - hives (raised bumps), rash, or redness all over your body
4. **Your body may hold too much fluid (severe fluid retention)** during treatment with TAXOTERE. This can be life threatening. To decrease the chance of this happening, you must take another medicine, a corticosteroid, before each TAXOTERE treatment. You must take the corticosteroid exactly as your doctor tells you. Tell your doctor or nurse before your TAXOTERE treatment if you forget to take corticosteroid dose or do not take it as your doctor tells you.

What is TAXOTERE?
TAXOTERE is a prescription anti-cancer medicine used to treat certain people with:
- breast cancer

- non-small cell lung cancer
- prostate cancer
- stomach cancer
- head and neck cancer

The effectiveness of TAXOTERE in children has not been established.

Who should not take TAXOTERE?
Do not take TAXOTERE if you:
- have had a severe allergic reaction to:
  - docetaxel, the active ingredient in TAXOTERE, **or**
  - any other medicines that contain polysorbate 80. Ask your doctor or pharmacist if you are not sure.
  See "What is the most important information I should know about TAXOTERE?" for the signs and symptoms of a severe allergic reaction.
- have a low white blood cell count.

What should I tell my doctor before receiving TAXOTERE?
Before you receive TAXOTERE, tell your doctor if you:
- are allergic to any medicines. See "Who should not take TAXOTERE?" Also, see the end of this leaflet for a list of the ingredients in TAXOTERE.
- have liver problems
- have any other medical conditions
- are pregnant or plan to become pregnant. TAXOTERE can harm your unborn baby.
- are breast-feeding or plan to breast-feed. It is not known if TAXOTERE passes into your breast milk. You and your doctor should decide if you will take TAXOTERE or breast-feed.

Tell your doctor about all the medicines you take including prescription and non-prescription medicines, vitamins, and herbal supplements. TAXOTERE may affect the way other medicines work, and other medicines may affect the way TAXOTERE works.
Know the medicines you take. Keep a list of them and show it to your doctor and pharmacist when you get a new medicine.

How will I receive TAXOTERE?
- TAXOTERE will be given to you as an intravenous (IV) injection into your vein, usually over 1 hour.
- TAXOTERE is usually given every 3 weeks.
- Your doctor will decide how long you will receive treatment with TAXOTERE.
- Your doctor will check your blood cell counts and other blood tests during your treatment with TAXOTERE to check for side effects of TAXOTERE.
- Your doctor may stop your treatment, change the timing of your treatment, or change the dose of your treatment if you have certain side effects while taking TAXOTERE.

What are the possible side effects of TAXOTERE?
TAXOTERE may cause serious side effects including death.
- See "What is the most important information I should know about TAXOTERE?"
- **Acute Myeloid Leukemia (AML),** a type of blood cancer, can happen in people who take TAXOTERE along with certain other medicines. Tell your doctor about all the medicines you take.
- **Other Blood Disorders** – Changes in blood counts due to leukemia and other blood disorders may occur years after treatment with Taxotere.
- **Skin Reactions** including redness and swelling of your arms and legs with peeling of your skin.
- **Neurologic Symptoms** including numbness, tingling, or burning in your hands and feet.

The most common side effects of TAXOTERE include:
- changes in your sense of taste
- feeling short of breath
- constipation
- decreased appetite
- changes in your fingernails or toenails
- swelling of your hands, face or feet
- feeling weak or tired
- joint and muscle pain
- nausea and vomiting
- diarrhea
- mouth or lips sores
- hair loss
- rash
- redness of the eye, excess tearing
- skin reactions at the site of TAXOTERE administration such as increased skin pigmentation, redness, tenderness, swelling, warmth or dryness of the skin.
- tissue damage if TAXOTERE leaks out of the vein into the tissues

Tell your doctor if you have any side effect that bothers you or does not go away.
These are not all the possible side effects of TAXOTERE. For more information ask your doctor or pharmacist.
Call your doctor or for medical advice about side effects. You may report side effects to FDA at 1-800-FDA-1088.

General information about TAXOTERE
Medicines are sometimes prescribed for purposes other than those listed in a Patient Information leaflet. This Patient Information leaflet summarizes the most important infor-

mation about TAXOTERE. If you would like more information, talk with your doctor. You can ask your pharmacist or doctor for information about TAXOTERE that is written for healthcare professionals.
For more information contact 1-800-633-1610

What are the ingredients in TAXOTERE?
Active ingredient: docetaxel
Inactive ingredients include: ethanol and polysorbate 80

Every three-week injection of TAXOTERE for breast, non-small cell lung and stomach, and head and neck cancers
Take your oral corticosteroid medicine as your doctor tells you.
Oral corticosteroid dosing:
Day 1   Date: _____ Time: _____ AM _____ PM
Day 2   Date: _____ Time: _____ AM _____ PM
(Taxotere Treatment Day)
Day 3   Date: _____ Time: _____ AM _____ PM

Every three-week injection of TAXOTERE for prostate cancer
Take your oral corticosteroid medicine as your doctor tells you.
Oral corticosteroid dosing:
Date: _____ Time: _____
Date: _____ Time: _____
(Taxotere Treatment Day)
Time: _____

---

sanofi-aventis U.S. LLC
Bridgewater, NJ 08807
© 2010 sanofi-aventis U.S. LLC

UROXATRAL®   ℞
[ŭr-ŏks-ă-tral]
(alfuzosin HCl)
Extended-Release Tablets for Oral Use

HIGHLIGHTS OF PRESCRIBING INFORMATION
These highlights do not include all the information needed to use UROXATRAL safely and effectively. See full prescribing information for UROXATRAL.
UROXATRAL® (alfuzosin HCl) Extended-Release Tablets for Oral use
Initial U.S. Approval: 2003

——————RECENT MAJOR CHANGES——————

Warnings and Precautions (5.4)	April 2010
Adverse Reactions (6.2)	May 2010
Drug Interactions (7.4)	April 2010

——————INDICATIONS AND USAGE——————
UROXATRAL, an alpha₁-adrenoreceptor-antagonist, is indicated for the treatment of signs and symptoms of benign prostatic hyperplasia.
UROXATRAL is not indicated for the treatment of hypertension. (1)

——————DOSAGE AND ADMINISTRATION——————
10 mg once daily taken immediately after the same meal each day.
Tablets should not be chewed or crushed (2, 12.3)

——————DOSAGE FORMS AND STRENGTHS——————
Extended-release tablet: 10 mg (3)

——————CONTRAINDICATIONS——————
- Moderate or severe hepatic impairment (4, 8.7, 12.3)
- Co-administration with potent CYP3A4 inhibitors (e.g. ketoconazole, itraconazole, ritonavir) (4, 7.1, 12.3)
- Hypersensitivity to alfuzosin or any of the ingredients (4)

——————WARNINGS AND PRECAUTIONS——————
- Postural hypotension/syncope: Care should be taken in patients with symptomatic hypotension or who have had a hypotensive response to other medications or are concomitantly treated with antihypertensive medication or nitrates (5.1)
- Use with caution in patients with severe renal impairment (5.2, 8.6, 12.3)
- Should not be used in combination with other alpha-blockers (5.4, 7.2)
- Prostate carcinoma should be ruled out prior to treatment (5.6)
- Intraoperative Floppy Iris Syndrome (IFIS) during cataract surgery may require modifications to the surgical technique (5.7)
- Discontinue UROXATRAL if symptoms of angina pectoris appear or worsen (5.8)
- Use with caution in patients with a history of QT prolongation or who are taking medications which prolong the QT interval (5.9)

ADVERSE REACTIONS

Most common adverse reactions in clinical studies (incidence ≥2%): dizziness, upper respiratory infection, headache, fatigue. (6.1)

Adverse reactions reported during post-marketing experience include: angina pectoris in patients with pre-existing coronary artery disease, hepatocellular and cholestatic liver injury, priapism, angioedema (6.2)

Other adverse reactions have also been reported (6)

To report SUSPECTED ADVERSE REACTIONS, contact sanofi-aventis at 1-800-633-1610 or FDA at 1-800-FDA-1088 or www.fda.gov/medwatch.

DRUG INTERACTIONS

• Contraindicated for co-administration with potent CYP3A4 inhibitors (4, 7.1, 12.3)
• Should not be used in combination with other alpha-blockers (5.4, 7.2)
• Concomitant use of PDE5 inhibitors with alpha-blockers, including UROXATRAL, can potentially cause symptomatic hypotension (5.4, 7.4)

USE IN SPECIFIC POPULATIONS

• Use with caution in patients with severe renal impairment (creatinine clearance ≤ 30 mL/min) (5.2, 8.6, 12.3)
• Do not use in patients with moderate or severe hepatic impairment (4, 8.7, 12.3)

See 17 for PATIENT COUNSELING INFORMATION and FDA-approved patient labeling

Revised: 04/2010

FULL PRESCRIBING INFORMATION: CONTENTS*

FULL PRESCRIBING INFORMATION

1 INDICATIONS AND USAGE

UROXATRAL is indicated for the treatment of signs and symptoms of benign prostatic hyperplasia. UROXATRAL is not indicated for the treatment of hypertension.

2 DOSAGE AND ADMINISTRATION

The recommended dosage is one 10 mg UROXATRAL (alfuzosin HCl) extended-release tablet once daily. The extent of absorption of Uroxatral is 50% lower under fasting conditions. Therefore, Uroxatral should be taken immediately after the same meal each day. The tablets should not be chewed or crushed.

3 DOSAGE FORMS AND STRENGTHS

UROXATRAL (alfuzosin HCl) extended-release tablet 10 mg is available as a round, three-layer tablet: one white layer between two yellow layers, debossed with ×10.

4 CONTRAINDICATIONS

UROXATRAL is contraindicated for use in patients with moderate or severe hepatic impairment (Childs-Pugh categories B and C), since alfuzosin blood levels are increased in these patients. [see Clinical Pharmacology (12.3)].

UROXATRAL is contraindicated for use with potent CYP3A4 inhibitors such as ketoconazole, itraconazole, and ritonavir, since alfuzosin blood levels are increased. [see Clinical Pharmacology (12.3)].

UROXATRAL is contraindicated in patients known to be hypersensitive to alfuzosin hydrochloride or any component of UROXATRAL tablets.

5 WARNINGS AND PRECAUTIONS

5.1 Postural Hypotension

Postural hypotension with or without symptoms (e.g., dizziness) may develop within a few hours following administration of UROXATRAL. As with other alpha-blockers, there is a potential for syncope. Patients should be warned of the possible occurrence of such events and should avoid situations where injury could result should syncope occur. There may be an increased risk of hypotension/postural hypotension and syncope when taking UROXATRAL concomitantly with anti-hypertensive medication and nitrates. Care should be taken when UROXATRAL is administered to patients with symptomatic hypotension or patients who have had a hypotensive response to other medications.

5.2 Renal Impairment

Caution should be exercised when UROXATRAL is administered in patients with severe renal impairment [see Use in Specific Populations (8.6) and Clinical Pharmacology (12.3)].

5.3 Hepatic Impairment

UROXATRAL is contraindicated for use in patients with moderate or severe hepatic impairment [see Use in Specific Populations (8.7) and Contraindications (4)]. The pharmacokinetics of UROXATRAL have not been studied in patients with mild hepatic impairment [see Clinical Pharmacology (12.3)].

5.4 Pharmacodynamic Drug-Drug Interactions

UROXATRAL is a selective alpha-blocker and should not be used in combination with other alpha-blockers [see Drug Interactions (7.2)].

Caution is advised when alpha adrenergic blocking agents, including UROXATRAL, are co-administered with PDE5 inhibitors. Alpha-adrenergic blockers and PDE5 inhibitors are both vasodilators that can lower blood pressure. Concomitant use of these two drug classes can potentially cause symptomatic hypotension [see Drug Interactions (7.4)].

5.5 Pharmacokinetic Drug-Drug Interactions

UROXATRAL is contraindicated for use with potent CYP3A4 inhibitors (e.g. ketoconazole, itraconazole, ritonavir) since alfuzosin blood levels are increased [see Contraindications (4), Drug Interactions (7.1) and Clinical Pharmacology (12.3)].

5.6 Prostatic Carcinoma

Carcinoma of the prostate and benign prostatic hyperplasia (BPH) cause many of the same symptoms. These two diseases frequently coexist. Therefore, patients thought to have BPH should be examined prior to starting treatment with UROXATRAL to rule out the presence of carcinoma of the prostate.

5.7 Intraoperative Floppy Iris Syndrome (IFIS)

IFIS has been observed during cataract surgery in some patients on or previously treated with alpha-1 blockers. This variant of small pupil syndrome is characterized by the combination of a flaccid iris that billows in response to intraoperative irrigation currents, progressive intraoperative miosis despite preoperative dilation with standard mydriatic drugs, and potential prolapse of the iris toward the phacoemulsification incisions. The patient's ophthalmologist should be prepared for possible modifications to their surgical technique, such as the utilization of iris hooks, iris dilator rings, or viscoelastic substances.

There does not appear to be a benefit of stopping alpha-1 blocker therapy prior to cataract surgery.

5.8 Coronary Insufficiency

If symptoms of angina pectoris should appear or worsen, UROXATRAL should be discontinued.

5.9 Patients with Congenital or Acquired QT Prolongation

Use with caution in patients with acquired or congenital QT prolongation or who are taking medications that prolong the QT interval [see Clinical Pharmacology (12.2)].

5.10 Laboratory Test Interactions

No laboratory test interactions with UROXATRAL tablets are known.

6 ADVERSE REACTIONS

6.1 Clinical Studies Experience

Because clinical studies are conducted under widely varying conditions, adverse reaction rates observed in the clinical studies of a drug cannot be directly compared to rates in the clinical studies of another drug and may not reflect the rates observed in practice.

The incidence of treatment-emergent adverse events has been ascertained from 3 placebo-controlled clinical trials involving 1,608 men where daily doses of 10 and 15 mg alfuzosin were evaluated. In these 3 trials, 473 men received UROXATRAL (alfuzosin HCl) 10 mg extended-release tablets. In these studies, 4% of patients taking UROXATRAL (alfuzosin HCl) 10 mg extended-release tablets withdrew from the study due to adverse events, compared with 3% in the placebo group.

Table 1 summarizes the treatment-emergent adverse events that occurred in ≥2% of patients receiving UROXATRAL, and at an incidence numerically higher than that of the placebo group. In general, the adverse events seen in long-term use were similar in type and frequency to the events described below for the 3-month trials.

Table 1—Treatment-Emergent Adverse Events Occurring in ≥2% of UROXATRAL-Treated Patients and More Frequently than with Placebo in 3-Month Placebo-Controlled Clinical Studies

Adverse Event	Placebo (n=678)	UROXATRAL (n=473)
Dizziness	19 (2.8%)	27 (5.7%)
Upper respiratory tract infection	4 (0.6%)	14 (3.0%)
Headache	12 (1.8%)	14 (3.0%)
Fatigue	12 (1.8%)	13 (2.7%)

The following adverse events, reported by between 1% and 2% of patients receiving UROXATRAL and occurring more frequently than with placebo, are listed alphabetically by body system and by decreasing frequency within body system:

Body as a whole: pain
Gastrointestinal system: abdominal pain, dyspepsia, constipation, nausea
Reproductive system: impotence
Respiratory system: bronchitis, sinusitis, pharyngitis
Signs and Symptoms of Orthostasis in Clinical Studies: The adverse reactions related to orthostasis that occurred in the double-blind phase 3 studies with alfuzosin 10 mg are summarized in Table 2. Approximately 20% to 30% of patients in these studies were taking antihypertensive medication.

Table 2—Number (%) of Patients with Symptoms Possibly Associated with Orthostasis in 3-Month Placebo-Controlled Clinical Studies

Symptoms	Placebo (n=678)	UROXATRAL (n=473)
Dizziness	19 (2.8%)	27 (5.7%)
Hypotension or postural hypotension	0	2 (0.4%)
Syncope	0	1 (0.2%)

Testing for blood pressure changes or orthostatic hypotension was conducted in three controlled studies. Decreased systolic blood pressure (≤90 mm Hg, with a decrease ≥20 mm Hg from baseline) was observed in none of the 674 placebo patients and 1 (0.2%) of the 469 UROXATRAL patients. Decreased diastolic blood pressure (≤50 mm Hg, with a decrease ≥15 mm Hg from baseline) was observed in 3 (0.4%) of the placebo patients and 4 (0.9%) of the UROXATRAL patients. A positive orthostatic test (decrease in systolic blood pressure of ≥20 mm Hg upon standing from the supine position) was seen in 52 (7.7%) of placebo patients and in 31 (6.6%) of the UROXATRAL patients.

6.2 Post-Marketing Experience

The following adverse reactions have been identified during post approval use of UROXATRAL. Because these reactions are reported voluntarily from a population of uncertain size, it is not always possible to reliably estimate their frequency.

General disorders: edema
Cardiac disorders: tachycardia, chest pain, angina pectoris in patients with pre-existing coronary artery disease, atrial fibrillation
Gastrointestinal disorders: diarrhea
Hepatobiliary disorders: hepatocellular and cholestatic liver injury (including cases with jaundice leading to drug discontinuation)
Respiratory system disorders: rhinitis
Reproductive system disorders: priapism
Skin and subcutaneous tissue disorders: rash, pruritis, urticaria, angioedema
Vascular disorders: flushing

During cataract surgery, a variant of small pupil syndrome known as Intraoperative Floppy Iris Syndrome (IFIS) has

Table 3. Mean QT and QTc changes in msec (95% CI) from baseline at T_{max} (relative to placebo) with different methodologies to correct for effect of heart rate.

Drug/Dose	QT	Fridericia method	Population-specific method	Subject-specific method
Alfuzosin 10 mg	-5.8 (-10.2, -1.4)	4.9 (0.9, 8.8)	1.8 (-1.4, 5.0)	1.8 (-1.3, 5.0)
Alfuzosin 40 mg	-4.2 (-8.5, 0.2)	7.7 (1.9, 13.5)	4.2 (-0.6, 9.0)	4.3 (-0.5, 9.2)
Moxifloxacin* 400 mg	6.9 (2.3, 11.5)	12.7 (8.6, 16.8)	11.0 (7.0, 15.0)	11.1 (7.2, 15.0)

* Active control

been reported in some patients on or previously treated with alpha-1 blockers [see Warnings and Precautions (5.7)].

7 DRUG INTERACTIONS

7.1 CYP3A4 Inhibitors
UROXATRAL is contraindicated for use with potent CYP3A4 inhibitors such as ketoconazole, itraconazole, or ritonavir, since alfuzosin blood levels are increased. [see Contraindications (4), Warnings and Precautions (5.5) and Clinical Pharmacology (12.3)].

7.2 Alpha-blockers
The pharmacokinetic and pharmacodynamic interactions between UROXATRAL and other alpha-blockers have not been determined. However, interactions may be expected, and UROXATRAL should NOT be used in combination with other alpha-blockers [see Warnings and Precautions (5.4)].

7.3 Antihypertensive Medication and Nitrates
There may be an increased risk of hypotension/postural hypotension and syncope when taking UROXATRAL concomitantly with anti-hypertensive medication and nitrates [see Warnings and Precautions (5.1)].

7.4 PDE5 Inhibitors
Caution is advised when alpha adrenergic blocking agents, including UROXATRAL, are co-administered with PDE5 inhibitors. Alpha-adrenergic blockers and PDE5 inhibitors are both vasodilators that can lower blood pressure. Concomitant use of these two drug classes can potentially cause symptomatic hypotension [see Warnings and Precautions (5.4)].

8 USE IN SPECIFIC POPULATIONS

8.1 Pregnancy
Pregnancy Category B. UROXATRAL is not indicated for use in women.

There was no evidence of teratogenicity or embryotoxicity in rats at maternal (oral gavage) doses up to 250 mg/kg/day, corresponding to systemic exposure levels 1,200-fold higher than in humans. In rabbits, up to the dose of 100 mg/kg/day (approximately 3 times the clinical dose by body surface area) given orally (via gavage), no evidence of fetal toxicity or teratogenicity was seen.

Gestation was slightly prolonged in rats with a maternal dose >5 mg/kg/day (oral gavage), which corresponds to systemic exposure levels (based on AUC of unbound drug) 12 times higher than human exposure levels, but there were no difficulties with parturition.

8.4 Pediatric Use
UROXATRAL is not indicated for use in children.

8.5 Geriatric Use
Of the total number of subjects in clinical studies of UROXATRAL, 48% were 65 years of age and over, whereas 11% were 75 and over. No overall differences in safety or effectiveness were observed between these subjects and younger subjects [see Clinical Pharmacology (12.3)]

8.6 Renal Impairment
Systemic exposure was increased by approximately 50% in pharmacokinetic studies of patients with mild, moderate, and severe renal impairment [see Clinical Pharmacology (12.3)]. In phase 3 studies, the safety profile of patients with mild (n=172) or moderate (n=56) renal impairment was similar to the patients with normal renal function in those studies. Safety data are available in only a limited number of patients (n=6) with creatinine clearance below 30 mL/min; therefore, caution should be exercised when UROXATRAL is administered in patients with severe renal impairment [see Warnings and Precautions (5.2)].

8.7 Hepatic Impairment
The pharmacokinetics of UROXATRAL have not been studied in patients with mild hepatic impairment. UROXATRAL is contraindicated for use in patients with moderate or severe hepatic impairment [see Contraindications (4), Warnings and Precautions (5.3) and Clinical Pharmacology (12.3)].

10 OVERDOSAGE
Should overdose of UROXATRAL lead to hypotension, support of the cardiovascular system is of first importance. Restoration of blood pressure and normalization of heart rate may be accomplished by keeping the patient in the supine position. If this measure is inadequate, then the adminis-

tration of intravenous fluids should be considered. If necessary, vasopressors should then be used, and the renal function should be monitored and supported as needed. Alfuzosin is 82% to 90% protein bound; therefore, dialysis may not be of benefit.

11 DESCRIPTION
Each UROXATRAL extended-release tablet contains 10 mg alfuzosin hydrochloride as the active ingredient. Alfuzosin hydrochloride is a white to off-white crystalline powder that melts at approximately 240°C. It is freely soluble in water, sparingly soluble in alcohol, and practically insoluble in dichloromethane.

Alfuzosin hydrochloride is (R,S)-N-[3-[(4-amino-6,7-dimethoxy-2-quinazolinyl) methylamino] propyl] tetrahydro-2-furancarboxamide hydrochloride. The empirical formula of alfuzosin hydrochloride is $C_{19}H_{27}N_5O_4 \cdot HCl$. The molecular weight of alfuzosin hydrochloride is 425.9. Its structural formula is:

The tablet also contains the following inactive ingredients: colloidal silicon dioxide (NF), ethylcellulose (NF), hydrogenated castor oil (NF), hydroxypropyl methylcellulose (USP), magnesium stearate (NF), mannitol (USP), microcrystalline cellulose (NF), povidone (USP), and yellow ferric oxide (NF).

12 CLINICAL PHARMACOLOGY

12.1 Mechanism of Action
Alfuzosin is a selective antagonist of post-synaptic alpha$_1$-adrenoreceptors, which are located in the prostate, bladder base, bladder neck, prostatic capsule, and prostatic urethra.

12.2 Pharmacodynamics
The symptoms associated with benign prostatic hyperplasia (BPH) such as urinary frequency, nocturia, weak stream, hesitancy and incomplete emptying are related to two components, anatomical (static) and functional (dynamic). The static component is related to the prostate size. Prostate size alone does not correlate with symptom severity. The dynamic component is a function of the smooth muscle tone in the prostate and its capsule, the bladder neck, and the bladder base as well as the prostatic urethra. The smooth muscle tone is regulated by alpha-adrenergic receptors. Alfuzosin exhibits selectivity for alpha$_1$-adrenergic receptors in the lower urinary tract. Blockade of these adrenoreceptors can cause smooth muscle in the bladder neck and prostate to relax, resulting in an improvement in urine flow and a reduction in symptoms of BPH.

Cardiac Electrophysiology
The effect of 10 mg and 40 mg alfuzosin on QT interval was evaluated in a double-blind, randomized, placebo and active-controlled (moxifloxacin 400 mg), 4-way crossover single dose study in 45 healthy white male subjects aged 19 to 45 years. The QT interval was measured at the time of peak alfuzosin plasma concentrations. The 40 mg dose of alfuzosin was chosen because this dose achieves higher blood levels than those achieved with the co-administration of UROXATRAL and ketoconazole 400 mg. Table 3 summarizes the effect on uncorrected QT and mean corrected QT interval (QTc) with different methods of correction (Fridericia, population-specific and subject-specific correction methods) at the time of peak alfuzosin plasma concentrations. No single one of these correction methodologies is known to be more valid. The mean change of heart rate associated with a 10 mg dose of alfuzosin in this study was 5.2 beats/minute and 5.8 beats/minute with 40 mg alfuzosin. The change in heart rate with moxifloxacin was 2.8 beats/minute.

[See table 3 above]

The QT effect appeared greater for 40 mg compared to 10 mg alfuzosin. The effect of the highest alfuzosin dose (four times the therapeutic dose) studied did not appear as large as that of the active control moxifloxacin at its therapeutic dose. This study, however, was not designed to make

direct statistical comparisons between the drugs or the dose levels. There was no signal of Torsade de Pointes in the extensive post-marketing experience with alfuzosin outside the United States.

A separate post-marketing QT study evaluated the effect of the co-administration of 10 mg alfuzosin with a drug of similar QT effect size. In this study, the mean placebo-subtracted QTcF increase of alfuzosin 10 mg alone was 1.9 msec (upperbound 95% CI, 5.5 msec). The concomitant administration of the two drugs showed an increased QT effect when compared with either drug alone. This QTcF increase [5.9 msec (UB 95% CI, 9.4 msec)] was not more than additive. Although this study was not designed to make direct statistical comparisons between drugs, the QT increase with both drugs given together appeared to be lower than the QTcF increase seen with the positive control moxifloxacin 400 mg [10.2 msec (UB 95% CI, 13.8 msec)]. The clinical impact of these QTc changes is unknown.

12.3 Pharmacokinetics
The pharmacokinetics of UROXATRAL have been evaluated in adult healthy male volunteers after single and/or multiple administration with daily doses ranging from 7.5 mg to 30 mg, and in patients with BPH at doses from 7.5 mg to 15 mg.

Absorption
The absolute bioavailability of UROXATRAL 10 mg tablets under fed conditions is 49%. Following multiple dosing of 10 mg UROXATRAL under fed conditions, the time to maximum concentration is 8 hours. C_{max} and AUC_{0-24} are 13.6 (SD = 5.6) ng/mL and 194 (SD = 75) ng•h/mL, respectively. UROXATRAL exhibits linear kinetics following single and multiple dosing up to 30 mg. Steady-state plasma levels are reached with the second dose of UROXATRAL administration. Steady-state alfuzosin plasma concentrations are 1.2-to 1.6-fold higher than those observed after a single administration.

Effect of Food
As illustrated in Figure 1, the extent of absorption is 50% lower under fasting conditions. Therefore, UROXATRAL should be taken immediately following a meal [see Dosage and Administration (2)].

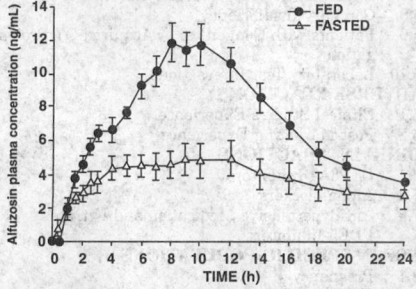

Figure 1 – Mean (SEM) Alfuzosin Plasma Concentration-Time Profiles after a Single Administration of UROXATRAL 10 mg tablets to 8 Healthy Middle-Aged Male Volunteers in Fed and Fasted States

Distribution
The volume of distribution following intravenous administration in healthy male middle-aged volunteers was 3.2 L/kg. Results of in vitro studies indicate that alfuzosin is moderately bound to human plasma proteins (82% to 90%), with linear binding over a wide concentration range (5 to 5,000 ng/mL).

Metabolism
Alfuzosin undergoes extensive metabolism by the liver, with only 11% of the administered dose excreted unchanged in the urine. Alfuzosin is metabolized by three metabolic pathways: oxidation, O-demethylation, and N-dealkylation. The metabolites are not pharmacologically active. CYP3A4 is the principal hepatic enzyme isoform involved in its metabolism.

Excretion
Following oral administration of ^{14}C-labeled alfuzosin solution, the recovery of radioactivity after 7 days (expressed as a percentage of the administered dose) was 69% in feces and 24% in urine. Following oral administration of UROXATRAL 10 mg tablets, the apparent elimination half-life is 10 hours.

Specific Populations
Elderly: In a pharmacokinetic assessment during phase 3 clinical studies in patients with BPH, there was no relationship between peak plasma concentrations of alfuzosin and age. However, trough levels were positively correlated with age. The concentrations in subjects ≥75 years of age were approximately 35% greater than in those below 65 years of age.

Renal Impairment: The Pharmacokinetic profiles of UROXATRAL 10 mg tablets in subjects with normal renal function (CL_{CR}>80 mL/min), mild impairment (CL_{CR} 60 to 80 mL/min), moderate impairment (CL_{CR} 30 to 59 mL/min),

Table 4—Mean Change (SD) from Baseline to week 12 in International Prostate Symptom Score in Three Randomized, Controlled, Double Blind Studies

Symptom Score	Study 1		Study 2		Study 3	
	Placebo (n=167)	UROXATRAL 10 mg (n=170)	Placebo (n=152)	UROXATRAL 10 mg (n=137)	Placebo (n=150)	UROXATRAL 10 mg (n=151)
Total symptom score						
Baseline	18.2 (6.4)	18.2 (6.3)	17.7 (4.1)	17.3 (3.5)	17.7 (5.0)	18.0 (5.4)
Change*	-1.6 (5.8)	-3.6 (4.8)	-4.9 (5.9)	-6.9 (4.9)	-4.6 (5.8)	-6.5 (5.2)
p-value	0.001		0.002		0.007	

* Difference between baseline and week 12.

Table 5—Mean (SD) Change from Baseline to Week 12 in Peak Urine Flow Rate (mL/sec) in Three Randomized, Controlled, Double-Blind Studies

	Study 1		Study 2		Study 3	
	Placebo (n=167)	UROXATRAL 10 mg (n=170)	Placebo (n=147)	UROXATRAL 10 mg (n=136)	Placebo (n=150)	UROXATRAL 10 mg (n=151)
Mean Peak flow rate						
Baseline	10.2 (4.0)	9.9 (3.9)	9.2 (2.0)	9.4 (1.9)	9.3 (2.6)	9.5 (3.0)
Change*	0.2 (3.5)	1.7 (4.2)	1.4 (3.2)	2.3 (3.6)	0.9 (3.0)	1.5 (3.3)
p-value	0.0004		0.03		0.22	

* Difference between baseline and week 12.

and severe impairment (CL_{CR} <30 mL/min) were compared. These clearances were calculated by the Cockcroft-Gault formula. Relative to subjects with normal renal function, the mean C_{max} and AUC values were increased by approximately 50% in patients with mild, moderate, or severe renal impairment *[see Warnings and Precautions (5.2) and Use in Specific Populations (8.6)].*

Hepatic Impairment: The pharmacokinetics of UROXATRAL have not been studied in patients with mild hepatic impairment. In patients with moderate or severe hepatic insufficiency (Child-Pugh categories B and C), the plasma apparent clearance (CL/F) was reduced to approximately one-third to one-fourth that observed in healthy subjects. This reduction in clearance results in three to four-fold higher plasma concentrations of alfuzosin in these patients compared to healthy subjects. Therefore, UROXATRAL is contraindicated in patients with moderate to severe hepatic impairment *[see Contraindications (4), Warnings and Precautions (5.3) and Use in Specific Populations (8.7)].*

Drug-Drug Interactions
Metabolic Interactions
CYP3A4 is the principal hepatic enzyme isoform involved in the metabolism of alfuzosin.
Potent CYP3A4 Inhibitors
Repeated oral administration of 400 mg/day of ketoconazole, a potent inhibitor of CYP3A4, increased alfuzosin C_{max} by 2.3-fold and AUClast by 3.2-fold, following a single 10 mg dose of alfuzosin.

In another study, repeated oral administration of a lower (200 mg/day) dose of ketoconazole increased alfuzosin C_{max} by 2.1-fold and AUClast by 2.5-fold, following a single 10 mg dose of alfusion.

Therefore, UROXATRAL is contraindicated for co-administration with potent inhibitors of CYP3A4 because exposure is increased, (e.g., ketoconazole, itraconazole, or ritonavir) *[see Contraindications (4), Warnings and Precautions (5.5) and Drug Interactions (7.1)].*
Moderate CYP3A4 Inhibitors
Diltiazem: Repeated co-administration of 240 mg/day of diltiazem, a moderately-potent inhibitor of CYP3A4, with 7.5 mg/day (2.5 mg three times daily) alfuzosin (equivalent to the exposure with UROXATRAL) increased the C_{max} and AUC_{0-24} of alfuzosin 1.5- and 1.3-fold, respectively. Alfuzosin increased the C_{max} and AUC_{0-12} of diltiazem 1.4-fold. Although no changes in blood pressure were observed in this study, diltiazem is an antihypertensive medication and the combination of UROXATRAL and antihypertensive medications has the potential to cause hypotension in some patients *[see Warnings and Precautions (5.1)].*

In human liver microsomes, at concentrations that are achieved at the therapeutic dose, alfuzosin did not inhibit CYP1A2, 2A6, 2C9, 2C19, 2D6 or 3A4 isoenzymes. In primary culture of human hepatocytes, alfuzosin did not induce CYP1A, 2A6 or 3A4 isoenzymes.

Other Interactions
Warfarin: Multiple dose administration of an immediate release tablet formulation of alfuzosin 5 mg twice daily for six days to six healthy male volunteers did not affect the pharmacological response to a single 25 mg oral dose of warfarin.
Digoxin: Repeated co-administration of UROXATRAL 10 mg tablets and digoxin 0.25 mg/day for 7 days did not influence the steady-state pharmacokinetics of either drug.
Cimetidine: Repeated administration of 1 g/day cimetidine increased both alfuzosin C_{max} and AUC values by 20%.
Atenolol: Single administration of 100 mg atenolol with a single dose of 2.5 mg of an immediate release alfuzosin tablet in eight healthy young male volunteers increased alfuzosin C_{max} and AUC values by 28% and 21%, respectively. Alfuzosin increased atenolol C_{max} and AUC values by 26% and 14%, respectively. In this study, the combination of alfuzosin with atenolol caused significant reductions in mean blood pressure and in mean heart rate. *[see Warnings and Precautions (5.1)].*
Hydrochlorothiazide: Single administration of 25 mg hydrochlorothiazide did not modify the pharmacokinetic parameters of alfuzosin. There was no evidence of pharmacodynamic interaction between alfuzosin and hydrochlorothiazide in the 8 patients in this study.

13 NONCLINICAL TOXICOLOGY
13.1 Carcinogenesis, Mutagenesis, Impairment of Fertility
There was no evidence of a drug-related increase in the incidence of tumors in mice following dietary administration of 100 mg/day alfuzosin for 98 weeks (13 and 15 times the level of exposure to humans based on AUC of unbound drug) in females and males, respectively. The highest dose tested in female mice may not have constituted a maximally tolerated dose. Likewise, there was no evidence of a drug-related increase in the incidence of tumors in rats following dietary administration of 100 mg/kg/day alfuzosin for 104 weeks (53 and 37 times the level of exposure to humans based on AUC of unbound drug) in females and males, respectively.
Alfuzosin showed no evidence of mutagenic effect in the Ames and mouse lymphoma assays, and was free of any clastogenic effects in the Chinese hamster ovary cell and *in vivo* mouse micronucleus assays. Alfuzosin treatment did not induce DNA repair in a human cell line.
There was no evidence of reproductive organ toxicity when male rats were given alfuzosin at daily oral (gavage) doses of up to 250 mg/kg/day for 26 weeks, which corresponds to levels of exposure several hundred times that in humans. No impairment of fertility was observed following oral (gavage) administration to male rats at doses of up to 125 mg/kg/day for 70 days. Estrous cycling was inhibited in rats and dogs at doses of 25 mg/kg and 20 mg/kg, respectively, corresponding to levels of systemic exposure (based on AUC of unbound drug) 12- and 18-fold higher, respectively, than in humans, although this did not result in impaired fertility in rats.

14 CLINICAL STUDIES
Three randomized placebo-controlled, double-blind, parallel-arm, 12-week studies were conducted with the 10 mg daily dose of alfuzosin. In these three studies, 1,608 patients [mean age 64.2 years, range 49–92 years; Caucasian (96.1%), Black (1.6%), Asian (1.1%), Other (1.2%)] were randomized and 473 patients received UROXATRAL 10 mg daily. Table 4 provides the results of the three studies that evaluated the 10 mg dose.
There were two primary efficacy variables in these three studies. The International Prostate Symptom Score (IPSS, or AUA Symptom Score) consists of seven questions that assess the severity of both irritative (frequency, urgency, nocturia) and obstructive (incomplete emptying, stopping and starting, weak stream, and pushing or straining) symptoms, with possible scores ranging from 0 to 35. The second efficacy variable was peak urinary flow rate. The peak flow rate was measured just prior to the next dose in study 2 and on average at 16 hours post-dosing in studies 1 and 3.
There was a statistically significant reduction from baseline to last assessment (Week 12) in the IPSS versus placebo in all three studies, indicating a reduction in symptom severity (Table 5 and Figures 2, 3, and 4).
[See table 4 above]

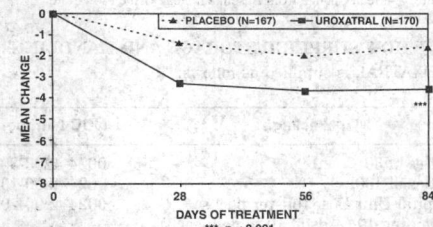

Figure 2—Mean Change from Baseline in Total Symptom Score: Study 1

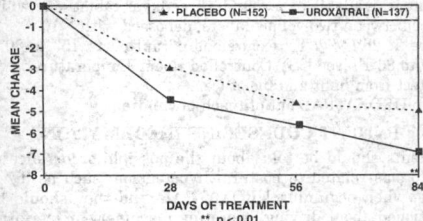

Figure 3—Mean Change from Baseline in Total Symptom Score: Study 2

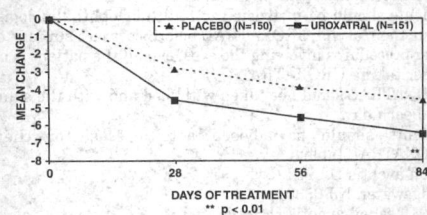

Figure 4—Mean Change from Baseline in Total Symptom Score: Study 3

Peak urinary flow rate was increased statistically significantly from baseline to last assessment (Week 12) versus placebo in studies 1 and 2 (Table 5 and Figures 5, 6, and 7).
[See table 5 above]

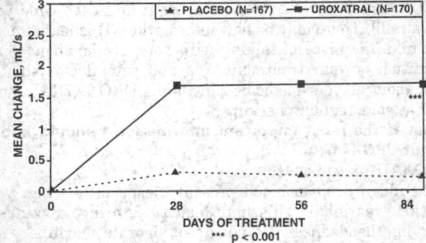

Figure 5—Mean Change from Baseline in Peak Urine Flow Rate (mL/s): Study 1

[See figure 6 at top of next page]
[See figure 7 on next page]
Mean total IPSS decreased at the first scheduled observation at Day 28 and mean peak flow rate increased starting at the first scheduled observation at Day 14 in studies 2 and 3 and Day 28 in study 1.

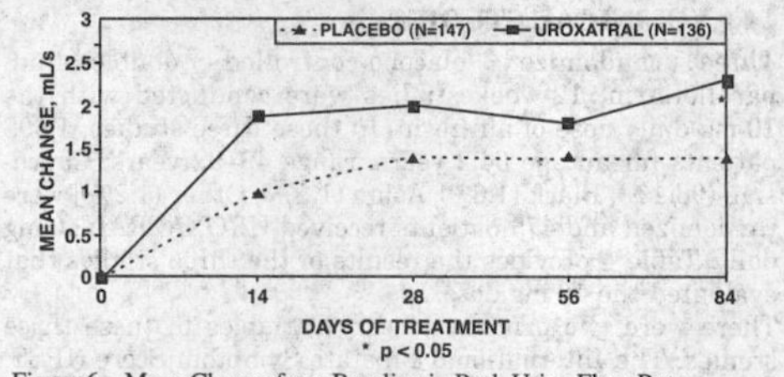

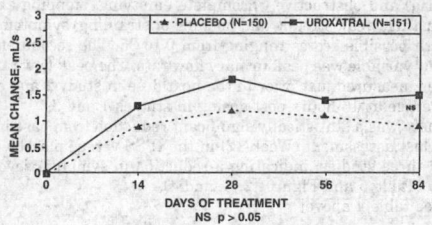

Figure 6—Mean Change from Baseline in Peak Urine Flow Rate (mL/s): Study 2

Figure 7—Mean Change from Baseline in Peak Urine Flow Rate (mL/s): Study 3

16 HOW SUPPLIED/STORAGE AND HANDLING

UROXATRAL is supplied as follows:

Package	NDC Number
Bottles of 30	0024-4200-30
Bottles of 100	0024-4200-10
Hospital Unit Dose (blister packs containing 10 cards of 10 tablets each)	0024-4200-20

UROXATRAL (alfuzosin HCl) extended-release tablet 10 mg is available as a round, three-layer tablet: one white layer between two yellow layers, debossed with ×10.
Store at 25°C (77°F); excursions permitted to 15° to 30°C (59° to 86°F) [see USP Controlled Room Temperature].
Protect from light and moisture.
Keep UROXATRAL out of reach of children.

17 PATIENT COUNSELING INFORMATION

Patients should be told about the possible occurrence of symptoms related to postural hypotension, such as dizziness, when beginning UROXATRAL, and they should be cautioned about driving, operating machinery, or performing hazardous tasks during this period. This is important for those with low blood pressure or who are taking antihypertensive medications or nitrates.
Patients should be instructed to tell their ophthalmologist about their use of UROXATRAL before cataract surgery or other procedures involving the eyes, even if the patient is no longer taking UROXATRAL.
UROXATRAL should be taken with food and with the same meal each day.
Patients should be advised not to crush or chew UROXATRAL tablets.
sanofi-aventis U.S. LLC
Bridgewater, NJ 08807
© 2010 sanofi-aventis U.S. LLC
FDA-APPROVED PATIENT LABELING
Patient Information
UROXATRAL®
(Alfuzosin hydrochloride
extended-release tablets)
Read the Patient Information that comes with UROXATRAL before you start using it and each time you get a refill. There may be new information. This leaflet does not take the place of talking with your doctor about your condition or your treatment. You and your doctor should talk about all your medicines, including UROXATRAL, now and at your regular checkups.
What is the most important information I should know about UROXATRAL?
UROXATRAL can cause:
• a sudden drop in blood pressure, especially when you start treatment. This may lead to fainting, dizziness, or lightheadedness. Do not drive, operate machinery, or do any dangerous activities until you know how UROXATRAL affects you. This is especially important if you already have a problem with low blood pressure or take medicines to treat high blood pressure. If you begin to feel dizzy or lightheaded, lie down with your legs and feet up, and if your symptoms do not improve call your doctor.
What is UROXATRAL?
UROXATRAL is a prescription medicine that is called an "alpha-blocker". UROXATRAL is used in adult men to treat the symptoms of benign prostatic hyperplasia (BPH). UROXATRAL may help to relax the muscles in the prostate and the bladder which may lessen the symptoms of BPH and improve urine flow.
Before prescribing UROXATRAL, your doctor may examine your prostate gland and do a blood test called a prostate specific antigen (PSA) test to check for prostate cancer. Prostate cancer and BPH can cause the same symptoms. Prostate cancer needs a different treatment.
UROXATRAL is not for use in women or children.
Some medicines called "alpha-blockers" are used to treat high blood pressure. UROXATRAL has not been studied for the treatment of high blood pressure.
Who should not take UROXATRAL?
Do not take UROXATRAL if you:
• have liver problems
• are taking antifungal drugs like ketoconazole or HIV drugs called protease inhibitors
• are already taking an alpha-blocker for either high blood pressure or prostate problems
• are a woman
• are a child under the age of 18
• are allergic to UROXATRAL. The active ingredient is alfuzosin hydrochloride. See the end of this leaflet for a complete list of ingredients in UROXATRAL.
Before taking UROXATRAL, tell your doctor:
• if you have liver problems
• if you have kidney problems
• if you or any family members have a rare heart condition known as congenital prolongation of the QT interval.
• about all the medicines you take, including prescription and non-prescription medicines, vitamins and herbal supplements. Some of your other medicines may affect the way you respond or react to UROXATRAL.
• if you have had low blood pressure, especially after taking another medicine. Signs of low blood pressure are fainting, dizziness, and lightheadedness.
• if you have a heart problem called angina (pain in your chest, jaw, or arm).
What you need to know while taking UROXATRAL (alfuzosin HCl) tablets
• If you have an eye surgery for cataract (clouding of the eye) planned, tell your ophthalmologist that you are using UROXATRAL or have previously been treated with an alpha-blocker.
How do I take UROXATRAL?
• Take UROXATRAL exactly as your doctor prescribes it.
• Take one UROXATRAL tablet after the same meal each day. UROXATRAL should be taken just after eating food. Do not take it on an empty stomach.
• Swallow the UROXATRAL tablet whole. Do not crush, split, or chew UROXATRAL tablets.
• If you take too much UROXATRAL call your local poison control center or emergency room right away.
What are the possible side effects of UROXATRAL?
The most common side effects with UROXATRAL are:
• dizziness
• headache
• tiredness
Call your doctor if you get any side effect that bothers you. These are not all the side effects of UROXATRAL. For more information ask your doctor or pharmacist.
How do I store UROXATRAL?
Store UROXATRAL between 59°F and 86°F (15°C and 30°C).
Protect from light and moisture.
Keep UROXATRAL and all medicines out of the reach of children.
General information about UROXATRAL:
Medicines are sometimes prescribed for conditions that are not mentioned in patient information leaflets. Do not use UROXATRAL for a condition for which it was not prescribed. Do not give UROXATRAL to other people, even if they have the same symptoms you have. It may harm them. This leaflet summarizes the most important information about UROXATRAL. If you would like more information, talk with your doctor. You can ask your doctor or pharmacist for information about UROXATRAL that is written for health professionals.
You may also visit our website at www.UROXATRAL.com or call 1-800-446-6267.
What are the ingredients of UROXATRAL?
Active Ingredient: alfuzosin hydrochloride
Inactive Ingredients: colloidal silicon dioxide (NF), ethylcellulose (NF), hydrogenated castor oil (NF), hydroxypropyl methylcellulose (USP), magnesium stearate (NF), mannitol (USP), microcrystalline cellulose (NF), povidone (USP), and yellow ferric oxide (NF).
sanofi-aventis U.S. LLC
Bridgewater, NJ 08807
© 2010 sanofi-aventis U.S. LLC

XYZAL®
℞

[zy' zall]
(levocetirizine dihydrochloride)
5 mg tablets
2.5 mg/5 mL (0.5 mg/mL) oral solution

HIGHLIGHTS OF PRESCRIBING INFORMATION

These highlights do not include all the information needed to use XYZAL safely and effectively. See full prescribing information for XYZAL.
XYZAL (levocetirizine dihydrochloride)
5 mg tablets
2.5 mg/5 mL (0.5 mg/mL) oral solution
Initial U.S. Approval: 1995

——————RECENT MAJOR CHANGES——————

Indications and Usage, Seasonal Allergic Rhinitis (1.1)	08/2009
Indications and Usage, Perennial Allergic Rhinitis (1.2)	08/2009
Indications and Usage, Chronic Idiopathic Urticaria (1.3)	08/2009
Dosage and Administration, Children 6 months to 5 Years (2.3)	08/2009

——————INDICATIONS AND USAGE——————

XYZAL is a histamine H_1-receptor antagonist indicated for:
• The relief of symptoms associated with seasonal and perennial allergic rhinitis (1.1, 1.2)
• The treatment of the uncomplicated skin manifestations of chronic idiopathic urticaria (1.3)

——————DOSAGE AND ADMINISTRATION——————

• Adults and children 12 years of age and older: 5 mg once daily in the evening (2.1)
• Children 6 to 11 years of age: 2.5 mg once daily in the evening (2.2)
• Children 6 months to 5 years of age: 1.25 mg (1/2 teaspoon oral solution) [2.5mL] once daily in the evening (2.3)
• Renal Impairment
Adjust the dose in patients 12 years of age and older with decreased renal function (2.4, 12.3)

——————DOSAGE FORMS AND STRENGTHS——————

• Immediate release breakable (scored) tablets, 5 mg (3)
• Immediate release oral solution, 2.5 mg per 5 mL (0.5 mg per mL) (3)

——————CONTRAINDICATIONS——————

• Patients with a known hypersensitivity to levocetirizine or any of the ingredients of XYZAL or to cetirizine (4)
• Patients with end-stage renal disease at less than 10 mL/min creatinine clearance or patients undergoing hemodialysis (4)
• Children 6 months to 11 years of age with renal impairment (4)

——————WARNINGS AND PRECAUTIONS——————

• Avoid engaging in hazardous occupations requiring complete mental alertness such as driving or operating machinery when taking XYZAL (5.1).
• Avoid concurrent use of alcohol or other central nervous system depressants with XYZAL (5.1).

——————ADVERSE REACTIONS——————

The most common adverse reactions (rate ≥2% and > placebo) were somnolence, nasopharyngitis, fatigue, dry mouth, and pharyngitis in subjects 12 years of age and older, and pyrexia, somnolence, cough, and epistaxis in children 6 to 12 years of age. In subjects 1 to 5 years of age, the most common adverse reactions (rate ≥2% and > placebo) were pyrexia, diarrhea, vomiting, and otitis media. In subjects 6 to 11 months of age, the most common adverse reactions (rate ≥3% and > placebo) were diarrhea and constipation. (6.1).
To report SUSPECTED ADVERSE REACTIONS, contact UCB, Inc. at 866-822-0068 or FDA at 1-800-FDA-1088 or www.fda.gov/medwatch.

——————USE IN SPECIFIC POPULATIONS——————

• Renal Impairment
Because XYZAL is substantially excreted by the kidneys, the risk of adverse reactions to this drug may be greater in patients with impaired renal function (8.6 and 12.3).
• Pediatric Use
Do not exceed the recommended doses of 2.5 mg and 1.25 mg once daily in children 6 to 11 years and 6 months to 5 years of age, respectively. Systemic exposure with these doses in respective pediatric age groups is comparable to that from a 5 mg once daily dose in adults. (12.3).
See 17 for PATIENT COUNSELING INFORMATION
Revised: 08/2009

FULL PRESCRIBING INFORMATION

1 INDICATIONS AND USAGE

1.1 Seasonal Allergic Rhinitis

XYZAL® is indicated for the relief of symptoms associated with seasonal allergic rhinitis in adults and children 2 years of age and older.

1.2 Perennial Allergic Rhinitis

XYZAL is indicated for the relief of symptoms associated with perennial allergic rhinitis in adults and children 6 months of age and older.

1.3 Chronic Idiopathic Urticaria

XYZAL is indicated for the treatment of the uncomplicated skin manifestations of chronic idiopathic urticaria in adults and children 6 months of age and older.

2 DOSAGE AND ADMINISTRATION

XYZAL is available as 2.5 mg/5 mL (0.5 mg/mL) oral solution and as 5 mg breakable (scored) tablets, allowing for the administration of 2.5 mg, if needed. XYZAL can be taken without regard to food consumption.

2.1 Adults and Children 12 Years of Age and Older

The recommended dose of XYZAL is 5 mg (1 tablet or 2 teaspoons [10 mL] oral solution) once daily in the evening. Some patients may be adequately controlled by 2.5 mg (1/2 tablet or 1 teaspoon [5 mL] oral solution) once daily in the evening.

2.2 Children 6 to 11 Years of Age

The recommended dose of XYZAL is 2.5 mg (1/2 tablet or 1 teaspoon [5 mL] oral solution) once daily in the evening. The 2.5 mg dose should not be exceeded because the systemic exposure with 5 mg is approximately twice that of adults [see Clinical Pharmacology (12.3)].

2.3 Children 6 Months to 5 Years of Age

The recommended initial dose of XYZAL is 1.25 mg (1/2 teaspoon oral solution) [2.5 mL] once daily in the evening. The 1.25 mg once daily dose should not be exceeded based on comparable exposure to adults receiving 5 mg [see Clinical Pharmacology (12.3)].

2.4 Dose Adjustment for Renal and Hepatic Impairment

In adults and children 12 years of age and older with:
• Mild renal impairment (creatinine clearance [CL_{CR}] = 50-80 mL/min): a dose of 2.5 mg once daily is recommended;
• Moderate renal impairment (CL_{CR} = 30-50 mL/min): a dose of 2.5 mg once every other day is recommended;
• Severe renal impairment (CL_{CR} = 10-30 mL/min): a dose of 2.5 mg twice weekly (administered once every 3-4 days) is recommended;

• End-stage renal disease patients (CL_{CR} < 10 mL/min) and patients undergoing hemodialysis should not receive XYZAL.

No dose adjustment is needed in patients with solely hepatic impairment. In patients with both hepatic impairment and renal impairment, adjustment of the dose is recommended.

3 DOSAGE FORMS AND STRENGTHS

XYZAL oral solution is a clear, colorless liquid containing 0.5 mg of levocetirizine dihydrochloride per mL.

XYZAL tablets are white, film-coated, oval-shaped, scored, imprinted (with the letter Y in red color on both halves of the scored tablet) and contain 5 mg levocetirizine dihydrochloride.

4 CONTRAINDICATIONS

The use of XYZAL is contraindicated in:

4.1 Patients with Known Hypersensitivity

Patients with known hypersensitivity to levocetirizine or any of the ingredients of XYZAL, or to cetirizine. Observed reactions range from urticaria to anaphylaxis [see Adverse Reactions (6.2)].

4.2 Patients with End-Stage Renal Disease

Patients with end-stage renal disease (CL_{CR} < 10 mL/min) and patients undergoing hemodialysis

4.3 Pediatric Patients with Impaired Renal Function

Children 6 months to 11 years of age with impaired renal function

5 WARNINGS AND PRECAUTIONS

5.1 Activities Requiring Mental Alertness

In clinical trials the occurrence of somnolence, fatigue, and asthenia has been reported in some patients under therapy with XYZAL. Patients should be cautioned against engaging in hazardous occupations requiring complete mental alertness, and motor coordination such as operating machinery or driving a motor vehicle after ingestion of XYZAL. Concurrent use of XYZAL with alcohol or other central nervous system depressants should be avoided because additional reductions in alertness and additional impairment of central nervous system performance may occur.

6 ADVERSE REACTIONS

Use of XYZAL has been associated with somnolence, fatigue, and asthenia [see Warnings and Precautions (5.1)].

6.1 Clinical Trials Experience

The safety data described below reflect exposure to XYZAL in 2708 patients with seasonal or perennial allergic rhinitis or chronic idiopathic urticaria in 14 controlled clinical trials of 1 week to 6 months duration.

The short-term (exposure up to 6 weeks) safety data for adults and adolescents are based upon eight clinical trials in which 1896 patients (825 males and 1071 females aged 12 years and older) were treated with XYZAL 2.5, 5, or 10 mg once daily in the evening.

The short-term safety data from pediatric patients are based upon two clinical trials in which 243 children with seasonal or perennial allergic rhinitis (162 males and 81 females 6 to 12 years of age) were treated with XYZAL 5 mg once daily for 4 to 6 weeks, one clinical trial in which 114 children (65 males and 49 females 1 to 5 years of age) with allergic rhinitis or chronic idiopathic urticaria were treated with XYZAL 1.25 mg twice daily for 2 weeks, and one clinical trial in which 45 children (28 males and 17 females 6 to 11 months of age) with symptoms of allergic rhinitis or chronic urticaria were treated with XYZAL 1.25 mg once daily for 2 weeks.

The long-term (exposure of 4 or 6 months) safety data in adults and adolescents are based upon two clinical trials in which 428 patients (190 males and 238 females) with allergic rhinitis were exposed to treatment with XYZAL 5 mg once daily. Long term safety data are also available from an 18-month trial in 255 XYZAL-treated subjects 12-24 months of age.

Because clinical trials are conducted under widely varying conditions, adverse reaction rates observed in the clinical trials of a drug cannot be directly compared to rates in the clinical trial of another drug and may not reflect the rates observed in practice.

Adults and Adolescents 12 years of Age and Older

In studies up to 6 weeks in duration, the mean age of the adult and adolescent patients was 32 years, 44% of the patients were men and 56% were women, and the large majority (more than 90%) was Caucasian.

In these trials 43% and 42% of the subjects in the XYZAL 2.5 mg and 5 mg groups, respectively, had at least one adverse event compared to 43% in the placebo group.

In placebo-controlled trials of 1-6 weeks in duration, the most common adverse reactions were somnolence, nasopharyngitis, fatigue, dry mouth, and pharyngitis, and most were mild to moderate in intensity. Somnolence with XYZAL showed dose ordering between tested doses of 2.5, 5 and 10 mg and was the most common adverse reaction leading to discontinuation (0.5%).

Table 1 lists adverse reactions that were reported in greater than or equal to 2% of subjects aged 12 years and older exposed to XYZAL 2.5 mg or 5 mg in eight placebo-controlled clinical trials and that were more common with XYZAL than placebo.

Table 1 Adverse Reactions Reported in ≥ 2%* of Subjects Aged 12 Years and Older Exposed to XYZAL 2.5 mg or 5 mg Once Daily in Placebo-Controlled Clinical Trials 1-6 Weeks in Duration

Adverse Reactions	XYZAL 2.5 mg (n = 421)	XYZAL 5 mg (n = 1070)	Placebo (n = 912)
Somnolence	22 (5%)	61 (6%)	16 (2%)
Nasopharyngitis	25 (6%)	40 (4%)	28 (3%)
Fatigue	5 (1%)	46 (4%)	20 (2%)
Dry Mouth	12 (3%)	26 (2%)	11 (1%)
Pharyngitis	10 (2%)	12 (1%)	9 (1%)

* Rounded to the closest unit percentage

Additional adverse reactions of medical significance observed at a higher incidence than in placebo in adults and adolescents aged 12 years and older exposed to XYZAL are syncope (0.2%) and weight increased (0.5%).

Pediatric Patients 6 to 12 Years of Age

A total of 243 pediatric patients 6 to 12 years of age received XYZAL 5 mg once daily in two short-term placebo controlled double-blind trials. The mean age of the patients was 9.8 years, 79 (32%) were 6 to 8 years of age, and 50% were Caucasian. Table 2 lists adverse reactions that were reported in greater than or equal to 2% of subjects aged 6 to 12 years exposed to XYZAL 5 mg in placebo-controlled clinical trials and that were more common with XYZAL than placebo.

Table 2 Adverse Reactions Reported in ≥2%* of Subjects Aged 6-12 Years Exposed to XYZAL 5 mg Once Daily in Placebo-Controlled Clinical Trials 4 and 6 Weeks in Duration

Adverse Reactions	XYZAL 5 mg (n = 243)	Placebo (n = 240)
Pyrexia	10 (4%)	5 (2%)
Cough	8 (3%)	2 (<1%)
Somnolence	7 (3%)	1 (<1%)
Epistaxis	6 (2%)	1 (<1%)

* Rounded to the closest unit percentage

Pediatric Patients 1 to 5 Years of Age

A total of 114 pediatric patients 1 to 5 years of age received XYZAL 1.25 mg twice daily in a two week placebo-controlled double-blind safety trial. The mean age of the patients was 3.8 years, 32% were 1 to 2 years of age, 71% were Caucasian and 18% were Black. Table 3 lists adverse reactions that were reported in greater than or equal to 2% of subjects aged 1 to 5 years exposed to XYZAL 1.25 mg twice daily in the placebo-controlled safety trial and that were more common with XYZAL than placebo.

Table 3 Adverse Reactions Reported in ≥2%* of Subjects Aged 1-5 Years Exposed to XYZAL 1.25 mg Twice Daily in a 2-Week Placebo-Controlled Clinical Trial

Adverse Reactions	XYZAL 1.25 mg Twice Daily (n = 114)	Placebo (n = 59)
Pyrexia	5 (4%)	1 (2%)
Diarrhea	4 (4%)	2 (3%)
Vomiting	4 (4%)	2 (3%)
Otitis Media	3 (3%)	0 (0%)

* Rounded to the closest unit percentage

Pediatric Patients 6 to 11 Months of Age

A total of 45 pediatric patients 6 to 11 months of age received XYZAL 1.25 mg once daily in a two week placebo-controlled double-blind safety trial. The mean age of the patients was 9 months, 51% were Caucasian and 31% were

Black. Adverse reactions that were reported in more than 1 subject (i.e. greater than or equal to 3% of subjects) aged 6 to 11 months exposed to XYZAL 1.25 mg once daily in the placebo-controlled safety trial and that were more common with XYZAL than placebo included diarrhea and constipation which were reported in 6 (13%) and 1 (4%) and 3 (7%) and 1 (4%) children in the XYZAL and placebo-treated groups, respectively.

Long-Term Clinical Trials Experience

In two controlled clinical trials, 428 patients (190 males and 238 females) aged 12 years and older were treated with XYZAL 5 mg once daily for 4 or 6 months. The patient characteristics and the safety profile were similar to that seen in the short-term studies. Ten (2.3%) patients treated with XYZAL discontinued because of somnolence, fatigue or asthenia compared to 2 (<1%) in the placebo group.

There are no long term clinical trials in children below 12 years of age with allergic rhinitis or chronic idiopathic urticaria.

Laboratory Test Abnormalities

Elevations of blood bilirubin and transaminases were reported in <1% of patients in the clinical trials. The elevations were transient and did not lead to discontinuation in any patient.

6.2 Post-Marketing Experience

In addition to the adverse reactions reported during clinical trials and listed above, adverse events have also been identified during post-approval use of XYZAL in other countries. Because these events are reported voluntarily from a population of uncertain size, it is not always possible to reliably estimate their frequency or establish a causal relationship to drug exposure. Adverse events of hypersensitivity and anaphylaxis, angioneurotic edema, fixed drug eruption, pruritus, rash, and urticaria, convulsion, aggression and agitation, visual disturbances, palpitations, dyspnea, nausea, hepatitis, and myalgia have been reported.

Besides these events reported under treatment with XYZAL, other potentially severe adverse events have been reported from the post-marketing experience with cetirizine. Since levocetirizine is the principal pharmacologically active component of cetirizine, one should take into account the fact that the following adverse events could also potentially occur under treatment with XYZAL: hallucinations, suicidal ideation, orofacial dyskinesia, severe hypotension, cholestasis, glomerulonephritis, and still birth.

7 DRUG INTERACTIONS

In vitro data indicate that levocetirizine is unlikely to produce pharmacokinetic interactions through inhibition or induction of liver drug-metabolizing enzymes. No *in vivo* drug-drug interaction studies have been performed with levocetirizine. Drug interaction studies have been performed with racemic cetirizine.

7.1 Antipyrine, Azithromycin, Cimetidine, Erythromycin, Ketoconazole, Theophylline, and Pseudoephedrine

Pharmacokinetic interaction studies performed with racemic cetirizine demonstrated that cetirizine did not interact with antipyrine, pseudoephedrine, erythromycin, azithromycin, ketoconazole, and cimetidine. There was a small decrease (~16%) in the clearance of cetirizine caused by a 400 mg dose of theophylline. It is possible that higher theophylline doses could have a greater effect.

7.2 Ritonavir

Ritonavir increased the plasma AUC of cetirizine by about 42% accompanied by an increase in half-life (53%) and a decrease in clearance (29%) of cetirizine. The disposition of ritonavir was not altered by concomitant cetirizine administration.

8 USE IN SPECIFIC POPULATIONS

8.1 Pregnancy

Pregnancy Category B

There are no adequate and well-controlled studies in pregnant women. Because animal reproduction studies are not always predictive of human response, XYZAL should be used during pregnancy only if clearly needed.

Teratogenic Effects:

In rats and rabbits, levocetirizine was not teratogenic at oral doses approximately 320 and 390, respectively, times the maximum recommended daily oral dose in adults on a mg/m^2 basis.

8.3 Nursing Mothers

No peri- and post-natal animal studies have been conducted with levocetirizine. In mice, cetirizine caused retarded pup weight gain during lactation at an oral dose in dams that was approximately 40 times the maximum recommended daily oral dose in adults on a mg/m^2 basis. Studies in beagle dogs indicated that approximately 3% of the dose of cetirizine was excreted in milk. Cetirizine has been reported to be excreted in human breast milk. Because levocetirizine is also expected to be excreted in human milk, use of XYZAL in nursing mothers is not recommended.

8.4 Pediatric Use

The recommended dose of XYZAL for the treatment of the uncomplicated skin manifestations of chronic idiopathic urticaria in patients 6 months to 17 years of age is based on extrapolation of efficacy from adults 18 years of age and older [see *Clinical Studies (14)*].

The recommended dose of XYZAL in patients 6 months to 11 years of age for the treatment of the symptoms of perennial allergic rhinitis and chronic idiopathic urticaria and in patients 2 to 11 years of age for the treatment of the symptoms of seasonal allergic rhinitis is based on cross-study comparisons of the systemic exposure of XYZAL in adults and pediatric patients and on the safety profile of XYZAL in both adult and pediatric patients at doses equal to or higher than the recommended dose for patients 6 months to 11 years of age.

The safety of XYZAL 5 mg once daily was evaluated in 243 pediatric patients 6 to 12 years of age in two placebo-controlled clinical trials lasting 4 and 6 weeks. The safety of XYZAL 1.25 mg twice daily was evaluated in one 2-week clinical trial in 114 pediatric patients 1 to 5 years of age and the safety of XYZAL 1.25 mg once daily was evaluated in one 2-week clinical trial in 45 pediatric patients 6 to 11 months of age [see *Adverse Reactions (6.1)*].

The effectiveness of XYZAL 1.25 mg once daily (6 months to 5 years of age) and 2.5 mg once daily (6 to 11 years of age) for the treatment of the symptoms of seasonal and perennial allergic rhinitis and chronic idiopathic urticaria is supported by the extrapolation of demonstrated efficacy of XYZAL 5 mg once daily in patients 12 years of age and older and based on the pharmacokinetic comparison between adults and children.

Cross-study comparisons indicate that administration of a 5 mg dose of XYZAL to 6 to 12 year old pediatric seasonal allergic rhinitis patients resulted in about 2-fold the systemic exposure (AUC) observed when 5 mg of XYZAL was administered to healthy adults. Therefore, in children 6 to 11 years of age the recommended dose of 2.5 mg once daily should not be exceeded. In a population pharmacokinetics study the administration of 1.25 mg once daily in children 6 months to 5 years of age resulted in systemic exposure comparable to 5 mg once daily in adults. [see *Dosage and Administration (2.2); Clinical Studies (14);* and *Clinical Pharmacology (12.3)*].

8.5 Geriatric Use

Clinical studies of XYZAL for each approved indication did not include sufficient numbers of patients aged 65 years and older to determine whether they respond differently than younger patients. Other reported clinical experience has not identified differences in responses between the elderly and younger patients. In general, dose selection for an elderly patient should be cautious, usually starting at the low end of the dosing range reflecting the greater frequency of decreased hepatic, renal, or cardiac function and of concomitant disease or other drug therapy.

8.6 Renal Impairment

XYZAL is known to be substantially excreted by the kidneys and the risk of adverse reactions to this drug may be greater in patients with impaired renal function. Because elderly patients are more likely to have decreased renal function, care should be taken in dose selection and it may be useful to monitor renal function [see *Dosage and Administration (2)* and *Clinical Pharmacology (12.3)*].

8.7 Hepatic Impairment

As levocetirizine is mainly excreted unchanged by the kidneys, it is unlikely that the clearance of levocetirizine is significantly decreased in patients with solely hepatic impairment [see *Clinical Pharmacology (12.3)*].

10 OVERDOSAGE

Overdosage has been reported with XYZAL.

Symptoms of overdose may include drowsiness in adults and initially agitation and restlessness, followed by drowsiness in children. There is no known specific antidote to XYZAL. Should overdose occur, symptomatic or supportive treatment is recommended. XYZAL is not effectively removed by dialysis, and dialysis will be ineffective unless a dialyzable agent has been concomitantly ingested.

The acute maximal non-lethal oral dose of levocetirizine was 240 mg/kg in mice (approximately 190 times the maximum recommended daily oral dose in adults, approximately 230 times the maximum recommended daily oral dose in children 6 to 11 years of age, and approximately 180 times the maximum recommended daily oral dose in children 6 months to 5 years of age on a mg/m^2 basis). In rats the maximal non-lethal oral dose was 240 mg/kg (approximately 390 times the maximum recommended daily oral dose in adults, approximately 460 times the maximum recommended daily oral dose in children 6 to 11 years of age, and approximately 370 times the maximum recommended daily oral dose in children 6 months to 5 years of age on a mg/m^2 basis).

11 DESCRIPTION

Levocetirizine dihydrochloride, the active component of XYZAL tablets and oral solution, is an orally active H_1-receptor antagonist. The chemical name is (R)-[2-[4-[(4-chlorophenyl) phenylmethyl]-1-piperazinyl] ethoxy] acetic acid dihydrochloride. Levocetirizine dihydrochloride is the R enantiomer of cetirizine hydrochloride, a racemic compound with antihistaminic properties. The empirical formula of levocetirizine dihydrochloride is $C_{21}H_{25}ClN_2O_3 \bullet 2HCl$. The molecular weight is 461.82 and the chemical structure is shown below:

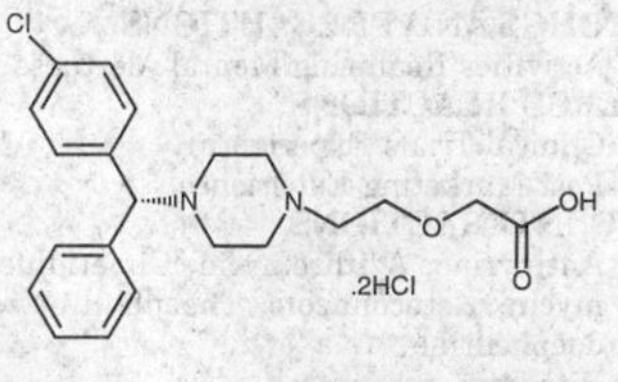

Levocetirizine dihydrochloride is a white, crystalline powder and is water soluble.

XYZAL 5 mg tablets are formulated as immediate release, white, film-coated, oval-shaped scored tablets for oral administration. The tablets are imprinted on both halves of the scored line with the letter Y in red (Opacode® Red). Inactive ingredients are: microcrystalline cellulose, lactose monohydrate, colloidal anhydrous silica, and magnesium stearate. The film coating contains hypromellose, titanium dioxide, and macrogol 400.

XYZAL 0.5 mg/mL oral solution is formulated as an immediate release, clear, colorless liquid. Inactive ingredients are: sodium acetate trihydrate, glacial acetic acid, maltitol solution, glycerin, methylparaben, propylparaben, saccharin, flavoring (consisting of triacetin, natural & artificial flavors, dl-alpha-tocopherol), purified water.

12 CLINICAL PHARMACOLOGY

12.1 Mechanism of Action

Levocetirizine, the active enantiomer of cetirizine, is an anti-histamine; its principal effects are mediated via selective inhibition of H_1 receptors. The antihistaminic activity of levocetirizine has been documented in a variety of animal and human models. *In vitro* binding studies revealed that levocetirizine has an affinity for the human H_1-receptor 2-fold higher than that of cetirizine (Ki = 3 nmol/L *vs.* 6 nmol/L, respectively). The clinical relevance of this finding is unknown.

12.2 Pharmacodynamics

Studies in adult healthy subjects showed that levocetirizine at doses of 2.5 mg and 5 mg inhibited the skin wheal and flare caused by the intradermal injection of histamine. In contrast, dextrocetirizine exhibited no clear change in the inhibition of the wheal and flare reaction. Levocetirizine at a dose of 5 mg inhibited the wheal and flare caused by intradermal injection of histamine in 14 pediatric subjects (aged 6 to 11 years) and the activity persisted for at least 24 hours. The clinical relevance of histamine wheal skin testing is unknown.

A QT/QTc study using a single dose of 30 mg of levocetirizine did not demonstrate an effect on the QTc interval. While a single dose of levocetirizine had no effect, the effects of levocetirizine may not be at steady state following single dose. The effect of levocetirizine on the QTc interval following multiple dose administration is unknown. Levocetirizine is not expected to have QT/QTc effects because of the results of QTc studies with cetirizine and the long post-marketing history of cetirizine without reports of QT prolongation.

12.3 Pharmacokinetics

Levocetirizine exhibited linear pharmacokinetics over the therapeutic dose range in adult healthy subjects.

• Absorption

Levocetirizine is rapidly and extensively absorbed following oral administration. In adults, peak plasma concentrations are achieved 0.9 hour after administration of the oral tablet. The accumulation ratio following daily oral administration is 1.12 with steady state achieved after 2 days. Peak concentrations are typically 270 ng/mL and 308 ng/mL following a single and a repeated 5 mg once daily dose, respectively. Food had no effect on the extent of exposure (AUC) of the levocetirizine tablet, but T_{max} was delayed by about 1.25 hours and C_{max} was decreased by about 36% after administration with a high fat meal; therefore, levocetirizine can be administered with or without food.

A dose of 5 mg (10 mL) of XYZAL oral solution is bioequivalent to a 5 mg dose of XYZAL tablets. Following oral administration of a 5 mg dose of XYZAL oral solution to healthy adult subjects, the mean peak plasma concentrations were achieved approximately 0.5 hour post-dose.

• Distribution

The mean plasma protein binding of levocetirizine *in vitro* ranged from 91 to 92%, independent of concentration in the range of 90-5000 ng/mL, which includes the therapeutic plasma levels observed. Following oral dosing, the average apparent volume of distribution is approximately 0.4 L/kg, representative of distribution in total body water.

• **Metabolism**
The extent of metabolism of levocetirizine in humans is less than 14% of the dose and therefore differences resulting from genetic polymorphism or concomitant intake of hepatic drug metabolizing enzyme inhibitors are expected to be negligible. Metabolic pathways include aromatic oxidation, N- and O-dealkylation, and taurine conjugation. Dealkylation pathways are primarily mediated by CYP 3A4 while aromatic oxidation involves multiple and/or unidentified CYP isoforms.

• **Elimination**
The plasma half-life in adult healthy subjects was about 8 to 9 hours after administration of oral tablets and oral solution, and the mean oral total body clearance for levocetirizine was approximately 0.63 mL/kg/min. The major route of excretion of levocetirizine and its metabolites is via urine, accounting for a mean of 85.4% of the dose. Excretion via feces accounts for only 12.9% of the dose. Levocetirizine is excreted both by glomerular filtration and active tubular secretion. Renal clearance of levocetirizine correlates with that of creatinine clearance. In patients with renal impairment the clearance of levocetirizine is reduced [see *Dosage and Administration* (2.3)].

• **Drug Interaction Studies**
In vitro data on metabolite interaction indicate that levocetirizine is unlikely to produce, or be subject to metabolic interactions. Levocetirizine at concentrations well above C_{max} level achieved within the therapeutic dose ranges is not an inhibitor of CYP isoenzymes 1A2, 2C9, 2C19, 2A1, 2D6, 2E1, and 3A4, and is not an inducer of UGT1A or CYP isoenzymes 1A2, 2C9 and 3A4.
No formal *in vivo* drug interaction studies have been performed with levocetirizine. Studies have been performed with the racemic cetirizine [see *Drug Interactions (7)*].

• **Pediatric Patients**
Data from a pediatric pharmacokinetic study with oral administration of a single dose of 5 mg levocetirizine in 14 children age 6 to 11 years with body weight ranging between 20 and 40 kg show that C_{max} and AUC values are about 2-fold greater than that reported in healthy adult subjects in a cross-study comparison. The mean C_{max} was 450 ng/mL, occurring at a mean time of 1.2 hours, weight-normalized, total body clearance was 30% greater, and the elimination half-life 24% shorter in this pediatric population than in adults.
Dedicated pharmacokinetic studies have not been conducted in pediatric patients younger than 6 years of age. A retrospective population pharmacokinetic analysis was conducted in 324 subjects (181 children 1 to 5 years of age, 18 children 6 to 11 years of age, and 124 adults 18 to 55 years of age) who received single or multiple doses of levocetirizine ranging from 1.25 mg to 30 mg. Data generated from this analysis indicated that administration of 1.25 mg once daily to children 6 months to 5 years of age results in plasma concentrations similar to those of adults receiving 5 mg once daily.

• **Geriatric Patients**
Limited pharmacokinetic data are available in elderly subjects. Following once daily repeat oral administration of 30 mg levocetirizine for 6 days in 9 elderly subjects (65–74 years of age), the total body clearance was approximately 33% lower compared to that in younger adults. The disposition of racemic cetirizine has been shown to be dependent on renal function rather than on age. This finding would also be applicable for levocetirizine, as levocetirizine and cetirizine are both predominantly excreted in urine. Therefore, the XYZAL dose should be adjusted in accordance with renal function in elderly patients [see *Dosage and Administration (2)*].

• **Gender**
Pharmacokinetic results for 77 patients (40 men, 37 women) were evaluated for potential effect of gender. The half-life was slightly shorter in women (7.08 ± 1.72 hr) than in men (8.62 ± 1.84 hr); however, the body weight-adjusted oral clearance in women (0.67 ± 0.16 mL/min/kg) appears to be comparable to that in men (0.59 ± 0.12 mL/min/kg). The same daily doses and dosing intervals are applicable for men and women with normal renal function.

• **Race**
The effect of race on levocetirizine has not been studied. As levocetirizine is primarily renally excreted, and there are no important racial differences in creatinine clearance, pharmacokinetic characteristics of levocetirizine are not expected to be different across races. No race-related differences in the kinetics of racemic cetirizine have been observed.

• **Renal Impairment**
Levocetirizine exposure (AUC) exhibited 1.8-, 3.2-, 4.3-, and 5.7-fold increase in mild, moderate, severe, renal impaired, and end-stage renal disease patients, respectively, compared to healthy subjects. The corresponding increases of half-life estimates were 1.4-, 2.0-, 2.9-, and 4-fold, respectively.

Table 4 Mean Reflective Total Symptom Score* in Allergic Rhinitis Dose-Ranging Trials

Treatment	N	Baseline	On Treatment Adjusted Mean	Difference from Placebo		
				Estimate	95% CI	p-value
Seasonal Allergic Rhinitis Trial – Reflective total symptom score						
XYZAL 2.5 mg	116	7.83	4.27	0.91	(0.37, 1.45)	0.001
XYZAL 5 mg	115	7.45	4.06	1.11	(0.57, 1.65)	<0.001
XYZAL 10 mg	118	7.15	3.57	1.61	(1.07, 2.15)	<0.001
Placebo	118	7.94	5.17			
Perennial Allergic Rhinitis Trial – Reflective total symptom score						
XYZAL 2.5 mg	133	7.14	4.12	1.17	(0.71, 1.63)	<0.001
XYZAL 5 mg	127	7.18	4.07	1.22	(0.76, 1.69)	<0.001
XYZAL 10 mg	129	7.58	4.19	1.10	(0.64, 1.57)	<0.001
Placebo	128	7.22	5.29			

* Total symptom score is the sum of individual symptoms of sneezing, rhinorrhea, nasal pruritus, and ocular pruritus as assessed by patients on a 0-3 categorical severity scale.

The total body clearance of levocetirizine after oral dosing was correlated to the creatinine clearance and was progressively reduced based on severity of renal impairment. Therefore, it is recommended to adjust the dose and dosing intervals of levocetirizine based on creatinine clearance in patients with mild, moderate, or severe renal impairment. In end-stage renal disease patients (CL_{CR} < 10 mL/min) levocetirizine is contraindicated. The amount of levocetirizine removed during a standard 4-hour hemodialysis procedure was <10%.
The dosage of XYZAL should be reduced in patients with mild renal impairment. Both the dosage and frequency of administration should be reduced in patients with moderate or severe renal impairment [see *Dosage and Administration (2.4)*].

• **Hepatic Impairment**
XYZAL has not been studied in patients with hepatic impairment. The non-renal clearance (indicative of hepatic contribution) was found to constitute about 28% of the total body clearance in healthy adult subjects after oral administration.
As levocetirizine is mainly excreted unchanged by the kidney, it is unlikely that the clearance of levocetirizine is significantly decreased in patients with solely hepatic impairment [see *Dosage and Administration (2)*].

13 NONCLINICAL TOXICOLOGY

13.1 Carcinogenesis, Mutagenesis, Impairment of Fertility

No carcinogenicity studies have been performed with levocetirizine. However, evaluation of cetirizine carcinogenicity studies are relevant for determination of the carcinogenic potential of levocetirizine. In a 2-year carcinogenicity study, in rats, cetirizine was not carcinogenic at dietary doses up to 20 mg/kg (approximately 15 times the maximum recommended daily oral dose in adults, approximately 10 times the maximum recommended daily oral dose in children 6 to 11 years of age and approximately 15 times the maximum recommended daily oral dose in children 6 months to 5 years of age on a mg/m^2 basis). In a 2-year carcinogenicity study in mice, cetirizine caused an increased incidence of benign hepatic tumors in males at a dietary dose of 16 mg/kg (approximately 6 times the maximum recommended daily oral dose in adults, approximately 4 times the maximum recommended daily oral dose in children 6 to 11 years of age, and approximately 6 times the maximum recommended daily oral dose in children 6 months to 5 years of age on a mg/m^2 basis). No increased incidence of benign tumors was observed at a dietary dose of 4 mg/kg (approximately 2 times the maximum recommended daily oral dose in adults, equivalent to the maximum recommended daily oral dose in children 6 to 11 years of age and approximately 2 times the maximum recommended daily oral dose in children 6 months to 5 years of age on a mg/m^2 basis). The clinical significance of these findings during long-term use of XYZAL is not known.
Levocetirizine was not mutagenic in the Ames test, and not clastogenic in the human lymphocyte assay, the mouse lymphoma assay, and *in vivo* micronucleus test in mice.
In a fertility and general reproductive performance study in mice, cetirizine did not impair fertility at an oral dose of 64 mg/kg (approximately 25 times the recommended daily oral dose in adults on a mg/m^2 basis).

13.2 Animal Toxicology

Reproductive Toxicology Studies
In rats and rabbits, levocetirizine was not teratogenic at oral doses up to 200 and 120 mg/kg, respectively, (approximately 320 and 390, respectively, times the maximum recommended daily oral dose in adults on a mg/m^2 basis).
In mice, cetirizine caused retarded pup weight gain during lactation at an oral dose in dams of 96 mg/kg (approximately 40 times the maximum recommended daily oral dose in adults on a mg/m^2 basis).

14 CLINICAL STUDIES

14.1 Seasonal and Perennial Allergic Rhinitis

Adults and Adolescents 12 Years of Age and Older
The efficacy of XYZAL was evaluated in six randomized, placebo-controlled, double-blind clinical trials in adult and adolescent patients 12 years and older with symptoms of seasonal allergic rhinitis or perennial allergic rhinitis. The six clinical trials include three dose-ranging trials of 2 to 4 weeks duration, one 2-week efficacy trial in patients with seasonal allergic rhinitis, and two efficacy trials (one 6-week and one 6-month) in patients with perennial allergic rhinitis.
These trials included a total of 2412 patients (1068 males and 1344 females) of whom 265 were adolescents 12 to 17 years of age. Efficacy was assessed using a total symptom score from patient recording of 4 symptoms (sneezing, rhinorrhea, nasal pruritus, and ocular pruritus) in five studies and 5 symptoms (sneezing, rhinorrhea, nasal pruritus, ocular pruritus, and nasal congestion) in one study. Patients recorded symptoms using a 0-3 categorical severity scale (0 = absent, 1 = mild, 2 = moderate, 3 = severe) once daily in the evening reflective of the 24 hour treatment period. In one study, patients also recorded these symptoms in an instantaneous (1 hour before the next dose) manner. The primary endpoint was the mean total symptom score averaged over the first week and over 2 weeks for seasonal allergic rhinitis trials, and 4 weeks for perennial allergic rhinitis trials.
The three dose-ranging trials were conducted to evaluate the efficacy of XYZAL 2.5, 5, and 10 mg once daily in the evening. One trial was 2 weeks in duration conducted in patients with seasonal allergic rhinitis, and two trials were 4 weeks in duration conducted in patients with perennial allergic rhinitis. In these trials, each of the three doses of XYZAL demonstrated greater decrease in the reflective total symptom score than placebo and the difference was statistically significant for all three doses in two of the studies. Results for two of these trials are shown in Table 4.
[See table 4 above]
One clinical trial was designed to evaluate the efficacy of XYZAL 5 mg once daily in the evening compared with placebo in patients with seasonal allergic rhinitis over a 2-week treatment period. In this trial, XYZAL 5 mg demonstrated a greater decrease from baseline in the reflective and instantaneous total symptom score than placebo, and the difference was statistically significant (see Table 5). The results of the instantaneous total symptom score support efficacy at the end of the dosing interval.
One clinical trial evaluated the efficacy of XYZAL 5 mg once daily in the evening compared to placebo in patients with perennial allergic rhinitis over a 6-week treatment period. Another trial conducted over a 6-month treatment period

Table 5   Mean Reflective Total Symptom Score* and Instantaneous Total Symptom Score in Allergic Rhinitis Trials

Treatment	N	Baseline	On Treatment Adjusted Mean	Difference from Placebo		
				Estimate	95% CI	p-value
Seasonal Allergic Rhinitis Trial – Reflective total symptom score						
XYZAL 5 mg	118	8.40	5.20	0.89	(0.30, 1.47)	0.003
Placebo	117	8.50	6.09			
Seasonal Allergic Rhinitis Trial – Instantaneous total symptom score						
XYZAL 5 mg	118	7.24	4.58	0.73	(0.17, 1.28)	0.011
Placebo	117	7.48	5.30			
Perennial Allergic Rhinitis Trial – Reflective total symptom score						
XYZAL 5 mg	150	7.69	3.93	1.17	(0.70, 1.64)	<0.001
Placebo	142	7.44	5.10			

*Total symptom score is the sum of individual symptoms of sneezing, rhinorrhea, nasal pruritus, and ocular pruritus as assessed by patients on a 0-3 categorical severity scale.

Table 6   Mean Reflective Pruritus Severity Score in Chronic Idiopathic Urticaria Trials

Treatment	N	Baseline	On Treatment Adjusted Mean	Difference from Placebo		
				Estimate	95% CI	p-value
Dose-Ranging Trial – Reflective pruritus severity score						
XYZAL 2.5 mg	69	2.08	1.02	0.82	(0.58, 1.06)	<0.001
XYZAL 5 mg	62	2.07	0.92	0.91	(0.66, 1.16)	<0.001
XYZAL 10 mg	55	2.04	0.73	1.11	(0.85, 1.37)	<0.001
Placebo	60	2.25	1.84			
Chronic Idiopathic Urticaria Trial – Reflective pruritus severity score						
XYZAL 5 mg	80	2.07	0.94	0.62	(0.38, 0.86)	<0.001
Placebo	82	2.06	1.56			

assessed efficacy at 4 weeks. XYZAL 5 mg demonstrated a greater decrease from baseline in the reflective total symptom score than placebo and the difference from placebo was statistically significant. Results of one of these trials are shown in Table 5.

[See table 5 above]

Onset of action was evaluated in two environmental exposure unit studies in allergic rhinitis patients with a single dose of XYZAL 2.5 or 5 mg. XYZAL 5 mg was found to have an onset of action 1 hour after oral intake. Onset of action was also assessed from the daily recording of symptoms in the evening before dosing in the seasonal and perennial allergic rhinitis trials. In these trials, onset of effect was seen after 1 day of dosing.

Pediatric Patients Less than 12 Years of Age

There are no clinical efficacy trials with XYZAL 2.5 mg once daily in pediatric patients under 12 years of age, and no clinical efficacy trials with XYZAL 1.25 mg once daily in pediatric patients 6 months to 5 years of age. The clinical efficacy of XYZAL in pediatric patients under 12 years of age has been extrapolated from adult clinical efficacy trials based on pharmacokinetic comparisons [see *Use in Specific Populations (8.4)*].

14.2   Chronic Idiopathic Urticaria

Adult Patients 18 Years of Age and Older

The efficacy of XYZAL for the treatment of the uncomplicated skin manifestations of chronic idiopathic urticaria was evaluated in two multi-center, randomized, placebo-controlled, double-blind clinical trials of 4 weeks duration in adult patients 18 to 85 years of age with chronic idiopathic urticaria. The two trials included one 4-week dose-ranging trial and one 4-week single-dose level efficacy trial. These trials included 423 patients (139 males and 284 females). Most patients (>90%) were Caucasian and the mean age was 41. Of these patients, 146 received XYZAL 5 mg once daily in the evening. Efficacy was assessed based on patient recording of pruritus severity on a severity score of 0-3 (0 = none to 3 = severe). The primary efficacy endpoint was the mean reflective pruritus severity score over the first week and over the entire treatment period. Additional efficacy variables were the instantaneous pruritus severity score, the number and size of wheals, and duration of pruritus.

The dose-ranging trial was conducted to evaluate the efficacy of XYZAL 2.5, 5, and 10 mg once daily in the evening. In this trial, each of the three doses of XYZAL demonstrated greater decrease in the reflective pruritus severity score than placebo and the difference was statistically significant for all three doses (see Table 6).

The single dose level trial evaluated the efficacy of XYZAL 5 mg once daily in the evening compared to placebo in patients with chronic idiopathic urticaria over a 4-week treatment period. XYZAL 5 mg demonstrated a greater decrease from baseline in the reflective pruritus severity score than placebo and the difference from placebo was statistically significant.

Duration of pruritus, number and size of wheals, and instantaneous pruritus severity score also showed significant improvement over placebo. The significant improvement in the instantaneous pruritus severity score over placebo confirmed end of dosing interval efficacy (see Table 6).

[See table 6 above]

Pediatric Patients

There are no clinical efficacy trials in pediatric patients with chronic idiopathic urticaria [see *Use in Specific Populations (8.4)*].

16   HOW SUPPLIED/STORAGE AND HANDLING

XYZAL tablets are white, film-coated, oval-shaped, scored, imprinted (with the letter Y in red color on both halves of the scored tablet) and contain 5 mg levocetirizine dihydrochloride. They are supplied in unit of use HDPE bottles and unit of use blisters.

90 Tablets (NDC 0024-5800-90)

30 count box, 3 cards of 10 (NDC 0024-5800-32)

XYZAL oral solution is a clear, colorless liquid containing 0.5 mg of levocetirizine dihydrochloride per mL.

Oral solution in 5 oz glass bottles (NDC 0024-5801-20)

Storage:

Store at 20-25°C (68-77°F); excursions permitted to 15-30°C (59-86°F) [see USP Controlled Room Temperature].

17   PATIENT COUNSELING INFORMATION

17.1   Activities Requiring Mental Alertness

Patients should be cautioned against engaging in hazardous occupations requiring complete mental alertness, and motor coordination such as operating machinery or driving a motor vehicle after ingestion of XYZAL.

17.2   Concomitant Use of Alcohol and other Central Nervous System Depressants

Concurrent use of XYZAL with alcohol or other central nervous system depressants should be avoided because additional reduction in mental alertness may occur.

17.3   Dosing of XYZAL

The daily dose in adults and adolescents 12 years of age and older should not exceed 5 mg once daily in the evening. In children 6 to 11 years of age the recommended dose is 2.5 mg once daily in the evening. In children 6 months to 5 years of age, the recommended dose is 1.25 mg once daily in the evening. Patients should be advised to not ingest more than the recommended dose of XYZAL because of the increased risk of somnolence at higher doses.

Manufactured for:

UCB, Inc.

Smyrna, GA 30080

and

Co-marketed by sanofi-aventis U.S. LLC

Bridgewater, NJ 08807

XYZAL is a registered trademark of the UCB Group of companies.

©2009 UCB, Inc. All rights reserved.

Shown in Product Identification Guide, page 319

Scandipharm, Inc.
(See AXCAN PHARMA U.S., INC.)

Schering Corporation
for product information, please see Merck

Schering-Plough HealthCare Products, Inc.
for product information, please see Merck

G.D. Searle & Co.
A Division of Pfizer
235 EAST 42ND STREET
NEW YORK, NY 10017-5755

For updates to the product information listed below, please check the Pfizer Web site, http://www.pfizerpro.com, or call (800) 438-1985. For complete product listing, please see the Manufacturers' Index.

For Medical Information, Contact:
(800) 438-1985
24 hours a day, 7 days a week

Distribution:
1855 Shelby Oaks Drive North
Memphis, TN 38134
(901) 387-5200

Customer Service:
(800) 533-4535

CELEBREX®   ℞
[sell-e-brecks]
(celecoxib)
Capsules

HIGHLIGHTS OF PRESCRIBING INFORMATION
These highlights do not include all the information needed to use CELEBREX safely and effectively. See full prescribing information for CELEBREX.
CELEBREX® (celecoxib) capsules
Initial U.S. Approval: 1998

WARNING: CARDIOVASCULAR AND GASTRO-INTESTINAL RISKS
See full prescribing information for complete boxed warning
Cardiovascular Risk
• CELEBREX, may cause an increased risk of serious cardiovascular thrombotic events, myocardial infarction, and stroke, which can be fatal. All NSAIDs may have a similar risk. This risk may increase with

duration of use. Patients with cardiovascular disease or risk factors for cardiovascular disease may be at greater risk. *(5.1, 14.7)*
- CELEBREX is contraindicated for the treatment of perioperative pain in the setting of coronary artery bypass graft (CABG) surgery. *(4, 5.1)*

Gastrointestinal Risk
- NSAIDs, including CELEBREX, cause an increased risk of serious gastrointestinal adverse events including bleeding, ulceration, and perforation of the stomach or intestines, which can be fatal. These events can occur at any time during use and without warning symptoms. Elderly patients are at greater risk for serious gastrointestinal (GI) events. *(5.4)*

---INDICATIONS AND USAGE---
CELEBREX is a nonsteroidal anti-inflammatory drug indicated for:
- Osteoarthritis (OA) (1.1)
- Rheumatoid Arthritis (RA) (1.2)
- Juvenile Rheumatoid Arthritis (JRA) in patients 2 years and older (1.3)
- Ankylosing Spondylitis (AS) (1.4)
- Acute Pain (AP) (1.5)
- Primary Dysmenorrhea (PD) (1.6)
- Familial Adenomatous Polyposis (FAP)-adjunct to usual care (1.7)

---DOSAGE AND ADMINISTRATION---
Use lowest effective dose for the shortest duration consistent with treatment goals for the individual patient. (1, 5.1, 5.4)
- OA: 200 mg once daily or 100 mg twice daily (2.1, 14.1)
- RA: 100 to 200 mg twice daily (2.2, 14.2)
- JRA: 50 mg twice daily in patients 10-25 kg. 100 mg twice daily in patients more than 25 kg (2.3, 14.3)
- AS: 200 mg once daily single dose or 100 mg twice daily. If no effect is observed after 6 weeks, a trial of 400 mg (single or divided doses) may be of benefit (2.4, 14.4)
- AP and PD: 400 mg initially, followed by 200 mg dose if needed on first day. On subsequent days, 200 mg twice daily as needed (2.5, 14.5)
- FAP: 400 mg twice daily with food, as an adjunct to usual care (2.6, 14.6)

Reduce daily dose by 50% in patients with moderate hepatic impairment (Child-Pugh Class B).
Consider a dose reduction by 50% (or alternative management for JRA) in patients who are known or suspected to be CYP2C9 poor metabolizers, (2.7, 8.4, 8.8, 12.3).

---DOSAGE FORMS AND STRENGTHS---
Capsules: 50 mg, 100 mg, 200 mg and 400 mg (3)

---CONTRAINDICATIONS---
- Known hypersensitivity to celecoxib or sulfonamides (4)
- History of asthma, urticaria, or other allergic-type reactions after taking aspirin or other NSAIDs (4, 5.7, 5.8, 5.13)
- Use during the perioperative period in the setting of coronary artery bypass graft (CABG) surgery (4, 5.1)

---WARNINGS AND PRECAUTIONS---
- Serious and potentially fatal cardiovascular (CV) thrombotic events, myocardial infarction, and stroke. Patients with known CV disease/risk factors may be at greater risk (5.1, 14.7, 17.2).
- Serious gastrointestinal (GI) adverse events, which can be fatal. The risk is greater in patients with a prior history of ulcer disease or GI bleeding, and in patients at high risk for GI events, especially the elderly. CELEBREX should be used with caution in these patients (5.4, 8.5, 14.7, 17.3).
- Elevated liver enzymes and, rarely, severe hepatic reactions. Discontinue use of CELEBREX immediately if abnormal liver enzymes persist or worsen (5.5, 17.4).
- New onset or worsening of hypertension. Blood pressure should be monitored closely during treatment with CELEBREX (5.2, 7.4, 17.2).
- Fluid retention and edema. CELEBREX should be used with caution in patients with fluid retention or heart failure (5.3, 17.6).
- Renal papillary necrosis and other renal injury with long term use. Use CELEBREX with caution in the elderly, those with impaired renal function, heart failure, liver dysfunction, and those taking diuretics, ACE-inhibitors, or angiotensin II antagonists (5.6, 7.4, 8.7, 17.6).
- Anaphylactoid reactions. Do not use CELEBREX in patients with the aspirin triad (5.7, 10, 17.7).
- Serious skin adverse events such as exfoliative dermatitis, Stevens-Johnson syndrome (SJS), and toxic epidermal necrolysis (TEN), which can be fatal and can occur without warning even without known prior sulfa allergy. Discontinue CELEBREX at first appearance of rash or skin reactions (5.8, 17.5).

---ADVERSE REACTIONS---
Most common adverse reactions in arthritis trials (>2% and >placebo): abdominal pain, diarrhea, dyspepsia, flatulence,

peripheral edema, accidental injury, dizziness, pharyngitis, rhinitis, sinusitis, upper respiratory tract infection, rash (6.1).

To report SUSPECTED ADVERSE REACTIONS, contact Pfizer at 1-800-438-1985 or FDA at 1-800-FDA-1088 or www.fda.gov/medwatch

---DRUG INTERACTIONS---
- Concomitant use of CELEBREX and warfarin may result in increased risk of bleeding complications. (7.1)
- Concomitant use of CELEBREX increases lithium plasma levels. (7.2)
- Concomitant use of CELEBREX may reduce the antihypertensive effect of ACE Inhibitors and angiotensin II antagonists (7.4)
- Use caution with drugs known to inhibit P450 2C9 or metabolized by 2D6 due to the potential for increased plasma levels (2.7, 8.4, 8.8, 12.3).

---USE IN SPECIFIC POPULATIONS---
- Pregnancy Category C prior to 30 weeks gestation; Category D starting at 30 weeks gestation (5.9, 8.1, 17.8)

See 17 for PATIENT COUNSELING INFORMATION and Medication Guide
Revised: June 2009

FULL PRESCRIBING INFORMATION: CONTENTS*
BOXED WARNING
* Sections or subsections omitted from the Full Prescribing Information are not listed.

FULL PRESCRIBING INFORMATION

WARNING: CARDIOVASCULAR AND GASTROINTESTINAL RISKS
Cardiovascular Risk
- CELEBREX may cause an increased risk of serious cardiovascular thrombotic events, myocardial infarction, and stroke, which can be fatal. All nonsteroidal anti-inflammatory drugs (NSAIDs) may have a similar risk. This risk may increase with duration of use. Patients with cardiovascular disease or risk factors for cardiovascular disease may be at greater risk. *(5.1, 14.7)*
- CELEBREX is contraindicated for the treatment of perioperative pain in the setting of coronary artery bypass graft (CABG) surgery. *(4, 5.1)*

Gastrointestinal Risk
- NSAIDs, including CELEBREX, cause an increased risk of serious gastrointestinal adverse events including bleeding, ulceration, and perforation of the stomach or intestines, which can be fatal. These events can occur at any time during use and without warning symptoms. Elderly patients are at greater risk for serious gastrointestinal events. *(5.4)*

1. INDICATIONS AND USAGE
Carefully consider the potential benefits and risks of CELEBREX and other treatment options before deciding to use CELEBREX. Use the lowest effective dose for the shortest duration consistent with individual patient treatment goals [*see Warnings and Precautions (5)*]

1.1 Osteoarthritis (OA)
CELEBREX is indicated for relief of the signs and symptoms of OA [*see Clinical Studies (14.1)*]

1.2 Rheumatoid Arthritis (RA)
CELEBREX is indicated for relief of the signs and symptoms of RA [*see Clinical Studies (14.2)*]

1.3 Juvenile Rheumatoid Arthritis (JRA)
CELEBREX is indicated for relief of the signs and symptoms of JRA in patients 2 years and older [*see Clinical Studies (14.3)*]

1.4 Ankylosing Spondylitis (AS)
CELEBREX is indicated for the relief of signs and symptoms of AS [*see Clinical Studies (14.4)*]

1.5 Acute Pain (AP)
CELEBREX is indicated for the management of AP in adults [*see Clinical Studies (14.5)*]

1.6 Primary Dysmenorrhea (PD)
CELEBREX is indicated for the treatment of PD [*see Clinical Studies (14.5)*]

1.7 Familial Adenomatous Polyposis (FAP)
CELEBREX is indicated to reduce the number of adenomatous colorectal polyps in FAP, as an adjunct to usual care (e.g., endoscopic surveillance, surgery). It is not known whether there is a clinical benefit from a reduction in the number of colorectal polyps in FAP patients. It is also not known whether the effects of CELEBREX treatment will persist after CELEBREX is discontinued. The efficacy and safety of CELEBREX treatment in patients with FAP beyond six months have not been studied [*see Warnings and Precautions (5.15), Clinical Studies (14.6)*] •

2. DOSAGE AND ADMINISTRATION
Use lowest effective dose for the shortest duration consistent with treatment goals for the individual patient.
These doses can be given without regard to timing of meals.

2.1 Osteoarthritis
For relief of the signs and symptoms of OA the recommended oral dose is 200 mg per day administered as a single dose or as 100 mg twice daily.

2.2 Rheumatoid Arthritis
For relief of the signs and symptoms of RA the recommended oral dose is 100 to 200 mg twice daily.

2.3 Juvenile Rheumatoid Arthritis
For the relief of the signs and symptoms of JRA the recommended oral dose for pediatric patients (age 2 years and older) is based on weight. For patients ≥10 kg to ≤25 kg the recommended dose is 50 mg twice daily. For patients >25 kg the recommended dose is 100 mg twice daily.
For patients who have difficulty swallowing capsules, the contents of a CELEBREX capsule can be added to applesauce. The entire capsule contents are carefully emptied onto a level teaspoon of cool or room temperature applesauce and ingested immediately with water. The sprinkled capsule contents on applesauce are stable for up to 6 hours under refrigerated conditions (2-8° C/35-45° F).

2.4 Ankylosing Spondylitis
For the management of the signs and symptoms of AS, the recommended dose of Celebrex is 200 mg daily in single (once per day) or divided (twice per day) doses. If no effect is observed after 6 weeks, a trial of 400 mg daily may be worthwhile. If no effect is observed after 6 weeks on 400 mg daily, a response is not likely and consideration should be given to alternate treatment options.

2.5 Management of Acute Pain and Treatment of Primary Dysmenorrhea
The recommended dose of Celebrex is 400 mg initially, followed by an additional 200 mg dose if needed on the first day. On subsequent days, the recommended dose is 200 mg twice daily as needed.

2.6 Familial Adenomatous Polyposis
Usual medical care for FAP patients should be continued while on Celebrex. To reduce the number of adenomatous colorectal polyps in patients with FAP, the recommended oral dose is 400 mg twice per day to be taken with food.

2.7 Special Populations
Hepatic insufficiency: The daily recommended dose of Celebrex capsules in patients with moderate hepatic impairment (Child-Pugh Class B) should be reduced by 50%. The use of Celebrex in patients with severe hepatic impairment is not recommended [*see Warnings and Precautions (5.5), Use in Specific Populations (8.6) and Clinical Pharmacology (12.3)*].
Poor Metabolizers of CYP2C9 Substrates: Patients who are known or suspected to be poor CYP2C9 metabolizers based on previous history/experience with other CYP2C9 substrates (such as warfarin, phenytoin) should be administered celecoxib with caution. Consider starting treatment at half the lowest recommended dose in poor metabolizers. Consider using alternative management in JRA patients who are poor metabolizers. [*see Use in Specific populations (8.8), and Clinical Pharmacology (12.3)*].

3. DOSAGE FORMS AND STRENGTHS
Capsules: 50 mg, 100 mg, 200 mg and 400 mg

4. CONTRAINDICATIONS
Celebrex is contraindicated:
- In patients with known hypersensitivity to celecoxib, aspirin, or other NSAIDs.
- In patients who have demonstrated allergic-type reactions to sulfonamides.
- In patients who have experienced asthma, urticaria, or allergic-type reactions after taking aspirin or other NSAIDs. Severe anaphylactoid reactions to NSAIDs, some of them fatal, have been reported in such patients [*see Warnings and Precautions (5.7, 5.13)*].
- For the treatment of peri-operative pain in the setting of coronary artery bypass graft (CABG) surgery [*see Warnings and Precautions (5.1)*].

5. WARNINGS AND PRECAUTIONS

5.1 Cardiovascular Thrombotic Events
Chronic use of Celebrex may cause an increased risk of serious adverse cardiovascular thrombotic events, myocardial infarction, and stroke, which can be fatal. In the APC (Adenoma Prevention with Celecoxib) trial, the hazard ratio for the composite endpoint of cardiovascular death, MI, or stroke was 3.4 (95% CI 1.4–8.5) for Celebrex 400 mg twice daily and 2.8 (95% CI 1.1–7.2) with Celebrex 200 mg twice daily compared to placebo. Cumulative rates for this composite endpoint over 3 years were 3.0% (20/671 subjects) and 2.5% (17/685 subjects), respectively, compared to 0.9% (6/679 subjects) with placebo treatment. The increases in both celecoxib dose groups versus placebo-treated patients were mainly due to an increased incidence of myocardial infarction [*see Clinical Studies (14.7)*].
All NSAIDs, both COX-2 selective and non-selective, may have a similar risk. Patients with known CV disease or risk factors for CV disease may be at greater risk. To minimize the potential risk for an adverse CV event in patients treated with Celebrex, the lowest effective dose should be used for the shortest duration consistent with individual patient treatment goals. Physicians and patients should remain alert for the development of such events, even in the absence of previous CV symptoms. Patients should be informed about the signs and/or symptoms of serious CV toxicity and the steps to take if they occur.
There is no consistent evidence that concurrent use of aspirin mitigates the increased risk of serious CV thrombotic events associated with NSAID use. The concurrent use of aspirin and Celebrex does increase the risk of serious GI events [*see Warnings and Precautions (5.4)*].
Two large, controlled, clinical trials of a different COX-2 selective NSAID for the treatment of pain in the first 10-14 days following CABG surgery found an increased incidence of myocardial infarction and stroke [*see Contraindications (4)*].

5.2 Hypertension
As with all NSAIDs, Celebrex can lead to the onset of new hypertension or worsening of preexisting hypertension, either of which may contribute to the increased incidence of CV events. Patients taking thiazides or loop diuretics may have impaired response to these therapies when taking NSAIDs. NSAIDs, including Celebrex, should be used with caution in patients with hypertension. Blood pressure should be monitored closely during the initiation of therapy with Celebrex and throughout the course of therapy. The rates of hypertension from the CLASS trial in the Celebrex, ibuprofen and diclofenac-treated patients were 2.4%, 4.2% and 2.5%, respectively [*see Clinical Studies (14.7)*].

5.3 Congestive Heart Failure and Edema
Fluid retention and edema have been observed in some patients taking NSAIDs, including Celebrex [*see Adverse Reactions (6.1)*]. In the CLASS study [*see Clinical Studies (14.7)*], the Kaplan-Meier cumulative rates at 9 months of peripheral edema in patients on Celebrex 400 mg twice daily (4-fold and 2-fold the recommended OA and RA doses, respectively, and the approved dose for FAP), ibuprofen 800 mg three times daily and diclofenac 75 mg twice daily were 4.5%, 6.9% and 4.7%, respectively. Celebrex should be used with caution in patients with fluid retention or heart failure.

5.4 Gastrointestinal (GI) Effects

Risk of GI Ulceration, Bleeding, and Perforation
NSAIDs, including Celebrex, can cause serious gastrointestinal events including bleeding, ulceration, and perforation of the stomach, small intestine or large intestine, which can be fatal. These serious adverse events can occur at any time, with or without warning symptoms, in patients treated with NSAIDs. Only one in five patients who develop a serious upper GI adverse event on NSAID therapy is symptomatic. Complicated and symptomatic ulcer rates were 0.78% at nine months for all patients in the CLASS trial, and 2.19% for the subgroup on low-dose ASA. Patients 65 years of age and older had an incidence of 1.40% at nine months, 3.06% when also taking ASA [*see Clinical Studies (14.7)*]. With longer duration of use of NSAIDs, there is a trend for increasing the likelihood of developing a serious GI event at some time during the course of therapy. However, even short-term therapy is not without risk.
NSAIDs should be prescribed with extreme caution in patients with a prior history of ulcer disease or gastrointestinal bleeding. Patients with a prior history of peptic ulcer disease and/or gastrointestinal bleeding who use NSAIDs have a greater than 10-fold increased risk for developing a GI bleed compared to patients with neither of these risk factors. Other factors that increase the risk of GI bleeding in patients treated with NSAIDs include concomitant use of oral corticosteroids or anticoagulants, longer duration of NSAID therapy, smoking, use of alcohol, older age, and poor general health status. Most spontaneous reports of fatal GI events are in elderly or debilitated patients and therefore special care should be taken in treating this population.
To minimize the potential risk for an adverse GI event, the lowest effective dose should be used for the shortest duration consistent with individual patient treatment goals. Physicians and patients should remain alert for signs and symptoms of GI ulceration and bleeding during Celebrex therapy and promptly initiate additional evaluation and treatment if a serious GI adverse event is suspected. For high-risk patients, alternate therapies that do not involve NSAIDs should be considered.

5.5 Hepatic Effects
Borderline elevations of one or more liver-associated enzymes may occur in up to 15% of patients taking NSAIDs, and notable elevations of ALT or AST (approximately 3 or more times the upper limit of normal) have been reported in approximately 1% of patients in clinical trials with NSAIDs. These laboratory abnormalities may progress, may remain unchanged, or may be transient with continuing therapy. Rare cases of severe hepatic reactions, including jaundice and fatal fulminant hepatitis, liver necrosis and hepatic failure (some with fatal outcome) have been reported with NSAIDs, including Celebrex [*see Adverse Reactions (6.1)*]. In controlled clinical trials of Celebrex, the incidence of borderline elevations (greater than or equal to 1.2 times and less than 3 times the upper limit of normal) of liver associated enzymes was 6% for Celebrex and 5% for placebo, and approximately 0.2% of patients taking Celebrex and 0.3% of patients taking placebo had notable elevations of ALT and AST.
A patient with symptoms and/or signs suggesting liver dysfunction, or in whom an abnormal liver test has occurred, should be monitored carefully for evidence of the development of a more severe hepatic reaction while on therapy with Celebrex. If clinical signs and symptoms consistent with liver disease develop, or if systemic manifestations occur (e.g., eosinophilia, rash, etc.), Celebrex should be discontinued.

5.6 Renal Effects
Long-term administration of NSAIDs has resulted in renal papillary necrosis and other renal injury. Renal toxicity has also been seen in patients in whom renal prostaglandins have a compensatory role in the maintenance of renal perfusion. In these patients, administration of an NSAID may cause a dose-dependent reduction in prostaglandin formation and, secondarily, in renal blood flow, which may precipitate overt renal decompensation. Patients at greatest risk of this reaction are those with impaired renal function, heart failure, liver dysfunction, those taking diuretics, ACE-inhibitors, angiotensin II receptor antagonists, and the elderly. Discontinuation of NSAID therapy is usually followed by recovery to the pretreatment state. Clinical trials with Celebrex have shown renal effects similar to those observed with comparator NSAIDs.
No information is available from controlled clinical studies regarding the use of Celebrex in patients with advanced renal disease. Therefore, treatment with Celebrex is not recommended in these patients with advanced renal disease. If CELEBREX therapy must be initiated, close monitoring of the patient's renal function is advisable.

5.7 Anaphylactoid Reactions
As with NSAIDs in general, anaphylactoid reactions have occurred in patients without known prior exposure to Celebrex. In post-marketing experience, rare cases of anaphylactic reactions and angioedema have been reported in patients receiving Celebrex. Celebrex should not be given to patients with the aspirin triad. This symptom complex typically occurs in asthmatic patients who experience rhinitis with or without nasal polyps, or who exhibit severe, potentially fatal bronchospasm after taking aspirin or other NSAIDs [*see Contraindications (4), Warnings and Precautions (5.7)*]. Emergency help should be sought in cases where an anaphylactoid reaction occurs.

5.8 Skin Reactions
Celebrex is a sulfonamide and can cause serious skin adverse events such as exfoliative dermatitis, Stevens-Johnson syndrome (SJS), and toxic epidermal necrolysis (TEN), which can be fatal. These serious events can occur without warning and in patients without prior known sulfa allergy. Patients should be informed about the signs and symptoms of serious skin manifestations and use of the drug should be discontinued at the first appearance of skin rash or any other sign of hypersensitivity.

5.9 Pregnancy
In late pregnancy, starting at 30 weeks gestation, Celebrex should be avoided because it may cause premature closure of the ductus arteriosus [*see Use in Specific Populations (8.1)*].

5.10 Corticosteroid Treatment
Celebrex cannot be expected to substitute for corticosteroids or to treat corticosteroid insufficiency. Abrupt discontinuation of corticosteroids may lead to exacerbation of corticosteroid-responsive illness. Patients on prolonged corticosteroid therapy should have their therapy tapered slowly if a decision is made to discontinue corticosteroids.

5.11 Hematological Effects
Anemia is sometimes seen in patients receiving Celebrex. In controlled clinical trials the incidence of anemia was 0.6% with Celebrex and 0.4% with placebo. Patients on long-term treatment with Celebrex should have their hemoglobin or hematocrit checked if they exhibit any signs or symptoms of anemia or blood loss. Celebrex does not generally affect platelet counts, prothrombin time (PT), or partial thromboplastin time (PTT), and does not inhibit platelet aggregation at indicated dosages [*see Clinical Pharmacology (12.2)*].

5.12 Disseminated Intravascular Coagulation (DIC)
Celebrex should be used only with caution in pediatric patients with systemic onset JRA due to the risk of disseminated intravascular coagulation.

5.13 Preexisting Asthma
Patients with asthma may have aspirin-sensitive asthma. The use of aspirin in patients with aspirin-sensitive asthma has been associated with severe bronchospasm, which can be fatal. Since cross reactivity, including bronchospasm, between aspirin and other nonsteroidal anti-inflammatory drugs has been reported in such aspirin-sensitive patients,

CELEBREX should not be administered to patients with this form of aspirin sensitivity and should be used with caution in patients with preexisting asthma.

5.14 Laboratory Tests

Because serious GI tract ulcerations and bleeding can occur without warning symptoms, physicians should monitor for signs or symptoms of GI bleeding. Patients on long-term treatment with NSAIDs should have a CBC and a chemistry profile checked periodically. If abnormal liver tests or renal tests persist or worsen, CELEBREX should be discontinued.

In controlled clinical trials, elevated BUN occurred more frequently in patients receiving CELEBREX compared with patients on placebo. This laboratory abnormality was also seen in patients who received comparator NSAIDs in these studies. The clinical significance of this abnormality has not been established.

5.15 GI Cancer in Familial Adenomatous Polyposis

Treatment with CELEBREX in FAP has not been shown to reduce the risk of gastrointestinal cancer or the need for prophylactic colectomy or other FAP-related surgeries. Therefore, the usual care of FAP patients should not be altered because of the concurrent administration of CELEBREX. In particular, the frequency of routine endoscopic surveillance should not be decreased and prophylactic colectomy or other FAP-related surgeries should not be delayed.

5.16 Inflammation

The pharmacological activity of CELEBREX in reducing inflammation, and possibly fever, may diminish the utility of these diagnostic signs in detecting infectious complications of presumed noninfectious, painful conditions.

5.17 Concomitant NSAID Use

The concomitant use of CELEBREX with any dose of a non-aspirin NSAID should be avoided due to the potential for increased risk of adverse reactions.

6. ADVERSE REACTIONS

Of the CELEBREX-treated patients in the pre-marketing controlled clinical trials, approximately 4,250 were patients with OA, approximately 2,100 were patients with RA, and approximately 1,050 were patients with post-surgical pain. More than 8,500 patients received a total daily dose of CELEBREX of 200 mg (100 mg twice daily or 200 mg once daily) or more, including more than 400 treated at 800 mg (400 mg twice daily). Approximately 3,900 patients received CELEBREX at these doses for 6 months or more; approximately 2,300 of these have received it for 1 year or more and 124 of these have received it for 2 years or more.

Because clinical trials are conducted under widely varying conditions, adverse reaction rates observed in the clinical trials of a drug cannot be directly compared to rates in the clinical trials of another drug and may not reflect the rates observed in practice. The adverse reaction information from clinical trials does, however, provide a basis for identifying the adverse events that appear to be related to drug use and for approximating rates.

6.1 Pre-marketing Controlled Arthritis Trials

Table 1 lists all adverse events, regardless of causality, occurring in ≥2% of patients receiving CELEBREX from 12 controlled studies conducted in patients with OA or RA that included a placebo and/or a positive control group. Since these 12 trials were of different durations, and patients in the trials may not have been exposed for the same duration of time, these percentages do not capture cumulative rates of occurrence.

[See table 1 above]

In placebo- or active-controlled clinical trials, the discontinuation rate due to adverse events was 7.1% for patients receiving CELEBREX and 6.1% for patients receiving placebo. Among the most common reasons for discontinuation due to adverse events in the CELEBREX treatment groups were dyspepsia and abdominal pain (cited as reasons for discontinuation in 0.8% and 0.7% of CELEBREX patients, respectively). Among patients receiving placebo, 0.6% discontinued due to dyspepsia and 0.6% withdrew due to abdominal pain.

The following adverse reactions occurred in 0.1-1.9% of patients treated with CELEBREX (100-200 mg twice daily or 200 mg once daily):

Gastrointestinal:	Constipation, diverticulitis, dysphagia, eructation, esophagitis, gastritis, gastroenteritis, gastroesophageal reflux, hemorrhoids, hiatal hernia, melena, dry mouth, stomatitis, tenesmus, vomiting
Cardiovascular:	Aggravated hypertension, angina pectoris, coronary artery disorder, myocardial infarction

General:	Allergy aggravated, allergic reaction, chest pain, cyst NOS, edema generalized, face edema, fatigue, fever, hot flushes, influenza-like symptoms, pain, peripheral pain
Central, peripheral nervous system:	Leg cramps, hypertonia, hypoesthesia, migraine, paresthesia, vertigo
Hearing and vestibular:	Deafness, tinnitus
Heart rate and rhythm:	Palpitation, tachycardia
Liver and biliary:	Hepatic function abnormal, SGOT increased, SGPT increased
Metabolic and nutritional:	BUN increased, CPK increased, hypercholesterolemia, hyperglycemia, hypokalemia, NPN increased, creatinine increased, alkaline phosphatase increased, weight increased
Musculoskeletal:	Arthralgia, arthrosis, myalgia, synovitis, tendinitis
Platelets (bleeding or clotting):	Ecchymosis, epistaxis, thrombocythemia,
Psychiatric:	Anorexia, anxiety, appetite increased, depression, nervousness, somnolence
Hemic:	Anemia
Respiratory:	Bronchitis, bronchospasm, bronchospasm aggravated, coughing, dyspnea, laryngitis, pneumonia
Skin and appendages:	Alopecia, dermatitis, photosensitivity reaction, pruritus, rash erythematous, rash maculopapular, skin disorder, skin dry, sweating increased, urticaria
Application site disorders:	Cellulitis, dermatitis contact
Urinary:	Albuminuria, cystitis, dysuria, hematuria, micturition frequency, renal calculus

The following serious adverse events (causality not evaluated) occurred in <0.1% of patients (cases reported only in post-marketing experience are indicated *in italics*):

Cardiovascular:	Syncope, congestive heart failure, ventricular fibrillation, pulmonary embolism, cerebrovascular accident, peripheral gangrene, thrombophlebitis, *vasculitis, deep venous thrombosis*

Table 1: Adverse Events Occurring in ≥2% of CELEBREX Patients from Pre-marketing Controlled Arthritis Trials

	CBX N=4146	Placebo N=1864	NAP N=1366	DCF N=387	IBU N=345
Gastrointestinal					
Abdominal Pain	4.1%	2.8%	7.7%	9.0%	9.0%
Diarrhea	5.6%	3.8%	5.3%	9.3%	5.8%
Dyspepsia	8.8%	6.2%	12.2%	10.9%	12.8%
Flatulence	2.2%	1.0%	3.6%	4.1%	3.5%
Nausea	3.5%	4.2%	6.0%	3.4%	6.7%
Body as a whole					
Back Pain	2.8%	3.6%	2.2%	2.6%	0.9%
Peripheral Edema	2.1%	1.1%	2.1%	1.0%	3.5%
Injury-Accidental	2.9%	2.3%	3.0%	2.6%	3.2%
Central, Peripheral Nervous System					
Dizziness	2.0%	1.7%	2.6%	1.3%	2.3%
Headache	15.8%	20.2%	14.5%	15.5%	15.4%
Psychiatric					
Insomnia	2.3%	2.3%	2.9%	1.3%	1.4%
Respiratory					
Pharyngitis	2.3%	1.1%	1.7%	1.6%	2.6%
Rhinitis	2.0%	1.3%	2.4%	2.3%	0.6%
Sinusitis	5.0%	4.3%	4.0%	5.4%	5.8%
Upper Respiratory Infection	8.1%	6.7%	9.9%	9.8%	9.9%
Skin					
Rash	2.2%	2.1%	2.1%	1.3%	1.2%

CBX = CELEBREX 100–200 mg twice daily or 200 mg once daily;
NAP = Naproxen 500 mg twice daily;
DCF = Diclofenac 75 mg twice daily;
IBU = Ibuprofen 800 mg three times daily.

Gastrointestinal:	Intestinal obstruction, intestinal perforation, gastrointestinal bleeding, colitis with bleeding, esophageal perforation, pancreatitis, ileus
Liver and biliary:	Cholelithiasis, *hepatitis, jaundice, liver failure*
Hemic and lymphatic:	Thrombocytopenia, *agranulocytosis, aplastic anemia, pancytopenia, leucopenia*
Metabolic:	Hypoglycemia, *hyponatremia*
Nervous:	Ataxia, suicide, *aseptic meningitis, ageusia, anosmia, fatal intracranial hemorrhage [see Drug Interactions (7.1)]*
Renal:	Acute renal failure, *interstitial nephritis*
Skin:	*Erythema multiforme, exfoliative dermatitis, Stevens-Johnson syndrome, toxic epidermal necrolysis*
General:	Sepsis, sudden death, *anaphylactoid reaction, angioedema*

6.2 The Celecoxib Long-Term Arthritis Safety Study [see *Special Studies* (14.7)]

Hematological Events: The incidence of clinically significant decreases in hemoglobin (>2 g/dL) was lower in patients on CELEBREX 400 mg twice daily (0.5%) compared to patients on either diclofenac 75 mg twice daily (1.3%) or ibuprofen 800 mg three times daily 1.9%. The lower incidence of events with CELEBREX was maintained with or without ASA use [see *Clinical Pharmacology (12.2)*].

Withdrawals/Serious Adverse Events: Kaplan-Meier cumulative rates at 9 months for withdrawals due to adverse events for CELEBREX, diclofenac and ibuprofen were 24%, 29%, and 26%, respectively. Rates for serious adverse events (i.e., causing hospitalization or felt to be life-threatening or otherwise medically significant), regardless of causality, were not different across treatment groups (8%, 7%, and 8%, respectively).

6.3 Juvenile Rheumatoid Arthritis Study

In a 12-week, double-blind, active-controlled study, 242 JRA patients 2 years to 17 years of age were treated with celecoxib or naproxen; 77 JRA patients were treated with celecoxib 3 mg/kg BID, 82 patients were treated with celecoxib 6 mg/kg BID, and 83 patients were treated with naproxen 7.5 mg/kg BID. The most commonly occurring (≥5%) adverse events in celecoxib treated patients were headache, fever (pyrexia), upper abdominal pain, cough, nasopharyngitis, abdominal pain, nausea, arthralgia, diarrhea and vomiting. The most commonly occurring (≥5%) adverse experiences for naproxen-treated patients were headache, nausea, vomiting, fever, upper abdominal pain, diarrhea, cough, abdominal pain, and dizziness (Table 2). Compared with naproxen, celecoxib at doses of 3 and 6 mg/kg BID had no observable deleterious effect on growth and development during the course of the 12-week double-blind study. There was no substantial difference in the number of clinical exacerbations of uveitis or systemic features of JRA among treatment groups.

In a 12-week, open-label extension of the double-blind study described above, 202 JRA patients were treated with celecoxib 6 mg/kg BID. The incidence of adverse events was similar to that observed during the double-blind study; no unexpected adverse events of clinical importance emerged.

Table 2: Adverse Events Occurring in ≥5% of JRA Patients in Any Treatment Group, by System Organ Class (% of patients with events)

System Organ Class Preferred Term	All Doses Twice Daily		
	Celecoxib 3 mg/kg N=77	Celecoxib 6 mg/kg N=82	Naproxen 7.5 mg/kg N=83
Any Event	64	70	72
Eye Disorders	5	5	5
Gastrointestinal	26	24	36
Abdominal pain NOS	4	7	7
Abdominal pain upper	8	6	10
Vomiting NOS	3	6	11
Diarrhea NOS	5	4	8
Nausea	7	4	11
General	13	11	18
Pyrexia	8	9	11
Infections	25	20	27
Nasopharyngitis	5	6	5
Injury and Poisoning	4	6	5
Investigations*	3	11	7
Musculoskeletal	8	10	17
Arthralgia	3	7	4
Nervous System	17	11	21
Headache NOS	13	10	16
Dizziness (excl vertigo)	1	1	7
Respiratory	8	15	15
Cough	7	7	8
Skin & Subcutaneous	10	7	18

*Abnormal laboratory tests, which include: Prolonged activated partial thromboplastin time, Bacteriuria NOS present, Blood creatine phosphokinase increased, Blood culture positive, Blood glucose increased, Blood pressure increased, Blood uric acid increased, Hematocrit decreased, Hematuria present, Hemoglobin decreased, Liver function tests NOS abnormal, Proteinuria present, Transaminase NOS increased, Urine analysis abnormal NOS

6.4   Other Pre-Approval Studies
Adverse Events from Ankylosing Spondylitis Studies: A total of 378 patients were treated with CELEBREX in placebo- and active-controlled AS studies. Doses up to 400 mg once daily were studied. The types of adverse events reported in the AS studies were similar to those reported in the OA/RA studies.
Adverse Events from Analgesia and Dysmenorrhea Studies: Approximately 1,700 patients were treated with CELEBREX in analgesia and dysmenorrhea studies. All patients in post-oral surgery pain studies received a single dose of study medication. Doses up to 600 mg/day of CELEBREX were studied in primary dysmenorrhea and post-orthopedic surgery pain studies. The types of adverse events in the analgesia and dysmenorrhea studies were similar to those reported in arthritis studies. The only additional adverse event reported was post-dental extraction alveolar osteitis (dry socket) in the post-oral surgery pain studies.
Adverse Events from the Familial Adenomatous Polyposis Study: The adverse event profile reported for the 83 pa-

tients with familial adenomatous polyposis enrolled in the randomized, controlled clinical trial was similar to that reported for patients in the arthritis-controlled trials. Intestinal anastomotic ulceration was the only new adverse event reported in the FAP trial, regardless of causality, and was observed in 3 of 58 patients (one at 100 mg twice daily, and two at 400 mg twice daily) who had prior intestinal surgery.

6.5   The APC and PreSAP Trials
Adverse reactions from long-term, placebo-controlled polyp prevention studies: Exposure to CELEBREX in the APC and PreSAP trials was 400 to 800 mg daily for up to 3 years [*see Special Studies Adenomatous Polyp Prevention Studies (14.7)*].
Some adverse reactions occurred in higher percentages of patients than in the arthritis pre-marketing trials (treatment durations up to 12 weeks; see *Adverse events from* CELEBREX *pre-marketing controlled arthritis trials*, above). The adverse reactions for which these differences in patients treated with CELEBREX were greater as compared to the arthritis pre-marketing trials were as follows:

	CELEBREX (400 to 800 mg daily) N = 2285	Placebo N=1303
Diarrhea	10.5%	7.0%
Gastroesophageal reflux disease	4.7%	3.1%
Nausea	6.8%	5.3%
Vomiting	3.2%	2.1%
Dyspnea	2.8%	1.6%
Hypertension	12.5%	9.8%

The following additional adverse reactions occurred in ≥0.1% and <1% of patients taking CELEBREX, at an incidence greater than placebo in the long-term polyp prevention studies and were either not reported during the controlled arthritis pre-marketing trials or occurred with greater frequency in the long-term, placebo-controlled polyp prevention studies:

Nervous system disorders:	Cerebral infarction
Eye disorders:	Vitreous floaters, conjunctival hemorrhage
Ear and labyrinth:	Labyrinthitis
Cardiac disorders:	Angina unstable, aortic valve incompetence, coronary artery atherosclerosis, sinus bradycardia, ventricular hypertrophy
Vascular disorders:	Deep vein thrombosis
Reproductive system and breast disorders:	Ovarian cyst
Investigations:	Blood potassium increased, blood sodium increased, blood testosterone decreased
Injury, poisoning and procedural complications:	Epicondylitis, tendon rupture

7.   DRUG INTERACTIONS

General: Celecoxib metabolism is predominantly mediated via cytochrome P450 (CYP) 2C9 in the liver. Co-administration of celecoxib with drugs that are known to inhibit CYP2C9 should be done with caution. Significant interactions may occur when celecoxib is administered together with drugs that inhibit CYP2C9.
In vitro studies indicate that celecoxib, although not a substrate, is an inhibitor of CYP2D6. Therefore, there is a potential for an *in vivo* drug interaction with drugs that are metabolized by CYP2D6.

7.1   Warfarin
Anticoagulant activity should be monitored, particularly in the first few days, after initiating or changing CELEBREX therapy in patients receiving warfarin or similar agents, since these patients are at an increased risk of bleeding complications. The effect of celecoxib on the anticoagulant effect of warfarin was studied in a group of healthy subjects receiving daily 2-5 mg doses of warfarin. In these subjects, celecoxib did not alter the anticoagulant effect of warfarin as determined by prothrombin time. However, in post-marketing experience, serious bleeding events, some of which were fatal, have been reported, predominantly in the elderly, in association with increases in prothrombin time in patients receiving CELEBREX concurrently with warfarin.

7.2   Lithium
In a study conducted in healthy subjects, mean steady-state lithium plasma levels increased approximately 17% in subjects receiving lithium 450 mg twice daily with CELEBREX 200 mg twice daily as compared to subjects receiving lithium alone. Patients on lithium treatment should be closely monitored when CELEBREX is introduced or withdrawn.

7.3   Aspirin
CELEBREX can be used with low-dose aspirin. However, concomitant administration of aspirin with CELEBREX increases the rate of GI ulceration or other complications, compared to use of CELEBREX alone [*see Warnings and Precautions (5.1, 5.4) and Clinical Studies (14.7)*]. Because of its lack of platelet effects, CELEBREX is not a substitute for aspirin for cardiovascular prophylaxis [*see Clinical Pharmacology (12.2)*].

7.4   ACE-inhibitors and Angiotensin II Antagonists
Reports suggest that NSAIDs may diminish the antihypertensive effect of Angiotensin Converting Enzyme (ACE) inhibitors and angiotensin II antagonists. This interaction should be given consideration in patients taking CELEBREX concomitantly with ACE-inhibitors and angiotensin II antagonists [*see Clinical Pharmacology (12.2)*].

7.5   Fluconazole
Concomitant administration of fluconazole at 200 mg once daily resulted in a two-fold increase in celecoxib plasma concentration. This increase is due to the inhibition of celecoxib metabolism via P450 2C9 by fluconazole [*see Clinical Pharmacology (12.3)*]. CELEBREX should be introduced at the lowest recommended dose in patients receiving fluconazole.

7.6   Furosemide
Clinical studies, as well as post-marketing observations, have shown that NSAIDs can reduce the natriuretic effect of furosemide and thiazides in some patients. This response has been attributed to inhibition of renal prostaglandin synthesis.

7.7   Methotrexate
In an interaction study of rheumatoid arthritis patients taking methotrexate, CELEBREX did not have an effect on the pharmacokinetics of methotrexate [*see Clinical Pharmacology (12.3)*].

7.8   Concomitant NSAID Use
The concomitant use of CELEBREX with any dose of a non-aspirin NSAID should be avoided due to the potential for increased risk of adverse reactions.

8.   USE IN SPECIFIC POPULATIONS

8.1   Pregnancy
Pregnancy Category C. Pregnancy category D from 30 weeks of gestation onward.
Teratogenic effects: Celecoxib at oral doses ≥150 mg/kg/day (approximately 2-fold human exposure at 200 mg twice daily as measured by AUC_{0-24}), caused an increased incidence of ventricular septal defects, a rare event, and fetal alterations, such as ribs fused, sternebrae fused and sternebrae misshapen when rabbits were treated throughout organogenesis. A dose-dependent increase in diaphragmatic hernias was observed when rats were given celecoxib at oral doses ≥30 mg/kg/day (approximately 6-fold human exposure based on the AUC_{0-24} at 200 mg twice daily) throughout organogenesis. There are no studies in pregnant women. CELEBREX should be used during pregnancy only if the potential benefit justifies the potential risk to the fetus.
Nonteratogenic effects: Celecoxib produced pre-implantation and post-implantation losses and reduced embryo/fetal survival in rats at oral dosages ≥50 mg/kg/day (approximately 6-fold human exposure based on the AUC_{0-24} at 200 mg twice daily). These changes are expected with inhibition of prostaglandin synthesis and are not the result of permanent alteration of female reproductive function, nor are they expected at clinical exposures. No studies have been conducted to evaluate the effect of celecoxib on the closure of the ductus arteriosus in humans. Therefore, use of CELEBREX during the third trimester of pregnancy should be avoided.

8.2   Labor and Delivery
Celecoxib produced no evidence of delayed labor or parturition at oral doses up to 100 mg/kg in rats (approximately 7-fold human exposure as measured by the AUC_{0-24} at 200 mg BID). The effects of CELEBREX on labor and delivery in pregnant women are unknown.

8.3   Nursing Mothers
Limited data from 3 published reports that included a total of 12 breastfeeding women showed low levels of CELEBREX in breast milk. The calculated average daily infant dose was 10-40 mcg/kg/day, less than 1% of the weight-based therapeutic dose for a two-year old-child. A report of two breastfed infants 17 and 22 months of age did not show any adverse events. Caution should be exercised when CELEBREX is administered to a nursing woman.

8.4   Pediatric Use
CELEBREX is approved for relief of the signs and symptoms of Juvenile Rheumatoid Arthritis in patients 2 years and older. Safety and efficacy have not been studied beyond six months in children. The long-term cardiovascular toxicity in children exposed to CELEBREX has not been evaluated and it is unknown if long-term risks may be similar to that seen in adults exposed to CELEBREX or other COX-2 selective and non-selective NSAIDs [(*see Boxed Warning, Warnings and Precautions (5.12), and Clinical Studies (14.3)*].

The use of celecoxib in patients 2 years to 17 years of age with pauciarticular, polyarticular course JRA or in patients with systemic onset JRA was studied in a 12-week, double-blind, active controlled, pharmacokinetic, safety and efficacy study, with a 12-week open-label extension. Celecoxib has not been studied in patients under the age of 2 years, in patients with body weight less than 10 kg (22 lbs), and in patients with active systemic features. Patients with systemic onset JRA (without active systemic features) appear to be at risk for the development of abnormal coagulation laboratory tests. In some patients with systemic onset JRA, both celecoxib and naproxen were associated with mild prolongation of activated partial thromboplastin time (APTT) but not prothrombin time (PT). NSAIDs including celecoxib should be used only with caution in patients with systemic onset JRA, due to the risk of disseminated intravascular coagulation. Patients with systemic onset JRA should be monitored for the development of abnormal coagulation tests [*see Dosage and Administration (2.3), Warnings and Precautions (5.12), Adverse Reactions (6.3), Animal Toxicology (13.2), Clinical Studies (14.3)*].

Alternative therapies for treatment of JRA should be considered in pediatric patients identified to be CYP2C9 poor metabolizers [see *Poor Metabolizers of CYP2C9 substrates (8.8)*].

8.5 Geriatric Use

Of the total number of patients who received CELEBREX in pre-approval clinical trials, more than 3,300 were 65-74 years of age, while approximately 1,300 additional patients were 75 years and over. No substantial differences in effectiveness were observed between these subjects and younger subjects. In clinical studies comparing renal function as measured by the GFR, BUN and creatinine, and platelet function as measured by bleeding time and platelet aggregation, the results were not different between elderly and young volunteers. However, as with other NSAIDs, including those that selectively inhibit COX-2, there have been more spontaneous post-marketing reports of fatal GI events and acute renal failure in the elderly than in younger patients [*see Warnings and Precautions (5.4, 5.6)*].

8.6 Hepatic Insufficiency

The daily recommended dose of CELEBREX capsules in patients with moderate hepatic impairment (Child-Pugh Class B) should be reduced by 50%. The use of CELEBREX in patients with severe hepatic impairment is not recommended [*see Dosage and Administration (2.7) and Clinical Pharmacology (12.3)*].

8.7 Renal Insufficiency

CELEBREX is not recommended in patients with severe renal insufficiency [*see Warnings and Precautions (5.6) and Clinical Pharmacology (12.3)*].

8.8 Poor Metabolizers of CYP2C9 Substrates

Patients who are known or suspected to be poor CYP2C9 metabolizers based on previous history/experience with other CYP2C9 substrates (such as warfarin, phenytoin) should be administered celecoxib with caution. Consider starting treatment at half the lowest recommended dose. Alternative management should be considered in JRA patients identified to be CYP2C9 poor metabolizers. [*see Dosage and Administration (2.7) and Clinical Pharmacology (12.3)*].

10. OVERDOSAGE

No overdoses of CELEBREX were reported during clinical trials. Doses up to 2400 mg/day for up to 10 days in 12 patients did not result in serious toxicity. Symptoms following acute NSAID overdoses are usually limited to lethargy, drowsiness, nausea, vomiting, and epigastric pain, which are generally reversible with supportive care. Gastrointestinal bleeding can occur.

Hypertension, acute renal failure, respiratory depression and coma may occur, but are rare. Anaphylactoid reactions have been reported with therapeutic ingestion of NSAIDs, and may occur following an overdose.

Patients should be managed by symptomatic and supportive care following an NSAID overdose. There are no specific antidotes. No information is available regarding the removal of celecoxib by hemodialysis, but based on its high degree of plasma protein binding (>97%) dialysis is unlikely to be useful in overdose. Emesis and/or activated charcoal (60 to 100 g in adults, 1 to 2 g/kg in children) and/or osmotic cathartic may be indicated in patients seen within 4 hours of ingestion with symptoms or following a large overdose. Forced diuresis, alkalinization of urine, hemodialysis, or hemoperfusion may not be useful due to high protein binding.

11. DESCRIPTION

CELEBREX (celecoxib) is chemically designated as 4-[5-(4-methylphenyl)- 3-(trifluoromethyl)-1H-pyrazol-1-yl] benzenesulfonamide and is a diaryl-substituted pyrazole. The empirical formula is $C_{17}H_{14}F_3N_3O_2S$, and the molecular weight is 381.38; the chemical structure is as follows:

Table 3
Summary of Single Dose (200 mg) Disposition Kinetics of Celecoxib in Healthy Subjects[1]

Mean (%CV) PK Parameter Values				
C_{max}, ng/mL	T_{max}, hr	Effective $t_{1/2}$, hr	V_{ss}/F, L	CL/F, L/hr
705 (38)	2.8 (37)	11.2 (31)	429 (34)	27.7 (28)

[1] Subjects under fasting conditions (n=36, 19-52 yrs.)

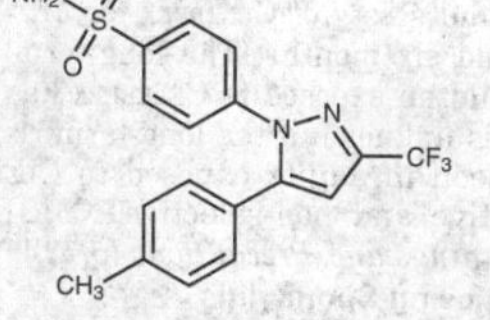

CELEBREX oral capsules contain either 50 mg, 100 mg, 200 mg or 400 mg of celecoxib, together with inactive ingredients including: croscarmellose sodium, edible inks, gelatin, lactose monohydrate, magnesium stearate, povidone and sodium lauryl sulfate.

12. CLINICAL PHARMACOLOGY

12.1 Mechanism of Action

CELEBREX is a nonsteroidal anti-inflammatory drug that exhibits anti-inflammatory, analgesic, and antipyretic activities in animal models. The mechanism of action of CELEBREX is believed to be due to inhibition of prostaglandin synthesis, primarily via inhibition of cyclooxygenase-2 (COX-2), and at therapeutic concentrations in humans, CELEBREX does not inhibit the cyclooxygenase-1 (COX-1) isoenzyme. In animal colon tumor models, CELEBREX reduced the incidence and multiplicity of tumors.

12.2 Pharmacodynamics

Platelets: In clinical trials using normal volunteers, CELEBREX at single doses up to 800 mg and multiple doses of 600 mg twice daily for up to 7 days duration (higher than recommended therapeutic doses) had no effect on reduction of platelet aggregation or increase in bleeding time. Because of its lack of platelet effects, CELEBREX is not a substitute for aspirin for cardiovascular prophylaxis. It is not known if there are any effects of CELEBREX on platelets that may contribute to the increased risk of serious cardiovascular thrombotic adverse events associated with the use of CELEBREX.

Fluid Retention: Inhibition of PGE2 synthesis may lead to sodium and water retention through increased reabsorption in the renal medullary thick ascending loop of Henle and perhaps other segments of the distal nephron. In the collecting ducts, PGE2 appears to inhibit water reabsorption by counteracting the action of antidiuretic hormone.

12.3 Pharmacokinetics

Absorption: Peak plasma levels of celecoxib occur approximately 3 hrs after an oral dose. Under fasting conditions, both peak plasma levels (C_{max}) and area under the curve (AUC) are roughly dose-proportional up to 200 mg BID; at higher doses there are less than proportional increases in C_{max} and AUC [*see Food Effects*]. Absolute bioavailability studies have not been conducted. With multiple dosing, steady-state conditions are reached on or before Day 5. The pharmacokinetic parameters of celecoxib in a group of healthy subjects are shown in Table 3.

[See table 3 above]

Food Effects: When CELEBREX capsules were taken with a high fat meal, peak plasma levels were delayed for about 1 to 2 hours with an increase in total absorption (AUC) of 10% to 20%. Under fasting conditions, at doses above 200 mg, there is less than a proportional increase in C_{max} and AUC, which is thought to be due to the low solubility of the drug in aqueous media.

Coadministration of CELEBREX with an aluminum- and magnesium-containing antacids resulted in a reduction in plasma celecoxib concentrations with a decrease of 37% in C_{max} and 10% in AUC. CELEBREX, at doses up to 200 mg twice daily, can be administered without regard to timing of meals. Higher doses (400 mg twice daily) should be administered with food to improve absorption.

In healthy adult volunteers, the overall systemic exposure (AUC) of celecoxib was equivalent when celecoxib was administered as intact capsule or capsule contents sprinkled on applesauce. There were no significant alterations in Cmax, Tmax or $t_{1/2}$ after administration of capsule contents on applesauce [*see Dosage and Administration (2)*].

Distribution: In healthy subjects, celecoxib is highly protein bound (~97%) within the clinical dose range. *In vitro* studies indicate that celecoxib binds primarily to albumin and, to a lesser extent, α_1-acid glycoprotein. The apparent volume of distribution at steady state (V_{ss}/F) is approximately 400 L, suggesting extensive distribution into the tissues. Celecoxib is not preferentially bound to red blood cells.

Metabolism: Celecoxib metabolism is primarily mediated via CYP2C9. Three metabolites, a primary alcohol, the corresponding carboxylic acid and its glucuronide conjugate, have been identified in human plasma. These metabolites are inactive as COX-1 or COX-2 inhibitors.

CYP2C9 activity is reduced in individuals with genetic polymorphisms that lead to reduced enzyme activity, such as those homozygous for the CYP2C9*2 and CYP2C9*3 polymorphisms. Limited data from 4 published reports that included a total of 8 subjects with the homozygous CYP2C9*3/*3 genotype showed celecoxib systemic levels that were 3- to 7-fold higher in these subjects compared to subjects with CYP2C9*1/*1 or *I/*3 genotypes. The pharmacokinetics of celecoxib have not been evaluated in subjects with other CYP2C9 polymorphisms, such as *2, *5, *6, *9 and *11. It is estimated that the frequency of the homozygous *3/*3 genotype is 0.3% to 1.0% in various ethnic groups. [*see Dosage and Administration (2.7), Use in Specific Populations (8.8)*].

Excretion: Celecoxib is eliminated predominantly by hepatic metabolism with little (<3%) unchanged drug recovered in the urine and feces. Following a single oral dose of radiolabeled drug, approximately 57% of the dose was excreted in the feces and 27% was excreted into the urine. The primary metabolite in both urine and feces was the carboxylic acid metabolite (73% of dose) with low amounts of the glucuronide also appearing in the urine. It appears that the low solubility of the drug prolongs the absorption process making terminal half-life ($t_{1/2}$) determinations more variable. The effective half-life is approximately 11 hours under fasted conditions. The apparent plasma clearance (CL/F) is about 500 mL/min.

Geriatric: At steady state, elderly subjects (over 65 years old) had a 40% higher C_{max} and a 50% higher AUC compared to the young subjects. In elderly females, celecoxib C_{max} and AUC are higher than those for elderly males, but these increases are predominantly due to lower body weight in elderly females. Dose adjustment in the elderly is not generally necessary. However, for patients of less than 50 kg in body weight, initiate therapy at the lowest recommended dose [*see Dosage and Administration (2.7) and Use in Specific Populations (8.5)*].

Pediatric: The steady state pharmacokinetics of celecoxib administered as an investigational oral suspension was evaluated in 152 JRA patients 2 years to 17 years of age weighing ≥10 kg with pauciarticular or polyarticular course JRA and in patients with systemic onset JRA. Population pharmacokinetic analysis indicated that the oral clearance (unadjusted for body weight) of celecoxib increases less than proportionally to increasing weight, with 10 kg and 25 kg patients predicted to have 40% and 24% lower clearance, respectively, compared with a 70 kg adult RA patient.

Twice-daily administration of 50 mg capsules to JRA patients weighing ≥12 to ≤25 kg and 100 mg capsules to JRA patients weighing >25 kg should achieve plasma concentrations similar to those observed in a clinical trial that demonstrated the non-inferiority of celecoxib to naproxen 7.5 mg/kg twice daily (*see Dosage and Administration (2.3)*. Celecoxib has not been studied in JRA patients under the age of 2 years, in patients with body weight less than 10 kg (22 lbs), or beyond 24 weeks.

Race: Meta-analysis of pharmacokinetic studies has suggested an approximately 40% higher AUC of celecoxib in Blacks compared to Caucasians. The cause and clinical significance of this finding is unknown.

Hepatic Insufficiency: A pharmacokinetic study in subjects with mild (Child-Pugh Class A) and moderate (Child-Pugh Class B) hepatic impairment has shown that steady-state celecoxib AUC is increased about 40% and 180%, respectively, above that seen in healthy control subjects. Therefore, the daily recommended dose of CELEBREX capsules should be reduced by approximately 50% in patients with moderate (Child-Pugh Class B) hepatic impairment. Patients with severe hepatic impairment (Child-Pugh Class C) have not been studied. The use of CELEBREX in patients with severe hepatic impairment is not recommended [*see Dosage and Administration (2.7) and Use in Specific Populations (8.6)*].

Renal Insufficiency: In a cross-study comparison, celecoxib AUC was approximately 40% lower in patients with chronic renal insufficiency (GFR 35-60 mL/min) than that seen in subjects with normal renal function. No significant relationship was found between GFR and celecoxib clearance. Patients with severe renal insufficiency have not been studied. Similar to other NSAIDs, Celebrex is not recommended in patients with severe renal insufficiency [*see Warnings and Precautions (5.6)*].

Drug interactions:

In vitro studies indicate that celecoxib is not an inhibitor of cytochrome P450 2C9, 2C19 or 3A4.

In vivo studies have shown the following:

Lithium: In a study conducted in healthy subjects, mean steady-state lithium plasma levels increased approximately 17% in subjects receiving lithium 450 mg twice daily with Celebrex 200 mg twice daily as compared to subjects receiving lithium alone [*see Drug Interactions (7.2)*].

Fluconazole: Concomitant administration of fluconazole at 200 mg once daily resulted in a two-fold increase in celecoxib plasma concentration. This increase is due to the inhibition of celecoxib metabolism via P450 2C9 by fluconazole [*see Drug Interactions (7.5)*].

Other Drugs: The effects of celecoxib on the pharmacokinetics and/or pharmacodynamics of glyburide, ketoconazole, methotrexate [*see Drug Interactions (7.7)*], phenytoin, and tolbutamide have been studied *in vivo* and clinically important interactions have not been found.

13. NONCLINICAL TOXICOLOGY

13.1 Carcinogenesis, Mutagenesis, Impairment of Fertility

Celecoxib was not carcinogenic in rats given oral doses up to 200 mg/kg for males and 10 mg/kg for females (approximately 2-to 4-fold the human exposure as measured by the $AUC_{0\text{-}24}$ at 200 mg twice daily) or in mice given oral doses up to 25 mg/kg for males and 50 mg/kg for females (approximately equal to human exposure as measured by the $AUC_{0\text{-}24}$ at 200 mg twice daily) for two years.

Celecoxib was not mutagenic in an Ames test and a mutation assay in Chinese hamster ovary (CHO) cells, nor clastogenic in a chromosome aberration assay in CHO cells and an *in vivo* micronucleus test in rat bone marrow.

Celecoxib did not impair male and female fertility in rats at oral doses up to 600 mg/kg/day (approximately 11-fold human exposure at 200 mg twice daily based on the $AUC_{0\text{-}24}$).

13.2 Animal Toxicology

An increase in the incidence of background findings of spermatocele with or without secondary changes such as epididymal hypospermia as well as minimal to slight dilation of the seminiferous tubules was seen in the juvenile rat. These reproductive findings while apparently treatment-related did not increase in incidence or severity with dose and may indicate an exacerbation of a spontaneous condition. Similar reproductive findings were not observed in studies of juvenile or adult dogs or in adult rats treated with celecoxib. The clinical significance of this observation is unknown.

14. CLINICAL STUDIES

14.1 Osteoarthritis

Celebrex has demonstrated significant reduction in joint pain compared to placebo. Celebrex was evaluated for treatment of the signs and the symptoms of OA of the knee and hip in placebo- and active-controlled clinical trials of up to 12 weeks duration. In patients with OA, treatment with Celebrex 100 mg twice daily or 200 mg once daily resulted in improvement in WOMAC (Western Ontario and McMaster Universities) osteoarthritis index, a composite of pain, stiffness, and functional measures in OA. In three 12-week studies of pain accompanying OA flare, Celebrex doses of 100 mg twice daily and 200 mg twice daily provided significant reduction of pain within 24-48 hours of initiation of dosing. At doses of 100 mg twice daily or 200 mg twice daily the effectiveness of Celebrex was shown to be similar to that of naproxen 500 mg twice daily. Doses of 200 mg twice daily provided no additional benefit above that seen with 100 mg twice daily. A total daily dose of 200 mg has been shown to be equally effective whether administered as 100 mg twice daily or 200 mg once daily.

14.2 Rheumatoid Arthritis

Celebrex has demonstrated significant reduction in joint tenderness/pain and joint swelling compared to placebo. Celebrex was evaluated for treatment of the signs and symptoms of RA in placebo- and active-controlled clinical trials of up to 24 weeks in duration. Celebrex was shown to be superior to placebo in these studies, using the ACR20 Responder Index, a composite of clinical, laboratory, and functional measures in RA. Celebrex doses of 100 mg twice daily and 200 mg twice daily were similar in effectiveness and both were comparable to naproxen 500 mg twice daily.

Although Celebrex 100 mg twice daily and 200 mg twice daily provided similar overall effectiveness, some patients derived additional benefit from the 200 mg twice daily dose. Doses of 400 mg twice daily provided no additional benefit above that seen with 100-200 mg twice daily.

14.3 Juvenile Rheumatoid Arthritis

In a 12-week, randomized, double-blind active-controlled, parallel-group, multicenter, non-inferiority study, patients from 2 years to 17 years of age with pauciarticular, polyarticular course JRA or systemic onset JRA (with currently inactive systemic features), received one of the following treatments: celecoxib 3 mg/kg (to a maximum of 150 mg) twice daily; celecoxib 6 mg/kg (to a maximum of 300 mg) twice daily; or naproxen 7.5 mg/kg (to a maximum of 500 mg) twice daily. The response rates were based upon the JRA Definition of Improvement greater than or equal to 30% (JRA DOI 30) criterion, which is a composite of clinical, laboratory, and functional measures of JRA. The JRA DOI 30 response rates at week 12 were 69%, 80% and 67% in the celecoxib 3 mg/kg BID, celecoxib 6 mg/kg BID, and naproxen 7.5 mg/kg BID treatment groups, respectively.

The efficacy and safety of Celebrex for JRA have not been studied beyond six months. The long-term cardiovascular toxicity in children exposed to Celebrex has not been evaluated and it is unknown if the long-term risk may be similar to that seen in adults exposed to Celebrex or other COX-2 selective and non-selective NSAIDs [(*see Boxed Warning, Warnings and Precautions (5.12)*].

14.4 Ankylosing Spondylitis

Celebrex was evaluated in AS patients in two placebo- and active-controlled clinical trials of 6 and 12 weeks duration. Celebrex at doses of 100 mg twice daily, 200 mg once daily and 400 mg once daily was shown to be statistically superior to placebo in these studies for all three co-primary efficacy measures assessing global pain intensity (Visual Analogue Scale), global disease activity (Visual Analogue Scale) and functional impairment (Bath Ankylosing Spondylitis Functional Index). In the 12-week study, there was no difference in the extent of improvement between the 200 mg and 400 mg Celebrex doses in a comparison of mean change from baseline, but there was a greater percentage of patients who responded to Celebrex 400 mg, 53%, than to Celebrex 200 mg, 44%, using the Assessment in Ankylosing Spondylitis response criteria (ASAS 20). The ASAS 20 defines a responder as improvement from baseline of at least 20% and an absolute improvement of at least 10 mm, on a 0 to 100 mm scale, in at least three of the four following domains: patient global pain, Bath Ankylosing Spondylitis Functional Index, and inflammation. The responder analysis also demonstrated no change in the responder rates beyond 6 weeks.

14.5 Analgesia, including Primary Dysmenorrhea

In acute analgesic models of post-oral surgery pain, post-orthopedic surgical pain, and primary dysmenorrhea, Celebrex relieved pain that was rated by patients as moderate to severe. Single doses [*see Dosage and Administration (2.5)*] of Celebrex provided pain relief within 60 minutes.

14.6 Familial Adenomatous Polyposis

Celebrex was evaluated to reduce the number of adenomatous colorectal polyps. A randomized, double-blind, placebo-controlled study was conducted in patients with FAP. The study population included 58 patients with a prior subtotal or total colectomy and 25 patients with an intact colon. Thirteen patients had the attenuated FAP phenotype.

One area in the rectum and up to four areas in the colon were identified at baseline for specific follow-up, and polyps were counted at baseline and following six months of treatment. The mean reduction in the number of colorectal polyps was 28% for Celebrex 400 mg twice daily, 12% for Celebrex 100 mg twice daily and 5% for placebo. The reduction in polyps observed with Celebrex 400 mg twice daily was statistically superior to placebo at the six-month timepoint (p=0.003). (See Figure 1)

Figure 1
Percent Change from Baseline in Number of Colorectal Polyps (FAP Patients)

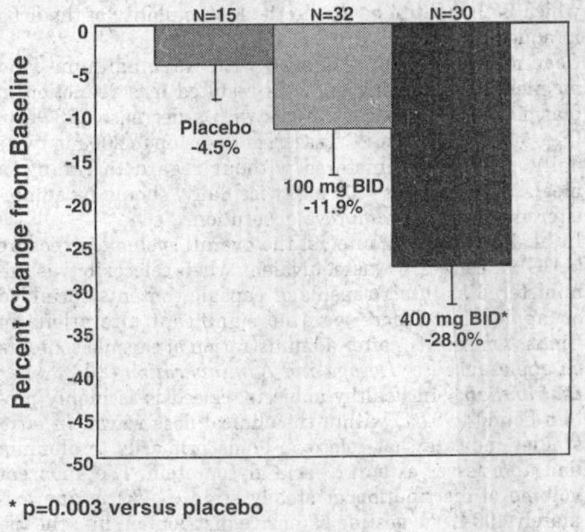
N=15
N=32
N=30
0
-5
-10
-15
-20
-25
-30
-35
-40
-45
-50
Percent Change from Baseline
Placebo
-4.5%
100 mg BID
-11.9%
400 mg BID*
-28.0%

* p=0.003 versus placebo

14.7 Special Studies

Adenomatous Polyp Prevention Studies:

Cardiovascular safety was evaluated in two randomized, double-blind, placebo-controlled, three year studies involving patients with Sporadic Adenomatous Polyps treated with Celebrex: the APC trial (Adenoma Prevention with Celecoxib) and the PreSAP trial (Prevention of Spontaneous Adenomatous Polyps). In the APC trial, there was a dose-related increase in the composite endpoint (adjudicated) of cardiovascular death, myocardial infarction, or stroke with celecoxib compared to placebo over 3 years of treatment. The PreSAP trial did not demonstrate a statistically significant increased risk for the same composite endpoint (adjudicated):

- In the APC trial, the hazard ratios compared to placebo for a composite endpoint (adjudicated) of cardiovascular death, myocardial infarction, or stroke were 3.4 (95% CI 1.4-8.5) with celecoxib 400 mg twice daily and 2.8 (95% CI 1.1-7.2) with celecoxib 200 mg twice daily. Cumulative rates for this composite endpoint over 3 years were 3.0% (20/671 subjects) and 2.5% (17/685 subjects), respectively, compared to 0.9% (6/679 subjects) with placebo treatment. The increases in both celecoxib dose groups versus placebo-treated patients were mainly due to an increased incidence of myocardial infarction.
- In the PreSAP trial, the hazard ratio for this same composite endpoint (adjudicated) was 1.2 (95% CI 0.6-2.4) with celecoxib 400 mg once daily compared to placebo. Cumulative rates for this composite endpoint over 3 years were 2.3% (21/933 subjects) and 1.9% (12/628 subjects), respectively.

Clinical trials of other COX-2 selective and non-selective NSAIDs of up to three-years duration have shown an increased risk of serious cardiovascular thrombotic events, myocardial infarction, and stroke, which can be fatal. As a result, all NSAIDs are considered potentially associated with this risk.

Celecoxib Long-Term Arthritis Safety Study (CLASS):

This was a prospective, long-term, safety outcome study conducted post-marketing in approximately 5,800 OA patients and 2,200 RA patients. Patients received Celebrex 400 mg twice daily (4-fold and 2-fold the recommended OA and RA doses, respectively, and the approved dose for FAP), ibuprofen 800 mg three times daily or diclofenac 75 mg twice daily (common therapeutic doses). Median exposures for Celebrex (n = 3,987) and diclofenac (n = 1,996) were 9 months while ibuprofen (n = 1,985) was 6 months. The primary endpoint of this outcome study was the incidence of complicated ulcers (gastrointestinal bleeding, perforation or obstruction). Patients were allowed to take concomitant low-dose (≤ 325 mg/day) aspirin (ASA) for cardiovascular prophylaxis (ASA subgroups: Celebrex, n = 882; diclofenac, n = 445; ibuprofen, n = 412). Differences in the incidence of complicated ulcers between Celebrex and the combined group of ibuprofen and diclofenac were not statistically significant.

Patients on Celebrex and concomitant low-dose ASA (N=882) experienced 4-fold higher rates of complicated ulcers compared to those not on ASA (N=3105). The Kaplan-Meier rate for complicated ulcers at 9 months was 1.12% versus 0.32% for those on low-dose ASA and those not on ASA, respectively [*see Warnings and Precautions (5.4)*].

The estimated cumulative rates at 9 months of complicated and symptomatic ulcers for patients treated with Celebrex 400 mg twice daily are described in Table 4. Table 4 also displays results for patients less than or greater than 65 years of age. The difference in rates between Celebrex alone and Celebrex with ASA groups may be due to the higher risk for GI events in ASA users.

Table 4: Complicated and Symptomatic Ulcer Rates in Patients Taking Celebrex 400 mg Twice Daily (Kaplan-Meier Rates at 9 months [%]) Based on Risk Factors

All Patients	
Celebrex alone (n=3105)	0.78
Celebrex with ASA (n=882)	2.19
Patients <65 Years	
Celebrex alone (n=2025)	0.47
Celebrex with ASA (n=403)	1.26
Patients ≥65 Years	
Celebrex alone (n=1080)	1.40
Celebrex with ASA (n=479)	3.06

In a small number of patients with a history of ulcer disease, the complicated and symptomatic ulcer rates in patients taking Celebrex alone or Celebrex with ASA were, respectively, 2.56% (n=243) and 6.85% (n=91) at 48 weeks. These results are to be expected in patients with a prior history of ulcer disease [*see Warnings and Precautions (5.4) and Adverse Reactions (6.1)*].

Cardiovascular safety outcomes were also evaluated in the CLASS trial. Kaplan-Meier cumulative rates for investigator-reported serious cardiovascular thromboembolic adverse events (including MI, pulmonary embolism, deep venous thrombosis, unstable angina, transient ischemic attacks, and ischemic cerebrovascular accidents) demonstrated no differences between the CELEBREX, diclofenac, or ibuprofen treatment groups. The cumulative rates in all patients at nine months for CELEBREX, diclofenac, and ibuprofen were 1.2%, 1.4%, and 1.1%, respectively. The cumulative rates in non-ASA users at nine months in each of the three treatment groups were less than 1%. The cumulative rates for myocardial infarction in non-ASA users at nine months in each of the three treatment groups were less than 0.2%. There was no placebo group in the CLASS trial, which limits the ability to determine whether the three drugs tested had no increased risk of CV events or if they all increased the risk to a similar degree.

Endoscopic Studies: The correlation between findings of short-term endoscopic studies with CELEBREX and the relative incidence of clinically significant serious upper GI events with long-term use has not been established. Serious clinically significant upper GI bleeding has been observed in patients receiving CELEBREX in controlled and open-labeled trials [*see Warnings and Precautions (5.4) and Clinical Studies (14.7)*].

A randomized, double-blind study in 430 RA patients was conducted in which an endoscopic examination was performed at 6 months. The incidence of endoscopic ulcers in patients taking CELEBREX 200 mg twice daily was 4% vs. 15% for patients taking diclofenac SR 75 mg twice daily. However, CELEBREX was not statistically different than diclofenac for clinically relevant GI outcomes in the CLASS trial [*see Clinical Studies (14.7)*].

The incidence of endoscopic ulcers was studied in two 12-week, placebo-controlled studies in 2157 OA and RA patients in whom baseline endoscopies revealed no ulcers. There was no dose relationship for the incidence of gastroduodenal ulcers and the dose of CELEBREX (50 mg to 400 mg twice daily). The incidence for naproxen 500 mg twice daily was 16.2 and 17.6% in the two studies, for placebo was 2.0 and 2.3%, and for all doses of CELEBREX the incidence ranged between 2.7%-5.9%. There have been no large, clinical outcome studies to compare clinically relevant GI outcomes with CELEBREX and naproxen.

In the endoscopic studies, approximately 11% of patients were taking aspirin (≤ 325 mg/day). In the CELEBREX groups, the endoscopic ulcer rate appeared to be higher in aspirin users than in non-users. However, the increased rate of ulcers in these aspirin users was less than the endoscopic ulcer rates observed in the active comparator groups, with or without aspirin.

16. HOW SUPPLIED/STORAGE AND HANDLING

CELEBREX 50 mg capsules are white, with reverse printed white on red band of body and cap with markings of 7767 on the cap and 50 on the body, supplied as:

NDC Number	Size
0025-1515-01	bottle of 60

CELEBREX 100 mg capsules are white, with reverse printed white on blue band of body and cap with markings of 7767 on the cap and 100 on the body, supplied as:

NDC Number	Size
0025-1520-31	bottle of 100
0025-1520-51	bottle of 500
0025-1520-34	carton of 100 unit dose

CELEBREX 200 mg capsules are white, with reverse printed white on gold band with markings of 7767 on the cap and 200 on the body, supplied as:

NDC Number	Size
0025-1525-31	bottle of 100
0025-1525-51	bottle of 500
0025-1525-34	carton of 100 unit dose

CELEBREX 400 mg capsules are white, with reverse printed white on green band with markings of 7767 on the cap and 400 on the body, supplied as:

NDC Number	Size
0025-1530-02	bottle of 60
0025-1530-01	carton of 100 unit dose

Storage: Store at 25°C (77°F); excursions permitted to 15-30°C (59-86°F) [see USP Controlled Room Temperature]

17. PATIENT COUNSELING INFORMATION

Patients should be informed of the following information before initiating therapy with CELEBREX and periodically during the course of ongoing therapy.

17.1 Medication Guide

Patients should be informed of the availability of a Medication Guide for NSAIDs that accompanies each prescription dispensed, and should be instructed to read the Medication Guide prior to using CELEBREX.

Serious side effects include:

- heart attack
- stroke
- high blood pressure
- heart failure from body swelling (fluid retention)
- kidney problems including kidney failure
- bleeding and ulcers in the stomach and intestine
- low red blood cells (anemia)
- life-threatening skin reactions
- life-threatening allergic reactions
- liver problems including liver failure
- asthma attacks in people who have asthma

17.2 Cardiovascular Effects

Patients should be informed that CELEBREX may cause serious CV side effects such as MI or stroke, which may result in hospitalization and even death. Patients should be informed of the the signs and symptoms of chest pain, shortness of breath, weakness, slurring of speech, and to seek immediate medical advice if they observe any of these signs or symptoms. [*see Warnings and Precautions (5.1)*].

Patients should be informed that CELEBREX can lead to the onset of new hypertension or worsening of preexisting hypertension, and that CELEBREX may impair the response of some antihypertensive agents. Patients should be instructed on the proper follow up for monitoring of blood pressure. [*see Warnings and Precautions (5.2) and Drug Interactions (7.4)*].

17.3 Gastrointestinal Effects

Patients should be informed that CELEBREX can cause gastrointestinal discomfort and more serious side effects, such as ulcers and bleeding, which may result in hospitalization and even death. Patients should be informed of the signs and symptoms of ulcerations and bleeding, and to seek immediate medical advice if they observe any signs or symptoms that are indicative of these disorders, including epigastric pain, dyspepsia, melena, and hematemesis. [*see Warnings and Precautions (5.4)*].

17.4 Hepatic Effects

Patients should be informed of the warning signs and symptoms of hepatotoxicity (e.g., nausea, fatigue, lethargy, pruritus, jaundice, right upper quadrant tenderness, and "flu-like" symptoms). Patients should be instructed that they should stop therapy and seek immediate medical therapy if these signs and symptoms occur [*see Warnings and Precautions (5.5), Use in Specific Populations (8.6)*].

17.5 Adverse Skin Reactions

Patients should be informed that CELEBREX is a sulfonamide and can cause serious skin side effects such as exfoliative dermatitis, SJS, and TEN, which may result in hospitalizations and even death. Although serious skin reactions may occur without warning, patients should be informed of the signs and symptoms of skin rash and blisters, fever, or other signs of hypersensitivity such as itching, and seek immediate medical advice when observing any indicative signs or symptoms.

Patients should be advised to stop CELEBREX immediately if they develop any type of rash and contact their physician as soon as possible.

Patients with prior history of sulfa allergy should not take CELEBREX [*see Warnings and Precautions (5.8)*].

17.6 Weight Gain and Edema

Long-term administration of NSAIDs including CELEBREX has resulted in renal injury. Patients at greatest risk are those taking diuretics, ACE-inhibitors, angiotensin II antagonists, or with renal or liver dysfunction, heart failure, and the elderly [*see Warnings and Precautions (5.3, 5.6), Use in Specific Populations (8)*].

Patients should be instructed to promptly report to their physicians signs or symptoms of unexplained weight gain or edema following treatment with CELEBREX [*see Warnings and Precautions (5.3)*].

17.7 Anaphylactoid Reactions

Patients should be informed of the signs and symptoms of an anaphylactoid reaction (e.g., difficulty breathing, swelling of the face or throat). Patients should be instructed to seek immediate emergency assistance if they develop any of these signs and symptoms [*see Warnings and Precautions (5.7)*].

17.8 Effects During Pregnancy

Patients should be informed that in late pregnancy CELEBREX should be avoided because it may cause premature closure of the ductus arteriosus [*see Warnings and Precautions (5.9), Use in Specific Populations (8.1)*].

17.9 Preexisting Asthma

Patients should be instructed to tell their physicians if they have a history of asthma or aspirin-sensitive asthma because the use of NSAIDs in patients with aspirin-sensitive asthma has been associated with severe bronchospasm, which can be fatal. Patients with this form of aspirin sensitivity should be instructed not to take Celebrex. Patients

---

Other side effects include:

- stomach pain
- constipation
- diarrhea
- gas
- heartburn
- nausea
- vomiting
- dizziness

with preexisting asthma should be instructed to seek immediate medical attention if their asthma worsens after taking Celebrex [*see Warnings and Precautions (5.13)*].

17.10 GI Cancer in Familial Adenomatous Polyposis

Patients with FAP should be informed that CELEBREX has not been shown to reduce colorectal, duodenal or other FAP-related cancers, or the need for endoscopic surveillance, prophylactic or other FAP-related surgery. Therefore, all patients with FAP should be instructed to continue their usual care while receiving CELEBREX [*see Warnings and Precautions (5.15)*].

Distributed by
G.D. Searle LLC
Division of Pfizer Inc, NY, NY 10017
LAB-0036-13.0
June 2009

Medication Guide
for
Non-Steroidal Anti-Inflammatory Drugs (NSAIDs)
(See the end of this Medication Guide for a list of prescription NSAID medicines.)

What is the most important information I should know about medicines called Non-Steroidal Anti-Inflammatory Drugs (NSAIDs)?

NSAID medicines may increase the chance of a heart attack or stroke that can lead to death.

This chance increases:
- with longer use of NSAID medicines
- in people who have heart disease

NSAID medicines should never be used right before or after a heart surgery called a "coronary artery bypass graft (CABG)."

NSAID medicines can cause ulcers and bleeding in the stomach and intestines at any time during treatment. Ulcers and bleeding:
- can happen without warning symptoms
- may cause death

The chance of a person getting an ulcer or bleeding increases with:
- taking medicines called "corticosteroids" and "anticoagulants"
- longer use
- smoking
- drinking alcohol
- older age
- having poor health

NSAID medicines should only be used:
- exactly as prescribed
- at the lowest dose possible for your treatment
- for the shortest time needed

What are Non-Steroidal Anti-Inflammatory Drugs (NSAIDs)?

NSAID medicines are used to treat pain and redness, swelling, and heat (inflammation) from medical conditions such as:
- different types of arthritis
- menstrual cramps and other types of short-term pain

Who should not take a Non-Steroidal Anti-Inflammatory Drug (NSAID)?

Do not take an NSAID medicine:
- if you had an asthma attack, hives, or other allergic reaction with aspirin or any other NSAID medicine
- for pain right before or after heart bypass surgery

Tell your healthcare provider:
- about all of your medical conditions.
- about all of the medicines you take. NSAIDs and some other medicines can interact with each other and cause serious side effects. **Keep a list of your medicines to show to your healthcare provider and pharmacist.**
- if you are pregnant. **NSAID medicines should not be used by pregnant women late in their pregnancy.**
- if you are breastfeeding. **Talk to your doctor.**

What are the possible side effects of Non-Steroidal Anti-Inflammatory Drugs (NSAIDs)?
[See table at top of previous page]

Get emergency help right away if you have any of the following symptoms:
- shortness of breath or trouble breathing
- chest pain
- weakness in one part or side of your body
- slurred speech
- swelling of the face or throat

Stop your NSAID medicine and call your healthcare provider right away if you have any of the following symptoms:
- nausea
- more tired or weaker than usual
- itching
- your skin or eyes look yellow
- stomach pain
- flu-like symptoms
- vomit blood
- there is blood in your bowel movement or it is black and sticky like tar
- skin rash or blisters with fever
- unusual weight gain
- swelling of the arms and legs, hands and feet

These are not all the side effects with NSAID medicines. Talk to your healthcare provider or pharmacist for more information about NSAID medicines.

Call your doctor for medical advice about side effects. You may report side effects to FDA at 1-800-FDA-1088.

Other information about Non-Steroidal Anti-Inflammatory Drugs (NSAIDs)
- Aspirin is an NSAID medicine but it does not increase the chance of a heart attack. Aspirin can cause bleeding in the brain, stomach, and intestines. Aspirin can also cause ulcers in the stomach and intestines.
- Some of these NSAID medicines are sold in lower doses without a prescription (over–the–counter). Talk to your healthcare provider before using over–the–counter NSAIDs for more than 10 days.

NSAID medicines that need a prescription

Generic Name	Tradename
Celecoxib	Celebrex
Diclofenac	Cataflam, Voltaren, Arthrotec (combined with misoprostol)
Diflunisal	Dolobid
Etodolac	Lodine, Lodine XL
Fenoprofen	Nalfon, Nalfon 200
Flurbiprofen	Ansaid
Ibuprofen	Motrin, Tab-Profen, Vicoprofen* (combined with hydrocodone), Combunox (combined with oxycodone)
Indomethacin	Indocin, Indocin SR, Indo-Lemmon, Indomethagan
Ketoprofen	Oruvail
Ketorolac	Toradol
Mefenamic Acid	Ponstel
Meloxicam	Mobic
Nabumetone	Relafen
Naproxen	Naprosyn, Anaprox, Anaprox DS, EC-Naproxyn, Naprelan, Naprapac (copackaged with lansoprazole)
Oxaprozin	Daypro
Piroxicam	Feldene
Sulindac	Clinoril
Tolmetin	Tolectin, Tolectin DS, Tolectin 600

* Vicoprofen contains the same dose of ibuprofen as over-the-counter (OTC) NSAIDs, and is usually used for less than 10 days to treat pain. The OTC NSAID label warns that long term continuous use may increase the risk of heart attack or stroke.

This Medication Guide has been approved by the U.S. Food and Drug Administration.

Shionogi Pharma, Inc.
FIVE CONCOURSE PARKWAY
SUITE 1800
ATALANTA, GA 30328

Telephone: 800-461-3696

CUVPOSA ℞
[cuv-posa]
(glycopyrrolate)
oral solution

HIGHLIGHTS OF PRESCRIBING INFORMATION
These highlights do not include all the information needed to use CUVPOSA safely and effectively. See full prescribing information for CUVPOSA.
CUVPOSA (glycopyrrolate) oral solution
Initial U.S. Approval: 1961

———INDICATIONS AND USAGE———
CUVPOSA is an anticholinergic indicated to reduce chronic severe drooling in patients aged 3-16 with neurologic conditions associated with problem drooling (e.g., cerebral palsy). (1)

———DOSAGE AND ADMINISTRATION———
- Initiate dosing at 0.02 mg/kg three times daily and titrate in increments of 0.02 mg/kg every 5-7 days, based on therapeutic response and adverse reactions. (2)
- Maximum recommended dose is 0.1 mg/kg three times daily, not to exceed 1.5-3 mg per dose based upon weight. (2)
- Administer at least one hour before or two hours after meals. (2)

———DOSAGE FORMS AND STRENGTHS———
1 mg/5 mL, oral solution in 16 ounce bottles. (3)

———CONTRAINDICATIONS———
- Medical conditions that preclude anticholinergic therapy. (4)
- Concomitant use of solid oral dosage forms of potassium chloride. (4)

———WARNINGS AND PRECAUTIONS———
- Constipation or intestinal pseudo-obstruction: May present as abdominal distention, pain, nausea, or vomiting. Assess patients for constipation, particularly within 4-5 days of initial dosing or after a dose increase. (5.1)
- Incomplete mechanical intestinal obstruction: May present as diarrhea. If obstruction is suspected, discontinue CUVPOSA and evaluate. (5.2)
- High ambient temperature: To reduce risk of heat prostration, avoid high temperatures. (5.3)

———ADVERSE REACTIONS———
The most common adverse reactions (incidence ≥30%) are dry mouth, vomiting, constipation, flushing, and nasal congestion. (6)

To report SUSPECTED ADVERSE REACTIONS, contact Shionogi Drug Safety Department at 1-800-849-9707 ext. 1454 or FDA at 1-800-FDA-1088 or www.fda.gov/medwatch

———DRUG INTERACTIONS———
- Digoxin tablets: Use with glycopyrrolate can increase digoxin serum levels. Monitor patients and consider use of alternative dosage forms of digoxin. (7)
- Amantadine: Effects of glycopyrrolate may be increased with concomitant administration of amantadine. Consider decreasing the dose of glycopyrrolate during concomitant use. (7)
- Atenolol or metformin: Glycopyrrolate may increase serum levels of atenolol or metformin. Consider dose reduction when used with glycopyrrolate. (7)
- Haloperidol or levodopa: Glycopyrrolate may decrease serum levels of haloperidol or levodopa. Consider a dose increase when used with glycopyrrolate. (7)

———USE IN SPECIFIC POPULATIONS———
- Pediatric use: The safety and effectiveness of glycopyrrolate has not been established in patients under 3 years of age. (8.4)
- Renal Impairment: Use CUVPOSA with caution in patients with renal impairment. (8.6)

See 17 for PATIENT COUNSELING INFORMATION and FDA-approved patient labeling

Revised: 07/2010

FULL PRESCRIBING INFORMATION

1   INDICATIONS AND USAGE

CUVPOSA is indicated to reduce chronic severe drooling in patients aged 3 to 16 years with neurologic conditions associated with problem drooling (e.g. cerebral palsy).

2   DOSAGE AND ADMINISTRATION

CUVPOSA must be measured and administered with accurate measuring device [see Patient Counseling Information (17)].

Initiate dosing at 0.02 mg/kg orally three times daily and titrate in increments of 0.02 mg/kg every 5-7 days based on therapeutic response and adverse reactions. The maximum recommended dosage is 0.1 mg/kg three times daily not to exceed 1.5-3 mg per dose based upon weight. For greater detail, see Table 1.

During the four-week titration period, dosing can be increased consistent with the recommended dose titration schedule while ensuring that the anticholinergic adverse events are tolerable. Prior to each increase in dose, review the tolerability of the current dose level with the patient's caregiver.

CUVPOSA should be dosed at least one hour before or two hours after meals.

The presence of high fat food reduces the oral bioavailability of CUVPOSA if taken shortly after a meal [see Clinical Pharmacology (12.3)].

[See table at top of next page]

3   DOSAGE FORMS AND STRENGTHS

CUVPOSA is available as a 1 mg/5 mL clear, cherry-flavored solution for oral administration in 16 ounce bottles.

4   CONTRAINDICATIONS

CUVPOSA is contraindicated in:
- Patients with medical conditions that preclude anticholinergic therapy (e.g., glaucoma, paralytic ileus, unstable cardiovascular status in acute hemorrhage, severe ulcerative colitis, toxic megacolon complicating ulcerative colitis, myasthenia gravis).
- Patients taking solid oral dosage forms of potassium chloride. The passage of potassium chloride tablets through the gastrointestinal (GI) tract may be arrested or delayed with coadministration of CUVPOSA.

5   WARNINGS AND PRECAUTIONS

5.1   Constipation or Intestinal Pseudo-obstruction

Constipation is a common dose-limiting adverse reaction which sometimes leads to glycopyrrolate discontinuation [see Adverse Reactions (6.1)]. Assess patients for constipation, particularly within 4-5 days of initial dosing or after a dose increase. Intestinal pseudo-obstruction has been reported and may present as abdominal distention, pain, nausea or vomiting.

5.2   Incomplete Mechanical Intestinal Obstruction

Diarrhea may be an early symptom of incomplete mechanical intestinal obstruction, especially in patients with ileostomy or colostomy. If incomplete mechanical intestinal obstruction is suspected, discontinue treatment with CUVPOSA and evaluate for intestinal obstruction.

5.3   High Ambient Temperatures

In the presence of high ambient temperature, heat prostration (fever and heat stroke due to decreased sweating) can occur with use of anticholinergic drugs such as CUVPOSA. Advise parents/caregivers to avoid exposure of the patient to hot or very warm environmental temperatures.

5.4   Operating Machinery or an Automobile

CUVPOSA may produce drowsiness or blurred vision. As appropriate for a given age, warn the patient not to engage

Table 1: Recommended Dose Titration Schedule (each dose to be given three times daily)

Weight		Dose Level 1		Dose Level 2		Dose Level 3		Dose Level 4		Dose Level 5	
Kg	lb	(∼0.02 mg/kg)		(∼0.04 mg/kg)		(∼0.06 mg/kg)		(∼0.08 mg/kg)		(∼0.1 mg/kg)	
13-17	27-38	0.3 mg	1.5 mL	0.6 mg	3 mL	0.9 mg	4.5 mL	1.2 mg	6 mL	1.5 mg	7.5 mL
18-22	39-49	0.4 mg	2 mL	0.8 mg	4 mL	1.2 mg	6 mL	1.6 mg	8 mL	2.0 mg	10 mL
23-27	50-60	0.5 mg	2.5 mL	1.0 mg	5 mL	1.5 mg	7.5 mL	2.0 mg	10 mL	2.5 mg	12.5 mL
28-32	61-71	0.6 mg	3 mL	1.2 mg	6 mL	1.8 mg	9 mL	2.4 mg	12 mL	3.0 mg	15 mL
33-37	72-82	0.7 mg	3.5 mL	1.4 mg	7 mL	2.1 mg	10.5 mL	2.8 mg	14 mL	3.0 mg	15 mL
38-42	83-93	0.8 mg	4 mL	1.6 mg	8 mL	2.4 mg	12 mL	3.0 mg	15 mL	3.0 mg	15 mL
43-47	94-104	0.9 mg	4.5 mL	1.8 mg	9 mL	2.7 mg	13.5 mL	3.0 mg	15 mL	3.0 mg	15 mL
≥48	≥105	1.0 mg	5 mL	2.0 mg	10 mL	3.0 mg	15 mL	3.0 mg	15 mL	3.0 mg	15 mL

in activities requiring mental alertness such as operating a motor vehicle or other machinery, or performing hazardous work while taking CUVPOSA.

5.5   Anticholinergic Drug Effects
Use CUVPOSA with caution in patients with conditions that are exacerbated by anticholinergic drug effects including:
- Autonomic neuropathy
- Renal disease
- Ulcerative colitis – Large doses may suppress intestinal motility to the point of producing a paralytic ileus and for this reason may precipitate or aggravate "toxic megacolon," a serious complication of the disease.
- Hyperthyroidism
- Coronary heart disease, congestive heart failure, cardiac tachyarrhythmias, tachycardia, and hypertension
- Hiatal hernia associated with reflux esophagitis, since anticholinergic drugs may aggravate this condition

6   ADVERSE REACTIONS
The following serious adverse reactions are described elsewhere in the labeling:
- Constipation or intestinal pseudo-obstruction *[see Warnings and Precautions (5.1)]*
- Incomplete mechanical intestinal obstruction *[see Warnings and Precautions (5.2)]*

The most common adverse reactions reported with CUVPOSA are dry mouth, vomiting, constipation, flushing, and nasal congestion.

6.1   Clinical Trials Experience
Because clinical trials are conducted under widely varying conditions, adverse reaction rates observed in the clinical trials of a drug cannot be directly compared to rates in the clinical trials of another drug and may not reflect the rates observed in practice.

The data described below reflect exposure to CUVPOSA in 151 subjects, including 20 subjects who participated in a 8-week placebo-controlled study (Study 1) and 137 subjects who participated in a 24-week open-label study (six subjects who received CUVPOSA in the placebo-controlled study and 131 new subjects).

Table 2 presents adverse reactions reported by ≥ 15% of CUVPOSA-treated subjects from the placebo-controlled clinical trial.

Table 2: Adverse Reactions Occurring in ≥ 15% of CUVPOSA-Treated Subjects and at a Greater Frequency than Placebo in Study 1

	CUVPOSA (N=20) n (%)	Placebo (N=18) n (%)
Dry Mouth	8 (40%)	2 (11%)
Vomiting	8 (40%)	2 (11%)
Constipation	7 (35%)	4 (22%)
Flushing	6 (30%)	3 (17%)
Nasal Congestion	6 (30%)	2 (11%)
Headache	3 (15%)	1 (6%)
Sinusitis	3 (15%)	1 (6%)
Upper Respiratory Tract Infection	3 (15%)	0
Urinary Retention	3 (15%)	0

The following adverse reactions occurred at a rate of <2% of patients receiving CUVPOSA in the open-label study.
- Gastrointestinal: Abdominal distention, abdominal pain, stomach discomfort, chapped lips, flatulence, retching, dry tongue
- General Disorders: Irritability, pain
- Infections: Pneumonia, sinusitis, tracheostomy infection, upper respiratory tract infection, urinary tract infection
- Investigations: Heart rate increased
- Metabolism and Nutrition: Dehydration
- Nervous System: Headache, convulsion, dysgeusia, nystagmus
- Psychiatric: Agitation, restlessness, abnormal behavior, aggression, crying, impulse control disorder, moaning, mood altered
- Respiratory: Increased viscosity of bronchial secretion, nasal congestion, nasal dryness
- Skin: Dry skin, pruritus, rash
- Vascular: Pallor

6.2   Postmarketing Experience
The following adverse reactions have been identified during postapproval use of other formulations of glycopyrrolate for other indications. Because these reactions are reported voluntarily from a population of uncertain size, it is not always possible to reliably estimate their frequency or establish a causal relationship to drug exposure.

Additional adverse reactions identified during postapproval use of glycopyrrolate tablets include: loss of taste and suppression of lactation.

7   DRUG INTERACTIONS
Drugs Affected by Reduced GI Transit Time
Glycopyrrolate reduces GI transit time, which may result in altered release of certain drugs when formulated in delayed- or controlled-release dosage forms.
- The passage of potassium chloride tablets through the GI tract may be arrested or delayed with coadministration of glycopyrrolate. Solid dosage forms of potassium chloride are contraindicated *[see Contraindications (4)].*
- Digoxin administered as slow dissolution oral tablets may have increased serum levels and enhanced action when administered with glycopyrrolate. Monitor patients receiving slow dissolution digoxin for increased action if glycopyrrolate is coadministered regularly. Consider the use of other oral dosage forms of digoxin (e.g., elixir or capsules).

Amantadine
The anticholinergic effects of glycopyrrolate may be increased with concomitant administration of amantadine. Consider decreasing the dose of glycopyrrolate during coadministration of amantadine.

Drugs Whose Plasma Levels May be Increased by Glycopyrrolate
Coadministration of glycopyrrolate may result in increased levels of certain drugs.
- Atenolol's bioavailability may be increased with coadministration of glycopyrrolate. A reduction in the atenolol dose may be needed.
- Metformin plasma levels may be elevated with coadministration of glycopyrrolate, increasing metformin's pharmacologic and toxic effects. Monitor clinical response to metformin with concomitant glycopyrrolate administration; consider a dose reduction of metformin if warranted.

Drugs Whose Plasma Levels May be Decreased by Glycopyrrolate
Coadministration of glycopyrrolate may result in decreased levels of certain drugs.
- Haloperidol's serum levels may be decreased when coadministered with glycopyrrolate, resulting in worsening of

schizophrenic symptoms, and development of tardive dyskinesia. Closely monitor patients if coadministration cannot be avoided.
- Levodopa's therapeutic effect may be reduced with glycopyrrolate administration. Consider increasing the dose of levodopa.

8   USE IN SPECIFIC POPULATIONS
8.1   Pregnancy
Pregnancy Category C
There are no adequate and well-controlled studies in pregnant women. Animal reproduction studies have not been conducted with glycopyrrolate. It is also not known whether glycopyrrolate can cause fetal harm when administered to a pregnant woman or can affect reproduction capacity. CUVPOSA should be given to a pregnant woman only if clearly needed.

8.3   Nursing Mothers
It is not known whether this drug is excreted in human milk. Because many drugs are excreted in human milk, caution should be exercised when CUVPOSA is administered to a nursing woman.

8.4   Pediatric Use
CUVPOSA was evaluated for chronic severe drooling in patients aged 3 to 16 years with neurologic conditions associated with problem drooling. CUVPOSA has not been studied in subjects under the age of 3 years.

8.5   Geriatric Use
Clinical studies of CUVPOSA did not include subjects aged 65 and over.

8.6   Renal Impairment
Because glycopyrrolate is largely renally eliminated, CUVPOSA should be used with caution in patients with renal impairment (see Clinical Pharmacology 12.3).

10   OVERDOSAGE
Because glycopyrrolate is a quaternary amine which does not easily cross the blood-brain barrier, symptoms of glycopyrrolate overdosage are generally more peripheral in nature rather than central compared to other anticholinergic agents. In case of accidental overdose, therapy may include:
- Maintaining an open airway, providing ventilation as necessary.
- Managing any acute conditions such as hyperthermia, coma and or seizures as applicable, and managing any jerky myoclonic movements or choreoathetosis which may lead to rhabdomyolysis in some cases of anticholinergic overdosage.
- Administering a quaternary ammonium anticholinesterase such as neostigmine to help alleviate peripheral anticholinergic effects such as anticholinergic induced ileus.
- Administering activated charcoal orally as appropriate.

11   DESCRIPTION
CUVPOSA is an anticholinergic drug available as an oral solution containing 1 mg glycopyrrolate per 5 mL. The chemical name for glycopyrrolate is pyrrolidinium, 3-[(cyclopentylhydroxyphenylacetyl)oxy]-1,1-dimethyl-, bromide. The chemical structure is:

The empirical formula for CUVPOSA is $C_{19}H_{28}BrNO_3$ and the molecular weight is 398.33. The inactive ingredients in CUVPOSA are: citric acid, glycerin, natural and artificial

Table 3: Pharmacokinetic Parameters (mean ± SD) for CUVPOSA, Fasting and Fed, in Healthy Adults

	Cmax (ng/mL)	Tmax (hrs)	AUC$_{0-T}$ (ng·hr/mL)	AUC$_{0-Inf}$ (ng·hr/mL)	T½ (hrs)
Fasting (n=37)	0.318 ± 0.190	3.10 ± 1.08	1.74 ± 1.07	1.81 ± 1.09	3.0 ± 1.2
Fed (n=36)	0.084 ± 0.081	2.60 ± 1.12	0.38 ± 0.14	0.46 ± 0.13*	3.2 ±1.1*

* n=35

cherry flavor, methylparaben, propylene glycol, propylparaben, saccharin sodium, sodium citrate, sorbitol solution, and purified water.

12 CLINICAL PHARMACOLOGY

12.1 Mechanism of Action
Glycopyrrolate is a competitive inhibitor of acetylcholine receptors that are located on certain peripheral tissues, including salivary glands. Glycopyrrolate indirectly reduces the rate of salivation by preventing the stimulation of these receptors.

12.2 Pharmacodynamics
Glycopyrrolate inhibits the action of acetylcholine on salivary glands thereby reducing the extent of salivation.

12.3 Pharmacokinetics
Absorption
In a parallel study of children (n=6 per group) aged 7-14 years undergoing intraocular surgery receiving either intravenous (IV) or oral glycopyrrolate as a premedication, the mean absolute bioavailability of glycopyrrolate tablets was low (approximately 3%) and highly variable among subjects (range 1.3 to 13.3%). A similar pattern of low and variable relative bioavailability is seen in adults.
Analysis of population pharmacokinetic data from normal adults and children with cerebral palsy associated chronic moderate to severe drooling failed to demonstrate linear pharmacokinetics across the dose range. In the same analysis, population estimates of the apparent oral clearance (scaled by weight in children and adults) ranged from 5.28 ~ 38.95 L/hr/kg for healthy adults and 8.07 ~ 25.65 L/hr/kg for patients with cerebral palsy, a reflection of the low and highly variable oral bioavailability of glycopyrrolate.
Absorption of CUVPOSA (fasting) was compared to that of a marketed glycopyrrolate oral tablet. The Cmax after oral solution administration was 23% lower compared to tablet administration and the AUC$_{0-inf}$ was 28% lower after oral solution administration. Mean Cmax after oral solution administration in the fasting state was 0.318 ng/mL, and mean AUC$_{0-24}$ was 1.74 ng.hr/mL. Mean time to maximum plasma concentration for CUVPOSA was 3.1 hours, and mean plasma half-life was 3.0 hours.
In healthy adults, a high fat meal was shown to significantly affect the absorption of glycopyrrolate oral solution (10 mL, 1 mg/5 mL). The mean Cmax under fed high fat meal conditions was approximately 74% lower than the Cmax observed under fasting conditions. Similarly, mean AUC$_{0-T}$ was reduced by about 78% by the high fat meal compared with the fasting AUC$_{0-T}$. A high fat meal markedly reduces the oral bioavailability of CUVPOSA. Therefore, CUVPOSA should be dosed at least one hour before or two hours after meals. Pharmacokinetic results (mean ± SD) are described in Table 3.
[See table above]
Distribution
After IV administration, glycopyrrolate has a mean volume of distribution in children aged 1 to 14 years of approximately 1.3 to 1.8 L/kg, with a range from 0.7 to 3.9 L/kg. In adults aged 60-75 years, the volume of distribution was lower (0.42 L/kg +/- 0.22).
Metabolism
In adult patients who underwent surgery for cholelithiasis and were given a single IV dose of tritiated glycopyrrolate, approximately 85% of total radioactivity was excreted in urine and < 5% was present in T-tube drainage of bile. In both urine and bile, > 80% of the radioactivity corresponded to unchanged drug. These data suggest a small proportion of IV glycopyrrolate is excreted as one or more metabolites.
Elimination
Approximately 65-80% of an IV glycopyrrolate dose was eliminated unchanged in urine in adults. In two studies, after IV administration to pediatric patients ages 1-14 years, mean clearance values ranged from 1.01-1.41 L/kg/hr (range 0.32–2.22 L/kg/ hr). In adults, IV clearance values were 0.54 ± 0.14 L/kg/hr.
Pediatrics
The estimated apparent clearance of glycopyrrolate from a population pharmacokinetic analysis (scaled by weight in children and adults) of oral and IV data was found to be 13.2 L/hr/Kg or 92 7L/hr for a typical 70 kg subject. In the

same population based analysis, gender was not identified as having an effect on either glycopyrrolate clearance or systemic exposure.
Gender
Population pharmacokinetic evaluation of adults and children administered IV or oral glycopyrrolate identified no effect of gender on glycopyrrolate clearance or systemic exposure.
Race
The pharmacokinetics of glycopyrrolate by race has not been characterized.
Elderly
Glycopyrrolate pharmacokinetics have not been characterized in the elderly.
Renal Impairment
In one study, glycopyrrolate 4 mcg/kg was administered intravenously in uremic patients undergoing renal transplantation surgery. Mean AUC (10.6 mcg•h/L), mean plasma clearance (0.43 L/hr/kg) and mean 3-hour urinary excretion (0.7%) for glycopyrrolate were significantly different than those of control patients (3.73 µg•h/L, 1.14 L/hr/kg, and 50%, respectively). These results suggest that elimination of glycopyrrolate is severely impaired in patients with renal failure.
Hepatic Impairment
Glycopyrrolate is largely renally eliminated. The pharmacokinetics of glycopyrrolate has not been evaluated in patients with hepatic impairment.

13 NONCLINICAL TOXICOLOGY

13.1 Carcinogenesis, Mutagenesis, Impairment of Fertility
Long-term animal studies have not been performed to evaluate the carcinogenic potential of glycopyrrolate.
Glycopyrrolate did not elicit any genotoxic effects in the Ames mutagenicity assay, the human lymphocyte chromosome aberration assay, or the micronucleus assay.
Glycopyrrolate has not been evaluated for potential to impair fertility.

14 CLINICAL STUDIES
CUVPOSA was evaluated in a multi-center, randomized, double-blind, placebo-controlled, parallel, eight-week study for the control of pathologic drooling in children (Study 1). The study enrolled 38 subjects aged 3-23 years; thirty-six subjects were aged 3-16 years and two patients were greater than 16 years. The subjects were male or female, weighed at least 13 kg (27 lbs), and had cerebral palsy, mental retardation, or another neurologic condition associated with problem drooling defined as drooling in the absence of treatment so that clothing became damp on most days (approximately five to seven days per week). Subjects were randomized in a 1:1 fashion to receive CUVPOSA or placebo. Doses of study medication were titrated over a 4-week period to optimal response beginning at 0.02 mg/kg given three times a day increasing doses in increments of approximately 0.02 mg/kg three times per day every 5-7 days, not to exceed the lesser of approximately 0.1 mg/kg three times per day or 3 mg three times per day.
Subjects were evaluated on the 9-point modified Teacher's Drooling Scale (mTDS), which is presented below. The mTDS evaluations were recorded by parents/caregivers 3 times daily approximately two hours post-dose on evaluation days during pre-treatment baseline and at Weeks 2, 4, 6 and 8 of therapy.
Modified Teacher's Drooling Scale
1 = Dry: never drools
2 = Mild: only the lips are wet; occasionally
3 = Mild: only the lips are wet; frequently
4 = Moderate: wet on lips and chin; occasionally
5 = Moderate: wet on the lips and chin; frequently
6 = Severe: drools to the extent that clothing becomes damp; occasionally
7 = Severe: drools to the extent that clothing becomes damp; frequently
8 = Profuse: clothing, hands, tray and objects become wet; occasionally
9 = Profuse: clothing, hands, tray and objects become wet; frequently

Responders were defined as subjects with at least a 3-point reduction in mean daily mTDS scores from baseline to Week 8. Table 4 presents the proportion of responders at Week 8 and Figure 1 presents mean mTDS values from baseline through Week 8.

Table 4: Percentage of Responders at Week 8

CUVPOSA Group (N=20)	Placebo Group (N=18)
15/20 (75%)	2/18 (11%)

Figure 1. Mean (± 2 Standard Errors) mTDS Scores

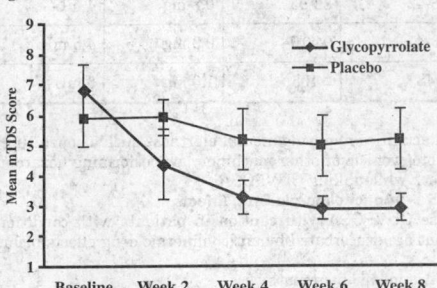

16 HOW SUPPLIED/STORAGE AND HANDLING
NDC 59630-206-16: 1 mg/5 mL clear, cherry-flavored solution; 16 oz. bottle.
Store at room temperature 20°-25°C (68°-77°F); excursions permitted to 15°-30°C (59°-86°F) [See USP Controlled Room Temperature].

17 PATIENT COUNSELING INFORMATION
See FDA-Approved Patient Labeling.
- Advise parent/caregivers to measure CUVPOSA with an accurate measuring device. A household teaspoon is not an accurate measuring device. Parents/caregivers should use a dosing cup available in pharmacies to accurately measure the correct milliliter dose for the patient. An oral syringe, also available in pharmacies, should be used to dispense CUVPOSA into the child's mouth from the cup. A pharmacist can recommend an appropriate measuring device and can provide instructions for measuring the correct dose.
- Administering CUVPOSA with a high fat meal substantially reduces the amount of glycopyrrolate absorbed. Administer CUVPOSA at least one hour before or two hours after meals.
- CUVPOSA is started at a low dose and gradually titrated over a period of weeks based on therapeutic response and adverse reactions. Parents/caregivers should not increase the dose without the physician's permission.
- Common adverse reactions from CUVPOSA include overly dry mouth, constipation, vomiting, flushing of the skin or face, and urinary retention. Side effects can sometimes be difficult to detect in some patients with neurologic problems who cannot adequately communicate how they feel. If side effects become troublesome after increasing a dose, decrease the dose to the prior one and contact your physician.
- Constipation is the most common side effect of glycopyrrolate, and if constipation occurs, stop administering glycopyrrolate to the patient and call a healthcare practitioner.
- Inability of the patient to urinate, dry diapers or undergarments, irritability or crying may be signs of urinary retention, and if urinary retention occurs, parents/caregivers should stop administering glycopyrrolate and call their healthcare practitioner.
- If the patient develops a skin rash, hives or an allergic reaction, parents/caregivers should stop administering glycopyrrolate and call their healthcare practitioner as this could be a sign of hypersensitivity to this product.
- Drugs like glycopyrrolate can reduce sweating, and if the patient is in a hot environment and flushing of the skin occurs, this may be due to overheating. Parents/caregivers should be advised to avoid exposure of the patient to hot or very warm environmental temperatures to avoid overheating and the possibility of heat exhaustion or heat stroke.
Manufactured by:
Mikart, Inc.
Atlanta, GA 30318
Manufactured for:
SHIONOGI PHARMA, INC.
Atlanta, GA 30328
GLY-PI-01

PATIENT and CAREGIVER INFORMATION

CUVPOSA (glycopyrrolate) Oral Solution

Please read the Patient and Caregiver Information that comes with CUVPOSA before you start giving it to your child, and each time you get a refill. This leaflet does not take the place of talking with your doctor about your child's medical condition or treatment.

What is CUVPOSA?

CUVPOSA is a prescription medicine used in children with medical conditions that cause too much (abnormal) drooling.

Who should not take CUVPOSA?

Do not give CUVPOSA to anyone who:
• has problems urinating
• has a bowel problem called paralytic ileus
• lacks normal bowel tone or tension
• has severe ulcerative colitis or certain other serious bowel problems with severe ulcerative colitis
• has myasthenia gravis

What should I tell the doctor before giving CUVPOSA to my child?

Tell your doctor if your child:
• has any allergies
• has any stomach or bowel problems, including ulcerative colitis
• has any problems with constipation
• has thyroid problems
• has high blood pressure
• has heart problems or abnormal heart beats
• has a hiatal hernia with gastroesophageal reflux disease (GERD)
• has any eye problems
• has any problems urinating
• has any other medical conditions
• is pregnant or plans to become pregnant. It is not known if CUVPOSA can harm an unborn baby.
• is breastfeeding or plans to breastfeed. It is not known if CUVPOSA passes into breast milk and if it can harm the baby.

Tell your doctor about all the medicines that your child takes, including prescription and non-prescription medicines, vitamins, and herbal supplements. Some medicine may affect the way CUVPOSA works, and CUVPOSA may affect how some other medicines work.

How should I give CUVPOSA?

• Give CUVPOSA exactly as prescribed by your child's doctor.
• Give CUVPOSA 1 hour before or 2 hours after meals.
• Your doctor will tell you how much (milliliters or mLs) of CUVPOSA to give your child.
• Do not change the dose of CUVPOSA unless your doctor tells you to.
• You must measure the dose of CUVPOSA before giving it to your child. Use a specially marked dose measuring cup (available at most pharmacies) to measure the right dose of CUVPOSA.
• To help make sure that your child swallows the dose, you should use an oral syringe to give the child each dose of CUVPOSA, after you measure the dose needed with a dose measuring cup. Oral syringes are also available at most pharmacies.
• If you have questions about how to measure the dose or how to use an oral syringe, ask your pharmacist or doctor.
• The dose of CUVPOSA that is needed to control drooling may be different for each child. CUVPOSA is usually started at a low dose, and slowly increased as directed by your doctor. This slow increase in dose continues until the best dose for your child is reached, to control drooling.
• During this time it is important to stay in close contact with your child's doctor, and tell the doctor about any side effects that your child has. See "What are the possible side effects of CUVPOSA?"

What should I avoid while taking CUVPOSA?

• CUVPOSA may cause sleepiness or blurred vision. Do not drive a car, operate heavy machinery, or do other dangerous activities while taking CUVPOSA.
• Avoid overheating. See "What are the possible side effects of CUVPOSA?"

What are the possible side effects of CUVPOSA?

CUVPOSA can cause serious side effects including:
• **Constipation.** Constipation is common with CUVPOSA. Tell your doctor if your child strains with bowel movements, goes longer between bowel movements, can not have a bowel movement, or their stomach is firm and large. The dose of CUVPOSA may need to be decreased or stopped.
• **Diarrhea and intestinal blockage.** Diarrhea can be an early symptom of a blockage in the intestine. This is especially true if your child has a colostomy or ileostomy. Tell your doctor if your child has any diarrhea while taking CUVPOSA.
• **Problems with control of body temperature (overheating or heat stroke).** CUVPOSA can cause your child to sweat

less. Your child can become overheated, and develop heat stroke if they are in an area that is very hot. Avoid overheating. Call your doctor right away if your child becomes sick and has any of these symptoms of heatstroke:
• hot, red skin
• decreased alertness or passing out (unconsciousness)
• fast, weak pulse
• fast, shallow breathing
• increased body temperature (fever)

The most common side effects of CUVPOSA include:
• dry mouth
• vomiting
• flushing of the face or skin
• nasal congestion
• headache
• swollen sinuses (sinusitis)
• upper respiratory tract infection
• problems urinating, difficulty starting urination

Tell your doctor if your child has any side effect that concerns you or that does not go away. These are not all the possible side effects of CUVPOSA.

Call your doctor for medical advice about side effects. You may report side effects to FDA at 1-800-FDA-1088.

How should I store CUVPOSA?

Store CUVPOSA between 68°F to 77°F (20°C to 25°C).

Keep CUVPOSA out of the reach of children.

General information about CUVPOSA:

Medicines are sometimes prescribed for purposes other than those listed in a Patient Information leaflet. Do not use CUVPOSA for a condition for which it was not prescribed. Do not give CUVPOSA to other people even if they have the same condition. It may harm them.

This leaflet summarizes the most important information about CUVPOSA. If you would like more information, talk with your doctor. You can ask your doctor or pharmacist for information about CUVPOSA that is written for health professionals.

For more information, go to: www.cuvposa.com or call 1-800-849-9707 ext.1454.

What are the ingredients in CUVPOSA?

Active Ingredient: glycopyrrolate

Inactive Ingredients: citric acid glycerin, natural and artificial cherry flavor, methylparaben, propylene glycol, propylparaben, saccharin sodium, sodium citrate, sorbitol solution, and purified water

Issued July 2010
Manufactured by:
Mikart, Inc.
Atlanta, GA 30318
Manufactured for:
SHIONOGI PHARMA, INC.
Atlanta, GA 30328
GLY-PPI-01 Rev 07/2010

Distributed by: Shionogi Pharma, Inc.

KAPVAY   ℞

(clonidine hydrochloride)
extended-release tablets, oral

HIGHLIGHTS OF PRESCRIBING INFORMATION

These highlights do not include all the information needed to use KAPVAY safely and effectively. See full prescribing information for KAPVAY.

KAPVAY (clonidine hydrochloride) extended-release tablets, oral

Initial U.S. Approval: 1974

————INDICATIONS AND USAGE————

KAPVAY™ is a centrally acting alpha$_2$-adrenergic agonist indicated for the treatment of attention deficit hyperactivity disorder (ADHD) as monotherapy or as adjunctive therapy to stimulant medications. (1)

The efficacy of KAPVAY is based on the results of two clinical trials in children and adolescents. (14) Maintenance efficacy has not been systematically evaluated, and patients who are continued on longer-term treatment require periodic reassessment. (1)

This extended-release formulation of clonidine hydrochloride is also approved for the treatment of hypertension under the trade name JENLOGA. (1)

————DOSAGE AND ADMINISTRATION————

Dosing should be initiated with one 0.1 mg tablet at bedtime, and the daily dosage should be adjusted in increments of 0.1 mg/day at weekly intervals until desired response is achieved. Doses should be taken twice a day, with either an equal or higher split dosage being given at bedtime, as depicted below (2.1)

Total Daily Dose	Morning Dose	Bedtime Dose
0.1 mg/day		0.1 mg
0.2 mg/day	0.1 mg	0.1 mg
0.3 mg/day	0.1 mg	0.2 mg
0.4 mg/day	0.2 mg	0.2 mg

• Tablets should not be crushed, chewed or broken before swallowing. (2.1)
• Do not substitute for other clonidine products on a mg-per-mg basis, because of differing pharmacokinetic profiles. (2.1)
• When discontinuing, taper the dose in decrements of no more than 0.1 mg every 3 to 7 days. (2.4)

————DOSAGE FORMS AND STRENGTHS————

Extended-release tablets: 0.1 mg and 0.2 mg, not scored. (3)

————CONTRAINDICATIONS————

Clonidine hydrochloride tablets should not be used in patients with known hypersensitivity to clonidine. (4)

————WARNINGS AND PRECAUTIONS————

• Hypotension/bradycardia: Use KAPVAY with caution in patients at risk for hypotension, bradycardia, and heart block. Measure heart rate and blood pressure prior to initiation of therapy, following dose increases, and periodically while on therapy. Advise patients to avoid becoming dehydrated or overheated. (5.1)
• Somnolence/Sedation: Has been observed with KAPVAY. Consider the potential for additive sedative effects with CNS depressant drugs. Caution patients against operating heavy equipment or driving until they know how they respond to KAPVAY. (5.2)
• Abrupt Discontinuation: Patients should be instructed not to discontinue KAPVAY therapy without consulting their physician due to the potential risk of withdrawal effects. KAPVAY should be discontinued slowly in decrements of no more than 0.1 mg every 3 to 7 days. (5.3)
• Allergic Reactions: In patients who have developed localized contact sensitization or other allergic reaction to clonidine in a transdermal system, substitution of oral clonidine hydrochloride therapy may be associated with the development of a generalized skin rash, urticaria, or angioedema. (5.4)
• Use in patients with vascular disease, cardiac conduction disease, or chronic renal failure: Monitor carefully and uptitrate slowly. (5.5)
• Other clonidine containing products: Do not use KAPVAY concomitantly with other products containing clonidine, (e.g. Catapres®). (5.6)

————ADVERSE REACTIONS————

Common and drug related adverse reactions (incidence at least 5% and twice the rate of placebo) reported with the use of KAPVAY include (6.1):

Somnolence, fatigue, upper respiratory tract infection (cough, rhinitis, sneezing), irritability, throat pain (sore throat), insomnia, nightmares, emotional disorder, constipation, nasal congestion, increased body temperature, dry mouth, and ear pain.

To report SUSPECTED ADVERSE REACTIONS, contact Shionogi Pharma, Inc. at 1-800-849-9707 ext. 1454 or FDA at 1-800-FDA-1088 or www.fda.gov/medwatch.

————DRUG INTERACTIONS————

• Sedating Drugs: Clonidine may potentiate the CNS-depressive effects of alcohol, barbiturates or other sedating drugs. (7.1)
• Tricyclic Antidepressants: May reduce the hypotensive effect of clonidine. (7.2)
• Drugs Known to Affect Sinus Node Function or AV Nodal Conduction: Caution is warranted in patients receiving clonidine concomitantly with agents known to affect sinus node function or AV nodal conduction (e.g., digitalis, calcium channel blockers and beta-blockers) due to a potential for additive effects such as bradycardia and AV block. (7.3)
• Use with other products containing clonidine: Do not use KAPVAY concomitantly with other products containing clonidine (e.g. Catapres®). (7.4)
• Antihypertensive drugs: Use caution when coadministered with KAPVAY. (7.5)

————USE IN SPECIFIC POPULATIONS————

• Since clonidine hydrochloride is excreted in human milk, caution should be exercised when KAPVAY is administered to a nursing woman. (8.3)
• KAPVAY has not been studied in children less than 6 years old. (8.4)
• Renal Insufficiency: The dosage of KAPVAY must be adjusted according to the degree of impairment, and patients should be carefully monitored. (8.6)

See Section 17 for Patient Counseling Information

FULL PRESCRIBING INFORMATION: CONTENTS*
1   **INDICATIONS AND USAGE**
2   **DOSAGE AND ADMINISTRATION**
    2.1   General Dosing Information
    2.2   Dose Selection
    2.3   Maintenance Treatment

FULL PRESCRIBING INFORMATION

1. INDICATIONS AND USAGE

KAPVAY ™ (clonidine hydrochloride) extended-release is indicated for the treatment of attention deficit hyperactivity disorder (ADHD) as monotherapy and as adjunctive therapy to stimulant medications.

The efficacy of KAPVAY in the treatment of ADHD is based on two controlled trials (one monotherapy and one adjunctive to stimulant medication) in children and adolescents ages 6-17 who met DSM-IV criteria for ADHD hyperactive or combined hyperactive/inattentive subtypes [see Clinical Studies (14)]. In the adjunctive study, KAPVAY was administered to patients who had been on a stable regimen of either methylphenidate or amphetamine (or their derivatives) and who had not achieved an optimal response. The effectiveness of KAPVAY for longer-term use (more than 5 weeks) has not been systematically evaluated in controlled trials.

A diagnosis of ADHD implies the presence of hyperactive-impulsive and/or inattentive symptoms that cause impairment and were present before the age of 7 years. The symptoms must cause clinically significant impairment, e.g., in social, academic, or occupational functioning, and be present in two or more settings, e.g., school (or work) and at home. The symptoms must not be better accounted for by another mental disorder. For the Inattentive Type, at least six of the following symptoms must have persisted for at least 6 months: lack of attention to details/careless mistakes; lack of sustained attention; poor listener; failure to follow through on tasks; poor organization; avoids tasks requiring sustained mental effort; loses things; easily distracted; forgetful. For the Hyperactive-Impulsive Type, at least six of the following symptoms must have persisted for at least 6 months: fidgeting/squirming; leaving seat; inappropriate running/climbing; difficulty with quiet activities; "on the go"; excessive talking; blurting answers; can't wait turn; intrusive. The Combined Type requires both inattentive and hyperactive-impulsive criteria to be met.

Special Diagnostic Considerations

Specific etiology of this syndrome is unknown, and there is no single diagnostic test. Adequate diagnosis requires the use not only of medical but also of special psychological, educational, and social resources. Learning may or may not be impaired. The diagnosis must be based upon a complete history and evaluation of the patient and not solely on the presence of the required number of DSM-IV® characteristics.

Need for Comprehensive Treatment program

KAPVAY is indicated as an integral part of a total treatment program for ADHD that may include other measures (psychological, educational, and social) for patients with this syndrome. Drug treatment may not be indicated for all patients with this syndrome. KAPVAY is not intended for use in patients who exhibit symptoms secondary to environmental factors and/or other primary psychiatric disorders, including psychosis. Appropriate educational/vocational placement is essential and psychosocial intervention is often helpful. When remedial measures alone are insufficient, the decision to prescribe KAPVAY will depend upon the physician's assessment of the chronicity and severity of the patient's symptoms and on the level of functional impairment. NOTE: This extended-release formulation of clonidine hydrochloride is also approved for the treatment of hypertension in adults under the trade name JENLOGA.

2. DOSAGE AND ADMINISTRATION

KAPVAY is an extended-release tablet formulation of clonidine hydrochloride. While it is dosed twice a day, the same as the immediate-release clonidine formulation, it is not to be used interchangeably with the immediate-release formulation.

2.1 General Dosing Information

KAPVAY is an extended-release tablet and, therefore, must be swallowed whole and never crushed, cut or chewed. KAPVAY may be taken with or without food.

Due to the lack of controlled clinical trial data and differing pharmacokinetic profiles, substitution of KAPVAY for other clonidine products on a mg-per-mg basis is not recommended.

2.2 Dose Selection

The dose of KAPVAY, administered either as monotherapy or as adjunctive therapy to a psychostimulant, should be individualized according to the therapeutic needs and response of the patient. Dosing should be initiated with one 0.1 mg tablet at bedtime, and the daily dosage should be adjusted in increments of 0.1 mg/day at weekly intervals until the desired response is achieved. Doses should be taken twice a day, with either an equal or higher split dosage being given at bedtime (see Table 1).

Table 1 KAPVAY Dosing Guidance

Total Daily Dose	Morning Dose	Bedtime Dose
0.1 mg/day		0.1 mg
0.2 mg/day	0.1 mg	0.1 mg
0.3 mg/day	0.1 mg	0.2 mg
0.4 mg/day	0.2 mg	0.2 mg

Doses of KAPVAY higher than 0.4 mg/day (0.2 mg twice daily) were not evaluated in clinical trials for ADHD and are not recommended.

When KAPVAY is being added-on to a psychostimulant, the dose of the psychostimulant can be adjusted depending on the patient's response to KAPVAY.

2.3 Maintenance Treatment

The effectiveness of KAPVAY for longer-term use (more than 5 weeks) has not been systematically evaluated in controlled trials. Therefore the physician electing to use KAPVAY for extended periods should periodically re-evaluate the long-term usefulness of the drug for the individual patient.

2.4 Discontinuation

When discontinuing KAPVAY, the total daily dose should be tapered in decrements of no more than 0.1 mg every 3 to 7 days.

3. DOSAGE FORM AND STRENGTHS

KAPVAY tablets are available in two strengths, 0.1 mg and 0.2 mg as an extended-release formulation. Both the 0.1 mg and 0.2 mg tablets are white, non-scored, standard convex with debossing on one side. The 0.1 mg tablets are round and the 0.2 mg tablets are oval. KAPVAY tablets must be swallowed whole and never crushed, cut or chewed.

4. CONTRAINDICATIONS

KAPVAY should not be used in patients with known hypersensitivity to clonidine.

5. WARNINGS AND PRECAUTIONS

5.1 Hypotension/Bradycardia

Treatment with KAPVAY can cause dose related decreases in blood pressure and heart rate. In patients that completed 5 weeks of treatment in a controlled, fixed-dose monotherapy study in pediatric patients, during the treatment period the maximum placebo-subtracted mean change in systolic blood pressure was -4.0 mmHg on KAPVAY 0.2 mg/day and -8.8 mmHg on KAPVAY 0.4 mg/day. The maximum placebo-subtracted mean change in diastolic blood pressure was -4.0 mmHg on KAPVAY 0.2 mg/day and -7.3 mmHg on KAPVAY 0.4 mg/day. The maximum placebo-subtracted mean change in heart rate was -4.0 beats per minute on KAPVAY 0.2 mg/day and -7.7 beats per minute on KAPVAY 0.4 mg/day.

During the taper period of the fixed-dose monotherapy study the maximum placebo-subtracted mean change in systolic blood pressure was +3.4 mmHg on KAPVAY 0.2 mg/day and -5.6 mmHg on KAPVAY 0.4 mg/day. The maximum placebo-subtracted mean change in diastolic blood pressure was +3.3 mmHg on KAPVAY 0.2 mg/day and -5.4 mmHg on KAPVAY 0.4 mg/day. The maximum placebo-subtracted mean change in heart rate was -0.6 beats per minute on KAPVAY 0.2 mg/day and -3.0 beats per minute on KAPVAY 0.4 mg/day.

Measure heart rate and blood pressure prior to initiation of therapy, following dose increases, and periodically while on therapy. Use KAPVAY with caution in patients with a history of hypotension, heart block, bradycardia, or cardiovascular disease, because it can decrease blood pressure and heart rate. Use caution in treating patients who have a history of syncope or may have a condition that predisposes them to syncope, such as hypotension, orthostatic hypotension, bradycardia, or dehydration. Use KAPVAY with caution in patients treated concomitantly with antihypertensives or other drugs that can reduce blood pressure or heart rate or increase the risk of syncope. Advise patients to avoid becoming dehydrated or overheated.

5.2 Sedation and Somnolence

Somnolence and sedation were commonly reported adverse reactions in clinical studies. In patients that completed 5 weeks of therapy in a controlled fixed dose pediatric monotherapy study, 31% of patients treated with 0.4 mg/day and 38% treated with 0.2 mg/day vs 7% of placebo treated patients reported somnolence as an adverse event. In patients that completed 5 weeks of therapy in a controlled flexible dose pediatric adjunctive to stimulants study, 19% of patients treated with KAPVAY+stimulant vs 8% treated with placebo+stimulant reported somnolence. Before using KAPVAY with other centrally active depressants (such as phenothiazines, barbiturates, or benzodiazepines), consider the potential for additive sedative effects. Caution patients against operating heavy equipment or driving until they know how they respond to treatment with KAPVAY. Advise patients to avoid use with alcohol.

5.3 Abrupt Discontinuation

No studies evaluating abrupt discontinuation of KAPVAY in children with ADHD have been conducted. In children and adolescents with ADHD, physicians should gradually reduce the dose of KAPVAY in decrements of no more than 0.1 mg every 3 to 7 days. Patients should be instructed not to discontinue KAPVAY therapy without consulting their physician due to the potential risk of withdrawal effects.

In adults with hypertension, sudden cessation of clonidine hydrochloride extended-release formulation treatment in the 0.2 to 0.6 mg/day range resulted in reports of headache, tachycardia, nausea, flushing, warm feeling, brief lightheadedness, tightness in chest, and anxiety.

In adults with hypertension, sudden cessation of treatment with immediate-release clonidine has, in some cases, resulted in symptoms such as nervousness, agitation, headache, and tremor accompanied or followed by a rapid rise in blood pressure and elevated catecholamine concentrations in the plasma.

5.4 Allergic Reactions

In patients who have developed localized contact sensitization to clonidine transdermal system, continuation of clonidine transdermal system or substitution of oral clonidine hydrochloride therapy may be associated with the development of a generalized skin rash.

In patients who develop an allergic reaction from clonidine transdermal system, substitution of oral clonidine hydrochloride may also elicit an allergic reaction (including generalized rash, urticaria, or angioedema).

5.5 Patients with Vascular Disease, Cardiac Conduction Disease, or Renal Failure

Clonidine hydrochloride should be used with caution in patients with severe coronary insufficiency, conduction disturbances, recent myocardial infarction, cerebrovascular disease or chronic renal failure.

5.6 Other Clonidine-Containing Products

Clonidine, the active ingredient in KAPVAY, is also approved as an antihypertensive. Do not use KAPVAY in patients concomitantly taking other clonidine-containing products, (e.g. Catapres®).

6. ADVERSE REACTIONS

6.1 Clinical Trial Experience

Two KAPVAY ADHD clinical studies evaluated 256 patients who received active therapy, in one of the two placebo-controlled studies (Studies 1 and 2) with primary efficacy end-points at 5-weeks.

Study 1: Fixed-dose KAPVAY Monotherapy

Study 1 was a multi-center, randomized, double-blind, placebo-controlled study with primary efficacy endpoint at 5 weeks, of two fixed doses (0.2 mg/day or 0.4 mg/day) of KAPVAY in children and adolescents (6 to 17 years of age) who met DSM-IV criteria for ADHD hyperactive or combined inattentive/hyperactive subtypes.

Commonly observed adverse reactions (incidence of ≥ 2% in either active treatment group and greater than the rate on placebo) during the treatment period are listed in Table 2. [See table 2 at right]

Commonly observed adverse reactions (incidence of ≥ 2% in either active treatment group and greater than the rate on placebo) during the taper period are listed in Table 3. [See table 3 at top of next page]

Study 2: Flexible-dose KAPVAY as Adjunctive Therapy to Psychostimulants

Study 2 was a multi-center, randomized, double-blind, placebo-controlled study, with primary efficacy endpoint at 5 weeks, of a flexible dose of KAPVAY as adjunctive therapy to a psychostimulant in children and adolescents (6 to 17 years) who met DSM-IV criteria for ADHD hyperactive or combined inattentive/hyperactive subtypes. KAPVAY was initiated at 0.1 mg/day and titrated up to 0.4 mg/day over a 3-week period. Most KAPVAY treated patients (75.5%) were escalated to the maximum dose of 0.4 mg/day.

Commonly observed adverse reactions (incidence of ≥ 2% in the treatment group and greater than the rate on placebo) during the treatment period are listed in Table 4. [See table 4 on next page]

Commonly observed adverse reactions (incidence of ≥ 2% in the treatment group and greater than the rate on placebo) during the taper period are listed in Table 5. [See table 5 on next page]

Most common adverse reactions, defined as events that were reported in at least 5% of drug-treated patients and at least twice the rate as in placebo patients, during the treatment period were somnolence, fatigue, upper respiratory tract infection, irritability, throat pain, insomnia, nightmares, emotional disorder, constipation, nasal congestion, increased body temperature, dry mouth, and ear pain. The most common adverse reactions that were reported during the taper phase were upper abdominal pain and gastrointestinal virus.

Adverse Reactions Leading to Discontinuation

Thirteen percent (13%) of patients receiving KAPVAY discontinued from the pediatric monotherapy study due to adverse events, compared to 1% in the placebo group. The most common adverse reactions leading to discontinuation of KAPVAY monotherapy treated patients were from somnolence/sedation (5%) and fatigue (4%). Less common adverse reactions leading to discontinuation (occurring in approximately 1% of patients) included: formication, vomiting, prolonged QT, increased heart rate, and rash. In the pediatric adjunctive treatment to stimulants study, one patient discontinued from KAPVAY + stimulant group because of bradyphrenia.

Effects on Laboratory Tests, Vital Signs, and Electrocardiograms

KAPVAY treatment was not associated with any clinically important effects on any laboratory parameters in either of the placebo-controlled studies.

Mean decreases in blood pressure and heart rate were seen [see Warnings and Precautions (5.1)].

There were no changes on ECGs to suggest a drug-related effect.

7. DRUG INTERACTIONS

No drug interaction studies have been conducted with KAPVAY in children. The following have been reported with other oral immediate release formulations of clonidine.

7.1 Interactions with CNS-depressant Drugs

Clonidine may potentiate the CNS-depressive effects of alcohol, barbiturates or other sedating drugs.

7.2 Interactions with Tricyclic Antidepressants

If a patient is receiving clonidine hydrochloride and also taking tricyclic antidepressants the hypotensive effects of clonidine may be reduced.

7.3 Interactions with Drugs Known to Affect Sinus Node Function or AV Nodal Conduction

Due to a potential for additive effects such as bradycardia and AV block, caution is warranted in patients receiving clonidine concomitantly with agents known to affect sinus node function or AV nodal conduction (e.g., digitalis, calcium channel blockers and beta-blockers).

7.4 Use with other products containing clonidine

Do not use KAPVAY concomitantly with other products containing clonidine (e.g. Catapres®).

Table 2 Common Adverse Reactions in the Fixed-Dose Monotherapy Trial- Treatment period (Study 1)

Preferred Term	Percentage of Patients Reporting Event		
	KAPVAY 0.4 mg/day N=78	KAPVAY 0.2 mg/day N=76	Placebo (N=76)
Somnolence[1]	31%	38%	5%
Headache	19%	29%	18%
Upper Abdominal Pain	13%	20%	17%
Fatigue[2]	13%	16%	1%
Upper Respiratory Tract Infection	6%	11%	4%
Irritability	6%	9%	3%
Throat Pain	6%	8%	3%
Nausea	8%	5%	4%
Nightmare	9%	3%	0
Dizziness	3%	7%	5%
Insomnia	6%	4%	1%
Emotional Disorder	5%	4%	1%
Constipation	6%	1%	0
Dry Mouth	5%	0	1%
Nasal Congestion	5%	3%	1%
Body Temperature Increased	1%	5%	3%
Gastrointestinal Viral	0%	7%	4%
Diarrhea	1%	4%	3%
Ear Pain	0	5%	1%
Nasopharyngitis	3%	3%	1%
Abnormal Sleep-Related Event	1%	3%	0
Aggression	1%	3%	1%
Asthma	1%	3%	1%
Bradycardia	4%	0	0
Enuresis	4%	0	0
Influenza like Illness	3%	1%	1%
Tearfulness	3%	1%	0
Thirst	3%	1%	0
Tremor	3%	1%	0
Epistaxis	0	3%	0
Lower Respiratory Tract Infection	0	3%	1%
Pollakiuria	0	3%	0
Sleep Terror	0	3%	0

1. Somnolence includes the terms "somnolence" and "sedation".
2. Fatigue includes the terms "fatigue" and "lethargy".

7.5 Antihypertensive Drugs

Use caution when KAPVAY is administered concomitantly with antihypertensive drugs, due to the potential for additive pharmacodynamic effects (e.g., hypotension, syncope) [see Warnings and Precautions (5.2)].

8. USE IN SPECIFIC POPULATIONS

8.1 Pregnancy

Pregnancy Category C: Oral administration of clonidine hydrochloride to pregnant rabbits during the period of embryo/fetal organogenesis at doses of up to 80 mcg/kg/day (approximately 3 times the oral maximum recommended daily dose [MRHD] of 0.4 mg/day on a mg/m² basis) produced no evidence of teratogenic or embryotoxic potential. In pregnant rats, however, doses as low as 15 mcg/kg/day (1/3 the MRHD on a mg/m² basis) were associated with increased resorptions in a study in which dams were treated continuously from 2 months prior to mating and throughout gestation. Increased resorptions were not associated with treatment at the same or at higher dose levels (up to 3 times the MRHD) when treatment of the dams was restricted to gestation days 6-15. Increases in resorptions were observed in both rats and mice at 500 mcg/kg/day (10 and 5 times the MRHD in rats and mice, respectively) or higher when the animals were treated on gestation days 1-14; 500 mcg/kg/day was the lowest dose employed in this study. No adequate and well-controlled studies have been conducted in pregnant women. Because animal reproduction studies are not always predictive of human response, this drug should not be used during pregnancy unless clearly needed.

8.3 Nursing Mothers

Since clonidine hydrochloride is excreted in human milk, caution should be exercised when KAPVAY is administered to a nursing woman.

8.4 Pediatric Use

A study was conducted in which young rats were treated orally with clonidine hydrochloride from day 21 of age to adulthood at doses of up to 300 mcg/kg/day, which is approximately 3 times the maximum recommended human dose (MRHD) of 0.4 mg/day on a mg/m² basis. A slight delay in onset of preputial separation was seen in males treated with the highest dose (with a no-effect dose of 100 mcg/kg/day, which is approximately equal to the MRHD), but there were no drug effects on fertility or on other measures of sexual or neurobehavioral development.

KAPVAY has not been studied in children with ADHD less than 6 years old.

8.6 Patients with Renal Impairment

The impact of renal impairment on the pharmacokinetics of clonidine in children has not been assessed. The initial dosage of KAPVAY should be based on degree of impairment. Monitor patients carefully for hypotension and bradycardia, and titrate to higher doses cautiously. Since only a minimal amount of clonidine is removed during routine hemodialysis, there is no need to give supplemental KAPVAY following dialysis.

8.7 Adult Use in ADHD

KAPVAY has not been studied in adult patients with ADHD.

9.0 DRUG ABUSE AND DEPENDENCE

9.1 Controlled Substance

KAPVAY is not a controlled substance and has no known potential for abuse or dependence.

10. OVERDOSAGE

Symptoms

Clonidine overdose: hypertension may develop early and may be followed by hypotension, bradycardia, respiratory depression, hypothermia, drowsiness, decreased or absent reflexes, weakness, irritability and miosis. The frequency of CNS depression may be higher in children than adults. Large overdoses may result in reversible cardiac conduction defects or dysrhythmias, apnea, coma and seizures. Signs and symptoms of overdose generally occur within 30 minutes to two hours after exposure.

Treatment

Consult with a Certified Poison Control Center for up-to-date guidance and advice.

11. DESCRIPTION

KAPVAY (clonidine hydrochloride) extended-release is a centrally acting alpha₂-adrenergic agonist available as 0.1 mg or 0.2 mg extended-release tablets for oral administration. Each 0.1 mg and 0.2 mg tablet is equivalent to 0.087 mg and 0.174 mg, respectively, of the free base.

The inactive ingredients are sodium lauryl sulfate, lactose monohydrate, hypromellose type 2208, partially pregelatinized starch, colloidal silicon dioxide, and magnesium stearate. The formulation is designed to delay the absorption of active drug in order to decrease peak to trough plasma concentration differences. Clonidine hydrochloride is an imidazoline derivative and exists as a mesomeric compound. The chemical name is 2-(2,6-dichlorophenylamino)-2-imidazoline hydrochloride. The following is the structural formula:

$C_9H_9Cl_2N_3 \cdot HCl$ Mol. Wt. 266.56

Clonidine hydrochloride is an odorless, bitter, white, crystalline substance soluble in water and alcohol.

12 CLINICAL PHARMACOLOGY

12.1 Mechanism of Action

Clonidine stimulates alpha₂-adrenergic receptors in the brain. Clonidine is not a central nervous system stimulant. The mechanism of action of clonidine in ADHD is not known.

12.2 Pharmacodynamics

Clonidine is a known antihypertensive agent. By stimulating alpha₂-adrenergic receptors in the brain stem, clonidine reduces sympathetic outflow from the central nervous system and decreases peripheral resistance, renal vascular resistance, heart rate, and blood pressure.

12.3 Pharmacokinetics

Single-dose Pharmacokinetics in Adults

Immediate-release clonidine hydrochloride and KAPVAY have different pharmacokinetic characteristics; dose substitution on a milligram for milligram basis will result in differences in exposure. A comparison across studies suggests that the Cmax is 50% lower for KAPVAY compared to immediate-release clonidine hydrochloride.

Following oral administration of an immediate release formulation, plasma clonidine concentration peaks in approximately 3 to 5 hours and the plasma half-life ranges from 12 to 16 hours. The half-life increases up to 41 hours in patients with severe impairment of renal function. Following oral administration about 40-60% of the absorbed dose is

Table 3 Common Adverse Reactions in the Fixed-Dose Monotherapy Trial- Taper period* (Study 1)

Preferred Term	Percentage of Patients Reporting Event		
	KAPVAY 0.4 mg/day N=78	KAPVAY 0.2 mg/day N=76	Placebo (N=76)
Abdominal Pain Upper	6%	0	3%
Headache	2%	5%	3%
Gastrointestinal Viral	5%	0	0
Somnolence	3%	2%	0
Heart Rate Increased	3%	0	0
Otitis Media Acute	0	3%	0

*Taper Period: 0.2 mg dose, week 8; 0.4 mg dose, weeks 6-8; Placebo dose, weeks 6-8

Table 4 Common Adverse Reactions in the Flexible-Dose Adjunctive to Stimulant Therapy Trial- Treatment Period (Study 2)

Preferred Term	Percentage of Patients Reporting Event	
	KAPVAY+STM (N=102)	PBO+STM (N=96)
Somnolence[1]	19%	8%
Fatigue[2]	16%	4%
Abdominal Pain Upper	12%	7%
Nasal Congestion	6%	5%
Throat Pain	6%	3%
Decreased Appetite	5%	4%
Body Temperature Increased	4%	2%
Dizziness	4%	2%
Insomnia	4%	2%
Epistaxis	3%	0
Rhinorrhea	3%	0
Abdominal Pain	2%	1%
Anxiety	2%	0
Pain in Extremity	2%	0

1. Somnolence includes the terms: "somnolence" and "sedation".
2. Fatigue includes the terms "fatigue" and "lethargy".

Table 5 Common Adverse Reactions in the Flexible-Dose Adjunctive to Stimulant Therapy Trial- Taper Period* (Study 2)

Preferred Term	Percentage of Patients Reporting Event	
	KAPVAY+STM (N=102)	PBO+STM (N=96)
Nasal Congestion	4%	2%
Headache	3%	1%
Irritability	3%	2%
Throat Pain	3%	1%
Gastroenteritis Viral	2%	0
Rash	2%	0

*Taper Period: weeks 6-8

recovered in the urine as unchanged drug in 24 hours. About 50% of the absorbed dose is metabolized in the liver. Although studies of the effect of renal impairment and studies of clonidine excretion have not been performed with KAPVAY, results are likely to be similar to those of the immediate release formulation.

The pharmacokinetic profile of KAPVAY administration was evaluated in an open-label, three-period, randomized, crossover study of 15 healthy adult subjects who received three single dose regimens of clonidine: 0.1 mg of KAPVAY under fasted conditions, 0.1 mg of KAPVAY following a high fat meal, and 0.1 mg of clonidine immediate-release (Catapres®) under fasted conditions. Treatments were separated by one-week washout periods.

Mean concentration-time data from the 3 treatments are shown in Table 6 and Figure 1. After administration of KAPVAY, maximum clonidine concentrations were approximately 50% of the Catapres maximum concentrations and occurred approximately 5 hours later relative to Catapres. Similar elimination half-lives were observed and total systemic bioavailability following KAPVAY was approximately 89% of that following Catapres.

Food had no effect on plasma concentrations, bioavailability, or elimination half-life.

[See table 6 at right]

Figure 1   Mean Clonidine Concentration-Time Profiles after Single Dose Administration

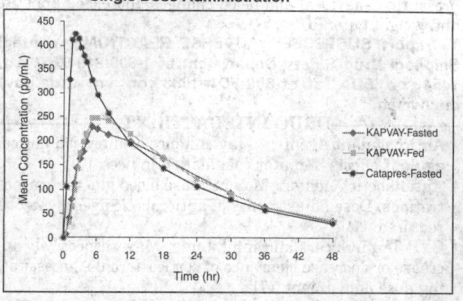

Multiple-dose Pharmacokinetics in Children and Adolescents

Plasma clonidine concentrations in children and adolescents (0.1 mg bid and 0.2 mg bid) with ADHD are greater than those of adults with hypertension with children and adolescents receiving higher doses on a mg/kg basis. Body weight normalized clearance (CL/F) in children and adolescents was higher than CL/F observed in adults with hypertension. Clonidine concentrations in plasma increased with increases in dose over the dose range of 0.2 to 0.4 mg/day. Clonidine CL/F was independent of dose administered over the 0.2 to 0.4 mg/day dose range. Clonidine CL/F appeared to decrease slightly with increases in age over the range of 6 to 17 years, and females had a 23% lower CL/F than males. The incidence of "sedation-like" AEs (somnolence and fatigue) appeared to be independent of clonidine dose or concentration within the studied dose range in the titration study. Results from the add-on study showed that clonidine CL/F was 11% higher in patients who were receiving methylphenidate and 44% lower in those receiving amphetamine compared to subjects not on adjunctive therapy.

13   NONCLINICAL TOXICOLOGY

13.1   Carcinogenesis, Mutagenesis and Impairment of Fertility

Clonidine HCl was not carcinogenic when administered in the diet of rats (for up to 132 weeks) or mice (for up to 78 weeks) at doses of up to 1620 (male rats), 2040 (female rats), or 2500 (mice) mcg/kg/day. These doses are approximately 20, 25, and 15 times, respectively, the maximum recommended human dose (MRHD) of 0.4 mg/day on a mg/m^2 basis.

There was no evidence of genotoxicity in the Ames test for mutagenicity or mouse micronucleus test for clastogenicity. Fertility of male or female rats was unaffected by clonidine HCl doses as high as 150 mcg/kg/day (approximately 3 times the MRDHD on a mg/m^2 basis). In a separate experiment, fertility of female rats appeared to be adversely affected at dose levels of 500 and 2000 mcg/kg/day (10 and 40 times the MRHD on a mg/m^2 basis).

13.2   Ocular Toxicity

In several studies with oral clonidine hydrochloride, a dose-dependent increase in the incidence and severity of spontaneous retinal degeneration was seen in albino rats treated for six months or longer. Tissue distribution studies in dogs and monkeys showed a concentration of clonidine in the choroid. In combination with amitriptyline, clonidine hydrochloride administration led to the development of corneal lesions in rats within 5 days.

In view of the retinal degeneration seen in rats, eye examinations were performed during clinical trials in 908 adult patients before, and periodically after, the start of clonidine therapy for hypertension. In 353 of these 908 patients, the eye examinations were carried out over periods of 24 months or longer. Except for some dryness of the eyes, no drug-related abnormal ophthalmological findings were recorded and, according to specialized tests such as electroretinography and macular dazzle, retinal function was unchanged.

14.   CLINICAL STUDIES

The efficacy of KAPVAY in the treatment of ADHD was established in 2 (one monotherapy *and one adjunctive therapy*) placebo-controlled trials in pediatric patients aged 6 to 17, who met DSM-IV criteria of ADHD hyperactive or combined hyperactive/inattentive subtypes. Signs and symptoms of ADHD were evaluated using the investigator administered and scored ADHD Rating Scale-IV-Parent Version (ADHDRS-IV) total score including hyperactive/impulsivity and inattentive subscales.

Study 1 was an 8-week randomized, double-blind, placebo-controlled, fixed dose study of children and adolescents aged 6 to 17 (N=236) with a 5-week primary efficacy endpoint. Patients were randomly assigned to one of the following three treatment groups: KAPVAY (CLON) 0.2 mg/day (N=78), KAPVAY 0.4 mg/day (N=80), or placebo (N=78). Dosing for the KAPVAY groups started at 0.1 mg/day and was titrated in increments of 0.1 mg/week to their respective dose (as divided doses). Patients were maintained at their dose for a minimum of 2 weeks before being gradually tapered down to 0.1 mg/day at the last week of treatment. At both doses, improvements in ADHD symptoms were statistically significantly superior in KAPVAY-treated patients compared with placebo-treated patients at the end of 5 weeks as measured by the ADHDRS-IV total score.

Study 2 was an 8-week randomized, double-blind, placebo-controlled, flexible dose study in children and adolescents aged 6 to 17 (N=198) with a 5-week primary efficacy end point. Patients had been treated with a psychostimulant (methylphenidate or amphetamine) for four weeks with inadequate response. Patients were randomly assigned to one of two treatment groups: KAPVAY adjunct to a psychostimulant (N=102) or psychostimulant alone (N=96). The KAPVAY dose was initiated at 0.1 mg/day and doses were titrated in increments of 0.1 mg/week up to 0.4 mg/day, as divided doses, over a 3-week period based on tolerability and clinical response. The dose was maintained for a minimum of 2 weeks before being gradually tapered to 0.1 mg/day at the last week of treatment. ADHD symptoms were statistically significantly improved in KAPVAY plus stimulant group compared with the stimulant alone group at the end of 5 weeks as measured by the ADHDRS-IV total score.

16   HOW SUPPLIED/STORAGE AND HANDLING

KAPVAY extended-release tablets are white, non-scored, standard convex with debossing ("651" for 0.1 mg and "652" for 0.2 mg) on one side.

The 0.1 mg are round tablets supplied in bottles containing 60 (NDC 59630-658-60) or 180 tablets (NDC 59630-658-18). The 0.2 mg are oval tablets supplied in bottles containing 60 (NDC 59630-659-60) or 180 tablets (NDC 59630-659-18). Store at 20°-25°C (68°-77°F) [see USP Controlled Room Temperature].

Dispense in a tight, light-resistant container.

17   PATIENT COUNSELING INFORMATION

See FDA-approved Patient Labeling

17.1   General Information

Prescribers or other health professionals should inform patients, their families, and their caregivers about the benefits and risks associated with treatment with KAPVAY and should counsel them in its appropriate use. The prescriber or health professional should instruct patients, their families, and their caregivers to read the Patient Information and should assist them in understanding its contents. Patients should be given the opportunity to discuss the contents of the Patient Information and to obtain answers to any questions they may have. The complete text of the Patient Information is attached to the package insert.

17.2   Abrupt Discontinuation

Patients should be advised not to discontinue KAPVAY abruptly. In order to minimize potential withdrawal effects (see Warnings and Precautions), when discontinuing KAPVAY therapy, patients should be instructed to decrease their total daily dose of KAPVAY in decrements of no more than 0.1 mg every 3 to 7 days.

17.3   Allergic Reactions

In patients who have developed an allergic reaction from clonidine transdermal system, substitution of oral clonidine hydrochloride may also elicit an allergic reaction (including generalized rash, urticaria, or angioedema).

17.4   Dosing

If the total daily dose of KAPVAY does not allow equal doses to be given in the morning and at bedtime (e.g., if the total daily dose is 0.3 mg/day), the higher of the two doses should be taken at bedtime (e.g., in a patient on 0.3 mg/day, a 0.1 mg dose should be taken in the morning and a 0.2 mg dose should be taken at bedtime). KAPVAY must be swallowed whole and never crushed, cut, or chewed.

17.5   Pregnancy

Patients should be instructed to consult a physician if they are nursing, pregnant, or thinking of becoming pregnant while taking KAPVAY.

17.6   Food

Patients may take KAPVAY with or without food.

17.7   Missed Dose

If patients miss a dose of KAPVAY, they should skip the dose and take the next dose as scheduled. Do not take more than the prescribed total daily amount of KAPVAY in any 24-hour period.

17.8   Impairment in Ability to Operate Machinery or Vehicles

No evaluation of the effects of KAPVAY on the ability to drive or operate machinery was performed during the development program. However, given the observed incidence of somnolence with KAPVAY, patients should be instructed to use caution when driving a car or operating hazardous machinery until they know how they will respond to treatment with KAPVAY.

PATIENT INFORMATION

KAPVAY™ (KAP-vay)

(clonidine hydrochloride) Extended-Release Tablets

Read the Patient Information that comes with KAPVAY before you start taking it and each time you get a refill. There may be new information. This Patient Information leaflet does not take the place of talking to your doctor about your medical condition or treatment.

What is KAPVAY?

KAPVAY is a prescription medicine used for the treatment of Attention-Deficit Hyperactivity Disorder (ADHD). Your doctor may prescribe KAPVAY alone or together with certain other ADHD medicines.
• KAPVAY is not a central nervous system (CNS) stimulant.
• KAPVAY should be used as part of a total treatment program for ADHD that may include counseling or other therapies.

Who should not take KAPVAY?

• Do not take KAPVAY if you are allergic to clonidine in KAPVAY. See the end of this leaflet for a complete list of ingredients in KAPVAY.

What should I tell my doctor before taking KAPVAY?

Before you take KAPVAY, tell your doctor if you:
• have kidney problems
• have low or high blood pressure
• have a history of passing out (syncope)
• have heart problems, including history of heart attack
• have had a stroke or have stroke symptoms
• had a skin reaction (such as a rash) after taking clonidine in a transdermal form (skin patch)
• have any other medical conditions
• are pregnant or plan to become pregnant. It is not known if KAPVAY will harm your unborn baby. Talk to your doctor if you are pregnant or plan to become pregnant.
• are breastfeeding or plan to breastfeed. KAPVAY can pass into your breast milk. Talk to your doctor about the best way to feed your baby if you take KAPVAY.

Tell your doctor about all of the medicines that you take, including prescription and non-prescription medicines, vitamins, and herbal supplements.

KAPVAY and certain other medicines may affect each other causing serious side effects. Sometimes the doses of other medicines may need to be changed while taking KAPVAY.

Especially tell your doctor if you take:
• anti-depression medicines
• heart or blood pressure medicine
• other medicines that contain clonidine
• a medicine that makes you sleepy (sedation)

Ask your doctor or pharmacist for a list of these medicines, if you are not sure if your medicine is listed above.

Table 6   Pharmacokinetic Parameters of Clonidine in Healthy Adult Volunteers

Parameter	CATAPRES-Fasted n=15		KAPVAY-Fed n=15		KAPVAY-Fasted n=14	
	Mean	SD	Mean	SD	Mean	SD
C$_{max}$ (pg/mL)	443	59.6	235	34.7	258	33.3
AUC$_{inf}$ (hr*pg/mL)	7313	1812	6505	1728	6729	1650
hT$_{max}$ (hr)	2.07	0.5	6.80	3.61	6.50	1.23
T$_{1/2}$ (hr)	12.57	3.11	12.67	3.76	12.65	3.56

Know the medicines that you take. Keep a list of your medicines with you to show your doctor and pharmacist when you get a new medicine.

How should I take KAPVAY?

- Take KAPVAY exactly as your doctor tells you to take it.
- Your doctor will tell you how many KAPVAY tablets to take and when to take them. Your doctor may change your dose of KAPVAY. Do not change your dose of KAPVAY without talking to your doctor.
- Do not stop taking KAPVAY without talking to your doctor.
- KAPVAY can be taken with or without food
- KAPVAY should be taken 2 times a day (in the morning and at bedtime).
- If you miss a dose of KAPVAY, skip the missed dose. Just take the next dose at your regular time. Do not take two doses at the same time.
- Take KAPVAY tablets whole. Do not chew, crush or break KAPVAY tablets. Tell your doctor if you cannot swallow KAPVAY tablets whole. You may need a different medicine.
- If you take too much KAPVAY, call your Poison Control Center or go to the nearest hospital emergency room right away.

What should I avoid while taking KAPVAY?

- Do not drink alcohol or take other medicines that make you sleepy or dizzy while taking KAPVAY until you talk with your doctor. KAPVAY taken with alcohol or medicines that cause sleepiness or dizziness may make your sleepiness or dizziness worse.
- Do not drive, operate heavy machinery or do other dangerous activities until you know how KAPVAY will affect you.
- Avoid becoming dehydrated or overheated.

What are possible side effects of KAPVAY?

KAPVAY may cause serious side effects, including:
- Low blood pressure and low heart rate. Your doctor should check your heart rate and blood pressure before starting treatment and regularly during treatment with KAPVAY.
- Sleepiness.
- Withdrawal symptoms. Suddenly stopping KAPVAY may cause withdrawal symptoms including: increased blood pressure, headache, increased heart rate, lightheadedness, tightness in your chest and nervousness.

The most common side effects of KAPVAY include:
- sleepiness
- tiredness
- upper respiratory tract infection, symptoms may include:
  - cough
  - runny nose
  - sneezing
- irritability
- sore throat
- trouble sleeping (insomnia)
- nightmares
- change in mood
- constipation
- stuffy nose
- increased body temperature
- dry mouth
- ear pain

Tell your doctor if you have any side effects that bother you or that does not go away.
These are not all of the possible side effects of KAPVAY. For more information, ask your doctor or pharmacist.
Call your doctor for medical advice about side effects. You may report side effects to FDA at 1-800-FDA-1088.

How should I store KAPVAY?

- Store KAPVAY between 68°-77°F (20°-25°C).
- Keep KAPVAY in a tightly closed container and keep KAPVAY out of the light.

Keep KAPVAY and all medicines out of the reach of children.

General information about the safe and effective use of KAPVAY

Medicines are sometimes prescribed for purposes other than those listed in a Patient Information leaflet. Do not use KAPVAY for a condition for which it was not prescribed. Do not give KAPVAY to other people, even if they have the same symptoms that you have. It may harm them.

This Patient Information leaflet summarizes the most important information about KAPVAY. If you would like more information, talk with your doctor. You can also ask your doctor or pharmacist for information about KAPVAY that is written for healthcare professionals.
For more information about KAPVAY, go to www.KAPVAY.com or call 1-800-849-9707 ext. 1454.

What are the ingredients in KAPVAY?

- Active Ingredient: clonidine hydrochloride
- Inactive Ingredients: sodium lauryl sulfate, lactose monohydrate, hypromellose type 2208, partially pregelatinized starch, colloidal silicon dioxide, and magnesium stearate

Issued: 09/2010
Distributed by:
Shionogi Pharma, Inc.
Atlanta, GA 30328

ORAPRED ODT® ℞
[OR-a-pred]
(prednisolone sodium phosphate orally disintegrating tablets)

HIGHLIGHTS OF PRESCRIBING INFORMATION
These highlights do not include all the information needed to use Orapred ODT® safely and effectively. See full prescribing information for Orapred ODT.
Orapred ODT® (prednisolone sodium phosphate orally disintegrating tablets)
Initial U.S. Approval: 1955

INDICATIONS AND USAGE
Orapred ODT is a corticosteroid indicated
- as an anti-inflammatory or immunosuppressive agent for certain allergic, dermatologic, gastrointestinal, hematologic, ophthalmologic, nervous system, renal, respiratory, rheumatologic, specific infectious diseases or conditions and organ transplantation (1)
- for the treatment of certain endocrine conditions (1)
- for palliation of certain neoplastic conditions (1)

DOSAGE AND ADMINISTRATION
Individualize dosing based on disease severity and patient response (2):
- Initial Dose: 10 mg to 60 mg of prednisolone (as 13.4 mg to 80.6 mg of prednisolone sodium phosphate)
- Maintenance Dose: Use lowest dosage that will maintain an adequate clinical response
- Discontinuation: Withdraw gradually if discontinuing long-term or high-dose therapy
- Take with food to avoid gastrointestinal (GI) irritation
DO NOT BREAK OR USE PARTIAL ORAPRED ODT TABLETS. USE AN APPROPRIATE FORMULATION OF PREDNISOLONE IF INDICATED DOSE CANNOT BE OBTAINED USING ORAPRED ODT.

DOSAGE FORMS AND STRENGTHS
Orally Disintegrating Tablets:
- 10 mg Tablets (as 13.4 mg prednisolone sodium phosphate) (3)
- 15 mg Tablets (as 20.2 mg prednisolone sodium phosphate) (3)
- 30 mg Tablets (as 40.3 mg prednisolone sodium phosphate) (3)

CONTRAINDICATIONS
- Hypersensitivity to prednisolone or any components of this product. (4)

WARNINGS AND PRECAUTIONS
- Hypothalamic-pituitary-adrenal (HPA) axis suppression, Cushing's syndrome and hyperglycemia: Monitor patients for these conditions with chronic use taper doses gradually for withdrawal after chronic use. (5.1)
- Infections: Increased susceptibility to new infection and increased risk of exacerbation, dissemination, or reactivation of latent infection. Signs and symptoms of infection may be masked. (5.2)
- Elevated blood pressure, salt and water retention and hypokalemia: Monitor blood pressure and sodium, potassium serum levels. (5.3)
- GI perforation: increased risk in patients with certain GI disorders. Signs and symptoms may be masked. (5.4)
- Behavioral and mood disturbances: May include euphoria, insomnia, mood swings, personality changes, severe depression, and psychosis. Existing conditions may be aggravated. (5.5)
- Decreases in bone density: Monitor bone density in patients receiving long term corticosteroid therapy. (5.6)
- Ophthalmic effects: May include cataracts, infections and glaucoma. Monitor intraocular pressure if corticosteroid therapy is continued for more than 6 weeks. (5.7)
- Live or live attenuated vaccines: Do not administer to patients receiving immunosuppressive doses of corticosteroids. (5.8)

- Negative effects on growth and development: Monitor pediatric patients on long-term corticosteroid therapy. (5.9)
- Use in pregnancy: Fetal harm can occur with first trimester use. Apprise women of potential harm to the fetus. (5.10)

ADVERSE REACTIONS
Common adverse reactions for corticosteroids include fluid retention, alteration in glucose tolerance, elevation in blood pressure, behavioral and mood changes, increased appetite and weight gain. (6)
To report SUSPECTED ADVERSE REACTIONS, contact Shionogi Drug Safety Department at 1-800-849-9707 ext. 1454 or FDA at 1-800-FDA-1088 or www.fda.gov/medwatch.

DRUG INTERACTIONS
- Anticoagulant Agents: May enhance or diminish anticoagulant effects. Monitor coagulation indices. (7)
- Antidiabetic Agents: May increase blood glucose concentrations. Dose adjustments of antidiabetic agents may be required. (7)
- CYP 3A4 inducers and inhibitors: May, respectively, increase or decrease clearance of corticosteroids, necessitating dose adjustment. (7)
- Cyclosporine: Increase in activity of both, cyclosporine and corticosteroid when administered concurrently. Convulsions have been reported with concurrent use. (7)
- NSAIDS including aspirin and salicylates: Increased risk of gastrointestinal side effects. (7)

See 17 for PATIENT COUNSELING INFORMATION
Revised: 08/2010

FULL PRESCRIBING INFORMATION: CONTENTS*
1 INDICATIONS AND USAGE
  1.1 Allergic Conditions
  1.2 Dermatologic Diseases
  1.3 Endocrine Conditions
  1.4 Gastrointestinal Diseases
  1.5 Hematologic Diseases
  1.6 Neoplastic Conditions
  1.7 Nervous System Conditions
  1.8 Ophthalmic Conditions
  1.9 Conditions Related to Organ Transplantation
  1.10 Pulmonary Diseases
  1.11 Renal Conditions
  1.12 Rheumatologic Conditions
  1.13 Specific Infectious Diseases
2 DOSAGE AND ADMINISTRATION
  2.1 Recommended Dosing
  2.2 Recommended Monitoring
  2.3 Corticosteroid Comparison Chart
3 DOSAGE FORMS AND STRENGTHS
4 CONTRAINDICATIONS
5 WARNINGS AND PRECAUTIONS
  5.1 Alterations in Endocrine Function
  5.2 Increased Risks Related to Infections
  5.3 Alterations in Cardiovascular/Renal Function
  5.4 Use in Patients with Gastrointestinal Disorders
  5.5 Behavioral and Mood Disturbances
  5.6 Decrease in Bone Density
  5.7 Ophthalmic Effects
  5.8 Vaccination
  5.9 Effect on Growth and Development
  5.10 Use in Pregnancy
  5.11 Neuromuscular Effects
  5.12 Kaposi's Sarcoma
6 ADVERSE REACTIONS
7 DRUG INTERACTIONS
8 USE IN SPECIFIC POPULATIONS
  8.1 Pregnancy
  8.3 Nursing Mothers
  8.4 Pediatric Use
  8.5 Geriatric Use
10 OVERDOSAGE
11 DESCRIPTION
12 CLINICAL PHARMACOLOGY
  12.1 Mechanism of Action
  12.3 Pharmacokinetics
13 NONCLINICAL TOXICOLOGY
  13.1 Carcinogenesis, Mutagenesis, Impairment of Fertility
16 HOW SUPPLIED/STORAGE AND HANDLING
17 PATIENT COUNSELING INFORMATION
* Sections or subsections omitted from the full prescribing information are not listed

FULL PRESCRIBING INFORMATION

1 INDICATIONS AND USAGE
Orapred ODT (prednisolone sodium phosphate orally disintegrating tablet) is indicated in the treatment of the following diseases or conditions:

1.1 Allergic Conditions

Control of severe or incapacitating allergic conditions intractable to adequate trials of conventional treatment in adult and pediatric populations with:
- Atopic dermatitis
- Drug hypersensitivity reactions
- Seasonal or perennial allergic rhinitis
- Serum sickness

1.2 Dermatologic Diseases
- Bullous dermatitis herpetiformis
- Contact dermatitis
- Exfoliative erythroderma
- Mycosis fungoides
- Pemphigus
- Severe erythema multiforme (Stevens-Johnson syndrome)

1.3 Endocrine Conditions
- Congenital adrenal hyperplasia
- Hypercalcemia of malignancy
- Nonsuppurative thyroiditis
- Primary or secondary adrenocortical insufficiency: hydrocortisone or cortisone is the first choice; synthetic analogs may be used in conjunction with mineralocorticoids where applicable.

1.4 Gastrointestinal Diseases

During acute episodes in:
- Crohn's Disease
- Ulcerative colitis

1.5 Hematologic Diseases
- Acquired (autoimmune) hemolytic anemia
- Diamond-Blackfan anemia
- Idiopathic thrombocytopenic purpura in adults
- Pure red cell aplasia
- Secondary thrombocytopenia in adults

1.6 Neoplastic Conditions

For the treatment of:
- Acute leukemia
- Aggressive lymphomas

1.7 Nervous System Conditions
- Acute exacerbations of multiple sclerosis
- Cerebral edema associated with primary or metastatic brain tumor, craniotomy or head injury

1.8 Ophthalmic Conditions
- Sympathetic ophthalmia
- Uveitis and ocular inflammatory conditions unresponsive to topical corticosteroids

1.9 Conditions Related to Organ Transplantation
- Acute or chronic solid organ rejection

1.10 Pulmonary Diseases
- Acute exacerbations of chronic obstructive pulmonary disease (COPD)
- Allergic bronchopulmonary aspergillosis
- Aspiration pneumonitis
- Asthma
- Fulminating or disseminated pulmonary tuberculosis when used concurrently with appropriate chemotherapy
- Hypersensitivity pneumonitis
- Idiopathic bronchiolitis obliterans with organizing pneumonia
- Idiopathic eosinophilic pneumonias
- Idiopathic pulmonary fibrosis Pneumocystis carinii pneumonia (PCP) associated with hypoxemia occurring in an HIV (+) individual who is also under treatment with appropriate anti-PCP antibiotics
- Symptomatic sarcoidosis

1.11 Renal Conditions

To induce a diuresis or remission of proteinuria in nephrotic syndrome, without uremia, of the idiopathic type or that due to lupus erythematosus

1.12 Rheumatologic Conditions

As adjunctive therapy for short term administration (to tide the patient over an acute episode or exacerbation) in:
- Acute gouty arthritis

During an exacerbation or as maintenance therapy in selected cases of:
- Ankylosing spondylitis
- Dermatomyositis /polymyositis
- Polymyalgia rheumatica/temporal arteritis
- Psoriatic arthritis
- Relapsing polychondritis
- Rheumatoid arthritis, including juvenile rheumatoid arthritis (selected cases may require low dose maintenance therapy)
- Sjogren's syndrome
- Systemic lupus erythematosus
- Vasculitis

1.13 Specific Infectious Diseases
- Trichinosis with neurologic or myocardial involvement
- Tuberculous meningitis with subarachnoid block or impending block, (used concurrently with appropriate antituberculous chemotherapy

2 DOSAGE AND ADMINISTRATION

2.1 Recommended Dosing

Dosage of Orapred ODT should be individualized according to the severity of the disease and the response of the patient. For pediatric patients, the recommended dosage should be governed by the same considerations rather than strict adherence to the ratio indicated by age or body weight.

Do not break or use partial Orapred ODT tablets. Use an appropriate formulation of prednisolone if indicated dose cannot be obtained using Orapred ODT. This may become important in the treatment of conditions that require tapering doses that cannot be adequately accommodated by Orapred ODT, e.g., tapering the dose below 10 mg.

The initial dose of Orapred ODT may vary from 10 to 60 mg (prednisolone base) per day, depending on the specific disease entity being treated. In situations of less severity, lower doses will generally suffice while in selected patients higher initial doses may be required. The initial dosage should be maintained or adjusted until a satisfactory response is noted. If after a reasonable period of time, there is a lack of satisfactory clinical response, Orapred should be discontinued and the patient placed on other appropriate therapy. **IT SHOULD BE EMPHASIZED THAT DOSAGE REQUIREMENTS ARE VARIABLE AND MUST BE INDIVIDUALIZED ON THE BASIS OF THE DISEASE UNDER TREATMENT AND THE RESPONSE OF THE PATIENT.** After a favorable response is noted, the proper maintenance dosage should be determined by decreasing the initial drug dosage in small decrements at appropriate time intervals until the lowest dosage that will maintain an adequate clinical response is reached. It should be kept in mind that constant monitoring is needed in regard to drug dosage. Included in the situations which may make dosage adjustments necessary are changes in clinical status secondary to remissions or exacerbations in the disease process, the patient's individual drug responsiveness, and the effect of patient exposure to stressful situations not directly related to the disease entity under treatment; in this latter situation it may be necessary to increase the dosage of Orapred ODT for a period of time consistent with the patient's condition. If after long term therapy the drug is to be stopped, it is recommended that it be withdrawn gradually rather than abruptly.

Orapred ODT are packaged in a blister. Patients should be instructed not to remove the tablet from the blister until just prior to dosing. The blister pack should then be peeled open, and the orally disintegrating tablet placed on the tongue, where tablets may be swallowed whole as any conventional tablet, or allowed to dissolve in the mouth, with or without the assistance of water. Orally disintegrating tablet dosage forms are friable and are not intended to be cut, split, or broken.

Multiple Sclerosis

In the treatment of acute exacerbations of multiple sclerosis, daily doses of 200 mg of prednisolone for a week followed by 80 mg every other day for one month have been shown to be effective.

Pediatric

In pediatric patients, the initial dose of Orapred may vary depending on the specific disease entity being treated. The range of initial doses is 0.14 to 2 mg/kg/day in three or four divided doses (4 to 60 mg/m²bsa/day).

Nephrotic Syndrome

The standard regimen used to treat nephrotic syndrome in pediatric patients is 60 mg/m²/day given in three divided doses for 4 weeks, followed by 4 weeks of single dose alternate-day therapy at 40 mg/m²/day.

Asthma

The National Heart, Lung, and Blood Institute (NHLBI) recommended dosing for systemic *prednisone, prednisolone or methylprednisolone* in children whose asthma is uncontrolled by inhaled corticosteroids and long-acting bronchodilators is 1-2 mg/kg/ day in single or divided doses.

It is further recommended that short course, or "burst" therapy, be continued until a child achieves a peak expiratory flow rate of 80% of his or her personal best or symptoms resolve. This usually requires 3 to 10 days of treatment, although it can take longer. There is no evidence that tapering the dose after improvement will prevent a relapse.

2.2 Recommended Monitoring

Blood pressure, body weight, routine laboratory studies, including serum potassium and fasting blood glucose, should be obtained at regular intervals during prolonged therapy. Appropriate diagnostic studies should be performed in patients with known or suspected peptic ulcer disease and in patients at risk for reactivation of latent tuberculosis infections.

2.3 Corticosteroid Comparison Chart

For the purpose of comparison, one 10 mg Orapred ODT tablet (13.4 mg prednisolone sodium phosphate) is equivalent to the following milligram dosage of the various glucocorticoids:

Betamethasone 1.75 mg	Paramethasone 4 mg
Cortisone 50 mg	Prednisolone 10 mg
Dexamethasone 1.75 mg	Prednisone 10 mg
Hydrocortisone 40 mg	Triamcinolone 8 mg
Methylprednisolone 8 mg	

These dose relationships apply only to oral or intravenous administration of these compounds. When these substances or their derivatives are injected intramuscularly or into joint spaces, their relative properties may be greatly altered.

3 DOSAGE FORMS AND STRENGTHS

Orally disintegrating tablets:
- 10 mg prednisolone (as 13.4 mg prednisolone sodium phosphate)
- 15 mg prednisolone (as 20.2 mg prednisolone sodium phosphate)
- 30 mg prednisolone (as 40.3 mg prednisolone sodium phosphate)

4 CONTRAINDICATIONS

Orapred ODT is contraindicated in patients who are hypersensitive to corticosteroids such as prednisolone or any components of this product. Rare instances of anaphylactoid reactions have occurred in patients receiving corticosteroid therapy.

5 WARNINGS AND PRECAUTIONS

5.1 Alterations in Endocrine Function

Hypothalamic-pituitary-adrenal (HPA) axis suppression, Cushing's syndrome, and hyperglycemia. Monitor patients for these conditions with chronic use.

Corticosteroids can produce reversible HPA axis suppression with the potential for glucocorticosteroid insufficiency after withdrawal of treatment. Drug induced secondary adrenocortical insufficiency may be minimized by gradual reduction of dosage. This type of relative insufficiency may persist for months after discontinuation of therapy; therefore, in any situation of stress occurring during that period, hormone therapy should be reinstituted.

Since mineralocorticoid secretion may be impaired, salt and/or a mineralocorticoid should be administered concurrently.

Mineralocorticoid supplementation is of particular importance in infancy.

Metabolic clearance of corticosteroids is decreased in hypothyroid patients and increased in hyperthyroid patients. Changes in thyroid status of the patient may necessitate adjustment in dosage.

5.2 Increased Risks Related to Infections

Corticosteroids may increase the risks related to infections with any pathogen, including viral, bacterial, fungal, protozoan, or helminthic infections. The degree to which the dose, route and duration of corticosteroid administration correlates with the specific risks of infection is not well characterized, however, with increasing doses of corticosteroids, the rate of occurrence of infectious complications increases. Corticosteroids may mask some signs of infection and may reduce resistance to new infections.

Corticosteroids may exacerbate infections and increase risk of disseminated infection.

The use of Orapred in active tuberculosis should be restricted to those cases of fulminating or disseminated tuberculosis in which the corticosteroid is used for the management of the disease in conjunction with an appropriate antituberculous regimen.

Chickenpox and measles can have a more serious or even fatal course in non-immune children or adults on corticosteroids. In children or adults who have not had these diseases, particular care should be taken to avoid exposure. If a patient is exposed to chickenpox, prophylaxis with varicella zoster immune globulin (VZIG) may be indicated. If patient is exposed to measles, prophylaxis with pooled intramuscular immunoglobulin (IG) may be indicated. If chickenpox develops, treatment with antiviral agents may be considered. Corticosteroids should be used with great care in patients with known or suspected Strongyloides (threadworm) infestation. In such patients, corticosteroid-induced immunosuppression may lead to Strongyloides hyperinfection and dissemination with widespread larval migration, often accompanied by severe enterocolitis and potentially fatal gram-negative septicemia.

Corticosteroids may exacerbate systemic fungal infections and therefore should not be used in the presence of such infections unless they are needed to control drug reactions. *Corticosteroids may increase risk of reactivation or exacerbation of latent infection.*

If corticosteroids are indicated in patients with latent tuberculosis or tuberculin reactivity, close observation is necessary as reactivation of the disease may occur. During prolonged corticosteroid therapy, these patients should receive chemoprophylaxis.

Corticosteroids may activate latent amebiasis. Therefore, it is recommended that latent or active amebiasis be ruled out before initiating corticosteroid therapy in any patient who has spent time in the tropics or in any patient with unexplained diarrhea.

Corticosteroids should not be used in cerebral malaria.

5.3 Alterations in Cardiovascular/Renal Function

Corticosteroids can cause elevation of blood pressure, salt and water retention, and increased excretion of potassium and calcium. These effects are less likely to occur with the synthetic derivatives except when used in large doses. Dietary salt restriction and potassium supplementation may be necessary. These agents should be used with caution in patients with hypertension, congestive heart failure, or renal insufficiency.

Literature reports suggest an association between use of corticosteroids and left ventricular free wall rupture after a recent myocardial infarction; therefore, therapy with corticosteroids should be used with caution in these patients

5.4 Use in Patients with Gastrointestinal Disorders

There is an increased risk of gastrointestinal (GI) perforation in patients with certain GI disorders. Signs of GI perforation, such as peritoneal irritation, may be masked in patients receiving corticosteroids.

Corticosteroids should be used with caution if there is a probability of impending perforation, abscess or other pyogenic infections; diverticulitis; fresh intestinal anastomoses; and active or latent peptic ulcer.

5.5 Behavioral and Mood Disturbances

Corticosteroid use may be associated with central nervous system effects ranging from euphoria, insomnia, mood swings, personality changes, and severe depression, to frank psychotic manifestations. Also, existing emotional instability or psychotic tendencies may be aggravated by corticosteroids.

5.6 Decrease in Bone Density

Corticosteroids decrease bone formation and increase bone resorption both through their effect on calcium regulation (i.e., decreasing absorption and increasing excretion) and inhibition of osteoblast function. This, together with a decrease in the protein matrix of the bone secondary to an increase in protein catabolism, and reduced sex hormone production, may lead to inhibition of bone growth in children and adolescents and the development of osteoporosis at any age. Special consideration should be given to patients at increased risk of osteoporosis (e.g., postmenopausal women) before initiating corticosteroid therapy and bone density should be monitored in patients on long term corticosteroid therapy.

5.7 Ophthalmic Effects

Prolonged use of corticosteroids may produce posterior subcapsular cataracts, glaucoma with possible damage to the optic nerves, and may enhance the establishment of secondary ocular infections due to fungi or viruses.

The use of oral corticosteroids is not recommended in the treatment of optic neuritis and may lead to an increase in the risk of new episodes.

Intraocular pressure may become elevated in some individuals. If steroid therapy is continued for more than 6 weeks, intraocular pressure should be monitored.

Patients with Ocular Herpes Simplex

Corticosteroids should be used cautiously in patients with ocular herpes simplex because of possible corneal perforation.

Corticosteroids **should not be used in active** ocular herpes simplex.

5.8 Vaccination

Administration of live or live attenuated vaccines is contraindicated in patients receiving immunosuppressive doses of corticosteroids. Killed or inactivated vaccines may be administered; however, the response to such vaccines cannot be predicted. Immunization procedures may be undertaken in patients who are receiving corticosteroids as replacement therapy, e.g., for Addison's disease.

While on corticosteroid therapy, patients should not be vaccinated against smallpox. Other immunization procedures should not be undertaken in patients who are on corticosteroids, especially on high dose, because of possible hazards of neurological complications and a lack of antibody response.

5.9 Effect on Growth and Development

Long-term use of corticosteroids can have negative effects on growth and development in children. Growth and development of pediatric patients on prolonged corticosteroid therapy should be carefully monitored.

5.10 Use in Pregnancy

Prednisolone can cause fetal harm when administered to a pregnant woman. Human and animal studies suggest that use of corticosteroids during the first trimester of pregnancy is associated with an increased risk of orofacial clefts, intrauterine growth restriction and decreased birth weight. If this drug is used during pregnancy, or if the patient be-

comes pregnant while using this drug, the patient should be apprised of the potential hazard to the fetus. [see *Use in Specific Populations (8.1)*].

5.11 Neuromuscular Effects

Although controlled clinical trials have shown corticosteroids to be effective in speeding the resolution of acute exacerbations of multiple sclerosis, they do not show that they affect the ultimate outcome or natural history of the disease. The studies do show that relatively high doses of corticosteroids are necessary to demonstrate a significant effect. [see *Dosage and Administration (3)*].

An acute myopathy has been observed with the use of high doses of corticosteroids, most often occurring in patients with disorders of neuromuscular transmission (e.g., myasthenia gravis), or in patients receiving concomitant therapy with neuromuscular blocking drugs (e.g., pancuronium). This acute myopathy is generalized, may involve ocular and respiratory muscles, and may result in quadriparesis. Elevation of creatinine kinase may occur. Clinical improvement or recovery after stopping corticosteroids may require weeks to years.

5.12 Kaposi's Sarcoma

Kaposi's sarcoma has been reported to occur in patients receiving corticosteroid therapy, most often for chronic conditions. Discontinuation of corticosteroids may result in clinical improvement.

6 ADVERSE REACTIONS

Common adverse reactions for corticosteroids include fluid retention, alteration in glucose tolerance, elevation in blood pressure, behavioral and mood changes, increased appetite and weight gain.

Allergic Reactions: Anaphylactoid reaction, anaphylaxis, angioedema

Cardiovascular: Bradycardia, cardiac arrest, cardiac arrhythmias, cardiac enlargement, circulatory collapse, congestive heart failure, fat embolism, hypertension, hypertrophic cardiomyopathy in premature infants, myocardial rupture following recent myocardial infarction, pulmonary edema, syncope, tachycardia, thromboembolism, thrombophlebitis, vasculitis

Dermatologic: Acne, allergic dermatitis, cutaneous and subcutaneous atrophy, dry scalp, edema, facial erythema, hyper or hypopigmentation, impaired wound healing, increased sweating, petechiae and ecchymoses, rash, sterile abscess, striae, suppressed reactions to skin tests, thin fragile skin, thinning scalp hair, urticaria

Endocrine: Abnormal fat deposits, decreased carbohydrate tolerance, development of Cushingoid state, hirsutism, manifestations of latent diabetes mellitus and increased requirements for insulin or oral hypoglycemic agents in diabetics, menstrual irregularities, moon facies, secondary adrenocortical and pituitary unresponsiveness (particularly in times of stress, as in trauma, surgery or illness), suppression of growth in children

Fluid and Electrolyte Disturbances: Fluid retention, potassium loss, hypertension, hypokalemic alkalosis, sodium retention

Gastrointestinal: Abdominal distention; elevation in serum liver enzyme levels (usually reversible upon discontinuation); hepatomegaly, hiccups, malaise, nausea, pancreatitis; peptic ulcer with possible perforation and hemorrhage; ulcerative esophagitis

General: Increased appetite and weight gain

Metabolic: Negative nitrogen balance due to protein catabolism

Musculoskeletal: Aseptic necrosis of femoral and humeral heads; charcot-like arthropathy, loss of muscle mass; muscle weakness; osteoporosis; pathologic fracture of long bones; steroid myopathy; tendon rupture; vertebral compression fractures

Neurological: Arachnoiditis, convulsions; depression, emotional instability, euphoria, headache; increased intracranial pressure with papilledema (pseudotumor cerebri) usually following discontinuation of treatment; insomnia, meningitis, mood swings, neuritis, neuropathy, paraparesis/paraplegia, paresthesia, personality changes, sensory disturbances, vertigo

Ophthalmic: Exophthalmos; glaucoma; increased intraocular pressure; posterior subcapsular cataracts

Reproductive: Alteration in motility and number of spermatozoa

7 DRUG INTERACTIONS

• **Aminoglutethimide:** Aminoglutethimide may lead to loss of corticosteroid-induced adrenal suppression.

• **Amphotericin B:** There have been cases reported in which concomitant use of Amphotericin B and hydrocortisone was followed by cardiac enlargement and congestive heart failure (see also Potassium depleting agents).

• **Anticholinesterase agents:** Concomitant use of anticholinesterase agents and corticosteroids may produce severe weakness in patients with myasthenia gravis. If possible, anticholinesterase agents should be withdrawn at least 24 hours before initiating corticosteroid therapy.

• **Anticoagulant agents:** Co-administration of corticosteroids and warfarin usually results in inhibition of response to warfarin, although there have been some conflicting reports. Therefore, coagulation indices should be monitored frequently to maintain the desired anticoagulant effect.

• **Antidiabetic Agents:** Because corticosteroids may increase blood glucose concentrations, dosage adjustments of antidiabetic agents may be required.

• **Antitubercular drugs:** Serum concentrations of isoniazid may be decreased.

• **CYP 3A4 inducers (e.g. barbiturates, phenytoin, carbamazepine, and rifampin):** Drugs such as barbiturates, phenytoin, ephedrine, and rifampin, which induce hepatic microsomal drug metabolizing enzyme activity may enhance metabolism of prednisolone and require that the dosage of Orapred be increased.

• **CYP 3A4 inhibitors (e.g., ketoconazole, macrolide antibiotics):** Ketoconazole has been reported to decrease the metabolism of certain corticosteroids by up to 60% leading to an increased risk of corticosteroid side effects.

• **Cholestyramine:** Cholestyramine may increase the clearance of corticosteroids.

• **Cyclosporine:** Increased activity of both cyclosporine and corticosteroids may occur when the two are used concurrently. Convulsions have been reported with this concurrent use.

• **Digitalis:** Patients on digitalis glycosides may be at increased risk of arrhythmias due to hypokalemia.

• **Estrogens, including oral contraceptives:** Estrogens may decrease the hepatic metabolism of certain corticosteroids thereby increasing their effect.

• **NSAIDS, including aspirin and salicylates:** Concomitant use of aspirin or other non-steroidal anti-inflammatory agents and corticosteroids increases the risk of gastrointestinal side effects. Aspirin should be used cautiously in conjunction with corticosteroids in hypoprothrombinemia. The clearance of salicylates may be increased with concurrent use of corticosteroids.

• **Potassium-depleting agents (e.g., diuretics, Amphotericin B):** When corticosteroids are administered concomitantly with potassium-depleting agents, patients should be observed closely for development of hypokalemia.

• **Skin Tests:** Corticosteroids may suppress reactions to skin tests.

• **Toxoids and live or inactivated Vaccines:** Due to inhibition of antibody response, patients on prolonged corticosteroid therapy may exhibit a diminished response to toxoids and live or inactivated vaccines. Corticosteroids may also potentiate the replication of some organisms contained in live attenuated vaccines.

8 USE IN SPECIFIC POPULATIONS

8.1 Pregnancy

Pregnancy Category D [see *Warnings and Precautions (5.10)*]

Orapred has not been formally evaluated in clinical or nonclinical studies for effects on pregnancy and fetal development. Multiple cohort and case controlled studies in humans suggest that maternal corticosteroid use during the first trimester increases the incidence of cleft lip with or without cleft palate from about 1/1000 infants to 3-5/1000 infants. Two prospective case control studies showed decreased birth weight in infants exposed to maternal corticosteroids in utero. In humans, the risk of decreased birth weight appears to be dose related and may be minimized by administering lower corticosteroid doses. It is likely that underlying maternal conditions contribute to intrauterine growth restriction and decreased birth weight, but it is unclear to what extent these maternal conditions contribute to the increased risk of orofacial clefts.

Thus, prednisolone can cause fetal harm when used during pregnancy. Orapred should be used during pregnancy only if the potential benefit justifies the potential risk to the fetus. If this drug is used during pregnancy, or if the patient becomes pregnant while using this drug, the patient should be apprised of the potential hazard to the fetus. Infants born to mothers who have received corticosteroids during pregnancy should be carefully observed for signs of hypoadrenalism.

Published literature indicates prednisolone has been shown to be teratogenic in rats, rabbits, hamsters, and mice with increased incidence of cleft palate in offspring, supportive of the clinical data. In teratogenicity studies, cleft palate along with an elevation of fetal lethality (or increase in resorptions) and reductions in fetal body weight was seen in rats at maternal doses of 30 mg/kg (equivalent to 290 mg in a 60 kg individual based on mg/m^2 body surface comparison) and higher. Cleft palate was observed in mice at a maternal dose of 20 mg/kg (equivalent to 100 mg in a 60 kg individual based on mg/m^2 comparison). Additionally, constriction of the ductus arteriosus was observed in fetuses of pregnant rats exposed to prednisolone.

8.3 Nursing Mothers

Prednisolone is secreted in human milk. Reports suggest that prednisolone concentrations in human milk are 5 to 25% of maternal serum levels, and that total infant daily doses are small, about 0.14% of the maternal daily dose. Therefore, caution should be exercised when prednisolone is administered to a nursing woman. High doses of corticosteroids for long periods could potentially produce problems in infant growth and development and interfere with endogenous corticosteroid production. The risk of infant exposure to prednisolone through breast milk should be weighed against the known benefits of breastfeeding for both the mother and baby. If prednisolone must be prescribed to a breastfeeding mother, the lowest dose should be prescribed to achieve the desired clinical effect.

8.4 Pediatric Use

The efficacy and safety of prednisolone in the pediatric population are based on the well-established course of effect of corticosteroids, which is similar in pediatric and adult populations. Published studies provide evidence of efficacy and safety in pediatric patients for the treatment of nephrotic syndrome (>2 years of age), and aggressive lymphomas and leukemias (>1 month of age). However, some of these conclusions and other indications for pediatric use of corticosteroid, e.g., severe asthma and wheezing, are based on adequate and well-controlled trials conducted in adults, on the premises that the course of the diseases and their pathophysiology are considered to be substantially similar in both populations.

The adverse effects of prednisolone in pediatric patients are similar to those in adults [*see Adverse Reactions (6.2)*]. Like adults, pediatric patients should be carefully observed with frequent measurements of blood pressure, weight, height, intraocular pressure, and clinical evaluation for the presence of infection, psychosocial disturbances, thromboembolism, peptic ulcers, cataracts, and osteoporosis. Children, who are treated with corticosteroids by any route, including systemically administered corticosteroids, may experience a decrease in their growth velocity. This negative impact of corticosteroids on growth has been observed at low systemic doses and in the absence of laboratory evidence of HPA axis suppression (i.e., cosyntropin stimulation and basal cortisol plasma levels).

Growth velocity may therefore be a more sensitive indicator of systemic corticosteroid exposure in children than some commonly used tests of HPA axis function. The linear growth of children treated with corticosteroids by any route should be monitored, and the potential growth effects of prolonged treatment should be weighed against clinical benefits obtained and the availability of other treatment alternatives. In order to minimize the potential growth effects of corticosteroids, children should be *titrated* to the lowest effective dose.

8.5 Geriatric Use

No overall differences in safety or effectiveness were observed between elderly subjects and younger subjects, and other reported clinical experience with prednisolone has not identified differences in responses between the elderly and younger patients. However, the incidence of corticosteroid-induced side effects may be increased in geriatric patients and appear to be dose-related. Osteoporosis is the most frequently encountered complication, which occurs at a higher incidence rate in corticosteroid-treated geriatric patients as compared to younger populations and in age-matched controls. Losses of bone mineral density appear to be greatest early on in the course of treatment and may recover over time after steroid withdrawal or use of lower doses (i.e., ≤5 mg/day). Prednisolone doses of 7.5 mg/day or higher, have been associated with an increased relative risk of both vertebral and nonvertebral fractures, even in the presence of higher bone density compared to patients with involutional osteoporosis.

Routine screening of geriatric patients, including regular assessments of bone mineral density and institution of fracture prevention strategies, along with regular review of Orapred indication should be undertaken to minimize complications and keep the Orapred dose at the lowest acceptable level. Co-administration of bisphosphonates has been shown to retard the rate of bone loss in corticosteroid-treated males and postmenopausal females, and these agents are recommended in the prevention and treatment of corticosteroid-induced osteoporosis.

It has been reported that equivalent weight-based doses yield higher total and unbound prednisolone plasma concentrations and reduced renal and non-renal clearance in elderly patients compared to younger populations. However, it is not clear whether dosing reductions would be necessary in elderly patients, since these pharmacokinetic alterations may be offset by age-related differences in responsiveness of target organs and/or less pronounced suppression of adrenal release of cortisol. Dose selection for an elderly patient should be cautious, usually starting at the low end of the dosing range, reflecting the greater frequency of decreased hepatic, renal, or cardiac function, and of concomitant disease or other drug therapy.

This drug is known to be substantially excreted by the kidney, and the risk of toxic reactions to this drug may be greater in patients with impaired renal function. Because elderly patients are more likely to have decreased renal function, care should be taken in dose selection, and it may be useful to monitor renal function.

10 OVERDOSAGE

The effects of accidental ingestion of large quantities of prednisolone over a very short period of time have not been reported, but prolonged use of the drug can produce mental symptoms, moon face, abnormal fat deposits, fluid retention, excessive appetite, weight gain, hypertrichosis, acne, striae, ecchymosis, increased sweating, pigmentation, dry scaly skin, thinning scalp hair, increased blood pressure, tachycardia, thrombophlebitis, decreased resistance to infection, negative nitrogen balance with delayed bone and wound healing, headache, weakness, menstrual disorders, accentuated menopausal symptoms, neuropathy, fractures, osteoporosis, peptic ulcer, decreased glucose tolerance, hypokalemia, and adrenal insufficiency. Hepatomegaly and abdominal distention have been observed in children.

Treatment of acute overdosage is by immediate gastric lavage or emesis followed by supportive and symptomatic therapy. For chronic overdosage in the face of severe disease requiring continuous steroid therapy, the dosage of prednisolone may be reduced only temporarily, or alternate day treatment may be introduced.

11 DESCRIPTION

Orapred ODT (prednisolone sodium phosphate disintegrating tablets) is a sodium salt of the phosphoester of the glucocorticoid prednisolone. Glucocorticoids are adrenocortical steroids, both naturally occurring and synthetic, which are readily absorbed from the gastrointestinal tract. Prednisolone sodium phosphate occurs as white or slightly yellow, friable granules or powder. It is freely soluble in water; soluble in methanol; slightly soluble in alcohol and in chloroform; and very slightly soluble in acetone and in dioxane.

The chemical name of prednisolone sodium phosphate is pregna-1, 4-diene-3, 20-dione, 11, 17-dihydroxy-21-(phosphonooxy)-, disodium salt, (11ß)-. The empirical formula is $C_{21}H_{27}Na_2O_8P$; the molecular weight is 484.39. Its chemical structure is:

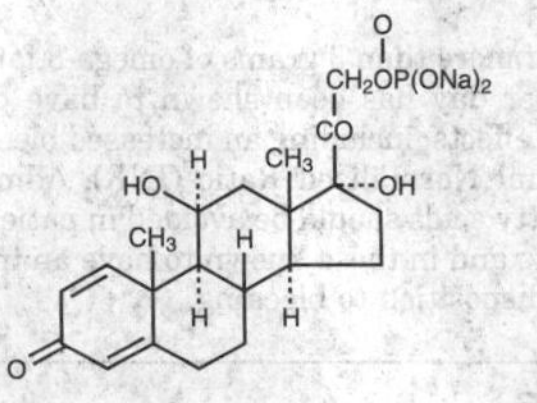

Each orally disintegrating tablet also contains the following inactive ingredients: citric acid, colloidal silicon dioxide, crospovidone, grape flavor, hypromellose, magnesium stearate, mannitol, methacrylate copolymer, microcrystalline cellulose, sodium bicarbonate, sucralose, and sucrose.

12 CLINICAL PHARMACOLOGY

12.1 Mechanism of Action

Prednisolone is a synthetic adrenocortical steroid drug with predominantly glucocorticoid properties. Some of these properties reproduce the physiological actions of endogenous glucocorticosteroids, but others do not necessarily reflect any of the adrenal hormones' normal functions; they are seen only after administration of large therapeutic doses of the drug. The pharmacological effects of prednisolone which are due to its glucocorticoid properties include: promotion of gluconeogenesis; increased deposition of glycogen in the liver; inhibition of the utilization of glucose; anti-insulin activity; increased catabolism of protein; increased lipolysis; stimulation of fat synthesis and storage; increased glomerular filtration rate and resulting increase in urinary excretion of urate (creatinine excretion remains unchanged); and increased calcium excretion. Depressed production of eosinophils and lymphocytes occurs, but erythropoiesis and production of polymorphonuclear leukocytes are stimulated. Inflammatory processes (edema, fibrin deposition, capillary dilatation, migration of leukocytes and phagocytosis) and the later stages of wound healing (capillary proliferation, deposition of collagen, cicatrization) are inhibited. Prednisolone can stimulate secretion of various components of gastric juice. Suppression of the production of corticotropin may lead to suppression of endogenous corticosteroids. Prednisolone has slight mineralocorticoid activity, whereby entry of sodium into cells and loss of intracellular potassium is stimulated. This is particularly evident in the kidney, where rapid ion exchange leads to sodium retention and hypertension.

12.3 Pharmacokinetics

Absorption:

Oral administration of single doses of 30 mg prednisolone base equivalent of Orapred ODT, and Pediapred Solution to 21 adult volunteers yielded comparable pharmacokinetic data:

Table 1. Comparison of Mean Pharmacokinetic Parameters (%CV) in Healthy Volunteers Following a Single Dose of 30 mg Orapred ODT and Pediapred Solution,

Dose* (30 mg prednisolone base equivalent)	$AUC_{0-\infty}$ (ng·hr/mL) (± S.D.)	C_{max} (ng·hr/mL)† (± S.D.)
Pediapred Solution	2426.1 (360.0)	461.33 (77.94)
Orapred ODT	2408.1 (361.5)	420.91 (78.28)

*Administered under fasting conditions.
†Mean values of 21 normal volunteers

Distribution:

Prednisolone is 70-90% protein-bound in the plasma and the volume of distribution is reported as 0.22-0.7 L/kg.

Metabolism:

Prednisolone is reported to be metabolized mainly in the liver and excreted in the urine as sulfate and glucuronide conjugates.

Excretion:

Prednisolone is eliminated from the plasma with a mean (± SD) half-life of 2.6 (± 0.27) hours.

Special Populations

The systemic availability, metabolism and elimination of prednisolone after administration of single weight-based doses (0.8 mg/kg) of intravenous (IV) prednisolone and oral prednisone were reported in a small study of 19 younger (23 to 34 years) and 12 geriatric (65 to 89 years) subjects. Results showed that the systemic availability of total and unbound prednisolone, as well as interconversion between prednisolone and prednisone were independent of age. The mean unbound fraction of prednisolone was higher, and the steady-state volume of distribution (V_{ss}) of unbound prednisolone was reduced in elderly patients. Plasma prednisolone concentrations were higher in elderly subjects, and the higher AUCs of total and unbound prednisolone were most likely reflective of an impaired metabolic clearance, evidenced by reduced fractional urinary clearance of 6b-hydroxyprednisolone. Despite these findings of higher total and unbound prednisolone concentrations, elderly subjects had higher AUCs of cortisol, suggesting that the elderly population is less sensitive to suppression of endogenous cortisol or their capacity for hepatic inactivation of cortisol is diminished.

13 NONCLINICAL TOXICOLOGY

13.1 Carcinogenesis, Mutagenesis, Impairment of Fertility

Orapred was not formally evaluated in carcinogenicity studies. Review of the published literature identified the potential for malignancy at doses within the therapeutic range. In a 2-year study, male Sprague-Dawley rats administered prednisolone in drinking water at an estimated continuous daily prednisolone consumption of 368 mcg/kg/day (equivalent to 3.5 mg/day in a 60 kg individual based on an mg/m^2 body surface area comparison) developed increased incidences of hepatic adenomas. However infrequent administration of prednisolone did not result in malignancy. In an 18-month study, intermittent (1, 2, 4.5 or 9 times per month) oral gavage of 3 mg/kg prednisolone did not induce tumors in female Sprague-Dawley rats (equivalent to 29 mg in a 60 kg individual based on a mg/m^2 body surface area comparison).

Orapred was not formally evaluated for genotoxicity. However, in published studies prednisolone was not mutagenic with or without metabolic activation in the Ames bacterial reverse mutation assay using *Salmonella typhimurium* and *Escherichia coli*, or in a mammalian cell gene mutation assay using mouse lymphoma L5178Y cells, according to current evaluation standards. In a published chromosomal aberration study in Chinese Hamster Lung (CHL) cells, a slight increase was seen in the incidence of structural chromosomal aberrations with metabolic activation at the highest concentration tested, however, the effect appears to be equivocal.

Orapred was not formally evaluated in fertility studies. However, alterations in motility and numbers of spermatozoa, and menstrual irregularities have been described with clinical use [see *Adverse Reactions (6)*].

16 HOW SUPPLIED/STORAGE AND HANDLING

Orapred ODT (prednisolone sodium phosphate orally disintegrating tablets) 13.4 mg prednisolone sodium

phosphate (equivalent to 10 mg prednisolone base) are white, flat faced, bevelled tablet, debossed with ORA on one side and 10 on the other. Supplied as:
• NDC 59630-700-48: 48 tablets per carton. Each carton has 8 cards containing 6 tablets.

Oraprod ODT (prednisolone sodium phosphate orally disintegrating tablets) 20.2 mg prednisolone sodium phosphate (equivalent to 15 mg prednisolone base) are white, flat faced, bevelled tablet, debossed with ORA on one side and 15 on the other. Supplied as:
• NDC 59630-701-48: 48 tablets per carton. Each carton has 8 cards containing 6 tablets.

Oraprod ODT: (prednisolone sodium phosphate orally disintegrating tablets) 40.3 mg prednisolone sodium phosphate (equivalent to 30 mg prednisolone base) are white, flat faced, beveled tablets, debossed with ORA on one side and 30 on the other. Supplied as:
• NDC 59630-702-48: 48 tablets per carton. Each carton has 8 cards containing 6 tablets.

Store at 20 to 25°C (68 to 77°F); excursions permitted to 15 to 30°C (59 to 86°F). [See USP controlled Room Temperature]. Protect from moisture.
Do not break or use partial Oraprod ODT tablets. Keep out of the reach of children.

17   PATIENT COUNSELING INFORMATION

Advise patients not to discontinue the use of Oraprod abruptly or without medical supervision, to advise any healthcare provider that they are taking it, and to seek medical advice at once should they develop fever or other signs of infection. Inform patients to take Oraprod exactly as prescribed, follow the instructions on the prescription label, and not stop taking Oraprod without first checking with their health-care providers, as there may be a need for gradual dose reduction.

Patients should discuss with their physician if they have had recent or ongoing infections or if they have recently received a vaccine.

Warn patients who are on immunosuppressant doses of corticosteroids to avoid exposure to chickenpox or measles. Advise patients that if they are exposed, to seek medical advice without delay.

There are a number of medicines that can interact with Oraprod. Patients should inform their healthcare provider of all the medicines they are taking, including over-the-counter and prescription medicines (such as phenytoin, diuretics, digitalis or digoxin, rifampin, amphotericin B, cyclosporine, insulin or diabetes medicines, ketoconazole, estrogens including birth control pills and hormone replacement therapy, blood thinners such as warfarin, aspirin or other NSAIDS, barbiturates, dietary supplements, and herbal products. If patients are taking any of these drugs, alternate therapy, dosage adjustment, and/or special test may be needed during the treatment.

For missed doses, inform patients to take the missed dose as soon as they remember. If it is almost time for the next dose, the missed dose should be skipped and the medicine taken at the next regularly scheduled time. Advise patients not to take an extra dose to make up for the missed dose.

Inform patients to take Oraprod with food to avoid GI irritation.

Advise patients of common adverse reactions that could occur with Oraprod use to include fluid retention, alteration in glucose tolerance, elevation in blood pressure, behavioral and mood changes, increased appetite and weight gain.

Oraprod ODT tablets are packaged in a blister. Patients should be instructed not to remove the tablet from the blister until just prior to dosing. The blister pack should then be peeled open, and the orally disintegrating tablet placed on the tongue, where the tablets may be swallowed whole as any conventional tablet, or allowed to dissolve in the mouth, with or without the assistance of water. Orally disintegrating tablet dosage forms are friable and are not intended to be cut, split, or broken.

ORP-PI-04
Revised 07/2010
Manufactured for:
Shionogi Pharma, Inc.
Atlanta, GA 30328
For Inquiries call 1-800-849-9707 ext. 1454
U.S. Patent No. 6,740,341

PRENATE® ESSENTIAL™   ℞
[PRE-Nate]
Rx prenatal vitamin & DHA

DESCRIPTION
PRENATE ESSENTIAL™ is a prescription prenatal/postnatal multivitamin/mineral/ essential fatty acid softgel. Each softgel is blue- green in color, opaque, and imprinted with "Prenate" on one side.
[See table above]

Supplement Facts
Serving Size 1 Softgel

Amount Per Serving:		% DV For Adults	% DV for Pregnant and Lactating Women
Vitamin C	85 mg	142%	142%
Vitamin D$_3$	200 IU	50%	50%
Vitamin E	10 IU	33%	33%
Vitamin B$_6$	25 mg	1250%	1000%
Folate	1 mg	250%	125%
(L-methylfolate as Metafolin 600 mcg)			
(folic acid, USP 400mcg)			
Vitamin B$_{12}$	12 mcg	200%	150%
Biotin	250 mcg	83%	83%
Calcium	140 mg	14%	11%
(calcium carbonate)			
Iron (ferrous fumarate)	28 mg	156%	156%
Iodine (potassium iodide)	150 mcg	100%	100%
Magnesium	45 mg	11%	10%
(magnesium oxide)			
Docosahexaenoic Acid (DHA)	300 mg	*	*
Eicosapentaenoic Acid (EPA)	40mg	*	*
(from 340 mg omega-3 fatty acids from fish oil)			

Percent Daily Values are based on a 2,000 calorie diet
*Daily Value (DV) not established

Other Ingredients: fish oil, gelatin, hydrogenated vegetable oil, glycerin, sorbitol, beeswax, soy lecithin, titanium dioxide, vanillin, FD&C blue No. 1, propylene glycol, hypromellose.

INDICATIONS
PRENATE ESSENTIAL is a multivitamin/mineral/essential fatty acid nutritional supplement indicated for use in improving the nutritional status of women throughout pregnancy and in the postnatal period for both lactating and non-lactating mothers. PRENATE ESSENTIAL can also be beneficial in improving the nutritional status of women prior to conception.

CONTRAINDICATIONS
PRENATE ESSENTIAL is contraindicated in patients with a known hypersensitivity to any of the ingredients.

WARNING
Ingestion of more than 3 grams of omega-3 fatty acids (such as DHA) per day has been shown to have potential antithrombotic effects, including an increased bleeding time and International Normalized Ratio (INR). Administration of omega-3 fatty acids should be avoided in patients taking anticoagulants and in those known to have an inherited or acquired predisposition to bleeding.

> **WARNING**
> Accidental overdose of iron-containing products is a leading cause of fatal poisoning in children under 6. Keep this product out of reach of children. In case of accidental overdose, call a doctor or poison control center immediately.

PRECAUTIONS
Folic acid alone is improper therapy in the treatment of pernicious anemia and other megaloblastic anemias where vitamin B$_{12}$ is deficient. Folic acid in doses above 1 mg daily may obscure pernicious anemia in that hematologic remission can occur while neurological manifestations progress.

ADVERSE REACTIONS
Allergic sensitization has been reported following both oral and parenteral administration of folic acid.

DOSAGE AND ADMINISTRATION
Before, during, and/or after pregnancy, one softgel daily or as directed by a physician.

HOW SUPPLIED
Unit-dose packs of 30 softgels
• NDC # 59630-419-30
KEEP THIS AND ALL DRUGS OUT OF THE REACH OF CHILDREN.
Store at 20°-25°C (68°-77°F). Excursions permitted to 15°-30°C (59°-86°F).
[See USP Controlled Room Temperature]
For inquiries call 1-800-849-9707 extension 1454.
PNE-PI-1
Rev. 02/10
U.S. Patents #5,997,915; #6,254,904; #6,011,040; #6,451,360; #6,673,381; #6,808,725; #6,441,168
Prenate Essential® is a registered trademark of Shionogi Pharma, Inc. Metafolin® is a registered trademark of Merck KGaA, Darmstadt Germany. ©2010 Shionogi Pharma, Inc. Atlanta, GA

All rights reserved.
Manufactured for:
SHIONOGI PHARMA, INC.
Atlanta, Georgia USA 30328 Manufactured by:
Catalent Pharma Solutions, Swindon, UK.
Made in the United Kingdom
Prenate® Essential™
Rx prenatal vitamin & DHA
With
META FOLIN®

ULESFIA LOTION   ℞
[Yoo-Les-fee-ah]
(benzyl alcohol)
Lotion

HIGHLIGHTS OF PRESCRIBING INFORMATION
These highlights do not include all the information needed to use Ulesfia® Lotion safely and effectively. See full prescribing information for Ulesfia Lotion.
Ulesfia (benzyl alcohol) Lotion
For topical use only
Initial U.S. Approval: 2009

──────INDICATIONS AND USAGE──────
Ulesfia Lotion is a pediculocide indicated for the topical treatment of head lice infestation in patients 6 months of age and older. (1.1)
Ulesfia Lotion does not have ovicidal activity. (1.2)

──────DOSAGE AND ADMINISTRATION──────
• Apply Ulesfia Lotion to dry hair, using enough to completely saturate the scalp and hair. (2)
• Rinse off with water after 10 minutes. (2)
• Repeat treatment in 7 days. (2)

Table 1: Ulesfia Lotion Usage Guideline

Hair Length		Amount of Ulesfia Lotion per Application
Short	0-2 inches	4-6 oz (½-¾ bottle)
	2-4 inches	6-8 oz (¾-1 bottle)
Medium	4-8 inches	8-12 oz (1-1½ bottles)
	8-16 inches	12-24 oz (1½-3 bottles)
Long	16-22 inches	24-32 oz (3-4 bottles)
	Over 22 inches	32-48 oz (4-6 bottles)

──────DOSAGE FORMS AND STRENGTHS──────
Ulesfia Lotion, 5% in 8 oz. bottles (3)

──────CONTRAINDICATIONS──────
None. (4)

──────WARNINGS AND PRECAUTIONS──────
• Neonatal toxicity: Risk of gasping syndrome if benzyl alcohol is used in neonates. (5.1)
• Eye irritation: Avoid eye exposure. Flush immediately with water if Ulesfia Lotion comes into contact with eyes. (5.2)
• Contact dermatitis: May occur with Ulesfia Lotion. (5.3)
• Use in children: Ulesfia Lotion should only be used on children under the direct supervision of an adult. Keep out of reach of children. (5.4)

IMPORTANT NOTICE: Updated drug information is sent bi-monthly via the PDR® Update Insert. For *monthly* email updates, register at PDR.net.

ADVERSE REACTIONS

Most common adverse reactions (> 1% and more common than with placebo): ocular irritation, application site irritation, and application site anesthesia and hypoesthesia. (6)

To report SUSPECTED ADVERSE REACTIONS, contact Shionogi Pharma, Inc. Drug Safety at 1-800-849-9707 ext. 1454 or FDA at 1-800-FDA-1088 or www.fda.gov/medwatch.

DRUG INTERACTIONS

Drug interaction studies were not conducted. (7)

USE IN SPECIFIC POPULATIONS

Pediatric Use: Safety in pediatric patients under six months of age has not been established. (8.4)

See 17 for PATIENT COUNSELING INFORMATION and FDA-approved patient labeling

Revised: 05/2010

FULL PRESCRIBING INFORMATION

1 INDICATIONS AND USAGE

1.1 Indication

Ulesfia Lotion is indicated for the topical treatment of head lice infestation in patients 6 months of age and older.

1.2 Limitation of Use

Ulesfia Lotion does not have ovicidal activity.

1.3 Adjunctive Measures

Ulesfia Lotion should be used in the context of an overall lice management program:

- Wash (in hot water) or dry-clean all recently worn clothing, hats, used bedding, and towels.
- Wash personal care items such as combs, brushes and hair clips in hot water.
- A fine-tooth comb or special nit comb may be used to remove dead lice and nits.

2 DOSAGE AND ADMINISTRATION

Ulesfia Lotion is not for oral, ophthalmic, or intravaginal use.

Using the guideline in Table 1, apply sufficient Ulesfia Lotion to dry hair to completely saturate the scalp and hair; leave on for 10 minutes, then thoroughly rinse off with water. Repeat treatment after 7 days. Avoid contact with eyes.

Table 1: Ulesfia Lotion Usage Guideline

Hair Length		Amount of Ulesfia Lotion per Application
Short	0-2 inches	4-6 oz (½-¾ bottle)
	2-4 inches	6-8 oz (¾-1 bottle)
Medium	4-8 inches	8-12 oz (1-1½ bottles)
	8-16 inches	12-24 oz (1½-3 bottles)
Long	16-22 inches	24-32 oz (3-4 bottles)
	Over 22 inches	32-48 oz (4-6 bottles)

3 DOSAGE FORM AND STRENGTH

Ulesfia Lotion contains 5% benzyl alcohol and is supplied in 8 ounce polypropylene bottles.

4 CONTRAINDICATIONS

None.

5 WARNINGS AND PRECAUTIONS

5.1 Neonatal Toxicity

Intravenous administration of products containing benzyl alcohol has been associated with neonatal gasping syndrome consisting of severe metabolic acidosis, gasping respirations, progressive hypotension, seizures, central nervous system depression, intraventricular hemorrhage, and death in preterm, low birth weight infants. Neonates (i.e. patients less than 1 month of age or preterm infants with a corrected age of less than 44 weeks) could be at risk for gasping syndrome if treated with Ulesfia Lotion [see Use in Specific Populations (8.4)].

5.2 Eye Irritation

Avoid eye exposure. Ulesfia Lotion may cause eye irritation. If Ulesfia Lotion comes in contact with the eyes, flush them immediately with water. If irritation persists, consult a physician.

5.3 Contact Dermatitis

Ulesfia Lotion may cause allergic or irritant dermatitis.

5.4 Use in Children

Ulesfia Lotion should only be used on children (6 months of age and older) under the direct supervision of an adult. Keep out of reach of children.

6 ADVERSE REACTIONS

6.1 Clinical Studies Experience

Because clinical studies are conducted under widely varying conditions, adverse reaction rates observed in the clinical studies of a drug cannot be directly compared to rates in the clinical studies of another drug and may not reflect the rates observed in practice. The rates of adverse reactions below were derived from two randomized, multi-center, vehicle-controlled clinical trials and one open-label study in subjects with head lice infestation.

Skin, scalp, and ocular irritation were monitored in the clinical trials. All subjects were queried about the presence of skin and scalp symptoms; the results are presented in Table 2.

Table 2: Monitored Adverse Reactions - Application Site Symptoms

Event	Ulesfia Lotion	Vehicle
Application site Irritation	2% (11/478)	1% (2/336)
Application site anesthesia & hypoesthesia	2% (10/478)	0% (0/336)
Pain	1% (5/478)	0% (1/336)

The subset of subjects who did not have pruritus, erythema, edema or pyoderma of skin and scalp, or ocular irritation prior to treatment were assessed for these signs and symptoms after treatment; the results are presented in Table 3.

Table 3: Monitored Adverse Reactions - Pruritus, Erythema, Pyoderma and Ocular Irritation with Onset After Treatment

Signs/Symptoms	Ulesfia Lotion	Vehicle
Pruritus	12% (14/116)	4% (3/67)
Erythema	10% (32/309)	9% (19/217)
Pyoderma	7% (22/308)	4% (10/230)
Ocular irritation	6% (26/428)	1% (3/313)

Other less common reactions (less than 1% but more than 0.1%) were, in decreasing order of incidence: application site dryness, application site excoriation, paraesthesia, application site dermatitis, excoriation, thermal burn, dandruff, erythema, rash, and skin exfoliation.

7 DRUG INTERACTIONS

Drug interaction studies were not conducted with Ulesfia Lotion.

8 USE IN SPECIFIC POPULATIONS

8.1 Pregnancy

Pregnancy Category B

There are no adequate and well-controlled studies with topical benzyl alcohol in pregnant women. Reproduction studies conducted in rats and rabbits were negative. Because animal reproduction studies are not always predictive of human response, this drug should be used during pregnancy only if clearly needed.

No comparisons of animal exposure with human exposure are provided in this labeling due to the low systemic exposure noted in the clinical pharmacokinetic study [see Clinical Pharmacology (12.3)] which did not allow for the determination of human AUC values that could be used for this calculation.

Pregnant rats were dosed with benzyl alcohol via subcutaneous injection at 100, 250, and 500 mg/kg/day. No teratogenic effects were noted at any dose. Maternal toxicity and decreased fetal weight occurred at 500 mg/kg/day. When pregnant rabbits received subcutaneous injections of benzyl alcohol at 100, 250, and 400 mg/kg/day, there were no teratogenic effects in offspring at any dose. In rabbits, maternal toxicity occurred at the two higher doses and was associated with decreased fetal weight at the highest dose.

8.3 Nursing Mothers

It is not known whether benzyl alcohol is excreted into human milk. Because some systemic absorption of topical benzyl alcohol may occur and because many drugs are excreted in human milk, caution should be exercised when Ulesfia Lotion is administered to a nursing woman.

8.4 Pediatric Use

The safety and effectiveness of Ulesfia Lotion was evaluated in two multicenter, randomized, double-blind, vehicle-controlled studies which were conducted in 628 subjects 6 months of age and older with active head lice infestation [see Clinical Studies (14)].

Rates of adverse events in younger children (6 months to 12 years) were similar to those of older children and adults.

Safety in pediatric patients below the age of 6 months has not been established. Ulesfia Lotion is not recommended in pediatric patients under six months of age because of the potential for increased systemic absorption due to a high ratio of skin surface area to body mass and the potential for an immature skin barrier.

Neonates could be at risk for gasping syndrome if treated with Ulesfia Lotion [see Warnings and Precautions (5.1)]. Intravenous administration of products containing benzyl alcohol has been associated with neonatal gasping syndrome. The gasping syndrome (characterized by central nervous depression, metabolic acidosis, gasping respirations, and high levels of benzyl alcohol and its metabolites found in the blood and urine) has been associated with benzyl alcohol dosages > 99 mg/kg/day in preterm neonates. Additional symptoms may include gradual neurological deterioration, seizures, intracranial hemorrhage, hemotologic abnormalities, skin breakdown, hepatic and renal failure, hypotension, bradycardia, and cardiovascular collapse. Although expected systemic exposure of benzyl alcohol from proper use of Ulesfia Lotion is substantially lower than those reported in association with the gasping syndrome, the minimum amount of benzyl alcohol at which toxicity may occur is not known.

8.5 Geriatric Use

The safety of Ulesfia Lotion in patients over 60 years of age has not been established.

10 OVERDOSAGE

If oral ingestion occurs, seek medical advice immediately.

11 DESCRIPTION

Ulesfia Lotion is supplied as a white topical lotion containing benzyl alcohol, 5%. Inactive ingredients in this formulation are water, mineral oil, sorbitan monooleate, polysorbate 80, carbomer 934P and trolamine.

The active ingredient, benzyl alcohol, is a clear, colorless liquid with a mild aromatic odor. Benzyl alcohol has a molecular mass of 108.14 g/mol. The molecular formula is C_7H_8O.

The chemical structure of benzyl alcohol is

Benzyl Alcohol

12 CLINICAL PHARMACOLOGY

12.1 Mechanism of Action

In vitro studies of the effect of Ulesfia Lotion on native, captured lice suggest that benzyl alcohol inhibits lice from closing their respiratory spiracles, allowing the vehicle to obstruct the spiracles and causing the lice to asphyxiate.

12.3 Pharmacokinetics

The absorption of benzyl alcohol from Ulesfia Lotion was evaluated in 19 subjects with head lice infestation. Subjects were divided into two age groups: 6 months to 3 years and 4 to 11 years. Ulesfia Lotion was applied for an exaggerated exposure period (3 times the normal exposure period). Benzyl alcohol was quantified in a single plasma sample in 4 out of 19 subjects (21%): three subjects in the 6 months to 3 years age group at 0.5 hour post-treatment (ranging from 1.97 to 2.99 mcg/mL) and one subject in the 4 to 11 year age group (1.63 mcg/mL) at 1 hour post-treatment out of a total of 102 samples analyzed.

13 NONCLINICAL TOXICOLOGY

13.1 Carcinogenesis, Mutagenesis, Impairment of Fertility

Long-term studies in animals to evaluate carcinogenic potential of Ulesfia Lotion have not been conducted. No evidence of carcinogenic activity was noted for benzyl alcohol in 2 year oral carcinogenicity studies in rats (doses up to 400 mg/kg benzyl alcohol) or mice (doses up to 200 mg/kg benzyl alcohol) conducted by the National Toxicology Program.

Benzyl alcohol has produced mixed results in genetic testing. Benzyl alcohol was negative in the Ames test with and without metabolic activation, sex-linked recessive lethal assay, and a replicative DNA synthesis assay (conducted in male rats). Negative results were obtained in the mouse lymphoma assay with metabolic activation, but a positive response was noted in the mouse lymphoma assay without metabolic activation at a concentration producing a high level of cellular toxicity. Benzyl alcohol was positive in the Chinese hamster ovary chromosomal aberration assay with metabolic activation.

No fertility studies have been conducted with benzyl alcohol.

14 CLINICAL STUDIES

Two multicenter, randomized, double-blind, vehicle-controlled studies were conducted in 628 subjects 6 months of age and older with active head lice infestation. For the evaluation of efficacy, the youngest subject from each household was enrolled in the Primary Treatment Cohort with Ulesfia Lotion or vehicle. Other infested household members were enrolled in a Secondary Treatment Cohort and received the same treatment as the youngest subjects. The Secondary Treatment Cohort was not included in the efficacy analysis, but was evaluated for all safety parameters. In Study One, 125 Primary Treatment Cohort Subjects were randomized to Ulesfia Lotion (N=63) and vehicle (N=62). Study Two enrolled 125 Primary Treatment Cohort Subjects: 64 randomized to Ulesfia Lotion and 61 to vehicle. Treatment was applied two times separated by one week. Efficacy was assessed as the proportion of subjects who were free of live lice 14 days after the final treatment. Subjects with live lice present at any time after first treatment were considered to be treatment failures. Table 4 contains the proportion of subjects who were free of live lice in each of the two trials.

Table 4: Proportion of Subjects Free of Live Lice 14 Days After Last Treatment

	Ulesfia LOTION	Vehicle
Study 1	(N=63) 48 (76.2%)	(N=62) 3 (4.8%)
Study 2	(N=64) 48 (75.0%)	(N=61) 16 (26.2%)

16 HOW SUPPLIED/STORAGE AND HANDLING

Ulesfia Lotion 5% is supplied as 8 fl oz (227 g) polypropylene bottles (NDC 59630-780-08).
Store at 20°-25° C (68°-77° F); excursions permitted to 15°-30° C (59°-86° F) [See USP controlled room temperature]. Do not freeze. Keep out of reach of children.

17 PATIENT COUNSELING INFORMATION

See 17.3 for FDA-approved patient labeling.

17.1 Instructions to Patients

This medication is to be used as directed by the physician. Use only on scalp and scalp hair. Avoid contact with eyes. As with any topical medication, patients should wash hands after application.

Instruct patients on proper use of Ulesfia Lotion, including the amount to apply, how long to leave it on the hair, and the importance of a second treatment 1 week (7 days) after the initial application.

17.2 Adverse Reactions

Inform patients that Ulesfia Lotion may cause eye irritation, skin irritation, and contact sensitization.

Instruct patients to inform a physician if the area of the application shows signs of irritation and any signs of adverse reactions.

17.3 FDA-Approved Patient Labeling

Patient Information
Ulesfia (Yoo-Les-fee-ah)
(benzyl alcohol 5%)
Lotion

Read the Patient Information that comes with Ulesfia Lotion before you start using it and each time you get a refill. There may be new information. This leaflet does not take the place of talking to your healthcare provider about your medical condition or treatment.

> **Note: For use on scalp hair and scalp only**

What is Ulesfia Lotion?
Ulesfia Lotion is a prescription medicine used to get rid of lice in scalp hair of children and adults.
It is not known if Ulesfia Lotion is safe for children under 6 months of age or in people over age 60.
Once Ulesfia Lotion is washed off, a fine-tooth comb may be used to remove treated lice and nits from the hair and scalp. All personal items exposed to the hair or lice should be washed in hot water or dry-cleaned. See "How do I stop the spread of lice?" at the end of this leaflet.

What should I tell my healthcare provider before I use Ulesfia Lotion?
Tell your healthcare provider if your baby was born early so your healthcare provider can decide if your infant is old enough for Ulesfia Lotion.

Tell your healthcare provider about all of your medical conditions, including if you:
• have any skin conditions or sensitivities,
• are pregnant or planning to become pregnant. It is not known if Ulesfia Lotion can harm your unborn baby,
• are breastfeeding. It is not known if Ulesfia Lotion passes into your breast milk or if it can harm your baby. You should choose to breastfeed or use Ulesfia Lotion, but not both. Talk to your healthcare provider about other ways to feed your baby while using Ulesfia Lotion.

How should I use Ulesfia Lotion?
• Use Ulesfia Lotion exactly as prescribed. Your healthcare provider will prescribe the treatment that is right for you. Do not change your treatment unless you talk to your healthcare provider.
• Use Ulesfia Lotion in two Applications that are one week apart. Ulesfia Lotion gets rid of lice but does not get rid of lice eggs so a second treatment is needed one week (7 days) after the first treatment.
• Ulesfia Lotion coats the lice on your scalp and scalp hair. It is important to use enough Ulesfia Lotion to coat completely every single louse and to leave it on your scalp for the full 10 minutes. See the detailed Patient Instructions for Use at the end of this leaflet.
• Because you need to completely cover all of the lice with Ulesfia Lotion, you may need help in applying Ulesfia Lotion to your scalp and hair. Make sure that you and anyone who helps you apply Ulesfia Lotion reads and understands this leaflet and the Patient Instructions for Use.
• Children need adult help in applying Ulesfia Lotion.
• Do not get into eyes. If Ulesfia Lotion gets in the eye, flush with water right away.
• Do not swallow Ulesfia Lotion. If swallowed, call your healthcare provider right away.
• Wash your hands after you apply Ulesfia Lotion.

What are the possible side effects of Ulesfia Lotion?
People using Ulesfia Lotion may have skin or eye:
• itching,
• redness,
• irritation. If skin or eye irritation happens, rinse with water right away, then call your healthcare provider or go to the emergency department.
These are not all the side effects of Ulesfia Lotion. For more information, ask your healthcare provider.
Call your doctor for medical advice about side effects. You may report side effects to FDA at 1-800-FDA-1088.

How should I store Ulesfia Lotion?
• Store Ulesfia Lotion in a dry place at room temperature, (59 °to 86° F or 15°to 30° C).
• Do not freeze Ulesfia Lotion.

Keep Ulesfia Lotion and all medicines out of the reach of children.

What are the ingredients in Ulesfia Lotion?
Active ingredient: benzyl alcohol, 5%
Inactive ingredients: purified water, mineral oil, sorbitan monooleate, polysorbate 80, carbomer 934P and trolamine

General Information about Ulesfia Lotion
Medicines are sometimes prescribed for conditions other than those described in the patient information leaflets. Do not use Ulesfia Lotion for any condition for which it was not prescribed by your healthcare provider. Do not give Ulesfia Lotion to other people, even if they have the same symptoms as you. It may harm them.
This leaflet summarizes the most important information about Ulesfia Lotion. If you would like more information, talk to your healthcare provider. You can also ask your healthcare provider for information about Ulesfia Lotion that is written for healthcare professionals.

Patient Instructions for Use
Apply the full amount of Ulesfia Lotion prescribed by your healthcare provider for each of your 2 treatments one week apart. Ulesfia Lotion gets rid of lice but does not get rid of lice eggs so a second treatment is needed one week (7 days) after the first treatment. For different hair lengths, use the following as a guide for the amount of Ulesfia Lotion you may need to cover the hair and scalp completely.

Hair Length	Amount of Ulesfia Lotion to apply each time
Short- up to 2 inches	up to ¾ the bottle
Short- 2-4 inches	up to 1 bottle
Medium- 4-8 inches	up to 1½ bottles
Medium- 8-16 inches	up to 3 bottles
Long- 16-22 inches	up to 4 bottles
Long- 22 inches or more	up to 6 bottles

Step 1

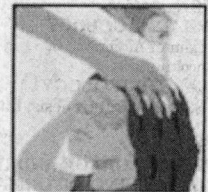

• Cover your face and eyes with a towel and keep your eyes closed tightly.
• Apply Ulesfia Lotion directly to dry hair.
• Ulesfia Lotion must cover your entire scalp and all scalp hair. Have an adult help you apply Ulesfia Lotion.

Step 2

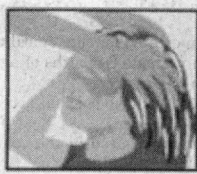

• Massage Ulesfia Lotion into your hair and scalp.
• When your head is completely covered with enough Ulesfia Lotion, *dripping* will happen. Protect your eyes and skin from these drips with your towel.

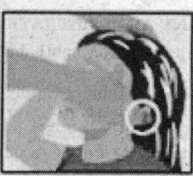

• Be sure to apply Ulesfia Lotion to the area behind your ears

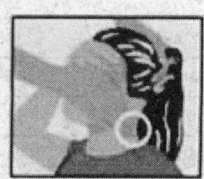

• Be sure to apply Ulesfia Lotion to the back of your neck. If not enough Ulesfia Lotion is used, some lice may escape treatment. It is important to use the full amount of Ulesfia Lotion prescribed by your doctor.

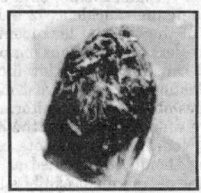

Correct application of Ulesfia Lotion
Step 3

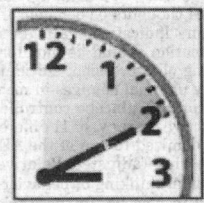

• Allow Ulesfia Lotion to stay on your hair for 10 minutes. Use a timer or clock.
• Start timing after you have completely covered your hair and scalp with Ulesfia Lotion.
Step 4

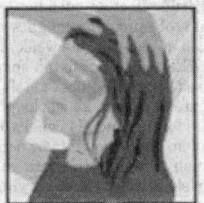

• After 10 minutes, completely rinse Ulesfia Lotion from your hair and scalp with water.
• You or anyone who helps you apply Ulesfia Lotion should wash your hands after application.
• You can shampoo your hair right after the treatment.
• A lice comb may be used to remove the dead lice after both treatments.
Step 5
One week (7 days) after your first treatment, repeat the steps above to help get rid of lice that hatched from eggs.
How do I stop the spread of lice?
To help prevent the spread of lice from one person to another, here are some steps you can take.

• Avoid head-to-head contact at school, on the playground, in physical education classes, during sports activities, and while playing with other children.
• Do not share combs, brushes, hats, scarves, bandannas, ribbons, barrettes, hair bands, towels, helmets, or other hair-related personal items with anyone else, whether they have lice or not.
• Avoid sleepovers and slumber parties during lice outbreaks. Lice can live in bedding, pillows, and carpets that have recently been used by someone with lice.
• After finishing treatment with lice medicine, check everyone in your family for lice after one week. Be sure to talk to your healthcare provider about treatments for those who have lice.
• Machine-wash any bedding and clothing used by anyone having lice or thought to have been exposed to lice. Machine wash at high temperatures (150°F) and tumble in a hot dryer for 20 minutes.

This Patient Leaflet has been approved by the U.S. Food and Drug Administration.
DISTRIBUTED BY:
Shionogi Pharma, Inc.
Atlanta, GA 30328
MANUFACTURED BY:
Contract Pharmaceuticals Limited
Mississauga, ON L5N 6L6
Canada
BNZ-PI-10 Rev. 05/10

Shire US Inc.
725 CHESTERBROOK BOULEVARD
WAYNE, PA 19087

Direct Inquiries to:
Customer Service
(800) 828-2088
For Medical Information Contact:
(800) 828-2088

CARBATROL®
[căr-bŏ'trŏl]
(carbamazepine) Extended-Release Capsules
100 mg • 200 mg • 300 mg
Prescribing information

℞

> **WARNING**
> **SERIOUS DERMATOLOGIC REACTIONS AND HLA-B*1502 ALLELE**
> SERIOUS AND SOMETIMES FATAL DERMATOLOGIC REACTIONS, INCLUDING TOXIC EPIDERMAL NECROLYSIS (TEN) AND STEVENS-JOHNSON SYNDROME (SJS), HAVE BEEN REPORTED DURING TREATMENT WITH CARBAMAZEPINE. THESE REACTIONS ARE ESTIMATED TO OCCUR IN 1 TO 6 PER 10,000 NEW USERS IN COUNTRIES WITH MAINLY CAUCASIAN POPULATIONS, BUT THE RISK IN SOME ASIAN COUNTRIES IS ESTIMATED TO BE ABOUT 10 TIMES HIGHER. STUDIES IN PATIENTS OF CHINESE ANCESTRY HAVE FOUND A STRONG ASSOCIATION BETWEEN THE RISK OF DEVELOPING SJS/TEN AND THE PRESENCE OF HLA-B*1502, AN INHERITED ALLELIC VARIANT OF THE HLA-B GENE. HLA-B*1502 IS FOUND ALMOST EXCLUSIVELY IN PATIENTS WITH ANCESTRY ACROSS BROAD AREAS OF ASIA. PATIENTS WITH ANCESTRY IN GENETICALLY AT-RISK POPULATIONS SHOULD BE SCREENED FOR THE PRESENCE OF HLA-B*1502 PRIOR TO INITIATING TREATMENT WITH CARBATROL. PATIENTS TESTING POSITIVE FOR THE ALLELE SHOULD NOT BE TREATED WITH CARBATROL UNLESS THE BENEFIT CLEARLY OUTWEIGHS THE RISK (SEE WARNINGS AND PRECAUTIONS/LABORATORY TESTS).
> **APLASTIC ANEMIA AND AGRANULOCYTOSIS**
> APLASTIC ANEMIA AND AGRANULOCYTOSIS HAVE BEEN REPORTED IN ASSOCIATION WITH THE USE OF CARBAMAZEPINE. DATA FROM A POPULATION-BASED CASE-CONTROL STUDY DEMONSTRATE THAT THE RISK OF DEVELOPING THESE REACTIONS IS 5-8 TIMES GREATER THAN IN THE GENERAL POPULATION. HOWEVER, THE OVERALL RISK OF THESE REACTIONS IN THE UNTREATED GENERAL POPULATION IS LOW, APPROXIMATELY SIX PATIENTS PER ONE MILLION POPULATION PER YEAR FOR AGRANULOCYTOSIS AND TWO PATIENTS PER ONE MILLION POPULATION PER YEAR FOR APLASTIC ANEMIA.
> ALTHOUGH REPORTS OF TRANSIENT OR PERSISTENT DECREASED PLATELET OR WHITE BLOOD CELL COUNTS ARE NOT UNCOMMON IN ASSOCIATION WITH THE USE OF CARBAMAZEPINE, DATA ARE NOT AVAILABLE TO ESTIMATE ACCURATELY THEIR INCIDENCE OR OUTCOME. HOWEVER, THE VAST MAJORITY OF THE CASES OF LEUKOPENIA HAVE NOT PROGRESSED TO THE MORE SERIOUS CONDITIONS OF APLASTIC ANEMIA OR AGRANULOCYTOSIS.
> BECAUSE OF THE VERY LOW INCIDENCE OF AGRANULOCYTOSIS AND APLASTIC ANEMIA, THE VAST MAJORITY OF MINOR HEMATOLOGIC CHANGES OBSERVED IN MONITORING OF PATIENTS ON CARBAMAZEPINE ARE UNLIKELY TO SIGNAL THE OCCURRENCE OF EITHER ABNORMALITY. NONETHELESS, COMPLETE PRETREATMENT HEMATOLOGICAL TESTING SHOULD BE OBTAINED AS A BASELINE. IF A PATIENT IN THE COURSE OF TREATMENT EXHIBITS LOW OR DECREASED WHITE BLOOD CELL OR PLATELET COUNTS, THE PATIENT SHOULD BE MONITORED CLOSELY. DISCONTINUATION OF THE DRUG SHOULD BE CONSIDERED IF ANY EVIDENCE OF SIGNIFICANT BONE MARROW DEPRESSION DEVELOPS.

Before prescribing Carbatrol, the physician should be thoroughly familiar with the details of this prescribing information, particularly regarding use with other drugs, especially those which accentuate toxicity potential.

DESCRIPTION
CARBATROL®* is an anticonvulsant and specific analgesic for trigeminal neuralgia, available for oral administration as 100 mg, 200 mg and 300 mg extended-release capsules of

---

Carbamazepine, USP. Carbamazepine is a white to off-white powder, practically insoluble in water and soluble in alcohol and in acetone. Its molecular weight is 236.27. Its chemical name is 5H-dibenz[b,f]azepine-5-carboxamide, and its structural formula is:

CARBAMAZEPINE

Carbatrol is a multi-component capsule formulation consisting of three different types of beads: immediate-release beads, extended-release beads, and enteric-release beads. The three bead types are combined in a specific ratio to provide twice daily dosing of Carbatrol.
Inactive ingredients: citric acid, colloidal silicon dioxide, lactose monohydrate, microcrystalline cellulose, polyethylene glycol, povidone, sodium lauryl sulfate, talc, triethyl citrate and other ingredients.
The 100 mg capsule shells contain gelatin-NF, FD&C Blue #2, Yellow Iron Oxide, and titanium dioxide and are imprinted with white ink; the 200 mg capsule shells contain gelatin-NF, FD&C Red #3, FD&C Yellow #6, Yellow Iron Oxide, FD&C Blue #2, and titanium dioxide, and are imprinted with white ink; and the 300 mg capsule shells contain gelatin-NF, FD&C Blue #2, FD&C Yellow #6, Red Iron Oxide, Yellow Iron Oxide, and titanium dioxide, and are imprinted with white ink.

CLINICAL PHARMACOLOGY
In controlled clinical trials, carbamazepine has been shown to be effective in the treatment of psychomotor and grand mal seizures, as well as trigeminal neuralgia.
Mechanism of Action
Carbamazepine has demonstrated anticonvulsant properties in rats and mice with electrically and chemically induced seizures. It appears to act by reducing polysynaptic responses and blocking the post-tetanic potentiation. Carbamazepine greatly reduces or abolishes pain induced by stimulation of the infraorbital nerve in cats and rats. It depresses thalamic potential and bulbar and polysynaptic reflexes, including the linguomandibular reflex in cats. Carbamazepine is chemically unrelated to other anticonvulsants or other drugs used to control the pain of trigeminal neuralgia. The mechanism of action remains unknown.
The principal metabolite of carbamazepine, carbamazepine-10,11-epoxide, has anticonvulsant activity as demonstrated in several *in vivo* animal models of seizures. Though clinical activity for the epoxide has been postulated, the significance of its activity with respect to the safety and efficacy of carbamazepine has not been established.
Pharmacokinetics
Carbamazepine (CBZ): Taken every 12 hours, carbamazepine extended-release capsules provide steady state plasma levels comparable to immediate-release carbamazepine tablets given every 6 hours, when administered at the same total mg daily dose.
Following a single 200 mg oral extended-release dose of carbamazepine, peak plasma concentration was 1.9 ± 0.3 µg/mL and the time to reach the peak was 19 ± 7 hours. Following chronic administration (800 mg every 12 hours), the peak levels were 11.0 ± 2.5 µg/mL and the time to reach the peak was 5.9 ± 1.8 hours. The pharmacokinetics of extended-release carbamazepine is linear over the single dose range of 200-800 mg.
Carbamazepine is 76% bound to plasma proteins. Carbamazepine is primarily metabolized in the liver. Cytochrome P450 3A4 was identified as the major isoform responsible for the formation of carbamazepine-10,11-epoxide. Since carbamazepine induces its own metabolism, the half-life is also variable. Following a single extended-release dose of carbamazepine, the average half-life range from 35-40 hours and 12-17 hours on repeated dosing. The apparent oral clearance following a single dose was 25 ± 5 mL/min and following multiple dosing was 80 ± 30 mL/min.
After oral administration of ^{14}C-carbamazepine, 72% of the administered radioactivity was found in the urine and 28% in the feces. This urinary radioactivity was composed largely of hydroxylated and conjugated metabolites, with only 3% of unchanged carbamazepine.
Carbamazepine-10,11-epoxide (CBZ-E): Carbamazepine-10,11-epoxide is considered to be an active metabolite of carbamazepine. Following a single 200 mg oral extended-release dose of carbamazepine, the peak plasma concentration of carbamazepine-10,11-epoxide was 0.11 ± 0.012 µg/mL and the time to reach the peak was 36 ± 6 hours. Following chronic administration of an extended-release dose of carbamazepine (800 mg every 12 hours), the peak levels of carbamazepine-10,11-epoxide were 2.2 ± 0.9 µg/mL and the time to reach the peak was 14 ± 8 hours. The plasma half-life of carbamazepine-10,11-epoxide

following administration of carbamazepine is 34 ± 9 hours. Following a single oral dose of extended-release carbamazepine (200-800 mg) the AUC and C_{max} of carbamazepine-10,11-epoxide were less than 10% of carbamazepine. Following multiple dosing of extended-release carbamazepine (800-1600 mg daily for 14 days), the AUC and C_{max} of carbamazepine-10,11-epoxide were dose related, ranging from 15.7 µg.hr/mL and 1.5 µg/mL at 800 mg/day to 32.6 µg.hr/mL and 3.2 µg/mL at 1600 mg/day, respectively, and were less than 30% of carbamazepine. Carbamazepine-10,11-epoxide is 50% bound to plasma proteins.

Food Effect: A high fat meal diet increased the rate of absorption of a single 400 mg dose (mean T_{max} was reduced from 24 hours, in the fasting state, to 14 hours and C_{max} increased from 3.2 to 4.3 µg/mL) but not the extent (AUC) of absorption. The elimination half-life remains unchanged between fed and fasting state. The multiple dose study conducted in the fed state showed that the steady-state C_{max} values were within the therapeutic concentration range. The pharmacokinetic profile of extended-release carbamazepine was similar when given by sprinkling the beads over applesauce compared to the intact capsule administered in the fasted state.

Special Populations

Hepatic Dysfunction: The effect of hepatic impairment on the pharmacokinetics of carbamazepine is not known. However, given that carbamazepine is primarily metabolized in the liver, it is prudent to proceed with caution in patients with hepatic dysfunction.

Renal Dysfunction: The effect of renal impairment on the pharmacokinetics of carbamazepine is not known.

Gender: No difference in the mean AUC and C_{max} of carbamazepine and carbamazepine-10,11-epoxide was found between males and females.

Age: Carbamazepine is more rapidly metabolized to carbamazepine-10,11-epoxide in young children than adults. In children below the age of 15, there is an inverse relationship between CBZ-E/CBZ ratio and increasing age.

Race: No information is available on the effect of race on the pharmacokinetics of carbamazepine.

INDICATIONS AND USAGE

Epilepsy

Carbatrol is indicated for use as an anticonvulsant drug. Evidence supporting efficacy of carbamazepine as an anticonvulsant was derived from active drug-controlled studies that enrolled patients with the following seizure types:

1. Partial seizures with complex symptomatology (psychomotor, temporal lobe). Patients with these seizures appear to show greater improvements than those with other types.
2. Generalized tonic-clonic seizures (grand mal).
3. Mixed seizure patterns which include the above, or other partial or generalized seizures. Absence seizures (petit mal) do not appear to be controlled by carbamazepine (see PRECAUTIONS, General).

Trigeminal Neuralgia

Carbatrol is indicated in the treatment of the pain associated with true trigeminal neuralgia. Beneficial results have also been reported in glossopharyngeal neuralgia. This drug is not a simple analgesic and should not be used for the relief of trivial aches or pains.

CONTRAINDICATIONS

Carbamazepine should not be used in patients with a history of previous bone marrow depression, hypersensitivity to the drug, or known sensitivity to any of the tricyclic compounds, such as amitriptyline, desipramine, imipramine, protriptyline and nortriptyline. Likewise, on theoretical grounds its use with monoamine oxidase inhibitors is not recommended. Before administration of carbamazepine, MAO inhibitors should be discontinued for a minimum of 14 days, or longer if the clinical situation permits.

WARNINGS

Serious Dermatologic Reactions

Serious and sometimes fatal dermatologic reactions, including toxic epidermal necrolysis (TEN) and Stevens-Johnson syndrome (SJS), have been reported with carbamazepine

treatment. The risk of these events is estimated to be about 1 to 6 per 10,000 new users in countries with mainly Caucasian populations. However, the risk in some Asian countries is estimated to be about 10 times higher. Carbatrol should be discontinued at the first sign of a rash, unless the rash is clearly not drug-related. If signs or symptoms suggest SJS/TEN, use of this drug should not be resumed and alternative therapy should be considered.

SJS/TEN and HLA-B*1502 Allele

Retrospective case-control studies have found that in patients of Chinese ancestry there is a strong association between the risk of developing SJS/TEN with carbamazepine treatment and the presence of an inherited variant of the HLA-B gene, HLA-B*1502. The occurrence of higher rates of these reactions in countries with higher frequencies of this allele suggests that the risk may be increased in allele-positive individuals of any ethnicity. Across Asian populations, notable variation exists in the prevalence of HLA-B*1502. Greater than 15% of the population is reported positive in Hong Kong, Thailand, Malaysia, and parts of the Philippines, compared to about 10% in Taiwan and 4% in North China. South Asians, including Indians, appear to have intermediate prevalence of HLA-B*1502, averaging 2 to 4%, but higher in some groups. HLA-B*1502 is present in <1% of the population in Japan and Korea. HLA-B*1502 is largely absent in individuals not of Asian origin (e.g., Caucasians, African-Americans, Hispanics, and Native Americans).

Prior to initiating Carbatrol therapy, testing for HLA-B*1502 should be performed in patients with ancestry in populations in which HLA-B*1502 may be present. In deciding which patients to screen, the rates provided above for the prevalence of HLA-B*1502 may offer a rough guide, keeping in mind the limitations of these figures due to wide variability in rates even within ethnic groups, the difficulty in ascertaining ethnic ancestry, and the likelihood of mixed ancestry. Carbatrol should not be used in patients positive for HLA-B*1502 unless the benefits clearly outweigh the risks. Tested patients who are found to be negative for the allele are thought to have a low risk of SJS/TEN (see **WARNINGS** and **PRECAUTIONS/Laboratory Tests**).

Over 90% of carbamazepine treated patients who will experience SJS/TEN have this reaction within the first few months of treatment. This information may be taken into consideration in determining the need for screening of genetically at-risk patients currently on Carbatrol.

The HLA-B*1502 allele has not been found to predict risk of less severe adverse cutaneous reactions from carbamazepine, such as anticonvulsant hypersensitivity syndrome or non-serious rash (maculopapular eruption [MPE]).

Limited evidence suggests that HLA-B*1502 may be a risk factor for the development of SJS/TEN in patients of Chinese ancestry taking other anti-epileptic drugs associated with SJS/TEN. Consideration should be given to avoiding use of other drugs associated with SJS/TEN in HLA-B*1502 positive patients, when alternative therapies are otherwise equally acceptable. Application of HLA-B*1502 genotyping as a screening tool has important limitations and must never substitute for appropriate clinical vigilance and patient management. Many HLA-B*1502-positive Asian patients treated with carbamazepine will not develop SJS/TEN, and these reactions can still occur infrequently in HLA-B*1502-negative patients of any ethnicity. The role of other possible factors in the development of, and morbidity from, SJS/TEN, such as AED dose, compliance, concomitant medications, co-morbidities, and the level of dermatologic monitoring have not been studied.

Patients should be made aware that Carbatrol contains carbamazepine and should not be used in combination with any other medications containing carbamazepine.

Aplastic anemia and agranulocytosis

Aplastic anemia and agranulocytosis have been reported in association with the use of carbamazepine. Data from a population-based case-control study demonstrate that the risk of developing these reactions is 5-8 times greater than in the general population. However, the overall risk of these reactions in the untreated general population is low, ap-

proximately six patients per one million population per year for agranulocytosis and two patients per one million population per year for aplastic anemia.

Although reports of transient or persistent decreased platelet or white blood cell counts are not uncommon in association with the use of carbamazepine, data are not available to estimate accurately their incidence or outcome. However, the vast majority of the cases of leukopenia have not progressed to the more serious conditions of aplastic anemia or agranulocytosis. Because of the very low incidence of agranulocytosis and aplastic anemia, the vast majority of minor hematologic changes observed in monitoring of patients on carbamazepine are unlikely to signal the occurrence of either abnormality. Nonetheless, complete pretreatment hematological testing should be obtained as a baseline. If a patient in the course of treatment exhibits low or decreased white blood cell or platelet counts, the patient should be monitored closely. Discontinuation of the drug should be considered if any evidence of significant bone marrow depression develops.

Suicidal behavior and Ideation

Antiepileptic drugs (AEDs), including Carbatrol, increase the risk of suicidal thoughts or behavior in patients taking these drugs for any indication. Patients treated with any AED for any indication should be monitored for the emergence or worsening of depression, suicidal thoughts or behavior, and/or any unusual changes in mood or behavior. Pooled analyses of 199 placebo-controlled clinical trials (mono- and adjunctive therapy) of 11 different AEDs showed that patients randomized to one of the AEDs had approximately twice the risk (adjusted Relative Risk 1.8, 95% CI:1.2, 2.7) of suicidal thinking or behavior compared to patients randomized to placebo. In these trials, which had a median treatment duration of 12 weeks, the estimated incidence rate of suicidal behavior or ideation among 27,863 AED-treated patients was 0.43%, compared to 0.24% among 16,029 placebo-treated patients, representing an increase of approximately one case of suicidal thinking or behavior for every 530 patients treated. There were four suicides in drug-treated patients in the trials and none in placebo-treated patients, but the number is too small to allow any conclusion about drug effect on suicide.

The increased risk of suicidal thoughts or behavior with AEDs was observed as early as one week after starting drug treatment with AEDs and persisted for the duration of treatment assessed. Because most trials included in the analysis did not extend beyond 24 weeks, the risk of suicidal thoughts or behavior beyond 24 weeks could not be assessed. The risk of suicidal thoughts or behavior was generally consistent among drugs in the data analyzed. The finding of increased risk with AEDs of varying mechanisms of action and across a range of indications suggests that the risk applies to all AEDs used for any indication. The risk did not vary substantially by age (5-100 years) in the clinical trials analyzed.

Table 1 shows absolute and relative risk by indication for all evaluated AEDs.

[See table 1 below]

The relative risk for suicidal thoughts or behavior was higher in clinical trials for epilepsy than in clinical trials for psychiatric or other conditions, but the absolute risk differences were similar for the epilepsy and psychiatric indications.

Anyone considering prescribing Carbatrol or any other AED must balance the risk of suicidal thoughts or behavior with the risk of untreated illness. Epilepsy and many other illnesses for which AEDs are prescribed are themselves associated with morbidity and mortality and an increased risk of suicidal thoughts or behavior. Should suicidal thoughts and behavior emerge during treatment, the prescriber needs to consider whether the emergence of these symptoms in any given patient may be related to the illness being treated.

Patients, their caregivers, and families should be informed that AEDs increase the risk of suicidal thoughts and behavior and should be advised of the need to be alert for the emergence or worsening of the signs and symptoms of depression, any unusual changes in mood or behavior, or the emergence of suicidal thoughts, behavior, or thoughts about self-harm. Behaviors of concern should be reported immediately to healthcare providers.

Usage in Pregnancy

Carbamazepine can cause fetal harm when administered to a pregnant woman.

Epidemiological data suggest that there may be an association between the use of carbamazepine during pregnancy and congenital malformations, including spina bifida. The prescribing physician will wish to weigh the benefits of therapy against the risks in treating or counseling women of childbearing potential. If this drug is used during pregnancy, or if the patient becomes pregnant while taking this drug, the patient should be apprised of the potential hazard to the fetus.

Retrospective case reviews suggest that, compared with monotherapy, there may be a higher prevalence of teratogenic effects associated with the use of anticonvulsants in combination therapy.

Table 1 – Risk by indication for antiepileptic drugs in the pooled analysis

Indication	Placebo Patients with Events Per 1000 Patients	Drug Patients with Events Per 1000 Patients	Relative Risk: Incidence of Events in Drug Patients/ Incidence in Placebo Patients	Risk Difference: Additional Drug Patients with Events Per 1000 Patients
Epilepsy	1.0	3.4	3.5	2.4
Psychiatric	5.7	8.5	1.5	2.9
Other	1.0	1.8	1.9	0.9
Total	2.4	4.3	1.8	1.9

IMPORTANT NOTICE: Updated drug information is sent bi-monthly via the PDR® Update Insert. For *monthly* email updates, register at PDR.net.

In humans, transplacental passage of carbamazepine is rapid (30-60 minutes), and the drug is accumulated in the fetal tissues, with higher levels found in liver and kidney than in brain and lung.

Carbamazepine has been shown to have adverse effects in reproduction studies in rats when given orally in dosages 10-25 times the maximum human daily dosage (MHDD) of 1200 mg on a mg/kg basis or 1.5-4 times the MHDD on a mg/m^2 basis. In rat teratology studies, 2 of 135 offspring showed kinked ribs at 250 mg/kg and 4 of 119 offspring at 650 mg/kg showed other anomalies (cleft palate, 1; talipes, 1; anophthalmos, 2). In reproduction studies in rats, nursing offspring demonstrated a lack of weight gain and an unkempt appearance at a maternal dosage level of 200 mg/kg.

Antiepileptic drugs should not be discontinued abruptly in patients in whom the drug is administered to prevent major seizures because of the strong possibility of precipitating status epilepticus with attendant hypoxia and threat to life. In individual cases where the severity and frequency of the seizure disorder are such that removal of medication does not pose a serious threat to the patient, discontinuation of the drug may be considered prior to and during pregnancy, although it cannot be said with any confidence that even minor seizures do not pose some hazard to the developing embryo or fetus.

Tests to detect defects using current accepted procedures should be considered a part of routine prenatal care in childbearing women receiving carbamazepine.

To provide information regarding the effects of in utero exposure to Carbatrol, physicians are advised to recommend that pregnant patients taking Carbatrol enroll in the North American Antiepileptic Drug (NAAED) Pregnancy Registry. This can be done by calling the toll free number 1-888-233-2334, and must be done by patients themselves. Information on the registry can also be found at the website http://www.aedpregnancyregistry.org/.

General

Patients with a history of adverse hematologic reaction to any drug may be particularly at risk of bone marrow depression.

In patients with seizure disorder, carbamazepine should not be discontinued abruptly because of the strong possibility of precipitating status epilepticus with attendant hypoxia and threat to life.

Carbamazepine has shown mild anticholinergic activity; therefore, patients with increased intraocular pressure should be closely observed during therapy.

Because of the relationship of the drug to other tricyclic compounds, the possibility of activation of a latent psychosis and, in elderly patients, of confusion or agitation should be considered.

Co-administration of carbamazepine and delavirdine may lead to loss of virologic response and possible resistance to PRESCRIPTOR or to the class of non-nucleoside reverse transcriptase inhibitors.

PRECAUTIONS

General

Before initiating therapy, a detailed history and physical examination should be made.

Carbamazepine should be used with caution in patients with a mixed seizure disorder that includes atypical absence seizures, since in these patients carbamazepine has been associated with increased frequency of generalized convulsions (see INDICATIONS AND USAGE).

Therapy should be prescribed only after critical benefit-to-risk appraisal in patients with a history of cardiac, hepatic, or renal damage; adverse hematologic reaction to other drugs; or interrupted courses of therapy with carbamazepine.

Information for Patients

Patients should be made aware of the early toxic signs and symptoms of a potential hematologic problem, such as fever, sore throat, rash, ulcers in the mouth, easy bruising, petechial or purpuric hemorrhage, and should be advised to report to the physician immediately if any such signs or symptoms appear.

Patients, their caregivers, and families should be counseled that AEDs, including Carbatrol, may increase the risk of suicidal thoughts and behavior and should be advised of the need to be alert for the emergence or worsening of symptoms of depression, any unusual changes in mood or behavior, or the emergence of suicidal thoughts, behavior, or thoughts about self-harm. Behaviors of concern should be reported immediately to healthcare providers.

Since dizziness and drowsiness may occur, patients should be cautioned about the hazards of operating machinery or automobiles or engaging in other potentially dangerous tasks.

Patients should be encouraged to enroll in the NAAED Pregnancy Registry if they become pregnant. This registry is collecting information about the safety of antiepileptic drugs during pregnancy. To enroll, patients can call the toll free number 1-888-233-2334 (see Warnings - Usage in Pregnancy)

If necessary, the Carbatrol capsules can be opened and the contents sprinkled over food, such as a teaspoon of applesauce or other similar food products. Carbatrol capsules or their contents should not be crushed or chewed.

Carbatrol may interact with some drugs. Therefore, patients should be advised to report to their doctors the use of any other prescription or non-prescription medication or herbal products.

Laboratory Tests

For genetically at-risk patients [See WARNINGS], high-resolution *'HLA-B*1502 typing'* is recommended. The test is positive if either one or two HLA-B*1502 alleles are detected and negative if no HLA-B*1502 alleles are detected.

Complete pretreatment blood counts, including platelets and possibly reticulocytes and serum iron, should be obtained as a baseline. If a patient in the course of treatment exhibits low or decreased white blood cell or platelet counts, the patient should be monitored closely. Discontinuation of the drug should be considered if any evidence of significant bone marrow depression develops.

Baseline and periodic evaluations of liver function, particularly in patients with a history of liver disease, must be performed during treatment with this drug since liver damage may occur. The drug should be discontinued immediately in cases of aggravated liver dysfunction or active liver disease.

Baseline and periodic eye examinations, including slit-lamp, funduscopy, and tonometry, are recommended since many phenothiazines and related drugs have been shown to cause eye changes.

Baseline and periodic complete urinalysis and BUN determinations are recommended for patients treated with this agent because of observed renal dysfunction.

Increases in total cholesterol, LDL and HDL have been observed in some patients taking anticonvulsants. Therefore, periodic evaluation of these parameters is also recommended. Monitoring of blood levels (see CLINICAL PHARMACOLOGY) has increased the efficacy and safety of anticonvulsants. This monitoring may be particularly useful in cases of dramatic increase in seizure frequency and for verification of compliance. In addition, measurement of drug serum levels may aid in determining the cause of toxicity when more than one medication is being used.

Thyroid function tests have been reported to show decreased values with carbamazepine administered alone.

Hyponatremia has been reported in association with carbamazepine use, either alone or in combination with other drugs.

Interference with some pregnancy tests has been reported.

Drug Interactions

Clinically meaningful drug interactions have occurred with concomitant medications and include, but are not limited to the following:

Agents Highly Bound to Plasma Protein:

Carbamazepine is not highly bound to plasma proteins; therefore, administration of Carbatrol® to a patient taking another drug that is highly protein bound should not cause increased free concentrations of the other drug.

Agents that Inhibits Cytochrome P450 Isoenzymes and/or Epoxide Hydrolase:

Carbamazepine is metabolized mainly by cytochrome P450 (CYP) 3A4 to the active carbamazepine 10,11-epoxide, which is further metabolized to the trans-diol by epoxide hydrolase. Therefore, the potential exists for interaction between carbamazepine and any agent that inhibits CYP3A4 and/or epoxide hydrolase. Agents that are CYP3A4 inhibitors that have been found, or are expected, to increase plasma levels of Carbatrol® are the following:

Acetazolamide, azole antifungals, cimetidine, clarithromycin[(1)]*, dalfopristin, danazol, delavirdine, diltiazem, erythromycin*[(1)]*, fluoxetine, fluvoxamine, grapefruit juice, isoniazid, itraconazole, ketoconazole, loratadine, nefazadone, niacinamide, nicotinamide, protease inhibitors, propoxyphene, quinine, quinupristin, troleandomycin, valproate*[(1)]*, verapamil, zileuton.*

[(1)]also inhibits epoxide hydrolase resulting in increased levels of the active metabolite carbamazepine 10,11-epoxide

Thus, if a patient has been titrated to a stable dosage of Carbatrol®, and then begins a course of treatment with one of these CYP3A4 or epoxide hydrolase inhibitors, it is reasonable to expect that a dose reduction for Carbatrol® may be necessary.

Agents that Induce Cytochrome P450 Isoenzymes:

Carbamazepine is metabolized by CYP3A4. Therefore, the potential exists for interaction between carbamazepine and any agent that induces CYP3A4. Agents that are CYP inducers that have been found, or are expected, to decrease plasma levels of Carbatrol® are the following:

Cisplatin, doxorubicin HCL, felbamate, rifampin, phenobarbital, phenytoin[(2)]*, primidone, methsuximide, and theophylline*

[(2)]Phenytoin plasma levels have also been reported to increase and decrease in the presence of carbamazepine, see below.

Thus, if a patient has been titrated to a stable dosage on Carbatrol®, and then begins a course of treatment with one of these CYP3A4 inducers, it is reasonable to expect that a dose increase for Carbatrol® may be necessary.

Agents with Decreased Levels in the Presence of Carbamazepine due to Induction of Cytochrome P450 Enzymes:

Carbamazepine is known to induce CYP1A2 and CYP3A4. Therefore, the potential exists for interaction between carbamazepine and any agent metabolized by one (or more) of these enzymes. Agents that have been found, or are expected to have decreased plasma levels in the presence of Carbatrol® due to induction of CYP enzymes are the following:

Acetaminophen, alprazolam, amitriptyline, bupropion, buspirone, citalopram, clobazam, clonazepam, clozapine, cyclosporin, delavirdine, desipramine, diazepam, dicumarol, doxycycline, ethosuximide, felbamate, felodipine, glucocorticoids, haloperidol, itraconazole, lamotrigine, levothyroxine, lorazepam, methadone, midazolam, mirtazapine, nortriptyline, olanzapine, oral contraceptives[(3)]*, oxcarbazepine, phenytoin*[(4)]*, praziquantel, protease inhibitors, quetiapine, risperidone, theophylline, topiramate, tiagabine, tramadol, triazolam, trazodone*[(5)]*, valproate, warfarin*[(6)]*, ziprasidone, and zonisamide.*

[(3)]Break through bleeding has been reported among patients receiving concomitant oral contraceptives and their reliability may be adversely affected.

[(4)]Phenytoin has also been reported to increase in the presence of carbamazepine. Careful monitoring of phenytoin plasma levels following co-medication with carbamazepine is advised.

[(5)]Following co-administration of carbamazepine 400 mg/day with trazodone 100 mg to 300 mg daily, carbamazepine reduced trough plasma concentrations of trazodone (as well as meta-chlorophenylpiperazine [mCPP]) by 76 and 60% respectively, compared to precarbamazepine values.

[(6)]Warfarin's anticoagulant effect can be reduced in the presence of carbamazepine.

Thus, if a patient has been titrated to a stable dosage on one of the agents in this category, and then begins a course of treatment with Carbatrol®, it is reasonable to expect that a dose increase for the concomitant agent may be necessary.

Agents with Increased Levels in the Presence of Carbamazepine:

Carbatrol® increases the plasma levels of the following agents:

Clomipramine HCl, phenytoin[(7)]*, and primidone*

[(7)]Phenytoin has also been reported to decrease in the presence of carbamazepine. Careful monitoring of phenytoin plasma levels following co-medication with carbamazepine is advised.

Thus, if a patient has been titrated to a stable dosage on one of the agents in this category, and then begins a course of the treatment with Carbatrol®, it is reasonable to expect that a dose decrease for the concomitant agent may be necessary.

Pharmacological/Pharmacodynamic Interactions with Carbamazepine:

Concomitant administration of carbamazepine and lithium may increase the risk of neurotoxic side effects.

Given the anticonvulsant properties of carbamazepine, Carbatrol® may reduce the thyroid function as has been reported with other anticonvulsants. Additionally, antimalarial drugs, such as chloroquine and mefloquine, may antagonize the activity of carbamazepine.

Thus if a patient has been titrated to a stable dosage on one of the agents in this category, and then begins a course of treatment with Carbatrol®, it is reasonable to expect that a dose adjustment may be necessary.

Because of its primary CNS effect, caution should be used when Carbatrol® is taken with other centrally acting drugs and alcohol.

Carcinogenesis, Mutagenesis, Impairment of Fertility:

Administration of carbamazepine to Sprague-Dawley rats for two years in the diet at doses of 25, 75, and 250 mg/kg/day (low dose approximately 0.2 times the maximum human daily dose of 1200 mg on a mg/m^2 basis), resulted in a dose-related increase in the incidence of hepatocellular tumors in females and of benign interstitial cell adenomas in the testes of males.

Carbamazepine must, therefore, be considered to be carcinogenic in Sprague-Dawley rats. Bacterial and mammalian mutagenicity studies using carbamazepine produced negative results. The significance of these findings relative to the use of carbamazepine in humans is, at present, unknown.

Usage in Pregnancy

Pregnancy Category D (See WARNINGS)

Labor and Delivery

The effect of carbamazepine on human labor and delivery is unknown.

Nursing Mothers

Carbamazepine and its epoxide metabolite are transferred to breast milk and during lactation. The concentrations of carbamazepine and its epoxide metabolite are approximately 50% of the maternal plasma concentration. Because of the potential for serious adverse reactions in nursing infants from carbamazepine, a decision should be made whether to discontinue nursing or to discontinue the drug, taking into account the importance of the drug to the mother.

Pediatric Use

Substantial evidence of carbamazepine effectiveness for use in the management of children with epilepsy (see INDICATIONS for specific seizure types) is derived from clinical investigations performed in adults and from studies in several *in vitro* systems which support the conclusion that (1) the pathogenic mechanisms underlying seizure propagation are essentially identical in adults and children, and (2) the mechanism of action of carbamazepine in treating seizures is essentially identical in adults and children. Taken as a whole, this information supports a conclusion that the generally acceptable therapeutic range of total carbamazepine in plasma (i.e., 4-12 µg/mL) is the same in children and adults.

The evidence assembled was primarily obtained from short-term use of carbamazepine. The safety of carbamazepine in children has been systematically studied up to 6 months. No longer term data from clinical trials is available.

Geriatric Use

No systematic studies in geriatric patients have been conducted.

ADVERSE REACTIONS

General: If adverse reactions are of such severity that the drug must be discontinued, the physician must be aware that abrupt discontinuation of any anticonvulsant drug in a responsive patient with epilepsy may lead to seizures or even status epilepticus with its life-threatening hazards.

The most severe adverse reactions previously observed with carbamazepine were reported in the hemopoietic system and skin (see BOX WARNING), and the cardiovascular system.

The most frequently observed adverse reactions, particularly during the initial phases of therapy, are dizziness, drowsiness, unsteadiness, nausea, and vomiting. To minimize the possibility of such reactions, therapy should be initiated at the lowest dosage recommended. The following additional adverse reactions were previously reported with carbamazepine:

Hemopoietic System: Aplastic anemia, agranulocytosis, pancytopenia, bone marrow depression, thrombocytopenia, leukopenia, leukocytosis, eosinophilia, acute intermittent porphyria.

Skin: Toxic epidermal necrolysis (TEN) and Stevens-Johnson syndrome (SJS) (see BOXED WARNING), pruritic and erythematous rashes, urticaria, photosensitivity reactions, alterations in skin pigmentation, exfoliative dermatitis, erythema multiforme and nodosum, purpura, aggravation of disseminated lupus erythematosus, alopecia, and diaphoresis. In certain cases, discontinuation of therapy may be necessary. Isolated cases of hirsutism have been reported, but a causal relationship is not clear.

Cardiovascular System: Congestive heart failure, edema, aggravation of hypertension, hypotension, syncope and collapse, aggravation of coronary artery disease, arrhythmias and AV block, thrombophlebitis, thromboembolism, and adenopathy or lymphadenopathy. Some of these cardiovascular complications have resulted in fatalities. Myocardial infarction has been associated with other tricyclic compounds.

Liver: Abnormalities in liver function tests, cholestatic and hepatocellular jaundice, hepatitis.

Respiratory System: Pulmonary hypersensitivity characterized by fever, dyspnea, pneumonitis, or pneumonia.

Genitourinary System: Urinary frequency, acute urinary retention, oliguria with elevated blood pressure, azotemia, renal failure, and impotence. Albuminuria, glycosuria, elevated BUN, and microscopic deposits in the urine have also been reported.

Testicular atrophy occurred in rats receiving carbamazepine orally from 4-52 weeks at dosage levels of 50-400 mg/kg/day. Additionally, rats receiving carbamazepine in the diet for 2 years at dosage levels of 25, 75, and 250 mg/kg/day had a dose-related incidence of testicular atrophy and aspermatogenesis. In dogs, it produced a brownish discoloration, presumably a metabolite, in the urinary bladder at dosage levels of 50 mg/kg/day and higher. Relevance of these findings to humans is unknown.

Nervous System: Dizziness, drowsiness, disturbances of coordination, confusion, headache, fatigue, blurred vision, visual hallucinations, transient diplopia, oculomotor disturbances, nystagmus, speech disturbances, abnormal involuntary movements, peripheral neuritis and paresthesias, depression with agitation, talkativeness, tinnitus, and hyperacusis.

There have been reports of associated paralysis and other symptoms of cerebral arterial insufficiency, but the exact relationship of these reactions to the drug has not been established.

Isolated cases of neuroleptic malignant syndrome have been reported with concomitant use of psychotropic drugs.

Digestive System: Nausea, vomiting, gastric distress and abdominal pain, diarrhea, constipation, anorexia, and dryness of the mouth and pharynx, including glossitis and stomatitis.

Eyes: Scattered punctate cortical lens opacities, as well as conjunctivitis, have been reported. Although a direct causal relationship has not been established, many phenothiazines and related drugs have been shown to cause eye changes.

Musculoskeletal System: Aching joints and muscles, and leg cramps.

Metabolism: Fever and chills, inappropriate antidiuretic hormone (ADH) secretion syndrome has been reported. Cases of frank water intoxication, with decreased serum sodium (hyponatremia) and confusion have been reported in association with carbamazepine use (see PRECAUTIONS, Laboratory Tests). Decreased levels of plasma calcium have been reported.

Other: Isolated cases of a lupus erythematosus-like syndrome have been reported. There have been occasional reports of elevated levels of cholesterol, HDL cholesterol, and triglycerides in patients taking anticonvulsants.

A case of aseptic meningitis, accompanied by myoclonus and peripheral eosinophilia, has been reported in a patient taking carbamazepine in combination with other medications. The patient was successfully dechallenged, and the meningitis reappeared upon rechallenge with carbamazepine.

DRUG ABUSE AND DEPENDENCE

No evidence of abuse potential has been associated with carbamazepine, nor is there evidence of psychological or physical dependence in humans.

OVERDOSAGE

Acute Toxicity

Lowest known lethal dose: adults, >60 g (39-year-old man). Highest known doses survived: adults, 30 g (31-year-old woman); children, 10 g (6-year-old boy); small children, 5 g (3-year-old girl).

Oral LD_{50} in animals (mg/kg): mice, 1100-3750; rats, 3850-4025; rabbits, 1500-2680; guinea pigs, 920.

Signs and Symptoms

The first signs and symptoms appear after 1-3 hours. Neuromuscular disturbances are the most prominent. Cardiovascular disorders are generally milder, and severe cardiac complications occur only when very high doses (>60 g) have been ingested.

Respiration: Irregular breathing, respiratory depression.

Cardiovascular System: Tachycardia, hypotension or hypertension, shock, conduction disorders.

Nervous System and Muscles: Impairment of consciousness ranging in severity to deep coma. Convulsions, especially in small children. Motor restlessness, muscular twitching, tremor, athetoid movements, opisthotonos, ataxia, drowsiness, dizziness, mydriasis, nystagmus, adiadochokinesia, ballism, psychomotor disturbances, dysmetria. Initial hyperreflexia, followed by hyporeflexia.

Gastrointestinal Tract: Nausea, vomiting.

Kidneys and Bladder: Anuria or oliguria, urinary retention.

Laboratory Findings: Isolated instances of overdosage have included leukocytosis, reduced leukocyte count, glycosuria, and acetonuria. ECG may show dysrhythmias.

Combined Poisoning: When alcohol, tricyclic antidepressants, barbiturates, or hydantoins are taken at the same time, the signs and symptoms of acute poisoning with carbamazepine may be aggravated or modified.

Treatment

For the most up to date information on management of carbamazepine overdose, please contact the poison center for your area by calling 1-800-222-1222. The prognosis in cases of carbamazepine poisoning is generally favorable. Of 5,645 cases of carbamazepine exposures reported to US poison centers in 2002, a total of 8 deaths (0.14% mortality rate) occurred. Over 39% of the cases reported to these poison centers were managed safely at home with conservative care. Successful management of large or intentional carbamazepine exposures requires implementation of supportive care, frequent monitoring of serum drug concentrations, as well as aggressive but appropriate gastric decontamination.

Elimination of the Drug: The primary method for gastric decontamination of carbamazepine overdose is use of activated charcoal. For substantial recent ingestions, gastric lavage may also be considered. Administration of activated charcoal prior to hospital assessment has the potential to significantly reduce drug absorption. There is no specific antidote. In overdose, absorption of carbamazepine may be prolonged and delayed. More than one dose of activated charcoal may be beneficial in patients that have evidence of continued absorption (e.g., rising serum carbamazepine levels).

Measures to Accelerate Elimination: The data on use of dialysis to enhance elimination in carbamazepine is scarce. Dialysis, particularly high flux or high efficiency hemodialysis, may be considered in patients with severe carbamazepine poisoning associated with renal failure or in cases of status epilepticus, or where there are rising serum drug levels and worsening clinical status despite appropriate supportive care and gastric decontamination. For severe cases of carbamazepine overdose unresponsive to other measures, charcoal hemoperfusion may be used to enhance drug clearance.

Respiratory Depression: Keep the airways free; resort, if necessary, to endotracheal intubation, artificial respiration, and administration of oxygen.

Hypotension, Shock: Keep the patient's legs raised and administer a plasma expander. If blood pressure fails to rise despite measures taken to increase plasma volume, use of vasoactive substances should be considered.

Convulsions: Diazepam or barbiturates.

Warning: Diazepam or barbiturates may aggravate respiratory depression (especially in children), hypotension, and coma. However, barbiturates should not be used if drugs that inhibit monoamine oxidase have also been taken by the patient either in overdosage or in recent therapy (within 1 week).

Surveillance: Respiration, cardiac function (ECG monitoring), blood pressure, body temperature, pupillary reflexes, and kidney and bladder function should be monitored for several days.

Treatment of Blood Count Abnormalities: If evidence of significant bone marrow depression develops, the following recommendations are suggested: (1) stop the drug, (2) perform daily CBC, platelet, and reticulocyte counts, (3) do a bone marrow aspiration and trephine biopsy immediately and repeat with sufficient frequency to monitor recovery. Special periodic studies might be helpful as follows: (1) white cell and platelet antibodies, (2) ^{59}Fe-ferrokinetic studies, (3) peripheral blood cell typing, (4) cytogenetic studies on marrow and peripheral blood, (5) bone marrow culture studies for colony-forming units, (6) hemoglobin electrophoresis for A_2 and F hemoglobin, and (7) serum folic acid and B_{12} levels.

A fully developed aplastic anemia will require appropriate, intensive monitoring and therapy, for which specialized consultation should be sought.

DOSAGE AND ADMINISTRATION

Monitoring of blood levels has increased the efficacy and safety of anticonvulsants (see PRECAUTIONS, Laboratory Tests). Dosage should be adjusted to the needs of the individual patients. A low initial daily dosage with gradual increase is advised. As soon as adequate control is achieved, the dosage may be reduced very gradually to the minimum effective level. The Carbatrol capsules may be opened and the beads sprinkled over food, such as a teaspoon of applesauce or other similar food products if this method of administration is preferred. Carbatrol capsules or their contents should not be crushed or chewed. Carbatrol can be taken with or without meals.

Carbatrol is an extended-release formulation for twice a day administration. When converting patients from immediate release carbamazepine to Carbatrol extended-release capsules, the same total daily mg dose of carbamazepine should be administered.

Epilepsy (see INDICATIONS AND USAGE)

Adults and children over 12 years of age. Initial: 200 mg twice daily. Increase at weekly intervals by adding up to 200 mg/day until the optimal response is obtained. Dosage generally should not exceed 1000 mg per day in children 12-15 years of age, and 1200 mg daily in patients above 15 years of age. Doses up to 1600 mg daily have been used in adults. **Maintenance:** Adjust dosage to the minimum effective level, usually 800-1200 mg daily.

Children under 12 years of age: Children taking total daily dosages of immediate-release carbamazepine of 400 mg or greater may be converted to the same total daily dosage of Carbatrol extended-release capsules, using a twice daily regimen. Ordinarily, optimal clinical response is achieved at daily doses below 35 mg/kg. If satisfactory clinical response has not been achieved, plasma levels should be measured to determine whether or not they are in the therapeutic range. No recommendation regarding the safety of Carbatrol for use at doses above 35 mg/kg/24 hours can be made.

Combination Therapy: Carbatrol may be used alone or with other anticonvulsants. When added to existing anticonvulsant therapy, the drug should be added gradually while the other anticonvulsants are maintained or gradually decreased, except phenytoin, which may have to be increased (see PRECAUTIONS, Drug Interactions, and Pregnancy Category D).

Trigeminal Neuralgia (see INDICATIONS AND USAGE)

Initial: On the first day, start with one 200 mg capsule. This daily dose may be increased by up to 200 mg/day every 12 hours only as needed to achieve freedom from pain. Do not exceed 1200 mg daily.

Maintenance: Control of pain can be maintained in most patients with 400-800 mg daily. However, some patients may be maintained on as little as 200 mg daily, while others may require as much as 1200 mg daily. At least once every 3 months throughout the treatment period, attempts should be made to reduce the dose to the minimum effective level or even to discontinue the drug.

HOW SUPPLIED

Carbatrol (carbamazepine) extended-release capsules is supplied in three dosage strengths.

100 mg-Two-piece hard gelatin capsule (bluish green opaque body and cap) printed with the Shire logo in white ink.

Supplied in bottles of 120 .... NDC 54092-171-12

200 mg-Two-piece hard gelatin capsule (light gray opaque body with bluish green opaque cap) printed with the Shire logo in white ink.

Supplied in bottles of 120 .... NDC 54092-172-12

300 mg-Two-piece hard gelatin capsule (black opaque body with bluish green opaque cap) printed with the Shire logo in white ink.

Supplied in bottles of 120 .... NDC 54092-173-12

Store at 25°C (77°F); excursions permitted to 15-30°C (59-86°F) [see USP controlled room temperature]. PROTECT FROM LIGHT AND MOISTURE.

Manufactured for:

Shire US Inc.

725 Chesterbrook Blvd., Wayne PA 19087

1-800-828-2088, Made in U.S.A. © 2009 Shire US Inc.

006618   172 1207 012   (Rev 04/09)

Registered in the US Patent and Trade Office

CAR-00182

Shown in Product Identification Guide, page 319

INTUNIV™

℞

[*in-TOO-niv*]

(guanfacine)

extended-release tablets

HIGHLIGHTS OF PRESCRIBING INFORMATION

These highlights do not include all the information needed to use INTUNIV™ safely and effectively. See full prescribing information for INTUNIV™.

INTUNIV™ (guanfacine) extended-release tablets

Initial U.S. Approval: 1986

————————INDICATIONS AND USAGE————————

INTUNIV™ is a selective alpha-$_{2A}$-adrenergic receptor agonist indicated for the treatment of Attention Deficit Hyperactivity Disorder (ADHD). The efficacy of INTUNIV™ is based on results of two 8 to 9 week studies in children and adolescents (14.1). Maintenance treatment has not been systematically evaluated, and patients who are continued on longer-term treatment require periodic reassessment (1).

————————DOSAGE AND ADMINISTRATION————————

For all patients (2.1):

• Dose once daily.

• Tablets should not be crushed, chewed or broken before swallowing.

• Do not administer with high-fat meals, because of increased exposure.

• Do not substitute for immediate-release guanfacine tablets on a mg-per-mg basis, because of differing pharmacokinetic profiles.

Dose Selection (2.2):

• If switching from immediate-release guanfacine, discontinue that treatment and titrate with INTUNIV™ as directed.

• Begin at a dose of 1 mg once daily and adjust in increments of no more than 1 mg/week.

• Maintain the dose within the range of 1-4 mg/day, depending on clinical response and tolerability.

• Consider dosing on a mg/kg basis. Improvements observed at starting doses of 0.05-0.08 mg/kg once daily. Doses up to 0.12 mg/kg once daily may provide additional benefit.

• Doses above 4 mg/day have not been studied.

Discontinuation (2.4):

• When discontinuing, taper the dose in decrements of no more than 1 mg every 3 to 7 days.

————————DOSAGE FORMS AND STRENGTHS————————

• Extended-release tablets: 1 mg, 2 mg, 3 mg and 4 mg (3)

————————CONTRAINDICATIONS————————

History of hypersensitivity to INTUNIV™, its inactive ingredients, or other products containing guanfacine (e.g. TENEX®) (4).

————————WARNINGS AND PRECAUTIONS————————

• Hypotension, bradycardia, and syncope: Use INTUNIV™ with caution in patients at risk for hypotension, bradycardia, heart block, or syncope (e.g., those taking antihypertensives). Measure heart rate and blood pressure prior to initiation of therapy, following dose increases, and periodically while on therapy. Advise patients to avoid becoming dehydrated or overheated (5.1).

• Sedation and somnolence: Occur commonly with INTUNIV™. Consider the potential for additive sedative effects with CNS depressant drugs. Caution patients against operating heavy equipment or driving until they know how they respond to INTUNIV™ (5.2).

• Other guanfacine-containing products: Do not use INTUNIV™ concomitantly with other products containing guanfacine (e.g., Tenex) (5.3).

————————ADVERSE REACTIONS————————

Most common and dose-related adverse reactions: somnolence, sedation, abdominal pain, dizziness, hypotension/decreased blood pressure, dry mouth and constipation. (6).

To report SUSPECTED ADVERSE REACTIONS, contact Shire US Inc. at 1-800-828-2088 or FDA at 1-800-FDA-1088 or www.fda.gov/medwatch.

————————DRUG INTERACTIONS————————

• CYP3A4/5 inhibitors (e.g., ketoconazole): Coadministration may increase rate and extent of guanfacine exposure. Use concomitantly with caution (7.1).

• CYP3A4 inducers (e.g., rifampin): Coadministration may decrease rate and extent of guanfacine exposure. Consider dose increase of INTUNIV™ (7.2).

• Valproic acid: Coadministration may increase serum valproic acid concentrations (7.3).

• Antihypertensive drugs: Use caution when coadministered with INTUNIV™ (5.1, 7.4).

• CNS depressants: Use caution when coadministered with INTUNIV™ (5.2, 7.5).

————————USE IN SPECIFIC POPULATIONS————————

• Hepatic or Renal Impairment: dose reduction may be required in patients with clinically significant impairment of hepatic or renal function (8.6).

See 17 for PATIENT COUNSELING INFORMATION and FDA-approved Patient Labeling.

Revised: 08/2009

FULL PRESCRIBING INFORMATION: CONTENTS*

1   INDICATIONS AND USAGE

2   DOSAGE AND ADMINISTRATION

2.1   General Dosing Information

2.2   Dose Selection

2.3   Maintenance Treatment

2.4   Discontinuation

2.5   Missed Doses

3   DOSAGE FORMS AND STRENGTHS

4   CONTRAINDICATIONS

5   WARNINGS AND PRECAUTIONS

5.1   Hypotension, Bradycardia, and Syncope

5.2   Sedation and Somnolence

5.3   Other Guanfacine-Containing Products

6   ADVERSE REACTIONS

6.1   Clinical Trial Experience

7   DRUG INTERACTIONS

7.1   CYP3A4/5 Inhibitors

7.2   CYP3A4 Inducers

7.3   Valproic Acid

7.4   Antihypertensive Drugs

7.5   CNS Depressant Drugs

8   USE IN SPECIFIC POPULATIONS

8.1   Pregnancy

8.3   Nursing Mothers

8.4   Pediatric Use

8.5   Geriatric Use

8.6   Use in Patients with Renal or Hepatic Impairment

9   DRUG ABUSE AND DEPENDENCE

9.1   Controlled Substance

10   OVERDOSAGE

11   DESCRIPTION

12   CLINICAL PHARMACOLOGY

12.1   Mechanism of Action

12.2   Pharmacodynamics

12.3   Pharmacokinetics

13   NONCLINICAL TOXICOLOGY

13.1   Carcinogenesis, Mutagenesis, Impairment of Fertility

14   CLINICAL STUDIES

14.1   Safety and Efficacy Studies

16   HOW SUPPLIED/STORAGE AND HANDLING

17   PATIENT COUNSELING INFORMATION

17.1   Dosing and Administration

17.2   Adverse Reactions

*Sections or subsections omitted from full prescribing information are not listed.

FULL PRESCRIBING INFORMATION

1   INDICATIONS AND USAGE

INTUNIV™ is indicated for the treatment of Attention Deficit Hyperactivity Disorder (ADHD). The efficacy of INTUNIV™ was studied for the treatment of ADHD in two controlled clinical trials (8 and 9 weeks in duration) in children and adolescents ages 6-17 who met DSM-IV® criteria for ADHD [*see Clinical Studies (14)*]. The effectiveness of INTUNIV™ for longer-term use (more than 9 weeks) has not been systematically evaluated in controlled trials.

A diagnosis of ADHD implies the presence of hyperactive-impulsive and/or inattentive symptoms that cause impairment and were present before the age of 7 years. The symptoms must cause clinically significant impairment, e.g., in social, academic, or occupational functioning, and be present in two or more settings, e.g., school (or work) and at home. The symptoms must not be better accounted for by another mental disorder. For the Inattentive Type, at least six of the following symptoms must have persisted for at least 6 months: lack of attention to details/careless mistakes; lack of sustained attention; poor listener; failure to follow through on tasks; poor organization; avoids tasks requiring sustained mental effort; loses things; easily distracted; forgetful. For the Hyperactive-Impulsive Type, at least six of the following symptoms must have persisted for at least 6 months: fidgeting/squirming; leaving seat; inappropriate running/climbing; difficulty with quiet activities; "on the go"; excessive talking; blurting answers; can't wait turn; intrusive. The Combined Type requires both inattentive and hyperactive-impulsive criteria to be met.

Special Diagnostic Considerations

Specific etiology of this syndrome is unknown, and there is no single diagnostic test. Adequate diagnosis requires the use not only of medical but also of special psychological, educational, and social resources. Learning may or may not be impaired. The diagnosis must be based upon a complete history and evaluation of the patient and not solely on the presence of the required number of DSM-IV® characteristics.

Need for Comprehensive Treatment Program

INTUNIV™ is indicated as an integral part of a total treatment program for ADHD that may include other measures (psychological, educational, and social) for patients with this syndrome. Drug treatment may not be indicated for all patients with this syndrome. INTUNIV™ is not intended for use in patients who exhibit symptoms secondary to environmental factors and/or other primary psychiatric disorders, including psychosis. Appropriate educational/vocational placement is essential and psychosocial intervention is often helpful. When remedial measures alone are insufficient, the decision to prescribe INTUNIV™ will depend upon the physician's assessment of the chronicity and severity of the patient's symptoms and on the level of functional impairment.

2   DOSAGE AND ADMINISTRATION

2.1   General Dosing Information

INTUNIV™ is an extended-release tablet and should be dosed once daily. **Tablets should not be crushed, chewed or broken before swallowing because this will increase the rate of guanfacine release.** Do not administer with high fat meals, due to increased exposure.

Do not substitute for immediate-release guanfacine tablets on a mg-mg basis, because of differing pharmacokinetic profiles. INTUNIV™ has a delayed T_{max}, reduced C_{max} and lower bioavailability compared to those of the same dose of immediate-release guanfacine [*see Clinical Pharmacology (12.3)*].

2.2   Dose Selection

If switching from immediate-release guanfacine, discontinue that treatment, and titrate with INTUNIV™ according to the following recommended schedule.

Begin at a dose of 1 mg/day, and adjust in increments of no more than 1 mg/week.

Maintain the dose within the range of 1-4 mg once daily, depending on clinical response and tolerability. In clinical trials, patients were randomized to doses of 1 mg, 2 mg, 3 mg or 4 mg and received INTUNIV™ once daily in the morning [*see Clinical Studies (14.1)*].

Clinically relevant improvements were observed beginning at doses in the range 0.05-0.08 mg/kg once daily. Efficacy increased with increasing weight-adjusted dose (mg/kg). If well tolerated, doses up to 0.12 mg/kg once daily may provide additional benefit. Doses above 4 mg/day have not been studied.

In clinical trials, there were dose-related and exposure-related risks for several clinically significant adverse reactions (hypotension, bradycardia, sedative events). Thus, consideration should be given to dosing INTUNIV™ on a mg/kg basis, in order to balance the exposure-related potential benefits and risks of treatment.

2.3 Maintenance Treatment

The effectiveness of INTUNIV™ for longer-term use (more than 9 weeks) has not been systematically evaluated in controlled trials. Therefore the physician electing to use INTUNIV™ for extended periods should periodically re-evaluate the long-term usefulness of the drug for the individual patient.

2.4 Discontinuation

In a pharmacodynamic study in healthy young adult volunteers receiving INTUNIV™ (4 mg once daily) or placebo, the effects of abrupt discontinuation were compared to tapering. There were greater mean increases in systolic and diastolic blood pressure and heart rate after abrupt discontinuation of INTUNIV™, but these changes generally reflected a return to original baseline and were not meaningfully different for the two discontinuation strategies. However, infrequent, transient elevations in blood pressure above original baseline (i.e., rebound) have been reported to occur upon abrupt discontinuation of guanfacine. To minimize these effects, the dose should generally be tapered in decrements of no more than 1 mg every 3 to 7 days.

2.5 Missed Doses

When reinitiating patients to the previous maintenance dose after two or more missed consecutive doses, physicians should consider titration based on patient tolerability.

3 DOSAGE FORMS AND STRENGTHS

1 mg, 2 mg, 3 mg and 4 mg extended-release tablets

	1 mg	2 mg	3 mg	4 mg
Color	White/ off-white	White/ off-white	Green	Green
Shape	Round	Caplet	Round	Caplet
Debossment (top/bottom)	503 / 1mg	503 / 2mg	503 / 3mg	503 / 4mg

4 CONTRAINDICATIONS

Patients with a history of hypersensitivity to INTUNIV™, its inactive ingredients [see Description (11)], or other products containing guanfacine (e.g. TENEX®) should not take INTUNIV™.

5 WARNINGS AND PRECAUTIONS

5.1 Hypotension, Bradycardia, and Syncope

Treatment with INTUNIV™ can cause decreases in blood pressure and heart rate. In the pediatric, short-term (8-9 weeks), controlled trials, the maximum mean changes from baseline in systolic blood pressure, diastolic blood pressure, and pulse were −5 mm Hg, −3 mm Hg, and −6 bpm, respectively, for all dose groups combined (generally one week after reaching target doses of 1 mg/day, 2 mg/day, 3 mg/day or 4 mg/day). These changes were dose dependent. Decreases in blood pressure and heart rate were usually modest and asymptomatic; however, hypotension and bradycardia can occur. Hypotension was reported as an adverse event for 6% of the INTUNIV™ group and 4% of the placebo group. Orthostatic hypotension was reported for 1% of the INTUNIV™ group and none in the placebo group. In long-term, open label studies, (mean exposure of approximately 10 months), maximum decreases in systolic and diastolic blood pressure occurred in the first month of therapy. Decreases were less pronounced over time. Syncope occurred in 1% of pediatric subjects in the clinical program. The majority of these cases occurred in the long-term, open-label studies.

Measure heart rate and blood pressure prior to initiation of therapy, following dose increases, and periodically while on therapy. Use INTUNIV™ with caution in patients with a history of hypotension, heart block, bradycardia, or cardiovascular disease, because it can decrease blood pressure and heart rate. Use caution in treating patients who have a history of syncope or may have a condition that predisposes them to syncope, such as hypotension, orthostatic hypotension, bradycardia, or dehydration. Use INTUNIV™ with caution in patients treated concomitantly with antihypertensives or other drugs that can reduce blood pressure or heart rate or increase the risk of syncope. Advise patients to avoid becoming dehydrated or overheated.

5.2 Sedation and Somnolence

Somnolence and sedation were commonly reported adverse reactions in clinical studies (38% for INTUNIV™ vs. 12% for placebo) in children and adolescents with ADHD, especially during initial use [see Adverse Reactions (6.1)]. Before using INTUNIV™ with other centrally active depressants (such as phenothiazines, barbiturates, or benzodiazepines), consider the potential for additive sedative effects. Caution patients against operating heavy equipment or driving until they know how they respond to treatment with INTUNIV™. Advise patients to avoid use with alcohol.

5.3 Other Guanfacine-Containing Products

Guanfacine, the active ingredient in INTUNIV™, is also approved as an antihypertensive. Do not use INTUNIV™ in patients concomitantly taking other guanfacine-containing products (e.g., Tenex).

6 ADVERSE REACTIONS

The following serious adverse reactions are described elsewhere in the labelling:

- Hypotension, bradycardia, and syncope [see Warnings and Precautions (5.1)]
- Sedation and somnolence [see Warnings and Precautions (5.2)]

The most common adverse reactions with INTUNIV™ are: somnolence/sedation, abdominal pain, dizziness, hypotension/decreased blood pressure, dry mouth, and constipation.

Twelve percent (12%) of patients receiving INTUNIV™ discontinued from the clinical studies due to adverse events, compared to 4% in the placebo group. The most common adverse reactions leading to discontinuation of INTUNIV™-treated patients from the studies were somnolence/sedation (6%) and fatigue (2%). Less common adverse reactions leading to discontinuation (occurring in approximately 1% of patients) included: hypotension/decreased blood pressure, headache, and dizziness.

6.1 Clinical Trial Experience

Short Term Clinical Studies

Common Adverse Reactions—Two short-term, placebo-controlled, double-blind pivotal studies (Studies 1 and 2) were conducted in children and adolescents with ADHD, using fixed doses of INTUNIV™ (1, 2, 3, and 4 mg/day). The most commonly reported adverse reactions (occurring in ≥ 2% of patients) that were considered drug-related and reported in a greater percentage of patients taking INTUNIV™ compared to patients taking placebo are shown in Table 1. Adverse reactions that are dose-related include: somnolence, sedation, abdominal pain, dizziness, hypotension/decreased blood pressure, dry mouth and constipation.

Table 1: Percentage of Patients Experiencing Common (≥ 2%) Adverse Reactions in Short-Term Studies 1 and 2

Adverse Reaction Term	Placebo	All Doses
	(N=149)	of INTUNIV™ (N=513)
Somnolence[a]	12%	38%
Headache	19%	24%
Fatigue	3%	14%
Abdominal pain (upper)	7%	10%
Nausea	2%	6%
Lethargy	3%	6%
Dizziness	4%	6%
Irritability	4%	6%
Hypotension/Decreased blood pressure	4%	6%
Decreased appetite	3%	5%
Dry mouth	1%	4%
Constipation	1%	4%

a: The somnolence term includes somnolence, sedation, and hypersomnia.

Less Common Adverse Reactions—Less common adverse reactions (< 2%) reported in pivotal Studies 1 and 2 that occurred in more than one patient taking INTUNIV™ and were more common than in the placebo group are listed below.

Table 2: Less Common Adverse Reactions (< 2%) in Short-Term Studies 1 and 2

Body System	Adverse Reaction
Cardiac	Atrioventricular block, bradycardia, sinus arrhythmia
Gastrointestinal	Dyspepsia
General	Asthenia, chest pain
Investigations	Increased alanine aminotransferase, increased blood pressure, increased weight
Nervous system	Postural dizziness
Renal	Increased urinary frequency, enuresis
Respiratory	Asthma
Vascular	Orthostatic hypotension, pallor

In addition, the following less common (< 2%) psychiatric disorders occurred in more than one patient receiving INTUNIV™ and were more common than in the placebo group. The relationship to INTUNIV™ could not be determined because these events may also occur as symptoms in pediatric patients with ADHD: agitation, anxiety, depression, emotional lability, nightmares or interrupted sleep.

Long Term Clinical Studies

Common Adverse Reactions

Patients from the two short-term, placebo-controlled studies 1 and 2 were eligible to participate in one of two long-term, flexible-dose, open-label studies. The mean duration of exposure of the 446 patients who received open-label treatment was approximately 10 months. The distribution of patients among the doses prior to tapering off upon completion of the study was 37%, 33%, 27% and 3% on 4 mg, 3 mg, 2 mg and 1 mg, respectively.

The most common adverse reactions (≥ 5%) reported during open label treatment are shown in Table 3.

Table 3: Percentage of Patients Experiencing Common (≥ 5%) Adverse Reactions during Long-Term (Up to 10 months), Flexible-dose, Open-Label Follow-up from Studies 1 and 2

Adverse Reaction Term	All Doses of INTUNIV™ (N=446)
Somnolence[a]	45%
Headache	26%
Fatigue	15%
Abdominal pain (upper)	11%
Hypotension / Decreased Blood Pressure	10%
Vomiting	9%
Dizziness	7%
Nausea	7%
Weight increased	7%
Irritability	6%

a: The somnolence term includes somnolence, sedation, and hypersomnia.

Adverse Reactions Leading to Discontinuation-Eighteen percent (18%) of patients receiving INTUNIV™ discontinued from long-term studies due to adverse events. The most frequent adverse reactions leading to discontinuation (≥ 2%) were somnolence (3%), syncopal events (2%), increased weight (2%), depression (2%), and fatigue (2%). Other adverse reactions leading to discontinuation in the long-term studies (occurring in approximately 1% of patients) included: hypotension/decreased blood pressure, sedation, headache, and lethargy.

Serious Adverse Reactions-In long-term open label studies, serious adverse reactions occurring in more than one patient were syncope (2%) and convulsion (0.4%).

Less Common Adverse Reactions-Adverse reactions that occurred in < 5% of patients but ≥ 2% in open-label, long-term studies that are considered possibly related to INTUNIV™ include: syncopal events, constipation, stomach discomfort, hypertension/increased blood pressure, decreased appetite, diarrhea, dry mouth, lethargy, and insomnia.

Effects on Height, Weight, and Body Mass Index (BMI)

Patients taking INTUNIV™ demonstrated similar growth compared to normative data. Patients taking INTUNIV™ had a mean increase in weight of 1 kg (2 lbs) compared to those receiving placebo over a comparative treatment period. Patients receiving INTUNIV™ for at least 12 months in open-label studies gained an average of 8 kg (17 lbs) in weight and 8 cm (3 in) in height. The height, weight, and BMI percentile remained stable in patients at 12 months in the long-term studies compared to when they began receiving INTUNIV™.

Laboratory Tests

In short and long-term studies, no clinically important effects were identified on any laboratory parameters.

Effects on Heart Rate and QT Interval

The effect of two dose levels of immediate-release guanfacine (4 mg and 8 mg) on the QT interval was evaluated in a double-blind, randomized, placebo- and active-controlled, cross-over study in healthy adults.

A dose-dependent decrease in heart rate was observed during the first 12 hours, at time of maximal concentrations. The mean change in heart rate was -13 bpm at 4 mg and -22 bpm at 8 mg.

An apparent increase in mean QTc was observed for both doses. However, guanfacine does not appear to interfere with cardiac repolarization of the form associated with proarrhythmic drugs. This finding has no known clinical relevance.

7 DRUG INTERACTIONS

7.1 CYP3A4/5 Inhibitors

Use caution when INTUNIV™ is administered to patients taking ketoconazole and other strong CYP3A4/5 inhibitors, since elevation of plasma guanfacine concentration increases the risk of adverse events such as hypotension, bradycardia, and sedation. There was a substantial increase in the rate and extent of guanfacine exposure when administered with ketoconazole; the guanfacine exposure increased 3-fold (AUC).

7.2 CYP3A4 Inducers

When patients are taking INTUNIV™ concomitantly with a CYP3A4 inducer, an increase in the dose of INTUNIV™ within the recommended dose range may be considered. There was a significant decrease in the rate and extent of guanfacine exposure when co-administered with rifampin, a CYP3A4 inducer. The exposure to guanfacine decreased by 70% (AUC).

7.3 Valproic Acid

Co-administration of guanfacine and valproic acid can result in increased concentrations of valproic acid. The mechanism of this interaction is unknown, although both guanfacine (via a Phase I metabolite, 3-hydroxy guanfacine) and valproic acid are metabolized by glucuronidation, possibly resulting in competitive inhibition. When INTUNIV™ is co-administered with valproic acid, monitor patients for potential additive CNS effects, and consider monitoring serum valproic acid concentrations. Adjustments in the dose of valproic acid may be indicated when co-administered with INTUNIV™.

7.4 Antihypertensive Drugs

Use caution when INTUNIV™ is administered concomitantly with antihypertensive drugs, due to the potential for additive pharmacodynamic effects (e.g., hypotension, syncope) *[see Warnings and Precautions (5.1)]*.

7.5 CNS Depressant Drugs

Caution should be exercised when INTUNIV™ is administered concomitantly with CNS depressant drugs (e.g. alcohol, sedative/hypnotics, benzodiazepines, barbiturates, and antipsychotics) due to the potential for additive pharmacodynamic effects (e.g., sedation, somnolence) *[see Warnings and Precautions (5.2)]*.

8 USE IN SPECIFIC POPULATIONS

8.1 Pregnancy

Pregnancy Category B

Rat experiments have shown that guanfacine crosses the placenta. However, administration of guanfacine to rats and rabbits at 6 and 4 times, respectively, the maximum recommended human dose of 4 mg/day on a mg/m^2 basis resulted in no evidence of harm to the fetus. Higher doses (20 times the maximum recommended human dose in both rabbits and rats) were associated with reduced fetal survival and maternal toxicity. There are no adequate and well-controlled studies of guanfacine in pregnant women. Because animal reproduction studies are not always predictive of human response, this drug should be used during pregnancy only if clearly needed.

8.3 Nursing Mothers

It is not known whether guanfacine is excreted in human milk. Because many drugs are excreted in human milk, caution should be exercised when INTUNIV™ is administered to a nursing woman. Experiments with rats have shown that guanfacine is excreted in the milk.

8.4 Pediatric Use

The safety and efficacy of INTUNIV™ in pediatric patients less than 6 years of age have not been established. For children and adolescents 6 years and older, efficacy beyond 9 weeks and safety beyond 2 years of treatment have not been established *[see Adverse Reactions (6) and Clinical Studies (14)]*.

8.5 Geriatric Use

The safety and efficacy of INTUNIV™ in geriatric patients have not been established.

8.6 Use in Patients with Renal or Hepatic Impairment

Renal Impairment

The impact of renal impairment on the pharmacokinetics of guanfacine in children was not assessed. In adult patients with impaired renal function, the cumulative urinary excretion of guanfacine and the renal clearance diminished as renal function decreased. In patients on hemodialysis, the dialysis clearance was about 15% of the total clearance. The low dialysis clearance suggests that the hepatic elimination (metabolism) increases as renal function decreases. It may be necessary to adjust the dose in patients with significant impairment of renal function.

Hepatic Impairment

The impact of hepatic impairment on PK of guanfacine in children was not assessed. Guanfacine in adults is cleared both by the liver and the kidney, and approximately 50% of the clearance of guanfacine is hepatic. It may be necessary to adjust the dose in patients with significant impairment of hepatic function.

9 DRUG ABUSE AND DEPENDENCE

9.1 Controlled Substance

INTUNIV™ is not a controlled substance and has no known potential for abuse or dependence.

10 OVERDOSAGE

Symptoms

Two cases of accidental overdose of INTUNIV™ were reported in clinical trials in pediatric ADHD patients. These reports included adverse reactions of sedation and bradycardia in one patient and somnolence and dizziness in the other patient.

During post-marketing surveillance of guanfacine as an antihypertensive treatment for adults, drowsiness, lethargy, bradycardia and hypotension have been observed following overdose. Similar symptoms have been described in voluntary reports to the American Association of Poison Control Center's National Poison Data System. Miosis of the pupils may be noted on examination. No fatal overdoses of guanfacine have been reported in published literature.

Treatment

Consult a Certified Poison Control Center for up to date guidance and advice. Gastric lavage may be indicated if performed soon after ingestion. Activated charcoal may be useful in limiting absorption. Guanfacine is not dialyzable in clinically significant amounts (2.4%).

Management of INTUNIV™ overdose should include monitoring for and the treatment of hypotension, bradycardia, lethargy and respiratory depression. Children and adolescents who develop lethargy should be observed for the development of more serious toxicity including coma, bradycardia and hypotension for up to 24 hours, due to the possibility of delayed onset hypotension.

11 DESCRIPTION

INTUNIV™ is a once-daily, extended-release formulation of guanfacine hydrochloride (HCl) in a matrix tablet formulation for oral administration only. The chemical designation is N-amidino-2-(2,6-dichlorophenyl) acetamide monohydrochloride. The molecular formula is $C_9H_9Cl_2N_3O$•HCl corresponding to a molecular weight of 282.55. The chemical structure is:

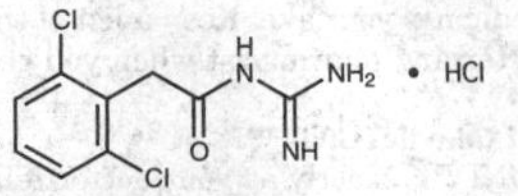

Guanfacine HCl is a white to off-white crystalline powder, sparingly soluble in water (approximately 1 mg/mL) and alcohol and slightly soluble in acetone. The only organic solvent in which it has relatively high solubility is methanol (>30 mg/mL). Each tablet contains guanfacine HCl equivalent to 1 mg, 2 mg, 3 mg, or 4 mg of guanfacine base. The tablets also contain hypromellose, methacrylic acid copolymer, lactose, povidone, crospovidone, microcrystalline cellulose, fumaric acid, and glyceryl behenate. In addition, the 3mg and 4mg tablets also contain green pigment blend PB-1763.

12 CLINICAL PHARMACOLOGY

12.1 Mechanism of Action

Guanfacine is a selective alpha$_{2A}$-adrenergic receptor agonist. Guanfacine is not a central nervous system (CNS) stimulant. The mechanism of action of guanfacine in ADHD is not known.

12.2 Pharmacodynamics

Guanfacine is a selective alpha$_{2A}$-adrenergic receptor agonist in that it has a 15-20 times higher affinity for this receptor subtype than for the alpha$_{2B}$ or alpha$_{2C}$ subtypes.

Guanfacine is a known antihypertensive agent. By stimulating alpha$_{2A}$-adrenergic receptors, guanfacine reduces sympathetic nerve impulses from the vasomotor center to the heart and blood vessels. This results in a decrease in peripheral vascular resistance and a reduction in heart rate.

12.3 Pharmacokinetics

Absorption and Distribution

Guanfacine is readily absorbed and approximately 70% bound to plasma proteins independent of drug concentration. After oral administration of INTUNIV™ the time to peak plasma concentration is approximately 5 hours in children and adolescents with ADHD.

Immediate-release guanfacine and INTUNIV™ have different pharmacokinetic characteristics; dose substitution on a milligram for milligram basis will result in differences in exposure.

A comparison across studies suggests that the C_{max} is 60% lower and $AUC_{0-\infty}$ 43% lower, respectively, for INTUNIV™ compared to immediate-release guanfacine. Therefore, the relative bioavailability of INTUNIV™ to immediate-release guanfacine is 58%. The mean pharmacokinetic parameters in adults following the administration of INTUNIV™ 1 mg once daily and immediate-release guanfacine 1mg once daily are summarized in Table 4.

Table 4: Pharmacokinetic Parameters in Adults

Parameter	INTUNIV™ 1 mg once daily (n=52)	Immediate-release guanfacine 1 mg once daily (n=12)
C_{max} (ng/mL)	1.0 ± 0.3	2.5 ± 0.6
$AUC_{0-\infty}$ (ng.h/mL)	32 ± 9	56 ± 15
t_{max} (h)	6.0 (4.0-8.0)	3.0 (1.5-4.0)
$t_{1/2}$ (h)	18 ± 4	16 ± 3

Note: Values are mean +/- SD, except for t_{max} which is median (range)

Exposure to guanfacine was higher in children (ages 6-12) compared to adolescents (ages 13-17) and adults. After oral administration of multiple doses of INTUNIV™ 4 mg, the C_{max} was 10 ng/mL compared to 7 ng/mL and the AUC was 162 ng h/mL compared to 116 ng h/mL in children (ages 6-12) and adolescents (ages 13-17), respectively. These differences are probably attributable to the lower body weight of children compared to adolescents and adults.

The pharmacokinetics were affected by intake of food when a single dose of INTUNIV™ 4 mg was administered with a high-fat breakfast. The mean exposure increased (C_{max} ~75% and AUC ~40%) compared to dosing in a fasted state.

Dose Proportionality

Following administration of INTUNIV™ in single doses of 1 mg, 2 mg, 3 mg, and 4 mg to adults, C_{max} and $AUC_{0-\infty}$ of guanfacine were proportional to dose.

Metabolism and Elimination

In vitro studies with human liver microsomes and recombinant CYP's demonstrated that guanfacine was primarily metabolized by CYP3A4. In pooled human hepatic microsomes, guanfacine did not inhibit the activities of the major cytochrome P450 isoenzymes (CYP1A2, CYP2C8, CYP2C9, CYP2C19, CYP2D6 or CYP3A4/5). Guanfacine is a substrate of CYP3A4/5 and exposure is affected by CYP3A4/5 inducers/inhibitors.

Renal and Hepatic Impairment

The impact of renal impairment on PK of guanfacine in children was not assessed *[see Use in Specific Populations (8.6)]*.

13 NONCLINICAL TOXICOLOGY

13.1 Carcinogenesis, Mutagenesis, Impairment of Fertility

No carcinogenic effect of guanfacine was observed in studies of 78 weeks in mice or 102 weeks in rats at doses up to 6-7 times the maximum recommended human dose of 4 mg/day on a mg/m^2 basis.

Guanfacine was not genotoxic in a variety of test models, including the Ames test and an *in vitro* chromosomal aberration test; however, a marginal increase in numerical aberrations (polyploidy) was observed in the latter study.

No adverse effects were observed in fertility studies in male and female rats at doses up to 30 times the maximum recommended human dose on a mg/m^2 basis.

14 CLINICAL STUDIES

14.1 Safety and Efficacy Studies

The efficacy of INTUNIV™ in the treatment of ADHD was established in 2 placebo-controlled trials in children and adolescents ages 6-17. Study 1 evaluated 2 mg, 3 mg and 4 mg of INTUNIV™ dosed once daily in an 8-week, double-blind, placebo-controlled, parallel-group, fixed dose design (n=345). Study 2 evaluated 1 mg, 2 mg, 3 mg and 4 mg of INTUNIV™ dosed once daily in a 9-week, double-blind, placebo-controlled, parallel-group, fixed-dose design (n=324). In Studies 1 and 2, patients were randomized to a fixed dose of INTUNIV™ . Doses were titrated in increments of up to 1 mg/week. The lowest dose of 1 mg used in Study 2 was assigned only to patients less than 50 kg (110 lbs). Patients who weighed less than 25 kg (55 lbs) were not included in either study.

	1 mg	2 mg	3 mg	4 mg
Color	White/off-white	White/off-white	Green	Green
Shape	Round	Caplet	Round	Caplet
Debossment (top/bottom)	503 / 1mg	503 / 2mg	503 / 3mg	503 / 4mg
NDC number	54092-513-02	54092-515-02	54092-517-02	54092-519-02

Signs and symptoms of ADHD were evaluated on a once weekly basis using the clinician administered and scored ADHD Rating Scale-IV (ADHD-RS), which includes both hyperactive/impulsive and inattentive subscales. In both studies, the primary outcome was the change from baseline to endpoint in mean ADHD-RS scores.

The mean reductions in ADHD-RS scores at endpoint were statistically significantly greater for INTUNIV™ compared to placebo for Studies 1 and 2. Placebo-adjusted changes from baseline were statistically significant for each of the 2 mg, 3 mg, and 4 mg INTUNIV™ randomized treatment groups in both studies, as well as the 1 mg INTUNIV™ treatment group (for patients 55-110 lbs) that was included only in Study 2.

Dose-responsive efficacy was evident, particularly when data were examined on a weight-adjusted (mg/kg) basis. When evaluated over the dose range of 0.01-0.17 mg/kg/day, clinically relevant improvements were observed beginning at doses in the range 0.05-0.08 mg/kg/day. Doses up to 0.12 mg/kg/day were shown to provide additional benefit. Controlled, long-term efficacy studies (>9 weeks) have not been conducted.

Subgroup analyses were performed to identify any differences in response based on gender or age (6-12 vs. 13-17). Analyses of the primary outcome did not suggest any differential responsiveness on the basis of gender. Analyses by age subgroup revealed a statistically significant treatment effect only in the 6-12 age subgroup. Due to the relatively small proportion of adolescent patients (ages 13-17) enrolled into these studies (approximately 25%), these data may not be sufficient to demonstrate efficacy in the adolescent subgroup. In these studies, patients were randomized to a fixed dose of INTUNIV™ rather than optimized by body weight. Therefore, it is likely that some adolescent patients were randomized to a dose that resulted in relatively low plasma guanfacine concentrations compared to the younger subgroup. Over half (55%) of the adolescent patients received doses of 0.01-0.04mg/kg. In studies in which systematic pharmacokinetic data were obtained, there was a strong inverse correlation between body weight and plasma guanfacine concentrations.

16   HOW SUPPLIED/STORAGE AND HANDLING

INTUNIV™ is supplied in 1 mg, 2 mg, 3 mg, and 4 mg strength extended-release tablets in 100 count bottles. [See table above]
Storage -Store at 25°C (77°F); excursions permitted to 15° to 30°C (59° to 86°F). See USP Controlled Room Temperature.

17   PATIENT COUNSELING INFORMATION
[See FDA-Approved Patient Labeling.]
17.1   Dosing and Administration
Instruct patients to swallow INTUNIV™ whole with water, milk or other liquid. **Tablets should not be crushed, chewed or broken prior to administration because this may increase the rate of release of the active drug.** Patients should not take INTUNIV™ together with a high-fat meal, since this can raise blood levels of INTUNIV™. Instruct the parent or caregiver to supervise the child or adolescent taking INTUNIV™ and to keep the bottle of tablets out of reach of children.

Instruct patients on how to properly taper the medication, if the physician decides to discontinue treatment.

17.2   Adverse Reactions
Advise patients that sedation can occur, particularly early in treatment or with dose increases. Caution against operating heavy equipment or driving until they know how they respond to treatment with INTUNIV™. Headache and abdominal pain can also occur. If any of these symptoms persist, or other symptoms occur, the patient should be advised to discuss the symptoms with the physician.

Advise patients to avoid becoming dehydrated or overheated, and to avoid use with alcohol.

Patient Information
INTUNIV™ (in-TOO-niv)
(guanfacine)
Extended-Release Tablets
Read the Patient Information that comes with INTUNIV™ before you start taking it and each time you get a refill. There may be new information. **This leaflet does not take the place of talking with your doctor about your medical condition or your treatment.**

What is INTUNIV™?
INTUNIV™ is a prescription medicine used to treat the symptoms of attention deficit/hyperactivity disorder (ADHD).
INTUNIV™ is not a central nervous system (CNS) stimulant.
INTUNIV™ should be used as a part of a total treatment program for ADHD that may include counselling or other therapies.
It is not known if INTUNIV™ is effective:
• for use longer than 9 weeks
It is not known if INTUNIV™ is safe or effective:
• in children younger than 6 years old
• in adults

What should I tell my doctor before taking INTUNIV™?
Before you take INTUNIV™, tell your doctor if you:
• have heart problems or a low heart rate
• have fainted
• have low blood pressure
• have liver or kidney problems
• have any other medical conditions
• are pregnant or plan to become pregnant. It is not known if INTUNIV™ will harm your unborn baby. Talk to your doctor if you are pregnant or plan to become pregnant.
• are breast-feeding or plan to breast-feed. It is not known if INTUNIV™ passes into your breast milk. You and your doctor should decide if you will take INTUNIV™ or breastfeed.

Tell your doctor about all of the medicines you take, including prescription and non-prescription medicines, vitamins, and herbal supplements.
INTUNIV™ may affect the way other medicines work, and other medicines may affect how INTUNIV™ works.
Especially tell your doctor if you take:
• ketoconazole
• medicines that can affect enzyme metabolism
• valproic acid
• high blood pressure medicine
• sedatives
• benzodiazepines
• barbiturates
• antipsychotics
Ask your doctor or pharmacist for a list of these medicines, if you are not sure.
Know the medicines you take. Keep a list of them and show it to your doctor and pharmacist when you get a new medicine.

How should I take INTUNIV™?
• Take INTUNIV™ exactly as your doctor tells you.
• Your doctor may change your dose. Do not change your dose of INTUNIV™ without talking to your doctor.
• Do not stop taking INTUNIV™ without talking to your doctor.
• INTUNIV™ should be taken 1 time a day.
• INTUNIV™ should be swallowed whole with a small amount of water, milk, or other liquid.
• Do not crush, chew, or break INTUNIV™. Tell your doctor if you can not swallow INTUNIV™ whole.
• Do not take INTUNIV™ with a high-fat meal.
• Your doctor will check your blood pressure and heart rate while you take INTUNIV™.
• If you take too much INTUNIV™, call your local Poison Control Center or go to the nearest emergency room right away.

What should I avoid while taking INTUNIV™?
• Do not drive, operate heavy machinery, or do other dangerous activities until you know how INTUNIV™ affects you. INTUNIV™ can slow your thinking and motor skills.
• Do not drink alcohol or take other medicines that make you sleepy or dizzy while taking INTUNIV™ until you talk with your doctor. INTUNIV™ taken with alcohol or medicines that cause sleepiness or dizziness may make your sleepiness or dizziness worse.

What are the possible side effects of INTUNIV™?
INTUNIV™ may cause serious side effects including:
• low blood pressure
• low heart rate
• fainting
• sleepiness
• tiredness
• drowsiness

Get medical help right away, if you have any of the symptoms listed above.
The most common side effects of INTUNIV™ include:
• sleepiness
• drowsiness
• low blood pressure
• headache
• nausea
• stomach pain
• dry mouth
• dizziness
• irritability
• constipation
• not hungry (decreased appetite)
Tell the doctor if you have any side effect that bothers you or that does not go away.
These are not all the possible side effects of INTUNIV™. For more information, ask your doctor or pharmacist.
Call your doctor for medical advice about side effects. You may report side effects to FDA at 1-800-FDA-1088.
How should I store INTUNIV™?
• Store INTUNIV™ between 59°F to 86°F (15°C to 30°C)
Keep INTUNIV™ and all medicines out of the reach of children.
General Information about INTUNIV™
Medicines are sometimes prescribed for purposes other than those listed in a Patient Information Leaflet. Do not use INTUNIV™ for a condition for which it was not prescribed. Do not give INTUNIV™ to other people, even if they have the same symptoms that you have. It may harm them.
This leaflet summarizes the most important information about INTUNIV™. If you would like more information, talk with your doctor. You can ask your pharmacist or doctor for information about INTUNIV™ that is written for health professionals.
For more information, go to **www.INTUNIV.com** or call **1-800-828-2088.**
What are the ingredients in INTUNIV™?
Active ingredient: guanfacine hydrochloride
Inactive ingredients: hypromellose, methacrylic acid copolymer, lactose, povidone, crospovidone, microcrystalline cellulose, fumaric acid, and glycerol behenate. In addition, the 3mg and 4mg tablets also contain green pigment blend PB-1763.
Manufactured for Shire US Inc., Wayne, PA 19087.
INTUNIV™ is a trademark of Shire LLC.
©2009 Shire Pharmaceuticals Inc.
This product is covered by US patents including 5,854,290; 6,287,599; 6,811,794.
Version: August 2009
Shown in Product Identification Guide, page 319

LIALDA™   ℞
[li-al-da]
(mesalamine)
Delayed Release Tablets
Prescribing Information

DESCRIPTION

Each **LIALDA** delayed release tablet for oral administration contains 1.2g 5-aminosalicylic acid (5-ASA; mesalamine), an anti-inflammatory agent. Mesalamine also has the chemical name 5-amino-2-hydroxybenzoic acid and its structural formula is:

Molecular formula: $C_7H_7NO_3$
Molecular weight: 153.14
The tablet is coated with a gastro-resistant pH dependent polymer film, which breaks down at or above pH 7, normally in the terminal ileum where mesalamine then begins to be released from the tablet core. The tablet core contains mesalamine with hydrophilic and lipophilic excipients.
The inactive ingredients of **LIALDA** tablets are sodium carboxymethylcellulose, carnauba wax, stearic acid, silica (colloidal hydrated), sodium starch glycolate (type A), talc, magnesium stearate, methacrylic acid copolymer types A and B, triethylcitrate, titanium dioxide, red ferric oxide and polyethyleneglycol 6000.

CLINICAL PHARMACOLOGY
The mechanism of action of mesalamine is not fully understood, but appears to be topical. Mucosal production of arachidonic acid metabolites, both through the cyclooxygenase and lipoxygenase pathways, is increased in patients with chronic inflammatory bowel disease, and it is possible that mesalamine diminishes inflammation by blocking cyclooxygenase and inhibiting prostaglandin production in the

colon. Recent data also suggest that mesalamine can inhibit the activation of NFκB, a nuclear transcription factor that regulates the transcription of many genes for pro-inflammatory proteins.

Pharmacokinetics

Absorption: The total absorption of mesalamine from **LIALDA** 2.4g or 4.8g given once daily for 14 days to healthy volunteers was found to be approximately 21-22% of the administered dose.

Gamma-scintigraphy studies have shown that a single dose of **LIALDA** 1.2g (one tablet) passed intact through the upper gastrointestinal tract of fasted healthy volunteers. Scintigraphic images showed a trail of radio-labeled tracer in the colon, suggesting that mesalamine had distributed throughout this region of the gastrointestinal tract.

In a single dose study, **LIALDA** 1.2g, 2.4g and 4.8g were administered in the fasted state to healthy subjects. Plasma concentrations of mesalamine were detectable after 2 hours and reached a maximum by 9-12 hours on average for the doses studied. The pharmacokinetic parameters are highly variable among subjects (Table 1). Mesalamine systemic exposure in terms of area under the plasma concentration-time curve (AUC) was slightly more than dose proportional between 1.2g and 4.8g **LIALDA**. Maximum plasma concentrations (C_{max}) of mesalamine increased approximately dose proportionately between 1.2g and 2.4g and subproportionately between 2.4g and 4.8g **LIALDA,** with the dose normalized value at 4.8g representing, on average, 74% of that at 2.4g based on geometric means.

[See table 1 above]

Table 1: Mean (SD) PK Parameters for Mesalamine Following Single Dose Administration of LIALDA Under Fasting Conditions

Parameter[1] of Mesalamine	LIALDA 1.2g (N=47)	LIALDA 2.4g (N=48)	LIALDA 4.8g (N=48)
AUC_{0-t} (ng.h/mL)	9039^{+} (5054)	20538 (12980)	41434 (26640)
$AUC_{0-\infty}$ (ng.h/mL)	9578• (5214)	21084 (13185)	44775$^{\#}$ (30302)
C_{max} (ng/mL)	857 (638)	1595 (1484)	2154 (1140)
T_{max}* (h)	9.0** (4.0-32.1)	12.0 (4.0-34.1)	12.0 (4.0-34.0)
T_{lag}* (h)	2.0** (0-8.0)	2.0 (1.0-4.0)	2.0 (1.0-4.0)
$T_{½}$ (h) (Terminal Phase)	8.56 (6.38)	7.05§ (5.54)	7.25$^{\#}$ (8.32)

[1] Arithmetic mean of parameter values are presented except for T_{max} and T_{lag}.
*Median (min, max); $^{+}$N=43, • N=27, §N=33, $^{\#}$N=36, **N=46

Administration of a single dose of **LIALDA** 4.8g with a high fat meal resulted in further delay in absorption and plasma concentrations of mesalamine were detectable 4 hours following dosing. However, high fat meal increased systemic exposure of mesalamine (mean C_{max}: ↑ 91%; mean AUC: ↑ 16%) compared to results in the fasted state. **LIALDA** was administered with food in the Phase 3 trials.

In a single and multiple dose pharmacokinetic study of **LIALDA** 2.4g or 4.8g was administered once daily with standard meals to 28 healthy volunteers per dose group. Plasma concentrations of mesalamine were detectable after 4 hours and were maximal by 8 hours after the single dose. Steady state was achieved generally by 2 days after dosing. Mean AUC at steady state was only modestly greater (1.1- to 1.4-fold) than predictable from single dose pharmacokinetics.

Distribution: Mesalamine is approximately 43% bound to plasma proteins at the concentration of 2.5 μg/mL.

Metabolism: The major metabolite of mesalamine (5-aminosalicylic acid) is N-acetyl-5-aminosalicylic acid. Its formation is brought about by N-acetyltransferase activity in the liver and intestinal mucosa.

Elimination: Elimination of mesalamine is mainly via the renal route following metabolism to N-acetyl-5-aminosalicylic acid (acetylation). However, there is also limited excretion of the parent drug in urine. Of the approximately 21-22% of the dose absorbed, less than 8% of the dose was excreted unchanged in the urine, compared with greater than 13% for N-acetyl-5-aminosalicylic acid. The apparent terminal half-lives for mesalamine and its major metabolite after administration of **LIALDA** 2.4g and 4.8g were, on average, 7-9 hours and 8-12 hours, respectively.

Special Populations

Geriatrics: No pharmacokinetic information is available in patients who are 65 years or older (see **PRECAUTIONS**).

Pediatrics: No pharmacokinetic information is available in patients who are less than 18 years of age (see **PRECAUTIONS**).

Gender: No consistent trend on gender effect was observed in the clinical trials.

Renal Insufficiency: No information is available in patients with mild, moderate, and severe renal impairment (see **PRECAUTIONS**).

Hepatic Insufficiency: No information is available for patients with hepatic impairment (see **PRECAUTIONS**).

Race: No pharmacokinetic information is available which examines **LIALDA** in different races.

Drug-Drug Interaction

There are no data available on interactions between **LIALDA** and other drugs. However, there have been reports of interaction between other mesalamine medications and other drugs (see **PRECAUTIONS**).

CLINICAL TRIALS

Active, Mild to Moderate Ulcerative Colitis

Two similarly designed, randomized, double blind, placebo-controlled trials were conducted in 517 adult patients with active, mild to moderate ulcerative colitis. The study population was primarily Caucasian (80%), had a mean age of 42 years (6% age 65 years or older), and was approximately 50% male. Both studies used **LIALDA** doses of 2.4g/day and 4.8g/day administered once daily for 8 weeks except for the 2.4g/day group in Study 1, which was given in two divided doses (1.2g BID). The primary efficacy end-point in both trials was to compare the percentage of patients in remission after 8 weeks of treatment for the **LIALDA** treatment groups vs placebo. Remission was defined as an Ulcerative Colitis Disease Activity Index (UC-DAI) of ≤ 1, with scores of zero for rectal bleeding and for stool frequency, and a sigmoidoscopy score reduction of 1 point or more from baseline.

In both studies, the **LIALDA** doses of 2.4g/day and 4.8g/day demonstrated superiority over placebo in the primary efficacy endpoint (Table 2). Both **LIALDA** doses also provided consistent benefit in secondary efficacy parameters, including clinical improvement, treatment failure, clinical remission, and sigmoidoscopic improvement. **LIALDA** 2.4g/day and 4.8g/day had similar efficacy profiles.

Table 2: Patients in Remission at Week 8

Dose	Study 1	Study 2
	(n=262)	(n=255)
	n/N (%)	n/N (%)
LIALDA 2.4g/day	30/88 (34.1)	34/84 (40.5)
LIALDA 4.8g/day	26/89 (29.2)	35/85 (41.2)
Placebo	11/85 (12.9)	19/86 (22.1)

INDICATIONS AND USAGE

LIALDA tablets are indicated for the induction of remission in patients with active, mild to moderate ulcerative colitis. Safety and effectiveness of **LIALDA** beyond 8 weeks has not been established.

CONTRAINDICATIONS

LIALDA is contraindicated in patients with hypersensitivity to salicylates (including mesalamine) or to any of the components of **LIALDA**.

PRECAUTIONS

General: Patients with pyloric stenosis may have prolonged gastric retention of **LIALDA**, which could delay mesalamine release in the colon.

The majority of patients who are intolerant or hypersensitive to sulfasalazine can take mesalamine medications without risk of similar reactions. However, caution should be exercised when treating patients allergic to sulfasalazine.

Mesalamine has been associated with an acute intolerance syndrome that may be difficult to distinguish from a flare of inflammatory bowel disease. Although the exact frequency of occurrence has not been determined, it has occurred in 3% of patients in controlled clinical trials of mesalamine or sulfasalazine. Symptoms include cramping, acute abdominal pain and bloody diarrhea, sometimes fever, headache and rash. If acute intolerance syndrome is suspected, prompt withdrawal is required.

Mesalamine-induced cardiac hypersensitivity reactions (myocarditis and pericarditis) have been reported with LIALDA and other mesalamine medications. Caution should be taken in prescribing this medication to patients with conditions predisposing to the development of myocarditis or pericarditis.

Renal: Reports of renal impairment, including minimal change nephropathy, and acute or chronic interstitial nephritis have been associated with mesalamine medications and prodrugs of mesalamine. For any patient with known renal dysfunction, caution should be exercised and **LIALDA** should be used only if the benefits outweigh the risks. It is recommended that all patients have an evaluation of renal function prior to initiation of therapy and periodically while on treatment. In animal studies with mesalamine, a 13-week oral toxicity study in mice and 13-week and 52-week oral toxicity studies in rats and cynomolgus monkeys have shown the kidney to be the major target organ of mesalamine toxicity. Oral daily doses of 2400 mg/kg in mice and 1150 mg/kg in rats produced renal lesions including granular and hyaline casts, tubular degeneration, tubular dilation, renal infarct, papillary necrosis, tubular necrosis, and interstitial nephritis. In cynomolgus monkeys, oral daily doses of 250 mg/kg or higher produced nephrosis, papillary edema, and interstitial fibrosis.

Information for Patients: Patients should be instructed to swallow **LIALDA** tablets whole, taking care not to break the outer coating. The outer coating is designed to remain intact to protect the active ingredient, mesalamine, and ensure its availability throughout the colon.

Hepatic Impairment: No information is available on patients with hepatic impairment, and therefore, caution is recommended in these patients.

Drug Interaction: No investigations have been performed between **LIALDA** and other drugs. However, the following are reports of interactions between mesalamine medications and other drugs. The concurrent use of mesalamine with known nephrotoxic agents, including non-steroidal anti-inflammatory drugs (NSAIDs) may increase the risk of renal reactions. In patients receiving azathioprine or 6-mercaptopurine, concurrent use of mesalamine can increase the potential for blood disorders.

Carcinogenesis, Mutagenesis, Impairment of Fertility: In a 104-week dietary carcinogenicity study in CD-1 mice, mesalamine at doses up to 2500 mg/kg/day was not tumorigenic. This dose is 2.2 times the maximum recommended human dose (based on a body surface area comparison) of **LIALDA**. Furthermore, in a 104-week dietary carcinogenicity study in Wistar rats, mesalamine up to a dose of 800 mg/kg/day was not tumorigenic. This dose is 1.4 times the recommended human dose (based on a body surface area comparison) of **LIALDA**.

No evidence of mutagenicity was observed in an *in vitro* Ames test or an *in vivo* mouse micronucleus test.

No effects on fertility or reproductive performance were observed in male or female rats at oral doses of mesalamine up to 400 mg/kg/day (0.7 times the maximum recommended human dose based on a body surface area comparison). Semen abnormalities and infertility in men, which have been reported in association with sulfasalazine, have not been seen with other mesalamine products during controlled clinical trials.

Pregnancy:

Teratogenic Effects: Pregnancy Category B

Reproduction studies with mesalamine have been performed in rats at doses up to 1000 mg/kg/day (1.8 times the maximum recommended human dose based on a body surface area comparison) and rabbits at doses up to 800 mg/kg/day (2.9 times the maximum recommended human dose based on a body surface area comparison) and have revealed no evidence of impaired fertility or harm to the fetus due to mesalamine. There are, however, no adequate and well-controlled studies in pregnant women. Because animal reproduction studies are not always predictive of human response, this drug should be used during pregnancy only if clearly needed. Mesalamine is known to cross the placental barrier.

Nursing Mothers: Low concentrations of mesalamine and higher concentrations of its N-acetyl metabolite have been detected in human breast milk. While there is limited experience of lactating women using mesalamine, caution should be exercised if **LIALDA** is administered to a nursing mother, and used only if the benefits outweigh the risks.

Pediatric Use: Safety and effectiveness of **LIALDA** tablets in pediatric patients who are less than 18 years of age have not been studied.

Geriatric Use: Clinical trials of **LIALDA** did not include sufficient numbers of patients aged 65 and over to determine whether they respond differently from younger patients. Other reported clinical experience has not identified differences in responses between the elderly and younger patients. In general, dose selection for an elderly patient should be cautious, usually starting at the low end of the dosing range, reflecting the greater frequency of decreased hepatic, renal, or cardiac function, and of concurrent disease or other drug therapy.

ADVERSE REACTIONS

LIALDA tablets have been evaluated in 655 ulcerative colitis patients in controlled and open-label trials.

In two 8-week placebo-controlled clinical trials involving 535 ulcerative colitis patients, 356 received 2.4g/day or 4.8g/day **LIALDA** tablets and 179 received placebo. More treatment emergent adverse events occurred in the placebo group (119) than in each of the **LIALDA** treatment groups (109 in 2.4g/day, 92 in 4.8g/day). A lower percentage of **LIALDA** patients discontinued therapy due to adverse events compared to placebo (2.2% vs 7.3%). The most frequent adverse event leading to discontinuation from **LIALDA** therapy was exacerbation of ulcerative colitis (0.8%).

The majority of adverse events in the double blind, placebo-controlled trials were mild or moderate in severity. The percentage of patients with severe adverse events was higher in the placebo group (6.1% in placebo; 1.1% in 2.4g/day; 2.2% in 4.8g/day). The most common severe adverse events were gastrointestinal disorders which were mainly symptoms associated with ulcerative colitis. Pancreatitis occurred in less than 1% of patients during clinical trials and resulted in discontinuation of therapy with **LIALDA** in patients experiencing this event.

Overall, the percentage of patients who experienced any adverse event was similar across treatment groups. Treatment related adverse events occurring in **LIALDA** or placebo groups at a frequency of at least 1% in two Phase 3, 8-week, double blind, placebo-controlled trials are listed in Table 3. The most common treatment related adverse events with **LIALDA** 2.4g/day and 4.8g/day were headache (5.6% and 3.4%, respectively) and flatulence (4% and 2.8%, respectively).

Table 3. Treatment Related Adverse Events in Two Phase 3 Trials Experienced by at Least 1% of the LIALDA Group and at a Rate Greater than Placebo

Event	LIALDA 2.4g/day (n = 177)	LIALDA 4.8g/day (n = 179)	Placebo (n = 179)
Headache	10 (5.6%)	6 (3.4%)	1 (0.6%)
Flatulence	7 (4%)	5 (2.8%)	5 (2.8%)
Increased alanine aminotransferase	1 (0.6%)	2 (1.1%)	0
Alopecia	0	2 (1.1%)	0
Pruritis	1 (0.6%)	2 (1.1%)	0

The following treatment-related adverse events, presented by body system, were reported infrequently (less than 1%) by **LIALDA**-treated ulcerative colitis patients in controlled trials.

Cardiovascular and Vascular: tachycardia, hypertension, hypotension

Dermatological: acne, prurigo, rash, urticaria

Gastrointestinal Disorders: abdominal distention, diarrhea, pancreatitis, rectal polyp, vomiting

Hematologic: decreased platelet count

Hepatobiliary Disorders: elevated total bilirubin

Musculoskeletal and Connective Tissue Disorders: arthralgia, back pain

Nervous System Disorders: somnolence, tremor

Respiratory, Thoracic and Mediastinal Disorders: pharyngolaryngeal pain

General Disorders and Administrative Site Disorders: asthenia, face edema, fatigue, pyrexia

Special Senses: ear pain

Post Marketing Experience

The following adverse reactions have been identified during post-approval use of Lialda in clinical practice. Because these reactions are reported voluntarily from a population of uncertain size, it is not always possible to reliably estimate their frequency or establish a causal relationship to drug exposure.

Cardiac Disorders: Myocarditis and pericarditis.

Hepatobiliary Disorders: Hepatitis

Renal Disorders: Interstitial nephritis

Respiratory, Thoracic and Mediastinal Disorders: Hypersensitivity pneumonitis (including interstitial pneumonitis, allergic alveolitis, eosinophilic pneumonitis).

DRUG ABUSE AND DEPENDENCY

Abuse: None reported.

Dependency: Drug dependence has not been reported with chronic administration of mesalamine.

OVERDOSAGE

LIALDA is an aminosalicylate, and symptoms of salicylate toxicity may include tinnitus, vertigo, headache, confusion, drowsiness, sweating, hyperventilation, vomiting, and diarrhea. Severe intoxication may lead to disruption of electrolyte balance and blood-pH, hyperthermia, and dehydration. Conventional therapy for salicylate toxicity may be beneficial in the event of acute overdosage. This includes prevention of further gastrointestinal tract absorption by emesis and, if necessary, by gastric lavage. Fluid and electrolyte imbalance should be corrected by the administration of appropriate intravenous therapy. Adequate renal function should be maintained.

DOSAGE AND ADMINISTRATION

The recommended dosage for the induction of remission in adult patients with active, mild to moderate ulcerative colitis is two to four 1.2g tablets to be taken once daily with meal for a total daily dose of 2.4g or 4.8g. Treatment duration in controlled clinical trials was up to 8 weeks.

HOW SUPPLIED

LIALDA tablets are available as red-brown ellipsoidal film coated tablets containing 1.2g mesalamine, and debossed on one side with S476.

NDC 54092-476-12 Bottle of 120 tablets

Store at room temperature 15°C to 25°C (59°F to 77°F); excursions permitted to 30°C (86°F). See USP Controlled Room Temperature.

Manufactured for **Shire US Inc.**,
725 Chesterbrook Blvd., Wayne, PA 19087, USA.

U.S. Patent No. 6,773,720. by license of Giuliani S.p.A., Milan, Italy.

476 1207 002B N7600A Rev. 6/09 GIPI1

Shown in Product Identification Guide, page 319

PENTASA® ℞

[*pĕn-tā-să*]
(mesalamine)
Controlled-Release Capsules 250 mg and 500 mg
Rx only

Prescribing Information as of June 2008

DESCRIPTION

PENTASA (mesalamine) for oral administration is a controlled-release formulation of mesalamine, an aminosalicylate anti-inflammatory agent for gastrointestinal use. Chemically, mesalamine is 5-amino-2-hydroxybenzoic acid. It has a molecular weight of 153.14.

The structural formula is:

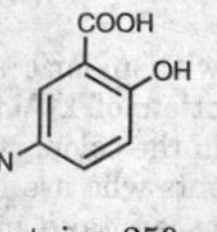

Each 250 mg capsule contains 250 mg of mesalamine. It also contains the following inactive ingredients: acetylated monoglyceride, castor oil, colloidal silicon dioxide, ethylcellulose, hydroxypropyl methylcellulose, starch, stearic acid, sugar, talc, and white wax. The capsule shell contains D&C Yellow #10, FD&C Blue #1, FD&C Green #3, gelatin, titanium dioxide, and other ingredients.

Each 500 mg capsule contains 500 mg of mesalamine. It also contains the following inactive ingredients: acetylated monoglyceride, castor oil, colloidal silicon dioxide, ethylcellulose, hydroxypropyl methylcellulose, starch, stearic acid, sugar, talc, and white wax. The capsule shell contains FD&C Blue #1, gelatin, titanium dioxide, and other ingredients.

CLINICAL PHARMACOLOGY

Sulfasalazine is split by bacterial action in the colon into sulfapyridine (SP) and mesalamine (5-ASA). It is thought that the mesalamine component is therapeutically active in ulcerative colitis. The usual oral dose of sulfasalazine for active ulcerative colitis in adults is 2 to 4 g per day in divided doses. Four grams of sulfasalazine provide 1.6 g of free mesalamine to the colon.

The mechanism of action of mesalamine (and sulfasalazine) is unknown, but appears to be topical rather than systemic. Mucosal production of arachidonic acid (AA) metabolites, both through the cyclooxygenase pathways, ie, prostanoids, and through the lipoxygenase pathways, ie, leukotrienes (LTs) and hydroxyeicosatetraenoic acids (HETEs), is increased in patients with chronic inflammatory bowel disease, and it is possible that mesalamine diminishes inflammation by blocking cyclooxygenase and inhibiting prostaglandin (PG) production in the colon.

Human Pharmacokinetics and Metabolism

Absorption. PENTASA is an ethylcellulose-coated, controlled-release formulation of mesalamine designed to release therapeutic quantities of mesalamine throughout the gastrointestinal tract. Based on urinary excretion data, 20% to 30% of the mesalamine in PENTASA is absorbed. In contrast, when mesalamine is administered orally as an unformulated 1-g aqueous suspension, mesalamine is approximately 80% absorbed.

Plasma mesalamine concentration peaked at approximately 1 µg/mL 3 hours following a 1-g PENTASA dose and declined in a biphasic manner. The literature describes a mean terminal half-life of 42 minutes for mesalamine following intravenous administration. Because of the continuous release and absorption of mesalamine from PENTASA throughout the gastrointestinal tract, the true elimination half-life cannot be determined after oral administration. N-acetylmesalamine, the major metabolite of mesalamine, peaked at approximately 3 hours at 1.8 µg/mL, and its concentration followed a biphasic decline. Pharmacological activities of N-acetylmesalamine are unknown, and other metabolites have not been identified.

Oral mesalamine pharmacokinetics were nonlinear when PENTASA capsules were dosed from 250 mg to 1 g four times daily, with steady-state mesalamine plasma concentrations increasing about nine times, from 0.14 µg/mL to 1.21 µg/mL, suggesting saturable first-pass metabolism. N-acetylmesalamine pharmacokinetics were linear.

Elimination. About 130 mg free mesalamine was recovered in the feces following a single 1-g PENTASA dose, which was comparable to the 140 mg of mesalamine recovered from the molar equivalent sulfasalazine tablet dose of 2.5 g. Elimination of free mesalamine and salicylates in feces increased proportionately with PENTASA dose. N-acetylmesalamine was the primary compound excreted in the urine (19% to 30%) following PENTASA dosing.

CLINICAL TRIALS

In two randomized, double-blind, placebo-controlled, dose-response trials (UC-1 and UC-2) of 625 patients with active mild to moderate ulcerative colitis, PENTASA, at an oral dose of 4 g/day given 1 g four times daily, produced consistent improvement in prospectively identified primary efficacy parameters, PGA, Tx F, and SI as shown in the table below.

The 4-g dose of PENTASA also gave consistent improvement in secondary efficacy parameters, namely the frequency of trips to the toilet, stool consistency, rectal bleeding, abdominal/rectal pain, and urgency. The 4-g dose of PENTASA induced remission as assessed by endoscopic and symptomatic endpoints.

In some patients, the 2-g dose of PENTASA was observed to improve efficacy parameters measured. However, the 2-g dose gave inconsistent results in primary efficacy parameters across the two adequate and well-controlled trials.

[See first table at top of next page]

INDICATIONS AND USAGE

PENTASA is indicated for the induction of remission and for the treatment of patients with mildly to moderately active ulcerative colitis.

CONTRAINDICATIONS

PENTASA is contraindicated in patients who have demonstrated hypersensitivity to mesalamine, any other components of this medication, or salicylates.

PRECAUTIONS

General

Caution should be exercised if PENTASA is administered to patients with impaired hepatic function.

Mesalamine has been associated with an acute intolerance syndrome that may be difficult to distinguish from a flare of inflammatory bowel disease. Although the exact frequency of occurrence cannot be ascertained, it has occurred in 3% of patients in controlled clinical trials of mesalamine or sulfasalazine. Symptoms include cramping, acute abdominal pain and bloody diarrhea, sometimes fever, headache, and rash. If acute intolerance syndrome is suspected, prompt withdrawal is required. If a rechallenge is performed later in order to validate the hypersensitivity, it should be carried out under close medical supervision at reduced dose and only if clearly needed.

Renal

Caution should be exercised if PENTASA is administered to patients with impaired renal function. Single reports of nephrotic syndrome and interstitial nephritis associated with mesalamine therapy have been described in the foreign literature. There have been rare reports of interstitial nephritis in patients receiving PENTASA. In animal studies, a 13-week oral toxicity study in mice and 13-week and 52-week oral toxicity studies in rats and cynomolgus monkeys have shown the kidney to be the major target organ of mesalamine toxicity. Oral daily doses of 2400 mg/kg in mice and 1150 mg/kg in rats produced renal lesions including granular and hyaline casts, tubular degeneration, tubular dilation, renal infarct, papillary necrosis, tubular necrosis, and interstitial nephritis. In cynomolgus monkeys, oral daily doses of 250 mg/kg or higher produced nephrosis, papillary edema, and interstitial fibrosis. Patients with pre-existing renal disease, increased BUN or serum creatinine, or proteinuria should be carefully monitored, especially during the initial phase of treatment. Mesalamine-induced nephrotoxicity should be suspected in patients developing renal dysfunction during treatment.

Drug Interactions
There are no data on interactions between PENTASA and other drugs.

Carcinogenesis, Mutagenesis, Impairment of Fertility
In a 104-week dietary carcinogenicity study of mesalamine, CD-1 mice were treated with doses up to 2500 mg/kg/day and it was not tumorigenic. For a 50 kg person of average height (1.46 m² body surface area), this represents 2.5 times the recommended human dose on a body surface area basis (2960 mg/m²/day). In a 104-week dietary carcinogenicity study in Wistar rats, mesalamine up to a dose of 800 mg/kg/day was not tumorigenic. This dose represents 1.5 times the recommended human dose on a body surface area basis.

No evidence of mutagenicity was observed in an in vitro Ames test and an in vivo mouse micronucleus test.

No effects on fertility or reproductive performance were observed in male or female rats at oral doses of mesalamine up to 400 mg/kg/day (0.8 times the recommended human dose based on body surface area).

Semen abnormalities and infertility in men, which have been reported in association with sulfasalazine, have not been seen with PENTASA capsules during controlled clinical trials.

Pregnancy
Category B. Reproduction studies have been performed in rats at doses up to 1000 mg/kg/day (5900 mg/M²) and rabbits at doses of 800 mg/kg/day (6856 mg/M²) and have revealed no evidence of teratogenic effects or harm to the fetus due to mesalamine. There are, however, no adequate and well-controlled studies in pregnant women. Because animal reproduction studies are not always predictive of human response, PENTASA should be used during pregnancy only if clearly needed.

Mesalamine is known to cross the placental barrier.

Nursing Mothers
Minute quantities of mesalamine were distributed to breast milk and amniotic fluid of pregnant women following sulfasalazine therapy. When treated with sulfasalazine at a dose equivalent to 1.25 g/day of mesalamine, 0.02 μg/mL to 0.08 μg/mL and trace amounts of mesalamine were measured in amniotic fluid and breast milk, respectively. N-acetylmesalamine, in quantities of 0.07 μg/mL to 0.77 μg/mL and 1.13 μg/mL to 3.44 μg/mL, was identified in the same fluids, respectively.

Caution should be exercised when PENTASA is administered to a nursing woman.

No controlled studies with PENTASA during breast-feeding have been carried out. Hypersensitivity reactions like diarrhea in the infant cannot be excluded.

Pediatric Use
Safety and efficacy of PENTASA in pediatric patients have not been established.

ADVERSE REACTIONS
In combined domestic and foreign clinical trials, more than 2100 patients with ulcerative colitis or Crohn's disease received PENTASA therapy. Generally, PENTASA therapy was well tolerated. The most common events (ie, greater than or equal to 1%) were diarrhea (3.4%), headache (2.0%), nausea (1.8%), abdominal pain (1.7%), dyspepsia (1.6%), vomiting (1.5%), and rash (1.0%).

In two domestic placebo-controlled trials involving over 600 ulcerative colitis patients, adverse events were fewer in PENTASA-treated patients than in the placebo group (PENTASA 14% vs placebo 18%) and were not dose-related. Events occurring at 1% or more are shown in the table below. Of these, only nausea and vomiting were more frequent in the PENTASA group. Withdrawal from therapy due to adverse events was more common on placebo than PENTASA (7% vs 4%).

[See table 1 above]

Clinical laboratory measurements showed no significant abnormal trends for any test, including measurement of hematological, liver, and kidney function.

The following adverse events, presented by body system, were reported infrequently (ie, less than 1%) during domestic ulcerative colitis and Crohn's disease trials. In many cases, the relationship to PENTASA has not been established.

Parameter Evaluated	Clinical Trial UC-1			Clinical Trial UC-2		
		PENTASA			PENTASA	
	PL (n=90)	4 g/day (n=95)	2 g/day (n=97)	PL (n=83)	4 g/day (n=85)	2 g/day (n = 83)
PGA	36%	59%*	57%*	31%	55%*	41%
Tx F	22%	9%*	18%	31%	9%*	17%*
SI	−2.5	−5.0*	−4.3*	−1.6	−3.8*	−2.6
Remission†	12%	26%*	24%*	12%	27%*	12%

* p <0.05 vs placebo.
PGA: Physician Global Assessment: proportion of patients with complete or marked improvement.
Tx F: Treatment Failure: proportion of patients developing severe or fulminant UC requiring steroid therapy or hospitalization or worsening of the disease at 7 days of therapy, or lack of significant improvement by 14 days of therapy.
SI: Sigmoidoscopic Index: an objective measure of disease activity rated by a standard (15-point) scale that includes mucosal vascular pattern, erythema, friability, granularity/ulcerations, and mucopus: improvement over baseline.
† Defined as complete resolution of symptoms plus improvement of endoscopic endpoints. To be considered in remission, patients had a "1" score for one of the endoscopic components (mucosal vascular pattern, erythema, granularity, or friability) and "0" for the others.

Table 1.　Adverse Events Occurring in More Than 1% of Either Placebo or PENTASA Patients in Domestic Placebo-controlled Ulcerative Colitis Trials. (PENTASA Comparison to Placebo)

Event	PENTASA n=451		Placebo n=173	
Diarrhea	16	(3.5%)	13	(7.5%)
Headache	10	(2.2%)	6	(3.5%)
Nausea	14	(3.1%)	—	
Abdominal Pain	5	(1.1%)	7	(4.0%)
Melena (Bloody Diarrhea)	4	(0.9%)	6	(3.5%)
Rash	6	(1.3%)	2	(1.2%)
Anorexia	5	(1.1%)	2	(1.2%)
Fever	4	(0.9%)	2	(1.2%)
Rectal Urgency	1	(0.2%)	4	(2.3%)
Nausea and Vomiting	5	(1.1%)	—	
Worsening of Ulcerative Colitis	2	(0.4%)	2	(1.2%)
Acne	1	(0.2%)	2	(1.2%)

Gastrointestinal: abdominal distention, anorexia, constipation, duodenal ulcer, dysphagia, eructation, esophageal ulcer, fecal incontinence, GGTP increase, GI bleeding, increased alkaline phosphatase, LDH increase, mouth ulcer, oral moniliases, pancreatitis, rectal bleeding, SGOT increase, SGPT increase, stool abnormalities (color or texture change), thirst
Dermatological: acne, alopecia, dry skin, eczema, erythema nodosum, nail disorder, photosensitivity, pruritus, sweating, urticaria
Nervous System: depression, dizziness, insomnia, somnolence, paresthesia
Cardiovascular: palpitations, pericarditis, vasodilation
Other: albuminuria, amenorrhea, amylase increase, arthralgia, asthenia, breast pain, conjunctivitis, ecchymosis, edema, fever, hematuria, hypomenorrhea, Kawasaki-like syndrome, leg cramps, lichen planus, lipase increase, malaise, menorrhagia, metrorrhagia, myalgia, pulmonary infiltrates, thrombocythemia, thrombocytopenia, urinary frequency

One week after completion of an 8-week ulcerative colitis study, a 72-year-old male, with no previous history of pulmonary problems, developed dyspnea. The patient was subsequently diagnosed with interstitial pulmonary fibrosis without eosinophilia by one physician and bronchiolitis obliterans with organizing pneumonitis by a second physician. A causal relationship between this event and mesalamine therapy has not been established.

Published case reports and/or spontaneous postmarketing surveillance have described infrequent instances of pericarditis, fatal myocarditis, chest pain and T-wave abnormalities, hypersensitivity pneumonitis, pancreatitis, nephrotic syndrome, interstitial nephritis, hepatitis, aplastic anemia, pancytopenia, leukopenia, agranulocytosis, or anemia while receiving mesalamine therapy. Anemia can be a part of the clinical presentation of inflammatory bowel disease. Allergic reactions, which could involve eosinophilia, can be seen in connection with PENTASA therapy.

Postmarketing Reports
The following events have been identified during post-approval use of the PENTASA brand of mesalamine in clinical practice. Because they are reported voluntarily from a population of unknown size, estimates of frequency cannot be made. These events have been chosen for inclusion due to a combination of seriousness, frequency of reporting, or potential causal connection to mesalamine:

Gastrointestinal: Reports of hepatotoxicity, including elevated liver enzymes (SGOT/AST, SGPT/ALT, GGT, LDH, alkaline phosphatase, bilirubin), hepatitis, jaundice, cholestatic jaundice, cirrhosis, and possible hepatocellular damage including liver necrosis and liver failure. Some of these cases were fatal. One case of Kawasaki-like syndrome which included hepatic function changes was also reported.
Other: Postmarketing reports of pneumonitis, granulocytopenia, systemic lupus erythematosus, acute renal failure, chronic renal failure and angioedema have been received in patients taking PENTASA.

OVERDOSAGE
Single oral doses of mesalamine up to 5 g/kg in pigs or a single intravenous dose of mesalamine at 920 mg/kg in rats were not lethal.

There is no clinical experience with PENTASA overdosage. PENTASA is an aminosalicylate, and symptoms of salicylate toxicity may be possible, such as: tinnitus, vertigo, headache, confusion, drowsiness, sweating, hyperventilation, vomiting, and diarrhea. Severe intoxication with salicylates can lead to disruption of electrolyte balance and blood-pH, hyperthermia, and dehydration.

Treatment of Overdosage. Since PENTASA is an aminosalicylate, conventional therapy for salicylate toxicity may be beneficial in the event of acute overdosage. This includes prevention of further gastrointestinal tract absorption by emesis and, if necessary, by gastric lavage. Fluid and electrolyte imbalance should be corrected by the administration of appropriate intravenous therapy. Adequate renal function should be maintained.

DOSAGE AND ADMINISTRATION
The recommended dosage for the induction of remission and the symptomatic treatment of mildly to moderately active ulcerative colitis is 1g (4 PENTASA 250 mg capsules or 2 PENTASA 500 mg capsules) 4 times a day for a total daily dosage of 4g. Treatment duration in controlled trials was up to 8 weeks.

HOW SUPPLIED
PENTASA controlled-release 250 mg capsules are supplied in bottles of 240 capsules (NDC 54092-189-81). Each green and blue capsule contains 250 mg of mesalamine in controlled-release beads. PENTASA controlled-release capsules are identified with a pentagonal starburst logo and the number 2010 on the green portion and PENTASA 250 mg or S429 250 mg on the blue portion of the capsules.

PENTASA controlled-release 500 mg capsules are supplied in bottles of 120 capsules (NDC 54092-191-12). Each blue capsule contains 500 mg of mesalamine in controlled-release beads. PENTASA controlled-release capsules are identified with a pentagonal starburst logo and PENTASA 500 mg or S429 500 mg on the capsules.

Store at 25°C (77°F) excursions permitted to 15-30°C (59-86°F) [see USP Controlled Room Temperature].

Manufactured for **Shire US Inc.** 725 Chesterbrook Blvd., Wayne, PA 19087, USA

Licensed U.S. Patent Nos. B1 4,496,553 and 4,980,173

189 0107 009

Licensed from Ferring A/S, Denmark

© 2008 Shire US Inc.

Rev. 06/2008

PEN-00042

Shown in Product Identification Guide, page 319

VYVANSE® ⓒ ℞

[VI-van-se]

(lisdexamfetamine dimesylate)

Capsules

HIGHLIGHTS OF PRESCRIBING INFORMATION

These highlights do not include all the information needed to use Vyvanse safely and effectively. See full prescribing information for Vyvanse.

Vyvanse® (lisdexamfetamine dimesylate) Capsules, CII

Initial U.S. Approval: 2007

WARNING: POTENTIAL FOR ABUSE
See full prescribing information for complete boxed warning
• **Amphetamines have a high potential for abuse; prolonged administration may lead to dependence (9)**
• **Misuse of amphetamines may cause sudden death and serious cardiovascular adverse events**

————————RECENT MAJOR CHANGES————————

None

————————INDICATIONS AND USAGE————————

Vyvanse, a prodrug of the stimulant dextroamphetamine, is indicated for the treatment of Attention Deficit Hyperactivity Disorder (ADHD). (1)

• Children: Efficacy was established in two trials in 6-12 year olds with ADHD. (14)

• Adults: Efficacy was established in two trials in adults with ADHD. (14)

————————DOSAGE AND ADMINISTRATION————————

• Recommended dose: Adults and pediatric patients ages (6-12); 30 mg once daily in the morning (2)

• Maximum dose: 70 mg once daily in the morning (2)

————————DOSAGE FORMS AND STRENGTHS————————

• Capsules: 20 mg, 30 mg, 40 mg, 50 mg, 60 mg, 70 mg (3)

————————CONTRAINDICATIONS————————

• Advanced arteriosclerosis (4)

• Symptomatic cardiovascular disease (4)

• Moderate to severe hypertension (4)

• Hyperthyroidism (4)

• Known hypersensitivity or idiosyncrasy to sympathomimetic amines (4)

• Glaucoma (4)

• Agitated states (4)

• History of drug abuse (4)

• During or within 14 days following the administration of monoamine oxidase inhibitors (MAOI) (4, 7.2)

————————WARNINGS AND PRECAUTIONS————————

• Serious Cardiovascular Events: Sudden death has been reported in association with CNS stimulant treatment at usual doses in children and adolescents with structural cardiac abnormalities or other serious heart problems. Sudden death, stroke, and myocardial infarction have been reported in adults taking stimulant drugs at usual doses for ADHD. Stimulant products generally should not be used in patients with known structural cardiac abnormalities, cardiomyopathy, serious heart rhythm abnormalities, coronary artery disease, or other serious heart problems. (5.1)

• Increase in Blood Pressure: Monitor blood pressure and pulse at appropriate intervals in patients taking Vyvanse. Use with caution in patients for whom blood pressure increases may be problematic. (5.1)

• Psychiatric Adverse Events: Use of stimulants may cause treatment-emergent psychotic or manic symptoms in patients with no prior history, or exacerbation of symptoms in patients with pre-existing psychosis. Clinical evaluation for bipolar disorder is recommended prior to stimulant use. Monitor for aggressive behavior. (5.2)

• Seizures: may lower the convulsive threshold, and in the presence of seizures, should be discontinued. (5.3)

• Visual Disturbance: difficulties with accommodation and blurring of vision have been reported with stimulant treatment. (5.4)

• Tics: may exacerbate tics. Clinical evaluation for tics and Tourette's syndrome is recommended prior to stimulant administration. (5.5)

• Long-Term Suppression of Growth: monitor height and weight at appropriate intervals in pediatric patients taking Vyvanse. (5.6)

————————ADVERSE REACTIONS————————

• Children ages 6 to 12: Most common adverse reactions (incidence ≥5% and at a rate at least twice placebo) were decreased appetite, dizziness, dry mouth, irritability, insomnia, upper abdominal pain, nausea, vomiting, and decreased weight. (6.1)

• Adults: Most common adverse reactions (incidence ≥5% and at a rate at least twice placebo) were upper abdominal pain, diarrhea, nausea, fatigue, feeling jittery, irritability, anorexia, decreased appetite, headaches, anxiety, and insomnia. (6.1)

To report SUSPECTED ADVERSE REACTIONS, contact Shire US Inc. at 1-800-828-2088 or FDA at 1-800-FDA-1088 or www.fda.gov/medwatch.

————————DRUG INTERACTIONS————————

• Urinary acidifying agents may reduce blood levels of amphetamine. (7.1)

• Urinary alkalinizing agents may increase blood levels of amphetamine. (7.2)

• MAOI antidepressants are contraindicated. (4; 7.2)

• The effects of adrenergic blockers, antihistamines, antihypertensives, phenobarbital, and phenytoin may be reduced by amphetamines. (7.3)

• The effects of tricyclic antidepressants, meperidine, phenobarbital and phenytoin may be potentiated by amphetamines. (7.4)

• Norepinephrine may potentiate the effects of amphetamines. (7.6)

————————USE IN SPECIFIC POPULATIONS————————

• Pregnancy: Use only if the potential benefit justifies the potential risk to the fetus. Based on animal data, may cause fetal harm. (8.1)

• Nursing Mothers: should refrain from breastfeeding. (8.3)

• Pediatric Use: has not been studied in children under 6 years of age or in adolescents over 12 years of age. (8.4)

• Geriatric Use: has not been studied in geriatric patients. (8.5)

See 17 for PATIENT COUNSELING INFORMATION and Medication Guide

Revised: 08/2010

FULL PRESCRIBING INFORMATION

WARNING: POTENTIAL FOR ABUSE
AMPHETAMINES HAVE A HIGH POTENTIAL FOR ABUSE. ADMINISTRATION OF AMPHETAMINES FOR PROLONGED PERIODS OF TIME MAY LEAD TO DRUG DEPENDENCE. PARTICULAR ATTENTION SHOULD BE PAID TO THE POSSIBILITY OF SUBJECTS OBTAINING AMPHETAMINES FOR NON-THERAPEUTIC USE OR DISTRIBUTION TO OTHERS AND THE DRUGS SHOULD BE PRESCRIBED OR DISPENSED SPARINGLY.
MISUSE OF AMPHETAMINES MAY CAUSE SUDDEN DEATH AND SERIOUS CARDIOVASCULAR ADVERSE EVENTS.

1 INDICATIONS AND USAGE

1.1 Attention Deficit Hyperactivity Disorder

Vyvanse® is indicated for the treatment of Attention Deficit Hyperactivity Disorder (ADHD).

The efficacy of Vyvanse in the treatment of ADHD was established on the basis of two controlled trials in children aged 6 to 12 and two controlled trials in adults who met DSM-IV-TR® criteria for ADHD [*see CLINICAL STUDIES (14)*].

A diagnosis of Attention Deficit Hyperactivity Disorder (ADHD; DSM-IV®) implies the presence of hyperactive-impulsive and/or inattentive symptoms that cause impairment and were present before the age of 7 years. The symptoms must cause clinically significant impairment, e.g. in social, academic, or occupational functioning, and be present in two or more settings, e.g. school (or work) and at home. The symptoms must not be better accounted for by another mental disorder. For the Inattentive Type, at least 6 of the following symptoms must have persisted for at least 6 months: lack of attention to details/careless mistakes; lack of sustained attention; poor listener; failure to follow through on tasks; poor organization; avoids tasks requiring sustained mental effort; loses things; easily distracted; forgetful. For the Hyperactive-Impulsive Type, at least 6 of the following symptoms (or adult equivalent symptoms) must have persisted for at least 6 months: fidgeting/squirming; leaving seat; inappropriate running/climbing; difficulty with quiet activities; "on the go"; excessive talking; blurting answers; can't wait turn; intrusive. The Combined Type requires both inattentive and hyperactive-impulsive criteria to be met.

Special Diagnostic Considerations

Specific etiology of this syndrome is unknown, and there is no single diagnostic test. Adequate diagnosis requires the use not only of medical but also of special psychological, educational, and social resources. Learning may or may not be impaired. The diagnosis must be based upon a complete history and evaluation of the patient and not solely on the presence of the required number of DSM-IV characteristics.

Need for Comprehensive Treatment Program

Vyvanse is indicated as an integral part of a total treatment program for ADHD that may include other measures (psychological, educational, social) for patients with this syndrome. Drug treatment may not be indicated for all patients with this syndrome. Stimulants are not intended for use in patients who exhibit symptoms secondary to environmental factors and/or other primary psychiatric disorders, including psychosis. Appropriate educational/vocational placement is essential and psychosocial intervention is often helpful. When remedial measures alone are insufficient, the decision to prescribe stimulant medication will depend upon the physician's assessment of the chronicity and severity of the patient's symptoms and on the level of functional impairment.

Long-Term Use

The effectiveness of Vyvanse for long-term use, i.e., for more than 4 weeks, has not been systematically evaluated in controlled trials. Therefore, the physician who elects to use Vyvanse for extended periods should periodically re-evaluate the long-term usefulness of the drug for the individual patient.

2   DOSAGE AND ADMINISTRATION

Dosage should be individualized according to the therapeutic needs and response of the patient. Vyvanse should be administered at the lowest effective dosage.

In children 6 to 12 years of age or adults who are either starting treatment for the first time or switching from another medication, 30 mg once daily in the morning is the recommended dose. If the decision is made in the judgment of the clinician to increase the dose beyond 30 mg/day, daily dosage may be adjusted in increments of 10 mg or 20 mg at approximately weekly intervals. The maximum recommended dose is 70 mg/day; doses greater than 70 mg/day of Vyvanse have not been studied. Amphetamines are not recommended for children under 3 years of age. Vyvanse has not been studied in children under 6 years of age or over 12 years of age.

Vyvanse should be taken in the morning. Afternoon doses should be avoided because of the potential for insomnia.

Vyvanse may be taken with or without food.

Vyvanse capsules may be taken whole, or the capsule may be opened and the entire contents dissolved in a glass of water. The solution should be consumed immediately and should not be stored. The dose of a single capsule should not be divided. The contents of the entire capsule should be taken, and patients should not take anything less than one capsule per day.

Where possible, drug administration should be interrupted occasionally to determine if there is a recurrence of behavioral symptoms sufficient to require continued treatment.

3   DOSAGE FORM AND STRENGTHS

Vyvanse capsules 20 mg: ivory body/ivory cap (imprinted with NRP104 or S489 and 20 mg)

Vyvanse capsules 30 mg: white body/orange cap (imprinted with NRP104 or S489 and 30 mg)

Vyvanse capsules 40 mg: white body/blue green cap (imprinted with NRP104 or S489 and 40 mg)

Vyvanse capsules 50 mg: white body/blue cap (imprinted with NRP104 or S489 and 50 mg)

Vyvanse capsules 60 mg: aqua blue body/aqua blue cap (imprinted with NRP104 or S489 and 60 mg)

Vyvanse capsules 70 mg: blue body/orange cap (imprinted with NRP104 or S489 and 70 mg)

4   CONTRAINDICATIONS

- Advanced arteriosclerosis, symptomatic cardiovascular disease, moderate to severe hypertension, hyperthyroidism, known hypersensitivity or idiosyncratic reaction to sympathomimetic amines, glaucoma
- Agitated states
- Patients with a history of drug abuse
- During or within 14 days following the administration of monoamine oxidase inhibitors (hypertensive crises may result) [See Drug Interactions (7.2)]

5   WARNINGS AND PRECAUTIONS

5.1   Serious Cardiovascular Events

Sudden Death and Pre-existing Structural Cardiac Abnormalities or Other Serious Heart Problems

Children and Adolescents

Sudden death has been reported in association with CNS stimulant treatment at usual doses in children and adolescents with structural cardiac abnormalities or other serious heart problems. Although some serious heart problems alone carry an increased risk of sudden death, stimulant products generally should not be used in children or adolescents with known serious structural cardiac abnormalities, cardiomyopathy, serious heart rhythm abnormalities, or other serious cardiac problems that may place them at increased vulnerability to the sympathomimetic effects of a stimulant drug [see CONTRAINDICATIONS (4)].

Adults

Sudden death, stroke, and myocardial infarction have been reported in adults taking stimulant drugs at usual doses for ADHD. Although the role of stimulants in these adult cases is unknown, adults have a greater likelihood than children of having *serious structural* cardiac abnormalities, cardiomyopathy, serious heart rhythm abnormalities, coronary artery disease, or other serious cardiac problems. Adults with such abnormalities should also generally not be treated with stimulant drugs [see CONTRAINDICATIONS (4)].

Hypertension and Other Cardiovascular Conditions

Stimulant medications cause a modest increase in average blood pressure (about 2-4 mm Hg) and average heart rate (about 3-6 bpm) and individuals may have larger increases.

Table 1 Adverse Reactions Reported by 2% or More of Pediatric Patients Taking Vyvanse in a 4-Week Clinical Trial

Body System	Preferred Term	Vyvanse (n=218)	Placebo (n=72)
Gastrointestinal Disorders	Abdominal Pain Upper	12%	6%
	Vomiting	9%	4%
	Nausea	6%	3%
	Dry Mouth	5%	0%
General Disorder and Administration Site Conditions	Pyrexia	2%	1%
Investigations	Weight Decreased	9%	1%
Metabolism and Nutrition	Decreased Appetite	39%	4%
Nervous System Disorders	Dizziness	5%	0%
	Somnolence	2%	1%
Psychiatric Disorders	Insomnia	19%	3%
	Irritability	10%	0%
	Initial Insomnia	4%	0%
	Affect lability	3%	0%
	Tic	2%	0%
Skin and Subcutaneous Tissue Disorders	Rash	3%	0%

Note: This table includes those reactions for which the incidence in patients taking Vyvanse is at least twice the incidence in patients taking placebo.

While the mean changes alone would not be expected to have short-term consequences, all patients should be monitored for larger changes in heart rate and blood pressure. Caution is indicated in treating patients whose underlying medical conditions might be compromised by increases in blood pressure or heart rate, e.g. those with pre-existing hypertension, heart failure, recent myocardial infarction, or ventricular arrhythmia [see CONTRAINDICATIONS (4)].

Assessing Cardiovascular Status in Patients Being Treated with Stimulant Medications

Children, adolescents, or adults who are being considered for treatment with stimulant medications should have a careful history (including assessment for a family history of sudden death or ventricular arrhythmia) and physical exam to assess for the presence of cardiac disease, and should receive further cardiac evaluation if findings suggest such disease (e.g. electrocardiogram and echocardiogram). Patients who develop symptoms such as exertional chest pain, unexplained syncope, or other symptoms suggestive of cardiac disease during stimulant treatment should undergo a prompt cardiac evaluation.

5.2   Psychiatric Adverse Events

Pre-existing Psychosis

Administration of stimulants may exacerbate symptoms of behavior disturbance and thought disorder in patients with a pre-existing psychotic disorder.

Bipolar Illness

Particular care should be taken in using stimulants to treat ADHD in patients with comorbid bipolar disorder because of concern for possible induction of a mixed/manic episode in such patients. Prior to initiating treatment with a stimulant, patients with comorbid depressive symptoms should be adequately screened to determine if they are at risk for bipolar disorder. Such screening should include a detailed psychiatric history, including a family history of suicide, bipolar disorder, and depression.

Emergence of New Psychotic or Manic Symptoms

Treatment-emergent psychotic or manic symptoms, e.g. hallucinations, delusional thinking, or mania in children and adolescents without a prior history of psychotic illness or mania, can be caused by stimulants at usual doses. If such symptoms occur, consideration should be given to a possible causal role of the stimulant, and discontinuation of treatment may be appropriate. In a pooled analysis of multiple short-term, placebo-controlled studies, such symptoms occurred in about 0.1% (4 patients with events out of 3482 exposed to methylphenidate or amphetamine for several weeks at usual doses) of stimulant-treated patients compared to 0 in placebo-treated patients.

Aggression

Aggressive behavior or hostility is often observed in children and adolescents with ADHD, and has been reported in clinical trials and the postmarketing experience of some medications indicated for the treatment of ADHD. Although there is no systematic evidence that stimulants cause aggressive behavior or hostility, patients beginning treatment of ADHD should be monitored for the appearance of, or worsening of, aggressive behavior or hostility.

5.3   Seizures

There is some clinical evidence that stimulants may lower the convulsive threshold in patients with prior history of seizures, in patients with prior EEG abnormalities in absence of seizures, and, very rarely, in patients without a history of seizures and no prior EEG evidence of seizures. In the presence of seizures, the drug should be discontinued.

5.4   Visual Disturbance

Difficulties with accommodation and blurring of vision have been reported with stimulant treatment.

5.5   Tics

Amphetamines have been reported to exacerbate motor and phonic tics and Tourette's syndrome. Therefore, clinical evaluation for tics and Tourette's syndrome should precede use of stimulant medications.

5.6   Long-Term Suppression of Growth

Careful follow-up of weight and height in children ages 7 to 10 years who were randomized to either methylphenidate or non-medication treatment groups over 14 months, as well as in naturalistic subgroups of newly methylphenidate-treated and non-medication treated children over 36 months (to the ages of 10 to 13 years), suggests that consistently medicated children (i.e. treatment for 7 days per week throughout the year) have a temporary slowing in growth rate (on average, a total of about 2 cm less growth in height and 2.7 kg less growth in weight over 3 years), without evidence of growth rebound during this period of development. In a controlled trial of amphetamine (d- to l-enantiomer ratio of 3:1) in adolescents, mean weight change from baseline within the initial 4 weeks of therapy was -1.1 lbs. and -2.8 lbs., respectively, for patients receiving 10 mg and 20 mg of amphetamine. Higher doses were associated with greater weight loss within the initial 4 weeks of treatment. In a controlled trial of Vyvanse in children ages 6 to 12 years, mean weight loss from baseline after 4 weeks of therapy was -0.9, -1.9, and -2.5 lbs., respectively, for patients receiving 30 mg, 50 mg, and 70 mg of Vyvanse, compared to a 1 lb weight gain for patients receiving placebo. Higher doses were associated with greater weight loss with 4 weeks of treatment. Careful follow-up for weight in children ages 6 to 12 years who received Vyvanse over 12 months suggests that consistently medicated children (i.e. treatment for 7 days per week throughout the year) have a slowing in growth rate, measured by body weight as demonstrated by an age- and sex-normalized mean change from baseline in percentile, of -13.4 over 1 year (average percentiles at baseline and 12 months were 60.6 and 47.2, respectively). Therefore, growth should be monitored during treatment with stimulants, and patients who are not growing or gaining weight as expected may need to have their treatment interrupted.

Table 2 Adverse Reactions Reported by 2% or More of Adult Patients Taking Vyvanse in a 4-Week Clinical Trial

Body System	Preferred Term	Vyvanse (n=358)	Placebo (n=62)
Gastrointestinal Disorders	Dry Mouth	26%	3%
	Diarrhea	7%	0%
	Nausea	7%	0%
General Disorder and Administration Site Conditions	Feeling Jittery	4%	0%
Investigations	Blood Pressure Increased	3%	0%
	Heart Rate Increased	2%	0%
Metabolism and Nutrition Disorders	Decreased Appetite	27%	3%
	Anorexia	5%	0%
Nervous System Disorders	Tremor	2%	0%
Psychiatric Disorders	Insomnia	27%	8%
	Anxiety	6%	0%
	Agitation	3%	0%
	Restlessness	3%	0%
Respiratory, Thoracic, and Mediastinal Disorders	Dyspnea	2%	0%
Skin and Subcutaneous Tissue Disorders	Hyperhidrosis	3%	0%

Note: This table includes those events for which the incidence in patients taking Vyvanse is at least twice the incidence in patients taking placebo.

5.7 Prescribing and Dispensing

The least amount of amphetamine feasible should be prescribed or dispensed at one time in order to minimize the possibility of overdosage. Vyvanse should be used with caution in patients who use other sympathomimetic drugs.

6 ADVERSE REACTIONS

6.1 Clinical Studies Experience

The premarketing development program for Vyvanse included exposures in a total of 762 participants in clinical trials (348 pediatric patients, 358 adult patients and 56 healthy adult subjects). Of these, 348 pediatric (aged 6 to 12) patients were evaluated in two controlled clinical studies (one parallel-group and one crossover), one open-label extension study, and one single-dose clinical pharmacology study, and 358 adult patients were evaluated in one controlled clinical study and one open-label extension study. The information included in this section is based on data from the 4-week parallel-group controlled clinical studies in pediatric and adult patients with ADHD. Adverse reactions were assessed by collecting adverse events, results of physical examinations, vital signs, weights, laboratory analyses, and ECGs.

Adverse reactions during exposure were obtained primarily by general inquiry and recorded by clinical investigators using terminology of their own choosing. Consequently, it is not possible to provide a meaningful estimate of the proportion of individuals experiencing adverse reactions without first grouping similar types of reactions into a smaller number of standardized reactions categories. In the tables and listings that follow, MedDRA terminology has been used to classify reported adverse reactions.

The stated frequencies of adverse reactions represent the proportion of individuals who experienced a treatment-emergent adverse reaction of the type listed at least once.

Adverse Reactions Associated with Discontinuation of Treatment in Clinical Trials

In the controlled pediatric (aged 6 to 12) trial, 10% (21/218) of Vyvanse-treated patients discontinued due to adverse reactions compared to 1% (1/72) who received placebo. The most frequent adverse events leading to discontinuation and considered to be drug-related (i.e. leading to discontinuation in at least 1% of Vyvanse-treated patients and at a rate at least twice that of placebo) were ECG voltage criteria for ventricular hypertrophy, tic, vomiting, psychomotor hyperactivity, insomnia, and rash (2/218 each; 1%).

In the controlled adult trial, 6% (21/358) of Vyvanse-treated patients discontinued due to adverse events compared to 2% (1/62) who received placebo. The most frequent adverse events leading to discontinuation and considered to be drug-related (i.e. leading to discontinuation in at least 1% of Vyvanse-treated patients and at a rate at least twice that of placebo) were insomnia (8/358; 2%), tachycardia (3/358; 1%), irritability (2/358; 1%), hypertension (4/358; 1%), headache (2/358; 1%), anxiety (2/358; 1%), and dyspnea (3/358; 1%).

Adverse Reactions Occurring at an Incidence of 2% or More Among Vyvanse Treated Patients in Clinical Trials

Adverse reactions reported in the controlled trials in pediatric and adult patients treated with Vyvanse or placebo are presented in Tables 1 and 2 below. The prescriber should be aware that these figures cannot be used to predict the incidence of adverse reactions in the course of usual medical practice where patient characteristics and other factors differ from those which prevailed in the clinical trials. Similarly, the cited frequencies cannot be compared with figures obtained from other clinical investigations involving different treatment uses and investigators. The cited figures, however, do provide the prescribing physician with some basis for estimating the relative contribution of drug and non-drug factors to the adverse reaction incidence rate in the population studied.

Pediatric
[See table 1 at top of previous page]

Adult
[See table 2 above]
In addition, adverse reactions observed at a rate of less than 2% included decreased libido and erectile dysfunction.

Vital Signs
Weight Loss—In the controlled adult trial, mean weight loss after 4 weeks of therapy was 2.8 lbs, 3.1 lbs, and 4.3 lbs, for patients receiving final doses of 30 mg, 50 mg, and 70 mg of Vyvanse, respectively, compared to a mean weight gain of 0.5 lbs for patients receiving placebo.

6.2 Postmarketing Reports

The following adverse reactions have been identified during post approval use of Vyvanse. Because these reactions are reported voluntarily from a population of uncertain size, it is not possible to reliably estimate their frequency or establish a causal relationship to drug exposure.

Cardiac Disorders—Palpitation
Eye Disorders—Vision blurred, mydriasis, diplopia
General Disorders and Administration Site Conditions—Fatigue
Hepatobiliary Disorders—Eosinophilic Hepatitis
Immune System Disorders—Anaphylactic reaction, hypersensitivity
Nervous System Disorders—Somnolence, seizure, dyskinesia
Psychiatric Disorder—Psychotic episodes, mania, hallucination, depression, aggression, dysphoria, euphoria, logorrhea
Skin and Subcutaneous Tissue Disorder—Stevens-Johnson Syndrome, angioedema, urticaria

6.3 Adverse Reactions Associated with the Use of Amphetamine

Cardiovascular
Palpitations, tachycardia, elevation of blood pressure, sudden death, myocardial infarction. There have been isolated reports of cardiomyopathy associated with chronic amphetamine use.

Central Nervous System
Psychotic episodes at recommended doses, overstimulation, restlessness, dizziness, insomnia, euphoria, dyskinesia, dysphoria, depression, tremor, headache, exacerbation of motor and phonic tics and Tourette's syndrome, seizures, stroke.

Gastrointestinal
Dryness of the mouth, unpleasant taste, diarrhea, constipation, other gastrointestinal disturbances.

Allergic
Urticaria, rashes, and hypersensitivity reactions, including angioedema and anaphylaxis. Serious skin reactions, including Stevens-Johnson Syndrome and Toxic Epidermal Necrolysis have been reported.

Endocrine
Impotence, changes in libido.

7 DRUG INTERACTIONS

7.1 Agents that Lower Blood Levels of Amphetamines

Urinary Acidifying Agents
These agents (ammonium chloride, sodium acid phosphate, etc.) increase the concentration of the ionized species of the amphetamine molecule, thereby increasing urinary excretion.

Methenamine Therapy
Urinary excretion of amphetamines is increased, and efficacy is reduced, by acidifying agents used in methenamine therapy.

7.2 Agents that Increase Blood Levels of Amphetamines

Urinary Alkalinizing Agents
These agents (acetazolamide, some thiazides) increase the concentration of the non-ionized species of the amphetamine molecule, thereby decreasing urinary excretion.

Monoamine Oxidase Inhibitors
MAOI antidepressants, as well as a metabolite of furazolidone, slow amphetamine metabolism. This slowing potentiates amphetamines, increasing their effect on the release of norepinephrine and other monoamines from adrenergic nerve endings; this can cause headaches and other signs of hypertensive crisis. A variety of toxic neurological effects and malignant hyperpyrexia can occur, sometimes with fatal results.

7.3 Agents Whose Effects May be Reduced by Amphetamines

Adrenergic Blockers
Adrenergic blockers are inhibited by amphetamines.

Antihistamines
Amphetamines may counteract the sedative effect of antihistamines.

Antihypertensives
Amphetamines may antagonize the hypotensive effects of antihypertensives.

Veratrum Alkaloids
Amphetamines inhibit the hypotensive effect of veratrum alkaloids.

Ethosuximide
Amphetamines may delay intestinal absorption of ethosuximide.

7.4 Agents Whose Effects May be Potentiated by Amphetamines

Antidepressants, Tricyclic
Amphetamines may enhance the activity of tricyclic antidepressants or sympathomimetic agents; d-amphetamine with desipramine or protriptyline and possibly other tricyclics cause striking and sustained increases in the concentration of d-amphetamine in the brain; cardiovascular effects can be potentiated.

Meperidine
Amphetamines potentiate the analgesic effect of meperidine.

Phenobarbital
Amphetamines may delay intestinal absorption of phenobarbital; co-administration of phenobarbital may produce a synergistic anticonvulsant action.

Phenytoin
Amphetamines may delay intestinal absorption of phenytoin; co-administration of phenytoin may produce a synergistic anticonvulsant action.

7.5 Agents that May Reduce the Effects of Amphetamines

Chlorpromazine
Chlorpromazine blocks dopamine and norepinephrine receptors, thus inhibiting the central stimulant effects of amphetamines, and can be used to treat amphetamine poisoning.

Haloperidol
Haloperidol blocks dopamine receptors, thus inhibiting the central stimulant effects of amphetamines.

Lithium Carbonate
The anorectic and stimulatory effects of amphetamines may be inhibited by lithium carbonate.

7.6 Agents that May Potentiate the Effects of Amphetamines

Norepinephrine

Amphetamines enhance the adrenergic effect of norepinephrine.

Propoxyphene Overdosage

In cases of propoxyphene overdosage, amphetamine CNS stimulation is potentiated and fatal convulsions can occur.

7.7 Drug/Laboratory Test Interactions

Amphetamines can cause a significant elevation in plasma corticosteroid levels. This increase is greatest in the evening. Amphetamine may interfere with urinary steroid determinations.

8 USE IN SPECIFIC POPULATIONS

8.1 Pregnancy

Animal reproduction studies of lisdexamfetamine dimesylate have not been performed. Studies have been performed with the active metabolite of lisdexamfetamine, d-amphetamine, either alone or in combination with l-amphetamine, as noted below.

Teratogenic Effects

Pregnancy Category C

Amphetamine (d- to l-enantiomer ratio of 3:1) had no apparent effects on embryofetal morphological development or survival when orally administered to pregnant rats and rabbits throughout the period of organogenesis at doses of up to 6 and 16 mg/kg/day, respectively. Fetal malformations and death have been reported in mice following parenteral administration of d-amphetamine doses of 50 mg/kg/day or greater to pregnant animals. Administration of these doses was also associated with severe maternal toxicity.

A number of studies in rodents indicate that prenatal or early postnatal exposure to amphetamine (d- or d,l-) at doses similar to those used clinically can result in longterm neurochemical and behavioral alterations. Reported behavioral effects include learning and memory deficits, altered locomotor activity, and changes in sexual function.

There are no adequate and well-controlled studies in pregnant women. There has been one report of severe congenital bony deformity, tracheo-esophageal fistula, and anal atresia (vater association) in a baby born to a woman who took dextroamphetamine sulfate with lovastatin during the first trimester of pregnancy. Amphetamines should be used during pregnancy only if the potential benefit justifies the potential risk to the fetus.

Nonteratogenic Effects

Infants born to mothers dependent on amphetamines have an increased risk of premature delivery and low birth weight. Also, these infants may experience symptoms of withdrawal as demonstrated by dysphoria, including agitation, and significant lassitude.

8.2 Labor and Delivery

The effects of Vyvanse on labor and delivery in humans is unknown.

8.3 Nursing Mothers

Amphetamines are excreted into human milk. Mothers taking amphetamines should be advised to refrain from nursing.

8.4 Pediatric Use

Vyvanse is indicated for use in children with ADHD aged 6 to 12 years. Vyvanse has not been studied in children under 6 years of age or adolescents. Long-term effects of amphetamines in children have not been well established. Amphetamines are not recommended for use in children under 3 years of age.

A study was conducted in which juvenile rats received oral doses of 4, 10, or 40 mg/kg/day of lisdexamfetamine dimesylate from day 7 to day 63 of age. These doses are approximately 0.3, 0.7, and 3 times the maximum recommended human daily dose of 70 mg on a mg/m^2 basis. Dose-related decreases in food consumption, bodyweight gain, and crown-rump length were seen; after a four-week drug-free recovery period, bodyweights and crown-rump lengths had significantly recovered in females but were still substantially reduced in males. Time to vaginal opening was delayed in females at the highest dose, but there were no drug effects on fertility when the animals were mated beginning on day 85 of age.

In a study in which juvenile dogs received lisdexamfetamine dimesylate for 6 months beginning at 10 weeks of age, decreased bodyweight gain was seen at all doses tested (2, 5, and 12 mg/kg/day, which are approximately 0.5, 1, and 3 times the maximum recommended human daily dose on a mg/m^2 basis). This effect partially or fully reversed during a four-week drug-free recovery period.

8.5 Geriatric Use

Vyvanse has not been studied in the geriatric population.

9 DRUG ABUSE AND DEPENDENCE

9.1 Controlled Substance

Vyvanse is classified as a Schedule II controlled substance.

9.2 Abuse and Dependence

Amphetamines have been extensively abused. Tolerance, extreme psychological dependence, and severe social disability have occurred. There are reports of patients who have increased the dosage to levels many times higher than recommended. Abrupt cessation following prolonged high-dosage administration results in extreme fatigue and mental depression; changes are also noted on the sleep EEG. Manifestations of chronic intoxication with amphetamines may include severe dermatoses, marked insomnia, irritability, hyperactivity, and personality changes. The most severe manifestation of chronic intoxication is psychosis, often clinically indistinguishable from schizophrenia.

Human Studies

In a human abuse liability study, when equivalent oral doses of 100 mg lisdexamfetamine dimesylate and 40 mg immediate-release d-amphetamine sulfate were administered to individuals with a history of drug abuse, lisdexamfetamine dimesylate 100 mg produced subjective responses on a scale of "Drug Liking Effects" (primary endpoint) that were significantly less than d-amphetamine immediate-release 40 mg. However, oral administration of 150 mg lisdexamfetamine dimesylate produced increases in positive subjective responses on this scale that were statistically indistinguishable from the positive subjective responses produced by 40 mg of oral immediate-release d-amphetamine and 200 mg of diethylpropion (C-IV).[1]

Intravenous administration of 50 mg lisdexamfetamine dimesylate to individuals with a history of drug abuse produced positive subjective responses on scales measuring "Drug Liking", "Euphoria", "Amphetamine Effects", and "Benzedrine Effects" that were greater than placebo but less than those produced by an equivalent dose (20 mg) of intravenous d-amphetamine.

Animal Studies

In animal studies, lisdexamfetamine dimesylate produced behavioral effects qualitatively similar to those of the CNS stimulant d-amphetamine. In monkeys trained to self-administer cocaine, intravenous lisdexamfetamine dimesylate maintained self-administration at a rate that was statistically less than that for cocaine, but greater than that of placebo.

10 OVERDOSAGE

Individual patient response to amphetamines varies widely. Toxic symptoms may occur idiosyncratically at low doses.

Symptoms: Manifestations of acute overdosage with amphetamines include restlessness, tremor, hyperreflexia, rapid respiration, confusion, assaultiveness, hallucinations, panic states, hyperpyrexia, and rhabdomyolysis. Fatigue and depression usually follow the central nervous system stimulation. Cardiovascular effects include arrhythmias, hypertension or hypotension, and circulatory collapse. Gastrointestinal symptoms include nausea, vomiting, diarrhea, and abdominal cramps. Fatal poisoning is usually preceded by convulsions and coma.

Treatment: Consult with a Certified Poison Control Center for up-to-date guidance and advice. Management of acute amphetamine intoxication is largely symptomatic and includes gastric lavage, administration of activated charcoal, administration of a cathartic, and sedation. Experience with hemodialysis or peritoneal dialysis is inadequate to permit recommendation in this regard. Acidification of the urine increases amphetamine excretion but is believed to increase risk of acute renal failure if myoglobinuria is present. If acute severe hypertension complicates amphetamine overdosage, administration of intravenous phentolamine has been suggested. However, a gradual drop in blood pressure will usually result when sufficient sedation has been achieved. Chlorpromazine antagonizes the central stimulant effects of amphetamines and can be used to treat amphetamine intoxication.

The prolonged release of Vyvanse in the body should be considered when treating patients with overdose.

11 DESCRIPTION

Vyvanse (lisdexamfetamine dimesylate) is designed as a capsule for once-a-day oral administration. The chemical designation for lisdexamfetamine dimesylate is (2S)-2,6-diamino-*N*-[(1*S*)-1-methyl-2-phenylethyl] hexanamide dimethanesulfonate. The molecular formula is $C_{15}H_{25}N_3O{\bullet}(CH_4O_3S)_2$, which corresponds to a molecular weight of 455.60. The chemical structure is:

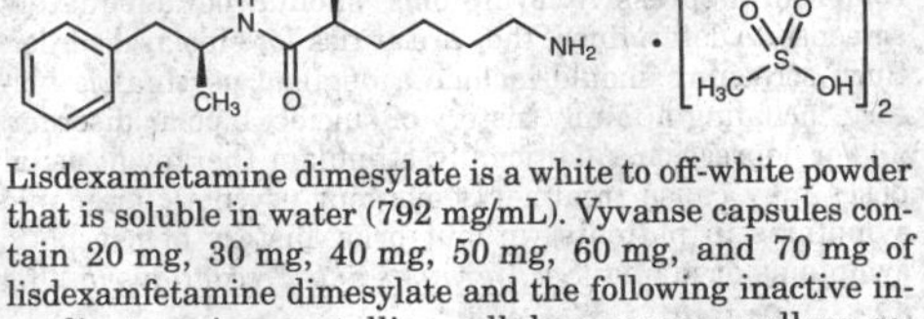

Lisdexamfetamine dimesylate is a white to off-white powder that is soluble in water (792 mg/mL). Vyvanse capsules contain 20 mg, 30 mg, 40 mg, 50 mg, 60 mg, and 70 mg of lisdexamfetamine dimesylate and the following inactive ingredients: microcrystalline cellulose, croscarmellose sodium, and magnesium stearate. The capsule shells contain gelatin, titanium dioxide, and one or more of the following: D&C Red #28, D&C Yellow #10, FD&C Blue #1, FD&C Green #3, and FD&C Red #40.

12 CLINICAL PHARMACOLOGY

12.1 Mechanism of Action

Lisdexamfetamine is a prodrug of dextroamphetamine. After oral administration, lisdexamfetamine is rapidly absorbed from the gastrointestinal tract and converted to dextroamphetamine, which is responsible for the drug's activity. Amphetamines are non-catecholamine sympathomimetic amines with CNS stimulant activity. The mode of therapeutic action in Attention Deficit Hyperactivity Disorder (ADHD) is not known. Amphetamines are thought to block the reuptake of norepinephrine and dopamine into the presynaptic neuron and increase the release of these monoamines into the extraneuronal space. The parent drug, lisdexamfetamine, does not bind to the sites responsible for the reuptake of norepinephrine and dopamine *in vitro*.

12.3 Pharmacokinetics

Pharmacokinetic studies of dextroamphetamine after oral administration of lisdexamfetamine have been conducted in healthy adult and pediatric (aged 6 to 12) patients with ADHD.

In 18 pediatric patients (aged 6 to 12) with ADHD, the T_{max} of dextroamphetamine was approximately 3.5 hours following single-dose oral administration of lisdexamfetamine dimesylate either 30 mg, 50 mg, or 70 mg after an 8-hour overnight fast. The T_{max} of lisdexamfetamine was approximately 1 hour. Linear pharmacokinetics of dextroamphetamine after single-dose oral administration of lisdexamfetamine dimesylate was established over the dose range of 30 mg to 70 mg in children aged 6 to 12 years.

There is no unexpected accumulation of dextroamphetamine AUC at steady state in healthy adults and no accumulation of lisdexamfetamine after once-daily dosing for 7 consecutive days.

Food does not affect the observed AUC and C_{max} of dextroamphetamine in healthy adults after single-dose oral administration of 70 mg of Vyvanse capsules but prolongs T_{max} by approximately 1 hour (from 3.8 hrs at fasted state to 4.7 hrs after a high fat meal). After an 8-hour fast, the AUCs for dextroamphetamine following oral administration of lisdexamfetamine dimesylate in solution and as intact capsules were equivalent.

Weight/Dose normalized AUC and C_{max} were 22% and 12% lower, respectively, in adult females than in males on day 7 following a 70 mg/day dose of lisdexamfetamine dimesylate for 7 days. Weight/Dose normalized AUC and C_{max} values were the same in girls and boys following single doses of 30-70 mg.

Metabolism and Excretion

After oral administration, lisdexamfetamine is rapidly absorbed from the gastrointestinal tract. Lisdexamfetamine is converted to dextroamphetamine and l-lysine, which is believed to occur by first-pass intestinal and/or hepatic metabolism. Lisdexamfetamine is not metabolized by cytochrome P450 enzymes. Following the oral administration of a 70 mg dose of radiolabeled lisdexamfetamine dimesylate to 6 healthy subjects, approximately 96% of the oral dose radioactivity was recovered in the urine and only 0.3% recovered in the feces over a period of 120 hours. Of the radioactivity recovered in the urine, 42% of the dose was related to amphetamine, 25% to hippuric acid, and 2% to intact lisdexamfetamine. Plasma concentrations of unconverted lisdexamfetamine are low and transient, generally becoming non-quantifiable by 8 hours after administration. The plasma elimination half-life of lisdexamfetamine typically averaged less than one hour in studies of lisdexamfetamine dimesylate in volunteers.

Dextroamphetamine is known to inhibit monoamine oxidase. The ability of dextroamphetamine and its metabolites to inhibit various P450 isozymes and other enzymes has not been adequately elucidated. *In vitro* experiments with human microsomes indicate minor inhibition of CYP2D6 by amphetamine and minor inhibition of CYP1A2, 2D6, and 3A4 by one or more metabolites, but there are no *in vivo* studies of p450 enzyme inhibition.

Special Populations

Age

The pharmacokinetics of dextroamphetamine is similar in pediatric (aged 6 to 12) and adolescent (aged 13 to 17) ADHD patients, and healthy adult volunteers. Any differences in kinetics seen after oral administration are a result of differences in mg/kg dosing.

Gender

Systemic exposure to dextroamphetamine is similar for men and women given the same mg/kg dose.

Race

Formal pharmacokinetic studies for race have not been conducted.

13 NONCLINICAL TOXICOLOGY

13.1 Carcinogenesis/Mutagenesis and Impairment of Fertility

Carcinogenicity studies of lisdexamfetamine dimesylate have not been performed.

No evidence of carcinogenicity was found in studies in which d-, l-amphetamine (enantiomer ratio of 1:1) was administered to mice and rats in the diet for 2 years at doses of up to 30 mg/kg/day in male mice, 19 mg/kg/day in female mice, and 5 mg/kg/day in male and female rats. Lisdexamfetamine dimesylate was not clastogenic in the mouse bone marrow micronucleus test *in vivo* and was negative when tested in the *E. coli* and *S. typhimurium* components of the Ames test and in the L5178Y/TK$^+$ mouse lymphoma assay *in vitro*.

Amphetamine (d- to l-enantiomer ratio of 3:1) did not adversely affect fertility or early embryonic development in the rat at doses of up to 20 mg/kg/day.

13.2   Animal Toxicology

Acute administration of high doses of amphetamine (d- or d,l-) has been shown to produce long-lasting neurotoxic effects, including irreversible nerve fiber damage, in rodents. The significance of these findings to humans is unknown.

14   CLINICAL STUDIES

The efficacy of Vyvanse in the treatment of ADHD was established on the basis of two controlled trials in children aged 6 to 12 and two controlled trials in adults who met Diagnostic and Statistical Manual of Mental Disorders, 4th edition (DSM-IV-TR) criteria for ADHD [*see INDICATIONS AND USAGE (1)*].

Pediatric

A double-blind, randomized, placebo-controlled, parallel-group study was conducted in children aged 6 to 12 (N=290) who met DSM-IV criteria for ADHD (either the combined type or the hyperactive-impulsive type). Patients were randomized to fixed dose treatment groups receiving final doses of 30, 50, or 70 mg of Vyvanse or placebo once daily in the morning for four weeks. All subjects receiving Vyvanse were initiated on 30 mg for the first week of treatment. Subjects assigned to the 50 and 70 mg dose groups were titrated by 20 mg per week until they achieved their assigned dose. Significant improvements in ADHD symptoms, based upon investigator ratings on the ADHD Rating Scale (ADHD-RS), were observed at endpoint for all Vyvanse doses compared to patients who received placebo. Mean effects at all doses were fairly similar, although the highest dose (70 mg/day) was numerically superior to both lower doses (30 and 50 mg/day). The effects were maintained throughout the day based on parent ratings (Conners' Parent Rating Scale) in the morning (approximately 10 am), afternoon (approximately 2 pm), and early evening (approximately 6 pm).

A double-blind, placebo-controlled, randomized, crossover design, analog classroom study was conducted in children aged 6 to 12 (N=52) who met DSM-IV criteria for ADHD (either the combined type or the hyperactive-impulsive type). Following a 3-week open-label dose titration with Adderall XR®, patients were both randomly assigned to continue the same dose of Adderall XR (10, 20, or 30 mg), Vyvanse (30, 50, or 70 mg), or placebo once daily in the morning for 1 week each treatment. A significant difference in patient behavior, based upon the average of investigator ratings on the Swanson, Kotkin, Agler, M.Flynn, and Pelham (SKAMP)-Deportment scores across 8 assessments conducted at 2, 3, 4, 5, 6, 8, 10, and 12 hours post-dose were observed between patients who received Vyvanse compared to patients who received placebo. The drug effect was similar for all 8 sessions.

A second double-blind, placebo-controlled, randomized, crossover design, analog classroom study was conducted in children aged 6 to 12 (N=129) who met DSM-IV criteria for ADHD (either the combined type or the hyperactive-impulsive type). Following a 4-week open-label dose titration with Vyvanse (30, 50, 70 mg), patients were randomly assigned to continue Vyvanse or placebo once daily in the morning for 1 week each treatment. A significant difference in patient behavior, based upon the average of investigator ratings on the SKAMP-Deportment scores across all 7 assessments conducted at 1.5, 2.5, 5.0, 7.5, 10.0, 12.0, and 13.0 hours post-dose, were observed between patients who received Vyvanse compared to patients who received placebo.

Adult

A double-blind, randomized, placebo-controlled, parallel-group study was conducted in adults (N=420) who met DSM-IV criteria for ADHD. In this four-week study, patients were randomized to fixed dose treatment groups receiving final doses of 30, 50, or 70 mg of Vyvanse or placebo. All subjects receiving Vyvanse were initiated on 30 mg for the first week of treatment. Subjects assigned to the 50 and 70 mg dose groups were titrated by 20 mg per week until they achieved their assigned dose. Significant improvements in ADHD symptoms, based upon investigator ratings on the ADHD Rating Scale (ADHD-RS), were observed at end point for all Vyvanse doses compared to placebo.

The second study was a multi-center, randomized, double-blind, placebo-controlled, crossover design, modified analog classroom study of Vyvanse to simulate a workplace environment in 142 adults who met DSM-IV-TR criteria for ADHD. There was a 4-week open-label, dose optimization

phase with Vyvanse (30, 50, or 70 mg/day in the morning). Subjects were then randomized to one of two treatment sequences: 1) Vyvanse (optimized dose) followed by placebo, each for one week, or 2) placebo followed by Vyvanse, each for one week. Efficacy assessments occurred at the end of each week, using the Permanent Product Measure of Performance (PERMP). The PERMP is a skill-adjusted math test that measures attention in ADHD. Vyvanse treatment, compared to placebo, resulted in a statistically significant improvement in attention across all post-dose time points, as measured by average PERMP total scores over the course of one assessment day, as well as at each time point measured. The PERMP assessments were administered at pre-dose (-0.5 hours) and at 2, 4, 8, 10, 12, and 14 hours post-dose.

15   REFERENCES

[1] Jasinski DR, Krishnan S. Abuse liability and safety of oral lisdexamfetamine dimesylate in individuals with a history of stimulant abuse. *Journal of Psychopharmacology*. 2009.

16   HOW SUPPLIED/STORAGE AND HANDLING

Vyvanse capsules 20 mg: ivory body/ivory cap (imprinted with NRP104 or S489 and 20 mg), bottles of 100, NDC 59417-102-10

Vyvanse capsules 30 mg: white body/orange cap (imprinted with NRP104 or S489 and 30 mg), bottles of 100, NDC 59417-103-10

Vyvanse capsules 40 mg: white body/blue green cap (imprinted with NRP104 or S489 and 40 mg), bottles of 100, NDC 59417-104-10

Vyvanse capsules 50 mg: white body/blue cap (imprinted with NRP104 or S489 and 50 mg), bottles of 100, NDC 59417-105-10

Vyvanse capsules 60 mg: aqua blue body/aqua blue cap (imprinted with NRP104 or S489 and 60 mg), bottles of 100, NDC 59417-106-10

Vyvanse capsules 70 mg: blue body/orange cap (imprinted with NRP104 or S489 and 70 mg), bottles of 100, NDC 59417-107-10

Dispense in a tight, light-resistant container as defined in the USP.

Store at 25° C (77° F). Excursions permitted to 15-30° C (59-86° F) [see USP Controlled Room Temperature]

17   PATIENT COUNSELING INFORMATION

See Medication Guide

17.1   Information on Medication Guide

Prescribers or other health professionals should inform patients, their families, and their caregivers about the benefits and risks associated with treatment with Vyvanse and should counsel them in its appropriate use. A patient Medication Guide is available for Vyvanse. The prescriber or health professional should instruct patients, their families, and their caregivers to read the Medication Guide and should assist them in understanding its contents. Patients should be given the opportunity to discuss the contents of the Medication Guide and to obtain answers to any questions they may have. The complete text of the Medication Guide is attached to the package insert.

17.2   Controlled Substance Status/Potential for Abuse, Misuse, and Dependence

Patients should be advised that Vyvanse is a federally controlled substance because it can be abused or lead to dependence. Additionally, it should be emphasized that Vyvanse should be stored in a safe place to prevent misuse and/or abuse. Patient history (including family history) of abuse or dependence on alcohol, prescription medicines, or illicit drugs should be evaluated [*See Drug Abuse and Dependence (9)*].

17.3   Serious Cardiovascular Risks

Patients should be advised of serious cardiovascular risk (including sudden death, myocardial infarction, stroke, and hypertension) with Vyvanse. Patients who develop symptoms such as exertional chest pain, unexplained syncope, or other symptoms suggestive of cardiac disease during treatment should undergo a prompt cardiac evaluation [*See Warning and Precautions (5.1)*].

17.4   Psychiatric Risks

Prior to initiating treatment with a stimulant, patients with comorbid depressive symptoms should be adequately screened to determine if they are at risk for bipolar disorder. Such screening should include a detailed psychiatric history, including a family history of suicide, bipolar disorder, and/or depression. Additionally, stimulant therapy at usual doses may cause treatment-emergent psychotic or manic symptoms in patients without prior history of psychotic symptoms or mania [*See Warnings and Precautions (5.2)*].

17.5   Growth

Growth should be monitored during treatment with stimulants, and patients who are not growing or gaining weight as expected may need to have their treatment interrupted. [*See Warnings and Precautions (5.6)*].

17.6   Pregnancy

Patients should be advised to notify their physicians if they become pregnant or intend to become pregnant during treatment [*see Dosage and Administration (2)* and *Use in Specific Populations (8.1)*].

17.7   Nursing

Patients should be advised not to breast feed if they are taking Vyvanse [*see Use in Specific Populations (8.3)*].

17.8   Impairment in Ability to Operate Machinery or Vehicles

Amphetamines may impair the ability of the patient to engage in potentially hazardous activities such as operating machinery or vehicles; the patient should therefore be cautioned accordingly.

Pharmacist: Medication Guide to be dispensed to patients

Manufactured for: Shire US Inc., Wayne, PA 19087
Made in USA
For more information call 1-800-828-2088
Vyvanse® is a trademark of Shire LLC
©2010 Shire US Inc.
US Pat No. 7,105,486 and US Pat No. 7,223,735
Last Modified: 08/2010

MEDICATION GUIDE

VYVANSE®
(LISDEXAMFETAMINE DIMESYLATE) CII

Read the Medication Guide that comes with Vyvanse before you or your child starts taking it and each time you get a refill. There may be new information. This Medication Guide does not take the place of talking to your doctor about you or your child's treatment with Vyvanse.

What is the most important information I should know about Vyvanse?

Vyvanse is a stimulant medicine. The following have been reported with use of stimulant medicines.

1. Heart-related problems:

- **sudden death in patients who have heart problems or heart defects**
- **stroke and heart attack in adults**
- **increased blood pressure and heart rate**

Tell your doctor if you or your child have any heart problems, heart defects, high blood pressure, or a family history of these problems.

Your doctor should check you or your child carefully for heart problems before starting Vyvanse.

Your doctor should check you or your child's blood pressure and heart rate regularly during treatment with Vyvanse.

Call your doctor right away if you or your child has any signs of heart problems such as chest pain, shortness of breath, or fainting while taking Vyvanse.

2. Mental (Psychiatric) problems:

All Patients

- **new or worse behavior and thought problems**
- **new or worse bipolar illness**
- **new or worse aggressive behavior or hostility**

Children and Teenagers

- **new psychotic symptoms (such as hearing voices, believing things that are not true, are suspicious) or new manic symptoms**

Tell your doctor about any mental problems you or your child have, or about a family history of suicide, bipolar illness, or depression.

Call your doctor right away if you or your child have any new or worsening mental symptoms or problems while taking Vyvanse, especially seeing or hearing things that are not real, believing things that are not real, or are suspicious.

What Is Vyvanse?

Vyvanse is a central nervous system stimulant prescription medicine. **It is used for the treatment of Attention-Deficit Hyperactivity Disorder (ADHD).** Vyvanse may help increase attention and decrease impulsiveness and hyperactivity in patients with ADHD.

Vyvanse should be used as a part of a total treatment program for ADHD that may include counseling or other therapies.

Vyvanse is a federally controlled substance (CII) because it can be abused or lead to dependence. Keep Vyvanse in a safe place to prevent misuse and abuse. Selling or giving away Vyvanse may harm others, and is against the law.

Tell your doctor if you or your child have (or have a family history of) ever abused or been dependent on alcohol, prescription medicines or street drugs.

Who should not take Vyvanse?
Vyvanse should not be taken if you or your child:

- have heart disease or hardening of the arteries

- have moderate to severe high blood pressure
- have hyperthyroidism
- have an eye problem called glaucoma
- are very anxious, tense, or agitated
- have a history of drug abuse
- are taking or have taken within the past 14 days an anti-depression medicine called a monoamine oxidase inhibitor or MAOI.
- is sensitive to, allergic to, or had a reaction to other stimulant medicines

Vyvanse has not been studied in children less than 6 years old. Vyvanse is not recommended for use in children less than 3 years old.

Vyvanse may not be right for you or your child. Before starting Vyvanse tell your or your child's doctor about all health conditions (or a family history of) including:

- heart problems, heart defects, high blood pressure
- mental problems including psychosis, mania, bipolar illness, or depression
- tics or Tourette's syndrome
- liver or kidney problems
- thyroid problems
- seizures or have had an abnormal brain wave test (EEG)

Tell your doctor if you or your child is pregnant, planning to become pregnant, or breastfeeding.

Can Vyvanse be taken with other medicines?

Tell your doctor about all of the medicines that you or your child take including prescription and non-prescription medicines, vitamins, and herbal supplements. Vyvanse and some medicines may interact with each other and cause serious side effects. Sometimes the doses of other medicines will need to be adjusted while taking Vyvanse.

Your doctor will decide whether Vyvanse can be taken with other medicines.

Especially tell your doctor if you or your child takes:

- anti-depression medicines including MAOIs
- anti-psychotic medicines
- lithium
- blood pressure medicines
- seizure medicines
- narcotic pain medicines

Know the medicines that you or your child takes. Keep a list of your medicines with you to show your doctor and pharmacist.

Do not start any new medicine while taking Vyvanse without talking to your doctor first.

How should Vyvanse be taken?

- **Take Vyvanse exactly as prescribed.** Vyvanse comes in 6 different strength capsules. Your doctor may adjust the dose until it is right for you or your child.
- Take Vyvanse once a day in the morning.
- Vyvanse can be taken with or without food.
- From time to time, your doctor may stop Vyvanse treatment for a while to check ADHD symptoms.
- Your doctor may do regular checks of the blood, heart, and blood pressure while taking Vyvanse. Children should have their height and weight checked often while taking Vyvanse. Vyvanse treatment may be stopped if a problem is found during these check-ups.
- **If you or your child takes too much Vyvanse or overdoses, call your doctor or poison control center right away, or get emergency treatment.**

What are possible side effects of Vyvanse?

See "What is the most important information I should know about Vyvanse?" for information on reported heart and mental problems.

Other serious side effects include:

- slowing of growth (height and weight) in children
- seizures, mainly in patients with a history of seizures
- eyesight changes or blurred vision

Common side effects include:

- upper belly pain
- dizziness
- irritability
- nausea
- weight loss
- decreased appetite
- dry mouth
- trouble sleeping
- vomiting

Vyvanse may affect your or your child's ability to drive or do other dangerous activities.

Talk to your doctor if you or your child has side effects that are bothersome or do not go away.

This is not a complete list of possible side effects. Ask your doctor or pharmacist for more information.

Call your doctor for medical advice about side effects. You may report side effects to FDA at 1-800-FDA-1088.

How should I store Vyvanse?

- Store Vyvanse in a safe place at room temperature, 59 to 86° F (15 to 30° C). Protect from light.
- **Keep Vyvanse and all medicines out of the reach of children.**

General information about Vyvanse

Medicines are sometimes prescribed for purposes other than those listed in a Medication Guide. Do not use Vyvanse for a condition for which it was not prescribed. Do not give Vyvanse to other people, even if they have the same condition. It may harm them and it is against the law.

This Medication Guide summarizes the most important information about Vyvanse. If you would like more information, talk with your doctor. You can ask your doctor or pharmacist for information about Vyvanse that was written for healthcare professionals. For more information about Vyvanse, please contact Shire US Inc. at 1-800-828-2088.

What are the ingredients in Vyvanse?

Active Ingredient: lisdexamfetamine dimesylate

Inactive Ingredients: microcrystalline cellulose, croscarmellose sodium, and magnesium stearate. The capsule shells contain gelatin, titanium dioxide, and one or more of the following: D&C Red #28, D&C Yellow #10, FD&C Blue #1, FD&C Green #3, and FD&C Red #40.

This Medication Guide has been approved by the U.S. Food and Drug Administration.

©2010 Shire US Inc.

US Pat No. 7,105,486 and US Pat No. 7,223,735

Last Modified: 08/2010

Shown in Product Identification Guide, page 319

Sigma-Tau Pharmaceuticals, Inc.
9841 WASHINGTONIAN BLVD. SUITE 500
GAITHERSBURG, MD 20878

Phone: 1 (800) 447-0169
1 (301) 948-1041
FAX: 1 (301) 948-1862
E-mail: sigmatauinfo@sigmatau.com

ABELCET® ℞
[AB-el-cet]
(Amphotericin B Lipid Complex Injection)

DESCRIPTION

ABELCET® is a sterile, pyrogen-free suspension for intravenous infusion. ABELCET® consists of amphotericin B complexed with two phospholipids in a 1:1 drug-to-lipid molar ratio. The two phospholipids, L-α-dimyristoylphosphatidylcholine (DMPC) and L-α-dimyristoylphosphatidylglycerol (DMPG), are present in a 7:3 molar ratio. ABELCET® is yellow and opaque in appearance, with a pH of 5-7.

NOTE: Liposomal encapsulation or incorporation in a lipid complex can substantially affect a drug's functional properties relative to those of the unencapsulated or nonlipid-associated drug. In addition, different liposomal or lipid-complexed products with a common active ingredient may vary from one another in the chemical composition and physical form of the lipid component. Such differences may affect functional properties of these drug products.

Amphotericin B is a polyene, antifungal antibiotic produced from a strain of *Streptomyces nodosus*. Amphotericin B is designated chemically as [1R-(1R*, 3S*, 5R*, 6R*, 9R*, 11R*, 15S*, 16R*, 17R*, 18S*, 19E, 21E, 23E, 25E, 27E, 29E, 31E, 33R*, 35S*, 36R*, 37S*)]-33-[(3-Amino-3, 6-dideoxy-β-D-mannopyranosyl) oxy]-1,3,5,6,9,11,17, 37-octahydroxy-15,16,18-trimethyl-13-oxo-14,39-dioxabicyclo[33.3.1] nonatriaconta-19, 21, 23, 25, 27, 29, 31-heptaene-36-carboxylic acid.

It has a molecular weight of 924.09 and a molecular formula of $C_{47}H_{73}NO_{17}$. The structural formula is:

ABELCET® is provided as a sterile, opaque suspension in 20 mL glass, single-use vials. Each 20 mL vial contains 100 mg of amphotericin B (see DOSAGE AND ADMINISTRATION), and each mL of ABELCET® contains:

Amphotericin B USP	5 mg
L-α-dimyristoylphosphatidylcholine (DMPC)	3.4 mg
L-α-dimyristoylphosphatidylglycerol (DMPG)	1.5 mg
Sodium Chloride USP	9 mg
Water for Injection USP, q.s. 1 mL	

MICROBIOLOGY

Mechanism of Action

The active component of ABELCET®, amphotericin B, acts by binding to sterols in the cell membrane of susceptible fungi, with a resultant change in the permeability of the membrane. Mammalian cell membranes also contain sterols, and damage to human cells is believed to occur through the same mechanism of action.

Activity *in vitro* and *in vivo*

ABELCET® shows *in vitro* activity against *Aspergillus* sp. (n=3) and *Candida* sp, (n=10), with MICs generally <1 µg/mL. Depending upon the species and strain of *Aspergillus* and *Candida* tested, significant *in vitro* differences in susceptibility to amphotericin B have been reported (MICs ranging from 0.1 to >10 µg/mL). However, standardized techniques for susceptibility testing for antifungal agents have not been established, and results of susceptibility studies do not necessarily correlate with clinical outcome. ABELCET® is active in animal models against *Aspergillus fumigatus, Candida albicans, C. guillermondii, C. stellatoideae,* and *C. tropicalis, Cryptococcus sp., Coccidioidomyces sp., Histoplasma sp.,* and *Blastomyces sp.* in which endpoints were clearance of microorganisms from target organ(s) and/or prolonged survival of infected animals.

Drug Resistance

Fungal species with decreased susceptibility to amphotericin B have been isolated after serial passage in culture media containing the drug, and from some patients receiving prolonged therapy. Although the relevance of drug resistance to clinical outcome has not been established, fungal species which are resistant to amphotericin B may also be resistant to ABELCET®.

CLINICAL PHARMACOLOGY

Pharmacokinetics

The assay used to measure amphotericin B in the blood after the administration of ABELCET® does not distinguish amphotericin B that is complexed with the phospholipids of ABELCET® from amphotericin B that is uncomplexed.

The pharmacokinetics of amphotericin B after the administration of ABELCET® are nonlinear. Volume of distribution and clearance from blood increase with increasing dose of ABELCET®, resulting in less than proportional increases in blood concentrations of amphotericin B over a dose range of 0.6-5 mg/kg/day. The pharmacokinetics of amphotericin B in whole blood after the administration of ABELCET® and amphotericin B desoxycholate are:

[See table below]

Pharmacokinetic Parameters of Amphotericin B in Whole Blood in Patients Administered Multiple Doses of ABELCET® or Amphotericin B Desoxycholate

Pharmacokinetic Parameter	ABELCET® 5 mg/kg/day for 5-7 days Mean ± SD	Amphotericin B 0.6 mg/kg/day for 42 days[a] Mean ± SD
Peak Concentration (µg/mL)	1.7 ± 0.8 (n=10)[b]	1.1 ± 0.2 (n=5)
Concentration at End of Dosing Interval (µg/mL)	0.6 ± 0.3 (n=10)[b]	0.4 ± 0.2 (n=5)
Area Under Blood Concentration-Time Curve (AUC_{0-24h}) (µg*h/mL)	14 ± 7 (n=14)[b,c]	17.1 ± 5 (n=5)
Clearance (mL/h*kg)	436 ± 188.5 (n=14)[b,c]	38 ± 15 (n=5)
Apparent Volume of Distribution (Vd_{area}) (L/kg)	131 ± 57.7 (n=8)[c]	5 ± 2.8 (n=5)
Terminal Elimination Half-Life (h)	173.4 ± 78 (n=8)[c]	91.1 ± 40.9 (n=5)
Amount Excreted in Urine Over 24 h After Last Dose (% of dose)[d]	0.9 ± 0.4 (n=8)[c]	9.6 ± 2.5 (n=8)

[a] Data from patients with mucocutaneous leishmaniasis. Infusion rate was 0.25 mg/kg/h.
[b] Data from studies in patients with cytologically proven cancer being treated with chemotherapy or neutropenic patients with presumed or proven fungal infection. Infusion rate was 2.5 mg/kg/h.
[c] Data from patients with mucocutaneous leishmaniasis. Infusion rate was 4 mg/kg/h.
[d] Percentage of dose excreted in 24 hours after last dose.

The large volume of distribution and high clearance from blood of amphotericin B after the admistration of ABELCET® probably reflect uptake by tissues. The long terminal elimination half-life probably reflects a slow redistribution from tissues. Although amphotericin B is excreted slowly, there is little accumulation in the blood after repeated dosing. AUC of amphotericin B increased approximately 34% from day 1 after the administration of ABELCET® 5 mg/kg/day for 7 days. The effect of gender or ethnicity on the pharmacokinetics of ABELCET® has not been studied.

Tissue concentrations of amphotericin B have been obtained at autopsy from one heart transplant patient who received three doses of ABELCET® at 5.3 mg/kg/day:

Concentration in Human Tissues

Organ	Amphotericin B Tissue Concentration (μg/g)
Spleen	290
Lung	222
Liver	196
Lymph Node	7.6
Kidney	6.9
Heart	5
Brain	1.6

This pattern of distribution is consistent with that observed in preclinical studies in dogs in which greatest concentrations of amphotericin B after ABELCET® administration were observed in the liver, spleen, and lung; however, the relationship of tissue concentrations of amphotericin B to its biological activity when administered as ABELCET® is unknown.

Special Populations

Hepatic Impairment: The effect of hepatic impairment on the disposition of ABELCET® is not known.

Renal Impairment: The effect of renal impairment on the disposition of ABELCET® is not known. The effect of dialysis on the elimination of ABELCET® has not been studied; however, amphotericin B is not removed by hemodialysis when administered as amphotericin B desoxycholate.

Pediatric and Elderly Patients: The pharmacokinetics and pharmacodynamics of pediatric patients (≤16 years of age) and elderly patients (≥65 years of age) have not been studied.

INDICATIONS AND USAGE

ABELCET® is indicated for the treatment of invasive fungal infections in patients who are refractory to or intolerant of conventional amphotericin B therapy. This is based on open-label treatment of patients judged by their physicians to be intolerant to or failing conventional amphotericin B therapy (See DESCRIPTION OF CLINICAL STUDIES).

DESCRIPTION OF CLINICAL STUDIES

Fungal Infections

Data from 473 patients were pooled from three open-label studies in which ABELCET® was provided for the treatment of patients with invasive fungal infections who were judged by their physicians to be refractory to or intolerant of conventional amphotericin B, or who had preexisting nephrotoxicity. Results of these studies demonstrated effectiveness of ABELCET® in the treatment of invasive fungal infections as a second line therapy.

Patients were defined by their individual physician as being refractory to or failing conventional amphotericin B therapy based on overall clinical judgement after receiving a minimum total dose of 500 mg of amphotericin B. Nephrotoxicity was defined as a serum creatinine that had increased to >2.5 mg/dL in adults and >1.5 mg/dL in pediatric patients, or a creatinine clearance of <25 mL/min while receiving conventional amphotericin B therapy.

Of the 473 patients, four were enrolled more than once; each enrollment contributed separately to the denominator. The median age was 39 years (range of <1 to 93 years); 307 patients were male and 166 female. Patients were Caucasian (381, 81%), African-American (41, 9%), Hispanic (27, 6%), Asian (10, 2%), and various other races (14, 3%). The median baseline neutrophil count was 4,000 PMN/mm^3; of these, 101 (21%) had a baseline neutrophil count <500/mm^3.

Two-hundred eighty-two patients of the 473 patients were considered evaluable for response to therapy; the other 191 patients were excluded on the basis of unconfirmed diagnosis, confounding factors, concomitant systemic antifungal therapy, or receiving 4 doses or less of ABELCET®. For evaluable patients, the following fungal infections were treated (n=282): aspergillosis (n=111), candidiasis (n=87), zygomycosis (n=25), cryptococcosis (n=16), and fusariosis (n=11). There were fewer than 10 evaluable patients for each of several other fungal species treated.

For each type of fungal infection listed above there were some patients successfully treated. However, in the absence of controlled studies it is unknown how response would have compared to either continuing conventional amphotericin B therapy or the use of alternative antifungal agents.

Renal Function: Patients with aspergillosis who initiated treatment with ABELCET® when serum creatinine was above 2.5 mg/dL experienced a decline in serum creatinine during treatment (Figure 1). Serum creatinine levels were also lower during treatment with ABELCET® when compared to the serum creatinine levels of patients treated with conventional amphotericin B in a retrospective historical control study. Meaningful statistical testing of the differences between these two groups is precluded since these data were obtained from two separate studies.

Figure 1
Changes in Mean Serum Creatinine Over Time
Patients with Aspergillosis and Serum Creatinine >2.5 mg/dL at Baseline

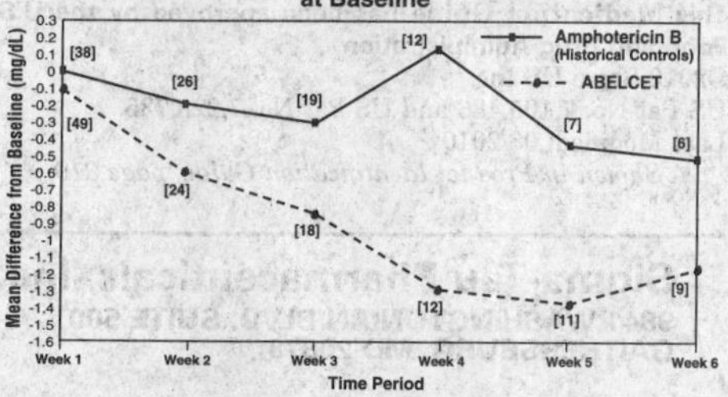

[ ]= Number of patients at each time point.
Note: These curves do not represent the clinical course of a given patient, but that of an open-label cohort of patients.

Figure 2
Changes in Mean Serum Creatinine Over Time
Patients with Fungal Infections and Serum Creatinine >2.5 mg/dL at Baseline

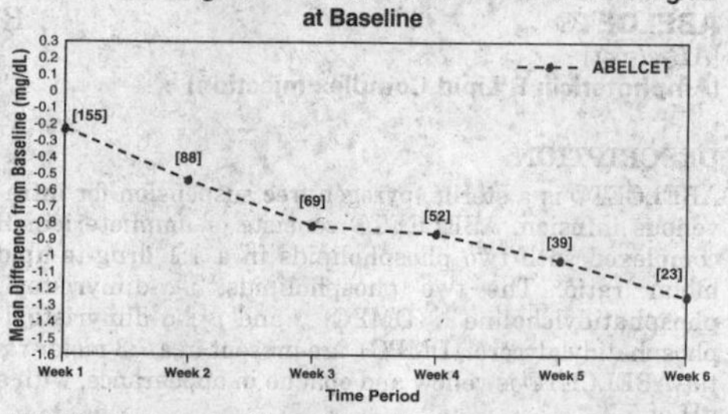

[ ]= Number of patients at each time point.
Note: These curves do not represent the clinical course of a given patient, but that of an open-label cohort of patients.

In a randomized study of ABELCET® for the treatment of invasive candidiasis in patients with normal baseline renal function, the incidence of nephrotoxicity was significantly less for ABELCET® at a dose of 5 mg/kg/day than for conventional amphotericin B at a dose of 0.7 mg/kg/day.

Despite generally less nephrotoxicity of ABELCET® observed at a dose of 5 mg/kg/day compared with conventional amphotericin B therapy at a dose range of 0.6-1 mg/kg/day, dose-limiting renal toxicity may still be observed with ABELCET®. Renal toxicity of doses greater than 5 mg/kg/day of ABELCET® has not been formally studied.

CONTRAINDICATIONS

ABELCET® is contraindicated in patients who have shown hypersensitivity to amphotericin B or any other component in the formulation.

WARNINGS

Anaphylaxis has been reported with amphotericin B desoxycholate and other amphotericin B-containing drugs. Anaphylaxis has been reported with ABELCET® with an incidence rate of <0.1%. If severe respiratory distress occurs, the infusion should be immediately discontinued. The patient should not receive further infusions of ABELCET®.

PRECAUTIONS

General: As with any amphotericin B-containing product, during the initial dosing of ABELCET®, the drug should be administered under close clinical observation by medically trained personnel.

Acute reactions including fever and chills may occur 1 to 2 hours after starting an intravenous infusion of ABELCET®. These reactions are usually more common with the first few doses of ABELCET® and generally diminish with subsequent doses. Infusion has been rarely associated with hypotension, bronchospasm, arrhythmias, and shock.

Laboratory Tests: Serum creatinine should be monitored frequently during ABELCET® therapy (see ADVERSE REACTIONS). It is also advisable to regularly monitor liver function, serum electrolytes (particularly magnesium and potassium), and complete blood counts.

Drug Interactions: No formal clinical studies of drug interactions have been conducted with ABELCET®. However, when administered concomitantly, the following drugs are known to interact with amphotericin B; therefore, the following drugs may interact with ABELCET®:

Antineoplastic agents: Concurrent use of antineoplastic agents and amphotericin B may enhance the potential for renal toxicity, bronchospasm, and hypotension. Antineoplastic agents should be given concomitantly with ABELCET® with great caution.

Corticosteroids and corticotropin (ACTH): Concurrent use of corticosteroids and corticotropin (ACTH) with amphotericin B may potentiate hypokalemia which could predispose the patient to cardiac dysfunction. If used concomitantly with ABELCET®, serum electrolytes and cardiac function should be closely monitored.

Cyclosporin A: Data from a prospective study of prophylactic ABELCET® in 22 patients undergoing bone marrow transplantation suggested that concurrent initiation of cyclosporin A and ABELCET® within several days of bone marrow ablation may be associated with increased nephrotoxicity.

Digitalis glycosides: Concurrent use of amphotericin B may induce hypokalemia and may potentiate digitalis toxicity. When administered concomitantly with ABELCET®, serum potassium levels should be closely monitored.

Flucytosine: Concurrent use of flucytosine with amphotericin B-containing preparations may increase the toxicity of flucytosine by possibly increasing its cellular uptake and/or impairing its renal excretion. Flucytosine should be given concomitantly with ABELCET® with caution.

Imidazoles (e.g., ketoconazole, miconazole, clotrimazole, fluconazole, etc.): Antagonism between amphotericin B and imidazole derivatives such as miconazole and ketoconazole, which inhibit ergosterol synthesis, has been reported in both *in vitro* and *in vivo* animal studies. The clinical significance of these findings has not been determined.

Leukocyte transfusions: Acute pulmonary toxicity has been reported in patients receiving intravenous amphotericin B and leukocyte transfusions. Leukocyte transfusions and ABELCET® should not be given concurrently.

Other nephrotoxic medications: Concurrent use of amphotericin B and agents such as aminoglycosides and pentamidine may enhance the potential for drug-induced renal toxicity. Aminoglycosides and pentamidine should be used concomitantly with ABELCET® only with great caution. Intensive monitoring of renal function is recommended in patients requiring any combination of nephrotoxic medications.

Skeletal muscle relaxants: Amphotericin B-induced hypokalemia may enhance the curariform effect of skeletal muscle relaxants (e.g., tubocurarine) due to hypokalemia. When administered concomitantly with ABELCET®, serum potassium levels should be closely monitored.

Zidovudine: Increased myelotoxicity and nephrotoxicity were observed in dogs when either ABELCET® (at doses 0.16 or 0.5 times the recommended human dose) or amphotericin B desoxycholate (at 0.5 times the recommended human dose) were administered concomitantly with zidovudine for 30 days. If zidovudine is used concomitantly with ABELCET®, renal and hematologic function should be closely monitored.

Carcinogenesis, Mutagenesis, and Impairment of Fertility: No long-term studies in animals have been performed to evaluate the carcinogenic potential of ABELCET®. The following *in vitro* (with and without metabolic activation) and *in vivo* studies to assess ABELCET® for mutagenic potential were conducted: bacterial reverse mutation assay, mouse lymphoma forward mutation assay, chromosomal aberration assay in CHO cells, and *in vivo* mouse micronucleus assay. ABELCET® was found to be without mutagenic effects in all assay systems. Studies demonstrated that ABELCET® had no impact on fertility in male and female rats at doses up to 0.32 times the recommended human dose (based on body surface area considerations).

Pregnancy: There are no reports of pregnant women having been treated with ABELCET®. Teratogenic Effects. Pregnancy Category B: Reproductive studies in rats and rabbits at doses of ABELCET® up to 0.64 times the human dose revealed no harm to the fetus. Because animal reproductive studies are not always predictive of human response, and adequate and well-controlled studies have not been conducted in pregnant women, ABELCET® should be used during pregnancy only after taking into account the importance of the drug to the mother.

Nursing Mothers: It is not known whether ABELCET® is excreted in human milk. Because many drugs are excreted in human milk, and because of the potential for serious adverse reactions in breast-fed infants from ABELCET®, a decision should be made whether to discontinue nursing or to discontinue the drug, taking into account the importance of the drug to the mother.

Pediatric Use: One hundred eleven children (2 were enrolled twice and counted as separate patients), age 16 years and under, of whom 11 were less than 1 year, have been treated with ABELCET® at 5 mg/kg/day in two open-label studies and one small, prospective, single-arm study. In one single-center study, 5 children with hepatosplenic candidiasis were effectively treated with 2.5 mg/kg/day of ABELCET®. No serious unexpected adverse events have been reported.

Geriatric Use: Forty-nine elderly patients, age 65 years or over, have been treated with ABELCET® at 5 mg/kg/day in two open-label studies and one small, prospective, single-arm study. No serious unexpected adverse events have been reported.

ADVERSE REACTIONS

The total safety data base is composed of 921 patients treated with ABELCET® (5 patients were enrolled twice and counted as separate patients), of whom 775 were treated with 5 mg/kg/day. Of these 775 patients, 194 patients were treated in four comparative studies; 25 were treated in open-label, non-comparative studies; and 556 patients were treated in an open-label, emergency-use program. Most had underlying hematologic neoplasms, and many were receiving multiple concomitant medications. Of the 556 patients treated with ABELCET®, 9% discontinued treatment due to adverse events regardless of presumed relationship to study drug.

In general, the adverse events most commonly reported with ABELCET® were transient chills and/or fever during infusion of the drug.

Adverse Events[a] with an Incidence of ≥3% (N=556)

Adverse Event	Percentage (%) of Patients
Chills	18
Fever	14
Increased Serum Creatinine	11
Multiple Organ Failure	11
Nausea	9
Hypotension	8
Respiratory Failure	8
Vomiting	8
Dyspnea	7
Sepsis	7
Diarrhea	6
Headache	6
Heart Arrest	6
Hypertension	5
Hypokalemia	5
Infection	5
Kidney Failure	5
Pain	5
Thrombocytopenia	5
Abdominal Pain	4
Anemia	4
Bilirubinemia	4
Gastrointestinal Hemorrhage	4
Leukopenia	4
Rash	4
Respiratory Disorder	4
Chest Pain	3
Nausea and Vomiting	3

[a] The causal association between these adverse events and ABELCET® is uncertain.

The following adverse events have also been reported in patients using ABELCET® in open-label, uncontrolled clinical studies. The causal association between these adverse events and ABELCET® is uncertain.

Body as a whole: malaise, weight loss, deafness, injection site reaction including inflammation

Allergic: bronchospasm, wheezing, asthma, anaphylactoid and other allergic reactions

Cardiopulmonary: cardiac failure, pulmonary edema, shock, myocardial infarction, hemoptysis, tachypnea, thrombophlebitis, pulmonary embolus, cardiomyopathy, pleural effusion, arrhythmias including ventricular fibrillation.

Dermatological: maculopapular rash, pruritus, exfoliative dermatitis, erythema multiforme

Gastrointestinal: acute liver failure, hepatitis, jaundice, melena, anorexia, dyspepsia, cramping, epigastric pain, veno-occlusive liver disease, diarrhea, hepatomegaly, cholangitis, cholecystitis

Hematologic: coagulation defects, leukocytosis, blood dyscrasias including eosinophilia

Musculoskeletal: myasthenia, including bone, muscle, and joint pains

Neurologic: convulsions, tinnitus, visual impairment, hearing loss, peripheral neuropathy, transient vertigo, diplopia, encephalopathy, cerebral vascular accident, extrapyramidal syndrome and other neurologic symptoms

Urogenital: oliguria, decreased renal function, anuria, renal tubular acidosis, impotence, dysuria

Serum electrolyte abnormalities: hypomagnesemia, hyperkalemia, hypocalcemia, hypercalcemia

Liver function test abnormalities: increased AST, ALT, alkaline phosphatase, LDH

Renal function test abnormalities: increased BUN

Other test abnormalities: acidosis, hyperamylasemia, hypoglycemia, hyperglycemia, hyperuricemia, hypophosphatemia

To report SUSPECTED ADVERSE REACTIONS, contact Sigma-Tau Pharmaceuticals, Inc. at 1-888-393-4584 or by email at drugsafety@sigmatau.com or contact the FDA at 1-800-FDA-1088 or www.fda.gov/safety/medwatch.

OVERDOSAGE

Amphotericin B desoxycholate overdose has been reported to result in cardio-respiratory arrest. Fifteen patients have been reported to have received one or more doses of ABELCET® between 7-13 mg/kg. None of these patients had a serious acute reaction to ABELCET®. If an overdose is suspected, discontinue therapy, monitor the patient's clinical status, and administer supportive therapy as required. ABELCET® is not hemodialyzable.

DOSAGE AND ADMINISTRATION

The recommended daily dosage for adults and children is 5 mg/kg given as a single infusion. ABELCET® should be administered by intravenous infusion at a rate of 2.5 mg/kg/h. If the infusion time exceeds 2 hours, mix the contents by shaking the infusion bag every 2 hours.

Renal toxicity of ABELCET®, as measured by serum creatinine levels, has been shown to be dose dependent. Decisions about dose adjustments should be made only after taking into account the overall clinical condition of the patient.

Preparation of Admixture for Infusion: Shake the vial gently until there is no evidence of any yellow sediment at the bottom. Withdraw the appropriate dose of ABELCET® from the required number of vials into one or more sterile syringes using an 18-gauge needle. Remove the needle from each syringe filled with ABELCET® and replace with the 5-micron filter needle supplied with each vial. Each filter needle may be used to filter the contents of up to four 100 mg vials. Insert the filter needle of the syringe into an IV bag containing 5% Dextrose Injection USP, and empty the contents of the syringe into the bag. The final infusion concentration should be 1 mg/mL. For pediatric patients and patients with cardiovascular disease the drug may be diluted with 5% Dextrose Injection to a final infusion concentration of 2 mg/mL. Before infusion, shake the bag until the contents are thoroughly mixed. Do not use the admixture after dilution with 5% Dextrose Injection if there is any evidence of foreign matter. Vials are for single use. Unused material should be discarded. Aseptic technique must be strictly observed throughout handling of ABELCET®, since no bacteriostatic agent or preservative is present.

DO NOT DILUTE WITH SALINE SOLUTIONS OR MIX WITH OTHER DRUGS OR ELECTROLYTES as the compatibility of ABELCET® with these materials has not been established. An existing intravenous line should be flushed with 5% Dextrose Injection before infusion of ABELCET®, or a separate infusion line should be used. DO NOT USE AN IN-LINE FILTER.

The diluted ready-for-use admixture is stable for up to 48 hours at 2° to 8°C (36° to 46°F) and an additional 6 hours at room temperature.

HOW SUPPLIED

Single-use vials along with 5-micron filter needles are individually packaged.

100 mg of ABELCET® in 20 mL of suspension NDC 57665-101-41

STORAGE

Prior to admixture, ABELCET® should be stored at 2° to 8°C (36° to 46°F) and protected from exposure to light. Do not freeze. ABELCET® should be retained in the carton until time of use.

The admixed ABELCET® and 5% Dextrose Injection may be stored for up to 48 hours at 2° to 8°C (36° to 46°F) and an additional 6 hours at room temperature. Do not freeze. Any unused material should be discarded.

U.S. Patent Nos. 4,973,465
                5,616,334
                6,406,713

                      I-101-41-US-M

SIGMA-TAU PHARMACEUTICALS, INC.
Manufactured by Sigma-Tau PharmaSource, Inc., Indianapolis, IN 46268. Distributed by Sigma-Tau Pharmaceuticals, Inc., Gaithersburg, MD 20878.
Revised 05/2010

Solvay Pharmaceuticals, Inc./ Abbott Laboratories
Pharmaceutical Products Division
NORTH CHICAGO, IL 60064 U.S.A.

Pharmaceutical Products Division—
Direct Inquiries to:
Customer Service:
(800) 255-5162
Patient Access Program:
(800) 441-4987
For Medical Information Contact:
(800) 633-9110 or www.abbottmedinfo.com
Adverse experiences or side effects
(for all Abbott drug products):
(800) 633-9110 or rxabbott.com
Sales and Ordering:
(800) 255-5162

CREON®   ℞
[krē 'ŏn]
(pancrelipase)
delayed-release capsules

HIGHLIGHTS OF PRESCRIBING INFORMATION
These highlights do not include all the information needed to use CREON safely and effectively. See full prescribing information for CREON.
CREON (pancrelipase) delayed-release capsules
Initial U.S. Approval: 2009

————**RECENT MAJOR CHANGES**————
Indications and Usage, Chronic Pancreatitis, Pancreatectomy (1) 4/2010
Dosage and Administration, Chronic Pancreatitis or Pancreatectomy (2.1) 4/2010

————**INDICATIONS AND USAGE**————
CREON is a combination of porcine-derived lipases, proteases, and amylases indicated for the treatment of exocrine pancreatic insufficiency due to cystic fibrosis, chronic pancreatitis, pancreatectomy, or other conditions. (1)

————**DOSAGE AND ADMINISTRATION**————
Dosage
CREON is not interchangeable with any other pancrelipase product.
Infants (up to 12 months)
• Infants may be given 2,000 to 4,000 lipase units per 120 mL of formula or per breast-feeding. (2.1)
• Do not mix CREON capsule contents directly into formula or breast milk prior to administration. (2.2)
Children Older than 12 Months and Younger than 4 Years
• Enzyme dosing should begin with 1,000 lipase units/kg of body weight per meal for children less than age 4 years to a maximum of 2,500 lipase units/kg of body weight per meal (or less than or equal to 10,000 lipase units/kg of body weight per day), or less than 4,000 lipase units/g fat ingested per day. (2.1)
Children 4 Years and Older and Adults
• Enzyme dosing should begin with 500 lipase units/kg of body weight per meal for those older than age 4 years to a maximum of 2,500 lipase units/kg of body weight per meal (or less than or equal to 10,000 lipase units/kg of body weight per day), or less than 4,000 lipase units/g fat ingested per day. (2.1)
Adults with Exocrine Pancreatic Insufficiency Due to Chronic Pancreatitis or Pancreatectomy
• In one clinical trial, patients received CREON at a dose of 72,000 lipase units per meal while consuming at least 100 g of fat per day. Lower starting doses recommended in the literature are consistent with the 500 lipase units/kg of body weight per meal lowest starting dose recommended for adults in the Cystic Fibrosis Foundation Consensus Conferences Guidelines. Dosage should be individualized based on clinical symptoms, the degree of steatorrhea present and the fat content of the diet. (2.1)
Limitations on Dosing
• Dosing should not exceed the recommended maximum dosage set forth by the Cystic Fibrosis Foundation Consensus Conferences Guidelines. (2.1)
Administration
CREON should be swallowed whole. For infants or patients unable to swallow intact capsules, the contents may be sprinkled on soft acidic food, e.g., applesauce. (2.2)

Information on the Solvay/Abbott Pharmaceutical Products listed on these pages is from the prescribing information in use as of June 1, 2010. For more information, please visit rxabbott.com or call 1-800-633-9110.

DOSAGE FORMS AND STRENGTHS

- Capsules: 6,000 USP units of lipase; 19,000 USP units of protease; 30,000 USP units of amylase capsules have an orange opaque cap with imprint "CREON 1206" and a blue opaque body. (3)
- Capsules: 12,000 USP units of lipase; 38,000 USP units of protease; 60,000 USP units of amylase capsules have a brown opaque cap with imprint "CREON 1212" and a colorless transparent body. (3)
- Capsules: 24,000 USP units of lipase; 76,000 USP units of protease; 120,000 USP units of amylase capsules have an orange opaque cap with imprint "CREON 1224" and a colorless transparent body. (3)

CONTRAINDICATIONS

None (4)

WARNINGS AND PRECAUTIONS

- Fibrosing colonopathy is associated with high-dose use of pancreatic enzyme replacement in the treatment of cystic fibrosis patients. Exercise caution when doses of CREON exceed 2,500 lipase units/kg of body weight per meal (or greater than 10,000 lipase units/kg of body weight per day). (5.1)
- To avoid irritation of oral mucosa, do not chew CREON or retain in the mouth.. (5.2)
- Exercise caution when prescribing CREON to patients with gout, renal impairment, or hyperuricemia. (5.3)
- There is theoretical risk of viral transmission with all pancreatic enzyme products including CREON. (5.4)
- Exercise caution when administering pancrelipase to a patient with a known allergy to proteins of porcine origin. (5.5)

ADVERSE REACTIONS

- Treatment-emergent adverse events occurring in at least 2 cystic fibrosis patients (greater than or equal to 6%) receiving CREON or placebo are abdominal pain, abdominal pain upper, abnormal feces, cough, dizziness, flatulence, headache, and weight decreased. (6.1)
- Treatment-emergent adverse events that occurred in at least 1 chronic pancreatitis or pancreatectomy patient (greater than or equal to 4%) receiving CREON were abdominal pain, abnormal feces, diabetes mellitus inadequate control, flatulence, frequent bowel movements, hyperglycemia, hypoglycemia, and nasopharyngitis. (6.1)

To report SUSPECTED ADVERSE REACTIONS, contact Abbott Laboratories at 1-800-241-1643 or FDA at 1-800-FDA-1088 or www.fda.gov/medwatch.

USE IN SPECIFIC POPULATIONS

Pediatric Patients

- The safety and effectiveness of CREON were assessed in pediatric cystic fibrosis patients, aged 12 to 17 years old. (8.4)
- The safety and efficacy of pancreatic enzyme products with different formulations of pancrelipase in pediatric patients have been described in the medical literature and through clinical experience. (8.4)

See 17 for PATIENT COUNSELING INFORMATION and Medication Guide

Revised: 04/2010

FULL PRESCRIBING INFORMATION: CONTENTS*

17 PATIENT COUNSELING INFORMATION

* Sections or subsections omitted from the full prescribing information are not listed

FULL PRESCRIBING INFORMATION

1 INDICATIONS AND USAGE

CREON® (pancrelipase) is indicated for the treatment of exocrine pancreatic insufficiency due to cystic fibrosis, chronic pancreatitis, pancreatectomy, or other conditions.

2 DOSAGE AND ADMINISTRATION

2.1 Dosage

CREON is not interchangeable with other pancrelipase products.

CREON is orally administered. Therapy should be initiated at the lowest recommended dose and gradually increased. The dosage of CREON should be individualized based on clinical symptoms, the degree of steatorrhea present, and the fat content of the diet [see Limitations on Dosing below and see Warnings and Precautions (5.1)].

Dosage recommendations for pancreatic enzyme replacement therapy were published following the Cystic Fibrosis Foundation Consensus Conferences.[1, 2, 3] CREON should be administered in a manner consistent with the recommendations of the Conferences provided in the following paragraphs. Patients may be dosed on a fat ingestion-based or actual body weight-based dosing scheme.

Additional recommendations for pancreatic enzyme therapy in patients with exocrine pancreatic insufficiency due to chronic pancreatitis or pancreatectomy are based on a clinical trial conducted in these populations.

Infants (up to 12 months)
Infants may be given 2,000 to 4,000 lipase units per 120 mL of formula or per breast-feeding. Do not mix CREON capsule contents directly into formula or breast milk prior to administration [see Dosage and Administration (2.2)].

Children Older than 12 Months and Younger than 4 Years
Enzyme dosing should begin with 1,000 lipase units/kg of body weight per meal for children less than age 4 years to a maximum of 2,500 lipase units/kg of body weight per meal (or less than or equal to 10,000 lipase units/kg of body weight per day), or less than 4,000 lipase units/g fat ingested per day.

Children 4 Years and Older and Adults
Enzyme dosing should begin with 500 lipase units/kg of body weight per meal for those older than age 4 years to a maximum of 2,500 lipase units/kg of body weight per meal (or less than or equal to 10,000 lipase units/kg of body weight per day), or less than 4,000 lipase units/g fat ingested per day.

Usually, half of the prescribed CREON dose for an individualized full meal should be given with each snack. The total daily dose should reflect approximately three meals plus two or three snacks per day.

Enzyme doses expressed as lipase units/kg of body weight per meal should be decreased in older patients because they weigh more but tend to ingest less fat per kilogram of body weight.

Adults with Exocrine Pancreatic Insufficiency Due to Chronic Pancreatitis or Pancreatectomy
In one clinical trial, patients received CREON at a dose of 72,000 lipase units per meal while consuming at least 100 g of fat per day [see Clinical Studies (14.2)]. Lower starting doses recommended in the literature are consistent with the 500 lipase units/kg of body weight per meal lowest starting dose recommended for adults in the Cystic Fibrosis Foundation Consensus Conferences Guidelines.[1, 2, 3, 4] The initial starting dose and increases in the dose per meal should be individualized based on clinical symptoms, the degree of steatorrhea present, and the fat content of the diet.

Usually, half of the prescribed CREON dose for an individualized full meal should be given with each snack.

Limitations on Dosing
Dosing should not exceed the recommended maximum dosage set forth by the Cystic Fibrosis Foundation Consensus Conferences Guidelines.[1, 2, 3] If symptoms and signs of steatorrhea persist, the dosage may be increased by the healthcare professional. Patients should be instructed not to increase the dosage on their own. There is great interindividual variation in response to enzymes; thus, a range of doses is recommended. Changes in dosage may require an adjustment period of several days. If doses are to exceed 2,500 lipase units/kg of body weight per meal, further investigation is warranted. Doses greater than 2,500 lipase units/kg of body weight per meal (or greater than 10,000 lipase units/kg of body weight per day) should be used with caution and only if they are documented to be effective by 3-day fecal fat measures that indicate a significantly improved coefficient of fat absorption. Doses greater than 6,000 lipase units/kg of body weight per meal have been associated with colonic stricture, indicative of fibrosing

colonopathy, in children less than 12 years of age [see Warnings and Precautions (5.1)]. Patients currently receiving higher doses than 6,000 lipase units/kg of body weight per meal should be examined and the dosage either immediately decreased or titrated downward to a lower range.

2.2 Administration

CREON should always be taken as prescribed by a healthcare professional.

Infants (up to 12 months)
CREON should be administered to infants immediately prior to each feeding, using a dosage of 2,000 to 4,000 lipase units per 120 mL of formula or per breast-feeding. Contents of the capsule may be administered directly to the mouth or with a small amount of applesauce. Administration should be followed by breast milk or formula. Contents of the capsule should not be mixed directly into formula or breast milk as this may diminish efficacy. Care should be taken to ensure that CREON is not crushed or chewed or retained in the mouth, to avoid irritation of the oral mucosa.

Children and Adults
CREON should be taken during meals or snacks, with sufficient fluid. CREON capsules and capsule contents should not be crushed or chewed. Capsules should be swallowed whole.

For patients who are unable to swallow intact capsules, the capsules may be carefully opened and the contents added to a small amount of acidic soft food with a pH of 4 or less, such as applesauce, at room temperature. The CREON-soft food mixture should be swallowed immediately without crushing or chewing, and followed with water or juice to ensure complete ingestion. Care should be taken to ensure that no drug is retained in the mouth.

3 DOSAGE FORMS AND STRENGTHS

The active ingredient in CREON evaluated in clinical trials is lipase. CREON is dosed by lipase units.

Other active ingredients include protease and amylase. Each CREON capsule strength contains the specified amounts of lipase, protease, and amylase as follows:

- 6,000 USP units of lipase; 19,000 USP units of protease; 30,000 USP units of amylase capsules have an orange opaque cap with imprint "CREON 1206" and a blue opaque body.
- 12,000 USP units of lipase; 38,000 USP units of protease; 60,000 USP units of amylase capsules have a brown opaque cap with imprint "CREON 1212" and a colorless transparent body.
- 24,000 USP units of lipase; 76,000 USP units of protease; 120,000 USP units of amylase capsules have an orange opaque cap with imprint "CREON 1224" and a colorless transparent body.

4 CONTRAINDICATIONS

None.

5 WARNINGS AND PRECAUTIONS

5.1 Fibrosing Colonopathy

Fibrosing colonopathy has been reported following treatment with different pancreatic enzyme products.[5, 6] Fibrosing colonopathy is a rare, serious adverse reaction initially described in association with high-dose pancreatic enzyme use, usually over a prolonged period of time and most commonly reported in pediatric patients with cystic fibrosis. The underlying mechanism of fibrosing colonopathy remains unknown. Doses of pancreatic enzyme products exceeding 6,000 lipase units/kg of body weight per meal have been associated with colonic stricture in children less than 12 years of age.[1] Patients with fibrosing colonopathy should be closely monitored because some patients may be at risk of progressing to stricture formation. It is uncertain whether regression of fibrosing colonopathy occurs.[1] It is generally recommended, unless clinically indicated, that enzyme doses should be less than 2,500 lipase units/kg of body weight per meal (or less than 10,000 lipase units/kg of body weight per day) or less than 4,000 lipase units/g fat ingested per day [see Dosage and Administration (2.1)].

Doses greater than 2,500 lipase units/kg of body weight per meal (or greater than 10,000 lipase units/kg of body weight per day) should be used with caution and only if they are documented to be effective by 3-day fecal fat measures that indicate a significantly improved coefficient of fat absorption. Patients receiving higher doses than 6,000 lipase units/kg of body weight per meal should be examined and the dosage either immediately decreased or titrated downward to a lower range.

5.2 Potential for Irritation to Oral Mucosa

Care should be taken to ensure that no drug is retained in the mouth. CREON should not be crushed or chewed or mixed in foods having a pH greater than 4. These actions can disrupt the protective enteric coating resulting in early release of enzymes, irritation of oral mucosa, and/or loss of enzyme activity [see Dosage and Administration (2.2) and Patient Counseling Information (17.1)]. For patients who are unable to swallow intact capsules, the capsules may be carefully opened and the contents added to a small amount of acidic soft food with a pH of 4 or less, such as applesauce, at room temperature. The CREON-soft food mixture should be swallowed immediately and followed with water or juice to ensure complete ingestion.

5.3 Potential for Risk of Hyperuricemia

Caution should be exercised when prescribing CREON to patients with gout, renal impairment, or hyperuricemia. Porcine-derived pancreatic enzyme products contain purines that may increase blood uric acid levels.

5.4 Potential Viral Exposure from the Product Source

CREON is sourced from pancreatic tissue from swine used for food consumption. Although the risk that CREON will transmit an infectious agent to humans has been reduced by testing for certain viruses during manufacturing and by inactivating certain viruses during manufacturing, there is a theoretical risk for transmission of viral disease, including diseases caused by novel or unidentified viruses. Thus, the presence of porcine viruses that might infect humans cannot be definitely excluded. However, no cases of transmission of an infectious illness associated with the use of porcine pancreatic extracts have been reported.

5.5 Allergic Reactions

Caution should be exercised when administering pancrelipase to a patient with a known allergy to proteins of porcine origin. Rarely, severe allergic reactions including anaphylaxis, asthma, hives, and pruritus, have been reported with other pancreatic enzyme products with different formulations of the same active ingredient (pancrelipase). The risks and benefits of continued CREON treatment in patients with severe allergy should be taken into consideration with the overall clinical needs of the patient.

6 ADVERSE REACTIONS

The most serious adverse reactions reported with different pancreatic enzyme products of the same active ingredient (pancrelipase) include fibrosing colonopathy, hyperuricemia and allergic reactions *[see Warnings and Precautions (5)]*.

6.1 Clinical Trials Experience

Because clinical trials are conducted under widely varying conditions, adverse reaction rates observed in the clinical trials of a drug cannot be directly compared to the rates in the clinical trials of another drug and may not reflect the rates observed in practice.

The short-term safety of CREON was assessed in two clinical trials conducted in 86 patients with exocrine pancreatic insufficiency (EPI). Study 1 was conducted in 32 patients with EPI due to cystic fibrosis (CF); Study 2 was conducted in 54 patients with EPI due to chronic pancreatitis or pancreatectomy.

Cystic Fibrosis

Study 1 was a randomized, double-blind, placebo-controlled, crossover study of 32 patients, ages 12 to 43 years, with EPI due to CF. In this study, patients were randomized to receive CREON at a dose of 4,000 lipase units/g fat ingested per day or matching placebo for 5 to 6 days of treatment, followed by crossover to the alternate treatment for an additional 5 to 6 days. The mean exposure to CREON during this study was 5 days.

One patient experienced duodenitis and gastritis of moderate severity reported as a serious adverse event 16 days after completing treatment with CREON.

Transient neutropenia without clinical sequelae was observed as an abnormal laboratory finding in one patient receiving CREON and a macrolide antibiotic.

The incidence of adverse events (regardless of causality) was higher during placebo treatment (71%) than during CREON treatment (50%). Adverse events reported during the study were predominantly gastrointestinal complaints, and the type and incidence of adverse events were similar in adolescents (12 to 18 years) and adults (greater than 18 years).

Because clinical trials are conducted under controlled conditions, the observed adverse event rates may not reflect the rates observed in clinical practice.

Table 1 enumerates treatment-emergent adverse events that occurred in at least 2 patients (greater than or equal to 6%) treated with either CREON or placebo in Study 1.

Table 1: Treatment-Emergent Adverse Events Occurring in at least 2 Patients (greater than or equal to 6%) in Either Treatment Group of the Placebo-Controlled, Crossover Clinical Study of CREON in Cystic Fibrosis (Study 1)

MedDRA Primary System Organ Class Preferred Term	CREON Capsules n = 32 (%)	Placebo n = 31 (%)
Gastrointestinal Disorders		
Abnormal Feces	1 (3)	6 (19)
Flatulence	3 (9)	8 (26)
Abdominal Pain	3 (9)	8 (26)
Abdominal Pain Upper	0	3 (10)
Investigations		
Weight Decreased	1 (3)	2 (6)
Nervous System Disorders		
Headache	2 (6)	8 (26)
Dizziness	2 (6)	0
Respiratory, Thoracic and Mediastinal Disorders		
Cough	2 (6)	0

Chronic Pancreatitis or Pancreatectomy

Study 2 was a randomized, double-blind, placebo-controlled, parallel group study of 54 adult patients, ages 32 to 75 years, with EPI due to chronic pancreatitis or pancreatectomy. Patients received single-blind placebo treatment during a 5-day run-in period followed by an intervening period of up to 16 days of investigator-directed treatment with no restrictions on pancreatic enzyme replacement therapy. Patients were then randomized to receive CREON or matching placebo for 7 days. The CREON dose was 72,000 lipase units per main meal (3 main meals) and 36,000 lipase units per snack (2 snacks). The mean exposure to CREON during this study was 6.8 days.

The incidence of treatment-emergent adverse events (regardless of causality) was 20% with CREON treatment and 21% with placebo treatment. The most common adverse events reported during the study were related to glycemic control and were reported more commonly during CREON treatment (12%) than during placebo treatment (7%).

Because clinical trials are conducted under controlled conditions, the observed adverse event rates may not reflect the rates observed in clinical practice.

Table 2 enumerates treatment-emergent adverse events that occurred in at least 1 patient (greater than or equal to 4%) in the CREON group.

Table 2: Treatment-Emergent Adverse Events Reported During the Randomized Period in at least 1 Patient (greater than or equal to 4%) in the CREON Group in Chronic Pancreatitis or Pancreatectomy (Study 2)

MedDRA Primary System Organ Class Preferred Term	CREON Capsules n = 25 (%)	Placebo n = 29 (%)
Gastrointestinal Disorders		
Abdominal Pain	1 (4)	1 (3)
Abnormal Feces	1 (4)	0
Flatulence	1 (4)	0
Frequent Bowel Movements	1 (4)	0
Infections and Infestations		
Nasopharyngitis	1 (4)	0
Metabolism and Nutritional Disorders		
Diabetes Mellitus Inadequate Control	1 (4)	0
Hyperglycemia	1 (4)	2 (7)
Hypoglycemia	1 (4)	1 (3)

6.2 Postmarketing Experience

Postmarketing data from this formulation of CREON has been available since 2009. The following adverse events have been reported with this formulation of CREON in spontaneous postmarketing reports: gastrointestinal disorders (including abdominal pain, diarrhea, flatulence, constipation and nausea), skin disorders (including pruritus, urticaria and rash), blurred vision, myalgia, muscle spasm, and asymptomatic elevations of liver enzymes.

Delayed- and immediate-release pancreatic enzyme products with different formulations of the same active ingredient (pancrelipase) have been used for the treatment of patients with exocrine pancreatic insufficiency due to cystic fibrosis and other conditions, such as chronic pancreatitis. The long-term safety profile of these products has been described in the medical literature. The most serious adverse events included fibrosing colonopathy, distal intestinal obstruction syndrome (DIOS), recurrence of pre-existing carcinoma, and severe allergic reactions including anaphylaxis, asthma, hives, and pruritus. In general, these products have a well defined and favorable risk-benefit profile in exocrine pancreatic insufficiency.

Because these reactions are reported voluntarily from a population of uncertain size, it is not always possible to reliably estimate their frequency or establish a causal relationship to drug exposure.

7 DRUG INTERACTIONS

No drug interactions have been identified. No formal interaction studies have been conducted.

8 USE IN SPECIFIC POPULATIONS

8.1 Pregnancy

Teratogenic effects

Pregnancy Category C: Animal reproduction studies have not been conducted with pancrelipase. It is also not known whether pancrelipase can cause fetal harm when administered to a pregnant woman or can affect reproduction capacity. The risk and benefit of pancrelipase should be considered in the context of the need to provide adequate nutritional support to a pregnant woman with exocrine pancreatic insufficiency. Adequate caloric intake during pregnancy is important for normal maternal weight gain and fetal growth. Reduced maternal weight gain and malnutrition can be associated with adverse pregnancy outcomes. Patients should notify their healthcare professional if they are pregnant or are thinking of becoming pregnant during treatment with CREON.

8.3 Nursing Mothers

It is not known whether this drug is excreted in human milk. Because many drugs are excreted in human milk, caution should be exercised when CREON is administered to a nursing woman. The risk and benefit of pancrelipase should be considered in the context of the need to provide adequate nutritional support to a nursing mother with exocrine pancreatic insufficiency.

8.4 Pediatric Use

The short-term safety and efficacy of CREON were assessed in a single, randomized, double-blind, placebo-controlled, crossover study of 32 patients with exocrine pancreatic insufficiency due to cystic fibrosis, including 12 patients between 12 and 18 years of age. The safety and efficacy in 12 to 18 year old patients in this study were similar to adult patients *[see Adverse Reactions (6.1) and Clinical Studies (14)]*.

The safety and efficacy of pancreatic enzyme products with different formulations of pancrelipase consisting of the same active ingredient (lipases, proteases, and amylases) for treatment of children with exocrine pancreatic insufficiency due to cystic fibrosis have been described in the medical literature and through clinical experience.

Dosing of pediatric patients should be in accordance with recommended guidance from the Cystic Fibrosis Foundation Consensus Conferences *[see Dosage and Administration (2.1)]*. Doses of other pancreatic enzyme products exceeding 6,000 lipase units/kg of body weight per meal have been associated with fibrosing colonopathy and colonic strictures in children less than 12 years of age *[see Warnings and Precautions (5.1)]*.

10 OVERDOSAGE

There have been no reports of overdose in clinical trials with CREON, or in clinical trials or postmarketing surveillance with other pancreatic enzyme products. Chronic high doses of pancreatic enzyme products have been associated with fibrosing colonopathy and colonic strictures *[see Dosage and Administration (2.1) and Warnings and Precautions (5.1)]*. High doses of pancreatic enzyme products have been associated with hyperuricosuria and hyperuricemia, and should be used with caution in patients with a history of hyperuricemia, gout, or renal impairment *[see Warnings and Precautions (5.3)]*.

11 DESCRIPTION

CREON is a pancreatic enzyme preparation consisting of pancrelipase, an extract derived from porcine pancreatic glands. Pancrelipase contains multiple enzyme classes, including porcine-derived lipases, proteases, and amylases.

Pancrelipase is a beige-white amorphous powder. It is miscible in water and practically insoluble or insoluble in alcohol and ether.

Each delayed-release capsule for oral administration contains enteric-coated spheres (0.71–1.60 mm in diameter).

The active ingredient evaluated in clinical trials is lipase. CREON is dosed by lipase units.

Other active ingredients include protease and amylase.

CREON contains the following inactive ingredients: cetyl alcohol, dimethicone, hypromellose phthalate, polyethylene glycol, and triethyl citrate. The imprinting ink on the capsule contains dimethicone, 2-ethoxyethanol, shellac, soya lecithin, and titanium dioxide.

Information on the Solvay/Abbott Pharmaceutical Products listed on these pages is from the prescribing information in use as of June 1, 2010. For more information, please visit rxabbott.com or call 1-800-633-9110.

6,000 USP units of lipase; 19,000 USP units of protease; 30,000 USP units of amylase capsules have a Swedish-orange opaque cap with imprint "CREON 1206" and a blue opaque body. The shells contain FD&C Blue No. 2, gelatin, red iron oxide, sodium lauryl sulfate, titanium dioxide, and yellow iron oxide.

12,000 USP units of lipase; 38,000 USP units of protease; 60,000 USP units of amylase capsules have a brown opaque cap with imprint "CREON 1212" and a colorless transparent body. The shells contain black iron oxide, gelatin, red iron oxide, sodium lauryl sulfate, titanium dioxide, and yellow iron oxide.

24,000 USP units of lipase; 76,000 USP units of protease; 120,000 USP units of amylase capsules have a Swedish-orange opaque cap with imprint "CREON 1224" and a colorless transparent body. The shells contain gelatin, red iron oxide, sodium lauryl sulfate, titanium dioxide, and yellow iron oxide.

12 CLINICAL PHARMACOLOGY

12.1 Mechanism of Action

The pancreatic enzymes in CREON catalyze the hydrolysis of fats to monoglyceride, glycerol and free fatty acids, proteins into peptides and amino acids, and starches into dextrins and short chain sugars such as maltose and maltriose in the duodenum and proximal small intestine, thereby acting like digestive enzymes physiologically secreted by the pancreas.

12.3 Pharmacokinetics

The pancreatic enzymes in CREON are enteric-coated to minimize destruction or inactivation in gastric acid. CREON is expected to release most of the enzymes *in vivo* at a pH greater than 5.5. Pancreatic enzymes are not absorbed from the gastrointestinal tract in appreciable amounts.

13 NONCLINICAL TOXICOLOGY

13.1 Carcinogenesis, Mutagenesis, Impairment of Fertility

Carcinogenicity, genetic toxicology, and animal fertility studies have not been performed.

14 CLINICAL STUDIES

The short-term safety and efficacy of CREON were evaluated in two studies conducted in 86 patients with exocrine pancreatic insufficiency (EPI). Study 1 was conducted in 32 patients with EPI due to cystic fibrosis (CF); Study 2 was conducted in 54 patients with EPI due to chronic pancreatitis or pancreatectomy.

14.1 Cystic Fibrosis

Study 1 was a randomized, double-blind, placebo-controlled, crossover study in 32 patients, ages 12 to 43 years, with exocrine pancreatic insufficiency due to cystic fibrosis. The final analysis population was limited to 29 patients; 3 patients were excluded due to protocol deviations. Patients were randomized to receive CREON at a dose of 4,000 lipase units/g fat ingested per day or matching placebo for 5 to 6 days of treatment, followed by crossover to the alternate treatment for an additional 5 to 6 days. All patients consumed a high-fat diet (greater than or equal to 100 grams of fat per day) during the treatment periods.

The primary efficacy endpoint was the mean difference in the coefficient of fat absorption (CFA) between CREON and placebo treatment. The CFA was determined by a 72-hour stool collection during both treatments, when both fat excretion and fat ingestion were measured. Each patient's CFA during placebo treatment was used as their no-treatment CFA value.

Mean CFA was 89% with CREON treatment compared to 49% with placebo treatment. The mean difference in CFA was 41 percentage points in favor of CREON treatment with 95% CI: (34, 47) and p<0.001.

Subgroup analyses of the CFA results showed that mean change in CFA with CREON treatment was greater in patients with lower no-treatment (placebo) CFA values than in patients with higher no-treatment (placebo) CFA values. There were no differences in response to CREON by age or gender, with similar responses to CREON observed in male and female patients, and in younger (under 18 years of age) and older patients.

14.2 Chronic Pancreatitis or Pancreatectomy

Study 2 was a randomized, double-blind, placebo-controlled, parallel group study of 54 adult patients, ages 32 to 75 years, with EPI due to chronic pancreatitis or pancreatectomy. The final analysis population was limited to 52 patients; 2 patients were excluded due to protocol violations. Ten patients had a history of pancreatectomy (7 were treated with CREON). In this study, patients received placebo for 5 days (run-in period), followed by pancreatic enzyme replacement therapy as directed by the investigator for 16 days; this was followed by randomization to CREON or matching placebo for 7 days of treatment (double-blind period). Only patients with CFA less than 80% in the run-in period were randomized to the double-blind period. The dose of CREON during the double-blind period was 72,000 lipase units per main meal (3 main meals) and 36,000 lipase units per snack (2 snacks). All patients consumed a high-fat diet (greater than or equal to 100 grams of fat per day) during the treatment period.

The primary efficacy endpoint was the mean change in CFA from the run-in period to the end of the double-blind period. The CFA was determined by a 72-hour stool collection during the run-in and double-blind treatment periods, when both fat excretion and fat ingestion were measured (Table 3).

Table 3: Percent Change in CFA in Study 2 (Run-in Period to End of Double-Blind Period)

	CREON n = 24	Placebo n = 28
CFA [%]		
Run-in Period (Mean, SD)	54 (19)	57 (21)
End of Double-Blind Period (Mean, SD)	86 (6)	66 (20)
Change in CFA * [%]		
Run-in Period to End of Double-Blind Period (Mean, SD)	32 (18)	9 (13)
Treatment Difference (95% CI)	21 (14, 28)	

* p<0.0001

The mean percent change in CFA from the run-in period to the end of the double-blind period was 32% for CREON and 9% for placebo (p<0.0001). Subgroup analyses of the CFA results showed that mean change in CFA was greater in patients with lower run-in period CFA values than in patients with higher run-in period CFA values. Only 1 of the patients with a history of total pancreatectomy was treated with CREON in the study. That patient had a CFA of 26% during the run-in period and a CFA of 73% at the end of the double-blind period. The remaining 6 patients with a history of partial pancreatectomy treated with CREON on the study had a mean CFA of 42% during the run-in period and a mean CFA of 84% at the end of the double-blind period.

15 REFERENCES

1. Borowitz DS, Grand RJ, Durie PR, et al. Use of pancreatic enzyme supplements for patients with cystic fibrosis in the context of fibrosing colonopathy. *Journal of Pediatrics*. 1995; 127: 681-684.
2. Borowitz DS, Baker RD, Stallings V. Consensus report on nutrition for pediatric patients with cystic fibrosis. *Journal of Pediatric Gastroenterology Nutrition*. 2002 Sep; 35: 246-259.
3. Stallings VA, Stark LJ, Robinson KA, et al. Evidence-based practice recommendations for nutrition-related management of children and adults with cystic fibrosis and pancreatic insufficiency: results of a systematic review. *Journal of the American Dietetic Association*. 2008; 108: 832-839.
4. Dominguez-Munoz JE. Pancreatic enzyme therapy for pancreatic exocrine insufficiency. *Current Gastroenterology Reports*. 2007; 9: 116-122.
5. Smyth RL, Ashby D, O'Hea U, et al. Fibrosing colonopathy in cystic fibrosis: results of a case-control study. *Lancet*. 1995; 346: 1247-1251.
6. FitzSimmons SC, Burkhart GA, Borowitz DS, et al. High-dose pancreatic-enzyme supplements and fibrosing colonopathy in children with cystic fibrosis. *New England Journal of Medicine*. 1997; 336: 1283-1289.

16 HOW SUPPLIED/STORAGE AND HANDLING

CREON (pancrelipase) Delayed-Release Capsules
6,000 USP units of lipase; 19,000 USP units of protease; 30,000 USP units of amylase
Each CREON capsule is available as a two-piece gelatin capsule with orange opaque cap with imprint "CREON 1206" and a blue opaque body that contains tan-colored, delayed-release pancrelipase supplied in bottles of:
• 100 capsules (NDC 0032-1206-01)
• 250 capsules (NDC 0032-1206-07)
CREON (pancrelipase) Delayed-Release Capsules
12,000 USP units of lipase; 38,000 USP units of protease; 60,000 USP units of amylase
Each CREON capsule is available as a two-piece gelatin capsule with a brown opaque cap with imprint "CREON 1212" and a colorless transparent body that contains tan-colored, delayed-release pancrelipase supplied in bottles of:
• 100 capsules (NDC 0032-1212-01)
• 250 capsules (NDC 0032-1212-07)
CREON (pancrelipase) Delayed-Release Capsules
24,000 USP units of lipase; 76,000 USP units of protease; 120,000 USP units of amylase
Each CREON capsule is available as a two-piece gelatin capsule with orange opaque cap with imprint "CREON 1224" and a colorless transparent body that contains tan-colored, delayed-release pancrelipase supplied in bottles of:
• 100 capsules (NDC 0032-1224-01)
• 250 capsules (NDC 0032-1224-07)

Storage and Handling

CREON must be stored at room temperature up to 25°C (77°F) and protected from moisture. Temperature excursions are permitted between 25°C to 40°C (77°F and 104°F) for up to 30 days. Product should be discarded if exposed to higher temperature and moisture conditions higher than 70%. AFTER OPENING, KEEP BOTTLE TIGHTLY CLOSED between uses to PROTECT FROM MOISTURE. Keep out of reach of children.
DO NOT CRUSH CREON delayed-release capsules or the capsule contents.

17 PATIENT COUNSELING INFORMATION

See Medication Guide
CREON is available in capsule strengths of:
• 6,000 USP units of lipase; 19,000 USP units of protease; 30,000 USP units of amylase
• 12,000 USP units of lipase; 38,000 USP units of protease; 60,000 USP units of amylase
• 24,000 USP units of lipase; 76,000 USP units of protease; 120,000 USP units of amylase
Healthcare professionals should inform patients of the following important information about CREON.

17.1 Dosing and Administration

• Instruct patients and caregivers that CREON should only be taken as directed by their healthcare professional *[see Dosage and Administration (2)]*.
• Instruct patients and caregivers that CREON should always be taken with food *[see Dosage and Administration (2)]*.
• Instruct patients who are unable to swallow intact capsules to sprinkle the contents of CREON on a small amount of acidic soft food, such as applesauce, at room temperature. Instruct these patients to swallow the CREON-soft food mixture immediately without crushing or chewing, and follow with water or juice to ensure complete ingestion and to avoid irritation of the oral mucosa *[see Dosage and Administration (2)]*.
• Tell patients that CREON or their contents should not be crushed or chewed as doing so could cause early release of enzymes and/or loss of enzymatic activity *[see Dosage and Administration (2)]*.
• Instruct patients to notify their healthcare professional if they are pregnant or are thinking of becoming pregnant during treatment with CREON *[see Use in Specific Populations (8.1)]*.
• Instruct patients to notify their healthcare professional if they are breast feeding or are thinking of breast feeding during treatment with CREON *[see Use in Specific Populations (8.3)]*.

17.2 Fibrosing Colonopathy

Advise patients and caregivers to follow dosing instructions carefully, as doses of pancreatic enzyme products exceeding 6,000 lipase units/kg of body weight per meal have been associated with colonic strictures in children below the age of 12 years *[see Dosage and Administration (2)]*.

17.3 Allergic Reactions

Advise patients and caregivers to contact their healthcare professional immediately if allergic reactions to CREON develop *[see Warnings and Precautions (5.5)]*.

Manufactured by:
Abbott Products GmbH
Hannover, Germany
Marketed By:
Abbott Laboratories
North Chicago, IL 60064, U.S.A.
1055216 6E
© 2010 Abbott Laboratories
MEDICATION GUIDE
CREON® (krē 'ŏn)
(pancrelipase)
Delayed-Release Capsules
Read this Medication Guide before you or your child start taking CREON and each time you or your child get a prescription refilled. There may be new information. This information does not take the place of talking with your healthcare professional about your medical condition or your treatment.

What is the most important information I should know about CREON?
• CREON may increase your chance of having a rare bowel disorder called fibrosing colonopathy. This condition is serious and may require surgery. The risk of having this condition may be reduced by following the dosing instructions that your healthcare professional gave you. Call your healthcare professional right away if you have any unusual or severe stomach area (abdominal) pain.
• **Take CREON exactly as prescribed. Do not take more or less CREON than directed by your healthcare professional.**

What is CREON?

CREON is a prescription pancreatic enzyme medicine used to improve food digestion in people who cannot digest food properly because they have exocrine pancreatic insufficiency. CREON contains a mixture of digestive enzymes (including lipases, proteases, and amylases) from pig pancreas. CREON is safe and effective in children.

What should I tell my healthcare professional before taking CREON?

Tell your healthcare professional if you:
- are allergic to pork (pig) products.
- have a history of intestinal blockage or a condition called fibrosing colonopathy.
- have gout, kidney disease, or a condition called high blood uric acid (hyperuricemia).
- have trouble swallowing capsules.
- are pregnant or planning to become pregnant. It is not known if CREON will harm your unborn baby.
- are breast-feeding or plan to breast-feed. It is not known if CREON passes into your breast milk. **Tell your healthcare professional about all the medicines you take,** including prescription and nonprescription medicines, vitamins, and dietary or herbal supplements.

Know the medicines you take. Keep a list of them and show it to your healthcare professional and pharmacist when you get a new medicine.

How should I take CREON?

- **Take CREON exactly as instructed by your healthcare professional.**

Infants (up to 12 months)

Contents of the capsule may be put directly in the infant's mouth or in a small amount of applesauce and administered (or given) just prior to feeding the infant breast milk or formula. Do not mix CREON capsule contents directly into formula or breast milk prior to administration. Care should be taken to ensure that the entire administered dose is swallowed and not retained in the mouth, to avoid irritation of the mouth.

Children and Adults

- Always take CREON during a meal or a snack and follow it with sufficient fluid.
- If you forget to take CREON, call your healthcare professional or wait until your next meal and take your usual number of capsules. **Do not make up for missed doses.** Take your next dose at the usual time.
- If you or your child takes more CREON than directed, call your healthcare professional right away.
- Swallow CREON whole. Do not crush or chew the contents of the capsules.

If you have trouble swallowing capsules, you can add the contents of an open capsule directly onto your food. To do so, carefully open the capsules and sprinkle the contents on a small amount of applesauce at room temperature as described below. Swallow the soft food right away without chewing and follow with water or juice.

A. Hold the capsule upright so that you can read the word CREON on the capsule.

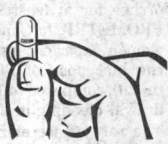

B. Carefully twist off the top portion of the capsule over the food you plan to eat.

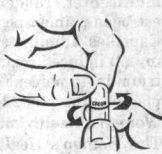

C. Sprinkle the contents of the capsule onto the soft food. Do not crush the contents of the capsules.

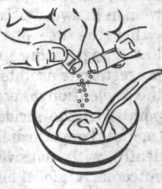

D. Swallow the CREON-soft food right away without chewing and follow with water or juice to make sure the contents of the *capsules* are swallowed completely.

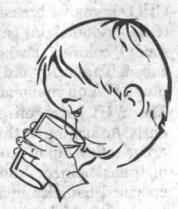

What are the possible side effects of CREON?

CREON may cause serious side effects, including:
- CREON may increase your chance of having a rare bowel disorder called fibrosing colonopathy. See "What is the most important information I should know about CREON?"
- increase in blood uric acid levels, for example, worsening of gout, or painful, swollen joints. Call your healthcare professional right away if you have any of these symptoms.
- allergic reactions. For example, symptoms of an allergic reaction include: trouble with breathing, skin rashes, or swollen lips. Call your healthcare professional right away if you have any of these symptoms.

The most common side effects include:
- gassiness (flatulence)
- stomach area (abdominal) pain
- headache
- dizziness

Tell your healthcare professional if you have any side effect that bothers you or that does not go away.

These are not all the side effects of CREON. Call your doctor for medical advice about side effects. You may report side effects to the FDA at 1-800-FDA-1088 or www.fda.gov/medwatch. You may also report side effects to Solvay Pharmaceuticals, Inc. at 1-800-241-1643.

How should I store CREON?

- Store CREON at room temperature (up to 25°C or 77°F) for up to 12 weeks after the bottle is opened.
- If you store CREON at temperatures greater than room temperature (up to 40°C or 104°F), throw away after 30 days.
- Store CREON in the container you were given by the pharmacy.
- Keep the bottle closed tightly.
- Protect the bottle from moisture.
- **Keep CREON and all medicines out of reach of children.**

General information about the safe and effective use of CREON

Medicines are sometimes prescribed for purposes other than those listed in a Medication Guide. Do not use CREON for a condition for which it was not prescribed. Do not give CREON to other people to take, even if they have the same symptoms you have. It may harm them.

This Medication Guide summarizes the most important information about CREON. If you would like more information, talk to your healthcare professional. You can ask your healthcare professional or pharmacist for information about CREON that is written for healthcare professionals. For more information, go to www.creon-us.com or call toll-free [1-800-241-1643].

What are the ingredients in CREON?

Active Ingredient: pancrelipase

Inactive Ingredients: cetyl alcohol, dimethicone, gelatin, hypromellose phthalate, polyethylene glycol, red iron oxide, sodium lauryl sulfate, titanium dioxide, triethyl citrate, and yellow iron oxide. In addition, the 6,000 strength contains FD&C Blue No. 2 and the 12,000 strength contains black iron oxide. The imprinting ink on the capsule contains dimethicone, 2-ethoxyethanol, shellac, soya lecithin, and titanium dioxide.

Additional information about pancreatic enzymes

CREON and other pancreatic enzyme products are made from pancreatic organs of pigs used for food. There is a theoretical risk of contracting a viral infection from pig-derived medicines, but no human illness has been reported.

The risk of fibrosing colonopathy, increased blood uric acid levels, and the theoretical risk of viral transmission is present with all pancreatic enzyme products including CREON. You should report any change in condition or illness to your healthcare professional.

© 2009 Solvay Pharmaceuticals, Inc.

Manufactured for Solvay Pharmaceuticals, Inc., Marietta, GA 30062, U.S.A.

1055216 1E Rev Apr 2009

This Medication Guide has been approved by the U.S. Food and Drug Administration.

Issued April 2009

Revised: 04/2010

PROMETRIUM®   ℞
[pro-mē-trē-um]
(progesterone, USP)
Capsules 100 mg
Capsules 200 mg

> **WARNING: CARDIOVASCULAR DISORDERS, BREAST CANCER AND PROBABLE DEMENTIA FOR ESTROGEN PLUS PROGESTIN THERAPY**
> Estrogens plus progestin therapy should not be used for the prevention of cardiovascular disease or dementia. (See CLINICAL STUDIES and WARNINGS, Cardiovascular disorders and Dementia.)

The Women's Health Initiative (WHI) estrogen plus progestin substudy reported increased risks of stroke, deep vein thrombosis (DVT), pulmonary embolism, and myocardial infarction in postmenopausal women (50 to 79 years of age) during 5.6 years of treatment with daily oral conjugated estrogens (CE) [0.625 mg] combined with medroxyprogesterone acetate (MPA) [2.5 mg], relative to placebo. (See CLINICAL STUDIES and WARNINGS, Cardiovascular disorders.)

The WHI estrogen plus progestin substudy also demonstrated an increased risk of invasive breast cancer. (See CLINICAL STUDIES and WARNINGS, Malignant neoplasms, *Breast Cancer*.)

The Women's Health Initiative Memory Study (WHIMS) estrogen plus progestin ancillary study of the WHI reported an increased risk of probable dementia in postmenopausal women 65 years of age or older.

DESCRIPTION

PROMETRIUM (progesterone, USP) Capsules contain micronized progesterone for oral administration. Progesterone has a molecular weight of 314.47 and a molecular formula of $C_{21}H_{30}O_2$. Progesterone (pregn-4-ene-3, 20-dione) is a white or creamy white, odorless, crystalline powder practically insoluble in water, soluble in alcohol, acetone and dioxane and sparingly soluble in vegetable oils, stable in air, melting between 126° and 131°C. The structural formula is:

Progesterone is synthesized from a starting material from a plant source and is chemically identical to progesterone of human ovarian origin. PROMETRIUM Capsules are available in multiple strengths to afford dosage flexibility for optimum management. PROMETRIUM Capsules contain 100 mg or 200 mg micronized progesterone.

The inactive ingredients for PROMETRIUM Capsules 100 mg include: peanut oil NF, gelatin NF, glycerin USP, lecithin NF, titanium dioxide USP, D&C Yellow No. 10, and FD&C Red No. 40.

The inactive ingredients for PROMETRIUM Capsules 200 mg include: peanut oil NF, gelatin NF, glycerin USP, lecithin NF, titanium dioxide USP, D&C Yellow No. 10, and FD&C Yellow No. 6.

CLINICAL PHARMACOLOGY

PROMETRIUM Capsules are an oral dosage form of micronized progesterone which is chemically identical to progesterone of ovarian origin. The oral bioavailability of progesterone is increased through micronization.

Pharmacokinetics

A. Absorption

After oral administration of progesterone as a micronized soft-gelatin capsule formulation, maximum serum concentrations were attained within 3 hours. The absolute bioavailability of micronized progesterone is not known. Table 1 summarizes the mean pharmacokinetic parameters in postmenopausal women after five oral daily doses of PROMETRIUM Capsules 100 mg as a micronized soft-gelatin capsule formulation.

[See table 1 at top of next page]

Serum progesterone concentrations appeared linear and dose proportional following multiple dose administration of PROMETRIUM Capsules 100 mg over the dose range 100 mg/day to 300 mg/day in postmenopausal women. Although doses greater than 300 mg/day were not studied in females, serum concentrations from a study in male volunteers appeared linear and dose proportional between 100 mg/day and 400 mg/day. The pharmacokinetic parameters in male volunteers were generally consistent with those seen in postmenopausal women.

B. Distribution

Progesterone is approximately 96 percent to 99 percent bound to serum proteins, primarily to serum albumin (50 to 54 percent) and transcortin (43 to 48 percent).

C. Metabolism

Progesterone is metabolized primarily by the liver largely to pregnanediols and pregnanolones. Pregnanediols and

---

TABLE 1. Pharmacokinetic Parameters of PROMETRIUM

Parameter	PROMETRIUM Capsules Daily Dose		
	100 mg	200 mg	300 mg
Cmax (ng/mL)	17.3 ± 21.9[a]	38.1 ± 37.8	60.6 ± 72.5
Tmax (hr)	1.5 ± 0.8	2.3 ± 1.4	1.7 ± 0.6
AUC (0-10) (ng × hr/mL)	43.3 ± 30.8	101.2 ± 66.0	175.7 ± 170.3

[a] Mean ± S.D.

TABLE 2. Mean (± S.D.) Pharmacokinetic Parameters for Estradiol, Estrone, and Equilin Following Coadministration of Conjugated Estrogens 0.625 mg and PROMETRIUM Capsules 200 mg for 12 Days to Postmenopausal Women

Drug	Conjugated Estrogens			Conjugated Estrogens plus PROMETRIUM Capsules		
	Cmax (ng/mL)	Tmax (hr)	AUC(0-24h) (ng × h/mL)	Cmax (ng/mL)	Tmax (hr)	AUC(0-24h) (ng × h/mL)
Estradiol	0.037 ± 0.048	12.7 ± 9.1	0.676 ± 0.737	0.030 ± 0.032	17.32 ± 1.21	0.561 ± 0.572
Estrone Total[a]	3.68 ± 1.55	10.6 ± 6.8	61.3 ± 26.36	4.93 ± 2.07	7.5 ± 3.8	85.9 ± 41.2
Equilin Total[a]	2.27 ± 0.95	6.0 ± 4.0	28.8 ± 13.0	3.22 ± 1.13	5.3 ± 2.6	38.1 ± 20.2

[a] Total estrogens is the sum of conjugated and unconjugated estrogen.

TABLE 3. Incidence of Endometrial Hyperplasia in Women Receiving 3 Years of Treatment

Endometrial Diagnosis	Treatment Group					
	Conjugated Estrogens 0.625 mg + PROMETRIUM Capsules 200 mg (cyclical)		Conjugated Estrogens 0.625 mg alone		Placebo	
	Number of patients	% of patients	Number of patients	% of patients	Number of patients	% of patients
	n=117		n=115		n=116	
HYPERPLASIA[a]	7	6	74	64	3	3
Adenocarcinoma	0	0	0	0	1	1
Atypical hyperplasia	1	1	14	12	0	0
Complex hyperplasia	0	0	27	23	1	1
Simple hyperplasia	6	5	33	29	1	1

[a] Most advanced result to least advanced result:
Adenocarcinoma > atypical hyperplasia > complex hyperplasia > simple hyperplasia

pregnanolones are conjugated in the liver to glucuronide and sulfate metabolites. Progesterone metabolites which are excreted in the bile may be deconjugated and may be further metabolized in the gut via reduction, dehydroxylation, and epimerization.

D. Excretion
The glucuronide and sulfate conjugates of pregnanediol and pregnanolone are excreted in the bile and urine. Progesterone metabolites are eliminated mainly by the kidneys. Progesterone metabolites which are excreted in the bile may undergo enterohepatic recycling or may be excreted in the feces.

E. Special Populations
The pharmacokinetics of PROMETRIUM Capsules have not been assessed in low body weight or obese patients.
Race: There is insufficient information available from trials conducted with PROMETRIUM Capsules to compare progesterone pharmacokinetics in different racial groups.
Hepatic Insufficiency: The effects of hepatic impairment on PROMETRIUM Capsule pharmacokinetics have not been studied.
Renal Insufficiency: The effects of renal impairment on PROMETRIUM Capsule pharmacokinetics have not been studied.

F. Food–Drug Interaction
Concomitant food ingestion increased the bioavailability of PROMETRIUM Capsules relative to a fasting state when administered to postmenopausal women at a dose of 200 mg.

G. Drug Interactions
The metabolism of progesterone by human liver microsomes was inhibited by ketoconazole (IC$_{50}$ <0.1 μM). Ketoconazole is a known inhibitor of cytochrome P450 3A4, hence these data suggest that ketoconazole or other known inhibitors of this enzyme may increase the bioavailability of progesterone. The clinical relevance of the *in vitro* findings is unknown.

Coadministration of conjugated estrogens and PROMETRIUM Capsules to 29 postmenopausal women over a 12-day period resulted in an increase in total estrone concentrations (Cmax 3.68 ng/mL to 4.93 ng/mL) and total equilin concentrations (Cmax 2.27 ng/mL to 3.22 ng/mL) and a decrease in circulating 17β estradiol concentrations (Cmax 0.037 ng/mL to 0.030 ng/mL). The half-life of the conjugated estrogens was similar with coadministration of PROMETRIUM Capsules. Table 2 summarizes the pharmacokinetic parameters.
[See table 2 above]

CLINICAL STUDIES

Effects on the endometrium
In a randomized, double-blind clinical trial, 358 postmenopausal women, each with an intact uterus, received treatment for up to 36 months. The treatment groups were: PROMETRIUM Capsules at the dose of 200 mg/day for 12 days per 28-day cycle in combination with conjugated estrogens 0.625 mg/day (n=120); conjugated estrogens 0.625 mg/day only (n=119); or placebo (n=119). The subjects in all three treatment groups were primarily Caucasian women (87 percent or more of each group). The results for the incidence of endometrial hyperplasia in women receiving up to 3 years of treatment are shown in Table 3. A comparison of the PROMETRIUM Capsules plus conjugated estrogens treatment group to the conjugated estrogens only group showed a significantly lower rate of hyperplasia (6 percent combination product versus 64 percent estrogen alone) in the PROMETRIUM Capsules plus conjugated estrogens treatment group throughout 36 months of treatment.
[See table 3 at left]

The times to diagnosis of endometrial hyperplasia over 36 months of treatment are shown in Figure 1. This figure illustrates graphically that the proportion of patients with hyperplasia was significantly greater for the conjugated estrogens group (64 percent) compared to the conjugated estrogens plus PROMETRIUM Capsules group (6 percent).

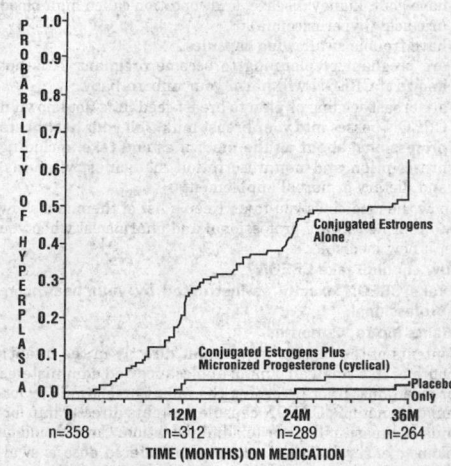

n= total number of patients left at each time interval

Figure 1. Time to Hyperplasia in Women Receiving up to 36 Months of Treatment

The discontinuation rates due to hyperplasia over the 36 months of treatment are as shown in Table 4. For any degree of hyperplasia, the discontinuation rate for patients who received conjugated estrogens plus PROMETRIUM Capsules was similar to that of the placebo only group, while the discontinuation rate for patients who received conjugated estrogens alone was significantly higher. Women who permanently discontinued treatment due to hyperplasia were similar in demographics to the overall study population.
[See table 4 at top of next page]

Effects on secondary amenorrhea
In a single-center, randomized, double-blind clinical study that included premenopausal women with secondary amenorrhea for at least 90 days, administration of 10 days of PROMETRIUM Capsules therapy resulted in 80 percent of women experiencing withdrawal bleeding within 7 days of the last dose of PROMETRIUM Capsules, 300 mg/day (n=20), compared to 10 percent of women experiencing withdrawal bleeding in the placebo group (n=21).

The rate of secretory transformation was evaluated in a multicenter, randomized, double-blind clinical study in estrogen-primed postmenopausal women. PROMETRIUM Capsules administered orally for 10 days at 400 mg/day (n=22) induced complete secretory changes in the endometrium in 45 percent of women compared to 0 percent in the placebo group (n=23).

Women's Health Initiative Studies
The Women's Health Initiative (WHI) enrolled approximately 27,000 predominantly healthy postmenopausal women in two substudies to assess the risks and benefits of either the use of daily oral conjugated estrogens (CE) [0.625 mg] alone or in combination with medroxyprogesterone acetate (MPA) [2.5 mg] compared to placebo in the prevention of certain chronic diseases. The primary endpoint was the incidence of coronary heart disease (CHD) (nonfatal myocardial infarction [MI], silent MI and CHD death), with invasive breast cancer as the primary adverse outcome. A "global index" included the earliest occurrence of CHD, invasive breast cancer, stroke, pulmonary embolism (PE), endometrial cancer (only in the CE plus MPA substudy), colorectal cancer, hip fracture, or death due to other cause. The study did not evaluate the effects of CE or CE plus MPA on menopausal symptoms.

The WHI estrogen plus progestin substudy was stopped early. According to the predefined stopping rule, after an average follow-up of 5.6 years of treatment, the increased risk of breast cancer and cardiovascular events exceeded the specified benefits included in the "global index." The absolute excess risk of events in the "global index" was 19 per 10,000 women-years. For those outcomes included in the

WHI "global index" that reached statistical significance after 5.6 years of follow-up, the absolute excess risks per 10,000 women-years in the group treated with CE plus MPA were 7 more CHD events, 8 more strokes, 10 more PEs, and 8 more invasive breast cancers, while the absolute risk reductions per 10,000 women-years were 6 fewer colorectal cancers and 5 fewer hip fractures.

Results of the estrogen plus progestin substudy, which included 16,608 women (average age of 63 years, range 50 to 79; 83.9 percent White, 6.8 percent Black, 5.4 percent Hispanic, 3.9 percent Other) are presented in Table 5. These results reflect centrally adjudicated data after an average follow-up of 5.6 years.

[See table 5 at right]

Women's Health Initiative Memory Study

The estrogen plus progestin Women's Health Initiative Memory Study (WHIMS), an ancillary study of WHI, enrolled 4,532 predominantly healthy postmenopausal women 65 years of age and older (47 percent were 65 to 69 years of age; 35 percent were 70 to 74 years of age; and 18 percent were 75 years of age and older) to evaluate the effects of daily CE (0.625 mg) plus MPA (2.5 mg) on the incidence of probable dementia (primary outcome) compared with placebo.

After an average follow-up of 4 years, the relative risk of probable dementia for CE (0.625 mg) plus MPA (2.5 mg) versus placebo was 2.05 (95 percent CI 1.21–3.48). The absolute risk of probable dementia for CE plus MPA versus placebo was 45 versus 22 per 10,000 women-years. The most common classification of probable dementia in the treatment group and placebo group was Alzheimer's disease. Since the ancillary study was conducted in women 65 to 79 years of age, it is unknown whether these findings apply to younger postmenopausal women. (See **BOXED WARNING, WARNINGS,** Dementia and **PRECAUTIONS,** Geriatric Use.)

INDICATIONS AND USAGE

PROMETRIUM Capsules are indicated for use in the prevention of endometrial hyperplasia in nonhysterectomized postmenopausal women who are receiving conjugated estrogens tablets. They are also indicated for use in secondary amenorrhea.

CONTRAINDICATIONS

PROMETRIUM Capsules should not be used in women with any of the following conditions:

1. **PROMETRIUM Capsules should not be used in patients with known hypersensitivity to its ingredients. PROMETRIUM Capsules contain peanut oil and should never be used by patients allergic to peanuts.**
2. Undiagnosed abnormal genital bleeding.
3. Known, suspected, or history of breast cancer.
4. Active deep vein thrombosis, pulmonary embolism or history of these conditions.
5. Active arterial thromboembolic disease (for example, stroke and myocardial infarction), or a history of these conditions.
6. Known liver dysfunction or disease.
7. Known or suspected pregnancy.

WARNINGS

See **BOXED WARNING.**

1. Cardiovascular disorders

An increased risk of pulmonary embolism, deep vein thrombosis (DVT), stroke, and myocardial infarction has been reported with estrogen plus progestin therapy. Should any of these occur or be suspected, estrogen with progestin should be discontinued immediately.

Risk factors for arterial vascular disease (for example, hypertension, diabetes mellitus, tobacco use, hypercholesterolemia, and obesity) and/or venous thromboembolism (for example, personal history or family history of venous thromboembolism [VTE], obesity, and systemic lupus erythematosus) should be managed appropriately.

a. Stroke

In the Women's Health Initiative (WHI) estrogen plus progestin substudy, a statistically significant increased risk of stroke was reported in all women receiving daily conjugated estrogens (CE 0.625 mg) plus medroxyprogesterone acetate (MPA 2.5 mg) compared to placebo (33 versus 25 per 10,000 women-years). The increase in risk was demonstrated after the first year and persisted. (See **CLINICAL STUDIES.**) Should a stroke occur or be suspected, estrogen plus progestin therapy should be discontinued immediately.

b. Coronary Heart Disease

In the WHI estrogen plus progestin substudy, there was a statistically non-significant increased risk of CHD events (defined as nonfatal MI, silent MI, or CHD death) reported in women receiving daily CE/MPA compared to women receiving placebo (41 versus 34 per 10,000 women-years). An

TABLE 4. Discontinuation Rate Due to Hyperplasia Over 36 Months of Treatment

Most Advanced Biopsy Result Through 36 Months of Treatment	Treatment Group					
	Conjugated Estrogens + PROMETRIUM Capsules (cyclical)		Conjugated Estrogens (alone)		Placebo	
	n=120		n=119		n=119	
	Number of patients	% of patients	Number of patients	% of patients	Number of patients	% of patients
Adenocarcinoma	0	0	0	0	1	1
Atypical hyperplasia	1	1	10	8	0	0
Complex hyperplasia	0	0	21	18	1	1
Simple hyperplasia	1	1	13	11	0	0

TABLE 5. Relative and Absolute Risk Seen in the Estrogen Plus Progestin Substudy of WHI at an Average of 5.6 Years[a]

Event[c]	Relative Risk CE/MPA versus Placebo (95% nCI[b])	Placebo n = 8,102	CE/MPA n = 8,506
		Absolute Risk per 10,000 Women-years	
CHD events	1.23 (0.99-1.53)	34	41
Non-fatal MI [b]	*1.28 (1.00-1.63)*	*25*	*31*
CHD death	*1.10 (0.70-1.75)*	*8*	*8*
All stroke	1.31 (1.03-1.88)	25	33
Ischemic stroke	*1.44 (1.09-1.90)*	*18*	*26*
Deep vein thrombosis[c]	1.95 (1.43-2.67)	13	26
Pulmonary embolism	2.13 (1.45-3.11)	8	18
Invasive breast cancer[d]	1.24 (1.01-1.54)	33	41
Colorectal cancer	0.61 (0.42-0.87)	16	10
Endometrial cancer[c]	0.82 (0.48-1.36)	7	6
Cervical cancer[c]	1.44 (0.47-4.42)	1	2
Hip fracture	0.67 (0.47-0.96)	16	11
Vertebral fractures[c]	0.68 (0.48-0.96)	17	12
Lower arm/wrist fractures[c]	0.71 (0.59-0.85)	62	44
Total fractures[c]	0.76 (0.69-0.83)	199	152
Overall mortality[c, e]	1.00 (0.83-1.19)	52	52
Global Index[f]	1.13 (1.02-1.25)	165	184

[a] Results are based on centrally adjudicated data.
[b] Nominal confidence intervals unadjusted for multiple looks and multiple comparisons.
[c] Not included in Global Index.
[d] Includes metastatic and non-metastatic breast cancer with the exception of *in situ* breast cancer.
[e] All deaths, except from breast or colorectal cancer, definite/probable CHD, PE, or cerebrovascular disease.
[f] A subset of the events was combined in a "global index" defined as the earliest occurrence of CHD events, invasive breast cancer, stroke, pulmonary embolism, endometrial cancer, colorectal cancer, hip fracture, or death due to other causes.

increase in relative risk was demonstrated in year 1 and a trend toward decreasing relative risk was reported in years 2 through 5. (See **CLINICAL STUDIES.**)

In postmenopausal women with documented heart disease (n = 2,763, average age 66.7 years), in a controlled clinical trial of secondary prevention of cardiovascular disease (Heart and Estrogen/Progestin Replacement Study [HERS]), treatment with daily CE (0.625 mg) plus MPA (2.5 mg) demonstrated no cardiovascular benefit. During an average follow-up of 4.1 years, treatment with CE plus MPA did not reduce the overall rate of CHD events in postmenopausal women with established coronary heart disease. There were more CHD events in the CE plus MPA-treated group than in the placebo group in year 1, but not during the subsequent years. Two thousand three hundred and twenty-one (2,321) women from the original HERS trial agreed to participate in an open-label extension of HERS, HERS II. Average follow-up in HERS II was an additional 2.7 years, for a total of 6.8 years overall. Rates of CHD events were comparable among women in the CE plus MPA

group and the placebo group in HERS, HERS II, and overall.

c. Venous Thromboembolism (VTE)

In the WHI estrogen plus progestin substudy, a statistically significant 2-fold greater rate of VTE (DVT and pulmonary embolism [PE]), was reported in women receiving daily CE (0.625 mg) plus MPA (2.5 mg) compared to women receiving placebo (35 versus 17 per 10,000 women-years) and PE. Statistically significant increases in risk for both DVT (26 versus 13 per 10,000 women-years) and PE (18 versus 8 per 10,000 women-years) were also demonstrated. The increase in VTE risk was observed during the first year and persisted. (See **CLINICAL STUDIES.**) Should a VTE occur or

---

Information on the Solvay/Abbott Pharmaceutical Products listed on these pages is from the prescribing information in use as of June 1, 2010. For more information, please visit rxabbott.com or call 1-800-633-9110.

be suspected, estrogen plus progestin therapy should be discontinued immediately.

If feasible, estrogens with progestins should be discontinued at least 4 to 6 weeks before surgery of the type associated with an increased risk of thromboembolism, or during periods of prolonged immobilization.

2. Malignant neoplasms

a. Breast Cancer

The most important randomized clinical trial providing information about breast cancer is the Women's Health Initiative (WHI) substudy of daily CE (0.625 mg) plus MPA (2.5 mg). In the estrogen plus progestin substudy, after a mean follow-up of 5.6 years, the WHI substudy reported an increased risk of breast cancer in women who took daily CE plus MPA. In this substudy, prior use of estrogen alone or estrogen plus progestin therapy was reported by 26 percent of the women. The relative risk of invasive breast cancer was 1.24 (95 percent nCI 1.01-1.54), and the absolute risk was 41 versus 33 cases per 10,000 women-years, for estrogen plus progestin compared with placebo.

Among women who reported prior use of hormone therapy, the relative risk of invasive breast cancer was 1.86, and the absolute risk was 46 versus 25 cases per 10,000 women-years, for estrogen plus progestin compared with placebo. Among women who reported no prior use of hormone therapy, the relative risk of invasive breast cancer was 1.09, and the absolute risk was 40 versus 36 cases per 10,000 women-years for estrogen plus progestin compared with placebo. In the same substudy, invasive breast cancers were larger and diagnosed at a more advanced stage in the CE (0.625 mg) plus MPA (2.5 mg) group compared with the placebo group. Metastatic disease was rare with no apparent difference between the two groups. Other prognostic factors such as histologic subtype, grade and hormone receptor status did not differ between the groups.

The use of estrogen plus progestin has been reported to result in an increase in abnormal mammograms requiring further evaluation. All women should receive yearly breast examinations by a healthcare provider and perform monthly breast self-examinations. In addition, mammography examinations should be scheduled based on patient age, risk factors, and prior mammogram results.

b. Endometrial Cancer

An increased risk of endometrial cancer has been reported with the use of unopposed estrogen therapy in a woman with a uterus. The reported endometrial cancer risk among unopposed estrogen users is about 2 to 12 times greater than in nonusers, and appears dependent on duration of treatment and on estrogen dose. Most studies show no significant increased risk associated with the use of estrogens for less than 1 year. The greatest risk appears associated with prolonged use, with increased risks of 15- to 24-fold for 5 to 10 years or more and this risk has been shown to persist for at least 8 to 15 years after estrogen therapy is discontinued.

Clinical surveillance of all women using estrogen plus progestin therapy is important. Adequate diagnostic measures, including directed or random endometrial sampling when indicated, should be undertaken to rule out malignancy in all cases of undiagnosed persistent or recurring abnormal vaginal bleeding. There is no evidence that the use of natural estrogens results in a different endometrial risk profile than synthetic estrogens of equivalent estrogen dose. Adding a progestin to estrogen therapy in postmenopausal women has been shown to reduce the risk of endometrial hyperplasia, which may be a precursor to endometrial cancer.

c. Ovarian Cancer

The WHI estrogen plus progestin substudy reported a statistically non-significant increased risk of ovarian cancer. After an average follow-up of 5.6 years, the relative risk for ovarian cancer for CE plus MPA versus placebo was 1.58 (95 percent nCI 0.77–3.24). The absolute risk for CE plus MPA versus placebo was 4 versus 3 cases per 10,000 women-years. In some epidemiologic studies, the use of estrogen-only products, in particular for 5 or more years, has been associated with an increased risk of ovarian cancer. However, the duration of exposure associated with increased risk is not consistent across all epidemiologic studies and some report no association.

3. Probable Dementia

In the estrogen plus progestin Women's Health Initiative Memory Study (WHIMS), an ancillary study of WHI, a population of 4,532 postmenopausal women 65 to 79 years of age was randomized to daily CE (0.625 mg) plus MPA (2.5 mg) or placebo.

In the WHIMS estrogen plus progestin ancillary study, after an average follow-up of 4 years, 40 women in the CE plus MPA group and 21 women in the placebo group were diagnosed with probable dementia. The relative risk of probable dementia for estrogen plus progestin versus placebo was 2.05 (95 percent CI 1.21-3.48). The absolute risk of probable dementia for CE plus MPA versus placebo was 45 versus 22 cases per 10,000 women-years. It is unknown whether these findings apply to younger postmenopausal women. (See **CLINICAL STUDIES** and **PRECAUTIONS, Geriatric Use.**)

4. Vision abnormalities

Discontinue medication pending examination if there is sudden partial or complete loss of vision, or if there is a sudden onset of proptosis, diplopia or migraine. If examination reveals papilledema or retinal vascular lesions, medication should be permanently discontinued.

PRECAUTIONS

A. General

1. Addition of a progestin when a woman has not had a hysterectomy

Studies of the addition of a progestin for 10 or more days of a cycle of estrogen administration, or daily with estrogen in a continuous regimen, have reported a lowered incidence of endometrial hyperplasia than would be induced by estrogen treatment alone. Endometrial hyperplasia may be a precursor to endometrial cancer.

There are, however, possible risks that may be associated with the use of progestins with estrogens compared with estrogen-alone regimens. These include a possible increased risk of breast cancer.

2. Fluid Retention

Progesterone may cause some degree of fluid retention. Women with conditions that might be influenced by this factor, such as cardiac or renal dysfunction, warrant careful observation.

3. Dizziness and Drowsiness

PROMETRIUM Capsules may cause transient dizziness and drowsiness and should be used with caution when driving a motor vehicle or operating machinery. PROMETRIUM Capsules should be taken as a single daily dose at bedtime.

B. Patient Information

General: **This product contains peanut oil and should not be used if you are allergic to peanuts.**

Physicians are advised to discuss the contents of the Patient Information leaflet with patients for whom they prescribe PROMETRIUM Capsules.

C. Drug-Laboratory Test Interactions

The following laboratory results may be altered by the use of estrogen-progestin combination drugs:

• Increased sulfobromophthalein retention and other hepatic function tests.
• Coagulation tests: increase in prothrombin factors VII, VIII, IX and X.
• Pregnanediol determination.
• Thyroid function: increase in PBI, and butanol extractable protein bound iodine and decrease in T3 uptake values.

D. Carcinogenesis, Mutagenesis, Impairment of Fertility

Progesterone has not been tested for carcinogenicity in animals by the oral route of administration. When implanted into female mice, progesterone produced mammary carcinomas, ovarian granulosa cell tumors and endometrial stromal sarcomas. In dogs, long-term intramuscular injections produced nodular hyperplasia and benign and malignant mammary tumors. Subcutaneous or intramuscular injections of progesterone decreased the latency period and increased the incidence of mammary tumors in rats previously treated with a chemical carcinogen.

Progesterone did not show evidence of genotoxicity in in vitro studies for point mutations or for chromosomal damage. In vivo studies for chromosome damage have yielded positive results in mice at oral doses of 1000 mg/kg and 2000 mg/kg. Exogenously administered progesterone has been shown to inhibit ovulation in a number of species and it is expected that high doses given for an extended duration would impair fertility until the cessation of treatment.

E. Pregnancy

PROMETRIUM Capsules should not be used during pregnancy. (See **CONTRAINDICATIONS**.)

Pregnancy Category B: Reproductive studies have been performed in mice at doses up to 9 times the human oral dose, in rats at doses up to 44 times the human oral dose, in rabbits at a dose of 10 mcg/day delivered locally within the uterus by an implanted device, in guinea pigs at doses of approximately one-half the human oral dose and in rhesus monkeys at doses approximately the human dose, all based on body surface area, and have revealed little or no evidence of impaired fertility or harm to the fetus due to progesterone.

F. Nursing Mothers

Detectable amounts of progestin have been identified in the milk of nursing mothers receiving progestins. Caution should be exercised when PROMETRIUM Capsules are administered to a nursing woman.

G. Pediatric Use

PROMETRIUM Capsules are not indicated for pediatric use and no clinical data have been collected in children.

H. Geriatric Use

Clinical studies of PROMETRIUM Capsules did not include sufficient numbers of subjects aged 65 and over to determine whether they respond differently from younger subjects.

The Women's Health Initiative Study

In the Women's Health Initiative (WHI) estrogen plus progestin substudy, there was a higher relative risk of nonfatal stroke and invasive breast cancer in women greater than 65 years of age. (See **WARNINGS, Cardiovascular disorders** and **Malignant neoplasms**.)

The Women's Health Initiative Memory Study

In the Women's Health Initiative Memory Study (WHIMS) of postmenopausal women 65 to 79 years of age, there was an increased risk of developing probable dementia in the estrogen plus progestin ancillary study when compared to placebo. (See **WARNINGS, Probable Dementia**.)

ADVERSE REACTIONS

See **BOXED WARNING, WARNINGS** and **PRECAUTIONS**.

Because clinical trials are conducted under widely varying conditions, adverse reaction rates observed in the clinical trials of a drug cannot be directly compared to rates in the clinical trials of another drug and may not reflect the rates observed in practice.

In a multicenter, randomized, double-blind, placebo-controlled clinical trial, the effects of PROMETRIUM Capsules on the endometrium was studied in a total of 875 postmenopausal women. Table 6 lists adverse experiences greater than or equal to 2 percent of women who received cyclic PROMETRIUM Capsules 200 mg daily (12 days per calendar month cycle) with 0.625 mg conjugated estrogens or placebo.

TABLE 6. Adverse Experiences (≥ 2%) Reported in an 875 Patient Placebo-Controlled Trial in Postmenopausal Women Over a 3-Year Period [Percentage (%) of Patients Reporting]

	PROMETRIUM Capsules 200 mg with Conjugated Estrogens 0.625 mg	Placebo
	(n=178)	(n=174)
Headache	31	27
Breast Tenderness	27	6
Joint Pain	20	29
Depression	19	12
Dizziness	15	9
Abdominal Bloating	12	5
Hot Flashes	11	35
Urinary Problems	11	9
Abdominal Pain	10	10
Vaginal Discharge	10	3
Nausea/Vomiting	8	7
Worry	8	4
Chest Pain	7	5
Diarrhea	7	4
Night Sweats	7	17
Breast Pain	6	2
Swelling of Hands and Feet	6	9
Vaginal Dryness	6	10
Constipation	3	2
Breast Carcinoma	2	<1
Breast Excisional Biopsy	2	<1
Cholecystectomy	2	<1

Effects on Secondary Amenorrhea

In a multicenter, randomized, double-blind, placebo-controlled clinical trial, the effects of PROMETRIUM on secondary amenorrhea was studied in 49 estrogen-primed postmenopausal women. Table 7 lists adverse experiences greater than or equal to 5 percent of women who received PROMETRIUM or placebo.

TABLE 7. Adverse Experiences (≥ 5%) Reported in Patients Using 400 mg/day in a Placebo-Controlled Trial in Estrogen-Primed Postmenopausal Women

Adverse Experience	PROMETRIUM Capsules 400 mg	Placebo
	n=25	n=24
	Percentage (%) of Patients	
Fatigue	8	4
Headache	16	8
Dizziness	24	4
Abdominal Distention (Bloating)	8	8
Abdominal Pain (Cramping)	20	13
Diarrhea	8	4
Nausea	8	0
Back Pain	8	8
Musculoskeletal Pain	12	4
Irritability	8	4
Breast Pain	16	8
Infection Viral	12	0
Coughing	8	0

In an open label, multicenter, parallel group, postmarketing dosing study consisting of three consecutive 28-day treatment cycles, 220 women with secondary amenorrhea were randomized to PROMETRIUM 300 mg/day (n = 113) or PROMETRIUM 400 mg/day (n = 107). They received daily estrogen therapy (0.625 mg conjugated estrogen). Eight (8) patients (5 at 400 mg/day; 3 at 300 mg/day) were found to have abnormal PAP smears classified by the investigator as clinically significant. Further evaluation found that 6 of the 8 results were infectious in nature (i.e., Candida, HPV, bacterial vaginosis, Trichomonas).

Postmarketing Experience:
The following additional adverse reactions have been reported with PROMETRIUM Capsules. Because these reactions are reported voluntarily from a population of uncertain size, it is not always possible to reliably estimate the frequency or establish a causal relationship to drug exposure.

Genitourinary System: endometrial carcinoma, hypospadia, intra-uterine death, menorrhagia, menstrual disorder, metrorrhagia, ovarian cyst, spontaneous abortion.

Cardiovascular: circulatory collapse, congenital heart disease (including ventricular septal defect and patent ductus arteriosus), hypertension, hypotension, tachycardia.

Gastrointestinal: acute pancreatitis, cholestasis, cholestatic hepatitis, dysphagia, hepatic failure, hepatic necrosis, hepatitis, increased liver function tests (including alanine aminotransferase increased, aspartate aminotransferase increased, gamma-glutamyl transferase increased), jaundice, swollen tongue.

Skin: alopecia, pruritus, urticaria.

Eyes: blurred vision, diplopia, visual disturbance.

Central Nervous System: aggression, convulsion, depersonalization, depressed consciousness, disorientation, dysarthria, loss of consciousness, paresthesia, sedation, stupor, syncope (with and without hypotension), transient ischemic attack, suicidal ideation.

During initial therapy, a few women have experienced a constellation of many or all of the following symptoms: extreme dizziness and/or drowsiness, blurred vision, slurred speech, difficulty walking, loss of consciousness, vertigo, confusion, disorientation, feeling drunk, and shortness of breath.

Miscellaneous: abnormal gait, anaphylactic reaction, arthralgia, blood glucose increased, choking, cleft lip, cleft palate, difficulty walking, dyspnea, face edema, feeling abnormal, feeling drunk, hypersensitivity, asthma, muscle cramp, throat tightness, tinnitus, vertigo, weight decreased, weight increased.

OVERDOSAGE
No studies on overdosage have been conducted in humans. In the case of overdosage, PROMETRIUM Capsules should be discontinued and the patient should be treated symptomatically.

DOSAGE AND ADMINISTRATION
Prevention of Endometrial Hyperplasia
PROMETRIUM Capsules should be given as a single daily dose at bedtime, 200 mg orally for 12 days sequentially per 28-day cycle, to postmenopausal women with a uterus who are receiving daily conjugated estrogens tablets.
Treatment of Secondary Amenorrhea
PROMETRIUM Capsules may be given as a single daily dose of 400 mg at bedtime for 10 days.
Some women may experience difficulty swallowing PROMETRIUM Capsules. For these women, PROMETRIUM Capsules should be taken with a glass of water while in the standing position.

HOW SUPPLIED
PROMETRIUM (progesterone, USP) Capsules 100 mg are round, peach-colored capsules branded with black imprint "SV."
NDC 0032-1708-01 (Bottle of 100)
PROMETRIUM (progesterone, USP) Capsules 200 mg are oval, pale yellow-colored capsules branded with black imprint "SV2."
NDC 0032-1711-01 (Bottle of 100)
Store at 25°C (77°F); excursions permitted to 15° to 30°C (59° to 86°F) [See USP Controlled Room Temperature].
Protect from excessive moisture.
Dispense in tight, light-resistant container as defined in USP/NF, accompanied by a Patient Insert.
Keep out of reach of children.
Manufactured by:
Catalent Pharma Solutions
St. Petersburg, FL 33716
Marketed by:
Abbott Laboratories
North Chicago, IL 60064, U.S.A.
© 2010 Abbott Laboratories
All rights reserved.
500032 3E Rev Mar 2010

PATIENT INFORMATION
PROMETRIUM® (progesterone, USP)
Capsules 100 mg
Capsules 200 mg
Read this PATIENT INFORMATION before you start taking PROMETRIUM® Capsules and read what you get each time you refill your PROMETRIUM Capsules prescription. There may be new information. This information does not take the place of talking to your healthcare provider about your medical condition or your treatment.

WHAT IS THE MOST IMPORTANT INFORMATION I SHOULD KNOW ABOUT PROMETRIUM CAPSULES (A Progesterone Hormone)?
• Progesterone with or without estrogens should not be used to prevent heart disease, heart attacks, strokes, or dementia.
• Using estrogens with or without progestins may increase your chance of getting heart attacks, strokes, breast cancer, and blood clots. Using estrogens with or without progestins may increase your chance of getting dementia, based on a study of women age 65 and older. You and your healthcare provider should talk regularly about whether you still need treatment with PROMETRIUM Capsules.

THIS PRODUCT CONTAINS PEANUT OIL AND SHOULD NOT BE USED IF YOU ARE ALLERGIC TO PEANUTS.

What is PROMETRIUM Capsules?
PROMETRIUM Capsules contain the female hormone called progesterone.
What is PROMETRIUM Capsules used for?
Treatment of Menstrual Irregularities
PROMETRIUM Capsules are used for the treatment of secondary amenorrhea (absence of menstrual periods in women who have previously had a menstrual period) due to a decrease in progesterone. When you do not produce enough progesterone, menstrual irregularities can occur. If your healthcare provider has determined your body does not produce enough progesterone on its own, PROMETRIUM Capsules may be prescribed to provide the progesterone you need.
Protection of the Endometrium (Lining of the Uterus)
PROMETRIUM Capsules are used in combination with estrogen-containing medications in postmenopausal women with a uterus. Taking estrogens alone increases the chance of developing a condition called endometrial hyperplasia, that may lead to cancer of the lining of the uterus. The ad-

dition of a progestin is generally recommended for women with a uterus to reduce the chance of getting cancer of the uterus.
Who should not take PROMETRIUM Capsules?
Do not start taking PROMETRIUM Capsules if you:
• **Are allergic to peanuts.**
• **Have unusual vaginal bleeding.**
• **Currently have or have had certain cancers.** Estrogens/progestins may increase the chance of getting certain types of cancers, including cancer of the breast or uterus. If you have or have had cancer, talk with your healthcare provider about whether you should take PROMETRIUM Capsules.
• **Had a stroke or heart attack.**
• **Currently have or have had blood clots.**
• **Currently have or have had liver problems.**
• **Are allergic to any of the ingredients in PROMETRIUM Capsules.** See the list of ingredients at the end of this leaflet.
• **Think you may be pregnant.**
Tell your healthcare provider:
• **If you are breastfeeding.** The hormones in PROMETRIUM Capsules can pass into your milk.
• **About all of your medical problems.** Your healthcare provider may need to check you more carefully if you have certain conditions, such as diabetes, asthma (wheezing), epilepsy (seizures), migraine, endometriosis, lupus, problems with your heart, liver, thyroid, kidneys, or have high calcium levels in your blood.
• **About all the medicines you take.** This includes prescription and nonprescription medicines, vitamins, and herbal supplements. Some medicines may affect how PROMETRIUM Capsules works. PROMETRIUM Capsules may also affect how your other medicines work.
• **If you have an abnormal PAP smear:** Your healthcare provider should be told that you are taking progesterone.
How should I take PROMETRIUM Capsules?
1. Prevention of Endometrial Hyperplasia: Postmenopausal women with a uterus who are taking estrogens should take a single daily dose of 200 mg PROMETRIUM Capsules at bedtime for 12 continuous days per 28-day cycle.
2. Secondary Amenorrhea: PROMETRIUM Capsules may be given as a single daily dose of 400 mg at bedtime for 10 days.
3. **PROMETRIUM Capsules are to be taken at bedtime as some women become very drowsy and/or dizzy after taking PROMETRIUM Capsules. In a small percentage of these women, these effects may be increased including blurred vision, difficulty speaking, difficulty walking, and feeling abnormal. If you experience these symptoms, discuss them with your healthcare provider immediately. Taking PROMETRIUM Capsules at bedtime may minimize the impact of these symptoms.**
If you experience difficulty in swallowing PROMETRIUM Capsules, it is recommended that you take your daily dose at bedtime with a glass of water while in the standing position.
What are the possible side effects of PROMETRIUM Capsules?
The following side effects are grouped by how serious they are and how often they happen when you are treated:
Serious but less common side effects include:
• *Risk to the Fetus:* Rare cases of cleft palate, cleft lip, hypospadias, ventricular septal defect, patent ductus arteriosus, and other congenital heart defects.
• *Abnormal Blood Clotting:* stroke (cutting off blood to part of the brain), heart attack (cutting off blood to part of the heart), pulmonary embolus (cutting off blood to part of the lungs), visual loss or blindness (cutting off blood vessels in the eye).
Less serious but common side effects include:
• Headaches
• Breast pain
• Irregular vaginal bleeding or spotting
• Stomach/abdominal cramps, bloating
• Nausea and vomiting
• Hair loss
• Fluid retention
• Vaginal yeast infection
These are not all the possible side effects of PROMETRIUM Capsules. For more information, ask your healthcare provider or pharmacist.
Some of the warning signs of serious side effects include:
• Breast lumps (Ask your healthcare provider to show you how to examine your breasts monthly.)
• Unusual bleeding from the vagina

Information on the Solvay/Abbott Pharmaceutical Products listed on these pages is from the prescribing information in use as of June 1, 2010. For more information, please visit rxabbott.com or call 1-800-633-9110.

- Dizziness and faintness
- Changes in speech
- Severe headaches
- Chest pain
- Shortness of breath
- Pains in your legs
- Changes in vision
- Vomiting
- Yellowing of the skin, eyes or nail beds

Call your healthcare provider right away if you get any of these warning signs, or any other unusual symptoms that concern you.

What can I do to lower my chances of getting a serious side effect with PROMETRIUM Capsules?

- Talk with your healthcare provider regularly about whether you should continue taking PROMETRIUM Capsules.
- See your healthcare provider right away if you get unusual vaginal bleeding while taking PROMETRIUM Capsules.
- Have a pelvic exam, breast exam, and mammogram (breast X-ray) every year unless your healthcare provider tells you something else. If members of your family have had breast cancer or if you have ever had breast lumps or an abnormal mammogram, you may need to have breast exams more often.
- If you have high blood pressure, high cholesterol (fat in the blood), diabetes, are overweight, or if you use tobacco, you may have higher chances for getting heart disease. Ask your healthcare provider for ways to lower your chances for getting heart disease.

General information about safe and effective use of PROMETRIUM Capsules

- Medicines are sometimes prescribed for conditions that are not mentioned in patient information leaflets. Do not take PROMETRIUM Capsules for conditions for which it was not prescribed.
- Your healthcare provider has prescribed this drug for you and you alone. Do not give PROMETRIUM Capsules to other people, even if they have the same symptoms you have. It may harm them.
- PROMETRIUM Capsules should be taken as a single daily dose at bedtime. Some women may experience extreme dizziness and/or drowsiness during initial therapy. In a small percentage of women, these effects may be increased including blurred vision, difficulty speaking, difficulty walking, and feeling abnormal. If you experience these symptoms, discuss them with your healthcare provider immediately. A single bedtime dose may reduce the impact of these symptoms.
- Use caution when driving a motor vehicle or operating machinery as dizziness or drowsiness may occur.

Keep PROMETRIUM Capsules out of the reach of children.

This leaflet provides a summary of the most important information about PROMETRIUM Capsules. If you would like more information, talk with your healthcare provider or pharmacist. You can ask for information about PROMETRIUM Capsules that is written for health professionals. You can get more information by calling the toll free number 1-800-241-1643.

What are the ingredients in PROMETRIUM Capsules?

Active ingredient: 100 mg or 200 mg micronized progesterone

The inactive ingredients for PROMETRIUM Capsules 100 mg include: peanut oil NF, gelatin NF, glycerin USP, lecithin NF, titanium dioxide USP, D&C Yellow No. 10, and FD&C Red No. 40.

The inactive ingredients for PROMETRIUM Capsules 200 mg include: peanut oil NF, gelatin NF, glycerin USP, lecithin NF, titanium dioxide USP, D&C Yellow No. 10, and FD&C Yellow No. 6.

HOW SUPPLIED

PROMETRIUM Capsules 100 mg are round, peach-colored capsules branded with black imprint "SV."
PROMETRIUM Capsules 200 mg are oval, pale yellow-colored capsules branded with black imprint "SV2."
Store at 25°C (77°F); excursions permitted to 15° to 30°C (59° to 86°F) [See USP Controlled Room Temperature].
Protect from excessive moisture.
Manufactured by:
Catalent Pharma Solutions
St. Petersburg, FL 33716
Marketed by:
Abbott Laboratories
North Chicago, IL 60064, U.S.A.
© 2010 Abbott Laboratories.
All rights reserved.
500033 3E Rev Mar 2010

Somerset Pharmaceuticals, Inc.
781 CHESTNUT RIDGE ROAD
MORGANTOWN, WEST VIRGINIA 26505

For Medical Information Contact:
Generally:
Professional Services Department
(800) 892-8889
In Emergencies:
(800) 892-8889

ELDEPRYL® ℞
(selegiline hydrochloride)
Capsules
5 mg
℞ only

DESCRIPTION

ELDEPRYL (selegiline hydrochloride) is a levorotatory acetylenic derivative of phenethylamine. It is commonly referred to in the clinical and pharmacological literature as l-deprenyl.

The chemical name is: (R)-(-)-N,2-dimethyl-N-2-propynylphenethylamine hydrochloride. It is a white to near white crystalline powder, freely soluble in water, chloroform, and methanol, and has a molecular weight of 223.75. The structural formula is as follows:

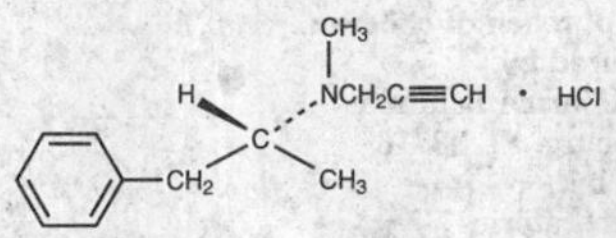

Each aqua blue capsule is band imprinted with the Somerset logo on the cap and "Eldepryl 5 mg" on the body. Each capsule contains 5 mg selegiline hydrochloride. Inactive ingredients are anhydrous citric acid, lactose, magnesium stearate, and microcrystalline cellulose.

CLINICAL PHARMACOLOGY

The mechanisms accounting for selegiline's beneficial adjunctive action in the treatment of Parkinson's disease are not fully understood. Inhibition of monoamine oxidase, type B, activity is generally considered to be of primary importance; in addition, there is evidence that selegiline may act through other mechanisms to increase dopaminergic activity.

Selegiline is best known as an irreversible inhibitor of monoamine oxidase (MAO), an intracellular enzyme associated with the outer membrane of mitochondria. Selegiline inhibits MAO by acting as a 'suicide' substrate for the enzyme; that is, it is converted by MAO to an active moiety which combines irreversibly with the active site and/or the enzyme's essential FAD cofactor. Because selegiline has greater affinity for type B rather than for type A active sites, it can serve as a selective inhibitor of MAO type B if it is administered at the recommended dose.

MAOs are widely distributed throughout the body; their concentration is especially high in liver, kidney, stomach, intestinal wall, and brain. MAOs are currently subclassified into two types, A and B, which differ in their substrate specificity and tissue distribution. In humans, intestinal MAO is predominantly type A, while most of that in brain is type B. In CNS neurons, MAO plays an important role in the catabolism of catecholamines (dopamine, norepinephrine and epinephrine) and serotonin. MAOs are also important in the catabolism of various exogenous amines found in a variety of foods and drugs. MAO in the GI tract and liver (primarily type A), for example, is thought to provide vital protection from exogenous amines (e.g., tyramine) that have the capacity, if absorbed intact, to cause a 'hypertensive crisis,' the so-called 'cheese reaction.' (If large amounts of certain exogenous amines gain access to the systemic circulation - e.g., from fermented cheese, red wine, herring, over-the-counter cough/cold medications, etc. - they are taken up by adrenergic neurons and displace norepinephrine from storage sites within membrane bound vesicles. Subsequent release of the displaced norepinephrine causes the rise in systemic blood pressure, etc.)

In theory, since MAO-A of the gut is not inhibited, patients treated with selegiline at a dose of 10 mg a day should be able to take medications containing pharmacologically active amines and consume tyramine-containing foods without risk of uncontrolled hypertension. Although rare, a few reports of hypertensive reactions have occurred in patients receiving ELDEPRYL at the recommended dose, with

---

tyramine-containing foods. In addition, one case of hypertensive crisis has been reported in a patient taking the recommended dose of selegiline and a sympathomimetic medication, ephedrine. The pathophysiology of the 'cheese reaction' is complicated and, in addition to its ability to inhibit MAO-B selectively, selegiline's relative freedom from this reaction has been attributed to an ability to prevent tyramine and other indirect acting sympathomimetics from displacing norepinephrine from adrenergic neurons. However, until the pathophysiology of the cheese reaction is more completely understood, it seems prudent to assume that selegiline can ordinarily only be used safely without dietary restrictions at doses where it presumably selectively inhibits MAO-B (e.g., 10 mg/day).

In short, attention to the dose dependent nature of selegiline's selectivity is critical if it is to be used without elaborate restrictions being placed on diet and concomitant drug use although, as noted above, a few cases of hypertensive reactions have been reported at the recommended dose. (See WARNINGS and PRECAUTIONS.)

It is important to be aware that selegiline may have pharmacological effects unrelated to MAO-B inhibition. As noted above, there is some evidence that it may increase dopaminergic activity by other mechanisms, including interfering with dopamine re-uptake at the synapse. Effects resulting from selegiline administration may also be mediated through its metabolites. Two of its three principal metabolites, amphetamine and methamphetamine, have pharmacological actions of their own; they interfere with neuronal uptake and enhance release of several neurotransmitters (e.g., norepinephrine, dopamine, serotonin). However, the extent to which these metabolites contribute to the effects of selegiline are unknown.

Rationale for the Use of a Selective Monoamine Oxidase Type B Inhibitor in Parkinson's Disease: Many of the prominent symptoms of Parkinson's disease are due to a deficiency of striatal dopamine that is the consequence of a progressive degeneration and loss of a population of dopaminergic neurons which originate in the substantia nigra of the midbrain and project to the basal ganglia or striatum. Early in the course of Parkinson's Disease, the deficit in the capacity of these neurons to synthesize dopamine can be overcome by administration of exogenous levodopa, usually given in combination with a peripheral decarboxylase inhibitor (carbidopa).

With the passage of time, due to the progression of the disease and/or the effect of sustained treatment, the efficacy and quality of the therapeutic response to levodopa diminishes. Thus, after several years of levodopa treatment, the response, for a given dose of levodopa, is shorter, has less predictable onset and offset (i.e., there is 'wearing off'), and is often accompanied by side effects (e.g., dyskinesia, akinesias, on-off phenomena, freezing, etc.).

This deteriorating response is currently interpreted as a manifestation of the inability of the ever decreasing population of intact nigrostriatal neurons to synthesize and release adequate amounts of dopamine.

MAO-B inhibition may be useful in this setting because, by blocking the catabolism of dopamine, it would increase the net amount of dopamine available (i.e., it would increase the pool of dopamine). Whether or not this mechanism or an alternative one actually accounts for the observed beneficial effects of adjunctive selegiline is unknown.

Selegiline's benefit in Parkinson's disease has only been documented as an adjunct to levodopa/carbidopa. Whether or not it might be effective as a sole treatment is unknown, but past attempts to treat Parkinson's disease with non-selective MAOI monotherapy are reported to have been unsuccessful. It is important to note that attempts to treat Parkinsonian patients with combinations of levodopa and currently marketed non-selective MAO inhibitors were abandoned because of multiple side effects including hypertension, increase in involuntary movement, and toxic delirium.

Pharmacokinetic Information (Absorption, Distribution, Metabolism and Elimination—ADME):

The absolute bioavailability of selegiline following oral dosing is not known; however, selegiline undergoes extensive metabolism (presumably attributable to presystemic clearance in gut and liver). The major plasma metabolites are N-desmethylselegiline, L-amphetamine and L-methamphetamine. Only N-desmethylselegiline has MAO-B inhibiting activity. The peak plasma levels of these metabolites following a single oral dose of 10 mg are from 4 to almost 20 times greater than that of the maximum plasma concentration of selegiline [1 ng/mL]. The maximum concentrations of amphetamine and methamphetamine, however, are far below those ordinarily expected to produce clinically important effects.

Single oral dose studies do not predict multiple dose kinetics, however, at steady state the peak plasma level of

---

selegiline is 4 fold that obtained following a single dose. Metabolite concentrations increase to a lesser extent, averaging 2 fold that seen after a single dose.

The bioavailability of selegiline is increased 3 to 4 fold when it is taken with food.

The extent of systemic exposure to selegiline at a given dose varies considerably among individuals. Estimates of systemic clearance of selegiline are not available. Following a single oral dose, the mean elimination half-life of selegiline is two hours. Under steady state conditions the elimination half-life increases to ten hours.

Because selegiline's inhibition of MAO-B is irreversible, it is impossible to predict the extent of MAO-B inhibition from steady state plasma levels. For the same reason, it is not possible to predict the rate of recovery of MAO-B activity as a function of plasma levels. The recovery of MAO-B activity is a function of de novo protein synthesis; however, information about the rate of de novo protein synthesis is not yet available. Although platelet MAO-B activity returns to the normal range within 5 to 7 days of selegiline discontinuation, the linkage between platelet and brain MAO-B inhibition is not fully understood nor is the relationship of MAO-B inhibition to the clinical effect established (see CLINICAL PHARMACOLOGY).

Special Populations:

Renal Impairment: No pharmacokinetic information is available on selegiline or its metabolites in renally impaired subjects.

Hepatic Impairment: No pharmacokinetic information is available on selegiline or its metabolites in hepatically impaired subjects.

Age: Although a general conclusion about the effects of age on the pharmacokinetics of selegiline is not warranted because of the size of the sample evaluated (12 subjects greater than 60 years of age, 12 subjects between the ages of 18 to 30), systemic exposure was about twice as great in older as compared to a younger population given a single oral dose of 10 mg.

Gender: No information is available on the effects of gender on the pharmacokinetics of selegiline.

INDICATIONS AND USAGE

ELDEPRYL is indicated as an adjunct in the management of Parkinsonian patients being treated with levodopa/carbidopa who exhibit deterioration in the quality of their response to this therapy. There is no evidence from controlled studies that selegiline has any beneficial effect in the absence of concurrent levodopa therapy.

Evidence supporting this claim was obtained in randomized controlled clinical investigations that compared the effects of added selegiline or placebo in patients receiving levodopa/carbidopa. Selegiline was significantly superior to placebo on all three principal outcome measures employed: change from baseline in daily levodopa/carbidopa dose, the amount of 'off' time, and patient self-rating of treatment success. Beneficial effects were also observed on other measures of treatment success (e.g., measures of reduced end of dose akinesia, decreased tremor and sialorrhea, improved speech and dressing ability and improved overall disability as assessed by walking and comparison to previous state).

CONTRAINDICATIONS

ELDEPRYL is contraindicated in patients with a known hypersensitivity to this drug.

ELDEPRYL is contraindicated for use with meperidine (DEMEROL & other trade names). This contraindication is often extended to other opioids. (See **Drug Interactions**.)

WARNINGS

Selegiline should not be used at daily doses exceeding those recommended (10 mg/day) because of the risks associated with non-selective inhibition of MAO. (See CLINICAL PHARMACOLOGY.)

The selectivity of selegiline for MAO-B may not be absolute even at the recommended daily dose of 10 mg a day. Rare cases of hypertensive reactions associated with ingestion of tyramine-containing foods have been reported in patients taking the recommended daily dose of selegiline. The selectivity is further diminished with increasing daily doses. The precise dose at which selegiline becomes a non-selective inhibitor of all MAO is unknown, but may be in the range of 30 to 40 mg a day.

Severe CNS toxicity associated with hyperpyrexia and death have been reported with the combination of tricyclic antidepressants and non-selective MAOIs (NARDIL, PARNATE). A similar reaction has been reported for a patient on amitriptyline and ELDEPRYL. Another patient receiving protriptyline and ELDEPRYL developed tremors, agitation, and restlessness followed by unresponsiveness and death two weeks after ELDEPRYL was added. Related adverse events including hypertension, syncope, asystole, diaphoresis, seizures, changes in behavioral and mental status, and muscular rigidity have also been reported in some patients receiving ELDEPRYL and various tricyclic antidepressants.

Serious, sometimes fatal, reactions with signs and symptoms that may include hyperthermia, rigidity, myoclonus, autonomic instability with rapid fluctuations of the vital signs, and mental status changes that include extreme agitation progressing to delirium and coma have been reported with patients receiving a combination of fluoxetine hydrochloride (PROZAC) and non-selective MAOIs. Similar signs have been reported in some patients on the combination of ELDEPRYL (10 mg a day) and selective serotonin re-uptake inhibitors including fluoxetine, sertraline and paroxetine.

Since the mechanisms of these reactions are not fully understood, it seems prudent, in general, to avoid this combination of ELDEPRYL and tricyclic antidepressants as well as ELDEPRYL and selective serotonin re-uptake inhibitors. At least 14 days should elapse between discontinuation of ELDEPRYL and initiation of treatment with a tricyclic antidepressant or selective serotonin re-uptake inhibitors. Because of the long half-lives of fluoxetine and its active metabolite, at least five weeks (perhaps longer, especially if fluoxetine has been prescribed chronically and/or at higher doses) should elapse between discontinuation of fluoxetine and initiation of treatment with ELDEPRYL.

PRECAUTIONS

General: Some patients given selegiline may experience an exacerbation of levodopa associated side effects, presumably due to the increased amounts of dopamine reaction with super sensitive, post-synaptic receptors. These effects may often be mitigated by reducing the dose of levodopa/carbidopa by approximately 10 to 30%.

The decision to prescribe selegiline should take into consideration that the MAO system of enzymes is complex and incompletely understood and there is only a limited amount of carefully documented clinical experience with selegiline. Consequently, the full spectrum of possible responses to selegiline may not have been observed in pre-marketing evaluation of the drug. It is advisable, therefore, to observe patients closely for atypical responses.

Melanoma: Epidemiological studies have shown that patients with Parkinson's disease have a higher risk (2- to approximately 6-fold higher) of developing melanoma than the general population. Whether the increased risk observed was due to Parkinson's disease or other factors, such as drugs used to treat Parkinson's disease, is unclear.

For the reasons stated above, patients and providers are advised to monitor for melanomas frequently and on a regular basis when using ELDEPRYL for any indication. Ideally, periodic skin examinations should be performed by appropriately qualified individuals (e.g., dermatologists).

Information for Patients: Patients should be advised of the possible need to reduce levodopa dosage after the initiation of ELDEPRYL therapy.

Patients (or their families if the patient is incompetent) should be advised not to exceed the daily recommended dose of 10 mg. The risk of using higher daily doses of selegiline should be explained, and a brief description of the 'cheese reaction' provided. Rare hypertensive reactions with selegiline at recommended doses associated with dietary influences have been reported.

Consequently, it may be useful to inform patients (or their families) about the signs and symptoms associated with MAOI induced hypertensive reactions. In particular, patients should be urged to report, immediately, any severe headache or other atypical or unusual symptoms not previously experienced.

There have been reports of patients experiencing intense urges to gamble, increased sexual urges, and other intense urges, and the inability to control these urges while taking one or more of the medications that increase central dopaminergic tone, and that are generally used for the treatment of Parkinson's disease, including ELDEPRYL. Although it is not proven that the medications caused these events, these urges were reported to have stopped in some cases when the dose was reduced or the medication was stopped. Prescribers should ask patients about the development of new or increased gambling urges, sexual urges or other urges while being treated with ELDEPRYL. Patients should inform their physician if they experience new or increased gambling urges, increased sexual urges or other intense urges while taking ELDEPRYL. Physicians should consider dose reduction or stopping the medication if a patient develops such urges while taking ELDEPRYL.

Laboratory Tests: No specific laboratory tests are deemed essential for the management of patients on ELDEPRYL. Periodic routine evaluation of all patients, however, is appropriate.

Drug Interactions: The occurrence of stupor, muscular rigidity, severe agitation, and elevated temperature has been reported in some patients receiving the combination of selegiline and meperidine. Symptoms usually resolve over days when the combination is discontinued. This is typical of the interaction of meperidine and MAOIs. Other serious reactions (including severe agitation, hallucinations, and

death) have been reported in patients receiving this combination (see **CONTRAINDICATIONS**). Severe toxicity has also been reported in patients receiving the combination of tricyclic antidepressants and ELDEPRYL and selective serotonin re-uptake inhibitors and ELDEPRYL. (See **WARNINGS** for details.) One case of hypertensive crisis has been reported in a patient taking the recommended doses of selegiline and a sympathomimetic medication (ephedrine).

Carcinogenesis, Mutagenesis, and Impairment of Fertility: Assessment of the carcinogenic potential of selegiline in mice and rats is ongoing.

Selegiline did not induce mutations or chromosomal damage when tested in the bacterial mutation assay in Salmonella typhimurium and in an *in vivo* chromosomal aberration assay. While these studies provide some reassurance that selegiline is not mutagenic or clastogenic, they are not definitive because of methodological limitations. No definitive *in vitro* chromosomal aberration or *in vitro* mammalian gene mutation assays have been performed.

The effect of selegiline on fertility has not been adequately assessed.

Pregnancy: *Pregnancy Category C:* No teratogenic effects were observed in a study of embryo-fetal development in Sprague-Dawley rats at oral doses of 4, 12, and 36 mg/kg or 4, 12 and 35 times the human therapeutic dose on a mg/m[2] basis. No teratogenic effects were observed in a study of embryo-fetal development in New Zealand White rabbits at oral doses of 5, 25, and 50 mg/kg or 10, 48, and 95 times the human therapeutic dose on a mg/m[2] basis; however, in this study, the number of litters produced at the two higher doses was less than recommended for assessing teratogenic potential. In the rat study, there was a decrease in fetal body weight at the highest dose tested. In the rabbit study, increases in total resorptions and % post-implantation loss, and a decrease in the number of live fetuses per dam occurred at the highest dose tested. In a peri- and postnatal development study in Sprague-Dawley rats (oral doses of 4, 16, and 64 mg/kg or 4, 15, and 62 times the human therapeutic dose on a mg/m[2] basis), an increase in the number of stillbirths and decreases in the number of pups per dam, pup survival, and pup body weight (at birth and throughout the lactation period) were observed at the two highest doses. At the highest dose tested, no pups born alive survived to Day 4 postpartum. Postnatal development at the highest dose tested in dams could not be evaluated because of the lack of surviving pups. The reproductive performance of the untreated offspring was not assessed.

There are no adequate and well-controlled studies in pregnant women. Selegiline should be used during pregnancy only if the potential benefit justifies the potential risk to the fetus.

Nursing Mothers: It is not known whether selegiline hydrochloride is excreted in human milk. Because many drugs are excreted in human milk, consideration should be given to discontinuing the use of all but absolutely essential drug treatments in nursing women.

Pediatric Use: The effects of selegiline hydrochloride in children have not been evaluated.

ADVERSE REACTIONS

Introduction: The number of patients who received selegiline in prospectively monitored pre-marketing studies is limited. While other sources of information about the use of selegiline are available (e.g., literature reports, foreign post-marketing reports, etc.) they do not provide the kind of information necessary to estimate the incidence of adverse events. Thus, overall incidence figures for adverse reactions associated with the use of selegiline cannot be provided. Many of the adverse reactions seen have also been reported as symptoms of dopamine excess.

Moreover, the importance and severity of various reactions reported often cannot be ascertained. One index of relative importance, however, is whether or not a reaction caused treatment discontinuation. In prospective pre-marketing studies, the following events led, in decreasing order of frequency, to discontinuation of treatment with selegiline: nausea, hallucinations, confusion, depression, loss of balance, insomnia, orthostatic hypotension, increased akinetic involuntary movements, agitation, arrhythmia, bradykinesia, chorea, delusions, hypertension, new or increased angina pectoris, and syncope. Events reported only once as a cause of discontinuation are ankle edema, anxiety, burning lips/mouth, constipation, drowsiness/lethargy, dystonia, excess perspiration, increased freezing, gastrointestinal bleeding, hair loss, increased tremor, nervousness, weakness, and weight loss.

Experience with ELDEPRYL obtained in parallel, placebo controlled, randomized studies provides only a limited basis for estimates of adverse reaction rates. The following reactions that occurred with greater frequency among the 49 patients assigned to selegiline as compared to the 50 patients assigned to placebo in the only parallel, placebo controlled trial performed in patients with Parkinson's disease are shown in the following Table. None of these adverse reactions led to a discontinuation of treatment.

INCIDENCE OF TREATMENT-EMERGENT ADVERSE EXPERIENCES IN THE PLACEBO-CONTROLLED CLINICAL TRIAL

Adverse Event	Number of Patients Reporting Events	
	selegiline hydrochloride N = 49	Placebo N = 50
Nausea	10	3
Dizziness/Lightheaded/Fainting	7	1
Abdominal Pain	4	2
Confusion	3	0
Hallucinations	3	1
Dry mouth	3	1
Vivid Dreams	2	0
Dyskinesias	2	5
Headache	2	1

The following events were reported once in either or both groups:

Ache, generalized	1	0
Anxiety/Tension	1	1
Anemia	0	1
Diarrhea	1	0
Hair Loss	0	1
Insomnia	1	1
Lethargy	1	0
Leg pain	1	0
Low back pain	1	0
Malaise	0	1
Palpitations	1	0
Urinary Retention	1	0
Weight Loss	1	0

In all prospectively monitored clinical investigations, enrolling approximately 920 patients, the following adverse events, classified by body system, were reported.

Central Nervous System: *Motor/Coordination/Extrapyramidal:* increased tremor, chorea, loss of balance, restlessness, blepharospasm, increased bradykinesia, facial grimace, falling down, heavy leg, muscle twitch*, myoclonic jerks*, stiff neck, tardive dyskinesia, dystonic symptoms, dyskinesia, involuntary movements, freezing, festination, increased apraxia, muscle cramps.

Mental Status/Behavioral/Psychiatric: hallucinations, dizziness, confusion, anxiety, depression, drowsiness, behavior/mood change, dreams/nightmares, tiredness, delusions, disorientation, lightheadedness, impaired memory*, increased energy*, transient high*, hollow feeling, lethargy/malaise, apathy, overstimulation, vertigo, personality change, sleep disturbance, restlessness, weakness, transient irritability.

Pain/Altered Sensation: headache, back pain, leg pain, tinnitus, migraine, supraorbital pain, throat burning, generalized ache, chills, numbness of toes/fingers, taste disturbance.

Autonomic Nervous System: dry mouth, blurred vision, sexual dysfunction.

Cardiovascular: orthostatic hypotension, hypertension, arrhythmia, palpitations, new or increased angina pectoris, hypotension, tachycardia, peripheral edema, sinus bradycardia, syncope.

Gastrointestinal: nausea/vomiting, constipation, weight loss, anorexia, poor appetite, dysphagia, diarrhea, heartburn, rectal bleeding, bruxism*, gastrointestinal bleeding (exacerbation of preexisting ulcer disease).

Genitourinary/Gynecologic/Endocrine: slow urination, transient anorgasmia*, nocturia, prostatic hypertrophy, urinary hesitancy, urinary retention, decreased penile*, urinary frequency.

Skin and Appendages: increased sweating, diaphoresis, facial hair, hair loss, hematoma, rash, photosensitivity.

Miscellaneous: asthma, diplopia, shortness of breath, speech affected.

Post-marketing Reports: The following experiences were described in spontaneous post-marketing reports. These reports do not provide sufficient information to establish a clear causal relationship with the use of ELDEPRYL.

CNS: Seizure in dialyzed chronic renal failure patient on concomitant medications.

* indicates events reported only at doses greater than 10 mg/day.

OVERDOSAGE

Selegiline: No specific information is available about clinically significant overdoses with ELDEPRYL. However, experience gained during selegiline's development reveals that some individuals exposed to doses of 600 mg of d,l-selegiline suffered severe hypotension and psychomotor agitation.

Since the selective inhibition of MAO-B by selegiline hydrochloride is achieved only at doses in the range recommended for the treatment of Parkinson's disease (e.g., 10 mg/day), overdoses are likely to cause significant inhibition of both MAO-A and MAO-B. Consequently, the signs and symptoms of overdose may resemble those observed with marketed non-selective MAO inhibitors [e.g., tranylcypromine (PARNATE), isocarboxazide (MARPLAN), and phenelzine (NARDIL)].

Overdose with Non-Selective MAO Inhibition: NOTE: This section is provided for reference; it does not describe events that have actually been observed with selegiline in overdose.

Characteristically, signs and symptoms of non-selective MAOI overdose may not appear immediately. Delays of up to 12 hours between ingestion of drug and the appearance of signs may occur. Importantly, the peak intensity of the syndrome may not be reached for upwards of a day following the overdose. Death has been reported following overdosage. Therefore, immediate hospitalization, with continuous patient observation and monitoring for a period of at least two days following the ingestion of such drugs in overdose, is strongly recommended.

The clinical picture of MAOI overdose varies considerably; its severity may be a function of the amount of drug consumed. The central nervous and cardiovascular systems are prominently involved.

Signs and symptoms of overdosage may include, alone or in combination, any of the following: drowsiness, dizziness, faintness, irritability, hyperactivity, agitation, severe headache, hallucinations, trismus, opisthotonos, convulsions, and coma; rapid and irregular pulse, hypertension, hypotension and vascular collapse; precordial pain, respiratory depression and failure, hyperpyrexia, diaphoresis, and cool, clammy skin.

Treatment Suggestions For Overdose: NOTE: Because there is no recorded experience with selegiline overdose, the following suggestions are offered based upon the assumption that selegiline overdose may be modeled by non-selective MAOI poisoning. In any case, up-to-date information about the treatment of overdose can often be obtained from a certified Regional Poison Control Center. Telephone numbers of certified Poison Control Centers are listed in the Physicians' Desk Reference (PDR).

Treatment of overdose with non-selective MAOIs is symptomatic and supportive. Induction of emesis or gastric lavage with instillation of charcoal slurry may be helpful in early poisoning, provided the airway has been protected against aspiration. Signs and symptoms of central nervous system stimulation, including convulsions, should be treated with diazepam, given slowly intravenously. Phenothiazine derivatives and central nervous system stimulants should be avoided. Hypotension and vascular collapse should be treated with intravenous fluids and, if necessary, blood pressure titration with an intravenous infusion of a dilute pressor agent. It should be noted that adrenergic agents may produce a markedly increased pressor response.

Respiration should be supported by appropriate measures, including management of the airway, use of supplemental oxygen, and mechanical ventilatory assistance, as required. Body temperature should be monitored closely. Intensive management of hyperpyrexia may be required. Maintenance of fluid and electrolyte balance is essential.

DOSAGE AND ADMINISTRATION

ELDEPRYL is intended for administration to Parkinsonian patients receiving levodopa/carbidopa therapy who demonstrate a deteriorating response to this treatment. The recommended regimen for the administration of ELDEPRYL is 10 mg per day administered as divided doses of 5 mg each taken at breakfast and lunch. There is no evidence that additional benefit will be obtained from the administration of higher doses. Moreover, higher doses should ordinarily be avoided because of the increased risk of side effects.

After two to three days of selegiline treatment, an attempt may be made to reduce the dose of levodopa/carbidopa. A reduction of 10 to 30% was achieved with the typical participant in the domestic placebo controlled trials who was assigned to selegiline treatment. Further reductions of levodopa/carbidopa may be possible during continued selegiline therapy.

HOW SUPPLIED

ELDEPRYL Capsules are available containing 5 mg of selegiline hydrochloride. Each aqua blue capsule is band imprinted with the Somerset logo on the cap and "Eldepryl 5 mg" on the body.
They are available as:
NDC 39506-022-60
bottles of 60 capsules
Store at 20° to 25°C (68° to 77°F). [See USP for Controlled Room Temperature.]

Somerset
PHARMACEUTICALS, INC.
Morgantown, WV 26505

Literature issued MARCH 2009
ELD:R20C
Shown in Product Identification Guide, page 319

Spectrum Pharmaceuticals, Inc.
157 TECHNOLOGY DRIVE
IRVINE, CA 92618

Phone (949) 788-6700
Fax (949) 788-6706

ZEVALIN® ℞
(ibritumomab tiuxetan)
Injection for intravenous use

HIGHLIGHTS OF PRESCRIBING INFORMATION
These highlights do not include all the information needed to use Zevalin safely and effectively. See full prescribing information for Zevalin.
ZEVALIN® (ibritumomab tiuxetan)
Injection for intravenous use
Initial U.S. Approval: 2002

> **WARNING: SERIOUS INFUSION REACTIONS, PROLONGED AND SEVERE CYTOPENIAS, and SEVERE CUTANEOUS AND MUCOCUTANEOUS REACTIONS**
> *See full prescribing information for complete boxed warning.*
> - **Serious Infusion Reactions, some fatal, may occur within 24 hours of rituximab infusion. (5.1)**
> - **Prolonged and Severe Cytopenias occur in most patients. (5.2)**
> - **Severe Cutaneous and Mucocutaneous Reactions, some fatal, reported with Zevalin therapeutic regimen. (5.3, 6.3)**
> - **Do not administer Y-90 Zevalin to patients with altered biodistribution. (5.4)**
> - **Do not exceed 32 mCi (1184 MBq) of Y-90 Zevalin. (2.2)**

RECENT MAJOR CHANGES
Indications and Usage (1) 9/2009
Dosage and Administration (2) 9/2009
Warnings and Precautions (5) 9/2009

INDICATIONS AND USAGE
Zevalin is a CD20-directed radiotherapeutic antibody administered as part of the Zevalin therapeutic regimen indicated for the treatment of patients with:
- relapsed or refractory, low-grade or follicular B-cell non-Hodgkin's lymphoma (NHL) (1.1).
- previously untreated follicular NHL who achieve a partial or complete response to first-line chemotherapy (1.2).

DOSAGE AND ADMINISTRATION
- **Day 1:** Administer rituximab 250 mg/m² IV. Within 4 hours after rituximab infusion, administer 5 mCi In-111 Zevalin IV. (2.2)
- **Day 7, 8, or 9:**
Administer rituximab 250 mg/m² IV infusion. (2.2)
  - If platelets ≥ 150,000/mm³: Within 4 hours after rituximab infusion, administer 0.4 mCi/kg (14.8 MBq per kg) Y-90 Zevalin IV.
  - If platelets ≥ 100,000 but ≤ 149,000/mm³ in relapsed or refractory patients: Within 4 hours after rituximab infusion, administer 0.3 mCi/kg (11.1 MBq per kg) Y-90 Zevalin IV.

DOSAGE FORMS AND STRENGTHS
- 3.2 mg per 2 mL, single-use vial. (3)

CONTRAINDICATIONS
None.

WARNINGS AND PRECAUTIONS
- **Serious Infusion Reactions:** Immediately stop and permanently discontinue rituximab, In-111 Zevalin, and Y-90 Zevalin. (5.1, 6.1)
- **Prolonged and Severe Cytopenias:** Do not administer Zevalin to patients with ≥ 25% lymphoma marrow involvement or impaired bone marrow reserve. (5.2, 6.1)
- **Severe Cutaneous and Mucocutaneous Reactions:** Discontinue rituximab, or Zevalin infusions if patients develop severe cutaneous or mucocutaneous reactions. (5.3, 6.3)
- **Leukemia and Myelodysplastic Syndrome** (5.5, 6.1)
- **Embryo-fetal Toxicity:** May cause fetal harm if given during pregnancy. (5.6, 8.1)
- **Extravasation:** Monitor for extravasation and terminate infusion if it occurs. Resume infusion in another limb. (5.7, 6.3)
- **Immunization:** Do not administer live viral vaccines to patients who recently received Zevalin. (5.8)

- **Laboratory Monitoring:** Obtain complete blood counts (CBC) and platelet counts at least weekly. (5.9)

---ADVERSE REACTIONS---

Common adverse reactions (≥ 40%) in clinical trials were: neutropenia, leukopenia, thrombocytopenia, anemia, infection, asthenia, musculoskeletal symptoms and gastrointestinal symptoms. (6)

To report SUSPECTED ADVERSE REACTIONS, contact Spectrum Pharmaceuticals, Inc. at 1-866-298-8433 or FDA at 1-800-FDA-1088 or www.fda.gov/medwatch

---DRUG INTERACTIONS---

- Monitor patients receiving medications that interfere with platelet function or coagulation more frequently for thrombocytopenia and bleeding. (7)

---USE IN SPECIFIC POPULATIONS---

- **Nursing Mother:** Discontinue nursing. (8.3)

See 17 for PATIENT COUNSELING INFORMATION

Revised: 05/2010

FULL PRESCRIBING INFORMATION: CONTENTS*
WARNING: SERIOUS INFUSION REACTIONS, PROLONGED AND SEVERE CYTOPENIAS, AND SEVERE CUTANEOUS AND MUCOCUTANEOUS REACTIONS

FULL PRESCRIBING INFORMATION

> **WARNING: SERIOUS INFUSION REACTIONS, PROLONGED AND SEVERE CYTOPENIAS, AND SEVERE CUTANEOUS AND MUCOCUTANEOUS REACTIONS**
>
> **Serious Infusion Reactions: Deaths have occurred within 24 hours of rituximab infusion, an essential component of the Zevalin therapeutic regimen. These fatalities were associated with hypoxia, pulmonary infiltrates, acute respiratory distress syndrome, myocardial infarction, ventricular fibrillation, or cardiogenic shock.**

Most (80%) fatalities occurred with the first rituximab infusion [see *Warnings and Precautions (5.1)* and *Adverse Reactions (6.1)*]. **Discontinue rituximab, In-111 Zevalin, and Y-90 Zevalin infusions in patients who develop severe infusion reactions.**

Prolonged and Severe Cytopenias: Y-90 Zevalin administration results in severe and prolonged cytopenias in most patients. Do not administer the Zevalin therapeutic regimen to patients with ≥ 25% lymphoma marrow involvement and/or impaired bone marrow reserve [see *Warnings and Precautions (5.2)* and *Adverse Reactions (6.1)*].

Severe Cutaneous and Mucocutaneous Reactions: Severe cutaneous and mucocutaneous reactions, some fatal, can occur with the Zevalin therapeutic regimen. Discontinue rituximab, In-111 Zevalin, and Y-90 Zevalin infusions in patients experiencing severe cutaneous or mucocutaneous reactions [see *Warnings and Precautions (5.3)* and *Adverse Reactions (6.3)*].

Dosing: The dose of Y-90 Zevalin should not exceed 32.0 mCi (1184 MBq). Do not administer Y-90 Zevalin to patients with altered biodistribution as determined by imaging with In-111 Zevalin [see *Dosage and Administration (2.2)*].

---

1   INDICATIONS AND USAGE

1.1   Relapsed or Refractory, Low-grade or Follicular NHL

Zevalin is indicated for the treatment of relapsed or refractory, low-grade or follicular B-cell non-Hodgkin's lymphoma (NHL).

1.2   Previously Untreated Follicular NHL

Zevalin is indicated for the treatment of previously untreated follicular NHL in patients who achieve a partial or complete response to first-line chemotherapy.

2   DOSAGE AND ADMINISTRATION

Recommended Dosing Schedule:

- Administer the Zevalin therapeutic regimen as outlined in Section 2.1.
- Initiate the Zevalin therapeutic regimen following recovery of platelet counts to ≥150,000/mm³ at least 6 weeks, but no more than 12 weeks, following the last dose of first-line chemotherapy.

2.1   Overview of Dosing Schedule

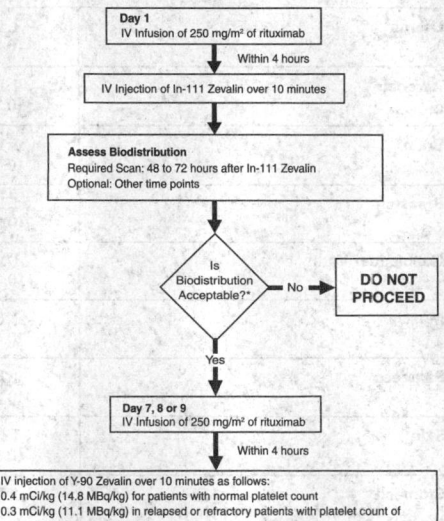

Day 1
IV Infusion of 250 mg/m² of rituximab

Within 4 hours

IV Injection of In-111 Zevalin over 10 minutes

Assess Biodistribution
Required Scan: 48 to 72 hours after In-111 Zevalin
Optional: Other time points

Is Biodistribution Acceptable?* — No → **DO NOT PROCEED**

Yes

Day 7, 8 or 9
IV Infusion of 250 mg/m² of rituximab

Within 4 hours

IV injection of Y-90 Zevalin over 10 minutes as follows:
0.4 mCi/kg (14.8 MBq/kg) for patients with normal platelet count
0.3 mCi/kg (11.1 MBq/kg) in relapsed or refractory patients with platelet count of 100,000 - 149,000 cells/mm³

| **DO NOT TREAT PATIENTS WITH <100,000 PLATELETS/mm³** | **THE MAXIMUM ALLOWABLE DOSE OF Y-90 ZEVALIN IS 32.0 mCi (1184) MBq** |

* See IMAGE ACQUISITION AND INTERPRETATION

2.2   Zevalin Therapeutic Regimen Dosage and Administration

Day 1:

- Premedicate with acetaminophen 650 mg orally and diphenhydramine 50 mg orally prior to rituximab infusion.
- Administer rituximab 250 mg/m² intravenously at an initial rate of 50 mg/hr. In the absence of infusion reactions, escalate the infusion rate in 50 mg/hr increments every 30 minutes to a maximum of 400 mg/hr. Do not mix or dilute rituximab with other drugs.
- Immediately stop the rituximab infusion for serious infusion reactions and discontinue the Zevalin therapeutic regimen [see *Boxed Warning* and *Warnings and Precautions (5.1)*].
- Temporarily slow or interrupt the rituximab infusion for less severe infusion reactions. If symptoms improve, continue the infusion at one-half the previous rate.

- Administer 5 mCi In-111 Zevalin over 10 minutes as an intravenous injection within 4 hours following completion of the rituximab infusion. Use a 0.22 micron low-protein-binding in-line filter between the syringe and the infusion port. After injection, flush the line with at least 10 mL of normal saline.

Day 7, 8 or 9:

Verify that expected biodistribution is present [see *Dosage and Administration (2.5)*].

- Premedicate with acetaminophen 650 mg orally and diphenhydramine 50 mg orally prior to rituximab infusion.
- Administer rituximab 250 mg/m² intravenously at an initial rate of 100 mg/hr. Increase rate by 100 mg/hr increments at 30 minute intervals, to a maximum of 400 mg/hr, as tolerated. If infusion reactions occurred during rituximab infusion on Day 1 of treatment, administer rituximab at an initial rate of 50 mg/hr and escalate the infusion rate in 50 mg/hr increments every 30 minutes to a maximum of 400 mg/hr.
- Administer Y-90 Zevalin injection through a free flowing intravenous line within 4 hours following completion of rituximab infusion. Use a 0.22 micron low-protein-binding in-line filter between the syringe and the infusion port. After injection, flush the line with at least 10 mL of normal saline.
- **If platelet count ≥150,000/mm³,** administer Y-90 Zevalin over 10 minutes as an intravenous injection at a dose of Y-90 0.4 mCi per kg (14.8 MBq per kg) actual body weight.
- **If platelet count 100,000-149,000/mm³,** in relapsed or refractory patients, administer Y-90 Zevalin over 10 minutes as an intravenous injection at a dose of Y-90 0.3 mCi per kg (11.1 MBq per kg) actual body weight.
- **Do not administer more than 32 mCi (1184 MBq) Y-90 Zevalin dose regardless of the patient's body weight.**
- Monitor patients closely for evidence of extravasation during the injection of Y-90 Zevalin. Immediately stop infusion and restart in another limb if any signs or symptoms of extravasation occur [see *Warnings and Precautions (5.7)*].

2.3   Directions for Preparation of Radiolabeled In-111 and Y-90 Zevalin Doses

Two separate and distinctly-labeled kits are required for preparation of Indium-111 (In-111) Zevalin and Yttrium-90 (Y-90) Zevalin. Follow the detailed instructions for the preparation of radiolabeled Zevalin [see *Dosage and Administration (2.4)*]. The procedures are different for the preparation of In-111 Zevalin and of Y-90 Zevalin.

Directions for Preparation of Radiolabeled In-111 Zevalin Dose

Required materials not supplied in the kit:

1. Indium-111 Chloride Sterile Solution (In-111 Chloride) from GE Healthcare, or Mallinckrodt/Covidien
2. Three sterile 1 mL plastic syringes
3. One sterile 3 mL plastic syringe
4. Two sterile 10 mL plastic syringes with 18-20 G needles
5. Instant thin-layer chromatographic (ITLC) silica gel strips
6. 0.9% Sodium Chloride aqueous solution for the chromatography solvent
7. Developing chamber for chromatography
8. Suitable radioactivity counting apparatus
9. Filter, 0.22 micrometer, low-protein-binding
10. Appropriate lead shielding for reaction vial and syringe for In-111

Method:

1. Allow contents of the refrigerated In-111 Zevalin kit (Zevalin vial, 50 mM sodium acetate vial, formulation buffer vial, and empty reaction vial) to reach room temperature.
2. Place the empty reaction vial in an appropriate lead shield.
3. Determine the amount of each component needed:
   i. Calculate volume of In-111 Chloride equivalent to 5.5 mCi based on the activity concentration of the In-111 Chloride stock.
   ii. The volume of 50 mM Sodium Acetate solution needed is 1.2 times the volume of In-111 Chloride solution determined in step 3.a, above.
   iii. Calculate volume of formulation buffer needed to bring the reaction vial contents to a final volume of 10 mL.
4. Transfer the calculated volume of 50 mM of Sodium Acetate to the empty reaction vial. Coat the entire inner surface of the reaction vial by gentle inversion or rolling.
5. Transfer 5.5 mCi of In-111 Chloride to the reaction vial using a lead shielded syringe. Mix the two solutions by gentle inversion or rolling.
6. Transfer 1 mL of Zevalin (ibritumomab tiuxetan) to the reaction vial. **Do not shake or agitate the vial contents.**
7. Allow the labeling reaction to proceed at room temperature for 30 minutes. A shorter or longer reaction time may adversely alter the final labeled product.

8. **Immediately** after the 30-minute incubation period, transfer the calculated volume of formulation buffer from step 3.c. to the reaction vial. Gently add the formulation buffer down the side of the reaction vial. If necessary, withdraw an equal volume of air to normalize pressure.

9. Measure the final product for total activity using a radioactivity calibration system suitable for the measurement of In-111.

10. Using supplied labels, record the date and time of preparation, total activity and volume, date and time of expiration, and affix these labels to the shielded reaction vial container.

11. Patient Dose: Calculate the volume required for an In-111 Zevalin dose of 5 mCi. Withdraw the required volume from the reaction vial into a sterile syringe. Assay the syringe in a dose calibrator suitable for the measurement of In-111. Using the supplied labels, record patient identifier, total activity and volume and the date and time of expiration, and affix these labels to the syringe and shielded unit dose container.

12. Determine Radiochemical Purity [see *Dosage and Administration (2.4)*].

13. Store Indium-111 Zevalin at 2-8°C (36-46°F) until use and administer within 12 hours of radiolabeling. Immediately prior to administration, assay the syringe and contents using an appropriate radioactivity calibration system.

Directions for Preparation of Radiolabeled Y-90 Zevalin Dose

Required materials not supplied in the kit:
1. Yttrium-90 Chloride Sterile Solution
2. Three sterile 1 mL plastic syringes
3. One sterile 3 mL plastic syringe
4. Two sterile 10 mL plastic syringes with 18-20 G needles
5. ITLC silica gel strips
6. 0.9% Sodium Chloride aqueous solution for the chromatography solvent
7. Developing chamber for chromatography
8. Suitable radioactivity counting apparatus
9. Filter, 0.22 micrometer, low-protein-binding
10. Appropriate acrylic shielding for reaction vial and syringe for Y-90

Method:
1. Allow contents of the refrigerated Y-90 Zevalin kit (Zevalin vial, 50 mM sodium acetate vial, and formulation buffer vial) to reach room temperature.
2. Place the empty reaction vial in an appropriate acrylic shield.
3. Determine the amount of each component needed:
   i. Calculate volume of Y-90 Chloride equivalent to 40 mCi based on the activity concentration of the Y-90 Chloride stock.
   ii. The volume of 50 mM Sodium Acetate solution needed is 1.2 times the volume of Y-90 Chloride solution determined in step 3.a, above.
   iii. Calculate the volume of formulation buffer needed to bring the reaction vial contents to a final volume of 10 mL.
4. Transfer the calculated volume of 50 mM Sodium Acetate to the empty reaction vial. Coat the entire inner surface of the reaction vial by gentle inversion or rolling.
5. Transfer 40 mCi of Y-90 Chloride to the reaction vial using an acrylic shielded syringe. Mix the two solutions by gentle inversion or rolling.
6. Transfer 1.3 mL of Zevalin (ibritumomab tiuxetan) to the reaction vial. **Do not shake or agitate the vial contents.**
7. Allow the labeling reaction to proceed at room temperature for 5 minutes. A shorter or longer reaction time may adversely alter the final labeled product.
8. **Immediately** after the 5-minute incubation period, transfer the calculated volume of formulation buffer from step 3.c. to the reaction vial. Gently add the formulation buffer down the side of the reaction vial. If necessary, withdraw an equal volume of air to normalize pressure.
9. Measure the final product for total activity using a radioactivity calibration system suitable for the measurement of Y-90.
10. Using the supplied labels, record the date and time of preparation, the total activity and volume, and the date and time of expiration, and affix these labels to the shielded reaction vial container.
11. Patient Dose: Calculate the volume required for a Y-90 Zevalin dose [see *Dosage and Administration (2.2)*]. Withdraw the required volume from the reaction vial. Assay the syringe in the dose calibrator suitable for the measurement of Y-90. The measured dose must be within 10% of the prescribed dose of Y-90 Zevalin and **must not exceed 32 mCi (1184 MBq)**. Using the supplied labels, record the patient identifier, total activity and volume and the date and time of expiration, and affix these labels to the syringe and shielded unit dose container.

12. Determine Radiochemical Purity [see *Dosage and Administration (2.4)*].
13. Store Yttrium-90 Zevalin at 2-8°C (36-46°F) until use and administer within 8 hours of radiolabeling. Immediately prior to administration, assay the syringe and contents using a radioactivity calibration system suitable for the measurement of Y-90.

Table 1. Estimated Radiation Absorbed Doses from Y-90 Zevalin and In-111 Zevalin

Organ	Y-90 Zevalin cGy/mCi (mGy/MBq) Median	Range	In-111 Zevalin cGy/mCi (mGy/MBq) Median	Range
Spleen*	34.78 (9.4)	6.66-74.00 (1.8-20.0)	3.33 (0.9)	0.74-6.66 (0.2-1.8)
Liver*	17.76 (4.8)	10.73-29.97 (2.9-8.1)	2.59 (0.7)	1.48-4.07 (0.4-1.1)
Lower Large Intestinal Wall*	17.39 (4.7)	11.47-30.34 (3.1-8.2)	1.48 (0.4)	0.74-2.22 (0.2-0.6)
Upper Large Intestinal Wall*	13.32 (3.6)	7.40-24.79 (2.0-6.7)	1.11 (0.3)	0.74-2.22 (0.2-0.6)
Heart Wall*	10.73 (2.9)	5.55-11.84 (1.5-3.2)	1.48 (0.4)	0.74-1.85 (0.2-0.5)
Lungs*	7.4 (2)	4.44-12.58 (1.2-3.4)	0.74 (0.2)	0.74-1.48 (0.2-0.4)
Testes*	5.55 (1.5)	3.70-15.91 (1.0-4.3)	0.37 (0.1)	0.37-1.11 (0.1-0.3)
Small Intestine*	5.18 (1.4)	2.96-7.77 (0.8-2.1)	0.74 (0.2)	0.74-1.11 (0.2-0.3)
Red Marrow†	4.81 (1.3)	2.22-6.66 (0.6-1.8)	0.74 (0.2)	0.37-0.74 (0.1-0.2)
Urinary Bladder Wall‡	3.33 (0.9)	2.59-4.81 (0.7-1.3)	0.74 (0.2)	0.37-0.74 (0.1-0.2)
Bone Surfaces†	3.33 (0.9)	1.85-4.44 (0.5-1.2)	0.74 (0.2)	0.37-0.74 (0.1-0.2)
Total Body‡	1.85 (0.5)	1.48-2.59 (0.4-0.7)	0.37 (0.1)	0.37-0.74 (0.1-0.2)
Ovaries‡	1.48 (0.4)	1.11-1.85 (0.3-0.5)	0.74 (0.2)	0.74-0.74 (0.2-0.2)
Uterus‡	1.48 (0.4)	1.11-1.85 (0.3-0.5)	0.74 (0.2)	0.37-0.74 (0.1-0.2)
Adrenals‡	1.11 (0.3)	0.74-1.85 (0.2-0.5)	0.74 (0.2)	0.74-1.11 (0.2-0.3)
Brain‡	1.11 (0.3)	0.74-1.85 (0.2-0.5)	0.37 (0.1)	0.00-0.37 (0.0-0.1)
Breasts‡	1.11 (0.3)	0.74-1.85 (0.2-0.5)	0.37 (0.1)	0.37-0.37 (0.1-0.1)
Gallbladder Wall‡	1.11 (0.3)	0.74-1.85 (0.2-0.5)	1.11 (0.3)	0.74-1.48 (0.2-0.4)
Muscle‡	1.11 (0.3)	0.74-1.85 (0.2-0.5)	0.37 (0.1)	0.37-0.37 (0.1-0.1)
Pancreas‡	1.11 (0.3)	0.74-1.85 (0.2-0.5)	0.74 (0.2)	0.74-1.11 (0.2-0.3)
Skin‡	1.11 (0.3)	0.74-1.85 (0.2-0.5)	0.37 (0.1)	0.00-0.37 (0.0-0.1)
Stomach‡	1.11 (0.3)	0.74-1.85 (0.2-0.5)	0.74 (0.2)	0.37-0.74 (0.1-0.2)
Thymus‡	1.11 (0.3)	0.74-1.85 (0.2-0.5)	0.37 (0.1)	0.37-0.74 (0.1-0.2)
Thyroid‡	1.11 (0.3)	0.74-1.85 (0.2-0.5)	0.37 (0.1)	0.00-0.37 (0.0-0.1)
Kidneys*	0.37 (0.1)	0.00-1.11 (0.0-0.3)	0.74 (0.2)	0.37-0.74 (0.1-0.2)

*Organ region of interest
†Sacrum region of interest
‡Whole body region of interest

2.4   Procedure for Determining Radiochemical Purity
Use the following procedures for radiolabeling both In-111 Zevalin and Y-90 Zevalin:
1. Place a small drop of either In-111 Zevalin or Y-90 Zevalin at the origin of an ITLC silica gel strip.
2. Place the ITLC silica gel strip into a chromatography chamber with the origin at the bottom and the solvent

front at the top. Allow the solvent (0.9% NaCl) to migrate at least 5 cm from the bottom of the strip. Remove the strip from the chamber and cut the strip in half. Count each half of the ITLC silica gel strip for one minute (CPM) with a suitable counting apparatus.

3. Calculate the percent RCP as follows:

$$\% \text{ RCP} = \frac{\text{CPM bottom half}}{\text{CPM bottom half} + \text{CPM top half}} \times 100$$

4. Repeat the ITLC procedure if the radiochemical purity is <95%. If repeat testing confirms that radiochemical purity is <95%, do not administer the In-111 or Y-90 Zevalin dose.

2.5 Image Acquisition and Interpretation of Biodistribution

Assess the biodistribution of In-111 Zevalin by a visual evaluation of whole body planar view anterior and posterior gamma images obtained at 48-72 hours after injection. Images at additional time points may be necessary to resolve ambiguities. Acquire whole body anterior/posterior planar images using a large field-of-view gamma camera and medium energy collimators. Suggested gamma camera settings: 256×1024 matrix; dual energy photopeaks set at 172 and 247 keV; 15% symmetric window; scan speed of 10 cm/min for the 48-72 hour scan, and 7-10 cm/min for subsequent scans.

Expected Biodistribution
- Activity in the blood pool areas (heart, abdomen, neck, and extremities) may be faintly visible.
- Moderately high to high uptake in normal liver and spleen.
- Moderately low or very low uptake in normal kidneys, urinary bladder, and normal (uninvolved) bowel.
- Non-fixed areas within the bowel lumen that change position with time; delayed imaging as described above may be necessary to confirm gastrointestinal clearance.
- Focal fixed areas of uptake in the bowel wall (localization to lymphoid aggregates in bowel wall).

Tumor uptake may be visualized however tumor visualization on the In-111 Zevalin scan is not required for Y-90 Zevalin therapy.

Altered Biodistribution
The criteria for altered biodistribution are met if any of the following is detected on visual inspection of the required gamma images:
- Intense localization of radiotracer in the liver and spleen and bone marrow indicative of reticuloendothelial system uptake.
- Increased uptake in normal organs (not involved by tumor) such as:
  - Diffuse uptake in normal lung more intense than the liver.
  - Kidneys have greater intensity than the liver on the posterior view.
  - Fixed areas (unchanged with time) of uptake in the normal bowel greater than uptake in the liver.
  - In less than 0.5% of patients receiving In-111 Zevalin, prominent bone marrow uptake was observed, characterized by clear visualization of the long bones and ribs.

Consider bone marrow involvement by lymphoma, increased marrow activity due to recent hematopoietic growth factor administration, and increased reticuloendothelial uptake in patients with HAMA and HACA, as possible causes of prominent bone marrow uptake. Re-assess biodistribution after correction of underlying factors.

2.6 Radiation Dosimetry

Estimations of radiation-absorbed doses for In-111 Zevalin and Y-90 Zevalin were performed using sequential whole body images and the MIRDOSE 3 software program. The estimated radiation absorbed doses to organs and marrow from a course of the Zevalin therapeutic regimen are summarized in Table 1. Absorbed dose estimates for the lower large intestine, upper large intestine, and small intestine have been modified from the standard MIRDOSE 3 output to account for the assumption that activity is within the intestine wall rather than the intestine contents.
[See table 1 at top of previous page]

3 DOSAGE FORMS AND STRENGTHS

3.2 mg ibritumomab tiuxetan per 2 mL, single-use vial.

4 CONTRAINDICATIONS

None.

5 WARNINGS AND PRECAUTIONS

5.1 Serious Infusion Reactions

See also prescribing information for rituximab.
Rituximab, alone or as a component of the Zevalin therapeutic regimen, can cause severe, including fatal, infusion reactions. These reactions typically occur during the first rituximab infusion with time to onset of 30 to 120 minutes. Signs and symptoms of severe infusion reactions may in-

Table 2. Per-Patient Incidence (%) of Selected* Adverse Reactions Occurring in ≥ 5% of Patients with Previously Untreated Follicular NHL Treated with the Zevalin Therapeutic Regimen

	Zevalin (n=206)		Observation (n=203)	
	All Grades[†]	Grade[†] 3-4	All Grades[†]	Grade[†] 3-4
	%	%	%	%
Gastrointestinal Disorders				
Abdominal pain	17	2	13	<1
Diarrhea	11	0	3	0
Nausea	18	0	2	0
Body as a Whole				
Asthenia	15	1	8	<1
Fatigue	33	1	9	0
Influenza-like illness	8	0	3	0
Pyrexia	10	3	4	0
Musculoskeletal				
Myalgia	9	0	3	0
Metabolism				
Anorexia	8	0	2	0
Respiratory, Thoracic & Media				
Cough	11	<1	5	0
Pharyngolaryngeal pain	7	0	2	0
Epistaxis	5	2	<1	0
Nervous System				
Dizziness	7	0	2	0
Vascular				
Hypertension	7	3	2	<1
Skin & Subcutaneous				
Night sweats	8	0	2	0
Petechiae	8	2	0	0
Pruritus	7	0	1	0
Rash	7	0	<1	0
Infections & Infestations				
Bronchitis	8	0	3	0
Nasopharyngitis	19	0	10	0
Rhinitis	8	0	2	0
Sinusitis	7	<1	<1	0
Urinary tract infection	7	<1	3	0
Blood and Lymphatic System				
Thrombocytopenia	62	51	1	0
Neutropenia	45	41	3	2
Anemia	22	5	4	0
Leukopenia	43	36	4	1
Lymphopenia	26	18	9	5

*Between-group difference of ≥5%
†NCI CTCAE version 2.0

clude urticaria, hypotension, angioedema, hypoxia, bronchospasm, pulmonary infiltrates, acute respiratory distress syndrome, myocardial infarction, ventricular fibrillation, and cardiogenic shock. Temporarily slow or interrupt the rituximab infusion for less severe infusion reactions. Immediately stop rituximab, In-111 Zevalin, or Y-90 Zevalin administration for severe infusion reactions [*see Boxed Warning and Dosage and Administration (2.2)*].

5.2 Prolonged and Severe Cytopenias

Cytopenias with delayed onset and prolonged duration, some complicated by hemorrhage and severe infection, are the most common severe adverse reactions of the Zevalin therapeutic regimen. When used according to recommended doses, the incidences of severe thrombocytopenia and neutropenia are greater in patients with mild baseline thrombocytopenia (100,000 to 149,000/mm³) compared to those with normal pretreatment platelet counts. Severe cytopenias persisting more than 12 weeks following administration can occur [see Boxed Warning and Adverse Reactions (6.1)].

Do not administer the Zevalin therapeutic regimen to patients with ≥ 25% lymphoma marrow involvement and/or impaired bone marrow reserve. Monitor patients for cytopenias and their complications (e.g., febrile neutropenia, hemorrhage) for up to 3 months after use of the Zevalin therapeutic regimen. Avoid using drugs which interfere with platelet function or coagulation following the Zevalin therapeutic regimen.

5.3 Severe Cutaneous and Mucocutaneous Reactions
Erythema multiforme, Stevens-Johnson syndrome, toxic epidermal necrolysis, bullous dermatitis, and exfoliative dermatitis, some fatal, were reported in post-marketing experience. The time to onset of these reactions was variable, ranging from a few days to 4 months after administration of the Zevalin therapeutic regimen. Discontinue the Zevalin therapeutic regimen in patients experiencing a severe cutaneous or mucocutaneous reaction [see Boxed Warning and Adverse Reactions (6.3)].

5.4 Altered Biodistribution
Do not administer Y-90 Zevalin to patients with altered biodistribution of In-111 Zevalin. In a post-marketing registry designed to collect biodistribution images and other information in reported cases of altered biodistribution, there were 12 (1.3%) patients reported to have altered biodistribution among 953 patients registered. For descriptions of expected and altered biodistribution image characteristics [see Dosage and Administration (2.5)].

5.5 Leukemia and Myelodysplastic Syndrome
Myelodysplastic syndrome (MDS) and/or acute myelogenous leukemia (AML) were reported in 5.2% (11/211) of patients with relapsed or refractory NHL enrolled in clinical studies and 1.5% (8/535) of patients included in the expanded-access trial, with median follow-up of 6.5 and 4.4 years, respectively. Among the 19 reported cases, the median time to the diagnosis of MDS or AML was 1.9 years following treatment with the Zevalin therapeutic regimen; however, the cumulative incidence continues to increase [see Adverse Reactions (6.1)].

Among 204 patients receiving Y-90 Zevalin following first-line chemotherapy, two patients (1%) were diagnosed with AML within 3 years of receiving Zevalin.

5.6 Embryo-Fetal Toxicity
Based on its radioactivity, Y-90 Zevalin may cause fetal harm when administered to a pregnant woman. If the Zevalin therapeutic regimen is administered during pregnancy, the patient should be apprised of the potential hazard to a fetus [see Use in Specific Populations (8.1)].

5.7 Extravasation
Monitor patents closely for evidence of extravasation during Zevalin infusion. Immediately terminate the infusion if signs or symptoms of extravasation occur and restart in another limb [see Dosage and Administration (2.2)].

5.8 Immunization
The safety of immunization with live viral vaccines following the Zevalin therapeutic regimen has not been studied. Do not administer live viral vaccines to patients who have recently received Zevalin. The ability to generate an immune response to any vaccine following the Zevalin therapeutic regimen has not been studied.

5.9 Laboratory Monitoring
Monitor complete blood counts (CBC) and platelet counts following the Zevalin therapeutic regimen weekly until levels recover or as clinically indicated.

5.10 Radionuclide Precautions
During and after radiolabeling Zevalin with In-111 or Y-90, minimize radiation exposure to patients and to medical personnel, consistent with institutional good radiation safety practices and patient management procedures.

5.11 Creutzfeldt-Jakob Disease (CJD)
The Zevalin therapeutic regimen contains albumin, a derivative of human blood. Based on effective donor screening and product manufacturing processes, Zevalin carries an extremely remote risk for transmission of viral diseases. A theoretical risk for transmission of Creutzfeldt-Jakob disease (CJD) also is considered extremely remote. No cases of transmission of viral diseases or CJD have ever been identified for albumin.

6 ADVERSE REACTIONS
The following serious adverse reactions are discussed in greater detail in other sections of the label:
- Serious Infusion Reactions [see Boxed Warning and Warnings and Precautions (5.1)].
- Prolonged and Severe Cytopenias [see Boxed Warning and Warnings and Precautions (5.2)].
- Severe Cutaneous and Mucocutaneous Reactions [see Boxed Warning and Warnings and Precautions (5.3)].
- Leukemia and Myelodysplastic Syndrome [see Warnings and Precautions (5.5)].

The most common adverse reactions of Zevalin are cytopenias, fatigue, abdominal pain, nausea, nasopharyngitis, asthenia, diarrhea, cough and pyrexia.

The most serious adverse reactions of Zevalin are prolonged and severe cytopenias (thrombocytopenia, anemia, lymphopenia, neutropenia) and secondary malignancies.

Because the Zevalin therapeutic regimen includes the use of rituximab, see prescribing information for rituximab.

6.1 Clinical Trials Experience
Because clinical trials are conducted under widely varying conditions, adverse reaction rates observed in the clinical trials of a drug cannot be directly compared to rates in the clinical trials of another drug and may not reflect the rates observed in practice.

The reported safety data reflects exposure to Zevalin in 349 patients with relapsed or refractory, low-grade, follicular or transformed NHL across 5 trials (4 single arm and 1 randomized) and in 206 patients with previously untreated follicular NHL in a randomized trial (Study 4) who received any portion of the Zevalin therapeutic regimen. The safety data reflect exposure to Zevalin in 270 patients with relapsed or refractory NHL with platelet counts ≥150,000/ mm³ who received 0.4 mCi/kg (14.8 MBq/kg) of Y-90 Zevalin (Group 1 in Table 4), 65 patients with relapsed or refractory NHL with platelet counts of 100,000 to 149,000/mm³ who received 0.3 mCi/kg (11.1 MBq/kg) of Y-90 Zevalin (Group 2 in Table 4), and 204 patients with previously untreated NHL with platelet counts ≥150,000/mm³ who received 0.4 mCi/kg (14.8 MBq/kg) of Y-90 Zevalin; all patients received a single course of Zevalin.

Table 2 displays selected adverse reaction incidence rates in patients who received any portion of the Zevalin therapeutic regimen (n=206) or no further therapy (n=203) following first-line chemotherapy (Study 4).

[See table 2 at top of previous page]

Table 3 shows hematologic toxicities in 349 Zevalin-treated patients with relapsed or refractory, low-grade, follicular or transformed B-cell NHL. Grade 2-4 hematologic toxicity occurred in 86% of Zevalin-treated patients.

Table 3. Per-Patient Incidence (%) of Hematologic Adverse Reactions in Patients with Relapsed or Refractory Low-grade, Follicular or Transformed B-cell NHL* (N = 349)

	All Grades %	Grade 3-4 %
Thrombocytopenia	95	63
Neutropenia	77	60
Anemia	61	17
Ecchymosis	7	<1

*Occurring within the 12 weeks following the first rituximab infusion of the Zevalin therapeutic regimen

Prolonged and Severe Cytopenias
Patients in clinical studies were not permitted to receive hematopoietic growth factors beginning 2 weeks prior to administration of the Zevalin therapeutic regimen.

The incidence and duration of severe hematologic toxicity in previously treated NHL patients (N=335) and in previously untreated patients (Study 4) receiving Y-90 Zevalin are shown in Table 4.

[See table 4 at left]

Cytopenias were more severe and more prolonged among eleven (5%) patients who received Zevalin after first-line fludarabine or a fludarabine-containing chemotherapy regimen as compared to patients receiving non-fludarabine-containing regimens. Among these eleven patients, the median platelet nadir was 13,000/mm³ with a median duration of platelets below 50,000/mm³ of 56 days and the median time for platelet recovery from nadir to Grade 1 toxicity or baseline was 35 days. The median ANC was 355/mm³, with a median duration of ANC below 1,000/mm³ of 37 days and the median time for ANC recovery from nadir to Grade 1 toxicity or baseline was 20 days.

The median time to cytopenia was similar across patients with relapsed/refractory NHL and those completing first-line chemotherapy, with median ANC nadir at 61-62 days, platelet nadir at 49-53 days, and hemoglobin nadir at 68-69 days after Y-90-Zevalin administration.

Information on hematopoietic growth factor use and platelet transfusions is based on 211 patients with relapsed/refractory NHL and 206 patients following first-line chemotherapy. Filgrastim was given to 13% of patients and erythropoietin to 8% with relapsed or refractory disease; 14% of patients receiving Zevalin following first-line chemotherapy received granulocyte-colony stimulating factors and 5% received erythropoiesis-stimulating agents. Platelet transfusions were given to approximately 22% of all Zevalin-treated patients. Red blood cell transfusions were given to 20% of patients with relapsed or refractory NHL and 2% of patients receiving Zevalin following first-line chemotherapy.

Infections
In relapsed or refractory NHL patients, infections occurred in 29% of 349 patients during the first 3 months after initiating the Zevalin therapeutic regimen and 3% developed serious infections (urinary tract infection, febrile neutropenia, sepsis, pneumonia, cellulitis, colitis, diarrhea, osteomyelitis, and upper respiratory tract infection). Life-threatening

Table 4. Severe Hematologic Toxicity in Patients Receiving Zevalin

Baseline Platelet Count	Group 1 (n=270) ≥ 150,000/mm³	Group 2 (n=65) 100,000 to 149,000/mm³	Study 4 (n=204) ≥ 150,000/mm³
Y-90 Zevalin Dose	0.4 mCi/kg (14.8 MBq/kg)	0.3 mCi/kg (11.1 MBq/kg)	0.4 mCi/kg (14.8 MBq/kg)
ANC			
Median nadir (per mm³)	800	600	721
Per Patient Incidence ANC <1000/mm³	57%	74%	65%
Per Patient Incidence ANC <500/mm³	30%	35%	26%
Median Duration (Days)* ANC <1000/mm³	22	29	29
Median Time to Recovery†	12	13	15
Platelets			
Median nadir (per mm³)	41,000	24,000	42,000
Per Patient Incidence Platelets <50,000/mm³	61%	78%	61%
Per Patient Incidence Platelets <10,000/mm³	10%	14%	4%
Median Duration (Days)‡ Platelets <50,000/mm³	24	35	26
Median Time to Recovery†	13	14	14

* Day from last ANC ≥1000/mm³ to first ANC ≥1000/mm³ following nadir, censored at next treatment or death
†Day from nadir to first count at level of Grade 1 toxicity or baseline
‡Day from last platelet count ≥50,000/mm³ to day of first platelet count ≥50,000/mm³ following nadir, censored at next treatment or death

infections were reported in 2% (sepsis, empyema, pneumonia, febrile neutropenia, fever, and biliary stent-associated cholangitis). From 3 months to 4 years after Zevalin treatment, 6% of patients developed infections; 2% were serious (urinary tract infection, bacterial or viral pneumonia, febrile neutropenia, perihilar infiltrate, pericarditis, and intravenous drug-associated viral hepatitis) and 1% were life-threatening infections (bacterial pneumonia, respiratory disease, and sepsis).

When administered following first-line chemotherapy (Table 2), Grade 3-4 infections occurred in 8% of Zevalin treated patients and in 2% of controls and included neutropenic sepsis (1%), bronchitis, catheter sepsis, diverticulitis, herpes zoster, influenza, lower respiratory tract infection, sinusitis, and upper respiratory tract infection.

Leukemia and Myelodysplastic Syndrome

Among 746 patients with relapsed/refractory NHL, 19 (2.6%) patients developed MDS/AML with a median follow-up of 4.4 years. The overall incidence of MDS/AML among the 211 patients included in the clinical studies was 5.2% (11/211), with a median follow-up of 6.5 years and median time to development of MDS/AML of 2.9 years. The cumulative Kaplan-Meier estimated incidence of MDS/secondary leukemia in this patient population was 2.2% at 2 years and 5.9% at 5 years. The incidence of MDS/AML among the 535 patients in the expanded access programs was 1.5% (8/535) with a median follow-up of 4.4 years and median time to development of MDS/AML of 1.5 years. Multiple cytogenetic abnormalities were described, most commonly involving chromosomes 5 and/or 7. The risk of MDS/AML was not associated with the number of prior treatments (0-1 versus 2-10).

Among 204 patients receiving Y-90-Zevalin following first-line treatment, 2 (1%) developed AML at approximately 2 and 3.3 years after Zevalin administration, respectively.

6.2 Immunogenicity

As with all therapeutic proteins, there is a potential for immunogenicity. The incidence of antibody formation is highly dependent on the sensitivity and specificity of the assay. Additionally, the observed incidence of antibody (including neutralizing antibody) positivity in an assay may be influenced by several factors including assay methodology, sample handling, timing of sample collection, concomitant medications, and underlying disease. For these reasons, comparisons of the incidence of HAMA/HACA to the Zevalin therapeutic regimen with the incidence of antibodies to other products may be misleading.

HAMA and HACA response data on 446 patients from 8 clinical studies conducted over a 10-year time period are available. Overall, 11/446 (2.5%) had evidence of either HAMA formation (N=8) or HACA formation (N=4). Six of these patients developed HAMA/HACA after treatment with Zevalin and 5 were HAMA/HACA positive at baseline. Of the 6 who were HAMA/HACA positive, only one was positive for both. Furthermore, in 6 of the 11 patients, the HAMA/HACA reverted to negative within 2 weeks to 3 months. No patients had increasing levels of HAMA/HACA at the end of the studies.

Only 6/446 patients (1.3%) had developed evidence of antibody formation after treatment with Zevalin, and of these, many either reverted to negative or decreased over time. This data demonstrates that HAMA/HACA develop infrequently, are typically transient, and do not increase with time.

6.3 Post-Marketing Experience

The following adverse reactions have been identified during post-approval use of the Zevalin therapeutic regimen in hematologic malignancies. Because these reactions are reported voluntarily from a population of uncertain size, it is not always possible to reliably estimate their frequency or establish a causal relationship to drug exposure. Decisions to include these reactions in labeling are typically based on one or more of the following factors: (1) seriousness of the reaction, (2) frequency of reporting, or (3) strength of causal connection to the Zevalin therapeutic regimen.

- Cutaneous and mucocutaneous reactions: erythema multiforme, Stevens-Johnson syndrome, toxic epidermal necrolysis, bullous dermatitis, and exfoliative dermatitis [*see Boxed Warning and Warnings and Precautions (5.3)*].
- Infusion site erythema and ulceration following extravasation [*see Warnings and Precautions (5.7)*].
- Radiation injury in tissues near areas of lymphomatous involvement within a month of Zevalin administration.

7 DRUG INTERACTIONS

No formal drug interaction studies have been performed with Zevalin. Patients receiving medications that interfere with platelet function or coagulation should have more frequent laboratory monitoring for thrombocytopenia.

8 USE IN SPECIFIC POPULATIONS

8.1 Pregnancy

Teratogenic Effects: Category D [*see Warnings and Precautions (5.6)*]: Based on its radioactivity, Y-90 Zevalin may cause fetal harm when administered to a pregnant woman.

Immunoglobulins are known to cross the placenta. There are no adequate and well-controlled studies in pregnant women. Animal reproductive toxicology studies of Zevalin have not been conducted.

Advise women of childbearing potential to use adequate contraception. Inform women who become pregnant while receiving Zevalin of the potential fetal risks [*see Patient Counseling Information (17)*].

8.3 Nursing Mothers

Because human IgG is excreted in human milk, it is expected that Zevalin would be present in human milk. Because of the potential for adverse reactions in nursing infants from Y-90 or In-111 Zevalin, a decision should be made to discontinue nursing or not administer the Zevalin therapeutic regimen, taking into account the importance of the drug to the mother.

8.4 Pediatric Use

The safety and effectiveness of Zevalin have not been established in pediatric patients.

8.5 Geriatric Use

Of 349 patients with relapsed/refractory NHL treated with the Zevalin therapeutic regimen in clinical studies, 38% (132 patients) were age 65 years and over, while 12% (41 patients) were age 75 years and over.

Of 414 patients enrolled in Study 4 (Zevalin following first-line chemotherapy) 206 patients received Zevalin. Of these patients 14% (29 patients) were 65 years and over, while 2% (4 patients) were 75 years and older. In the control arm, 10% (21 patients) were 65 years or over and 0% (0 patients) were 75 years or older.

No overall differences in safety or effectiveness were observed between these subjects and younger subjects, but greater sensitivity of some older individuals cannot be ruled out.

10 OVERDOSAGE

Severe cytopenias which may require stem cell support have occurred at doses higher than the recommended maximum total dose of 32 mCi (1184 MBq).

11 DESCRIPTION

Zevalin (ibritumomab tiuxetan) is the immunoconjugate resulting from a stable thiourea covalent bond between the monoclonal antibody ibritumomab and the linker-chelator tiuxetan [N-[2-bis(carboxymethyl)amino]-3-(p-isothiocyanatophenyl)-propyl]-[N-[2-bis(carboxymethyl)amino]-2-(methyl)-ethyl]glycine. This linker-chelator provides a high affinity, conformationally restricted chelation site for Indium-111 or Yttrium-90. The approximate molecular weight of ibritumomab tiuxetan is 148 kD. The antibody moiety of Zevalin is ibritumomab, a murine IgG$_1$ kappa monoclonal antibody directed against the CD20 antigen.

Ibritumomab tiuxetan is a clear, colorless, sterile, pyrogen-free, preservative-free solution that may contain translucent particles. Each single-use vial includes 3.2 mg of ibritumomab tiuxetan in 2 mL of 0.9% Sodium Chloride.

Physical / Radiochemical Characteristics of In-111

Indium-111 decays by electron capture, with a physical half-life of 67.3 hours (2.81 days). The product of radioactive decay is non-radioactive Cadmium-111. Radiation emission data for In-111 are summarized in Table 5.

Table 5. Principal In-111 Radiation Emission Data

Radiation	Mean % per Disintegration	Mean Energy (keV)
Gamma-2	90.2	171.3
Gamma-3	94.0	245.4

External Radiation

The exposure rate constant for 1 mCi (37 MBq) of In-111 is 8.3×10^{-4} C/kg/hr (3.2 R/hr) at 1 cm.

To allow correction for physical decay of In-111, the fractions that remain at selected intervals before and after the time of calibration are shown in Table 6.

Table 6. Physical Decay Chart: In-111 Half-life 2.81 Days (67.3 Hours)

Calibration Time (Hrs.)	Fraction Remaining
-48	1.64
-42	1.54
-36	1.45
-24	1.28
-12	1.13

-6	1.06
0	1.00
6	0.94
12	0.88
24	0.78
36	0.69
42	0.65
48	0.61

Physical / Radiochemical Characteristics of Y-90

Yttrium-90 decays by emission of beta particles, with a physical half-life of 64.1 hours (2.67 days). The product of radioactive decay is non-radioactive Zirconium-90. The range of beta particles in soft tissue (χ_{90}) is 5 mm. Radiation emission data for Y-90 are summarized in Table 7.

Table 7. Principal Y-90 Radiation Emission Data

Radiation	Mean % per Disintegration	Mean Energy (keV)
Beta minus	100	750-935

External Radiation

The exposure rate for 1 mCi (37 MBq) of Y-90 is 8.3×10^{-3} C/kg/hr (32 R/hr) at the mouth of an open Y-90 vial.

To allow correction for physical decay of Y-90, the fractions that remain at selected intervals before and after the time of calibration are shown in Table 8.

Table 8. Physical Decay Chart: Y-90 Half-life 2.67 Days (64.1 Hours)

Calibration Time (Hrs.)	Fraction Remaining	Calibration Time (Hrs.)	Fraction Remaining
-36	1.48	0	1.00
-24	1.30	1	0.99
-12	1.14	2	0.98
-8	1.09	3	0.97
-7	1.08	4	0.96
-6	1.07	5	0.95
-5	1.06	6	0.94
-4	1.04	7	0.93
-3	1.03	8	0.92
-2	1.02	12	0.88
-1	1.01	24	0.77
0	1.00	36	0.68

12 CLINICAL PHARMACOLOGY

12.1 Mechanism of Action

Ibritumomab tiuxetan binds specifically to the CD20 antigen (human B-lymphocyte-restricted differentiation antigen, Bp35). The apparent affinity (K_D) of ibritumomab tiuxetan for the CD20 antigen ranges between approximately 14 to 18 nM. The CD20 antigen is expressed on pre-B and mature B lymphocytes and on > 90% of B-cell non-Hodgkin's lymphomas (NHL). The CD20 antigen is not shed from the cell surface and does not internalize upon antibody binding.

The chelate tiuxetan, which tightly binds In-111 or Y-90, is covalently linked to ibritumomab. The beta emission from Y-90 induces cellular damage by the formation of free radicals in the target and neighboring cells.

Ibritumomab tiuxetan binding was observed *in vitro* on lymphoid cells of the bone marrow, lymph node, thymus, red and white pulp of the spleen, and lymphoid follicles of the tonsil, as well as lymphoid nodules of other organs such as the large and small intestines.

12.2 Pharmacodynamics

In clinical studies, administration of the Zevalin therapeutic regimen resulted in sustained depletion of circulating B

Table 9. Summary of Efficacy Data*

	Study 1	Study 2	
	Zevalin therapeutic regimen N = 54	Zevalin therapeutic regimen N = 64	Rituximab N = 66
Overall Response Rate (%)	74	83	55
Complete Response Rate[†] (%)	15	38	18
Median DR[‡,§] (Months) [Range[¶]]	6.4 [0.5-49.9+]	14.3 [1.8-47.6+]	11.5 [1.2-49.7+]
Median TTP[‡,#] (Months) [Range[¶]]	6.8 [1.1-50.9+]	12.1 [2.1-49.0+]	10.1 [0.7-51.3+]

*IWRC: International Workshop Response Criteria
[†]CRu and CR: Unconfirmed and confirm complete response
[‡]Estimated with observed range
[§]Duration of response: interval from the onset of response to disease progression
[¶]"+" indicates an ongoing response
[#]Time to Disease Progression: interval from the first infusion to disease progression

cells. At four weeks, the median number of circulating B cells was zero (range, 0-1084/mm³). B-cell recovery began at approximately 12 weeks following treatment, and the median level of B cells was within the normal range (32 to 341/mm³) by 9 months after treatment. Median serum levels of IgG and IgA remained within the normal range throughout the period of B-cell depletion. Median IgM serum levels dropped below normal (median 49 mg/dL, range 13-3990 mg/dL) after treatment and recovered to normal values by 6-months post therapy.

12.3 Pharmacokinetics
Pharmacokinetic and biodistribution studies were performed using In-111 Zevalin (5 mCi [185 MBq] In-111, 1.6 mg ibritumomab tiuxetan). In an early study designed to assess the need for pre-administration of unlabeled antibody, only 18% of known sites of disease were imaged when In-111 Zevalin was administered without unlabeled ibritumomab. When preceded by unlabeled ibritumomab (1.0 mg/kg or 2.5 mg/kg), In-111 Zevalin detected 56% and 92% of known disease sites, respectively. These studies were conducted with a Zevalin therapeutic regimen that included unlabeled ibritumomab.
In pharmacokinetic studies of patients receiving the Zevalin therapeutic regimen, the mean effective half-life for Y-90 activity in blood was 30 hours, and the mean area under the fraction of injected activity (FIA) vs. time curve in blood was 39 hours. Over 7 days, a median of 7.2% of the injected activity was excreted in urine.

13 NONCLINICAL TOXICOLOGY
13.1 Carcinogenesis, Mutagenesis, Impairment of Fertility
Carcinogenicity and mutogenicity studies have not been conducted. However, radiation is a potential carcinogen and mutagen. No animal studies have been performed to determine the effects of Zevalin on fertility in males or females. In clinical studies, the Zevalin therapeutic regimen results in a significant radiation dose to the testes: the radiation dose to the ovaries has not been established [see Dosage and Administration (2.6)]. There is a potential risk that the Zevalin therapeutic regimen could cause toxic effects on the male and female gonads. Effective contraceptive methods should be used during treatment and for up to 12 months following the Zevalin therapeutic regimen [see Patient Counseling Information (17)].

13.2 Animal Toxicology and/or Pharmacology
Animal reproductive toxicology studies of the Zevalin therapeutic regimen have not been conducted. Because the Zevalin therapeutic regimen includes the use of rituximab, also see prescribing information for rituximab.

14 CLINICAL STUDIES
14.1 Relapsed or Refractory, Low-grade or Follicular Lymphoma
Study 1 was a single arm study of 54 patients with relapsed follicular lymphoma, who were refractory to rituximab treatment. Patients had a World Health Organization (WHO) Performance Status (PS) 0-2, <25% bone marrow involvement by NHL, no prior bone marrow transplantation, and acceptable hematologic, renal, and hepatic function. Refractoriness to rituximab was defined as failure to achieve a complete or partial response or time-to-disease-progression

(TTP) of < 6 months. The main efficacy outcome measure of the study was the overall response rate (ORR) using the International Workshop Response Criteria (IWRC). Other efficacy outcome measures included time-to-disease-progression (TTP) and duration of response (DR). Table 9 summarizes efficacy data from Study 1.
Study 2 was a randomized (1:1), open-label, multicenter study comparing the Zevalin therapeutic regimen with rituximab. The trial was conducted in 130 patients with relapsed or refractory low-grade or follicular non-Hodgkin's lymphoma (NHL); no patient had received prior rituximab. Patients had histologically confirmed NHL requiring therapy, a WHO PS 0-2, <25% bone marrow involvement by NHL, no prior bone marrow transplantation, and acceptable hematologic function. Sixty-four patients received the Zevalin therapeutic regimen, and 66 patients received rituximab given as an IV infusion at 375 mg per m² weekly times 4 doses. The main efficacy outcome measure of the study was ORR using the IWRC. The ORR was significantly higher for patients receiving the Zevalin therapeutic regimen (83% vs. 55%, p<0.001). Time-to-disease-progression was not significantly different between study arms. Table 9 summarizes efficacy data from Study 2.
[See table 9 above]
Study 3 was a single arm study of 30 patients of whom 27 had relapsed or refractory low-grade, follicular NHL and a platelet count 100,000 to 149,000/mm³. Patients with ≥ 25% lymphomatous marrow involvement, prior myeloablative therapy with stem cell support, prior external beam radiation to > 25% of active marrow or neutrophil count <1,500/mm³ were ineligible for Study 3. All patients received Y-90 Zevalin [0.3 mCi per kg (11.1 MBq per kg)]. Objective, durable clinical responses were observed [89% ORR (95% CI: 70-97%) with a median duration of response of 11.6 months (range: 1.0-42.4+ months)].

14.2 Follicular, B-Cell NHL Upon Completion of First-Line Chemotherapy
Study 4 was a multi-center, randomized, open-label study conducted in patients with follicular NHL with a partial (PR) or complete response (CR/CRu) upon completion of first-line chemotherapy. Randomization was stratified by center and response to first-line therapy (CR or PR). Key eligibility criteria were <25% bone marrow involvement, no prior external beam radiation or myeloablative therapy, and recovery of platelets to normal levels. Patients were randomized to receive Zevalin (n=208) or no further therapy (n=206). Y-90 Zevalin was administered at least 6 weeks but no more than 12 weeks following the last dose of chemotherapy. The main efficacy outcome measure was progression-free survival (PFS) assessed by study investigators using the International Workshop to Standardize Response Criteria for non-Hodgkin's Lymphoma (1999).
Among the 414 patients, 49% were male, 99% were Caucasian, 12% were ≥65 years old, 83% had a WHO performance status of 0, and 65% had Stage IV disease. Thirty-nine (9.5%) patients received single agent chlorambucil, 22 (5%) patients received fludarabine or a fludarabine-containing regimen, 294 (71%) patients received cyclophosphamide-containing combination chemotherapy [CHOP (31%); CHOP-like (15%); CVP/COP (26%)] and 59 (14%) patients received rituximab-containing combination chemotherapy as first-line treatment.

Progression-free survival was significantly prolonged among Zevalin-treated patients compared to those receiving no further treatment [median PFS 38 months vs. 18 months; HR 0.46 (95% CI: 0.35, 0.60) p<0.0001 Cox model stratified by response to first-line therapy and initial treatment strategy (immediate vs. watch-and-wait)]. The number of patients who died was too small to permit a reliable comparison on survival.
The results for PFS are presented in Figure 1.

Figure 1. Study 4: Kaplan-Meier Estimator for Investigator-Assessed Progression Free Survival Time

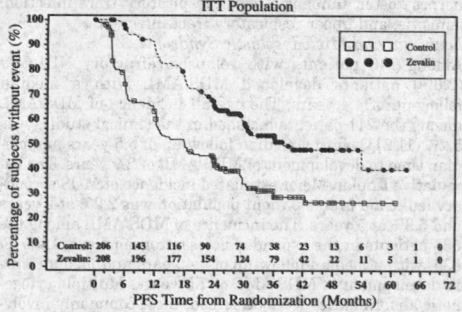

16 HOW SUPPLIED/STORAGE AND HANDLING
There are two kits necessary for preparation of the Zevalin therapeutic regimen: one for preparation of In-111 radiolabeled Zevalin (NDC 68152-104-04) and one for preparation of Y-90 radiolabeled Zevalin (NDC 68152-103-03). The contents of all vials are sterile, pyrogen-free, contain no preservatives, and are not radioactive. Each kit contains four identification labels and the following four vials:
1. One (1) Zevalin vial containing 3.2 mg ibritumomab tiuxetan in 2 mL 0.9% Sodium Chloride as a clear, colorless solution.
2. One (1) 50 mM Sodium Acetate Vial containing 13.6 mg Sodium Acetate trihydrate in 2 mL Water for Injection, USP as a clear, colorless solution.
3. One (1) Formulation Buffer Vial containing 750 mg Albumin (Human), 76 mg Sodium Chloride, 28 mg Sodium Phosphate Dibasic Dodecahydrate, 4 mg Pentetic Acid, 2 mg Potassium Phosphate Monobasic and 2 mg Potassium Chloride in 10 mL Water for Injection, pH 7.1 as a clear yellow to amber colored solution.
4. One (1) empty Reaction Vial.
Indium-111 Chloride Sterile Solution (In-111 Chloride) must be ordered separately from either GE Healthcare, or Mallinckrodt/Covidien.
Yttrium-90 Chloride Sterile Solution is shipped directly from the supplier upon placement of an order for the Y-90 Zevalin kit.
Rituximab (Rituxan®, Biogen Idec and Genentech USA) must be ordered separately.
Storage
Store kits at 2-8°C (36-46°F). Do not freeze.

17 PATIENT COUNSELING INFORMATION
Advise patients:
• To contact a healthcare professional for severe signs and symptoms of infusion reactions.
• To take premedications as prescribed [see Dosage and Administration (2.2) and Warnings and Precautions (5.1)].
• To report any signs or symptoms of cytopenias (bleeding, easy bruising, petechiae or purpura, pallor, weakness or fatigue).
• To avoid medications that interfere with platelet function, except as directed by a healthcare professional [see Warnings and Precautions (5.2)].
• To seek prompt medical evaluation for diffuse rash, bullae, or desquamation of the skin or oral mucosa.
• To immediately report symptoms of infection (e.g. pyrexia) [see Adverse Reactions (6.3)].
• That immunization with live viral vaccines is not recommended for 12 months following the Zevalin therapeutic regimen [see Warnings and Precautions (5.8)].
• To use effective contraceptive methods during treatment and for a minimum of 12 months following Zevalin therapy.
• To discontinue nursing during and after Zevalin treatment [see Use In Special Populations (8.3)].

© 2009 Spectrum Pharmaceuticals, Inc.
Irvine, CA 92618
U.S. License No. 1832
Protected by U.S. Patent Nos. 5,736,137, 5,776,456, 5,843,439, 6,207,858, 6,399,061, 6,682,734, 6,994,840, 7,229,620, 7,381,560, 7,422,739 and other patents and patents pending.

Stiefel Laboratories, Inc.
Research Triangle Park, NC 27709

Direct Inquiries to:
Professional Services Department
1-888-STIEFEL

DUAC® TOPICAL GEL
[dū-ăk]
(clindamycin phosphate, 1% - benzoyl peroxide, 5%)
For Dermatological Use Only.
Not for Ophthalmic Use.
Rx Only

℞

DESCRIPTION
Duac® Topical Gel contains clindamycin phosphate, (7(S)-chloro-7-deoxylincomycin-2-phosphate), equivalent to 1% clindamycin, and 5% benzoyl peroxide.
Clindamycin phosphate is a water soluble ester of the semi-synthetic antibiotic produced by a 7(S)-chloro-substitution of the 7(R)-hydroxyl group of the parent antibiotic lincomycin.
Clindamycin phosphate is $C_{18}H_{34}ClN_2O_8PS$. The structural formula for clindamycin phosphate is represented below:

Clindamycin phosphate has a molecular weight of 504.97 and its chemical name is methyl 7-chloro-6,7,8-trideoxy-6-(1-methyl-*trans*-4-propyl-L-2-pyrrolidinecarboxamido)-1-thio-L-*threo*-α-D-*galacto*-octopyranoside 2-(dihydrogen phosphate).
Benzoyl peroxide is $C_{14}H_{10}O_4$. It has the following structural formula:

Benzoyl peroxide has a molecular weight of 242.23.
Each gram of Duac® Topical Gel contains 10 mg (1%) clindamycin, as phosphate, and 50 mg (5%) benzoyl peroxide in a base consisting of carbomer 940, dimethicone, disodium lauryl sulfosuccinate, edetate disodium, glycerin, methylparaben, poloxamer 182, purified water, silicon dioxide, and sodium hydroxide.

CLINICAL PHARMACOLOGY
A comparative study of the pharmacokinetics of Duac® Topical Gel and 1% clindamycin solution alone in 78 patients indicated that mean plasma clindamycin levels during the four week dosing period were < 0.5 ng/ml for both treatment groups.
Benzoyl peroxide has been shown to be absorbed by the skin where it is converted to benzoic acid. Less than 2% of the dose enters systemic circulation as benzoic acid.
Microbiology
Mechanism of Action
Clindamycin binds to the 50S ribosomal subunits of susceptible bacteria and prevents elongation of peptide chains by interfering with peptidyl transfer, thereby suppressing protein synthesis.
Benzoyl peroxide is a potent oxidizing agent.
In Vivo Activity
No microbiology studies were conducted in the clinical trials with this product.
In Vitro Activity
The clindamycin and benzoyl peroxide components individually have been shown to have *in vitro* activity against *Propionibacterium acnes*, an organism which has been associated with acne vulgaris; however, the clinical significance of this is not known.
Drug Resistance
There are reports of an increase of *P. acnes* resistance to clindamycin in the treatment of acne. In patients with *P. acnes* resistant to clindamycin, the clindamycin component may provide no additional benefit beyond benzoyl peroxide alone.

Mean percent reduction in inflammatory lesion counts

	Study 1 (n=120)	Study 2 (n=273)	Study 3 (n=280)	Study 4 (n=288)	Study 5 (n=358)
Duac® Topical Gel	65%	56%	42%	57%	52%
Benzoyl Peroxide	36%	37%	32%	57%	41%
Clindamycin	34%	30%	38%	49%	33%
Vehicle	19%	-0.4%	29%		29%

Local reactions with use of Duac® Topical Gel % of patients using Duac® Topical Gel with symptom present Combined results from 5 studies (n=397)

	Before Treatment (Baseline)			During Treatment		
	Mild	Moderate	Severe	Mild	Moderate	Severe
Erythema	28%	3%	0	26%	5%	0
Peeling	6%	<1%	0	17%	2%	0
Burning	3%	<1%	0	5%	<1%	0
Dryness	6%	<1%	0	15%	1%	0

CLINICAL STUDIES
In five randomized, double-blind clinical studies of 1,319 patients, 397 used Duac® Topical Gel, 396 used benzoyl peroxide, 349 used clindamycin and 177 used vehicle. Duac® Topical Gel applied once daily for 11 weeks was significantly more effective than vehicle, benzoyl peroxide, and clindamycin in the treatment of inflammatory lesions of moderate to moderately severe facial acne vulgaris in three of the five studies (Studies 1, 2, and 5).
Patients were evaluated and acne lesions counted at each clinical visit: weeks 2, 5, 8, 11. The primary efficacy measures were the lesion counts and the investigator's global assessment evaluated at week 11. Patients were instructed to wash the face, wait 10 to 20 minutes, and then apply medication to the entire face, once daily, in the evening before retiring. Percent reductions in inflammatory lesion counts after treatment for 11 weeks in these five studies are shown in the following table:
[See first table above]
The Duac® Topical Gel group showed greater overall improvement in the investigator's global assessment than the benzoyl peroxide, clindamycin and vehicle groups in three of the five studies (Studies 1, 2, and 5).
Clinical studies have not adequately demonstrated the effectiveness of Duac® Topical Gel versus benzoyl peroxide alone in the treatment of non-inflammatory lesions of acne.

INDICATIONS AND USAGE
Duac® Topical Gel is indicated for the topical treatment of inflammatory acne vulgaris.
Duac® Topical Gel has not been demonstrated to have any additional benefit when compared to benzoyl peroxide alone in the same vehicle when used for the treatment of non-inflammatory acne.

CONTRAINDICATIONS
Duac® Topical Gel is contraindicated in those individuals who have shown hypersensitivity to any of its components or to lincomycin. It is also contraindicated in those having a history of regional enteritis, ulcerative colitis, pseudomembranous colitis, or antibiotic-associated colitis.

WARNINGS
ORALLY AND PARENTERALLY ADMINISTERED CLINDAMYCIN HAS BEEN ASSOCIATED WITH SEVERE COLITIS WHICH MAY RESULT IN PATIENT DEATH. USE OF THE TOPICAL FORMULATION OF CLINDAMYCIN RESULTS IN ABSORPTION OF THE ANTIBIOTIC FROM THE SKIN SURFACE. DIARRHEA, BLOODY DIARRHEA, AND COLITIS (INCLUDING PSEUDOMEMBRANOUS COLITIS) HAVE BEEN REPORTED WITH THE USE OF TOPICAL AND SYSTEMIC CLINDAMYCIN. STUDIES INDICATE A TOXIN(S) PRODUCED BY CLOSTRIDIA IS ONE PRIMARY CAUSE OF ANTIBIOTIC-ASSOCIATED COLITIS. THE COLITIS IS USUALLY CHARACTERIZED BY SEVERE PERSISTENT DIARRHEA AND SEVERE ABDOMINAL CRAMPS AND MAY BE ASSOCIATED WITH THE PASSAGE OF BLOOD AND MUCUS. ENDOSCOPIC EXAMINATION MAY REVEAL PSEUDOMEMBRANOUS COLITIS. STOOL CULTURE FOR *Clostridium difficile* AND STOOL ASSAY FOR *Clostridium difficile* TOXIN MAY BE HELPFUL DIAGNOSTICALLY. WHEN SIGNIFICANT DIARRHEA OCCURS, THE DRUG SHOULD BE DISCONTINUED. LARGE BOWEL ENDOSCOPY SHOULD BE CONSIDERED TO ESTABLISH A DEFINITIVE DIAGNOSIS IN CASES OF SEVERE DIARRHEA. ANTIPERISTALTIC AGENTS SUCH AS OPIATES AND DIPHENOXYLATE WITH ATROPINE MAY PROLONG AND/OR WORSEN THE CONDITION. DIARRHEA, COLITIS AND PSEUDOMEMBRANOUS COLITIS HAVE BEEN OBSERVED TO BEGIN UP TO SEVERAL WEEKS FOLLOWING CESSATION OF ORAL AND PARENTERAL THERAPY WITH CLINDAMYCIN.
Mild cases of pseudomembranous colitis usually respond to drug discontinuation alone. In moderate to severe cases, consideration should be given to management with fluids and electrolytes, protein supplementation and treatment with an antibacterial drug clinically effective against *Clostridium difficile* colitis.

PRECAUTIONS
General
For dermatological use only; not for ophthalmic use. Concomitant topical acne therapy should be used with caution because a possible cumulative irritancy effect may occur, especially with the use of peeling, desquamating, or abrasive agents.
The use of antibiotic agents may be associated with the overgrowth of nonsusceptible organisms, including fungi. If this occurs, discontinue use of this medication and take appropriate measures.
Avoid contact with eyes and mucous membranes.
Clindamycin and erythromycin containing products should not be used in combination. *In vitro* studies have shown antagonism between these two antimicrobials. The clinical significance of this *in vitro* antagonism is not known.
Information for Patients
Patients using Duac® Topical Gel should receive the following information and instructions:
1. Duac® Topical Gel is to be used as directed by the physician. It is for external use only. Avoid contact with eyes, and inside the nose, mouth, and all mucous membranes, as this product may be irritating.
2. This medication should not be used for any disorder other than that for which it was prescribed.
3. Patients should not use any other topical acne preparation unless otherwise directed by their physician.
4. Patients should report any signs of local adverse reactions to their physician. Patients who develop allergic symptoms such as severe swelling or shortness of breath should discontinue use and contact their physician immediately.
5. Duac® Topical Gel may bleach hair or colored fabric.
6. Duac® Topical Gel can be stored at room temperature up to 25°C (77°F) for up to 2 months. Do not freeze. Keep tube tightly closed. Keep out of the reach of small children. Discard any unused product after 2 months.
7. Before applying Duac® Topical Gel to affected areas, wash the skin gently, rinse with warm water, and pat dry.
8. Excessive or prolonged exposure to sunlight should be limited. To minimize exposure to sunlight, a hat or other clothing should be worn.
Carcinogenesis, Mutagenesis, Impairment of Fertility
Benzoyl peroxide has been shown to be a tumor promoter and progression agent in a number of animal studies. The clinical significance of this is unknown.
Benzoyl peroxide in acetone at doses of 5 and 10 mg administered twice per week induced squamous cell skin tumors in transgenic TgAC mice in a study using 20 weeks of topical treatment.
Genotoxicity studies were not conducted with Duac® Topical Gel. Clindamycin phosphate was not genotoxic in *Salmonella typhimurium* or in a rat micronucleus test.

Benzoyl peroxide has been found to cause DNA strand breaks in a variety of mammalian cell types, to be mutagenic in *Salmonella typhimurium* tests by some but not all investigators, and to cause sister chromatid exchanges in Chinese hamster ovary cells. Studies have not been performed with Duac® Topical Gel or benzoyl peroxide to evaluate the effect on fertility. Fertility studies in rats treated orally with up to 300 mg/kg/day of clindamycin (approximately 120 times the amount of clindamycin in the highest recommended adult human dose of 2.5 g Duac® Topical Gel, based on mg/m^2) revealed no effects on fertility or mating ability.

Pregnancy
Teratogenic Effects
Pregnancy Category C
Animal reproduction studies have not been conducted with Duac® Topical Gel or benzoyl peroxide. It is also not known whether Duac® Topical Gel can cause fetal harm when administered to a pregnant woman or can affect reproduction capacity. Duac® Topical Gel should be given to a pregnant woman only if clearly needed.
Developmental toxicity studies performed in rats and mice using oral doses of clindamycin up to 600 mg/kg/day (240 and 120 times the amount of clindamycin in the highest recommended adult human dose based on mg/m^2, respectively) or subcutaneous doses of clindamycin up to 250 mg/kg/day (100 and 50 times the amount of clindamycin in the highest recommended adult human dose based on mg/m^2, respectively) revealed no evidence of teratogenicity.

Nursing Women
It is not known whether Duac® Topical Gel is secreted into human milk after topical application. However, orally and parenterally administered clindamycin has been reported to appear in breast milk. Because of the potential for serious adverse reactions in nursing infants, a decision should be made whether to discontinue nursing or to discontinue the drug, taking into account the importance of the drug to the mother.

Pediatric Use
Safety and effectiveness of this product in pediatric patients below the age of 12 have not been established.

ADVERSE REACTIONS
During clinical trials, all patients were graded for facial erythema, peeling, burning, and dryness on the following scale: 0 = absent, 1 = mild, 2 = moderate, and 3 = severe. The percentage of patients that had symptoms present before treatment (at baseline) and during treatment were as follows:
[See second table on previous page]
(Percentages derived by # subjects with symptom score/# enrolled Duac® Topical Gel subjects, n = 397).
Anaphylaxis, as well as allergic reactions leading to hospitalization, has been reported in post-marketing use with Duac® Topical Gel. Because these reactions are reported voluntarily from a population of uncertain size, it is not always possible to reliably estimate their frequency or establish a causal relationship to a drug exposure.

DOSAGE AND ADMINISTRATION
Duac® Topical Gel should be applied once daily, in the evening or as directed by the physician, to affected areas after the skin is gently washed, rinsed with warm water and patted dry.

HOW SUPPLIED
Duac® (clindamycin, 1% - benzoyl peroxide, 5%) Topical Gel is available in:
• 45 gram tube   NDC 0145-2371-05
• Care System (CS) Convenience Kit   NDC 0145-2367-01 includes Duac® Topical Gel (clindamycin, 1% - benzoyl peroxide, 5%) 45 grams and SFC™ Lotion 106.6 mL (3.6 Fl Oz)
Prior to Dispensing: Store in a cold place, preferably in a refrigerator, between 2°C and 8°C (36°F and 46°F). Do not freeze.
Dispensing Instructions for the Pharmacist: Dispense Duac® Topical Gel with a 60 day expiration date and specify "Store at room temperature up to 25°C (77°F). Do not freeze."
Keep tube tightly closed. Keep out of the reach of small children.
U.S. Patent No. 5,466,446
Patent Pending
©2008 Stiefel Laboratories, Inc.
Stiefel Laboratories, Inc.
255 Alhambra Circle
Coral Gables, FL 33134-7412 USA
301135
Rev. July 2008
DUAC, STIEFEL and STIEFEL and the "S" logo are registered trademarks and SFC is a trademark of Stiefel Laboratories, Inc.

EVOCLIN®
[ĕ-vō-klĭn]
(clindamycin phosphate) Foam, 1%
Rx Only
FOR TOPICAL USE ONLY.
NOT FOR OPHTHALMIC, ORAL, OR INTRAVAGINAL USE.

R̞

DESCRIPTION
Evoclin Foam contains clindamycin phosphate, USP, a topical antibiotic for topical dermatologic use.
Clindamycin phosphate is a water-soluble ester of the semisynthetic antibiotic produced by a 7 (S)-chloro-substitution of the 7(R)-hydroxyl group of the parent antibiotic, lincomycin.
The chemical name for clindamycin phosphate is methyl 7-chloro-6,7,8-trideoxy-6-(1-methyl-*trans*-4-propyl-L-2-pyrrolidinecarboxamido)-1-thio-L-*threo*-α-D-*galacto*-octopyranoside 2-(dihydrogen phosphate), with the empirical formula $C_{18}H_{34}ClN_2O_8PS$, a molecular weight of 504.97. The following is the chemical structure:

clindamycin phosphate

Evoclin® (clindamycin phosphate) Foam, 1%, contains clindamycin phosphate, USP, at a concentration equivalent to 10 mg clindamycin per gram in a thermolabile hydroethanolic foam vehicle consisting of cetyl alcohol, ethanol (58%), polysorbate 60, potassium hydroxide, propylene glycol, purified water, and stearyl alcohol pressurized with a hydrocarbon (propane/butane) propellant.

CLINICAL PHARMACOLOGY
Pharmacokinetics
In an open label, parallel group study in 24 patients with acne vulgaris, 12 patients (3 male and 9 female) applied 4 grams of Evoclin Foam once-daily for five days, and 12 patients (7 male and 5 female) applied 4 grams of Clindagel® (clindamycin phosphate) Topical Gel, 1%, once daily for five days. On Day 5, the mean C_{max} and AUC(0-12) were 23% and 9% lower, respectively, for Evoclin Foam than for Clindagel®.
Following multiple applications of Evoclin Foam less than 0.024% of the total dose was excreted unchanged in the urine over 12 hours on Day 5.

Microbiology
The clindamycin component has been shown to have in vitro activity against *Propionibacterium acnes*, an organism which is associated with acne vulgaris; however, the clinical significance of this activity against *P. acnes* was not examined in clinical trials with this product. Cross-resistance between clindamycin and erythromycin has been demonstrated.

CLINICAL STUDIES
In one multicenter, randomized, double-blind, vehicle-controlled clinical trial patients with mild to moderate acne vulgaris used Evoclin (clindamycin phosphate) Foam, 1% or the vehicle foam once daily for twelve weeks. Treatment response, defined as the proportion of patients clear or almost clear, based on the Investigator Static Global Assessment (ISGA), and the mean percent reductions in lesion counts at the end of treatment in this study are shown in the following table:

Efficacy Parameters	Evoclin Foam	Vehicle Foam
	n=386	n=127
Treatment response (ISGA)	31%	18%*
Percent reduction in lesion counts		
Inflammatory Lesions	49%	35%*
Noninflammatory Lesions	38%	27%*
Total Lesions	43%	31%*

*P<0.05

INDICATIONS AND USAGE
Evoclin is indicated for topical application in the treatment of acne vulgaris. In view of the potential for diarrhea, bloody diarrhea and pseudomembranous colitis, the physician should consider whether other agents are more appropriate. (See CONTRAINDICATIONS, WARNINGS, and ADVERSE REACTIONS.)

CONTRAINDICATIONS
Evoclin is contraindicated in individuals with a history of hypersensitivity to preparations containing clindamycin or lincomycin, a history of regional enteritis or ulcerative colitis, or a history of antibiotic-associated colitis.

WARNINGS
Orally and parenterally administered clindamycin has been associated with severe colitis, which may result in patient death. Use of the topical formulation of clindamycin results in absorption of the antibiotic from the skin surface. Diarrhea, bloody diarrhea, and colitis (including pseudomembranous colitis) have been reported with the use of topical and systemic clindamycin.
Studies indicate a toxin(s) produced by *Clostridia* is one primary cause of antibiotic-associated colitis. The colitis is usually characterized by severe persistent diarrhea and severe abdominal cramps and may be associated with the passage of blood and mucus. Endoscopic examination may reveal pseudomembranous colitis. Stool culture for *Clostridium difficile* and stool assay for *C. difficile* toxin may be helpful diagnostically.
When significant diarrhea occurs, the drug should be discontinued. Large bowel endoscopy should be considered to establish a definitive diagnosis in cases of severe diarrhea. Antiperistaltic agents, such as opiates and diphenoxylate with atropine, may prolong and/or worsen the condition.
Diarrhea, colitis, and pseudomembranous colitis have been observed to begin up to several weeks following cessation of oral and parenteral therapy with clindamycin.
Mild cases of pseudomembranous colitis usually respond to drug discontinuation alone. In moderate to severe cases, consideration should be given to management with fluids and electrolytes, protein supplementation and treatment with an antibacterial drug clinically effective against *C. difficile* colitis.
Avoid contact of Evoclin with eyes. If contact occurs, rinse eyes thoroughly with water.

PRECAUTIONS
General
Evoclin should be prescribed with caution in atopic individuals.
Drug Interactions
Clindamycin has been shown to have neuromuscular blocking properties that may enhance the action of other neuromuscular blocking agents. Therefore, it should be used with caution in patients receiving such agents.
Carcinogenesis, Mutagenesis, Impairment of Fertility
The carcinogenicity of a 1% clindamycin phosphate gel similar to Evoclin was evaluated by daily application to mice for two years. The daily doses used in this study were approximately 3 and 15 times higher than the human dose of clindamycin phosphate from 5 milliliters of Evoclin, assuming complete absorption and based on a body surface area comparison. No significant increase in tumors was noted in the treated animals.
A 1% clindamycin phosphate gel similar to Evoclin caused a statistically significant shortening of the median time to tumor onset in a study in hairless mice in which tumors were induced by exposure to simulated sunlight.
Genotoxicity tests performed included a rat micronucleus test and an Ames Salmonella revision test. Both tests were negative.
Reproduction studies in rats using oral doses of clindamycin hydrochloride and clindamycin palmitate hydrochloride have revealed no evidence of impaired fertility.
Pregnancy
Teratogenic effects - Pregnancy Category B
Reproduction studies have been performed in rats and mice using subcutaneous and oral doses of clindamycin phosphate, clindamycin hydrochloride and clindamycin palmitate hydrochloride. These studies revealed no evidence of fetal harm. The highest dose used in the rat and mouse teratogenicity studies was equivalent to a clindamycin phosphate dose of 432 mg/kg. For a rat, that dose is 84 fold higher, and for a mouse 42 fold higher, than the anticipated human dose of clindamycin phosphate from Evoclin based on a mg/m^2 comparison. There are, however, no adequate and well-controlled studies in pregnant women. Because animal reproduction studies are not always predictive of human response, this drug should be used during pregnancy only if clearly needed.
Nursing Mothers
It is not known whether clindamycin is excreted in human milk following use of Evoclin. However, orally and parenterally administered clindamycin has been reported to appear in breast milk. Because of the potential for serious adverse reactions in nursing infants, a decision should be made whether to discontinue nursing or to discontinue the drug, taking into account the importance of the drug to the mother.

Pediatric Use
Safety and effectiveness of Evoclin in children under the age of 12 have not been studied.
Geriatric Use
The clinical study with Evoclin did not include sufficient numbers of patients aged 65 and over to determine if they respond differently than younger patients.

ADVERSE REACTIONS

The incidence of adverse events occurring in ≥1% of the patients in clinical studies comparing Evoclin and its vehicle is presented below:

Selected Adverse Events Occurring in ≥1% of Subjects

Adverse Event	Number (%) of Subjects	
	Evoclin Foam	Vehicle Foam
	N = 439	N = 154
Headache	12 (3%)	1 (1%)
Application site burning	27 (6%)	14 (9%)
Application site pruritus	5 (1%)	5 (3%)
Application site dryness	4 (1%)	5 (3%)
Application site reaction, not otherwise specified	3 (1%)	4 (3%)

In a contact sensitization study, none of the 203 subjects developed evidence of allergic contact sensitization to Evoclin. Orally and parenterally administered clindamycin has been associated with severe colitis, which may end fatally. Cases of diarrhea, bloody diarrhea, and colitis (including pseudomembranous colitis) have been reported as adverse reactions in patients treated with oral and parenteral formulations of clindamycin and rarely with topical clindamycin (see WARNINGS). Abdominal pain and gastrointestinal disturbances, as well as gram-negative folliculitis, have also been reported in association with the use of topical formulations of clindamycin.

OVERDOSAGE

Topically applied Evoclin may be absorbed in sufficient amounts to produce systemic effects (see WARNINGS).

DOSAGE AND ADMINISTRATION

Apply Evoclin once daily to affected areas after the skin is washed with mild soap and allowed to fully dry. Use enough to cover the entire affected area.
To Use Evoclin:
1. Do not dispense Evoclin directly onto your hands or face, because the foam will begin to melt on contact with warm skin.
2. Remove the clear cap. Align the black mark with the nozzle of the actuator.
3. Hold the can at an upright angle and then press firmly to dispense. Dispense an amount directly into the cap or onto a cool surface. Dispense an amount of Evoclin that will cover the affected area(s). If the can seems warm or the foam seems runny, run the can under cold water.
4. Pick up small amounts of Evoclin with your fingertips and gently massage into the affected areas until the foam disappears.

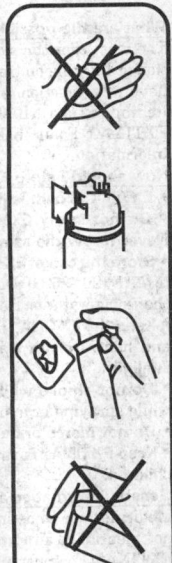

Throw away any of the unused medicine that you dispensed out of the can.
Avoid contact of Evoclin with eyes. If contact occurs, rinse eyes thoroughly with water.

HOW SUPPLIED

Evoclin containing clindamycin phosphate equivalent to 10 mg clindamycin per gram, is available in the following sizes: 100 gram can - NDC 63032-061-00 and 50 gram can – NDC 63032-061-50

STORAGE AND HANDLING

Store at controlled room temperature, 68°-77°F (20°-25°C).
FLAMMABLE. AVOID FIRE, FLAME OR SMOKING DURING AND IMMEDIATELY FOLLOWING APPLICATION.
Contents under pressure. Do not puncture or incinerate. Do not expose to heat or store at temperature above 120°F (49°C).
Keep out of reach of children.
Manufactured for
Stiefel Laboratories, Inc.
Coral Gables, FL 33134
USA
For additional information:
1-888-500-DERM or visit
www.evoclin.com
AW No: AW-0668 P/N: 128598-0807
U.S. Patent No. 7,141,237
The wisp logo and VersaFoam-HF are trademarks, and Evoclin, the V logo and Stiefel are registered trademarks of Stiefel Laboratories, Inc.
© 2007 Stiefel Laboratories, Inc.
Printed in USA
February 2007

EXTINA®   Rx

[ex-TEEN-ah]
(ketoconazole)
Foam, 2%
For topical use only

HIGHLIGHTS OF PRESCRIBING INFORMATION

These highlights do not include all the information needed to use EXTINA® Foam safely and effectively. See full prescribing information for EXTINA® Foam.
EXTINA® (ketoconazole) Foam, 2%
For topical use only
Initial U.S. Approval: 1981

———INDICATIONS AND USAGE———
EXTINA® Foam is indicated for topical treatment of seborrheic dermatitis in immunocompetent patients 12 years of age and older (1).
Safety and efficacy of EXTINA® Foam for treatment of fungal infections have not been established.

———DOSAGE AND ADMINISTRATION———
• EXTINA® Foam should be applied to the affected area(s) twice daily for four weeks (2).
• EXTINA® Foam is not for ophthalmic, oral, or intravaginal use (2).

———DOSAGE FORMS AND STRENGTHS———
EXTINA® Foam contains 2% ketoconazole in a thermolabile hydroethanolic foam in 50 g and 100 g containers (3).

———CONTRAINDICATIONS———
None

———WARNINGS AND PRECAUTIONS———
• EXTINA® Foam may result in contact sensitization, including photoallergenicity (5.1, 6.2).
• The contents of EXTINA® Foam are flammable (5.2).

———ADVERSE REACTIONS———
The most common adverse reactions observed in clinical studies (incidence > 1%) were application site burning and application site reaction (6.1).
To report SUSPECTED ADVERSE REACTIONS, contact Stiefel Laboratories, Inc. at 1-888-500-DERM or adverse.event@stiefel.com and FDA at 1-800-FDA-1088 or www.fda.gov/medwatch.
See 17 for PATIENT COUNSELING INFORMATION and FDA-approved patient labeling

Revised: 05/2010

FULL PRESCRIBING INFORMATION: CONTENTS*

FULL PRESCRIBING INFORMATION

1   INDICATIONS AND USAGE

EXTINA® (ketoconazole) Foam, 2% is indicated for the topical treatment of seborrheic dermatitis in immunocompetent patients 12 years of age and older. Safety and efficacy of EXTINA® Foam for treatment of fungal infections have not been established.

2   DOSAGE AND ADMINISTRATION

EXTINA® Foam should be applied to the affected area(s) twice daily for four weeks.
Hold the container upright, and dispense EXTINA® Foam into the cap of the can or other cool surface in an amount sufficient to cover the affected area(s). Dispensing directly onto hands is not recommended, as the foam will begin to melt immediately upon contact with warm skin. Pick up small amounts of EXTINA® Foam with the fingertips, and gently massage into the affected area(s) until the foam disappears. For hair-bearing areas, part the hair, so that EXTINA® Foam may be applied directly to the skin (rather than on the hair).
Avoid contact with the eyes and other mucous membranes. EXTINA® Foam is not for ophthalmic, oral or intravaginal use.

3   DOSAGE FORMS AND STRENGTHS

EXTINA® Foam contains 2% ketoconazole in a thermolabile hydroethanolic foam, and is provided in 50 g and 100 g aluminum containers.

4   CONTRAINDICATIONS

None

5   WARNINGS AND PRECAUTIONS

5.1   Contact Sensitization
EXTINA® Foam may result in contact sensitization, including photoallergenicity. *[See Adverse Reactions (6.2)]*
5.2   Flammable Contents
The contents of EXTINA® Foam include alcohol and propane/butane, which are flammable. Avoid fire, flame and/or smoking during and immediately following application. Do not puncture and/or incinerate the containers. Do not expose containers to heat and/or store at temperatures above 120°F (49°C).
5.3   Systemic Effects
Hepatitis has been seen with orally administered ketoconazole (1:10,000 reported incidence). Lowered testosterone and ACTH–induced corticosteroid serum levels have been seen with high doses of orally administered ketoconazole. These effects have not been seen with topical ketoconazole.

6   ADVERSE REACTIONS

6.1   Adverse Reactions in Clinical Trials
Because clinical trials are conducted under widely varying conditions, adverse reaction rates observed in the clinical trials of a drug cannot be directly compared to rates in the clinical trials of another drug, and may not reflect the rates observed in practice. The adverse reaction information from clinical trials does, however, provide a basis for identifying the adverse reactions that appear to be related to drug use and for approximating rates.
The safety data presented in Table 1 (below) reflect exposure to EXTINA® Foam in 672 subjects, 12 years and older with seborrheic dermatitis. Subjects applied EXTINA® Foam or vehicle foam twice daily for 4 weeks to affected areas on the face, scalp, and/or chest. Adverse reactions occurring in > 1% of subjects are presented in Table 1.

Table 1: Adverse Reactions Reported by > 1% Subjects in Clinical Trials

Adverse Reactions	EXTINA® Foam N = 672 n (%)	Vehicle Foam N = 497 n (%)
Subjects with an Adverse Reaction	188 (28%)	122 (25%)
Application site burning	67 (10%)	49 (10%)
Application site reaction	41 (6%)	24 (5%)

Application site reactions that were reported in ≤ 1% of subjects were dryness, erythema, irritation, paresthesia, pruritus, rash and warmth.

6.2 Dermal Safety Studies

In a photoallergenicity study, 9 of 53 subjects (17%) had reactions during the challenge period at both the irradiated and non-irradiated sites treated with EXTINA® Foam. EXTINA® Foam may cause contact sensitization.

8 USE IN SPECIFIC POPULATIONS

8.1 Pregnancy

Teratogenic Effects, Pregnancy Category C:

Ketoconazole has been shown to be teratogenic (syndactylia and oligodactylia) in the rat when given orally in the diet at 80 mg/kg/day (4.8 times the maximum expected human topical dose based on a mg/m^2 comparison, assuming 100% absorption from 8 g of foam). However, these effects may be partly related to maternal toxicity, which was also observed at this dose level. *[See Pharmacokinetics (12.3)]*

No reproductive studies in animals have been performed with EXTINA® Foam. There are no adequate and well-controlled studies of EXTINA® Foam in pregnant women. EXTINA® Foam should be used during pregnancy only if the potential benefit justifies the potential risk to the fetus.

8.3 Nursing Mothers

It is not known whether EXTINA® Foam administered topically could result in sufficient systemic absorption to produce detectable quantities in breast milk. Because many drugs are excreted in human milk, caution should be exercised when EXTINA® Foam is administered to women who are breastfeeding.

8.4 Pediatric Use

The safety and effectiveness of EXTINA® Foam in pediatric patients less than 12 years of age have not been established. Of the 672 subjects treated with EXTINA® Foam in the clinical trials, 44 (7%) were from 12 to 17 years of age. *[See Clinical Studies (14)]*

8.5 Geriatric Use

Of the 672 subjects treated with EXTINA® Foam in the clinical trials, 107 (16%) were 65 years and over.

11 DESCRIPTION

EXTINA® Foam contains 2% ketoconazole USP, an antifungal agent, in a thermolabile hydroethanolic foam for topical application.

The chemical name for ketoconazole is piperazine, 1-acetyl-4-[4-[[2-(2,4-dichlorophenyl)-2-(1*H*-imidazol-1-ylmethyl)-1,3-dioxolan-4-yl]methoxy]phenyl]-, *cis*- with the molecular formula $C_{26}H_{28}Cl_2N_4O_4$ and a molecular weight of 531.43. The following is the chemical structure:

EXTINA® Foam contains 20 mg ketoconazole per gram in a thermolabile hydroethanolic foam vehicle consisting of cetyl alcohol, citric acid, ethanol (denatured with *tert*-butyl alcohol and brucine sulfate) 58%, polysorbate 60, potassium citrate, propylene glycol, purified water, and stearyl alcohol pressurized with a hydrocarbon (propane/butane) propellant.

12 CLINICAL PHARMACOLOGY

12.1 Mechanism of Action

The mechanism of action of ketoconazole in the treatment of seborrheic dermatitis is not known.

12.2 Pharmacodynamics

The pharmacodynamics of EXTINA® Foam has not been established.

12.3 Pharmacokinetics

In a bioavailability study, 12 subjects with moderate to severe seborrheic dermatitis applied 3 g of EXTINA® Foam twice daily for 4 weeks. Circulating plasma levels of ketoconazole were < 6 ng/mL for a majority of subjects (75%), with a maximum level of 11 ng/mL observed in one subject.

12.4 Microbiology

Ketoconazole is an antifungal agent which inhibits the *in vitro* synthesis of ergosterol, a key sterol in the cell membrane of *Malassezia furfur*. The clinical significance of antifungal activity in the treatment of seborrheic dermatitis is not known.

13 NONCLINICAL TOXICOLOGY

13.1 Carcinogenesis, Mutagenesis, Impairment of Fertility

Long-term animal studies have not been performed to evaluate the carcinogenic or photo-carcinogenic potential of EXTINA® Foam.

In oral carcinogenicity studies in mice (18-months) and rats (24-months) at dose levels of 5, 20 and 80 mg/kg/day

ketoconazole was not carcinogenic. The high dose in these studies was approximately 2.4 to 4.8 times the expected topical dose in humans based on a mg/m^2 comparison. In a bacterial reverse mutation assay, ketoconazole did not express any mutagenic potential. In three *in vivo* assays (sister chromatid exchange in humans, dominant lethal and micronucleus tests in mice), ketoconazole did not exhibit any genotoxic potential.

At oral dose levels of 75 mg/kg/day (4.5 times the expected topical human dose in mg/m^2), ketoconazole impaired reproductive performance and fertility when administered to male rats (increased abnormal sperm, decreased sperm mobility and decreased pregnancy in mated females).

14 CLINICAL STUDIES

The safety and efficacy of EXTINA® Foam were evaluated in a randomized, double-blind, vehicle-controlled study in subjects 12 years and older with mild to severe seborrheic dermatitis. In the study, 427 subjects received EXTINA® Foam and 420 subjects received vehicle foam. Subjects applied EXTINA® Foam or vehicle foam twice daily for 4 weeks to affected areas on the face, scalp, and/or chest. The overall disease severity in terms of erythema, scaling, and induration was assessed at Baseline and week 4 on a 5-point Investigator's Static Global Assessment (ISGA) scale.

Treatment success was defined as achieving a Week 4 (end of treatment) ISGA score of 0 (clear) or 1 (majority of lesions have individual scores for scaling, erythema, and induration that averages 1 [minimal or faint]) and at least two grades of improvement from baseline. The results are presented in Table 2. The database was not large enough to assess whether there were differences in effects in age, gender, or race subgroups.

Table 2: Efficacy Results

Number of Subjects	EXTINA® Foam N = 427 n (%)	Vehicle Foam N = 420 n (%)
Subjects Achieving Treatment Success	239 (56%)	176 (42%)

16 HOW SUPPLIED/STORAGE AND HANDLING

EXTINA® Foam, 2% is supplied in 50 g (NDC 63032-051-50) and 100 g (NDC 63032-051-00) aluminum containers. Store at controlled room temperature 68°–77°F (20°-25°C). Do not store under refrigerated conditions. **Do not expose containers to heat, and/or store at temperatures above 120°F (49°C).** Do not store in direct sunlight. **Contents are flammable.**

Contents under pressure. Do not puncture and/or incinerate container.

Keep out of reach of children.

17 PATIENT COUNSELING INFORMATION

See FDA-approved patient labeling. (17.3)

17.1 Instructions for Use

• **Avoid fire, flame and/or smoking during and immediately following application.**

• Do not apply EXTINA® Foam directly to hands. Dispense onto a cool surface, and apply to the affected areas using the fingertips.

17.2 Local Reactions

• EXTINA® Foam may cause skin irritation (application site burning and/or reactions)

• EXTINA® Foam may cause contact sensitization.

• As with any topical medication, patients should wash their hands after application.

• Inform a physician if the area of application shows signs of increased irritation and report any signs of adverse reactions.

17.3 Patient Package Insert

-See below-

PATIENT INFORMATION

EXTINA® (ex-TEEN-ah) Foam (ketoconazole, 2%)

IMPORTANT: For skin use only. Do not use in the eyes, mouth or vagina.

Read the Patient Information that comes with EXTINA® Foam before you start using it and each time you get a refill. There may be new information. This leaflet does not take the place of talking with your doctor about your condition or treatment.

What is EXTINA® Foam?

EXTINA® Foam is used on the skin (topical) to treat a skin condition called seborrheic dermatitis in patients 12 years and older. Seborrheic dermatitis can cause areas of flaky skin (scales) on the scalp, face, ears, chest or upper back. EXTINA® Foam has not been studied in children less than 12 years old.

What should I tell my doctor before using EXTINA® Foam?

For female patients, tell your doctor if you:

• **are pregnant or become pregnant.** It is not known if EXTINA® Foam can harm a fetus (unborn baby).

• **breastfeeding.** It is not known if EXTINA® Foam passes into breast milk.

How should I use EXTINA® Foam?

• **Apply EXTINA® Foam exactly as prescribed.** EXTINA® Foam is usually applied to the affected skin areas two times a day (once in the morning and once at night) for 4 weeks. Talk to your doctor if your skin does not improve after 4 weeks of treatment with EXTINA® Foam.

• **Keep the EXTINA® Foam can away from and do not spray it near fire, open flame, or direct heat. EXTINA® Foam is flammable. Never throw the EXTINA® Foam can into a fire, even if the can is empty.**

Instructions for applying EXTINA® Foam

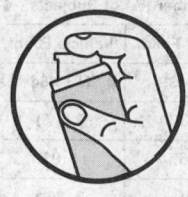

1. Hold the can at an upright angle.
2. Push the button to spray EXTINA® Foam directly into the cap of the can or other cool surface. Spray only the amount of EXTINA® Foam that you will need to cover your affected skin. **Do not spray EXTINA® Foam directly onto your affected skin or your hands** because the foam will begin to melt right away when it touches your skin.

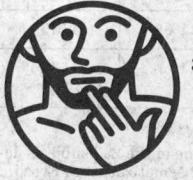

3. If your fingers are warm, rinse them in cold water first. Be sure to dry them well before handling the EXTINA® Foam. If the EXTINA® Foam can seems warm or the foam seems runny, place the can under cool running water for a few minutes.
4. Using your fingertips, gently massage EXTINA® Foam into the affected areas until the foam disappears.
5. If you are treating skin areas with hair such as your scalp, move any hair away so that the foam can be applied to the affected skin.

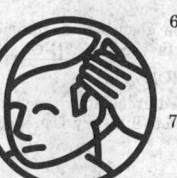

6. **Do not get EXTINA® Foam in your eyes, mouth or vagina. If any EXTINA® Foam gets in your eyes, mouth or vagina, rinse areas well with water.**
7. Wash your hands well after applying EXTINA® Foam.

What are the possible side effects of EXTINA® Foam?

The most common side effects of EXTINA® Foam are reaction or burning on treated skin areas. Tell your doctor if you have any reaction on your treated skin such as redness, itching, or a rash. These are not all the side effects of EXTINA® Foam. Ask your doctor or pharmacist for more information.

How should I store EXTINA® Foam?

• EXTINA® Foam is flammable.

• **Do not spray EXTINA® Foam near fire or direct heat.** Never throw the can into a fire, even if the can is empty.

• **Store the can of EXTINA® Foam at room temperature, 68° to 77°F (20°-25°C).** Do not place the EXTINA® Foam can in the refrigerator or freezer.

• **Keep the EXTINA® Foam can away from all sources of fire and heat. Do not leave the EXTINA® Foam can in direct sunlight.**

• **Do not smoke while holding the EXTINA® Foam can** or while spraying or applying the foam.

• **Do not pierce or burn the EXTINA® Foam can.**

• **Keep EXTINA® Foam and all medicines out of the reach of children.**

General information about EXTINA® Foam

Medicines are sometimes prescribed for conditions that are not mentioned in Patient Information leaflets. Do not use EXTINA® Foam for any other condition for which it was not prescribed. Do not give EXTINA® Foam to other people, even if they have the same condition that you have. It may harm them.

This leaflet summarizes the most important information about EXTINA® Foam. If you would like more information, talk with your doctor. You can ask your doctor or pharmacist for information about EXTINA® Foam that is written for health professionals.

If you have questions about EXTINA® Foam you can also call: 1-888-500-DERM (this is a toll-free number) between 6:00 a.m. and 4:00 p.m. Pacific Standard Time, Monday through Friday.

What are the ingredients in EXTINA® Foam?

Active ingredients: ketoconazole

Inactive Ingredients: cetyl alcohol, citric acid, ethanol (denatured with tert-butyl alcohol and brucine sulfate) 58%, polysorbate 60, potassium citrate, propylene glycol, purified water, and stearyl alcohol pressurized with a hydrocarbon (propane/butane) propellant.

Rx Only

This Patient Information leaflet has been approved by the U.S. Food and Drug Administration.

The Patient Information leaflet was last revised: November 2008

Manufactured for

Stiefel Laboratories, Inc., Coral Gables, FL 33134 USA

VERSAFOAM-HF, VERSAFOAM-HF and Design, EXTINA®, and V Design, STIEFEL, and STIEFEL and Design are registered trademarks of Stiefel Laboratories, Inc. U.S. Patent Pending

©2008 Stiefel Laboratories, Inc.

302418

AW No.: AW-0854

LUXIQ®   ℞

[lŭk-sēk]

(betamethasone valerate) Foam, 0.12%

Rx Only

For Dermatologic Use Only

Not for Ophthalmic Use

DESCRIPTION

Luxíq Foam contains betamethasone valerate, USP, a synthetic corticosteroid, for topical dermatologic use. The corticosteroids constitute a class of primarily synthetic steroids used topically as anti-inflammatory agents.

Betamethasone valerate is 9-fluoro11β,17, 21-trihydroxy-16β-methylpregna-1, 4-diene-3, 20-dione 17-valerate, with the empirical formula $C_{27}H_{37}FO_6$, a molecular weight of 476.58. The following is the chemical structure:

Betamethasone valerate

Betamethasone valerate is a white to practically white, odorless crystalline powder, and is practically insoluble in water, freely soluble in acetone and in chloroform, soluble in alcohol, and slightly soluble in benzene and in ether.

Luxíq® (betamethasone valerate) Foam, 0.12%, contains 1.2 mg betamethasone valerate, USP, per gram in a thermolabile hydroethanolic foam vehicle consisting of cetyl alcohol, citric acid, ethanol (60.4%), polysorbate 60, potassium citrate, propylene glycol, purified water, and stearyl alcohol pressurized with a hydrocarbon (propane/butane) propellant.

CLINICAL PHARMACOLOGY

Like other topical corticosteroids, betamethasone valerate foam has anti-inflammatory, antipruritic, and vasoconstrictive properties. The mechanism of the anti-inflammatory activity of the topical steroids, in general, is unclear. However, corticosteroids are thought to act by the induction of phospholipase A_2 inhibitory proteins, collectively called lipocortins. It is postulated that these proteins control the biosynthesis of potent mediators of inflammation such as prostaglandins and leukotrienes by inhibiting the release of their common precursor arachidonic acid. Arachidonic acid is released from membrane phospholipids by phospholipase A_2.

Pharmacokinetics

Topical corticosteroids can be absorbed from intact healthy skin. The extent of percutaneous absorption of topical corticosteroids is determined by many factors, including the vehicle and the integrity of the epidermal barrier. Occlusion, inflammation and/or other disease processes in the skin may also increase percutaneous absorption.

The use of pharmacodynamic endpoints for assessing the systemic exposure of topical corticosteroids is necessary due to the fact that circulating levels are well below the level of detection. Once absorbed through the skin, topical corticosteroids are handled through pharmacokinetic pathways similar to systemically administered corticosteroids. They are metabolized, primarily in the liver, and are then excreted by the kidneys. In addition, some corticosteroids and their metabolites are also excreted in the bile.

CLINICAL STUDIES

The safety and efficacy of Luxíq has been demonstrated in a four-week trial. An adequate and well-controlled clinical trial was conducted in 190 patients with moderate to severe scalp psoriasis. Patients were treated twice daily for four weeks with Luxíq Foam, Placebo foam, a commercially available betamethasone valerate lotion 0.12% (formerly expressed as 0.1% betamethasone), or Placebo lotion. At four weeks of treatment, study results of 159 patients demonstrated that the efficacy of Luxíq Foam in treating scalp psoriasis is superior to that of Placebo foam, and is comparable to that of a currently marketed BMV lotion (see Table below).

[See table above]

Subjects with Target Lesion Parameter Clear at Endpoint	Luxíq Foam n (%)	BMV lotion n (%)	Placebo foam n (%)
Scaling	30 (47%)	22 (35%)	2 (6%)
Erythema	26 (41%)	16 (25%)	2 (6%)
Plaque Thickness	42 (66%)	25 (40%)	5 (16%)
Investigator's Global: Subjects Completely Clear or Almost Clear at Endpoint	43 (67%)	29 (46%)	6 (19%)

INDICATIONS AND USAGE

Luxíq is a medium potency topical corticosteroid indicated for relief of the inflammatory and pruritic manifestations of corticosteroid-responsive dermatoses of the scalp.

CONTRAINDICATIONS

Luxíq is contraindicated in patients who are hypersensitive to betamethasone valerate, to other corticosteroids, or to any ingredient in this preparation.

PRECAUTIONS

General

Systemic absorption of topical corticosteroids has caused reversible hypothalamic-pituitary-adrenal (HPA) axis suppression with the potential for glucocorticosteroid insufficiency after withdrawal of treatment. Manifestations of Cushing's syndrome, hyperglycemia, and glucosuria can also be produced in some patients by systemic absorption of topical corticosteroids while on treatment.

Conditions which augment systemic absorption include the application of the more potent steroids, use over large surface areas, prolonged use, and the addition of occlusive dressings.

Therefore, patients applying a topical steroid to a large surface area or to areas under occlusion should be evaluated periodically for evidence of HPA axis suppression. If HPA axis suppression is noted, an attempt should be made to withdraw the drug, to reduce the frequency of application, or to substitute a less potent steroid.

Recovery of HPA axis function is generally prompt upon discontinuation of topical corticosteroids. Infrequently, signs and symptoms of glucocorticosteroid insufficiency may occur requiring supplemental systemic corticosteroids. For information on systemic supplementation, see prescribing information for those products.

Pediatric patients may be more susceptible to systemic toxicity from equivalent doses due to their larger skin surface to body mass ratios. (See **PRECAUTIONS-Pediatric Use.**)

If irritation develops, Luxíq should be discontinued and appropriate therapy instituted. Allergic contact dermatitis with corticosteroids is usually diagnosed by observing a failure to heal rather than noting a clinical exacerbation, as with most topical products not containing corticosteroids. Such an observation should be corroborated with appropriate diagnostic patch testing.

In the presence of dermatological infections, the use of an appropriate antifungal or antibacterial agent should be instituted. If a favorable response does not occur promptly, use of Luxíq should be discontinued until the infection has been adequately controlled.

Information for Patients

Patients using topical corticosteroids should receive the following information and instructions:

1. This medication is to be used as directed by the physician. It is for external use only. Avoid contact with the eyes.

2. This medication should not be used for any disorder other than that for which it was prescribed.

3. The treated scalp area should not be bandaged or otherwise covered or wrapped so as to be occlusive unless directed by the physician.

4. Patients should report to their physician any signs of local adverse reactions.

5. As with other corticosteroids, therapy should be discontinued when control is achieved. If no improvement is seen within 2 weeks, contact the physician.

Laboratory Tests

The following tests may be helpful in evaluating patients for HPA axis suppression:

ACTH stimulation test

A.M. plasma cortisol test

Urinary free cortisol test

Carcinogenesis, Mutagenesis, and Impairment of Fertility

Long-term animal studies have not been performed to evaluate the carcinogenic potential or the effect on fertility of betamethasone valerate.

Betamethasone was genotoxic in the *in vitro* human peripheral blood lymphocyte chromosome aberration assay with metabolic activation and in the *in vivo* mouse bone marrow micronucleus assay.

Pregnancy Category C

Corticosteroids have been shown to be teratogenic in laboratory animals when administered systemically at relatively low dosage levels. Some corticosteroids have been shown to be teratogenic after dermal application in laboratory animals. There are no adequate and well-controlled studies in pregnant women. Therefore, Luxíq should be used during pregnancy only if the potential benefit justifies the potential risk to the fetus.

Drugs of this class should not be used extensively on pregnant patients, in large amounts, or for prolonged periods of time.

Nursing Mothers

Systemically administered corticosteroids appear in human milk and could suppress growth, interfere with endogenous corticosteroid production, or cause other untoward effects. It is not known whether topical administration of corticosteroids could result in sufficient systemic absorption to produce detectable quantities in breast milk. Because many drugs are excreted in human milk, caution should be exercised when Luxíq is administered to a nursing woman.

Pediatric Use

Safety and effectiveness in pediatric patients have not been established. Because of a higher ratio of skin surface area to body mass, pediatric patients are at a greater risk than adults of HPA axis suppression and Cushing's syndrome when they are treated with topical corticosteroids. They are therefore also at greater risk of adrenal insufficiency during and/or after withdrawal of treatment. Adverse effects including striae have been reported with inappropriate use of topical corticosteroids in infants and children. Hypothalamic-pituitary-adrenal (HPA) axis suppression, Cushing's syndrome, linear growth retardation, delayed weight gain, and intracranial hypertension have been reported in children receiving topical corticosteroids. Manifestations of adrenal suppression in children include low plasma cortisol levels and an absence of response to ACTH stimulation. Manifestations of intracranial hypertension include bulging fontanelles, headaches, and bilateral papilledema.

Administration of topical corticosteroids to children should be limited to the least amount compatible with an effective therapeutic regimen. Chronic corticosteroid therapy may interfere with the growth and development of children.

ADVERSE REACTIONS

The most frequent adverse event was burning/itching/stinging at the application site; the incidence and severity of this event were as follows:

[See table at top of next page]

Other adverse events which were considered to be possibly, probably, or definitely related to Luxíq occurred in 1 patient each; these were paresthesia, pruritus, acne, alopecia, and conjunctivitis.

The following additional local adverse reactions have been reported with topical corticosteroids, and they may occur more frequently with the use of occlusive dressings. These reactions are listed in an approximately decreasing order of occurrence: irritation; dryness; folliculitis; acneiform eruptions; hypopigmentation; perioral dermatitis; allergic contact dermatitis; secondary infection; skin atrophy; striae; and miliaria.

Systemic absorption of topical corticosteroids has produced reversible hypothalamic-pituitary-adrenal (HPA) axis suppression, manifestations of Cushing's syndrome, hyperglycemia, and glucosuria in some patients.

Incidence and severity of burning/itching/stinging

Product	Total incidence	Maximum severity		
		Mild	Moderate	Severe
Luxíq Foam n=63	34 (54%)	28 (44%)	5 (8%)	1 (2%)
Betamethasone valerate lotion n=63	33 (52%)	26 (41%)	6 (10%)	1 (2%)
Placebo Foam n=32	24 (75%)	13 (41%)	7 (22%)	4 (12%)
Placebo Lotion n=30	20 (67%)	12 (40%)	5 (17%)	3 (10%)

OVERDOSAGE

Topically applied Luxíq can be absorbed in sufficient amounts to produce systemic effects. (See **PRECAUTIONS**)

DOSAGE AND ADMINISTRATION

Note: For proper dispensing of foam, can must be inverted. For application to the scalp invert can and dispense a small amount of Luxíq onto a saucer or other cool surface. Do not dispense directly onto hands as foam will begin to melt immediately upon contact with warm skin. Pick up small amounts of foam with fingers and gently massage into affected area until foam disappears. Repeat until entire affected scalp area is treated. Apply twice daily, once in the morning and once at night.

As with other corticosteroids, therapy should be discontinued when control is achieved. If no improvement is seen within 2 weeks, reassessment of the diagnosis may be necessary.

Luxíq should not be used with occlusive dressings unless directed by a physician.

HOW SUPPLIED

Luxíq is supplied in 100 gram (NDC 63032-021-00) and 50 gram (NDC 63032-021-50) aluminum cans.

Store at controlled room temperature 68–77°F (20–25°C).

WARNING

FLAMMABLE. AVOID FIRE, FLAME OR SMOKING DURING AND IMMEDIATELY FOLLOWING APPLICATION. Keep out of reach of children. Contents under pressure. Do not puncture or incinerate container. Do not expose to heat or store at temperatures above 120°F (49°C).

Manufactured for
Stiefel Laboratories, Inc.
Coral Gables, FL 33134
USA

For additional information visit www.luxiq.com
Questions? Call 1-888-500-DERM (3376). Side effects may be reported to this number.

303203

P/N: xxxxxxxx

Luxíq, VersaFoam-HF, VersaFoam-HF & Design, Stiefel, and Stiefel & Design are registered trademarks of Stiefel Laboratories, Inc.

©2009 Stiefel Laboratories, Inc.

PATIENT INFORMATION

Luxíq®

(betamethasone valerate) Foam, 0.12%

About Luxíq

Your doctor has prescribed Luxíq (betamethasone valerate) Foam, 0.12%, for the relief of corticosteroid-responsive skin conditions of the scalp. Luxíq works because its active ingredient is betamethasone valerate, 0.12%. Betamethasone belongs to a group of medicines known as topical corticosteroids. These agents are used to reduce the inflammation, redness, swelling, itching, and tenderness associated with dermatologic conditions.

Other ingredients in Luxíq include cetyl alcohol, citric acid, ethanol, polysorbate 60, potassium citrate, propylene glycol, purified water, and stearyl alcohol. The foam is dispensed from an aluminum can that is pressurized by a hydrocarbon propellant (propane and butane).

If you answer YES to one or more of the following questions, tell your doctor (or pharmacist) before using this medicine, so you can get advice about what to do.

• Are you allergic to any of the ingredients contained in Luxíq?
• Are you pregnant? Planning on becoming pregnant while using Luxíq? Or are you breastfeeding?
• Do you think you have an infection on your scalp?

How to apply Luxíq

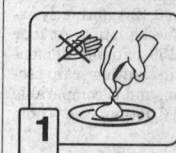

Turn the can upside down and dispense a small amount of Luxíq onto a clean saucer or other cool, clean surface. Do not dispense directly onto hands, as foam will begin to melt immediately upon contact with warm skin.

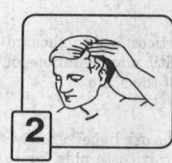

Pick up small amounts of foam with fingers and gently massage into affected area until foam disappears. Repeat until entire affected scalp area is treated. Apply twice daily, once in the morning and once at night. Use sparingly—only enough to cover the affected areas. Gently massage the foam in until it is absorbed and allow the areas to dry naturally. When applying to the scalp, move the hair away so that the foam can be applied directly to each affected area.

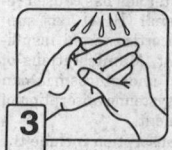

Wash your hands immediately after applying Luxíq, and discard any unused medication.

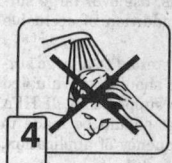

Do not wash or rinse the treated areas immediately after applying Luxíq.

• Do not use this medication for any condition other than the one for which it was prescribed.
• **Luxíq is for external use only.**
• **Keep the foam away from your eyes,** as it will sting. If the foam gets into your eyes, rinse well with cold water. If the stinging continues, contact your doctor immediately.

WHAT YOU SHOULD KNOW ABOUT LUXÍQ:

What to do if you miss an application

If you forget to apply Luxíq at the scheduled time, use it as soon as you remember, and then go back to your regular schedule. If you remember at or about the time of your next daily application, apply that dose and continue with your normal application schedule. If you miss several doses, tell your doctor at your next appointment.

About side effects

As with all medications, there may be some side effects. The most frequent side effects associated with the use of Luxíq include mild burning, stinging, or itching at the site of application. These side effects typically disappear shortly after application. Let your doctor know if you notice any of the following:

• Any unusual effects that you do not understand.
• Affected areas that do not seem to be healing after several weeks of using the foam.

Important safety notes

• The treated areas should not be bandaged or covered unless directed by your doctor.
• Keep this and all medicines out of the reach of children.
• Store the can at controlled room temperature 68-77° F (20-25° C) and protect it from direct sunlight, as this is a pressurized container.
• **Keep away from and do not spray near fire, open flame, or direct heat—this product is flammable.** Do not smoke while using or holding the can. Keep the can away from all sources of ignition. Do not pierce or burn the can, and never throw the can in a fire, even if empty.
• When you have finished your treatment, dispose of the can safely. A completely empty can is recyclable.

• Do not use the foam after the expiration date shown on the bottom of the can.
• Do not give Luxíq to anyone else. Your doctor has prescribed this medicine for your use only.

Manufactured for
Stiefel Laboratories, Inc.
Coral Gables, FL 33134
USA

For additional information visit www.luxiq.com
Questions? Call 1-888-500-DERM (3376), Serious side effects may be reported to this number.

303203

P/N: xxxxxxxx

Printed in: U.S.A.

November 2009

Luxiq, VersaFoam-HF, VersaFoam-HF & Design, Stiefel, and Stiefel & Design are registered trademarks of Stiefel Laboratories, Inc.

©2009 Stiefel Laboratories, Inc.

OLUX-E   ℞

[ō-lŭks]

(clobetasol propionate)

Foam, 0.05%

Rx Only

For Topical Use Only

Not For Ophthalmic, Oral, Or Intravaginal Use

DESCRIPTION

Olux-E (clobetasol propionate) Foam, an emulsion aerosol foam, contains the active ingredient clobetasol propionate, USP, a synthetic corticosteroid for topical dermatologic use. Clobetasol, an analog of prednisolone, has a high degree of glucocorticoid activity and a slight degree of mineralocorticoid activity.

Clobetasol propionate is 21-chloro-9-fluoro-11β, 17-dihydroxy-16β-methylpregna-1,4-diene-3,20-dione 17-propionate, with the empirical formula $C_{25}H_{32}ClFO_5$, and a molecular weight of 466.97. The following is the chemical structure:

Figure 1: Structural Formula

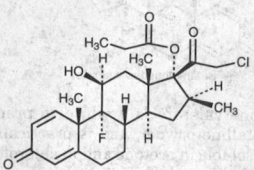

Clobetasol Propionate, USP

Clobetasol propionate is a white to cream-colored crystalline powder, practically insoluble in water.

Each gram of Olux-E Foam contains 0.5 mg clobetasol propionate, USP. The foam also contains anhydrous citric acid USP, cetyl alcohol NF, cyclomethicone NF, isopropyl myristate NF, light mineral oil NF, polyoxyl 20 cetostearyl ether NF, potassium citrate monohydrate USP, propylene glycol USP, purified water USP, sorbitan monolaurate NF, white petrolatum USP, and phenoxyethanol NF as a preservative.

Olux-E Foam is dispensed from an aluminum can pressurized with a hydrocarbon (propane/butane) propellant.

CLINICAL PHARMACOLOGY

The contribution to efficacy by individual components of the vehicle has not been established.

Topical corticosteroids share anti-inflammatory, antipruritic, and vasoconstrictive properties.

The mechanism of the anti-inflammatory activity of topical steroids is unclear. However, corticosteroids are thought to act by the induction of phospholipase A_2 inhibitory proteins, collectively called lipocortins. It is postulated that these proteins control the biosynthesis of potent mediators of inflammation such as prostaglandins and leukotrienes by inhibiting the release of their common precursor, arachidonic acid. Arachidonic acid is released from membrane phospholipids by phospholipase A_2.

Pharmacokinetics

Topical corticosteroids can be absorbed from intact healthy skin. The extent of percutaneous absorption of topical corticosteroids is determined by many factors, including the product formulation and the integrity of the epidermal barrier. Occlusion, inflammation and/or other disease processes in the skin may increase percutaneous absorption. The use of pharmacodynamic endpoints for assessing the systemic exposure of topical corticosteroids may be necessary due to the fact that circulating levels are often below the level of detection. Once absorbed through the skin, topical corticosteroids are metabolized, primarily in the liver, and are then excreted by the kidneys. Some corticosteroids and their metabolites are also excreted in the bile.

Following twice daily application of Olux-E Foam for one week to 32 adult patients with mild to moderate plaque-type psoriasis, mean peak plasma concentrations (±SD) of 59 ± 36 pg/mL of clobetasol were observed at around 5 hours post-dose on day 8.

CLINICAL STUDIES

In a randomized study of subjects 12 years of age and older with moderate to severe atopic dermatitis, 251 subjects were treated with Olux-E Foam and 126 subjects were treated with Vehicle Foam. Subjects were treated twice daily for two weeks. At the end of treatment, 131 of 251 subjects (52%) treated with Olux-E Foam compared with 18 of 126 (14%) treated with Vehicle Foam achieved treatment success. Treatment success was defined by an Investigator's Static Global Assessment (ISGA) score of clear (0) or almost clear (1) with at least 2 grades improvement from baseline, and scores of absent or minimal (0 or 1) for erythema and induration/papulation.

In an additional randomized study of subjects 12 years of age and older with mild to moderate plaque-type psoriasis, 253 subjects were treated with Olux-E Foam and 123 subjects were treated with Vehicle Foam. Subjects were treated twice daily for two weeks. At the end of treatment, 41 of 253 subjects (16%) treated with Olux-E Foam compared with 5 of 123 (4%) treated with Vehicle Foam achieved treatment success. Treatment success was defined by an Investigator's Static Global Assessment (ISGA) score of clear (0) or almost clear (1) with at least 2 grades improvement from baseline, scores of none or faint/minimal (0 or 1) for erythema and scaling, and a score of none (0) for plaque thickness.

INDICATIONS AND USAGE

Olux-E Foam is indicated for the treatment of inflammatory and pruritic manifestations of corticosteroid-responsive dermatoses in patients 12 years of age or older (see **PRECAUTIONS**). Treatment should be limited to 2 consecutive weeks and patients should not use greater than 50 grams per week (see **DOSAGE AND ADMINISTRATION**).

Patients should be instructed to use Olux-E Foam for the minimum amount of time necessary to achieve the desired results (see **PRECAUTIONS**).

Use in pediatric patients under 12 years of age is not recommended because of numerically high rates of hypothalamic-pituitary-adrenal (HPA) axis suppression seen in patients under 12 years of age (see **PRECAUTIONS**: Pediatric Use).

CONTRAINDICATIONS

Olux-E Foam is contraindicated in patients who are hypersensitive to clobetasol propionate or to any ingredient in this preparation.

WARNINGS

The propellant in Olux-E Foam is flammable. Avoid fire, flame or smoking during and immediately following application.

PRECAUTIONS

General

Olux-E Foam has been shown to suppress the HPA axis.

Systemic absorption of topical corticosteroids has caused reversible adrenal suppression with the potential for glucocorticosteroid insufficiency after withdrawal from treatment. Manifestations of Cushing's syndrome, hyperglycemia, and glucosuria can also be produced in some patients by systemic absorption of topical corticosteroids while on treatment.

Pediatric patients may be more susceptible to systemic toxicity from equivalent doses because of their larger skin surface to body mass ratios (see **PRECAUTIONS**: Pediatric Use).

Conditions which increase systemic absorption include the application of more potent steroids, use over large surface areas, prolonged use, and the addition of occlusive dressings. Therefore, patients applying a topical steroid to a large surface area or to areas under occlusion should be evaluated periodically for evidence of adrenal suppression (see laboratory tests below). If adrenal suppression is noted, an attempt should be made to withdraw the drug, to reduce the frequency of application, or to substitute a less potent steroid.

Recovery of HPA axis function is generally prompt upon discontinuation of topical corticosteroids. Infrequently, signs and symptoms of glucocorticosteroid insufficiency may occur, requiring supplemental systemic corticosteroids.

In a study evaluating the potential for HPA axis suppression, using the cosyntropin stimulation test, Olux-E Foam demonstrated adrenal suppression after two weeks of twice daily use in patients with atopic dermatitis of at least 30% body surface area (BSA). The proportion of subjects twelve years of age and older demonstrating HPA axis suppression was 16.2% (6 out of 37). In this study HPA axis suppression was defined as serum cortisol level ≤18 mcg/dL 30-min post cosyntropin stimulation. The laboratory suppression was transient; in all subjects serum cortisol levels returned to normal when tested 4 weeks post treatment.

Patients with acute illness or injury may have increased morbidity and mortality with intermittent HPA axis suppression. Patients should be instructed to use Olux-E Foam for the minimum amount of time necessary to achieve the desired results (see **INDICATIONS AND USAGE**).

If irritation develops, Olux-E Foam should be discontinued and appropriate therapy instituted. Allergic contact dermatitis with corticosteroids is usually diagnosed by observing a *failure to heal* rather than noting a clinical exacerbation as with most topical products not containing corticosteroids. Such an observation should be corroborated with appropriate diagnostic patch testing.

If concomitant skin infections are present or develop, an appropriate antifungal or antibacterial agent should be used. If a favorable response does not occur promptly, use of Olux-E Foam should be discontinued until the infection has been adequately controlled.

Olux-E Foam should not be used in the treatment of rosacea or perioral dermatitis, and should not be used on the face or the groin, axillae, or other intertriginous areas.

Information for Patients

Patients using topical corticosteroids should receive the following information and instructions:

1. This medication is to be used as directed by the physician. It is for external use only. Unless directed by the prescriber, it should not be used on the face, or in skinfold areas, such as the underarms or groin. Avoid contact with the eyes or other mucous membranes. Wash hands after use.
2. This medication should not be used for any disorder other than that for which it was prescribed.
3. The treated skin area should not be bandaged, wrapped, or otherwise covered so as to be occlusive unless directed by the physician.
4. Patients should report any signs of local or systemic adverse reactions to the physician.
5. Patients should inform their physicians that they are using Olux-E Foam if surgery is contemplated.
6. As with other corticosteroids, therapy should be discontinued when control is achieved. If no improvement is seen within 2 weeks, contact the physician.
7. Patients should not use more than 50 grams per week of Olux-E Foam, or an amount greater than 21 capfuls per week (see **DOSAGE AND ADMINISTRATION**).

Laboratory Tests

The cosyntropin ($ACTH_{1-24}$) stimulation test may be helpful in evaluating patients for HPA axis suppression.

Carcinogenesis, Mutagenesis, Impairment of Fertility

Long-term animal studies have not been performed to evaluate the carcinogenic potential of clobetasol propionate.

Clobetasol propionate was non-mutagenic in four different test systems: the Ames test, the mouse lymphoma test, the *Saccharomyces cerevisiae* gene conversion assay, and the *E. coli* B WP2 fluctuation test. In the *in vivo* mouse micronucleus test a positive finding was observed at 24 hours, but not at 48 hours, following oral administration at a dose of 2000 mg/kg.

Studies in the rat following subcutaneous administration of clobetasol propionate at dosage levels up to 0.05 mg/kg per day revealed that the females exhibited an increase in the number of resorbed embryos and a decrease in the number of living fetuses at the highest dose.

Pregnancy

Teratogenic effects

Pregnancy Category C

Corticosteroids have been shown to be teratogenic in laboratory animals when administered systemically at relatively low dosage levels. Some corticosteroids have been shown to be teratogenic after dermal application to laboratory animals.

Clobetasol propionate has not been tested for teratogenicity when applied topically; however, it is absorbed percutaneously, and when administered subcutaneously, it was a significant teratogen in both the rabbit and the mouse. Clobetasol propionate has greater teratogenic potential than steroids that are less potent.

Teratogenicity studies in mice using the subcutaneous route resulted in fetotoxicity at the highest dose tested (1 mg/kg) and teratogenicity at all dose levels tested down to 0.03 mg/kg. These doses are approximately 1.4 and 0.04 times, respectively, the human topical dose of Olux-E Foam based on body surface area comparisons. Abnormalities seen included cleft palate and skeletal abnormalities.

In rabbits, clobetasol propionate was teratogenic at doses of 0.003 and 0.01 mg/kg. These doses are approximately 0.02 and 0.05 times, respectively, the human topical dose of Olux-E Foam based on body surface area comparisons. Abnormalities seen included cleft palate, cranioschisis, and other skeletal abnormalities.

There are no adequate and well-controlled studies of the teratogenic potential of clobetasol propionate in pregnant women. Olux-E Foam should be used during pregnancy only if the potential benefit justifies the potential risk to the fetus.

Nursing Mothers

Systemically administered corticosteroids appear in human milk and could suppress growth, interfere with endogenous corticosteroid production, or cause other untoward effects. It is not known whether topical administration of corticosteroids could result in sufficient systemic absorption to produce detectable quantities in breast milk. Because many drugs are excreted in human milk, caution should be exercised when Olux-E Foam is administered to a nursing woman.

Pediatric Use

Use in pediatric patients under 12 years of age is not recommended.

After two weeks of twice daily treatment with Olux-E Foam, 7 of 15 patients (47%) aged 6 to 11 years of age demonstrated HPA axis suppression. The laboratory suppression was transient; in all subjects serum cortisol levels returned to normal when tested 4 weeks post treatment.

In 92 patients from 12 to 17 years of age, safety was similar to that observed in the adult population. Based on this data, no adjustment of dosage of Olux-E Foam in adolescent patients 12 to 17 years of age is warranted.

Because of a higher ratio of skin surface area to body mass, pediatric patients are at a greater risk than adults of HPA axis suppression and Cushing's syndrome when they are treated with topical corticosteroids. They are therefore also at greater risk of adrenal insufficiency during and/or after withdrawal of treatment. Adverse effects including striae have been reported with inappropriate use of topical corticosteroids in infants and children.

HPA axis suppression, Cushing's syndrome, linear growth retardation, delayed weight gain, and intracranial hypertension have been reported in children receiving topical corticosteroids. Manifestations of adrenal suppression in children include low plasma cortisol levels and an absence of response to ACTH stimulation. Manifestations of intracranial hypertension include bulging fontanelles, headaches, and bilateral papilledema. Administration of topical corticosteroids to children should be limited to the least amount compatible with an effective therapeutic regimen. Chronic corticosteroid therapy may interfere with the growth and development of children.

Geriatric Use

A limited number of patients at or above 65 years of age have been treated with Olux-E Foam (n = 58) in US clinical trials. While the number of patients is too small to permit separate analysis of efficacy and safety, the adverse reactions reported in this population were similar to those reported by younger patients. Based on available data, no adjustment of dosage of Olux-E Foam in geriatric patients is warranted.

ADVERSE REACTIONS

In controlled clinical trials involving 821 subjects exposed to Olux-E Foam and Vehicle Foam, the pooled incidence of local adverse reactions in trials for atopic dermatitis and psoriasis with Olux-E Foam was 1.9% for application site atrophy and 1.6% for application site reaction. Most local adverse events were rated as mild to moderate and they were not affected by age, race or gender. Because clinical trials are conducted under widely varying conditions, adverse reaction rates observed in the clinical trials of a drug cannot be directly compared to rates in the clinical trials of another drug and may not reflect the rates observed in clinical practice.

The following additional local adverse reactions have been reported with topical corticosteroids: folliculitis, acneiform eruptions, hypopigmentation, perioral dermatitis, allergic contact dermatitis, secondary infection, irritation, striae, and miliaria. They may occur more frequently with the use of occlusive dressings and higher potency corticosteroids, such as clobetasol propionate.

Cushing's syndrome has been reported in infants and adults as a result of prolonged use of topical clobetasol propionate formulations.

OVERDOSAGE

Topically applied Olux-E Foam can be absorbed in sufficient amounts to produce systemic effects (see **PRECAUTIONS**).

DOSAGE AND ADMINISTRATION

Apply a thin layer of Olux-E Foam to the affected area(s) twice daily, morning and evening. For proper dispensing of foam, shake the can, hold it upside down, and depress the actuator. Dispense a small amount of foam (not more than a dollop the size of a golf ball) and gently massage the medication into the affected areas (excluding the face, groin, and axillae) until the foam is absorbed. Avoid contact with the eyes.

Treatment should be limited to 2 consecutive weeks and patients should not use greater than 50 grams per week or an amount greater than 21 capfuls per week.

Therapy should be discontinued when control has been achieved. If no improvement is seen within 2 weeks, reassessment of diagnosis may be necessary. Unless directed by a physician, Olux-E Foam should not be used with occlusive dressings.

HOW SUPPLIED

Olux-E (clobetasol propionate) Foam, 0.05% is supplied in 100 gram (NDC 63032-101-00) and 50 gram (NDC 63032-101-50) aluminum cans.

Store at controlled room temperature 68–77°F (20–25°C).

FLAMMABLE. AVOID FIRE, FLAME OR SMOKING DURING AND IMMEDIATELY FOLLOWING APPLICATION.

Contents under pressure. Do not puncture or incinerate. Do not expose to heat or store at temperatures above 120°F (49°C).

Avoid contact with eyes or other mucous membranes.

Keep out of reach of children.

Manufactured for
Stiefel Laboratories, Inc.
Coral Gables, FL 33134
USA
For additional information:
1-888-500-DERM or visit
www.olux-e.com
U.S. Patent No. 6,730,288
U.S. Patent No. 7,029,659
March 2007

SORIATANE® ℞

[sōr-ī-ă-tēn]
(acitretin)
CAPSULES

CAUSES BIRTH DEFECTS

DO NOT GET PREGNANT

Rx Only

CONTRAINDICATIONS AND WARNINGS:

Soriatane must not be used by females who are pregnant, or who intend to become pregnant during therapy or at any time for at least 3 years following discontinuation of therapy. Soriatane also must not be used by females who may not use reliable contraception while undergoing treatment and for at least 3 years following discontinuation of treatment.

Acitretin is a metabolite of etretinate (Tegison®), and major human fetal abnormalities have been reported with the administration of acitretin and etretinate. Potentially, any fetus exposed can be affected.

Clinical evidence has shown that concurrent ingestion of acitretin and ethanol has been associated with the formation of etretinate, which has a significantly longer elimination half-life than acitretin. Because the longer elimination half-life of etretinate would increase the duration of teratogenic potential for female patients, ethanol must not be ingested by female patients either during treatment with Soriatane or for 2 months after cessation of therapy. This allows for elimination of acitretin, thus removing the substrate for transesterification to etretinate. The mechanism of the metabolic process for conversion of acitretin to etretinate has not been fully defined. It is not known whether substances other than ethanol are associated with transesterification.

Acitretin has been shown to be embryotoxic and/or teratogenic in rabbits, mice, and rats at oral doses of 0.6, 3 and 15 mg/kg, respectively. These doses are approximately 0.2, 0.3 and 3 times the maximum recommended therapeutic dose, respectively, based on a mg/m^2 comparison.

Major human fetal abnormalities associated with acitretin and/or etretinate administration have been reported including meningomyelocele, meningoencephalocele, multiple synostoses, facial dysmorphia, syndactyly, absence of terminal phalanges, malformations of hip, ankle and forearm, low-set ears, high palate, decreased cranial volume, cardiovascular malformation and alterations of the skull and cervical vertebrae.

Soriatane should be prescribed only by those who have special competence in the diagnosis and treatment of severe psoriasis, are experienced in the use of systemic retinoids, and understand the risk of teratogenicity.

Because of Soriatane's teratogenicity, a program called the *Do Your P.A.R.T* program, Pregnancy Prevention Actively Required During and After Treatment, has been developed to educate women of childbearing potential and their healthcare providers about the serious risks associated with acitretin and to help prevent pregnancies from occurring with the use of this drug and for 3 years after its discontinuation. The *Do Your P.A.R.T.* program requirements are described below (see also PRECAUTIONS section).

Important Information for Women of Childbearing Potential:

Soriatane should be considered only for women with severe psoriasis unresponsive to other therapies or whose clinical condition contraindicates the use of other treatments.

Females of reproductive potential must not be given a prescription for Soriatane until pregnancy is excluded. Soriatane is contraindicated in females of reproductive potential unless the patient meets ALL of the following conditions:

- **Must have had 2 negative urine or serum pregnancy tests with a sensitivity of at least 25 mIU/mL before receiving the initial Soriatane prescription. The first test (a screening test) is obtained by the prescriber when the decision is made to pursue Soriatane therapy. The second pregnancy test (a confirmation test) should be done during the first 5 days of the menstrual period immediately preceding the beginning of Soriatane therapy. For patients with amenorrhea, the second test should be done at least 11 days after the last act of unprotected sexual intercourse (without using 2 effective forms of contraception [birth control] simultaneously).**
- **Must have a pregnancy test repeated every month during Soriatane treatment. The patient must have a negative result from a urine or serum pregnancy test before receiving a Soriatane prescription. To encourage compliance with this recommendation, a limited supply of the drug should be prescribed. For at least 3 years after discontinuing Soriatane therapy, a pregnancy test must be repeated every 3 months.**
- **Must have selected and have committed to use 2 effective forms of contraception (birth control) simultaneously, at least 1 of which must be a primary form, unless absolute abstinence is the chosen method, or the patient has undergone a hysterectomy or is clearly postmenopausal.**
- **Patients must use 2 effective forms of contraception (birth control) simultaneously for at least 1 month prior to initiation of Soriatane therapy, during Soriatane therapy, and for at least 3 years after discontinuing Soriatane therapy. A Soriatane Patient Referral Form is available so that patients can receive an initial free contraceptive counseling session and pregnancy testing. Counseling about contraception and behaviors associated with an increased risk of pregnancy must be repeated on a monthly basis by the prescriber during Soriatane therapy and every 3 months for at least 3 years following discontinuation of Soriatane therapy. Effective forms of contraception include both primary and secondary forms of contraception. Primary forms of contraception include: tubal ligation, partner's vasectomy, intrauterine devices, birth control pills, and injectable/implantable/insertable/topical hormonal birth control products. Secondary forms of contraception include latex condoms (with or without spermicide), diaphragms and cervical caps (which must be used with a spermicide).**

Any birth control method can fail. Therefore, it is critically important that women of childbearing potential use 2 effective forms of contraception (birth control) simultaneously. It has not been established if there is a pharmacokinetic interaction between acitretin and combined oral contraceptives. However, it has been established that acitretin interferes with the contraceptive effect of microdosed progestin preparations.[1] Microdosed "minipill" progestin preparations are not recommended for use with Soriatane. *It is not known whether other progestational contraceptives, such as implants and injectables, are adequate methods of contraception during acitretin therapy.*

Prescribers are advised to consult the package insert of any medication administered concomitantly with hormonal contraceptives, since some medications may decrease the effectiveness of these birth control products. Patients should be prospectively cautioned not to self-medicate with the herbal supplement St. John's Wort because a possible interaction has been suggested with hormonal contraceptives based on reports of breakthrough bleeding on oral contraceptives shortly after starting St. John's Wort. Pregnancies have been reported by users of combined hormonal contraceptives who also used some form of St. John's Wort (see PRECAUTIONS).

- **Must have signed a Patient Agreement/Informed Consent for Female Patients that contains warnings about the risk of potential birth defects if the fetus is exposed to Soriatane, about contraceptive failure, about the fact that they must not ingest beverages or products containing ethanol while taking Soriatane and for 2 months after Soriatane treatment has been discontinued, and about preventing pregnancy while taking Soriatane and for at least 3 years after discontinuing Soriatane therapy.**

If pregnancy does occur during Soriatane therapy or at any time for at least 3 years following discontinuation of Soriatane therapy, the prescriber and patient should discuss the possible effects on the pregnancy. The available information is as follows:

Acitretin, the active metabolite of etretinate, is teratogenic and is contraindicated during pregnancy. The risk of severe fetal malformations is well established when systemic retinoids are taken during pregnancy. Pregnancy must also be prevented after stopping acitretin therapy, while the drug is being eliminated to below a threshold blood concentration that would be associated with an increased incidence of birth defects. Because this threshold has not been established for acitretin in humans and because elimination rates vary among patients, the duration of posttherapy contraception to achieve adequate elimination cannot be calculated precisely. It is strongly recommended that contraception be continued for at least 3 years after stopping treatment with acitretin, based on the following considerations:

- **In the absence of transesterification to form etretinate, greater than 98% of the acitretin would be eliminated within 2 months, assuming a mean elimination half-life of 49 hours.**
- **In cases where etretinate is formed, as has been demonstrated with concomitant administration of acitretin and ethanol,**
- **greater than 98% of the etretinate formed would be eliminated in 2 years, assuming a mean elimination half-life of 120 days.**
  - **greater than 98% of the etretinate formed would be eliminated in 3 years, based on the longest demonstrated elimination half-life of 168 days.**

However, etretinate was found in plasma and subcutaneous fat in one patient reported to have had sporadic alcohol intake, 52 months after she stopped acitretin therapy.[2]

- **Severe birth defects have been reported where conception occurred during the time interval when the patient was being treated with acitretin and/or etretinate. In addition, severe birth defects have also been reported when conception occurred after the mother completed therapy. These cases have been reported both prospectively (before the outcome was known) and retrospectively (after the outcome was known). The events below are listed without distinction as to whether the reported birth defects are consistent with retinoid-induced embryopathy or not.**
  - **There have been 318 prospectively reported cases involving pregnancies and the use of etretinate, acitretin or both. In 238 of these cases, the conception occurred after the last dose of etretinate (103 cases), acitretin (126) or both (9). Fetal outcome remained unknown in approximately one-half of these cases, of which 62 were terminated and 14 were spontaneous abortions. Fetal outcome is known for the other 118 cases and 15 of the outcomes were abnormal (including cases of absent hand/wrist, clubfoot, GI malformation, hypocalcemia, hypotonia, limb malformation, neonatal apnea/anemia, neonatal ichthyosis, placental disorder/death, undescended testicle and 5 cases of premature birth). In the 126 prospectively reported cases where conception occurred after the last dose of acitretin only, 43 cases involved conception at least 1 year but less than 2 years after the last dose. There were 3 reports of abnormal outcomes out of these 43 cases (involving limb malformation, GI tract malformations and premature birth). There were only 4 cases where conception occurred at least 2 years after the last dose but there were no reports of birth defects in these cases.**
  - **There is also a total of 35 retrospectively reported cases where conception occurred at least one year after the last dose of etretinate, acitretin or both. From these cases there are 3 reports of birth defects when the conception occurred at least 1 year but less than 2 years after the last dose of acitretin (including heart malformations, Turner's Syndrome, and unspecified congenital malformations) and 4 reports of birth defects when conception occurred 2 or more years after the last dose of acitretin (including foot malformation, cardiac malformations [2 cases] and unspecified neonatal and infancy disorder). There were 3 additional**

abnormal outcomes in cases where conception occurred 2 or more years after the last dose of etretinate (including chromosome disorder, forearm aplasia, and stillbirth).

- Females who have taken Tegison (etretinate) must continue to follow the contraceptive recommendations for Tegison. Tegison is no longer marketed in the US; for information, call Stiefel at 1-888-500-DERM (3376).
- Patients should not donate blood during and for at least 3 years following the completion of Soriatane therapy because women of childbearing potential must not receive blood from patients being treated with Soriatane.

Important Information For Males Taking Soriatane:

- Patients should not donate blood during and for at least 3 years following Soriatane therapy because women of childbearing potential must not receive blood from patients being treated with Soriatane.
- Samples of seminal fluid from 3 male patients treated with acitretin and 6 male patients treated with etretinate have been assayed for the presence of acitretin. The maximum concentration of acitretin observed in the seminal fluid of these men was 12.5 ng/mL. Assuming an ejaculate volume of 10 mL, the amount of drug transferred in semen would be 125 ng, which is 1/200,000 of a single 25 mg capsule. Thus, although it appears that residual acitretin in seminal fluid poses little, if any, risk to a fetus while a male patient is taking the drug or after it is discontinued, the no-effect limit for teratogenicity is unknown and there is no registry for birth defects associated with acitretin. The available data are as follows:

There have been 25 cases of reported conception when the male partner was taking acitretin. The pregnancy outcome is known in 13 of these 25 cases. Of these, 9 reports were retrospective and 4 were prospective (meaning the pregnancy was reported prior to knowledge of the outcome)[3]

[See first table at top right]

For All Patients: A SORIATANE MEDICATION GUIDE MUST BE GIVEN TO THE PATIENT EACH TIME SORIATANE IS DISPENSED, AS A REQUIRED BY LAW.

DESCRIPTION

Soriatane (acitretin), a retinoid, is available in 10 mg, 17.5 mg, 22.5 mg, and 25 mg gelatin capsules for oral administration. Chemically, acitretin is all-trans-9-(4-methoxy-2,3,6-trimethylphenyl)-3,7-dimethyl-2,4,6,8-nonatetraenoic acid. It is a metabolite of etretinate and is related to both retinoic acid and retinol (vitamin A). It is a yellow to greenish-yellow powder with a molecular weight of 326.44. The structural formula is:

Each capsule contains acitretin, microcrystalline cellulose, sodium ascorbate, gelatin, black monogramming ink and maltodextrin (a mixture of polysaccharides).
Gelatin capsule shells contain gelatin, iron oxide (yellow, black, and red), and titanium dioxide. They may also contain benzyl alcohol, carboxymethylcellulose sodium, edetate calcium disodium.

CLINICAL PHARMACOLOGY

The mechanism of action of Soriatane is unknown.

Pharmacokinetics:
Absorption:
Oral absorption of acitretin is optimal when given with food. For this reason, acitretin was given with food in all of the following studies. After administration of a single 50 mg oral dose of acitretin to 18 healthy subjects, maximum plasma concentrations ranged from 196 to 728 ng/mL (mean 416 ng/mL) and were achieved in 2 to 5 hours (mean 2.7 hours). The oral absorption of acitretin is linear and proportional with increasing doses from 25 to 100 mg. Approximately 72% (range 47% to 109%) of the administered dose was absorbed after a single 50 mg dose of acitretin was given to 12 healthy subjects.
Distribution:
Acitretin is more than 99.9% bound to plasma proteins, primarily albumin.
Metabolism:
(see *Pharmacokinetic Drug Interactions: Ethanol*):
Following oral absorption, acitretin undergoes extensive metabolism and interconversion by simple isomerization to its 13-cis form (cis-acitretin). The formation of cis-acitretin relative to parent compound is not altered by dose or fed/fast conditions of oral administration of acitretin. Both par-

ent compound and isomer are further metabolized into chain-shortened breakdown products and conjugates, which are excreted. Following multiple-dose administration of acitretin, steady-state concentrations of acitretin and cis-acitretin in plasma are achieved within approximately 3 weeks.
Elimination:
The chain-shortened metabolites and conjugates of acitretin and cis-acitretin are ultimately excreted in the feces (34% to 54%) and urine (16% to 53%). The terminal elimination half-life of acitretin following multiple-dose administration is 49 hours (range 33 to 96 hours), and that of cis-acitretin under the same conditions is 63 hours (range 28 to 157 hours). The accumulation ratio of the parent compound is 1.2; that of cis-acitretin is 6.6.
Special Populations:
Psoriasis:
In an 8-week study of acitretin pharmacokinetics in patients with psoriasis, mean steady-state trough concentrations of acitretin increased in a dose proportional manner with dosages ranging from 10 to 50 mg daily. Acitretin plasma concentrations were nonmeasurable (<4 ng/mL) in all patients 3 weeks after cessation of therapy.
Elderly:
In a multiple-dose study in healthy young (n=6) and elderly (n=8) subjects, a two-fold increase in acitretin plasma concentrations were seen in elderly subjects, although the elimination half-life did not change.
Renal Failure:
Plasma concentrations of acitretin were significantly (59.3%) lower in end-stage renal failure subjects (n=6) when compared to age-matched controls, following single 50 mg oral doses. Acitretin was not removed by hemodialysis in these subjects.

Pharmacokinetic Drug Interactions
(see also boxed CONTRAINDICATIONS AND WARNINGS and *PRECAUTIONS: Drug Interactions*): In studies of in

vivo pharmacokinetic drug interactions, no interaction was seen between acitretin and cimetidine, digoxin, phenprocoumon or glyburide.
Ethanol:
Clinical evidence has shown that etretinate (a retinoid with a much longer half-life, see below) can be formed with concurrent ingestion of acitretin and ethanol. In a two-way crossover study, all 10 subjects formed etretinate with concurrent ingestion of a single 100 mg oral dose of acitretin during a 3-hour period of ethanol ingestion (total ethanol, approximately 1.4 g/kg body weight). A mean peak etretinate concentration of 59 ng/mL (range 22 to 105 ng/mL) was observed, and extrapolation of AUC values indicated that the formation of etretinate in this study was comparable to a single 5 mg oral dose of etretinate. There was no detectable formation of etretinate when a single 100 mg oral dose of acitretin was administered without concurrent ethanol ingestion, although the formation of etretinate without concurrent ethanol ingestion cannot be excluded (see boxed CONTRAINDICATIONS AND WARNINGS). Of 93 evaluable psoriatic patients on acitretin therapy in several foreign studies (10 to 80 mg/day), 16% had measurable etretinate levels (>5 ng/mL).
Etretinate has a much longer elimination half-life compared to that of acitretin. In one study the apparent mean terminal half-life after 6 months of therapy was approximately 120 days (range 84 to 168 days). In another study of 47 patients treated chronically with etretinate, 5 had detectable serum drug levels (in the range of 0.5 to 12 ng/mL) 2.1 to 2.9 years after therapy was discontinued. The long half-life appears to be due to storage of etretinate in adipose tissue.
Progestin-only Contraceptives:
It has not been established if there is a pharmacokinetic interaction between acitretin and combined oral contraceptives. However, it has been established that acitretin interferes with the contraceptive effect of microdosed progestin preparations.[1] Microdosed "minipill" progestin preparations

Timing of Paternal Acitretin Treatment Relative to Conception

	Delivery of Healthy Neonate	Spontaneous Abortion	Induced Abortion	Total
At time of conception	5*	5	1	11
Discontinued ~4 weeks prior	0	0	1**	1
Discontinued ~6 to 8 months prior	0	1	0	1

* Four of 5 cases were prospective.
** With malformation pattern not typical of retinoid embryopathy (bilateral cystic hygromas of neck, hypoplasia of lungs bilateral, pulmonary atresia, VSD with overriding truncus arteriosus).

Table 1. Summary of the Soriatane Efficacy Results of the 8-Week Double-Blind Phase of Studies A and B

Efficacy Variables	Study A		Study B		
	Total daily dose		Total daily dose		
	Placebo (N=29)	50 mg (N=29)	Placebo (N=72)	25 mg (N=74)	50 mg (N=71)
Physician's Global Evaluation					
Baseline	4.62	4.55	4.43	4.37	4.49
Mean Change After 8 Weeks	−0.29	−2.00*	−0.06	−1.06*	−1.57*
Scaling					
Baseline	4.10	3.76	3.97	4.11	4.10
Mean Change After 8 Weeks	−0.22	−1.62*	−0.21	−1.50*	−1.78*
Thickness					
Baseline	4.10	4.10	4.03	4.11	4.20
Mean Change After 8 Weeks	−0.39	−2.10*	−0.18	−1.43*	−2.11*
Erythema					
Baseline	4.21	4.59	4.42	4.24	4.45
Mean Change After 8 Weeks	−0.33	−2.10*	−0.37	−1.12*	−1.65*

* Values were statistically significantly different from placebo and from baseline (p ≤ 0.05). No adjustment for multiplicity was done for Study B.
The efficacy variables consisted of: the mean severity rating of scale, lesion thickness, erythema, and the physician's global evaluation of the current status of the disease. Ratings of scaling, erythema, and lesion thickness, and the ratings of the global assessments were made using a seven-point scale (0=none, 1=trace, 2=mild, 3=mild-moderate, 4=moderate, 5=moderate-severe, 6=severe).

are *not* recommended for use with Soriatane. *It is not known whether other progestational contraceptives, such as implants and injectables, are adequate methods of contraception during acitretin therapy.*

CLINICAL STUDIES

In two double-blind placebo controlled studies, Soriatane was administered once daily to patients with severe psoriasis (ie, covering at least 10% to 20% of the body surface area). At 8 weeks (see Table 1) patients treated in Study A with 50 mg Soriatane per day showed significant improvements ($p \leq 0.05$) relative to baseline and to placebo in the physician's global evaluation and in the mean ratings of severity of psoriasis (scaling, thickness, and erythema). In Study B, differences from baseline and from placebo were statistically significant ($p \leq 0.05$) for all variables at both the 25 mg and 50 mg doses; it should be noted for Study B that no statistical adjustment for multiplicity was carried out.

[See table 1 on previous page]

A subset of 141 patients from both pivotal Studies A and B continued to receive Soriatane in an open fashion for up to 24 weeks. At the end of the treatment period, all efficacy variables, as indicated in Table 2, were significantly improved ($p \leq 0.01$) from baseline, including extent of psoriasis, mean ratings of psoriasis severity and physician's global evaluation.

Table 2. Summary of the First Course of Soriatane Therapy (24 Weeks)

Variables	Study A	Study B
Mean Total Daily Soriatane Dose (mg)	42.8	43.1
Mean Duration of Therapy (Weeks)	21.1	22.6
Physician's Global Evaluation	N=39	N=98
Baseline	4.51	4.43
Mean Change From Baseline	-2.26*	-2.60*
Scaling	N=59	N=132
Baseline	3.97	4.07
Mean Change From Baseline	−2.15*	−2.42*
Thickness	N=59	N=132
Baseline	4.00	4.12
Mean Change From Baseline	−2.44*	−2.66*
Erythema	N=59	N=132
Baseline	4.35	4.33
Mean Change From Baseline	−2.31*	−2.29*

* Indicates that the difference from baseline was statistically significant ($p \leq 0.01$).

The efficacy variables consisted of: the mean severity rating of scale, lesion thickness, erythema, and the physician's global evaluation of the current status of the disease. Ratings of scaling, erythema, and lesion thickness, and the ratings of the global assessments were made using a seven-point scale (0=none, 1=trace, 2=mild, 3=mild-moderate, 4=moderate, 5=moderate-severe, 6=severe).

All efficacy variables improved significantly in a subset of 55 patients from Study A treated for a second, 6-month maintenance course of therapy (for a total of 12 months of treatment); a small subset of patients (n=4) from Study A continued to improve after a third 6-month course of therapy (for a total of 18 months of treatment).

INDICATIONS AND USAGE

Soriatane is indicated for the treatment of severe psoriasis in adults. Because of significant adverse effects associated with its use, Soriatane should be prescribed only by those knowledgeable in the systemic use of retinoids. In females of reproductive potential, Soriatane should be reserved for non-pregnant patients who are unresponsive to other therapies or whose clinical condition contraindicates the use of other treatments (see boxed CONTRAINDICATIONS AND WARNINGS — Soriatane can cause severe birth defects).

Most patients experience relapse of psoriasis after discontinuing therapy. Subsequent courses, when clinically indicated, have produced efficacy results similar to the initial course of therapy.

CONTRAINDICATIONS

Pregnancy Category X
(see boxed CONTRAINDICATIONS AND WARNINGS).
Soriatane is contraindicated in patients with severely impaired liver or kidney function and in patients with chronic abnormally elevated blood lipid values (see boxed WARNINGS: *Hepatotoxicity*, WARNINGS: *Lipids and Possible Cardiovascular Effects*, and PRECAUTIONS).

An increased risk of hepatitis has been reported to result from combined use of methotrexate and etretinate. Consequently, the combination of methotrexate with Soriatane is also contraindicated (see PRECAUTIONS: *Drug Interactions*).

Since both Soriatane and tetracyclines can cause increased intracranial pressure, their combined use is contraindicated (see WARNINGS: *Pseudotumor Cerebri*).

Soriatane is contraindicated in cases of hypersensitivity to the preparation (acitretin or excipients) or to other retinoids.

WARNINGS

(see also boxed CONTRAINDICATIONS AND WARNINGS)

> ***Hepatotoxicity:*** Of the 525 patients treated in US clinical trials, 2 had clinical jaundice with elevated serum bilirubin and transaminases considered related to Soriatane treatment. Liver function test results in these patients returned to normal after Soriatane was discontinued. Two of the 1289 patients treated in European clinical trials developed biopsy-confirmed toxic hepatitis. A second biopsy in one of these patients revealed nodule formation suggestive of cirrhosis. One patient in a Canadian clinical trial of 63 patients developed a three-fold increase of transaminases. A liver biopsy of this patient showed mild lobular disarray, multifocal hepatocyte loss and mild triaditis of the portal tracts compatible with acute reversible hepatic injury. The patient's transaminase levels returned to normal 2 months after Soriatane was discontinued.
>
> The potential of Soriatane therapy to induce hepatotoxicity was prospectively evaluated using liver biopsies in an open-label study of 128 patients. Pretreatment and posttreatment biopsies were available for 87 patients. A comparison of liver biopsy findings before and after therapy revealed 49 (58%) patients showed no change, 21 (25%) improved and 14 (17%) patients had a worsening of their liver biopsy status. For 6 patients, the classification changed from class 0 (no pathology) to class I (normal fatty infiltration; nuclear variability and portal inflammation; both mild); for 7 patients, the change was from class I to class II (fatty infiltration, nuclear variability, portal inflammation and focal necrosis; all moderate to severe); and for 1 patient, the change was from class II to class IIIb (fibrosis, moderate to severe). No correlation could be found between liver function test result abnormalities and the change in liver biopsy status, and no cumulative dose relationship was found.
>
> Elevations of AST (SGOT), ALT (SGPT), GGT (GGTP) or LDH have occurred in approximately 1 in 3 patients treated with Soriatane. Of the 525 patients treated in clinical trials in the US, treatment was discontinued in 20 (3.8%) due to elevated liver function test results. If hepatotoxicity is suspected during treatment with Soriatane, the drug should be discontinued and the etiology further investigated.
>
> Ten of 652 patients treated in US clinical trials of etretinate, of which acitretin is the active metabolite, had clinical or histologic hepatitis considered to be possibly or probably related to etretinate treatment. There have been reports of hepatitis-related deaths worldwide; a few of these patients had received etretinate for a month or less before presenting with hepatic symptoms or signs.

Hyperostosis:
In adults receiving long-term treatment with Soriatane, appropriate examinations should be periodically performed in view of possible ossification abnormalities (see ADVERSE REACTIONS). Because the frequency and severity of iatrogenic bony abnormality in adults is low, periodic radiography is only warranted in the presence of symptoms or long-term use of Soriatane. If such disorders arise, the continuation of therapy should be discussed with the patient on the basis of a careful risk/benefit analysis. In clinical trials with Soriatane, patients were prospectively evaluated for evidence of development or change in bony abnormalities of the vertebral column, knees and ankles.
Vertebral Results:
Of 380 patients treated with Soriatane, 15% had preexisting abnormalities of the spine which showed new changes or progression of preexisting findings. Changes included de-

generative spurs, anterior bridging of spinal vertebrae, diffuse idiopathic skeletal hyperostosis, ligament calcification and narrowing and destruction of a cervical disc space. De novo changes (formation of small spurs) were seen in 3 patients after 1½ to 2½ years.
Skeletal Appendicular Results:
Six of 128 patients treated with Soriatane showed abnormalities in the knees and ankles before treatment that progressed during treatment. In 5, these changes involved the formation of additional spurs or enlargement of existing spurs. The sixth patient had degenerative joint disease which worsened. No patients developed spurs de novo. Clinical complaints did not predict radiographic changes.
Lipids and Possible Cardiovascular Effects:
Blood lipid determinations should be performed before Soriatane is administered and again at intervals of 1 to 2 weeks until the lipid response to the drug is established, usually within 4 to 8 weeks. In patients receiving Soriatane during clinical trials, 66% and 33% experienced elevation in triglycerides and cholesterol, respectively. Decreased high density lipoproteins (HDL) occurred in 40% of patients. These effects of Soriatane were generally reversible upon cessation of therapy.
Patients with an increased tendency to develop hypertriglyceridemia included those with disturbances of lipid metabolism, diabetes mellitus, obesity, increased alcohol intake or a familial history of these conditions. Because of the risk of hypertriglyceridemia, serum lipids must be more closely monitored in high-risk patients and during long-term treatment.
Hypertriglyceridemia and lowered HDL may increase a patient's cardiovascular risk status. Although no causal relationship has been established, there have been post-marketing reports of acute myocardial infarction or thromboembolic events in patients on Soriatane therapy. In addition, elevation of serum triglycerides to greater than 800 mg/dL has been associated with fatal fulminant pancreatitis. Therefore, dietary modifications, reduction in Soriatane dose, or drug therapy should be employed to control significant elevations of triglycerides. If, despite these measures, hypertriglyceridemia and low HDL levels persist, the discontinuation of Soriatane should be considered.
Ophthalmologic Effects:
The eyes and vision of 329 patients treated with Soriatane were examined by ophthalmologists. The findings included dry eyes (23%), irritation of eyes (9%) and brow and lash loss (5%). The following were reported in less than 5% of patients: Bell's Palsy, blepharitis and/or crusting of lids, blurred vision, conjunctivitis, corneal epithelial abnormality, cortical cataract, decreased night vision, diplopia, itchy eyes or eyelids, nuclear cataract, pannus, papilledema, photophobia, posterior subcapsular cataract, recurrent sties and subepithelial corneal lesions.
Any patient treated with Soriatane who is experiencing visual difficulties should discontinue the drug and undergo ophthalmologic evaluation.
Pancreatitis:
Lipid elevations occur in 25% to 50% of patients treated with Soriatane. Triglyceride increases sufficient to be associated with pancreatitis are much less common, although fatal fulminant pancreatitis has been reported. There have been rare reports of pancreatitis during Soriatane therapy in the absence of hypertriglyceridemia.
Pseudotumor Cerebri:
Soriatane and other retinoids administered orally have been associated with cases of pseudotumor cerebri (benign intracranial hypertension). Some of these events involved concomitant use of isotretinoin and tetracyclines. However, the event seen in a single Soriatane patient was not associated with tetracycline use. Early signs and symptoms include papilledema, headache, nausea and vomiting and visual disturbances. Patients with these signs and symptoms should be examined for papilledema and, if present, should discontinue Soriatane immediately and be referred for neurological evaluation and care. Since both Soriatane and tetracyclines can cause increased intracranial pressure, their combined use is contraindicated (see CONTRAINDICATIONS).

PRECAUTIONS

A description of the *Do Your P.A.R.T.* materials is provided below. The main goals of the materials are to explain the program requirements, to reinforce the educational messages, and to assess program effectiveness.
The *Do Your P.A.R.T.* booklet includes:
*The *Do Your P.A.R.T. Patient Brochure:* information on the program requirements, risks of acitretin, and the types of contraceptive methods
*The *Contraceptive Counseling Referral Form* for female patients who want to receive free contraception counseling reimbursed by the manufacturer
*The *Patient Agreement/Informed Consent Form* for female patients
*Medication Guide

The *Do Your P.A.R.T.* program also includes a voluntary patient survey for women of childbearing potential to assess the effectiveness of the Soriatane Pregnancy Prevention Program *Do Your P.A.R.T.*

Information for Patients:

(see Medication Guide for all patients and Patient Agreement/Informed Consent for Female Patients at end of professional labeling):

Patients should be instructed to read the Medication Guide supplied as required by law when Soriatane is dispensed.

Females of reproductive potential:

Soriatane can cause severe birth defects. Female patients must not be pregnant when Soriatane therapy is initiated, they must not become pregnant while taking Soriatane, and for at least 3 years after stopping Soriatane, so that the drug can be eliminated to below a blood concentration that would be associated with an increased incidence of birth defects. Because this threshold has not been established for acitretin in humans and because elimination rates vary among patients, the duration of posttherapy contraception to achieve adequate elimination cannot be calculated precisely (see boxed **CONTRAINDICATIONS AND WARNINGS**).

Females of reproductive potential should also be advised that they must not ingest beverages or products containing ethanol while taking Soriatane and for 2 months after Soriatane treatment has been discontinued. This allows for elimination of the acitretin which can be converted to etretinate in the presence of alcohol.

Female patients should be advised that any method of birth control can fail, including tubal ligation, and that microdosed progestin "minipill" preparations are not recommended for use with Soriatane (see *CLINICAL PHARMACOLOGY: Pharmacokinetic Drug Interactions*). Data from one patient who received a very low-dosed progestin contraceptive (levonorgestrel 0.03 mg) had a significant increase of the progesterone level after three menstrual cycles during acitretin treatment.[2]

Female patients should sign a consent form prior to beginning Soriatane therapy (see boxed **CONTRAINDICATIONS AND WARNINGS**).

Nursing Mothers:

Studies on lactating rats have shown that etretinate is excreted in the milk. There is one prospective case report where acitretin is reported to be excreted in human milk. Therefore, nursing mothers should not receive Soriatane prior to or during nursing because of the potential for serious adverse reactions in nursing infants.

All Patients:

Depression and/or other psychiatric symptoms such as aggressive feelings or thoughts of self-harm have been reported. These events, including self-injurious behavior, have been reported in patients taking other systemically administered retinoids, as well as in patients taking Soriatane. Since other factors may have contributed to these events, it is not known if they are related to Soriatane. Patients should be counseled to stop taking Soriatane and notify their prescriber immediately if they experience psychiatric symptoms.

Patients should be advised that a transient worsening of psoriasis is sometimes seen during the initial treatment period. Patients should be advised that they may have to wait 2 to 3 months before they get the full benefit of Soriatane, although some patients may achieve significant improvements within the first 8 weeks of treatment as demonstrated in clinical trials.

Decreased night vision has been reported with Soriatane therapy. Patients should be advised of this potential problem and warned to be cautious when driving or operating any vehicle at night. Visual problems should be carefully monitored (see WARNINGS and ADVERSE REACTIONS).

Patients should be advised that they may experience decreased tolerance to contact lenses during the treatment period and sometimes after treatment has stopped.

Patients should not donate blood during and for at least 3 years following therapy because Soriatane can cause birth defects and women of childbearing potential must not receive blood from patients being treated with Soriatane.

Because of the relationship of Soriatane to vitamin A, patients should be advised against taking vitamin A supplements in excess of minimum recommended daily allowances to avoid possible additive toxic effects.

Patients should avoid the use of sun lamps and excessive exposure to sunlight (non-medical UV exposure) because the effects of UV light are enhanced by retinoids.

Patients should be advised that they must not give their Soriatane to any other person.

For Prescribers:

Soriatane has not been studied in and is not indicated for treatment of acne.

Phototherapy:

Significantly lower doses of phototherapy are required when Soriatane is used because Soriatane-induced effects on the stratum corneum can increase the risk of erythema (burning) (see DOSAGE AND ADMINISTRATION).

Drug Interactions:

Ethanol:

Clinical evidence has shown that etretinate can be formed with concurrent ingestion of acitretin and ethanol (see boxed CONTRAINDICATIONS AND WARNINGS and CLINICAL PHARMACOLOGY: *Pharmacokinetics*).

Glibenclamide:

In a study of 7 healthy male volunteers, acitretin treatment potentiated the blood glucose lowering effect of glibenclamide (a sulfonylurea similar to chlorpropamide) in 3 of the 7 subjects. Repeating the study with 6 healthy male volunteers in the absence of glibenclamide did not detect an effect of acitretin on glucose tolerance. Careful supervision of diabetic patients under treatment with Soriatane is recommended (see CLINICAL PHARMACOLOGY: *Pharmacokinetics* and DOSAGE AND ADMINISTRATION).

Hormonal Contraceptives:

It has not been established if there is a pharmacokinetic interaction between acitretin and combined oral contraceptives. However, it has been established that acitretin interferes with the contraceptive effect of microdosed progestin "minipill" preparations. Microdosed "minipill" progestin preparations are not recommended for use with Soriatane (see CLINICAL PHARMACOLOGY: *Pharmacokinetic Drug Interactions). It is not known whether other progestational contraceptives, such as implants and injectables, are adequate methods of contraception during acitretin therapy.*

Methotrexate:

An increased risk of hepatitis has been reported to result from combined use of methotrexate and etretinate. Consequently, the combination of methotrexate with acitretin is also contraindicated (see CONTRAINDICATIONS).

Phenytoin:

If acitretin is given concurrently with phenytoin, the protein binding of phenytoin may be reduced.

Tetracyclines:

Since both acitretin and tetracyclines can cause increased intracranial pressure, their combined use is contraindicated (see *CONTRAINDICATIONS and WARNINGS: Pseudotumor Cerebri*).

Vitamin A and oral retinoids:

Concomitant administration of vitamin A and/or other oral retinoids with acitretin must be avoided because of the risk of hypervitaminosis A.

Other:

There appears to be no pharmacokinetic interaction between acitretin and cimetidine, digoxin, or glyburide. Investigations into the effect of acitretin on the protein binding of anticoagulants of the coumarin type (warfarin) revealed no interaction.

Laboratory Tests:

If significant abnormal laboratory results are obtained, either dosage reduction with careful monitoring or treatment discontinuation is recommended, depending on clinical judgment.

Blood Sugar:

Some patients receiving retinoids have experienced problems with blood sugar control. In addition, new cases of diabetes have been diagnosed during retinoid therapy, including diabetic ketoacidosis. In diabetics, blood-sugar levels should be monitored very carefully.

Lipids:

In clinical studies, the incidence of hypertriglyceridemia was 66%, hypercholesterolemia was 33% and that of decreased HDL was 40%. Pretreatment and follow-up measurements should be obtained under fasting conditions. It is recommended that these tests be performed weekly or every other week until the lipid response to Soriatane has stabilized (see WARNINGS).

Liver Function Tests:

Elevations of AST (SGOT), ALT (SGPT) or LDH were experienced by approximately 1 in 3 patients treated with Soriatane. It is recommended that these tests be performed prior to initiation of Soriatane therapy, at 1- to 2-week intervals until stable and thereafter at intervals as clinically indicated (see CONTRAINDICATIONS and boxed WARNINGS).

Carcinogenesis, Mutagenesis, Impairment of Fertility:

Carcinogenesis:

A carcinogenesis study of acitretin in Wistar rats, at doses up to 2 mg/kg/day administered 7 days/week for 104 weeks, has been completed. There were no neoplastic lesions observed that were considered to have been related to treatment with acitretin. An 80-week carcinogenesis study in mice has been completed with etretinate, the ethyl ester of acitretin. Blood level data obtained during this study demonstrated that etretinate was metabolized to acitretin and that blood levels of acitretin exceeded those of etretinate at all times studied. In the etretinate study, an increased incidence of blood vessel tumors (hemangiomas and hemangiosarcomas at several different sites) was noted in male, but not female, mice at doses approximately one-half the maximum recommended human therapeutic dose based on a mg/m^2 comparison.

Mutagenesis:

Acitretin was evaluated for mutagenic potential in the Ames test, in the Chinese hamster (V79/HGPRT) assay, in unscheduled DNA synthesis assays using rat hepatocytes and human fibroblasts and in an in vivo mouse micronucleus assay. No evidence of mutagenicity of acitretin was demonstrated in any of these assays.

Impairment of Fertility:

In a fertility study in rats, the fertility of treated animals was not impaired at the highest dosage of acitretin tested, 3 mg/kg/day (approximately one-half the maximum recommended therapeutic dose based on a mg/m^2 comparison). Chronic toxicity studies in dogs revealed testicular changes (reversible mild to moderate spermatogenic arrest and appearance of multinucleated giant cells) in the highest dosage group (50 then 30 mg/kg/day).

No decreases in sperm count or concentration and no changes in sperm motility or morphology were noted in 31 men (17 psoriatic patients, 8 patients with disorders of keratinization and 6 healthy volunteers) given 30 to 50 mg/day of acitretin for at least 12 weeks.

In these studies, no deleterious effects were seen on either testosterone production, LH or FSH in any of the 31 men.[4-6] No deleterious effects were seen on the hypothalamic-pituitary axis in any of the 18 men where it was measured.[4,5]

Pregnancy:

Teratogenic Effects:

Pregnancy Category X

(see boxed CONTRAINDICATIONS AND WARNINGS).

In a study in which acitretin was administered to male rats only at a dosage of 5 mg/kg/day for 10 weeks (approximate duration of one spermatogenic cycle) prior to and during mating with untreated female rats, no teratogenic effects were observed in the progeny (see boxed CONTRAINDICATIONS AND WARNINGS for information about male use of Soriatane).

Nonteratogenic Effects:

In rats dosed at 3 mg/kg/day (approximately one-half the maximum recommended therapeutic dose based on a mg/m^2 comparison), slightly decreased pup survival and delayed incisor eruption were noted. At the next lowest dose tested, 1 mg/kg/day, no treatment-related adverse effects were observed.

Pediatric Use:

Safety and effectiveness in pediatric patients have not been established. No clinical studies have been conducted in pediatric patients. Ossification of interosseous ligaments and tendons of the extremities, skeletal hyperostoses, decreases in bone mineral density, and premature epiphyseal closure have been reported in children taking other systemic retinoids, including etretinate, a metabolite of Soriatane. A causal relationship between these effects and Soriatane has not been established. While it is not known that these occurrences are more severe or more frequent in children, there is special concern in pediatric patients because of the implications for growth potential (see WARNINGS: Hyperostosis).

Geriatric Use:

Clinical studies of Soriatane did not include sufficient numbers of subjects aged 65 and over to determine whether they respond differently than younger subjects. Other reported clinical experience has not identified differences in responses between the elderly and younger patients. In general, dose selection for an elderly patient should be cautious, usually starting at the low end of the dosing range, reflecting the greater frequency of decreased hepatic, renal, or cardiac function, and of concomitant disease or other drug therapy. A twofold increase in acitretin plasma concentrations was seen in healthy elderly subjects compared with young subjects, although the elimination half-life did not change (see CLINICAL PHARMACOLOGY: Special Populations).

ADVERSE REACTIONS

Hypervitaminosis A produces a wide spectrum of signs and symptoms primarily of the mucocutaneous, musculoskeletal, hepatic, neuropsychiatric, and central nervous systems. Many of the clinical adverse reactions reported to date with Soriatane administration resemble those of the hypervitaminosis A syndrome.

Adverse Events/Postmarketing Reports:

In addition to the events listed in the tables for the clinical trials, the following adverse events have been identified during postapproval use of Soriatane. Because these events are reported voluntarily from a population of uncertain size, it is not always possible to reliably estimate their frequency or establish a causal relationship to drug exposure.

Cardiovascular:

Acute myocardial infarction, thromboembolism (see WARNINGS), stroke.

Nervous System:

Myopathy with peripheral neuropathy has been reported during Soriatane therapy. Both conditions improved with discontinuation of the drug.

Table 3. Adverse Events Frequently Reported During Clinical Trials Percent of Patients Reporting (N=525)

BODY SYSTEM	> 75%	50% to 75%	25% to 50%	10% to 25%
CNS				Rigors
Eye Disorders				Xerophthalmia
Mucous Membranes	Cheilitis		Rhinitis	Dry mouth Epistaxis
Musculoskeletal				Arthralgia Spinal hyperostosis (progression of existing lesions)
Skin and Appendages		Alopecia Skin peeling	Dry skin Nail disorder Pruritus	Erythematous rash Hyperesthesia Paresthesia Paronychia Skin atrophy Sticky skin

Psychiatric:
Aggressive feelings and/or suicidal thoughts have been reported. These events, including self-injurious behavior, have been reported in patients taking other systemically administered retinoids, as well as in patients taking Soriatane. Since other factors may have contributed to these events, it is not known if they are related to Soriatane (see PRECAUTIONS).

Reproductive:
Vulvo-vaginitis due to Candida albicans

Skin and Appendages:
Thinning of the skin, skin fragility and scaling may occur all over the body, particularly on the palms and soles; nail fragility is frequently observed.

Clinical Trials:
During clinical trials with Soriatane, 513/525 (98%) of patients reported a total of 3545 adverse events. One-hundred sixteen patients (22%) left studies prematurely, primarily because of adverse experiences involving the mucous membranes and skin. Three patients died. Two of the deaths were not drug related (pancreatic adenocarcinoma and lung cancer); the other patient died of an acute myocardial infarction, considered remotely related to drug therapy. In clinical trials, Soriatane was associated with elevations in liver function test results or triglyceride levels and hepatitis.
The tables below list by body system and frequency the adverse events reported during clinical trials of 525 patients with psoriasis.
[See table 3 above]
[See table 4 at top of next page]

Laboratory:
Soriatane therapy induces changes in liver function tests in a significant number of patients. Elevations of AST (SGOT), ALT (SGPT) or LDH were experienced by approximately 1 in 3 patients treated with Soriatane. In most patients, elevations were slight to moderate and returned to normal either during continuation of therapy or after cessation of treatment. In patients receiving Soriatane during clinical trials, 66% and 33% experienced elevation in triglycerides and cholesterol, respectively. Decreased high density lipoproteins (HDL) occurred in 40% (see WARNINGS). Transient, usually reversible elevations of alkaline phosphatase have been observed.
Table 5 lists the laboratory abnormalities reported during clinical trials.
[See table 5 at top of page 3144]

OVERDOSAGE
In the event of acute overdosage, Soriatane must be withdrawn at once. Symptoms of overdose are identical to acute hypervitaminosis A, ie, headache and vertigo. The acute oral toxicity (LD$_{50}$) of acitretin in both mice and rats was greater than 4000 mg/kg.
In one reported case of overdose, a 32-year-old male with Darier's disease took 21 × 25 mg capsules (525 mg single dose). He vomited several hours later but experienced no other ill effects.
All female patients of childbearing potential who have taken an overdose of Soriatane must:
1) Have a pregnancy test at the time of overdose; 2) Be counseled as per the boxed CONTRAINDICATIONS AND WARNINGS and PRECAUTIONS sections regarding birth defects and contraceptive use for at least 3 years' duration after the overdose.

DOSAGE AND ADMINISTRATION
There is intersubject variation in the pharmacokinetics, clinical efficacy and incidence of side effects with Soriatane. A number of the more common side effects are dose related. Individualization of dosage is required to achieve sufficient therapeutic response while minimizing side effects. Soriatane therapy should be initiated at 25 to 50 mg per day, given as a single dose with the main meal. Maintenance doses of 25 to 50 mg per day may be given dependent upon an individual patient's response to initial treatment. Relapses may be treated as outlined for initial therapy.
When Soriatane is used with phototherapy, the prescriber should decrease the phototherapy dose, dependent on the patient's individual response (see PRECAUTIONS: General).
Females who have taken Tegison (etretinate) must continue to follow the contraceptive recommendations for Tegison. Tegison is no longer marketed in the US; for information, call Stiefel at 1-888-500-DERM (3376).

Information for Pharmacists:
A Soriatane Medication Guide must be given to the patient each time Soriatane is dispensed, as required by law.

HOW SUPPLIED
Brown and white capsules, 10 mg, imprinted "A-10 mg"; bottles of 30 (NDC 0145-0090-25).
Rich yellow capsules, 17.5 mg, imprinted "A-17.5 mg"; bottles of 30 (NDC 0145-3817-03).
Brown capsules, 22.5 mg, imprinted "A-22.5 mg"; bottles of 30 (NDC 0145-3821-03).
Brown and yellow capsules, 25 mg, imprinted "A-25 mg"; bottles of 30 (NDC 0145-0091-25).
Store between 15° and 25°C (59° and 77°F). Protect from light. Avoid exposure to high temperatures and humidity after the bottle is opened.

REFERENCES
1. Berbis Ph, et al.: *Arch Dermatol Res* (1988) 280: 388-389. **2.** Maier H, Honigsmann H: Concentration of etretinate in plasma and subcutaneous fat after long-term acitretin. *Lancet* 348:1107, 1996. **3.** Geiger JM, Walker M: Is there a reproductive safety risk in male patients treated with acitretin (Neotigason®/Soriatane®)? *Dermatology* 205: 105-107, 2002. **4.** Sigg C, et al.: Andrological investigations in patients treated with etretin. *Dermatologica* 175:48-49, 1987. **5.** Parsch EM, et al.: Andrological investigation in men treated with acitretin (Ro 10-1670). *Andrologia* 22: 479-482, 1990. **6.** Kadar L, et al.: Spermatological investigations in psoriatic patients treated with acitretin. In: Pharmacology of Retinoids in the Skin; Reichert U. et al., ed, KARGER, Basel, vol. 3, pp 253-254, 1988.

PATIENT AGREEMENT/INFORMED CONSENT FOR FEMALE PATIENTS
To be completed by the patient* and signed by her prescriber

CAUSES BIRTH DEFECTS

DO NOT GET PREGNANT

*Must also be initialed by the parent or guardian of a minor patient (under age 18)
Read each item below and initial in the space provided to show that you understand each item. **Do not sign this consent and do not take SORIATANE® (acitretin) if there is anything that you do not understand.**

(Patient's name)
1. I understand that there is a very high risk that my unborn baby could have severe birth defects if I am pregnant or become pregnant while taking SORIATANE in any amount even for short periods of time. Birth defects have also happened in babies of women who became pregnant after stopping SORIATANE treatment.
INITIAL: _____
2. I understand that I must not become pregnant while taking SORIATANE and for at least 3 years after the end of my treatment with SORIATANE.
INITIAL: _____
3. I know that I must avoid all alcohol, including drinks, food, medicines, and over-the-counter products that contain alcohol. I understand that the risk of birth defects may last longer than 3 years if I swallow any form of alcohol during SORIATANE therapy, and for 2 months after I stop taking SORIATANE.
INITIAL: _____
4. I understand that I must not have sexual intercourse, or I must use 2 separate, effective forms of birth control **at the same time**. The only exceptions are if I have had surgery to remove the womb (a hysterectomy) or my prescriber has told me I have gone completely through menopause.
INITIAL: _____
5. I understand that I have to use 2 effective forms of birth control (contraception) at the same time for at least 1 month before starting SORIATANE, for the entire time of SORIATANE therapy, and for at least 3 years after SORIATANE treatment has stopped.
INITIAL: _____
6. I understand that any form of birth control can fail. Therefore, I must use 2 different methods at the same time, every time I have sexual intercourse.
INITIAL: _____
7. I understand that the following are considered effective forms of birth control: Primary: Tubal ligation (having my tubes tied), partner's vasectomy, birth control pills, injectable/implantable/insertable/topical (patch) hormonal birth control products, and IUDs (intrauterine devices). Secondary: Latex condoms (with or without spermicide, which is a special cream or jelly that kills sperm), diaphragms and cervical caps (which must be used with a spermicide). I understand that at least 1 of my 2 methods of birth control must be a primary method.
INITIAL: _____
8. I will talk with my prescriber about any medicines or dietary supplements I plan to take during my SORIATANE treatment because certain birth control methods may not work if I am taking certain medicines or herbal products (for example, Saint John's wort).
INITIAL: _____
9. Unless I have had a hysterectomy or my prescriber says I have gone completely through menopause, I understand that I must have 2 negative pregnancy test results before I can get a prescription to start SORIATANE. I will then have pregnancy tests on a monthly basis during my SORIATANE therapy as instructed by my prescriber. In addition, for at least 3 years after the end of my treatment with SORIATANE, I will have a pregnancy test every 3 months.
INITIAL: _____
10. I understand that I should not start taking SORIATANE until I am *sure* that I am not pregnant and have negative results from 2 pregnancy tests.
INITIAL: _____
11. I have received information on emergency contraception (birth control).
INITIAL: _____
12. I understand that my prescriber can give me a referral for a free contraceptive (birth control) counseling session and pregnancy testing.
INITIAL: _____
13. I understand that on a monthly basis during SORIATANE therapy and every 3 months for at least 3 years after stopping SORIATANE treatment that I should receive counseling from my prescriber about contraception (birth control) and behaviors associated with an increased risk of pregnancy.
INITIAL: _____
14. I understand that I must stop taking SORIATANE right away and call my prescriber if I get pregnant, miss my menstrual period, stop birth control, or have sexual intercourse without using my 2 birth control methods during and at least 3 years after stopping SORIATANE treatment.
INITIAL: _____
15. If I do become pregnant while on SORIATANE or at any time within 3 years of stopping SORIATANE, I understand that I should report my pregnancy to Stiefel at 1-888-500-DERM (3376) or to the Food and Drug Administration (FDA) MedWatch program at 1-800-FDA-1088. The information I share will be kept confidential (private) and will help the company and the FDA evaluate the pregnancy prevention program to prevent birth defects.
INITIAL: _____

I have received a copy of the Do Your P.A.R.T™ brochure. My prescriber has answered all my questions about SORIATANE. I understand that it is my responsibility to follow my doctor's instructions, and not to get pregnant during SORIATANE treatment or for at least 3 years after I stop taking SORIATANE.

I now authorize my prescriber, _____, to begin my treatment with SORIATANE.

Patient signature: _____
Date: _____
Parent/guardian signature (if under age 18): _____
Date: _____
Please print: Patient name and address:
_____
_____
Telephone: _____

I have fully explained to the patient, _____, the nature and purpose of the treatment described above and the risks to females of childbearing potential. I have asked the patient if she has any questions regarding her treatment with SORIATANE and have answered those questions to the best of my ability.

Prescriber signature: _____
Date: _____

MEDICATION GUIDE FOR PATIENTS

SORIATANE®
[sor-RYE-uh-tane]
(acitretin)
CAPSULES

Read this Medication Guide carefully before you start taking Soriatane and read it each time you get more Soriatane. There may be new information.

The first information in this Guide is about birth defects and how to avoid pregnancy. **After this section there is important safety information about possible effects for any patient taking Soriatane.** ALL patients should read this entire Medication Guide carefully.

This information does not take the place of talking with your prescriber about your medical condition or treatment.

What is the most important information I should know about Soriatane?

Soriatane can cause severe birth defects. If you are a female who can get pregnant, you should use Soriatane only if you are not pregnant now, can avoid becoming pregnant for at least 3 years, and other medicines do not work for your severe psoriasis or you cannot use other psoriasis medicines. Information about effects on unborn babies and about how to avoid pregnancy is found in the next section: "What are the important warnings and instructions for females taking Soriatane?".

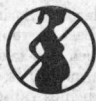

CAUSES BIRTH DEFECTS

DO NOT GET PREGNANT

What are the important warnings and instructions for females taking Soriatane?

- Before you receive your Soriatane prescription, you should have discussed and signed a Patient Information/Consent form with your prescriber. This is to help make sure you understand the risk of birth defects and how to avoid getting pregnant. If you did not talk to your prescriber about this and sign the form, contact your prescriber.

- You must not take Soriatane if you are pregnant or might become pregnant during treatment or at any time for at least 3 years after you stop treatment because Soriatane can cause severe birth defects.

- During Soriatane treatment and for 2 months after you stop Soriatane treatment, you must avoid drinks, foods, and all medicines that contain alcohol. This includes over-the-counter products that contain alcohol. Avoiding alcohol is very important, because alcohol changes Soriatane into a drug that may take longer than 3 years to leave your body. The chance of birth defects may last longer than 3 years if you swallow any form of alcohol during Soriatane therapy and for 2 months after you stop taking Soriatane.

- You and your prescriber must be sure you are not pregnant before you start Soriatane therapy. You must have negative results from 2 pregnancy tests before you start Soriatane treatment. A negative result shows you are not pregnant. Because it takes a few days after pregnancy begins for a test to show that you are pregnant, the first neg-

ative test may not ensure you are not pregnant. Do not start Soriatane until you have negative results from 2 pregnancy tests.

- The **first pregnancy test** will be done at the time you and your prescriber decide if Soriatane might be right for you.

- The **second pregnancy test** will usually be done during the first 5 days of your menstrual period, right before you plan to start Soriatane. Your prescriber may suggest another time.

- After you start Soriatane therapy, you must have a pregnancy test repeated each month that you are taking Soriatane. This is to be sure that you are not pregnant during treatment because Soriatane can cause birth defects.

- For at least 3 years after stopping Soriatane treatment, you must have a pregnancy test repeated every three months to make sure that you are not pregnant.

- **Discuss effective birth control (contraception)** with your prescriber. You must use 2 effective forms of birth control

Table 4. Adverse Events Less Frequently Reported During Clinical Trials (Some of Which May Bear No Relationship to Therapy) Percent of Patients Reporting (N=525)

BODY SYSTEM	1% to 10%		< 1%	
Body as a Whole	Anorexia Edema Fatigue Hot flashes Increased appetite		Alcohol intolerance Dizziness Fever Influenza-like symptoms	Malaise Moniliasis Muscle weakness Weight increase
Cardiovascular	Flushing		Chest pain Cyanosis Increased bleeding time	Intermittent claudication Peripheral ischemia
CNS (also see Psychiatric)	Headache Pain		Abnormal gait Migraine Neuritis	Pseudotumor cerebri (intracranial hypertension)
Eye Disorders	Abnormal/blurred vision Blepharitis Conjunctivitis/ irritation Corneal epithelial abnormality	Decreased night vision/night blindness Eye abnormality Eye pain Photophobia	Abnormal lacrimation Chalazion Conjunctival hemorrhage Corneal ulceration Diplopia Ectropion	Itchy eyes and lids Papilledema Recurrent sties Subepithelial corneal lesions
Gastrointestinal	Abdominal pain Diarrhea Nausea Tongue disorder		Constipation Dyspepsia Esophagitis Gastritis Gastroenteritis	Glossitis Hemorrhoids Melena Tenesmus Tongue ulceration
Liver and Biliary			Hepatic function abnormal Hepatitis Jaundice	
Mucous Membranes	Gingival bleeding Gingivitis Increased saliva	Stomatitis Thirst Ulcerative stomatitis	Altered saliva Anal disorder Gum hyperplasia	Hemorrhage Pharyngitis
Musculoskeletal	Arthritis Arthrosis Back pain Hypertonia Myalgia	Osteodynia Peripheral joint hyperostosis (progression of existing lesions)	Bone disorder Olecranon bursitis Spinal hyperostosis (new lesions) Tendonitis	
Psychiatric	Depression Insomnia Somnolence		Anxiety Dysphonia Libido decreased Nervousness	
Reproductive			Atrophic vaginitis Leukorrhea	
Respiratory	Sinusitis		Coughing Increased sputum Laryngitis	
Skin and Appendages	Abnormal skin odor Abnormal hair texture Bullous eruption Cold/clammy skin Dermatitis Increased sweating Infection	Psoriasiform rash Purpura Pyogenic granuloma Rash Seborrhea Skin fissures Skin ulceration Sunburn	Acne Breast pain Cyst Eczema Fungal infection Furunculosis Hair discoloration Herpes simplex Hyperkeratosis Hypertrichosis Hypoesthesia Impaired healing Otitis media	Otitis externa Photosensitivity reaction Psoriasis aggravated Scleroderma Skin nodule Skin hypertrophy Skin disorder Skin irritation Sweat gland disorder Urticaria Verrucae
Special Senses/Other	Earache Taste perversion Tinnitus		Ceruminosis Deafness Taste loss	
Urinary			Abnormal urine Dysuria Penis disorder	

Table 5. Abnormal Laboratory Test Results Reported During Clinical Trials Percent of Patients Reporting

BODY SYSTEM	50% to 75%	25% to 50%	10% to 25%	1% to 10%
Electrolytes			Increased: – Phosphorus – Potassium – Sodium	Decreased: – Phosphorus – Potassium – Sodium
			Increased and decreased: –Magnesium	Increased and decreased: – Calcium – Chloride
Hematologic		Increased: – Reticulocytes	Decreased: – Hematocrit – Hemoglobin – WBC Increased: – Haptoglobin – Neutrophils – WBC	Increased: – Bands – Basophils – Eosinophils – Hematocrit – Hemoglobin – Lymphocytes – Monocytes
				Decreased: – Haptoglobin – Lymphocytes – Neutrophils – Reticulocytes Increased or decreased: – Platelets – RBC
Hepatic		Increased: – Cholesterol – LDH – SGOT – SGPT Decreased: – HDL cholesterol	Increased: – Alkaline phosphatase – Direct bilirubin – GGTP	Increased: – Globulin – Total bilirubin – Total protein Increased and decreased: – Serum albumin
Miscellaneous	Increased: – Triglycerides	Increased: – CPK – Fasting blood sugar	Decreased: – Fasting blood sugar – High occult blood	Increased and decreased: – Iron
Renal			Increased: – Uric acid	Increased: – BUN – Creatinine
Urinary		WBC in urine	Acetonuria Hematuria RBC in urine	Glycosuria Proteinuria

(contraception) at the same time during all of the following:

• for at least 1 month before beginning Soriatane treatment
• during treatment with Soriatane
• for at least 3 years after stopping Soriatane treatment

• If you are sexually active, you must use 2 effective forms of birth control (contraception) at the same time even if you think you cannot become pregnant, unless 1 of the following is true for you:
   • You had your womb (uterus) removed during an operation (a hysterectomy).
   • Your prescriber said you have gone completely through menopause (the "change of life").

• **You can get a free birth control counseling session and pregnancy testing from a prescriber or family planning expert. Your prescriber can give you a Soriatane Patient Referral Form for this free session.**

• **You must use 2 effective forms of birth control (contraception) at the same time while you are on Soriatane treatment. You must use birth control for at least 1 month before you start Soriatane, during treatment, and at least 3 years after you stop Soriatane treatment.**

The following are considered effective forms of birth control:

Primary Forms:
• having your tubes tied (tubal ligation)
• partner's vasectomy
• IUD (intrauterine device)
• birth control pills that contain both estrogen and progestin (combination oral contraceptives)
• hormonal birth control products that are injected, implanted, or inserted in your body
• birth control patch

Secondary Forms (use with a Primary Form):
• diaphragms with spermicide
• latex condoms (with or without spermicide)
• cervical caps with spermicide

At least 1 of your 2 methods of birth control must be a primary form.

• **If you have sex at any time without using 2 effective forms of birth control (contraception) at the same time,** or if you get pregnant or miss your period, stop using Soriatane and call your prescriber right away.

• **Consider "Emergency Contraception" (EC) if you have sex with a male without correctly using 2 effective forms of birth control (contraception) at the same time.** EC is also called "emergency birth control" or the "morning after" pill. Contact your prescriber **as soon as possible** if you have sex without using 2 effective forms of birth control (contraception) at the same time, because EC works best if it is used within 1 or 2 days after sex. EC is not a replacement for your usual 2 effective forms of birth control (contraception) because it is not as effective as regular birth control methods.

You can get EC from private doctors or nurse practitioners, women's health centers, or hospital emergency rooms. You can get the name and phone number of EC providers nearest you by calling the free Emergency Contraception Hotline at 1-888-NOT-2-LATE (1-888-668-2528).

• **Stop taking Soriatane right away and contact your prescriber if you get pregnant while taking Soriatane or at any time for at least 3 years after treatment has stopped. You need to discuss the possible effects on the unborn baby with your prescriber.**

• **If you do become pregnant while taking Soriatane or at any time for at least 3 years after stopping Soriatane, you should report your pregnancy to Stiefel Laboratories, Inc. at 1-888-500-DERM (3376) or directly to the Food and Drug Administration (FDA) MedWatch program (1-800-FDA-1088).** Your name will be kept in private (confidential). The information you share will help the FDA and the manufacturer evaluate the Pregnancy Prevention Program for Soriatane.

• **Do not take Soriatane if you are breast feeding.** Soriatane can pass into your milk and may harm your baby. You will need to choose either to breast feed or take Soriatane, but not both.

What should males know before taking Soriatane?

Small amounts of Soriatane are found in the semen of males taking Soriatane. Based upon available information, it ap-

pears that these small amounts of Soriatane in semen pose little, if any, risk to an unborn child while a male patient is taking the drug or after it is discontinued. Discuss any concerns you have about this with your prescriber.

All patients should read the rest of this Medication Guide.

What is Soriatane?

Soriatane is a medicine used to treat severe forms of psoriasis in adults. Psoriasis is a skin disease that causes cells in the outer layer of the skin to grow faster than normal and pile up on the skin's surface. In the most common type of psoriasis, the skin becomes inflamed and produces red, thickened areas, often with silvery scales. **Because Soriatane can have serious side effects,** you should talk with your prescriber about whether Soriatane's possible benefits outweigh its possible risks.

Soriatane may not work right away. You may have to wait 2 to 3 months before you get the full benefit of Soriatane. Psoriasis gets worse for some patients when they first start Soriatane treatment.

Soriatane has not been studied in children.

Who should not take Soriatane?

• **Do NOT take Soriatane if you can get pregnant.** Do not take Soriatane if you are pregnant or might get pregnant during Soriatane treatment or at any time for **at least 3 years** after you stop Soriatane treatment (see "What are the important warnings and instructions for females taking Soriatane?").

• **Do NOT take Soriatane if you are breast feeding.** Soriatane can pass into your milk and may harm your baby. You will need to choose either to breast feed or take Soriatane, but not both.

• **Do NOT take Soriatane if you have severe liver or kidney disease.**

• **Do NOT take Soriatane if you have repeated high blood lipids** (fat in the blood).

• **Do NOT take Soriatane if you take these medicines:**
   • methotrexate
   • tetracyclines
   The use of these medicines with Soriatane may cause serious side effects.

• **Do NOT take Soriatane if you are allergic to acitretin,** the active ingredient in Soriatane, to any of the other ingredients (see the end of this Medication Guide for a list of all the ingredients in Soriatane), or to any similar drugs (ask your prescriber or pharmacist whether any drugs you are allergic to are related to Soriatane).

Tell your prescriber if you have or ever had:
• diabetes or high blood sugar
• liver problems
• kidney problems
• high cholesterol or high triglycerides (fat in the blood)
• heart disease
• depression
• alcoholism
• an allergic reaction to a medication

Your prescriber needs this information to decide if Soriatane is right for you and to know what dose is best for you.

Tell your prescriber about all the medicines you take, including prescription and non-prescription medicines, vitamins, and herbal supplements. Some medicines can cause serious side effects if taken while you also take Soriatane. Some medicines may affect how Soriatane works, or Soriatane may affect how your other medicines work. **Be especially sure to tell your prescriber if you are taking the following medicines:**
• methotrexate
• tetracyclines
• phenytoin
• vitamin A supplements
• progestin-only oral contraceptives ("minipills")
• Tegison® or Tigason (etretinate). Tell your prescriber if you have ever taken this medicine in the past.
• St. John's Wort herbal supplement

Tell your prescriber if you are getting phototherapy treatment. Your doses of phototherapy may need to be changed to prevent a burn.

How should I take Soriatane?

• Take Soriatane with food.
• Be sure to take your medicine as prescribed by your prescriber. The dose of Soriatane varies from patient to patient. The number of capsules you must take is chosen specially for you by your prescriber. This dose may change during treatment.
• If you miss a dose, do not double the next dose. Skip the missed dose and resume your normal schedule.
• If you take too much Soriatane (overdose), call your local poison control center or emergency room.

You should have blood tests for liver function, cholesterol and triglycerides before starting treatment and during treatment to check your body's response to Soriatane. Your prescriber may also do other tests.

IMPORTANT NOTICE: Updated drug information is sent bi-monthly via the PDR® Update Insert. For *monthly* email updates, register at PDR.net.

Once you stop taking Soriatane, your psoriasis may return. Do *not* treat this new psoriasis with leftover Soriatane. It is important to see your prescriber again for treatment recommendations because your situation may have changed.

What should I avoid while taking Soriatane?
- **Avoid pregnancy.** See "What is the most important information I should know about Soriatane?", and "What are the important warnings and instructions for females taking Soriatane?".
- **Avoid breast feeding.** See "What are the important warnings and instructions for females taking Soriatane?"
- **Avoid alcohol.** Females must avoid drinks, foods, medicines, and over-the-counter products that contain alcohol. The risk of birth defects may continue for longer than 3 years if you swallow any form of alcohol during Soriatane treatment and for 2 months after stopping Soriatane (see "What are the important warnings and instructions for females taking Soriatane?").
- **Avoid giving blood. Do not donate blood** while you are taking Soriatane and **for at least 3 years after stopping** Soriatane treatment. Soriatane in your blood can harm an unborn baby if your blood is given to a pregnant woman. Soriatane does not affect your ability to receive a blood transfusion.
- **Avoid progestin-only birth control pills ("minipills").** This type of birth control pill may not work while you take Soriatane. Ask your prescriber if you are not sure what type of pills you are using.
- **Avoid night driving if you develop any sudden vision problems.** Stop taking Soriatane and call your prescriber if this occurs (see "Serious side effects").
- **Avoid non-medical ultraviolet (UV) light.** Soriatane can make your skin more sensitive to UV light. Do not use sunlamps, and avoid sunlight as much as possible. If you are taking light treatment (phototherapy), your prescriber may need to change your light dosages to avoid burns.
- **Avoid dietary supplements containing vitamin A.** Soriatane is related to vitamin A. Therefore, do not take supplements containing vitamin A, because they may add to the unwanted effects of Soriatane. Check with your prescriber or pharmacist if you have any questions about vitamin supplements.
- **DO NOT SHARE Soriatane with anyone else, even if they have the same symptoms.** Your medicine may harm them or their unborn child.

What are the possible side effects of Soriatane?
- **Soriatane can cause birth defects.** See "What is the most important information I should know about Soriatane?" and "What are the important warnings and instructions for females taking Soriatane?"
- Psoriasis gets worse for some patients when they first start Soriatane treatment. Some patients have more redness or itching. If this happens, tell your prescriber. These symptoms usually get better as treatment continues, but your prescriber may need to change the amount of your medicine.

Serious side effects.
These do not happen often, but they can lead to permanent harm, or rarely, to death. Stop taking Soriatane and call your prescriber right away if you get the following signs or symptoms:
- **Bad headaches, nausea, vomiting, blurred vision.** These symptoms can be signs of increased brain pressure that can lead to blindness or even death.
- **Decreased vision in the dark** (night blindness). Since this can start suddenly, you should be very careful when driving at night. This problem usually goes away when Soriatane treatment stops. If you develop any vision problems or eye pain stop taking Soriatane and call your prescriber.
- **Depression.** There have been some reports of patients developing mental problems including a depressed mood, aggressive feelings, or thoughts of ending their own life (suicide). These events, including suicidal behavior, have been reported in patients taking other drugs similar to Soriatane as well as patients taking Soriatane. Since other things may have contributed to these problems, it is not known if they are related to Soriatane. It is very important to stop taking Soriatane and call your prescriber right away if you develop such problems.
- **Yellowing of your skin or the whites of your eyes, nausea and vomiting, loss of appetite, or dark urine.** These can be signs of serious liver damage.
- **Aches or pains in your bones, joints, muscles, or back; trouble moving; loss of feeling in your hands or feet.** These can be signs of abnormal changes to your bones or muscles.
- **Frequent urination, great thirst or hunger.** Soriatane can affect blood sugar control, even if you do not already have diabetes. These are some of the signs of high blood sugar.
- **Shortness of breath, dizziness, nausea, chest pain, weakness, trouble speaking, or swelling of a leg.** These may be signs of a heart attack, blood clots, or stroke.

Soriatane can cause serious changes in blood fats (lipids). It is possible for these changes to cause blood vessel blockages that lead to heart attacks, strokes, or blood clots.

Common side effects.
If you develop any of these side effects or any unusual reaction, check with your prescriber to find out if you need to change the amount of Soriatane you take. These side effects usually get better if the Soriatane dose is reduced or Soriatane is stopped.
- **Chapped lips; peeling fingertips, palms, and soles; itching; scaly skin all over; weak nails; sticky or fragile (weak) skin; runny or dry nose, or nosebleeds.** Your prescriber or pharmacist can recommend a lotion or cream to help treat drying or chapping.
- **Dry mouth**
- **Joint pain**
- **Tight muscles**
- **Hair loss.** Most patients have some hair loss, but this condition varies among patients. No one can tell if you will lose hair, how much hair you may lose or if and when it may grow back.
- **Dry eyes.** Soriatane may dry your eyes. Wearing **contact lenses** may be uncomfortable during and after treatment with Soriatane because of the dry feeling in your eyes. If this happens, remove your contact lenses and call your prescriber. Also read the section about vision under "Serious side effects".
- **Rise in blood fats (lipids).** Soriatane can cause your blood fats (lipids) to rise. Most of the time this is not serious. But sometimes the increase can become a serious problem (see information under "Serious side effects"). You should have blood tests as directed by your prescriber.

These are not all the possible side effects of Soriatane. For more information, ask your prescriber or pharmacist.

How should I store Soriatane?
Keep Soriatane away from sunlight, high temperature, and humidity. **Keep Soriatane away from children.**

What are the ingredients in Soriatane?
Active ingredient: acitretin
Inactive ingredients: microcrystalline cellulose, sodium ascorbate, gelatin, black monogramming ink and maltodextrin (a mixture of polysaccharides). Gelatin capsule shells contain gelatin, iron oxide (yellow, black, and red), and titanium dioxide. They may also contain benzyl alcohol, carboxymethylcellulose sodium, edetate calcium disodium.

General information about the safe and effective use of Soriatane
Medicines are sometimes prescribed for purposes other than those listed in a Medication Guide. Do not use Soriatane for a condition for which it was not prescribed. Do not give Soriatane to other people, even if they have the same symptoms that you have.

This Medication Guide summarizes the most important information about Soriatane. If you would like more information, talk with your prescriber. You can ask your pharmacist or prescriber for information about Soriatane that is written for health professionals.

This Medication Guide has been approved by the U.S. Food and Drug Administration.

Tegison® is a registered trademark of Hoffmann-La Roche Inc.

Do Your P.A.R.T. is a trademark, SORIATANE, STIEFEL, and STIEFEL & Design are registered trademarks of Stiefel Laboratories, Inc.
©2009 Stiefel Laboratories, Inc.
STIEFEL®
Manufactured for
Stiefel Laboratories, Inc.
Coral Gables, FL 33134 USA
July 2009
303795

Shown in Product Identification Guide, page 319

VELTIN™   ℞
[*vel-tin*]
(clindamycin phosphate and tretinoin)
Gel 1.2%/0.025%
For topical use only

HIGHLIGHTS OF PRESCRIBING INFORMATION
These highlights do not include all the information needed to use VELTIN Gel safely and effectively. See full prescribing information for VELTIN Gel.

VELTIN™ (clindamycin phosphate and tretinoin) Gel 1.2%/0.025%
For topical use only
Initial U.S. Approval: 2006
——————**INDICATIONS AND USAGE**——————
- VELTIN Gel is a lincosamide antibiotic and retinoid combination product indicated for the topical treatment of acne vulgaris in patients 12 years or older. (1)

——————**DOSAGE AND ADMINISTRATION**——————
- Apply a pea size amount once daily in the evening lightly covering the entire affected area. Avoid the eyes, lips, and mucous membranes. (2)
- Not for oral, ophthalmic, or intravaginal use. (2)
——————**DOSAGE FORMS AND STRENGTHS**——————
- Topical gel: clindamycin phosphate 1.2% and tretinoin 0.025% in 30 gram and 60 gram tubes. (3)
——————**CONTRAINDICATIONS**——————
- VELTIN Gel is contraindicated in patients with regional enteritis, ulcerative colitis, or history of antibiotic-associated colitis. (4)
——————**WARNINGS AND PRECAUTIONS**——————
- Colitis: Clindamycin can cause severe colitis, which may result in death. Diarrhea, bloody diarrhea, and colitis (including pseudomembranous colitis) have been reported with the use of clindamycin. VELTIN Gel should be discontinued if significant diarrhea occurs. (5.1)
- Ultraviolet Light and Environmental Exposure: Avoid exposure to sunlight, sunlamps, and weather extremes. Wear sunscreen daily. (5.2)
——————**ADVERSE REACTIONS**——————
- Observed local treatment-related adverse reactions (≥ 1%) in clinical studies with VELTIN Gel were application site reactions, including dryness, irritation, exfoliation, erythema, pruritus, and dermatitis. Sunburn was also reported. (6.1)

To report SUSPECTED ADVERSE REACTIONS, contact Stiefel Laboratories, Inc. at 1-888-784-3335 or FDA at 1-800-FDA-1088 or www.fda.gov/medwatch.
——————**DRUG INTERACTIONS**——————
- VELTIN Gel should not be used in combination with erythromycin-containing products because of its clindamycin component. (7.1)
——————**USE IN SPECIFIC POPULATIONS**——————
- Pediatric Use: The efficacy and safety have not been established in pediatric patients below the age of 12 years. (8.4)

See 17 for PATIENT COUNSELING INFORMATION
Revised: 07/2010

FULL PRESCRIBING INFORMATION

1   INDICATIONS AND USAGE

VELTIN™ (clindamycin phosphate and tretinoin) Gel, 1.2%/0.025% is indicated for the topical treatment of acne vulgaris in patients 12 years or older.

2   DOSAGE AND ADMINISTRATION

VELTIN Gel should be applied once daily in the evening, gently rubbing the medication to lightly cover the entire affected area. Approximately a pea sized amount will be needed for each application. Avoid the eyes, lips, and mucous membranes.

VELTIN Gel is not for oral, ophthalmic, or intravaginal use.

3   DOSAGE FORMS AND STRENGTHS

VELTIN Gel, containing clindamycin phosphate 1.2% and tretinoin 0.025%, is a yellow, opaque topical gel. Each gram

Table 1: Treatment-Related Adverse Reactions Reported by ≥1% of Subjects

	VELTIN Gel N=1104 n (%)	Clindamycin Gel N=1091 n (%)	Tretinoin Gel N=1084 n (%)	Vehicle Gel N=552 n (%)
Patients with at least one adverse reaction	140 (13)	38 (3)	141 (13)	17 (3)
Application site dryness	64 (6)	12 (1)	62 (6)	3 (1)
Application site irritation	50 (5)	4 (<1)	57 (5)	5 (1)
Application site exfoliation	50 (5)	2 (<1)	56 (5)	2 (<1)
Application site erythema	40 (4)	6 (1)	39 (4)	3 (1)
Application site pruritus	26 (2)	7 (1)	23 (2)	6 (1)
Sunburn	11 (1)	6 (1)	7 (1)	3 (1)
Application site dermatitis	6 (1)	0 (0)	8 (1)	1 (<1)

Table 2: VELTIN GEL-Treated Patients with Local Skin Reactions

	VELTIN GEL		VEHICLE GEL	
Local Reaction	Baseline N= 476 N (%)	End of Treatment N= 409 N (%)	Baseline N= 219 N (%)	End of Treatment N= 209 N (%)
Erythema	24%	21%	31%	35%
Scaling	8%	19%	14%	12%
Dryness	11%	22%	18%	13%
Burning	8%	13%	8%	4%
Itching	17%	15%	22%	14%

of VELTIN Gel contains, as dispensed, 10 mg (1%) clindamycin as clindamycin phosphate, and 0.25 mg (0.025%) tretinoin solubilized in an aqueous based gel.

4 CONTRAINDICATIONS

VELTIN Gel is contraindicated in patients with regional enteritis, ulcerative colitis, or history of antibiotic-associated colitis.

5 WARNINGS AND PRECAUTIONS
5.1 Colitis

Systemic absorption of clindamycin has been demonstrated following topical use. Diarrhea, bloody diarrhea, and colitis (including pseudomembranous colitis) have been reported with the use of topical clindamycin. If significant diarrhea occurs, VELTIN Gel should be discontinued.

Severe colitis has occurred following oral or parenteral administration of clindamycin with an onset of up to several weeks following cessation of therapy. Antiperistaltic agents such as opiates and diphenoxylate with atropine may prolong and/or worsen severe colitis. Severe colitis may result in death.

Studies indicate a toxin(s) produced by clostridia is one primary cause of antibiotic-associated colitis. The colitis is usually characterized by severe persistent diarrhea and severe abdominal cramps and may be associated with the passage of blood and mucus. Stool cultures for *Clostridium difficile* and stool assay for *C. difficile* toxin may be helpful diagnostically.

5.2 Ultraviolet Light and Environmental Exposure

Exposure to sunlight, including sunlamps, should be avoided during the use of VELTIN Gel, and patients with sunburn should be advised not to use the product until fully recovered because of heightened susceptibility to sunlight as a result of the use of tretinoin. Patients who may be required to have considerable sun exposure due to occupation and those with inherent sensitivity to the sun should exercise particular caution. Daily use of sunscreen products and protective apparel (e.g., a hat) are recommended. Weather extremes, such as wind or cold, also may be irritating to patients under treatment with VELTIN Gel.

6 ADVERSE REACTIONS
6.1 Adverse Reactions in Clinical Studies

Because clinical studies are conducted under widely varying conditions, adverse reaction rates observed in clinical studies of a drug cannot be directly compared to rates in the clinical studies of another drug and may not reflect the rates observed in clinical practice.

The safety data reflect exposure to VELTIN Gel in 1,104 patients with acne vulgaris. Patients were 12 years or older

and were treated once daily in the evening for 12 weeks. Adverse reactions that were reported in ≥1% of patients treated with VELTIN Gel are presented in Table 1.
[See table 1 above]
Local skin reactions actively assessed at baseline and end of treatment with a score > 0 are presented in Table 2.
[See table 2 above]
During the twelve weeks of treatment, each local skin reaction peaked at week 2 and gradually reduced thereafter.

7 DRUG INTERACTIONS
7.1 Erythromycin

VELTIN Gel should not be used in combination with erythromycin-containing products due to possible antagonism to the clindamycin component. *In vitro* studies have shown antagonism between these 2 antimicrobials. The clinical significance of this *in vitro* antagonism is not known.

7.2 Neuromuscular Blocking Agents

Clindamycin has been shown to have neuromuscular blocking properties that may enhance the action of other neuromuscular blocking agents. Therefore, VELTIN Gel should be used with caution in patients receiving such agents.

8 USE IN SPECIFIC POPULATIONS
8.1 Pregnancy

Pregnancy Category C. There are no well-controlled studies in pregnant women treated with VELTIN Gel. VELTIN Gel should be used during pregnancy only if the potential benefit justifies the potential risk to the fetus. A limit teratology study performed in Sprague Dawley rats treated topically with VELTIN Gel or 0.025% tretinoin gel at a dose of 2 mL/kg during gestation days 6 to 15 did not result in teratogenic effects. Although no systemic levels of tretinoin were detected, craniofacial and heart abnormalities were described in drug-treated groups. These abnormalities are consistent with retinoid effects and occurred at 16 times the recommended clinical dose assuming 100% absorption and based on body surface area comparison. For purposes of comparison of the animal exposure to human exposure, the recommended clinical dose is defined as 1 g of VELTIN Gel applied daily to a 50 kg person.

Clindamycin
Reproductive developmental toxicity studies performed in rats and mice using oral doses of clindamycin up to 600 mg/kg/day (480 and 240 times the recommended clinical dose based on body surface area comparison, respectively) or subcutaneous doses of clindamycin up to 180 mg/kg/day (140 and 70 times the recommended clinical dose based on body surface area comparison, respectively) revealed no evidence of teratogenicity.

Tretinoin
Oral tretinoin has been shown to be teratogenic in mice, rats, hamsters, rabbits, and primates. It was teratogenic and fetotoxic in Wistar rats when given orally at doses greater than 1 mg/kg/day (32 times the recommended clinical dose based on body surface area comparison). However, variations in teratogenic doses among various strains of rats have been reported. In the cynomologous monkey, a species in which tretinoin metabolism is closer to humans than in other species examined, fetal malformations were reported at oral doses of 10 mg/kg/day or greater, but none were observed at 5 mg/kg/day (324 times the recommended clinical dose based on body surface area comparison), although increased skeletal variations were observed at all doses. Dose-related teratogenic effects and increased abortion rates were reported in pigtail macaques.

With widespread use of any drug, a small number of birth defect reports associated temporally with the administration of the drug would be expected by chance alone. Thirty cases of temporally associated congenital malformations have been reported during two decades of clinical use of another formulation of topical tretinoin. Although no definite pattern of teratogenicity and no causal association have been established from these cases, 5 of the reports describe the rare birth defect category, holoprosencephaly (defects associated with incomplete midline development of the forebrain). The significance of these spontaneous reports in terms of risk to fetus is not known.

8.3 Nursing Mothers

It is not known whether clindamycin is excreted in human milk following use of VELTIN Gel. However, orally and parenterally administered clindamycin has been reported to appear in breast milk. Because of the potential for serious adverse reactions in nursing infants, a decision should be made whether to discontinue nursing or to discontinue the drug, taking into account the importance of the drug to the mother. It is not known whether tretinoin is excreted in human milk. Because many drugs are excreted in human milk, caution should be exercised when VELTIN Gel is administered to a nursing woman.

8.4 Pediatric Use

Safety and effectiveness of VELTIN Gel in pediatric patients below the age of 12 years have not been established. Clinical trials of VELTIN Gel included 2,086 patients 12-17 years of age with acne vulgaris. [See Clinical Studies (14).]

8.5 Geriatric Use

Clinical studies of VELTIN Gel did not include sufficient numbers of subjects aged 65 and over to determine whether they respond differently from younger subjects.

11 DESCRIPTION

VELTIN (clindamycin phosphate and tretinoin) Gel, 1.2%/0.025%, is a fixed combination of two solubilized active ingredients in an aqueous based gel. Clindamycin phosphate is a water soluble ester of the semi-synthetic antibiotic produced by a 7(S)-chloro-substitution of the 7(R)-hydroxyl group of the parent antibiotic lincomycin.

The chemical name for clindamycin phosphate is methyl 7-chloro-6,7,8-trideoxy-6-(1-methyl-*trans*-4-propyl-L-2-pyrrolidinecarboxamido)-1-thio-L-*threo*-α-D-*galacto*-octopyranoside 2-(dihydrogen phosphate). The structural formula for clindamycin phosphate is represented below:
Clindamycin phosphate:

Molecular Formula: $C_{18}H_{34}ClN_2O_8PS$
Molecular Weight: 504.97
The chemical name for tretinoin is all-*trans* 3,7-dimethyl-9-(2,6,6-trimethyl-1-cyclohexen-1-yl)-2,4,6,8-nonatetraenoic acid. It is a member of the retinoid family of compounds. The structural formula for tretinoin is represented below:
Tretinoin:

Molecular Formula: $C_{20}H_{28}O_2$
Molecular Weight: 300.44
VELTIN Gel contains the following inactive ingredients: butylated hydroxytoluene, carbomer 940, anhydrous citric acid, edetate disodium, methylparaben, laureth 4, propylene glycol, tromethamine, and purified water.

12 CLINICAL PHARMACOLOGY
12.1 Mechanism of Action

Clindamycin
[See Microbiology (12.4).]

Tretinoin

Although the exact mode of action of tretinoin is unknown, current evidence suggests that topical tretinoin decreases cohesiveness of follicular epithelial cells with decreased microcomedone formation. Additionally, tretinoin stimulates mitotic activity and increased turnover of follicular epithelial cells causing extrusion of the comedones.

12.3 Pharmacokinetics

In an open-label study of 17 patients with moderate-to-severe acne vulgaris, topical administration of approximately 3 grams of VELTIN Gel once daily for 5 days, clindamycin concentrations were quantifiable in all 17 patients starting from 1 hour post dose. All plasma clindamycin concentrations were ≤5.56 ng/mL on day 5, with the exception of one subject who had a maximum clindamycin concentration of 8.73 ng/mL at 4 hours post-dose. There was no appreciable increase in systemic exposure to tretinoin, as compared to the baseline value. The average tretinoin concentration across all sampling times on day 5 ranged from 1.19 to 1.23 ng/mL compared with the corresponding baseline mean tretinoin concentration range of 1.16 to 1.30 ng/mL.

12.4 Microbiology

No microbiology studies were conducted in the clinical trials with this product.

Mechanism of Action

Clindamycin binds to the 50S ribosomal subunit of susceptible bacteria and prevents elongation of peptide chains by interfering with peptidyl transfer, thereby suppressing protein synthesis. Clindamycin has been shown to have *in vitro* activity against *Propionibacterium acnes (P. acnes)*, an organism that has been associated with acne vulgaris; however, the clinical significance of this activity against *P. acnes* was not examined in clinical studies with VELTIN Gel. *P. acnes* resistance to clindamycin has been documented.

Inducible Clindamycin Resistance

The treatment of acne with antimicrobials is associated with the development of antimicrobial resistance in *P. acnes* as well as other bacteria (e.g. *Staphylococcus aureus*, *Streptococcus pyogenes*). The use of clindamycin may result in developing inducible resistance in these organisms. This resistance is not detected by routine susceptibility testing.

Cross Resistance

Resistance to clindamycin is often associated with resistance to erythromycin.

13 NONCLINICAL TOXICOLOGY

13.1 Carcinogenesis, Mutagenesis, Impairment of Fertility

Long-term animal studies have not been performed to evaluate the carcinogenic potential of VELTIN Gel or the effect of VELTIN Gel on fertility. VELTIN Gel was negative for mutagenic potential when evaluated in an *in vitro* Ames *Salmonella* reversion assay. VELTIN Gel was equivocal for clastogenic potential in the absence of metabolic activation when tested in an *in vitro* chromosomal aberration assay.

Clindamycin

Once daily dermal administration of 1% clindamycin as clindamycin phosphate in the VELTIN Gel vehicle (32 mg/kg/day, 13 times the recommended clinical dose based on body surface area comparison) to mice for up to 2 years did not produce evidence of tumorigenicity.

Fertility studies in rats treated orally with up to 300 mg/kg/day of clindamycin (240 times the recommended clinical dose based on body surface area comparison) revealed no effects on fertility or mating ability.

Tretinoin

In two independent mouse studies where tretinoin was administered topically (0.025% or 0.1%) three times per week for up to two years no carcinogenicity was observed, with maximum effects of dermal amyloidosis. However, in a dermal carcinogenicity study in mice, tretinoin applied at a dose of 5.1 µg (1.4 times the recommended clinical dose based on body surface area comparison) three times per week for 20 weeks acted as a weak promoter of skin tumor formation following a single application of dimethylbenz[α]anthracene (DMBA).

In a study in female SENCAR mice, papillomas were induced by topical exposure to DMBA followed by promotion with 12-O-tetradecanoyl-phorbol 13-acetate or mezerein for up to 20 weeks. Topical application of tretinoin prior to each application of promoting agent resulted in a reduction in the number of papillomas per mouse. However, papillomas resistant to topical tretinoin suppression were at higher risk for pre-malignant progression.

Tretinoin has been shown to enhance photoco-carcinogenicity in properly performed specific studies, employing concurrent or intercurrent exposure to tretinoin and UV radiation. The photoco-carcinogenic potential of the clindamycin tretinoin combination is unknown. Although the significance of these studies to humans is not clear, patients should avoid exposure to sun.

The genotoxic potential of tretinoin was evaluated in an *in vitro* Ames *Salmonella* reversion test and an *in vitro* chromosomal aberration assay in Chinese hamster ovary cells. Both tests were negative.

In oral fertility studies in rats treated with tretinoin, the no-observed-effect-level was 2 mg/kg/day (64 times the recommended clinical dose based on body surface area comparison).

14 CLINICAL STUDIES

The safety and efficacy of VELTIN Gel, applied once daily for the treatment of acne vulgaris, was evaluated in 12-week multicenter, randomized, blinded studies in subjects 12 years and older.

Treatment response was defined as the percent of subjects who had a two grade improvement from baseline to Week 12 based on the Investigator's Global Assessment (IGA) and a mean absolute change from baseline to Week 12 in two out of three (total, inflammatory and non-inflammatory) lesion counts. The IGA scoring scale used in all the clinical trials for VELTIN Gel is as follows:

[See first table above]

In Study 1, 1649 subjects were randomized to VELTIN Gel, Clindamycin gel, Tretinoin gel, and vehicle gel. The median age of subjects was 17 years old and 58% were females. At baseline, subjects had an average of 71 total lesions of which the mean number of inflammatory lesions was 25.5 lesions and the mean number of non-inflammatory lesions was 45.1 lesions. The majority of subjects enrolled with a baseline IGA score of 3. The efficacy results at week 12 are presented in Table 3.

[See table 3 above]

The safety and efficacy of clindamycin-tretinoin gel was also evaluated in two additional 12-week, multi-centered, randomized, blinded, studies in patients 12 years and older. A total of 2219 subjects with mild-to-moderate acne vulgaris were treated once daily for 12 weeks. Of the 2219 subjects, 634 subjects were treated with clindamycin-tretinoin gel. These studies demonstrated consistent outcomes.

0	Clear	Normal, clear skin with no evidence of acne vulgaris.
1	Almost Clear	Skin almost clear; rare non-inflammatory lesions present, with rare non-inflamed papules (papules must be resolving and may be hyperpigmented, though not pink-red) requiring no further treatment in the Investigator's opinion.
2	Mild	Some non-inflammatory lesions are present, with few inflammatory lesions (papules/pustules only, no nodulo-cystic lesions).
3	Moderate	Non-inflammatory lesions predominate, with multiple inflammatory lesions evident; several to many comedones and papules/pustules, and there may or may not be 1 small nodulo-cystic lesion.
4	Severe	Inflammatory lesions are more apparent; many comedones and papules/pustules, there may or may not be a few nodulo-cystic lesions.
5	Very Severe	Highly inflammatory lesions predominate; variable numbers of comedones, many papules/pustules and nodulo-cystic lesions.

Table 3: Efficacy Results at Week 12

Study 1	VELTIN Gel N=476	Clindamycin Gel N=467	Tretinoin Gel N=464	Vehicle Gel N=242
Investigator's Global Assessment				
Percentage of subjects achieving Two Grade Improvement	36.3%	26.6%	26.1%	20.2%
Percentage of subjects achieving an IGA of 0 or 1 with a Two Grade Improvement	33.2%	24.0%	22.6%	17.8%
Inflammatory Lesions:				
Mean absolute reduction	15.5	14.5	13.9	11.1
Mean percentage (%) reduction	60.4%	56.5%	54.5%	43.3%
Non-inflammatory Lesions:				
Mean absolute reduction	23.2	19.5	22.1	17.0
Mean percentage (%) reduction	51.0%	42.9%	47.3%	36.0%
Total Lesions:				
Mean absolute reduction	38.7	34.0	36.0	28.1
Mean percentage (%) reduction	55.0%	49.0%	50.5%	39.1%

16 HOW SUPPLIED/STORAGE AND HANDLING

How Supplied

VELTIN Gel is supplied as follows:
30 g aluminum tubes NDC 0145-0071-30
60 g aluminum tubes NDC 0145-0071-60

Storage and Handling

- Store at 25°C (77°F); excursions permitted to 15–30°C (59–86°F).
- Protect from heat.
- Protect from light.
- Protect from freezing.
- Keep out of reach of children.
- Keep tube tightly closed.

17 PATIENT COUNSELING INFORMATION

[See FDA-approved Patient Labeling].

17.1 Instructions for Use

- At bedtime, the face should be gently washed with a mild soap and water. After patting the skin dry, apply VELTIN Gel as a thin layer over the entire affected area (excluding the eyes and lips).
- Patients should be advised not to use more than a pea sized amount to cover the face and not to apply more often than once daily (at bedtime) as this will not make for faster results and may increase irritation.
- A sunscreen should be applied every morning and reapplied over the course of the day as needed. Patients should be advised to avoid exposure to sunlight, sunlamp, ultraviolet light, and other medicines that may increase sensitivity to sunlight.
- Other topical products with a strong drying effect, such as abrasive soaps or cleansers, may cause an increase in skin irritation with VELTIN Gel.

17.2 Skin Irritation

VELTIN Gel may cause irritation such as erythema, scaling, itching, burning, or stinging.

17.3 Colitis

In the event a patient treated with VELTIN Gel experiences severe diarrhea or gastrointestinal discomfort, VELTIN Gel should be discontinued and a physician should be contacted.

VEL:PI2

PATIENT INFORMATION
VELTIN (vel-tin)
(clindamycin phosphate and tretinoin) Gel

IMPORTANT: For use on skin only (topical use). Do not get VELTIN Gel in your mouth, eyes, or vagina.

Read the Patient Information that comes with VELTIN Gel before you start using it and each time you get a refill. There may be new information. This leaflet does not take the place of talking with your doctor about your medical condition or your treatment.

What is VELTIN Gel?
VELTIN Gel is prescription medicine used on the skin to treat acne in people 12 years and older.
It is not known if VELTIN Gel is safe and effective in children under 12 years of age.

Who should not use VELTIN Gel?
Do not use VELTIN Gel if you have:
• Crohn's disease
• ulcerative colitis
• had inflammation of the colon (colitis) with past antibiotic use
Talk to your doctor if you are not sure if you have one of these conditions.

What should I tell my doctor before using VELTIN Gel?
Before using VELTIN Gel, tell your doctor if you:
• have any allergies
• **Plan to have surgery with general anesthesia.** One of the medicines in VELTIN Gel can affect how certain anesthesia medicines work.
• have any other medical conditions
• **are pregnant or plan to become pregnant.** It is not known if VELTIN Gel may harm your unborn baby.
• **are breast-feeding or plan to breast-feed.** It is not known if VELTIN Gel passes into your breast milk. One of the medicines in VELTIN Gel contains clindamycin. When clindamycin is taken by mouth or injection, it may pass into breast milk. You and your doctor should decide if you will take VELTIN Gel or breast feed. You should not do both.
Tell your doctor about all the medicines and skin products you use. Especially tell your doctor if you take medicine that contains erythromycin. VELTIN Gel should not be used with products that contain erythromycin.
Know the medicines you take. Keep a list of your medicines and show it to your doctor and pharmacist when you get a new medicine.

How should I use VELTIN Gel?
• Use VELTIN Gel exactly as prescribed.
• Your doctor will tell you how long to use VELTIN Gel.
• **Do not** apply VELTIN Gel more than one time each day.
• **Do not** use too much VELTIN Gel, because it may irritate your skin.
Instructions for applying VELTIN Gel:
1. At bedtime, wash your face gently with a mild soap, rinse with water.
2. Pat the skin dry.
3. Squeeze a pea sized amount of medication onto one fingertip. Then, gently rub over the entire affected area. **Do not get VELTIN Gel in your eyes, mouth, or on your lips.**

What should I avoid while using VELTIN Gel?
• Limit your time in sunlight. Avoid using tanning beds or sun lamps. If you have to be in sunlight, wear a wide-brimmed hat or other protective clothing. Apply a sunscreen every morning and re-apply during the day as needed.
• Avoid wind and cold weather during treatment with VELTIN Gel. These may be irritating to your skin.
• Avoid using abrasive soaps and cleansers. These may cause increased skin irritation with VELTIN Gel.

What are the possible side effects of VELTIN Gel?
VELTIN Gel may cause serious side effects, including:
• **Inflammation of the colon (colitis).** Clindamycin, one of the ingredients in VELTIN Gel, can cause severe colitis that may lead to death. Stop taking VELTIN Gel and call your doctor if you develop severe watery diarrhea, or bloody diarrhea.
• **Sunburn.** VELTIN Gel may cause your skin to become sunburned more easily. If your face is sunburned, do not use VELTIN Gel until your sunburn is completely healed. Tretinoin, one of the medicines in VELTIN Gel, makes your skin more sensitive to sunlight. See "What should I avoid while using VELTIN Gel?"

Common side effects of VELTIN Gel include:
• **Skin irritation.** VELTIN Gel may cause skin irritation such as dryness, peeling, burning, or itching.
Talk to your doctor about any side effect that bothers you or that does not go away.
These are not all the side effects with VELTIN Gel. Ask your doctor or pharmacist for more information.
Call your doctor for medical advice about side effects. You may report side effects to FDA at 1-800-FDA-1088.

How should I store VELTIN Gel?
• **Store VELTIN Gel** at room temperature, between 59°F to 86°F (15°C to 30°C).
• Protect from freezing.
• Keep VELTIN Gel away from heat and light.
• **Keep VELTIN Gel and all medicines out of the reach of children.**

General information about VELTIN Gel
Medicines are sometimes prescribed for purposes other than those listed in the patient information leaflet. Do not use VELTIN Gel for a condition for which it was not prescribed. **Do not give VELTIN Gel to other people, even if they have the same symptoms you have. It may harm them.**
This patient information leaflet summarizes the most important information about VELTIN Gel. If you would like more information, talk with your doctor. You can also ask your pharmacist or doctor for information about VELTIN Gel that is written for healthcare professionals. For more information call 1-888-784-3335.

What are the ingredients in VELTIN Gel?
Active Ingredients: clindamycin phosphate and tretinoin
Inactive Ingredients: butylated hydroxytoluene, carbomer 940, anhydrous citric acid, edetate disodium, methylparaben, laureth 4, propylene glycol, tromethamine, and purified water.
Manufactured for:
Stiefel Laboratories, Inc.
Research Triangle Park, NC 27709
Manufactured by:
DPT Laboratories, Ltd.
307 E. Josephine Street
San Antonio, TX 78215
Issued July 2010
VEL:PIL1
STIEFEL and STIEFEL & Design are registered trademarks of Stiefel Laboratories, Inc.
VELTIN is a trademark of Astellas Pharma Europe B.V.
©2010 Stiefel Laboratories, Inc.

VERDESO® ℞
[ver-de-sō]
(desonide)
Foam, 0.05%
For topical use only

HIGHLIGHTS OF PRESCRIBING INFORMATION
These highlights do not include all the information needed to use Verdeso Foam safely and effectively. See full prescribing information for Verdeso Foam.
Verdeso® (desonide) Foam, 0.05%
For topical use only
Initial U.S. Approval: 1972

————INDICATIONS AND USAGE————
• Verdeso Foam is a corticosteroid indicated for the topical treatment of mild to moderate atopic dermatitis in patients 3 months of age and older. (1)

————DOSAGE AND ADMINISTRATION————
• Verdeso Foam should be applied to the affected area(s) twice daily. (2)
• Discontinue therapy when control has been achieved. (2)
• If no improvement is seen within 4 weeks, reassess diagnosis. (2)
• Unless directed by a physician, do not use with occlusive dressings. (2)
• Verdeso Foam is not for oral, ophthalmic, or intravaginal use. (2)
• The safety and efficacy of Verdeso Foam has not been established beyond 4 weeks of use. (2)

————DOSAGE FORMS AND STRENGTHS————
• White to off-white petroleum-based emulsion aerosol foam containing 0.05% desonide. (3)

————CONTRAINDICATIONS————
• None. (4)

————WARNINGS AND PRECAUTIONS————
• Verdeso Foam has been shown to product reversible HPA axis suppression. (5.1, 8.4, 14)
• Systemic effects of topical corticosteroids may also include manifestations of Cushing's syndrome, hyperglycema, facial swelling, glycosuria, withdrawal syndrome, and growth retardation in children. (5.1)
• Systemic absorption may require evaluation for HPA axis suppression. (5.1, 5.5)
• Modify use should HPA axis suppression develop. (5.1)
• Potent corticosteroids, use on large areas, prolonged use or occlusive use may increase systemic absorption. (5.1)
• Pediatric patients may be more susceptible to systemic toxicity. (5.1, 8.4, 12.2)
• Concomitant therapy with topical corticosteroids should be used with caution because a cumulative effect may occur. (5.1)
• Discontinue use if irritation develops. (5.2)
• Initiate appropriate therapy if concomitant skin infections develop. (5.3)

• The propellant in Verdeso Foam is flammable. Avoid fire, flame, or smoking during and immediately following application. (5.4)

————ADVERSE REACTIONS————
• The most common adverse reactions (>1%) are upper respiratory tract infection, cough, application site burning, headache, viral infection, and increased blood pressure. (6.1)
• In post-marketing reports, the most common adverse reactions were application site irritation followed by application site erythema. (6.2)
To report SUSPECTED ADVERSE REACTIONS, contact Stiefel Laboratories, Inc. at 1-888-500-DERM (3376) or FDA at 1-800-FDA-1088 or www.fda.gov/medwatch.

————USE IN SPECIFIC POPULATIONS————
• Administration of topical corticosteroids to children should be limited to the least amount compatible with an effective therapeutic regimen since these patients are at a greater risk than adults of HPA axis suppression and Cushing's syndrome when they are treated with topical corticosteroids. (8.4)
See 17 for PATIENT COUNSELING INFORMATION and FDA-approved patient labeling

Revised: 05/2010

FULL PRESCRIBING INFORMATION: CONTENTS*
* Sections or subsections omitted from the full prescribing information are not listed

FULL PRESCRIBING INFORMATION

1 INDICATIONS AND USAGE

Verdeso® (desonide) Foam, 0.05% is indicated for the treatment of mild to moderate atopic dermatitis in patients 3 months of age and older.
Patients should be instructed to use Verdeso Foam for the minimum amount of time necessary to achieve the desired results because of the potential for Verdeso Foam to suppress the hypothalamic-pituitary-adrenal (HPA) axis. Treatment should not exceed 4 consecutive weeks.

2 DOSAGE AND ADMINISTRATION

Verdeso Foam is not for oral, ophthalmic, or intravaginal use.
A thin layer of Verdeso Foam should be applied to the affected area(s) twice daily. Shake the can before use. Verdeso Foam should be dispensed by inverting the can (upright actuation will cause loss of the propellant which may affect product delivery). Dispense the smallest amount of foam necessary to adequately cover the affected area(s) with a thin layer.
The medication should not be dispensed directly on the face. Dispense in hands and gently massage into affected areas of the face until the medication disappears. For areas other than the face, the medication may be dispensed directly onto the affected area. Take care to avoid contact with the eyes or other mucous membranes.
Patients should dispense the smallest amount of foam as necessary to adequately cover the affected area with a thin layer. Therapy should be discontinued when control is

achieved. If no improvement is seen within 4 weeks, reassessment of diagnosis may be necessary. The safety and efficacy of Verdeso Foam has not been established beyond 4 weeks of use. Treatment should not exceed 4 consecutive weeks.
Unless directed by a physician, Verdeso Foam should not be used with occlusive dressings.

3 DOSAGE FORMS AND STRENGTHS

White to off-white petrolatum-based emulsion aerosol foam containing 0.05% desonide.

4 CONTRAINDICATIONS

None.

5 WARNINGS AND PRECAUTIONS

5.1 Hypothalamic-pituitary-adrenal Axis Suppression

Verdeso Foam has been shown to reversibly suppress the HPA axis.
Topical application of Verdeso Foam may result in systemic absorption and effects including HPA axis suppression, manifestations of Cushing's syndrome, hyperglycemia, facial swelling, glycosuria, withdrawal, and growth retardation in children.
Conditions that augment systemic absorption include the application of topical corticosteroids over large body surface areas, prolonged use, or the addition of occlusive dressings.
Because of the potential for systemic absorption, use of topical corticosteroids may require that patients be periodically evaluated for HPA axis suppression.
An ACTH stimulation test may be helpful in evaluating patients for HPA axis suppression. If HPA axis suppression is documented, an attempt should be made to gradually withdraw the drug, to reduce the frequency of application, or to substitute a less potent steroid. Manifestations of adrenal insufficiency may require supplemental systemic corticosteroids. Recovery of HPA axis function is generally prompt and complete upon discontinuation of topical corticosteroids.
The effect of Verdeso Foam on HPA axis function was investigated in pediatric patients in one study. In this study, patients with atopic dermatitis covering at least 25% of their body applied Verdeso Foam twice daily for 4 weeks. Three out of 75 patients (4%) displayed adrenal suppression after 4 weeks of use based on the cosyntropin stimulation test. The laboratory suppression was transient; all subjects had returned to normal when tested 4 weeks post treatment.
Pediatric patients may be more susceptible than adults to systemic toxicity from equivalent doses of Verdeso Foam due to their larger skin surface to body mass ratios. [see *Use in Specific Populations (8.4)*].
Concomitant therapy with topical corticosteroids should be used with caution because a cumulative effect may occur.

5.2 Skin Irritation

Verdeso Foam may cause local skin adverse reactions [see *Adverse Reactions (6)*]. If irritation develops, Verdeso Foam should be discontinued and appropriate therapy instituted. Allergic contact dermatitis with corticosteroids is usually diagnosed by observing a failure to heal rather than noticing a clinical exacerbation. Such an observation should be corroborated with appropriate diagnostic patch testing.

5.3 Concomitant Skin Infections

If concomitant skin infections are present or develop, the use of an appropriate antifungal, antibacterial or antiviral agent should be instituted. If a favorable response does not occur promptly, use of Verdeso Foam should be discontinued until the infection has been adequately controlled.

5.4 Flammable Contents

The contents of Verdeso Foam include alcohol and propane/butane, which are flammable. Avoid fire, flame and/or smoking during and immediately following application. Do not puncture and/or incinerate the containers. Do not expose containers to heat and/or store at temperatures above 120°F (49°C).

5.5 Laboratory Tests

The cosyntropin ($ACTH_{1-24}$) stimulation test may be helpful in evaluating patients for HPA axis suppression.

6 ADVERSE REACTIONS

6.1 Clinical Trial Experience

Because clinical trials are conducted under widely varying conditions, adverse reaction rate observed in the clinical trials of a drug cannot be directly compared to rates in the clinical trials of another drug and may not reflect the rates observed in clinical practice. In a controlled clinical study of 581 patients 3 months to 17 years of age, adverse reactions occurred at the application site in 6% of subjects treated with Verdeso Foam and 14% of subjects treated with Vehicle Foam. Other commonly reported adverse reactions for Verdeso Foam and Vehicle Foam are noted in Table 1.

Table 1—Adverse Reactions in the Clinical Trial

Adverse Reaction	*Verdeso Foam*	*Vehicle Foam*
	(N=387)	*(N=194)*
Upper respiratory tract infection	37 (10%)	12 (6%)
Cough	14 (4%)	3 (2%)
Application site burning	11 (3%)	15 (8%)
Viral infection	6 (2%)	0 (0%)
Elevated blood pressure	6 (2%)	1 (1%)
Headache	7 (2%)	1 (1%)
Asthma	3 (1%)	0 (0%)
Irritability	2 (1%)	0 (0%)
Pharyngitis	2 (1%)	0 (0%)
Application site atrophy	5 (1%)	0 (0%)
Application site reactions (including atrophy, striae, telangiectasia and pigmentation changes)	3 (1%)	6 (3%)

Other local adverse events occurred at rates less than 1.0%. The majority of adverse reactions were transient and mild to moderate in severity, and they were not affected by age, race, or gender.
The following additional local adverse reactions have been reported with topical corticosteroids. They may occur more frequently with the use of occlusive dressings and higher potency corticosteroids. These reactions are listed in an approximate decreasing order of occurrence: folliculitis, acneiform eruptions, hypopigmentation, perioral dermatitis, allergic contact dermatitis, secondary infection, striae, and miliaria.

6.2 Post-marketing Experience

The following adverse reactions have been identified during post approval use of Verdeso Foam: application site irritation, application site erythema, application site reactions, skin reactions, and swelling face. Because these reactions are reported voluntarily from a population of uncertain size, it is not always possible to reliably estimate their frequency or establish a causal relationship to drug exposure.

8 USE IN SPECIFIC POPULATIONS

8.1 Pregnancy

Teratogenic Effects: Pregnancy Category C:
There are no adequate and well-controlled studies of Verdeso Foam in pregnant women. Therefore, Verdeso Foam should be used during pregnancy only if the potential benefit justifies the potential risk to the fetus.
Corticosteroids have been shown to be teratogenic in laboratory animals when administered systemically at relatively low dosage levels. Some corticosteroids have been shown to be teratogenic after dermal application in laboratory animals.
No long-term reproductive studies in animals have been performed with Verdeso Foam. Dermal embryofetal development studies were conducted in rats and rabbits with a desonide cream, 0.05% formulation. Topical doses of 0.2, 0.6, and 2.0 g cream/kg/day of a desonide cream, 0.05% formulation or 2.0 g/kg of the cream base were administered topically to pregnant rats (gestational days 6–15) and pregnant rabbits (gestational days 6–18). Maternal body weight loss was noted at all dose levels of the desonide cream, 0.05% formulation in rats and rabbits. Teratogenic effects characteristic of corticosteroids were noted in both species. The desonide cream, 0.05% formulation was teratogenic in rats at topical doses of 0.6 and 2.0 g cream/kg/day and in rabbits at a topical dose of 2.0 g cream/kg/day. No teratogenic effects were noted for the desonide cream, 0.05% formulation at a topical dose of 0.2 g cream/kg/day in rats and at a topical dose of 0.6 g cream/kg/day in rabbits. These doses (0.2 g cream/kg/day in rats and 0.6 g cream/kg/day in rabbits) are similar to the maximum recommended human dose based on body surface area comparisons.

8.3 Nursing Mothers

Systemically administered corticosteroids appear in human milk and could suppress growth, interfere with endogenous corticosteroid production, or cause other untoward effects. It is not known whether topical administration of corticosteroids could result in sufficient systemic absorption to produce detectable quantities in human milk. Because many drugs are excreted in human milk, caution should be exercised when Verdeso Foam is administered to a nursing woman.
If used during lactation, Verdeso Foam should not be applied on the chest to avoid accidental ingestion by the infant.

8.4 Pediatric Use

Safety and efficacy in pediatric patients below 3 months of age have not been established and therefore the use of Verdeso Foam is not recommended.
Because of a higher ratio of skin surface area to body mass, pediatric patients are at a greater risk than adults of HPA axis suppression and Cushing's syndrome when they are treated with topical corticosteroids. They are therefore also at greater risk of adrenal insufficiency during and/or after withdrawal of treatment. Adverse effects including striae have been reported with inappropriate use of topical corticosteroids in infants and children. HPA axis suppression, Cushing's syndrome, linear growth retardation, delayed weight gain, and intracranial hypertension have been reported in children receiving topical corticosteroids. Manifestations of adrenal suppression in children include low plasma cortisol levels and an absence of response to ACTH stimulation. Manifestations of intracranial hypertension include bulging fontanelles, headaches, and bilateral papilledema. Administration of topical corticosteroids to children should be limited to the least amount compatible with an effective therapeutic regimen. Chronic corticosteroid therapy may interfere with the growth and development of children.
The effect of Verdeso Foam on HPA axis function was investigated in pediatric patients, ages 6 months to 17 years, in one study. In this study, patients with atopic dermatitis covering at least 25% of their body applied Verdeso Foam twice daily for 4 weeks. Three out of 75 patients (4%) displayed adrenal suppression after 4 weeks of use based on the ACTH stimulation test. The suppression was transient; all subjects' cortisol levels had returned to normal when tested 4 weeks post treatment.

8.5 Geriatric Use

Clinical studies of Verdeso Foam did not include any subjects aged 65 or over to determine whether they respond differently from younger subjects. In general, dose selection for an elderly patient should be cautious, usually starting at the low end of the dosing range, reflecting the greater frequency of decreased hepatic, renal, or cardiac function, and of concomitant disease or other drug therapy.

10 OVERDOSAGE

Topically applied Verdeso Foam can be absorbed in sufficient amounts to produce systemic effects.
Because of a higher ratio of skin surface area to body mass, pediatric patients are at a greater risk than adults of HPA axis suppression and Cushing's syndrome when they are treated with topical corticosteroids.

11 DESCRIPTION

Verdeso Foam is a petrolatum-based emulsion aerosol foam containing the active ingredient desonide, a low-potency topical corticosteroid.
Chemically, desonide is (11β,16α)-11,21-dihydroxy-16, 17-[(1-methylethylidene)-bis(oxy)]-pregna-1,4-diene-3,20-dione. The structural formula of desonide is represented below:

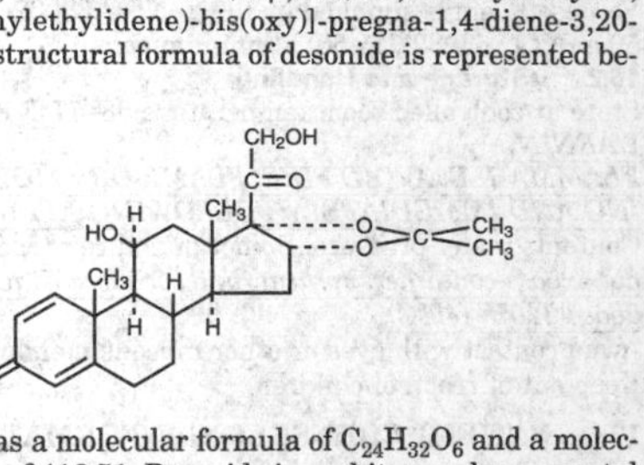

Desonide has a molecular formula of $C_{24}H_{32}O_6$ and a molecular weight of 416.51. Desonide is a white powder or crystal that is practically insoluble in water, sparingly soluble in ethanol and in acetone, and soluble in chloroform. Each gram of Verdeso Foam contains 0.5 mg desonide. The foam also contains anhydrous citric acid, cetyl alcohol, cyclomethicone, isopropyl myristate, light mineral oil, white petrolatum, polyoxyl 20 cetostearyl ether, potassium citrate (monohydrate), propylene glycol, purified water, sorbitan monolaurate, and phenoxyethanol as a preservative.
Verdeso Foam is dispensed from an aluminum can pressurized with a hydrocarbon (propane/butane) propellant.

12 CLINICAL PHARMACOLOGY

12.1 Mechanism of Action

Topical corticosteroids share anti-inflammatory, antipruritic, and vasoconstrictive actions.
The mechanism of anti-inflammatory activity of the topical corticosteroids is unclear. However, corticosteroids are thought to act by the induction of phospholipase A2 inhibitory proteins, collectively called lipocortins. It is postulated

that these proteins control the biosynthesis of potent mediators of inflammation such as prostaglandins and leukotrienes by inhibiting the release of their common precursor arachidonic acid. Arachidonic acid is released from membrane phospholipids by phospholipase A2.

12.2 Pharmacodynamics
In an HPA axis suppression study, 3 of 75 (4%) pediatric patients with mild to moderate atopic dermatitis covering at least 25% body surface area, who applied Verdeso Foam twice daily, experienced reversible suppression of the adrenal glands (as indicated by a 30-minute post-stimulation cortisol level (18 mcg/dL) following 4 weeks of therapy. [See also *Warnings and Precautions (5.1), Pediatric Use (8.4) and Clinical Studies (14)*].

12.3 Pharmacokinetics
The extent of percutaneous absorption of topical corticosteroids is determined by many factors, including the product formulation, the integrity of the epidermal barrier, and age. Occlusion, inflammation and/or other disease processes in the skin may also increase percutaneous absorption. Once absorbed through the skin, topical corticosteroids are handled through pharmacokinetic pathways similar to systemically administered corticosteroids. They are metabolized, primarily in the liver, and are then excreted by the kidneys. Some corticosteroids and their metabolites are also excreted in the bile.

13 NONCLINICAL TOXICOLOGY
13.1 Carcinogenesis, Mutagenesis, Impairment of Fertility
Long-term animal studies have not been performed to evaluate the carcinogenic or photo co-carcinogenic potential of Verdeso Foam or the effect on fertility of desonide.
Desonide revealed no evidence of mutagenic potential based on the results of two in vitro genotoxicity tests (Ames assay, mouse lymphoma cell assay) and an in vivo genotoxicity test (mouse micronucleus assay).

14 CLINICAL STUDIES
In a double-blind, randomized study of 581 patients ages 3 months to 17 years old, with mild to moderate atopic dermatitis, Verdeso Foam was applied twice daily for 4 weeks. Success was defined as the proportion of patients who had all of the following: an Investigator's Static Global Assessment (ISGA) score of clear or almost clear, a minimum improvement in the 5 point ISGA score of 2 grades from Baseline to Week 4, and a score of absent or minimal for both erythema and induration/papulation at Week 4. The results of this study are presented in the following table.

	Verdeso Foam	Vehicle Foam
Number of Patients	387	194
Patients Achieving Success	152 (39%)	18 (9%)

16 HOW SUPPLIED/STORAGE AND HANDLING
16.1 How Supplied
Verdeso Foam is supplied in 100 g (NDC 63032-111-00) and 50 g (NDC 63032-111-50) aluminum cans.
16.2 Storage and Handling
Store at controlled room temperature 68–77°F (20–25°C).
WARNING
FLAMMABLE. AVOID FIRE, FLAME OR SMOKING DURING AND IMMEDIATELY FOLLOWING APPLICATION.
Contents under pressure. Do not puncture or incinerate. *Do not expose containers to heat, and/or store at temperatures above 120°F (49°C).*
Avoid contact with eyes or other mucous membranes.
Keep out of reach of children.

17 PATIENT COUNSELING INFORMATION
See FDA-Approved Patient Labeling
17.1 Information for Patients
Patients using topical corticosteroids should receive the following information and instructions:
1. This medication is to be used as directed by the physician. It is for external use only. Avoid contact with the eyes or other mucous membranes. The medication should not be dispensed directly onto the face. Dispense in hands and gently massage into affected areas of the face until the medication disappears. For areas other than the face, the medication may be dispensed directly on the affected area. Wash hands after use.
2. This medication should not be used for any disorder other than that for which it was prescribed.
3. The treated skin area should not be bandaged, otherwise covered, or wrapped so as to be occlusive unless directed by the physician.
4. Patients should report any signs of local or systemic adverse reactions to the physician.

5. Patients should inform their physicians that they are using Verdeso Foam if surgery is contemplated.
6. Therapy should be discontinued when control is achieved. If no improvement is seen within 4 weeks, contact the physician.
7. Do not use other corticosteroid-containing products while using Verdeso Foam without first consulting your physician.
8. The propellant in Verdeso Foam is flammable. Avoid fire, flame or smoking during and immediately following application.
VDS:1PI

FDA-Approved Patient Labeling
PATIENT INFORMATION
Verdeso (ver-DES-o) (desonide) Foam 0.05%
Read the Patient Information that comes with Verdeso Foam before you start using it and each time you get a refill. There may be new information. This leaflet does not take the place of talking with your doctor about your condition or treatment.

What is Verdeso Foam?
Verdeso Foam is a prescription medicine used on the skin (topical) to treat mild or moderate atopic dermatitis in people 3 months of age and older.
It is not known if Verdeso Foam is safe and effective when used for longer than 4 weeks in a row. You should not use Verdeso Foam for more than 4 weeks in a row without talking with your doctor.
It is not know if Verdeso Foam is safe and effective in children younger than 3 months of age.

What should I tell my doctor before using Verdeso Foam?
Before using Verdeso Foam, tell your doctor if you:
- have a skin infection that is not healing
- have had irritation or other skin reaction to a steroid medicine in the past
- plan to have surgery
- are pregnant or plan to become pregnant. It is not known if Verdeso Foam will harm your unborn baby.
- are breastfeeding or plan to breast feed. It is not know if Verdeso Foam passes into your breast milk. If you use Verdeso Foam while breast-feeding, do not apply it to your chest area. This will help prevent your baby from swallowing Verdeso Foam.
Tell your doctor about all the medicines you take, including prescription and non-prescription medicines, vitamins, and herbal supplements. Especially tell your doctor if you use another medicine on your skin for your atopic dermatitis. Know the medicines you take. Keep a list of them to show your doctor and pharmacist when you get a new medicine.

How should I use Verdeso Foam?
- Use Verdeso Foam exactly as prescribed. Do not use more Verdeso Foam than is needed to cover the affected areas.
- Do not get Verdeso Foam in your eyes, mouth, or vagina.
- Verdeso Foam is usually applied to the affected skin areas 2 times each day.
- Talk to your doctor if your skin does not improve after using Verdeso Foam for 4 weeks.
- You should not use Verdeso Foam for more than 4 weeks in a row without talking with your doctor.
- Verdeso Foam contains alcohol. Alcohol based products are flammable. Avoid fire, flames or smoking while applying Verdeso Foam to your skin and right after you apply it.
- Applying Verdeso Foam.
1. Before applying Verdeso Foam for the first time, break the tiny plastic seal at the base of the nozzle by gently pushing it back away from the seal. Shake the can before use. Remove the cap.
2. Turn the can upside down. Depress the button to dispense a small amount of Verdeso Foam into the palm of your hand or directly onto the affected skin area. Do not apply Verdeso Foam directly to your face. Use the smallest amount of Verdeso Foam needed to cover the affected areas with a thin layer.
3. Gently massage the Verdeso Foam into the affected areas until it disappears. Avoid getting the medicine in your eyes.
4. Do not apply directly on the face. Place in hands and gently massage affected areas of face. Take care to avoid eyes and lips. Remember to wash hands after use.
5. Do not apply a bandage over Verdeso Foam unless your doctor tells you to.
What are the possible side effects of Verdeso Foam?
Common side effects of Verdeso Foam include:
- upper respiratory tract infection
- burning where you apply Verdeso Foam
- cough
- headache
- increased blood pressure
Tell your doctor if you have any side effects that bother you or that do not go away.
These are not all the possible side effects of Verdeso Foam. Ask your doctor or pharmacist for more information.

Call your doctor for medical advice about side effects. You may report side effects to FDA at 1-800-FDA-1088 or to Stiefel at 1-888-500-DERM (3376).
How should I store Verdeso Foam?
- Store the can of Verdeso Foam at room temperature, 68° to 77°F (20°-25°C). Do not place the Verdeso Foam can in the refrigerator or freezer.
- Do not break through (puncture) the Verdeso Foam can.
- Do not throw the can into fire. Verdeso Foam is flammable.
- Keep Verdeso Foam and all medicines out of the reach of children.
General information about Verdeso Foam
Do not use Verdeso Foam for a condition for which it was not prescribed. Do not give Verdeso Foam to other people, even if they have the same symptoms that you have. It may harm them.
This leaflet summarizes the most important information about Verdeso Foam. If you would like more information, talk with your doctor. You can ask your doctor or pharmacist for information about Verdeso Foam that is written for health professionals.
What are the ingredients in Verdeso Foam?
Active ingredient: desonide
Inactive Ingredients: anhydrous citric acid, cetyl alcohol, cyclomethicone, isopropyl myristate, light mineral oil, white petrolatum, polyoxyl 20 cetostearyl ether, potassium citrate (monohydrate), propylene glycol, purified water, sorbitan monolaurate, and phenoxyethanol as a preservative. The can is, pressurized with a hydrocarbon (propane/butane) propellant.
Manufactured for
Stiefel Laboratories, Inc.
Coral Gables, FL 33134
USA
April 2010
VDS:1PIL
VERDESO, VERSAFOAM-EF, VERSAFOAM-EF & Design, STIEFEL, and STIEFEL & DESIGN are registered trademarks of Stiefel Laboratories, Inc.
© 2010 Stiefel Laboratories, Inc.

VUSION®   ℞
[Vu-sion]
(miconazole nitrate, zinc oxide, and white petrolatum) Ointment, for Topical Use Only

HIGHLIGHTS OF PRESCRIBING INFORMATION
These highlights do not include all the information needed to use VUSION Ointment safely and effectively. See full prescribing information for VUSION Ointment.
VUSION® (miconazole nitrate, zinc oxide, and white petrolatum)
Ointment, for topical use only
Initial U.S. Approval: 2006
————————INDICATIONS AND USAGE————————
- VUSION Ointment is indicated for adjunctive treatment of diaper dermatitis when complicated by documented candidiasis (microscopic evidence of pseudohyphae and/or budding yeast) in immunocompetent pediatric patients 4 weeks and older. (1)
- VUSION Ointment should not be used as a substitute for frequent diaper changes. (1)
- VUSION Ointment should not be used to prevent the occurrence of diaper dermatitis, since preventative use may result in the development of drug resistance. (1)
————————DOSAGE AND ADMINISTRATION————————
- VUSION Ointment is for topical use only. VUSION Ointment is not for oral, ophthalmic, or intravaginal use. (2)
- VUSION Ointment should be applied as a thin layer to the affected area at each diaper change for 7 days. (2)
- VUSION Ointment should be used as part of a treatment regimen that includes gentle cleansing of the diaper area and frequent diaper changes. (2)
————————DOSAGE FORMS AND STRENGTHS————————
- Ointment with 0.25% miconazole nitrate, 15% zinc oxide, and 81.35% white petrolatum. (3)
————————CONTRAINDICATIONS————————
- None
————————WARNINGS AND PRECAUTIONS————————
- If irritation occurs or if the disease worsens, discontinue use of the medication, and contact the health care provider. (5)
————————ADVERSE REACTIONS————————
To report SUSPECTED ADVERSE REACTIONS, contact Stiefel Laboratories, Inc. at 1-866-440-5508 or FDA at 1-800-FDA-1088 or www.fda.gov/medwatch.
See 17 for PATIENT COUNSELING INFORMATION
Revised: 04/2010

FULL PRESCRIBING INFORMATION

1   INDICATIONS AND USAGE

1.1   Indication

VUSION Ointment is indicated for the adjunctive treatment of diaper dermatitis only when complicated by documented candidiasis (microscopic evidence of pseudohyphae and/or budding yeast), in immunocompetent pediatric patients 4 weeks and older. A positive fungal culture for *Candida albicans* is not adequate evidence of candidal infection since colonization with *C. albicans* can result in a positive culture. The presence of candidal infection should be established by microscopic evaluation prior to initiating treatment. VUSION should be used as part of a treatment regimen that includes measures directed at the underlying diaper dermatitis, including gentle cleansing of the diaper area and frequent diaper changes.

VUSION should not be used as a substitute for frequent diaper changes. VUSION should not be used to prevent the occurrence of diaper dermatitis, since preventative use may result in the development of drug resistance.

1.2   Limitations of Use

The safety and efficacy of VUSION have not been demonstrated in immunocompromised patients, or in infants less than 4 weeks of age (premature or term).

The safety and efficacy of VUSION have not been evaluated in incontinent adult patients. **VUSION should not be used to prevent the occurrence of diaper dermatitis, such as in an adult institutional setting, since preventative use may result in the development of drug resistance.**

2   DOSAGE AND ADMINISTRATION

VUSION is not for oral, ophthalmic, or intravaginal use. Before applying VUSION, gently cleanse the skin with lukewarm water and pat dry with a soft towel. Avoid using any scented soaps, shampoos, or lotions on the diaper area.

Apply VUSION to the affected area at each diaper change for 7 days. Continue treatment for the full 7 days, even if there is improvement. The safety of VUSION when used for longer than 7 days is not known. Do not use VUSION for longer than 7 days. If symptoms have not improved by day 7, see your health care provider.

Gently apply a thin layer of VUSION to the diaper area with the fingertips. Do not rub VUSION into the skin as this may cause additional irritation. Thoroughly wash hands after applying VUSION.

3   DOSAGE FORMS AND STRENGTHS

White ointment containing 0.25% miconazole nitrate, 15% *zinc oxide*, and 81.35% white petrolatum.

4   CONTRAINDICATIONS

None

5   WARNINGS AND PRECAUTIONS

If irritation occurs or if the disease worsens, discontinue use of the medication, and contact the health care provider.
The safety and efficacy of VUSION have not been evaluated in incontinent adult patients. **VUSION should not be used to prevent the occurrence of diaper dermatitis, such as in an adult institutional setting, since preventative use may result in the development of drug resistance.**

6   ADVERSE REACTIONS

6.1   Clinical Trials Experience

Because clinical trials are conducted under widely varying conditions, adverse reaction rate observed in the clinical trials of a drug cannot be directly compared to rates in the clinical trials of another drug and may not reflect the rates observed in clinical practice.

A total of 835 infants and young children were evaluated in the clinical development program. Of 418 subjects in the VUSION group, 58 (14%) reported one or more adverse events. Of 417 subjects in the zinc oxide/white petrolatum control group, 85 (20%) reported one or more adverse events. Adverse events that occurred at a rate of ≥ 1% for subjects who were treated with VUSION were approximately the same in type and frequency as for subjects who were treated with zinc oxide/white petrolatum ointment.

6.2   Post-marketing Experience

The following adverse reactions have been identified during post approval use of VUSION.

GASTROINTESTINAL DISORDERS: vomiting
GENERAL DISORDERS AND ADMINISTRATION SITE CONDITIONS: burning sensation, condition aggravated, inflammation, pain
INJURY, POISONING AND PROCEDURAL COMPLICATIONS: accidental exposure
SKIN AND SUBCUTANEOUS TISSUE DISORDERS: blister, dermatitis contact, diaper dermatitis, dry skin, erythema, pruritus, rash, skin exfoliation

Because these reactions are reported voluntarily from a population of uncertain size, it is not always possible to reliably estimate their frequency or establish a causal relationship to drug exposure.

7   DRUG INTERACTIONS

Drug-drug interaction studies were not conducted. Women who take a warfarin anticoagulant and use a miconazole intravaginal cream or suppository may be at risk for developing an increased prothrombin time, international normalized ratio (INR), and bleeding. The potential for this interaction between warfarin and VUSION is unknown.

8   USE IN SPECIFIC POPULATIONS

8.1   Pregnancy

Pregnancy Category C

There are no adequate and well-controlled studies of VUSION in pregnant women. Therefore, VUSION should be used during pregnancy only if the potential benefit justifies the potential risk to the fetus.

Miconazole nitrate administration has been shown to result in prolonged gestation and decreased numbers of live young in rats and in increased number of resorptions and decreased number of live young in rabbits at oral doses of 100 mg/kg/day and 80 mg/kg/day, which are 28 and 45 times the maximum possible topical exposure of caregivers, respectively, assuming 100% absorption.

8.3   Nursing Mothers

Safety and efficacy of VUSION have not been established in nursing mothers. It is not known if the active components of VUSION may be present in milk.

8.4   Pediatric Use

Efficacy was not demonstrated in infants less than 4 weeks of age. Safety and efficacy have not been established in very-low-birth-weight infants.

VUSION should not be used to prevent diaper dermatitis. The safety of VUSION when used for longer than 7 days is not known. Do not use more than 7 days.

8.5   Geriatric Use

Safety and efficacy in a geriatric population have not been evaluated.

11   DESCRIPTION

VUSION contains the synthetic antifungal agent, miconazole nitrate (0.25%) USP, zinc oxide (15%) USP, and white petrolatum (81.35%) USP.

The chemical name of miconazole nitrate is 1-[2, 4-dichloro-ß-[(2,4-dichlorobenzyl)oxy] phenethyl] imidazole mononitrate with empirical formula $C_{18}H_{14}Cl_4N_2O \cdot HNO_3$ and molecular weight of 479.15. The structural formula of miconazole nitrate is as follows:

and enantiomer, HNO$_3$

The zinc oxide has an empirical formula of ZnO and a molecular weight of 81.39.

The white petrolatum, which is obtained from petroleum and is wholly or nearly decolorized, is a purified mixture of semisolid saturated hydrocarbons having the general chemical formula C_nH_{2n+2}. The hydrocarbons consist mainly of branched and unbranched chains. White petrolatum contains butylated hydroxytoluene (BHT) as stabilizer.

Each gram of VUSION contains 2.5 mg of miconazole nitrate USP, 150 mg of zinc oxide USP, and 813.5 mg of white petrolatum USP containing butylated hydroxytoluene, trihydroxystearin, and Chemoderm® 1001/B fragrance.[1]

VUSION is a smooth, uniform, white ointment.

12   CLINICAL PHARMACOLOGY

12.1   Mechanism of Action

The miconazole component of VUSION is an antifungal agent [see Clinical Pharmacology (12.4)]. The mechanism of action of white petrolatum and zinc oxide for the adjunctive treatment of diaper dermatitis is unknown.

12.2   Pharmacodynamics

The human pharmacodynamics of Vusion is unknown [see Clinical Pharmacology (12.4) for fungal pharmacodynamics].

12.3   Pharmacokinetics

The topical absorption of miconazole from VUSION was studied in immunocompetent male and female infants and children (n=17) with diaper dermatitis complicated by documented candidiasis (microscopic evidence of pseudohyphae and/or budding yeast) ranging in age from 1 month to 21 months. After multiple daily applications to the affected area at every diaper change (approximately 5-12 times per day) for 7 days, the plasma concentrations of miconazole were below the lower limit of quantitation (LOQ) of 0.5 ng/mL in 15 out of 17 (88%) subjects. In the other 2 remaining subjects, the plasma concentrations of miconazole were 0.57 and 0.58 ng/mL, respectively at a single timepoint (4 hours after the last application) on Day 7.

12.4   Microbiology

The miconazole nitrate component in this product has been shown to have *in vitro* activity against *Candida albicans*, an organism that is associated with diaper dermatitis. The activity of miconazole nitrate against *C. albicans* is based on the inhibition of the ergosterol biosynthesis in the cell membrane. The accumulation of ergosterol precursors and toxic peroxides results in cytolysis of the cell. *In vitro* minimal inhibitory concentration (MIC) test results for *C. albicans* isolates obtained from treatment failures in Clinical Study 1 (*see Clinical Studies (14)*) does not appear to indicate that resistance to miconazole nitrate was the reason for treatment failure. The clinical significance of the *in vitro* activity of miconazole nitrate against *C. albicans* in the setting of diaper dermatitis is unclear.

13   NONCLINICAL TOXICOLOGY

13.1   Carcinogenesis, Mutagenesis, Impairment of Fertility

The carcinogenic potential of VUSION in animals has not been evaluated.

Miconazole nitrate was negative in a bacterial reverse mutation test, a chromosome aberration test in mice, and micronucleus assays in mice and rats.

Miconazole nitrate had no adverse effect on fertility in a study in rats at oral doses of up to 320 mg/kg/day, which is 89 times the maximum possible topical exposure of caregivers, assuming 100% absorption.

14   CLINICAL STUDIES

Study 1 was a double-blind, multicenter study in which VUSION was compared to the zinc oxide and white petrolatum combination treatment and included 236 infants and toddlers with diaper dermatitis, complicated by candidiasis as documented by KOH tests that demonstrated psuedohyphae and/or budding yeasts. Study medication was applied at every diaper change for 7 days.

The primary endpoint was "Overall Cure" and required that subjects be both clinically cured (total resolution of all signs and symptoms of infection) and microbiologically cured (eradication of candidiasis). Primary efficacy was assessed 1 week following the end of treatment, at Day 14.

Study results are shown in the following table.

Overall Cure at Day 14	
VUSION n=112	Zinc Oxide/White Petrolatum n=124
26 (23%)	12 (10%)

Two additional studies provided supportive evidence of the clinical efficacy of VUSION in infants and toddlers with diaper dermatitis, some of whom cultured positive for *C. albicans*. However, candidal infection was not documented in the culture-positive subjects, as microscopic testing (e.g. KOH) was not done. Therefore, the positive culture results may have reflected colonization rather than infection.

16 HOW SUPPLIED/STORAGE AND HANDLING

16.1 How Supplied

VUSION is a smooth, uniform, white ointment supplied in an aluminum tube, as follows:

50g (NDC 0145-0002-04)

16.2 Storage Conditions

Store at controlled room temperature between 20°C and 25°C (68°F and 77°F); with excursions permitted between 15°C and 30°C (59°F and 86°F).

Keep out of reach of children.

17 PATIENT COUNSELING INFORMATION

See FDA-Approved Patient Labeling

Patients using VUSION should be informed about the following information:

- VUSION is to be used only for diaper dermatitis that is complicated by documented candidiasis (i.e. documented by microscopic testing).
- VUSION should not be used as a substitute for frequent diaper changes.
- VUSION should not be used to prevent diaper dermatitis.
- VUSION should not be used long term.
- VUSION should be used only as directed by the health care provider.
- VUSION is for external use only. It is not for oral, ophthalmic, or intravaginal use.
- Gently cleanse the diaper area with lukewarm water or a very mild soap and pat the area dry with a soft towel before applying VUSION.
- Gently apply VUSION to the diaper area with the fingertips after each diaper change. Do not rub VUSION into the skin as this may cause additional irritation.
- Thoroughly wash hands after applying VUSION.
- Treatment should be continued for 7 days, even if there is improvement. Do not use VUSION for longer than 7 days. If symptoms have not improved by day 7, see your health care provider.
- VUSION should not be used on children for whom it is not prescribed.

VSN:2PI

FDA-APPROVED PATIENT LABELING

VUSION® (Vu-sion) Ointment

(0.25% miconazole nitrate, 15% zinc oxide and 81.35% white petrolatum)

IMPORTANT: For Skin Use Only. Do not use in the mouth, eyes, or vagina.

Read the Patient Information that comes with VUSION before you use it on your child. This leaflet does not take the place of talking to your health care provider about your child's medical condition or treatment. If you have any questions or if you are not sure about any of the information on VUSION, ask your health care provider, or pharmacist.

What is VUSION?

VUSION is a prescription skin medicine used to treat diaper rash that also has a yeast infection in children who are at least 4 weeks old and who have a normal immune system. VUSION contains medicines that will help treat the yeast infection and the diaper rash, *but you must also change your child's diapers very often so that your child is not wearing a wet or soiled diaper. Even if you use VUSION, diaper rash will not go away if you do not keep your child's diaper area clean and dry.* You should use water or a very mild cleanser to clean your child's diaper area. VUSION is not to be used to prevent diaper rash or to be used for more than 7 days.

Your health care provider will need to do a special test to tell if your child's diaper rash also has a yeast infection. Do not use VUSION on your child's diaper rash unless your health care provider tells you that there is also a yeast infection.

Who should not use VUSION?

VUSION is not for treatment of all cases of diaper rash. VUSION is only for diaper rash that also has a yeast infection. Most cases of diaper rash do not need the yeast medicine that is in VUSION because most cases of diaper rash do not also have a yeast infection.

Do not use VUSION on any other children or other family member.

Do not use VUSION on your child's diaper rash if they are allergic to anything in it. See the end of this leaflet for a list of ingredients in VUSION.

Do not use on infants less than 4 weeks of age.

Do not use in infants or children who do not have a normal immune system.

How should I use VUSION on my child?

VUSION is applied to the skin on your child's diaper area at each diaper change.

Apply VUSION for the full 7 days even if the diaper rash starts to go away. Call your child's health care provider if the diaper rash gets worse or does not go away with 7 days of treatment with VUSION. *VUSION should not be used for more than 7 days.*

To apply VUSION:

- Gently, clean the skin on your child's diaper area with warm (*not hot*) water. You may also use a very mild soap. Pat the area dry with a soft towel.
- Use your fingertips and gently apply a thin layer of VUSION to your child's diaper area at each diaper change. Do not rub VUSION into your child's skin. Rubbing the skin can cause more irritation.
- Wash your hands after applying VUSION on your child.

VUSION is for skin use only.

Call your child's health care provider or poison control center right away if any VUSION is swallowed. Call your child's health care provider if VUSION gets in the eye.

Keep out of reach of children.

What other steps will help diaper rash go away?

- Check your child's diaper often. Change the diaper at the first sign of wetness.
- Clean your child's diaper area after each diaper change. Gently wipe the diaper area from the front to back using warm (*not hot*) water. You may also use a mild soap. Rinse the diaper area well. Pat dry with a soft towel.
- Keep the diaper area open to air when possible.
- Even if you use VUSION, *diaper rash will not go away if you do not keep your child's diaper area clean and dry.*

What are the possible side effects of VUSION?

VUSION may cause irritation. You should call your child's health care provider if irritation appears or if the diaper rash gets worse.

How should I store VUSION?

- *Keep VUSION out of the reach of children to avoid the risk of accidental ingestion.*
- Store VUSION at room temperature between 68°F to 77°F (20°C to 25°C).

General information about VUSION

Medicines are sometimes prescribed for conditions that are not mentioned in patient information leaflets.

Do not use VUSION for a condition for which it was not prescribed. Do not give VUSION to other children or family members, even if they have the same symptoms your child has. It may harm them.

This leaflet summarizes the most important information about VUSION. If you would like more information, talk to your child's health care provider. You can ask your child's health care provider or pharmacist for information about VUSION that is written for healthcare professionals.

Side effects may be reported to Stiefel Laboratories, Inc. at 1-866-440-5508 or the FDA at 1-800-FDA-1088.

What are the ingredients in VUSION?

Active Ingredients: miconazole nitrate, zinc oxide, and white petrolatum

Inactive Ingredients: trihydroxystearin, butylated hydroxyltoluene (BHT), and Chemoderm® 1001/B fragrance

This Patient Information leaflet has been approved by the U.S. Food and Drug Administration.

The Patient Information leaflet was last revised: January 2010

VSN:2PIL

Manufactured for:

Stiefel Laboratories, Inc.

Coral Gables, FL 33134 USA

Manufactured by:

DSM Pharmaceuticals, Inc.

Greenville, NC 27834

VUSION, STIEFEL, and STIEFEL & Design are registered trademarks of Stiefel Laboratories, Inc.

[1]Chemoderm is a registered trademark of Firmenich Inc.

©2010 Stiefel Laboratories, Inc.

Revised March 2010

SAP#

P/N#

XOLEGEL®

[*Xol-a-gel*]

(ketoconazole) Gel

For Topical Use Only

℞

HIGHLIGHTS OF PRESCRIBING INFORMATION

These highlights do not include all the information needed to use XOLEGEL safely and effectively. See full prescribing information for XOLEGEL.

XOLEGEL® (ketoconazole) Gel

For Topical Use Only

Initial U.S. Approval: 1981

INDICATIONS AND USAGE

- XOLEGEL is an azole antifungal indicated for topical treatment of seborrheic dermatitis in immunocompetent adults and children 12 years of age and older. (1, 12.1)
- Safety and efficacy of XOLEGEL for treatment of fungal infections have not been established. (1)

DOSAGE AND ADMINISTRATION

- XOLEGEL should be applied once daily to the affected area for 2 weeks. (2)
- XOLEGEL is for topical use only, and not for oral, ophthalmic, or intravaginal use. (2)

DOSAGE FORMS AND STRENGTHS

- XOLEGEL is a translucent to clear amber colored gel containing 2% ketoconazole. (3)

CONTRAINDICATIONS

- None.

WARNINGS AND PRECAUTIONS

- Hepatitis and, at high doses, lowered testosterone and ACTH induced corticosteroid serum levels have been seen with orally administered ketoconazole; these effects have not been seen with topically administered ketoconazole. (5.1)
- XOLEGEL is flammable. Avoid using near fire, flame, or smoking during and immediately following application of XOLEGEL. (5.2)

ADVERSE REACTIONS

- The most common treatment-related adverse reaction was application site burning (4%). (6)
- Treatment-related application site reactions that were reported in <1% of subjects were: dermatitis discharge, dryness, erythema, irritation, pain, pruritus, and pustules. (6)
- Treatment-related adverse reactions that were reported in < 1% of subjects were: eye irritation, eye swelling, keratoconjunctivitis sicca, impetigo, pyogenic granuloma, dizziness, headache, paresthesia, acne, nail discoloration, facial swelling. (6)

To report SUSPECTED ADVERSE REACTIONS, contact Stiefel Laboratories, Inc. at 1-866-440-5508 or FDA at 1-800-FDA-1088 or www.fda.gov/medwatch.

USE IN SPECIFIC POPULATIONS

- Based on animal data, XOLEGEL may cause fetal harm. (8.1)

See 17 for PATIENT COUNSELING INFORMATION and FDA-approved patient labeling

Revised: 04/2010

FULL PRESCRIBING INFORMATION: CONTENTS*

* Sections or subsections omitted from the full prescribing information are not listed

---

FULL PRESCRIBING INFORMATION

1 INDICATIONS AND USAGE

XOLEGEL is indicated for the topical treatment of seborrheic dermatitis in immunocompetent adults and children 12 years of age and older.

Safety and efficacy of XOLEGEL for treatment of fungal infections have not been established.

2 DOSAGE AND ADMINISTRATION

XOLEGEL should be applied once daily to the affected area for 2 weeks.

XOLEGEL is for topical use only, and not for oral, ophthalmic, or intravaginal use.

3 DOSAGE FORMS AND STRENGTHS

XOLEGEL is a translucent to clear amber colored gel containing 2% ketoconazole.

4 CONTRAINDICATIONS

None.

5 WARNINGS AND PRECAUTIONS

5.1 Systemic Effects

Hepatitis and, at high doses, lowered testosterone and ACTH induced corticosteroid serum levels have been seen with orally administered ketoconazole; these effects have not been seen with topically administered ketoconazole.

If irritation occurs or if the disease worsens, use of the medication should be discontinued and the health care provider should be contacted.

5.2 Flammable Contents

XOLEGEL is flammable. Avoid being near fire, flame, or smoking during and immediately following application of XOLEGEL.

6 ADVERSE REACTIONS

Because clinical trials are conducted under widely varying conditions, adverse reaction rates observed in the clinical trials of a drug cannot be directly compared to rates in the clinical trials of another drug and may not reflect the rates observed in clinical practice.

In the 3 safety and efficacy trials, 65 of 933 subjects (7%) experienced at least one treatment-related adverse event. The most common treatment-related adverse reaction was application site burning (4%). Treatment-related application site reactions that were reported in < 1% of subjects were: dermatitis, discharge, dryness, erythema, irritation, pain, pruritus, and pustules. Other treatment-related adverse reactions that were reported in < 1% of subjects were: eye irritation, eye swelling, keratoconjunctivitis sicca, impetigo, pyogenic granuloma, dizziness, headache, paresthesia, acne, nail discoloration, facial swelling.

7 DRUG INTERACTIONS

Formal drug interaction studies with XOLEGEL have not been performed.

8 USE IN SPECIFIC POPULATIONS

8.1 Pregnancy

Pregnancy Category C

There are no adequate and well controlled trials in pregnant women. XOLEGEL should be used during pregnancy only if the potential benefit justifies the potential risk to the fetus.

Reproductive toxicity studies have not been performed with XOLEGEL. Ketoconazole was tested for its effects on offspring in the rat at oral doses of 10, 20, 40, 80, and 160 mg/kg. Ketoconazole was teratogenic (syndactylia and oligodactylia) at 80 mg/kg/day and embryotoxic at 160 mg/kg/day (76 and 152 times the human dose, respectively). However, these effects may be related to maternal toxicity, which was also seen at these dose levels.

Oral doses of 10, 20, 40, 80, and 160 mg/kg were studied in pre- and postnatal development studies in rats. Doses of 40 mg/kg (38 times the human dose) and above were associated with maternal toxicity, an increase in the length of gestation, and an increase in the number of stillborn fetuses. These doses of ketoconazole were also toxic to the offspring, resulting in a decrease in fetal/pup weights and viability.

8.3 Nursing Mothers

It is not known whether XOLEGEL is excreted in human milk. Because many drugs are excreted in human milk, caution should be exercised when XOLEGEL is administered to a nursing woman.

If used during lactation and XOLEGEL is applied to the chest, care should be taken to avoid accidental ingestion by the infant.

8.4 Pediatric Use

Safety and effectiveness in pediatric subjects below the age of 12 have not been established.

8.5 Geriatric Use

Of the 933 subjects in the three safety and efficacy trials, 193 (20.7%) were 65 and older, while 61 (6.5%) were 75 and older. No overall differences in safety or effectiveness were observed between these subjects and younger subjects but greater sensitivity of some older individuals cannot be ruled out.

10 OVERDOSAGE

XOLEGEL is intended for topical use only.

There has been no experience of overdose with XOLEGEL. No incidents of accidental ingestion have been reported. A health care provider or poison control center should be contacted in the event of accidental ingestion.

11 DESCRIPTION

XOLEGEL contains the antifungal agent ketoconazole USP at 2% in a topical anhydrous gel vehicle for topical administration. Chemically, ketoconazole is (±)-cis-1-Acetyl-4-[p-[[2-(2,4-dichlorophenyl)-2-(1H-imidazol-1-ylmethyl)-1,3-dioxolan-4-yl]methoxy]phenyl]piperazine, with the molecular formula $C_{26}H_{28}Cl_2N_4O_4$ and a molecular weight of 531.43.

[See chemical structure at top of next column]

Each gram contains: 20 mg ketoconazole USP, dehydrated alcohol (34%), ascorbic acid, butylated hydroxytoluene, citric acid monohydrate, glycerin, hydroxypropyl cellulose, polyethylene glycol 400, PPG-15 stearyl ether, propylene glycol, FD&C yellow No. 6, and FD&C yellow No. 10.

XOLEGEL is a smooth, translucent to clear, amber gel.

Figure 1

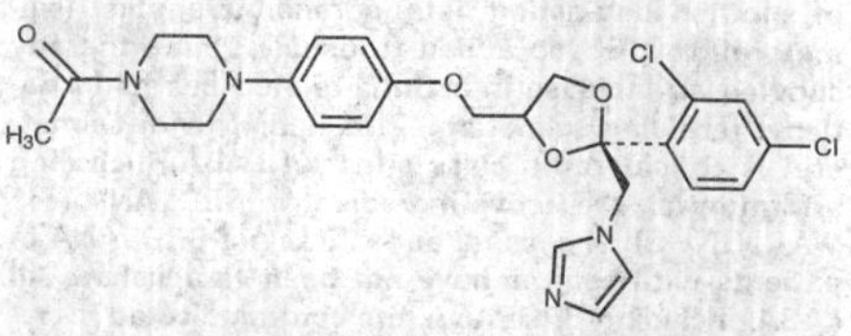

12 CLINICAL PHARMACOLOGY

12.1 Mechanism of Action

The mechanism of action of ketoconazole in the treatment of seborrheic dermatitis is unknown.

12.2 Pharmacodynamics

Pharmacodynamic markers for seborrheic dermatitis have not been identified.

12.3 Pharmacokinetics

In a pharmacokinetic absorption trial, eighteen subjects, both males and females, with severe seborrheic dermatitis (range 1-14% of body surface area) applied XOLEGEL once daily for 2 weeks. The median total amount of gel applied was 4.6 g (range 1.65–46.3 g). Daily doses ranged from 0.05 to 3.47 g. Mean (± standard deviation [SD]) peak plasma levels were 1.35 (± 3.18) ng/mL on Day 7 (range from <0.1 ng/mL, to 13.9 ng/mL), and 0.80 (± 1.22) ng/mL on Day 14 (range from <0.1 ng/mL to 5.4 ng/mL). Median T_{max} was 8 hours on Day 7 and 7 hours on Day 14. Mean (± SD) AUC_{0-24} values were 20.8 (± 44.7) ng•h/mL and 15.6 (± 26.4) ng•h/mL on Day 7 and 14, respectively.

The plasma levels from an oral dose of 200 mg ketoconazole taken with a meal are approximately 250 times higher than the resulting plasma levels of ketoconazole following topical application of XOLEGEL.

13 NONCLINICAL TOXICOLOGY

13.1 Carcinogenesis, Mutagenesis, Impairment of Fertility

Long-term studies to assess the carcinogenic potential of XOLEGEL have not been conducted. A long-term feeding study in Swiss Albino mice and in Wistar rats showed no evidence of oncogenic activity. Ketoconazole gel at a dosage up to 5 mg/kg/dose is not photocarcinogenic when topically applied to hairless mice five days per week for a period of 40 weeks. Ketoconazole produced no evidence of mutagenicity in the dominant lethal mutation test in male and female mice at single oral doses up to 80 mg/kg. When tested in the Ames assay, ketoconazole was found to be non-mutagenic to *Salmonella typhimurium* in the presence and absence of metabolic activation. Ketoconazole, in combination with another drug, gave equivocal results in the mouse micronucleus test. At oral doses of 75 to 80 mg/kg/day (71 to 76 times the human dose) ketoconazole impaired the reproductive performance in female (decreased pregnancy and implantation rates) and male (increased abnormal sperm and decreased sperm motility) rats.

14 CLINICAL STUDIES

Study 1 was a multicenter, double-blind, randomized, vehicle-controlled trial which enrolled 459 subjects 12 years of age and older with moderate to severe seborrheic dermatitis. A total of 229 subjects were treated with XOLEGEL, and 230 subjects were treated with vehicle. All subjects were treated once daily for 14 days, and efficacy was assessed at Day 28 (i.e., 2 weeks after end of treatment). Effective Treatment was defined as:

- an Investigator's Global Assessment score of ≤ 1 (completely clear or almost clear) and
- erythema and scaling scores of 0 (none) if the baseline score was 2, or 1 (mild) if the baseline score was 3.

The proportion of subjects effectively treated is shown in Table 1.

Table 1: Trial Results

	XOLEGEL N=229	*Vehicle N=230*
Number and proportion of subjects effectively treated	58 (25.3%)	32 (13.9%)

Two additional double-blind, randomized, vehicle-controlled, parallel, and multi-center trials that included a total of 316 subjects treated with XOLEGEL provided supportive evidence of the efficacy of XOLEGEL for treatment of seborrheic dermatitis. Subjects applied either XOLEGEL or vehicle study treatment to the affected area(s) once daily for 14 days and were followed through Day 28.

Efficacy was assessed by the proportion of subjects who were completely clear at Day 28. The contribution to efficacy of individual components of the vehicle has not been established.

16 HOW SUPPLIED/STORAGE AND HANDLING

16.1 How Supplied

XOLEGEL® (ketoconazole, USP) Gel, 2% is supplied in 45-gram (NDC 0145-0003-05) white-coated aluminum tubes with white caps, and is dispensed with FDA-Approved Patient Labeling. (17.2)

16.2 Storage and Handling

Store at 25°C (77°F); excursions permitted to 15°-30°C (59°-86°F).

Contents are flammable.

Keep out of reach of children.

17 PATIENT COUNSELING INFORMATION

See FDA-Approved Patient Labeling. (17.2)

17.1 Information for Patients

- This medication is to be used as directed by the health care provider. It is for external use only.
- XOLEGEL may be irritating to mucus membranes. Contact with the eyes, nostrils, and mouth should be avoided.
- As with any topical medication, patients should wash their hands after application.
- This medication should not be used for any disorder other than that for which it has been prescribed.
- Patients should report any signs of adverse reactions to their health care provider.

17.2 Patient Package Insert

PATIENT INFORMATION

XOLEGEL® (Xol-a-gel)

(Ketoconazole, USP) Gel, 2%

Read the Patient Information that comes with XOLEGEL carefully before you start using it and each time you get a refill. There may be new information. This leaflet does not take the place of talking with your health care provider. If you have any questions about XOLEGEL, ask your health care provider.

What is XOLEGEL?

XOLEGEL is a prescription medicine used on the skin to treat a skin condition called seborrheic dermatitis.

Patients with seborrheic dermatitis can have areas of dry, flaky skin on the scalp, face, ears, chest, or upper back.

XOLEGEL is only to be used in adults and in children older than 12 years of age who have a normal (healthy) immune system. XOLEGEL has not been studied in children below the age of 12.

It is not know whether XOLEGEL can be used to treat fungal infections.

XOLEGEL is a translucent to clear, amber colored gel.

What should I tell my health care provider before using XOLEGEL?

- Tell your health care provider about all of your medical conditions, including if you are pregnant or planning to become pregnant, or are breastfeeding or planning to breastfeed. XOLEGEL should be used during pregnancy and breastfeeding only if needed.
- Tell your health care provider about all of the medicines you take, including prescription and non-prescription medicines, vitamins, and herbal supplements. Keep a list of your medicines and show it to your health care provider and pharmacist. Tell your health care provider and pharmacist when you get a new medicine. It is not known if XOLEGEL and other medicines can interact with each other.

How should I use XOLEGEL?

- Use XOLEGEL exactly as prescribed. Talk to your health care provider if your condition gets worse or does not get better by the end of your treatment.
- Wash your hands before and after applying XOLEGEL.
- Spread a thin layer of XOLEGEL evenly on the affected skin with your fingertips. Be sure to cover all affected areas.
- Do not wash the areas where you applied XOLEGEL for at least 3 hours after you apply it.
- Wait at least 20 minutes after you spread XOLEGEL on your skin before you put makeup or sunscreens on the affected areas.
- Use XOLEGEL once daily for 2 weeks.

What should I avoid while using XOLEGEL?

- XOLEGEL is only to be used on the skin. It is not for eye, mouth, or vaginal use.
- Do not touch your eyes, nose, or mouth while you are applying XOLEGEL. Wash your hands well after you apply it. Irritation may occur if you get XOLEGEL in your eyes, nose, or mouth.
- If used during breastfeeding and XOLEGEL is applied on the chest, take care to avoid accidental ingestion of XOLEGEL by the baby.
- XOLEGEL is flammable (it can catch fire). Stay away from heat, flame, or smoking while you are applying XOLEGEL and right after you apply it.
- This medication should be not be used for any disorder other than that for which it has been prescribed.

What are the possible side effects of XOLEGEL?

- The effects of XOLEGEL during pregnancy, including whether XOLOGEL can harm your unborn baby, are not known.

- It is not know if XOLEGEL can pass into your breastmilk or if it can harm your breastfed baby.
- Stop using XOLEGEL and talk to your health care provider if you develop itching, a rash, or any skin irritation after using XOLEGEL.
- Stop using XOLEGEL and talk to your health care provider if your skin condition (seborrheic dermatitis) gets worse.
- The most common side effect is a burning feeling where XOLEGEL is applied.
- Report any side effects to your health care provider to receive immediate medical attention. You can also report suspected side effects by calling the US Food and Drug Administration at 1-800-FDA-1088, or reporting via the internet at www.fda.gov/medwatch.

These are not all of the side effects of XOLEGEL. For more information, ask your health care provider or pharmacist.

How should I store XOLEGEL?

- Store XOLEGEL at 59°F to 86°F (15° to 30°C).
- Keep XOLEGEL and all medicines out of the reach of children.
- Contents are flammable. Avoid storing XOLEGEL near heat or flame.

General information about XOLEGEL

Medicines are sometimes prescribed for conditions that are not mentioned in Patient Information leaflets. Do not use XOLEGEL for a condition for which it was not prescribed. Do not give XOLEGEL to other people, even if they have the same symptoms that you have. It may harm them.

This Patient Information leaflet summarizes the most important information about XOLEGEL. If you would like more information, talk with your health care provider. You can also ask your pharmacist or health care provider for information about XOLEGEL that is written for health professionals.

What are the ingredients in XOLEGEL?

Active ingredient: ketoconazole, USP

Inactive ingredients: dehydrated alcohol, ascorbic acid, butylated hydroxytoluene, citric acid monohydrate, glycerin, hydroxypropyl cellulose, polyethylene glycol 400, PPG-15 stearyl ether, propylene glycol, FD&C yellow No. 6, and FD&C Yellow No. 10.

This Patient Information leaflet has been approved by the U.S. Food and Drug Administration.

The Patient Information leaflet was last revised: January 2010.

MANUFACTURED BY:
DPT Laboratories, Ltd.
307 E. Josephine Street
San Antonio, TX 78215

FOR:
Stiefel Laboratories, Inc.
255 Alhambra Circle
Coral Gables, FL 33134

US Patent Number 7,179,475 and application 10,722,134 (Patent Pending)
Revised January 2010
XGL:1PI
SAP
FG No
P/N

XOLEGEL, STIEFEL, and STIEFEL & Design are registered trademarks of Stiefel Laboratories, Inc.
© 2010 Stiefel Laboratories, Inc.
STIEFEL®

Sunovion Pharmaceuticals Inc.
84 WATERFORD DR.
MARLBOROUGH, MA 01752
(508) 481-6700

For Medical Information Inquiries:
Medical Information
(800) 739-0565
minfo@sunovion.com
www.SunovionMedical.com
For Adverse Event Reporting
(877) 737-7226
For Customer Service
(888) 394-7377
CAC@sunovion.com

BROVANA® ℞
(arformoterol tartrate)
Inhalation Solution
15 mcg*/2 mL
*potency expressed as arformoterol
For oral inhalation only

WARNING: ASTHMA RELATED DEATH
Long-acting beta$_2$-adrenergic agonists (LABA) increase the risk of asthma-related death. Data from a large placebo-controlled US study that compared the safety of another long-acting beta$_2$-adrenergic agonist (salmeterol) or placebo added to usual asthma therapy showed an increase in asthma-related deaths in patients receiving salmeterol. This finding with salmeterol is considered a class effect of LABA, including arformoterol, the active ingredient in BROVANA (see WARNINGS). The safety and efficacy of BROVANA in patients with asthma have not been established. All LABA, including BROVANA, are contraindicated in patients with asthma without use of a long-term asthma control medication (see CONTRAINDICATIONS).

DESCRIPTION

BROVANA (arformoterol tartrate) Inhalation Solution is a sterile, clear, colorless, aqueous solution of the tartrate salt of arformoterol, the (R,R)-enantiomer of formoterol.

Arformoterol is a selective beta$_2$-adrenergic bronchodilator. The chemical name for arformoterol tartrate is formamide, N-[2-hydroxy-5-[(1R)-1-hydroxy-2-[[(1R)-2-(4-methoxyphenyl)-1-methylethyl]amino]ethyl]phenyl]-, (2R, 3R)-2,3-dihydroxybutanedioate (1:1 salt), and its established structural formula is as follows:

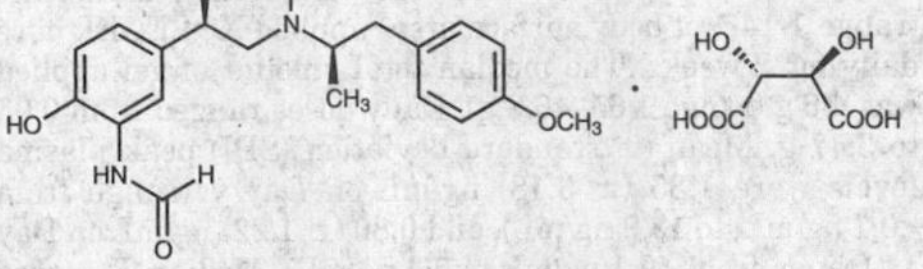

The molecular weight of *arformoterol tartrate* is 494.5 g/mol, and its empirical formula is $C_{19}H_{24}N_2O_4 \cdot C_4H_6O_6$ (1:1 salt). It is a white to off-white solid that is slightly soluble in water.

Arformoterol tartrate is the United States Adopted Name (USAN) for (R,R)-formoterol L-tartrate.

BROVANA is supplied as 2 mL of arformoterol tartrate solution packaged in 2.1 mL unit-dose, low-density polyethylene (LDPE) ready-to-use vials. Each ready-to-use vial contains 15 mcg of arformoterol (equivalent to 22 mcg of arformoterol tartrate) in a sterile, isotonic saline solution, pH-adjusted to 5.0 with citric acid and sodium citrate.

BROVANA requires no dilution before administration by nebulization. Like all other nebulized treatments, the amount delivered to the lungs will depend upon patient factors, the nebulizer used, and compressor performance. Using the PARI LC PLUS® nebulizer (with mouthpiece) connected to a PARI DURA-NEB® 3000 compressor under *in vitro* conditions, the mean delivered dose from the mouthpiece (% nominal) was approximately 4.1 mcg (27.6%) at a mean flow rate of 3.3 L/min. The mean nebulization time was 6 minutes or less. BROVANA should be administered from a standard jet nebulizer at adequate flow rates via face mask or mouthpiece (see **Dosage and Administration**).

Patients should be carefully instructed on the correct use of this drug product (please refer to the accompanying **Medication Guide**).

CLINICAL PHARMACOLOGY

Mechanism of Action

Arformoterol, the (R,R)-enantiomer of formoterol, is a selective long-acting beta$_2$-adrenergic receptor agonist (beta$_2$-agonist) that has two-fold greater potency than racemic formoterol (which contains both the (S,S) and (R,R)-enantiomers). The (S,S)-enantiomer is about 1,000-fold less potent as a beta$_2$-agonist than the (R,R)-enantiomer. While it is recognized that beta$_2$-receptors are the predominant adrenergic receptors in bronchial smooth muscle and beta$_1$-receptors are the predominant receptors in the heart, data indicate that there are also beta$_2$-receptors in the human heart comprising 10% to 50% of the total beta-adrenergic receptors. The precise function of these receptors has not been established, but they raise the possibility that even highly selective beta$_2$-agonists may have cardiac effects.

The pharmacologic effects of beta$_2$-adrenoceptor agonist drugs, including arformoterol, are at least in part attributable to stimulation of intracellular adenyl cyclase, the enzyme that catalyzes the conversion of adenosine triphosphate (ATP) to cyclic-3′,5′-adenosine monophosphate (cyclic AMP). Increased intracellular cyclic AMP levels cause relaxation of bronchial smooth muscle and inhibition of release of mediators of immediate hypersensitivity from cells, especially from mast cells.

In vitro tests show that arformoterol is an inhibitor of the release of mast cell mediators, such as histamine and leukotrienes, from the human lung. Arformoterol also inhibits histamine-induced plasma albumin extravasation in anesthetized guinea pigs and inhibits allergen-induced eosinophil influx in dogs with airway hyper-responsiveness. The relevance of these *in vitro* and animal findings to humans is unknown.

Animal Pharmacology

In animal studies investigating its cardiovascular effects, arformoterol induced dose-dependent increases in heart rate and decreases in blood pressure consistent with its pharmacology as a beta-adrenergic agonist. In dogs, at systemic exposures higher than anticipated clinically, arformoterol also induced exaggerated pharmacologic effects of a beta-adrenergic agonist on cardiac function as measured by electrocardiogram (sinus tachycardia, atrial premature beats, ventricular escape beats, PVCs).

Studies in laboratory animals (minipigs, rodents, and dogs) have demonstrated the occurrence of arrhythmias and sudden death (with histologic evidence of myocardial necrosis) when beta-agonists and methylxanthines are administered concurrently. The clinical significance of these findings is unknown.

Pharmacokinetics

The pharmacokinetics (PK) of arformoterol have been investigated in healthy subjects, elderly subjects, renally and hepatically impaired subjects, and chronic obstructive pulmonary disease (COPD) patients following the nebulization of the recommended therapeutic dose and doses up to 96 mcg.

Absorption

In COPD patients administered 15 mcg arformoterol every 12 hours for 14 days, the mean steady-state peak (R,R)-formoterol plasma concentration (C_{max}) and systemic exposure ($AUC_{0\text{-}12h}$) were 4.3 pg/mL and 34.5 pg*hr/mL, respectively. The median steady-state peak (R,R)-formoterol plasma concentration time (t_{max}) was observed approximately one half hour after drug administration.

Systemic exposure to (R,R)-formoterol increased linearly with dose in COPD patients following arformoterol doses of 5 mcg, 15 mcg, or 25 mcg twice daily for 2 weeks or 15 mcg, 25 mcg, or 50 mcg once daily for 2 weeks.

In a crossover study in patients with COPD, when arformoterol 15 mcg inhalation solution and 12 and 24 mcg formoterol fumarate inhalation powder (Foradil® Aerolizer™) was administered twice daily for 2 weeks, the accumulation index was approximately 2.5 based on the plasma (R,R)-formoterol concentrations in all three treatments. At steady state, geometric means of systemic exposure ($AUC_{0\text{-}12h}$) to (R,R)-formoterol following 15 mcg of arformoterol inhalation solution and 12 mcg of formoterol fumarate inhalation powder were 39.33 pg*hr/mL and 33.93 pg*hr/mL, respectively (ratio 1.16; 90% CI 1.00, 1.35), while the geometric means of the C_{max} were 4.30 pg/mL and 4.75 pg/mL, respectively (ratio 0.91; 90% CI 0.76, 1.09).

In a study in patients with asthma, treatment with arformoterol 50 mcg with pre- and post-treatment with activated charcoal resulted in a geometric mean decrease in (R,R)-formoterol $AUC_{0\text{-}6h}$ by 27% and C_{max} by 23% as compared to treatment with arformoterol 50 mcg alone. This suggests that a substantial portion of systemic drug exposure is due to pulmonary absorption.

Distribution

The binding of arformoterol to human plasma proteins *in vitro* was 52-65% at concentrations of 0.25, 0.5 and 1.0 ng/mL of radiolabeled arformoterol. The concentrations of arformoterol used to assess the plasma protein binding were higher than those achieved in plasma following inhalation of multiple doses of 50 mcg arformoterol.

Metabolism

In vitro profiling studies in hepatocytes and liver microsomes have shown that arformoterol is primarily metabolized by direct conjugation (glucuronidation) and secondarily by O-demethylation. At least five human uridine diphosphoglucuronosyltransferase (UGT) isozymes catalyze arformoterol glucuronidation *in vitro*. Two cytochrome P450 isozymes (CYP2D6 and secondarily CYP2C19) catalyze the O-demethylation of arformoterol.

Arformoterol did not inhibit CYP1A2, CYP2A6, CYP2C9/10, CYP2C19, CYP2D6, CYP2E1, CYP3A4/5, or CYP4A9/11 enzymes at >1,000-fold higher concentrations than the expected peak plasma concentrations following a therapeutic dose.

Arformoterol was almost entirely metabolized following oral administration of 35 mcg of radiolabeled arformoterol in eight healthy subjects. Direct conjugation of arformoterol with glucuronic acid was the major metabolic pathway. Most of the drug-related material in plasma and urine was in the form of glucuronide or sulfate conjugates of arformoterol. O-Desmethylation and conjugates of the O-desmethyl metabolite were relatively minor metabolites accounting for less than 17% of the dose recovered in urine and feces.

Elimination

After administration of a single oral dose of radiolabeled arformoterol to eight healthy male subjects, 63% of the total radioactive dose was recovered in urine and 11% in feces within 48 hours. A total of 89% of the total radioactive dose was recovered within 14 days, with 67% in urine and 22% in feces. Approximately 1% of the dose was recovered as unchanged arformoterol in urine over 14 days. Renal clearance was 8.9 L/hr for unchanged arformoterol in these subjects.

In COPD patients given 15 mcg inhaled arformoterol twice a day for 14 days, the mean terminal half-life of arformoterol was 26 hours.

IMPORTANT NOTICE: Updated drug information is sent bi-monthly via the PDR® Update Insert. For *monthly* email updates, register at PDR.net.

Special Populations

Gender

A population PK analysis indicated that there was no effect of gender upon the pharmacokinetics of arformoterol.

Race

The influence of race on arformoterol pharmacokinetics was assessed using a population PK analysis and data from healthy subjects. There was no clinically significant impact of race upon the pharmacokinetic profile of arformoterol.

Geriatric

The pharmacokinetic profile of arformoterol in 24 elderly subjects (aged 65 years or older) was compared to a younger cohort of 24 subjects (18-45 years) that were matched for body weight and gender. No significant differences in systemic exposure (AUC and C_{max}) were observed when the two groups were compared.

Pediatric

The pharmacokinetics of arformoterol have not been studied in pediatric subjects.

Hepatic Impairment

The pharmacokinetic profile of arformoterol was assessed in 24 subjects with mild, moderate, and severe hepatic impairment. The systemic exposure (C_{max} and AUC) to arformoterol increased 1.3 to 2.4-fold in subjects with hepatic impairment compared to 16 demographically matched healthy control subjects. No clear relationship between drug exposure and the severity of hepatic impairment was observed. BROVANA should be used cautiously in patients with hepatic impairment.

Renal Impairment

The impact of renal disease upon the pharmacokinetics of arformoterol was studied in 24 subjects with mild, moderate, or severe renal impairment. Systemic exposure (AUC and C_{max}) to arformoterol was similar in renally impaired patients compared with demographically matched healthy control subjects.

Pharmacogenetics

Arformoterol is eliminated through the action of multiple drug metabolizing enzymes. Direct glucuronidation of arformoterol is mediated by several UGT enzymes and is the primary elimination route. O-Desmethylation is a secondary route catalyzed by the CYP enzymes CYP2D6 and CYP2C19. In otherwise healthy subjects with reduced CYP2D6 and/or UGT1A1 enzyme activity, there was no impact on systemic exposure to arformoterol compared to subjects with normal CYP2D6 and/or UGT1A1 enzyme activities.

Pharmacodynamics

Systemic Safety and Pharmacokinetic/Pharmacodynamic Relationships

The predominant adverse effects of inhaled $beta_2$-agonists occur as a result of excessive activation of systemic beta-adrenergic receptors. The most common adverse effects may include skeletal muscle tremor and cramps, insomnia, tachycardia, decreases in plasma potassium, and increases in plasma glucose.

Effects on Serum Potassium and Serum Glucose Levels

Changes in serum potassium and serum glucose were evaluated in a dose ranging study of twice daily (5 mcg, 15 mcg, or 25 mcg; 215 patients with COPD) and once daily (15 mcg, 25 mcg, or 50 mcg; 191 patients with COPD) BROVANA in COPD patients. At 2 and 6 hours post dose at week 0 (after the first dose), mean changes in serum potassium ranging from 0 to –0.3 mEq/L were observed in the BROVANA groups with similar changes observed after 2 weeks of treatment. Changes in mean serum glucose levels, ranging from a decrease of 1.2 mg/dL to an increase of 32.8 mg/dL were observed for BROVANA dose groups at both 2 and 6 hours post dose, both after the first dose and 14 days of daily treatment.

Electrophysiology

The effect of BROVANA on QT interval was evaluated in a dose ranging study following multiple doses of BROVANA 5 mcg, 15 mcg, or 25 mcg twice daily or 15 mcg, 25 mcg, or 50 mcg once daily for 2 weeks in patients with COPD. ECG assessments were performed at baseline, time of peak plasma concentration and throughout the dosing interval. Different methods of correcting for heart rate were employed, including a subject-specific method and the Fridericia method.

Relative to placebo, the mean change in subject-specific QT_c averaged over the dosing interval ranged from -1.8 to 2.7 msec, indicating little effect of BROVANA on cardiac repolarization after 2 weeks of treatment. The maximum mean change in subject-specific QT_c for the BROVANA 15 mcg twice daily dose was 17.3 msec, compared with 15.4 msec in the placebo group. No apparent correlation of QT_c with arformoterol plasma concentration was observed.

Electrocardiographic Monitoring in Patients with COPD

The effect of different doses of BROVANA on cardiac rhythm was assessed using 24-hour Holter monitoring in two 12-week double-blind, placebo-controlled studies of 1,456 patients with COPD (873 received BROVANA at 15 or 25 mcg twice daily or 50 mcg once daily doses; 293 received placebo; 290 received salmeterol). The 24-hour Holter monitoring occurred once at baseline, and up to 3 times during the 12-week treatment period. The rates of new-onset cardiac arrhythmias not present at baseline over the double-blind 12-week treatment period were similar (approximately 33-34%) for patients who received BROVANA 15 mcg twice daily to those who received placebo. There was a dose-related increase in new, treatment emergent arrhythmias seen in patients who received BROVANA 25 mcg twice daily and 50 mcg once daily, 37.6% and 40.1 %, respectively. The frequencies of new treatment emergent events of non-sustained (3-10 beat run) and sustained (>10 beat run) ventricular tachycardia were 7.4% and 1.1% in BROVANA 15 mcg twice daily and 6.9% and 1.0% in placebo. In patients who received BROVANA 25 mcg twice daily and 50 mcg once daily the frequencies of non-sustained (6.2% and 8.2%, respectively) and sustained ventricular tachycardia (1.0% and 1.0%, respectively) were similar. Five cases of ventricular tachycardia were reported as adverse events (1 in BROVANA 15 mcg twice daily and 4 in placebo), with two of these events leading to discontinuation of treatment (2 in placebo).

There were no baseline occurrences of atrial fibrillation/flutter observed on 24-hour Holter monitoring in patients treated with BROVANA 15 mcg twice daily or placebo. New, treatment emergent atrial fibrillation/flutter occurred in 0.4% of patients who received BROVANA 15 mcg twice daily and 0.3% of patients who received placebo. There was a dose-related increase in the frequency of atrial fibrillation/flutter reported in the BROVANA 25 mcg twice daily and 50 mcg once daily dose groups of 0.7% and 1.4%, respectively. Two cases of atrial fibrillation/flutter were reported as adverse events (1 in BROVANA 15 mcg twice daily and 1 in placebo).

Dose-related increases in mean maximum change in heart rate in the 12 hours after dosing were also observed following 12 weeks of dosing with BROVANA 15 mcg twice daily (8.8 bpm), 25 mcg twice daily (9.9 bpm) and 50 mcg once daily (12 bpm) versus placebo (8.5 bpm).

Tachyphylaxis/Tolerance

In two placebo-controlled clinical trials in patients with COPD involving approximately 725 patients in each, the overall efficacy of BROVANA was maintained throughout the 12-week trial duration. However, tolerance to the bronchodilator effect of BROVANA was observed after 6 weeks of dosing, evidenced by a decrease in bronchodilator effect as measured by FEV_1. FEV_1 improvement at the end of the 12-hour dosing interval decreased by approximately one third (22.1% mean improvement after the first dose compared to 14.6% at week 12). Tolerance to the FEV_1 bronchodilator effect of BROVANA was not accompanied by other clinical manifestations of tolerance in these trials.

CLINICAL TRIALS

Adult COPD Trials

BROVANA (arformoterol tartrate) Inhalation Solution was studied in two identical, 12-week, double-blind, placebo- and active-controlled, randomized, multi-center, parallel group trials conducted in the United States (Clinical Trial A and Clinical Trial B). A total of 1,456 adult patients (age range: 34 to 89 years; mean age: 63 years) with COPD who had a mean FEV_1 of 1.3 L (42% of predicted) were enrolled in the two clinical trials. The diagnosis of COPD was based on a prior clinical diagnosis of COPD, a smoking history (greater than 15 pack-years), age (at least 35 years), spirometry results (baseline $FEV_1 \leq 65\%$ of predicted value and >0.70 L, and a FEV_1/forced vital capacity (FVC) ratio ≤70%). About 80% of patients in these studies had bronchodilator reversibility, defined as a 10% or greater increase in FEV_1 after inhalation of 2 actuations (180 mcg racemic albuterol from a metered dose inhaler). Both trials compared BROVANA 15 mcg twice daily (288 patients), 25 mcg twice daily (292 patients), 50 mcg once daily (293 patients) with placebo (293 subjects). Both trials included salmeterol inhalation aerosol, 42 mcg twice daily as an active comparator (290 patients).

In both 12-week trials, BROVANA 15 mcg twice daily resulted in significantly greater post-dose bronchodilation (as measured by percent change from study baseline FEV_1 at the end of the dosing interval over the 12 weeks of treatment, the primary efficacy endpoint) compared to placebo. Compared to BROVANA 15 mcg twice daily, BROVANA 25 mcg twice daily and 50 mcg once daily did not provide sufficient additional benefit on a variety of endpoints, including FEV_1, to support the use of higher doses. Plots of the mean change in FEV_1 values obtained over the 12 hours after dosing for the BROVANA 15 mcg twice daily dose group and for the placebo group are provided in Figures 1 and 2 for Clinical Trial A, below. The plots include mean FEV_1 change observed after the first dose and after 12 weeks of treatment. The results from Clinical Trial B were similar.

Figure 1 Mean Change in FEV_1 Over Time for Clinical Trial A at Week 0 (Day 1)

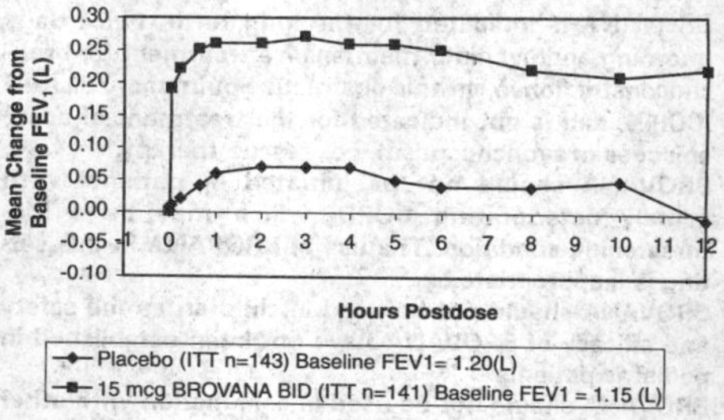
Mean Change from Baseline FEV, (L)
Hours Postdose
Placebo (ITT n=143) Baseline FEV1= 1.20(L)
15 mcg BROVANA BID (ITT n=141) Baseline FEV1 = 1.15 (L)

Figure 2 Mean Change in FEV_1 Over Time for Clinical Trial A at Week 12

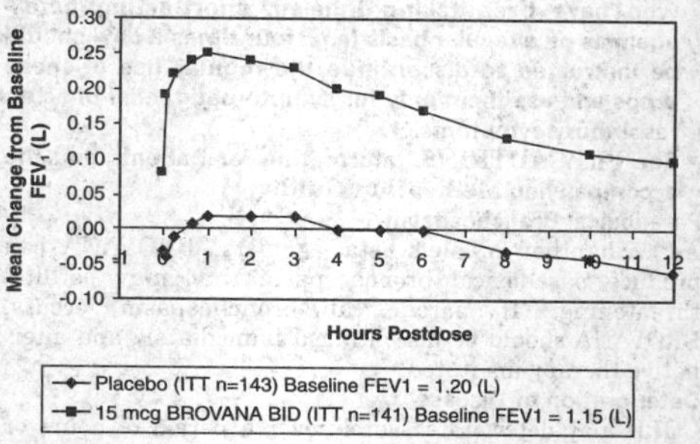
Mean Change from Baseline FEV, (L)
Hours Postdose
Placebo (ITT n=143) Baseline FEV1 = 1.20 (L)
15 mcg BROVANA BID (ITT n=141) Baseline FEV1 = 1.15 (L)

BROVANA 15 mcg twice daily significantly improved bronchodilation compared to placebo over the 12 hours after dosing (FEV_1 AUC_{0-12h}). This improvement was maintained over the 12 week study period.

Following the first dose of BROVANA 15 mcg, the median time to onset of bronchodilation, defined by an FEV_1 increase of 15%, occurred at 6.7 min. When defined as an increase in FEV_1 of 12% and 200 mL, the time to onset of bronchodilation was 20 min after dosing. Peak bronchodilator effect was generally seen within 1-3 hours of dosing. In both clinical trials, compared to placebo, patients treated with BROVANA demonstrated improvements in peak expiratory flow rates, supplemental ipratropium and rescue albuterol use.

INDICATIONS AND USAGE

BROVANA (arformoterol tartrate) Inhalation Solution is indicated for the long term, twice daily (morning and evening) maintenance treatment of bronchoconstriction in patients with chronic obstructive pulmonary disease (COPD), including chronic bronchitis and emphysema. BROVANA is for use by nebulization only.

CONTRAINDICATIONS

BROVANA (arformoterol tartrate) Inhalation Solution is contraindicated in patients with a history of hypersensitivity to arformoterol, racemic formoterol or to any other components of this product.

All LABA, including BROVANA, are contraindicated in patients with asthma without use of a long-term asthma control medication (see **WARNINGS**).

WARNINGS

- **ASTHMA RELATED DEATH**

  Long-acting $beta_2$-adrenergic agonists increase the risk of asthma-related death. The safety and efficacy of BROVANA in patients with asthma have not been established. All LABA, including BROVANA, are contraindicated in patients with asthma without use of a long-term asthma control medication (see CONTRAINDICATIONS).

  - A 28-week, placebo-controlled US study comparing the safety of salmeterol with placebo, each added to usual asthma therapy, showed an increase in asthma-related deaths in patients receiving salmeterol (13/13,176 in patients treated with salmeterol vs. 3/13,179 in patients treated with placebo; RR 4.37, 95% CI 1.25, 15.34). The increased risk of asthma-related death is considered a class effect of the long-acting $beta_2$-adrenergic agonists, including BROVANA. No study adequate to determine whether the rate of asthma related death is increased in patients treated with BROVANA has been conducted.
  - Clinical studies with racemic formoterol (Foradil® Aerolizer™) suggested a higher incidence of serious asthma exacerbations in patients who received racemic formoterol than in those who received placebo. The sizes of these studies were not adequate to precisely quantify the differences in serious asthma exacerbation rates between treatment groups.

- The studies described above enrolled patients with asthma. Data are not available to determine whether the rate of death in patients with COPD is increased by long-acting beta₂-adrenergic agonists.
- BROVANA is indicated for the long term, twice daily (morning and evening) maintenance treatment for bronchoconstriction in chronic obstructive pulmonary disease (COPD), and is not indicated for the treatment of acute episodes of bronchospasm, i.e., rescue therapy.
- BROVANA should not be initiated in patients with acutely deteriorating COPD, which may be a life-threatening condition. The use of BROVANA in this setting is inappropriate.
- BROVANA should not be used in children as the safety and efficacy of BROVANA have not been established in pediatric patients.
- BROVANA should not be used in conjunction with other inhaled, long-acting beta₂-agonists. BROVANA should not be used with other medications containing long-acting beta₂-agonists.
- When beginning treatment with BROVANA, patients who have been taking inhaled, short-acting beta₂-agonists on a regular basis (e.g., four times a day) should be instructed to discontinue the regular use of these drugs and use them only for symptomatic relief of acute respiratory symptoms.
- See PRECAUTIONS, Information for Patients and the accompanying Medication Guide.

Paradoxical Bronchospasm
As with other inhaled beta₂-agonists, BROVANA can produce paradoxical bronchospasm that may be life-threatening. If paradoxical bronchospasm occurs, BROVANA should be discontinued immediately and alternative therapy instituted.

Deterioration of Disease
COPD may deteriorate acutely over a period of hours or chronically over several days or longer. If BROVANA no longer controls the symptoms of bronchoconstriction, or the patient's inhaled, short-acting beta₂-agonist becomes less effective or the patient needs more inhalation of short-acting beta₂-agonist than usual, these may be markers of deterioration of disease. In this setting, a re-evaluation of the patient and the COPD treatment regimen should be undertaken at once. Increasing the daily dosage of BROVANA beyond the recommended 15 mcg twice daily dose is not appropriate in this situation.

Cardiovascular Effects
BROVANA, like other beta₂-agonists, can produce a clinically significant cardiovascular effect in some patients as measured by increases in pulse rate, blood pressure, and/or symptoms. Although such effects are uncommon after administration of BROVANA at the recommended dose, if they occur, the drug may need to be discontinued. In addition, beta-agonists have been reported to produce ECG changes, such as flattening of the T wave, prolongation of the QT_c interval, and ST segment depression. The clinical significance of these findings is unknown. BROVANA, as with other sympathomimetic amines, should be used with caution in patients with cardiovascular disorders, especially coronary insufficiency, cardiac arrhythmias, and hypertension (see PRECAUTIONS, General).

Immediate Hypersensitivity Reactions
Immediate hypersensitivity reactions may occur after administration of BROVANA as demonstrated by cases of anaphylactic reaction, urticaria, angioedema, rash and bronchospasm.

Do Not Exceed Recommended Dose
Fatalities have been reported in association with excessive use of inhaled sympathomimetic drugs. As with other inhaled beta₂-adrenergic drugs, BROVANA should not be used more often, at higher doses than recommended, or with other long-acting beta-agonists.

PRECAUTIONS
General
BROVANA (arformoterol tartrate) Inhalation Solution should not be used to treat acute symptoms of COPD. BROVANA has not been studied in the relief of acute symptoms and extra doses should not be used for that purpose. When prescribing BROVANA, the physician should also provide the patient with an inhaled, short-acting beta₂-agonist for treatment of COPD symptoms that occur acutely, despite regular twice-daily (morning and evening) use of BROVANA. Patients should also be cautioned that increasing inhaled beta₂-agonist use is a signal of deteriorating disease for which prompt medical attention is indicated (see Information for Patients and the accompanying Medication Guide).
BROVANA, like other sympathomimetic amines, should be used with caution in patients with cardiovascular disorders, especially coronary insufficiency, cardiac arrhythmias, and hypertension; in patients with convulsive disorders or thyrotoxicosis; and in patients who are unusually responsive to sympathomimetic amines. Clinically significant changes in

systolic and/or diastolic blood pressure, pulse rate and electrocardiograms have been seen infrequently in individual patients in controlled clinical studies with arformoterol tartrate. Doses of the related beta₂-agonist albuterol, when administered intravenously, have been reported to aggravate preexisting diabetes mellitus and ketoacidosis.
Beta-agonist medications may produce significant hypokalemia in some patients, possibly though intracellular shunting, which has the potential to produce adverse cardiovascular effects. The decrease in serum potassium is usually transient, not requiring supplementation.
Clinically significant changes in blood glucose and/or serum potassium were infrequent during clinical studies with long-term administration of BROVANA at the recommended dose.

Information for Patients
Patients should be instructed to read the accompanying Medication Guide with each new prescription and refill. The complete text of the Medication Guide is reprinted at the end of this document. Patients should be given the following information:
1. Patients should be informed that long-acting beta₂-adrenergic agonists, such as BROVANA, increase the risk of asthma-related death. All LABA, including BROVANA, should not be used in patients with asthma without use of a long-term asthma control medication (see CONTRAINDICATIONS).
2. BROVANA is not indicated to relieve acute respiratory symptoms and extra doses should not be used for that purpose. Acute symptoms should be treated with an inhaled, short-acting, beta₂-agonist (the health-care provider should prescribe the patient with such medication and instruct the patient in how it should be used). Patients should be instructed to seek medical attention if their symptoms worsen, if BROVANA treatment becomes less effective, or if they need more inhalations of a short-acting beta₂-agonist than usual. Patients should not inhale more than one dose at any one time. The daily dosage of BROVANA should not exceed one ready-to-use vial (15 mcg) by inhalation twice daily (30 mcg total daily dose).
3. Patients should be informed that treatment with beta₂-agonists may lead to adverse events which include palpitations, chest pain, rapid heart rate, tremor, or nervousness.
4. Patients should be instructed to use BROVANA by nebulizer only and not to inject or swallow this inhalation solution.
5. Patients should protect BROVANA ready-to-use vials from light and excessive heat. The protective foil pouches should be stored under refrigeration between 2°C and 8°C (36°–46°F). They should not be used after the expiration date stamped on the container. After opening the pouch, unused ready-to-use vials should be returned to, and stored in, the pouch. An opened ready-to-use vial should be used right away. Discard any ready-to-use vial if the solution is not colorless.
6. The drug compatibility (physical and chemical), efficacy and safety of BROVANA when mixed with other drugs in a nebulizer have not been established.
7. Women should be advised to contact their physician if they become pregnant or if they are nursing.
8. It is important that patients understand how to use BROVANA appropriately and how it should be used in relation to other medications to treat COPD they are taking (see the accompanying Medication Guide and the Instructions for Using BROVANA).

Drug Interactions
If additional adrenergic drugs are to be administered by any route, they should be used with caution because the pharmacologically predictable sympathetic effects of BROVANA may be potentiated.
When paroxetine, a potent inhibitor of CYP2D6, was co-administered with BROVANA at steady-state, exposure to either drug was not altered. Dosage adjustments of BROVANA are not necessary when the drug is given concomitantly with potent CYP2D6 inhibitors.
Concomitant treatment with methylxanthines (aminophylline, theophylline), steroids, or diuretics may potentiate any hypokalemic effect of adrenergic agonists.
The ECG changes and/or hypokalemia that may result from the administration of non-potassium sparing diuretics (such as loop or thiazide diuretics) can be acutely worsened by beta-agonists, especially when the recommended dose of the beta-agonist is exceeded. Although the clinical significance of these effects is not known, caution is advised in the co-administration of beta-agonists with non-potassium sparing diuretics.
BROVANA, as with other beta₂-agonists, should be administered with extreme caution to patients being treated with monoamine oxidase inhibitors, tricyclic antidepressants, or drugs known to prolong the QT_c interval because the action of adrenergic agonists on the cardiovascular system may be potentiated by these agents. Drugs that are known to pro-

long the QT_c interval have an increased risk of ventricular arrhythmias. The concurrent use of intravenously or orally administered methylxanthines (e.g., aminophylline, theophylline) by patients receiving BROVANA has not been completely evaluated. In two combined 12-week placebo controlled trials that included BROVANA doses of 15 mcg twice daily, 25 mcg twice daily, and 50 mcg once daily, 54 of 873 BROVANA-treated subjects received concomitant theophylline at study entry. In a 12-month controlled trial that included a 50 mcg once daily BROVANA dose, 30 of the 528 BROVANA-treated subjects received concomitant theophylline at study entry. In these trials, heart rate and systolic blood pressure were approximately 2-3 bpm and 6-8 mm Hg higher, respectively, in subjects on concomitant theophylline compared with the overall population.
Beta-adrenergic receptor antagonists (beta-blockers) and BROVANA may interfere with the effect of each other when administered concurrently. Beta-blockers not only block the therapeutic effects of beta-agonists, but may produce severe bronchospasm in COPD patients. Therefore, patients with COPD should not normally be treated with beta-blockers. However, under certain circumstances, e.g., as prophylaxis after myocardial infarction, there may be no acceptable alternatives to the use of beta-blockers in patients with COPD. In this setting, cardioselective beta-blockers could be considered, although they should be administered with caution.

Carcinogenesis, Mutagenesis, Impairment of Fertility
Long-term studies were conducted in mice using oral administration and rats using inhalation administration to evaluate the carcinogenic potential of arformoterol.
In a 24-month carcinogenicity study in CD-1 mice, arformoterol caused a dose-related increase in the incidence of uterine and cervical endometrial stromal polyps and stromal cell sarcoma in female mice at oral doses of 1 mg/kg and above (AUC exposure approximately 70 times adult exposure at the maximum recommended daily inhalation dose). In a 24-month carcinogenicity study in Sprague-Dawley rats, arformoterol caused a statistically significant increase in the incidence of thyroid gland c-cell adenoma and carcinoma in female rats at an inhalation dose of 200 mcg/kg (AUC exposure approximately 130 times adult exposure at the maximum recommended daily inhalation dose). There were no tumor findings with an inhalation dose of 40 mcg/kg (AUC exposure approximately 55 times adult exposure at the maximum recommended daily inhalation dose).
Arformoterol was not mutagenic or clastogenic in the following tests: mutagenicity tests in bacteria, chromosome aberration analyses in mammalian cells, and micronucleus test in mice.
Arformoterol had no effects on fertility and reproductive performance in rats at oral doses up to 10 mg/kg (approximately 2700 times the maximum recommended daily inhalation dose in adults on a mg/m² basis).
Pregnancy: Teratogenic Effects
Pregnancy Category C
Arformoterol has been shown to be teratogenic in rats based upon findings of omphalocele (umbilical hernia), a malformation, at oral doses of 1 mg/kg and above (AUC exposure approximately 370 times adult exposure at the maximum recommended daily inhalation dose). Increased pup loss at birth and during lactation and decreased pup weights were observed in rats at oral doses of 5 mg/kg and above (AUC exposure approximately 1100 times adult exposure at the maximum recommended daily inhalation dose). Delays in development were evident with an oral dose of 10 mg/kg (AUC exposure approximately 2400 times adult exposure at the maximum recommended daily inhalation dose).
Arformoterol has been shown to be teratogenic in rabbits based upon findings of malpositioned right kidney, a malformation, at oral doses of 20 mg/kg and above (AUC exposure approximately 8400 times adult exposure at the maximum recommended daily inhalation dose). Malformations including brachydactyly, bulbous aorta, and liver cysts were observed at doses of 40 mg/kg and above (approximately 22,000 times the maximum recommended daily inhalation dose in adults on a mg/m² basis). Malformation including adactyly, lobular dysgenesis of the lung, and interventricular septal defect were observed at 80 mg/kg (approximately 43,000 times the maximum recommended daily inhalation dose in adults on a mg/m² basis). Embryolethality was observed at 80 mg/kg/day (approximately 43,000 times the maximum recommended daily inhalation dose in adults on a mg/m² basis). Decreased pup body weights were observed at doses of 40 mg/kg/day and above (approximately 22,000 times the maximum recommended daily inhalation dose in adults on a mg/m² basis). There were no teratogenic findings in rabbits with oral dose of 10 mg/kg and lower (AUC exposure approximately 4900 times adult exposure at the maximum recommended daily inhalation dose).
There are no adequate and well-controlled studies in pregnant women. BROVANA should be used during pregnancy only if the potential benefit justifies the potential risk to the fetus.

Use in Labor and Delivery

There are no human studies that have investigated the effects of BROVANA on preterm labor or labor at term. Because beta-agonists may potentially interfere with uterine contractility, BROVANA should be used during labor and delivery only if the potential benefit justifies the potential risk.

Nursing Mothers

In reproductive studies in rats, arformoterol was excreted in the milk. It is not known whether arformoterol is excreted in human milk. Because many drugs are excreted in human milk, caution should be exercised when BROVANA is administered to a nursing woman.

Pediatric

BROVANA is approved for use in the long term maintenance treatment of bronchoconstriction associated with chronic obstructive pulmonary disease, including chronic bronchitis and emphysema. This disease does not occur in children. The safety and effectiveness of BROVANA in pediatric patients have not been established.

Geriatric

Of the 873 patients who received BROVANA in two placebo-controlled clinical studies in adults with COPD, 391 (45%) were 65 years of age or older while 96 (11%) were 75 years of age or older. No overall differences in safety or effectiveness were observed between these subjects and younger subjects. Among subjects age 65 years and older, 129 (33%) received BROVANA at the recommended dose of 15 mcg twice daily, while the remainder received higher doses. ECG alerts for ventricular ectopy in patients 65 to ≤ 75 years of age were comparable among patients receiving 15 mcg twice daily, 25 mcg twice daily, and placebo (3.9%, 5.2%, and 7.1%, respectively). A higher frequency (12.4%) was observed when BROVANA was dosed at 50 mcg once daily. The clinical significance of this finding is not known. Other reported clinical experience has not identified differences in responses between the elderly and younger patients, but greater sensitivity of some older individuals cannot be ruled out.

ADVERSE REACTIONS

Experience in Adult Patients with COPD

Of the 1,456 COPD patients in the two 12-week, placebo-controlled trials, 288 were treated with BROVANA (arformoterol tartrate) Inhalation Solution 15 mcg twice daily and 293 were treated with placebo. Doses of 25 mcg twice daily and 50 mcg once daily were also evaluated. The numbers and percent of patients who reported adverse events were comparable in the 15 mcg twice daily and placebo groups.

The following table shows adverse events where the frequency was greater than or equal to 2% in the BROVANA 15 mcg twice daily group and where the rates of adverse events in the BROVANA 15 mcg twice daily group exceeded placebo. Ten adverse events demonstrated a dose relationship: asthenia, fever, bronchitis, COPD, headache, vomiting, hyperkalemia, leukocytosis, nervousness, and tremor.

Table 1: Number of Patients Experiencing Adverse Events from Two 12-Week, Double-Blind, Placebo Controlled Clinical Trials

	BROVANA 15 mcg twice daily		Placebo	
	n	(%)	n	(%)
Total Patients	288	(100)	293	(100)
Pain	23	(8)	16	(5)
Chest Pain	19	(7)	19	(6)
Back Pain	16	(6)	6	(2)
Diarrhea	16	(6)	13	(4)
Sinusitis	13	(5)	11	(4)
Leg Cramps	12	(4)	6	(2)
Dyspnea	11	(4)	7	(2)
Rash	11	(4)	5	(2)
Flu Syndrome	10	(3)	4	(1)
Peripheral Edema	8	(3)	7	(2)
Lung Disorder*	7	(2)	2	(1)

* Reported terms coded to "Lung Disorder" were predominantly pulmonary or chest congestion.

Adverse events occurring in patients treated with BROVANA 15 mcg twice daily with a frequency of <2%, but greater than placebo were as follows:

Body as a Whole: abscess, allergic reaction, digitalis intoxication, fever, hernia, injection site pain, neck rigidity, neoplasm, pelvic pain, retroperitoneal hemorrhage

Cardiovascular: arteriosclerosis, atrial flutter, AV block, congestive heart failure, heart block, myocardial infarct, QT interval prolonged, supraventricular tachycardia, inverted T-wave

Digestive: constipation, gastritis, melena, oral moniliasis, periodontal abscess, rectal hemorrhage

Metabolic and Nutritional Disorders: dehydration, edema, glucose tolerance decreased, gout, hyperglycemia, hyperlipemia, hypoglycemia, hypokalemia

Musculoskeletal: arthralgia, arthritis, bone disorder, rheumatoid arthritis, tendinous contracture

Nervous: agitation, cerebral infarct, circumoral paresthesia, hypokinesia, paralysis, somnolence, tremor

Respiratory: carcinoma of the lung, respiratory disorder, voice alteration

Skin and Appendages: dry skin, herpes simplex, herpes zoster, skin discoloration, skin hypertrophy

Special Senses: abnormal vision, glaucoma

Urogenital: breast neoplasm, calcium crystalluria, cystitis, glycosuria, hematuria, kidney calculus, nocturia, PSA increase, pyuria, urinary tract disorder, urine abnormality. Overall, the frequency of all cardiovascular adverse events for BROVANA in the two placebo controlled trials was low and comparable to placebo (6.9% in BROVANA 15 mcg twice daily and 13.3% in the placebo group). There were no frequently occurring specific cardiovascular adverse events for BROVANA (frequency ≥1% and greater than placebo). The rate of COPD exacerbations was also comparable between the BROVANA 15 mcg twice daily and placebo groups, 12.2% and 15.1%, respectively.

Other adverse reactions which may occur with selective beta$_2$-adrenoceptor agonists such as BROVANA include: angina, hypertension or hypotension, tachycardia, arrhythmias, nervousness, headache, tremor, dry mouth, palpitation, muscle cramps, nausea, dizziness, fatigue, malaise, hypokalemia, hyperglycemia, metabolic acidosis and insomnia.

Drug Abuse and Dependence

There were no reported cases of abuse or evidence of drug dependence with the use of BROVANA in the clinical trials.

OVERDOSAGE

The expected signs and symptoms associated with overdosage of BROVANA (arformoterol tartrate) Inhalation Solution are those of excessive beta-adrenergic stimulation and/or occurrence or exaggeration of any of the signs and symptoms listed under **ADVERSE REACTIONS**, e.g., angina, hypertension or hypotension, tachycardia, with rates up to 200 bpm, arrhythmias, nervousness, headache, tremor, dry mouth, palpitation, muscle cramps, nausea, dizziness, fatigue, malaise, hypokalemia, hyperglycemia, metabolic acidosis and insomnia. As with all inhaled sympathomimetic medications, cardiac arrest and even death may be associated with an overdose of BROVANA.

Treatment of overdosage consists of discontinuation of BROVANA together with institution of appropriate symptomatic and/or supportive therapy. The judicious use of a cardioselective beta-receptor blocker may be considered, bearing in mind that such medication can produce bronchospasm. There is insufficient evidence to determine if dialysis is beneficial for overdosage of BROVANA. Cardiac monitoring is recommended in cases of overdosage.

Clinical signs in dogs included flushing of the body surface and facial area, reddening of the ears and gums, tremor, and increased heart rate. A death was reported in dogs after a single oral dose of 5 mg/kg (approximately 4500 times the maximum recommended daily inhalation dose in adults on a mg/m^2 basis). Death occurred for a rat that received arformoterol at a single inhalation dose of 1600 mcg/kg (approximately 430 times the maximum recommended daily inhalation dose in adults on a mg/m^2 basis).

DOSAGE AND ADMINISTRATION

The recommended dose of BROVANA (arformoterol tartrate) Inhalation Solution for COPD patients is 15 mcg administered twice a day (morning and evening) by nebulization. A total daily dose greater than 30 mcg (15 mcg twice daily) is not recommended. BROVANA should be administered by the inhaled route via a standard jet nebulizer connected to an air compressor (see the accompanying **Medication Guide**). BROVANA should not be swallowed. BROVANA should be stored refrigerated in foil pouches. After opening the pouch, unused ready-to-use vials should be returned to, and stored in, the pouch. An opened ready-to-use vial should be used right away.

If the recommended maintenance treatment regimen fails to provide the usual response, medical advice should be sought immediately, as this is often a sign of destabilization

of COPD. Under these circumstances, the therapeutic regimen should be re-evaluated and additional therapeutic options should be considered.

No dose adjustment is required for patients with renal or hepatic impairment. However, since the clearance of BROVANA is prolonged in patients with hepatic impairment, they should be monitored closely.

The drug compatibility (physical and chemical), efficacy, and safety of BROVANA when mixed with other drugs in a nebulizer have not been established.

The safety and efficacy of BROVANA have been established in clinical trials when administered using the PARI LC PLUS® nebulizers and PARI DURA-NEB® 3000 compressors. The safety and efficacy of BROVANA when administered using other nebulizer systems has not been established.

HOW SUPPLIED

BROVANA (arformoterol tartrate) Inhalation Solution is supplied in a single strength (15 mcg of arformoterol, equivalent to 22 mcg of arformoterol tartrate) as 2 mL of a sterile solution in low-density polyethylene (LDPE) ready-to-use vials overwrapped in foil. BROVANA is available in a shelf-carton containing 30 or 60 ready-to-use vials.

NDC 63402-911-30: carton of 30 individually pouched ready-to-use vials.

NDC 63402-911-64: carton of 60 ready-to-use vials (15×4 ready-to-use vial pouches).

CAUTION: Federal law (U.S.) prohibits dispensing without prescription.

Storage

Store BROVANA in the protective foil pouch under refrigeration at 36°-46°F (2°-8°C). Protect from light and excessive heat. After opening the pouch, unused ready-to-use vials should be returned to, and stored in, the pouch. An opened ready-to-use vial should be used right away. Discard any ready-to-use vial if the solution is not colorless. Unopened foil pouches of BROVANA can also be stored at room temperature 68°-77°F, (20°-25°C) for up to 6 weeks. If stored at room temperature, discard if not used after 6 weeks or if past the expiration date, whichever is sooner.

SEPRACOR

Manufactured for:

Sepracor Inc.

Marlborough, MA 01752 USA

For customer service, call 1-888-394-7377.

To report adverse events, call 1-877-737-7226.

For medical information, call 1-800-739-0565.

June 2010

MEDICATION GUIDE

BROVANA [Brō vă´ -nah]

(arformoterol tartrate) Inhalation Solution

BROVANA is only for use with a nebulizer.

Read the Medication Guide that comes with BROVANA before you start using it and each time you get a refill. There may be new information. This Medication Guide does not take the place of talking to your healthcare provider about your medical condition or treatment.

What is the most important information I should know about BROVANA?

BROVANA can cause serious side effects, including:

* **People with asthma, who take long-acting beta$_2$ adrenergic agonist (LABA) medicines, such as BROVANA, have an increased risk of death from asthma problems.**
* It is not known if LABA medicines, such as BROVANA, increase the risk of death in people with chronic obstructive pulmonary disease (COPD).
* **Get emergency medical care if:**
  * **breathing problems worsen quickly**
  * **you use your rescue inhaler medicine, but it does not relieve your breathing problems**

What is BROVANA?

BROVANA is used long term, 2 times each day (morning and evening), in controlling symptoms of chronic obstructive pulmonary disease (COPD) in adults with COPD.

BROVANA is only for use with a nebulizer.

LABA medicines such as BROVANA help the muscles around the airways in your lungs stay relaxed to prevent symptoms, such as wheezing, cough, chest tightness, and shortness of breath.

BROVANA should not be used in children. **It is not known if BROVANA is safe and effective in children.**

It is not known if BROVANA is safe and effective in people with asthma.

Who should not use BROVANA?

Do not use BROVANA if you:

* have had a serious allergic reaction to arformoterol, formoterol, or any of the ingredients in BROVANA. Ask your healthcare provider if you are not sure. See the end of this Medication Guide for a complete list of ingredients in BROVANA.
* have asthma without using a long-term asthma control medicine.

What should I tell my healthcare provider before using BROVANA?

Tell your healthcare provider about all of your health conditions, including if you:

- have heart problems
- have high blood pressure
- have seizures
- have thyroid problems
- have diabetes
- have liver problems
- are pregnant or planning to become pregnant. It is not known if BROVANA can harm your unborn baby.
- are breastfeeding. It is not known if BROVANA passes into your milk and if it can harm your baby.

Tell your healthcare provider about all the medicines you take including prescription and non-prescription medicines, vitamins and herbal supplements. BROVANA and certain other medicines may interact with each other. This may cause serious side effects.

Know the medicines you take. Keep a list of them to show your healthcare provider and pharmacist each time you get a new medicine.

How should I use BROVANA?

Read the step-by-step instructions for using BROVANA at the end of this Medication Guide.

- Use BROVANA exactly as prescribed. One ready-to-use vial of BROVANA is one dose. The usual dose of BROVANA is 1 ready-to-use vial, twice a day (morning and evening) breathed in through your nebulizer machine. The 2 doses should be about 12 hours apart. **Do not use more than 2 ready-to-use vials of BROVANA a day.**
- Do not swallow or inject BROVANA.
- BROVANA is for use with a standard jet nebulizer machine connected to an air compressor. Read the complete instructions for use at the end of this Medication Guide before starting BROVANA.
- Do not mix other medicines with BROVANA in your nebulizer machine.
- If you miss a dose of BROVANA. Just skip that dose. Take your next dose at your usual time. Do not take 2 doses at one time.
- While you are using BROVANA 2 times each day:
  - **do not use** other medicines that contain a long-acting beta$_2$-agonist (LABA) for any reason.
  - **do not use** your short-acting beta$_2$-agonist medicine on a regular basis (four times a day).
- **BROVANA does not relieve sudden symptoms of COPD.** Always have a rescue inhaler medicine with you to treat sudden symptoms. If you do not have a rescue inhaler medicine, call your healthcare provider to have one prescribed for you.
- Do not stop using BROVANA or other medicines to control or treat your COPD unless told to do so by your healthcare provider because your symptoms might get worse. Your healthcare provider will change your medicines as needed.
- **Do not use BROVANA:**
  - **more often than prescribed**
  - **more medicine than prescribed for you**
  - **with other LABA medicines**

Call your healthcare provider or get emergency medical care right away if:

- your breathing problems worsen with BROVANA
- you need to use your rescue inhaler medicine more often than usual
- your rescue inhaler medicine does not work as well for you at relieving symptoms

What are the possible side effects with BROVANA?

BROVANA can cause serious side effects, including:

- See "What is the most important information I should know about BROVANA?"
- Sudden shortness of breath immediately after use of Brovana
- If your COPD symptoms worsen over time do not increase your dose of Brovana, instead call your healthcare provider.
- Increased blood pressure
- Fast or irregular heartbeat
- **serious allergic reactions including rash, hives, swelling of the face, mouth, and tongue, and breathing problems.** Call your healthcare provider or get emergency medical care if you get any symptoms of a serious allergic reaction.

Common side effects of BROVANA include:

- **chest or back pain**
- **diarrhea**
- **sinus congestion**
- **headache**
- **tremor**
- **nervousness**
- **leg cramps**
- **high blood potassium**
- **shortness of breath**
- **rash**
- **fever**

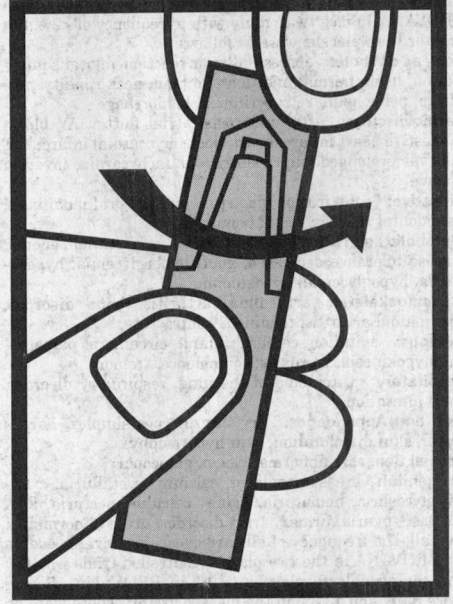

Figure 1

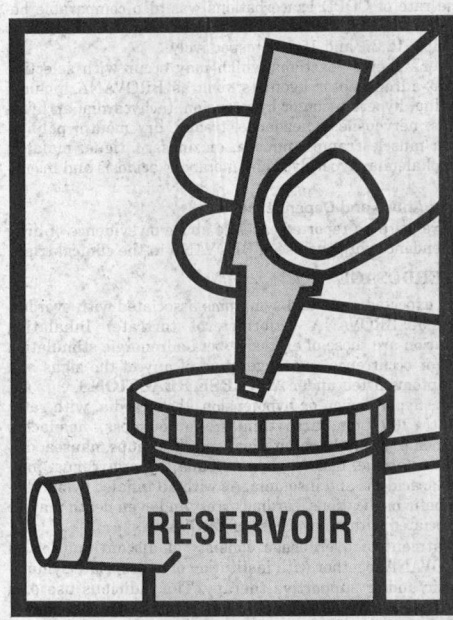

Figure 2

- **increased white blood cells**
- **vomiting**
- **tiredness**
- **leg swelling**
- **chest congestion or bronchitis**

Tell your healthcare provider if you get any side effect that bothers you or that does not go away.

These are not all the side effects with BROVANA. Ask your healthcare provider or pharmacist for more information. Call your doctor for medical advice about side effects. You may report side effects to FDA at 1-800-FDA-1088.

How should I store BROVANA?

- Store BROVANA in a refrigerator between 36° to 46°F (2° to 8°C) in the protective foil pouch. Protect from light and excessive heat. **Do not open a sealed pouch until you are ready to use a dose of BROVANA. After opening the pouch, unused ready-to-use vials should be returned to, and stored in, the pouch. An opened ready-to-use vial should be used right away.** BROVANA may be used directly from the refrigerator.
- BROVANA may also be stored at room temperature between 68°F to 77°F (20°C to 25°C) for up to 6 weeks (42 days). If stored at room temperature, discard BROVANA if it is not used after 6 weeks or if past the expiration date, whichever is sooner. Space is provided on the packaging to record room temperature storage times.
- Do not use BROVANA after the expiration date provided on the foil pouch and ready-to-use vial.

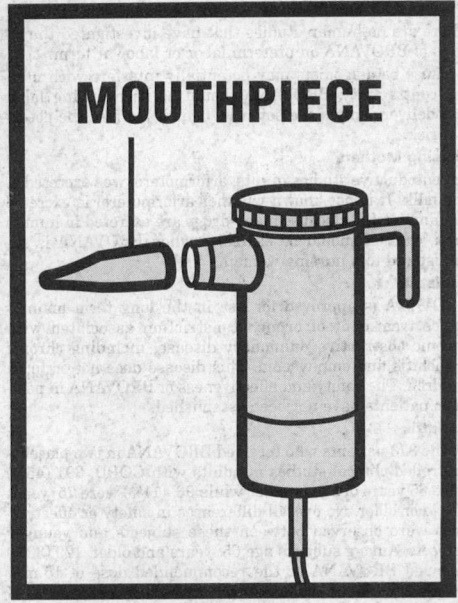

Figure 3

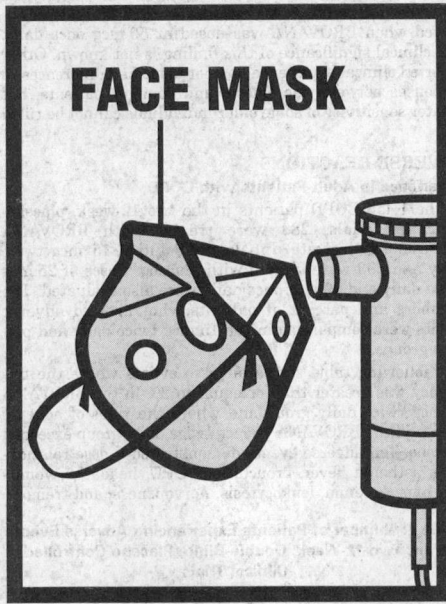

Figure 4

- BROVANA should be colorless. Discard BROVANA if it is not colorless.
- **Keep BROVANA and all medicines out of the reach of children.**

General Information about BROVANA

Medicines are sometimes prescribed for purposes not mentioned in a Medication Guide. Do not use BROVANA for a condition for which it was not prescribed. Do not give BROVANA to other people, even if they have the same condition. It may harm them.

This Medication Guide summarizes the most important information about BROVANA. If you would like more information, talk with your healthcare provider. You can ask your healthcare provider or pharmacist for information about BROVANA that was written for healthcare professionals.

- For customer service, call 1-888-394-7377.
- To report side effects, call 1-877-737-7226.
- For medical information, call 1-800-739-0565.

Instructions for Using BROVANA (arformoterol tartrate) Inhalation Solution

BROVANA is used only in a standard jet nebulizer machine connected to an air compressor. Make sure you know how to use your nebulizer machine before you use it to breathe-in BROVANA or other medicines.

Do not mix BROVANA with other medicines in your nebulizer machine.

BROVANA comes sealed in a foil pouch. Do not open a sealed pouch until you are ready to use a dose of BROVANA. After opening the pouch, unused ready-to-use vials should be returned to, and stored in, the pouch. An opened ready-to-use vial should be used right away.

1. Open the foil pouch by tearing on the rough edge along the seam of the pouch. Remove a ready-to-use vial of BROVANA.
2. Carefully twist open the top of the ready-to-use vial and use it right away (**Figure 1**).
[See figure 1 at top of previous page]
3. Squeeze all of the medicine from the ready-to-use vial into the nebulizer medicine cup (reservoir) (**Figure 2**).
[See figure 2 on previous page]
4. Connect the nebulizer reservoir to the mouthpiece (**Figure 3**) or face mask (**Figure 4**).
[See figure 3 at top of previous page]
[See figure 4 on previous page]
5. Connect the nebulizer to the compressor (**Figure 5**).

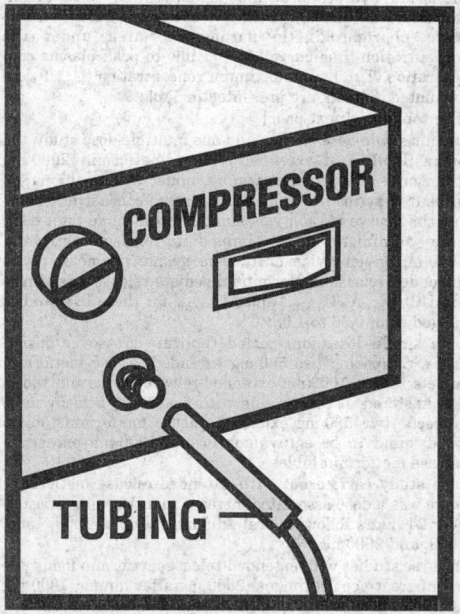

Figure 5

6. Sit in a comfortable, upright position. Place the mouthpiece in your mouth (**Figure 6**) (or put on the face mask) and turn on the compressor.

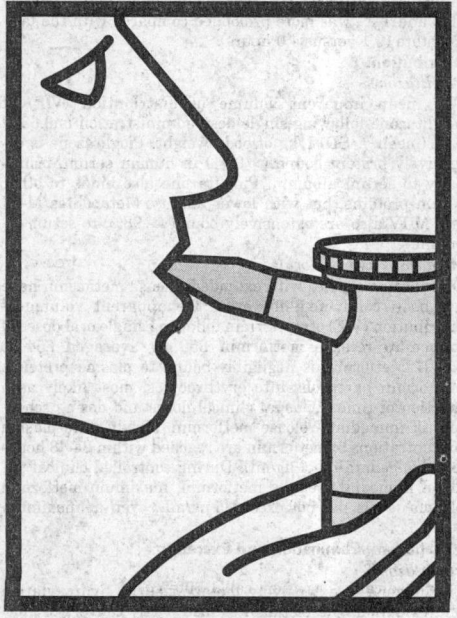

Figure 6

7. Breathe as calmly, deeply, and evenly as possible until no more mist is formed in the nebulizer reservoir. It takes about 5 to 10 minutes for each treatment.
8. Clean the nebulizer (see manufacturer's instructions).

Rx Only

This Medication Guide has been approved by the Food and Drug Administration.

SEPRACOR
Manufactured for:
Sepracor Inc.
Marlborough, MA 01752 USA
June 2010
Shown in Product Identification Guide, page 319

Takeda Pharmaceuticals America, Inc.
**ONE TAKEDA PARKWAY
DEERFIELD, IL 60015**

Direct Inquiries to:
Sales and Ordering:
Customer Service
(877) 5TAKEDA
(877) 582-5332
For Medical Information:
(877) TAKEDA7
(877) 825-3327
To Report Adverse Drug Experiences:
(877) TAKEDA7
(877) 825-3327

ACTOPLUS MET®   ℞
[ak-TO-plus-mĕt]
**(pioglitazone hydrochloride and metformin hydrochloride)
tablets**

ACTOPLUS MET® XR
**(pioglitazone hydrochloride and metformin hydrochloride extended-release)
tablets**

WARNING: CONGESTIVE HEART FAILURE AND LACTIC ACIDOSIS
Congestive Heart Failure
- Thiazolidinediones, including pioglitazone, which is a component of ACTOPLUS MET and ACTOPLUS MET XR, cause or exacerbate congestive heart failure in some patients (see **WARNINGS, Pioglitazone**). After initiation of ACTOPLUS MET or ACTOPLUS MET XR, and after dose increases, observe patients carefully for signs and symptoms of heart failure (including excessive, rapid weight gain, dyspnea, and/or edema). If these signs and symptoms develop, the heart failure should be managed according to the current standards of care. Furthermore, discontinuation or dose reduction of ACTOPLUS MET or ACTOPLUS MET XR must be considered.
- ACTOPLUS MET and ACTOPLUS MET XR are not recommended in patients with symptomatic heart failure. Initiation of ACTOPLUS MET or ACTOPLUS MET XR in patients with established NYHA Class III or IV heart failure is contraindicated (see **CONTRAINDICATIONS** and **WARNINGS, Pioglitazone**).
Lactic Acidosis
- Lactic acidosis is a rare, but serious complication that can occur due to metformin accumulation. The risk increases with conditions such as sepsis, dehydration, excess alcohol intake, hepatic insufficiency, renal impairment, and acute congestive heart failure.
- The onset is often subtle, accompanied only by nonspecific symptoms such as malaise, myalgias, respiratory distress, increasing somnolence, and nonspecific abdominal distress.
- Laboratory abnormalities include low pH, increased anion gap and elevated blood lactate.
- If acidosis is suspected, ACTOPLUS MET or ACTOPLUS MET XR should be discontinued and the patient hospitalized immediately (see **WARNINGS, Metformin Hydrochloride**).

DESCRIPTION
ACTOPLUS MET® tablets are formulated with pioglitazone hydrochloride and immediate-release metformin hydrochloride. ACTOPLUS MET® XR tablets are formulated with pioglitazone hydrochloride and extended-release metformin hydrochloride. Both ACTOPLUS MET® and ACTOPLUS MET® XR contain two oral antihyperglycemic drugs used in the management of type 2 diabetes: pioglitazone and metformin. ACTOPLUS MET® is available in 15 mg pioglitazone/500 mg metformin hydrochloride and 15 mg pioglitazone/850 mg metformin

---

hydrochloride tablets. ACTOPLUS MET® XR is available in 15 mg pioglitazone/1000 mg extended-release metformin hydrochloride and 30 mg pioglitazone/1000 mg extended-release metformin hydrochloride tablets.

Pioglitazone is an oral antihyperglycemic agent that acts primarily by decreasing insulin resistance. Pioglitazone is used in the management of type 2 diabetes. Pharmacological studies indicate that pioglitazone improves sensitivity to insulin in muscle and adipose tissue and inhibits hepatic gluconeogenesis. Pioglitazone improves glycemic control while reducing circulating insulin levels.

Pioglitazone (±)-5-[[4-[2-(5-ethyl-2-pyridinyl)ethoxy]phenyl]methyl]-2,4-thiazolidinedione monohydrochloride belongs to a different chemical class and has a different pharmacological action than the sulfonylureas, biguanides, or the α-glucosidase inhibitors. The molecule contains one asymmetric center, and the synthetic compound is a racemate. The two enantiomers of pioglitazone interconvert *in vivo*. The structural formula is as shown:

pioglitazone hydrochloride

Pioglitazone hydrochloride is an odorless white crystalline powder that has a molecular formula of $C_{19}H_{20}N_2O_3S \cdot HCl$ and a molecular weight of 392.90. It is soluble in N,N-dimethylformamide, slightly soluble in anhydrous ethanol, very slightly soluble in acetone and acetonitrile, practically insoluble in water, and insoluble in ether.

Metformin hydrochloride (N,N-dimethylimidodicarbonimidic diamide hydrochloride) is not chemically or pharmacologically related to any other classes of oral antihyperglycemic agents. Metformin hydrochloride is a white crystalline powder with a molecular formula of $C_4H_{11}N_5 \cdot HCl$ and a molecular weight of 165.62. Metformin hydrochloride is freely soluble in water and is practically insoluble in acetone, ether, and chloroform. The pKa of metformin is 12.4. The pH of a 1% aqueous solution of metformin hydrochloride is 6.68. The structural formula is as shown:

metformin hydrochloride

ACTOPLUS MET is available as a tablet for oral administration containing pioglitazone hydrochloride and metformin hydrochloride equivalent to 15 mg pioglitazone and 500 mg metformin hydrochloride (ACTOPLUS MET 15 mg/500 mg) or 850 mg metformin hydrochloride (ACTOPLUS MET 15 mg/850 mg). ACTOPLUS MET is formulated with the following excipients: povidone, microcrystalline cellulose, croscarmellose sodium, magnesium stearate, hypromellose 2910, polyethylene glycol 8000, titanium dioxide, and talc.

ACTOPLUS MET XR is available as a tablet for once-a-day oral administration containing pioglitazone hydrochloride and metformin hydrochloride equivalent to 15 mg pioglitazone and 1000 mg metformin hydrochloride (ACTOPLUS MET XR 15 mg/1000 mg) or 30 mg pioglitazone and 1000 mg metformin hydrochloride (ACTOPLUS MET XR 30 mg/1000 mg). ACTOPLUS MET XR is formulated with the following excipients: candelilla wax, cellulose acetate, povidone, hydroxypropyl cellulose, lactose monohydrate, magnesium stearate, hypromellose, polyethylene glycols (PEG 400, PEG 8000), sodium lauryl sulfate, titanium dioxide, and triacetin. Tablets are imprinted with ink containing shellac, iron oxide red (15 mg/1000 mg strength only), FD&C Blue No. 2 Lake (30 mg/1000 mg strength only), propylene glycol, and ammonium hydroxide.

ACTOPLUS MET XR: SYSTEM COMPONENTS AND PERFORMANCE
ACTOPLUS MET XR consists of an extended-release metformin core coated tablet with an immediate-release pioglitazone layer. The metformin core tablet is an extended-release formulation using the patented single composition osmotic technology (SCOT™) for once-daily (q.d.) oral administration. The tablet is similar in appearance to other film-coated oral administered tablets but it consists of an osmotically active core formulation that is surrounded by a semipermeable membrane and coated with a pioglitazone drug layer. Two laser drilled exit ports exist in the membrane, one on either side of the tablet. The core formulation is composed primarily of drug with small concentrations of excipients. The semipermeable membrane is permeable to water but not to higher molecular weight components of biological fluids. Upon ingestion, the pioglitazone

Table 1. Mean (SD) Pharmacokinetic Parameters for ACTOPLUS MET®

Regimen	N	AUC(0-inf) (ng·h/mL)	N	C_{max} (ng/mL)	N	T_{max} (h)	N	$T_{1/2}$ (h)
pioglitazone								
15 mg/500 mg ACTOPLUS MET®	51	5984 (1599)	63	585 (198)	63	1.8 (0.9)	51	8.7 (3.9)
15 mg pioglitazone and 500 mg immediate-release metformin	54	5810 (1472)	63	608 (204)	63	1.7 (0.9)	54	7.9 (3.1)
15 mg/850 mg ACTOPLUS MET®	52	5671 (1585)	60	569 (222)	60	1.9 (0.8)	52	7.2 (1.8)
15 mg pioglitazone and 850 mg immediate-release metformin	55	5957 (1680)	61	603 (239)	61	2.0 (1.5)	55	7.2 (1.8)
metformin								
15 mg/500 mg ACTOPLUS MET®	59	7783 (2266)	63	1203 (325)	63	2.3 (0.9)	59	8.6 (14.3)
15 mg pioglitazone and 500 mg immediate-release metformin	59	7599 (2385)	63	1215 (329)	63	2.5 (0.9)	59	6.7 (5.9)
15 mg/850 mg ACTOPLUS MET®	47	11927 (3311)	60	1827 (536)	60	2.4 (0.9)	47	17.6 (20.1)
15 mg pioglitazone and 850 mg immediate-release metformin	52	11569 (3494)	61	1797 (525)	61	2.3 (0.8)	52	17.0 (18.1)

layer is dissolved, water is then taken up through the membrane, which in turn dissolves the metformin and excipients in the core formulation. The dissolved metformin and excipients exit through the laser drilled ports in the membrane. The rate of drug delivery is constant and dependent upon the maintenance of a constant osmotic gradient across the membrane. This situation exists so long as there is undissolved metformin present in the core tablet. Following the dissolution of the core materials, the rate of drug delivery slowly decreases until the osmotic gradient across the membrane falls to zero at which time delivery ceases. The membrane coating remains intact during the transit of the dosage form through the gastrointestinal tract and is excreted in the feces.

CLINICAL PHARMACOLOGY

Mechanism of Action

ACTOPLUS MET and ACTOPLUS MET XR

ACTOPLUS MET and ACTOPLUS MET XR combine two antihyperglycemic agents with complementary mechanisms of action to improve glycemic control in patients with type 2 diabetes: pioglitazone, a member of the thiazolidinedione class, and metformin hydrochloride, a member of the biguanide class. Thiazolidinediones are insulin-sensitizing agents that act primarily by enhancing peripheral glucose utilization, whereas biguanides act primarily by decreasing endogenous hepatic glucose production.

Pioglitazone

Pioglitazone depends on the presence of insulin for its mechanism of action. Pioglitazone decreases insulin resistance in the periphery and in the liver resulting in increased insulin-dependent glucose disposal and decreased hepatic glucose output. Unlike sulfonylureas, pioglitazone is not an insulin secretagogue. Pioglitazone is a potent and highly selective agonist for peroxisome proliferator-activated receptor-gamma (PPARγ). PPAR receptors are found in tissues important for insulin action such as adipose tissue, skeletal muscle, and liver. Activation of PPARγ nuclear receptors modulates the transcription of a number of insulin responsive genes involved in the control of glucose and lipid metabolism.

In animal models of diabetes, pioglitazone reduces the hyperglycemia, hyperinsulinemia, and hypertriglyceridemia characteristic of insulin-resistant states such as type 2 diabetes. The metabolic changes produced by pioglitazone result in increased responsiveness of insulin-dependent tissues and are observed in numerous animal models of insulin resistance.

Since pioglitazone enhances the effects of circulating insulin (by decreasing insulin resistance), it does not lower blood glucose in animal models that lack endogenous insulin.

Metformin hydrochloride

Metformin hydrochloride improves glucose tolerance in patients with type 2 diabetes, lowering both basal and postprandial plasma glucose. Metformin decreases hepatic glucose production, decreases intestinal absorption of glucose and improves insulin sensitivity by increasing peripheral glucose uptake and utilization. Unlike sulfonylureas, metformin does not produce hypoglycemia in either patients with type 2 diabetes or normal subjects (except in special circumstances, see **PRECAUTIONS, General:** *Metformin*

hydrochloride) and does not cause hyperinsulinemia. With metformin therapy, insulin secretion remains unchanged while fasting insulin levels and day-long plasma insulin response may actually decrease.

Pharmacokinetics and Drug Metabolism

Absorption and Bioavailability:

ACTOPLUS MET

In bioequivalence studies of ACTOPLUS MET 15 mg/500 mg and 15 mg/850 mg, the area under the curve (AUC) and maximum concentration (C_{max}) of both the pioglitazone and the immediate-release metformin component following a single dose of the combination tablet were bioequivalent to pioglitazone (ACTOS®) 15 mg concomitantly administered with immediate-release metformin (Glucophage®) 500 mg or 850 mg tablets, respectively, under fasted conditions in healthy subjects (Table 1).
[See table 1 above]

Administration of ACTOPLUS MET 15 mg/850 mg with food resulted in no change in overall exposure of pioglitazone. With metformin there was no change in AUC; however, mean peak serum concentration of metformin was decreased by 28% when administered with food. A delayed time to peak serum concentration was observed for both components (1.9 hours for pioglitazone and 0.8 hours for metformin) under fed conditions. These changes are not likely to be clinically significant.

ACTOPLUS MET XR

In bioequivalence studies of ACTOPLUS MET XR 15 mg/1000 mg and 30 mg/1000 mg, the area under the curve (AUC) and maximum concentration (C_{max}) of both the pioglitazone and the extended-release metformin components following a single dose of the combination tablet were bioequivalent to pioglitazone (ACTOS®) 15 mg and 30 mg concomitantly administered with extended-release metformin hydrochloride (FORTAMET®) 1000 mg tablets under fed conditions in healthy subjects (**Table 2**).
[See table 2 at top of next page]

Administration of ACTOPLUS MET® XR 30 mg/1000 mg with food resulted in no change in total (AUC) exposure of pioglitazone; however, a decrease in C_{max} by approximately 18% was observed. With the extended-release metformin component there was an increase in C_{max} by approximately 98% and AUC exposure by approximately 85% when administered with food. These levels are comparable to exposures obtained with extended release metformin when administered with food. Time to peak serum concentration was prolonged by approximately 3 and 2 hours for pioglitazone and extended-release metformin respectively, under fed conditions.

Pioglitazone

Following oral administration, in the fasting state, pioglitazone is first measurable in serum within 30 minutes, with peak concentrations observed within 2 hours. Food slightly delays the time to peak serum concentration to 3 to 4 hours, but does not alter the extent of absorption.

Metformin hydrochloride

The absolute bioavailability of a 500 mg immediate-release metformin tablet given under fasting conditions is approximately 50%-60%. Studies using single oral doses of immediate-release metformin tablets of 500 mg to 1500 mg,

and 850 mg to 2550 mg, indicate that there is a lack of dose proportionality with increasing doses, which is due to decreased absorption rather than an alteration in elimination. Food decreases the extent of and slightly delays the absorption of immediate-release metformin, as shown by approximately a 40% lower mean peak plasma concentration, a 25% lower AUC in plasma concentration versus time curve, and a 35 minute prolongation of time to peak plasma concentration following administration of a single 850 mg tablet of immediate-release metformin with food, compared to the same tablet strength administered fasting. The clinical relevance of these decreases is unknown.

The appearance of metformin in plasma from an extended-release metformin tablet is slower and more prolonged compared to immediate-release metformin (see FORTAMET prescribing information). In a multiple-dose crossover study, 23 patients with type 2 diabetes mellitus were administered either extended-release metformin hydrochloride 2000 mg once a day (after dinner) or immediate-release (IR) metformin hydrochloride 1000 mg twice a day (after breakfast and after dinner). After 4 weeks of treatment, steady-state pharmacokinetic parameters, area under the concentration-time curve (AUC), time to peak plasma concentration (T_{max}), and maximum concentration (C_{max}) were evaluated. Results are presented in **Table 3**.
[See table 3 on next page]

In four single-dose studies and one multiple-dose study, the bioavailability of extended-release metformin 2000 mg given once daily, in the evening, under fed conditions [as measured by the area under the plasma concentration versus time curve (AUC)] was similar to the same total daily dose administered as immediate-release metformin 1000 mg given twice daily. The geometric mean ratios (extended-release metformin/immediate-release metformin) of AUC_{0-24hr}, AUC_{0-72hr}, and $AUC_{0-inf.}$ for these five studies ranged from 0.96 to 1.08.

In a single-dose, four-period replicate crossover design study, comparing two 500 mg extended-release metformin tablets to one 1000 mg extended-release metformin tablet administered in the evening with food to 29 healthy male subjects, two 500 mg extended-release metformin tablets were found to be equivalent to one 1000 mg extended-release metformin tablet.

In a study carried out with extended-release metformin, there was a dose-associated increase in metformin exposure over 24 hours following oral administration of 1000, 1500, 2000, and 2500 mg.

In three studies with extended-release metformin using different treatment regimens (2000 mg after dinner, 1000 mg after breakfast and after dinner, and 2500 mg after dinner), the pharmacokinetics of metformin as measured by AUC appeared linear following multiple-dose administration.

The extent of absorption (as measured by AUC) of extended-release metformin increased by approximately 60% when given with food. When extended-release metformin was administered with food, C_{max} was increased by approximately 30% and T_{max} was more prolonged compared with the fasting state (6.1 versus 4.0 hours).

Distribution:

Pioglitazone

The mean apparent volume of distribution (V/F) of pioglitazone following single-dose administration is 0.63 ± 0.41 (mean ± SD) L/kg of body weight. Pioglitazone is extensively protein bound (> 99%) in human serum, principally to serum albumin. Pioglitazone also binds to other serum proteins, but with lower affinity. Metabolites M-III and M-IV also are extensively bound (> 98%) to serum albumin.

Metformin hydrochloride

Distribution studies with extended-release metformin have not been conducted; however, the apparent volume of distribution (V/F) of metformin following single oral doses of immediate-release metformin 850 mg averaged 654 ± 358 L. Metformin is negligibly bound to plasma proteins. Metformin partitions into erythrocytes, most likely as a function of time. At usual clinical doses and dosing schedules of immediate-release metformin, steady-state plasma concentrations of metformin are reached within 24-48 hours and are generally <1 µg/mL. During controlled clinical trials of immediate-release metformin, maximum metformin plasma levels did not exceed 5 µg/mL, even at maximum doses.

Metabolism, Elimination and Excretion:

Pioglitazone

Pioglitazone is extensively metabolized by hydroxylation and oxidation; the metabolites also partly convert to glucuronide or sulfate conjugates. Metabolites M-II and M-IV (hydroxy derivatives of pioglitazone) and M-III (keto derivative of pioglitazone) are pharmacologically active in animal models of type 2 diabetes. In addition to pioglitazone, M-III and M-IV are the principal drug-related species found in human serum following multiple dosing. At steady-state, in both healthy volunteers and in patients with type 2 diabetes, pioglitazone comprises approximately 30% to 50% of the total peak serum concentrations and 20% to 25% of the total AUC.

In vitro data demonstrate that multiple CYP isoforms are involved in the metabolism of pioglitazone. The cytochrome P450 isoforms involved are CYP2C8 and, to a lesser degree, CYP3A4 with additional contributions from a variety of other isoforms including the mainly extrahepatic CYP1A1. *In vivo* studies of pioglitazone in combination with P450 inhibitors and substrates have been performed (see **PRECAUTIONS, Drug Interactions,** *Pioglitazone*). Urinary 6ß-hydroxycortisol/cortisol ratios measured in patients treated with pioglitazone showed that pioglitazone is not a strong CYP3A4 enzyme inducer.

Following oral administration, approximately 15% to 30% of the pioglitazone dose is recovered in the urine. Renal elimination of pioglitazone is negligible and the drug is excreted primarily as metabolites and their conjugates. It is presumed that most of the oral dose is excreted into the bile either unchanged or as metabolites and eliminated in the feces.

The mean serum half-life of pioglitazone and total pioglitazone ranges from 3 to 7 hours and 16 to 24 hours, respectively. Pioglitazone has an apparent clearance, CL/F, calculated to be 5 to 7 L/hr.

Metformin hydrochloride

Intravenous single-dose studies in normal subjects demonstrate that metformin is excreted unchanged in the urine and does not undergo hepatic metabolism (no metabolites have been identified in humans) nor biliary excretion. Renal clearance is approximately 3.5 times greater than creatinine clearance which indicates that tubular secretion is the major route of metformin elimination. Following oral administration, approximately 90% of the absorbed drug is eliminated via the renal route within the first 24 hours, with a plasma elimination half-life of approximately 6.2 hours. In blood, the elimination half-life is approximately 17.6 hours, suggesting that the erythrocyte mass may be a compartment of distribution.

Metabolism studies with extended-release metformin tablets have not been conducted.

In healthy nondiabetic adults (N=18) receiving extended-release metformin 2500 mg daily, the percent of the metformin dose excreted in urine over 24 hours was 40.9% and the renal clearance was 542 ± 310 mL/min. After repeated administration of extended-release metformin, there is little or no accumulation of metformin in plasma, with most of the drug being eliminated via renal excretion over a 24-hour dosing interval.

Special Populations

Renal Insufficiency:

Pioglitazone

The serum elimination half-life of pioglitazone, M-III and M-IV remains unchanged in patients with moderate (creatinine clearance 30 to 60 mL/min) to severe (creatinine clearance < 30 mL/min) renal impairment when compared to normal subjects.

Metformin hydrochloride

In patients with decreased renal function (based on creatinine clearance), the plasma and blood half-life of metformin is prolonged and the renal clearance is decreased in proportion to the decrease in creatinine clearance (see **CONTRAINDICATIONS** and **WARNINGS,** *Metformin hydrochloride*, also see GLUCOPHAGE® prescribing information, CLINICAL PHARMACOLOGY, Pharmacokinetics). Since metformin is contraindicated in patients with renal impairment, ACTOPLUS MET and ACTOPLUS MET XR are also contraindicated in these patients.

Hepatic Insufficiency:

Pioglitazone

Compared with normal controls, subjects with impaired hepatic function (Child-Pugh Grade B/C) have an approximate 45% reduction in pioglitazone and total pioglitazone mean peak concentrations but no change in the mean AUC values. Therapy with ACTOPLUS MET or ACTOPLUS MET XR should not be initiated if the patient exhibits clinical evidence of active liver disease or serum transaminase levels (ALT) exceed 2.5 times the upper limit of normal (see **PRECAUTIONS, General:** *Pioglitazone*).

Metformin hydrochloride

No pharmacokinetic studies of metformin have been conducted in subjects with hepatic insufficiency.

Elderly:

Pioglitazone

In healthy elderly subjects, peak serum concentrations of pioglitazone and total pioglitazone are not significantly different, but AUC values are slightly higher and the terminal half-life values slightly longer than for younger subjects. These changes were not of a magnitude that would be considered clinically relevant.

Metformin hydrochloride

Limited data from controlled pharmacokinetic studies of immediate-release metformin in healthy elderly subjects suggest that total plasma clearance of metformin is de-

Table 2. Mean (SD) Pharmacokinetic Parameters for ACTOPLUS MET® XR

Regimen	N	AUC(0-inf) (ng·h/mL)	N	C_max (ng/mL)	N	T_max (h)	N	T_{1/2} (h)
pioglitazone								
15 mg/1000 mg ACTOPLUS MET® XR	59	5113 (1598)	60	487 (126)	60	3.0 (1.0)	60	5.8 (1.4)
15 mg pioglitazone and 1000 mg extended-release metformin	59	5979 (1726)	60	560 (130)	60	3.1 (1.1)	60	6.3 (2.0)
30 mg/1000 mg ACTOPLUS MET® XR	55	8242 (2587)	57	777 (250)	57	3.5 (1.4)	55	6.7 (3.8)
30 mg pioglitazone and 1000 mg extended-release metformin	55	9177 (2200)	57	866 (243)	57	3.1 (1.3)	55	7.6 (3.3)
metformin								
15 mg/1000 mg ACTOPLUS MET® XR	50	14454 (3579)	60	1551 (404)	60	7.2 (1.9)	50	11.7 (7.0)
15 mg pioglitazone and 1000 mg extended-release metformin	50	14787 (3313)	60	1590 (361)	60	6.9 (1.8)	50	11.0 (5.0)
30 mg/1000 mg ACTOPLUS MET® XR	54	12705 (3577)	58	1322 (335)	58	8.0 (2.0)	54	11.1 (5.0)
30 mg pioglitazone and 1000 mg extended-release metformin	54	12796 (3882)	58	1332 (414)	58	7.4 (2.0)	54	11.4 (5.5)

Table 3. Extended-Release Metformin vs. Immediate-Release Metformin Steady-State Pharmacokinetic Parameters at 4 Weeks

Pharmacokinetic Parameters (mean ± SD)	Extended-Release Metformin 2000 mg (administered daily with dinner)	Immediate-Release Metformin 2000 mg (administered as 1000 mg twice daily)
AUC_{0-24 hrs} (ng • hr/mL)	26,811 ± 7055	27,371 ± 5,781
T_max (hr)	6 (3-10)	3 (1-8)
C_max (ng/mL)	2849 ± 797	1820 ± 370

creased, the half-life is prolonged, and C_max is increased, compared to healthy young subjects. From these data, it appears that the change in metformin pharmacokinetics with aging is primarily accounted for by a change in renal function (see GLUCOPHAGE® prescribing information, CLINICAL PHARMACOLOGY, Special Populations, Geriatrics). ACTOPLUS MET or ACTOPLUS MET XR treatment should not be initiated in patients ≥ 80 years of age unless measurement of creatinine clearance demonstrates that renal function is not reduced (see **WARNINGS,** *Metformin hydrochloride* and **DOSAGE AND ADMINISTRATION**; also see GLUCOPHAGE® prescribing information).

Pediatrics:

Pioglitazone

Pharmacokinetic data in the pediatric population are not available. Use in pediatric patients is not recommended for the treatment of diabetes due to lack of long-term safety data. Risks including fractures and other adverse effects associated with pioglitazone, one of the components of ACTOPLUS MET and ACTOPLUS MET XR, have not been determined in this population (see **WARNINGS** and **PRECAUTIONS**).

Metformin hydrochloride

After administration of a single oral immediate-release metformin 500 mg tablet with food, geometric mean metformin C_max and AUC differed less than 5% between pediatric type 2 diabetic patients (12 to 16 years of age) and gender- and weight-matched healthy adults (20 to 45 years of age), and all with normal renal function.

Pharmacokinetic data for extended-release metformin tablets in the pediatric population are not available.

Gender:

Pioglitazone

As monotherapy and in combination with sulfonylurea, metformin, or insulin, pioglitazone improved glycemic control in both males and females. The mean C_max and AUC values were increased 20% to 60% in females. In controlled clinical trials, decreases from baseline in HbA1c were generally greater for females than for males (average mean difference in HbA1c 0.5%). Since therapy should be individualized for each patient to achieve glycemic control, no dose adjustment is recommended based on gender alone.

Metformin hydrochloride

Metformin pharmacokinetic parameters did not differ significantly between normal subjects and patients with type 2 diabetes when analyzed according to gender (males = 19, females = 16). Similarly, in controlled clinical studies in pa-

tients with type 2 diabetes, the antihyperglycemic effect of immediate-release metformin was comparable in males and females.

Five studies indicated that with extended-release metformin treatment, the pharmacokinetic results for males and females were comparable.

Ethnicity:

Pioglitazone

Pharmacokinetic data among various ethnic groups are not available.

Metformin hydrochloride

No studies of metformin pharmacokinetic parameters according to race have been performed. In controlled clinical studies of immediate-release metformin in patients with type 2 diabetes, the antihyperglycemic effect was comparable in whites (n=249), blacks (n=51), and Hispanics (n=24).

Drug-Drug Interactions

Co-administration of a single dose of immediate-release metformin (1000 mg) and pioglitazone after 7 days of pioglitazone (45 mg) did not alter the pharmacokinetics of the single dose of metformin. Specific pharmacokinetic drug interaction studies with ACTOPLUS MET or ACTOPLUS MET XR have not been performed, although such studies have been conducted with the individual pioglitazone and metformin components.

Pioglitazone

The following drugs were studied in healthy volunteers with co-administration of pioglitazone 45 mg once daily. Results are listed below:

Oral Contraceptives: Co-administration of pioglitazone (45 mg once daily) and an oral contraceptive (1 mg norethindrone plus 0.035 mg ethinyl estradiol once daily) for 21 days, resulted in 11% and 11-14% decrease in ethinyl estradiol AUC (0-24h) and C_max respectively. There were no significant changes in norethindrone AUC (0-24h) and C_max. In view of the high variability of ethinyl estradiol pharmacokinetics, the clinical significance of this finding is unknown.

Midazolam: Administration of pioglitazone for 15 days followed by a single 7.5 mg dose of midazolam syrup resulted in a 26% reduction in midazolam C_max and AUC.

Nifedipine ER: Co-administration of pioglitazone for 7 days with 30 mg nifedipine ER administered orally once daily for 4 days to male and female volunteers resulted in a ratio of least square mean (90% CI) values for unchanged nifedipine of 0.83 (0.73-0.95) for C_max and 0.88 (0.80-0.96) for AUC. In view of the high variability of nifedipine pharmacokinetics, the clinical significance of this finding is unknown.

Ketoconazole: Co-administration of pioglitazone for 7 days with ketoconazole 200 mg administered twice daily resulted in a ratio of least square mean (90% CI) values for unchanged pioglitazone of 1.14 (1.06-1.23) for C_{max}, 1.34 (1.26-1.41) for AUC and 1.87 (1.71-2.04) for C_{min}.

Atorvastatin Calcium: Co-administration of pioglitazone for 7 days with atorvastatin calcium (LIPITOR®) 80 mg once daily resulted in a ratio of least square mean (90% CI) values for unchanged pioglitazone of 0.69 (0.57-0.85) for C_{max}, 0.76 (0.65-0.88) for AUC and 0.96 (0.87-1.05) for C_{min}. For unchanged atorvastatin the ratio of least square mean (90% CI) values were 0.77 (0.66-0.90) for C_{max}, 0.86 (0.78-0.94) for AUC and 0.92 (0.82-1.02) for C_{min}.

Cytochrome P450: See **PRECAUTIONS, Drug Interactions,** *Pioglitazone*

Gemfibrozil: Concomitant administration of gemfibrozil (oral 600 mg twice daily), an inhibitor of CYP2C8, with pioglitazone (oral 30 mg) in 10 healthy volunteers pretreated for 2 days prior with gemfibrozil (oral 600 mg twice daily) resulted in pioglitazone exposure (AUC_{0-24}) being 226% of the pioglitazone exposure in the absence of gemfibrozil (see **PRECAUTIONS, Drug Interactions,** *Pioglitazone*).[1]

Rifampin: Concomitant administration of rifampin (oral 600 mg once daily), an inducer of CYP2C8 with pioglitazone (oral 30 mg) in 10 healthy volunteers pre-treated for 5 days prior with rifampin (oral 600 mg once daily) resulted in a decrease in the AUC of pioglitazone by 54% (see **PRECAUTIONS, Drug Interactions,** *Pioglitazone*).[2]

In other drug-drug interaction studies, pioglitazone had no significant effect on the pharmacokinetics of fexofenadine, glipizide, digoxin, warfarin, ranitidine HCl or theophylline.

Metformin hydrochloride

See **PRECAUTIONS, Drug Interactions,** *Metformin hydrochloride*

Pharmacodynamics and Clinical Effects

Pioglitazone

Clinical studies demonstrate that pioglitazone improves insulin sensitivity in insulin-resistant patients. Pioglitazone enhances cellular responsiveness to insulin, increases insulin-dependent glucose disposal, improves hepatic sensitivity to insulin, and improves dysfunctional glucose homeostasis. In patients with type 2 diabetes, the decreased insulin resistance produced by pioglitazone results in lower plasma glucose concentrations, lower plasma insulin levels, and lower HbA1c values. Based on results from an open-label extension study, the glucose-lowering effects of pioglitazone appear to persist for at least one year. In controlled clinical studies, pioglitazone in combination with metformin had an additive effect on glycemic control.

Patients with lipid abnormalities were included in placebo-controlled monotherapy clinical studies with pioglitazone. Overall, patients treated with pioglitazone had mean decreases in triglycerides, mean increases in HDL cholesterol, and no consistent mean changes in LDL cholesterol and total cholesterol compared to the placebo group. A similar pattern of results was seen in 16-week and 24-week combination therapy studies of pioglitazone with metformin.

Clinical Studies

There have been no clinical efficacy studies conducted with ACTOPLUS MET or ACTOPLUS MET XR. However, the efficacy and safety of the separate components have been previously established and the co-administration of the separate components has been evaluated for efficacy and safety in two clinical studies. These clinical studies established an added benefit of pioglitazone in patients with inadequately controlled type 2 diabetes while on metformin therapy. Bioequivalence of ACTOPLUS MET with co-administered pioglitazone and immediate-release metformin tablets and ACTOPLUS MET XR with co-administered pioglitazone and extended-release metformin tablets was demonstrated for both tablet strengths of ACTOPLUS MET and ACTOPLUS MET XR, respectively (see **CLINICAL PHARMACOLOGY, Pharmacokinetics and Drug Metabolism**).

Clinical Trials of Pioglitazone Add-on Therapy in Patients Not Adequately Controlled on Metformin

Two treatment-randomized, controlled clinical studies in patients with type 2 diabetes were conducted to evaluate the safety and efficacy of pioglitazone plus metformin. Both studies included patients receiving metformin, either alone or in combination with another antihyperglycemic agent, who had inadequate glycemic control. All other antihyperglycemic agents were discontinued prior to starting study treatment. In the first study, 328 patients received either 30 mg of pioglitazone or placebo once daily for 16 weeks in addition to their established metformin regimen. In the second study, 827 patients received either 30 mg or 45 mg of pioglitazone once daily for 24 weeks in addition to their established metformin regimen.

In the first study, the addition of pioglitazone 30 mg once daily to metformin treatment significantly reduced the mean HbA1c by 0.8% and the mean fasting plasma glucose (FPG) by 38 mg/dL at Week 16 compared to that observed with metformin alone. In this 16 week study, patients randomized to either pioglitazone or placebo treatment received a median metformin daily dose of 1500 mg with doses ranging from 500 mg to 3400 mg. In the second study, the mean reductions from Baseline at Week 24 in HbA1c were 0.8% and 1.0% for the 30 mg and 45 mg doses, respectively. Mean reductions from Baseline in FPG were 38 mg/dL and 51 mg/dL, respectively. In this 24 week study, patients randomized to either pioglitazone 30 mg or pioglitazone 45 mg treatment received a median metformin daily dose of 1700 mg with doses ranging from 500 mg to 3000 mg. Based on these reductions in HbA1c and FPG (Table 4), the addition of pioglitazone to metformin resulted in significant improvements in glycemic control irrespective of the metformin dose.

[See table 4 below]

INDICATIONS AND USAGE

ACTOPLUS MET and ACTOPLUS MET XR are indicated as an adjunct to diet and exercise to improve glycemic control in adults with type 2 diabetes mellitus who are already treated with pioglitazone and metformin or who have inadequate glycemic control on pioglitazone alone or metformin alone.

Management of type 2 diabetes should also include nutritional counseling, weight reduction as needed, and exercise. These efforts are important not only in the primary treatment of type 2 diabetes, but also to maintain the efficacy of drug therapy. Prior to initiation or escalation of oral antidiabetic therapy in patients with type 2 diabetes mellitus, secondary causes of poor glycemic control, e.g., infection, should be investigated and treated.

CONTRAINDICATIONS

Initiation of ACTOPLUS MET and ACTOPLUS MET XR in patients with established New York Heart Association (NYHA) Class III or IV heart failure is contraindicated (see **BOXED WARNING**).

In addition, ACTOPLUS MET and ACTOPLUS MET XR are contraindicated in patients with:

1. Renal disease or renal dysfunction (e.g., as suggested by serum creatinine levels ≥ 1.5 mg/dL [males], ≥ 1.4 mg/dL [females], or abnormal creatinine clearance) which may also result from conditions such as cardiovascular collapse (shock), acute myocardial infarction, and septicemia (see **WARNINGS, Metformin hydrochloride** and **PRECAUTIONS, General: Metformin hydrochloride**).
2. Known hypersensitivity to pioglitazone, metformin or any other component of ACTOPLUS MET or ACTOPLUS MET XR.
3. Acute or chronic metabolic acidosis, including diabetic ketoacidosis, with or without coma. Diabetic ketoacidosis should be treated with insulin.

ACTOPLUS MET or ACTOPLUS MET XR should be temporarily discontinued in patients undergoing radiologic studies involving intravascular administration of iodinated contrast materials, because use of such products may result in acute alteration of renal function (see **PRECAUTIONS, General: Metformin hydrochloride**).

WARNINGS

Metformin hydrochloride

Lactic Acidosis: Lactic acidosis is a rare, but serious, metabolic complication that can occur due to metformin accumulation during treatment with ACTOPLUS MET (pioglitazone hydrochloride and metformin hydrochloride) or ACTOPLUS MET XR (pioglitazone hydrochloride and metformin hydrochloride extended-release) tablets; when it occurs, it is fatal in approximately 50% of cases. Lactic acidosis may also occur in association with a number of pathophysiologic conditions, including diabetes mellitus, and whenever there is significant tissue hypoperfusion and hypoxemia. Lactic acidosis is characterized by elevated blood lactate levels (> 5 mmol/L), decreased blood pH, electrolyte disturbances with an increased anion gap, and an increased lactate/pyruvate ratio. When metformin is implicated as the cause of lactic acidosis, metformin plasma levels > 5 µg/mL are generally found.

The reported incidence of lactic acidosis in patients receiving metformin hydrochloride is very low (approximately 0.03 cases/1000 patient-years, with approximately 0.015 fatal cases/1000 patient-years). In more than 20,000 patient-years exposure to metformin in clinical trials, there were no reports of lactic acidosis. Reported cases have occurred primarily in diabetic patients with significant renal insufficiency, including both intrinsic renal disease and renal hypoperfusion, often in the setting of multiple concomitant medical/surgical problems and multiple concomitant medications. Patients with congestive heart failure requiring pharmacologic management, in particular those with unstable or acute congestive heart failure who are at risk of hypoperfusion and hypoxemia, are at increased risk of lactic acidosis. The risk of lactic acidosis increases with the degree of renal dysfunction and the patient's age. The risk of lactic acidosis may, therefore, be significantly decreased by

Table 4. Glycemic Parameters in 16-Week and 24-Week Pioglitazone + Metformin Hydrochloride Combination Studies

Parameter	Placebo + metformin	Pioglitazone 30 mg + metformin
16-Week Study		
HbA1c (%)	**N=153**	**N=161**
Baseline mean	9.8	9.9
Mean change from Baseline at 16 Weeks	0.2	-0.6*, †
Difference in change from placebo + metformin		-0.8
Responder rate (%)‡	**22**	**54**
Fasting Plasma Glucose (FPG) (mg/dL)	**N=157**	**N=165**
Baseline mean	260	254
Mean change from Baseline at 16 Weeks	-5	-43*, †
Difference in change from placebo + metformin		-38
Responder rate (%)§	**24**	**59**

Parameter	Pioglitazone 30 mg + metformin	Pioglitazone 45 mg + metformin
24-Week Study		
HbA1c (%)	**N=400**	**N=398**
Baseline mean	9.9	9.8
Mean Change from Baseline at 24 Weeks	-0.8*	-1.0*
Responder rate (%)‡	**56**	**63**
Fasting Plasma Glucose (FPG) (mg/dL)	**N=398**	**N=399**
Baseline mean	233	232
Mean Change from Baseline at 24 Weeks	-38*	-51*, ¶
Responder rate (%)§	**52**	**64**

* significant change from Baseline p ≤ 0.050.
† significant difference from placebo plus metformin, p ≤ 0.050.
‡ patients who achieved HbA1c ≤ 6.1% or ≥ 0.6% decrease from Baseline.
§ patients who achieved a decrease in FPG by ≥ 30 mg/dL.
¶ significant difference from 30 mg pioglitazone, p ≤ 0.050.

regular monitoring of renal function in patients taking metformin and by use of the minimum effective dose of metformin. In particular, treatment of the elderly should be accompanied by careful monitoring of renal function. Metformin treatment should not be initiated in patients ≥ 80 years of age unless measurement of creatinine clearance demonstrates that renal function is not reduced, as these patients are more susceptible to developing lactic acidosis. In addition, metformin should be promptly withheld in the presence of any condition associated with hypoxemia, dehydration, or sepsis. Because impaired hepatic function may significantly limit the ability to clear lactate, metformin should generally be avoided in patients with clinical or laboratory evidence of hepatic disease. Patients should be cautioned against excessive alcohol intake, either acute or chronic, when taking metformin, since alcohol potentiates the effects of metformin hydrochloride on lactate metabolism. In addition, metformin should be temporarily discontinued prior to any intravascular radiocontrast study and for any surgical procedure (see **PRECAUTIONS, General: *Metformin hydrochloride***).

The onset of lactic acidosis often is subtle, and accompanied only by nonspecific symptoms such as malaise, myalgias, respiratory distress, increasing somnolence, and nonspecific abdominal distress. There may be associated hypothermia, hypotension, and resistant bradyarrhythmias with more marked acidosis. The patient and the patient's physician must be aware of the possible importance of such symptoms and the patient should be instructed to notify the physician immediately if they occur (see **PRECAUTIONS, General: *Metformin hydrochloride***). Metformin should be withdrawn until the situation is clarified. Serum electrolytes, ketones, blood glucose, and, if indicated, blood pH, lactate levels, and even blood metformin levels may be useful. Once a patient is stabilized on any dose level of metformin, gastrointestinal symptoms, which are common during initiation of therapy, are unlikely to be drug related. Later occurrence of gastrointestinal symptoms could be due to lactic acidosis or other serious disease.

Levels of fasting venous plasma lactate above the upper limit of normal but less than 5 mmol/L in patients taking metformin do not necessarily indicate impending lactic acidosis and may be explainable by other mechanisms, such as poorly controlled diabetes or obesity, vigorous physical activity, or technical problems in sample handling (see **PRECAUTIONS, General: *Metformin hydrochloride***).

Lactic acidosis should be suspected in any diabetic patient with metabolic acidosis lacking evidence of ketoacidosis (ketonuria and ketonemia).

Lactic acidosis is a medical emergency that must be treated in a hospital setting. In a patient with lactic acidosis who is taking metformin, the drug should be discontinued immediately and general supportive measures promptly instituted. Because metformin hydrochloride is dialyzable (with a clearance of up to 170 mL/min under good hemodynamic conditions), prompt hemodialysis is recommended to correct the acidosis and remove the accumulated metformin. Such management often results in prompt reversal of symptoms and recovery (see **CONTRAINDICATIONS** and **PRECAUTIONS, General: *Metformin hydrochloride***).

Pioglitazone

Cardiac Failure and Other Cardiac Effects: Pioglitazone, like other thiazolidinediones, can cause fluid retention when used alone or in combination with other antihyperglycemic agents, including insulin. Fluid retention may lead to or exacerbate heart failure. Patients should be observed for signs and symptoms of heart failure. If these signs and symptoms develop, the heart failure should be managed according to current standards of care. Furthermore, discontinuation or dose reduction of pioglitazone must be considered. Patients with NYHA Class III and IV cardiac status were not studied during pre-approval clinical trials and pioglitazone is not recommended in these patients (see **BOXED WARNING** and **CONTRAINDICATIONS**).

In one 16-week U.S. double-blind, placebo-controlled clinical trial involving 566 patients with type 2 diabetes, pioglitazone at doses of 15 mg and 30 mg in combination with insulin was compared to insulin therapy alone. This trial included patients with long-standing diabetes and a high prevalence of pre-existing medical conditions as follows: arterial hypertension (57.2%), peripheral neuropathy (22.6%), coronary heart disease (19.6%), retinopathy (13.1%), myocardial infarction (8.8%), vascular disease (6.4%), angina pectoris (4.4%), stroke and/or transient ischemic attack (4.1%), and congestive heart failure (2.3%).

In this study, two of the 191 patients receiving 15 mg pioglitazone plus insulin (1.1%) and two of the 188 patients receiving 30 mg pioglitazone plus insulin (1.1%) developed congestive heart failure compared with none of the 187 patients on insulin therapy alone. All four of these patients had previous histories of cardiovascular conditions including coronary artery disease, previous CABG procedures, and myocardial infarction. In a 24-week dose-controlled study in which pioglitazone was co-administered with insulin, 0.3% of patients (1/345) on 30 mg and 0.9% (3/345) of patients on 45 mg reported CHF as a serious adverse event.

Table 5. Weight Changes (kg) from Baseline during Double-Blind Clinical Trials with Pioglitazone

		Control Group (Placebo)	pioglitazone 15 mg	pioglitazone 30 mg	pioglitazone 45 mg
		Median (25th/75th percentile)	Median (25th/75th percentile)	Median (25th/75th percentile)	Median (25th/75th percentile)
Monotherapy		-1.4 (-2.7/0.0) n=256	0.9 (-0.5/3.4) n = 79	1.0 (-0.9/3.4) n=188	2.6 (0.2/5.4) n = 79
Combination Therapy	Sulfonylurea	-0.5 (-1.8/0.7) n=187	2.0 (0.2/3.2) n=183	3.1 (1.1/5.4) n=528	4.1 (1.8/7.3) n=333
	Metformin	-1.4 (-3.2/0.3) n=160	N/A	0.9 (-0.3/3.2) n=567	1.8 (-0.9/5.0) n=407
	Insulin	0.2 (-1.4/1.4) n=182	2.3 (0.5/4.3) n=190	3.3 (0.9/6.3) n=522	4.1 (1.4/6.8) n=338

Note: Trial durations of 16 to 26 weeks

Analysis of data from these studies did not identify specific factors that predict increased risk of congestive heart failure on combination therapy with insulin.

In type 2 diabetes and congestive heart failure (systolic dysfunction)

A 24-week post-marketing safety study was performed to compare pioglitazone (n=262) to glyburide (n=256) in uncontrolled diabetic patients (mean HbA1c 8.8% at baseline) with NYHA Class II and III heart failure and ejection fraction less than 40% (mean EF 30% at baseline). Over the course of the study, overnight hospitalization for congestive heart failure was reported in 9.9% of patients on pioglitazone compared to 4.7% of patients on glyburide with a treatment difference observed from 6 weeks. This adverse event associated with pioglitazone was more marked in patients using insulin at baseline and in patients over 64 years of age. No difference in cardiovascular mortality between the treatment groups was observed.

Pioglitazone should be initiated at the lowest approved dose if it is prescribed for patients with type 2 diabetes and systolic heart failure (NYHA Class II). If subsequent dose escalation is necessary, the dose should be increased gradually only after several months of treatment with careful monitoring for weight gain, edema, or signs and symptoms of congestive heart failure exacerbation.

Prospective Pioglitazone Clinical Trial In Macrovascular Events (PROactive)

In PROactive, 5238 patients with type 2 diabetes and a prior history of macrovascular disease were treated with ACTOS (n=2605), force-titrated up to 45 mg once daily, or placebo (n=2633) (see **ADVERSE REACTIONS**). The percentage of patients who had an event of serious heart failure was higher for patients treated with ACTOS (5.7%, n=149) than for patients treated with placebo (4.1%, n=108). The incidence of death subsequent to a report of serious heart failure was 1.5% (n=40) in patients treated with ACTOS and 1.4% (n=37) in placebo-treated patients. In patients treated with an insulin-containing regimen at baseline, the incidence of serious heart failure was 6.3% (n=54/864) with ACTOS and 5.2% (n=47/896) with placebo. For those patients treated with a sulfonylurea-containing regimen at baseline, the incidence of serious heart failure was 5.8% (n=94/1624) with ACTOS and 4.4% (n=71/1626) with placebo.

PRECAUTIONS

Macrovascular Outcomes: There have been no clinical studies establishing conclusive evidence of macrovascular risk reduction with ACTOPLUS MET, ACTOPLUS MET XR, or any other anti-diabetic drug.

General: *Pioglitazone*

Pioglitazone exerts its antihyperglycemic effect only in the presence of insulin. Therefore, ACTOPLUS MET and ACTOPLUS MET XR should not be used in patients with type 1 diabetes or for the treatment of diabetic ketoacidosis.

Hypoglycemia: Patients receiving pioglitazone in combination with insulin or oral hypoglycemic agents may be at risk for hypoglycemia, and a reduction in the dose of the concomitant agent may be necessary.

Cardiovascular: In U.S. placebo-controlled clinical trials that excluded patients with New York Heart Association (NYHA) Class III and IV cardiac status, the incidence of serious cardiac adverse events related to volume expansion was not increased in patients treated with pioglitazone as monotherapy or in combination with sulfonylureas or metformin vs. placebo-treated patients. In insulin combination studies, a small number of patients with a history of previously existing cardiac disease developed congestive heart failure when treated with pioglitazone in combination with insulin (see **WARNINGS, *Pioglitazone***). Patients with NYHA Class III and IV cardiac status were not studied in pre-approval pioglitazone clinical trials. Pioglitazone is not indicated in patients with NYHA Class III or IV cardiac status.

In postmarketing experience with pioglitazone, cases of congestive heart failure have been reported in patients both with and without previously known heart disease.

Edema: In all U.S. clinical trials with pioglitazone, edema was reported more frequently in patients treated with pioglitazone than in placebo-treated patients and appears to be dose related (see **ADVERSE REACTIONS**). In postmarketing experience, reports of initiation or worsening of edema have been received. Since thiazolidinediones, including pioglitazone, can cause fluid retention, which can exacerbate or lead to congestive heart failure, ACTOPLUS MET or ACTOPLUS MET XR should be used with caution in patients at risk for heart failure. Patients should be monitored for signs and symptoms of heart failure (see **BOXED WARNING, WARNINGS, *Pioglitazone***, and **PRECAUTIONS, Information for Patients**).

Weight Gain: Dose related weight gain was observed with pioglitazone alone and in combination with other hypoglycemic agents (**Table 5**). The mechanism of weight gain is unclear but probably involves a combination of fluid retention and fat accumulation.

[See table 5 above]

Ovulation: Therapy with pioglitazone, like other thiazolidinediones, may result in ovulation in some premenopausal anovulatory women. Thus, adequate contraception in premenopausal women should be recommended while taking ACTOPLUS MET or ACTOPLUS MET XR. This possible effect has not been investigated in clinical studies so the frequency of this occurrence is not known.

Hematologic: Across all clinical studies with pioglitazone, mean hemoglobin values declined by 2% to 4% in patients treated with pioglitazone. These changes primarily occurred within the first 4 to 12 weeks of therapy and remained relatively constant thereafter. These changes may be related to increased plasma volume and have rarely been associated with any significant hematologic clinical effects (see **ADVERSE REACTIONS, Laboratory Abnormalities**). ACTOPLUS MET or ACTOPLUS MET XR may cause decreases in hemoglobin and hematocrit.

Hepatic Effects: In pre-approval clinical studies worldwide, over 4500 subjects were treated with pioglitazone. In U.S. clinical studies, over 4700 patients with type 2 diabetes received pioglitazone. There was no evidence of drug-induced hepatotoxicity or elevation of ALT levels in the clinical studies.

During pre-approval placebo-controlled clinical trials in the U.S., a total of 4 of 1526 (0.26%) patients treated with pioglitazone and 2 of 793 (0.25%) placebo-treated patients had ALT values ≥ 3 times the upper limit of normal. The ALT elevations in patients treated with pioglitazone were reversible and were not clearly related to therapy with pioglitazone.

In postmarketing experience with pioglitazone, reports of hepatitis and of hepatic enzyme elevations to 3 or more times the upper limit of normal have been received. Very rarely, these reports have involved hepatic failure with and without fatal outcome, although causality has not been established.

Pending the availability of the results of additional large, long-term controlled clinical trials and additional postmarketing safety data on pioglitazone, it is recommended that patients treated with ACTOPLUS MET or ACTOPLUS MET XR undergo periodic monitoring of liver enzymes.

Serum ALT (alanine aminotransferase) levels should be evaluated prior to the initiation of therapy with ACTOPLUS MET or ACTOPLUS MET XR in all patients and periodically thereafter per the clinical judgment of the health care professional. Liver function tests should also be obtained for patients if symptoms suggestive of hepatic dysfunction occur, e.g., nausea, vomiting, abdominal pain, fatigue, anorexia, or dark urine. The decision whether to continue the patient on therapy with ACTOPLUS MET or ACTOPLUS MET XR should be guided by clinical judgment pending laboratory evaluations. If jaundice is observed, drug therapy should be discontinued.

Therapy with ACTOPLUS MET or ACTOPLUS MET XR should not be initiated if the patient exhibits clinical evidence of active liver disease or the ALT levels exceed 2.5 times the upper limit of normal. Patients with mildly elevated liver enzymes (ALT levels at 1 to 2.5 times the upper limit of normal) at baseline or any time during therapy with ACTOPLUS MET or ACTOPLUS MET XR should be evaluated to determine the cause of the liver enzyme elevation. Initiation or continuation of therapy with ACTOPLUS MET or ACTOPLUS MET XR in patients with mildly elevated liver enzymes should proceed with caution and include appropriate clinical follow-up which may include more frequent liver enzyme monitoring. If serum transaminase levels are increased (ALT > 2.5 times the upper limit of normal), liver function tests should be evaluated more frequently until the levels return to normal or pretreatment values. If ALT levels exceed 3 times the upper limit of normal, the test should be repeated as soon as possible. If ALT levels remain > 3 times the upper limit of normal or if the patient is jaundiced, ACTOPLUS MET or ACTOPLUS MET XR therapy should be discontinued.

Macular Edema: Macular edema has been reported in postmarketing experience in diabetic patients who were taking pioglitazone or another thiazolidinedione. Some patients presented with blurred vision or decreased visual acuity, but some patients appear to have been diagnosed on routine ophthalmologic examination. Some patients had peripheral edema at the time macular edema was diagnosed. Some patients had improvement in their macular edema after discontinuation of their thiazolidinedione. It is unknown whether or not there is a causal relationship between pioglitazone and macular edema. Patients with diabetes should have regular eye exams by an ophthalmologist, per the Standards of Care of the American Diabetes Association. Additionally, any diabetic who reports any kind of visual symptom should be promptly referred to an ophthalmologist, regardless of the patient's underlying medications or other physical findings (see **ADVERSE REACTIONS**).

Fractures: In a randomized trial (PROactive) in patients with type 2 diabetes (mean duration of diabetes 9.5 years), an increased incidence of bone fracture was noted in female patients taking pioglitazone. During a mean follow-up of 34.5 months, the incidence of bone fracture in females was 5.1% (44/870) for pioglitazone versus 2.5% (23/905) for placebo. This difference was noted after the first year of treatment and remained during the course of the study. The majority of fractures observed in female patients were nonvertebral fractures including lower limb and distal upper limb. No increase in fracture rates was observed in men treated with pioglitazone 1.7% (30/1735) versus placebo 2.1% (37/1728). The risk of fracture should be considered in the care of patients, especially female patients, treated with pioglitazone and attention should be given to assessing and maintaining bone health according to current standards of care.

General: *Metformin hydrochloride*
Monitoring of renal function: Metformin is known to be substantially excreted by the kidney, and the risk of metformin accumulation and lactic acidosis increases with the degree of impairment of renal function. Thus, patients with serum creatinine levels above the upper limit of normal for their age should not receive ACTOPLUS MET or ACTOPLUS MET XR. In patients with advanced age, ACTOPLUS MET or ACTOPLUS MET XR should be carefully titrated to establish the minimum dose for adequate glycemic effect, because aging is associated with reduced renal function. In elderly patients, particularly those ≥ 80 years of age, renal function should be monitored regularly and, generally, ACTOPLUS MET or ACTOPLUS MET XR should not be titrated to the maximum dose of the metformin component (see **WARNINGS**, *Metformin hydrochloride* and **DOSAGE AND ADMINISTRATION**). Before initiation of therapy with ACTOPLUS MET or ACTOPLUS MET XR and at least annually thereafter, renal function should be assessed and verified as normal. In patients in whom development of renal dysfunction is anticipated, renal function should be assessed more frequently and ACTOPLUS MET or ACTOPLUS MET XR discontinued if evidence of renal impairment is present.

Use of concomitant medications that may affect renal function or metformin disposition: Concomitant medication(s) that may affect renal function or result in significant hemo-

dynamic change or may interfere with the disposition of metformin, such as cationic drugs that are eliminated by renal tubular secretion (see **PRECAUTIONS, Drug Interactions,** *Metformin hydrochloride*), should be used with caution.

Radiologic studies involving the use of intravascular iodinated contrast materials (for example, intravenous urogram, intravenous cholangiography, angiography, and computed tomography (CT) scans with intravascular contrast materials): Intravascular contrast studies with iodinated materials can lead to acute alteration of renal function and have been associated with lactic acidosis in patients receiving metformin (see **CONTRAINDICATIONS**). Therefore, in patients in whom any such study is planned, ACTOPLUS MET or ACTOPLUS MET XR should be temporarily discontinued at the time of or prior to the procedure, and withheld for 48 hours subsequent to the procedure and reinstituted only after renal function has been re-evaluated and found to be normal.

Hypoxic states: Cardiovascular collapse (shock) from whatever cause, acute congestive heart failure, acute myocardial infarction and other conditions characterized by hypoxemia have been associated with lactic acidosis and may also cause prerenal azotemia. When such events occur in patients receiving ACTOPLUS MET or ACTOPLUS MET XR therapy, the drug should be promptly discontinued.

Surgical procedures: Use of ACTOPLUS MET or ACTOPLUS MET XR should be temporarily suspended for any surgical procedure (except minor procedures not associated with restricted intake of food and fluids) and should not be restarted until the patient's oral intake has resumed and renal function has been evaluated as normal.

Alcohol intake: Alcohol is known to potentiate the effect of metformin on lactate metabolism. Patients, therefore, should be warned against excessive alcohol intake, acute or chronic, while receiving ACTOPLUS MET or ACTOPLUS MET XR.

Impaired hepatic function: Since impaired hepatic function has been associated with some cases of lactic acidosis, ACTOPLUS MET and ACTOPLUS MET XR should generally be avoided in patients with clinical or laboratory evidence of hepatic disease.

Vitamin B_{12} levels: In controlled clinical trials of metformin at 29 weeks' duration, a decrease to subnormal levels of previously normal serum vitamin B_{12} levels, without clinical manifestations, was observed in approximately 7% of patients. Such decrease, possibly due to interference with B_{12} absorption from the B_{12}-intrinsic factor complex, is, however, very rarely associated with anemia and appears to be rapidly reversible with discontinuation of metformin or vitamin B_{12} supplementation. Measurement of hematologic parameters on an annual basis is advised in patients on ACTOPLUS MET or ACTOPLUS MET XR and any apparent abnormalities should be appropriately investigated and managed (see **PRECAUTIONS, General:** *Metformin hydrochloride* and **Laboratory Tests**). Certain individuals (those with inadequate vitamin B_{12} or calcium intake or absorption) appear to be predisposed to developing subnormal vitamin B_{12} levels. In these patients, routine serum vitamin B_{12} measurements at two- to three-year intervals may be useful.

Change in clinical status of patients with previously controlled type 2 diabetes: A patient with type 2 diabetes previously well controlled on ACTOPLUS MET or ACTOPLUS MET XR who develops laboratory abnormalities or clinical illness (especially vague and poorly defined illness) should be evaluated promptly for evidence of ketoacidosis or lactic acidosis. Evaluation should include serum electrolytes and ketones, blood glucose and, if indicated, blood pH, lactate, pyruvate and metformin levels. If acidosis of either form occurs, ACTOPLUS MET and ACTOPLUS MET XR must be stopped immediately and other appropriate corrective measures initiated (see **WARNINGS,** *Metformin hydrochloride*).

Hypoglycemia: Hypoglycemia does not occur in patients receiving metformin alone under usual circumstances of use, but could occur when caloric intake is insufficient, when strenuous exercise is not compensated by caloric supplementation, or during concomitant use with hypoglycemic agents (such as sulfonylureas or insulin) or ethanol. Elderly, debilitated or malnourished patients and those with adrenal or pituitary insufficiency or alcohol intoxication are particularly susceptible to hypoglycemic effects. Hypoglycemia may be difficult to recognize in the elderly and in people who are taking beta-adrenergic blocking drugs.

Loss of control of blood glucose: When a patient stabilized on any diabetic regimen is exposed to stress such as fever, trauma, infection, or surgery, a temporary loss of glycemic control may occur. At such times, it may be necessary to withhold ACTOPLUS MET or ACTOPLUS MET XR and temporarily administer insulin. ACTOPLUS MET or ACTOPLUS MET XR may be reinstituted after the acute episode is resolved.

Laboratory Tests
FPG and HbA1c measurements should be performed periodically to monitor glycemic control and therapeutic response to ACTOPLUS MET or ACTOPLUS MET XR.

Liver enzyme monitoring is recommended prior to initiation of therapy with ACTOPLUS MET or ACTOPLUS MET XR in all patients and periodically thereafter per the clinical judgment of the health care professional (see **PRECAUTIONS, General:** *Pioglitazone* and **ADVERSE REACTIONS,** Serum Transaminase Levels).

Initial and periodic monitoring of hematologic parameters (e.g., hemoglobin/hematocrit and red blood cell indices) and renal function (serum creatinine) should be performed, at least on an annual basis. While megaloblastic anemia has rarely been seen with metformin therapy, if this is suspected, Vitamin B_{12} deficiency should be excluded.

Information for Patients
Patients should be instructed regarding the importance of adhering to dietary instructions, a regular exercise program, and regular testing of blood glucose and HbA1c. During periods of stress such as fever, trauma, infection, or surgery, medication requirements may change and patients should be reminded to seek medical advice promptly.

The risks of lactic acidosis, its symptoms and conditions that predispose to its development, as noted in the **WARNINGS,** *Metformin hydrochloride* and **PRECAUTIONS, General:** *Metformin hydrochloride* sections, should be explained to patients. Patients should be advised to discontinue ACTOPLUS MET or ACTOPLUS MET XR immediately and to promptly notify their health care professional if unexplained hyperventilation, myalgia, malaise, unusual somnolence or other nonspecific symptoms occur. Gastrointestinal symptoms are common during initiation of metformin treatment and may occur during initiation of ACTOPLUS MET or ACTOPLUS MET XR therapy; however, patients should consult with their physician if they develop unexplained symptoms. Although gastrointestinal symptoms that occur after stabilization are unlikely to be drug related, such an occurrence of symptoms should be evaluated to determine if it may be due to lactic acidosis or other serious disease.

Patients should be counseled against excessive alcohol intake, either acute or chronic, while receiving ACTOPLUS MET or ACTOPLUS MET XR.

Patients who experience an unusually rapid increase in weight or edema or who develop shortness of breath or other symptoms of heart failure while on ACTOPLUS MET or ACTOPLUS MET XR should immediately report these symptoms to their physician.

Patients should be told that blood tests for liver function will be performed prior to the start of therapy and periodically thereafter per the clinical judgment of the health care professional. Patients should be told to seek immediate medical advice for unexplained nausea, vomiting, abdominal pain, fatigue, anorexia, or dark urine.

Patients should be informed about the importance of regular testing of renal function and hematologic parameters when receiving treatment with ACTOPLUS MET or ACTOPLUS MET XR.

Therapy with a thiazolidinedione, which is the active pioglitazone component of the ACTOPLUS MET and ACTOPLUS MET XR tablets, may result in ovulation in some premenopausal anovulatory women. As a result, these patients may be at an increased risk for pregnancy while taking ACTOPLUS MET or ACTOPLUS MET XR. Thus, adequate contraception in premenopausal women should be recommended. This possible effect has not been investigated in clinical studies so the frequency of this occurrence is not known.

Combination antihyperglycemic therapy may cause hypoglycemia. When initiating ACTOPLUS MET or ACTOPLUS MET XR, the risks of hypoglycemia, its symptoms and treatment, and conditions that predispose to its development should be explained to patients.

Patients should be told to take ACTOPLUS MET or ACTOPLUS MET XR as prescribed and instructed that any change in dosing should only be done if directed by their physician. Patients should be informed that if they miss a dose, to take the next dose as prescribed unless directed otherwise by their physician. Patients should be informed that ACTOPLUS MET XR must be swallowed whole and not chewed, cut, or crushed, and that the inactive ingredients may occasionally be eliminated in the feces as a soft mass that may resemble the original tablet.

Drug Interactions
Pioglitazone
In vivo drug-drug interaction studies have suggested that pioglitazone may be a weak inducer of CYP450 isoform 3A4 substrate.

An enzyme inhibitor of CYP2C8 (such as gemfibrozil) may significantly increase the AUC of pioglitazone and an enzyme inducer of CYP2C8 (such as rifampin) may significantly decrease the AUC of pioglitazone. Therefore, if an inhibitor or inducer of CYP2C8 is started or stopped during treatment with pioglitazone, changes in diabetes treatment may be needed based on clinical response (see **CLINICAL PHARMACOLOGY, Drug-Drug Interactions,** *Pioglitazone*).

Metformin hydrochloride (Clinical Evaluation of Drug Interactions Conducted with Immediate-Release Metformin)

Glyburide: In a single-dose interaction study in type 2 diabetes patients, co-administration of metformin and glyburide did not result in any changes in either metformin pharmacokinetics or pharmacodynamics. Decreases in glyburide AUC and C_{max} were observed, but were highly variable. The single-dose nature of this study and the lack of correlation between glyburide blood levels and pharmacodynamic effects, makes the clinical significance of this interaction uncertain.

Furosemide: A single-dose, metformin-furosemide drug interaction study in healthy subjects demonstrated that pharmacokinetic parameters of both compounds were affected by co-administration. Furosemide increased the metformin plasma and blood C_{max} by 22% and blood AUC by 15%, without any significant change in metformin renal clearance. When administered with metformin, the C_{max} and AUC of furosemide were 31% and 12% smaller, respectively, than when administered alone and the terminal half-life was decreased by 32%, without any significant change in furosemide renal clearance. No information is available about the interaction of metformin and furosemide when co-administered chronically.

Nifedipine: A single-dose, metformin-nifedipine drug interaction study in normal healthy volunteers demonstrated that co-administration of nifedipine increased plasma metformin C_{max} and AUC by 20% and 9%, respectively and increased the amount excreted in the urine. T_{max} and half-life were unaffected. Nifedipine appears to enhance the absorption of metformin. Metformin had minimal effects on nifedipine.

Cationic Drugs: Cationic drugs (e.g., amiloride, digoxin, morphine, procainamide, quinidine, quinine, ranitidine, triamterene, trimethoprim, and vancomycin) that are eliminated by renal tubular secretion theoretically have the potential for interaction with metformin by competing for common renal tubular transport systems. Such interaction between metformin and oral cimetidine has been observed in normal healthy volunteers in both single- and multiple-dose, metformin-cimetidine drug interaction studies with a 60% increase in peak metformin plasma and whole blood concentrations and a 40% increase in plasma and whole blood metformin AUC. There was no change in elimination half-life in the single-dose study. Metformin had no effect on cimetidine pharmacokinetics. Although such interactions remain theoretical (except for cimetidine), careful patient monitoring and dose adjustment of ACTOPLUS MET or ACTOPLUS MET XR and/or the interfering drug is recommended in patients who are taking cationic medications that are excreted via the proximal renal tubular secretory system.

Other: Certain drugs tend to produce hyperglycemia and may lead to loss of glycemic control. These drugs include thiazides and other diuretics, corticosteroids, phenothiazines, thyroid products, estrogens, oral contraceptives, phenytoin, nicotinic acid, sympathomimetics, calcium channel blocking drugs, and isoniazid. When such drugs are administered to a patient receiving ACTOPLUS MET or ACTOPLUS MET XR, the patient should be closely observed to maintain adequate glycemic control. When such drugs are withdrawn from a patient receiving ACTOPLUS MET or ACTOPLUS MET XR, the patient should be observed closely for hypoglycemia.

In healthy volunteers, the pharmacokinetics of metformin and propranolol and metformin and ibuprofen were not affected when co-administered in single-dose interaction studies.

Metformin is negligibly bound to plasma proteins and is therefore, less likely to interact with highly protein-bound drugs such as salicylates, sulfonamides, chloramphenicol and probenecid.

Carcinogenesis, Mutagenesis, Impairment of Fertility

ACTOPLUS MET and ACTOPLUS MET XR

No animal studies have been conducted with ACTOPLUS MET or ACTOPLUS MET XR. The following data are based on findings in studies performed with pioglitazone or metformin individually.

Pioglitazone

A two-year carcinogenicity study was conducted in male and female rats at oral doses up to 63 mg/kg (approximately 14 times the maximum recommended human oral dose of 45 mg based on mg/m^2). Drug-induced tumors were not observed in any organ except for the urinary bladder. Benign and/or malignant transitional cell neoplasms were observed in male rats at 4 mg/kg/day and above (approximately equal to the maximum recommended human oral dose based on mg/m^2). A two-year carcinogenicity study was conducted in male and female mice at oral doses up to 100 mg/kg/day (approximately 11 times the maximum recommended human oral dose based on mg/m^2). No drug-induced tumors were observed in any organ.

During prospective evaluation of urinary cytology involving more than 1800 patients receiving pioglitazone in clinical trials up to one year in duration, no new cases of bladder tumors were identified. In two 3-year studies in which pioglitazone was compared to placebo or glyburide, there were 16/3656 (0.44%) reports of bladder cancer in patients taking pioglitazone compared to 5/3679 (0.14%) in patients not taking pioglitazone. After excluding patients in whom exposure to study drug was less than one year at the time of diagnosis of bladder cancer, there were six (0.16%) cases on pioglitazone and two (0.05%) on placebo.

Pioglitazone HCl was not mutagenic in a battery of genetic toxicology studies, including the Ames bacterial assay, a mammalian cell forward gene mutation assay (CHO/HPRT and AS52/XPRT), an *in vitro* cytogenetics assay using CHL cells, an unscheduled DNA synthesis assay, and an *in vivo* micronucleus assay.

No adverse effects upon fertility were observed in male and female rats at oral doses up to 40 mg/kg pioglitazone HCl daily prior to and throughout mating and gestation (approximately 9 times the maximum recommended human oral dose based on mg/m^2).

Metformin hydrochloride

Long-term carcinogenicity studies have been performed in rats (dosing duration of 104 weeks) and mice (dosing duration of 91 weeks) at doses up to and including 900 mg/kg/day and 1500 mg/kg/day, respectively. These doses are both approximately four times a human daily dose of 2000 mg of the metformin component of ACTOPLUS MET and ACTOPLUS MET XR based on body surface area comparisons. No evidence of carcinogenicity with metformin was found in either male or female mice. Similarly, there was no tumorigenic potential observed with metformin in male rats. There was, however, an increased incidence of benign stromal uterine polyps in female rats treated with 900 mg/kg/day.

There was no evidence of mutagenic potential of metformin in the following *in vitro* tests: Ames test (*S. typhimurium*), gene mutation test (mouse lymphoma cells), or chromosomal aberrations test (human lymphocytes). Results in the *in vivo* mouse micronucleus test were also negative.

Fertility of male or female rats was unaffected by metformin when administered at doses as high as 600 mg/kg/day, which is approximately three times the maximum recommended human daily dose of the metformin component of ACTOPLUS MET and ACTOPLUS MET XR based on body surface area comparisons.

Animal Toxicology

Pioglitazone

Heart enlargement has been observed in mice (100 mg/kg), rats (4 mg/kg and above) and dogs (3 mg/kg) treated orally with the pioglitazone HCl component of ACTOPLUS MET and ACTOPLUS MET XR (approximately 11, 1, and 2 times the maximum recommended human oral dose for mice, rats, and dogs, respectively, based on mg/m^2). In a one-year rat study, drug-related early death due to apparent heart dysfunction occurred at an oral dose of 160 mg/kg/day (approximately 35 times the maximum recommended human oral dose based on mg/m^2). Heart enlargement was seen in a 13-week study in monkeys at oral doses of 8.9 mg/kg and above (approximately 4 times the maximum recommended human oral dose based on mg/m^2), but not in a 52-week study at oral doses up to 32 mg/kg (approximately 13 times the maximum recommended human oral dose based on mg/m^2).

Pregnancy: Pregnancy Category C

ACTOPLUS MET and ACTOPLUS MET XR

Because current information strongly suggests that abnormal blood glucose levels during pregnancy are associated with a higher incidence of congenital anomalies, as well as increased neonatal morbidity and mortality, most experts recommend that insulin be used during pregnancy to maintain blood glucose levels as close to normal as possible. ACTOPLUS MET and ACTOPLUS MET XR should not be used during pregnancy unless the potential benefit justifies the potential risk to the fetus.

There are no adequate and well-controlled studies in pregnant women with ACTOPLUS MET or ACTOPLUS MET XR or their individual components. No animal studies have been conducted with the combined products in ACTOPLUS MET or ACTOPLUS MET XR. The following data are based on findings in studies performed with pioglitazone or metformin individually.

Pioglitazone

Pioglitazone was not teratogenic in rats at oral doses up to 80 mg/kg or in rabbits given up to 160 mg/kg during organogenesis (approximately 17 and 40 times the maximum recommended human oral dose based on mg/m^2, respectively). Delayed parturition and embryotoxicity (as evidenced by increased postimplantation losses, delayed development and reduced fetal weights) were observed in rats at oral doses of 40 mg/kg/day and above (approximately 10 times the maximum recommended human oral dose based on mg/m^2). No functional or behavioral toxicity was observed in offspring of rats. In rabbits, embryotoxicity was observed at an oral dose of 160 mg/kg (approximately 40 times the maximum recommended human oral dose based on mg/m^2). Delayed postnatal development, attributed to decreased body weight, was observed in offspring of rats at oral doses of 10 mg/kg and above during late gestation and lactation periods (approximately 2 times the maximum recommended human oral dose based on mg/m^2).

Metformin hydrochloride

Metformin was not teratogenic in rats and rabbits at doses up to 600 mg/kg/day. This represents an exposure of about two and six times a human daily dose of 2000 mg based on body surface area comparisons for rats and rabbits, respectively. Determination of fetal concentrations demonstrated a partial placental barrier to metformin.

Nursing Mothers

No studies have been conducted with the combined components of ACTOPLUS MET or ACTOPLUS MET XR. In studies performed with the individual components, both pioglitazone and metformin are secreted in the milk of lactating rats. It is not known whether pioglitazone and/or metformin is secreted in human milk. Because many drugs are excreted in human milk, ACTOPLUS MET and ACTOPLUS MET XR should not be administered to a breastfeeding woman. If ACTOPLUS MET or ACTOPLUS MET XR is discontinued, and if diet alone is inadequate for controlling blood glucose, insulin therapy should be considered.

Pediatric Use

Safety and effectiveness of ACTOPLUS MET or ACTOPLUS MET XR in pediatric patients have not been established. Use in pediatric patients is not recommended for the treatment of diabetes due to lack of long-term safety data. Risks including fractures and other adverse effects associated with pioglitazone, one of the components of ACTOPLUS MET and ACTOPLUS MET XR, have not been determined in this population (see **WARNINGS** and **PRECAUTIONS**).

Elderly Use

Pioglitazone

Approximately 500 patients in placebo-controlled clinical trials of pioglitazone were 65 and over. No significant differences in effectiveness and safety were observed between these patients and younger patients.

Metformin hydrochloride

Controlled clinical studies of immediate-release metformin did not include sufficient numbers of elderly patients to determine whether they respond differently from younger patients, although other reported clinical experience has not identified differences in responses between the elderly and young patients.

Of the 389 patients who received extended-release metformin in controlled Phase III clinical studies, 26.5% [103/389] were 65 years and older. No overall differences in effectiveness or safety were observed between these patients and younger patients.

Metformin is known to be substantially excreted by the kidney and because the risk of serious adverse reactions to the drug is greater in patients with impaired renal function, ACTOPLUS MET and ACTOPLUS MET XR should only be used in patients with normal renal function (see **CONTRAINDICATIONS**, **WARNINGS,** ***Metformin hydrochloride*** and **CLINICAL PHARMACOLOGY, Special Populations**). Because aging is associated with reduced renal function, ACTOPLUS MET and ACTOPLUS MET XR should be used with caution as age increases. Care should be taken in dose selection and should be based on careful and regular monitoring of renal function. Generally, elderly patients should not be titrated to the maximum dose of ACTOPLUS MET or ACTOPLUS MET XR (see **WARNINGS,** ***Metformin hydrochloride*** and **DOSAGE AND ADMINISTRATION**).

ADVERSE REACTIONS

Over 8500 patients with type 2 diabetes have been treated with pioglitazone in randomized, double-blind, controlled clinical trials. This includes 2605 high-risk patients with type 2 diabetes treated with pioglitazone from the PROactive clinical trial. Over 6000 patients have been treated for 6 months or longer, and over 4500 patients for one year or longer. Over 3000 patients have received pioglitazone for at least 2 years.

The most common adverse events reported in at least 5% of patients in the controlled 16-week clinical trial between placebo plus metformin and pioglitazone 30 mg plus metformin were upper respiratory tract infection (15.6% and 15.5%), diarrhea (6.3% and 4.8%), combined edema/peripheral edema (2.5% and 6.0%) and headache (1.9% and 6.0%), respectively.

The incidence and type of adverse events reported in at least 5% of patients in any combined treatment group from the 24-week study comparing pioglitazone 30 mg plus metformin and pioglitazone 45 mg plus metformin are shown in Table 6; the rate of adverse events resulting in study discontinuation between the two treatment groups was 7.8% and 7.7%, respectively.

Table 6. Adverse Events That Occurred in ≥ 5% of Patients in Any Treatment Group During the 24-Week Study

Adverse Event Preferred Term	Pioglitazone 30 mg + metformin N=411 n (%)	Pioglitazone 45 mg + metformin N=416 n (%)
Upper Respiratory Tract Infection	51 (12.4)	56 (13.5)
Diarrhea	24 (5.8)	20 (4.8)
Nausea	24 (5.8)	15 (3.6)
Headache	19 (4.6)	22 (5.3)
Urinary Tract Infection	24 (5.8)	22 (5.3)
Sinusitis	18 (4.4)	21 (5.0)
Dizziness	22 (5.4)	20 (4.8)
Edema Lower Limb	12 (2.9)	47 (11.3)
Weight Increased	12 (2.9)	28 (6.7)

Most clinical adverse events were similar between groups treated with pioglitazone in combination with metformin and those treated with pioglitazone monotherapy. Other adverse events reported in at least 5% of patients in controlled clinical trials between placebo and pioglitazone monotherapy included myalgia (2.7% and 5.4%), tooth disorder (2.3% and 5.3%), diabetes mellitus aggravated (8.1% and 5.1%) and pharyngitis (0.8% and 5.1%), respectively.

In U.S. double-blind studies, anemia was reported in ≤ 2% of patients treated with pioglitazone plus metformin (see **PRECAUTIONS, General: Pioglitazone**).

In monotherapy studies, edema was reported for 4.8% (with doses from 7.5 mg to 45 mg) of patients treated with pioglitazone versus 1.2% of placebo-treated patients. Most of these events were considered mild or moderate in intensity (see **PRECAUTIONS, General: Pioglitazone**).

Prospective Pioglitazone Clinical Trial In Macrovascular Events (PROactive)

In PROactive, 5238 patients with type 2 diabetes and a prior history of macrovascular disease were treated with ACTOS (n=2605), force-titrated up to 45 mg daily, or placebo (n=2633), in addition to standard of care. Almost all subjects (95%) were receiving cardiovascular medications (beta blockers, ACE inhibitors, ARBs, calcium channel blockers, nitrates, diuretics, aspirin, statins, fibrates). Patients had a mean age of 61.8 years, mean duration of diabetes 9.5 years, and mean HbA1c of 8.1%. Average duration of follow-up was 34.5 months. The primary objective of this trial was to examine the effect of ACTOS on mortality and macrovascular morbidity in patients with type 2 diabetes mellitus who were at high risk for macrovascular events. The primary efficacy variable was the time to the first occurrence of any event in the cardiovascular composite endpoint (see Table 7 below). Although there was no statistically significant difference between ACTOS and placebo for the 3-year incidence of a first event within this composite, there was no increase in mortality or in total macrovascular events with ACTOS.

Table 7. Number of First and Total Events for Each Component within the Cardiovascular Composite Endpoint

Cardiovascular Events	Placebo N=2633 First Events (N)	Placebo N=2633 Total events (N)	ACTOS N=2605 First Events (N)	ACTOS N=2605 Total events (N)
Any event	572	900	514	803
All-cause mortality	122	186	110	177
Non-fatal MI	118	157	105	131
Stroke	96	119	76	92
ACS	63	78	42	65
Cardiac intervention	101	240	101	195
Major leg amputation	15	28	9	28
Leg revascularization	57	92	71	115

Postmarketing reports of new onset or worsening diabetic macular edema with decreased visual acuity have also been received (see **PRECAUTIONS, General: Pioglitazone**).

Laboratory Abnormalities

Hematologic: Pioglitazone may cause decreases in hemoglobin and hematocrit. The fall in hemoglobin and hematocrit with pioglitazone appears to be dose related. Across all clinical studies, mean hemoglobin values declined by 2% to 4% in patients treated with pioglitazone. These changes generally occurred within the first 4 to 12 weeks of therapy and remained relatively stable thereafter. These changes may be related to increased plasma volume associated with pioglitazone therapy and have rarely been associated with any significant hematologic clinical effects (see **PRECAUTIONS, General: Pioglitazone**).

In controlled clinical trials of metformin at 29 weeks' duration, a decrease to subnormal levels of previously normal serum vitamin B_{12} levels, without clinical manifestations, was observed in approximately 7% of patients. Such decrease, possibly due to interference with B_{12} absorption from the B_{12}-intrinsic factor complex, is, however, very rarely associated with anemia and appears to be rapidly reversible with discontinuation of metformin or vitamin B_{12} supplementation (see **PRECAUTIONS, General: Metformin hydrochloride**).

Serum Transaminase Levels: During all clinical studies in the U.S., 14 of 4780 (0.30%) patients treated with pioglitazone had alanine aminotransferase (ALT) values ≥ 3 times the upper limit of normal during treatment. All patients with follow-up values had reversible elevations in ALT. In the population of patients treated with pioglitazone, mean values for bilirubin, aspartate aminotransferase (AST), ALT, alkaline phosphatase, and γ-glutamyl transferase (GGT) were decreased at the final visit compared with baseline. Fewer than 0.9% of patients treated with pioglitazone were withdrawn from clinical trials in the U.S. due to abnormal liver function tests.

In pre-approval clinical trials, there were no cases of idiosyncratic drug reactions leading to hepatic failure (see **PRECAUTIONS, General: Pioglitazone**).

CPK Levels: During required laboratory testing in clinical trials with pioglitazone, sporadic, transient elevations in creatine phosphokinase levels (CPK) were observed. An isolated elevation to greater than 10 times the upper limit of

normal was noted in 9 patients (values of 2150 to 11400 IU/L). Six of these patients continued to receive pioglitazone, two patients had completed receiving study medication at the time of the elevated value and one patient discontinued study medication due to the elevation. These elevations resolved without any apparent clinical sequelae. The relationship of these events to pioglitazone therapy is unknown.

OVERDOSAGE

Pioglitazone

During controlled clinical trials, one case of overdose with pioglitazone was reported. A male patient took 120 mg per day for four days, then 180 mg per day for seven days. The patient denied any clinical symptoms during this period.

In the event of overdosage, appropriate supportive treatment should be initiated according to patient's clinical signs and symptoms.

Metformin hydrochloride

Overdose of metformin hydrochloride has occurred, including ingestion of amounts greater than 50 grams. Hypoglycemia was reported in approximately 10% of cases, but no causal association with metformin hydrochloride has been established. Lactic acidosis has been reported in approximately 32% of metformin overdose cases (see **WARNINGS, Metformin hydrochloride**). Metformin is dialyzable with a clearance of up to 170 mL/min under good hemodynamic conditions. Therefore, hemodialysis may be useful for removal of accumulated metformin from patients in whom metformin overdosage is suspected.

DOSAGE AND ADMINISTRATION

General

The use of ACTOPLUS MET or ACTOPLUS MET XR in the management of type 2 diabetes should be individualized on the basis of effectiveness and tolerability.

• The starting doses of ACTOPLUS MET or ACTOPLUS MET XR should be based on the patient's current regimen of pioglitazone and/or metformin and the starting doses of these two drugs. The usual starting dose of pioglitazone is 15 to 30 mg daily. The usual starting dose of metformin is 850 to 1000 mg daily.

• To reduce the gastrointestinal side effects associated with metformin, ACTOPLUS MET and ACTOPLUS MET XR should be administered with a meal.

• After initiation of ACTOPLUS MET or ACTOPLUS MET XR or with dose increase, patients should be carefully monitored for adverse events related to fluid retention (see **BOXED WARNING** and **WARNINGS, Pioglitazone**).

• The dosage of ACTOPLUS MET or ACTOPLUS MET XR should be gradually titrated, as needed, based on the adequacy of the therapeutic response.

• The total daily doses of ACTOPLUS MET or ACTOPLUS MET XR should not exceed the maximum recommended total daily doses of pioglitazone (45 mg) or metformin (2550 mg for immediate-release metformin and 2000 mg for extended-release metformin.)

No studies have been performed specifically examining the safety and efficacy of ACTOPLUS MET or ACTOPLUS MET XR in patients previously treated with other oral hypoglycemic agents and switched to ACTOPLUS MET or ACTOPLUS MET XR. Any change in therapy of type 2 diabetes should be undertaken with care and appropriate monitoring as changes in glycemic control can occur.

Sufficient time should be given to assess adequacy of therapeutic response. Ideally, the response to therapy should be evaluated using HbA1c, which is a better indicator of long-term glycemic control than FPG alone. HbA1c reflects glycemia over the past two to three months. In clinical use, it is recommended that patients be treated with ACTOPLUS MET or ACTOPLUS MET XR for a period of time adequate to evaluate change in HbA1c (8-12 weeks) unless glycemic control as measured by FPG deteriorates.

Dosage Recommendations

The dosage recommendations for ACTOPLUS MET and ACTOPLUS MET XR are summarized in Table 8.

[See table 8 at left]

ACTOPLUS MET

The usual **starting dose of ACTOPLUS MET** is 15 mg/500 mg or 15 mg/850 mg tablet strength of pioglitazone/immediate-release metformin administered once or twice daily with food to reduce the gastrointestinal side effects associated with metformin.

The **maximal total daily dose of ACTOPLUS MET** is 45 mg/2550 mg of pioglitazone/immediate-release metformin. This maximal dosage should be administered in divided doses with meals.

ACTOPLUS MET XR

The usual **starting dose of ACTOPLUS MET XR** is 15 mg/1000 mg or 30 mg/1000 mg tablet strength of pioglitazone/extended-release metformin administered once daily with the evening meal.

The **maximal total daily dose of ACTOPLUS MET XR** is 45 mg/2000 mg of pioglitazone/extended-release metformin administered once daily with the evening meal.

Table 8. ACTOPLUS MET and ACTOPLUS MET XR Dosage Recommendations

	ACTOPLUS MET Pioglitazone/immediate-release metformin hydrochloride	ACTOPLUS MET XR Pioglitazone/extended-release metformin hydrochloride
Tablet Strengths	15 mg/500 mg 15 mg/850 mg	15 mg/1000 mg 30 mg/1000 mg
Starting Dose	15 mg/500 mg or 15 mg/850 mg tablets once or twice daily with food	15 mg/1000 mg or 30 mg/1000 mg tablets once daily with evening meal
Maximum Recommended Daily Dose	45 mg/2550 mg administered in divided doses with food	45 mg/2000 mg administered once daily with evening meal

Patients should be informed that ACTOPLUS MET XR must be swallowed whole and not chewed, cut, or crushed, and that the inactive ingredients may occasionally be eliminated in the feces as a soft mass that may resemble the original tablet.

Special Patient Populations

Pregnancy: ACTOPLUS MET and ACTOPLUS MET XR are not recommended for use during pregnancy, or in breastfeeding women.

Geriatric: The initial and maintenance dosing of ACTOPLUS MET or ACTOPLUS MET XR should be conservative in patients with advanced age, due to the potential for decreased renal function in this population. Any dosage adjustment should be based on a careful assessment of renal function. Generally, elderly, debilitated, and malnourished patients should not be titrated to the maximum dose of ACTOPLUS MET or ACTOPLUS MET XR. Monitoring of renal function is necessary to aid in prevention of metformin-associated lactic acidosis, particularly in the elderly (see **WARNINGS, *Metformin hydrochloride*** and **PRECAUTIONS, General: *Metformin hydrochloride***).

Renal Impairment: Metformin is substantially excreted by the kidney. ACTOPLUS MET and ACTOPLUS MET XR should only be used in patients with normal renal function (see **CONTRAINDICATIONS, WARNINGS, *Metformin hydrochloride*, PRECAUTIONS** and **CLINICAL PHARMACOLOGY, Special Populations**). Any dosage adjustment in ACTOPLUS MET or ACTOPLUS MET XR should be based on a careful assessment of renal function.

Hepatic Impairment: Therapy with ACTOPLUS MET or ACTOPLUS MET XR should not be initiated if the patient exhibits clinical evidence of active liver disease or increased serum transaminase levels (ALT greater than 2.5 times the upper limit of normal) at start of therapy (see **PRECAUTIONS, General: *Pioglitazone*** and **CLINICAL PHARMACOLOGY, Special Populations, Hepatic Insufficiency**). Liver enzyme monitoring is recommended in all patients prior to initiation of therapy with ACTOPLUS MET or ACTOPLUS MET XR and periodically thereafter (see **PRECAUTIONS, General: *Pioglitazone*** and **PRECAUTIONS, Laboratory Tests**).

Pediatric: Use in pediatric patients is not recommended for the treatment of diabetes due to lack of long-term safety data. Risks including fractures and other adverse effects associated with pioglitazone, one of the components of ACTOPLUS MET and ACTOPLUS MET XR, have not been determined in this population (see **WARNINGS** and **PRECAUTIONS**).

HOW SUPPLIED

ACTOPLUS MET is available in 15 mg pioglitazone/500 mg metformin hydrochloride and 15 mg pioglitazone/850 mg metformin hydrochloride tablets as follows:

15 mg/500 mg tablet: white to off-white, oblong, film-coated tablet with "4833M" on one side, and "15/500" on the other, available in:

Bottles of 60	NDC 64764-155-60
Bottles of 180	NDC 64764-155-18

15 mg/850 mg tablet: white to off-white, oblong, film-coated tablet with "4833M" on one side, and "15/850" on the other, available in:

Bottles of 60	NDC 64764-158-60
Bottles of 180	NDC 64764-158-18

ACTOPLUS MET XR is available in 15 mg pioglitazone/1000 mg metformin hydrochloride extended-release and 30 mg pioglitazone/1000 mg metformin hydrochloride extended-release tablets as follows:

15 mg/1000 mg tablet: round, white to off-white, film-coated tablet imprinted with "4833X" and "15/1000" in red on one side, available in:

Bottles of 30	NDC 64764-510-30
Bottles of 60	NDC 64764-510-60
Bottles of 90	NDC 64764-510-90

30 mg/1000 mg tablet: round, white to off-white, film-coated tablet imprinted with "4833X" and "30/1000" in light blue on one side, available in:

Bottles of 30	NDC 64764-310-30
Bottles of 60	NDC 64764-310-60
Bottles of 90	NDC 64764-310-90

STORAGE

ACTOPLUS MET

Store at 25°C (77°F); excursions permitted to 15-30°C (59-86°F) [see USP Controlled Room Temperature]. Keep container tightly closed, and protect from moisture and humidity.

ACTOPLUS MET XR

Store at 25°C (77°F); excursions permitted to 15-30°C (59-86°F). Avoid excessive heat and humidity. Dispense in a tightly closed, light-resistant container.

REFERENCES

1. Deng, LJ, et al. Effect of gemfibrozil on the pharmacokinetics of pioglitazone. *Eur J Clin Pharmacol* 2005; 61: 831-836, Table 1.
2. Jaakkola, T, et al. Effect of rifampicin on the pharmacokinetics of pioglitazone. *Br J Clin Pharmacol* 2006; 61:1 70-78.

ACTOS®, ACTOPLUS MET®, and ACTOPLUS MET® XR are registered trademarks of Takeda Pharmaceutical Company Limited and used under license by Takeda Pharmaceuticals America, Inc.

All other trademark names are the property of their respective owners.

Distributed by:

Takeda Pharmaceuticals America, Inc.

Deerfield, IL 60015

© 2009 Takeda Pharmaceuticals America, Inc.

05-1122 Revised: March 2009

MEDICATION GUIDE

ACTOPLUS MET® (ak-TŌ-plus-met)

(pioglitazone hydrochloride and metformin hydrochloride) Tablets

and

ACTOPLUS MET® XR

(ak-TŌ-plus-met eX-R)

(pioglitazone hydrochloride and metformin hydrochloride extended-release) Tablets

Read this Medication Guide carefully before you start taking ACTOPLUS MET or ACTOPLUS MET XR and each time you get a refill. There may be new information. This information does not take the place of talking with your doctor about your medical condition or your treatment. If you have any questions about ACTOPLUS MET or ACTOPLUS MET XR, ask your doctor or pharmacist.

What is the most important information I should know about ACTOPLUS MET and ACTOPLUS MET XR?

ACTOPLUS MET and ACTOPLUS MET XR can cause serious side effects, including **new or worse heart failure.**

- Pioglitazone, one of the medicines in ACTOPLUS MET and ACTOPLUS MET XR, can cause your body to keep extra fluid (fluid retention), which leads to swelling (edema) and weight gain. Extra body fluid can make some heart problems worse or lead to heart failure. Heart failure means your heart does not pump blood well enough.
- If you have severe heart failure, you cannot start ACTOPLUS MET or ACTOPLUS MET XR.
- If you have heart failure with symptoms (such as shortness of breath or swelling), even if these symptoms are not severe, ACTOPLUS MET or ACTOPLUS MET XR may not be right for you.

Call your doctor right away if you have any of the following:

- swelling or fluid retention, especially in the ankles or legs.
- shortness of breath or trouble breathing, especially when you lie down.
- an unusually fast increase in weight.
- unusual tiredness.

Metformin, one of the medicines in ACTOPLUS MET and ACTOPLUS MET XR, can cause a rare but serious condition called lactic acidosis (a buildup of an acid in the blood) that can cause death. Lactic acidosis is a medical emergency and must be treated in the hospital.

Most people who have had lactic acidosis with metformin have other things that, combined with the metformin, led to the lactic acidosis. Tell your doctor if you have any of the following, because you have a higher chance for getting lactic acidosis with ACTOPLUS MET or ACTOPLUS MET XR if you:

- have kidney problems or your kidneys are affected by certain x-ray tests that use injectable dye. People whose kidneys are not working properly should not take ACTOPLUS MET or ACTOPLUS MET XR.
- have liver problems.
- drink alcohol very often, or drink a lot of alcohol in short-term "binge" drinking.
- get dehydrated (lose a large amount of body fluids). This can happen if you are sick with a fever, vomiting, or diarrhea. Dehydration can also happen when you sweat a lot with activity or exercise and do not drink enough fluids.
- have surgery.
- have a heart attack, severe infection, or stroke.
- are 80 years of age or older, and your kidneys are not working properly.

The best way to keep from having a problem with lactic acidosis from metformin is to tell your doctor if you have any of the problems in the list above. Your doctor may decide to stop your ACTOPLUS MET or ACTOPLUS MET XR for a while if you have any of these things.

Lactic acidosis can be hard to diagnose early, because the early symptoms could seem like the symptoms of many other health problems besides lactic acidosis. You should call your doctor right away if you get the following symptoms, which could be signs of lactic acidosis:

- You feel very weak or tired.
- You have unusual (not normal) muscle pain.
- You have stomach pains, nausea or vomiting.
- You have trouble breathing.
- You feel dizzy or lightheaded.
- You have a slow or irregular heartbeat.

ACTOPLUS MET and ACTOPLUS MET XR can have other serious side effects. See "What are the possible side effects of ACTOPLUS MET and ACTOPLUS MET XR?"

What are ACTOPLUS MET and ACTOPLUS MET XR?

ACTOPLUS MET and ACTOPLUS MET XR are prescription medicines used with diet and exercise to improve blood sugar (glucose) control in adults with type 2 diabetes.

ACTOPLUS MET contains 2 prescription diabetes medicines called pioglitazone hydrochloride (ACTOS) and metformin hydrochloride (GLUCOPHAGE).

ACTOPLUS MET XR contains 2 prescription diabetes medicines called pioglitazone hydrochloride (ACTOS) and metformin hydrochloride extended-release (FORTAMET).

ACTOPLUS MET XR works longer in your body than ACTOPLUS MET so it can be taken once a day instead of two or three times a day.

Your doctor will decide if you should take ACTOPLUS MET or ACTOPLUS MET XR.

ACTOPLUS MET or ACTOPLUS MET XR can be used for adults with type 2 diabetes who:

- are taking pioglitazone alone and do not have good enough blood sugar control,
- are taking metformin alone and do not have good enough blood sugar control, or
- are already taking both pioglitazone and metformin

If you are taking pioglitazone or metformin, check with your healthcare provider and make sure you understand exactly how your healthcare provider wants you to switch over to ACTOPLUS MET or ACTOPLUS MET XR.

It is important to eat the right foods, lose weight if needed, and exercise regularly in order to manage your type 2 diabetes. Diet, weight loss, and exercise are the main treatment for type 2 diabetes and they also help your diabetes medicines work better for you.

ACTOPLUS MET and ACTOPLUS MET XR have not been studied in children and are not recommended for children under the age of 18. The risks of giving ACTOPLUS MET or ACTOPLUS MET XR to a child are not known. See "What are some other possible side effects of ACTOPLUS MET and ACTOPLUS MET XR?"

Who should not take ACTOPLUS MET and ACTOPLUS MET XR?

Do not take ACTOPLUS MET or ACTOPLUS MET XR if you:

- are allergic to any of the ingredients in ACTOPLUS MET or ACTOPLUS MET XR. See the end of this Medication Guide for a complete list of ingredients in ACTOPLUS MET and ACTOPLUS MET XR.
- have kidneys which are not working properly.
- have a condition called metabolic acidosis, including diabetic ketoacidosis. Diabetic ketoacidosis should be treated with insulin.
- are going to have an x-ray procedure with an injection of dyes (contrast agents) in your vein with a needle. Talk to your doctor about when to stop ACTOPLUS MET or ACTOPLUS MET XR and when to start it again.

People with severe heart failure should not start taking ACTOPLUS MET or ACTOPLUS MET XR. See "What is the most important information I should know about ACTOPLUS MET and ACTOPLUS MET XR?".

What should I tell my doctor before taking ACTOPLUS MET and ACTOPLUS MET XR?

Before starting ACTOPLUS MET or ACTOPLUS MET XR, ask your doctor about what the choices are for diabetes medicines and what the expected benefits and possible risks are for you in particular.

Tell your doctor about all of your medical conditions, especially if you:

- **have heart failure.**
- **have kidney problems.**
- **are going to have dye injected into a vein for an x-ray, CAT scan, heart study, or other type of scanning.**
- **drink a lot of alcohol** (all the time or short binge drinking).
- **have type 1 ("juvenile") diabetes or had diabetic ketoacidosis.** These conditions should be treated with insulin.
- **are 80 years old or older.** People over 80 years should not take ACTOPLUS MET or ACTOPLUS MET XR unless their kidney function is checked and it is normal.
- **have a type of diabetic eye disease called macular edema** (swelling of the back of the eye).
- **have liver problems.** Your doctor should do blood tests to check your liver before you start taking ACTOPLUS MET or ACTOPLUS MET XR and during treatment as needed.
- **are pregnant or planning to become pregnant.** ACTOPLUS MET and ACTOPLUS MET XR should not be

used during pregnancy. It is not known if ACTOPLUS MET and ACTOPLUS MET XR can harm your unborn baby. Talk to your doctor about the best way to control your blood glucose levels while pregnant.

- **are a premenopausal woman (before the "change of life"), who does not have periods regularly or at all.** ACTOPLUS MET and ACTOPLUS MET XR may increase your chance of becoming pregnant. Talk to your doctor about birth control choices while taking ACTOPLUS MET or ACTOPLUS MET XR. Tell your doctor right away if you become pregnant while taking ACTOPLUS MET or ACTOPLUS MET XR.
- **are breastfeeding or plan to breastfeed.** It is not known if ACTOPLUS MET and ACTOPLUS MET XR pass into your milk and if they can harm your baby. You should not take ACTOPLUS MET or ACTOPLUS MET XR if you breastfeed your baby. Talk to your doctor about the best way to control your blood glucose levels while breastfeeding.

Tell your doctor about all the medicines you take including prescription and non-prescription medicines, vitamins, and herbal supplements. ACTOPLUS MET or ACTOPLUS MET XR and some of your other medicines can affect each other. You may need to have your dose of ACTOPLUS MET or ACTOPLUS MET XR or certain other medicines adjusted. Certain other medicines can affect your blood sugar (glucose) control.

Know the medicines you take. Keep a list of your medicines and show it to your doctor and pharmacist before you start a new medicine. They will tell you if it is okay to take ACTOPLUS MET or ACTOPLUS MET XR with other medicines.

How should I take ACTOPLUS MET or ACTOPLUS MET XR?

- Take ACTOPLUS MET or ACTOPLUS MET XR exactly as prescribed. Your doctor will tell you how many ACTOPLUS MET or ACTOPLUS MET XR tablets to take and how often you should take them. Your doctor may need to change your dose of ACTOPLUS MET or ACTOPLUS MET XR to control your blood glucose. Do not change your dose unless told to do so by your doctor.
- Take ACTOPLUS MET with meals to lower your chance of an upset stomach.
- Take ACTOPLUS MET XR once a day with the evening meal to lower your chance of an upset stomach.
- If you take ACTOPLUS MET XR, swallow the **ACTOPLUS MET XR tablets whole. Do not chew, cut, or crush the tablets.** If you cannot swallow ACTOPLUS MET XR whole, tell your doctor. You may need a different medicine.
- If you take ACTOPLUS MET XR, you may see something that looks like the ACTOPLUS MET XR tablet in your stools. This is normal.
- If you miss a dose of ACTOPLUS MET or ACTOPLUS MET XR, take your next dose as prescribed unless your doctor tells you differently. Do not take two doses at one time the next day.
- If you take too much ACTOPLUS MET or ACTOPLUS MET XR, call your doctor or poison control center right away.
- If your body is under stress, for example: due to fever, infection, trauma (such as a car accident), or surgery, the dose of your diabetes medicines may need to be changed. Call your doctor right away.
- Stay on your diet and exercise programs and test your blood sugar regularly while taking ACTOPLUS MET or ACTOPLUS MET XR.
- Your doctor should do blood tests before starting ACTOPLUS MET or ACTOPLUS MET XR and from time to time to check your liver, kidneys, and blood cells.
- Your doctor should also do regular blood tests (for example, hemoglobin A1C) to check how well your blood sugar is controlled with ACTOPLUS MET or ACTOPLUS MET XR.
- Your doctor should check your eyes regularly. Some people have had vision changes due to swelling in the back of the eye, called macular edema, while taking ACTOPLUS MET or ACTOPLUS MET XR.
- It may take 2-3 months to see the full effect on your blood sugar level.

You may need to stop ACTOPLUS MET or ACTOPLUS MET XR for a short time. Call your doctor for instructions if you:

- are sick with severe vomiting, diarrhea, or fever or if you drink a much lower amount of liquid than normal.
- plan to have surgery.
- are having an x-ray procedure with injection of dye.

What are other possible side effects of ACTOPLUS MET and ACTOPLUS MET XR?

ACTOPLUS MET and ACTOPLUS MET XR can cause other serious side effects including:

- **Weight gain.** Pioglitazone, one of the medicines in ACTOPLUS MET and ACTOPLUS MET XR, can cause weight gain that may be due to fluid retention or extra body fat. Weight gain due to fluid retention can be a serious problem for people with certain conditions, including

heart problems. See "What is the most important information I should know about ACTOPLUS MET and ACTOPLUS MET XR?"

- **Liver problems.** It is important for your liver to be working normally when you take ACTOPLUS MET or ACTOPLUS MET XR. Your doctor should do blood tests to check your liver before you start taking ACTOPLUS MET or ACTOPLUS MET XR and during treatment as needed. Call your doctor right away if you have unexplained symptoms such as:
  - nausea or vomiting.
  - stomach pain.
  - unusual or unexplained tiredness.
  - loss of appetite.
  - dark urine.
  - yellowing of your skin or the whites of your eyes.
- **Macular edema** (diabetic eye disease with swelling in the back of the eye). Tell your doctor right away if you have any changes in your vision. Your doctor should check your eyes regularly.
- **Fractures (broken bones),** usually in the hand, upper arm, or foot in women. Talk to your doctor for advice on how to keep your bones healthy. It is not known if ACTOPLUS MET and ACTOPLUS MET XR can affect the bones of children.
- **Low red blood cell count (anemia).**
- **Low blood sugar (hypoglycemia).** Lightheadedness, dizziness, shakiness, or hunger may indicate that your blood sugar is too low. This can happen if you skip meals, if you use another medicine that lowers blood sugar, or if you have certain medical problems. Call your doctor if low blood sugar levels are a problem for you.
- **Ovulation** (release of an egg from an ovary in a woman) leading to pregnancy. Ovulation may happen when premenopausal women who do not have regular monthly periods take ACTOPLUS MET or ACTOPLUS MET XR. This can increase the chance of pregnancy. See "What should I tell my doctor before taking ACTOPLUS MET and ACTOPLUS MET XR?".

In studies of pioglitazone (one of the medicines in ACTOPLUS MET and ACTOPLUS MET XR), bladder cancer occurred in a few more people who were taking pioglitazone than in people who were taking other diabetes medicines. There were too few cases to know if the bladder cancer was related to pioglitazone.

The most common side effects of ACTOPLUS MET and ACTOPLUS MET XR reported in clinical trials included diarrhea, nausea, and upset stomach. These side effects usually happen during the first few weeks of treatment. Taking ACTOPLUS MET or ACTOPLUS MET XR with meals can help lessen these side effects. However, if you have unusual or unexpected stomach problems, talk with your doctor. Stomach problems that start up later during treatment may be a sign of something more serious.

Other common side effects of ACTOPLUS MET and ACTOPLUS MET XR are cold-like symptoms (upper respiratory infection), headache, urinary tract infection, dizziness, sinus infection, and anemia.

Tell your doctor if you have any side effect that bothers you or that does not go away. These are not all the side effects of ACTOPLUS MET and ACTOPLUS MET XR. For more information, ask your doctor or pharmacist.

Call your doctor for medical advice about side effects. You may report side effects to FDA at 1-800-FDA-1088.

How should I store ACTOPLUS MET and ACTOPLUS MET XR?

- Store ACTOPLUS MET and ACTOPLUS MET XR at 59° to 86°F (15° to 30°C). Keep ACTOPLUS MET and ACTOPLUS MET XR in the original container to protect from light.
- Keep the ACTOPLUS MET and ACTOPLUS MET XR bottle tightly closed and protect from getting wet (away from moisture and humidity).

Keep ACTOPLUS MET and ACTOPLUS MET XR and all medicines out of the reach of children.

General information about ACTOPLUS MET and ACTOPLUS MET XR

Medicines are sometimes prescribed for purposes other than those listed in a Medication Guide. Do not use ACTOPLUS MET or ACTOPLUS MET XR for a condition for which it is not prescribed. Do not give ACTOPLUS MET or ACTOPLUS MET XR to other people, even if they have the same symptoms you have. It may harm them.

This Medication Guide summarizes the most important information about ACTOPLUS MET and ACTOPLUS MET XR. If you would like more information, talk with your doctor. You can ask your doctor or pharmacist for information about ACTOPLUS MET and ACTOPLUS MET XR that is written for healthcare professionals. For more information, go to www.actoplusmetxr.com or call 1-877-825-3327.

What are the ingredients in ACTOPLUS MET and ACTOPLUS MET XR?

Active Ingredients: pioglitazone hydrochloride and metformin hydrochloride

Inactive Ingredients for ACTOPLUS MET: povidone, microcrystalline cellulose, croscarmellose sodium, magnesium stearate, hypromellose 2910, polyethylene glycol 8000, titanium dioxide, and talc.

Inactive Ingredients for ACTOPLUS MET XR: candelilla wax, cellulose acetate, povidone, hydroxypropyl cellulose, lactose monohydrate, magnesium stearate, hypromellose, polyethylene glycols (PEG 400, PEG 8000), sodium lauryl sulfate, titanium dioxide, and triacetin. Ink contains shellac, iron-oxide red (15 mg/1000 mg tablet strength), FD&C Blue No. 2 Lake (30 mg/1000 mg tablet strength), propylene glycol, and ammonium hydroxide.

Always check to make sure that the medicine you are taking is the correct one. ACTOPLUS MET tablets look like this:

- 15 mg/500 mg strength tablets—white to off-white, oblong tablet with "15/500" on one side and "4833M" on the other.
- 15 mg/850 mg strength tablets—white to off-white, oblong tablet with "15/850" on one side and "4833M" on the other.

ACTOPLUS MET XR tablets look like this:

- 15 mg/1000 mg strength tablets—white to off-white, round tablet imprinted with "15/1000" and "4833X" in red on one side.
- 30 mg/1000 mg strength tablets—white to off-white, round tablet imprinted with "30/1000" and "4833X" in light blue on one side.

ACTOS®, ACTOPLUS MET®, and ACTOPLUS MET® XR are registered trademarks of Takeda Pharmaceutical Company Limited and used under license by Takeda Pharmaceuticals America, Inc.

All other trademarks are the property of their respective owners.

This Medication Guide has been approved by the U.S. Food and Drug Administration.

Distributed by:

Takeda Pharmaceuticals America, Inc.

Deerfield, IL 60015

© 2009 Takeda Pharmaceuticals America, Inc.

05-1122-MG   Revised: March 2009

Shown in Product Identification Guide, page 320

ACTOS® ℞

[ăk'tōs]

(pioglitazone hydrochloride)

Tablets

WARNING: CONGESTIVE HEART FAILURE

- Thiazolidinediones, including ACTOS, cause or exacerbate congestive heart failure in some patients (see **WARNINGS**). After initiation of ACTOS, and after dose increases, observe patients carefully for signs and symptoms of heart failure (including excessive, rapid weight gain, dyspnea, and/or edema). If these signs and symptoms develop, the heart failure should be managed according to the current standards of care. Furthermore, discontinuation or dose reduction of ACTOS must be considered.
- ACTOS is not recommended in patients with symptomatic heart failure. Initiation of ACTOS in patients with established NYHA Class III or IV heart failure is contraindicated (see **CONTRAINDICATIONS** and **WARNINGS**).

DESCRIPTION

ACTOS (pioglitazone hydrochloride) is an oral antidiabetic agent that acts primarily by decreasing insulin resistance. ACTOS is used in the management of type 2 diabetes mellitus (also known as non-insulin-dependent diabetes mellitus [NIDDM] or adult-onset diabetes). Pharmacological studies indicate that ACTOS improves sensitivity to insulin in muscle and adipose tissue and inhibits hepatic gluconeogenesis. ACTOS improves glycemic control while reducing circulating insulin levels.

Pioglitazone [(±)-5-[[4-[2-(5-ethyl-2-pyridinyl)ethoxy] phenyl]methyl]-2,4-] thiazolidinedione monohydrochloride belongs to a different chemical class and has a different pharmacological action than the sulfonylureas, metformin, or the α-glucosidase inhibitors. The molecule contains one asymmetric carbon, and the compound is synthesized and used as the racemic mixture. The two enantiomers of pioglitazone interconvert *in vivo*. No differences were found in the pharmacologic activity between the two enantiomers. The structural formula is as shown:

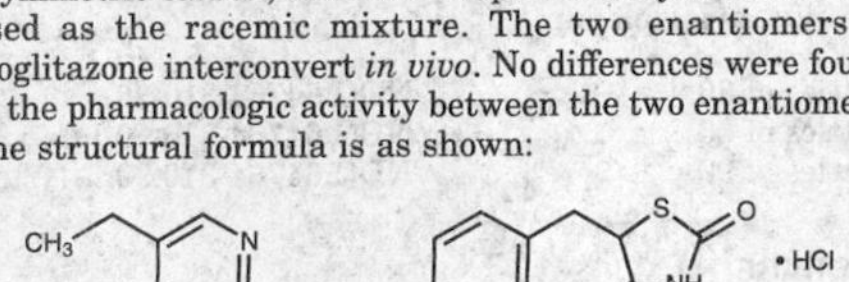

Pioglitazone hydrochloride is an odorless white crystalline powder that has a molecular formula of $C_{19}H_{20}N_2O_3S \cdot HCl$ and a molecular weight of 392.90 daltons. It is soluble in

N,N-dimethylformamide, slightly soluble in anhydrous ethanol, very slightly soluble in acetone and acetonitrile, practically insoluble in water, and insoluble in ether.
ACTOS is available as a tablet for oral administration containing 15 mg, 30 mg, or 45 mg of pioglitazone (as the base) formulated with the following excipients: lactose monohydrate NF, hydroxypropylcellulose NF, carboxymethylcellulose calcium NF, and magnesium stearate NF.

CLINICAL PHARMACOLOGY

Mechanism of Action

ACTOS is a thiazolidinedione antidiabetic agent that depends on the presence of insulin for its mechanism of action. ACTOS decreases insulin resistance in the periphery and in the liver resulting in increased insulin-dependent glucose disposal and decreased hepatic glucose output. Unlike sulfonylureas, pioglitazone is not an insulin secretagogue. Pioglitazone is a potent agonist for peroxisome proliferator-activated receptor-gamma (PPARγ). PPAR receptors are found in tissues important for insulin action such as adipose tissue, skeletal muscle, and liver. Activation of PPARγ nuclear receptors modulates the transcription of a number of insulin responsive genes involved in the control of glucose and lipid metabolism.
In animal models of diabetes, pioglitazone reduces the hyperglycemia, hyperinsulinemia, and hypertriglyceridemia characteristic of insulin-resistant states such as type 2 diabetes. The metabolic changes produced by pioglitazone result in increased responsiveness of insulin-dependent tissues and are observed in numerous animal models of insulin resistance.
Since pioglitazone enhances the effects of circulating insulin (by decreasing insulin resistance), it does not lower blood glucose in animal models that lack endogenous insulin.

Pharmacokinetics and Drug Metabolism

Serum concentrations of total pioglitazone (pioglitazone plus active metabolites) remain elevated 24 hours after once daily dosing. Steady-state serum concentrations of both pioglitazone and total pioglitazone are achieved within 7 days. At steady-state, two of the pharmacologically active metabolites of pioglitazone, Metabolites III (M-III) and IV (M-IV), reach serum concentrations equal to or greater than pioglitazone. In both healthy volunteers and in patients with type 2 diabetes, pioglitazone comprises approximately 30% to 50% of the peak total pioglitazone serum concentrations and 20% to 25% of the total area under the serum concentration-time curve (AUC).
Maximum serum concentration (C_{max}), AUC, and trough serum concentrations (C_{min}) for both pioglitazone and total pioglitazone increase proportionally at doses of 15 mg and 30 mg per day. There is a slightly less than proportional increase for pioglitazone and total pioglitazone at a dose of 60 mg per day.
Absorption: Following oral administration, in the fasting state, pioglitazone is first measurable in serum within 30 minutes, with peak concentrations observed within 2 hours. Food slightly delays the time to peak serum concentration to 3 to 4 hours, but does not alter the extent of absorption.
Distribution: The mean apparent volume of distribution (Vd/F) of pioglitazone following single-dose administration is 0.63 ± 0.41 (mean ± SD) L/kg of body weight. Pioglitazone is extensively protein bound (> 99%) in human serum, principally to serum albumin. Pioglitazone also binds to other serum proteins, but with lower affinity. Metabolites M-III and M-IV also are extensively bound (> 98%) to serum albumin.
Metabolism: Pioglitazone is extensively metabolized by hydroxylation and oxidation; the metabolites also partly convert to glucuronide or sulfate conjugates. Metabolites M-II and M-IV (hydroxy derivatives of pioglitazone) and M-III (keto derivative of pioglitazone) are pharmacologically active in animal models of type 2 diabetes. In addition to pioglitazone, M-III and M-IV are the principal drug-related species found in human serum following multiple dosing. At steady-state, in both healthy volunteers and in patients with type 2 diabetes, pioglitazone comprises approximately 30% to 50% of the total peak serum concentrations and 20% to 25% of the total AUC.
In vitro data demonstrate that multiple CYP isoforms are involved in the metabolism of pioglitazone. The cytochrome P450 isoforms involved are CYP2C8 and, to a lesser degree, CYP3A4 with additional contributions from a variety of other isoforms including the mainly extrahepatic CYP1A1. *In vivo* studies of *pioglitazone in* combination with P450 inhibitors and substrates have been performed (see **Drug Interactions**). Urinary 6β-hydroxycortisol/cortisol ratios measured in patients treated with ACTOS showed that pioglitazone is not a strong CYP3A4 enzyme inducer.
Excretion and Elimination: Following oral administration, approximately 15% to 30% of the pioglitazone dose is recovered in the urine. Renal elimination of pioglitazone is negligible, and the drug is excreted primarily as metabolites and their conjugates. It is presumed that most of the oral dose is excreted into the bile either unchanged or as metabolites and eliminated in the feces.
The mean serum half-life of pioglitazone and total pioglitazone ranges from 3 to 7 hours and 16 to 24 hours, respectively. Pioglitazone has an apparent clearance, CL/F, calculated to be 5 to 7 L/hr.

Table 1 Lipids in a 26-Week Placebo-Controlled Monotherapy Dose-Ranging Study

	Placebo	ACTOS 15 mg Once Daily	ACTOS 30 mg Once Daily	ACTOS 45 mg Once Daily
Triglycerides (mg/dL)	N=79	N=79	N=84	N=77
Baseline (mean)	262.8	283.8	261.1	259.7
Percent change from baseline (mean)	4.8%	-9.0%	-9.6%	-9.3%
HDL Cholesterol (mg/dL)	N=79	N=79	N=83	N=77
Baseline (mean)	41.7	40.4	40.8	40.7
Percent change from baseline (mean)	8.1%	14.1%	12.2%	19.1%
LDL Cholesterol (mg/dL)	N=65	N=63	N=74	N=62
Baseline (mean)	138.8	131.9	135.6	126.8
Percent change from baseline (mean)	4.8%	7.2%	5.2%	6.0%
Total Cholesterol (mg/dL)	N=79	N=79	N=84	N=77
Baseline (mean)	224.6	220.0	222.7	213.7
Percent change from baseline (mean)	4.4%	4.6%	3.3%	6.4%

Special Populations

Renal Insufficiency: The serum elimination half-life of pioglitazone, M-III, and M-IV remains unchanged in patients with moderate (creatinine clearance 30 to 60 mL/min) to severe (creatinine clearance < 30 mL/min) renal impairment when compared to normal subjects. No dose adjustment in patients with renal dysfunction is recommended (see **DOSAGE AND ADMINISTRATION**).
Hepatic Insufficiency: Compared with normal controls, subjects with impaired hepatic function (Child-Pugh Grade B/C) have an approximate 45% reduction in pioglitazone and total pioglitazone mean peak concentrations but no change in the mean AUC values.
ACTOS therapy should not be initiated if the patient exhibits clinical evidence of active liver disease or serum transaminase levels (ALT) exceed 2.5 times the upper limit of normal (see **PRECAUTIONS**, Hepatic Effects).
Elderly: In healthy elderly subjects, peak serum concentrations of pioglitazone and total pioglitazone are not significantly different, but AUC values are slightly higher and the terminal half-life values slightly longer than for younger subjects. These changes were not of a magnitude that would be considered clinically relevant.
Pediatrics: Pharmacokinetic data in the pediatric population are not available.
Gender: The mean C_{max} and AUC values were increased 20% to 60% in females. As monotherapy and in combination with sulfonylurea, metformin, or insulin, ACTOS improved glycemic control in both males and females. In controlled clinical trials, hemoglobin A_{1c} (HbA_{1c}) decreases from baseline were generally greater for females than for males (average mean difference in HbA_{1c} 0.5%). Since therapy should be individualized for each patient to achieve glycemic control, no dose adjustment is recommended based on gender alone.
Ethnicity: Pharmacokinetic data among various ethnic groups are not available.

Drug-Drug Interactions

The following drugs were studied in healthy volunteers with a co-administration of ACTOS 45 mg once daily. Listed below are the results:
Oral Contraceptives: Co-administration of ACTOS (45 mg once daily) and an oral contraceptive (1 mg norethindrone plus 0.035 mg ethinyl estradiol once daily) for 21 days, resulted in 11% and 11-14% decrease in ethinyl estradiol AUC (0-24h) and C_{max} respectively. There were no significant changes in norethindrone AUC (0-24h) and C_{max}. In view of the high variability of ethinyl estradiol pharmacokinetics, the clinical significance of this finding is unknown.
Fexofenadine HCl: Co-administration of ACTOS for 7 days with 60 mg fexofenadine administered orally twice daily resulted in no significant effect on pioglitazone pharmacokinetics. ACTOS had no significant effect on fexofenadine pharmacokinetics.
Glipizide: Co-administration of ACTOS and 5 mg glipizide administered orally once daily for 7 days did not alter the steady-state pharmacokinetics of glipizide.
Digoxin: Co-administration of ACTOS with 0.25 mg digoxin administered orally once daily for 7 days did not alter the steady-state pharmacokinetics of digoxin.
Warfarin: Co-administration of ACTOS for 7 days with warfarin did not alter the steady-state pharmacokinetics of warfarin. ACTOS has no clinically significant effect on prothrombin time when administered to patients receiving chronic warfarin therapy.
Metformin: Co-administration of a single dose of metformin (1000 mg) and ACTOS after 7 days of ACTOS did not alter the pharmacokinetics of the single dose of metformin.
Midazolam: Administration of ACTOS for 15 days followed by a single 7.5 mg dose of midazolam syrup resulted in a 26% reduction in midazolam C_{max} and AUC.
Ranitidine HCl: Co-administration of ACTOS for 7 days with ranitidine administered orally twice daily for either 4 or 7 days resulted in no significant effect on pioglitazone pharmacokinetics. ACTOS showed no significant effect on ranitidine pharmacokinetics.
Nifedipine ER: Co-administration of ACTOS for 7 days with 30 mg nifedipine ER administered orally once daily for 4 days to male and female volunteers resulted in least square mean (90% CI) values for unchanged nifedipine of 0.83 (0.73-0.95) for C_{max} and 0.88 (0.80-0.96) for AUC. In view of the high variability of nifedipine pharmacokinetics, the clinical significance of this finding is unknown.
Ketoconazole: Co-administration of ACTOS for 7 days with ketoconazole 200 mg administered twice daily resulted in least square mean (90% CI) values for unchanged pioglitazone of 1.14 (1.06-1.23) for C_{max}, 1.34 (1.26-1.41) for AUC and 1.87 (1.71-2.04) for C_{min}.
Atorvastatin Calcium: Co-administration of ACTOS for 7 days with atorvastatin calcium (LIPITOR®) 80 mg once daily resulted in least square mean (90% CI) values for unchanged pioglitazone of 0.69 (0.57-0.85) for C_{max}, 0.76 (0.65-0.88) for AUC and 0.96 (0.87-1.05) for C_{min}. For unchanged atorvastatin the least square mean (90% CI) values were 0.77 (0.66-0.90) for C_{max}, 0.86 (0.78-0.94) for AUC and 0.92 (0.82-1.02) for C_{min}.
Theophylline: Co-administration of ACTOS for 7 days with theophylline 400 mg administered twice daily resulted in no change in the pharmacokinetics of either drug.
Cytochrome P450: See **PRECAUTIONS**
Gemfibrozil: Concomitant administration of gemfibrozil (oral 600 mg twice daily), an inhibitor of CYP2C8, with pioglitazone (oral 30 mg) in 10 healthy volunteers pre-treated for 2 days prior with gemfibrozil (oral 600 mg twice daily) resulted in pioglitazone exposure (AUC_{0-24}) being 226% of the pioglitazone exposure in the absence of gemfibrozil (see **PRECAUTIONS**).[1]
Rifampin: Concomitant administration of rifampin (oral 600 mg once daily), an inducer of CYP2C8 with pioglitazone (oral 30 mg) in 10 healthy volunteers pre-treated for 5 days prior with rifampin (oral 600 mg once daily) resulted in a decrease in the AUC of pioglitazone by 54% (see **PRECAUTIONS**).[2]

Pharmacodynamics and Clinical Effects

Clinical studies demonstrate that ACTOS improves insulin sensitivity in insulin-resistant patients. ACTOS enhances cellular responsiveness to insulin, increases insulin-dependent glucose disposal, improves hepatic sensitivity to insulin, and improves dysfunctional glucose homeostasis. In patients with type 2 diabetes, the decreased insulin resistance produced by ACTOS results in lower plasma glucose concentrations, lower plasma insulin levels, and lower HbA_{1c} values. Based on results from an open-label extension study, the glucose lowering effects of ACTOS appear to persist for at least one year. In controlled clinical trials, ACTOS in combination with sulfonylurea, metformin, or insulin had an additive effect on glycemic control.
Patients with lipid abnormalities were included in clinical trials with ACTOS. Overall, patients treated with ACTOS had mean decreases in triglycerides, mean increases in HDL cholesterol, and no consistent mean changes in LDL and total cholesterol.

Figure 1 Mean Change from Baseline for FPG and HbA₁c in a 26-Week Placebo-Controlled Dose-Ranging Study

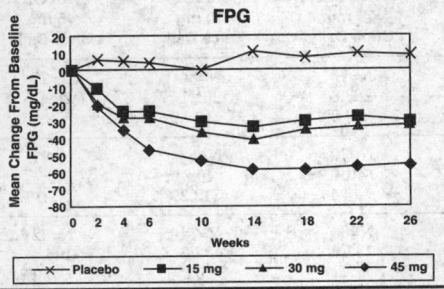

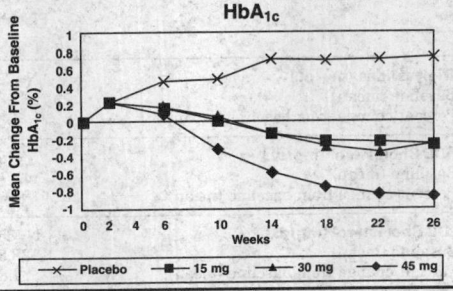

and 45 mg of ACTOS produced statistically significant improvements in HbA₁c and fasting plasma glucose (FPG) at endpoint compared to placebo (**Figure 1, Table 2**).

Figure 1 shows the time course for changes in FPG and HbA₁c for the entire study population in this 26-week study.
[See figure 1 at left]

Table 2 shows HbA₁c and FPG values for the entire study population.
[See table 2 at left]

The study population included patients not previously treated with antidiabetic medication (naïve; 31%) and patients who were receiving antidiabetic medication at the time of study enrollment (previously treated; 69%). The data for the naïve and previously-treated patient subsets are shown in **Table 3**. All patients entered an 8 week washout/run-in period prior to double-blind treatment. This run-in period was associated with little change in HbA₁c and FPG values from screening to baseline for the naïve patients; however, for the previously-treated group, washout from previous antidiabetic medication resulted in deterioration of glycemic control and increases in HbA₁c and FPG. Although most patients in the previously-treated group had a decrease from baseline in HbA₁c and FPG with ACTOS, in many cases the values did not return to screening levels by the end of the study. The study design did not permit the evaluation of patients who switched directly to ACTOS from another antidiabetic agent.
[See table 3 at left]

In a 24-week, placebo-controlled study, 260 patients with type 2 diabetes were randomized to one of two forced-titration ACTOS treatment groups or a mock titration placebo group. Therapy with any previous antidiabetic agent was discontinued 6 weeks prior to the double-blind treatment. In one ACTOS treatment group, patients received an initial dose of 7.5 mg once daily. After four weeks, the dose was increased to 15 mg once daily and after four weeks, the dose was increased to 30 mg once daily for the remainder of the study (16 weeks). In the second ACTOS treatment group, patients received an initial dose of 15 mg once daily and were titrated to 30 mg once daily and 45 mg once daily in a similar manner. Treatment with ACTOS, as described, produced statistically significant improvements in HbA₁c and FPG at endpoint compared to placebo (**Table 4**).
[See table 4 at top of next page]

For patients who had not been previously treated with antidiabetic medication (24%), mean values at screening were 10.1% for HbA₁c and 238 mg/dL for FPG. At baseline, mean HbA₁c was 10.2% and mean FPG was 243 mg/dL. Compared with placebo, treatment with ACTOS titrated to a final dose of 30 mg and 45 mg resulted in reductions from baseline in mean HbA₁c of 2.3% and 2.6% and mean FPG of 63 mg/dL and 95 mg/dL, respectively. For patients who had been previously treated with antidiabetic medication (76%), this medication was discontinued at screening. Mean values at screening were 9.4% for HbA₁c and 216 mg/dL for FPG. At baseline, mean HbA₁c was 10.7% and mean FPG was 290 mg/dL. Compared with placebo, treatment with ACTOS titrated to a final dose of 30 mg and 45 mg resulted in reductions from baseline in mean HbA₁c of 1.3% and 1.4% and mean FPG of 55 mg/dL and 60 mg/dL, respectively. For many previously-treated patients, HbA₁c and FPG had not returned to screening levels by the end of the study.

In a 16-week study, 197 patients with type 2 diabetes were randomized to treatment with 30 mg of ACTOS or placebo once daily. Therapy with any previous antidiabetic agent was discontinued 6 weeks prior to the double-blind period. Treatment with 30 mg of ACTOS produced statistically significant improvements in HbA₁c and FPG at endpoint compared to placebo (**Table 5**).

Table 2 Glycemic Parameters in a 26-Week Placebo-Controlled Dose-Ranging Study

	Placebo	ACTOS 15 mg Once Daily	ACTOS 30 mg Once Daily	ACTOS 45 mg Once Daily
TOTAL POPULATION				
HbA₁c (%)	N=79	N=79	N=85	N=76
Baseline (mean)	10.4	10.2	10.2	10.3
Change from baseline (adjusted mean⁺)	0.7	-0.3	-0.3	-0.9
Difference from placebo (adjusted mean⁺)		-1.0*	-1.0*	-1.6*
FPG (mg/dL)	N=79	N=79	N=84	N=77
Baseline (mean)	268	267	269	276
Change from baseline (adjusted mean⁺)	9	-30	-32	-56
Difference from placebo (adjusted mean⁺)		-39*	-41*	-65*

⁺ Adjusted for baseline, pooled center, and pooled center by treatment interaction
*p ≤ 0.050 vs. placebo

Table 3 Glycemic Parameters in a 26-Week Placebo-Controlled Dose-Ranging Study

	Placebo	ACTOS 15 mg Once Daily	ACTOS 30 mg Once Daily	ACTOS 45 mg Once Daily
Naïve to Therapy	N=25	N=26	N=26	N=21
HbA₁c (%)				
Screening (mean)	9.3	10.0	9.5	9.8
Baseline (mean)	9.0	9.9	9.3	10.0
Change from baseline (adjusted mean*)	0.6	-0.8	-0.6	-1.9
Difference from placebo (adjusted mean*)		-1.4	-1.3	-2.6
FPG (mg/dL)	N=25	N=26	N=26	N=21
Screening (mean)	223	245	239	239
Baseline (mean)	229	251	225	235
Change from baseline (adjusted mean*)	16	-37	-41	-64
Difference from placebo (adjusted mean*)		-52	-56	-80
Previously Treated	N=54	N=53	N=59	N=55
HbA₁c (%)				
Screening (mean)	9.3	9.0	9.1	9.0
Baseline (mean)	10.9	10.4	10.4	10.6
Change from baseline (adjusted mean*)	0.8	-0.1	-0.0	-0.6
Difference from placebo (adjusted mean*)		-1.0	-0.9	-1.4
FPG (mg/dL)	N=54	N=53	N=58	N=56
Screening (mean)	222	209	230	215
Baseline (mean)	285	275	286	292
Change from baseline (adjusted mean*)	4	-32	-27	-55
Difference from placebo (adjusted mean*)		-36	-31	-59

* Adjusted for baseline and pooled center

Table 5 Glycemic Parameters in a 16-Week Placebo-Controlled Study

	Placebo	ACTOS 30 mg Once Daily
Total Population	N=93	N=100
HbA₁c (%)		
Baseline (mean)	10.3	10.5
Change from baseline (adjusted mean⁺)	0.8	-0.6
Difference from placebo (adjusted mean⁺)		-1.4*
FPG (mg/dL)	N=91	N=99
Baseline (mean)	270	273
Change from baseline (adjusted mean⁺)	8	-50
Difference from placebo (adjusted mean⁺)		-58*

⁺ Adjusted for baseline, pooled center, and pooled center by treatment interaction
*p ≤ 0.050 vs. placebo

In a 26-week, placebo-controlled, dose-ranging study, mean triglyceride levels decreased in the 15 mg, 30 mg, and 45 mg ACTOS dose groups compared to a mean increase in the placebo group. Mean HDL levels increased to a greater extent in patients treated with ACTOS than in the placebo-treated patients. There were no consistent differences for LDL and total cholesterol in patients treated with ACTOS compared to placebo (**Table 1**).
[See table 1 at top of previous page]
In the two other monotherapy studies (24 weeks and 16 weeks) and in combination therapy studies with sulfonylurea (24 weeks and 16 weeks) and metformin (24 weeks and 16 weeks), the results were generally consistent with the data above. In placebo-controlled trials, the placebo-corrected mean changes from baseline decreased 5% to 26% for triglycerides and increased 6% to 13% for HDL in patients treated with ACTOS. A similar pattern of results was seen in 24-week combination therapy studies of ACTOS with sulfonylurea or metformin.
In a combination therapy study with insulin (16 weeks), the placebo-corrected mean percent change from baseline in tri-

glyceride values for patients treated with ACTOS was also decreased. A placebo-corrected mean change from baseline in LDL cholesterol of 7% was observed for the 15 mg dose group. Similar results to those noted above for HDL and total cholesterol were observed. A similar pattern of results was seen in a 24-week combination therapy study with ACTOS with insulin.

Clinical Studies
Monotherapy
In the U.S., three randomized, double-blind, placebo-controlled trials with durations from 16 to 26 weeks were conducted to evaluate the use of ACTOS as monotherapy in patients with type 2 diabetes. These studies examined ACTOS at doses up to 45 mg or placebo once daily in 865 patients.
In a 26-week, dose-ranging study, 408 patients with type 2 diabetes were randomized to receive 7.5 mg, 15 mg, 30 mg, or 45 mg of ACTOS, or placebo once daily. Therapy with any previous antidiabetic agent was discontinued 8 weeks prior to the double-blind period. Treatment with 15 mg, 30 mg,

For patients who had not been previously treated with antidiabetic medication (40%), mean values at screening were 10.3% for HbA1c and 240 mg/dL for FPG. At baseline, mean HbA1c was 10.4% and mean FPG was 254 mg/dL. Compared with placebo, treatment with ACTOS 30 mg resulted in reductions from baseline in mean HbA1c of 1.0% and mean FPG of 62 mg/dL. For patients who had been previously treated with antidiabetic medication (60%), this medication was discontinued at screening. Mean values at screening were 9.4% for HbA1c and 216 mg/dL for FPG. At baseline, mean HbA1c was 10.6% and mean FPG was 287 mg/dL. Compared with placebo, treatment with ACTOS 30 mg resulted in reductions from baseline in mean HbA1c of 1.3% and mean FPG of 46 mg/dL. For many previously-treated patients, HbA1c and FPG had not returned to screening levels by the end of the study.

Combination Therapy

Three 16-week, randomized, double-blind, placebo-controlled clinical studies and three 24-week, randomized, double-blind, dose-controlled clinical studies were conducted to evaluate the effects of ACTOS on glycemic control in patients with type 2 diabetes who were inadequately controlled (HbA1c ≥ 8%) despite current therapy with a sulfonylurea, metformin, or insulin. Previous diabetes treatment may have been monotherapy or combination therapy.

ACTOS Plus Sulfonylurea Studies

Two clinical studies were conducted with ACTOS in combination with a sulfonylurea. Both studies included patients with type 2 diabetes on a sulfonylurea, either alone or in combination with another antidiabetic agent. All other antidiabetic agents were withdrawn prior to starting study treatment. In the first study, 560 patients were randomized to receive 15 mg or 30 mg of ACTOS or placebo once daily for 16 weeks in addition to their current sulfonylurea regimen. When compared to placebo at Week 16, the addition of ACTOS to the sulfonylurea significantly reduced the mean HbA1c by 0.9% and 1.3% and mean FPG by 39 mg/dL and 58 mg/dL for the 15 mg and 30 mg doses, respectively.

In the second study, 702 patients were randomized to receive 30 mg or 45 mg of ACTOS once daily for 24 weeks in addition to their current sulfonylurea regimen. The mean reductions from baseline at Week 24 in HbA1c were 1.55% and 1.67% for the 30 mg and 45 mg doses, respectively. Mean reductions from baseline in FPG were 51.5 mg/dL and 56.1 mg/dL.

The therapeutic effect of ACTOS in combination with sulfonylurea was observed in patients regardless of whether the patients were receiving low, medium, or high doses of sulfonylurea.

ACTOS Plus Metformin Studies

Two clinical studies were conducted with ACTOS in combination with metformin. Both studies included patients with type 2 diabetes on metformin, either alone or in combination with another antidiabetic agent. All other antidiabetic agents were withdrawn prior to starting study treatment. In the first study, 328 patients were randomized to receive either 30 mg of ACTOS or placebo once daily for 16 weeks in addition to their current metformin regimen. When compared to placebo at Week 16, the addition of ACTOS to metformin significantly reduced the mean HbA1c by 0.8% and decreased the mean FPG by 38 mg/dL.

In the second study, 827 patients were randomized to receive either 30 mg or 45 mg of ACTOS once daily for 24 weeks in addition to their current metformin regimen. The mean reductions from baseline at Week 24 in HbA1c were 0.80% and 1.01% for the 30 mg and 45 mg doses, respectively. Mean reductions from baseline in FPG were 38.2 mg/dL and 50.7 mg/dL.

The therapeutic effect of ACTOS in combination with metformin was observed in patients regardless of whether the patients were receiving lower or higher doses of metformin.

ACTOS Plus Insulin Studies

Two clinical studies were conducted with ACTOS in combination with insulin. Both studies included patients with type 2 diabetes on insulin, either alone or in combination with another antidiabetic agent. All other antidiabetic agents were withdrawn prior to starting study treatment. In the first study, 566 patients receiving a median of 60.5 units per day of insulin were randomized to receive either 15 mg or 30 mg of ACTOS or placebo once daily for 16 weeks in addition to their insulin regimen. When compared to placebo at Week 16, the addition of ACTOS to insulin significantly reduced both HbA1c by 0.7% and 1.0% and FPG by 35 mg/dL and 49 mg/dL for the 15 mg and 30 mg dose, respectively.

In the second study, 690 patients receiving a median of 60.0 units per day of insulin received either 30 mg or 45 mg of ACTOS once daily for 24 weeks in addition to their current insulin regimen. The mean reductions from baseline at Week 24 in HbA1c were 1.17% and 1.46% for the 30 mg and 45 mg doses, respectively. Mean reductions from baseline in FPG were 31.9 mg/dL and 45.8 mg/dL. Improved glycemic control was accompanied by mean decreases from baseline in insulin dose requirements of 6.0% and 9.4% per day for the 30 mg and 45 mg dose, respectively.

Table 4 Glycemic Parameters in a 24-Week Placebo-Controlled Forced-Titration Study

	Placebo	ACTOS 30 mg+ Once Daily	ACTOS 45 mg+ Once Daily
Total Population			
HbA1c (%)	N=83	N=85	N=85
Baseline (mean)	10.8	10.3	10.8
Change from baseline (adjusted mean++)	0.9	-0.6	-0.6
Difference from placebo (adjusted mean++)		-1.5*	-1.5*
FPG (mg/dL)	N=78	N=82	N=85
Baseline (mean)	279	268	281
Change from baseline (adjusted mean++)	18	-44	-50
Difference from placebo (adjusted mean++)		-62*	-68*

+ Final dose in forced titration
++ Adjusted for baseline, pooled center, and pooled center by treatment interaction
* p ≤ 0.050 vs. placebo

Table 6 Weight Changes (kg) from Baseline during Double-Blind Clinical Trials with ACTOS

		Control Group (Placebo) Median (25th/75th percentile)	ACTOS 15 mg Median (25th/75th percentile)	ACTOS 30 mg Median (25th/75th percentile)	ACTOS 45 mg Median (25th/75th percentile)
Monotherapy		-1.4 (-2.7/0.0) n=256	0.9 (-0.5/3.4) n=79	1.0 (-0.9/3.4) n=188	2.6 (0.2/5.4) n=79
Combination Therapy	Sulfonylurea	-0.5 (-1.8/0.7) n=187	2.0 (0.2/3.2) n=183	3.1 (1.1/5.4) n=528	4.1 (1.8/7.3) n=333
	Metformin	-1.4 (-3.2/0.3) n=160	N/A	0.9 (-0.3/3.2) n=567	1.8 (-0.9/5.0) n=407
	Insulin	0.2 (-1.4/1.4) n=182	2.3 (0.5/4.3) n=190	3.3 (0.9/6.3) n=522	4.1 (1.4/6.8) n=338

Note: Trial durations of 16 to 26 weeks

The therapeutic effect of ACTOS in combination with insulin was observed in patients regardless of whether the patients were receiving lower or higher doses of insulin.

INDICATIONS AND USAGE

ACTOS is indicated as an adjunct to diet and exercise to improve glycemic control in adults with type 2 diabetes mellitus.

CONTRAINDICATIONS

Initiation of ACTOS in patients with established New York Heart Association (NYHA) Class III or IV heart failure is contraindicated (see **BOXED WARNING**).

ACTOS is contraindicated in patients with known hypersensitivity to this product or any of its components.

WARNINGS

Cardiac Failure and Other Cardiac Effects

ACTOS, like other thiazolidinediones, can cause fluid retention when used alone or in combination with other antidiabetic agents, including insulin. Fluid retention may lead to or exacerbate heart failure. Patients should be observed for signs and symptoms of heart failure. If these signs and symptoms develop, the heart failure should be managed according to current standards of care. Furthermore, discontinuation or dose reduction of ACTOS must be considered (see **BOXED WARNING**). Patients with NYHA Class III and IV cardiac status were not studied during pre-approval clinical trials and ACTOS is not recommended in these patients (see **BOXED WARNING** and **CONTRAINDICATIONS**).

In one 16-week, U.S. double-blind, placebo-controlled clinical trial involving 566 patients with type 2 diabetes, ACTOS at doses of 15 mg and 30 mg in combination with insulin was compared to insulin therapy alone. This trial included patients with long-standing diabetes and a high prevalence of pre-existing medical conditions as follows: arterial hypertension (57.2%), peripheral neuropathy (22.6%), coronary heart disease (19.6%), retinopathy (13.1%), myocardial infarction (8.8%), vascular disease (6.4%), angina pectoris (4.4%), stroke and/or transient ischemic attack (4.1%), and congestive heart failure (2.3%).

In this study, two of the 191 patients receiving 15 mg ACTOS plus insulin (1.1%) and two of the 188 patients receiving 30 mg ACTOS plus insulin (1.1%) developed congestive heart failure compared with none of the 187 patients on insulin therapy alone. All four of these patients had previous histories of cardiovascular conditions including coronary artery disease, previous CABG procedures, and myocardial infarction. In a 24-week, dose-controlled study in which ACTOS was coadministered with insulin, 0.3% of patients (1/345) on 30 mg and 0.9% (3/345) of patients on 45 mg reported CHF as a serious adverse event.

Analysis of data from these studies did not identify specific factors that predict increased risk of congestive heart failure on combination therapy with insulin.

In type 2 diabetes and congestive heart failure (systolic dysfunction)

A 24-week post-marketing safety study was performed to compare ACTOS (n=262) to glyburide (n=256) in uncontrolled diabetic patients (mean HbA1c 8.8% at baseline) with NYHA Class II and III heart failure and ejection fraction less than 40% (mean EF 30% at baseline). Over the course of the study, overnight hospitalization for congestive heart failure was reported in 9.9% of patients on ACTOS compared to 4.7% of patients on glyburide with a treatment difference observed from 6 weeks. This adverse event associated with ACTOS was more marked in patients using insulin at baseline and in patients over 64 years of age. No difference in cardiovascular mortality between the treatment groups was observed.

ACTOS should be initiated at the lowest approved dose if it is prescribed for patients with type 2 diabetes and systolic heart failure (NYHA Class II). If subsequent dose escalation is necessary, the dose should be increased gradually only after several months of treatment with careful monitoring for weight gain, edema, or signs and symptoms of CHF exacerbation.

Prospective Pioglitazone Clinical Trial In Macrovascular Events (PROactive)

In PROactive, 5238 patients with type 2 diabetes and a prior history of macrovascular disease were treated with ACTOS (n=2605), force-titrated up to 45 mg once daily, or placebo (n=2633) (see **ADVERSE REACTIONS**). The percentage of patients who had an event of serious heart failure was higher for patients treated with ACTOS (5.7%, n=149) than for patients treated with placebo (4.1%, n=108). The incidence of death subsequent to a report of serious heart failure was 1.5% (n=40) in patients treated with ACTOS and 1.4% (n=37) in placebo-treated patients. In patients treated with an insulin-containing regimen at baseline, the incidence of serious heart failure was 6.3% (n=54/864) with ACTOS and 5.2% (n=47/896) with placebo. For those patients treated with a sulfonylurea-containing regimen at baseline, the incidence of serious heart failure was 5.8% (n=94/1624) with ACTOS and 4.4% (n=71/1626) with placebo.

PRECAUTIONS

General

ACTOS exerts its antihyperglycemic effect only in the presence of insulin. Therefore, ACTOS should not be used in patients with type 1 diabetes or for the treatment of diabetic ketoacidosis.

Hypoglycemia: Patients receiving ACTOS in combination with insulin or oral hypoglycemic agents may be at risk for hypoglycemia, and a reduction in the dose of the concomitant agent may be necessary.

Cardiovascular: In U.S. placebo-controlled clinical trials that excluded patients with New York Heart Association (NYHA) Class III and IV cardiac status, the incidence of serious cardiac adverse events related to volume expansion was not increased in patients treated with ACTOS as monotherapy or in combination with sulfonylureas or metformin vs. placebo-treated patients. In insulin combination studies, a small number of patients with a history of previously existing cardiac disease developed congestive heart failure when treated with ACTOS in combination with insulin (see WARNINGS). Patients with NYHA Class III and IV cardiac status were not studied in these ACTOS clinical trials. ACTOS is not indicated in patients with NYHA Class III or IV cardiac status.

In postmarketing experience with ACTOS, cases of congestive heart failure have been reported in patients both with and without previously known heart disease.

Edema: ACTOS should be used with caution in patients with edema. In all U.S. clinical trials, edema was reported more frequently in patients treated with ACTOS than in placebo-treated patients and appears to be dose related (see ADVERSE REACTIONS). In postmarketing experience, reports of initiation or worsening of edema have been received. Since thiazolidinediones, including ACTOS, can cause fluid retention, which can exacerbate or lead to congestive heart failure, ACTOS should be used with caution in patients at risk for heart failure. Patients should be monitored for signs and symptoms of heart failure (see BOXED WARNING, WARNINGS, and PRECAUTIONS, Information for Patients).

Weight Gain: Dose related weight gain was seen with ACTOS alone and in combination with other hypoglycemic agents (Table 6). The mechanism of weight gain is unclear but probably involves a combination of fluid retention and fat accumulation.

[See table 6 on previous page]

Ovulation: Therapy with ACTOS, like other thiazolidinediones, may result in ovulation in some premenopausal anovulatory women. As a result, these patients may be at an increased risk for pregnancy while taking ACTOS. Thus, adequate contraception in premenopausal women should be recommended. This possible effect has not been investigated in clinical studies so the frequency of this occurrence is not known.

Hematologic: ACTOS may cause decreases in hemoglobin and hematocrit. Across all clinical studies, mean hemoglobin values declined by 2% to 4% in patients treated with ACTOS. These changes primarily occurred within the first 4 to 12 weeks of therapy and remained relatively constant thereafter. These changes may be related to increased plasma volume and have rarely been associated with any significant hematologic clinical effects (see ADVERSE REACTIONS, Laboratory Abnormalities).

Hepatic Effects: In pre-approval clinical studies worldwide, over 4500 subjects were treated with ACTOS. In U.S. clinical studies, over 4700 patients with type 2 diabetes received ACTOS. There was no evidence of drug-induced hepatotoxicity or elevation of ALT levels in the clinical studies.

During pre-approval placebo-controlled clinical trials in the U.S., a total of 4 of 1526 (0.26%) patients treated with ACTOS and 2 of 793 (0.25%) placebo-treated patients had ALT values ≥ 3 times the upper limit of normal. The ALT elevations in patients treated with ACTOS were reversible and were not clearly related to therapy with ACTOS.

In postmarketing experience with ACTOS, reports of hepatitis and of hepatic enzyme elevations to 3 or more times the upper limit of normal have been received. Very rarely, these reports have involved hepatic failure with and without fatal outcome, although causality has not been established.

Pending the availability of the results of additional large, long-term controlled clinical trials and additional postmarketing safety data, it is recommended that patients treated with ACTOS undergo periodic monitoring of liver enzymes.

Serum ALT (alanine aminotransferase) levels should be evaluated prior to the initiation of therapy with ACTOS in all patients and periodically thereafter per the clinical judgment of the health care professional. Liver function tests should also be obtained for patients if symptoms suggestive of hepatic dysfunction occur, e.g., nausea, vomiting, abdominal pain, fatigue, anorexia, or dark urine. The decision whether to continue the patient on therapy with ACTOS should be guided by clinical judgment pending laboratory evaluations. If jaundice is observed, drug therapy should be discontinued.

Therapy with ACTOS should not be initiated if the patient exhibits clinical evidence of active liver disease or the ALT levels exceed 2.5 times the upper limit of normal. Patients with mildly elevated liver enzymes (ALT levels at 1 to 2.5 times the upper limit of normal) at baseline or any time during therapy with ACTOS should be evaluated to determine the cause of the liver enzyme elevation. Initiation or continuation of therapy with ACTOS in patients with mildly elevated liver enzymes should proceed with caution and include appropriate clinical follow-up which may include more frequent liver enzyme monitoring. If serum transaminase levels are increased (ALT > 2.5 times the upper limit of normal), liver function tests should be evaluated more frequently until the levels return to normal or pretreatment values. If ALT levels exceed 3 times the upper limit of normal, the test should be repeated as soon as possible. If ALT levels remain > 3 times the upper limit of normal or if the patient is jaundiced, ACTOS therapy should be discontinued.

Macular Edema: Macular edema has been reported in post-marketing experience in diabetic patients who were taking pioglitazone or another thiazolidinedione. Some patients presented with blurred vision or decreased visual acuity, but some patients appear to have been diagnosed on routine ophthalmologic examination. Some patients had peripheral edema at the time macular edema was diagnosed. Some patients had improvement in their macular edema after discontinuation of their thiazolidinedione. It is unknown whether or not there is a causal relationship between pioglitazone and macular edema. Patients with diabetes should have regular eye exams by an ophthalmologist, per the Standards of Care of the American Diabetes Association. Additionally, any diabetic who reports any kind of visual symptom should be promptly referred to an ophthalmologist, regardless of the patient's underlying medications or other physical findings (see ADVERSE REACTIONS).

Fractures: In a randomized trial (PROactive) in patients with type 2 diabetes (mean duration of diabetes 9.5 years), an increased incidence of bone fracture was noted in female patients taking pioglitazone. During a mean follow-up of 34.5 months, the incidence of bone fracture in females was 5.1% (44/870) for pioglitazone versus 2.5% (23/905) for placebo. This difference was noted after the first year of treatment and remained during the course of the study. The majority of fractures observed in female patients were nonvertebral fractures including lower limb and distal upper limb. No increase in fracture rates was observed in men treated with pioglitazone 1.7% (30/1735) versus placebo 2.1% (37/1728). The risk of fracture should be considered in the care of patients, especially female patients, treated with pioglitazone and attention should be given to assessing and maintaining bone health according to current standards of care.

Macrovascular Outcomes: There have been no clinical studies establishing conclusive evidence of macrovascular risk reduction with ACTOS or any other anti-diabetic drug.

Laboratory Tests

FPG and HbA$_{1c}$ measurements should be performed periodically to monitor glycemic control and the therapeutic response to ACTOS.

Liver enzyme monitoring is recommended prior to initiation of therapy with ACTOS in all patients and periodically thereafter per the clinical judgment of the health care professional (see PRECAUTIONS, General, Hepatic Effects and ADVERSE REACTIONS, Serum Transaminase Levels).

Information for Patients

It is important to instruct patients to adhere to dietary instructions and to have blood glucose and glycosylated hemoglobin tested regularly. During periods of stress such as fever, trauma, infection, or surgery, medication requirements may change and patients should be reminded to seek medical advice promptly.

Patients who experience an unusually rapid increase in weight or edema or who develop shortness of breath or other symptoms of heart failure while on ACTOS should immediately report these symptoms to their physician.

Patients should be told that blood tests for liver function will be performed prior to the start of therapy and periodically thereafter per the clinical judgment of the health care professional. Patients should be told to seek immediate medical advice for unexplained nausea, vomiting, abdominal pain, fatigue, anorexia, or dark urine.

Patients should be told to take ACTOS once daily. ACTOS can be taken with or without meals. If a dose is missed on one day, the dose should not be doubled the following day. When using combination therapy with insulin or oral hypoglycemic agents, the risks of hypoglycemia, its symptoms and treatment, and conditions that predispose to its development should be explained to patients and their family members.

Therapy with ACTOS, like other thiazolidinediones, may result in ovulation in some premenopausal anovulatory women. As a result, these patients may be at an increased risk for pregnancy while taking ACTOS. Thus, adequate contraception in premenopausal women should be recommended. This possible effect has not been investigated in clinical studies so the frequency of this occurrence is not known.

Drug Interactions

In vivo drug-drug interaction studies have suggested that pioglitazone may be a weak inducer of CYP 450 isoform 3A4 substrate (see CLINICAL PHARMACOLOGY, Metabolism and Drug-Drug Interactions).

An enzyme inhibitor of CYP2C8 (such as gemfibrozil) may significantly increase the AUC of pioglitazone and an enzyme inducer of CYP2C8 (such as rifampin) may significantly decrease the AUC of pioglitazone. Therefore, if an inhibitor or inducer of CYP2C8 is started or stopped during treatment with pioglitazone, changes in diabetes treatment may be needed based on clinical response (see CLINICAL PHARMACOLOGY, Drug-Drug Interactions).

Carcinogenesis, Mutagenesis, Impairment of Fertility

A two-year carcinogenicity study was conducted in male and female rats at oral doses up to 63 mg/kg (approximately 14 times the maximum recommended human oral dose of 45 mg based on mg/m^2). Drug-induced tumors were not observed in any organ except for the urinary bladder. Benign and/or malignant transitional cell neoplasms were observed in male rats at 4 mg/kg/day and above (approximately equal to the maximum recommended human oral dose based on mg/m^2). A two-year carcinogenicity study was conducted in male and female mice at oral doses up to 100 mg/kg/day (approximately 11 times the maximum recommended human oral dose based on mg/m^2). No drug-induced tumors were observed in any organ.

During prospective evaluation of urinary cytology involving more than 1800 patients receiving ACTOS in clinical trials up to one year in duration, no new cases of bladder tumors were identified. In two 3-year studies in which pioglitazone was compared to placebo or glyburide, there were 16/3656 (0.44%) reports of bladder cancer in patients taking pioglitazone compared to 5/3679 (0.14%) in patients not taking pioglitazone. After excluding patients in whom exposure to study drug was less than one year at the time of diagnosis of bladder cancer, there were six (0.16%) cases on pioglitazone and two (0.05%) on placebo.

Pioglitazone HCl was not mutagenic in a battery of genetic toxicology studies, including the Ames bacterial assay, a mammalian cell forward gene mutation assay (CHO/HPRT and AS52/XPRT), an in vitro cytogenetics assay using CHL cells, an unscheduled DNA synthesis assay, and an in vivo micronucleus assay.

No adverse effects upon fertility were observed in male and female rats at oral doses up to 40 mg/kg pioglitazone HCl daily prior to and throughout mating and gestation (approximately 9 times the maximum recommended human oral dose based on mg/m^2).

Animal Toxicology

Heart enlargement has been observed in mice (100 mg/kg), rats (4 mg/kg and above) and dogs (3 mg/kg) treated orally with pioglitazone HCl (approximately 11, 1, and 2 times the maximum recommended human oral dose for mice, rats, and dogs, respectively, based on mg/m^2). In a one-year rat study, drug-related early death due to apparent heart dysfunction occurred at an oral dose of 160 mg/kg/day (approximately 35 times the maximum recommended human oral dose based on mg/m^2). Heart enlargement was seen in a 13-week study in monkeys at oral doses of 8.9 mg/kg and above (approximately 4 times the maximum recommended human oral dose based on mg/m^2), but not in a 52-week study at oral doses up to 32 mg/kg (approximately 13 times the maximum recommended human oral dose based on mg/m^2).

Pregnancy

Pregnancy Category C. Pioglitazone was not teratogenic in rats at oral doses up to 80 mg/kg or in rabbits given up to 160 mg/kg during organogenesis (approximately 17 and 40 times the maximum recommended human oral dose based on mg/m^2, respectively). Delayed parturition and embryotoxicity (as evidenced by increased postimplantation losses, delayed development and reduced fetal weights) were observed in rats at oral doses of 40 mg/kg/day and above (approximately 10 times the maximum recommended human oral dose based on mg/m^2). No functional or behavioral toxicity was observed in offspring of rats. In rabbits, embryotoxicity was observed at an oral dose of 160 mg/kg (approximately 40 times the maximum recommended human oral dose based on mg/m^2). Delayed postnatal development, attributed to decreased body weight, was observed in offspring of rats at oral doses of 10 mg/kg and above during late gestation and lactation periods (approximately 2 times the maximum recommended human oral dose based on mg/m^2). There are no adequate and well-controlled studies in pregnant women. ACTOS should be used during pregnancy only if the potential benefit justifies the potential risk to the fetus.

Because current information strongly suggests that abnormal blood glucose levels during pregnancy are associated with a higher incidence of congenital anomalies, as well as increased neonatal morbidity and mortality, most experts recommend that insulin be used during pregnancy to maintain blood glucose levels as close to normal as possible.

Nursing Mothers

Pioglitazone is secreted in the milk of lactating rats. It is not known whether ACTOS is secreted in human milk. Because many drugs are excreted in human milk, ACTOS should not be administered to a breastfeeding woman.

Pediatric Use

Safety and effectiveness of ACTOS in pediatric patients have not been established.

Elderly Use

Approximately 500 patients in placebo-controlled clinical trials of ACTOS were 65 and over. No significant differences in effectiveness and safety were observed between these patients and younger patients.

ADVERSE REACTIONS

Over 8500 patients with type 2 diabetes have been treated with ACTOS in randomized, double-blind, controlled clinical trials. This includes 2605 high-risk patients with type 2 diabetes treated with ACTOS from the PROactive clinical trial. Over 6000 patients have been treated for 6 months or longer, and over 4500 patients for one year or longer. Over 3000 patients have received ACTOS for at least 2 years. The overall incidence and types of adverse events reported in placebo-controlled clinical trials of ACTOS monotherapy at doses of 7.5 mg, 15 mg, 30 mg, or 45 mg once daily are shown in **Table 7**.

Table 7 Placebo-Controlled Clinical Studies of ACTOS Monotherapy: Adverse Events Reported at a Frequency ≥ 5% of Patients Treated with ACTOS

	(% of Patients)	
	Placebo N=259	ACTOS N=606
Upper Respiratory Tract Infection	8.5	13.2
Headache	6.9	9.1
Sinusitis	4.6	6.3
Myalgia	2.7	5.4
Tooth Disorder	2.3	5.3
Diabetes Mellitus Aggravated	8.1	5.1
Pharyngitis	0.8	5.1

For most clinical adverse events the incidence was similar for groups treated with ACTOS monotherapy and those treated in combination with sulfonylureas, metformin, and insulin. There was an increase in the occurrence of edema in the patients treated with ACTOS and insulin compared to insulin alone.

In a 16-week, placebo-controlled ACTOS plus insulin trial (n=379), 10 patients treated with ACTOS plus insulin developed dyspnea and also, at some point during their therapy, developed either weight change or edema. Seven of these 10 patients received diuretics to treat these symptoms. This was not reported in the insulin plus placebo group.

The incidence of withdrawals from placebo-controlled clinical trials due to an adverse event other than hyperglycemia was similar for patients treated with placebo (2.8%) or ACTOS (3.3%).

In controlled combination therapy studies with either a sulfonylurea or insulin, mild to moderate hypoglycemia, which appears to be dose related, was reported (see **PRECAUTIONS, General**, Hypoglycemia and **DOSAGE and ADMINISTRATION, Combination Therapy**).

In U.S. double-blind studies, anemia was reported in ≤ 2% of patients treated with ACTOS plus sulfonylurea, metformin or insulin (see **PRECAUTIONS, General**, Hematologic).

In monotherapy studies, edema was reported for 4.8% (with doses from 7.5 mg to 45 mg) of patients treated with ACTOS versus 1.2% of placebo-treated patients. In combination therapy studies, edema was reported for 7.2% of patients treated with ACTOS and sulfonylureas compared to 2.1% of patients on sulfonylureas alone. In combination therapy studies with metformin, edema was reported in 6.0% of patients on combination therapy compared to 2.5% of patients on metformin alone. In combination therapy studies with insulin, edema was reported in 15.3% of patients on combination therapy compared to 7.0% of patients on insulin alone. Most of these events were considered mild or moderate in intensity (see **PRECAUTIONS, General**, Edema).

In one 16-week clinical trial of insulin plus ACTOS combination therapy, more patients developed congestive heart

Table 8 Number of First and Total Events for Each Component within the Cardiovascular Composite Endpoint

Cardiovascular Events	Placebo N=2633		ACTOS N=2605	
	First Events (N)	Total events (N)	First Events (N)	Total events (N)
Any event	572	900	514	803
All-cause mortality	122	186	110	177
Non-fatal MI	118	157	105	131
Stroke	96	119	76	92
ACS	63	78	42	65
Cardiac intervention	101	240	101	195
Major leg amputation	15	28	9	28
Leg revascularization	57	92	71	115

failure on combination therapy (1.1%) compared to none on insulin alone (see **WARNINGS, Cardiac Failure and Other Cardiac Effects**).

Prospective Pioglitazone Clinical Trial In Macrovascular Events (PROactive)

In PROactive, 5238 patients with type 2 diabetes and a prior history of macrovascular disease were treated with ACTOS (n=2605), force-titrated up to 45 mg daily or placebo (n=2633) in addition to standard of care. Almost all subjects (95%) were receiving cardiovascular medications (beta blockers, ACE inhibitors, ARBs, calcium channel blockers, nitrates, diuretics, aspirin, statins, fibrates). Patients had a mean age of 61.8 years, mean duration of diabetes 9.5 years, and mean HbA$_{1c}$ 8.1%. Average duration of follow-up was 34.5 months. The primary objective of this trial was to examine the effect of ACTOS on mortality and macrovascular morbidity in patients with type 2 diabetes mellitus who were at high risk for macrovascular events. The primary efficacy variable was the time to the first occurrence of any event in the cardiovascular composite endpoint (see **table 8** below). Although there was no statistically significant difference between ACTOS and placebo for the 3-year incidence of a first event within this composite, there was no increase in mortality or in total macrovascular events with ACTOS.

[See table 8 above]

Postmarketing reports of new onset or worsening diabetic macular edema with decreased visual acuity have also been received (see **PRECAUTIONS, General**, Macular Edema).

Laboratory Abnormalities

Hematologic: ACTOS may cause decreases in hemoglobin and hematocrit. The fall in hemoglobin and hematocrit with ACTOS appears to be dose related. Across all clinical studies, mean hemoglobin values declined by 2% to 4% in patients treated with ACTOS. These changes generally occurred within the first 4 to 12 weeks of therapy and remained relatively stable thereafter. These changes may be related to increased plasma volume associated with ACTOS therapy and have rarely been associated with any significant hematologic clinical effects.

Serum Transaminase Levels: During all clinical studies in the U.S., 14 of 4780 (0.30%) patients treated with ACTOS had ALT values ≥ 3 times the upper limit of normal during treatment. All patients with follow-up values had reversible elevations in ALT. In the population of patients treated with ACTOS, mean values for bilirubin, AST, ALT, alkaline phosphatase, and GGT were decreased at the final visit compared with baseline. Fewer than 0.9% of patients treated with ACTOS were withdrawn from clinical trials in the U.S. due to abnormal liver function tests.

In pre-approval clinical trials, there were no cases of idiosyncratic drug reactions leading to hepatic failure (see **PRECAUTIONS, General**, Hepatic Effects).

CPK Levels: During required laboratory testing in clinical trials, sporadic, transient elevations in creatine phosphokinase levels (CPK) were observed. An isolated elevation to greater than 10 times the upper limit of normal was noted in 9 patients (values of 2150 to 11400 IU/L). Six of these patients continued to receive ACTOS, two patients had completed receiving study medication at the time of the elevated value and one patient discontinued study medication due to the elevation. These elevations resolved without any apparent clinical sequelae. The relationship of these events to ACTOS therapy is unknown.

OVERDOSAGE

During controlled clinical trials, one case of overdose with ACTOS was reported. A male patient took 120 mg per day for four days, then 180 mg per day for seven days. The patient denied any clinical symptoms during this period.

In the event of overdosage, appropriate supportive treatment should be initiated according to patient's clinical signs and symptoms.

DOSAGE AND ADMINISTRATION

ACTOS should be taken once daily without regard to meals. The management of antidiabetic therapy should be individualized. Ideally, the response to therapy should be evaluated using HbA$_{1c}$ which is a better indicator of long-term glycemic control than FPG alone. HbA$_{1c}$ reflects glycemia over the past two to three months. In clinical use, it is recommended that patients be treated with ACTOS for a period of time adequate to evaluate change in HbA$_{1c}$ (three months) unless glycemic control deteriorates. After initiation of ACTOS or with dose increase, patients should be carefully monitored for adverse events related to fluid retention (see **BOXED WARNING** and **WARNINGS**).

Monotherapy

ACTOS monotherapy in patients not adequately controlled with diet and exercise may be initiated at 15 mg or 30 mg once daily. For patients who respond inadequately to the initial dose of ACTOS, the dose can be increased in increments up to 45 mg once daily. For patients not responding adequately to monotherapy, combination therapy should be considered.

Combination Therapy

Sulfonylureas: ACTOS in combination with a sulfonylurea may be initiated at 15 mg or 30 mg once daily. The current sulfonylurea dose can be continued upon initiation of ACTOS therapy. If patients report hypoglycemia, the dose of the sulfonylurea should be decreased.

Metformin: ACTOS in combination with metformin may be initiated at 15 mg or 30 mg once daily. The current metformin dose can be continued upon initiation of ACTOS therapy. It is unlikely that the dose of metformin will require adjustment due to hypoglycemia during combination therapy with ACTOS.

Insulin: ACTOS in combination with insulin may be initiated at 15 mg or 30 mg once daily. The current insulin dose can be continued upon initiation of ACTOS therapy. In patients receiving ACTOS and insulin, the insulin dose can be decreased by 10% to 25% if the patient reports hypoglycemia or if plasma glucose concentrations decrease to less than 100 mg/dL. Further adjustments should be individualized based on glucose-lowering response.

Maximum Recommended Dose

The dose of ACTOS should not exceed 45 mg once daily in monotherapy or in combination with sulfonylurea, metformin, or insulin.

Dose adjustment in patients with renal insufficiency is not recommended (see **CLINICAL PHARMACOLOGY, Pharmacokinetics and Drug Metabolism**).

Therapy with ACTOS should not be initiated if the patient exhibits clinical evidence of active liver disease or increased serum transaminase levels (ALT greater than 2.5 times the upper limit of normal) at start of therapy (see **PRECAUTIONS, General**, Hepatic Effects and **CLINICAL PHARMACOLOGY, Special Populations**, Hepatic Insufficiency). Liver enzyme monitoring is recommended in all patients prior to initiation of therapy with ACTOS and periodically thereafter (see **PRECAUTIONS, General**, Hepatic Effects). There are no data on the use of ACTOS in patients under 18 years of age; therefore, use of ACTOS in pediatric patients is not recommended.

No data are available on the use of ACTOS in combination with another thiazolidinedione.

HOW SUPPLIED

ACTOS is available in 15 mg, 30 mg, and 45 mg tablets as follows:

15 mg Tablet: white to off-white, round, convex, non-scored tablet with "ACTOS" on one side, and "15" on the other, available in:
NDC 64764-151-04 Bottles of 30
NDC 64764-151-05 Bottles of 90
NDC 64764-151-06 Bottles of 500

30 mg Tablet: white to off-white, round, flat, non-scored tablet with "ACTOS" on one side, and "30" on the other, available in:
NDC 64764-301-14 Bottles of 30
NDC 64764-301-15 Bottles of 90
NDC 64764-301-16 Bottles of 500

45 mg Tablet: white to off-white, round, flat, non-scored tablet with "ACTOS" on one side, and "45" on the other, available in:
NDC 64764-451-24 Bottles of 30
NDC 64764-451-25 Bottles of 90
NDC 64764-451-26 Bottles of 500

STORAGE
Store at 25°C (77°F); excursions permitted to 15-30°C (59-86°F) [see USP Controlled Room Temperature]. Keep container tightly closed, and protect from moisture and humidity.

REFERENCES
1. Deng, LJ, et al. Effect of gemfibrozil on the pharmacokinetics of pioglitazone. *Eur J Clin Pharmacol* 2005; 61: 831-836, Table 1.
2. Jaakkola, T, et al. Effect of rifampicin on the pharmacokinetics of pioglitazone. *Clin Pharmacol Brit Jour* 2006; 61:1 70-78.

Rx only
Manufactured by:
Takeda Pharmaceutical Company Limited
Osaka, Japan
Marketed by:
Takeda Pharmaceuticals America, Inc.
One Takeda Parkway
Deerfield, IL 60015
ACTOS® is a registered trademark of Takeda Pharmaceutical Company Limited and used under license by Takeda Pharmaceuticals America, Inc.
All other trademark names are the property of their respective owners.
August 2008
ACT0808-R14

MEDICATION GUIDE
ACTOS® (ak-TŌS)
(pioglitazone hydrochloride) tablets
Read this Medication Guide carefully before you start taking ACTOS and each time you get a refill. There may be new information. This information does not take the place of talking with your doctor about your medical condition or your treatment. If you have any questions about ACTOS, ask your doctor or pharmacist.

What is the most important information I should know about ACTOS?
ACTOS can cause serious side effects, including **new or worse heart failure.**

• ACTOS can cause your body to keep extra fluid (fluid retention), which leads to swelling (edema) and weight gain. Extra body fluid can make some heart problems worse or lead to heart failure. Heart failure means your heart does not pump blood well enough.
• If you have severe heart failure, you cannot start ACTOS.
• If you have heart failure with symptoms (such as shortness of breath or swelling), even if these symptoms are not severe, ACTOS may not be right for you.
Call your doctor right away if you have any of the following:
• swelling or fluid retention, especially in the ankles or legs.
• shortness of breath or trouble breathing, especially when you lie down.
• an unusually fast increase in weight.
• unusual tiredness.
ACTOS can have other serious side effects. See "What are the possible side effects of ACTOS?"

What is ACTOS?
ACTOS is a prescription medicine used with diet and exercise to improve blood sugar (glucose) control in adults with type 2 diabetes. ACTOS is a diabetes medicine called pioglitazone hydrochloride that may be taken alone or with other diabetes medicines.
Your doctor will decide if you should take ACTOS.
It is important to eat the right foods, lose weight if needed, and exercise regularly in order to manage your type 2 diabetes. Diet, weight loss, and exercise are the main treatments for type 2 diabetes and they also help your diabetes medicines work better for you.
ACTOS has not been studied in children and is not recommended for children under the age of 18. The risks of giving ACTOS to a child are not known. See "What are some other possible side effects of ACTOS?"

Who should not take ACTOS?
Do not take ACTOS if you:

• are allergic to any of the ingredients in ACTOS. See the end of this Medication Guide for a complete list of ingredients in ACTOS.
People with severe heart failure should not start taking ACTOS. See "What is the most important information I should know about ACTOS?"

What should I tell my doctor before taking ACTOS?
Before starting ACTOS, ask your doctor about what the choices are for diabetes medicines and what the expected benefits and possible risks are for you in particular.
Tell your doctor about all of your medical conditions, especially if you:
• **have heart failure.**
• **have type 1 ("juvenile") diabetes or had diabetic ketoacidosis.** These conditions should be treated with insulin.
• **have a type of diabetic eye disease called macular edema** (swelling of the back of the eye).
• **have liver problems.** Your doctor should do blood tests to check your liver before you start taking ACTOS and during treatment as needed.
• **are pregnant or planning to become pregnant.** ACTOS should not be used during pregnancy. It is not known if ACTOS can harm your unborn baby. Talk to your doctor about the best way to control your blood glucose levels while pregnant.
• **are a premenopausal woman (before the "change of life"), who does not have periods regularly or at all.** ACTOS may increase your chance of becoming pregnant. Talk to your doctor about birth control choices while taking ACTOS. Tell your doctor right away if you become pregnant while taking ACTOS.
• **are breastfeeding or plan to breastfeed.** It is not known if ACTOS passes into your milk and if it can harm your baby. You should not take ACTOS if you breastfeed your baby. Talk to your doctor about the best way to control your blood glucose levels while breastfeeding.
Tell your doctor about all the medicines you take including prescription and non-prescription medicines, vitamins, and herbal supplements. ACTOS and some of your other medicines can affect each other. You may need to have your dose of ACTOS or certain other medicines adjusted. Certain other medicines can affect your blood sugar (glucose) control.
Know the medicines you take. Keep a list of your medicines and show it to your doctor and pharmacist before you start a new medicine. They will tell you if it is okay to take ACTOS with other medicines.

How should I take ACTOS?
• Take ACTOS exactly as prescribed.
• Your doctor may need to change your dose of ACTOS to control your blood glucose. Do not change your dose unless told to do so by your doctor.
• ACTOS may be prescribed alone or with other diabetes medicines. This will depend on how well your blood sugar is controlled.
• Take ACTOS one time each day, with or without food.
• If you miss a dose of ACTOS, take your next dose as prescribed unless your doctor tells you differently. Do not take two doses at one time the next day.
• If you take too much ACTOS, call your doctor or poison control center right away.
• If your body is under stress, for example: due to fever, infection, trauma (such as a car accident), or surgery, the dose of your diabetes medicines may need to be changed. Call your doctor right away.
• Stay on your diet and exercise programs and test your blood sugar regularly while taking ACTOS.
• Your doctor should do blood tests before starting ACTOS and from time to time to check your liver, kidneys, and blood cells.
• Your doctor should also do regular blood tests (for example, hemoglobin A1C) to check how well your blood sugar is controlled with ACTOS.
• Your doctor should check your eyes regularly. Some people have had vision changes due to swelling in the back of the eye, called macular edema, while taking ACTOS.
• It may take 2-3 months to see the full effect on your blood sugar level.

What are other possible side effects of ACTOS?
ACTOS can cause other serious side effects including:
• **Weight gain.** Pioglitazone, the medicine in ACTOS can cause weight gain that may be due to fluid retention or extra body fat. Weight gain due to fluid retention can be a serious problem for people with certain conditions, including heart problems. See "What is the most important information I should know about ACTOS?".
• **Liver problems.** It is important for your liver to be working normally when you take ACTOS. Your doctor should do blood tests to check your liver before you start taking ACTOS and during treatment as needed. Call your doctor right away if you have unexplained symptoms such as:
  ○ nausea or vomiting.
  ○ stomach pain.
  ○ unusual or unexplained tiredness.

○ loss of appetite.
○ dark urine.
○ yellowing of your skin or the whites of your eyes.
• **Macular edema** (diabetic eye disease with swelling in the back of the eye). Tell your doctor right away if you have any changes in your vision. Your doctor should check your eyes regularly.
• **Fractures (broken bones),** usually in the hand, upper arm, or foot in women. Talk to your doctor for advice on how to keep your bones healthy. It is not known if ACTOS can affect the bones of children.
• **Low red blood cell count (anemia).**
• **Low blood sugar (hypoglycemia).** Lightheadedness, dizziness, shakiness, or hunger may indicate that your blood sugar is too low. This can happen if you skip meals, if you use another medicine that lowers blood sugar, or if you have certain medical problems. Call your doctor if low blood sugar levels are a problem for you.
• **Ovulation** (release of an egg from an ovary in a woman) leading to pregnancy. Ovulation may happen when premenopausal women who do not have regular monthly periods take ACTOS. This can increase the chance of pregnancy. See "What should I tell my doctor before taking ACTOS?".
In studies of pioglitazone (the medicine in ACTOS), bladder cancer occurred in a few more people who were taking pioglitazone than in people who were taking other diabetes medicines. There were too few cases to know if the bladder cancer was related to pioglitazone.
Other common side effects of ACTOS are:
• cold-like symptoms (respiratory tract infection),
• headache,
• sinus infection,
• muscle pain,
• tooth disorder,
• sore throat.
Tell your doctor if you have any side effect that bothers you or that does not go away. These are not all the side effects of ACTOS. For more information, ask your doctor or pharmacist.
Call your doctor for medical advice about side effects. You may report side effects to FDA at 1-800-FDA-1088.

How should I store ACTOS?
• Store ACTOS at 59° to 86°F (15° to 30°C). Keep ACTOS in the original container to protect from light.
• Keep the ACTOS bottle tightly closed and protect from getting wet (away from moisture and humidity).
Keep ACTOS and all medicines out of the reach of children.

General information about ACTOS
Medicines are sometimes prescribed for purposes other than those listed in a Medication Guide. Do not use ACTOS for a condition for which it is not prescribed. Do not give ACTOS to other people, even if they have the same symptoms you have. It may harm them.
This Medication Guide summarizes the most important information about ACTOS. If you would like more information, talk with your doctor. You can ask your doctor or pharmacist for information about ACTOS that is written for healthcare professionals. For more information, go to www.actos.com or call 1-877-825-3327.

What are the ingredients in ACTOS?
Active Ingredient: pioglitazone hydrochloride
Inactive Ingredients: lactose monohydrate, hydroxypropylcellulose, carboxymethylcellulose calcium, and magnesium stearate.
Always check to make sure that the medicine you are taking is the correct one. ACTOS tablets look like this:

• 15 mg strength tablets – white to off-white, round, convex, non-scored with "ACTOS" on one side, and "15" on the other.
• 30 mg strength tablets – white to off-white, round, flat, non-scored with "ACTOS" on one side, and "30" on the other.
• 45 mg strength tablets – white to off-white, round, flat, non-scored with "ACTOS" on one side, and "45" on the other.

ACTOS® is a registered trademark of Takeda Pharmaceutical Company Limited and used under license by Takeda Pharmaceuticals America, Inc.
All other trademarks are the property of their respective owners.
This Medication Guide has been approved by the U.S. Food and Drug Administration.
Distributed by:
Takeda Pharmaceuticals America, Inc.
Deerfield, IL 60015
© 2009 Takeda Pharmaceuticals America, Inc.
September 2009
ACT0909-R2/MG

Shown in Product Identification Guide, page 319

AMITIZA® ℞
[ahm-i-TEE-za]
(lubiprostone)
capsules

HIGHLIGHTS OF PRESCRIBING INFORMATION
These highlights do not include all the information needed to use AMITIZA safely and effectively. See full prescribing information for AMITIZA.
AMITIZA (lubiprostone) Capsules
Initial U.S. Approval: 2006

————————INDICATIONS AND USAGE————————
Amitiza is a chloride channel activator indicated for:
• Treatment of chronic idiopathic constipation in adults (1.1)
• Treatment of irritable bowel syndrome with constipation in women ≥ 18 years old (1.2)

————————DOSAGE AND ADMINISTRATION————————
Chronic idiopathic constipation
• 24 mcg taken twice daily orally with food and water (2.1)
Irritable bowel syndrome with constipation
• 8 mcg taken twice daily orally with food and water (2.2)

————————DOSAGE FORMS AND STRENGTHS————————
• Gelatin capsules: 8 mcg and 24 mcg (3)

————————CONTRAINDICATIONS————————
• Patients with known or suspected mechanical gastrointestinal obstruction should not receive Amitiza (4)

————————WARNINGS AND PRECAUTIONS————————
• Women who could become pregnant should have a negative pregnancy test prior to beginning therapy and should be capable of complying with effective contraceptive measures (8.1)
• Use during pregnancy only if the potential benefit justifies the potential risk to the fetus (5.1)
• Patients may experience nausea; concomitant administration of food may reduce this symptom (5.2)
• Do not prescribe for patients that have severe diarrhea (5.3)
• Patients taking Amitiza may experience dyspnea within an hour of first dose. This symptom generally resolves within 3 hours, but may recur with repeat dosing (5.4)
• Evaluate patients with symptoms suggestive of mechanical gastrointestinal obstruction prior to initiating treatment with Amitiza (5.5)

————————ADVERSE REACTIONS————————
• Most common adverse reactions (incidence > 4%) in chronic idiopathic constipation are nausea, diarrhea, headache, abdominal pain, abdominal distension, and flatulence (6.1)
• Most common adverse reactions (incidence > 4%) in irritable bowel syndrome with constipation are nausea, diarrhea, and abdominal pain (6.1)
To report SUSPECTED ADVERSE REACTIONS, contact Takeda Pharmaceuticals North America, Inc., at 1-877-825-3327 or FDA at 1-800-FDA-1088 or www.fda.gov/medwatch.
See 17 for PATIENT COUNSELING INFORMATION
Revised: May/2009

Table 1: Percent of Patients with Adverse Reactions (Chronic Idiopathic Constipation)

System/Adverse Reaction[1]	Placebo N = 316 %	Amitiza 24 mcg Once Daily N = 29 %	Amitiza 24 mcg Twice Daily N = 1113 %
Gastrointestinal disorders			
Nausea	3	17	29
Diarrhea	< 1	7	12
Abdominal pain	3	3	8
Abdominal distension	2	-	6
Flatulence	2	3	6
Vomiting	-	-	3
Loose stools	-	-	3
Abdominal discomfort[2]	< 1	3	3
Dyspepsia	< 1	-	2
Dry mouth	< 1	-	1
Stomach discomfort	< 1	-	1
Nervous system disorders			
Headache	5	3	11
Dizziness	< 1	3	3
General disorders and site administration conditions			
Edema	< 1	-	3
Fatigue	< 1	-	2
Chest discomfort/pain	-	3	2
Respiratory, thoracic, and mediastinal disorders			
Dyspnea	-	3	2

[1]Includes only those events associated with treatment (possibly, probably, or definitely related, as assessed by the investigator).
[2]This term combines "abdominal tenderness," "abdominal rigidity," "gastrointestinal discomfort," and "abdominal discomfort."

FULL PRESCRIBING INFORMATION

1 INDICATIONS AND USAGE
1.1 Chronic Idiopathic Constipation
Amitiza® is indicated for the treatment of chronic idiopathic constipation in adults.
1.2 Irritable Bowel Syndrome with Constipation
Amitiza is indicated for the treatment of irritable bowel syndrome with constipation (IBS-C) in women ≥ 18 years old.

2 DOSAGE AND ADMINISTRATION
Amitiza should be taken twice daily orally with food and water. Physicians and patients should periodically assess the need for continued therapy.
2.1 Chronic Idiopathic Constipation
24 mcg twice daily orally with food and water.
2.2 Irritable Bowel Syndrome with Constipation
8 mcg twice daily orally with food and water.

3 DOSAGE FORMS AND STRENGTHS
Amitiza is available as an oval, gelatin capsule containing 8 mcg or 24 mcg of lubiprostone.
• 8-mcg capsules are pink and are printed with "SPI" on one side
• 24-mcg capsules are orange and are printed with "SPI" on one side

4 CONTRAINDICATIONS
Amitiza is contraindicated in patients with known or suspected mechanical gastrointestinal obstruction.

5 WARNINGS AND PRECAUTIONS
5.1 Pregnancy
The safety of Amitiza in pregnancy has not been evaluated in humans. In guinea pigs, lubiprostone has been shown to have the potential to cause fetal loss. Amitiza should be used during pregnancy only if the potential benefit justifies the potential risk to the fetus. Women who could become pregnant should have a negative pregnancy test prior to beginning therapy with Amitiza and should be capable of complying with effective contraceptive measures. See *Use in Specific Populations* (8.1).
5.2 Nausea
Patients taking Amitiza may experience nausea. If this occurs, concomitant administration of food with Amitiza may reduce symptoms of nausea. See *Adverse Reactions* (6.1).
5.3 Diarrhea
Amitiza should not be prescribed to patients that have severe diarrhea. Patients should be aware of the possible occurrence of diarrhea during treatment. Patients should be instructed to inform their physician if severe diarrhea occurs. See *Adverse Reactions* (6.1).

5.4 Dyspnea
In clinical trials conducted to study Amitiza in treatment of chronic idiopathic constipation and IBS-C there were reports of dyspnea. This was reported at 2.5% of the treated chronic idiopathic constipation population and at 0.4% in the treated IBS-C population. Although not classified as serious adverse events, some patients discontinued treatment on study because of this event. There have been postmarketing reports of dyspnea when using Amitiza 24 mcg. Most have not been characterized as serious adverse events, but some patients have discontinued therapy because of dyspnea. These events have usually been described as a sensation of chest tightness and difficulty taking in a breath, and generally have an acute onset within 30–60 minutes after taking the first dose. They generally resolve within a few hours after taking the dose, but recurrence has been frequently reported with subsequent doses.
5.5 Bowel Obstruction
In patients with symptoms suggestive of mechanical gastrointestinal obstruction, the treating physician should perform a thorough evaluation to confirm the absence of such an obstruction prior to initiating therapy with Amitiza.

6 ADVERSE REACTIONS
6.1 Clinical Studies Experience
Because clinical studies are conducted under widely varying conditions, adverse reaction rates observed in the clinical studies of a drug cannot be directly compared to rates in the clinical studies of another drug and may not reflect the rates observed in practice.
Chronic Idiopathic Constipation
Adverse reactions in dose-finding, efficacy, and long-term clinical studies: The data described below reflect exposure to Amitiza in 1175 patients with chronic idiopathic constipation (29 at 24 mcg once daily, 1113 at 24 mcg twice daily, and 33 at 24 mcg three times daily) over 3- or 4-week, 6-month, and 12-month treatment periods; and from 316 patients receiving placebo over short-term exposure (≤ 4 weeks). The total population (N = 1491) had a mean age of 49.7 (range 19–86) years; was 87.1% female; 84.8% Caucasian, 8.5% African American, 5.0% Hispanic, 0.9% Asian; and 15.5% elderly (≥ 65 years of age). Table 1 presents data for the adverse reactions that occurred in at least 1% of patients who received Amitiza 24 mcg twice daily and that occurred more frequently with study drug than placebo. In addition, corresponding adverse reaction incidences in patients receiving Amitiza 24 mcg once daily is shown.
[See table 1 above]
Nausea: Approximately 29% of patients who received Amitiza 24 mcg twice daily experienced an adverse reaction of nausea; 4% of patients had severe nausea while 9% of patients discontinued treatment due to nausea. The rate of nausea associated with Amitiza (any dosage) was substantially lower among male (7%) and elderly patients (18%). Further analysis of the safety data revealed that long-term exposure to Amitiza does not appear to place patients at an elevated risk for experiencing nausea. The incidence of

nausea increased in a dose-dependent manner with the lowest overall incidence for nausea reported at the 24 mcg once daily dosage (17%). In open-labeled, long-term studies, patients were allowed to adjust the dosage of Amitiza down to 24 mcg once daily from 24 mcg twice daily if experiencing nausea. Nausea decreased when Amitiza was administered with food. No patients in the clinical studies were hospitalized due to nausea.

Diarrhea: Approximately 12% of patients who received Amitiza 24 mcg twice daily experienced an adverse reaction of diarrhea; 2% of patients had severe diarrhea while 2% of patients discontinued treatment due to diarrhea.

Electrolytes: No serious adverse reactions of electrolyte imbalance were reported in clinical studies, and no clinically significant changes were seen in serum electrolyte levels in patients receiving Amitiza.

Less common adverse reactions: The following adverse reactions (assessed by investigator as probably or definitely related to treatment) occurred in less than 1% of patients receiving Amitiza 24 mcg twice daily in clinical studies, occurred in at least two patients, and occurred more frequently in patients receiving study drug than those receiving placebo: fecal incontinence, muscle cramp, defecation urgency, frequent bowel movements, hyperhidrosis, pharyngolaryngeal pain, intestinal functional disorder, anxiety, cold sweat, constipation, cough, dysgeusia, eructation, influenza, joint swelling, myalgia, pain, syncope, tremor, decreased appetite.

Irritable Bowel Syndrome with Constipation

Adverse reactions in dose-finding, efficacy, and long-term clinical studies: The data described below reflect exposure to Amitiza 8 mcg twice daily in 1011 patients with IBS-C for up to 12 months and from 435 patients receiving placebo twice daily for up to 16 weeks. The total population (N = 1267) had a mean age of 46.5 (range 18–85) years; was 91.6% female; 77.5% Caucasian, 12.9% African American, 8.6% Hispanic, 0.4% Asian; and 8.0% elderly (≥ 65 years of age). Table 2 presents data for the adverse reactions that occurred in at least 1% of patients who received Amitiza 8 mcg twice daily and that occurred more frequently with study drug than placebo.

Table 2: Percent of Patients with Adverse Reactions (IBS-C Studies)

System/Adverse Reaction[1]	Placebo N = 435 %	Amitiza 8 mcg Twice Daily N = 1011 %
Gastrointestinal disorders		
Nausea	4	8
Diarrhea	4	7
Abdominal pain	5	5
Abdominal distension	2	3

[1]Includes only those events associated with treatment (possibly or probably related, as assessed by the investigator).

Less common adverse reactions: The following adverse reactions (assessed by investigator as probably related to treatment) occurred in less than 1% of patients receiving Amitiza 8 mcg twice daily in clinical studies, occurred in at least two patients, and occurred more frequently in patients receiving study drug than those receiving placebo: dyspepsia, loose stools, vomiting, fatigue, dry mouth, edema, increased alanine aminotransferase, increased aspartate aminotransferase, constipation, eructation, gastroesophageal reflux disease, dyspnea, erythema, gastritis, increased weight, palpitations, urinary tract infection, anorexia, anxiety, depression, fecal incontinence, fibromyalgia, hard feces, lethargy, rectal hemorrhage, pollakiuria.

One open-labeled, long-term clinical study was conducted in patients with IBS-C receiving Amitiza 8 mcg twice daily. This study comprised 476 intent-to-treat patients (mean age 47.5 [range 21–82] years; 93.5% female; 79.2% Caucasian, 11.6% African American, 8.6% Hispanic, 0.2% Asian; 7.8% ≥ 65 years of age) who were treated for an additional 36 weeks following an initial 12–16-week, double-blinded treatment period. The adverse reactions that were reported during this study were similar to those observed in the two double-blinded, controlled studies.

6.2 Postmarketing Experience

The following adverse reactions have been identified during post-approval use of Amitiza 24 mcg for the treatment of chronic idiopathic constipation. Because these reactions are reported voluntarily from a population of uncertain size, it is not always possible to reliably estimate their frequency or establish a causal relationship to drug exposure.

Voluntary reports of adverse reactions occurring with the use of Amitiza include the following: syncope, allergic-type reactions (including rash, swelling, and throat tightness), malaise, increased heart rate, muscle cramps or muscle spasms, rash, and asthenia.

7 DRUG INTERACTIONS

Based upon the results of *in vitro* human microsome studies, there is low likelihood of drug–drug interactions. *In vitro* studies using human liver microsomes indicate that cytochrome P450 isoenzymes are not involved in the metabolism of lubiprostone. Further *in vitro* studies indicate microsomal carbonyl reductase may be involved in the extensive biotransformation of lubiprostone to the metabolite M3 (See *Pharmacokinetics* [12.3].). Additionally, *in vitro* studies in human liver microsomes demonstrate that lubiprostone does not inhibit cytochrome P450 isoforms 3A4, 2D6, 1A2, 2A6, 2B6, 2C9, 2C19, or 2E1, and *in vitro* studies of primary cultures of human hepatocytes show no induction of cytochrome P450 isoforms 1A2, 2B6, 2C9, and 3A4 by lubiprostone. No drug–drug interaction studies have been performed. Based on the available information, no protein binding–mediated drug interactions of clinical significance are anticipated.

8 USE IN SPECIFIC POPULATIONS

8.1 Pregnancy

Teratogenic effects: Pregnancy Category C. [See *Warnings and Precautions* (5.1).]

Teratology studies with lubiprostone have been conducted in rats at oral doses up to 2000 mcg/kg/day (approximately 332 times the recommended human dose, based on body surface area), and in rabbits at oral doses of up to 100 mcg/kg/day (approximately 33 times the recommended human dose, based on body surface area). Lubiprostone was not teratogenic in rats or rabbits. In guinea pigs, lubiprostone caused fetal loss at repeated doses of 10 and 25 mcg/kg/day (approximately 2 and 6 times the highest recommended human dose, respectively, based on body surface area) administered on days 40 to 53 of gestation.

There are no adequate and well-controlled studies in pregnant women. However, during clinical testing of Amitiza, six women became pregnant. Per protocol, Amitiza was discontinued upon pregnancy detection. Four of the six women delivered healthy babies. The fifth woman was monitored for 1 month following discontinuation of study drug, at which time the pregnancy was progressing as expected; the patient was subsequently lost to follow-up. The sixth pregnancy was electively terminated.

Amitiza should be used during pregnancy only if the potential benefit justifies the potential risk to the fetus. If a woman is or becomes pregnant while taking the drug, the patient should be apprised of the potential hazard to the fetus.

8.3 Nursing Mothers

It is not known whether lubiprostone is excreted in human milk. Because many drugs are excreted in human milk and because of the potential for serious adverse reactions in nursing infants from lubiprostone, a decision should be made whether to discontinue nursing or to discontinue the drug, taking into account the importance of the drug to the mother.

8.4 Pediatric Use

Safety and effectiveness in pediatric patients have not been studied.

8.5 Geriatric Use

Chronic Idiopathic Constipation

The efficacy of Amitiza in the elderly (≥ 65 years of age) subpopulation was consistent with the efficacy in the overall study population. Of the total number of constipated patients treated in the dose-finding, efficacy, and long-term studies of Amitiza, 15.5% were ≥ 65 years of age, and 4.2% were ≥ 75 years of age. Elderly patients taking Amitiza (any dosage) experienced a lower incidence rate of associated nausea compared to the overall study population taking Amitiza (18% vs. 29%, respectively).

Irritable Bowel Syndrome with Constipation

The safety profile of Amitiza in the elderly (≥ 65 years of age) subpopulation (8.0% were ≥ 65 years of age and 1.8% were ≥ 75 years of age) was consistent with the safety profile in the overall study population. Clinical studies of Amitiza did not include sufficient numbers of patients aged 65 years and over to determine whether they respond differently from younger patients.

8.6 Renal Impairment

Amitiza has not been studied in patients who have renal impairment.

8.7 Hepatic Impairment

Amitiza has not been studied in patients who have hepatic impairment.

10 OVERDOSAGE

There have been two confirmed reports of overdosage with Amitiza. The first report involved a 3-year-old child who accidentally ingested 7 or 8 capsules of 24 mcg of Amitiza and fully recovered. The second report was a study patient who self-administered a total of 96 mcg of Amitiza per day for 8 days. The patient experienced no adverse reactions during this time. Additionally, in a Phase 1 cardiac repolarization study, 38 of 51 patients given a single oral dose of 144 mcg of Amitiza (6 times the highest recommended dose) experienced an adverse event that was at least possibly related to the study drug. Adverse reactions that occurred in at least 1% of these patients included the following: nausea (45%), diarrhea (35%), vomiting (27%), dizziness (14%), headache (12%), abdominal pain (8%), flushing/hot flash (8%), retching (8%), dyspnea (4%), pallor (4%), stomach discomfort (4%), anorexia (2%), asthenia (2%), chest discomfort (2%), dry mouth (2%), hyperhidrosis (2%), and syncope (2%).

11 DESCRIPTION

Amitiza (lubiprostone) is chemically designated as (–)-7-[(2*R*,4a*R*,5*R*,7a*R*)-2-(1,1-difluoropentyl)-2-hydroxy-6-oxooctahydrocyclopenta[*b*]pyran-5-yl]heptanoic acid. The molecular formula of lubiprostone is $C_{20}H_{32}F_2O_5$ with a molecular weight of 390.46 and a chemical structure as follows:

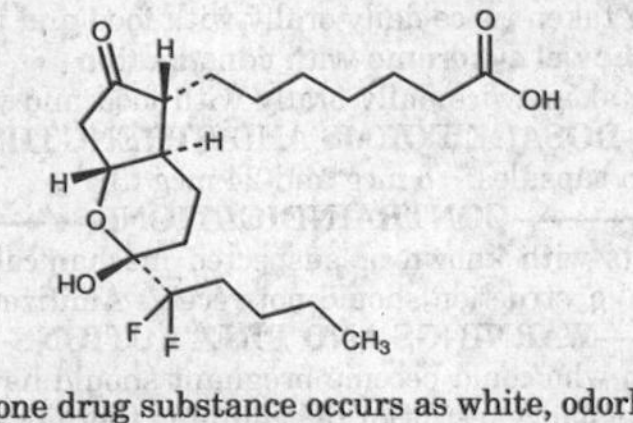

Lubiprostone drug substance occurs as white, odorless crystals or crystalline powder, is very soluble in ether and ethanol, and is practically insoluble in hexane and water. Amitiza is available as an imprinted, oval, soft gelatin capsule in two strengths. Pink capsules contain 8 mcg of lubiprostone and the following inactive ingredients: medium-chain triglycerides, gelatin, sorbitol, ferric oxide, titanium dioxide, and purified water. Orange capsules contain 24 mcg of lubiprostone and the following inactive ingredients: medium-chain triglycerides, gelatin, sorbitol, FD&C Red #40, D&C Yellow #10, and purified water.

12 CLINICAL PHARMACOLOGY

12.1 Mechanism of Action

Lubiprostone is a locally acting chloride channel activator that enhances a chloride-rich intestinal fluid secretion without altering sodium and potassium concentrations in the serum. Lubiprostone acts by specifically activating ClC-2, which is a normal constituent of the apical membrane of the human intestine, in a protein kinase A–independent fashion. By increasing intestinal fluid secretion, lubiprostone increases motility in the intestine, thereby facilitating the passage of stool and alleviating symptoms associated with chronic idiopathic constipation. Patch clamp cell studies in human cell lines have indicated that the majority of the beneficial biological activity of lubiprostone and its metabolites is observed only on the apical (luminal) portion of the gastrointestinal epithelium. Additionally, activation of ClC-2 by lubiprostone has been shown to stimulate recovery of mucosal barrier function via the restoration of tight junction protein complexes in *ex vivo* studies of ischemic porcine intestine.

12.2 Pharmacodynamics

Although the pharmacologic effects of lubiprostone in humans have not been fully evaluated, animal studies have shown that oral administration of lubiprostone increases chloride ion transport into the intestinal lumen, enhances fluid secretion into the bowels, and improves fecal transit.

12.3 Pharmacokinetics

Lubiprostone has low systemic availability following oral administration and concentrations of lubiprostone in plasma are below the level of quantitation (10 pg/mL). Therefore, standard pharmacokinetic parameters such as area under the curve (AUC), maximum concentration (C_{max}), and half-life ($t_{1/2}$) cannot be reliably calculated. However, the pharmacokinetic parameters of M3 (only measurable active metabolite of lubiprostone) have been characterized. Gender has no effect on the pharmacokinetics of M3 following the oral administration of lubiprostone.

Absorption

Concentrations of lubiprostone in plasma are below the level of quantitation (10 pg/mL) because lubiprostone has a low systemic availability following oral administration. Peak plasma levels of M3, after a single oral dose with 24 mcg of lubiprostone, occurred at approximately 1.10 hours. The C_{max} was 41.5 pg/mL and the mean $AUC_{0\text{-}t}$ was 57.1 pg•hr/mL. The $AUC_{0\text{-}t}$ of M3 increases dose proportionally after single 24-mcg and 144-mcg doses of lubiprostone.

Distribution

In vitro protein binding studies indicate lubiprostone is approximately 94% bound to human plasma proteins. Studies in rats given radiolabeled lubiprostone indicate minimal distribution beyond the gastrointestinal tissues. Concentrations of radiolabeled lubiprostone at 48 hours post-administration were minimal in all tissues of the rats.

Metabolism

The results of both human and animal studies indicate that lubiprostone is rapidly and extensively metabolized by 15-position reduction, α-chain β-oxidation, and ω-chain ω-oxidation. These biotransformations are not mediated by the hepatic cytochrome P450 system but rather appear to be mediated by the ubiquitously expressed carbonyl reductase. M3, a metabolite of lubiprostone found in both humans and animals, is formed by the reduction of the carbonyl group at the 15-hydroxy moiety that consists of both α-hydroxy and β-hydroxy epimers. M3 makes up less than 10% of the dose of radiolabeled lubiprostone. Animal studies have shown that metabolism of lubiprostone rapidly occurs within the stomach and jejunum, most likely in the absence of any systemic absorption. This is presumed to be the case in humans as well.

Elimination

Lubiprostone could not be detected in plasma; however, M3 has a $t_{1/2}$ ranging from 0.9 to 1.4 hours. After a single oral dose of 72 mcg of ^{3}H-labeled lubiprostone, 60% of total administered radioactivity was recovered in the urine within 24 hours and 30% of total administered radioactivity was recovered in the feces by 168 hours. Lubiprostone and M3 are only detected in trace amounts in human feces.

Food Effect

A study was conducted with a single 72-mcg dose of ^{3}H-labeled lubiprostone to evaluate the potential of a food effect on lubiprostone absorption, metabolism, and excretion. Pharmacokinetic parameters of total radioactivity demonstrated that C_{max} decreased by 55% while $AUC_{0-\infty}$ was unchanged when lubiprostone was administered with a high-fat meal. The clinical relevance of the effect of food on the pharmacokinetics of lubiprostone is not clear. However, lubiprostone was administered with food and water in a majority of clinical trials.

13 NONCLINICAL TOXICOLOGY

13.1 Carcinogenesis, Mutagenesis, Impairment of Fertility

Carcinogenesis

Two 2-year oral (gavage) carcinogenicity studies (one in Crl:B6C3F1 mice and one in Sprague-Dawley rats) were conducted with lubiprostone. In the 2-year carcinogenicity study in mice, lubiprostone doses of 25, 75, 200, and 500 mcg/kg/day (approximately 2, 6, 17, and 42 times the highest recommended human dose, respectively, based on body surface area) were used. In the 2-year rat carcinogenicity study, lubiprostone doses of 20, 100, and 400 mcg/kg/day (approximately 3, 17, and 68 times the highest recommended human dose, respectively, based on body surface area) were used. In the mouse carcinogenicity study, there was no significant increase in any tumor incidences. There was a significant increase in the incidence of interstitial cell adenoma of the testes in male rats at the 400 mcg/kg/day dose. In female rats, treatment with lubiprostone produced hepatocellular adenoma at the 400 mcg/kg/day dose.

Mutagenesis

Lubiprostone was not genotoxic in the in vitro Ames reverse mutation assay, the in vitro mouse lymphoma (L5178Y TK$^{+/-}$) forward mutation assay, the in vitro Chinese hamster lung (CHL/IU) chromosomal aberration assay, and the in vivo mouse bone marrow micronucleus assay.

Impairment of Fertility

Lubiprostone, at oral doses of up to 1000 mcg/kg/day, had no effect on the fertility and reproductive function of male and female rats. However, the number of implantation sites and live embryos were significantly reduced in rats at the 1000 mcg/kg/day dose as compared to control. The number of dead or resorbed embryos in the 1000 mcg/kg/day group was higher compared to the control group, but was not statistically significant. The 1000 mcg/kg/day dose in rats is approximately 166 times the highest recommended human dose of 48 mcg/day, based on body surface area.

14 CLINICAL STUDIES

14.1 Chronic Idiopathic Constipation

Dose-finding Study

A dose-finding, double-blinded, parallel-group, placebo-controlled, Phase 2 study was conducted in patients with chronic idiopathic constipation. Following a 2-week baseline/washout period, patients (N = 127) were randomized to receive placebo (n = 33), Amitiza 24 mcg/day (24 mcg once daily; n = 29), Amitiza 48 mcg/day (24 mcg twice daily; n = 32), or Amitiza 72 mcg/day (24 mcg three times daily; n = 33) for 3 weeks. Patients were chosen for participation based on their need for relief of constipation, which was defined as less than 3 spontaneous bowel movements (SBMs) per week. The primary efficacy variable was the daily average number of SBMs.

The study demonstrated that all patients who took Amitiza experienced a noticeable improvement in clinical response. Based on the efficacy analysis, there was no statistically significant improvement in the clinical response beyond a total

daily dose of 24 mcg during treatment weeks 2 and 3 (Figure 1).

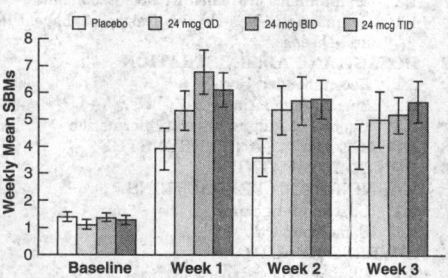

Figure 1: Weekly Mean (± Standard Error) Spontaneous Bowel Movements (Dose-finding Study)

Efficacy Studies

Two double-blinded, placebo-controlled studies of identical design were conducted in patients with chronic idiopathic constipation. Chronic idiopathic constipation was defined as, on average, less than 3 SBMs per week along with one or more of the following symptoms of constipation for at least 6 months prior to randomization: 1) very hard stools for at least a quarter of all bowel movements; 2) sensation of incomplete evacuation following at least a quarter of all bowel movements; and 3) straining with defecation at least a quarter of the time.

Following a 2-week baseline/washout period, a total of 479 patients (mean age 47.2 [range 20–81] years; 88.9% female; 80.8% Caucasian, 9.6% African American, 7.3% Hispanic, 1.5% Asian; 10.9% ≥ 65 years of age) were randomized and received Amitiza 24 mcg twice daily (48 mcg/day) or placebo twice daily for 4 weeks. The primary endpoint of the studies was SBM frequency. The studies demonstrated that patients treated with Amitiza had a higher frequency of SBMs during Week 1 than the placebo patients. In both studies, results similar to those in Week 1 were also observed in Weeks 2, 3, and 4 of therapy (Table 3).

[See table 3 above]

In both studies, Amitiza demonstrated increases in the percentage of patients who experienced SBMs within the first 24 hours after administration when compared to placebo (56.7% vs. 36.9% in Study 1 and 62.9% vs. 31.9% in Study 2, respectively). Similarly, the time to first SBM was shorter for patients receiving Amitiza than for those receiving placebo.

Signs and symptoms related to constipation, including abdominal bloating, abdominal discomfort, stool consistency, and straining, as well as constipation severity ratings, were also improved with Amitiza versus placebo. The results were consistent in subpopulation analyses for gender, race, and elderly patients (≥ 65 years of age).

Following 4 weeks of treatment with Amitiza 24 mcg twice daily, withdrawal of Amitiza did not result in a rebound effect.

Long-term Studies

Three open-labeled, long-term clinical safety and efficacy studies were conducted in patients with chronic idiopathic constipation receiving Amitiza 24 mcg twice daily. These

studies comprised 871 patients (mean age 51.0 [range 19–86] years; 86.1% female; 86.9% Caucasian, 7.3% African American, 4.5% Hispanic, 0.7% Asian; 18.4% ≥ 65 years of age) who were treated for 6–12 months (24–48 weeks). Patients provided regular assessments of abdominal bloating, abdominal discomfort, and constipation severity. These studies demonstrated that Amitiza decreased abdominal bloating, abdominal discomfort, and constipation severity over the 6–12-month treatment periods.

14.2 Irritable Bowel Syndrome with Constipation

Efficacy Studies

Two double-blinded, placebo-controlled studies of similar design were conducted in patients with IBS-C. IBS was defined as abdominal pain or discomfort occurring over at least 6 months with two or more of the following: 1) relieved with defecation; 2) onset associated with a change in stool frequency; and 3) onset associated with a change in stool form. Patients were sub-typed as having IBS-C if they also experienced two of three of the following: 1) < 3 spontaneous bowel movements per week, 2) > 25% hard stools, and 3) > 25% spontaneous bowel movements associated with straining.

Following a 4-week baseline/washout period, a total of 1154 patients (mean age 46.6 [range 18–85] years; 91.6% female; 77.4% Caucasian, 13.2% African American, 8.5% Hispanic, 0.4% Asian; 8.3% ≥ 65 years of age) were randomized and received Amitiza 8 mcg twice daily (16 mcg/day) or placebo twice daily for 12 weeks. The primary efficacy endpoint was assessed weekly utilizing the patient's response to a global symptom relief question based on a 7-point, balanced scale ("significantly worse" to "significantly relieved"): "How would you rate your relief of IBS symptoms (abdominal discomfort/pain, bowel habits, and other IBS symptoms) over the past week compared to how you felt before you entered the study?"

The primary efficacy analysis was a comparison of the proportion of "overall responders" in each arm. A patient was considered an "overall responder" if the criteria for being designated a "monthly responder" were met in at least 2 of the 3 months on study. A "monthly responder" was defined as a patient who had reported "significantly relieved" for at least 2 weeks of the month or at least "moderately relieved" in all 4 weeks of that month. During each monthly evaluation period, patients reporting "moderately worse" or "significantly worse" relief, an increase in rescue medication use, or those who discontinued due to lack of efficacy, were deemed non-responders.

The percentage of patients in Study 1 qualifying as an "overall responder" was 13.8% in the group receiving Amitiza 8 mcg twice daily compared to 7.8% of patients receiving placebo twice daily. In Study 2, 12.1% of patients in the Amitiza 8 mcg group were "overall responders" versus 5.7% of patients in the placebo group. In both studies, the treatment differences between the placebo and Amitiza groups were statistically significant.

Results in men: The two randomized, placebo-controlled, double-blinded studies comprised 97 (8.4%) male patients, which is insufficient to determine whether men with IBS-C respond differently to Amitiza from women.

Study 1 also assessed the rebound effect from the withdrawal of Amitiza. Following 12 weeks of treatment with Amitiza 8 mcg twice daily, withdrawal of Amitiza did not result in a rebound effect.

Table 3: Spontaneous Bowel Movement Frequency Rates[1] (Efficacy Studies)

Trial	Study Arm	Baseline Mean ± SD Median	Week 1 Mean ± SD Median	Week 2 Mean ± SD Median	Week 3 Mean ± SD Median	Week 4 Mean ± SD Median	Week 1 Change from Baseline Mean ± SD Median	Week 4 Change from Baseline Mean ± SD Median
Study 1	Placebo	1.6 ± 1.3 1.5	3.5 ± 2.3 3.0	3.2 ± 2.5 3.0	2.8 ± 2.2 2.0	2.9 ± 2.4 2.3	1.9 ± 2.2 1.5	1.3 ± 2.5 1.0
	Amitiza 24 mcg Twice Daily	1.4 ± 0.8 1.5	5.7 ± 4.4 5.0	5.1 ± 4.1 4.0	5.3 ± 4.9 5.0	5.3 ± 4.7 4.0	4.3 ± 4.3 3.5	3.9 ± 4.6 3.0
Study 2	Placebo	1.5 ± 0.8 1.5	4.0 ± 2.7 3.5	3.6 ± 2.7 3.0	3.4 ± 2.8 3.0	3.5 ± 2.9 3.0	2.5 ± 2.6 1.5	1.9 ± 2.7 1.5
	Amitiza 24 mcg Twice Daily	1.3 ± 0.9 1.5	5.9 ± 4.0 5.0	5.0 ± 4.2 4.0	5.6 ± 4.6 5.0	5.4 ± 4.8 4.3	4.6 ± 4.1 3.8	4.1 ± 4.8 3.0

[1] Frequency rates are calculated as 7 times (number of SBMs) / (number of days observed for that week).

16 HOW SUPPLIED/STORAGE AND HANDLING

Amitiza is available as an oval, soft gelatin capsule containing 8 mcg or 24 mcg of lubiprostone with "SPI" printed on one side. Amitiza is available as follows:

8-mcg pink capsule
• Bottles of 60 (NDC 64764-080-60)
24-mcg orange capsule
• Bottles of 60 (NDC 64764-240-60)
• Bottles of 100 (NDC 64764-240-10)
Store at 25°C (77°F); excursions permitted to 15°–30°C (59°–86°F).
PROTECT FROM EXTREME TEMPERATURES.

17 PATIENT COUNSELING INFORMATION
17.1 Dosing Instructions
Amitiza should be taken twice daily with food and water to reduce potential symptoms of nausea. The capsule should be taken once in the morning and once in the evening daily as prescribed. The capsule should be swallowed whole and should not be broken apart or chewed. Physicians and patients should periodically assess the need for continued therapy.
Patients on treatment who experience severe nausea, diarrhea, or dyspnea should inform their physician. Patients taking Amitiza may experience dyspnea within an hour of the first dose. This symptom generally resolves within 3 hours, but may recur with repeat dosing.
Chronic Idiopathic Constipation
Patients should take a single 24 mcg capsule of Amitiza twice daily with food and water.
Irritable Bowel Syndrome with Constipation
Patients should take a single 8 mcg capsule of Amitiza twice daily with food and water.
Marketed by:
Sucampo Pharma Americas, Inc.
Bethesda, MD 20814
and
Takeda Pharmaceuticals America, Inc.
Deerfield, IL 60015
Amitiza® is a registered trademark of Sucampo Pharmaceuticals, Inc.
©2009 Sucampo Pharma Americas, Inc.
750-04412-1 05/09
Shown in Product Identification Guide, page 320

DEXILANT ℞
[*decks-ĭ-launt*]
(dexlansoprazole)
delayed release capsules

HIGHLIGHTS OF PRESCRIBING INFORMATION
These highlights do not include all the information needed to use DEXILANT safely and effectively. See full prescribing information for DEXILANT.
DEXILANT (dexlansoprazole) delayed release capsules
Initial U.S. Approval: 1995 (lansoprazole)

——RECENT MAJOR CHANGES——
Dosage and Administration
• Important Administration Information (2.3) 06/2010
  Warnings and Precautions
• Bone Fracture (5.2) 08/2010

——INDICATIONS AND USAGE——
DEXILANT is a proton pump inhibitor (PPI) indicated for:
• Healing of all grades of erosive esophagitis (EE). (1.1)
• Maintaining healing of EE. (1.2)
• Treating heartburn associated with symptomatic non-erosive gastroesophageal reflux disease (GERD). (1.3)

——DOSAGE AND ADMINISTRATION——
• Healing of EE: 60 mg once daily for up to 8 weeks. (2.1)
• Maintenance of healed EE: 30 mg once daily for up to 6 months. (2.1)
• Symptomatic non-erosive GERD: 30 mg once daily for 4 weeks. (2.1)
• Hepatic impairment: Consider 30 mg maximum daily dose for patients with moderate hepatic impairment (Child-Pugh Class B). No studies were conducted in patients with severe hepatic impairment (Child-Pugh Class C). (2.2, 8.7)
• DEXILANT can be taken without regard to food. (2.3)
• DEXILANT should be swallowed whole. Alternatively, capsules can be opened, sprinkled on one tablespoon of applesauce, and swallowed immediately. (2.3)

——DOSAGE FORMS AND STRENGTHS——
Capsules: 30 mg and 60 mg. (3)

——CONTRAINDICATIONS——
Patients with known hypersensitivity to any component of the formulation. (4)

——WARNINGS AND PRECAUTIONS——
Gastric malignancy: Symptomatic response with DEXILANT does not preclude the presence of gastric malignancy. (5.1)
Bone Fracture: Long-term and multiple daily dose PPI therapy may be associated with an increased risk for osteoporosis-related fractures of the hip, wrist or spine. (5.2)

——ADVERSE REACTIONS——
Most commonly reported adverse reactions (≥2%): diarrhea, abdominal pain, nausea, upper respiratory tract infection, vomiting, and flatulence. (6.1)
To report SUSPECTED ADVERSE REACTIONS, contact Takeda Pharmaceuticals America, Inc. at 1-877-TAKEDA-7 (1-877-825-3327) or FDA at 1-800-FDA-1088 or www.fda.gov/medwatch.

——DRUG INTERACTIONS——
• Atazanavir: Do not co-administer with DEXILANT because atazanavir systemic concentrations may be substantially decreased. (7.1)
• Drugs with pH-dependent absorption (e.g., ampicillin esters, digoxin, iron salts, ketoconazole): DEXILANT may interfere with absorption of drugs for which gastric pH is important for bioavailability. (7.1)
• Warfarin: Patients taking concomitant warfarin may require monitoring for increases in international normalized ratio (INR) and prothrombin time. (7.2)
• Tacrolimus: Concomitant tacrolimus use may increase tacrolimus whole blood concentrations. (7.3)

——USE IN SPECIFIC POPULATIONS——
• Nursing mothers: Discontinue drug or nursing, taking into consideration importance of drug to mother. (8.3)
See 17 for PATIENT COUNSELING INFORMATION and FDA-approved patient labeling.

Revised: 08/2010

FULL PRESCRIBING INFORMATION: CONTENTS*
1 INDICATIONS AND USAGE
  1.1 Healing of Erosive Esophagitis
  1.2 Maintenance of Healed Erosive Esophagitis
  1.3 Symptomatic Non-Erosive Gastroesophageal Reflux Disease
2 DOSAGE AND ADMINISTRATION
  2.1 Recommended Dose
  2.2 Special Populations
  2.3 Important Administration Information
3 DOSAGE FORMS AND STRENGTHS
4 CONTRAINDICATIONS
5 WARNINGS AND PRECAUTIONS
  5.1 Gastric Malignancy
  5.2 Bone Fracture
6 ADVERSE REACTIONS
  6.1 Clinical Trials Experience
  6.2 Postmarketing Experience
7 DRUG INTERACTIONS
  7.1 Drugs with pH-Dependent Absorption Pharmacokinetics
  7.2 Warfarin
  7.3 Tacrolimus
8 USE IN SPECIFIC POPULATIONS
  8.1 Pregnancy
  8.3 Nursing Mothers
  8.4 Pediatric Use
  8.5 Geriatric Use
  8.6 Renal Impairment
  8.7 Hepatic Impairment
10 OVERDOSAGE
11 DESCRIPTION
12 CLINICAL PHARMACOLOGY
  12.1 Mechanism of Action
  12.2 Pharmacodynamics
  12.3 Pharmacokinetics
  12.4 Effect of Food on Pharmacokinetics and Pharmacodynamics
  12.5 Special Populations
  12.6 Drug-Drug Interactions
13 NONCLINICAL TOXICOLOGY
  13.1 Carcinogenesis, Mutagenesis, Impairment of Fertility
  13.2 Animal Toxicology and/or Pharmacology
14 CLINICAL STUDIES
  14.1 Healing of Erosive Esophagitis
  14.2 Maintenance of Healed Erosive Esophagitis
  14.3 Symptomatic Non-Erosive GERD
16 HOW SUPPLIED/STORAGE AND HANDLING
17 PATIENT COUNSELING INFORMATION
* Sections or subsections omitted from the full prescribing information are not listed.

FULL PRESCRIBING INFORMATION

1 INDICATIONS AND USAGE
1.1 Healing of Erosive Esophagitis
DEXILANT is indicated for healing of all grades of erosive esophagitis (EE) for up to 8 weeks.
1.2 Maintenance of Healed Erosive Esophagitis
DEXILANT is indicated to maintain healing of EE for up to 6 months.

1.3 Symptomatic Non-Erosive Gastroesophageal Reflux Disease
DEXILANT is indicated for the treatment of heartburn associated with symptomatic non-erosive gastroesophageal reflux disease (GERD) for 4 weeks.

2 DOSAGE AND ADMINISTRATION
2.1 Recommended Dose
DEXILANT is available as capsules in 30 mg and 60 mg strengths for adult use. Directions for use in each indication are summarized in Table 1.

Table 1: DEXILANT Dosing Recommendations

Indication	Recommended Dose	Frequency
Healing of EE	60 mg	Once daily for up to 8 weeks
Maintenance of Healed EE	30 mg	Once daily*
Symptomatic Non-Erosive GERD	30 mg	Once daily for 4 weeks

* Controlled studies did not extend beyond 6 months.

2.2 Special Populations
No adjustment for DEXILANT is necessary for patients with mild hepatic impairment (Child-Pugh Class A). Consider a maximum daily dose of 30 mg for patients with moderate hepatic impairment (Child-Pugh Class B). No studies have been conducted in patients with severe hepatic impairment (Child-Pugh Class C) [see Use in Specific Populations (8.7) and Clinical Pharmacology (12.5)].
No dosage adjustment is necessary for elderly patients or for patients with renal impairment [see Clinical Pharmacology (12.5)].
2.3 Important Administration Information
DEXILANT can be taken without regard to food.
DEXILANT should be swallowed whole.
• Alternatively, DEXILANT capsules can be opened and administered as follows
  –Open capsule;
  –Sprinkle intact granules on one tablespoon of applesauce;
  –Swallow immediately. Granules should not be chewed.

3 DOSAGE FORMS AND STRENGTHS
• 30 mg capsules are opaque, blue and gray with TAP and "30" imprinted on the capsule.
• 60 mg capsules are opaque, blue with TAP and "60" imprinted on the capsule.

4 CONTRAINDICATIONS
DEXILANT is contraindicated in patients with known hypersensitivity to any component of the formulation [see Description (11)]. Hypersensitivity and anaphylaxis have been reported with DEXILANT use [see Adverse Reactions (6.1)].

5 WARNINGS AND PRECAUTIONS
5.1 Gastric Malignancy
Symptomatic response with DEXILANT does not preclude the presence of gastric malignancy.
5.2 Bone Fracture
Several published observational studies suggest that proton pump inhibitor (PPI) therapy may be associated with an increased risk for osteoporosis-related fractures of the hip, wrist or spine. The risk of fracture was increased in patients who received high-dose, defined as multiple daily doses, and long-term PPI therapy (a year or longer). Patients should use the lowest dose and shortest duration of PPI therapy appropriate to the condition being treated. Patients at risk for osteoporosis-related fractures should be managed according to established treatment guidelines [see Dosage and Administration (2) and Adverse Reactions (6)].

6 ADVERSE REACTIONS
6.1 Clinical Trials Experience
The safety of DEXILANT was evaluated in 4548 patients in controlled and uncontrolled clinical studies, including 863 patients treated for at least 6 months and 203 patients treated for one year. Patients ranged in age from 18 to 90 years (median age 48 years), with 54% female, 85% Caucasian, 8% Black, 4% Asian, and 3% other races. Six randomized controlled clinical trials were conducted for the treatment of EE, maintenance of healed EE, and symptomatic GERD, which included 896 patients on placebo, 455 patients on DEXILANT 30 mg, 2218 patients on DEXILANT 60 mg, and 1363 patients on lansoprazole 30 mg once daily. As clinical trials are conducted under widely varying conditions, adverse reaction rates observed in the clinical trials of a drug cannot be directly compared to rates in the clinical trials of another drug and may not reflect the rates observed in practice.
Most Commonly Reported Adverse Reactions
The most common adverse reactions (≥2%) that occurred at a higher incidence for DEXILANT than placebo in the controlled studies are presented in Table 2.

[See table below]

Adverse Reactions Resulting in Discontinuation

In controlled clinical studies, the most common adverse reaction leading to discontinuation from DEXILANT therapy was diarrhea (0.7%).

Other Adverse Reactions

Other adverse reactions that were reported in controlled studies at an incidence of less than 2% are listed below by body system:

Blood and Lymphatic System Disorders: anemia, lymphadenopathy

Cardiac Disorders: angina, arrhythmia, bradycardia, chest pain, edema, myocardial infarction, palpitation, tachycardia

Ear and Labyrinth Disorders: ear pain, tinnitus, vertigo

Endocrine Disorders: goiter

Eye Disorders: eye irritation, eye swelling

Gastrointestinal Disorders: abdominal discomfort, abdominal tenderness, abnormal feces, anal discomfort, Barrett's esophagus, bezoar, bowel sounds abnormal, breath odor, colitis microscopic, colonic polyp, constipation, dry mouth, duodenitis, dyspepsia, dysphagia, enteritis, eructation, esophagitis, gastric polyp, gastritis, gastroenteritis, gastrointestinal disorders, gastrointestinal hypermotility disorders, GERD, GI ulcers and perforation, hematemesis, hematochezia, hemorrhoids, impaired gastric emptying, irritable bowel syndrome, mucus stools, nausea and vomiting, oral mucosal blistering, painful defecation, proctitis, paresthesia oral, rectal hemorrhage

General Disorders and Administration Site Conditions: adverse drug reaction, asthenia, chest pain, chills, feeling abnormal, inflammation, mucosal inflammation, nodule, pain, pyrexia

Hepatobiliary Disorders: biliary colic, cholelithiasis, hepatomegaly

Immune System Disorders: hypersensitivity

Infections and Infestations: candida infections, influenza, nasopharyngitis, oral herpes, pharyngitis, sinusitis, viral infection, vulvo-vaginal infection

Injury, Poisoning and Procedural Complications: falls, fractures, joint sprains, overdose, procedural pain, sunburn

Laboratory Investigations: ALP increased, ALT increased, AST increased, bilirubin decreased/increased, blood creatinine increased, blood gastrin increased, blood glucose increased, blood potassium increased, liver function test abnormal, platelet count decreased, total protein increased, weight increase

Metabolism and Nutrition Disorders: appetite changes, hypercalcemia, hypokalemia

Musculoskeletal and Connective Tissue Disorders: arthralgia, arthritis, muscle cramps, musculoskeletal pain, myalgia

Nervous System Disorders: altered taste, convulsion, dizziness, headaches, migraine, memory impairment, paresthesia, psychomotor hyperactivity, tremor, trigeminal neuralgia

Psychiatric Disorders: abnormal dreams, anxiety, depression, insomnia, libido changes

Renal and Urinary Disorders: dysuria, micturition urgency

Reproductive System and Breast Disorders: dysmenorrhea, dyspareunia, menorrhagia, menstrual disorder

Respiratory, Thoracic and Mediastinal Disorders: aspiration, asthma, bronchitis, cough, dyspnoea, hiccups, hyperventilation, respiratory tract congestion, sore throat

Skin and Subcutaneous Tissue Disorders: acne, dermatitis, erythema, pruritis, rash, skin lesion, urticaria

Vascular Disorders: deep vein thrombosis, hot flush, hypertension

Additional adverse reactions that were reported in a long-term uncontrolled study and were considered related to DEXILANT by the treating physician included: anaphylaxis, auditory hallucination, B-cell lymphoma, bursitis, central obesity, cholecystitis acute, decreased hemoglobin, dehydration, diabetes mellitus, dysphonia, epistaxis, folliculitis, gastrointestinal pain, gout, herpes zoster, hyperglycemia, hyperlipidemia, hypothyroidism, increased neutrophils, MCHC decrease, neutropenia, oral soft tissue disorder, rectal tenesmus, restless legs syndrome, somnolence, thrombocythemia, tonsillitis.

Other adverse reactions not observed with DEXILANT, but occurring with the racemate lansoprazole can be found in the lansoprazole package insert, ADVERSE REACTIONS section.

6.2 Postmarketing Experience

Adverse reactions have been identified during post-approval of DEXILANT. As these reactions are reported voluntarily from a population of uncertain size, it is not always possible to reliably estimate their frequency or establish a causal relationship to drug exposure.

Eye Disorders: blurred vision

Gastrointestinal Disorders: oral edema

General Disorders and Administration Site Conditions: facial edema

Immune System Disorders: anaphylactic shock (requiring emergency intervention), Stevens-Johnson syndrome, toxic epidermal necrolysis (some fatal)

Musculoskeletal System Disorders: bone fracture

Respiratory, Thoracic and Mediastinal Disorders: pharyngeal edema, throat tightness

Skin and Subcutaneous Tissue Disorders: generalized rash, leucocytoclastic vasculitis

7 DRUG INTERACTIONS

7.1 Drugs with pH-Dependent Absorption Pharmacokinetics

DEXILANT causes inhibition of gastric acid secretion. DEXILANT is likely to substantially decrease the systemic concentrations of the HIV protease inhibitor atazanavir, which is dependent upon the presence of gastric acid for absorption, and may result in a loss of therapeutic effect of atazanavir and the development of HIV resistance. Therefore, DEXILANT should not be co-administered with atazanavir.

It is theoretically possible that DEXILANT may interfere with the absorption of other drugs where gastric pH is an important determinant of oral bioavailability (e.g., ampicillin esters, digoxin, iron salts, ketoconazole).

7.2 Warfarin

Co-administration of DEXILANT 90 mg and warfarin 25 mg did not affect the pharmacokinetics of warfarin or INR *[see Clinical Pharmacology (12.6)]*. However, there have been reports of increased INR and prothrombin time in patients receiving PPIs and warfarin concomitantly. Increases in INR and prothrombin time may lead to abnormal bleeding and even death. Patients treated with DEXILANT and warfarin concomitantly may need to be monitored for increases in INR and prothrombin time.

7.3 Tacrolimus

Concomitant administration of dexlansoprazole and tacrolimus may increase whole blood levels of tacrolimus, especially in transplant patients who are intermediate or poor metabolizers of CYP2C19.

8 USE IN SPECIFIC POPULATIONS

8.1 Pregnancy

Teratogenic Effects

Pregnancy Category B. There are no adequate and well-controlled studies with dexlansoprazole in pregnant women. There were no adverse fetal effects in animal reproduction studies of dexlansoprazole in rabbits. Because animal reproduction studies are not always predictive of human response, DEXILANT should be used during pregnancy only if clearly needed.

A reproduction study conducted in rabbits at oral dexlansoprazole doses up to approximately 9 times the maximum recommended human dexlansoprazole dose (60 mg per day) revealed no evidence of impaired fertility or harm to the fetus due to dexlansoprazole. In addition, reproduction studies performed in pregnant rats with oral lansoprazole at doses up to 40 times the recommended human lansoprazole dose and in pregnant rabbits at oral lansoprazole doses up to 16 times the recommended human lansoprazole dose revealed no evidence of impaired fertility or harm to the fetus due to lansoprazole *[see Nonclinical Toxicology (13.2)]*.

Table 2: Incidence of Treatment-Emergent Adverse Reactions in Controlled Studies

Adverse Reaction	Placebo (N=896) %	DEXILANT 30 mg (N=455) %	DEXILANT 60 mg (N=2218) %	DEXILANT Total (N=2621) %	Lansoprazole 30 mg (N=1363) %
Diarrhea	2.9	5.1	4.7	4.8	3.2
Abdominal Pain	3.5	3.5	4.0	4.0	2.6
Nausea	2.6	3.3	2.8	2.9	1.8
Upper Respiratory Tract Infection	0.8	2.9	1.7	1.9	0.8
Vomiting	0.8	2.2	1.4	1.6	1.1
Flatulence	0.6	2.6	1.4	1.6	1.2

8.3 Nursing Mothers

It is not known whether dexlansoprazole is excreted in human milk. However, lansoprazole and its metabolites are present in rat milk following the administration of lansoprazole. As many drugs are excreted in human milk, and because of the potential for tumorigenicity shown for lansoprazole in rat carcinogenicity studies *[see Carcinogenesis, Mutagenesis, Impairment of Fertility (13.1)]*, a decision should be made whether to discontinue nursing or to discontinue the drug, taking into account the importance of the drug to the mother.

8.4 Pediatric Use

Safety and effectiveness of DEXILANT in pediatric patients (less than 18 years of age) have not been established.

8.5 Geriatric Use

In clinical studies of DEXILANT, 11% of patients were aged 65 years and over. No overall differences in safety or effectiveness were observed between these patients and younger patients, and other reported clinical experience has not identified significant differences in responses between geriatric and younger patients, but greater sensitivity of some older individuals cannot be ruled out *[see Clinical Pharmacology (12.5)]*.

8.6 Renal Impairment

No dosage adjustment of DEXILANT is necessary in patients with renal impairment. The pharmacokinetics of dexlansoprazole in patients with renal impairment are not expected to be altered since dexlansoprazole is extensively metabolized in the liver to inactive metabolites, and no parent drug is recovered in the urine following an oral dose of dexlansoprazole *[see Clinical Pharmacology (12.5)]*.

8.7 Hepatic Impairment

No dosage adjustment for DEXILANT is necessary for patients with mild hepatic impairment (Child-Pugh Class A). DEXILANT 30 mg should be considered for patients with moderate hepatic impairment (Child-Pugh Class B). No studies have been conducted in patients with severe hepatic impairment (Child-Pugh Class C) *[see Clinical Pharmacology (12.5)]*.

10 OVERDOSAGE

There have been no reports of significant overdose of DEXILANT. Multiple doses of DEXILANT 120 mg and a single dose of DEXILANT 300 mg did not result in death or other severe adverse events. Dexlansoprazole is not expected to be removed from the circulation by hemodialysis. If an overdose occurs, treatment should be symptomatic and supportive.

11 DESCRIPTION

The active ingredient in DEXILANT (dexlansoprazole) delayed release capsules is (+)-2-[(*R*)-{[3-methyl-4-(2,2,2-trifluoroethoxy)pyridin-2-yl] methyl} sulfinyl]-*1H*-benzimidazole, a compound that inhibits gastric acid secretion. Dexlansoprazole is the *R*-enantiomer of lansoprazole (a racemic mixture of the *R*- and *S*-enantiomers). Its empirical formula is: $C_{16}H_{14}F_3N_3O_2S$, with a molecular weight of 369.36. The structural formula is:

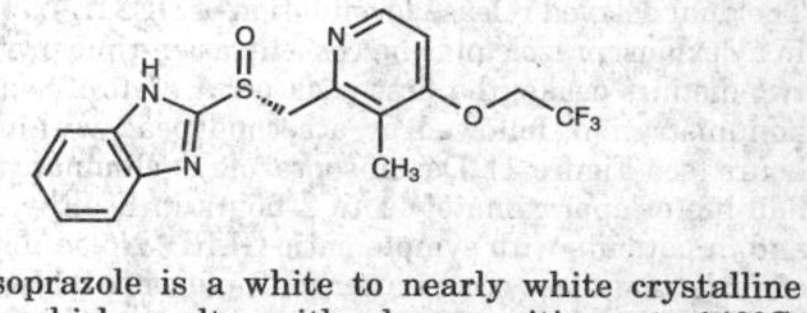

Dexlansoprazole is a white to nearly white crystalline powder which melts with decomposition at 140°C. Dexlansoprazole is freely soluble in dimethylformamide, methanol, dichloromethane, ethanol, and ethyl acetate; and soluble in acetonitrile; slightly soluble in ether; and very slightly soluble in water; and practically insoluble in hexane.

Dexlansoprazole is stable when exposed to light. Dexlansoprazole is more stable in neutral and alkaline conditions than acidic conditions.

DEXILANT is supplied as a dual delayed release formulation in capsules for oral administration. The capsules contain dexlansoprazole in a mixture of two types of enteric-coated granules with different pH-dependent dissolution profiles *[see Clinical Pharmacology (12.3)]*.

DEXILANT is available in two dosage strengths: 30 mg and 60 mg, per capsule. Each capsule contains enteric-coated granules consisting of dexlansoprazole (active ingredient) and the following inactive ingredients: sugar spheres, magnesium carbonate, sucrose, low-substituted hydroxypropyl cellulose, titanium dioxide, hydroxypropyl cellulose, hypromellose 2910, talc, methacrylic acid copolymers, polyethylene glycol 8000, triethyl citrate, polysorbate 80, and colloidal silicon dioxide. The components of the capsule shell include the following inactive ingredients: hypromellose, carrageenan and potassium chloride. Based on the capsule shell color, blue contains FD&C Blue No. 2 and aluminum lake; gray contains ferric oxide and aluminum lake; and both contain titanium dioxide.

12 CLINICAL PHARMACOLOGY

12.1 Mechanism of Action

Dexlansoprazole is a PPI that suppresses gastric acid secretion by specific inhibition of the (H^+,K^+)-ATPase in the gastric parietal cell. By acting specifically on the proton pump, dexlansoprazole blocks the final step of acid production.

12.2 Pharmacodynamics

Antisecretory Activity

The effects of DEXILANT 60 mg (n=20) or lansoprazole 30 mg (n=23) once daily for five days on 24-hour intragastric pH were assessed in healthy subjects in a multiple-dose crossover study. The results are summarized in Table 3.

Table 3: Effect on 24-hour Intragastric pH on Day 5 After Administration of DEXILANT or Lansoprazole

DEXILANT 60 mg	Lansoprazole 30 mg
Mean Intragastric pH	
4.55	4.13
% Time Intragastric pH > 4 (hours)	
71 (17 hours)	60 (14 hours)

Serum Gastrin Effects

The effect of DEXILANT on serum gastrin concentrations was evaluated in approximately 3460 patients in clinical trials up to 8 weeks and in 1023 patients for up to 6 to 12 months. The mean fasting gastrin concentrations increased from baseline during treatment with DEXILANT 30 mg and 60 mg doses. In patients treated for more than 6 months, mean serum gastrin levels increased during approximately the first 3 months of treatment and were stable for the remainder of treatment. Mean serum gastrin levels returned to pre-treatment levels within one month of discontinuation of treatment.

Enterochromaffin-Like Cell (ECL) Effects

There were no reports of ECL cell hyperplasia in gastric biopsy specimens obtained from 653 patients treated with DEXILANT 30 mg, 60 mg or 90 mg for up to 12 months.

During lifetime exposure of rats dosed daily with up to 150 mg per kg per day of lansoprazole, marked hypergastrinemia was observed followed by ECL cell proliferation and formation of carcinoid tumors, especially in female rats *[see Nonclinical Toxicology (13.1)]*.

Effect on Cardiac Repolarization

A study was conducted to assess the potential of DEXILANT to prolong the QT/QT_c interval in healthy adult subjects. DEXILANT doses of 90 mg or 300 mg did not delay cardiac repolarization compared to placebo. The positive control (moxifloxacin) produced statistically significantly greater mean maximum and time-averaged QT/QT_c intervals compared to placebo.

12.3 Pharmacokinetics

The dual delayed release formulation of DEXILANT results in a dexlansoprazole plasma concentration-time profile with two distinct peaks; the first peak occurs 1 to 2 hours after administration, followed by a second peak within 4 to 5 hours (see Figure 1). Dexlansoprazole is eliminated with a half-life of approximately 1 to 2 hours in healthy subjects and in patients with symptomatic GERD. No accumulation of dexlansoprazole occurs after multiple, once daily doses of DEXILANT 30 mg or 60 mg, although mean AUC_t and C_{max} values of dexlansoprazole were slightly higher (less than 10%) on day 5 than on day 1.

Figure 1: Mean Plasma Dexlansoprazole Concentration – Time Profile Following Oral Administration of 30 or 60 mg DEXILANT Once Daily for 5 Days in Healthy Subjects

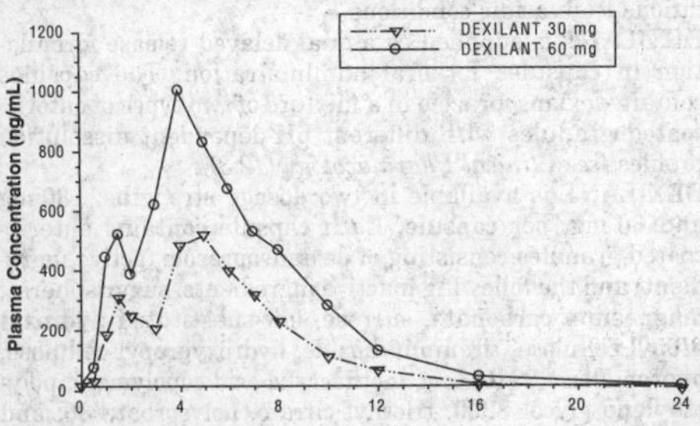

The pharmacokinetics of dexlansoprazole are highly variable, with percent coefficient of variation (CV%) values for C_{max}, AUC, and CL/F of greater than 30% (see Table 4).

Table 4: Mean (CV%) Pharmacokinetic Parameters for Subjects on Day 5 After Administration of DEXILANT

Dose (mg)	C_{max} (ng/mL)	AUC_{24} (ng·h/mL)	CL/F (L/h)
30	658 (40%) (N=44)	3275 (47%) (N=43)	11.4 (48%) (N=43)
60	1397 (51%) (N=79)	6529 (60%) (N=73)	11.6 (46%) (N=41)

Absorption

After oral administration of DEXILANT 30 mg or 60 mg to healthy subjects and symptomatic GERD patients, mean C_{max} and AUC values of dexlansoprazole increased approximately dose proportionally (see Figure 1).

Distribution

Plasma protein binding of dexlansoprazole ranged from 96.1% to 98.8% in healthy subjects and was independent of concentration from 0.01 to 20 mcg per mL. The apparent volume of distribution (V_z/F) after multiple doses in symptomatic GERD patients was 40.3 L.

Metabolism

Dexlansoprazole is extensively metabolized in the liver by oxidation, reduction, and subsequent formation of sulfate, glucuronide and glutathione conjugates to inactive metabolites. Oxidative metabolites are formed by the cytochrome P450 (CYP) enzyme system including hydroxylation mainly by CYP2C19, and oxidation to the sulfone by CYP3A4.

CYP2C19 is a polymorphic liver enzyme which exhibits three phenotypes in the metabolism of CYP2C19 substrates; extensive metabolizers (*1/*1), intermediate metabolizers (*1/mutant) and poor metabolizers (mutant/mutant). Dexlansoprazole is the major circulating component in plasma regardless of CYP2C19 metabolizer status. In CYP2C19 intermediate and extensive metabolizers, the major plasma metabolites are 5-hydroxy dexlansoprazole and its glucuronide conjugate, while in CYP2C19 poor metabolizers dexlansoprazole sulfone is the major plasma metabolite.

Elimination

Following the administration of DEXILANT, no unchanged dexlansoprazole is excreted in urine. Following the administration of $[^{14}C]$dexlansoprazole to 6 healthy male subjects, approximately 50.7% (standard deviation (SD): 9.0%) of the administered radioactivity was excreted in urine and 47.6% (SD: 7.3%) in the feces. Apparent clearance (CL/F) in healthy subjects was 11.4 to 11.6 L/h, respectively, after 5-days of 30 or 60 mg once daily administration.

Effect of CYP2C19 Polymorphism on Systemic Exposure of Dexlansoprazole

Systemic exposure of dexlansoprazole is generally higher in intermediate and poor metabolizers. In male Japanese subjects who received a single dose of DEXILANT 30 mg or 60 mg (N=2 to 6 subjects/group), mean dexlansoprazole C_{max} and AUC values were up to 2 times higher in intermediate compared to extensive metabolizers; in poor metabolizers, mean C_{max} was up to 4 times higher and mean AUC was up to 12 times higher compared to extensive metabolizers. Though such study was not conducted in Caucasians and African Americans, it is expected dexlansoprazole exposure in these races will be affected by CYP2C19 phenotypes as well.

12.4 Effect of Food on Pharmacokinetics and Pharmacodynamics

In food-effect studies in healthy subjects receiving DEXILANT under various fed conditions compared to fasting, increases in C_{max} ranged from 12% to 55%, increases in AUC ranged from 9% to 37%, and t_{max} varied (ranging from a decrease of 0.7 hours to an increase of 3 hours). No significant differences in mean intragastric pH were observed between fasted and various fed conditions. However, the percentage of time intragastric pH exceeded 4 over the 24-hour dosing interval decreased slightly when DEXILANT was administered after a meal (57%) relative to fasting (64%), primarily due to a decreased response in intragastric pH during the first 4 hours after dosing. Because of this, while DEXILANT can be taken without regard to food, some patients may benefit from administering the dose prior to a meal if post-meal symptoms do not resolve under post-fed conditions.

12.5 Special Populations

Pediatric Use

The pharmacokinetics of dexlansoprazole in patients under the age of 18 years have not been studied.

Geriatric Use

The terminal elimination half-life of dexlansoprazole is significantly increased in geriatric subjects compared to younger subjects (2.23 and 1.5 hours, respectively); this difference is not clinically relevant. Dexlansoprazole exhibited higher systemic exposure (AUC) in geriatric subjects (34.5% higher) than younger subjects. No dosage adjustment is needed in geriatric patients *[see Use in Specific Populations (8.5)]*.

Renal Impairment

Dexlansoprazole is extensively metabolized in the liver to inactive metabolites, and no parent drug is recovered in the urine following an oral dose of dexlansoprazole. Therefore, the pharmacokinetics of dexlansoprazole are not expected to be altered in patients with renal impairment, and no studies were conducted in subjects with renal impairment *[see Use in Specific Populations (8.6)]*. In addition, the pharmacokinetics of lansoprazole were studied in patients with mild, moderate or severe renal impairment; results demonstrated no need for a dose adjustment for this patient population.

Hepatic Impairment

In a study of 12 patients with moderately impaired hepatic function who received a single oral dose of DEXILANT 60 mg, plasma exposure (AUC) of bound and unbound dexlansoprazole in the hepatic impairment group was approximately 2 times greater compared to subjects with normal hepatic function. This difference in exposure was not due to a difference in protein binding between the two liver function groups. No adjustment for DEXILANT is necessary for patients with mild hepatic impairment (Child-Pugh Class A). DEXILANT 30 mg should be considered for patients with moderate hepatic impairment (Child-Pugh Class B). No studies have been conducted in patients with severe hepatic impairment (Child-Pugh Class C) *[see Use in Specific Populations (8.7)]*.

Gender

In a study of 12 male and 12 female healthy subjects who received a single oral dose of DEXILANT 60 mg, females had higher systemic exposure (AUC) (42.8% higher) than males. No dosage adjustment is necessary in patients based on gender.

12.6 Drug-Drug Interactions

Warfarin

In a study of 20 healthy subjects, co-administration of DEXILANT 90 mg once daily for 11 days with a single 25 mg oral dose of warfarin on day 6 did not result in any significant differences in the pharmacokinetics of warfarin or INR compared to administration of warfarin with placebo. However, there have been reports of increased INR and prothrombin time in patients receiving PPIs and warfarin concomitantly *[see Drug Interactions (7.2)]*.

Cytochrome P 450 Interactions

Dexlansoprazole is metabolized, in part, by CYP2C19 and CYP3A4 *[see Clinical Pharmacology (12.3)]*.

In vitro studies have shown that DEXILANT is not likely to inhibit CYP isoforms 1A1, 1A2, 2A6, 2B6, 2C8, 2C9, 2C19, 2D6, 2E1 or 3A4. As such, no clinically relevant interactions with drugs metabolized by these CYP enzymes would be expected. Furthermore, clinical drug-drug interaction studies in mainly CYP2C19 extensive and intermediate metabolizers have shown that DEXILANT does not affect the pharmacokinetics of diazepam, phenytoin, or theophylline. The subjects' CYP1A2 genotypes in the drug-drug interaction study with theophylline were not determined.

13 NONCLINICAL TOXICOLOGY

13.1 Carcinogenesis, Mutagenesis, Impairment of Fertility

The carcinogenic potential of dexlansoprazole was assessed using lansoprazole studies. In two 24-month carcinogenicity studies, Sprague-Dawley rats were treated orally with lansoprazole at doses of 5 to 150 mg per kg per day, about 1 to 40 times the exposure on a body surface (mg/m^2) basis of a 50 kg person of average height [1.46 m^2 body surface area (BSA)] given the recommended human dose of lansoprazole 30 mg per day.

Lansoprazole produced dose-related gastric ECL cell hyperplasia and ECL cell carcinoids in both male and female rats *[see Clinical Pharmacology (12.2)]*.

In rats, lansoprazole also increased the incidence of intestinal metaplasia of the gastric epithelium in both sexes. In male rats, lansoprazole produced a dose-related increase of testicular interstitial cell adenomas. The incidence of these adenomas in rats receiving doses of 15 to 150 mg per kg per day (4 to 40 times the recommended human lansoprazole dose based on BSA) exceeded the low background incidence (range = 1.4 to 10%) for this strain of rat.

In a 24-month carcinogenicity study, CD-1 mice were treated orally with lansoprazole doses of 15 mg to 600 mg per kg per day, 2 to 80 times the recommended human lansoprazole dose based on BSA. Lansoprazole produced a dose-related increased incidence of gastric ECL cell hyperplasia. It also produced an increased incidence of liver tumors (hepatocellular adenoma plus carcinoma). The tumor incidences in male mice treated with 300 mg and 600 mg lansoprazole per kg per day (40 to 80 times the recommended human lansoprazole dose based on BSA) and female mice treated with 150 mg to 600 mg lansoprazole per kg per day (20 to 80 times the recommended human

Table 5: EE Healing Rates*: All Grades

Study	Number of Patients (N)[†]	Treatment Group (daily)	Week 4 % Healed	Week 8[‡] % Healed	(95% CI) for the Treatment Difference (DEXILANT–Lansoprazole) by Week 8
1	657	DEXILANT 60 mg	70	87	(-1.5, 6.1)[§]
	648	Lansoprazole 30 mg	65	85	
2	639	DEXILANT 60 mg	66	85	(2.2, 10.5)[§]
	656	Lansoprazole 30 mg	65	79	

CI = Confidence interval

* Based on crude rate estimates, patients who did not have endoscopically documented healed EE and prematurely discontinued were considered not healed.
† Patients with at least one post baseline endoscopy
‡ Primary efficacy endpoint
§ Demonstrated non-inferiority to lansoprazole

lansoprazole dose based on BSA) exceeded the ranges of background incidences in historical controls for this strain of mice. Lansoprazole treatment produced adenoma of rete testis in male mice receiving 75 to 600 mg per kg per day (10 to 80 times the recommended human lansoprazole dose based on BSA).

A 26-week p53 (+/-) transgenic mouse carcinogenicity study of lansoprazole was not positive.

Lansoprazole was negative in the Ames test, the *ex vivo* rat hepatocyte unscheduled DNA synthesis (UDS) test, the *in vivo* mouse micronucleus test and the rat bone marrow cell chromosomal aberration test. Lansoprazole was positive in *in vitro* human lymphocyte chromosomal aberration tests. Dexlansoprazole was positive in the Ames test and in the *in vitro* chromosome aberration test using Chinese hamster lung cells. Dexlansoprazole was negative in the *in vivo* mouse micronucleus test.

The potential effects of dexlansoprazole on fertility and reproductive performance were assessed using lansoprazole studies. Lansoprazole at oral doses up to 150 mg per kg per day (40 times the recommended human lansoprazole dose based on BSA) was found to have no effect on fertility and reproductive performance of male and female rats.

13.2 Animal Toxicology and/or Pharmacology
Reproductive Toxicology Studies
A reproduction study conducted in rabbits at oral dexlansoprazole doses up to 30 mg per kg per day (approximately 9 times the maximum recommended human dexlansoprazole dose [60 mg per day] based on BSA) revealed no evidence of impaired fertility or harm to the fetus due to dexlansoprazole. In addition, reproduction studies performed in pregnant rats with oral lansoprazole at doses up to 150 mg per kg per day (40 times the recommended human lansoprazole dose based on BSA) and in pregnant rabbits at oral lansoprazole doses up to 30 mg per kg per day (16 times the recommended human lansoprazole dose based on BSA) revealed no evidence of impaired fertility or harm to the fetus due to lansoprazole.

14 CLINICAL STUDIES
14.1 Healing of Erosive Esophagitis
Two multi-center, double-blind, active-controlled, randomized, 8-week studies were conducted in patients with endoscopically confirmed EE. Severity of the disease was classified based on the Los Angeles Classification Grading System (Grades A-D). Patients were randomized to one of the following three treatment groups: DEXILANT 60 mg daily, DEXILANT 90 mg daily or lansoprazole 30 mg daily. Patients who were *H. pylori* positive or who had Barrett's Esophagus and/or definite dysplastic changes at baseline were excluded from these studies. A total of 4092 patients were enrolled and ranged in age from 18 to 90 years (median age 48 years) with 54% male. Race was distributed as follows: 87% Caucasian, 5% Black and 8% other. Based on the Los Angeles Classification, 71% of patients had mild EE (Grades A and B) and 29% of patients had moderate to severe EE (Grades C and D) before treatment.

The studies were designed to test non-inferiority. If non-inferiority was demonstrated then superiority would be tested. Although non-inferiority was demonstrated in both studies, the finding of superiority in one study was not replicated in the other.

The proportion of patients with healed EE at week 4 or 8 is presented below in Table 5.
[See table above]
DEXILANT 90 mg was studied and did not provide additional clinical benefit over DEXILANT 60 mg.

14.2 Maintenance of Healed Erosive Esophagitis
A multi-center, double-blind, placebo-controlled, randomized study was conducted in patients who successfully completed an EE study and showed endoscopically confirmed healed EE. Maintenance of healing and symptom resolution over a six-month period were evaluated with DEXILANT

30 mg or 60 mg once daily compared to placebo. A total of 445 patients were enrolled and ranged in age from 18 to 85 years (median age 49 years), with 52% female. Race was distributed as follows: 90% Caucasian, 5% Black and 5% other.

Sixty-six percent of patients treated with 30 mg of DEXILANT remained healed over the six-month time period as confirmed by endoscopy (see Table 6).

Table 6: Maintenance Rates* of Healed EE at Month 6

Number of Patients (N)[†]	Treatment Group (daily)	Maintenance Rate (%)
125	DEXILANT 30 mg	66.4[‡]
119	Placebo	14.3

* Based on crude rate estimates, patients who did not have endoscopically documented relapse and prematurely discontinued were considered to have relapsed.
† Patients with at least one post baseline endoscopy
‡ Statistically significant vs placebo

DEXILANT 60 mg was studied and did not provide additional clinical benefit over DEXILANT 30 mg.
DEXILANT 30 mg demonstrated a higher median percent of 24-hour heartburn-free days compared to placebo over the 6-month treatment period.

14.3 Symptomatic Non-Erosive GERD
A multi-center, double-blind, placebo-controlled, randomized, 4-week study was conducted in patients with a diagnosis of symptomatic non-erosive GERD made primarily by presentation of symptoms. These patients who identified heartburn as their primary symptom, had a history of heartburn for 6 months or longer, had heartburn on at least 4 of 7 days immediately prior to randomization and had no esophageal erosions as confirmed by endoscopy. However, patients with symptoms which were not acid-related may not have been excluded using these inclusion criteria. Patients were randomized to one of the following treatment groups: DEXILANT 30 mg daily, 60 mg daily, or placebo. A total of 947 patients were enrolled and ranged in age from 18 to 86 years (median age 48 years) with 71% female. Race was distributed as follows: 82% Caucasian, 14% Black and 4% other.

DEXILANT 30 mg provided statistically significantly greater percent of days with heartburn-free 24-hour periods over placebo as assessed by daily diary over 4 weeks (see Table 7). DEXILANT 60 mg was studied and provided no additional clinical benefit over DEXILANT 30 mg.

Table 7: Median Percentages of 24-Hour Heartburn-Free Periods During the 4 Week Treatment Period of the Symptomatic Non-Erosive GERD Study

N	Treatment Group (daily)	Heartburn-Free 24-hour Periods (%)
312	DEXILANT 30 mg	54.9*
310	Placebo	18.5

*Statistically significant vs placebo

A higher percentage of patients on DEXILANT 30 mg had heartburn-free 24-hour periods compared to placebo as early as the first three days of treatment and this was sustained throughout the treatment period (percentage of pa-

tients on Day 3: DEXILANT 38% versus placebo 15%; on Day 28: DEXILANT 63% versus placebo 40%).

16 HOW SUPPLIED/STORAGE AND HANDLING
DEXILANT delayed release capsules, 30 mg, are opaque, blue and gray with TAP and "30" imprinted on the capsule and supplied as:

NDC Number	Size
64764-171-11	Unit dose package of 100
64764-171-30	Bottle of 30
64764-171-90	Bottle of 90
64764-171-19	Bottle of 1000

DEXILANT delayed release capsules, 60 mg, are opaque, blue with TAP and "60" imprinted on the capsule and supplied as:

NDC Number	Size
64764-175-11	Unit dose package of 100
64764-175-30	Bottle of 30
64764-175-90	Bottle of 90
64764-175-19	Bottle of 1000

Store at 25°C (77°F); excursions permitted to 15-30°C (59-86°F). [See USP Controlled Room Temperature]

17 PATIENT COUNSELING INFORMATION
To ensure the safe and effective use of DEXILANT, this information and instructions provided in the FDA-approved Patient Information Leaflet should be discussed with the patient. Inform patients of the following:
Tell your patients to watch for signs of an allergic reaction as these could be serious and may require that DEXILANT be discontinued. Advise your patients to tell you if they take atazanavir, tacrolimus, warfarin and drugs that are affected by gastric pH changes [see Drug Interactions (7)].
Advise patients to follow the dosing instructions in the Patient Information Leaflet.
DEXILANT is available as a delayed release capsule.
DEXILANT may be taken without regard to food.
DEXILANT should be swallowed whole.
• Alternatively, DEXILANT capsules can be opened and administered as follows:
  –Open capsule;
  –Sprinkle intact granules on one tablespoon of applesauce;
  –Swallow immediately. Granules should not be chewed.
  –Do not store for later use.

FDA-Approved Patient Labeling
Patient Information
DEXILANT (decks-ĭ-launt)
(dexlansoprazole)
delayed release capsules
Read the information that comes with DEXILANT before you start taking it and each time you get a refill. There may be new information. This information does not take the place of talking with your doctor about your medical condition or your treatment.

What is DEXILANT?
DEXILANT is a prescription medicine called a proton pump inhibitor (PPI). DEXILANT reduces the amount of acid in your stomach.
DEXILANT is used in adults:
• for 4 weeks to treat heartburn related to gastroesophageal reflux disease (GERD).
• for up to 8 weeks to heal acid-related damage to the lining of the esophagus (called erosive esophagitis or EE).
• for up to 6 months to stop erosive esophagitis from coming back.
GERD happens when acid from your stomach enters the tube (esophagus) that connects your mouth to your stomach. This may cause a burning feeling in your chest or throat, sour taste or burping.
In some cases, acid can damage the lining of your esophagus. This damage is called erosive esophagitis or EE.
DEXILANT may help your acid-related symptoms, but you could still have serious stomach problems. Talk with your doctor.
It is not known if DEXILANT is safe and effective in children under 18 years of age.
Who should not take DEXILANT?
Do not take DEXILANT if you are allergic to DEXILANT or any of its ingredients. See the end of this leaflet for a complete list of ingredients in DEXILANT.
What should I tell my doctor before taking DEXILANT?
Before you take DEXILANT, tell your doctor if you:
• have liver problems
• have any other medical conditions
• are pregnant or plan to become pregnant. It is not known if DEXILANT will harm your unborn baby. Talk to your doctor if you are pregnant or plan to become pregnant.

- are breast-feeding or planning to breast-feed. You and your doctor should decide if you will take DEXILANT or breast-feed. You should not do both without first talking with your doctor.

Tell your doctor about all the medicines you take, including prescription and non-prescription medicines, vitamins, and herbal supplements. DEXILANT may affect how other medicines work, and other medicines may affect how DEXILANT works. Especially tell your doctor if you take:

- ampicillin sodium (Unasyn) or ampicillin trihydrate (Principen)
- atazanavir (Reyataz)
- digoxin (Lanoxicaps, Lanoxin)
- a product that contains iron
- ketoconazole (Nizoral)
- warfarin (Coumadin, Jantoven)
- tacrolimus (Prograf)

Ask your doctor or pharmacist if you are not sure if your medicine is listed above.

How should I take DEXILANT?

- Take DEXILANT exactly as prescribed by your doctor.
- Do not change your dose or stop taking DEXILANT without talking to your doctor first.
- You can take DEXILANT with or without food.
- Swallow DEXILANT capsules whole.
- If you have trouble swallowing DEXILANT capsules whole, you can open the capsules and sprinkle the contents on a tablespoon of applesauce. Be sure to swallow the applesauce mixture right away. Do not chew the mixture. Do not store for later use.
- If you miss a dose, take it as soon as you remember. If it is almost time for your next dose, skip the missed dose. Just take the next dose at your regular time. Do not take 2 doses at the same time. If you are not sure about dosing, call your doctor.
- If you take too much DEXILANT, call your doctor right away.

What are the possible side effects of DEXILANT?

Serious allergic reactions. Tell your doctor if you get any of the following symptoms with DEXILANT.

- rash
- face swelling
- throat tightness
- difficulty breathing

Your doctor may stop DEXILANT if these symptoms happen.

The most common side effects of DEXILANT include:

- diarrhea
- stomach pain
- nausea
- common cold
- vomiting
- gas

People who are taking multiple daily doses of proton pump inhibitor medicines for a long period of time may have an increased risk of fractures of the hip, wrist or spine.

Tell your doctor if you have any side effect that bothers you or that does not go away. These are not all the possible side effects of DEXILANT. For more information, ask your doctor or pharmacist. Call your doctor for medical advice about side effects. You may report side effects to the FDA at 1-800-FDA-1088.

How should I store DEXILANT?

- Store DEXILANT at room temperature between 59° to 86°F (15° to 30°C).

Keep DEXILANT and all medicines out of the reach of children.

General information about DEXILANT

Medicines are sometimes prescribed for conditions other than those listed in a Patient Information Leaflet. Do not use DEXILANT for conditions for which it was not prescribed. Do not give DEXILANT to other people, even if they have the same symptoms you have. It may harm them.

This Patient Information Leaflet provides a summary of the most important information about DEXILANT. For more information, ask your doctor. You can ask your doctor or pharmacist for information that is written for healthcare professionals. For more information, go to www.DEXILANT.com or call 1-877-825-3327.

What is in DEXILANT?

Active ingredient: dexlansoprazole.

Inactive ingredients: sugar spheres, magnesium carbonate, sucrose, low-substituted hydroxypropyl cellulose, titanium dioxide, hydroxypropyl cellulose, hypromellose 2910, talc, methacrylic acid copolymers, polyethylene glycol 8000, triethyl citrate, polysorbate 80, and colloidal silicon dioxide. The capsule shell is made of hypromellose, carrageenan and potassium chloride. Based on the capsule shell color, blue contains FD&C Blue No. 2 and aluminum lake; gray contains ferric oxide and aluminum lake; and both contain titanium dioxide.

Distributed by
Takeda Pharmaceuticals America, Inc.
Deerfield, IL 60015

DEXILANT is a trademark of Takeda Pharmaceuticals North America, Inc. and used under license by Takeda Pharmaceuticals America, Inc. Trademark registered with the U.S. Patent and Trademark office.
All other trademark names are the property of their respective owners.
©2009, 2010 Takeda Pharmaceuticals America, Inc.

DEX006 R8
August 2010

Shown in Product Identification Guide, page 320

DUETACT® ℞

[doo-et'-ăct]

(pioglitazone hydrochloride and glimepiride)
Tablets

> **WARNING: CONGESTIVE HEART FAILURE**
> - Thiazolidinediones, including pioglitazone, which is a component of DUETACT, cause or exacerbate congestive heart failure in some patients (see **WARNINGS, *Pioglitazone hydrochloride***). After initiation of DUETACT, observe patients carefully for signs and symptoms of heart failure (including excessive, rapid weight gain, dyspnea, and/or edema). If these signs and symptoms develop, the heart failure should be managed according to the current standards of care. Furthermore, discontinuation of DUETACT must be considered.
> - DUETACT is not recommended in patients with symptomatic heart failure. Initiation of DUETACT in patients with established NYHA Class III or IV heart failure is contraindicated (see **CONTRAINDICATIONS** and **WARNINGS, *Pioglitazone hydrochloride***).

DESCRIPTION

DUETACT® (pioglitazone hydrochloride and glimepiride) tablets contain two oral antihyperglycemic agents used in the management of type 2 diabetes: pioglitazone hydrochloride and glimepiride. The concomitant use of pioglitazone and a sulfonylurea, the class of drugs that includes glimepiride, has been previously approved based on clinical trials in patients with type 2 diabetes inadequately controlled on a sulfonylurea. Additional efficacy and safety information about pioglitazone and glimepiride monotherapies may be found in the prescribing information for each individual drug.

Pioglitazone hydrochloride is an oral antihyperglycemic agent that acts primarily by decreasing insulin resistance. Pioglitazone is used in the management of type 2 diabetes. Pharmacological studies indicate that pioglitazone improves sensitivity to insulin in muscle and adipose tissue and inhibits hepatic gluconeogenesis. Pioglitazone improves glycemic control while reducing circulating insulin levels. Pioglitazone (±)-5-[[4-[2-(5-ethyl-2-pyridinyl)ethoxy] phenyl]methyl]-2,4-thiazolidinedione monohydrochloride belongs to a different chemical class and has a different pharmacological action than the sulfonylureas, biguanides, or the α-glucosidase inhibitors. The molecule contains one asymmetric center, and the synthetic compound is a racemate. The two enantiomers of pioglitazone interconvert *in vivo*. The structural formula is as shown:

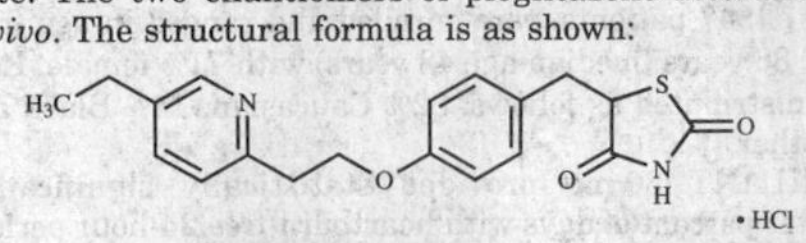

pioglitazone hydrochloride

Pioglitazone hydrochloride is an odorless, white crystalline powder that has a molecular formula of $C_{19}H_{20}N_2O_3S \cdot HCl$ and a molecular weight of 392.90. It is soluble in *N,N*-dimethylformamide, slightly soluble in anhydrous ethanol, very slightly soluble in acetone and acetonitrile, practically insoluble in water, and insoluble in ether.

Glimepiride 1-[[*p*-[2-(3-ethyl-4-methyl-2-oxo-3-pyrroline-1-carboxamido)ethyl]phenyl] sulfonyl]-3-(*trans*-4-methylcyclohexyl)-urea is an oral blood glucose-lowering drug of the sulfonylurea class and is used in the management of type 2 diabetes. The molecule is the trans-isomer with respect to the cyclohexyl substituents. The chemical structure is as shown:

[See chemical structure at top of next column]

Glimepiride is a white to yellowish-white crystalline, odorless, to practically odorless powder, that has a molecular formula of $C_{24}H_{34}N_4O_5S$ and a molecular weight of 490.62. It is soluble in dimethylsulfoxide, slightly soluble in acetone, very slightly soluble in acetonitrile and methanol, and practically insoluble in water.

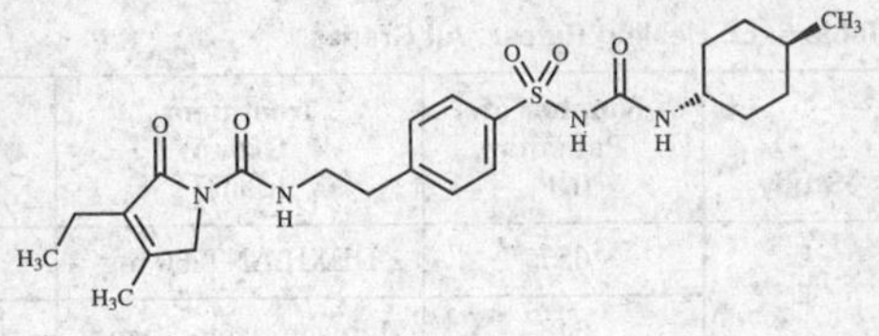

glimepiride

DUETACT is available as a tablet for oral administration containing 30 mg pioglitazone hydrochloride (as the base) with 2 mg glimepiride (30 mg/2 mg) or 30 mg pioglitazone hydrochloride (as the base) with 4 mg glimepiride (30 mg/4 mg) formulated with the following excipients: croscarmellose sodium NF, lactose monohydrate NF, magnesium stearate NF, hydroxypropyl cellulose NF, polysorbate 80 NF, and microcrystalline cellulose NF.

CLINICAL PHARMACOLOGY

Mechanism of Action

DUETACT

DUETACT combines two antihyperglycemic agents with different mechanisms of action to improve glycemic control in patients with type 2 diabetes: pioglitazone hydrochloride, a member of the thiazolidinedione class, and glimepiride, a member of the sulfonylurea class. Thiazolidinediones are insulin-sensitizing agents that act primarily by enhancing peripheral glucose utilization, whereas sulfonylureas are insulin secretogogues that act primarily by stimulating release of insulin from functioning pancreatic beta cells.

Pioglitazone hydrochloride

Pioglitazone depends on the presence of insulin for its mechanism of action. Pioglitazone decreases insulin resistance in the periphery and in the liver resulting in increased insulin-dependent glucose disposal and decreased hepatic glucose output. Pioglitazone is a potent and highly selective agonist for peroxisome proliferator-activated receptor-gamma (PPARγ). PPAR receptors are found in tissues important for insulin action such as adipose tissue, skeletal muscle, and liver. Activation of PPARγ nuclear receptors modulates the transcription of a number of insulin responsive genes involved in the control of glucose and lipid metabolism.

In animal models of diabetes, pioglitazone reduces the hyperglycemia, hyperinsulinemia, and hypertriglyceridemia characteristic of insulin-resistant states such as type 2 diabetes. The metabolic changes produced by pioglitazone result in increased responsiveness of insulin-dependent tissues and are observed in numerous animal models of insulin resistance.

Since pioglitazone enhances the effects of circulating insulin (by decreasing insulin resistance), it does not lower blood glucose in animal models that lack endogenous insulin.

Glimepiride

The primary mechanism of action of glimepiride in lowering blood glucose appears to be dependent on stimulating the release of insulin from functioning pancreatic beta cells. In addition, extrapancreatic effects may also play a role in the activity of sulfonylureas such as glimepiride. This is supported by both preclinical and clinical studies demonstrating that glimepiride administration can lead to increased sensitivity of peripheral tissues to insulin. These findings are consistent with the results of a long-term, randomized, placebo-controlled trial in which glimepiride therapy improved postprandial insulin/C-peptide responses and overall glycemic control without producing clinically meaningful increases in fasting insulin/C-peptide levels. However, as with other sulfonylureas, the mechanism by which glimepiride lowers blood glucose during long-term administration has not been clearly established.

Pharmacokinetics and Drug Metabolism

Absorption and Bioavailability

DUETACT

Bioequivalence studies were conducted following a single dose of the DUETACT 30 mg/2 mg and 30 mg/4 mg tablets and concomitant administration of ACTOS (30 mg) and glimepiride (2 mg or 4 mg) under fasting conditions in healthy subjects.

Based on the area under the curve (AUC) and maximum concentration (C_{max}) of both pioglitazone and glimepiride, DUETACT 30 mg/2 mg and 30 mg/4 mg were bioequivalent to ACTOS 30 mg concomitantly administered with glimepiride (2 mg or 4 mg, respectively) (**Table 1**).

[See table 1 at top of next page]

Food did not change the systemic exposures of glimepiride or pioglitazone following administration of DUETACT. The presence of food did not significantly alter the time to peak serum concentration of glimepiride or pioglitazone or peak exposure (C_{max}) of pioglitazone. However, for glimepiride, there was a 22% increase in C_{max} when DUETACT was administered with food.

Pioglitazone hydrochloride
Following oral administration, in the fasting state, pioglitazone is first measurable in serum within 30 minutes, with peak concentrations observed within 2 hours.
Glimepiride
After oral administration, glimepiride is completely (100%) absorbed from the GI tract. Studies with single oral doses in normal subjects and with multiple oral doses in patients with type 2 diabetes have shown significant absorption of glimepiride within 1 hour after administration and C_{max} at 2 to 3 hours.

Distribution
Pioglitazone hydrochloride
The mean apparent volume of distribution (Vd/F) of pioglitazone following single-dose administration is 0.63 ± 0.41 (mean $\pm$ SD) L/kg of body weight. Pioglitazone is extensively protein bound (> 99%) in human serum, principally to serum albumin. Pioglitazone also binds to other serum proteins, but with lower affinity. Metabolites M-III and M-IV also are extensively bound (> 98%) to serum albumin.
Glimepiride
After intravenous (IV) dosing in normal subjects, Vd/F was 8.8 L (113 mL/kg), and the total body clearance (CL) was 47.8 mL/min. Protein binding was greater than 99.5%.

Metabolism
Pioglitazone hydrochloride
Pioglitazone is extensively metabolized by hydroxylation and oxidation; the metabolites also partly convert to glucuronide or sulfate conjugates. Metabolites M-II and M-IV (hydroxy derivatives of pioglitazone) and M-III (keto derivative of pioglitazone) are pharmacologically active in animal models of type 2 diabetes. In addition to pioglitazone, M-III and M-IV are the principal drug-related species found in human serum following multiple dosing. At steady-state, in both healthy volunteers and in patients with type 2 diabetes, pioglitazone comprises approximately 30% to 50% of the total peak serum concentrations and 20% to 25% of the total AUC.

In vitro data demonstrate that multiple CYP isoforms are involved in the metabolism of pioglitazone. The cytochrome P450 isoforms involved are CYP2C8 and, to a lesser degree, CYP3A4 with additional contributions from a variety of other isoforms including the mainly extrahepatic CYP1A1. *In vivo* studies of pioglitazone in combination with P450 inhibitors and substrates have been performed (see **PRECAUTIONS, Drug Interactions,** *Pioglitazone hydrochloride*). Urinary 6β-hydroxycortisol/cortisol ratios measured in patients treated with pioglitazone showed that pioglitazone is not a strong CYP3A4 enzyme inducer.
Glimepiride
Glimepiride is completely metabolized by oxidative biotransformation after either an IV or oral dose. The major metabolites are the cyclohexyl hydroxy methyl derivative (M1) and the carboxyl derivative (M2). CYP2C9 has been shown to be involved in the biotransformation of glimepiride to M1. M1 is further metabolized to M2 by one or several cytosolic enzymes. M1, but not M2, possesses about 1/3 of the pharmacological activity as compared to its parent in an animal model; however, whether the glucose-lowering effect of M1 is clinically meaningful is not clear.

Excretion and Elimination
Pioglitazone hydrochloride
Following oral administration, approximately 15% to 30% of the pioglitazone dose is recovered in the urine. Renal elimination of pioglitazone is negligible and the drug is excreted primarily as metabolites and their conjugates. It is presumed that most of the oral dose is excreted into the bile either unchanged or as metabolites and eliminated in the feces.

The mean serum half-life of pioglitazone and total pioglitazone ranges from 3 to 7 hours and 16 to 24 hours, respectively. Pioglitazone has an apparent clearance, CL/f, calculated to be 5 to 7 L/hr.
Glimepiride
When ^{14}C-glimepiride was given orally, approximately 60% of the total radioactivity was recovered in the urine in 7 days and M1 (predominant) and M2 accounted for 80-90% of that recovered in the urine. Approximately 40% of the total radioactivity was recovered in feces and M1 and M2 (predominant) accounted for about 70% of that recovered in feces. No parent drug was recovered from urine or feces. After IV dosing in patients, no significant biliary excretion of glimepiride or its M1 metabolite has been observed.

Special Populations
Renal Insufficiency
Pioglitazone hydrochloride
The serum elimination half-life of pioglitazone, M-III and M-IV remains unchanged in patients with moderate (creatinine clearance 30 to 60 mL/min) to severe (creatinine clearance < 30 mL/min) renal impairment when compared to normal subjects. No dose adjustment in patients with renal dysfunction is recommended.

Table 1. Mean (SD) Pharmacokinetic Parameters for DUETACT

Regimen		N	AUC(0-inf) (ng·h/mL)	N	C_{max} (ng/mL)	N	T_{max} (h)	N	$T_{1/2}$ (h)
30 mg/2 mg DUETACT	pioglitazone	58	11414 (2704)	66	910 (336)	66	1.81 (1.11)	65	14.02 (6.23)
	glimepiride	62	651 (239)	66	156 (52.5)	66	1.39 (0.29)	63	7.05 (4.32)
30 mg pioglitazone + 2 mg glimepiride tablets	pioglitazone	58	11496 (2926)	66	975 (367)	66	1.48 (1.13)	65	12.71 (5.60)
	glimepiride	62	635 (240)	66	165 (53.1)	66	1.36 (0.35)	63	5.54 (4.21)
30 mg/4 mg DUETACT	pioglitazone	55	11119 (3399)	67	1062 (333)	67	1.53 (0.81)	67	10.88 (4.71)
	glimepiride	64	1645 (576)	67	319 (95.3)	67	1.45 (0.39)	64	10.52 (3.49)
30 mg pioglitazone + 4 mg glimepiride tablets	pioglitazone	55	10674 (2895)	67	1026 (346)	67	1.52 (1.95)	67	12.21 (6.30)
	glimepiride	64	1590 (554)	67	313 (97.8)	67	1.76 (1.13)	64	9.07 (3.47)

Glimepiride
A single-dose, open-label study was conducted in 15 patients with renal impairment. Glimepiride (3 mg) was administered to 3 groups of patients with different levels of mean creatinine clearance (CLcr); (Group I, CLcr = 77.7 mL/min, n = 5), (Group II, CLcr = 27.7 mL/min, n = 3), and (Group III, CLcr = 9.4 mL/min, n = 7). Glimepiride was found to be well tolerated in all 3 groups. The results showed that glimepiride serum levels decreased as renal function decreased. However, M1 and M2 serum levels (mean AUC values) increased 2.3 and 8.6 times from Group I to Group III. The apparent terminal half-life ($T_{1/2}$) for glimepiride did not change, while the half-lives for M1 and M2 increased as renal function decreased. Mean urinary excretion of M1 plus M2 as percent of dose, however, decreased (44.4%, 21.9%, and 9.3% for Groups I to III).
A multiple-dose titration study was also conducted in 16 patients with type 2 diabetes and with renal impairment using doses ranging from 1-8 mg daily for 3 months. The results were consistent with those observed after single doses. All patients with a CLcr less than 22 mL/min had adequate control of their glucose levels with a dosage regimen of only 1 mg daily. The results from this study suggested that a starting dose of 1 mg glimepiride may be given to patients with type 2 diabetes and kidney disease, and the dose may be titrated based on fasting blood glucose levels (see **DOSAGE AND ADMINISTRATION, Special Patient Populations**).

Hepatic Insufficiency
Pioglitazone hydrochloride
Compared with normal controls, subjects with impaired hepatic function (Child-Pugh Grade B/C) have an approximate 45% reduction in pioglitazone and total pioglitazone mean peak concentrations but no change in the mean AUC values. Therapy with DUETACT should not be initiated if the patient exhibits clinical evidence of active liver disease or serum transaminase levels (ALT) exceed 2.5 times the upper limit of normal (see **PRECAUTIONS, General:** *Pioglitazone hydrochloride*, Hepatic Effects).
Glimepiride
No studies were performed in patients with hepatic insufficiency.

Elderly
Pioglitazone hydrochloride
In healthy elderly subjects, peak serum concentrations of pioglitazone and total pioglitazone are not significantly different, but AUC values are slightly higher and the terminal half-life values slightly longer than for younger subjects. These changes were not of a magnitude that would be considered clinically relevant.
Glimepiride
Comparison of glimepiride pharmacokinetics in patients with type 2 diabetes ≤65 years and those >65 years was performed in a study using a dosing regimen of 6 mg daily. There were no significant differences in glimepiride pharmacokinetics between the two age groups. The mean AUC at steady-state for the older patients was about 13% lower than that for the younger patients; the mean weight-adjusted clearance for the older patients was about 11% higher than that for the younger patients.

Pediatrics
No pharmacokinetic studies of DUETACT were performed in pediatric patients.
Gender
Pioglitazone hydrochloride
As monotherapy and in combination with sulfonylurea, metformin, or insulin, pioglitazone improved glycemic control in both males and females. The mean C_{max} and AUC values were increased 20% to 60% in females. In controlled clinical trials, hemoglobin A1C (A1C) decreases from baseline were generally greater for females than for males (average mean difference in A1C 0.5%). Since therapy should be individualized for each patient to achieve glycemic control, no dose adjustment is recommended based on gender alone.
Glimepiride
There were no differences between males and females in the pharmacokinetics of glimepiride when adjustment was made for differences in body weight.
Ethnicity
Pioglitazone hydrochloride
Pharmacokinetic data among various ethnic groups are not available.
Glimepiride
No pharmacokinetic studies to assess the effects of race have been performed, but in placebo-controlled studies of glimepiride in patients with type 2 diabetes, the antihyperglycemic effect was comparable in whites (n = 536), blacks (n = 63), and Hispanics (n = 63).
Other Populations
Glimepiride
There were no important differences in glimepiride metabolism in subjects identified as phenotypically different drug-metabolizers by their metabolism of sparteine. The pharmacokinetics of glimepiride in morbidly obese patients were similar to those in the normal weight group, except for a lower C_{max} and AUC. However, since neither C_{max} nor AUC values were normalized for body surface area, the lower values of C_{max} and AUC for the obese patients were likely the result of their excess weight and not due to a difference in the kinetics of glimepiride.
Drug-Drug Interactions
Co-administration of pioglitazone (45 mg) and a sulfonylurea (5 mg glipizide) administered orally once daily for 7 days did not alter the steady-state pharmacokinetics of glipizide. Glimepiride and glipizide have similar metabolic pathways and are mediated by CYP2C9; therefore, drug-drug interaction between pioglitazone and glimepiride is considered unlikely. Specific pharmacokinetic drug interaction studies with DUETACT have not been performed, although such studies have been conducted with the individual pioglitazone and glimepiride components.
Pioglitazone hydrochloride
The following drugs were studied in healthy volunteers with co-administration of pioglitazone 45 mg once daily. Results are listed below:
Oral Contraceptives: Co-administration of pioglitazone (45 mg once daily) and an oral contraceptive (1 mg norethindrone plus 0.035 mg ethinyl estradiol once daily) for 21 days, resulted in 11% and 11-14% decrease in ethinyl estradiol AUC (0-24h) and C_{max} respectively. There were no significant changes in norethindrone AUC (0-24h) and C_{max}. In view of the high variability of ethinyl estradiol pharmacokinetics, the clinical significance of this finding is unknown.

Table 2. Glycemic Parameters in 16-Week and 24-Week Pioglitazone Hydrochloride + Sulfonylurea Combination Studies

Parameter	Placebo + sulfonylurea	Pioglitazone 15 mg + sulfonylurea	Pioglitazone 30 mg + sulfonylurea
16-Week Study			
A1C (%)	N=181	N=176	N=182
Baseline mean	9.86	10.01	9.93
Mean change from baseline at 16 weeks	0.06	-0.82*[†]	-1.22*[†]
Difference in change from placebo + sulfonylurea		-0.88	-1.28
Responder rate (%) (a)	23.8	56.8	74.2
FPG (mg/dL)	N=182	N=179	N=186
Baseline mean	236	246.8	238.9
Mean change from baseline at 16 weeks	5.6	-33.8*[†]	-52.3*[†]
Difference in change from placebo + sulfonylurea		-39.4	-57.9
Responder rate (%) (b)	22.0	55.3	67.7

Parameter		Pioglitazone 30 mg + sulfonylurea	Pioglitazone 45 mg + sulfonylurea
24-Week Study			
A1C (%)		N=340	N=332
Baseline mean		9.77	9.85
Mean change from baseline at 24 weeks		-1.55*	-1.67*
Responder rate (%) (a)		77.4	79.5
FPG (mg/dL)		N=338	N=329
Baseline mean		214.4	217.2
Mean change from baseline at 24 weeks		-51.5*	-56.1*
Responder rate (%) (b)		63.6	71.1

* significant change from baseline $p \leq 0.050$
[†] significant difference from placebo plus sulfonylurea, $p \leq 0.050$
(a) patients who achieved an A1C $\leq 6.1\%$ or $\geq 0.6\%$ decrease from baseline
(b) patients who achieved a decrease in FPG by ≥ 30 mg/dL

Midazolam: Administration of pioglitazone for 15 days followed by a single 7.5 mg dose of midazolam syrup resulted in a 26% reduction in midazolam C_{max} and AUC.

Nifedipine ER: Co-administration of pioglitazone for 7 days with 30 mg nifedipine ER administered orally once daily for 4 days to male and female volunteers resulted in a ratio of least square mean (90% CI) values for unchanged nifedipine of 0.83 (0.73-0.95) for C_{max} and 0.88 (0.80-0.96) for AUC. In view of the high variability of nifedipine pharmacokinetics, the clinical significance of this finding is unknown.

Ketoconazole: Co-administration of pioglitazone for 7 days with ketoconazole 200 mg administered twice daily resulted in a ratio of least square mean (90% CI) values for unchanged pioglitazone of 1.14 (1.06-1.23) for C_{max}, 1.34 (1.26-1.41) for AUC and 1.87 (1.71-2.04) for C_{min}.

Atorvastatin Calcium: Co-administration of pioglitazone for 7 days with atorvastatin calcium (LIPITOR®) 80 mg once daily resulted in a ratio of least square mean (90% CI) values for unchanged pioglitazone of 0.69 (0.57-0.85) for C_{max}, 0.76 (0.65-0.88) for AUC and 0.96 (0.87-1.05) for C_{min}. For unchanged atorvastatin, the ratio of least square mean (90% CI) values were 0.77 (0.66-0.90) for C_{max}, 0.86 (0.78-0.94) for AUC and 0.92 (0.82-1.02) for C_{min}.

Cytochrome P450: See **PRECAUTIONS, Drug Interactions,** *Pioglitazone hydrochloride.*

Gemfibrozil: Concomitant administration of gemfibrozil (oral 600 mg twice daily), an inhibitor of CYP2C8, with pioglitazone (oral 30 mg) in 10 healthy volunteers pretreated for 2 days prior with gemfibrozil (oral 600 mg twice daily) resulted in pioglitazone exposure (AUC_{0-24}) being 226% of the pioglitazone exposure in the absence of gemfibrozil (see **PRECAUTIONS, Drug Interactions,** *Pioglitazone hydrochloride*).[1]

Rifampin: Concomitant administration of rifampin (oral 600 mg once daily), an inducer of CYP2C8 with pioglitazone (oral 30 mg) in 10 healthy volunteers pre-treated for 5 days prior with rifampin (oral 600 mg once daily) resulted in a decrease in the AUC of pioglitazone by 54% (see **PRECAUTIONS, Drug Interactions,** *Pioglitazone hydrochloride*).[2]

In other drug-drug interaction studies, pioglitazone had no significant effect on the pharmacokinetics of fexofenadine, metformin, digoxin, warfarin, ranitidine, or theophylline.

Glimepiride

The hypoglycemic action of sulfonylureas may be potentiated by certain drugs, including nonsteroidal anti-inflammatory drugs and other drugs that are highly protein bound, such as salicylates, sulfonamides, chloramphenicol, coumarins, probenecid, monoamine oxidase inhibitors, and beta adrenergic blocking agents. Due to the potential drug interaction between these drugs and glimepiride, the patient should be observed closely for hypoglycemia when these drugs are co-administered. Conversely, when these drugs are withdrawn, the patient should be observed closely for loss of glycemic control.

Certain drugs tend to produce hyperglycemia and may lead to loss of control. These drugs include the thiazides and other diuretics, corticosteroids, phenothiazines, thyroid products, estrogens, oral contraceptives, phenytoin, nicotinic acid, sympathomimetics, and isoniazid. Due to the potential drug interaction between these drugs and glimepiride, the patient should be observed closely for loss of glycemic control when these drugs are co-administered. Conversely, when these drugs are withdrawn, the patient should be observed closely for hypoglycemia.

Aspirin: Co-administration of aspirin (1 g three times daily) and glimepiride led to a 34% decrease in the mean glimepiride AUC and, therefore, a 34% increase in the mean CL/f. The mean C_{max} had a decrease of 4%. Blood glucose and serum C-peptide concentrations were unaffected and no hypoglycemic symptoms were reported. Pooled data from clinical trials showed no evidence of clinically significant adverse interactions with uncontrolled concurrent administration of aspirin and other salicylates.

Cimetidine/Ranitidine: Co-administration of either cimetidine (800 mg once daily) or ranitidine (150 mg twice daily) with a single 4-mg oral dose of glimepiride did not significantly alter the absorption and disposition of glimepiride, and no differences were seen in hypoglycemic symptomatology. Pooled data from clinical trials showed no evidence of clinically significant adverse interactions with uncontrolled concurrent administration of H2-receptor antagonists.

Propranolol: Concomitant administration of propranolol (40 mg three times daily) and glimepiride significantly increased C_{max}, AUC, and $T_{1/2}$ of glimepiride by 23%, 22%, and 15%, respectively, and it decreased CL/f by 18%. The recovery of M1 and M2 from urine, however, did not change. The pharmacodynamic responses to glimepiride were nearly identical in normal subjects receiving propranolol and placebo. Pooled data from clinical trials in patients with type 2 diabetes showed no evidence of clinically significant adverse interactions with uncontrolled concurrent administration of beta-blockers. However, if beta-blockers are used, caution should be exercised and patients should be warned about the potential for hypoglycemia.

Warfarin: Concomitant administration of glimepiride (4 mg once daily) did not alter the pharmacokinetic characteristics of R- and S-warfarin enantiomers following administration of a single dose (25 mg) of racemic warfarin to healthy subjects. No changes were observed in warfarin plasma protein binding. Glimepiride treatment did result in a slight, but statistically significant, decrease in the pharmacodynamic response to warfarin. The reductions in mean area under the prothrombin time (PT) curve and maximum PT values during glimepiride treatment were very small (3.3% and 9.9%, respectively) and are unlikely to be clinically important.

Ramipril: The responses of serum glucose, insulin, C-peptide, and plasma glucagon to 2 mg glimepiride were unaffected by co-administration of ramipril (an ACE inhibitor) 5 mg once daily in normal subjects. No hypoglycemic symptoms were reported. Pooled data from clinical trials in patients with type 2 diabetes showed no evidence of clinically significant adverse interactions with uncontrolled concurrent administration of ACE inhibitors.

Miconazole: A potential interaction between oral miconazole and oral hypoglycemic agents leading to severe hypoglycemia has been reported. Whether this interaction also occurs with the intravenous, topical, or vaginal preparations of miconazole is not known. There is a potential interaction of glimepiride with inhibitors (e.g. fluconazole) and inducers (e.g. rifampicin) of cytochrome P450 2C9.

Although no specific interaction studies were performed with glimepiride, pooled data from clinical trials showed no evidence of clinically significant adverse interactions with uncontrolled concurrent administration of calcium-channel blockers, estrogens, fibrates, NSAIDS, HMG CoA reductase inhibitors, sulfonamides, or thyroid hormone.

Pharmacodynamics and Clinical Effects

Pioglitazone hydrochloride

Clinical studies demonstrate that pioglitazone improves insulin sensitivity in insulin-resistant patients. Pioglitazone enhances cellular responsiveness to insulin, increases insulin-dependent glucose disposal, improves hepatic sensitivity to insulin, and improves dysfunctional glucose homeostasis. In patients with type 2 diabetes, the decreased insulin resistance produced by pioglitazone results in lower plasma glucose concentrations, lower plasma insulin levels, and lower A1C values. Based on results from an open-label extension study, the glucose-lowering effects of pioglitazone appear to persist for at least one year. In controlled clinical studies, pioglitazone in combination with a sulfonylurea had an additive effect on glycemic control.

Patients with lipid abnormalities were included in placebo-controlled monotherapy clinical studies with pioglitazone. Overall, patients treated with pioglitazone had mean decreases in triglycerides, mean increases in HDL cholesterol, and no consistent mean changes in LDL cholesterol and total cholesterol compared to the placebo group. A similar pattern of results was seen in 16-week and 24-week combination therapy studies of pioglitazone with a sulfonylurea.

Glimepiride

A mild glucose-lowering effect first appeared following single oral doses as low as 0.5-0.6 mg in healthy subjects. The time required to reach the maximum effect (i.e., minimum blood glucose level $[T_{min}]$) was about 2 to 3 hours. In patients with type 2 diabetes, both fasting and 2-hour postprandial glucose levels were significantly lower with glimepiride (1, 2, 4, and 8 mg once daily) than with placebo after 14 days of oral dosing. The glucose-lowering effect in all active treatment groups was maintained over 24 hours.

In larger dose-ranging studies, blood glucose and A1C were found to respond in a dose-dependent manner over the range of 1 to 4 mg/day of glimepiride. Some patients, particularly those with higher fasting plasma glucose (FPG) levels, may benefit from doses of glimepiride up to 8 mg once daily. No difference in response was found when glimepiride was administered once or twice daily.

In two 14-week, placebo-controlled studies in 720 subjects, the average net reduction in A1C for patients treated with 8 mg of glimepiride once daily was 2.0% in absolute units compared with placebo-treated patients. In a long-term, randomized, placebo-controlled study of patients with type 2 diabetes unresponsive to dietary management, glimepiride therapy improved postprandial insulin/C-peptide responses, and 75% of patients achieved and maintained control of blood glucose and A1C. Efficacy results were not affected by age, gender, weight, or race. In long-term extension trials with previously-treated patients, no meaningful deterioration in mean fasting plasma glucose (FPG) or A1C levels was seen after 2 1/2 years of glimepiride therapy.

Glimepiride therapy is effective in controlling blood glucose without deleterious changes in the plasma lipoprotein profiles of patients treated for type 2 diabetes.

Clinical Studies

There have been no clinical efficacy studies conducted with DUETACT. However, the efficacy and safety of the separate components have been previously established. The co-administration of pioglitazone and a sulfonylurea, including glimepiride, has been evaluated for efficacy and safety in two clinical studies. These clinical studies established an added benefit of pioglitazone in glycemic control of patients with inadequately controlled type 2 diabetes while on sulfonylurea therapy. Bioequivalence of DUETACT with co-administered pioglitazone and glimepiride tablets was demonstrated at the 30 mg/2 mg and 30 mg/4 mg dosage strengths (see **CLINICAL PHARMACOLOGY, Pharmacokinetics and Drug Metabolism, Absorption and Bioavailability**).

Clinical Studies of Pioglitazone Add-On Therapy in Patients Not Adequately Controlled on a Sulfonylurea

Two treatment-randomized, controlled clinical studies in patients with type 2 diabetes were conducted to evaluate the safety and efficacy of pioglitazone plus a sulfonylurea. Both studies included patients receiving a sulfonylurea, either alone or in combination with another antihyperglycemic agent, who had inadequate glycemic control. Excluding the sulfonylurea agent, all other antihyperglycemic agents were discontinued prior to starting study treatment. In the first study, 560 patients were randomized to receive 15 mg or 30 mg of pioglitazone or placebo once daily in addition to their current sulfonylurea regimen for 16 weeks. In the second study, 702 patients were randomized to receive 30 mg or 45 mg of pioglitazone once daily in addition to their current sulfonylurea regimen for 24 weeks.

In the first study, the addition of pioglitazone 15 mg or 30 mg once daily to treatment with a sulfonylurea after 16 weeks significantly reduced the mean A1C by 0.88% and 1.28% and the mean FPG by 39.4 mg/dL and 57.9 mg/dL, respectively, from that observed with sulfonylurea treatment alone. In the second study, the mean reductions from baseline at Week 24 in A1C were 1.55% and 1.67% for the 30 mg and 45 mg doses, respectively. Mean reductions from baseline in FPG were 51.5 mg/dL and 56.1 mg/dL, respectively. Based on these reductions in A1C and FPG (**Table 2**), the addition of pioglitazone to sulfonylurea resulted in significant improvements in glycemic control irrespective of the sulfonylurea dosage.

[See table 2 at top of previous page]

INDICATIONS AND USAGE

DUETACT is a thiazolidinedione and sulfonylurea combination product indicated as an adjunct to diet and exercise to improve glycemic control in adults with type 2 diabetes mellitus who are already treated with a thiazolidinedione and a sulfonylurea or who have inadequate glycemic control on a thiazolidinedione alone or a sulfonylurea alone.

CONTRAINDICATIONS

Initiation of DUETACT in patients with established New York Heart Association (NYHA) Class III or IV heart failure is contraindicated (see **BOXED WARNING**).

In addition, DUETACT is contraindicated in patients with:
1. Known hypersensitivity to pioglitazone, glimepiride or any other component of DUETACT.
2. Diabetic ketoacidosis, with or without coma. This condition should be treated with insulin.

WARNINGS

Glimepiride

SPECIAL WARNING ON INCREASED RISK OF CARDIOVASCULAR MORTALITY

The administration of oral hypoglycemic drugs has been reported to be associated with increased cardiovascular mortality as compared to treatment with diet alone or diet plus insulin. This warning is based on the study conducted by the University Group Diabetes Program (UGDP), a long-term, prospective clinical trial designed to evaluate the effectiveness of glucose-lowering drugs in preventing or delaying vascular complications in patients with non-insulin-dependent diabetes. The study involved 823 patients who were randomly assigned to one of four treatment groups (Diabetes, 19 supp. 2: 747-830, 1970).

UGDP reported that patients treated for 5 to 8 years with diet plus a fixed dose of tolbutamide (1.5 grams per day) had a rate of cardiovascular mortality approximately 2-1/2 times that of patients treated with diet alone. A significant increase in total mortality was not observed, but the use of tolbutamide was discontinued based on the increase in cardiovascular mortality, thus limiting the opportunity for the study to show an increase in overall mortality. Despite controversy regarding the interpretation of these results, the findings of the UGDP study provide an adequate basis for this warning. The patient should be informed of the potential risks and advantages of glimepiride tablets and of alternative modes of therapy.

Although only one drug in the sulfonylurea class (tolbutamide) was included in this study, it is prudent from a safety standpoint to consider that this warning may also apply to other oral hypoglycemic drugs in this class, in view of their close similarities in mode of action and chemical structure.

Table 3. Weight Changes (kg) from Baseline During Double-Blind Clinical Trials with Pioglitazone

		Control Group (Placebo)	pioglitazone 15 mg	pioglitazone 30 mg	pioglitazone 45 mg
		Median (25th/75th percentile)	Median (25th/75th percentile)	Median (25th/75th percentile)	Median (25th/75th percentile)
Monotherapy		-1.4 (-2.7/0.0) n=256	0.9 (-0.5/3.4) n=79	1.0 (-0.9/3.4) n=188	2.6 (0.2/5.4) n=79
Combination Therapy	Sulfonylurea	-0.5 (-1.8/0.7) n=187	2.0 (0.2/3.2) n=183	3.1 (1.1/5.4) n=528	4.1 (1.8/7.3) n=333
	Metformin	-1.4 (-3.2/0.3) n=160	N/A	0.9 (-0.3/3.2) n=567	1.8 (-0.9/5.0) n=407
	Insulin	0.2 (-1.4/1.4) n=182	2.3 (0.5/4.3) n=190	3.3 (0.9/6.3) n=522	4.1 (1.4/6.8) n=338

Note: Trial durations of 16 to 26 weeks

Pioglitazone hydrochloride
Cardiac Failure and Other Cardiac Effects

Pioglitazone, like other thiazolidinediones, can cause fluid retention when used alone or in combination with other antidiabetic agents, including insulin. Fluid retention may lead to or exacerbate heart failure. Patients should be observed for signs and symptoms of heart failure. If these signs and symptoms develop, the heart failure should be managed according to current standards of care. Furthermore, discontinuation or dose reduction of pioglitazone must be considered. Patients with NYHA Class III and IV cardiac status were not studied during pre-approval clinical trials and pioglitazone is not recommended in these patients (see **BOXED WARNING** and **CONTRAINDICATIONS**).

In one 16-week U.S. double-blind, placebo-controlled clinical trial involving 566 patients with type 2 diabetes, pioglitazone at doses of 15 mg and 30 mg in combination with insulin was compared to insulin therapy alone. This trial included patients with long-standing diabetes and a high prevalence of pre-existing medical conditions as follows: arterial hypertension (57.2%), peripheral neuropathy (22.6%), coronary heart disease (19.6%), retinopathy (13.1%), myocardial infarction (8.8%), vascular disease (6.4%), angina pectoris (4.4%), stroke and/or transient ischemic attack (4.1%), and congestive heart failure (2.3%).

In this study, two of the 191 patients receiving 15 mg pioglitazone plus insulin (1.1%) and two of the 188 patients receiving 30 mg pioglitazone plus insulin (1.1%) developed congestive heart failure compared with none of the 187 patients on insulin therapy alone. All four of these patients had previous histories of cardiovascular conditions including coronary artery disease, previous CABG procedures, and myocardial infarction. In a 24-week dose-controlled study in which pioglitazone was coadministered with insulin, 0.3% of patients (1/345) on 30 mg and 0.9% (3/345) of patients on 45 mg reported CHF as a serious adverse event. Analysis of data from these studies did not identify specific factors that predict increased risk of congestive heart failure on combination therapy with insulin.

In type 2 diabetes and congestive heart failure (systolic dysfunction)

A 24-week post-marketing safety study was performed to compare pioglitazone (n=262) to glyburide (n=256) in uncontrolled diabetic patients (mean A1C 8.8% at baseline) with NYHA Class II and III heart failure and ejection fraction less than 40% (mean EF 30% at baseline). Over the course of the study, overnight hospitalization for congestive heart failure was reported in 9.9% of patients on pioglitazone compared to 4.7% of patients on glyburide with a treatment difference observed from 6 weeks. This adverse event associated with pioglitazone was more marked in patients using insulin at baseline and in patients over 64 years of age. No difference in cardiovascular mortality between the treatment groups was observed.

Pioglitazone should be initiated at the lowest approved dose if it is prescribed for patients with type 2 diabetes and systolic heart failure (NYHA Class II). If subsequent dose escalation is necessary, the dose should be increased gradually only after several months of treatment with careful monitoring for weight gain, edema, or signs and symptoms of CHF exacerbation (see **DOSAGE AND ADMINISTRATION, Special Patient Populations**).

Prospective Pioglitazone Clinical Trial In Macrovascular Events (PROactive)

In PROactive, 5238 patients with type 2 diabetes and a prior history of macrovascular disease were treated with ACTOS (n=2605), force-titrated up to 45 mg once daily, or placebo (n=2633) (see **ADVERSE REACTIONS**). The percentage of patients who had an event of serious heart failure was higher for patients treated with ACTOS (5.7%, n=149) than for patients treated with placebo (4.1%, n=108). The incidence of death subsequent to a report of serious heart failure was 1.5% (n=40) in patients treated with ACTOS and 1.4% (n=37) in placebo-treated patients. In patients treated with an insulin-containing regimen at baseline, the incidence of serious heart failure was 6.3% (n=54/864) with ACTOS and 5.2% (n=47/896) with placebo. For those patients treated with a sulfonylurea-containing regimen at baseline, the incidence of serious heart failure was 5.8% (n=94/1624) with ACTOS and 4.4% (n=71/1626) with placebo.

PRECAUTIONS

General
Pioglitazone hydrochloride

Pioglitazone exerts its antihyperglycemic effect only in the presence of insulin. Therefore, DUETACT should not be used in patients with type 1 diabetes or for the treatment of diabetic ketoacidosis.

Hypoglycemia: Patients receiving pioglitazone in combination with insulin or oral hypoglycemic agents may be at risk for hypoglycemia, and a reduction in the dose of the concomitant agent may be necessary.

Cardiovascular: In U.S. placebo-controlled clinical trials that excluded patients with New York Heart Association (NYHA) Class III and IV cardiac status, the incidence of serious cardiac adverse events related to volume expansion was not increased in patients treated with pioglitazone as monotherapy or in combination with sulfonylureas or metformin vs. placebo-treated patients. In insulin combination studies, a small number of patients with a history of previously existing cardiac disease developed congestive heart failure when treated with pioglitazone in combination with insulin (see **WARNINGS, Pioglitazone hydrochloride, Cardiac Failure and Other Cardiac Effects**). Patients with NYHA Class III and IV cardiac status were not studied in pre-approval pioglitazone clinical trials. Pioglitazone is not indicated in patients with NYHA Class III or IV cardiac status.

In postmarketing experience with pioglitazone, cases of congestive heart failure have been reported in patients both with and without previously known heart disease.

Edema: In all U.S. clinical trials with pioglitazone, edema was reported more frequently in patients treated with pioglitazone than in placebo-treated patients and appears to be dose related (see **ADVERSE REACTIONS, Pioglitazone hydrochloride**). In postmarketing experience, reports of initiation or worsening of edema have been received. Since thiazolidinediones, including pioglitazone, can cause fluid retention, which can exacerbate or lead to congestive heart failure, DUETACT should be used with caution in patients at risk for heart failure. Patients should be monitored for signs and symptoms of heart failure (see **BOXED WARNING, WARNINGS, Pioglitazone hydrochloride**, and **PRECAUTIONS, Information for Patients**).

Weight Gain: Dose related weight gain was observed with pioglitazone alone and in combination with other hypoglycemic agents (**Table 3**). The mechanism of weight gain is unclear but probably involves a combination of fluid retention and fat accumulation.

[See table 3 above]

Ovulation: Therapy with pioglitazone, like other thiazolidinediones, may result in ovulation in some premenopausal anovulatory women. Thus, adequate contraception in premenopausal women should be recommended while taking DUETACT. This possible effect has not been investigated in clinical studies so the frequency of this occurrence is not known.

Hematologic: Across all clinical studies with pioglitazone, mean hemoglobin values declined by 2% to 4% in patients treated with pioglitazone. These changes primarily occurred within the first 4 to 12 weeks of therapy and remained relatively constant thereafter. These changes may be related to increased plasma volume and have rarely been associated with any significant hematologic clinical effects (see **ADVERSE REACTIONS, Laboratory Abnormalities,** *Pioglitazone hydrochloride,* Hematologic). DUETACT may cause decreases in hemoglobin and hematocrit.

Hepatic Effects: In pre-approval clinical studies worldwide, over 4500 subjects were treated with pioglitazone. In U.S. clinical studies, over 4700 patients with type 2 diabetes received pioglitazone. There was no evidence of drug-induced hepatotoxicity or elevation of ALT levels in the clinical studies.

During pre-approval placebo-controlled clinical trials in the U.S., a total of 4 of 1526 (0.26%) patients treated with pioglitazone and 2 of 793 (0.25%) placebo-treated patients had ALT values ≥ 3 times the upper limit of normal. The ALT elevations in patients treated with pioglitazone were reversible and were not clearly related to therapy with pioglitazone.

In postmarketing experience with pioglitazone, reports of hepatitis and of hepatic enzyme elevations to 3 or more times the upper limit of normal have been received. Very rarely, these reports have involved hepatic failure with and without fatal outcome, although causality has not been established.

Pending the availability of the results of additional large, long-term controlled clinical trials and additional postmarketing safety data on pioglitazone, it is recommended that patients treated with DUETACT undergo periodic monitoring of liver enzymes.

Serum ALT (alanine aminotransferase) levels should be evaluated prior to the initiation of therapy with DUETACT in all patients and periodically thereafter per the clinical judgment of the health care professional. Liver function tests should also be obtained for patients if symptoms suggestive of hepatic dysfunction occur, e.g., nausea, vomiting, abdominal pain, fatigue, anorexia, or dark urine. The decision whether to continue the patient on therapy with DUETACT should be guided by clinical judgment pending laboratory evaluations. If jaundice is observed, drug therapy should be discontinued.

Therapy with DUETACT should not be initiated if the patient exhibits clinical evidence of active liver disease or the ALT levels exceed 2.5 times the upper limit of normal. Patients with mildly elevated liver enzymes (ALT levels at 1 to 2.5 times the upper limit of normal) at baseline or any time during therapy with DUETACT should be evaluated to determine the cause of the liver enzyme elevation. Initiation or continuation of therapy with DUETACT in patients with mildly elevated liver enzymes should proceed with caution and include appropriate clinical follow-up which may include more frequent liver enzyme monitoring. If serum transaminase levels are increased (ALT > 2.5 times the upper limit of normal), liver function tests should be evaluated more frequently until the levels return to normal or pretreatment values. If ALT levels exceed 3 times the upper limit of normal, the test should be repeated as soon as possible. If ALT levels remain > 3 times the upper limit of normal or if the patient is jaundiced, DUETACT therapy should be discontinued.

Macular Edema: Macular edema has been reported in post-marketing experience in diabetic patients who were taking pioglitazone or another thiazolidinedione. Some patients presented with blurred vision or decreased visual acuity, but some patients appear to have been diagnosed on routine ophthalmologic examination. Some patients had peripheral edema at the time macular edema was diagnosed. Some patients had improvement in their macular edema after discontinuation of their thiazolidinedione. It is unknown whether or not there is a causal relationship between pioglitazone and macular edema. Patients with diabetes should have regular eye exams by an ophthalmologist, per the Standards of Care of the American Diabetes Association. Additionally, any diabetic who reports any kind of visual symptom should be promptly referred to an ophthalmologist, regardless of the patient's underlying medications or other physical findings (see **ADVERSE REACTIONS**).

Fractures: In a randomized trial (PROactive) in patients with type 2 diabetes (mean duration of diabetes 9.5 years), an increased incidence of bone fracture was noted in female patients taking pioglitazone. During a mean follow-up of 34.5 months, the incidence of bone fracture in females was 5.1% (44/870) for pioglitazone versus 2.5% (23/905) for placebo. This difference was noted after the first year of treatment and remained during the course of the study. The majority of fractures observed in female patients were nonvertebral fractures including lower limb and distal upper limb. No increase in fracture rates was observed in men treated with pioglitazone 1.7% (30/1735) versus placebo 2.1% (37/1728). The risk of fracture should be considered in

the care of patients, especially female patients, treated with pioglitazone and attention should be given to assessing and maintaining bone health according to current standards of care.

Macrovascular Outcomes: There have been no clinical studies establishing conclusive evidence of macrovascular risk reduction with DUETACT or any other anti-diabetic drug.

General

Glimepiride

Hypoglycemia: All sulfonylurea drugs are capable of producing severe hypoglycemia. Proper patient selection, dosage, and instructions are important to avoid hypoglycemic episodes. Patients with impaired renal function may be more sensitive to the glucose-lowering effect of glimepiride. A starting dose of 1 mg of glimepiride once daily followed by appropriate dose titration is recommended in those patients (see **DOSAGE AND ADMINISTRATION, Special Patient Populations**). Debilitated or malnourished patients, and those with adrenal, pituitary, or hepatic insufficiency are particularly susceptible to the hypoglycemic action of glucose-lowering drugs. Hypoglycemia may be difficult to recognize in the elderly and in people who are taking beta-adrenergic blocking drugs or other sympatholytic agents. Hypoglycemia is more likely to occur when caloric intake is deficient, after severe or prolonged exercise, when alcohol is ingested, or when more than one glucose-lowering drug is used. Combined use of glimepiride with insulin or metformin may increase the potential for hypoglycemia.

Loss of control of blood glucose: When a patient stabilized on any diabetic regimen is exposed to stress such as fever, trauma, infection, or surgery, a loss of control may occur. The effectiveness of any oral hypoglycemic drug, including DUETACT, in lowering blood glucose to a desired level decreases in many patients over a period of time, which may be due to progression of the severity of the diabetes or to diminished responsiveness to the drug.

Hemolytic Anemia: Treatment of patients with glucose-6-phosphate dehydrogenase (G6PD) deficiency with sulfonylurea agents can lead to hemolytic anemia. Because DUETACT contains glimepiride which belongs to the class of sulfonylurea agents, caution should be used in patients with G6PD deficiency and a non-sulfonylurea alternative should be considered. In postmarketing reports, hemolytic anemia has also been reported in patients who did not have known G6PD deficiency.

Laboratory Tests

FPG and A1C measurements should be performed periodically to monitor glycemic control and therapeutic response to DUETACT.

Liver enzyme monitoring is recommended prior to initiation of therapy with DUETACT in all patients and periodically thereafter per the clinical judgment of the health care professional (see **PRECAUTIONS, General: *Pioglitazone hydrochloride,* Hepatic Effects** and **ADVERSE REACTIONS, Laboratory Abnormalities,** *Pioglitazone hydrochloride,* Serum Transaminase Levels).

Information for Patients

Patients should be instructed regarding the importance of adhering to dietary instructions, a regular exercise program, and regular testing of blood glucose and A1C. During periods of stress such as fever, trauma, infection, or surgery, medication requirements may change and patients should be reminded to seek medical advice promptly. Patients should also be informed of the potential risks and advantages of DUETACT and of alternative modes of therapy.

Prior to initiation of DUETACT therapy, the risks of hypoglycemia, its symptoms and treatment, and conditions that predispose to its development should be explained to patients and responsible family members (see **PRECAUTIONS, General: *Pioglitazone hydrochloride* and *Glimepiride,* Hypoglycemia**). Combination therapy of DUETACT with other antihyperglycemic agents may also cause hypoglycemia.

Patients who experience an unusually rapid increase in weight or edema or who develop shortness of breath or other symptoms of heart failure while on DUETACT should immediately report these symptoms to their physician.

Patients should be told that blood tests for liver function will be performed prior to the start of therapy and periodically thereafter per the clinical judgment of the health care professional. Patients should be told to seek immediate medical advice for unexplained nausea, vomiting, abdominal pain, fatigue, anorexia, or dark urine.

Therapy with a thiazolidinedione, including the active pioglitazone component of the DUETACT tablet, may result in ovulation in some premenopausal anovulatory women. As a result, these patients may be at an increased risk for pregnancy while taking DUETACT. This possible effect has not been investigated in clinical studies so the frequency of this occurrence is not known. Thus, adequate contraception in premenopausal women should be recommended. Patients who become pregnant while on DUETACT or are planning a pregnancy should be advised to discuss with their physician

a regimen appropriate for maintaining adequate glycemic control (see **PRECAUTIONS, Pregnancy: Pregnancy Category C**).

Patients should be told to take a single dose of DUETACT once daily with the first main meal and instructed that any change in dosing should be made only if directed by their physician (see **DOSAGE AND ADMINISTRATION, Maximum Recommended Dose**).

Drug Interactions

Pioglitazone hydrochloride

In vivo drug-drug interaction studies have suggested that pioglitazone may be a weak inducer of CYP 450 isoform 3A4 substrate.

An enzyme inhibitor of CYP2C8 (such as gemfibrozil) may significantly increase the AUC of pioglitazone and an enzyme inducer of CYP2C8 (such as rifampin) may significantly decrease the AUC of pioglitazone. Therefore, if an inhibitor or inducer of CYP2C8 is started or stopped during treatment with pioglitazone, changes in diabetes treatment may be needed based on clinical response (see **CLINICAL PHARMACOLOGY, Drug-Drug Interactions,** *Pioglitazone hydrochloride*).

Glimepiride

(See **CLINICAL PHARMACOLOGY, Drug-Drug Interactions,** *Glimepiride*)

Carcinogenesis, Mutagenesis, Impairment of Fertility

DUETACT

No animal studies have been conducted with DUETACT. The following data are based on findings in studies performed with pioglitazone or glimepiride individually.

Pioglitazone hydrochloride

A two-year carcinogenicity study was conducted in male and female rats at oral doses up to 63 mg/kg (approximately 14 times the maximum recommended human oral dose of 45 mg based on mg/m^2). Drug-induced tumors were not observed in any organ except for the urinary bladder. Benign and/or malignant transitional cell neoplasms were observed in male rats at 4 mg/kg/day and above (approximately equal to the maximum recommended human oral dose based on mg/m^2). A two-year carcinogenicity study was conducted in male and female mice at oral doses up to 100 mg/kg/day (approximately 11 times the maximum recommended human oral dose based on mg/m^2). No drug-induced tumors were observed in any organ.

During prospective evaluation of urinary cytology involving more than 1800 patients receiving pioglitazone in clinical trials up to one year in duration, no new cases of bladder tumors were identified. In two 3 year studies in which pioglitazone was compared to placebo or glyburide, there were 16/3656 (0.44%) reports of bladder cancer in patients taking pioglitazone compared to 5/3679 (0.14%) in patients not taking pioglitazone. After excluding patients in whom exposure to study drug was less than one year at the time of diagnosis of bladder cancer, there were six cases (0.16%) on pioglitazone and two (0.05%) on placebo.

Pioglitazone hydrochloride was not mutagenic in a battery of genetic toxicology studies, including the Ames bacterial assay, a mammalian cell forward gene mutation assay (CHO/HPRT and AS52/XPRT), an *in vitro* cytogenetics assay using CHL cells, an unscheduled DNA synthesis assay, and an *in vivo* micronucleus assay.

No adverse effects upon fertility were observed in male and female rats at oral doses up to 40 mg/kg pioglitazone hydrochloride daily prior to and throughout mating and gestation (approximately 9 times the maximum recommended human oral dose based on mg/m^2).

Glimepiride

Studies in rats at doses of up to 5000 ppm in complete feed (approximately 340 times the maximum recommended human dose, based on surface area) for 30 months showed no evidence of carcinogenesis. In mice, administration of glimepiride for 24 months resulted in an increase in benign pancreatic adenoma formation which was dose related and is thought to be the result of chronic pancreatic stimulation. The no-effect dose for adenoma formation in mice in this study was 320 ppm in complete feed, or 46-54 mg/kg body weight/day. This is about 35 times the maximum human recommended dose of 8 mg once daily based on surface area. Glimepiride was non-mutagenic in a battery of *in vitro* and *in vivo* mutagenicity studies (Ames test, somatic cell mutation, chromosomal aberration, unscheduled DNA synthesis, mouse micronucleus test).

There was no effect of glimepiride on male mouse fertility in animals exposed up to 2500 mg/kg body weight (>1,700 times the maximum recommended human dose based on surface area). Glimepiride had no effect on the fertility of male and female rats administered up to 4000 mg/kg body weight (approximately 4,000 times the maximum recommended human dose based on surface area).

Animal Toxicology

Pioglitazone hydrochloride

Heart enlargement has been observed in mice (100 mg/kg), rats (4 mg/kg and above) and dogs (3 mg/kg) treated orally with pioglitazone hydrochloride (approximately 11, 1, and 2 times the maximum recommended human oral dose for mice, rats, and dogs, respectively, based on mg/m^2). In a one-year rat study, drug-related early death due to apparent heart dysfunction occurred at an oral dose of 160 mg/kg/day (approximately 35 times the maximum recommended human oral dose based on mg/m^2). Heart enlargement was seen in a 13-week study in monkeys at oral doses of 8.9 mg/kg and above (approximately 4 times the maximum recommended human oral dose based on mg/m^2), but not in a 52-week study at oral doses up to 32 mg/kg (approximately 13 times the maximum recommended human oral dose based on mg/m^2).

Glimepiride

Reduced serum glucose values and degranulation of the pancreatic beta cells were observed in beagle dogs exposed to 320 mg glimepiride/kg/day for 12 months (approximately 1,000 times the recommended human dose based on surface area). No evidence of tumor formation was observed in any organ. One female and one male dog developed bilateral subcapsular cataracts. Non-GLP studies indicated that glimepiride was unlikely to exacerbate cataract formation. Evaluation of the co-cataractogenic potential of glimepiride in several diabetic and cataract rat models was negative and there was no adverse effect of glimepiride on bovine ocular lens metabolism in organ culture.

Pregnancy

Pregnancy Category C

DUETACT

Because current information strongly suggests that abnormal blood glucose levels during pregnancy are associated with a higher incidence of congenital anomalies, as well as increased neonatal morbidity and mortality, most experts recommend that insulin be used during pregnancy to maintain blood glucose levels as close to normal as possible. DUETACT should not be used during pregnancy unless the potential benefit justifies the potential risk to the fetus.

There are no adequate and well-controlled studies in pregnant women with DUETACT or its individual components. No animal studies have been conducted with the combined products in DUETACT. The following data are based on findings in studies performed with pioglitazone or glimepiride individually.

Pioglitazone hydrochloride

Pioglitazone was not teratogenic in rats at oral doses up to 80 mg/kg or in rabbits given up to 160 mg/kg during organogenesis (approximately 17 and 40 times the maximum recommended human oral dose based on mg/m^2, respectively). Delayed parturition and embryotoxicity (as evidenced by increased postimplantation losses, delayed development and reduced fetal weights) were observed in rats at oral doses of 40 mg/kg/day and above (approximately 10 times the maximum recommended human oral dose based on mg/m^2). No functional or behavioral toxicity was observed in offspring of rats. In rabbits, embryotoxicity was observed at an oral dose of 160 mg/kg (approximately 40 times the maximum recommended human oral dose based on mg/m^2). Delayed postnatal development, attributed to decreased body weight, was observed in offspring of rats at oral doses of 10 mg/kg and above during late gestation and lactation periods (approximately 2 times the maximum recommended human oral dose based on mg/m^2).

Glimepiride

Teratogenic Effects: Glimepiride did not produce teratogenic effects in rats exposed orally up to 4000 mg/kg body weight (approximately 4,000 times the maximum recommended human dose based on surface area) or in rabbits exposed up to 32 mg/kg body weight (approximately 60 times the maximum recommended human dose based on surface area). Glimepiride has been shown to be associated with intrauterine fetal death in rats when given in doses as low as 50 times the human dose based on surface area and in rabbits when given in doses as low as 0.1 times the human dose based on surface area. This fetotoxicity, observed only at doses inducing maternal hypoglycemia, has been similarly noted with other sulfonylureas, and is believed to be directly related to the pharmacologic (hypoglycemic) action of glimepiride.

Nonteratogenic Effects: In some studies in rats, offspring of dams exposed to high levels of glimepiride during pregnancy and lactation developed skeletal deformities consisting of shortening, thickening, and bending of the humerus during the postnatal period. Significant concentrations of glimepiride were observed in the serum and breast milk of the dams as well as in the serum of the pups. These skeletal deformations were determined to be the result of nursing from mothers exposed to glimepiride.

Prolonged severe hypoglycemia (4 to 10 days) has been reported in neonates born to mothers who were receiving a sulfonylurea drug at the time of delivery. This has been reported more frequently with the use of agents with prolonged half-lives. Patients who are planning a pregnancy should consult their physician, and it is recommended that they change over to insulin for the entire course of pregnancy and lactation.

Nursing Mothers

No studies have been conducted with the combined components of DUETACT. In studies performed with the individual components, pioglitazone was secreted in the milk of lactating rats and significant concentrations of glimepiride were observed in the serum and breast milk of the dams and serum of the pups. It is not known whether pioglitazone or glimepiride are secreted in human milk. However, other sulfonylureas are excreted in human milk. Because the potential for hypoglycemia in nursing infants may exist, and because of the effects on nursing animals, DUETACT should not be administered to a woman breastfeeding. If DUETACT is discontinued, and if diet alone is inadequate for controlling blood glucose, insulin therapy should be considered (see **PRECAUTIONS, Pregnancy: Pregnancy Category C,** *Glimepiride*, Nonteratogenic Effects).

Pediatric Use

Safety and effectiveness of DUETACT in pediatric patients have not been established.

Elderly Use

Pioglitazone hydrochloride

Approximately 500 patients in placebo-controlled clinical trials of pioglitazone were 65 and over. No significant differences in effectiveness and safety were observed between these patients and younger patients.

Glimepiride

In U.S. clinical studies of glimepiride, 608 of 1986 patients were 65 and over. No overall differences in safety or effectiveness were observed between these subjects and younger subjects, but greater sensitivity of some older individuals cannot be ruled out.

Comparison of glimepiride pharmacokinetics in patients with type 2 diabetes ≤65 years (n=49) and those >65 years (n=42) was performed in a study using a dosing regimen of 6 mg daily. There were no significant differences in glimepiride pharmacokinetics between the two age groups (see **CLINICAL PHARMACOLOGY, Special Populations, Elderly:** *Glimepiride*).

Glimepiride is known to be substantially excreted by the kidney, and the risk of toxic reactions to this drug may be greater in patients with impaired renal function. Because elderly patients are more likely to have decreased renal function, care should be taken in dose selection, and it may be useful to monitor renal function.

Elderly patients are particularly susceptible to hypoglycemic action of glucose-lowering drugs. In elderly, debilitated, or malnourished patients, or in patients with renal and hepatic insufficiency, the initial dosing, dose increments, and maintenance dosage should be conservative based upon blood glucose levels prior to and after initiation of treatment to avoid hypoglycemic reactions. Hypoglycemia may be difficult to recognize in the elderly and in people who are taking beta-adrenergic blocking drugs or other sympatholytic agents (see **CLINICAL PHARMACOLOGY, Special Populations, Renal Insufficiency:** *Glimepiride*; **PRECAUTIONS, General:** ***Glimepiride***, Hypoglycemia and **DOSAGE AND ADMINISTRATION, Special Patient Populations**).

ADVERSE REACTIONS

The adverse events reported in at least 5% of patients in the controlled 16-week clinical studies between placebo plus a sulfonylurea and pioglitazone (15 mg and 30 mg combined) plus sulfonylurea-treatment arms were upper respiratory tract infection (15.5% and 16.6%), accidental injury (8.6% and 3.5%) and combined edema/peripheral edema (2.1% and 7.2%), respectively.

The incidence and type of adverse events reported in at least 5% of patients in any combined treatment group from the 24-week study comparing pioglitazone 30 mg plus a sulfonylurea and pioglitazone 45 mg plus a sulfonylurea are shown in Table 4; the rate of adverse events resulting in study discontinuation between the two treatment groups was 6.0% and 9.7%, respectively.

Table 4. Adverse Events That Occurred in ≥ 5% of Patients in Any Treatment Group During the 24-Week Study

Adverse Event	Pioglitazone 30 mg + sulfonylurea N=351 n (%)	Pioglitazone 45 mg + sulfonylurea N=351 n (%)
Hypoglycemia	47 (13.4)	55 (15.7)
Upper Respiratory Tract Infection	43 (12.3)	52 (14.8)
Weight Increased	32 (9.1)	47 (13.4)
Edema Lower Limb	20 (5.7)	43 (12.3)
Headache	25 (7.1)	14 (4.0)
Urinary Tract Infection	20 (5.7)	24 (6.8)
Diarrhea	21 (6.0)	15 (4.3)
Nausea	18 (5.1)	14 (4.0)
Pain in Limb	19 (5.4)	14 (4.0)

In U.S. double-blind studies, anemia was reported in ≤ 2% of patients treated with pioglitazone plus a sulfonylurea (see **PRECAUTIONS, General:** ***Pioglitazone hydrochloride***).

Pioglitazone hydrochloride

Over 8500 patients with type 2 diabetes have been treated with pioglitazone in randomized, double-blind, controlled clinical trials. This includes 2605 high-risk patients with type 2 diabetes treated with pioglitazone from the PROactive clinical trial. Over 6000 patients have been treated for 6 months or longer, and over 4500 patients for one year or longer. Over 3000 patients have received pioglitazone for at least 2 years.

Most clinical adverse events were similar between groups treated with pioglitazone in combination with a sulfonylurea and those treated with pioglitazone monotherapy. Other adverse events reported in at least 5% of patients in controlled clinical studies between placebo and pioglitazone monotherapy included myalgia (2.7% and 5.4%), tooth disorder (2.3% and 5.3%), diabetes mellitus aggravated (8.1% and 5.1%) and pharyngitis (0.8% and 5.1%), respectively.

In monotherapy studies, edema was reported for 4.8% (with doses from 7.5 mg to 45 mg) of patients treated with pioglitazone versus 1.2% of placebo-treated patients. Most of these events were considered mild or moderate in intensity (see **PRECAUTIONS, General:** ***Pioglitazone hydrochloride***, Edema).

Prospective Pioglitazone Clinical Trial In Macrovascular Events (PROactive)

In PROactive, 5238 patients with type 2 diabetes and a prior history of macrovascular disease were treated with ACTOS (n=2605), force-titrated up to 45 mg daily, or placebo (n=2633), in addition to standard of care. Almost all subjects (95%) were receiving cardiovascular medications (beta blockers, ACE inhibitors, ARBs, calcium channel blockers, nitrates, diuretics, aspirin, statins, fibrates). Patients had a mean age of 61.8 years, mean duration of diabetes 9.5 years, and mean A1C 8.1%. Average duration of follow-up was 34.5 months. The primary objective of this trial was to examine the effect of ACTOS on mortality and macrovascular morbidity in patients with type 2 diabetes mellitus who were at high risk for macrovascular events. The primary efficacy variable was the time to the first occurrence of any event in the cardiovascular composite endpoint (see table 5 below). Although there was no statistically significant difference between ACTOS and placebo for the 3-year incidence of a first event within this composite, there was no increase in mortality or in total macrovascular events with ACTOS.

[See table 5 at top of next page]

Postmarketing reports of new onset or worsening diabetic macular edema with decreased visual acuity have also been received (see **PRECAUTIONS, General:** ***Pioglitazone hydrochloride***).

Glimepiride

Adverse events that occurred in controlled clinical trials with placebo and glimepiride monotherapy, other than hypoglycemia, headache and nausea, also included dizziness (0.3% and 1.7%) and asthenia (1.0% and 1.6%), respectively.

Gastrointestinal Reactions: Vomiting, gastrointestinal pain, and diarrhea have been reported with glimepiride, but the incidence in placebo-controlled trials was less than 1%. In rare cases, there may be an elevation of liver enzyme levels. In isolated instances, impairment of liver function (e.g. with cholestasis and jaundice), as well as hepatitis, which may also lead to liver failure have been reported with sulfonylureas, including glimepiride.

Dermatologic Reactions: Allergic skin reactions, e.g., pruritus, erythema, urticaria, and morbilliform or maculopapular eruptions, occur in less than 1% of glimepiride-treated patients. These may be transient and may disappear despite continued use of glimepiride. If those hypersensitivity reactions persist or worsen, the drug should be discontinued. Porphyria cutanea tarda, photosensitivity reactions, and allergic vasculitis have been reported with sulfonylureas.

Metabolic Reactions: Hepatic porphyria reactions and disulfiram-like reactions have been reported with sulfonylureas; however, no cases have yet been reported with glimepiride tablets. Cases of hyponatremia have been reported with glimepiride and all other sulfonylureas, most often in patients who are on other medications or have medical conditions known to cause hyponatremia or increase release of antidiuretic hormone. The syndrome of inappropriate antidiuretic hormone (SIADH) secretion has been reported with certain other sulfonylureas, and it has been suggested that these sulfonylureas may augment the peripheral (antidiuretic) action of ADH and/or increase release of ADH.

Hematologic Reactions: Leukopenia, agranulocytosis, thrombocytopenia, hemolytic anemia, aplastic anemia, and pancytopenia have been reported with sulfonylureas.

Other Reactions: Changes in accommodation and/or blurred vision may occur with the use of glimepiride. In placebo-controlled trials of glimepiride, the incidence of blurred vision with placebo was 0.7%, and with glimepiride, 0.4%. This is thought to be due to changes in blood glucose, and may be more pronounced when treatment is initiated. This condition is also seen in untreated diabetic patients, and may actually be reduced by treatment.

Laboratory Abnormalities

Pioglitazone hydrochloride

Hematologic: Pioglitazone may cause decreases in hemoglobin and hematocrit. The fall in hemoglobin and hematocrit with pioglitazone appears to be dose related. Across all clinical studies, mean hemoglobin values declined by 2% to 4% in patients treated with pioglitazone. These changes generally occurred within the first 4 to 12 weeks of therapy and remained relatively stable thereafter. These changes may be related to increased plasma volume associated with pioglitazone therapy and have rarely been associated with any significant hematologic clinical effects (see **PRECAUTIONS, General:** ***Pioglitazone hydrochloride***, Hematologic).

Serum Transaminase Levels: During all clinical studies in the U.S., 14 of 4780 (0.30%) patients treated with pioglitazone had ALT values ≥ 3 times the upper limit of normal during treatment. All patients with follow-up values had reversible elevations in ALT. In the population of patients treated with pioglitazone, mean values for bilirubin, AST, ALT, alkaline phosphatase, and GGT were decreased at the final visit compared with baseline. Fewer than 0.9% of patients treated with pioglitazone were withdrawn from clinical trials in the U.S. due to abnormal liver function tests.

In pre-approval clinical trials, there were no cases of idiosyncratic drug reactions leading to hepatic failure (see **PRECAUTIONS, General:** ***Pioglitazone hydrochloride***, Hepatic Effects).

CPK Levels: During required laboratory testing in clinical trials with pioglitazone, sporadic, transient elevations in creatine phosphokinase levels (CPK) were observed. An isolated elevation to greater than 10 times the upper limit of normal was noted in 9 patients (values of 2150 to 11400 IU/L). Six of these patients continued to receive pioglitazone, two patients had completed receiving study medication at the time of the elevated value and one patient discontinued study medication due to the elevation. These elevations resolved without any apparent clinical sequelae. The relationship of these events to pioglitazone therapy is unknown.

OVERDOSAGE

Pioglitazone hydrochloride

During controlled clinical trials, one case of overdose with pioglitazone was reported. A male patient took 120 mg per day for four days, then 180 mg per day for seven days. The patient denied any clinical symptoms during this period.

In the event of overdosage, appropriate supportive treatment should be initiated according to patient's clinical signs and symptoms.

Glimepiride

Overdosage of sulfonylureas, including glimepiride, can produce hypoglycemia. Mild hypoglycemic symptoms without loss of consciousness or neurologic findings should be treated aggressively with oral glucose and adjustments in drug dosage and/or meal patterns. Close monitoring should continue until the physician is assured that the patient is out of danger. Severe hypoglycemic reactions with coma, seizure, or other neurological impairment occur infrequently, but constitute medical emergencies requiring immediate hospitalization. If hypoglycemic coma is diagnosed or suspected, the patient should be given a rapid intravenous injection of concentrated (50%) glucose solution. This should be followed by a continuous infusion of a more dilute (10%) glucose solution at a rate that will maintain the blood glucose at a level above 100 mg/dL. Patients should be closely monitored for a minimum of 24 to 48 hours, because hypoglycemia may recur after apparent clinical recovery.

DOSAGE AND ADMINISTRATION

General

The use of antihyperglycemic therapy in the management of type 2 diabetes should be individualized on the basis of effectiveness and tolerability. Failure to follow an appropriate dosage regimen may precipitate hypoglycemia.

Dosage Recommendations

Selecting the starting dose of DUETACT should be based on the patient's current regimen of pioglitazone and/or sulfonylurea. Those patients who may be more sensitive to antihyperglycemic drugs should be monitored carefully during dose adjustment. After initiation of DUETACT, patients should be carefully monitored for adverse events related to fluid retention (see **BOXED WARNING** and **WARNINGS,** ***Pioglitazone hydrochloride***). It is recommended that a single dose of DUETACT be administered once daily with the first main meal.

Table 5. Number of First and Total Events for Each Component within the Cardiovascular Composite Endpoint

Cardiovascular Events	Placebo N=2633		ACTOS N=2605	
	First Events (N)	Total events (N)	First Events (N)	Total events (N)
Any event	572	900	514	803
All-cause mortality	122	186	110	177
Non-fatal MI	118	157	105	131
Stroke	96	119	76	92
ACS	63	78	42	65
Cardiac intervention	101	240	101	195
Major leg amputation	15	28	9	28
Leg revascularization	57	92	71	115

Starting dose for patients currently on glimepiride monotherapy

Based on the usual starting dose of pioglitazone (15 mg or 30 mg daily), DUETACT may be initiated at 30 mg/2 mg or 30 mg/4 mg tablet strengths once daily, and adjusted after assessing adequacy of therapeutic response.

For patients with type 2 diabetes and systolic dysfunction, see **DOSAGE AND ADMINISTRATION, Special Patient Populations.**

Starting dose for patients currently on pioglitazone monotherapy

Based on the usual starting doses of glimepiride (1 mg or 2 mg once daily), and pioglitazone 15 mg or 30 mg, DUETACT may be initiated at 30 mg/2 mg once daily, and adjusted after assessing adequacy of therapeutic response.

For patients who are not currently on glimepiride and may be more sensitive to hypoglycemia, see **DOSAGE AND ADMINISTRATION, Special Patient Populations.**

Starting dose for patients switching from combination therapy of pioglitazone plus glimepiride as separate tablets

DUETACT may be initiated with 30 mg/2 mg or 30 mg/4 mg tablet strengths based on the dose of pioglitazone and glimepiride already being taken. Patients who are not controlled with 15 mg of pioglitazone in combination with glimepiride should be carefully monitored when switched to DUETACT.

Starting dose for patients currently on a different sulfonylurea monotherapy or switching from combination therapy of pioglitazone plus a different sulfonylurea (e.g. glyburide, glipizide, chlorpropamide, tolbutamide, acetohexamide)

No exact dosage relationship exists between glimepiride and the other sulfonylurea agents. Therefore, based on the maximum starting dose of 2 mg glimepiride, DUETACT should be limited initially to a starting dose of 30 mg/2 mg once daily, and adjusted after assessing adequacy of therapeutic response.

Any change in diabetic therapy should be undertaken with care and appropriate monitoring as changes in glycemic control can occur. Patients should be observed carefully for hypoglycemia (1-2 weeks) when being transferred to DUETACT, especially from longer half-life sulfonylureas (e.g. chlorpropamide) due to potential overlapping of drug effect.

Sufficient time should be given to assess adequacy of therapeutic response. Ideally, the response to therapy should be evaluated using A1C, which is a better indicator of long-term glycemic control than FPG alone. A1C reflects glycemia over the past two to three months. In clinical use, it is recommended that patients be treated with DUETACT for a period of time adequate to evaluate change in A1C (8-12 weeks) unless glycemic control as measured by FPG deteriorates.

Special Patient Populations

DUETACT is not recommended for use in pregnancy, nursing mothers or for use in pediatric patients.

In elderly, debilitated, or malnourished patients, or in patients with renal or hepatic insufficiency, the initial dosing, dose increments, and maintenance dosage of DUETACT should be conservative to avoid hypoglycemic reactions. These patients should be started at 1 mg of glimepiride prior to prescribing DUETACT. During initiation of DUETACT therapy and any subsequent dose adjustment, patients should be observed carefully for hypoglycemia (see **PRECAUTIONS, General:** ***Glimepiride***, Hypoglycemia).

Therapy with DUETACT should not be initiated if the patient exhibits clinical evidence of active liver disease or increased serum transaminase levels (ALT greater than 2.5 times the upper limit of normal) at start of therapy (see **PRECAUTIONS, General:** ***Pioglitazone hydrochloride***, Hepatic Effects and **CLINICAL PHARMACOLOGY, Special Populations, Hepatic Insufficiency:** *Pioglitazone hydrochloride*). Liver enzyme monitoring is recommended in all patients prior to initiation of therapy with DUETACT and periodically thereafter (see **PRECAUTIONS, General:** ***Pioglitazone hydrochloride***, Hepatic Effects and **PRECAUTIONS, Laboratory Tests**).

The lowest approved dose of DUETACT therapy should be prescribed to patients with type 2 diabetes and systolic dysfunction only after titration from 15 mg to 30 mg of pioglitazone has been safely tolerated. If subsequent dose adjustment is necessary, patients should be carefully monitored for weight gain, edema, or signs and symptoms of CHF exacerbation (see **WARNINGS,** ***Pioglitazone hydrochloride*****, Cardiac Failure and Other Cardiac Effects**).

Maximum Recommended Dose

DUETACT tablets are available as a 30 mg pioglitazone plus 2 mg glimepiride or a 30 mg pioglitazone plus 4 mg glimepiride formulation for oral administration. The maximum recommended daily dose for pioglitazone is 45 mg and the maximum recommended daily dose for glimepiride is 8 mg.

DUETACT should therefore not be given more than once daily at any of the tablet strengths.

HOW SUPPLIED

DUETACT is available in 30 mg pioglitazone plus 2 mg glimepiride or 30 mg pioglitazone plus 4 mg glimepiride tablets as follows:

30 mg/2 mg tablet: white to off-white, round, convex, uncoated tablet, debossed with 30/2 on one side and 4833G on the other, available in:

NDC 64764-302-30 Bottles of 30

NDC 64764-302-90 Bottles of 90

30 mg/4 mg tablet: white to off-white, round, convex, uncoated tablet, debossed with 30/4 on one side and 4833G on the other, available in:

NDC 64764-304-30 Bottles of 30

NDC 64764-304-90 Bottles of 90

STORAGE

Store at 25°C (77°F); excursions permitted to 15-30°C (59-86°F) [see USP Controlled Room Temperature]. Keep container tightly closed and protect from moisture and humidity.

REFERENCES

1. Deng, LJ, et al. Effect of gemfibrozil on the pharmacokinetics of pioglitazone. Eur J Clin Pharmacol 2005; 61: 831-836, Table 1.
2. Jaakkola, T, et al. Effect of rifampicin on the pharmacokinetics of pioglitazone. Br J Clin Pharmacol 2006; 61:1 70-78.

HUMAN OPHTHALMOLOGY DATA

Glimepiride

Ophthalmic examinations were carried out in over 500 subjects during long-term studies using the methodology of Taylor and West and Laties et al. No significant differences were seen between glimepiride and glyburide in the number of subjects with clinically important changes in visual acuity, intraocular tension, or in any of the five lens-related variables examined.

Ophthalmic examinations were carried out during long-term studies using the method of Chylack et al. No significant or clinically meaningful differences were seen between glimepiride and glipizide with respect to cataract progression by subjective LOCS II grading and objective image analysis systems, visual acuity, intraocular pressure, and general ophthalmic examination.

Rx only

ACTOS® and DUETACT® are registered trademarks of Takeda Pharmaceutical Company Limited and used under license by Takeda Pharmaceuticals America, Inc.

Distributed by:
Takeda Pharmaceuticals America, Inc.
Deerfield, IL 60015
© 2006, 2009 Takeda Pharmaceuticals America, Inc.
July 2009
DTA0709-R2

MEDICATION GUIDE

DUETACT® (doo-et' -ăct)
(pioglitazone hydrochloride and glimepiride) tablets

Read this Medication Guide carefully before you start taking DUETACT and each time you get a refill. There may be new information. This information does not take the place of talking with your doctor about your medical condition or your treatment. If you have any questions about DUETACT, ask your doctor or pharmacist.

What is the most important information I should know about DUETACT?

DUETACT can cause serious side effects, including **new or worse heart failure.**

- Pioglitazone, one of the medicines in DUETACT, can cause your body to keep extra fluid (fluid retention), which leads to swelling (edema) and weight gain. Extra body fluid can make some heart problems worse or lead to heart failure. Heart failure means your heart does not pump blood well enough.
- If you have severe heart failure, you cannot start DUETACT.
- If you have heart failure with symptoms (such as shortness of breath or swelling), even if these symptoms are not severe, DUETACT may not be right for you.

Call your doctor right away if you have any of the following:

- swelling or fluid retention, especially in the ankles or legs.
- shortness of breath or trouble breathing, especially when you lie down.
- an unusually fast increase in weight.
- unusual tiredness.

DUETACT can have other serious side effects. See "What are the possible side effects of DUETACT?"

What is DUETACT?

DUETACT is a prescription medicine used with diet and exercise to improve blood sugar (glucose) control in adults with type 2 diabetes.

DUETACT contains 2 prescription diabetes medicines called, pioglitazone hydrochloride (ACTOS) and glimepiride, a sulfonylurea.

Your doctor will decide if you should take DUETACT.

It is important to eat the right foods, lose weight if needed, and exercise regularly in order to manage your type 2 diabetes. Diet, weight loss, and exercise are the main treatments for type 2 diabetes and they also help your diabetes medicines work better for you.

DUETACT has not been studied in children and is not recommended for children under the age of 18. The risks of giving DUETACT to a child are not known. See "What are some other possible side effects of DUETACT?"

Who should not take DUETACT?

Do not take DUETACT if you:

- are allergic to any of the ingredients in DUETACT. See the end of this Medication Guide for a complete list of ingredients in DUETACT.
- have a condition called diabetic ketoacidosis. Diabetic ketoacidosis should be treated with insulin.

People with severe heart failure should not start taking DUETACT. See "What is the most important information I should know about DUETACT?".

What should I tell my doctor before taking DUETACT?

Before starting DUETACT, ask your doctor about what the choices are for diabetes medicines and what the expected benefits and possible risks are for you in particular.

Tell your doctor about all of your medical conditions, especially if you:

- **have heart failure.**
- **have kidney problems.**
- **have type 1 ("juvenile") diabetes or had diabetic ketoacidosis.** These conditions should be treated with insulin.
- **have a type of diabetic eye disease called macular edema** (swelling of the back of the eye).
- **have liver problems.** Your doctor should do blood tests to check your liver before you start taking DUETACT and during treatment as needed.
- **are pregnant or planning to become pregnant.** DUETACT should not be used during pregnancy. It is not known if DUETACT can harm your unborn baby. Talk to your doctor about the best way to control your blood glucose levels while pregnant.
- **are a premenopausal woman (before the "change of life"), who does not have periods regularly or at all.** DUETACT may increase your chance of becoming pregnant. Talk to your doctor about birth control choices while taking DUETACT. Tell your doctor right away if you become pregnant while taking DUETACT.
- **are breastfeeding or plan to breastfeed.** It is not known if DUETACT passes into your milk and if it can harm your baby. You should not take DUETACT if you breastfeed your baby. Talk to your doctor about the best way to control your blood glucose levels while breastfeeding.
- **have G6PD deficiency** (an inherited condition where you don't produce enough of the enzyme (G6PD). Taking glimepiride, one of the medicines in DUETACT, with this condition may cause your red blood cells to be destroyed too quickly (hemolytic anemia).

Tell your doctor about all the medicines you take including prescription and non-prescription medicines, vitamins, and herbal supplements. DUETACT and some of your other medicines can affect each other. You may need to have your dose of DUETACT or certain other medicines adjusted. Certain other medicines can affect your blood sugar (glucose) control.

Know the medicines you take. Keep a list of your medicines and show it to your doctor and pharmacist before you start a new medicine. They will tell you if it is okay to take DUETACT with other medicines.

How should I take DUETACT?

- Take DUETACT exactly as prescribed.
- Your doctor may need to change your dose of DUETACT to control your blood glucose. Do not change your dose unless told to do so by your doctor.
- DUETACT may be prescribed alone or with other diabetes medicines. This will depend on how well your blood sugar is controlled.
- Take DUETACT one time each day with the first meal.
- If you miss a dose of DUETACT, take your next dose as prescribed unless your doctor tells you differently. Do not take two doses at one time the next day.
- If you take too much DUETACT, call your doctor or poison control center right away.
- If your body is under stress, for example: due to fever, infection, trauma (such as a car accident), or surgery, the dose of your diabetes medicines may need to be changed. Call your doctor right away.
- Stay on your diet and exercise programs and test your blood sugar regularly while taking DUETACT.
- Your doctor should do blood tests before starting DUETACT and from time to time to check your liver, kidneys, and blood cells.
- Your doctor should also do regular blood tests (for example, hemoglobin A1C) to check how well your blood sugar is controlled with DUETACT.
- Your doctor should check your eyes regularly. Some people have had vision changes due to swelling in the back of the eye, called macular edema, while taking DUETACT.
- It may take 2-3 months to see the full effect on your blood sugar level.

What are other possible side effects of DUETACT?

DUETACT can cause other serious side effects including:

- **The chance of death from serious heart or blood vessel problems may be higher** when using a sulfonylurea, an ingredient in DUETACT. The risk may be higher when compared to using diet alone or diet and insulin to control blood sugar levels.
- **Low blood sugar (hypoglycemia).** Lightheadedness, dizziness, shakiness, or hunger may indicate that your blood sugar is too low. This can happen if you skip meals, if you use another medicine that lowers blood sugar, or if you have certain medical problems. Call your doctor if low blood sugar levels are a problem for you.
- **Weight gain.** Pioglitazone, one of the medicines in DUETACT, can cause weight gain that may be due to fluid retention or extra body fat. Weight gain due to fluid retention can be a serious problem for people with certain heart problems. See "What is the most important information I should know about DUETACT?".
- **Liver problems.** It is important for your liver to be working normally when you take DUETACT. Your doctor should do blood tests to check your liver before you start taking DUETACT and during treatment as needed. Call your doctor right away if you have unexplained symptoms such as:
  - nausea or vomiting.
  - stomach pain.
  - unusual or unexplained tiredness.
  - loss of appetite.
  - dark urine.
  - yellowing of your skin or the whites of your eyes.
- **Macular edema** (diabetic eye disease with swelling in the back of the eye). Tell your doctor right away if you have any changes in your vision. Your doctor should check your eyes regularly.
- **Fractures (broken bones),** usually in the hand, upper arm, or foot in women. Talk to your doctor for advice on how to keep your bones healthy. It is not known if DUETACT can affect the bones of children.
- **Low red blood cell count (anemia).**
- **Ovulation** (release of an egg from an ovary in a woman) leading to pregnancy. Ovulation may happen when premenopausal women who do not have regular monthly periods take DUETACT. This can increase the chance of pregnancy. See "What should I tell my doctor before taking DUETACT?".

In studies of pioglitazone (one of the medicines in DUETACT), bladder cancer occurred in a few more people who were taking pioglitazone than in people who were taking other diabetes medicines. There were too few cases to know if the bladder cancer was related to pioglitazone.

Other common side effects of DUETACT are:

- cold-like symptoms (upper respiratory infection),
- headache,
- urinary tract infection,
- diarrhea,
- nausea,
- arm or leg pain.

Tell your doctor if you have any side effect that bothers you or that does not go away. These are not all the side effects of DUETACT. For more information, ask your doctor or pharmacist.

Call your doctor for medical advice about side effects. You may report side effects to FDA at 1-800-FDA-1088.

How should I store DUETACT?

- Store DUETACT at 59° to 86°F (15° to 30°C). Keep DUETACT in the original container to protect from light.
- Keep the DUETACT bottle tightly closed and protect from getting wet (away from moisture and humidity).

Keep DUETACT and all medicines out of the reach of children.

General information about DUETACT

Medicines are sometimes prescribed for purposes other than those listed in a Medication Guide. Do not use DUETACT for a condition for which it is not prescribed. Do not give DUETACT to other people, even if they have the same symptoms you have. It may harm them.

This Medication Guide summarizes the most important information about DUETACT. If you would like more information, talk with your doctor. You can ask your doctor or pharmacist for information about DUETACT that is written for healthcare professionals. For more information, go to www.duetact.com or call 1-877-825-3327.

What are the ingredients in DUETACT?

Active Ingredients: pioglitazone hydrochloride and glimepiride

Inactive Ingredients: croscarmellose sodium, lactose monohydrate, magnesium stearate, hydroxypropyl cellulose, polysorbate 80, and microcrystalline cellulose.

Always check to make sure that the medicine you are taking is the correct one. DUETACT tablets look like this:

- 30 mg/2 mg strength tablets—white to off-white, round tablet with "30/2" on one side and "4833G" on the other.
- 30 mg/4 mg strength tablets—white to off-white, round tablet with "30/4" on one side and "4833G" on the other.

DUETACT® is a registered trademark of Takeda Pharmaceutical Company Limited and used under license by Takeda Pharmaceuticals America, Inc.

All other trademarks are the property of their respective owners.

This Medication Guide has been approved by the U.S. Food and Drug Administration.

Distributed by:
Takeda Pharmaceuticals America, Inc.
Deerfield, IL 60015
© 2009 Takeda Pharmaceuticals America, Inc.
September 2009
DTA0509-R1/MG

Shown in Product Identification Guide, page 320

ROZEREM® ℞
(ramelteon)
tablet, film coated for oral use

HIGHLIGHTS OF PRESCRIBING INFORMATION

These highlights do not include all the information needed to use ROZEREM safely and effectively. See full prescribing information for ROZEREM.

ROZEREM (ramelteon) tablet, film coated for oral use
Initial U.S. Approval: 2005

RECENT MAJOR CHANGES

Indications and Usage (1) 10/2008
Warnings and Precautions
Severe anaphylactic/anaphylactoid reactions (5.1) 10/2008
Abnormal thinking and behavioral changes (5.3) 10/2008

---INDICATIONS AND USAGE---

ROZEREM is indicated for the treatment of insomnia characterized by difficulty with sleep onset. (1)

---DOSAGE AND ADMINISTRATION---

- Adult dose: 8 mg taken within 30 minutes of going to bed (2.1)
- Should not be taken with or immediately after a high-fat meal (2.1)
- Total daily dose should not exceed 8 mg (2.1)

---DOSAGE FORMS AND STRENGTHS---

8 mg tablets (3)

---CONTRAINDICATIONS---

- History of angioedema while taking ROZEREM (4)
- Fluvoxamine (strong CYP1A2 inhibitor): Increases AUC for ramelteon and should not be used in combination (7.1)

---WARNINGS AND PRECAUTIONS---

- Severe anaphylactic/anaphylactoid reactions: Angioedema and anaphylaxis have been reported. Do not rechallenge if such reactions occur. (5.1)
- Need to evaluate for co-morbid diagnoses: Reevaluate if insomnia persists after 7 to 10 days of treatment. (5.2)
- Abnormal thinking, behavioral changes, complex behaviors: May include "sleep-driving" and hallucinations. Immediately evaluate any new onset behavioral changes. (5.3)
- Depression: Worsening of depression or suicidal thinking may occur. (5.3)
- CNS effects: Potential impairment of activities requiring complete mental alertness such as operating machinery or driving a motor vehicle, after ingesting the drug. (5.4)
- Reproductive effects: Include decreased testosterone and increased prolactin levels. Effect on reproductive axis in developing humans is unknown. (5.5)
- Patients with severe sleep apnea: Rozerem is not recommended for use in this population. (5.6)

---ADVERSE REACTIONS---

- Most common adverse reactions (≥3% and more common than with placebo) are: somnolence, dizziness, fatigue, nausea, and exacerbated insomnia. (6.1)

To report SUSPECTED ADVERSE REACTIONS, contact Takeda Pharmaceuticals America, Inc. at 1-877-TAKEDA-7 or FDA at 1-800-FDA-1088 or www.fda.gov/medwatch

---DRUG INTERACTIONS---

- Rifampin (strong CYP enzyme inducer): Decreases exposure to and effects of ramelteon. (7.1)
- Ketoconazole (strong CYP3A4 inhibitor): Increases AUC for ramelteon; administer with caution. (7.1)
- Fluconazole (strong CYP2C9 inhibitor): Increases systemic exposure of ramelteon; administer with caution. (7.1)
- Alcohol: Causes additive psychomotor impairment; should not be used in combination. (7.2)

---USE IN SPECIFIC POPULATIONS---

- Pregnancy: Based on animal data may cause fetal harm. Do not use unless the potential benefit justifies the potential risk. (8.1)
- Nursing mothers: Use with caution. (8.3)
- Pediatric use: Safety and effectiveness not established. (8.4)
- Geriatric use: No overall differences in safety and efficacy between elderly and younger adult subjects. (8.5)
- Hepatic impairment: Is not recommended in patients with severe impairment; use with caution in moderate impairment. (8.8)

See 17 for PATIENT COUNSELING INFORMATION and Medication Guide

Revised: 07/2009

FULL PRESCRIBING INFORMATION: CONTENTS*

* Sections or subsections omitted from the full prescribing information are not listed

FULL PRESCRIBING INFORMATION

1   INDICATIONS AND USAGE

ROZEREM is indicated for the treatment of insomnia characterized by difficulty with sleep onset.

The clinical trials performed in support of efficacy were up to 6 months in duration. The final formal assessments of sleep latency were performed after 2 days of treatment during the crossover study (elderly only), at 5 weeks in the 6-week study (adults and elderly), and at the end of the 6-month study (adults and elderly) [see Clinical Studies (14)].

2   DOSAGE AND ADMINISTRATION

2.1   Dosage in Adults

The recommended dose of ROZEREM is 8 mg taken within 30 minutes of going to bed. It is recommended that ROZEREM not be taken with or immediately after a high-fat meal.

The total ROZEREM dose should not exceed 8 mg per day.

2.2   Dosing in Patients with Hepatic Impairment

ROZEREM is not recommended in patients with severe hepatic impairment. ROZEREM should be used with caution in patients with moderate hepatic impairment [see Warnings and Precautions (5.6), Clinical Pharmacology (12.4)].

2.3   Administration with Other Medications

ROZEREM should not be used in combination with fluvoxamine. ROZEREM should be used with caution in patients taking other CYP1A2 inhibiting drugs [see Drug Interactions (7), Clinical Pharmacology (12.5)].

3   DOSAGE FORMS AND STRENGTHS

ROZEREM is available in an 8 mg strength tablet for oral administration.

ROZEREM 8 mg tablets are round, pale orange-yellow, film-coated, with "TAK" and "RAM-8" printed on one side.

4   CONTRAINDICATIONS

Patients who develop angioedema after treatment with ROZEREM should not be rechallenged with the drug. Patients should not take ROZEREM in conjunction with fluvoxamine (Luvox) [see Drug Interactions (7)].

5   WARNINGS AND PRECAUTIONS

5.1   Severe Anaphylactic and Anaphylactoid Reactions

Rare cases of angioedema involving the tongue, glottis or larynx have been reported in patients after taking the first or subsequent doses of ROZEREM. Some patients have had additional symptoms such as dyspnea, throat closing, or nausea and vomiting that suggest anaphylaxis. Some patients have required medical therapy in the emergency department. If angioedema involves the tongue, glottis or larynx, airway obstruction may occur and be fatal. Patients who develop angioedema after treatment with ROZEREM should not be rechallenged with the drug.

5.2   Need to Evaluate for Co-morbid Diagnoses

Since sleep disturbances may be the presenting manifestation of a physical and/or psychiatric disorder, symptomatic treatment of insomnia should be initiated only after a careful evaluation of the patient. The failure of insomnia to remit after 7 to 10 days of treatment may indicate the presence of a primary psychiatric and/or medical illness that should be evaluated. Worsening of insomnia, or the emergence of new cognitive or behavioral abnormalities, may be the result of an unrecognized underlying psychiatric or physical disorder and requires further evaluation of the patient. Exacerbation of insomnia and emergence of cognitive and behavioral abnormalities were seen with ROZEREM during the clinical development program.

5.3   Abnormal Thinking and Behavioral Changes

A variety of cognitive and behavior changes have been reported to occur in association with the use of hypnotics. In primarily depressed patients, worsening of depression (including suicidal ideation and completed suicides) has been reported in association with the use of hypnotics.

Hallucinations, as well as behavioral changes such as bizarre behavior, agitation and mania have been reported with ROZEREM use. Amnesia, anxiety and other neuro-psychiatric symptoms may also occur unpredictably.

Complex behaviors such as "sleep-driving" (i.e., driving while not fully awake after ingestion of a hypnotic) and other complex behaviors (e.g., preparing and eating food, making phone calls, or having sex), with amnesia for the event, have been reported in association with hypnotic use. The use of alcohol and other CNS depressants may increase the risk of such behaviors. These events can occur in hypnotic-naïve as well as in hypnotic-experienced persons. Complex behaviors have been reported with the use of ROZEREM. Discontinuation of ROZEREM should be strongly considered for patients who report any complex sleep behavior.

5.4   CNS Effects

Patients should avoid engaging in hazardous activities that require concentration (such as operating a motor vehicle or heavy machinery) after taking ROZEREM.

After taking ROZEREM, patients should confine their activities to those necessary to prepare for bed.

Patients should be advised not to consume alcohol in combination with ROZEREM as alcohol and ROZEREM may have additive effects when used in conjunction.

5.5   Reproductive Effects

Use in Adolescents and Children

ROZEREM has been associated with an effect on reproductive hormones in adults, e.g., decreased testosterone levels and increased prolactin levels. It is not known what effect chronic or even chronic intermittent use of ROZEREM may have on the reproductive axis in developing humans [see Clinical Trials (14.3)].

5.6   Use in Patients with Concomitant Illness

ROZEREM has not been studied in subjects with severe sleep apnea and is not recommended for use in this population [see Use in Specific Populations (8.7)].

ROZEREM should not be used by patients with severe hepatic impairment [see Clinical Pharmacology (12.4)].

5.7   Laboratory Tests

Monitoring

No standard monitoring is required.

For patients presenting with unexplained amenorrhea, galactorrhea, decreased libido, or problems with fertility, assessment of prolactin levels and testosterone levels should be considered as appropriate.

Interference with laboratory tests

ROZEREM is not known to interfere with commonly used clinical laboratory tests. In addition, in vitro data indicate that ramelteon does not cause false-positive results for benzodiazepines, opiates, barbiturates, cocaine, cannabinoids, or amphetamines in two standard urine drug screening methods in vitro.

6   ADVERSE REACTIONS

The following serious adverse reactions are discussed in greater detail in other sections:

- Severe anaphylactic and anaphylactoid reactions [see Warnings and Precautions (5.1)]
- Abnormal thinking, behavior changes, and complex behaviors [see Warnings and Precautions (5.3)]
- CNS effects [see Warnings and Precautions (5.4)]

6.1   Clinical Trials Experience

Adverse Reactions Resulting in Discontinuation of Treatment

The data described in this section reflect exposure to ROZEREM in 5373 subjects, including 722 exposed for 6 months or longer, and 448 subjects for one year.

Six percent of the 5373 individual subjects exposed to ROZEREM in clinical studies discontinued treatment owing to an adverse event, compared with 2% of the 2279 subjects receiving placebo. The most frequent adverse events leading to discontinuation in subjects receiving ROZEREM were somnolence, dizziness, nausea, fatigue, headache, and insomnia; all of which occurred in 1% of the patients or less.

ROZEREM Most Commonly Observed Adverse Events

Table 1 displays the incidence of adverse events reported by the 2861 patients with chronic insomnia who participated in placebo-controlled trials of ROZEREM.

Because clinical trials are conducted under widely varying conditions, adverse reaction rates observed in the clinical trials of a drug cannot be directly compared to rates in clinical trials of other drugs, and may not reflect the rates observed in practice. The adverse reaction information from clinical trials does, however, provide a basis for identifying the adverse events that appear to be related to drug use and for approximating rates.

Table 1. Incidence (% of subjects) of Treatment-Emergent Adverse Events

MedDRA Preferred Term	Placebo (n=1456)	Ramelteon 8 mg (n=1405)
Somnolence	2%	3%
Fatigue	2%	3%
Dizziness	3%	4%
Nausea	2%	3%
Insomnia exacerbated	2%	3%

7 DRUG INTERACTIONS

7.1 Effects of Other Drugs on ROZEREM

Fluvoxamine (strong CYP1A2 inhibitor): $AUC_{0\text{-}inf}$ for ramelteon increased approximately 190-fold, and the C_{max} increased approximately 70-fold upon coadministration of fluvoxamine and ROZEREM, compared to ROZEREM administered alone. ROZEREM should not be used in combination with fluvoxamine *[see Contraindications (4), Clinical Pharmacology (12.5)]*. Other less strong CYP1A2 inhibitors have not been adequately studied. ROZEREM should be administered with caution to patients taking less strong CYP1A2 inhibitors.

Rifampin (strong CYP enzyme inducer): Administration of multiple doses of rifampin once daily for 11 days resulted in a mean decrease of approximately 80% (40% to 90%) in total exposure to ramelteon. Efficacy may be reduced when ROZEREM is used in combination with strong CYP enzyme inducers such as rifampin *[see Clinical Pharmacology (12.5)]*.

Ketoconazole (strong CYP3A4 inhibitor): The $AUC_{0\text{-}inf}$ and C_{max} of ramelteon increased by approximately 84% and 36% upon coadministration of ketoconazole with ROZEREM. ROZEREM should be administered with caution in subjects taking strong CYP3A4 inhibitors such as ketoconazole *[see Clinical Pharmacology (12.5)]*.

Fluconazole (strong CYP2C9 inhibitor): The $AUC_{0\text{-}inf}$ and C_{max} of ramelteon was increased by approximately 150% when ROZEREM was coadministered with fluconazole. ROZEREM should be administered with caution in subjects taking strong CYP2C9 inhibitors such as fluconazole *[see Clinical Pharmacology (12.5)]*.

7.2 Effect of Alcohol on ROZEREM

Alcohol by itself impairs performance and can cause sleepiness. Since the intended effect of ROZEREM is to promote sleep, patients should be cautioned not to consume alcohol when using ROZEREM *[see Clinical Pharmacology (12.5)]*. Use of the products in combination may have an additive effect.

7.3 Drug/Laboratory Test Interactions

ROZEREM is not known to interfere with commonly used clinical laboratory tests. In addition, *in vitro* data indicate that ramelteon does not cause false-positive results for benzodiazepines, opiates, barbiturates, cocaine, cannabinoids, or amphetamines in two standard urine drug screening methods *in vitro*.

8 USE IN SPECIFIC POPULATIONS

8.1 Pregnancy

Pregnancy Category C

In animal studies, ramelteon produced evidence of developmental toxicity, including teratogenic effects, in rats at doses much greater than the recommended human dose (RHD) of 8 mg/day. There are no adequate and well-controlled studies in pregnant women. ROZEREM should be used during pregnancy only if the potential benefit justifies the potential risk to the fetus.

Oral administration of ramelteon (10, 40, 150 or 600 mg/kg/day) to pregnant rats during the period of organogenesis was associated with increased incidences of fetal structural abnormalities (malformations and variations) at doses greater than 40 mg/kg/day. The no-effect dose is approximately 50 times the RHD on a body surface area (mg/m^2) basis. Treatment of pregnant rabbits during the period of organogenesis produced no evidence of embryo-fetal toxicity at oral doses of up to 300 mg/kg/day (or up to 720 times the RHD on a mg/m^2 basis).

When rats were orally administered ramelteon (30, 100, or 300 mg/kg/day) throughout gestation and lactation, growth retardation, developmental delay, and behavioral changes were observed in the offspring at doses greater than 30 mg/kg/day. The no-effect dose is 36 times the RHD on a mg/m^2 basis. Increased incidences of malformation and death among offspring were seen at the highest dose.

8.2 Labor and delivery

The potential effects of ROZEREM on the duration of labor and/or delivery, for either the mother or the fetus, have not been studied. ROZEREM has no established use in labor and delivery.

8.3 Nursing Mothers

It is not known whether ramelteon is secreted into human milk; however ramelteon is secreted into the milk of lactating rats. Because many drugs are excreted into human milk, caution should be exercised when administered to a nursing woman.

8.4 Pediatric Use

Safety and effectiveness of ROZEREM in pediatric patients have not been established. Further study is needed prior to determining that this product may be used safely in prepubescent and pubescent patients.

8.5 Geriatric Use

A total of 654 subjects in double-blind, placebo-controlled, efficacy trials who received ROZEREM were at least 65 years of age; of these, 199 were 75 years of age or older. No overall differences in safety or efficacy were observed between elderly and younger adult subjects.

A double-blind, randomized, placebo-controlled study in elderly subjects with insomnia (n=33) evaluated the effect of a single dose of ROZEREM on balance, mobility, and memory functions after middle of the night awakening. There is no information on the effect of multiple dosing. Night time dosing of ROZEREM 8 mg did not impair middle of the night balance, mobility, or memory functions relative to placebo. The effects on night balance in the elderly cannot be definitively known from this study.

8.6 Chronic Obstructive Pulmonary Disease

The respiratory depressant effect of ROZEREM was evaluated in a crossover design study of subjects (n=26) with mild to moderate COPD after administering a single 16 mg dose or placebo, and in a separate study (n=25), the effects of ROZEREM on respiratory parameters were evaluated after administering an 8 mg dose or placebo in a crossover design to patients with moderate to severe COPD, defined as patients who had forced expiratory volume at one second (FEV_1)/forced vital capacity ratio of <70%, and a FEV_1 <80% of predicted with <12% reversibility to albuterol. Treatment with a single dose of ROZEREM has no demonstrable respiratory depressant effects in subjects with mild to severe COPD, as measured by arterial O2 saturation (SaO2). There is no available information on the respiratory effects of multiple doses of ROZEREM in patients with COPD. The respiratory depressant effects in patients with COPD cannot be definitively known from this study.

8.7 Sleep Apnea

The effects of ROZEREM were evaluated after administering a 16 mg dose or placebo in a crossover design to subjects (n=26) with mild to moderate obstructive sleep apnea. Treatment with ROZEREM 16 mg for one night showed no difference compared with placebo on the Apnea/Hypopnea Index (the primary outcome variable), apnea index, hypopnea index, central apnea index, mixed apnea index, and obstructive apnea index. Treatment with a single dose of ROZEREM does not exacerbate mild to moderate obstructive sleep apnea. There is no available information on the respiratory effects of multiple doses of ROZEREM in patients with sleep apnea. The effects on exacerbation in patients with mild to moderate sleep apnea cannot be definitively known from this study.

ROZEREM has not been studied in subjects with severe obstructive sleep apnea; use of ROZEREM is not recommended in such patients.

8.8 Hepatic Impairment

Exposure to ROZEREM was increased by 4-fold in subjects with mild hepatic impairment and by more than 10-fold in subjects with moderate hepatic impairment. ROZEREM should be used with caution in patients with moderate hepatic impairment *[see Clinical Pharmacology (12.4)]*. ROZEREM is not recommended in patients with severe hepatic impairment.

8.9 Renal Impairment

No effects on C_{max} and $AUC_{0\text{-}t}$ of parent drug or M-II were seen. No adjustment of ROZEREM dosage is required in patients with renal impairment *[see Clinical Pharmacology (12.4)]*.

9 DRUG ABUSE AND DEPENDENCE

ROZEREM is not a controlled substance.

Discontinuation of ramelteon in animals or in humans after chronic administration did not produce withdrawal signs. Ramelteon does not appear to produce physical dependence.

Human Data: A laboratory abuse potential study was performed with ROZEREM *[see Clinical Studies (14.2)]*.

Animal Data: Ramelteon did not produce any signals from animal behavioral studies indicating that the drug produces rewarding effects. Monkeys did not self-administer ramelteon and the drug did not induce a conditioned place preference in rats. There was no generalization between ramelteon and midazolam. Ramelteon did not affect rotorod performance, an indicator of disruption of motor function, and it did not potentiate the ability of diazepam to interfere with rotorod performance.

10 OVERDOSAGE

General symptomatic and supportive measures should be used, along with immediate gastric lavage where appropriate. Intravenous fluids should be administered as needed. As in all cases of drug overdose, respiration, pulse, blood pressure, and other appropriate vital signs should be monitored, and general supportive measures employed.

Hemodialysis does not effectively reduce exposure to ROZEREM. Therefore, the use of dialysis in the treatment of overdosage is not appropriate.

Poison Control Center: As with the management of all overdosage, the possibility of multiple drug ingestion should be considered. Contact a poison control center for current information on the management of overdosage.

11 DESCRIPTION

ROZEREM (ramelteon) is an orally active hypnotic chemically designated as *(S)-N*-[2-(1,6,7,8-tetrahydro-2*H*-indeno-[5,4-*b*]furan-8-yl)ethyl]propionamide and containing one chiral center. The compound is produced as the (*S*)-enantiomer, with an empirical formula of $C_{16}H_{21}NO_2$, molecular weight of 259.34, and the following chemical structure:

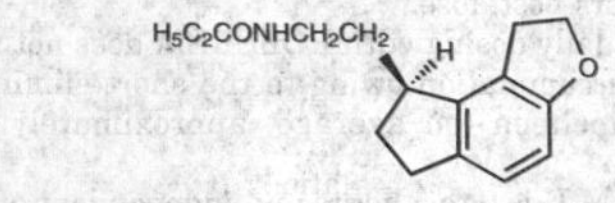

Ramelteon is freely soluble in organic solvents, such as methanol, ethanol, and dimethyl sulfoxide; soluble in 1-octanol and acetonitrile; and very slightly soluble in water and in aqueous buffers from pH 3 to pH 11.

Each ROZEREM tablet includes the following inactive ingredients: lactose monohydrate, starch, hydroxypropyl cellulose, magnesium stearate, hypromellose, copovidone, titanium dioxide, yellow ferric oxide, polyethylene glycol 8000, and ink containing shellac and synthetic iron oxide black.

12 CLINICAL PHARMACOLOGY

12.1 Mechanism of Action

ROZEREM (ramelteon) is a melatonin receptor agonist with both high affinity for melatonin MT_1 and MT_2 receptors and selectivity over the MT_3 receptor. Ramelteon demonstrates full agonist activity *in vitro* in cells expressing human MT_1 or MT_2 receptors.

The activity of ramelteon at the MT_1 and MT_2 receptors is believed to contribute to its sleep-promoting properties, as these receptors, acted upon by endogenous melatonin, are thought to be involved in the maintenance of the circadian rhythm underlying the normal sleep-wake cycle.

Ramelteon has no appreciable affinity for the GABA receptor complex or for receptors that bind neuropeptides, cytokines, serotonin, dopamine, noradrenaline, acetylcholine, and opiates. Ramelteon also does not interfere with the activity of a number of selected enzymes in a standard panel.

The major metabolite of ramelteon, M-II, is active and has approximately one tenth and one fifth the binding affinity of the parent molecule for the human MT_1 and MT_2 receptors, respectively, and is 17- to 25-fold less potent than ramelteon in *in vitro* functional assays. Although the potency of M-II at MT_1 and MT_2 receptors is lower than the parent drug, M-II circulates at higher concentrations than the parent producing 20- to 100-fold greater mean systemic exposure when compared to ramelteon. M-II has weak affinity for the serotonin $5\text{-}HT_{2B}$ receptor, but no appreciable affinity for other receptors or enzymes. Similar to ramelteon, M-II does not interfere with the activity of a number of endogenous enzymes.

All other known metabolites of ramelteon are inactive.

12.3 Pharmacokinetics

The pharmacokinetic profile of ROZEREM has been evaluated in healthy subjects as well as in subjects with hepatic or renal impairment. When administered orally to humans in doses ranging from 4 to 64 mg, ramelteon undergoes rapid, high first-pass metabolism, and exhibits linear pharmacokinetics. Maximal serum concentration (C_{max}) and area under the concentration-time curve (AUC) data show substantial intersubject variability, consistent with the high first-pass effect; the coefficient of variation for these values is approximately 100%. Several metabolites have been identified in human serum and urine.

Absorption

Ramelteon is absorbed rapidly, with median peak concentrations occurring at approximately 0.75 hour (range, 0.5 to 1.5 hours) after fasted oral administration. Although the total absorption of ramelteon is at least 84%, the absolute oral bioavailability is only 1.8% due to extensive first-pass metabolism.

Distribution

In vitro protein binding of ramelteon is approximately 82% in human serum, independent of concentration. Binding to albumin accounts for most of that binding, since 70% of the drug is bound in human serum albumin. Ramelteon is not distributed selectively to red blood cells.

Ramelteon has a mean volume of distribution after intravenous administration of 73.6 L, suggesting substantial tissue distribution.

Metabolism

Metabolism of ramelteon consists primarily of oxidation to hydroxyl and carbonyl derivatives, with secondary metabolism producing glucuronide conjugates. CYP1A2 is the major isozyme involved in the hepatic metabolism of ramelteon; the CYP2C subfamily and CYP3A4 isozymes are also involved to a minor degree.

The rank order of the principal metabolites by prevalence in human serum is M-II, M-IV, M-I, and M-III. These metabolites are formed rapidly and exhibit a monophasic decline and rapid elimination. The overall mean systemic exposure of M-II is approximately 20- to 100-fold higher than parent drug.

Elimination

Following oral administration of radiolabeled ramelteon, 84% of total radioactivity was excreted in urine and approximately 4% in feces, resulting in a mean recovery of 88%. Less than 0.1% of the dose was excreted in urine and feces as the parent compound. Elimination was essentially complete by 96 hours post-dose.

Repeated once daily dosing with ROZEREM does not result in significant accumulation owing to the short elimination half-life of ramelteon (on average, approximately 1-2.6 hours).

The half-life of M-II is 2 to 5 hours and independent of dose. Serum concentrations of the parent drug and its metabolites in humans are at or below the lower limits of quantitation within 24 hours.

Effect of Food

When administered with a high-fat meal, the $AUC_{0\text{-}inf}$ for a single 16 mg dose of ROZEREM was 31% higher and the C_{max} was 22% lower than when given in a fasted state. Median T_{max} was delayed by approximately 45 minutes when ROZEREM was administered with food. Effects of food on the AUC values for M-II were similar. It is therefore recommended that ROZEREM not be taken with or immediately after a high-fat meal *[see Dosage and Administration (2.1)]*.

12.4 Pharmacokinetics in Special Populations

Age: In a group of 24 elderly subjects aged 63 to 79 years administered a single ROZEREM 16 mg dose, the mean C_{max} and $AUC_{0\text{-}inf}$ values were 11.6 ng/mL (SD, 13.8) and 18.7 ng·hr/mL (SD, 19.4), respectively. The elimination half-life was 2.6 hours (SD, 1.1). Compared with younger adults, the total exposure ($AUC_{0\text{-}inf}$) and C_{max} of ramelteon were 97% and 86% higher, respectively, in elderly subjects. The $AUC_{0\text{-}inf}$ and C_{max} of M-II were increased by 30% and 13%, respectively, in elderly subjects.

Gender: There are no clinically meaningful gender-related differences in the pharmacokinetics of ROZEREM or its metabolites.

Hepatic Impairment: Exposure to ROZEREM was increased almost 4-fold in subjects with mild hepatic impairment after 7 days of dosing with 16 mg/day; exposure was further increased (more than 10-fold) in subjects with moderate hepatic impairment. Exposure to M-II was only marginally increased in mildly and moderately impaired subjects relative to healthy matched controls. The pharmacokinetics of ROZEREM have not been evaluated in subjects with severe hepatic impairment (Child-Pugh Class C). ROZEREM should be used with caution in patients with moderate hepatic impairment *[see Warnings and Precautions (5.6)]*.

Renal Impairment: The pharmacokinetic characteristics of ROZEREM were studied after administering a 16 mg dose to subjects with mild, moderate, or severe renal impairment based on pre-dose creatinine clearance (53 to 95, 35 to 49, or 15 to 30 mL/min/1.73 m^2, respectively), and in subjects who required chronic hemodialysis. Wide intersubject variability was seen in ROZEREM exposure parameters. However, no effects on C_{max} or $AUC_{0\text{-}t}$ of parent drug or M-II were seen in any of the treatment groups; the incidence of adverse events was similar across groups. These results are consistent with the negligible renal clearance of ramelteon, which is principally eliminated via hepatic metabolism. No adjustment of ROZEREM dosage is required in patients with renal impairment, including patients with severe renal impairment (creatinine clearance of ≤ 30 mL/min/1.73 m^2) and patients who require chronic hemodialysis.

12.5 Drug-Drug Interactions

ROZEREM has a highly variable intersubject pharmacokinetic profile (approximately 100% coefficient of variation in C_{max} and AUC). As noted above, CYP1A2 is the major isozyme involved in the metabolism of ROZEREM; the CYP2C subfamily and CYP3A4 isozymes are also involved to a minor degree.

Effects of Other Drugs on ROZEREM Metabolism

Fluvoxamine (strong CYP1A2 inhibitor): When fluvoxamine 100 mg twice daily was administered for 3 days prior to single-dose co-administration of ROZEREM 16 mg and fluvoxamine, the $AUC_{0\text{-}inf}$ for ramelteon increased approximately 190-fold, and the C_{max} increased approximately 70-fold, compared to ROZEREM administered alone. ROZEREM should not be used in combination with fluvoxamine. Other less strong CYP1A2 inhibitors have not been adequately studied. ROZEREM should be administered with caution to patients taking less strong CYP1A2 inhibitors [see *Contraindications*].

Rifampin (strong CYP enzyme inducer): Administration of rifampin 600 mg once daily for 11 days resulted in a mean decrease of approximately 80% (40% to 90%) in total exposure to ramelteon and metabolite M-II, (both $AUC_{0\text{-}inf}$ and C_{max}) after a single 32 mg dose of ROZEREM. Efficacy may be reduced when ROZEREM is used in combination with strong CYP enzyme inducers such as rifampin.

Ketoconazole (strong CYP3A4 inhibitor): The $AUC_{0\text{-}inf}$ and C_{max} of ramelteon increased by approximately 84% and 36%, respectively, when a single 16 mg dose of ROZEREM was administered on the fourth day of ketoconazole 200 mg twice daily administration, compared to administration of ROZEREM alone. Similar increases were seen in M-II pharmacokinetic variables. ROZEREM should be administered with caution in subjects taking strong CYP3A4 inhibitors such as ketoconazole.

Fluconazole (strong CYP2C9 inhibitor): The total and peak systemic exposure ($AUC_{0\text{-}inf}$ and C_{max}) of ramelteon after a single 16 mg dose of ROZEREM was increased by approximately 150% when administered with fluconazole. Similar increases were also seen in M-II exposure. ROZEREM should be administered with caution in subjects taking strong CYP2C9 inhibitors such as fluconazole.

Interaction studies of concomitant administration of ROZEREM with fluoxetine (CYP2D6 inhibitor), omeprazole (CYP1A2 inducer/CYP2C19 inhibitor), theophylline (CYP1A2 substrate), and dextromethorphan (CYP2D6 substrate) did not produce clinically meaningful changes in either peak or total exposures to ramelteon or the M-II metabolite.

Effects of ROZEREM on Metabolism of Other Drugs

Concomitant administration of ROZEREM with omeprazole (CYP2C19 substrate), dextromethorphan (CYP2D6 substrate), midazolam (CYP3A4 substrate), theophylline (CYP1A2 substrate), digoxin (p-glycoprotein substrate) and warfarin (CYP2C9 [S]/CYP1A2 [R] substrate) did not produce clinically meaningful changes in peak and total exposures to these drugs.

Effect of Alcohol on ROZEREM

With single-dose, daytime co-administration of ROZEREM 32 mg and alcohol (0.6 g/kg), there were no clinically meaningful or statistically significant effects on peak or total exposure to ROZEREM. However, an additive effect was seen on some measures of psychomotor performance (i.e., the Digit Symbol Substitution Test, the Psychomotor Vigilance Task Test, and a Visual Analog Scale of Sedation) at some post-dose time points. No additive effect was seen on the Delayed Word Recognition Test. Because alcohol by itself impairs performance, and the intended effect of ROZEREM is to promote sleep, patients should be cautioned not to consume alcohol when using ROZEREM.

13 NONCLINICAL TOXICOLOGY

13.1 Carcinogenesis, Mutagenesis, Impairment of Fertility

Carcinogenesis

Ramelteon was administered to mice and rats at oral doses of 0, 30, 100, 300, or 1000 mg/kg/day (mice) and 0, 15, 60, 250, or 1000 mg/kg/day (rats). Mice and rats were dosed for two years, except at the high dose (94 weeks for male and female mice and female rats). In mice, dose-related increases in the incidence of hepatic tumors (adenomas, carcinomas, hepatoblastomas) were observed in males and females. The no-effect dose for hepatic tumors in mice (30 mg/kg/day) is approximately 20 times the recommended human dose (RHD) of 8 mg/day on a body surface area (mg/m^2) basis.

In rats, the incidence of hepatic adenoma and benign Leydig cell tumors of the testis was increased in males at doses ≥ 250 mg/kg/day. In females, the incidence of hepatic adenoma was increased at doses ≥ 60 mg/kg/day. The incidence of hepatic carcinoma was increased in males and female rats at 1000 mg/kg/day. The no-effect dose for tumors in rats (15 mg/kg/day) is approximately 20 times the RHD on a mg/m^2 basis.

Mutagenesis

Ramelteon was not genotoxic in the *in vitro* bacterial reverse mutation (Ames) assay, the *in vitro* mouse lymphoma $TK^{+/-}$ assay, and in *in vivo* oral micronucleus assays in mouse and rat. Ramelteon was clastogenic in the *in vitro* chromosomal aberration assay in Chinese hamster lung cells.

Separate studies indicated that the concentration of the M-II metabolite formed in the presence of metabolic activation exceeded the concentration of ramelteon; therefore, the genotoxic potential of the M-II metabolite was also assessed in the *in vitro* studies.

Impairment of Fertility

When ramelteon (doses of 6 to 600 mg/kg/day) was administered orally to male and female rats prior to and during mating and early gestation, alterations in estrus cyclicity and decreased numbers of corpora lutea, implantations, and live embryos were observed at doses greater than 20 mg/kg/day. The no-effect dose is approximately 24 times the recommended human dose of 8 mg/day on a body surface area (mg/m^2) basis. Oral administration of ramelteon (up to 600 mg/kg/day) to male rats had no effects on sperm quality or reproductive performance.

14 CLINICAL STUDIES

14.1 Controlled Clinical Trials

Chronic Insomnia

Three randomized, double-blind trials in subjects with chronic insomnia employing polysomnography (PSG) were provided as objective support of Rozerem's effectiveness in sleep initiation.

One study enrolled younger adults (aged 18 to 64 years, inclusive) with chronic insomnia and employed a parallel design in which the subjects received a single, nightly dose of ROZEREM (8 mg or 16 mg) or matching placebo for 35 days. PSG was performed on the first two nights in each of Weeks 1, 3, and 5 of treatment. ROZEREM reduced the average latency to persistent sleep at each of the time points when compared to placebo. The 16 mg dose conferred no additional benefit for sleep initiation.

The second study employing PSG was a three-period crossover trial performed in subjects aged 65 years and older with a history of chronic insomnia. Subjects received ROZEREM (4 mg or 8 mg) or placebo and underwent PSG assessment in a sleep laboratory for two consecutive nights in each of the three study periods. Both doses of ROZEREM reduced latency to persistent sleep when compared to placebo.

The third study evaluated long term efficacy and safety in adults with chronic insomnia. Subjects received a single, nightly dose of ROZEREM 8 mg or matching placebo for 6 months. PSG was performed on the first two nights of Week 1 and Months 1, 3, 5, and 6. ROZEREM reduced sleep latency at each time point when compared to placebo. In this study, when the PSG results from nights 1 and 2 of Month 7 were compared to the results from nights 22 and 23 of Month 6, there was a statistically significant increase in LPS of 33% (9.5 minutes) in the ramelteon group. There was no increase in LPS in the placebo group when the same time periods were compared.

A randomized, double-blind, parallel group study was conducted in outpatients aged 65 years and older with chronic insomnia and employed subjective measures of efficacy (sleep diaries). Subjects received ROZEREM (4 mg or 8 mg) or placebo for 35 nights. ROZEREM reduced patient-reported sleep latency compared to placebo. A similarly designed study performed in younger adults (aged 18-64 years) using 8 mg and 16 mg of ramelteon did not replicate this finding of reduced patient-reported sleep latency compared to placebo.

While the 16 mg dose was evaluated as a potential treatment for adults, it was shown to confer no additional benefit for sleep initiation and was associated with higher incidences of fatigue, headache and next-day somnolence.

Transient Insomnia

In a randomized, double-blind, parallel-group trial using a first-night-effect model, healthy adults received placebo or ROZEREM before spending one night in a sleep laboratory and being evaluated with PSG. ROZEREM demonstrated a decrease in mean latency to persistent sleep as compared to placebo.

14.2 Studies Pertinent to Safety Concerns for Sleep-promoting Drugs

Results from Human Laboratory Abuse Liability Studies

A human laboratory abuse potential study was performed in 14 subjects with a history of sedative/hypnotic or anxiolytic drug abuse. Subjects received single oral doses of ROZEREM (16, 80, or 160 mg), triazolam (0.25, 0.50, or 0.75 mg) or placebo. All subjects received each of the 7 treatments separated by a wash-out period and underwent multiple standard tests of abuse potential. No differences in subjective responses indicative of abuse potential were found between ROZEREM and placebo at doses up to 20 times the recommended therapeutic dose. The positive control drug, triazolam, consistently showed a dose-response effect on these subjective measures, as demonstrated by the differences from placebo in peak effect and overall 24-hour effect.

Residual Pharmacological Effect in Insomnia Trials
In order to evaluate potential next-day residual effects, the following scales were used: a Memory Recall Test, a Word List Memory Test, a Visual Analog Mood and Feeling Scale, the Digit-Symbol Substitution Test, and a post-sleep questionnaire to assess alertness and ability to concentrate. There was no evidence of next-day residual effect seen after 2 nights of ramelteon use during the crossover studies.
In a 35-night, double-blind, placebo-controlled, parallel-group study in adults with chronic insomnia, measures of residual effects were performed at three time points. Overall, the magnitudes of any observed differences were small. At Week 1, patients who received 8 mg of ROZEREM had a mean VAS score (46 mm on a 100 mm scale) indicating more fatigue in comparison to patients who received placebo (42 mm). At Week 3, patients who received 8 mg of ROZEREM had a lower mean score for immediate recall (7.5 out of 16 words) compared to patients who received placebo (8.2 words); and the patients treated with ROZEREM had a mean VAS score indicating more sluggishness (27 mm on a 100 mm VAS) in comparison to the placebo-treated patients (22 mm). Patients who received ROZEREM did not have next-morning residual effects that were different from placebo at Week 5.
Rebound Insomnia / Withdrawal
Potential rebound insomnia and withdrawal effects were assessed in four studies in which subjects received ROZEREM or placebo for up to 6 months; 3 were 35-day studies, one was a 6 month study. These studies included a total of 2533 subjects, of whom 854 were elderly.
Tyrer Benzodiazepine Withdrawal Symptom Questionnaire (BWSQ): The BWSQ is a self-report questionnaire that solicits specific information on 20 symptoms commonly experienced during withdrawal from benzodiazepine receptor agonists; ROZEREM is not a benzodiazepine receptor agonist.
In two of the three 35-day insomnia studies, the questionnaire was administered one week after completion of treatment; in the third study, the questionnaire was administered on Days 1 and 2 after completion. In all three of the 35-day studies, subjects receiving ROZEREM 4 mg, 8 mg, or 16 mg daily reported BWSQ scores similar to those of subjects receiving placebo.
In the 6 month study, there was no evidence of withdrawal from the 8 mg dose as measured by the BWSQ.
Rebound Insomnia: Rebound insomnia was assessed in the 35-day studies by measuring sleep latency after abrupt treatment discontinuation. One of these studies employed PSG in younger adult subjects receiving ROZEREM 8 mg or 16 mg; the other two studies employed subjective measures of sleep-onset insomnia in elderly subjects receiving ROZEREM 4 mg or 8 mg, and in younger adult subjects receiving ROZEREM 8 mg or 16 mg. There was no evidence that ROZEREM caused rebound insomnia during the post-treatment period.

14.3 Studies to Evaluate Effects on Endocrine Function
Two controlled studies evaluated the effects of ROZEREM on endocrine function.
In the first trial, ROZEREM 16 mg once daily or placebo was administered to 99 healthy volunteer subjects for 4 weeks. This study evaluated the thyroid axis, adrenal axis and reproductive axis. No clinically significant endocrinopathies were demonstrated in this study. However, the study was limited in its ability to detect such abnormalities due to its limited duration.
In the second trial, ROZEREM 16 mg once daily or placebo was administered to 122 subjects with chronic insomnia for 6 months. This study evaluated the thyroid axis, adrenal axis and reproductive axis.
There were no significant abnormalities seen in either the thyroid or the adrenal axes. Abnormalities were, however, noted within the reproductive axis. Overall, the mean serum prolactin level change from baseline was 4.9 µg/L (34% increase) for women in the ROZEREM group compared with −0.6 µg/L (4% decrease) for women in the placebo group (p=0.003). No differences between active- and placebo-treated groups occurred among men. Thirty-two percent of all patients who were treated with ramelteon in this study (women and men) had prolactin levels that increased from normal baseline levels compared to 19% of patients who were treated with placebo. Subject-reported menstrual patterns were similar between the two treatment groups.
In a 12-month, open-label study in adult and elderly patients, there were two patients who were noted to have abnormal morning cortisol levels, and subsequent abnormal ACTH stimulation tests. A 29-year-old female patient was diagnosed with a prolactinoma. The relationship of these events to ROZEREM therapy is not clear.

16 HOW SUPPLIED/STORAGE AND HANDLING
ROZEREM is available as round, pale orange-yellow, film-coated, 8 mg tablets, with "TAK" and "RAM-8" printed on one side, in the following quantities:

NDC 64764-805-30	Bottles of 30
NDC 64764-805-10	Bottles of 100
NDC 64764-805-50	Bottles of 500

Store at 25°C (77°F); excursions permitted to 15° to 30°C (59° to 86°F) [see USP controlled room temperature]. Keep container tightly closed and protected from moisture and humidity.

17 PATIENT COUNSELING INFORMATION
Prescribers or other healthcare professionals should inform patients, their families, and their caregivers about the benefits and risks associated with treatment with hypnotics, should counsel them in their appropriate use and should instruct them to read the accompanying Medication Guide *[see Medication Guide (17.5)].*

17.1 Severe Anaphylactic and Anaphylactoid Reactions
Inform patients that severe anaphylactic and anaphylactoid reactions have occurred with ramelteon. Describe the relevant signs/symptoms and advise seeking immediate medical attention if any such things occur.

17.2 Sleep-driving and other Complex Behaviors
There have been reports of people getting out of bed after taking a sleep medication and driving their cars while not fully awake, often with no memory of the event. If a patient experiences such an episode, it should be reported to his or her doctor immediately, since "sleep-driving" can be dangerous. This behavior is more likely to occur when sleep medications are taken with alcohol or other central nervous system depressants. Other complex behaviors (e.g., preparing and eating food, making phone calls, or having sex) have been reported in patients who are not fully awake after taking a sleep medication. As with sleep-driving, patients usually do not remember these events.

17.3 Endocrine Effects
Patients should consult their health care providers if they experience one of the following: cessation of menses or galactorrhea in females, decreased libido, or problems with fertility. Describe the relevant signs/symptoms and advise seeking medical attention if any such things occur.

17.4 Administration Instructions
• Patients should be advised to take ROZEREM within 30 minutes prior to going to bed and should confine their activities to those necessary to prepare for bed.
• Patients should be advised that they should not take ROZEREM with or immediately after a high-fat meal.
• Do not break the tablet; it should be swallowed whole.

17.5 Medication Guide
See attached leaflet.
Manufactured by:
Takeda Pharmaceutical Company Limited
540-8645 Osaka, JAPAN
Manufactured in:
Takeda Ireland Ltd.
Kilruddery, County Wicklow, Republic of Ireland
Distributed by:
Takeda Pharmaceuticals America, Inc.
Deerfield, IL 60015
ROZEREM® is a registered trademark of Takeda Pharmaceutical Company Limited and used under license by Takeda Pharmaceuticals America, Inc.
©2005, 2008 Takeda Pharmaceuticals America, Inc.
05-1143 Revised: 10/2008

MEDICATION GUIDE
ROZEREM® (rō-Zair-em)
(ramelteon)
Read the Medication Guide that comes with ROZEREM before you start taking it and each time you get a refill. There may be new information. This Medication Guide does not take the place of talking to your doctor about your medical condition or treatment.
What is the most important information I should know about ROZEREM?
ROZEREM may cause severe allergic reactions. Symptoms include swelling of the tongue or throat, trouble breathing, and nausea and vomiting. Get emergency medical help if you get these symptoms after taking ROZEREM.
After taking ROZEREM, you may get up out of bed while not being fully awake and do an activity that you do not know you are doing. The next morning, you may not remember that you did anything during the night. You have a higher chance for doing these activities if you drink alcohol or take other medicines that make you sleepy with ROZEREM. Activities may include:
• driving a car ("sleep-driving")
• making and eating food
• talking on the phone
• having sex
• sleep-walking
Call your doctor right away if you find out that you have done any of the above activities after taking ROZEREM.
Important:
1. Take ROZEREM exactly as prescribed
  • Do not take more ROZEREM than prescribed.

• Take ROZEREM within 30 minutes of going to bed, not sooner.
2. Do not take ROZEREM if you:
  • drink alcohol
  • take other medicines that can make you sleepy. Talk to your doctor about all of your medicines. Your doctor will tell you if you can take ROZEREM with your other medicines.
  • cannot get a full night's sleep
WHAT IS ROZEREM?
ROZEREM is a hypnotic (sleep) medicine. ROZEREM is used in adults for the treatment of the symptom of trouble falling asleep from insomnia.
ROZEREM is not for children.
Who should not take ROZEREM?
Do not take ROZEREM if you are allergic to anything in it. See the end of this Medication Guide for a complete list of ingredients in ROZEREM.
Do not take ROZEREM if you are currently taking Luvox (fluvoxamine).
ROZEREM may not be right for you. Before starting ROZEREM, tell your doctor about all of your health conditions, including if you:
• have a history of depression, mental illness, or suicidal thoughts
• have liver disease
• have a lung disease or breathing problems
• are pregnant, planning to become pregnant, or breastfeeding
Tell your doctor about all of the medicines you take including prescription and nonprescription medicines, vitamins and herbal supplements. Medicines can interact with each other, sometimes causing serious side effects.
Do not take ROZEREM with:
• other medicines that can make you sleepy
• Luvox® (fluvoxamine)
Know the medicines you take. Keep a list of your medicines with you to show your doctor and pharmacist each time you get a new medicine.
How should I take ROZEREM?
• Take ROZEREM exactly as prescribed. Do not take more ROZEREM than prescribed for you.
• Do not break the tablets. They should be swallowed whole.
• **Take ROZEREM within 30 minutes of going to bed.** After taking ROZEREM only do activities to get ready for bed.
• Do not take ROZEREM with or right after a meal.
• **Do not take ROZEREM unless you are able to get a full night's sleep before you must be active again.**
• **Call your doctor if your insomnia worsens or is not better within 7-10 days.** This may mean that there is another condition causing your sleep problems.
• If you take too much ROZEREM or overdose, call your doctor or poison control center right away, or get emergency treatment.
What are the possible side effects of ROZEREM?
Possible serious side effects of ROZEREM include:
• **severe allergic reactions.** Symptoms include swelling of the tongue or throat, trouble breathing, and nausea and vomiting. Get emergency medical help if you get these symptoms after taking ROZEREM.
• **getting out of bed while not being fully awake and do an activity that you do not know you are doing.** (See "What is the most important information I should know about ROZEREM?")
• **abnormal thoughts and behavior.** Symptoms include worsening of depression, suicidal thoughts or actions, nightmares, and hallucinations.
• **hormone effects.** ROZEREM can decrease testosterone levels and increase prolactin levels in the blood. Symptoms of low testosterone or high prolactin levels are:
  ○ **decreased interest in sex**
  ○ **problems getting pregnant**
  ○ **irregular menstrual periods or no menstrual periods**
  ○ **leakage of milk from the nipples of a person who is not breastfeeding**
Call your doctor right away if you have any of the above side effects or any other side effects that worry you while using ROZEREM. Call your doctor for medical advice about side effects. You may report side effects to the FDA at 1-800-FDA-1088.
The most common side effects of ROZEREM are:
• drowsiness
• tiredness
• dizziness
• You may still feel drowsy the next day after taking ROZEREM. **Do not drive or do other dangerous activities after taking ROZEREM until you feel fully awake.**
These are not all the side effects of ROZEREM. Ask your doctor or pharmacist for more information.
How should I Store ROZEREM?
• Store ROZEREM tablets at room temperature, 59° to 86° F (15° to 30°C). Keep the container tightly closed and protected from moisture and humidity.

- Keep ROZEREM and all medicines out of reach of children.

General Information about ROZEREM

- Medicines are sometimes prescribed for purposes other than those listed in a Medication Guide.
- Do not use ROZEREM for a condition for which it was not prescribed.
- Do not share ROZEREM with other people, even if you think they have the same symptoms that you have. It may harm them.

This Medication Guide summarizes the most important information about ROZEREM. If you would like more information, talk with your doctor. You can ask your doctor or pharmacist for information about ROZEREM that is written for healthcare professionals. For more information about ROZEREM, please call Takeda Pharmaceuticals America, Inc. at 1-877-TAKEDA-7 or visit www.rozerem.com.

What are the ingredients in ROZEREM?

Active Ingredient: ramelteon

Inactive Ingredients: lactose monohydrate, starch, hydroxypropyl cellulose, magnesium stearate, hypromellose, copovidone, titanium dioxide, yellow ferric oxide, polyethylene glycol 8000, and ink containing shellac and synthetic iron oxide black.

Rx Only

This Medication Guide has been approved by the U.S. Food and Drug Administration.

05-1143-MG   Revised: 10/2008

Shown in Product Identification Guide, page 320

ULORIC®
(febuxostat)
tablet for oral use

R

HIGHLIGHTS OF PRESCRIBING INFORMATION
These HIGHLIGHTS do not include all the information needed to use ULORIC safely and effectively. See full prescribing information for ULORIC.
ULORIC (febuxostat) tablet for oral use
Initial U.S. Approval: 2009

─────────INDICATIONS AND USAGE─────────

ULORIC is a xanthine oxidase (XO) inhibitor indicated for the chronic management of hyperuricemia in patients with gout. (1)
ULORIC is not recommended for the treatment of asymptomatic hyperuricemia. (1)

───────DOSAGE AND ADMINISTRATION───────

- ULORIC is recommended at 40 mg or 80 mg once daily. The recommended starting dose of ULORIC is 40 mg once daily. For patients who do not achieve a serum uric acid (sUA) less than 6 mg per dL after 2 weeks with 40 mg, ULORIC 80 mg is recommended. (2.1)
- ULORIC can be administered without regard to food or antacid use. (2.1)
- No dose adjustment is necessary when administering ULORIC to patients with mild to moderate renal or hepatic impairment. (2.2)

───────DOSAGE FORMS AND STRENGTHS───────

Tablet: 40 mg, 80 mg. (3)

─────────────CONTRAINDICATIONS─────────────

ULORIC is contraindicated in patients being treated with azathioprine, mercaptopurine, or theophylline. (4)

───────WARNINGS AND PRECAUTIONS───────

- Gout Flare: An increase in gout flares is frequently observed during initiation of anti-hyperuricemic agents, including ULORIC. If a gout flare occurs during treatment, ULORIC need not be discontinued. Prophylactic therapy (i.e., non-steroidal anti-inflammatory drug (NSAID) or colchicine upon initiation of treatment) may be beneficial for up to six months. (2.4, 5.1)
- Cardiovascular Events: A higher rate of cardiovascular thromboembolic events was observed in patients treated with ULORIC than allopurinol in clinical trials. Monitor for signs and symptoms of MI and stroke. (5.2)
- Liver Enzyme Elevation: Transaminase elevations have been observed in ULORIC-treated patients. Monitor liver function tests periodically. (5.3)

─────────────ADVERSE REACTIONS─────────────

Adverse reactions occurring in at least 1% of ULORIC-treated patients, and, at least 0.5% greater than placebo, are liver function abnormalities, nausea, arthralgia, and rash. (6.1)
To report SUSPECTED ADVERSE REACTIONS, contact Takeda Pharmaceuticals at 1.877.825.3327 or FDA at 1-800-FDA-1088 or www.fda.gov/medwatch

─────────────DRUG INTERACTIONS─────────────

Concomitant administration of ULORIC with XO substrate drugs, azathioprine, mercaptopurine, or theophylline could increase plasma concentrations of these drugs resulting in severe toxicity. (7)

───────USE IN SPECIFIC POPULATIONS───────

- There is insufficient data in patients with severe renal impairment. No studies have been conducted in patients with severe hepatic impairment. Caution should be exercised in these patients. (8.6, 8.7)
- No studies have been conducted in patients with secondary hyperuricemia (including patients being treated for Lesch-Nyhan syndrome or malignant disease, or in organ transplant recipients); therefore, ULORIC is not recommended for use in these patients. (8.8)

See 17 for PATIENT COUNSELING INFORMATION and FDA-approved patient labeling

Revised: 02/2009

FULL PRESCRIBING INFORMATION: CONTENTS*

FULL PRESCRIBING INFORMATION

1   INDICATIONS AND USAGE

ULORIC® is a xanthine oxidase (XO) inhibitor indicated for the chronic management of hyperuricemia in patients with gout.
ULORIC is not recommended for the treatment of asymptomatic hyperuricemia.

2   DOSAGE AND ADMINISTRATION
2.1   Recommended Dose
For treatment of hyperuricemia in patients with gout, ULORIC is recommended at 40 mg or 80 mg once daily.
The recommended starting dose of ULORIC is 40 mg once daily. For patients who do not achieve a serum uric acid (sUA) less than 6 mg per dL after 2 weeks with 40 mg, ULORIC 80 mg is recommended.
ULORIC can be taken without regard to food or antacid use [see Clinical Pharmacology (12.3)].

2.2   Special Populations
No dose adjustment is necessary when administering ULORIC in patients with mild to moderate renal impairment [see Use in Specific Populations (8.6) and Clinical Pharmacology (12.3)]. The recommended starting dose of ULORIC is 40 mg once daily. For patients who do not achieve a sUA less than 6 mg per dL after 2 weeks with 40 mg, ULORIC 80 mg is recommended.
No dose adjustment is necessary in patients with mild to moderate hepatic impairment [see Use in Specific Populations (8.7) and Clinical Pharmacology (12.3)].

2.3   Uric Acid Level
Testing for the target serum uric acid level of less than 6 mg per dL may be performed as early as 2 weeks after initiating ULORIC therapy.

2.4   Gout Flares
Gout flares may occur after initiation of ULORIC due to changing serum uric acid levels resulting in mobilization of urate from tissue deposits. Flare prophylaxis with a non-steroidal anti-inflammatory drug (NSAID) or colchicine is recommended upon initiation of ULORIC. Prophylactic therapy may be beneficial for up to six months [see Clinical Studies (14.1)].
If a gout flare occurs during ULORIC treatment, ULORIC need not be discontinued. The gout flare should be managed concurrently, as appropriate for the individual patient [see Warnings and Precautions (5.1)].

3   DOSAGE FORMS AND STRENGTHS
- 40 mg tablets, light green to green, round shaped, debossed with "TAP" and "40"
- 80 mg tablets, light green to green, teardrop shaped, debossed with "TAP" and "80"

4   CONTRAINDICATIONS
ULORIC is contraindicated in patients being treated with azathioprine, mercaptopurine, or theophylline [see Drug Interactions (7)].

5   WARNINGS AND PRECAUTIONS
5.1   Gout Flare
After initiation of ULORIC, an increase in gout flares is frequently observed. This increase is due to reduction in serum uric acid levels resulting in mobilization of urate from tissue deposits.
In order to prevent gout flares when ULORIC is initiated, concurrent prophylactic treatment with an NSAID or colchicine is recommended [see Dosage and Administration (2.4)].
5.2   Cardiovascular Events
In the randomized controlled studies, there was a higher rate of cardiovascular thromboembolic events (cardiovascular deaths, non-fatal myocardial infarctions, and non-fatal strokes) in patients treated with ULORIC [0.74 per 100 P-Y (95% CI 0.36-1.37)] than allopurinol [0.60 per 100 P-Y (95% CI 0.16-1.53)] [see Adverse Reactions (6.1)]. A causal relationship with ULORIC has not been established. Monitor for signs and symptoms of myocardial infarction (MI) and stroke.
5.3   Liver Enzyme Elevations
During randomized controlled studies, transaminase elevations greater than 3 times the upper limit of normal (ULN) were observed (AST: 2%, 2%, and ALT: 3%, 2% in ULORIC and allopurinol-treated patients, respectively). No dose-effect relationship for these transaminase elevations was noted. Laboratory assessment of liver function is recommended at, for example, 2 and 4 months following initiation of ULORIC and periodically thereafter.

6   ADVERSE REACTIONS
6.1   Clinical Trials Experience
Because clinical trials are conducted under widely varying conditions, adverse reaction rates observed in the clinical trials of a drug cannot be directly compared to rates in the clinical trials of another drug and may not reflect the rates observed in practice.
A total of 2757 subjects with hyperuricemia and gout were treated with ULORIC 40 mg or 80 mg daily in clinical studies. For ULORIC 40 mg, 559 patients were treated for ≥ 6 months. For ULORIC 80 mg, 1377 subjects were treated for ≥ 6 months, 674 patients were treated for ≥ 1 year and 515 patients were treated for ≥ 2 years.
Most Common Adverse Reactions
In three randomized, controlled clinical studies (Studies 1, 2 and 3), which were 6 to 12 months in duration, the following adverse reactions were reported by the treating physician as related to study drug. Table 1 summarizes adverse reactions reported at a rate of at least 1% in ULORIC treatment groups and at least 0.5% greater than placebo.
[See table 1 at top of next page]
The most common adverse reaction leading to discontinuation from therapy was liver function abnormalities in 1.8% of ULORIC 40 mg, 1.2% of ULORIC 80 mg, and in 0.9% of allopurinol-treated subjects.
In addition to the adverse reactions presented in Table 1, dizziness was reported in more than 1% of ULORIC-treated subjects although not at a rate more than 0.5% greater than placebo.
Less Common Adverse Reactions
In phase 2 and 3 clinical studies the following adverse reactions occurred in less than 1% of subjects and in more than one subject treated with doses ranging from 40 mg to 240 mg of ULORIC. This list also includes adverse reactions (less than 1% of subjects) associated with organ systems from Warnings and Precautions.
Blood and Lymphatic System Disorders: anemia, idiopathic thrombocytopenic purpura, leukocytosis/leukopenia, neutropenia, pancytopenia, splenomegaly, thrombocytopenia.
Cardiac Disorders: angina pectoris, atrial fibrillation/flutter, cardiac murmur, ECG abnormal, palpitations, sinus bradycardia, tachycardia.
Ear and Labyrinth Disorders: deafness, tinnitus, vertigo.
Eye Disorders: vision blurred.

IMPORTANT NOTICE: Updated drug information is sent bi-monthly via the PDR® Update Insert. For *monthly* email updates, register at PDR.net.

Gastrointestinal Disorders: abdominal distention, abdominal pain, constipation, dry mouth, dyspepsia, flatulence, frequent stools, gastritis, gastroesophageal reflux disease, gastrointestinal discomfort, gingival pain, haematemesis, hyperchlorhydria, hematochezia, mouth ulceration, pancreatitis, peptic ulcer, vomiting.
General Disorders and Administration Site Conditions: asthenia, chest pain/discomfort, edema, fatigue, feeling abnormal, gait disturbance, influenza-like symptoms, mass, pain, thirst.
Hepatobiliary Disorders: cholelithiasis/cholecystitis, hepatic steatosis, hepatitis, hepatomegaly.
Immune System Disorder: hypersensitivity.
Infections and Infestations: herpes zoster.
Procedural Complications: contusion.
Metabolism and Nutrition Disorders: anorexia, appetite decreased/increased, dehydration, diabetes mellitus, hypercholesterolemia, hyperglycemia, hyperlipidemia, hypertriglyceridemia, hypokalemia, weight decreased/increased.
Musculoskeletal and Connective Tissue Disorders: arthritis, joint stiffness, joint swelling, muscle spasms/twitching/tightness/weakness, musculoskeletal pain/stiffness, myalgia.
Nervous System Disorders: altered taste, balance disorder, cerebrovascular accident, Guillain-Barré syndrome, headache, hemiparesis, hypoesthesia, hyposmia, lacunar infarction, lethargy, mental impairment, migraine, paresthesia, somnolence, transient ischemic attack, tremor.
Psychiatric Disorders: agitation, anxiety, depression, insomnia, irritability, libido decreased, nervousness, panic attack, personality change.
Renal and Urinary Disorders: hematuria, nephrolithiasis, pollakiuria, proteinuria, renal failure, renal insufficiency, urgency, incontinence.
Reproductive System and Breast Changes: breast pain, erectile dysfunction, gynecomastia.
Respiratory, Thoracic and Mediastinal Disorders: bronchitis, cough, dyspnea, epistaxis, nasal dryness, paranasal sinus hypersecretion, pharyngeal edema, respiratory tract congestion, sneezing, throat irritation, upper respiratory tract infection.
Skin and Subcutaneous Tissue Disorders: alopecia, angioedema, dermatitis, dermographism, ecchymosis, eczema, hair color changes, hair growth abnormal, hyperhidrosis, peeling skin, petechiae, photosensitivity, pruritus, purpura, skin discoloration/altered pigmentation, skin lesion, skin odor abnormal, urticaria.
Vascular Disorders: flushing, hot flush, hypertension, hypotension.
Laboratory Parameters: activated partial thromboplastin time prolonged, creatine increased, bicarbonate decreased, sodium increased, EEG abnormal, glucose increased, cholesterol increased, triglycerides increased, amylase increased, potassium increased, TSH increased, platelet count decreased, hematocrit decreased, hemoglobin decreased, MCV increased, RBC decreased, creatinine increased, blood urea increased, BUN/creatinine ratio increased, creatine phosphokinase (CPK) increased, alkaline phosphatase increased, LDH increased, PSA increased, urine output increased/decreased, lymphocyte count decreased, neutrophil count decreased, WBC increased/decreased, coagulation test abnormal, low density lipoprotein (LDL) increased, prothrombin time prolonged, urinary casts, urine positive for white blood cells and protein.

Cardiovascular Safety

Cardiovascular events and deaths were adjudicated to one of the pre-defined endpoints from the Anti-Platelet Trialists' Collaborations (APTC) (cardiovascular death, non-fatal myocardial infarction, and non-fatal stroke) in the randomized controlled and long-term extension studies. In the Phase 3 randomized controlled studies, the incidences of adjudicated APTC events per 100 patient-years of exposure were: Placebo 0 (95% CI 0.00-6.16), ULORIC 40 mg 0 (95% CI 0.00-1.08), ULORIC 80 mg 1.09 (95% CI 0.44-2.24), and allopurinol 0.60 (95% CI 0.16-1.53).

In the long-term extension studies, the incidences of adjudicated APTC events were: ULORIC 80 mg 0.97 (95% CI 0.57-1.56), and allopurinol 0.58 (95% CI 0.02-3.24).

Overall, a higher rate of APTC events was observed in ULORIC than in allopurinol-treated patients. A causal relationship with ULORIC has not been established. Monitor for signs and symptoms of MI and stroke.

7 DRUG INTERACTIONS

7.1 Xanthine Oxidase Substrate Drugs

ULORIC is an XO inhibitor. Drug interaction studies of ULORIC with drugs that are metabolized by XO (e.g., theophylline, mercaptopurine, azathioprine) have not been conducted. Inhibition of XO by ULORIC may cause increased plasma concentrations of these drugs leading to toxicity *[see Clinical Pharmacology (12.3)]*. ULORIC is contraindicated in patients being treated with azathioprine, mercaptopurine, or theophylline *[see Contraindications (4)]*.

Table 1: Adverse Reactions Occurring in ≥ 1% of ULORIC-Treated Patients and at Least 0.5% Greater than Seen in Patients Receiving Placebo in Controlled Studies

Adverse Reactions	Placebo (N=134)	ULORIC 40 mg daily (N=757)	ULORIC 80 mg daily (N=1279)	allopurinol* (N=1277)
Liver Function Abnormalities	0.7%	6.6%	4.6%	4.2%
Nausea	0.7%	1.1%	1.3%	0.8%
Arthralgia	0%	1.1%	0.7%	0.7%
Rash	0.7%	0.5%	1.6%	1.6%

*Of the subjects who received allopurinol, 10 received 100 mg, 145 received 200 mg, and 1122 received 300 mg, based on level of renal impairment.

7.2 Cytotoxic Chemotherapy Drugs

Drug interaction studies of ULORIC with cytotoxic chemotherapy have not been conducted. No data are available regarding the safety of ULORIC during cytotoxic chemotherapy.

7.3 *In Vivo* Drug Interaction Studies

Based on drug interaction studies in healthy subjects, ULORIC does not have clinically significant interactions with colchicine, naproxen, indomethacin, hydrochlorothiazide, warfarin or desipramine *[see Clinical Pharmacology (12.3)]*. Therefore, ULORIC may be used concomitantly with these medications.

8 USE IN SPECIFIC POPULATIONS

8.1 Pregnancy

Pregnancy Category C: There are no adequate and well-controlled studies in pregnant women. ULORIC should be used during pregnancy only if the potential benefit justifies the potential risk to the fetus.

Febuxostat was not teratogenic in rats and rabbits at oral doses up to 48 mg per kg (40 and 51 times the human plasma exposure at 80 mg per day for equal body surface area, respectively) during organogenesis. However, increased neonatal mortality and a reduction in the neonatal body weight gain were observed when pregnant rats were treated with oral doses up to 48 mg per kg (40 times the human plasma exposure at 80 mg per day) during organogenesis and through lactation period.

8.3 Nursing Mothers

Febuxostat is excreted in the milk of rats. It is not known whether this drug is excreted in human milk. Because many drugs are excreted in human milk, caution should be exercised when ULORIC is administered to a nursing woman.

8.4 Pediatric Use

Safety and effectiveness in pediatric patients under 18 years of age have not been established.

8.5 Geriatric Use

No dose adjustment is necessary in elderly patients. Of the total number of subjects in clinical studies of ULORIC, 16 percent were 65 and over, while 4 percent were 75 and over. Comparing subjects in different age groups, no clinically significant differences in safety or effectiveness were observed but greater sensitivity of some older individuals cannot be ruled out. The C_{max} and AUC_{24} of febuxostat following multiple oral doses of ULORIC in geriatric subjects (≥ 65 years) were similar to those in younger subjects (18-40 years) *[see Clinical Pharmacology (12.3)]*.

8.6 Renal Impairment

No dose adjustment is necessary in patients with mild or moderate renal impairment (Cl_{cr} 30-89 mL per min). The recommended starting dose of ULORIC is 40 mg once daily. For patients who do not achieve a sUA less than 6 mg per dL after 2 weeks with 40 mg, ULORIC 80 mg is recommended.

There are insufficient data in patients with severe renal impairment (Cl_{cr} less than 30 mL per min); therefore, caution should be exercised in these patients *[see Clinical Pharmacology (12.3)]*.

8.7 Hepatic Impairment

No dose adjustment is necessary in patients with mild or moderate hepatic impairment (Child-Pugh Class A or B). No studies have been conducted in patients with severe hepatic impairment (Child-Pugh Class C); therefore, caution should be exercised in these patients *[see Clinical Pharmacology (12.3)]*.

8.8 Secondary Hyperuricemia

No studies have been conducted in patients with secondary hyperuricemia (including organ transplant recipients); ULORIC is not recommended for use in patients whom the rate of urate formation is greatly increased (e.g., malignant disease and its treatment, Lesch-Nyhan syndrome). The concentration of xanthine in urine could, in rare cases, rise sufficiently to allow deposition in the urinary tract.

10 OVERDOSAGE

ULORIC was studied in healthy subjects in doses up to 300 mg daily for seven days without evidence of dose-limiting toxicities. No overdose of ULORIC was reported in clinical studies. Patients should be managed by symptomatic and supportive care should there be an overdose.

11 DESCRIPTION

ULORIC (febuxostat) is a xanthine oxidase inhibitor. The active ingredient in ULORIC is 2-[3-cyano-4-(2-methylpropoxy) phenyl]-4-methylthiazole-5-carboxylic acid, with a molecular weight of 316.38. The empirical formula is $C_{16}H_{16}N_2O_3S$.

The chemical structure is:

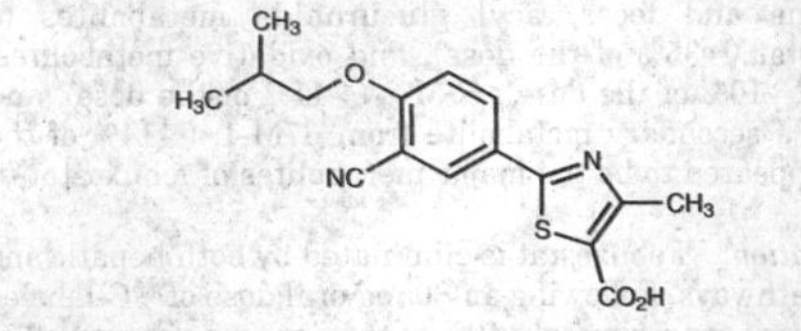

Febuxostat is a non-hygroscopic, white crystalline powder that is freely soluble in dimethylformamide; soluble in dimethylsulfoxide; sparingly soluble in ethanol; slightly soluble in methanol and acetonitrile; and practically insoluble in water. The melting range is 205°C to 208°C.

ULORIC tablets for oral use contain the active ingredient, febuxostat, and are available in two dosage strengths, 40 mg and 80 mg. Inactive ingredients include lactose monohydrate, microcrystalline cellulose, hydroxypropyl cellulose, sodium croscarmellose, silicon dioxide and magnesium stearate. ULORIC tablets are coated with Opadry II, green.

12 CLINICAL PHARMACOLOGY

12.1 Mechanism of Action

ULORIC, a xanthine oxidase inhibitor, achieves its therapeutic effect by decreasing serum uric acid. ULORIC is not expected to inhibit other enzymes involved in purine and pyrimidine synthesis and metabolism at therapeutic concentrations.

12.2 Pharmacodynamics

Effect on Uric Acid and Xanthine Concentrations: In healthy subjects, ULORIC resulted in a dose dependent decrease in 24-hour mean serum uric acid concentrations, and an increase in 24-hour mean serum xanthine concentrations. In addition, there was a decrease in the total daily urinary uric acid excretion. Also, there was an increase in total daily urinary xanthine excretion. Percent reduction in 24-hour mean serum uric acid concentrations was between 40% to 55% at the exposure levels of 40 mg and 80 mg daily doses.

Effect on Cardiac Repolarization: The effect of ULORIC on cardiac repolarization as assessed by the QTc interval was evaluated in normal healthy subjects and in patients with gout. ULORIC in doses up to 300 mg daily, at steady state, did not demonstrate an effect on the QTc interval.

12.3 Pharmacokinetics

In healthy subjects, maximum plasma concentrations (C_{max}) and AUC of febuxostat increased in a dose proportional manner following single and multiple doses of 10 mg to 120 mg. There is no accumulation when therapeutic doses are administered every 24 hours. Febuxostat has an apparent mean terminal elimination half-life ($t_{1/2}$) of approximately 5 to 8 hours. Febuxostat pharmacokinetic parameters for patients with hyperuricemia and gout estimated by population pharmacokinetic analyses were similar to those estimated in healthy subjects.

Absorption: The absorption of radiolabeled febuxostat following oral dose administration was estimated to be at least 49% (based on total radioactivity recovered in urine). Maximum plasma concentrations of febuxostat occurred between 1 to 1.5 hours post-dose. After multiple oral 40 mg and 80 mg once daily doses, C_{max} is approximately 1.6 ± 0.6 mcg per mL (N=30), and 2.6 ± 1.7 mcg per mL (N=227), respectively. Absolute bioavailability of the febuxostat tablet has not been studied.

Following multiple 80 mg once daily doses with a high fat meal, there was a 49% decrease in C_{max} and an 18% decrease in AUC, respectively. However, no clinically significant change in the percent decrease in serum uric acid concentration was observed (58% fed vs. 51% fasting). Thus, ULORIC may be taken without regard to food.

Concomitant ingestion of an antacid containing magnesium hydroxide and aluminum hydroxide with an 80 mg single dose of ULORIC has been shown to delay absorption of febuxostat (approximately 1 hour) and to cause a 31% decrease in C_{max} and a 15% decrease in AUC_∞. As AUC rather than C_{max} was related to drug effect, change observed in AUC was not considered clinically significant. Therefore, ULORIC may be taken without regard to antacid use.

Distribution: The mean apparent steady state volume of distribution (V_{ss}/F) of febuxostat was approximately 50 L (CV ~40%). The plasma protein binding of febuxostat is approximately 99.2%, (primarily to albumin), and is constant over the concentration range achieved with 40 mg and 80 mg doses.

Metabolism: Febuxostat is extensively metabolized by both conjugation via uridine diphosphate glucuronosyltransferase (UGT) enzymes including UGT1A1, UGT1A3, UGT1A9, and UGT2B7 and oxidation via cytochrome P450 (CYP) enzymes including CYP1A2, 2C8 and 2C9 and non-P450 enzymes. The relative contribution of each enzyme isoform in the metabolism of febuxostat is not clear. The oxidation of the isobutyl side chain leads to the formation of four pharmacologically active hydroxy metabolites, all of which occur in plasma of humans at a much lower extent than febuxostat.

In urine and feces, acyl glucuronide metabolites of febuxostat (~35% of the dose), and oxidative metabolites, 67M-1 (~10% of the dose), 67M-2 (~11% of the dose), and 67M-4, a secondary metabolite from 67M-1, (~14% of the dose) appeared to be the major metabolites of febuxostat *in vivo*.

Elimination: Febuxostat is eliminated by both hepatic and renal pathways. Following an 80 mg oral dose of ^{14}C-labeled febuxostat, approximately 49% of the dose was recovered in the urine as unchanged febuxostat (3%), the acyl glucuronide of the drug (30%), its known oxidative metabolites and their conjugates (13%), and other unknown metabolites (3%). In addition to the urinary excretion, approximately 45% of the dose was recovered in the feces as the unchanged febuxostat (12%), the acyl glucuronide of the drug (1%), its known oxidative metabolites and their conjugates (25%), and other unknown metabolites (7%).

The apparent mean terminal elimination half-life ($t_{1/2}$) of febuxostat was approximately 5 to 8 hours.

Special Populations

Pediatric Use: The pharmacokinetics of ULORIC in patients under the age of 18 years have not been studied.

Geriatric Use: The C_{max} and AUC of febuxostat and its metabolites following multiple oral doses of ULORIC in geriatric subjects (≥ 65 years) were similar to those in younger subjects (18-40 years). In addition, the percent decrease in serum uric acid concentration was similar between elderly and younger subjects. No dose adjustment is necessary in geriatric patients *[see Use in Specific Populations (8.5)]*.

Renal Impairment: Following multiple 80 mg doses of ULORIC in healthy subjects with mild (Cl_{cr} 50-80 mL per min), moderate (Cl_{cr} 30-49 mL per min) or severe renal impairment (Cl_{cr} 10-29 mL per min), the C_{max} of febuxostat did not change relative to subjects with normal renal function (Cl_{cr} greater than 80 mL per min). AUC and half-life of febuxostat increased in subjects with renal impairment in comparison to subjects with normal renal function, but values were similar among three renal impairment groups. Mean febuxostat AUC values were up to 1.8 times higher in subjects with renal impairment compared to those with normal renal function. Mean C_{max} and AUC values for 3 active metabolites increased up to 2- and 4-fold, respectively. However, the percent decrease in serum uric acid concentration for subjects with renal impairment was comparable to those with normal renal function (58% in normal renal function group and 55% in the severe renal function group).

No dose adjustment is necessary in patients with mild to moderate renal impairment *[see Dosage and Administration (2) and Use in Specific Populations (8.6)]*. The recommended starting dose of ULORIC is 40 mg once daily. For patients who do not achieve a sUA less than 6 mg per dL after 2 weeks with 40 mg, ULORIC 80 mg is recommended. There is insufficient data in patients with severe renal impairment; caution should be exercised in those patients *[see Use in Specific Populations (8.6)]*.

ULORIC has not been studied in end stage renal impairment patients who are on dialysis.

Hepatic Impairment: Following multiple 80 mg doses of ULORIC in patients with mild (Child-Pugh Class A) or moderate (Child-Pugh Class B) hepatic impairment, an average of 20-30% increase was observed for both C_{max} and AUC_{24} (total and unbound) in hepatic impairment groups compared to subjects with normal hepatic function. In addition, the percent decrease in serum uric acid concentration was comparable between different hepatic groups (62% in healthy group, 49% in mild hepatic impairment group, and 48% in moderate hepatic impairment group). No dose adjustment is necessary in patients with mild or moderate hepatic impairment. No studies have been conducted in subjects with severe hepatic impairment (Child-Pugh Class C); caution should be exercised in those patients *[see Use in Specific Populations (8.7)]*.

Gender: Following multiple oral doses of ULORIC, the C_{max} and AUC_{24} of febuxostat were 30% and 14% higher in females than in males, respectively. However, weight-corrected C_{max} and AUC were similar between the genders. In addition, the percent decrease in serum uric acid concentrations was similar between genders. No dose adjustment is necessary based on gender.

Race: No specific pharmacokinetic study was conducted to investigate the effects of race.

Drug-Drug Interactions

Effect of ULORIC on Other Drugs

Xanthine Oxidase Substrate Drugs-Azathioprine, Mercaptopurine, and Theophylline: Febuxostat is an XO inhibitor. Drug interaction studies of ULORIC with drugs that are metabolized by XO (e.g., theophylline, mercaptopurine, azathioprine) have not been conducted. Inhibition of XO by ULORIC may cause increased plasma concentrations of these drugs leading to toxicity. ULORIC is contraindicated in patients being treated with azathioprine, mercaptopurine, and theophylline *[see Contraindications (4) and Drug Interactions (7)]*.

Azathioprine and mercaptopurine undergo metabolism via three major metabolic pathways, one of which is mediated by XO. Although ULORIC drug interaction studies with azathioprine and mercaptopurine have not been conducted, concomitant administration of allopurinol [a xanthine oxidase inhibitor] with azathioprine or mercaptopurine has been reported to substantially increase plasma concentrations of these drugs. Because ULORIC is a xanthine oxidase inhibitor, it could inhibit the XO-mediated metabolism of azathioprine and mercaptopurine leading to increased plasma concentrations of azathioprine or mercaptopurine that could result in severe toxicity.

Theophylline is a CYP1A2 and XO substrate. Although no ULORIC drug interaction study with theophylline has been conducted, concomitant administration of theophylline with allopurinol, a xanthine oxidase inhibitor at doses ≥ 600 mg per day, has been reported to increase theophylline plasma concentrations. Because ULORIC is a xanthine oxidase inhibitor and theophylline is a low therapeutic index drug, ULORIC could inhibit the XO-mediated metabolism of theophylline leading to increased plasma concentrations of theophylline that could induce severe theophylline toxicity.

P450 Substrate Drugs: In vitro studies have shown that febuxostat does not inhibit P450 enzymes CYP1A2, 2C9, 2C19, 2D6, or 3A4 and it also does not induce CYP1A2, 2B6, 2C9, 2C19, or 3A4 at clinically relevant concentrations. As such, pharmacokinetic interactions between ULORIC and drugs metabolized by these CYP enzymes are unlikely.

Effect of Other Drugs on ULORIC

Febuxostat is metabolized by conjugation and oxidation via multiple metabolizing enzymes. The relative contribution of each enzyme isoform is not clear. Drug interactions between ULORIC and a drug that inhibits or induces one particular enzyme isoform is in general not expected.

In Vivo Drug Interaction Studies

Colchicine: No dose adjustment is necessary for either ULORIC or colchicine when the two drugs are co-administered. Administration of ULORIC (40 mg once daily) with colchicine (0.6 mg twice daily) resulted in an increase of 12% in C_{max} and 7% in AUC_{24} of febuxostat. In addition, administration of colchicine (0.6 mg twice daily) with ULORIC (120 mg daily) resulted in less than 11% change in C_{max} or AUC of colchicine for both AM and PM doses. These changes were not considered clinically significant.

Naproxen: No dose adjustment is necessary for ULORIC or naproxen when the two drugs are co-administered. Administration of ULORIC (80 mg once daily) with naproxen (500 mg twice daily) resulted in a 28% increase in C_{max} and a 40% increase in AUC of febuxostat. The increases were not considered clinically significant. In addition, there were no significant changes in the C_{max} or AUC of naproxen (less than 2%).

Indomethacin: No dose adjustment is necessary for either ULORIC or indomethacin when these two drugs are co-administered. Administration of ULORIC (80 mg once daily) with indomethacin (50 mg twice daily) did not result in any significant changes in C_{max} or AUC of febuxostat or indomethacin (less than 7%).

Hydrochlorothiazide: No dose adjustment is necessary for ULORIC when co-administered with hydrochlorothiazide. Administration of ULORIC (80 mg) with hydrochlorothiazide (50 mg) did not result in any clinically significant changes in C_{max} or AUC of febuxostat (less than 4%), and serum uric acid concentrations were not substantially affected.

Warfarin: No dose adjustment is necessary for warfarin when co-administered with ULORIC. Administration of ULORIC (80 mg once daily) with warfarin had no effect on the pharmacokinetics of warfarin in healthy subjects. INR and Factor VII activity were also not affected by the co-administration of ULORIC.

Desipramine: Co-administration of drugs that are CYP2D6 substrates (such as desipramine) with ULORIC are not expected to require dose adjustment. Febuxostat was shown to be a weak inhibitor of CYP2D6 *in vitro* and *in vivo*. Administration of ULORIC (120 mg once daily) with desipramine (25 mg) resulted in an increase in C_{max} (16%) and AUC (22%) of desipramine, which was associated with a 17% decrease in the 2-hydroxydesipramine to desipramine metabolic ratio (based on AUC).

13 NONCLINICAL TOXICOLOGY

13.1 Carcinogenesis, Mutagenesis, Impairment of Fertility

Carcinogenesis: Two-year carcinogenicity studies were conducted in F344 rats and B6C3F1 mice. Increased transitional cell papilloma and carcinoma of urinary bladder was observed at 24 mg per kg (25 times the human plasma exposure at maximum recommended human dose of 80 mg per day) and 18.75 mg per kg (12.5 times the human plasma exposure at 80 mg per day) in male rats and female mice, respectively. The urinary bladder neoplasms were secondary to calculus formation in the kidney and urinary bladder.

Mutagenesis: Febuxostat showed a positive mutagenic response in a chromosomal aberration assay in a Chinese hamster lung fibroblast cell line with and without metabolic activation *in vitro*. Febuxostat was negative in the *in vitro* Ames assay and chromosomal aberration test in human peripheral lymphocytes, and L5178Y mouse lymphoma cell line, and *in vivo* tests in mouse micronucleus, rat unscheduled DNA synthesis and rat bone marrow cells.

Impairment of Fertility: Febuxostat at oral doses up to 48 mg per kg per day (approximately 35 times the human plasma exposure at 80 mg per day) had no effect on fertility and reproductive performance of male and female rats.

13.2 Animal Toxicology

A 12-month toxicity study in beagle dogs showed deposition of xanthine crystals and calculi in kidneys at 15 mg per kg (approximately 4 times the human plasma exposure at 80 mg per day). A similar effect of calculus formation was noted in rats in a six-month study due to deposition of xanthine crystals at 48 mg per kg (approximately 35 times the human plasma exposure at 80 mg per day).

14 CLINICAL STUDIES

A serum uric acid level of less than 6 mg per dL is the goal of anti-hyperuricemic therapy and has been established as appropriate for the treatment of gout.

14.1 Management of Hyperuricemia in Gout

The efficacy of ULORIC was demonstrated in three randomized, double-blind, controlled trials in patients with hyperuricemia and gout. Hyperuricemia was defined as a baseline serum uric acid level ≥ 8 mg per dL.

Study 1 randomized patients to: ULORIC 40 mg daily, ULORIC 80 mg daily, or allopurinol (300 mg daily for patients with estimated creatinine clearance (Cl_{cr}) ≥ 60 mL per min or 200 mg daily for patients with estimated Cl_{cr} ≥ 30 mL per min and ≤ 59 mL per min). The duration of Study 1 was 6 months.

Study 2 randomized patients to: placebo, ULORIC 80 mg daily, ULORIC 120 mg daily, ULORIC 240 mg daily or allopurinol (300 mg daily for patients with a baseline serum creatinine ≤ 1.5 mg per dL or 100 mg daily for patients with a baseline serum creatinine greater than 1.5 mg per dL and ≤ 2 mg per dL). The duration of Study 2 was 6 months.

Study 3, a 1-year study, randomized patients to: ULORIC 80 mg daily, ULORIC 120 mg daily, or allopurinol 300 mg daily. Subjects who completed Study 2 and Study 3 were eligible to enroll in a phase 3 long-term extension study in which subjects received treatment with ULORIC for over three years.

In all three studies, subjects received naproxen 250 mg twice daily or colchicine 0.6 mg once or twice daily for gout flare prophylaxis. In Study 1 the duration of prophylaxis was 6 months; in Study 2 and Study 3 the duration of prophylaxis was 8 weeks.

The efficacy of ULORIC was also evaluated in a 4 week dose ranging study which randomized patients to: placebo, ULORIC 40 mg daily, ULORIC 80 mg daily, or ULORIC 120 mg daily. Subjects who completed this study were eligible to enroll in a long-term extension study in which subjects received treatment with ULORIC for up to five years.

Patients in these studies were representative of the patient population for which ULORIC use is intended. Table 2 summarizes the demographics and baseline characteristics for the subjects enrolled in the studies.

Table 2: Patient Demographics and Baseline Characteristics in Study 1, Study 2 and Study 3

Male	95%
Race: Caucasian	80%
African American	10%
Ethnicity: Hispanic or Latino	7%
Alcohol User	67%
Mild to Moderate Renal Insufficiency [percent with estimated Cl_{cr} less than 90 mL per min]	59%
History of Hypertension	49%
History of Hyperlipidemia	38%
BMI $\geq$ 30 kg per m^2	63%
Mean BMI	33 kg per m^2
Baseline sUA $\geq$ 10 mg per dL	36%
Mean baseline sUA	9.7 mg per dL
Experienced a gout flare in previous year	85%

Serum Uric Acid Level less than 6 mg per dL at Final Visit:
ULORIC 80 mg was superior to allopurinol in lowering serum uric acid to less than 6 mg per dL at the final visit. ULORIC 40 mg daily, although not superior to allopurinol, was effective in lowering serum uric acid to less than 6 mg per dL at the final visit (Table 3).
[See table 3 above]
In 76% of ULORIC 80 mg patients, reduction in serum uric acid levels to less than 6 mg per dL was noted by the Week 2 visit. Average serum uric acid levels were maintained at 6 mg per dL or below throughout treatment in 83% of these patients.
In all treatment groups, fewer subjects with higher baseline serum urate levels ($\geq$ 10 mg per dL) and/or tophi achieved the goal of lowering serum uric acid to less than 6 mg per dL at the final visit; however, a higher proportion achieved a serum uric acid less than 6 mg per dL with ULORIC 80 mg than with ULORIC 40 mg or allopurinol.
Study 1 evaluated efficacy in patients with mild to moderate renal impairment (i.e., baseline estimated CL_{cr} less than 90 mL per minute). The results in this sub-group of patients are shown in Table 4.
[See table 4 at right]

16   HOW SUPPLIED/STORAGE AND HANDLING

ULORIC 40 mg tablets are light green to green in color, round shaped, debossed with "TAP" on one side and "40" on the other side and supplied as:

NDC Number	Size
64764-918-11	Hospital Unit Dose Pack of 100 Tablets
64764-918-30	Bottle of 30 Tablets
64764-918-90	Bottle of 90 Tablets
64764-918-18	Bottle of 500 Tablets

ULORIC 80 mg tablets are light green to green in color, teardrop shaped, debossed with "TAP" on one side and "80" on the other side and supplied as:

NDC Number	Size
64764-677-11	Hospital Unit Dose Pack of 100 Tablets
64764-677-30	Bottle of 30 Tablets
64764-677-13	Bottle of 100 Tablets
64764-677-19	Bottle of 1000 Tablets

Protect from light. Store at 25°C (77°F); excursions permitted to 15°–30°C (59°–86°F) [See USP Controlled Room Temperature]

17   PATIENT COUNSELING INFORMATION

[see FDA-Approved Patient Labeling (17.2)]

17.1   General Information

Patients should be advised of the potential benefits and risks of ULORIC. Patients should be informed about the potential for gout flares, elevated liver enzymes and adverse cardiovascular events after initiation of ULORIC therapy. Concomitant prophylaxis with an NSAID *or colchicine for* gout flares should be considered.
Patients should be instructed to inform their healthcare professional if they develop a rash, chest pain, shortness of breath or neurologic symptoms suggesting a stroke. Patients should be instructed to inform their healthcare professional of any other medications they are currently taking with ULORIC, including over-the-counter medications.

Table 3: Proportion of Patients with Serum Uric Acid Levels Less Than 6 mg per dL at Final Visit

Study*	ULORIC 40 mg daily	ULORIC 80 mg daily	allopurinol	Placebo	Difference in Proportion (95% CI) ULORIC 40 mg vs allopurinol	Difference in Proportion (95% CI) ULORIC 80 mg vs allopurinol
Study 1 (6 months) (N=2268)	45%	67%	42%		3% (-2%, 8%)	25% (20%, 30%)
Study 2 (6 months) (N=643)		72%	39%	1%		33% (26%, 42%)
Study 3 (12 months) (N=491)		74%	36%			38% (30%, 46%)

*Randomization was balanced between treatment groups, except in Study 2 in which twice as many patients were randomized to each of the active treatment groups compared to placebo.

Table 4: Proportion of Patients with Serum Uric Acid Levels Less Than 6 mg per dL in Patients with Mild or Moderate Renal Impairment at Final Visit

ULORIC 40 mg daily (N=479)	ULORIC 80 mg daily (N=503)	allopurinol* 300 mg daily (N=501)	Difference in Proportion (95% CI) ULORIC 40 mg vs allopurinol	Difference in Proportion (95% CI) ULORIC 80 mg vs allopurinol
50%	72%	42%	7% (1%, 14%)	29% (23%, 35%)

*Allopurinol patients (n=145) with estimated $Cl_{cr} \geq 30$ mL per min and $Cl_{cr} \leq 59$ mL per min were dosed at 200 mg daily.

17.2   FDA-Approved Patient Labeling

Patient Information
ULORIC® (Ū – 'lor – ik)
(febuxostat) tablets
Read the Patient Information that comes with ULORIC before you start taking it and each time you get a refill. There may be new information. This information does not take the place of talking with your healthcare provider about your medical condition or your treatment.
What is ULORIC?
ULORIC is a prescription medicine called a xanthine oxidase (XO) inhibitor, used to lower blood uric acid levels in adults with gout.
It is not known if ULORIC is safe and effective in children under 18 years of age.
Who should not take ULORIC?
Do not take ULORIC if you:
• take Azathioprine (Azasan®, Imuran®)
• take Mercaptopurine (Purinethol®)
• take Theophylline (Theo-24®, Elixophyllin®, Theochron®, Theolair®, Uniphyl®)
It is not known if ULORIC is safe and effective in children under 18 years of age.
What should I tell my healthcare provider before taking ULORIC?
Before taking ULORIC tell your healthcare provider about all of your medical conditions, including if you:
• have liver or kidney problems
• have a history of heart disease or stroke
• are pregnant or plan to become pregnant. It is not known if ULORIC will harm your unborn baby. Talk with your healthcare provider if you are pregnant or plan to become pregnant.
• are breast-feeding or plan to breast-feed. It is not known if ULORIC passes into your breast milk. You and your healthcare provider should decide if you should take ULORIC while breast-feeding.
Tell your healthcare provider about all the medicines you take, including prescription and non-prescription medicines, vitamins, and herbal supplements. ULORIC may affect the way other medicines work, and other medicines may affect how ULORIC works.
Know the medicines you take. Keep a list of them and show it to your healthcare provider and pharmacist when you get a new medicine.
How should I take ULORIC?
• Take ULORIC exactly as your healthcare provider tells you to take it.
• ULORIC can be taken with or without food.
• ULORIC can be taken with antacids.
• Your gout may flare up when you start taking ULORIC,

do not stop taking your ULORIC even if you have a flare. Your healthcare provider may give you other medicines to help prevent your gout flares.
• Your healthcare provider may do certain tests while you take ULORIC.
What are the possible side effects of ULORIC?
Heart problems. A small number of heart attacks, strokes and heart-related deaths were seen in clinical studies. It is not certain that ULORIC caused these events.
The most common side effects of ULORIC include:
• liver problems
• nausea
• gout flares
• joint pain
• rash
Tell your healthcare provider if you have any side effect that bothers you or that does not go away. These are not all of the possible side effects of ULORIC. For more information, ask your healthcare provider or pharmacist.
Call your doctor for medical advice about side effects. You may report side effects to the FDA at 1-800-FDA-1088.
How should I store ULORIC?
Store ULORIC between 59°F-86°F (15°C-30°C).
Keep ULORIC out of the light.
Keep ULORIC and all medicines out of the reach of children.
General information about the safe and effective use of ULORIC
Medicines are sometimes prescribed for purposes other than those listed in a patient information leaflet. Do not use ULORIC for a condition for which it was not prescribed. Do not give ULORIC to other people, even if they have the same symptoms that you have. It may harm them.
This patient information leaflet summarizes the most important information about ULORIC. If you would like more information about ULORIC talk with your healthcare provider. You can ask your healthcare provider or pharmacist for information about ULORIC that is written for health professionals. For more information go to www.uloric.com, or call 1-877-825-3327.
What are the ingredients in ULORIC?
Active Ingredient: febuxostat
Inactive ingredients include: lactose monohydrate, microcrystalline cellulose, hydroxypropyl cellulose, sodium croscarmellose, silicon dioxide, magnesium stearate, and Opadry II, green
Distributed by
Takeda Pharmaceuticals America, Inc.
Deerfield, IL 60015
U.S. Patent Nos. - 6,225,474; 7,361,676; 5,614,520.

ULORIC® is a registered trademark of Teijin Pharma Limited and used under license by Takeda Pharmaceuticals America, Inc.

All other trademark names are the property of their respective owners

©2009 Takeda Pharmaceuticals America, Inc.

PI1114 R1; February 2009

Shown in Product Identification Guide, page 320

Talecris Biotherapeutics, Inc.

79 T.W. ALEXANDER DRIVE
RESEARCH TRIANGLE PARK, NC 27709

Direct Inquiries to:
For Clinical and Technical Information Contact:
1-800-520-2807
For Customer Service Contact:
1-800-243-4153

GAMUNEX®

[găm-ew-nĕks]   ℞

Immune Globulin Intravenous (Human), 10% Caprylate/Chromatography Purified
FOR INTRAVENOUS USE ONLY

HIGHLIGHTS OF PRESCRIBING INFORMATION

These highlights do not include all the information needed to use GAMUNEX safely and effectively. See full prescribing information for GAMUNEX.

GAMUNEX (Immune Globulin Intravenous [Human], 10% Caprylate/Chromatography Purified) 10% Liquid Preparation

Initial U.S. Approval: 2003

WARNING: ACUTE RENAL DYSFUNCTION and FAILURE

See full prescribing information for complete boxed warning.

- **Renal dysfunction, acute renal failure, osmotic nephrosis, and death may be associated with Immune Globulin Intravenous (Human) (IGIV) products in predisposed patients.**
- **Renal dysfunction and acute renal failure occur more commonly in patients receiving IGIV products containing sucrose. GAMUNEX does not contain sucrose.**
- **Administer IGIV products at the minimum concentration available and the minimum infusion rate practicable.**

RECENT MAJOR CHANGES

- Indications and Usage, Chronic Inflammatory Demyelinating Polyneuropathy (CIDP) (1.3)   09/2008
- Dosage and Administration, Chronic Inflammatory Demyelinating Polyneuropathy (CIDP) (2.4)   09/2008
- Dosage and Administration, Primary Humoral Immunodeficiency (2.2)   10/2008

INDICATIONS AND USAGE

GAMUNEX is an immune globulin intravenous (human), 10% liquid indicated for treatment of:
- Primary Humoral Immunodeficiency (PI) (1.1)
- Idiopathic Thrombocytopenic Purpura (ITP) (1.2)
- Chronic Inflammatory Demyelinating Polyneuropathy (CIDP) (1.3)

DOSAGE AND ADMINISTRATION

- Intravenous Use Only

Indication	Dose	Initial Infusion rate	Maintenance infusion rate (if tolerated)
PI (2.2)	300-600 mg/kg	1 mg/kg/min	8 mg/kg/min Every 3-4 weeks
ITP (2.3)	2 g/kg	1 mg/kg/min	8 mg/kg/min
CIDP (2.4)	loading dose: 2 g/kg maintenance dose: 1 g/kg	2 mg/kg/min	8 mg/kg/min Every 3 weeks

- Ensure that patients with pre-existing renal insufficiency are not volume depleted; discontinue GAMUNEX if renal function deteriorates. (5.2)
- For patients at risk of renal dysfunction or thrombotic events, administer GAMUNEX at the minimum infusion rate practicable. (5.2)

DOSAGE FORMS AND STRENGTHS

GAMUNEX is supplied in 1 g, 2.5 g, 5 g, 10 g, or 20 g single use bottles. (3)

1 g	10 mL
2.5 g	25 mL
5 g	50 mL
10 g	100 mL
20 g	200 mL

CONTRAINDICATIONS

- Anaphylactic or severe systemic reactions to human immunoglobulin (4)
- IgA deficient patients with antibodies against IgA and a history of hypersensitivity (4)

WARNINGS AND PRECAUTIONS

- IgA deficient patients with antibodies against IgA are at greater risk of developing severe hypersensitivity and anaphylactic reactions. Epinephrine should be available immediately to treat any acute severe hypersensitivity reactions. (5.1)
- Monitor renal function, including blood urea nitrogen, serum creatinine, and urine output in patients at risk of developing acute renal failure. (5.2)
- Hyperproteinemia, increased serum viscosity and hyponatremia occur in patients receiving IGIV therapy. (5.3)
- Thrombotic events have occurred in patients receiving IGIV therapy. Monitor patients with known risk factors for thrombotic events; consider baseline assessment of blood viscosity for those at risk of hyperviscosity. (5.4)
- Aseptic Meningitis Syndrome has been reported with GAMUNEX and other IGIV treatments, especially with high doses or rapid infusion. (5.5)
- Hemolytic anemia can develop subsequent to IGIV therapy due to enhanced RBC sequestration. (5.6)
- IGIV recipients should be monitored for pulmonary adverse reactions (TRALI). (5.7)
- The product is made from human plasma and may contain infectious agents, e.g., viruses and, theoretically, the Creutzfeldt-Jakob disease agent. (5.9)

ADVERSE REACTIONS

- **PI** - Most common drug related adverse reactions during clinical trials were headache and cough. (6.1)
- **ITP** - Most common drug related adverse reactions during clinical trials were headache, vomiting, fever, and nausea. (6.1)
- **CIDP** - Most common drug related adverse reactions during clinical trials were headache and fever. (6.1)

To report SUSPECTED ADVERSE REACTIONS, contact Talecris Biotherapeutics at 1-800-520-2807 or FDA at 1-800-FDA-1088 or www.fda.gov/medwatch.

DRUG INTERACTIONS

- The passive transfer of antibodies may interfere with the response to live viral vaccines. (7)
- The passive transfer of antibodies may confound the results of serological testing. (7)

USE IN SPECIFIC POPULATIONS

- In patients over age 65 or in any patient at risk of developing renal insufficiency, do not exceed the recommended dose, and infuse GAMUNEX at the minimum infusion rate practicable. (8.5)
- Pregnancy: no human or animal data. Use only if clearly needed. (8.1)

See 17 for PATIENT COUNSELING INFORMATION

Revised: 10/2008

FULL PRESCRIBING INFORMATION: CONTENTS*

1 **INDICATIONS AND USAGE**
    1.1   Primary Humoral Immunodeficiency (PI)
    1.2   Idiopathic Thrombocytopenic Purpura (ITP)
    1.3   Chronic Inflammatory Demyelinating Polyneuropathy (CIDP)
2 **DOSAGE AND ADMINISTRATION**
    2.1   Preparation and Handling
    2.2   Treatment of Primary Humoral Immunodeficiency
    2.3   Treatment of Idiopathic Thrombocytopenic Purpura
    2.4   Treatment of Chronic Inflammatory Demyelinating Polyneuropathy
    2.5   Administration
3 **DOSAGE FORMS AND STRENGTH**
4 **CONTRAINDICATIONS**
5 **WARNINGS AND PRECAUTIONS**
    5.1   Sensitivity
    5.2   Renal Failure
    5.3   Hyperproteinemia
    5.4   Thrombotic Events
    5.5   Aseptic Meningitis Syndrome (AMS)
    5.6   Hemolysis
    5.7   Transfusion-related Acute Lung Injury (TRALI)
    5.8   Volume Overload
    5.9   General
    5.10 Laboratory Tests
6 **ADVERSE REACTIONS**
    6.1   Adverse Drug Reaction Overview
    6.2   Clinical Trials Adverse Drug Reactions
    6.3   Postmarketing Experience
7 **DRUG INTERACTIONS**
8 **USE IN SPECIFIC POPULATIONS**
    8.1   Pregnancy
    8.3   Nursing Mothers
    8.4   Pediatric Use
    8.5   Geriatric Use
11 **DESCRIPTION**
12 **CLINICAL PHARMACOLOGY**
    12.1 Mechanism of Action
    12.3 Pharmacokinetics
14 **CLINICAL STUDIES**
    14.1 Treatment of Primary Humoral Immunodeficiency
    14.2 Treatment of Idiopathic Thrombocytopenic Purpura
    14.3 Treatment of Chronic Inflammatory Demyelinating Polyneuropathy
15 **REFERENCES**
16 **HOW SUPPLIED/STORAGE AND HANDLING**
17 **PATIENT COUNSELING INFORMATION**
* Sections or subsections omitted from the full prescribing information are not listed.

FULL PRESCRIBING INFORMATION

WARNING: ACUTE RENAL DYSFUNCTION AND ACUTE RENAL FAILURE

Immune Globulin Intravenous (Human) products have been reported to be associated with renal dysfunction, acute renal failure, osmotic nephrosis and death.(1) Patients predisposed to acute renal failure include patients with any degree of pre-existing renal insufficiency, diabetes mellitus, age greater than 65, volume depletion, sepsis, paraproteinemia, or patients receiving known nephrotoxic drugs. Especially in such patients, IGIV products should be administered at the minimum concentration available and the minimum rate of infusion practicable. While these reports of renal dysfunction and acute renal failure have been associated with the use of many of the licensed IGIV products, those containing sucrose as a stabilizer accounted for a disproportionate share of the total number. GAMUNEX does not contain sucrose. Glycine, a natural amino acid, is used as a stabilizer. (See Dosage and Administration [2.5] and Warnings and Precautions [5.2] for important information intended to reduce the risk of acute renal failure.)

---

1   INDICATIONS AND USAGE

Gamunex is an immune globulin intravenous (human) 10% liquid indicated for the treatment of:

1.1   Primary Humoral Immunodeficiency (PI)

GAMUNEX is indicated as replacement therapy of primary humoral immunodeficiency. This includes, but is not limited to, congenital agammaglobulinemia, common variable immunodeficiency, X-linked agammaglobulinemia, Wiskott-Aldrich syndrome, and severe combined immunodeficiencies.(2-9)

1.2   Idiopathic Thrombocytopenic Purpura (ITP)

GAMUNEX is indicated in Idiopathic Thrombocytopenic Purpura to rapidly raise platelet counts to prevent bleeding or to allow a patient with ITP to undergo surgery.(10-15)

1.3   Chronic Inflammatory Demyelinating Polyneuropathy (CIDP)

GAMUNEX is indicated for the treatment of CIDP to improve neuromuscular disability and impairment and for maintenance therapy to prevent relapse.

2   DOSAGE AND ADMINISTRATION

For intravenous use only.

GAMUNEX consists of 9%-11% protein in 0.16-0.24 M glycine. The buffering capacity of GAMUNEX is 35.0 mEq/L (0.35 mEq/g protein). A dose of 1 g/kg body weight therefore represents an acid load of 0.35 mEq/kg body weight. The total buffering capacity of whole blood in a normal individual is 45-50 mEq/L of blood, or 3.6 mEq/kg body weight.(16) Thus, the acid load delivered with a dose of 1 g/kg of GAMUNEX would be neutralized by the buffering capacity of whole blood alone, even if the dose was infused instantaneously.

2.1   Preparation and Handling

- GAMUNEX should be inspected visually for particulate

matter and discoloration prior to administration, whenever solution and container permit. Do not use if turbid.

- Do not freeze. Solutions that have been frozen should not be used.
- The GAMUNEX vial is for single use only. GAMUNEX contains no preservative. Any vial that has been entered should be used promptly. Partially used vials should be discarded.
- GAMUNEX should be infused using a separate line by itself, without mixing with other intravenous fluids or medications the subject might be receiving.
- GAMUNEX is not compatible with saline. If dilution is required, GAMUNEX may be diluted with 5% dextrose in water (D5/W). No other drug interactions or compatibilities have been evaluated.
- Content of vials may be pooled under aseptic conditions into sterile infusion bags and infused within 8 hours after pooling.
- Do not mix with immune globulin intravenous (IGIV) products from other manufacturers.
- Do not use after expiration date.

2.2 Treatment of Primary Humoral Immunodeficiency

As there are significant differences in the half-life of IgG among patients with primary immunodeficiencies, the frequency and amount of immunoglobulin therapy may vary from patient to patient. The proper amount can be determined by monitoring clinical response.

The dose of GAMUNEX for replacement therapy in primary immune deficiency diseases is 300 to 600 mg/kg body weight (3-6 mL/kg) administered every 3 to 4 weeks. The dosage may be adjusted over time to achieve the desired trough levels and clinical responses.

If a patient routinely receives a dose of less than 400 mg/kg of GAMUNEX every 3 to 4 weeks (less than 4 mL/kg), and is at risk of measles exposure (i.e., traveling to a measles endemic area), administer a dose of at least 400 mg/kg (4 mL/kg) just prior to the expected measles exposure. If a patient has been exposed to measles, a dose of 400 mg/kg (4 mL/kg) should be administered as soon as possible after exposure.

2.3 Treatment of Idiopathic Thrombocytopenic Purpura

GAMUNEX may be administered at a total dose of 2 g/kg, divided in two doses of 1 g/kg (10 mL/kg) given on two consecutive days or into five doses of 0.4 g/kg (4 mL/kg) given on five consecutive days. If after administration of the first of two daily 1 g/kg (10 mL/kg) doses, an adequate increase in the platelet count is observed at 24 hours, the second dose of 1g/kg body weight may be withheld.

Forty-eight ITP subjects were treated with 2 g/kg GAMUNEX, divided in two 1 g/kg doses (10 mL/kg) given on two successive days. With this dose regimen 35/39 subjects (90%) responded with a platelet count from less than or equal to 20 $\times 10^9$/L to more than or equal to 50 $\times 10^9$/L within 7 days after treatment.(17)

The high dose regimen (1 g/kg $\times$ 1-2 days) is not recommended for individuals with expanded fluid volumes or where fluid volume may be a concern.

2.4 Treatment of Chronic Inflammatory Demyelinating Polyneuropathy

GAMUNEX may be initially administered as a total loading dose of 2 g/kg (20 mL/kg) given in divided doses over two to four consecutive days. GAMUNEX may be administered as a maintenance infusion of 1 g/kg (10 mL/kg) administered over 1 day or divided into two doses of 0.5 g/kg (5 mL/kg) given on two consecutive days, every 3 weeks.

2.5 Administration

GAMUNEX should be inspected visually for particulate matter and discoloration prior to administration, whenever solution and container permit. Do not use if turbid and/or if discoloration is observed.

Only administer intravenously. GAMUNEX should be at room temperature during administration.

Only 18 gauge needles should be used to penetrate the stopper for dispensing product from the 10 mL vial; 16 gauge needles or dispensing pins should only be used with 25 mL vial sizes and larger. Needles or dispensing pins should only be inserted once and be within the stopper area delineated by the raised ring. The stopper should be penetrated perpendicular to the plane of the stopper within the ring.

GAMUNEX® vial size	Gauge of needle to penetrate stopper
10 mL	18 gauge
25, 50, 100, 200 mL	16 gauge

Any vial that has been opened should be used promptly. Partially used vials should be discarded.

If dilution is required, GAMUNEX may be diluted with 5% dextrose in water (D5/W).

Table 1: Reasons for Discontinuation Due to Adverse Events: All PI Studies

Study Number	Number of Subjects Treated with GAMUNEX®	Number of Subjects Discontinued Due to Adverse Events	Adverse Event
100152	18	0	—
100174	20	1	Coombs negative hypochromic anemia*
100175	87	1	Autoimmune pure red cell aplasia*

*Both events were considered unrelated to study drug as per the investigator.

Rate of Administration

It is recommended that GAMUNEX should initially be infused at a rate of 0.01 mL/kg per minute (1 mg/kg per minute) for the first 30 minutes.

If well-tolerated, the rate may be gradually increased to a maximum of 0.08 mL/kg per minute (8 mg/kg per minute).

Indication	Initial infusion rate (first 30 minutes)	Maximum infusion rate (if tolerated)
PI	1 mg/kg/min	8 mg/kg/min
ITP	1 mg/kg/min	8 mg/kg/min
CIDP	2 mg/kg/min	8 mg/kg/min

Certain severe adverse drug reactions may be related to the rate of infusion. Slowing or stopping the infusion usually allows the symptoms to disappear promptly.

Ensure that patients with pre-existing renal insufficiency are not volume depleted; discontinue GAMUNEX if renal function deteriorates.

For patients at risk of renal dysfunction or thromboembolic events, administer GAMUNEX at the minimum infusion rate practicable.

Incompatibilities

GAMUNEX is not compatible with saline. If dilution is required, GAMUNEX may be diluted with 5% dextrose in water (D5/W). No other drug interactions or compatibilities have been evaluated.

Shelf Life

GAMUNEX may be stored for 36 months at 2-8ºC (36-46ºF) from the date of manufacture AND product may be stored at temperatures not to exceed 25ºC (77ºF) for up to 6 months any time during the 36 month shelf life, after which the product must be immediately discarded.

Special Precautions for Storage

Do not freeze. Frozen product should not be used.

Do not use after expiration date.

3 DOSAGE FORMS AND STRENGTH

GAMUNEX is supplied in 1 g, 2.5 g, 5 g, 10 g, or 20 g single use bottles.

- 1 g in 10 mL solution
- 2.5 g in 25 mL solution
- 5 g in 50 mL solution
- 10 g in 100 mL solution
- 20 g in 200 mL solution

4 CONTRAINDICATIONS

- GAMUNEX is contraindicated in individuals with acute severe hypersensitivity reactions to Immune Globulin (Human).
- GAMUNEX contains trace amounts of IgA. It is contraindicated in IgA deficient patients with antibodies against IgA and history of hypersensitivity. *(See Description [11])*

5 WARNINGS AND PRECAUTIONS

5.1 Sensitivity

Severe hypersensitivity reactions may occur. In case of hypersensitivity, IGIV infusion should be immediately discontinued and appropriate treatment instituted. Epinephrine should be immediately available for treatment of acute severe hypersensitivity reaction. *(See Patient Counseling Information [17])*

GAMUNEX contains trace amounts of IgA (average 46 micrograms/mL). It is contraindicated in IgA deficient patients with antibodies against IgA and history of hypersensitivity. *(See Patient Counseling Information [17])*

5.2 Renal Failure

Assure that patients are not volume depleted prior to the initiation of the infusion of IGIV. Periodic monitoring of renal function and urine output is particularly important in patients judged to have a potential increased risk for developing acute renal failure. Renal function, including measurement of blood urea nitrogen (BUN)/serum creatinine, should be assessed prior to the initial infusion of GAMUNEX and again at appropriate intervals thereafter. If renal function deteriorates, discontinuation of the product should be considered. *(See Patient Counseling Information [17])* For patients judged to be at risk for developing renal dysfunction and/or at risk of developing thrombotic events, it may be prudent to reduce the amount of product infused per unit time by infusing GAMUNEX at a rate less than 8 mg IG/kg/min (0.08 mL/kg/min). *(See Boxed Warning) (See Dosage and Administration [2.5])*

5.3 Hyperproteinemia

Hyperproteinemia, increased serum viscosity and hyponatremia may occur in patients receiving IGIV therapy. The hyponatremia is likely to be a pseudohyponatremia as demonstrated by a decreased calculated serum osmolality or elevated osmolar gap. Distinguishing true hyponatremia from pseudohyponatremia is clinically critical, as treatment aimed at decreasing serum free water in patients with pseudohyponatremia may lead to volume depletion, a further increase in serum viscosity and a disposition to thromboembolic events.(18)

5.4 Thrombotic Events

Thrombotic events have been reported in association with IGIV.(19-21) Patients at risk may include those with a history of atherosclerosis, multiple cardiovascular risk factors, advanced age, impaired cardiac output, coagulation disorders, prolonged periods of immobilization and/or known or suspected hyperviscosity. The potential risks and benefits of IGIV should be weighed against those of alternative therapies for all patients for whom IGIV administration is being considered. Baseline assessment of blood viscosity should be considered in patients at risk for hyperviscosity, including those with cryoglobulins, fasting chylomicronemia/markedly high triacylglycerols (triglycerides), or monoclonal gammopathies.

5.5 Aseptic Meningitis Syndrome (AMS)

An aseptic meningitis syndrome (AMS) has been reported to occur infrequently in association with Immune Globulin Intravenous (Human) treatment. Discontinuation of IGIV treatment has resulted in remission of AMS within several days without sequelae.(22-24) The syndrome usually begins within several hours to two days following IGIV treatment. It is characterized by symptoms and signs including severe headache, nuchal rigidity, drowsiness, fever, photophobia, painful eye movements, nausea and vomiting. Cerebrospinal fluid (CSF) studies are frequently positive with pleocytosis up to several thousand cells per cu mm, predominantly from the granulocytic series, and elevated protein levels up to several hundred mg/dl. Patients exhibiting such symptoms and signs should receive a thorough neurological examination, including CSF studies, to rule out other causes of meningitis. It appears that patients with a history of migraine may be more susceptible. *(See Patient Counseling Information [17])*

5.6 Hemolysis

Immune Globulin Intravenous (Human) (IGIV) products can contain blood group antibodies which may act as hemolysins and induce in vivo coating of red blood cells with immunoglobulin, causing a positive direct antiglobulin reaction and, rarely, hemolysis.(25–27) Hemolytic anemia can develop subsequent to IGIV therapy due to enhanced RBC sequestration. IGIV recipients should be monitored for clinical signs and symptoms of hemolysis.(28) If signs and/or symptoms of hemolysis are present after IGIV infusion, appropriate confirmatory laboratory testing should be done. *(See Patient Counseling Information [17])*

5.7 Transfusion-related Acute Lung Injury (TRALI)

There have been reports of noncardiogenic pulmonary edema [Transfusion-Related Acute Lung Injury (TRALI)] in patients administered IGIV.(29) TRALI is characterized by severe respiratory distress, pulmonary edema, hypoxemia, normal left ventricular function, and fever and typically occurs within 1-6 hrs after transfusion. Patients with TRALI may be managed using oxygen therapy with adequate ventilatory support.

IGIV recipients should be monitored for pulmonary adverse reactions. *(See Patient Counseling Information [17])* If TRALI is suspected, appropriate tests should be performed for the presence of anti-neutrophil antibodies in both the product and patient serum.

5.8 Volume Overload

The high dose regimen (1 g/kg $\times$ 1-2 days) is not recommended for individuals with expanded fluid volumes or where fluid volume may be a concern.

5.9 General

Because this product is made from human blood, it may carry a risk of transmitting infectious agents, e.g., viruses, and, theoretically, the Creutzfeldt-Jakob (CJD) agent. ALL infections thought by a physician possibly to have been transmitted by this product should be reported by the physician or other healthcare provider to Talecris Biotherapeutics, Inc. [1-800-520-2807]. The physician should discuss the risks and benefits of this product with the patient, before prescribing or administering it to the patient. *(See Patient Counseling Information [17])*

5.10 Laboratory Tests

If signs and/or symptoms of hemolysis are present after IGIV infusion, appropriate confirmatory laboratory testing should be done.

If TRALI is suspected, appropriate tests should be performed for the presence of anti-neutrophil antibodies in both the product and patient serum.

Because of the potentially increased risk of thrombosis, baseline assessment of blood viscosity should be considered in patients at risk for hyperviscosity, including those with cryoglobulins, fasting chylomicronemia/markedly high triacylglycerols (triglycerides), or monoclonal gammopathies.

6 ADVERSE REACTIONS

6.1 Adverse Drug Reaction Overview

The most serious adverse reaction observed in clinical study subjects receiving GAMUNEX for PI was an exacerbation of autoimmune pure red cell aplasia in one subject.

The most serious adverse reaction observed in clinical study subjects receiving GAMUNEX for ITP was myocarditis in one subject that occurred 50 days post study drug infusion and was not considered drug related.

The most serious adverse reaction observed in clinical study subjects receiving GAMUNEX for CIDP was pulmonary embolism (PE) in one subject with a history of PE.

The most common drug related adverse reactions observed at a rate ≥5% in subjects with PI were headache, cough, injection site reaction, nausea, pharyngitis and urticaria.

The most common drug related adverse reactions observed at a rate ≥5% in subjects with ITP were headache, vomiting, fever, nausea, back pain and rash.

The most common drug related adverse reactions observed at a rate ≥5% in subjects with CIDP were headache, fever, chills, hypertension, rash, nausea and asthenia.

6.2 Clinical Trials Adverse Drug Reactions

Because clinical studies are conducted under widely varying conditions, adverse reaction rates observed cannot be directly compared to rates in other clinical trials and may not reflect the rates observed in practice.

Adverse events similar to those previously reported with the administration of intravenous and intramuscular immunoglobulin products may occur. Cases of reversible aseptic meningitis, migraine, isolated cases of reversible hemolytic anemia and reversible increases in liver function tests have been observed with GAMUNEX. Immediate anaphylactic reactions can possibly occur (<0.01%). Epinephrine should be available for treatment of any acute anaphylactoid reaction. *(see Warnings and Precautions [5.1])*

Treatment of Primary Humoral Immunodeficiency

The following table shows the number of subjects treated with GAMUNEX in clinical trials to study PI, and the reason for discontinuation due to adverse events:

[See table 1 at top of previous page]

In study 100175, 9 subjects in each treatment group were pretreated with non-steroidal medication prior to infusion. Generally, diphenhydramine and acetaminophen were used. Any adverse events in trial 100175, irrespective of the causality assessment, are given in the following table.

Table 2: Subjects with At Least One Adverse Event Irrespective of Causality (Study 100175)

Adverse Event	GAMUNEX® No. of subjects: 87 No. of subjects with AE (percentage of all subjects)	GAMIMUNE® N, 10% No. of subjects: 85 No. of subjects with AE (percentage of all subjects)
Cough increased	47 (54%)	46 (54%)
Rhinitis	44 (51%)	45 (53%)
Pharyngitis	36 (41%)	39 (46%)
Headache	22 (25%)	28 (33%)
Fever	24 (28%)	27 (32%)
Diarrhea	24 (28%)	27 (32%)
Asthma	25 (29%)	17 (20%)
Nausea	17 (20%)	22 (26%)
Ear Pain	16 (18%)	12 (14%)
Asthenia	9 (10%)	13 (15%)

The subset of drug related adverse events in trial 100175 reported by at least 5% of subjects during the 9-month treatment are given in the following table.

Table 3: Subjects with At Least One Drug Related Adverse Event (Study 100175)

Drug Related Adverse Event	GAMUNEX® No. of subjects: 87 No. of subjects with drug related AE (percentage of all subjects)	GAMIMUNE® N, 10% No. of subjects: 85 No. of subjects with drug related AE (percentage of all subjects)
Headache	7 (8%)	8 (9%)
Cough increased	6 (7%)	4 (5%)
Injection site reaction	4 (5%)	7 (8%)
Nausea	4 (5%)	4 (5%)
Pharyngitis	4 (5%)	3 (4%)
Urticaria	4 (5%)	1 (1%)

Adverse events, which were reported by at least 5% of subjects were also analyzed by frequency and in relation to infusions administered. The analysis is displayed in the following table.

[See table 4 above]

The mean number of adverse events per infusion that occurred during or on the same day as an infusion was 0.21 in both the GAMUNEX and GAMIMUNE® N, Immune Globulin Intravenous (Human), 10%, treatment groups.

In all three trials in primary humoral immundeficiencies, the maximum infusion rate was 0.08 mL/kg/ min (8 mg/kg/min). The infusion rate was reduced for 11 of 222 exposed subjects (7 GAMUNEX, 4 GAMIMUNE N, 10%) at 17 occasions. In most instances, mild to moderate hives/urticaria, itching, pain or reaction at infusion site, anxiety or headache was the main reason. There was one case of severe chills. There were no anaphylactic or anaphylactoid reactions to GAMUNEX or GAMIMUNE N, 10%.

Table 4: Adverse Event Frequency (Study 100175)

Adverse Event		GAMUNEX® No. of infusions: 825 No. of AE (percentage of all infusions)	GAMIMUNE® N, 10% No. of infusions: 865 No. of AE (percentage of all infusions)
Cough increased	All	154 (18.7%)	148 (17.1%)
	Drug related	*14 (1.7%)*	*11 (1.3%)*
Pharyngitis	All	96 (11.6%)	99 (11.4%)
	Drug related	*7 (0.8%)*	*9 (1.0%)*
Headache	All	57 (6.9%)	69 (8.0%)
	Drug related	*7 (0.8%)*	*11 (1.3%)*
Fever	All	41 (5.0%)	65 (7.5%)
	Drug related	*1 (0.1%)*	*9 (1.0%)*
Nausea	All	31 (3.8%)	43 (5.0%)
	Drug related	*4 (0.5%)*	*4 (0.5%)*
Urticaria	All	5 (0.6%)	8 (0.9%)
	Drug related	*4 (0.5%)*	*5 (0.6%)*

Table 5: Reasons for Discontinuation Due to Adverse Events: All ITP Studies

Study Number	Number of Subjects Treated with GAMUNEX®	Number of Subjects Discontinued Due to Adverse Events	Adverse Event
100213	28	1	Hives
100176	48	1	Headache, Fever, Vomiting

In trial 100175, serum samples were drawn to monitor the viral safety at baseline and one week after the first infusion (for parvovirus B19), eight weeks after first and fifth infusion, and 16 weeks after the first and fifth infusion of IGIV (for hepatitis C) and at any time of premature discontinuation of the study. Viral markers of hepatitis C, hepatitis B, HIV-1, and parvovirus B19 were monitored by nucleic acid testing (NAT, Polymerase Chain Reaction (PCR)), and serological testing. There were no treatment emergent findings of viral transmission for either GAMUNEX or GAMIMUNE N, 10%.(30-32)

Treatment of Idiopathic Thrombocytopenic Purpura

The following table shows the number of subjects treated with GAMUNEX in clinical trials to study ITP, and the reason for discontinuation due to adverse events:

[See table 5 above]

One subject, a 10-year-old boy, died suddenly from myocarditis 50 days after his second infusion of GAMUNEX. The death was judged to be unrelated to GAMUNEX.

No pre-medication with corticosteroids was permitted by the protocol. Twelve (12) ITP subjects treated in each treatment group were pretreated with medication prior to infusion. Generally, diphenhydramine and/or acetaminophen were used. More than 90% of the observed drug related adverse events were of mild to moderate severity and of transient nature.

The infusion rate was reduced for 4 of the 97 exposed subjects (1 GAMUNEX, 3 GAMIMUNE N, 10%) on 4 occasions. Mild to moderate headache, nausea, and fever were the reported reasons. There were no anaphylactic or anaphylactoid reactions to GAMUNEX or GAMIMUNE N, 10%.

Any adverse events in trial 100176, irrespective of the causality assessment, reported by at least 5% of subjects during the 3-month trial are given in the following table.

Table 6: Subjects with At Least One Adverse Event Irrespective of Causality (Study 100176)

Adverse Event	GAMUNEX® No. of subjects: 48 No. of subjects with AE (percentage of all subjects)	GAMIMUNE® N, 10% No. of subjects: 49 No. of subjects with AE (percentage of all subjects)
Headache	28 (58%)	30 (61%)
Ecchymosis, Purpura	19 (40%)	25 (51%)
Hemorrhage (All systems)	14 (29%)	16 (33%)
Epistaxis	11 (23%)	12 (24%)
Petechiae	10 (21%)	15 (31%)

Fever	10 (21%)	7 (14%)
Vomiting	10 (21%)	10 (20%)
Nausea	10 (21%)	7 (14%)
Thrombocyto-penia	7 (15%)	8 (16%)
Accidental injury	6 (13%)	8 (16%)
Rhinitis	6 (13%)	6 (12%)
Pharyngitis	5 (10%)	5 (10%)
Rash	5 (10%)	6 (12%)
Pruritis	4 (8%)	1 (2%)
Asthenia	3 (6%)	5 (10%)
Abdominal Pain	3 (6%)	4 (8%)
Arthralgia	3 (6%)	6 (12%)
Back Pain	3 (6%)	3 (6%)
Dizziness	3 (6%)	3 (6%)
Flu Syndrome	3 (6%)	3 (6%)
Neck Pain	3 (6%)	1 (2%)
Anemia	3 (6%)	0 (0%)
Dyspepsia	3 (6%)	0 (0%)

The subset of drug related adverse events in trial 100176 reported by at least 5% of subjects during the 3-month trial are given in the following table.

Table 7: Subjects with At Least One Drug Related Adverse Event (Study 100176)

Drug Related Adverse Event	GAMUNEX® No. of subjects: 48 No. of subjects with drug related AE (percentage of all subjects)	GAMIMUNE® N, 10% No. of subjects: 49 No. of subjects with drug related AE (percentage of all subjects)
Headache	24 (50%)	24 (49%)
Vomiting	6 (13%)	8 (16%)
Fever	5 (10%)	5 (10%)
Nausea	5 (10%)	4 (8%)
Back Pain	3 (6%)	2 (4%)
Rash	3 (6%)	0 (0%)

Serum samples were drawn to monitor the viral safety of the ITP subjects at baseline, nine days after the first infusion (for parvovirus B19), and 3 months after the first infusion of IGIV and at any time of premature discontinuation of the study. Viral markers of hepatitis C, hepatitis B, HIV-1, and parvovirus B19 were monitored by nucleic acid testing (NAT, PCR), and serological testing. There were no treatment related emergent findings of viral transmission for either GAMUNEX®, Immune Globulin Intravenous (Human), 10% Caprylate/Chromatography Purified, or GAMIMUNE® N, Immune Globulin Intravenous (Human), 10%.(17)

Treatment of Chronic Inflammatory Demyelinating Polyneuropathy

In study 100538, 113 subjects were exposed to GAMUNEX and 95 were exposed to Placebo. (See Clinical Studies [14.3]) As a result of the study design, the drug exposure with GAMUNEX was almost twice that of Placebo, with 1096 GAMUNEX infusions versus 575 Placebo infusions. Therefore, adverse reactions are reported per infusion (represented as frequency) to correct for differences in drug exposure between the 2 groups. The majority of loading-doses were administered over 2 days. The majority of maintenance-doses were administered over 1 day. Infusions were administered in the mean over 2.7 hours.

The following table shows the numbers of subjects per treatment group in the CIDP clinical trial, and the reason for discontinuation due to adverse events:

Table 9: Subjects with At Least One Adverse Event Irrespective of Causality (Study 100538)

MedDRA Preferred Term*	GAMUNEX® No. of subjects: 113			Placebo No. of subjects: 95		
	No. of Subjects (%)	No. of Adverse Events	Incidence density†	No. of Subjects (%)	No. of Adverse Events	Incidence density†
Any Adverse Event	85 (75)	377	0.344	45 (47)	120	0.209
Headache	36 (32)	57	0.052	8 (8)	15	0.026
Pyrexia (fever)	15 (13)	27	0.025	0	0	0
Hypertension	10 (9)	20	0.018	4 (4)	6	0.010
Rash	8 (7)	13	0.012	1 (1)	1	0.002
Arthralgia	8 (7)	11	0.010	1 (1)	1	0.002
Asthenia	9 (8)	10	0.009	3 (3)	4	0.007
Chills	9 (8)	10	0.009	0	0	0
Back pain	9 (8)	10	0.009	3 (3)	3	0.005
Nausea	7 (6)	9	0.008	3 (3)	3	0.005
Dizziness	7 (6)	3	0.006	1 (1)	1	0.002
Influenza	6 (5)	6	0.005	2 (2)	2	0.003

* Reported in ≥5% of subjects in any treatment group irrespective of causality.
† Calculated by the total number of adverse events divided by the number of infusions received (1096 for GAMUNEX and 575 for Placebo)

Table 8: Reasons for Discontinuation Due to Adverse Events: CIDP

Number of Subjects		Number of Subjects Discontinued due to Adverse Events	Adverse Event
GAMUNEX®	113	3 (2.7%)	Urticaria, Dyspnea, Bronchopneumonia
Placebo	95	2 (2.1%)	Cerebrovascular Accident, Deep Vein Thrombosis

Adverse events reported by at least 5% of subjects in any treatment group irrespective of causality are shown in the following table.
[See table 9 above]

Drug-related adverse events reported by at least 5% of subjects in any treatment group are reported in the table below. The most common drug-related events with GAMUNEX were headache and pyrexia:
[See table 10 at top of next page]

Laboratory Abnormalities

During the course of the clinical program, ALT and AST elevations were identified in some subjects.

• For ALT, in the primary humoral immunodeficiency (PI) study (100175) treatment emergent elevations above the upper limit of normal were transient and observed among 14/80 (18%) of subjects in the GAMUNEX group versus 5/88 (6%) of subjects in the GAMIMUNE N, 10% group (p = 0.026).

• In the ITP study which employed a higher dose per infusion, but a maximum of only two infusions, the reverse finding was observed among 3/44 (7%) of subjects in the GAMUNEX group versus 8/43 (19%) of subjects in the GAMIMUNE N, 10% group (p = 0.118).

• In the CIDP study (100538), 15/113 (13%) of subjects in the GAMUNEX group and 7/95 (7%) in the Placebo group (p=0.168) had a treatment emergent transient elevation of ALT.

Elevations of ALT and AST were generally mild (<3 times upper limit of normal), transient, and were not associated with obvious symptoms of liver dysfunction.

GAMUNEX may contain low levels of anti-Blood Group A and B antibodies primarily of the IgG₄ class. Direct antiglobulin tests (DAT or direct Coombs tests), which are carried out in some centers as a safety check prior to red blood cell transfusions, may become positive temporarily. Hemolytic events not associated with positive DAT findings were observed in clinical trials.(17, 30-33)

6.3 Postmarketing Experience
Because postmarketing reporting of adverse reactions is voluntary and from a population of uncertain size, it is not always possible to reliably estimate the frequency of these reactions or establish a causal relationship to product exposure.

GAMUNEX Postmarketing Experience
The following adverse reactions have been identified and reported during the post marketing use of GAMUNEX:
• *Hematologic:* Hemolytic anemia
• *Infections and Infestations:* Aseptic meningitis

General
The following adverse reactions have been identified and reported during the post marketing use of IGIV products (34):
• *Respiratory:* Apnea, Acute Respiratory Distress Syndrome (ARDS), TRALI, cyanosis, hypoxemia, pulmonary edema, dyspnea, bronchospasm
• *Cardiovascular:* Cardiac arrest, thromboembolism, vascular collapse, hypotension
• *Neurological:* Coma, loss of consciousness, seizures/convulsions, tremor
• *Integumentary:* Stevens-Johnson syndrome, epidermolysis, erythema multiforme, bullous dermatitis
• *Hematologic:* Pancytopenia, leukopenia, hemolysis, positive direct antiglobulin (Coombs test)
• *General/Body as a Whole:* Pyrexia, rigors
• *Musculoskeletal:* Back pain
• *Gastrointestinal:* Hepatic dysfunction, abdominal pain

7 DRUG INTERACTIONS
GAMUNEX may be diluted with 5% dextrose in water (D5/W). Admixtures of GAMUNEX with other drugs and intravenous solutions have not been evaluated. It is recommended that GAMUNEX be administered separately from other drugs or medications which the patient may be receiving. The product should not be mixed with IGIVs from other manufacturers.
The infusion line may be flushed before and after administration of GAMUNEX with 5% dextrose in water.
Various passively transferred antibodies in immunoglobulin preparations can confound the results of serological testing. Antibodies in GAMUNEX may interfere with the response to live viral vaccines such as measles, mumps and rubella. Physicians should be informed of recent therapy with IGIVs, so that administration of live viral vaccines, if indicated, can be appropriately delayed 3 or more months from the time of IGIV administration. (See Patient Counseling Information [17])

8 USE IN SPECIFIC POPULATIONS
8.1 Pregnancy
Pregnancy Category C. Animal reproduction studies have not been conducted with GAMUNEX. It is not known whether GAMUNEX can cause fetal harm when administered to a pregnant woman or can affect reproduction capacity. GAMUNEX should be given to a pregnant woman only if clearly needed.
8.3 Nursing Mothers
GAMUNEX has not been evaluated in nursing mothers.

Table 10: Subjects with At Least One Drug Related Adverse Event (Study 100538)

MedDRA Preferred Term*	GAMUNEX® No. of subjects: 113			Placebo No. of subjects: 95		
	No. of Subjects (%)	No. of Adverse Events	Incidence density[†]	No. of Subjects (%)	No. of Adverse Events	Incidence density[†]
Any drug-related adverse event	62 (55)	194	0.177	16 (17)	25	0.043
Headache	31 (27)	44	0.040	6 (6)	7	0.012
Pyrexia (fever)	15 (13)	26	0.024	0	0	0
Chills	8 (7)	9	0.008	0	0	0
Hypertension	7 (6)	16	0.015	3 (3)	3	0.005
Rash	6 (5)	8	0.007	1 (1)	1	0.002
Nausea	6 (5)	7	0.006	3 (3)	3	0.005
Asthenia	6 (5)	6	0.005	0	0	0

* Reported in ≥5% of subjects in any treatment group.
† Calculated by the total number of adverse events divided by the number of infusions received (1096 for GAMUNEX and 575 for Placebo)

Table 12: Log₁₀ Virus Reduction

Process Step	Log_{10} Virus Reduction					
	Enveloped Viruses			Non-enveloped Viruses		
	HIV	PRV	BVDV	Reo	HAV	PPV
Caprylate Precipitation/Depth Filtration	C/I *	C/I	2.7	≥ 3.5	≥ 3.6	4.0
Caprylate Incubation	≥ 4.5	≥ 4.6	≥ 4.5	NA[†]	NA	NA
Depth Filtration[‡]	CAP[§]	CAP	CAP	≥ 4.3	≥ 2.0	3.3
Column Chromatography	≥ 3.0	≥ 3.3	4.0	≥ 4.0	≥ 1.4	4.2
Low pH Incubation (21 days)	≥ 6.5	≥ 4.3	≥ 5.1	NA	NA	NA
Global Reduction	≥ 14.0	≥ 12.2	≥ 16.3	≥ 7.5	≥ 5.0	8.2

* C/I - Interference by caprylate precluded determination of virus reduction for this step. Although removal of viruses is likely to occur at the caprylate precipitation/depth filtration step, BVDV is the only enveloped virus for which reduction is claimed. The presence of caprylate prevents detection of other, less resistant enveloped viruses and therefore their removal cannot be assessed.
† Not Applicable - This step has no effect on non-enveloped viruses.
‡ Some mechanistic overlap occurs between depth filtration and other steps. Therefore, Talecris Biotherapeutics, Inc. has chosen to exclude this step from the global virus reduction calculations.
§ CAP - The presence of caprylate in the process at this step prevents detection of enveloped viruses, and their removal cannot be assessed.

8.4 Pediatric Use
Treatment of Primary Immunodeficiency
GAMUNEX was evaluated in 18 pediatric subjects (age range 0-16 years). Twenty-one percent of PI subjects (Study 100175) exposed to GAMUNEX were children. Pharmacokinetics, safety and efficacy were similar to those in adults with the exception that vomiting was more frequently reported in pediatrics (3 of 18 subjects). No pediatric-specific dose requirements were necessary to achieve serum IgG levels.
One subject, a 10-year-old boy, died suddenly from myocarditis 50 days after his second infusion of GAMUNEX. The death was judged to be unrelated to GAMUNEX.
Treatment of Idiopathic Thrombocytopenic Purpura
GAMUNEX was evaluated in 12 pediatric subjects with acute ITP. Twenty-five percent of the acute ITP subjects (Study 100176) exposed to GAMUNEX were children. Pharmacokinetics, safety and efficacy were similar to those in adults with the exception that fever was more frequently reported in pediatrics (6 of 12 subjects). No pediatric-specific dose requirements were necessary to achieve serum IgG levels.
Treatment of Chronic Inflammatory Demyelinating Polyneuropathy
The safety and effectiveness of GAMUNEX has not been established in pediatric subjects with CIDP.

8.5 Geriatric Use
Patients > 65 years of age may be at increased risk for developing certain adverse reactions such as thromboembolic events and acute renal failure. (See Boxed Warning, Warnings and Precautions [5.2]) Clinical studies of GAMUNEX did not include sufficient numbers of subjects aged 65 and over to determine whether they respond differently from younger subjects.

Table 11: Clinical Studies of GAMUNEX® by Age Group

Clinical Study	Indication	Number of Subjects	
		< 65 years	≥ 65 years
100175	PI	78	9
100152	PI	18	0
100174	PI	20	0
10039	PI	19	0
100213	ITP	22	6
100176	ITP	44	4
10038	ITP	18	3
100538	CIDP	44	15

11 DESCRIPTION
GAMUNEX is a ready-to-use sterile solution of human immune globulin protein for intravenous administration. GAMUNEX consists of 9%–11% protein in 0.16–0.24 M glycine. Not less than 98% of the protein has the electrophoretic mobility of gamma globulin. GAMUNEX contains trace levels of fragments, IgA (average 0.046 mg/mL), and IgM. The distribution of IgG subclasses is similar to that found in normal serum. GAMUNEX doses of 1 g/kg correspond to a glycine dose of 0.15 g/kg. While toxic effects of glycine administration have been reported,(35) the doses and rates of administration were 3–4 fold greater than those for GAMUNEX. In another study, it was demonstrated that intravenous bolus doses of 0.44 g/kg glycine were not associated with serious adverse effects.(36) Caprylate is a saturated medium-chain (C8) fatty acid of plant origin. Medium chain fatty acids are considered to be essentially non-toxic. Human subjects receiving medium chain fatty acids parenterally have tolerated doses of 3.0 to 9.0 g/kg/day for periods of several months without adverse effects.(37) Residual caprylate concentrations in the final container are no more than 0.216 g/L (1.3 mmol/L).The measured buffer capacity is 35 mEq/L and the osmolality is 258 mOsmol/kg solvent, which is close to physiological osmolality (285-295 mOsmol/kg). The pH of GAMUNEX is 4.0–4.5. GAMUNEX contains no preservative and is latex-free.
GAMUNEX is made from large pools of human plasma by a combination of cold ethanol fractionation, caprylate precipitation and filtration, and anion-exchange chromatography. Isotonicity is achieved by the addition of glycine. GAMUNEX is incubated in the final container (at the low pH of 4.0–4.3), for a minimum of 21 days at 23° to 27°C. The product is intended for intravenous administration.
The capacity of the manufacturing process to remove and/or inactivate enveloped and non-enveloped viruses has been validated by laboratory spiking studies on a scaled down process model, using the following enveloped and non-enveloped viruses: human immunodeficiency virus, type I (HIV-1) as the relevant virus for HIV-1 and HIV–2; bovine viral diarrhea virus (BVDV) as a model for hepatitis C virus; pseudorabies virus (PRV) as a model for large DNA viruses (e.g., herpes viruses); Reo virus type 3 (Reo) as a model for non-enveloped viruses and for its resistance to physical and chemical inactivation; hepatitis A virus (HAV) as relevant non-enveloped virus, and porcine parvovirus (PPV) as a model for human parvovirus B19.
Overall virus reduction was calculated only from steps that were mechanistically independent from each other and truly additive. In addition, each step was verified to provide robust virus reduction across the production range for key operating parameters.
[See table 12 at left]
Additionally, the manufacturing process was investigated for its capacity to decrease the infectivity of an experimental agent of transmissible spongiform encephalopathy (TSE), considered as a model for the vCJD and CJD agents.(38-42)
Several of the individual production steps in the GAMUNEX manufacturing process have been shown to decrease TSE infectivity of that experimental model agent. TSE reduction steps include two depth filtrations (in sequence, a total of ≥ 6.6 logs). These studies provide reasonable assurance that low levels of CJD/vCJD agent infectivity, if present in the starting material, would be removed.

12 CLINICAL PHARMACOLOGY
12.1 Mechanism of Action
Treatment of Primary Humoral Immunodeficiency
GAMUNEX supplies a broad spectrum of opsonic and neutralizing IgG antibodies against bacteria or their toxins. The mechanism of action in PI has not been fully elucidated.
Treatment of Idiopathic Thrombocytopenic Purpura
The mechanism of action of high doses of immunoglobulins in the treatment of Idiopathic Thrombocytopenic Purpura (ITP) has not been fully elucidated.
Treatment of Chronic Inflammatory Demyelinating Polyneuropathy
The precise mechanism of action in CIDP has not been fully elucidated.

12.3 Pharmacokinetics
Two randomized pharmacokinetic crossover trials were carried out with GAMUNEX in 38 subjects with Primary Humoral Immunodeficiencies given 3 infusions 3 or 4 weeks apart of test product at a dose of 100-600 mg/kg body weight per infusion. One trial compared the pharmacokinetic characteristics of GAMUNEX to GAMIMUNE N, 10% (study 100152), and the other trial compared the pharmacokinetics of GAMUNEX (10% strength) with a 5% concentration of this product (study 100174). The ratio of the geometric least square means for dose-normalized IgG peak levels of GAMUNEX and GAMIMUNE N, 10% was 0.996. The corresponding value for the dose-normalized area under the curve (AUC) of IgG levels was 0.990. The results of both PK parameters were within the pre-established limits of 0.080 and 1.25. Similar results were obtained in the comparison of GAMUNEX 10% to a 5% concentration of GAMUNEX. (31,32)
The main pharmacokinetic parameters of GAMUNEX, measured as total IgG in study 100152 are displayed below:
[See table 13 at top of next page]
The two pharmacokinetic trials with GAMUNEX show the IgG concentration/time curve follows a biphasic slope with a distribution phase of about 5 days characterized by a fall in serum IgG levels to about 65-75% of the peak levels achieved immediately post-infusion. This phase is followed

by the elimination phase with a half-life of approximately 35 days.(31, 32) IgG trough levels were measured over nine months in the therapeutic equivalence trial (100175). Mean trough levels were 7.8 +/- 1.9 mg/mL for the GAMUNEX treatment group and 8.2 +/- 2.0 mg/mL for the GAMIMUNE N, 10% control group.(30)

14   CLINICAL STUDIES

14.1   Treatment of Primary Humoral Immunodeficiency

In a randomized, double-blind, parallel group clinical trial with 172 subjects with primary humoral immunodeficiencies (study 100175) GAMUNEX was demonstrated to be at least as efficacious as GAMIMUNE N, 10% in the prevention of any infection, i.e. validated plus clinically defined, non-validated infections of any organ system, during a nine month treatment period. Twenty six subjects were excluded from the Per Protocol analysis (2 due to non-compliance and 24 due to protocol violations). The endpoint was the proportion of subjects with at least one of the following validated infections: pneumonia, acute sinusitis and acute exacerbations of chronic sinusitis.

[See table 14 at right]

The annual rate of validated infections (Number of Infections/year/subject) was 0.18 in the group treated with GAMUNEX and 0.43 in the group treated with GAMIMUNE N, 10% (p=0.023). The annual rates for any infection (validated plus clinically-defined, non-validated infections of any organ system) were 2.88 and 3.38, respectively (p=0.300).(30, 43)

14.2   Treatment of Idiopathic Thrombocytopenic Purpura

A double-blind, randomized, parallel group clinical trial with 97 ITP subjects was carried out to prove the hypothesis that GAMUNEX was at least as effective as GAMIMUNE N, 10% in raising platelet counts from less than or equal to 20×10^9/L to more than 50 $\times 10^9$/L within 7 days after treatment with 2 g/kg IGIV (study 100176). Twenty-four percent of the subjects were less than or equal to 16 years of age. GAMUNEX was demonstrated to be at least as effective as GAMIMUNE N, 10% in the treatment of adults and children with acute or chronic ITP.(11)

[See table 15 at right]

A trial was conducted to evaluate the clinical response to rapid infusion of GAMUNEX in patients with ITP. The study involved 28 chronic ITP subjects, wherein the subjects received 1 g/kg GAMUNEX on three occasions for treatment of relapses. The infusion rate was randomly assigned to 0.08, 0.11, or 0.14 mL/kg/min (8, 11 or 14 mg/min). Premedication with corticosteroids to alleviate infusion-related intolerability was not permitted. Pre-treatment with antihistamines, anti-pyretics and analgesics was permitted. The average dose was approximately 1 g/kg body weight at all three prescribed rates of infusion (0.08, 0.11 and 0.14 mL/kg/min). All patients were administered each of the three planned infusions except seven subjects. Based on 21 patients per treatment group, the a posteriori power to detect twice as many drug-related adverse events between groups was 23%. Of the seven subjects that did not complete the study, five did not require additional treatment, one withdrew because he refused to participate without concomitant medication (prednisone) and one experienced an adverse event (hives); however, this was at the lowest dose rate level (0.08 mL/kg/ min).

14.3   Treatment of Chronic Inflammatory Demyelinating Polyneuropathy

A multi-center, randomized, double-blind Placebo-controlled trial (study 100538, The Immune Globulin Intravenous (Human), 10% Caprylate/Chromatography Purified CIDP Efficacy or ICE study) was conducted with GAMUNEX.(44) This study included two separately randomized study periods to assess whether GAMUNEX was more effective than Placebo for the treatment of CIDP (assessed in the Efficacy Period for up to 24 weeks) and whether long-term administration of GAMUNEX could maintain long-term benefit (assessed in the 24 week Randomized Withdrawal Period).

In the Efficacy Period, there was a requirement for Rescue (crossover) to the alternate study drug if the subject did not improve and maintain this improvement until the end of the 24 week treatment period. Subjects entering the Rescue phase followed the same dosing and schedule as in the Efficacy period. Any subject who was Rescued (crossed over) and did not improve and maintain this improvement was withdrawn from the study.

Subjects who completed 24 weeks treatment in the Efficacy period or Rescue phase and responded to therapy were eligible for entry into a double-blind Randomized Withdrawal Period. Eligible subjects were re-randomized to GAMUNEX *or Placebo. Any subject who relapsed was withdrawn from the study.*

The Efficacy Period and the Rescue treatment started with a loading dose of 2 g/kg bw of GAMUNEX or equal volume of Placebo given over 2-4 consecutive days. All other infusions (including the first infusion of the Randomized Withdrawal Period) were given as maintenance doses of 1 g/kg bw (or equivalent volume of Placebo) every three weeks.

Table 13: PK Parameters of GAMUNEX® and GAMIMUNE® N, 10% (Study 100152)

	GAMUNEX®				GAMIMUNE® N, 10%			
	N	Mean	SD	Median	N	Mean	SD	Median
Cmax (mg/mL)	17	19.04	3.06	19.71	17	19.31	4.17	19.30
Cmax-norm (kg/mL)	17	0.047	0.007	0.046	17	0.047	0.008	0.047
AUC(0-tn)* (mg*hr/mL)	17	6746.48	1348.13	6949.47	17	6854.17	1425.08	7119.86
AUC(0-tn) norm* (kg*hr/mL)	17	16.51	1.83	16.95	17	16.69	2.04	16.99
T 1/2† (days)	16	35.74	8.69	33.09	16	34.27	9.28	31.88

* Partial AUC: defined as pre-dose concentration to the last concentration common across both treatment periods in the same patient.
† only 15 subjects were valid for the analysis of $T_{1/2}$

Table 14: Primary Endpoint Per Protocol Analysis (Study 100175)

	GAMUNEX® (n=73) No. of subjects with at least one infection	GAMIMUNE® N, 10% (n=73) No. of subjects with at least one infection	Mean Difference (90% confidence interval)	p-Value
Validated Infections	9 (12%)	17 (23%)	-0.117 (-0.220, -0.015)	0.06
Acute Sinusitis	4 (5%)	10 (14%)		
Exacerbation of Chronic Sinusitis	5 (7%)	6 (8%)		
Pneumonia	0 (0%)	2 (3%)		
Any Infection (Validated plus Clinically defined non-validated Infections)	56 (77%)	57 (78%)	-0.020 (-0.135, 0.096)	0.78

Table 15: Platelet Response of Per Protocol Analysis (Study 100176)

	GAMUNEX® (n=39)	GAMIMUNE® N, 10% (n=42)	Mean Difference (90% confidence interval)
By Day 7	35 (90%)	35 (83%)	0.075 (-0.037, 0.186)
By Day 23	35 (90%)	36 (86%)	0.051 (-0.058, 0.160)
Sustained for 7 days	29 (74%)	25 (60%)	0.164 (0.003, 0.330)

The Responder rates of the GAMUNEX and Placebo treatment groups was measured by the INCAT score. The INCAT (Inflammatory Neuropathy Cause and Treatment) scale is used to assess functional disability of both upper and lower extremities in demyelinating polyneuropathy. The INCAT scale has upper and lower extremity components (maximum of 5 points for upper (arm disability) and maximum of 5 points for lower (leg disability)) that add up to a maximum of 10-points (0 is normal and 10 is severely incapacitated).(45) At the start of the efficacy portion of the study, the INCAT scores were as follows: Upper Extremity mean was 2.2 ± 1.0, and median was 2.0 with a range of 0 to 5; Lower Extremity mean was 1.9 ± 0.9, and median was 2.0 with a range of 1 to 5; Total Overall Score mean was 4.2 ± 1.4, and median was 4.0 with a range of 2 to 9. A Responder was defined as a subject with at least 1-point improvement from baseline in the adjusted INCAT score that was maintained through 24 weeks.

Significantly more subjects with CIDP responded to GAMUNEX: 28 of 59 subjects (47.5%) responded to GAMUNEX compared with 13 of 58 subjects (22.4%) administered Placebo (25% difference; [95% CI: 7%-43%]; p=0.006). The study included both subjects who were IGIV naive and subjects who had previous IGIV experience. The outcome was influenced by the group of subjects who experienced prior therapy with IGIV, as shown by the outcomes table, below.

Time to relapse for the subset of 57 subjects who previously responded to GAMUNEX was evaluated: 31 were randomly reassigned to continue to receive GAMUNEX and 26 subjects were randomly reassigned to Placebo in the Randomized Withdrawal Period. Subjects who continued to receive GAMUNEX experienced a significantly longer time to relapse versus subjects treated with Placebo (p=0.011). The probability of relapse was 13% with GAMUNEX versus 45% with Placebo (hazard ratio, 0.19 [95% confidence interval, 0.05, 0.70]).

[See table 16 at top of next page]

The following table shows outcomes for the Rescue Phase (which are supportive data):

[See table 17 on next page]

The following Kaplan-Meier curves show the outcomes for the Randomized Withdrawal Period:

Figure 1: Outcome for Randomized Withdrawal Period

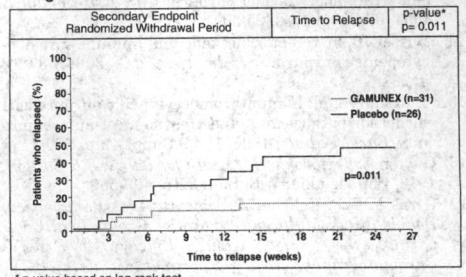

* p-value based on log-rank test

15   REFERENCES

1. Cayco AV, Perazella MA, Hayslett JP. Renal insufficiency after intravenous immune globulin therapy: a report of two cases and an analysis of the literature. *J Am Soc Nephrol*, 1997. 8 (11): p. 1788-94.

Table 16: Outcomes in Intent-to-Treat Population Efficacy Period

Efficacy Period	GAMUNEX®		Placebo		p-value*
	Responder	Non-Responder	Responder	Non-Responder	
All Subjects	28/59 (47.5%)	31/59 (52.5%)	13/58 (22.4%)	45/58 (77.6%)	0.006
IGIV - Naïve Subjects	17/39 (43.6%)	22/39 (56.4%)	13/46 (28.3%)	33/46 (71.7%)	0.174
IGIV - Experienced Subjects	11/20 (55.0%)	9/20 (45.0%)	0/12 (0%)	12/12 (100%)	0.002

*p-value based on Fisher's exact method

Table 17: Outcomes in Rescue Phase

Rescue Phase	GAMUNEX®		Placebo		p-value*
	Success	Failure	Success	Failure	
All Subjects	25/45 (55.6%)	20/45 (44.4%)	6/23 (26.1%)	17/23 (73.9%)	0.038
IGIV - Naïve Subjects	19/33 (57.6%)	14/33 (42.4%)	6/18 (33.3%)	12/18 (66.7%)	0.144
IGIV - Experienced Subjects	6/12 (50%)	6/12 (50%)	0/5 (0%)	5/5 (100%)	0.102

*p-value based on Fisher's exact method

2. Ammann AJ, et al. Use of intravenous gamma-globulin in antibody immunodeficiency: results of a multicenter controlled trial. *Clin Immunol Immunopathol*, 1982. 22(1): p. 60-7.
3. Buckley RH, Schiff RI. The use of intravenous immune globulin in immunodeficiency diseases. *N Engl J Med*, 1991. 325(2): p. 110-7.
4. Cunningham-Rundles C, Bodian C. Common variable immunodeficiency: clinical and immunological features of 248 patients. *Clin Immunol*, 1999. 92(1): p. 34-48.
5. Nolte MT, et al. Intravenous immunoglobulin therapy for antibody deficiency. *Clin Exp Immunol*, 1979. 36(2): p. 237-43.
6. Pruzanski W, et al. Relationship of the dose of intravenous gammaglobulin to the prevention of infections in adults with common variable immunodeficiency. *Inflammation*, 1996. 20(4): p. 353-9.
7. Roifman CM, Levison H, Gelfand EW. High-dose versus low-dose intravenous immunoglobulin in hypogamma-globulinaemia and chronic lung disease. *Lancet*, 1987. 1(8541): p. 1075-7.
8. Sorensen RU, Polmar SH. Efficacy and safety of high-dose intravenous immune globulin therapy for antibody deficiency syndromes. *Am J Med*, 1984. 76(3A): p. 83-90.
9. Stephan JL, et al. Severe combined immunodeficiency: a retrospective single-center study of clinical presentation and outcome in 117 patients. *J Pediatr*, 1993. 123(4): p. 564-72.
10. Blanchette VS, Kirby MA, and Turner C. Role of intravenous immunoglobulin G in autoimmune hematologic disorders. *Semin Hematol*, 1992. 29(3 Suppl 2): p. 72-82.
11. Lazarus AH, Freedman J, Semple JW. Intravenous immunoglobulin and anti-D in idiopathic thrombocytopenic purpura (ITP): mechanisms of action. *Transfus Sci*, 1998. 19(3): p. 289-94.
12. Semple JW, Lazarus AH, Freedman J. The cellular immunology associated with autoimmune thrombocytopenic purpura: an update. *Transfus Sci*, 1998. 19(3): p. 245-51.
13. Imbach PA. Harmful and beneficial antibodies in immune thrombocytopenic purpura. *Clin Exp Immunol*, 1994. 97(Suppl 1): p. 25-30.
14. Bussel JB. Fc receptor blockade and immune thrombocytopenic purpura. *Semin Hematol*, 2000. 37(3): p. 261-6.
15. Imbach P, et al. Immunthrombocytopenic purpura as a model for pathogenesis and treatment of auto immunity. *Eur J Pediatr*, 1995. 154(9 Suppl 4): p. S60-4.
16. Guyton A. *Textbook of Medical Physiology. 5th Edition.* 1976, Philadelphia: W.B. Saunders. 499-500.
17. Cyrus P, F.G., Kelleher J, Schwartz L. *A Randomized, Double-Blind, Multicenter, Parallel Group Trial Comparing the Safety, and Efficacy of IGIV-Chromatography, 10% (Experimental) with IGIV-Solvent Detergent Treated, 10% (Control) in Patients with Idiopathic (Immune) Thrombocytopenic Purpura (ITP), 2000. Report on file.*
18. Steinberger BA, Ford SM, Coleman TA. Intravenous Immunoglobulin Therapy Results in Post-infusional Hyperproteinemia, Increased Serum Viscosity, and Pseudohyponatremia. *Am J Hematol* 73:97-100 (2003).
19. Dalakas MC. High-dose intravenous Immunoglobulin and serum viscosity: risk of precipitating thromboembolic events. *Neurology*, 44:223-226.
20. Woodruff RK, Grigg AP, Firkin FC, Smith IL. Fatal thrombotic events during treatment of autoimmune thrombocytopenia with intravenous immunoglobulin in elderly patients. *Lancet* 1986;2:217-218.
21. Wolberg AS, Kon RH, Monroe DM, Hoffman M. Coagulation factor XI is a contaminant in intravenous immunoglobulin preparations. *Am J Hematol* 2000; 65,30-34.
22. Casteels-Van Daele M, et al. Intravenous immune globulin and acute aseptic meningitis [letter]. *N Engl J Med*, 1990. 323(9): p. 614-5.
23. Kato E, et al. Administration of immune globulin associated with aseptic meningitis [letter]. *Jama*, 1988. 259(22): p. 3269-71.
24. Scribner CL, et al. Aseptic meningitis and intravenous immunoglobulin therapy [editorial; comment]. *Ann Intern Med*, 1994. 121(4): p. 305-6.
25. Copelan EA, Strohm PL, Kennedy MS, Tutschka PJ. Hemolysis following intravenous immune globulin therapy. *Transfusion* 1986;26: 410-412.
26. Thomas MJ, Misbah SA, Chapel HM, Jones M, Elrington G, Newsom-Davis J. Hemolysis after high-dose intravenous Ig. *Blood* 1993;15:3789.
27. Wilson JR, Bhoopalam N, Fisher M. Hemolytic anemia associated with intravenous immunoglobulin. *Muscle & Nerve* 1997;20:1142-1145.
28. Kessary-Shoham H, Levy Y, Shoenfeld Y, Lorber M, Gershon H. In vivo administration of intravenous immunoglobulin (IVIg) can lead to enhanced erythrocyte sequestration. *J Autoimmune* 1999;13:129-135.
29. Rizk A, Gorson KC, Kenney L, Weinstein R. Transfusion-related acute lung injury after the infusion of IVIG. *Transfusion* 2001:41:264-268.
30. Kelleher J, F.G., Cyrus P, Schwartz L. *A Randomized, Double-Blind, Multicenter, Parallel Group Trial Comparing the Safety and Efficacy of IGIV-Chromatography, 10% (Experimental) with IGIV-Solvent Detergent Treated, 10% (Control) in Patients with Primary Immune Deficiency (PID), 2000. Report on file.*
31. Bayever E, M.F., Sundaresan P, Collins S. Randomized, Double-Blind, Multicenter, Repeat Dosing, Cross-Over Trial Comparing the Safety, Pharmacokinetics, and Clinical Outcomes of IGIV-Chromatography, 10% (Experimental) with IGIV-Solvent Detergent Treated, 10% (Control) in Patients with Primary Humoral Immune Deficiency (BAY-41-1000-100152). *MMRR-1512/1*, 1999.
32. Lathia C, E.B., Sundaresan PR, Schwartz L. *A Randomized, Open-Label, Multicenter, Repeat Dosing, Cross-Over Trial Comparing the Safety, Pharmacokinetics, and Clinical Outcomes of IGIV-Chromatography, 5% with IGIV-Chromatography 10% in Patients with Primary Humoral Immune Deficiency (BAY-41-1000-100174). 2000.*
33. Kelleher J, S.L. *IGIV-C 10% Rapid Infusion Trial in Idiopathic (Immune) Thrombocytopenic Purpura (ITP), 2001. Report on file.*
34. Pierce LR, Jain N. Risks associated with the use of intravenous immunoglobulin. *Trans Med Rev* 2003; 17,241-251.
35. Hahn RG, Stalberg HP, Gustafsson SA. Intravenous infusion of irrigating fluids containing glycine or mannitol with and without ethanol. *J Urol*, 1989. 142(4): p. 1102-5.
36. Tai VM, M.E., Lee-Brotherton V, Manley JJ, Nestmann ER, Daniels JM. Safety Evaluation of Intravenous Glycine in Formulation Development. in *J Pharm Pharmaceut Sci*. 2000.
37. Traul KA, et al. Review of the toxicologic properties of medium-chain triglycerides. *Food Chem Toxicol*, 2000. 38(1): p. 79-98.
38. Stenland CJ, Lee DC, Brown P, et al. Partitioning of human and sheep forms of the pathogenic prion protein during the purification of therapeutic proteins from human plasma. *Transfusion* 2002. 42(11):1497-500.
39. Lee DC, Stenland CJ, Miller JL, et al. A direct relationship between the partitioning of the pathogenic prion protein and transmissible spongiform encephalopathy infectivity during the purification of plasma proteins. *Transfusion* 2001. 41(4):449-55.
40. Lee DC, Stenland CJ, Hartwell RC, et al. Monitoring plasma processing steps with a sensitive Western blot assay for the detection of the prion protein. *J Virol Methods* 2000. 84(1):77-89.
41. Cai K, Miller JL, Stenland CJ, et al. Solvent-dependent precipitation of prion protein. *Biochim Biophys Acta* 2002. 1597(1):28-35.
42. Trejo SR, Hotta JA, Lebing W, et al. Evaluation of virus and prion reduction in a new intravenous immunoglobulin manufacturing process. *Vox Sang* 2003. 84(3): 176-87.
43. *Data on File.*
44. Hughes RAC, Donofrio P, Bril V, et al. Intravenous immune globulin (10% caprylate/chromatography purified) for the treatment of chronic inflammatory demyelinating polyradiculoneuropathy (ICE study): a randomized Placebo-controlled trial. *Lancet Neurol* 2008. 7:136-144.
45. Hughes R, Bensa S, Willison H, Van den BP, Comi G, Illa I, et al. Randomized controlled trial of intravenous immunoglobulin versus oral prednisolone in chronic inflammatory demyelinating polyradiculoneuropathy. *Ann Neurol* 2001 Aug;50(2):195-201.

16   HOW SUPPLIED/STORAGE AND HANDLING

GAMUNEX is supplied in single-use, tamper evident vials (shrink band) containing the labeled amount of functionally active IgG. The three larger vial size labels incorporate integrated hangers. The components used in the packaging for GAMUNEX are latex-free. GAMUNEX is supplied in the following sizes:

NDC Number	Size	Grams Protein
13533-645-12	10 mL	1.0
13533-645-15	25 mL	2.5
13533-645-20	50 mL	5.0
13533-645-71	100 mL	10.0
13533-645-24	200 mL	20.0

GAMUNEX may be stored for 36 months at 2-8°C (36-46°F), AND product may be stored at temperatures not to exceed 25°C (77°F) for up to 6 months anytime during the 36 month shelf life, after which the product must be immediately used or discarded. Do not freeze. Do not use after expiration date.

17   PATIENT COUNSELING INFORMATION

(See Boxed Warning and Warnings and Precautions Sections)

Inform patients to immediately report the following to their physician:
- signs and symptoms of renal failures, such as decreased urine output, sudden weight gain, fluid retention/edema, and/or shortness of breath
- signs and symptoms of aseptic meningitis, such as headache, neck stiffness, drowsiness, fever, sensitivity to light, painful eye movements, nausea, and vomiting
- signs and symptoms of hemolysis, such as fatigue, increased heart rate, yellowing of the skin or eyes, and dark-colored urine
- signs and symptoms of TRALI, such as severe respiratory distress, pulmonary edema, hypoxemia, normal left ventricular function, and fever. TRALI typically occurs within 1 to 6 hours following transfusion.

Inform patients that GAMUNEX is made from human plasma and may contain infectious agents that can cause disease (e.g., viruses, and, theoretically, the CJD agent). Inform patients that the risk GAMUNEX may transmit an infectious agent has been reduced by screening plasma donors for prior exposure to certain viruses, by testing the donated plasma for certain virus infections and by inactivating and/or removing certain viruses during manufacturing.

Inform patients that administration of IgG may interfere with the response to live viral vaccines such as measles, mumps and rubella. Inform patients to notify their immunizing physician of therapy with GAMUNEX.

Rx only
Manufactured by:
Talecris Biotherapeutics, Inc.
Research Triangle Park, NC 27709 USA
U.S. License No. 1716
08939392/08939393
October 2008

Teva Biologics & Specialty Products

Division of Teva Pharmaceuticals USA
425 Privet Road
Horsham, PA 19044

For all Inquiries Call:
800-292-4283

ADIPEX-P® C IV R
(Phentermine Hydrochloride USP 37.5 mg)

DESCRIPTION

Phentermine hydrochloride USP has the chemical name of α,α-Dimethylphenethylamine hydrochloride. The structural formula is as follows:

$$CH_2C-NH_2 \cdot HCl$$ with two CH_3 groups

$C_{10}H_{15}N \cdot HCl$ M.W. 185.7

Phentermine hydrochloride is a white, odorless, hygroscopic, crystalline powder which is soluble in water and lower alcohols, slightly soluble in chloroform and insoluble in ether.
ADIPEX-P®, an anorectic agent for oral administration, is available as a capsule or tablet containing 37.5 mg of phentermine hydrochloride (equivalent to 30 mg of phentermine base).
ADIPEX-P® Capsules contain the inactive ingredients Corn Starch, Gelatin, Lactose Monohydrate, Magnesium Stearate, Titanium Dioxide, Black Iron Oxide, FD&C Blue #1, FD&C Red #40 and D&C Red #33.
ADIPEX-P® Tablets contain the inactive ingredients Corn Starch, Lactose (Anhydrous), Magnesium Stearate, Microcrystalline Cellulose, Pregelatinized Starch, Sucrose, and FD&C Blue #1.

CLINICAL PHARMACOLOGY

ADIPEX-P® is a sympathomimetic amine with pharmacologic activity similar to the prototype drugs of this class used in obesity, the amphetamines. Actions include central nervous system stimulation and elevation of blood pressure. Tachyphylaxis and tolerance have been demonstrated with all drugs of this class in which these phenomena have been looked for.
Drugs of this class used in obesity are commonly known as "anorectics" or "anorexigenics." It has not been established that the action of such drugs in treating obesity is primarily one of appetite suppression. Other central nervous system actions, or metabolic effects, may be involved, for example. Adult obese subjects instructed in dietary management and treated with "anorectic" drugs lose more weight on the average than those treated with placebo and diet, as determined in relatively short-term clinical trials.
The magnitude of increased weight loss of drug-treated patients over placebo-treated patients is only a fraction of a pound a week. The rate of weight loss is greatest in the first weeks of therapy for both drug and placebo subjects and tends to decrease in succeeding weeks. The possible origins of the increased weight loss due to the various drug effects are not established. The amount of weight loss associated with the use of an "anorectic" drug varies from trial to trial, and the increased weight loss appears to be related in part to variables other than the drugs prescribed, such as the physician-investigator, the population treated and the diet prescribed. Studies do not permit conclusions as to the relative importance of the drug and non-drug factors on weight loss.
The natural history of obesity is measured in years, whereas the studies cited are restricted to a few weeks' duration; thus, the total impact of drug-induced weight loss over that of diet alone must be considered clinically limited.

INDICATIONS AND USAGE

ADIPEX-P® (phentermine hydrochloride) is indicated as a short-term (a few weeks) adjunct in a regimen of weight reduction based on exercise, behavioral modification and caloric restriction in the management of exogenous obesity for patients with an initial body mass index ≥ 30 kg/m^2, or ≥ 27 kg/m^2 in the presence of other risk factors (e.g., hypertension, diabetes, hyperlipidemia).
Below is a chart of Body Mass Index (BMI) based on various heights and weights.
BMI is calculated by taking the patient's weight, in kilograms (kg), divided by the patient's height, in meters (m), squared. Metric conversions are as follows: pounds ÷ 2.2 = kg; inches × 0.0254 = meters.

BODY MASS INDEX (BMI), kg/m^2

Weight (pounds)	Height (feet, inches)					
	5'0"	5'3"	5'6"	5'9"	6'0"	6'3"
140	27	25	23	21	19	18
150	29	27	24	22	20	19
160	31	28	26	24	22	20
170	33	30	28	25	23	21
180	35	32	29	27	25	23
190	37	34	31	28	26	24
200	39	36	32	30	27	25
210	41	37	34	31	29	26
220	43	39	36	33	30	28
230	45	41	37	34	31	29
240	47	43	39	36	33	30
250	49	44	40	37	34	31

The limited usefulness of agents of this class (see **CLINICAL PHARMACOLOGY**) should be measured against possible risk factors inherent in their use such as those described below.

CONTRAINDICATIONS

Advanced arteriosclerosis, cardiovascular disease, moderate to severe hypertension, hyperthyroidism, known hypersensitivity or idiosyncrasy to the sympathomimetic amines, glaucoma.
Agitated states.
Patients with a history of drug abuse.
During or within 14 days following the administration of monoamine oxidase inhibitors (hypertensive crises may result).

WARNINGS

ADIPEX-P® is indicated only as short-term monotherapy for the management of exogenous obesity. The safety and efficacy of combination therapy with phentermine and any other drug products for weight loss, including selective serotonin reuptake inhibitors (e.g., fluoxetine, sertraline, fluvoxamine, paroxetine), have not been established. Therefore, coadministration of these drug products for weight loss is not recommended.
Primary Pulmonary Hypertension (PPH)-a rare, frequently fatal disease of the lungs-has been reported to occur in patients receiving a combination of phentermine with fenfluramine or dexfenfluramine. The possibility of an association between PPH and the use of phentermine alone cannot be ruled out; there have been rare cases of PPH in patients who reportedly have taken phentermine alone. The initial symptom of PPH is usually dyspnea. Other initial symptoms include: angina pectoris, syncope or lower extremity edema. Patients should be advised to report immediately any deterioration in exercise tolerance. Treatment should be discontinued in patients who develop new, unexplained symptoms of dyspnea, angina pectoris, syncope or lower extremity edema.
Valvular Heart Disease: Serious regurgitant cardiac valvular disease, primarily affecting the mitral, aortic and/or tricuspid valves, has been reported in otherwise healthy persons who had taken a combination of phentermine with fenfluramine or dexfenfluramine for weight loss. The etiology of these valvulopathies has not been established and their course in individuals after the drugs are stopped is not known. The possibility of an association between valvular heart disease and the use of phentermine alone cannot be ruled out; there have been rare cases of valvular heart disease in patients who reportedly have taken phentermine alone.
Tolerance to the anorectic effect usually develops within a few weeks. When this occurs, the recommended dose should not be exceeded in an attempt to increase the effect; rather, the drug should be discontinued.
ADIPEX-P® may impair the ability of the patient to engage in potentially hazardous activities such as operating machinery or driving a motor vehicle; the patient should therefore be cautioned accordingly.

DRUG ABUSE AND DEPENDENCE: ADIPEX-P® is related chemically and pharmacologically to the amphetamines. Amphetamines and related stimulant drugs have been extensively abused, and the possibility of abuse of ADIPEX-P® should be kept in mind when evaluating the desirability of including a drug as part of a weight reduction program. Abuse of amphetamines and related drugs may be associated with intense psychological dependence and severe social dysfunction. There are reports of patients who have increased the dosage to many times that recommended. Abrupt cessation following prolonged high dosage administration results in extreme fatigue and mental depression; changes are also noted on the sleep EEG. Manifestations of chronic intoxication with anorectic drugs include severe dermatoses, marked insomnia, irritability, hyperactivity and personality changes. The most severe manifestation of chronic intoxications is psychosis, often clinically indistinguishable from schizophrenia.
Usage with Alcohol: Concomitant use of alcohol with ADIPEX-P® may result in an adverse drug interaction.

PRECAUTIONS

General
Caution is to be exercised in prescribing ADIPEX-P® (phentermine hydrochloride) for patients with even mild hypertension.
Insulin requirements in diabetes mellitus may be altered in association with the use of ADIPEX-P® and the concomitant dietary regimen.
ADIPEX-P® may decrease the hypotensive effect of guanethidine.
The least amount feasible should be prescribed or dispensed at one time in order to minimize the possibility of overdosage.
Carcinogenesis, Mutagenesis, Impairment of Fertility: Studies have not been performed with ADIPEX-P® (phentermine hydrochloride) to determine the potential for carcinogenesis, mutagenesis or impairment of fertility.
Pregnancy—Teratogenic Effects: Pregnancy Category C. Animal reproduction studies have not been conducted with ADIPEX-P®. It is also not known whether ADIPEX-P® can cause fetal harm when administered to a pregnant woman or can affect reproductive capacity. ADIPEX-P® should be given to a pregnant woman only if clearly needed.
Nursing Mothers
Because of the potential for serious adverse reactions in nursing infants, a decision should be made whether to discontinue nursing or to discontinue the drug, taking into account the importance of the drug to the mother.
Pediatric Use
Safety and effectiveness in pediatric patients have not been established.

ADVERSE REACTIONS

Cardiovascular: Primary pulmonary hypertension and/or regurgitant cardiac valvular disease (see **WARNINGS**), palpitation, tachycardia, elevation of blood pressure.
Central Nervous System: Overstimulation, restlessness, dizziness, insomnia, euphoria, dysphoria, tremor, headache; rarely psychotic episodes at recommended doses.
Gastrointestinal: Dryness of the mouth, unpleasant taste, diarrhea, constipation, other gastrointestinal disturbances.
Allergic: Urticaria.
Endocrine: Impotence, changes in libido.

OVERDOSAGE

Manifestations of acute overdosage with phentermine include restlessness, tremor, hyperreflexia, rapid respiration, confusion, assaultiveness, hallucinations, panic states. Fatigue and depression usually follow the central stimulation. Cardiovascular effects include arrhythmia, hypertension or hypotension, and circulatory collapse. Gastrointestinal symptoms include nausea, vomiting, diarrhea and abdominal cramps. Fatal poisoning usually terminates in convulsions and coma.
Management of acute phentermine intoxication is largely symptomatic and includes lavage and sedation with a barbiturate. Experience with hemodialysis or peritoneal dialysis is inadequate to permit recommendations in this regard. Acidification of the urine increases phentermine excretion. Intravenous phentolamine (Regitine®, CIBA) has been suggested for possible acute, severe hypertension, if this complicates phentermine overdosage.

DOSAGE AND ADMINISTRATION

Exogenous Obesity: Dosage should be individualized to obtain an adequate response with the lowest effective dose. The usual adult dose is one capsule or tablet (37.5 mg) daily, administered before breakfast or 1–2 hours after breakfast. For tablets, the dosage may be adjusted to the patient's need. For some patients ½ tablet (18.75 mg) daily may be adequate, while in some cases it may be desirable to give ½ tablet (18.75 mg) two times a day.
Late evening medication should be avoided because of the possibility of resulting insomnia.

Phentermine is not recommended for use in patients sixteen (16) years of age and under.

HOW SUPPLIED

Available in tablets and capsules containing 37.5 mg phentermine hydrochloride (equivalent to 30 mg phentermine base). Each blue and white, oblong, scored tablet is debossed with "ADIPEX-P" and "9"-"9". The #3 capsule has an opaque white body and an opaque bright blue cap. Each capsule is imprinted with "ADIPEX-P" - "37.5" on the cap and two stripes on the body using dark blue ink.
Tablets are packaged in bottles of 30 (NDC 57844-009-56); 100 (NDC 57844-009-01); and 1000 (NDC 57844-009-10).
Capsules are packaged in bottles of 100 (NDC 57844-019-01).
Store at 20° to 25°C (86° to 77°F)
[See USP Controlled Room Temperature].
Dispense in a tight container as defined in the USP, with a child-resistant closure (as required).
Manufactured for:
GATE PHARMACEUTICALS
Div. of Teva Pharmaceuticals USA
Sellersville, PA 18960
Manufactured by:
TEVA PHARMACEUTICALS USA
Sellersville, PA 18960 Rev. S 7/2005

PROGLYCEM® ℞

[*pro-glī-cem*]
brand of diazoxide
Capsules
Suspension, USP
FOR ORAL ADMINISTRATION

DESCRIPTION

PROGLYCEM® (diazoxide) is a nondiuretic benzothiadiazine derivative taken orally for the management of symptomatic hypoglycemia. PROGLYCEM® **Capsules** contain 50 mg diazoxide, USP. The **Suspension** contains 50 mg of diazoxide, USP in each milliliter and has a chocolate-mint flavor; alcohol content is approximately 7.25%. Other ingredients: Sorbitol solution, chocolate cream flavor, propylene glycol, magnesium aluminum silicate, carboxymethycellulose sodium, mint flavor, sodium benzoate, methylparaben, hydrochloric acid to adjust pH, poloxamer 188, propylparaben, purified water.
Diazoxide has the following structural formula:

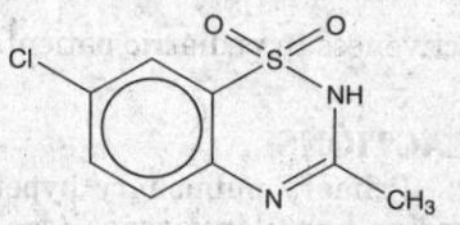

Diazoxide is 7-chloro-3-methyl-2*H*-1,2,4-benzothiadiazine 1,1-dioxide with the empirical formula $C_8H_7ClN_2O_2S$ and the molecular weight 230.7. It is a white powder practically insoluble to sparingly soluble in water.

CLINICAL PHARMACOLOGY

Diazoxide administered orally produces a prompt dose-related increase in blood glucose level, due primarily to an inhibition of insulin release from the pancreas, and also to an extrapancreatic effect.
The hyperglycemic effect begins within an hour and generally lasts no more than eight hours in the presence of normal renal function.
PROGLYCEM® decreases the excretion of sodium and water, resulting in fluid retention which may be clinically significant.
The hypotensive effect of diazoxide on blood pressure is usually not marked with the oral preparation. This contrasts with the intravenous preparation of diazoxide (see ADVERSE REACTIONS).
Other pharmacologic actions of PROGLYCEM® include increased pulse rate; increased serum uric acid levels due to decreased excretion; increased serum levels of free fatty acids' decreased chloride excretion; decreased para-aminohippuric acid; (PAH) clearance with no appreciable effect on glomerular filtration rate.
The concomitant administration of a benzothiazide diuretic may intensify the hyperglycemic and hyperuricemic effects of PROGLYCEM®. In the presence of hypokalemia, hyperglycemic effects are also potentiated.
PROGLYCEM®-induced hyperglycemia is reversed by the administration of insulin or tolbutamide. The inhibition of insulin release by PROGLYCEM® is antagonized by alpha-adrenergic blocking agents.
PROGLYCEM® is extensively bound (more than 90%) to serum proteins, and is excreted in the kidneys. The plasma half-life following I.V. administration is 28 ± 8.3 hours. Limited data on oral administration revealed a half-life of 24 and 36 hours in two adults. In four children aged four months to six years, the plasma half-life varied from 9.5 to 24 hours on long-term oral administration. The half-life may be prolonged following overdosage, and in patients with impaired renal function.

INDICATIONS AND USAGE

PROGLYCEM® (ORAL DIAZOXIDE) is useful in the management of hypoglycemia due to hyperinsulinism associated with the following conditions:
Adults: Inoperable islet cell adenoma or carcinoma, or extrapancreatic malignancy.
Infants and Children: Leucine sensitivity, islet cell hyperplasia, nesidioblastosis, extrapancreatic malignancy, islet cell adenoma, or adenomatosis. PROGLYCEM® may be used preoperatively as a temporary measure, and postoperatively, if hypoglycemia persists.
PROGLYCEM® should be used only after a diagnosis of hypoglycemia due to one of the above conditions has been definitely established. When other specific medical therapy or surgical management either has been unsuccessful or is not feasible, treatment with PROGLYCEM® should be considered.

CONTRAINDICATIONS

The use of PROGLYCEM® for functional hypoglycemia is contraindicated. The drug should not be used in patients hypersensitive to diazoxide or to other thiazides unless the potential benefits outweigh the possible risks.

WARNINGS

The antidiuretic property of diazoxide may lead to significant fluid retention, which in patients with compromised cardiac reserve, may precipitate congestive heart failure. The fluid retention will respond to conventional therapy with diuretics.
It should be noted that concomitantly administered thiazides may potentiate the hyperglycemic and hyperuricemic actions of diazoxide (See DRUG INTERACTIONS and ANIMAL PHARMACOLOGY AND/OR TOXICOLOGY).
Ketoacidosis and nonketotic hyperosmolar coma have been reported in patients treated with recommended doses of PROGLYCEM® usually during intercurrent illness. Prompt recognition and treatment are essential (See OVERDOSAGE), and prolonged surveillance following the acute episode is necessary because of the long drug half-life of approximately 30 hours. The occurrence of these serious events may be reduced by careful education of patients regarding the need for monitoring the urine for sugar and ketones and for prompt reporting of abnormal findings and unusual symptoms to the physician. Transient cataracts occurred in association with hyperosmolar coma in an infant, and subsided on correction of the hyper-osmolarity. Cataracts have been observed in several animals receiving daily doses of intravenous or oral diazoxide.
The development of abnormal facial features in four children treated chronically (>4 years) with PROGLYCEM® for hypoglycemia hyperinsulinism in the same clinic has been reported.

PRECAUTIONS

General: Treatment with PROGLYCEM® should be initiated under close clinical supervision, with careful monitoring of blood glucose and clinical response until the patient's condition has stabilized. This usually requires several days. If not effective in two to three weeks, the drug should be discontinued.
Prolonged treatment requires regular monitoring of the urine for sugar and ketones, especially under stress conditions, with prompt reporting of any abnormalities to the physician. Additionally, blood sugar levels should be monitored periodically by the physician to determine the need for dose adjustment.
The effects of diazoxide on the hematopoietic system and the level of serum uric acid should be kept in mind; the latter should be considered particularly in patients with hyperuricemia or a history of gout.
In some patients, higher blood levels have been observed with the oral suspension than with the capsule formulation of PROGLYCEM®. Dosage should be adjusted as necessary in individual patients if changed from one formulation to the other.
Since the plasma half-life of diazoxide is prolonged in patients with impaired renal function, a reduced dosage should be considered. Serum electrolyte levels should also be evaluated for such patients.
The antihypertensive effect of other drugs may be enhanced by PROGLYCEM®, and this should be kept in mind when administering it concomitantly with antihypertensive agents.
Because of the protein binding, administration of PROGLYCEM® with coumarin or its derivatives may require reduction in the dosage of the anticoagulant, although there has been no reported evidence of excessive anticoagulant effect. In addition, PROGLYCEM® may possibly displace bilirubin from albumin; this should be kept in mind particularly when treating newborns with increased bilirubinemia.
Information for Patients: During treatment with PROGLYCEM® the patient should be advised to consult regularly with the physician and to cooperate in the periodic monitoring of his condition by laboratory tests. In addition, the patient should be advised:
- to take the drug on a regular schedule as prescribed, not to skip doses, not to take extra doses;
- not to use this drug with other medications unless this is done with the physician's advice;
- not to allow anyone else to take this medication;
- to follow dietary instructions;
- to report promptly any adverse effects (i.e., increased urinary frequency, increased thirst, fruity breath odor);
- to report pregnancy or to discuss plans for pregnancy.

Laboratory tests: The following procedures may be especially important in patient monitoring (not necessarily inclusive); blood glucose determinations (recommended at periodic intervals in patients taking diazoxide orally for treatment of hypoglycemia, until stabilized); blood urea nitrogen (BUN) determinations and creatinine clearance determinations; hematocrit determinations; platelet count determinations; total and differential leukocyte counts; serum aspartate aminotransferase (AST) level determinations; serum uric acid level determinations; and urine testing for glucose and ketones (in patients being treated with diazoxide for hypoglycemia, semi-quantitative estimation of sugar and ketones in serum performed by the patient and reported to the physician provides frequent and relatively inexpensive monitoring of the condition).
Drug Interactions: Since diazoxide is highly bound to serum proteins, it may displace other substances which are also bound to protein, such as bilirubin or coumarin and its derivatives, resulting in higher blood levels of these substances. Concomitant administration of oral diazoxide and diphenylhydantoin may result in a loss of seizure control. These potential interactions must be considered when administering PROGLYCEM® **Capsules** or **Suspension**.
The concomitant administration of thiazides or other commonly used diuretics may potentiate the hyperglycemic and hyperuricemic effects of diazoxide.
Drug/Laboratory Test Interactions: The hyperglycemic and hyperuricemic effects of diazoxide preclude proper assessment of these metabolic states. Increased renin secretion, IgG concentrations and decreased cortisol secretions have also been noted. Diazoxide inhibits glucagon-stimulated insulin release and causes a false-negative insulin response to glucagon.
Carcinogenesis, mutagenesis, impairment of fertility: No long-term animal dosing study has been done to evaluate the carcinogenic potential of diazoxide. No laboratory study of mutagenic potential or animal study of effects on fertility has been done.
Pregnancy Category C: Reproduction studies using the oral preparation in rats have revealed increased fetal resorptions and delayed parturition, as well as fetal skeletal anomalies; evidence of skeletal and cardiac teratogenic effects in rabbits has been noted with intravenous administration. The drug has also been demonstrated to cross the placental barrier in animals and to cause degeneration of the fetal pancreatic beta cells (See ANIMAL PHARMACOLOGY AND/OR TOXICOLOGY). Since there are no adequate data on fetal effects of this drug when given to pregnant women, safety in pregnancy has not been established. When the use of PROGLYCEM® is considered, the indications should be limited to those specified above for adults (See INDICATIONS AND USAGE), and the potential benefits to the mother must be weighed against possible harmful effects to the fetus.
Non-teratogenic effects: Diazoxide crosses the placental barrier and appears in cord blood. When given to the mother prior to delivery of the infant, the drug may produce fetal or neonatal hyperbilirubinemia, thrombocytopenia, altered carbohydrate metabolism, and possibly other side effects that have occurred in adults.
Alopecia and hypertrichosis lanuginosa have occurred in infants whose mothers received oral diazoxide during the last 19 to 60 days of pregnancy.
Labor and delivery: Since intravenous administration of the drug during labor may cause cessation of uterine contractions, and administration of oxytocic agents may be required to reinstate labor, caution is advised in administering PROGLYCEM® at that time.
Nursing mothers: Information is not available concerning the passage of diazoxide in breast milk. Because many drugs are excreted in human milk and because of the potential for adverse reactions from diazoxide in nursing infants, a decision should be made whether to discontinue nursing or to discontinue the drug, taking into account the importance of the drug to the mother.
Pediatric use: (See INDICATIONS AND USAGE).

IMPORTANT NOTICE: Updated drug information is sent bi-monthly via the PDR® Update Insert. For *monthly* email updates, register at PDR.net.

ADVERSE REACTIONS

Frequent and Serious: Sodium and fluid retention is most common in young infants and in adults and may precipitate congestive heart failure in patients with compromised cardiac reserve. It usually responds to diuretic therapy (See DRUG INTERACTIONS).

Infrequent but Serious: Diabetic ketoacidosis and hyperosmolar nonketotic coma may develop very rapidly. Conventional therapy with insulin and restoration of fluid and electrolyte balance is usually effective if instituted promptly. Prolonged surveillance is essential in view of the long half-life of PROGLYCEM® (See OVERDOSAGE).

Other frequent adverse reactions: Hirsutism of the lanugo type, mainly on the forehead, back and limbs, occurs most commonly in children and women and may be cosmetically unacceptable. It subsides on discontinuation of the drug.

Hyperglycemia or glycosuria may require reduction in dosage in order to avoid progression to ketoacidosis or hyperosmolar coma.

Gastrointestinal intolerance may include anorexia, nausea, vomiting, abdominal pain, ileus, diarrhea, transient loss of taste.

Tachycardia, palpitations, increased levels of serum uric acid are common.

Thrombocytopenia with or without purpura may require discontinuation of the drug. Neutropenia is transient, is not associated with increased susceptibility to infection, and ordinarily does not require discontinuation of the drug. Skin rash, headache, weakness, and malaise may also occur.

Other adverse reactions which have been observed are:

Cardiovascular: hypotension occurs occasionally, which may be augmented by thiazide diuretics given concurrently. A few cases of transient hypertension, for which no explanation is apparent, have been noted. Chest pain has been reported rarely.

Hematologic: eosinophilia; decreased hemoglobin/hematocrit; excessive bleeding, decreased IgG.

Hepato-renal: increased AST, alkaline phosphatase; azotemia, decreased creatinine clearance, reversible nephrotic syndrome, decreased urinary output, hematuria, albuminuria. *Neurologic:* anxiety, dizziness, insomnia, polyneuritis, paresthesia, pruritus, extrapyramidal signs. *Ophthalmologic:* transient cataracts, subconjunctival hemorrhage, ring scotoma, blurred vision, diplopia, lacrimation. *Skeletal, integumentary:* monilial dermatitis, herpes, advance in bone age; loss of scalp hair. *Systemic:* fever, lymphadenopathy. *Other:* gout acute pancreatitis/pancreatic necrosis, galactorrhea, enlargement of lump in breast.

OVERDOSAGE

An overdosage of PROGLYCEM® causes marked hyperglycemia which may be associated with ketoacidosis. It will respond to prompt insulin administration and restoration of fluid and electrolyte balance. Because of the drug's long half-life (approximately 30 hours), the symptoms of overdosage require prolonged surveillance for periods up to seven days until the blood sugar level stabilizes within the normal range. One investigator reported successful lowering of diazoxide blood levels by peritoneal dialysis in one patient and by hemodialysis in another.

DOSAGE AND ADMINISTRATION

Patients should be under close clinical observation when treatment with PROGLYCEM® is initiated. The clinical response and blood glucose level should be carefully monitored until the patient's condition has stabilized satisfactory; in most instances, this may be accomplished in several days. If administration of PROGLYCEM® is not effective after two or three weeks, the drug should be discontinued.

The dosage of PROGLYCEM® must be individualized based on the severity of the hypoglycemic condition and the blood glucose level and clinical response of the patient. The dosage should be adjusted until the desired clinical and laboratory effects are produced with the least amount of the drug. Special care should be taken to assure accuracy of dosage in infants and young children.

Adults and children: The usual daily dosage is 3 to 8 mg/kg, divided into two or three equal doses every 8 or 12 hours. In certain instances, patients with refractory hypoglycemia may require higher dosages. Ordinarily, an appropriate starting dosage is 3 mg/kg/day, divided into three equal doses every 8 hours. Thus an average adult would receive a starting dosage of approximately 200 mg daily.

Infants and newborns: The usual daily dosage is 8 to 15 mg/kg divided into two or three equal doses every 8 to 12 hours. An appropriate starting dosage is 10 mg/kg/day, divided into three equal doses every 8 hours.

ANIMAL PHARMACOLOGY AND/OR TOXICOLOGY

Oral diazoxide in the mouse, rat, rabbit, dog, pig, and monkey produces a rapid and transient rise in blood glucose levels. In dogs, increased blood glucose is accompanied by increased free fatty acids, lactate, and pyruvate in the serum. In mice, a marked decrease in liver glycogen and an increase in the blood urea nitrogen level occur.

In acute toxicity studies the LD_{50} for oral diazoxide suspension is >5000 mg/kg in the rat, >522 mg/kg in the neonatal rat, between 1900 and 2572 mg/kg in the mouse, and 219 mg/kg in the guinea pig. Although the oral LD_{50} was not determined in the dog, a dosage of up to 500 mg/kg was well tolerated.

In subacute oral toxicity studies, diazoxide at 400 mg/kg in the rat produced growth retardation, edema, increases in liver and kidney weights, and adrenal hypertrophy. Daily dosages up to 1080 mg/kg for three months produced hyperglycemia, an increase in liver weight and an increase in mortality. In dogs given oral diazoxide at approximately 40 mg/kg/day for one month, no biologically significant gross or microscopic abnormalities were observed. Cataracts, attributed to markedly disturbed carbohydrate metabolism, have been observed in a few dogs given repeated daily doses of oral or intravenous diazoxide. The lenticular changes resembled those which occur experimentally in animals with increased blood glucose levels. In chronic toxicity studies, rats given a daily dose of 200 mg/kg diazoxide for 52 weeks had a decrease in weight gain and an increase in heart, liver, adrenal and thyroid weights. Mortality in drug-treated and control groups was not different. Dogs treated with diazoxide at dosages of 50, 100, and 200 mg/kg/day for 82 weeks had higher blood glucose levels than controls. Mild bone marrow stimulation and increased pancreas weights were evident in the drug-treated dogs; several developed inguinal hernias, one had a testicular seminoma, and another had a mass near the penis. Two females had inguinal mammary swellings. The etiology of these changes was not established. There was no difference in mortality between drug-treated and control groups. In a second chronic oral toxicity study, dogs given milled diazoxide at 50, 100, and 200 mg/kg/day had anorexia and severe weight loss, causing death in a few. Hematologic, biochemical, and histologic examination did not indicate any cause of death other than inanition. After one year of treatment, there is no evidence of herniation or tissue swelling in any of the dogs.

When diazoxide was administered at high dosages concomitantly with either chlorothiazide to rats or trichlormethiazide to dogs, increased toxicity was observed. In rats, the combination was nephrotoxic; epithelial hyperplasia was observed in the collecting tubules. In dogs, a diabetic syndrome was produced which resulted in ketosis and death. Neither of the drugs given alone produced these effects. Although the data are inconclusive, reproduction and teratology studies in several species of animals indicate that diazoxide, when administered during the critical period of embryo formation, may interfere with normal fetal development, possibly through altered glucose metabolism. Parturition was occasionally prolonged in animals treated at term. Intravenous administration of diazoxide to pregnant sheep, goats, and swine produced in the fetus an appreciable increase in blood glucose level and degeneration of the beta cells of the Islets of Langerhans. The reversibility of these effects was not studied.

HOW SUPPLIED

PROGLYCEM® (diazoxide capsules, USP), 50 mg, half opaque orange and half clear capsules, branded in black with BNP 6000: bottle of 100 (NDC 0575-6000-01).

PROGLYCEM® suspension, 50 mg/mL, a chocolate-mint flavored suspension; bottle of 30 ml (NDC 0575-6200-30), with dropper calibrated to deliver 10, 20, 30, 40 and 50 mg diazoxide. **Shake well before each use. Protect from light. Store in carton until contents are used. Store in light resistant container as defined in the USP. Store PROGLYCEM® Capsules and Suspension at 25°C (77°F) excursions permitted 15°-30°C (59-86°F). [See USP Controlled Room Temperature].**

PROGLYCEM® (diazoxide capsules, USP), manufactured by IVAX Pharmaceuticals, Inc., Miami, Florida 33137

PROGLYCEM® (diazoxide USP), Oral Suspension, manufactured by TEVA PHARMACEUTICALS USA, Sellersville, PA 18960

Capsules Manufactured by:
IVAX Pharmaceuticals, Inc.
Miami, Fl 33137

Suspension Manufactured for:
GATE PHARMACEUTICALS
Div. of Teva Pharmaceuticals USA
Sellersville, PA 18960

Suspension Manufactured by:
TEVA PHARMACEUTICALS USA
Sellersville, PA 18960

Iss. 2/2008
I22481

TEV-TROPIN® ℞
[tĕv-trōpĭn]
[somatropin (rDNA origin) forinjection]
5 mg (15 IU)
℞ only

DESCRIPTION

TEV-TROPIN® (somatropin, rDNA origin, for injection), a polypeptide of recombinant DNA origin, has 191 amino acid residues and a molecular weight of about 22,124 daltons. It has an amino acid sequence identical to that of human growth hormone of pituitary origin. TEV-TROPIN® is a strain of *Escherichia coli* modified by insertion of the human growth hormone gene.

TEV-TROPIN® is a sterile, white, lyophilized powder, intended for subcutaneous administration, after reconstitution with bacteriostatic 0.9% sodium chloride injection, USP, (normal saline) (benzyl alcohol preserved). The quantitative composition of the lyophilized drug per vial is:

5 mg (15 IU) vial:

Somatropin	5 mg (15 IU)
Mannitol	30 mg

The diluent contains bacteriostatic 0.9% sodium chloride injection, USP, (normal saline), 0.9% benzyl alcohol as a preservative, and water for injection. A 5 mL vial of the diluent will be supplied with each dispensed vial of TEV-TROPIN®. TEV-TROPIN® is a highly-purified preparation. Reconstituted solutions have a pH in the range of 7.0 to 9.0.

CLINICAL PHARMACOLOGY

Clinical trials have demonstrated that TEV-TROPIN® is equivalent in its therapeutic effectiveness and in its pharmacokinetic profile to those of human growth hormone of pituitary origin (somatropin). TEV-TROPIN® stimulates linear growth in children who lack adequate levels of endogenous growth hormone. Treatment of growth hormone-deficient children with TEV-TROPIN® produces increased growth rates and IGF-1 (Insulin-Like Growth Factor-1) concentrations that are similar to those seen after therapy with human growth hormone of pituitary origin.

Both TEV-TROPIN® and somatropin have also been shown to have other actions including:

A. *Tissue Growth*

1. Skeletal Growth. TEV-TROPIN® stimulates skeletal growth in patients with growth hormone deficiency. The measurable increase in body length after administration of TEV-TROPIN® results from its effect on the epiphyseal growth plates of long bones. Concentration of IGF-1, which may play a role in skeletal growth, are low in the serum of growth hormone-deficient children but increase during treatment with TEV-TROPIN®. Mean serum alkaline phosphatase concentrations are increased.

2. Cell Growth. It has been shown that there are fewer skeletal muscle cells in short statured children who lack endogenous growth hormone as compared with normal children. Treatment with somatropin results in an increase in both the number and size of muscle cells.

3. Organ Growth. Somatropin influences the size of internal organs and it also increases red cell mass.

B. *Protein Metabolism*

Linear growth is facilitated, in part, by increased cellular protein synthesis. Nitrogen retention, as demonstrated by decreased urinary nitrogen excretion and serum urea nitrogen, results from treatment with somatropin.

C. *Carbohydrate Metabolism*

Children with hypopituitarism sometimes experience fasting hypoglycemia that is improved by treatment with somatropin. Large doses of somatropin may impair glucose tolerance.

D. *Lipid Metabolism*

Administration of somatropin to growth hormone-deficient patients mobilizes lipid, reduces body fat stores, and increases plasma fatty acids.

E. *Mineral Metabolism*

Sodium, potassium, and phosphorous are conserved by somatropin. Serum concentrations of inorganic phosphates increased in patients with growth hormone deficiency after therapy with TEV-TROPIN® or somatropin. Serum calcium concentrations are not significantly altered in patients treated with either somatropin or TEV-TROPIN®.

F. *Connective Tissue Metabolism*

Somatropin stimulates the synthesis of chondroitin sulfate and collagen as well as the urinary excretion of hydroxyproline.

PHARMACOKINETICS

Following intravenous administration of 0.1 mg/kg of TEV-TROPIN®, the elimination half-life was about 0.42 hours (approximately 25 minutes) and the mean plasma clearance (±SD) was 133 (±16) mL/min in healthy male volunteers.

In the same volunteers, after a subcutaneous injection of 0.1 mg/kg TEV-TROPIN® to the forearm, the mean peak serum concentration (±SD) was 80 (±50) ng/mL which occurred approximately 7 hours post-injection and the apparent elimination half-life was approximately 2.7 hours. Compared to intravenous administration, the extent of systemic availability from subcutaneous administration was approximately 70%.

INDICATION AND USAGE

TEV-TROPIN® is indicated for the treatment of children who have growth failure due to an inadequate secretion of normal endogenous growth hormone.

CONTRAINDICATIONS

TEV-TROPIN® reconstituted with bacteriostatic 0.9% sodium chloride injection, USP (normal saline) (benzyl alcohol preserved) should not be administered to patients with a known sensitivity to benzyl alcohol (see **WARNINGS**).

Somatropin should not be used for growth promotion in pediatric patients with closed epiphyses.

Somatropin is contraindicated in patients with active proliferative or severe non-proliferative diabetic retinopathy.

In general, somatropin is contraindicated in the presence of active malignancy. Any preexisting malignancy should be inactive and its treatment complete prior to instituting therapy with somatropin. Somatropin should be discontinued if there is evidence of recurrent activity. Since growth hormone deficiency may be an early sign of the presence of a pituitary tumor (or, rarely, other brain tumors), the presence of such tumors should be ruled out prior to initiation of treatment. Somatropin should not be used in patients with any evidence of progression or recurrence of an underlying intracranial tumor.

Treatment with pharmacologic amounts of somatropin is contraindicated in patients with acute critical illness due to complications following open heart surgery, abdominal surgery or multiple accidental trauma, or those with acute respiratory failure. Two placebo-controlled clinical trials in non-growth hormone deficient adult patients (n = 522) with these conditions in intensive care units revealed a significant increase in mortality (41.9% vs. 19.3%) among somatropin-treated patients (doses 5.3 to 8 mg/day) compared to those receiving placebo (see **WARNINGS**).

Somatropin is contraindicated in patients with Prader-Willi syndrome who are severely obese or have severe respiratory impairment (see **WARNINGS**). TEV-TROPIN® is not indicated for the treatment of pediatric patients who have growth failure due to genetically confirmed Prader-Willi syndrome.

WARNINGS

Increased mortality in patients with acute critical illness due to complications following open heart surgery, abdominal surgery or multiple accidental trauma, or those with acute respiratory failure has been reported after treatment with pharmacologic doses of somatropin (see **CONTRAINDICATIONS**). The safety of continuing somatropin treatment in patients receiving replacement doses for approved indications who concurrently develop these illnesses has not been established. Therefore, the potential benefit of treatment continuation with somatropin in patients experiencing acute critical illnesses should be weighed against the potential risk.

There have been reports of fatalities after initiating therapy with somatropin in pediatric patients with Prader-Willi syndrome who had one or more of the following risk factors: severe obesity, history of upper airway obstructions or sleep apnea, or unidentified respiratory infection. Male patients with one or more of these factors may be at greater risk than females. Patients with Prader-Willi syndrome should be evaluated for signs of upper airway obstruction and sleep apnea before initiation of treatment with somatropin. If during treatment with somatropin, patients show signs of upper airway obstruction (including onset of or increased snoring) and/or new onset sleep apnea, treatment should be interrupted. All patients with Prader-Willi syndrome treated with somatropin should also have effective weight control and be monitored for signs of respiratory infection, which should be diagnosed as early as possible and treated aggressively (see **CONTRAINDICATIONS**). TEV-TROPIN® is not indicated for the treatment of pediatric patients who have growth failure due to genetically confirmed Prader-Willi syndrome.

Benzyl alcohol as a preservative in bacteriostatic normal saline, USP, has been associated with toxicity in newborns. When administering TEV-TROPIN® to newborns, reconstitute with sterile normal saline for injection, USP. WHEN RECONSTITUTING WITH STERILE NORMAL SALINE, USE ONLY ONE DOSE PER VIAL AND DISCARD THE UNUSED PORTION.

PRECAUTIONS

General

TEV-TROPIN® therapy should be carried out under the regular guidance of a physician who is experienced in the diagnosis and management of pediatric patients with growth hormone deficiency.

Patients with preexisting tumors or growth hormone deficiency secondary to an intracranial lesion should be examined routinely for progression or recurrence of the underlying disease process. In pediatric patients, clinical literature has not revealed a relationship between somatropin replacement therapy and recurrence of CNS tumors. However, in childhood cancer survivors, an increased risk of a second neoplasm has been reported in patients treated with somatropin after their first neoplasm. Intracranial tumors, in particular meningiomas, in patients treated with radiation to the head for their first neoplasm, were the most common of these second neoplasms. In adults, it is unknown whether there is any relationship between somatropin replacement therapy and CNS tumor recurrence.

Treatment with somatropin may decrease insulin sensitivity, particularly at higher doses in susceptible patients. As a result, previously undiagnosed impaired glucose tolerance and overt diabetes mellitus may be unmasked during somatropin treatment. Therefore, glucose levels should be monitored periodically in all patients treated with somatropin, especially in those with risk factors for diabetes mellitus, such as obesity, Turner syndrome, or a family history of diabetes mellitus. Patients with preexisting type 1 or type 2 diabetes mellitus or impaired glucose tolerance should be monitored closely during somatropin therapy. The doses of antihyperglycemic drugs (i.e., insulin or oral agents) may require adjustment when somatropin therapy is instituted in these patients.

In patients with hypopituitarism (multiple hormone deficiencies), standard hormonal replacement therapy should be monitored closely when somatropin therapy is administered. Undiagnosed/untreated hypothyroidism may prevent an optimal response to somatropin, in particular, the growth response in children. Patients with Turner syndrome have an inherently increased risk of developing autoimmune thyroid disease and primary hypothyroidism. In patients with growth hormone deficiency, central (secondary) hypothyroidism may first become evident or worsen during somatropin treatment. Therefore, patients treated with somatropin should have periodic thyroid function tests and thyroid hormone replacement therapy should be initiated or appropriately adjusted when indicated.

Patients with endocrine disorders, including growth hormone deficiency, may have an increased incidence of slipped capital femoral epiphysis. Any child who develops a limp or complains of hip or knee pain during somatropin therapy should be evaluated.

Intracranial hypertension (IH) with papilledema, visual changes, headache, nausea and/or vomiting has been reported in a small number of patients treated with growth hormone products. IH has been reported more frequently after treatment with IGF-I. Symptoms usually occur within the first eight weeks after the initiation of growth hormone therapy. In all reported cases, IH-associated signs and symptoms resolved rapidly after temporary suspension or termination of therapy. Funduscopic examination should be performed routinely before initiating treatment with somatropin to exclude preexisting papilledema and periodically during the course of somatropin therapy. If papilledema is observed by funduscopy during somatropin treatment, treatment should be stopped. If somatropin induced idiopathic IH is diagnosed, treatment with somatropin can be restarted at a lower dose after IH-associated signs and symptoms have resolved.

Progression of scoliosis can occur in children who experience rapid growth. Because somatropin increases growth rate, patients with a history of scoliosis who are treated with somatropin should be monitored for progression of scoliosis. Bone age should be monitored periodically during somatropin administration, especially in patients who are pubertal and/or receiving concomitant thyroid hormone replacement therapy. Under these circumstances, epiphyseal maturation may progress rapidly.

When somatropin is administered subcutaneously at the same site over a long period of time, tissue atrophy may result. This can be avoided by rotating the injection site. As is the case with any protein, local or systemic allergic reactions may occur. Parents/Patient should be informed that such reactions are possible and that prompt medical attention should be sought if allergic reactions occur.

Information for Patients

Patients being treated with TEV-TROPIN® and/or their caregivers should be informed about the potential benefits and risks associated with treatment. See the patient information included with the product and/or injection device. This information is intended to aid in the safe and effective administration of the medication. It is not a disclosure of all possible adverse or intended effects.

Patients and caregivers who will administer TEV-TROPIN® should receive appropriate training and instruction on the proper use of TEV-TROPIN® from the physician or other suitable qualified health care professional. A puncture-resistant container for the disposal of used needles and syringes should be strongly recommended. Patients and/or caregivers should be thoroughly instructed in the importance of proper disposal, and cautioned against any reuse of needles and syringes.

Laboratory Tests

Serum levels of inorganic phosphorus, alkaline phosphatase, and IGF-I may increase after somatropin therapy.

Drug Interactions

The microsomal enzyme 11β-hydroxysteroid dehydrogenase type 1 (11βHSD-1) is required for conversion of cortisone to its active metabolite, cortisol, in hepatic and adipose tissue. Growth hormone and somatropin inhibit 11βHSD-1. Consequently, individuals with untreated GH deficiency have relative increases in 11βHSD-1 and serum cortisol. Introduction of somatropin treatment may result in inhibition of 11βHSD-1 and reduced serum cortisol concentrations. As a consequence, previously undiagnosed central (secondary) hypoadrenalism may be unmasked and glucocorticoid replacement may be required in patients treated with somatropin. In addition, patients treated with glucocorticoid replacement for previously diagnosed hypoadrenalism may require an increase in their maintenance or stress doses following initiation of somatropin treatment; this may be especially true for patients treated with cortisone acetate and prednisone since conversion of these drugs to their biologically active metabolites is dependent on the activity of 11βHSD-1.

Pharmacologic glucocorticoid therapy and supraphysiologic glucocorticoid treatment may attenuate the growth promoting effects of somatropin in children. Therefore, glucocorticoid replacement dosing should be carefully adjusted in children receiving concomitant somatropin and glucocorticoid treatments to avoid both hypoadrenalism and an inhibitory effect on growth.

Limited published data indicate that somatropin treatment increases cytochrome P450 (CP450) mediated antipyrine clearance in man. These data suggest that somatropin administration may alter the clearance of compounds known to be metabolized by CP450 liver enzymes (e.g., corticosteroids, sex steroids, anticonvulsants, cyclosporine). Careful monitoring is advisable when somatropin is administered in combination with other drugs known to be metabolized by CP450 liver enzymes.

Carcinogenesis, Mutagenesis, Impairment of Fertility

Carcinogenesis, mutagenesis and reproduction studies have not been conducted with TEV-TROPIN®.

Pregnancy

Pregnancy Category C. Animal reproduction studies have not been conducted with TEV-TROPIN®. It is also not known whether TEV-TROPIN® can cause fetal harm when administered to a pregnant woman or can affect reproductive capacity. TEV-TROPIN® should be given to a pregnant woman only if clearly needed.

Nursing Mothers

It is not known whether this drug is excreted in human milk. Because many drugs are excreted in human milk, caution should be exercised when TEV-TROPIN® is administered to a nursing woman.

Geriatric Use

The safety and effectiveness of somatropin in patients aged 65 and over has not been evaluated in clinical studies. Elderly patients may be more sensitive to the action of somatropin, and may be more prone to develop adverse reactions.

ADVERSE REACTIONS

Utilizing a double-antibody immunoassay, no antibodies to growth hormone could be detected in a group of 164 naïve and previously treated clinical trial patients after treatment with TEV-TROPIN® for up to 40 months. However, utilizing the less specific polyethelene glycol (PEG) precipitation immunoassay, 27 of the 164 patient group were tested after treatment with TEV-TROPIN® for 4 to 6 months and antibodies to growth hormone were detected in two patients (7.4%). The binding capacity of the antibodies from the two antibody positive patients was not determined.

None of the patients with anti-GH antibodies in the clinical studies experienced decreased linear growth response to TEV-TROPIN® or any other associated adverse event. Growth hormone antibody binding capacities below 2 mg/L have not been associated with growth attenuation. In some cases, when binding capacity exceeds 2 mg/L, growth attenuation has been observed.

In studies of growth hormone-deficient children, headaches occurred infrequently. Injection site reactions (e.g., pain, bruise) occurred in 8 of the 164 treated patients.

Leukemia has been reported in a small number of patients treated with other growth hormone products. It is uncertain whether this risk is related to the pathology of growth hormone deficiency itself, growth hormone therapy, or other associated treatments such as radiation therapy for intracranial tumors.

OVERDOSAGE

The recommended dosage of up to 0.1 mg/kg (0.3 IU/kg) of body weight 3 times per week should not be exceeded. Acute overdose could cause initial hypoglycemia and subsequent hyperglycemia. Repeated use of doses in excess of those recommended could result in signs and symptoms of gigantism and/or acromegaly consistent with the known effects of excess human growth hormone.

DOSAGE AND ADMINISTRATION

A dosage of up to 0.1 mg/kg (0.3 IU/kg) of body weight administered 3 times per week by subcutaneous injection is recommended. TEV-TROPIN® should be reconstituted with 1-5mL of bacteriostatic 0.9% sodium chloride for injection, USP (benzyl alcohol preserved).* The stream of normal saline should be aimed against the side of the vial to prevent foaming. Swirl the vial with a GENTLE rotary motion until the contents are completely dissolved and the solution is clear. DO NOT SHAKE. Since TEV-TROPIN® is a protein, shaking or vigorous mixing will cause the solution to be cloudy. If the resulting solution is cloudy or contains particulate matter, the contents MUST NOT be injected.

*Benzyl alcohol as a preservative in bacteriostatic normal saline, USP, has been associated with toxicity in newborns. When administering TEV-TROPIN® to newborns, reconstitute with sterile normal saline for injection, USP.

Occasionally, after refrigeration, some cloudiness may occur. This is not unusual for proteins like TEV-TROPIN®. Allow the product to warm to room temperature. If cloudiness persists or particulate matter is noted, the contents MUST NOT be used.

Before and after injection, the septum of the vial should be wiped with rubbing alcohol or an alcoholic antiseptic solution to prevent contamination of the contents by repeated needle insertions.

TEV-TROPIN® can be administered using (1) a standard sterile disposable syringe or (2) using a Tjet Needle-Free injection device. For proper use, please refer to the **User's Manual** provided with the administration device.

STABILITY AND STORAGE

Before Reconstitution—Vials of TEV-TROPIN® are stable when refrigerated at 36° to 46°F (2° to 8°C). Expiration dates are stated on the labels.

After Reconstitution—Vials of TEV-TROPIN® are stable for up to 14 days when reconstituted with 0.9% sodium chloride (normal saline), USP, and stored in a refrigerator at 36° to 46°F (2° to 8°C). Do not freeze the reconstituted solution.

HOW SUPPLIED

TEV-TROPIN® (somatropin, rDNA origin, for injection) is supplied as .5 mg (15 IU) of lyophilized, sterile somatropin per vial.

Each 5 mg carton contains one vial of TEV-TROPIN® (5 mg per vial) and one vial of diluent [5-mL of bacteriostatic 0.9% sodium chloride for injection, USP (benzyl alcohol preserved)], and is supplied in single cartons or cartons of six.

Manufactured In Israel By:
BIO-TECHNOLOGY GENERAL (ISRAEL) LTD.
Be'er Tuvia, Israel
Distributed By:
GATE PHARMACEUTICALS
div. of Teva Pharmaceuticals USA
Sellersville, PA 18960

Rev. K 10/2009
0082-5008v6

Teva Neuroscience, Inc.
**901 E. 104TH STREET, SUITE 900
KANSAS CITY, MO 64131**

For Company Inquiries Contact:
1-800-221-4026
For Medical Information Contact:
1-888-4-TEVA-RX
(1-888-483-8279)

AZILECT®
[az-il-ect]
(rasagiline mesylate)
Tablets for Oral Use

℞

HIGHLIGHTS OF PRESCRIBING INFORMATION

These highlights do not include all the information needed to use AZILECT® safely and effectively. See full prescribing information for AZILECT®.
AZILECT® (rasagiline mesylate) Tablets for Oral Use
Initial U.S. Approval: 2006

———RECENT MAJOR CHANGES———

Dosage and Administration	12/2009
Contraindications	12/2009
Warnings and Precautions	12/2009

———INDICATIONS AND USAGE———

AZILECT is indicated for the treatment of the signs and symptoms of idiopathic Parkinson's disease as initial monotherapy and as adjunct therapy to levodopa. (1)

———DOSAGE AND ADMINISTRATION———

• Monotherapy: AZILECT 1 mg once daily (2.1)
• As adjunct to levodopa: AZILECT 0.5 mg once daily. Dose increase to 1 mg daily as required for sufficient clinical response. (2.2)
• Patients with mild hepatic impairment: AZILECT 0.5 mg once daily should not be exceeded. AZILECT should not be used in patients with moderate or severe hepatic impairment (2.3)
• AZILECT has not been studied in patients with severe renal impairment (2.4)
• Patients taking ciprofloxacin or other CYP1A2 inhibitors: AZILECT 0.5 mg once daily should not be exceeded. (2.5)

———DOSAGE FORMS AND STRENGTHS———

• AZILECT 0.5 mg tablets (containing, as the active ingredient, rasagiline mesylate equivalent to 0.5 mg of rasagiline base) (3)
• AZILECT 1 mg tablets (containing, as the active ingredient, rasagiline mesylate equivalent to 1 mg of rasagiline base) (3)

———CONTRAINDICATIONS———

• Concomitant use of:
- meperidine, tramadol, methadone or propoxyphene (4.1)
- dextromethorphan, St. John's wort or cyclobenzaprine (4.2)
- other MAO inhibitors (selective or non-selective) (4.3)

———WARNINGS AND PRECAUTIONS———

• Risk of severe CNS toxicity (serotonin syndrome) when AZILECT is combined with antidepressants. (5.1)
• Concomitant use of ciprofloxacin or other CYP1A2 inhibitors: Increase in rasagiline plasma concentrations. 0.5 mg rasagiline once daily should not be exceeded (5.2)
• Patients with hepatic impairment: Increase in rasagiline plasma concentrations. Limit dose to 0.5 mg rasagiline in mild hepatic impairment. AZILECT should not be used in patients with moderate or severe hepatic impairment (5.3)
• Risk for Hypertensive Crisis and nonselective MAO inhibition above the recommended Doses (5.4)
• Melanoma (5.4)
• AZILECT may cause lower blood pressure, especially postural hypotension (5.7) or increase blood pressure in different patients (5.8)
• AZILECT may cause or exacerbate hallucinations or potentially other manifestations of psychotic-like behavior (5.9)

———ADVERSE REACTIONS———

• Most common adverse reactions (treatment difference ≥ 3% greater than placebo); with monotherapy: flu syndrome, arthralgia, depression, dyspepsia. (6.1)
• Most common adverse reactions (treatment difference ≥ 3% greater than placebo); when used as adjunct to levodopa: dyskinesia, accidental injury, weight loss, postural hypotension, vomiting, anorexia, arthralgia, abdominal pain, nausea, constipation, dry mouth, rash, abnormal dreams, fall. (6.1)

To report SUSPECTED ADVERSE REACTIONS, contact TEVA at 1-800-221-4026 or FDA at 1-800-FDA-1088 or www.fda.gov/medwatch.

———DRUG INTERACTIONS———

• Meperidine: Risk of serious, sometimes fatal reactions from serotonin syndrome. See also Contraindications. (7.1)
• Dextromethorphan: Risk of psychosis episodes or bizarre behavior. See also Contraindications. (7.2)
• MAO inhibitors: Risk of non-selective MAO inhibition and hypertensive crisis. See also Contraindications. (7.4)
• Antidepressants (SSRIs, SNRIs, tricyclic, tetracyclic, or triazolopyridine): Concomitant use not recommended. (7.5)
• Levodopa: See also Warnings and Precautions. (7.6)
• Ciprofloxacin and Other CYP1A2 Inhibitors: Increased rasagiline plasma levels possible. Increased risk of adverse events. See also Dosage and Administration and Warnings and Precautions.(7.7)

———USE IN SPECIFIC POPULATIONS———

• Pregnancy: AZILECT should be used only if the potential benefit justifies the potential risk to the fetus. (8.1)
• Nursing mothers: Rasagiline inhibits prolactin secretion and may inhibit milk secretion. It is not known whether rasagiline is excreted in human milk. Use with caution. (8.3)
• Hepatic impairment: Rasagiline plasma concentrations may be increased. See also Dosage and Administration and Warnings and Precautions. (8.6)

See 17 for PATIENT COUNSELING INFORMATION.
Revised: 12/2009

———

FULL PRESCRIBING INFORMATION: CONTENTS*

*Sections or subsections omitted from the full prescribing information are not listed.

FULL PRESCRIBING INFORMATION
AZILECT® (rasagiline tablets)

1 INDICATIONS AND USAGE

AZILECT (rasagiline tablets) is indicated for the treatment of the signs and symptoms of idiopathic Parkinson's disease as initial monotherapy and as adjunct therapy to levodopa. The effectiveness of AZILECT was demonstrated in patients with early Parkinson's disease who were receiving AZILECT as monotherapy and who were not receiving any concomitant dopaminergic therapy. The effectiveness of AZILECT as adjunct therapy was demonstrated in patients with Parkinson's disease who were treated with levodopa.

2 DOSAGE AND ADMINISTRATION

AZILECT is a selective inhibitor of monoamine oxidase (MAO)-B at recommended doses of 0.5 or 1 mg daily. Dietary tyramine restriction is not ordinarily required with recommended doses of AZILECT. However, certain foods (e.g., aged cheeses, such as Stilton cheese) may contain very high amounts (i.e., > 150 mg) of tyramine and could potentially cause a hypertensive "cheese" reaction in patients taking AZILECT even at the recommended dose due to mild increased sensitivity to tyramine. The selectivity for inhibiting MAO-B diminishes in a dose-related manner as the dose is progressively increased above the recommended daily dose [see Warnings and Precautions (5.4), Clinical Pharmacology (12.3, and Information for Patients (17.3))].

2.1 Monotherapy

The recommended AZILECT dose for the treatment of Parkinson's disease patients is 1 mg administered orally once daily.

2.2 Adjunctive Therapy

The recommended initial dose is 0.5 mg administered orally once daily. If a sufficient clinical response is not achieved, the dose may be increased to 1 mg administered once daily.

Change of Levodopa Dose in Adjunct Therapy

When AZILECT is used in combination with levodopa, a reduction of the levodopa dosage may be considered based upon individual response. During the controlled trials of AZILECT as adjunct therapy to levodopa, levodopa dosage was reduced in some patients. In clinical studies, dosage reduction of levodopa was allowed within the first 6 weeks if dopaminergic side effects, including dyskinesia and hallucinations, emerged. In Study 1, levodopa dosage reduction occurred in 8% of patients in the placebo group and in 16% and 17% of patients in the 0.5 mg/day and 1 mg/day rasagiline groups, respectively. In those patients who had levodopa dosage reduced, the dose was reduced on average by about 7%, 9%, and 13% in the placebo, 0.5 mg/day, and 1 mg/day groups, respectively. In Study 2, levodopa dosage reduction occurred in 6% of patients in the placebo group and in 9% in the rasagiline 1 mg/day group. In patients who had their levodopa dosage reduced, the dose was reduced on average by about 13% and 11% in the placebo and the rasagiline groups, respectively.

2.3 Patients with Hepatic Impairment

AZILECT plasma concentrations will increase in patients with hepatic impairment. Patients with mild hepatic impairment should use 0.5 mg daily of AZILECT. AZILECT should not be used in patients with moderate or severe hepatic impairment [see Warnings and Precautions (5.3), Use in Specific Populations (8.6), and Clinical Pharmacology (12.3)].

2.4 Patients with Renal Impairment

Dose adjustment of AZILECT is not required for patients with mild or moderate renal impairment because AZILECT plasma concentrations are not increased in patients with moderate renal impairment. Rasagiline has not been studied in patients with severe renal impairment.

2.5 Patients Taking Ciprofloxacin or Other CYP1A2 Inhibitors

Rasagiline plasma concentrations are expected to double in patients taking concomitant ciprofloxacin and other CYP1A2 inhibitors. Therefore, patients taking concomitant ciprofloxacin or other CYP1A2 inhibitors should use 0.5 mg daily of AZILECT [see Warnings and Precautions (5.2), Drug Interactions (7.7), and Clinical Pharmacology (12.3)].

3 DOSAGE FORMS AND STRENGTHS

AZILECT 0.5 mg Tablets: White to off-white, round, flat, beveled tablets, debossed with "GIL 0.5" on one side and plain on the other side containing, as the active ingredient, rasagiline mesylate equivalent to 0.5 mg of rasagiline base. AZILECT 1 mg Tablets: White to off-white, round, flat, beveled tablets, debossed with "GIL 1" on one side and plain on the other side containing, as the active ingredient, rasagiline mesylate equivalent to 1 mg of rasagiline base.

4 CONTRAINDICATIONS

4.1 Meperidine and Certain Other Analgesics

AZILECT is contraindicated for use with meperidine. Serious adverse reactions have been precipitated with concomitant use of meperidine (e.g., Demerol and other tradenames) and MAO inhibitors (MAOIs) including selective MAO-B inhibitors. These adverse reactions are often described as "serotonin syndrome", a potentially serious condition, which can result in death. Typical clinical signs and symptoms include behavioral and cognitive/mental status changes (e.g., confusion, hypomania, hallucinations, agitation, delirium, headache, and coma), autonomic effects (e.g., syncope, shivering, sweating, high fever/hyperthermia, hypertension, hypotension, tachycardia, nausea, diarrhea), and somatic effects (e.g., muscular rigidity, myoclonus, muscle twitching, hyperreflexia manifested by clonus, and tremor). At least 14 days should elapse between discontinuation of AZILECT and initiation of treatment with meperidine.

For similar reasons, AZILECT should not be administered with the analgesic agents tramadol, methadone, and propoxyphene.

In the post-marketing period, serotonin syndrome has been reported in a patient erroneously treated with a higher than recommended dose of AZILECT (4 mg daily) and tramadol.

4.2 Other Drugs

AZILECT should not be used with the antitussive agent dextromethorphan. The combination of MAO inhibitors and dextromethorphan has been reported to cause brief episodes of psychosis or bizarre behavior. AZILECT is also contraindicated for use with St. John's wort, and cyclobenzaprine (a tricyclic muscle relaxant).

4.3 MAO Inhibitors

AZILECT should not be administered along with any other MAO inhibitor (selective or non-selective) because of the increased risk of non-selective MAO inhibition that may lead to a hypertensive crisis. At least 14 days should elapse between discontinuation of AZILECT and initiation of treatment with any MAO inhibitor.

5 WARNINGS AND PRECAUTIONS

5.1 Coadministration with Antidepressants

Severe CNS toxicity associated with hyperpyrexia has been reported with the combined treatment of an antidepressant (e.g., selective serotonin reuptake inhibitors-SSRIs, serotonin-norepinephrine reuptake inhibitors-SNRIs, tricyclic antidepressants, tetracyclic antidepressants, triazolopyridine antidepressants) and a non-selective MAOI (e.g., phenelzine, tranylcypromine) or selective MAO-B inhibitors, such as selegiline (Eldepryl) and rasagiline (AZILECT). These adverse reactions are often described as "serotonin syndrome" which can result in death. In the post-marketing period, non-fatal cases of serotonin syndrome have been reported in patients treated with antidepressants concomitantly with AZILECT.

The symptoms of serotonin syndrome have included behavioral and cognitive/mental status changes (e.g., confusion, hypomania, hallucinations, agitation, delirium, headache, and coma), autonomic effects (e.g., syncope, shivering, sweating, high fever/hyperthermia, hypertension, tachycardia, nausea, diarrhea), and somatic effects (e.g., muscular rigidity, myoclonus, muscle twitching, hyperreflexia manifested by clonus, and tremor).

AZILECT clinical trials did not allow concomitant use of fluoxetine or fluvoxamine with AZILECT, but the following antidepressants and doses were allowed in the AZILECT trials: amitriptyline ≤ 50 mg/daily, trazodone ≤ 100 mg/daily, citalopram ≤ 20 mg/daily, sertraline ≤ 100 mg/daily and paroxetine ≤ 30 mg/daily.

Although a small number of rasagiline-treated patients were concomitantly exposed to antidepressants (tricyclics n=115; SSRIs n=141), the exposure, both in dose and number of subjects, was not adequate to rule out the possibility of an untoward reaction from combining these agents. Furthermore, because the mechanisms of these reactions are not fully understood, it seems prudent, in general, to avoid the combination of AZILECT with any antidepressant. At least 14 days should elapse between discontinuation of AZILECT and initiation of treatment with a SSRI, SNRI, tricyclic, tetracyclic, or triazolopyridine antidepressant. Because of the long half lives of certain antidepressants (e.g., fluoxetine and its active metabolite), at least five weeks (perhaps longer, especially if fluoxetine has been prescribed chronically and/or at higher doses) should elapse between discontinuation of fluoxetine and initiation of AZILECT [see Drug Interactions (7.5)].

5.2 Ciprofloxacin and Other CYP1A2 Inhibitors

Rasagiline plasma concentrations may increase up to 2 fold in patients using concomitant ciprofloxacin and other CYP1A2 inhibitors [see Dosage and Administration (2.5), Drug Interactions (7.7), and Clinical Pharmacology (12.3)].

5.3 Hepatic Impairment

Rasagiline plasma concentration may increase in patients with mild (up to 2 fold, Child-Pugh score 5-6), moderate (up to 7 fold, Child-Pugh score 7-9), and severe (Child-Pugh score 10-15) hepatic impairment. Patients with mild hepatic impairment should be given the dose of 0.5 mg/day. AZILECT should not be used in patients with moderate or severe hepatic impairment [see Dosage and Administration (2.3) and Clinical Pharmacology (12.3)].

5.4 Risk for Hypertensive Crisis and Nonselective Monoamine Oxidase Inhibition Above The Recommended Doses

AZILECT is a selective inhibitor of monoamine oxidase (MAO)-B at the recommended doses of 0.5 or 1 mg daily. AZILECT should not be used at daily doses exceeding 1 mg/day (or 0.5 mg/day for patients with mild hepatic impairment or in patients using concomitant ciprofloxacin or another CYP1A2 inhibitor) because of the risks of hypertensive crisis and other adverse reactions associated with non-selective inhibition of MAO [see Dosage and Administration (2), Drug Interactions (7.9), and Clinical Pharmacology (12.3)].

Dietary tyramine restriction is not ordinarily required with ingestion of most foods and beverages that may contain tyramine, during treatment with recommended doses of AZILECT. However, certain foods (e.g., aged cheeses, such as Stilton cheese) may contain very high amounts (i.e., > 150 mg) of tyramine and could potentially cause a hypertensive "cheese" reaction in patients taking AZILECT even at the recommended doses due to mild increased sensitivity to tyramine. Patients should be advised to avoid foods (e.g., aged cheese) containing a very large amount of tyramine while taking recommended doses of AZILECT because of the potential for large increases in blood pressure. Selectivity for inhibiting MAO-B diminishes in a dose-related manner as the dose is progressively increased above the recommended daily doses.

There were no cases of hypertensive crisis in the clinical development program associated with 1 mg daily rasagiline treatment, in which most patients did not follow dietary tyramine restriction.

Rare cases of hypertensive crisis have been reported in the post-marketing period in patients after ingesting unknown amounts of tyramine-rich foods while taking recommended doses of AZILECT.

5.5 Melanoma

Epidemiological studies have shown that patients with Parkinson's disease have a higher risk (2- to approximately 6-fold higher) of developing melanoma than the general population. Whether the increased risk observed was due to Parkinson's disease or other factors, such as drugs used to treat Parkinson's disease, is unclear.

For the reasons stated above, patients and providers are advised to monitor for melanomas frequently and on a regular basis. Ideally, periodic skin examinations should be performed by appropriately qualified individuals (e.g., dermatologists).

5.6 Dyskinesia

When used as an adjunct to levodopa, AZILECT may cause dyskinesia or potentiate dopaminergic side effects and exacerbate pre-existing dyskinesia (treatment-emergent dyskinesia occurred in about 18% of patients treated with 0.5 mg or 1 mg rasagiline as an adjunct to levodopa, and 10% of patients who received placebo as an adjunct to levodopa). Decreasing the dose of levodopa may ameliorate this side effect.

5.7 Lowering of Blood Pressure and Postural/Orthostatic Hypotension

In placebo controlled studies of AZILECT given in combination with levodopa, the incidence of postural hypotension consisting of a systolic blood pressure decrease (≥ 30 mm Hg) or a diastolic blood pressure decrease (≥ 20 mm Hg) after standing was 13.4 % with AZILECT (1 mg/day) compared to 8.5 % with placebo.

At the 1 mg dose, the frequency of orthostatic hypotension at any time during the study was approximately 44 % for AZILECT vs 33% for placebo for mild to moderate systolic blood pressure decrements (≥ 20 mm Hg), 40 % for AZILECT vs 33 % for placebo for mild to moderate diastolic blood pressure decrements (≥ 10 mm Hg), 7 % for AZILECT vs 3 % for placebo for severe systolic blood pressure decrements (≥ 40 mm Hg), and 9 % for AZILECT vs 6 % for placebo for severe diastolic blood pressure decrements (≥ 20 mm Hg). There was also an increased risk for some of these abnormalities at the lower 0.5 mg daily dose and for an individual patient having mild to moderate or severe postural hypotension for both systolic and diastolic blood pressure.

Clinical trial data further suggest that postural hypotension occurs most frequently in the first two months of AZILECT treatment and tends to decrease over time.

Some patients treated with AZILECT experienced a mildly increased risk for significant decreases in blood pressure unrelated to standing but while supine.

The risk for post-treatment hypotension (e.g., systolic < 90 or diastolic < 50 mm Hg) combined with a significant decrease from baseline (e.g., systolic > 30 or diastolic > 20 mm Hg) was higher for AZILECT 1 mg (3.2 %) compared to placebo (1.3 %).

There was no clear increased risk for lowering of blood pressure or postural hypotension associated with AZILECT 1 mg/day as monotherapy.

When used as an adjunct to levodopa, postural hypotension was also reported as an adverse reaction in approximately 6% of patients treated with 0.5 mg rasagiline, 9% of patients treated with 1 mg rasagiline and 3% of patients treated with placebo. Postural hypotension led to drug discontinuation and premature withdrawal from clinical trials in one (0.7%) patient treated with rasagiline 1 mg/day, no patients treated with rasagiline 0.5 mg/day and no placebo-treated patients.

5.8 Elevation of Blood Pressure

In studies in which AZILECT (1 mg/day) was given in conjunction with levodopa, AZILECT produced an increased incidence of a significant, high blood pressure (e.g., systolic > 180 or diastolic > 100 mm Hg) of 4% compared to 3% for placebo.

The risk for developing post-treatment high blood pressure (e.g., systolic > 180 or diastolic >100 mm Hg) combined with a significant increase from baseline (e.g., systolic > 30 or diastolic > 20 mm Hg) was higher for AZILECT (2 %) compared to placebo (1 %).

There was no increased frequency of the incidence of hypertension as an adverse reaction in the adjunctive treatment pivotal trials for AZILECT treatment vs placebo.

There was no observed increased risk for increasing blood pressure or high blood pressure (based upon various measurements and analyses) or for the development of hypertension as an adverse reaction in the monotherapy study for 1 mg daily AZILECT treatment (vs placebo).

5.9 Hallucinations/Psychotic-Like Behavior

In the monotherapy study, hallucinations were reported as an adverse event in 1.3% of patients treated with 1 mg rasagiline and in 0.7% of patients treated with placebo. In the monotherapy trial, hallucinations led to drug discontinuation and premature withdrawal from clinical trials in 1.3% of the 1 mg rasagiline-treated patients and in none of the placebo-treated patients.

When used as an adjunct to levodopa, hallucinations were reported as an adverse reaction in approximately 5% of patients treated with 0.5 mg/day AZILECT, 4% of patients treated with 1 mg/day AZILECT and 3% of patients treated with placebo. Hallucinations led to drug discontinuation and premature withdrawal from clinical trials in about 1% of patients treated with 0.5 mg/day or 1 mg/day rasagiline and none of the placebo-treated patients.

Patients should be informed of the possibility of developing hallucinations and instructed to report them to their health care provider promptly should they develop.

Patients with a major psychotic disorder should ordinarily not be treated with AZILECT because of the risk of exacerbating the psychosis with an increase in central dopaminergic tone. In addition, many treatments for psychosis that decrease in central dopaminergic tone may decrease the effectiveness of AZILECT.

AZILECT administration may cause or exacerbate psychotic-like behavior based upon post-marketing reports. This adverse reaction has been reported with many anti-Parkinsonian drugs that increase central dopaminergic tone. This abnormal behavior has been exhibited by one or more of a variety of manifestations including paranoia, confusional state/confusion, psychotic disorder, agitation, delusion, and hallucinations.

5.10 Withdrawal-Emergent Hyperpyrexia and Confusion

A symptom complex resembling neuroleptic malignant syndrome (characterized by elevated temperature, muscular rigidity, altered consciousness, and autonomic instability), with no other obvious etiology, has been reported in association with rapid dose reduction, withdrawal of, or changes in drugs that increase central dopaminergic tone. *[see Dosage and Administration (2.2)].*

Withdrawal emergent hyperpyrexia was not reported in the AZILECT clinical development program.

5.11 Laboratory Tests

No specific laboratory tests are required for the treatment of patients on AZILECT.

6 ADVERSE REACTIONS

6.1 Clinical Studies Experience

During the clinical development of AZILECT, 1361 Parkinson's disease patients received rasagiline as initial monotherapy or as adjunct therapy to levodopa. As these two populations differ, not only in the adjunct use of levodopa during rasagiline treatment, but also in the severity and duration of their disease, they may have differential risks for various adverse reactions. Therefore, most of the adverse reactions data in this section are presented separately for each population.

Because clinical trials are conducted under widely varying conditions, adverse reaction rates observed in the clinical trials of a drug cannot be directly compared to rates in the clinical trials of another drug and may not reflect the rates of adverse reactions observed in practice.

Patients Receiving AZILECT as Initial Monotherapy Treatment

Adverse Reactions Leading to Discontinuation in Controlled Clinical Studies

In the double-blind, placebo-controlled trials conducted in patients receiving AZILECT as monotherapy, approximately 5% of the 149 patients treated with rasagiline discontinued treatment due to adverse reactions compared to 2% of the 151 patients who received placebo.

The only adverse reaction that led to the discontinuation of more than one patient was hallucinations.

Adverse Reaction Incidence in Controlled Clinical Studies

The most commonly observed adverse reactions were those in which the treatment difference for the incidence in

AZILECT-treated patients was ≥ 3 % greater than the incidence in the placebo-treated patients and included flu syndrome, arthralgia, depression, and dyspepsia. Table 1 lists treatment-emergent adverse reactions that occurred in ≥ 2% of patients receiving AZILECT as monotherapy participating in the double-blind, placebo-controlled trial and were numerically more frequent than in the placebo group.

Table 1. Treatment-Emergent* Adverse Reactions in AZILECT 1 mg-Treated Monotherapy Patients

Placebo-Controlled Studies Without Levodopa Treatment	AZILECT 1 mg (N=149)	Placebo (N=151)
	% of Patients	% of Patients
Headache	14	12
Arthralgia	7	4
Dyspepsia	7	4
Depression	5	2
Fall	5	3
Flu syndrome	5	1
Conjunctivitis	3	1
Fever	3	1
Gastroenteritis	3	1
Rhinitis	3	1
Arthritis	2	1
Ecchymosis	2	0
Malaise	2	0
Neck Pain	2	0
Paresthesia	2	1
Vertigo	2	1

*Incidence ≥ 2% in AZILECT 1 mg group and numerically more frequent than in placebo group

Other events of potential clinical importance reported by 1% or more of patients receiving AZILECT as monotherapy, and at least as frequent as in the placebo group, in descending order of frequency include: dizziness, diarrhea, chest pain, albuminuria, allergic reaction, alopecia, angina pectoris, anorexia, asthma, hallucinations, impotence, leukopenia, libido decreased, liver function tests abnormal, skin carcinoma, syncope, vesiculobullous rash, vomiting.

There were no significant differences in the safety profile based on age or gender.

Patients Receiving AZILECT as Adjunct to Levodopa Therapy

Adverse Reactions Leading to Discontinuation in Controlled Clinical Studies

In a double-blind, placebo-controlled trial (Study 1) conducted in patients treated with AZILECT as adjunct to levodopa therapy, approximately 9% of the 164 patients treated with AZILECT 0.5 mg/day and 7% of the 149 patients treated with AZILECT 1 mg/day discontinued treatment due to adverse reactions compared to 6% of the 159 patients who received placebo. The adverse reactions that led to discontinuation of more than one rasagiline-treated patient were: diarrhea, weight loss, hallucination, and rash. Adverse event reporting was considered more reliable for Study 1 than for the second controlled trial (Study 2); therefore only the adverse event data from Study 1 are presented in this section of labeling.

Adverse Reactions: Incidence in Controlled Clinical Studies

The most commonly observed adverse reactions were those in which the treatment difference for the incidence in AZILECT-treated patients (n=149) was ≥ 3 % greater than the incidence in the placebo-treated patients (n=159) and included dyskinesia, accidental injury, weight loss, postural hypotension, vomiting, anorexia, arthralgia, abdominal pain, nausea, constipation, dry mouth, rash, abnormal dreams, and fall.

Table 2 lists treatment-emergent adverse reactions that occurred in ≥ 2% of patients treated with AZILECT 1 mg/day as adjunct to levodopa therapy participating in the double-blind, placebo-controlled trial (Study 1) and that were numerically more frequent than the placebo group. The table also shows the rates for the 0.5 mg group in Study 1.

Table 2. Incidence of Treatment-Emergent* Adverse Reactions in Patients Receiving AZILECT as Adjunct to Levodopa Therapy in Study 1

	AZILECT 1 mg + Levodopa (N=149)	AZILECT 0.5 mg + Levodopa (N=164)	Placebo + Levodopa (N=159)
	% of patients	% of patients	% of patients
Dyskinesia	18	18	10
Accidental injury	12	8	5
Nausea	12	10	8
Headache	11	8	10
Fall	11	12	8
Weight loss	9	2	3
Constipation	9	4	5
Postural hypotension	9	6	3
Arthralgia	8	6	4
Vomiting	7	4	1
Dry mouth	6	2	3
Rash	6	3	3
Somnolence	6	4	4
Abdominal pain	5	2	1
Anorexia	5	2	1
Diarrhea	5	7	4
Ecchymosis	5	2	3
Dyspepsia	5	4	4
Paresthesia	5	2	3
Abnormal dreams	4	1	1
Hallucinations	4	5	3
Ataxia	3	6	1
Dyspnea	3	5	2
Infection	3	2	2
Neck pain	3	1	1
Sweating	3	2	1
Tenosynovitis	3	1	0
Dystonia	3	2	1
Gingivitis	2	1	1
Hemorrhage	2	1	1
Hernia	2	1	1
Myasthenia	2	2	1

*Incidence ≥ 2% in AZILECT 1 mg group and numerically more frequent than in placebo group

Several of the more common adverse reactions seemed dose-related, including weight loss, postural hypotension, and dry mouth.

Other adverse reactions of potential clinical importance reported in Study 1 by 1% or more of patients treated with rasagiline 1 mg/day as adjunct to levodopa therapy, and at least as frequent as in the placebo group, in descending order of frequency include: skin carcinoma, anemia, albuminuria, amnesia, arthritis, bursitis, cerebrovascular accident, confusion, dysphagia, epistaxis, leg cramps, pruritus, skin ulcer.

There were no significant differences in the safety profile based on age or gender.

Other Adverse Reactions Observed During All Phase 2/3 Clinical Trials

Rasagiline was administered to approximately 1361 patients during all PD phase 2/3 clinical trials. About 283 patients received rasagiline for at least one year, approximately 410 patients received rasagiline for at least two years, 116 patients received rasagiline for at least 3 years, and 245 patients received rasagiline for more than 3 years, with some patients treated for more than 5 years. The long-term safety profile was similar to that observed with shorter duration exposure.

The frequencies listed below represent the proportion of the 1361 individuals exposed to rasagiline who experienced events of the type cited.

All events that occurred at least twice (or once for serious or potentially serious events), except those already listed above, trivial events, terms too vague to be meaningful, adverse events with no plausible relation to treatment, and events that would be expected in patients of the age studied, were reported without regard to determination of a causal relationship to rasagiline.

Events are further classified within body system categories and enumerated in order of decreasing frequency using the following definitions: frequent adverse events are defined as those occurring in at least 1/100 patients, infrequent adverse events are defined as those occurring in at least 1/100 to 1/1000 patients and rare adverse events are defined as those occurring in fewer than 1/1000 patients.

Body as a whole: Frequent: asthenia *Infrequent:* chills, face edema, flank pain, photosensitivity reaction
Cardiovascular system: Frequent: bundle branch block *Infrequent:* deep thrombophlebitis, heart failure, migraine, myocardial infarct, phlebitis, ventricular tachycardia *Rare:* arterial thrombosis, atrial arrhythmia, AV block complete, AV block second degree, bigeminy, cerebral hemorrhage, cerebral ischemia, ventricular fibrillation
Digestive system: Frequent: gastrointestinal hemorrhage *Infrequent:* colitis, esophageal ulcer, esophagitis, fecal incontinence, intestinal obstruction, mouth ulceration, stomach ulcer, stomatitis, tongue edema *Rare:* hematemesis, hemorrhagic gastritis, intestinal perforation, intestinal stenosis, jaundice, large intestine perforation, megacolon, melena
Hemic and Lymphatic system: Infrequent: macrocytic anemia *Rare:* purpura, thrombocythemia
Metabolic and Nutritional disorders: Infrequent: hypocalcemia
Musculoskeletal system: Infrequent: bone necrosis, muscle atrophy *Rare:* arthrosis
Nervous system: Frequent: abnormal gait, anxiety, hyperkinesia, hypertonia, neuropathy, tremor *Infrequent:* agitation, aphasia, circumoral paresthesia, convulsion, delusions, dementia, dysarthria, dysautonomia, dysesthesia, emotional lability, facial paralysis, foot drop, hemiplegia, hypesthesia, incoordination, manic reaction, myoclonus, neuritis, neurosis, paranoid reaction, personality disorder, psychosis, wrist drop *Rare:* apathy, delirium, hostility, manic depressive reaction, myelitis, neuralgia, psychotic depression, stupor
Respiratory system: Frequent: cough increased *Infrequent:* apnea, emphysema, laryngismus, pleural effusion, pneumothorax *Rare:* interstitial pneumonia, larynx edema, lung fibrosis
Skin and Appendages: Infrequent: eczema, urticaria *Rare:* exfoliative dermatitis, leukoderma
Special senses: Infrequent: blepharitis, deafness, diplopia, eye hemorrhage, eye pain, glaucoma, keratitis, ptosis, retinal degeneration, taste perversion, visual field defect *Rare:* blindness, parosmia, photophobia, retinal detachment, retinal hemorrhage, strabismus, taste loss, vestibular disorder
Urogenital system: Frequent: hematuria, urinary incontinence *Infrequent:* acute kidney failure, dysmenorrhea, dysuria, kidney calculus, nocturia, polyuria, scrotal edema, sexual function abnormal, urinary retention, urination impaired, vaginal hemorrhage, vaginal moniliasis, vaginitis *Rare:* abnormal ejaculation, amenorrhea, anuria, epididymitis, gynecomastia, hydroureter, leukorrhea, priapism

6.2 Post-marketing Experience

The following adverse events not described in sections 4 and 5 have been identified during the post-marketing/post-approval use of AZILECT. Because these adverse events are reported voluntarily from a population of uncertain size, it is not possible to reliably estimate their frequency nor to establish unequivocally a causal relationship to drug exposure: Increased libido including hypersexuality, impulse control symptoms, pathological gambling *[see Patient Counseling Information (17.11)]*

7 DRUG INTERACTIONS

7.1 Meperidine

Serious, sometimes fatal reactions have been precipitated with concomitant use of meperidine (e.g., Demerol and other tradenames) and MAO inhibitors including selective MAO-B inhibitors *[see Contraindications (4.1)].*

7.2 Dextromethorphan

The concomitant use of AZILECT and dextromethorphan was not allowed in clinical studies. The combination of MAO inhibitors and dextromethorphan has been reported to cause brief episodes of psychosis or bizarre behavior. Therefore, in view of AZILECT's MAO inhibitory activity, dextromethorphan should not be used concomitantly with AZILECT *[see Contraindications (4.2)].*

7.3 Sympathomimetic Medications

The concomitant use of AZILECT and sympathomimetic medications was not allowed in clinical studies. Severe hypertensive reactions have followed the administration of sympathomimetics and non-selective MAO inhibitors. One case of hypertensive crisis has been reported in a patient taking the recommended dose of a selective MAO-B inhibitor and a sympathomimetic medication (ephedrine). Elevated blood pressure was reported in another patient taking the recommended dose of AZILECT and ophthalmic drops with a sympathomimetic medication (tetrahydrozoline).

Because AZILECT is a selective MAOI, hypertensive reactions are not ordinarily expected with the concomitant use of sympathomimetic medications. Nevertheless, caution should be exercised when concomitantly using recommended doses of AZILECT with any sympathomimetic medications including nasal, oral, and ophthalmic decongestants and cold remedies.

7.4 MAO Inhibitors

AZILECT should not be administered along with other MAO inhibitors because of the increased risk of non-selective MAO inhibition that may lead to a hypertensive crisis *[see Contraindications (4.3)].*

7.5 Antidepressants

Concomitant use of AZILECT with one of many classes of antidepressants (e.g., SSRIs, SNRIs, triazolopyridine, tricyclic or tetracyclic antidepressants) is not recommended *[see Warnings and Precautions (5.1)].*

7.6 Levodopa/Carbidopa

[see Warnings and Precautions (5.6) and Clinical Pharmacology (12.3)].

7.7 Ciprofloxacin and Other CYP1A2 Inhibitors

Rasagiline plasma concentrations may increase up to 2 fold in patients using concomitant ciprofloxacin and other CYP1A2 inhibitors. This could result in increased adverse events *[see Warnings and Precautions (5.2) and Clinical Pharmacology (12.3)].*

7.8 Theophylline

[see Clinical Pharmacology (12.3)].

7.9 Tyramine/Rasagiline Interaction

MAO in the gastrointestinal tract and liver (primarily type A) is thought to provide vital protection from exogenous amines (e.g., tyramine) that have the capacity, if absorbed intact, to cause a "hypertensive crisis," the so-called "cheese reaction". If large amounts of certain exogenous amines (e.g., from fermented cheese, herring, over-the-counter cough/cold medications) gain access to the systemic circulation because MAO-A has been inhibited, they cause release of norepinephrine which may result in a rise in systemic blood pressure. MAOIs that selectively inhibit MAO-B are largely devoid of the potential to cause tyramine-induced hypertensive crisis.

Results of a special tyramine challenge study indicate that rasagiline is selective for MAO-B at recommended doses and can ordinarily be used without dietary tyramine restriction. However, certain foods (e.g., aged cheeses, such as Stilton cheese) may contain very high amounts (i.e., > 150 mg) of tyramine and could potentially cause a hypertensive cheese reaction in patients taking AZILECT due to mild increased sensitivity to tyramine. Patients should be advised to avoid foods (e.g., aged cheese) containing a very large amount of tyramine while taking recommended doses of AZILECT because of the potential for large increases in blood pressure. Selectivity for inhibiting MAO-B diminishes in a dose-related manner as the dose is progressively increased above the recommended daily doses.

There were no cases of hypertensive crisis in the clinical development program associated with 1 mg daily rasagiline treatment, in which most patients did not follow dietary tyramine restriction.

Despite the selective inhibition of MAO-B at recommended doses of AZILECT, there have been post-marketing reports of patients who experienced significantly elevated blood pressure (including rare cases of hypertensive crisis) after ingestion of unknown amounts of tyramine-rich foods while taking recommended doses of AZILECT *[see Dosing and Administration (2), and Warnings and Precautions 5.4)].*

8 USE IN SPECIFIC POPULATIONS

8.1 Pregnancy

Category C

No effect on embryo-fetal development was observed in a combined mating/fertility and embryo-fetal development study in female rats at doses up to 3 mg/kg/day (approximately 30 times the expected plasma rasagiline exposure (AUC) at the maximum recommended human dose [MRHD, 1 mg/day]). Effects on embryo-fetal development in rabbit have not been adequately assessed.

In a study in which pregnant rats were dosed with rasagiline (0.1, 0.3, 1 mg/kg/day) orally, from the beginning of organogenesis to day 20 post-partum, offspring survival was decreased and offspring body weight was reduced at doses of 0.3 mg/kg/day and 1 mg/kg/day (10 and 16 times the expected plasma rasagiline exposure [AUC] at the MRHD). No plasma data were available at the no-effect dose (0.1 mg/kg); however, that dose is 1 times the MRHD on a mg/m² basis. Rasagiline's effect on physical and behavioral development was not adequately assessed in this study.

Rasagiline may be given as an adjunct therapy to levodopa/carbidopa treatment. In a study in which pregnant rats were dosed with rasagiline (0.1, 0.3, 1 mg/kg/day) and levodopa/carbidopa (80/20 mg/kg/day) (alone and in combination) throughout the period of organogenesis, there was an increased incidence of wavy ribs in fetuses from rats treated with rasagiline in combination with levodopa/carbidopa at 1/80/20 mg/kg/day (approximately 8 times the plasma AUC expected in humans at the MRHD and 1/1 times the MRHD of levodopa/carbidopa [800/200 mg/day] on a mg/m² basis). In a study in which pregnant rabbits were dosed throughout the period of organogenesis with rasagiline alone (3 mg/kg) or in combination with levodopa/carbidopa (rasagiline: 0.1, 0.6, 1.2 mg/kg, levodopa/carbidopa: 80/20 mg/kg/day), an increase in embryo-fetal death was noted at rasagiline doses of 0.6 and 1.2 mg/kg/day when administered in combination with levodopa/carbidopa (approximately 7 and 13 times, respectively, the plasma rasagiline AUC at the MRHD). There was an increase in cardiovascular abnormalities with levodopa/carbidopa alone (1/1 times the MRHD on a mg/m² basis) and to a greater extent when rasagiline (at all doses; 1-13 times the plasma rasagiline AUC at the MRHD) was administered in combination with levodopa/carbidopa.

There are no adequate and well-controlled studies of rasagiline in pregnant women. Therefore, AZILECT should be used during pregnancy only if the potential benefit justifies the potential risk to the fetus.

8.3 Nursing Mothers

In rats rasagiline was shown to inhibit prolactin secretion and it may inhibit milk secretion in females.

It is not known whether rasagiline is excreted in human milk. Because many drugs are excreted in human milk, caution should be exercised when AZILECT is administered to a nursing woman.

8.4 Pediatric Use

The safety and effectiveness of AZILECT in the pediatric population have not been studied.

8.5 Geriatric Use

Approximately half of patients in clinical trials were 65 years and over. There were no significant differences in the safety profile of the geriatric and non-geriatric patients.

8.6 Hepatic Impairment

Rasagiline plasma concentration may be increased in patients with mild (up to 2 fold, Child-Pugh score 5-6), moderate (up to 7 fold, Child-Pugh score 7-9), and severe (Child-Pugh score 10-15) hepatic impairment. Patients with mild hepatic impairment should be given the dose of 0.5 mg/day. AZILECT should not be used in patients with moderate or severe hepatic impairment *[see Dosage and Administration (2.3), Warnings and Precautions (5.3) and Clinical Pharmacology (12.3)].*

8.7 Renal Impairment

Dose adjustment of AZILECT is not required for patients with mild or moderate renal impairment because AZILECT plasma concentrations are not increased in patients with moderate renal impairment. Rasagiline has not been studied in patients with severe renal impairment.

9 DRUG ABUSE AND DEPENDENCE

9.1 Controlled Substance

AZILECT is not a controlled substance.

9.2 Abuse

Studies conducted in mice and rats did not reveal any potential for drug abuse and dependence. Clinical trials have not revealed any evidence of the potential for abuse, tolerance or physical dependence; however, systematic studies in humans designed to evaluate these effects have not been performed.

9.3 Dependence

Studies conducted in mice and rats did not reveal any potential for drug abuse and dependence. Clinical trials have not revealed any evidence of the potential for abuse, tolerance or physical dependence; however, systematic studies in humans designed to evaluate these effects have not been performed.

10 OVERDOSE

No cases of AZILECT overdose were reported in clinical trials.

Rasagiline was well tolerated in a single-dose study in healthy volunteers receiving 20 mg/day and in a ten-day study in healthy volunteers receiving 10 mg/day. Adverse events were mild or moderate. In a dose escalation study in patients on chronic levodopa therapy treated with 10 mg of rasagiline there were three reports of cardiovascular side effects (including hypertension and postural hypotension) which resolved following treatment discontinuation.

Symptoms of overdosage, although not observed with rasagiline during clinical development, may resemble those observed with non-selective MAO inhibitors (MAOIs).

Although no cases of overdose have been observed with rasagiline during the clinical development program, the following description of presenting symptoms and clinical course is based upon overdose descriptions of non-selective MAO inhibitors.

Characteristically, signs and symptoms of non-selective MAOI overdose may not appear immediately. Delays of up to 12 hours between ingestion of drug and the appearance of signs may occur. Importantly, the peak intensity of the syndrome may not be reached for upwards of a day following the overdose. Death has been reported following overdosage. Therefore, immediate hospitalization, with continuous patient observation and monitoring for a period of at least two days following the ingestion of such drugs in overdose, is strongly recommended.

The clinical picture of MAOI overdose varies considerably; its severity may be a function of the amount of drug consumed. The central nervous and cardiovascular systems are prominently involved.

Signs and symptoms of overdosage may include, alone or in combination, any of the following: drowsiness, dizziness, faintness, irritability, hyperactivity, agitation, severe headache, hallucinations, trismus, opisthotonos, convulsions, and coma; rapid and irregular pulse, hypertension, hypotension and vascular collapse; precordial pain, respiratory depression and failure, hyperpyrexia, diaphoresis, and cool, clammy skin.

There is no specific antidote for rasagiline overdose. The following suggestions are offered based upon the assumption that rasagiline overdose may be modeled after non-selective MAO inhibitor poisoning. Treatment of overdose with non-selective MAO inhibitors is symptomatic and supportive. Respiration should be supported by appropriate measures, including management of the airway, use of supplemental oxygen, and mechanical ventilatory assistance, as required. Body temperature should be monitored closely. Intensive management of hyperpyrexia may be required. Maintenance of fluid and electrolyte balance is essential. For this reason, in cases of overdose with AZILECT, dietary tyramine restriction should be observed for several weeks to avoid the risk of a hypertensive/cheese reaction.

A poison control center should be called for the most current treatment guidelines.

A post-marketing report described a single patient who developed a non-fatal serotonin syndrome after ingesting 100 mg of AZILECT in a suicide attempt. Another patient who was treated in error with 4 mg AZILECT daily and tramadol also developed a serotonin syndrome. One patient who was treated in error with 3 mg AZILECT daily experienced alternating episodes of vascular fluctuations consisting of hypertension and orthostatic hypotension.

11 DESCRIPTION

AZILECT® tablets contain rasagiline (as the mesylate), a propargylamine-based drug indicated for the treatment of idiopathic Parkinson's disease. It is designated chemically as: 1H-Inden-1-amine, 2, 3-dihydro-N-2-propynyl-, (1R)-, methanesulfonate. The empirical formula of rasagiline mesylate is $(C_{12}H_{13}N)CH_4SO_3$ and its molecular weight is 267.34.

Its structural formula is:

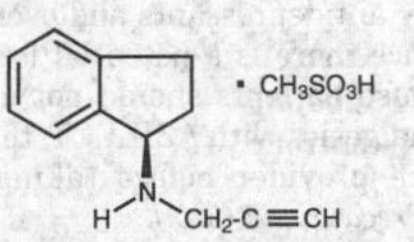

Rasagiline mesylate is a white to off-white powder, freely soluble in water or ethanol and sparingly soluble in isopropanol. Each AZILECT tablet for oral administration contains rasagiline mesylate equivalent to 0.5 mg or 1 mg of rasagiline base.

Each AZILECT tablet also contains the following inactive ingredients: mannitol, starch, pregelatinized starch, colloidal silicon dioxide, stearic acid and talc.

12 CLINICAL PHARMACOLOGY

12.1 Mechanism of Action

AZILECT functions as a selective, irreversible MAO-B inhibitor indicated for the treatment of idiopathic Parkinson's disease. The results of a clinical trial designed to examine the effects of Azilect on blood pressure when it is administered with increasing doses of tyramine indicates the functional selectivity can be incomplete when healthy subjects ingest large amounts of tyramine while receiving recommended doses of AZILECT. The selectivity for inhibiting MAO-B diminishes in a dose-related manner.

MAO, a flavin-containing enzyme, is classified into two major molecular species, A and B, and is localized in mitochondrial membranes throughout the body in nerve terminals, brain, liver and intestinal mucosa. MAO regulates the metabolic degradation of catecholamines and serotonin in the CNS and peripheral tissues. MAO-B is the major form in the human brain. In *ex vivo* animal studies in brain, liver and intestinal tissues, rasagiline was shown to be a potent, irreversible monoamine oxidase type B (MAO-B) selective inhibitor. Rasagiline at the recommended therapeutic dose was also shown to be a potent and irreversible inhibitor of MAO-B in platelets. The precise mechanisms of action of rasagiline are unknown. One mechanism is believed to be related to its MAO-B inhibitory activity, which causes an increase in extracellular levels of dopamine in the striatum. The elevated dopamine level and subsequent increased dopaminergic activity are likely to mediate rasagiline's beneficial effects seen in models of dopaminergic motor dysfunction.

12.2 Pharmacodynamics

Platelet MAO Activity in Clinical Studies

Studies in healthy subjects and in Parkinson's disease patients have shown that rasagiline inhibits platelet MAO-B irreversibly. The inhibition lasts at least 1 week after last dose. Almost 25-35% MAO-B inhibition was achieved after a single rasagiline dose of 1 mg/day and more than 55% of MAO-B inhibition was achieved after a single rasagiline dose of 2 mg/day. Over 90% inhibition was achieved 3 days after rasagiline daily dosing at 2 mg/day and this inhibition level was maintained 3 days post-dose. Multiple doses of rasagiline of 0.5, 1 and 2 mg per day resulted in complete MAO-B inhibition.

12.3 Pharmacokinetics

Rasagiline in the range of 1-6 mg demonstrated a more than proportional increase in AUC, while Cmax was dose proportional. Rasagiline mean steady-state half life is 3 hours but there is no correlation of pharmacokinetics with its pharmacological effect because of its irreversible inhibition of MAO-B.

Absorption

Rasagiline is rapidly absorbed, reaching peak plasma concentration (Cmax) in approximately 1 hour. The absolute bioavailability of rasagiline is about 36%.

Food does not affect the Tmax of rasagiline, although Cmax and exposure (AUC) are decreased by approximately 60% and 20%, respectively, when the drug is taken with a high fat meal. Because AUC is not significantly affected, AZILECT can be administered with or without food *[see Dosage and Administration (2)]*.

Distribution

The mean volume of distribution at steady-state is 87 L, indicating that the tissue binding of rasagiline is in excess of plasma protein binding. Plasma protein binding ranges from 88-94% with mean extent of binding of 61-63% to human albumin over the concentration range of 1-100 ng/mL.

Metabolism and Elimination

Rasagiline undergoes almost complete biotransformation in the liver prior to excretion. The metabolism of rasagiline proceeds through two main pathways: N-dealkylation and/or hydroxylation to yield 1-aminoindan (AI), 3-hydroxy-N-propargyl-1 aminoindan (3-OH-PAI) and 3-hydroxy-1-aminoindan (3-OH-AI). *In vitro* experiments indicate that both routes of rasagiline metabolism are dependent on the cytochrome P450 (CYP) system, with CYP1A2 being the major isoenzyme involved in rasagiline metabolism. Glucuronide conjugation of rasagiline and its metabolites, with subsequent urinary excretion, is the major elimination pathway.

After oral administration of ^{14}C-labeled rasagiline, elimination occurred primarily via urine and secondarily via feces (62% of total dose in urine and 7% of total dose in feces over 7 days), with a total calculated recovery of 84% of the dose over a period of 38 days. Less than 1% of rasagiline was excreted as unchanged drug in urine.

Special Populations

Hepatic Impairment

Following repeat dose administration (7 days) of rasagiline (1 mg/day) in subjects with mild hepatic impairment (Child-Pugh score 5-6), AUC and Cmax were increased by 2 fold and 1.4 fold, respectively, compared to healthy subjects. In subjects with moderate hepatic impairment (Child-Pugh score 7-9), AUC and Cmax were increased by 7 fold and 2 fold, respectively, compared to healthy subjects *[see Dosage and Administration (2.3) and Warnings and Precautions (5.3)]*.

Renal Impairment

Following repeat dose administration (8 days) of rasagiline (1 mg/day) in subjects with moderate renal impairment, rasagiline exposure (AUC) was similar to rasagiline exposure in healthy subjects, while the major metabolite 1-AI exposure (AUC) was increased 1.5-fold in subjects with moderate renal impairment, compared to healthy subjects. Because 1-AI is not an MAO inhibitor, no dose adjustment is needed for patients with mild and moderate renal impairment. Data are not available for patients with severe renal impairment.

Elderly

Since age has little influence on rasagiline pharmacokinetics, it can be administered at the recommended dose in the elderly (≥ 65 years).

Pediatric

AZILECT has not been investigated in patients below 18 years of age.

Gender

The pharmacokinetic profile of rasagiline is similar in men and women.

Drug-Drug Interactions

Tyramine Effect

[see Dosage and Administration (2), Warnings and Precautions (5.4), and Drug Interactions (7.9)].

Levodopa

Data from population pharmacokinetic studies comparing rasagiline clearance in the presence and absence of levodopa have given conflicting results. Although there may be some increase in rasagiline blood levels in the presence of levodopa, the effect is modest and rasagiline dosing need not be modified in the presence of levodopa.

Effect of Other Drugs on the Metabolism of AZILECT

In vitro metabolism studies showed that CYP1A2 was the major enzyme responsible for the metabolism of rasagiline. There is the potential for inhibitors of this enzyme to alter AZILECT clearance when coadministered *[see Dosage and Administration (2.5) and Warnings and Precautions (5.2)]*.

Ciprofloxacin: When ciprofloxacin, an inhibitor of CYP1A2, was administered to healthy volunteers (n=12) at 500 mg (BID) with rasagiline at 2 mg/day, the AUC of rasagiline increased by 83% and there was no change in the elimination half life *[see Dosage and Administration (2.5) and Warnings and Precautions (5.2)]*.

Theophylline: Coadministration of rasagiline 1 mg/day and theophylline, a substrate of CYP1A2, up to 500 mg twice daily to healthy subjects (n=24) did not affect the pharmacokinetics of either drug.

Antidepressants: Severe CNS toxicity (occasionally fatal) associated with hyperpyrexia as part of a serotonin syndrome, has been reported with combined treatment of an antidepressant (e.g., from one of many classes including tricyclic or tetracyclic antidepressants, SSRIs, SNRIs, triazolopyridine antidepressants) and non-selective MAOI or a selective MAO-B inhibitor *[see Warnings and Precautions (5.1)]*.

Effect of AZILECT on Other Drugs

No additional *in vivo* trials have investigated the effect of AZILECT on other drugs metabolized by the cytochrome P450 enzyme system. *In vitro* studies showed that rasagiline at a concentration of 1mcg/ml (equivalent to a level that is 160 times the average Cmax ~ 5.9-8.5 ng/mL in Parkinson's disease patients after 1 mg rasagiline multiple dosing) did not inhibit cytochrome P450 isoenzymes, CYP1A2, CYP2A6, CYP2C9, CYP2C19, CYP2D6, CYP2E1, CYP3A4 and CYP4A. These results indicate that rasagiline is unlikely to cause any clinically significant interference with substrates of these enzymes.

13 NONCLINICAL TOXICOLOGY

13.1 Carcinogenesis, Mutagenesis, Impairment of Fertility

Carcinogenesis

Two year carcinogenicity studies were conducted in CD-1 mice at oral (gavage) doses of 1, 15, and 45 mg/kg and in Sprague-Dawley rats at oral (gavage) doses of 0.3, 1, and 3 mg/kg (males) or 0.5, 2, 5, and 17 mg/kg (females). In rats, there was no increase in tumors at any dose tested. Plasma exposures at the highest dose tested were approximately 33 and 260 times, in male and female rats, respectively, the expected plasma exposures in humans at the maximum recommended dose (MRD) of 1 mg/day.

In mice, there was an increase in lung tumors (combined adenomas/carcinomas) at 15 and 45 mg/kg males and females. Plasma exposures associated with the no-effect dose (1 mg/kg) were approximately 5 times those expected in humans at the MRD.

The carcinogenic potential of rasagiline administered in combination with levodopa/carbidopa has not been examined.

Mutagenesis

Rasagiline was reproducibly clastogenic in *in vitro* chromosomal aberration assays in human lymphocytes in the presence of metabolic activation and was mutagenic and clastogenic in the *in vitro* mouse lymphoma tk assay in the absence and presence of metabolic activation. Rasagiline was negative in the *in vitro* bacterial reverse mutation (Ames) assay, the *in vivo* unscheduled DNA synthesis assay, and the *in vivo* micronucleus assay in CD-1 mice. Rasagiline was also negative in the *in vivo* micronucleus assay in CD-1 mice when administered in combination with levodopa/carbidopa.

Impairment of Fertility

Rasagiline had no effect on mating performance or fertility in male rats treated prior to and throughout the mating period, or in female rats treated from prior to mating through day 17 of gestation at oral doses up to 3 mg/kg/day (approximately 30 times the expected plasma rasagiline exposure (AUC) at the maximum recommended human dose [1 mg/day]). The effect of rasagiline administered in combination with levodopa/carbidopa on mating and fertility has not been examined.

14 CLINICAL TRIALS

The effectiveness of AZILECT for the treatment of Parkinson's disease was established in three 18- to 26-week, randomized, placebo-controlled trials. In one of these trials AZILECT was given as initial monotherapy and in the other two as adjunctive therapy to levodopa.

14.1 Monotherapy Use of AZILECT

The monotherapy trial was a double-blind, randomized, fixed-dose parallel group, 26-week study in early Parkinson's disease patients not receiving any concomitant dopaminergic therapy at the start of the study. The majority of the patients were not treated with any anti-Parkinson's disease medication before receiving rasagiline treatment.

In this trial, 404 patients were randomly assigned to receive placebo (138 patients), rasagiline 1 mg/day (134 patients) or rasagiline 2 mg/day (132 patients). Patients were not allowed to take levodopa, dopamine agonists, selegiline or amantadine, but if necessary, could take stable doses of anticholinergic medication. The average Parkinson's disease duration was approximately 1 year (range 0 to 11 years).

The primary measure of effectiveness was the change from baseline in the total score of the Unified Parkinson's Disease Rating Scale (UPDRS), [mentation (Part I) + activities of daily living (ADL) (Part II) + motor function (Part III)]. The UPDRS is a multi-item rating scale that measures the ability of a patient to perform mental and motor tasks as well as activities of daily living. A reduction in the score represents improvement and a beneficial change from baseline appears as a negative number.

Rasagiline (1 or 2 mg once daily) had a significant beneficial effect relative to placebo on the primary measure of effectiveness in patients receiving six months of treatment and not on dopaminergic therapy. Patients who received rasagiline had significantly less worsening in the UPDRS score, compared to those who received placebo. The effectiveness of rasagiline 1 mg and 2 mg was comparable. Table 3 displays the results of the monotherapy trial.

Table 3. Parkinson's Disease Patients not on Dopaminergic Therapy (Monotherapy)

Primary Measure of Effectiveness: Change in total UPDRS score			
	Baseline score	Change from baseline to termination score	p-value vs. placebo
Placebo	24.5	3.9	—
1.0 mg/day	24.7	0.1	0.0001
2.0 mg/day	25.9	0.7	0.0001

For the comparison between rasagiline 1 mg/day and placebo, no differences in effectiveness based on age or gender were detected.

14.2 Adjunctive Use of AZILECT

Two multicenter, randomized, multinational trials were conducted in more advanced Parkinson's disease patients treated chronically with levodopa and experiencing motor fluctuations (including but not limited to, end of dose "wearing off," sudden or random "off," etc.). The first (Study 1) was conducted in North America (U.S. and Canada) and compared two doses (0.5 mg and 1 mg daily) of rasagiline and placebo while the second (Study 2) was conducted outside of North America (several European countries, Argentina, Israel) and studied only a single dose (1 mg daily) of rasagiline and placebo. Patients had had Parkinson's disease for an average of 9 years (range 5 months to 33 years), had been taking levodopa for an average of 8 years (range 5 months to 32 years), and had been experiencing motor fluctuations for approximately 3 to 4 years (range 1 month to 23 years). Patients kept home diaries just prior to baseline and at specified intervals during the trial. Diaries recorded one of the following four conditions for each half-hour interval over a 24-hour period: "ON" (period of relatively good function and mobility) as either "ON" with no dyskinesia or

without troublesome dyskinesia, or "ON" with troublesome dyskinesia, "OFF" (period of relatively poor function and mobility) or asleep. "Troublesome" dyskinesia is defined as that which interferes with the patient's daily activity. All patients had been inadequately controlled and were experiencing motor fluctuations typical of advanced stage disease despite receiving levodopa/decarboxylase inhibitor. The average dose of levodopa/decarboxylase inhibitor was approximately 700 to 800 mg (range 150 to 3000 mg/day). Patients were also allowed to take stable doses of additional anti-PD medications at entry into the trials. In both trials, approximately 65% of patients were on dopamine agonists and in the North American study (Study 1) approximately 35% were on entacapone. The majority of patients taking entacapone were taking a dopamine agonist as well.

In both trials the primary measure of effectiveness was the change in the mean number of hours that were spent in the "OFF" state at baseline compared to the mean number of hours that were spent in the "OFF" state during the treatment period.

The first adjunct study (Study 1) was a double-blind, randomized, fixed-dose, parallel group trial conducted in 472 levodopa-treated Parkinson's disease patients who were experiencing motor fluctuations. Patients were randomly assigned to receive placebo (159 patients), rasagiline 0.5 mg/day (164 patients), or rasagiline 1 mg/day (149 patients), and were treated for 26 weeks. Patients averaged approximately 6 hours daily in the "OFF" state at baseline, as confirmed by home diaries.

The second adjunct study (Study 2) was a double-blind, randomized, parallel group trial conducted in 687 levodopa-treated Parkinson's disease patients who were experiencing motor fluctuations. Patients were randomly assigned to receive placebo (229 patients), rasagiline 1 mg/day (231 patients) or an active comparator, a COMT inhibitor taken along with scheduled doses of levodopa/decarboxylase inhibitor (227 patients). Patients were treated for 18 weeks. Patients averaged approximately 5.6 hours daily in the "OFF" state at baseline as confirmed by home diaries.

In both studies, rasagiline 1 mg once daily reduced "OFF" time compared to placebo when added to levodopa in patients experiencing motor fluctuations (Tables 4 and 5). The lower dose (0.5 mg) of rasagiline also significantly reduced "OFF" time (Table 4), but had a numerically smaller effect than the 1 mg dose of rasagiline. In Study 2, the active comparator also reduced "OFF" time when compared to placebo.

Table 4. Parkinson's Disease Patients Receiving AZILECT as Adjunct Therapy (Study 1)

Primary Measure of Effectiveness: Change in mean total daily "OFF" time			
	Baseline (hours)	Change from baseline to treatment period (hours)	p-value vs. placebo
Placebo	6.0	-0.9	—
0.5 mg/day	6.0	-1.4	0.0199
1.0 mg/day	6.3	-1.9	<0.0001

Table 5. Parkinson's Disease Patients Receiving AZILECT as Adjunct Therapy (Study 2)

Primary Measure of Effectiveness: Change in mean total daily "OFF" time			
	Baseline (hours)	Change from baseline to treatment period (hours)	p-value vs. placebo
Placebo	5.5	-0.40	—
1.0 mg/day	5.6	-1.2	0.0001

In both studies, dosage reduction of levodopa was allowed within the first 6 weeks if dopaminergic side effects, including dyskinesia and hallucinations, emerged. In Study 1, levodopa dosage reduction occurred in 8% of patients in the placebo group and in 16% and 17% of patients in the 0.5 mg/day and 1 mg/day rasagiline groups, respectively. In those patients who had levodopa dosage reduced, the dose was reduced on average by about 7%, 9%, and 13% in the placebo, 0.5 mg/day, and 1 mg/day groups, respectively. In Study 2, levodopa dosage reduction occurred in 6% of patients in the placebo group and in 9% in the rasagiline 1 mg/day group. In patients who had their levodopa dosage reduced, the dose was reduced on average by about 13% and 11% in the placebo and the rasagiline groups, respectively.

For the comparison between rasagiline 1 mg/day and placebo in both studies, no differences in effectiveness based on age or gender were detected.

Several secondary outcome assessments in the two studies showed statistically significant improvements with rasagiline. These included effects on the activities of daily living (ADL) subscale of the UPDRS performed during an "OFF" period and the motor subscale of the UPDRS performed during an "ON" period. In both scales, a negative response represents improvement. Tables 6 and 7 show these results for Studies 1 and 2.

Table 6. Secondary Measures of Effectiveness (Study 1)

	Baseline (score)	Change from baseline to last value
UPDRS ADL (Activities of Daily Living) subscale score while "OFF"		
Placebo	15.5	0.68
0.5 mg/day	15.8	-0.60
1.0 mg/day	15.5	-0.68
UPDRS Motor subscale score while "ON"		
Placebo	20.8	1.21
0.5 mg/day	21.5	-1.43
1.0 mg/day	20.9	-1.30

Table 7. Secondary Measures of Effectiveness (Study 2)

	Baseline (score)	Change from baseline to last value
UPDRS ADL (Activities of Daily Living) subscale score while "OFF"		
Placebo	18.7	-0.89
1.0 mg/day	19.0	-2.61
UPDRS Motor subscale score while "ON"		
Placebo	23.5	-0.82
1.0 mg/day	23.8	-3.87

16 HOW SUPPLIED

AZILECT 0.5 mg Tablets:
White to off-white, round, flat, beveled tablets, debossed with "GIL 0.5" on one side and plain on the other side. Supplied as bottles of 30 tablets (NDC 68546-142-56).
AZILECT 1 mg Tablets:
White to off-white, round, flat, beveled tablets, debossed with "GIL 1" on one side and plain on the other side. Supplied as bottles of 30 tablets (NDC 68546-229-56).
Storage:
Store at 25°C (77°F) with excursions permitted to 15°-30°C (59°-86°F).

17 INFORMATION FOR PATIENTS

17.1 Coadministration of Antidepressants and Other Drugs

Patients should inform their physician if they are taking, or planning to take, any prescription or over-the-counter drugs, especially antidepressants and over-the-counter cold medications, since there is a potential for interaction with AZILECT. Because patients should not use meperidine or certain other analgesics with AZILECT, they should contact their healthcare provider before taking analgesics *[see Warnings and Precautions (5.1)]*.

17.2 Ciprofloxacin or Other CYP1A2 Inhibitors

Patients should be informed that they should contact their healthcare provider of AZILECT if they take ciprofloxacin or a similar drug that could increase blood levels of rasagiline because of the need to adjust the dose of AZILECT *[see Warnings and Precautions (5.2)]*.

17.3 Risk of Hypertensive Crisis and Nonselective Monoamine Oxidase Inhibition Above the Recommended Doses

Patients should be advised not to exceed the maximum recommended daily dose of 1 mg/day (0.5 mg/day for subjects with mild hepatic impairment and subjects using concomitant ciprofloxacin and other CYP1A2 inhibitors).
The risk of using higher than recommended daily doses of AZILECT should be explained, and a brief description of the hypertensive/cheese reaction provided.

The possibility exists that very tyramine-rich foods (e.g., aged cheese such as Stilton) could possibly cause an increase in blood pressure. Patients should be advised to avoid certain foods (e.g., aged cheese) containing a very large amount of tyramine while taking recommended doses of AZILECT because of the potential for large increases in blood pressure. If patients eat foods very rich in tyramine and do not feel well soon after eating, they should contact their healthcare provider *[see Warnings and Precautions (5.4)]*.

17.4   Melanoma
It is not known if melanoma is associated with Parkinson's disease or the medicines used to treat Parkinson's disease. Patients being treated with AZILECT should be advised to have periodic skin examinations. *[see Warnings and Precautions (5.5)]*.

17.5   Dyskinesia
Patients taking AZILECT as adjunct to levodopa should be advised that there is a possibility of dyskinesia or increased dyskinesia *[see Warnings and Precautions (5.6)]*.

17.6   Lowering of Blood Pressure and Postural/Orthostatic Hypotension
Patients should be advised that they may develop postural (orthostatic) hypotension with or without symptoms such as dizziness, nausea, syncope, and sometimes sweating. Hypotension and/or orthostatic symptoms may occur more frequently during initial therapy or with an increase in dose at any time (cases have been seen after weeks of treatment). Accordingly, patients should be cautioned against standing up rapidly after sitting or lying down, especially if they have been doing so for prolonged periods, and especially, at the initiation of treatment with AZILECT *[see Warnings and Precautions (5.7)]*.

17.7   Elevation of Blood Pressure
Patients should be alerted to the possibility of increases in blood pressure during treatment with AZILECT. Exacerbation of hypertension may occur. Medication dose adjustment may be necessary if elevation of blood pressure is sustained over multiple evaluations *[see Warnings and Precautions (5.8)]*.

17.8   Hallucinations/Psychotic-Like Behavior
Patients should be informed that hallucinations or other manifestations of psychotic-like behavior can occur when taking AZILECT. Patients should also be advised that, if they have a major psychotic disorder, that AZILECT should not ordinarily be used because of the risk of exacerbating the psychosis. Patients with a major psychotic disorder should also be aware that many treatments for psychosis may decrease the effectiveness of AZILECT *[see Warnings and Precautions (5.9)]*.

17.9   Withdrawal-Emergent Hyperpyrexia and Confusion
Patients should be told to contact their healthcare provider if they wish to discontinue Azilect.

17.10   Missing Dose
Patients should be instructed to take AZILECT as prescribed. If a dose is missed, the patient should not double-up the dose of AZILECT. The next dose should be taken at the usual time on the following day.

17.11   Impulse Control/Compulsive Behaviors
There have been reports of patients experiencing intense urges to gamble, increased sexual urges, other intense urges, and the inability to control these urges while taking one or more of the medications that increase central dopaminergic tone and that are generally used for the treatment of Parkinson's disease (including AZILECT). Although it is not proven that the medications caused these events, these urges were reported to have stopped in some cases when the dose was reduced or the medication was stopped. Prescribers should ask patients about the development of new or increased gambling urges, sexual urges, or other urges while being treated with rasagiline. Patients should inform their physician if they experience new or increased gambling urges, increased sexual urges, or other intense urges while taking rasagiline. Physicians should consider dose reduction or stopping the medication if a patient develops such urges while taking rasagiline.

U.S. Patent Nos. 5387612, 5453446, 5457133, 5532415, 5786390, 6126968

Marketed by: TEVA Neuroscience, Inc., Kansas City, MO 64131

Distributed by: TEVA Pharmaceuticals USA, Inc., North Wales, PA 19454

Product of Israel

Shown in Product Identification Guide, page 320

COPAXONE®
[co-PAX-own]
(glatiramer acetate injection)
solution for subcutaneous injection   ℞

HIGHLIGHTS OF PRESCRIBING INFORMATION
These highlights do not include all the information needed to use COPAXONE safely and effectively. See full prescribing information for COPAXONE.

COPAXONE (glatiramer acetate injection) solution for subcutaneous injection
Initial U.S. Approval: 1996

——————RECENT MAJOR CHANGES——————
Indications and Usage (1) 2/2009

——————INDICATIONS AND USAGE——————
COPAXONE is indicated for reduction of the frequency of relapses in patients with Relapsing-Remitting Multiple Sclerosis, including patients who have experienced a first clinical episode and have MRI features consistent with multiple sclerosis.

——————DOSAGE AND ADMINISTRATION——————
- For subcutaneous injection only (2.1)
- Recommended dose: 20 mg/day (2.1)
- Before use, allow the solution to warm to room temperature (2.2)

——————DOSAGE FORMS AND STRENGTHS——————
- Prefilled syringe containing 1 mL solution with 20 mg of glatiramer acetate (3)

——————CONTRAINDICATIONS——————
Known hypersensitivity to glatiramer acetate or mannitol (4)

——————WARNINGS AND PRECAUTIONS——————
- Immediate Post-Injection Reaction (flushing, chest pain, palpitations, anxiety, dyspnea, throat constriction, and/or urticaria), generally transient and self-limiting (5.1)
- Chest pain, usually transient (5.2)
- Lipoatrophy and skin necrosis may occur. Instruct patient in proper injection technique and to rotate injection sites daily (5.3)
- COPAXONE can modify immune response (5.4)

——————ADVERSE REACTIONS——————
- In controlled studies, most common adverse reactions (≥10% and ≥1.5 times higher than placebo) were: injection site reactions, vasodilatation, rash, dyspnea, and chest pain (6.1)

To report SUSPECTED ADVERSE REACTIONS, contact TEVA at 1-800-221-4026 or FDA at 1-800-FDA-1088 or www.fda.gov/medwatch

——————USE IN SPECIFIC POPULATIONS——————
- Nursing Mothers: It is not known if COPAXONE is excreted in human milk (8.3)
- Pediatric Use: The safety and effectiveness of COPAXONE have not been established in patients under 18 years of age (8.4)

See 17 for PATIENT COUNSELING INFORMATION and FDA-approved patient labeling

Revised: 03/2009

FULL PRESCRIBING INFORMATION: CONTENTS*

*Sections or subsections omitted from the full prescribing information are not listed

FULL PRESCRIBING INFORMATION
COPAXONE (glatiramer acetate injection)

1   INDICATIONS AND USAGE
COPAXONE is indicated for reduction of relapses in patients with Relapsing-Remitting Multiple Sclerosis (RRMS), including patients who have experienced a first clinical episode and have MRI features consistent with multiple sclerosis.

2   DOSAGE AND ADMINISTRATION
2.1   Recommended Dose
COPAXONE is for subcutaneous use only. Do not administer intravenously. The recommended dose of COPAXONE is 20 mg/day.

2.2   Instructions for Use
Remove one blister that contains the syringe from the COPAXONE prefilled syringes package. Since this product should be refrigerated, let the prefilled syringe stand at room temperature for 20 minutes to allow the solution to warm to room temperature. Inspect the COPAXONE syringe visually for particulate matter and discoloration prior to administration, whenever solution and container permit. The solution in the syringe should appear clear, colorless to slightly yellow. If particulate matter or discoloration is observed, discard the COPAXONE syringe.

Areas for self-injection include arms, abdomen, hips, and thighs. The prefilled syringe is for single use only. Discard unused portions.

3   DOSAGE FORMS AND STRENGTHS
Single-use prefilled syringe containing 1 mL solution with 20 mg of glatiramer acetate and 40 mg of mannitol.

4   CONTRAINDICATIONS
COPAXONE is contraindicated in patients with known hypersensitivity to glatiramer acetate or mannitol.

5   WARNINGS AND PRECAUTIONS
5.1   Immediate Post-Injection Reaction
Approximately 16% of patients exposed to COPAXONE in the 5 placebo-controlled trials compared to 4% of those on placebo experienced a constellation of symptoms immediately after injection that included at least two of the following: flushing, chest pain, palpitations, anxiety, dyspnea, constriction of the throat, and urticaria. The symptoms were generally transient and self-limited and did not require treatment. In general, these symptoms have their onset several months after the initiation of treatment, although they may occur earlier, and a given patient may experience one or several episodes of these symptoms. Whether or not any of these symptoms actually represent a specific syndrome is uncertain. During the postmarketing period, there have been reports of patients with similar symptoms who received emergency medical care.

Whether an immunologic or nonimmunologic mechanism mediates these episodes, or whether several similar episodes seen in a given patient have identical mechanisms, is unknown.

5.2   Chest Pain
Approximately 13% of COPAXONE patients in the 5 placebo-controlled studies compared to 6% of placebo patients experienced at least one episode of what was described as transient chest pain. While some of these episodes occurred in the context of the Immediate Post-Injection Reaction described above, many did not. The temporal relationship of this chest pain to an injection of COPAXONE was not always known. The pain was transient (usually lasting only a few minutes), often unassociated with other symptoms, and appeared to have no clinical sequelae. Some patients experienced more than one such episode, and episodes usually began at least 1 month after the initiation of treatment. The pathogenesis of this symptom is unknown.

5.3   Lipoatrophy and Skin Necrosis
At injection sites, localized lipoatrophy and, rarely, injection site skin necrosis have been reported during the postmarketing experience. Lipoatrophy may occur at various times after treatment onset (sometimes after several months) and is thought to be permanent. There is no known therapy for lipoatrophy. To assist in possibly minimizing these events, the patient should be advised to follow proper injection technique and to rotate injection sites daily.

5.4   Potential Effects on Immune Response
Because COPAXONE can modify immune response, it may interfere with immune functions. For example, treatment with COPAXONE may interfere with the recognition of foreign antigens in a way that would undermine the body's tumor surveillance and its defenses against infection. There is no evidence that COPAXONE does this, but there has not been a systematic evaluation of this risk. Because

Table 1: Adverse reactions in controlled clinical trials with an incidence ≥2% of patients and more frequent with COPAXONE than with placebo

		GA 20 mg (N=563)	Placebo (N=564)
Blood And Lymphatic System Disorders	Lymphadenopathy	7%	3%
Cardiac Disorders	Palpitations	9%	4%
	Tachycardia	5%	2%
Eye Disorders	Eye Disorder	3%	1%
	Diplopia	3%	2%
Gastrointestinal Disorders	Nausea	15%	11%
	Vomiting	7%	4%
	Dysphagia	2%	1%
General Disorders And Administration Site Conditions	Injection Site Erythema	43%	10%
	Injection Site Pain	40%	20%
	Injection Site Pruritus	27%	4%
	Injection Site Mass	26%	6%
	Asthenia	22%	21%
	Pain	20%	17%
	Injection Site Edema	19%	4%
	Chest Pain	13%	6%
	Injection Site Inflammation	9%	1%
	Edema	8%	2%
	Injection Site Reaction	8%	1%
	Pyrexia	6%	5%
	Injection Site Hypersensitivity	4%	0%
	Local Reaction	3%	1%
	Chills	3%	1%
	Face Edema	3%	1%
	Edema Peripheral	3%	2%
	Injection Site Fibrosis	2%	1%
	Injection Site Atrophy*	2%	0%
Immune System Disorders	Hypersensitivity	3%	2%
Infections And Infestations	Infection	30%	28%
	Influenza	14%	13%
	Rhinitis	7%	5%
	Bronchitis	6%	5%
	Gastroenteritis	6%	4%
	Vaginal Candidiasis	4%	2%
Metabolism And Nutrition Disorders	Weight Increased	3%	1%
Musculoskeletal And Connective Tissue Disorders	Back Pain	12%	10%
Neoplasms Benign, Malignant And Unspecified (Incl Cysts And Polyps)	Benign Neoplasm of Skin	2%	1%

(Table continued on next page)

COPAXONE is an antigenic material, it is possible that its use may lead to the induction of host responses that are untoward, but systematic surveillance for these effects has not been undertaken.

Although COPAXONE is intended to minimize the autoimmune response to myelin, there is the possibility that continued alteration of cellular immunity due to chronic treatment with COPAXONE may result in untoward effects. Glatiramer acetate-reactive antibodies are formed in most patients exposed to daily treatment with the recommended dose. Studies in both the rat and monkey have suggested that immune complexes are deposited in the renal glomeruli. Furthermore, in a controlled trial of 125 RRMS patients given COPAXONE, 20 mg, subcutaneously every day for 2 years, serum IgG levels reached at least 3 times baseline values in 80% of patients by 3 months of initiation of treatment. By 12 months of treatment, however, 30% of patients still had IgG levels at least 3 times baseline values, and 90% had levels above baseline by 12 months. The antibodies are exclusively of the IgG subtype and predominantly of the IgG-1 subtype. No IgE type antibodies could be detected in any of the 94 sera tested; nevertheless, anaphylaxis can be associated with the administration of most any foreign substance, and therefore, this risk cannot be excluded.

6 ADVERSE REACTIONS
6.1 Clinical Trials Experience
Because clinical trials are conducted under widely varying conditions, adverse reaction rates observed in the clinical trials of a drug cannot be directly compared to rates in the clinical trials of another drug and may not reflect the rates observed in clinical practice.

Incidence in Controlled Clinical Trials
Among 563 patients treated with COPAXONE in blinded placebo controlled trials, approximately 5% of the subjects discontinued treatment because of an adverse reaction. The adverse reactions most commonly associated with discontinuation were: injection site reactions, dyspnea, urticaria, vasodilatation, and hypersensitivity. The most common adverse reactions were: injection site reactions, vasodilatation, rash, dyspnea, and chest pain.

Table 1 lists treatment-emergent signs and symptoms that occurred in at least 2% of patients treated with COPAXONE in the placebo-controlled trials. These signs and symptoms were numerically more common in patients treated with COPAXONE than in patients treated with placebo. Adverse reactions were usually mild in intensity.

[See table 1 at left and on next page]

Adverse reactions which occurred only in 4-5 more subjects in the COPAXONE group than in the placebo group (less than 1% difference), but for which a relationship to COPAXONE could not be excluded, were arthralgia and herpes simplex.

Laboratory analyses were performed on all patients participating in the clinical program for COPAXONE. Clinically significant laboratory values for hematology, chemistry, and urinalysis were similar for both COPAXONE and placebo groups in blinded clinical trials. In controlled trials one patient discontinued treatment due to thrombocytopenia (16×10^9/L), which resolved after discontinuation of treatment.

Data on adverse reactions occurring in the controlled clinical trials were analyzed to evaluate differences based on sex. No clinically significant differences were identified. Ninety-six percent of patients in these clinical trials were Caucasian. The majority of patients treated with COPAXONE were between the ages of 18 and 45. Consequently, data are inadequate to perform an analysis of the adverse reaction incidence related to clinically relevant age subgroups.

Other Adverse Reactions
In the paragraphs that follow, the frequencies of less commonly reported adverse clinical reactions are presented. Because the reports include reactions observed in open and uncontrolled premarketing studies (n= 979), the role of COPAXONE in their causation cannot be reliably determined. Furthermore, variability associated with adverse reaction reporting, the terminology used to describe adverse reactions, etc., limit the value of the quantitative frequency estimates provided. Reaction frequencies are calculated as the number of patients who used COPAXONE and reported a reaction divided by the total number of patients exposed to COPAXONE. All reported reactions are included except those already listed in the previous table, those too general to be informative, and those not reasonably associated with the use of the drug. Reactions are further classified within body system categories and enumerated in order of decreasing frequency using the following definitions: *Frequent* adverse reactions are defined as those occurring in at least 1/100 patients and *infrequent* adverse reactions are those occurring in 1/100 to 1/1,000 patients.

Body as a Whole:
Frequent: Abscess
Infrequent: Injection site hematoma, injection site fibrosis, moon face, cellulitis, generalized edema, hernia, injection site abscess, serum sickness, suicide attempt, injection site hypertrophy, injection site melanosis, lipoma, and photosensitivity reaction.

Cardiovascular:
Frequent: Hypertension.
Infrequent: Hypotension, midsystolic click, systolic murmur, atrial fibrillation, bradycardia, fourth heart sound, postural hypotension, and varicose veins.

Digestive:
Infrequent: Dry mouth, stomatitis, burning sensation on tongue, cholecystitis, colitis, esophageal ulcer, esophagitis, gastrointestinal carcinoma, gum hemorrhage, hepatomegaly, increased appetite, melena, mouth ulceration, pancreas disorder, pancreatitis, rectal hemorrhage, tenesmus, tongue discoloration, and duodenal ulcer.

Endocrine:
Infrequent: Goiter, hyperthyroidism, and hypothyroidism.

Gastrointestinal:
Frequent: Bowel urgency, oral moniliasis, salivary gland enlargement, tooth caries, and ulcerative stomatitis.

Hemic and Lymphatic:
Infrequent: Leukopenia, anemia, cyanosis, eosinophilia, hematemesis, lymphedema, pancytopenia, and splenomegaly.

Metabolic and Nutritional:
Infrequent: Weight loss, alcohol intolerance, Cushing's syndrome, gout, abnormal healing, and xanthoma.

Musculoskeletal:
Infrequent: Arthritis, muscle atrophy, bone pain, bursitis, kidney pain, muscle disorder, myopathy, osteomyelitis, tendon pain, and tenosynovitis.

Nervous:
Frequent: Abnormal dreams, emotional lability, and stupor.
Infrequent: Aphasia, ataxia, convulsion, circumoral paresthesia, depersonalization, hallucinations, hostility, hypokinesia, coma, concentration disorder, facial paralysis, decreased libido, manic reaction, memory impairment, myoclonus, neuralgia, paranoid reaction, paraplegia, psychotic depression, and transient stupor.

Respiratory:
Frequent: Hyperventilation and hay fever.
Infrequent: Asthma, pneumonia, epistaxis, hypoventilation, and voice alteration.

Skin and Appendages:
Frequent: Eczema, herpes zoster, pustular rash, skin atrophy, and warts.
Infrequent: Dry skin, skin hypertrophy, dermatitis, furunculosis, psoriasis, angioedema, contact dermatitis, erythema nodosum, fungal dermatitis, maculopapular rash, pigmentation, benign skin neoplasm, skin carcinoma, skin striae, and vesiculobullous rash.

Special Senses:
Frequent: Visual field defect.
Infrequent: Dry eyes, otitis externa, ptosis, cataract, corneal ulcer, mydriasis, optic neuritis, photophobia, and taste loss.

Urogenital:
Frequent: Amenorrhea, hematuria, impotence, menorrhagia, suspicious papanicolaou smear, urinary frequency, and vaginal hemorrhage.
Infrequent: Vaginitis, flank pain (kidney), abortion, breast engorgement, breast enlargement, carcinoma *in situ* cervix, fibrocystic breast, kidney calculus, nocturia, ovarian cyst, priapism, pyelonephritis, abnormal sexual function, and urethritis.

6.2 Postmarketing Experience
Reports of adverse events occurring under treatment with COPAXONE not mentioned above that have been received since market introduction and may or may not have causal relationship to COPAXONE are listed below. Because these events are reported voluntarily from a population of uncertain size, it is not always possible to reliably estimate their frequency or establish a causal relationship to drug exposure.

Body as a Whole: sepsis; SLE syndrome; hydrocephalus; enlarged abdomen; injection site hypersensitivity; allergic reaction; anaphylactoid reaction

Cardiovascular System: thrombosis; peripheral vascular disease; pericardial effusion; myocardial infarct; deep thrombophlebitis; coronary occlusion; congestive heart failure; cardiomyopathy; cardiomegaly; arrhythmia; angina pectoris

Digestive System: tongue edema; stomach ulcer; hemorrhage; liver function abnormality; liver damage; hepatitis; eructation; cirrhosis of the liver; cholelithiasis

Hemic and Lymphatic System: thrombocytopenia; lymphoma-like reaction; acute leukemia

Metabolic and Nutritional Disorders: hypercholesterolemia

Musculoskeletal System: rheumatoid arthritis; generalized spasm

Nervous System: myelitis; meningitis; CNS neoplasm; cerebrovascular accident; brain edema; abnormal dreams; aphasia; convulsion; neuralgia

Respiratory System: pulmonary embolus; pleural effusion; carcinoma of lung; hay fever

Special Senses: glaucoma; blindness; visual field defect

Urogenital System: urogenital neoplasm; urine abnormality; ovarian carcinoma; nephrosis; kidney failure; breast carcinoma; bladder carcinoma; urinary frequency

7 DRUG INTERACTIONS
Interactions between COPAXONE and other drugs have not been fully evaluated. Results from existing clinical trials do not suggest any significant interactions of COPAXONE with therapies commonly used in MS patients, including the concurrent use of corticosteroids for up to 28 days. COPAXONE has not been formally evaluated in combination with interferon beta.

Table 1 *(cont.)*: Adverse reactions in controlled clinical trials with an incidence ≥2% of patients and more frequent with COPAXONE than with placebo

		GA 20 mg (N=563)	Placebo (N=564)
Nervous System Disorders	Tremor	4%	2%
	Migraine	4%	2%
	Syncope	3%	2%
	Speech Disorder	2%	1%
Psychiatric Disorders	Anxiety	13%	10%
	Nervousness	2%	1%
Renal And Urinary Disorders	Micturition Urgency	5%	4%
Respiratory, Thoracic And Mediastinal Disorders	Dyspnea	14%	4%
	Cough	6%	5%
	Laryngospasm	2%	1%
Skin And Subcutaneous Tissue Disorders	Rash	19%	11%
	Hyperhidrosis	7%	5%
	Pruritus	5%	4%
	Urticaria	3%	1%
	Skin Disorder	3%	1%
Vascular Disorders	Vasodilatation	20%	5%

*Injection site atrophy comprises terms relating to localized lipoatrophy at injection site

8 USE IN SPECIFIC POPULATIONS
8.1 Pregnancy
Pregnancy Category B.
Administration of glatiramer acetate by subcutaneous injection to pregnant rats and rabbits resulted in no adverse effects on offspring development. There are no adequate and well-controlled studies in pregnant women. Because animal reproduction studies are not always predictive of human response, COPAXONE should be used during pregnancy only if clearly needed.
In rats or rabbits receiving glatiramer acetate by subcutaneous injection during the period of organogenesis, no adverse effects on embryo-fetal development were observed at doses up to 37.5 mg/kg/day (18 and 36 times, respectively, the therapeutic human dose of 20 mg/day on a mg/m² basis).
In rats receiving subcutaneous glatiramer acetate at doses of up to 36 mg/kg from day 15 of pregnancy throughout lactation, no significant effects on delivery or on offspring growth and development were observed.

8.2 Labor and Delivery
The effects of COPAXONE on labor and delivery in pregnant women are unknown.

8.3 Nursing Mothers
It is not known if glatiramer acetate is excreted in human milk. Because many drugs are excreted in human milk, caution should be exercised when COPAXONE is administered to a nursing woman.

8.4 Pediatric Use
The safety and effectiveness of COPAXONE have not been established in patients under 18 years of age.

8.5 Geriatric Use
COPAXONE has not been studied in elderly patients.

8.6 Use in Patients with Impaired Renal Function
The pharmacokinetics of glatiramer acetate in patients with impaired renal function have not been determined.

11 DESCRIPTION
COPAXONE is the brand name for glatiramer acetate (formerly known as copolymer-1). Glatiramer acetate, the active ingredient of COPAXONE, consists of the acetate salts of synthetic polypeptides, containing four naturally occurring amino acids: L-glutamic acid, L-alanine, L-tyrosine, and L-lysine with an average molar fraction of 0.141, 0.427, 0.095, and 0.338, respectively. The average molecular weight of glatiramer acetate is 5,000–9,000 daltons. Glatiramer acetate is identified by specific antibodies.
Chemically, glatiramer acetate is designated L-glutamic acid polymer with L-alanine, L-lysine and L-tyrosine, acetate (salt). Its structural formula is:

$$(Glu, Ala, Lys, Tyr)_x \cdot xCH_3COOH$$
$$(C_5H_9NO_4 \cdot C_3H_7NO_2 \cdot C_6H_{14}N_2O_2 \cdot C_9H_{11}NO_3)_x \cdot xC_2H_4O_2$$
CAS - 147245-92-9

COPAXONE is a clear, colorless to slightly yellow, sterile, nonpyrogenic solution for subcutaneous injection. Each 1 mL of solution contains 20 mg of glatiramer acetate and 40 mg of mannitol. The pH range of the solution is approximately 5.5 to 7.0. The biological activity of COPAXONE is determined by its ability to block the induction of experimental autoimmune encephalomyelitis (EAE) in mice.

12 CLINICAL PHARMACOLOGY
12.1 Mechanism of Action
The mechanism(s) by which glatiramer acetate exerts its effects in patients with MS are not fully understood. However, glatiramer acetate is thought to act by modifying immune processes that are believed to be responsible for the pathogenesis of MS. This hypothesis is supported by findings of studies that have been carried out to explore the pathogenesis of experimental autoimmune encephalomyelitis, a condition induced in animals through immunization against central nervous system derived material containing myelin and often used as an experimental animal model of MS. Studies in animals and *in vitro* systems suggest that upon its administration, glatiramer acetate-specific suppressor T-cells are induced and activated in the periphery.
Because glatiramer acetate can modify immune functions, concerns exist about its potential to alter naturally occurring immune responses. There is no evidence that glatiramer acetate does this, but this has not been systematically evaluated *[see Warnings and Precautions (5.4)].*

12.3 Pharmacokinetics
Results obtained in pharmacokinetic studies performed in humans (healthy volunteers) and animals support that a substantial fraction of the therapeutic dose delivered to patients subcutaneously is hydrolyzed locally. Larger fragments of glatiramer acetate can be recognized by glatiramer acetate-reactive antibodies. Some fraction of the injected material, either intact or partially hydrolyzed, is presumed to enter the lymphatic circulation, enabling it to reach regional lymph nodes, and some may enter the systemic circulation intact.

13 NONCLINICAL TOXICOLOGY
13.1 Carcinogenesis, Mutagenesis, Impairment of Fertility
In a 2-year carcinogenicity study, mice were administered up to 60 mg/kg/day glatiramer acetate by subcutaneous injection (up to 15 times the human therapeutic dose of 20 mg/day on a mg/m² basis). No increase in systemic neoplasms was observed. In males receiving the 60-mg/kg/day dose, there was an increased incidence of fibrosarcomas at the injection sites. These sarcomas were associated with skin damage precipitated by repetitive injections of an irritant over a limited skin area.
In a 2-year carcinogenicity study, rats were administered up to 30 mg/kg/day glatiramer acetate by subcutaneous injection (up to 15 times the human therapeutic dose on a mg/m² basis). No increase in neoplasms was observed.
Glatiramer acetate was not mutagenic in *in vitro* (Ames

Table 2: Study 1 Efficacy Results

	COPAXONE (N=25)	Placebo (N=25)	P-Value
% Relapse-Free Patients	14/25 (56%)	7/25 (28%)	0.085
Mean Relapse Frequency	0.6/2 years	2.4/2 years	0.005
Reduction in Relapse Rate Compared to Prestudy	3.2	1.6	0.025
Median Time to First Relapse (days)	>700	150	0.03
% of Progression-Free* Patients	20/25 (80%)	13/25 (52%)	0.07

*Progression was defined as an increase of at least 1 point on the DSS, persisting for at least 3 consecutive months.

Table 3: Study 2 Efficacy Results

	COPAXONE (N=125)	Placebo (N=126)	P-Value
Mean No. of Relapses	1.19/2 years	1.68/2 years	0.055
% Relapse-Free Patients	42/125 (34%)	34/126 (27%)	0.25
Median Time to First Relapse (days)	287	198	0.23
% of Progression-Free Patients	98/125 (78%)	95/126 (75%)	0.48
Mean Change in DSS	-0.05	+0.21	0.023

test, mouse lymphoma tk) assays. Glatiramer acetate was clastogenic in two separate *in vitro* chromosomal aberration assays in cultured human lymphocytes but not clastogenic in an *in vivo* mouse bone marrow micronucleus assay.

When glatiramer acetate was administered by subcutaneous injection prior to and during mating (males and females) and throughout gestation and lactation (females) at doses up to 36 mg/kg/day (18 times the human therapeutic dose on a mg/m² basis) no adverse effects were observed on reproductive or developmental parameters.

14 CLINICAL STUDIES
14.1 Relapsing-Remitting Multiple Sclerosis (RRMS)
Evidence supporting the effectiveness of COPAXONE in decreasing the frequency of relapses derives from 3 placebo-controlled trials, all of which used a COPAXONE dose of 20 mg/day.

Study 1 was performed at a single center. Fifty patients were enrolled and randomized to receive daily doses of either COPAXONE, 20 mg subcutaneously, or placebo (COPAXONE: n=25; placebo: n=25). Patients were diagnosed with RRMS by standard criteria, and had had at least 2 exacerbations during the 2 years immediately preceding enrollment. Patients were ambulatory, as evidenced by a score of no more than 6 on the Kurtzke Disability Scale Score (DSS), a standard scale ranging from 0–Normal to 10–Death due to MS. A score of 6 is defined as one at which a patient is still ambulatory with assistance; a score of 7 means the patient must use a wheelchair.

Patients were examined every 3 months for 2 years, as well as within several days of a presumed exacerbation. To confirm an exacerbation, a blinded neurologist had to document objective neurologic signs, as well as document the existence of other criteria (e.g., the persistence of the neurological signs for at least 48 hours).

The protocol-specified primary outcome measure was the proportion of patients in each treatment group who remained exacerbation free for the 2 years of the trial, but two other important outcomes were also specified as endpoints: the frequency of attacks during the trial, and the change in the number of attacks compared with the number which occurred during the previous 2 years.

Table 2 presents the values of the three outcomes described above, as well as several protocol specified secondary measures. These values are based on the intent-to-treat population (i.e., all patients who received at least 1 dose of treatment and who had at least 1 on-treatment assessment):
[See table 2 above]

Study 2 was a multicenter trial of similar design which was performed in 11 US centers. A total of 251 patients (COPAXONE: n=125; placebo: n=126) were enrolled. The primary outcome measure was the Mean 2-Year Relapse Rate. Table 3 presents the values of this outcome for the intent-to-treat population, as well as several secondary measures:
[See table 3 above]

In both studies, COPAXONE exhibited a clear beneficial effect on relapse rate, and it is based on this evidence that COPAXONE is considered effective.

In Study 3, 481 patients who had recently (within 90 days) experienced an isolated demyelinating event and who had lesions typical of multiple sclerosis on brain MRI were randomized to receive either COPAXONE 20 mg/day (n=243) or placebo (n=238). The primary outcome measure was time to development of a second exacerbation. Patients were followed for up to three years or until they reached the primary endpoint. Secondary outcomes were brain MRI measures, including number of new T2 lesions and T2 lesion volume.

Time to development of a second exacerbation was significantly delayed in patients treated with COPAXONE compared to placebo (Hazard Ratio = 0.55; 95% confidence interval 0.40 to 0.77; Figure 1). The Kaplan-Meier estimates of the percentage of patients developing a relapse within 36 months were 42.9% in the placebo group and 24.7% in the COPAXONE group.

Figure 1: Time to Second Exacerbation

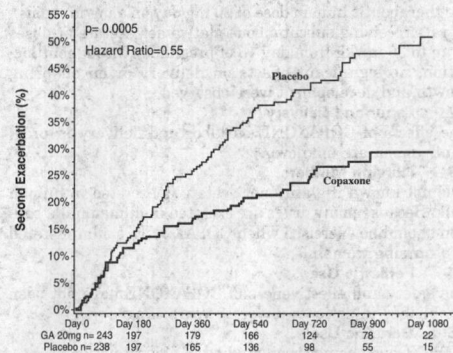

Patients treated with COPAXONE demonstrated fewer new T2 lesions at the last observation (rate ratio 0.41; confidence interval 0.28 to 0.59; p < 0.0001). Additionally, baseline-adjusted T2 lesion volume at the last observation was lower for patients treated with COPAXONE (ratio of 0.89; confidence interval 0.84 to 0.94; p = 0.0001).

Study 4 was a multinational study in which MRI parameters were used both as primary and secondary endpoints. A total of 239 patients with RRMS (COPAXONE: n=119; and placebo: n=120) were randomized. Inclusion criteria were similar to those in the second study with the additional criterion that patients had to have at least one Gd-enhancing lesion on the screening MRI. The patients were treated in a double-blind manner for nine months, during which they underwent monthly MRI scanning. The primary endpoint for the double-blind phase was the total cumulative number of T1 Gd-enhancing lesions over the nine months. Table 4 summarizes the results for the primary outcome measure monitored during the trial for the intent-to-treat cohort.

Table 4: Study 4 MRI Results

	COPAXONE (N=119)	Placebo (N=120)	P-Value
Medians of the Cumulative Number of T1 Gd-Enhancing Lesions	11	17	0.0030

Figure 2 displays the results of the primary outcome on a monthly basis.

Figure 2: Median Cumulative Number of Gd-Enhancing Lesions

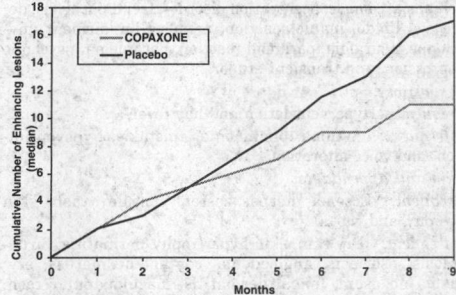

16 HOW SUPPLIED/STORAGE AND HANDLING
COPAXONE is supplied as a single-use prefilled syringe containing 1 mL of a clear, colorless to slightly yellow, sterile, nonpyrogenic solution containing 20 mg of glatiramer acetate and 40 mg of mannitol in cartons of 30 single-use prefilled syringes with 33 alcohol preps (NDC 68546-317-30).

The recommended storage condition for the COPAXONE is refrigeration (2°C to 8°C / 36°F to 46°F). However, excursions from recommended storage conditions (15°C to 30°C / 59°F to 86° F) for up to one month have been shown to have no adverse impact on the product. Exposure to higher temperatures or intense light should be avoided. COPAXONE should not be frozen. If a COPAXONE syringe freezes, it should be discarded.

COPAXONE contains no preservative. Do not use if the solution contains any particulate matter.

17 PATIENT COUNSELING INFORMATION
[See FDA-Approved Patient Labeling (17.7)]
17.1 Pregnancy
Instruct patients that if they are pregnant or plan to become pregnant while taking COPAXONE they should inform their physician.

17.2 Immediate Post-Injection Reaction
Advise patients that COPAXONE may cause various symptoms after injection, include flushing, chest pain, palpitations, anxiety, dyspnea, constriction of the throat, and urticaria. These symptoms are generally transient and self-limited and do not require specific treatment. Inform patients that these symptoms may occur early or may have their onset several months after the initiation of treatment. A patient may experience one or several episodes of these symptoms.

17.3 Chest Pain
Advise patients that they may experience transient chest pain either as part of the Immediate Post-Injection Reaction or in isolation. Inform patients that the pain should be transient (usually only lasting a few minutes). Some patients may experience more than one such episode, usually beginning at least one month after the initiation of treatment. Patient should be advised to seek medical attention if they experience chest pain of unusual duration or intensity.

17.4 Lipoatrophy and Skin Necrosis at Injection Site
Advise patients that localized lipoatrophy, and rarely, injection site necrosis may occur at injections sites. Instruct patients to follow proper injection technique and to rotate injection areas and sites on a daily basis.

17.5 Instructions for Use
Instruct patients to read the COPAXONE Patient Information leaflet carefully. Caution patients to use aseptic technique. The first injection should be performed under the supervision of a health care professional. Instruct patients to rotate injection areas and sites on a daily basis. Caution patients against the reuse of needles or syringes. Instruct patients in safe disposal procedures.

17.6 Storage Conditions
Advise patients that the recommended storage condition for COPAXONE is refrigeration (36-46° F /2-8°C), although COPAXONE can be stored at room temperature (59-86°F /15-30°C) for up to one month. COPAXONE should not be exposed to higher temperatures or intense light.

17.7 FDA-Approved Patient Labeling

Read this information carefully before you use COPAXONE. Read the information you get when you refill your COPAXONE prescriptions because there may be new information. This information does not take the place of your doctor's advice. Ask your doctor or pharmacist if you do not understand some of this information or if you want to know more about this medicine.

What is COPAXONE?

COPAXONE (co-PAX-own) is a medicine you inject to treat Relapsing-Remitting Multiple Sclerosis. Although COPAXONE is not a cure; patients treated with COPAXONE have fewer relapses.

Who should not use COPAXONE?

• Do not use COPAXONE if you are allergic to glatiramer acetate or mannitol.

What are the possible side effects of COPAXONE?

• **Call your doctor right away if you develop any of the following symptoms: hives, skin rash with irritation, dizziness, sweating, chest pain, trouble breathing, or severe pain at the injection site.** Do not give yourself any more injections until your doctor tells you to begin again.

• The most common side effects of COPAXONE are redness, pain, swelling, itching, or a lump at the injection site. These reactions are usually mild and seldom require medical care.

• Some patients report a short-term reaction right after injecting COPAXONE. This reaction can involve flushing (feeling of warmth and/or redness), chest tightness or pain with heart palpitations, anxiety, and trouble breathing. These symptoms generally appear within minutes after an injection, last a few minutes, and then go away by themselves without further problems.

• A permanent depression under the skin at the injection site may occur, due to a local destruction of fat tissue.

• **If symptoms become severe, call the emergency phone number in your area.** Do not give yourself any more injections until your doctor tells you to begin again.

These are not all the possible side effects of COPAXONE. For a complete list, ask your doctor or pharmacist. Tell your doctor about any side effects you have while taking COPAXONE.

Information for pregnant and nursing women

• COPAXONE has not been studied in pregnant women. Talk to your doctor about the risks and benefits of COPAXONE if you are pregnant or planning a pregnancy.

• It is not known if COPAXONE passes into breastmilk. Talk to your baby's doctor about the risks and benefits of breastfeeding while using COPAXONE.

How should I use COPAXONE?

• The recommended dose of COPAXONE for the treatment of Relapsing-Remitting Multiple Sclerosis is 20 mg once a day injected subcutaneously (in the fatty layer under the skin).

• Look at the medicine in the prefilled syringe. If the medicine is cloudy or has particles in it, do not use it. Instead, call Shared Solutions® at 1-800-887-8100 for assistance.

• Have a friend or relative with you if you need help, especially when you first start giving yourself injections.

• Each prefilled syringe should be used for only one injection. Do not reuse the prefilled syringe. After use, throw it away properly.

• Do not change the dose or dosing schedule or stop taking the medicine without talking with your doctor.

How do I inject COPAXONE?

There are 3 basic steps for injecting COPAXONE prefilled syringes:
1. Gather the materials.
2. Choose the injection site.
3. Give yourself the injection.

Step 1: Gather the materials

1. First, place each of the items you will need on a clean, flat surface in a well-lit area:
   • 1 blister pack with COPAXONE Prefilled Syringe Remove only 1 blister pack from the COPAXONE Prefilled Syringe carton. Keep all unused syringes in the Prefilled Syringe carton and store them in the refrigerator.
   • Alcohol prep (wipe)
   • Dry cotton ball (not supplied)
2. Let the blister pack with the syringe inside warm up to room temperature for 20 minutes.
3. To prevent infection, wash and dry your hands. Do not touch your hair or skin after washing.
4. There may be small air bubbles in the syringe. To avoid loss of medicine when using COPAXONE prefilled syringes, do not expel (or do not attempt to expel) the air bubble from the syringe before injecting the medicine.

Step 2: Choose the injection site

• There are 7 possible injection areas on your body: arms, thighs, hips and lower stomach area (abdomen) (See Figure 1).

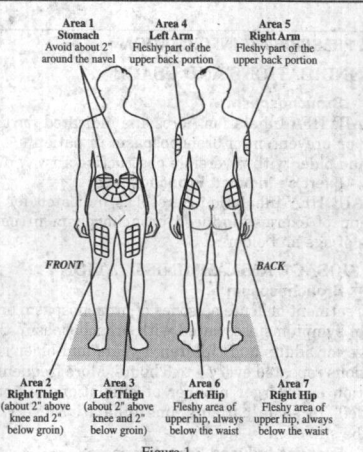

Area 1
Stomach
Avoid about 2"
around the navel

Area 4
Left Arm
Fleshy part of the
upper back portion

Area 5
Right Arm
Fleshy part of the
upper back portion

FRONT   BACK

Area 2
Right Thigh
(about 2" above
knee and 2"
below groin)

Area 3
Left Thigh
(about 2" above
knee and 2"
below groin)

Area 6
Left Hip
Fleshy area of
upper hip, always
below the waist

Area 7
Right Hip
Fleshy area of
upper hip, always
below the waist

Figure 1

• Each day, pick a different injection area from one of the 7 areas. **Do not inject in the same area more than once a week.**

• Within each injection area there are multiple injection sites. Have a plan for rotating your injection sites. Keep a record of your injection sites, so you know where you have injected.

• There are some sites in your body that may be hard to reach for self-injection (like the back of your arm), and you may need help.

• Do not inject in sites where skin depression has occurred, because further injections in these sites may make the depression deeper.

Step 3: Give yourself the injection

1. Remove the syringe from its protective blister pack by peeling back the paper label. Before use, look at the liquid in the syringe. If it is cloudy or contains any particles, do not use it and call Shared Solutions® at 1-800-887-8100 for assistance. If the liquid is clear, place the syringe on the clean, flat surface.
2. Choose an injection site on your body. Clean the injection site with a new alcohol prep and let the site air dry to reduce stinging.
3. Pick up the syringe as you would a pencil. Remove the needle shield from the needle.
4. With your other hand, pinch about a 2-inch fold of skin between your thumb and index finger (See Figure 2).
5. Insert the needle at a 90-degree angle (straight in), resting the heel of your hand against your body. When the needle is all the way in release the fold of skin (See Figure 3).

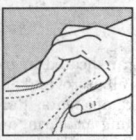

Figure 2

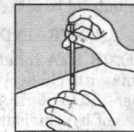

Figure 3

6. To inject the medicine, hold the syringe steady and push down the plunger.
7. When you have injected all of the medicine, pull the needle straight out.
8. Press a dry cotton ball on the injection site for a few seconds. **Do not rub the injection site.**
9. Throw away the syringe in a safe hard-walled plastic container.

What is the proper use and disposal of prefilled syringes?

Each prefilled syringe should be used for only 1 injection. Throw away all used prefilled syringes in a hard-walled plastic container, such as an empty liquid laundry detergent bottle. Keep the container closed tightly and out of the reach of children. When the container is full, check with your doctor, pharmacist, or nurse about proper disposal, as laws vary from state to state.

How should I store COPAXONE prefilled syringes?

Keep the COPAXONE prefilled syringe carton in the refrigerator, out of the reach of children.
The COPAXONE package should be refrigerated at 36-46°F (2-8°C). You can store it at room temperature, 59-86°F (15-30°C), for up to one month. Do not store COPAXONE at room temperature for longer than one month. **Do not freeze COPAXONE.** If a COPAXONE prefilled syringe freezes, throw it away in a proper container.
COPAXONE is light sensitive. Protect it from light when not injecting. Do not use the prefilled syringe if the solution contains particles or is cloudy.

General advice about prescription medicines

Medicines are sometimes prescribed for conditions that are not mentioned in patient information leaflets. Do not use COPAXONE for a condition for which it was not prescribed. Do not give COPAXONE to other people, even if they have the same condition you have. It may harm them.
This leaflet summarizes the most important information about COPAXONE. If you would like more information, talk with your doctor. You can ask your pharmacist or doctor for information about COPAXONE that is written for health professionals. Also, you can call Shared Solutions® for any questions about COPAXONE and its use. The phone number for Shared Solutions® is 1-800-887-8100.
U.S. Patent Nos. 5981589, 6054430, 6342476, 6362161, 6620847, 6939539, 7199098.
Marketed by: TEVA Neuroscience, Inc., Kansas City, MO 64131
Distributed by: TEVA Pharmaceuticals USA, Inc., North Wales, PA 19454
Product of Israel
Revised: 03/2009   TEVA Neuroscience, Inc.
Shown in Product Identification Guide, page 320

Teva Respiratory, LLC.
425 PRIVET ROAD
HORSHAM, PA 19044

For All Inquiries Call:
1-888-482-9522

PROAIR® HFA   ℞
(albuterol sulfate)
Inhalation aerosol

HIGHLIGHTS OF PRESCRIBING INFORMATION
These highlights do not include all the information needed to use PROAIR HFA safely and effectively. See full prescribing information for PROAIR HFA.
PROAIR HFA (albuterol sulfate) aerosol, metered for respiratory (inhalation) use
Initial U.S. Approval: 1981

————————**RECENT MAJOR CHANGES**————————
Indications and Usage 9/2008
Dosage and Administration 9/2008
————————**INDICATIONS AND USAGE**————————
PROAIR HFA inhalation aerosol is a beta$_2$-adrenergic agonist indicated for:
• Treatment or prevention of bronchospasm in patients 4 years of age and older with reversible obstructive airway disease (1.1)
• Prevention of exercise-induced bronchospasm in patients 4 years of age and older. (1.2)
————————**DOSAGE AND ADMINISTRATION**————————
For oral inhalation only
• Treatment or prevention of bronchospasm in adults and children 4 years of age and older: 2 inhalations every 4 to 6 hours. In some patients, one inhalation every 4 hours may be sufficient. (2.1)
• Prevention of exercise-induced bronchospasm in adults and children 4 years of age and older: 2 inhalations 15 to 30 minutes before exercise. (2.2)
• Priming information: Prime PROAIR HFA before using for the first time, or when the inhaler has not been used for more than 2 weeks. To prime PROAIR HFA, release 3 sprays into the air away from the face. Shake well before each spray. (2.3)
• Cleaning information: At least once a week, wash the actuator with warm water, shake off excess, and air dry thoroughly. (2.3)
————————**DOSAGE FORMS AND STRENGTHS**————————
Inhalation Aerosol: Each actuation delivers 108 mcg of albuterol sulfate from the actuator mouthpiece (equivalent to 90 mcg of albuterol base). Supplied in 8.5-g canister containing 200 actuations. (3)
————————**CONTRAINDICATIONS**————————
Hypersensitivity to albuterol and any other PROAIR HFA Inhalation Aerosol Components. (4)
————————**WARNINGS AND PRECAUTIONS**————————
• Life-threatening paradoxical bronchospasm may occur. Discontinue PROAIR HFA immediately and treat with alternative therapy. (5.1)
• Need for more doses of PROAIR HFA than usual may be a sign of deterioration of asthma and requires reevaluation of treatment. (5.2)
• PROAIR HFA is not a substitute for corticosteroids. (5.3)
• Cardiovascular effects may occur. Use with caution in patients sensitive to sympathomimetic drugs and patients with cardiovascular or convulsive disorders. (5.4, 5.7)
• Excessive use may be fatal. Do not exceed recommended dose. (5.5)

- Immediate hypersensitivity reactions may occur. Discontinue PROAIR HFA immediately. (5.6)
- Hypokalemia and changes in blood glucose may occur. (5.7, 5.8)

---ADVERSE REACTIONS---

Most common adverse reactions (≥3.0% and >placebo) are headache, tachycardia, pain, dizziness, pharyngitis, and rhinitis. (6.1)

To report SUSPECTED ADVERSE REACTIONS, contact Teva Specialty Pharmaceuticals LLC at 1-888-482-9522 or FDA at 1-800-FDA-1088 or www.fda.gov/medwatch

---DRUG INTERACTIONS---

- Other short-acting sympathomimetic aerosol bronchodilators and adrenergic drugs: May potentiate effect. (7)
- Beta-blockers: May decrease effectiveness of PROAIR HFA and produce severe bronchospasm. Patients with asthma should not normally be treated with beta-blockers. (7.1)
- Diuretics, or non-potassium sparing diuretics: May potentiate hypokalemia or ECG changes. Consider monitoring potassium levels. (7.2)
- Digoxin: May decrease serum digoxin levels. Consider monitoring digoxin levels. (7.3)
- Monoamine oxidase (MAO) inhibitors and tricyclic antidepressants: May potentiate effect of albuterol on the cardiovascular system. Consider alternative therapy in patients taking MAOs or tricyclic antidepressants. (7.4)

See 17 for PATIENT COUNSELING INFORMATION and FDA-approved patient labeling

FULL PRESCRIBING INFORMATION: CONTENTS*

* Sections or subsections omitted from the full prescribing information are not listed.

FULL PRESCRIBING INFORMATION

1 INDICATIONS AND USAGE

1.1 Bronchospasm

PROAIR HFA Inhalation Aerosol is indicated for the treatment or prevention of bronchospasm in patients 4 years of age and older with reversible obstructive airway disease.

1.2 Exercise-Induced Bronchospasm

PROAIR HFA Inhalation Aerosol is indicated for the prevention of exercise-induced bronchospasm in patients 4 years of age and older.

2 DOSAGE AND ADMINISTRATION

2.1 Bronchospasm

For treatment of acute episodes of bronchospasm or prevention of symptoms associated with bronchospasm, the usual dosage for adults and children 4 years and older is two inhalations repeated every 4 to 6 hours. More frequent administration or a larger number of inhalations is not recommended. In some patients, one inhalation every 4 hours may be sufficient.

2.2 Exercise-Induced Bronchospasm

The usual dosage for adults and children 4 years of age or older is two inhalations 15 to 30 minutes before exercise.

2.3 Administration Information

Administer PROAIR HFA by oral inhalation only. Shake well before each spray. To maintain proper use of this product and to prevent medication build-up and blockage, it is important to follow the cleaning directions carefully.

Priming: Prime the inhaler before using for the first time and in cases where the inhaler has not been used for more than 2 weeks by releasing three sprays into the air, away from the face.

Cleaning: As with all HFA-containing albuterol inhalers, to maintain proper use of this product and to prevent medication build-up and blockage, it is important to keep the plastic mouthpiece clean. The inhaler may cease to deliver medication if the plastic actuator mouthpiece is not properly cleaned and dried. To clean: Wash the plastic mouthpiece with warm running water for 30 seconds, shake off excess water, and air dry thoroughly at least once a week. If the mouthpiece becomes blocked, washing the mouthpiece will remove the blockage. If it is necessary to use the inhaler before it is completely dry, shake off excess water, replace canister, spray twice into the air away from face, and take the prescribed dose. After such use, the mouthpiece should be rewashed and allowed to air dry thoroughly [see Patient Counseling Information (17.8)].

3 DOSAGE FORMS & STRENGTHS

PROAIR HFA is an inhalation aerosol. PROAIR HFA is supplied as an 8.5 g/200 actuations pressurized aluminum canister with a red plastic actuator and white dust cap each in boxes of one. Each actuation delivers 120 mcg of albuterol sulfate from the canister valve and 108 mcg of albuterol sulfate from the actuator mouthpiece (equivalent to 90 mcg of albuterol base).

4 CONTRAINDICATIONS

PROAIR HFA Inhalation Aerosol is contraindicated in patients with a history of hypersensitivity to albuterol and any other PROAIR HFA Inhalation Aerosol components. Rare cases of hypersensitivity reactions, including urticaria, angioedema, and rash have been reported after the use of albuterol sulfate [see Warnings and Precautions (5.6)].

5 WARNINGS & PRECAUTIONS

5.1 Paradoxical Bronchospasm

PROAIR HFA Inhalation Aerosol can produce paradoxical bronchospasm that may be life threatening. If paradoxical bronchospasm occurs, PROAIR HFA Inhalation Aerosol should be discontinued immediately and alternative therapy instituted. It should be recognized that paradoxical bronchospasm, when associated with inhaled formulations, frequently occurs with the first use of a new canister.

5.2 Deterioration of Asthma

Asthma may deteriorate acutely over a period of hours or chronically over several days or longer. If the patient needs more doses of PROAIR HFA Inhalation Aerosol than usual, this may be a marker of destabilization of asthma and requires re-evaluation of the patient and treatment regimen, giving special consideration to the possible need for anti-inflammatory treatment, e.g., corticosteroids.

5.3 Use of Anti-inflammatory Agents

The use of beta-adrenergic-agonist bronchodilators alone may not be adequate to control asthma in many patients. Early consideration should be given to adding anti-inflammatory agents, e.g., corticosteroids, to the therapeutic regimen.

5.4 Cardiovascular Effects

PROAIR HFA Inhalation Aerosol, like other beta-adrenergic agonists, can produce clinically significant cardiovascular effects in some patients as measured by pulse rate, blood pressure, and/or symptoms. Although such effects are uncommon after administration of PROAIR HFA Inhalation Aerosol at recommended doses, if they occur, the drug may need to be discontinued. In addition, beta-agonists have been reported to produce ECG changes, such as flattening of the T wave, prolongation of the QTc interval, and ST segment depression. The clinical significance of these findings is unknown. Therefore, PROAIR HFA Inhalation Aerosol, like all sympathomimetic amines, should be used with caution in patients with cardiovascular disorders, especially coronary insufficiency, cardiac arrhythmias, and hypertension.

5.5 Do Not Exceed Recommended Dose

Fatalities have been reported in association with excessive use of inhaled sympathomimetic drugs in patients with asthma. The exact cause of death is unknown, but cardiac arrest following an unexpected development of a severe acute asthmatic crisis and subsequent hypoxia is suspected.

5.6 Immediate Hypersensitivity Reactions

Immediate hypersensitivity reactions may occur after administration of albuterol sulfate, as demonstrated by rare cases of urticaria, angioedema, rash, bronchospasm, anaphylaxis, and oropharyngeal edema. The potential for hypersensitivity must be considered in the clinical evaluation of patients who experience immediate hypersensitivity reactions while receiving PROAIR HFA Inhalation Aerosol.

5.7 Coexisting Conditions

PROAIR HFA Inhalation Aerosol, like all sympathomimetic amines, should be used with caution in patients with cardiovascular disorders, especially coronary insufficiency, cardiac arrhythmias, and hypertension; in patients with convulsive disorders, hyperthyroidism, or diabetes mellitus; and in patients who are unusually responsive to sympathomimetic amines. Clinically significant changes in systolic and diastolic blood pressure have been seen in individual patients and could be expected to occur in some patients after use of any beta-adrenergic bronchodilator. Large doses of intravenous albuterol have been reported to aggravate pre-existing diabetes mellitus and ketoacidosis.

5.8 Hypokalemia

As with other beta-agonists, PROAIR HFA Inhalation Aerosol may produce significant hypokalemia in some patients, possibly through intracellular shunting, which has the potential to produce adverse cardiovascular effects. The decrease is usually transient, not requiring supplementation.

6 ADVERSE REACTIONS

Use of PROAIR HFA may be associated with the following:
- Paradoxical bronchospasm [see Warnings and Precautions (5.1)]
- Cardiovascular Effects [see Warnings and Precautions (5.4)]
- Immediate hypersensitivity reactions [see Warnings and Precautions (5.6)]
- Hypokalemia [see Warnings and Precautions (5.8)]

6.1 Clinical Trials Experience

A total of 1090 subjects were treated with PROAIR HFA Inhalation Aerosol, or with the same formulation of albuterol as in PROAIR HFA Inhalation Aerosol, during the worldwide clinical development program.

Because clinical trials are conducted under widely varying conditions, adverse reaction rates observed in the clinical trials of a drug cannot be directly compared to rates in the clinical trials of another drug and may not reflect the rates observed in practice.

Adult and Adolescent Patients 12 Years of Age and Older: The adverse reaction information presented in the table below concerning PROAIR HFA Inhalation Aerosol is derived from a 6-week, blinded study which compared PROAIR HFA Inhalation Aerosol (180 mcg four times daily) with a double-blinded matched placebo HFA-Inhalation Aerosol and an evaluator-blinded marketed active comparator HFA-134a albuterol inhaler in 172 asthmatic patients 12 to 76 years of age.

The table lists the incidence of all adverse events (whether considered by the investigator drug related or unrelated to drug) from this study which occurred at a rate of 3% or greater in the PROAIR HFA Inhalation Aerosol treatment group and more frequently in the PROAIR HFA Inhalation Aerosol treatment group than in the matched placebo group. Overall, the incidence and nature of the adverse events reported for PROAIR HFA Inhalation Aerosol and the marketed active comparator HFA-134a albuterol inhaler were comparable.

[See table at top of next page]

Adverse events reported by less than 3% of the patients receiving PROAIR HFA Inhalation Aerosol but by a greater proportion of PROAIR HFA Inhalation Aerosol patients than the matched placebo patients, which have the potential to be related to PROAIR HFA Inhalation Aerosol, included chest pain, infection, diarrhea, glossitis, accidental injury (nervous system), anxiety, dyspnea, ear disorder, ear pain, and urinary tract infection.

In small cumulative dose studies, tremor, nervousness, and headache were the most frequently occurring adverse events.

Pediatric Patients 4 to 11 Years of Age: Adverse events reported in a 3-week pediatric clinical trial comparing the same formulation of albuterol as in PROAIR HFA Inhalation Aerosol (180 mcg albuterol four times daily) to a matching placebo HFA inhalation aerosol occurred at a low incidence rate (no greater than 2% in the active treatment group) and were similar to those seen in adult and adolescent trials.

6.2 Postmarketing Experience

The following adverse reactions have been identified during postapproval use of PROAIR HFA. Because these reactions are reported voluntarily from a population of uncertain size, it is not always possible to reliably estimate their frequency or establish a causal relationship to drug exposure. Reports have included rare cases of aggravated bronchospasm, lack of efficacy, asthma exacerbation (reported fatal in one case), muscle cramps, and various oropharyngeal side effects such as throat irritation, altered taste, glossitis, tongue ulceration, and gagging.

The following adverse events have been observed in postapproval use of inhaled albuterol: urticaria, angioedema, rash, bronchospasm, hoarseness, oropharyngeal edema, and arrhythmias (including atrial fibrillation, supraventricular tachycardia, extrasystoles). In addition, albuterol, like other sympathomimetic agents, can cause adverse reactions such as: angina, hypertension or hypotension, palpitations, central nervous system stimulation, insomnia, headache, nervousness, tremor, muscle cramps, drying or irritation of the oropharynx, hypokalemia, hyperglycemia, and metabolic acidosis.

Adverse Experience Incidences (% of Patients) in a Six Week Clinical Trial*

Body System/ Adverse Event (as Preferred Term)		PROAIR HFA Inhalation Aerosol (N=58)	Marketed active comparator HFA-134a albuterol inhaler (N=56)	Matched Placebo HFA-134a Inhalation Aerosol (N=58)
Body as a Whole	Headache	7	5	2
Cardiovascular	Tachycardia	3	2	0
Musculoskeletal	Pain	3	0	0
Nervous System	Dizziness	3	0	0
Respiratory System	Pharyngitis	14	7	9
	Rhinitis	5	4	2

* This table includes all adverse events (whether considered by the investigator drug related or unrelated to drug) which occurred at an incidence rate of at least 3.0% in the PROAIR HFA Inhalation Aerosol group and more frequently in the PROAIR HFA Inhalation Aerosol group than in the placebo HFA Inhalation Aerosol group.

7 DRUG INTERACTIONS

Other short-acting sympathomimetic aerosol bronchodilators should not be used concomitantly with PROAIR HFA Inhalation Aerosol. If additional adrenergic drugs are to be administered by any route, they should be used with caution to avoid deleterious cardiovascular effects.

7.1 Beta-Blockers

Beta-adrenergic-receptor blocking agents not only block the pulmonary effect of beta-agonists, such as PROAIR HFA Inhalation Aerosol, but may produce severe bronchospasm in asthmatic patients. Therefore, patients with asthma should not normally be treated with beta-blockers. However, under certain circumstances, e.g., as prophylaxis after myocardial infarction, there may be no acceptable alternatives to the use of beta-adrenergic-blocking agents in patients with asthma. In this setting, consider cardioselective beta-blockers, although they should be administered with caution.

7.2 Diuretics

The ECG changes and/or hypokalemia which may result from the administration of non-potassium sparing diuretics (such as loop or thiazide diuretics) can be acutely worsened by beta-agonists, especially when the recommended dose of the beta-agonist is exceeded. Although the clinical significance of these effects is not known, caution is advised in the coadministration of beta-agonists with non-potassium sparing diuretics. Consider monitoring potassium levels.

7.3 Digoxin

Mean decreases of 16% and 22% in serum digoxin levels were demonstrated after single dose intravenous and oral administration of albuterol, respectively, to normal volunteers who had received digoxin for 10 days. The clinical significance of these findings for patients with obstructive airway disease who are receiving albuterol and digoxin on a chronic basis is unclear. Nevertheless, it would be prudent to carefully evaluate the serum digoxin levels in patients who are currently receiving digoxin and PROAIR HFA Inhalation Aerosol.

7.4 Monoamine Oxidase Inhibitors or Tricyclic Antidepressants

PROAIR HFA Inhalation Aerosol should be administered with extreme caution to patients being treated with monoamine oxidase inhibitors or tricyclic antidepressants, or within 2 weeks of discontinuation of such agents, because the action of albuterol on the cardiovascular system may be potentiated. Consider alternative therapy in patients taking MAO inhibitors or tricyclic antidepressants.

8 USE IN SPECIFIC POPULATIONS

8.1 Pregnancy

Teratogenic Effects: Pregnancy Category C:

There are no adequate and well-controlled studies of PROAIR HFA Inhalation Aerosol or albuterol sulfate in pregnant women. During worldwide marketing experience, various congenital anomalies, including cleft palate and limb defects, have been reported in the offspring of patients treated with albuterol. Some of the mothers were taking multiple medications during their pregnancies. No consistent pattern of defects can be discerned, and a relationship between albuterol use and congenital anomalies has not been established. Animal reproduction studies in mice and rabbits revealed evidence of teratogenicity. PROAIR HFA Inhalation Aerosol should be used during pregnancy only if the potential benefit justifies the potential risk to the fetus.

In a mouse reproduction study, subcutaneously administered albuterol sulfate produced cleft palate formation in 5 of 111 (4.5%) fetuses at an exposure approximately eight-tenths of the maximum recommended human dose (MRHD) for adults on a mg/m^2 basis and in 10 of 108 (9.3%) fetuses at approximately 8 times the MRHD. Similar effects were not observed at approximately one-thirteenth of the MRHD. Cleft palate also occurred in 22 of 72 (30.5%) fetuses from females treated subcutaneously with isoproterenol (positive control).

In a rabbit reproduction study, orally administered albuterol sulfate induced cranioschisis in 7 of 19 fetuses (37%) at approximately 630 times the MRHD.

In a rat reproduction study, an albuterol sulfate/HFA-134a formulation administered by inhalation did not produce any teratogenic effects at exposures approximately 65 times the MRHD *[see Nonclinical Toxicology (13.2)]*.

8.2 Labor and Delivery

Because of the potential for beta-agonist interference with uterine contractility, use of PROAIR HFA Inhalation Aerosol for relief of bronchospasm during labor should be restricted to those patients in whom the benefits clearly outweigh the risk. PROAIR HFA Inhalation Aerosol has not been approved for the management of pre-term labor. The benefit:risk ratio when albuterol is administered for tocolysis has not been established. Serious adverse reactions, including pulmonary edema, have been reported during or following treatment of premature labor with beta$_2$-agonists, including albuterol.

8.3 Nursing Mothers

Plasma levels of albuterol sulfate and HFA-134a after inhaled therapeutic doses are very low in humans, but it is not known whether the components of PROAIR HFA Inhalation Aerosol are excreted in human milk.

Caution should be exercised when PROAIR HFA Inhalation Aerosol is administered to a nursing woman. Because of the potential for tumorigenicity shown for albuterol in animal studies and lack of experience with the use of PROAIR HFA Inhalation Aerosol by nursing mothers, a decision should be made whether to discontinue nursing or to discontinue the drug, taking into account the importance of the drug to the mother.

8.4 Pediatric Use

The safety and effectiveness of PROAIR HFA Inhalation Aerosol for the treatment or prevention of bronchospasm in children 12 years of age and older with reversible obstructive airway disease is based on one 6-week clinical trial in 116 patients 12 years of age and older with asthma comparing doses of 180 mcg four times daily with placebo, and one single-dose crossover study comparing doses of 90, 180, and 270 mcg with placebo in 58 patients *[see Clinical Studies (14.1)]*. The safety and effectiveness of PROAIR HFA Inhalation Aerosol for treatment of exercise-induced bronchospasm in children 12 years of age and older is based on one single-dose crossover study in 24 adults and adolescents with exercise-induced bronchospasm comparing doses of 180 mcg with placebo *[see Clinical Studies (14.2)]*.

The safety of PROAIR HFA Inhalation Aerosol in children 4 to 11 years of age is based on one 3-week clinical trial in 50 patients 4 to 11 years of age with asthma using the same formulation of albuterol as in PROAIR HFA Inhalation *Aerosol comparing doses of* 180 mcg four times daily with placebo. The effectiveness of PROAIR HFA Inhalation Aerosol in children 4 to 11 years of age is extrapolated from clinical trials in patients 12 years of age and older with asthma and exercise-induced bronchospasm, based on data from a single-dose study comparing the bronchodilatory effect of PROAIR HFA 90 mcg and 180 mcg with placebo in 55 patients with asthma and a 3-week clinical trial using the same formulation of albuterol as in PROAIR HFA Inhalation Aerosol in 95 asthmatic children 4 to 11 years of age comparing a dose of 180 mcg albuterol four times daily with placebo *[see Clinical Studies (14.1)]*.

The safety and effectiveness of PROAIR HFA Inhalation Aerosol in pediatric patients below the age of 4 years have not been established.

8.5 Geriatric Use

Clinical studies of PROAIR HFA Inhalation Aerosol did not include sufficient numbers of patients aged 65 and over to determine whether they respond differently from younger patients. Other reported clinical experience has not identified differences in responses between elderly and younger patients. In general, dose selection for an elderly patient should be cautious, usually starting at the low end of the dosing range, reflecting the greater frequency of decreased hepatic, renal, or cardiac function, and of concomitant disease or other drug therapy *[see Warnings and Precautions (5.4, 5.7)]*.

All beta$_2$-adrenergic agonists, including albuterol, are known to be substantially excreted by the kidney, and the risk of toxic reactions may be greater in patients with impaired renal function. Because elderly patients are more likely to have decreased renal function, care should be taken in dose selection, and it may be useful to monitor renal function.

10 OVERDOSAGE

The expected symptoms with overdosage are those of excessive beta-adrenergic stimulation and/or occurrence or exaggeration of any of the symptoms listed under ADVERSE REACTIONS, e.g., seizures, angina, hypertension or hypotension, tachycardia with rates up to 200 beats per minute, arrhythmias, nervousness, headache, tremor, dry mouth, palpitation, nausea, dizziness, fatigue, malaise, and insomnia.

Hypokalemia may also occur. As with all sympathomimetic medications, cardiac arrest and even death may be associated with abuse of PROAIR HFA Inhalation Aerosol.

Treatment consists of discontinuation of PROAIR HFA Inhalation Aerosol together with appropriate symptomatic therapy. The judicious use of a cardioselective beta-receptor blocker may be considered, bearing in mind that such medication can produce bronchospasm. There is insufficient evidence to determine if dialysis is beneficial for overdosage of PROAIR HFA Inhalation Aerosol.

The oral median lethal dose of albuterol sulfate in mice is greater than 2,000 mg/kg (approximately 6,800 times the maximum recommended daily inhalation dose for adults on a mg/m^2 basis and approximately 3,200 times the maximum recommended daily inhalation dose for children on a mg/m^2 basis). In mature rats, the subcutaneous median lethal dose of albuterol sulfate is approximately 450 mg/kg (approximately 3,000 times the maximum recommended daily inhalation dose for adults on a mg/m^2 basis and approximately 1,400 times the maximum recommended daily inhalation dose for children on a mg/m^2 basis). In young rats, the subcutaneous median lethal dose is approximately 2,000 mg/kg (approximately 14,000 times the maximum recommended daily inhalation dose for adults on a mg/m^2 basis and approximately 6,400 times the maximum recommended daily inhalation dose for children on a mg/m^2 basis). The inhalation median lethal dose has not been determined in animals.

11 DESCRIPTION

The active ingredient of PROAIR HFA (albuterol sulfate) Inhalation Aerosol is albuterol sulfate, a racemic salt, of albuterol. Albuterol sulfate has the chemical name α^1-[(*tert*-butylamino) methyl]-4-hydroxy-*m*-xylene-α,α'-diol sulfate (2:1) (salt), and has the following chemical structure:

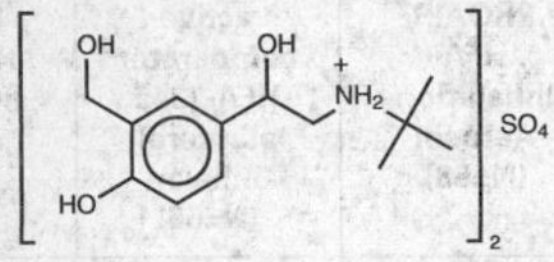

The molecular weight of albuterol sulfate is 576.7, and the empirical formula is $(C_{13}H_{21}NO_3)_2 \bullet H_2SO_4$. Albuterol sulfate is a white to off-white crystalline powder. It is soluble in water and slightly soluble in ethanol. Albuterol sulfate is the official generic name in the United States, and salbutamol sulfate is the World Health Organization recommended generic name. PROAIR HFA Inhalation Aerosol is a pressurized metered-dose aerosol unit for oral inhalation. It contains a microcrystalline suspension of albuterol sulfate in propellant HFA-134a (1, 1, 1, 2-tetrafluoroethane) and ethanol.

Prime the inhaler before using for the first time and in cases where the inhaler has not been used for more than 2 weeks by releasing three sprays into the air, away from the face. After priming, each actuation delivers 108 mcg albuterol sulfate, from the actuator mouthpiece (equivalent to 90 mcg of albuterol base). Each canister provides 200 actuations (inhalations).

This product does not contain chlorofluorocarbons (CFCs) as the propellant.

12 CLINICAL PHARMACOLOGY

12.1 Mechanism of Action

Albuterol sulfate is a beta$_2$-adrenergic agonist. The pharmacologic effects of albuterol sulfate are attributable to activation of beta$_2$-adrenergic receptors on airway smooth muscle. Activation of beta$_2$-adrenergic receptors leads to the activation of adenylcyclase and to an increase in the intracellular concentration of cyclic-3′, 5′ adenosine monophosphate (cyclic AMP). This increase of cyclic AMP is associated with the activation of protein kinase A, which in turn inhibits the phosphorylation of myosin and lowers intracellular ionic calcium concentrations, resulting in muscle relaxation. Albuterol relaxes the smooth muscle of all airways, from the trachea to the terminal bronchioles. Albuterol acts as a functional antagonist to relax the airway irrespective of the spasmogen involved, thus protecting against all bronchoconstrictor challenges. Increased cyclic AMP concentrations are also associated with the inhibition of release of mediators from mast cells in the airway. While it is recognized that beta$_2$-adrenergic receptors are the predominant receptors on bronchial smooth muscle, data indicate that there are beta-receptors in the human heart, 10% to 50% of which are cardiac beta$_2$-adrenergic receptors. The precise function of these receptors has not been established *[see Warnings and Precautions (5.4)]*.

Albuterol has been shown in most controlled clinical trials to have more effect on the respiratory tract, in the form of bronchial smooth muscle relaxation, than isoproterenol at comparable doses while producing fewer cardiovascular effects. However, inhaled albuterol, like other beta-adrenergic agonist drugs, can produce a significant cardiovascular effect in some patients, as measured by pulse rate, blood pressure, symptoms, and/or electrocardiographic changes *[see Warnings and Precautions (5.4)]*.

12.2 Pharmacokinetics

The systemic levels of albuterol are low after inhalation of recommended doses. In a crossover study conducted in healthy male and female volunteers, high cumulative doses of PROAIR HFA Inhalation Aerosol (1,080 mcg of albuterol base administered over one hour) yielded mean peak plasma concentrations (C_{max}) and systemic exposure (AUC_{inf}) of approximately 4,100 pg/mL and 28,426 pg/mL*hr, respectively compared to approximately 3,900 pg/mL and 28,395 pg/mL*hr, respectively following the same dose of an active HFA-134a albuterol inhaler comparator. The terminal plasma half-life of albuterol delivered by PROAIR HFA Inhalation Aerosol was approximately 6 hours. Comparison of the pharmacokinetic parameters demonstrated no differences between the products.

The pharmacokinetic profile of PROAIR HFA Inhalation Aerosol was evaluated in a two-way cross-over study in 11 healthy pediatric volunteers, 4 to 11 years of age. A single dose administration of PROAIR HFA Inhalation Aerosol (180 mcg albuterol base) yielded a least square mean (SE) C_{max} and $AUC_{0-\infty}$ of 1,100 (1.18) pg/mL and 5,120 (1.15) pg/mL*hr, respectively. The least square mean (SE) terminal plasma half-life of albuterol delivered by PROAIR HFA Inhalation Aerosol was 166 (7.8) minutes.

Metabolism and Elimination: Information available in the published literature suggests that the primary enzyme responsible for the metabolism of albuterol in humans is SULTIA3 (sulfotransferase). When racemic albuterol was administered either intravenously or via inhalation after oral charcoal administration, there was a 3- to 4-fold difference in the area under the concentration-time curves between the (R)- and (S)-albuterol enantiomers, with (S)-albuterol concentrations being consistently higher. However, without charcoal pretreatment, after either oral or inhalation administration the differences were 8- to 24-fold, suggesting that the (R)-albuterol is preferentially metabolized in the gastrointestinal tract, presumably by SULTIA3.

The primary route of elimination of albuterol is through renal excretion (80% to 100%) of either the parent compound or the primary metabolite. Less than 20% of the drug is detected in the feces. Following intravenous administration of racemic albuterol, between 25% and 46% of the (R)-albuterol fraction of the dose was excreted as unchanged (R)-albuterol in the urine.

Geriatric, Pediatric, Hepatic/Renal Impairment: No pharmacokinetic studies for PROAIR HFA Inhalation Aerosol have been conducted in neonates or elderly subjects.

The effect of hepatic impairment on the pharmacokinetics of PROAIR HFA Inhalation Aerosol has not been evaluated.

The effect of renal impairment on the pharmacokinetics of albuterol was evaluated in 5 subjects with creatinine clearance of 7 to 53 mL/min, and the results were compared with those from healthy volunteers. Renal disease had no effect on the half-life, but there was a 67% decline in albuterol clearance. Caution should be used when administering high doses of PROAIR HFA Inhalation Aerosol to patients with renal impairment *[see Use in Specific Populations (8.5)]*.

13 NONCLINICAL TOXICOLOGY

13.1 Carcinogenesis, Mutagenesis, Impairment of Fertility

In a 2-year study in Sprague-Dawley rats, albuterol sulfate caused a dose-related increase in the incidence of benign leiomyomas of the mesovarium at and above dietary doses of 2 mg/kg (approximately 15 times the maximum recommended daily inhalation dose for adults on a mg/m^2 basis and approximately 6 times the maximum recommended daily inhalation dose for children on a mg/m^2 basis). In another study this effect was blocked by the coadministration of propranolol, a non-selective beta-adrenergic antagonist.

In an 18-month study in CD-1 mice, albuterol sulfate showed no evidence of tumorigenicity at dietary doses of up to 500 mg/kg (approximately 1,600 times the maximum recommended daily inhalation dose for adults on a mg/m^2 basis and approximately 740 times the maximum recommended daily inhalation dose for children on a mg/m^2 basis). In a 22-month study in Golden Hamsters, albuterol sulfate showed no evidence of tumorigenicity at dietary doses of up to 50 mg/kg (approximately 210 times the maximum recommended daily inhalation dose for adults on a mg/m^2 basis and approximately 100 times the maximum recommended daily inhalation dose for children on a mg/m^2 basis).

Albuterol sulfate was not mutagenic in the Ames test or a mutation test in yeast. Albuterol sulfate was not clastogenic in a human peripheral lymphocyte assay or in an AH1 strain mouse micronucleus assay.

Reproduction studies in rats demonstrated no evidence of impaired fertility at oral doses up to 50 mg/kg (approximately 310 times the maximum recommended daily inhalation dose for adults on a mg/m^2 basis).

13.2 Animal Toxicology and/or Pharmacology

Preclinical: Intravenous studies in rats with albuterol sulfate have demonstrated that albuterol crosses the blood-brain barrier and reaches brain concentrations amounting to approximately 5% of the plasma concentrations. In structures outside the blood-brain barrier (pineal and pituitary glands), albuterol concentrations were found to be 100 times those in the whole brain.

Studies in laboratory animals (minipigs, rodents, and dogs) have demonstrated the occurrence of cardiac arrhythmias and sudden death (with histologic evidence of myocardial necrosis) when β-agonists and methylxanthines were administered concurrently. The clinical significance of these findings is unknown.

Propellant HFA-134a is devoid of pharmacological activity except at very high doses in animals (380–1300 times the maximum human exposure based on comparisons of AUC values), primarily producing ataxia, tremors, dyspnea, or salivation. These are similar to effects produced by the structurally related chlorofluorocarbons (CFCs), which have been used extensively in metered-dose inhalers.

In animals and humans, propellant HFA-134a was found to be rapidly absorbed and rapidly eliminated, with an elimination half-life of 3–27 minutes in animals and 5–7 minutes in humans. Time to maximum plasma concentration (T_{max}) and mean residence time are both extremely short leading to a transient appearance of HFA-134a in the blood with no evidence of accumulation.

Reproductive Toxicology Studies: A study in CD-1 mice given albuterol sulfate subcutaneously showed cleft palate formation in 5 of 111 (4.5%) fetuses at 0.25 mg/kg (less than the maximum recommended daily inhalation dose for adults on a mg/m^2 basis) and in 10 of 108 (9.3%) fetuses at 2.5 mg/kg (approximately 8 times the maximum recommended daily inhalation dose for adults on a mg/m^2 basis). The drug did not induce cleft palate formation at a dose of 0.025 mg/kg (less than the maximum recommended daily inhalation dose for adults on a mg/m^2 basis). Cleft palate also occurred in 22 of 72 (30.5%) fetuses from females treated subcutaneously with 2.5 mg/kg of isoproterenol (positive control).

A reproduction study in Stride Dutch rabbits revealed cranioschisis in 7 of 19 fetuses (37%) when albuterol sulfate was administered orally at 50 mg/kg (approximately 630 times the maximum recommended daily inhalation dose for adults on a mg/m^2 basis).

In an inhalation reproduction study in Sprague-Dawley rats, the albuterol sulfate/HFA-134a did not exhibit any teratogenic effects at 10.5 mg/kg (approximately 65 times the maximum recommended daily inhalation dose for adults on a mg/m^2 basis).

A study in which pregnant rats were dosed with radiolabeled albuterol sulfate demonstrated that drug-related material is transferred from the maternal circulation to the fetus.

14 CLINICAL STUDIES

14.1 Bronchospasm Associated with Asthma

Adult and Adolescent Patients 12 Years of Age and Older: In a 6-week, randomized, double-blind, placebo-controlled trial, PROAIR HFA Inhalation Aerosol (58 patients) was compared to a matched placebo HFA inhalation aerosol (58 patients) in asthmatic patients 12 to 76 years of age at a dose of 180 mcg albuterol four times daily. An evaluator-blind marketed active comparator HFA-134a albuterol inhaler arm (56 patients) was included.

Serial FEV$_1$ measurements, shown below as percent change from test-day baseline at Day 1 and at Day 43, demonstrated that two inhalations of PROAIR HFA Inhalation Aerosol produced significantly greater improvement in FEV$_1$ over the pre-treatment value than the matched placebo, as well as a comparable bronchodilator effect to the marketed active comparator HFA-134a albuterol inhaler.

FEV$_1$ as Mean Percent Change from Test-Day Pre-Dose in a 6-Week Clinical Trial

Day 1

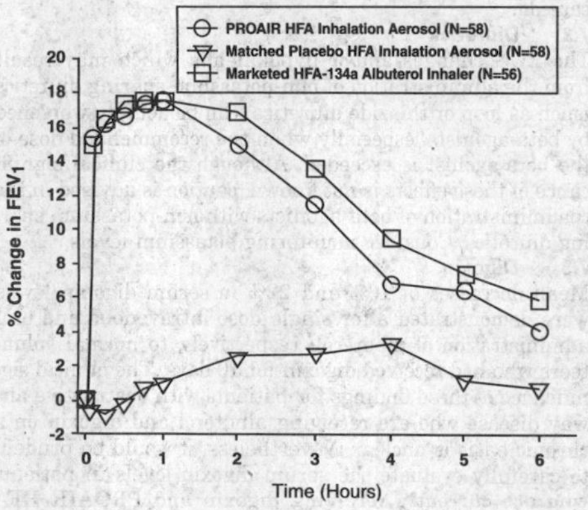

Day 43

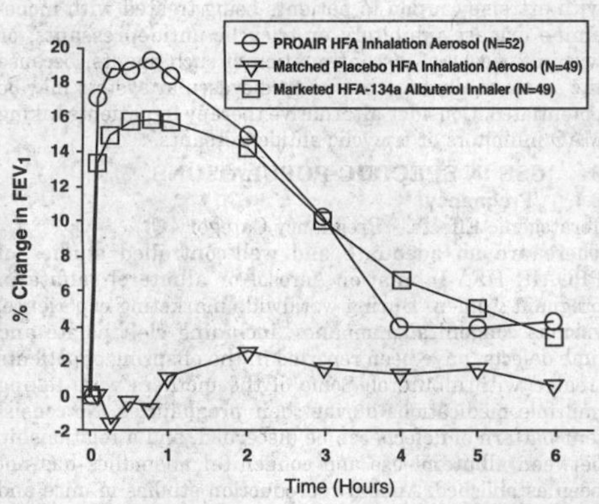

In this study, 31 of 58 patients treated with PROAIR HFA Inhalation Aerosol achieved a 15% increase in FEV$_1$ within 30 minutes post-dose on Day 1. In these patients, the median time to onset, median time to peak effect, and median duration of effect were 8.2 minutes, 47 minutes, and approximately 3 hours, respectively. In some patients, the duration of effect was as long as 6 hours.

In a placebo-controlled, single-dose, crossover study, PROAIR HFA Inhalation Aerosol, administered at albuterol doses of 90, 180 and 270 mcg, produced bronchodilator responses significantly greater than those observed with a matched placebo HFA inhalation aerosol and comparable to a marketed active comparator HFA-134a albuterol inhaler.

Pediatric Patients 4 to 11 Years of Age: In a 3-week, randomized, double-blind, placebo-controlled trial, the same formulation of albuterol as in PROAIR HFA Inhalation Aerosol (50 patients) was compared to a matched placebo HFA inhalation aerosol (45 patients) in asthmatic children 4 to 11 years of age at a dose of 180 mcg albuterol four times daily. Serial FEV_1 measurements, expressed as the maximum percent change from test-day baseline in percent predicted FEV_1 at Day 1 and at Day 22 observed within two hours post-dose, demonstrated that two inhalations of HFA albuterol sulfate produced significantly greater improvement in FEV_1 over the pre-treatment value than the matched placebo.

In this study, 21 of 50 pediatric patients treated with the same formulation of albuterol as in PROAIR HFA Inhalation Aerosol achieved a 15% increase in FEV_1 within 30 minutes post-dose on Day 1. In these patients, the median time to onset, median time to peak effect and median duration of effect were 10 minutes, 31 minutes, and approximately 4 hours, respectively. In some pediatric patients, the duration of effect was as long as 6 hours.

In a placebo-controlled, single-dose, crossover study in 55 pediatric patients 4 to 11 years of age, PROAIR HFA Inhalation Aerosol, administered at albuterol doses of 90 and 180 mcg, was compared with a matched placebo HFA inhalation aerosol. Serial FEV_1 measurements, expressed as the baseline-adjusted percent predicted FEV_1 observed over 6 hours post-dose, demonstrated that one and two inhalations of PROAIR HFA Inhalation Aerosol produced significantly greater bronchodilator responses than the matched placebo.

14.2 Exercise-Induced Bronchospasm

In a randomized, single-dose, crossover study in 24 adults and adolescents with exercise-induced bronchospasm (EIB), two inhalations of PROAIR HFA taken 30 minutes before exercise prevented EIB for the hour following exercise (defined as maintenance of FEV_1 within 80% of post-dose, pre-exercise baseline values) in 83% (20 of 24) of patients as compared to 25% (6 of 24) of patients when they received placebo.

Some patients who participated in these clinical trials were using concomitant steroid therapy.

16 HOW SUPPLIED/STORAGE & HANDLING

PROAIR HFA (albuterol sulfate) Inhalation Aerosol is supplied as a pressurized aluminum canister with a red plastic actuator and white dust cap each in boxes of one. Each canister contains 8.5 g of the formulation and provides 200 actuations (NDC 59310-579-20). Each actuation delivers 120 mcg of albuterol sulfate from the canister valve and 108 mcg of albuterol sulfate from the actuator mouthpiece (equivalent to 90 mcg of albuterol base).

SHAKE WELL BEFORE USE. Store between 15° and 25°C (59° and 77°F). Contents under pressure. Do not puncture or incinerate. Protect from freezing temperatures and prolonged exposure to direct sunlight. Exposure to temperatures above 120°F may cause bursting. For best results, canister should be at room temperature before use. Avoid spraying in eyes. Keep out of reach of children.

See FDA-Approved Patient Labeling (17.8) for priming and cleaning instructions.

The red actuator supplied with PROAIR HFA Inhalation Aerosol should not be used with the canister from any other inhalation aerosol products. The PROAIR HFA Inhalation Aerosol canister should not be used with the actuator from any other inhalation aerosol products.

The labeled amount of medication in each actuation cannot be assured after 200 actuations, even though the canister may not be completely empty. Discard the inhaler (canister plus actuator) after 200 actuations have been used. Never immerse the canister into water to determine how full the canister is ("float test").

PROAIR HFA Inhalation Aerosol does not contain chlorofluorocarbons (CFCs) as the propellant.

17 PATIENT COUNSELING INFORMATION

See FDA-Approved Patient Labeling (17.8)

Patients should be given the following information:

17.1 Frequency of Use

The action of PROAIR HFA Inhalation Aerosol should last for 4 to 6 hours. Do not use PROAIR HFA Inhalation Aerosol more frequently than recommended. Instruct patients to not increase the dose or frequency of doses of PROAIR HFA Inhalation Aerosol without consulting the physician. If patients find that treatment with PROAIR HFA Inhalation Aerosol becomes less effective for symptomatic relief, symptoms become worse, and/or they need to use the product more frequently than usual, they should seek medical attention immediately.

17.2 Priming and Cleaning

Priming: Priming is essential to ensure appropriate albuterol content in each actuation. Instruct patients to prime the inhaler before using for the first time and in cases where the inhaler has not been used for more than 2 weeks by releasing three sprays into the air, away from the face.

Cleaning: To ensure proper dosing and prevent actuator orifice blockage, instruct patients to wash the red plastic actuator mouthpiece and dry thoroughly at least once a week. Detailed cleaning instructions are included in the illustrated Information for the Patient leaflet.

17.3 Paradoxical Bronchospasm

Inform patients that PROAIR HFA Inhalation Aerosol can produce paradoxical bronchospasm. Instruct patients to discontinue PROAIR HFA Inhalation Aerosol if paradoxical bronchospasm occurs.

17.4 Concomitant Drug Use

While patients are taking PROAIR HFA Inhalation Aerosol, other inhaled drugs and asthma medications should be taken only as directed by a physician.

17.5 Common Adverse Events

Common adverse effects of treatment with inhaled albuterol include palpitations, chest pain, rapid heart rate, tremor, or nervousness.

17.6 Pregnancy

Patients who are pregnant or nursing should contact their physician about the use of PROAIR HFA Inhalation Aerosol.

17.7 General Information on Use

Effective and safe use of PROAIR HFA Inhalation Aerosol includes an understanding of the way that it should be administered.

Shake well before each spray.

Use PROAIR HFA Inhalation Aerosol only with the actuator supplied with the product. Discard the canister after 200 sprays have been used. Never immerse the canister in water to determine how full the canister is ("float test").

In general, the technique for administering PROAIR HFA Inhalation Aerosol to children is similar to that for adults. Children should use PROAIR HFA Inhalation Aerosol under adult supervision, as instructed by the patient's physician.

17.8 FDA-Approved Patient Labeling

See tear-off illustrated Information for the Patient leaflet below.

Mktd by: Teva Specialty Pharmaceuticals LLC
Horsham, PA 19044
Mfd by: IVAX Pharmaceuticals Ireland
Waterford, Ireland

Copyright ©2008, Teva Specialty Pharmaceuticals LLC
All rights reserved.
PROAIR® HFA is a registered trademark of Teva Specialty Pharmaceuticals LLC

Manufactured In Ireland PE 2015 Rev. 09/08

Attention Pharmacist:
Detach Patient's Instructions for use from package insert and dispense with the product.

Information for the Patient

PROAIR® HFA (albuterol sulfate) Inhalation Aerosol

Read this leaflet carefully before you start to use PROAIR HFA.

Keep this leaflet because it has important summary information about PROAIR HFA. Your healthcare provider has more information or advice.

Read the new leaflet that comes with each refill of your prescription because there may be new information.

What is PROAIR HFA?

PROAIR HFA is a kind of medicine called a fast-acting bronchodilator. Fast-acting bronchodilators help to quickly open the airways in your lungs so that you can breathe more easily.

Each dose of PROAIR HFA should last up to 4 to 6 hours.

Take PROAIR HFA as directed by your doctor. Do not take extra doses or take more often without asking your doctor.

Get medical help right away if PROAIR HFA no longer helps your symptoms. Also get medical help if your symptoms get worse or if you need to use your inhaler more often.

While you are using PROAIR HFA, use other inhaled medicines and asthma medicines only as directed by your doctor.

Tell your doctor if you are pregnant or nursing, and ask about the use of PROAIR HFA.

Possible side effects of taking PROAIR HFA include fast or irregular heartbeat, chest pain, shakiness, and nervousness. With the first use of a new canister, worsening of wheezing may occur.

The parts of your PROAIR HFA inhaler:

[See figure 1 at top of next column]

There are 2 main parts to your PROAIR HFA inhaler—the metal canister that holds the medicine and the red plastic actuator that sprays the medicine from the canister (see Figure 1).

Figure 1

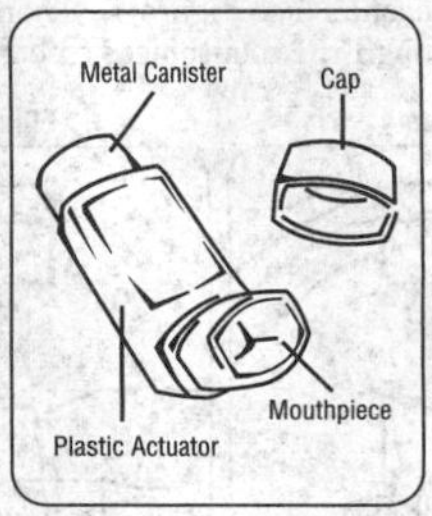
Metal Canister
Cap
Mouthpiece
Plastic Actuator

The inhaler also has a cap that covers the mouthpiece of the actuator.

Do not use the PROAIR HFA actuator with a canister of medicine from any other inhaler. And do not use a PROAIR HFA canister with an actuator from any other inhaler.

How to Use Your PROAIR HFA

Before using your PROAIR HFA:

If a child needs help using the inhaler, an adult should help the child use the inhaler. An adult should watch a child use the inhaler to be sure it is used correctly.

The inhaler should be at room temperature before you use it.

Check each time to make sure the canister fits firmly in the plastic actuator. Also look into the mouthpiece to make sure there are no foreign objects there, especially if the cap is not being used to cover the mouthpiece.

Priming your PROAIR HFA:

You must prime the inhaler to get the right amount of medicine. Prime the inhaler before you use it for the first time or if you have not used it for more than 14 days. To prime the inhaler, take the cap off the mouthpiece of the actuator. Then shake the inhaler well, and spray it into the air away from your face. Shake and spray the inhaler like this 2 more times to finish priming it.

Instructions for taking a dose from your PROAIR HFA:

Read through the 6 steps below before using PROAIR HFA. If you have any questions, ask your doctor or pharmacist.

1. Take the cap off the mouthpiece of the actuator. **Shake the inhaler well** before each spray.
2. Hold the inhaler with the mouthpiece down (see Figure 2). **Breathe out through your mouth** and push as much air from your lungs as you can. Put the mouthpiece in your mouth and close your lips around it.
3. **Push the top of the canister all the way down while you breathe in deeply and slowly through your mouth** (see Figure 3). Right after the spray comes out, take your finger off the canister. After you have breathed in all the way, take the inhaler out of your mouth and close your mouth.

Figure 2

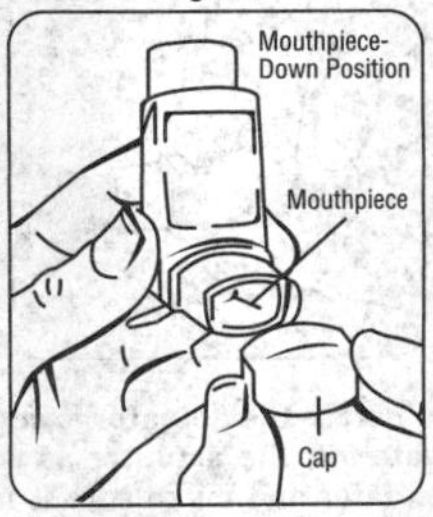
Mouthpiece-
Down Position
Mouthpiece
Cap

Figure 3

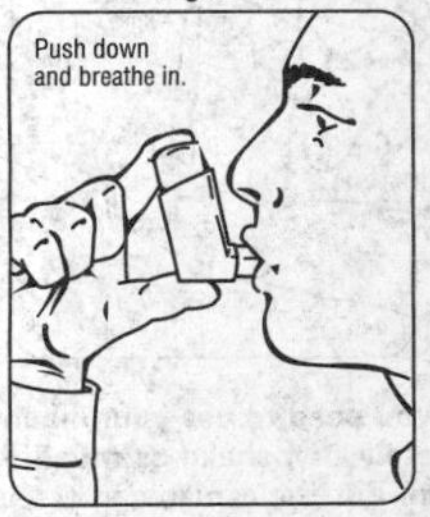
Push down
and breathe in.

4. **Hold your breath as long as you can**, up to 10 seconds, then breathe normally.
5. If your doctor has prescribed more sprays, wait 1 minute and **shake** the inhaler again. Repeat steps 2 through 4.
6. Put the cap back on the mouthpiece after every time you use the inhaler, and make sure it snaps firmly into place.

When to Replace Your PROAIR HFA

- **Before you reach 200 sprays**, you should refill your prescription or ask your doctor if you need another prescription for PROAIR HFA.
- **Throw the inhaler away** when you have used 200 sprays. You should not keep using the inhaler after 200 sprays even though the canister may not be completely empty because you cannot be sure you will receive any medicine.
- **Do not use the inhaler** after the expiration date, which is on the packaging it comes in.

How to Clean Your PROAIR HFA

It is very important to keep the plastic actuator clean so the medicine will not build-up and block the spray. Do not try to clean the metal canister or let it get wet. The inhaler may stop spraying if it is not cleaned correctly.

Wash the actuator at least once a week.

Cleaning instructions:

- Take the canister out of the actuator, and take the cap off the mouthpiece.

- Wash the actuator through the top with warm running water for 30 seconds (see Figure 4). Then wash the actuator again through the mouthpiece (see Figure 5).

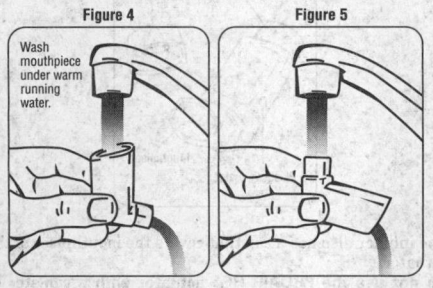

Figure 4   **Figure 5**

Wash mouthpiece under warm running water.

- Shake off as much water from the actuator as you can. Look into the mouthpiece to make sure any medicine build-up has been completely washed away. If there is any build-up, repeat steps in Figures 4 and 5.
- Let the actuator air-dry completely, such as overnight (see Figure 6).

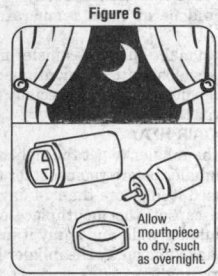

Figure 6

Allow mouthpiece to dry, such as overnight.

- When the actuator is dry, put the canister in the actuator and make sure it fits firmly. Shake the inhaler well and spray it twice into the air away from your face. Put the cap back on the mouthpiece.

If your actuator becomes blocked:

Blockage from medicine build-up is more likely to happen if you do not let the actuator air-dry completely. If the actuator gets blocked so that little or no medicine comes out of the mouthpiece (see Figures 7 and 8), wash the actuator as described in the "Cleaning Instructions" section above.

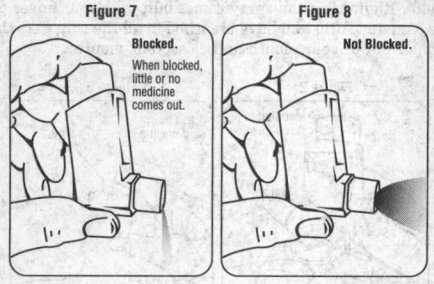

Figure 7   **Figure 8**

Blocked. When blocked, little or no medicine comes out.

Not Blocked.

If you need to use your inhaler before the actuator is completely dry, shake as much water off the actuator as you can. Put the canister in the actuator and make sure it fits firmly. Shake the inhaler well and spray it twice into the air away from your face. Then take your dose as prescribed. Then clean and air-dry it completely.

Storing Your PROAIR HFA

Store between 15° and 25° C (59° and 77° F). Avoid exposure to extreme heat and cold. For best results, canister should be at room temperature.

Shake well before use.

Contents Under Pressure. Do not puncture. Do not store near heat or open flame. Exposure to temperatures above 120°F may cause bursting. Never throw container into fire or incinerator. Avoid spraying in eyes. Keep out of reach of children.

For questions related to proper use and maintenance of your PROAIR HFA inhaler, please call Teva Specialty Pharmaceuticals customer service at 1-888-482-9522.

Mktd by: Teva Specialty Pharmaceuticals LLC
Horsham, PA 19044
Mfd by: IVAX Pharmaceuticals Ireland
Waterford, Ireland
Copyright ©2008, Teva Specialty Pharmaceuticals LLC
All rights reserved.
PROAIR® HFA is a registered trademark of Teva Specialty Pharmaceuticals LLC
Manufactured In Ireland   PE 2015 Rev. 09/08
Shown in Product Identification Guide, page 320

QVAR® 40 mcg
(beclomethasone dipropionate HFA, 40 mcg)
INHALATION AEROSOL
For Oral Inhalation Only   ℞

QVAR® 80 mcg
(beclomethasone dipropionate HFA, 80 mcg)
INHALATION AEROSOL
For Oral Inhalation Only

DESCRIPTION

The active component of QVAR 40 mcg Inhalation Aerosol and QVAR 80 mcg Inhalation Aerosol is beclomethasone dipropionate, USP, an anti-inflammatory corticosteroid having the chemical name 9-chloro-11β,17,21-trihydroxy-16β-methylpregna-1,4-diene-3,20-dione 17,21-dipropionate. Beclomethasone dipropionate (BDP) is a diester of beclomethasone, a synthetic corticosteroid chemically related to dexamethasone. Beclomethasone differs from dexamethasone in having a chlorine at the 9-alpha carbon in place of a fluorine, and in having a 16 beta-methyl group instead of a 16 alpha-methyl group. Beclomethasone dipropionate is a white to creamy white, odorless powder with a molecular formula of $C_{28}H_{37}ClO_7$ and a molecular weight of 521.1. Its chemical structure is:

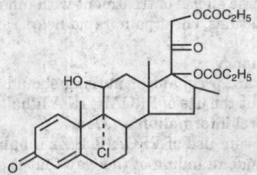

QVAR is a pressurized, metered-dose aerosol intended for oral inhalation only. Each unit contains a solution of beclomethasone dipropionate in propellant HFA-134a (1,1,1,2 tetrafluoroethane) and ethanol. QVAR 40 mcg delivers 40 mcg of beclomethasone dipropionate from the actuator and 50 mcg from the valve. QVAR 80 mcg delivers 80 mcg of beclomethasone dipropionate from the actuator and 100 mcg from the valve. Both products deliver 50 microliters (59 milligrams) of solution formulation from the valve with each actuation. Each canister provides 100 inhalations. QVAR should be "primed" or actuated twice prior to taking the first dose from a new canister, or when the inhaler has not been used for more than ten days. Avoid spraying in the eyes or face while priming QVAR. This product does not contain chlorofluorocarbons (CFCs).

CLINICAL PHARMACOLOGY

Airway inflammation is known to be an important component in the pathogenesis of asthma. Inflammation occurs in both large and small airways. Corticosteroids have multiple anti-inflammatory effects, inhibiting both inflammatory cells (e.g., mast cells, eosinophils, basophils, lymphocytes, macrophages, and neutrophils) and release of inflammatory mediators (e.g., histamine, eicosanoids, leukotrienes, and cytokines). These anti-inflammatory actions of corticosteroids such as beclomethasone dipropionate contribute to their efficacy in asthma.

Beclomethasone dipropionate is a prodrug that is rapidly activated by hydrolysis to the active monoester, 17 monopropionate (17-BMP). Beclomethasone 17 monopropionate has been shown *in vitro* to exhibit a binding affinity for the human glucocorticoid receptor which is approximately 13 times that of dexamethasone, 6 times that of triamcinolone acetonide, 1.5 times that of budesonide and 25 times that of beclomethasone dipropionate. The clinical significance of these findings is unknown.

Studies in patients with asthma have shown a favorable ratio between topical anti-inflammatory activity and systemic corticosteroid effects with recommended doses of QVAR.

Pharmacokinetics

Beclomethasone dipropionate (BDP) undergoes rapid and extensive conversion to beclomethasone-17-monopropionate (17-BMP) during absorption. The pharmacokinetics of 17-BMP has been studied in asthmatics given single doses.

Absorption

The mean peak plasma concentration (C_{max}) of BDP was 88 pg/ml at 0.5 hour after inhalation of 320 mcg using QVAR (four actuations of the 80 mcg/actuation strength). The mean peak plasma concentration of the major and most active metabolite, 17-BMP, was 1419 pg/ml at 0.7 hour after inhalation of 320 mcg of QVAR. When the same nominal dose is provided by the two QVAR strengths (40 and 80 mcg/actuation), equivalent systemic pharmacokinetics can be expected. The C_{max} of 17-BMP increased dose proportionally in the dose range of 80 and 320 mcg.

Metabolism

Three major metabolites are formed via cytochrome P450 3A catalyzed biotransformation - beclomethasone-17-monopropionate (17-BMP), beclomethasone-21-mono-propionate (21-BMP) and beclomethasone (BOH). Lung slices metabolize BDP rapidly to 17-BMP and more slowly to BOH. 17-BMP is the most active metabolite.

Distribution

The *in vitro* protein binding for 17-BMP was reported to be 94-96% over the concentration range of 1000 to 5000 pg/mL. Protein binding was constant over the concentration range evaluated. There is no evidence of tissue storage of BDP or its metabolites.

Elimination

The major route of elimination of inhaled BDP appears to be via hydrolysis. More than 90% of inhaled BDP is found as 17-BMP in the systemic circulation. The mean elimination half-life of 17-BMP is 2.8 hours. Irrespective of the route of administration (injection, oral or inhalation), BDP and its metabolites are mainly excreted in the feces. Less than 10% of the drug and its metabolites are excreted in the urine.

Special Populations

Formal pharmacokinetic studies using QVAR were not conducted in any special populations.

Pediatrics

The pharmacokinetics of 17-BMP, including dose and strength proportionalities, is similar in children and adults, although the exposure is highly variable. In 17 children (mean age 10 years), the C_{max} of 17-BMP was 787 pg/ml at 0.6 hour after inhalation of 160 mcg (four actuations of the 40 mcg/actuation strength of HFA beclomethasone dipropionate). The systemic exposure to 17-BMP from 160 mcg of HFA-BDP administered without a spacer was comparable to the systemic exposure to 17-BMP from 336 mcg CFC-BDP administered with a large volume spacer in 14 children (mean age 12 years). This implies that approximately twice the systemic exposure to 17-BMP would be expected for comparable mg doses of HFA-BDP without a spacer and CFC-BDP with a large volume spacer.

Pharmacodynamics

Improvement in asthma control following inhalation can occur within 24 hours of beginning treatment in some patients, although maximum benefit may not be achieved for 1 to 2 weeks, or longer. The effects of QVAR on the hypothalamic-pituitary-adrenal (HPA) axis were studied in 40 corticosteroid naive patients. QVAR, at doses of 80, 160 or 320 mcg twice daily was compared with placebo and 336 mcg twice daily of beclomethasone dipropionate in a CFC propellant based formulation (CFC-BDP). Active treatment groups showed an expected dose-related reduction in 24-hour urinary free cortisol (a sensitive marker of adrenal production of cortisol). Patients treated with the highest recommended dose of QVAR (320 mcg twice daily) had a 37.3% reduction in 24-hour urinary free cortisol compared to a reduction of 47.3% produced by treatment with 336 mcg twice daily of CFC-BDP. There was a 12.2% reduction in 24 hour urinary free cortisol seen in the group of patients that received 80 mcg twice daily of QVAR and a 24.6% reduction in the group of patients that received 160 mcg twice daily. An open label study of 354 asthma patients given QVAR at recommended doses for one year assessed the effect of QVAR treatment on the HPA axis (as measured by both morning and stimulated plasma cortisol). Less than 1% of patients treated for one year with QVAR had an abnormal response (peak less than 18 mcg/dL) to short-cosyntropin test.

CLINICAL TRIALS

Blinded, randomized, parallel, placebo-controlled and active-controlled clinical studies were conducted in 940 adult asthma patients to assess the efficacy and safety of QVAR in the treatment of asthma. Fixed doses ranging from 40 mcg to 160 mcg twice daily were compared to placebo, and doses ranging from 40 mcg to 320 mcg twice daily were compared with doses of 42 mcg to 336 mcg twice daily of an active CFC-BDP comparator. These studies provided information about appropriate dosing through a range of asthma severity. A blinded, randomized, parallel, placebo-controlled study was conducted in 353 pediatric patients (age 5–12 years) to assess the efficacy and safety of HFA beclomethasone dipropionate in the treatment of asthma. Fixed doses of 40 mcg and 80 mcg twice daily were compared to placebo in this study. In these adult and pediatric efficacy trials, at the doses studied, measures of pulmonary function [forced expiratory volume in 1 second (FEV_1) and morning peak expiratory flow (AM PEF)] and asthma symptoms were significantly improved with QVAR treatment when compared to placebo.

In controlled clinical trials with adult patients not adequately controlled with beta-agonist alone, QVAR was effective at improving asthma control at doses as low as 40 mcg twice daily (80 mcg/day). Comparable asthma control was achieved at lower daily doses of QVAR than with CFC-BDP. Treatment with increasing doses of both QVAR and CFC-BDP generally resulted in increased improvement in FEV_1. In this trial the improvement in FEV_1 across doses was greater for QVAR than for CFC-BDP, indicating a shift in the dose response curve for QVAR.

Patients Not Previously Receiving Corticosteroid Therapy

In a 6 week clinical trial, 270 steroid naive patients with symptomatic asthma being treated with as-needed beta-agonist bronchodilators, were randomized to receive either 40 mcg twice daily of QVAR, 80 mcg twice daily of QVAR, or placebo. Both doses of QVAR were effective in improving asthma control with significantly greater improvements in FEV_1, AM PEF, and asthma symptoms than with placebo. Shown below is the change from baseline in AM PEF during this trial.

A 6-Week Clinical Trial in Patients with Mild to Moderate Asthma Not on Corticosteriod Therapy Prior to Study Entry: Mean Change in AM PEF

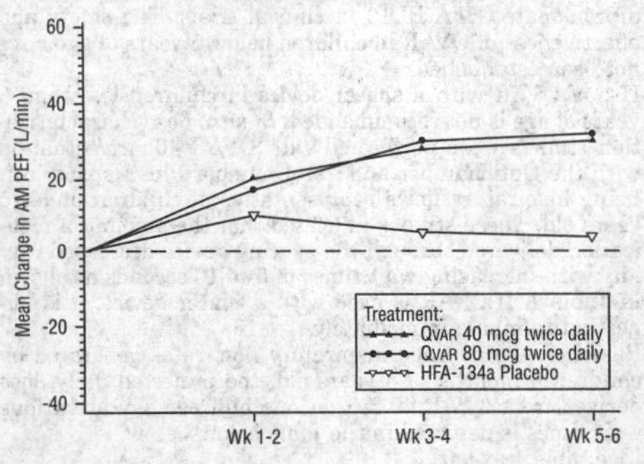

In a 6-week clinical trial, 256 patients with symptomatic asthma being treated with as-needed beta-agonist bronchodilators, were randomized to receive either 160 mcg twice daily of QVAR (delivered as either 40 mcg/actuation or 80 mcg/actuation) or placebo. Treatment with QVAR significantly improved asthma control, as assessed by FEV_1, AM PEF, and asthma symptoms, when compared to treatment with placebo. Comparable improvement in AM PEF was seen for patients receiving 160 mcg twice daily QVAR from the 40 mcg and 80 mcg strength products.

Patients Responsive to a Short Course of Oral Corticosteroids

In another clinical trial, 347 patients with symptomatic asthma, being treated with as-needed inhaled beta-agonist bronchodilators and, in some cases, inhaled corticosteroids, were given a 7–12 day course of oral corticosteroids and then randomized to receive either 320 mcg daily of QVAR, 672 mcg of CFC-BDP, or placebo. Patients treated with either QVAR or CFC-BDP had significantly better asthma control, as assessed by AM PEF, FEV_1 and asthma symptoms, and fewer study withdrawals due to asthma symptoms, than those treated with placebo over 12 weeks of treatment. A daily dose of 320 mcg QVAR administered in divided doses provided comparable control of AM PEF and FEV_1 as 672 mcg of CFC-BDP. Shown below are the mean AM PEF results from this trial.

A 12-Week Clinical Trial in Moderate Symptomatic Patients with Asthma Responding to Oral Corticosteroid Therapy: Mean AM PEF by Study Week

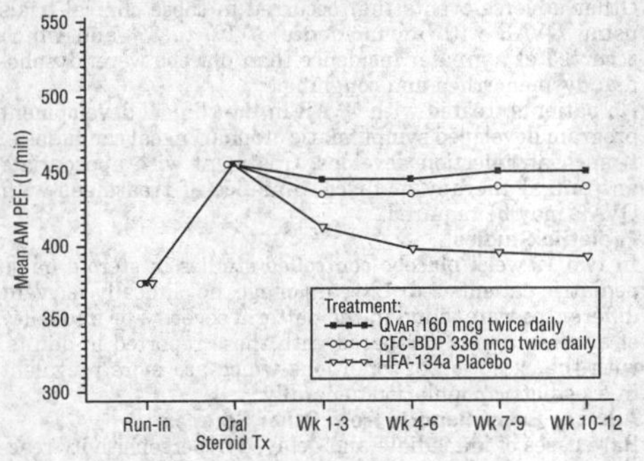

Patients Previously on Inhaled Corticosteroids

In a 6-week clinical trial, 323 patients, who exhibited a deterioration in asthma control during an inhaled corticosteroid washout period, were randomized to daily treatment with either 40, 160, or 320 mcg twice daily QVAR or 42, 168, or 336 mcg twice daily CFC-BDP. Treatment with increasing doses of both QVAR and CFC-BDP resulted in increased improvement in FEV_1, $FEF_{25-75\%}$ *(forced expiratory flow over 25–75% of the vital capacity), and asthma symptoms.* Shown below is the change from baseline in FEV_1 as percent predicted after 6 weeks of treatment.

[See figure at top of next column]

Patients Previously Maintained on Oral Corticosteroids

Clinical experience has shown that some patients with asthma who require oral corticosteroid therapy for control of symptoms can be partially or completely withdrawn from

A 6-Week Dose Response Clinical Trial in Patients with Inhaled Corticosteroid Dependent Asthma: Mean Change in FEV_1 as Percent of Predicted

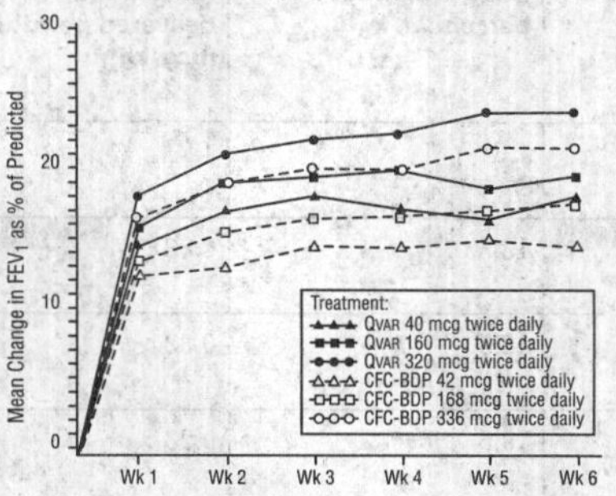

oral corticosteroids if therapy with beclomethasone dipropionate aerosol is substituted. Inhaled corticosteroids may not be effective for all patients with asthma or at all stages of the disease in a given patient.

Pediatric Experience

In one 12-week clinical trial, pediatric patients (age 5–12 years) with symptomatic asthma (N=353) being treated with as-needed beta-agonist bronchodilators were randomized to receive either 40 mcg or 80 mcg twice daily of HFA beclomethasone dipropionate or placebo. Both doses were effective in improving asthma control with significantly greater improvements in FEV_1 (9% and 10% predicted change from baseline at week 12 in FEV_1 percent predicted, respectively) than with placebo (4% predicted change).

INDICATIONS AND USAGE

QVAR is indicated in the maintenance treatment of asthma as prophylactic therapy in patients 5 years of age and older. QVAR is also indicated for asthma patients who require systemic corticosteroid administration, where adding QVAR may reduce or eliminate the need for the systemic corticosteroids.

Beclomethasone dipropionate is NOT indicated for the relief of acute bronchospasm.

CONTRAINDICATIONS

QVAR is contraindicated in the primary treatment of status asthmaticus or other acute episodes of asthma where intensive measures are required. Hypersensitivity to any of the ingredients of this preparation contraindicates its use.

WARNINGS

Particular care is needed in patients who are transferred from systemically active corticosteroids to QVAR because deaths due to adrenal insufficiency have occurred in asthmatic patients during and after transfer from systemic corticosteroids to less systemically available inhaled corticosteroids. After withdrawal from systemic corticosteroids, a number of months are required for recovery of hypothalamic-pituitary-adrenal (HPA) function.

Patients who have been previously maintained on 20 mg or more per day of prednisone (or its equivalent) may be most susceptible, particularly when their systemic corticosteroids have been almost completely withdrawn. During this period of HPA suppression, patients may exhibit signs and symptoms of adrenal insufficiency when exposed to trauma, surgery, or infections (particularly gastroenteritis) or other conditions with severe electrolyte loss. Although QVAR may provide control of asthmatic symptoms during these episodes, in recommended doses it supplies less than normal physiological amounts of glucocorticoid systemically and does NOT provide the mineralocorticoid that is necessary for coping with these emergencies.

During periods of stress or a severe asthmatic attack, patients who have been withdrawn from systemic corticosteroids should be instructed to resume oral corticosteroids (in large doses) immediately and to contact their physician for further instruction. These patients should also be instructed to carry a warning card indicating that they may need supplementary systemic steroids during periods of stress or a severe asthma attack.

Transfer of patients from systemic steroid therapy to QVAR may unmask allergic conditions previously suppressed by the systemic steroid therapy, e.g., rhinitis, conjunctivitis, and eczema.

Persons who are on drugs which suppress the immune system are more susceptible to infections than healthy individuals. Chickenpox and measles, for example, can have a more serious or even fatal course in non-immune children or adults on corticosteroids. In such children or adults who have not had these diseases or been properly immunized, particular care should be taken to avoid exposure. It is not known how the dose, route and duration of corticosteroid administration affects the risk of developing a disseminated infection. Nor is the contribution of the underlying disease and/or prior corticosteroid treatment known. If exposed to chickenpox, prophylaxis with varicella-zoster immune globulin (VZIG) may be indicated. If exposed to measles, prophylaxis with pooled intramuscular immunoglobulin (IG) may be indicated. (See the respective package inserts for complete VZIG and IG prescribing information.) If chickenpox develops, treatment with antiviral agents may be considered.

QVAR is not a bronchodilator and is not indicated for rapid relief of bronchospasm.

As with other inhaled asthma medications, bronchospasm, with an immediate increase in wheezing, may occur after dosing. If bronchospasm occurs following dosing with QVAR, it should be treated immediately with a short acting inhaled bronchodilator. Treatment with QVAR should be discontinued and alternate therapy instituted. Patients should be instructed to contact their physician immediately when episodes of asthma, which are not responsive to bronchodilators, occur during the course of treatment with QVAR. During such episodes, patients may require therapy with oral corticosteroids.

PRECAUTIONS

General

During withdrawal from oral corticosteroids, some patients may experience symptoms of systemically active corticosteroid withdrawal, e.g., joint and/or muscular pain, lassitude and depression, despite maintenance or even improvement of respiratory function. Although suppression of HPA function below the clinical normal range did not occur with doses of QVAR up to and including 640 mcg/day, a dose dependent reduction of adrenal cortisol production was observed. Since inhaled beclomethasone dipropionate is absorbed into the circulation and can be systemically active, HPA axis suppression by QVAR could occur when recommended doses are exceeded or in particularly sensitive individuals. Since individual sensitivity to effects on cortisol production exist, physicians should consider this information when prescribing QVAR. Because of the possibility of systemic absorption of inhaled corticosteroids, patients treated with these drugs should be observed carefully for any evidence of systemic corticosteroid effect. Particular care should be taken in observing patients postoperatively or during periods of stress for evidence of inadequate adrenal response.

It is possible that systemic corticosteroid effects, such as hypercorticism and adrenal suppression, may appear in a small number of patients, particularly at higher doses. If such changes occur, QVAR should be reduced slowly, consistent with accepted procedures for management of asthma symptoms and for tapering of systemic steroids.

A 12 month randomized controlled clinical trial evaluated the effects of HFA beclomethasone dipropionate without spacer versus CFC beclomethasone dipropionate with large volume spacer on growth in children age 5–11. A total of 520 patients were enrolled, of whom 394 received HFA-BDP (100–400 mcg/day ex-valve) and 126 received CFC-BDP (200–800 mcg/day ex-valve). Similar control of asthma was noted in each treatment arm. When comparing results at month 12 to baseline, the mean growth velocity in children treated with HFA-BDP was approximately 0.5 cm/year less than that noted with children treated with CFC-BDP via large volume spacer.

A reduction in growth velocity in growing children may occur as a result of inadequate control of chronic diseases such as asthma or from use of corticosteroids for treatment. Physicians should closely follow the growth of all pediatric patients taking corticosteroids by any route and weigh the benefits of corticosteroid therapy and asthma control against the possibility of growth suppression.

The long-term and systemic effects of QVAR in humans are still not fully known. In particular, the effects resulting from chronic use of the agent on developmental or immunologic processes in the mouth, pharynx, trachea, and lung are unknown.

Inhaled corticosteroids should be used with caution, if at all, in patients with active or quiescent tuberculosis infection of the respiratory tract; untreated systemic fungal, bacterial, parasitic or viral infections; or ocular herpes simplex.

Rare instances of glaucoma, increased intraocular pressure, and cataracts have been reported following the inhaled administration of corticosteroids.

Information for Patients

Patients being treated with QVAR should receive the following information and instructions. This information is intended to aid them in the safe and effective use of this medication. It is not a disclosure of all possible adverse or intended effects.

Persons who are on immunosuppressant doses of corticosteroids should be warned to avoid exposure to chickenpox or measles. Patients should also be advised that if they are exposed to these diseases, medical advice should be sought without delay.

Patients should use QVAR at regular intervals as directed. Results of clinical trials indicated significant improvements

TABLE 1

	Wait time, seconds	Mean medication delivery through AeroChamber, mcg/actuation*	Body Weight 50th percentile, kg†	Medication delivered per dose, mcg/kg‡,§
Age 6 months, Flow rate 4.8 L/min	0	11.5	7.6	1.2
Age 2 years, Flow rate 8.2 L/min	0	14.1	13.5	0.83
Age 2 years, Flow rate 8.2 L/min	5	5.4	13.5	0.32
Age 2 years, Flow rate 8.2 L/min	10	3.9	13.5	0.23
Age 5 years, Flow rate 11.0 L/min	0	17.5	18	0.78

* Summary Report; Pediatric Dose Characterization of QVAR with Spacer; 3M Pharmaceutical Development, July 21, 2004.
† CDC Growth charts, developed by the National Center for Health Statistics in collaboration with the National Center for Chronic Disease Prevention and Health Promotion (2000).
‡ Includes an estimated 20% loss in the masks
§ QVAR 40mcg in an average adult without using a spacer delivers approximately 0.4 mcg/kg, or bid, 0.8 mcg/kg/day.

Adverse Events Reported by at Least 3% of the Patients for Either QVAR or CFC-BDP by Treatment and Daily Dose

Adverse Events	Placebo (N = 289) %	QVAR				CFC-BDP			
		Total (N = 624) %	80–160 mcg (N = 233) %	320 mcg (N = 335) %	640 mcg (N = 56) %	Total (N = 283) %	84 mcg (N = 59) %	336 mcg (N = 55) %	672 mcg (N = 169) %
HEADACHE	9	12	15	8	25	15	14	11	17
PHARYNGITIS	4	8	6	5	27	10	12	9	10
UPPER RESP TRACT INFECTION	11	9	7	11	5	12	3	9	17
RHINITIS	9	6	8	3	7	11	15	9	10
INCREASED ASTHMA SYMPTOMS	18	3	3	4	0	8	14	5	7
ORAL SYMPTOMS INHALATION ROUTE	2	3	3	3	2	6	7	5	5
SINUSITIS	2	3	3	3	0	4	7	2	4
PAIN	<1	2	1	2	5	3	3	5	2
BACK PAIN	1	1	2	<1	4	4	2	4	4
NAUSEA	0	1	<1	1	2	3	5	5	1
DYSPHONIA	2	<1	1	0	4	4	0	0	6

may occur within the first 24 hours of treatment in some patients; however, the full benefit may not be achieved until treatment has been administered for 1 to 2 weeks, or longer. The patient should not increase the prescribed dosage but should contact their physician if symptoms do not improve or if the condition worsens.

Patients should be advised that QVAR is not intended for use in the treatment of acute asthma. The patient should be instructed to contact their physician immediately if there is any deterioration of their asthma.

Patients should be instructed on the proper use of their inhaler. Patients may wish to rinse their mouth after QVAR use. The patient should be advised that QVAR may have a different taste and inhalation sensation than that of an inhaler containing CFC propellant.

QVAR use should not be stopped abruptly. The patient should contact their physician immediately if use of QVAR is discontinued.

For the proper use of QVAR, the patient should read and carefully follow the accompanying Patient's Instructions.

Carcinogenesis, Mutagenesis, Impairment of Fertility
The carcinogenicity of beclomethasone dipropionate was evaluated in rats which were exposed for a total of 95 weeks, 13 weeks at inhalation doses up to 0.4 mg/kg/day and the remaining 82 weeks at combined oral and inhalation doses up to 2.4 mg/kg/day. There was no evidence of carcinogenicity in this study at the highest dose, which is approximately 30 and 55 times the maximum recommended daily inhalation dose in adults and children, respectively, on a mg/m² basis.
Beclomethasone dipropionate did not induce gene mutation in the bacterial cells or mammalian Chinese Hamster ovary

(CHO) cells in vitro. No significant clastogenic effect was seen in cultured CHO cells in vitro or in the mouse micronucleus test in vivo.

In rats, beclomethasone dipropionate caused decreased conception rates at an oral dose of 16 mg/kg/day (approximately 200 times the maximum recommended daily inhalation dose in adults on a mg/m² basis). Impairment of fertility, as evidence by inhibition of the estrous cycle in dogs, was observed following treatment by the oral route at a dose of 0.5 mg/kg/day (approximately 20 times the maximum recommended daily inhalation dose in adults on a mg/m² basis). No inhibition of the estrous cycle in dogs was seen following 12 months of exposure to beclomethasone dipropionate by the Inhalation route at an estimated daily dose of 0.33 mg/kg (approximately 15 times the maximum recommended daily inhalation dose in adults on a mg/m² basis).

Pregnancy
Teratogenic Effects
Pregnancy Category C
Like other corticosteroids, parenteral (subcutaneous) beclomethasone dipropionate was teratogenic and embryocidal in the mouse and rabbit when given at a dose of 0.1 mg/kg/day in mice or at a dose of 0.025 mg/kg/day in rabbits. These doses in mice and rabbits were approximately one-half the maximum recommended daily inhalation dose in adults on a mg/m² basis. No teratogenicity or embryocidal effects were seen in rats when exposed to an inhalation dose of 15 mg/kg/day (approximately 190 times the maximum recommended daily inhalation dose in adults on a mg/m² basis). There are no adequate and well controlled studies in pregnant women. Beclomethasone dipropionate should be used during pregnancy only if the potential benefit justifies the potential risk to the fetus.

Non-teratogenic Effects
Findings of drug-related adrenal toxicity in fetuses following administration of beclomethasone dipropionate to rats suggest that infants born of mothers receiving substantial doses of QVAR during pregnancy should be observed for adrenal suppression.
Nursing Mothers
Corticosteroids are secreted in human milk. Because of the potential for serious adverse reactions in nursing infants from QVAR, a decision should be made whether to discontinue nursing or to discontinue the drug, taking into account the importance of the drug to the mother.
Pediatric Use
Eight-hundred and thirty-four children between the ages of 5 and 12 were treated with HFA beclomethasone dipropionate (HFA BDP) in clinical trials. The safety and effectiveness of QVAR in children below 5 years of age have not been established.
Use of QVAR with a spacer device in children less than 5 years of age is not recommended. In vitro dose characterization studies were performed with QVAR 40 mcg/actuation with the Optichamber and AeroChamber Plus® spacer utilizing inspiratory flows representative of children under 5 years old. These studies indicated that the amount of medication delivered through the spacing device decreased rapidly with increasing wait times of 5 to 10 seconds as shown in Table 1. If QVAR is used with a spacer device, it is important to inhale immediately.
Based on the average inspiratory flow rates generated by children 6 months to 5 years old, the projected daily dose derived from QVAR 40 mcg at one puff per day at various wait times is depicted in the table below:
[See table 1 at left]
Oral inhaled corticosteroids have been shown to cause a reduction in growth velocity in children and teenagers with extended use. If a child or teenager on any corticosteroid appears to have growth suppression, the possibility that they are particularly sensitive to this effect of corticosteroids should be considered (see PRECAUTIONS, General).
Geriatric Use
Clinical studies of QVAR did not include sufficient numbers of subjects aged 65 and over to determine whether they respond differently from younger subjects. Other reported clinical experience has not identified differences in responses between the elderly and younger patients. In general, dose selection for an elderly patient should be cautious, usually starting at the low end of the dosing range, reflecting the greater frequency of decreased hepatic, renal, or cardiac function, and of concomitant disease or other drug therapy.

ADVERSE REACTIONS

The following reporting rates of common adverse experiences are based upon four clinical trials in which 1196 Patients (671 female and 525 male adults previously treated with as-needed bronchodilators and/or inhaled corticosteroids) were treated with QVAR (doses of 40, 80, 160, or 320 mcg twice daily) or CFC-BDP (doses of 42, 168, or 336 mcg twice daily) or placebo. The table below includes all events reported by patients taking QVAR (whether considered drug related or not) that occurred at a rate over 3% for either QVAR or CFC-BDP. In considering these data, difference in average duration of exposure and clinical trial design should be taken into account.
[See second table at left]
Other adverse events that occurred in these clinical trials using QVAR with an incidence of 1% to 3% and which occurred at a greater incidence than placebo were: dysphonia, dysmenorrhea and coughing.
No patients treated with QVAR in the clinical development program developed symptomatic oropharyngeal candidiasis. If such an infection develops, treatment with appropriate antifungal therapy or discontinuance of treatment with QVAR may be required.
Pediatric Studies
In two 12-week placebo controlled studies in steroid naive pediatric patients 5 to 12 years of age, no clinically relevant differences were found in the pattern, severity, or frequency of adverse events compared with those reported in adults, with the exception of conditions which are more prevalent in a pediatric population generally.
Adverse Event Reports from Other Sources
Rare cases of immediate and delayed hypersensitivity reactions, including urticaria, angioedema, rash, and bronchospasm, have been reported following the oral and intranasal inhalation of beclomethasone dipropionate.

OVERDOSAGE

There were no deaths over 15 days following the oral administration of a single dose of 3000 mg/kg in mice, 2000 mg/kg in rats, and 1000 mg/kg in rabbits. The doses in mice, rats, and rabbits were 19,000, 25,000, and 25,000 times, respectively, the maximum recommended daily inhalation in adults or 36,000, 48,000, and 48,000 times, respectively the maximum recommended daily inhalation dose in children on a mg/m² basis.

DOSAGE AND ADMINISTRATION

Patients should prime QVAR by actuating into the air twice before using for the first time or if QVAR has not been used for over ten days. Avoid spraying in the eyes or face when priming QVAR. QVAR is a solution aerosol, which does not require shaking. Consistent dose delivery is achieved, whether using the 40 or 80 mcg strengths, due to proportionality of the two products (i.e., two actuations of 40 mcg strength should provide a dose comparable to one actuation of the 80 mcg strength).

QVAR should be administered by the oral inhaled route in patients 5 years of age and older. Use of QVAR with a spacer device in children less than 5 years of age is not recommended (see PRECAUTIONS, Pediatric Use). The onset and degree of symptom relief will vary in individual patients. Improvement in asthma symptoms should be expected within the first or second week of starting treatment, but maximum benefit should not be expected until 3–4 weeks of therapy. For patients who do not respond adequately to the starting dose after 3–4 weeks of therapy, higher doses may provide additional asthma control. The safety and efficacy of QVAR when administered in excess of recommended doses has not been established.

[See table at top right]

As with any inhaled corticosteroid, physicians are advised to titrate the dose of QVAR downward over time to the lowest level that maintains proper asthma control. This is particularly important in children since a controlled study has shown that QVAR has the potential to affect growth in children. Patients should be instructed on the proper use of their inhaler.

Patients Not Receiving Systemic Corticosteroids

Patients who require maintenance therapy of their asthma may benefit from treatment with QVAR at the doses recommended above. In patients who respond to QVAR, improvement in pulmonary function is usually apparent within 1 to 4 weeks after the start of therapy. Once the desired effect is achieved, consideration should be given to tapering to the lowest effective dose.

Patients Maintained on Systemic Corticosteroids

QVAR may be effective in the management of asthmatics maintained on systemic corticosteroids and may permit replacement or significant reduction in the dosage of systemic corticosteroids.

The patient's asthma should be reasonably stable before treatment with QVAR is started. Initially, QVAR should be used concurrently with the patient's usual maintenance dose of systemic corticosteroids. After approximately one week, gradual withdrawal of the systemic corticosteroids is started by reducing the daily or alternate daily dose. Reductions may be made after an interval of one or two weeks, depending on the response of the patient. A slow rate of withdrawal is strongly recommended. Generally these decrements should not exceed 2.5 mg of prednisone or its equivalent. During withdrawal, some patients may experience symptoms of systemic corticosteroid withdrawal, e.g. joint and/or muscular pain, lassitude and depression, despite maintenance or even improvement in pulmonary function. Such patients should be encouraged to continue with the inhaler but should be monitored for objective signs of adrenal insufficiency. If evidence of adrenal insufficiency occurs, the systemic corticosteroid doses should be increased temporarily and thereafter withdrawal should continue more slowly. During periods of stress or a severe asthma attack, transfer patients may require supplementary treatment with systemic corticosteroids.

DIRECTIONS FOR USE

Illustrated Patient's Instructions for proper use accompany each package of QVAR.

HOW SUPPLIED

QVAR is supplied in two strengths:

QVAR 40 mcg is supplied in a 7.3 g canister containing 100 actuations with a beige plastic actuator and gray dust cap, and Patient's Instructions; box of one; 100 Actuations – NDC 59310-175-40

QVAR 80 mcg is supplied in a 7.3 g canister containing 100 actuations with a dark mauve plastic actuator and gray dust cap, and Patient's Instructions; box of one; 100 Actuations – NDC 59310-177-80

The correct amount of medication in each inhalation cannot be assured after 100 actuations from the 7.3 g canister even though the canister is not completely empty. The canister should be discarded when the labeled number of actuations have been used.

Store QVAR Inhalation Aerosol when not being used, so that the product rests on the concave end of the canister with the plastic actuator on top.

Store at 25°C (77°F).

Excursions between 15° and 30°C (59° and 86°F) are permitted (see USP). For optimal results, the canister should be at room temperature when used. QVAR Inhalation Aerosol canister should only be used with the QVAR Inhalation Aerosol actuator and the actuator should not be used with any other inhalation drug product.

Recommended Dosage for QVAR:

Previous Therapy	Recommended Starting Dose	Highest Recommended Dose
Adults and Adolescents:		
Bronchodilators Alone	40 to 80 mcg twice daily	320 mcg twice daily
Inhaled Corticosteroids	40 to 160 mcg twice daily	320 mcg twice daily
Children 5 to 11 years:		
Bronchodilators Alone	40 mcg twice daily	80 mcg twice daily
Inhaled Corticosteroids	40 mcg twice daily	80 mcg twice daily

CONTENTS UNDER PRESSURE

Do not puncture. Do not use or store near heat or open flame. Exposure to temperatures above 49°C (120°F) may cause bursting. Never throw container into fire or incinerator.

Keep out of reach of children.

Rx only

Mktd by:
Teva Specialty Pharmaceuticals LLC– Horsham, PA 19044
Developed and
Manufactured by:
3M Drug Delivery Systems
Northridge, CA 91324
OR
3M Health Care, Ltd.
Loughborough, UK
August 2008
© 2008 Teva Specialty Pharmaceuticals LLC
634600
QVAR® is a registered trademark of the IVAX Corporation, a member of the TEVA Group.
Rev. 08/08
OptiChamber is a registered trademark of Respironics Healthscan, Inc. and AeroChamber Plus is a registered trademark of Trudell Medical International Trudell Partnership Holdings Limited and Packard Medical Supply Centre Ltd.

PATIENT'S INSTRUCTIONS

QVAR®

(beclomethasone dipropionate HFA)

INHALATION AEROSOL

Attention Pharmacist: Detach "Patient's Instructions for Use" from package insert and dispense with the product.

PATIENT'S INSTRUCTIONS

It is important that you read these instructions before using QVAR.

Correct and regular use of the inhaler will prevent or lessen the severity of asthma attacks.

1. Remove the plastic cap (see Figure 1) and be sure there are no foreign objects in the mouthpiece.

Figure 1

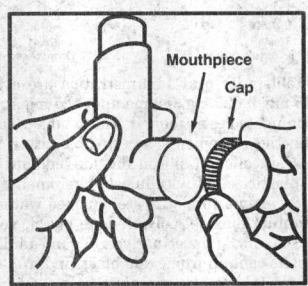

Mouthpiece
Cap

2. As with all aerosol medications, it is recommended to prime the QVAR inhaler before using for the very first time after purchase, and in cases where the inhaler has not been used for more than ten days. Prime by releasing two actuations into the air, away from your eyes and face. Be sure the canister is firmly seated in the plastic mouthpiece adapter before each use.

3. BREATHE OUT AS FULLY AS YOU COMFORTABLY CAN. Hold the inhaler as shown in Figure 2. Close your lips around the mouthpiece, keeping your tongue below it. [See figure 2 at top of next column]

4. WHILE BREATHING IN DEEPLY AND SLOWLY, PRESS DOWN ON THE CAN WITH YOUR FINGER. When you have finished breathing in, hold your breath as long as you comfortably can (i.e., 5–10 seconds).

5. TAKE YOUR FINGER OFF THE CAN and remove the inhaler from your mouth. Breathe out gently.

6. If your physician has told you to take more than one inhalation per treatment repeat steps 3 through 5.

7. You should rinse your mouth with water after treatment.

8. For normal hygiene, the mouthpiece of your inhaler should be cleaned weekly with a clean, dry tissue or cloth. DO NOT WASH OR PUT ANY PART OF YOUR INHALER IN WATER.

Figure 2

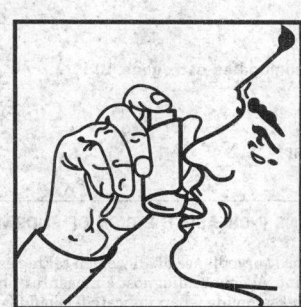

9. DISCARD THE CANISTER AFTER the date calculated by your physician or pharmacist. The correct amount of medication in each inhalation cannot be assured after 100 actuations from the 7.3 g canister even though the canister is not completely empty. The canister should be discarded when the labeled number of actuations have been used. Before the discard date you should consult your physician to determine whether a refill is needed. It is advisable to keep track of the number of doses taken from the canister to better predict when a refill is necessary. Just as you should not take extra doses without consulting your physician, you also should not stop taking QVAR without consulting your physician.

IMPORTANT QVAR is preventive therapy for asthma and must be used regularly and at the times your physician has prescribed.

DO NOT CONFUSE QVAR WITH OTHER ASTHMA MEDICATION. QVAR WILL NOT PROVIDE IMMEDIATE RELIEF IF YOU ARE HAVING AN ASTHMA ATTACK.

Your physician will decide whether other medication is needed should you require immediate relief. If you also use another medicine by inhalation, you should consult your physician for instructions on when to use it in relation to using QVAR. If this is the first time you will be using QVAR, it may take from 1 to 4 weeks before you feel the full benefits.

QVAR Inhalation Aerosol canister should only be used with the QVAR Inhalation Aerosol mouthpiece and the mouthpiece should not be used with any other inhalation drug product.

DOSAGE

Use only as directed by your physician.

CONTENTS UNDER PRESSURE

Do not puncture. Do not use or store near heat or open flame. Exposure to temperatures above 49°C (120°F) may cause bursting. Never throw container into fire or incinerator.

Keep out of reach of children.

Avoid spraying in eyes.

Store at 25°C (77°F). For optimal results, the canister should be at room temperature when used. Store QVAR Inhalation Aerosol when not being used, so that the product rests on the concave end of the canister with the plastic actuator on top.

Mktd by:
Teva Specialty Pharmaceuticals LLC
Horsham, PA 19044
Developed and
Manufactured by:
3M Drug Delivery Systems
Northridge, CA 91324
OR
3M Health Care, Ltd.
Loughborough, UK
© 2008 Teva Specialty Pharmaceuticals LLC
QVAR® is a registered trademark of the IVAX Corporation, a member of the TEVA Group.
634600
Rev. 08/08

Shown in Product Identification Guide, page 320

Teva Women's Health, Inc.
400 CHESTNUT RIDGE ROAD
WOODCLIFF LAKE, NJ 07677

Direct Inquiries for ParaGard to:
877-727-2427
Direct Inquiries for Plan B and Plan B One-Step to:
800-330-1271
All Other Inquiries to:
800-222-0190

ENJUVIA®
[ĕn-jew-vē-ă]
(synthetic conjugated estrogens, B)
Tablets
11001651
R̥ only
Package Insert

R̥

ESTROGENS INCREASE THE RISK OF ENDOMETRIAL CANCER

Close clinical surveillance of all women taking estrogens is important. Adequate diagnostic measures, including endometrial sampling when indicated, should be undertaken to rule out malignancy in all cases of undiagnosed persistent or recurring abnormal vaginal bleeding. There is no evidence that the use of "natural" estrogens results in a different endometrial risk profile than synthetic estrogens at equivalent estrogen doses. (See **WARNINGS, Malignant neoplasms, *Endometrial cancer*.**)

CARDIOVASCULAR AND OTHER RISKS

Estrogens with or without progestins should not be used for the prevention of cardiovascular disease or dementia. (See **CLINICAL STUDIES** and **WARNINGS, Cardiovascular disorders** and **Dementia**.)

The estrogen alone substudy of the Women's Health Initiative (WHI) reported increased risks of stroke and deep vein thrombosis (DVT) in postmenopausal women (50 to 79 years of age) during 6.8 years and 7.1 years, respectively, of treatment with oral conjugated estrogens (CE 0.625 mg) alone per day, relative to placebo. (See **CLINICAL STUDIES** and **WARNINGS, Cardiovascular disorders**.)

The estrogen-plus-progestin substudy of the WHI reported increased risks of myocardial infarction, stroke, invasive breast cancer, pulmonary emboli, and deep vein thrombosis in postmenopausal women (50 to 79 years of age) during 5.6 years of treatment with oral conjugated estrogens (CE 0.625 mg) combined with medroxyprogesterone acetate (MPA 2.5 mg) per day, relative to placebo. (See **CLINICAL STUDIES**, and **WARNINGS, Cardiovascular disorders** and **Malignant neoplasms, *Breast cancer*.**)

The Women's Health Initiative Memory Study (WHIMS), a substudy of WHI study, reported increased risk of developing probable dementia in postmenopausal women 65 years of age or older during 5.2 years of treatment with CE 0.625 mg alone and during 4 years of treatment with CE 0.625 mg combined with MPA 2.5 mg, relative to placebo. It is unknown whether this finding applies to younger postmenopausal women. (See **CLINICAL STUDIES**, **WARNINGS, Dementia** and **PRECAUTIONS, Geriatric Use**.)

Other doses of conjugated estrogens and medroxyprogesterone acetate, and other combinations and dosage forms of estrogens and progestins, were not studied in the WHI clinical trials, and in the absence of comparable data, these risks should be assumed to be similar. Because of these risks, estrogens with or without progestins should be prescribed at the lowest effective doses and for the shortest duration consistent with treatment goals and risks for the individual woman.

DESCRIPTION

ENJUVIA® (synthetic conjugated estrogens, B) tablets contain a blend of ten (10) synthetic estrogenic substances. The estrogenic substances are: sodium estrone sulfate, sodium equilin sulfate, sodium 17α-dihydroequilin sulfate, sodium 17α-estradiol sulfate, sodium 17β-dihydroequilin sulfate, sodium 17α-dihydroequilenin sulfate, sodium 17β-dihydroequilenin sulfate, sodium equilenin sulfate, sodium 17β-estradiol sulfate, and sodium $\Delta^{8,9}$-dehydroestrone sulfate.

The structural formulae for these estrogens are:

$C_{18}H_{21}NaO_5S$
372.42
Sodium Estrone Sulfate

$C_{18}H_{19}NaO_5S$
370.41
Sodium Equilin Sulfate

$C_{18}H_{21}NaO_5S$
372.42
Sodium 17α-Dihydroequilin Sulfate

$C_{18}H_{23}NaO_5S$
374.44
Sodium 17α-Estradiol Sulfate

$C_{18}H_{21}NaO_5S$
372.42
Sodium 17β-Dihydroequilin Sulfate

$C_{18}H_{19}NaO_5S$
370.41
Sodium 17α-Dihydroequilenin Sulfate

$C_{18}H_{19}NaO_5S$
370.41
Sodium 17β-Dihydroequilenin Sulfate

$C_{18}H_{17}NaO_5S$
368.39
Sodium Equilenin Sulfate

$C_{18}H_{23}NaO_5S$
374.44
Sodium 17β-Estradiol Sulfate

$C_{18}H_{19}NaO_5S$
371.41
Sodium $\Delta^{8,9}$ dehydroestrone Sulfate

ENJUVIA tablets for oral administration are available in 0.3 mg, 0.45 mg, 0.625 mg, 0.9 mg and 1.25 mg strengths of synthetic conjugated estrogens, B. These tablets contain the following inactive ingredients: ascorbyl palmitate, butylated hydroxyanisole, colloidal silicon dioxide, edetate disodium dehydrate, plasticized ethylcellulose, hypromellose, lactose monohydrate, magnesium stearate, purified water, iron oxide red, titanium dioxide, polyethylene glycol, polysorbate 80, triacetate and triacetin/glycerol. In addition, the 0.45 mg tablets contain iron oxide black and iron oxide yellow; the 0.9 mg tablets also contain D&C yellow no. 10 aluminum lake, FD&C blue no. 1 aluminum lake and FD&C yellow no. 6 aluminum lake; and the 1.25 mg tablets contain iron oxide yellow.

CLINICAL PHARMACOLOGY

Endogenous estrogens are largely responsible for the development and maintenance of the female reproductive system and secondary sexual characteristics. Although circulating estrogens exist in a dynamic equilibrium of metabolic interconversions, estradiol is the principal intracellular human estrogen and is substantially more potent than its metabolites, estrone and estriol, at the receptor level.

The primary source of estrogen in normally cycling adult women is the ovarian follicle, which secretes 70 to 500 mcg of estradiol daily, depending on the phase of the menstrual cycle. After menopause, most endogenous estrogen is produced by conversion of androstenedione, secreted by the adrenal cortex, to estrone by peripheral tissues. Thus, estrone and the sulfate-conjugated form, estrone sulfate, are the most abundant circulating estrogens in postmenopausal women.

Estrogens act through binding to nuclear receptors in estrogen-responsive tissues. To date, two estrogen receptors have been identified. These vary in proportion from tissue to tissue.

Circulating estrogens modulate the pituitary secretion of the gonadotropins, luteinizing hormone (LH) and follicle-stimulating hormone (FSH), through a negative feedback mechanism. Estrogens act to reduce the elevated levels of these hormones in postmenopausal women.

A. Absorption

Synthetic conjugated estrogens, B are soluble in water and are well absorbed from the gastrointestinal tract after release from the drug formulation. ENJUVIA tablets release synthetic conjugated estrogens, B slowly over a period of several hours. Table 1 and Table 2 summarize the mean pharmacokinetic parameters for unconjugated (free) and conjugated (total) estrogens following single administration of two 0.625 mg tablets to 21 healthy postmenopausal women under fasting conditions. The effect of food on the bioavailability of synthetic conjugated estrogens, B following administration of ENJUVIA tablets has not been studied. However, the presence of food did not significantly affect the pharmacokinetics of a similar formulation of synthetic conjugated estrogens, B.

[See table 1 below]
[See table 2 at top of next page]

B. Distribution

The distribution of exogenous estrogens is similar to that of endogenous estrogens. Estrogens are widely distributed in the body and are generally found in higher concentrations in the sex hormone target organs. Estrogens circulate in the blood largely bound to sex hormone binding globulin (SHBG) and albumin.

C. Metabolism

Exogenous estrogens are metabolized in the same manner as endogenous estrogens. Circulating estrogens exist in a dynamic equilibrium of metabolic interconversions. These transformations take place mainly in the liver. Estradiol is converted reversibly to estrone, and both can be converted to estriol, which is the major urinary metabolite. Estrogens also undergo enterohepatic recirculation via sulfate and glucuronide conjugation in the liver, biliary secretion of conjugates into the intestine, and hydrolysis in the intestine followed by reabsorption. In postmenopausal women, a significant portion of the circulating estrogens exists as sulfate conjugates, especially estrone sulfate, which serves as a circulating reservoir for the formation of more active estrogens.

D. Excretion

Estradiol, estrone, and estriol are excreted in the urine along with glucuronide and sulfate conjugates. The mean (SD) apparent terminal elimination half-life ($t_{1/2}$) of conjugated estrone is 14 ($\pm$ 6) hours and conjugated equilin is 11 ($\pm$ 6) hours.

E. Special Populations

No pharmacokinetic studies were conducted in special populations, including patients with renal or hepatic impairment.

F. Drug Interactions

In vitro and *in vivo* studies have shown that estrogens are metabolized partially by cytochrome P450 3A4 (CYP3A4). Therefore, inducers or inhibitors of CYP3A4 may affect estrogen drug metabolism. Inducers of CYP3A4, such as St. John's Wort preparations (Hypericum perforatum), phenobarbital, carbamazepine, and rifampin, may reduce plasma concentrations of estrogens, possibly resulting in a decrease in therapeutic effects and/or changes in the uterine bleeding profile. Inhibitors of CYP3A4, such as erythromycin, clarithromycin, ketoconazole, itraconazole, ritonavir, and grapefruit juice, may increase plasma concentrations of estrogens and may result in side effects.

CLINICAL STUDIES

Effects on Vasomotor Symptoms

A randomized, double-blind, placebo-controlled, dose-ranging, multi-center clinical study was conducted to evaluate the safety and effectiveness of ENJUVIA tablets for the treatment of vasomotor symptoms in 281 naturally or surgically postmenopausal women aged 26 to 65 years who were experiencing a minimum of seven moderate to severe

Table 1. Mean Pharmacokinetic Parameters of Unconjugated (Free) Estrogens Following a Single Dose of 2 × 0.625 mg ENJUVIA Tablets Under Fasting Conditions*

	C_{max} (pg/mL)	t_{max} (hr)	$t_{1/2}$ (hr)	AUC_{0-48h} (pg·hr/mL)
Baseline-corrected estrone (% CV)	75.87 (39)	9.29 (25)	23.46 (59)	1601.59 (41)
Equilin (% CV)	41.94 (49)	8.38 (27)	15.09 (55)	707.21 (46)

C_{max} = peak plasma concentration; t_{max} = time peak concentration occurs; $t_{1/2}$ = apparent terminal-phase disposition half-life. AUC_{0-48h} = total area under the concentration-time curve from time zero to time of last quantifiable concentration (48h); * $\Delta^{8,9}$ Dehydroestrone (free) levels were below the assay limit of quantitation; CV = Coefficient of Variance

hot flushes per day or 50 per week at randomization. The majority (81%) of patients were Caucasian (n=228) and 17.4% were Black (n=49). Patients were randomized to receive ENJUVIA tablets 0.3 mg, 0.625 mg, 1.25 mg, or placebo once daily for 12 weeks.

ENJUVIA (0.3 mg, 0.625 mg and 1.25 mg tablets) was shown to be statistically better than placebo at weeks 4 and 12 for relief of both the frequency and severity of moderate to severe vasomotor symptoms (Table 3 and 4).

[See table 3 at right]

[See table 4 below]

Effects on Vulvar and Vaginal Atrophy

A randomized, double-blind, placebo-controlled, multi-center clinical study was conducted to evaluate the safety and effectiveness of ENJUVIA 0.3 mg tablets for the treatment of symptoms of vulvar and vaginal atrophy in 248 naturally or surgically postmenopausal women between 32 to 81 years of age (mean 58.6 years) who at baseline had ≤ 5% superficial cells on a vaginal smear, a vaginal pH > 5.0, and who identified their most bothersome moderate to severe symptom of vulvar and vaginal atrophy. The majority (82%) of the women were Caucasian (n=203), 11% were Hispanic (n=26), 4% were Black (n=9) and 3% were Asian (n=6). All patients were assessed for improvement in the mean change from baseline to Week 12 for three co-primary efficacy variables: most bothersome symptom of vulvar and vaginal atrophy (defined as the moderate to severe symptom that had been identified by the patient as most bothersome to her at baseline); percentage of vaginal superficial cells and percentage of vaginal parabasal cells; and vaginal pH.

In this study, a statistically significant mean change between baseline and week 12 for the group treated with ENJUVIA 0.3 mg tablets compared to placebo was observed for the symptoms, vaginal dryness and pain with intercourse. See Table 5. ENJUVIA 0.3 mg tablets increased superficial cells by a mean of 17.1% as compared to 2.0% for placebo (statistically significant). A corresponding statistically significant mean reduction from baseline in parabasal cells (41.7% for ENJUVIA 0.3 mg tablets and 6.8% for placebo) was observed at week 12. The mean reduction between baseline and week 12 in the pH was 1.69 in the ENJUVIA 0.3 mg tablets group and 0.45 in the placebo group (statistically significant).

Table 5. Change from Baseline to Week 12 in the Severity of Vaginal Dryness and Pain with Intercourse, Symptoms That Were Identified by the Menopausal Study Patient as Her Most Bothersome Symptom of Vulvar and Vaginal Atrophy at Baseline

Most Bothersome Symptom at Baseline*	ENJUVIA 0.3 mg	Placebo
Vaginal Dryness		
n	56	54
Baseline Severity	2.52	2.54
Mean Severity at Week 12	0.80	1.81
Mean Change in Severity from Baseline (s.d.)	-1.71 (0.85)	-0.72 (0.66)
p-value vs. placebo	<0.001	—
Pain With Intercourse		
n	35	40
Baseline Severity	2.74	2.70
Mean Severity at Week 12	0.94	1.95
Mean Change in Severity from Baseline (s.d.)	-1.80 (1.02)	-0.75 (0.95)
p-value vs. placebo	<0.001	—

* Treatment differences assessed by ANCOVA or rank ANCOVA (% cell data) with baseline as covariate for the modified intent-to-treat population, last-observation-carried-forward data set.

Women's Health Initiative Studies

The WHI enrolled approximately 27,000 predominantly healthy postmenopausal women in two substudies to assess the risks and benefits of either the use of oral conjugated estrogens (CE 0.625 mg) alone per day or in combination with medroxyprogesterone acetate (CE 0.625 mg/MPA 2.5 mg) per day compared to placebo in the prevention of certain chronic diseases. The primary endpoint was the incidence of coronary heart disease (CHD) (nonfatal myocardial infarction (MI), silent MI and CHD death), with invasive breast cancer as the primary adverse outcome studied.

Table 2. Mean Pharmacokinetic Parameters of Conjugated (Total) Estrogens Following a Single Dose of 2 × 0.625 mg ENJUVIA Tablets Under Fasting Conditions

	C_{max} (ng/mL)	t_{max} (h)	$t_{1/2}$ (h)	AUC_{0-48h} (ng·h/mL)
Baseline-corrected estrone (% CV)	3.74 (29)	8.00 (27)	14.26 (26)	62.03 (34)
Equilin (% CV)	3.69 (44)	8.05 (36)	11.28 (28)	58.25 (53)
$\Delta^{8,9}$ Dehydroestrone (% CV)	0.74 (32)	7.55 (37)	14.14 (26)	12.93 (39)

C_{max} = peak plasma concentration; t_{max} = time peak concentration occurs; $t_{1/2}$ = apparent terminal-phase disposition half-life; AUC_{0-48h} = total area under the concentration-time curve from time zero to time of last quantifiable concentration (48h); CV = Coefficient of Variance

Table 3. Mean Number and Mean Change in Number of Moderate to Severe Hot Flushes Per Week ITT Population With LOCF

	0.3 mg n=66	0.625 mg n=71	1.25 mg n=69	Placebo n=70
Baseline				
Mean (SD)	104.3 (57.7)	97.3 (82.1)	86.8 (42.1)	96.4 (58.2)
Week 4				
Mean (SD)	47.0 (52.9)	23.3 (26.9)	24.6 (47.0)	57.8 (47.5)
Mean Change from Baseline (SE)	-49.8 (5.2)	-72.8 (5.0)	-68.3 (5.1)	-37.2 (5.0)
p-value versus placebo	0.005	<0.001	<0.001	—
Week 12				
Mean (SD)	30.7 (47.7)	12.2 (18.7)	12.4 (26.3)	47.5 (49.8)
Mean Change from Baseline (SE)	-66.3 (4.6)	-84.6 (4.4)	-82.6 (4.5)	-48.3 (4.5)
p-value versus placebo	<0.001	<0.001	<0.001	—

ITT = Intent to treat; LOCF = Last Observation Carried Forward, SD = Standard Deviation; SE = Standard Error

Table 4. Mean Change in Severity of Moderate to Severe Hot Flushes Per Week, ITT Population with LOCF

	0.3 mg n=66	0.625 mg n=71	1.25 mg n=69	Placebo n=70
Baseline				
Mean (SD)	2.5 (0.3)	2.5 (0.3)	2.5 (0.3)	2.5 (0.3)
Week 4				
Mean (SD)	2.1 (0.8)	1.9 (1.0)	1.5 (1.1)	2.2 (0.8)
Mean Change from Baseline (SE)	-0.5 (0.1)	-0.6 (0.1)	-1.0 (0.1)	-0.3 (0.1)
p-value versus placebo	0.036	0.002	<0.001	—
Week 12				
Mean (SD)	1.5 (1.2)	1.1 (1.2)	1.0 (1.1)	1.9 (1.1)
Mean Change from Baseline (SE)	-1.0 (0.1)	-1.4 (0.1)	-1.5 (0.1)	-0.6 (0.1)
p-value versus placebo	0.023	<0.001	<0.001	—

ITT = Intent to treat; LOCF = Last Observation Carried Forward; SD = Standard Deviation; SE = Standard Error

A "global index" included the earliest occurrence of CHD, invasive breast cancer, stroke, pulmonary embolism (PE), endometrial cancer (only in the estrogen plus progestin substudy), colorectal cancer, hip fracture, or death due to other causes. The study did not evaluate the effects of CE or CE/MPA on menopausal symptoms.

The estrogen-alone substudy was stopped early because an increased risk of stroke was observed and it was deemed that no further information would be obtained regarding the risks and benefits of estrogen alone in predetermined primary endpoints. Results of the estrogen-alone substudy, which included 10,739 women (average age of 63 years, range 50 to 79; 75.3% White, 15.1% Black, 6.1% Hispanic, 3.6% Other), after an average follow-up of 6.8 years are presented in Table 6.

[See table 6 at top of next page]

For those outcomes included in the WHI "global index" that reached statistical significance, the absolute excess risk per 10,000 women-years in the group treated with estrogen-alone was 12 more strokes, while the absolute risk reduction per 10,000 women-years was 6 fewer hip fractures. The absolute excess risk of events included in the "global index" was a nonsignificant 2 events per 10,000 women-years. There was no difference between the groups in terms of all-cause mortality. (See BOXED WARNINGS, WARNINGS, and PRECAUTIONS.)

Final centrally adjudicated results for CHD events and centrally adjudicated results for invasive breast cancer incidence from the estrogen-alone substudy, after an average follow-up of 7.1 years, reported no overall difference for primary CHD events (nonfatal MI, silent MI and CHD death) and invasive breast cancer incidence in women receiving CE alone compared with placebo (see Table 6).

The estrogen-plus-progestin substudy was also stopped early because, according to the predefined stopping rule, after an average follow-up of 5.2 years of treatment, the

Table 6: Relative And Absolute Risk Seen In The Estrogen-Alone Substudy Of WHI[a]

Event	Relative Risk CE vs. Placebo (95% nCI[a])	Placebo n = 5,429	CE n = 5,310
		Absolute Risk per 10,000 Women-Years	
CHD events[b]	0.95 (0.79-1.16)	56	53
Nonfatal MI[b]	*0.91 (0.73-1.14)*	*43*	*40*
CHD death[b]	*1.01 (0.71-1.43)*	*16*	*16*
Stroke[c]	1.39 (1.10-1.77)	32	44
Deep vein thrombosis[b,d]	1.47 (1.06-2.06)	15	23
Pulmonary embolism[b]	1.37 (0.90-2.07)	10	14
Invasive breast cancer[b]	0.80 (0.62-1.04)	34	28
Colorectal cancer[c]	1.08 (0.75-1.55)	16	17
Hip fracture[c]	0.61 (0.41-0.91)	17	11
Vertebral fractures[c,d]	0.62 (0.42-0.93)	17	11
Total fractures[c,d]	0.70 (0.63-0.79)	195	139
Death due to other causes[c,e]	1.08 (0.88-1.32)	50	53
Overall mortality[c,d]	1.04 (0.88-1.32)	78	81
Global index[c,f]	1.01 (0.91-1.12)	190	192

[a] Nominal confidence intervals unadjusted for multiple looks and multiple comparisons
[b] Results are based on centrally adjudicated data for an average follow-up of 7.1 years
[c] Results are based on an average follow-up of 6.8 years
[d] Not included in Global Index
[e] All deaths, except from breast or colorectal cancer, definite/probable CHD, PE or cerebrovascular disease
[f] A subset of the events was combined in a "global index", defined as the earliest occurrence of CHD events, invasive breast cancer, stroke, pulmonary embolism, colorectal cancer, hip fracture, or death due to other causes

Table 7. Relative And Absolute Risk Seen in the Estrogen-Plus Progestin Substudy of WHI at an Average of 5.6 Years[a]

Event	Relative Risk CE/MPA vs. Placebo (95% nCI[b])	Placebo n = 8102	CE/MPA n = 8506
		Absolute Risk per 10,000 Women-Years	
CHD events	1.24 (1.00-1.54)	33	39
Non-fatal MI	*1.28 (1.00-1.63)*	*25*	*31*
CHD death	*1.10 (0.70-1.75)*	*8*	*8*
All strokes	1.31 (1.02-1.68)	24	31
Ischemic stroke	*1.44 (1.09-1.90)*	*18*	*26*
Deep vein thrombosis	1.95 (1.43–2.67)	13	26
Pulmonary embolism	2.13 (1.45-3.11)	8	18
Invasive breast cancer[c]	1.24 (1.01-1.54)	33	41
Invasive colorectal cancer	0.56 (0.38-0.81)	16	9
Endometrial cancer	0.81 (0.48-1.36)	7	6
Cervical cancer	1.44 (0.47-4.42)	1	2
Hip fracture	0.67 (0.47-0.96)	16	11
Vertebral fractures	0.65 (0.46-0.92)	17	11
Lower arm/wrist fractures	0.71 (0.59-0.85)	62	44
Total fractures	0.76 (0.69-0.83)	199	152

[a] Results are based on centrally adjudicated data. Mortality data was not part of the adjudicated data; however, data at 5.2 years of follow-up showed no difference between the groups in terms of all-cause mortality (RR 0.98, 95% nCI 0.82-1.18)
[b] Nominal confidence intervals unadjusted for multiple looks and multiple comparisons
[c] Includes metastatic and non-metastatic breast cancer, with the exception of *in situ* breast cancer

increased risk of breast cancer and cardiovascular events exceeded the specified benefits included in the "global index." The absolute excess risk of events included in the "global index" was 19 per 10,000 women-years (RR 1.15, 95% nCI 1.03-1.28).

For those outcomes included in the WHI "global index" that reached statistical significance after 5.6 years of follow-up, the absolute excess risks per 10,000 women-years in the group treated with CE/MPA were 6 more CHD events, 7 more strokes, 10 more PEs, and 8 more invasive breast cancers, while the absolute risk reductions per 10,000 women-years were 7 fewer colorectal cancers and 5 fewer hip fractures. (See BOXED WARNINGS, WARNINGS, and PRECAUTIONS.)

Results of the estrogen-plus-progestin substudy, which included 16,608 women (average age of 63 years, range 50 to 79; 83.9% White, 6.8% Black, 5.4% Hispanic, 3.9% Other) are presented in Table 7 below.

[See table 7 below]

Women's Health Initiative Memory Study

The estrogen-alone Women's Health Initiative Memory Study (WHIMS), a substudy of WHI study, enrolled 2,947 predominantly healthy postmenopausal women 65 years of age and older (45% were age 65 to 69 years, 36% were 70 to 74 years, and 19% were 75 years of age and older) to evaluate the effects of conjugated estrogens (CE 0.625 mg) on the incidence of probable dementia (primary outcome) compared with placebo.

After an average follow-up of 5.2 years, 28 women in the estrogen-alone group (37 per 10,000 women-years) and 19 in the placebo group (25 per 10,000 women-years) were diagnosed with probable dementia. The relative risk of probable dementia in the estrogen-alone group was 1.49 (95% CI 0.83-2.66) compared to placebo. It is unknown whether these findings apply to younger postmenopausal women. (See BOXED WARNING, WARNINGS, Dementia and PRECAUTIONS, Geriatric Use.)

The estrogen-plus-progestin WHIMS substudy enrolled 4,532 predominantly healthy postmenopausal women 65 years of age and older (47% were aged 65 to 69 years, 35% were 70 to 74 years, and 18% were 75 years of age and older) to evaluate the effects of CE 0.625 mg plus MPA 2.5 mg on the incidence of probable dementia (primary outcome) compared with placebo.

After an average follow-up of 4 years, 40 women in the estrogen plus progestin group (45 per 10,000 women-years) and 21 in the placebo group (22 per 10,000 women-years) were diagnosed with probable dementia. The relative risk of probable dementia in the hormone therapy group was 2.05 (95% CI 1.21-3.48) compared to placebo. Differences between groups became apparent in the first year of treatment. It is unknown whether these findings apply to younger postmenopausal women. (See BOXED WARNING, WARNINGS, Dementia, and PRECAUTIONS, Geriatric Use.)

When data from the two populations were pooled as planned in the WHIMS protocol, the reported overall relative risk for probable dementia was 1.76 (95% CI 1.19-2.60). It is unknown whether these findings apply to younger postmenopausal women. (See BOXED WARNING, WARNINGS, Dementia, and PRECAUTIONS, Geriatric Use.)

INDICATIONS AND USAGE

ENJUVIA tablets are indicated in the:
1. Treatment of moderate to severe vasomotor symptoms associated with menopause.
2. Treatment of moderate to severe vaginal dryness and pain with intercourse, symptoms of vulvar and vaginal atrophy, associated with menopause. When prescribing solely for the treatment of moderate to severe vaginal dryness and pain with intercourse, topical vaginal products should be considered.

CONTRAINDICATIONS

ENJUVIA tablets should not be used in women with any of the following conditions:
1. Undiagnosed abnormal genital bleeding.
2. Known, suspected, or history of cancer of the breast.
3. Known or suspected estrogen-dependent neoplasia.
4. Active deep vein thrombosis, pulmonary embolism or a history of these conditions.
5. Active or recent (e.g., within the past year) arterial thromboembolic disease (e.g., stroke, myocardial infarction).
6. Liver dysfunction or disease.
7. Known hypersensitivity to the ingredients of ENJUVIA Tablets.
8. Known or suspected pregnancy. There is no indication for ENJUVIA in pregnancy. There appears to be little or no increased risk of birth defects in children born to women who have used estrogens and progestins from oral contraceptives inadvertently during early pregnancy. (See PRECAUTIONS.)

WARNINGS

See BOXED WARNINGS.

1. Cardiovascular disorders

Estrogen and estrogen/progestin therapies have been associated with an increased risk of cardiovascular events such as myocardial infarction and stroke, as well as venous thrombosis and pulmonary embolism (venous thromboembolism (VTE)). Should any of these occur or be suspected, estrogens should be discontinued immediately.

Risk factors for arterial vascular disease (e.g., hypertension, diabetes mellitus, tobacco use, hypercholesterolemia, and obesity) and/or venous thromboembolism (e.g., personal history or family history of VTE, obesity, and systemic lupus erythematosus) should be managed appropriately.

a. Stroke

In the estrogen-alone substudy of the Women's Health Initiative (WHI) study, statistically significant increased risk of stroke was reported in women receiving CE 0.625 mg daily compared to women receiving placebo (44 versus 32 per 10,000 women-years). The increase in risk was demonstrated in year 1 and persisted. (See CLINICAL STUDIES).

In the estrogen-plus-progestin substudy of WHI study, a statistically significant increased risk of stroke was reported in women receiving CE/MPA 0.625 mg/2.5 mg daily compared to women receiving placebo (31 vs. 24 per 10, 000 women-years). The increase in risk was demonstrated after the first year and persisted. (See CLINICAL PHARMACOLOGY, CLINICAL STUDIES.)

b. Coronary heart disease

In the estrogen-alone substudy of WHI, no overall effect on coronary heart disease (CHD) events (defined as non-fatal MI, silent MI or death due to CHD) was reported in women receiving estrogen alone compared to placebo. (See CLINICAL STUDIES.)

In the estrogen-plus-progestin substudy of the WHI study, no statistically significant increase of CHD events was reported in women receiving CE/MPA compared to women receiving placebo (39 versus 33 per 10,000 women-years). An increase in relative risk was demonstrated in year 1, and a trend toward decreasing relative risk was reported in years 2 through 5.

In postmenopausal women with documented heart disease (n = 2,763, average age 66.7 years), a controlled clinical trial of secondary prevention of cardiovascular disease (Heart and Estrogen/Progestin Replacement Study (HERS)) treatment with CE/MPA (0.625 mg/2.5 mg per day) demonstrated no cardiovascular benefit. During an average follow-up of 4.1 years, treatment with CE/MPA did not reduce the overall rate of CHD events in postmenopausal women with established coronary heart disease. There were more CHD events in the CE/MPA-treated group than in the placebo group in year 1, but not during the subsequent years. Participation in an open label extension of the original HERS trial (HERS II) was agreed to by 2,321 women. Average follow-up in HERS II was an additional 2.7 years, for a total of 6.8 years overall. Rates of CHD events were comparable among women in the CE/MPA group and the placebo group in HERS, HERS II, and overall. Large doses of estrogen (5 mg conjugated estrogens per day), comparable to those used to treat cancer of the prostate and breast, have been shown in a large prospective clinical trial in men to increase the risks of nonfatal myocardial infarction, pulmonary embolism, and thrombophlebitis.

c. Venous thromboembolism

In the estrogen-alone substudy of WHI the risk of VTE (DVT and pulmonary embolism [PE]), was reported to be increased for women taking conjugated equine estrogens (30 vs. 22 per 10,000 women-years), although only the increased risk of DVT reached statistical significance (23 vs. 15 per 10,000 women years). The increase in VTE risk was demonstrated during the first year. (See CLINICAL STUDIES.)

In the estrogen-plus-progestin substudy of WHI, a statistically significant 2-fold greater rate of VTE was reported in women receiving CE/MPA compared to women receiving placebo (35 vs. 17 per 10,000 women-years). Statistically significant increases in risk for both DVT (26 vs. 13 per 10,000 women-years) and PE (18 vs. 8 per 10,000 women-years) were also demonstrated. The increase in VTE risk was demonstrated during the first year and persisted.

If feasible, estrogens should be discontinued at least 4 to 6 weeks before surgery of the type associated with an increased risk of thromboembolism, or during periods of prolonged immobilization.

2. Malignant neoplasms

a. Endometrial cancer

The use of unopposed estrogens in women with intact uteri has been associated with an increased risk of endometrial cancer. The reported endometrial cancer risk among unopposed estrogen users is about 2- to 12-times greater than in non-users, and appears dependent on duration of treatment and on estrogen dose. Most studies show no significant increased risk associated with use of estrogens for less than 1 year. The greatest risk appears associated with prolonged use, with increased risks of 15- to 24-fold for 5 to 10 years or more. This risk has been shown to persist for at least 8 to 15 years after estrogen therapy is discontinued.

Clinical surveillance of all women taking estrogen/progestin combinations is important. Adequate diagnostic measures, including endometrial sampling when indicated, should be undertaken to rule out malignancy in all cases of undiagnosed persistent or recurring abnormal vaginal bleeding. There is no ev-

idence that the use of natural estrogens results in a different endometrial risk profile than synthetic estrogens of equivalent estrogen dose. Adding a progestin to estrogen therapy has been shown to reduce the risk of endometrial hyperplasia, which may be a precursor to endometrial cancer.

b. Breast cancer

In some studies, the use of estrogens and progestins by postmenopausal women has been reported to increase the risk of breast cancer. The most important randomized clinical trial providing information about this issue is the Women's Health Initiative (WHI) (see CLINICAL STUDIES). The results from observational studies are generally consistent with those of the WHI clinical trial.

Observational studies have also reported an increased risk of breast cancer for estrogen-plus-progestin combination therapy, and a smaller increased risk for estrogen-alone therapy, after several years of use. For both findings, the excess risk increased with duration of use, and appeared to return to baseline over about five years after stopping treatment (only the observational studies have substantial data on risk after stopping). In these studies, the risk of breast cancer was greater, and became apparent earlier, with estrogen-plus-progestin combination therapy as compared to estrogen-alone therapy. However, these studies have not found significant variation in the risk of breast cancer among different estrogens or among different estrogen-plus-progestin combinations, doses, or routes of administration.

In the estrogen-alone substudy of WHI, after an average of 7.1 years of follow-up, CE (0.625 mg daily) was not associated with an increased risk of invasive breast cancer (RR 0.80, 95% nCI 0.62-1.04).

In the estrogen-plus-progestin substudy, after a mean follow-up of 5.6 years, the WHI substudy reported an increased risk of breast cancer. In this substudy, prior use of estrogen alone or estrogen-plus-progestin combination hormone therapy was reported by 26% of the women. The relative risk of invasive breast cancer was 1.24 (95% nCI 1.01-1.54), and the absolute risk was 41 vs. 33 cases per 10,000 women-years, for estrogen plus progestin compared with placebo, respectively. Among women who reported prior use of hormone therapy, the relative risk of invasive breast cancer was 1.86, and the absolute risk was 46 vs. 25 cases per 10,000 women-years, for estrogen plus progestin compared with placebo. Among women who reported no prior use of hormone therapy, the relative risk of invasive breast cancer was 1.09, and the absolute risk was 40 vs. 36 cases per 10,000 women-years for estrogen plus progestin compared with placebo. In the WHI trial, invasive breast cancers were larger and diagnosed at a more advanced stage in the estrogen-plus-progestin group compared with the placebo group. Metastatic disease was rare, with no apparent difference between the two groups. Other prognostic factors, such as histologic subtype, grade and hormone receptor status did not differ between the groups.

The use of estrogen alone and estrogen plus progestin has been reported to result in an increase in abnormal mammograms requiring further evaluation. All women should receive yearly breast examinations by a healthcare provider and perform monthly breast self-examinations. In addition, mammography examinations should be scheduled based on patient age, risk factors, and prior mammogram results.

3. Dementia

In the estrogen-alone Women's Health Initiative Memory Study (WHIMS), a substudy of WHI, a population of 2,947 hysterectomized women aged 65 to 79 years was randomized to CE (0.625 mg daily) or placebo. In the estrogen-plus-progestin WHIMS substudy, a population of 4,532 postmenopausal women aged 65 to 79 years was randomized to CE/MPA (0.625 mg/2.5 mg daily) or placebo.

In the estrogen-alone substudy, after an average follow-up of 5.2 years, 28 women in the estrogen-alone group and 19 women in the placebo group were diagnosed with probable dementia. The relative risk of probable dementia for CE alone vs. placebo was 1.49 (95% CI 0.83-2.66). The absolute risk of probable dementia for CE alone vs. placebo was 37 vs. 25 cases per 10,000 women-years.

In the estrogen-plus-progestin substudy, after an average follow-up of four years, 40 women in the estrogen-plus-progestin group and 21 women in the placebo group were diagnosed with probable dementia. The relative risk of probable dementia for estrogen plus progestin vs. placebo was 2.05 (95% CI 1.21-3.48). The absolute risk of probable dementia for CE/MPA vs. placebo was 45 vs. 22 cases per 10,000 women-years.

When data from the two populations were pooled as planned in the WHIMS protocol, the reported overall relative risk for probable dementia was 1.76 (95% CI 1.19-2.60). Since both substudies were conducted in women aged 65 to 79 years, it is unknown whether these findings apply to younger postmenopausal women. (See BOXED WARNINGS and PRECAUTIONS, and Geriatric Use.)

4. Gallbladder disease

A two- to four-fold increase in the risk of gallbladder disease requiring surgery in postmenopausal women receiving estrogens has been reported.

5. Hypercalcemia

Estrogen administration may lead to severe hypercalcemia in patients with breast cancer and bone metastases. If hypercalcemia occurs, use of the drug should be stopped and appropriate measures taken to reduce the serum calcium level.

6. Visual abnormalities

Retinal vascular thrombosis has been reported in patients receiving estrogens. Discontinue medication pending examination if there is sudden partial or complete loss of vision, or a sudden onset of proptosis, diplopia, or migraine. If examination reveals papilledema or retinal vascular lesions, estrogens should be permanently discontinued.

PRECAUTIONS

A. General

1. Addition of a progestin when a woman has not had a hysterectomy

Studies of the addition of a progestin for 10 or more days of a cycle of estrogen administration, or daily with estrogen in a continuous regimen, have reported a lowered incidence of endometrial hyperplasia than would be induced by estrogen treatment alone. Endometrial hyperplasia may be a precursor to endometrial cancer.

There are, however, possible risks that may be associated with the use of progestins with estrogens compared to estrogen-alone regimens. These include: a possible increased risk of breast cancer, adverse effects on lipoprotein metabolism (e.g., lowering HDL, raising LDL) and impairment of glucose tolerance.

2. Elevated blood pressure

In a small number of case reports, substantial increases in blood pressure have been attributed to idiosyncratic reactions to estrogens. In a large, randomized, placebo-controlled clinical trial, a generalized effect of estrogens on blood pressure was not seen. Blood pressure should be monitored at regular intervals with estrogen use.

3. Hypertriglyceridemia

In patients with pre-existing hypertriglyceridemIa, estrogen therapy may be associated with elevations of plasma triglycerides leading to pancreatitis and other complications.

4. Impaired liver function and past history of cholestatic jaundice

Estrogens may be poorly metabolized in patients with impaired liver function. For patients with a history of cholestatic jaundice associated with past estrogen use or with pregnancy, caution should be exercised and in the case of recurrence, medication should be discontinued.

5. Hypothyroidism

Estrogen administration leads to increased thyroid-binding globulin (TBG) levels. Patients with normal thyroid function can compensate for the increased TBG by making more thyroid hormone, thus maintaining free T_4 and T_3 serum concentrations in the normal range. Patients dependent on thyroid hormone replacement therapy who are also receiving estrogens may require increased doses of their thyroid replacement therapy. These patients should have their thyroid function monitored to maintain their free thyroid hormone levels in an acceptable range.

6. Fluid retention

Estrogens may cause some degree of fluid retention. Because of this, patients who have conditions that might be influenced by this factor, such as a cardiac or renal dysfunction, warrant careful observation when estrogens are prescribed.

7. Hypocalcemia

Estrogens should be used with caution in individuals with severe hypocalcemia.

8. Ovarian cancer

The estrogen-plus-progestin substudy of WHI reported that after an average follow-up of 5.6 years, the relative risk for ovarian cancer for estrogen plus progestin vs. placebo was 1.58 (95% nCI 0.77–3.24), but was not statistically significant. The absolute risk for estrogen plus progestin vs. placebo was 4.2 vs. 2.7 cases per 10,000 women-years. In some epidemiologic studies, the use of estrogen only products, in particular for 10 or more years, has been associated with an increased risk of ovarian cancer. Other epidemiologic studies have not found these associations.

9. **Exacerbation of endometriosis**
Endometriosis may be exacerbated with administration of estrogens. Malignant transformation of residual endometrial implants has been reported in women treated post-hysterectomy with estrogen-alone therapy. For patients known to have residual endometriosis post-hysterectomy, the addition of progestin should be considered.

10. **Exacerbation of other conditions**
Estrogens may cause an exacerbation of asthma, diabetes mellitus, epilepsy, migraine, porphyria, systemic lupus erythematosus, and hepatic hemangiomas and should be used with caution in women with these conditions.

B. **Information for Patients**
Physicians are advised to discuss the **PATIENT INFORMATION** leaflet with patients for whom they prescribe ENJUVIA tablets.

C. **Laboratory Tests**
Estrogen administration should be initiated at the lowest dose approved for the indication and then guided by clinical response rather than by serum hormone levels (e.g., estradiol, FSH).

D. **Drug/Laboratory Test Interactions**
1. Accelerated prothrombin time, partial thromboplastin time, and platelet aggregation time; increased platelet count; increased factors II, VII antigen, VIII antigen, VIII coagulant activity, IX, X, XII, VII-X complex, II-VII-X complex, and beta-thromboglobulin; decreased levels of anti-factor Xa and antithrombin III, decreased antithrombin III activity; increased levels of fibrinogen and fibrinogen activity; increased plasminogen antigen and activity.
2. Increased thyroid-binding globulin (TBG) levels leading to increased circulating total thyroid hormone levels as measured by protein-bound iodine (PBI), T_4 levels (by column or by radioimmunoassay) or T_3 levels by radioimmunoassay. T_3 resin uptake is decreased, reflecting the elevated TBG. Free T_4 and free T_3 concentrations are unaltered. Patients on thyroid replacement therapy may require higher doses of thyroid hormone.
3. Other binding proteins may be elevated in serum, (i.e., corticosteroid binding globulin (CBG), sex hormone binding globulin (SHBG)) leading to increased total circulating corticosteroids and sex steroids, respectively. Free hormone concentrations may be decreased. Other plasma proteins may be increased (angiotensinogen/renin substrate, alpha-1-antitrypsin, ceruloplasmin).
4. Increased plasma HDL and HDL_2 cholesterol subfraction concentrations, reduced LDL cholesterol concentration, increased triglyceride levels.
5. Impaired glucose tolerance.
6. Reduced response to metyrapone test.

E. **Carcinogenesis, Mutagenesis, Impairment of Fertility**
See **BOXED WARNINGS**, **WARNINGS** and **PRECAUTIONS**.
Long-term continuous administration of natural and synthetic estrogens in certain animal species increases the frequency of carcinomas of the breast, uterus, cervix, vagina, testis, and liver.

F. **Pregnancy**
ENJUVIA tablets should not be used during pregnancy. (See **CONTRAINDICATIONS**.)

G. **Nursing Mothers**
Estrogen administration to nursing mothers has been shown to decrease the quantity and quality of the milk. Detectable amounts of estrogens have been identified in the milk of mothers receiving this drug. Caution should be exercised when ENJUVIA is administered to a nursing woman.

H. **Pediatric Use**
The safety and efficacy of ENJUVIA tablets in pediatric patients has not been established.

I. **Geriatric Use**
Clinical studies of ENJUVIA did not include sufficient numbers of subjects aged 65 and over to determine whether they respond differently from younger subjects. Of the total number of subjects in the estrogen-alone substudy of the WHI study, 46 percent (n = 4,943) were 65 years and older, while 7.1 percent (n = 767) were 75 years and older. There was a higher relative risk (CE versus placebo) of stroke in women less than 75 years of age compared to women 75 years and over.
In the estrogen-alone substudy of WHIMS, a substudy of WHI, a population of 2,947 hysterectomized women, aged 65 to 79 years, was randomized to CE (0.625 per day) or placebo. After an average follow-up of 5.2 years, the relative risk (CE vs. placebo) of probable dementia was 1.49 (95% CI 0.83-2.66). The absolute risk of developing probable dementia with estrogen alone was 37 vs. 25 cases per 10,000 women-years with placebo.
Of the total number of subjects in the estrogen-plus-progestin substudy of the WHI study, 44 percent (n = 7,320) were 65-74 years of age, while 6.6 percent (n = 1,095) were 75 years and older. There was a higher relative risk (CE/MPA versus placebo) of non-fatal stroke and invasive breast cancer in women 75 and older compared to women less than 75 years of age. In women greater than 75, the increased risk of non-fatal stroke and invasive breast cancer observed in the estrogen-plus-progestin combination group compared to the placebo group was 75 vs. 24 per 10,000 women-years and 52 vs. 12 per 10,000 women-years, respectively.
In the estrogen-plus-progestin substudy of WHIMS, a population of 4,532 postmenopausal women, aged 65 to 79 years, was randomized to CE/MPA (CE 0.625 mg/2.5 mg). In the estrogen-plus-progestin group, after an average follow-up of 4 years, the relative risk (CE/MPA versus placebo) of probable dementia was 2.05 (95% CI 1.21-3.48). The absolute risk of developing probable dementia with CE/MPA was 45 vs. 22 cases per 10,000 women-years with placebo.
Seventy-nine percent of the cases of probable dementia occurred in women that were older than 70 for the CE group, and 82 percent of the cases of probable dementia occurred in women who were older than 70 in the CE/MPA group. The most common classification of probable dementia in both the treatment groups and placebo groups was Alzheimer's disease.
When data from the two populations were pooled as planned in the WHIMS protocol, the reported overall relative risk for probable dementia was 1.76 (95% CI 1.19-2.60). Since both substudies were conducted in women aged 65 to 79 years, it is unknown whether these findings apply to younger postmenopausal women. (See BOXED WARNINGS and WARNINGS, Dementia.)

ADVERSE REACTIONS
See **BOXED WARNINGS**, **WARNINGS** and **PRECAUTIONS**.
Because clinical trials are conducted under widely varying conditions, adverse reaction rates observed in the clinical trials of a drug cannot be directly compared to rates in the clinical trials of another drug and may not reflect the rates observed in practice. The adverse reaction information from clinical trials does, however, provide a basis for identifying the adverse events that appear to be related to drug use and for approximating rates.
In a 12-week clinical trial, 209 postmenopausal women with vasomotor symptoms were treated with ENJUVIA. Adverse events that occurred in the study at a rate greater than or equal to 5% and greater than placebo, regardless of relationship to study drug, are summarized in Table 8.
[See table 8 at left]
In a second 12-week clinical trial, 310 women with symptoms of vulvar and vaginal atrophy were treated (154 women with ENJUVIA 0.3 mg tablets and 156 women with placebo). The only adverse event that occurred at a rate of >5% was headache; seven patients (4.55%) with ENJUVIA and twelve patients (7.69%) with placebo.
The following additional adverse reactions have been reported with estrogen and/or progestin therapy:
1. **Genitourinary system**
Changes in vaginal bleeding pattern and abnormal withdrawal bleeding or flow; breakthrough bleeding; spotting; dysmenorrhea; increase in size of uterine leiomyomata; vaginitis, including vaginal candidiasis; change in amount of cervical secretion; changes in cervical ectropion; ovarian cancer; endometrial hyperplasia; endometrial cancer.
2. **Breasts**
Tenderness, enlargement, pain, nipple discharge, galactorrhea; fibrocystic breast changes; breast cancer.
3. **Cardiovascular**
Deep and superficial venous thrombosis; pulmonary embolism; thrombophlebitis; myocardial infarction; stroke; increase in blood pressure.

Table 8. ENJUVIA Tablets – Number (%) of Patients Reporting Adverse Events* with ≥ 5% Occurrence Rate by Body System

Body System/Adverse Events*	0.3 mg n=68	0.625 mg n=72	1.25 mg n=69	Placebo n=72
Number of Patients in Safety Sample (%)	68 (100)	72 (100)	69 (100)	72 (100)
Number of Patients with Adverse Events (%)	49 (72)	55 (76)	56 (81)	51 (71)
Number of Patients without Adverse Events (%)	19 (28)	17 (24)	13 (19)	21 (29)
Body as a Whole				
Abdominal Pain	3 (4)	11 (15)	3 (4)	7 (10)
Accidental Injury	6 (8)	2 (3)	3 (4)	5 (7)
Flu Syndrome	4 (6)	3 (4)	5 (7)	3 (4)
Headache	10 (15)	18 (25)	11 (16)	15 (21)
Pain	10 (15)	14 (19)	7 (10)	6 (8)
Digestive System				
Flatulence	3 (4)	5 (7)	3 (4)	2 (3)
Nausea	5 (7)	7 (10)	8 (12)	6 (8)
Nervous System				
Dizziness	5 (7)	3 (4)	1 (1)	3 (4)
Paresthesia	0	4 (6)	1 (1)	0
Respiratory System				
Bronchitis	0	3 (4)	5 (7)	3 (4)
Rhinitis	3 (4)	4 (6)	5 (7)	4 (6)
Sinusitis	2 (3)	3 (4)	5 (7)	2 (3)
Urogenital System				
Breast Pain	0	9 (12)	10 (14)	3 (4)
Dysmenorrhea	1 (2)	6 (8)	1 (1)	2 (3)
Vaginitis	1 (2)	5 (7)	2 (3)	3 (4)

*Treatment-emergent adverse events, regardless of relationship to study drug

4. Gastrointestinal

Nausea, vomiting; abdominal cramps, bloating; cholestatic jaundice; increased incidence of gallbladder disease; pancreatitis, enlargement of hepatic hemangiomas.

5. Skin

Chloasma or melasma that may persist when drug is discontinued; erythema multiforme; erythema nodosum; hemorrhagic eruption; loss of scalp hair; hirsutism; pruritus, rash.

6. Eyes

Retinal vascular thrombosis, intolerance to contact lenses.

7. Central Nervous System

Headache; migraine; dizziness; mental depression; chorea; nervousness; mood disturbances; irritability; exacerbation of epilepsy, dementia.

8. Miscellaneous

Increase or decrease in weight; reduced carbohydrate tolerance; aggravation of porphyria; edema; arthralgias; leg cramps; changes in libido; urticaria, angioedema, anaphylactoid/anaphylactic reactions; hypocalcemia; exacerbation of asthma; increased triglycerides.

OVERDOSAGE

Serious ill effects have not been reported following acute ingestion of large doses of estrogen-containing products by young children. Overdosage of estrogen may cause nausea and vomiting, and withdrawal bleeding may occur in females.

DOSAGE AND ADMINISTRATION

When estrogen is prescribed for a postmenopausal woman with a uterus, a progestin should also be initiated to reduce the risk of endometrial cancer. A woman without a uterus does not need progestin. Use of estrogen, alone or in combination with a progestin, should be with the lowest effective dose and for the shortest duration consistent with treatment goals and risks for the individual woman. Patients should be re-evaluated periodically as clinically appropriate (e.g., 3-month to 6-month intervals) to determine if treatment is still necessary (see BOXED WARNINGS and WARNINGS). For women who have a uterus, adequate diagnostic measures, such as endometrial sampling, when indicated, should be undertaken to rule out malignancy in cases of undiagnosed persistent or recurring abnormal vaginal bleeding.

ENJUVIA tablets are taken orally, once daily for:

1. The treatment of moderate to severe vasomotor symptoms, associated with menopause.
   - ENJUVIA 0.3 mg
   - ENJUVIA 0.45 mg
   - ENJUVIA 0.625 mg
   - ENJUVIA 0.9 mg
   - ENJUVIA 1.25 mg
2. The treatment of moderate to severe vaginal dryness and pain with intercourse, symptoms of vulvar and vaginal atrophy, associated with menopause. When prescribing solely for the treatment of moderate to severe vaginal dryness and pain during intercourse, topical vaginal products should be considered.
   - ENJUVIA 0.3 mg

Patients should be started at the lowest approved dose of 0.3 mg ENJUVIA daily. Subsequent dosage adjustment (which will differ depending on the indication) may be made based upon the individual patient response. This dose should be periodically reassessed by the healthcare provider.

HOW SUPPLIED

ENJUVIA®

(synthetic conjugated estrogens, B) Tablets

0.3 mg:
The tablets are oval, white, film-coated, and debossed with "E" on one side and "1" on the reverse and are available in bottles of:
100 Tablets   NDC 51285-406-02

0.45 mg:
The tablets are oval, mauve, film-coated, and debossed with "E" on one side and "2" on the reverse and are available in bottles of:
100 Tablets   NDC 51285-407-02

0.625 mg:
The tablets are oval, pink, film-coated, and debossed with "E" on one side and "3" on the reverse and are available in bottles of:
100 Tablets   NDC 51285-408-02

0.9 mg:
The tablets are oval, light blue-green, film-coated, and debossed with "E" on one side and "5" on the reverse and are available in bottles of:
100 Tablets   NDC 51285-409-02

1.25 mg:
The tablets are oval, yellow, film-coated, and debossed with "E" on one side and "4" on the reverse and are available in bottles of:

---

100 Tablets   NDC 51285-410-02
Store at 20° to 25°C (68° to 77°F) [See USP Controlled Room Temperature].
Keep this and all drugs out of the reach of children.
Dispense in a tight container with a child-resistant closure.
Pharmacist: Include one "Patient Information" leaflet with each prescription.
Iss. 3/2010

Shown in Product Identification Guide, page 320

LOSEASONIQUE   ℞

[lo-sea-son-ique]

(levonorgestrel/ethinyl estradiol tablets and ethinyl estradiol tablets)
For Oral Use

HIGHLIGHTS OF PRESCRIBING INFORMATION

These highlights do not include all the information needed to use LoSeasonique tablets safely and effectively. See full prescribing information for LoSeasonique.

LoSeasonique (levonorgestrel/ethinyl estradiol tablets and ethinyl estradiol tablets) for oral use

Initial U.S. Approval: 1982

> **WARNING: CIGARETTE SMOKING AND SERIOUS CARDIOVASCULAR EVENTS**
> *See full prescribing information for complete boxed warning.*
> - **Women who are over 35 years old and smoke should not use LoSeasonique. (4)**
> - **Cigarette smoking increases the risk of serious cardiovascular events from combination oral contraceptive (COC) use.**

——————INDICATIONS AND USAGE——————
LoSeasonique is an estrogen/progestin COC indicated for use by women to prevent pregnancy. (1)

————DOSAGE AND ADMINISTRATION————
Take one tablet daily by mouth at the same time every day for 91 days. (2)

————DOSAGE FORMS AND STRENGTHS————
LoSeasonique consists of 84 orange tablets containing 0.1 mg levonorgestrel and 0.02 mg ethinyl estradiol, and 7 yellow tablets containing 0.01 mg ethinyl estradiol. (3)

——————CONTRAINDICATIONS——————
- A high risk of arterial or venous thrombotic diseases (4)
- Breast cancer or other estrogen- or progestin-sensitive cancer (4)
- Liver tumors or liver disease (4)
- Pregnancy (4)

————WARNINGS AND PRECAUTIONS————
- Vascular risks: Stop LoSeasonique if a thrombotic event occurs. Stop LoSeasonique at least 4 weeks before and through 2 weeks after major surgery. Start LoSeasonique no earlier than 4 weeks after delivery, in women who are not breastfeeding. (5.1)
- Liver disease: Discontinue LoSeasonique if jaundice occurs. (5.3)
- High blood pressure: Do not prescribe LoSeasonique for women with uncontrolled hypertension or hypertension with vascular disease. (5.4)
- Carbohydrate and lipid metabolic effects: Monitor prediabetic and diabetic women taking LoSeasonique. Consider an alternate contraceptive method for women with uncontrolled dyslipidemias. (5.6)
- Headache: Evaluate significant change in headaches and discontinue LoSeasonique if indicated. (5.7)
- Uterine bleeding: Evaluate irregular bleeding or amenorrhea. (5.8)

——————ADVERSE REACTIONS——————
The most common adverse reactions for COCs are irregular uterine bleeding, nausea, breast tenderness, and headaches. (6)

To report SUSPECTED ADVERSE REACTIONS, contact Duramed Pharmaceuticals Inc. at 1-800-222-0190 or FDA at 1-800-FDA-1088 or www.fda.gov/medwatch.

——————DRUG INTERACTIONS——————
Drugs or herbal products that induce certain enzymes, including CYP3A4, may decrease the effectiveness of COCs or increase breakthrough bleeding. Counsel patients to use a back-up method or alternative method of contraception when enzyme inducers are used with COCs. (7)

————USE IN SPECIFIC POPULATIONS————
- Nursing: Not recommended for nursing mothers; can decrease milk production (8.3)

See 17 for PATIENT COUNSELING INFORMATION and FDA-approved Patient Labeling.

Revised: 10/2008

FULL PRESCRIBING INFORMATION: CONTENTS*
WARNING: CIGARETTE SMOKING AND SERIOUS CARDIOVASCULAR EVENTS
1   INDICATIONS AND USAGE

---

* Sections or subsections omitted from the full prescribing information are not listed.

FULL PRESCRIBING INFORMATION

> **WARNING: CIGARETTE SMOKING AND SERIOUS CARDIOVASCULAR EVENTS**
> Cigarette smoking increases the risk of serious cardiovascular events from combination oral contraceptives (COC) use. This risk increases with age, particularly in women over 35 years of age, and with the number of cigarettes smoked. For this reason, COCs should not be used by women who are over 35 years of age and smoke. [See CONTRAINDICATIONS (4).]

1   INDICATIONS AND USAGE

LoSeasonique™ (levonorgestrel/ethinyl estradiol tablets and ethinyl estradiol tablets) is indicated for use by women to prevent pregnancy.

2   DOSAGE AND ADMINISTRATION

Take one tablet by mouth at the same time every day. The dosage of LoSeasonique is one orange tablet containing levonorgestrel and ethinyl estradiol daily for 84 consecutive days, followed by one yellow ethinyl estradiol tablet for 7 days. To achieve maximum contraceptive effectiveness, LoSeasonique must be taken exactly as directed and at intervals not exceeding 24 hours.

Instruct the patient to begin taking LoSeasonique on the first Sunday after the onset of menstruation. If menstruation begins on a Sunday, the first orange tablet is taken that day. One orange tablet should be taken daily for 84 consecutive days, followed by one yellow tablet for 7 consecutive days. A non-hormonal back-up method of contraception (such as condoms or spermicide) should be used until an orange tablet has been taken daily for 7 consecutive days. A scheduled period should occur during the 7 days that the yellow tablets are taken.

Begin the next and all subsequent 91-day cycles without interruption on the same day of the week (Sunday) on which the patient began her first dose of LoSeasonique, following the same schedule: 84 days taking an orange tablet followed by 7 days taking a yellow tablet. If the patient does not immediately start her next pill pack, she should protect herself from pregnancy by using a non-hormonal back-up method of contraception until she has taken an orange tablet daily for 7 consecutive days.

If unscheduled spotting or bleeding occurs, instruct the patient to continue on the same regimen. If the bleeding is persistent or prolonged, advise the patient to consult her healthcare provider.

For patient instructions regarding missed pills, *see PATIENT COUNSELING INFORMATION (17.2).*

For postpartum women who are not breastfeeding, start LoSeasonique no earlier than four to six weeks postpartum. If the patient starts on LoSeasonique postpartum and has not yet had a period, evaluate for possible pregnancy, and instruct her to use an additional method of contraception until she has taken an orange tablet for 7 consecutive days.

3 DOSAGE FORMS AND STRENGTHS

LoSeasonique tablets are available in Extended-Cycle Tablet Dispensers, each containing a 13-week supply of tablets: 84 orange tablets, each containing 0.1 mg of levonorgestrel and 0.02 mg ethinyl estradiol, and 7 yellow tablets each containing 0.01 mg of ethinyl estradiol. The orange tablets are round, film-coated, unscored tablets with a debossed stylized **b** on one side and **28** on the other side. The yellow tablets are round, film-coated, unscored tablet with a debossed stylized **b** on one side and **556** on the other side.

4 CONTRAINDICATIONS

Do not prescribe LoSeasonique to women who are known to have the following conditions:
- A high risk of arterial or venous thrombotic diseases. Examples include women who are known to:
  - Smoke, if over age 35
  - Have deep vein thrombosis or pulmonary embolism, now or in the past
  - Have cerebrovascular disease
  - Have coronary artery disease
  - Have thrombogenic valvular or thrombogenic rhythm diseases of the heart (for example, subacute bacterial endocarditis with valvular disease, or atrial fibrillation)
  - Have hypercoagulopathies
  - Have uncontrolled hypertension
  - Have diabetes with vascular disease
  - Have headaches with focal neurological symptoms or have migraine headaches with or without aura if over age 35
- Breast cancer or other estrogen- or progestin-sensitive cancer, now or in the past
- Liver tumors, benign or malignant, or liver disease
- Pregnancy, because there is no reason to use OCs during pregnancy

5 WARNINGS AND PRECAUTIONS

5.1 Vascular Events

Stop COCs if an arterial or deep venous thrombotic event occurs. Although use of COCs increases the risk of venous thromboembolism, pregnancy increases the risk of venous thromboembolism as much or more than the use of COCs. The risk of venous thromboembolism in women using COCs is 3 to 9 per 10,000 woman-years. Use of COCs also increases the risk of arterial thromboses such as strokes and myocardial infarctions, especially in women with other risk factors for these events.

Use of LoSeasonique provides women with more hormonal exposure on a yearly basis than conventional monthly oral contraceptives containing the same strength synthetic estrogens and progestins (an additional 9 and 13 weeks of exposure to progestin and estrogen, respectively, per year.) If feasible, stop COCs at least 4 weeks before and through 2 weeks after major surgery or other surgeries known to have an elevated risk of thromboembolism.

Start COCs no earlier than 4 weeks after delivery, in women who are not breastfeeding. The risk of postpartum thromboembolism decreases after the third postpartum week, whereas the risk of ovulation increases after the third postpartum week.

Stop COCs if there is unexplained loss of vision, proptosis, diplopia, papilledema, or retinal vascular lesions. Evaluate for retinal vein thrombosis immediately.

5.2 Carcinoma of the Breast and Cervix

Women who currently have or have had breast cancer should not use COCs because breast cancer may be hormonally sensitive.

There is substantial evidence that COCs do not increase the incidence of breast cancer. Although some past studies have suggested that COCs might increase the incidence of breast cancer, more recent studies have not confirmed such findings.

Some studies suggest that COCs are associated with an increase in the risk of cervical cancer or intraepithelial neoplasia. However, there is controversy about the extent to which these findings are due to differences in sexual behavior and other factors.

5.3 Liver Disease

Discontinue COCs if jaundice develops. Steroid hormones may be poorly metabolized in patients with impaired liver function.

Hepatic adenomas are associated with COC use. An estimate of the attributable risk is 3.3 cases/100,000 COC users. Rupture of hepatic adenomas may cause death through intra-abdominal hemorrhage.

Studies have shown an increased risk of developing hepatocellular carcinoma in long-term (> 8 years) COC users. However, the attributable risk of liver cancers in COC users is less than one case per million users.

Oral contraceptive-related cholestasis may occur in women with a history of pregnancy-related cholestasis. Women with a history of COC-related cholestasis may have the condition recur with subsequent COC use.

5.4 High Blood Pressure

For women with well-controlled hypertension, monitor blood pressure and stop COCs if blood pressure rises significantly. Women with uncontrolled hypertension or hypertension with vascular disease should not use COCs.

An increase in blood pressure has been reported in women taking COCs, and this increase is more likely in older women and with extended duration of use. The incidence of hypertension increases with increasing concentration of progestin.

5.5 Gallbladder Disease

Studies suggest a small increased relative risk of developing gallbladder disease among COC users.

5.6 Carbohydrate and Lipid Metabolic Effects

Carefully monitor prediabetic and diabetic women who are taking COCs. COCs may decrease glucose tolerance in a dose-related fashion.

Consider alternative contraception for women with uncontrolled dyslipidemias. A small proportion of women will have adverse lipid changes while on COCs.

5.7 Headache

If a woman taking COCs develops new headaches that are recurrent, persistent, or severe, evaluate the cause and discontinue COCs if indicated.

5.8 Bleeding Irregularities

Unscheduled (breakthrough) bleeding and spotting sometimes occur in patients on COCs, especially during the first 3 months of use. If bleeding persists, check for causes such as pregnancy or malignancy. If pathology and pregnancy are excluded, bleeding irregularities may resolve over time or with a change to a different COC product.

When prescribing LoSeasonique, the convenience of fewer planned menses (4 per year instead of 13 per year) should be weighed against the inconvenience of increased unscheduled bleeding and/or spotting. The clinical trial that evaluated the efficacy of LoSeasonique also assessed unscheduled bleeding. The participants in this 12-month clinical trial (N=2,185) completed the equivalent of over 20,000 28-day cycles of exposure and were composed primarily of women who had used OCs previously (89%), as opposed to new users (11%). A total of 209 subjects (9.6%) discontinued LoSeasonique, at least in part, due to bleeding and/or spotting.

Scheduled (withdrawal) bleeding and/or spotting remained fairly constant over time, with an average of 2-3 days of bleeding and/or spotting per each 91-day cycle. Unscheduled bleeding and unscheduled spotting decreased over successive 91-day cycles. Table 1 below presents the number of days with unscheduled bleeding in treatment cycles 1 and 4. Table 2 presents the number of days with unscheduled spotting in treatment cycles 1 and 4.

Table 1: Total Number of Days with Unscheduled Bleeding

91-Day Treatment Cycle	Days per 84-Day Interval				Days per 28-Day Interval
	Q1	Median	Q3	Mean	Mean
1st	0	5	11	7.5	2.5
4th	0	0	5	3.5	1.2

Q1=Quartile 1: 25% of women had this number of days of unscheduled bleeding
Median: 50% of women had ≤ this number of days of unscheduled bleeding
Q3=Quartile 3: 75% of women had ≤ this number of days of unscheduled bleeding

Table 2: Total Number of Days with Unscheduled Spotting

91-Day Treatment Cycle	Days per 84-Day Interval				Days per 28-Day Interval
	Q1	Median	Q3	Mean	Mean
1st	3	10	19	14.0	4.7
4th	0	3	10	6.5	2.2

Q1=Quartile 1: 25% of women had ≤ this number of days of unscheduled spotting
Median: 50% of women had ≤ this number of days of unscheduled spotting
Q3=Quartile 3: 75% of women had ≤ this number of days of unscheduled spotting

Figure 1 shows the percentage of LoSeasonique subjects participating in the primary clinical trial with ≥ 7 days or ≥ 20 days of unscheduled bleeding and/or spotting, or just unscheduled bleeding, during each 91-day treatment cycle.

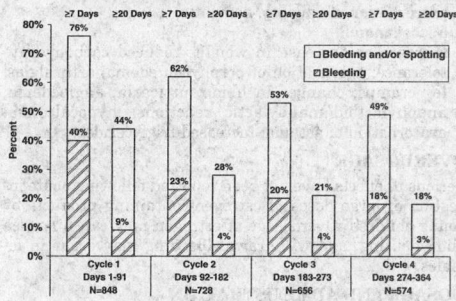

Figure 1. Percent of Women Taking LoSeasonique who Reported Unscheduled Bleeding and/or Spotting (Based on Daily Diaries)

Amenorrhea sometimes occurs in women who are using COCs. Pregnancy should be ruled out in the event of amenorrhea. Some women may encounter amenorrhea or oligomenorrhea after stopping COCs, especially when such a condition was pre-existent.

5.9 Interference with Laboratory Tests

The use of COCs may change the results of some laboratory tests, such as coagulation factors, lipids, glucose tolerance, and binding proteins. Women on thyroid hormone replacement therapy may need increased doses of thyroid hormone because serum concentrations of thyroid binding globulin increase with use of COCs.

5.10 Monitoring

A woman who is taking COCs should have a yearly visit with her healthcare provider for a blood pressure check and for other indicated healthcare.

6 ADVERSE REACTIONS

The following serious adverse reactions with the use of COCs are discussed elsewhere in the labeling:
- Serious cardiovascular events and smoking *[see BOXED WARNING]*
- Vascular events *[see WARNINGS AND PRECAUTIONS (5.1)]*
- Liver disease *[see WARNINGS AND PRECAUTIONS (5.3)]*

Adverse reactions commonly reported by COC users are:
- Irregular uterine bleeding
- Nausea
- Breast tenderness
- Headache

6.1 Clinical Trial Experience

Because clinical trials are conducted under widely varying conditions, adverse reaction rates observed in the clinical trials of a drug cannot be directly compared to the rates in the clinical trials of another drug and may not reflect the rates observed in practice.

The clinical trial that evaluated the safety and efficacy of LoSeasonique was a 12-month, multicenter, non-comparative open-label study, which enrolled women aged 18-41, of whom 2,185 took at least one dose of LoSeasonique.

Adverse Reactions Leading to Study Discontinuation: 11% of the women discontinued from the clinical trial due to an adverse reaction; the most common adverse reactions leading to discontinuation were irregular and/or heavy uterine bleeding, headache, mood changes, nausea, acne, and weight gain.

Common Treatment-Emergent Adverse Reactions (≥ 5% of women): headaches (33%); irregular and/or heavy uterine bleeding (13%), dysmenorrhea (11%), nausea and/or vomiting (11%), back pain (8%).

7 DRUG INTERACTIONS

No formal drug-drug interaction studies were conducted with LoSeasonique.

7.1 Changes in Contraceptive Effectiveness Associated with Co-Administration of Other Products

If a woman on hormonal contraceptives takes a drug or herbal product that induces enzymes, including CYP3A4, that metabolize contraceptive hormones, counsel her to use additional contraception or a different method of contraception. Drugs or herbal products that induce such enzymes may decrease the plasma concentrations of contraceptive

hormones, and may decrease the effectiveness of hormonal contraceptives or increase breakthrough bleeding. Some drugs or herbal products that may decrease the effectiveness of hormonal contraceptives include:
• barbiturates
• bosentan
• carbamazepine
• felbamate
• griseofulvin
• oxcarbazepine
• phenytoin
• rifampin
• St. John's wort
• topiramate

HIV protease inhibitors: Significant changes (increase or decrease) in the plasma levels of the estrogen and progestin have been noted in some cases of co-administration of HIV protease inhibitors.

Antibiotics: There have been reports of pregnancy while taking hormonal contraceptives and antibiotics, but clinical pharmacokinetic studies have not shown consistent effects of antibiotics on plasma concentrations of synthetic steroids.

Consult the labeling of all concurrently-used drugs to obtain further information about interactions with hormonal contraceptives or the potential for enzyme alterations.

7.2 Increase in Plasma Levels of Estradiol Associated with Co-Administered Drugs

Co-administration of atorvastatin and certain COCs containing ethinyl estradiol increase AUC values for ethinyl estradiol by approximately 20%. Ascorbic acid and acetaminophen may increase plasma ethinyl estradiol levels, possibly by inhibition of conjugation. CYP3A4 inhibitors such as itraconazole or ketoconazole may increase plasma hormone levels.

7.3 Changes in Plasma Levels of Co-Administered Drugs

Combination OCs containing some synthetic estrogens (e.g., ethinyl estradiol) may inhibit the metabolism of other compounds. Combination OCs have been shown to significantly decrease plasma concentrations of lamotrigine likely due to induction of lamotrigine glucuronidation. This may reduce seizure control; therefore, dosage adjustments of lamotrigine may be necessary. Consult the labeling of the concurrently-used drug to obtain further information about interactions with COCs or the potential for enzyme alterations.

8 USE IN SPECIFIC POPULATIONS

8.1 Pregnancy

There is little or no increased risk of birth defects in women who inadvertently use COCs during early pregnancy. Epidemiologic studies and meta-analyses have not found an increased risk of genital or non-genital birth defects (including cardiac anomalies and limb reduction defects) following exposure to low dose COCs prior to conception or during early pregnancy.

The administration of COCs to induce withdrawal bleeding should not be used as a test for pregnancy. Combination OCs should not be used during pregnancy to treat threatened or habitual abortion.

Women who do not breastfeed may start COCs no earlier than four to six weeks postpartum.

8.3 Nursing Mothers

When possible, advise the nursing mother to use other forms of contraception until she has weaned her child. Estrogen-containing OCs can reduce milk production in breastfeeding mothers. This is less likely to occur once breastfeeding is well established; however, it can occur at any time in some women. Small amounts of estrogen and progestin from low dose COCs are present in breast milk, but these doses have not produced adverse effects in breastfeeding infants.

8.4 Pediatric Use

Safety and efficacy of LoSeasonique have been established in women of reproductive age. Safety and efficacy are expected to be the same for postpubertal adolescents under the age of 18 as for users 18 years and older. Use of this product before menarche is not indicated.

8.5 Geriatric Use

This product has not been studied in postmenopausal women and is not indicated in this population.

10 OVERDOSAGE

There have been no reports of serious ill effects from overdose, including ingestion by children. Overdosage may cause withdrawal bleeding in females and nausea.

11 DESCRIPTION

LoSeasonique (levonorgestrel/ethinyl estradiol and ethinyl estradiol) tablets provide an oral contraceptive regimen of 84 orange tablets each containing 0.1 mg levonorgestrel and 0.02 mg ethinyl estradiol, followed by 7 yellow tablets each containing 0.01 mg ethinyl estradiol.

Table 3: Mean (SD) Pharmacokinetic Parameters Following a Single Dose Administration of Three Tablets of LoSeasonique in 30 Healthy Women under Fasting Conditions

	$AUC_{0-\infty}$	C_{max}	T_{max}	$T_{1/2}$
Levonorgestrel	76.5 ± 24.9 ng*hr/mL	6.0 ± 1.6 ng/mL	1.6 ± 0.6 hours	28.5 ± 8.7 hours
Ethinyl estradiol	1335.8 ± 365.3 pg*hr/mL	122.8 ± 39.5 pg/mL	1.8 ± 0.7 hours	17.5 ± 7.4 hours

$AUC_{0-\infty}$ = area under the drug concentration curve from time 0 to infinity
C_{max} = maximum concentration
T_{max} = time to maximum concentration

The structural formulas for the active components are:

Levonorgestrel
$C_{21}H_{28}O_2$ MW: 312.4

Levonorgestrel is chemically 18,19-Dinorpregn-4-en-20-yn-3-one, 13-ethyl-17-hydroxy-, (17α)-, (-)-.

Ethinyl Estradiol
$C_{20}H_{24}O_2$ MW: 296.4

Ethinyl Estradiol is 19-Norpregna-1,3,5(10)-trien-20-yne-3,17-diol, (17α)-.

Inactive ingredients for the orange tablets include FD&C Yellow # 6 (Sunset Yellow) aluminum lake, hypromellose, lactose, magnesium stearate, microcrystalline cellulose, corn starch, titanium dioxide and triacetin.

Inactive ingredients for the yellow tablets include anhydrous lactose, FD&C Yellow # 10 aluminum lake, FD&C Yellow # 6 (Sunset Yellow) aluminum lake, hypromellose, magnesium stearate, microcrystalline cellulose, polacrilin potassium, polyethylene glycol, polysorbate 80 and titanium dioxide.

12 CLINICAL PHARMACOLOGY

12.1 Mechanism of Action

Combination OCs lower the risk of becoming pregnant primarily by suppressing ovulation. Other possible mechanisms may include cervical mucus changes that inhibit sperm penetration and endometrial changes that reduce the likelihood of implantation.

12.3 Pharmacokinetics

Absorption

No specific investigation of the absolute bioavailability of LoSeasonique in humans has been conducted. However, literature indicates that levonorgestrel is rapidly and completely absorbed after oral administration (bioavailability nearly 100%) and is not subject to first-pass metabolism. Ethinyl estradiol is rapidly and almost completely absorbed from the gastrointestinal tract but, due to first-pass metabolism in gut mucosa and liver, the systemic bioavailability of ethinyl estradiol is approximately 43%.

The mean plasma pharmacokinetic parameters of LoSeasonique following a single oral dose of three levonorgestrel/ethinyl estradiol combination tablets in normal healthy women under fasting conditions are reported in Table 3.

[See table 3 above]

The effect of food on the rate and the extent of levonorgestrel and ethinyl estradiol absorption following oral administration of LoSeasonique has not been evaluated.

Distribution

The apparent volume of distribution of levonorgestrel and ethinyl estradiol is reported to be approximately 1.8 L/kg and 4.3 L/kg, respectively. Levonorgestrel is about 97.5 to 99% protein-bound, principally to sex hormone-binding globulin (SHBG) and, to a lesser extent, serum albumin. Ethinyl estradiol is about 95 to 97% bound to serum albumin. Ethinyl estradiol does not bind to SHBG, but induces SHBG synthesis, which leads to decreased levonorgestrel clearance. Following repeated daily dosing of combination levonorgestrel/ethinyl estradiol OCs, levonorgestrel plasma concentrations accumulate more than predicted based on single-dose pharmacokinetics, due in part, to increased SHBG levels that are induced by ethinyl estradiol, and a possible reduction in hepatic metabolic capacity.

Metabolism

Following absorption, levonorgestrel is conjugated at the 17β-OH position to form sulfate conjugates and, to a lesser extent, glucuronide conjugates in plasma. Significant amounts of conjugated and unconjugated 3α, 5β-tetrahydrolevonorgestrel are also present in plasma, along with much smaller amounts of 3α, 5α-tetrahydrolevonorgestrel and 16β-hydroxylevonorgestrel. Levonorgestrel and its phase I metabolites are excreted primarily as glucuronide conjugates. Metabolic clearance rates may differ among individuals by several-fold, and this may account in part for the wide variation observed in levonorgestrel concentrations among users.

First-pass metabolism of ethinyl estradiol involves formation of ethinyl estradiol-3-sulfate in the gut wall, followed by 2-hydroxylation of a portion of the remaining untransformed ethinyl estradiol by hepatic cytochrome P-450 3A4 (CYP3A4). Levels of CYP3A4 vary widely among individuals and can explain the variation in rates of ethinyl estradiol hydroxylation. Hydroxylation at the 4-, 6-, and 16-positions may also occur, although to a much lesser extent than 2-hydroxylation. The various hydroxylated metabolites are subject to further methylation and/or conjugation.

Excretion

About 45% of levonorgestrel and its metabolites are excreted in the urine and about 32% are excreted in feces, mostly as glucuronide conjugates. Ethinyl estradiol is excreted in the urine and feces as glucuronide and sulfate conjugates, and then undergoes enterohepatic recirculation.

Race

The effect of race on the pharmacokinetics of LoSeasonique has not been evaluated.

Renal and Hepatic Impairment

No formal studies were conducted to evaluate the effect of hepatic or renal disease on the disposition of LoSeasonique. However, steroid hormones may be poorly metabolized in patients with impaired liver function.

13 NONCLINICAL TOXICOLOGY

13.1 Carcinogenesis, Mutagenesis, Impairment of Fertility

[See *WARNINGS AND PRECAUTIONS (5.2, 5.3)*.]

14 CLINICAL STUDIES

In a 12-month multicenter open-label clinical trial, 2,185 women aged 18-41 were studied to assess the safety and efficacy of LoSeasonique, completing the equivalent of 20,937 28-day cycles of exposure. The racial demographic of those enrolled was: Caucasian (75%), African-American (12%), Hispanic (10%), Asian (2%), and Other (2%). There were no exclusions for body mass index (BMI) or weight. The weight range for those women treated was 87 to 381 lbs., with a mean weight of 159 lbs. Among the women in the trial, 59% were current or recent hormonal contraceptive users, 30% were prior users (had used hormonal contraceptives in the past but not in the 6 months prior to enrollment) and 11% were new starts. Of treated women, 14.2% were lost to follow-up, 11.6% discontinued due to an adverse event, and 10.3% discontinued by withdrawing their consent.

The pregnancy rate (Pearl Index [PI]) in women aged 18 to 35 years was 2.74 pregnancies per 100 women-years of use (95% confidence interval 1.92–3.78), based on 36 pregnancies that occurred after the onset of treatment and within 14 days after the last combination pill. Cycles in which conception did not occur, but which included the use of backup contraception, were not included in the calculation of the PI. The PI includes patients who did not take the drug correctly.

16 HOW SUPPLIED/STORAGE AND HANDLING

Lo Seasonique (levonorgestrel/ethinyl estradiol tablets and ethinyl estradiol tablets) are available in an Extended-Cycle Tablet Dispenser that contains 84 round, orange tablets and 7 round, yellow tablets. Each orange tablet (debossed stylized **b** on one side and **28** on the other side) contains 0.1 mg levonorgestrel and 0.02 mg ethinyl estradiol. Each yellow tablet (debossed stylized **b** on one side and **556** on the other side) contains 0.01 mg ethinyl estradiol. The tablets should not be removed from the protective blister packaging and outer plastic dispenser to avoid damage to the product. The plastic dispenser should be kept in the foil pouch until dispensed to the patient.

Box of 2 Extended-Cycle Tablet Dispensers NDC 51285-092-87

Storage
Store at 20 to 25°C [68 to 77°F] [See USP Controlled Room Temperature].

17 PATIENT COUNSELING INFORMATION
See FDA-APPROVED PATIENT LABELING (17.2)

17.1 Information for Patients
- Counsel patients that cigarette smoking increases the risk of serious cardiovascular events from COC use, and that women who are over 35 years old and smoke should not use COCs.
- Counsel patients that this product does not protect against HIV-infection (AIDS) and other sexually transmitted diseases.
- Counsel patients to take one tablet daily by mouth at the same time every day. Instruct patients what to do in the event pills are missed.
- Counsel patients to use a back-up or alternative method of contraception when enzyme inducers are used with COCs.
- Counsel patients who are breastfeeding or who desire to breastfeed that COCs may reduce breast milk production. This is less likely to occur if breastfeeding is well established.
- Counsel any patient who starts COCs postpartum, and who has not yet had a period, to use an additional method of contraception until she has taken an orange tablet for 7 consecutive days.

17.2 FDA Approved Patient Labeling
Guide for Using LoSeasonique

> **WARNING TO WOMEN WHO SMOKE**
> Do not use LoSeasonique if you smoke cigarettes and are over 35 years old. Smoking increases your risk of serious cardiovascular side effects from birth control pills, including death from heart attack, blood clots or stroke. This risk increases with age and the number of cigarettes you smoke.

Birth control pills help to lower the chances of becoming pregnant. They do not protect against HIV infection (AIDS) and other sexually transmitted diseases.

WHAT IS LoSeasonique?
LoSeasonique is a birth control pill. It contains two female hormones, an estrogen called ethinyl estradiol, and a progestin called levonorgestrel.

HOW WELL DOES LoSeasonique WORK?
Your chance of getting pregnant depends on how well you follow the directions for taking your birth control pills. The more carefully you follow the directions, the less chance you have of getting pregnant.

Based on the results of a single clinical study lasting 12 months, 2 to 4 women, out of 100 women, may get pregnant during the first year they use LoSeasonique.

The following chart shows the chance of getting pregnant for women who use different methods of birth control. Each box on the chart contains a list of birth control methods that are similar in effectiveness. The most effective methods are at the top of the chart. The box on the bottom of the chart shows the chance of getting pregnant for women who do not use birth control and are trying to get pregnant.

[See figure at top of next column]

HOW DO I TAKE LoSeasonique?
1. Take one pill every day at the same time. If you miss pills you could get pregnant. This includes starting the pack late. The more pills you miss, the more likely you are to get pregnant.
2. Many women have spotting or light bleeding, or may feel sick to their stomach during the first few months of taking LoSeasonique. If you feel sick to your stomach, do not stop taking the pill. The problem will usually go away. If it doesn't go away, check with your healthcare provider.
3. Missing pills can also cause spotting or light bleeding, even when you take the missed pills later. On the days you take 2 pills to make up for missed pills, you could also feel a little sick to your stomach.
4. If you have trouble remembering to take LoSeasonique, talk to your healthcare provider about how to make pill-taking easier or about using another method of birth control.

Before you start taking LoSeasonique
1. Decide what time of day you want to take your pill. It is important to take it at about the same time every day.
2. Look at your Extended-Cycle Tablet Dispenser. Your Tablet Dispenser consists of 3 trays with cards that hold 91 individually sealed pills (a 13-week or 91-day cycle). The

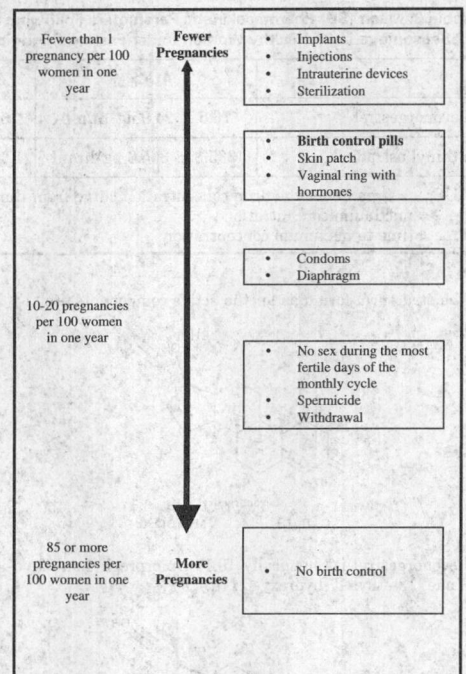

91 pills consist of 84 orange and 7 yellow pills. Trays 1 and 2 each contain 28 orange pills (4 rows of 7 pills). Tray 3 contains 35 pills consisting of 28 orange pills (4 rows of 7 pills) and 7 yellow pills (1 row of 7 pills).

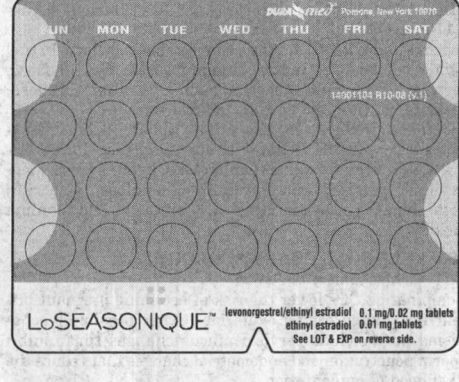

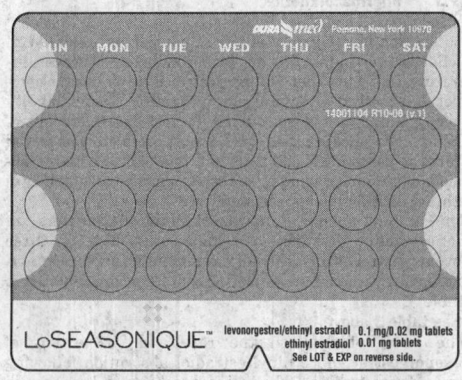

[See figure at top of next column]
3. Also find:
- Where on the first tray in the pack to start taking pills (upper left corner at the start arrow) and
- In what order to take the pills (follow the weeks and arrow).
4. Be sure you have ready at all times another kind of birth control (such as condoms or spermicides), to use as a back-up in case you miss pills.

When to Start LoSeasonique
1. Take the first orange pill on the Sunday after your period starts, even if you are still bleeding. If your period begins on Sunday, start the first orange pill that same day.

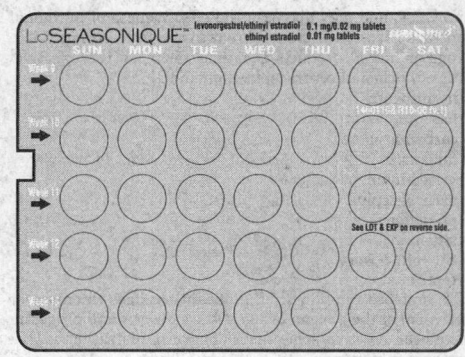

2. Use another method of birth control (such as condoms or spermicides) as a back-up method if you have sex anytime from the Sunday you start your first orange pill until the next Sunday (first 7 days). If you have been using a different hormonal method of birth control (such as a different pill, the "patch," or the "vaginal ring"), you need to use another method of birth control (such as condoms or spermicides) each time you have sex after stopping your old method of birth control until you have taken LoSeasonique for 7 days.

How to Take LoSeasonique
1. Take one pill at the same time every day until you have taken the last pill in the tablet dispenser.
- Do not skip pills even if you are experiencing spotting or bleeding or feel sick to your stomach (nausea).
- Do not skip pills even if you do not have sex very often.
2. When you finish a tablet dispenser
- After taking the last yellow pill, start taking the first orange pill from a new Extended-Cycle Tablet Dispenser the very next day (this should be on a Sunday) regardless of when your period started.
3. If you miss your scheduled period when you are taking the yellow pills, contact your healthcare provider because you may be pregnant. If you are pregnant, you should stop taking LoSeasonique.

WHAT TO DO IF YOU MISS PILLS
If you **MISS 1** orange pill:
1. Take it as soon as you remember. Take the next pill at your regular time. This means you may take 2 pills in 1 day.
2. You do not need to use a back-up birth control method if you have sex.
If you **MISS 2** orange pills in a row:
1. Take 2 pills on the day you remember, and 2 pills the next day.
2. Then take 1 pill a day until you finish the pack.
3. You could become pregnant if you have sex in the **7 days** after you miss two pills. You MUST use another birth control method (such as condoms or spermicide) as a back up for the 7 days after you restart your pills.
If you **MISS 3 OR MORE** orange pills in a row:
1. Do not take the missed pills. Keep taking 1 pill every day as indicated on the pack until you have completed all of the remaining pills in the pack. For example: If you resume taking the pill on Thursday, take the pill under "Thursday" and do not take the missed pills. You may experience bleeding during the week following the missed pills.
2. You could become pregnant if you have sex during the days of missed pills or during the first **7 days** after restarting your pills.
3. You MUST use a non-hormonal birth control method (such as condoms or spermicide) as a back-up when you miss pills and for the first 7 days after you restart your pills. If you do not have your period when you are taking the yellow pills, call your healthcare provider because you may be pregnant.
If you **MISS ANY** of the 7 yellow pills:
1. Throw away the missed pills.
2. Keep taking the scheduled pills until the pack is finished.
3. You do not need a back-up method of birth control.

Finally, if you are still not sure what to do about the pills you have missed
1. Use a back-up method anytime you have sex.
2. Keep taking one pill each day until you contact your healthcare provider.

WHO SHOULD NOT TAKE LOSEASONIQUE?
Your healthcare provider will not give you LoSeasonique if you have:
- Ever had breast cancer or any cancer that is sensitive to female hormones
- Liver disease, including liver tumors
- Ever had blood clots in your arms, legs, or lungs
- Ever had a stroke
- Ever had a heart attack
- Certain heart valve problems or heart rhythm abnormalities that can cause blood clots to form in the heart
- An inherited problem with your blood that makes it clot more than normal
- High blood pressure that medicine can't control

- Diabetes with kidney, eye, or blood vessel damage
- Certain kinds of severe migraine headaches with aura, numbness, weakness or changes in vision

Also, do not take birth control pills if you:
- Smoke and are over 35 years old
- Are pregnant

Birth control pills may not be a good choice for you if you have ever had jaundice (yellowing of the skin or eyes) caused by pregnancy.

WHAT ELSE SHOULD I KNOW ABOUT TAKING LoSeasonique?

Birth control pills do **not** protect you against any sexually transmitted disease, including HIV, the virus that causes AIDS.

Do not skip any pills, even if you do not have sex often.

Birth control pills should not be taken during pregnancy. However, birth control pills taken by accident during pregnancy are not known to cause birth defects.

If you are breastfeeding, consider another birth control method until you are ready to stop breastfeeding. Birth control pills that contain estrogen, like LoSeasonique, may decrease the amount of milk you make. A small amount of the pill's hormones pass into breast milk, but this has not caused harmful effects in breastfeeding infants.

Tell your health care provider about all medicines and herbal products that you take. Some medicines and herbal products may make birth control pills less effective, including:
- barbiturates
- bosentan
- carbamazepine
- felbamate
- griseofulvin
- oxcarbazepine
- phenytoin
- rifampin
- St. John's wort
- topiramate

Consider using another birth control method when you take medicines that may make birth control pills less effective. Birth control pills may interact with lamotrigine, an anticonvulsant used for epilepsy. This may increase the risk of seizures, so your physician may need to adjust the dose of lamotrigine.

If you have vomiting or diarrhea, your birth control pills may not work as well. Use another birth control method, like condoms or a spermicide, until you check with your health care provider.

WHAT ARE THE MOST SERIOUS RISKS OF TAKING BIRTH CONTROL PILLS?

Like pregnancy, birth control pills increase the risk of serious blood clots, especially in women who have other risk factors, such as smoking, obesity, or age > 35. It is possible to die from a problem caused by a blood clot, such as a heart attack or a stroke. Some examples of serious blood clots are blood clots in the:
- Legs (thrombophlebitis)
- Lungs (pulmonary embolus)
- Eyes (loss of eyesight)
- Heart (heart attack)
- Brain (stroke)

A few women who take birth control pills may get:
- High blood pressure
- Gallbladder problems
- Rare cancerous or noncancerous liver tumors

All of these events are uncommon in healthy women.

Call your health care provider right away if you have:
- Persistent leg pain
- Sudden shortness of breath
- Sudden blindness, partial or complete
- Severe pain in your chest
- Sudden, severe headache unlike your usual headaches
- Weakness or numbness in an arm or leg, or trouble speaking
- Yellowing of the skin or eyeballs

WHAT ARE COMMON SIDE EFFECTS OF BIRTH CONTROL PILLS?

The most common side effects of birth control pills are:
- Spotting or bleeding between menstrual periods
- Nausea
- Breast tenderness
- Headache

These side effects are usually mild and usually disappear with time.

Less common side effects are:
- Acne
- Less sexual desire
- Bloating or fluid retention
- Blotchy darkening of the skin, especially on the face
- High blood sugar, especially in women who already have diabetes
- High fat levels in the blood.

- Depression, especially if you have had depression in the past. Call your health care provider immediately if you have any thoughts of harming yourself.
- Problems tolerating contact lenses
- Weight changes

This is not a complete list of possible side effects. Talk to your health care provider if you develop any side effects that concern you.

No serious problems have been reported from a birth control pill overdose, even when accidentally taken by children.

DO BIRTH CONTROL PILLS CAUSE CANCER?

Birth control pills do not appear to cause breast cancer. However, if you have breast cancer now, or have had it in the past, do not use birth control pills because some breast cancers are sensitive to hormones.

Women who use birth control pills may have a slightly higher chance of getting cervical cancer. However, this may be due to other reasons such as having more sexual partners.

WHAT SHOULD I KNOW ABOUT MY PERIOD WHEN TAKING LoSeasonique?

When you take LoSeasonique, which has a 91-day extended dosing cycle, you should expect to have 4 scheduled periods per year (bleeding when you are taking the 7 yellow pills). Each period is likely to last about 2 to 3 days. However, you will probably have more bleeding or spotting between your scheduled periods than if you were using a birth control pill with a 28-day dosing cycle. This bleeding or spotting tends to decrease with time. Do not stop taking LoSeasonique because of this bleeding or spotting. If the spotting continues for more than 7 consecutive days or if the bleeding is heavy, call your healthcare provider.

WHAT IF I MISS MY SCHEDULED PERIOD WHEN TAKING LoSeasonique?

You should consider the possibility that you are pregnant if you miss your scheduled period (no bleeding on the days that you are taking yellow tablets). Since scheduled periods are less frequent when you are taking LoSeasonique, notify your healthcare provider that you have missed your period and that you are taking LoSeasonique. Also notify your healthcare provider if you have symptoms of pregnancy such as morning sickness or unusual breast tenderness. It is important that your healthcare provider evaluates you to determine if you are pregnant. Stop taking LoSeasonique if it is determined that you are pregnant.

WHAT IF I WANT TO BECOME PREGNANT?

You may stop taking the pill whenever you wish. Consider a visit with your health care provider for a pre-pregnancy checkup before you stop taking the pill.

Rx only

DURAMED PHARMACEUTICALS, INC.
Subsidiary of Barr Pharmaceuticals, Inc. Pomona, New York 10970
Issued October 2008
11001294
Revised 10/24/2008
Shown in Product Identification Guide, page 320

PARAGARD® T380A

[pa-ra'gard]
intrauterine copper contraceptive

PRESCRIBING INFORMATION

ParaGard® T 380A Intrauterine Copper Contraceptive Patients should be counseled that this product does not protect against HIV infection (AIDS) and other sexually transmitted diseases.

ParaGard® T 380A Intrauterine Copper Contraceptive should be placed and removed only by healthcare professionals who are experienced with these procedures.

DESCRIPTION

[See figure below]

ParaGard® T 380A Intrauterine Copper Contraceptive (ParaGard®) is a T-shaped intrauterine device (IUD), measuring 32 mm horizontally and 36 mm vertically, with a 3 mm diameter bulb at the tip of the vertical stem. A mono-

filament polyethylene thread is tied through the tip, resulting in two white threads, each at least 10.5 cm in length, to aid in detection and removal of the device. The T-frame is made of polyethylene with barium sulfate to aid in detecting the device under x-ray. ParaGard® also contains copper: approximately 176 mg of wire coiled along the vertical stem and a 68.7 mg collar on each side of the horizontal arm. The total exposed copper surface area is 380 ± 23 mm². One ParaGard® weighs less than one (1) gram. No component of ParaGard® or its packaging contains latex.

ParaGard® is packaged together with an insertion tube and solid white rod in a Tyvek® polyethylene pouch that is then sterilized. A moveable flange on the insertion tube aids in gauging the depth of insertion through the cervical canal and into the uterine cavity.

CLINICAL PHARMACOLOGY

The contraceptive effectiveness of ParaGard® is enhanced by copper continuously released into the uterine cavity. Possible mechanism(s) by which copper enhances contraceptive efficacy include interference with sperm transport or fertilization, and prevention of implantation.

INDICATIONS AND USAGE

ParaGard® is indicated for intrauterine contraception for up to 10 years. The pregnancy rate in clinical studies has been less than 1 pregnancy per 100 women each year.

Table 1: Percentage of women experiencing an unintended pregnancy during the first year of typical use and first year of perfect use of contraception and the percentage continuing use at the end of the first year: United States

Method (1)	% of Women Experiencing an Accidental Pregnancy within the First Year of Use		% of Women Continuing Use at One Year[a]
	Typical Use[b] (2)	Perfect Use[c] (3)	(4)
Chance[d]	85	85	
Spermicides[e]	26	6	40
Periodic Abstinence	25		63
Calendar		9	
Ovulation Method		3	
Sympto-thermal[f]		2	
Post-ovulation		1	
Cap[g]			
Parous women	40	26	42
Nulliparous women	20	9	56
Sponge			
Parous women	40	20	42
Nulliparous women	20	9	56
Diaphragm[g]	20	6	56
Withdrawal	19	4	
Condom[h]			
Female (Reality)	21	5	56
Male	14	3	61
Pill	5		71
Progestin only		0.5	
Combined		0.1	
IUD			
Progesterone T	2.0	1.5	81
Copper T 380A	0.8	0.6	78
LNg 20	0.1	0.1	81

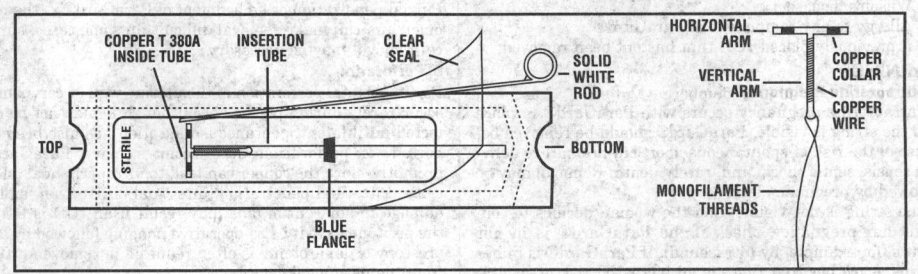

Depo Provera	0.3	0.3	70
Norplant and Norplant-2	0.05	0.05	88
Female sterilization	0.5	0.5	100
Male sterilization	0.15	0.10	100

Emergency Contraceptive Pills: Treatment initiated within 72 hours after unprotected intercourse reduces the risk of pregnancy by at least 75%.[i]

Lactational Amenorrhea Method: LAM is a highly effective temporary method of contraception.[j]

Footnotes to Table 1

Source: Trussel J. Contraceptive efficacy. In Hatcher RA, Trussel J. Stewart F, Cates W, Stewart GK, Kowal D, Guest F, Contraceptive Technology: Seventeenth Revised Edition. New York NY: Irvington Publishers, 1998.

a) Among couples attempting to avoid pregnancy, the percentage who continue to use a method for one year.
b) Among typical couples who initiate use of a method (not necessarily for the first time), the percentage who experience an accidental pregnancy during the first year if they do not stop use for any other reason.
c) Among couples who initiate use of a method (not necessarily for the first time) and who use it perfectly (both consistently and correctly), the percentage who experience an accidental pregnancy during the first year if they do not stop use for any reason.
d) The percents becoming pregnant in columns (2) and (3) are based on data from populations where contraception is not used and from women who cease using contraception in order to become pregnant. Among such populations, about 89% become pregnant within one year. This estimate was lowered slightly (to 85%) to represent the percentage who would become pregnant within one year among women now relying on reversible methods of contraception if they abandoned contraception altogether.
e) Foams, creams, gels, vaginal suppositories, and vaginal film.
f) Cervical mucus (ovulation) method supplemented by calendar in the pre-ovulatory and basal body temperature in the post-ovulatory phases.
g) With spermicidal cream or jelly.
h) Without spermicides.
i) The treatment schedule is one dose within 72 hours after unprotected intercourse, and a second dose 12 hours after the first dose. Preven is the only dedicated product specifically marketed for emergency contraception. The Food and Drug Administration has also declared the following brands of oral contraceptive to be safe and effective for emergency contraception: Ovral (1 dose is 2 white pills), Alesse (1 dose is 5 pink pills), Nordette or Levlen (1 dose is 4 light-orange pills), Lo/Ovral (1 dose is 4 white pills), Triphasil or Tri-Levlen (1 dose is 4 yellow pills).
j) However, to maintain effective protection against pregnancy, another method of contraception must be used as soon as menstruation resumes, the frequency or duration of breastfeeds is reduced, bottle feeds are introduced or the baby reaches 6 months of age.

CONTRAINDICATIONS

ParaGard® should not be placed when one or more of the following conditions exist:

1. Pregnancy or suspicion of pregnancy
2. Abnormalities of the uterus resulting in distortion of the uterine cavity
3. Acute pelvic inflammatory disease, or current behavior suggesting a high risk for pelvic inflammatory disease
4. Postpartum endometritis or postabortal endometritis in the past 3 months
5. Known or suspected uterine or cervical malignancy
6. Genital bleeding of unknown etiology
7. Mucopurulent cervicitis
8. Wilson's disease
9. Allergy to any component of ParaGard®
10. A previously placed IUD that has not been removed

WARNINGS

1. Intrauterine Pregnancy

If intrauterine pregnancy occurs with ParaGard® in place and the string is visible, ParaGard® should be removed because of the risk of spontaneous abortion, premature delivery, sepsis, septic shock, and, rarely, death. Removal may be followed by pregnancy loss.

If the string is not visible, and the woman decides to continue her pregnancy, check if the ParaGard® is in her uterus (for example, by ultrasound). If ParaGard® is in her uterus, warn her that there is an increased risk of spontaneous abortion and sepsis, septic shock, and rarely, death.[1] In addition, the risk of premature labor and delivery is increased.[1]

Human data about risk of birth defects from copper exposure are limited. However, studies have not detected a pattern of abnormalities, and published reports do not suggest a risk that is higher than the baseline risk for birth defects.

2. Ectopic Pregnancy

Women who become pregnant while using ParaGard® should be evaluated for ectopic pregnancy. A pregnancy that occurs with ParaGard® in place is more likely to be ectopic than a pregnancy in the general population. However, because ParaGard® prevents most pregnancies, women who use ParaGard® have a lower risk of an ectopic pregnancy than sexually active women who do not use any contraception.[2-3]

3. Pelvic Infection

Although pelvic inflammatory disease (PID) in women using IUDs is uncommon, IUDs may be associated with an increased relative risk of PID compared to other forms of contraception and to no contraception. The highest incidence of PID occurs within 20 days following insertion. Therefore, the visit following the first post-insertion menstrual period is an opportunity to assess the patient for infection, as well as to check that the IUD is in place. (See **INSTRUCTIONS FOR USE, Continuing Care.**) Since pelvic infection is most frequently associated with sexually transmitted organisms, IUDs are not recommended for women at high risk for sexual infection. Prophylactic antibiotics at the time of insertion do not appear to lower the incidence of PID.[4]

PID can have serious consequences, such as tubal damage (leading to ectopic pregnancy or infertility), hysterectomy, sepsis, and, rarely, death. It is therefore important to promptly assess and treat any woman who develops signs or symptoms of PID.

Guidelines for treatment of PID are available from the Centers for Disease Control and Prevention (CDC), Atlanta, Georgia at www.cdc.gov or 1-800-311-3435. Antibiotics are the mainstay of therapy. Most healthcare professionals also remove the IUD.

The significance of actinomyces-like organisms on Papanicolaou smear in an asymptomatic IUD user is unknown,[5-6] and so this finding alone does not always require IUD removal and treatment. However, because pelvic actinomycosis is a serious infection, a woman who has *symptoms* of pelvic infection possibly due to actinomyces should be treated and have her IUD removed.

4. Immunocompromise

Women with AIDS should not have IUDs inserted unless they are clinically stable on antiretroviral therapy. Limited data suggest that asymptomatic women infected with human immunodeficiency virus may use intrauterine devices. Little is known about the use of IUDs in women who have illnesses causing serious immunocompromise. Therefore these women should be carefully monitored for infection if they choose to use an IUD. The risk of pregnancy should be weighed against the theoretical risk of infection.

5. Embedment

Partial penetration or embedment of ParaGard® in the myometrium can make removal difficult. In some cases, surgical removal may be necessary.

6. Perforation

Partial or total perforation of the uterine wall or cervix may occur rarely during placement, although it may not be detected until later. Spontaneous migration has also been reported. If perforation does occur, remove ParaGard® promptly, since the copper can lead to intraperitoneal adhesions. Intestinal penetration, intestinal obstruction, and/or damage to adjacent organs may result if an IUD is left in the peritoneal cavity. Pre-operative imaging followed by laparoscopy or laparotomy is often required to remove an IUD from the peritoneal cavity.

Table 2. Summary of Rates (No. per 100 Subjects) by Year for Adverse Events Causing Discontinuation

Adverse Event	Year									
	1	2	3	4	5	6	7	8	9	10
Pregnancy	0.7	0.3	0.6	0.2	0.3	0.2	0.0	0.4	0.0	0.0
Expulsion	5.7	2.5	1.6	1.2	0.3	0.0	0.6	1.7	0.2	0.4
Bleeding/Pain	11.9	9.8	7.0	3.5	3.7	2.7	3.0	2.5	2.2	3.7
Other Medical Event	2.5	2.1	1.6	1.7	0.1	0.3	1.0	0.4	0.7	0.3
No. of Women at Start of Year	4932	3149	2018	1121	872	621	563	483	423	325

* Rates were calculated by weighting the annual rates by the number of subjects starting each year for each of the Population Council (3,536 subjects) and the World Health Organization (1,396 subjects) trials.

7. Expulsion

Expulsion can occur, usually during the menses and usually in the first few months after insertion. There is an increased risk of expulsion in the nulliparous patient. If unnoticed, an unintended pregnancy could occur.

8. Wilson's Disease

Theoretically, ParaGard® can exacerbate Wilson's disease, a rare genetic disease affecting copper excretion.

PRECAUTIONS

Patients should be counseled that this product does not protect against HIV infection (AIDS) and other sexually transmitted diseases.

1. Information for patients

Before inserting ParaGard® discuss the Patient Package Insert with the patient, and give her time to read the information. Discuss any questions she may have concerning ParaGard® as well as other methods of contraception. Instruct her to promptly report symptoms of infection, pregnancy, or missing strings.

2. Insertion precautions, continuing care, and removal.

(See **INSTRUCTIONS FOR USE.**)

3. Vaginal bleeding

In the 2 largest clinical trials with ParaGard® (see ADVERSE REACTIONS, Table 2), menstrual changes were the most common medical reason for discontinuation of ParaGard®. Discontinuation rates for pain and bleeding combined are highest in the first year of use and diminish thereafter. The percentage of women who discontinued ParaGard® because of bleeding problems or pain during these studies ranged from 11.9% in the first year to 2.2 % in year 9. Women complaining of heavy vaginal bleeding should be evaluated and treated, and may need to discontinue ParaGard®. (See **ADVERSE REACTIONS.**)

4. Vasovagal reactions, including fainting

Some women have vasovagal reactions immediately after insertion. Hence, patients should remain supine until feeling well and should be cautious when getting up.

5. Expulsion following placement after a birth or abortion

ParaGard® has been placed immediately after delivery, although risk of expulsion may be higher than when ParaGard® is placed at times unrelated to delivery.[7] However, unless done immediately postpartum, insertion should be delayed to the second postpartum month because insertion during the first postpartum month (except for immediately after delivery) has been associated with increased risk of perforation.[8]

ParaGard® can be placed immediately after abortion, although immediate placement has a slightly higher risk of expulsion than placement at other times.[9] Placement after second trimester abortion is associated with a higher risk of expulsion than placement after the first trimester abortion.[9]

6. Magnetic resonance imaging (MRI)

Limited data suggest that MRI at the level of 1.5 Tesla is acceptable in women using ParaGard®. One study examined the effect of MRI on the CU-7® Intrauterine Copper Contraceptive and Lippes Loop™ intrauterine devices. Neither device moved under the influence of the magnetic field or heated during the spin-echo sequences usually employed for pelvic imaging.[10] An in vitro study did not detect movement or temperature change when ParaGard® was subjected to MRI.[11]

7. Medical diathermy

Theoretically, medical (non-surgical) diathermy (short-wave and microwave heat therapy) in a patient with a metal-containing IUD may cause heat injury to the surrounding tissue. However, a small study of eight women did not detect a significant elevation of intrauterine temperature when diathermy was performed in the presence of a copper IUD.[12]

8. Pregnancy

ParaGard® is contraindicated during pregnancy. (See CONTRAINDICATIONS and WARNINGS.)

9. Nursing mothers

Nursing mothers may use ParaGard®. No difference has been detected in concentration of copper in human milk before and after insertion of copper IUDs. The literature is conflicting, but limited data suggest that there may be an increased risk of perforation and expulsion if a woman is lactating. [13]

10. Pediatric use

ParaGard® is not indicated before menarche. Safety and efficacy have been established in women over 16 years old.

ADVERSE REACTIONS

The most serious adverse events associated with intrauterine contraception are discussed in **WARNINGS** and **PRECAUTIONS**. These include:

Intrauterine pregnancy	Pelvic infection
Septic abortion	Perforation
Ectopic pregnancy	Embedment

Table 2 shows discontinuation rates from two clinical studies by adverse event and year.

[See table at top of previous page]

The following adverse events have also been observed. These are listed alphabetically and not by order of frequency or severity.

Anemia	Menstrual flow, prolonged
Backache	Menstrual spotting
Dysmenorrhea	Pain and cramping
Dyspareunia	Urticarial allergic skin reaction
Expulsion, complete or partial	Vaginitis
Leukorrhea	

INSTRUCTIONS FOR USE

The placement technique for ParaGard® is different from that used for other IUDs. Therefore, the clinician should be familiar with the following instructions.

ParaGard® may be placed at any time during the cycle when the clinician is reasonably certain the patient is not pregnant. For information about timing of postpartum and postabortion insertions, see **PRECAUTIONS**.

A single ParaGard® should be placed at the fundus of the uterine cavity. ParaGard® should be removed on or before 10 years from the date of insertion.

Before Placement:

1. Make sure that the patient is an appropriate candidate for ParaGard® and that she has read the Patient Package Insert.
2. Use of an analgesic before insertion is at the discretion of the patient and the clinician.
3. Establish the size and position of the uterus by pelvic examination.
4. Insert a speculum and cleanse the vagina and cervix with an antiseptic solution.
5. Apply a tenaculum to the cervix and use gentle traction to align the cervical canal with the uterine cavity.
6. Gently insert a sterile sound to measure the depth of the uterine cavity.
7. The uterus should sound to a depth of 6 to 9 cm except when inserting ParaGard® immediately post-abortion or post-partum. Insertion of ParaGard® into a uterine cavity measuring less than 6 cm may increase the incidence of expulsion, bleeding, pain, and perforation. If you encounter cervical stenosis, avoid undue force. Dilators may be helpful in this situation.

How to Load and Place ParaGard®:

Do not bend the arms of ParaGard® earlier than 5 minutes before it is to be placed in the uterus. Use aseptic technique when handling ParaGard® and the part of the insertion tube that will enter the uterus.

STEP 1

Load ParaGard® into the insertion tube by folding the two horizontal arms of ParaGard® against the stem and push the tips of the arms securely into the insertion tube.

If you do not have sterile gloves, you can do STEPS 1 and 2 while ParaGard® is in the sterile package. First, place the package face up on a clean surface. Next, open at the bottom end (where arrow says OPEN). Pull the solid white rod partially from the package so it will not interfere with assem-

bly. Place thumb and index finger on top of package on ends of the horizontal arms. Use other hand to push insertion tube against arms of ParaGard® (shown by arrow in Fig. 1). This will start bending the T arms.

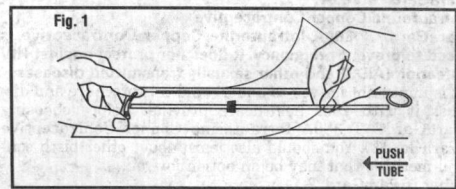

Fig. 1

PUSH TUBE

STEP 2

Bring the thumb and index finger closer together to continue bending the arms until they are alongside the stem. Use the other hand to withdraw the insertion tube just enough so that the insertion tube can be pushed and rotated onto the tips of the arms. Your goal is to secure the tips of the arms inside the tube (Fig. 2). Insert the arms no further than necessary to insure retention. Introduce the solid white rod into the insertion tube from the bottom, alongside the threads, **until it touches the bottom of the ParaGard®**.

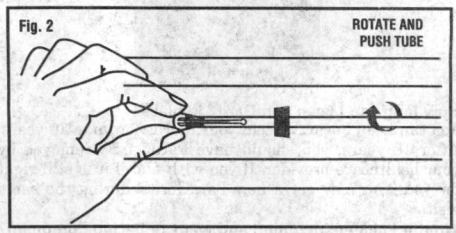

Fig. 2

ROTATE AND PUSH TUBE

STEP 3

Grasp the insertion tube at the open end of the package; adjust the blue flange so that the distance from the top of the ParaGard® (where it protrudes from the inserter) to the blue flange is the same as the uterine depth that you measured with the sound. Rotate the insertion tube so that the horizontal arms of the T and the long axis of the blue flange lie in the same horizontal plane (Fig. 3). Now pass the loaded insertion tube through the cervical canal until ParaGard® just touches the fundus of the uterus. The blue flange should be at the cervix in the horizontal plane.

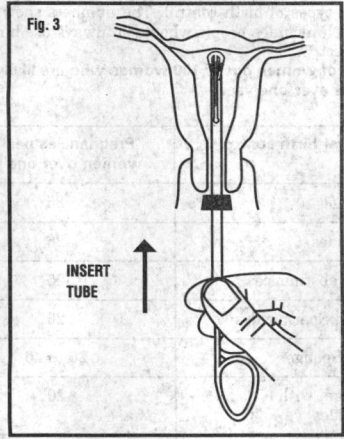

Fig. 3

INSERT TUBE

STEP 4

To release the arms of ParaGard®, hold the solid white rod steady and withdraw the insertion tube no more than one centimeter This releases the arms of ParaGard® high in the uterine fundus (Fig. 4).

[See figure 4 at top of next column]

STEP 5

Gently and carefully move the insertion tube upward toward the top of the uterus, until slight resistance is felt. This will ensure placement of the T at the highest possible position within the uterus (Fig. 5).

[See figure 5 on next column]

STEP 6

Hold the insertion tube steady and withdraw the solid white rod (Fig. 6).

[See figure 6 on next column]

STEP 7

Gently and slowly withdraw the insertion tube from the cervical canal. Only the threads should be visible protruding

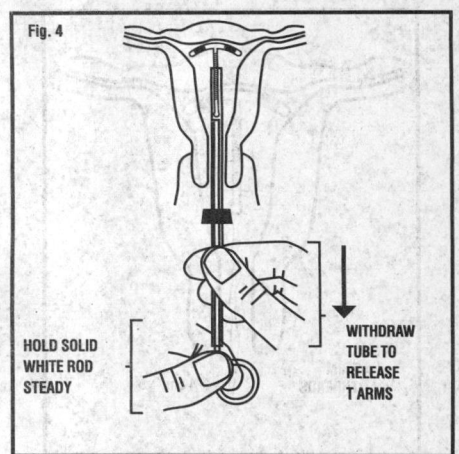

Fig. 4

HOLD SOLID WHITE ROD STEADY

WITHDRAW TUBE TO RELEASE T ARMS

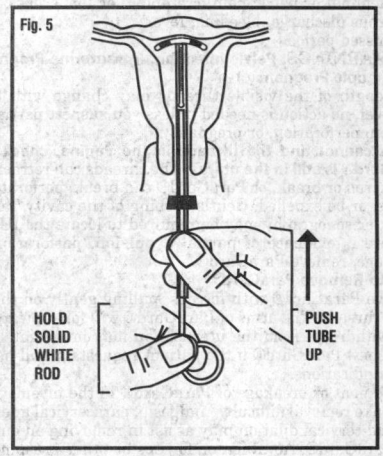

Fig. 5

HOLD SOLID WHITE ROD

PUSH TUBE UP

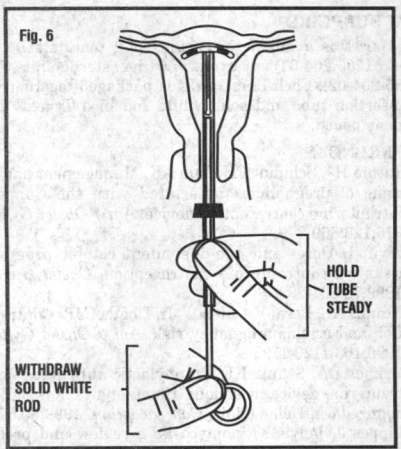

Fig. 6

HOLD TUBE STEADY

WITHDRAW SOLID WHITE ROD

from the cervix. (Fig. 7). Trim the threads so that 3 to 4 cm protrude into the vagina. Note the length of the threads in the patient's records.

If you suspect that ParaGard® is not in the correct position, check placement (with ultrasound, if necessary). If ParaGard® is not positioned completely within the uterus, remove it and replace it with a new ParaGard®. Do not reinsert an expelled or partially expelled ParaGard®.

[See figure 7 at top of next page]

CAUTION

Instrumentation of the cervical os may result in vasovagal reactions, including fainting. Have the patient remain supine until she feels well, and have her get up with caution.

Continuing Care:

Following placement, examine the patient after her first menses to confirm that ParaGard® is still in place. **You should be able to see or feel only the threads.** If ParaGard® has been partially or completely expelled, remove it. You can place a new ParaGard® if the patient desires and if she is not pregnant. Do not reinsert a used ParaGard®.

Evaluate the patient promptly if she complains of any of the following:

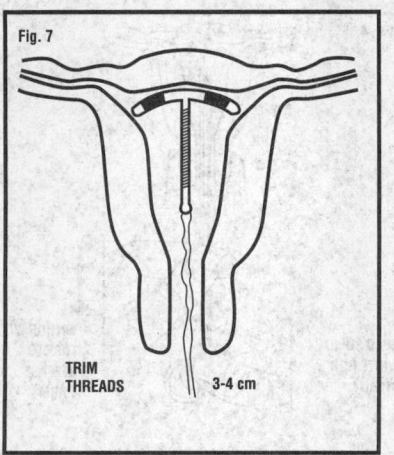

Fig. 7

TRIM THREADS   3-4 cm

- Abdominal or pelvic pain, cramping, or tenderness; malodorous discharge; bleeding; fever
- A missed period

(See **WARNINGS, Pelvic Infection, Intrauterine Pregnancy** and **Ectopic Pregnancy**.)

The length of the visible threads may change with time. However, no action is needed unless you suspect partial expulsion, perforation, or pregnancy.

If you cannot find the threads in the vagina, check that ParaGard® is still in the uterus. The threads can retract into the uterus or break, or ParaGard® can break, perforate the uterus, or be expelled. Gentle probing of the cavity, radiography, or sonography may be required to locate the IUD.

If there is evidence of partial expulsion, perforation, or breakage, remove ParaGard®.

How to Remove ParaGard®

Remove ParaGard® with forceps, pulling gently on the exposed threads. The arms of ParaGard® will fold upwards as it is withdrawn from the uterus. You may immediately insert a new ParaGard® if the patient requests it and has no contraindications.

Embedment or breakage of ParaGard® in the myometrium can make removal difficult. Analgesia, paracervical anesthesia, and cervical dilation may assist in removing an embedded ParaGard®. An alligator forceps or other grasping instrument may be helpful. Hysteroscopy may also be helpful.

HOW SUPPLIED

ParaGard® is available in cartons of 1 (one) sterile unit (NDC 51285-204-01) or cartons of 5 (five) sterile units (NDC 51285-204-02). Each ParaGard® is packaged together with an insertion tube and solid white rod in a Tyvek® polyethylene pouch.

REFERENCES

1. Tatum HJ, Schmidt FH, Jain AK. Management and outcome of pregnancies associated with the Copper T intrauterine contraceptive device. *Am J Obstet Gynecol.* 976;126:869-879.
2. Sivin I. Dose- and age-dependent ectopic pregnancy risks with intrauterine contraception. *Obstet Gynecol.* 1999;78:291-298.
3. Franks AL, Beral V, Cates W Jr, Hogue CJR. Contraception and ectopic pregnancy risk. *Am J Obstet Gynecol.* 1990;163:1120-1123.
4. Grimes DA, Schulz KF. Prophylactic antibiotics for intrauterine device insertion: a metaanalysis of the randomized controlled trials. *Contraception.* 1999;60:57-63.
5. Lippes J. Pelvic actinomycosis: a review and preliminary look at prevalence. *Am J Obstet Gynecol.* 1999;180:265-269.
6. Petitti DB, Yamamoto D, Morgenstern N. Factors associated with actinomyces-like organisms on Papanicolaou smear in users of intrauterine contraceptive devices. *Am J Obstet Gynecol.* 1983;145:338-341.
7. Grimes D, Schulz K, van Vliet H, Stanwood N. Immediate post-partum insertion of intrauterine devices: a Cochrane review. *Hum Reprod.* 2002;17:549-554.
8. Cole LP, Edelman DA, Potts DM, Wheeler RG, Laufe LE. Postpartum insertion of modified intrauterine devices. *J Reprod Med.* 1984;29:677-682.
9. Grimes DA, Schulz KF, Stanwood N. Immediate post-abortal insertion of intrauterine devices. (Cochrane Review). In: *The Cochrane Library,* Issue 2, 2003. Oxford: Update Software.
10. Hess T, Stepanow B, Knopp MV. Magnetic resonance imaging: safety of intrauterine contraceptive devices during MR imaging. *Eur Radiol.* 1996;6:66-68.
11. Mark AS, Hricak H. Intrauterine devices. MR imaging. *Radiology.* 1987;162:311-314.
12. Heick A., Espersen T., Pedersen HL, Raahauge J: Is diathermy safe in women with copper-bearing IUDs? *Acta Obstet Gynecol Scand.* 1991;70(2):153-5.
13. Rodrigues da Cunha AC, Dorea JG, Cantuaria AA. Intrauterine device and maternal copper metabolism during lactation. Contraception 2001;63:37-9.

INFORMATION FOR PATIENTS

ParaGard® T 380A
Intrauterine Copper Contraceptive
ParaGard® T 380A Intrauterine Copper Contraceptive is used to prevent pregnancy. It does not protect against HIV infection (AIDS) and other sexually transmitted diseases.

It is important for you to understand this brochure and discuss it with your healthcare provider before choosing ParaGard® T 380A Intrauterine Copper Contraceptive (ParaGard®). You should also learn about other birth control methods that may be an option for you.

What is ParaGard®?

ParaGard® is a copper-releasing device that is placed in your uterus to prevent pregnancy for up to 10 years. ParaGard® is made of white plastic in the shape of a "T." Copper is wrapped around the stem and arms of the "T". Two white threads are attached to the stem of the "T". The threads are the only part of ParaGard® that you can feel when ParaGard® is in your uterus. ParaGard® and its components do not contain latex.

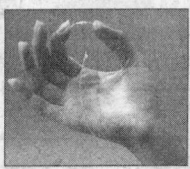

How long can I keep ParaGard® in place?

You can keep ParaGard® in your uterus for up to 10 years. After 10 years, you should have ParaGard® removed by your healthcare provider. If you wish and if it is still right for you, you may get a new ParaGard® during the same visit.

What if I change my mind and want to become pregnant?

Your healthcare provider can remove ParaGard® at any time. After discontinuation of ParaGard®, its contraceptive effect is reversed.

How does ParaGard® work?

Ideas about how ParaGard® works include preventing sperm from reaching the egg, preventing sperm from fertilizing the egg, and preventing the egg from advanced (implanting) in the uterus. ParaGard® does not stop your ovaries from making an egg (ovulating) each month.

How well does ParaGard® work?

Fewer than 1 in 100 women become pregnant each year while using ParaGard®.

The table below shows the chance of getting pregnant using different types of birth control. The numbers show *typical* use, which includes people who don't always use birth control correctly.

Number of women out of 100 women who are likely to get pregnant over one year

Method of birth control	Pregnancies per 100 women over one year
No Method	85
Spermicides	26
Periodic abstinence	25
Cap with Spermicides	20
Vaginal Sponge	20 to 40
Diaphragm with Spermicides	20
Withdrawal	19
Condom without spermicides (female)	21
Condom without spermicides (male)	14
Oral Contraceptives	5
IUDs, Depo-Provera, implants, sterilization	less than 1

Who might use ParaGard®?

You might choose ParaGard® if you
- need birth control that is very effective
- need birth control that stops working when you stop using it
- need birth control that is easy to use

Who should not use ParaGard®?

You should not use ParaGard® if you
- Might be pregnant
- Have a uterus that is abnormally shaped inside
- Have a pelvic infection called pelvic inflammatory disease (PID) or have current behavior that puts you at high risk of PID (for example, because you are having sex with several men, or your partner is having sex with other women)
- Have had an infection in your uterus after a pregnancy or abortion in the past 3 months
- Have cancer of the uterus or cervix
- Have unexplained bleeding from your vagina
- Have an infection in your cervix
- Have Wilson's disease (a disorder in how the body handles copper)
- Are allergic to anything in ParaGard®
- Already have an intrauterine contraceptive in your uterus

How is ParaGard® placed in the uterus?

ParaGard® is placed in your uterus during an office visit. Your healthcare provider first examines you to find the position of your uterus. Next, he or she will cleanse your vagina and cervix, measure your uterus, and then slide a plastic tube containing ParaGard® into your uterus. The tube is removed, leaving ParaGard® inside your uterus. Two white threads extend into your vagina. The threads are trimmed so they are just long enough for you to feel with your fingers when doing a self-check. As ParaGard® goes in, you may feel cramping or pinching. Some women feel faint, nauseated, or dizzy for a few minutes afterwards. Your healthcare provider may ask you to lie down for a while and to get up slowly.

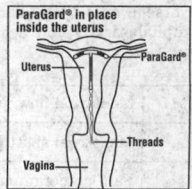

ParaGard® in place inside the uterus

Uterus — ParaGard®

Threads

Vagina

How do I check that ParaGard® is in my uterus?

Visit your healthcare provider for a check-up about one month after placement to make sure ParaGard® is still in your uterus.

You can also check to make sure that ParaGard® is still in your uterus by reaching up to the top of your vagina with clean fingers to feel the two threads. Do not pull on the threads. If you cannot feel the threads, ask your healthcare provider to check if ParaGard® is in the right place. If you can feel more of ParaGard® than just the threads, ParaGard® is *not* in the right place. If you can't see your healthcare provider right away, use an additional birth control method. If ParaGard® is in the wrong place, your chances of getting pregnant are increased. It is a good habit for you to check that ParaGard® is in place once a month. You may use tampons when you are using ParaGard®.

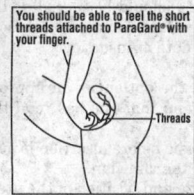

You should be able to feel the short threads attached to ParaGard® with your finger.

Threads

What if I become pregnant while using ParaGard®?

If you think you are pregnant, contact your healthcare professional *right away*. If you are pregnant and ParaGard® is in your uterus, you may get a severe infection or shock, have a miscarriage or premature labor and delivery, or even die. Because of these risks, your healthcare provider will recommend that you have ParaGard® removed, even though removal may cause miscarriage.

If you continue a pregnancy with ParaGard® in place, see your healthcare provider regularly. Contact your healthcare provider right away if you get fever, chills, cramping, pain, bleeding, flu-like symptoms, or an unusual, bad smelling vaginal discharge.

A pregnancy with ParaGard® in place has a greater than usual chance of being ectopic (outside your uterus). Ectopic pregnancy is an emergency that may require surgery. An ectopic pregnancy can cause internal bleeding, infertility, and death. Unusual vaginal bleeding or abdominal pain may be signs of an ectopic pregnancy.

Copper in ParaGard® does not seem to cause birth defects.

What side effects can I expect with ParaGard®?

The most common side effects of ParaGard® are heavier, longer periods and spotting between periods; most of these side effects diminish after 2-3 months. However, if your menstrual flow continues to be heavy or long, or spotting continues, contact your healthcare provider.

Infrequently, serious side effects may occur:

- Pelvic inflammatory disease (PID): Uncommonly, ParaGard® and other IUDs are associated with PID. PID is an infection of the uterus, tubes, and nearby organs. PID is most likely to occur in the first 20 days after placement. You have a higher chance of getting PID if you or your partner have sex with more than one person. PID is treated with antibiotics. However, PID can cause serious problems such as infertility, ectopic pregnancy, and chronic pelvic pain. Rarely, PID may even cause death. More serious cases of PID require surgery or a hysterectomy (removal of the uterus). Contact your healthcare provider right away if you have any of the signs of PID: abdominal or pelvic pain, painful sex, unusual or bad smelling vaginal discharge, chills, heavy bleeding, or fever.
- Difficult removals: Occasionally ParaGard® may be hard to remove because it is stuck in the uterus. Surgery may sometimes be needed to remove ParaGard®.
- Perforation: Rarely, ParaGard® goes through the wall of the uterus, especially during placement. This is called perforation. If ParaGard® perforates the uterus, it should be removed. Surgery may be needed. Perforation can cause infection, scarring, or damage to other organs. If ParaGard® perforates the uterus, you are not protected from pregnancy.
- Expulsion: ParaGard® may partially or completely fall out of the uterus. This is called expulsion. Women who have never been pregnant may be more likely to expel ParaGard® than women who have been pregnant before. If you think that ParaGard® has partly or completely fallen out, use an additional birth control method, such as a condom and call your healthcare provider.

You may have other side effects with ParaGard®. For example, you may have anemia (low blood count), backache, pain during sex, menstrual cramps, allergic reaction, vaginal infection, vaginal discharge, faintness, or pain. This is not a complete list of possible side effects. If you have questions about a side effect, check with your healthcare provider.

When should I call my healthcare provider?

Call your healthcare provider if you have any concerns about ParaGard®. Be sure to call if you

- Think you are pregnant
- Have pelvic pain or pain during sex
- Have unusual vaginal discharge or genital sores
- Have unexplained fever
- Might be exposed to sexually transmitted diseases (STDs)
- Cannot feel ParaGard®'s threads or can feel the threads are much longer
- Can feel any other part of the ParaGard® besides the threads
- Become HIV positive or your partner becomes HIV positive
- Have severe or prolonged vaginal bleeding
- Miss a menstrual period

General advice about prescription medicines

This brochure summarizes the most important information about ParaGard®. If you would like more information, talk with your healthcare provider. You can ask your healthcare provider for information about ParaGard® that is written for healthcare professionals.

Checklist

This checklist will help you and your healthcare provider discuss the pros and cons of ParaGard® for you. Do you have any of the following conditions?

	Yes	No	Don't know
Abnormal Pap smear	☐	☐	☐
Abnormalities of the uterus	☐	☐	☐
Allergy to copper	☐	☐	☐
Anemia or blood clotting problems	☐	☐	☐
Bleeding between periods	☐	☐	☐
Cancer of the uterus or cervix	☐	☐	☐
Fainting attacks	☐	☐	☐
Genital sores	☐	☐	☐
Heavy menstrual flow	☐	☐	☐
HIV or AIDS	☐	☐	☐
Infection of the uterus or cervix	☐	☐	☐
IUD in place now or in the past	☐	☐	☐
More than one sexual partner	☐	☐	☐

Pelvic infection (PID)	☐	☐	☐
Possible pregnancy	☐	☐	☐
Repeated episodes of pelvic infection (PID)	☐	☐	☐
Serious infection following a pregnancy or abortion in the past 3 months	☐	☐	☐
Severe menstrual cramps	☐	☐	☐
Sexual transmitted disease (STD) such as gonorrhea or chlamydia	☐	☐	☐
Wilson's disease	☐	☐	☐

DURAMED PHARMACEUTICALS, INC.
Subsidiary of Barr Pharmaceuticals, Inc.
Pomona, New York 10970
©2006 Duramed Pharmaceuticals, Inc.
Revision: MAY 2006 (v.1)
P/N 11001035

PLAN B ONE-STEP   ℞
[plăn b]
(levonorgestrel)
Tablet, 1.5 mg, For Oral Use

HIGHLIGHTS OF PRESCRIBING INFORMATION

These highlights do not include all the information needed to use Plan B One-Step safely and effectively. See full prescribing information for Plan B One-Step.

Plan B One-Step (levonorgestrel) tablet, 1.5 mg, for oral use
Initial U.S. Approval: 1982

————————INDICATIONS AND USAGE————————

Plan B One-Step is a progestin-only emergency contraceptive indicated for prevention of pregnancy following unprotected intercourse or a known or suspected contraceptive failure. Plan B One-Step is available only by prescription for women younger than age 17 years, and available over the counter for women 17 years and older. Plan B One-Step is not intended for routine use as a contraceptive. (1)

———————DOSAGE AND ADMINISTRATION———————

One tablet taken orally as soon as possible within 72 hours after unprotected intercourse. Efficacy is better if the tablet is taken as soon as possible after unprotected intercourse. (2)

—————DOSAGE FORMS AND STRENGTHS—————

1.5 mg tablet (3)

————————CONTRAINDICATIONS————————

Known or suspected pregnancy (4)

—————WARNINGS AND PRECAUTIONS—————

- Ectopic pregnancy: Women who become pregnant or complain of lower abdominal pain after taking Plan B One-Step should be evaluated for ectopic pregnancy. (5.1)
- Plan B One-Step is not effective in terminating an existing pregnancy. (5.2)
- Effect on menses: Plan B One-Step may alter the next expected menses. If menses is delayed beyond 1 week, pregnancy should be considered. (5.3)
- STI/HIV: Plan B One-Step does not protect against STI/HIV. (5.4)

————————ADVERSE REACTIONS————————

The most common adverse reactions (≥10%) in clinical trials included heavier menstrual bleeding (31%), nausea (14%), lower abdominal pain (13%), fatigue (13%), headache (10%), and dizziness (10%). (6.1)

To report SUSPECTED ADVERSE REACTIONS, contact Barr Laboratories at 1-800-330-1271 or FDA at 1-800-FDA-1088 or www.fda.gov/medwatch

————————DRUG INTERACTIONS————————

Drugs or herbal products that induce certain enzymes, such as CYP3A4, may decrease the effectiveness of progestin-only pills. (7)

—————USE IN SPECIFIC POPULATIONS—————

- Nursing Mothers: Small amounts of progestin pass into the breast milk of nursing women taking progestin-only pills for long-term contraception, resulting in detectable steroid levels in infant plasma. (8.3)
- Plan B One-Step is not intended for use in premenarcheal (8.4) or postmenopausal females (8.5).

See 17 for PATIENT COUNSELING INFORMATION.

Revised 8/2009

FULL PRESCRIBING INFORMATION: CONTENTS*

1   **INDICATIONS AND USAGE**
2   **DOSAGE AND ADMINISTRATION**
3   **DOSAGE FORMS AND STRENGTHS**
4   **CONTRAINDICATIONS**

5   **WARNINGS AND PRECAUTIONS**
    5.1   Ectopic Pregnancy
    5.2   Existing Pregnancy
    5.3   Effect on Menses
    5.4   STI/HIV
    5.5   Physical Examination and Follow-up
    5.6   Fertility Following Discontinuation
6   **ADVERSE REACTIONS**
    6.1   Clinical Trial Experience
    6.2   Postmarketing Experience
7   **DRUG INTERACTIONS**
8   **USE IN SPECIFIC POPULATIONS**
    8.1   Pregnancy
    8.3   Nursing Mothers
    8.4   Pediatric Use
    8.5   Geriatric Use
    8.6   Race
    8.7   Hepatic Impairment
    8.8   Renal Impairment
9   **DRUG ABUSE AND DEPENDENCE**
10 **OVERDOSAGE**
11 **DESCRIPTION**
12 **CLINICAL PHARMACOLOGY**
    12.1   Mechanism of Action
    12.3   Pharmacokinetics
13 **NONCLINICAL TOXICOLOGY**
    13.1   Carcinogenesis, Mutagenesis, Impairment of Fertility
14 **CLINICAL STUDIES**
16 **HOW SUPPLIED/STORAGE AND HANDLING**
17 **PATIENT COUNSELING INFORMATION**
    17.1   Information for Patients
*Sections or subsections omitted from the full prescribing information are not listed

—————————————————————————————

FULL PRESCRIBING INFORMATION

1   INDICATIONS AND USAGE

Plan B® One-Step is a progestin-only emergency contraceptive indicated for prevention of pregnancy following unprotected intercourse or a known or suspected contraceptive failure. To obtain optimal efficacy, the tablet should be taken as soon as possible within 72 hours of intercourse.

Plan B One-Step is available only by prescription for women younger than age 17 years, and available over the counter for women 17 years and older.

Plan B One-Step is not indicated for routine use as a contraceptive.

2   DOSAGE AND ADMINISTRATION

Take Plan B One-Step orally as soon as possible within 72 hours after unprotected intercourse or a known or suspected contraceptive failure. Efficacy is better if the tablet is taken as soon as possible after unprotected intercourse. Plan B One-Step can be used at any time during the menstrual cycle.

If vomiting occurs within two hours of taking the tablet, consideration should be given to repeating the dose.

3   DOSAGE FORMS AND STRENGTHS

The Plan B One-Step tablet is supplied as an almost white, round tablet containing 1.5 mg of levonorgestrel and is marked G00 on one side.

4   CONTRAINDICATIONS

Plan B One-Step is contraindicated for use in the case of known or suspected pregnancy.

5   WARNINGS AND PRECAUTIONS

5.1   Ectopic Pregnancy

Ectopic pregnancies account for approximately 2% of all reported pregnancies. Up to 10% of pregnancies reported in clinical studies of routine use of progestin-only contraceptives are ectopic.

A history of ectopic pregnancy is not a contraindication to use of this emergency contraceptive method. Healthcare providers, however, should consider the possibility of an ectopic pregnancy in women who become pregnant or complain of lower abdominal pain after taking Plan B One-Step. A follow-up physical or pelvic examination is recommended if there is any doubt concerning the general health or pregnancy status of any woman after taking Plan B One-Step.

5.2   Existing Pregnancy

Plan B One-Step is not effective in terminating an existing pregnancy.

5.3   Effects on Menses

Some women may experience spotting a few days after taking Plan B One-Step. Menstrual bleeding patterns are often irregular among women using progestin-only oral contraceptives and women using levonorgestrel for postcoital and emergency contraception.

If there is a delay in the onset of expected menses beyond 1 week, consider the possibility of pregnancy.

5.4   STI/HIV

Plan B One-Step does not protect against HIV infection (AIDS) or other sexually transmitted infections (STIs).

5.5 Physical Examination and Follow-up

A physical examination is not required prior to prescribing Plan B One-Step. A follow-up physical or pelvic examination is recommended if there is any doubt concerning the general health or pregnancy status of any woman after taking Plan B One-Step.

5.6 Fertility Following Discontinuation

A rapid return of fertility is likely following treatment with Plan B One-Step for emergency contraception; therefore, routine contraception should be continued or initiated as soon as possible following use of Plan B One-Step to ensure ongoing prevention of pregnancy.

6 ADVERSE REACTIONS

6.1 Clinical Trials Experience

Because clinical trials are conducted under widely varying conditions, adverse reaction rates observed in the clinical trials of a drug cannot be directly compared to rates in the clinical trials of another drug and may not reflect the rates observed in clinical practice.

Plan B One-Step was studied in a randomized, double-blinded multicenter clinical trial. In this study, all women who had received at least one dose of study medication were included in the safety analysis: 1,379 women in the Plan B One-Step group, and 1,377 women in the Plan B group (2 doses of 0.75 mg levonorgestrel taken 12 hours apart). The mean age of women given Plan B One-Step was 27 years. The racial demographic of those enrolled was 54% Chinese, 12% Other Asian or Black, and 34% were Caucasian in each treatment group. 1.6% of women in the Plan B One-Step group and 1.4% in Plan B group were lost to follow-up.

The most common adverse events (>10%) in the clinical trial for women receiving Plan B One-Step included heavier menstrual bleeding (30.9%), nausea (13.7%), lower abdominal pain (13.3%), fatigue (13.3%), and headache (10.3%). Table 1 lists those adverse events that were reported in > 4% of Plan B One-Step users.

Table 1. Adverse Events in > 4% of Women, by % Frequency

Most Common Adverse Events (MedDRA)	Plan B One-Step N = 1359 (%)
Heavier menstrual bleeding	30.9
Nausea	13.7
Lower abdominal pain	13.3
Fatigue	13.3
Headache	10.3
Dizziness	9.6
Breast tenderness	8.2
Delay of menses (> 7 days)	4.5

6.2 Postmarketing Experience

The following adverse reactions have been identified during post-approval use of Plan B (2 doses of 0.75 mg levonorgestrel taken 12 hours apart). Because these reactions are reported voluntarily from a population of uncertain size, it is not always possible to reliably estimate their frequency or establish a causal relationship to drug exposure.

Gastrointestinal Disorders
Abdominal Pain, Nausea, Vomiting
General Disorders and Administration Site Conditions
Fatigue
Nervous System Disorders
Dizziness, Headache
Reproductive System and Breast Disorders
Dysmenorrhea, Irregular Menstruation, Oligomenorrhea, Pelvic Pain

7 DRUG INTERACTIONS

Drugs or herbal products that induce enzymes, including CYP3A4, that metabolize progestins may decrease the plasma concentrations of progestins, and may decrease the effectiveness of progestin-only pills. Some drugs or herbal products that may decrease the effectiveness of progestin-only pills include:

- barbiturates
- bosentan
- carbamazepine
- felbamate
- griseofulvin
- oxcarbazepine
- phenytoin
- rifampin
- St. John's wort
- topiramate

Table 2. Pharmacokinetic Parameter Values Following Single Dose Administration of Plan B One-Step (levonorgestrel) tablet 1.5 mg to 30 Healthy Female Volunteers under Fasting Conditions

	Mean (± SD)				
	C_{max} (ng/mL)	AUC_t (ng•hr/mL)*	AUC_{inf} (ng•hr/mL)*	T_{max} (hr)**	$t_{1/2}$ (hr)
Levonorgestrel	19.1 (9.7)	294.8 (208.8)	307.5 (218.5)	1.7 (1.0-4.0)	27.5 (5.6)

C_{max} = maximum concentration
AUC_t = area under the drug concentration curve from time 0 to time of last determinable concentration
AUC_{inf} = area under the drug concentration curve from time 0 to infinity
T_{max} = time to maximum concentration
$t_{1/2}$ = elimination half life
* N=29
**median (range)

Significant changes (increase or decrease) in the plasma levels of the progestin have been noted in some cases of co-administration with HIV protease inhibitors or with non-nucleoside reverse transcriptase inhibitors.

Consult the labeling of all concurrently used drugs to obtain further information about interactions with progestin-only pills or the potential for enzyme alterations.

8 USE IN SPECIFIC POPULATIONS

8.1 Pregnancy

Many studies have found no harmful effects on fetal development associated with long-term use of contraceptive doses of oral progestins. The few studies of infant growth and development that have been conducted with progestin-only pills have not demonstrated significant adverse effects.

8.3 Nursing Mothers

In general, no adverse effects of progestin-only pills have been found on breastfeeding performance or on the health, growth, or development of the infant. However, isolated post-marketing cases of decreased milk production have been reported. Small amounts of progestins pass into the breast milk of nursing mothers taking progestin-only pills for long-term contraception, resulting in detectable steroid levels in infant plasma.

8.4 Pediatric Use

Safety and efficacy of progestin-only pills for long-term contraception have been established in women of reproductive age. Safety and efficacy are expected to be the same for postpubertal adolescents less than 17 years and for users 17 years and older. Use of Plan B One-Step emergency contraception before menarche is not indicated.

8.5 Geriatric Use

This product is not intended for use in postmenopausal women.

8.6 Race

No formal studies have evaluated the effect of race. However, clinical trials demonstrated a higher pregnancy rate in Chinese women with both Plan B and the Yuzpe regimen (another form of emergency contraception). There was a non-statistically significant increased rate of pregnancy among Chinese women in the Plan B One-Step trial. The reason for this apparent increase in the pregnancy rate with emergency contraceptives in Chinese women is unknown.

8.7 Hepatic Impairment

No formal studies were conducted to evaluate the effect of hepatic disease on the disposition of Plan B One-Step.

8.8 Renal Impairment

No formal studies were conducted to evaluate the effect of renal disease on the disposition of Plan B One-Step.

9 DRUG ABUSE AND DEPENDENCE

Levonorgestrel is not a controlled substance. There is no information about dependence associated with the use of Plan B One-Step.

10 OVERDOSAGE

There are no data on overdosage of Plan B One-Step, although the common adverse event of nausea and associated vomiting may be anticipated.

11 DESCRIPTION

The Plan B One-Step tablet contains 1.5 mg of a single active steroid ingredient, levonorgestrel [18,19-Dinorpregn-4-en-20-yn-3-one-13-ethyl-17-hydroxy-, (17 α)-(-)-], a totally synthetic progestogen. The inactive ingredients are colloidal silicon dioxide, corn starch, lactose monohydrate, magnesium stearate, potato starch, and talc.

Levonorgestrel has a molecular weight of 312.45, and the following structural and molecular formulas:
[See chemical structure at top of next column]

12 CLINICAL PHARMACOLOGY

12.1 Mechanism of Action

Emergency contraceptive pills are not effective if a woman is already pregnant. Plan B One-Step is believed to act as an emergency contraceptive principally by preventing ovulation or fertilization (by altering tubal transport of sperm

$C_{21}H_{28}O_2$

and/or ova). In addition, it may inhibit implantation (by altering the endometrium). It is not effective once the process of implantation has begun.

12.3 Pharmacokinetics

Absorption

Following a single dose administration of Plan B One-Step in 30 women under fasting conditions, maximum plasma concentrations of levonorgestrel of 19.1 ng/mL were reached at 1.7 hours. See Table 2.

[See table above]

Effect of Food: The effect of food on the rate and the extent of levonorgestrel absorption following single oral administration of Plan B One-Step has not been evaluated.

Distribution

The apparent volume of distribution of levonorgestrel is reported to be approximately 1.8 L/kg. It is about 97.5 to 99% protein-bound, principally to sex hormone binding globulin (SHBG) and, to a lesser extent, serum albumin.

Metabolism

Following absorption, levonorgestrel is conjugated at the 17β-OH position to form sulfate conjugates and, to a lesser extent, glucuronide conjugates in plasma. Significant amounts of conjugated and unconjugated 3α, 5β-tetrahydrolevonorgestrel are also present in plasma, along with much smaller amounts of 3α, 5α-tetrahydrolevonorgestrel and 16βhydroxylevonorgestrel. Levonorgestrel and its phase I metabolites are excreted primarily as glucuronide conjugates. Metabolic clearance rates may differ among individuals by several-fold, and this may account in part for the wide variation observed in levonorgestrel concentrations among users.

Excretion

About 45% of levonorgestrel and its metabolites are excreted in the urine and about 32% are excreted in feces, mostly as glucuronide conjugates.

Specific Populations

Pediatric

This product is not intended for use in the premenarcheal population, and pharmacokinetic data are not available for this population.

Geriatric

This product is not intended for use in postmenopausal women, and pharmacokinetic data are not available for this population.

Race

No formal studies have evaluated the effect of race. However, clinical trials demonstrated a higher pregnancy rate in Chinese women with both Plan B and the Yuzpe regimen (another form of emergency contraception). There was a non-statistically significant increased rate of pregnancy among Chinese women in the Plan B One-Step trial. The reason for this apparent increase in the pregnancy rate with emergency contraceptives in Chinese women is unknown [see USE IN SPECIFIC POPULATIONS (8.6)].

Hepatic Impairment

No formal studies were conducted to evaluate the effect of hepatic disease on the disposition of Plan B One-Step.

Renal Impairment

No formal studies were conducted to evaluate the effect of renal disease on the disposition of Plan B One-Step.

Drug-Drug Interactions

No formal drug-drug interaction studies were conducted with Plan B One-Step [see DRUG INTERACTIONS (7)].

13 NONCLINICAL TOXICOLOGY

13.1 Carcinogenesis, Mutagenesis, Impairment of Fertility

Carcinogenicity: There is no evidence of increased risk of cancer with short-term use of progestins. There was no increase in tumorgenicity following administration of levonorgestrel to rats for 2 years at approximately 5 μg/day, to dogs for 7 years at up to 0.125 mg/kg/day, or to rhesus monkeys for 10 years at up to 250 μg/kg/day. In another 7 year dog study, administration of levonorgestrel at 0.5 mg/kg/day did increase the number of mammary adenomas in treated dogs compared to controls. There were no malignancies.

Genotoxicity: Levonorgestrel was not found to be mutagenic or genotoxic in the Ames Assay, in vitro mammalian culture assays utilizing mouse lymphoma cells and Chinese hamster ovary cells, and in an in vivo micronucleus assay in mice.

Fertility: There are no irreversible effects on fertility following cessation of exposures to levonorgestrel or progestins in general.

14 CLINICAL STUDIES

A double-blind, randomized, multicenter, multinational study evaluated and compared the efficacy and safety of three different regimens for emergency contraception. Subjects were enrolled at 15 sites in 10 countries; the racial/ethnic characteristics of the study population overall were 54% Chinese, 34% Caucasian, and 12% Black or Asian (other than Chinese). 2,381 healthy women with a mean age of 27 years, who needed emergency contraception within 72 hours of unprotected intercourse were involved and randomly allocated into one of the two levonorgestrel groups. A single dose of 1.5 mg of levonorgestrel (Plan B One-Step) was administered to women allocated into group 1. Two doses of 0.75 mg levonorgestrel 12 hours apart (Plan B) were administered to women in group 2. In the Plan B One-Step group, 16 pregnancies occurred in 1,198 women and in the Plan B group, 20 pregnancies occurred in 1,183 women. The number of pregnancies expected in each group was calculated based on the timing of intercourse with regard to each woman's menstrual cycle. Among women receiving Plan B One-Step, 84% of expected pregnancies were prevented and among those women taking Plan B, 79% of expected pregnancies were prevented. The expected pregnancy rate of 8% (with no contraceptive use) was reduced to approximately 1% with Plan B One-Step.

Emergency contraceptives are not as effective as routine contraception since their failure rate, while low based on a single use, would accumulate over time with repeated use [see INDICATIONS AND USAGE (1)].

In the clinical study, bleeding disturbances were the most common adverse event reported after taking the levonorgestrel-containing regimens. More than half of the women had menses within two days of the expected time; however, 31% of women experienced change in their bleeding pattern during the study period; 4.5% of women had menses more than 7 days after the expected time.

16 HOW SUPPLIED/STORAGE AND HANDLING

The Plan B One-Step (levonorgestrel) tablet 1.5 mg is available in a PVC/aluminum foil blister package. The tablet is almost white, round, and marked G00 on one side.
NDC 51285-942-88 (1 tablet unit of use package)
Store Plan B One-Step at 20° to 25°C (68° to 77°F) [see USP Controlled Room Temperature].

17 PATIENT COUNSELING INFORMATION

17.1 Information for Patients

• Take Plan B One-Step as soon as possible and not more than 72 hours after unprotected intercourse or a known or suspected contraceptive failure.
• If you vomit within two hours of taking the tablet, immediately contact your healthcare provider to discuss whether to take another tablet.
• Seek medical attention if you experience severe lower abdominal pain 3 to 5 weeks after taking Plan B One-Step, in order to be evaluated for an ectopic pregnancy.
• After taking Plan B One-Step, consider the possibility of pregnancy if your period is delayed more than one week beyond the date you expected your period.
• Do not use Plan B One-Step as routine contraception.
• Plan B One-Step is not effective in terminating an existing pregnancy.
• Plan B One-Step does not protect against HIV-infection (AIDS) and other sexually transmitted diseases/infections.
• For women younger than age 17 years, Plan B One-Step is available only by prescription.
Mfg. by Gedeon Richter, Ltd., Budapest, Hungary
for Duramed Pharmaceuticals, Inc.
Subsidiary of Barr Pharmaceuticals, Inc.
Pomona, New York 10970
Phone: 1-800-330-1271
Website: www.PlanBOneStep.com

Revised: August 2009
11001524
Shown in Product Identification Guide, page 320

SEASONIQUE® ℞
[see-son-eek]
(levonorgestrel/ethinyl estradiol tablets and ethinyl estradiol tablets)
For Oral Use

HIGHLIGHTS OF PRESCRIBING INFORMATION
These highlights do not include all the information needed to use Seasonique safely and effectively. See full prescribing information for Seasonique.
Seasonique (levonorgestrel/ethinyl estradiol tablets and ethinyl estradiol tablets) for oral use
Initial U.S. Approval: 1982

> **WARNING: CIGARETTE SMOKING AND SERIOUS CARDIOVASCULAR EVENTS**
> *See full prescribing information for complete boxed warning.*
> • **Women who are over 35 years old and smoke should not use Seasonique.**
> • **Cigarette smoking increases the risk of serious cardiovascular events from combination oral contraceptive (COC) use.**

——————INDICATIONS AND USAGE——————
Seasonique is an estrogen/progestin COC indicated for use by women to prevent pregnancy. (1)
————DOSAGE AND ADMINISTRATION————
Take one tablet daily by mouth at the same time every day for 91 days. (2)
————DOSAGE FORMS AND STRENGTHS————
Seasonique consists of 84 light blue-green tablets containing 0.15 mg levonorgestrel and 0.03 mg ethinyl estradiol, and 7 yellow tablets containing 0.01 mg ethinyl estradiol. (3)
——————CONTRAINDICATIONS——————
• A high risk of arterial or venous thrombotic diseases (4)
• Undiagnosed abnormal genital bleeding (4)
• Breast cancer or other estrogen- or progestin-sensitive cancer (4)
• Liver tumors or liver disease (4)
• Pregnancy (4)
————WARNINGS AND PRECAUTIONS————
• Vascular risks: Stop Seasonique if a thrombotic event occurs. Stop Seasonique at least 4 weeks before and through 2 weeks after major surgery. Start Seasonique no earlier than 4 weeks after delivery, in women who are not breastfeeding. (5.1)
• Liver disease: Discontinue Seasonique if jaundice occurs. (5.3)
• High blood pressure: Do not prescribe Seasonique for women with uncontrolled hypertension or hypertension with vascular disease. (5.4)
• Carbohydrate and lipid metabolic effects: Monitor prediabetic and diabetic women taking Seasonique. Consider an alternate contraceptive method for women with uncontrolled dyslipidemias. (5.6)
• Headache: Evaluate significant change in headaches and discontinue Seasonique if indicated. (5.7)
• Uterine bleeding: Evaluate irregular bleeding or amenorrhea. (5.8)
——————ADVERSE REACTIONS——————
The most common adverse reactions (≥5%) in clinical trials for Seasonique are irregular and/or heavy uterine bleeding, weight gain, and acne. (6)
To report SUSPECTED ADVERSE REACTIONS, contact Duramed Pharmaceuticals at 1-800-222-0190 or FDA at 1-800-FDA-1088 or *www.fda.gov/medwatch*.
——————DRUG INTERACTIONS——————
Drugs or herbal products that induce certain enzymes, including CYP3A4, may decrease the effectiveness of COCs or increase breakthrough bleeding. Counsel patients to use a back-up method or alternative method of contraception when enzyme inducers are used with COCs. (7.1)
————USE IN SPECIFIC POPULATIONS————
Nursing Mothers: Not recommended for nursing mothers; can decrease milk production. (8.3)
See 17 for PATIENT COUNSELING INFORMATION and FDA-Approved Patient Labeling
Revised: July 2010

FULL PRESCRIBING INFORMATION: CONTENTS*

*Sections or subsections omitted from the full prescribing information are not listed.

FULL PRESCRIBING INFORMATION

> **WARNING: CIGARETTE SMOKING AND SERIOUS CARDIOVASCULAR EVENTS**
> Cigarette smoking increases the risk of serious cardiovascular events from combination oral contraceptives (COC) use. This risk increases with age, particularly in women over 35 years of age, and with the number of cigarettes smoked. For this reason, COCs should not be used by women who are over 35 years of age and smoke. *[See Contraindications (4).]*

1. INDICATIONS AND USAGE

Seasonique® (levonorgestrel/ethinyl estradiol tablets and ethinyl estradiol tablets) is indicated for use by women to prevent pregnancy.

2. DOSAGE AND ADMINISTRATION

Take one tablet by mouth at the same time every day. The dosage of Seasonique is one light blue-green tablet containing levonorgestrel and ethinyl estradiol daily for 84 consecutive days, followed by one yellow ethinyl estradiol tablet for 7 days. To achieve maximum contraceptive effectiveness, Seasonique must be taken exactly as directed and at intervals not exceeding 24 hours.

Instruct the patient to begin taking Seasonique on the first Sunday after the onset of menstruation. If menstruation begins on a Sunday, the first light blue-green tablet is taken that day. One light blue-green tablet should be taken daily for 84 consecutive days, followed by one yellow tablet for 7 consecutive days. A non-hormonal back-up method of contraception (such as condoms or spermicide) should be used until a light blue-green tablet has been taken daily for 7 consecutive days. A scheduled period should occur during the 7 days that the yellow tablets are taken.

Begin the next and all subsequent 91-day cycles without interruption on the same day of the week (Sunday) on which the patient began her first dose of Seasonique, following the same schedule: 84 days taking a light blue-green tablet followed by 7 days taking a yellow tablet. If the patient does not immediately start her next pill pack, she should protect herself from pregnancy by using a non-hormonal back-up method of contraception until she has taken a light blue-green tablet daily for 7 consecutive days. If unscheduled spotting or bleeding occurs, instruct the patient to continue on the same regimen. If the bleeding is persistent or prolonged, advise the patient to consult her healthcare provider.

For patient instructions regarding missed pills, *see FDA-Approved Patient Labeling*.

For postpartum women who are not breastfeeding, start Seasonique no earlier than four to six weeks postpartum due to increased risk of thromboembolism. If the patient starts on Seasonique postpartum and has not yet had a period, evaluate for possible pregnancy, and instruct her to use an additional method of contraception until she has taken a light blue-green tablet for 7 consecutive days.

3. DOSAGE FORMS AND STRENGTHS

Seasonique tablets (levonorgestrel/ethinyl estradiol tablets and ethinyl estradiol tablets) are available in Extended-Cycle Tablet Dispensers, each containing a 13-week supply of tablets: 84 light blue-green tablets, each containing 0.15 mg of levonorgestrel and 0.03 mg ethinyl estradiol, and 7 yellow tablets each containing 0.01 mg of ethinyl estradiol. The light blue-green tablets are round, film-coated, biconvex, unscored tablets debossed with stylized **b** on one side and **555** on the other side. The yellow tablets are round, biconvex, film-coated, unscored tablets debossed with stylized **b** on one side and **556** on the other side.

4. CONTRAINDICATIONS

Do not prescribe Seasonique to women who are known to have the following:

- A high risk of arterial or venous thrombotic diseases. Examples include women who are known to:
  - Smoke, if over age 35 *[see Boxed Warning and Warnings and Precautions (5.1)]*.
  - Have deep vein thrombosis or pulmonary embolism, now or in the past *[see Warnings and Precautions (5.1)]*.
  - Have cerebrovascular disease *[see Warnings and Precautions (5.1)]*
  - Have coronary artery disease *[see Warnings and Precautions (5.1)]*.
  - Have thrombogenic valvular or thrombogenic rhythm diseases of the heart (for example, subacute bacterial endocarditis with valvular disease, or atrial fibrillation) *[see Warnings and Precautions (5.1)]*.
  - Have inherited or acquired hypercoagulopathies *[see Warnings and Precautions (5.1)]*.
  - Have uncontrolled hypertension *[see Warnings and Precautions (5.4)]*.
  - Have diabetes with vascular disease *[see Warnings and Precautions (5.6)]*.
  - Have headaches with focal neurological symptoms or have migraine headaches with or without aura if over age 35 *[see Warnings and Precautions (5.7)]*.
- Undiagnosed abnormal genital bleeding *[see Warnings and Precautions (5.8)]*.
- Breast cancer or other estrogen- or progestin-sensitive cancer, now or in the past *[see Warnings and Precautions (5.2)]*.
- Liver tumors, benign or malignant, or liver disease *[see Warnings and Precautions (5.3) and Use in Specific Populations (8.6)]*.
- Pregnancy, because there is no reason to use COCs during pregnancy *[see Warnings and Precautions (5.9) and Use in Specific Populations (8.1)]*.

5. WARNINGS AND PRECAUTIONS

5.1 Thrombotic and Other Vascular Events

Stop Seasonique if an arterial or deep venous thrombotic event occurs. Although the use of COCs increases the risk of venous thromboembolism, pregnancy increases the risk of venous thromboembolism as much or more than the use of COCs. The risk of venous thromboembolism in women using COCs is 3 to 9 per 10,000 woman-years. The excess risk is highest during the first year of use of a COC. Use of COCs also increases the risk of arterial thromboses such as strokes and myocardial infarctions, especially in women with other risk factors for these events. The risk of thromboembolic disease due to COCs gradually disappears after COC use is discontinued.

Use of Seasonique provides women with more hormonal exposure on a yearly basis than conventional monthly oral contraceptives containing the same strength synthetic estrogens and progestins (an additional 9 and 13 weeks of exposure to progestin and estrogen, respectively, per year).

If feasible, stop Seasonique at least 4 weeks before and through 2 weeks after major surgery or other surgeries known to have an elevated risk of thromboembolism.

Start Seasonique no earlier than 4-6 weeks after delivery, in women who are not breastfeeding. The risk of postpartum thromboembolism decreases after the third postpartum week, whereas the risk of ovulation increases after the third postpartum week.

COCs have been shown to increase both the relative and attributable risks of cerebrovascular events (thrombotic and hemorrhagic strokes), although, in general, the risk is greatest among older (>35 years of age), and hypertensive women who also smoke. COCs also increase the risk for stroke in women with other underlying risk factors.

Oral contraceptives must be used with caution in women with cardiovascular disease risk factors.

Stop Seasonique if there is unexplained loss of vision, proptosis, diplopia, papilledema, or retinal vascular lesions. Evaluate for retinal vein thrombosis immediately.

5.2 Carcinoma of the Breast and Cervix

Women who currently have or have had breast cancer should not use Seasonique because breast cancer may be hormonally sensitive.

There is substantial evidence that COCs do not increase the incidence of breast cancer. Although some past studies have suggested that COCs might increase the incidence of breast cancer, more recent studies have not confirmed such findings.

Some studies suggest that COCs are associated with an increase in the risk of cervical cancer or intraepithelial neoplasia. However, there is controversy about the extent to which these findings are due to differences in sexual behavior and other factors.

5.3 Liver Disease

Discontinue Seasonique if jaundice develops. Steroid hormones may be poorly metabolized in patients with impaired liver function. Acute or chronic disturbances of liver function may necessitate the discontinuation of COC use until markers of liver function return to normal and COC causation has been excluded.

Hepatic adenomas are associated with COC use. An estimate of the attributable risk is 3.3 cases/100,000 COC users. Rupture of hepatic adenomas may cause death through intra-abdominal hemorrhage.

Studies have shown an increased risk of developing hepatocellular carcinoma in long-term (> 8 years) COC users. However, the attributable risk of liver cancers in COC users is less than one case per million users.

Oral contraceptive-related cholestasis may occur in women with a history of pregnancy-related cholestasis. Women with a history of COC-related cholestasis may have the condition recur with subsequent COC use.

5.4 High Blood Pressure

For women with well-controlled hypertension, monitor blood pressure and stop Seasonique if blood pressure rises significantly. Women with uncontrolled hypertension or hypertension with vascular disease should not use COCs.

An increase in blood pressure has been reported in women taking COCs, and this increase is more likely in older women and with extended duration of use. The incidence of hypertension increases with increasing concentration of progestin.

5.5 Gallbladder Disease

Studies suggest a small increased relative risk of developing gallbladder disease among COC users.

5.6 Carbohydrate and Lipid Metabolic Effects

Carefully monitor prediabetic and diabetic women who are taking Seasonique. COCs may decrease glucose tolerance in a dose-related fashion.

Consider alternative contraception for women with uncontrolled dyslipidemias. A small proportion of women will have adverse lipid changes while on COCs.

Women with hypertriglyceridemia, or a family history thereof, may be at an increased risk of pancreatitis when using COCs.

5.7 Headache

If a woman taking Seasonique develops new headaches that are recurrent, persistent, or severe, evaluate the cause and discontinue Seasonique if indicated.

An increase in frequency or severity of migraine during COC use (which may be prodromal of a cerebrovascular event) may be a reason for immediate discontinuation of the COC.

5.8 Bleeding Irregularities

Unscheduled (breakthrough) bleeding and spotting sometimes occur in patients on COCs, especially during the first 3 months of use. If bleeding persists, check for causes such as pregnancy or malignancy. If pathology and pregnancy are excluded, bleeding irregularities may resolve over time or with a change to a different COC.

When prescribing Seasonique, the convenience of fewer planned menses (4 per year instead of 13 per year) should be weighed against the inconvenience of increased unscheduled bleeding and/or spotting. The primary clinical trial (PSE-301) that evaluated the efficacy of Seasonique also assessed unscheduled bleeding. The participants in the 12-month clinical trial (N=1,006) completed the equivalent of 8,681 28-day cycles of exposure and were composed primarily of women who had used oral contraceptives previously (89%) as opposed to new users (11%). A total of 82 (8.2%) of the women discontinued Seasonique, at least in part, due to bleeding or spotting.

Scheduled (withdrawal) bleeding and/or spotting remained fairly constant over time, with an average of 3 days of bleeding and/or spotting per each 91-day cycle. Unscheduled bleeding and unscheduled spotting decreased over successive 91-day cycles. Table 1 below presents the number of days with unscheduled bleeding in treatment cycles 1 and 4. Table 2 presents the number of days with unscheduled spotting in treatment cycles 1 and 4.

Table 1: Total Number of Days with Unscheduled Bleeding

91-Day Treatment Cycle	Days per 84-Day Interval				Days per 28-Day Interval
	Q1	Median	Q3	Mean	Mean
1st	1	4	10	6.9	1.7
4th	0	1	4	3.2	0.8

Q1=Quartile 1: 25% of women had this number of days of unscheduled bleeding

Median: 50% of women had ≤ this number of days of unscheduled bleeding

Q3=Quartile 3: 75% of women had ≤ this number of days of unscheduled bleeding

Table 2: Total Number of Days with Unscheduled Spotting

91-Day Treatment Cycle	Days per 84-Day Interval				Days per 28-Day Interval
	Q1	Median	Q3	Mean	Mean
1st	1	4	11	7.4	1.9
4th	0	2	7	4.4	1.1

Q1=Quartile 1: 25% of women had ≤ this number of days of unscheduled spotting

Median: 50% of women had ≤ this number of days of unscheduled spotting

Q3=Quartile 3: 75% of women had ≤ this number of days of unscheduled spotting

Figure 1 shows the percentage of Seasonique subjects participating in trial PSE-301 with ≥ 7 days or ≥ 20 days of unscheduled bleeding and/or spotting, or only unscheduled bleeding, during each 91-day treatment cycle.

Figure 1. Percent of Women Taking Seasonique who Reported Unscheduled Bleeding and/or Spotting or only Unscheduled Bleeding

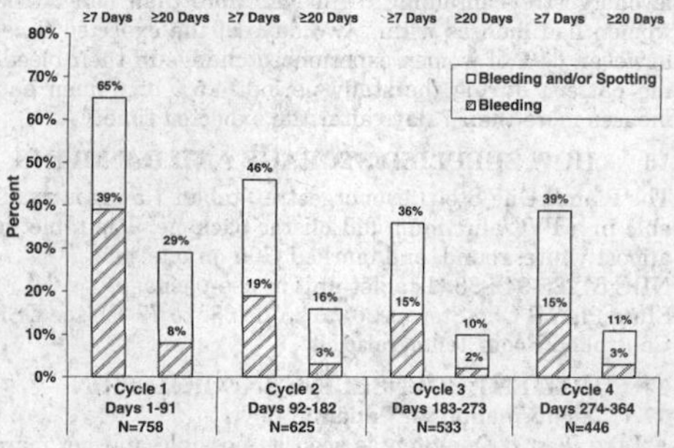

Amenorrhea sometimes occurs in women who are using COCs. Pregnancy should be ruled out in the event of amenorrhea. Some women may encounter amenorrhea or oligomenorrhea after stopping COCs, especially when such a condition was pre-existent.

5.9 COC Use Before or During Early Pregnancy

Extensive epidemiological studies have revealed no increased risk of birth defects in women who have used oral contraceptives prior to pregnancy. Studies also do not suggest a teratogenic effect, particularly in so far as cardiac anomalies and limb-reduction defects are concerned, when taken inadvertently during early pregnancy. Oral contraceptive use should be discontinued if pregnancy is confirmed.

The administration of oral contraceptives to induce withdrawal bleeding should not be used as a test for pregnancy *[see Use in Specific Populations (8.1)]*.

5.10 Emotional Disorders

Women with a history of depression should be carefully observed and Seasonique discontinued if depression recurs to a serious degree.

5.11 Interference with Laboratory Tests

The use of COCs may change the results of some laboratory tests, such as coagulation factors, lipids, glucose tolerance, and binding proteins. Women on thyroid hormone replacement therapy may need increased doses of thyroid hormone because serum concentrations of thyroid binding globulin increase with use of COCs.

5.12 Monitoring

A woman who is taking COCs should have a yearly visit with her healthcare provider for a blood pressure check and for other indicated health care.

5.13 Other Conditions

In women with hereditary angioedema, exogenous estrogens may induce or exacerbate symptoms of angioedema. Chloasma may occasionally occur, especially in women with a history of chloasma gravidarum. Women with a tendency to chloasma should avoid exposure to the sun or ultraviolet radiation while taking COCs.

6. ADVERSE REACTIONS

The following serious adverse reactions with the use of COCs are discussed elsewhere in the labeling:

- Serious cardiovascular events and smoking *[see Boxed Warning and Warnings and Precautions (5.1)]*
- Vascular events *[see Warnings and Precautions (5.1)]*
- Liver disease *[see Warnings and Precautions (5.3)]*

Adverse reactions commonly reported by COC users are:

- Irregular uterine bleeding
- Nausea
- Breast tenderness
- Headache

6.1 Clinical Trial Experience

Because clinical trials are conducted under widely varying conditions, adverse reaction rates observed in the clinical trials of a drug cannot be directly compared to the rates in the clinical trials of another drug and may not reflect the rates observed in practice.

The clinical trial that evaluated the safety and efficacy of Seasonique was a 12-month, randomized, multicenter, open-label study, which enrolled women aged 18-40, of whom 1,006 took at least one dose of Seasonique.

Adverse Reactions Leading to Study Discontinuation: 16.3% of the women discontinued from the clinical trial due to an adverse reaction; the most common adverse reactions (≥ 1% of women) leading to discontinuation were irregular and/or heavy uterine bleeding (5.9%), weight gain (2.4%), mood changes (1.5%), and acne (1.0%).

Common Treatment-Emergent Adverse Reactions (≥ 5% of women): irregular and/or heavy uterine bleeding (17%), weight gain (5%), acne (5%).

Serious Adverse Reactions: migraine, cholecystitis, cholelithiasis, pancreatitis, abdominal pain, and major depressive disorder.

6.2 Postmarketing Experience

The following adverse reactions have been identified during post-approval use of Seasonique. Because these reactions are reported voluntarily from a population of uncertain size, it is not possible to reliably estimate their frequency of establish a causal relationship to drug exposure.

Gastrointestinal disorders: abdominal distension, vomiting

General disorders and administration site conditions: chest pain, fatigue, malaise, edema peripheral, pain

Immune system disorders: hypersensitivity reaction

Investigations: blood pressure increased

Musculoskeletal and connective tissue disorders: muscle spasms, pain in extremity

Nervous system disorders: dizziness, loss of consciousness

Psychiatric disorders: insomnia

Reproductive and breast disorders: dysmenorrhea

Respiratory, thoracic and mediastinal disorders: pulmonary embolism, pulmonary thrombosis

Skin and subcutaneous tissue disorders: alopecia

Vascular disorders: thrombosis

7. DRUG INTERACTIONS

No drug-drug interaction studies were conducted with Seasonique.

7.1 Changes in Contraceptive Effectiveness Associated with Co-Administration of Other Products

If a woman on hormonal contraceptives takes a drug or herbal product that induces enzymes, including CYP3A4, that metabolize contraceptive hormones, counsel her to use additional contraception or a different method of contraception. Drugs or herbal products that induce such enzymes may decrease the plasma concentrations of contraceptive hormones, and may decrease the effectiveness of hormonal contraceptives or increase breakthrough bleeding. Some drugs or herbal products that may decrease the effectiveness of hormonal contraceptives include:

- barbiturates
- bosentan
- carbamazepine
- felbamate
- griseofulvin
- oxcarbazepine
- phenytoin
- rifampin
- St. John's wort
- topiramate

HIV protease inhibitors and non-nucleoside reverse transcriptase inhibitors: Significant changes (increase or decrease) in the plasma levels of the estrogen and progestin have been noted in some cases of co-administration of HIV protease inhibitors or with non-nucleoside reverse transcriptase inhibitors.

Antibiotics: There have been reports of pregnancy while taking hormonal contraceptives and antibiotics, but clinical pharmacokinetic studies have not shown consistent effects of antibiotics on plasma concentrations of synthetic steroids.

Consult the labeling of all concurrently-used drugs to obtain further information about interactions with hormonal contraceptives or the potential for enzyme alterations.

7.2 Increase in Plasma Levels of Estradiol Associated with Co-Administered Drugs

Co-administration of atorvastatin and certain COCs containing ethinyl estradiol increase AUC values for ethinyl estradiol by approximately 20%. Ascorbic acid and acetaminophen may increase plasma ethinyl estradiol levels, possibly by inhibition of conjugation. CYP3A4 inhibitors such as itraconazole or ketoconazole may increase plasma hormone levels.

7.3 Changes in Plasma Levels of Co-Administered Drugs

COCs containing some synthetic estrogens (e.g., ethinyl estradiol) may inhibit the metabolism of other compounds. COCs have been shown to significantly decrease plasma concentrations of lamotrigine likely due to induction of lamotrigine glucuronidation. This may reduce seizure control; therefore, dosage adjustments of lamotrigine may be necessary. Consult the labeling of the concurrently-used drug to obtain further information about interactions with COCs or the potential for enzyme alterations.

8. USE IN SPECIFIC POPULATIONS

8.1. Pregnancy

There is little or no increased risk of birth defects in women who inadvertently use COCs during early pregnancy. Epidemiologic studies and meta-analyses have not found an increased risk of genital or non-genital birth defects (including cardiac anomalies and limb-reduction defects) following exposure to low dose COCs prior to conception or during early pregnancy.

The administration of COCs to induce withdrawal bleeding should not be used as a test for pregnancy. COCs should not be used during pregnancy to treat threatened or habitual abortion.

Women who do not breastfeed may start COCs no earlier than four to six weeks postpartum.

8.3. Nursing Mothers

When possible, advise the nursing mother to use other forms of contraception until she has weaned her child. Estrogen-containing COCs can reduce milk production in breastfeeding mothers. This is less likely to occur once breastfeeding is well established; however, it can occur at any time in some women. Small amounts of oral contraceptive steroids and/or metabolites are present in breast milk.

8.4. Pediatric Use

Safety and efficacy of Seasonique have been established in women of reproductive age. Safety and efficacy are expected to be the same for postpubertal adolescents under the age of 18 as for users 18 years and older. Use of Seasonique before menarche is not indicated.

8.5. Geriatric Use

Seasonique has not been studied in women who have reached menopause and is not indicated in this population.

8.6 Hepatic Impairment

No studies have been conducted to evaluate the effect of hepatic disease on the disposition of Seasonique. However, steroid hormones may be poorly metabolized in patients with impaired liver function. Acute or chronic disturbances of liver function may necessitate the discontinuation of COC use until markers of liver function return to normal. *[See Contraindications (4) and Warnings and Precautions (5.3)]*.

8.7 Renal Impairment

No studies have been conducted to evaluate the effect of renal disease on the disposition of Seasonique.

10. OVERDOSAGE

There have been no reports of serious ill effects from overdose of oral contraceptives, including ingestion by children. Overdosage may cause withdrawal bleeding in females and nausea.

11. DESCRIPTION

Seasonique (levonorgestrel/ethinyl estradiol tablets and ethinyl estradiol tablets) is an extended-cycle oral contraceptive consisting of 84 light blue-green tablets each containing 0.15 mg of levonorgestrel, a synthetic progestogen and 0.03 mg of ethinyl estradiol, and 7 yellow tablets containing 0.01 mg of ethinyl estradiol.

The structural formulas for the active components are:

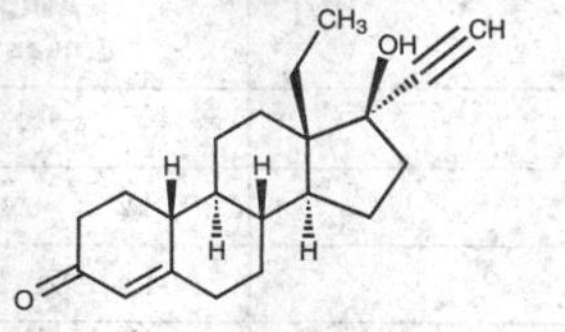

Levonorgestrel

$C_{21}H_{28}O_2$ MW: 312.4

Levonorgestrel is chemically 18,19-Dinorpregn-4-en-20-yn-3-one, 13-ethyl-17-hydroxy-, 17α)-, (-)-.

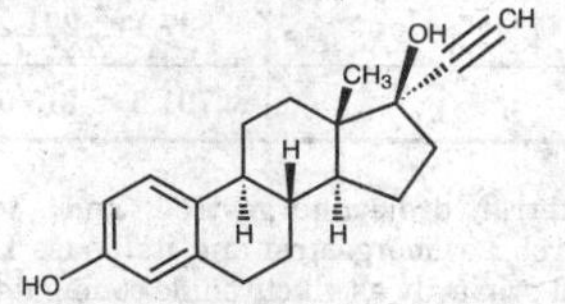

Ethinyl Estradiol

$C_{20}H_{24}O_2$ MW: 296.4

Ethinyl Estradiol is 19-Norpregna-1,3,5(10)-trien-20-yne-3,17-diol, (17α)-.

Each light blue-green tablet contains the following inactive ingredients: anhydrous lactose, D&C yellow no. 10 aluminum lake, FD&C blue no. 1 aluminum lake, FD&C yellow no. 6/Sunset yellow aluminum lake, hypromellose, lactose monohydrate, magnesium stearate, microcrystalline cellulose, titanium dioxide and triacetin.

Each yellow tablet contains the following inactive ingredients: anhydrous lactose, D&C yellow no. 10 aluminum lake, FD&C yellow no. 6/Sunset yellow aluminum lake, hypromellose, magnesium stearate, microcrystalline cellulose, polacrilin potassium, polyethylene glycol, polysorbate 80 and titanium dioxide.

12. CLINICAL PHARMACOLOGY

12.1. Mechanism of action

COCs lower the risk of becoming pregnant primarily by suppressing ovulation. Other possible mechanisms may include cervical mucus changes that inhibit sperm penetration and endometrial changes that reduce the likelihood of implantation.

12.3. Pharmacokinetics

Absorption

Ethinyl estradiol and levonorgestrel are absorbed with maximum plasma concentrations occurring within 2 hours after Seasonique administration. Levonorgestrel is completely absorbed after oral administration (bioavailability nearly 100%) and is not subject to first-pass metabolism. Ethinyl estradiol is absorbed from the gastrointestinal tract but, due to first-pass metabolism in gut mucosa and liver, the bioavailability of ethinyl estradiol is approximately 43%.

The daily exposure to levonorgestrel and ethinyl estradiol on Day 21, corresponding to the end of a typical 3-week contraceptive regimen, and on Day 84, at the end of an extended cycle regimen, were similar. There was no additional accumulation of ethinyl estradiol after dosing a 0.03 mg ethinyl estradiol tablet during Days 84-91. The mean plasma pharmacokinetic parameters of Seasonique following a single dose of one levonorgestrel/ethinyl estradiol combination tablet, for 84 days, in normal healthy women are reported in Table 3.

[See table 3 at top of next page]

The effect of food on the rate and the extent of levonorgestrel and ethinyl estradiol absorption following oral administration of Seasonique has not been evaluated.

Distribution

The apparent volume of distribution of levonorgestrel and ethinyl estradiol are reported to be approximately 1.8 L/kg and 4.3 L/kg, respectively. Levonorgestrel is about 97.5 - 99% protein-bound, principally to sex hormone binding globulin (SHBG) and, to a lesser extent, serum albumin. Ethinyl estradiol is about 95 - 97% bound to serum albumin. Ethinyl estradiol does not bind to SHBG, but induces SHBG synthesis, which leads to decreased levonorgestrel clearance. Following repeated daily dosing of levonorgestrel/ethinyl estradiol oral contraceptives, levonorgestrel plasma concentrations accumulate more than predicted based on single-dose pharmacokinetics, due in part, to increased SHBG levels that are induced by ethinyl estradiol, and a possible reduction in hepatic metabolic capacity.

Metabolism

Following absorption, levonorgestrel is conjugated at the 17β-OH position to form sulfate and to a lesser extent, glucuronide conjugates in plasma. Significant amounts of conjugated and unconjugated 3α,5β-tetrahydrolevonorgestrel are also present in plasma, along with much smaller amounts

Table 3: Mean Pharmacokinetic Parameters for Seasonique during Daily One Tablet Dosing for 84 Days

	$AUC_{0-24\ hr}$ (mean ± SD)	C_{max} (mean ± SD)	T_{max} (mean ± SD)
Levonorgestrel			
Day 1	18.2 ± 6.1 ng•hr/mL	3.0 ± 1.0 ng/mL	1.3 ± 0.4 hours
Day 21	64.4 ± 25.1 ng•hr/mL	6.2 ± 1.6 ng/mL	1.3 ± 0.4 hours
Day 84	60.2 ± 24.6 ng•hr/mL	5.5 ± 1.6 ng/mL	1.3± 0.3 hours
Ethinyl Estradiol			
Day 1	509.3 ± 172.0 pg•hr/mL	69.8 ± 26 pg/mL	1.5 ± 0.3 hours
Day 21	837.1 ± 271.2 pg•hr/mL	99.6± 31 pg/mL	1.5 ± 0.3 hours
Day 84	791.5 ± 215.0 pg•hr/mL	91.3 ± 32 pg/mL	1.6 ± 0.3 hours

of 3α,5α-tetrahydrolevonorgestrel and 16β-hydroxy-levonorgestrel. Levonorgestrel and its phase I metabolites are excreted primarily as glucuronide conjugates. Metabolic clearance rates may differ among individuals by several-fold, and this may account in part for the wide variation observed in levonorgestrel concentrations among users.

First-pass metabolism of ethinyl estradiol involves formation of ethinyl estradiol-3-sulfate in the gut wall, followed by 2-hydroxylation of a portion of the remaining untransformed ethinyl estradiol by hepatic cytochrome P-450 3A4 (CYP3A4). Levels of CYP3A4 vary widely among individuals and can explain the variation in rates of ethinyl estradiol hydroxylation. Hydroxylation at the 4-, 6-, and 16-positions may also occur, although to a much lesser extent than 2-hydroxylation. The various hydroxylated metabolites are subject to further methylation and/or conjugation.

Excretion
About 45% of levonorgestrel and its metabolites are excreted in the urine and about 32% are excreted in feces, mostly as glucuronide conjugates. The terminal elimination half-life for levonorgestrel after a single dose of Seasonique was about 34 hours.
Ethinyl estradiol is excreted in the urine and feces as glucuronide and sulfate conjugates, and it undergoes enterohepatic recirculation. The terminal elimination half-life of ethinyl estradiol after a single dose of Seasonique was found to be about 18 hours.
Race
The effect of race on the pharmacokinetics of Seasonique has not been evaluated.

13. NONCLINICAL TOXICOLOGY

13.1. Carcinogenesis, Mutagenesis, Impairment of Fertility
[See Warnings and Precautions (5.2, 5.3)].

14. CLINICAL STUDIES

In a 12-month, multicenter, randomized, open-label clinical trial, 1,006 women aged 18-40 were studied to assess the safety and efficacy of Seasonique, completing the equivalent of 8,681 28-day cycles of exposure. The racial demographic of those enrolled was: Caucasian (80%), African-American (11%), Hispanic (5%), Asian (2%), and Other (2%). There were no exclusions for body mass index (BMI) or weight. The weight range of those women treated was 91 to 360 lbs., with a mean weight of 156 lbs. Among the women in the trial, 63% were current or recent hormonal contraceptive users, 26% were prior users (who had used hormonal contraceptives in the past but not in the 6 months prior to enrollment), and 11% were new starts. Of treated women, 14.8% were lost to follow-up, 16.3% discontinued due to an adverse event, and 12.9% discontinued by withdrawing their consent.
The pregnancy rate (Pearl Index [PI]) in women aged 18-35 years was 1.34 pregnancies per 100 women-years of use (95% confidence interval 0.54-2.75), based on 7 pregnancies that occurred after the onset of treatment and within 14 days after the last combination pill. Cycles in which conception did not occur, but which included the use of backup contraception, were not included in the calculation of the PI. The PI includes patients who did not take the drug correctly.

16. HOW SUPPLIED/STORAGE AND HANDLING

16.1 How Supplied
Seasonique tablets (levonorgestrel/ethinyl estradiol tablets and ethinyl estradiol tablets) are available in Extended-Cycle Tablet Dispensers (NDC 51285-087-87), each containing a 13-week supply of tablets: 84 light blue-green tablets, each containing 0.15 mg of levonorgestrel and 0.03 mg ethinyl estradiol, and 7 yellow tablets each containing 0.01 mg of ethinyl estradiol. The light blue-green tablets are round, film-coated, biconvex, unscored tablets debossed with stylized **b** on one side and **555** on the other side. The

yellow tablets are round, biconvex, film-coated, unscored tablets debossed with stylized **b** on one side and **556** on the other side.
Box of 2 Extended-Cycle Tablet
Dispensers NDC 51285-087-87

16.2 Storage Conditions
Store at 20° to 25° C (68° to 77° F) [See USP Controlled Room Temperature].

17. PATIENT COUNSELING INFORMATION

See FDA-Approved Patient Labeling
- Counsel patients that cigarette smoking increases the risk of serious cardiovascular events from COC use, and that women who are over 35 years old and smoke should not use COCs.
- Counsel patients that this product does not protect against HIV-infection (AIDS) and other sexually transmitted diseases.
- Counsel patients on Warnings and Precautions associated with COCs.
- Counsel patients to take one tablet daily by mouth at the same time every day. Instruct patients what to do in the event pills are missed. See **WHAT TO DO IF YOU MISS PILLS** section of FDA-Approved Patient Labeling.
- Counsel patients to use a back-up or alternative method of contraception when enzyme inducers are used with COCs.
- Counsel patients who are breastfeeding or who desire to breastfeed that COCs may reduce breast milk production. This is less likely to occur if breastfeeding is well established.
- Counsel any patient who starts COCs postpartum, and who has not yet had a period, to use an additional method of contraception until she has taken a light blue-green tablet for 7 consecutive days.
- Counsel patients that amenorrhea may occur. Pregnancy should be considered in the event of amenorrhea, and should be ruled out if amenorrhea is associated with symptoms of pregnancy, such as morning sickness or unusual breast tenderness.

DURAMED PHARMACEUTICALS, INC.
Subsidiary of Barr Pharmaceuticals, Inc. Pomona, New York 10970
11001500

FDA-APPROVED PATIENT LABELING
Guide for Using Seasonique

WARNING TO WOMEN WHO SMOKE
Do not use Seasonique if you smoke cigarettes and are over 35 years old. Smoking increases your risk of serious cardiovascular side effects from birth control pills, including death from heart attack, blood clots or stroke. This risk increases with age and the number of cigarettes you smoke.

Birth control pills help to lower the chances of becoming pregnant. They do not protect against HIV infection (AIDS) and other sexually transmitted diseases.
What Is Seasonique?
Seasonique is a birth control pill. It contains two female hormones, an estrogen called ethinyl estradiol, and a progestin called levonorgestrel.
How Well Does Seasonique Work?
Your chance of getting pregnant depends on how well you follow the directions for taking your birth control pills. The more carefully you follow the directions, the less chance you have of getting pregnant.
Based on the results of a single clinical study lasting 12 months, 1 to 3 women, out of 100 women, may get pregnant during the first year they use Seasonique.
The following chart shows the chance of getting pregnant for women who use different methods of birth control. Each box on the chart contains a list of birth control methods that

are similar in effectiveness. The most effective methods are at the top of the chart. The box on the bottom of the chart shows the chance of getting pregnant for women who do not use birth control and are trying to get pregnant.

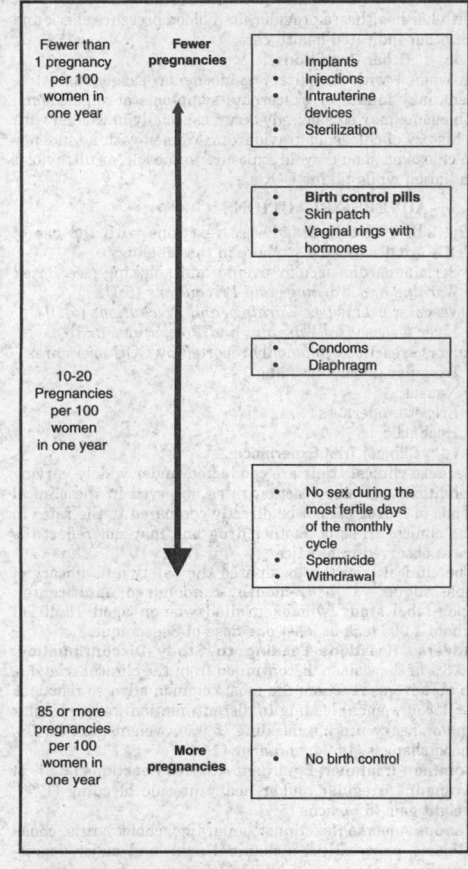

How Do I Take Seasonique?
1. Take one pill every day at the same time. If you miss pills you could get pregnant. This includes starting the pack late. The more pills you miss, the more likely you are to get pregnant.
2. Many women have spotting or light bleeding, or may feel sick to their stomach during the first few months of taking Seasonique. If you feel sick to your stomach, do not stop taking the pill. The problem will usually go away. If it doesn't go away, check with your healthcare provider.
3. Missing pills can also cause spotting or light bleeding, even when you take the missed pills later. On the days you take 2 pills to make up for missed pills, you could also feel a little sick to your stomach.
4. If you have trouble remembering to take Seasonique, talk to your healthcare provider about how to make pill-taking easier or about using another method of birth control.
Before you start taking Seasonique
1. Decide what time of day you want to take your pill. It is important to take it at about the same time every day.
2. Look at your Extended-Cycle Tablet Dispenser. Your Tablet Dispenser consists of 3 trays with cards that hold 91 individually sealed pills (a 13-week or 91-day cycle). The 91 pills consist of 84 light blue-green and 7 yellow pills. Trays 1 and 2 each contain 28 light blue-green pills (4 rows of 7 pills). Tray 3 contains 35 pills consisting of 28 light blue-green pills (4 rows of 7 pills) and 7 yellow pills (1 row of 7 pills).
[See first figure at top of next page]
[See second figure on next page]
[See third figure on next page]
3. Also find:
- Where on the first tray in the pack to start taking pills (upper left corner at the start arrow) and
- In what order to take the pills (follow the weeks and arrow).
4. Be sure you have ready at all times another kind of birth control (such as condoms or spermicides), to use as a back-up in case you miss pills.
When to Start Seasonique
1. Take the first light blue-green pill on the Sunday after your period starts, even if you are still bleeding. If your period begins on Sunday, start the first light blue-green pill that same day.
2. Use another method of birth control (such as condoms or spermicides) as a back-up method if you have sex anytime

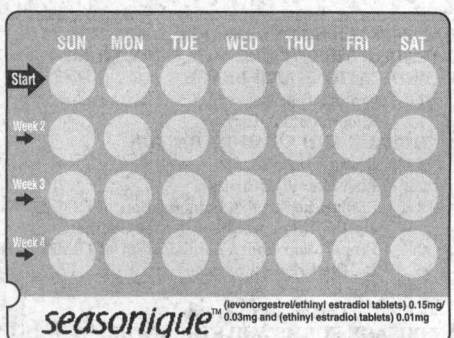

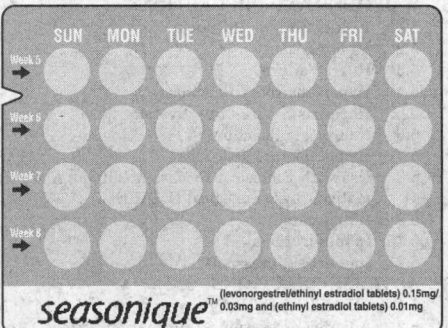

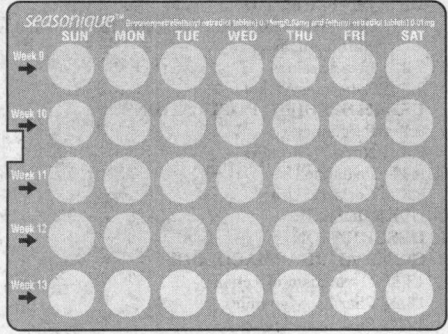

from the Sunday you start your first light blue-green pill until the next Sunday (first 7 days). If you have been using a different hormonal method of birth control (such as a different pill, the "patch," or the "vaginal ring"), you need to use another method of birth control (such as condoms or spermicides) each time you have sex after stopping your old method of birth control until you have taken Seasonique for 7 days.

How to Take Seasonique

1. Take one pill at the same time every day until you have taken the last pill in the tablet dispenser.
- Do not skip pills even if you are experiencing spotting or bleeding or feel sick to your stomach (nausea).
- Do not skip pills even if you do not have sex very often.

2. When you finish a tablet dispenser
- After taking the last yellow pill, start taking the first light blue-green pill from a new Extended-Cycle Tablet Dispenser the very next day (this should be on a Sunday) regardless of when your period started.

3. If you miss your scheduled period when you are taking the yellow pills, contact your healthcare provider because you may be pregnant. If you are pregnant, you should stop taking Seasonique.

What To Do If You Miss Pills

If you MISS 1 light blue-green pill:
1. Take it as soon as you remember. Take the next pill at your regular time. This means you may take 2 pills in 1 day.
2. You do not need to use a back-up birth control method if you have sex.

If you MISS 2 light blue-green pills in a row:
1. Take 2 pills on the day you remember, and 2 pills the next day.
2. Then take 1 pill a day until you finish the pack.
3. You could become pregnant if you have sex in the 7 days after you miss two pills. You MUST use another birth control method (such as condoms or spermicide) as a back up for the 7 days after you restart your pills.

If you MISS 3 OR MORE light blue-green pills in a row:
1. Do not take the missed pills. Keep taking 1 pill every day as indicated on the pack until you have completed all of the remaining pills in the pack. For example: If you resume taking the pill on Thursday, take the pill under "Thursday" and do not take the missed pills. You may experience bleeding during the week following the missed pills.

2. You could become pregnant if you have sex during the days of missed pills or during the first 7 days after restarting your pills.

3. You MUST use a non-hormonal birth control method (such as condoms or spermicide) as a back-up when you miss pills and for the first 7 days after you restart your pills. If you do not have your period when you are taking the yellow pills, call your healthcare provider because you may be pregnant.

If you MISS ANY of the 7 yellow pills:
1. Throw away the missed pills.
2. Keep taking the scheduled pills until the pack is finished.
3. You do not need a back-up method of birth control.

Finally, if you are still not sure what to do about the pills you have missed

1. Use a back-up method anytime you have sex.
2. Keep taking one pill each day until you contact your healthcare provider.

Who Should Not Take Seasonique?

Your healthcare provider will not give you Seasonique if you have:
- Ever had breast cancer or any cancer that is sensitive to female hormones
- Liver disease, including liver tumors
- Ever had blood clots in your arms, legs, or lungs
- Ever had a stroke
- Ever had a heart attack
- Certain heart valve problems or heart rhythm abnormalities that can cause blood clots to form in the heart
- An inherited problem with your blood that makes it clot more than normal
- High blood pressure that medicine can't control
- Diabetes with kidney, eye, or blood vessel damage
- Certain kinds of severe migraine headaches with aura, numbness, weakness or changes in vision

Also, do not take birth control pills if you:
- Smoke and are over 35 years old
- Are pregnant

Birth control pills may not be a good choice for you if you have ever had jaundice (yellowing of the skin or eyes) caused by pregnancy.

What Else Should I Know About Taking Seasonique?

Birth control pills do **not** protect you against any sexually transmitted disease, including HIV, the virus that causes AIDS.

Do not skip any pills, even if you do not have sex often.

Birth control pills should not be taken during pregnancy. However, birth control pills taken by accident during pregnancy are not known to cause birth defects.

If you are breastfeeding, consider another birth control method until you are ready to stop breastfeeding. Birth control pills that contain estrogen, like Seasonique, may decrease the amount of milk you make. A small amount of the pill's hormones pass into breast milk.

Tell your healthcare provider about all medicines and herbal products that you take. Some medicines and herbal products may make birth control pills less effective, including:
- barbiturates
- bosentan
- carbamazepine
- felbamate
- griseofulvin
- oxcarbazepine
- phenytoin
- rifampin
- St. John's wort
- topiramate

Consider using another birth control method when you take medicines that may make birth control pills less effective.

Birth control pills may interact with lamotrigine, an anticonvulsant used for epilepsy. This may increase the risk of seizures, so your physician may need to adjust the dose of lamotrigine.

If you have vomiting or diarrhea, your birth control pills may not work as well. Use another birth control method, like condoms or a spermicide, until you check with your healthcare provider.

What Are The Most Serious Risks Of Taking Birth Control Pills?

Like pregnancy, birth control pills increase the risk of serious blood clots, especially in women who have other risk factors, such as smoking, obesity, or age > 35. It is possible to die from a problem caused by a blood clot, such as a heart attack or a stroke. Some examples of serious blood clots are blood clots in the:
- Legs (thrombophlebitis)
- Lungs (pulmonary embolus)
- Eyes (loss of eyesight)
- Heart (heart attack)
- Brain (stroke)

Women who take birth control pills may get:
- High blood pressure
- Gallbladder problems
- Rare cancerous or noncancerous liver tumors

All of these events are uncommon in healthy women. Call your healthcare provider right away if you have:
- Persistent leg pain
- Sudden shortness of breath
- Sudden blindness, partial or complete
- Severe pain in your chest
- Sudden, severe headache unlike your usual headaches
- Weakness or numbness in an arm or leg, or trouble speaking
- Yellowing of the skin or eyeballs

What Are Common Side Effects Of Birth Control Pills?

The most common side effects of birth control pills are:
- Spotting or bleeding between menstrual periods
- Nausea
- Breast tenderness
- Headache

These side effects are usually mild and usually disappear with time.

Less common side effects are:
- Acne
- Less sexual desire
- Bloating or fluid retention
- Blotchy darkening of the skin, especially on the face
- High blood sugar, especially in women who already have diabetes
- High fat levels in the blood
- Depression, especially if you have had depression in the past. Call your healthcare provider immediately if you have any thoughts of harming yourself.
- Problems tolerating contact lenses
- Weight changes

This is not a complete list of possible side effects. Talk to your healthcare provider if you develop any side effects that concern you. You may report side effects to the FDA at 1-800-FDA-1088.

No serious problems have been reported from a birth control pill overdose, even when accidentally taken by children.

Do Birth Control Pills Cause Cancer?

Birth control pills do not appear to cause breast cancer. However, if you have breast cancer now, or have had it in the past, do not use birth control pills because some breast cancers are sensitive to hormones.

Women who use birth control pills may have a slightly higher chance of getting cervical cancer. However, this may be due to other reasons such as having more sexual partners.

What Should I Know About My Period When Taking Seasonique?

When you take Seasonique, which has a 91-day extended dosing cycle, you should expect to have 4 scheduled periods per year (bleeding when you are taking the 7 yellow pills). Each period is likely to last about 3 days. However, you will probably have more bleeding or spotting between your scheduled periods than if you were using a birth control pill with a 28-day dosing cycle. During the first Seasonique 91-day treatment cycle, about 3 in 10 women may have 20 or more days of unplanned bleeding or spotting. This bleeding or spotting tends to decrease with time. Do not stop taking Seasonique because of this bleeding or spotting. If the spotting continues for more than 7 consecutive days or if the bleeding is heavy, call your healthcare provider.

What If I Miss My Scheduled Period When Taking Seasonique?

You should consider the possibility that you are pregnant if you miss your scheduled period (no bleeding on the days that you are taking yellow tablets). Since scheduled periods are less frequent when you are taking Seasonique, notify your healthcare provider that you have missed your period and that you are taking Seasonique. Also notify your healthcare provider if you have symptoms of pregnancy such as morning sickness or unusual breast tenderness. It is important that your healthcare provider evaluates you to determine if you are pregnant. Stop taking Seasonique if it is determined that you are pregnant.

What If I Want To Become Pregnant?

You may stop taking the pill whenever you wish. Consider a visit with your healthcare provider for a pre-pregnancy checkup before you stop taking the pill.

General Advice About Seasonique

Your healthcare provider prescribed Seasonique for you. Do not share Seasonique with anyone else. Keep Seasonique out of the reach of children.

If you have concerns or questions, ask your healthcare provider. You may also ask your healthcare providers for a more detailed label written for medical professionals.

DURAMED PHARMACEUTICALS, INC.
Subsidiary of Barr Pharmaceuticals, Inc. Pomona, New York 10970
11001500
Revised July 2010
Shown in Product Identification Guide, page 320

Topical BioMedics, Inc.

PO BOX 494
RHINEBECK, NY 12572-0494

Direct Inquiries to:
Professional Services at Topricin
Phone: (845) 871-4900 ext. 1115
Fax: (845) 876-0818
E-mail: info@topicalbiomedics.com for Free samples and
prescription pads

TOPRICIN®   OTC
[toe-pri-sin]

KEY FACTS

Topricin® is an odorless, non-irritating, Pain Relief and
Healing cream that provides superior relief of all trauma
injuries and excellent adjunctive support in medical treatment protocols such as: post surgical trauma, physical and
occupational therapy, physiatry, physical and sports medicine. Greaseless and contains no chemical preservatives, or
menthol, camphor, capsaicin, methyl salicylates or fra-
grances. Topricin is the ideal topical treatment that is safe
for the entire family, and the best alternative option for patients who cannot tolerate oral pain medications.

ACTIVE INGREDIENTS (HPUS)

Arnica Montana 6X, Echinacea 6X, Aesculus 6X, Ruta
Graveolens 6X, Lachesis 8X, Rhus Tox 6X Belladonna 6X,
Crotalus 8X, Heloderma 8X, Naja 8X, Graphites 6X.

MAJOR USES

Superior topical relief of pain edema and a healing treatment for all soft tissue neuropathic pain, repetitive motion
and cumulative trauma work/sports injuries.

BENEFITS

Rapidly relieves: stiffness, soreness, numbness, tingling
pain/burning pain associated with these soft tissue ail-
ments: carpal tunnel syndrome, other peripheral neuropathic pain, arthritis, lower back pain, muscle spasm of the
back, neck, legs, and feet, muscle soreness, strains, sprains.
First aid: bruises, minor burns. Use before and after exercise.

DIRECTIONS

Apply generously 3–4 times a day or more often if needed.
Be sure the application covers the entire joint or area of
pain. Massage in until absorbed. Reapply before bed and at
the start of the day for best results. Can be used with hot
and cold therapy or Phonophoresis. For further information
go to www.topicalbiomedics.com

SAFETY INFORMATION

For external use only, use only as directed, if pain persists
for more than 7 days or worsens, Consult a doctor. This homeopathic medicine has no known side effects or contraindications. This medicine complies with all FDA regulations
as an OTC medicine, safe to use for children over 2 years,
adults, pregnant women and the elderly. Paraben and Petroleum free

INACTIVE INGREDIENTS

Purified water, purified coconut oil, glycerin, medium chain
triglyceride.

HOW SUPPLIED

Consumer size: 2oz tube, 4oz jar, and 8oz flip top bottle.
For Professionals only: 16oz and 32oz pump bottle.
Other products: Topricin Junior 1.5oz tube, Topricin Foot
Therapy Cream 2oz, 4oz and 8oz flip top bottle.
Countertop Display available for medical office or pharmacy
shelf.

Shown in Product Identification Guide, page 320

UCB, Inc.

**1950 LAKE PARK DRIVE
SMYRNA, GA 30080**

Direct Inquiries to:
UCB, Inc.
1950 Lake Park Drive
Smyrna, GA 30080
(800) 477–7877
For Medical Information Contact:
Medical Affairs Department
(866) 822–0068
FAX: 770-970-8859

CIMZIA®   ℞
[CIM-zee-uh]
(certolizumab pegol)
Lyophilized powder for solution and solution for
subcutaneous injection

HIGHLIGHTS OF PRESCRIBING INFORMATION
These highlights do not include all the information needed
to use CIMZIA® safely and effectively. See full prescribing
information for CIMZIA.
CIMZIA (certolizumab pegol)
Lyophilized powder for solution and solution for
subcutaneous injection
Initial U.S. Approval: 2008

WARNING: RISK OF SERIOUS INFECTIONS
*See full prescribing information for complete boxed
warning.*
- Increased risk of serious infections leading to hospitalization or death including tuberculosis (TB), bacterial sepsis, invasive fungal infections (such as histoplasmosis), and infections due to other opportunistic
pathogens.
- CIMZIA should be discontinued if a patient develops
a serious infection or sepsis.
- Perform test for latent TB; if positive, start treatment
for TB prior to starting CIMZIA.
- Monitor all patients for active TB during treatment,
even if initial latent TB test is negative (5.1)
- Lymphoma and other malignancies, some fatal, have
been reported in children and adolescent patients
treated with TNF blockers, of which CIMZIA is a
member (5.2). CIMZIA is not indicated for use in pediatric patients.

—————RECENT MAJOR CHANGES—————

Warnings and Precautions, Neurologic Reactions	07/2010
Boxed Warning, Risk of Malignancy	11/2009
Warnings and Precautions, Malignancies (5.2)	11/2009

————INDICATIONS AND USAGE————
CIMZIA is a tumor necrosis factor (TNF) blocker indicated
for:
- Reducing signs and symptoms of Crohn's disease and
maintaining clinical response in adult patients with moderately to severely active disease who have had an inadequate response to conventional therapy (1.1)
- Treatment of adults with moderately to severely active
rheumatoid arthritis (1.2)

————DOSAGE AND ADMINISTRATION————
CIMZIA is administered by subcutaneous injection. The initial dose of CIMZIA is 400 mg (given as two subcutaneous
injections of 200 mg).
Crohn's Disease (2.1)
- 400 mg initially and at Weeks 2 and 4. If response occurs,
follow with 400 mg every four weeks
Rheumatoid Arthritis (2.2)
- 400 mg initially and at Weeks 2 and 4, followed by 200 mg
every other week; for maintenance dosing, 400 mg every 4
weeks can be considered

————DOSAGE FORMS AND STRENGTHS————
- 200 mg lyophilized powder for reconstitution with 1 mL of
sterile Water for Injection, USP (3)
- 200 mg/mL in a single-use prefilled glass syringe (3)

————————CONTRAINDICATIONS————————
- None (4)

————WARNINGS AND PRECAUTIONS————
- Serious infections – do not start CIMZIA during an active
infection. If an infection develops, monitor carefully, and
stop CIMZIA if infection becomes serious (5.1)
- Cases of lymphoma and other malignancies have been observed among patients receiving TNF blockers (5.2)
- Heart failure, worsening or new onset may occur (5.3)
- Anaphylaxis or serious allergic reactions may occur (5.4)
- Hepatitis B virus reactivation – monitor HBV carriers
during and several months after therapy. If reactivation
occurs, stop CIMZIA and begin anti-viral therapy (5.5)
- Demyelinating disease, exacerbation or new onset, may
occur (5.6)
- Cytopenias, pancytopenia – advise patients to seek immediate medical attention if symptoms develop, and consider
stopping CIMZIA (5.7)
- Lupus-like syndrome – stop CIMZIA if syndrome develops
(5.9)

————————ADVERSE REACTIONS————————
The most common adverse reactions (incidence ≥7% and
higher than placebo): upper respiratory tract infection,
rash, and urinary tract infection (6.1)
**To report SUSPECTED ADVERSE REACTIONS, contact
UCB, Inc. at 1-866-822-0068 or FDA at 1-800-FDA-1088 or
www.fda.gov/medwatch**

————————DRUG INTERACTIONS————————
- Use with Biological DMARDs – increased risk of serious
infections (5.8, 7.1)
- Live vaccines – do not give with CIMZIA (5.10, 7.2)
- Laboratory tests – may interfere with aPTT tests (7.3)
See 17 for PATIENT COUNSELING INFORMATION
and MEDICATION GUIDE

                     Revised: 07/2010

FULL PRESCRIBING INFORMATION: CONTENTS*
WARNING: RISK OF SERIOUS INFECTIONS
1 INDICATIONS AND USAGE
  1.1 Crohn's Disease
  1.2 Rheumatoid Arthritis
2 DOSAGE AND ADMINISTRATION
  2.1 Crohn's Disease
  2.2 Rheumatoid Arthritis
  2.3 Preparation and Administration of CIMZIA Us-
     ing the Lyophilized Powder for Solution
  2.4 Preparation and Administration of CIMZIA Us-
     ing the Prefilled Syringe
  2.5 Monitoring to Assess Safety
  2.6 Concomitant Medications
3 DOSAGE FORMS AND STRENGTHS
4 CONTRAINDICATIONS
5 WARNINGS AND PRECAUTIONS
  5.1 Risk of Serious Infections
  5.2 Malignancies
  5.3 Heart Failure
  5.4 Hypersensitivity Reactions
  5.5 Hepatitis B Virus Reactivation
  5.6 Neurologic Reactions
  5.7 Hematological Reactions
  5.8 Use with Biological Disease-Modifying Antirheu-
     matic Drugs (Biological DMARDs)
  5.9 Autoimmunity
  5.10 Immunizations
  5.11 Immunosuppression
6 ADVERSE REACTIONS
  6.1 Clinical Trials Experience
  6.2 Adverse Reaction Information from Other
     Sources
7 DRUG INTERACTIONS
  7.1 Use with Anakinra, Abatacept, Rituximab, and
     Natalizumab
  7.2 Live Vaccines
  7.3 Laboratory Tests
8 USE IN SPECIFIC POPULATIONS
  8.1 Pregnancy
  8.3 Nursing Mothers
  8.4 Pediatric Use
  8.5 Geriatric Use
10 OVERDOSAGE
11 DESCRIPTION
12 CLINICAL PHARMACOLOGY
  12.1 Mechanism of Action
  12.2 Pharmacodynamics
  12.3 Pharmacokinetics
13 NONCLINICAL TOXICOLOGY
  13.1 Carcinogenesis, Mutagenesis, and Impairment of
     Fertility
14 CLINICAL STUDIES
  14.1 Crohn's Disease
  14.2 Rheumatoid Arthritis
15 REFERENCES
16 HOW SUPPLIED/STORAGE AND HANDLING
17 PATIENT COUNSELING INFORMATION
  17.1 Patient Counseling
  17.2 Instruction on Prefilled Syringe Self-Injection
     Technique
  17.3 Medication Guide
* Sections or subsections omitted from the full prescribing
information are not listed.

FULL PRESCRIBING INFORMATION

**WARNINGS:
SERIOUS INFECTIONS**
Patients treated with CIMZIA are at increased risk for
developing serious infections that may lead to hospitalization or death [see Warnings and Precautions
(5.1) and Adverse Reactions (6.1)]. Most patients who
developed these infections were taking concomitant
immunosuppressants such as methotrexate or
corticosteroids.
CIMZIA should be discontinued if a patient develops a
serious infection or sepsis.
Reported infections include:
- Active tuberculosis, including reactivation of latent
tuberculosis. Patients with tuberculosis have frequently presented with disseminated or extrapulmonary disease. Patients should be tested for latent tuberculosis before CIMZIA use and during therapy.
Treatment for latent infection should be initiated
prior to CIMZIA use.
- Invasive fungal infections, including histoplasmosis,
coccidioidomycosis, candidiasis, aspergillosis, blas-

---

tomycosis, and pneumocystosis. Patients with histoplasmosis or other invasive fungal infections may present with disseminated, rather than localized disease. Antigen and antibody testing for histoplasmosis may be negative in some patients with active infection. Empiric anti-fungal therapy should be considered in patients at risk for invasive fungal infections who develop severe systemic illness.

• Bacterial, viral and other infections due to opportunistic pathogens.

The risks and benefits of treatment with CIMZIA should be carefully considered prior to initiating therapy in patients with chronic or recurrent infection.

Patients should be closely monitored for the development of signs and symptoms of infection during and after treatment with CIMZIA, including the possible development of tuberculosis in patients who tested negative for latent tuberculosis infection prior to initiating therapy. *[see Warnings and Precautions (5.1) and Adverse Reactions (6.1)]*.

MALIGNANCY

Lymphoma and other malignancies, some fatal, have been reported in children and adolescent patients treated with TNF blockers, of which CIMZIA is a member *[see Warnings and Precautions (5.2)]*. CIMZIA is not indicated for use in pediatric patients.

1 INDICATIONS AND USAGE

1.1 Crohn's Disease

CIMZIA is indicated for reducing signs and symptoms of Crohn's disease and maintaining clinical response in adult patients with moderately to severely active disease who have had an inadequate response to conventional therapy.

1.2 Rheumatoid Arthritis

CIMZIA is indicated for the treatment of adults with moderately to severely active rheumatoid arthritis (RA).

2 DOSAGE AND ADMINISTRATION

CIMZIA is administered by subcutaneous injection. Injection sites should be rotated and injections should not be given into areas where the skin is tender, bruised, red or hard. When a 400 mg dose is needed (given as two subcutaneous injections of 200 mg), injections should occur at separate sites in the thigh or abdomen.

The solution should be carefully inspected visually for particulate matter and discoloration prior to administration. The solution should be a clear colorless to yellow liquid, essentially free from particulates and should not be used if cloudy or if foreign particulate matter is present. CIMZIA does not contain preservatives; therefore, unused portions of drug remaining in the syringe or vial should be discarded.

2.1 Crohn's Disease

The recommended initial adult dose of CIMZIA is 400 mg (given as two subcutaneous injections of 200 mg) initially, and at Weeks 2 and 4. In patients who obtain a clinical response, the recommended maintenance regimen is 400 mg every four weeks.

2.2 Rheumatoid Arthritis

The recommended dose of CIMZIA for adult patients with rheumatoid arthritis is 400 mg (given as two subcutaneous injections of 200 mg) initially and at Weeks 2 and 4, followed by 200 mg every other week. For maintenance dosing, CIMZIA 400 mg every 4 weeks can be considered *[see Clinical Studies (14.2)]*.

2.3 Preparation and Administration of CIMZIA Using the Lyophilized Powder for Solution

The lyophilized powder should be prepared and administered by a health care professional. CIMZIA is provided in a package that contains everything required to reconstitute and inject the drug as described below. CIMZIA should be brought to room temperature before reconstituting to facilitate dissolution.

Reconstitute each lyophilized vial of CIMZIA using appropriate aseptic technique, with 1 mL of sterile Water for Injection, USP, and a syringe with a 20 gauge needle. Gently swirl each vial of CIMZIA without shaking so that all of the lyophilized powder comes into contact with the sterile Water for Injection. Leave the vials undisturbed to fully reconstitute (this may take as long as 30 minutes). Reconstituted CIMZIA has a concentration of approximately 200 mg/mL. Once reconstituted, CIMZIA is a clear to opalescent, colorless to pale yellow liquid essentially free from particulates. Prior to injecting, reconstituted CIMZIA should be at room temperature. Do not leave reconstituted CIMZIA at room temperature for more than 2 hours prior to administration. Using a new 20 gauge (reconstitution) needle for each vial, withdraw the reconstituted solution into a separate syringe for each vial, so that each syringe contains 1 mL of CIMZIA (200 mg of certolizumab pegol). Switch each 20 gauge needle to a 23 gauge (dosing) needle and inject the full contents of each syringe subcutaneously into the thigh or abdomen.

Where a 400 mg dose is required, separate sites should be used for each 200 mg injection.

Once reconstituted, CIMZIA can be stored in the vials for up to 24 hours at 2 to 8°C (36 to 46 °F) prior to injection. Do not freeze.

2.4 Preparation and Administration of CIMZIA Using the Prefilled Syringe

A patient may self-inject CIMZIA if a physician determines that it is appropriate, with medical follow-up, as necessary, after proper training in subcutaneous injection technique. Patients using CIMZIA should be instructed to inject the full amount in the syringe (1 mL), according to the directions provided in the Patient Instructions for Use *[see FDA approved Medication Guide (17.3)]*.

2.5 Monitoring to Assess Safety

Before initiation of therapy with CIMZIA, all patients must be evaluated for both active and inactive (latent) tuberculosis infection. The possibility of undetected latent tuberculosis should be considered in patients who have immigrated from or traveled to countries with a high prevalence of tuberculosis or had close contact with a person with active tuberculosis. Appropriate screening tests (e.g. tuberculin skin test and chest x-ray) should be performed in all patients.

2.6 Concomitant Medications

CIMZIA may be used as monotherapy or concomitantly with non-biological disease modifying anti-rheumatic drugs (DMARDs). In rheumatoid arthritis clinical studies, patients on CIMZIA therapy also took concomitant methotrexate (MTX) with the recommended CIMZIA dose of 200 mg every other week. CIMZIA should not be used in combination with biological DMARDs or other tumor necrosis factor (TNF) blocker therapy.

3 DOSAGE FORMS AND STRENGTHS

• **Lyophilized Powder for Reconstitution**

Sterile, white, lyophilized powder for reconstitution and then subcutaneous administration. Each single-use vial provides approximately 200 mg of CIMZIA.

• **Prefilled Syringe**

A single-use, 1 mL prefilled glass syringe with a fixed 25 gauge ½ inch thin wall needle, providing 200 mg (1 mL) of CIMZIA.

4 CONTRAINDICATIONS

None.

5 WARNINGS AND PRECAUTIONS

5.1 Risk of Serious Infections

(see also Boxed Warning)

Serious and sometimes fatal infection due to bacterial, mycobacterial, invasive fungal, viral, or other opportunistic pathogens has been reported in patients receiving TNF-blocking agents. Among opportunistic infections, tuberculosis, histoplasmosis, aspergillosis, candidiasis, coccidioidomycosis, listeriosis, and pneumocystosis were the most common. Patients have frequently presented with disseminated rather than localized disease, and are often taking concomitant immunosuppressants such as methotrexate or corticosteroids with CIMZIA.

Treatment with CIMZIA should not be initiated in patients with an active infection, including clinically important localized infections. The risks and benefits of treatment should be considered prior to initiating therapy in patients:

• with chronic or recurrent infection
• who have been exposed to tuberculosis
• who have resided or traveled in areas of endemic tuberculosis or endemic mycoses, such as histoplasmosis, coccidioidomycosis, or blastomycosis
• with underlying conditions that may predispose them to infection

Cases of reactivation of tuberculosis or new tuberculosis infections have been observed in patients receiving CIMZIA, including patients who have previously received treatment for latent or active tuberculosis. Patients should be evaluated for tuberculosis risk factors and tested for latent infection prior to initiating CIMZIA and periodically during therapy.

Treatment of latent tuberculosis infection prior to therapy with TNF-blocking agents has been shown to reduce the risk of tuberculosis reactivation during therapy. Induration of 5 mm or greater with tuberculin skin testing should be considered a positive test result when assessing if treatment for latent tuberculosis is needed prior to initiating CIMZIA, even for patients previously vaccinated with Bacille Calmette-Guerin (BCG).

Anti-tuberculosis therapy should also be considered prior to initiation of CIMZIA in patients with a past history of latent or active tuberculosis in whom an adequate course of treatment cannot be confirmed, and for patients with a negative test for latent tuberculosis but having risk factors for tuberculosis infection. Consultation with a physician with expertise in the treatment of tuberculosis is recommended to aid in the decision of whether initiating anti-tuberculosis therapy is appropriate for an individual patient.

Tuberculosis should be strongly considered in patients who develop a new infection during CIMZIA treatment, especially in patients who have previously or recently traveled to countries with a high prevalence of tuberculosis, or who have had close contact with a person with active tuberculosis.

Patients should be closely monitored for the development of signs and symptoms of infection during and after treatment with CIMZIA, including the development of tuberculosis in patients who tested negative for latent tuberculosis infection prior to initiating therapy. Tests for latent tuberculosis infection may also be falsely negative while on therapy with CIMZIA.

CIMZIA should be discontinued if a patient develops a serious infection or sepsis. A patient who develops a new infection during treatment with CIMZIA should be closely monitored, undergo a prompt and complete diagnostic workup appropriate for an immunocompromised patient, and appropriate antimicrobial therapy should be initiated.

For patients who reside or travel in regions where mycoses are endemic, invasive fungal infection should be suspected if they develop a serious systemic illness. Appropriate empiric antifungal therapy should be considered while a diagnostic workup is being performed. Antigen and antibody testing for histoplasmosis may be negative in some patients with active infection. When feasible, the decision to administer empiric antifungal therapy in these patients should be made in consultation with a physician with expertise in the diagnosis and treatment of invasive fungal infections and should take into account both the risk for severe fungal infection and risks of antifungal therapy.

5.2 Malignancies

In the controlled portions of clinical studies of some TNF blockers, more cases of malignancies have been observed among patients receiving TNF blockers compared to control patients. During controlled and open-labeled portions of CIMZIA studies of Crohn's disease and other diseases, malignancies (excluding non-melanoma skin cancer) were observed at a rate (95% confidence interval) of 0.5 (0.4, 0.7) per 100 patient-years among 4,650 CIMZIA-treated patients versus a rate of 0.6 (0.1, 1.7) per 100 patient-years among 1,319 placebo-treated patients. The size of the control group and limited duration of the controlled portions of the studies precludes the ability to draw firm conclusions.

Malignancies, some fatal, have been reported among children, adolescents, and young adults who received treatment with TNF-blocking agents (initiation of therapy ≤ 18 years of age), of which CIMZIA is a member. Approximately half the cases were lymphomas, including Hodgkin's and non-Hodgkin's lymphoma. The other cases represented a variety of different malignancies and included rare malignancies usually associated with immunosuppression and malignancies that are not usually observed in children and adolescents. The malignancies occurred after a median of 30 months of therapy (range 1 to 84 months). Most of the patients were receiving concomitant immunosuppressants. These cases were reported post-marketing and are derived from a variety of sources including registries and spontaneous post-marketing reports.

In the controlled portions of clinical trials of all the TNF blockers, more cases of lymphoma have been observed among patients receiving TNF blockers compared to control patients. In controlled studies of CIMZIA for Crohn's disease and other investigational uses, there was one case of lymphoma among 2,657 Cimzia-treated patients and one case of Hodgkin's lymphoma among 1,319 placebo-treated patients.

In the CIMZIA RA clinical trials (placebo-controlled and open label) a total of three cases of lymphoma were observed among 2,367 patients. This is approximately 2-fold higher than expected in the general population. Patients with RA, particularly those with highly active disease, are at a higher risk for the development of lymphoma.

Rates in clinical studies for CIMZIA cannot be compared to the rates of clinical trials of other TNF blockers and may not predict the rates observed when CIMZIA is used in a broader patient population. Patients with Crohn's disease that require chronic exposure to immunosuppressant therapies may be at higher risk than the general population for the development of lymphoma, even in the absence of TNF blocker therapy *[see Adverse Reactions (6.1)]*. The potential role of TNF blocker therapy in the development of malignancies in adults is not known.

Cases of acute and chronic leukemia have been reported in association with post-marketing TNF-blocker use in RA and other indications. Even in the absence of TNF-blocker therapy, patients with RA may be at a higher risk (approximately 2-fold) than the general population for the development of leukemia.

5.3 Heart Failure

Cases of worsening congestive heart failure (CHF) and new onset CHF have been reported with TNF blockers, including

CIMZIA. CIMZIA has not been formally studied in patients with CHF; however, in clinical studies in patients with CHF with another TNF blocker, worsening congestive heart failure (CHF) and increased mortality due to CHF were observed. Exercise caution in patients with heart failure and monitor them carefully *[see Adverse Reactions (6.1)]*.

5.4 Hypersensitivity Reactions

The following symptoms that could be compatible with hypersensitivity reactions have been reported rarely following CIMZIA administration to patients: angioedema, dyspnea, hypotension, rash, serum sickness, and urticaria. If such reactions occur, discontinue further administration of CIMZIA and institute appropriate therapy. There are no data on the risks of using CIMZIA in patients who have experienced a severe hypersensitivity reaction towards another TNF blocker; in these patients caution is needed *[see Adverse Reactions (6.1)]*.

5.5 Hepatitis B Virus Reactivation

Use of TNF blockers, including CIMZIA, may increase the risk of reactivation of hepatitis B virus (HBV) in patients who are chronic carriers of this virus. In some instances, HBV reactivation occurring in conjunction with TNF blocker therapy has been fatal. The majority of reports have occurred in patients concomitantly receiving other medications that suppress the immune system, which may also contribute to HBV reactivation.

Evaluate patients at risk for HBV infection for prior evidence of HBV infection before initiating CIMZIA therapy. Exercise caution in prescribing CIMZIA for patients identified as carriers of HBV. Adequate data are not available on the safety or efficacy of treating patients who are carriers of HBV with anti-viral therapy in conjunction with TNF blocker therapy to prevent HBV reactivation.

Patients who are carriers of HBV and require treatment with CIMZIA should be closely monitored for clinical and laboratory signs of active HBV infection throughout therapy and for several months following termination of therapy.

In patients who develop HBV reactivation, discontinue CIMZIA and initiate effective anti-viral therapy with appropriate supportive treatment. The safety of resuming TNF blocker therapy after HBV reactivation is controlled is not known. Therefore, exercise caution when considering resumption of CIMZIA therapy in this situation and monitor patients closely.

5.6 Neurologic Reactions

Use of TNF blockers, of which CIMZIA is a member, has been associated with rare cases of new onset or exacerbation of clinical symptoms and/or radiographic evidence of central nervous system demyelinating disease, including multiple sclerosis, and with peripheral demyelinating disease, including Guillain-Barré syndrome. Exercise caution in considering the use of CIMZIA in patients with pre-existing or recent-onset central or peripheral nervous system demyelinating disorders. Rare cases of neurological disorders, including seizure disorder, optic neuritis, and peripheral neuropathy have been reported in patients treated with CIMZIA *[see Adverse Reactions (6.1)]*.

5.7 Hematological Reactions

Rare reports of pancytopenia, including aplastic anemia, have been reported with TNF blockers. Adverse reactions of the hematologic system, including medically significant cytopenia (e.g., leukopenia, pancytopenia, thrombocytopenia) have been infrequently reported with CIMZIA *[see Adverse Reactions (6.1)]*. The causal relationship of these events to CIMZIA remains unclear.

Although no high risk group has been identified, exercise caution in patients being treated with CIMZIA who have ongoing, or a history of, significant hematologic abnormalities. Advise all patients to seek immediate medical attention if they develop signs and symptoms suggestive of blood dyscrasias or infection (e.g., persistent fever, bruising, bleeding, pallor) while on CIMZIA. Consider discontinuation of CIMZIA therapy in patients with confirmed significant hematologic abnormalities.

5.8 Use with Biological Disease-Modifying Antirheumatic Drugs (Biological DMARDs)

Serious infections were seen in clinical studies with concurrent use of anakinra (an interleukin-1 antagonist) and another TNF blocker, etanercept, with no added benefit compared to entanercept alone. A higher risk of serious infections was also observed in combination use of TNF blockers with abatacept and rituximab. Because of the nature of the adverse events seen with this combination therapy, similar toxicities may also result from the use of CIMZIA in this combination. Therefore, the use of CIMZIA in combination with other biological DMARDs is not recommended *[see Drug Interactions (7.1)]*.

5.9 Autoimmunity

Treatment with CIMZIA may result in the formation of autoantibodies and rarely, in the development of a lupus-like syndrome. If a patient develops symptoms suggestive of a lupus-like syndrome following treatment with CIMZIA, discontinue treatment *[see Adverse Reactions (6.1)]*.

5.10 Immunizations

No data are available on the response to vaccinations or the secondary transmission of infection by live vaccines in patients receiving CIMZIA. Do not administer live vaccines or attenuated vaccines concurrently with CIMZIA.

5.11 Immunosuppression

Since TNF mediates inflammation and modulates cellular immune responses, the possibility exists for TNF blockers, including CIMZIA, to affect host defenses against infections and malignancies. The impact of treatment with CIMZIA on the development and course of malignancies, as well as active and/or chronic infections, is not fully understood *[see Warnings and Precautions (5.1, 5.2, 5.5) and Adverse Reactions (6.1)]*. The safety and efficacy of CIMZIA in patients with immunosuppression has not been formally evaluated.

6 ADVERSE REACTIONS

6.1 Clinical Trials Experience

The most serious adverse reactions were:

- Serious Infections *[see Warnings and Precautions (5.1)]*
- Malignancies *[see Warnings and Precautions (5.2)]*
- Heart Failure *[see Warnings and Precautions (5.3)]*

In premarketing controlled trials of all patient populations combined the most common adverse reactions (≥ 8%) were upper respiratory infections (18%), rash (9%) and urinary tract infections (8%).

Adverse Reactions Most Commonly Leading to Discontinuation of Treatment in Premarketing Controlled Trials

The proportion of patients with Crohn's disease who discontinued treatment due to adverse reactions in the controlled clinical studies was 8% for CIMZIA and 7% for placebo. The most common adverse reactions leading to the discontinuation of CIMZIA (for at least 2 patients and with a higher incidence than placebo) were abdominal pain (0.4% CIMZIA, 0.2% placebo), diarrhea (0.4% CIMZIA, 0% placebo), and intestinal obstruction (0.4% CIMZIA, 0% placebo).

The proportion of patients with rheumatoid arthritis who discontinued treatment due to adverse reactions in the controlled clinical studies was 5% for CIMZIA and 2.5% for placebo. The most common adverse reactions leading to discontinuation of CIMZIA were tuberculosis infections (0.5%); and pyrexia, urticaria, pneumonia, and rash (0.3%).

Because clinical studies are conducted under widely varying and controlled conditions, adverse reaction rates observed in clinical studies of a drug cannot be directly compared to rates in the clinical studies of another drug, and may not predict the rates observed in a broader patient population in clinical practice.

Controlled Studies with Crohn's Disease

The data described below reflect exposure to CIMZIA at 400 mg subcutaneous dosing in studies of patients with Crohn's disease. In the safety population in controlled studies, a total of 620 patients with Crohn's disease received CIMZIA at a dose of 400 mg, and 614 subjects received placebo (including subjects randomized to placebo in Study CD2 following open label dosing of CIMZIA at Weeks 0, 2, 4). In controlled and uncontrolled studies, 1,564 patients received CIMZIA at some dose level, of whom 1,350 patients received 400 mg CIMZIA. Approximately 55% of subjects were female, 45% were male, and 94% were Caucasian. The majority of patients in the active group were between the ages of 18 and 64.

During controlled clinical studies, the proportion of patients with serious adverse reactions was 10% for CIMZIA and 9% for placebo. The most common adverse reactions (occurring in ≥ 5% of CIMZIA-treated patients, and with a higher incidence compared to placebo) in controlled clinical studies with CIMZIA were upper respiratory infections (e.g. nasopharyngitis, laryngitis, viral infection) in 20% of CIMZIA-treated patients and 13% of placebo-treated patients, urinary tract infections (e.g. bladder infection, bacteriuria, cystitis) in 7% of CIMZIA-treated patients and in 6% of placebo-treated patients, and arthralgia (6% CIMZIA, 4% placebo).

Other Adverse Reactions

The most commonly occurring adverse reactions in controlled trials of Crohn's disease were described above. Other serious or significant adverse reactions reported in controlled and uncontrolled studies in Crohn's disease and other diseases, occurring in patients receiving CIMZIA at doses of 400 mg or other doses include:

Blood and lymphatic system disorders: Anemia, leukopenia, lymphadenopathy, pancytopenia, and thrombophilia.

Cardiac disorders: Angina pectoris, arrhythmias, atrial fibrillation, cardiac failure, hypertensive heart disease, myocardial infarction, myocardial ischemia, pericardial effusion, pericarditis, stroke and transient ischemic attack.

Eye disorders: Optic neuritis, retinal hemorrhage, and uveitis.

General disorders and administration site conditions: Bleeding and injection site reactions.

Hepatobiliary disorders: Elevated liver enzymes and hepatitis.

Immune system disorders: Alopecia totalis.

Psychiatric disorders: Anxiety, bipolar disorder, and suicide attempt.

Renal and urinary disorders: Nephrotic syndrome and renal failure.

Reproductive system and breast disorders: Menstrual disorder.

Skin and subcutaneous tissue disorders: Dermatitis, erythema nodosum, and urticaria.

Vascular disorders: Thrombophlebitis, vasculitis.

Controlled Studies with Rheumatoid Arthritis

CIMZIA was studied primarily in placebo-controlled trials and in long-term follow-up studies. The data described below reflect the exposure to CIMZIA in 2,367 RA patients, including 2,030 exposed for at least 6 months, 1,663 exposed for at least one year and 282 for at least 2 years; and 1,774 in adequate and well-controlled studies. In placebo-controlled studies, the population had a median age of 53 years at entry; approximately 80% were females, 93% were Caucasian and all patients were suffering from active rheumatoid arthritis, with a median disease duration of 6.2 years. Most patients received the recommended dose of CIMZIA or higher.

Table 1 summarizes the reactions reported at a rate of at least 3% in patients treated with CIMZIA 200 mg every other week compared to placebo (saline formulation), given concomitantly with methotrexate.

Table 1: Adverse Reactions Reported by ≥3% of Patients Treated with CIMZIA Dosed Every Other Week during Placebo-Controlled Period of Rheumatoid Arthritis Studies, with Concomitant Methotrexate.

Adverse Reaction (Preferred Term)	Placebo + MTX# (%) N =324	CIMZIA 200 mg EOW + MTX (%) N =640
Upper respiratory tract infection	2	6
Headache	4	5
Hypertension	2	5
Nasopharyngitis	1	5
Back pain	1	4
Pyrexia	2	3
Pharyngitis	1	3
Rash	1	3
Acute bronchitis	1	3
Fatigue	2	3

EOW = Every other Week, MTX = Methotrexate.

Hypertensive adverse reactions were observed more frequently in patients receiving CIMZIA than in controls. These adverse reactions occurred more frequently among patients with a baseline history of hypertension and among patients receiving concomitant corticosteroids and non-steroidal anti-inflammatory drugs.

Patients receiving CIMZIA 400 mg as monotherapy every 4 weeks in rheumatoid arthritis controlled clinical trials had similar adverse reactions to those patients receiving CIMZIA 200 mg every other week.

Other Adverse Reactions

Other infrequent adverse reactions (occurring in less than 3% of RA patients) were similar to those seen in Crohn's disease patients.

Infections

The incidence of infections in controlled studies in Crohn's disease was 38% for CIMZIA-treated patients and 30% for placebo-treated patients. The infections consisted primarily of upper respiratory infections (20% for CIMZIA, 13% for placebo). The incidence of serious infections during the controlled clinical studies was 3% per patient-year for CIMZIA-treated patients and 1% for placebo-treated patients. Serious infections observed included bacterial and viral infections, pneumonia, and pyelonephritis.

The incidence of new cases of infections in controlled clinical studies in rheumatoid arthritis was 0.91 per patient-year for all CIMZIA-treated patients and 0.72 per patient-year for placebo-treated patients. The infections consisted primarily of upper respiratory tract infections, herpes infections, urinary tract infections, and lower respiratory tract infections. In the controlled rheumatoid arthritis studies, there were more new cases of serious infection adverse reactions in the CIMZIA treatment groups, compared to the placebo groups (0.06 per patient-year for all CIMZIA doses vs. 0.02 per patient-year for placebo). Rates of serious infections in the 200 mg every other week dose group were 0.06 per patient-year and in the 400 mg every 4 weeks dose group were 0.04 per patient-year. Serious infections included tuberculosis, pneumonia, cellulitis, and pyelonephritis. In the placebo group, no serious infection occurred in more than one subject. There is no evidence of increased risk of infections with continued exposure over time *[see Warnings and Precautions (5.1)]*.

Tuberculosis and Opportunistic Infections
In completed and ongoing global clinical studies in all indications including 5,118 CIMZIA-treated patients, the overall rate of tuberculosis is approximately 0.61 per 100 patient-years across all indications.
The majority of cases occurred in countries with high endemic rates of TB. No cases of TB (0/980) have been reported in the US or Canada across all indications. Reports include cases of miliary, lymphatic, peritoneal, as well as pulmonary TB. The median time to onset of TB for all patients exposed to CIMZIA across all indications was 345 days. In the studies with CIMZIA in RA, there were 36 cases of TB among 2,367 exposed patients, including some fatal cases. Rare cases of opportunistic infections have also been reported in these clinical trials. *[see Warnings and Precautions (5.1)].*
Malignancies
In clinical studies of CIMZIA, the overall incidence rate of malignancies was similar for CIMZIA-treated and control patients. For some TNF blockers, more cases of malignancies have been observed among patients receiving those TNF blockers compared to control patients. *[see Warnings and Precautions (5.2)]*
Heart Failure
In placebo-controlled and open-label rheumatoid arthritis studies, cases of new or worsening heart failure have been reported for CIMZIA-treated patients. The majority of these cases were mild to moderate and occurred during the first year of exposure. *[see Warnings and Precautions (5.3)].*
Autoantibodies
In clinical studies in Crohn's disease, 4% of patients treated with CIMZIA and 2% of patients treated with placebo that had negative baseline ANA titers developed positive titers during the studies. One of the 1,564 Crohn's disease patients treated with CIMZIA developed symptoms of a lupus-like syndrome.
In clinical trials of TNF blockers, including CIMZIA, in patients with RA, some patients have developed ANA. Four patients out of 2,367 patients treated with CIMZIA in RA clinical studies developed clinical signs suggestive of a lupus-like syndrome. The impact of long-term treatment with CIMZIA on the development of autoimmune diseases is unknown *[see Warnings and Precautions (5.9)].*
Immunogenicity
Patients were tested at multiple time points for antibodies to certolizumab pegol during Studies CD1 and CD2. The overall percentage of antibody positive patients was 8% in patients continuously exposed to CIMZIA, approximately 6% were neutralizing *in vitro*. No apparent correlation of antibody development to adverse events or efficacy was observed. Patients treated with concomitant immunosuppressants had a lower rate of antibody development than patients not taking immunosuppressants at baseline (3% and 11%, respectively). The following adverse events were reported in Crohn's disease patients who were antibody-positive (N = 100) at an incidence at least 3% higher compared to antibody-negative patients (N = 1,242): abdominal pain, arthralgia, edema peripheral, erythema nodosum, injection site erythema, injection site pain, pain in extremity, and upper respiratory tract infection.
The overall percentage of patients with antibodies to certolizumab pegol detectable on at least one occasion was 7% (105 of 1,509) in the rheumatoid arthritis placebo-controlled trials. Approximately one third (3%, 39 of 1,509) of these patients had antibodies with neutralizing activity *in vitro*. Patients treated with concomitant immunosuppressants (MTX) had a lower rate of antibody development than patients not taking immunosuppressants at baseline. Patients treated with concomitant immunosuppressant therapy (MTX) in RA-I, RA-II, RA-III had a lower rate of neutralizing antibody formation overall than patients treated with CIMZIA monotherapy in RA-IV (2% vs. 8%). Both the loading dose of 400 mg every other week at Weeks 0, 2 and 4 and concomitant use of MTX were associated with reduced immunogenicity.
Antibody formation was associated with lowered drug plasma concentration and reduced efficacy. In patients receiving the recommended CIMZIA dosage of 200 mg every other week with concomitant MTX, the ACR20 response was lower among antibody positive patients than among antibody-negative patients (Study RA-I, 48% versus 60%; Study RA-II 35% versus 59%, respectively). In Study RA-III, too few patients developed antibodies to allow for meaningful analysis of ACR20 response by antibody status. In Study RA-IV (monotherapy), the ACR20 response was 33% versus 56%, antibody-positive versus antibody-negative status, respectively. *[see Clinical Pharmacology (12.3)].* No association was seen between antibody development and the development of adverse events.
The data reflect the percentage of patients whose test results were considered positive for antibodies to certolizumab pegol in an ELISA, and are highly dependent on the sensitivity and specificity of the assay. The observed incidence of antibody (including neutralizing antibody) positivity in an assay is highly dependent on several factors, including assay sensitivity and specificity, assay methodology, sample handling, timing of sample collection, concomitant medications, and underlying disease. For these reasons, comparison of the incidence of antibodies to certolizumab pegol with the incidence of antibodies to other products may be misleading.
Hypersensitivity Reactions
The following symptoms that could be compatible with hypersensitivity reactions have been reported rarely following CIMZIA administration to patients: angioedema, dermatitis allergic, dizziness (postural), dyspnea, hot flush, hypotension, injection site reactions, malaise, pyrexia, rash, serum sickness, and (vasovagal) syncope *[see Warnings and Precautions (5.4)].*

6.2 Adverse Reaction Information from Other Sources
Because these reactions are reported voluntarily from a population of uncertain size, it is not always possible to estimate reliably their frequency or establish a causal relationship to drug exposure.
Skin: case of severe skin reactions, including Stevens-Johnson syndrome, toxic epidermal necrolysis, erythema multiforme, and new or worsening psoriasis (all sub-types including pustular and palmoplantar) have been identified during post-approval use of TNF blockers.

7 DRUG INTERACTIONS

7.1 Use with Anakinra, Abatacept, Rituximab, and Natalizumab
An increased risk of serious infections has been seen in clinical studies of other TNF-blocking agents used in combination with anakinra or abatacept, with no added benefit. Formal drug interaction studies have not been performed with rituximab or natalizumab. Because of the nature of the adverse events seen with these combinations with TNF blocker therapy, similar toxicities may also result from the use of CIMZIA in these combinations. There is not enough information to assess the safety and efficacy of such combination therapy. Therefore, the use of CIMZIA in combination with anakinra, abatacept, rituximab, or natalizumab is not recommended *[see Warnings and Precautions (5.8)].*

7.2 Live Vaccines
Do not give live (including attenuated) vaccines concurrently with CIMZIA *[see Warnings and Precautions (5.10)].*

7.3 Laboratory Tests
Interference with certain coagulation assays has been detected in patients treated with CIMZIA. Certolizumab pegol may cause erroneously elevated activated partial thromboplastin time (aPTT) assay results in patients without coagulation abnormalities. This effect has been observed with the PTT-Lupus Anticoagulant (LA) test and Standard Target Activated Partial Thromboplastin time (STA-PTT) Automate tests from Diagnostica Stago, and the HemosIL APTT-SP liquid and HemosIL lyophilized silica tests from Instrumentation Laboratories. Other aPTT assays may be affected as well. Interference with thrombin time (TT) and prothrombin time (PT) assays has not been observed. There is no evidence that CIMZIA therapy has an effect on *in vivo* coagulation.

8 USE IN SPECIFIC POPULATIONS

8.1 Pregnancy
Pregnancy Category B – Because certolizumab pegol does not cross-react with mouse or rat TNFα, reproduction studies were performed in rats using a rodent anti-murine TNFα pegylated Fab′ fragment (cTN3 PF) similar to certolizumab pegol. Reproduction studies have been performed in rats at doses up to 100 mg/kg and have revealed no evidence of impaired fertility or harm to the fetus due to cTN3 PF. There are, however, no adequate and well-controlled studies of CIMZIA in pregnant women. Because animal reproduction studies are not always predictive of human response, this drug should be used during pregnancy only if clearly needed.

8.3 Nursing Mothers
It is not known whether this drug is excreted in human milk. Because many drugs are excreted in human milk and because of the potential for serious adverse reactions in nursing infants from CIMZIA, a decision should be made whether to discontinue nursing or discontinue the drug, taking into account the importance of the drug to the mother.

8.4 Pediatric Use
Safety and effectiveness in pediatric patients have not been established.

8.5 Geriatric Use
Clinical studies of CIMZIA did not include sufficient numbers of patients aged 65 and over to determine whether they respond differently from younger subjects. Other reported clinical experience has not identified differences in responses between the elderly and younger patients. Population pharmacokinetic analyses of patients enrolled in CIMZIA clinical studies concluded that there was no apparent difference in drug concentration regardless of age. Because there is a higher incidence of infections in the elderly population in general, use caution when treating the elderly with CIMZIA *[see Warnings and Precautions (5.1)].*

10 OVERDOSAGE

The maximum tolerated dose of certolizumab pegol has not been established. Doses of up to 800 mg subcutaneous and 20 mg/kg intravenous have been administered without evidence of dose-limiting toxicities. In cases of overdosage, it is recommended that patients be monitored closely for any adverse reactions or effects, and appropriate symptomatic treatment instituted immediately.

11 DESCRIPTION

CIMZIA (certolizumab pegol) is a TNF blocker. CIMZIA is a recombinant, humanized antibody Fab′ fragment, with specificity for human tumor necrosis factor alpha (TNFα), conjugated to an approximately 40kDa polyethylene glycol (PEG2MAL40K). The Fab′ fragment is manufactured in *E. coli* and is subsequently subjected to purification and conjugation to PEG2MAL40K, to generate certolizumab pegol. The Fab′ fragment is composed of a light chain with 214 amino acids and a heavy chain with 229 amino acids. The molecular weight of certolizumab pegol is approximately 91 kiloDaltons.
CIMZIA is supplied as either a sterile, white, lyophilized powder for solution or as a sterile, solution in a single-use prefilled 1 mL glass syringe for subcutaneous injection. After reconstitution of the lyophilized powder with 1 mL sterile Water for Injection, USP, the resulting pH is approximately 5.2. Each single-use vial provides approximately 200 mg certolizumab pegol, 100 mg sucrose, 0.9 mg lactic acid, and 0.1 mg polysorbate.
Each prefilled syringe delivers 1 mL (200 mg) of drug product with a pH of approximately 4.7. Each 1 mL syringe of CIMZIA contains 200 mg of certolizumab pegol, 1.36 mg of sodium acetate, 7.31 mg sodium chloride, and Water for Injection, USP.
CIMZIA is a clear to opalescent solution that is colorless to pale yellow and essentially free from particulates. No preservatives are present.

12 CLINICAL PHARMACOLOGY

12.1 Mechanism of Action
Certolizumab pegol binds to human TNFα with a KD of 90pM. TNFα is a key pro-inflammatory cytokine with a central role in inflammatory processes. Certolizumab pegol selectively neutralizes TNFα (IC_{90} of 4 ng/mL for inhibition of human TNFα in the *in vitro* L929 murine fibrosarcoma cytotoxicity assay) but does not neutralize lymphotoxin α (TNFβ). Certolizumab pegol cross-reacts poorly with TNF from rodents and rabbits, therefore *in vivo* efficacy was evaluated using animal models in which human TNFα was the physiologically active molecule.
Certolizumab pegol was shown to neutralize membrane-associated and soluble human TNFα in a dose-dependent manner. Incubation of monocytes with certolizumab pegol resulted in a dose-dependent inhibition of LPS-induced TNFα and IL-1β production in human monocytes.
Certolizumab pegol does not contain a fragment crystallizable (Fc) region, which is normally present in a complete antibody, and therefore does not fix complement or cause antibody-dependent cell-mediated cytotoxicity *in vitro*. It does not induce apoptosis *in vitro* in human peripheral blood-derived monocytes or lymphocytes, nor does certolizumab pegol induce neutrophil degranulation.
A tissue reactivity study was carried out *ex vivo* to evaluate potential cross-reactivity of certolizumab pegol with cryosections of normal human tissues. Certolizumab pegol showed no reactivity with a designated standard panel of normal human tissues.

12.2 Pharmacodynamics
Biological activities ascribed to TNFα include the upregulation of cellular adhesion molecules and chemokines, upregulation of major histocompatibility complex (MHC) class I and class II molecules, and direct leukocyte activation. TNFα stimulates the production of downstream inflammatory mediators, including interleukin-1, prostaglandins, platelet activating factor, and nitric oxide. Elevated levels of TNFα have been implicated in the pathology of Crohn's disease and rheumatoid arthritis. Certolizumab pegol binds to TNFα, inhibiting its role as a key mediator of inflammation. TNFα is strongly expressed in the bowel wall in areas involved by Crohn's disease and fecal concentrations of TNFα in patients with Crohn's disease have been shown to reflect clinical severity of the disease. After treatment with certolizumab pegol, patients with Crohn's disease demonstrated a decrease in the levels of C-reactive protein (CRP). Increased TNFα levels are found in the synovial fluid of rheumatoid arthritis patients and play an important role in the joint destruction that is a hallmark of this disease.

12.3 Pharmacokinetics
- **Absorption**

A total of 126 healthy subjects received doses of up to 800 mg certolizumab pegol subcutaneously (sc) and up to

Table 2 Study CD1 – Clinical Response and Remission, Overall Study Population

Timepoint	% Response or Remission (95% CI)	
	Placebo (N = 328)	CIMZIA 400 mg (N = 331)
Week 6		
Clinical Response#	27% (22%, 32%)	35% (30%, 40%)*
Clinical Remission#	17% (13%, 22%)	22% (17%, 26%)
Week 26		
Clinical Response	27% (22%, 31%)	37% (32%, 42%)*
Clinical Remission	18% (14%, 22%)	29% (25%, 34%)*
Both Weeks 6 & 26		
Clinical Response	16% (12%, 20%)	23% (18%, 28%)*
Clinical Remission	10% (7%, 13%)	14% (11%, 18%)

* p-value < 0.05 logistic regression test
\# Clinical response is defined as decrease in CDAI of at least 100 points, and clinical remission is defined as CDAI ≤ 150 points

Table 3 Study CD2 - Clinical Response and Clinical Remission

	% Response or Remission (95% CI)	
	CIMZIA 400 mg ×3 + Placebo N = 210	CIMZIA 400 mg N = 215
Week 26		
Clinical Response#	36% (30%, 43%)	63% (56%, 69%)*
Clinical Remission#	29% (22%, 35%)	48% (41%, 55%)*

* p < 0.05
\# Clinical response is defined as decrease in CDAI of at least 100 points, and clinical remission is defined as CDAI ≤ 150 points

10 mg/kg intravenously (IV) in four pharmacokinetic studies. Data from these studies demonstrate that single intravenous and subcutaneous doses of certolizumab pegol have predictable dose-related plasma concentrations with a linear relationship between the dose administered and the maximum plasma concentration (C_{max}), and the Area Under the certolizumab pegol plasma concentration versus time Curve (AUC). A mean C_{max} of approximately 43 to 49 mcg/mL occurred at Week 5 during the initial loading dose period using the recommended dose regimen for the treatment of patients with rheumatoid arthritis (400 mg sc at Weeks 0, 2 and 4 followed by 200 mg every other week). Certolizumab pegol plasma concentrations were broadly dose-proportional and pharmacokinetics observed in patients with rheumatoid arthritis and Crohn's disease were consistent with those seen in healthy subjects.

Following subcutaneous administration, peak plasma concentrations of certolizumab pegol were attained between 54 and 171 hours post-injection. Certolizumab pegol has bioavailability (F) of approximately 80% (ranging from 76% to 88%) following subcutaneous administration compared to intravenous administration.

• **Distribution**
The steady state volume of distribution (Vss) was estimated as 6 to 8 L in the population pharmacokinetic analysis for patients with Crohn's disease and patients with rheumatoid arthritis.

• **Metabolism**
The metabolism of certolizumab pegol has not been studied in human subjects. Data from animals indicate that once cleaved from the Fab′ fragment the PEG moiety is mainly excreted in urine without further metabolism.

• **Elimination**
PEGylation, the covalent attachment of PEG polymers to peptides, delays the metabolism and elimination of these entities from the circulation by a variety of mechanisms, including decreased renal clearance, proteolysis, and immunogenicity. Accordingly, certolizumab pegol is an antibody Fab′ fragment conjugated with PEG in order to extend the terminal plasma elimination half-life ($t_{1/2}$) of the Fab′. The terminal elimination phase half-life ($t_{1/2}$) was approximately 14 days for all doses tested. The clearance following IV administration to healthy subjects ranged from 9.21 mL/h to 14.38 mL/h. The clearance following sc dosing was estimated 17 mL/h in the Crohn's disease population PK analysis with an inter-subject variability of 38% (CV) and an inter-occasion variability of 16%. Similarly, the clearance following sc dosing was estimated as 21.0 mL/h in the RA population PK analysis, with an inter-subject variability of 30.8% (%CV) and inter-occasion variability 22.0%. The route of elimination of certolizumab pegol has not been studied in human subjects. Studies in animals indicate that the major route of elimination of the PEG component is via urinary excretion.

• **Special Populations**
Population pharmacokinetic analysis was conducted on data from patients with rheumatoid arthritis and patients with Crohn's disease, to evaluate the effect of age, race, gender, methotrexate use, concomitant medication, creatinine clearance and presence of anti-certolizumab antibodies on pharmacokinetics of certolizumab pegol.

Only bodyweight and presence of anti-certolizumab antibodies significantly affected certolizumab pegol pharmacokinetics. Pharmacokinetic exposure was inversely related to body weight but pharmacodynamic exposure-response analysis showed that no additional therapeutic benefit would be expected from a weight-adjusted dose regimen. The presence of anti-certolizumab antibodies was associated with a 3.6-fold increase in clearance.

Age: Pharmacokinetics of certolizumab pegol was not different in elderly compared to young adults.
Gender: Pharmacokinetics of certolizumab pegol was similar in male and female subjects.
Renal Impairment: Specific clinical studies have not been performed to assess the effect of renal impairment on the pharmacokinetics of CIMZIA. The pharmacokinetics of the PEG (polyethylene glycol) fraction of certolizumab pegol is expected to be dependent on renal function but has not been assessed in renal impairment. There are insufficient data to provide a dosing recommendation in moderate and severe renal impairment.
Race: A specific clinical study showed no difference in pharmacokinetics between Caucasian and Japanese subjects.

• **Drug Interaction Studies**
Methotrexate pharmacokinetics is not altered by concomitant administration with CIMZIA in patients with rheumatoid arthritis. The effect of methotrexate on CIMZIA pharmacokinetics was not studied. However, methotrexate-treated patients have lower incidence of antibodies to CIMZIA. Thus, therapeutic plasma levels are more likely to be sustained when CIMZIA is administered with methotrexate in patients with rheumatoid arthritis.

Formal drug-drug interaction studies have not been conducted with CIMZIA upon concomitant administration with corticosteroids, nonsteroidal anti-inflammatory drugs, analgesics or immunosupressants.

13 NONCLINICAL TOXICOLOGY
13.1 Carcinogenesis, Mutagenesis, and Impairment of Fertility
Long-term animal studies of CIMZIA have not been conducted to assess its carcinogenic potential. Certolizumab pegol was not genotoxic in the Ames test, the human peripheral blood lymphocytes chromosomal aberration assay, or the mouse bone marrow micronucleus assay.

Since certolizumab pegol does not cross-react with mouse or rat TNFα, reproduction studies were performed in rats using a rodent anti-murine TNFα pegylated Fab fragment (cTN3 PF), similar to certolizumab pegol. The cTN3 PF had no effects on the fertility and general reproductive performance of male and female rats at intravenous doses up 100 mg/kg, administered twice weekly.

14 CLINICAL STUDIES
14.1 Crohn's Disease
The efficacy and safety of CIMZIA were assessed in two double-blind, randomized, placebo-controlled studies in patients aged 18 years and older with moderately to severely active Crohn's disease, as defined by a Crohn's Disease Activity Index (CDAI[1]) of 220 to 450 points, inclusive. CIMZIA was administered subcutaneously at a dose of 400 mg in both studies. Stable concomitant medications for Crohn's disease were permitted.

Study CD1
Study CD1 was a randomized placebo-controlled study in 662 patients with active Crohn's disease. CIMZIA or placebo was administered at Weeks 0, 2, and 4 and then every four weeks to Week 24. Assessments were done at Weeks 6 and 26. Clinical response was defined as at least a 100-point reduction in CDAI score compared to baseline, and clinical remission was defined as an absolute CDAI score of 150 points or lower.

The results for Study CD1 are provided in Table 2. At Week 6, the proportion of clinical responders was statistically significantly greater for CIMZIA-treated patients compared to controls. The difference in clinical remission rates was not statistically significant at Week 6. The difference in the proportion of patients who were in clinical response at both Weeks 6 and 26 was also statistically significant, demonstrating maintenance of clinical response.
[See table 2 above]

Study CD2
Study CD2 was a randomized treatment-withdrawal study in patients with active Crohn's disease. All patients who entered the study were dosed initially with CIMZIA 400 mg at Weeks 0, 2, and 4 and then assessed for clinical response at Week 6 (as defined by at least a 100-point reduction in CDAI score). At Week 6, a group of 428 clinical responders was randomized to receive either CIMZIA 400 mg or placebo, every four weeks starting at Week 8, as maintenance therapy through Week 24. Non-responders at Week 6 were withdrawn from the study. Final evaluation was based on the CDAI score at Week 26. Patients who withdrew or who received rescue therapy were considered not to be in clinical response. Three randomized responders received no study injections, and were excluded from the ITT analysis.

The results for clinical response and remission are shown in Table 3. At Week 26, a statistically significantly greater proportion of Week 6 responders were in clinical response and in clinical remission in the CIMZIA-treated group compared to the group treated with placebo.
[See table 3 above]

Baseline use of immunosuppressants or corticosteroids had no impact on the clinical response to CIMZIA.

14.2 Rheumatoid Arthritis
The efficacy and safety of CIMZIA were assessed in four randomized, placebo-controlled, double-blind studies (RA-I, RA-II, RA-III, and RA-IV) in patients ≥ 18 years of age with moderately to severely active rheumatoid arthritis diagnosed according to the American College of Rheumatology (ACR) criteria. Patients had ≥ 9 swollen and tender joints and had active RA for at least 6 months prior to baseline. CIMZIA was administered subcutaneously in combination with MTX at stable doses of at least 10 mg weekly in Studies RA-I, RA-II, and RA-III. CIMZIA was administered as monotherapy in Study RA-IV.

Study RA-I and Study RA-II evaluated patients who had received MTX for at least 6 months prior to study medication, but had an incomplete response to MTX alone. Patients were treated with a loading dose of 400 mg at Weeks 0, 2 and 4 (for both treatment arms) or placebo followed by either 200 mg or 400 mg of CIMZIA or placebo every other week, in combination with MTX for 52 weeks in Study RA-I and for 24 weeks in Study RA-II. Patients were evaluated for signs and symptoms and structural damage using the ACR20 response at Week 24 (RA-I and RA-II) and modified

Table 4: ACR Responses in Studies RA-I, and RA-IV (Percent of Patients)

Response	Study RA-I Methotrexate Combination (24 and 52 weeks)			Study RA-IV Monotherapy (24 weeks)		
	Placebo + MTX N=199	CIMZIA* 200 mg + MTX q 2 weeks N=393	CIMZIA* 200 mg + MTX - Placebo + MTX (95% CI)‡	Placebo N=109	CIMZIA† 400 mg q 4 weeks N=111	CIMZIA† 400 mg - Placebo (95% CI)‡
ACR20						
Week 24	14%	59%	45% (38%, 52%)	9%	46%	36% (25%, 47%)
Week 52	13%	53%	40% (33%, 47%)	NA	NA	
ACR50						
Week 24	8%	37%	30% (24%, 36%)	4%	23%	19% (10%, 28%)
Week 52	8%	38%	30% (24%, 37%)	NA	NA	
ACR70						
Week 24	3%	21%	18% (14%, 23%)	0%	6%	6% (1%, 10%)
Week 52	4%	21%	18% (13%, 22%)	NA	NA	
Major Clinical Response§	1%	13%	12% (8%, 15%)			

* CIMZIA administered every 2 weeks preceded by a loading dose of 400 mg at Weeks 0, 2 and 4
† CIMZIA administered every 4 weeks not preceded by a loading dose regimen
‡ 95% Confidence Intervals constructed using the large sample approximation to the Normal Distribution.
§ Major clinical response is defined as achieving ACR70 response over a continuous 6-month period

Table 5: Components of ACR Response in Studies RA-I and RA-IV

Parameter*	Study RA-I				Study RA-IV			
	Placebo + MTX N=199		CIMZIA† 200 mg + MTX q 2 weeks N=393		Placebo + MTX N=109		CIMZIA‡ 400 mg q 4 weeks Monotheraphy N=111	
	Baseline	Week 24	Baseline	Week 24	Baseline	Week 24	Baseline	Week 24
Number of tender joints (0-68)	28	27	29	9	28 (12.5)	24 (15.4)	30 (13.7)	16 (15.8)
Number of swollen joints (0-66)	20	19	20	4	20 (9.3)	16 (12.5)	21 (10.1)	12 (11.2)
Physician global assessment§	66	56	65	25	4 (0.6)	3 (1.0)	4 (0.7)	3 (1.1)
Patient global assessment§	67	60	64	32	3 (0.8)	3 (1.0)	3 (0.8)	3 (1.0)
Pain§¶	65	60	65	32	55 (20.8)	60 (26.7)	58 (21.9)	39 (29.6)
Disability index (HAQ)#	1.75	1.63	1.75	1.00	1.55 (0.65)	1.62 (0.68)	1.43 (0.63)	1.04 (0.74)
CRP (mg/L)	16.0	14.0	16.0	4.0	11.3	13.5	11.6	6.4

* For Study RA-I, median is presented. For Study RA-IV, mean (SD) is presented except for CRP which presents geometric mean
† CIMZIA administered every 2 weeks preceded by a loading dose of 400 mg at Weeks 0, 2 and 4
‡ CIMZIA administered every 4 weeks not preceded by a loading dose regimen
§ Study RA-I - Visual Analog Scale: 0 = best, 100 = worst. Study RA-IV - Five Point Scale: 1 = best, 5 = worst
¶ Patient Assessment of Arthritis Pain. Visual Analog Scale: 0=best, 100=worst
# Health Assessment Questionnaire Disability Index; 0 = best, 3 = worst, measures the patient's ability to perform the following: dress/groom, arise, eat, walk, reach, grip, maintain hygiene, and maintain daily activity
All values are last observation carried forward.

Total Sharp Score (mTSS) at Week 52 (RA-I). The open-label extension follow-up study enrolled 846 patients who received 400 mg of CIMZIA every other week.
Study RA-III evaluated 247 patients who had active disease despite receiving MTX for at least 6 months prior to study enrollment. Patients received 400 mg of CIMZIA every four weeks for 24 weeks without a prior loading dose. Patients were evaluated for signs and symptoms of RA using the ACR20 at Week 24.
Study RA-IV (monotherapy) evaluated 220 patients who had failed at least one DMARD use prior to receiving CIMZIA. Patients were treated with CIMZIA 400 mg or placebo every 4 weeks for 24 weeks. Patients were evaluated for signs and symptoms of active RA using the ACR20 at Week 24.

Clinical Response
The percent of CIMZIA-treated patients achieving ACR20, 50, and 70 responses in Studies RA-I and RA-IV are shown in Table 4. CIMZIA-treated patients had higher ACR20, 50 and 70 response rates at 6 months compared to placebo-treated patients. The results in study RA-II (619 patients) were similar to the results in RA-I at Week 24. The results in study RA-III (247 patients) were similar to those seen in study RA-IV. Over the one-year Study RA-I, 13% of CIMZIA-treated patients achieved a major clinical response, defined as achieving an ACR70 response over a continuous 6-month period, compared to 1% of placebo-treated patients.
[See table 4 above]
[See table 5 above]
The percent of patients achieving ACR20 responses by visit for Study RA-I is shown in Figure 1. Among patients receiving CIMZIA, clinical responses were seen in some patients within one to two weeks after initiation of therapy.

[See figure 1 at top of next column]
Radiographic Response
In Study RA-I, inhibition of progression of structural damage was assessed radiographically and expressed as the change in modified Total Sharp Score (mTSS) and its components, the Erosion Score (ES) and Joint Space Narrowing (JSN) score, at Week 52, compared to baseline. CIMZIA inhibited the progression of structural damage compared to placebo plus MTX after 12 months of treatment as shown in Table 6. In the placebo group, 52% of patients experienced no radiographic progression (mTSS ≤0.0) at Week 52 compared to 69% in the CIMZIA 200 mg every other week treatment group. Study RA-II showed similar results at Week 24.

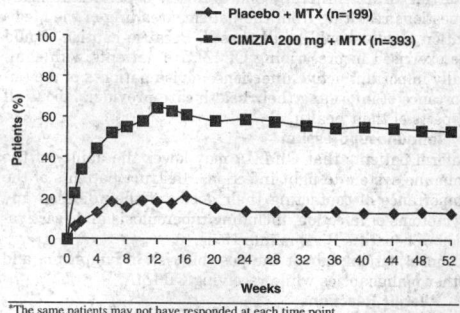

Figure 1 Study RA-I ACR20 Response Over 52 Weeks*

Legend: Placebo + MTX (n=199); CIMZIA 200 mg + MTX (n=393)

*The same patients may not have responded at each time point

Table 6: Radiographic Changes at 6 and 12 months in Study RA-I

	Placebo + MTX N=199 Mean (SD)	CIMZIA 200 mg + MTX N=393 Mean (SD)	CIMZIA 200 mg + MTX – Placebo + MTX Mean Difference
mTSS			
Baseline	40 (45)	38 (49)	—
Week 24	1.3 (3.8)	0.2 (3.2)	-1.1
Week 52	2.8 (7.8)	0.4 (5.7)	-2.4
Erosion Score			
Baseline	14 (21)	15 (24)	—
Week 24	0.7 (2.1)	0.0 (1.5)	-0.7
Week 52	1.5 (4.3)	0.1 (2.5)	-1.4
JSN Score			
Baseline	25 (27)	24 (28)	—
Week 24	0.7 (2.4)	0.2 (2.5)	-0.5
Week 52	1.4 (5.0)	0.4 (4.2)	-1.0

An ANCOVA was fitted to the ranked change from baseline for each measure with region and treatment as factors and rank baseline as a covariate.

Physical Function Response
In studies RA-I, RA-II, RA-III, and RA-IV, CIMZIA-treated patients achieved greater improvements from baseline than placebo-treated patients in physical function as assessed by the Health Assessment Questionnaire – Disability Index (HAQ-DI) at Week 24 (RA-II, RA-III and RA-IV) and at Week 52 (RA-I).

15 REFERENCES
1. Best WR, Becktel JM, Singleton JW, Kern F: Development of a Crohn's Disease Activity Index, National Cooperative Crohn's Disease Study. Gastroenterology 1976; 70(3): 439-444

16 HOW SUPPLIED/STORAGE AND HANDLING
Storage and Stability
Refrigerate intact carton at 2 to 8 °C (36 to 46 °F). Do not freeze. Do not separate contents of carton prior to use. Do not use beyond expiration date, which is located on the drug label and carton. Protect solution from light.
• Lyophilized Powder for Reconstitution:
NDC 50474-700-62

Pack Content

Qty.	Item
2	Type I glass vials with rubber stopper and overseals each containing 200 mg of lyophilized CIMZIA for reconstitution.
2	2 mL Type I glass vials containing 1 mL sterile Water for Injection
2	3 mL plastic syringes
4	20 gauge luer-lock needles (1 inch)
2	23 gauge luer-lock needles (1 inch)
8	Alcohol swabs

• Prefilled Syringe
NDC 50474-710-79
2 alcohol swabs and 2 single use prefilled glass syringes with a fixed 25 ½ gauge thin-wall needle, each containing 200 mg (1 mL) of CIMZIA.

17 PATIENT COUNSELING INFORMATION
See Medication Guide (17.3).
17.1 Patient Counseling
Advise patients of the potential risks and benefits of CIMZIA therapy. Be sure that patients receive the

Medication Guide and allow them time to read it prior to starting CIMZIA therapy and to review it periodically. Any questions resulting from the patient's reading of the Medication Guide should be discussed. Because caution should be exercised in prescribing CIMZIA to patients with clinically important active infections, advise patients of the importance of informing their health care providers about all aspects of their health.

- **Immunosuppression**

Inform patients that CIMZIA may lower the ability of the immune system to fight infections. Instruct patients of the importance of contacting their doctor if they develop any symptoms of infection, including tuberculosis and reactivation of hepatitis B virus infections.

Counsel patients about the possible risk of lymphoma and other malignancies while receiving CIMZIA.

- **Allergic Reactions**

Advise patients to seek immediate medical attention if they experience any symptoms of severe allergic reactions. The prefilled syringe components do not contain any latex or dry natural rubber.

- **Other Medical Conditions**

Advise patients to report any signs of new or worsening medical conditions such as heart disease, neurological disease, or autoimmune disorders. Advise patients to report promptly any symptoms suggestive of a cytopenia such as bruising, bleeding, or persistent fever.

17.2 Instruction on Prefilled Syringe Self-Injection Technique

In the event that the patient or caregiver is giving the CIMZIA injection, they need to be instructed by a qualified healthcare professional in proper injection technique, and their ability to administer CIMZIA subcutaneous injections should be checked to ensure correct administration. Suitable sites for injection include the thigh or abdomen. CIMZIA should be injected when the liquid is at room temperature *[see FDA-approved Medication Guide (17.3)]*

To avoid needle-stick injury, patients and healthcare providers should not attempt to place the needle cover back on the syringe or otherwise recap the needle. Be sure to properly dispose of needles and syringes in a puncture-proof container, and instruct patients and caregivers in proper syringe and needle disposal technique. Actively discourage any reuse of the injection materials.

17.3 Medication Guide

MEDICATION GUIDE
CIMZIA® (CIM-zee-uh)
(certolizumab pegol)

Read the Medication Guide that comes with CIMZIA before you start using it, and before each injection of CIMZIA. This Medication Guide does not take the place of talking with your doctor about your medical condition or treatment.

What is the most important information I should know about CIMZIA?

CIMZIA is a medicine that affects your immune system. CIMZIA can lower the ability of the immune system to fight infections. Serious infections have happened in patients taking CIMZIA. These infections include tuberculosis (TB) and infections caused by viruses, fungi or bacteria that have spread throughout the body. Some patients have died from these infections.

- Your doctor should test you for TB before starting CIMZIA.
- Your doctor should monitor you closely for signs and symptoms of TB during treatment with CIMZIA.

Before starting CIMZIA, tell your doctor if you:

- think you have an infection. You should not start taking CIMZIA if you have any kind of infection.
- are being treated for an infection
- have signs of an infection, such as a fever, cough, flu-like symptoms
- have any open cuts or sores on your body
- get a lot of infections or have infections that keep coming back
- have diabetes
- have HIV
- have tuberculosis (TB), or have been in close contact with someone with TB
- were born in, lived in, or traveled to countries where there is more risk for getting TB. Ask your doctor if you are not sure.
- live or have lived in certain parts of the country (such as the Ohio and Mississippi River valleys) where there is an increased risk for getting certain kinds of fungal infections (histoplasmosis, coccidioidomycosis, blastomycosis). These infections may develop or become more severe if you take CIMZIA. If you do not know if you have lived in an area where histoplasmosis, coccidioidomycosis, or blastomycosis is common, ask your doctor.
- have or have had hepatitis B
- use the medicine Kineret® (anakinra), Orencia® (abatacept), Rituxan® (rituximab), or Tysabri® (natalizumab)

After starting CIMZIA, if you get an infection, any sign of an infection including a fever, cough, flu-like symptoms, or have open cuts or sores on your body, call your doctor right away. CIMZIA can make you more likely to get infections or make any infection that you may have worse.

Certain types of Cancer

- There have been cases of unusual cancers in children and teenage patients using TNF-blocking agents.
- For people taking TNF-blocker medicines, including CIMZIA, the chances of getting lymphoma or other cancers may increase.
- People with RA, especially more serious RA, may have a higher chance for getting a kind of cancer called lymphoma.

See the section "What are the possible side effects of CIMZIA?" for more information.

What is CIMZIA?

CIMZIA is a medicine called a Tumor Necrosis Factor (TNF) blocker. CIMZIA is used in adult patients to:

- Lessen the signs and symptoms of moderately to severely active Crohn's disease (CD) in adults who have not been helped enough by usual treatments.
- Treat moderately to severely active rheumatoid arthritis (RA).

It is not known whether CIMZIA is safe and effective in children.

What should I tell my doctor before starting treatment with CIMZIA?

CIMZIA may not be right for you. Before starting CIMZIA, tell your doctor about all of your medical conditions, including if you:

- **have an infection**. (See, 'What is the most important information I should know about CIMZIA?")
- **have or have had any type of cancer.**
- **have congestive heart failure.**
- **have seizures, any numbness or tingling, or a disease that affects your nervous system such as multiple sclerosis.**
- **are scheduled to receive a vaccine.** Do not receive a live vaccine while taking CIMZIA.
- **are allergic to any of the ingredients in CIMZIA.** See the end of this Medication Guide for a list of the ingredients in CIMZIA.

Tell your doctor if you are pregnant, planning to become pregnant, or breastfeeding. CIMZIA has not been studied in pregnant or nursing women.

Tell your doctor about all the medicines you take including prescription and nonprescription medicines, vitamins and herbal supplements. Your doctor will tell you if it is okay to take your other medicines while taking CIMZIA. Especially, tell your doctor if you take:

- Kineret® (anakinra), Orencia® (abatacept), Rituxan® (rituximab), Tysabri® (natalizumab). You have a higher chance for serious infections when taking CIMZIA with Kineret®, Orencia®, Rituxan®, or Tysabri®.
- A TNF blocker: Remicade® (infliximab), Humira® (adalimumab), Enbrel® (etanercept), Simponi™ (golimumab).

You should not take CIMZIA while you take one of these medicines.

How should I use CIMZIA?

Lyophilized Powder for Reconstitution:

- If your doctor prescribes the CIMZIA lyophilized pack, CIMZIA should be injected by a healthcare provider. Each dose of CIMZIA will be given as two separate injections under the skin in your stomach area (abdomen) or upper leg (thigh).
- Make sure to keep all of your injection and follow-up appointments with your doctor.

Prefilled Syringe:

- If your doctor prescribes the CIMZIA prefilled syringe, see the section **"Patient Instructions for Use"** at the end of the Medication Guide for complete instructions for use.
- Do not give yourself an injection of CIMZIA unless you have been shown by your doctor or nurse. Call your doctor if you have questions. Someone you know can also help you with your injection after they have been trained by your doctor or nurse.
- CIMZIA is given by an injection under the skin. Your doctor will tell you how much CIMZIA to inject and how often to inject CIMZIA, based on your condition to be treated. Do not use more CIMZIA or inject more often than prescribed.
- Depending on the amount of CIMZIA prescribed by your doctor, you may need more than one injection at a time.
- If you are prescribed to take 400 mg of CIMZIA, you will need two injections. You will need to use two CIMZIA prefilled syringes.
- CIMZIA may be injected into your abdomen or thigh area. If you are prescribed to have more than one injection, each injection should be given at a different site in your abdomen or thigh.
- Make sure the solution in the prefilled syringe is clear and colorless to light yellow. The solution should be essentially free from particles. **Do not use the CIMZIA prefilled syringe if the medicine looks cloudy or if there are large or colored particles.**
- Do not miss any doses of CIMZIA. If you forget to take CIMZIA, inject a dose as soon as you remember. Then, take your next dose at your regularly scheduled time.
- Make sure to keep all follow-up appointments with your doctor.

What are the possible side effects of CIMZIA?

CIMZIA can cause serious side effects including:

See "What is the most important information I should know about CIMZIA?"

- **Heart Failure** including new heart failure or worsening of heart failure you already have. Symptoms include shortness of breath, swelling of your ankles or feet, or sudden weight gain.
- **Nervous System Problems** such as multiple sclerosis, seizures, or inflammation of the nerves of the eyes. Symptoms include dizziness, numbness or tingling, problems with your vision, and weakness in your arms or legs.
- **Allergic Reactions.** Signs of an allergic reaction include a skin rash, swelling of the face, tongue, lips, or throat, or trouble breathing.
- **Hepatitis B virus reactivation in patients who carry the virus in their blood.** In some cases patients have died as a result of hepatitis B virus being reactivated. Your doctor should monitor you carefully during treatment with CIMZIA if you carry the hepatitis B virus in your blood. Tell your doctor if you have any of the following symptoms:
  - feel unwell
  - poor appetite
  - tiredness (fatigue)
  - fever, skin rash, or joint pain
- **Blood Problems.** Your body may not make enough of the blood cells that help fight infections or help stop bleeding. Symptoms include a fever that doesn't go away, bruising or bleeding very easily, or looking very pale.
- **Immune reactions including a lupus-like syndrome.** Symptoms include shortness of breath, joint pain, or a rash on the cheeks or arms that worsens with sun exposure.

Call your doctor right away if you develop any of the above side effects or symptoms.

The most common side effects in people taking CIMZIA are:

- upper respiratory infections (flu, cold)
- rash
- urinary tract infections (bladder infections)

Other side effects with CIMZIA include:

- **Psoriasis.** Some people using CIMZIA had new psoriasis or worsening of psoriasis they already had. Tell your doctor if you develop red scaly patches or raised bumps that are filled with pus. Your doctor may decide to stop your treatment with CIMZIA.
- **Injection site reactions.** Redness, rash, swelling, itching or bruising can happen in some people. These symptoms will usually go away within a few days. If you have pain, redness, or swelling around the injection site that doesn't go away within a few days or gets worse, call your doctor right away.

Tell your doctor about any side effect that bothers you or does not go away.

These are not all of the side effects with CIMZIA. Ask your doctor or pharmacist for more information.

Call your doctor for medical advice about side effects. You may report side effects to FDA at 1-800-FDA-1088.

General information about CIMZIA

Medicines are sometimes prescribed for purposes that are not mentioned in Medication Guides. Do not use CIMZIA for a condition for which it was not prescribed. Do not give CIMZIA to other people, even if they have the same condition. It may harm them.

This Medication Guide summarizes the most important information about CIMZIA. If you would like more information, talk with your doctor. You can ask your doctor or pharmacist for information about CIMZIA that is written for health professionals.

For more information go to www.CIMZIA.com or you can enroll in a patient support program by calling 1-866-4CIMZIA (424-6942).

How should I store CIMZIA?

- Keep CIMZIA in the refrigerator at 36°F-46°F (2°C-8°C)
- Let CIMZIA come to room temperature before injecting it.
- **Do not freeze** CIMZIA.
- **Protect** CIMZIA **from light**. Store CIMZIA in the carton.
- Do not use CIMZIA if the medication is expired (today's date is past the date printed on the vial, prefilled syringe or carton), or if the liquid looks cloudy or discolored.

The vials and prefilled syringe are glass. Do not drop or crush them.

Always keep CIMZIA, injection supplies, puncture-proof container, and all other medicines out of the reach of children.

What are the ingredients in CIMZIA?

CIMZIA lyophilized powder:

Active ingredient: certolizumab pegol.

Inactive ingredients: sucrose, lactic acid, polysorbate.

The pack contains Water for Injection, for reconstitution of the lyophilized powder.

CIMZIA prefilled syringe:

Active ingredient: certolizumab pegol
Inactive ingredients: sodium acetate, sodium chloride, and Water for Injection.
CIMZIA has no preservatives.

Patient Instructions for Use
The instructions below are only to be used with CIMZIA in Prefilled Syringes.

What do I need to do to prepare and give an injection of CIMZIA?
Do not use the CIMZIA prefilled syringe if:
• any name other than "CIMZIA" is on the package and prefilled syringe label
• the expiration date on the container has passed
• the packaging is torn or if the tamper evident seals are missing or broken on the top and bottom of carton when you receive it. If this is the case, contact your pharmacist
• the prefilled syringe is frozen or has been left in direct sunlight
• the medicine in the prefilled syringe is not clear to pale yellow, or has large, colored particles in it.

Preparing to use the CIMZIA prefilled syringe
Each CIMZIA prefilled syringe package comes with these items in a tray:
• 2 glass prefilled syringes of CIMZIA. Each has a fixed needle.
• 2 alcohol swabs

For each injection you will use-
• 1 prefilled syringe of CIMZIA with needle
• 1 alcohol swab

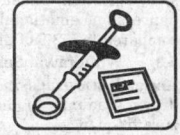

For each injection you will also need:
• 1 clean cotton ball or gauze pads. These are not included in CIMZIA prefilled syringe package.
• a puncture-proof container for disposing of used needles and syringes. (See the section entitled "How do I dispose of needles and syringes?")
If you do not have all the supplies you need, talk to your pharmacist.
• Each prefilled syringe contains the right dose of medicine for one injection (200 mg).
• Depending on the amount of CIMZIA prescribed by your doctor, you may need to take more than one injection.
• If you are prescribed to take 400 mg of CIMZIA, you will need to take two injections. You will need to use two CIMZIA prefilled syringes.
• CIMZIA may be injected into your abdomen or thigh area. If you are prescribed to take more than one injection, each injection should be given at a different injection site, in your abdomen and thigh.

1. Take either one or two CIMZIA prefilled syringes and alcohol swabs out of the refrigerator for injection, depending on your prescribed dose. If there is still a prefilled syringe in the carton, put it back in the refrigerator right away. If both prefilled syringes are used, throw away the empty carton after you finish your injection.
2. Let the medicine in the syringe come to room temperature before injection. This will take about 30 minutes.
For your protection, it's important that you carefully follow these instructions:

Choosing and preparing an injection site
• 3.Wash your hands thoroughly.

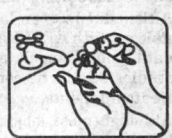

• 4.Choose a different site on your abdomen or thigh for each injection. Each new injection should be given at least one inch from a site you used before. If you choose the abdomen, avoid the 2 inches around your navel. Do not inject into areas where the skin is tender, bruised, red or hard or where you have scars or stretch marks. Change injection sites between your abdomen and thighs to reduce the risk of reaction. You may find it helpful to keep notes on the locations of injection sites you use.
5.Use an alcohol swab to wipe over the site where you will inject CIMZIA. Do not touch the clean area again until you are ready for the injection.

Using the CIMZIA prefilled syringe
6.Remove the needle cover by pulling straight up on the plastic ring. Take care not to touch the needle and do not allow the needle to touch any surface. Place the needle cover to the side.

7.Hold the syringe so the needle is pointing up. Lightly tap the syringe to push any air bubbles to the top. Push the plunger slowly to remove any bubbles. Stop pushing the plunger once all of the air bubbles are gone. If a small drop of liquid comes out of the needle that is okay.
8.Hold the syringe with the needle facing down. Do not touch the needle with your fingers or let it touch any surface.
9.Hold the syringe in one hand. Use the other hand to gently pinch a fold of cleaned area of skin. Insert the needle at about a 45 degree angle with a quick, short, "dart-like" motion.

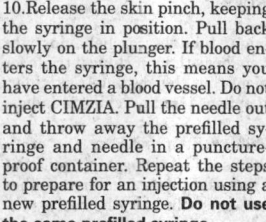

10.Release the skin pinch, keeping the syringe in position. Pull back slowly on the plunger. If blood enters the syringe, this means you have entered a blood vessel. Do not inject CIMZIA. Pull the needle out and throw away the prefilled syringe and needle in a puncture-proof container. Repeat the steps to prepare for an injection using a new prefilled syringe. **Do not use the same prefilled syringe.**
11.If no blood appears, inject all of the medicine in the prefilled syringe under the skin.
12.When the syringe is empty, remove the needle from the skin and press the clean cotton ball or gauze pad over the injection site for ten seconds. Do not rub the injection site. You may have a slight amount of bleeding. This is normal.
13.To avoid needle-stick injury, do not try to recap the needle. Throw away the used prefilled syringe and needle in a special puncture-proof container **(see the section entitled "How should I dispose of needles and syringes?")**

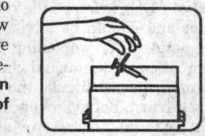

14.Repeat steps 5-13 above if you are prescribed to take a second injection of CIMZIA (total 400 mg dose).

How should I throw away (dispose of) needles and syringes?
To avoid needle-stick injury, do not try to recap the needle. Before you start injecting CIMZIA at home, check with your doctor for instructions on the right way to throw away your used needles and used prefilled syringes. There may be special state or local laws about throwing away used needles and syringes.
Ask your doctor or pharmacist about how to get a puncture-proof container ("sharps" container) that will meet the requirements of your particular state or town.
When the container is about two-thirds full, tape the lid closed. Dispose of the container as instructed by your doctor, nurse or pharmacist. Do not throw away the container in the trash or recycle.
Alcohol swabs may be placed in the trash, unless you are instructed otherwise.
Always keep CIMZIA, injection supplies, puncture-proof container, and all other medicines out of the reach of children.
This Medication Guide has been approved by the U.S. Food and Drug Administration.

Product developed and manufactured for:
UCB, Inc.
1950 Lake Park Drive
Smyrna, GA 30080
US License No. 1736
Revised 11/2009
Shown in Product Identification Guide, page 320

KEPPRA XR®
[*KEPP-ruh XR*]
(levetiracetam)
extended-release tablets

℞

HIGHLIGHTS OF PRESCRIBING INFORMATION
These highlights do not include all the information needed to use KEPPRA XR® safely and effectively. See full prescribing information for KEPPRA XR.

KEPPRA XR (levetiracetam) extended-release tablets
Initial U.S. Approval: 1999

─────────INDICATIONS AND USAGE─────────
KEPPRA XR is an antiepileptic drug indicated for adjunctive therapy in the treatment of partial onset seizures in patients ≥16 years of age with epilepsy (1)

─────DOSAGE AND ADMINISTRATION─────
Treatment should be initiated with a dose of 1000 mg once daily. The daily dosage may be adjusted in increments of 1000 mg every 2 weeks to a maximum recommended daily dose of 3000 mg (2).
See full prescribing information for use in patients with impaired renal function. (2.1).

─────DOSAGE FORMS AND STRENGTHS─────
• 500 mg white, film-coated extended-release tablet (3)
• 750 mg white, film-coated extended-release tablet (3)

─────────CONTRAINDICATIONS─────────
• None (4)

─────WARNINGS AND PRECAUTIONS─────
• Suicidal Behavior and Ideation. (5.1)
• Neuropsychiatric Adverse Reactions: KEPPRA XR causes somnolence, dizziness, and behavioral abnormalities. The adverse reactions that may be seen in patients receiving KEPPRA XR tablets are expected to be similar to those seen in patients receiving immediate-release KEPPRA tablets. (5.2)
• In controlled trials of immediate-release KEPPRA tablets in patients experiencing partial onset seizures, immediate-release KEPPRA causes somnolence and fatigue, coordination difficulties, and behavioral abnormalities (e.g., psychotic symptoms, suicidal ideation, and other abnormalities). (5.2)
• Withdrawal Seizures: KEPPRA XR must be gradually withdrawn. (5.3)

─────────ADVERSE REACTIONS─────────
• Most common adverse reactions (difference in incidence rate is ≥5% between KEPPRA XR-treated patients and placebo-treated patients and occurred more frequently in KEPPRA XR-treated patients) include: somnolence and irritability (6.1).

To report SUSPECTED ADVERSE REACTIONS, contact UCB, Inc. at 866-822-0068 or FDA at 1-800-FDA-1088 or www.fda.gov/medwatch.

─────USE IN SPECIFIC POPULATIONS─────
• To enroll in the UCB AED Pregnancy Registry call 888-537-7734 (toll free). To enroll in the North American Antiepileptic Drug Pregnancy Registry call (888) 233-2334 (toll free). (8.1)
• A dose adjustment is recommended for patients with impaired renal function, based on the patient's estimated creatinine clearance (8.6).

See 17 for PATIENT COUNSELING INFORMATION
Revised: 08/2010

* Sections or subsections omitted from the Full Prescribing Information are not listed.

FULL PRESCRIBING INFORMATION

1 INDICATIONS AND USAGE

KEPPRA XR® is indicated as adjunctive therapy in the treatment of partial onset seizures in patients ≥16 years of age with epilepsy.

2 DOSAGE AND ADMINISTRATION

Treatment should be initiated with a dose of 1000 mg once daily. The daily dosage may be adjusted in increments of 1000 mg every 2 weeks to a maximum recommended daily dose of 3000 mg.

2.1 Adult Patients With Impaired Renal Function

KEPPRA XR dosing must be individualized according to the patient's renal function status. Recommended doses and adjustment for dose for adults are shown in Table 1. To use this dosing table, an estimate of the patient's creatinine clearance (CLcr) in mL/min is needed. CLcr in mL/min may be estimated from serum creatinine (mg/dL) determination using the following formula:

$$CLcr = \frac{[140\text{-age (years)}] \times weight\ (kg)}{72 \times serum\ creatinine\ (mg/dL)} \times^1 0.85$$

1. For female patients

Then CLcr is adjusted for body surface area (BSA) as follows:

$$CLcr\ (mL/min/1.73m^2) = \frac{CLcr\ (mL/min)}{BSA\ subject\ (m^2)} \times 1.73$$

Table 1: Dosing Adjustment Regimen For Adult Patients With Impaired Renal Function

Group	Creatinine Clearance (mL/min/1.73m²)	Dosage (mg)	Frequency
Normal	> 80	1000 to 3000	Every 24 h
Mild	50–80	1000 to 2000	Every 24 h
Moderate	30–50	500 to 1500	Every 24 h
Severe	< 30	500 to 1000	Every 24 h

3 DOSAGE FORMS AND STRENGTHS

KEPPRA XR tablets are white, oblong-shaped, film-coated extended-release tablets imprinted in red with "UCB 500XR" on one side and contain 500 mg levetiracetam. KEPPRA XR tablets are white, oblong-shaped, film-coated extended-release tablets imprinted in red with "UCB 750XR" on one side and contain 750 mg levetiracetam.

4 CONTRAINDICATIONS

None

5 WARNINGS AND PRECAUTIONS

5.1 Suicidal Behavior and Ideation

Antiepileptic drugs (AEDs), including Keppra XR, increase the risk of suicidal thoughts or behavior in patients taking these drugs for any indication. Patients treated with any AED for any indication should be monitored for the emergence or worsening of depression, suicidal thoughts or behavior, and/or any unusual changes in mood or behavior. Pooled analyses of 199 placebo-controlled clinical trials (mono- and adjunctive therapy) of 11 different AEDs showed that patients randomized to one of the AEDs had approximately twice the risk (adjusted Relative Risk 1.8, 95% CI:1.2, 2.7) of suicidal thinking or behavior compared to patients randomized to placebo. In these trials, which had a median treatment duration of 12 weeks, the estimated incidence rate of suicidal behavior or ideation among 27,863 AED-treated patients was 0.43%, compared to 0.24% among 16,029 placebo-treated patients, representing an increase of approximately one case of suicidal thinking or behavior for every 530 patients treated. There were four suicides in drug-treated patients in the trials and none in placebo-treated patients, but the number is too small to allow any conclusion about drug effect on suicide.

The increased risk of suicidal thoughts or behavior with AEDs was observed as early as one week after starting drug treatment with AEDs and persisted for the duration of treatment assessed. Because most trials included in the analysis did not extend beyond 24 weeks, the risk of suicidal thoughts or behavior beyond 24 weeks could not be assessed.

The risk of suicidal thoughts or behavior was generally consistent among drugs in the data analyzed. The finding of increased risk with AEDs of varying mechanisms of action and across a range of indications suggests that the risk applies to all AEDs used for any indication. The risk did not vary substantially by age (5-100 years) in the clinical trials analyzed. Table 2 shows absolute and relative risk by indication for all evaluated AEDs.

[See table 2 below]

The relative risk for suicidal thoughts or behavior was higher in clinical trials for epilepsy than in clinical trials for psychiatric or other conditions, but the absolute risk differences were similar for the epilepsy and psychiatric indications.

Anyone considering prescribing Keppra XR or any other AED must balance the risk of suicidal thoughts or behavior with the risk of untreated illness. Epilepsy and many other illnesses for which AEDs are prescribed are themselves associated with morbidity and mortality and an increased risk of suicidal thoughts and behavior. Should suicidal thoughts and behavior emerge during treatment, the prescriber needs to consider whether the emergence of these symptoms in any given patient may be related to the illness being treated.

Patients, their caregivers, and families should be informed that AEDs increase the risk of suicidal thoughts and behavior and should be advised of the need to be alert for the emergence or worsening of the signs and symptoms of depression, any unusual changes in mood or behavior, or the emergence of suicidal thoughts, behavior, or thoughts about self-harm. Behaviors of concern should be reported immediately to healthcare providers.

5.2 Neuropsychiatric Adverse Reactions

KEPPRA XR Tablets

In some patients experiencing partial onset seizures, KEPPRA XR causes somnolence, dizziness, and behavioral abnormalities.

In the KEPPRA XR double-blind, controlled trial in patients experiencing partial onset seizures, 7.8% of KEPPRA XR-treated patients experienced somnolence compared to 2.5% of placebo-treated patients. Dizziness was reported in 5.2% of KEPPRA XR-treated patients compared to 2.5% of placebo-treated patients.

A total of 6.5% of KEPPRA XR-treated patients experienced non-psychotic behavioral disorders (reported as irritability and aggression) compared to 0% of placebo-treated patients. Irritability was reported in 6.5% of KEPPRA XR-treated patients. Aggression was reported in 1.3% of KEPPRA XR-treated patients.

No patient discontinued treatment or had a dose reduction as a result of these adverse reactions.

The number of patients exposed to KEPPRA XR was considerably smaller than the number of patients exposed to immediate-release KEPPRA tablets in controlled trials. Therefore, certain adverse reactions observed in the immediate-release KEPPRA controlled trials may also occur in patients receiving KEPPRA XR.

Immediate-Release KEPPRA Tablets

In controlled trials of immediate-release KEPPRA tablets in patients experiencing partial onset seizures, immediate-release KEPPRA causes the occurrence of central nervous system adverse reactions that can be classified into the following categories: 1) somnolence and fatigue, 2) coordination difficulties, and 3) behavioral abnormalities.

In controlled trials of adult patients with epilepsy experiencing partial onset seizures, 14.8% of immediate-release KEPPRA-treated patients reported somnolence, compared to 8.4% of placebo patients. There was no clear dose response up to 3000 mg/day.

In controlled trials of adult patients with epilepsy experiencing partial onset seizures, 14.7% of treated patients reported asthenia, compared to 9.1% of placebo patients.

A total of 3.4% of immediate-release KEPPRA-treated patients experienced coordination difficulties, (reported as either ataxia, abnormal gait, or incoordination) compared to 1.6% of placebo patients.

Somnolence, asthenia and coordination difficulties occurred most frequently within the first 4 weeks of treatment.

In controlled trials of patients with epilepsy experiencing partial onset seizures, 5 (0.7%) immediate-release KEPPRA-treated patients experienced psychotic symptoms compared to 1 (0.2%) placebo patient.

A total of 13.3% of immediate-release KEPPRA patients experienced other behavioral symptoms (reported as aggression, agitation, anger, anxiety, apathy, depersonalization, depression, emotional lability, hostility, irritability, etc.) compared to 6.2% of placebo patients.

5.3 Withdrawal Seizures

Antiepileptic drugs, including KEPPRA XR, should be withdrawn gradually to minimize the potential of increased seizure frequency.

5.4 Hematologic Abnormalities

Although there were no obvious hematologic abnormalities observed in treated patients in the KEPPRA XR controlled study, the limited number of patients makes any conclusion tentative. The data from the partial seizure patients in the immediate-release KEPPRA controlled studies should be considered to be relevant for KEPPRA XR-treated patients.

In controlled trials of immediate-release KEPPRA tablets in patients experiencing partial onset seizures, minor, but statistically significant, decreases compared to placebo in total mean RBC count ($0.03 \times 10^6/mm^3$), mean hemoglobin (0.09 g/dL), and mean hematocrit (0.38%), were seen in immediate-release KEPPRA-treated patients. A total of 3.2% of treated and 1.8% of placebo patients had at least one possibly significant ($\leq 2.8 \times 10^9/L$) decreased WBC, and 2.4% of treated and 1.4% of placebo patients had at least one possibly significant ($\leq 1.0 \times 10^9/L$) decreased neutrophil count. Of the treated patients with a low neutrophil count, all but one rose towards or to baseline with continued treatment. No patient was discontinued secondary to low neutrophil counts.

5.5 Hepatic Abnormalities

There were no meaningful changes in mean liver function tests (LFT) in the KEPPRA XR controlled trial. No patients were discontinued from the controlled trial for LFT abnormalities.

There were no meaningful changes in mean liver function tests (LFT) in controlled trials of immediate-release KEPPRA tablets in adult patients; lesser LFT abnormalities were similar in drug and placebo-treated patients in controlled trials (1.4%). No patients were discontinued from controlled trials for LFT abnormalities except for 1 (0.07%) adult epilepsy patient receiving open treatment.

5.6 Laboratory Tests

Although effects on laboratory tests were not clinically significant with KEPPRA XR treatment, it is expected that the data from immediate-release KEPPRA tablets controlled studies would be considered relevant for KEPPRA XR-treated patients.

Although most laboratory tests are not systematically altered with immediate-release KEPPRA treatment, there have been relatively infrequent abnormalities seen in hematologic parameters and liver function tests.

6 ADVERSE REACTIONS

6.1 Clinical Studies Experience

Because clinical trials are conducted under widely varying conditions, adverse reaction rates observed in the clinical trials of a drug cannot be directly compared to rates in the clinical trials of another drug and may not reflect the rates observed in practice.

The prescriber should be aware that the adverse reaction incidence figures in the following table, obtained when KEPPRA XR was added to concurrent AED therapy, cannot be used to predict the frequency of adverse experiences in the course of usual medical practice where patient characteristics and other factors may differ from those prevailing during clinical studies. Similarly, the cited frequencies cannot be directly compared with figures obtained from other clinical investigations involving different treatments, uses, or investigators. An inspection of these frequencies,

Table 2 Risk by indication for antiepileptic drugs in the pooled analysis

Indication	Placebo Patients with Events Per 1000 Patients	Drug Patients with Events Per 1000 Patients	Relative Risk: Incidence of Events in Drug Patients/ Incidence in Placebo Patients	Risk Difference: Additional Drug Patients with Events Per 1000 Patients
Epilepsy	1.0	3.4	3.5	2.4
Psychiatric	5.7	8.5	1.5	2.9
Other	1.0	1.8	1.9	0.9
Total	2.4	4.3	1.8	1.9

however, does provide the prescriber with one basis to estimate the relative contribution of drug and non-drug factors to the adverse reaction incidences in the population studied.

KEPPRA XR Tablets

In the well-controlled clinical study using KEPPRA XR in patients with partial onset seizures, the most frequently reported adverse reactions in patients receiving KEPPRA XR in combination with other AEDs, not seen at an equivalent frequency among placebo-treated patients, were irritability and somnolence.

Table 3 lists treatment-emergent adverse reactions that occurred in at least 5% of epilepsy patients treated with KEPPRA XR participating in the placebo-controlled study and were numerically more common than in patients treated with placebo. In this study, either KEPPRA XR or placebo was added to concurrent AED therapy. Adverse reactions were usually mild to moderate in intensity.

Table 3: Incidence (%) Of Treatment-Emergent Adverse Reactions In The Placebo-Controlled, Add-On Study By Body System (Adverse Reactions Occurred In At Least 5% Of KEPPRA XR-Treated Patients And Occurred More Frequently Than Placebo-Treated Patients)

Body System/ Adverse Reaction	KEPPRA XR (N=77) %	Placebo (N=79) %
Gastrointestinal Disorders		
Nausea	5	3
Infections and Infestations		
Influenza	8	4
Nasopharyngitis	7	5
Nervous System Disorders		
Somnolence	8	3
Dizziness	5	3
Psychiatric Disorders		
Irritability	7	0

Discontinuation Or Dose Reduction In The KEPPRA XR Well-Controlled Clinical Study

In the well-controlled clinical study using KEPPRA XR, 5.2% of patients receiving KEPPRA XR and 2.5% receiving placebo discontinued as a result of an adverse event. The adverse reactions that resulted in discontinuation and that occurred more frequently in KEPPRA XR-treated patients than in placebo-treated patients were asthenia, epilepsy, mouth ulceration, rash and respiratory failure. Each of these adverse reactions led to discontinuation in a KEPPRA XR-treated patient and no placebo-treated patients.

Comparison Of Gender, Age And Race

There are insufficient data for KEPPRA XR to support a statement regarding the distribution of adverse experience reports by gender, age and race.

Table 4 lists the adverse reactions seen in the well-controlled studies of immediate-release KEPPRA tablets in adult patients experiencing partial onset seizures. Although the pattern of adverse reactions in the KEPPRA XR study seems somewhat different from that seen in partial onset seizure well-controlled studies for immediate-release KEPPRA tablets, this is possibly due to the much smaller number of patients in this study compared to the immediate-release tablet studies. The adverse reactions for KEPPRA XR are expected to be similar to those seen with immediate-release KEPPRA tablets.

Immediate-Release KEPPRA Tablets

In well-controlled clinical studies of immediate-release KEPPRA tablets as adjunctive therapy to other AEDs in adults with partial onset seizures, the most frequently reported adverse reactions, not seen at an equivalent frequency among placebo-treated patients, were somnolence, asthenia, infection and dizziness.

Table 4 lists treatment-emergent adverse reactions that occurred in at least 1% of adult epilepsy patients treated with immediate-release KEPPRA tablets participating in placebo-controlled studies and were numerically more common than in patients treated with placebo. In these studies, either immediate-release KEPPRA tablets or placebo was added to concurrent AED therapy. Adverse reactions were usually mild to moderate in intensity.

Table 4: Incidence (%) Of Treatment-Emergent Adverse Reactions In Placebo-Controlled, Add-On Studies In Adults Experiencing Partial Onset Seizures By Body System (Adverse Reactions Occurred In At Least 1% Of Immediate-Release KEPPRA-Treated Patients And Occurred More Frequently Than Placebo-Treated Patients)

Body System/ Adverse Reaction	Immediate- release KEPPRA (N=769) %	Placebo (N=439) %
Body as a Whole		
Asthenia	15	9
Headache	14	13
Infection	13	8
Pain	7	6
Digestive System		
Anorexia	3	2
Nervous System		
Somnolence	15	8
Dizziness	9	4
Depression	4	2
Nervousness	4	2
Ataxia	3	1
Vertigo	3	1
Amnesia	2	1
Anxiety	2	1
Hostility	2	1
Paresthesia	2	1
Emotional Lability	2	0
Respiratory System		
Pharyngitis	6	4
Rhinitis	4	3
Cough Increased	2	1
Sinusitis	2	1
Special Senses		
Diplopia	2	1

In addition, the following adverse reactions were seen in other well-controlled studies of immediate-release KEPPRA tablets: balance disorder, disturbance in attention, eczema, hyperkinesia, memory impairment, myalgia, personality disorders, pruritus, and vision blurred.

6.2 Postmarketing Experience

In addition to the adverse reactions listed above for immediate-release KEPPRA tablets *[see Adverse Reactions (6.1)]*, the following adverse events have been identified during postapproval use of immediate-release KEPPRA tablets. Because these events are reported voluntarily from a population of uncertain size, it is not always possible to reliably estimate their frequency or establish a causal relationship to drug exposure. The listing is alphabetized: abnormal liver function test, erythema multiforme, hepatic failure, hepatitis, leukopenia, neutropenia, pancreatitis, pancytopenia (with bone marrow suppression identified in some of these cases), Stevens-Johnson syndrome, thrombocytopenia, toxic epidermal necrolysis, and weight loss. Alopecia has been reported with immediate-release KEPPRA use; recovery was observed in majority of cases where immediate-release KEPPRA was discontinued.

7 DRUG INTERACTIONS

7.1 General Information

In vitro data on metabolic interactions indicate that KEPPRA XR is unlikely to produce, or be subject to, pharmacokinetic interactions. Levetiracetam and its major metabolite, at concentrations well above C_{max} levels achieved within the therapeutic dose range, are neither inhibitors of nor high affinity substrates for human liver cytochrome P450 isoforms, epoxide hydrolase or UDP-glucuronidation enzymes. In addition, levetiracetam does not affect the *in vitro* glucuronidation of valproic acid. Levetiracetam circulates largely unbound (<10% bound) to plasma proteins; clinically significant interactions with other drugs through competition for protein binding sites are therefore unlikely.

Potential pharmacokinetic interactions were assessed in clinical pharmacokinetic studies (phenytoin, valproate, oral contraceptive, digoxin, warfarin, probenecid) and through pharmacokinetic screening with immediate-release KEPPRA tablets in the placebo-controlled clinical studies in epilepsy patients. The following are the results of these studies. The potential for drug interactions for KEPPRA XR is expected to be essentially the same as that with immediate-release KEPPRA tablets.

7.2 Phenytoin

Immediate-release KEPPRA tablets (3000 mg daily) had no effect on the pharmacokinetic disposition of phenytoin in patients with refractory epilepsy. Pharmacokinetics of levetiracetam were also not affected by phenytoin.

7.3 Valproate

Immediate-release KEPPRA tablets (1500 mg twice daily) did not alter the pharmacokinetics of valproate in healthy volunteers. Valproate 500 mg twice daily did not modify the rate or extent of levetiracetam absorption or its plasma clearance or urinary excretion. There also was no effect on exposure to and the excretion of the primary metabolite, ucb L057.

7.4 Other Antiepileptic Drugs

Potential drug interactions between immediate-release KEPPRA tablets and other AEDs (carbamazepine, gabapentin, lamotrigine, phenobarbital, phenytoin, primidone and valproate) were also assessed by evaluating the serum concentrations of levetiracetam and these AEDs during placebo-controlled clinical studies. These data indicate that levetiracetam does not influence the plasma concentration of other AEDs and that these AEDs do not influence the pharmacokinetics of levetiracetam.

7.5 Oral Contraceptives

Immediate-release KEPPRA tablets (500 mg twice daily) did not influence the pharmacokinetics of an oral contraceptive containing 0.03 mg ethinyl estradiol and 0.15 mg levonorgestrel, or of the luteinizing hormone and progesterone levels, indicating that impairment of contraceptive efficacy is unlikely. Coadministration of this oral contraceptive did not influence the pharmacokinetics of levetiracetam.

7.6 Digoxin

Immediate-release KEPPRA tablets (1000 mg twice daily) did not influence the pharmacokinetics and pharmacodynamics (ECG) of digoxin given as a 0.25 mg dose every day. Coadministration of digoxin did not influence the pharmacokinetics of levetiracetam.

7.7 Warfarin

Immediate-release KEPPRA tablets (1000 mg twice daily) did not influence the pharmacokinetics of R and S warfarin. Prothrombin time was not affected by levetiracetam. Coadministration of warfarin did not affect the pharmacokinetics of levetiracetam.

7.8 Probenecid

Probenecid, a renal tubular secretion blocking agent, administered at a dose of 500 mg four times a day, did not change the pharmacokinetics of levetiracetam 1000 mg twice daily. C^{ss}_{max} of the metabolite, ucb L057, was approximately doubled in the presence of probenecid while the fraction of drug excreted unchanged in the urine remained the same. Renal clearance of ucb L057 in the presence of probenecid decreased 60%, probably related to competitive inhibition of tubular secretion of ucb L057. The effect of immediate-release KEPPRA tablets on probenecid was not studied.

8 USE IN SPECIFIC POPULATIONS

8.1 Pregnancy

Pregnancy Category C

There are no adequate and well-controlled studies in pregnant women. In animal studies, levetiracetam produced evidence of developmental toxicity, including teratogenic effects, at doses similar to or greater than human therapeutic doses. KEPPRA XR should be used during pregnancy only if the potential benefit justifies the potential risk to the fetus. As with other antiepileptic drugs, physiological changes during pregnancy may affect levetiracetam concentration. There have been reports of decreased levetiracetam concentration during pregnancy. Discontinuation of antiepileptic treatments may result in disease worsening, which can be harmful to the mother and the fetus.

Oral administration of levetiracetam to female rats throughout pregnancy and lactation led to increased incidences of minor fetal skeletal abnormalities and retarded offspring growth pre- and/or postnatally at doses ≥350 mg/kg/day (approximately equivalent to the maximum recommended human dose of 3000 mg [MRHD] on a mg/m² basis) and with increased pup mortality and offspring behavioral alterations at a dose of 1800 mg/kg/day (6 times the MRHD on a mg/m^2 basis). The developmental no effect dose was 70 mg/kg/day (0.2 times the MRHD on a mg/m^2 basis). There was no overt maternal toxicity at the doses used in this study.

Oral administration of levetiracetam to pregnant rabbits during the period of organogenesis resulted in increased embryofetal mortality and increased incidences of minor fetal skeletal abnormalities at doses ≥600 mg/kg/day (approximately 4 times MRHD on a mg/m^2 basis) and in decreased fetal weights and increased incidences of fetal malformations at a dose of 1800 mg/kg/day (12 times the MRHD on a mg/m^2 basis). The developmental no effect dose was 200 mg/kg/day (1.3 times the MRHD on a mg/m^2 basis). Maternal toxicity was also observed at 1800 mg/kg/day.

When levetiracetam was administered orally to pregnant rats during the period of organogenesis, fetal weights were decreased and the incidence of fetal skeletal variations was increased at a dose of 3600 mg/kg/day (12 times the MRHD). 1200 mg/kg/day (4 times the MRHD) was a developmental no effect dose. There was no evidence of maternal toxicity in this study.

Treatment of rats with levetiracetam during the last third of gestation and throughout lactation produced no adverse developmental or maternal effects at oral doses of up to 1800 mg/kg/day (6 times the MRHD on a mg/m^2 basis).

Pregnancy Registries

To provide information regarding the effects of in utero exposure to KEPPRA XR, physicians are advised to recommend that pregnant patients taking KEPPRA XR enroll in the North American Antiepileptic Drug (NAAED) pregnancy registry. This can be done by calling the toll free number 1-888-233-2334, and must be done by the patients themselves. Information on the registry can also be found at the website http://www.aedpregnancyregistry.org/.

UCB, Inc. has established the UCB AED Pregnancy Registry to advance scientific knowledge about safety and outcomes in pregnant women being treated with all UCB antiepileptic drugs including KEPPRA XR. To ensure broad program access and reach, either a healthcare provider or the patient can initiate enrollment in the UCB AED Pregnancy Registry by calling (888) 537-7734 (toll free).

8.2 Labor And Delivery

The effect of KEPPRA XR on labor and delivery in humans is unknown.

8.3 Nursing Mothers

Levetiracetam is excreted in breast milk. Because of the potential for serious adverse reactions in nursing infants from KEPPRA XR, a decision should be made whether to discontinue nursing or discontinue the drug, taking into account the importance of the drug to the mother.

8.4 Pediatric Use

Safety and effectiveness of KEPPRA XR in patients below the age of 16 years have not been established.

8.5 Geriatric Use

There were insufficient numbers of elderly subjects in controlled trials of epilepsy to adequately assess the effectiveness of KEPPRA XR in these patients. It is expected that the safety of KEPPRA XR in elderly patients 65 and over would be comparable to the safety observed in clinical studies of immediate-release KEPPRA tablets.

Of the total number of subjects in clinical studies of immediate-release levetiracetam, 347 were 65 and over. No overall differences in safety were observed between these subjects and younger subjects. There were insufficient numbers of elderly subjects in controlled trials of epilepsy to adequately assess the effectiveness of immediate-release KEPPRA in these patients.

A study in 16 elderly subjects (age 61-88 years) with oral administration of single dose and multiple twice-daily doses of immediate-release KEPPRA tablets for 10 days showed no pharmacokinetic differences related to age alone.

Levetiracetam is known to be substantially excreted by the kidney, and the risk of adverse reactions to this drug may be greater in patients with impaired renal function. Because elderly patients are more likely to have decreased renal function, care should be taken in dose selection, and it may be useful to monitor renal function.

8.6 Use In Patients With Impaired Renal Function

The effect of KEPPRA XR on renally impaired patients was not assessed in the well-controlled study. However, it is expected that the effect on KEPPRA XR-treated patients would be similar to the effect seen in well-controlled studies of immediate-release KEPPRA tablets. Caution should be taken in dosing patients with moderate and severe renal impairment and in patients undergoing hemodialysis. The dosage should be reduced in patients with impaired renal function receiving KEPPRA XR [*see Clinical Pharmacology (12.3) and Dosage and Administration (2.1)*].

Clearance of immediate-release levetiracetam is decreased in patients with renal impairment and is correlated with creatinine clearance.

9 DRUG ABUSE AND DEPENDENCE

The abuse and dependence potential of KEPPRA XR has not been evaluated in human studies.

10 OVERDOSAGE

Signs, Symptoms And Laboratory Findings Of Acute Overdosage In Humans

The signs and symptoms for KEPPRA XR overdose are expected to be similar to those seen with immediate-release KEPPRA tablets.

The highest known dose of oral immediate-release KEPPRA received in the clinical development program was 6000 mg/day. Other than drowsiness, there were no adverse reactions in the few known cases of overdose in clinical trials. Cases of somnolence, agitation, aggression, depressed level of consciousness, respiratory depression and coma were observed with immediate-release KEPPRA overdoses in postmarketing use.

Treatment Or Management Of Overdose

There is no specific antidote for overdose with KEPPRA XR. If indicated, elimination of unabsorbed drug should be attempted by emesis or gastric lavage; usual precautions should be observed to maintain airway. General supportive care of the patient is indicated including monitoring of vital signs and observation of the patient's clinical status. A Certified Poison Control Center should be contacted for up to date information on the management of overdose with KEPPRA XR.

Hemodialysis

Standard hemodialysis procedures result in significant clearance of levetiracetam (approximately 50% in 4 hours) and should be considered in cases of overdose. Although hemodialysis has not been performed in the few known cases of overdose, it may be indicated by the patient's clinical state or in patients with significant renal impairment.

11 DESCRIPTION

KEPPRA XR is an antiepileptic drug available as 500 mg and 750 mg (white) extended-release tablets for oral administration.

The chemical name of levetiracetam, a single enantiomer, is (-)-(S)-α-ethyl-2-oxo-1-pyrrolidine acetamide, its molecular formula is $C_8H_{14}N_2O_2$ and its molecular weight is 170.21. Levetiracetam is chemically unrelated to existing antiepileptic drugs (AEDs). It has the following structural formula:

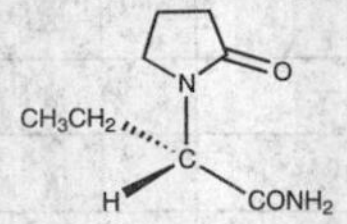

Levetiracetam is a white to off-white crystalline powder with a faint odor and a bitter taste. It is very soluble in water (104.0 g/100 mL). It is freely soluble in chloroform (65.3 g/100 mL) and in methanol (53.6 g/100 mL), soluble in ethanol (16.5 g/100 mL), sparingly soluble in acetonitrile (5.7 g/100 mL) and practically insoluble in n-hexane. (Solubility limits are expressed as g/100 mL solvent.)

KEPPRA XR tablets contain the labeled amount of levetiracetam. Inactive ingredients: colloidal anhydrous silica, hypromellose, magnesium stearate, polyethylene glycol 6000, polyvinyl alcohol-partially hydrolyzed, titanium dioxide (E171), Macrogol/PEG3350, and talc. The imprinting ink contains shellac, FD&C Red #40, n-butyl alcohol, propylene glycol, titanium dioxide, ethanol, and methanol.

12 CLINICAL PHARMACOLOGY

12.1 Mechanism Of Action

The precise mechanism(s) by which levetiracetam exerts its antiepileptic effect is unknown. The antiepileptic activity of levetiracetam was assessed in a number of animal models of epileptic seizures. Levetiracetam did not inhibit single seizures induced by maximal stimulation with electrical current or different chemoconvulsants and showed only minimal activity in submaximal stimulation and in threshold tests. Protection was observed, however, against secondarily generalized activity from focal seizures induced by pilocarpine and kainic acid, two chemoconvulsants that induce seizures that mimic some features of human complex partial seizures with secondary generalization. Levetiracetam also displayed inhibitory properties in the kindling model in rats, another model of human complex partial seizures, both during kindling development and in the fully kindled state. The predictive value of these animal models for specific types of human epilepsy is uncertain.

In vitro and *in vivo* recordings of epileptiform activity from the hippocampus have shown that levetiracetam inhibits burst firing without affecting normal neuronal excitability, suggesting that levetiracetam may selectively prevent hypersynchronization of epileptiform burst firing and propagation of seizure activity.

Levetiracetam at concentrations of up to 10 μM did not demonstrate binding affinity for a variety of known receptors, such as those associated with benzodiazepines, GABA (gamma-aminobutyric acid), glycine, NMDA (N-methyl-D-aspartate), re-uptake sites, and second messenger systems. Furthermore, *in vitro* studies have failed to find an effect of levetiracetam on neuronal voltage-gated sodium or T-type calcium currents and levetiracetam does not appear to directly facilitate GABAergic neurotransmission. However, *in vitro* studies have demonstrated that levetiracetam opposes the activity of negative modulators of GABA- and glycine-gated currents and partially inhibits N-type calcium currents in neuronal cells.

A saturable and stereoselective neuronal binding site in rat brain tissue has been described for levetiracetam. Experimental data indicate that this binding site is the synaptic vesicle protein SV2A, thought to be involved in the regulation of vesicle exocytosis. Although the molecular significance of levetiracetam binding to synaptic vesicle protein SV2A is not understood, levetiracetam and related analogs showed a rank order of affinity for SV2A which correlated with the potency of their antiseizure activity in audiogenic seizure-prone mice. These findings suggest that the interaction of levetiracetam with the SV2A protein may contribute to the antiepileptic mechanism of action of the drug.

12.3 Pharmacokinetics

Overview

Bioavailability of Keppra XR tablets is similar to that of the Keppra IR Tablets. The pharmacokinetics (AUC and C_{max}) were shown to be dose proportional after single dose administration of 1000 mg, 2000 mg, and 3000 mg extended-release levetiracetam. Plasma half-life of extended-release levetiracetam is approximately 7 hours.

Levetiracetam is almost completely absorbed after oral administration. The pharmacokinetics of levetiracetam are linear and time-invariant, with low intra- and inter-subject variability. Levetiracetam is not significantly protein-bound (<10% bound) and its volume of distribution is close to the volume of intracellular and extracellular water. Sixty-six percent (66%) of the dose is renally excreted unchanged. The major metabolic pathway of levetiracetam (24% of dose) is an enzymatic hydrolysis of the acetamide group. It is not liver cytochrome P450 dependent. The metabolites have no known pharmacological activity and are renally excreted. Plasma half-life of levetiracetam across studies is approximately 6-8 hours. The half-life is increased in the elderly (primarily due to impaired renal clearance) and in subjects with renal impairment.

Absorption and Distribution

Extended-release levetiracetam peak plasma concentrations occur in about 4 hours. The time to peak plasma concentrations is about 3 hours longer with extended-release levetiracetam than with immediate-release tablets.

Single administration of two 500 mg extended-release levetiracetam tablets once daily produced comparable maximal plasma concentrations and area under the plasma concentration versus time as did the administration of one 500 mg immediate-release tablet twice daily in fasting conditions. After multiple dose extended-release levetiracetam tablets intake, extent of exposure (AUC_{0-24}) was similar to extent of exposure after multiple dose immediate-release tablets intake. C_{max} and C_{min} were lower by 17% and 26% after multiple dose extended-release levetiracetam tablets intake in comparison to multiple dose immediate-release tablets intake. Intake of a high fat, high calorie breakfast before the administration of extended-release levetiracetam tablets resulted in a higher peak concentration, and longer median time to peak. The median time to peak (T_{max}) was 2 hours longer in the fed state.

Two 750 mg extended-release levetiracetam tablets were bioequivalent to a single administration of three 500 mg extended-release levetiracetam tablets.

Metabolism

Levetiracetam is not extensively metabolized in humans. The major metabolic pathway is the enzymatic hydrolysis of the acetamide group, which produces the carboxylic acid metabolite, ucb L057 (24% of dose) and is not dependent on any liver cytochrome P450 isoenzymes. The major metabolite is inactive in animal seizure models. Two minor metabolites were identified as the product of hydroxylation of the 2-oxo-pyrrolidine ring (2% of dose) and opening of the 2-oxo-pyrrolidine ring in position 5 (1% of dose). There is no enantiomeric interconversion of levetiracetam or its major metabolite.

Elimination

Levetiracetam plasma half-life in adults is 7 ± 1 hour and is unaffected by either dose or repeated administration. Levetiracetam is eliminated from the systemic circulation by renal excretion as unchanged drug which represents 66% of administered dose. The total body clearance is 0.96 mL/min/kg and the renal clearance is 0.6 mL/min/kg. The mechanism of excretion is glomerular filtration with subsequent partial tubular reabsorption. The metabolite ucb L057 is excreted by glomerular filtration and active tubular secretion with a renal clearance of 4 mL/min/kg. Levetiracetam elimination is correlated to creatinine clearance. Levetiracetam clearance is reduced in patients with impaired renal function [see Use in Specific Populations (8.6) and Dosage and Administration (2.1)].

Pharmacokinetic Interactions

In vitro data on metabolic interactions indicate that levetiracetam is unlikely to produce, or be subject to, pharmacokinetic interactions. Levetiracetam and its major metabolite, at concentrations well above C_{max} levels achieved within the therapeutic dose range, are neither inhibitors of, nor high affinity substrates for, human liver cytochrome P450 isoforms, epoxide hydrolase or UDP-glucuronidation enzymes. In addition, levetiracetam does not affect the *in vitro* glucuronidation of valproic acid. The pharmacokinetics of immediate-release levetiracetam are linear over the dose range of 500-5000 mg. Levetiracetam and its major metabolite are less than 10% bound to plasma proteins; clinically significant interactions with other drugs through competition for protein binding sites are therefore unlikely.

Potential pharmacokinetic interactions of or with immediate-release levetiracetam were assessed in clinical pharmacokinetic studies (phenytoin, valproate, warfarin, digoxin, oral contraceptive, probenecid) and through pharmacokinetic screening in the placebo-controlled clinical studies in epilepsy patients [see Drug Interactions (7)]. The potential for drug interactions for extended-release levetiracetam is expected to be similar to that with immediate-release levetiracetam.

Special Populations

Elderly

There are insufficient pharmacokinetic data to specifically address the use of extended-release levetiracetam in the elderly population.

Pharmacokinetics of immediate-release levetiracetam were evaluated in 16 elderly subjects (age 61-88 years) with creatinine clearance ranging from 30 to 74 mL/min. Following oral administration of twice-daily dosing for 10 days, total body clearance decreased by 38% and the half-life was 2.5 hours longer in the elderly compared to healthy adults. This is most likely due to the decrease in renal function in these subjects.

Pediatric Patients

Safety and effectiveness of KEPPRA XR in patients below the age of 16 years have not been established.

Gender

Extended-release levetiracetam C_{max} was 21-30% higher and AUC was 8-18% higher in women (N=12) compared to men (N=12). However, clearances adjusted for body weight were comparable.

Race

Formal pharmacokinetic studies of the effects of race have not been conducted with extended-release or immediate-release levetiracetam. Cross study comparisons involving Caucasians (N=12) and Asians (N=12), however, show that pharmacokinetics of immediate-release levetiracetam were comparable between the two races.

Renal Impairment

The effect of KEPPRA XR on renally impaired patients was not assessed in the well-controlled study. However, it is expected that the effect on KEPPRA XR-treated patients would be similar to that seen in well-controlled studies of immediate-release KEPPRA tablets. In patients with end stage renal disease on dialysis, it is recommended that immediate-release KEPPRA be used instead of KEPPRA XR.

The disposition of immediate-release levetiracetam was studied in adult subjects with varying degrees of renal function. Total body clearance of levetiracetam is reduced in patients with impaired renal function by 40% in the mild group (CLcr = 50-80 mL/min), 50% in the moderate group (CLcr = 30-50 mL/min) and 60% in the severe renal impairment group (CLcr <30 mL/min). Clearance of levetiracetam is correlated with creatinine clearance.

In anuric (end stage renal disease) patients, the total body clearance decreased 70% compared to normal subjects (CLcr >80mL/min). Approximately 50% of the pool of levetiracetam in the body is removed during a standard 4 hour hemodialysis procedure.

Dosage should be reduced in patients with impaired renal function receiving levetiracetam; immediate-release levetiracetam should be given to patients on dialysis [see Dosage and Administration (2.1)].

Hepatic Impairment

In subjects with mild (Child-Pugh A) to moderate (Child-Pugh B) hepatic impairment, the pharmacokinetics of levetiracetam were unchanged. In patients with severe hepatic impairment (Child-Pugh C), total body clearance was 50% that of normal subjects, but decreased renal clearance accounted for most of the decrease. No dose adjustment is needed for patients with hepatic impairment.

13 NONCLINICAL TOXICOLOGY

13.1 Carcinogenesis, Mutagenesis, Impairment Of Fertility

Carcinogenesis

Rats were dosed with levetiracetam in the diet for 104 weeks at doses of 50, 300 and 1800 mg/kg/day. The highest

dose corresponds to 6 times the maximum recommended daily human dose (MRHD) of 3000 mg on a mg/m² basis and it also provided systemic exposure (AUC) approximately 6 times that achieved in humans receiving the MRHD. There was no evidence of carcinogenicity. A study was conducted in which mice received levetiracetam in the diet for 80 weeks at doses of 60, 240 and 960 mg/kg/day (high dose is equivalent to 2 times the MRHD on a mg/m² or exposure basis). Although no evidence for carcinogenicity was seen, the potential for a carcinogenic response has not been fully evaluated in that species because adequate doses have not been studied.

Mutagenesis

Levetiracetam was not mutagenic in the Ames test or in mammalian cells *in vitro* in the Chinese hamster ovary/HGPRT locus assay. It was not clastogenic in an *in vitro* analysis of metaphase chromosomes obtained from Chinese hamster ovary cells or in an *in vivo* mouse micronucleus assay. The hydrolysis product and major human metabolite of levetiracetam (ucb L057) was not mutagenic in the Ames test or the *in vitro* mouse lymphoma assay.

Impairment Of Fertility

No adverse effects on male or female fertility or reproductive performance were observed in rats at oral doses up to 1800 mg/kg/day (approximately 6 times the maximum recommended human dose on a mg/m² or exposure basis).

13.2 Animal Toxicology And/Or Pharmacology

In animal studies, levetiracetam produced evidence of developmental toxicity at doses similar to or greater than human therapeutic doses.

14 CLINICAL STUDIES

The effectiveness of the immediate-release formulation of KEPPRA as adjunctive therapy (added to other antiepileptic drugs) in adults was established in three multicenter, randomized, double-blind, placebo controlled clinical studies in 904 patients who had refractory partial onset seizures with or without secondary generalization for at least two years and had taken two or more classical AEDs.

The effectiveness of KEPPRA XR as adjunctive therapy (added to other antiepileptic drugs) was established in one multicenter, randomized, double-blind, placebo-controlled clinical study across 7 countries in patients who had refractory partial onset seizures with or without secondary generalization. Patients enrolled had at least eight partial seizures with or without secondary generalization during the 8-week baseline period and at least two partial seizures in each 4-week interval of the baseline period. Patients were taking a stable dose regimen of at least one and could take a maximum of three AEDs. After a prospective baseline period of 8 weeks, 158 patients were randomized to placebo (N=79) or KEPPRA XR (2×500 mg tablets) (N=79) given once daily over a 12-week treatment period.

The primary efficacy endpoint was the percent reduction over placebo in mean weekly frequency of partial onset seizures. The median percent reduction in weekly partial onset seizure frequency from baseline over the treatment period was 46.1% in the KEPPRA XR 1000 mg treatment group (N=74) and 33.4% in the placebo group (N=78). The estimated percent reduction over placebo in weekly partial onset seizure frequency over the treatment period was 14.4% (statistically significant).

The relationship between the effectiveness of the same daily dose of KEPPRA XR and immediate-release KEPPRA has not been studied and is unknown.

16 HOW SUPPLIED/STORAGE AND HANDLING

16.1 How Supplied

KEPPRA XR 500 mg tablets are white, oblong-shaped, film-coated tablets imprinted with "UCB 500XR" in red on one side. They are supplied in white HDPE bottles containing 60 tablets (NDC 50474-598-66).

KEPPRA XR 750 mg tablets are white, oblong-shaped, film-coated tablets imprinted with "UCB 750XR" in red on one side. They are supplied in white HDPE bottles containing 60 tablets (NDC 50474-599-66).

16.2 Storage

Store at 25°C (77°F); excursions permitted to 15-30°C (59-86°F) [see USP Controlled Room Temperature].

17 PATIENT COUNSELING INFORMATION

Patients and caregivers should be informed of the availability of a Medication Guide, and they should be instructed to read the Medication Guide prior to taking KEPPRA XR. The Medication Guide may also be found in the full prescribing information for KEPPRA XR posted on http://www.ucb-usa.com or by calling 1-866-822-0068. Patients should be instructed to take KEPPRA XR only as prescribed.

Patients, their caregivers, and families should be counseled that AEDs, including KEPPRA XR, may increase the risk of suicidal thoughts and behavior and should be advised of the need to be alert for the emergence or worsening of symptoms of depression, any unusual changes in mood or behav-

ior, or the emergence of suicidal thoughts, behavior, or thoughts about self-harm. Behaviors of concern should be reported immediately to healthcare providers.

Patients should be advised that KEPPRA XR may cause irritability and aggression. In addition, patients should be advised that they may experience changes in behavior that have been seen with other formulations of KEPPRA, which include agitation, anger, anxiety, apathy, depression, hostility, irritability and, in rare cases, psychotic symptoms.

Patients should be instructed to only take KEPPRA XR as prescribed and to swallow the tablets whole. They should not be chewed, broken, or crushed.

Patients should be advised to notify their physician if they become pregnant or intend to become pregnant during therapy. Patients should be encouraged to enroll in the NAAED Pregnancy Registry if they become pregnant. This registry is collecting information about the safety of antiepileptic drugs during pregnancy. To enroll, patients can call the toll free number 1-888-233-2334. UCB, Inc. has established the UCB AED Pregnancy Registry to advance scientific knowledge about safety and outcomes in pregnant women being treated with all UCB antiepileptic drugs including KEPPRA XR. To ensure broad program access and reach, either a healthcare provider or the patient can initiate enrollment in the UCB AED Pregnancy Registry by calling (888) 537-7734 (toll free) [see Use In Specific Populations (8.1)].

Patients should be advised that KEPPRA XR may cause dizziness and somnolence. Accordingly, patients should be advised not to drive or operate heavy machinery or engage in other hazardous activities until they have gained sufficient experience on KEPPRA XR to gauge whether it adversely affects their performance of these activities.

KEPPRA XR manufactured for
UCB, Inc.
Smyrna, GA 30080
KEPPRA XR is a registered trademark of the UCB Group of companies
© 2010, UCB, Inc., Smyrna, GA 30080
All rights reserved.
Printed in the U.S.A.

MEDICATION GUIDE

KEPPRA XR® (KEPP-ruh XR) (levetiracetam) extended-release tablets

Read this Medication Guide before you start taking KEPPRA XR and each time you get a refill. There may be new information. This information does not take the place of talking to your healthcare provider about your medical condition or treatment.

What is the most important information I should know about KEPPRA XR?

Like other antiepileptic drugs, KEPPRA XR may cause suicidal thoughts or actions in a very small number of people, about 1 in 500 people taking it.

Call a healthcare provider right away if you have any of these symptoms, especially if they are new, worse, or worry you:

- thoughts about suicide or dying
- attempts to commit suicide
- new or worse depression
- new or worse anxiety
- feeling agitated or restless
- panic attacks
- trouble sleeping (insomnia)
- new or worse irritability
- acting aggressive, being angry, or violent
- acting on dangerous impulses
- an extreme increase in activity and talking (mania)
- other unusual changes in behavior or mood

Do not stop KEPPRA XR without first talking to a healthcare provider.

- Stopping KEPPRA XR suddenly can cause serious problems. Stopping a seizure medicine suddenly can cause seizures that will not stop (status epilepticus).
- Suicidal thoughts or actions can be caused by things other than medicines. If you have suicidal thoughts or actions, your healthcare provider may check for other causes.

How can I watch for early symptoms of suicidal thoughts and actions?

- Pay attention to any changes, especially sudden changes, in mood, behaviors, thoughts, or feelings.
- Keep all follow-up visits with your healthcare provider as scheduled.
- Call your healthcare provider between visits as needed, especially if you are worried about symptoms.

What is KEPPRA XR?

KEPPRA XR is a prescription medicine taken by mouth that is used with other medicines to treat partial onset seizures in people 16 years of age and older with epilepsy.

It is not known if KEPPRA XR is safe or effective in people under 16 years of age.

Before taking your medicine, make sure you have received the correct medicine. Compare the name above with the name on your bottle and the appearance of your medicine with the description of KEPPRA XR provided below. Tell your pharmacist immediately if you think you have been given the wrong medicine.

500 mg KEPPRA XR tablets are white, oblong-shaped, film-coated tablets marked with "UCB 500XR" in red on one side.

750 mg KEPPRA XR tablets are white, oblong-shaped, film-coated tablets marked with "UCB 750XR" in red on one side.

What should I tell my healthcare provider before starting KEPPRA XR?

Before taking KEPPRA XR, tell your healthcare provider about all of your medical conditions, including if you:

- have or have had depression, mood problems or suicidal thoughts or behavior
- have kidney problems
- are pregnant or planning to become pregnant. It is not known if KEPPRA XR will harm your unborn baby. You and your healthcare provider will have to decide if you should take KEPPRA XR while you are pregnant. If you become pregnant while taking KEPPRA XR, talk to your healthcare provider about registering with the North American Antiepileptic Drug Pregnancy Registry. You can enroll in this registry by calling 1-888-233-2334. You can also enroll in the UCB AED Pregnancy Registry by calling 1-888-537-7734. The purpose of these registries is to collect information about the safety of KEPPRA XR and other antiepileptic medicine during pregnancy.
- are breast feeding. KEPPRA XR can pass into your milk and may harm your baby. You and your healthcare provider should discuss whether you should take KEPPRA XR or breast feed; you should not do both.

Tell your healthcare provider about all the medicines you take, including prescription and nonprescription medicines, vitamins, and herbal supplements. Do not start a new medicine without first talking with your healthcare provider.

Know the medicines you take. Keep a list of them to show your healthcare provider and pharmacist each time you get a new medicine.

How should I take KEPPRA XR?

Take KEPPRA XR exactly as prescribed.

- Your healthcare provider will tell you how much KEPPRA XR to take and when to take it. KEPPRA XR is usually taken once a day. Take KEPPRA XR at the same time each day.
- Your healthcare provider may change your dose. Do not change your dose without talking to your healthcare provider.
- Take KEPPRA XR with or without food.
- Swallow the tablets whole. Do not chew, break, or crush tablets.
- If you miss a dose of KEPPRA XR, take it as soon as you remember. If it is almost time for your next dose, just skip the missed dose. Take the next dose at your regular time. **Do not take two doses at the same time.**
- If you take too much KEPPRA XR, call your local Poison Control Center or go to the nearest emergency room right away.

What should I avoid while taking KEPPRA XR?

Do not drive, operate machinery or do other dangerous activities until you know how KEPPRA XR affects you. KEPPRA XR may make you dizzy or sleepy.

What are the possible side effects of KEPPRA XR?

- See "What is the most important information I should know about KEPPRA XR?"

KEPPRA XR can cause serious side effects.

Call your healthcare provider right away if you have any of these symptoms:

- mood and behavior changes such as aggression, agitation, anger, anxiety, apathy, mood swings, depression, hostility, and irritability. A few people may get psychotic symptoms such as hallucinations (seeing or hearing things that are really not there), delusions (false or strange thoughts or beliefs) and unusual behavior.
- extreme sleepiness, tiredness, and weakness
- problems with muscle coordination (problems walking and moving)

Common side effects seen in people who take KEPPRA XR and other formulations of KEPPRA include:

- sleepiness
- weakness
- dizziness
- infection

These side effects can happen at any time but happen more often within the first 4 weeks of treatment.

Tell your healthcare provider if you have any side effect that bothers you or that does not go away.

These are not all the possible side effects of KEPPRA XR. For more information, ask your healthcare provider or pharmacist.

Call your doctor for medical advice about side effects. You may also report side effects to FDA at 1-800-FDA-1088.

How should I store KEPPRA XR?

- Store KEPPRA XR at room temperature, 59°F to 86°F (15°C to 30°C) away from heat and light.

- **Keep KEPPRA XR and all medicines out of the reach of children.**

General information about KEPPRA XR.

Medicines are sometimes prescribed for purposes other than those listed in a Medication Guide. Do not use KEPPRA XR for a condition for which it was not prescribed. Do not give KEPPRA XR to other people, even if they have the same symptoms that you have. It may harm them.

This Medication Guide summarizes the most important information about KEPPRA XR. If you would like more information, talk with your healthcare provider. You can ask your pharmacist or healthcare provider for information about KEPPRA XR that is written for health professionals. You can also get information about KEPPRA XR at www.keppraxr.com or call 1-866-822-0068.

What are the ingredients of KEPPRA XR?

KEPPRA XR tablet active ingredient: levetiracetam

Inactive ingredients: colloidal anhydrous silica, hypromellose, magnesium stearate, polyethylene glycol 6000, polyvinyl alcohol-partially hydrolyzed, titanium dioxide (E171), Macrogol/PEG3350, and talc. The imprinting ink contains shellac, FD&C Red #40, n-butyl alcohol, propylene glycol, titanium dioxide, ethanol, and methanol.

KEPPRA XR does not contain lactose or gluten.

Rx Only

This Medication Guide has been approved by the US Food and Drug Administration.

Distributed by
UCB, Inc.
Smyrna, GA 30080
KEPPRA XR is a registered trademark of the UCB Group of companies

Printed in the U.S.A.
Rev. 2E 02/2010

METADATE CD® Ⓒ ℞

[mĕt-ă-dāt]
(methylphenidate HCl, USP)
Extended-Release Capsules

Once Daily

DESCRIPTION

METADATE CD is a central nervous system (CNS) stimulant. The extended-release capsules comprise both immediate-release (IR) and extended-release (ER) beads such that 30% of the dose is provided by the IR component and 70% of the dose is provided by the ER component. METADATE CD is available in six capsule strengths containing 10 mg (3 mg IR; 7 mg ER), 20 mg (6 mg IR; 14 mg ER), 30 mg (9 mg IR; 21 mg ER), 40 mg (12 mg IR; 28 mg ER), 50 mg (15 mg IR; 35 mg ER), or 60 mg (18 mg IR; 42 mg ER) of methylphenidate hydrochloride for oral administration.

Chemically, methylphenidate HCl is d,l (racemic)-$threo$-methyl α-phenyl-2-piperidineacetate hydrochloride. Its empirical formula is $C_{14}H_{19}NO_2 \cdot HCl$. Its structural formula is:

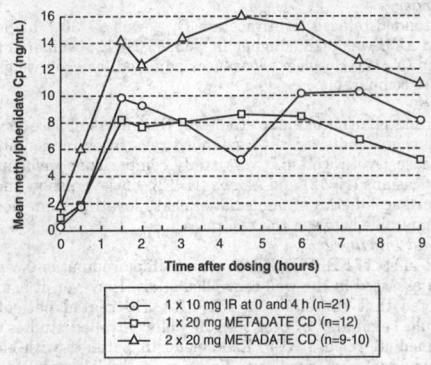

Methylphenidate HCl USP is a white, odorless, crystalline powder. Its solutions are acid to litmus. It is freely soluble in water and in methanol, soluble in alcohol, and slightly soluble in chloroform and in acetone. Its molecular weight is 269.77.

METADATE CD also contains the following inert ingredients: Sugar spheres, povidone, hydroxypropylmethylcellulose and polyethylene glycol, ethylcellulose aqueous dispersion, dibutyl sebacate, gelatin, and titanium dioxide.

The individual capsules contain the following color agents:

10 mg capsules: FD&C Blue No. 2, FDA/E172 Yellow Iron Oxide
20 mg capsules: FD&C Blue No. 2
30 mg capsules: FD&C Blue No. 2, FDA/E172 Red Iron Oxide
40 mg capsules: FDA/E172 Yellow Iron Oxide
50 mg capsules: FD&C Blue No. 2, FDA/E172 Red Iron Oxide

CLINICAL PHARMACOLOGY

Pharmacodynamics

Methylphenidate HCl is a central nervous system (CNS) stimulant. The mode of therapeutic action in Attention Deficit Hyperactivity Disorder (ADHD) is not known. Methylphenidate is thought to block the reuptake of norepinephrine and dopamine into the presynaptic neuron and increase the release of these monoamines into the extraneuronal space. Methylphenidate is a racemic mixture comprised of the d- and l-$threo$ enantiomers. The d-$threo$ enantiomer is more pharmacologically active than the l-$threo$ enantiomer.

Pharmacokinetics

The pharmacokinetics of the METADATE CD methylphenidate hydrochloride formulation have been studied in healthy adult volunteers and in children with Attention Deficit Hyperactivity Disorder (ADHD).

Absorption And Distribution

Methylphenidate is readily absorbed. METADATE CD has a plasma/time concentration profile showing two phases of drug release with a sharp, initial slope similar to a methylphenidate immediate-release tablet, and a second rising portion approximately three hours later, followed by a gradual decline. (See Figure 1 below.)

Comparison Of Immediate Release (IR) And METADATE CD Formulations After Repeated Doses Of Methylphenidate HCl In Children With ADHD

METADATE CD was administered as repeated once-daily doses of 20 mg or 40 mg to children aged 7-12 years with ADHD for one week. After a dose of 20 mg, the mean (±SD) early C_{max} was 8.6 (±2.2) ng/mL, the later C_{max} was 10.9 (±3.9)* ng/mL and AUC_{0-9h} was 63.0 (±16.8) ng•h/mL. The corresponding values after a 40 mg dose were 16.8 (±5.1) ng/mL, 15.1 (±5.8)* ng/mL and 120 (±39.6) ng•h/mL, respectively. The early peak concentrations (median) were reached about 1.5 hours after dose intake, and the second peak concentrations (median) were reached about 4.5 hours after dose intake. The means for C_{max} and AUC following a dose of 20 mg were slightly lower than those seen with 10 mg of the immediate-release formulation, dosed at 0 and 4 hours.

*25-30% of the subjects had only one observed peak (C_{max}) concentration of methylphenidate.

FIGURE 1

Comparison of Immediate Release (IR) and METADATE CD Formulations After Repeated Doses of Methylphenidate HCl in Children with ADHD

- ○— 1 × 10 mg IR at 0 and 4 h (n=21)
- □— 1 × 20 mg METADATE CD (n=12)
- △— 2 × 20 mg METADATE CD (n=9-10)

Dose Proportionality

Following single oral doses of 10-60 mg methylphenidate free base as a solution given to ten healthy male volunteers, C_{max} and AUC increased proportionally with increasing doses. After the 60 mg dose, t_{max} was reached 1.5 hours post-dose, with a mean C_{max} of 31.8 ng/mL (range 24.7-40.9 ng/mL).

Following one week of repeated once-daily doses of 20 mg or 40 mg METADATE CD to children aged 7-12 years with ADHD, C_{max} and AUC were proportional to the administered dose.

Food Effects

In a study in adult volunteers to investigate the effects of a high-fat meal on the bioavailability of a dose of 40 mg, the presence of food delayed the early peak by approximately 1 hour (range -2 to 5 hours delay). The plasma levels rose rapidly following the food-induced delay in absorption. Overall, a high-fat meal increased the C_{max} of METADATE CD by about 30% and AUC by about 17%, on average (see DOSAGE and ADMINISTRATION).

After a single dose, the bioavailability (C_{max} and AUC) of methylphenidate in 26 healthy adults was unaffected by sprinkling the capsule contents on applesauce as compared to the intact capsule. This finding demonstrates that a 20 mg METADATE CD Capsule, when opened and sprinkled on one tablespoon of applesauce, is bioequivalent to the intact capsule.

Metabolism And Excretion

In humans, methylphenidate is metabolized primarily via deesterification to alpha-phenyl-piperidine acetic acid (ritalinic acid). The metabolite has little or no pharmacologic activity.

In vitro studies showed that methylphenidate was not metabolized by cytochrome P450 isoenzymes, and did not inhibit cytochrome P450 isoenzymes at clinically observed plasma drug concentrations.

The mean terminal half-life ($t_{1/2}$) of methylphenidate following administration of METADATE CD ($t_{1/2}$=6.8h) is longer than the mean terminal ($t_{1/2}$) following administration of methylphenidate hydrochloride immediate-release tablets ($t_{1/2}$=2.9h) and methylphenidate hydrochloride sustained-release tablets ($t_{1/2}$=3.4h) in healthy adult volunteers. This suggests that the elimination process observed for METADATE CD is controlled by the release rate of methylphenidate from the extended-release formulation, and that the drug absorption is the rate-limiting process.

Special Populations

Gender

The pharmacokinetics of methylphenidate after a single dose of METADATE CD were similar between adult men and women.

Race

The influence of race on the pharmacokinetics of methylphenidate after METADATE CD administration has not been studied.

Age

The pharmacokinetics of methylphenidate after METADATE CD administration have not been studied in children less than 6 years of age.

Renal Insufficiency

There is no experience with the use of METADATE CD in patients with renal insufficiency. After oral administration of radiolabeled methylphenidate in humans, methylphenidate was extensively metabolized and approximately 80% of the radioactivity was excreted in the urine in the form of ritalinic acid. Since renal clearance is not an important route of methylphenidate clearance, renal insufficiency is expected to have little effect on the pharmacokinetics of METADATE CD.

Hepatic Insufficiency

There is no experience with the use of METADATE CD in patients with hepatic insufficiency.

CLINICAL STUDIES

METADATE CD was evaluated in a double-blind, parallel-group, placebo-controlled trial in which 321 untreated or previously treated pediatric patients with a DSM-IV diagnosis of Attention Deficit Hyperactivity Disorder (ADHD), 6 to 15 years of age, received a single morning dose for up to 3 weeks. Patients were required to have the combined or predominantly hyperactive-impulsive subtype of ADHD; patients with the predominantly inattentive subtype were excluded. Patients randomized to the METADATE CD group received 20 mg daily for the first week. Their dosage could be increased weekly to a maximum of 60 mg by the third week, depending on individual response to treatment.

The patient's regular school teacher completed the teachers' version of the Conners' Global Index Scale (TCGIS), a scale for assessing ADHD symptoms, in the morning and again in the afternoon on three alternate days of each treatment week. The change from baseline of the overall average (i.e., an average of morning and afternoon scores over 3 days) of the total TCGIS scores during the last week of treatment was analyzed as the primary efficacy parameter. Patients treated with METADATE CD showed a statistically significant improvement in symptom scores from baseline over patients who received placebo. (See Figure 2.) Separate analyses of TCGIS scores in the morning and afternoon revealed superiority in improvement with METADATE CD over placebo during both time periods. (See Figure 3.) This demonstrates that a single morning dose of METADATE CD exerts a treatment effect in both the morning and the afternoon.

FIGURE 2
Least Squares Mean Change from Baseline in TCGIS Scores*

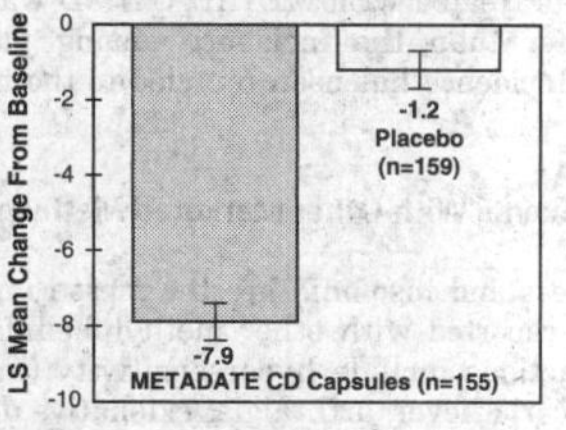

[See figure 3 at top of next column]

INDICATION AND USAGE

Attention Deficit Hyperactivity Disorder (ADHD)

METADATE CD (methylphenidate HCl, USP) Extended-Release Capsules are indicated for the treatment of Attention Deficit Hyperactivity Disorder (ADHD).

FIGURE 3
Least Squares Mean Change from Baseline in TCGIS Scores, Morning/Afternoon Groups*

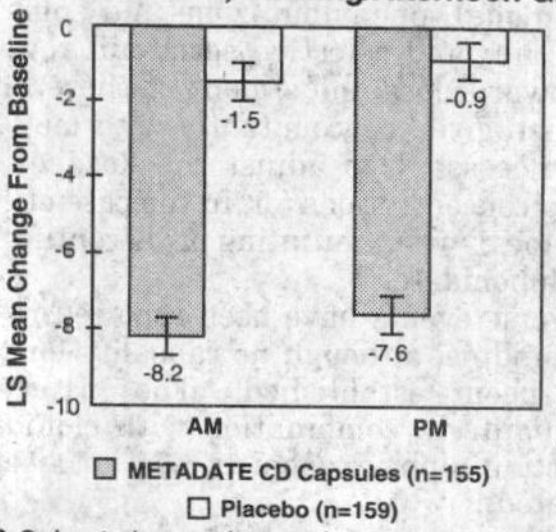

*FIGURES 2 & 3: Last observation carried forward analysis at week 3. Error bars represent the standard error of the mean.

The efficacy of METADATE CD in the treatment of ADHD was established in one controlled trial of children aged 6 to 15 who met DSM-IV criteria for ADHD (see CLINICAL PHARMACOLOGY).

A diagnosis of Attention Deficit Hyperactivity Disorder (ADHD; DSM-IV) implies the presence of hyperactive-impulsive or inattentive symptoms that caused impairment and were present before age 7 years. The symptoms must cause clinically significant impairment, e.g., in social, academic, or occupational functioning, and be present in two or more settings, e.g., school (or work) and at home. The symptoms must not be better accounted for by another mental disorder. For the Inattentive Type, at least six of the following symptoms must have persisted for at least 6 months: lack of attention to details/careless mistakes; lack of sustained attention; poor listener; failure to follow through on tasks; poor organization; avoids tasks requiring sustained mental effort; loses things; easily distracted; forgetful. For the Hyperactive-Impulsive Type, at least six of the following symptoms must have persisted for at least 6 months: fidgeting/squirming; leaving seat; inappropriate running/climbing; difficulty with quiet activities; "on the go;" excessive talking; blurting answers; can't wait turn; intrusive. The Combined Types requires both inattentive and hyperactive-impulsive criteria to be met.

Special Diagnostic Considerations

Specific etiology of this syndrome is unknown, and there is no single diagnostic test. Adequate diagnosis requires the use not only of medical but of special psychological, educational, and social resources. Learning may or may not be impaired. The diagnosis must be based upon a complete history and evaluation of the child and not solely on the presence of the required number of DSM-IV characteristics.

Need For Comprehensive Treatment Program

METADATE CD is indicated as an integral part of a total treatment program for ADHD that may include other measures (psychological, educational, social) for patients with this syndrome. Drug treatment may not be indicated for all children with this syndrome. Stimulants are not intended for use in the child who exhibits symptoms secondary to environmental factors and/or other primary psychiatric disorders, including psychosis. Appropriate educational placement is essential and psychosocial intervention is often helpful. When remedial measures alone are insufficient, the decision to prescribe stimulant medication will depend upon the physician's assessment of the chronicity and severity of the child's symptoms.

Long-Term Use

The effectiveness of METADATE CD for long-term use, i.e., for more than 3 weeks, has not been systematically evaluated in controlled trials. Therefore, the physician who elects to use METADATE CD for extended periods should periodically re-evaluate the long-term usefulness of the drug for the individual patient (see DOSAGE and ADMINISTRATION).

CONTRAINDICATIONS

Agitation

METADATE CD is contraindicated in patients with marked anxiety, tension and agitation, since the drug may aggravate these symptoms.

Hypersensitivity To Methylphenidate Or Other Excipients

METADATE CD is contraindicated in patients known to be hypersensitive to methylphenidate or other components of the product.

METADATE CD contains sucrose. Therefore, patients with rare hereditary problems of fructose intolerance, glucose-galactose malabsorption, or sucrase-isomaltase insufficiency should not take this medicine.

Glaucoma

METADATE CD is contraindicated in patients with glaucoma.

Tics

METADATE CD is contraindicated in patients with motor tics or with a family history or diagnosis of Tourette's syndrome (see ADVERSE REACTIONS).

Monoamine Oxidase Inhibitors

METADATE CD is contraindicated during treatment with monoamine oxidase inhibitors, and also within a minimum of 14 days following discontinuation of a monoamine oxidase inhibitor (hypertensive crises may result).

Hypertension And Other Cardiovascular Conditions

METADATE CD is contraindicated in patients with severe hypertension, angina pectoris, cardiac arrhythmias, heart failure, recent myocardial infarction, hyperthyroidism or thyrotoxicosis (see WARNINGS).

Halogenated Anesthetics

There is a risk of sudden blood pressure increase during surgery. If surgery is planned, METADATE CD should not be taken on the day of the surgery.

WARNINGS

Serious Cardiovascular Events

Sudden Death And Pre-existing Structural Cardiac Abnormalities Or Other Serious Heart Problems

Children And Adolescents

Sudden death has been reported in association with CNS stimulant treatment at usual doses in children and adolescents with structural cardiac abnormalities or other serious heart problems. Although some serious heart problems alone carry an increased risk of sudden death, stimulant products generally should not be used in children or adolescents with known serious structural cardiac abnormalities, cardiomyopathy, serious heart rhythm abnormalities, or other serious cardiac problems that may place them at increased vulnerability to the sympathomimetic effects of a stimulant drug (see CONTRAINDICATIONS).

Adults

Sudden deaths, stroke, and myocardial infarction have been reported in adults taking stimulant drugs at usual doses for ADHD. Although the role of stimulants in these adult cases is also unknown, adults have a greater likelihood than children of having serious structural cardiac abnormalities, cardiomyopathy, serious heart rhythm abnormalities, coronary artery disease, or other serious cardiac problems. Adults with such abnormalities should also generally not be treated with stimulant drugs (see CONTRAINDICATIONS).

Hypertension And Other Cardiovascular Conditions

Stimulant medications cause a modest increase in average blood pressure (about 2-4 mmHg) and average heart rate (about 3-6 bpm), and individuals may have larger increases. While the mean changes alone would not be expected to have short-term consequences, all patients should be monitored for larger changes in heart rate and blood pressure. Caution is indicated in treating patients whose underlying medical conditions might be compromised by increases in blood pressure or heart rate, e.g., those with pre-existing hypertension, heart failure, recent myocardial infarction, or ventricular arrhythmia (see CONTRAINDICATIONS).

Assessing Cardiovascular Status In Patients Being Treated With Stimulant Medications

Children, adolescents, or adults who are being considered for treatment with stimulant medications should have a careful history (including assessment for a family history of sudden death or ventricular arrhythmia) and physical exam to assess for the presence of cardiac disease, and should receive further cardiac evaluation if findings suggest such disease (e.g., electrocardiogram and echocardiogram). Patients who develop symptoms such as exertional chest pain, unexplained syncope, or other symptoms suggestive of cardiac disease during stimulant treatment should undergo a prompt cardiac evaluation.

Psychiatric Adverse Events

Pre-Existing Psychosis

Administration of stimulants may exacerbate symptoms of behavior disturbance and thought disorder in patients with a pre-existing psychotic disorder.

Bipolar Illness

Particular care should be taken in using stimulants to treat ADHD in patients with comorbid bipolar disorder because of concern for possible induction of a mixed/manic episode in such patients. Prior to initiating treatment with a stimulant, patients with comorbid depressive symptoms should be adequately screened to determine if they are at risk for bipolar disorder; such screening should include a detailed psychiatric history, including a family history of suicide, bipolar disorder, and depression.

Emergence Of New Psychotic Or Manic Symptoms

Treatment emergent psychotic or manic symptoms, e.g., hallucinations, delusional thinking, or mania in children and adolescents without prior history of psychotic illness or mania can be caused by stimulants at usual doses. If such symptoms occur, consideration should be given to a possible causal role of the stimulant, and discontinuation of treatment may be appropriate. In a pooled analysis of multiple short-term, placebo-controlled studies, such symptoms occurred in about 0.1% (4 patients with events out of 3482 exposed to methylphenidate or amphetamine for several weeks at usual doses) of stimulant-treated patients compared to 0 in placebo-treated patients.

Aggression

Aggressive behavior or hostility is often observed in children and adolescents with ADHD, and has been reported in clinical trials and the postmarketing experience of some medications indicated for the treatment of ADHD. Although there is no systematic evidence that stimulants cause aggressive behavior or hostility, patients beginning treatment for ADHD should be monitored for the appearance of or worsening of aggressive behavior or hostility.

Long-Term Suppression Of Growth

Careful follow-up of weight and height in children ages 7 to 10 years who were randomized to either methylphenidate or non-medication treatment groups over 14 months, as well as in naturalistic subgroups of newly methylphenidate-treated and non-medication treated children over 36 months (to the ages of 10 to 13 years), suggests that consistently medicated children (i.e., treatment for 7 days per week throughout the year) have a temporary slowing in growth rate (on average, a total of about 2 cm less growth in height and 2.7 kg less growth in weight over 3 years), without evidence of growth rebound during this period of development. Published data are inadequate to determine whether chronic use of amphetamines may cause a similar suppression of growth, however, it is anticipated that they likely have this effect as well. Therefore, growth should be monitored during treatment with stimulants, and patients who are not growing or gaining height or weight as expected may need to have their treatment interrupted.

Seizures

There is some clinical evidence that stimulants may lower the convulsive threshold in patients with prior history of seizures, in patients with prior EEG abnormalities in absence of seizures, and, very rarely, in patients without a history of seizures and no prior EEG evidence of seizures. In the presence of seizures, the drug should be discontinued.

Visual Disturbance

Difficulties with accommodation and blurring of vision have been reported with stimulant treatment.

Use In Children Under Six Years Of Age

METADATE CD should not be used in children under six years, since safety and efficacy in this age group have not been established.

Drug Dependence

METADATE CD should be given cautiously to patients with a history of drug dependence or alcoholism. Chronic abusive use can lead to marked tolerance and psychological dependence with varying degrees of abnormal behavior. Frank psychotic episodes can occur, especially with parenteral abuse. Careful supervision is required during withdrawal from abusive use since severe depression may occur. Withdrawal following chronic therapeutic use may unmask symptoms of the underlying disorder that may require follow-up.

PRECAUTIONS

Hematologic Monitoring

Periodic CBC, differential, and platelet counts are advised during prolonged therapy.

Drug Testing

METADATE CD contains methylphenidate which may result in a positive result during drug testing.

Information For Patients

Patients should be instructed to take one dose in the morning before breakfast. The patients should be instructed that the capsule may be swallowed whole, or alternatively, the capsule may be opened and the capsule contents sprinkled onto a small amount (tablespoon) of applesauce and given immediately, and not stored for future use. The capsules and the capsule contents must not be crushed or chewed.

Prescribers or other health professionals should inform patients, their families, and their caregivers about the benefits and risks associated with treatment with methylphenidate and should counsel them in its appropriate use. A patient Medication Guide is available for Metadate CD. The prescriber or healthcare professional should instruct patients, their families, and their caregivers to read the Medication Guide and should assist them in understanding its contents. Patients should be given the opportunity to discuss the contents of the Medication Guide and to obtain answers to any questions they may have. The complete text of the Medication Guide is reprinted at the end of this document. The Medication Guide may also be found in the full prescribing information for METADATE CD on http://ucb-group.com/products/cns/equasym-metadate/ or by calling 1-866-822-0068.

Drug Interactions

Because of possible effects on blood pressure, METADATE CD should be used cautiously with pressor agents.

Human pharmacologic studies have shown that methylphenidate may inhibit the metabolism of coumarin anticoagulants, anticonvulsants (e.g., phenobarbital, phenytoin, primidone), phenylbutazone and some antidepressants (tricyclics and selective serotonin reuptake inhibitors). Downward dose adjustment of these drugs may be required when given concomitantly with methylphenidate. It may be necessary to adjust the dosage and monitor plasma drug concentrations (or, in the case of coumarin, coagulation times), when initiating or discontinuing concomitant methylphenidate.

Serious adverse events have been reported in concomitant use with clonidine, although no causality for the combination has been established. The safety of using methylphenidate in combination with clonidine or other centrally acting alpha-2 agonists has not been systematically evaluated.

In theory, there is a possibility that the clearance of methylphenidate might be affected by urinary pH, either being increased with acidifying agents or decreased with alkalizing agents. This should be considered when methylphenidate is given in combination with agents that alter urinary pH.

Halogenated Anesthetics

There is a risk of sudden blood pressure increase during surgery. If surgery is planned, METADATE CD should not be taken the day of the surgery.

Carcinogenesis, Mutagenesis, And Impairment Of Fertility

In a lifetime carcinogenicity study carried out in B6C3F1 mice, methylphenidate caused an increase in hepatocellular adenomas and, in males only, an increase in hepatoblastomas, at a daily dose of approximately 60 mg/kg/day. This dose is approximately 30 times and 4 times the maximum recommended human dose of METADATE CD on a mg/kg and mg/m^2 basis, respectively. Hepatoblastoma is a relatively rare rodent malignant tumor type. There was no increase in total malignant hepatic tumors. The mouse strain used is sensitive to the development of hepatic tumors, and the significance of these results to humans is unknown.

Methylphenidate did not cause any increases in tumors in a lifetime carcinogenicity study carried out in F344 rats; the highest dose used was approximately 45 mg/kg/day, which is approximately 22 times and 5 times the maximum recommended human dose of METADATE CD on a mg/kg and mg/m^2 basis, respectively.

In a 24-week carcinogenicity study in the transgenic mouse strain p53+/-, which is sensitive to genotoxic carcinogens, there was no evidence of carcinogenicity. Male and female mice were fed diets containing the same concentration of methylphenidate as in the lifetime carcinogenicity study; the high-dose groups were exposed to 60 to 74 mg/kg/day of methylphenidate.

Methylphenidate was not mutagenic in the *in vitro* Ames reverse mutation assay or in the *in vitro* mouse lymphoma cell forward mutation assay. Sister chromatid exchanges and chromosome aberrations were increased, indicative of a weak clastogenic response, in an *in vitro* assay in cultured Chinese Hamster Ovary cells. Methylphenidate was negative *in vivo* in males and females in the mouse bone marrow micronucleus assay.

Methylphenidate did not impair fertility in male or female mice that were fed diets containing the drug in an 18-week Continuous Breeding study. The study was conducted at doses up to 160 mg/kg/day, approximately 80-fold and 8-fold the highest recommended human dose of METADATE CD on a mg/kg and mg/m^2 basis, respectively.

Pregnancy

Teratogenic Effects

Pregnancy Category C

Methylphenidate has been shown to have teratogenic effects in rabbits when given in doses of 200 mg/kg/day, which is approximately 100 times and 40 times the maximum recommended human dose on a mg/kg and mg/m^2 basis, respectively.

A reproduction study in rats revealed no evidence of teratogenicity at an oral dose of 58 mg/kg/day. However, this dose, which caused some maternal toxicity, resulted in decreased postnatal pup weights and survival when given to the dams from day one of gestation through the lactation period. This dose is approximately 30 fold and 6 fold the maximum recommended human dose of METADATE CD on a mg/kg and mg/m^2 basis, respectively.

There are no adequate and well-controlled studies in pregnant women. METADATE CD should be used during pregnancy only if the potential benefit justifies the potential risk to the fetus.

Nursing Mothers

It is not known whether methylphenidate is excreted in human milk. Because many drugs are excreted in human milk, caution should be exercised if METADATE CD is administered to a nursing woman.

Pediatric Use

The safety and efficacy of METADATE CD in children under 6 years old have not been established. Long-term effects of methylphenidate in children have not been well established (see WARNINGS).

ADVERSE REACTIONS

The premarketing development program for METADATE CD included exposures in a total of 228 participants in clinical trials (188 pediatric patients with ADHD, 40 healthy adult subjects). These participants received METADATE CD 20, 40, and/or 60 mg/day. The 188 patients (ages 6 to 15) were evaluated in one controlled clinical study, one controlled, crossover clinical study, and one uncontrolled clinical study. Safety data on all patients are included in the discussion that follows. Adverse reactions were assessed by collecting adverse events, results of physical examinations, vital signs, weights, laboratory analyses, and ECGs.

Adverse events during exposure were obtained primarily by general inquiry and recorded by clinical investigators using terminology of their own choosing. Consequently, it is not possible to provide a meaningful estimate of the proportion of individuals experiencing adverse events without first grouping similar types of events into a smaller number of standardized event categories. In the tables and listings that follow, COSTART terminology has been used to classify reported adverse events.

The stated frequencies of adverse events represent the proportion of individuals who experienced, at least once, a treatment-emergent adverse event of the type listed. An event was considered treatment emergent if it occurred for the first time or worsened while receiving therapy following baseline evaluation.

Adverse Findings In Clinical Trials With METADATE CD

Adverse Events Associated With Discontinuation Of Treatment

In the 3-week placebo-controlled, parallel-group trial, two METADATE CD-treated patients (1%) and no placebo-treated patients discontinued due to an adverse event (rash and pruritus; and headache, abdominal pain, and dizziness, respectively).

Adverse Events Occurring At An Incidence Of 5% Or More Among METADATE CD-Treated Patients

Table 1 enumerates, for a pool of the three studies in pediatric patients with ADHD, at METADATE CD doses of 20, 40, or 60 mg/day, the incidence of treatment-emergent adverse events. One study was a 3-week placebo-controlled, parallel-group trial, one study was a controlled, crossover trial, and the third study was an open titration trial. The table includes only those events that occurred in 5% or more of patients treated with METADATE CD where the incidence in patients treated with METADATE CD was greater than the incidence in placebo-treated patients.

The prescriber should be aware that these figures cannot be used to predict the incidence of adverse events in the course of usual medical practice where patient characteristics and other factors differ from those which prevailed in the clinical trials. Similarly, the cited frequencies cannot be compared with figures obtained from other clinical investigations involving different treatments, uses, and investigators. The cited figures, however, do provide the prescribing physician with some basis for estimating the relative contribution of drug and non-drug factors to the adverse event incidence rate in the population studied.

TABLE 1 Incidence of Treatment-Emergent Events[1] in a Pool of 3-4 Week Clinical Trials of METADATE CD

Body System	Preferred Term	METADATE CD (n=188)	Placebo (n=190)
General	Headache	12%	8%
	Abdominal pain (stomach ache)	7%	4%
Digestive System	Anorexia (loss of appetite)	9%	2%
Nervous System	Insomnia	5%	2%

[1] : Events, regardless of causality, for which the incidence for patients treated with METADATE CD was at least 5% and greater than the incidence among placebo-treated patients. Incidence has been rounded to the nearest whole number.

Adverse Events With Other Marketed Methylphenidate HCl Products

Nervousness and insomnia are the most common adverse reactions reported with other methylphenidate products. Other reactions include hypersensitivity (including skin rash, urticaria, fever, arthralgia, exfoliative dermatitis, erythema multiforme with histopathological findings of necrotizing vasculitis, and thrombocytopenic purpura); anorexia; nausea; dizziness; palpitations; headache; dyskinesia; drowsiness; blood pressure and pulse changes, both up and down; tachycardia; angina; cardiac arrhythmia; abdominal pain; weight loss during prolonged therapy. There have been rare reports of Tourette's Syndrome and obsessive-compulsive disorder. Toxic psychosis has been reported.

Although a definite causal relationship has not been established, the following have been reported in patients taking this drug: instances of abnormal liver function, ranging from transaminase elevation to hepatic coma; isolated cases of cerebral arteritis and/or occlusion; leucopenia and/or anemia; transient depressed mood; a few instances of scalp hair loss. Very rare reports of neuroleptic malignant syndrome (NMS) have been reported, and, in most of these, patients were concurrently receiving therapies associated with NMS. In a single report, a ten year old boy who had been taking methylphenidate for approximately 18 months experienced an NMS-like event within 45 minutes of ingesting his first dose of venlafaxine. It is uncertain whether this case represented a drug-drug interaction, a response to either drug alone, or some other cause.

In children, loss of appetite, abdominal pain, weight loss during prolonged therapy, insomnia and tachycardia may occur more frequently; however, any of the other adverse reactions listed above may also occur.

Postmarketing Experience

In addition to the adverse events listed above, the following have been reported in patients receiving METADATE CD worldwide. The list is alphabetized: abnormal behavior, aggression, anxiety, cardiac arrest, depression, fixed drug eruption, hyperactivity, irritability, migraine, obsessive-compulsive disorder, peripheral coldness, Raynaud's phenomenon, reversible ischaemic neurological deficit, sudden death, suicidal behavior (including completed suicide), and thrombocytopenia. Data are insufficient to support an estimation of incidence or establish causation.

DRUG ABUSE AND DEPENDENCE

Controlled Substance Class

METADATE CD, like other methylphenidate products, is classified as a Schedule II controlled substance by federal regulation.

Abuse, Dependence, And Tolerance

See WARNINGS for boxed warning containing drug abuse and dependence information.

OVERDOSAGE

Signs And Symptoms

Signs and symptoms of acute methylphenidate overdosage, resulting principally from overstimulation of the CNS and from excessive sympathomimetic effects, may include the following: vomiting, agitation, tremors, hyperreflexia, muscle twitching, convulsions (may be followed by coma), euphoria, confusion, hallucinations, delirium, sweating, flushing, headache, hyperpyrexia, tachycardia, palpitations, cardiac arrhythmias, hypertension, mydriasis, and dryness of mucous membranes.

Recommended Treatment

Treatment consists of appropriate supportive measures. The patient must be protected against self-injury and against external stimuli that would aggravate overstimulation already present. Gastric contents may be evacuated by gastric lavage as indicated. Before performing gastric lavage, control agitation and seizures if present and protect the airway. Other measures to detoxify the gut include administration of activated charcoal and a cathartic. Intensive care must be provided to maintain adequate circulation and respiratory exchange; external cooling procedures may be required for hyperpyrexia.

Efficacy of peritoneal dialysis or extracorporeal hemodialysis for METADATE CD overdosage has not been established.

The prolonged release of methylphenidate from METADATE CD should be considered when treating patients with overdose.

Poison Control Center

As with the management of all overdosage, the possibility of multiple drug ingestion should be considered. The physician may wish to consider contacting a poison control center for up-to-date information on the management of overdosage with methylphenidate.

DOSAGE AND ADMINISTRATION

METADATE CD is administered once daily in the morning, before breakfast.

METADATE CD may be swallowed whole with the aid of liquids, or alternatively, the capsule may be opened and the capsule contents sprinkled onto a small amount (tablespoon) of applesauce and given immediately, and not stored for future use. Drinking some fluids, e.g. water, should follow the intake of the sprinkles with applesauce. The capsules and the capsule contents must not be crushed or chewed (see PRECAUTIONS: Information for Patients).

Dosage should be individualized according to the needs and responses of the patient.

Initial Treatment

The recommended starting dose of METADATE CD is 20 mg once daily. Dosage may be adjusted in weekly 10-20 mg increments to a maximum of 60 mg/day taken once daily in the morning, depending upon tolerability and degree of efficacy observed. Daily dosage above 60 mg is not recommended.

Maintenance/Extended Treatment

There is no body of evidence available from controlled trials to indicate how long the patient with ADHD should be treated with METADATE CD. It is generally agreed, however, that pharmacological treatment of ADHD may be needed for extended periods. Nevertheless, the physician who elects to use METADATE CD for extended periods in patients with ADHD should periodically re-evaluate the long-term usefulness of the drug for the individual patient with trials off medication to assess the patient's functioning without pharmacotherapy. Improvement may be sustained when the drug is either temporarily or permanently discontinued.

Dose Reduction And Discontinuation

If paradoxical aggravation of symptoms or other adverse events occur, the dosage should be reduced, or, if necessary, the drug should be discontinued.

If improvement is not observed after appropriate dosage adjustment over a one-month period, the drug should be discontinued.

HOW SUPPLIED

METADATE CD (methylphenidate HCl, USP) Extended-Release Capsules are available in six strengths:

10 mg, green/white capsules, imprinted with "UCB 579" in white letters on the green cap, and "10 mg" in black letters on the white body of the capsule.
NDC 53014-579-07   Bottle of 100 Capsules
20 mg, blue/white capsules, imprinted with "UCB 580" in white letters on the blue cap, and "20 mg" in black letters on the white body of the capsule.
NDC 53014-580-07   Bottle of 100 Capsules
30 mg, reddish-brown/white capsules, imprinted with "UCB 581" in white letters on the reddish-brown cap, and "30 mg" in black letters on the white body of the capsule.
NDC 53014-581-07   Bottle of 100 Capsules
40 mg, yellow ivory/white capsules, imprinted with "UCB 582" in black letters on the yellow ivory cap, and "40 mg" in black letters on the white body of the capsule.
NDC 53014-582-07   Bottle of 100 Capsules
50 mg, purple/white capsules, imprinted with "UCB 583" in white letters on the purple cap, and "50 mg" in black letters on the white body of the capsule.
NDC 53014-583-07   Bottle of 100 Capsules
60 mg, white/white capsules, imprinted with "UCB 584" in black letters on the white cap, and "60 mg" in black letters on the white body of the capsule.
NDC 53014-584-07   Bottle of 100 Capsules
Store at 25°C (77°F); excursions permitted to 15°-30°C (59°-86°F) [See USP Controlled Room Temperature].
Keep out of the reach of children.

REFERENCE

American Psychiatric Association. *Diagnostic and Statistical Manual of Mental Disorders.* American Psychiatric Association 1994. 4th ed. Washington D.C.

For Medical Information

Contact: Medical Affairs Department
Phone: (866) 822-0068
Fax: (770) 970-8859
Marketed by UCB, Inc.
Smyrna, GA 30080
Manufactured by UCB Manufacturing, Inc.
Rochester, NY 14623
8E 08/2008
METADATE CD is a registered trademark of the UCB Group of companies
©2008, UCB, Inc., Smyrna, GA 30080
All rights reserved. Printed in U.S.A.

MEDICATION GUIDE

METADATE CD® (methylphenidate HCl, USP) Extended-Release Capsules CII

Read the Medication Guide that comes with METADATE CD before you or your child starts taking it and each time you get a refill. There may be new information. This Medication Guide does not take the place of talking to your doctor about your or your child's treatment with METADATE CD.

What is the most important information I should know about Metadate CD?
The following have been reported with use of methylphenidate HCl, USP and other stimulant medicines.
1. **Heart-related problems:**
   - **sudden death in patients who have heart problems or heart defects**
   - **stroke and heart attack in adults**
   - **increased blood pressure and heart rate**
Tell your doctor if you or your child have any heart problems, heart defects, high blood pressure, or a family history of these problems.

Your doctor should check you or your child carefully for heart problems before starting METADATE CD.
Your doctor should check your or your child's blood pressure and heart rate regularly during treatment with METADATE CD.
Call your doctor right away if you or your child has any signs of heart problems such as chest pain, shortness of breath, or fainting while taking METADATE CD.
2. **Mental (Psychiatric) problems:**
All Patients
   - **new or worse behavior and thought problems**
   - **new or worse bipolar illness**
   - **new or worse aggressive behavior or hostility**
Children and Teenagers
   - **new psychotic symptoms (such as hearing voices, believing things that are not true, are suspicious) or new manic symptoms**
Tell your doctor about any mental problems you or your child have, or about a family history of suicide, bipolar illness, or depression.
Call your doctor right away if you or your child have any new or worsening mental symptoms or problems while taking METADATE CD, especially seeing or hearing things that are not real, believing things that are not real, or are suspicious.

What Is METADATE CD?

METADATE CD is a central nervous system stimulant prescription medicine. **It is used for the treatment of Attention-Deficit Hyperactivity Disorder (ADHD).**
METADATE CD may help increase attention and decrease impulsiveness and hyperactivity in patients with ADHD.
METADATE CD should be used as a part of a total treatment program for ADHD that may include counseling or other therapies.

METADATE CD is a federally controlled substance (CII) because it can be abused or lead to dependence. Keep METADATE CD in a safe place to prevent misuse and abuse. Selling or giving away METADATE CD may harm others, and is against the law.
Tell your doctor if you or your child have (or have a family history of) ever abused or been dependent on alcohol, prescription medicines or street drugs.

Who should not take METADATE CD?

METADATE CD should not be taken if you or your child:
- are very anxious, tense, or agitated
- have an eye problem called glaucoma
- have tics or Tourette's syndrome, or a family history of Tourette's syndrome. Tics are hard to control repeated movements or sounds.
- have severe high blood pressure or a heart problem
- have hyperthyroidism
- are taking or have taken within the past 14 days an antidepression medicine called a monoamine oxidase inhibitor or MAOI.
- are allergic to anything in METADATE CD. See the end of this Medication Guide for a complete list of ingredients.
METADATE CD should not be used in children less than 6 years old because it has not been studied in this age group.
METADATE CD may not be right for you or your child. Before starting METADATE CD tell your or your child's doctor about all health conditions (or a family history of) including:
- heart problems, heart defects, high blood pressure
- mental problems including psychosis, mania, bipolar illness, or depression
- tics or Tourette's syndrome
- seizures or have had an abnormal brain wave test (EEG)
Tell your doctor if you or your child is pregnant, planning to become pregnant, or breastfeeding.
Can METADATE CD be taken with other medicines?
Tell your doctor about all of the medicines that you or your child take including prescription and nonprescription medicines, vitamins, and herbal supplements. METADATE CD and some medicines may interact with each other and cause serious side effects. Sometimes the doses of other medicines will need to be adjusted while taking METADATE CD.
Your doctor will decide whether METADATE CD can be taken with other medicines.
Especially tell your doctor if you or your child takes:
- anti-depression medicines including MAOIs
- seizure medicines
- blood thinner medicines
- blood pressure medicines
- cold or allergy medicines that contain decongestants
Know the medicines that you or your child takes. Keep a list of your medicines with you to show your doctor and pharmacist.

Do not start any new medicine while taking METADATE CD without talking to your doctor first.

How should METADATE CD be taken?

- **Take METADATE CD exactly as prescribed.** Your doctor may adjust the dose until it is right for you or your child.
- Take METADATE CD once each day in the morning before breakfast. METADATE CD is an extended release capsule. It releases medicine into your body throughout the day.
- METADATE CD can be taken with or without food.
- Swallow METADATE CD capsules whole with water or other liquids. If you cannot swallow the capsule, open it and sprinkle the medicine over a spoonful of applesauce. Swallow the applesauce and medicine mixture without chewing. Follow with a drink of water or other liquid. **Never chew or crush the capsule or the medicine inside the capsule.**
- From time to time, your doctor may stop METADATE CD treatment for a while to check ADHD symptoms.
- Your doctor may do regular checks of the blood, heart, and blood pressure while taking METADATE CD. Children should have their height and weight checked often while taking METADATE CD. METADATE CD treatment may be stopped if a problem is found during these check-ups.
- If you or your child takes too much METADATE CD or overdoses, call your doctor or poison control center right away, or get emergency treatment.

What are possible side effects of METADATE CD?

See "What is the most important information I should know about METADATE CD?" for information on reported heart and mental problems.

Other serious side effects include:
- slowing of growth (height and weight) in children
- seizures, mainly in patients with a history of seizures
- eyesight changes or blurred vision

Common side effects include:
- headache
- decreased appetite
- stomach ache
- nervousness
- trouble sleeping
- dizziness

Talk to your doctor if you or your child has side effects that are bothersome or do not go away.

This is not a complete list of possible side effects. Ask your doctor or pharmacist for more information

Call your doctor for medical advice about side effects. You may report side effects to FDA at 1-800-FDA-1088.

How should I store METADATE CD?

- Store METADATE CD in a safe place at room temperature, 59 to 86° F (15 to 30° C). Protect from moisture.
- **Keep METADATE CD and all medicines out of the reach of children.**

General information about METADATE CD

Medicines are sometimes prescribed for purposes other than those listed in a Medication Guide. Do not use METADATE CD for a condition for which it was not prescribed. Do not give METADATE CD to other people, even if they have the same condition. It may harm them and it is against the law.

This Medication Guide summarizes the most important information about METADATE CD. If you would like more information, talk with your doctor. You can ask your doctor or pharmacist for information about METADATE CD that was written for healthcare professionals. For more information about METADATE CD call 1-866-822-0068.

What are the ingredients in METADATE CD?

Active Ingredient: methylphenidate HCl

Inactive Ingredients: sugar spheres, povidone, hydroxypropylmethylcellulose and polyethylene glycol, ethylcellulose aqueous dispersion, dibutyl sebacate, gelatin, and titanium dioxide.

The individual capsules contain the following coloring agents:

10 mg capsules: FD&C Blue No. 2, FDA/E172 Yellow Iron Oxide

20 mg capsules: FD&C Blue No. 2

30 mg capsules: FD&C Blue No. 2, FDA/E172 Red Iron Oxide

40 mg capsules: FDA/E172 Yellow Iron Oxide

50 mg capsules: FD&C Blue No. 2, FDA/E172 Red Iron Oxide

This Medication Guide has been approved by the U.S. Food and Drug Administration.

Marketed by UCB, Inc.

Smyrna, GA 30080

Manufactured by UCB Manufacturing, Inc.

Rochester, NY 14623

METADATE CD is a registered trademark of the UCB Group of companies

2E 06/2009

TUSSIONEX® PENNKINETIC®   ℂⅢ ℞

[tu-sē-ō-něks pěn-kĭ-nětĭk]

(hydrocodone polistirex and chlorpheniramine polistirex) Extended-Release Suspension

DESCRIPTION

Each teaspoonful (5 mL) of TUSSIONEX Pennkinetic Extended-Release Suspension contains hydrocodone polistirex equivalent to 10 mg of hydrocodone bitartrate and chlorpheniramine polistirex equivalent to 8 mg of chlorpheniramine maleate. TUSSIONEX Pennkinetic Extended-Release Suspension provides up to 12-hour relief per dose. Hydrocodone is a centrally-acting narcotic antitussive. Chlorpheniramine is an antihistamine. TUSSIONEX Pennkinetic Extended-Release Suspension is for oral use only.

Hydrocodone Polistirex

Sulfonated styrene-divinylbenzene copolymer complex with $4,5\alpha$-epoxy-3-methoxy-17-methylmorphinan-6-one.

Chlorpheniramine Polistirex

Sulfonated styrene-divinylbenzene copolymer complex with 2-[p-chloro-α-[2-(dimethylamino)ethyl]-benzyl]pyridine.

Inactive Ingredients

Ascorbic acid, D&C Yellow No. 10, ethylcellulose, FD&C Yellow No. 6, flavor, high fructose corn syrup, methylparaben, polyethylene glycol 3350, polysorbate 80, pregelatinized starch, propylene glycol, propylparaben, purified water, sucrose, vegetable oil, xanthan gum.

CLINICAL PHARMACOLOGY

Hydrocodone is a semisynthetic narcotic antitussive and analgesic with multiple actions qualitatively similar to those of codeine. The precise mechanism of action of hydrocodone and other opiates is not known; however, hydrocodone is believed to act directly on the cough center. In excessive doses, hydrocodone, like other opium derivatives, will depress respiration. The effects of hydrocodone in therapeutic doses on the cardiovascular system are insignificant. Hydrocodone can produce miosis, euphoria, and physical and psychological dependence.

Chlorpheniramine is an antihistamine drug (H_1 receptor antagonist) that also possesses anticholinergic and sedative activity. It prevents released histamine from dilating capillaries and causing edema of the respiratory mucosa.

Hydrocodone release from TUSSIONEX Pennkinetic Extended-Release Suspension is controlled by the Pennkinetic System, an extended-release drug delivery system, which combines an ion-exchange polymer matrix with a diffusion rate-limiting permeable coating. Chlorpheniramine release is prolonged by use of an ion-exchange polymer system.

Following multiple dosing with TUSSIONEX Pennkinetic Extended-Release Suspension, hydrocodone mean (S.D.) peak plasma concentrations of 22.8 (5.9) ng/mL occurred at 3.4 hours. Chlorpheniramine mean (S.D.) peak plasma concentrations of 58.4 (14.7) ng/mL occurred at 6.3 hours following multiple dosing. Peak plasma levels obtained with an immediate-release syrup occurred at approximately 1.5 hours for hydrocodone and 2.8 hours for chlorpheniramine. The plasma half-lives of hydrocodone and chlorpheniramine have been reported to be approximately 4 and 16 hours, respectively.

INDICATIONS AND USAGE

TUSSIONEX Pennkinetic Extended-Release Suspension is indicated for relief of cough and upper respiratory symptoms associated with allergy or a cold in adults and children 6 years of age and older.

CONTRAINDICATIONS

TUSSIONEX Pennkinetic Extended-Release Suspension is contraindicated in patients with a known allergy or sensitivity to hydrocodone or chlorpheniramine.

The use of TUSSIONEX Pennkinetic Extended-Release Suspension is contraindicated in children less than 6 years of age due to the risk of fatal respiratory depression.

WARNINGS

Respiratory Depression

As with all narcotics, TUSSIONEX Pennkinetic Extended-Release Suspension produces dose-related respiratory depression by directly acting on brain stem respiratory centers. Hydrocodone affects the center that controls respiratory rhythm and may produce irregular and periodic breathing. Caution should be exercised when TUSSIONEX Pennkinetic Extended-Release Suspension is used postoperatively and in patients with pulmonary disease, or whenever ventilatory function is depressed. If respiratory depression occurs, it may be antagonized by the use of naloxone hydrochloride and other supportive measures when indicated (see OVERDOSAGE).

Head Injury and Increased Intracranial Pressure

The respiratory depressant effects of narcotics and their capacity to elevate cerebrospinal fluid pressure may be markedly exaggerated in the presence of head injury, other intracranial lesions, or a pre-existing increase in intracranial pressure. Furthermore, narcotics produce adverse reactions, which may obscure the clinical course of patients with head injuries.

Acute Abdominal Conditions

The administration of narcotics may obscure the diagnosis or clinical course of patients with acute abdominal conditions.

Obstructive Bowel Disease

Chronic use of narcotics may result in obstructive bowel disease especially in patients with underlying intestinal motility disorder.

Pediatric Use

The use of TUSSIONEX Pennkinetic Extended-Release Suspension is contraindicated in children less than 6 years of age (see CONTRAINDICATIONS).

In pediatric patients, as well as adults, the respiratory center is sensitive to the depressant action of narcotic cough suppressants in a dose-dependent manner. Caution should be exercised when administering TUSSIONEX Pennkinetic Extended-Release Suspension to pediatric patients 6 years of age and older. Overdose or concomitant administration of TUSSIONEX Pennkinetic Extended-Release Suspension with other respiratory depressants may increase the risk of respiratory depression in pediatric patients. Benefit to risk ratio should be carefully considered, especially in pediatric patients with respiratory embarrassment (e.g., croup) (see PRECAUTIONS).

PRECAUTIONS

General

Caution is advised when prescribing this drug to patients with narrow-angle glaucoma, asthma, or prostatic hypertrophy.

Special Risk Patients

As with any narcotic agent, TUSSIONEX Pennkinetic Extended-Release Suspension should be used with caution in elderly or debilitated patients and those with severe impairment of hepatic or renal function, hypothyroidism, Addison's disease, prostatic hypertrophy, or urethral stricture. The usual precautions should be observed and the possibility of respiratory depression should be kept in mind.

Information for Patients

As with all narcotics, TUSSIONEX Pennkinetic Extended-Release Suspension may produce marked drowsiness and impair the mental and/or physical abilities required for the performance of potentially hazardous tasks such as driving a car or operating machinery; patients should be cautioned accordingly. TUSSIONEX Pennkinetic Extended-Release Suspension must not be diluted with fluids or mixed with other drugs as this may alter the resin-binding and change the absorption rate, possibly increasing the toxicity.

Patients should be advised to measure TUSSIONEX Pennkinetic Extended-Release Suspension with an accurate measuring device. A household teaspoon is not an accurate measuring device and could lead to overdosage, especially when a half a teaspoon is measured. A pharmacist can recommend an appropriate measuring device and can provide instructions for measuring the correct dose.

Shake well before using.

Keep out of the reach of children.

Cough Reflex

Hydrocodone suppresses the cough reflex; as with all narcotics, caution should be exercised when TUSSIONEX Pennkinetic Extended-Release Suspension is used postoperatively, and in patients with pulmonary disease.

Drug Interactions

Patients receiving narcotics, antihistaminics, antipsychotics, antianxiety agents, or other CNS depressants (including alcohol) concomitantly with TUSSIONEX Pennkinetic Extended-Release Suspension may exhibit an additive CNS depression. When combined therapy is contemplated, the dose of one or both agents should be reduced.

The use of MAO inhibitors or tricyclic antidepressants with hydrocodone preparations may increase the effect of either the antidepressant or hydrocodone.

The concurrent use of other anticholinergics with hydrocodone may produce paralytic ileus.

Carcinogenesis, Mutagenesis, Impairment of Fertility

Carcinogenicity, mutagenicity, and reproductive studies have not been conducted with TUSSIONEX Pennkinetic Extended-Release Suspension.

Pregnancy

Teratogenic Effects – Pregnancy Category C

Hydrocodone has been shown to be teratogenic in hamsters when given in doses 700 times the human dose. There are no adequate and well-controlled studies in pregnant women. TUSSIONEX Pennkinetic Extended-Release Suspension should be used during pregnancy only if the potential benefit justifies the potential risk to the fetus.

Nonteratogenic Effects

Babies born to mothers who have been taking opioids regularly prior to delivery will be physically dependent. The withdrawal signs include irritability and excessive crying, tremors, hyperactive reflexes, increased respiratory rate, increased stools, sneezing, yawning, vomiting, and fever. The intensity of the syndrome does not always correlate with the duration of maternal opioid use or dose.

Labor and Delivery

As with all narcotics, administration of TUSSIONEX Pennkinetic Extended-Release Suspension to the mother shortly before delivery may result in some degree of respiratory depression in the newborn, especially if higher doses are used.

Nursing Mothers

It is not known whether this drug is excreted in human milk. Because many drugs are excreted in human milk and because of the potential for serious adverse reactions in nursing infants from TUSSIONEX Pennkinetic Extended-Release Suspension, a decision should be made whether to discontinue nursing or to discontinue the drug, taking into account the importance of the drug to the mother.

Pediatric Use

The use of TUSSIONEX Pennkinetic Extended-Release Suspension is contraindicated in children less than 6 years of age (see CONTRAINDICATIONS and ADVERSE REACTIONS, Respiratory, Thoracic and Mediastinal Disorders). TUSSIONEX Pennkinetic Extended-Release Suspension should be used with caution in pediatric patients 6 years of age and older (see WARNINGS, Pediatric Use).

Geriatric Use

Clinical studies of TUSSIONEX did not include sufficient numbers of subjects aged 65 and over to determine whether they respond differently from younger subjects. Other reported clinical experience has not identified differences in responses between the elderly and younger patients. In general, dose selection for an elderly patient should be cautious, usually starting at the low end of the dosing range, reflecting the greater frequency of decreased hepatic, renal, or cardiac function, and of concomitant disease or other drug therapy.

This drug is known to be substantially excreted by the kidney, and the risk of toxic reactions to this drug may be greater in patients with impaired renal function. Because elderly patients are more likely to have decreased renal function, care should be taken in dose selection, and it may be useful to monitor renal function.

ADVERSE REACTIONS

Gastrointestinal Disorders

Nausea and vomiting may occur; they are more frequent in ambulatory than in recumbent patients. Prolonged administration of TUSSIONEX Pennkinetic Extended-Release Suspension may produce constipation.

General Disorders and Administration Site Conditions

Death

Nervous System Disorders

Sedation, drowsiness, mental clouding, lethargy, impairment of mental and physical performance, anxiety, fear, dysphoria, euphoria, dizziness, psychic dependence, mood changes.

Renal and Urinary Disorders

Ureteral spasm, spasm of vesical sphincters, and urinary retention have been reported with opiates.

Respiratory, Thoracic and Mediastinal Disorders

Dryness of the pharynx, occasional tightness of the chest, and respiratory depression (see CONTRAINDICATIONS).

TUSSIONEX Pennkinetic Extended-Release Suspension may produce dose-related respiratory depression by acting directly on brain stem respiratory centers (see OVERDOSAGE). Use of TUSSIONEX Pennkinetic Extended-Release Suspension in children less than 6 years of age has been associated with fatal respiratory depression. Overdose with TUSSIONEX Pennkinetic Extended-Release Suspension in children 6 years of age and older, in adolescents, and in adults has been associated with fatal respiratory depression.

Skin and Subcutaneous Tissue Disorders

Rash, pruritus.

DRUG ABUSE AND DEPENDENCE

TUSSIONEX Pennkinetic Extended-Release Suspension is a Schedule III narcotic. Psychic dependence, physical dependence and tolerance may develop upon repeated administration of narcotics; therefore, TUSSIONEX Pennkinetic Extended-Release Suspension should be prescribed and administered with caution. However, psychic dependence is unlikely to develop when TUSSIONEX Pennkinetic Extended-Release Suspension is used for a short time for the treatment of cough. Physical dependence, the condition in which continued administration of the drug is required to prevent the appearance of a withdrawal syndrome, assumes clinically significant proportions only after several weeks of continued oral narcotic use, although some mild degree of physical dependence may develop after a few days of narcotic therapy.

OVERDOSAGE

Signs and Symptoms

Serious overdosage with hydrocodone is characterized by respiratory depression (a decrease in respiratory rate and/or tidal volume, Cheyne-Stokes respiration, cyanosis), extreme somnolence progressing to stupor or coma, skeletal muscle flaccidity, cold and clammy skin, and sometimes bradycardia and hypotension. Although miosis is characteristic of narcotic overdose, mydriasis may occur in terminal narcosis or severe hypoxia. In severe overdosage apnea, circulatory collapse, cardiac arrest and death may occur. The manifestations of chlorpheniramine overdosage may vary from central nervous system depression to stimulation.

Treatment

Primary attention should be given to the reestablishment of adequate respiratory exchange through provision of a patent airway and the institution of assisted or controlled ventilation. The narcotic antagonist naloxone hydrochloride is a specific antidote for respiratory depression which may result from overdosage or unusual sensitivity to narcotics including hydrocodone. Therefore, an appropriate dose of naloxone hydrochloride should be administered, preferably by the intravenous route, simultaneously with efforts at respiratory resuscitation. Since the duration of action of hydrocodone in this formulation may exceed that of the antagonist, the patient should be kept under continued surveillance and repeated doses of the antagonist should be administered as needed to maintain adequate respiration. For further information, see full prescribing information for naloxone hydrochloride. An antagonist should not be administered in the absence of clinically significant respiratory depression. Oxygen, intravenous fluids, vasopressors and other supportive measures should be employed as indicated. Gastric emptying may be useful in removing unabsorbed drug.

DOSAGE AND ADMINISTRATION

It is important that TUSSIONEX is measured with an accurate measuring device (see PRECAUTIONS, Information for Patients). A household teaspoon is not an accurate measuring device and could lead to overdosage, especially when half a teaspoon is to be measured. It is strongly recommended that an accurate measuring device be used. A pharmacist can provide an appropriate measuring device and can provide instructions for measuring the correct dose.

Shake well before using.

Adults and Children 12 Years and Older

5 mL (1 teaspoonful) every 12 hours; do not exceed 10 mL (2 teaspoonfuls) in 24 hours.

Children 6-11 Years of Age

2.5 mL (½ teaspoonful) every 12 hours; do not exceed 5 mL (1 teaspoonful) in 24 hours. This medicine is contraindicated in children under 6 years of age (see CONTRAINDICATIONS).

HOW SUPPLIED

TUSSIONEX Pennkinetic (hydrocodone polistirex and chlorpheniramine polistirex) Extended-Release Suspension is a gold-colored suspension.

NDC 53014-548-67 473 mL bottle

For Medical Information

Contact: Medical Affairs Department
Phone: (866) 822-0068
Fax: (770) 970-8859

Storage:

Shake well. Dispense in a well-closed container.

Store at 20-25°C (68-77°F); excursions permitted to 15-30°C (59-86°F)

[see USP Controlled Room Temperature].

TUSSIONEX Pennkinetic Extended-Release Suspension

Manufactured for:
UCB, Inc.
Smyrna, GA 30080

TUSSIONEX and PENNKINETIC are trademarks of the UCB Group of companies.

Printed in the U.S.A.
Rev. 01/2008

VIMPAT® Ⓒ℞
[*VIM-păt*]
(lacosamide)
Tablet, Film Coated for Oral use

VIMPAT® Ⓒ℞
(lacosamide)
Injection for Intravenous use

VIMPAT® Ⓒ℞
(lacosamide)
Oral Solution

HIGHLIGHTS OF PRESCRIBING INFORMATION

These highlights do not include all the information needed to use VIMPAT® safely and effectively. See full prescribing information for VIMPAT.

VIMPAT® (lacosamide) Tablet, Film Coated for Oral use, CV
VIMPAT® (lacosamide) Injection for Intravenous use, CV
VIMPAT® (lacosamide) Oral Solution, CV
Initial U.S. Approval: 2008

RECENT MAJOR CHANGES

Indications and Usage	04/2010
Dosage and Administration	04/2010
Warnings and Precautions	04/2010

INDICATIONS AND USAGE

VIMPAT is indicated for:

- **Partial-onset seizures (1.1):** Tablets and oral solution are indicated for adjunctive therapy in patients ≥17 years. Injection is indicated as short term replacement when oral administration is not feasible in these patients.

DOSAGE AND ADMINISTRATION

- **Partial-onset seizures (2.1):** Initially, give 50 mg twice daily (100 mg/day). The dose may be increased, based on clinical response and tolerability, at weekly intervals by 100 mg/day given as two divided doses to a daily dose of 200 to 400 mg/day. VIMPAT injection may be given without further dilution or mixed in compatible diluent and should be administered intravenously over a period of 30 to 60 minutes. **(2.1)**
- **Oral-Intravenous Replacement therapy (2.1):** When switching from oral VIMPAT, the initial total daily intravenous dosage of VIMPAT should be equivalent to the total daily dosage and frequency of oral VIMPAT. At the end of the intravenous treatment period, the patient may be switched to VIMPAT oral administration at the equivalent daily dosage and frequency of the intravenous administration.

  See full prescribing information for compatibility and stability **(2.1)** and dosing in patients with renal impairment **(2.2)** and hepatic impairment **(2.3)**.

DOSAGE FORMS AND STRENGTHS

- 50 mg (pink), 100 mg (dark yellow), 150 mg (salmon), 200 mg (blue) film-coated tablets **(3)**
- 200 mg/20 mL single-use vial for intravenous use **(3)**
- 10 mg/mL oral solution **(3)**

CONTRAINDICATIONS

- None

WARNINGS AND PRECAUTIONS

- Suicidal Behavior and Ideation **(5.1)**
- Patients should be advised that VIMPAT may cause dizziness and ataxia. **(5.2)**
- Caution is advised for patients with known cardiac conduction problems [e.g., second-degree atrioventricular (AV) block], who are taking drugs known to induce PR interval prolongation, or with severe cardiac disease such as myocardial ischemia or heart failure. **(5.3)**
- Patients should be advised that VIMPAT may cause syncope. **(5.4)**
- In patients with seizure disorders, VIMPAT should be gradually withdrawn to minimize the potential of increased seizure frequency. **(5.5)**
- Multiorgan Hypersensitivity Reactions **(5.6)**
- Phenylketonurics **(5.7)**

ADVERSE REACTIONS

Most common adverse reactions (≥10% and greater than placebo) are diplopia, headache, dizziness, nausea **(6.1)**

To report SUSPECTED ADVERSE REACTIONS, contact UCB, Inc. at 1-800-477-7877 or FDA at 1-800-FDA-1088 or www.fda.gov/medwatch

USE IN SPECIFIC POPULATIONS

- To enroll in the UCB AED Pregnancy Registry call 1-888-537-7734 (toll free). To enroll in the North American Antiepileptic Drug Pregnancy Registry call 1-888-233-2334 (toll free). **(8.1)**
- *Renal impairment:* Dose adjustment is recommended for patients with severe renal impairment (creatinine clearance ≤ 30 mL/min). Dose supplementation should be considered following hemodialysis. **(12.3)**
- *Hepatic impairment:* Dose adjustment is recommended for patients with mild or moderate hepatic impairment.

Use in severe hepatic impairment patients is not recommended. Patients with co-existing hepatic and renal impairment should be monitored closely during dose titration. (12.3)

See 17 for PATIENT COUNSELING INFORMATION and Medication Guide

Revised: 04/2010

FULL PRESCRIBING INFORMATION: CONTENTS*

* Sections or subsections omitted from the full prescribing information are not listed

FULL PRESCRIBING INFORMATION

1 INDICATIONS AND USAGE

1.1 Partial-Onset Seizures

VIMPAT (lacosamide) tablets are indicated as adjunctive therapy in the treatment of partial-onset seizures in patients with epilepsy aged 17 years and older.

VIMPAT (lacosamide) injection for intravenous use is indicated as adjunctive therapy in the treatment of partial-onset seizures in patients with epilepsy aged 17 years and older when oral administration is temporarily not feasible.

2 DOSAGE AND ADMINISTRATION

VIMPAT may be taken with or without food.

When using VIMPAT oral solution, it is recommended that a calibrated measuring device be obtained and used. A household teaspoon or tablespoon is not an adequate measuring device. Healthcare providers should recommend a device that can measure and deliver the prescribed dose accurately, and provide instructions for measuring the dosage.

2.1 Partial-Onset Seizures

VIMPAT can be initiated with either oral or intravenous administration. The initial dose should be 50 mg twice daily (100 mg per day). VIMPAT can be increased at weekly intervals by 100 mg/day given as two divided doses up to the recommended maintenance dose of 200 to 400 mg/day, based on individual patient response and tolerability. In clinical trials, the 600 mg daily dose was not more effective than the 400 mg daily dose, and was associated with a substantially higher rate of adverse reactions. [see *Clinical Studies (14.1)*]

Switching from Oral to Intravenous Dosing

When switching from oral VIMPAT, the initial total daily intravenous dosage of VIMPAT should be equivalent to the total daily dosage and frequency of oral VIMPAT and should be infused intravenously over a period of 30 to 60 minutes. There is experience with twice daily intravenous infusion for up to 5 days.

Switching from Intravenous to Oral Dosing

At the end of the intravenous treatment period, the patient may be switched to VIMPAT oral administration at the equivalent daily dosage and frequency of the intravenous administration.

Compatibility and Stability

VIMPAT injection can be administered intravenously without further dilution or may be mixed with diluents. VIMPAT injection was found to be physically compatible and chemically stable when mixed with the following diluents for at least 24 hours and stored in glass or polyvinyl chloride (PVC) bags at ambient room temperature 15-30°C (59-86°F).

Diluents:

Sodium Chloride Injection 0.9% (w/v)
Dextrose Injection 5% (w/v)
Lactated Ringer's Injection

The stability of VIMPAT injection in other infusion solutions has not been evaluated. Product with particulate matter or discoloration should not be used.

Any unused portion of VIMPAT injection should be discarded.

2.2 Patients with Renal Impairment

No dose adjustment is necessary in patients with mild to moderate renal impairment. A maximum dose of 300 mg/day VIMPAT is recommended for patients with severe renal impairment [creatinine clearance (CL_{CR}) $\leq$30mL/min] and in patients with endstage renal disease. VIMPAT is effectively removed from plasma by hemodialysis. Following a 4-hour hemodialysis treatment, dosage supplementation of up to 50% should be considered. In all renally impaired patients, the dose titration should be performed with caution. [see *Use in Specific Populations (8.6)*]

2.3 Patients with Hepatic Impairment

The dose titration should be performed with caution in patients with hepatic impairment. A maximum dose of 300 mg/day is recommended for patients with mild or moderate hepatic impairment.

VIMPAT use is not recommended in patients with severe hepatic impairment [see *Use in Specific Populations (8.7)*].

3 DOSAGE FORMS AND STRENGTHS

50 mg (pink), 100 mg (dark yellow), 150 mg (salmon), and 200 mg (blue) film-coated tablets
200 mg/20mL injection
10 mg/mL oral solution

4 CONTRAINDICATIONS

None.

5 WARNINGS AND PRECAUTIONS

5.1 Suicidal Behavior and Ideation

Antiepileptic drugs (AEDs), including VIMPAT, increase the risk of suicidal thoughts or behavior in patients taking these drugs for any indication. Patients treated with any AED for any indication should be monitored for the emergence or worsening of depression, suicidal thoughts or behavior, and/or any unusual changes in mood or behavior.

Pooled analyses of 199 placebo-controlled clinical trials (mono- and adjunctive therapy) of 11 different AEDs showed that patients randomized to one of the AEDs had approximately twice the risk (adjusted Relative Risk 1.8, 95% CI:1.2, 2.7) of suicidal thinking or behavior compared to patients randomized to placebo. In these trials, which had a median treatment duration of 12 weeks, the estimated incidence of suicidal behavior or ideation among 27,863 AED-treated patients was 0.43%, compared to 0.24% among 16,029 placebo-treated patients, representing an increase of approximately one case of suicidal thinking or behavior for every 530 patients treated. There were four suicides in drug-treated patients in the trials and none in placebo-treated patients, but the number of events is too small to allow any conclusion about drug effect on suicide.

The increased risk of suicidal thoughts or behavior with AEDs was observed as early as one week after starting treatment with AEDs and persisted for the duration of treatment assessed. Because most trials included in the analysis did not extend beyond 24 weeks, the risk of suicidal thoughts or behavior beyond 24 weeks could not be assessed.

The risk of suicidal thoughts or behavior was generally consistent among drugs in the data analyzed. The finding of increased risk with AEDs of varying mechanisms of action and across a range of indications suggests that the risk applies to all AEDs used for any indication. The risk did not vary substantially by age (5-100 years) in the clinical trials analyzed.

Table 1 shows absolute and relative risk by indication for all evaluated AEDs.

[See table 1 below]

The relative risk for suicidal thoughts or behavior was higher in clinical trials for epilepsy than in clinical trials for psychiatric or other conditions, but the absolute risk differences were similar.

Anyone considering prescribing VIMPAT or any other AED must balance this risk with the risk of untreated illness. Epilepsy and many other illnesses for which antiepileptics are prescribed are themselves associated with morbidity and mortality and an increased risk of suicidal thoughts and behavior. Should suicidal thoughts and behavior emerge during treatment, the prescriber needs to consider whether the emergence of these symptoms in any given patient may be related to the illness being treated.

Patients, their caregivers, and families should be informed that AEDs increase the risk of suicidal thoughts and behavior and should be advised of the need to be alert for the emergence or worsening of the signs and symptoms of depression, any unusual changes in mood or behavior, or the emergence of suicidal thoughts, behavior, or thoughts about self-harm. Behaviors of concern should be reported immediately to healthcare providers.

5.2 Dizziness and Ataxia

Patients should be advised that VIMPAT may cause dizziness and ataxia. Accordingly, they should be advised not to drive a car or to operate other complex machinery until they are familiar with the effects of VIMPAT on their ability to perform such activities.

In patients with partial-onset seizures taking 1 to 3 concomitant AEDs, dizziness was experienced by 25% of patients randomized to the recommended doses (200 to 400 mg/day) of VIMPAT (compared with 8% of placebo patients) and was the adverse event most frequently leading to discontinuation (3%). Ataxia was experienced by 6% of patients randomized to the recommended doses (200 to 400 mg/day) of VIMPAT (compared to 2% of placebo patients). The onset of dizziness and ataxia was most commonly observed during titration. There was a substantial increase in these adverse events at doses higher than 400 mg/day. [see *Adverse Reactions/Table 2 (6.1)*]

5.3 Cardiac Rhythm and Conduction Abnormalities
PR interval prolongation

Dose-dependent prolongations in PR interval with VIMPAT have been observed in clinical studies in patients and in healthy volunteers. [see *Clinical Pharmacology (12.2)*] In clinical trials in patients with partial-onset epilepsy, asymptomatic first-degree atrioventricular (AV) block was observed as an adverse reaction in 0.4% (4/944) of patients randomized to receive VIMPAT and 0% (0/364) of patients randomized to receive placebo. In clinical trials in patients with diabetic neuropathy, asymptomatic first-degree AV block was observed as an adverse reaction in 0.5% (5/1023) of patients receiving VIMPAT and 0% (0/291) of patients receiving placebo. When VIMPAT is given with other drugs that prolong the PR interval, further PR prolongation is possible.

VIMPAT should be used with caution in patients with known conduction problems (e.g. marked first-degree AV block, second-degree or higher AV block and sick sinus syndrome without pacemaker), or with severe cardiac disease such as myocardial ischemia or heart failure. In such

Table 1 Risk by indication for antiepileptic drugs in the pooled analysis

Indication	Placebo Patients with Events Per 1000 Patients	Drug Patients with Events Per 1000 Patients	Relative Risk: Incidence of Events in Drug Patients/Incidence in Placebo Patients	Risk Difference: Additional Drug Patients with Events Per 1000 Patients
Epilepsy	1.0	3.4	3.5	2.4
Psychiatric	5.7	8.5	1.5	2.9
Other	1.0	1.8	1.9	0.9
Total	2.4	4.3	1.8	1.9

patients, obtaining an ECG before beginning VIMPAT, and after VIMPAT is titrated to steady-state, is recommended.

Atrial fibrillation and Atrial flutter

In the short-term investigational trials of VIMPAT in epilepsy patients, there were no cases of atrial fibrillation or flutter. In patients with diabetic neuropathy, 0.5% of patients treated with VIMPAT experienced an adverse reaction of atrial fibrillation or atrial flutter, compared to 0% of placebo-treated patients. VIMPAT administration may predispose to atrial arrhythmias (atrial fibrillation or flutter), especially in patients with diabetic neuropathy and/or cardiovascular disease. Patients should be made aware of the symptoms of atrial fibrillation and flutter (e.g., palpitations, rapid pulse, shortness of breath) and told to contact their physician should any of these symptoms occur.

5.4   Syncope

In the short-term controlled trials of VIMPAT in epilepsy patients with no significant system illnesses, there was no increase in syncope compared to placebo. In the short-term controlled trials of VIMPAT in patients with diabetic neuropathy, 1.2% of patients who were treated with VIMPAT reported an adverse reaction of syncope or loss of consciousness, compared to 0% of placebo-treated patients with diabetic neuropathy. Most of the cases of syncope were observed in patients receiving doses above 400 mg/day. The cause of syncope was not determined in most cases. However, several were associated with either changes in orthostatic blood pressure, atrial flutter/fibrillation (and associated tachycardia), or bradycardia.

5.5   Withdrawal of Antiepileptic Drugs (AEDs)

As with all AEDs, VIMPAT should be withdrawn gradually (over a minimum of 1 week) to minimize the potential of increased seizure frequency in patients with seizure disorders.

5.6   Multiorgan Hypersensitivity Reactions

One case of symptomatic hepatitis and nephritis was observed among 4011 subjects exposed to VIMPAT during clinical development. The event occurred in a healthy volunteer, 10 days after stopping VIMPAT treatment. The subject was not taking any concomitant medication and potential known viral etiologies for hepatitis were ruled out. The subject fully recovered within a month, without specific treatment. The case is consistent with a delayed multiorgan hypersensitivity reaction. Additional potential cases included 2 with rash and elevated liver enzymes and 1 with myocarditis and hepatitis of uncertain etiology.

Multiorgan hypersensitivity reactions (also known as Drug Reaction with Eosinophilia and Systemic Symptoms, or DRESS) have been reported with other anticonvulsants and typically, although not exclusively, present with fever and rash associated with other organ system involvement, that may or may not include eosinophilia, hepatitis, nephritis, lymphadenopathy, and/or myocarditis. Because this disorder is variable in its expression, other organ system signs and symptoms not noted here may occur. If this reaction is suspected, VIMPAT should be discontinued and alternative treatment started.

5.7   Phenylketonurics

VIMPAT oral solution contains aspartame, a source of phenylalanine. A 200 mg dose of VIMPAT oral solution (equivalent to 20 mL) contains 0.32 mg of phenylalanine.

6   ADVERSE REACTIONS

Because clinical trials are conducted under widely varying conditions, adverse reaction rates observed in the clinical trials of a drug cannot be directly compared to rates in the clinical trials of another drug and may not reflect the rates observed in practice.

In all controlled and uncontrolled trials in patients with partial-onset seizures, 1327 patients have received VIMPAT of whom 1000 have been treated for longer than 6 months and 852 for longer than 12 months.

6.1   Clinical Trials Experience

Controlled Trials

Adverse reactions leading to discontinuation

In controlled clinical trials, the rate of discontinuation as a result of an adverse event was 8% and 17% in patients randomized to receive VIMPAT at the recommended doses of 200 and 400 mg/day, respectively, 29% at 600 mg/day, and 5% in patients randomized to receive placebo. The adverse events most commonly (>1% in the VIMPAT total group and greater than placebo) leading to discontinuation were dizziness, ataxia, vomiting, diplopia, nausea, vertigo, and vision blurred.

Most common adverse reactions

Table 2 gives the incidence of treatment-emergent adverse events that occurred in ≥2% of adult patients with partial-onset seizures in the total VIMPAT group and for which the incidence was greater than placebo. The majority of adverse events in the VIMPAT patients were reported with a maximum intensity of 'mild' or 'moderate'.

[See table 2 above]

Table 2: Treatment-Emergent Adverse Event Incidence in Double-Blind, Placebo-Controlled Partial-Onset Seizure Trials (Events ≥2% of Patients in VIMPAT Total and More Frequent Than in the Placebo Group)

System Organ Class/ Preferred Term	Placebo N=364 %	VIMPAT 200 mg/day N=270 %	VIMPAT 400 mg/day N=471 %	VIMPAT 600 mg/day N=203 %	VIMPAT Total N=944 %
Ear and labyrinth disorder					
Vertigo	1	5	3	4	4
Eye disorders					
Diplopia	2	6	10	16	11
Vision blurred	3	2	9	16	8
Gastrointestinal disorders					
Nausea	4	7	11	17	11
Vomiting	3	6	9	16	9
Diarrhea	3	3	5	4	4
General disorders and administration site conditions					
Fatigue	6	7	7	15	9
Gait disturbance	<1	<1	2	4	2
Asthenia	1	2	2	4	2
Injury, poisoning and procedural complications					
Contusion	3	3	4	2	3
Skin laceration	2	2	3	3	3
Nervous system disorders					
Dizziness	8	16	30	53	31
Headache	9	11	14	12	13
Ataxia	2	4	7	15	8
Somnolence	5	5	8	8	7
Tremor	4	4	6	12	7
Nystagmus	4	2	5	10	5
Balance disorder	0	1	5	6	4
Memory impairment	2	1	2	6	2
Psychiatric disorders					
Depression	1	2	2	2	2
Skin and subcutaneous disorders					
Pruritus	1	3	2	3	2

Laboratory abnormalities

Abnormalities in liver function tests have been observed in controlled trials with VIMPAT in adult patients with partial-onset seizures who were taking 1 to 3 concomitant anti-epileptic drugs. Elevations of ALT to ≥3× ULN occurred in 0.7% (7/935) of VIMPAT patients and 0% (0/356) of placebo patients. One case of hepatitis with transaminases >20× ULN was observed in one healthy subject 10 days after VIMPAT treatment completion, along with nephritis (proteinuria and urine casts). Serologic studies were negative for viral hepatitis. Transaminases returned to normal within one month without specific treatment. At the time of this event, bilirubin was normal. The hepatitis/nephritis was interpreted as a delayed hypersensitivity reaction to VIMPAT.

Other Adverse Reactions in Patients with Partial-Onset Seizures

The following is a list of treatment-emergent adverse events reported by patients treated with VIMPAT in all clinical trials in patients with partial-onset seizures, including controlled trials and long-term open-label extension trials. Events addressed in other tables or sections are not listed here. Events included in this list from the controlled trials occurred more frequently on drug than on placebo and were based on consideration of VIMPAT pharmacology, frequency above that expected in the population, seriousness, and likelihood of a relationship to VIMPAT. Events are further classified within system organ class.

Blood and lymphatic system disorders: neutropenia, anemia
Cardiac disorders: palpitations
Ear and labyrinth disorders: tinnitus
Gastrointestinal disorders: constipation, dyspepsia, dry mouth, oral hypoaesthesia
General disorders and administration site conditions: irritability, pyrexia, feeling drunk
Injury, poisoning, and procedural complications: fall
Musculoskeletal and connective tissue disorders: muscle spasms
Nervous system disorders: paresthesia, cognitive disorder, hypoaesthesia, dysarthria, disturbance in attention, cerebellar syndrome
Psychiatric disorders: confusional state, mood altered, depressed mood

Intravenous Adverse Reactions

Adverse reactions with intravenous administration generally appeared similar to those observed with the oral formulation, although intravenous administration was associated with local adverse events such as injection site pain or discomfort (2.5%), irritation (1%), and erythema (0.5%). One case of profound bradycardia (26 bpm: BP 100/60 mmHg) was observed in a patient during a 15 minute infusion of 150mg VIMPAT. This patient was on a beta-blocker. Infusion was discontinued and the patient experienced a rapid recovery.

Comparison of Gender and Race

The overall adverse event rate was similar in male and female patients. Although there were few non-Caucasian patients, no differences in the incidences of adverse events compared to Caucasian patients were observed.

6.2 Postmarketing Experience

The following adverse reactions have been identified during postapproval use of VIMPAT. Because these reactions are reported voluntarily from a population of uncertain size, it is not always possible to reliably estimate their frequency or establish a causal relationship to drug exposure.

Cardiac disorders: Bradycardia

Skin and subcutaneous tissue disorders: Rash

7 DRUG INTERACTIONS

Drug-drug interaction studies in healthy subjects showed no pharmacokinetic interactions between VIMPAT and carbamazepine, valproate, digoxin, metformin, omeprazole, or an oral contraceptive containing ethinylestradiol and levonorgestrel. There was no evidence for any relevant drug-drug interaction of VIMPAT with common AEDs in the placebo-controlled clinical trials in patients with partial-onset seizures [see *Clinical Pharmacology (12.3)*].

The lack of pharmacokinetic interaction does not rule out the possibility of pharmacodynamic interactions, particularly among drugs that affect the heart conduction system.

8 USE IN SPECIFIC POPULATIONS

8.1 Pregnancy

Pregnancy Category C

Lacosamide produced developmental toxicity (increased embryofetal and perinatal mortality, growth deficit) in rats following administration during pregnancy. Developmental neurotoxicity was observed in rats following administration during a period of postnatal development corresponding to the third trimester of human pregnancy. These effects were observed at doses associated with clinically relevant plasma exposures.

Lacosamide has been shown in vitro to interfere with the activity of collapsin response mediator protein-2 (CRMP-2), a protein involved in neuronal differentiation and control of axonal outgrowth. Potential adverse effects on CNS development can not be ruled out.

There are no adequate and well-controlled studies in pregnant women. VIMPAT should be used during pregnancy only if the potential benefit justifies the potential risk to the fetus.

Oral administration of lacosamide to pregnant rats (20, 75, or 200 mg/kg/day) and rabbits (6.25, 12.5, or 25 mg/kg/day) during the period of organogenesis did not produce any teratogenic effects. However, the maximum doses evaluated were limited by maternal toxicity in both species and embryofetal death in rats. These doses were associated with maternal plasma lacosamide exposures [area under the plasma-time concentration curve; (AUC)] ≈2 and 1 times (rat and rabbit, respectively) that in humans at the maximum recommended human dose (MRHD) of 400 mg/day.

When lacosamide (25, 70, or 200 mg/kg/day) was orally administered to rats throughout gestation, parturition, and lactation, increased perinatal mortality and decreased body weights were observed in the offspring at the highest dose. The no-effect dose for pre- and post-natal developmental toxicity in rats (70 mg/kg/day) was associated with a maternal plasma lacosamide AUC approximately equal to that in humans at the MRHD.

Oral administration of lacosamide (30, 90, or 180 mg/kg/day) to rats during the neonatal and juvenile periods of postnatal development resulted in decreased brain weights and long-term neurobehavioral changes (altered open field performance, deficits in learning and memory). The early postnatal period in rats is generally thought to correspond to late pregnancy in humans in terms of brain development. The no-effect dose for developmental neurotoxicity in rats was associated with a plasma lacosamide AUC approximately 0.5 times that in humans at the MRHD.

Pregnancy Registry

UCB, Inc. has established the UCB AED Pregnancy Registry to advance scientific knowledge about safety and outcomes in pregnant women being treated with VIMPAT. To ensure broad program access and reach, either a healthcare provider or the patient can initiate enrollment in the UCB AED Pregnancy Registry by calling 1-888-537-7734 (toll free).

Physicians are also advised to recommend that pregnant patients taking VIMPAT enroll in the North American Antiepileptic Drug Pregnancy Registry. This can be done by calling the toll free number 1-888-233-2334, and must be done by patients themselves. Information on the registry can also be found at the website http://www.aedpregnancyregistry.org/.

8.2 Labor and Delivery

The effects of VIMPAT on labor and delivery in pregnant women are unknown. In a pre- and post-natal study in rats, there was a tendency for prolonged gestation in all lacosamide treated groups at plasma exposures (AUC) at or below the plasma AUC in humans at the maximum recommended human dose of 400 mg/day.

8.3 Nursing Mothers

Studies in lactating rats have shown that lacosamide and/or its metabolites are excreted in milk. It is not known whether VIMPAT is excreted in human milk. Because many drugs are excreted into human milk, a decision should be made whether to discontinue nursing or to discontinue VIMPAT, taking into account the importance of the drug to the mother.

8.4 Pediatric Use

The safety and effectiveness of VIMPAT in pediatric patients <17 years have not been established.

Lacosamide has been shown in vitro to interfere with the activity of CRMP-2, a protein involved in neuronal differentiation and control of axonal outgrowth. Potential adverse effects on CNS development can not be ruled out. Administration of lacosamide to rats during the neonatal and juvenile periods of postnatal development resulted in decreased brain weights and long-term neurobehavioral changes (altered open field performance, deficits in learning and memory). The no-effect dose for developmental neurotoxicity in rats was associated with a plasma lacosamide exposure (AUC) approximately 0.5 times the human plasma AUC at the maximum recommended human dose of 400 mg/day.

8.5 Geriatric Use

There were insufficient numbers of elderly patients enrolled in partial-onset seizure trials (n=18) to adequately assess the effectiveness of VIMPAT in this population.

In healthy subjects, the dose and body weight normalized pharmacokinetic parameters AUC and C_{max} were approximately 20% higher in elderly subjects compared to young subjects. The slightly higher lacosamide plasma concentrations in elderly subjects are possibly caused by differences in total body water (lean body weight) and age-associated decreased renal clearance. No VIMPAT dose adjustment based on age is considered necessary. Caution should be exercised for dose titration in elderly patients.

8.6 Patients with Renal Impairment

A maximum dose of 300 mg/day is recommended for patients with severe renal impairment ($CL_{CR} \leq 30$mL/min) and in patients with endstage renal disease. VIMPAT is effectively removed from plasma by hemodialysis. Following a 4-hour hemodialysis treatment, AUC of VIMPAT is reduced by approximately 50%. Therefore dosage supplementation of up to 50% following hemodialysis should be considered. In all renal impaired patients, the dose titration should be performed with caution. [see *Dosage and Administration (2.2)* and *Clinical Pharmacology (12.3)*]

8.7 Patients with Hepatic Impairment

Patients with mild to moderate hepatic impairment should be observed closely during dose titration. A maximum dose of 300 mg/day is recommended for patients with mild to moderate hepatic impairment. The pharmacokinetics of lacosamide has not been evaluated in severe hepatic impairment. VIMPAT use is not recommended in patients with severe hepatic impairment. [see *Dosage and Administration (2.3)* and *Clinical Pharmacology (12.3)*] Patients with co-existing hepatic and renal impairment should be monitored closely during dose titration.

9 DRUG ABUSE AND DEPENDENCE

9.1 Controlled Substance

VIMPAT is a Schedule V controlled substance.

9.2 Abuse

In a human abuse potential study, single doses of 200 mg and 800 mg lacosamide produced euphoria-type subjective responses that differentiated statistically from placebo; at 800 mg, these euphoria-type responses were statistically indistinguishable from those produced by alprazolam, a Schedule IV drug. The duration of the euphoria-type responses following lacosamide was less than that following alprazolam. A high rate of euphoria was also reported as an adverse event in the human abuse potential study following single doses of 800 mg lacosamide (15% [5/34]) compared to placebo (0%) and in two pharmacokinetic studies following single and multiple doses of 300-800 mg lacosamide (ranging from 6% [2/33] to 25% [3/12]) compared to placebo (0%). However, the rate of euphoria reported as an adverse event in the VIMPAT development program at therapeutic doses was less than 1%.

9.3 Dependence

Abrupt termination of lacosamide in clinical trials with diabetic neuropathic pain patients produced no signs or symptoms that are associated with a withdrawal syndrome indicative of physical dependence. However, psychological dependence cannot be excluded due to the ability of lacosamide to produce euphoria-type adverse events in humans.

10 OVERDOSAGE

10.1 Signs, Symptoms, and Laboratory Findings of Acute Overdose in Humans

There is limited clinical experience with VIMPAT overdose in humans. The highest reported accidental overdose of VIMPAT during clinical development was 1200 mg/day which was non-fatal. The types of adverse events experienced by patients exposed to supratherapeutic doses during the trials were not clinically different from those of patients administered recommended doses of VIMPAT.

There has been a single case of intentional overdose by a patient who self-administered 12 grams VIMPAT along with large doses of zonisamide, topiramate, and gabapentin. The patient presented in a coma and was hospitalized. An EEG revealed epileptic waveforms. The patient recovered 2 days later.

10.2 Treatment or Management of Overdose

There is no specific antidote for overdose with VIMPAT. Standard decontamination procedures should be followed. General supportive care of the patient is indicated including monitoring of vital signs and observation of the clinical status of patient. A Certified Poison Control Center should be contacted for up to date information on the management of overdose with VIMPAT.

Standard hemodialysis procedures result in significant clearance of VIMPAT (reduction of systemic exposure by 50% in 4 hours). Hemodialysis has not been performed in the few known cases of overdose, but may be indicated based on the patient's clinical state or in patients with significant renal impairment.

11 DESCRIPTION

The chemical name of lacosamide, the single (R)-enantiomer, is (R)-2-acetamido-N-benzyl-3-methoxypropionamide (IUPAC). Lacosamide is a functionalized amino acid. Its molecular formula is $C_{13}H_{18}N_2O_3$ and its molecular weight is 250.30. The chemical structure is:

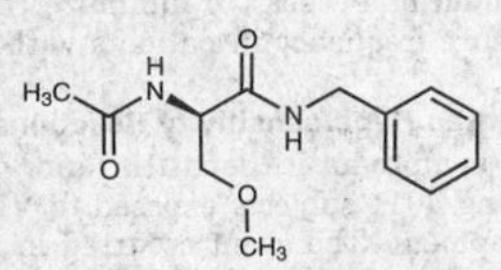

Lacosamide is a white to light yellow powder. It is sparingly soluble in water and slightly soluble in acetonitrile and ethanol.

11.1 VIMPAT Tablets

VIMPAT tablets contain the following inactive ingredients: colloidal silicon dioxide, crospovidone, hydroxypropylcellulose, hypromellose, lecithin, magnesium stearate, microcrystalline cellulose, polyethylene glycol, polyvinyl alcohol, talc, titanium dioxide, and dye pigments as specified below:

VIMPAT tablets are supplied as debossed tablets and contain the following coloring agents:

50 mg tablets: red iron oxide, black iron oxide, FD&C Blue #2/indigo carmine aluminum lake

100 mg tablets: yellow iron oxide

150 mg tablets: yellow iron oxide, red iron oxide, black iron oxide

200 mg tablets: FD&C Blue #2/indigo carmine aluminum lake

11.2 VIMPAT Injection

VIMPAT injection is a clear, colorless, sterile solution containing 10 mg lacosamide per mL for intravenous infusion. One 20-mL vial contains 200 mg of lacosamide drug substance. The inactive ingredients are sodium chloride and water for injection. Hydrochloric acid is used for pH adjustment. VIMPAT injection has a pH of 3.5 to 5.0.

11.3 VIMPAT Oral Solution

VIMPAT oral solution contains 10 mg of lacosamide per mL. The inactive ingredients are purified water, sorbitol solution, glycerin, polyethylene glycol, carboxymethylcellulose sodium, acesulfame potassium, methylparaben, flavoring (including natural and artificial flavors, propylene glycol, aspartame, and maltol), anhydrous citric acid and sodium chloride.

12 CLINICAL PHARMACOLOGY

12.1 Mechanism of Action

The precise mechanism by which VIMPAT exerts its antiepileptic effects in humans remains to be fully elucidated. *In vitro* electrophysiological studies have shown that lacosamide selectively enhances slow inactivation of voltage-gated sodium channels, resulting in stabilization of hyperexcitable neuronal membranes and inhibition of repetitive neuronal firing.

Lacosamide binds to collapsin response mediator protein-2 (CRMP-2), a phosphoprotein which is mainly expressed in the nervous system and is involved in neuronal differentiation and control of axonal outgrowth. The role of CRMP-2 binding in seizure control is unknown.

12.2 Pharmacodynamics

A pharmacokinetic-pharmacodynamic (efficacy) analysis was performed based on the pooled data from the 3 efficacy trials for partial-onset seizures. Lacosamide exposure is correlated with the reduction in seizure frequency. However, doses above 400 mg/day do not appear to confer additional benefit in group analyses.

Cardiac Electrophysiology

Electrocardiographic effects of VIMPAT were determined in a double-blind, randomized clinical pharmacology trial of 247 healthy subjects. Chronic oral doses of 400 and 800 mg/day were compared with placebo and a positive control (400 mg moxifloxacin). VIMPAT did not prolong QTc interval and did not have a dose-related or clinically important effect on QRS duration. VIMPAT produced a small, dose-related increase in mean PR interval. At steady-state, the time of the maximum observed mean PR interval corresponded with t_{max}. The placebo-subtracted maximum increase in PR interval (at t_{max}) was 7.3 ms for the 400 mg/day group and 11.9 ms for the 800 mg/day group. For patients who participated in the controlled trials, the placebo-subtracted mean maximum increase in PR interval for a 400 mg/day VIMPAT dose was 3.1 ms in patients with partial-onset seizures and 9.4 ms for patients with diabetic neuropathy.

12.3 Pharmacokinetics

The pharmacokinetics of VIMPAT have been studied in healthy adult subjects (age range 18 to 87), adults with partial-onset seizures, adults with diabetic neuropathy, and subjects with renal and hepatic impairment.

VIMPAT is completely absorbed after oral administration with negligible first-pass effect with a high absolute bioavailability of approximately 100%. The maximum lacosamide plasma concentrations occur approximately 1 to 4 hour post-dose after oral dosing, and elimination half-life is approximately 13 hours. Steady state plasma concentrations are achieved after 3 days of twice daily repeated administration. Pharmacokinetics of VIMPAT are dose proportional (100-800 mg) and time invariant, with low inter- and intra-subject variability. Compared to lacosamide the major metabolite, O-desmethyl metabolite, has a longer T_{max} (0.5 to 12 hours) and elimination half-life (15-23 hours).

Absorption and Bioavailability

VIMPAT is completely absorbed after oral administration. The oral bioavailability of VIMPAT tablets is approximately 100%. Food does not affect the rate and extent of absorption. After intravenous administration, C_{max} is reached at the end of infusion. The 30- and 60-minute intravenous infusions are bioequivalent to the oral tablet.

In a trial comparing the oral tablet with and an oral solution containing 10 mg/mL lacosamide, bioequivalence between both formulations was shown.

Distribution

The volume of distribution is approximately 0.6 L/kg and thus close to the volume of total body water. VIMPAT is less than 15% bound to plasma proteins.

Metabolism and Elimination

VIMPAT is primarily eliminated from the systemic circulation by renal excretion and biotransformation.

After oral and intravenous administration of 100 mg [14C]-lacosamide approximately 95% of radioactivity administered was recovered in the urine and less than 0.5% in the feces. The major compounds excreted were unchanged lacosamide (approximately 40% of the dose), its O-desmethyl metabolite (approximately 30%), and a structurally unknown polar fraction (~20%). The plasma exposure of the major human metabolite, O-desmethyl-lacosamide, is approximately 10% of that of lacosamide. This metabolite has no known pharmacological activity.

Lacosamide is a CYP2C19 substrate. The relative contribution of other CYP isoforms or non-CYP enzymes in the metabolism of lacosamide is not clear. The elimination half-life of the unchanged drug is approximately 13 hours and is not altered by different doses, multiple dosing or intravenous administration.

There is no enantiomeric interconversion of lacosamide.

Special Populations

Renal impairment

Lacosamide and its major metabolite are eliminated from the systemic circulation primarily by renal excretion.

The AUC of VIMPAT was increased approximately 25% in mildly (CL_{CR} 50-80 mL/min) and moderately (CL_{CR} 30-50 mL/min) and 60% in severely (CL_{CR}≤30mL/min) renally impaired patients compared to subjects with normal renal function (CL_{CR}>80mL/min), whereas C_{max} was unaffected. No dose adjustment is considered necessary in mildly and moderately renal impaired subjects. A maximum dose of 300 mg/day is recommended for patients with severe renal impairment (CL_{CR}≤30mL/min) and in patients with endstage renal disease. VIMPAT is effectively removed from plasma by hemodialysis. Following a 4-hour hemodialysis treatment, AUC of VIMPAT is reduced by approximately 50%. Therefore dosage supplementation of up to 50% following hemodialysis should be considered. In all renal impaired patients, the dose titration should be performed with caution. [see *Dosage and Administration (2.3)*]

Hepatic impairment

Lacosamide undergoes metabolism. Subjects with moderate hepatic impairment (Child-Pugh B) showed higher plasma concentrations of lacosamide (approximately 50-60% higher AUC compared to healthy subjects). The dose titration

should be performed with caution in patients with hepatic impairment. A maximum dose of 300 mg/day is recommended for patients with mild or moderate hepatic impairment.

Patients with mild to moderate hepatic impairment should be observed closely during dose titration. A maximum dose of 300 mg/day is recommended for patients with mild to moderate hepatic impairment. The pharmacokinetics of lacosamide have not been evaluated in severe hepatic impairment. VIMPAT use is not recommended in patients with severe hepatic impairment. [see *Dosage and Administration (2.3)*] Patients with co-existing hepatic and renal impairment should be monitored closely during dose titration.

Geriatric

In the elderly (>65 years), dose and body-weight normalized AUC and C_{max} is about 20% increased compared to young subjects (18-64 years). This may be related to body weight and decreased renal function in elderly subjects. Dose reduction is not considered to be necessary.

Pediatric Patients

Pharmacokinetics of VIMPAT have not been studied in pediatric patients.

Gender

VIMPAT clinical trials indicate that gender does not have a clinically relevant influence on the pharmacokinetics of VIMPAT.

Race

There are no clinically relevant differences in the pharmacokinetics of VIMPAT between Asian, Black, and Caucasian subjects.

CYP2C19 Polymorphism

There are no clinically relevant differences in the pharmacokinetics of VIMPAT between CYP2C19 poor metabolizers and extensive metabolizers. Results from a trial in poor metabolizers (PM) (N=4) and extensive metabolizers (EM) (N=8) of cytochrome P450 (CYP) 2C19 showed that lacosamide plasma concentrations were similar in PMs and EMs, but plasma concentrations and the amount excreted into urine of the O-desmethyl metabolite were about 70% reduced in PMs compared to EMs.

Drug interactions

In Vitro Assessment of Drug Interactions

In vitro metabolism studies indicate that lacosamide does not induce the enzyme activity of drug metabolizing cytochrome P450 isoforms CYP1A2, 2B6, 2C9, 2C19 and 3A4. Lacosamide did not inhibit CYP 1A1, 1A2, 2A6, 2B6, 2C8, 2C9, 2D6, 2E1, 3A4/5 at plasma concentrations observed in clinical studies.

In vitro data suggest that lacosamide has the potential to inhibit CYP2C19 at therapeutic concentrations. However, an in vivo study with omeprazole did not show an inhibitory effect on omeprazole pharmacokinetics.

Lacosamide was not a substrate or inhibitor for P-glycoprotein.

Lacosamide is a CYP2C19 substrate. The relative contribution of other CYP isoforms or non-CYP enzymes in the metabolism of lacosamide is not clear.

Since <15% of lacosamide is bound to plasma proteins, a clinically relevant interaction with other drugs through competition for protein binding sites is unlikely.

In Vivo Assessment of Drug Interactions

Drug interaction studies with AEDs

Effect of VIMPAT on concomitant AEDs: VIMPAT 400 mg/day had no influence on the pharmacokinetics of 600 mg/day valproic acid and 400 mg/day carbamazepine in healthy subjects.

The placebo-controlled clinical studies in patients with partial-onset seizures showed that steady-state plasma concentrations of levetiracetam, carbamazepine, carbamazepine epoxide, lamotrigine, topiramate, oxcarbazepine monohydroxy derivative (MHD), phenytoin, valproic acid, phenobarbital, gabapentin, clonazepam, and zonisamide were not affected by concomitant intake of VIMPAT at any dose.

Effect of concomitant AEDs on VIMPAT: Drug-drug interaction studies in healthy subjects showed that 600 mg/day valproic acid had no influence on the pharmacokinetics of 400 mg/day VIMPAT. Likewise, 400 mg/day carbamazepine had no influence on the pharmacokinetics of VIMPAT in a healthy subject study. Population pharmacokinetics results in patients with partial-onset seizures showed small reductions (15% to 20% lower) in lacosamide plasma concentrations when VIMPAT was coadministered with carbamazepine, phenobarbital or phenytoin.

Drug-drug interaction studies with other drugs

Digoxin

There was no effect of VIMPAT (400 mg/day) on the pharmacokinetics of digoxin (0.5 mg once daily) in a study in healthy subjects.

Metformin

There were no clinically relevant changes in metformin levels following coadministration of VIMPAT (400 mg/day). Metformin (500 mg three times a day) had no effect on the pharmacokinetics of VIMPAT (400 mg/day).

Omeprazole

Omeprazole is a CYP2C19 substrate and inhibitor.

There was no effect of VIMPAT (600 mg/day) on the pharmacokinetics of omeprazole (40 mg single dose) in healthy subjects. The data indicated that lacosamide had little in vivo inhibitory or inducing effect on CYP2C19.

Omeprazole at a dose of 40 mg once daily had no effect on the pharmacokinetics of VIMPAT (300 mg single dose). However, plasma levels of the O-desmethyl metabolite were reduced about 60% in the presence of omeprazole.

Oral Contraceptives

There was no influence of VIMPAT (400 mg/day) on the pharmacodynamics and pharmacokinetics of an oral contraceptive containing 0.03 mg ethinylestradiol and 0.15 mg levonorgestrel in healthy subjects, except that a 20% increase in ethinylestradiol Cmax was observed.

13 NONCLINICAL TOXICOLOGY

13.1 Carcinogenesis, Mutagenesis, Impairment of Fertility

There was no evidence of drug related carcinogenicity in mice or rats. Mice and rats received lacosamide once daily by oral administration for 104 weeks at doses producing plasma exposures (AUC) up to approximately 1 and 3 times, respectively, the plasma AUC in humans at the maximum recommended human dose (MRHD) of 400 mg/day.

Lacosamide was negative in an *in vitro* Ames test and an *in vivo* mouse micronucleus assay. Lacosamide induced a positive response in the *in vitro* mouse lymphoma assay.

No adverse effects on male or female fertility or reproduction were observed in rats at doses producing plasma exposures (AUC) up to approximately 2 times the plasma AUC in humans at the MRHD.

14 CLINICAL STUDIES

14.1 Effectiveness in Partial-Onset Seizures

The efficacy of VIMPAT as adjunctive therapy in partial-onset seizures was established in three 12-week, randomized, double-blind, placebo-controlled, multicenter trials in adult patients. Patients enrolled had partial-onset seizures with or without secondary generalization and were not adequately controlled with 1 to 3 concomitant AEDs. During an 8-week baseline period, patients were required to have an average of ≥4 partial-onset seizures per 28 days with no seizure-free period exceeding 21 days. In these 3 trials, patients had a mean duration of epilepsy of 24 years, and a median baseline seizure frequency ranging from 10 to 17 per 28 days. 84% of patients were taking 2 to 3 concomitant AEDs with or without concurrent vagal nerve stimulation. Study 1 compared doses of VIMPAT 200, 400, and 600 mg/day with placebo. Study 2 compared doses of VIMPAT 400 and 600 mg/day with placebo. Study 3 compared doses of VIMPAT 200 and 400 mg/day with placebo. In all three trials, following an 8-week Baseline Phase to establish baseline seizure frequency prior to randomization, subjects were randomized and titrated to the randomized dose (a 1-step back-titration of VIMPAT 100 mg/day or placebo was allowed in the case of intolerable adverse events at the end of the Titration Phase). During the Titration Phase in all 3 trials, treatment was initiated at 100 mg/day (50 mg given twice daily) and increased in weekly increments of 100 mg/day to the target dose. The Titration Phase lasted 6 weeks in Study 1 and Study 2 and 4 weeks in Study 3. In all three trials, the Titration Phase was followed by a Maintenance Phase that lasted 12 weeks, during which patients were to remain on a stable dose of VIMPAT.

A reduction in 28 day seizure frequency (Baseline to Maintenance Phase) as compared to the placebo group was the primary variable in all three trials. The criteria for statistical significance was p<0.05. A statistically significant effect was observed with VIMPAT treatment (Figure 1) at doses of 200 mg/day (Study 3), 400 mg/day (Studies 1, 2, and 3), and 600 mg/day (Studies 1 and 2).

Subset evaluations of VIMPAT demonstrate no important differences in seizure control as a function of gender or race, although data on race was limited (about 10% of patients were non-Caucasian).

[See figure 1 at top of next page]

Figure 2 presents the percentage of patients (X-axis) with a percent reduction in partial seizure frequency (responder rate) from Baseline to the Maintenance phase at least as great as that represented on the Y-axis. A positive value on the Y-axis indicates an improvement from Baseline (i.e., a decrease in seizure frequency), while a negative value indicates a worsening from Baseline (ie, an increase in seizure frequency). Thus, in a display of this type, a curve for an effective treatment is shifted to the left of the curve for placebo. The proportion of patients achieving any particular level of reduction in seizure frequency was consistently higher for the VIMPAT groups compared to the placebo group. For example, 40% of patients randomized to VIMPAT (400mg/day) experienced a 50% or greater reduction in seizure frequency, compared to 23% of patients randomized to placebo. Patients with an increase in seizure frequency

Figure 1 – Median Percent Reduction in Seizure Frequency per 28 days from Baseline to the Maintenance Phase by Dose

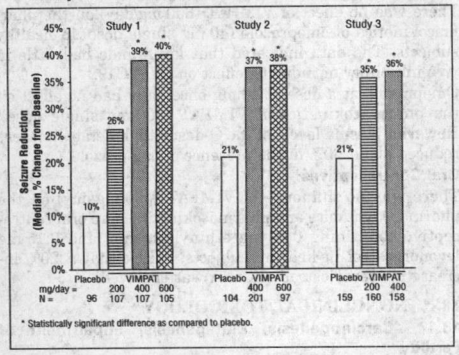

* Statistically significant difference as compared to placebo.

>100% are represented on the Y-axis as equal to or greater than -100%.

Figure 2 – Proportion of Patients by Responder Rate for VIMPAT and Placebo Groups in Studies 1, 2, and 3

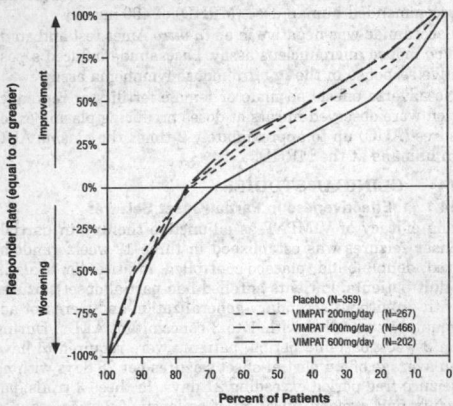

16 HOW SUPPLIED/STORAGE AND HANDLING

VIMPAT (lacosamide) Tablets 50 mg are pink, oval, film-coated tablets debossed with "SP" on one side and "50" on the other. They are supplied as follows:

Bottles of 60   NDC 0131-2477-35

VIMPAT (lacosamide) Tablets 100 mg are dark yellow, oval, film-coated tablets debossed with "SP" on one side and "100" on the other. They are supplied as follows:

Bottles of 60   NDC 0131-2478-35

VIMPAT (lacosamide) Tablets 150 mg are salmon, oval, film-coated tablets debossed with "SP" on one side and "150" on the other. They are supplied as follows:

Bottles of 60   NDC 0131-2479-35

VIMPAT (lacosamide) Tablets 200 mg are blue, oval, film-coated tablets debossed with "SP" on one side and "200" on the other. They are supplied as follows:

Bottles of 60   NDC 0131-2480-35

VIMPAT (lacosamide) injection 200 mg/20 mL is a clear, colorless sterile solution supplied in 20 mL colorless single-use glass vials.

200 mg/20 mL vial in   NDC 0131-1810-67
cartons of 10 vials

VIMPAT (lacosamide) oral solution 10 mg/mL is a clear, colorless to yellow or yellow-brown, strawberry-flavored liquid. It is supplied in PET bottles.

465 mL bottles   NDC 0131-5410-70

16.1 Storage

Store at 20° to 25°C (68° to 77°F); excursions permitted between 15° to 30°C (59° to 86°F). [See USP Controlled Room Temperature.]
Do not freeze Vimpat injection or oral solution. Discard any unused Vimpat oral solution remaining after seven (7) weeks of first opening the bottle.

17 PATIENT COUNSELING INFORMATION
[See Medication Guide]
Patients should be informed of the availability of a Medication Guide, and they should be instructed to read the Medication Guide prior to taking VIMPAT. Patients should be instructed to take VIMPAT only as prescribed.

17.1 Suicidal Thinking and Behavior
Patients, their caregivers, and families should be counseled that AEDs, including VIMPAT, may increase the risk of suicidal thoughts and behavior and should be advised of the need to be alert for the emergence or worsening of symptoms of depression, any unusual changes in mood or behavior, or the emergence of suicidal thoughts, behavior, or thoughts about self-harm. Behaviors of concern should be reported immediately to healthcare providers.

17.2 Dizziness and Ataxia
Patients should be counseled that VIMPAT use may cause dizziness, double vision, abnormal coordination and balance, and somnolence. Patients taking VIMPAT should be advised not to drive, operate complex machinery, or engage in other hazardous activities until they have become accustomed to any such effects associated with VIMPAT.

17.3 Cardiac Rhythm and Conduction Abnormalities
Patients should be counseled that VIMPAT is associated with electrocardiographic changes that may predispose to irregular beat and syncope, particularly in patients with underlying cardiovascular disease, with heart conduction problems or who are taking other medications that affect the heart. Patients who develop syncope should lay down with raised legs until recovered and contact their health care provider.

17.4 Multiorgan Hypersensitivity Reactions
Patients should be aware that VIMPAT may cause serious hypersensitivity reactions affecting multiple organs such as the liver and kidney. VIMPAT should be discontinued if a serious hypersensitivity reaction is suspected. Patients should also be instructed to report promptly to their physicians any symptoms of liver toxicity (e.g. fatigue, jaundice, dark urine).

17.5 Pregnancy Registry
UCB, Inc. has established the UCB AED Pregnancy Registry to advance scientific knowledge about safety and outcomes in pregnant women being treated with VIMPAT. To ensure broad program access and reach, either a healthcare provider or the patient can initiate enrollment in the UCB AED Pregnancy Registry by calling 1-888-537-7734 (toll free).
Patients should also be encouraged to enroll in the North American Antiepileptic Drug Pregnancy Registry if they become pregnant. This Registry is collecting information about the safety of AEDs during pregnancy. To enroll, patients can call the toll free number 1-888-233-2334 [see *Use in Specific Populations (8.1)*].

MEDICATION GUIDE
VIMPAT (VIM-păt) CV
(lacosamide)

Tablet, Oral Solution and Injection for Intravenous Use
Read this Medication Guide before you start taking VIMPAT and each time you get a refill. There may be new information. This Medication Guide describes important safety information about VIMPAT. This information does not take the place of talking to your healthcare provider about your medical condition or treatment.

What is the most important information I should know about VIMPAT?
Do not stop taking VIMPAT without first talking to your healthcare provider.
Stopping VIMPAT suddenly can cause serious problems.
VIMPAT can cause serious side effects, including:
1. Like other antiepileptic drugs, VIMPAT may cause suicidal thoughts or actions in a very small number of people, about 1 in 500.
Call a healthcare provider right away if you have any of these symptoms, especially if they are new, worse, or worry you:
- thoughts about suicide or dying
- attempt to commit suicide
- new or worse depression
- new or worse anxiety
- feeling agitated or restless
- panic attacks
- trouble sleeping (insomnia)
- new or worse irritability
- acting aggressive, being angry, or violent
- acting on dangerous impulses
- an extreme increase in activity and talking (mania)
- other unusual changes in behavior or mood

How can I watch for early symptoms of suicidal thoughts and actions?
- Pay attention to any changes, especially sudden changes, in mood, behaviors, thoughts, or feelings.
- Keep all follow-up visits with your healthcare provider as scheduled.

- Call your healthcare provider between visits as needed, especially if you are worried about symptoms.
- Suicidal thoughts or actions can be caused by things other than medicines. If you have suicidal thoughts or actions, your healthcare provider may check for other causes.
- **Do not stop VIMPAT without first talking to a healthcare provider.** Stopping VIMPAT suddenly can cause serious problems. Stopping seizure medicine suddenly in a patient who has epilepsy can cause seizures that will not stop (status epilepticus).
2. Vimpat may cause you to feel dizzy, have double vision, feel sleepy, or have problems with coordination and walking. Do not drive, operate heavy machinery, or do other dangerous activities until you know how VIMPAT affects you.
3. VIMPAT may cause you to have an irregular heartbeat or may cause you to faint. Call your healthcare provider if you have:
- fast, slow, or pounding heartbeat
- shortness of breath
- feel lightheaded
- fainted or if you feel like you are going to faint
If you have fainted or feel like you are going to faint you should lay down with your legs raised until you feel better.
4. VIMPAT is a federally controlled substance (C-V) because it can be abused or lead to drug dependence. Keep your VIMPAT in a safe place, to protect it from theft. Never give your VIMPAT to anyone else, because it may harm them. Selling or giving away this medicine is against the law.
What is VIMPAT?
VIMPAT is a prescription medicine used with other medicines to treat partial-onset seizures in people 17 years of age and older.
What should I tell my healthcare provider before taking VIMPAT?
Before you take VIMPAT, tell your healthcare provider, if you:
- have or have had depression, mood problems or suicidal thoughts or behavior
- have heart problems
- have kidney problems
- have liver problems
- have abused prescription medicines, street drugs or alcohol in the past
- have any other medical problems
- are pregnant or plan to become pregnant. It is not known if VIMPAT can harm your unborn baby. Tell your healthcare provider right away if you become pregnant while taking VIMPAT. You and your healthcare provider will decide if you should take VIMPAT while you are pregnant.
  - If you become pregnant while taking VIMPAT, talk to your healthcare provider about registering with the North American Antiepileptic Drug Pregnancy Registry. You can enroll in this registry by calling 1-888-233-2334. You can also enroll in the UCB AED Pregnancy Registry by calling 1-888-537-7734. The purpose of this registry is to collect information about the safety of antiepileptic medicine during pregnancy.
- are breastfeeding or plan to breastfeed. It is not known if VIMPAT passes into your breast milk or if it can harm your baby. Talk to your healthcare provider about the best way to feed your baby if you take VIMPAT.
Tell your healthcare provider about all the medicines you take, including prescription and non-prescription medicines, vitamins, and herbal supplements.
Taking VIMPAT with certain other medicines may cause side effects or affect how they work. Do not start or stop other medicines without talking to your healthcare provider. Know the medicines you take. Keep a list of them and show it to your healthcare provider and pharmacist each time you get a new medicine.
How should I take VIMPAT?
- Take VIMPAT exactly as your healthcare provider tells you.
- Your healthcare provider will tell you how much VIMPAT to take and when to take it.
- Your healthcare provider may change your dose if needed.
- Do not stop VIMPAT without first talking to a healthcare provider. Stopping VIMPAT suddenly in a patient who has epilepsy can cause seizures that will not stop (status epilepticus).
- VIMPAT may be taken with or without food..
- If your healthcare provider has prescribed VIMPAT oral solution, be sure to ask your pharmacist for a medicine dropper or medicine cup to help you measure the correct amount of VIMPAT oral solution. Do not use a household teaspoon. Ask your pharmacist for instructions on how to use the measuring device the right way.
- If you take too much VIMPAT, call your healthcare provider or local Poison Control Center right away.
What should I avoid while taking VIMPAT?
- Do not drive, operate heavy machinery, or do other dangerous activities until you know how VIMPAT affects you.

VIMPAT may cause you to feel dizzy, have double vision, feel sleepy, or have problems with coordination and walking.

What are the possible side effects of VIMPAT?
See "What is the most important information I should know about VIMPAT?".
VIMPAT may cause other serious side effects including:
VIMPAT may cause a serious allergic reaction that may affect your skin or other parts of your body such as your liver or blood cells.
Call your healthcare provider right away if you have:
• a skin rash, hives
• fever or swollen glands that do not go away
• shortness of breath, swelling of the legs, yellowing of the skin or whites of the eyes, or dark urine

The most common side effects of VIMPAT include:
• dizziness
• headache
• double vision
• nausea

These are not all of the possible side effects of VIMPAT. For more information ask your healthcare provider or pharmacist. Tell your healthcare provider about any side effect that bothers you or that does not go away. Call your healthcare provider for medical advice about side effects. You may report side effects to FDA at 1-800-FDA-1088.

How should I store VIMPAT?
• Store VIMPAT between 59° F to 86° F (15° C to 30° C)
Keep VIMPAT and all medicines out of the reach of children
General Information about VIMPAT
Medicines are sometimes prescribed for purposes other than those listed in a Medication Guide. Do not use VIMPAT for a condition for which it was not prescribed. Do not give VIMPAT to other people, even if they have the same symptoms you have. It may harm them.

This Medication Guide summarizes the most important information about VIMPAT. If you would like more information, talk with your healthcare provider. You can ask your pharmacist or healthcare provider for information about VIMPAT that is written for health professionals.

For more information, go to www.vimpat.com or call 1-800-477-7877.

What are the ingredients in VIMPAT?
Active ingredient: lacosamide
Tablet inactive ingredients: colloidal silicon dioxide, crospovidone, hydroxypropylcellulose, hypromellose, lecithin, magnesium stearate, microcrystalline cellulose, polyethylene glycol, polyvinyl alcohol, talc, titanium dioxide and additional ingredients listed below:
• **50 mg tablets:** red iron oxide, black iron oxide, FD&C Blue #2/indigo carmine aluminum lake
• **150 mg tablets:** yellow iron oxide, red iron oxide, black iron oxide
• **200 mg tablets:** FD&C Blue #2/indigo carmine aluminum lake
Oral solution inactive ingredients: purified water, sorbitol solution, glycerin, polyethylene glycol, carboxymethylcellulose sodium, acesulfame potassium, methylparaben, flavoring (including natural and artificial flavors, propylene glycol, aspartame, and maltol), anhydrous citric acid and sodium chloride.
Injection inactive ingredients: sodium chloride, water for injection, hydrochloric acid

Manufactured for
UCB, Inc.
Smyrna, GA 30080
Issued 04/2010
This Medication Guide has been approved by the U.S. Food and Drug Administration.

VIMPAT® is a registered trademark under license from Harris FRC Corporation and covered by one or more claims of U.S. Patent 38,551.
Shown in Product Identification Guide, page 320

Unimed Pharmaceuticals, Inc.
NORTH CHICAGO, IL 60064, U.S.A.

Pharmaceutical Products Division—
Direct Inquiries to:
Customer Service:
(800) 255-5162
Patient Access Program:
(800) 441-4987
For Medical Information Contact:
(800) 633-9110 or www.abbottmedinfo.com
Adverse experiences or side effects
(for all Abbott drug products):
(800) 633-9110 or rxabbott.com
Sales and Ordering:
(800) 255-5162

ANDROGEL® ℞
[ăn drō-jĕl]
(testosterone gel)
1% for topical use

HIGHLIGHTS OF PRESCRIBING INFORMATION
These highlights do not include all the information needed to use AndroGel safely and effectively. See full prescribing information for AndroGel.
AndroGel® (testosterone gel) 1% for topical use CIII
Initial U.S. Approval: 1953

> **WARNING: SECONDARY EXPOSURE TO TESTOSTERONE**
> **See full prescribing information for complete boxed warning**
> • Virilization has been reported in children who were secondarily exposed to testosterone gel (5.2, 6.2).
> • Children should avoid contact with unwashed or unclothed application sites in men using testosterone gel (5.2).
> • Healthcare providers should advise patients to strictly adhere to recommended instructions for use (5.2).

—————RECENT MAJOR CHANGES—————
• Boxed Warning 9/2009
• WARNINGS AND PRECAUTIONS (5.2) 9/2009
—————INDICATIONS AND USAGE—————
AndroGel is an androgen indicated for replacement therapy in males for conditions associated with a deficiency or absence of endogenous testosterone:
• Primary Hypogonadism (Congenital or Acquired) (1.1)
• Hypogonadotropic Hypogonadism (Congenital or Acquired) (1.1)
—————DOSAGE AND ADMINISTRATION—————
• Recommended starting dose: 5 g for adult males, applied topically once daily (2.1).
• Apply to clean, dry, intact skin of shoulders and upper arms and/or abdomen. Do NOT apply AndroGel to the genitals (2.1).
• Dose adjustment for adult males: If serum testosterone level is below the normal range, adjust dose from 5 g to 7.5 g and from 7.5 g to 10 g (2.3).
—————DOSAGE FORMS AND STRENGTHS—————
AndroGel (testosterone gel) 1% for topical use is available as:
• 2 × 75 g pumps (each pump dispenses 60 metered 1.25 g doses) (3)
• 2.5 g packet or 5 g packet (3)
—————CONTRAINDICATIONS—————
• Men with carcinoma of the breast or known or suspected prostate cancer (4, 5.1).
• Pregnant or breast feeding women. Testosterone may cause fetal harm (4).
—————WARNINGS AND PRECAUTIONS—————
• Patients with benign prostatic hyperplasia (BPH) treated with androgens are at an increased risk for worsening of signs and symptoms of BPH (5.1).
• Secondary exposure to testosterone in children and women can occur with use of testosterone gel (5.2). Cases of secondary exposure resulting in virilization of children have been reported (6.2).
• Children and women should avoid contact with unwashed or unclothed application site(s) in men using testosterone gel.
• To minimize the potential for transfer to others, patients using AndroGel should apply the product as directed and strictly adhere to the following (5.2):
  • Wash hands with soap and water after application.
  • Cover the application site with clothing after the gel has dried.
  • Wash the application site thoroughly with soap and water prior to any situation where skin-to-skin contact of the application site with another person is anticipated.
• Signs of virilization in children and women and the possibility of secondary exposure to testosterone gel should be brought to the attention of the healthcare provider. Testosterone gel should be promptly discontinued until the cause of the virilization is identified (5.2).
• Due to lack of controlled evaluations in women and potential virilizing effects, AndroGel is not indicated for use in women (5.3).
• Exogenous administration of androgens may lead to azoospermia (5.4).
• Edema may be a complication in patients with preexisting cardiac, renal, or hepatic disease (5.6, 6.2).
• Gynecomastia, enlargement of breast, may develop (5.7).
• Sleep apnea may occur in those with risk factors (5.8).
• Monitor serum testosterone, prostatic specific antigen, hemoglobin, hematocrit, liver function test, and lipid levels periodically (2.3, 5.1, 5.9).
• Alcohol-based gels are flammable until dry (5.10).

—————ADVERSE REACTIONS—————
Most common adverse reactions (incidence ≥ 5%) are acne, application site reaction, abnormal lab tests, and prostatic disorders (6).
Cases of testosterone secondary exposure resulting in virilization of children have been reported (6.2). Reported signs and symptoms have included enlargement of the penis or clitoris, premature development of pubic hair, increased erections and libido, aggressive behavior, and advanced bone age. In most cases with a reported outcome, these signs and symptoms were reported to have regressed with removal of the exposure to testosterone gel (5.2, 6.2). In a few cases, however, enlarged genitalia did not fully return to age-appropriate normal size and bone age remained modestly greater than chronological age.
To report SUSPECTED ADVERSE REACTIONS, contact Abbott Laboratories at 1-800-241-1643 or FDA at 1-800-FDA-1088 or www.fda.gov/medwatch.
—————DRUG INTERACTIONS—————
• Androgens may decrease blood glucose, and therefore insulin requirement in diabetic patients (7.1).
• Use of testosterone with ACTH or corticosteroids may result in increased fluid retention. Use with caution, particularly in patients with cardiac, renal, or hepatic disease (7.2).
• Changes in anticoagulant activity may be seen with androgens. More frequent monitoring of INR and prothrombin time is recommended (7.3).
—————USE IN SPECIFIC POPULATIONS—————
• Pregnancy: AndroGel may cause teratogenic effects. AndroGel should not be used in pregnant women (4, 8.1).
• Nursing mothers should not use AndroGel (4, 8.3).
• Safety and efficacy of AndroGel in males < 18 years old has not been established (8.4).
• There have not been sufficient numbers of geriatric patients involved in controlled clinical studies utilizing AndroGel to determine whether efficacy in those > 65 differs from younger subjects. Additionally, there is insufficient long-term safety data in geriatric patients to assess the potential risks of cardiovascular disease and prostate cancer (8.5).
• No formal studies were conducted involving patients with renal or hepatic insufficiencies (8.6).
See 17 for PATIENT COUNSELING INFORMATION and Medication Guide

Revised: 03/2010

FULL PRESCRIBING INFORMATION: CONTENTS*
1 INDICATIONS AND USAGE
   1.1 Testosterone Replacement Therapy
2 DOSAGE AND ADMINISTRATION
   2.1 General Dosing
   2.2 Administration
   2.3 Dose Adjustment and Patient Assessments
3 DOSAGE FORMS AND STRENGTHS
4 CONTRAINDICATIONS
5 WARNINGS AND PRECAUTIONS
   5.1 Benign Prostatic Hyperplasia and Potential Risk of Prostate Cancer
   5.2 Potential for Secondary Exposure to Testosterone
   5.3 Use in Women
   5.4 Potential for Adverse Effects on Spermatogenesis
   5.5 Hepatic Adverse Effects
   5.6 Edema
   5.7 Gynecomastia
   5.8 Sleep Apnea
   5.9 Laboratory Tests
   5.10 Flammable until Dry
6 ADVERSE REACTIONS
   6.1 Clinical Trial Experience
   6.2 Postmarketing Experience
7 DRUG INTERACTIONS
   7.1 Insulin
   7.2 Corticosteroids
   7.3 Oral Anticoagulants
8 USE IN SPECIFIC POPULATIONS
   8.1 Pregnancy
   8.3 Nursing Mothers
   8.4 Pediatric Use
   8.5 Geriatric Use
   8.6 Renal or Hepatic Impairment
9 DRUG ABUSE AND DEPENDENCE
   9.1 Controlled Substance
10 OVERDOSAGE
11 DESCRIPTION
12 CLINICAL PHARMACOLOGY
   12.1 Mechanism of Action
   12.3 Pharmacokinetics
13 NONCLINICAL TOXICOLOGY
   13.1 Carcinogenesis, Mutagenesis, Impairment of Fertility
14 CLINICAL STUDIES
   14.1 Clinical Trials in Adult Hypogonadal Males
   14.2 Phototoxicity in Humans

14.3 Testosterone Transfer from Male Patients to Female Partners

16 HOW SUPPLIED/STORAGE AND HANDLING

17 PATIENT COUNSELING INFORMATION

17.1 Men with known or suspected prostate or breast cancer should not use AndroGel.

17.2 Potential for Secondary Exposure to Testosterone and Steps to Prevent Secondary Exposure

17.3 Potential Adverse Reactions with Androgens

17.4 Patients Should Be Advised:

17.5 FDA-Approved Medication Guide

* Sections or subsections omitted from the full prescribing information are not listed

---

FULL PRESCRIBING INFORMATION

> **WARNING: SECONDARY EXPOSURE TO TESTOSTERONE**
> - Virilization has been reported in children who were secondarily exposed to testosterone gel (5.2, 6.2).
> - Children should avoid contact with any unwashed or unclothed application sites in men using testosterone gel (5.2).
> - Healthcare providers should advise patients to strictly adhere to recommended instructions for use (5.2).

---

1 INDICATIONS AND USAGE

1.1 Testosterone Replacement Therapy

AndroGel, an androgen, is indicated for replacement therapy in adult males for conditions associated with a deficiency or absence of endogenous testosterone:

- Primary Hypogonadism (Congenital or Acquired) - testicular failure due to cryptorchidism, bilateral torsion, orchitis, vanishing testis syndrome, orchiectomy, Klinefelter's syndrome, chemotherapy, or toxic damage from alcohol or heavy metals. These men usually have low serum testosterone levels and gonadotropins (FSH, LH) above the normal range.
- Hypogonadotropic Hypogonadism (Congenital or Acquired) - idiopathic gonadotropin or luteinizing hormone-releasing hormone (LHRH) deficiency or pituitary-hypothalamic injury from tumors, trauma, or radiation. These men have low testosterone serum levels but have gonadotropins in the normal or low range.

2 DOSAGE AND ADMINISTRATION

2.1 General Dosing

The recommended starting dose of AndroGel is 5 g once daily (preferably in the morning) to clean, dry, intact skin of the shoulders and upper arms and/or abdomen (area of application should be limited to the area that will be covered by the patient's short sleeve t-shirt). AndroGel must not be applied to the genitals. AndroGel is supplied as either a pump or in individual packets. After applying the gel, the application site should be allowed to dry for a few minutes prior to dressing. Avoid fire, flames or smoking until the gel has dried since alcohol based products, including AndroGel, are flammable. Hands should be washed with soap and water after AndroGel has been applied. *[see Warnings and Precautions (5.2, 5.10)].*

2.2 Administration

Multi-Dose Pump

Patients should be instructed to prime the pump before using it for the first time by fully depressing the pump mechanism (actuation) 3 times and discard this portion of the product to assure precise dose delivery. After the priming procedure, patients should completely depress the pump one time (actuation) for every 1.25 g (AndroGel Pump) of product required to achieve the daily prescribed dosage. The product may be delivered directly into the palm of the hand and then applied to the desired application sites, either one pump actuation at a time or upon completion of all pump actuations required for the daily dose. Alternatively, the product can be applied directly to the application sites. Application directly to the sites may prevent loss of product that may occur during transfer from the palm of the hand onto the application sites. Table 1 has specific dosing guidelines for adult males when the 75 g AndroGel Pump is used.

Table 1: Specific Dosing Guidelines for Using the Adult Multi-Dose Pump

Prescribed Daily Dose	Number of Pump Actuations in 75 g Pump
5 g	4 (once daily)
7.5 g	6 (once daily)
10 g	8 (once daily)

Packets

The entire contents should be squeezed into the palm of the hand and immediately applied to the application sites. Alternately, patients may squeeze a portion of the gel from the packet into the palm of the hand and apply to application sites. Repeat until entire contents have been applied.

2.3 Dose Adjustment and Patient Assessments

- To ensure proper dosing, serum testosterone levels should be measured at intervals and replaced to serum testosterone levels in the normal range. If the serum testosterone concentration is below the normal range, the daily AndroGel dose may be increased from 5 g to 7.5 g and from 7.5 g to 10 g for adult males as instructed by the physician. If the serum testosterone concentration exceeds the normal range, the daily AndroGel dose may be decreased. If the serum testosterone concentration consistently exceeds the normal range at a daily dose of 5 g, AndroGel therapy should be discontinued.

The following is general advice for treating and monitoring adult patients on AndroGel. No specific recommendations can be made.

- Prescribers should be aware that testosterone is contraindicated in men with known or suspected prostate cancer. Therefore, evaluation for prostate cancer prior to initiation of AndroGel therapy is appropriate *[see Contraindications (4)].*
- Based on results from controlled studies, serum PSA may rise when taking AndroGel. Therefore, periodic assessment of serum PSA is recommended in patients taking AndroGel *[see Adverse Reactions (6.1)].*
- Based on results from controlled studies, worsening of BPH may occur in patients taking AndroGel *[see Adverse Reactions (6.1)].* Therefore, periodic assessments for signs and symptoms of BPH are recommended in patients taking AndroGel.
- Hematocrit, serum lipid profile, and liver function test should be monitored in patients taking AndroGel *[see Warnings and Precautions (5.9)].*

3 DOSAGE FORMS AND STRENGTHS

AndroGel (testosterone gel) 1% for topical use is available in either unit-dose packets or multiple-dose pumps. The 75 g (60 metered-dose) pump delivers 1.25 g of product when the pump mechanism is fully depressed once.

AndroGel is available in the following three package containers:

- 2 × 75 g pumps (each pump dispenses 60 metered 1.25 g doses)
- 2.5 g packet
- 5 g packet

4 CONTRAINDICATIONS

AndroGel should not be used in any of the following patients:

- Men with carcinoma of the breast or known or suspected carcinoma of the prostate *[see Warnings and Precautions (5.1), Adverse Reactions (6.1), and Nonclinical Toxicology (13.1)].*
- Women who are or may become pregnant, or who are breastfeeding. AndroGel can cause fetal harm when administered to a pregnant woman. AndroGel may cause serious adverse reactions in nursing infants. Exposure of a female fetus or nursing infant to androgens may result in varying degrees of virilization. Pregnant women or those who may become pregnant need to be aware of the potential for transfer of testosterone from men treated with AndroGel *[see Warnings and Precautions (5.2) and Use in Specific Populations (8.1, 8.3)].*
- Men with known hypersensitivity to any of its ingredients, including alcohol and soy products.

5 WARNINGS AND PRECAUTIONS

5.1 Benign Prostatic Hyperplasia and Potential Risk of Prostate Cancer

- Patients with BPH treated with androgens are at an increased risk for worsening of signs and symptoms of BPH.
- Patients treated with androgens may be at increased risk for prostate cancer. Evaluation of the patient for prostate cancer prior to initiating and during treatment with androgens is appropriate.
- Increases in serum PSA from baseline values were seen in approximately 18% of individuals in an open label study of 162 hypogonadal men treated with AndroGel for up to 42 months. Most of these increases were seen within the first year of therapy *[see Contraindications (4), Warnings and Precautions (5.9), Adverse Reactions (6.1), and Nonclinical Toxicology (13.1)].*

5.2 Potential for Secondary Exposure to Testosterone

Secondary exposure to testosterone in children and women can occur with testosterone gel use in men *[see Clinical Studies (14.3)].* Cases of secondary exposure resulting in virilization of children have been reported in postmarketing surveillance. Signs and symptoms have included enlargement of the penis or clitoris, development of pubic hair, increased erections and libido, aggressive behavior, and advanced bone age. In most cases, these signs and symptoms regressed with removal of the exposure to testosterone gel. In a few cases, however, enlarged genitalia did not fully return to age-appropriate normal size, and bone age remained modestly greater than chronological age. The risk of transfer was increased in some of these cases by not adhering to precautions for the appropriate use of testosterone gel.

Inappropriate changes in genital size or development of pubic hair or libido in children, or changes in body hair distribution, significant increase in acne, or other signs of virilization in adult women should be brought to the attention of a physician and the possibility of secondary exposure to testosterone gel should also be brought to the attention of a physician. Testosterone gel should be promptly discontinued until the cause of virilization has been identified.

Testosterone may cause fetal harm in a pregnant woman due to virilization of a female fetus *[see Use in Specific Populations (8.1)].*

Strict adherence to the following precautions is advised in order to minimize the potential for secondary exposure to testosterone from AndroGel-treated skin:

- Children and women should avoid contact with unwashed or unclothed application site(s) of men using testosterone gel.
- AndroGel should only be applied to the shoulders, upper arms, and/or abdomen (area of application should be limited to the area that will be covered by the patient's short sleeve t-shirt).
- Patients should wash their hands immediately with soap and water after applying AndroGel.
- Patients should cover the application site(s) with clothing (e.g., a shirt) after the gel has dried.
- Prior to any situation in which skin-to-skin contact with the application site is anticipated, patients should wash the application site(s) thoroughly with soap and water to remove any testosterone residue.
- In the event that unwashed or unclothed skin to which AndroGel has been applied comes in direct contact with the skin of another person, the general area of contact on the other person should be washed with soap and water as soon as possible. Studies show that residual testosterone is removed from the skin surface by washing with soap and water.

5.3 Use in Women

Due to lack of controlled evaluations in women and potential virilizing effects, AndroGel is not indicated for use in women *[see Use in Specific Populations (8.1, 8.3)].*

5.4 Potential for Adverse Effects on Spermatogenesis

At large doses of exogenous androgens, spermatogenesis may be suppressed through feedback inhibition of pituitary follicle-stimulating hormone (FSH) which could possibly lead to adverse effects on semen parameters including sperm count.

5.5 Hepatic Adverse Effects

Prolonged use of high doses of orally active 17-alpha-alkyl androgens (e.g., methyltestosterone) has been associated with serious hepatic adverse effects (peliosis hepatis, hepatic neoplasms, cholestatic hepatitis, and jaundice). Peliosis hepatis can be a life-threatening or fatal complication. Long-term therapy with intramuscular testosterone enanthate has produced multiple hepatic adenomas. AndroGel is not known to produce these adverse effects.

There are rare reports of hepatocellular carcinoma in patients receiving long-term oral therapy with androgens in high doses. Withdrawal of the drugs did not lead to regression of the tumors in all cases.

5.6 Edema

Drugs in the androgen class may promote retention of sodium and water. Edema with or without congestive heart failure may be a serious complication in patients with pre-existing cardiac, renal, or hepatic disease *[see Adverse Reactions (6.2)].*

5.7 Gynecomastia

Gynecomastia may develop and may persist in patients being treated with androgens, including AndroGel, for hypogonadism.

5.8 Sleep Apnea

The treatment of hypogonadal men with testosterone products may potentiate sleep apnea in some patients, especially those with risk factors such as obesity or chronic lung diseases *[see Adverse Reactions (6.2)].*

5.9 Laboratory Tests

- Increases in hematocrit, reflective of increases in red blood cell mass, may require lowering or discontinuation of testosterone. Increase in red blood cell mass may increase the risk for a thromboembolic event.
- Changes in serum lipid profile may require dose adjustment or discontinuation of testosterone therapy.
- Androgens may decrease levels of thyroxin-binding globulin, resulting in decreased total T4 serum levels and increased resin uptake of T3 and T4. Free thyroid hormone levels remain unchanged, however, and there is no clinical evidence of thyroid dysfunction.
- Androgens should be used with caution in cancer patients at risk of hypercalcemia (and associated hypercalciuria).

Regular monitoring of serum calcium concentrations is recommended in these patients.

5.10 Flammable until Dry
- Alcohol Based Products including AndroGel are flammable; therefore avoid fire, flame or smoking until the gel has dried.

6 ADVERSE REACTIONS
6.1 Clinical Trial Experience
Because clinical trials are conducted under widely varying conditions, adverse reaction rates observed in the clinical trials of a drug cannot be directly compared to rates in the clinical trials of another drug and may not reflect the rates observed in practice.

Clinical Trials in Hypogonadal Men
Table 2 shows the incidence of all adverse events judged by the investigator to be at least possibly related to treatment with AndroGel and reported by >1% of patients in a 180 Day, Phase 3 study.

Table 2: Adverse Events Possibly, Probably or Definitely Related to Use of AndroGel in the 180-Day Controlled Clinical Trial

Adverse Event	Dose of AndroGel		
	5 g	7.5 g	10 g
	N = 77	N = 40	N = 78
Acne	1%	3%	8%
Alopecia	1%	0%	1%
Application Site Reaction	5%	3%	4%
Asthenia	0%	3%	1%
Depression	1%	0%	1%
Emotional Lability	0%	3%	3%
Gynecomastia	1%	0%	3%
Headache	4%	3%	0%
Hypertension	3%	0%	3%
Lab Test Abnormal*	6%	5%	3%
Libido Decreased	0%	3%	1%
Nervousness	0%	3%	1%
Pain Breast	1%	3%	1%
Prostate Disorder**	3%	3%	5%
Testis Disorder***	3%	0%	0%

Lab test abnormal occurred in nine patients with one or more of the following events reported: elevated hemoglobin or hematocrit, hyperlipidemia, elevated triglycerides, hypokalemia, decreased HDL, elevated glucose, elevated creatinine, elevated total bilirubin.
**Prostate disorders* included five patients with enlarged prostate, one with BPH, and one with elevated PSA results.
***Testis disorders* were reported in two patients: one with left varicocele and one with slight sensitivity of left testis.

Other less common adverse reactions, reported in fewer than 1% of patients included: amnesia, anxiety, discolored hair, dizziness, dry skin, hirsutism, hostility, impaired urination, paresthesia, penis disorder, peripheral edema, sweating, and vasodilation.
In this 180 day clinical trial, skin reactions at the site of application were reported with AndroGel, but none was severe enough to require treatment or discontinuation of drug.
Six patients (4%) in this trial had adverse events that led to discontinuation of AndroGel. These events included: cerebral hemorrhage, convulsion (neither of which were considered related to AndroGel administration), depression, sadness, memory loss, elevated prostate specific antigen, and hypertension. No AndroGel patient discontinued due to skin reactions.
In a separate uncontrolled pharmacokinetic study of 10 patients, two had adverse events associated with AndroGel; these were asthenia and depression in one patient and increased libido and hyperkinesia in the other.
In a 3 year, flexible dose, extension study, the incidence of all adverse events judged by the investigator to be at least possibly related to treatment with AndroGel and reported by > 1% of patients is shown in Table 3.

Table 3: Adverse Events Possibly, Probably or Definitely Related to Use of AndroGel in the 3 Year, Flexible Dose, Extension Study

Adverse Event	Percent of Subjects
	(N = 162)
Lab Test Abnormal+	9.3
Skin dry	1.9
Application Site Reaction	5.6
Acne	3.1

Pruritus	1.9
Enlarged Prostate	11.7
Carcinoma of Prostate	1.2
Urinary Symptoms*	3.7
Testis Disorder**	1.9
Gynecomastia	2.5
Anemia	2.5

+*Lab test abnormal* occurred in 15 patients with one or more of the following events reported: elevated AST, elevated ALT, elevated testosterone, elevated hemoglobin or hematocrit, elevated cholesterol, elevated cholesterol/LDL ratio, elevated triglycerides, elevated HDL, elevated serum creatinine.
Urinary symptoms included nocturia, urinary hesitancy, urinary incontinence, urinary retention, urinary urgency and weak urinary stream.
**Testis disorders* included three patients. There were two with a non-palpable testis and one with slight right testicular tenderness.

Two patients reported serious adverse events considered possibly related to treatment: deep vein thrombosis (DVT) and prostate disorder requiring a transurethral resection of the prostate (TURP).
Discontinuation for adverse events in this study included: two patients with application site reactions, one with kidney failure, and five with prostate disorders (including increase in serum PSA in 4 patients, and increase in PSA with prostate enlargement in a fifth patient).

Increases in Serum PSA Observed in Clinical Trials of Hypogonadal Men
During the initial 6-month study, the mean change in PSA values had a statistically significant increase of 0.26 ng/mL. Serum PSA was measured every 6 months thereafter in the 162 hypogonadal men on AndroGel in the 3-year extension study. There was no additional statistically significant increase observed in mean PSA from 6 months through 36 months. However, there were increases in serum PSA observed in approximately 18% of individual patients. The overall mean change from baseline in serum PSA values for the entire group from month 6 to 36 was 0.11 ng/mL.
Twenty-nine patients (18%) met the per-protocol criterion for increase in serum PSA, defined as >2× the baseline or any single serum PSA >6 ng/mL. Most of these (25/29) met this criterion by at least doubling of their PSA from baseline. In most cases where PSA at least doubled (22/25), the maximum serum PSA value was still <2 ng/mL. The first occurrence of a pre-specified, post-baseline increase in serum PSA was seen at or prior to Month 12 in most of the patients who met this criterion (23 of 29; 79%).
Four patients met this criterion by having a serum PSA >6 ng/mL and in these, maximum serum PSA values were 6.2 ng/mL, 6.6 ng/mL, 6.7 ng/mL, and 10.7 ng/mL. In two of these patients, prostate cancer was detected on biopsy. The first patient's PSA levels were 4.7 ng/mL and 6.2 ng/mL at baseline and at Month 6/Final, respectively. The second patient's PSA levels were 4.2 ng/mL, 5.2 ng/mL, 5.8 ng/mL, and 6.6 ng/mL at baseline, Month 6, Month 12, and Final, respectively.

6.2 Postmarketing Experience
The following adverse reactions have been identified during post approval use of AndroGel. Because the reactions are reported voluntarily from a population of uncertain size, it is not always possible to reliably estimate their frequency or establish a causal relationship to drug exposure.

Secondary Exposure to Testosterone in Children
Cases of secondary exposure to testosterone resulting in virilization of children have been reported in postmarket surveillance. Signs and symptoms of these reported cases have included enlargement of the clitoris (with surgical intervention) or the penis, development of pubic hair, increased erections and libido, aggressive behavior, and advanced bone age. In most cases with a reported outcome, these signs and symptoms were reported to have regressed with removal of the testosterone gel exposure. In a few cases, however, enlarged genitalia did not fully return to age appropriate normal size, and bone age remained modestly greater than chronological age. In some of the cases, direct contact with the sites of application on the skin of men using testosterone gel was reported. In at least one reported case, the reporter considered the possibility of secondary exposure from items such as the testosterone gel user's shirts and/or other fabric, such as towels and sheets [see *Warnings and Precautions (5.2)*].

Hypogonadal Men
Table 4 includes adverse reactions that have been identified postmarketing.

Table 4: Adverse Drug Reactions from Postmarketing Experience of AndroGel by MedDRA System Organ Class

Blood and the lymphatic system disorders:	Elevated Hgb, Hct (polycythemia)
Endocrine disorders:	Hirsutism
Gastrointestinal disorders:	Nausea
General disorders and administration site reactions:	Asthenia, edema, malaise
Genitourinary disorders:	Impaired urination
Hepatobiliary disorders:	Abnormal liver function tests (e.g. transaminases, elevated GCTP, bilirubin)
Investigations:	Elevated PSA, electrolyte changes (nitrogen, calcium, potassium, phosphorus, sodium), changes in serum lipids (hyperlipidemia, elevated triglycerides, decreased HDL), impaired glucose tolerance, fluctuating testosterone levels, weight increase
Neoplasms benign, malignant and unspecified (cysts and polyps):	Prostate cancer
Nervous system:	Headache, dizziness, sleep apnea, insomnia
Psychiatric disorders:	Depression, emotional lability, decreased libido, nervousness, hostility, amnesia, anxiety
Reproductive system and breast disorders:	Gynecomastia, mastodynia, prostatic enlargement, testicular atrophy, oligospermia, priapism (frequent or prolonged erections)
Respiratory disorders:	Dyspnea
Skin and subcutaneous tissue disorders:	Acne, alopecia, application site reaction (pruritus, dry skin, erythema, rash, discolored hair, paresthesia), sweating
Vascular disorders:	Hypertension, vasodilation (hot flushes)

7 DRUG INTERACTIONS
7.1 Insulin
Changes in insulin sensitivity or glycemic control may occur in patients treated with androgens. In diabetic patients, the metabolic effects of androgens may decrease blood glucose and, therefore, insulin requirements.
7.2 Corticosteroids
The concurrent use of testosterone with ACTH or corticosteroids may result in increased fluid retention and should be monitored cautiously, particularly in patients with cardiac, renal or hepatic disease.
7.3 Oral Anticoagulants
Changes in anticoagulant activity may be seen with androgens. More frequent monitoring of INR and prothrombin time are recommended in patients taking anticoagulants, especially at the initiation and termination of androgen therapy.

8 USE IN SPECIFIC POPULATIONS
8.1 Pregnancy
Pregnancy Category X: AndroGel is contraindicated during pregnancy or in women who may become pregnant. It is teratogenic and may cause fetal harm [see *Contraindications (4)*]. Exposure of a female fetus to androgens may result in varying degrees of virilization. If this drug is used during pregnancy, or if the patient becomes pregnant while taking this drug, the patient should be apprised of the potential hazard to a fetus.
8.3 Nursing Mothers
Although it is not known how much testosterone transfers into human milk, AndroGel is contraindicated in nursing women because of the potential for serious adverse reactions in nursing infants [see *Contraindications (4)*].

Testosterone and other androgens may adversely affect lactation.

8.4 Pediatric Use

Safety and efficacy of AndroGel in males < 18 years old has not been established. Improper use may result in acceleration of bone age and premature closure of epiphyses.

8.5 Geriatric Use

There have not been sufficient numbers of geriatric patients involved in controlled clinical studies utilizing AndroGel to determine whether efficacy in those over 65 years of age differs from younger subjects. Additionally, there is insufficient long-term safety data in geriatric patients to assess the potential risks of cardiovascular disease and prostate cancer.

8.6 Renal or Hepatic Impairment

No formal studies were conducted involving patients with renal or hepatic insufficiencies.

9 DRUG ABUSE AND DEPENDENCE

9.1 Controlled Substance

AndroGel contains testosterone, a Schedule III controlled substance as defined by the Anabolic Steroids Control Act. Oral ingestion of AndroGel will not result in clinically significant serum testosterone concentrations due to extensive first-pass metabolism.

10 OVERDOSAGE

There is one report of acute overdosage with use of an approved injectable testosterone product: this subject had serum testosterone levels of up to 11,400 ng/dL with a cerebrovascular accident. Treatment of overdosage would consist of discontinuation of AndroGel together with appropriate symptomatic and supportive care.

11 DESCRIPTION

AndroGel (testosterone gel) 1% is a clear, colorless hydroalcoholic gel containing 1% testosterone. Topical administration of AndroGel 5 g, 7.5 g, or 10 g contains 50 mg, 75 mg, or 100 mg of testosterone, respectively, is to be applied daily to the skin's surface. Approximately 10% of the applied testosterone dose is absorbed across skin of average permeability during a 24-hour period.

The active pharmacologic ingredient in AndroGel is testosterone. Testosterone USP is a white to practically white crystalline powder chemically described as 17-beta hydroxyandrost-4-en-3-one. The structural formula is:

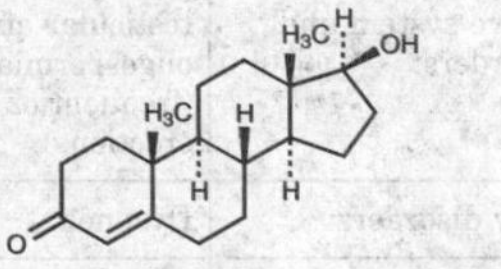

Testosterone

$C_{19}H_{28}O_2$ MW 288.42

Inactive ingredients in AndroGel are carbomer 980, ethanol 67.0%, isopropyl myristate, purified water, and sodium hydroxide. These ingredients are not pharmacologically active.

12 CLINICAL PHARMACOLOGY

12.1 Mechanism of Action

Endogenous androgens, including testosterone and dihydrotestosterone (DHT), are responsible for the normal growth and development of the male sex organs and for maintenance of secondary sex characteristics. These effects include the growth and maturation of prostate, seminal vesicles, penis and scrotum; the development of male hair distribution, such as facial, pubic, chest and axillary hair; laryngeal enlargement, vocal chord thickening, alterations in body musculature and fat distribution. Testosterone and DHT are necessary for the normal development of secondary sex characteristics. Male hypogonadism results from insufficient secretion of testosterone and is characterized by low serum testosterone concentrations. Signs/symptoms associated with male hypogonadism include erectile dysfunction and decreased sexual desire, fatigue and loss of energy, mood depression, regression of secondary sexual characteristics and osteoporosis.

Male hypogonadism has two main etiologies. Primary hypogonadism is caused by defects of the gonads, such as Klinefelter's Syndrome or Leydig cell aplasia, whereas secondary hypogonadism is the failure of the hypothalamus (or pituitary) to produce sufficient gonadotropins (FSH, LH).

12.3 Pharmacokinetics

Adult Males

Absorption

AndroGel delivers physiologic amounts of testosterone, producing circulating testosterone concentrations that approximate normal levels (298–1043 ng/dL) seen in healthy men. AndroGel provides continuous transdermal delivery of testosterone for 24 hours following a single application to intact, clean, dry skin of the shoulders, upper arms and/or abdomen.

AndroGel is a hydroalcoholic formulation that dries quickly when applied to the skin surface. The skin serves as a reservoir for the sustained release of testosterone into the systemic circulation. Approximately 10% of the testosterone dose applied on the skin surface from AndroGel is absorbed into systemic circulation. Therefore, 5 g and 10 g of AndroGel systemically deliver approximately 5 mg and 10 mg of testosterone, respectively. In a study with 10 g of AndroGel, all patients showed an increase in serum testosterone within 30 minutes, and eight of nine patients had a serum testosterone concentration within normal range by 4 hours after the initial application. Absorption of testosterone into the blood continues for the entire 24-hour dosing interval. Serum concentrations approximate the steady-state level by the end of the first 24 hours and are at steady state by the second or third day of dosing.

With single daily applications of AndroGel, follow-up measurements 30, 90 and 180 days after starting treatment have confirmed that serum testosterone concentrations are generally maintained within the eugonadal range. Figure 1 summarizes the 24-hour pharmacokinetic profiles of testosterone for hypogonadal men (<300 ng/dL) maintained on 5 g or 10 g of AndroGel for 30 days. The average (± SD) daily testosterone concentration produced by AndroGel 10 g on Day 30 was 792 (± 294) ng/dL and by AndroGel 5 g 566 (± 262) ng/dL.

Figure 1: Mean (± SD) Steady-State Serum Testosterone Concentrations on Day 30 in Patients Applying AndroGel Once Daily

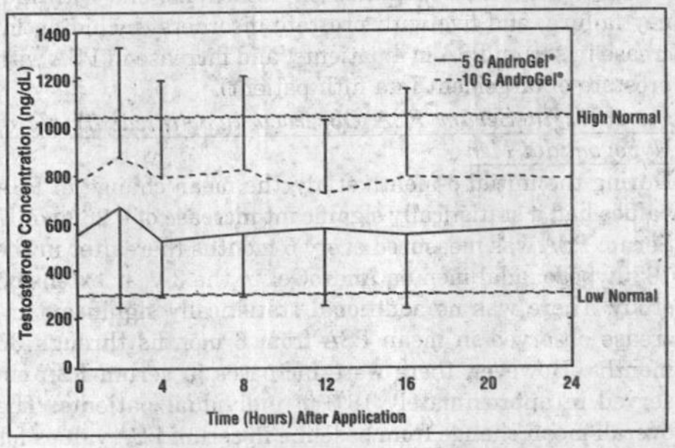

When AndroGel treatment is discontinued after achieving steady state, serum testosterone levels remain in the normal range for 24 to 48 hours but return to their pretreatment levels by the fifth day after the last application.

Distribution

Circulating testosterone is primarily bound in the serum to sex hormone-binding globulin (SHBG) and albumin. Approximately 40% of testosterone in plasma is bound to SHBG, 2% remains unbound (free) and the rest is bound to albumin and other proteins.

Metabolism

There is considerable variation in the half-life of testosterone as reported in the literature, ranging from 10 to 100 minutes. Testosterone is metabolized to various 17-keto steroids through two different pathways. The major active metabolites of testosterone are estradiol and DHT.

DHT concentrations increased in parallel with testosterone concentrations during AndroGel treatment. After 180 days of treatment in adult males, mean DHT concentrations were within the normal range with 5 g AndroGel and were about 7% above the normal range after a 10 g dose. The mean steady-state DHT/T ratio during 180 days of AndroGel treatment remained within normal limits and ranged from 0.23 to 0.29 (5 g/day) and from 0.27 to 0.33 (10 g/day).

Excretion

About 90% of a dose of testosterone given intramuscularly is excreted in the urine as glucuronic and sulfuric acid conjugates of testosterone and its metabolites; about 6% of a dose is excreted in the feces, mostly in the unconjugated form. Inactivation of testosterone occurs primarily in the liver.

13 NONCLINICAL TOXICOLOGY

13.1 Carcinogenesis, Mutagenesis, Impairment of Fertility

Testosterone has been tested by subcutaneous injection and implantation in mice and rats. In mice, the implant induced cervical-uterine tumors, which metastasized in some cases. There is suggestive evidence that injection of testosterone into some strains of female mice increases their susceptibility to hepatoma. Testosterone is also known to increase the number of tumors and decrease the degree of differentiation of chemically induced carcinomas of the liver in rats.

14 CLINICAL STUDIES

14.1 Clinical Trials in Adult Hypogonadal Males

AndroGel was evaluated in a multi-center, randomized, parallel-group, active-controlled, 180-day trial in 227 hypogonadal men. The study was conducted in 2 phases. During the Initial Treatment Period (Days 1-90), 73 patients were randomized to AndroGel 5 g daily, 78 patients to AndroGel 10 g daily, and 76 patients to a non-scrotal testosterone transdermal system. The study was double-blind for dose of AndroGel but open-label for active control. Patients who were originally randomized to AndroGel and who had single-sample serum testosterone levels above or below the normal range on Day 60 were titrated to 7.5 g daily on Day 91. During the Extended Treatment Period (Days 91-180), 51 patients continued on AndroGel 5 g daily, 52 patients continued on AndroGel 10 g daily, 41 patients continued on a non-scrotal testosterone transdermal system (5 mg daily), and 40 patients received AndroGel 7.5 g daily. Upon completion of the initial study, 163 enrolled and 162 patients received treatment in an open-label extension study of AndroGel for an additional period of up to 3 years.

Mean peak, trough and average serum testosterone concentrations within the normal range (298-1043 ng/dL) were achieved on the first day of treatment with doses of 5 g and 10 g. In patients continuing on AndroGel 5 g and 10 g, these mean testosterone levels were maintained within the normal range for the 180-day duration of the original study. Figure 2 summarizes the 24-hour pharmacokinetic profiles of testosterone administered as AndroGel for 30, 90 and 180 days. Testosterone concentrations were maintained as long as the patient continued to properly apply the prescribed AndroGel treatment.

Figure 2: Mean Steady-State Testosterone Concentrations in Patients with Once-Daily AndroGel Therapy

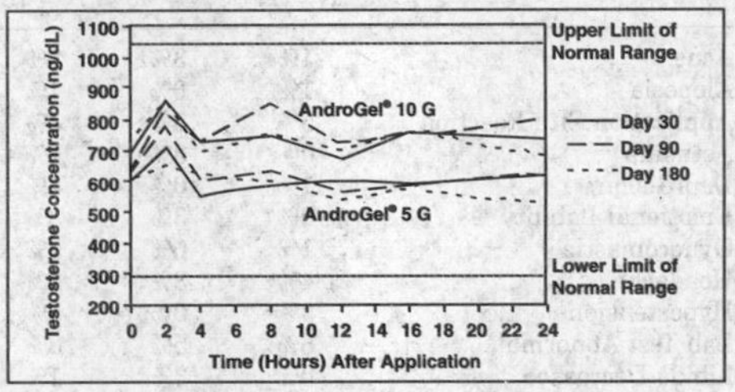

Table 5 summarizes the mean testosterone concentrations on Treatment Day 180 for patients receiving 5 g, 7.5 g, or 10 g of AndroGel. The 7.5 g dose produced mean concentrations intermediate to those produced by 5 g and 10 g of AndroGel.

Table 5: Mean (± SD) Steady-State Serum Testosterone Concentrations During Therapy (Day 180)

	5 g N = 44	7.5 g N = 37	10 g N = 48
Cavg	555 ± 225	601 ± 309	713 ± 209
Cmax	830 ± 347	901 ± 471	1083 ± 434
Cmin	371 ± 165	406 ± 220	485 ± 156

Of 129 hypogonadal men who were appropriately titrated with AndroGel and who had sufficient data for analysis, 87% achieved an average serum testosterone level within the normal range on Treatment Day 180.

In patients treated with AndroGel, there were no observed differences in the average daily serum testosterone concentrations at steady-state based on age, cause of hypogonadism, or body mass index.

AndroGel 5 g/day and 10 g/day resulted in significant increases over time in total body mass and total body lean mass, while total body fat mass and the percent body fat decreased significantly. These changes were maintained for 180 days of treatment during the original study. Changes in the 7.5 g dose group were similar. Bone mineral density in both hip and spine increased significantly from Baseline to Day 180 with 10 g AndroGel.

AndroGel treatment at 5 g/day and 10 g/day for 90 days produced significant improvement in libido (measured by sexual motivation, sexual activity and enjoyment of sexual activity as assessed by patient responses to a questionnaire). The degree of penile erection as subjectively estimated by the patients, increased with AndroGel treatment, as did the subjective score for "satisfactory duration of erection." AndroGel treatment at 5 g/day and 10 g/day produced positive effects on mood and fatigue. Similar changes were seen after 180 days of treatment and in the group treated with the 7.5 g dose. DHT concentrations increased in parallel with testosterone concentrations at AndroGel doses of 5 g/day and 10 g/day, but the DHT/T ratio stayed within the normal range, indicating enhanced availability of the major physiologically active androgen. Serum estradiol (E2) concentrations increased significantly within 30 days of starting treatment with AndroGel 5 or 10 g/day and remained elevated throughout the treatment period but remained within the normal range for eugonadal men. Serum levels of SHBG decreased very slightly (1 to 11%) during AndroGel treatment. In men with hypergonadotropic hypogonadism, serum levels of LH and FSH fell in a dose- and time-dependent manner during treatment with AndroGel.

14.2 Phototoxicity in Humans

The phototoxic potential of AndroGel was evaluated in a double-blind, single-dose study in 27 subjects with photosensitive skin types. The Minimal Erythema Dose (MED) of ultraviolet radiation was determined for each subject. A single 24 (+1) hour application of duplicate patches containing test articles (placebo gel, testosterone gel, or saline) was made to naive skin sites on Day 1. On Day 2, each subject received five exposure times of ultraviolet radiation, each exposure being 25% greater than the previous one. Skin evaluations were made on Days 2 to 5. Exposure of test and control article application sites to ultraviolet light did not produce increased inflammation relative to non-irradiated sites, indicating no phototoxic effect.

14.3 Testosterone Transfer from Male Patients to Female Partners

The potential for dermal testosterone transfer following AndroGel use was evaluated in a clinical study between males dosed with AndroGel and their untreated female partners. Two (2) to 12 hours after AndroGel (10 g) application by the male subjects, the couples (N = 38 couples) engaged in daily, 15-minute sessions of vigorous skin-to-skin contact so that the female partners gained maximum exposure to the AndroGel application sites. Under these study conditions, all unprotected female partners had a serum testosterone concentration >2 times the baseline value at some time during the study. When a shirt covered the application site(s), the transfer of testosterone from the males to the female partners was completely prevented.

16 HOW SUPPLIED/STORAGE AND HANDLING

AndroGel is supplied in non-aerosol, metered-dose pumps. The pump is composed of plastic and stainless steel and an LDPE/aluminum foil inner liner encased in rigid plastic with a polypropylene cap. Each 88 g AndroGel Pump in the twin package is capable of dispensing 75 g or 60 metered 1.25 g doses.

AndroGel is also supplied in unit-dose aluminum foil packets in cartons of 30. Each packet of 2.5 g or 5 g gel contains 25 mg or 50 mg testosterone, respectively.

NDC Number	Package Size
0051-8488-88	2 × 75 g pumps (each pump dispenses 60 metered 1.25 g doses)
0051-8425-30	30 packets (2.5 g per packet)
0051-8450-30	30 packets (5 g per packet)

Keep AndroGel out of the reach of children.

Storage

Store at 25°C (77°F); excursions permitted to 15° to 30°C (59° to 86°F) [see USP Controlled Room Temperature].

Disposal

Used AndroGel pumps or used AndroGel packets should be discarded in household trash in a manner that prevents accidental application or ingestion by children or pets.

17 PATIENT COUNSELING INFORMATION

See FDA-Approved Medication Guide (17.5)

17.1 Men with known or suspected prostate or breast cancer should not use AndroGel.

17.2 Potential for Secondary Exposure to Testosterone and Steps to Prevent Secondary Exposure

Secondary exposure to testosterone in children and women can occur with the use of testosterone gel in men. Cases of secondary exposure to testosterone have been reported in children with signs and symptoms including enlargement of the penis or clitoris, premature development of pubic hair, increased erections, and aggressive behavior.

- Physicians should advise patients of the reported signs and symptoms of secondary exposure which may include the following:
  - In children; unexpected sexual development including inappropriate enlargement of the penis or clitoris, premature development of pubic hair, increased erections, and aggressive behavior
  - In women; changes in hair distribution, increase in acne, or other signs of testosterone effects
- The possibility of secondary exposure to testosterone gel should be brought to the attention of a healthcare provider
- Testosterone gel should be promptly discontinued until the cause of virilization is identified

Strict adherence to the following precautions is advised to minimize the potential for secondary exposure to testosterone from testosterone gel in men *[see FDA-Approved Medication Guide (17.5)]*:

- **Children and women should avoid contact with unwashed or unclothed application site(s) of men using testosterone gel**

- **To minimize the potential for transfer** to others, patients using AndroGel should apply the product as directed and strictly adhere to the following:
  - **Wash hands** with soap and water after application
  - **Cover the application site(s)** with clothing after the gel has dried
  - **Wash the application site(s) thoroughly** with soap and water prior to any situation where skin-to-skin contact of the application site with another person is anticipated
  - In the event that unwashed or unclothed skin to which testosterone gel has been applied comes in contact with the skin of another person, the general area of contact on the other person should be washed with soap and water as soon as possible.

17.3 Potential Adverse Reactions with Androgens

Patients should be informed that treatment with androgens may lead to adverse reactions which include:

- Changes in urinary habits such as increased urination at night, trouble starting your urine stream, passing urine many times during the day, having an urge that you have to go to the bathroom right away, having a urine accident, being unable to pass urine and weak urine flow.
- Breathing disturbances, including those associated with sleep, or excessive daytime sleepiness.
- Too frequent or persistent erections of the penis.
- Nausea, vomiting, changes in skin color, or ankle swelling.

17.4 Patients Should Be Advised:

- **To read the Medication Guide before starting AndroGel therapy and to reread it each time the prescription is renewed**
- **Of the appropriate application and use of AndroGel to maximize the benefits and to minimize the risk of secondary exposure in children and women**
- To keep AndroGel out of the reach of children
- **That AndroGel is an alcohol based product and is flammable; therefore avoid fire, flame or smoking until the gel has dried**
- Of the importance of adhering to all recommended monitoring
- To report any changes in their state of health, such as changes in urinary habits, breathing, sleep, and mood

Marketed By:
Abbott Laboratories
North Chicago, IL 60064, U.S.A.
U.S. Patent No. 6,503,894
© 2010 Abbott Laboratories
500122/500127 2E Rev Mar 2010

17.5 FDA-Approved Medication Guide

MEDICATION GUIDE
AndroGel® (AN DROW JEL) CIII
(testosterone gel) 1%

Read the Medication Guide that comes with AndroGel before you start taking it and each time you get a refill. There may be new information. This Medication Guide does not take the place of talking to your healthcare provider about your medical condition or your treatment.

What is the most important information I should know about AndroGel?

Signs of puberty that are not expected (for example, pubic hair) have happened in young children who were accidentally exposed to testosterone through contact with men using AndroGel.

AndroGel can transfer from your body to others. This can happen if other people come into contact with the area where the AndroGel was applied to your skin.

- **Women and children should avoid contact with the unwashed or unclothed area where AndroGel has been applied.**
- **To lower the risk of transfer of AndroGel from your body to others, you should follow these important instructions:**
  - Apply AndroGel **only** to areas that will be covered by a short sleeve T-shirt. These areas are your shoulders and upper arms, or stomach area (abdomen), or shoulders, upper arms and stomach area.
  - Wash your hands **right away** with soap and water after applying AndroGel.
  - After the gel has dried, **cover the application area with clothing.** Keep the area covered until you have washed the application area well or have showered.
- **If you expect to have skin-to-skin contact with another person, first wash the application area well with soap and water.**
- **If a woman or child makes contact with the AndroGel application area, that area on the woman or child should be washed well with soap and water right away.**

Stop using AndroGel and call your healthcare provider right away if you see any signs and symptoms in a child or a woman that may have occurred through accidental exposure to AndroGel:

Signs and symptoms in **children** may include:
- enlarged penis or clitoris
- early development of pubic hair
- increased erections or sex drive
- aggressive behavior

Signs and symptoms in **women** may include:
- changes in body hair
- a large increase in acne

What is AndroGel?

AndroGel is a prescription medicine that contains testosterone. AndroGel is used to treat adult males who have low or no testosterone.

It is not known if AndroGel is safe or effective in children younger than 18 years old. Improper use of AndroGel may affect bone growth in children.

AndroGel is a controlled substance (CIII) because it contains testosterone that can be a target for people who abuse prescription medicines. Keep your AndroGel in a safe place to protect it. Never give your AndroGel to anyone else, even if they have the same symptoms you have. Selling or giving away this medicine may harm others and is against the law.

AndroGel is not meant for use in women.

Who should not use AndroGel?

Do not use AndroGel if you:

- have breast cancer
- have or might have prostate cancer
- are pregnant or may become pregnant or breast-feeding. AndroGel may harm your unborn or breast-feeding baby. Women who are pregnant or who may become pregnant should avoid contact with the area of skin where AndroGel has been applied.
- are allergic to testosterone or any of the ingredients in AndroGel including soy. See the end of this Medication Guide for a complete list of ingredients in AndroGel.

Talk to your healthcare provider before taking this medicine if you have any of the above conditions.

What should I tell my healthcare provider before using AndroGel?

Before you use AndroGel, tell your healthcare provider if you:

- have breast cancer or prostate cancer
- have urinary problems due to an enlarged prostate
- have heart problems
- have liver or kidney problems
- have problems breathing while you sleep (sleep apnea)
- have any other medical conditions

Tell your healthcare provider about all the medicines you take, including prescription and non-prescription medicines, vitamins, and herbal supplements.

Using AndroGel with certain other medicines can affect each other.

Especially, tell your healthcare provider if you take:

- insulin
- corticosteroids
- medicines that decrease blood clotting

Ask your healthcare provider or pharmacist for a list of these medicines, if you are not sure.

Know the medicines you take. Keep a list of them and show it to your healthcare provider and pharmacist when you get a new medicine.

How should I use AndroGel?

- It is important that you apply AndroGel exactly as prescribed by your healthcare provider. Your healthcare provider will tell you how much AndroGel to apply and when to apply it.
- Your healthcare provider may change your AndroGel dose. Do not change your AndroGel dose without talking to your healthcare provider.
- AndroGel is for skin use only.
- **Do not allow others to apply AndroGel to your body.**
- Applying AndroGel:
- AndroGel comes in a pump and in packets.
  - **If you are using the AndroGel pump:**
    - Before using the pump for the first time, you will need to prime the pump. To prime AndroGel, fully push down on the pump 3 times. Do not use any AndroGel that came out while priming. Wash it down the sink or throw it in the trash to avoid accidental exposure to others. Your AndroGel pump is ready to use now.
    - Your healthcare provider will tell you the number of times to press the pump for each dose.
  - **If you are using AndroGel packets:**
    - Tear open the packet completely at the dotted line.
    - Squeeze all of the AndroGel out of the packet into the palm of your hand. Squeeze from the bottom of the packet to the top.
    - Throw away the packet in the trash out of the reach of children to avoid accidental exposure.
- Squeeze the medicine into the palm of your hand and apply to clean dry, intact skin at the same time each day.
- You may also apply AndroGel from the pump or packet directly to your skin.
- Apply AndroGel only to areas that will be covered by a short sleeve t-shirt, as shown in the shaded areas in the figure below. These areas are your shoulders and upper arms, or stomach area, or shoulders, upper arm and stomach area.

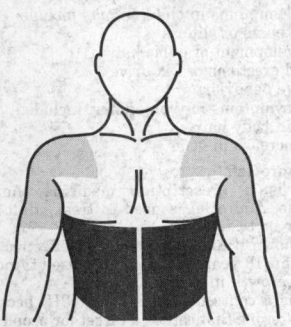

- **Do not apply AndroGel to your penis or scrotum.**
- **Wash your hands with soap and water right after you apply AndroGel.**
- Let the application areas dry for a few minutes before putting on a shirt.
- To prevent transfer of AndroGel to others, clothes (such as a t-shirt) should **always** be worn to cover the AndroGel application areas until you have washed the application areas well with soap and water.
- **AndroGel is flammable until dry. Let the gel dry before smoking or going near an open flame.**

Your healthcare provider will test your blood before you start and while you take AndroGel.

What are the possible side effects of AndroGel?
AndroGel can cause serious side effects including:
- See "**What is the most important information I should know about AndroGel?**"
  - **If you already have enlargement of your prostate gland your signs and symptoms can get worse** while using AndroGel. This can include:
    - increased urination at night
    - trouble starting your urine stream
    - having to pass urine many times during the day
    - having an urge that you have to go to the bathroom right away
    - having a urine accident
    - being unable to pass urine or weak urine flow
- **Possible increased risk of prostate cancer.** Your healthcare provider should check you for prostate cancer or any other prostate problems before you start and while you use AndroGel.
- **In large doses AndroGel may lower your sperm count.**
- **Swelling of your ankles, feet, or body, with or without heart failure.**
- **Enlarged or painful breasts.**
- **Have problems breathing while you sleep (sleep apnea).**
- **Blood clots in the legs.** This can include pain, swelling or redness of your legs.

Call your healthcare provider right away if you have any of the serious side effects listed above.

The most common side effects of AndroGel include:
- acne
- skin irritation where AndroGel is applied
- increased cholesterol levels
- increased prostate specific antigen (a test used to screen for prostate cancer)
- increased red blood cell count
- increased liver function tests

Other side effects include more erections than are normal for you or erections that last a long time.

Tell your healthcare provider if you have any side effect that bothers you or that does not go away.

These are not all the possible side effects of AndroGel. For more information, ask your healthcare provider or pharmacist.

Call your doctor for medical advice about side effects. You may report side effects to FDA at 1-800-FDA-1088.

How should I store AndroGel?
- Store AndroGel between 59°F to 86°F (15°C to 30°C).
- Safely throw away used AndroGel in household trash. Be careful to prevent accidental exposure of children or pets.
- Keep AndroGel away from fire.

Keep AndroGel and all medicines out of the reach of children.

General information about AndroGel
Medicines are sometimes prescribed for purposes other than those listed in a Medication Guide. Do not use AndroGel for a condition for which it was not prescribed. Do not give AndroGel to other people, even if they have the same symptoms you have. It may harm them.

This Medication Guide summarizes the most important information about AndroGel. If you would like more information, talk to your healthcare provider. You can ask your pharmacist or healthcare provider for information about AndroGel that is written for health professionals.

For more information, go to www.ANDROGEL.com or call 1-800-241-1643.

What are the ingredients in AndroGel?
Active ingredient: testosterone
Inactive ingredients: carbomer 980, ethyl alcohol 67.0%, isopropyl myristate, purified water and sodium hydroxide.
© 2010 Solvay Pharmaceuticals, Inc.
Marketed by:
Solvay Pharmaceuticals, Inc.
Marietta, GA 30062, U.S.A.
500122/500127 2E Rev Mar 2010
This Medication Guide has been approved by the U.S. Food and Drug Administration.
Issued March 2010
Revised: 03/2010

Upsher-Smith Laboratories, Inc.
6701 EVENSTAD DRIVE
MINNEAPOLIS, MN 55369

For Medical Information Contact:
Write: Medical Information Department
or call: (800) 654-2299
(during business hours-8:00 am to 5:00 pm CST)

AMLACTIN®   **OTC**
Moisturizing Body Lotion & Cream
[ăm-lăk-tĭn]

DESCRIPTION
AmLactin® Moisturizing Body Lotion and Cream are a special formulation of 12% lactic acid neutralized with ammonium hydroxide to provide a pH of 4.5-5.5. Lactic acid, an alpha-hydroxy acid, is a naturally occurring humectant for the skin. Both AmLactin® Moisturizing Body Lotion & Cream moisturize, exfoliate and soften rough, dry skin. Both formulas are fragrance free and available without a prescription. The cream formula is available in a tube to offer a choice in moisturizers.

DIRECTIONS
For best results, apply to dry skin twice a day.

CAUTION
For external use only.
Keep this product out of the reach of children.
Avoid contact with eyes, lips and mucous membranes. A mild irritation or rash may occur on sensitive skin with initial use. May cause transient stinging when applied to skin with fissures or abrasions. Irritation may occur when used on the face.
If irritation or rash continues, discontinue use and consult a physician.
Avoid unnecessary sun exposure and use a sunscreen.

AmLactin® Moisturizing Body Lotion & Cream Ingredients
Water, lactic acid neutralized with ammonium hydroxide, light mineral oil, glyceryl stearate, PEG-100 stearate, propylene glycol, glycerin, magnesium aluminum silicate, laureth-4, polyoxyl 40 stearate, cetyl alcohol, methylparaben, propylparaben and methylcellulose.
Store at 20-25°C (68-77°F). Avoid excessive heat.
Distributed by
UPSHER-SMITH LABORATORIES, INC.
Minneapolis, MN 55447
©2010 Upsher-Smith Laboratories, Inc.
All Rights Reserved
www.amlactin.com
MADE IN THE USA
*Most recommended moisturizing product for rough, dry skin: Omnibus Study, *Dermatology Times*, May 2009.
*Kloos Donoghue S. Podiatry management annual practice survey. *Podiatry Management*, February 2010.
QUESTIONS OR COMMENTS
Please call 1-800-654-2299
R0810
104638.01
Revised: 08/2010

DIVIGEL®   ℞
[div-e-gel]
(estradiol gel) 0.1%
Rx only

ESTROGENS INCREASE THE RISK OF ENDOMETRIAL CANCER
Close clinical surveillance of all women taking estrogens is important. Adequate diagnostic measures, including endometrial sampling when indicated, should be undertaken to rule out malignancy in all cases of undiagnosed persistent or recurring abnormal vaginal bleeding. There is no evidence that the use of "natural" estrogens results in a different endometrial risk profile than synthetic estrogens at equivalent estrogen doses. (See **WARNINGS, Malignant neoplasms,** *Endometrial cancer.*)

CARDIOVASCULAR AND OTHER RISKS
Estrogens with or without progestins should not be used for the prevention of cardiovascular disease or dementia. (See **CLINICAL STUDIES** and **WARNINGS, Cardiovascular disorders** and **Dementia.**)
The estrogen-alone substudy of the Women's Health Initiative (WHI) reported increased risks of stroke and deep vein thrombosis in postmenopausal women (50 to 79 years of age) during 6.8 years and 7.1 years, respectively, of treatment with oral conjugated estrogens (CE 0.625 mg) alone per day, relative to placebo. (See **CLINICAL STUDIES** and **WARNINGS, Cardiovascular disorders.**)
The estrogen-plus-progestin substudy of the WHI reported increased risk of myocardial infarction, stroke, invasive breast cancer, pulmonary emboli, and deep vein thrombosis in postmenopausal women (50 to 79 years of age) during 5.6 years of treatment with oral conjugated estrogens (CE 0.625 mg) combined with medroxyprogesterone acetate (MPA 2.5 mg) per day, relative to placebo. (See **CLINICAL STUDIES** and **WARNINGS, Cardiovascular disorders** and **Malignant neoplasms,** *Breast cancer.*)
The Women's Health Initiative Memory Study (WHIMS), a substudy of the WHI, reported an increased risk of developing probable dementia in postmenopausal women 65 years of age or older during 5.2 years of treatment with CE 0.625 mg alone and during 4 years of treatment with CE 0.625 mg combined with MPA 2.5 mg, relative to placebo. It is unknown whether this finding applies to younger postmenopausal women. (See **CLINICAL STUDIES, WARNINGS, Dementia,** and **PRECAUTIONS, Geriatric Use.**)
Other doses of oral conjugated estrogens with medroxyprogesterone acetate, and other combinations and dosage forms of estrogens and progestins were not studied in the WHI clinical trials and, in the absence of comparable data, these risks should be assumed to be similar. Because of these risks, estrogens with or without progestins should be prescribed at the lowest effective doses and for the shortest duration consistent with treatment goals and risks for the individual woman.

DESCRIPTION
Divigel® (estradiol gel) 0.1% is a clear, colorless gel, which is odorless when dry. It is designed to deliver sustained circulating concentrations of estradiol when applied once daily to the skin. The gel is applied to a small area (200 cm^2) of the thigh in a thin, quick-drying layer. Divigel® is available in three doses of 0.25, 0.5, and 1.0 g for topical application (corresponding to 0.25, 0.5, and 1.0 mg estradiol, respectively).
The active component of the topical gel is estradiol. Estradiol is a white crystalline powder, chemically described as estra-1,3,5(10)-triene-3,17ß-diol. It has an empirical formula of $C_{18}H_{24}O_2$ and molecular weight of 272.39. The structural formula is:

The remaining components of the gel (carbomer, ethanol, propylene glycol, purified water, and triethanolamine) are pharmacologically inactive.

CLINICAL PHARMACOLOGY
Divigel® provides estrogen therapy by delivering estradiol, the major estrogenic hormone secreted by the human ovary, to the systemic circulation following topical application.
Endogenous estrogens are largely responsible for the development and maintenance of the female reproductive system and secondary sexual characteristics. Although circulating estrogens exist in a dynamic equilibrium of metabolic interconversions, estradiol is the principal intracellular human estrogen and is substantially more potent than its metabolites, estrone and estriol, at the receptor level.
The primary source of estrogen in normally cycling adult women is the ovarian follicle, which secretes 70 to 500 mcg of estradiol daily, depending on the phase of the menstrual

cycle. After menopause, most endogenous estrogen is produced by conversion of androstenedione, secreted by the adrenal cortex, to estrone by peripheral tissues. Thus, estrone and the sulfate conjugated form, estrone sulfate, are the most abundant circulating estrogens in postmenopausal women.

Estrogens act through binding to nuclear receptors in estrogen-responsive tissues. To date, two estrogen receptors have been identified. These vary in proportion from tissue to tissue.

Circulating estrogens modulate the pituitary secretion of the gonadotropins, luteinizing hormone (LH) and follicle-stimulating hormone (FSH), through a negative feedback mechanism. Estrogens act to reduce the elevated levels of these hormones seen in postmenopausal women.

Pharmacokinetics

A. Absorption

Estradiol diffuses across intact skin and into the systemic circulation by a passive absorption process, with diffusion across the stratum corneum being the rate-limiting factor. In a 14-day, Phase 1, multiple-dose study, Divigel® demonstrated linear and approximately dose-proportional estradiol pharmacokinetics at steady state for both AUC_{0-24} and C_{max} following once daily dosing to the skin of either the right or left upper thigh (Table 1).

[See table 1 above]

Steady-state serum concentration of estradiol are achieved by day 12 following daily application of Divigel® to the skin of the upper thigh. The mean (SD) serum estradiol levels following once daily dosing at day 14 are shown in Figure 1.

Figure 1: Mean (SD) Serum Estradiol Concentrations (Values Uncorrected for Baseline) on Day 14 Following Multiple Daily Doses of Divigel 0.1%

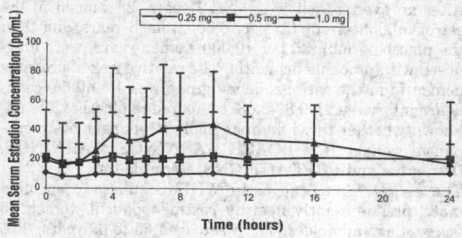

The effect of sunscreens and other topical lotions on the systemic exposure of Divigel® has not been evaluated. Studies conducted using topical estrogen gel approved products have shown that sunscreens have the potential for changing the systemic exposure of topically applied estrogen gels.

B. Distribution

The distribution of exogenous estrogens is similar to that of endogenous estrogens. Estrogens are widely distributed in the body and are generally found in higher concentrations in the sex hormone target organs. Estrogens circulate in the blood largely bound to sex hormone binding globulin (SHBG) and albumin.

C. Metabolism

Circulating estrogens exist in a dynamic equilibrium of metabolic interconversions. These transformations take place mainly in the liver. Estradiol is converted reversibly to estrone, and both can be converted to estriol, which is the major urinary metabolite. Estrogens also undergo enterohepatic recirculation via sulfate and glucuronide conjugation in the liver, biliary secretion of conjugates into the intestine, and hydrolysis in the intestine followed by reabsorption. In postmenopausal women, a significant proportion of the circulating estrogens exist as sulfate conjugates, especially estrone sulfate, which serves as a circulating reservoir for the formation of more active estrogens.

Estradiol from Divigel® avoids first pass metabolism and provides estradiol/estrone ratios at steady state in the range of 0.42 to 0.65.

D. Excretion

Estradiol, estrone, and estriol are excreted in the urine along with glucuronide and sulfate conjugates. The apparent terminal half-life for estradiol was about 10 hours following administration of Divigel®.

E. Special Populations

Divigel® has been studied only in postmenopausal women. No pharmacokinetic studies were conducted in special populations, including patients with renal or hepatic impairment.

F. Drug Interactions

In vitro and *in vivo* studies have shown that estrogens are metabolized partially by cytochrome P450 3A4 (CYP3A4). Therefore, inducers or inhibitors of CYP3A4 may affect estrogen drug metabolism. Inducers of CYP3A4, such as St. John's Wort preparations (Hypericum perforatum), phenobarbital, carbamazepine, and rifampin, may reduce plasma concentrations of estrogens, possibly resulting in a decrease in therapeutic effects and/or changes in the uterine bleeding profile. Inhibitors of CYP3A4, such as erythromycin, clarithromycin, ketoconazole, itraconazole, ritonavir, and grapefruit juice, may increase plasma concentrations of estrogens and result in side effects.

G. Potential for Estradiol Transfer and Effects of Washing

As with most topical products, there is a potential for estradiol transfer following physical contact with Divigel® application sites. The effect of estradiol transfer was evaluated in healthy postmenopausal women who topically applied 1.0 g of Divigel® (single dose) on one thigh. One and 8 hours after gel application, they engaged in direct thigh-to-arm contact with a partner for 15 minutes. While some elevation of estradiol levels over baseline was seen in the male subjects, the degree of transferability in this study was inconclusive.

The effect of application site washing on skin surface levels and serum concentrations of estradiol was determined in 16 healthy postmenopausal women after application of 1.0 g of Divigel® to a 200 cm² area on the thigh. Washing the application site with soap and water 1 hour after application removed all detectable amounts of estradiol from the surface of the skin, and resulted in a 30–38% decrease in the mean total 24-hour exposure to estradiol.

CLINICAL STUDIES

Effects on Vasomotor Symptoms

A randomized, double-blind, placebo-controlled trial evaluated the efficacy of 12-week treatment with three different daily doses of Divigel® (estradiol gel) 0.1% for vasomotor symptoms in 495 postmenopausal women (86.5% White; 10.1% Black) between 34 and 89 years of age (mean age 54.6) who had at least 50 moderate to severe hot flushes per week at baseline (2 week period prior to treatment). Subjects applied placebo, Divigel® 0.25 g (0.25 mg estradiol), Divigel® 0.5 g (0.5 mg estradiol) or Divigel® 1.0 g (1.0 mg estradiol) once daily to the thigh. Reductions in both the median daily frequency and the median daily severity of moderate to severe hot flushes were statistically significant for the 0.5 g/day and the 1.0 g/day Divigel® doses when compared to placebo at week 4. Statistically significant reductions in both the median daily frequency and the median daily severity of moderate to severe hot flushes for the Divigel® 0.25 g/day dose when compared to placebo were delayed to week 7. There were statistically significant reductions in median daily frequency and severity of hot flushes for all three Divigel® doses (0.25 g/day, 0.5 g/day and 1.0 g/day) compared to placebo at week 12. See Table 2 for results.

[See table 2 above]

Women's Health Initiative Studies

The Women's Health Initiative (WHI) enrolled a total of 27,000 predominantly healthy postmenopausal women in two substudies to assess the risks and benefits of either the use of oral conjugated estrogens (CE 0.625 mg) alone per day or in combination with medroxyprogesterone acetate (CE 0.625 mg/MPA 2.5 mg) per day compared to placebo in the prevention of certain chronic diseases. The primary endpoint was the incidence of coronary heart disease (CHD) (nonfatal myocardial infarction (MI), silent MI and CHD death), with invasive breast cancer as the primary adverse outcome studied. A "global index" included the earliest occurrence of CHD, invasive breast cancer, stroke, pulmonary embolism Time (hours) (PE), endometrial cancer (only in the estrogen-plus-progestin substudy), colorectal cancer, hip fracture, or death due to other cause. The study did not evaluate the effects of CE or CE/MPA on menopausal symptoms.

The estrogen-alone substudy was stopped early because an increased risk of stroke was observed and it was deemed that no further information would be obtained regarding the risks and benefits of estrogen alone in predetermined primary endpoints. Results of the estrogen-alone substudy, which included 10,739 women (average age of 63 years, range 50 to 79; 75.3% White, 15.1% Black, 6.1% Hispanic, 3.6% Other), after an average follow-up of 6.8 years are presented in Table 3.

[See table 3 at top of next page]

For those outcomes included in the WHI "global index" that reached statistical significance, the absolute excess risk per 10,000 women-years in the group treated with CE alone was

---

Table 1: Mean (%CV) Pharmacokinetic Parameters for Estradiol (uncorrected for baseline) on Day 14 Following Multiple Daily Doses of Divigel® 0.1%

Parameter (units)	Divigel® 0.25 g	Divigel® 0.5 g	Divigel® 1.0 g
AUC_{0-24} (pg•h/mL)	236 (94)	504 (149)	732 (81)
C_{max} (pg/mL)	14.7 (84)	28.4 (139)	51.5 (86)
C_{avg} (pg/mL)	9.8 (92)	21 (148)	30.5 (81)
t_{max}* (h)	16 (0, 72)	10 (0, 72)	8 (0, 48)
E2:E1 ratio	0.42	0.65	0.65

*Median (Min, Max).

Table 2: Summary of Change From Baseline in the Median Daily Frequency and Severity of Hot Flushes during Divigel® Treatment (ITT Population)

	Divigel®			Placebo
Evaluation	0.25 g/day N=121	0.5 g/day N=119	1.0 g/day N=124	N=124
Frequency of Daily Hot Flushes				
Baseline Median	9.72	9.24	9.64	9.32
Median Change: Week 4 p-value[†]	-5.00 0.132	-5.73 0.011	-7.20 <0.001	-3.63
Median Change: Week 7 p-value[†]	-6.62 <0.001	-7.14 <0.001	-7.71 <0.001	-4.37
Median Change: Week 12 p-value[†]	-6.88 <0.001	-7.29 <0.001	-8.35 <0.001	-4.48
Severity of Daily Hot Flushes				
Baseline Median	2.52	2.51	2.52	2.54
Median Change: Week 4 p-value[†]	-0.07 0.283	-0.18 <0.001	-0.47 <0.001	-0.04
Median Change: Week 7 p-value[†]	-0.24 <0.001	-0.46 <0.001	-1.06 <0.001	-0.06
Median Change: Week 12 p-value[†]	-0.33 0.021	-0.56 0.002	-1.69 <0.001	-0.13

[†]p-values from the van Elteren's test stratified by pooled center; comparison in median change was significant if $p<0.05$

Table 3: Relative And Absolute Risk Seen In The Estrogen-Alone Substudy Of WHI[a]

Event	Relative Risk CE vs. Placebo (95% nCI[a])	Placebo n = 5,429	CE n = 5,310
		Absolute Risk per 10,000 Women-Years	
CHD events[b]	0.95 (0.79-1.16)	56	53
Nonfatal MI[b]	*0.91 (0.73-1.14)*	*43*	*40*
CHD death[b]	*1.01 (0.71-1.43)*	*16*	*16*
Stroke[c]	1.39 (1.10-1.77)	32	44
Deep vein thrombosis[b,d]	1.47 (1.06-2.06)	15	23
Pulmonary embolism[b]	1.37 (0.90-2.07)	10	14
Invasive breast cancer[b]	0.80 (0.62-1.04)	34	28
Colorectal cancer[c]	1.08 (0.75-1.55)	16	17
Hip fracture[c]	0.61 (0.41-0.91)	17	11
Vertebral fractures[c,d]	0.62 (0.42-0.93)	17	11
Total fractures[c,d]	0.70 (0.63-0.79)	195	139
Death due to other causes[c,e]	1.08 (0.88-1.32)	50	53
Overall mortality[c,d]	1.04 (0.88-1.32)	78	81
Global index[c,f]	1.01 (0.91-1.12)	190	192

[a] Nominal confidence intervals unadjusted for multiple looks and multiple comparisons
[b] Results are based on centrally adjudicated data for an average follow-up of 7.1 years
[c] Results are based on an average follow-up of 6.8 years
[d] Not included in Global Index
[e] All deaths, except from breast or colorectal cancer, definite/probable CHD, PE or cerebrovascular disease
[f] A subset of the events was combined in a "global index", defined as the earliest occurrence of CHD events, invasive breast cancer, stroke, pulmonary embolism, colorectal cancer, hip fracture, or death due to other causes

Table 4: Relative And Absolute Risk Seen in the Estrogen-Plus-Progestin Substudy of WHI at an Average of 5.6 Years[a]

Event[c]	Relative Risk CE/MPA vs. Placebo (95% nCI[b])	Placebo n = 8102	CE/MPA n = 8506
		Absolute Risk per 10,000 Women-Years	
CHD events	1.24 (1.00-1.54)	33	39
Nonfatal MI	*1.28 (1.00-1.63)*	*25*	*31*
CHD death	*1.10 (0.70-1.75)*	*8*	*8*
All strokes	1.31 (1.02-1.68)	24	31
Ischemic stroke	*1.44 (1.09-1.90)*	*18*	*26*
Deep vein thrombosis	1.95 (1.43-2.67)	13	26
Pulmonary embolism	2.13 (1.45-3.11)	8	18
Invasive breast cancer[c]	1.24 (1.01-1.54)	33	41
Invasive colorectal cancer	0.56 (0.38-0.81)	16	9
Endometrial cancer	0.81 (0.48-1.36)	7	6
Cervical cancer	1.44 (0.47-4.42)	1	2
Hip fracture	0.67 (0.47-0.96)	16	11
Vertebral fractures	0.65 (0.46-0.92)	17	11
Lower arm/wrist fractures	0.71 (0.59-0.85)	62	44
Total fractures	0.76 (0.69-0.83)	199	152

[a] Results are based on centrally adjudicated data. Mortality data was not part of the adjudicated data; however, data at 5.2 years of follow-up showed no difference between the groups in terms of all-cause mortality (RR 0.98, 95% nCI 0.82-1.18)
[b] Nominal confidence intervals unadjusted for multiple looks and multiple comparisons.
[c] Includes metastatic and non-metastatic breast cancer, with the exception of in situ breast cancer

12 more strokes, while the absolute risk reduction per 10,000 women-years was 6 fewer hip fractures. The absolute excess risk of events included in the "global index" was a nonsignificant 2 events per 10,000 women-years. There was no difference between the groups in terms of all-cause mortality. (See **BOXED WARNINGS, WARNINGS,** and **PRECAUTIONS.**)

Final centrally adjudicated results for CHD events and centrally adjudicated results for invasive breast cancer incidence from the estrogen-alone substudy, after an average follow-up of 7.1 years, reported no overall difference for primary CHD events (nonfatal MI, silent MI and CHD death) and invasive breast cancer incidence in women receiving CE alone compared with placebo (see Table 3).

The estrogen-plus-progestin substudy was also stopped early because, according to the predefined stopping rule, after an average follow-up of 5.2 years of treatment, the increased risk of breast cancer and cardiovascular events exceeded the specified benefits included in the "global index." The absolute excess risk of events included in the "global index" was 19 per 10,000 women-years (RR 1.15, 95% nCI 1.03-1.28).

For those outcomes included in the WHI "global index" that reached statistical significance after 5.6 years of follow-up, the absolute excess risks per 10,000 women years in the group treated with CE/MPA were 6 more CHD events, 7 more strokes, 10 more PEs, and 8 more invasive breast cancers, while the absolute risk reductions per 10,000 women-years were 7 fewer colorectal cancers and 5 fewer hip fractures. (See **BOXED WARNINGS, WARNINGS,** and **PRECAUTIONS.**)

Results of the estrogen-plus-progestin substudy, which included 16,608 women (average age of 63 years, range 50 to 79; 83.9% White, 6.8% Black, 5.4% Hispanic, 3.9% Other), are presented in Table 4 below. These results reflect centrally adjudicated data after an average follow-up of 5.6 years.

[See table 4 below]

Women's Health Initiative Memory Study

The estrogen-alone Women's Health Initiative Memory Study (WHIMS), a substudy of the WHI, enrolled 2,947 predominantly healthy postmenopausal women 65 years of age and older (45% were aged 65 to 69 years, 36% were 70 to 74 years, and 19% were 75 years of age and older) to evaluate the effects of conjugated estrogens (CE 0.625 mg) on the incidence of probable dementia (primary outcome) compared with placebo.

After an average follow-up of 5.2 years, 28 women in the estrogen-alone group (37 per 10,000 women-years) and 19 in the placebo group (25 per 10,000 women-years) were diagnosed with probable dementia. The relative risk of probable dementia in the estrogen-alone group was 1.49 (95% confidence interval (CI), 0.83-2.66) compared to placebo. It is unknown whether these findings apply to younger postmenopausal women. (See **BOXED WARNINGS, WARNINGS, Dementia,** and **PRECAUTIONS, Geriatric Use.**)

The estrogen-plus-progestin WHIMS substudy enrolled 4,532 predominantly healthy postmenopausal women 65 years of age and older (47% were aged 65 to 69 years, 35% were 70 to 74 years, and 18% were 75 years of age and older) to evaluate the effects of conjugated estrogens (CE 0.625 mg) plus medroxyprogesterone acetate (MPA 2.5 mg) daily on the incidence of probable dementia (primary outcome) compared with placebo.

After an average follow-up of 4 years, 40 women in the estrogen-plus-progestin group (45 per 10,000 women-years) and 21 in the placebo group (22 per 10,000 women-years) were diagnosed with probable dementia. The relative risk of probable dementia in the hormone therapy group was 2.05 (95% CI, 1.21-3.48) compared to placebo.

When data from the two populations were pooled as planned in the WHIMS protocol, the reported overall relative risk for probable dementia was 1.76 (95% CI 1.19-2.60). It is unknown whether these findings apply to younger postmenopausal women. (See **BOXED WARNINGS, WARNINGS, Dementia,** and **PRECAUTIONS, Geriatric Use.**)

INDICATIONS AND USAGE

Divigel® (estradiol gel) 0.1% is indicated in the treatment of moderate to severe vasomotor symptoms associated with menopause.

CONTRAINDICATIONS

Estrogen products, including Divigel® (estradiol gel) 0.1% should not be used in women with any of the following conditions:

1. Undiagnosed abnormal genital bleeding.
2. Known, suspected, or history of cancer of the breast.
3. Known or suspected estrogen-dependent neoplasia.
4. Active deep vein thrombosis, pulmonary embolism, or history of these conditions.
5. Active or recent (e.g., within the past year) arterial thromboembolic disease (e.g., stroke, myocardial infarction).
6. Liver dysfunction or disease.
7. Known hypersensitivity to the ingredients of Divigel®.
8. Known or suspected pregnancy. There is no indication for Divigel® in pregnancy. There appears to be little or no increased risk of birth defects in children born to women who have used estrogens and progestins from oral contraceptives inadvertently during early pregnancy. (See **PRECAUTIONS.**)

WARNINGS

See **BOXED WARNINGS.**

1. Cardiovascular Disorders

Estrogen-alone therapy has been associated with an increased risk of stroke and deep vein thrombosis (DVT).

Estrogen-plus-progestin therapy has been associated with an increased risk of myocardial infarction as well as stroke, venous thrombosis and pulmonary embolism.

Should any of these occur or be suspected, estrogens should be discontinued immediately.

Risk factors for arterial vascular disease (e.g., hypertension, diabetes mellitus, tobacco use, hypercholesterolemia, and obesity) and/or venous thromboembolism (e.g., personal history or family history of VTE, obesity, and systemic lupus erythematosus) should be managed appropriately.

a. Stroke

In the estrogen-alone substudy of the Women's Health Initiative (WHI), a statistically significant increased risk of stroke was observed in women receiving CE 0.625 mg daily compared to placebo (44 versus 32 per 10,000 women-years). The increase in risk was observed in year 1 and persisted. (See **CLINICAL STUDIES**.)

In the estrogen-plus-progestin substudy of the WHI study, a statistically significant increased risk of stroke was reported in women receiving CE/MPA 0.625 mg/2.5 mg daily compared to women receiving placebo (31 versus 24 per 10,000 women-years). The increase in risk was demonstrated after the first year and persisted.

b. Coronary heart disease

In the estrogen-alone substudy of WHI, no overall effect on coronary heart disease (CHD) events (defined as non-fatal MI, silent MI, or death, due to CHD) was reported in women receiving estrogen-alone compared to placebo. (See **CLINICAL STUDIES**.)

In the estrogen-plus-progestin substudy of WHI, no statistically significant increase of CHD events was reported in women receiving CE/MPA compared to women receiving placebo (39 vs. 33 per 10,000 women-years). An increase in relative risk was demonstrated in year one and a trend toward decreasing relative risk was reported in years 2 through 5.

In postmenopausal women with documented heart disease (n=2,763, average age 66.7 years), a controlled clinical trial of secondary prevention of cardiovascular disease (Heart and Estrogen/Progestin Replacement Study (HERS)) treatment with CE/MPA (0.625 mg/2.5 mg per day) demonstrated no cardiovascular benefit. During an average follow-up of 4.1 years, treatment with CE/MPA did not reduce the overall rate of CHD events in postmenopausal women with established coronary heart disease. There were more CHD events in the CE/MPA-treated group than in the placebo group in year 1, but not during the subsequent years. Participation in an open label extension of the original HERS trial (HERS II) was agreed to by 2,321 women. Average follow-up in HERS II was an additional 2.7 years, for a total of 6.8 years overall. Rates of CHD events were comparable among women in the CE/MPA group and the placebo group in HERS, HERS II, and overall.

Large doses of estrogen (5 mg conjugated estrogens per day), comparable to those used to treat cancer of the prostate and breast, have been shown in a large prospective clinical trial in men to increase the risks of non-fatal myocardial infarction, pulmonary embolism, and thrombophlebitis.

c. Venous Thromboembolism

In the estrogen-alone substudy of WHI the risk of VTE (DVT and pulmonary embolism [PE]), was reported to be increased for women taking conjugated estrogens compared to placebo (30 versus 22 per 10,000 women-years), although only the increased risk of DVT reached statistical significance (23 vs. 15 per 10,000 women-years). The increase in VTE risk was demonstrated during the first two years. (See **CLINICAL STUDIES**.)

In the estrogen-plus-progestin substudy of WHI, a statistically significant two-fold greater rate of VTE, was reported in women receiving CE/MPA compared to women receiving placebo (35 vs. 17 per 10,000 women-years). Statistically significant increases in risk for both DVT (26 vs. 13 per 10,000 women-years) and PE (18 vs. 8 per 10,000 women-years) were also demonstrated. The increase in VTE risk was demonstrated during the first year and persisted. (See **CLINICAL STUDIES**.)

If feasible, estrogens should be discontinued at least 4 to 6 weeks before surgery of the type associated with an increased risk of thromboembolism, or during periods of prolonged immobilization.

2. Malignant Neoplasms

a. Endometrial Cancer

The use of unopposed estrogens in women with intact uteri has been associated with an increased risk of endometrial cancer. The reported endometrial cancer risk among unopposed estrogen users is about 2 to 12 times greater than in non-users, and appears dependent on duration of treatment and on estrogen dose. Most studies show no significant increased risk associated with use of estrogens for less than 1 year. The greatest risk appears associated with prolonged use, with increased risk of 15- to 24-fold for 5 to 10 years or more. This risk has been shown to persist for at least 8 to 15 years after estrogen therapy is discontinued.

Clinical surveillance of all women taking estrogen/progestin combinations is important. Adequate diagnostic measures, including endometrial sampling when indicated, should be undertaken to rule out malignancy in all cases of undiagnosed persistent or recurring abnormal vaginal bleeding. There is no evidence that the use of natural estrogens results in a different endometrial risk profile than synthetic estrogens of equivalent estrogen dose. Adding a progestin to estrogen therapy has been shown to reduce the risk of endometrial hyperplasia, which may be a precursor to endometrial cancer.

b. Breast Cancer

In some studies, the use of estrogens and progestins by postmenopausal women has been reported to increase the risk of breast cancer. The most important randomized clinical trial providing information about this issue is the Women's Health Initiative (WHI) (see **CLINICAL STUDIES**). The results from observational studies are generally consistent with those of the WHI clinical trial.

Observational studies have also reported an increased risk of breast cancer for estrogen-plus-progestin combination therapy, and a smaller increased risk for estrogen-alone therapy, after several years of use. For both findings, the excess risk increased with duration of use, and appeared to return to baseline over about five years after stopping treatment (only the observational studies have substantial data on risk after stopping). In these studies, the risk of breast cancer was greater, and became apparent earlier, with estrogen-plus-progestin combination therapy as compared to estrogen-alone therapy. However, these studies have not found significant variation in the risk of breast cancer among different estrogens or among different estrogen-plus-progestin combinations, doses, or routes of administration.

In the estrogen-alone substudy of WHI, after an average of 7.1 years of follow-up, CE (0.625 mg daily) was not associated with an increased risk of invasive breast cancer (RR 0.80, 95% nCI 0.62-1.04).

In the estrogen-plus-progestin substudy, after a mean follow-up of 5.6 years, the WHI substudy reported an increased risk of breast cancer.

In this substudy, prior use of estrogen-alone or estrogen/progestin combination hormone therapy was reported by 26% of the women. The relative risk of invasive breast cancer was 1.24 (95% nCI, 1.01-1.54), and the absolute risk was 41 versus 33 cases per 10,000 women-years, for estrogen-plus-progestin compared with placebo, respectively. Among women who reported prior use of hormone therapy, the relative risk of invasive breast cancer was 1.86, and the absolute risk was 46 versus 25 cases per 10,000 women-years, for estrogen-plus-progestin compared with placebo. Among women who reported no prior use of hormone therapy, the relative risk of invasive breast cancer was 1.09, and the absolute risk was 40 versus 36 cases per 10,000 women-years for estrogen-plus-progestin compared with placebo. In the WHI trial, invasive breast cancers were larger and diagnosed at a more advanced stage in the estrogen-plus-progestin group compared with the placebo group. Metastatic disease was rare with no apparent difference between the two groups. Other prognostic factors such as histologic subtype, grade and hormone receptor status did not differ between the groups.

The use of estrogen-alone and estrogen-plus-progestin has been reported to result in an increase in abnormal mammograms requiring further evaluation.

All women should receive yearly breast examinations by a healthcare provider and perform monthly breast self-examinations. In addition, mammography examinations should be scheduled based on patient age, risk factors, and prior mammogram results.

3. Dementia

In the estrogen-alone Women's Health Initiative Memory Study (WHIMS), a substudy of WHI, a population of 2,947 hysterectomized women aged 65 to 79 years was randomized to CE (0.625 mg daily) or placebo. In the estrogen-plus-progestin WHIMS, a population of 4,532 postmenopausal women aged 65 to 79 years was randomized to CE/MPA (0.625 mg/2.5 mg daily) or placebo.

In the estrogen-alone substudy, after an average follow-up of 5.2 years, 28 women in the estrogen-alone group and 19 women in the placebo group were diagnosed with probable dementia. The relative risk of probable dementia for CE alone versus placebo was 1.49 (95% CI, 0.83-2.66). The absolute risk of probable dementia for CE alone versus placebo was 37 versus 25 cases per 10,000 women-years.

In the estrogen-plus-progestin substudy, after an average follow-up of 4 years, 40 women in the estrogen-plus-progestin group and 21 women in the placebo group were diagnosed with probable dementia. The relative risk of probable dementia for estrogen-plus-progestin versus placebo was 2.05 (95% CI, 1.21-3.48). The absolute risk of probable dementia for CE/MPA versus placebo was 45 versus 22 cases per 10,000 women-years.

When data from the two populations were pooled as planned in the WHIMS protocol, the reported overall relative risk for probable dementia was 1.76 (95% CI 1.19-2.60). Since both substudies were conducted in women aged 65 to 79 years, it is unknown whether these findings apply to younger postmenopausal women. (See **BOXED WARNINGS** and **PRECAUTIONS**, and Geriatric Use.)

4. Gallbladder Disease

A two- to four-fold increase in the risk of gallbladder disease requiring surgery in postmenopausal women receiving estrogens has been reported.

5. Hypercalcemia

Estrogen administration may lead to severe hypercalcemia in patients with breast cancer and bone metastases. If hypercalcemia occurs, use of the drug should be stopped and appropriate measures taken to reduce the serum calcium level.

6. Visual Abnormalities

Retinal vascular thrombosis has been reported in patients receiving estrogens. Discontinue medication pending examination if there is sudden partial or complete loss of vision, or a sudden onset of proptosis, diplopia, or migraine. If examination reveals papilledema or retinal vascular lesions, estrogens should be permanently discontinued.

PRECAUTIONS

A. General

1. Addition of a progestin when a woman has not had a hysterectomy

Studies of the addition of a progestin for 10 or more days of a cycle of estrogen administration, or daily with estrogen in a continuous regimen, have reported a lowered incidence of endometrial hyperplasia than would be induced by estrogen treatment alone. Endometrial hyperplasia may be a precursor to endometrial cancer.

There are, however, possible risks that may be associated with the use of progestins with estrogens compared to estrogen-alone regimens. These include a possible increased risk of breast cancer, adverse effects on lipoprotein metabolism (e.g., lowering HDL, raising LDL), and impairment of glucose tolerance.

2. Elevated blood pressure

In a small number of case reports, substantial increases in blood pressure have been attributed to idiosyncratic reactions to estrogens. In a large, randomized, placebo-controlled clinical trial, a generalized effect of estrogens on blood pressure was not seen. Blood pressure should be monitored at regular intervals with estrogen use.

3. Hypertriglyceridemia

In patients with pre-existing hypertriglyceridemia, estrogen therapy may be associated with elevations of plasma triglycerides leading to pancreatitis and other complications.

4. Impaired liver function and past history of cholestatic jaundice

Estrogens may be poorly metabolized in patients with impaired liver function. For patients with a history of cholestatic jaundice associated with past estrogen use or with pregnancy, caution should be exercised, and in the case of recurrence, medication should be discontinued.

5. Hypothyroidism

Estrogen administration leads to increased thyroid-binding globulin (TBG) levels. Patients with normal thyroid function can compensate for the increased TBG by making more thyroid hormone, thus maintaining free T_4 and T_3 serum concentrations in the normal range. Patients dependent on thyroid hormone replacement therapy who are also receiving estrogens may require increased doses of their thyroid replacement therapy. These patients should have their thyroid function monitored to maintain their free thyroid hormone levels in an acceptable range.

6. Fluid retention

Estrogens may cause some degree of fluid retention. Because of this, patients who have conditions that might be influenced by this factor, such as a cardiac or renal dysfunction, warrant careful observation when estrogens are prescribed.

7. Hypocalcemia

Estrogens should be used with caution in individuals with severe hypocalcemia.

8. Ovarian cancer

The estrogen-plus-progestin substudy of the WHI reported that after an average follow-up of 5.6 years, the relative risk for ovarian cancer for estrogen-plus-progestin versus placebo was 1.58 (95% nCI, 0.77-3.24), but was not statistically significant. The absolute risk for estrogen-plus-progestin versus placebo was 4.2 versus 2.7 cases per 10,000 women-years. In some epidemiologic studies, the use of estrogen only products in particular for 10 or more years, has been associated with an increased risk of ovarian cancer. Other epidemiologic studies have not found these associations.

9. Exacerbation of endometriosis

Endometriosis may be exacerbated with administration of estrogens. Malignant transformation of residual endometrial implants have been reported in women treated post-hysterectomy with estrogen-alone therapy. For patients known to have residual endometriosis post-hysterectomy, the addition of progestin should be considered.

10. Exacerbation of other conditions

Estrogens may cause an exacerbation of asthma, diabetes mellitus, epilepsy, migraine or porphyria, systemic lupus erythematosus, and hepatic hemangiomas and should be used with caution in women with these conditions.

11. Photosensitivity/Photoallergy
The effects of direct sun exposure to Divigel® (estradiol gel) 0.1% application sites have not been evaluated in clinical trials. Nonclinical studies in guinea pigs showed no phototoxicity or photosensitivity. In addition, Divigel® has been shown to absorb light primarily at wavelengths below 290 nm. Therefore, Divigel® is not considered to have photosensitizing potential.

12. Sunscreen application
Studies conducted using other approved topical estrogen gel products have shown that sunscreens have the potential for changing the systemic exposure of topically applied estrogen gels. The effect of concomitant application of sunscreen and Divigel® to the same application site has not been clinically evaluated.

13. Miscellaneous
Alcohol based gels are flammable. Avoid fire, flame, or smoking until the gel has dried.
Occlusion of the area where the topical drug product is applied with clothing or other barriers is not recommended until the gel is completely dried.

14. Potential for Estradiol Transfer and Effects of Washing
There is a potential for drug transfer from one individual to the other following physical contact of Divigel® application sites. In a study to evaluate transferability to males from their female contacts, there was some elevation of estradiol levels over baseline in the male subjects, however, the degree of transferability in this study was inconclusive. Patients are advised to avoid skin contact with other subjects until the gel is completely dried. The site of application should be covered (clothed) after drying.
Washing the application site with soap and water 1 hour after the application resulted in a 30 to 38% decrease in the mean total 24-hour exposure to estradiol. Therefore, patients should refrain from washing the application site for at least one hour after application.

B. Information for Patients
Physicians and pharmacists are advised to discuss the **PATIENT INFORMATION** leaflet with patients for whom they prescribe or dispense Divigel®.

C. Laboratory Tests
Estrogen administration should be initiated at the lowest dose approved for the treatment of moderate-to-severe vasomotor symptoms associated with menopause and then guided by clinical response rather than by serum hormone levels (e.g., estradiol, FSH).

D. Drug and Laboratory Test Interactions
1. Accelerated prothrombin time, partial thromboplastin time, and platelet aggregation time; increased platelet count; increased factors II, VII antigen, VIII antigen, VIII coagulant activity, IX, X, XII, VII-X complex, II-VII-X complex, and beta-thromboglobulin; decreased levels of anti-factor Xa and antithrombin III, decreased antithrombin III activity; increased levels of fibrinogen and fibrinogen activity; increased plasminogen antigen and activity.
2. Increased thyroid binding globulin (TBG) levels leading to increased circulating total thyroid hormone levels, as measured by protein-bound iodine (PBI), T_4 levels (by column or by radioimmunoassay) or T_3 levels by radioimmunoassay. T_3 resin uptake is decreased, reflecting the elevated TBG. Free T_4 and free T_3 concentrations are unaltered. Patients on thyroid replacement therapy may require higher doses of thyroid hormone.
3. Other binding proteins may be elevated in serum (i.e., corticosteroid binding globulin (CBG), sex hormone binding globulin (SHBG) leading to increased total circulating corticosteroids and sex steroids, respectively. Free hormone concentrations may be decreased. Other plasma proteins may be increased (angiotensinogen/renin substrate, alpha-1-antitrypsin, ceruloplasmin).
4. Increased plasma HDL and HDL_2 cholesterol subfraction concentrations, reduced LDL cholesterol concentration, increased triglyceride levels.
5. Impaired glucose tolerance.
6. Reduced response to metyrapone test.

E. Carcinogenesis, Mutagenesis, Impairment of Fertility
See **BOXED WARNINGS, WARNINGS** and **PRECAUTIONS**.
Long-term continuous administration of natural and synthetic estrogens in certain animal species increases the frequency of carcinomas of the breast, uterus, cervix, vagina, testis and liver.

F. Pregnancy
Estrogen products, including Divigel®, should not be used in pregnancy. (See **CONTRAINDICATIONS**.)

G. Nursing Mothers
Estrogen administration to nursing mothers has been shown to decrease the quantity and quality of the milk. Detectable amounts of estrogens have been identified in the milk of mothers receiving estrogen therapy. Caution should be exercised when estrogen products, including Divigel® (estradiol gel) 0.1% are administered to a nursing woman.

H. Pediatric Use
Safety and efficacy of Divigel® in pediatric patients has not been established.

I. Geriatric Use
There have not been sufficient numbers of geriatric patients involved in studies utilizing Divigel® to determine whether those over 65 years of age differ from younger subjects in their response to Divigel®.
Of the total number of subjects in the estrogen-alone substudy of the Women's Health Initiative (WHI), 46% (n=4,943) were 65 years and older, while 7.1% (n=767) were 75 years and older. There was a higher relative risk (CE versus placebo) of stroke in women less than 75 years of age compared to women 75 years and older.
In the estrogen-alone substudy of the Women's Health Initiative Memory Study (WHIMS), a substudy of WHI, a population of 2,947 hysterectomized women, aged 65 to 79 years, was randomized to CE (0.625 mg per day) or placebo. After an average follow-up of 5.2 years, the relative risk (CE versus placebo) of probable dementia was 1.49 (95% CI, 0.83-2.66). The absolute risk of developing probable dementia with estrogen alone was 37 vs. 25 cases per 10,000 women-years with placebo.
Of the total number of subjects in the estrogen-plus-progestin substudy of the WHI, 44% (n=7,320) were 65 years and older, while 6.6% (n=1,095) were 75 years and older. There was a higher relative risk (CE/MPA versus placebo) of stroke and invasive breast cancer in women 75 and older compared to women less than 75 years of age. In women greater than 75, the increased risk of non-fatal stroke and invasive breast cancer observed in the estrogen-plus-progestin combination group compared to the placebo group was 75 vs. 24 per 10,000 women-years and 52 vs. 12 per 10,000 women years, respectively.
In the estrogen-plus-progestin substudy of WHIMS, a population of 4,532 postmenopausal women, aged 65 to 79 years, was randomized to CE/MPA (CE 0.625 mg/2.5 mg daily) or placebo. In the estrogen-plus-progestin group, after an average follow-up of 4 years, the relative risk (CE/MPA versus placebo) of probable dementia was 2.05 (95% CI, 1.21-3.48). The absolute risk of developing probable dementia with CE/MPA was 45 vs. 22 cases per 10,000 women-years with placebo.
Seventy-nine percent of the cases of probable dementia occurred in women that were older than 70 for the CE group, and 82 percent of the cases of probable dementia occurred in women who were older than 70 in the CE/MPA group. The most common classification of probable dementia in both the treatment groups and placebo groups was Alzheimer's disease.
When data from the two populations were pooled as planned in the WHIMS protocol, the reported overall risk of probable dementia was 1.76 (95% CI, 1.19-2.60). Since both substudies were conducted in women aged 65 to 79 years, it is unknown whether these findings apply to younger postmenopausal women. (See **BOXED WARNINGS**, and **WARNINGS, Dementia**.)

Table 5: Number (%) of Subjects with Common Adverse Events* in a 12-Week Placebo-Controlled Study of Divigel®

	Divigel®			Placebo
SYSTEM ORGAN CLASS Preferred Term	**0.25 g/day** **N=122** n (%)	**0.5 g/day** **N=123** n (%)	**1.0 g/day** **N=125** n (%)	**N=125** n (%)
INFECTIONS & INFESTATIONS				
Nasopharyngitis	7 (5.7)	5 (4.1)	6 (4.8)	5 (4.0)
Upper Respiratory Tract Infection	7 (5.7)	3 (2.4)	2 (1.6)	2 (1.6)
Vaginal mycosis	1 (0.8)	3 (2.4)	8 (6.4)	4 (3.2)
REPRODUCTIVE SYSTEM & BREAST DISORDERS				
Breast Tenderness	3 (2.5)	7 (5.7)	11 (8.8)	2 (1.6)
Metrorrhagia	5 (4.1)	7 (5.7)	12 (9.6)	2 (1.6)

*Adverse events reported by ≥5% of patients in any treatment group.

ADVERSE REACTIONS
See **BOXED WARNINGS, WARNINGS** and **PRECAUTIONS**.
Because clinical trials are conducted under widely varying conditions, adverse reaction rates observed in the clinical trials of a drug cannot be directly compared to rates in the clinical trials of another drug and may not reflect the rates observed in practice. The adverse reaction information from clinical trials does, however, provide a basis for identifying the adverse events that appear to be related to drug use and for approximating rates.
Divigel® was studied at doses of 0.25, 0.5 and 1.0 g/day in a 12-week, double-blind, placebo-controlled study that included a total of 495 postmenopausal women (86.5% Caucasian). The adverse events that occurred at a rate greater than 5% in any of the treatment groups are summarized in Table 5.
[See table 5 below]
In a 12-week placebo-controlled study of Divigel®, application site reactions were seen in <1% of subjects.
The following additional adverse reactions have been reported with estrogen and/or progestin therapy.
1. Genitourinary system: Changes in vaginal bleeding pattern and abnormal withdrawal bleeding or flow; breakthrough bleeding; spotting; dysmenorrhea; increase in size of uterine leiomyomata; vaginitis, including vaginal candidiasis; change in amount of cervical secretion; changes in cervical ectropion; ovarian cancer; endometrial hyperplasia; endometrial cancer; vaginal discharge.
2. Breasts: Tenderness; enlargement, pain, nipple discharge, galactorrhea, fibrocystic breast changes; breast cancer; nipple pain.
3. Cardiovascular: Deep and superficial venous thrombosis, pulmonary embolism; thrombophlebitis; myocardial infarction; stroke; increase in blood pressure.
4. Gastrointestinal: Nausea; vomiting; abdominal cramps; bloating; cholestatic jaundice; increased incidence of gallbladder disease; pancreatitis; enlargement of hepatic hemangiomas; abdominal pain.
5. Skin: Chloasma or melasma, which may persist when drug is discontinued; erythema multiforme; erythema nodosum; hemorrhagic eruption; loss of scalp hair; hirsutism; pruritus; rash.
6. Eyes: Retinal vascular thrombosis, intolerance to contact lenses.
7. Central Nervous System: Headache; migraine; dizziness; mental depression; chorea; nervousness; mood disturbances; irritability; exacerbation of epilepsy; dementia.
8. Miscellaneous: Increase or decrease in weight; reduced carbohydrate tolerance; aggravation of porphyria; edema; arthralgias; leg cramps; changes in libido; urticaria; angioedema; anaphylactoid/anaphylactic reactions; hypocalcemia; exacerbation of asthma; increased triglycerides; muscle cramps.

OVERDOSAGE
Serious ill effects have not been reported following acute ingestion of large doses of estrogen-containing drug products by young children. Overdosage of estrogen may cause nausea and vomiting, and withdrawal bleeding may occur in females.

DOSAGE AND ADMINISTRATION
When estrogen is prescribed for a postmenopausal woman with a uterus, a progestin should also be initiated to reduce the risk of endometrial cancer. A woman without a uterus does not need progestin. Use of estrogen, alone or in combination with a progestin, should be with the lowest effective dose and for the shortest duration consistent with treatment goals and risks for the individual woman. Patients should be re-evaluated periodically as clinically appropriate (e.g., 3-month to 6-month intervals) to determine if treatment is still necessary (see **BOXED WARNINGS** and **WARNINGS**). For women who have a uterus, adequate diagnostic measures, such as endometrial sampling, when indicated, should be undertaken to rule out malignancy in cases of undiagnosed persistent or recurring abnormal vaginal bleeding.
Divigel® (estradiol gel) 0.1%, at doses of 0.25, 0.5, and 1.0 g/day, is indicated for topical use in the treatment of moderate to severe vasomotor symptoms associated with menopause. Each gram of Divigel® contains 1 mg of estradiol.
Patients should be treated with the lowest effective dose of Divigel®. Generally, women should be started at 0.25 gram Divigel® daily. Subsequent dosage adjustments may be made based upon the individual patient response. This dose should be periodically reassessed by the healthcare provider.
Divigel® should be applied once daily on the skin of either the right or left upper thigh. The application surface area should be about 5 by 7 inches (approximately the size of two palm prints). The entire contents of a unit dose packet should be applied each day. To avoid potential skin irritation, Divigel® should be applied to the right or left upper

thigh on alternating days. Divigel® should not be applied on the face, breasts, or irritated skin or in or around the vagina. After application, the gel should be allowed to dry before dressing. The application site should not be washed within 1 hour after applying Divigel®. Contact of the gel with eyes should be avoided. Hands should be washed after application.

HOW SUPPLIED

Divigel® (estradiol gel), 0.1% is a clear, colorless, smooth, opalescent gel supplied in single-dose foil packets of 0.25, 0.5, and 1.0 g, corresponding to 0.25, 0.5, and 1.0 mg estradiol, respectively.

NDC 0245-0880-30, carton of 30 packets, 0.25 mg estradiol per single-dose foil packet

NDC 0245-0881-30, carton of 30 packets, 0.5 mg estradiol per single-dose foil packet

NDC 0245-0882-30, carton of 30 packets, 1.0 mg estradiol per single-dose foil packet

Keep out of the reach of children.

Store at 20 to 25°C (68 to 77°F). Excursions permitted to 15 to 30°C (59 to 86°F). [See USP Controlled Room Temperature.]

Manufactured by
Orion Corporation Orion Pharma
Tengströminkatu 8
FI-20360 Turku
Finland
Distributed by
UPSHER-SMITH LABORATORIES, INC.
Minneapolis, MN 55447
1-800-654-2299
Product of Finland
DVPI00   Revised 0607

PATIENT INFORMATION

(Updated June 2007)
Divigel®
(estradiol gel) 0.1%

Read this PATIENT INFORMATION leaflet before you start using Divigel® and read what you get each time you refill your Divigel® prescription. There may be new information. This information does not take the place of talking to your healthcare provider about your medical condition or your treatment.

WHAT IS THE MOST IMPORTANT INFORMATION I SHOULD KNOW ABOUT Divigel® (AN ESTROGEN HORMONE)?
- Estrogens increase the chance of getting cancer of the uterus. Report any unusual vaginal bleeding right away while you are taking estrogens. Vaginal bleeding after menopause may be a warning sign of cancer of the uterus (womb). Your healthcare provider should check any unusual vaginal bleeding to find out the cause.
- Do not use estrogens, with or without progestins, to prevent heart disease, heart attacks, or strokes. Using estrogens, with or without progestins, may increase your chance of getting heart attacks, strokes, breast cancer, and blood clots.
- Do not use estrogens, with or without progestins, to prevent dementia. Using estrogens, with or without progestins, may increase your risk of dementia.

You and your healthcare provider should talk regularly about whether you still need treatment with Divigel®.

What is Divigel®?
Divigel® is a medicine that contains an estrogen hormone (estradiol). Divigel® is a clear, colorless, smooth gel that is odorless when dry.

What is Divigel® used for?
Divigel® is used after menopause to:
- **Reduce moderate to severe hot flashes**
  Estrogens are hormones made by a woman's ovaries. The ovaries normally stop making estrogens when a woman is between 45 to 55 years old. This drop in body estrogen levels causes the "change of life" or menopause (the end of monthly menstrual periods). Sometimes, both ovaries are removed during an operation before natural menopause takes place. The sudden drop in estrogen levels causes "surgical menopause."
  When the estrogen levels begin dropping, some women develop very uncomfortable symptoms, such as feelings of warmth in the face, neck, and chest; or sudden strong feelings of heat and sweating ("hot flashes" or "hot flushes"). In some women, the symptoms are mild, and they will not need estrogens. In other women, symptoms can be more severe. You and your healthcare provider should talk regularly about whether you still need treatment with Divigel®.

Who should not use Divigel®?
Do not start using Divigel® if you:
- **Have unusual vaginal bleeding**

- **Currently have or have had certain cancers**
  Estrogens may increase the chances of getting certain types of cancers, including cancer of the breast and uterus. If you have or have had cancer, talk with your healthcare provider about whether you should use Divigel®.
- **Had a stroke or heart attack in the past year**
- **Currently have or have had blood clots**
- **Currently have or have had liver problems**
- **Are allergic to Divigel® or any of its ingredients**
  See the next section of this leaflet for a list of ingredients in Divigel®.
- **Think you may be pregnant**
  Tell your healthcare provider:
- **If you are breastfeeding**
  The hormone in Divigel® can pass into your milk.
- **About all of your medical problems**
  Your healthcare provider may need to check you more carefully if you have certain conditions, such as asthma (wheezing); epilepsy (seizures); migraine; endometriosis; lupus; problems with your heart, liver, thyroid, or kidneys; or have high calcium levels in your blood.
- **About all the medicines you take**
  This includes prescription and nonprescription medicines, vitamins, and herbal supplements. Some medicines may affect how Divigel® works. Divigel® may also affect how your other medicines work.
- **If you are going to have surgery or will be on bedrest**
  You may need to stop using Divigel®.

What are the ingredients in Divigel®?
The active ingredient in Divigel® is estradiol.
The inactive ingredients are carbomer, ethanol, propylene glycol, purified water, and triethanolamine.

How should I use Divigel®?
1. Divigel® should be used once daily.
2. Start at the lowest dose and talk to your healthcare provider about how well that dose is working for you
3. Divigel® should be used at the lowest dose possible for your treatment and only as long as needed. You and your healthcare provider should talk regularly (for example, every 3 to 6 months) about the dose you are taking and whether you still need treatment with Divigel®.

Important things to remember when using Divigel®
- **Wash your hands with soap and water after applying the gel to reduce the chance that the medicine will be spread from your hands to other people.**
- Allow the gel to dry before dressing. Try to keep the area dry for as long as possible.
- Do not allow others to come in contact with the area of skin where you applied the gel for at least one hour after you apply Divigel®.
- You should not allow others to apply the gel for you. However, if this is necessary, the individual should wear a disposable plastic glove to avoid direct contact with Divigel®.
- Do not apply Divigel® to your face, breast, or irritated skin
- Never apply Divigel® in or around the vagina
- **Divigel® contains alcohol. Alcohol based gels are flammable. Avoid fire, flame or smoking until the gel has dried.**

What should I do if I miss a dose?
If you miss a dose, do not double the dose on the next day to catch up. If your next dose is less than 12 hours away, it is best just to wait and apply your normal dose the next day. If it is more than 12 hours until the next dose, apply the dose you missed and resume your normal dosing the next day. Do not apply Divigel® more than once each day. If you accidentally spill some of the contents of a Divigel® packet, do not open a new packet. Wait and apply your normal dose the next day.

What should I do if someone else is exposed to Divigel®?
Once you have applied Divigel® (estradiol gel) 0.1%, it has dried, and you have washed your hands, there is little risk of transfer to another person. If someone else is exposed to Divigel® by direct contact with the wet gel, that person should wash the area of contact with soap and water as soon as possible. This is especially important for men and children. The longer the gel is in contact with the skin before washing, the chance is greater that the other person will absorb some of the estrogen hormone.

What should I do if I get Divigel® in my eyes?
If you get Divigel® in your eyes, flush your eyes right away with lukewarm tap water. If you have concerns, contact your healthcare provider.

What are the possible side effects of estrogens?
Less common but serious side effects include:
- Breast cancer
- Cancer of the uterus
- Stroke
- Heart attack
- Blood clots
- Dementia
- Gallbladder disease
- Ovarian cancer

Some of the warning signs of serious side effects include:
- Breast lumps
- Unusual vaginal bleeding
- Dizziness and faintness
- Changes in speech
- Severe headaches
- Chest pain
- Shortness of breath
- Pains in your legs
- Changes in vision
- Vomiting

Call your healthcare provider right away if you get any of these warning signs, or any other unusual symptom that concerns you.

Common side effects include:
- Headache
- Breast pain
- Irregular vaginal bleeding or spotting
- Stomach/abdominal cramps, bloating
- Nausea and vomiting
- Hair loss

Other side effects include:
- High blood pressure
- Liver problems
- High blood sugar
- Fluid retention
- Enlargement of benign tumors of the uterus ("fibroids")
- Vaginal yeast infection

These are not all the possible side effects of Divigel®. For more information, ask your healthcare provider or pharmacist

What can I do to lower my chances of a serious side effect with Divigel®?
Talk with your healthcare provider regularly about whether you should continue taking Divigel®. If you have a uterus, talk to your healthcare provider about whether the addition of a progestin is right for you. In general, the addition of a progestin is recommended for women with a uterus to reduce the chance of getting cancer of the uterus. See your healthcare provider right away if you get vaginal bleeding while taking Divigel®. Have a breast exam and mammogram (breast X-ray) every year unless your healthcare provider tells you otherwise. If members of your family have had breast cancer or if you have ever had breast lumps or an abnormal mammogram, you may need to have breast exams more often. If you have high blood pressure, high cholesterol (fat in the blood), diabetes, are overweight, or if you use tobacco, you may have higher chances of getting heart disease. Ask your healthcare provider for ways to lower your chances of getting heart disease.
Have an annual gynecological exam.

General information about safe and effective use of Divigel®
Medicines are sometimes prescribed for conditions that are not mentioned in patient information leaflets. Do not use Divigel® for conditions for which it was not prescribed. Do not give Divigel® to other people, even if they have the same symptoms you have. It may harm them.

Keep Divigel® out of the reach of children.

This leaflet provides a summary of the most important information about Divigel®. If you would like more information, talk with your healthcare provider or pharmacist. You can ask for information about Divigel® that is written for health professionals. You can get more information by calling the toll free number 1-800-654-2299.

How should Divigel® be applied?
- Divigel® should be applied once a day, around the same time each day.
- Apply Divigel® to clean, dry, and unbroken (without cuts or scrapes) skin. If you take a bath or shower, be sure to apply your Divigel® after your skin is dry. The application site should be completely dry before dressing or swimming.
- Apply Divigel® to either your left or right upper thigh. Change between your left and right upper thigh each day to help prevent skin irritation.

To Apply:
1. Wash and dry your hands thoroughly.
2. Sit in a comfortable position.
3. Cut or tear the Divigel® packet as shown in Diagram 1.

Diagram 1

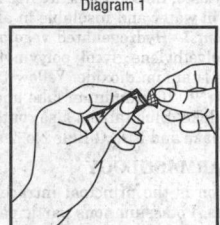

4. Using your thumb and index finger, squeeze the entire contents of the packet onto the skin of the upper thigh as shown in Diagram 2.

Diagram 2

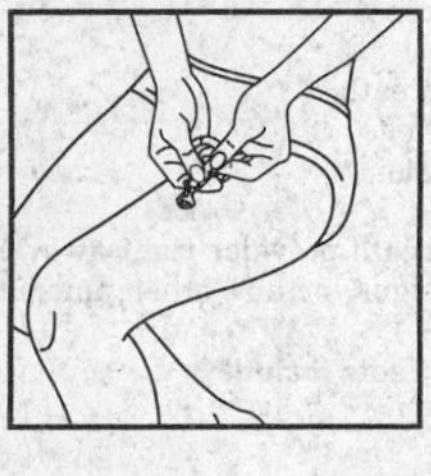

5. Gently spread the gel in a thin layer on your upper thigh over an area of about 5 by 7 inches, or two palm prints as shown in Diagram 3. It is not necessary to massage or rub in Divigel®.

Diagram 3

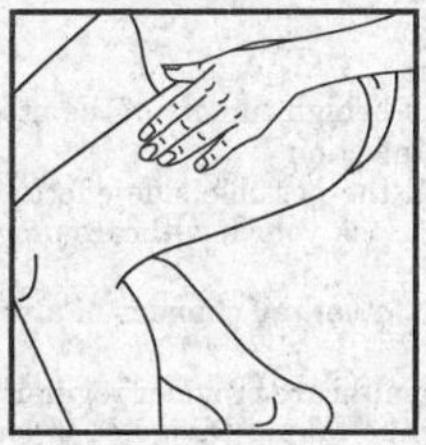

6. Allow the gel to dry completely before dressing.
7. Dispose of the empty Divigel® packet in the trash.
8. Wash your hands with soap and water immediately after applying Divigel® to remove any remaining gel and reduce the chance of transferring Divigel® to other people.

HOW IS Divigel® SUPPLIED?

Divigel® (estradiol gel) 0.1% is supplied in individual foil packets, each one containing a single day's dose.

Store Divigel® packets at 20 to 25°C (68 to 77°F). Excursions permitted to 15 to 30°C (59 to 86°F). [See USP Controlled Room Temperature.]

Manufactured by
Orion Corporation Orion Pharma
Tengströminkatu 8
FI-20360 Turku
Finland
Distributed by
UPSHER-SMITH LABORATORIES, INC
Minneapolis, MN 55447
1-800-654-2299
Product of Finland
DVPI00 Revised 0607

Shown in Product Identification Guide, page 321

KLOR-CON® ℞
[*klōr 'kon*]
Potassium Chloride
Extended-release Tablets, USP
8 mEq and 10 mEq

DESCRIPTION

Klor-Con® Extended-release Tablets, USP are a solid oral dosage form of potassium chloride. Each contains 600 mg or 750 mg of potassium chloride equivalent to 8 mEq or 10 mEq of potassium in a wax matrix tablet. This formulation is intended to provide an extended-release of potassium from the matrix to minimize the likelihood of producing high, localized concentrations of potassium within the gastrointestinal tract.

Klor-Con® Extended-release Tablets are an electrolyte replenisher. The chemical name is potassium chloride, and the structural formula is KCl. Potassium chloride, USP is a white, granular powder or colorless crystals. It is odorless and has a saline taste. Its solutions are neutral to litmus. It is freely soluble in water and insoluble in alcohol.

Inactive Ingredients: Hydrogenated vegetable oil, magnesium stearate, polyethylene glycol, polyvinyl alcohol, silicon dioxide, talc and titanium dioxide. Yellow tablets also contain D&C Yellow No. 10 aluminum lake and FD&C Yellow No. 6 aluminum lake. Blue tablets also contain FD&C Blue No. 1 aluminum lake and FD&C Blue No. 2 aluminum lake.

CLINICAL PHARMACOLOGY

The potassium ion is the principal intracellular cation of most body tissues. Potassium ions participate in a number of essential physiological processes including the maintenance of intracellular tonicity, the transmission of nerve impulses, the contraction of cardiac, skeletal and smooth muscle and the maintenance of normal renal function.

The intracellular concentration of potassium is approximately 150 to 160 mEq per liter. The normal adult plasma concentration is 3.5 to 5 mEq per liter. An active ion transport system maintains this gradient across the plasma membrane.

Potassium is a normal dietary constituent and under steady state conditions the amount of potassium absorbed from the gastrointestinal tract is equal to the amount excreted in the urine. The usual dietary intake of potassium is 50 to 100 mEq per day.

Potassium depletion will occur whenever the rate of potassium loss through renal excretion and/or loss from the gastrointestinal tract exceeds the rate of potassium intake. Such depletion usually develops slowly as a consequence of prolonged therapy with oral diuretics, primary or secondary hyperaldosteronism, diabetic ketoacidosis, severe diarrhea, or inadequate replacement of potassium in patients on prolonged parenteral nutrition. Depletion can develop rapidly with severe diarrhea, especially if associated with vomiting. Potassium depletion due to these causes is usually accompanied by a concomitant loss of chloride and is manifested by hypokalemia and metabolic alkalosis. Potassium depletion may produce weakness, fatigue, disturbances of cardiac rhythm (primarily ectopic beats), prominent U-waves in the electrocardiogram and, in advanced cases, flaccid paralysis and/or impaired ability to concentrate urine.

If potassium depletion associated with metabolic alkalosis cannot be managed by correcting the fundamental cause of the deficiency, e.g., where the patient requires long term diuretic therapy, supplemental potassium in the form of high potassium food or potassium chloride may be able to restore normal potassium levels.

In rare circumstances (e.g., patients with renal tubular acidosis) potassium depletion may be associated with metabolic acidosis and hyperchloremia. In such patients potassium replacement should be accomplished with potassium salts other than the chloride, such as potassium bicarbonate, potassium citrate, potassium acetate or potassium gluconate.

The potassium chloride in Klor-Con® Extended-release Tablets is completely absorbed before it leaves the small intestine. The wax matrix is not absorbed and is excreted in the feces; in some instances the empty matrices may be noticeable in the stool. When the bioavailability of the potassium ion from the Klor-Con® Extended-release Tablets is compared to that of a true solution the extent of absorption is similar.

The extended-release properties of Klor-Con® Extended-release Tablets are demonstrated by the finding that a significant increase in time is required for renal excretion of the first 50% of the Klor-Con® Extended-release Tablets dose as compared to the solution.

Increased urinary potassium excretion is first observed 1 hour after administration of Klor-Con® Extended-release Tablets, reaches a peak at 4 hours, and extends up to 8 hours. Mean daily steady-state plasma levels of potassium following daily administration of Klor-Con® Extended-release Tablets cannot be distinguished from those following administration of potassium chloride solution or from control plasma levels of potassium ion.

INDICATIONS AND USAGE

BECAUSE OF REPORTS OF INTESTINAL AND GASTRIC ULCERATION AND BLEEDING WITH EXTENDED-RELEASE POTASSIUM CHLORIDE PREPARATIONS, THESE DRUGS SHOULD BE RESERVED FOR THOSE PATIENTS WHO CANNOT TOLERATE OR REFUSE TO TAKE LIQUID OR EFFERVESCENT POTASSIUM PREPARATIONS OR FOR PATIENTS IN WHOM THERE IS A PROBLEM OF COMPLIANCE WITH THESE PREPARATIONS.

1. For the therapeutic use of patients with hypokalemia, with or without metabolic alkalosis; in digitalis intoxication; and in patients with hypokalemic familial periodic paralysis. If hypokalemia is the result of diuretic therapy, consideration should be given to the use of a lower dose of diuretic, which may be sufficient without leading to hypokalemia.
2. For the prevention of hypokalemia in patients who would be at particular risk if hypokalemia were to develop, e.g., digitalized patients or patients with significant cardiac arrhythmias.

The use of potassium salts in patients receiving diuretics for uncomplicated essential hypertension is often unnecessary when such patients have a normal dietary pattern and when low doses of the diuretic are used. Serum potassium should be checked periodically, however, and if hypokalemia occurs, dietary supplementation with potassium-containing foods may be adequate to control milder cases. In more severe cases, and if dose adjustment of the diuretic is ineffective or unwarranted, supplementation with potassium salts may be indicated.

CONTRAINDICATIONS

Potassium supplements are contraindicated in patients with hyperkalemia since a further increase in serum potassium concentration in such patients can produce cardiac arrest. Hyperkalemia may complicate any of the following conditions: chronic renal failure, systemic acidosis such as diabetic acidosis, acute dehydration, extensive tissue breakdown as in severe burns, adrenal insufficiency or the administration of a potassium-sparing diuretic (e.g., spironolactone, triamterene or amiloride) (see **OVERDOSAGE**).

Extended-release formulations of potassium chloride have produced esophageal ulceration in certain cardiac patients with esophageal compression due to an enlarged left atrium. Potassium supplementation, when indicated in such patients, should be given as a liquid preparation.

All solid oral dosage forms of potassium chloride are contraindicated in any patient in whom there is structural, pathological (e.g., diabetic gastroparesis) or pharmacologic (use of anticholinergic agents or other agents with anticholinergic properties at sufficient doses to exert anticholinergic effects) cause for arrest or delay in tablet passage through the gastrointestinal tract.

WARNINGS

Hyperkalemia (see **OVERDOSAGE**): In patients with impaired mechanisms for excreting potassium, the administration of potassium salts can produce hyperkalemia and cardiac arrest. This occurs most commonly in patients given potassium by the intravenous route but may also occur in patients given potassium orally. Potentially fatal hyperkalemia can develop rapidly and be asymptomatic.

The use of potassium salts in patients with chronic renal disease, or any other condition which impairs potassium excretion, requires particularly careful monitoring of the serum potassium concentration and appropriate dosage adjustment.

Interaction with Potassium-sparing Diuretics: Hypokalemia should not be treated by the concomitant administration of potassium salts and a potassium-sparing diuretic (e.g., spironolactone, triamterene or amiloride), since the simultaneous administration of these agents can produce severe hyperkalemia.

Interaction with Angiotensin Converting Enzyme Inhibitors: Angiotensin converting enzyme (ACE) inhibitors (e.g., captopril, enalapril) will produce some potassium retention by inhibiting aldosterone production. Potassium supplements should be given to patients receiving ACE inhibitors only with close monitoring.

Gastrointestinal Lesions: Solid oral dosage forms of potassium chloride can produce ulcerative and/or stenotic lesions of the gastrointestinal tract. Based on spontaneous adverse reaction reports, enteric-coated preparations of potassium chloride are associated with an increased frequency of small bowel lesions (40-50 per 100,000 patient years) compared to extended-release wax matrix formulations (less than one per 100,000 patient years). Because of the lack of extensive marketing experience with microencapsulated products, a comparison between such products and wax matrix or enteric-coated products is not available. Klor-Con® Extended-release Tablets are wax matrix tablets formulated to provide an extended rate of release of potassium chloride and thus to minimize the possibility of high local concentration of potassium near the gastrointestinal wall.

Prospective trials have been conducted in normal human volunteers in which the upper gastrointestinal tract was evaluated by endoscopic inspection before and after one week of solid oral potassium chloride therapy. The ability of this model to predict events occurring in usual clinical practice is unknown. Trials which approximated usual clinical practice did not reveal any clear differences between the wax matrix and microencapsulated dosage forms. In contrast, there was a higher incidence of gastric and duodenal lesions in subjects receiving a high dose of a wax matrix extended-release formulation under conditions which did not resemble usual or recommended clinical practice (i.e., 96 mEq per day in divided doses of potassium chloride administered to fasted patients, in the presence of an anticholinergic drug to delay gastric emptying). The upper gastrointestinal lesions observed by endoscopy were asymptomatic and were not accompanied by evidence of bleeding (hemoccult testing). The relevance of these findings to the usual conditions (i.e., non-fasting, no anticholinergic agent, smaller doses) under which extended-release potassium chloride products are used is uncertain; epidemiologic studies have not identified an elevated risk, compared to microencapsulated products, for upper gastrointestinal lesions in patients receiving wax matrix formulations. Klor-Con® Extended-release Tablets should be discontinued immediately and the possibility of ulceration, obstruction or perforation considered if severe vomiting, abdominal pain, distention or gastrointestinal bleeding occurs.

Metabolic Acidosis: Hypokalemia in patients with metabolic acidosis should be treated with an alkalinizing potassium salt such as potassium bicarbonate, potassium citrate, potassium acetate or potassium gluconate.

PRECAUTIONS

General: The diagnosis of potassium depletion is ordinarily made by demonstrating hypokalemia in a patient with a clinical history suggesting some cause for potassium depletion. In interpreting the serum potassium level, the physician should be aware that acute alkalosis *per se* can produce hypokalemia in the absence of a deficit in total body potassium while acute acidosis *per se* can increase the serum potassium concentration into the normal range even in the presence of a reduced total body potassium. The treatment of potassium depletion, particularly in the presence of cardiac disease, renal disease or acidosis requires careful attention to acid-base balance and appropriate monitoring of serum electrolytes, the electrocardiogram and the clinical status of the patient.

Information for Patients: Physicians should consider reminding the patient of the following:

- To take each dose with meals and with a full glass of water or other liquid.
- To take this medicine following the frequency and amount prescribed by the physician. This is especially important if the patient is also taking diuretics and/or digitalis preparations.
- To check with the physician if there is trouble swallowing the tablets or if the tablets seem to stick in the throat.
- To check with the physician at once if tarry stools or other evidence of gastrointestinal bleeding is noticed.
- To take each dose without crushing, chewing or sucking the tablets.

Laboratory Tests: When blood is drawn for analysis of plasma potassium it is important to recognize that artifactual elevations can occur after improper venipuncture technique or as a result of *in vitro* hemolysis of the sample.

Drug Interactions: Potassium-sparing diuretic, angiotensin converting enzyme inhibitors (see **WARNINGS**).

Carcinogenesis, Mutagenesis, Impairment of Fertility: Carcinogenicity, mutagenicity and fertility studies in animals have not been performed. Potassium is a normal dietary constituent.

Pregnancy: Pregnancy Category C. Animal reproduction studies have not been conducted with Klor-Con® Extended-release Tablets. It is unlikely that potassium supplementation that does not lead to hyperkalemia would have an adverse effect on the fetus or would affect reproductive capacity.

Nursing Mothers: The normal potassium ion content of human milk is about 13 mEq per liter. It is not known if Klor-Con® Extended-release Tablets have an effect on this content. Since oral potassium becomes part of the body potassium pool, so long as body potassium is not excessive, the contribution of potassium chloride supplementation should have little or no effect on the level in human milk.

Pediatric Use: Safety and effectiveness in the pediatric population have not been established.

Geriatric Use: Clinical studies of Klor-Con® Extended-release Tablets did not include sufficient numbers of subjects aged 65 and over to determine whether they respond differently from younger subjects. Other reported clinical experience has not identified differences in responses between the elderly and younger patients. In general, dose selection for an elderly patient should be cautious, usually starting at the low end of the dosing range, reflecting the greater frequency of decreased hepatic, renal or cardiac function, and of concomitant disease or other drug therapy. This drug is known to be substantially excreted by the kidney, and the risk of toxic reactions to this drug may be greater in patients with impaired renal function. Because elderly patients are more likely to have decreased renal function, care should be taken in dose selection, and it may be useful to monitor renal function.

ADVERSE REACTIONS

One of the most severe adverse effects is hyperkalemia (see **CONTRAINDICATIONS, WARNINGS** and **OVERDOSAGE**). There also have been reports of upper and lower gastrointestinal conditions including obstruction, bleeding, ulceration and perforation (see **CONTRAINDICATIONS** and **WARNINGS**).

The most common adverse reactions to oral potassium salts are nausea, vomiting, flatulence, abdominal pain/discomfort and diarrhea. These symptoms are due to irritation of the gastrointestinal tract and are best managed by taking the dose with meals or reducing the amount taken at one time. Skin rash has been reported rarely.

OVERDOSAGE

The administration of oral potassium salts to persons with normal excretory mechanisms for potassium rarely causes serious hyperkalemia. However, if excretory mechanisms are impaired, or if potassium is administered too rapidly intravenously, potentially fatal hyperkalemia can result (see **CONTRAINDICATIONS** and **WARNINGS**). It is important to recognize that hyperkalemia is usually asymptomatic and may be manifested only by an increased serum potassium concentration (6.5-8.0 mEq/L) and characteristic electrocardiographic changes (peaking of T-waves, loss of P-wave, depression of S-T segment and prolongation of the QT interval). Late manifestations include muscle paralysis and cardiovascular collapse from cardiac arrest (9-12 mEq/L).

Treatment measures for hyperkalemia include the following:

1. Elimination of foods and medications containing potassium and of any agents with potassium-sparing properties.
2. Intravenous administration of 300 to 500 mL/hr of 10% dextrose solution containing 10-20 units of crystalline insulin per 1,000 mL.
3. Correction of acidosis, if present, with intravenous sodium bicarbonate.
4. Use of exchange resins, hemodialysis or peritoneal dialysis.

In treating hyperkalemia, it should be recalled that in patients who have been stabilized on digitalis, too rapid a lowering of the serum potassium concentration can produce digitalis toxicity.

The extended release feature means that absorption and toxic effects may be delayed for hours. Consider standard measures to remove any unabsorbed drug.

DOSAGE AND ADMINISTRATION

The usual dietary potassium intake by the average adult is 50 to 100 mEq per day. Potassium depletion sufficient to cause hypokalemia usually requires the loss of 200 mEq or more of potassium from the total body store.

Dosage must be adjusted to the individual needs of each patient. The dose for the prevention of hypokalemia is typically in the range of 20 mEq per day. Doses of 40-100 mEq per day or more are used for the treatment of potassium depletion. Dosage should be divided if more than 20 mEq per day is given such that no more than 20 mEq is given in a single dose.

Each Klor-Con® Extended-release Tablet provides 8 mEq or 10 mEq of potassium chloride.

Klor-Con® Extended-release Tablets should be taken with meals and with a glass of water or other liquid. This product should not be taken on an empty stomach because of its potential for gastric irritation (see **WARNINGS**).

NOTE: Klor-Con® Extended-release Tablets must be swallowed whole and never crushed, chewed, or sucked.

HOW SUPPLIED

Film-coated Klor-Con® 8 (light blue, debossed with "KC 8"), Klor-Con® 10 (yellow, debossed with "KC 10"), round tablets containing:

- 600 mg potassium chloride (equivalent to 8 mEq) in bottles of 100 (NDC 0245-0040-11), bottles of 500 (NDC 0245-0040-15), unit dose packages of 100 (NDC 0245-0040-01), bulk packs of 5,000 for repack only (NDC 0245-0040-55), and bulk packs of 10,000 for repack only (NDC 0245-0040-00);
- 750 mg potassium chloride (equivalent to 10 mEq) in bottles of 100 (NDC 0245-0041-11), bottles of 500 (NDC 0245-0041-15), unit dose packages of 100 (NDC 0245-0041-01), bulk packs of 5,000 for repack only (NDC 0245-0041-55), and bulk packs of 10,000 for repack only (NDC 0245-0041-00).

Store at controlled room temperature, 15-30°C (59-86°F). Protect from light and moisture. Dispense in a tight container with child-resistant closure.

Manufactured by
UPSHER-SMITH LABORATORIES, INC.
Minneapolis, MN 55447
Revised 1008

Shown in Product Identification Guide, page 321

KLOR-CON® M ℞

[klōr'kŏn]

(Potassium Chloride Extended-releaseTablets, USP)
10 mEq, 15 mEq and 20 mEq
Micro-Dispersible Technology®
Rx only

DESCRIPTION

Klor-Con® M20 is an immediately dispersing extended-release oral dosage form of potassium chloride containing 1500 mg of microencapsulated potassium chloride, USP equivalent to 20 mEq of potassium in a tablet.

Klor-Con® M15 is an immediately dispersing extended-release oral dosage form of potassium chloride containing 1125 mg of microencapsulated potassium chloride, USP equivalent to 15 mEq of potassium in a tablet.

Klor-Con® M10 is an immediately dispersing extended-release oral dosage form of potassium chloride containing 750 mg of microencapsulated potassium chloride, USP equivalent to 10 mEq of potassium in a tablet.

These formulations are intended to slow the release of potassium so that the likelihood of a high localized concentration of potassium chloride within the gastrointestinal tract is reduced.

Klor-Con® M is an electrolyte replenisher. The chemical name of the active ingredient is potassium chloride, and the structural formula is KCl. Potassium chloride, USP occurs as a white, granular powder or as colorless crystals. It is odorless and has a saline taste. Its solutions are neutral to litmus. It is freely soluble in water and insoluble in alcohol.

Klor-Con® M is a tablet formulation (not enteric coated or wax matrix) containing individually microencapsulated potassium chloride crystals which disperse upon tablet disintegration. In simulated gastric fluid at 37°C and in the absence of outside agitation, Klor-Con® M begins disintegrating into microencapsulated crystals within seconds and completely disintegrates within one minute. The microencapsulated crystals are formulated to provide an extended release of potassium chloride.

Inactive Ingredients: croscarmellose sodium, ethylcellulose and microcrystalline cellulose.

CLINICAL PHARMACOLOGY

The potassium ion is the principal intracellular cation of most body tissues. Potassium ions participate in a number of essential physiological processes including the maintenance of intracellular tonicity; the transmission of nerve impulses; the contraction of cardiac, skeletal, and smooth muscle; and the maintenance of normal renal function.

The intracellular concentration of potassium is approximately 150 to 160 mEq per liter. The normal adult plasma concentration is 3.5 to 5 mEq per liter. An active ion transport system maintains this gradient across the plasma membrane.

Potassium is a normal dietary constituent and under steady-state conditions the amount of potassium absorbed from the gastrointestinal tract is equal to the amount excreted in the urine. The usual dietary intake of potassium is 50 to 100 mEq per day.

Potassium depletion will occur whenever the rate of potassium loss through renal excretion and/or loss from the gastrointestinal tract exceeds the rate of potassium intake. Such depletion usually develops as a consequence of therapy with diuretics, primary or secondary hyperaldosteronism, diabetic ketoacidosis or inadequate replacement of potassium in patients on prolonged parenteral nutrition. Depletion can develop rapidly with severe diarrhea, especially if associated with vomiting. Potassium depletion due to these causes is usually accompanied by a concomitant loss of chloride and is manifested by hypokalemia and metabolic alkalosis. Potassium depletion may produce weakness, fatigue, disturbances or cardiac rhythm (primarily ectopic beats), prominent U-waves in the electrocardiogram, and in advanced cases, flaccid paralysis and/or impaired ability to concentrate urine.

If potassium depletion associated with metabolic alkalosis cannot be managed by correcting the fundamental cause of the deficiency, e.g., where the patient requires long-term diuretic therapy, supplemental potassium in the form of high-potassium food or potassium chloride may be able to restore normal potassium levels.

In rare circumstances (e.g., patients with renal tubular acidosis) potassium depletion may be associated with metabolic acidosis and hyperchloremia. In such patients potassium replacement should be accomplished with potassium salts other than the chloride, such as potassium bicarbonate, potassium citrate, potassium acetate, or potassium gluconate.

INDICATIONS AND USAGE

BECAUSE OF REPORTS OF INTESTINAL AND GASTRIC ULCERATION AND BLEEDING WITH EXTENDED-RELEASE POTASSIUM CHLORIDE PREPARATIONS, THESE DRUGS SHOULD BE RESERVED FOR THOSE PATIENTS WHO CANNOT TOLERATE OR REFUSE TO TAKE LIQUID OR EFFERVESCENT POTASSIUM PREPARATIONS OR FOR PATIENTS IN WHOM THERE IS A PROBLEM OF COMPLIANCE WITH THESE PREPARATIONS.

1. For the treatment of patients with hypokalemia with or without metabolic alkalosis, in digitalis intoxication and in patients with hypokalemic familial periodic paralysis. If hypokalemia is the result of diuretic therapy, consideration should be given to the use of a lower dose of diuretic, which may be sufficient without leading to hypokalemia.
2. For the prevention of hypokalemia in patients who would be at particular risk if hypokalemia were to develop, e.g., digitalized patients or patients with significant cardiac arrhythmias.

The use of potassium salts in patients receiving diuretics for uncomplicated essential hypertension is often unnecessary when such patients have a normal dietary pattern and when low doses of the diuretic are used. Serum potassium should be checked periodically, however, and if hypokalemia occurs, dietary supplementation with potassium-containing foods may be adequate to control milder cases. In more severe cases, and if dose adjustment of the diuretic is ineffective or unwarranted, supplementation with potassium salts may be indicated.

CONTRAINDICATIONS

Potassium supplements are contraindicated in patients with hyperkalemia since a further increase in serum potassium concentration in such patients can produce cardiac arrest. Hyperkalemia may complicate any of the following conditions: chronic renal failure, systemic acidosis, such as diabetic acidosis, acute dehydration, extensive tissue breakdown as in severe burns, adrenal insufficiency, or the administration of a potassium-sparing diuretic (e.g., spironolactone, triamterene, or amiloride) (see **OVERDOSAGE**). Extended-release formulations of potassium chloride have produced esophageal ulceration in certain cardiac patients with esophageal compression due to enlarged left atrium. Potassium supplementation, when indicated in such patients, should be given as a liquid preparation or as an aqueous (water) suspension of Klor-Con® M (see **PRECAUTIONS: Information for Patients** and **DOSAGE AND ADMINISTRATION** sections).

All solid oral dosage forms of potassium chloride are contraindicated in any patient in whom there is structural, pathological (e.g., diabetic gastroparesis), or pharmacologic (use of anticholinergic agents or other agents with anticholinergic properties at sufficient doses to exert anticholinergic effects) cause for arrest or delay in tablet passage through the gastrointestinal tract.

WARNINGS

Hyperkalemia (see **OVERDOSAGE**)—In patients with impaired mechanisms for excreting potassium, the administration of potassium salts can produce hyperkalemia and cardiac arrest. This occurs most commonly in patients given potassium by the intravenous route but may also occur in patients given potassium orally. Potentially fatal hyperkalemia can develop rapidly and be asymptomatic. The use of potassium salts in patients with chronic renal disease, or any other condition which impairs potassium excretion, requires particularly careful monitoring of the serum potassium concentration and appropriate dosage adjustment.

Interaction with Potassium–Sparing Diuretics—Hypokalemia should not be treated by the concomitant administration of potassium salts and a potassium-sparing diuretic (e.g., spironolactone, triamterene, or amiloride) since the simultaneous administration of these agents can produce severe hyperkalemia.

Interaction with Angiotensin–Converting Enzyme Inhibitors—Angiotensin-converting enzyme (ACE) inhibitors (e.g., captopril, enalapril) will produce some potassium retention by inhibiting aldosterone production. Potassium supplements should be given to patients receiving ACE inhibitors only with close monitoring.

Gastrointestinal Lesions—Solid oral dosage forms of potassium chloride can produce ulcerative and/or stenotic lesions of the gastrointestinal tract. Based on spontaneous adverse reaction reports, enteric-coated preparations of potassium chloride are associated with an increased frequency of small bowel lesions (40-50 per 100,000 patient years) compared to extended-release wax matrix formulations (less than one per 100,000 patient years). Because of the lack of extensive marketing experience with microencapsulated products, a comparison between such products and wax matrix or enteric-coated products is not available. Klor-Con® M is a tablet formulated to provide an extended rate of release of microencapsulated potassium chloride and thus to minimize the possibility of a high local concentration of potassium near the gastrointestinal wall.

Prospective trials have been conducted in normal human volunteers in which the upper gastrointestinal tract was evaluated by endoscopic inspection before and after one week of solid oral potassium chloride therapy. The ability of this model to predict events occurring in usual clinical practice is unknown. Trials which approximated usual clinical practice did not reveal any clear differences between the wax matrix and microencapsulated dosage forms. In contrast, there was a higher incidence of gastric and duodenal lesions in subjects receiving a high dose of a wax matrix extended-release formulation under conditions which did not resemble usual or recommended clinical practice (i.e., 96 mEq per day in divided doses of potassium chloride administered to fasted patients, in the presence of an anticholinergic drug to delay gastric emptying). The upper gastrointestinal lesions observed by endoscopy were asymptomatic and were not accompanied by evidence of bleeding (Hemoccult testing). The relevance of these findings to the usual conditions (i.e., non-fasting, no anticholinergic agent,

smaller doses) under which extended-release potassium chloride products are used is uncertain; epidemiologic studies have not identified an elevated risk, compared to microencapsulated products, for upper gastrointestinal lesions in patients receiving wax matrix formulations. Klor-Con® M should be discontinued immediately and the possibility of ulceration, obstruction, or perforation should be considered if severe vomiting, abdominal pain, distention, or gastrointestinal bleeding occurs.

Metabolic Acidosis—Hypokalemia in patients with metabolic acidosis should be treated with an alkalinizing potassium salt such as potassium bicarbonate, potassium citrate, potassium acetate or potassium gluconate.

PRECAUTIONS

General: The diagnosis of potassium depletion is ordinarily made by demonstrating hypokalemia in a patient with a clinical history suggesting some cause for potassium depletion. In interpreting the serum potassium level, the physician should bear in mind that acute alkalosis *per se* can produce hypokalemia in the absence of a deficit in total body potassium while acute acidosis *per se* can increase the serum potassium concentration into the normal range even in the presence of a reduced total body potassium. The treatment of potassium depletion, particularly in the presence of cardiac disease, renal disease, or acidosis requires careful attention to acid-base balance and appropriate monitoring of serum electrolytes, the electrocardiogram, and the clinical status of the patient.

Information for Patients: Physicians should consider reminding the patient of the following:
To take each dose with meals and with a full glass of water or other liquid.
To take each dose without crushing, chewing or sucking the tablets. If those patients are having difficulty swallowing whole tablets, they may try one of the following alternate methods of administration:
a. Break the tablet in half, and take each half separately with a glass of water.
b. Prepare an aqueous (water) suspension as follows:
1. Place the whole tablet(s) in approximately one-half glass of water (4 fluid ounces).
2. Allow approximately 2 minutes for the tablet(s) to disintegrate.
3. Stir for about half a minute after the tablet(s) has disintegrated.
4. Swirl the suspension and consume the entire contents of the glass immediately by drinking or by the use of a straw.
5. Add another one fluid ounce of water, swirl, and consume immediately.
6. Then, add an additional one fluid ounce of water, swirl, and consume immediately.
Aqueous suspension of Klor-Con® M extended-release tablet that is not taken immediately should be discarded. The use of other liquids for suspending Klor-Con® M tablets is not recommended.
To take this medicine following the frequency and amount prescribed by the physician.
This is especially important if the patient is also taking diuretics and/or digitalis preparations.
To check with the physician at once if tarry stools or other evidence of gastrointestinal bleeding is noticed.

Laboratory Tests: When blood is drawn for analysis of plasma potassium it is important to recognize that artifactual elevations can occur after improper venipuncture technique or as a result of *in-vitro* hemolysis of the sample.

Drug Interactions: Potassium-sparing diuretics, angiotensin-converting enzyme inhibitors (see **WARNINGS**).

Carcinogenesis, Mutagenesis, Impairment of Fertility: Carcinogenicity, mutagenicity, and fertility studies in animals have not been performed.
Potassium is a normal dietary constituent.

Pregnancy Category C: Animal reproduction studies have not been conducted with Klor-Con® M. It is unlikely that potassium supplementation that does not lead to hyperkalemia would have an adverse effect on the fetus or would affect reproductive capacity.

Nursing Mothers: The normal potassium ion content of human milk is about 13 mEq per liter. Since oral potassium becomes part of the body potassium pool, so long as body potassium is not excessive, the contribution of potassium chloride supplementation should have little or no effect on the level in human milk.

Pediatric Use: Safety and effectiveness in pediatric patients have not been established.

Geriatric Use: Clinical studies of potassium chloride did not include sufficient numbers of subjects aged 65 and over to determine whether they respond differently from younger subjects. Other reported clinical experience has not identified differences in responses between the elderly and younger patients. In general, dose selection for an elderly patient should be cautious, usually starting at the low end

of the dosing range, reflecting the greater frequency of decreased hepatic, renal or cardiac function, and of concomitant disease or other drug therapy.
This drug is known to be substantially excreted by the kidney, and the risk of toxic reactions to this drug may be greater in patients with impaired renal function. Because elderly patients are more likely to have decreased renal function, care should be taken in dose selection; and it may be useful to monitor renal function.

ADVERSE REACTIONS

One of the most severe adverse effects is hyperkalemia (see **CONTRAINDICATIONS, WARNINGS** and **OVERDOSAGE**). There have also been reports of upper and lower gastrointestinal conditions including obstruction, bleeding, ulceration, and perforation (see **CONTRAINDICATIONS** and **WARNINGS**). The most common adverse reactions to oral potassium salts are nausea, vomiting, flatulence, abdominal pain/discomfort, and diarrhea. These symptoms are due to irritation of the gastrointestinal tract and are best managed by diluting the preparation further, taking the dose with meals or reducing the amount taken at one time.

OVERDOSAGE

The administration of oral potassium salts to persons with normal excretory mechanisms for potassium rarely causes serious hyperkalemia. However, if excretory mechanisms are impaired or if potassium is administered too rapidly intravenously, potentially fatal hyperkalemia can result (see **CONTRAINDICATIONS** and **WARNINGS**). It is important to recognize that hyperkalemia is usually asymptomatic and may be manifested only by an increased serum potassium concentration (6.5-8.0 mEq/L) and characteristic electrocardiographic changes (peaking of T-waves, loss of P-waves, depression of S-T segment, and prolongation of the QT-interval). Late manifestations include muscle paralysis and cardiovascular collapse from cardiac arrest (9-12 mEq/L).
Treatment measures for hyperkalemia include the following:
1. Patients should be closely monitored for arrythmias and electrolyte changes.
2. Elimination of foods and medications containing potassium and of any agents with potassium-sparing properties such as potassium-sparing diuretics, ARBS, ACE inhibitors, NSAIDs, certain nutritional supplements and many others.
3. Intravenous calcium gluconate if the patient is at no risk or low risk of developing digitalis toxicity.
4. Intravenous administration of 300 to 500 mL/hr of 10% dextrose solution containing 10-20 units of crystalline insulin per 1,000 mL.
5. Correction of acidosis, if present, with intravenous sodium bicarbonate.
6. Use of exchange resins, hemodialysis, or peritoneal dialysis.
In treating hyperkalemia, it should be recalled that in patients who have been stabilized on digitalis, too rapid a lowering of the serum potassium concentration can produce digitalis toxicity.
The extended release feature means that absorption and toxic effects may be delayed for hours. Consider standard measures to remove any unabsorbed drug.

DOSAGE AND ADMINISTRATION

The usual dietary intake of potassium by the average adult is 50 to 100 mEq per day. Potassium depletion sufficient to cause hypokalemia usually requires the loss of 200 or more mEq of potassium from the total body store.
Dosage must be adjusted to the individual needs of each patient. The dose for the prevention of hypokalemia is typically in the range of 20 mEq per day. Doses of 40-100 mEq per day or more are used for the treatment of potassium depletion. Dosage should be divided if more than 20 mEq per day is given such that no more than 20 mEq is given in a single dose.
Each Klor-Con® M20 tablet provides 1500 mg of potassium chloride equivalent to 20 mEq of potassium.
Each Klor-Con® M15 tablet provides 1125 mg of potassium chloride equivalent to 15 mEq of potassium.
Each Klor-Con® M10 tablet provides 750 mg of potassium chloride equivalent to 10 mEq of potassium.
Klor-Con® M tablets should be taken with meals and with a glass of water or other liquid. This product should not be taken on an empty stomach because of its potential for gastric irritation (see **WARNINGS**).
Patients having difficulty swallowing whole tablets may try one of the following alternate methods of administration:
a. Break the tablet in half and take each half separately with a glass of water.
b. Prepare an aqueous (water) suspension as follows:
1. Place the whole tablet(s) in approximately one-half glass of water (4 fluid ounces).

2. Allow approximately 2 minutes for the tablet(s) to disintegrate.
3. Stir for about half a minute after the tablet(s) has disintegrated.
4. Swirl the suspension and consume the entire contents of the glass immediately by drinking or by the use of a straw.
5. Add another one fluid ounce of water, swirl, and consume immediately.
6. Then, add an additional one fluid ounce of water, swirl, and consume immediately.

Aqueous suspension of Klor-Con® M extended-release tablet that is not taken immediately should be discarded. The use of other liquids for suspending Klor-Con® M tablets is not recommended.

HOW SUPPLIED

Klor-Con® M20 Extended-release Tablets, 1500 mg of potassium chloride (20 mEq of potassium) are available in bottles of 90 (NDC 0245-0058-90); bottles of 100 (NDC 0245-0058-11); bottles of 500 (NDC 0245-0058-15); bottles of 1000 (NDC 0245-0058-10); and cartons of 100 for unit dose dispensing (NDC 0245-0058-01). Klor-Con® M20 tablets are white, oblong, imprinted KC M20 and scored for flexibility of dosing.
Klor-Con® M15 Extended-release Tablets, 1125 mg of potassium chloride (15 mEq of potassium) are available in bottles of 100 (NDC 0245-0150-11); bottles of 1000 (NDC 0245-0150-10); and cartons of 100 for unit dose dispensing (NDC 0245-0150-01). Klor-Con® M15 tablets are white, oblong, imprinted M 15 and scored for flexibility of dosing.
Klor-Con® M10 Extended-release Tablets, 750 mg of potassium chloride (10 mEq of potassium) are available in bottles of 90 (NDC 0245-0057-90); bottles of 100 (NDC 0245-0057-11); bottles of 1000 (NDC 0245-0057-10); and cartons of 100 for unit dose dispensing (NDC 0245-0057-01). Klor-Con® M10 tablets are white, oblong and imprinted KC M10.
Keep tightly closed. Store at 20-25°C (68-77°F). Excursions permitted to 15-30°C (59-86°F). [See USP Controlled Room Temperature.]
Manufactured by
UPSHER-SMITH LABORATORIES, INC.
Minneapolis, MN 55447
US Patent 6,780,437
Certain manufacturing operations have been performed by other firms.
© 2005 Upsher-Smith Laboratories, Inc.
All rights reserved
103148
Revised 1208

PRENEXA PREMIER   ℞
[pre-nex-a]
Capsules
Rx only

Rx Prenatal Vitamin with Plant-Based DHA
• 1.25 mg Folic Acid and 310 mg DHA (key omega-3 fatty acid)
• Essential vitamins and minerals
• Gentle stool softener

DESCRIPTION

PreNexa® premier capsules are a prescription prenatal/postnatal multivitamin/mineral softgel capsule with plant-based DHA. PreNexa® premier capsules are available as opaque brown, oblong capsules imprinted "0179" and are available in 30-count bottles (NDC 0245-0179-30).

Each softgel capsule contains:

Vitamin C (ascorbic acid, USP)	28 mg
Calcium (tribasic calcium phosphate, NF)	160 mg
Iron (ferrous fumarate, USP)	27 mg
Vitamin D_3 (cholecalciferol, USP)	800 IU
Vitamin E (d-alpha tocopherol, USP)	30 IU
Vitamin B_6 (pyridoxine hydrochloride, USP)	25 mg
Folic Acid, USP	1.25 mg
DHA (docosahexaenoic acid, contained in the oil derived from microalgae)	310 mg
Docusate Sodium, USP	55 mg

Inactive Ingredients: Ethyl vanillin, FD&C blue #1, FD&C red #40, FD&C yellow #6, gelatin, glycerin, lecithin, palm kernel oil, sodium benzoate, soybean oil, sunflower oil, titanium dioxide, yellow beeswax, water and white ink (ammonium hydroxide, isopropyl alcohol, n-butyl alcohol, propylene glycol, shellac glaze in SD-45 alcohol, simethicone, titanium dioxide).
Contains: Soy

INDICATIONS

PreNexa® premier capsules are indicated to provide vitamin/mineral and plant-based DHA supplementation throughout pregnancy, during the postnatal period for both lactating and non-lactating mothers, and throughout the childbearing years. PreNexa® premier may be useful in improving the nutritional status of women prior to conception.

CONTRAINDICATIONS

PreNexa® premier capsules are contraindicated in patients with a known hypersensitivity to any of the ingredients. Do not take this product if you are presently taking mineral oil, unless directed by a doctor.

> **WARNING**
> Accidental overdose of iron-containing products is a leading cause of fatal poisoning in children under 6. KEEP THIS PRODUCT OUT OF THE REACH OF CHILDREN. In case of accidental overdose, call a doctor or poison control center immediately.

WARNING

Ingestion of more than 3 grams of omega-3 fatty acids (such as DHA) per day has been shown to have potential antithrombotic effects, including an increased bleeding time and International Normalized Ratio (INR). Administration of omega-3 fatty acids should be avoided in patients taking anticoagulants and in those known to have an inherited or acquired predisposition to bleeding.

PRECAUTION

Folic acid alone is improper therapy in the treatment of pernicious anemia and other megaloblastic anemias where vitamin B_{12} is deficient. Folic acid in doses above 1 mg daily may obscure pernicious anemia in that hematologic remission can occur while neurological manifestations progress.

ADVERSE REACTIONS

Allergic sensitization has been reported following both oral and parenteral administration of folic acid.
CAUTION
Exercise caution to ensure that the prescribed dosage of DHA does not exceed 1 gram (1000 mg) per day.

DOSAGE AND ADMINISTRATION

Before, during and/or after pregnancy, one softgel capsule daily or as directed by a physician.

HOW SUPPLIED

PreNexa® premier capsules are available as opaque brown, oblong capsules imprinted "0179" and are available in 30-count bottles (NDC 0245-0179-30).
KEEP THIS AND ALL DRUGS OUT OF REACH OF CHILDREN.
You may report side effects to FDA at 1-800-FDA-1088. You may also report side effects to Upsher-Smith Laboratories at 1-888-650-3789.
Store at 20-25°C (68-77°F). [See USP Controlled Room Temperature.]
Distributed by:
UPSHER-SMITH LABORATORIES, INC.
Minneapolis, MN 55447
MADE IN CANADA
1-800-654-2299   www.upsher-smith.com
US Patents 5,407,957; 5,492,938; 6,410,281; 7,163,811.
Other US Patents Pending.
PreNexa® premier capsules
Revised 0710
Shown in Product Identification Guide, page 321

ViiV Healthcare Company
FIVE MOORE DRIVE
RESEARCH TRIANGLE PARK, NC 27709

Direct Inquiries
1-877-ViiVUSA (1-877-844-8872)

COMBIVIR®   ℞
[kom' bə-vir]
(lamivudine and zidovudine)
Tablets 150 mg/300 mg

HIGHLIGHTS OF PRESCRIBING INFORMATION
These highlights do not include all the information needed to use COMBIVIR safely and effectively. See full prescribing information for COMBIVIR.
COMBIVIR (lamivudine and zidovudine) Tablets 150 mg/ 300 mg
Initial U.S. Approval: 1997

> **WARNING: RISK OF HEMATOLOGIC TOXICITY, MYOPATHY, LACTIC ACIDOSIS, EXACERBATIONS OF**

HEPATITIS B
See full prescribing information for complete boxed warning
• Hematologic toxicity including neutropenia and anemia have been associated with the use of zidovudine, one of the components of COMBIVIR (5.1)
• Symptomatic myopathy associated with prolonged use of zidovudine. (5.2)
• Lactic acidosis and hepatomegaly with steatosis, including fatal cases, have been reported with the use of nucleoside analogues including zidovudine. Suspend treatment if clinical or laboratory findings suggestive of lactic acidosis or pronounced hepatotoxicity occur. (5.3)
• Acute exacerbations of hepatitis B have been reported in patients who are co-infected with hepatitis B virus (HBV) and human immunodeficiency virus (HIV-1) and have discontinued lamivudine, a component of COMBIVIR. Monitor hepatic function closely in these patients and, if appropriate, initiate anti-hepatitis B treatment. (5.4)

——INDICATIONS AND USAGE——
COMBIVIR, a combination of two nucleoside analogue reverse transcriptase inhibitors, is indicated in combination with other antiretroviral agents for the treatment of HIV-1 infection. (1)

——DOSAGE AND ADMINISTRATION——
• Adults and Adolescents weighing ≥30 kg: 1 tablet twice daily. (2.1)
• Pediatrics: Dosage should be based on body weight not to exceed adult doses. (2.2)
• COMBIVIR, a fixed-dose product, should not be prescribed for pediatric patients weighing less than 30 kg or patients requiring dosage adjustment, such as those with renal or hepatic impairment, or patients experiencing dose-limiting adverse reactions. (2.3)

——DOSAGE FORMS AND STRENGTHS——
Tablets: Scored 150 mg lamivudine and 300 mg zidovudine (3)

——CONTRAINDICATIONS——
COMBIVIR Tablets are contraindicated in patients with previously demonstrated clinically significant hypersensitivity (e.g., anaphylaxis, Stevens-Johnson syndrome). (4)

——WARNINGS AND PRECAUTIONS——
• Hematologic toxicity/bone marrow suppression including neutropenia and anemia have been associated with the use of zidovudine, one of the components of COMBIVIR. (5.1)
• Symptomatic myopathy associated with prolonged use of zidovudine. (5.2)
• Lactic acidosis and hepatomegaly with steatosis, including fatal cases, have been reported with the use of nucleoside analogues including zidovudine. Suspend treatment if clinical or laboratory findings suggestive of lactic acidosis or pronounced hepatotoxicity occur. (5.3)
• Acute exacerbations of hepatitis B have been reported in patients who are co-infected with hepatitis B virus (HBV) and human immunodeficiency virus (HIV-1) and have discontinued lamivudine, a component of COMBIVIR. Monitor hepatic function closely in these patients and, if appropriate, initiate anti-hepatitis B treatment. (5.4)
• COMBIVIR should not be administered with other lamivudine- or zidovudine-containing products or emtricitabine-containing products. (5.5)
• Hepatic decompensation, some fatal, has occurred in HIV-1/HCV co-infected patients receiving combination antiretroviral therapy and interferon alfa with/without ribavirin. Discontinue COMBIVIR as medically appropriate and consider dose reduction or discontinuation of interferon alfa, ribavirin, or both. (5.6)
• Exacerbation of anemia has been reported in HIV-1/HCV co-infected patients receiving ribavirin and zidovudine. Co-administration of ribavirin and zidovudine is not advised. (5.6)
• Pancreatitis: Use with caution in pediatric patients with a history of pancreatitis or other significant risk factors for pancreatitis. Discontinue treatment as clinically appropriate. (5.7)
• Immune reconstitution syndrome (5.8) and redistribution/accumulation of body fat (5.9) have been reported in patients treated with combination antiretroviral therapy.

——ADVERSE REACTIONS——
• Most commonly reported adverse reactions (incidence greater than or equal to 15%) in adult and pediatric HIV-1 clinical studies of combination lamivudine and zidovudine were headache, nausea, malaise and fatigue, nasal signs and symptoms, diarrhea, and cough. (6.1)

To report SUSPECTED ADVERSE REACTIONS, contact GlaxoSmithKline at 1-888-825-5249 or FDA at 1-800-FDA-1088 or www.fda.gov/medwatch

DRUG INTERACTIONS

- Concomitant use with the following drugs should be avoided: stavudine (7.1), zalcitabine (7.1), doxorubicin (7.2).
- Bone marrow suppressive/cytotoxic agents: May increase the hematologic toxicity of zidovudine. (7.3)

USE IN SPECIFIC POPULATIONS

- Pregnancy: Physicians are encouraged to register patients in the Antiretroviral Pregnancy Registry by calling 1-800-258-4263. (8.1)
- Nursing Mothers: HIV-1 infected mothers in the United States should not breastfeed to avoid potential postnatal transmission of HIV-1. (8.3)

See 17 for PATIENT COUNSELING INFORMATION
Revised: 08/2010

FULL PRESCRIBING INFORMATION: CONTENTS*

WARNING: HEMATOLOGIC TOXICITY, MYOPATHY, LACTIC ACIDOSIS, EXACERBATIONS OF HEPATITIS B

FULL PRESCRIBING INFORMATION

> **WARNING: HEMATOLOGIC TOXICITY, MYOPATHY, LACTIC ACIDOSIS, EXACERBATIONS OF HEPATITIS B**
> Zidovudine, one of the 2 active ingredients in COMBIVIR® (lamivudine and zidovudine) Tablets, has been associated with hematologic toxicity including neutropenia and anemia, particularly in patients with advanced HIV-1 disease *[see Warnings and Precautions (5.1)].*
> Prolonged use of zidovudine has been associated with symptomatic myopathy *[see Warnings and Precautions (5.2)].*
> Lactic acidosis and hepatomegaly with steatosis, including fatal cases, have been reported with the use of nucleoside analogues alone or in combination, includ-

ing lamivudine, zidovudine, and other antiretrovirals. Suspend treatment if clinical or laboratory findings suggestive of lactic acidosis or pronounced hepatotoxicity occur *[see Warnings and Precautions (5.3)].*
> Acute exacerbations of hepatitis B have been reported in patients who are co-infected with hepatitis B virus (HBV) and HIV-1 and have discontinued lamivudine, which is one component of COMBIVIR. Hepatic function should be monitored closely with both clinical and laboratory follow-up for at least several months in patients who discontinue COMBIVIR and are co-infected with HIV-1 and HBV. If appropriate, initiation of anti-hepatitis B therapy may be warranted *[see Warnings and Precautions (5.4)].*

1 INDICATIONS AND USAGE

COMBIVIR, a combination of two nucleoside analogues, is indicated in combination with other antiretrovirals for the treatment of HIV-1 infection.

2 DOSAGE AND ADMINISTRATION

2.1 Adults and Adolescents Weighing ≥30 kg

The recommended oral dose of COMBIVIR in HIV-1-infected adults and adolescents weighing greater than or equal to 30 kg is 1 tablet (containing 150 mg of lamivudine and 300 mg of zidovudine) twice daily.

2.2 Pediatric Patients

The recommended oral dosage of scored COMBIVIR Tablets for pediatric patients who weigh greater than or equal to 30 kg and for whom a solid oral dosage form is appropriate is 1 tablet administered twice daily.

Before prescribing COMBIVIR Tablets, children should be assessed for the ability to swallow tablets. If a child is unable to reliably swallow a COMBIVIR tablet, the liquid oral formulations should be prescribed: EPIVIR® (lamivudine) Oral Solution and RETROVIR® (zidovudine) Syrup.

2.3 Patients Requiring Dosage Adjustment

Because COMBIVIR is a fixed-dose combination tablet, it should not be prescribed for pediatric patients weighing less than 30 kg or patients requiring dosage adjustment, such as those with reduced renal function (creatinine clearance less than 50 mL/min), patients with hepatic impairment, or patients experiencing dose-limiting adverse reactions. Liquid and solid oral formulations of the individual components of COMBIVIR are available for these populations.

3 DOSAGE FORMS AND STRENGTHS

COMBIVIR Tablets are white, scored, film-coated, modified capsule-shaped tablets, debossed on both tablet faces, such that when broken in half, the full "GX FC3" code is present on both halves of the tablet ("GX" on one face and "FC3" on the opposite face of the tablet).

4 CONTRAINDICATIONS

COMBIVIR Tablets are contraindicated in patients with previously demonstrated clinically significant hypersensitivity (e.g., anaphylaxis, Stevens-Johnson syndrome) to any of the components of the product.

5 WARNINGS AND PRECAUTIONS

5.1 Hemotologic Toxicity/Bone Marrow Suppression

Zidovudine, a component of COMBIVIR, has been associated with hematologic toxicity including neutropenia and anemia, particularly in patients with advanced HIV-1 disease. COMBIVIR should be used with caution in patients who have bone marrow compromise evidenced by granulocyte count less than 1,000 cells/mm^3 or hemoglobin less than 9.5 g/dL *[see Adverse Reactions (6.1)].*

Frequent blood counts are strongly recommended in patients with advanced HIV-1 disease who are treated with COMBIVIR. Periodic blood counts are recommended for other HIV-1-infected patients. If anemia or neutropenia develops, dosage interruption may be needed.

5.2 Myopathy

Myopathy and myositis, with pathological changes similar to that produced by HIV-1 disease, have been associated with prolonged use of zidovudine, and therefore may occur with therapy with COMBIVIR.

5.3 Lactic Acidosis/Hepatomegaly With Steatosis

Lactic acidosis and hepatomegaly with steatosis, including fatal cases, have been reported with the use of nucleoside analogues alone or in combination, including lamivudine, zidovudine, and other antiretrovirals. A majority of these cases have been in women. Obesity and prolonged nucleoside exposure may be risk factors. Particular caution should be exercised when administering COMBIVIR to any patient with known risk factors for liver disease; however, cases have also been reported in patients with no known risk factors. Treatment with COMBIVIR should be suspended in any patient who develops clinical or laboratory findings suggestive of lactic acidosis or pronounced hepatotoxicity (which may include hepatomegaly and steatosis even in the absence of marked transaminase elevations).

5.4 Patients With HIV-1 and Hepatitis B Virus Co-infection

Posttreatment Exacerbations of Hepatitis: In clinical trials in non-HIV-1-infected patients treated with lamivudine for chronic HBV, clinical and laboratory evidence of exacerbations of hepatitis have occurred after discontinuation of lamivudine. These exacerbations have been detected primarily by serum ALT elevations in addition to re-emergence of hepatitis B viral DNA (HBV DNA). Although most events appear to have been self-limited, fatalities have been reported in some cases. Similar events have been reported from post-marketing experience after changes from lamivudine-containing HIV-1 treatment regimens to non-lamivudine-containing regimens in patients infected with both HIV-1 and HBV. The causal relationship to discontinuation of lamivudine treatment is unknown. Patients should be closely monitored with both clinical and laboratory follow-up for at least several months after stopping treatment. There is insufficient evidence to determine whether re-initiation of lamivudine alters the course of posttreatment exacerbations of hepatitis.

Important Differences Among Lamivudine-Containing Products: COMBIVIR Tablets contain a higher dose of the same active ingredient (lamivudine) than EPIVIR-HBV® (lamivudine) Tablets and Oral Solution. EPIVIR-HBV was developed for treating chronic hepatitis B. Safety and efficacy of lamivudine have not been established for treatment of chronic hepatitis B in patients co-infected with HIV-1 and HBV.

Emergence of Lamivudine-Resistant HBV: In non-HIV-infected patients treated with lamivudine for chronic hepatitis B, emergence of lamivudine-resistant HBV has been detected and has been associated with diminished treatment response (see full prescribing information for EPIVIR-HBV for additional information). Emergence of hepatitis B virus variants associated with resistance to lamivudine has also been reported in HIV-1-infected patients who have received lamivudine-containing antiretroviral regimens in the presence of concurrent infection with hepatitis B virus.

5.5 Use With Other, Lamivudine-, Zidovudine-, and/or Emtricitabine-Containing Products

COMBIVIR is a fixed-dose combination of lamivudine and zidovudine. COMBIVIR should not be administered concomitantly with other lamivudine- or zidovudine-containing products including EPIVIR® (lamivudine) Tablets and Oral Solution, EPIVIR-HBV Tablets and Oral Solution, RETROVIR® (zidovudine) Tablets, Capsules, Syrup, and IV Infusion, EPZICOM® (abacavir sulfate and lamivudine) Tablets, or TRIZIVIR® (abacavir sulfate, lamivudine, and zidovudine) Tablets; or emtricitabine-containing products, including ATRIPLA® (efavirenz, emtricitabine, and tenofovir), EMTRIVA® (emtricitabine), or TRUVADA® (emtricitabine and tenofovir).

5.6 Use With Interferon- and Ribavirin-Based Regimens

In vitro studies have shown ribavirin can reduce the phosphorylation of pyrimidine nucleoside analogues such as lamivudine and zidovudine. Although no evidence of a pharmacokinetic or pharmacodynamic interaction (e.g., loss of HIV-1/HCV virologic suppression) was seen when ribavirin was coadministered with lamivudine or zidovudine in HIV-1/HCV co-infected patients *[see Clinical Pharmacology (12.3)]*, hepatic decompensation (some fatal) has occurred in HIV-1/HCV co-infected patients receiving combination antiretroviral therapy for HIV-1 and interferon alfa with or without ribavirin. Patients receiving interferon alfa with or without ribavirin and COMBIVIR should be closely monitored for treatment-associated toxicities, especially hepatic decompensation, neutropenia, and anemia. Discontinuation of COMBIVIR should be considered as medically appropriate. Dose reduction or discontinuation of interferon alfa, ribavirin, or both should also be considered if worsening clinical toxicities are observed, including hepatic decompensation (e.g., Child-Pugh greater than 6) (see the complete prescribing information for interferon and ribavirin). Exacerbation of anemia has been reported in HIV-1/HCV co-infected patients receiving ribavirin and zidovudine. Co-administration of ribavirin and zidovudine is not advised.

5.7 Pancreatitis

COMBIVIR should be used with caution in patients with a history of pancreatitis or other significant risk factors for the development of pancreatitis. Treatment with COMBIVIR should be stopped immediately if clinical signs, symptoms, or laboratory abnormalities suggestive of pancreatitis occur *[see Adverse Reactions (6.1)].*

5.8 Immune Reconstitution Syndrome

Immune reconstitution syndrome has been reported in patients treated with combination antiretroviral therapy, including COMBIVIR. During the initial phase of combination antiretroviral treatment, patients whose immune systems respond may develop an inflammatory response to indolent or residual opportunistic infections (such as *Mycobacterium avium* infection, cytomegalovirus, *Pneumocystis jirovecii* pneumonia [PCP], or tuberculosis), which may necessitate further evaluation and treatment.

5.9 Fat Redistribution

Redistribution/accumulation of body fat including central obesity, dorsocervical fat enlargement (buffalo hump), peripheral wasting, facial wasting, breast enlargement, and "cushingoid appearance" have been observed in patients receiving antiretroviral therapy. The mechanism and long-term consequences of these events are currently unknown. A causal relationship has not been established.

6   ADVERSE REACTIONS

The following adverse reactions are discussed in greater detail in other sections of the labeling.
* Hematologic toxicity, including neutropenia and anemia [see Boxed Warning, Warnings and Precautions (5.1)].
* Symptomatic myopathy [see Boxed Warning, Warnings and Precautions (5.2)].
* Lactic acidosis and hepatomegaly with steatosis [see Boxed Warning, Warnings and Precautions (5.3)].
* Acute exacerbations of hepatitis B [see Boxed Warning, Warnings and Precautions (5.4)].
* Hepatic decompensation in patients co-infected with HIV-1 and hepatitis C [see Warnings and Precautions (5.6)].
* Exacerbation of anemia in HIV-1/HCV co-infected patients receiving ribavirin and zidovudine [see Warnings and Precautions (5.6)].
* Pancreatitis [see Warnings and Precautions (5.7)].

6.1   Clinical Trials Experience

Because clinical trials are conducted under widely varying conditions, adverse reaction rates observed in the clinical trials of a drug cannot be directly compared to rates in the clinical trials of another drug and may not reflect the rates observed in practice.

Lamivudine Plus Zidovudine Administered As Separate Formulations: In 4 randomized, controlled trials of EPIVIR 300 mg per day plus RETROVIR 600 mg per day, the following selected adverse reactions and laboratory abnormalities were observed (see Tables 1 and 2).

Table 1. Selected Clinical Adverse Reactions (≥5% Frequency) in 4 Controlled Clinical Trials With EPIVIR 300 mg/day and RETROVIR 600 mg/day

Adverse Reaction	EPIVIR plus RETROVIR (n = 251)
Body as a whole	
Headache	35%
Malaise & fatigue	27%
Fever or chills	10%
Digestive	
Nausea	33%
Diarrhea	18%
Nausea & vomiting	13%
Anorexia and/or decreased appetite	10%
Abdominal pain	9%
Abdominal cramps	6%
Dyspepsia	5%
Nervous system	
Neuropathy	12%
Insomnia & other sleep disorders	11%
Dizziness	10%
Depressive disorders	9%
Respiratory	
Nasal signs & symptoms	20%
Cough	18%
Skin	
Skin rashes	9%
Musculoskeletal	
Musculoskeletal pain	12%
Myalgia	8%
Arthralgia	5%

Pancreatitis was observed in 9 of the 2,613 adult patients (0.3%) who received EPIVIR in controlled clinical trials [see Warnings and Precautions (5.7)].

Selected laboratory abnormalities observed during therapy are listed in Table 2.

Table 2. Frequencies of Selected Laboratory Abnormalities Among Adults in 4 Controlled Clinical Trials of EPIVIR 300 mg/day plus RETROVIR 600 mg/day[a]

Test (Abnormal Level)	EPIVIR plus RETROVIR % (n)
Neutropenia (ANC <750/mm³)	7.2% (237)
Anemia (Hgb<8.0 g/dL)	2.9% (241)
Thrombocytopenia (platelets<50,000/mm³)	0.4% (240)
ALT (>5.0 × ULN)	3.7% (241)
AST (>5.0 × ULN)	1.7% (241)
Bilirubin (>2.5 × ULN)	0.8% (241)
Amylase (>2.0 × ULN)	4.2% (72)

ULN = Upper limit of normal.
ANC = Absolute neutrophil count.
n = Number of patients assessed.
[a] Frequencies of these laboratory abnormalities were higher in patients with mild laboratory abnormalities at baseline.

6.2   Postmarketing Experience

In addition to adverse reactions reported from clinical trials, the following reactions have been identified during post-approval use of EPIVIR, RETROVIR, and/or COMBIVIR. Because they are reported voluntarily from a population of unknown size, estimates of frequency cannot be made. These events have been chosen for inclusion due to a combination of their seriousness, frequency of reporting, or potential causal connection to EPIVIR, RETROVIR, and/or COMBIVIR.

Body as a Whole: Redistribution/accumulation of body fat [see Warnings and Precautions (5.9)].
Cardiovascular: Cardiomyopathy.
Endocrine and Metabolic: Gynecomastia, hyperglycemia.
Gastrointestinal: Oral mucosal pigmentation, stomatitis.
General: Vasculitis, weakness.
Hemic and Lymphatic: Anemia, (including pure red cell aplasia and anemias progressing on therapy), lymphadenopathy, splenomegaly.
Hepatic and Pancreatic: Lactic acidosis and hepatic steatosis, pancreatitis, posttreatment exacerbation of hepatitis B [see Boxed Warning, Warnings and Precautions (5.3), (5.4), (5.7)].
Hypersensitivity: Sensitization reactions (including anaphylaxis), urticaria.
Musculoskeletal: Muscle weakness, CPK elevation, rhabdomyolysis.
Nervous: Paresthesia, peripheral neuropathy, seizures.
Respiratory: Abnormal breath sounds/wheezing.
Skin: Alopecia, erythema multiforme, Stevens-Johnson syndrome.

7   DRUG INTERACTIONS

No drug interaction studies have been conducted using COMBIVIR Tablets [see Clinical Pharmacology (12.3)].

7.1   Antiretroviral Agents

Lamivudine: Zalcitabine: Lamivudine and zalcitabine may inhibit the intracellular phosphorylation of one another. Therefore, use of COMBIVIR in combination with zalcitabine is not recommended.
Zidovudine: Stavudine: Concomitant use of COMBIVIR with stavudine should be avoided since an antagonistic relationship with zidovudine has been demonstrated in vitro.
Nucleoside Analogues Affecting DNA Replication: Some nucleoside analogues affecting DNA replication, such as ribavirin, antagonize the in vitro antiviral activity of zidovudine against HIV-1; concomitant use of such drugs should be avoided.

7.2   Doxorubicin

Zidovudine: Concomitant use of COMBIVIR with doxorubicin should be avoided since an antagonistic relationship with zidovudine has been demonstrated in vitro.

7.3   Hematologic/Bone Marrow Suppressive/Cytotoxic Agents

Zidovudine: Coadministration of ganciclovir, interferon alfa, ribavirin, and other bone marrow suppressive or cytotoxic agents may increase the hematologic toxicity of zidovudine.

7.4   Interferon- and Ribavirin-Based Regimens

Lamivudine: Although no evidence of a pharmacokinetic or pharmacodynamic interaction (e.g., loss of HIV-1/HCV virologic suppression) was seen when ribavirin was coadministered with lamivudine in HIV-1/HCV co-infected patients, hepatic decompensation (some fatal) has occurred in HIV-1/HCV co-infected patients receiving combination antiretroviral therapy for HIV-1 and interferon alfa with or without ribavirin [see Warnings and Precautions (5.5), Clinical Pharmacology (12.3)].

7.5   Trimethoprim/Sulfamethoxazole (TMP/SMX)

Lamivudine: No change in dose of either drug is recommended. There is no information regarding the effect on lamivudine pharmacokinetics of higher doses of TMP/SMX such as those used to treat PCP.

8   USE IN SPECIFIC POPULATIONS

8.1   Pregnancy

Pregnancy Category C.
Fetal Risk Summary: There are no adequate and well-controlled studies of COMBIVIR (lamivudine and zidovudine) in pregnant women. Clinical trial data demonstrate that maternal zidovudine treatment during pregnancy reduces vertical transmission of HIV-1 infection to the fetus. Animal reproduction studies performed with lamivudine and zidovudine showed increased embryotoxicity and fetal malformations (zidovudine), and increased embryolethality (lamivudine). COMBIVIR should be used during pregnancy only if the potential benefit justifies the potential risk to the fetus.

Antiretroviral Pregnancy Registry: To monitor maternal-fetal outcomes of pregnant women exposed to COMBIVIR and other antiretroviral agents, an Antiretroviral Pregnancy Registry has been established. Physicians are encouraged to register patients by calling 1-800-258-4263.

Clinical Considerations: Treatment of HIV during pregnancy optimizes the health of both mother and fetus. Clinical trial data reviewed by FDA demonstrate that maternal zidovudine treatment significantly reduces vertical transmission of HIV-1 infection to the fetus [see Clinical Studies (14.2)]. Published data suggest that combination antiretroviral regimens may reduce the rate of vertical transmission even further.

Pharmacokinetics of lamivudine and zidovudine in pregnant women are similar to the pharmacokinetics in nonpregnant women. No dose adjustments are needed during pregnancy.

In a clinical trial, adverse events among HIV-1-infected women were not different among untreated women and women treated with zidovudine. It is not known whether risks of adverse events associated with lamivudine are altered in pregnant women compared with other HIV-1-infected patients (see Human data below).

Data: Human Data: Lamivudine: Lamivudine pharmacokinetics were studied in pregnant women during 2 clinical studies conducted in South Africa. The study assessed pharmacokinetics in: 16 women at 36 weeks gestation using 150 mg lamivudine twice daily with zidovudine, 10 women at 38 weeks gestation using 150 mg lamivudine twice daily with zidovudine, and 10 women at 38 weeks gestation using lamivudine 300 mg twice daily without other antiretrovirals. Lamivudine pharmacokinetics in pregnant women were similar to those seen in nonpregnant adults and in postpartum women. Lamivudine concentrations were generally similar in maternal, neonatal, and umbilical cord serum samples.

Zidovudine: A randomized, double-blind, placebo-controlled trial was conducted in HIV-1-infected pregnant women to determine the utility of zidovudine for the prevention of maternal-fetal HIV-1 transmission. Zidovudine treatment during pregnancy reduced the rate of maternal-fetal HIV-1 transmission from 24.9% for infants born to placebo-treated mothers to 7.8% for infants born to mothers treated with zidovudine. There were no differences in pregnancy-related adverse events between the treatment groups. Congenital abnormalities occurred with similar frequency between neonates born to mothers who received zidovudine and neonates born to mothers who received placebo. The observed abnormalities included problems in embryogenesis (prior to 14 weeks) or were recognized on ultrasound before or immediately after initiation of study drug [see Clinical Studies (14.2)].

Zidovudine pharmacokinetics were studied in a Phase 1 study of 8 women during the last trimester of pregnancy. As pregnancy progressed, there was no evidence of drug accumulation. The pharmacokinetics of zidovudine were similar to that of nonpregnant adults. Consistent with passive transmission of the drug across the placenta, zidovudine concentrations in neonatal plasma at birth were essentially equal to those in maternal plasma at delivery.

Animal Data: Lamivudine: Animal reproduction studies performed at oral doses up to 130 and 60 times the adult dose in rats and rabbits, respectively, revealed no evidence of teratogenicity due to lamivudine. Increased early embryolethality occurred in rabbits at exposure levels similar to those in humans. However, there was no indication of this effect in rats at exposure levels up to 35 times those in humans. Based on animal studies, lamivudine crosses the placenta and is transferred to the fetus *[see Nonclinical Toxicology (13.2)]*.

Zidovudine: Increased fetal resorptions occurred in pregnant rats and rabbits treated with doses of zidovudine that produced drug plasma concentrations 66 to 226 times (rats) and 12 to 87 times (rabbits) the mean steady-state peak human plasma concentration following a single 100-mg dose of zidovudine. There were no other reported developmental anomalies. In another developmental toxicity study, pregnant rats received zidovudine up to near-lethal doses that produced peak plasma concentrations 350 times peak human plasma concentrations (300 times the daily exposure [AUC] in humans given 600 mg/day zidovudine). This dose was associated with marked maternal toxicity and an increased incidence of fetal malformations. However, there were no signs of teratogenicity at doses up to one fifth the lethal dose *[see Nonclinical Toxicology (13.2)]*.

8.3 Nursing Mothers

The Centers for Disease Control and Prevention recommend that HIV-1-infected mothers in the United States not breastfeed their infants to avoid risking postnatal transmission of HIV-1 infection. Because of both the potential for HIV-1 transmission and serious adverse reactions in nursing infants, mothers should be instructed not to breastfeed if they are receiving COMBIVIR.

Although no studies of COMBIVIR excretion in breast milk have been performed, lactation studies performed with lamivudine and zidovudine show that both drugs are excreted in human breast milk. Samples of breast milk obtained from 20 mothers receiving lamivudine monotherapy (300 mg twice daily) or combination therapy (150 mg lamivudine twice daily and 300 mg zidovudine twice daily) had measurable concentrations of lamivudine. In another study, after administration of a single dose of 200 mg zidovudine to 13 HIV-1-infected women, the mean concentration of zidovudine was similar in human milk and serum.

8.4 Pediatric Use

COMBIVIR should not be administered to pediatric patients weighing less than 30 kg, because it is a fixed-dose combination that cannot be adjusted for this patient population.

8.5 Geriatric Use

Clinical studies of COMBIVIR did not include sufficient numbers of subjects aged 65 and over to determine whether they respond differently from younger subjects. In general, dose selection for an elderly patient should be cautious, reflecting the greater frequency of decreased hepatic, renal, or cardiac function, and of concomitant disease or other drug therapy. COMBIVIR is not recommended for patients with impaired renal function (i.e., creatinine clearance less than 50 mL/min) because it is a fixed-dose combination that cannot be adjusted.

8.6 Renal Impairment

Reduction of the dosages of lamivudine and zidovudine is recommended for patients with impaired renal function. Patients with creatinine clearance less than 50 mL/min should not receive COMBIVIR because it is a fixed-dose combination that cannot be adjusted.

8.7 Hepatic Impairment

A reduction in the daily dose of zidovudine may be necessary in patients with mild to moderate impaired hepatic function or liver cirrhosis. COMBIVIR is not recommended for patients with impaired hepatic function because it is a fixed-dose combination that cannot be adjusted.

10 OVERDOSAGE

COMBIVIR: There is no known antidote for COMBIVIR.

Lamivudine: One case of an adult ingesting 6 grams of lamivudine was reported; there were no clinical signs or symptoms noted and hematologic tests remained normal. Because a negligible amount of lamivudine was removed via (4-hour) hemodialysis, continuous ambulatory peritoneal dialysis, and automated peritoneal dialysis, it is not known if continuous hemodialysis would provide clinical benefit in a lamivudine overdose event.

Zidovudine: Acute overdoses of zidovudine have been reported in pediatric patients and adults. These involved exposures up to 50 grams. The only consistent findings were nausea and vomiting. Other reported occurrences included headache, dizziness, drowsiness, lethargy, confusion, and 1 report of a grand mal seizure. Hematologic changes were transient. All patients recovered. Hemodialysis and peritoneal dialysis appear to have a negligible effect on the removal of zidovudine, while elimination of its primary metabolite, 3′-azido-3′-deoxy-5′-*O*-β-*D*-glucopyranuronosylthymidine (GZDV), is enhanced.

11 DESCRIPTION

COMBIVIR: COMBIVIR Tablets are combination tablets containing lamivudine and zidovudine. Lamivudine (EPIVIR) and zidovudine (RETROVIR, azidothymidine, AZT, or ZDV) are synthetic nucleoside analogues with activity against HIV-1.

COMBIVIR Tablets are for oral administration. Each film-coated tablet contains 150 mg of lamivudine, 300 mg of zidovudine, and the inactive ingredients colloidal silicon dioxide, hypromellose, magnesium stearate, microcrystalline cellulose, polyethylene glycol, polysorbate 80, sodium starch glycolate, and titanium dioxide.

Lamivudine: The chemical name of lamivudine is (2R, cis)-4-amino-1-(2-hydroxymethyl-1,3-oxathiolan-5-yl)-(1H)-pyrimidin-2-one. Lamivudine is the (-)enantiomer of a dideoxy analogue of cytidine. Lamivudine has also been referred to as (-)2′,3′-dideoxy, 3′-thiacytidine. It has a molecular formula of $C_8H_{11}N_3O_3S$ and a molecular weight of 229.3. It has the following structural formula:

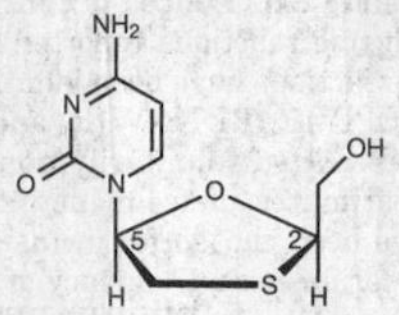

Lamivudine is a white to off-white crystalline solid with a solubility of approximately 70 mg/mL in water at 20°C.

Zidovudine: The chemical name of zidovudine is 3′-azido-3′-deoxythymidine. It has a molecular formula of $C_{10}H_{13}N_5O_4$ and a molecular weight of 267.24. It has the following structural formula:

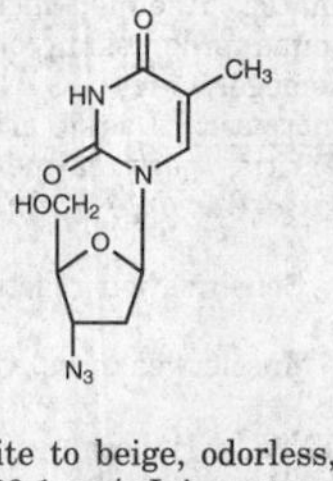

Zidovudine is a white to beige, odorless, crystalline solid with a solubility of 20.1 mg/mL in water at 25°C.

12 CLINICAL PHARMACOLOGY

12.1 Mechanism of Action

COMBIVIR is an antiviral agent *[see Clinical Pharmacology (12.4)]*.

Table 3. Pharmacokinetic Parameters[a] for Lamivudine and Zidovudine in Adults

Parameter	Lamivudine		Zidovudine	
Oral bioavailability (%)	86 ± 16	N = 12	64 ± 10	n = 5
Apparent volume of distribution (L/kg)	1.3 ± 0.4	N = 20	1.6 ± 0.6	n = 8
Plasma protein binding (%)	<36		<38	
CSF:plasma ratio[b]	0.12 [0.04 to 0.47]	n = 38[c]	0.60 [0.04 to 2.62]	N = 39[d]
Systemic clearance (L/hr/kg)	0.33 ± 0.06	N = 20	1.6 ± 0.6	n = 6
Renal clearance (L/hr/kg)	0.22 ± 0.06	N = 20	0.34 ± 0.05	n = 9
Elimination half-life (hr)[e]	5 to 7		0.5 to 3	

[a] Data presented as mean ± standard deviation except where noted.
[b] Median [range].
[c] Children.
[d] Adults.
[e] Approximate range.

12.3 Pharmacokinetics

Pharmacokinetics in Adults: *COMBIVIR:* One COMBIVIR Tablet was bioequivalent to 1 EPIVIR Tablet (150 mg) plus 1 RETROVIR Tablet (300 mg) following single-dose administration to fasting healthy subjects (n = 24).

Lamivudine: The pharmacokinetic properties of lamivudine in fasting patients are summarized in Table 3. Following oral administration, lamivudine is rapidly absorbed and extensively distributed. Binding to plasma protein is low. Approximately 70% of an intravenous dose of lamivudine is recovered as unchanged drug in the urine. Metabolism of lamivudine is a minor route of elimination. In humans, the only known metabolite is the trans-sulfoxide metabolite (approximately 5% of an oral dose after 12 hours).

Zidovudine: The pharmacokinetic properties of zidovudine in fasting patients are summarized in Table 3. Following oral administration, zidovudine is rapidly absorbed and extensively distributed. Binding to plasma protein is low. Zidovudine is eliminated primarily by hepatic metabolism. The major metabolite of zidovudine is GZDV. GZDV area under the curve (AUC) is about 3-fold greater than the zidovudine AUC. Urinary recovery of zidovudine and GZDV accounts for 14% and 74% of the dose following oral administration, respectively. A second metabolite, 3′-amino-3′-deoxythymidine (AMT), has been identified in plasma. The AMT AUC was one fifth of the zidovudine AUC.

[See table 3 below]

Effect of Food on Absorption of COMBIVIR: COMBIVIR may be administered with or without food. The lamivudine and zidovudine AUC following administration of COMBIVIR with food was similar when compared to fasting healthy subjects (n = 24).

Special Populations:

Pregnancy: See Use in Specific Populations (8.1).

COMBIVIR: No data are available.

Zidovudine: Zidovudine pharmacokinetics has been studied in a Phase 1 study of 8 women during the last trimester of pregnancy. As pregnancy progressed, there was no evidence of drug accumulation. The pharmacokinetics of zidovudine was similar to that of nonpregnant adults. Consistent with passive transmission of the drug across the placenta, zidovudine concentrations in neonatal plasma at birth were essentially equal to those in maternal plasma at delivery. Although data are limited, methadone maintenance therapy in 5 pregnant women did not appear to alter zidovudine pharmacokinetics. In a nonpregnant adult population, a potential for interaction has been identified.

Nursing Mothers: See Use in Specific Populations (8.3).

Pediatric Patients: COMBIVIR should not be administered to pediatric patients weighing less than 30 kg.

Geriatric Patients: The pharmacokinetics of lamivudine and zidovudine have not been studied in patients over 65 years of age.

Gender: A pharmacokinetic study in healthy male (n = 12) and female (n = 12) subjects showed no gender differences in zidovudine AUC_∞ or lamivudine AUC_∞ normalized for body weight.

Race: *Lamivudine:* There are no significant racial differences in lamivudine pharmacokinetics.

Zidovudine: The pharmacokinetics of zidovudine with respect to race have not been determined.

Drug Interactions: *See Drug Interactions (7).*

No drug interaction studies have been conducted using COMBIVIR Tablets. However, Table 4 presents drug interaction information for the individual components of COMBIVIR.

Lamivudine Plus Zidovudine: No clinically significant alterations in lamivudine or zidovudine pharmacokinetics were observed in 12 asymptomatic HIV-1-infected adult patients given a single dose of zidovudine (200 mg) in combination with multiple doses of lamivudine (300 mg q 12 hr).

[See table 4 at top of next page]

Ribavirin: In vitro data indicate ribavirin reduces phosphorylation of lamivudine, stavudine, and zidovudine. However, no pharmacokinetic (e.g., plasma concentrations or intracellular triphosphorylated active metabolite concentrations) or pharmacodynamic (e.g., loss of HIV-1/HCV virologic suppression) interaction was observed when ribavirin and lamivudine (n = 18), stavudine (n = 10), or zidovudine (n = 6) were coadministered as part of a multi-drug regimen to HIV-1/HCV co-infected patients *[see Warnings and Precautions (5.5)]*.

12.4 Microbiology

Mechanism of Action: *Lamivudine:* Intracellularly, lamivudine is phosphorylated to its active 5′-triphosphate metabolite, lamivudine triphosphate (3TC-TP). The principal mode of action of 3TC-TP is inhibition of reverse transcriptase (RT) via DNA chain termination after incorporation of the nucleotide analogue. 3TC-TP is a weak inhibitor of cellular DNA polymerases α, β, and γ.

Zidovudine: Intracellularly, zidovudine is phosphorylated to its active 5′-triphosphate metabolite, zidovudine triphosphate (ZDV-TP). The principal mode of action of ZDV-TP is inhibition of RT via DNA chain termination after incorporation of the nucleotide analogue. ZDV-TP is a weak inhibitor of the cellular DNA polymerases α and γ and has been reported to be incorporated into the DNA of cells in culture.

Antiviral Activity: *Lamivudine Plus Zidovudine:* In HIV-1–infected MT-4 cells, lamivudine in combination with zidovudine at various ratios exhibited synergistic antiretroviral activity.

Lamivudine: The antiviral activity of lamivudine against HIV-1 was assessed in a number of cell lines (including monocytes and fresh human peripheral blood lymphocytes) using standard susceptibility assays. EC_{50} values (50% effective concentrations) were in the range of 0.003 to 15 μM (1 μM = 0.23 mcg/mL). HIV-1 from therapy-naive subjects with no amino acid substitutions associated with resistance gave median EC_{50} values of 0.429 μM (range: 0.200 to 2.007 μM) from Virco (n = 92 baseline samples from COL40263) and 2.35 μM (1.37 to 3.68 μM) from Monogram Biosciences (n = 135 baseline samples from ESS30009). The EC_{50} values of lamivudine against different HIV-1 clades (A-G) ranged from 0.001 to 0.120 μM, and against HIV-2 isolates from 0.003 to 0.120 μM in peripheral blood mononuclear cells. Ribavirin (50 μM) decreased the anti-HIV-1 activity of lamivudine by 3.5 fold in MT-4 cells.

Zidovudine: The antiviral activity of zidovudine against HIV-1 was assessed in a number of cell lines (including monocytes and fresh human peripheral blood lymphocytes). The EC_{50} and EC_{90} values for zidovudine were 0.01 to 0.49 μM (1 μM = 0.27 mcg/mL) and 0.1 to 9 μM, respectively. HIV-1 from therapy-naive subjects with no amino acid substitutions associated with resistance gave median EC_{50} values of 0.011 μM (range: 0.005 to 0.110 μM) from Virco (n = 92 baseline samples from COL40263) and 0.0017 μM (0.006 to 0.0340 μM) from Monogram Biosciences (n = 135 baseline samples from ESS30009). The EC_{50} values of zidovudine against different HIV-1 clades (A-G) ranged from 0.00018 to 0.02 μM, and against HIV-2 isolates from 0.00049 to 0.004 μM. In cell culture drug combination studies, zidovudine demonstrates synergistic activity with the nucleoside reverse transcriptase inhibitors (NRTIs) abacavir, didanosine, lamivudine, and zalcitabine; the non-nucleoside reverse transcriptase inhibitors (NNRTIs) delavirdine and nevirapine; and the protease inhibitors (PIs) indinavir, nelfinavir, ritonavir, and saquinavir; and additive activity with interferon alfa. Ribavirin has been found to inhibit the phosphorylation of zidovudine in cell culture.

Resistance: *Lamivudine Plus Zidovudine Administered As Separate Formulations:* In patients receiving lamivudine monotherapy or combination therapy with lamivudine plus zidovudine, HIV-1 isolates from most patients became phenotypically and genotypically resistant to lamivudine within 12 weeks. In some patients harboring zidovudine-resistant virus at baseline, phenotypic sensitivity to zidovudine was restored by 12 weeks of treatment with lamivudine and zidovudine. Combination therapy with lamivudine plus zidovudine delayed the emergence of amino acid substitutions conferring resistance to zidovudine.

HIV-1 strains resistant to both lamivudine and zidovudine have been isolated from patients after prolonged lamivudine/zidovudine therapy. Dual resistance required the presence of multiple amino acid substitutions, the most essential of which may be G333E. The incidence of dual resistance and the duration of combination therapy required before dual resistance occurs are unknown.

Lamivudine: Lamivudine-resistant isolates of HIV-1 have been selected in cell culture and have also been recovered from patients treated with lamivudine or lamivudine plus zidovudine. Genotypic analysis of isolates selected in cell culture and recovered from lamivudine-treated patients showed that the resistance was due to a specific amino acid substitution in the HIV-1 reverse transcriptase at codon 184 changing the methionine to either isoleucine or valine (M184V/I).

Zidovudine: HIV-1 isolates with reduced susceptibility to zidovudine have been selected in cell culture and were also recovered from patients treated with zidovudine. Genotypic analyses of the isolates selected in cell culture and recovered from zidovudine-treated patients showed substitutions in the HIV-1 RT gene resulting in 6 amino acid substitutions (M41L, D67N, K70R, L210W, T215Y or F, and K219Q) that confer zidovudine resistance. In general, higher levels of resistance were associated with greater number of amino acid substitutions.

Cross-Resistance: Cross-resistance has been observed among NRTIs.

Lamivudine Plus Zidovudine: Cross-resistance between lamivudine and zidovudine has not been reported. In some patients treated with lamivudine alone or in combination with zidovudine, isolates have emerged with a substitution at codon 184, which confers resistance to lamivudine. Cross-resistance to abacavir, didanosine, tenofovir, and zalcitabine

has been observed in some patients harboring lamivudine-resistant HIV-1 isolates. In some patients treated with zidovudine plus didanosine or zalcitabine, isolates resistant to multiple drugs, including lamivudine, have emerged (see under Zidovudine below).

Lamivudine: See Lamivudine Plus Zidovudine (above).

Zidovudine: In a study of 167 HIV-1-infected patients, isolates (n = 2) with multi-drug resistance to didanosine, lamivudine, stavudine, zalcitabine, and zidovudine were recovered from patients treated for ≥1 year with zidovudine plus didanosine or zidovudine plus zalcitabine. The pattern of resistance-associated amino acid substitutions with such combination therapies was different (A62V, V75I, F77L, F116Y, Q151M) from the pattern with zidovudine monotherapy, with the Q151M substitution being most commonly associated with multi-drug resistance. The substitution at codon 151 in combination with substitutions at 62, 75, 77, and 116 results in a virus with reduced resistance to didanosine, lamivudine, stavudine, zalcitabine, and zidovudine. Thymidine analogue mutations (TAMs) are selected by zidovudine and confer cross-resistance to abacavir, didanosine, stavudine, tenofovir, and zalcitabine.

13 NONCLINICAL TOXICOLOGY
13.1 Carcinogenesis, Mutagenesis, Impairment of Fertility

Carcinogenicity: *Lamivudine:* Long-term carcinogenicity studies with lamivudine in mice and rats showed no evidence of carcinogenic potential at exposures up to 10 times (mice) and 58 times (rats) those observed in humans at the recommended therapeutic dose for HIV-1 infection.

Zidovudine: Zidovudine was administered orally at 3 dosage levels to separate groups of mice and rats (60 females and 60 males in each group). Initial single daily doses were 30, 60, and 120 mg/kg/day in mice and 80, 220, and 600 mg/kg/day in rats. The doses in mice were reduced to

20, 30, and 40 mg/kg/day after day 90 because of treatment-related anemia, whereas in rats only the high dose was reduced to 450 mg/kg/day on day 91 and then to 300 mg/kg/day on day 279.

In mice, 7 late-appearing (after 19 months) vaginal neoplasms (5 nonmetastasizing squamous cell carcinomas, 1 squamous cell papilloma, and 1 squamous polyp) occurred in animals given the highest dose. One late-appearing squamous cell papilloma occurred in the vagina of a middle-dose animal. No vaginal tumors were found at the lowest dose.

In rats, 2 late-appearing (after 20 months), nonmetastasizing vaginal squamous cell carcinomas occurred in animals given the highest dose. No vaginal tumors occurred at the low or middle dose in rats. No other drug-related tumors were observed in either sex of either species.

At doses that produced tumors in mice and rats, the estimated drug exposure (as measured by AUC) was approximately 3 times (mouse) and 24 times (rat) the estimated human exposure at the recommended therapeutic dose of 100 mg every 4 hours.

It is not known how predictive the results of rodent carcinogenicity studies may be for humans.

Mutagenicity: *Lamivudine:* Lamivudine was mutagenic in an L5178Y/TK$^{+/-}$ mouse lymphoma assay and clastogenic in a cytogenetic assay using cultured human lymphocytes. Lamivudine was negative in a microbial mutagenicity assay, in an in vitro cell transformation assay, in a rat micronucleus test, in a rat bone marrow cytogenetic assay, and in an assay for unscheduled DNA synthesis in rat liver.

Zidovudine: Zidovudine was mutagenic in an L5178Y/TK$^{+/-}$ mouse lymphoma assay, positive in an in vitro cell transformation assay, clastogenic in a cytogenetic assay using cultured human lymphocytes, and positive in mouse and rat micronucleus tests after repeated doses. It was negative in a cytogenetic study in rats given a single dose.

Table 4. Effect of Coadministered Drugs on Lamivudine and Zidovudine AUC[a]

Note: ROUTINE DOSE MODIFICATION OF LAMIVUDINE AND ZIDOVUDINE IS NOT WARRANTED WITH COADMINISTRATION OF THE FOLLOWING DRUGS.

Drugs That May Alter Lamivudine Blood Concentrations

Coadministered Drug and Dose	Lamivudine Dose	n	Lamivudine Concentrations AUC	Lamivudine Concentrations Variability	Concentration of Coadministered Drug
Nelfinavir 750 mg q 8 hr × 7 to 10 days	single 150 mg	11	↑AUC 10%	95% CI: 1% to 20%	↔
Trimethoprim 160 mg/ Sulfamethoxazole 800 mg daily × 5 days	single 300 mg	14	↑AUC 43%	90% CI: 32% to 55%	

Drugs That May Alter Zidovudine Blood Concentrations

Coadministered Drug and Dose	Zidovudine Dose	n	Zidovudine Concentrations AUC	Zidovudine Concentrations Variability	Concentration of Coadministered Drug
Atovaquone 750 mg q 12 hr with food	200 mg q 8 hr	14	↑AUC 31%	Range 23% to 78%[b]	↔
Clarithromycin 500 mg twice daily	100 mg q 4 hr × 7 days	4	↓AUC 12%	Range ↓34% to ↑14%	Not Reported
Fluconazole 400 mg daily	200 mg q 8 hr	12	↑AUC 74%	95% CI: 54% to 98%	Not Reported
Methadone 30 to 90 mg daily	200 mg q 4 hr	9	↑AUC 43%	Range 16% to 64%[b]	↔
Nelfinavir 750 mg q 8 hr × 7 to 10 days	single 200 mg	11	↓AUC 35%	Range 28% to 41%	↔
Probenecid 500 mg q 6 hr × 2 days	2 mg/kg q 8 hr × 3 days	3	↑AUC 106%	Range 100% to 170%[b]	Not Assessed
Rifampin 600 mg daily × 14 days	200 mg q 8 hr × 14 days	8	↓AUC 47%	90% CI: 41% to 53%	Not Assessed
Ritonavir 300 mg q 6 hr × 4 days	200 mg q 8 hr × 4 days	9	↓AUC 25%	95% CI: 15% to 34%	↔
Valproic acid 250 mg or 500 mg q 8 hr × 4 days	100 mg q 8 hr × 4 days	6	↑AUC 80%	Range 64% to 130%[b]	Not Assessed

↑ = Increase; ↓= Decrease; ↔ = no significant change; AUC = area under the concentration versus time curve; CI = confidence interval.
[a] This table is not all inclusive.
[b] Estimated range of percent difference.

Table 5. Number of Patients (%) With At Least 1 HIV-1 Disease-Progression Event or Death

Endpoint	Current Therapy (n = 460)	EPIVIR plus Current Therapy (n = 896)	EPIVIR plus a NNRTI[a] plus Current Therapy (n = 460)
HIV-1 progression or death	90 (19.6%)	86 (9.6%)	41 (8.9%)
Death	27 (5.9%)	23 (2.6%)	14 (3.0%)

[a] An investigational non-nucleoside reverse transcriptase inhibitor not approved in the United States.

Impairment of Fertility: *Lamivudine:* In a study of reproductive performance, lamivudine, administered to male and female rats at doses up to 130 times the usual adult dose based on body surface area considerations, revealed no evidence of impaired fertility (judged by conception rates) and no effect on the survival, growth, and development to weaning of the offspring.

Zidovudine: Zidovudine, administered to male and female rats at doses up to 7 times the usual adult dose based on body surface area considerations, had no effect on fertility judged by conception rates.

13.2 Reproductive and Developmental Toxicology Studies

Lamivudine: Reproduction studies have been performed in rats and rabbits at orally administered doses up to 4,000 mg/kg/day and 1,000 mg/kg/day, respectively, producing plasma levels up to approximately 35 times that for the adult HIV dose. No evidence of teratogenicity due to lamivudine was observed. Evidence of early embryolethality was seen in the rabbit at exposure levels similar to those observed in humans, but there was no indication of this effect in the rat at exposure levels up to 35 times those in humans. Studies in pregnant rats and rabbits showed that lamivudine is transferred to the fetus through the placenta.

Zidovudine: Oral teratology studies in the rat and in the rabbit at doses up to 500 mg/kg/day revealed no evidence of teratogenicity with zidovudine. Zidovudine treatment resulted in embryo/fetal toxicity as evidenced by an increase in the incidence of fetal resorptions in rats given 150 or 450 mg/kg/day and rabbits given 500 mg/kg/day. The doses used in the teratology studies resulted in peak zidovudine plasma concentrations (after one half of the daily dose) in rats 66 to 226 times, and in rabbits 12 to 87 times, mean steady-state peak human plasma concentrations (after one sixth of the daily dose) achieved with the recommended daily dose (100 mg every 4 hours). In an in vitro experiment with fertilized mouse oocytes, zidovudine exposure resulted in a dose-dependent reduction in blastocyst formation. In an additional teratology study in rats, a dose of 3,000 mg/kg/day (very near the oral median lethal dose in rats of 3,683 mg/kg) caused marked maternal toxicity and an increase in the incidence of fetal malformations. This dose resulted in peak zidovudine plasma concentrations 350 times peak human plasma concentrations. (Estimated AUC in rats at this dose level was 300 times the daily AUC in humans given 600 mg/day.) No evidence of teratogenicity was seen in this experiment at doses of 600 mg/kg/day or less.

14 CLINICAL STUDIES

There have been no clinical trials conducted with COMBIVIR. See *Clinical Pharmacology (12.3)* for information about bioequivalence. One COMBIVIR Tablet given twice daily is an alternative regimen to EPIVIR Tablets 150 mg twice daily plus RETROVIR 600 mg per day in divided doses.

14.1 Adults

Lamivudine Plus Zidovudine: The NUCB3007 (CAESAR) study was conducted using EPIVIR 150-mg Tablets (150 mg twice daily) and RETROVIR 100-mg Capsules (2 × 100 mg 3 times daily). CAESAR was a multi-center, double-blind, placebo-controlled study comparing continued current therapy (zidovudine alone [62% of patients] or zidovudine with didanosine or zalcitabine [38% of patients]) to the addition of EPIVIR or EPIVIR plus an investigational non-nucleoside reverse transcriptase inhibitor, randomized 1:2:1. A total of 1,816 HIV-1-infected adults with 25 to 250 (median 122) CD4 cells/mm³ at baseline were enrolled: median age was 36 years, 87% were male, 84% were nucleoside-experienced, and 16% were therapy-naive. The median duration on study was 12 months. Results are summarized in Table 5.

[See table 5 above]

14.2 Prevention of Maternal-Fetal HIV-1 Transmission

The utility of zidovudine alone for the prevention of maternal-fetal HIV-1 transmission was demonstrated in a randomized, double-blind, placebo-controlled trial conducted in HIV-1-infected pregnant women with CD4+ cell counts of 200 to 1,818 cells/mm³ (median in the treated group: 560 cells/mm³) who had little or no previous exposure to zidovudine. Oral zidovudine was initiated between 14 and 34 weeks of gestation (median 11 weeks of therapy) fol-

lowed by IV administration of zidovudine during labor and delivery. Following birth, neonates received oral zidovudine syrup for 6 weeks. The study showed a statistically significant difference in the incidence of HIV-1 infection in the neonates (based on viral culture from peripheral blood) between the group receiving zidovudine and the group receiving placebo. Of 363 neonates evaluated in the study, the estimated risk of HIV-1 infection was 7.8% in the group receiving zidovudine and 24.9% in the placebo group, a relative reduction in transmission risk of 68.7%. Zidovudine was well tolerated by mothers and infants. There was no difference in pregnancy-related adverse events between the treatment groups.

16 HOW SUPPLIED/STORAGE AND HANDLING

COMBIVIR Tablets, containing 150 mg lamivudine and 300 mg zidovudine, are white, scored, film-coated, modified-capsule-shaped tablets, debossed on both tablet faces, such that when broken in half, the full "GXFC3" code is present on both halves of the tablet ("GX" on one face and "FC3" on the opposite face of the tablet). They are available as follows:

60 Tablets/Bottle (NDC 0173-0595-00).
Unit Dose Pack of 120 (NDC 0173-0595-02).
Store between 2° and 30°C (36° and 86°F).

17 PATIENT COUNSELING INFORMATION

17.1 Advice for the Patient

Neutropenia and Anemia: Patients should be informed that the important toxicities associated with zidovudine are neutropenia and/or anemia. They should be told of the extreme importance of having their blood counts followed closely while on therapy, especially for patients with advanced HIV-1 disease *[see Warnings and Precautions (5.1)].*

Co-infection With HIV-1 and HBV: Patients co-infected with HIV-1 and HBV should be informed that deterioration of liver disease has occurred in some cases when treatment with lamivudine was discontinued. Patients should be advised to discuss any changes in regimen with their physician *[see Warnings and Precautions (5.4)].*

Drug Interactions: Patients should be cautioned about the use of other medications, including ganciclovir, interferon alfa, and ribavirin, which may exacerbate the toxicity of zidovudine *[see Drug Interactions (7.3)].*

Redistribution/Accumulation of Body Fat: Patients should be informed that redistribution or accumulation of body fat may occur in patients receiving antiretroviral therapy and that the cause and long-term health effects of these conditions are not known at this time *[see Warnings and Precautions (5.9)].*

Information About Therapy with COMBIVIR: COMBIVIR is not a cure for HIV-1 infection and patients may continue to experience illnesses associated with HIV-1 infection, including opportunistic infections. Patients should be advised that the use of COMBIVIR has not been shown to reduce the risk of transmission of HIV-1 to others through sexual contact or blood contamination. Patients should be advised of the importance of taking COMBIVIR exactly as it is prescribed.

COMBIVIR should not be coadministered with drugs containing lamivudine, zidovudine, or emtricitabine, including EPIVIR (lamivudine), EPIVIR-HBV (lamivudine), RETROVIR (zidovudine), EPZICOM (abacavir sulfate and lamivudine), TRIZIVIR (abacavir sulfate, lamivudine, and zidovudine), ATRIPLA (efavirenz, emtricitabine, and tenofovir), EMTRIVA (emtricitabine), or TRUVADA (emtricitabine and tenofovir) *[see Warnings and Precautions (5.5)].* EPIVIR, EPIVIR-HBV, RETROVIR, EPZICOM, and TRIZIVIR are registered trademarks of GlaxoSmithKline. The other brands listed are trademarks of their respective owners and are not trademarks of GlaxoSmithKline. The makers of these brands are not affiliated with and do not endorse GlaxoSmithKline or its products.

GlaxoSmithKline
Research Triangle Park, NC 27709
Lamivudine is manufactured under agreement from
Shire Pharmaceuticals Group plc
Basingstoke, UK
©2010, GlaxoSmithKline. All rights reserved.
August 2010
CMB:2PI

EPIVIR® ℞
[ĕp′ ə-vir]
(lamivudine)
Tablets and Oral Solution

HIGHLIGHTS OF PRESCRIBING INFORMATION
These highlights do not include all the information needed to use EPIVIR safely and effectively. See full prescribing information for EPIVIR.
EPIVIR (lamivudine) Tablets and Oral Solution
Initial U.S. Approval: 1995

WARNING: LACTIC ACIDOSIS, POSTTREATMENT EXACERBATIONS OF HEPATITIS B IN CO-INFECTED PATIENTS, DIFFERENT FORMULATIONS OF EPIVIR
See full prescribing information for complete boxed warning
- **Lactic acidosis and severe hepatomegaly with steatosis, including fatal cases, have been reported with the use of nucleoside analogues. Suspend treatment if clinical or laboratory findings suggestive of lactic acidosis or pronounced hepatotoxicity occur. (5.1)**
- **Severe acute exacerbations of hepatitis B have been reported in patients who are co-infected with hepatitis B virus (HBV) and human immunodeficiency virus (HIV-1) and have discontinued EPIVIR. Monitor hepatic function closely in these patients and, if appropriate, initiate anti-hepatitis B treatment. (5.2)**
- **Patients with HIV-1 infection should receive only dosage forms of EPIVIR appropriate for treatment of HIV-1. (5.2)**

———RECENT MAJOR CHANGES———
Dosage and Administration, Pediatric
Patients (2.2)   February 2008

———INDICATIONS AND USAGE———
EPIVIR is a nucleoside analogue reverse transcriptase inhibitor indicated in combination with other antiretroviral agents for the treatment of HIV-1 infection. Limitation of Use: The dosage of this product is for HIV-1 and not for HBV. (1)

———DOSAGE AND ADMINISTRATION———
- Adults and adolescents >16 years of age: 300 mg daily, administered as either 150 mg twice daily or 300 mg once daily. (2.1)
- Pediatric patients 3 months up to 16 years of age: Dosage should be based on body weight. (2.2)
- Patients With Renal Impairment: Doses of EPIVIR must be adjusted in accordance with renal function. (2.3)

———DOSAGE FORMS AND STRENGTHS———
- Tablets: 300 mg (3)
- Tablets: Scored 150 mg (3)
- Oral Solution: 10 mg/mL (3)

———CONTRAINDICATIONS———
EPIVIR Tablets and Oral Solution are contraindicated in patients with previously demonstrated clinically significant hypersensitivity (e.g., anaphylaxis) to any of the components of the products. (4)

———WARNINGS AND PRECAUTIONS———
- Lactic acidosis and severe hepatomegaly with steatosis: Reported with the use of nucleoside analogues. Suspend treatment if clinical or laboratory findings suggestive of lactic acidosis or pronounced hepatoxicity occur. (5.1)
- Severe acute exacerbations of hepatitis: Reported in patients who are co-infected with hepatitis B virus and HIV-1 and discontinued EPIVIR. Monitor hepatic function closely in these patients and, if appropriate, initiate anti-hepatitis B treatment. (5.2)
- Patients with HIV-1 infection should receive only dosage forms of EPIVIR appropriate for treatment of HIV-1. (5.2)
- Co-infected HIV-1/HBV Patients: Emergence of lamivudine-resistant HBV variants associated with lamivudine-containing antiretroviral regimens has been reported. (5.2)
- Emtricitabine should not be administered concomitantly with lamivudine-containing products. (5.3)
- Hepatic decompensation (some fatal) has occurred in HIV-1/HCV co-infected patients receiving interferon and ribavirin-based regimens. Monitor for treatment-associated toxicities. Discontinue EPIVIR as medically appropriate and consider dose reduction or discontinuation of interferon alfa, ribavirin, or both. (5.4)
- Pancreatitis: Use with caution in pediatric patients with a history of pancreatitis or other significant risk factors for pancreatitis. Discontinue treatment as clinically appropriate. (5.5)
- Immune reconstitution syndrome (5.6) and redistribution/accumulation of body fat (5.7) have been reported in patients treated with combination antiretroviral therapy.

———ADVERSE REACTIONS———
- The most common reported adverse reactions (incidence ≥15%) in adults were headache, nausea, malaise and fatigue, nasal signs and symptoms, diarrhea, and cough. (6.1)

• The most common reported adverse reactions (incidence ≥15%) in pediatric patients were fever and cough. (6.1)

To report SUSPECTED ADVERSE REACTIONS, contact GlaxoSmithKline at 1-888-825-5249 or FDA at 1-800-FDA-1088 or www.fda.gov/medwatch.

——————DRUG INTERACTIONS——————

Zalcitabine is not recommended for use in combination with EPIVIR. (7.2)

——————USE IN SPECIFIC POPULATIONS——————

• Pregnancy: Physicians are encouraged to register patients in the Antiretroviral Pregnancy Registry by calling 1-800-258-4263. (8.1)

Revised: April 2009

EPV:2PI

See 17 for PATIENT COUNSELING INFORMATION
Revised: 04/2010

FULL PRESCRIBING INFORMATION: CONTENTS*

WARNING: RISK OF LACTIC ACIDOSIS, EXACERBATIONS OF HEPATITIS B IN CO-INFECTED PATIENTS UPON DISCONTINUATION OF EPIVIR, DIFFERENT FORMULATIONS OF EPIVIR.

1 INDICATIONS AND USAGE
2 DOSAGE AND ADMINISTRATION
  2.1 Adults and Adolescents >16 years of age
  2.2 Pediatric Patients
  2.3 Patients With Renal Impairment
3 DOSAGE FORMS AND STRENGTHS
4 CONTRAINDICATIONS
5 WARNINGS AND PRECAUTIONS
  5.1 Lactic Acidosis/Severe Hepatomegaly With Steatosis
  5.2 Patients With HIV-1 and Hepatitis B Virus Co-infection
  5.3 Use With Other Lamivudine- and Emtricitabine-Containing Products
  5.4 Use With Interferon- and Ribavirin-Based Regimens
  5.5 Pancreatitis
  5.6 Immune Reconstitution Syndrome
  5.7 Fat Redistribution
6 ADVERSE REACTIONS
  6.1 Clinical Trials Experience
  6.2 Postmarketing Experience
7 DRUG INTERACTIONS
  7.1 Interferon- and Ribavirin-Based Regimens
  7.2 Zalcitabine
  7.3 Trimethoprim/Sulfamethoxazole (TMP/SMX)
  7.4 Drugs with No Observed Interactions With EPIVIR
8 USE IN SPECIFIC POPULATIONS
  8.1 Pregnancy
  8.3 Nursing Mothers
  8.4 Pediatric Use
  8.5 Geriatric Use
  8.6 Patients With Impaired Renal Function
10 OVERDOSAGE
11 DESCRIPTION
12 CLINICAL PHARMACOLOGY
  12.1 Mechanism of Action
  12.3 Pharmacokinetics
  12.4 Microbiology
13 NONCLINICAL TOXICOLOGY
  13.1 Carcinogenesis, Mutagenesis, Impairment of Fertility
  13.2 Reproductive Toxicology Studies
14 CLINICAL STUDIES
  14.1 Adults
  14.2 Pediatric Patients
16 HOW SUPPLIED/STORAGE AND HANDLING
17 PATIENT COUNSELING INFORMATION
  17.1 Advice for the Patient

* Sections or subsections omitted from the full prescribing information are not listed

FULL PRESCRIBING INFORMATION

WARNING: RISK OF LACTIC ACIDOSIS, EXACERBATIONS OF HEPATITIS B IN CO-INFECTED PATIENTS UPON DISCONTINUATION OF EPIVIR, DIFFERENT FORMULATIONS OF EPIVIR.

Lactic acidosis and severe hepatomegaly with steatosis, including fatal cases, have been reported with the use of nucleoside analogues alone or in combination, including lamivudine and other antiretrovirals. Suspend treatment if clinical or laboratory findings suggestive of lactic acidosis or pronounced hepatotoxicity occur [see Warnings and Precautions (5.1)].

Severe acute exacerbations of hepatitis B have been reported in patients who are co-infected with hepatitis B virus (HBV) and human immunodeficiency virus (HIV-1) and have discontinued EPIVIR. Hepatic function should be monitored closely with both clinical and lab- oratory follow-up for at least several months in patients who discontinue EPIVIR and are co-infected with HIV-1 and HBV. If appropriate, initiation of anti-hepatitis B therapy may be warranted [see Warnings and Precautions (5.2)].

EPIVIR Tablets and Oral Solution (used to treat HIV-1 infection) contain a higher dose of the active ingredient (lamivudine) than EPIVIR-HBV® Tablets and Oral Solution (used to treat chronic HBV infection). Patients with HIV-1 infection should receive only dosage forms appropriate for treatment of HIV-1 [see Warnings and Precautions (5.2)].

1 INDICATIONS AND USAGE

EPIVIR is a nucleoside analogue indicated in combination with other antiretroviral agents for the treatment of human immunodeficiency virus (HIV-1) infection. Limitation of use: The dosage of this product is for HIV-1 and not for HBV.

2 DOSAGE AND ADMINISTRATION

2.1 Adults and Adolescents >16 years of age

The recommended oral dose of EPIVIR in HIV-1-infected adults and adolescents >16 years of age is 300 mg daily, administered as either 150 mg twice daily or 300 mg once daily, in combination with other antiretroviral agents. If lamivudine is administered to a patient infected with HIV-1 and HBV, the dosage indicated for HIV-1 therapy should be used as part of an appropriate combination regimen [see Warnings and Precautions (5.2)].

2.2 Pediatric Patients

The recommended oral dose of EPIVIR Oral Solution in HIV-1-infected pediatric patients 3 months to 16 years of age is 4 mg/kg twice daily (up to a maximum of 150 mg twice a day), administered in combination with other antiretroviral agents.

EPIVIR is also available as a scored tablet for HIV-1-infected pediatric patients who weigh ≥14 kg and for whom a solid dosage form is appropriate. Before prescribing EPIVIR Tablets, children should be assessed for the ability to swallow tablets. If a child is unable to reliably swallow EPIVIR Tablets, the oral solution formulation should be prescribed. The recommended oral dosage of EPIVIR Tablets for HIV-1-infected pediatric patients is presented in Table 1.

[See table 1 above]

2.3 Patients With Renal Impairment

Dosing of EPIVIR is adjusted in accordance with renal function. Dosage adjustments are listed in Table 2 [see Clinical Pharmacology (12.3)].

Table 2. Adjustment of Dosage of EPIVIR in Adults and Adolescents (≥30 kg) in Accordance With Creatinine Clearance

Creatinine Clearance (mL/min)	Recommended Dosage of EPIVIR
≥50	150 mg twice daily or 300 mg once daily
30-49	150 mg once daily
15-29	150 mg first dose, then 100 mg once daily
5-14	150 mg first dose, then 50 mg once daily
<5	50 mg first dose, then 25 mg once daily

No additional dosing of EPIVIR is required after routine (4-hour) hemodialysis or peritoneal dialysis.

Although there are insufficient data to recommend a specific dose adjustment of EPIVIR in pediatric patients with renal impairment, a reduction in the dose and/or an increase in the dosing interval should be considered.

3 DOSAGE FORMS AND STRENGTHS

• **EPIVIR Scored Tablets**
150 mg, are white, diamond-shaped, scored, film-coated tablets debossed with "GX CJ7" on both sides.

• **EPIVIR Tablets**
300 mg, are gray, modified diamond-shaped, film-coated tablets engraved with "GX EJ7" on one side and plain on the reverse side.

• **EPIVIR Oral Solution**
A clear, colorless to pale yellow, strawberry-banana flavored liquid, containing 10 mg of lamivudine per 1 mL.

4 CONTRAINDICATIONS

EPIVIR Tablets and Oral Solution are contraindicated in patients with previously demonstrated clinically significant hypersensitivity (e.g., anaphylaxis) to any of the components of the products.

5 WARNINGS AND PRECAUTIONS

5.1 Lactic Acidosis/Severe Hepatomegaly With Steatosis

Lactic acidosis and severe hepatomegaly with steatosis, including fatal cases, have been reported with the use of nucleoside analogues alone or in combination, including lamivudine and other antiretrovirals. A majority of these cases have been in women. Obesity and prolonged nucleoside exposure may be risk factors. Particular caution should be exercised when administering EPIVIR to any patient with known risk factors for liver disease; however, cases also have been reported in patients with no known risk factors. Treatment with EPIVIR should be suspended in any patient who develops clinical or laboratory findings suggestive of lactic acidosis or pronounced hepatotoxicity (which may include hepatomegaly and steatosis even in the absence of marked transaminase elevations).

5.2 Patients With HIV-1 and Hepatitis B Virus Co-infection

Posttreatment Exacerbations of Hepatitis: In clinical trials in non-HIV-1-infected patients treated with lamivudine for chronic hepatitis B, clinical and laboratory evidence of exacerbations of hepatitis has occurred after discontinuation of lamivudine. These exacerbations have been detected primarily by serum ALT elevations in addition to re-emergence of HBV DNA. Although most events appear to have been self-limited, fatalities have been reported in some cases. Similar events have been reported from post-marketing experience after changes from lamivudine-containing HIV-1 treatment regimens to non-lamivudine-containing regimens in patients infected with both HIV-1 and HBV. The causal relationship to discontinuation of lamivudine treatment is unknown. Patients should be closely monitored with both clinical and laboratory follow-up for at least several months after stopping treatment. There is insufficient evidence to determine whether re-initiation of lamivudine alters the course of posttreatment exacerbations of hepatitis.

Important Differences Among Lamivudine-Containing Products: EPIVIR Tablets and Oral Solution contain a higher dose of the same active ingredient (lamivudine) than EPIVIR-HBV Tablets and EPIVIR-HBV Oral Solution. EPIVIR-HBV was developed for patients with chronic hepatitis B. The formulation and dosage of lamivudine in EPIVIR-HBV are not appropriate for patients co-infected with HIV-1 and HBV. Safety and efficacy of lamivudine have not been established for treatment of chronic hepatitis B in patients co-infected with HIV-1 and HBV. If treatment with EPIVIR-HBV is prescribed for chronic hepatitis B for a patient with unrecognized or untreated HIV-1 infection, rapid emergence of HIV-1 resistance is likely to result because of the subtherapeutic dose and the inappropriateness of monotherapy HIV-1 treatment. If a decision is made to administer lamivudine to patients co-infected with HIV-1 and HBV, EPIVIR Tablets, EPIVIR Oral Solution, COMBIVIR® (lamivudine/zidovudine) Tablets, EPZICOM® (abacavir sulfate and lamivudine) Tablets, or TRIZIVIR® (abacavir sulfate, lamivudine, and zidovudine) Tablets should be used as part of an appropriate combination regimen.

Emergence of Lamivudine-Resistant HBV: In non–HIV-1-infected patients treated with lamivudine for chronic hepatitis B, emergence of lamivudine-resistant HBV has been detected and has been associated with diminished treatment response (see full prescribing information for EPIVIR-HBV for additional information). Emergence of hepatitis B virus variants associated with resistance to lamivudine has also been reported in HIV-1-infected patients who have received lamivudine-containing antiretroviral regimens in the presence of concurrent infection with hepatitis B virus.

5.3 Use With Other Lamivudine- and Emtricitabine-Containing Products

EPIVIR should not be administered concomitantly with other lamivudine-containing products including EPIVIR-

Table 1. Dosing Recommendations for EPIVIR Tablets in Pediatric Patients

Weight (kg)	Dosage Regimen Using Scored 150-mg Tablet		Total Daily Dose
	AM Dose	PM Dose	
14 to 21	½ tablet (75 mg)	½ tablet (75 mg)	150 mg
>21 to <30	½ tablet (75 mg)	1 tablet (150 mg)	225 mg
≥30	1 tablet (150 mg)	1 tablet (150 mg)	300 mg

Table 3. Selected Clinical Adverse Reactions (≥5% Frequency) in Four Controlled Clinical Trials (NUCA3001, NUCA3002, NUCB3001, NUCB3002)

Adverse Reaction	EPIVIR 150 mg Twice Daily plus RETROVIR (n = 251)	RETROVIR[a] (n = 230)
Body as a Whole		
Headache	35%	27%
Malaise & fatigue	27%	23%
Fever or chills	10%	12%
Digestive		
Nausea	33%	29%
Diarrhea	18%	22%
Nausea & vomiting	13%	12%
Anorexia and/or decreased appetite	10%	7%
Abdominal pain	9%	11%
Abdominal cramps	6%	3%
Dyspepsia	5%	5%
Nervous System		
Neuropathy	12%	10%
Insomnia & other sleep disorders	11%	7%
Dizziness	10%	4%
Depressive disorders	9%	4%
Respiratory		
Nasal signs & symptoms	20%	11%
Cough	18%	13%
Skin		
Skin rashes	9%	6%
Musculoskeletal		
Musculoskeletal pain	12%	10%
Myalgia	8%	6%
Arthralgia	5%	5%

[a] Either zidovudine monotherapy or zidovudine in combination with zalcitabine.

Table 4. Frequencies of Selected Grade 3-4 Laboratory Abnormalities in Adults in Four 24-Week Surrogate Endpoint Studies (NUCA3001, NUCA3002, NUCB3001, NUCB3002) and a Clinical Endpoint Study (NUCB3007)

Test (Threshold Level)	24-Week Surrogate Endpoint Studies[a]		Clinical Endpoint Study[a]	
	EPIVIR plus RETROVIR	RETROVIR[b]	EPIVIR plus Current Therapy	Placebo plus Current Therapy[c]
Absolute neutrophil count (<750/mm³)	7.2%	5.4%	15%	13%
Hemoglobin (<8.0 g/dL)	2.9%	1.8%	2.2%	3.4%
Platelets (<50,000/mm³)	0.4%	1.3%	2.8%	3.8%
ALT (>5.0 × ULN)	3.7%	3.6%	3.8%	1.9%
AST (>5.0 × ULN)	1.7%	1.8%	4.0%	2.1%
Bilirubin (>2.5 × ULN)	0.8%	0.4%	ND	ND
Amylase (>2.0 × ULN)	4.2%	1.5%	2.2%	1.1%

[a] The median duration on study was 12 months.
[b] Either zidovudine monotherapy or zidovudine in combination with zalcitabine.
[c] Current therapy was either zidovudine, zidovudine plus didanosine, or zidovudine plus zalcitabine.
ULN = Upper limit of normal.
ND = Not done.

HBV Tablets, EPIVIR Oral Solution, COMBIVIR (lamivudine/zidovudine) Tablets, EPZICOM (abacavir sulfate and lamivudine) Tablets, or TRIZIVIR (abacavir sulfate, lamivudine, and zidovudine) or emtricitabine-containing products, including ATRIPLA® (efavirenz, emtricitabine, and tenofovir), EMTRIVA® (emtricitabine), or TRUVADA® (emtricitabine and tenofovir).

5.4   Use With Interferon- and Ribavirin-Based Regimens
In vitro studies have shown ribavirin can reduce the phosphorylation of pyrimidine nucleoside analogues such as lamivudine. Although no evidence of a pharmacokinetic or pharmacodynamic interaction (e.g., loss of HIV-1/HCV virologic suppression) was seen when ribavirin was coadministered with lamivudine in HIV-1/HCV co-infected patients *[see Clinical Pharmacology (12.3)]*, hepatic decompensation (some fatal) has occurred in HIV-1/HCV co-infected patients receiving combination antiretroviral therapy for HIV-1 and interferon alfa with or without ribavirin. Patients receiving interferon alfa with or without ribavirin and EPIVIR should be closely monitored for treatment-associated toxicities, especially hepatic decompensation. Discontinuation of EPIVIR should be considered as medically appropriate. Dose reduction or discontinuation of interferon alfa, ribavirin, or both should also be considered if worsening clinical toxicities are observed, including hepatic decompensation (e.g., Child-Pugh >6). See the complete prescribing information for interferon and ribavirin.

5.5   Pancreatitis
In pediatric patients with a history of prior antiretroviral nucleoside exposure, a history of pancreatitis, or other significant risk factors for the development of pancreatitis, EPIVIR should be used with caution. Treatment with EPIVIR should be stopped immediately if clinical signs, symptoms, or laboratory abnormalities suggestive of pancreatitis occur *[see Adverse Reactions (6.1)]*.

5.6   Immune Reconstitution Syndrome
Immune reconstitution syndrome has been reported in patients treated with combination antiretroviral therapy, including EPIVIR. During the initial phase of combination antiretroviral treatment, patients whose immune system responds may develop an inflammatory response to indolent or residual opportunistic infections (such as *Mycobacterium avium* infection, cytomegalovirus, *Pneumocystis jirovecii* pneumonia [PCP], or tuberculosis), which may necessitate further evaluation and treatment.

5.7   Fat Redistribution
Redistribution/accumulation of body fat including central obesity, dorsocervical fat enlargement (buffalo hump), peripheral wasting, facial wasting, breast enlargement, and "cushingoid appearance" have been observed in patients receiving antiretroviral therapy. The mechanism and long-term consequences of these events are currently unknown. A causal relationship has not been established.

6   ADVERSE REACTIONS
6.1   Clinical Trials Experience
The following adverse reactions are discussed in greater detail in other sections of the labeling:
• Lactic acidosis and severe hepatomegaly with steatosis *[see Boxed Warning, Warnings and Precautions (5.1)]*.

• Severe acute exacerbations of hepatitis B *[see Boxed Warning, Warnings and Precautions (5.2)]*.
• Hepatic decompensation in patients co-infected with HIV-1 and Hepatitis C *[see Warnings and Precautions (5.4)]*.
• Pancreatitis *[see Warnings and Precautions (5.5)]*.
Because clinical trials are conducted under widely varying conditions, adverse reaction rates observed in the clinical trials of a drug cannot be directly compared to rates in the clinical trials of another drug and may not reflect the rates observed in practice.
Adults - Clinical Trials in HIV-1:   The safety profile of EPIVIR in adults is primarily based on 3,568 HIV-1-infected patients in 7 clinical trials.
The most common adverse reactions are headache, nausea, malaise, fatigue, nasal signs and symptoms, diarrhea and cough.
Selected clinical adverse reactions in ≥5% of patients during therapy with EPIVIR 150 mg twice daily plus RETROVIR® 200 mg 3 times daily for up to 24 weeks are listed in Table 3.
[See table 3 at left]
Pancreatitis: Pancreatitis was observed in 9 out of 2,613 adult patients (0.3%) who received EPIVIR in controlled clinical trials EPV20001, NUCA3001, NUCB3001, NUCA3002, NUCB3002, and NUCB3007 *[see Warnings and Precautions (5.5)]*.
EPIVIR 300 mg Once Daily: The types and frequencies of clinical adverse reactions reported in patients receiving EPIVIR 300 mg once daily or EPIVIR 150 mg twice daily (in 3-drug combination regimens in EPV20001 and EPV40001) for 48 weeks were similar.
Selected laboratory abnormalities observed during therapy are summarized in Table 4.
[See table 4 at left]
The frequencies of selected laboratory abnormalities reported in patients receiving EPIVIR 300 mg once daily or EPIVIR 150 mg twice daily (in 3-drug combination regimens in EPV20001 and EPV40001) were similar.
Pediatric Patients – Clinical Trials in HIV-1:   EPIVIR Oral Solution has been studied in 638 pediatric patients 3 months to 18 years of age in 3 clinical trials.
Selected clinical adverse reactions and physical findings with a ≥5% frequency during therapy with EPIVIR 4 mg/kg twice daily plus RETROVIR 160 mg/m² 3 times daily in therapy-naive (≤56 days of antiretroviral therapy) pediatric patients are listed in Table 5.
[See table 5 at top of next page]
Pancreatitis: Pancreatitis, which has been fatal in some cases, has been observed in antiretroviral nucleoside-experienced pediatric patients receiving EPIVIR alone or in combination with other antiretroviral agents. In an open-label dose-escalation study (NUCA2002), 14 patients (14%) developed pancreatitis while receiving monotherapy with EPIVIR. Three of these patients died of complications of pancreatitis. In a second open-label study (NUCA2005), 12 patients (18%) developed pancreatitis. In Study ACTG300, pancreatitis was not observed in 236 patients randomized to EPIVIR plus RETROVIR. Pancreatitis was observed in 1 patient in this study who received open-label EPIVIR in combination with RETROVIR and ritonavir following discontinuation of didanosine monotherapy *[see Warnings and Precautions (5.5)]*.
Paresthesias and Peripheral Neuropathies: Paresthesias and peripheral neuropathies were reported in 15 patients (15%) in Study NUCA2002, 6 patients (9%) in Study NUCA2005, and 2 patients (<1%) in Study ACTG300.
Selected laboratory abnormalities experienced by therapy-naive (≤56 days of antiretroviral therapy) pediatric patients are listed in Table 6.
[See table 6 on next page]
Neonates - Clinical Trials in HIV-1:   Limited short-term safety information is available from 2 small, uncontrolled studies in South Africa in neonates receiving lamivudine with or without zidovudine for the first week of life following maternal treatment starting at Week 38 or 36 of gestation *[see Clinical Pharmacology (12.3)]*. Selected adverse reactions reported in these neonates included increased liver function tests, anemia, diarrhea, electrolyte disturbances, hypoglycemia, jaundice and hepatomegaly, rash, respiratory infections, and sepsis; 3 neonates died (1 from gastroenteritis with acidosis and convulsions, 1 from traumatic injury, and 1 from unknown causes). Two other nonfatal gastroenteritis or diarrhea cases were reported, including 1 with convulsions; 1 infant had transient renal insufficiency associated with dehydration. The absence of control groups limits assessments of causality, but it should be assumed that perinatally exposed infants may be at risk for adverse reactions comparable to those reported in pediatric and adult HIV-1-infected patients treated with lamivudine-containing combination regimens. Long-term effects of in utero and infant lamivudine exposure are not known.

6.2 Postmarketing Experience

In addition to adverse reactions reported from clinical trials, the following adverse reactions have been reported during postmarketing use of EPIVIR. Because these reactions are reported voluntarily from a population of unknown size, estimates of frequency cannot be made. These reactions have been chosen for inclusion due to a combination of their seriousness, frequency of reporting, or potential causal connection to lamivudine.

Body as a Whole: Redistribution/accumulation of body fat [see Warnings and Precautions (5.7)].

Endocrine and Metabolic: Hyperglycemia.

General: Weakness.

Hemic and Lymphatic: Anemia (including pure red cell aplasia and severe anemias progressing on therapy).

Hepatic and Pancreatic: Lactic acidosis and hepatic steatosis, posttreatment exacerbation of hepatitis B [see Boxed Warning, Warnings and Precautions (5.1, 5.2)].

Hypersensitivity: Anaphylaxis, urticaria.

Musculoskeletal: Muscle weakness, CPK elevation, rhabdomyolysis.

Skin: Alopecia, pruritus.

7 DRUG INTERACTIONS

Lamivudine is predominantly eliminated in the urine by active organic cationic secretion. The possibility of interactions with other drugs administered concurrently should be considered, particularly when their main route of elimination is active renal secretion via the organic cationic transport system (e.g., trimethoprim). No data are available regarding interactions with other drugs that have renal clearance mechanisms similar to that of lamivudine.

7.1 Interferon- and Ribavirin-Based Regimens

Although no evidence of a pharmacokinetic or pharmacodynamic interaction (e.g., loss of HIV-1/HCV virologic suppression) was seen when ribavirin was coadministered with lamivudine in HIV-1/HCV co-infected patients, hepatic decompensation (some fatal) has occurred in HIV-1/HCV co-infected patients receiving combination antiretroviral therapy for HIV-1 and interferon alfa with or without ribavirin [see Warnings and Precautions (5.4), Clinical Pharmacology (12.3)].

7.2 Zalcitabine

Lamivudine and zalcitabine may inhibit the intracellular phosphorylation of one another. Therefore, use of lamivudine in combination with zalcitabine is not recommended.

7.3 Trimethoprim/Sulfamethoxazole (TMP/SMX)

No change in dose of either drug is recommended. There is no information regarding the effect on lamivudine pharmacokinetics of higher doses of TMP/SMX such as those used to treat PCP.

7.4 Drugs with No Observed Interactions With EPIVIR

A drug interaction study showed no clinically significant interaction between EPIVIR and zidovudine.

8 USE IN SPECIFIC POPULATIONS

8.1 Pregnancy

Pregnancy Category C. There are no adequate and well-controlled studies of EPIVIR in pregnant women. Animal reproduction studies in rats and rabbits revealed no evidence of teratogenicity. Increased early embryolethality occurred in rabbits at exposure levels similar to those in humans. EPIVIR should be used during pregnancy only if the potential benefit justifies the potential risk to the fetus.

Lamivudine pharmacokinetics were studied in pregnant women during 2 clinical studies conducted in South Africa. The study assessed pharmacokinetics in: 16 women at 36 weeks gestation using 150 mg lamivudine twice daily with zidovudine, 10 women at 38 weeks gestation using 150 mg lamivudine twice daily with zidovudine, and 10 women at 38 weeks gestation using lamivudine 300 mg twice daily without other antiretrovirals. These studies were not designed or powered to provide efficacy information. Lamivudine pharmacokinetics in pregnant women were similar to those seen in non-pregnant adults and in postpartum women. Lamivudine concentrations were generally similar in maternal, neonatal, and umbilical cord serum samples. In a subset of subjects, lamivudine amniotic fluid specimens were collected following natural rupture of membranes. Amniotic fluid concentrations of lamivudine were typically 2 times greater than maternal serum levels and ranged from 1.2 to 2.5 mcg/mL (150 mg twice daily) and 2.1 to 5.2 mcg/mL (300 mg twice daily). It is not known whether risks of adverse events associated with lamivudine are altered in pregnant women compared with other HIV-1-infected patients.

Animal reproduction studies performed at oral doses up to 130 and 60 times the adult dose in rats and rabbits, respectively, revealed no evidence of teratogenicity due to lamivudine. Increased early embryolethality occurred in rabbits at exposure levels similar to those in humans. However, there was no indication of this effect in rats at exposure levels up to 35 times those in humans. Based on animal studies, lamivudine crosses the placenta and is transferred to the fetus [see Nonclinical Toxicology (13.2)].

Antiretroviral Pregnancy Registry: To monitor maternal-fetal outcomes of pregnant women exposed to lamivudine, a Pregnancy Registry has been established. Physicians are encouraged to register patients by calling 1-800-258-4263.

8.3 Nursing Mothers

The Centers for Disease Control and Prevention recommend that HIV-1-infected mothers in the United States not breastfeed their infants to avoid risking postnatal transmission of HIV-1 infection. Because of the potential for serious adverse reactions in nursing infants and HIV-1 transmission, mothers should be instructed not to breastfeed if they are receiving lamivudine.

Lamivudine is excreted into human milk. Samples of breast milk obtained from 20 mothers receiving lamivudine monotherapy (300 mg twice daily) or combination therapy (150 mg lamivudine twice daily and 300 mg zidovudine twice daily) had measurable concentrations of lamivudine.

8.4 Pediatric Use

The safety and effectiveness of twice-daily EPIVIR in combination with other antiretroviral agents have been established in pediatric patients 3 months and older [see Adverse Reactions (6.1), Clinical Pharmacology (12.3), Clinical Studies (14.2)].

8.5 Geriatric Use

Clinical studies of EPIVIR did not include sufficient numbers of subjects aged 65 and over to determine whether they respond differently from younger subjects. In general, dose selection for an elderly patient should be cautious, reflecting the greater frequency of decreased hepatic, renal, or cardiac function, and of concomitant disease or other drug therapy. In particular, because lamivudine is substantially excreted by the kidney and elderly patients are more likely to have decreased renal function, renal function should be monitored and dosage adjustments should be made accordingly [see Dosage and Administration (2.3), Clinical Pharmacology (12.3)].

8.6 Patients With Impaired Renal Function

Reduction of the dosage of EPIVIR is recommended for patients with impaired renal function [see Dosage and Administration (2.3), Clinical Pharmacology (12.3)].

10 OVERDOSAGE

There is no known antidote for EPIVIR. One case of an adult ingesting 6 g of EPIVIR was reported; there were no clinical signs or symptoms noted and hematologic tests remained normal. Two cases of pediatric overdose were reported in Study ACTG300. One case involved a single dose of 7 mg/kg of EPIVIR; the second case involved use of 5 mg/kg of EPIVIR twice daily for 30 days. There were no clinical signs or symptoms noted in either case. Because a negligible amount of lamivudine was removed via (4-hour) hemodialysis, continuous ambulatory peritoneal dialysis, and automated peritoneal dialysis, it is not known if continuous hemodialysis would provide clinical benefit in a lamivudine overdose event. If overdose occurs, the patient should be monitored, and standard supportive treatment applied as required.

11 DESCRIPTION

EPIVIR (also known as 3TC) is a brand name for lamivudine, a synthetic nucleoside analogue with activity against HIV-1 and HBV. The chemical name of lamivudine is (2R,cis)-4-amino-1-(2-hydroxymethyl-1,3-oxathiolan-5-yl)-(1H)-pyrimidin-2-one. Lamivudine is the (-)enantiomer of a dideoxy analogue of cytidine. Lamivudine has also been referred to as (-)2',3'-dideoxy, 3'-thiacytidine. It has a molecular formula of $C_8H_{11}N_3O_3S$ and a molecular weight of 229.3. It has the following structural formula:

Lamivudine is a white to off-white crystalline solid with a solubility of approximately 70 mg/mL in water at 20°C.

EPIVIR Tablets are for oral administration. Each scored 150-mg film-coated tablet contains 150 mg of lamivudine and the inactive ingredients hypromellose, magnesium stearate, microcrystalline cellulose, polyethylene glycol, polysorbate 80, sodium starch glycolate, and titanium dioxide.

Each 300-mg film-coated tablet contains 300 mg of lamivudine and the inactive ingredients black iron oxide, hypromellose, magnesium stearate, microcrystalline cellulose, polyethylene glycol, polysorbate 80, sodium starch glycolate, and titanium dioxide.

EPIVIR Oral Solution is for oral administration. One milliliter (1 mL) of EPIVIR Oral Solution contains 10 mg of lamivudine (10 mg/mL) in an aqueous solution and the inactive ingredients artificial strawberry and banana flavors, citric acid (anhydrous), methylparaben, propylene glycol, propylparaben, sodium citrate (dihydrate), and sucrose (200 mg).

Table 5. Selected Clinical Adverse Reactions and Physical Findings (≥5% Frequency) in Pediatric Patients in Study ACTG300

Adverse Reaction	EPIVIR plus RETROVIR (n = 236)	Didanosine (n = 235)
Body as a Whole		
Fever	25%	32%
Digestive		
Hepatomegaly	11%	11%
Nausea & vomiting	8%	7%
Diarrhea	8%	6%
Stomatitis	6%	12%
Splenomegaly	5%	8%
Respiratory		
Cough	15%	18%
Abnormal breath sounds/wheezing	7%	9%
Ear, Nose, and Throat		
Signs or symptoms of ears[a]	7%	6%
Nasal discharge or congestion	8%	11%
Other		
Skin rashes	12%	14%
Lymphadenopathy	9%	11%

[a] Includes pain, discharge, erythema, or swelling of an ear.

Table 6. Frequencies of Selected Grade 3-4 Laboratory Abnormalities in Pediatric Patients in Study ACTG300

Test (Threshold Level)	EPIVIR plus RETROVIR	Didanosine
Absolute neutrophil count (<400/mm³)	8%	3%
Hemoglobin (<7.0 g/dL)	4%	2%
Platelets (<50,000/mm³)	1%	3%
ALT (>10 × ULN)	1%	3%
AST (>10 × ULN)	2%	4%
Lipase (>2.5 × ULN)	3%	3%
Total Amylase (>2.5 × ULN)	3%	3%

ULN = Upper limit of normal.

Table 7. Pharmacokinetic Parameters (Mean ± SD) After a Single 300-mg Oral Dose of Lamivudine in 3 Groups of Adults With Varying Degrees of Renal Function

Parameter	Creatinine Clearance Criterion (Number of Subjects)		
	>60 mL/min (n = 6)	10-30 mL/min (n = 4)	<10 mL/min (n = 6)
Creatinine clearance (mL/min)	111 ± 14	28 ± 8	6 ± 2
C_{max} (mcg/mL)	2.6 ± 0.5	3.6 ± 0.8	5.8 ± 1.2
AUC_∞ (mcg•hr/mL)	11.0 ± 1.7	48.0 ± 19	157 ± 74
Cl/F (mL/min)	464 ± 76	114 ± 34	36 ± 11

Figure 1. Systemic Clearance (L/hr•kg) of Lamivudine in Relation to Age

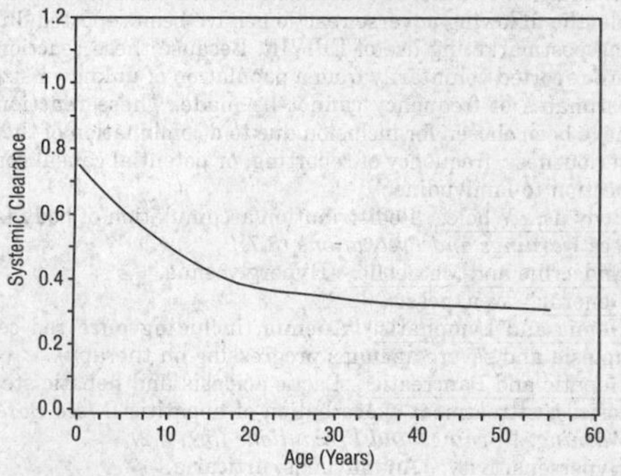

12 CLINICAL PHARMACOLOGY

12.1 Mechanism of Action

Lamivudine is an antiviral agent *[see Clinical Pharmacology (12.4)]*.

12.3 Pharmacokinetics

Pharmacokinetics in Adults: The pharmacokinetic properties of lamivudine have been studied in asymptomatic, HIV-1-infected adult patients after administration of single intravenous (IV) doses ranging from 0.25 to 8 mg/kg, as well as single and multiple (twice-daily regimen) oral doses ranging from 0.25 to 10 mg/kg.

The pharmacokinetic properties of lamivudine have also been studied as single and multiple oral doses ranging from 5 mg to 600 mg/day administered to HBV-infected patients.

The steady-state pharmacokinetic properties of the EPIVIR 300-mg tablet once daily for 7 days compared with the EPIVIR 150-mg tablet twice daily for 7 days were assessed in a crossover study in 60 healthy volunteers. EPIVIR 300 mg once daily resulted in lamivudine exposures that were similar to EPIVIR 150 mg twice daily with respect to plasma $AUC_{24,ss}$; however, $C_{max,ss}$ was 66% higher and the trough value was 53% lower compared with the 150-mg twice-daily regimen. Intracellular lamivudine triphosphate exposures in peripheral blood mononuclear cells were also similar with respect to $AUC_{24,ss}$ and $C_{max24,ss}$; however, trough values were lower compared with the 150-mg twice-daily regimen. Inter-subject variability was greater for intracellular lamivudine triphosphate concentrations versus lamivudine plasma trough concentrations. The clinical significance of observed differences for both plasma lamivudine concentrations and intracellular lamivudine triphosphate concentrations is not known.

Absorption and Bioavailability: Lamivudine was rapidly absorbed after oral administration in HIV-1-infected patients. Absolute bioavailability in 12 adult patients was 86% ± 16% (mean ± SD) for the 150-mg tablet and 87% ± 13% for the oral solution. After oral administration of 2 mg/kg twice a day to 9 adults with HIV-1, the peak serum lamivudine concentration (C_{max}) was 1.5 ± 0.5 mcg/mL (mean ± SD). The area under the plasma concentration versus time curve (AUC) and C_{max} increased in proportion to oral dose over the range from 0.25 to 10 mg/kg.

The accumulation ratio of lamivudine in HIV-1-positive asymptomatic adults with normal renal function was 1.50 following 15 days of oral administration of 2 mg/kg twice daily.

Effects of Food on Oral Absorption: An investigational 25-mg dosage form of lamivudine was administered orally to 12 asymptomatic, HIV-1-infected patients on 2 occasions, once in the fasted state and once with food (1,099 kcal; 75 grams fat, 34 grams protein, 72 grams carbohydrate). Absorption of lamivudine was slower in the fed state (T_{max}: 3.2 ± 1.3 hours) compared with the fasted state (T_{max}: 0.9 ± 0.3 hours); C_{max} in the fed state was 40% ± 23% (mean ± SD) lower than in the fasted state. There was no significant difference in systemic exposure (AUC_∞) in the fed and fasted states; therefore, EPIVIR Tablets and Oral Solution may be administered with or without food.

Distribution: The apparent volume of distribution after IV administration of lamivudine to 20 patients was 1.3 ± 0.4 L/kg, suggesting that lamivudine distributes into extravascular spaces. Volume of distribution was independent of dose and did not correlate with body weight.

Binding of lamivudine to human plasma proteins is low (<36%). In vitro studies showed that over the concentration range of 0.1 to 100 mcg/mL, the amount of lamivudine associated with erythrocytes ranged from 53% to 57% and was independent of concentration.

Metabolism: Metabolism of lamivudine is a minor route of elimination. In man, the only known metabolite of lamivudine is the trans-sulfoxide metabolite. Within 12 hours after a single oral dose of lamivudine in 6 HIV-1-infected adults, 5.2% ± 1.4% (mean ± SD) of the dose was excreted as the trans-sulfoxide metabolite in the urine. Serum concentrations of this metabolite have not been determined.

Elimination: The majority of lamivudine is eliminated unchanged in urine by active organic cationic secretion. In 9 healthy subjects given a single 300-mg oral dose of lamivudine, renal clearance was 199.7 ± 56.9 mL/min (mean ± SD). In 20 HIV-1-infected patients given a single IV dose, renal clearance was 280.4 ± 75.2 mL/min (mean ± SD), representing 71% ± 16% (mean ± SD) of total clearance of lamivudine.

In most single-dose studies in HIV-1-infected patients, HBV-infected patients, or healthy subjects with serum sampling for 24 hours after dosing, the observed mean elimination half-life ($t½$) ranged from 5 to 7 hours. In HIV-1-infected patients, total clearance was 398.5 ± 69.1 mL/min (mean ± SD). Oral clearance and elimination half-life were independent of dose and body weight over an oral dosing range of 0.25 to 10 mg/kg.

Special Populations: *Renal Impairment:* The pharmacokinetic properties of lamivudine have been determined in a small group of HIV-1-infected adults with impaired renal function (Table 7).

[See table 7 above]

Exposure (AUC_∞), C_{max}, and half-life increased with diminishing renal function (as expressed by creatinine clearance). Apparent total oral clearance (Cl/F) of lamivudine decreased as creatinine clearance decreased. T_{max} was not significantly affected by renal function. Based on these observations, it is recommended that the dosage of lamivudine be modified in patients with renal impairment *[see Dosage and Administration (2.3)]*.

Based on a study in otherwise healthy subjects with impaired renal function, hemodialysis increased lamivudine clearance from a mean of 64 to 88 mL/min; however, the length of time of hemodialysis (4 hours) was insufficient to significantly alter mean lamivudine exposure after a single-dose administration. Continuous ambulatory peritoneal dialysis and automated peritoneal dialysis have negligible effects on lamivudine clearance. Therefore, it is recommended, following correction of dose for creatinine clearance, that no additional dose modification be made after routine hemodialysis or peritoneal dialysis.

It is not known whether lamivudine can be removed by continuous (24-hour) hemodialysis.

The effects of renal impairment on lamivudine pharmacokinetics in pediatric patients are not known.

Hepatic Impairment: The pharmacokinetic properties of lamivudine have been determined in adults with impaired hepatic function. Pharmacokinetic parameters were not altered by diminishing hepatic function; therefore, no dose adjustment for lamivudine is required for patients with impaired hepatic function. Safety and efficacy of lamivudine have not been established in the presence of decompensated liver disease.

Pediatric Patients: In Study NUCA2002, pharmacokinetic properties of lamivudine were assessed in a subset of 57 HIV-1-infected pediatric patients (age range: 4.8 months to 16 years, weight range: 5 to 66 kg) after oral and IV administration of 1, 2, 4, 8, 12, and 20 mg/kg/day. In the 9 infants and children (range: 5 months to 12 years of age) receiving oral solution 4 mg/kg twice daily (the usual recommended pediatric dose), absolute bioavailability was 66% ± 26% (mean ± SD), which was less than the 86% ± 16% (mean ± SD) observed in adults. The mechanism for the diminished absolute bioavailability of lamivudine in infants and children is unknown.

Systemic clearance decreased with increasing age in pediatric patients, as shown in Figure 1.

[See figure 1 at top of next column]

After oral administration of lamivudine 4 mg/kg twice daily to 11 pediatric patients ranging from 4 months to 14 years of age, C_{max} was 1.1 ± 0.6 mcg/mL and half-life was 2.0 ± 0.6 hours. (In adults with similar blood sampling, the half-life was 3.7 ± 1 hours.) Total exposure to lamivudine, as reflected by mean AUC values, was comparable between pediatric patients receiving an 8-mg/kg/day dose and adults receiving a 4-mg/kg/day dose.

Distribution of lamivudine into cerebrospinal fluid (CSF) was assessed in 38 pediatric patients after multiple oral dosing with lamivudine. CSF samples were collected between 2 and 4 hours postdose. At the dose of 8 mg/kg/day, CSF lamivudine concentrations in 8 patients ranged from 5.6% to 30.9% (mean ± SD of 14.2% ± 7.9%) of the concentration in a simultaneous serum sample, with CSF lamivudine concentrations ranging from 0.04 to 0.3 mcg/mL.

Limited, uncontrolled pharmacokinetic and safety data are available from administration of lamivudine (and zidovudine) to 36 infants up to 1 week of age in 2 studies in South Africa. In these studies, lamivudine clearance was substantially reduced in 1-week-old neonates relative to pediatric patients (>3 months of age) studied previously. There is insufficient information to establish the time course of changes in clearance between the immediate neonatal period and the age-ranges >3 months old *[see Adverse Reactions (6.1)]*.

Geriatric Patients: The pharmacokinetics of lamivudine after administration of EPIVIR to patients over 65 years of age have not been studied *[see Use in Specific Populations (8.5)]*.

Gender: There are no significant gender differences in lamivudine pharmacokinetics.

Race: There are no significant racial differences in lamivudine pharmacokinetics.

Drug Interactions: *Interferon Alfa:* There was no significant pharmacokinetic interaction between lamivudine and interferon alfa in a study of 19 healthy male subjects *[see Warnings and Precautions (5.4)]*.

Ribavirin: In vitro data indicate ribavirin reduces phosphorylation of lamivudine, stavudine, and zidovudine. However, no pharmacokinetic (e.g., plasma concentrations or intracellular triphosphorylated active metabolite concentrations) or pharmacodynamic (e.g., loss of HIV-1/HCV virologic suppression) interaction was observed when ribavirin and lamivudine (n = 18), stavudine (n = 10), or zidovudine (n = 6) were coadministered as part of a multi-drug regimen to HIV-1/HCV co-infected patients *[see Warnings and Precautions (5.4)]*.

Trimethoprim/Sulfamethoxazole: Lamivudine and TMP/SMX were coadministered to 14 HIV-1-positive patients in a single-center, open-label, randomized, crossover study. Each patient received treatment with a single 300-mg dose of lamivudine and TMP 160 mg/SMX 800 mg once a day for 5 days with concomitant administration of lamivudine 300 mg with the fifth dose in a crossover design. Coadministration of TMP/SMX with lamivudine resulted in an increase of 43% ± 23% (mean ± SD) in lamivudine AUC_∞, a decrease of 29% ± 13% in lamivudine oral clearance, and a decrease of 30% ± 36% in lamivudine renal clearance. The pharmacokinetic properties of TMP and SMX were not altered by coadministration with lamivudine *[see Drug Interactions (7.3)]*.

Zidovudine: No clinically significant alterations in lamivudine or zidovudine pharmacokinetics were observed in 12 asymptomatic HIV-1-infected adult patients given a single dose of zidovudine (200 mg) in combination with multiple doses of lamivudine (300 mg q 12 hr) *[see Drug Interactions (7.4)]*.

12.4 Microbiology

Mechanism of Action: Intracellularly, lamivudine is phosphorylated to its active 5′-triphosphate metabolite, lamivudine triphosphate (3TC-TP). The principal mode of action of 3TC-TP is the inhibition of HIV-1 reverse transcriptase (RT) via DNA chain termination after incorporation of the nucleotide analogue into viral DNA. 3TC-TP is a weak inhibitor of mammalian DNA polymerases α, β, and γ.

Antiviral Activity: The antiviral activity of lamivudine against HIV-1 was assessed in a number of cell lines (including monocytes and fresh human peripheral blood lymphocytes) using standard susceptibility assays. EC_{50} values (50% effective concentrations) were in the range of 0.003 to 15 μM (1 μM = 0.23 mcg/mL). HIV-1 from therapy-naive subjects with no amino acid substitutions associated with resistance gave median EC_{50} values of 0.429 μM (range: 0.200 to 2.007 μM) from Virco (n = 92 baseline samples from COLA40263) and 2.35 μM (1.37 to 3.68 μM) from Monogram Biosciences (n = 135 baseline samples from

ESS30009). The EC_{50} values of lamivudine against different HIV-1 clades (A-G) ranged from 0.001 to 0.120 µM, and against HIV-2 isolates from 0.003 to 0.120 µM in peripheral blood mononuclear cells. Ribavirin (50 µM) decreased the anti-HIV-1 activity of lamivudine by 3.5 fold in MT-4 cells. In HIV-1-infected MT-4 cells, lamivudine in combination with zidovudine at various ratios exhibited synergistic antiretroviral activity. Please see the full prescribing information for EPIVIR-HBV for information regarding the inhibitory activity of lamivudine against HBV.

Resistance: Lamivudine-resistant variants of HIV-1 have been selected in cell culture. Genotypic analysis showed that the resistance was due to a specific amino acid substitution in the HIV-1 reverse transcriptase at codon 184 changing the methionine to either isoleucine or valine (M184V/I).

HIV-1 strains resistant to both lamivudine and zidovudine have been isolated from patients. Susceptibility of clinical isolates to lamivudine and zidovudine was monitored in controlled clinical trials. In patients receiving lamivudine monotherapy or combination therapy with lamivudine plus zidovudine, HIV-1 isolates from most patients became phenotypically and genotypically resistant to lamivudine within 12 weeks. In some patients harboring zidovudine-resistant virus at baseline, phenotypic sensitivity to zidovudine was restored by 12 weeks of treatment with lamivudine and zidovudine. Combination therapy with lamivudine plus zidovudine delayed the emergence of mutations conferring resistance to zidovudine.

Lamivudine-resistant HBV isolates develop substitutions (rtM204V/I) in the YMDD motif of the catalytic domain of the viral reverse transcriptase. rtM204V/I substitutions are frequently accompanied by other substitutions (rtV173L, rtL180M) which enhance the level of lamivudine resistance or act as compensatory mutations improving replication efficiency. Other substitutions detected in lamivudine-resistant HBV isolates include: rtL80I and rtA181T. Similar HBV mutants have been reported in HIV-1-infected patients who received lamivudine-containing antiretroviral regimens in the presence of concurrent infection with hepatitis B virus *[see Warnings and Precautions (5.2)]*.

Cross-Resistance: Lamivudine-resistant HIV-1 mutants were cross-resistant to didanosine (ddI) and zalcitabine (ddC). In some patients treated with zidovudine plus didanosine or zalcitabine, isolates resistant to multiple reverse transcriptase inhibitors, including lamivudine, have emerged.

Genotypic and Phenotypic Analysis of On-Therapy HIV-1 Isolates From Patients With Virologic Failure: *Study EPV20001:* Fifty-three of 554 (10%) patients enrolled in EPV20001 were identified as virological failures (plasma HIV-1 RNA level ≥400 copies/mL) by Week 48. Twenty-eight patients were randomized to the lamivudine once-daily treatment group and 25 to the lamivudine twice-daily treatment group. The median baseline plasma HIV-1 RNA levels of patients in the lamivudine once-daily group and lamivudine twice-daily group were 4.9 $\log_{10}$ copies/mL and 4.6 $\log_{10}$ copies/mL, respectively.

Genotypic analysis of on-therapy isolates from 22 patients identified as virologic failures in the lamivudine once-daily group showed that isolates from 0/22 patients contained treatment-emergent amino acid substitutions associated with zidovudine resistance (M41L, D67N, K70R, L210W, T215Y/F, or K219Q/E), isolates from 10/22 patients contained treatment-emergent amino acid substitutions associated with efavirenz resistance (L100I, K101E, K103N, V108I, or Y181C), and isolates from 8/22 patients contained a treatment-emergent lamivudine resistance-associated substitution (M184I or M184V).

Genotypic analysis of on-therapy isolates from patients (n = 22) in the lamivudine twice-daily treatment group showed that isolates from 1/22 patients contained treatment-emergent zidovudine resistance substitutions, isolates from 7/22 contained treatment-emergent efavirenz resistance substitutions, and isolates from 5/22 contained treatment-emergent lamivudine resistance substitutions.

Phenotypic analysis of baseline-matched on-therapy HIV-1 isolates from patients (n = 13) receiving lamivudine once daily showed that isolates from 12/13 patients were susceptible to zidovudine; isolates from 8/13 patients exhibited a 25- to 295-fold decrease in susceptibility to efavirenz, and isolates from 7/13 patients showed an 85- to 299-fold decrease in susceptibility to lamivudine.

Phenotypic analysis of baseline-matched on-therapy HIV-1 isolates from patients (n = 13) receiving lamivudine twice daily showed that isolates from all 13 patients were susceptible to zidovudine; isolates from 3/13 patients exhibited a 21- to 342-fold decrease in susceptibility to efavirenz, and isolates from 4/13 patients exhibited a 29- to 159-fold decrease in susceptibility to lamivudine.

Study EPV40001: Fifty patients received zidovudine 300 mg twice daily plus abacavir 300 mg twice daily plus lamivudine 300 mg once daily and 50 patients received zidovudine 300 mg plus abacavir 300 mg plus lamivudine

Table 8. Number of Patients (%) With at Least One HIV-1 Disease Progression Event or Death

Endpoint	Current Therapy (n = 460)	EPIVIR plus Current Therapy (n = 896)	EPIVIR plus an NNRTI[a] plus Current Therapy (n = 460)
HIV-1 progression or death	90 (19.6%)	86 (9.6%)	41 (8.9%)
Death	27 (5.9%)	23 (2.6%)	14 (3.0%)

[a] An investigational non-nucleoside reverse transcriptase inhibitor not approved in the United States.

Table 9. Outcomes of Randomized Treatment Through 48 Weeks (Intent-to-Treat)

Outcome	EPIVIR 300 mg Once Daily plus RETROVIR plus Efavirenz (n = 278)	EPIVIR 150 mg Twice Daily plus RETROVIR plus Efavirenz (n = 276)
Responder[a]	67%	65%
Virologic failure[b]	8%	8%
Discontinued due to clinical progression	<1%	0%
Discontinued due to adverse events	6%	12%
Discontinued due to other reasons[c]	18%	14%

[a]Achieved confirmed plasma HIV-1 RNA <400 copies/mL and maintained through 48 weeks.
[b]Achieved suppression but rebounded by Week 48, discontinued due to virologic failure, insufficient viral response according to the investigator, or never suppressed through Week 48.
[c]Includes consent withdrawn, lost to followup, protocol violation, data outside the study-defined schedule, and randomized but never initiated treatment.

150 mg all twice daily. The median baseline plasma HIV-1 RNA levels for patients in the 2 groups were 4.79 $\log_{10}$ copies/mL and 4.83 $\log_{10}$ copies/mL, respectively. Fourteen of 50 patients in the lamivudine once-daily treatment group and 9 of 50 patients in the lamivudine twice-daily group were identified as virologic failures.

Genotypic analysis of on-therapy HIV-1 isolates from patients (n = 9) in the lamivudine once-daily treatment group showed that isolates from 6 patients had an abacavir and/or lamivudine resistance-associated substitution M184V alone. On-therapy isolates from patients (n = 6) receiving lamivudine twice daily showed that isolates from 2 patients had M184V alone, and isolates from 2 patients harbored the M184V substitution in combination with zidovudine resistance-associated amino acid substitutions.

Phenotypic analysis of on-therapy isolates from patients (n = 6) receiving lamivudine once daily showed that HIV-1 isolates from 4 patients exhibited a 32- to 53-fold decrease in susceptibility to lamivudine. HIV-1 isolates from these 6 patients were susceptible to zidovudine.

Phenotypic analysis of on-therapy isolates from patients (n = 4) receiving lamivudine twice daily showed that HIV-1 isolates from 1 patient exhibited a 45-fold decrease in susceptibility to lamivudine and a 4.5-fold decrease in susceptibility to zidovudine.

13 NONCLINICAL TOXICOLOGY

13.1 Carcinogenesis, Mutagenesis, Impairment of Fertility

Long-term carcinogenicity studies with lamivudine in mice and rats showed no evidence of carcinogenic potential at exposures up to 10 times (mice) and 58 times (rats) those observed in humans at the recommended therapeutic dose for HIV-1 infection. Lamivudine was not active in a microbial mutagenicity screen or an in vitro cell transformation assay, but showed weak in vitro mutagenic activity in a cytogenetic assay using cultured human lymphocytes and in the mouse lymphoma assay. However, lamivudine showed no evidence of in vivo genotoxic activity in the rat at oral doses of up to 2,000 mg/kg, producing plasma levels of 35 to 45 times those in humans at the recommended dose for HIV-1 infection. In a study of reproductive performance, lamivudine administered to rats at doses up to 4,000 mg/kg/day, producing plasma levels 47 to 70 times those in humans, revealed no evidence of impaired fertility and no effect on the survival, growth, and development to weaning of the offspring.

13.2 Reproductive Toxicology Studies

Reproduction studies have been performed in rats and rabbits at orally administered doses up to 4,000 mg/kg/day and 1,000 mg/kg/day, respectively, producing plasma levels up to approximately 35 times that for the adult HIV dose. No evidence of teratogenicity due to lamivudine was observed. Evidence of early embryolethality was seen in the rabbit at exposure levels similar to those observed in humans, but there was no indication of this effect in the rat at exposure levels up to 35 times those in humans. Studies in pregnant rats and rabbits showed that lamivudine is transferred to the fetus through the placenta.

14 CLINICAL STUDIES

The use of EPIVIR is based on the results of clinical studies in HIV-1-infected patients in combination regimens with other antiretroviral agents. Information from trials with clinical endpoints or a combination of CD4+ cell counts and HIV-1 RNA measurements is included below as documentation of the contribution of lamivudine to a combination regimen in controlled trials.

14.1 Adults

Clinical Endpoint Study: NUCB3007 (CAESAR) was a multi-center, double-blind, placebo-controlled study comparing continued current therapy (zidovudine alone [62% of patients] or zidovudine with didanosine or zalcitabine [38% of patients]) to the addition of EPIVIR or EPIVIR plus an investigational non-nucleoside reverse transcriptase inhibitor (NNRTI), randomized 1:2:1. A total of 1,816 HIV-1-infected adults with 25 to 250 CD4+ cells/mm^3 (median = 122 cells/mm^3) at baseline were enrolled: median age was 36 years, 87% were male, 84% were nucleoside-experienced, and 16% were therapy-naive. The median duration on study was 12 months. Results are summarized in Table 8.

[See table 8 above]

Surrogate Endpoint Studies: *Dual Nucleoside Analogue Studies:* Principal clinical trials in the initial development of lamivudine compared lamivudine/zidovudine combinations with zidovudine monotherapy or with zidovudine plus zalcitabine. These studies demonstrated the antiviral effect of lamivudine in a 2-drug combination. More recent uses of lamivudine in treatment of HIV-1 infection incorporate it into multiple-drug regimens containing at least 3 antiretroviral drugs for enhanced viral suppression.

Dose Regimen Comparison Surrogate Endpoint Studies in Therapy-Naive Adults: EPV20001 was a multi-center, double-blind, controlled study in which patients were randomized 1:1 to receive EPIVIR 300 mg once daily or EPIVIR 150 mg twice daily, in combination with zidovudine 300 mg twice daily and efavirenz 600 mg once daily. A total of 554 antiretroviral treatment-naive HIV-1-infected adults enrolled: male (79%), Caucasian (50%), median age of 35 years, baseline CD4+ cell counts of 69 to 1,089 cells/mm^3 (median = 362 cells/mm^3), and median baseline plasma HIV-1 RNA of 4.66 $\log_{10}$ copies/mL. Outcomes of treatment through 48 weeks are summarized in Figure 2 and Table 9.

Figure 2. Virologic Response Through Week 48, EPV20001[a,b] (Intent-to-Treat)

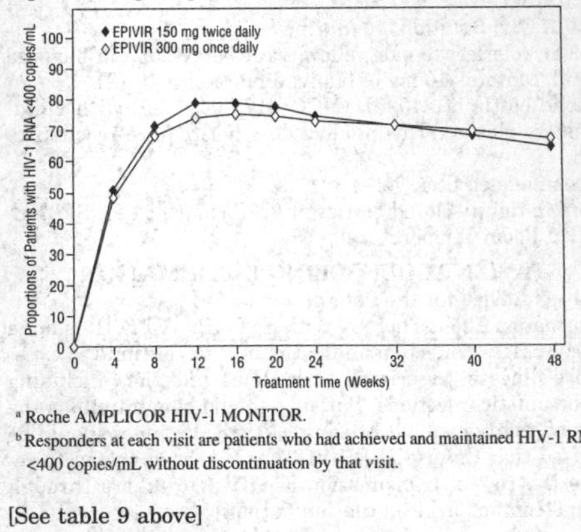

[a] Roche AMPLICOR HIV-1 MONITOR.
[b] Responders at each visit are patients who had achieved and maintained HIV-1 RNA <400 copies/mL without discontinuation by that visit.

[See table 9 above]

Table 10. Number of Patients (%) Reaching a Primary Clinical Endpoint (Disease Progression or Death)

Endpoint	EPIVIR plus RETROVIR (n = 236)	Didanosine (n = 235)
HIV disease progression or death (total)	15 (6.4%)	37 (15.7%)
Physical growth failure	7 (3.0%)	6 (2.6%)
Central nervous system deterioration	4 (1.7%)	12 (5.1%)
CDC Clinical Category C	2 (0.8%)	8 (3.4%)
Death	2 (0.8%)	11 (4.7%)

The proportions of patients with HIV-1 RNA <50 copies/mL (via Roche Ultrasensitive assay) through Week 48 were 61% for patients receiving EPIVIR 300 mg once daily and 63% for patients receiving EPIVIR 150 mg twice daily. Median increases in CD4+ cell counts were 144 cells/mm^3 at Week 48 in patients receiving EPIVIR 300 mg once daily and 146 cells/mm^3 for patients receiving EPIVIR 150 mg twice daily.

A small, randomized, open-label pilot study, EPV40001, was conducted in Thailand. A total of 159 treatment-naive adult patients (male 32%, Asian 100%, median age 30 years, baseline median CD4+ cell count 380 cells/mm^3, median plasma HIV-1 RNA 4.8 log$_{10}$ copies/mL) were enrolled. Two of the treatment arms in this study provided a comparison between lamivudine 300 mg once daily (n = 54) and lamivudine 150 mg twice daily (n = 52), each in combination with zidovudine 300 mg twice daily and abacavir 300 mg twice daily. In intent-to-treat analyses of 48-week data, the proportions of patients with HIV-1 RNA below 400 copies/mL were 61% (33/54) in the group randomized to once-daily lamivudine and 75% (39/52) in the group randomized to receive all 3 drugs twice daily; the proportions with HIV-1 RNA below 50 copies/mL were 54% (29/54) in the once-daily lamivudine group and 67% (35/52) in the all-twice-daily group; and the median increases in CD4+ cell counts were 166 cells/mm^3 in the once-daily lamivudine group and 216 cells/mm^3 in the all-twice-daily group.

14.2   Pediatric Patients

Clinical Endpoint Study: ACTG300 was a multi-center, randomized, double-blind study that provided for comparison of EPIVIR plus RETROVIR (zidovudine) with didanosine monotherapy. A total of 471 symptomatic, HIV-1-infected therapy-naive pediatric patients (≤56 days of antiretroviral therapy) were enrolled in these 2 treatment arms. The median age was 2.7 years (range: 6 weeks to 14 years), 58% were female, and 86% were non-Caucasian. The mean baseline CD4+ cell count was 868 cells/mm^3 (mean: 1,060 cells/mm^3 and range: 0 to 4,650 cells/mm^3 for patients ≤5 years of age; mean: 419 cells/mm^3 and range: 0 to 1,555 cells/mm^3 for patients >5 years of age) and the mean baseline plasma HIV-1 RNA was 5.0 log$_{10}$ copies/mL. The median duration on study was 10.1 months for the patients receiving EPIVIR plus RETROVIR and 9.2 months for patients receiving didanosine monotherapy. Results are summarized in Table 10.
[See table 10 above]

16   HOW SUPPLIED/STORAGE AND HANDLING

EPIVIR Scored Tablets, 150 mg

White, diamond-shaped, scored, film-coated tablets debossed with "GX CJ7" on both sides.
Bottle of 60 tablets (NDC 0173-0470-01) with child-resistant closure.

EPIVIR Tablets, 300 mg

Gray, modified diamond-shaped, film-coated tablets engraved with "GX EJ7" on one side and plain on the reverse side.
Bottle of 30 tablets (NDC 0173-0714-00) with child-resistant closure.

Recommended Storage:
Store EPIVIR Tablets at 25°C (77°F); excursions permitted to 15° to 30°C (59° to 86°F) [see USP Controlled Room Temperature].

EPIVIR Oral Solution, 10 mg/mL

A clear, colorless to pale yellow, strawberry-banana-flavored liquid, contains 10 mg of lamivudine in each 1 mL.
Plastic bottle of 240 mL (NDC 0173-0471-00) with child-resistant closure. This product does not require reconstitution.

Recommended Storage:
Store in tightly closed bottles at 25°C (77°F) [see USP Controlled Room Temperature].

17   PATIENT COUNSELING INFORMATION

17.1   Advice for the Patient

Information About Therapy With EPIVIR: EPIVIR is not a cure for HIV-1 infection and patients may continue to experience illnesses associated with HIV-1 infection, including opportunistic infections. Patients should remain under the care of a physician when using EPIVIR. Patients should be advised that the use of EPIVIR has not been shown to reduce the risk of transmission of HIV-1 to others through sexual contact or blood contamination.

Patients should be advised that the long-term effects of EPIVIR are unknown at this time.
Patients should be advised of the importance of taking EPIVIR with combination therapy on a regular dosing schedule and to avoid missing doses.
EPIVIR should not be coadministered with drugs containing lamivudine or emtricitabine, including COMBIVIR (lamivudine/zidovudine) Tablets, EPZICOM (abacavir sulfate and lamivudine) Tablets, TRIZIVIR (abacavir sulfate, lamivudine, and zidovudine), ATRIPLA (efavirenz, emtricitabine, and tenofovir), EMTRIVA (emtricitabine) or TRUVADA (emtricitabine and tenofovir) [see Warnings and Precautions (5.3)].
Redistribution/Accumulation of Body Fat: Patients should be informed that redistribution or accumulation of body fat may occur in patients receiving antiretroviral therapy, including EPIVIR, and that the cause and long-term health effects of these conditions are not known at this time [see Warnings and Precautions (5.7)].
Differences in Formulations of EPIVIR: Patients should be advised that EPIVIR Tablets and Oral Solution contain a higher dose of the same active ingredient (lamivudine) as EPIVIR-HBV Tablets and Oral Solution. If a decision is made to include lamivudine in the HIV-1 treatment regimen of a patient co-infected with HIV-1 and HBV, the formulation and dosage of lamivudine in EPIVIR (not EPIVIR-HBV) should be used [see Warnings and Precautions (5.2)].
Co-infection With HIV-1 and HBV: Patients co-infected with HIV-1 and HBV should be informed that deterioration of liver disease has occurred in some cases when treatment with lamivudine was discontinued. Patients should be advised to discuss any changes in regimen with their physician [see Warnings and Precautions (5.2)].
Risk of Pancreatitis: Parents or guardians should be advised to monitor pediatric patients for signs and symptoms of pancreatitis [see Warnings and Precautions (5.5)].
Sucrose Content of EPIVIR Oral Solution: Diabetic patients should be advised that each 15-mL dose of EPIVIR Oral Solution contains 3 grams of sucrose [see Description (11)].
COMBIVIR, EPIVIR, EPIVIR-HBV, EPZICOM, and TRIZIVIR are registered trademarks of GlaxoSmithKline. ATRIPLA, EMTRIVA, and TRUVADA are trademarks of their respective owners and are not trademarks of GlaxoSmithKline. The makers of these brands are not affiliated with and do not endorse GlaxoSmithKline or its products.

GlaxoSmithKline
Research Triangle Park, NC 27709
Manufactured under agreement from
Shire Pharmaceuticals Group plc
Basingstoke, UK

EPZICOM®   ℞

[ep' zih com]
**(abacavir sulfate and lamivudine)
Tablets**

WARNINGS

EPZICOM contains 2 nucleoside analogues (abacavir sulfate and lamivudine) and is intended only for patients whose regimen would otherwise include these 2 components.

Hypersensitivity Reactions: Serious and sometimes fatal hypersensitivity reactions have been associated with abacavir sulfate, a component of EPZICOM. Hypersensitivity to abacavir is a multi-organ clinical syndrome usually characterized by a sign or symptom in 2 or more of the following groups: (1) fever, (2) rash, (3) gastrointestinal (including nausea, vomiting, diarrhea, or abdominal pain), (4) constitutional (including generalized malaise, fatigue, or achiness), and (5) respiratory (including dyspnea, cough, or pharyngitis). Discontinue EPZICOM as soon as a hypersensitivity reaction is suspected.

Patients who carry the HLA-B*5701 allele are at high risk for experiencing a hypersensitivity reaction to

---

abacavir. Prior to initiating therapy with abacavir, screening for the HLA-B*5701 allele is recommended; this approach has been found to decrease the risk of hypersensitivity reaction. Screening is also recommended prior to reinitiation of abacavir in patients of unknown HLA-B*5701 status who have previously tolerated abacavir. HLA-B*5701-negative patients may develop a suspected hypersensitivity reaction to abacavir; however, this occurs significantly less frequently than in HLA-B*5701-positive patients.

Regardless of HLA-B*5701 status, permanently discontinue EPZICOM if hypersensitivity cannot be ruled out, even when other diagnoses are possible.

Following a hypersensitivity reaction to abacavir, NEVER restart EPZICOM or any other abacavir-containing product because more severe symptoms can occur within hours and may include life-threatening hypotension and death.

Reintroduction of EPZICOM or any other abacavir-containing product, even in patients who have no identified history or unrecognized symptoms of hypersensitivity to abacavir therapy, can result in serious or fatal hypersensitivity reactions. Such reactions can occur within hours (see WARNINGS and PRECAUTIONS: Information for Patients).

Lactic Acidosis and Severe Hepatomegaly: Lactic acidosis and severe hepatomegaly with steatosis, including fatal cases, have been reported with the use of nucleoside analogues alone or in combination, including abacavir, lamivudine, and other antiretrovirals (see WARNINGS).

Exacerbations of Hepatitis B: Severe acute exacerbations of hepatitis B have been reported in patients who are co-infected with hepatitis B virus (HBV) and human immunodeficiency virus (HIV-1) and have discontinued lamivudine, which is one component of EPZICOM. Hepatic function should be monitored closely with both clinical and laboratory follow-up for at least several months in patients who discontinue EPZICOM and are co-infected with HIV-1 and HBV. If appropriate, initiation of anti-hepatitis B therapy may be warranted (see WARNINGS).

DESCRIPTION

EPZICOM:

EPZICOM Tablets contain the following 2 synthetic nucleoside analogues: abacavir sulfate (ZIAGEN®, also a component of TRIZIVIR®) and lamivudine (also known as EPIVIR® or 3TC) with inhibitory activity against HIV-1.
EPZICOM Tablets are for oral administration. Each orange, film-coated tablet contains the active ingredients 600 mg of abacavir as abacavir sulfate and 300 mg of lamivudine, and the inactive ingredients magnesium stearate, microcrystalline cellulose, and sodium starch glycolate. The tablets are coated with a film (OPADRY® orange YS-1-13065-A) that is made of FD&C Yellow No. 6, hypromellose, polyethylene glycol 400, polysorbate 80, and titanium dioxide.

Abacavir Sulfate:

The chemical name of abacavir sulfate is (1S,cis)-4-[2-amino-6-(cyclopropylamino)-9H-purin-9-yl]-2-cyclopentene-1-methanol sulfate (salt) (2:1). Abacavir sulfate is the enantiomer with 1S, 4R absolute configuration on the cyclopentene ring. It has a molecular formula of $(C_{14}H_{18}N_6O)_2 \cdot H_2SO_4$ and a molecular weight of 670.76 daltons. It has the following structural formula:

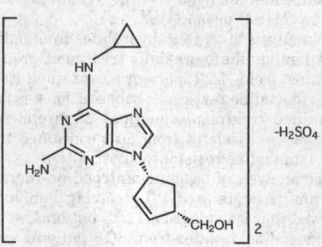

Abacavir sulfate is a white to off-white solid with a solubility of approximately 77 mg/mL in distilled water at 25°C.
In vivo, abacavir sulfate dissociates to its free base, abacavir. All dosages for abacavir sulfate are expressed in terms of abacavir.

Lamivudine:

The chemical name of lamivudine is (2R,cis)-4-amino-1-(2-hydroxymethyl-1,3-oxathiolan-5-yl)-(1H)-pyrimidin-2-one. Lamivudine is the (-)-enantiomer of a dideoxy analogue of cytidine. Lamivudine has also been referred to as (-)2′,3′-dideoxy, 3′-thiacytidine. It has a molecular formula of

---

$C_8H_{11}N_3O_3S$ and a molecular weight of 229.3 daltons. It has the following structural formula:

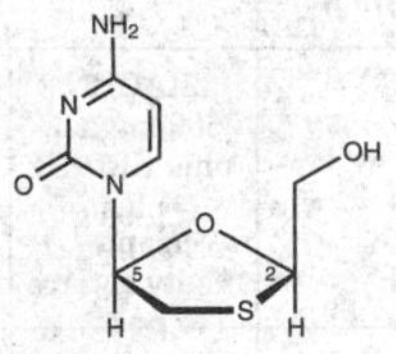

Lamivudine is a white to off-white crystalline solid with a solubility of approximately 70 mg/mL in water at 20°C.

MICROBIOLOGY

Mechanism of Action:

Abacavir is a carbocyclic synthetic nucleoside analogue. Abacavir is converted by cellular enzymes to the active metabolite, carbovir triphosphate (CBV-TP), an analogue of deoxyguanosine-5′-triphosphate (dGTP). CBV-TP inhibits the activity of HIV-1 reverse transcriptase (RT) both by competing with the natural substrate dGTP and by its incorporation into viral DNA. The lack of a 3′-OH group in the incorporated nucleotide analogue prevents the formation of the 5′ to 3′ phosphodiester linkage essential for DNA chain elongation, and therefore, the viral DNA growth is terminated. CBV-TP is a weak inhibitor of cellular DNA polymerases α, β, and γ.

Lamivudine is a synthetic nucleoside analogue. Intracellularly lamivudine is phosphorylated to its active 5′-triphosphate metabolite, lamivudine triphosphate (3TC-TP). The principal mode of action of 3TC-TP is inhibition of RT via DNA chain termination after incorporation of the nucleotide analogue. CBV-TP and 3TC-TP are weak inhibitors of cellular DNA polymerases α, β, and γ.

Antiviral Activity:

Abacavir:

The antiviral activity of abacavir against HIV-1 was evaluated against a T-cell tropic laboratory strain HIV-1_{IIIB} in lymphoblastic cell lines, a monocyte/macrophage tropic laboratory strain HIV-1_{BaL} in primary monocytes/macrophages, and clinical isolates in peripheral blood mononuclear cells. The concentration of drug necessary to effect viral replication by 50 percent (EC_{50}) ranged from 3.7 to 5.8 μM (1 μM = 0.28 mcg/mL) and 0.07 to 1.0 μM against HIV-1_{IIIB} and HIV-1_{BaL}, respectively, and was 0.26 ± 0.18 μM against 8 clinical isolates. The EC_{50} values of abacavir against different HIV-1 clades (A-G) ranged from 0.0015 to 1.05 μM, and against HIV-2 isolates, from 0.024 to 0.49 μM. Ribavirin (50 μM) had no effect on the anti–HIV-1 activity of abacavir in cell culture.

Lamivudine:

The antiviral activity of lamivudine against HIV-1 was assessed in a number of cell lines (including monocytes and fresh human peripheral blood lymphocytes) using standard susceptibility assays. EC_{50} values were in the range of 0.003 to 15 μM (1 μM = 0.23 mcg/mL). HIV-1 from therapy-naive subjects with no amino acid substitutions associated with resistance gave median EC_{50} values of 0.429 μM (range: 0.200 to 2.007 μM) from Virco (n = 92 baseline samples from COLA40263) and 2.35 μM (1.37 to 3.68 μM) from Monogram Biosciences (n = 135 baseline samples from ESS30009). The EC_{50} values of lamivudine against different HIV-1 clades (A-G) ranged from 0.001 to 0.120 μM, and against HIV-2 isolates from 0.003 to 0.120 μM in peripheral blood mononuclear cells. Ribavirin (50 μM) decreased the anti–HIV-1 activity of lamivudine by 3.5 fold in MT-4 cells.

The combination of abacavir and lamivudine has demonstrated antiviral activity in cell culture against non-subtype B isolates and HIV-2 isolates with equivalent antiviral activity as for subtype B isolates. Abacavir/lamivudine had additive to synergistic activity in cell culture in combination with the nucleoside reverse transcriptase inhibitors (NRTIs) emtricitabine, stavudine, tenofovir, zalcitabine, zidovudine; the non-nucleoside reverse transcriptase inhibitors (NNRTIs) delavirdine, efavirenz, nevirapine; the protease inhibitors (PIs) amprenavir, indinavir, lopinavir, nelfinavir, ritonavir, saquinavir; or the fusion inhibitor, enfuvirtide. Ribavirin, used in combination with interferon for the treatment of HCV infection, decreased the anti-HIV-1 potency of abacavir/lamivudine reproducibly by 2- to 6-fold in cell culture.

Resistance:

HIV-1 isolates with reduced susceptibility to the combination of abacavir and lamivudine have been selected in cell culture and have also been obtained from patients failing abacavir/lamivudine-containing regimens. Genotypic characterization of abacavir/lamivudine-resistant viruses selected in cell culture identified amino acid substitutions M184V/I, K65R, L74V, and Y115F in HIV-1 RT.

Table 1. Pharmacokinetic Parameters* for Abacavir and Lamivudine in Adults

Parameter	Abacavir		Lamivudine	
Oral bioavailability (%)	86 ± 25	n = 6	86 ± 16	n = 12
Apparent volume of distribution (L/kg)	0.86 ± 0.15	n = 6	1.3 ± 0.4	n = 20
Systemic clearance (L/hr/kg)	0.80 ± 0.24	n = 6	0.33 ± 0.06	n = 20
Renal clearance (L/hr/kg)	.007 ± .008	n = 6	0.22 ± 0.06	n = 20
Elimination half-life (hr)	1.45 ± 0.32	n = 20	5 to 7†	

* Data presented as mean ± standard deviation except where noted.
† Approximate range.

Genotypic analysis of isolates selected in cell culture and recovered from abacavir-treated patients demonstrated that amino acid substitutions K65R, L74V, Y115F, and M184V/I in HIV-1 RT contributed to abacavir resistance. Genotypic analysis of isolates selected in cell culture and recovered from lamivudine-treated patients showed that the resistance was due to a specific amino acid substitution in HIV-1 RT at codon 184 changing the methionine to either isoleucine or valine (M184V/I). In a study of therapy-naive adults receiving ZIAGEN 600 mg once daily (n = 384) or 300 mg twice daily (n = 386) in a background regimen of lamivudine 300 mg and efavirenz 600 mg once daily (Study CNA30021), the incidence of virologic failure at 48 weeks was similar between the 2 groups (11% in both arms). Genotypic (n = 38) and phenotypic analyses (n = 35) of virologic failure isolates from this study showed that the RT substitutions that emerged during abacavir/lamivudine once-daily and twice-daily therapy were K65R, L74V, Y115F, and M184V/I. The abacavir- and lamivudine-associated resistance substitution M184V/I was the most commonly observed substitution in virologic failure isolates from patients receiving abacavir/lamivudine once daily (56%, 10/18) and twice daily (40%, 8/20).

Thirty-nine percent (7/18) of the isolates from patients who experienced virologic failure in the abacavir once-daily arm had a >2.5-fold decrease in abacavir susceptibility with a median-fold decrease of 1.3 (range: 0.5 to 11) compared with 29% (5/17) of the failure isolates in the twice-daily arm with a median-fold decrease of 0.92 (range: 0.7 to 13). Fifty-six percent (10/18) of the virologic failure isolates in the once-daily abacavir group compared with 41% (7/17) of the failure isolates in the twice-daily abacavir group had a >2.5-fold decrease in lamivudine susceptibility with median-fold changes of 81 (range 0.79 to >116) and 1.1 (range 0.68 to >116) in the once-daily and twice-daily abacavir arms, respectively.

Cross-Resistance:

Cross-resistance has been observed among NRTIs. Viruses containing abacavir and lamivudine resistance-associated amino acid substitutions, namely, K65R, L74V, M184V, and Y115F, exhibit cross-resistance to didanosine, emtricitabine, lamivudine, tenofovir, and zalcitabine in cell culture and in patients. The K65R substitution can confer resistance to abacavir, didanosine, emtricitabine, lamivudine, stavudine, tenofovir, and zalcitabine; the L74V substitution can confer resistance to abacavir, didanosine, and zalcitabine; and the M184V substitution can confer resistance to abacavir, didanosine, emtricitabine, lamivudine, and zalcitabine.

The combination of abacavir/lamivudine has demonstrated decreased susceptibility to viruses with the substitutions K65R with or without the M184V/I substitution, viruses with L74V plus the M184V/I substitution, and viruses with thymidine analog mutations (TAMs: M41L, D67N, K70R, L210W, T215Y/F, K219 E/R/H/Q/N) plus M184V. An increasing number of TAMs is associated with a progressive reduction in abacavir susceptibility.

CLINICAL PHARMACOLOGY

Pharmacokinetics in Adults:

EPZICOM:

In a single-dose, 3-way crossover bioavailability study of 1 EPZICOM Tablet versus 2 ZIAGEN Tablets (2 × 300 mg) and 2 EPIVIR Tablets (2 × 150 mg) administered simultaneously in healthy subjects (n = 25), there was no difference in the extent of absorption, as measured by the area under the plasma concentration-time curve (AUC) and maximal peak concentration (C_{max}), of each component.

Abacavir:

Following oral administration, abacavir is rapidly absorbed and extensively distributed. After oral administration of a single dose of 600 mg of abacavir in 20 patients, C_{max} was 4.26 ± 1.19 mcg/mL (mean ± SD) and AUC_{∞} was 11.95 ± 2.51 mcg•hr/mL. Binding of abacavir to human plasma proteins is approximately 50% and was independent of concentration. Total blood and plasma drug-related radioactivity concentrations are identical, demonstrating that abacavir readily distributes into erythrocytes. The primary routes of elimination of abacavir are metabolism by alcohol dehydrogenase to form the 5′-carboxylic acid and glucuronyl transferase to form the 5′-glucuronide.

Lamivudine:

Following oral administration, lamivudine is rapidly absorbed and extensively distributed. After multiple-dose oral administration of lamivudine 300 mg once daily for 7 days to 60 healthy volunteers, steady-state C_{max} ($C_{max,ss}$) was 2.04 ± 0.54 mcg/mL (mean ± SD) and the 24-hour steady-state AUC ($AUC_{24,ss}$) was 8.87 ± 1.83 mcg•hr/mL. Binding to plasma protein is low. Approximately 70% of an intravenous dose of lamivudine is recovered as unchanged drug in the urine. Metabolism of lamivudine is a minor route of elimination. In humans, the only known metabolite is the trans-sulfoxide metabolite (approximately 5% of an oral dose after 12 hours).

The steady-state pharmacokinetic properties of the EPIVIR 300-mg Tablet once daily for 7 days compared with the EPIVIR 150-mg Tablet twice daily for 7 days were assessed in a crossover study in 60 healthy volunteers. EPIVIR 300 mg once daily resulted in lamivudine exposures that were similar to EPIVIR 150 mg twice daily with respect to plasma $AUC_{24,ss}$; however, $C_{max,ss}$ was 66% higher and the trough value was 53% lower compared with the 150-mg twice-daily regimen. Intracellular lamivudine triphosphate exposures in peripheral blood mononuclear cells were also similar with respect to $AUC_{24,ss}$ and $C_{max24,ss}$; however, trough values were lower compared with the 150-mg twice-daily regimen. Inter-subject variability was greater for intracellular lamivudine triphosphate concentrations versus lamivudine plasma trough concentrations. The clinical significance of observed differences for both plasma lamivudine concentrations and intracellular lamivudine triphosphate concentrations is not known.

In humans, abacavir and lamivudine are not significantly metabolized by cytochrome P450 enzymes.

The pharmacokinetic properties of abacavir and lamivudine in fasting patients are summarized in Table 1.

[See table 1 above]

Effect of Food on Absorption of EPZICOM:

EPZICOM may be administered with or without food. Administration with a high-fat meal in a single-dose bioavailability study resulted in no change in AUC_{last}, AUC_{∞}, and C_{max} for lamivudine. Food did not alter the extent of systemic exposure to abacavir (AUC∞), but the rate of absorption (C_{max}) was decreased approximately 24% compared with fasted conditions (n = 25). These results are similar to those from previous studies of the effect of food on abacavir and lamivudine tablets administered separately.

Special Populations:

Impaired Renal Function:

EPZICOM: Because lamivudine requires dose adjustment in the presence of renal insufficiency, EPZICOM is not recommended for use in patients with creatinine clearance <50 mL/min (see PRECAUTIONS).

Impaired Hepatic Function:

EPZICOM: Abacavir is contraindicated in patients with moderate to severe hepatic impairment and dose reduction is required in patients with mild hepatic impairment. Because EPZICOM is a fixed-dose combination and cannot be dose adjusted, EPZICOM is contraindicated for patients with hepatic impairment.

Pregnancy:

See PRECAUTIONS: Pregnancy.

Abacavir and Lamivudine: No data are available on the pharmacokinetics of abacavir or lamivudine during pregnancy.

Nursing Mothers:

See PRECAUTIONS: Nursing Mothers.

Abacavir: No data are available on the pharmacokinetics of abacavir in nursing mothers.

Table 2. Effect of Coadministered Drugs on Abacavir and Lamivudine AUC*

Note: ROUTINE DOSE MODIFICATION OF ABACAVIR AND LAMIVUDINE IS NOT WARRANTED WITH COADMINISTRATION OF THE FOLLOWING DRUGS.

Drugs That May Alter Abacavir Blood Concentrations

Coadministered Drug and Dose	Abacavir Dose	n	Abacavir Concentrations AUC	Abacavir Concentrations Variability	Concentration of Coadministered Drug
Ethanol 0.7 g/kg	Single 600 mg	24	↑41%	90% CI: 35% to 48%	↔

Drugs That May Alter Lamivudine Blood Concentrations

Coadministered Drug and Dose	Lamivudine Dose	n	Lamivudine Concentrations AUC	Lamivudine Concentrations Variability	Concentration of Coadministered Drug
Nelfinavir 750 mg q 8 hr × 7 to 10 days	Single 150 mg	11	↑10%	95% CI: 1% to 20%	↔
Trimethoprim 160 mg/ Sulfamethoxazole 800 mg daily × 5 days	Single 300 mg	14	↑43%	90% CI: 32% to 55%	↔

↑ = Increase; ↔ = no significant change; AUC = area under the concentration versus time curve; CI = confidence interval.
* See PRECAUTIONS: Drug Interactions for additional information on drug interactions.

Lamivudine: Samples of breast milk obtained from 20 mothers receiving lamivudine monotherapy (300 mg twice daily) or combination therapy (150 mg lamivudine twice daily and 300 mg zidovudine twice daily) had measurable concentrations of lamivudine.

Pediatric Patients:
EPZICOM: The pharmacokinetics of EPZICOM in pediatric patients are under investigation. There are insufficient data at this time to recommend a dose (see PRECAUTIONS: Pediatric Use).

Geriatric Patients:
The pharmacokinetics of abacavir and lamivudine have not been studied in patients over 65 years of age.

Gender:
Abacavir: A population pharmacokinetic analysis in HIV-1-infected male (n = 304) and female (n = 67) patients showed no gender differences in abacavir AUC normalized for lean body weight.
Lamivudine: A pharmacokinetic study in healthy male (n = 12) and female (n = 12) subjects showed no gender differences in lamivudine AUC∞ normalized for body weight.

Race:
Abacavir: There are no significant differences between blacks and Caucasians in abacavir pharmacokinetics.
Lamivudine: There are no significant racial differences in lamivudine pharmacokinetics.

Drug Interactions:
See PRECAUTIONS: Drug Interactions. The drug interactions described are based on studies conducted with the individual nucleoside analogues. In humans, abacavir and lamivudine are not significantly metabolized by cytochrome P450 enzymes nor do they inhibit or induce this enzyme system; therefore, it is unlikely that clinically significant drug interactions will occur with drugs metabolized through these pathways.

Abacavir:
Fifteen HIV-1-infected patients were enrolled in a crossover-designed drug interaction study evaluating single doses of abacavir (600 mg), lamivudine (150 mg), and zidovudine (300 mg) alone or in combination. Analysis showed no clinically relevant changes in the pharmacokinetics of abacavir with the addition of lamivudine or zidovudine or the combination of lamivudine and zidovudine. Lamivudine exposure (AUC decreased 15%) and zidovudine exposure (AUC increased 10%) did not show clinically relevant changes with concurrent abacavir.
In a study of 11 HIV-1-infected patients receiving methadone-maintenance therapy (40 mg and 90 mg daily), with 600 mg of ZIAGEN twice daily (twice the currently recommended dose), oral methadone clearance increased 22% (90% CI: 6% to 42%). This alteration will not result in a methadone dose modification in the majority of patients; however, an increased methadone dose may be required in a small number of patients.

Lamivudine:
No clinically significant alterations in lamivudine or zidovudine pharmacokinetics were observed in 12 asymptomatic HIV-1-infected adult patients given a single dose of zidovudine (200 mg) in combination with multiple doses of lamivudine (300 mg q 12 hr). Lamivudine pharmacokinetics are not significantly affected by abacavir.
[See table 2 above]

Ribavirin:
In vitro data indicate ribavirin reduces phosphorylation of lamivudine, stavudine, and zidovudine. However, no pharmacokinetic (e.g., plasma concentrations or intracellular triphosphorylated active metabolite concentrations) or pharmacodynamic (e.g., loss of HIV-1/HCV virologic suppression) interaction was observed when ribavirin and lamivudine (n = 18), stavudine (n = 10), or zidovudine (n = 6) were coadministered as part of a multi-drug regimen to HIV-1/HCV co-infected patients (see WARNINGS).

INDICATIONS AND USAGE
EPZICOM Tablets, in combination with other antiretroviral agents, are indicated for the treatment of HIV-1 infection.
Additional important information on the use of EPZICOM for treatment of HIV-1 infection:
• EPZICOM is one of multiple products containing abacavir. Before starting EPZICOM, review medical history for prior exposure to any abacavir-containing product in order to avoid reintroduction in a patient with a history of hypersensitivity to abacavir.
• In one controlled study (CNA30021), more patients taking ZIAGEN 600 mg once daily had severe hypersensitivity reactions compared with patients taking ZIAGEN 300 mg twice daily.
• As part of a triple-drug regimen, EPZICOM Tablets are recommended for use with antiretroviral agents from different pharmacological classes and not with other nucleoside/nucleotide reverse transcriptase inhibitors.
See WARNINGS, ADVERSE REACTIONS, and Description of Clinical Studies.

Description of Clinical Studies:
EPZICOM:
There have been no clinical trials conducted with EPZICOM (see CLINICAL PHARMACOLOGY for information about bioequivalence of EPZICOM). One EPZICOM Tablet given once daily is an alternative regimen to EPIVIR Tablets 300 mg once daily plus ZIAGEN Tablets 2 × 300 mg once daily as a component of antiretroviral therapy.
The following study was conducted with the individual components of EPZICOM.

Therapy-Naive Adults:
CNA30021 was an international, multi-center, double-blind, controlled study in which 770 HIV-1-infected, therapy-naive adults were randomized and received either ZIAGEN 600 mg once daily or ZIAGEN 300 mg twice daily, both in combination with EPIVIR 300 mg once daily and efavirenz 600 mg once daily. The double-blind treatment duration was at least 48 weeks. Study participants had a mean age of 37 years, were: male (81%), Caucasian (54%), black (27%), and American Hispanic (15%). The median baseline CD4+ cell count was 262 cells/mm³ (range: 21 to 918 cells/mm³) and the median baseline plasma HIV-1 RNA was 4.89 log₁₀ copies/mL (range: 2.60 to 6.99 log₁₀ copies/mL).

The outcomes of randomized treatment are provided in Table 3.

Table 3. Outcomes of Randomized Treatment Through Week 48 (CNA30021)

Outcome	ZIAGEN 600 mg q.d. plus EPIVIR plus Efavirenz (n = 384)	ZIAGEN 300 mg b.i.d. plus EPIVIR plus Efavirenz (n = 386)
Responder*	64% (71%)	65% (72%)
Virologic failure†	11% (5%)	11% (5%)
Discontinued due to adverse reactions	13%	11%
Discontinued due to other reasons‡	11%	13%

* Patients achieved and maintained confirmed HIV-1 RNA <50 copies/mL (<400 copies/mL) through Week 48 (Roche AMPLICOR Ultrasensitive HIV-1 MONITOR® standard test version 1.0).
† Includes viral rebound, failure to achieve confirmed <50 copies/mL (<400 copies/mL) by Week 48, and insufficient viral load response.
‡ Includes consent withdrawn, lost to follow-up, protocol violations, clinical progression, and other.

After 48 weeks of therapy, the median CD4+ cell count increases from baseline were 188 cells/mm³ in the group receiving ZIAGEN 600 mg once daily and 200 cells/mm³ in the group receiving ZIAGEN 300 mg twice daily. Through Week 48, 6 subjects (2%) in the group receiving ZIAGEN 600 mg once daily (4 CDC classification C events and 2 deaths) and 10 subjects (3%) in the group receiving ZIAGEN 300 mg twice daily (7 CDC classification C events and 3 deaths) experienced clinical disease progression. None of the deaths were attributed to study medications.

CONTRAINDICATIONS
EPZICOM Tablets are contraindicated in patients with previously demonstrated hypersensitivity to abacavir or to any other component of the product (see WARNINGS). NEVER restart EPZICOM or any other abacavir-containing product following a hypersensitivity reaction to abacavir, regardless of HLA-B*5701 status (see WARNINGS, PRECAUTIONS, and ADVERSE REACTIONS).
EPZICOM Tablets are contraindicated in patients with hepatic impairment (see CLINICAL PHARMACOLOGY).

WARNINGS
Hypersensitivity Reaction:
Serious and sometimes fatal hypersensitivity reactions have been associated with EPZICOM and other abacavir-containing products. Patients who carry the HLA-B*5701 allele are at high risk for experiencing a hypersensitivity reaction to abacavir. Prior to initiating therapy with abacavir, screening for the HLA-B*5701 allele is recommended; this approach has been found to decrease the risk of a hypersensitivity reaction. Screening is also recommended prior to reinitiation of abacavir in patients of unknown HLA-B*5701 status who have previously tolerated abacavir. For HLA-B*5701-positive patients, treatment with an abacavir-containing regimen is not recommended and should be considered only with close medical supervision and under exceptional circumstances when the potential benefit outweighs the risk.
HLA-B*5701-negative patients may develop a hypersensitivity reaction to abacavir; however, this occurs significantly less frequently than in HLA-B*5701-positive patients. Regardless of HLA-B*5701 status, permanently discontinue EPZICOM if hypersensitivity cannot be ruled out, even when other diagnoses are possible.
Important information on signs and symptoms of hypersensitivity, as well as clinical management, is presented below.
Signs and Symptoms of Hypersensitivity
Hypersensitivity to abacavir is a multi-organ clinical syndrome usually characterized by a sign or symptom in 2 or more of the following groups.
Group 1: Fever
Group 2: Rash
Group 3: Gastrointestinal (including nausea, vomiting, diarrhea, or abdominal pain)
Group 4: Constitutional (including generalized malaise, fatigue, or achiness)
Group 5: Respiratory (including dyspnea, cough, or pharyngitis)
Hypersensitivity to abacavir following the presentation of a single sign or symptom has been reported infrequently.
Hypersensitivity to abacavir was reported in approximately 8% of 2,670 patients (n = 206) in 9 clinical trials (range: 2% to 9%) with enrollment from November 1999 to February

2002. Data on time to onset and symptoms of suspected hypersensitivity were collected on a detailed data collection module. The frequencies of symptoms are shown in Figure 1. Symptoms usually appeared within the first 6 weeks of treatment with abacavir, although the reaction may occur at any time during therapy. Median time to onset was 9 days; 89% appeared within the first 6 weeks; 95% of patients reported symptoms from 2 or more of the 5 groups listed above.

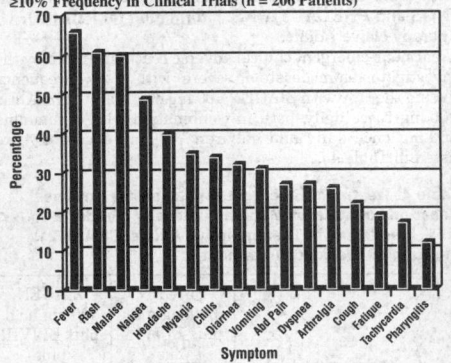

Figure 1: Hypersensitivity-Related Symptoms Reported with ≥10% Frequency in Clinical Trials (n = 206 Patients)

Other less common signs and symptoms of hypersensitivity include lethargy, myolysis, edema, abnormal chest x-ray findings (predominantly infiltrates, which can be localized), and paresthesia.

Anaphylaxis, liver failure, renal failure, hypotension, adult respiratory distress syndrome, respiratory failure, and death have occurred in association with hypersensitivity reactions. In one study, 4 patients (11%) receiving ZIAGEN 600 mg once daily experienced hypotension with a hypersensitivity reaction compared with 0 patients receiving ZIAGEN 300 mg twice daily.

Physical findings associated with hypersensitivity to abacavir in some patients include lymphadenopathy, mucous membrane lesions (conjunctivitis and mouth ulcerations), and rash. The rash usually appears maculopapular or urticarial, but may be variable in appearance. There have been reports of erythema multiforme. Hypersensitivity reactions have occurred without rash.

Laboratory abnormalities associated with hypersensitivity to abacavir in some patients include elevated liver function tests, elevated creatine phosphokinase, elevated creatinine, and lymphopenia.

Clinical Management of Hypersensitivity:

Discontinue EPZICOM as soon as a hypersensitivity reaction is suspected. To minimize the risk of a life-threatening hypersensitivity reaction, permanently discontinue EPZICOM if hypersensitivity cannot be ruled out, even when other diagnoses are possible (e.g., acute onset respiratory diseases such as pneumonia, bronchitis, pharyngitis, or influenza; gastroenteritis; or reactions to other medications).

Following a hypersensitivity reaction to abacavir, NEVER restart EPZICOM or any other abacavir-containing product because more severe symptoms can occur within hours and may include life-threatening hypotension and death.

When therapy with EPZICOM has been discontinued for reasons other than symptoms of a hypersensitivity reaction, and if reinitiation of EPZICOM or any other abacavir-containing product is under consideration, carefully evaluate the reason for discontinuation of EPZICOM to ensure that the patient did not have symptoms of a hypersensitivity reaction. If the patient is of unknown HLA-B*5701 status, screening for the allele is recommended prior to reinitiation of EPZICOM.

If hypersensitivity cannot be ruled out, DO NOT reintroduce EPZICOM or any other abacavir-containing product. Even in the absence of the HLA-B*5701 allele, it is important to permanently discontinue abacavir and not rechallenge with abacavir if a hypersensitivity reaction cannot be ruled out on clinical grounds, due to the potential for a severe or even fatal reaction.

If symptoms consistent with hypersensitivity are not identified, reintroduction can be undertaken with continued monitoring for symptoms of a hypersensitivity reaction. Make patients aware that a hypersensitivity reaction can occur with reintroduction of EPZICOM or any other abacavir-containing product and that reintroduction of EPZICOM or introduction of any other abacavir-containing product needs to be undertaken only if medical care can be readily accessed by the patient or others.

Risk Factor:

HLA-B*5701 Allele: Studies have shown that carriage of the HLA-B*5701 allele is associated with a significantly increased risk of a hypersensitivity reaction to abacavir.

CNA106030 (PREDICT-1), a randomized, double-blind study, evaluated the clinical utility of prospective HLA-B*5701 screening on the incidence of abacavir hypersensitivity reaction in abacavir-naive HIV-1-infected adults (n = 1,650). In this study, use of pre-therapy screening for the HLA-B*5701 allele and exclusion of subjects with this allele reduced the incidence of clinically suspected abacavir hypersensitivity reactions from 7.8% (66/847) to 3.4% (27/803). Based on this study, it is estimated that 61% of patients with the HLA-B*5701 allele will develop a clinically suspected hypersensitivity reaction during the course of abacavir treatment compared with 4% of patients who do not have the HLA-B*5701 allele.

Screening for carriage of the HLA-B*5701 allele is recommended prior to initiating treatment with abacavir. Screening is also recommended prior to reinitiation of abacavir in patients of unknown HLA-B*5701 status who have previously tolerated abacavir. For HLA-B*5701-positive patients, initiating or reinitiating treatment with an abacavir-containing regimen is not recommended and should be considered only with close medical supervision and under exceptional circumstances where potential benefit outweighs the risk.

Skin patch testing is used as a research tool and should not be used to aid in the clinical diagnosis of abacavir hypersensitivity.

In any patient treated with abacavir, the clinical diagnosis of hypersensitivity reaction must remain the basis of clinical decision-making. Even in the absence of the HLA-B*5701 allele, it is important to permanently discontinue abacavir and not rechallenge with abacavir if a hypersensitivity reaction cannot be ruled out on clinical grounds, due to the potential for a severe or even fatal reaction.

Abacavir Hypersensitivity Reaction Registry:

An Abacavir Hypersensitivity Registry has been established to facilitate reporting of hypersensitivity reactions and collection of information on each case. **Physicians should register patients by calling 1-800-270-0425.**

Lactic Acidosis/Severe Hepatomegaly With Steatosis:

Lactic acidosis and severe hepatomegaly with steatosis, including fatal cases, have been reported with the use of nucleoside analogues alone or in combination, including abacavir and lamivudine and other antiretrovirals. A majority of these cases have been in women. Obesity and prolonged nucleoside exposure may be risk factors. Particular caution should be exercised when administering EPZICOM to any patient with known risk factors for liver disease; however, cases have also been reported in patients with no known risk factors. Treatment with EPZICOM should be suspended in any patient who develops clinical or laboratory findings suggestive of lactic acidosis or pronounced hepatotoxicity (which may include hepatomegaly and steatosis even in the absence of marked transaminase elevations).

Posttreatment Exacerbations of Hepatitis:

In clinical trials in non-HIV-1-infected patients treated with lamivudine for chronic HBV, clinical and laboratory evidence of exacerbations of hepatitis have occurred after discontinuation of lamivudine. These exacerbations have been detected primarily by serum ALT elevations in addition to re-emergence of HBV DNA. Although most events appear to have been self-limited, fatalities have been reported in some cases. Similar events have been reported from postmarketing experience after changes from lamivudine-containing HIV-1 treatment regimens to non-lamivudine-containing regimens in patients infected with both HIV-1 and HBV. The causal relationship to discontinuation of lamivudine treatment is unknown. Patients should be closely monitored with both clinical and laboratory follow-up for at least several months after stopping treatment. There is insufficient evidence to determine whether re-initiation of lamivudine alters the course of posttreatment exacerbations of hepatitis.

Use With Interferon- and Ribavirin-Based Regimens:

In vitro studies have shown ribavirin can reduce the phosphorylation of pyrimidine nucleoside analogues such as lamivudine, a component of EPZICOM. Although no evidence of a pharmacokinetic or pharmacodynamic interaction (e.g., loss of HIV-1/HCV virologic suppression) was seen when ribavirin was coadministered with lamivudine in HIV-1/HCV co-infected patients (see CLINICAL PHARMACOLOGY: Drug Interactions), **hepatic decompensation (some fatal) has occurred in HIV-1/HCV co-infected patients receiving combination antiretroviral therapy for HIV-1 and interferon alfa with or without ribavirin.** Patients receiving interferon alfa with or without ribavirin and EPZICOM should be closely monitored for treatment-associated toxicities, especially hepatic decompensation. Discontinuation of EPZICOM should be considered as medically appropriate. Dose reduction or discontinuation of interferon alfa, ribavirin, or both should also be considered if worsening clinical toxicities are observed, including hepatic decompensation (e.g., Childs Pugh >6) (see the complete prescribing information for interferon and ribavirin).

Other:

EPZICOM contains fixed doses of 2 nucleoside analogues, abacavir and lamivudine, and should not be administered concomitantly with other abacavir-containing and/or lamivudine-containing products (ZIAGEN, EPIVIR, COMBIVIR®, or TRIZIVIR).

The complete prescribing information for all agents being considered for use with EPZICOM should be consulted before combination therapy with EPZICOM is initiated.

PRECAUTIONS

Therapy-Experienced Patients:

Abacavir:

In clinical trials, patients with prolonged prior NRTI exposure or who had HIV-1 isolates that contained multiple mutations conferring resistance to NRTIs had limited response to abacavir. The potential for cross-resistance between abacavir and other NRTIs should be considered when choosing new therapeutic regimens in therapy-experienced patients (see MICROBIOLOGY: Cross-Resistance).

Patients With HIV-1 and Hepatitis B Virus Co-infection:

Lamivudine:

Safety and efficacy of lamivudine have not been established for treatment of chronic hepatitis B in patients dually infected with HIV-1 and HBV. In non-HIV-1-infected patients treated with lamivudine for chronic hepatitis B, emergence of lamivudine-resistant HBV has been detected and has been associated with diminished treatment response (see EPIVIR-HBV package insert for additional information). Emergence of hepatitis B virus variants associated with resistance to lamivudine has also been reported in HIV-1-infected patients who have received lamivudine-containing antiretroviral regimens in the presence of concurrent infection with hepatitis B virus.

Patients With Impaired Renal Function:

EPZICOM:

Since EPZICOM is a fixed-dose tablet and the dosage of the individual components cannot be altered, patients with creatinine clearance <50 mL/min should not receive EPZICOM.

Patients With Impaired Hepatic Function:

EPZICOM:

EPZICOM is contraindicated in patients with hepatic impairment since it is a fixed-dose tablet and the dosage of the individual components cannot be altered.

Immune Reconstitution Syndrome:

Immune reconstitution syndrome has been reported in patients treated with combination antiretroviral therapy, including EPZICOM. During the initial phase of combination antiretroviral treatment, patients whose immune system responds may develop an inflammatory response to indolent or residual opportunistic infections (such as *Mycobacterium avium* infection, cytomegalovirus, *Pneumocystis jirovecii* pneumonia [PCP], or tuberculosis), which may necessitate further evaluation and treatment.

Fat Redistribution:

Redistribution/accumulation of body fat including central obesity, dorsocervical fat enlargement (buffalo hump), peripheral wasting, facial wasting, breast enlargement, and "cushingoid appearance" have been observed in patients receiving antiretroviral therapy. The mechanism and long-term consequences of these events are currently unknown. A causal relationship has not been established.

Myocardial Infarction:

In a published prospective, observational, epidemiological study designed to investigate the rate of myocardial infarction in patients on combination antiretroviral therapy, the use of abacavir within the previous 6 months was correlated with an increased risk of myocardial infarction (MI).[1] In a sponsor-conducted pooled analysis of clinical trials, no excess risk of MI was observed in abacavir-treated subjects as compared with control subjects. In totality, the available data from the observational cohort and from clinical trials are inconclusive.

As a precaution, the underlying risk of coronary heart disease should be considered when prescribing antiretroviral therapies, including abacavir, and action taken to minimize all modifiable risk factors (e.g., hypertension, hyperlipidemia, diabetes mellitus, and smoking).

Information for Patients:

Abacavir:

Hypersensitivity Reaction: Inform patients:

- that a Medication Guide and Warning Card summarizing the symptoms of the abacavir hypersensitivity reaction and other product information will be dispensed by the pharmacist with each new prescription and refill of EPZICOM, and encourage the patient to read the Medication Guide and Warning Card every time to obtain any new information that may be present about EPZICOM. (The complete text of the Medication Guide is reprinted at the end of this document.)
- to carry the Warning Card with them.
- how to identify a hypersensitivity reaction (see WARNINGS and MEDICATION GUIDE).
- that if they develop symptoms consistent with a hypersensitivity reaction they should call their doctor right away to determine if they should stop taking EPZICOM.

- that a hypersensitivity reaction can worsen and lead to hospitalization or death if EPZICOM is not immediately discontinued.
- **to not restart EPZICOM or any other abacavir-containing product following a hypersensitivity reaction because more severe symptoms can occur within hours and may include life-threatening hypotension and death.**
- that a hypersensitivity reaction is usually reversible if it is detected promptly and EPZICOM is stopped right away.
- that if they have interrupted EPZICOM for reasons other than symptoms of hypersensitivity (for example, those who have an interruption in drug supply), a serious or fatal hypersensitivity reaction may occur with reintroduction of abacavir.
- that in one study, more severe hypersensitivity reactions were seen when ZIAGEN was dosed 600 mg once daily.
- **to not restart EPZICOM or any other abacavir-containing product without medical consultation and that restarting abacavir needs to be undertaken only if medical care can be readily accessed by the patient or others.**

Lamivudine:
Patients co-infected with HIV-1 and HBV should be informed that deterioration of liver disease has occurred in some cases when treatment with lamivudine was discontinued. Patients should be advised to discuss any changes in regimen with their physician.

EPZICOM:
Inform patients that some HIV-1 medicines, including EPZICOM, can cause a rare, but serious condition called lactic acidosis with liver enlargement (hepatomegaly).
EPZICOM is not a cure for HIV-1 infection and patients may continue to experience illnesses associated with HIV-1 infection, including opportunistic infections. Patients should remain under the care of a physician when using EPZICOM. Advise patients that the use of EPZICOM has not been shown to reduce the risk of transmission of HIV-1 to others through sexual contact or blood contamination.
Inform patients that redistribution or accumulation of body fat may occur in patients receiving antiretroviral therapy and that the cause and long-term health effects of these conditions are not known at this time.
EPZICOM Tablets are for oral ingestion only.
Patients should be advised of the importance of taking EPZICOM exactly as it is prescribed.

Drug Interactions:
EPZICOM:
No clinically significant changes to pharmacokinetic parameters were observed for abacavir or lamivudine when administered together.

Abacavir:
Abacavir has no effect on the pharmacokinetic properties of ethanol. Ethanol decreases the elimination of abacavir causing an increase in overall exposure (see CLINICAL PHARMACOLOGY: Drug Interactions).
The addition of methadone has no clinically significant effect on the pharmacokinetic properties of abacavir. In a study of 11 HIV-1-infected patients receiving methadone-maintenance therapy (40 mg and 90 mg daily), with 600 mg of ZIAGEN twice daily (twice the currently recommended dose), oral methadone clearance increased 22% (90% CI: 6% to 42%). This alteration will not result in a methadone dose modification in the majority of patients; however, an increased methadone dose may be required in a small number of patients.

Lamivudine:
Trimethoprim (TMP) 160 mg/sulfamethoxazole (SMX) 800 mg once daily has been shown to increase lamivudine exposure (AUC). No change in dose of either drug is recommended. The effect of higher doses of TMP/SMX on lamivudine pharmacokinetics has not been investigated (see CLINICAL PHARMACOLOGY).
Lamivudine and zalcitabine may inhibit the intracellular phosphorylation of one another. Therefore, use of EPZICOM in combination with zalcitabine is not recommended.
See CLINICAL PHARMACOLOGY for additional drug interactions.

Carcinogenesis, Mutagenesis, Impairment of Fertility:
Carcinogenicity:
Abacavir: Abacavir was administered orally at 3 dosage levels to separate groups of mice and rats in 2-year carcinogenicity studies. Results showed an increase in the incidence of malignant and non-malignant tumors. Malignant tumors occurred in the preputial gland of males and the clitoral gland of females of both species, and in the liver of female rats. In addition, non-malignant tumors also occurred in the liver and thyroid gland of female rats. These observations were made at systemic exposures in the range of 6 to 32 times the human exposure at the recommended dose.
Lamivudine: Long-term carcinogenicity studies with lamivudine in mice and rats showed no evidence of carcinogenic potential at exposures up to 10 times (mice) and 58 times (rats) those observed in humans at the recommended therapeutic dose for HIV-1 infection.

It is not known how predictive the results of rodent carcinogenicity studies may be for humans.
Mutagenicity:
Abacavir: Abacavir induced chromosomal aberrations both in the presence and absence of metabolic activation in an in vitro cytogenetic study in human lymphocytes. Abacavir was mutagenic in the absence of metabolic activation, although it was not mutagenic in the presence of metabolic activation in an L5178Y mouse lymphoma assay. Abacavir was clastogenic in males and not clastogenic in females in an in vivo mouse bone marrow micronucleus assay. Abacavir was not mutagenic in bacterial mutagenicity assays in the presence and absence of metabolic activation.
Lamivudine: Lamivudine was mutagenic in an L5178Y mouse lymphoma assay and clastogenic in a cytogenetic assay using cultured human lymphocytes. Lamivudine was not mutagenic in a microbial mutagenicity assay, in an in vitro cell transformation assay, in a rat micronucleus test, in a rat bone marrow cytogenetic assay, and in an assay for unscheduled DNA synthesis in rat liver.
Impairment of Fertility:
Abacavir or lamivudine induced no adverse effects on the mating performance or fertility of male and female rats at doses producing systemic exposure levels approximately 8 or 130 times, respectively, higher than those in humans at the recommended dose based on body surface area comparisons.

Pregnancy:
Pregnancy Category C. There are no adequate and well-controlled studies of EPZICOM in pregnant women. Reproduction studies with abacavir and lamivudine have been performed in animals (see Abacavir and Lamivudine sections below). EPZICOM should be used during pregnancy only if the potential benefits outweigh the risks.
Abacavir:
Studies in pregnant rats showed that abacavir is transferred to the fetus through the placenta. Fetal malformations (increased incidences of fetal anasarca and skeletal malformations) and developmental toxicity (depressed fetal body weight and reduced crown-rump length) were observed in rats at a dose which produced 35 times the human exposure, based on AUC. Embryonic and fetal toxicities (increased resorptions, decreased fetal body weights) and toxicities to the offspring (increased incidence of stillbirth and lower body weights) occurred at half of the above-mentioned dose in separate fertility studies conducted in rats. In the rabbit, no developmental toxicity and no increases in fetal malformations occurred at doses that produced 8.5 times the human exposure at the recommended dose based on AUC.
Lamivudine:
Studies in pregnant rats showed that lamivudine is transferred to the fetus through the placenta. Reproduction studies with orally administered lamivudine have been performed in rats and rabbits at doses producing plasma levels up to approximately 35 times that for the recommended adult HIV dose. No evidence of teratogenicity due to lamivudine was observed. Evidence of early embryolethality was seen in the rabbit at exposure levels similar to those observed in humans, but there was no indication of this effect in the rat at exposure levels up to 35 times those in humans.

Antiretroviral Pregnancy Registry:
To monitor maternal-fetal outcomes of pregnant women exposed to EPZICOM or other antiretroviral agents, an Antiretroviral Pregnancy Registry has been established. Physicians are encouraged to register patients by calling 1-800-258-4263.

Nursing Mothers:
The Centers for Disease Control and Prevention recommend that HIV-1-infected mothers not breastfeed their infants to avoid risking postnatal transmission of HIV-1 infection.
Abacavir:
Abacavir is secreted into the milk of lactating rats.
Lamivudine:
Lamivudine is excreted in human breast milk and into the milk of lactating rats.
Because of both the potential for HIV-1 transmission and the potential for serious adverse reactions in nursing infants, **mothers should be instructed not to breastfeed if they are receiving EPZICOM.**

Pediatric Use:
Safety and effectiveness of EPZICOM in pediatric patients have not been established.

Geriatric Use:
Clinical studies of abacavir and lamivudine did not include sufficient numbers of patients aged 65 and over to determine whether they respond differently from younger patients. In general, dose selection for an elderly patient should be cautious, reflecting the greater frequency of decreased hepatic, renal, or cardiac function, and of concomitant disease or other drug therapy. EPZICOM is not recom-

mended for patients with impaired renal function or impaired hepatic function (see PRECAUTIONS and DOSAGE AND ADMINISTRATION).

ADVERSE REACTIONS
Abacavir:
Hypersensitivity Reaction:
Serious and sometimes fatal hypersensitivity reactions have been associated with abacavir sulfate, a component of EPZICOM.
In one study, once-daily dosing of ZIAGEN was associated with more severe hypersensitivity reactions (see WARNINGS and PRECAUTIONS: Information for Patients).
Therapy-Naive Adults:
Treatment-emergent clinical adverse reactions (rated by the investigator as moderate or severe) with a ≥5% frequency during therapy with ZIAGEN 600 mg once daily or ZIAGEN 300 mg twice daily, both in combination with lamivudine 300 mg once daily and efavirenz 600 mg once daily are listed in Table 4.

Table 4. Treatment-Emergent (All Causality) Adverse Reactions of at Least Moderate Intensity (Grades 2-4, ≥5% Frequency) in Therapy-Naive Adults (CNA30021) Through 48 Weeks of Treatment

Adverse Event	ZIAGEN 600 mg q.d. plus EPIVIR plus Efavirenz (n = 384)	ZIAGEN 300 mg b.i.d. plus EPIVIR plus Efavirenz (n = 386)
Drug hypersensitivity*†	9%	7%
Insomnia	7%	9%
Depression/Depressed mood	7%	7%
Headache/Migraine	7%	6%
Fatigue/Malaise	6%	8%
Dizziness/Vertigo	6%	6%
Nausea	5%	6%
Diarrhea*	5%	6%
Rash	5%	5%
Pyrexia	5%	3%
Abdominal pain/gastritis	4%	5%
Abnormal dreams	4%	5%
Anxiety	3%	5%

* Patients receiving ZIAGEN 600 mg once daily, experienced a significantly higher incidence of severe drug hypersensitivity reactions and severe diarrhea compared with patients who received ZIAGEN 300 mg twice daily. Five percent (5%) of patients receiving ZIAGEN 600 mg once daily had severe drug hypersensitivity reactions compared with 2% of patients receiving ZIAGEN 300 mg twice daily. Two percent (2%) of patients receiving ZIAGEN 600 mg once daily had severe diarrhea while none of the patients receiving ZIAGEN 300 mg twice daily had this event.
† **Study CNA30024 was a multi-center, double-blind, controlled study in which 649 HIV-1-infected, therapy-naive adults were randomized and received either ZIAGEN (300 mg twice daily), EPIVIR (150 mg twice daily), and efavirenz (600 mg once daily) or zidovudine (300 mg twice daily), EPIVIR (150 mg twice daily), and efavirenz (600 mg once daily). CNA30024 used double-blind ascertainment of suspected hypersensitivity reactions. During the blinded portion of the study, suspected hypersensitivity to abacavir was reported by investigators in 9% of 324 patients in the abacavir group and 3% of 325 patients in the zidovudine group.**

Laboratory Abnormalities:
Laboratory abnormalities observed in clinical studies of ZIAGEN were anemia, neutropenia, liver function test abnormalities, and elevations of CPK, blood glucose, and triglycerides. Additional laboratory abnormalities observed in clinical studies of EPIVIR were thrombocytopenia and elevated levels of bilirubin, amylase, and lipase.
The frequencies of treatment-emergent laboratory abnormalities were comparable between treatment groups in Study CNA30021.
Other Adverse Events:
In addition to adverse reactions listed above, other adverse events observed in the expanded access program for abacavir were pancreatitis and increased GGT.
Observed During Clinical Practice:
The following reactions have been identified during post-approval use of abacavir and lamivudine. Because they are reported voluntarily from a population of unknown size, estimates of frequency cannot be made. These events have been chosen for inclusion due to a combination of their seriousness, frequency of reporting, or potential causal connection to abacavir and/or lamivudine.

Abacavir:
Cardiovascular: Myocardial infarction.
Skin: Suspected Stevens-Johnson syndrome (SJS) and toxic epidermal necrolysis (TEN) have been reported in patients receiving abacavir primarily in combination with medications known to be associated with SJS and TEN, respectively. Because of the overlap of clinical signs and symptoms between hypersensitivity to abacavir and SJS and TEN, and the possibility of multiple drug sensitivities in some patients, abacavir should be discontinued and not restarted in such cases.
There have also been reports of erythema multiforme with abacavir use.
Abacavir and Lamivudine:
Body as a Whole: Redistribution/accumulation of body fat (see PRECAUTIONS: Fat Redistribution).
Digestive: Stomatitis.
Endocrine and Metabolic: Hyperglycemia.
General: Weakness.
Hemic and Lymphatic: Aplastic anemia, anemia (including pure red cell aplasia and severe anemias progressing on therapy), lymphadenopathy, splenomegaly.
Hepatic and Pancreatic: Lactic acidosis and hepatic steatosis, pancreatitis, posttreatment exacerbation of hepatitis B (see WARNINGS).
Hypersensitivity: Sensitization reactions (including anaphylaxis), urticaria.
Musculoskeletal: Muscle weakness, CPK elevation, rhabdomyolysis.
Nervous: Paresthesia, peripheral neuropathy, seizures.
Respiratory: Abnormal breath sounds/wheezing.
Skin: Alopecia, erythema multiforme, Stevens-Johnson syndrome.

OVERDOSAGE

Abacavir:
There is no known antidote for abacavir. It is not known whether abacavir can be removed by peritoneal dialysis or hemodialysis.
Lamivudine:
One case of an adult ingesting 6 grams of lamivudine was reported; there were no clinical signs or symptoms noted and hematologic tests remained normal. It is not known whether lamivudine can be removed by peritoneal dialysis or hemodialysis.

DOSAGE AND ADMINISTRATION

A Medication Guide and Warning Card that provide information about recognition of hypersensitivity reactions should be dispensed with each new prescription and refill. To facilitate reporting of hypersensitivity reactions and collection of information on each case, an Abacavir Hypersensitivity Registry has been established. **Physicians should register patients by calling 1-800-270-0425.**
The recommended oral dose of EPZICOM for adults is one tablet daily, in combination with other antiretroviral agents (see INDICATIONS AND USAGE: Description of Clinical Studies, PRECAUTIONS, MICROBIOLOGY, and CLINICAL PHARMACOLOGY).
EPZICOM can be taken with or without food.
Dose Adjustment:
Because it is a fixed-dose tablet, EPZICOM should not be prescribed for patients requiring dosage adjustment such as those with creatinine clearance <50 mL/min, those with hepatic impairment, or those experiencing dose-limiting adverse events. Use of EPIVIR Oral Solution and ZIAGEN Oral Solution may be considered.

HOW SUPPLIED

EPZICOM is available as tablets. Each tablet contains 600 mg of abacavir as abacavir sulfate and 300 mg of lamivudine. The tablets are orange, film-coated, modified capsule-shaped, and debossed with GS FC2 on one side with no markings on the reverse side. They are packaged as follows:
Bottles of 30 Tablets (NDC 0173-0742-00).
Store at 25°C (77°F); excursions permitted to 15° to 30°C (59° to 86°F) (see USP Controlled Room Temperature).

ANIMAL TOXICOLOGY

Myocardial degeneration was found in mice and rats following administration of abacavir for 2 years. The systemic exposures were equivalent to 7 to 24 times the expected systemic exposure in humans. The clinical relevance of this finding has not been determined.

REFERENCE

1. Data Collection on Adverse Events of Anti-HIV Drugs (D:A:D) Study Group. *Lancet.* 2008;371 (9622):1417-1426.

MEDICATION GUIDE

EPZICOM® (ep' zih com) Tablets
Generic name: abacavir (uH-BACK-ah-veer) sulfate and lamivudine (la-MIV-yoo-deen)
Read the Medication Guide that comes with EPZICOM before you start taking it and each time you get a refill because there may be new information. This information does not take the place of talking to your doctor about your medical condition or your treatment. Be sure to carry your EPZICOM Warning Card with you at all times.

What is the most important information I should know about EPZICOM?
• **Serious Allergic Reaction to Abacavir.** EPZICOM contains abacavir (also contained in ZIAGEN® and TRIZIVIR®). **Patients taking EPZICOM may have a serious allergic reaction (hypersensitivity reaction) that can cause death. Your risk of this allergic reaction is much higher if you have a gene variation called HLA-B*5701 than if you do not. Your doctor can determine with a blood test if you have this gene variation. If you get a symptom from 2 or more of the following groups while taking EPZICOM, call your doctor right away to determine if you should stop taking this medicine.**

	Symptom(s)
Group 1	Fever
Group 2	Rash
Group 3	Nausea, vomiting, diarrhea, abdominal (stomach area) pain
Group 4	Generally ill feeling, extreme tiredness, or achiness
Group 5	Shortness of breath, cough, sore throat

A list of these symptoms is on the Warning Card your pharmacist gives you. Carry this Warning Card with you.
If you stop EPZICOM because of an allergic reaction, NEVER take EPZICOM (abacavir sulfate and lamivudine) or any other abacavir-containing medicine (ZIAGEN and TRIZIVIR) again. If you take EPZICOM or any other abacavir-containing medicine again after you have had an allergic reaction, **WITHIN HOURS** you may get **life-threatening symptoms** that may include **very low blood pressure or death.**
If you stop EPZICOM for any other reason, even for a few days, and you are not allergic to EPZICOM, talk with your doctor before taking it again. Taking EPZICOM again can cause a serious allergic or life-threatening reaction, even if you never had an allergic reaction to it before. If your doctor tells you that you can take EPZICOM again, start taking it when you are around medical help or people who can call a doctor if you need one.
• **Lactic Acidosis.** Some human immunodeficiency virus (HIV) medicines, including EPZICOM, can cause a rare but serious condition called lactic acidosis with liver enlargement (hepatomegaly). Nausea and tiredness that don't get better may be symptoms of lactic acidosis. In some cases this condition can cause death. Women, overweight people, and people who have taken HIV medicines like EPZICOM for a long time have a higher chance of getting lactic acidosis and liver enlargement. Lactic acidosis is a medical emergency and must be treated in the hospital.
• **Worsening of hepatitis B virus (HBV) infection.** Patients with HBV infection, who take EPZICOM and then stop it, may get "flare-ups" of their hepatitis. "Flare-up" is when the disease suddenly returns in a worse way than before. If you have HBV infection, your doctor should closely monitor your liver function for several months after stopping EPZICOM. You may need to take anti-HBV medicines.
• **Use with interferon- and ribavirin-based regimens.** Worsening of liver disease (sometimes resulting in death) has occurred in patients infected with both HIV and hepatitis C virus who are taking anti-HIV medicines and are also being treated for hepatitis C with interferon with or without ribavirin. If you are taking EPZICOM as well as interferon with or without ribavirin and you experience side effects, be sure to tell your doctor.
EPZICOM can have other serious side effects. Be sure to read the section below entitled "What are the possible side effects of EPZICOM?"

What is EPZICOM?
EPZICOM is a prescription medicine used to treat HIV infection. EPZICOM includes 2 medicines: abacavir (ZIAGEN) and lamivudine or 3TC (EPIVIR®). See the end of this Medication Guide for a complete list of ingredients in EPZICOM. Both of these medicines are called nucleoside analogue reverse transcriptase inhibitors (NRTIs). When used together, they help lower the amount of HIV in your blood. This helps to keep your immune system as healthy as possible so that it can help fight infection.
Different combinations of medicines are used to treat HIV infection. You and your doctor should discuss which combination of medicines is best for you.

• **EPZICOM does not cure HIV infection or AIDS.** We do not know if EPZICOM will help you live longer or have fewer of the medical problems that people get with HIV or AIDS. It is very important that you see your doctor regularly while you are taking EPZICOM.
• **EPZICOM does not lower the risk of passing HIV to other people through sexual contact, sharing needles, or being exposed to your blood.** For your health and the health of others, it is important to always practice safe sex by using a latex or polyurethane condom or other barrier method to lower the chance of sexual contact with semen, vaginal secretions, or blood. Never use or share dirty needles.

Who should not take EPZICOM?
Do not take EPZICOM if you:
• **have ever had a serious allergic reaction (a hypersensitivity reaction) to EPZICOM or any other medicine that has abacavir as one of its ingredients (TRIZIVIR and ZIAGEN). See the end of this Medication Guide for a complete list of ingredients in EPZICOM.**
• **have a liver that does not function properly.**
• **are less than 18 years of age.**
Before starting EPZICOM tell your doctor about all of your medical conditions, including if you:
• **have been tested and know whether or not you have a particular gene variation called HLA-B*5701.**
• **are pregnant or planning to become pregnant.** We do not know if EPZICOM will harm your unborn child. You and your doctor will need to decide if EPZICOM is right for you. If you use EPZICOM while you are pregnant, talk to your doctor about how you can be on the Antiviral Pregnancy Registry for EPZICOM.
• **are breastfeeding.** Some of the ingredients in EPZICOM can be passed to your baby in your breast milk. It is not known if they could harm your baby. Also, mothers with HIV should not breastfeed because HIV can be passed to the baby in the breast milk.
• **have liver problems including hepatitis B virus infection.**
• **have kidney problems.**
• **have heart problems, smoke, or suffer from diseases that increase your risk of heart disease such as high blood pressure, high cholesterol, or diabetes.**
Tell your doctor about all the medicines you take, including prescription and nonprescription medicines, vitamins, and herbal supplements. Especially tell your doctor if you take any of the following medicines*:
• **methadone**
• **HIVID®** (zalcitabine, ddC)
• **EPIVIR** or **EPIVIR-HBV®** (lamivudine, 3TC), ZIAGEN (abacavir sulfate), COMBIVIR® (lamivudine and zidovudine), or TRIZIVIR (abacavir sulfate, lamivudine, and zidovudine).

How should I take EPZICOM?
• **Take EPZICOM by mouth exactly as your doctor prescribes it.** The usual dose is 1 tablet once a day. Do not skip doses.
• **You can take EPZICOM with or without food.**
• **If you miss a dose of EPZICOM, take the missed dose right away. Then, take the next dose at the usual time.**
• **Do not let your EPZICOM run out.**
• **Starting EPZICOM again can cause a serious allergic or life-threatening reaction, even if you never had an allergic reaction to it before.** If you run out of EPZICOM even for a few days, you must ask your doctor if you can start EPZICOM again. If your doctor tells you that you can take EPZICOM again, start taking it when you are around medical help or people who can call a doctor if you need one.
• **If you stop your anti-HIV drugs, even for a short time, the amount of virus in your blood may increase and the virus may become harder to treat.**
• **If you take too much EPZICOM, call your doctor or poison control center right away.**
What should I avoid while taking EPZICOM?
• Do not take **EPIVIR (lamivudine, 3TC), COMBIVIR (lamivudine and zidovudine), ZIAGEN (abacavir sulfate), or TRIZIVIR (abacavir sulfate, lamivudine, and zidovudine)** while taking EPZICOM. Some of these medicines are already in EPZICOM.
• Do not take zalcitabine (HIVID, ddC) while taking EPZICOM.
Avoid doing things that can spread HIV infection, as EPZICOM does not stop you from passing the HIV infection to others.
• **Do not share needles or other injection equipment.**
• **Do not share personal items that can have blood or body fluids on them, like toothbrushes and razor blades.**
• **Do not have any kind of sex without protection.** Always practice safe sex by using a latex or polyurethane condom or other barrier method to lower the chance of sexual contact with semen, vaginal secretions, or blood.
• **Do not breastfeed.** EPZICOM can be passed to babies in breast milk and could harm the baby. Also, mothers with HIV should not breastfeed because HIV can be passed to the baby in the breast milk.

What are the possible side effects of EPZICOM?

EPZICOM can cause the following serious side effects:

- **Serious allergic reaction that can cause death.** (See "What is the most important information I should know about EPZICOM?" at the beginning of this Medication Guide.)
- **Lactic acidosis with liver enlargement (hepatomegaly) that can cause death.** (See "What is the most important information I should know about EPZICOM?" at the beginning of this Medication Guide.)
- **Worsening of HBV infection.** (See "What is the most important information I should know about EPZICOM?" at the beginning of this Medication Guide.)
- **Changes in immune system.** When you start taking HIV medicines, your immune system may get stronger and could begin to fight infections that have been hidden in your body, such as pneumonia, herpes virus, or tuberculosis. If you have new symptoms after starting your HIV medicines, be sure to tell your doctor.
- **Changes in body fat.** These changes have happened in patients taking antiretroviral medicines like EPZICOM. The changes may include an increased amount of fat in the upper back and neck ("buffalo hump"), breast, and around the back, chest, and stomach area. Loss of fat from the legs, arms, and face may also happen. The cause and long-term health effects of these conditions are not known.

Some HIV medicines including EPZICOM may increase your risk of heart attack. If you have heart problems, smoke, or suffer from diseases that increase your risk of heart disease such as high blood pressure, high cholesterol, or diabetes, tell your doctor.

The most common side effects with EPZICOM are trouble sleeping, depression, headache, tiredness, dizziness, nausea, diarrhea, rash, fever, stomach pain, abnormal dreams, and anxiety. Most of these side effects did not cause people to stop taking EPZICOM.

This list of side effects is not complete. Call your doctor for medical advice about side effects. You may report side effects to FDA at 1-800-FDA-1088.

How should I store EPZICOM?

- Store EPZICOM at room temperature between 59° to 86°F (15° to 30°C).
- Keep EPZICOM and all medicines out of the reach of children.

General information for safe and effective use of EPZICOM

Medicines are sometimes prescribed for conditions that are not mentioned in Medication Guides. Do not use EPZICOM for a condition for which it was not prescribed. Do not give EPZICOM to other people, even if they have the same symptoms you have. It may harm them.

This Medication Guide summarizes the most important information about EPZICOM. If you would like more information, talk with your doctor. You can ask your doctor or pharmacist for the information that is written for healthcare professionals or call 1-888-825-5249.

What are the ingredients in EPZICOM?

Active ingredients: abacavir sulfate and lamivudine

Inactive ingredients: Each film-coated EPZICOM Tablet contains the inactive ingredients magnesium stearate, microcrystalline cellulose, and sodium starch glycolate. The tablets are coated with a film (OPADRY® orange YS-1-13065-A) that is made of FD&C Yellow No. 6, hypromellose, polyethylene glycol 400, polysorbate 80, and titanium dioxide.

This Medication Guide has been approved by the US Food and Drug Administration.

March 2009

EPZ:2MG

COMBIVIR, EPIVIR, EPZICOM, TRIZIVIR, and ZIAGEN are registered trademarks of GlaxoSmithKline.

* The brands listed are trademarks of their respective owners and are not trademarks of GlaxoSmithKline. The makers of these brands are not affiliated with and do not endorse GlaxoSmithKline or its products.

GlaxoSmithKline
Research Triangle Park, NC 27709
Lamivudine is manufactured under agreement from
Shire Pharmaceuticals Group plc
Basingstoke, UK
©2009, GlaxoSmithKline. All rights reserved.
March 2009
EPZ:2PI

LEXIVA® ℞

[lex-ē′ va]
(fosamprenavir calcium)
Tablets and Oral Suspension

HIGHLIGHTS OF PRESCRIBING INFORMATION

These highlights do not include all the information needed to use LEXIVA safely and effectively. See full prescribing information for LEXIVA.

LEXIVA (fosamprenavir calcium) Tablets and Oral Suspension
Initial U.S. Approval: 2003

————RECENT MAJOR CHANGES————

Warnings and Precautions (5.8) 9/2009
Warnings and Precautions, Nephrolithiasis (5.11) 9/2009
Contraindications (4) 4/2010
Warnings and Precautions (5.1) 4/2010

————INDICATIONS AND USAGE————

LEXIVA is an HIV protease inhibitor indicated in combination with other antiretroviral agents for the treatment of HIV-1 infection. (1)

————DOSAGE AND ADMINISTRATION————

- Therapy-Naive Adults: LEXIVA 1,400 mg twice daily; LEXIVA 1,400 mg once daily plus ritonavir 200 mg once daily; LEXIVA 1,400 mg once daily plus ritonavir 100 mg once daily; LEXIVA 700 mg twice daily plus ritonavir 100 mg twice daily. (2.1)
- Protease Inhibitor-Experienced Adults: LEXIVA 700 mg twice daily plus ritonavir 100 mg twice daily. (2.1)
- Pediatric Patients (2 to 18 years of age): Dosage should be calculated based on body weight (kg) and should not exceed adult dose. (2.2)
- Hepatic Impairment: Recommended adjustments for patients with mild, moderate, or severe hepatic impairment. (2.3)

Dosing Considerations
- LEXIVA Tablets may be taken with or without food. (2)
- LEXIVA Suspension: Adults should take without food; pediatric patients should take with food. (2)

————DOSAGE FORMS AND STRENGTHS————

700 mg tablets and 50 mg/mL oral suspension (3)

————CONTRAINDICATIONS————

- Hypersensitivity to LEXIVA or amprenavir (e.g., Stevens-Johnson syndrome). (4)
- Drugs highly dependent on CYP3A4 for clearance and for which elevated plasma levels may result in serious and/or life-threatening events. (4)
- Review ritonavir contraindications when used in combination. (4)

————WARNINGS AND PRECAUTIONS————

- Certain drugs should not be coadministered with LEXIVA due to risk of serious or life-threatening adverse reactions. (5.1)
- LEXIVA should be discontinued for severe skin reactions including Stevens-Johnson syndrome. (5.2) LEXIVA should be used with caution in patients with a known sulfonamide allergy. (5.3)
- Use of higher than approved doses may lead to transaminase elevations. Patients with hepatitis B or C are at increased risk of transaminase elevations. (5.4)
- Patients receiving LEXIVA may develop new onset or exacerbations of diabetes mellitus, hyperglycemia (5.5), immune reconstitution syndrome (5.6), redistribution/accumulation of body fat (5.7), and elevated triglyceride and cholesterol concentrations (5.8). Monitor cholesterol and triglycerides prior to therapy and periodically thereafter.
- Acute hemolytic anemia has been reported with amprenavir. (5.9)
- Hemophilia: Spontaneous bleeding may occur, and additional factor VIII may be required. (5.10)
- Nephrolithiasis: Cases of nephrolithiasis have been reported with fosamprenavir. (5.11)

————ADVERSE REACTIONS————

- In adults the most common adverse reactions (incidence ≥4%) are diarrhea, rash, nausea, vomiting, headache. (6.1)
- Vomiting was more frequent in pediatrics than in adults. (6.1)

To report SUSPECTED ADVERSE REACTIONS, contact GlaxoSmithKline at 1-888-825-5249 or FDA at 1-800-FDA-1088 or www.fda.gov/medwatch

————DRUG INTERACTIONS————

- Coadministration of LEXIVA with drugs that induce CYP3A4 may decrease amprenavir (active metabolite) concentrations leading to potential loss of virologic activity. (7, 12.3)
- Coadministration with drugs that inhibit CYP3A4 may increase amprenavir concentrations. (7, 12.3)
- Coadministration of LEXIVA and ritonavir may result in clinically significant interactions with drugs metabolized by CYP2D6. (7)

See 17 for PATIENT COUNSELING INFORMATION and FDA-approved patient labeling

Revised: 04/2010

FULL PRESCRIBING INFORMATION

1 INDICATIONS AND USAGE

LEXIVA® is indicated in combination with other antiretroviral agents for the treatment of human immunodeficiency virus (HIV-1) infection.

The following points should be considered when initiating therapy with LEXIVA plus ritonavir in protease inhibitor-experienced patients:

- The protease inhibitor-experienced patient study was not large enough to reach a definitive conclusion that LEXIVA plus ritonavir and lopinavir plus ritonavir are clinically equivalent [see Clinical Studies (14.2)].
- Once-daily administration of LEXIVA plus ritonavir is not recommended for adult protease inhibitor-experienced patients or any pediatric patients.

2 DOSAGE AND ADMINISTRATION

LEXIVA Tablets may be taken with or without food.
Adults should take LEXIVA Oral Suspension without food. Pediatric patients should take LEXIVA Oral Suspension with food [see Clinical Pharmacology (12.3)]. If emesis occurs within 30 minutes after dosing, re-dosing of LEXIVA Oral Suspension should occur.

Higher-than-approved dose combinations of LEXIVA plus ritonavir are not recommended due to an increased risk of transaminase elevations [see Overdosage (10)].

When LEXIVA is used in combination with ritonavir, prescribers should consult the full prescribing information for ritonavir.

2.1 Adults

Therapy-Naive Adults
- LEXIVA 1,400 mg twice daily (without ritonavir).
- LEXIVA 1,400 mg once daily plus ritonavir 200 mg once daily.
- LEXIVA 1,400 mg once daily plus ritonavir 100 mg once daily.

Dosing of LEXIVA 1,400 mg once daily plus ritonavir 100 mg once daily is supported by pharmacokinetic data [see Clinical Pharmacology (12.3)].
- LEXIVA 700 mg twice daily plus ritonavir 100 mg twice daily.

Dosing of LEXIVA 700 mg twice daily plus 100 mg ritonavir twice daily is supported by pharmacokinetic and safety data *[see Clinical Pharmacology (12.3)]*.

Protease Inhibitor-Experienced Adults
• LEXIVA 700 mg twice daily plus ritonavir 100 mg twice daily

2.2   Pediatric Patients (2 to 18 years of age)

The recommended dosage of LEXIVA in patients ≥2 years of age should be calculated based on body weight (kg) and should not exceed the recommended adult dose. The data are insufficient to recommend: (1) once-daily dosing of LEXIVA alone or in combination with ritonavir, and (2) any dosing of LEXIVA in therapy-experienced patients 2 to 5 years of age.

Therapy-Naive 2 to 5 Years of Age
• LEXIVA Oral Suspension 30 mg/kg twice daily, not to exceed the adult dose of LEXIVA 1,400 mg twice daily.

Therapy-Naive ≥6 Years of Age
• Either LEXIVA Oral Suspension 30 mg/kg twice daily not to exceed the adult dose of LEXIVA 1,400 mg twice daily or LEXIVA Oral Suspension 18 mg/kg plus ritonavir 3 mg/kg twice daily not to exceed the adult dose of LEXIVA 700 mg twice daily plus ritonavir 100 mg twice daily.

Therapy-Experienced ≥6 Years of Age
• LEXIVA Oral Suspension 18 mg/kg plus ritonavir 3 mg/kg administered twice daily not to exceed the adult dose of LEXIVA 700 mg twice daily plus ritonavir 100 mg twice daily.

Other Dosing Considerations
• When administered without ritonavir, the adult regimen of LEXIVA Tablets 1,400 mg twice daily may be used for pediatric patients weighing at least 47 kg.
• When administered in combination with ritonavir, LEXIVA Tablets may be used for pediatric patients weighing at least 39 kg; ritonavir capsules may be used for pediatric patients weighing at least 33 kg.

2.3   Patients With Hepatic Impairment

See Clinical Pharmacology (12.3).

Mild Hepatic Impairment (Child-Pugh score ranging from 5 to 6): LEXIVA should be used with caution at a reduced dosage of 700 mg twice daily without ritonavir (therapy-naive) or 700 mg twice daily plus ritonavir 100 mg once daily (therapy-naive or protease inhibitor-experienced).

Moderate Hepatic Impairment (Child-Pugh score ranging from 7 to 9): LEXIVA should be used with caution at a reduced dosage of 700 mg twice daily without ritonavir (therapy-naive), or 450 mg twice daily plus ritonavir 100 mg once daily (therapy-naive or protease inhibitor-experienced).

Severe Hepatic Impairment (Child-Pugh score ranging from 10 to 15): LEXIVA should be used with caution at a reduced dosage of 350 mg twice daily without ritonavir (therapy-naive) or 300 mg twice daily plus ritonavir 100 mg once daily (therapy-naive or protease inhibitor-experienced).

3   DOSAGE FORMS AND STRENGTHS

LEXIVA Tablets, 700 mg, are pink, film-coated, capsule-shaped, biconvex tablets with "GX LL7" debossed on one face.

LEXIVA Oral Suspension, 50 mg/mL, is a white to off-white suspension that has a characteristic grape-bubblegum-peppermint flavor.

4   CONTRAINDICATIONS

LEXIVA is contraindicated:
• in patients with previously demonstrated clinically significant hypersensitivity (e.g., Stevens-Johnson syndrome) to any of the components of this product or to amprenavir.
• when coadministered with drugs that are highly dependent on CYP3A4 for clearance and for which elevated plasma concentrations are associated with serious and/or life-threatening events (Table 1).

[See table 1 above]
• when coadministered with ritonavir in patients receiving the antiarrhythmic agents flecainide and propafenone. If LEXIVA is coadministered with ritonavir, reference should be made to the full prescribing information for ritonavir for additional contraindications.

5   WARNINGS AND PRECAUTIONS
5.1   Drug Interactions

See Table 1 for listings of drugs that are contraindicated due to potentially life-threatening adverse events, significant drug interactions, or due to loss of virologic activity *[see Contraindications (4), Drug Interactions (7.2)]*. See Table 6 for a listing of established and other potentially significant drug interactions *[see Drug Interactions (7.3)]*.

5.2   Skin Reactions

Severe and life-threatening skin reactions, including 1 case of Stevens-Johnson syndrome among 700 patients treated with LEXIVA in clinical studies. Treatment with LEXIVA should be discontinued for severe or life-threatening rashes and for moderate rashes accompanied by systemic symptoms *[see Adverse Reactions (6)]*.

Table 1. Drugs Contraindicated With LEXIVA. (Information in the table applies to LEXIVA with or without ritonavir, unless otherwise indicated.)

Drug Class/Drug Name	Clinical Comment
Alpha 1-adrenoreceptor antagonist: Alfuzosin	Potentially increased alfuzosin concentrations can result in hypotension.
Antiarrhythmics: Flecainide, propafenone	POTENTIAL for serious and/or life-threatening reactions such as cardiac arrhythmias secondary to increases in plasma concentrations of antiarrhythmics if LEXIVA is co-prescribed with **ritonavir**.
Antimycobacterials: Rifampin[a]	May lead to loss of virologic response and possible resistance to LEXIVA or to the class of protease inhibitors.
Ergot derivatives: Dihydroergotamine, ergonovine, ergotamine, methylergonovine	POTENTIAL for serious and/or life-threatening reactions such as acute ergot toxicity characterized by peripheral vasospasm and ischemia of the extremities and other tissues.
GI motility agents: Cisapride	POTENTIAL for serious and/or life-threatening reactions such as cardiac arrhythmias.
Herbal products: St. John's wort (*hypericum perforatum*)	May lead to loss of virologic response and possible resistance to LEXIVA or to the class of protease inhibitors.
HMG co-reductase inhibitors: Lovastatin, simvastatin	POTENTIAL for serious reactions such as risk of myopathy including rhabdomyolysis.
Neuroleptic: Pimozide	POTENTIAL for serious and/or life-threatening reactions such as cardiac arrhythmias.
Non-nucleoside reverse transcriptase inhibitor: Delavirdine[a]	May lead to loss of virologic response and possible resistance to delavirdine.
PDE5 inhibitor: Sildenafil (REVATIO®) (for treatment of pulmonary arterial hypertension)	A safe and effective dose has not been established when used with LEXIVA. There is increased potential for sildenafil-associated adverse events (which include visual disturbances, hypotension, prolonged erection, and syncope).
Sedative/hypnotics: Midazolam, triazolam	POTENTIAL for serious and/or life-threatening reactions such as prolonged or increased sedation or respiratory depression.

[a] *See Clinical Pharmacology (12.3) Tables 10, 11, 12, or 13 for magnitude of interaction.*

Table 2. Selected Moderate/Severe Clinical Adverse Reactions Reported in ≥2% of Antiretroviral-Naive Adult Patients

Adverse Reaction	APV30001[a]		APV30002[a]	
	LEXIVA 1,400 mg b.i.d. (n = 166)	Nelfinavir 1,250 mg b.i.d. (n = 83)	LEXIVA 1,400 mg q.d./ Ritonavir 200 mg q.d. (n = 322)	Nelfinavir 1,250 mg b.i.d. (n = 327)
Gastrointestinal				
Diarrhea	5%	18%	10%	18%
Nausea	7%	4%	7%	5%
Vomiting	2%	4%	6%	4%
Abdominal pain	1%	0%	2%	2%
Skin				
Rash	8%	2%	3%	2%
General disorders				
Fatigue	2%	1%	4%	2%
Nervous system				
Headache	2%	4%	3%	3%

[a] All patients also received abacavir and lamivudine twice daily.

5.3   Sulfa Allergy

LEXIVA should be used with caution in patients with a known sulfonamide allergy. Fosamprenavir contains a sulfonamide moiety. The potential for cross-sensitivity between drugs in the sulfonamide class and fosamprenavir is unknown. In a clinical study of LEXIVA used as the sole protease inhibitor, rash occurred in 2 of 10 patients (20%) with a history of sulfonamide allergy compared with 42 of 126 patients (33%) with no history of sulfonamide allergy. In 2 clinical studies of LEXIVA plus low-dose ritonavir, rash occurred in 8 of 50 patients (16%) with a history of sulfonamide allergy compared with 50 of 412 patients (12%) with no history of sulfonamide allergy.

5.4   Hepatic Toxicity

Use of LEXIVA with ritonavir at higher-than-recommended dosages may result in transaminase elevations and should not be used *[see Dosage and Administration (2), Overdosage (10)]*. Patients with underlying hepatitis B or C or marked elevations in transaminases prior to treatment may be at increased risk for developing or worsening of transaminase elevations. Appropriate laboratory testing should be conducted prior to initiating therapy with LEXIVA and patients should be monitored closely during treatment.

5.5   Diabetes/Hyperglycemia

New onset diabetes mellitus, exacerbation of pre-existing diabetes mellitus, and hyperglycemia have been reported

Table 3. Selected Moderate/Severe Clinical Adverse Reactions Reported in ≥2% of Protease Inhibitor-Experienced Adult Patients (Study APV30003)

Adverse Reaction	LEXIVA 700 mg b.i.d./ Ritonavir 100 mg b.i.d.[a] (n = 106)	Lopinavir 400 mg b.i.d./ Ritonavir 100 mg b.i.d.[a] (n = 103)
Gastrointestinal		
Diarrhea	13%	11%
Nausea	3%	9%
Vomiting	3%	5%
Abdominal pain	<1%	2%
Skin		
Rash	3%	0%
Nervous system		
Headache	4%	2%

[a]All patients also received 2 reverse transcriptase inhibitors.

Table 4. Grade 3/4 Laboratory Abnormalities Reported in ≥2% of Antiretroviral-Naive Adult Patients in Studies APV30001 and APV30002

Laboratory Abnormality	APV30001[a]		APV30002[a]	
	LEXIVA 1,400 mg b.i.d. (n = 166)	Nelfinavir 1,250 mg b.i.d. (n = 83)	LEXIVA 1,400 mg q.d./ Ritonavir 200 mg q.d. (n = 322)	Nelfinavir 1,250 mg b.i.d. (n = 327)
ALT (>5 × ULN)	6%	5%	8%	8%
AST (>5 × ULN)	6%	6%	6%	7%
Serum lipase (>2 × ULN)	8%	4%	6%	4%
Triglycerides[b] (>750 mg/dL)	0%	1%	6%	2%
Neutrophil count, absolute (<750 cells/mm³)	3%	6%	3%	4%

[a]All patients also received abacavir and lamivudine twice daily.
[b]Fasting specimens.
ULN = Upper limit of normal.

Table 5. Grade 3/4 Laboratory Abnormalities Reported in ≥2% of Protease Inhibitor-Experienced Adult Patients in Study APV30003

Laboratory Abnormality	LEXIVA 700 mg b.i.d./ Ritonavir 100 mg b.i.d.[a] (n = 104)	Lopinavir 400 mg b.i.d./ Ritonavir 100 mg b.i.d.[a] (n = 103)
Triglycerides[b] (>750 mg/dL)	11%[c]	6%[c]
Serum lipase (>2 × ULN)	5%	12%
ALT (>5 × ULN)	4%	4%
AST (>5 × ULN)	4%	2%
Glucose (>251 mg/dL)	2%[c]	2%[c]

[a]All patients also received 2 reverse transcriptase inhibitors.
[b]Fasting specimens.
[c]n = 100 for LEXIVA plus ritonavir, n = 98 for lopinavir plus ritonavir.
ULN = Upper limit of normal.

during postmarketing surveillance in HIV-infected patients receiving protease inhibitor therapy. Some patients required either initiation or dose adjustments of insulin or oral hypoglycemic agents for treatment of these events. In some cases, diabetic ketoacidosis has occurred. In those patients who discontinued protease inhibitor therapy, hyperglycemia persisted in some cases. Because these events have been reported voluntarily during clinical practice, estimates of frequency cannot be made and causal relationships between protease inhibitor therapy and these events have not been established.

5.6 Immune Reconstitution Syndrome
Immune reconstitution syndrome has been reported in patients treated with combination antiretroviral therapy, including LEXIVA. During the initial phase of combination antiretroviral treatment, patients whose immune system responds may develop an inflammatory response to indolent or residual opportunistic infections (such as *Mycobacterium avium* infection, cytomegalovirus, *Pneumocystis jirovecii* pneumonia [PCP], or tuberculosis), which may necessitate further evaluation and treatment.

5.7 Fat Redistribution
Redistribution/accumulation of body fat, including central obesity, dorsocervical fat enlargement (buffalo hump), peripheral wasting, facial wasting, breast enlargement, and "cushingoid appearance," have been observed in patients receiving antiretroviral therapy, including LEXIVA. The mechanism and long-term consequences of these events are currently unknown. A causal relationship has not been established.

5.8 Lipid Elevations
Treatment with LEXIVA plus ritonavir has resulted in increases in the concentration of triglycerides and cholesterol [see Adverse Reactions (6)]. Triglyceride and cholesterol testing should be performed prior to initiating therapy with LEXIVA and at periodic intervals during therapy. Lipid disorders should be managed as clinically appropriate [see Drug Interactions (7)].

5.9 Hemolytic Anemia
Acute hemolytic anemia has been reported in a patient treated with amprenavir.

5.10 Patients With Hemophilia
There have been reports of spontaneous bleeding in patients with hemophilia A and B treated with protease inhibitors. In some patients, additional factor VIII was required. In many of the reported cases, treatment with protease inhibitors was continued or restarted. A causal relationship between protease inhibitor therapy and these episodes has not been established.

5.11 Nephrolithiasis
Cases of nephrolithiasis were reported during postmarketing surveillance in HIV-infected patients receiving LEXIVA. Because these events were reported voluntarily during clinical practice, estimates of frequency cannot be made. If signs or symptoms of nephrolithiasis occur, temporary interruption or discontinuation of therapy may be considered.

5.12 Resistance/Cross-Resistance
Because the potential for HIV cross-resistance among protease inhibitors has not been fully explored, it is unknown what effect therapy with LEXIVA will have on the activity of subsequently administered protease inhibitors. LEXIVA has been studied in patients who have experienced treatment failure with protease inhibitors [see Clinical Studies (14.2)].

6 ADVERSE REACTIONS
- Severe or life-threatening skin reactions have been reported with the use of LEXIVA [see Warnings and Precautions (5.2)].
- The most common moderate to severe adverse reactions in clinical studies of LEXIVA were diarrhea, rash, nausea, vomiting, and headache.
- Treatment discontinuation due to adverse events occurred in 6.4% of patients receiving LEXIVA and in 5.9% of patients receiving comparator treatments. The most common adverse reactions leading to discontinuation of LEXIVA (incidence ≤1% of patients) included diarrhea, nausea, vomiting, AST increased, ALT increased, and rash.

6.1 Clinical Trials
Adults
The data for the 3 active-controlled clinical trials described below reflect exposure of 700 HIV-1 infected patients to LEXIVA Tablets, including 599 patients exposed to LEXIVA for >24 weeks, and 409 patients exposed for >48 weeks. The population age ranged from 17 to 72 years. Of these patients, 26% were female, 51% Caucasian, 31% black, 16% American Hispanic, and 70% were antiretroviral-naive. Sixty-one percent received LEXIVA 1,400 mg once daily plus ritonavir 200 mg once daily, 24% received LEXIVA 1,400 mg twice daily, and 15% received LEXIVA 700 mg twice daily plus ritonavir 100 mg twice daily.

Because clinical trials are conducted under widely varying conditions, adverse reaction rates observed in the clinical trials of a drug cannot be directly compared to rates in the clinical trials of another drug and may not reflect the rates observed in clinical practice.

Selected adverse reactions reported during the clinical efficacy studies of LEXIVA are shown in Tables 2 and 3. Each table presents adverse reactions of moderate or severe intensity in patients treated with combination therapy for up to 48 weeks.

[See table 2 on previous page]
[See table 3 above]

Skin rash (without regard to causality) occurred in approximately 19% of patients treated with LEXIVA in the pivotal efficacy studies. Rashes were usually maculopapular and of mild or moderate intensity, some with pruritus. Rash had a median onset of 11 days after initiation of LEXIVA and had a median duration of 13 days. Skin rash led to discontinuation of LEXIVA in <1% of patients. In some patients with mild or moderate rash, dosing with LEXIVA was often continued without interruption; if interrupted, reintroduction of LEXIVA generally did not result in rash recurrence.

The percentages of patients with Grade 3 or 4 laboratory abnormalities in the clinical efficacy studies of LEXIVA are presented in Tables 4 and 5.

[See table 4 above]

The incidence of Grade 3 or 4 hyperglycemia in antiretroviral-naive patients who received LEXIVA in the pivotal studies was <1%.

[See table 5 above]

Pediatric Patients: LEXIVA with and without ritonavir was studied in 144 pediatric patients 2 to 18 years of age in 2 open-label studies. Safety information from 75 pediatric patients receiving LEXIVA twice daily with or without ritonavir follows.

All adverse events regardless of causality, all drug-related adverse events, and all laboratory events occurred with similar frequency in pediatrics compared with adults, with the exception of vomiting. Vomiting, regardless of causality, occurred more frequently among pediatric patients receiving LEXIVA twice daily with ritonavir ([30%] all between 2 and 18 years of age) and without ritonavir ([56%] all between 2 and 5 years of age) compared with adults receiving LEXIVA twice daily with ritonavir (10%) and without ritonavir (16%). The median duration of drug-related vomiting episodes was 1 day (range: 1 to 62 days). Vomiting required temporary dose interruptions in 4 pediatric patients and was treatment-limiting in 1 pediatric patient, all of whom were receiving LEXIVA twice daily with ritonavir.

6.2 Postmarketing Experience

In addition to adverse reactions reported from clinical trials, the following reactions have been identified during post-approval use of LEXIVA. Because they are reported voluntarily from a population of unknown size, estimates of frequency cannot be made. These reactions have been chosen for inclusion due to a combination of their seriousness, frequency of reporting, or potential causal connection to LEXIVA.

Cardiac Disorders
Myocardial infarction.
Metabolism and Nutrition Disorders
Hypercholesterolemia.
Nervous System Disorders
Oral paresthesia.
Skin and Subcutaneous Tissue Disorders
Angioedema.
Urogenital
Nephrolithiasis.

7 DRUG INTERACTIONS

See also Contraindications (4), Clinical Pharmacology (12.3).

If LEXIVA is used in combination with ritonavir, see full prescribing information for ritonavir for additional information on drug interactions.

7.1 CYP Inhibitors and Inducers

Amprenavir, the active metabolite of fosamprenavir, is an inhibitor of cytochrome P450 3A4 metabolism and therefore should not be administered concurrently with medications with narrow therapeutic windows that are substrates of CYP3A4. Data also suggest that amprenavir induces CYP3A4.

Amprenavir is metabolized by CYP3A4. Coadministration of LEXIVA and drugs that induce CYP3A4, such as rifampin, may decrease amprenavir concentrations and reduce its therapeutic effect. Coadministration of LEXIVA and drugs that inhibit CYP3A4 may increase amprenavir concentrations and increase the incidence of adverse effects.

The potential for drug interactions with LEXIVA changes when LEXIVA is coadministered with the potent CYP3A4 inhibitor ritonavir. The magnitude of CYP3A4-mediated drug interactions (effect on amprenavir or effect on co-administered drug) may change when LEXIVA is coadministered with ritonavir. Because ritonavir is a CYP2D6 inhibitor, clinically significant interactions with drugs metabolized by CYP2D6 are possible when coadministered with LEXIVA plus ritonavir.

There are other agents that may result in serious and/or life-threatening drug interactions [see Contraindications (4)].

7.2 Drugs That Should Not Be Coadministered With LEXIVA

See Contraindications (4).

7.3 Established and Other Potentially Significant Drug Interactions

Table 6 provides a listing of established or potentially clinically significant drug interactions. Information in the table applies to LEXIVA with or without ritonavir, unless otherwise indicated.

[See table 6 at right and on pages 3306 and 3307]

8 USE IN SPECIFIC POPULATIONS

8.1 Pregnancy

Pregnancy Category C. Embryo/fetal development studies were conducted in rats (dosed from day 6 to day 17 of gestation) and rabbits (dosed from day 7 to day 20 of gestation). Administration of fosamprenavir to pregnant rats and rabbits produced no major effects on embryo-fetal development; however, the incidence of abortion was increased in rabbits that were administered fosamprenavir. Systemic exposures (AUC_{0-24hr}) to amprenavir at these dosages were 0.8 (rabbits) to 2 (rats) times the exposures in humans following administration of the maximum recommended human dose (MRHD) of fosamprenavir alone or 0.3 (rabbits) to 0.7 (rats)

Table 6. Established and Other Potentially Significant Drug Interactions

Concomitant Drug Class: Drug Name	Effect on Concentration of Amprenavir or Concomitant Drug	Clinical Comment
HIV-Antiviral Agents		
Non-nucleoside reverse transcriptase inhibitor: Efavirenz[a]	**LEXIVA:** ↓Amprenavir **LEXIVA/ritonavir:** ↓Amprenavir	Appropriate doses of the combinations with respect to safety and efficacy have not been established. An additional 100 mg/day (300 mg total) of ritonavir is recommended when efavirenz is administered with LEXIVA/ritonavir once daily. No change in the ritonavir dose is required when efavirenz is administered with LEXIVA plus ritonavir twice daily.
Non-nucleoside reverse transcriptase inhibitor: Nevirapine[a]	**LEXIVA:** ↓Amprenavir ↑Nevirapine **LEXIVA/ritonavir:** ↓Amprenavir ↑Nevirapine	Coadministration of nevirapine and LEXIVA without ritonavir is not recommended. No dosage adjustment required when nevirapine is administered with LEXIVA/ritonavir twice daily. The combination of nevirapine administered with LEXIVA/ritonavir once-daily regimen has not been studied.
HIV protease inhibitor: Atazanavir[a]	**LEXIVA:** Interaction has not been evaluated. **LEXIVA/ritonavir:** ↓Atazanavir ↔Amprenavir	Appropriate doses of the combinations with respect to safety and efficacy have not been established.
HIV protease inhibitors: Indinavir[a], nelfinavir[a]	**LEXIVA:** ↑Amprenavir Effect on indinavir and nelfinavir is not well established. **LEXIVA/ritonavir:** Interaction has not been evaluated.	Appropriate doses of the combinations with respect to safety and efficacy have not been established.
HIV protease inhibitors: Lopinavir/ritonavir[a]	↓Amprenavir ↓Lopinavir	An increased rate of adverse events has been observed. Appropriate doses of the combinations with respect to safety and efficacy have not been established.
HIV protease inhibitor: Saquinavir[a]	**LEXIVA:** ↓Amprenavir Effect on saquinavir is not well established. **LEXIVA/ritonavir:** Interaction has not been evaluated.	Appropriate doses of the combination with respect to safety and efficacy have not been established.
Other Agents		
Antiarrhythmics: Amiodarone, bepridil, lidocaine (systemic), and quinidine	↑Antiarrhythmics	Use with caution. Increased exposure may be associated with life-threatening reactions such as cardiac arrhythmias. Therapeutic concentration monitoring, if available, is recommended for antiarrhythmics.
Anticoagulant: Warfarin		Concentrations of warfarin may be affected. It is recommended that INR (international normalized ratio) be monitored.
Anticonvulsants: Carbamazepine, phenobarbital, phenytoin Phenytoin[a]	**LEXIVA:** ↓Amprenavir **LEXIVA/ritonavir:** ↑Amprenavir ↓Phenytoin	Use with caution. LEXIVA may be less effective due to decreased amprenavir plasma concentrations in patients taking these agents concomitantly. Plasma phenytoin concentrations should be monitored and phenytoin dose should be increased as appropriate. No change in LEXIVA/ritonavir dose is recommended.
Antidepressant: Paroxetine, trazodone	↓Paroxetine ↑Trazodone	Coadministration of paroxetine with LEXIVA/ritonavir significantly decreased plasma levels of paroxetine. Any paroxetine dose adjustment should be guided by clinical effect (tolerability and efficacy). Concomitant use of trazodone and LEXIVA with or without ritonavir may increase plasma concentrations of trazodone. Adverse events of nausea, dizziness, hypotension, and syncope have been observed following coadministration of trazodone and ritonavir. If trazodone is used with a CYP3A4 inhibitor such as LEXIVA, the combination should be used with caution and a lower dose of trazodone should be considered.

(Table continued on next page)

times the exposures in humans following administration of the MRHD of fosamprenavir in combination with ritonavir. In contrast, administration of amprenavir was associated with abortions and an increased incidence of minor skeletal variations resulting from deficient ossification of the femur, humerus, and trochlea, in pregnant rabbits at the tested dose; approximately one-twentieth the exposure seen at the recommended human dose.

The mating and fertility of the F_1 generation born to female rats given fosamprenavir was not different from control animals; however, fosamprenavir did cause a reduction in both pup survival and body weights. Surviving F_1 female rats showed an increased time to successful mating, an increased length of gestation, a reduced number of uterine implantation sites per litter, and reduced gestational body weights compared with control animals. Systemic exposure

Table 6 (cont.). Established and Other Potentially Significant Drug Interactions

Concomitant Drug Class: Drug Name	Effect on Concentration of Amprenavir or Concomitant Drug	Clinical Comment
Antifungals: Ketoconazole[a], itraconazole	↑Ketoconazole ↑Itraconazole	Increase monitoring for adverse events. **LEXIVA:** Dose reduction of ketoconazole or itraconazole may be needed for patients receiving more than 400 mg ketoconazole or itraconazole per day. **LEXIVA/ritonavir:** High doses of ketoconazole or itraconazole (>200 mg/day) are not recommended.
Anti-gout: Colchicine	↑Colchicine	Patients with renal or hepatic impairment should not be given colchicine with LEXIVA/ritonavir. **LEXIVA/ritonavir and coadministration of colchicine:** **Treatment of gout flares:** 0.6 mg (1 tablet) × 1 dose, followed by 0.3 mg (half tablet) 1 hour later. Dose to be repeated no earlier than 3 days. **Prophylaxis of gout flares:** If the original regimen was 0.6 mg twice a day, the regimen should be adjusted to 0.3 mg once a day. If the original regimen was 0.6 mg once a day, the regimen should be adjusted to 0.3 mg once every other day. **Treatment of familial Mediterranean fever (FMF):** Maximum daily dose of 0.6 mg (may be given as 0.3 mg twice a day). **LEXIVA and coadministration of colchicine:** **Treatment of gout flares:** 1.2 mg (2 tablets) × 1 dose. Dose to be repeated no earlier than 3 days. **Prophylaxis of gout flares:** If the original regimen was 0.6 mg twice a day, the regimen should be adjusted to 0.3 mg twice a day or 0.6 mg once a day. If the original regimen was 0.6 mg once a day, the regimen should be adjusted to 0.3 mg once a day. **Treatment of FMF:** Maximum daily dose of 1.2 mg (may be given as 0.6 mg twice a day).
Antimycobacterial: Rifabutin[a]	↑Rifabutin and rifabutin metabolite	A complete blood count should be performed weekly and as clinically indicated to monitor for neutropenia. **LEXIVA:** A dosage reduction of rifabutin by at least half the recommended dose is required. **LEXIVA/ritonavir:** Dosage reduction of rifabutin by at least 75% of the usual dose of 300 mg/day is recommended (a maximum dose of 150 mg every other day or 3 times per week).
Benzodiazepines: Alprazolam, clorazepate, diazepam, flurazepam	↑Benzodiazepines	Clinical significance is unknown. A decrease in benzodiazepine dose may be needed.
Calcium channel blockers: Diltiazem, felodipine, nifedipine, nicardipine, nimodipine, verapamil, amlodipine, nisoldipine, isradipine	↑Calcium channel blockers	Use with caution. Clinical monitoring of patients is recommended.
Corticosteroid: Dexamethasone	↓Amprenavir	Use with caution. LEXIVA may be less effective due to decreased amprenavir plasma concentrations.
Endothelin receptor antagonists: Bosentan	↑Bosentan	Coadministration of bosentan in patients on LEXIVA: In patients who have been receiving LEXIVA for at least 10 days, start bosentan at 62.5 mg once daily or every other day based upon individual tolerability. Coadministration of LEXIVA in patients on bosentan: Discontinue use of bosentan at least 36 hours prior to initiation of LEXIVA. After at least 10 days following the initiation of LEXIVA, resume bosentan at 62.5 mg once daily or every other day based upon individual tolerability.
Histamine H$_2$-receptor antagonists: Cimetidine, famotidine, nizatidine, ranitidine[a]	**LEXIVA:** ↓Amprenavir **LEXIVA/ritonavir:** Interaction not evaluated	Use with caution. LEXIVA may be less effective due to decreased amprenavir plasma concentrations.
HMG-CoA reductase inhibitors: Atorvastatin[a], rosuvastatin	↑Atorvastatin ↑Rosuvastatin	Use the lowest possible dose of atorvastatin or rosuvastatin with careful monitoring, or consider other HMG-CoA reductase inhibitors such as fluvastatin, or pravastatin.

(Table continued on next page)

(AUC$_{0-24hr}$) to amprenavir in the F$_0$ pregnant rats was approximately 2 times higher than exposures in humans following administration of the MRHD of fosamprenavir alone or approximately the same as those seen in humans following administration of the MRHD of fosamprenavir in combination with ritonavir.

There are no adequate and well-controlled studies in pregnant women. LEXIVA should be used during pregnancy only if the potential benefit justifies the potential risk to the fetus.

Antiretroviral Pregnancy Registry
To monitor maternal-fetal outcomes of pregnant women exposed to LEXIVA, an Antiretroviral Pregnancy Registry has been established. Physicians are encouraged to register patients by calling 1-800-258-4263.

8.3   Nursing Mothers
The Centers for Disease Control and Prevention recommend that HIV-infected mothers not breastfeed their infants to avoid risking postnatal transmission of HIV. Although it is not known if amprenavir is excreted in human milk, amprenavir is secreted into the milk of lactating rats. Because of both the potential for HIV transmission and the potential for serious adverse reactions in nursing infants, mothers should be instructed not to breastfeed if they are receiving LEXIVA.

8.4   Pediatric Use
The safety, pharmacokinetic profile, and virologic response of LEXIVA Oral Suspension and Tablets were evaluated in pediatric patients 2 to 18 years of age in 2 open-label studies [see Clinical Studies (14.3)]. No data are available for pediatric patients <2 years of age.
The adverse reaction profile seen in pediatrics was similar to that seen in adults. Vomiting, regardless of causality, was more frequent in pediatrics than in adults [see Adverse Reactions (6.1)].

8.5   Geriatric Use
Clinical studies of LEXIVA did not include sufficient numbers of patients aged 65 and over to determine whether they respond differently from younger adults. In general, dose selection for an elderly patient should be cautious, reflecting the greater frequency of decreased hepatic, renal, or cardiac function, and of concomitant disease or other drug therapy.

8.6   Hepatic Impairment
Amprenavir is principally metabolized by the liver; therefore, caution should be exercised when administering LEXIVA to patients with hepatic impairment because amprenavir concentrations may be increased [see Clinical Pharmacology (12.3)]. Patients with impaired hepatic function receiving LEXIVA with or without concurrent ritonavir require dose reduction [see Dosage and Administration (2.3)].

10   OVERDOSAGE
In a healthy volunteer repeat-dose pharmacokinetic study evaluating high-dose combinations of LEXIVA plus ritonavir, an increased frequency of Grade 2/3 ALT elevations (>2.5 × ULN) was observed with LEXIVA 1,400 mg twice daily plus ritonavir 200 mg twice daily (4 of 25 subjects). Concurrent Grade 1/2 elevations in AST (>1.25 × ULN) were noted in 3 of these 4 subjects. These transaminase elevations resolved following discontinuation of dosing. There is no known antidote for LEXIVA. It is not known whether amprenavir can be removed by peritoneal dialysis or hemodialysis. If overdosage occurs, the patient should be monitored for evidence of toxicity and standard supportive treatment applied as necessary.

11   DESCRIPTION
LEXIVA (fosamprenavir calcium) is a prodrug of amprenavir, an inhibitor of HIV protease. The chemical name of fosamprenavir calcium is (3S)-tetrahydrofuran-3-yl (1S,2R)-3-[[(4-aminophenyl) sulfonyl](isobutyl)amino]-1-benzyl-2-(phosphonooxy) propylcarbamate monocalcium salt. Fosamprenavir calcium is a single stereoisomer with the (3S)(1S,2R) configuration. It has a molecular formula of $C_{25}H_{34}CaN_3O_9PS$ and a molecular weight of 623.7. It has the following structural formula:

Fosamprenavir calcium is a white to cream-colored solid with a solubility of approximately 0.31 mg/mL in water at 25°C.

LEXIVA Tablets are available for oral administration in a strength of 700 mg of fosamprenavir as fosamprenavir calcium (equivalent to approximately 600 mg of amprenavir). Each 700-mg tablet contains the inactive ingredients colloidal silicon dioxide, croscarmellose sodium, magnesium stearate, microcrystalline cellulose, and povidone

IMPORTANT NOTICE: Updated drug information is sent bi-monthly via the PDR® Update Insert. For *monthly* email updates, register at PDR.net.

Table 6 (cont.). Established and Other Potentially Significant Drug Interactions

Concomitant Drug Class: Drug Name	Effect on Concentration of Amprenavir or Concomitant Drug	Clinical Comment
Immunosuppressants: Cyclosporine, tacrolimus, rapamycin	↑Immunosuppressants	Therapeutic concentration monitoring is recommended for immunosuppressant agents.
Inhaled beta agonist: Salmeterol	↑Salmeterol	Concurrent administration of salmeterol with LEXIVA is not recommended. The combination may result in increased risk of cardiovascular adverse events associated with salmeterol, including QT prolongation, palpitations, and sinus tachycardia.
Inhaled/nasal steroid: Fluticasone	**LEXIVA:** ↑Fluticasone **LEXIVA/ritonavir:** ↑Fluticasone	Use with caution. Consider alternatives to fluticasone, particularly for long-term use. May result in significantly reduced serum cortisol concentrations. Systemic corticosteroid effects including Cushings syndrome and adrenal suppression have been reported during postmarketing use in patients receiving ritonavir and inhaled or intranasally administered fluticasone. Coadministration of fluticasone and LEXIVA/ritonavir is not recommended unless the potential benefit to the patient outweighs the risk of systemic corticosteroid side effects.
Narcotic analgesic: Methadone	↓Methadone	Data suggest that the interaction is not clinically relevant; however, patients should be monitored for opiate withdrawal symptoms.
Oral contraceptives: Ethinyl estradiol/ norethin-drone[a]	**LEXIVA:** ↓Amprenavir ↓Ethinyl estradiol **LEXIVA/ritonavir:** ↓Ethinyl estradiol	Alternative methods of non-hormonal contraception are recommended. May lead to loss of virologic response.[a] Increased risk of transaminase elevations. No data are available on the use of LEXIVA/ritonavir with other hormonal therapies, such as hormone replacement therapy (HRT) for postmenopausal women.
PDE5 inhibitors: Sildenafil, tadalafil, vardenafil	↑Sildenafil ↑Tadalafil ↑Vardenafil	May result in an increase in PDE5 inhibitor-associated adverse events, including hypotension, syncope, visual disturbances, and priapism. <u>Use of PDE5 inhibitors for pulmonary arterial hypertension (PAH):</u> • Use of sildenafil (REVATIO) is contraindicated when used for the treatment of PAH *[see Contraindications (4)].* • The following dose adjustments are recommended for use of tadalafil (ADCIRCA™) with LEXIVA: <u>Coadministration of ADCIRCA in patients on LEXIVA:</u> In patients receiving LEXIVA for at least one week, start ADCIRCA at 20 mg once daily. Increase to 40 mg once daily based upon individual tolerability. <u>Coadministration of LEXIVA in patients on ADCIRCA:</u> Avoid use of ADCIRCA during the initiation of LEXIVA. Stop ADCIRCA at least 24 hours prior to starting LEXIVA. After at least one week following the initiation of LEXIVA, resume ADCIRCA at 20 mg once daily. Increase to 40 mg once daily based upon individual tolerability. <u>Use of PDE5 inhibitors for erectile dysfunction:</u> **LEXIVA:** Sildenafil: 25 mg every 48 hours. Tadalafil: no more than 10 mg every 72 hours. Vardenafil: no more than 2.5 mg every 24 hours. **LEXIVA/ritonavir:** Sildenafil: 25 mg every 48 hours. Tadalafil: no more than 10 mg every 72 hours. Vardenafil: no more than 2.5 mg every 72 hours. Use with increased monitoring for adverse events.
Proton pump inhibitors: Esomeprazole[a], lansoprazole, omeprazole, pantoprazole, rabeprazole	**LEXIVA:** ↔Amprenavir ↑Esomeprazole **LEXIVA/ritonavir:** ↔Amprenavir ↔Esomeprazole	Proton pump inhibitors can be administered at the same time as a dose of LEXIVA with no change in plasma amprenavir concentrations.
Tricyclic antidepressants: Amitriptyline, imipramine	↑Tricyclics	Therapeutic concentration monitoring is recommended for tricyclic antidepressants.

[a] See Clinical Pharmacology (12.3) Tables 10, 11, 12, or 13 for magnitude of interaction.

K30. The tablet film-coating contains the inactive ingredients hypromellose, iron oxide red, titanium dioxide, and triacetin.
LEXIVA Oral Suspension is available in a strength of 50 mg/mL of fosamprenavir as fosamprenavir calcium equivalent to approximately 43 mg of amprenavir. LEXIVA Oral Suspension is a white to off-white suspension with a grape-bubblegum-peppermint flavor. Each one milliliter (1 mL) contains the inactive ingredients artificial grape-

bubblegum flavor, calcium chloride dihydrate, hypromellose, methylparaben, natural peppermint flavor, polysorbate 80, propylene glycol, propylparaben, purified water, and sucralose.

12 CLINICAL PHARMACOLOGY
12.1 Mechanism of Action
Fosamprenavir is an antiviral agent *[see Clinical Pharmacology (12.4)].*

12.3 Pharmacokinetics
The pharmacokinetic properties of amprenavir after administration of LEXIVA, with or without ritonavir, have been evaluated in both healthy adult volunteers and in HIV-infected patients; no substantial differences in steady-state amprenavir concentrations were observed between the 2 populations.
The pharmacokinetic parameters of amprenavir after administration of LEXIVA (with and without concomitant ritonavir) are shown in Table 7.
[See table 7 at top of next page]
The mean plasma amprenavir concentrations of the dosing regimens over the dosing intervals are displayed in Figure 1.

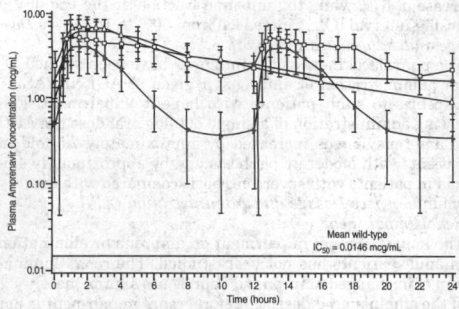

Figure 1. Mean (±SD) Steady-State Plasma Amprenavir Concentrations and Mean IC_{50} Values Against HIV from Protease Inhibitor-Naive Patients (in the Absence of Human Serum)

Absorption and Bioavailability
After administration of a single dose of LEXIVA to HIV-1-infected patients, the time to peak amprenavir concentration (T_{max}) occurred between 1.5 and 4 hours (median 2.5 hours). The absolute oral bioavailability of amprenavir after administration of LEXIVA in humans has not been established.
After administration of a single 1,400-mg dose in the fasted state, LEXIVA Oral Suspension (50 mg/mL) and LEXIVA Tablets (700 mg) provided similar amprenavir exposures (AUC), however, the C_{max} of amprenavir after administration of the suspension formulation was 14.5% higher compared with the tablet.
Effects of Food on Oral Absorption
Administration of a single 1,400-mg dose of LEXIVA Tablets in the fed state (standardized high-fat meal: 967 kcal, 67 grams fat, 33 grams protein, 58 grams carbohydrate) compared with the fasted state was associated with no significant changes in amprenavir C_{max}, T_{max}, or $AUC_{0-\infty}$ *[see Dosage and Administration (2)].*
Administration of a single 1,400-mg dose of LEXIVA Oral Suspension in the fed state (standardized high-fat meal: 967 kcal, 67 grams fat, 33 grams protein, 58 grams carbohydrate) compared with the fasted state was associated with a 46% reduction in C_{max}, a 0.72-hour delay in T_{max}, and a 28% reduction in amprenavir $AUC_{0-\infty}$.
Distribution
In vitro, amprenavir is approximately 90% bound to plasma proteins, primarily to alpha$_1$-acid glycoprotein. In vitro, concentration-dependent binding was observed over the concentration range of 1 to 10 mcg/mL, with decreased binding at higher concentrations. The partitioning of amprenavir into erythrocytes is low, but increases as amprenavir concentrations increase, reflecting the higher amount of unbound drug at higher concentrations.
Metabolism
After oral administration, fosamprenavir is rapidly and almost completely hydrolyzed to amprenavir and inorganic phosphate prior to reaching the systemic circulation. This occurs in the gut epithelium during absorption. Amprenavir is metabolized in the liver by the cytochrome P450 3A4 (CYP3A4) enzyme system. The 2 major metabolites result from oxidation of the tetrahydrofuran and aniline moieties. Glucuronide conjugates of oxidized metabolites have been identified as minor metabolites in urine and feces.
Elimination
Excretion of unchanged amprenavir in urine and feces is minimal. Unchanged amprenavir in urine accounts for approximately 1% of the dose; unchanged amprenavir was not detectable in feces. Approximately 14% and 75% of an administered single dose of ^{14}C-amprenavir can be accounted for as metabolites in urine and feces, respectively. Two metabolites accounted for >90% of the radiocarbon in fecal samples. The plasma elimination half-life of amprenavir is approximately 7.7 hours.

Special Populations
Hepatic Impairment
The pharmacokinetics of amprenavir have been studied after the administration of LEXIVA in combination with ritonavir to adult HIV-1-infected patients with mild, moderate, and severe hepatic impairment. Following 2 weeks of dosing with LEXIVA plus ritonavir, the AUC of amprenavir was increased by approximately 22% in patients with mild hepatic impairment, by approximately 70% in patients with moderate hepatic impairment, and by approximately 80% in patients with severe hepatic impairment compared with HIV-1-infected patients with normal hepatic function. Protein binding of amprenavir was decreased in patients with hepatic impairment. The unbound fraction at 2 hours (approximate C_{max}) ranged between a decrease of -7% to an increase of 57% while the unbound fraction at the end of the dosing interval (C_{min}) increased from 50% to 102% [see Dosage and Administration (2.3)].

The pharmacokinetics of amprenavir have been studied after administration of amprenavir given as AGENERASE® Capsules to adult patients with hepatic impairment. Following administration of a single 600-mg oral dose the AUC of amprenavir was increased by approximately 2.5-fold in patients with moderate cirrhosis and by approximately 4.5-fold in patients with severe cirrhosis compared with healthy volunteers [see Dosage and Administration (2.3)].

Renal Impairment
The impact of renal impairment on amprenavir elimination in adult patients has not been studied. The renal elimination of unchanged amprenavir represents approximately 1% of the administered dose; therefore, renal impairment is not expected to significantly impact the elimination of amprenavir.

Pediatric Patients
The pharmacokinetics of amprenavir after administration of LEXIVA Oral Suspension and LEXIVA Tablets, with or without ritonavir, have been evaluated in 124 patients 2 to 18 years of age. Pharmacokinetic parameters for LEXIVA administered with food and with or without ritonavir in this patient population are provided in Tables 8 and 9 below.

Table 8. Geometric Mean (95% CI) Steady-State Plasma Amprenavir Pharmacokinetic Parameters in Pediatric Patients Receiving LEXIVA 30 mg/kg Twice Daily

Parameter	n	2 to 5 Years LEXIVA 30 mg/kg b.i.d.
$AUC_{(24)}$ (mcg•hr/mL)	8	31.4 (13.7, 72.4)
C_{max} (mcg/mL)	8	5.00 (1.95, 12.8)
C_{min} (mcg/mL)	17	0.454 (0.342, 0.604)

[See table 9 above]
Geriatric Patients
The pharmacokinetics of amprenavir after administration of LEXIVA to patients over 65 years of age have not been studied [see Use in Specific Populations (8.5)].

Gender
The pharmacokinetics of amprenavir after administration of LEXIVA do not differ between males and females.

Race
The pharmacokinetics of amprenavir after administration of LEXIVA do not differ between blacks and non-blacks.

Drug Interactions
[See Contraindications (4), Warnings and Precautions (5.1), Drug Interactions (7).]

Amprenavir, the active metabolite of fosamprenavir, is metabolized in the liver by the cytochrome P450 enzyme system. Amprenavir inhibits CYP3A4. Data also suggest that amprenavir induces CYP3A4. Caution should be used when coadministering medications that are substrates, inhibitors, or inducers of CYP3A4, or potentially toxic medications that are metabolized by CYP3A4. Amprenavir does not inhibit CYP2D6, CYP1A2, CYP2C9, CYP2C19, CYP2E1, or uridine glucuronosyltransferase (UDPGT).

Drug interaction studies were performed with LEXIVA and other drugs likely to be coadministered or drugs commonly used as probes for pharmacokinetic interactions. The effects of coadministration on AUC, C_{max}, and C_{min} values are summarized in Table 10 (effect of other drugs on amprenavir) and Table 12 (effect of LEXIVA on other drugs). In addition, since LEXIVA delivers comparable amprenavir plasma concentrations as AGENERASE, drug interaction data derived from studies with AGENERASE are provided in Tables 11 and 13. For information regarding clinical recommendations, see Drug Interactions (7).

[See table 10 above and on next page]
[See table 11 at top of page 3310]
[See table 12 on pages 3310 and 3311]
[See table 13 at top of page 3312]

Table 7. Geometric Mean (95% CI) Steady-State Plasma Amprenavir Pharmacokinetic Parameters in Adults

Regimen	C_{max} (mcg/mL)	T_{max} (hours)[a]	AUC_{24} (mcg•hr/mL)	C_{min} (mcg/mL)
LEXIVA 1,400 mg b.i.d.	4.82 (4.06-5.72)	1.3 (0.8-4.0)	33.0 (27.6-39.2)	0.35 (0.27-0.46)
LEXIVA 1,400 mg q.d. plus Ritonavir 200 mg q.d.	7.24 (6.32-8.28)	2.1 (0.8-5.0)	69.4 (59.7-80.8)	1.45 (1.16-1.81)
LEXIVA 1,400 mg q.d. plus Ritonavir 100 mg q.d.	7.93 (7.25-8.68)	1.5 (0.75-5.0)	66.4 (61.1-72.1)	0.86 (0.74-1.01)
LEXIVA 700 mg b.i.d. plus Ritonavir 100 mg b.i.d.	6.08 (5.38-6.86)	1.5 (0.75-5.0)	79.2 (69.0-90.6)	2.12 (1.77-2.54)

[a]Data shown are median (range).

Table 9. Geometric Mean (95% CI) Steady-State Plasma Amprenavir Pharmacokinetic Parameters in Pediatric and Adolescent Patients Receiving LEXIVA Plus Ritonavir Twice Daily

Parameter	n	6 to 11 Years LEXIVA 18 mg/kg plus Ritonavir 3 mg/kg b.i.d.	n	12 to 18 Years LEXIVA 700 mg plus Ritonavir 100 mg b.i.d.
$AUC_{(0-24)}$ (mcg•hr/mL)	9	93.4 (67.8, 129)	8	58.8 (38.8, 89.0)
C_{max} (mcg/mL)	9	6.07 (4.40, 8.38)	8	4.33 (2.82, 6.65)
C_{min} (mcg/mL)	17	2.69 (2.15, 3.36)	24	1.61 (1.21, 2.15)

Table 10. Drug Interactions: Pharmacokinetic Parameters for Amprenavir After Administration of LEXIVA in the Presence of the Coadministered Drug(s)

Coadministered Drug(s) and Dose(s)	Dose of LEXIVA[a]	n	% Change in **Amprenavir** Pharmacokinetic Parameters (90% CI)		
			C_{max}	AUC	C_{min}
Antacid (MAALOX TC®) 30 mL single dose	1,400 mg single dose	30	↓35 (↓24 to ↓42)	↓18 (↓9 to ↓26)	↑14 (↓7 to ↑39)
Atazanavir 300 mg q.d. for 10 days	700 mg b.i.d. plus ritonavir 100 mg b.i.d. for 10 days	22	↔	↔	↔
Atorvastatin 10 mg q.d. for 4 days	1,400 mg b.i.d. for 2 weeks	16	↓18 (↓34 to ↑1)	↓27 (↓41 to ↓12)	↓12 (↓27 to ↓6)
Atorvastatin 10 mg q.d. for 4 days	700 mg b.i.d. plus ritonavir 100 mg b.i.d. for 2 weeks	16	↔	↔	↔
Efavirenz 600 mg q.d. for 2 weeks	1,400 mg q.d. plus ritonavir 200 mg q.d. for 2 weeks	16	↔	↓13 (↓30 to ↑7)	↓36 (↓8 to ↓56)
Efavirenz 600 mg q.d. plus additional ritonavir 100 mg q.d. for 2 weeks	1,400 mg q.d. plus ritonavir 200 mg q.d. for 2 weeks	16	↑18 (↑1 to ↑38)	↑11 (0 to ↑24)	↔
Efavirenz 600 mg q.d. for 2 weeks	700 mg b.i.d. plus ritonavir 100 mg b.i.d. for 2 weeks	16	↔	↔	↓17 (↓4 to ↓29)
Esomeprazole 20 mg q.d. for 2 weeks	1,400 mg b.i.d. for 2 weeks	25	↔	↔	↔

(Table continued on next page)

12.4 Microbiology
Mechanism of Action
Fosamprenavir is a prodrug that is rapidly hydrolyzed to amprenavir by cellular phosphatases in the gut epithelium as it is absorbed. Amprenavir is an inhibitor of HIV-1 protease. Amprenavir binds to the active site of HIV-1 protease and thereby prevents the processing of viral Gag and Gag-Pol polyprotein precursors, resulting in the formation of immature non-infectious viral particles.

Antiviral Activity
Fosamprenavir has little or no antiviral activity in vitro. The in vitro antiviral activity of amprenavir was evaluated against HIV-1 IIIB in both acutely and chronically infected lymphoblastic cell lines (MT-4, CEM-CCRF, H9) and in peripheral blood lymphocytes. The 50% effective concentration (EC_{50}) of amprenavir ranged from 0.012 to 0.08 μM in acutely infected cells and was 0.41 μM in chronically in-fected cells (1 μM = 0.50 mcg/mL). The median EC_{50} value of amprenavir against HIV-1 isolates from clades A to G was 0.00095 μM in peripheral blood mononuclear cells (PBMCs). Similarly, the EC_{50} values for amprenavir against monocytes/macrophage tropic HIV-1 isolates (clade B) ranged from 0.003 to 0.075 μM in monocyte/macrophage cultures. The EC_{50} values of amprenavir against HIV-2 isolates grown in PBMCs were higher than those for HIV-1 isolates, and ranged from 0.003 to 0.11 μM. Amprenavir exhibited synergistic anti–HIV-1 activity in combination with the nucleoside reverse transcriptase inhibitors (NRTIs) abacavir, didanosine, lamivudine, stavudine, tenofovir, and zidovudine; the non-nucleoside reverse transcriptase inhibitors (NNRTIs) delavirdine and efavirenz; and the protease inhibitors atazanavir and saquinavir. Amprenavir exhibited additive anti–HIV-1 activity in combination with the NNRTI nevirapine, the protease inhibitors indinavir,

lopinavir, nelfinavir, and ritonavir; and the fusion inhibitor enfuvirtide. These drug combinations have not been adequately studied in humans.

Resistance

HIV-1 isolates with decreased susceptibility to amprenavir have been selected in vitro and obtained from patients treated with fosamprenavir. Genotypic analysis of isolates from treatment-naive patients failing amprenavir-containing regimens showed mutations in the HIV-1 protease gene resulting in amino acid substitutions primarily at positions V32I, M46I/L, I47V, I50V, I54L/M, and I84V, as well as mutations in the p7/p1 and p1/p6 Gag and Gag-Pol polyprotein precursor cleavage sites. Some of these amprenavir resistance-associated mutations have also been detected in HIV-1 isolates from antiretroviral-naive patients treated with LEXIVA. Of the 488 antiretroviral-naive patients treated with LEXIVA 1,400 mg twice daily or LEXIVA 1,400 mg plus ritonavir 200 mg once daily in studies APV30001 and APV30002, respectively, 61 patients (29 receiving LEXIVA and 32 receiving LEXIVA/ritonavir) with virologic failure (plasma HIV-1 RNA >1,000 copies/mL on 2 occasions on or after Week 12) were genotyped. Five of the 29 antiretroviral-naive patients (17%) receiving LEXIVA without ritonavir in study APV30001 had evidence of genotypic resistance to amprenavir: I54L/M (n = 2), I54L + L33F (n = 1), V32I + I47V (n = 1), and M46I + I47V (n = 1). No amprenavir resistance-associated mutations were detected in antiretroviral-naive patients treated with LEXIVA/ritonavir for 48 weeks in study APV30002. However, the M46I and I50V mutations were detected in isolates from 1 virologic failure patient receiving LEXIVA/ritonavir once daily at Week 160 (HIV-1 RNA >500 copies/mL). Upon retrospective analysis of stored samples using an ultrasensitive assay, these resistant mutants were traced back to Week 84 (76 weeks prior to clinical virologic failure).

Cross-Resistance

Varying degrees of cross-resistance among HIV-1 protease inhibitors have been observed. An association between virologic response at 48 weeks (HIV-1 RNA level <400 copies/mL) and protease inhibitor-resistance mutations detected in baseline HIV-1 isolates from protease inhibitor-experienced patients receiving LEXIVA/ritonavir twice daily (n = 88), or lopinavir/ritonavir twice daily (n = 85) in study APV30003 is shown in Table 14. The majority of subjects had previously received either one (47%) or 2 protease inhibitors (36%), most commonly nelfinavir (57%) and indinavir (53%). Out of 102 subjects with baseline phenotypes receiving twice-daily LEXIVA/ritonavir, 54% (n = 55) had resistance to at least one protease inhibitor, with 98% (n = 54) of those having resistance to nelfinavir. Out of 97 subjects with baseline phenotypes in the lopinavir/ritonavir arm, 60% (n = 58) had resistance to at least one protease inhibitor, with 97% (n = 56) of those having resistance to nelfinavir.

Table 14. Responders at Study Week 48 by Presence of Baseline Protease Inhibitor Resistance-Associated Mutations[a]

PI-mutations[b]	LEXIVA/ Ritonavir b.i.d. (n = 88)		Lopinavir/ Ritonavir b.i.d. (n = 85)	
D30N	21/22	95%	17/19	89%
N88D/S	20/22	91%	12/12	100%
L90M	16/31	52%	17/29	59%
M46I/L	11/22	50%	12/24	50%
V82A/F/T/S	2/9	22%	6/17	35%
I54V	2/11	18%	6/11	55%
I84V	1/6	17%	2/5	40%

[a] Results should be interpreted with caution because the subgroups were small.
[b] Most patients had >1 protease inhibitor resistance-associated mutation at baseline.

The virologic response based upon baseline phenotype was assessed. Baseline isolates from protease inhibitor-experienced patients responding to LEXIVA/ritonavir twice daily had a median shift in susceptibility to amprenavir relative to a standard wild-type reference strain of 0.7 (range: 0.1 to 5.4, n = 62), and baseline isolates from individuals failing therapy had a median shift in susceptibility of 1.9 (range: 0.2 to 14, n = 29). Because this was a select patient population, these data do not constitute definitive clinical susceptibility break points. Additional data are needed to determine clinically relevant break points for LEXIVA. Isolates from 15 of the 20 patients receiving twice-daily LEXIVA/ritonavir up to Week 48 and experiencing virologic failure/ongoing replication were subjected to genotypic analysis. The following amprenavir resistance-associated mutations were found either alone or in combination: V32I, M46I/L, I47V, I50V, I54L/M, and I84V. Isolates from 4 of the 16 patients continuing to receive twice-daily LEXIVA/ritonavir up to Week 96 who experienced virologic failure

underwent genotypic analysis. Isolates from 2 patients contained amprenavir resistance-associated mutations: V32I, M46I, and I47V in 1 isolate and I84V in the other.

13 NONCLINICAL TOXICOLOGY

13.1 Carcinogenesis, Mutagenesis, Impairment of Fertility

In long-term carcinogenicity studies, fosamprenavir was administered orally for up to 104 weeks at doses of 250, 400, or 600 mg/kg/day in mice and at doses of 300, 825, or 2,250 mg/kg/day in rats. Exposures at these doses were 0.3- to 0.7-fold (mice) and 0.7- to 1.4-fold (rats) those in humans given 1,400 mg twice daily of fosamprenavir alone, and 0.2- to 0.3-fold (mice) and 0.3- to 0.7-fold (rats) those in humans given 1,400 mg once daily of fosamprenavir plus 200 mg ritonavir once daily. Exposures in the carcinogenicity studies were 0.1- to 0.3-fold (mice) and 0.3- to 0.6-fold (rats) those in humans given 700 mg of fosamprenavir plus 100 mg ritonavir twice daily. There was an increase in hepatocellular adenomas and hepatocellular carcinomas at all doses in male mice and at 600 mg/kg/day in female mice, and in hepatocellular adenomas and thyroid follicular cell adenomas at all doses in male rats, and at 835 mg/kg/day and 2,250 mg/kg/day in female rats. The relevance of the hepatocellular findings in the rodents for humans is uncertain. Repeat dose studies with fosamprenavir in rats produced effects consistent with enzyme induction, which predisposes rats, but not humans, to thyroid neoplasms. In addition, in rats only there was an increase in interstitial cell hyperplasia at

Table 10 *(cont.)*. **Drug Interactions: Pharmacokinetic Parameters for Amprenavir After Administration of LEXIVA in the Presence of the Coadministered Drug(s)**

Coadministered Drug(s) and Dose(s)	Dose of LEXIVA[a]	n	% Change in **Amprenavir** Pharmacokinetic Parameters (90% CI)		
			C_{max}	AUC	C_{min}
Esomeprazole 20 mg q.d. for 2 weeks	700 mg b.i.d. plus ritonavir 100 mg b.i.d. for 2 weeks	23	↔	↔	↔
Ethinyl estradiol/norethindrone 0.035 mg/0.5 mg q.d. for 21 days	700 mg b.i.d. plus ritonavir[b] 100 mg b.i.d. for 21 days	25	↔[c]	↔[c]	↔[c]
Ketoconazole[d] 200 mg q.d. for 4 days	700 mg b.i.d. plus ritonavir 100 mg b.i.d. for 4 days	15	↔	↔	↔
Lopinavir/ritonavir 533 mg/133 mg b.i.d.	1,400 mg b.i.d. for 2 weeks	18	↓13[e]	↓26[e]	↓42[e]
Lopinavir/ritonavir 400 mg/100 mg b.i.d. for 2 weeks	700 mg b.i.d. plus ritonavir 100 mg b.i.d. for 2 weeks	18	↓58 (↓42 to ↓70)	↓63 (↓51 to ↓72)	↓65 (↓54 to ↓73)
Methadone 70 to 120 mg q.d. for 2 weeks	700 mg b.i.d. plus ritonavir 100 mg b.i.d. for 2 weeks	19	↔[c]	↔[c]	↔[c]
Nevirapine 200 mg b.i.d. for 2 weeks[f]	1,400 mg b.i.d. for 2 weeks	17	↓25 (↓37 to ↓10)	↓33 (↓45 to ↓20)	↓35 (↓50 to ↓15)
Nevirapine 200 mg b.i.d. for 2 weeks[f]	700 mg b.i.d. plus ritonavir 100 mg b.i.d. for 2 weeks	17	↔	↓11 (↓23 to ↑3)	↓19 (↓32 to ↓4)
Phenytoin 300 mg q.d. for 10 days	700 mg b.i.d. plus ritonavir 100 mg b.i.d. for 10 days	13	↔	↑20 (↑8 to ↑34)	↑19 (↑6 to ↑33)
Ranitidine 300 mg single dose (administered 1 hour before fosamprenavir)	1,400 mg single dose	30	↓51 (↓43 to ↓58)	↓30 (↓22 to ↓37)	↔ (↓19 to ↑21)
Rifabutin 150 mg q.o.d. for 2 weeks	700 mg b.i.d. plus ritonavir 100 mg b.i.d. for 2 weeks	15	↑36[c] (↑18 to ↑55)	↑35[c] (↑17 to ↑56)	↑17[c] (↓1 to ↑39)
Tenofovir 300 mg q.d. for 4 to 48 weeks	700 mg b.i.d. plus ritonavir 100 mg b.i.d. for 4 to 48 weeks	45	NA	NA	↔[g]
Tenofovir 300 mg q.d. for 4 to 48 weeks	1,400 mg q.d. plus ritonavir 200 mg q.d. for 4 to 48 weeks	60	NA	NA	↔[g]

[a] Concomitant medication is also shown in this column where appropriate.
[b] Ritonavir C_{max}, AUC, and C_{min} increased by 63%, 45%, and 13%, respectively, compared with historical control.
[c] Compared with historical control.
[d] Patients were receiving LEXIVA/ritonavir for 10 days prior to the 4-day treatment period with both ketoconazole and LEXIVA/ritonavir.
[e] Compared with LEXIVA 700 mg/ritonavir 100 mg b.i.d. for 2 weeks.
[f] Patients were receiving nevirapine for at least 12 weeks prior to study.
[g] Compared with parallel control group.
↑ = Increase; ↓ = Decrease; ↔ = No change (↑ or ↓ ≤10%), NA = Not applicable.

Table 11. Drug Interactions: Pharmacokinetic Parameters for Amprenavir After Administration of AGENERASE in the Presence of the Coadministered Drug(s)

Coadministered Drug(s) and Dose(s)	Dose of AGENERASE[a]	n	% Change in **Amprenavir** Pharmacokinetic Parameters (90% CI)		
			C_{max}	AUC	C_{min}
Abacavir 300 mg b.i.d. for 2 to 3 weeks	900 mg b.i.d. for 2 to 3 weeks	4	↔[a]	↔[a]	↔[a]
Clarithromycin 500 mg b.i.d. for 4 days	1,200 mg b.i.d. for 4 days	12	↑15 (↑1 to ↑31)	↑18 (↑8 to ↑29)	↑39 (↑31 to ↑47)
Delavirdine 600 mg b.i.d. for 10 days	600 mg b.i.d. for 10 days	9	↑40[b]	↑130[b]	↑125[b]
Ethinyl estradiol/norethindrone 0.035 mg/1 mg for 1 cycle	1,200 mg b.i.d. for 28 days	10	↔	↓22 (↓35 to ↓8)	↓20 (↓41 to ↑8)
Indinavir 800 mg t.i.d. for 2 weeks (fasted)	750 or 800 mg t.i.d. for 2 weeks (fasted)	9	↑18 (↓13 to ↑58)	↑33 (↑2 to ↑73)	↑25 (↓27 to ↑116)
Ketoconazole 400 mg single dose	1,200 mg single dose	12	↓16 (↓25 to ↓6)	↑31 (↑20 to ↑42)	NA
Lamivudine 150 mg single dose	600 mg single dose	11	↔	↔	NA
Methadone 44 to 100 mg q.d. for >30 days	1,200 mg b.i.d. for 10 days	16	↓27[c]	↓30[c]	↓25[c]
Nelfinavir 750 mg t.i.d. for 2 weeks (fed)	750 or 800 mg t.i.d. for 2 weeks (fed)	6	↓14 (↓38 to ↑20)	↔	↑189 (↑52 to ↑448)
Rifabutin 300 mg q.d. for 10 days	1,200 mg b.i.d. for 10 days	5	↔	↓15 (↓28 to 0)	↓15 (↓38 to ↑17)
Rifampin 300 mg q.d. for 4 days	1,200 mg b.i.d. for 4 days	11	↓70 (↓76 to ↓62)	↓82 (↓84 to ↓78)	↓92 (↓95 to ↓89)
Saquinavir 800 mg t.i.d. for 2 weeks (fed)	750 or 800 mg t.i.d. for 2 weeks (fed)	7	↓37 (↓54 to ↓14)	↓32 (↓49 to ↓9)	↓14 (↓52 to ↑54)
Zidovudine 300 mg single dose	600 mg single dose	12	↔	↑13 (↓2 to ↑31)	NA

[a]Compared with parallel control group.
[b]Median percent change; confidence interval not reported.
[c]Compared with historical data.
↑ = Increase; ↓ = Decrease; ↔ = No change (↑ or ↓ <10%); NA = C_{min} not calculated for single-dose study.

Table 12. Drug Interactions: Pharmacokinetic Parameters for Coadministered Drug in the Presence of Amprenavir After Administration of LEXIVA

Coadministered Drug(s) and Dose(s)	Dose of LEXIVA[a]	n	% Change in Pharmacokinetic Parameters of **Coadministered Drug** (90% CI)		
			C_{max}	AUC	C_{min}
Atazanavir 300 mg q.d. for 10 days[b]	700 mg b.i.d. plus ritonavir 100 mg b.i.d. for 10 days	21	↓24 (↓39 to ↓6)	↓22 (↓34 to ↓9)	↔
Atorvastatin 10 mg q.d. for 4 days	1,400 mg b.i.d. for 2 weeks	16	↑304 (↑205 to ↑437)	↑130 (↑100 to ↑164)	↓10 (↓27 to ↑12)
Atorvastatin 10 mg q.d. for 4 days	700 mg b.i.d. plus ritonavir 100 mg b.i.d. for 2 weeks	16	↑184 (↑126 to ↑257)	↑153 (↑115 to ↑199)	↑73 (↑45 to ↑108)
Esomeprazole 20 mg q.d. for 2 weeks	1,400 mg b.i.d. for 2 weeks	25	↔	↑55 (↑39 to ↑73)	ND
Esomeprazole 20 mg q.d. for 2 weeks	700 mg b.i.d. plus ritonavir 100 mg b.i.d. for 2 weeks	23	↔	↔	ND

(Table continued on next page)

825 mg/kg/day and 2,250 mg/kg/day, and an increase in uterine endometrial adenocarcinoma at 2,250 mg/kg/day. The incidence of endometrial findings was slightly increased over concurrent controls, but was within background range for female rats. The relevance of the uterine endometrial adenocarcinoma findings in rats for humans is uncertain.

Fosamprenavir was not mutagenic or genotoxic in a battery of in vitro and in vivo assays. These assays included bacterial reverse mutation (Ames), mouse lymphoma, rat micronucleus, and chromosome aberrations in human lymphocytes.

The effects of fosamprenavir on fertility and general reproductive performance were investigated in male (treated for 4 weeks before mating) and female rats (treated for 2 weeks before mating through postpartum day 6). Systemic exposures (AUC_{0-24hr}) to amprenavir in these studies were 3 (males) to 4 (females) times higher than exposures in humans following administration of the MRHD of fosamprenavir alone or similar to those seen in humans following administration of fosamprenavir in combination with ritonavir. Fosamprenavir did not impair mating or fertility of male or female rats and did not affect the development and maturation of sperm from treated rats.

14   CLINICAL STUDIES
14.1   Therapy-Naive Adult Patients
Study APV30001

APV30001 was a randomized, open-label study, comparing treatment with LEXIVA Tablets (1,400 mg twice daily) versus nelfinavir (1,250 mg twice daily) in 249 antiretroviral treatment-naive patients. Both groups of patients also received abacavir (300 mg twice daily) and lamivudine (150 mg twice daily).

The mean age of the patients in this study was 37 years (range: 17 to 70 years), 69% of the patients were males, 20% were CDC Class C, 24% were Caucasian, 32% were black, and 44% were Hispanic. At baseline, the median CD4+ cell count was 212 cells/mm³ (range: 2 to 1,136 cells/mm³; 18% of patients had a CD4+ cell count of <50 cells/mm³ and 30% were in the range of 50 to <200 cells/mm³). Baseline median HIV-1 RNA was 4.83 log₁₀ copies/mL (range: 1.69 to 7.41 log₁₀ copies/mL; 45% of patients had >100,000 copies/mL).

The outcomes of randomized treatment are provided in Table 15.

[See table 15 on page 3312]

Treatment response by viral load strata is shown in Table 16.

[See table 16 on page 3312]

Through 48 weeks of therapy, the median increases from baseline in CD4+ cell counts were 201 cells/mm³ in the group receiving LEXIVA and 216 cells/mm³ in the nelfinavir group.

Study APV30002

APV30002 was a randomized, open-label study, comparing treatment with LEXIVA Tablets (1,400 mg once daily) plus ritonavir (200 mg once daily) versus nelfinavir (1,250 mg twice daily) in 649 treatment-naive patients. Both treatment groups also received abacavir (300 mg twice daily) and lamivudine (150 mg twice daily).

The mean age of the patients in this study was 37 years (range: 18 to 69 years), 73% of the patients were males, 22% were CDC Class C, 53% were Caucasian, 36% were black, and 8% were Hispanic. At baseline, the median CD4+ cell count was 170 cells/mm³ (range: 1 to 1,055 cells/mm³; 20% of patients had a CD4+ cell count of <50 cells/mm³ and 35% were in the range of 50 to <200 cells/mm³). Baseline median HIV-1 RNA was 4.81 log₁₀ copies/mL (range: 2.65 to 7.29 log₁₀ copies/mL; 43% of patients had >100,000 copies/mL).

The outcomes of randomized treatment are provided in Table 17.

[See table 17 at top of page 3313]

Treatment response by viral load strata is shown in Table 18.

[See page 18 on page 3313]

Through 48 weeks of therapy, the median increases from baseline in CD4+ cell counts were 203 cells/mm³ in the group receiving LEXIVA and 207 cells/mm³ in the nelfinavir group.

14.2   Protease Inhibitor-Experienced Adult Patients
Study APV30003

APV30003 was a randomized, open-label, multicenter study comparing 2 different regimens of LEXIVA plus ritonavir (LEXIVA Tablets 700 mg twice daily plus ritonavir 100 mg twice daily or LEXIVA Tablets 1,400 mg once daily plus ritonavir 200 mg once daily) versus lopinavir/ritonavir (400 mg/100 mg twice daily) in 315 patients who had experienced virologic failure to 1 or 2 prior protease inhibitor-containing regimens.

The mean age of the patients in this study was 42 years (range: 24 to 72 years), 85% were male, 33% were CDC Class C, 67% were Caucasian, 24% were black, and 9% were Hispanic. The median CD4+ cell count at baseline was 263 cells/mm³ (range: 2 to 1,171 cells/mm³). Baseline median plasma HIV-1 RNA level was 4.14 log₁₀ copies/mL (range: 1.69 to 6.41 log₁₀ copies/mL).

The median durations of prior exposure to NRTIs were 257 weeks for patients receiving LEXIVA/ritonavir twice daily (79% had ≥3 prior NRTIs) and 210 weeks for patients receiving lopinavir/ritonavir (64% had ≥3 prior NRTIs). The median durations of prior exposure to protease inhibitors were 149 weeks for patients receiving LEXIVA/ritonavir twice daily (49% received ≥2 prior protease inhibitors) and 130 weeks for patients receiving lopinavir/ritonavir (40% received ≥2 prior protease inhibitors).

The time-averaged changes in plasma HIV-1 RNA from baseline (AAUCMB) at 48 weeks (the endpoint on which the study was powered) were -1.4 $\log_{10}$ copies/mL for twice-daily LEXIVA/ritonavir and -1.67 $\log_{10}$ copies/mL for the lopinavir/ritonavir group.

The proportions of patients who achieved and maintained confirmed HIV-1 RNA <400 copies/mL (secondary efficacy endpoint) were 58% with twice-daily LEXIVA/ritonavir and 61% with lopinavir/ritonavir (95% CI for the difference: -16.6, 10.1). The proportions of patients with HIV-1 RNA <50 copies/mL with twice-daily LEXIVA/ritonavir and with lopinavir/ritonavir were 46% and 50%, respectively (95% CI for the difference: -18.3, 8.9). The proportions of patients who were virologic failures were 29% with twice-daily LEXIVA/ritonavir and 27% with lopinavir/ritonavir.

The frequency of discontinuations due to adverse events and other reasons, and deaths were similar between treatment arms.

Through 48 weeks of therapy, the median increases from baseline in CD4+ cell counts were 81 cells/mm³ with twice-daily LEXIVA/ritonavir and 91 cells/mm³ with lopinavir/ritonavir.

This study was not large enough to reach a definitive conclusion that LEXIVA/ritonavir and lopinavir/ritonavir are clinically equivalent.

Once-daily administration of LEXIVA plus ritonavir is not recommended for protease inhibitor-experienced patients. Through Week 48, 50% and 37% of patients receiving LEXIVA 1,400 mg plus ritonavir 200 mg once daily had plasma HIV-1 RNA <400 copies/mL and <50 copies/mL, respectively.

14.3 Pediatric Patients

Two open-label studies in pediatric patients 2 to 18 years of age were conducted. In one study, twice-daily dosing regimens (LEXIVA with or without ritonavir) were evaluated in combination with other antiretroviral agents. A second study evaluated once-daily dosing of LEXIVA with ritonavir; the data from this study were insufficient to support a once-daily dosing regimen in any pediatric patient population.

LEXIVA: Eighteen (16 therapy-naive and 2 therapy-experienced) pediatric patients received LEXIVA Oral Suspension without ritonavir twice daily. At Week 24, 67% (12/18) achieved HIV-1 RNA <400 copies/mL, and the median increase from baseline in CD4+ cell count was 353 cells/mm³.

LEXIVA plus ritonavir: Twenty-seven protease inhibitor-naive and 30 protease inhibitor-experienced pediatric patients received LEXIVA Oral Suspension or Tablets with ritonavir twice daily. At Week 24, 70% of protease inhibitor-naive (19/27) and 57% of protease inhibitor-experienced (17/30) patients achieved HIV-1 RNA <400 copies/mL; median increases from baseline in CD4+ cell counts were 131 cells/mm³ and 149 cells/mm³ in protease inhibitor-naive and experienced patients, respectively.

16 HOW SUPPLIED/STORAGE AND HANDLING

LEXIVA Tablets, 700 mg, are pink, film-coated, capsule-shaped, biconvex tablets, with "GX LL7" debossed on one face.

Bottle of 60 with child-resistant closure (NDC 0173-0721-00).

Store at controlled room temperature of 25°C (77°F); excursions permitted to 15° to 30°C (59° to 86°F) (see USP Controlled Room Temperature). Keep container tightly closed.

LEXIVA Oral Suspension, a white to off-white grape-bubblegum-peppermint-flavored suspension, contains 50 mg of fosamprenavir as fosamprenavir calcium equivalent to approximately 43 mg of amprenavir in each 1 mL. Bottle of 225 mL with child-resistant closure (NDC 0173-0727-00).

This product does not require reconstitution.

Store at 5° to 30°C (41° to 86°F). Shake vigorously before using. Do not freeze.

17 PATIENT COUNSELING INFORMATION

See FDA-approved Patient Labeling

17.1 Drug Interactions

A statement to patients and healthcare providers is included on the product's bottle label: ALERT: Find out about medicines that should NOT be taken with LEXIVA.

LEXIVA may interact with many drugs; therefore, patients should be advised to report to their healthcare provider the use of any other prescription or nonprescription medication or herbal products, particularly St. John's wort.

Patients receiving PDE5 inhibitors should be advised that they may be at an increased risk of PDE5 inhibitor-associated adverse events, including hypotension, visual changes, and priapism, and should promptly report any symptoms to their healthcare provider.

Patients receiving hormonal contraceptives should be instructed to use alternate contraceptive measures during therapy with LEXIVA because hormonal levels may be altered, and if used in combination with LEXIVA and ritonavir, liver enzyme elevations may occur.

17.2 Sulfa Allergy

Patients should inform their healthcare provider if they have a sulfa allergy. The potential for cross-sensitivity between drugs in the sulfonamide class and fosamprenavir is unknown.

17.3 Redistribution/Accumulation of Body Fat

Patients should be informed that redistribution or accumulation of body fat may occur in patients receiving antiretroviral therapy, including LEXIVA, and that the cause and long-term health effects of these conditions are not known at this time.

17.4 Information About Therapy With LEXIVA

Patients should be informed that LEXIVA is not a cure for HIV infection and that they may continue to develop opportunistic infections and other complications associated with HIV disease. The long-term effects of LEXIVA are unknown at this time. Patients should be told that there are currently no data demonstrating that therapy with LEXIVA can reduce the risk of transmitting HIV to others.

Patients should be told that sustained decreases in plasma HIV-1 RNA have been associated with a reduced risk of progression to AIDS and death. Patients should remain under the care of a physician while using LEXIVA. Patients should be advised to take LEXIVA every day as prescribed. LEXIVA must always be used in combination with other antiretroviral drugs. Patients should not alter the dose or discontinue therapy without consulting their physician. If a dose is missed, patients should take the dose as soon as possible and then return to their normal schedule. However, if a dose is skipped, the patient should not double the next dose.

17.5 Oral Suspension

Patients should be instructed to shake the bottle vigorously before each use and that refrigeration of the oral suspension may improve the taste for some patients.

Table 12 *(cont.)*. Drug Interactions: Pharmacokinetic Parameters for Coadministered Drug in the Presence of Amprenavir After Administration of LEXIVA

Coadministered Drug(s) and Dose(s)	Dose of LEXIVA[a]	n	% Change in Pharmacokinetic Parameters of Coadministered Drug (90% CI)		
			C_{max}	AUC	C_{min}
Ethinyl estradiol[c] 0.035 mg q.d. for 21 days	700 mg b.i.d. plus ritonavir 100 mg b.i.d. for 21 days	25	↓28 (↓21 to ↓35)	↓37 (↓30 to ↓42)	ND
Ketoconazole[d] 200 mg q.d. for 4 days	700 mg b.i.d. plus ritonavir 100 mg b.i.d. for 4 days	15	↑25 (↑0 to ↑56)	↑169 (↑108 to ↑248)	ND
Lopinavir/ritonavir[a] 533 mg/133 mg b.i.d. for 2 weeks	1,400 mg b.i.d. for 2 weeks	18	↔[f]	↔[f]	↔[f]
Lopinavir/ritonavir[e] 400 mg/100 mg b.i.d. for 2 weeks	700 mg b.i.d. plus ritonavir 100 mg b.i.d. for 2 weeks	18	↑30 (↓15 to ↑47)	↑37 (↓20 to ↑55)	↑52 (↓28 to ↑82)
Methadone 70 to 120 mg q.d. for 2 weeks	700 mg b.i.d. plus ritonavir 100 mg b.i.d. for 2 weeks	19	R-Methadone (active)		
			↓21[g] (↓30 to ↓12)	↓18[g] (↓27 to ↓8)	↓11[g] (↓21 to ↑1)
			S-Methadone (inactive)		
			↓43[g] (↓49 to ↓37)	↓43[g] (↓50 to ↓36)	↓41[g] (↓49 to ↓31)
Nevirapine 200 mg b.i.d. for 2 weeks[h]	1,400 mg b.i.d. for 2 weeks	17	↑25 (↑14 to ↑37)	↑29 (↑19 to ↑40)	↑34 (↑20 to ↑49)
Nevirapine 200 mg b.i.d. for 2 weeks[h]	700 mg b.i.d. plus ritonavir 100 mg b.i.d. for 2 weeks	17	↑13 (↑3 to ↑24)	↑14 (↑5 to ↑24)	↑22 (↑9 to ↑35)
Norethindrone[c] 0.5 mg q.d. for 21 days	700 mg b.i.d. plus ritonavir 100 mg b.i.d. for 21 days	25	↓38 (↓32 to ↓44)	↓34 (↓30 to ↓37)	↓26 (↓20 to ↓32)
Phenytoin 300 mg q.d. for 10 days	700 mg b.i.d. plus ritonavir 100 mg b.i.d. for 10 days	14	↓20 (↓12 to ↓27)	↓22 (↓17 to ↓27)	↓29 (↓23 to ↓34)
Rifabutin 150 mg every other day for 2 weeks[c]	700 mg b.i.d. plus ritonavir 100 mg b.i.d. for 2 weeks	15	↓14 (↓28 to ↑4)	↔	↑28 (↑12 to ↑46)
(25-O-desacetylrifabutin metabolite)			↑579 (↑479 to ↑698)	↑1,120 (↑965 to ↑1,300)	↑2,510 (↑1,910 to ↑3,300)
Rifabutin + 25-O-desacetylrifabutin metabolite			NA	↑64 (↑46 to ↑84)	NA

[a]Concomitant medication is also shown in this column where appropriate.
[b]Comparison arm of atazanavir 300 mg q.d. plus ritonavir 100 mg q.d. for 10 days.
[c]Administered as a combination oral contraceptive tablet: ethinyl estradiol 0.035 mg/norethindrone 0.5 mg.
[d]Patients were receiving LEXIVA/ritonavir for 10 days prior to the 4-day treatment period with both ketoconazole and LEXIVA/ritonavir.
[e]Data represent lopinavir concentrations.
[f]Compared with lopinavir 400 mg/ritonavir 100 mg b.i.d. for 2 weeks.
[g]Dose normalized to methadone 100 mg. The unbound concentration of the active moiety, R-methadone, was unchanged.
[h]Patients were receiving nevirapine for at least 12 weeks prior to study. [††]Comparison arm of rifabutin 300 mg q.d. for 2 weeks. AUC is $AUC_{(0-48hr)}$.
↑= Increase; ↓= Decrease; ↔ = No change (↑ or ↓ <10%); ND = Interaction cannot be determined as C_{min} was below the lower limit of quantitation.

Table 13. Drug Interactions: Pharmacokinetic Parameters for Coadministered Drug in the Presence of Amprenavir After Administration of AGENERASE

Coadministered Drug(s) and Dose(s)	Dose of AGENERASE	n	% Change in Pharmacokinetic Parameters of Coadministered Drug (90% CI)		
			C_{max}	AUC	C_{min}
Abacavir 300 mg b.i.d. for 2 to 3 weeks	900 mg b.i.d. for 2 to 3 weeks	4	↔[a]	↔[a]	↔[a]
Clarithromycin 500 mg b.i.d. for 4 days	1,200 mg b.i.d. for 4 days	12	↓10 (↓24 to ↑7)	↔	↔
Delavirdine 600 mg b.i.d. for 10 days	600 mg b.i.d. for 10 days	9	↓47[b]	↓61[b]	↓88[b]
Ethinyl estradiol 0.035 mg for 1 cycle	1,200 mg b.i.d. for 28 days	10	↔	↔	↑32 (↓3 to ↑79)
Indinavir 800 mg t.i.d. for 2 weeks (fasted)	750 mg or 800 mg t.i.d. for 2 weeks (fasted)	9	↓22[a]	↓38[a]	↑27[a]
Ketoconazole 400 mg single dose	1,200 mg single dose	12	↑19 (↑8 to ↑33)	↑44 (↑31 to ↑59)	NA
Lamivudine 150 mg single dose	600 mg single dose	11	↔	↔	NA
Methadone 44 to 100 mg q.d. for >30 days	1,200 mg b.i.d. for 10 days	16	R-Methadone (active)		
			↓25 (↓32 to ↓18)	↓13 (↓21 to ↓5)	↓21 (↓32 to ↓9)
			S-Methadone (inactive)		
			↓48 (↓55 to ↓40)	↓40 (↓46 to ↓32)	↓53 (↓60 to ↓43)
Nelfinavir 750 mg t.i.d. for 2 weeks (fed)	750 mg or 800 mg t.i.d. for 2 weeks (fed)	6	↑12[a]	↑15[a]	↑14[a]
Norethindrone 1 mg for 1 cycle	1,200 mg b.i.d. for 28 days	10	↔	↑18 (↑1 to ↑38)	↑45 (↑13 to ↑88)
Rifabutin 300 mg q.d. for 10 days	1,200 mg b.i.d. for 10 days	5	↑119 (↑82 to ↑164)	↑193 (↑156 to ↑235)	↑271 (↑171 to ↑409)
Rifampin 300 mg q.d. for 4 days	1,200 mg b.i.d. for 4 days	11	↔	↔	ND
Saquinavir 800 mg t.i.d. for 2 weeks (fed)	750 mg or 800 mg t.i.d. for 2 weeks (fed)	7	↑21[a]	↓19[a]	↓48[a]
Zidovudine 300 mg single dose	600 mg single dose	12	↑40 (↑14 to ↑71)	↑31 (↑19 to ↑45)	NA

[a] Compared with historical data.
[b] Median percent change; confidence interval not reported.
↑ = Increase; ↓ = Decrease; ↔ = No change (↑ or ↓ <10%); NA = C_{min} not calculated for single-dose study; ND = Interaction cannot be determined as C_{min} was below the lower limit of quantitation.

Table 15. Outcomes of Randomized Treatment Through Week 48 (APV30001)

Outcome (Rebound or discontinuation = failure)	LEXIVA 1,400 mg b.i.d. (n = 166)	Nelfinavir 1,250 mg b.i.d. (n = 83)
Responder[a]	66% (57%)	52% (42%)
Virologic failure	19%	32%
Rebound	16%	19%
Never suppressed through Week 48	3%	13%
Clinical progression	1%	1%
Death	0%	1%
Discontinued due to adverse reactions	4%	2%
Discontinued due to other reasons[b]	10%	10%

[a] Patients achieved and maintained confirmed HIV-1 RNA <400 copies/mL (<50 copies/mL) through Week 48 (Roche AMPLICOR HIV-1 MONITOR Assay Version 1.5).
[b] Includes consent withdrawn, lost to follow up, protocol violations, those with missing data, and other reasons.

Table 16. Proportions of Responders Through Week 48 by Screening Viral Load (APV30001)

Screening Viral Load HIV-1 RNA (copies/mL)	LEXIVA 1,400 mg b.i.d.		Nelfinavir 1,250 mg b.i.d.	
	<400 copies/mL	n	<400 copies/mL	n
≤100,000	65%	93	65%	46
>100,000	67%	73	36%	37

LEXIVA and AGENERASE are registered trademarks of GlaxoSmithKline.
GlaxoSmithKline Vertex Pharmaceuticals Incorporated Research Triangle Park, NC 27709 Cambridge, MA 02139
©2010, GlaxoSmithKline. All rights reserved.
April 2010
LXV:11PI
PHARMACIST-DETACH HERE AND GIVE INSTRUCTIONS TO PATIENT

PATIENT INFORMATION
LEXIVA®
(lex-EE-vah)
(fosamprenavir calcium)
Tablets and Oral Suspension
Read the Patient Information that comes with LEXIVA before you start taking it and each time you get a refill. There may be new information. This information does not take the place of talking with your healthcare provider about your medical condition or treatment. It is important to remain under a healthcare provider's care while taking LEXIVA. Do not change or stop treatment without first talking with your healthcare provider. Talk to your healthcare provider or pharmacist if you have any questions about LEXIVA.

What is the most important information I should know about LEXIVA?
LEXIVA can cause dangerous and life-threatening interactions if taken with certain other medicines. Tell your healthcare provider about all the medicines you take, including prescription and nonprescription medicines, vitamins, and herbal supplements.
• Some medicines cannot be taken at all with LEXIVA.
• Some medicines will require dose changes if taken with LEXIVA.
• Some medicines will require close monitoring if you take them with LEXIVA.
Know all the medicines you take, including prescription and nonprescription medicines, vitamins, and herbal supplements. Keep a list of the medicines you take. Show this list to all your healthcare providers and pharmacists anytime you get a new medicine or refill. Your healthcare providers and pharmacists must know all the medicines you take. They will tell you if you can take other medicines with LEXIVA. Do not start any new medicines while you are taking LEXIVA without talking with your healthcare provider or pharmacist. You can ask your healthcare provider or pharmacist for a list of medicines that can interact with LEXIVA.

What is LEXIVA?
LEXIVA is a medicine you take by mouth to treat HIV infection. HIV is the virus that causes AIDS (acquired immune deficiency syndrome). LEXIVA belongs to a class of anti-HIV medicines called protease inhibitors. LEXIVA is always used with other anti-HIV medicines. When used in combination therapy, LEXIVA may help lower the amount of HIV found in your blood, raise CD4+ (T) cell counts, and keep your immune system as healthy as possible, so it can help fight infection. However, LEXIVA does not work in all patients with HIV.

LEXIVA does not:
• cure HIV infection or AIDS. We do not know if LEXIVA will help you live longer or have fewer of the medical problems (opportunistic infections) that people get with HIV or AIDS. Opportunistic infections are infections that develop because the immune system is weak. Some of these conditions are pneumonia, herpes virus infections, and *Mycobacterium avium* complex (MAC) infections. It is very important that you see your healthcare provider regularly while you are taking LEXIVA. The long-term effects of LEXIVA are not known.
• lower the risk of passing HIV to other people through sexual contact, sharing needles, or being exposed to your blood. For your health and the health of others, it is important to always practice safer sex by using a latex or polyurethane condom to lower the chance of sexual contact with semen, vaginal secretions, or blood. Never use or share dirty needles.
LEXIVA has not been fully studied in children under the age of 2 or in adults over the age of 65.

Who should not take LEXIVA?
Do not take LEXIVA if you:
• are taking certain other medicines. Read the section "What is the most important information I should know about LEXIVA?" Do not take the following medicines* with LEXIVA. You could develop serious or life-threatening problems.
– HALCION® (triazolam; used for insomnia)
– Ergot medicines: dihydroergotamine, ergonovine, ergotamine, and methylergonovine such as CAFERGOT®, MIGRANAL®, D.H.E. 45®, ergotrate maleate, METHERGINE®, and others (used for migraine headaches)
• PROPULSID® (cisapride), used for certain stomach problems

IMPORTANT NOTICE: Updated drug information is sent bi-monthly via the PDR® Update Insert. For *monthly* email updates, register at PDR.net.

Table 17. Outcomes of Randomized Treatment Through Week 48 (APV30002)

Outcome (Rebound or discontinuation = failure)	LEXIVA 1,400 mg q.d./ Ritonavir 200 mg q.d. (n = 322)	Nelfinavir 1,250 mg b.i.d. (n = 327)
Responder[a]	69% (58%)	68% (55%)
Virologic failure	6%	16%
Rebound	5%	8%
Never suppressed through Week 48	1%	8%
Death	1%	0%
Discontinued due to adverse reactions	9%	6%
Discontinued due to other reasons[b]	15%	10%

[a] Patients achieved and maintained confirmed HIV-1 RNA <400 copies/mL (<50 copies/mL) through Week 48 (Roche AMPLICOR HIV-1 MONITOR Assay Version 1.5).
[b] Includes consent withdrawn, lost to follow up, protocol violations, those with missing data, and other reasons.

Table 18. Proportions of Responders Through Week 48 by Screening Viral Load (APV30002)

Screening Viral Load HIV-1 RNA (copies/mL)	LEXIVA 1,400 mg q.d./ Ritonavir 200 mg q.d. <400 copies/mL	n	Nelfinavir 1,250 mg b.i.d. <400 copies/mL	n
≤100,000	72%	197	73%	194
>100,000	66%	125	64%	133

- VERSED® (midazolam), used for sedation
- ORAP® (pimozide), used for Tourette's disorder
- REVATIO® (sildenafil), used for treatment of pulmonary arterial hypertension
- UROXATRAL® (alfuzosin), used for benign prostatic hyperplasia (BPH)
- are allergic to LEXIVA or any of its ingredients. The active ingredient is fosamprenavir calcium. See the end of this leaflet for a list of all the ingredients in LEXIVA.
- are allergic to AGENERASE (amprenavir).

You should not take AGENERASE (amprenavir) and LEXIVA at the same time.

There are other medicines you should not take if you are taking LEXIVA and NORVIR® (ritonavir) together. You could develop serious or life-threatening problems. Tell your healthcare provider about all medicines you are taking before you begin taking LEXIVA and NORVIR (ritonavir) together.

What should I tell my healthcare provider before taking LEXIVA?
Before taking LEXIVA, tell your healthcare provider about all of your medical conditions including if you:
- are pregnant or planning to become pregnant. It is not known if LEXIVA can harm your unborn baby. You and your healthcare provider will need to decide if LEXIVA is right for you. If you use LEXIVA while you are pregnant, talk to your healthcare provider about how you can be on the Antiretroviral Pregnancy Registry.
- are breastfeeding. You should not breastfeed if you are HIV-positive because of the chance of passing the HIV virus to your baby through your milk. Also, it is not known if LEXIVA can pass into your breast milk and if it can harm your baby. If you are a woman who has or will have a baby, talk with your healthcare provider about the best way to feed your baby.
- have liver problems. You may be given a lower dose of LEXIVA or LEXIVA may not be right for you.
- have kidney problems
- have diabetes. You may need dose changes in your insulin or other diabetes medicines.
- have hemophilia
- are allergic to sulfa medicines

Before taking LEXIVA, tell your healthcare provider about all the medicines you take, including prescription and non-prescription medicines, vitamins, and herbal supplements. LEXIVA can cause dangerous and life-threatening interactions if taken with certain other medicines. You may need dose changes in some of your medicines or closer monitoring with some medicines if you also take LEXIVA (see "What is the most important information I should know about LEXIVA."). Know all the medicines that you take and keep a list of them with you to show healthcare providers and pharmacists.

Women who use birth control pills should choose a different kind of contraception. The use of LEXIVA with NORVIR (ritonavir) in combination with birth control pills may be harmful to your liver. The use of LEXIVA with or without NORVIR may decrease the effectiveness of birth control pills. Talk to your healthcare provider about choosing an effective contraceptive.

How should I take LEXIVA?
- Take LEXIVA exactly as your healthcare provider prescribed.
- Do not take more or less than your prescribed dose of LEXIVA at any one time. Do not change your dose or stop taking LEXIVA without talking with your healthcare provider.
- You can take LEXIVA Tablets with or without food.
- Adults should take LEXIVA Oral Suspension without food.
- Pediatric patients should take LEXIVA Oral Suspension with food. If vomiting occurs within 30 minutes after dosing, the dose should be repeated.
- Shake LEXIVA Oral Suspension vigorously before each use.
- When your supply of LEXIVA or other anti-HIV medicine starts to run low, get more from your healthcare provider or pharmacy. The amount of HIV virus in your blood may increase if one or more of the medicines are stopped, even for a short time.
- Stay under the care of a healthcare provider while using LEXIVA.
- It is important that you do not miss any doses. If you miss a dose of LEXIVA by more than 4 hours, wait and take the next dose at the regular time. However, if you miss a dose by fewer than 4 hours, take your missed dose right away. Then take your next dose at the regular time.
- If you take too much LEXIVA, call your healthcare provider or poison control center right away.

What should I avoid while taking LEXIVA?
- Do not use certain medicines while you are taking LEXIVA. See "What is the most important information I should know about LEXIVA"and "Who should not take LEXIVA?"
- Do not breastfeed. See "Before taking LEXIVA, tell your healthcare provider". Talk with your healthcare provider about the best way to feed your baby.
- Avoid doing things that can spread HIV infection since LEXIVA doesn't stop you from passing the HIV infection to others.
- Do not share needles or other injection equipment.
- Do not share personal items that can have blood or body fluids on them, like toothbrushes or razor blades.
- Do not have any kind of sex without protection. Always practice safer sex by using a latex or polyurethane condom to lower the chance of sexual contact with semen, vaginal secretions, or blood.

What are the possible side effects of LEXIVA?
LEXIVA may cause the following side effects:
- skin rash. Skin rashes, some with itching, have happened in patients taking LEXIVA. Swelling of the face, lips, and tongue (angioedema) has also been reported. Tell your healthcare provider if you get a rash or develop facial swelling after starting LEXIVA.
- diabetes and high blood sugar (hyperglycemia). Some patients had diabetes before taking LEXIVA while others did not. Some patients may need changes in their diabetes medicine. Others may need a new diabetes medicine.
- increased bleeding problems in some patients with hemophilia.
- worse liver disease. Patients with liver problems, including hepatitis B or C, are more likely to get worse liver disease when they take anti-HIV medicines like LEXIVA.
- changes in blood tests. Some people have changes in blood tests while taking LEXIVA. These include increases seen in liver function tests and blood fat levels, and decreases in white blood cells. Your healthcare provider may do regular blood tests to see if LEXIVA is affecting your body.
- changes in body fat. These changes have happened in patients taking antiretroviral medicines like LEXIVA. The changes may include an increased amount of fat in the upper back and neck ("buffalo hump"), breast, and around the trunk. Loss of fat from the legs, arms, and face may also happen. The cause and long-term health effects of these conditions are not known at this time.
- kidney stones have been reported in some patients taking LEXIVA. If you develop signs or symptoms of kidney stones (pain in your side, blood in your urine, pain when you urinate) tell your healthcare provider right away.

Common side effects of LEXIVA are nausea, vomiting, and diarrhea. Tell your healthcare provider about any side effects that bother you or that won't go away.

This list of side effects of LEXIVA is not complete. Call your doctor for medical advice about side effects. You may report side effects to FDA at 1-800-FDA-1088.

How should I store LEXIVA?
- LEXIVA Tablets should be stored at room temperature between 59° and 86°F (15° to 30°C). Keep the container of LEXIVA Tablets tightly closed.
- LEXIVA Oral Suspension may be stored at room temperature or refrigerated. Refrigeration of LEXIVA Oral Suspension may improve taste for some patients. Do not freeze.
- Keep LEXIVA and all medicines out of the reach of children.
- Do not keep medicine that is out of date or that you no longer need. Be sure that if you throw any medicine away, it is out of the reach of children.

General information about LEXIVA
Medicines are sometimes prescribed for conditions that are not mentioned in patient information leaflets. Do not use LEXIVA for a condition for which it was not prescribed. Do not give LEXIVA to other people, even if they have the same symptoms you have. It may harm them.

This leaflet summarizes the most important information about LEXIVA. If you would like more information, talk with your healthcare provider. You can ask your pharmacist or healthcare provider for information about LEXIVA that is written for health professionals. For more information you can call toll-free 888-825-5249 or visit www.LEXIVA.com.

What are the ingredients in LEXIVA?
Tablets:
Active Ingredient: fosamprenavir calcium.
Inactive Ingredients: colloidal silicon dioxide, croscarmellose sodium, magnesium stearate, microcrystalline cellulose, and povidone K30. The tablet film-coating contains the inactive ingredients hypromellose, iron oxide red, titanium dioxide, and triacetin.
LEXIVA Tablets, 700 mg, are pink in color and are capsule-shaped, with the letters "GX LL7" printed on one side of the tablet.

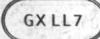

Oral Suspension:
Active Ingredient: fosamprenavir calcium
Inactive ingredients: artificial grape-bubblegum flavor, calcium chloride dihydrate, hypromellose, methylparaben, natural peppermint flavor, polysorbate 80, propylene glycol, propylparaben, purified water, and sucralose.
LEXIVA and AGENERASE are registered trademarks of GlaxoSmithKline.
* The brands listed are trademarks of their respective owners and are not trademarks of GlaxoSmithKline. The makers of these brands are not affiliated with and do not endorse GlaxoSmithKline or its products.
GlaxoSmithKline Vertex Pharmaceuticals Incorporated Research Triangle Park, NC 27709 Cambridge, MA 02139
©2010, GlaxoSmithKline. All rights reserved.
April 2010
LXV:8PIL

RESCRIPTOR®
[ree-SKRIP-tor]
brand of delavirdine mesylate
Tablets

℞

DESCRIPTION

RESCRIPTOR Tablets contain delavirdine mesylate, a synthetic non-nucleoside reverse transcriptase inhibitor of the human immunodeficiency virus type 1 (HIV-1). The chemical name of delavirdine mesylate is piperazine, 1-[3-[(1-methyl-ethyl)amino]-2-pyridinyl]-4-[[5-[(methylsulfonyl)amino]-1H-indol-2-yl]carbonyl]-, monomethanesulfonate. Its molecular formula is $C_{22}H_{28}N_6O_3S \cdot CH_4O_3S$, and its molecular weight is 552.68. The structural formula is:

· CH₃—SO₂—OH

Delavirdine mesylate is an odorless white-to-tan crystalline powder. The aqueous solubility of delavirdine free base at 23° C is 2942 µg/mL at pH 1.0, 295 µg/mL at pH 2.0, and 0.81 µg/mL at pH 7.4.

Each RESCRIPTOR Tablet, for oral administration, contains 100 or 200 mg of delavirdine mesylate (henceforth referred to as delavirdine). Inactive ingredients consist of lactose, microcrystalline cellulose, croscarmellose sodium, magnesium stearate, colloidal silicon dioxide, and carnauba wax. In addition, the 100 mg tablet contains Opadry White YS-1-7000-E and the 200 mg tablet contains hypromellose, Opadry White YS-1-18202-A and Pharmaceutical Ink Black.

MICROBIOLOGY
Mechanism of Action
Delavirdine is a non-nucleoside reverse transcriptase inhibitor (NNRTI) of HIV-1. Delavirdine binds directly to reverse transcriptase (RT) and blocks RNA-dependent and DNA-dependent DNA polymerase activities. Delavirdine does not compete with template: primer or deoxynucleoside triphosphates. HIV-2 RT and human cellular DNA polymerases α, γ, or δ are not inhibited by delavirdine. In addition, HIV-1 group O, a group of highly divergent strains that are uncommon in North America, may not be inhibited by delavirdine.

In Vitro HIV-1 Susceptibility
In vitro anti–HIV-1 activity of delavirdine was assessed by infecting cell lines of lymphoblastic and monocytic origin and peripheral blood lymphocytes with laboratory and clinical isolates of HIV-1. IC_{50} and IC_{90} values (50% and 90% inhibitory concentrations) for laboratory isolates (N=5) ranged from 0.005 to 0.030 µM and 0.04 to 0.10 µM, respectively. Mean IC_{50} of clinical isolates (N=74) was 0.038 µM (range 0.001 to 0.69 µM); 73 of 74 clinical isolates had an $IC_{50} \leq 0.18$ µM. The IC_{90} of 24 of these clinical isolates ranged from 0.05 to 0.10 µM. In drug combination studies of delavirdine with zidovudine, didanosine, zalcitabine, lamivudine, interferon-α, and protease inhibitors, additive to synergistic anti–HIV-1 activity was observed in cell culture. The relationship between the *in vitro* susceptibility of HIV-1 RT inhibitors and the inhibition of HIV replication in humans has not been established.

Drug Resistance
Phenotypic analyses of isolates from patients treated with RESCRIPTOR as monotherapy showed a 50-fold to 500-fold reduced susceptibility in 14 of 15 patients by week 8 of therapy. Genotypic analysis of HIV-1 isolates from patients receiving RESCRIPTOR plus zidovudine combination therapy (N=79) showed resistance conferring mutations in all isolates by week 24 of therapy. In RESCRIPTOR-treated patients the mutations in RT occurred predominantly at amino acid positions 103 and less frequently at positions 181 and 236. In a separate study, an average of 86-fold increase in the zidovudine susceptibility of patient isolates (N=24) was observed after 24 weeks of RESCRIPTOR and zidovudine combination therapy. The clinical relevance of the phenotypic and the genotypic changes associated with RESCRIPTOR therapy has not been established.

Cross-resistance
RESCRIPTOR may confer cross-resistance to other non-nucleoside RT inhibitors when used alone or in combination. Mutations at positions 103 and/or 181 have been found in resistant virus during treatment with RESCRIPTOR and other non-nucleoside RT inhibitors. These mutations have been associated with cross-resistance among non-nucleoside RT inhibitors *in vitro*.

CLINICAL PHARMACOLOGY
Pharmacokinetics
Absorption and Bioavailability
Delavirdine is rapidly absorbed following oral administration, with peak plasma concentrations occurring at approximately one hour. Following administration of delavirdine 400 mg tid (n=67, HIV-1–infected patients), the mean ± SD steady-state peak plasma concentration (C_{max}) was 35 ± 20 µM (range 2 to 100 µM), systemic exposure (AUC) was 180 ± 100 µM • hr (range 5 to 515 µM • hr) and trough concentration (C_{min}) was 15 ± 10 µM (range 0.1 to 45 µM). The single-dose bioavailability of delavirdine tablets relative to an oral solution was 85 ± 25% (n=16, non-HIV–infected subjects). The single-dose bioavailability of delavirdine tablets (100 mg strength) was increased by approximately 20% when a slurry of drug was prepared by allowing delavirdine tablets to disintegrate in water before administration (n=16, non-HIV–infected subjects). The bioavailability of the 200 mg strength delavirdine tablets has not been evaluated when administered as a slurry, because they are not readily dispersed in water (see DOSAGE AND ADMINISTRATION).

Delavirdine may be administered with or without food. In a multiple-dose, crossover study, delavirdine was administered every eight hours with food or every eight hours, one hour before or two hours after a meal (n=13, HIV-1–infected patients). Patients remained on their typical diet throughout the study; meal content was not standardized. When multiple doses of delavirdine were administered with food, geometric mean C_{max} was reduced by approximately 25%, but AUC and C_{min} were not altered.

Distribution
Delavirdine is extensively bound (approximately 98%) to plasma proteins, primarily albumin. The percentage of delavirdine that is protein-bound is constant over a delavirdine concentration range of 0.5 to 196 µM. In five HIV-1–infected patients whose total daily dose of delavirdine ranged from 600 to 1200 mg, cerebrospinal fluid concentrations of delavirdine averaged 0.4%± 0.07% of the corresponding plasma delavirdine concentrations; this represents about 20% of the fraction not bound to plasma proteins. Steady-state delavirdine concentrations in saliva (n=5, HIV-1–infected patients who received delavirdine 400 mg tid) and semen (n=5 healthy volunteers who received delavirdine 300 mg tid) were about 6% and 2%, respectively, of the corresponding plasma delavirdine concentrations collected at the end of a dosing interval.

Metabolism and Elimination
Delavirdine is extensively converted to several inactive metabolites. Delavirdine is primarily metabolized by cytochrome P450 3A (CYP3A), but *in vitro* data suggest that delavirdine may also be metabolized by CYP2D6. The major metabolic pathways for delavirdine are N-desalkylation and pyridine hydroxylation. Delavirdine exhibits nonlinear steady-state elimination pharmacokinetics, with apparent oral clearance decreasing by about 22-fold as the total daily dose of delavirdine increases from 60 to 1200 mg/day. In a study of ¹⁴C-delavirdine in six healthy volunteers who received multiple doses of delavirdine tablets 300 mg tid, approximately 44% of the radiolabeled dose was recovered in feces, and approximately 51% of the dose was excreted in urine. Less than 5% of the dose was recovered unchanged in urine. The parent plasma half-life of delavirdine increases with dose; mean half-life following 400 mg tid is 5.8 hours, with a range of 2 to 11 hours.

In vitro and *in vivo* studies have shown that delavirdine reduces CYP3A activity and inhibits its own metabolism. *In vitro* studies have also shown that delavirdine reduces CYP2C9, CYP2D6, and CYP2C19 activity. Inhibition of hepatic CYP3A activity by delavirdine is reversible within 1 week after discontinuation of drug.

Special Populations
Hepatic or Renal Impairment
The pharmacokinetics of delavirdine in patients with hepatic or renal impairment have not been investigated (see PRECAUTIONS).

Age
The pharmacokinetics of delavirdine have not been adequately studied in patients <16 years or >65 years of age.

Gender
Data from population pharmacokinetics suggest that the plasma concentrations of delavirdine tend to be higher in females than in males. However, this difference is not considered to be clinically significant.

Race
No significant differences in the mean trough delavirdine concentrations were observed between different racial or ethnic groups.

Drug Interactions
(see also PRECAUTIONS: Drug Interactions)
Specific drug interaction studies were performed with delavirdine and a number of drugs. Table 1 summarizes the effects of delavirdine on the geometric mean AUC, C_{max} and C_{min} of coadministered drugs. Table 2 shows the effects of coadministered drugs on the geometric mean AUC, C_{max} and C_{min} of delavirdine.

For information regarding clinical recommendations, see CONTRAINDICATIONS, WARNINGS, and PRECAUTIONS: Drug Interactions.

[See table 1 above]
[See table 2 at top of next page]

Table 1. Pharmacokinetic Parameters for Coadministered Drugs in the Presence of Delavirdine.

Coadministered Drug	Dose of Coadministered Drug	Dose of RESCRIPTOR	n	% Change in Pharmacokinetic Parameters of Coadministered Drug (90% CI)		
				C_{max}	AUC	C_{min}
HIV-Protease Inhibitors						
Indinavir	400 mg tid × 7 days	400 mg tid × 7 days	28	↓36* (↓52–↓14)	↔*	↑118* (↑16–↑312)
	600 mg tid × 7 days	400 mg tid × 7 days	28	↔	↑53* (↑7–↑120)	↑298* (↑104–↑678)
Nelfinavir†	750 mg tid × 14 days	400 mg tid × 7 days	12	↑88 (↑66–↑113)	↑107 (↑83–↑135)	↑136 (↑103–↑175)
Saquinavir	Soft gel capsule 1000 mg tid × 28 days	400 mg tid × 28 days	20	↑98‡ (↑4–↑277)	↑121‡ (↑14–↑340)	↑199‡ (↑37–↑553)
Nucleoside Reverse Transcriptase Inhibitors						
Didanosine (buffered tablets)	125 or 250 mg bid × 28 days	400 mg tid × 28 days	9	↓20§ (↓44–↑15)	↓21§ (↓40–↑5)	-
Zidovudine	200 mg tid for >38 days	100 mg qid to 400 mg tid for 8–10 days	34	↔	↔	-
Anti-infective Agents						
Clarithromycin	500 mg bid × 15 days	300 mg tid × 30 days	6	-	↑100	-
Rifabutin	300 mg qd for 15–99 days	400–1000 mg tid for 45–129 days	5	↑128 (↑71–↑203)	↑230 (↑119–↑396)	↑452 (↑246–↑781)

↑ Indicates increase
↓ Indicates decrease
↔ Indicates no significant change
- Indicates no data available
* Relative to indinavir 800 mg tid without RESCRIPTOR
† Plasma concentrations of the nelfinavir active metabolite (nelfinavir hydroxy-t-butylamide) were significantly reduced by delavirdine, which is more than compensated for by increased nelfinavir concentration
‡ Saquinavir soft gel capsule 1000 mg tid plus RESCRIPTOR 400 mg tid relative to saquinavir soft gel capsule 1200 mg tid without RESCRIPTOR
§ RESCRIPTOR taken with didanosine (buffered tablets) relative to doses of RESCRIPTOR and didanosine (buffered tablets) separated by at least 1 hr

Table 2. Pharmacokinetic Parameters for Delavirdine in the Presence of Coadministered Drugs

Coadministered Drug	Dose of Coadministered Drug	Dose of RESCRIPTOR	n	% Change in Delavirdine Pharmacokinetic Parameters (90% CI)		
				C_{max}	AUC	C_{min}
HIV-Protease Inhibitors						
Indinavir	400 or 600 mg tid × 7 days	400 mg tid × 7 days	81	No apparent changes based on a comparison to historical data		
Nelfinavir	750 mg tid × 7 days	400 mg tid × 14 days	7	↓27 (↓49–↑4)	↓31 (↓57–↑10)	↓33 (↓70–↑49)
Saquinavir	Soft gel capsule 1000 mg tid × 28 days	400 mg tid for 7–28 days	23	No apparent changes based on a comparison to historical data		
Nucleoside Reverse Transcriptase Inhibitors						
Didanosine (buffered tablets)	125 or 200 mg bid × 28 days	400 mg tid × 28 days	9	↓32* (↓48–↓11)	↓19* (↓37–↑6)	↔*
Zidovudine	200 mg tid for ≥ 7 days	400 mg tid for 7–14 days	42	No apparent changes based on a comparison to historical data		
Anti-infective Agents						
Clarithromycin	500 mg bid × 15 days	300 mg tid × 30 days	6	↔	↔	↔
Fluconazole	400 mg qd × 15 days	300 mg tid × 30 days	8	↔	↔	↔
Ketoconazole	Various	200–400 mg tid	26	-	-	↑50†
Rifabutin	300 mg qd × 14 days	400 mg tid × 28 days	7	↓72 (↓61–↓80)	↓82 (↓74–↓88)	↓94 (↓90–↓96)
Rifampin	600 mg qd × 15 days	400 mg tid × 30 days	7	↓90 (↓94–↓83)	↓97 (↓98–↓95)	↓100
Sulfamethoxazole or Trimethoprim & Sulfamethoxazole	Various	200–400 mg tid	311	-	-	↔†
Other						
Antacid (Maalox® TC)	20 mL	300 mg single dose	12	↓52 (↓68–↓29)	↓44 (↓58–↓27)	-
Fluoxetine	Various	200–400 mg tid	36	-	-	↑50†
Phenytoin, Phenobarbital, Carbamazepine	Various	300–400 mg tid	8	-	-	↓90†

↑ Indicates increase
↓ Indicates decrease
↔ Indicates no significant change
- Indicates no data available
* RESCRIPTOR taken with didanosine (buffered tablets) relative to doses of RESCRIPTOR and didanosine (buffered tablets) separated by at least 1 hr
† Population pharmacokinetic data from efficacy studies

Table 3: Outcomes of Randomized Treatment Through Week 52 for Protocol 21 Part 2

Outcome	ZDV + 3TC (N = 124) %	DLV + ZDV (N = 125) %	DLV + ZDV + 3TC (N = 124) %
HIV RNA <400 copies/mL*	14	2	45
HIV RNA ≥400 copies/mL†,‡	64	52	31
Discontinued due to adverse events‡	8	13	10
Discontinued due to other reasons†,§	14	33	14

* Corresponds to rates at Week 52 in proportion curve
† Virologic failures at or before Week 52
‡ Considered to be treatment failure in the analysis
§ Includes discontinuations due to consent withdrawn, loss to follow-up, protocol violations, non-compliance, pregnancy, never treated, and other reasons

INDICATIONS AND USAGE

RESCRIPTOR Tablets are indicated for the treatment of HIV-1 infection in combination with at least 2 other active antiretroviral agents when therapy is warranted.
The following should be considered before initiating therapy with RESCRIPTOR in treatment-naive patients. There are insufficient data directly comparing RESCRIPTOR-containing antiretroviral regimens with currently preferred 3-drug regimens for initial treatment of HIV. In studies comparing regimens consisting of 2 NRTIs (currently considered suboptimal) to RESCRIPTOR plus 2 NRTIs, the proportion of patients receiving the RESCRIPTOR regimen who achieved and sustained an HIV-1 RNA level <400 copies/mL over one year of therapy was relatively low (see DESCRIPTION OF CLINICAL STUDIES).
Resistant virus emerges rapidly when RESCRIPTOR is administered as monotherapy. Therefore, RESCRIPTOR should always be administered in combination with other antiretroviral agents.

DESCRIPTION OF CLINICAL STUDIES

For clinical Studies 21 Part II and 13C described below, efficacy was evaluated by the percentage of patients with a plasma HIV RNA level < 400 copies/mL as measured by the Roche Amplicor® HIV-1 Monitor (standard assay). An intent-to-treat analysis was performed where only subjects who achieved confirmed suppression and sustained it through Week 52 are regarded as responders. All other subjects (including never suppressed, discontinued, and those who rebounded after initial suppression of < 400 copies/mL) are considered failures at Week 52. Results of an interim analysis of efficacy conducted for studies 21 Part II and 13C by independent Data and Safety Monitoring Boards (DSMBs) revealed that the triple therapy arms in both studies produced significantly greater antiviral benefit than the dual therapy arms, and early termination of the studies was recommended.

Study 21 Part II

Study 21 Part II was a double-blind, randomized, placebo-controlled trial comparing treatment with RESCRIPTOR (DLV; 400 mg tid), zidovudine (ZDV; 200 mg tid), and lamivudine (3TC; 150 mg tid) versus RESCRIPTOR (400 mg tid) and zidovudine (200 mg tid) versus zidovudine (200 mg tid) and lamivudine (150 mg bid) in 373 HIV-1–infected patients (mean age 35 years [range 17 to 67], 87% male and 60% Caucasian) who were antiretroviral treatment naive (84%) or had limited nucleoside experience (16%). Mean baseline CD4 cell count was 359 cells/mm³ and mean baseline plasma HIV RNA was 4.4 $\log_{10}$ copies/mL.
Results showed that the mean increase from baseline in CD4 count at 52 weeks was 111 cells/mL for RESCRIPTOR + ZDV + 3TC, 27 cells/mL for RESCRIPTOR + ZDV, and 74 cells/mL for ZDV + 3TC.
The results of the intent-to-treat analysis of the percentage of patients with a plasma HIV RNA level <400 copies/mL are presented in Figure 1. HIV-1 RNA status and reasons for discontinuation of randomized treatment at 52 weeks are summarized in Table 3. Subjects who were never suppressed before discontinuation were placed in the discontinuation category.

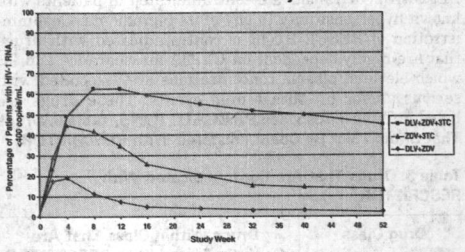

Figure 1
Percentage of Patients with HIV RNA Below 400 copies/mL
Standard PCR Assay
Protocol 21 Part 2
Intent-to-Treat Analysis

[See table 3 at left]

Study 13C

Study 13C was a double-blind, randomized, placebo-controlled trial comparing treatment with RESCRIPTOR (400 mg tid), zidovudine (200 mg tid or 300 mg bid) and either didanosine (ddI; 200 mg bid), zalcitabine (ddC; 0.75 mg tid) or lamivudine (150 mg bid) versus zidovudine (200 mg tid or 300 mg bid) and either didanosine (200 mg bid), zalcitabine (0.75 mg tid) or lamivudine (150 mg bid) in 345 HIV-1–infected patients (mean age 35.8 years [range 18 to 72], 66% male and 63% Caucasian) who were antiretroviral treatment naive (63%) or had limited antiretroviral experience (37%). Mean baseline CD4 cell count was 210 cells/mm³ and mean baseline plasma HIV RNA was 4.9 $\log_{10}$ copies/mL.
Results showed that the mean increase from baseline in CD4 count at 54 weeks was 102 cells/mL for RESCRIPTOR + ZDV + ddI or ddC or 3TC and 56 cells/mL for ZDV + ddI or ddC or 3TC.
The results of the intent-to-treat analysis of the percentage of patients with a plasma HIV RNA level <400 copies/mL are presented in Figure 2. HIV-1 RNA status and reasons for discontinuation of randomized treatment at 54 weeks are summarized in Table 4. Subjects who were never suppressed before discontinuation were placed in the discontinuation category.

Figure 2
Percentage of Patients with HIV RNA Below 400 copies/mL
Standard PCR Assay
Protocol 13C
Intent-to-Treat Analysis

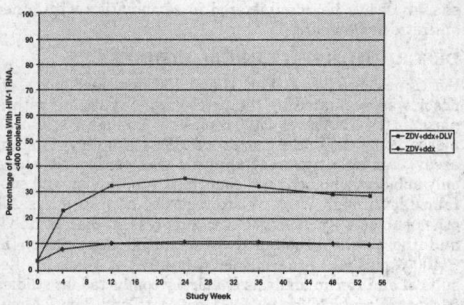

Table 4. Outcomes of Randomized Treatment Through Week 54 for Protocol 13C

Outcome	ZDV + ddx* (N = 173) %	ZDV + ddx + DLV (N = 172) %
HIV RNA <400 copies/mL†	10	29
HIV RNA ≥400 copies/mL‡,§	69	42
Discontinued due to adverse events‡	7	12
Discontinued due to other reasons‡¶	14	17

* ddx = ddI or ddC or 3TC
† Corresponds to rates at Week 54 in proportion curve
‡ Considered to be treatment failure in the analysis
§ Virologic failures at or before Week 54
¶ Includes discontinuations due to consent withdrawn, loss to follow-up, protocol violations, non-compliance, pregnancy, never treated, and other reasons

Results from several smaller supportive studies evaluating the use of RESCRIPTOR in treatment-naive patients suggest that it may have activity when used in combination with protease inhibitors and NRTIs in 3- or 4-drug combinations.

CONTRAINDICATIONS
RESCRIPTOR Tablets are contraindicated in patients with known hypersensitivity to any of its ingredients. Coadministration of RESCRIPTOR is contraindicated with drugs that are highly dependent on CYP3A for clearance and for which elevated plasma concentrations are associated with serious and/or life-threatening events. These drugs are listed in Table 5. **Also, see PRECAUTIONS, Table 6, Drugs That Should Not Be Coadministered With RESCRIPTOR.**

Table 5. Drugs That Are Contraindicated With RESCRIPTOR

Drug Class	Drugs Within Class That Are Contraindicated With RESCRIPTOR
Antihistamines	Astemizole, terfenadine
Ergot derivatives	Dihydroergotamine, ergonovine, ergotamine, methylergonovine
GI motility agent	Cisapride
Neuroleptic	Pimozide
Sedative/hypnotics	Alprazolam, midazolam, triazolam

WARNINGS
ALERT: Find out about medicines that should NOT be taken with RESCRIPTOR. This statement is included on the product's bottle label.
Drug Interactions
Because delavirdine may inhibit the metabolism of many different drugs (e.g., antiarrhythmics, calcium channel blockers, sedative hypnotics, and others), **serious and/or life-threatening drug interactions could result from inappropriate coadministration of some drugs with delavirdine.** In addition, some drugs may markedly reduce delavirdine plasma concentrations, resulting in suboptimal antiviral activity and subsequent emergence of drug resistance. All pre-

Table 6. Drugs That Should Not Be Coadministered With RESCRIPTOR

Drug Class: Drug Name	Clinical Comment
Anticonvulsant agents: phenytoin, phenobarbital, carbamazepine	May lead to loss of virologic response and possible resistance to RESCRIPTOR or to the class of non-nucleoside reverse transcriptase inhibitors.
Antihistamines: astemizole, terfenadine	CONTRAINDICATED due to potential for serious and/or life-threatening reactions such as cardiac arrhythmias.
Antimycobacterials: rifabutin,* rifampin*	May lead to loss of virologic response and possible resistance to RESCRIPTOR or to the class of non-nucleoside reverse transcriptase inhibitors or other coadministered antiviral agents.
Ergot Derivatives: dihydroergotamine, ergonovine, ergotamine, methylergonovine	CONTRAINDICATED due to potential for serious and/or life-threatening reactions such as acute ergot toxicity characterized by peripheral vasospasm and ischemia of the extremities and other tissues.
GI motility agent: cisapride	CONTRAINDICATED due to potential for serious and/or life-threatening reactions such as cardiac arrhythmias.
Herbal Products: St. John's wort (hypericum perforatum)	May lead to loss of virologic response and possible resistance to RESCRIPTOR or to the class of non-nucleoside reverse transcriptase inhibitors.
HMG-CoA reductase inhibitors: lovastatin, simvastatin	Potential for serious reactions such as risk of myopathy including rhabdomyolysis.
Neuroleptic: pimozide	CONTRAINDICATED due to potential for serious and/or life-threatening reactions such as cardiac arrhythmias.
Sedative/hypnotics: alprazolam, midazolam, triazolam	CONTRAINDICATED due to potential for serious and/or life-threatening reactions such as prolonged or increased sedation or respiratory depression.

*See **CLINICAL PHARMACOLOGY** for magnitude of interaction, Tables 1 and 2.

scribers should become familiar with the following tables in this package insert: **Table 5, Drugs That Are Contraindicated With RESCRIPTOR; Table 6, Drugs That Should Not Be Co-administered With RESCRIPTOR; and Table 7, Established and Other Potentially Significant Drug Interactions: Alteration in Dose or Regimen May Be Recommended Based on Drug Interaction Studies or Predicted Interaction.** Additional details on drug interactions can be found in Tables 1 and 2 under the **CLINICAL PHARMACOLOGY** section.

Concomitant use of lovastatin or simvastatin with RESCRIPTOR is not recommended. Caution should be exercised if RESCRIPTOR is used concurrently with other HMG-CoA reductase inhibitors that are also metabolized by the CYP3A4 pathway (e.g., atorvastatin or cerivastatin). The risk of myopathy including rhabdomyolysis may be increased when RESCRIPTOR is used in combination with these drugs.

Particular caution should be used when prescribing sildenafil in patients receiving RESCRIPTOR. Coadministration of sildenafil with RESCRIPTOR is expected to substantially increase sildenafil concentrations and may result in an increase in sildenafil-associated adverse events, including hypotension, visual changes, and priapism (see **PRECAUTIONS, Drug Interactions** and **Information for Patients,** and the complete prescribing information for sildenafil).

Concomitant use of St. John's Wort (hypericum perforatum) or St. John's wort containing products and RESCRIPTOR is not recommended. Coadministration of St. John's wort with non-nucleoside reverse transcriptase inhibitors (NNRTIs), including RESCRIPTOR, is expected to substantially decrease NNRTI concentrations and may result in suboptimal levels of RESCRIPTOR and lead to loss of virologic response and possible resistance to RESCRIPTOR or to the class of NNRTIs.

PRECAUTIONS
General
Delavirdine is metabolized primarily by the liver. Therefore, caution should be exercised when administering RESCRIPTOR Tablets to patients with impaired hepatic function.

Immune Reconstitution Syndrome
Immune reconstitution syndrome has been reported in patients treated with combination antiretroviral therapy, including RESCRIPTOR. During the initial phase of the combination antiretroviral treatment, patients whose immune system responds may develop an inflammatory response to indolent or residual opportunistic infections (such as *Mycobacterium avium* infection, cytomegalovirus, *Pneumocystis jirovecii* pneumonia (PCP), or tuberculosis), which may necessitate further evaluation and treatment.

Resistance/Cross-Resistance
Non-nucleoside reverse transcriptase inhibitors, when used alone or in combination, may confer cross-resistance to other non-nucleoside reverse transcriptase inhibitors.
Fat Redistribution
Redistribution/accumulation of body fat including central obesity, dorsocervical fat enlargement (buffalo hump), peripheral wasting, facial wasting, breast enlargement, and "cushingoid appearance" have been observed in patients receiving antiretroviral therapy. The mechanism and long-term consequences of these events are currently unknown. A causal relationship has not been established.
Skin Rash
Severe rash, including rare cases of erythema multiforme and Stevens-Johnson syndrome, has been reported in patients receiving RESCRIPTOR. Erythema multiforme and Stevens-Johnson syndrome were rarely seen in clinical trials and resolved after withdrawal of RESCRIPTOR. Any patient experiencing severe rash or rash accompanied by symptoms such as fever, blistering, oral lesions, conjunctivitis, swelling, and muscle or joint aches should discontinue RESCRIPTOR and consult a physician. Two cases of Stevens-Johnson syndrome have been reported through postmarketing surveillance out of a total of 339 surveillance reports.

In Studies 21 Part II and 13C (see **DESCRIPTION OF CLINICAL STUDIES**), rash (including maculopapular rash) was reported in more patients who were treated with RESCRIPTOR 400 mg tid (35% and 32%, respectively) than in those who were not treated with RESCRIPTOR (21% and 16%, respectively). The highest intensity of rash reported in these studies was severe (grade 3), which was observed in approximately 4% of patients treated with RESCRIPTOR in each study and in none of the patients who were not treated with RESCRIPTOR. Also in Studies 21 Part II and 13C, discontinuations due to rash were reported in more patients who received RESCRIPTOR 400 mg tid (3% and 4%, respectively) than in those who did not receive RESCRIPTOR (0% and 1%, respectively).

In most cases, the duration of the rash was less than two weeks and did not require dose reduction or discontinuation of RESCRIPTOR. Most patients were able to resume therapy after rechallenge with RESCRIPTOR following a treatment interruption due to rash. The distribution of the rash was mainly on the upper body and proximal arms, with decreasing intensity of the lesions on the neck and face, and progressively less on the rest of the trunk and limbs. Occurrence of a delavirdine-associated rash after one month is uncommon. Symptomatic relief has been obtained using diphenhydramine hydrochloride, hydroxyzine hydrochloride, and/or topical corticosteroids.
Information for Patients
A statement to patients and healthcare providers is included on the product's bottle label: **ALERT: Find out about**

medicines that should NOT be taken with RESCRIPTOR. A patient package insert (PPI) for RESCRIPTOR is available for patient information.

Patients should be informed that RESCRIPTOR is not a cure for HIV-1 infection and that they may continue to acquire illnesses associated with HIV-1 infection, including opportunistic infections. Treatment with RESCRIPTOR has not been shown to reduce the incidence or frequency of such illnesses, and patients should be advised to remain under the care of a physician when using RESCRIPTOR.

Patients should be advised that the use of RESCRIPTOR has not been shown to reduce the risk of transmission of HIV-1.

Patients should be instructed that the major toxicity of RESCRIPTOR is rash and should be advised to promptly notify their physician should rash occur. The majority of rashes associated with RESCRIPTOR occur within 1 to 3 weeks after initiating treatment with RESCRIPTOR. The rash normally resolves in 3 to 14 days and may be treated symptomatically while therapy with RESCRIPTOR is continued. Any patient experiencing severe rash or rash accompanied by symptoms such as fever, blistering, oral lesions, conjunctivitis, swelling, and muscle or joint aches should discontinue medication and consult a physician.

Patients should be informed that redistribution or accumulation of body fat may occur in patients receiving antiretroviral therapy and that the cause and long-term health effects of these conditions are not known at this time.

Patients should be informed to take RESCRIPTOR every day as prescribed. Patients should not alter the dose of RESCRIPTOR without consulting their doctor. If a dose is missed, patients should take the next dose as soon as possible. However, if a dose is skipped, the patient should not double the next dose.

Patients with achlorhydria should take RESCRIPTOR with an acidic beverage (e.g., orange or cranberry juice). However, the effect of an acidic beverage on the absorption of delavirdine in patients with achlorhydria has not been investigated.

Patients taking both RESCRIPTOR and antacids should be advised to take them at least 1 hour apart.

Because RESCRIPTOR may interact with certain drugs, patients should be advised to report to their doctor the use of any prescription, nonprescription medication or herbal products, particularly St. John's wort.

Patients receiving sildenafil and RESCRIPTOR should be advised that they may be at an increased risk of sildenafil-associated adverse events, including hypotension, visual changes, and prolonged penile erection, and should promptly report any symptoms to their doctor.

Drug Interactions
(see also CONTRAINDICATIONS, WARNINGS, and CLINICAL PHARMACOLOGY: Drug Interactions)

Delavirdine is an inhibitor of CYP3A isoform and other CYP isoforms to a lesser extent including CYP2C9, CYP2D6, and CYP2C19. Coadministration of RESCRIPTOR and drugs primarily metabolized by CYP3A (e.g., HMG-CoA reductase inhibitors, and sildenafil) may result in increased plasma concentrations of the coadministered drug that could increase or prolong both its therapeutic or adverse effects.

Delavirdine is metabolized primarily by CYP3A, but in vitro data suggest that delavirdine may also be metabolized by CYP2D6. Coadministration of RESCRIPTOR and drugs that induce CYP3A, such as rifampin, may decrease delavirdine plasma concentrations and reduce its therapeutic effect. Coadministration of RESCRIPTOR and drugs that inhibit CYP3A may increase delavirdine plasma concentrations. (See Table 6, Drugs That Should Not Be Coadministered With RESCRIPTOR, and Table 7, Established and Other Potentially Significant Drug Interactions: Alteration in Dose or Regimen May Be Recommended Based on Drug Interaction Studies or Predicted Interaction.)

[See table 6 at top of previous page]

[See table 7 above and on next page]

Carcinogenesis, Mutagenesis and Impairment of Fertility

Delavirdine was negative in a battery of genetic toxicology tests which included an Ames assay, an in vitro rat hepatocyte unscheduled DNA synthesis assay, an in vitro chromosome aberration assay in human peripheral lymphocytes, an in vitro mutation assay in Chinese hamster ovary cells, and an in vivo micronucleus test in mice.

Lifetime carcinogenicity studies were conducted in rats at doses of 10, 32 and 100 mg/kg/day and in mice at doses of 62.5, 250 and 500 mg/kg/day for males and 62.5, 125 and 250 mg/kg/day for females. In rats, delavirdine was noncarcinogenic at maximally tolerated doses that produced exposures (AUC) up to 12 (male rats) and 9 (female rats) times human exposure at the recommended clinical dose. In mice, delavirdine produced significant increases in the incidence of hepatocellular adenoma/adenocarcinoma in both males and females, hepatocellular adenoma in females, and mesenchymal urinary bladder tumors in males. The systemic drug exposures (AUC) in female mice were 0.5- to 3-fold and

in male mice 0.2- to 4-fold of those in humans at the recommended clinical dose. Given the lack of genotoxic activity of delavirdine, the relevance of urinary bladder and hepatocellular neoplasm in delavirdine-treated mice to humans is not known.

Delavirdine at doses of 20, 100, and 200 mg/kg/day did not cause impairment of fertility in rats when males were treated for 70 days and females were treated for 14 days prior to mating.

Pregnancy
Pregnancy Category C

Delavirdine has been shown to be teratogenic in rats. Delavirdine caused ventricular septal defects in rats at doses of 50, 100, and 200 mg/kg/day when administered during the period of organogenesis. The lowest dose of delavirdine that caused malformations produced systemic exposures in pregnant rats equal to or lower than the expected human exposure to RESCRIPTOR (C_{min} 15 μM) at the recommended dose. Exposure in rats approximately 5-fold higher than the expected human exposure resulted in marked maternal toxicity, embryotoxicity, fetal developmental delay, and reduced pup survival. Additionally, reduced

pup survival on postpartum day 0 occurred at an exposure (mean C_{min}) approximately equal to the expected human exposure. Delavirdine was excreted in the milk of lactating rats at a concentration three to five times that of rat plasma.

Delavirdine at doses of 200 and 400 mg/kg/day administered during the period of organogenesis caused maternal toxicity, embryotoxicity and abortions in rabbits. The lowest dose of delavirdine that resulted in these toxic effects produced systemic exposures in pregnant rabbits approximately 6-fold higher than the expected human exposure to RESCRIPTOR (C_{min} 15 μM) at the recommended dose. The no-observed-adverse-effect dose in the pregnant rabbit was 100 mg/kg/day. Various malformations were observed at this dose, but the incidence of such malformations was not statistically significantly different from those observed in the control group. Systemic exposures in pregnant rabbits at a dose of 100 mg/kg/day were lower than those expected in humans at the recommended clinical dose. Malformations were not apparent at 200 and 400 mg/kg/day; however, only a limited number of fetuses were available for examination as a result of maternal and embryo death.

Table 7. Established and Other Potentially Significant Drug Interactions: Alteration in Dose or Regimen May Be Recommended Based on Drug Interaction Studies or Predicted Interaction

Concomitant Drug Class: Drug Name	Effect on Concentration of delavirdine or Concomitant Drug	Clinical Comment
HIV-Antiviral Agents		
Amprenavir	↑ Amprenavir	Appropriate doses of this combination, with respect to safety, efficacy and pharmacokinetics, have not been established.
Didanosine*	↓ Delavirdine ↓ Didanosine	Administration of didanosine (buffered tablets) and RESCRIPTOR should be separated by at least one hour.
Indinavir*	↑ Indinavir	A dose reduction of indinavir to 600 mg tid should be considered when RESCRIPTOR and indinavir are coadministered.
Lopinavir/Ritonavir	↑ Lopinavir ↑ Ritonavir	Appropriate doses of this combination, with respect to safety, efficacy and pharmacokinetics, have not been established.
Nelfinavir*	↑ Nelfinavir ↓ Delavirdine	Appropriate doses of this combination, with respect to safety, efficacy and pharmacokinetics, have not been established. (See CLINICAL PHARMACOLOGY: Tables 1 and 2.)
Ritonavir	↑ Ritonavir	Appropriate doses of this combination, with respect to safety, efficacy and pharmacokinetics, have not been established.
Saquinavir*	↑ Saquinavir	A dose reduction of saquinavir (soft gelatin capsules) may be considered when RESCRIPTOR and saquinavir are coadministered. (See CLINICAL PHARMACOLOGY: Table 1.) Appropriate doses with respect to safety, efficacy and pharmacokinetics, have not been established.
Other Agents		
Acid blockers: antacids*	↓ Delavirdine	Doses of an antacid and RESCRIPTOR should be separated by at least one hour, because the absorption of delavirdine is reduced when coadministered with antacids.
H₂Receptor antagonists: cimetidine, famotidine, nizatidine, ranitidine Proton pump inhibitors: omeprazole, lansoprazole		These agents increase gastric pH and may reduce the absorption of delavirdine. Although the effect of these drugs on delavirdine absorption has not been evaluated, chronic use of these drugs with RESCRIPTOR is not recommended.
Amphetamines	↑ Amphetamines	Use with caution.
Antidepressant: trazodone	↑ trazodone	Concomitant use of trazodone and RESCRIPTOR may increase plasma concentrations of trazodone. Adverse events of nausea, dizziness, hypotension and syncope have been observed following coadministration of trazodone and ritonavir. If trazodone is used with a CYP3A4 inhibitor such as RESCRIPTOR, the combination should be used with caution and a lower dose of trazodone should be considered.
Antiarrhythmics: bepridil	↑ Antiarrhythmics	Use with caution. Increased bepridil exposure may be associated with life-threatening reactions such as cardiac arrhythmias.
Amiodarone, lidocaine (systemic), quinidine, flecainide, propafenone		Caution is warranted and therapeutic concentration monitoring is recommended, if available, for antiarrhythmics when coadministered with RESCRIPTOR.

(Table continued on next page)

Table 7 *(cont.).* **Established and Other Potentially Significant Drug Interactions: Alteration in Dose or Regimen May Be Recommended Based on Drug Interaction Studies or Predicted Interaction**

Concomitant Drug Class: Drug Name	Effect on Concentration of delavirdine or Concomitant Drug	Clinical Comment
Anticoagulant: warfarin	↑ Warfarin	It is recommended that INR (international normalized ratio) be monitored.
Anti-infective: clarithromycin*	↑ Clarithromycin	When coadministered with RESCRIPTOR, clarithromycin should be adjusted in patients with impaired renal function: • For patients with CL_{CR} 30 to 60 mL/min the dose of clarithromycin should be reduced by 50%. • For patients with CL_{CR}<30 mL/min the dose of clarithromycin should be reduced by 75%.
Calcium channel blockers: amlodipine, diltiazem, felodipine, isradipine, nifedipine, nicardipine, nimodipine, nisoldipine, verapamil	↑ Calcium channel blockers	Caution is warranted and clinical monitoring of patients is recommended.
Corticosteroid: dexamethasone	↓ Delavirdine	Use with caution. RESCRIPTOR may be less effective due to decreased delavirdine plasma concentrations in patients taking these agents concomitantly.
Erectile dysfunction agents: sildenafil	↑ Sildenafil	Sildenafil should not exceed a maximum single dose of 25 mg in a 48-hour period.
HMG-CoA reductase inhibitors: atorvastatin, cerivastatin, fluvastatin	↑ Atorvastatin ↑ Cerivastatin ↑ Fluvastatin	Use lowest possible dose of atorvastatin or cerivastatin, or fluvastatin with careful monitoring, or consider other HMG-CoA reductase inhibitors such as pravastatin in combination with RESCRIPTOR.
Immunosuppressants: cyclosporine, tacrolimus, rapamycin	↑ Immunosuppressants	Therapeutic concentration monitoring is recommended for immunosuppressant agents when coadministered with RESCRIPTOR.
Inhaled/nasal steroid: Fluticasone	↑ fluticasone	Concomitant use of fluticasone propionate and RESCRIPTOR may increase plasma concentrations of fluticasone propionate. Use with caution. Consider alternatives to fluticasone propionate, particularly for long-term use.
Narcotic analgesic: methadone	↑ Methadone	Dosage of methadone may need to be decreased when coadministered with RESCRIPTOR.
Oral contraceptives: ethinyl estradiol	↑ Ethinyl estradiol	Concentrations of ethinyl estradiol may increase. However, the clinical significance is unknown.

↑ Indicates increase
↓ Indicates decrease
* See **CLINICAL PHARMACOLOGY** for magnitude of interaction, Tables 1 and 2.

Table 8. Percent of Patients With Treatment-Emergent Rash in Pivotal Trials (Studies 21 Part II and 13C)*

Percent of Patients with:	Description of Rash Grade†	RESCRIPTOR 400 mg TID (N = 412)	Control Group Patients (N = 295)
Grade 1 Rash	Erythema, pruritus	69 (16.7%)	35 (11.9%)
Grade 2 Rash	Diffuse maculopapular rash, dry desquamation	59 (14.3%)	17 (5.8%)
Grade 3 Rash	Vesiculation, moist desquamation, ulceration	18 (4.4%)	0 (0.0%)
Grade 4 Rash	Erythema multiforme, Stevens-Johnson syndrome, toxic epidermal necrolysis, necrosis requiring surgery, exfoliative dermatitis	0 (0.0%)	0 (0.0%)
Rash of any Grade		146 (35.4%)	52 (17.6%)
Treatment discontinuation as a result of rash		13 (3.2%)	1 (0.3%)

* Includes events reported regardless of causality
† ACTG Toxicity Grading System; includes events reported as "rash", "maculopapular rash", and "urticaria"

No adequate and well-controlled studies in pregnant women have been conducted. RESCRIPTOR should be used during pregnancy only if the potential benefit justifies the potential risk to the fetus. Of 9 pregnancies reported in premarketing clinical studies and postmarketing experience, a total of 10 infants were born (including 1 set of twins). Eight of the infants were born healthy. One infant was born HIV-positive but was otherwise healthy and with no congenital abnor-

malities detected, and 1 infant was born prematurely (34 to 35 weeks) with a small muscular ventricular septal defect that spontaneously resolved. The patient received approximately six weeks of treatment with delavirdine and zidovudine early in the course of the pregnancy.
Antiretroviral Pregnancy Registry
To monitor maternal-fetal outcomes of pregnant women exposed to RESCRIPTOR and other antiretroviral agents, an

Antiretroviral Pregnancy Registry has been established. Physicians are encouraged to register patients by calling (800) 258-4263.
Nursing Mothers
The Centers for Disease Control and Prevention recommend that HIV-infected mothers not breastfeed their infants to avoid risking postnatal transmission of HIV. Because of both the potential for HIV transmission and any possible adverse reactions in nursing infants, **mothers should be instructed not to breastfeed if they are receiving RESCRIPTOR.**
Pediatric Use
Safety and effectiveness of delavirdine in combination with other antiretroviral agents have not been established in HIV-1–infected individuals younger than 16 years of age.
Geriatric Use
Clinical studies of RESCRIPTOR did not include sufficient numbers of subjects aged 65 and over to determine whether they respond differently from younger subjects. In general, caution should be taken when dosing RESCRIPTOR in elderly patients due to the greater frequency of decreased hepatic, renal or cardiac function and of concomitant disease or other drug therapy.

ADVERSE REACTIONS
The safety of RESCRIPTOR Tablets alone and in combination with other therapies has been studied in approximately 6,000 patients receiving RESCRIPTOR. The majority of adverse events were of mild or moderate (i.e., ACTG grade 1 or 2) intensity. The most frequently reported drug-related adverse event (i.e., events considered by the investigator to be related to the blinded study medication, or events with an unknown or missing causal relationship to the blinded medication) among patients receiving RESCRIPTOR was skin rash (see **Table 8** and **PRECAUTIONS: Skin Rash**).
[See table 8 below]
Adverse events of moderate to severe intensity reported by at least 5% of evaluable patients in any treatment group in the pivotal trials, which includes patients receiving RESCRIPTOR in combination with zidovudine and/or lamivudine in Study 21 Part II for up to 98 weeks and in combination with zidovudine and either lamivudine, didanosine, or zalcitabine in Study 13C for up to 72 weeks are summarized in Table 9.
[See table 9 at top of next page]
Other adverse events that occurred in patients receiving RESCRIPTOR (in combination treatment) in all phase II and III studies, and considered possibly related to treatment, and of at least ACTG grade 2 in intensity are listed below by body system.
Body as a Whole: Abdominal cramps, abdominal distention, abdominal pain (localized), abscess, allergic reaction, chills, edema (generalized or localized), epidermal cyst, fever, infection, infection viral, lip edema, malaise, Mycobacterium tuberculosis infection, neck rigidity, sebaceous cyst, and redistribution/accumulation of body fat (see **PRECAUTIONS, Fat Redistribution**).
Cardiovascular System: Abnormal cardiac rate and rhythm, cardiac insufficiency, cardiomyopathy, hypertension, migraine, pallor, peripheral vascular disorder, and postural hypotension.
Digestive System: Anorexia, bloody stool, colitis, constipation, decreased appetite, diarrhea (*Clostridium difficile*), diverticulitis, dry mouth, dyspepsia, dysphagia, enteritis at all levels, eructation, fecal incontinence, flatulence, gagging, gastroenteritis, gastroesophageal reflux, gastrointestinal bleeding, gastrointestinal disorder, gingivitis, gum hemorrhage, hepatomegaly, increased appetite, increased saliva, increased thirst, jaundice, mouth or tongue inflammation or ulcers, nonspecific hepatitis, oral/enteric moniliasis, pancreatitis, rectal disorder, sialadenitis, tooth abscess, and toothache.
Hemic and Lymphatic System: Adenopathy, bruising, eosinophilia, granulocytosis, leukopenia, pancytopenia, purpura, spleen disorder, thrombocytopenia, and prolonged prothrombin time.
Metabolic and Nutritional Disorders: Alcohol intolerance, amylase increased, bilirubinemia, hyperglycemia, hyperkalemia, hypertriglyceridemia, hyperuricemia, hypocalcemia, hyponatremia, hypophosphatemia, increased AST (SGOT), increased gamma glutamyl transpeptidase, increased lipase, increased serum alkaline phosphatase, increased serum creatinine, and weight increase or decrease.
Musculoskeletal System: Arthralgia or arthritis of single and multiple joints, bone disorder, bone pain, myalgia, tendon disorder, tenosynovitis, tetany, and vertigo.
Nervous System: Abnormal coordination, agitation, amnesia, change in dreams, cognitive impairment, confusion, decreased libido, disorientation, dizziness, emotional lability, euphoria, hallucination, hyperesthesia, hyperreflexia, hypertonia, hypesthesia, impaired concentration, manic symptoms, muscle cramp, nervousness, neuropathy, nystagmus, paralysis, paranoid symptoms, restlessness, sleep cycle disorder, somnolence, tingling, tremor, vertigo, and weakness.

Respiratory System: Chest congestion, dyspnea, epistaxis, hiccups, laryngismus, pneumonia, and rhinitis.

Skin and Appendages: Angioedema, dermal leukocytoclastic vasculitis, dermatitis, desquamation, diaphoresis, discolored skin, dry skin, erythema, erythema multiforme, folliculitis, fungal dermatitis, hair loss, herpes zoster or simplex, nail disorder, petechiae, non-application site pruritus, seborrhea, skin hypertrophy, skin disorder, skin nodule, Stevens-Johnson syndrome, urticaria, vesiculobullous rash, and wart.

Special Senses: Blepharitis, blurred vision, conjunctivitis, diplopia, dry eyes, ear pain, parosmia, otitis media, photophobia, taste perversion, and tinnitus.

Urogenital System: Amenorrhea, breast enlargement, calculi of the kidney, chromaturia, epididymitis, hematuria, hemospermia, impaired urination, impotence, kidney pain, metrorrhagia, nocturia, polyuria, proteinuria, testicular pain, urinary tract infection, and vaginal moniliasis.

Postmarketing Experience

Adverse event terms reported from postmarketing surveillance that were not reported in the phase II and III trials are presented below.

Digestive System: Hepatic failure.

Hemic and Lymphatic System: Hemolytic anemia.

Musculoskeletal System: Rhabdomyolysis.

Urogenital System: Acute kidney failure.

Laboratory Abnormalities

Marked laboratory abnormalities observed in at least 2% of patients during Studies 21 Part II and 13C are summarized in Table 10. Marked laboratory abnormalities are defined as any Grade 3 or 4 abnormality found in patients at any time during study.

[See table 10 at top of next page]

OVERDOSAGE

Human experience of acute overdose with RESCRIPTOR is limited.

Management of Overdosage

Treatment of overdosage with RESCRIPTOR should consist of general supportive measures, including monitoring of vital signs and observation of the patient's clinical status. There is no specific antidote for overdosage with RESCRIPTOR. If indicated, elimination of unabsorbed drug should be achieved by emesis or gastric lavage. Since delavirdine is extensively metabolized by the liver and is highly protein-bound, dialysis is unlikely to result in significant removal of the drug.

DOSAGE AND ADMINISTRATION

The recommended dosage for RESCRIPTOR Tablets is 400 mg (four 100 mg or two 200 mg tablets) three times daily. RESCRIPTOR should be used in combination with other antiretroviral therapy. The complete prescribing information for other antiretroviral agents should be consulted for information on dosage and administration.

The 100 mg RESCRIPTOR Tablets may be dispersed in water prior to consumption. To prepare a dispersion, add four 100 mg RESCRIPTOR Tablets to at least 3 ounces of water, allow to stand for a few minutes, and then stir until a uniform dispersion occurs (see **CLINICAL PHARMACOLOGY: Pharmacokinetics: Absorption and Bioavailability**). The dispersion should be consumed promptly. The glass should be rinsed with water and the rinse swallowed to insure the entire dose is consumed. **The 200 mg tablets should be taken as intact tablets, because they are not readily dispersed in water.** Note: The 200 mg tablets are approximately one-third smaller in size than the 100 mg tablets.

RESCRIPTOR Tablets may be administered with or without food (see **CLINICAL PHARMACOLOGY: Pharmacokinetics-Absorption and Bioavailability**). Patients with achlorhydria should take RESCRIPTOR with an acidic beverage (e.g., orange or cranberry juice). However, the effect of an acidic beverage on the absorption of delavirdine in patients with achlorhydria has not been investigated. Patients taking both RESCRIPTOR and antacids should be advised to take them at least one hour apart.

HOW SUPPLIED

RESCRIPTOR Tablets are available as follows:

100 mg: white, capsule-shaped tablets marked with "U 3761".

Bottles of 360 tablets NDC 63010-020-36

200 mg: white, capsule-shaped tablets marked with "RESCRIPTOR 200 mg".

Bottles of 180 tablets NDC 63010-021-18

Store at controlled room temperature 20° to 25°C (68° to 77°F) [see USP]. *Keep container tightly closed. Protect from high humidity.*

Rx only

ANIMAL TOXICOLOGY

Toxicities among various organs and organ systems in rats, mice, rabbits, dogs, and monkeys were observed following the administration of delavirdine. Necrotizing vasculitis

Table 9. Treatment-Emergent Events, Regardless of Causality, of Moderate-to-Severe or Life-Threatening Intensity Reported by at Least 5% of Evaluable* Patients in any Treatment Group

Adverse Events	Study 21 Part II			Study 13C	
	ZDV + 3TC (N = 123)	400 mg tid RESCRIPTOR + ZDV (N = 123)	400 mg tid RESCRIPTOR + ZDV + 3TC (N = 119)	ZDV + ddl, ddC, or 3TC (N = 172)	400 mg tid RESCRIPTOR + ZDV + ddl, ddC or 3TC (N = 170)
	% of pts. (N)	% of pts. (N)	% of pts. (N)	% of pts. (N)	% of pts. (N)
Body as a Whole					
Abdominal pain, generalized	2.4 (3)	3.3 (4)	5.0 (6)	1.7 (3)	2.4 (4)
Asthenia/fatigue	16.3 (20)	15.4 (19)	16.0 (19)	8.1 (14)	5.3 (9)
Fever	2.4 (3)	1.6 (2)	3.4 (4)	6.4 (11)	7.1 (12)
Flu syndrome	4.9 (6)	7.3 (9)	5.0 (6)	5.2 (9)	2.4 (4)
Headache	14.6 (18)	12.2 (15)	16.8 (20)	12.8 (22)	11.2 (19)
Localized pain	4.9 (6)	5.7 (7)	5.0 (6)	2.9 (5)	1.8 (3)
Digestive					
Diarrhea	8.1 (10)	2.4 (3)	4.2 (5)	8.1 (14)	5.9 (10)
Nausea	17.1 (21)	20.3 (25)	16.8 (20)	9.3 (16)	14.7 (25)
Vomiting	8.9 (11)	4.9 (6)	2.5 (3)	4.1 (7)	6.5 (11)
Nervous					
Anxiety	1.6 (2)	2.4 (3)	6.7 (8)	4.1 (7)	3.5 (6)
Depressive symptoms	6.5 (8)	4.9 (6)	12.6 (15)	3.5 (6)	5.9 (10)
Insomnia	4.9 (6)	4.9 (6)	5.0 (6)	2.9 (5)	1.2 (2)
Respiratory					
Bronchitis	4.1 (5)	6.5 (8)	6.7 (8)	3.5 (6)	3.5 (6)
Cough	9.8 (12)	4.1 (5)	5.0 (6)	5.2 (9)	3.5 (6)
Pharyngitis	6.5 (8)	1.6 (2)	5.0 (6)	4.1 (7)	3.5 (6)
Sinusitis	8.9 (11)	7.3 (9)	5.0 (6)	2.3 (4)	1.2 (2)
Upper respiratory infection	11.4 (14)	6.5 (8)	7.6 (9)	8.7 (15)	4.7 (8)
Skin					
Rashes	3.3 (4)	19.5 (24)	13.4 (16)	7.6 (13)	18.8 (32)

* Evaluable patients in Study 21 Part II were those who received at least 1 dose of study medication and returned for at least 1 clinic study visit. Evaluable patients in Study 13C were those who received at least 1 dose of study medication.

was the most significant toxicity that occurred in dogs when mean nadir serum concentrations of delavirdine were at least 7-fold higher than the expected human exposure to RESCRIPTOR (C_{min} 15 μM) at the recommended dose. Vasculitis in dogs was not reversible during a 2.5-month recovery period; however, partial resolution of the vascular lesion characterized by reduced inflammation, diminished necrosis, and intimal thickening occurred during this period. Other major target organs included the gastrointestinal tract, endocrine organs, liver, kidneys, bone marrow, lymphoid tissue, lung, and reproductive organs.

Distributed by
**Pharmacia & Upjohn Company
Division of Pfizer Inc, NY, NY 10017**
LAB-0059-6.0
May 2008

RESCRIPTOR®

(delavirdine mesylate) tablets
ALERT: Find out about medicines that should NOT be taken with RESCRIPTOR. Please also read the section "MEDICINES YOU SHOULD NOT TAKE WITH RESCRIPTOR."
Patient Information
RESCRIPTOR® (ree-SKRIP-tor)
Generic name: delavirdine mesylate (de-LAH-vur-deen MESS-ihl-ate)
Read this information carefully before taking RESCRIPTOR. Also, read this leaflet each time you renew the prescription, just in case anything has changed. This is a summary and not a replacement for a careful discussion with your healthcare provider (doctor, nurse, pharmacist). You and your healthcare provider should discuss RESCRIPTOR when you start taking this medication and at regular checkups. You should remain under a doctor's care when taking RESCRIPTOR and should not change or stop treatment without first talking with your healthcare provider.

What is RESCRIPTOR and how does it work?
RESCRIPTOR is a medicine used in combination with other anti-HIV medicines to treat people with HIV infection. Infection with HIV leads to the destruction of infection-fighting immune system cells (called CD_4 cells or T cells), which are important to the immune system. After a large number of CD_4 cells have been destroyed, the infected person develops acquired immune deficiency syndrome (AIDS). RESCRIPTOR helps to block HIV reverse transcriptase, a chemical the virus uses to make more copies of itself. The main goals of anti-HIV medicines like RESCRIPTOR are to decrease the amount of virus in your blood (called viral load) and to increase the number of CD_4 cells as much as possible for as long as possible.

RESCRIPTOR, when taken with other anti-HIV medicines, lowers the HIV viral load in patients. Patients who took RESCRIPTOR as part of combination therapy for HIV also had increases in their CD_4 cell count.

Does RESCRIPTOR cure HIV or AIDS?
RESCRIPTOR is not a cure for HIV infection or AIDS. People taking RESCRIPTOR may still develop opportunistic infections or other conditions associated with HIV infection. Opportunistic infections are infections that develop because the immune system is weak. Some of these conditions are pneumonia, herpes virus infections, *Mycobacterium avium* complex (MAC) infections, and Kaposi's sarcoma.

Table 10. Marked Laboratory Abnormalities Reported by ≥2% of Patients

Adverse Events	Toxicity Limit	Study 21 Part II			Study 13C	
		ZDV + 3TC N = 123	400 mg tid RESCRIPTOR + ZDV N = 123	400 mg tid RESCRIPTOR + ZDV + 3TC N = 119	ZDV + ddl, ddC or 3TC N = 172	400 mg tid RESCRIPTOR + ZDV + ddl, ddC or 3TC N = 170
		% pts.	% pts.	% pts.	% pts.	% pts.
Hematology						
Hemoglobin	<7 mg/dL	4.1	2.5	0.9	1.7	2.9
Neutrophils	<750/mm^3	5.7	4.9	3.4	10.4	7.6
Prothrombin time (PT)	>1.5 × ULN	0	0	1.7	2.9	2.4
Activated partial thromboplastin (APTT)	>2.33 × ULN	0	0.8	0	5.8	2.4
Chemistry						
Alananine aminotransferase (ALT/SGPT)	>5 × ULN	2.5	4.1	5.1	3.5	4.1
Amylase	>2 × ULN	0.8	2.5	2.6	3.5	2.9
Aspartate aminotransferase (AST/SGOT)	>5 × ULN	1.6	2.5	3.4	3.5	2.3
Bilirubin	>2.5 × ULN	0.8	2.5	1.7	1.2	0
Gamma glutamyl transferase (GGT)	>5 × ULN	N/A	N/A	N/A	4.1	1.8
Glucose (hypo-/ hyperglycemia)	>40 mg/dL >250 mg/dL	4.1	0.8	1.7	1.2	0.0

N/A = not applicable because no predose values were obtained for patients

Does RESCRIPTOR reduce the risk of passing HIV to others?
RESCRIPTOR does not reduce the risk of transmitting HIV to others through sexual contact or blood contamination. Continue to practice safe sex and do not use or share dirty needles.

How should I take RESCRIPTOR?
• You should stay under a healthcare provider's care when taking RESCRIPTOR. Do not change your treatment or stop treatment without first talking with your healthcare provider.
• You must take RESCRIPTOR every day exactly as your healthcare provider prescribed it. Follow the directions from your healthcare provider, exactly as written on the label.
• **The usual dose of RESCRIPTOR is two 200 mg tablets three times a day or four 100 mg tablets three times a day, in combination with other anti-HIV medicines. Either way, your total daily dose of RESCRIPTOR remains the same.**
• You can take RESCRIPTOR with or without food.
• If you have trouble swallowing tablets, the 100 mg RESCRIPTOR tablets may be dissolved in water. Place four tablets in at least 3 ounces of water and allow the tablets to sit in the water for a few minutes. Then, stir the water until the tablets have dissolved and drink the mixture right away. Add a little more water, swirl, and then drink the rest of the mixture to be sure that you get all the medicine. **The 200 mg tablets must be swallowed whole. They cannot be dissolved in water.**
• Many people find it easier to take their RESCRIPTOR with breakfast, lunch, and dinner, since food does not interfere with RESCRIPTOR. It is a good idea to get into the habit of taking RESCRIPTOR on a regular schedule to make it easier to remember. Figure out things that happen every day at pill-taking time and take your tablets then. By taking your medicine along with activities you do every day, such as getting up in the morning, brushing your teeth, eating lunch, coming home from work in the evening, or watching a favorite TV show, you will find it easier to remember to take every dose.
• When your RESCRIPTOR supply starts to run low, get more from your healthcare provider or pharmacy. This is very important because the amount of virus in your blood may increase if the medicine is stopped for even a short time. The virus may develop resistance to RESCRIPTOR and become harder to treat.

• Only take medicine that has been prescribed specifically for you. Do not give RESCRIPTOR to others or take medicine prescribed for someone else.

What should I do if I miss a dose of RESCRIPTOR?
If you forget to take a dose of RESCRIPTOR, take it as soon as possible. However, if you skip the dose entirely, do not double the next dose. If you forget a lot of doses, talk to your healthcare provider about how you should continue taking your medicine.

Who should not take RESCRIPTOR?
Together with your healthcare provider, you need to decide whether RESCRIPTOR is right for you.
• **Do not take RESCRIPTOR if you are taking certain medicines.** These could cause serious side effects that could cause death. Before you take RESCRIPTOR, you must tell your healthcare provider about all the medicines you are taking or are planning to take. These include other prescription and nonprescription medicines and herbal supplements.
For more information about medicines you should not take with RESCRIPTOR, please read the section titled **"MEDICINES YOU SHOULD NOT TAKE WITH RESCRIPTOR."**
• **Do not take RESCRIPTOR if you have an allergy to RESCRIPTOR.** Also tell your healthcare provider if you have any known allergies to other medicines, foods, preservatives, or dyes.
• **Tell your healthcare provider if you are pregnant or plan to become pregnant.** The effects of RESCRIPTOR on pregnant women or their unborn babies are not known.
• If you are breast-feeding, it is very important that you speak with your healthcare provider about the best way to feed your baby. If your baby does not already have HIV, there is a chance that it can be transmitted through breast-feeding. **The Centers for Disease Control and Prevention recommends that women with HIV do not breast-feed.**
• **Talk with your healthcare provider if you have liver or kidney disease.** RESCRIPTOR has not been studied in people with liver or kidney disease.
• **Certain medical problems may affect the use of RESCRIPTOR.** Be sure to tell your healthcare provider of any other medical problems you may have.

Can I take RESCRIPTOR with other medicines?
RESCRIPTOR may interact with other medicines, including those you take without a prescription. You must tell your healthcare provider about all medicines you are taking or

planning to take before you take RESCRIPTOR. It is a good idea to keep a complete list of all the medicines that you take, including nonprescription medicines, herbal remedies and supplements and street drugs. Update this list when medicines are added or stopped. Give copies of this list to all of your healthcare providers **every** time you visit or fill a prescription.

MEDICINES YOU SHOULD NOT TAKE WITH RESCRIPTOR
Do not take the following medicines with RESCRIPTOR because they can cause serious problems or death if taken with RESCRIPTOR:
• Versed® (midazolam) Injection and Syrup (for sedation)
• Halcion® (triazolam) Tablets (for sleep problems)
• Xanax® (alprazolam) Tablets (for anxiety)
• D.H.E. 45® Injection, Ergomar®, Migranal®, Wigraine® and Cafergot® (for migraine headaches)
• Methergine® (for bleeding after childbirth)
• Orap (pimozide) Tablets (for seizures)
• Propulsid (cisapride) Tablets and Suspension (for heartburn)
• Hismanal® (astemizole) Tablets (for allergies)
• Seldane® (terfenadine) Tablets (for allergies)
Do not take the following medicines when you take RESCRIPTOR. They may reduce the levels of RESCRIPTOR in the blood and make it less effective. Talk with your healthcare provider if you are currently taking these medicines because other medicines may have to be given to take their place:
• Rifampin (also known as Rimactane®, Rifadin®, Rifater®, Rifamate®) (to treat tuberculosis)
• Phenobarbital (for seizures)
• Dilantin® (phenytoin) (for seizures)
• Tegretol® (carbamazepine) (for seizures)
Do not take RESCRIPTOR with St. John's wort (hypericum perforatum), an herbal product sold as a dietary supplement, or products containing St. John's wort. Talk with your healthcare provider if you are taking or planning to take St. John's wort. Taking St. John's wort may decrease RESCRIPTOR levels and lead to increased viral load and possible resistance to RESCRIPTOR or cross-resistance to other anti-HIV medicines.
Do not take RESCRIPTOR with cholesterol-lowering medicines Mevacor® (lovastatin) or Zocor® (simvastatin) because of possible serious reactions. There is also an increased risk of drug interactions between RESCRIPTOR and Lipitor® (atorvastatin), Baycol® (cerivastatin) and Lescol® (fluvastatin); talk to your healthcare provider before you take any of these cholesterol-reducing medicines with RESCRIPTOR.
Medicines that require dosage adjustments:
It is possible that your healthcare provider may need to increase or decrease the dose of other medicines when you are taking RESCRIPTOR. Remember to tell your healthcare provider all the medicines you are taking or planning to take.
Before you take Viagra® (sildenafil) with RESCRIPTOR, talk to your healthcare provider about problems these two medicines can cause when taken together. You may get increased side effects of Viagra, such as low blood pressure, vision changes, and penis erection lasting more than 4 hours. If an erection lasts longer than 4 hours, get medical help right away to avoid permanent damage to your penis. Your healthcare provider can explain these symptoms to you.
• **If you are taking both Videx® (didanosine, ddl) and RESCRIPTOR:** Take Videx (buffered tablets) 1 hour before or 1 hour after you take RESCRIPTOR. Taking them together causes lower amounts of RESCRIPTOR in the blood, making both medicines less effective.
• **Protease inhibitors:** A number of healthy volunteers and HIV-infected patients were studied while taking RESCRIPTOR with one of these protease inhibitors: Crixivan® (indinavir), Invirase® and Fortovase® (saquinavir), Norvir® (ritonavir), or VIRACEPT® (nelfinavir). RESCRIPTOR was shown to increase the amount of these protease inhibitors in the blood. RESCRIPTOR is expected to increase the amount of Agenerase® (amprenavir) and Kaletra® (lopinavir + ritonavir) in the blood. **As a result, your healthcare provider may choose to lower the dose of these medicines or monitor certain lab tests if these protease inhibitors are taken in combination with RESCRIPTOR.**
• **Antacids** should be taken at least 1 hour before or 1 hour after you take RESCRIPTOR because they can slow the absorption of RESCRIPTOR.
Based on your history of taking other anti-HIV medicine, your healthcare provider will direct you on how to take RESCRIPTOR and other anti-HIV medicines. These drugs should be taken in a certain order or at specific times. This will depend on how many times a day each medicine should be taken. It will also depend on whether the medicines should be taken with or without food.

What are the possible side effects of RESCRIPTOR?
• This list of side effects is not complete. If you have questions about side effects, ask your doctor, nurse, or pharmacist. You should report any new or continuing symptoms to your healthcare provider right away. Your healthcare provider may be able to help you manage these side effects.

- The most important common side effect seen in people taking RESCRIPTOR has been a skin rash. The rash occurs mainly on the upper body and upper arms, and sometimes on the neck and face. The rash appears as a red area on the skin with slight bumps, and it can be itchy. The rash tends to occur early, usually within 1 to 3 weeks after you start taking RESCRIPTOR, and it usually lasts less than 2 weeks. Watch your rash carefully and talk to your healthcare provider about how to treat it. If the rash is going to be serious or severe (with fever, blistering, sores in the mouth, redness or swelling of the eyes, or muscle and joint aches), you and your healthcare provider will usually realize it during the first 3 days of the rash. If you have symptoms of a severe rash, you should stop taking RESCRIPTOR and speak with your healthcare provider as soon possible. Be prepared to explain where the rash is, your temperature, and whether or not you have other symptoms.
- Other side effects include headache, nausea, diarrhea, and tiredness. Of these, nausea was the most common.
- Changes in body fat have been seen in some patients taking antiretroviral therapy. These changes may include increased amount of fat in the upper back and neck ("buffalo hump"), breast, and around the trunk. Loss of fat from the legs, arms and face may also happen. The cause and long-term health effects of these conditions are not known at this time.
- Before you start using any medicine, talk with your healthcare provider about what to expect and discuss ways to reduce the side effects you may have.

How do I store RESCRIPTOR?
- Keep RESCRIPTOR and all other medicines out of the reach of children. Keep the bottle closed and store at room temperature (between 68°F and 77°F) away from sources of moisture such as a sink or other damp place. Heat and moisture may reduce the effectiveness of RESCRIPTOR.
- Do not keep medicine that is out of date or that you no longer need. Be sure that if you throw any medicine away, it is out of the reach of children.

General advice about prescription medicines:
Discuss all questions about your health with your healthcare provider. If you have questions about RESCRIPTOR or any other medicines you are taking, ask your healthcare provider. You can also call 1-888-847-2237 toll free.

Distributed by
Pharmacia & Upjohn Company
Division of Pfizer Inc, NY, NY 10017
LAB-0352-1.0
August 2006
Revised: 11/2008
Distributed by: Pharmacia and Upjohn Company

RETROVIR®   ℞
[re′trō-vir]
(zidovudine)
Tablets, Capsules, and Syrup

HIGHLIGHTS OF PRESCRIBING INFORMATION
These highlights do not include all the information needed to use RETROVIR safely and effectively. See full prescribing information for RETROVIR.
RETROVIR (zidovudine) Tablets, Capsules, and Syrup
Initial U.S. Approval: 1987

WARNING: RISK OF HEMATOLOGICAL TOXICITY, MYOPATHY, LACTIC ACIDOSIS
See full prescribing information for complete boxed warning.
- **Hematologic toxicity including neutropenia and severe anemia have been associated with the use of zidovudine. (5.1)**
- **Symptomatic myopathy associated with prolonged use of zidovudine. (5.2)**
- **Lactic acidosis and severe hepatomegaly with steatosis, including fatal cases, have been reported with the use of nucleoside analogues including RETROVIR. Suspend treatment if clinical or laboratory findings suggestive of lactic acidosis or pronounced hepatotoxicity occur. (5.3)**

RECENT MAJOR CHANGES
Dosage and Administration,
  Pediatric Patients (2.1)   November 2009
INDICATIONS AND USAGE
RETROVIR is a nucleoside analogue reverse transcriptase inhibitor indicated for:
- Treatment of Human Immunodeficiency Virus (HIV-1) infection in combination with other antiretroviral agents. (1.1)
- Prevention of maternal-fetal HIV-1 transmission. (1.2)

DOSAGE AND ADMINISTRATION
- Treatment of HIV-1 infection:

Adults: 600 mg/day in divided doses with other antiretroviral agents.
Pediatric patients (4 weeks to <18 years of age): Dosage should be calculated based on body weight not to exceed adult dose. (2.1)
- Prevention of maternal-fetal HIV-1 transmission: Specific dosage instructions for mother and infant. (2.2)
- Patients with severe anemia and/or neutropenia: Dosage interruption may be necessary. (2.3)
- Renal Impairment: Recommended dosage in hemodialysis or peritoneal dialysis patients is 100 mg every 6 to 8 hours. (2.4)

DOSAGE FORMS AND STRENGTHS
Tablets: 300 mg (3)
Capsules: 100 mg (3)
Syrup: 50 mg/5 mL (3)

CONTRAINDICATIONS
Hypersensitivity to zidovudine (e.g., anaphylaxis, Stevens-Johnson syndrome). (4)

WARNINGS AND PRECAUTIONS
- Hematologic toxicity/bone marrow suppression including neutropenia and severe anemia have been associated with the use of zidovudine. (5.1)
- Symptomatic myopathy associated with prolonged use of zidovudine. (5.2)
- Lactic acidosis and severe hepatomegaly with steatosis, including fatal cases, have been reported with the use of nucleoside analogues including RETROVIR. Suspend treatment if clinical or laboratory findings suggestive of lactic acidosis or pronounced hepatotoxicity occur. (5.3)
- Exacerbation of anemia has been reported in HIV-1/HCV co-infected patients receiving ribavirin and zidovudine. Coadministration of ribavirin and zidovudine is not advised. (5.4)
- Hepatic decompensation, (some fatal), has occurred in HIV-1/HCV co-infected patients receiving combination antiretroviral therapy and interferon alfa with/without ribavirin. Discontinue zidovudine as medically appropriate and consider dose reduction or discontinuation of interferon alfa, ribavirin, or both. (5.4)
- RETROVIR should not be administered with other zidovudine-containing combination products. (5.5)
- Immune reconstitution syndrome (5.6) and redistribution/accumulation of body fat (5.7) have been reported in patients treated with combination antiretroviral therapy.

ADVERSE REACTIONS
- Most commonly reported adverse reactions (incidence ≥15%) in adult HIV-1 clinical studies were headache, malaise, nausea, anorexia, and vomiting. (6.1)
- Most commonly reported adverse reactions (incidence ≥15%) in pediatric HIV-1 clinical studies were fever, cough, and digestive disorders. (6.1)
- Most commonly reported adverse reactions in neonates (incidence ≥15%) in the prevention of maternal-fetal transmission of HIV-1 clinical trial were anemia and neutropenia. (6.1)

To report SUSPECTED ADVERSE REACTIONS, contact GlaxoSmithKline at 1-888-825-5249 or FDA at 1-800-FDA-1088 or www.fda.gov/medwatch.

DRUG INTERACTIONS
- Stavudine: Concomitant use with zidovudine should be avoided. (7.1)
- Doxorubicin: Use with zidovudine should be avoided. (7.2)
- Bone marrow suppressive/cytotoxic agents: May increase the hematologic toxicity of zidovudine. (7.3)

USE IN SPECIFIC POPULATIONS
Pregnancy: Physicians are encouraged to register patients in the Antiretroviral Pregnancy Registry by calling 1-800-258-4263. (8.1)

See 17 for PATIENT COUNSELING INFORMATION
                                        Revised: 05/2010

FULL PRESCRIBING INFORMATION

WARNING: RISK OF HEMATOLOGICAL TOXICITY, MYOPATHY, LACTIC ACIDOSIS
RETROVIR® (zidovudine) Tablets, Capsules, and Syrup have been associated with hematologic toxicity including neutropenia and severe anemia, particularly in patients with advanced HIV-1 disease *[see Warnings and Precautions (5.1)].*
Prolonged use of RETROVIR has been associated with symptomatic myopathy *[see Warnings and Precautions (5.2)].*
Lactic acidosis and severe hepatomegaly with steatosis, including fatal cases, have been reported with the use of nucleoside analogues alone or in combination, including RETROVIR and other antiretrovirals. Suspend treatment if clinical or laboratory findings suggestive of lactic acidosis or pronounced hepatotoxicity occur *[see Warnings and Precautions (5.3)].*

---

1   INDICATIONS AND USAGE

1.1   Treatment of HIV-1
RETROVIR, a nucleoside reverse transcriptase inhibitor, is indicated in combination with other antiretroviral agents for the treatment of HIV-1 infection.

1.2   Prevention of Maternal-Fetal HIV-1 Transmission
RETROVIR is indicated for the prevention of maternal-fetal HIV-1 transmission *[see Dosage and Administration (2.2)].* The indication is based on a dosing regimen that included 3 components:
1. antepartum therapy of HIV-1 infected mothers
2. intrapartum therapy of HIV-1 infected mothers
3. post-partum therapy of HIV-1 exposed neonate.
Points to consider prior to initiating RETROVIR in pregnant women for the prevention of maternal-fetal HIV-1 transmission include:
- In most cases, RETROVIR for prevention of maternal-fetal HIV-1 transmission should be given in combination with other antiretroviral drugs.
- Prevention of HIV-1 transmission in women who have received RETROVIR for a prolonged period before pregnancy has not been evaluated.
- Because the fetus is most susceptible to the potential teratogenic effects of drugs during the first 10 weeks of gestation and the risks of therapy with RETROVIR during that period are not fully known, women in the first trimester of pregnancy who do not require immediate initiation of antiretroviral therapy for their own health may consider delaying use; this indication is based on use after 14 weeks gestation.

2 DOSAGE AND ADMINISTRATION

2.1 Treatment of HIV-1 Infection

Adults: The recommended oral dose of RETROVIR is 600 mg/day in divided doses in combination with other antiretroviral agents.

Pediatric Patients (4 Weeks to <18 Years of Age): Healthcare professionals should pay special attention to accurate calculation of the dose of RETROVIR, transcription of the medication order, dispensing information, and dosing instructions to minimize risk for medication dosing errors.

Prescribers should calculate the appropriate dose of RETROVIR for each child based on body weight (kg) and should not exceed the recommended adult dose.

Before prescribing RETROVIR Capsules or Tablets, children should be assessed for the ability to swallow capsules or tablets. If a child is unable to reliably swallow a RETROVIR Capsule or Tablet, the RETROVIR Syrup formulation should be prescribed.

The recommended dosage in pediatric patients 4 weeks of age and older and weighing ≥4 kg is provided in Table 1. RETROVIR Syrup should be used to provide accurate dosage when whole tablets or capsules are not appropriate.

Table 1: Recommended Pediatric Dosage of RETROVIR

Body Weight (kg)	Total Daily Dose	Dosage Regimen and Dose	
		b.i.d.	t.i.d.
4 to <9	24 mg/kg/day	12 mg/kg	8 mg/kg
≥9 to <30	18 mg/kg/day	9 mg/kg	6 mg/kg
≥30	600 mg/day	300 mg	200 mg

Alternatively, dosing for RETROVIR can be based on body surface area (BSA) for each child. The recommended oral dose of RETROVIR is 480 mg/m^2/day in divided doses (240 mg/m^2 twice daily or 160 mg/m^2 three times daily). In some cases the dose calculated by mg/kg will not be the same as that calculated by BSA.

2.2 Prevention of Maternal-Fetal HIV-1 Transmission

The recommended dosage regimen for administration to pregnant women (>14 weeks of pregnancy) and their neonates is:

Maternal Dosing: 100 mg orally 5 times per day until the start of labor *[see Clinical Studies (14.3)]*. During labor and delivery, intravenous RETROVIR should be administered at 2 mg/kg (total body weight) over 1 hour followed by a continuous intravenous infusion of 1 mg/kg/hour (total body weight) until clamping of the umbilical cord.

Neonatal Dosing: 2 mg/kg orally every 6 hours starting within 12 hours after birth and continuing through 6 weeks of age. Neonates unable to receive oral dosing may be administered RETROVIR intravenously at 1.5 mg/kg, infused over 30 minutes, every 6 hours.

2.3 Patients With Severe Anemia and/or Neutropenia

Significant anemia (hemoglobin <7.5 g/dL or reduction >25% of baseline) and/or significant neutropenia (granulocyte count <750 cells/mm^3 or reduction >50% from baseline) may require a dose interruption until evidence of marrow recovery is observed *[see Warnings and Precautions (5.1)]*. In patients who develop significant anemia, dose interruption does not necessarily eliminate the need for transfusion. If marrow recovery occurs following dose interruption, resumption in dose may be appropriate using adjunctive measures such as epoetin alfa at recommended doses, depending on hematologic indices such as serum erythropoetin level and patient tolerance.

2.4 Patients With Renal Impairment

End-Stage Renal Disease: In patients maintained on hemodialysis or peritoneal dialysis, the recommended dosage is 100 mg every 6 to 8 hours *[see Clinical Pharmacology (12.3)]*.

2.5 Patients With Hepatic Impairment

There are insufficient data to recommend dose adjustment of RETROVIR in patients with mild to moderate impaired hepatic function or liver cirrhosis.

3 DOSAGE FORMS AND STRENGTHS

RETROVIR Tablets 300 mg (biconvex, white, round, film-coated) containing 300 mg zidovudine, one side engraved "GX CW3" and "300" on the other side.

RETROVIR Capsules 100 mg (white, opaque cap and body) containing 100 mg zidovudine and printed with "Wellcome" and unicorn logo on cap and "Y9C" and "100" on body.

RETROVIR Syrup (colorless to pale yellow, strawberry-flavored) containing 50 mg zidovudine in each teaspoonful (5 mL).

4 CONTRAINDICATIONS

RETROVIR Tablets, Capsules, and Syrup are contraindicated in patients who have had potentially life-threatening allergic reactions (e.g., anaphylaxis, Stevens-Johnson syndrome) to any of the components of the formulations.

5 WARNINGS AND PRECAUTIONS

5.1 Hematologic Toxicity/Bone Marrow Suppression

RETROVIR should be used with caution in patients who have bone marrow compromise evidenced by granulocyte count <1,000 cells/mm^3 or hemoglobin <9.5 g/dL. Hematologic toxicities appear to be related to pretreatment bone marrow reserve and to dose and duration of therapy. In patients with advanced symptomatic HIV-1 disease, anemia and neutropenia were the most significant adverse events observed. In patients who experience hematologic toxicity, a reduction in hemoglobin may occur as early as 2 to 4 weeks, and neutropenia usually occurs after 6 to 8 weeks. There have been reports of pancytopenia associated with the use of RETROVIR, which was reversible in most instances after discontinuance of the drug. However, significant anemia, in many cases requiring dose adjustment, discontinuation of RETROVIR, and/or blood transfusions, has occurred during treatment with RETROVIR alone or in combination with other antiretrovirals.

Frequent blood counts are strongly recommended to detect severe anemia or neutropenia in patients with poor bone marrow reserve, particularly in patients with advanced HIV-1 disease who are treated with RETROVIR. For HIV-1-infected individuals and patients with asymptomatic or early HIV-1 disease, periodic blood counts are recommended. If anemia or neutropenia develops, dosage interruption may be needed *[see Dosage and Administration (2.3)]*.

5.2 Myopathy

Myopathy and myositis with pathological changes, similar to that produced by HIV-1 disease, have been associated with prolonged use of RETROVIR.

5.3 Lactic Acidosis/Severe Hepatomegaly With Steatosis

Lactic acidosis and severe hepatomegaly with steatosis, including fatal cases, have been reported with the use of nucleoside analogues alone or in combination, including zidovudine and other antiretrovirals. A majority of these cases have been in women. Obesity and prolonged exposure to antiretroviral nucleoside analogues may be risk factors. Particular caution should be exercised when administering RETROVIR to any patient with known risk factors for liver disease; however, cases have also been reported in patients with no known risk factors. Treatment with RETROVIR should be suspended in any patient who develops clinical or laboratory findings suggestive of lactic acidosis or pronounced hepatotoxicity (which may include hepatomegaly and steatosis even in the absence of marked transaminase elevations).

5.4 Use With Interferon- and Ribavirin-Based Regimens in HIV-1/HCV Co-Infected Patients

In vitro studies have shown ribavirin can reduce the phosphorylation of pyrimidine nucleoside analogues such as zidovudine. Although no evidence of a pharmacokinetic or pharmacodynamic interaction (e.g., loss of HIV-1/HCV virologic suppression) was seen when ribavirin was coadministered with zidovudine in HIV-1/HCV co-infected patients *[see Clinical Pharmacology (12.3)]*, exacerbation of anemia due to ribavirin has been reported when zidovudine is part of the HIV regimen. Coadministration of ribavirin and zidovudine is not advised. Consideration should be given to replacing zidovudine in established combination HIV-1/HCV therapy, especially in patients with a known history of zidovudine-induced anemia.

Hepatic decompensation (some fatal) has occurred in HIV-1/HCV co-infected patients receiving combination antiretroviral therapy for HIV-1 and interferon alfa with or without ribavirin. Patients receiving interferon alfa with or without ribavirin and zidovudine should be closely monitored for treatment-associated toxicities, especially hepatic decompensation, neutropenia, and anemia.

Discontinuation of zidovudine should be considered as medically appropriate. Dose reduction or discontinuation of interferon alfa, ribavirin, or both should also be considered if worsening clinical toxicities are observed, including hepatic decompensation (e.g., Child-Pugh >6) (see the complete prescribing information for interferon and ribavirin).

5.5 Use With Other Zidovudine-Containing Products

RETROVIR should not be administered with combination products that contain zidovudine as one of their components (e.g., COMBIVIR® [lamivudine and zidovudine] Tablets or TRIZIVIR® [abacavir sulfate, lamivudine, and zidovudine] Tablets).

5.6 Immune Reconstitution Syndrome

Immune reconstitution syndrome has been reported in patients treated with combination antiretroviral therapy, including RETROVIR. During the initial phase of combination antiretroviral treatment, patients whose immune systems respond may develop an inflammatory response to indolent or residual opportunistic infections (such as *Mycobacterium avium* infection, cytomegalovirus, *Pneumocystis jirovecii* pneumonia [PCP], or tuberculosis), which may necessitate further evaluation and treatment.

5.7 Fat Redistribution

Redistribution/accumulation of body fat, including central obesity, dorsocervical fat enlargement (buffalo hump), peripheral wasting, facial wasting, breast enlargement, and "cushingoid appearance," have been observed in patients receiving antiretroviral therapy. The mechanism and long-term consequences of these events are currently unknown. A causal relationship has not been established.

6 ADVERSE REACTIONS

6.1 Clinical Trials Experience

The following adverse reactions are discussed in greater detail in other sections of the labeling:

- Hematologic toxicity, including neutropenia and anemia *[see Boxed Warning, Warnings and Precautions (5.1)]*.
- Symptomatic myopathy *[see Boxed Warning, Warnings and Precautions (5.2)]*.
- Lactic acidosis and severe hepatomegaly with steatosis *[see Boxed Warning, Warnings and Precautions (5.3)]*.
- Hepatic decompensation in patients co-infected with HIV-1 and hepatitis C *[see Warnings and Precautions (5.4)]*.

Because clinical trials are conducted under widely varying conditions, adverse reaction rates observed in the clinical trials of a drug cannot be directly compared to rates in the clinical trials of another drug and may not reflect the rates observed in practice.

Adults: The frequency and severity of adverse reactions associated with the use of RETROVIR are greater in patients with more advanced infection at the time of initiation of therapy.

Table 2 summarizes events reported at a statistically significant greater incidence for patients receiving RETROVIR in a monotherapy study.

Table 2. Percentage (%) of Patients With Adverse Reactions[a] in Asymptomatic HIV-1 Infection (ACTG 019)

Adverse Reaction	RETROVIR 500 mg/day (n = 453)	Placebo (n = 428)
Body as a whole		
Asthenia	9%[b]	6%
Headache	63%	53%
Malaise	53%	45%
Gastrointestinal		
Anorexia	20%	11%
Constipation	6%[b]	4%
Nausea	51%	30%
Vomiting	17%	10%

[a]Reported in ≥5% of study population.
[b]Not statistically significant versus placebo.

In addition to the adverse reactions listed in Table 2, adverse reactions observed at an incidence of ≥5% in any treatment arm in clinical studies (NUCA3001, NUCA3002, NUCB3001, and NUCB3002) were abdominal cramps, abdominal pain, arthralgia, chills, dyspepsia, fatigue, insomnia, musculoskeletal pain, myalgia, and neuropathy. Additionally, in these studies hyperbilirubinemia was reported at an incidence of ≤0.8%.

Selected laboratory abnormalities observed during a clinical study of monotherapy with RETROVIR are shown in Table 3.

Table 3. Frequencies of Selected (Grade 3/4) Laboratory Abnormalities in Patients With Asymptomatic HIV-1 Infection (ACTG 019)

Test (Abnormal Level)	RETROVIR 500 mg/day (n = 453)	Placebo (n = 428)
Anemia (Hgb<8 g/dL)	1%	<1%
Granulocytopenia (<750 cells/mm^3)	2%	2%
Thrombocytopenia (platelets <50,000/mm^3)	0%	<1%
ALT (>5 × ULN)	3%	3%
AST (>5 × ULN)	1%	2%

ULN = Upper limit of normal.

Pediatrics: The clinical adverse reactions reported among adult recipients of RETROVIR may also occur in pediatric patients.

Study ACTG 300: Selected clinical adverse reactions and physical findings with a ≥5% frequency during therapy with EPIVIR® (lamivudine) Oral Suspension 4 mg/kg twice daily plus RETROVIR 160 mg/m^2 3 times daily compared with didanosine in therapy-naive (≤56 days of antiretroviral therapy) pediatric patients are listed in Table 4.

Table 4. Selected Clinical Adverse Reactions and Physical Findings (≥5% Frequency) in Pediatric Patients in Study ACTG 300

Adverse Reaction	EPIVIR plus RETROVIR (n = 236)	Didanosine (n = 235)
Body as a whole		
Fever	25%	32%
Digestive		
Hepatomegaly	11%	11%
Nausea & vomiting	8%	7%
Diarrhea	8%	6%
Stomatitis	6%	12%
Splenomegaly	5%	8%
Respiratory		
Cough	15%	18%
Abnormal breath sounds/wheezing	7%	9%
Ear, Nose, and Throat		
Signs or symptoms of ears[a]	7%	6%
Nasal discharge or congestion	8%	11%
Other		
Skin rashes	12%	14%
Lymphadenopathy	9%	11%

[a] Includes pain, discharge, erythema, or swelling of an ear.

Selected laboratory abnormalities experienced by therapy-naive (≤56 days of antiretroviral therapy) pediatric patients are listed in Table 5.

Table 5. Frequencies of Selected (Grade 3/4) Laboratory Abnormalities in Pediatric Patients in Study ACTG 300

Test (Abnormal Level)	EPIVIR plus RETROVIR	Didanosine
Neutropenia (ANC <400 cells/mm^3)	8%	3%
Anemia (Hgb<7.0 g/dL)	4%	2%
Thrombocytopenia (platelets<50,000/mm^3)	1%	3%
ALT (>10 × ULN)	1%	3%
AST (>10 × ULN)	2%	4%
Lipase (>2.5 × ULN)	3%	3%
Total amylase (>2.5 × ULN)	3%	3%

ULN = Upper limit of normal.
ANC = Absolute neutrophil count.

Macrocytosis was reported in the majority of pediatric patients receiving RETROVIR 180 mg/m^2 every 6 hours in open-label studies. Additionally, adverse reactions reported at an incidence of <6% in these studies were congestive heart failure, decreased reflexes, ECG abnormality, edema, hematuria, left ventricular dilation, nervousness/irritability, and weight loss.

Use for the Prevention of Maternal-Fetal Transmission of HIV-1: In a randomized, double-blind, placebo-controlled trial in HIV-1-infected women and their neonates conducted to determine the utility of RETROVIR for the prevention of maternal-fetal HIV-1 transmission, RETROVIR Syrup at 2 mg/kg was administered every 6 hours for 6 weeks to neonates beginning within 12 hours following birth. The most commonly reported adverse reactions were anemia (hemoglobin <9.0 g/dL) and neutropenia (<1,000 cells/mm^3). Anemia occurred in 22% of the neonates who received RETROVIR and in 12% of the neonates who received placebo. The mean difference in hemoglobin values was less than 1.0 g/dL for neonates receiving RETROVIR compared with neonates receiving placebo. No neonates with anemia required transfusion and all hemoglobin values spontaneously returned to normal within 6 weeks after completion of therapy with RETROVIR. Neutropenia in neonates was reported with similar frequency in the group that received RETROVIR (21%) and in the group that received placebo (27%). The long-term consequences of in utero and infant exposure to RETROVIR are unknown.

6.2 Postmarketing Experience
In addition to adverse reactions reported from clinical trials, the following reactions have been identified during postmarketing use of RETROVIR. Because they are reported voluntarily from a population of unknown size, estimates of frequency cannot be made. These reactions have been chosen for inclusion due to a combination of their seriousness, frequency of reporting, or potential causal connection to RETROVIR.

Body as a Whole: Back pain, chest pain, flu-like syndrome, generalized pain, redistribution/accumulation of body fat [see Warnings and Precautions (5.7)].
Cardiovascular: Cardiomyopathy, syncope.
Endocrine: Gynecomastia.
Eye: Macular edema.
Gastrointestinal: Dysphagia, flatulence, oral mucosa pigmentation, mouth ulcer.
General: Sensitization reactions including anaphylaxis and angioedema, vasculitis.
Hemic and Lymphatic: Aplastic anemia, hemolytic anemia, leukopenia, lymphadenopathy, pancytopenia with marrow hypoplasia, pure red cell aplasia.
Hepatobiliary Tract and Pancreas: Hepatitis, hepatomegaly with steatosis, jaundice, lactic acidosis, pancreatitis.
Musculoskeletal: Increased CPK, increased LDH, muscle spasm, myopathy and myositis with pathological changes (similar to that produced by HIV-1 disease), rhabdomyolysis, tremor.
Nervous: Anxiety, confusion, depression, dizziness, loss of mental acuity, mania, paresthesia, seizures, somnolence, vertigo.
Respiratory: Dyspnea, rhinitis, sinusitis.
Skin: Changes in skin and nail pigmentation, pruritus, Stevens-Johnson syndrome, toxic epidermal necrolysis, sweat, urticaria.
Special Senses: Amblyopia, hearing loss, photophobia, taste perversion.
Urogenital: Urinary frequency, urinary hesitancy.

7 DRUG INTERACTIONS
7.1 Antiretroviral Agents
Stavudine: Concomitant use of zidovudine with stavudine should be avoided since an antagonistic relationship has been demonstrated in vitro.
Nucleoside Analogues Affecting DNA Replication: Some nucleoside analogues affecting DNA replication, such as ribavirin, antagonize the in vitro antiviral activity of RETROVIR against HIV-1; concomitant use of such drugs should be avoided.
7.2 Doxorubicin
Concomitant use of zidovudine with doxorubicin should be avoided since an antagonistic relationship has been demonstrated in vitro.
7.3 Hematologic/Bone Marrow Suppressive/Cytotoxic Agents
Coadministration of ganciclovir, interferon alfa, ribavirin, and other bone marrow suppressive or cytotoxic agents may increase the hematologic toxicity of zidovudine.

8 USE IN SPECIFIC POPULATIONS
8.1 Pregnancy
Pregnancy Category C.
In humans, treatment with RETROVIR during pregnancy reduced the rate of maternal-fetal HIV-1 transmission from 24.9% for infants born to placebo-treated mothers to 7.8% for infants born to mothers treated with RETROVIR [see Clinical Studies (14.3)]. There were no differences in pregnancy-related adverse events between the treatment groups. Animal reproduction studies in rats and rabbits showed evidence of embryotoxicity and increased fetal malformations.

A randomized, double-blind, placebo-controlled trial was conducted in HIV-1-infected pregnant women to determine the utility of RETROVIR for the prevention of maternal-fetal HIV-1-transmission [see Clinical Studies (14.3)]. Congenital abnormalities occurred with similar frequency between neonates born to mothers who received RETROVIR and neonates born to mothers who received placebo. The observed abnormalities included problems in embryogenesis (prior to 14 weeks) or were recognized on ultrasound before or immediately after initiation of study drug.

Increased fetal resorptions occurred in pregnant rats and rabbits treated with doses of zidovudine that produced drug plasma concentrations 66 to 226 times (rats) and 12 to 87 times (rabbits) the mean steady-state peak human plasma concentration following a single 100-mg dose of zidovudine. There were no other reported developmental anomalies. In another developmental toxicity study, pregnant rats received zidovudine up to near-lethal doses that produced peak plasma concentrations 350 times peak human plasma concentrations (300 times the daily exposure [AUC] in humans given over 600 mg/day zidovudine). This dose was associated with marked maternal toxicity and an increased incidence of fetal malformations. However, there were no signs of teratogenicity at doses up to one fifth the lethal dose [see Nonclinical Toxicology (13.2)].

Antiretroviral Pregnancy Registry: To monitor maternal-fetal outcomes of pregnant women exposed to RETROVIR, an Antiretroviral Pregnancy Registry has been established. Physicians are encouraged to register patients by calling 1-800-258-4263.

8.3 Nursing Mothers
Zidovudine is excreted in human milk [see Clinical Pharmacology (12.3)].
The Centers for Disease Control and Prevention recommend that HIV-1-infected mothers in the United States not breastfeed their infants to avoid risking postnatal transmission of HIV-1 infection. Because of both the potential for HIV-1 transmission and the potential for serious adverse reactions in nursing infants, mothers should be instructed not to breastfeed if they are receiving RETROVIR.

8.4 Pediatric Use
RETROVIR has been studied in HIV-1-infected pediatric patients ≥6 weeks of age who had HIV-1-related symptoms or who were asymptomatic with abnormal laboratory values indicating significant HIV-1-related immunosuppression. RETROVIR has also been studied in neonates perinatally exposed to HIV-1 [see Dosage and Administration (2.1), Adverse Reactions (6.1), Clinical Pharmacology (12.3), Clinical Studies (14.2), (14.3)].

8.5 Geriatric Use
Clinical studies of RETROVIR did not include sufficient numbers of subjects aged 65 and over to determine whether they respond differently from younger subjects. Other reported clinical experience has not identified differences in responses between the elderly and younger patients. In general, dose selection for an elderly patient should be cautious, reflecting the greater frequency of decreased hepatic, renal, or cardiac function, and of concomitant disease or other drug therapy.

8.6 Renal Impairment
In patients with severely impaired renal function (CrCl<15 mL/min), dosage reduction is recommended [see Dosage and Administration (2.4), Clinical Pharmacology (12.3)].

8.7 Hepatic Impairment
Zidovudine is eliminated from the body primarily by renal excretion following metabolism in the liver (glucuronidation). Although the data are limited, zidovudine concentrations appear to be increased in patients with severely impaired hepatic function, which may increase the risk of hematologic toxicity [see Dosage and Administration (2.5), Clinical Pharmacology (12.3)].

10 OVERDOSAGE
Acute overdoses of zidovudine have been reported in pediatric patients and adults. These involved exposures up to 50 grams. No specific symptoms or signs have been identified following acute overdosage with zidovudine apart from those listed as adverse events such as fatigue, headache, vomiting, and occasional reports of hematological disturbances. All patients recovered without permanent sequelae. Hemodialysis and peritoneal dialysis appear to have a negligible effect on the removal of zidovudine while elimination of its primary metabolite, 3′-azido-3′-deoxy-5′-O-β-D-glucopyranuronosylthymidine (GZDV), is enhanced.

11 DESCRIPTION
RETROVIR is the brand name for zidovudine (formerly called azidothymidine [AZT]), a pyrimidine nucleoside analogue active against HIV-1. The chemical name of zidovudine is 3′-azido-3′-deoxythymidine; it has the following structural formula:

Zidovudine is a white to beige, odorless, crystalline solid with a molecular weight of 267.24 and a solubility of 20.1 mg/mL in water at 25°C. The molecular formula is $C_{10}H_{13}N_5O_4$.
RETROVIR Tablets are for oral administration. Each film-coated tablet contains 300 mg of zidovudine and the inactive ingredients hypromellose, magnesium stearate, microcrystalline cellulose, polyethylene glycol, sodium starch glycolate, and titanium dioxide.
RETROVIR Capsules are for oral administration. Each capsule contains 100 mg of zidovudine and the inactive ingredients corn starch, magnesium stearate, microcrystalline cellulose, and sodium starch glycolate. The 100-mg empty hard gelatin capsule, printed with edible black ink, consists of black iron oxide, dimethylpolysiloxane, gelatin, pharmaceutical shellac, soya lecithin, and titanium dioxide.
RETROVIR Syrup is for oral administration. Each teaspoonful (5 mL) of RETROVIR Syrup contains 50 mg of zidovudine and the inactive ingredients sodium benzoate 0.2% (added as a preservative), citric acid, flavors, glycerin, and liquid sucrose. Sodium hydroxide may be added to adjust pH.

12 CLINICAL PHARMACOLOGY

12.1 Mechanism of Action

Zidovudine is an antiviral agent *[see Clinical Pharmacology (12.4)]*.

12.3 Pharmacokinetics

Absorption and Bioavailability: In adults, following oral administration, zidovudine is rapidly absorbed and extensively distributed, with peak serum concentrations occurring within 0.5 to 1.5 hours. The AUC was equivalent when zidovudine was administered as RETROVIR Tablets or Syrup compared with RETROVIR Capsules. The pharmacokinetic properties of zidovudine in fasting adult patients are summarized in Table 6.

Table 6. Zidovudine Pharmacokinetic Parameters in Fasting Adult Patients

Parameter	Mean ± SD (except where noted)
Oral bioavailability (%)	64 ± 10 (n = 5)
Apparent volume of distribution (L/kg)	1.6 ± 0.6 (n = 8)
Plasma protein binding (%)	<38
CSF:plasma ratio[a]	0.6 [0.04 to 2.62] (n = 39)
Systemic clearance (L/hr/kg)	1.6 ± 0.6 (n = 6)
Renal clearance (L/hr/kg)	0.34 ± 0.05 (n = 9)
Elimination half-life (hr)[b]	0.5 to 3 (n = 19)

[a] Median [range].
[b] Approximate range.

Distribution: The apparent volume of distribution of zidovudine, following oral administration, is 1.6 ± 0.6 L/kg; and binding to plasma protein is low, <38% (Table 6).

Metabolism and Elimination: Zidovudine is primarily eliminated by hepatic metabolism. The major metabolite of zidovudine is GZDV. GZDV AUC is about 3-fold greater than the zidovudine AUC. Urinary recovery of zidovudine and GZDV accounts for 14% and 74%, respectively, of the dose following oral administration. A second metabolite, 3'-amino-3'-deoxythymidine (AMT), has been identified in the plasma following single-dose intravenous (IV) administration of zidovudine. The AMT AUC was one fifth of the zidovudine AUC. Pharmacokinetics of zidovudine were dose independent at oral dosing regimens ranging from 2 mg/kg every 8 hours to 10 mg/kg every 4 hours.

Effect of Food on Absorption: RETROVIR may be administered with or without food. The zidovudine AUC was similar when a single dose of zidovudine was administered with food.

Special Populations: *Renal Impairment:* Zidovudine clearance was decreased resulting in increased zidovudine and GZDV half-life and AUC in patients with impaired renal function (n = 14) following a single 200-mg oral dose (Table 7). Plasma concentrations of AMT were not determined. A dose adjustment should not be necessary for patients with creatinine clearance (CrCl) ≥15 mL/min.

Table 7. Zidovudine Pharmacokinetic Parameters in Patients With Severe Renal Impairment[a]

Parameter	Control Subjects (Normal Renal Function) (n = 6)	Patients With Renal Impairment (n = 14)
CrCl (mL/min)	120 ± 8	18 ± 2
Zidovudine AUC (ng•hr/mL)	1,400 ± 200	3,100 ± 300
Zidovudine half-life (hr)	1.0 ± 0.2	1.4 ± 0.1

[a] Data are expressed as mean ± standard deviation.

Hemodialysis and Peritoneal Dialysis: The pharmacokinetics and tolerance of zidovudine were evaluated in a multiple-dose study in patients undergoing hemodialysis (n = 5) or peritoneal dialysis (n = 6) receiving escalating doses up to 200 mg 5 times daily for 8 weeks. Daily doses of 500 mg or less were well tolerated despite significantly elevated GZDV plasma concentrations. Apparent zidovudine oral clearance was approximately 50% of that reported in patients with normal renal function. Hemodialysis and peritoneal dialysis appeared to have a negligible effect on the removal of zidovudine, whereas GZDV elimination was enhanced. A dosage adjustment is recommended for patients undergoing hemodialysis or peritoneal dialysis *[see Dosage and Administration (2.4)]*.

Hepatic Impairment: Data describing the effect of hepatic impairment on the pharmacokinetics of zidovudine are limited. However, because zidovudine is eliminated primarily by hepatic metabolism, it is expected that zidovudine clearance would be decreased and plasma concentrations would be increased following administration of the recommended adult doses to patients with hepatic impairment *[see Dosage and Administration (2.5)]*.

Pediatric Patients: Zidovudine pharmacokinetics have been evaluated in HIV-1-infected pediatric patients (Table 8).

Patients 3 Months to 12 Years of Age: Overall, zidovudine pharmacokinetics in pediatric patients greater than 3 months of age are similar to those in adult patients. Proportional increases in plasma zidovudine concentrations were observed following administration of oral solution from 90 to 240 mg/m² every 6 hours. Oral bioavailability, terminal half-life, and oral clearance were comparable to adult values. As in adult patients, the major route of elimination was by metabolism to GZDV. After intravenous dosing, about 29% of the dose was excreted in the urine unchanged, and about 45% of the dose was excreted as GZDV *[see Dosage and Administration (2.1)]*.

Patients <3 Months of Age: Zidovudine pharmacokinetics have been evaluated in pediatric patients from birth to 3 months of life. Zidovudine elimination was determined immediately following birth in 8 neonates who were exposed to zidovudine in utero. The half-life was 13.0 ± 5.8 hours. In neonates ≤14 days old, bioavailability was greater, total body clearance was slower, and half-life was longer than in pediatric patients >14 days old. For dose recommendations for neonates *[see Dosage and Administration (2.2)]*. [See table 8 below]

Pregnancy: Zidovudine pharmacokinetics have been studied in a Phase I study of 8 women during the last trimester of pregnancy. Zidovudine pharmacokinetics were similar to those of nonpregnant adults. Consistent with passive transmission of the drug across the placenta, zidovudine concen-

trations in neonatal plasma at birth were essentially equal to those in maternal plasma at delivery *[see Use in Specific Populations (8.1)]*.

Although data are limited, methadone maintenance therapy in 5 pregnant women did not appear to alter zidovudine pharmacokinetics.

Nursing Mothers: The Centers for Disease Control and Prevention recommend that HIV-1-infected mothers not breastfeed their infants to avoid risking postnatal transmission of HIV-1. After administration of a single dose of 200 mg zidovudine to 13 HIV-1-infected women, the mean concentration of zidovudine was similar in human milk and serum *[see Use in Specific Populations (8.3)]*.

Geriatric Patients: Zidovudine pharmacokinetics have not been studied in patients over 65 years of age.

Gender: A pharmacokinetic study in healthy male (n = 12) and female (n = 12) subjects showed no differences in zidovudine AUC when a single dose of zidovudine was administered as the 300-mg RETROVIR Tablet.

Drug Interactions: [See Drug Interactions (7)].
[See table 9 at top of next page]

Phenytoin: Phenytoin plasma levels have been reported to be low in some patients receiving RETROVIR, while in one case a high level was documented. However, in a pharmacokinetic interaction study in which 12 HIV-1-positive volunteers received a single 300-mg phenytoin dose alone and during steady-state zidovudine conditions (200 mg every 4 hours), no change in phenytoin kinetics was observed. Although not designed to optimally assess the effect of phenytoin on zidovudine kinetics, a 30% decrease in oral zidovudine clearance was observed with phenytoin.

Ribavirin: In vitro data indicate ribavirin reduces phosphorylation of lamivudine, stavudine, and zidovudine. However, no pharmacokinetic (e.g., plasma concentrations or intracellular triphosphorylated active metabolite concentrations) or pharmacodynamic (e.g., loss of HIV-1/HCV virologic suppression) interaction was observed when ribavirin and lamivudine (n = 18), stavudine (n = 10), or zidovudine (n = 6) were coadministered as part of a multi-drug regimen to HIV-1/HCV co-infected patients *[see Warnings and Precautions (5.4)]*.

12.4 Microbiology

Mechanism of Action: Zidovudine is a synthetic nucleoside analogue. Intracellularly, zidovudine is phosphorylated to its active 5'-triphosphate metabolite, zidovudine triphosphate (ZDV-TP). The principal mode of action of ZDV-TP is inhibition of reverse transcriptase (RT) via DNA chain termination after incorporation of the nucleotide analogue. ZDV-TP is a weak inhibitor of the cellular DNA polymerases α and γ and has been reported to be incorporated into the DNA of cells in culture.

Antiviral Activity: The antiviral activity of zidovudine against HIV-1 was assessed in a number of cell lines (including monocytes and fresh human peripheral blood lymphocytes). The EC_{50} and EC_{90} values for zidovudine were 0.01 to 0.49 µM (1 µM = 0.27 mcg/mL) and 0.1 to 9 µM, respectively. HIV-1 from therapy-naive subjects with no mutations associated with resistance gave median EC_{50} values of 0.011 µM (range: 0.005 to 0.110 µM) from Virco (n = 92 baseline samples from COL40263) and 0.0017 µM (0.006 to 0.0340 µM) from Monogram Biosciences (n = 135 baseline samples from ESS30009). The EC_{50} values of zidovudine against different HIV-1 clades (A-G) ranged from 0.00018 to 0.02 µM, and against HIV-2 isolates from 0.00049 to 0.004 µM. In cell culture drug combination studies, zidovudine demonstrates synergistic activity with the nucleoside reverse transcriptase inhibitors abacavir, didanosine, and lamivudine; the non-nucleoside reverse transcriptase inhibitors delavirdine and nevirapine; and the protease inhibitors indinavir, nelfinavir, ritonavir, and saquinavir; and additive activity with interferon alfa. Ribavirin has been found to inhibit the phosphorylation of zidovudine in cell culture.

Resistance: Genotypic analyses of the isolates selected in cell culture and recovered from zidovudine-treated patients showed mutations in the HIV-1 RT gene resulting in 6 amino acid substitutions (M41L, D67N, K70R, L210W, T215Y or F, and K219Q) that confer zidovudine resistance. In general, higher levels of resistance were associated with greater number of amino acid substitutions. In some patients harboring zidovudine-resistant virus at baseline, phenotypic sensitivity to zidovudine was restored by 12 weeks of treatment with lamivudine and zidovudine. Combination therapy with lamivudine plus zidovudine delayed the emergence of substitutions conferring resistance to zidovudine.

Cross-Resistance: In a study of 167 HIV-1-infected patients, isolates (n = 2) with multi-drug resistance to didanosine, lamivudine, stavudine, zalcitabine, and zidovudine were recovered from patients treated for ≥1 year with zidovudine plus didanosine or zidovudine plus zalcitabine. The pattern of resistance-associated amino acid substitutions with such combination therapies was different (A62V, V75I, F77L, F116Y, Q151M) from the pattern with zidovudine monotherapy, with the Q151M substitution

Table 8. Zidovudine Pharmacokinetic Parameters in Pediatric Patients[a]

Parameter	Birth to 14 Days of Age	14 Days to 3 Months of Age	3 Months to 12 Years of Age
Oral bioavailability (%)	89 ± 19 (n = 15)	61 ± 19 (n = 17)	65 ± 24 (n = 18)
CSF:plasma ratio	no data	no data	0.68 [0.03 to 3.25][b] (n = 38)
CL (L/hr/kg)	0.65 ± 0.29 (n = 18)	1.14 ± 0.24 (n = 16)	1.85 ± 0.47 (n = 20)
Elimination half-life (hr)	3.1 ± 1.2 (n = 21)	1.9 ± 0.7 (n = 18)	1.5 ± 0.7 (n = 21)

[a] Data presented as mean ± standard deviation except where noted.
[b] Median [range].

Table 9. Effect of Coadministered Drugs on Zidovudine AUC[a]

Note: ROUTINE DOSE MODIFICATION OF ZIDOVUDINE IS NOT WARRANTED WITH COADMINISTRATION OF THE FOLLOWING DRUGS.

Coadministered Drug and Dose	Zidovudine Dose	n	Zidovudine Concentrations AUC	Zidovudine Concentrations Variability	Concentration of Coadministered Drug
Atovaquone 750 mg q 12 hr with food	200 mg q 8 hr	14	↑AUC 31%	Range 23% to 78%[b]	↔
Clarithromycin 500 mg twice daily	100 mg q 4 hr × 7 days	4	↓AUC 12%	Range ↓34% to ↑14%	Not Reported
Fluconazole 400 mg daily	200 mg q 8 hr	12	↑AUC 74%	95% CI: 54% to 98%	Not Reported
Lamivudine 300 mg q 12 hr	single 200 mg	12	↑AUC 13%	90% CI: 2% to 27%	↔
Methadone 30 to 90 mg daily	200 mg q 4 hr	9	↑AUC 43%	Range 16% to 64%[b]	↔
Nelfinavir 750 mg q 8 hr × 7 to 10 days	single 200 mg	11	↓AUC 35%	Range 28% to 41%	↔
Probenecid 500 mg q 6 hr × 2 days	2 mg/kg q 8 hr × 3 days	3	↑AUC 106%	Range 100% to 170%[b]	Not Assessed
Rifampin 600 mg daily × 14 days	200 mg q 8 hr × 14 days	8	↓AUC 47%	90% CI: 41% to 53%	Not Assessed
Ritonavir 300 mg q 6 hr × 4 days	200 mg q 8 hr × 4 days	9	↓AUC 25%	95% CI: 15% to 34%	↔
Valproic acid 250 mg or 500 mg q 8 hr × 4 days	100 mg q 8 hr × 4 days	6	↑AUC 80%	Range 64% to 130%[b]	Not Assessed

↑ = Increase; ↓ = Decrease; ↔ = no significant change; AUC = area under the concentration versus time curve; CI = confidence interval.
[a] This table is not all inclusive.
[b] Estimated range of percent difference.

being most commonly associated with multi-drug resistance. The substitution at codon 151 in combination with substitutions at 62, 75, 77, and 116 results in a virus with reduced susceptibility to didanosine, lamivudine, stavudine, zalcitabine, and zidovudine. Thymidine analogue mutations (TAMs) are selected by zidovudine and confer cross-resistance to abacavir, didanosine, stavudine, tenofovir, and zalcitabine.

13 NONCLINICAL TOXICOLOGY

13.1 Carcinogenesis, Mutagenesis, Impairment of Fertility

Zidovudine was administered orally at 3 dosage levels to separate groups of mice and rats (60 females and 60 males in each group). Initial single daily doses were 30, 60, and 120 mg/kg/day in mice and 80, 220, and 600 mg/kg/day in rats. The doses in mice were reduced to 20, 30, and 40 mg/kg/day after day 90 because of treatment-related anemia, whereas in rats only the high dose was reduced to 450 mg/kg/day on day 91 and then to 300 mg/kg/day on day 279.

In mice, 7 late-appearing (after 19 months) vaginal neoplasms (5 nonmetastasizing squamous cell carcinomas, 1 squamous cell papilloma, and 1 squamous polyp) occurred in animals given the highest dose. One late-appearing squamous cell papilloma occurred in the vagina of a middle-dose animal. No vaginal tumors were found at the lowest dose.

In rats, 2 late-appearing (after 20 months), nonmetastasizing vaginal squamous cell carcinomas occurred in animals given the highest dose. No vaginal tumors occurred at the low or middle dose in rats. No other drug-related tumors were observed in either sex of either species.

At doses that produced tumors in mice and rats, the estimated drug exposure (as measured by AUC) was approximately 3 times (mouse) and 24 times (rat) the estimated human exposure at the recommended therapeutic dose of 100 mg every 4 hours.

It is not known how predictive the results of rodent carcinogenicity studies may be for humans.

Zidovudine was mutagenic in a 5178Y/TK[+/−] mouse lymphoma assay, positive in an in vitro cell transformation assay, clastogenic in a cytogenetic assay using cultured human lymphocytes, and positive in mouse and rat micronucleus tests after repeated doses. It was negative in a cytogenetic study in rats given a single dose.

Zidovudine, administered to male and female rats at doses up to 7 times the usual adult dose based on body surface area, had no effect on fertility judged by conception rates. Two transplacental carcinogenicity studies were conducted in mice. One study administered zidovudine at doses of 20 mg/kg/day or 40 mg/kg/day from gestation day 10 through parturition and lactation with dosing continuing in offspring for 24 months postnatally. The doses of zidovudine administered in this study produced zidovudine exposures approximately 3 times the estimated human exposure at recommended doses. After 24 months, an increase in incidence of vaginal tumors was noted with no increase in tumors in the liver or lung or any other organ in either gender. These findings are consistent with results of the standard oral carcinogenicity study in mice, as described earlier. A second study administered zidovudine at maximum tolerated doses of 12.5 mg/day or 25 mg/day (~1,000 mg/kg nonpregnant body weight or ~450 mg/kg of term body weight) to pregnant mice from days 12 through 18 of gestation. There was an increase in the number of tumors in the lung, liver, and female reproductive tracts in the offspring of mice receiving the higher dose level of zidovudine.

13.2 Reproductive and Developmental Toxicology Studies

Oral teratology studies in the rat and in the rabbit at doses up to 500 mg/kg/day revealed no evidence of teratogenicity with zidovudine. Zidovudine treatment resulted in embryo/fetal toxicity as evidenced by an increase in the incidence of fetal resorptions in rats given 150 or 450 mg/kg/day and rabbits given 500 mg/kg/day. The doses used in the teratology studies resulted in peak zidovudine plasma concentrations (after one half of the daily dose) in rats 66 to 226 times, and in rabbits 12 to 87 times, mean steady-state peak human plasma concentrations (after one sixth of the daily dose) achieved with the recommended daily dose (100 mg every 4 hours). In an in vitro experiment with fertilized mouse oocytes, zidovudine exposure resulted in a dose-dependent reduction in blastocyst formation. In an additional teratology study in rats, a dose of 3,000 mg/kg/day (very near the oral median lethal dose in rats of 3,683 mg/kg) caused marked maternal toxicity and an increase in the incidence of fetal malformations. This dose resulted in peak zidovudine plasma concentrations 350 times peak human plasma concentrations. (Estimated AUC in rats at this dose level was 300 times the daily AUC in humans given 600 mg/day.) No evidence of teratogenicity was seen in this experiment at doses of 600 mg/kg/day or less.

14 CLINICAL STUDIES

Therapy with RETROVIR has been shown to prolong survival and decrease the incidence of opportunistic infections in patients with advanced HIV-1 disease and to delay disease progression in asymptomatic HIV-1-infected patients.

14.1 Adults

Combination Therapy: RETROVIR in combination with other antiretroviral agents has been shown to be superior to monotherapy for one or more of the following endpoints: delaying death, delaying development of AIDS, increasing CD4+ cell counts, and decreasing plasma HIV-1 RNA.

The clinical efficacy of a combination regimen that includes RETROVIR was demonstrated in study ACTG 320. This study was a multi-center, randomized, double-blind, placebo-controlled trial that compared RETROVIR 600 mg/day plus EPIVIR 300 mg/day to RETROVIR plus EPIVIR plus indinavir 800 mg t.i.d. The incidence of AIDS-defining events or death was lower in the triple-drug–containing arm compared with the 2-drug–containing arm (6.1% versus 10.9%, respectively).

Monotherapy: In controlled studies of treatment-naive patients conducted between 1986 and 1989, monotherapy with RETROVIR, as compared with placebo, reduced the risk of HIV-1 disease progression, as assessed using endpoints that included the occurrence of HIV-1-related illnesses, AIDS-defining events, or death. These studies enrolled patients with advanced disease (BW 002), and asymptomatic or mildly symptomatic disease in patients with CD4+ cell counts between 200 and 500 cells/mm³ (ACTG 016 and ACTG 019). A survival benefit for monotherapy with RETROVIR was not demonstrated in the latter 2 studies. Subsequent studies showed that the clinical benefit of monotherapy with RETROVIR was time limited.

14.2 Pediatric Patients

ACTG 300 was a multi-center, randomized, double-blind study that provided for comparison of EPIVIR plus RETROVIR to didanosine monotherapy. A total of 471 symptomatic, HIV-1-infected therapy-naive pediatric patients were enrolled in these 2 treatment arms. The median age was 2.7 years (range: 6 weeks to 14 years), the mean baseline CD4+ cell count was 868 cells/mm³, and the mean baseline plasma HIV-1 RNA was 5.0 $\log_{10}$ copies/mL. The median duration that patients remained on study was approximately 10 months. Results are summarized in Table 10.

Table 10. Number of Patients (%) Reaching a Primary Clinical Endpoint (Disease Progression or Death)

Endpoint	EPIVIR plus RETROVIR (n = 236)	Didanosine (n = 235)
HIV disease progression or death (total)	15 (6.4%)	37 (15.7%)
Physical growth failure	7 (3.0%)	6 (2.6%)
Central nervous system deterioration	4 (1.7%)	12 (5.1%)
CDC Clinical Category C	2 (0.8%)	8 (3.4%)
Death	2 (0.8%)	11 (4.7%)

14.3 Prevention of Maternal-Fetal HIV-1 Transmission

The utility of RETROVIR for the prevention of maternal-fetal HIV-1 transmission was demonstrated in a randomized, double-blind, placebo-controlled trial (ACTG 076) conducted in HIV-1-infected pregnant women with CD4+ cell counts of 200 to 1,818 cells/mm³ (median in the treated group: 560 cells/mm³) who had little or no previous exposure to RETROVIR. Oral RETROVIR was initiated between 14 and 34 weeks of gestation (median 11 weeks of therapy) followed by IV administration of RETROVIR during labor and delivery. Following birth, neonates received oral RETROVIR Syrup for 6 weeks. The study showed a statistically significant difference in the incidence of HIV-1 infection in the neonates (based on viral culture from peripheral blood) between the group receiving RETROVIR and the group receiving placebo. Of 363 neonates evaluated in the study, the estimated risk of HIV-1 infection was 7.8% in the group receiving RETROVIR and 24.9% in the placebo group, a relative reduction in transmission risk of 68.7%. RETROVIR was well tolerated by mothers and infants. There was no difference in pregnancy-related adverse events between the treatment groups.

16 HOW SUPPLIED/STORAGE AND HANDLING

RETROVIR Tablets 300 mg (biconvex, white, round, film-coated) containing 300 mg zidovudine, one side engraved "GX CW3" and "300" on the other side.
Bottle of 60 (NDC 0173-0501-00).
Store at 15° to 25°C (59° to 77°F).
RETROVIR Capsules 100 mg (white, opaque cap and body) containing 100 mg zidovudine and printed with "Wellcome" and unicorn logo on cap and "Y9C" and "100" on body.
Bottles of 100 (NDC 0173-0108-55).
Store at 15° to 25°C (59° to 77°F) and protect from moisture.

RETROVIR Syrup (colorless to pale yellow, strawberry-flavored) containing 50 mg zidovudine in each teaspoonful (5 mL).

Bottle of 240 mL (NDC 0173-0113-18) with child-resistant cap.

Store at 15° to 25°C (59° to 77°F).

17 PATIENT COUNSELING INFORMATION

17.1 Information About Therapy With RETROVIR

Neutropenia and Anemia: Patients should be informed that the major toxicities of RETROVIR are neutropenia and/or anemia. The frequency and severity of these toxicities are greater in patients with more advanced disease and in those who initiate therapy later in the course of their infection. Patients should be informed that if toxicity develops, they may require transfusions or drug discontinuation. Patients should be informed of the extreme importance of having their blood counts followed closely while on therapy, especially for patients with advanced symptomatic HIV-1 disease *[see Boxed Warning, Warnings and Precautions (5.1)]*.

Myopathy: Patients should be informed that myopathy and myositis with pathological changes, similar to that produced by HIV-1 disease, have been associated with prolonged use of RETROVIR *[see Boxed Warning, Warnings and Precautions (5.2)]*.

Lactic Acidosis/Hepatomegaly: Patients should be informed that some HIV medicines, including RETROVIR, can cause a rare, but serious condition called lactic acidosis with liver enlargement (hepatomegaly) *[see Boxed Warning, Warnings and Precautions (5.3)]*.

HIV-1/HCV Co-Infection: Patients with HIV-1/HCV co-infection should be informed that hepatic decompensation (some fatal) has occurred in HIV-1/HCV co-infected patients receiving combination antiretroviral therapy for HIV-1 and interferon alfa with or without ribavirin *[see Warnings and Precautions (5.4)]*.

Redistribution/Accumulation of Body Fat: Patients should be informed that redistribution or accumulation of body fat may occur in patients receiving antiretroviral therapy and that the cause and long-term health effects of these conditions are not known at this time *[see Warnings and Precautions (5.7)]*.

Common Adverse Reactions: Patients should be informed that the most commonly reported adverse reactions in adult patients being treated with RETROVIR were headache, malaise, nausea, anorexia, and vomiting. The most commonly reported adverse reactions in pediatric patients receiving RETROVIR were fever, cough, and digestive disorders. Patients also should be encouraged to contact their physician if they experience muscle weakness, shortness of breath, symptoms of hepatitis or pancreatitis, or any other unexpected adverse events while being treated with RETROVIR *[see Adverse Reactions (6)]*.

Drug Interactions: Patients should be cautioned about the use of other medications, including ganciclovir, interferon alfa, and ribavirin, which may exacerbate the toxicity of RETROVIR *[see Drug Interactions (7)]*.

Pregnancy: Pregnant women considering the use of RETROVIR during pregnancy for prevention of HIV-1 transmission to their infants should be informed that transmission may still occur in some cases despite therapy. The long-term consequences of in utero and infant exposure to RETROVIR are unknown, including the possible risk of cancer *[see Use in Specific Populations (8.1)]*.

HIV-1-infected pregnant women should be informed not to breastfeed to avoid postnatal transmission of HIV to a child who may not yet be infected *[see Use in Specific Populations (8.3)]*.

Information About Therapy With RETROVIR: RETROVIR is not a cure for HIV-1 infection, and patients may continue to acquire illnesses associated with HIV-1 infection, including opportunistic infections. Therefore, patients should be informed to seek medical care for any significant change in their health status.

Patients should be informed of the importance of taking RETROVIR exactly as prescribed. They should be informed not to share medication and not to exceed the recommended dose. Patients should be informed that the long-term effects of RETROVIR are unknown at this time.

Patients should be informed that therapy with RETROVIR has not been shown to reduce the risk of transmission of HIV-1 to others through sexual contact or blood contamination.

RETROVIR, COMBIVIR, EPIVIR, and TRIZIVIR are registered trademarks of GlaxoSmithKline.

GlaxoSmithKline
Research Triangle Park, NC 27709
©2010, GlaxoSmithKline. All rights reserved.
May 2010
RTT:3PI

RETROVIR®
[re'trō-vir]
(zidovudine)
IV Infusion

FOR INTRAVENOUS INFUSION ONLY

℞

> **WARNING**
> **RETROVIR (ZIDOVUDINE) HAS BEEN ASSOCIATED WITH HEMATOLOGIC TOXICITY, INCLUDING NEUTROPENIA AND SEVERE ANEMIA, PARTICULARLY IN PATIENTS WITH ADVANCED HUMAN IMMUNODEFICIENCY VIRUS (HIV) DISEASE (SEE WARNINGS). PROLONGED USE OF RETROVIR HAS BEEN ASSOCIATED WITH SYMPTOMATIC MYOPATHY.**
> **LACTIC ACIDOSIS AND SEVERE HEPATOMEGALY WITH STEATOSIS, INCLUDING FATAL CASES, HAVE BEEN REPORTED WITH THE USE OF NUCLEOSIDE ANALOGUES ALONE OR IN COMBINATION, INCLUDING RETROVIR AND OTHER ANTIRETROVIRALS (SEE WARNINGS).**

DESCRIPTION

RETROVIR is the brand name for zidovudine (formerly called azidothymidine [AZT]), a pyrimidine nucleoside analogue active against HIV. RETROVIR IV Infusion is a sterile solution for intravenous infusion only. Each mL contains 10 mg zidovudine in Water for Injection. Hydrochloric acid and/or sodium hydroxide may have been added to adjust the pH to approximately 5.5. RETROVIR IV Infusion contains no preservatives.

The chemical name of zidovudine is 3′-azido-3′-deoxythymidine.

Zidovudine is a white to beige, odorless, crystalline solid with a molecular weight of 267.24 and a solubility of 20.1 mg/mL in water at 25° C. The molecular formula is $C_{10}H_{13}N_5O_4$.

MICROBIOLOGY

Mechanism of Action: Zidovudine is a synthetic nucleoside analogue. Intracellularly, zidovudine is phosphorylated to its active 5′-triphosphate metabolite, zidovudine triphosphate (ZDV-TP). The principal mode of action of ZDV-TP is inhibition of reverse transcriptase (RT) via DNA chain termination after incorporation of the nucleotide analogue. ZDV-TP is a weak inhibitor of the cellular DNA polymerases α and γ and has been reported to be incorporated into the DNA of cells in culture.

Antiviral Activity: Activity of zidovudine against HIV-1 was assessed in a number of cell lines (including monocytes and fresh human peripheral blood lymphocytes). The EC_{50} and EC_{90} values for zidovudine were 0.01 to 0.49 μM (1 μM = 0.27 mcg/mL) and 0.1 to 9 μM, respectively. HIV from therapy-naive subjects with no mutations associated with resistance gave median EC_{50} values of 0.011 μM (range: 0.005 to 0.110 μM) from Virco (n = 93 baseline samples from COLA40263) and 0.02 μM (0.01 to 0.03 μM) from Monogram Biosciences (n = 135 baseline samples from ESS30009). The EC_{50} values of zidovudine against different HIV-1 clades (A-G) ranged from 0.00018 to 0.02 μM, and against HIV-2 isolates from 0.00049 to 0.004 μM. In cell culture drug combination studies, zidovudine demonstrates synergistic activity with the nucleoside reverse transcriptase inhibitors (NRTIs) abacavir, didanosine, lamivudine, and zalcitabine; the non-nucleoside reverse transcriptase inhibitors (NNRTIs) delavirdine and nevirapine; and the protease inhibitors (PIs) indinavir, nelfinavir, ritonavir, and saquinavir; and additive activity with interferon alfa. Ribavirin has been found to inhibit the phosphorylation of zidovudine in cell culture.

Resistance: Genotypic analyses of the isolates selected in cell culture and recovered from zidovudine-treated patients showed mutations in the HIV-1 RT gene resulting in 6 amino acid substitutions (M41L, D67N, K70R, L210W, T215Y or F, and K219Q) that confer zidovudine resistance. In general, higher levels of resistance were associated with greater number of mutations. In some patients harboring zidovudine-resistant virus at baseline, phenotypic sensitiv-

---

ity to zidovudine was restored by 12 weeks of treatment with lamivudine and zidovudine. Combination therapy with lamivudine plus zidovudine delayed the emergence of mutations conferring resistance to zidovudine.

Cross-Resistance: In a study of 167 HIV-infected patients, isolates (n = 2) with multi-drug resistance to didanosine, lamivudine, stavudine, zalcitabine, and zidovudine were recovered from patients treated for ≥1 year with zidovudine plus didanosine or zidovudine plus zalcitabine. The pattern of resistance-associated mutations with such combination therapies was different (A62V, V75I, F77L, F116Y, Q151M) from the pattern with zidovudine monotherapy, with the Q151M mutation being most commonly associated with multi-drug resistance. The mutation at codon 151 in combination with mutations at 62, 75, 77, and 116 results in a virus with reduced susceptibility to didanosine, lamivudine, stavudine, zalcitabine, and zidovudine. Thymidine analogue mutations (TAMs) are selected by zidovudine and confer cross-resistance to abacavir, didanosine, stavudine, tenofovir, and zalcitabine.

CLINICAL PHARMACOLOGY

Pharmacokinetics: *Adults:* The pharmacokinetics of zidovudine have been evaluated in 22 adult HIV-infected patients in a Phase 1 dose-escalation study. Following intravenous (IV) dosing, dose-independent kinetics was observed over the range of 1 to 5 mg/kg. The major metabolite of zidovudine is 3′-azido-3′-deoxy-5′-O-β-D-glucopyranuronosylthymidine (GZDV). GZDV area under the curve (AUC) is about 3-fold greater than the zidovudine AUC. Urinary recovery of zidovudine and GZDV accounts for 18% and 60%, respectively, following IV dosing. A second metabolite, 3′-amino-3′-deoxythymidine (AMT), has been identified in the plasma following single-dose IV administration of zidovudine. The AMT AUC was one fifth of the zidovudine AUC.

The mean steady-state peak and trough concentrations of zidovudine at 2.5 mg/kg every 4 hours were 1.06 and 0.12 mcg/mL, respectively.

The zidovudine cerebrospinal fluid (CSF)/plasma concentration ratio was determined in 39 patients receiving chronic therapy with RETROVIR. The median ratio measured in 50 paired samples drawn 1 to 8 hours after the last dose of RETROVIR was 0.6.

Table 1. Zidovudine Pharmacokinetic Parameters Following Intravenous Administration in HIV-Infected Patients

Parameter	Mean ± SD (except where noted)
Apparent volume of distribution (L/kg)	1.6 ± 0.6 (n = 11)
Plasma protein binding (%)	<38
CSF:plasma ratio*	0.6 [0.04 to 2.62] (n = 39)
Systemic clearance (L/hr/kg)	1.6 (0.8 to 2.7) (n =18)
Renal clearance (L/hr/kg)	0.34 ± 0.05 (n = 16)
Elimination half-life (hr)†	1.1 (0.5 to 2.9) (n = 19)

*Median [range].
†Approximate range.

Adults With Impaired Renal Function: Zidovudine clearance was decreased resulting in increased zidovudine and GZDV half-life and AUC in patients with impaired renal function (n = 14) following a single 200-mg oral dose (Table 2). Plasma concentrations of AMT were not determined. A dose adjustment should not be necessary for patients with creatinine clearance (CrCl) ≥15 mL/min.

[See table 2 below]

Table 2. Zidovudine Pharmacokinetic Parameters in Patients With Severe Renal Impairment*

Parameter	Control Subjects (Normal Renal Function) (n = 6)	Patients With Renal Impairment (n = 14)
CrCl (mL/min)	120 ± 8	18 ± 2
Zidovudine AUC (ng•hr/mL)	1,400 ± 200	3,100 ± 300
Zidovudine half-life (hr)	1.0 ± 0.2	1.4 ± 0.1

*Data are expressed as mean ± standard deviation.

The pharmacokinetics and tolerance of oral zidovudine were evaluated in a multiple-dose study in patients undergoing hemodialysis (n = 5) or peritoneal dialysis (n = 6) receiving escalating doses up to 200 mg 5 times daily for 8 weeks. Daily doses of 500 mg or less were well tolerated despite significantly elevated GZDV plasma concentrations. Apparent zidovudine oral clearance was approximately 50% of that reported in patients with normal renal function. Hemodialysis and peritoneal dialysis appeared to have a negligible effect on the removal of zidovudine, whereas GZDV elimination was enhanced. A dosage adjustment is recommended for patients undergoing hemodialysis or peritoneal dialysis (see DOSAGE AND ADMINISTRATION: Dose Adjustment).

Adults With Impaired Hepatic Function: Data describing the effect of hepatic impairment on the pharmacokinetics of zidovudine are limited. However, because zidovudine is eliminated primarily by hepatic metabolism, it is expected that zidovudine clearance would be decreased and plasma concentrations would be increased following administration of the recommended adult doses to patients with hepatic impairment (see DOSAGE AND ADMINISTRATION: Dose Adjustment).

Pediatrics: Zidovudine pharmacokinetics have been evaluated in HIV-infected pediatric patients (Table 3).

Patients From 3 Months to 12 Years of Age: Overall, zidovudine pharmacokinetics in pediatric patients >3 months of age are similar to those in adult patients. Proportional increases in plasma zidovudine concentrations were observed following administration of oral solution from 90 to 240 mg/m² every 6 hours. Oral bioavailability, terminal half-life, and oral clearance were comparable to adult values. As in adult patients, the major route of elimination was by metabolism to GZDV. After intravenous dosing, about 29% of the dose was excreted in the urine unchanged and about 45% of the dose was excreted as GZDV (see DOSAGE AND ADMINISTRATION: Pediatrics).

Patients Younger Than 3 Months of Age: Zidovudine pharmacokinetics have been evaluated in pediatric patients from birth to 3 months of life. Zidovudine elimination was determined immediately following birth in 8 neonates who were exposed to zidovudine in utero. The half-life was 13.0 ± 5.8 hours. In neonates ≤14 days old, bioavailability was greater, total body clearance was slower, and half-life was longer than in pediatric patients >14 days old. For dose recommendations for neonates, see DOSAGE AND ADMINISTRATION: Neonatal Dosing.

[See table 3 above]

Pregnancy: Zidovudine pharmacokinetics have been studied in a Phase 1 study of 8 women during the last trimester of pregnancy. As pregnancy progressed, there was no evidence of drug accumulation. Zidovudine pharmacokinetics were similar to those of nonpregnant adults. Consistent with passive transmission of the drug across the placenta, zidovudine concentrations in neonatal plasma at birth were essentially equal to those in maternal plasma at delivery. Although data are limited, methadone maintenance therapy in 5 pregnant women did not appear to alter zidovudine pharmacokinetics. However, in another patient population, a potential for interaction has been identified (see PRECAUTIONS).

Nursing Mothers: The Centers for Disease Control and Prevention recommend that HIV-infected mothers not breastfeed their infants to avoid risking postnatal transmission of HIV. After administration of a single dose of 200 mg zidovudine to 13 HIV-infected women, the mean concentration of zidovudine was similar in human milk and serum (see PRECAUTIONS: Nursing Mothers).

Geriatric Patients: Zidovudine pharmacokinetics have not been studied in patients over 65 years of age.

Gender: A pharmacokinetic study in healthy male (n = 12) and female (n = 12) subjects showed no differences in zidovudine exposure (AUC) when a single dose of zidovudine was administered as the 300-mg RETROVIR Tablet.

Drug Interactions: See Table 4 and PRECAUTIONS: Drug Interactions.

Zidovudine Plus Lamivudine: No clinically significant alterations in lamivudine or zidovudine pharmacokinetics were observed in 12 asymptomatic HIV-infected adult patients given a single oral dose of zidovudine (200 mg) in combination with multiple oral doses of lamivudine (300 mg every 12 hours).

[See table 4 above]

Ribavirin: In vitro data indicate ribavirin reduces phosphorylation of lamivudine, stavudine, and zidovudine. However, no pharmacokinetic (e.g., plasma concentrations or intracellular triphosphorylated active metabolite concentrations) or pharmacodynamic (e.g., loss of HIV/HCV virologic suppression) interaction was observed when ribavirin and lamivudine (n = 18), stavudine (n = 10), or zidovudine (n = 6) were coadministered as part of a multi-drug regimen to HIV/HCV co-infected patients (see WARNINGS).

INDICATIONS AND USAGE

RETROVIR IV Infusion in combination with other antiretroviral agents is indicated for the treatment of HIV infection.

Table 3. Zidovudine Pharmacokinetic Parameters in Pediatric Patients*

Parameter	Birth to 14 Days of Age	14 Days to 3 Months of Age	3 Months to 12 Years of Age
Oral bioavailability (%)	89 ± 19 (n = 15)	61 ± 19 (n = 17)	65 ± 24 (n = 18)
CSF:plasma ratio	no data	no data	0.26 ± 0.17[†] (n = 28)
CL (L/hr/kg)	0.65 ± 0.29 (n = 18)	1.14 ± 0.24 (n = 16)	1.85 ± 0.47 (n = 20)
Elimination half-life (hr)	3.1 ± 1.2 (n = 21)	1.9 ± 0.7 (n = 18)	1.5 ± 0.7 (n = 21)

*Data presented as mean ± standard deviation except where noted.
[†]CSF ratio determined at steady-state on constant intravenous infusion.

Table 4. Effect of Coadministered Drugs on Zidovudine AUC*
Note: ROUTINE DOSE MODIFICATION OF ZIDOVUDINE IS NOT WARRANTED WITH COADMINISTRATION OF THE FOLLOWING DRUGS.

Coadministered Drug and Dose	Zidovudine Oral Dose	n	Zidovudine Concentrations AUC	Zidovudine Concentrations Variability	Concentration of Coadministered Drug
Atovaquone 750 mg q 12 hr with food	200 mg q 8 hr	14	↑AUC 31%	Range 23% to 78%[†]	↔
Fluconazole 400 mg daily	200 mg q 8 hr	12	↑AUC 74%	95% CI: 54% to 98%	Not Reported
Methadone 30 to 90 mg daily	200 mg q 4 hr	9	↑AUC 43%	Range 16% to 64%[†]	↔
Nelfinavir 750 mg q 8 hr × 7 to 10 days	single 200 mg	11	↓AUC 35%	Range 28% to 41%	↔
Probenecid 500 mg q 6 hr × 2 days	2 mg/kg q 8 hr × 3 days	3	↑AUC 106%	Range 100% to 170%[†]	Not Assessed
Rifampin 600 mg daily × 14 days	200 mg q 8 hr × 14 days	8	↓AUC 47%	90% CI: 41% to 53%	Not Assessed
Ritonavir 300 mg q 6 hr × 4 days	200 mg q 8 hr × 4 days	9	↓AUC 25%	95% CI: 15% to 34%	↔
Valproic acid 250 mg or 500 mg q 8 hr × 4 days	100 mg q 8 hr × 4 days	6	↑AUC 80%	Range 64% to 130%[†]	Not Assessed

↑ = Increase; ↓ = Decrease; ↔ = no significant change; AUC = area under the concentration versus time curve; CI = confidence interval.
* This table is not all inclusive.
[†] Estimated range of percent difference.

Maternal-Fetal HIV Transmission: RETROVIR is also indicated for the prevention of maternal-fetal HIV transmission as part of a regimen that includes oral RETROVIR beginning between 14 and 34 weeks of gestation, intravenous RETROVIR during labor, and administration of RETROVIR Syrup to the neonate after birth. The efficacy of this regimen for preventing HIV transmission in women who have received RETROVIR for a prolonged period before pregnancy has not been evaluated. The safety of RETROVIR for the mother or fetus during the first trimester of pregnancy has not been assessed (see Description of Clinical Studies).

Description of Clinical Studies: Therapy with RETROVIR has been shown to prolong survival and decrease the incidence of opportunistic infections in patients with advanced HIV disease at the initiation of therapy and to delay disease progression in asymptomatic HIV-infected patients. RETROVIR in combination with other antiretroviral agents has been shown to be superior to monotherapy in one or more of the following endpoints: delaying death, delaying development of AIDS, increasing CD4+ cell counts, and decreasing plasma HIV-1 RNA. The complete prescribing information for each drug should be consulted before combination therapy that includes RETROVIR is initiated.

Pregnant Women and Their Neonates: The utility of RETROVIR for the prevention of maternal-fetal HIV transmission was demonstrated in a randomized, double-blind, placebo-controlled trial (ACTG 076) conducted in HIV-infected pregnant women with CD4+ cell counts of 200 to 1,818 cells/mm³ (median in the treated group: 560 cells/mm³) who had little or no previous exposure to RETROVIR. Oral RETROVIR was initiated between 14 and 34 weeks of gestation (median 11 weeks of therapy) followed by intravenous administration of RETROVIR during labor and delivery. Following birth, neonates received oral RETROVIR Syrup for 6 weeks. The study showed a statistically significant difference in the incidence of HIV infection in the neonates (based on viral culture from peripheral blood) between the group receiving RETROVIR and the group receiving placebo. Of 363 neonates evaluated in the study, the estimated risk of HIV infection was 7.8% in the group receiving RETROVIR and 24.9% in the placebo group, a relative reduction in transmission risk of 68.7%. RETROVIR was well tolerated by mothers and infants. There was no difference in pregnancy-related adverse events between the treatment groups.

CONTRAINDICATIONS

RETROVIR IV Infusion is contraindicated for patients who have potentially life-threatening allergic reactions to any of the components of the formulation.

WARNINGS

COMBIVIR® and TRIZIVIR® are combination product tablets that contain zidovudine as one of their components. RETROVIR should not be administered concomitantly with COMBIVIR or TRIZIVIR.

The incidence of adverse reactions appears to increase with disease progression; patients should be monitored carefully, especially as disease progression occurs.

Bone Marrow Suppression: RETROVIR should be used with caution in patients who have bone marrow compromise evidenced by granulocyte count <1,000 cells/mm^3 or hemoglobin <9.5 g/dL. In patients with advanced symptomatic HIV disease, anemia and neutropenia were the most significant adverse events observed. There have been reports of pancytopenia associated with the use of RETROVIR, which was reversible in most instances, after discontinuance of the drug. However, significant anemia, in many cases requiring dose adjustment, discontinuation of RETROVIR, and/or blood transfusions, has occurred during treatment with RETROVIR alone or in combination with other antiretrovirals.

Frequent blood counts are strongly recommended in patients with advanced HIV disease who are treated with RETROVIR. For HIV-infected individuals and patients with asymptomatic or early HIV disease, periodic blood counts are recommended. If anemia or neutropenia develops, dosage adjustments may be necessary (see DOSAGE AND ADMINISTRATION).

Myopathy: Myopathy and myositis with pathological changes, similar to that produced by HIV disease, have been associated with prolonged use of RETROVIR.

Lactic Acidosis/Severe Hepatomegaly with Steatosis: Lactic acidosis and severe hepatomegaly with steatosis, including fatal cases, have been reported with the use of nucleoside analogues alone or in combination, including zidovudine and other antiretrovirals. A majority of these cases have been in women. Obesity and prolonged exposure to antiretroviral nucleoside analogues may be risk factors. Particular caution should be exercised when administering RETROVIR to any patient with known risk factors for liver disease; however, cases have also been reported in patients with no known risk factors. Treatment with RETROVIR should be suspended in any patient who develops clinical or laboratory findings suggestive of lactic acidosis or pronounced hepatotoxicity (which may include hepatomegaly and steatosis even in the absence of marked transaminase elevations).

Use With Interferon- and Ribavirin-Based Regimens: In vitro studies have shown ribavirin can reduce the phosphorylation of pyrimidine nucleoside analogues such as zidovudine. Although no evidence of a pharmacokinetic or pharmacodynamic interaction (e.g., loss of HIV/HCV virologic suppression) was seen when ribavirin was coadministered with zidovudine in HIV/HCV co-infected patients (see CLINICAL PHARMACOLOGY: Drug Interactions), **hepatic decompensation (some fatal) has occurred in HIV/HCV co-infected patients receiving combination antiretroviral therapy for HIV and interferon alfa with or without ribavirin.** Patients receiving interferon alfa with or without ribavirin and RETROVIR should be closely monitored for treatment-associated toxicities, especially hepatic decompensation, neutropenia, and anemia. Discontinuation of RETROVIR should be considered as medically appropriate. Dose reduction or discontinuation of interferon alfa, ribavirin, or both should also be considered if worsening clinical toxicities are observed, including hepatic decompensation (e.g., Childs Pugh >6) (see the complete prescribing information for interferon and ribavirin).

PRECAUTIONS

General: Zidovudine is eliminated from the body primarily by renal excretion following metabolism in the liver (glucuronidation). In patients with severely impaired renal function (CrCl<15 mL/min), dosage reduction is recommended. Although the data are limited, zidovudine concentrations appear to be increased in patients with severely impaired hepatic function, which may increase the risk of hematologic toxicity (see CLINICAL PHARMACOLOGY: Pharmacokinetics and DOSAGE AND ADMINISTRATION).

Immune Reconstitution Syndrome: Immune reconstitution syndrome has been reported in patients treated with combination antiretroviral therapy, including RETROVIR. During the initial phase of combination antiretroviral treatment, patients whose immune system responds may develop an inflammatory response to indolent or residual opportunistic infections (such as *Mycobacterium avium* infection, cytomegalovirus, *Pneumocystis jirovecii* pneumonia [PCP], or tuberculosis), which may necessitate further evaluation and treatment.

Information for Patients: RETROVIR is not a cure for HIV infection, and patients may continue to acquire illnesses associated with HIV infection, including opportunistic infections. Therefore, patients should be advised to seek medical care for any significant change in their health status.

The safety and efficacy of RETROVIR in treating women, intravenous drug users, and racial minorities is not significantly different than that observed in white males.

Patients should be informed that the major toxicities of RETROVIR are neutropenia and/or anemia. The frequency and severity of these toxicities are greater in patients with more advanced disease and in those who initiate therapy later in the course of their infection. They should be told

that if toxicity develops, they may require transfusions or drug discontinuation. They should be told of the extreme importance of having their blood counts followed closely while on therapy, especially for patients with advanced symptomatic HIV disease. They should be cautioned about the use of other medications, including ganciclovir and interferon alfa, which may exacerbate the toxicity of RETROVIR (see PRECAUTIONS: Drug Interactions). Patients should be informed that other adverse effects of RETROVIR include nausea and vomiting. Patients should also be encouraged to contact their physician if they experience muscle weakness, shortness of breath, symptoms of hepatitis or pancreatitis, or any other unexpected adverse events while being treated with RETROVIR.

Pregnant women considering the use of RETROVIR during pregnancy for prevention of HIV transmission to their infants should be advised that transmission may still occur in some cases despite therapy. The long-term consequences of in utero and neonatal exposure to RETROVIR are unknown, including the possible risk of cancer.

HIV-infected pregnant women should be advised not to breastfeed to avoid postnatal transmission of HIV to a child who may not yet be infected.

Patients should be advised that therapy with RETROVIR has not been shown to reduce the risk of transmission of HIV to others through sexual contact or blood contamination.

Drug Interactions: See CLINICAL PHARMACOLOGY section (Table 4) for information on zidovudine concentrations when coadministered with other drugs. For patients experiencing pronounced anemia or other severe zidovudine-associated events while receiving chronic administration of zidovudine and some of the drugs (e.g., fluconazole, valproic acid) listed in Table 4, zidovudine dose reduction may be considered.

Antiretroviral Agents: Concomitant use of zidovudine with stavudine should be avoided since an antagonistic relationship has been demonstrated in vitro.

Some nucleoside analogues affecting DNA replication, such as ribavirin, antagonize the in vitro antiviral activity of RETROVIR against HIV; concomitant use of such drugs should be avoided.

Doxorubicin: Concomitant use of zidovudine with doxorubicin should be avoided since an antagonistic relationship has been demonstrated in vitro (see CLINICAL PHARMACOLOGY for additional drug interactions).

Phenytoin: Phenytoin plasma levels have been reported to be low in some patients receiving RETROVIR, while in 1 case a high level was documented. However, in a pharmacokinetic interaction study in which 12 HIV-positive volunteers received a single 300-mg phenytoin dose alone and during steady-state zidovudine conditions (200 mg every 4 hours), no change in phenytoin kinetics was observed. Although not designed to optimally assess the effect of phenytoin on zidovudine kinetics, a 30% decrease in oral zidovudine clearance was observed with phenytoin.

Overlapping Toxicities: Coadministration of ganciclovir, interferon alfa, and other bone marrow suppressive or cytotoxic agents may increase the hematologic toxicity of zidovudine.

Carcinogenesis, Mutagenesis, Impairment of Fertility: Zidovudine was administered orally at 3 dosage levels to separate groups of mice and rats (60 females and 60 males in each group). Initial single daily doses were 30, 60, and 120 mg/kg/day in mice and 80, 220, and 600 mg/kg/day in rats. The doses in mice were reduced to 20, 30, and 40 mg/kg/day after day 90 because of treatment-related anemia, whereas in rats only the high dose was reduced to 450 mg/kg/day on day 91, and then to 300 mg/kg/day on day 279. In mice, 7 late-appearing (after 19 months) vaginal neoplasms (5 nonmetastasizing squamous cell carcinomas, 1 squamous cell papilloma, and 1 squamous polyp) occurred in animals given the highest dose. One late-appearing squamous cell papilloma occurred in the vagina of a middle-dose animal. No vaginal tumors were found at the lowest dose. In rats, 2 late-appearing (after 20 months), nonmetastasizing vaginal squamous cell carcinomas occurred in animals given the highest dose. No vaginal tumors occurred at the low or middle dose in rats. No other drug-related tumors were observed in either sex of either species.

At doses that produced tumors in mice and rats, the estimated drug exposure (as measured by AUC) was approximately 3 times (mouse) and 24 times (rat) the estimated human exposure at the recommended therapeutic dose of 100 mg every 4 hours.

Two transplacental carcinogenicity studies were conducted in mice. One study administered zidovudine at doses of 20 mg/kg/day or 40 mg/kg/day from gestation day 10 through parturition and lactation with dosing continuing in offspring for 24 months postnatally. The doses of zidovudine employed in this study produced zidovudine exposures approximately 3 times the estimated human exposure at recommended doses. After 24 months, an increase in incidence of vaginal tumors was noted with no increase in tumors in

the liver or lung or any other organ in either gender. These findings are consistent with results of the standard oral carcinogenicity study in mice, as described earlier. A second study administered zidovudine at maximum tolerated doses of 12.5 mg/day or 25 mg/day (~1,000 mg/kg nonpregnant body weight or ~450 mg/kg of term body weight) to pregnant mice from days 12 through 18 of gestation. There was an increase in the number of tumors in the lung, liver, and female reproductive tracts in the offspring of mice receiving the higher dose level of zidovudine. It is not known how predictive the results of rodent carcinogenicity studies may be for humans.

Zidovudine was mutagenic in a 5178Y/TK$^{+/-}$ mouse lymphoma assay, positive in an in vitro cell transformation assay, clastogenic in a cytogenetic assay using cultured human lymphocytes, and positive in mouse and rat micronucleus tests after repeated doses. It was negative in a cytogenetic study in rats given a single dose.

Zidovudine, administered to male and female rats at doses up to 7 times the usual adult dose based on body surface area considerations, had no effect on fertility judged by conception rates.

Pregnancy: Pregnancy Category C. Oral teratology studies in the rat and in the rabbit at doses up to 500 mg/kg/day revealed no evidence of teratogenicity with zidovudine. Zidovudine treatment resulted in embryo/fetal toxicity as evidenced by an increase in the incidence of fetal resorptions in rats given 150 or 450 mg/kg/day and rabbits given 500 mg/kg/day. The doses used in the teratology studies resulted in peak zidovudine plasma concentrations (after one half of the daily dose) in rats 66 to 226 times, and in rabbits 12 to 87 times, mean steady-state peak human plasma concentrations (after one sixth of the daily dose) achieved with the recommended daily dose (100 mg every 4 hours). In an in vitro experiment with fertilized mouse oocytes, zidovudine exposure resulted in a dose-dependent reduction in blastocyst formation. In an additional teratology study in rats, a dose of 3,000 mg/kg/day (very near the oral median lethal dose in rats of 3,683 mg/kg) caused marked maternal toxicity and an increase in the incidence of fetal malformations. This dose resulted in peak zidovudine plasma concentrations 350 times peak human plasma concentrations. (Estimated area under the curve [AUC] in rats at this dose level was 300 times the daily AUC in humans given 600 mg per day.) No evidence of teratogenicity was seen in this experiment at doses of 600 mg/kg/day or less.

Two rodent transplacental carcinogenicity studies were conducted (see Carcinogenesis, Mutagenesis, Impairment of Fertility).

A randomized, double-blind, placebo-controlled trial was conducted in HIV-infected pregnant women to determine the utility of RETROVIR for the prevention of maternal-fetal HIV transmission (see INDICATIONS AND USAGE: Description of Clinical Studies). Congenital abnormalities occurred with similar frequency between neonates born to mothers who received RETROVIR and neonates born to mothers who received placebo. Abnormalities were either problems in embryogenesis (prior to 14 weeks) or were recognized on ultrasound before or immediately after initiation of study drug.

Antiretroviral Pregnancy Registry: To monitor maternal-fetal outcomes of pregnant women exposed to RETROVIR, an Antiretroviral Pregnancy Registry has been established. Physicians are encouraged to register patients by calling 1-800-258-4263.

Nursing Mothers: The Centers for Disease Control and Prevention recommend that HIV-infected mothers not breastfeed their infants to avoid risking postnatal transmission of HIV.

Zidovudine is excreted in human milk (see CLINICAL PHARMACOLOGY: Pharmacokinetics: Nursing Mothers). Because of both the potential for HIV transmission and the potential for serious adverse reactions in nursing infants, mothers should be instructed not to breastfeed if they are receiving RETROVIR (see Pediatric Use and INDICATIONS AND USAGE: Maternal-Fetal HIV Transmission).

Pediatric Use: RETROVIR has been studied in HIV-infected pediatric patients over 3 months of age who had HIV-related symptoms or who were asymptomatic with abnormal laboratory values indicating significant HIV-related immunosuppression. RETROVIR has also been studied in neonates perinatally exposed to HIV (see ADVERSE REACTIONS, DOSAGE AND ADMINISTRATION, INDICATIONS AND USAGE: Description of Clinical Studies, and CLINICAL PHARMACOLOGY: Pharmacokinetics).

Geriatric Use: Clinical studies of RETROVIR did not include sufficient numbers of subjects aged 65 and over to determine whether they respond differently *from younger subjects*. Other reported clinical experience has not identified differences in responses between the elderly and younger patients. In general, dose selection for an elderly patient should be cautious, reflecting the greater frequency of decreased hepatic, renal, or cardiac function, and of concomitant disease or other drug therapy.

ADVERSE REACTIONS

The adverse events reported during intravenous administration of RETROVIR IV Infusion are similar to those reported with oral administration; neutropenia and anemia were reported most frequently. Long-term intravenous administration beyond 2 to 4 weeks has not been studied in adults and may enhance hematologic adverse events. Local reaction, pain, and slight irritation during intravenous administration occur infrequently.

Adults: The frequency and severity of adverse events associated with the use of RETROVIR are greater in patients with more advanced infection at the time of initiation of therapy.

Table 5 summarizes events reported at a statistically significantly greater incidence for patients receiving RETROVIR orally in a monotherapy study:

Table 5. Percentage (%) of Patients with Adverse Events* in Asymptomatic HIV Infection (ACTG 019)

Adverse Event	RETROVIR 500 mg/day (n = 453)	Placebo (n = 428)
Body as a whole		
Asthenia	8.6%[†]	5.8%
Headache	62.5%	52.6%
Malaise	53.2%	44.9%
Gastrointestinal		
Anorexia	20.1%	10.5%
Constipation	6.4%[†]	3.5%
Nausea	51.4%	29.9%
Vomiting	17.2%	9.8%

*Reported in ≥5% of study population.
[†]Not statistically significant versus placebo.

In addition to the adverse events listed in Table 5, other adverse events observed in clinical studies were abdominal cramps, abdominal pain, arthralgia, chills, dyspepsia, fatigue, hyperbilirubinemia, insomnia, musculoskeletal pain, myalgia, and neuropathy.

Selected laboratory abnormalities observed during a clinical study of monotherapy with oral RETROVIR are shown in Table 6.

[See table 6 above]

Pediatrics: *Study ACTG300:* Selected clinical adverse events and physical findings with a ≥5% frequency during therapy with EPIVIR 4 mg/kg twice daily plus RETROVIR 160 mg/m^2 orally 3 times daily compared with didanosine in therapy-naive (≤56 days of antiretroviral therapy) pediatric patients are listed in Table 7.

[See table 7 above]

Selected laboratory abnormalities experienced by therapy-naive (≤56 days of antiretroviral therapy) pediatric patients are listed in Table 8.

[See table 8 at right]

Additional adverse events reported in open-label studies in pediatric patients receiving RETROVIR 180 mg/m^2 every 6 hours were congestive heart failure, decreased reflexes, ECG abnormality, edema, hematuria, left ventricular dilation, macrocytosis, nervousness/irritability, and weight loss. The clinical adverse events reported among adult recipients of RETROVIR may also occur in pediatric patients.

Use for the Prevention of Maternal-Fetal Transmission of HIV: In a randomized, double-blind, placebo-controlled trial in HIV-infected women and their neonates conducted to determine the utility of RETROVIR for the prevention of maternal-fetal HIV transmission, RETROVIR Syrup at 2 mg/kg was administered every 6 hours for 6 weeks to neonates beginning within 12 hours following birth. The most commonly reported adverse experiences were anemia (hemoglobin <9.0 g/dL) and neutropenia (<1,000 cells/mm^3). Anemia occurred in 22% of the neonates who received RETROVIR and in 12% of the neonates who received placebo. The mean difference in hemoglobin values was less than 1.0 g/dL for neonates receiving RETROVIR compared to neonates receiving placebo. No neonates with anemia required transfusion and all hemoglobin values spontaneously returned to normal within 6 weeks after completion of therapy with RETROVIR. Neutropenia was reported with similar frequency in the group that received RETROVIR (21%) and in the group that received placebo (27%). The long-term consequences of in utero and infant exposure to RETROVIR are unknown.

Observed During Clinical Practice: In addition to adverse events reported from clinical trials, the following events have been identified during use of RETROVIR in clinical practice. Because they are reported voluntarily from a population of unknown size, estimates of frequency cannot be made. These events have been chosen for inclusion due to either their seriousness, frequency of reporting, potential causal connection to RETROVIR, or a combination of these factors.

Table 6. Frequencies of Selected (Grade 3/4) Laboratory Abnormalities in Patients with Asymptomatic HIV Infection (ACTG 019)

Adverse Event	RETROVIR 500 mg/day (n = 453)	Placebo (n = 428)
Anemia (Hgb<8 g/dL)	1.1%	0.2%
Granulocytopenia (<750 cells/mm^3)	1.8%	1.6%
Thrombocytopenia (platelets<50,000/mm^3)	0%	0.5%
ALT (>5 × ULN)	3.1%	2.6%
AST (>5 × ULN)	0.9%	1.6%
Alkaline phosphatase (>5 × ULN)	0%	0%

ULN = Upper limit of normal.

Table 7. Selected Clinical Adverse Events and Physical Findings (≥5% Frequency) in Pediatric Patients in Study ACTG300

Adverse Event	EPIVIR plus RETROVIR (n = 236)	Didanosine (n = 235)
Body as a Whole		
Fever	25%	32%
Digestive		
Hepatomegaly	11%	11%
Nausea & vomiting	8%	7%
Diarrhea	8%	6%
Stomatitis	6%	12%
Splenomegaly	5%	8%
Respiratory		
Cough	15%	18%
Abnormal breath sounds/wheezing	7%	9%
Ear, Nose, and Throat		
Signs or symptoms of ears*	7%	6%
Nasal discharge or congestion	8%	11%
Other		
Skin rashes	12%	14%
Lymphadenopathy	9%	11%

*Includes pain, discharge, erythema, or swelling of an ear.

Table 8. Frequencies of Selected (Grade 3/4) Laboratory Abnormalities in Pediatric Patients in Study ACTG300

Test (Abnormal Level)	EPIVIR plus RETROVIR	Didanosine
Neutropenia (ANC<400 cells/mm^3)	8%	3%
Anemia (Hgb<7.0 g/dL)	4%	2%
Thrombocytopenia (platelets<50,000/mm^3)	1%	3%
ALT (>10 × ULN)	1%	3%
AST (>10 × ULN)	2%	4%
Lipase (>2.5 × ULN)	3%	3%
Total amylase (>2.5 × ULN)	3%	3%

ULN = Upper limit of normal.
ANC = Absolute neutrophil count.

Body as a Whole: Back pain, chest pain, flu-like syndrome, generalized pain.
Cardiovascular: Cardiomyopathy, syncope.
Endocrine: Gynecomastia.
Eye: Macular edema.
Gastrointestinal: Constipation, dysphagia, flatulence, oral mucosal pigmentation, mouth ulcer.
General: Sensitization reactions including anaphylaxis and angioedema, vasculitis.
Hemic and Lymphatic: Aplastic anemia, hemolytic anemia, leukopenia, lymphadenopathy, pancytopenia with marrow hypoplasia, pure red cell aplasia.
Hepatobiliary Tract and Pancreas: Hepatitis, hepatomegaly with steatosis, jaundice, lactic acidosis, pancreatitis.
Musculoskeletal: Increased CPK, increased LDH, muscle spasm, myopathy and myositis with pathological changes (similar to that produced by HIV disease), rhabdomyolysis, tremor.
Nervous: Anxiety, confusion, depression, dizziness, loss of mental acuity, mania, paresthesia, seizures, somnolence, vertigo.
Respiratory: Cough, dyspnea, rhinitis, sinusitis.
Skin: Changes in skin and nail pigmentation, pruritus, rash, Stevens-Johnson syndrome, toxic epidermal necrolysis, sweat, urticaria.
Special Senses: Amblyopia, hearing loss, photophobia, taste perversion.
Urogenital: Urinary frequency, urinary hesitancy.

OVERDOSAGE

Acute overdoses of zidovudine have been reported in pediatric patients and adults. These involved exposures up to 50 grams. No specific symptoms or signs have been identified following acute overdosage with zidovudine apart from those listed as adverse events such as fatigue, headache, vomiting, and occasional reports of hematological disturbances. All patients recovered without permanent sequelae. Hemodialysis and peritoneal dialysis appear to have a negligible effect on the removal of zidovudine, while elimination of its primary metabolite, GZDV, is enhanced.

DOSAGE AND ADMINISTRATION

Adults: The recommended intravenous dose is 1 mg/kg infused over 1 hour. This dose should be administered 5 to 6 times daily (5 to 6 mg/kg daily). The effectiveness of this dose compared to higher dosing regimens in improving the neurologic dysfunction associated with HIV disease is unknown. A small randomized study found a greater effect of higher doses of RETROVIR on improvement of neurological symptoms in patients with pre-existing neurological disease.

Patients should receive RETROVIR IV Infusion only until oral therapy can be administered. The intravenous dosing regimen equivalent to the oral administration of 100 mg every 4 hours is approximately 1 mg/kg intravenously every 4 hours.

Maternal-Fetal HIV Transmission: The recommended dosing regimen for administration to pregnant women (>14 weeks of pregnancy) and their neonates is:

Maternal Dosing: 100 mg orally 5 times per day until the start of labor. During labor and delivery, intravenous RETROVIR should be administered at 2 mg/kg (total body weight) over 1 hour followed by a continuous intravenous infusion of 1 mg/kg/hour (total body weight) until clamping of the umbilical cord.

Neonatal Dosing: 2 mg/kg orally every 6 hours starting within 12 hours after birth and continuing through 6 weeks of age. Neonates unable to receive oral dosing may be administered RETROVIR intravenously at 1.5 mg/kg, infused over 30 minutes, every 6 hours. (See PRECAUTIONS if hepatic disease or renal insufficiency is present.)

Monitoring of Patients: Hematologic toxicities appear to be related to pretreatment bone marrow reserve and to dose and duration of therapy. In patients with poor bone marrow reserve, particularly in patients with advanced symptomatic HIV disease, frequent monitoring of hematologic indices is recommended to detect serious anemia or neutropenia (see WARNINGS). In patients who experience hematologic toxicity, reduction in hemoglobin may occur as early as 2 to 4 weeks, and neutropenia usually occurs after 6 to 8 weeks.

Dose Adjustment: *Anemia:* Significant anemia (hemoglobin of <7.5 g/dL or reduction of >25% of baseline) and/or significant neutropenia (granulocyte count of <750 cells/mm^3 or reduction of >50% from baseline) may require a dose interruption until evidence of marrow recovery is observed (see WARNINGS). In patients who develop significant anemia, dose interruption does not necessarily eliminate the need for transfusion. If marrow recovery occurs following dose interruption, resumption in dose may be appropriate using adjunctive measures such as epoetin alfa at recommended doses, depending on hematologic indices such as serum erythropoetin level and patient tolerance.

For patients experiencing pronounced anemia while receiving chronic coadministration of zidovudine and some of the drugs (e.g., fluconazole, valproic acid) listed in Table 4, zidovudine dose reduction may be considered.

End-Stage Renal Disease: In patients maintained on hemodialysis or peritoneal dialysis (CrCl <15 mL/min), recommended dosing is 1 mg/kg every 6 to 8 hours (see CLINICAL PHARMACOLOGY: Pharmacokinetics).

Hepatic Impairment: There are insufficient data to recommend dose adjustment of RETROVIR in patients with mild to moderate impaired hepatic function or liver cirrhosis. Since RETROVIR is primarily eliminated by hepatic metabolism, a reduction in the daily dose may be necessary in these patients. Frequent monitoring of hematologic toxicities is advised (see CLINICAL PHARMACOLOGY: Pharmacokinetics and PRECAUTIONS: General).

Method of Preparation: RETROVIR IV Infusion must be diluted prior to administration. The calculated dose should be removed from the 20-mL vial and added to 5% Dextrose Injection solution to achieve a concentration no greater than 4 mg/mL. Admixture in biologic or colloidal fluids (e.g., blood products, protein solutions, etc.) is not recommended. After dilution, the solution is physically and chemically stable for 24 hours at room temperature and 48 hours if refrigerated at 2° to 8°C (36° to 46°F). Care should be taken during admixture to prevent inadvertent contamination. As an additional precaution, the diluted solution should be administered within 8 hours if stored at 25°C (77°F) or 24 hours if refrigerated at 2° to 8°C to minimize potential administration of a microbially contaminated solution.

Parenteral drug products should be inspected visually for particulate matter and discoloration prior to administration whenever solution and container permit. Should either be observed, the solution should be discarded and fresh solution prepared.

Administration: RETROVIR IV Infusion is administered intravenously at a constant rate over 1 hour. Rapid infusion or bolus injection should be avoided. RETROVIR IV Infusion should not be given intramuscularly.

HOW SUPPLIED

RETROVIR IV Infusion, 10 mg zidovudine in each mL. 20-mL Single-Use Vial, Tray of 10 (NDC 0173-0107-93).
Store vials at 15° to 25°C (59° to 77°F) and protect from light.
GlaxoSmithKline, Research Triangle Park, NC 27709
©2006, GlaxoSmithKline. All rights reserved.
October 2006   RL-2308

SELZENTRY®
[sell-ZEN-tree]
(maraviroc)
Tablets

℞

HIGHLIGHTS OF PRESCRIBING INFORMATION
These highlights do not include all the information needed to use SELZENTRY safely and effectively. See full prescribing information for SELZENTRY.
SELZENTRY (maraviroc) Tablets
Initial U.S. Approval: 2007

WARNING: HEPATOTOXICITY
See full prescribing information for complete boxed warning
- Hepatotoxicity has been reported which may be preceded by evidence of a systemic allergic reaction (e.g., pruritic rash, eosinophilia or elevated IgE).

Table 1 Recommended Dosing Regimen

Concomitant Medications	SELZENTRY Dose
Potent CYP3A inhibitors (with or without a potent CYP3A inducer) including: • protease inhibitors (except tipranavir/ritonavir) • delavirdine • ketoconazole, itraconazole, clarithromycin • other potent CYP3A inhibitors (e.g., nefazodone, telithromycin)	150 mg twice daily
Other concomitant medications, including tipranavir/ritonavir, nevirapine, raltegravir all NRTIs and enfuvirtide	300 mg twice daily
Potent CYP3A inducers (without a potent CYP3A inhibitor) including: • efavirenz • rifampin • etravirine • carbamazepine, phenobarbital, and phenytoin	600 mg twice daily

Table 2 Recommended Dosing Regimens Based on Renal Function

Concomitant Medications*	SELZENTRY Dose Based on Renal Function				
	Normal	Mild	Moderate	Severe	End Stage Renal Disease (ESRD)
	CrCl >80 mL/min	CrCl >50 and ≤80 mL/min	CrCl ≥30 and ≤50 mL/min	CrCl <30 mL/min	On Regular Hemodialysis
Potent CYP3A inhibitors (with or without a CYP3A inducer)*	150 mg twice daily	150 mg twice daily	150 mg twice daily	NR	NR
Other concomitant medications*	300 mg twice daily	300 mg twice daily	300 mg twice daily	300 mg twice daily†	300 mg twice daily†
Potent CYP3A inducers (without a potent CYP3A inhibitor)*	600 mg twice daily	600 mg twice daily	600 mg twice daily	NR	NR

NR = not recommended
* See Table 1 for the list of concomitant medications.
† The SELZENTRY dose should be reduced to 150 mg twice daily if there are any symptoms of postural hypotension [see *Warnings and Precautions (5.2)*].

- Immediately evaluate patients with signs or symptoms of hepatitis or allergic reaction. (5.1)

RECENT MAJOR CHANGES

Indication and Usage (1)	11/2009
Dosage and Administration (2.2)	05/2010
Contraindications (4)	05/2010
Warnings and Precautions (5.2)	05/2010
Warnings and Precautions (5.1), (5.2), (5.4) (5.5)	11/2009

INDICATIONS AND USAGE
SELZENTRY is a CCR5 co-receptor antagonist indicated for combination antiretroviral treatment of adults infected with only CCR5-tropic HIV-1.
- In treatment-naïve subjects, more subjects treated with SELZENTRY experienced virologic failure and developed lamivudine resistance compared to efavirenz [see *Microbiology (12.4) Clinical Studies (14.3)*].
- Tropism testing with a highly sensitive tropism assay is required for the appropriate use of SELZENTRY (1).

DOSAGE AND ADMINISTRATION

When given with potent CYP3A inhibitors (with or without potent CYP3A inducers) including PIs (except tipranavir/ritonavir), delavirdine (2, 7.1)	150 mg twice daily
With NRTIs, tipranavir/ritonavir, nevirapine, raltegravir, and other drugs that are not potent CYP3A inhibitors or CYP3A inducers (2, 7.1)	300 mg twice daily
With potent CYP3A inducers including efavirenz (without a potent CYP3A inhibitor) (2, 7.1)	600 mg twice daily

A more complete list of coadministered drugs is listed in *Dosage and Administration (2)*.
Dose adjustment may be necessary in patients with renal impairment. (2.2).

DOSAGE FORMS AND STRENGTHS
Tablets: 150 mg and 300 mg (3)

CONTRAINDICATIONS
- SELZENTRY should not be used in patients with severe renal impairment or end-stage renal disease (ESRD) (CrCl < 30 mL/min) who are taking potent CYP3A inhibitors or inducers (4).

WARNINGS AND PRECAUTIONS
- Use caution when administering SELZENTRY to patients with pre-existing liver dysfunction or who are co-infected with viral hepatitis B or C (5.1).
- More cardiovascular events including myocardial ischemia and/or infarction were observed in treatment-experienced subjects who received SELZENTRY. Use with caution in patients at increased risk of cardiovascular events (5.2).
- If patients with severe renal impairment or end-stage renal disease (ESRD) receiving SELZENTRY (without concomitant CYP3A inducers or inhibitors) experience postural hypotension the SELZENTRY dose should be reduced from 300 mg twice daily to 150 mg twice daily (5.2).

ADVERSE REACTIONS
The most common adverse events in treatment-experienced subjects (>8% incidence) which occurred at a higher frequency compared to placebo are upper respiratory tract infections, cough, pyrexia, rash, and dizziness (6).
To report SUSPECTED ADVERSE REACTIONS, contact Pfizer at 1-800-438-1985 or FDA at 1-800-FDA-1088 or www.fda.gov/medwatch

DRUG INTERACTIONS
- Coadministration with CYP3A inhibitors, including protease inhibitors (except tipranavir/ritonavir) and delavirdine, will increase the concentration of SELZENTRY (7.1).
- Coadministration with CYP3A inducers, including efavirenz, may decrease the concentration of SELZENTRY (7.1).

USE IN SPECIFIC POPULATIONS
- SELZENTRY should only be used in pregnant women if the potential benefit justifies the potential risk to the fetus (8.1).
- There are no data available in pediatric patients; therefore, SELZENTRY should not be used in patients <16 years of age (8.4).

See 17 for PATIENT COUNSELING INFORMATION and Medication Guide

Revised: 05/2010

FULL PRESCRIBING INFORMATION: CONTENTS*

FULL PRESCRIBING INFORMATION

> **WARNING: HEPATOTOXICITY**
> Hepatotoxicity has been reported with SELZENTRY use. Evidence of a systemic allergic reaction (e.g., pruritic rash, eosinophilia or elevated IgE) prior to the development of hepatotoxicity may occur. Patients with signs or symptoms of hepatitis or allergic reaction following use of SELZENTRY should be evaluated immediately [*see Warnings and Precautions (5.1)*].

1   INDICATIONS AND USAGE

SELZENTRY, in combination with other antiretroviral agents, is indicated for adult patients infected with only CCR5-tropic HIV-1.

This indication is based on analyses of plasma HIV-1 RNA levels in two controlled studies of SELZENTRY in treatment-experienced subjects and one study in treatment-naïve subjects. Both studies in treatment-experienced subjects were conducted in clinically advanced, 3-class antiretroviral-experienced (NRTI, NNRTI, PI, or enfuvirtide) adults with evidence of HIV-1 replication despite ongoing antiretroviral therapy.

The following points should be considered when initiating therapy with SELZENTRY:

- Adult patients infected with only CCR5-tropic HIV-1 should use SELZENTRY.
- Tropism testing must be conducted with a highly sensitive tropism assay that has demonstrated the ability to identify patients appropriate for SELZENTRY use. Outgrowth of pre-existing low-level CXCR4- or dual/mixed-tropic HIV-1 not detected by tropism testing at screening has been associated with virologic failure on SELZENTRY. [see *Microbiology (12.4) Clinical Studies (14.3)*].

- Use of SELZENTRY is not recommended in subjects with dual/mixed or CXCR4-tropic HIV-1 as efficacy was not demonstrated in a phase 2 study of this patient group.
- The safety and efficacy of SELZENTRY have not been established in pediatric patients.
- In treatment-naïve subjects, more subjects treated with SELZENTRY experienced virologic failure and developed lamivudine resistance compared to efavirenz. [see *Microbiology (12.4) Clinical Studies (14.3)*]

2   DOSAGE AND ADMINISTRATION

2.1   Dose Recommendations for Patients with Normal Renal Function

The recommended dose of SELZENTRY differs based on concomitant medications due to drug interactions (see Table 1). SELZENTRY can be taken with or without food. SELZENTRY must be given in combination with other antiretroviral medications.

Table 1 gives the recommended dose adjustments [*see Drug Interactions (7.1)*].

[See table 1 at top of previous page]

2.2   Dose Recommendations for Patients with Renal Impairment

Table 2 provides dosing recommendations for patients based on renal function and concomitant medications.

[See table 2 on previous page]

3   DOSAGE FORMS AND STRENGTHS

- 150 mg blue, oval film-coated tablets debossed with "Pfizer" on one side and "MVC 150" on the other

Table 3 Percentage of Subjects with Selected Treatment-Emergent Adverse Events (All Causality) (≥2% on SELZENTRY and at a higher rate compared to placebo) Studies A4001027 and A4001028 (Pooled Analysis, 48 Weeks)

	SELZENTRY Twice Daily*	Exposure-adjusted rate (per 100 pt-yrs) PYE=309**	Placebo	Exposure-adjusted rate (per 100 pt-yrs) PYE=111**
	N=426 (%)		N=209 (%)	
EYE DISORDERS				
Conjunctivitis	2	3	1	3
Ocular infections, inflammations and associated manifestations	2	3	1	2
GASTROINTESTINAL DISORDERS				
Constipation	6	9	3	6
GENERAL DISORDERS AND ADMINISTRATION SITE CONDITIONS				
Pyrexia	13	20	9	17
Pain and discomfort	4	5	3	5
INFECTIONS AND INFESTATIONS				
Upper respiratory tract infection	23	37	13	27
Herpes infection	8	11	4	8
Sinusitis	7	10	3	6
Bronchitis	7	9	5	9
Folliculitis	4	5	2	4
Pneumonia	2	3	5	10
Anogenital warts	2	3	1	3
Influenza	2	3	0.5	1
Otitis media	2	3	0.5	1
METABOLISM AND NUTRITION DISORDERS				
Appetite disorders	8	11	7	13
MUSCULOSKELETAL AND CONNECTIVE TISSUE DISORDERS				
Joint related signs and symptoms	7	10	3	5
Muscle pains	3	4	0.5	1
NEOPLASMS BENIGN, MALIGNANT AND UNSPECIFIED				
Skin neoplasms benign	3	4	1	3
NERVOUS SYSTEM DISORDERS				
Dizziness/postural dizziness	9	13	8	17
Paresthesias and dysesthesias	5	7	3	6
Sensory abnormalities	4	6	1	3
Disturbances in consciousness	4	5	3	6
Peripheral neuropathies	4	5	3	6

(Table continued on next page)

Table 3 *(cont.)* **Percentage of Subjects with Selected Treatment-Emergent Adverse Events (All Causality) (≥2% on SELZENTRY and at a higher rate compared to placebo) Studies A4001027 and A4001028 (Pooled Analysis, 48 Weeks)**

	SELZENTRY Twice Daily*	Exposure-adjusted rate (per 100 pt-yrs) PYE=309**	Placebo	Exposure-adjusted rate (per 100 pt-yrs) PYE=111**
	N=426 (%)		N=209 (%)	
PSYCHIATRIC DISORDERS				
Disturbances in initiating and maintaining sleep	8	11	5	10
Depressive disorders	4	6	3	5
Anxiety symptoms	4	5	3	7
RENAL AND URINARY DISORDERS				
Bladder and urethral symptoms	5	7	1	3
Urinary tract signs and symptoms	3	4	1	3
RESPIRATORY, THORACIC AND MEDIASTINAL DISORDERS				
Coughing and associated symptoms	14	21	5	10
Upper respiratory tract signs and symptoms	6	9	3	6
Nasal congestion and inflammations	4	6	3	5
Breathing abnormalities	4	5	2	5
Paranasal sinus disorders	3	4	0.5	1
SKIN AND SUBCUTANEOUS TISSUE DISORDERS				
Rash	11	16	5	11
Apocrine and eccrine gland disorders	5	7	4	7.5
Pruritus	4	5	2	4
Lipodystrophies	3	5	0.5	1
Erythemas	2	3	1	2
VASCULAR DISORDERS				
Vascular hypertensive disorders	3	4	2	4

* 300 mg dose equivalent
** PYE = patient years of exposure

- 300 mg blue, oval film-coated tablets debossed with "Pfizer" on one side and "MVC 300" on the other

4 CONTRAINDICATIONS

SELZENTRY should not be used in patients with severe renal impairment or end-stage renal disease (ESRD) (CrCl < 30 mL/min) who are taking potent CYP3A inhibitors or inducers.

5 WARNINGS AND PRECAUTIONS

5.1 Hepatotoxicity

A case of possible SELZENTRY-induced hepatotoxicity with allergic features has been reported in a study of healthy volunteers. Discontinuation of SELZENTRY should be considered in any patient with signs or symptoms of hepatitis, or with increased liver transaminases combined with rash or other systemic symptoms.

The safety and efficacy of SELZENTRY have not been specifically studied in patients with significant underlying liver disorders. In studies of treatment-experienced HIV-infected subjects, approximately 6% of subjects were co-infected with hepatitis B and approximately 6% were co-infected with hepatitis C. Due to the small number of co-infected subjects studied, no conclusions can be drawn regarding whether they are at an increased risk for hepatic adverse events with SELZENTRY administration. However, caution should be used when administering SELZENTRY to patients with pre-existing liver dysfunction or who are co-infected with viral hepatitis B or C.

5.2 Cardiovascular Events

Use with caution in patients at increased risk for cardiovascular events. Eleven subjects (1.3%) who received SELZENTRY had cardiovascular events including myocardial ischemia and/or infarction during the Phase 3 studies in treatment-experienced studies [total exposure 609 patient-years (300 on once daily + 309 on twice daily SELZENTRY)], while no subjects who received placebo had such events (total exposure 111 patient-years). These subjects generally had cardiac disease or cardiac risk factors prior to SELZENTRY use, and the relative contribution of SELZENTRY to these events is not known.

In the Phase 2b/3 study in treatment-naïve subjects, 3 subjects (0.8%) who received SELZENTRY had events related to ischemic heart diseases and 5 subjects (1.4%) who received efavirenz had such events (total exposure 506 and 508 patient-years for SELZENTRY and efavirenz, respectively).

When SELZENTRY was administered to healthy volunteers at doses higher than the recommended dose, symptomatic postural hypotension was seen at a greater frequency than in placebo. However, when SELZENTRY was given at the recommended dose in HIV subjects in Phase 3 studies, postural hypotension was seen at a rate similar to placebo (approximately 0.5%). Caution should be used when administering SELZENTRY in patients with a history of postural hypotension or on concomitant medication known to lower blood pressure.

Postural Hypotension in Patients with Renal Impairment

Patients with impaired renal function may have cardiovascular co-morbidities and could be at increased risk of cardiovascular adverse events triggered by postural hypotension. An increased risk of postural hypotension may occur in patients with severe renal insufficiency or in those with end-stage renal disease (ESRD) due to increased maraviroc exposure in some patients. SELZENTRY should be used in patients with severe renal impairment or ESRD only if they are not receiving a concomitant potent CYP3A inhibitor or inducer. However, the use of SELZENTRY in these patients should only be considered when no alternative treatment options are available. If patients with severe renal impairment or ESRD experience any symptoms of postural hypotension while taking 300 mg twice daily the dose should be reduced to 150 mg twice daily [see *Dosage and Administration (2.2)*].

5.3 Immune Reconstitution Syndrome

Immune reconstitution syndrome has been reported in patients treated with combination antiretroviral therapy, including maraviroc. During the initial phase of combination antiretroviral treatment, patients whose immune system responds may develop an inflammatory response to indolent or residual opportunistic infections (such as infection with *Mycobacterium* avium, cytomegalovirus, *Pneumocystis* jirovecii, *Mycobacterium* tuberculosis, or reactivation of *Herpes* simplex and *Herpes* zoster), which may necessitate further evaluation and treatment.

5.4 Potential Risk of Infection

SELZENTRY antagonizes the CCR5 co-receptor located on some immune cells, and therefore could potentially increase the risk of developing infections. The overall incidence and severity of infection, as well as AIDS-defining category C infections, was comparable in the treatment groups during the Phase 3 treatment-experienced studies of SELZENTRY. While there was a higher rate of certain upper respiratory tract infections reported in the SELZENTRY arm compared to placebo (23% versus 13%), there was a lower rate of pneumonia (2% vs 5%) reported in subjects receiving SELZENTRY. A higher incidence of Herpes virus infections (11 per 100 patient-years) was also reported in the SELZENTRY arm when adjusted for exposure compared to placebo (8 per 100 patient-years).

In the Phase 2b/3 study in treatment-naïve subjects, the incidence of AIDS-defining Category C events when adjusted for exposure was 1.8 for SELZENTRY compared to 2.4 for efavirenz per 100 patient-years of exposure.

Patients should be monitored closely for evidence of infections while receiving SELZENTRY.

5.5 Potential Risk of Malignancy

While no increase in malignancy has been observed with SELZENTRY, due to this drug's mechanism of action it could affect immune surveillance and lead to an increased risk of malignancy.

The exposure-adjusted rate for malignancies per 100 patient-years of exposure in treatment-experienced studies was 4.6 for SELZENTRY compared to 9.3 on placebo. In treatment-naïve subjects, the rates were 1.0 and 2.4 per 100 patient-years of exposure for SELZENTRY and efavirenz, respectively.

Long-term follow-up is needed to more fully assess this risk.

6 ADVERSE REACTIONS

The following adverse reactions are discussed in other sections of the labeling:

- Hepatotoxicity [see *Boxed Warning, Warnings and Precautions (5.1)*]
- Cardiovascular events [see *Warnings and Precautions (5.2)*]

6.1 Clinical Trials Experience

Because clinical trials are conducted under widely varying conditions, adverse reaction rates observed in the clinical trials of a drug cannot be directly compared to rates in the clinical trials of another drug and may not reflect the rates observed in practice.

Studies in Treatment-Experienced Subjects

The safety profile of SELZENTRY is primarily based on 840 HIV-infected subjects who received at least one dose of SELZENTRY during two Phase 3 trials. A total of 426 of these subjects received the indicated twice daily dosing regimen.

Assessment of treatment-emergent adverse events is based on the pooled data from two studies in subjects with CCR5-tropic HIV-1 (A4001027 and A4001028). The median duration of maraviroc therapy for subjects in these studies was 48 weeks, with the total exposure on SELZENTRY twice daily at 309 patient-years versus 111 patient-years on placebo + OBT. The population was 89% male and 84% white, with mean age of 46 years (range 17–75 years). Subjects received dose equivalents of 300 mg maraviroc once or twice daily.

The most common adverse events reported with SELZENTRY twice daily therapy with frequency rates higher than placebo, regardless of causality, were upper respiratory tract infections, cough, pyrexia, rash, and dizziness. Additional adverse events that occurred with once daily dosing at a higher rate than both placebo and twice daily dosing were diarrhea, edema, influenza, esophageal candidiasis, sleep disorders, rhinitis, parasomnias, and urinary abnormalities. In these two studies, the rate of discontinuation due to adverse events was 5% for subjects who received SELZENTRY twice daily + optimized background therapy (OBT) as well as those who received placebo + OBT. Most of the adverse events reported were judged to be mild to moderate in severity. The data described below occurred with SELZENTRY twice daily dosing.

The total number of subjects reporting infections were 233 (55%) and 84 (40%) in the SELZENTRY twice daily and placebo groups, respectively. Correcting for the longer duration of exposure on SELZENTRY compared to placebo, the exposure-adjusted frequency (rate per 100 subject-years) of these events was 133 for both SELZENTRY twice daily and placebo.

Dizziness or postural dizziness occurred in 8% of subjects on either SELZENTRY or placebo, with 2 subjects (0.5%) on SELZENTRY permanently discontinuing therapy (1 due to syncope, 1 due to orthostatic hypotension) versus 1 subject on placebo (0.5%) permanently discontinuing therapy due to dizziness.

Treatment-emergent adverse events, regardless of causality, from A4001027 and A4001028 are summarized in Table 3. Selected events occurring at ≥2% of subjects and at a numerically higher rate in subjects treated with SELZENTRY are included; events that occurred at the same or higher rate on placebo are not displayed.

[See table 3 on pages 3331 and 3332]

Laboratory Abnormalities
Table 4 shows the treatment-emergent Grade 3–4 laboratory abnormalities that occurred in >2% of subjects receiving SELZENTRY.

[See table 4 at right]

Study in Treatment-Naïve Subjects
Treatment-Emergent Adverse Events
Treatment-emergent adverse events, regardless of causality, from Study A4001026, a double-blind comparative controlled study in which 721 treatment-naïve subjects received SELZENTRY 300 mg BID (N=360) or efavirenz (N=361) in combination with zidovudine/lamivudine for 96 weeks, are summarized in Table 5. Selected events occurring at ≥ 2% of subjects and at a numerically higher rate in subjects treated with SELZENTRY are included; events that occurred at the same or higher rate on efavirenz are not displayed.

[See table 5 at top of next page]

Laboratory Abnormalities
[See table 6 at top of page 3335]

Less Common Adverse Events in Clinical Trials
The following adverse events occurred in <2% of SELZENTRY-treated subjects. These events have been included because of their seriousness and either increased frequency on SELZENTRY or are potential risks due to the mechanism of action. Events attributed to the patient's underlying HIV infection are not listed.

Blood and Lymphatic System: marrow depression and hypoplastic anemia
Cardiac Disorders: unstable angina, acute cardiac failure, coronary artery disease, coronary artery occlusion, myocardial infarction, myocardial ischemia
Hepatobiliary Disorders: hepatic cirrhosis, hepatic failure, cholestatic jaundice, portal vein thrombosis, hypertransaminasemia, jaundice
Infections and Infestations: endocarditis, infective myositis, viral meningitis, pneumonia, treponema infections, septic shock, *Clostridium difficile* colitis, meningitis
Musculoskeletal and Connective Tissue Disorders: myositis, osteonecrosis, rhabdomyolysis, blood CK increased
Neoplasms benign, Malignant and Unspecified (including Cysts and Polyps): abdominal neoplasm, anal cancer, basal cell carcinoma, Bowen's disease, cholangiocarcinoma, diffuse large B-cell lymphoma, lymphoma, metastases to liver, esophageal carcinoma, nasopharyngeal carcinoma, squamous cell carcinoma, squamous cell carcinoma of skin, tongue neoplasm (malignant stage unspecified), anaplastic large cell lymphomas T- and null-cell types, bile duct neoplasms malignant, endocrine neoplasms malignant and unspecified
Nervous System Disorders: cerebrovascular accident, convulsions and epilepsy, tremor (excluding congenital), facial palsy, hemianopia, loss of consciousness, visual field defect

6.2 Postmarketing Experience
The following events have been identified during postapproval use of SELZENTRY. Because these reactions are reported voluntarily from a population of unknown size, it is not possible to estimate their frequency or establish a causal relationship to SELZENTRY exposure.
Skin and Subcutaneous Tissue Disorders
Stevens-Johnson syndrome.

7 DRUG INTERACTIONS
7.1 Effect of Concomitant Drugs on the Pharmacokinetics of Maraviroc
Maraviroc is a substrate of CYP3A and Pgp and hence its pharmacokinetics are likely to be modulated by inhibitors and inducers of these enzymes/transporters. Therefore, a dose adjustment may be required when maraviroc is coadministered with those drugs [see *Dosage and Administration (2)*].
Concomitant use of maraviroc and St. John's wort (hypericum perforatum) or products containing St. John's wort is not recommended. Coadministration of maraviroc with St. John's wort is expected to substantially decrease maraviroc concentrations and may result in suboptimal levels of maraviroc and lead to loss of virologic response and possible resistance to maraviroc.

Table 4 Maximum Shift in Laboratory Test Values (Without Regard to Baseline) Incidence ≥2% of Grade 3–4 Abnormalities (ACTG Criteria) Studies A4001027 and A4001028 (Pooled Analysis, 48 Weeks)

Laboratory Parameter Preferred Term	Limit	SELZENTRY Twice daily + OBT N =421* %	Placebo + OBT N =207* %
Aspartate aminotransferase	>5.0× ULN	4.8	2.9
Alanine aminotransferase	>5.0× ULN	2.6	3.4
Total bilirubin	>5.0× ULN	5.5	5.3
Amylase	>2.0× ULN	5.7	5.8
Lipase	>2.0× ULN	4.9	6.3
Absolute neutrophil count	<750/mm^3	4.3	2.4

*Percentages based on total subjects evaluated for each laboratory parameter

For additional drug interaction information see *Clinical Pharmacology (12.3)*.

8 USE IN SPECIFIC POPULATIONS
8.1 Pregnancy
Pregnancy Category B
The incidence of fetal variations and malformations was not increased in embryofetal toxicity studies performed with maraviroc in rats at exposures (AUC) approximately 20-fold higher and in rabbits at approximately 5-fold higher than human exposures at the recommended daily dose (up to 1000 mg/kg/day in rats and 75 mg/kg/day in rabbits). During the pre- and postnatal development studies in the offspring, development of the offspring, including fertility and reproductive performance, was not affected by the maternal administration of maraviroc.
However, there are no adequate and well-controlled studies in pregnant women. Because animal reproduction studies are not always predictive of human response, SELZENTRY should be used during pregnancy only if clearly needed.
Antiretroviral Pregnancy Registry
To monitor maternal-fetal outcomes of pregnant women exposed to SELZENTRY and other antiretroviral agents, an Antiretroviral Pregnancy Registry has been established. Physicians are encouraged to register patients by calling 1-800-258-4263.

8.3 Nursing Mothers
The Centers for Disease Control and Prevention recommend that HIV-infected mothers not breastfeed their infants to avoid risking postnatal transmission of HIV infection. Studies in lactating rats indicate that maraviroc is extensively secreted into rat milk. It is not known whether maraviroc is secreted into human milk. Because of the potential for both HIV transmission and serious adverse reactions in nursing infants, mothers should be instructed not to breastfeed if they are receiving SELZENTRY.

8.4 Pediatric Use
The pharmacokinetics, safety and efficacy of maraviroc in patients <16 years of age have not been established. Therefore, maraviroc should not be used in this patient population.

8.5 Geriatric Use
There were insufficient numbers of subjects aged 65 and over in the clinical studies to determine whether they respond differently from younger subjects. In general, caution should be exercised when administering SELZENTRY in elderly patients, also reflecting the greater frequency of decreased hepatic and renal function, of concomitant disease and other drug therapy.

8.6 Renal Impairment
Recommended doses of SELZENTRY for patients with impaired renal function (CrCl ≤ 80 mL/min) are based on the results of a pharmacokinetic study conducted in healthy subjects with various degrees of renal impairment. The pharmacokinetics of maraviroc in subjects with mild and moderate renal impairment was similar to that in subjects with normal renal function [see *Clinical Pharmacology (12.3)*]. A limited number of subjects with mild and moderate renal impairment in the Phase 3 clinical trials (n= 131 and n= 12, respectively) received the same dose of SELZENTRY as that administered to subjects with normal renal function. In these subjects there was no apparent difference in the adverse event profile for maraviroc compared to subjects with normal renal function.
If patients with severe renal impairment or end-stage renal disease (ESRD) not receiving a concomitant potent CYP3A inhibitor or inducer experience any symptoms of postural hypotension while taking SELZENTRY 300 mg twice daily, the dose should be reduced to 150 mg twice daily. No studies have been performed in subjects with severe renal impairment or ESRD co-treated with potent CYP3A inhibitors or

inducers. Hence, no dose of SELZENTRY can be recommended, and SELZENTRY is contraindicated for these patients. [see *Dosage and Administration (2.2)*, *Contraindications (4)*, *Warnings and Precautions (5.2)*, and *Clinical Pharmacology (12.3)*].

8.7 Hepatic Impairment
Maraviroc is principally metabolized by the liver; therefore, caution should be exercised when administering this drug to patients with hepatic impairment, because maraviroc concentrations may be increased. Maraviroc concentrations are higher when SELZENTRY 150 mg is administered with a potent CYP3A inhibitor compared to following administration of 300 mg without a CYP3A inhibitor, so patients with moderate hepatic impairment who receive SELZENTRY 150 mg with a potent CYP3A inhibitor should be monitored closely for maraviroc-associated adverse events. Maraviroc has not been studied in subjects with severe hepatic impairment [see *Warnings and Precautions (5.1)* and *Clinical Pharmacology (12.3)*].

8.8 Gender
Population pharmacokinetic analysis of pooled Phase 1/2a data indicated gender (female: n=96, 23.2% of the total population) does not affect maraviroc concentrations. Dosage adjustment based on gender is not necessary.

8.9 Race
Population pharmacokinetic analysis of pooled Phase 1/2a data indicated exposure was 26.5% higher in Asians (N=95) as compared to non-Asians (n=318). However, a study designed to evaluate pharmacokinetic differences between Caucasians (n=12) and Singaporeans (n=12) showed no difference between these two populations. No dose adjustment based on race is needed.

10 OVERDOSAGE
The highest dose administered in clinical studies was 1200 mg. The dose-limiting adverse event was postural hypotension, which was observed at 600 mg. While the recommended dose for SELZENTRY in patients receiving a CYP3A inducer without a CYP3A inhibitor is 600 mg twice daily, this dose is appropriate due to enhanced metabolism. Prolongation of the QT interval was seen in dogs and monkeys at plasma concentrations 6 and 12 times, respectively, those expected in humans at the intended exposure of 300 mg equivalents twice daily. However, no significant QT prolongation was seen in the studies in treatment-experienced subjects with HIV using the recommended doses of maraviroc or in a specific pharmacokinetic study to evaluate the potential of maraviroc to prolong the QT interval [see *Clinical Pharmacology (12.3)*].
There is no specific antidote for overdose with maraviroc. Treatment of overdose should consist of general supportive measures including keeping the patient in a supine position, careful assessment of patient vital signs, blood pressure and ECG.
If indicated, elimination of unabsorbed active maraviroc should be achieved by emesis or gastric lavage. Administration of activated charcoal may also be used to aid in removal of unabsorbed drug. Since maraviroc is moderately protein-bound, dialysis may be beneficial in removal of this medicine.

11 DESCRIPTION
SELZENTRY (maraviroc) is a selective, slowly reversible, small molecule antagonist of the interaction between human CCR5 and HIV-1 gp120. Blocking this interaction prevents CCR5-tropic HIV-1 entry into cells.
SELZENTRY is available as film-coated tablets for oral administration containing either 150 or 300 mg of maraviroc and the following inactive ingredients: microcrystalline cellulose, dibasic calcium phosphate (anhydrous), sodium starch glycolate, and magnesium stearate. The film coat

[Opadry® II Blue (85G20583)] contains FD&C blue #2 aluminum lake, soya lecithin, polyethylene glycol (macrogol 3350), polyvinyl alcohol, talc and titanium dioxide. Maraviroc is chemically described as 4,4-difluoro-N-[(1S)-3-[exo-3-(3-isopropyl-5-methyl-4H-1,2,4-triazol-4-yl)-8-azabicyclo[3.2.1]oct-8-yl]-1-phenylpropyl]cyclohexane-carboxamide.

The molecular formula is $C_{29}H_{41}F_2N_5O$ and the structural formula is:

Maraviroc is a white to pale colored powder with a molecular weight of 513.67. It is highly soluble across the physiological pH range (pH 1.0 to 7.5).

12 CLINICAL PHARMACOLOGY

12.1 Mechanism of Action

Maraviroc is an antiviral drug [see *Clinical Pharmacology (12.4)*].

12.2 Pharmacodynamics

Exposure Response Relationship in Treatment-Experienced Subjects

The relationship between maraviroc, modeled plasma trough concentration (C_{min}) (1–9 samples per patient taken on up to 7 visits), and virologic response was evaluated in 973 treatment-experienced HIV-1-infected subjects with varied optimized background antiretroviral regimens in studies A4001027 and A4001028. The C_{min}, baseline viral load, baseline CD4$^+$ cell count and overall sensitivity score (OSS) were found to be important predictors of virologic success (defined as viral load < 400 copies/mL at 24 weeks). Table 7 illustrates the proportion of subjects with virologic success (%) within each C_{min} quartile for 150 mg twice daily and 300 mg twice daily groups.
[See table 7 on next page]

Exposure Response Relationship in Treatment-Naïve Subjects

The relationship between maraviroc, modeled plasma trough concentration (C_{min}) (1–12 samples per patient taken on up to 8 visits), and virologic response was evaluated in 294 treatment-naive HIV-1-infected subjects receiving maraviroc 300 mg twice daily in combination with zidovudine/lamivudine in study A4001026. Table 8 illustrates the proportion (%) of subjects with virologic success < 50 copies/mL at 48 weeks within each C_{min} quartile for the 300 mg twice daily dose.

Table 8 Treatment-Naïve Subjects with Virologic Success by C_{min} Quartile (Q1–Q4)

		300 mg BID	
	n	Median C_{min}	% subjects with virologic success
Q1	75	23	57.3
Q2	72	39	72.2
Q3	73	56	74.0
Q4	74	81	83.8

Eighteen of 75 (24%) subjects in Q1 had no measurable maraviroc concentration on at least one occasion vs. 1 of 73 and 1 of 74 in quartiles 3 and 4 respectively.

Effects on Electrocardiogram

A placebo-controlled, randomized, crossover study to evaluate the effect on the QT interval of healthy male and female volunteers was conducted with three single oral doses of maraviroc and moxifloxacin. The placebo-adjusted mean maximum (upper 1-sided 95% CI) increases in QTc from baseline after 100, 300 and 900 mg of maraviroc were −2 (0), -1 (1), and 1 (3) msec, respectively, and 13 (15) msec for moxifloxacin 400 mg. No subject in any group had an increase in QTc of ≥60 msec from baseline. No subject experienced an interval exceeding the potentially clinically relevant threshold of 500 msec.

12.3 Pharmacokinetics

[See table 9 on next page]

Absorption

Peak maraviroc plasma concentrations are attained 0.5–4h following single oral doses of 1–1200 mg administered to uninfected volunteers. The pharmacokinetics of oral maraviroc are not dose-proportional over the dose range. The absolute bioavailability of a 100 mg dose is 23% and is predicted to be 33% at 300 mg. Maraviroc is a substrate for the efflux transporter P-glycoprotein.

Effect of Food on Oral Absorption

Coadministration of a 300mg tablet with a high fat breakfast reduced maraviroc C_{max} and AUC by 33% in healthy volunteers. There were no food restrictions in the studies that demonstrated the efficacy and safety of maraviroc [see

Table 5 Percentage of Subjects with Selected Treatment-Emergent Adverse Events (All Causality) (≥2% on SELZENTRY and at a higher rate compared to efavirenz) Study A4001026 (96 Weeks)

	SELZENTRY + zidovudine/lamivudine 300 mg BID N = 360 (%)	EFAVIRENZ + zidovudine/lamivudine 600 mg QD N = 361 (%)
BLOOD AND LYMPHATIC SYSTEM DISORDERS		
Anemias NEC	8	5
Neutropenias	4	3
EAR AND LABYRINTH DISORDERS		
Ear disorders NEC	3	2
GASTROINTESTINAL DISORDERS		
Flatulence, bloating and distention	10	7
Gastrointestinal atonic and hypomotility disorders NEC	9	5
Gastrointestinal signs and symptoms NEC	3	2
GENERAL DISORDERS AND ADMINISTRATION SITE CONDITIONS		
Body Temperature perception	3	1
INFECTIONS AND INFESTATIONS		
Bronchitis	13	9
Herpes Infection	7	6
Upper Respiratory Tract Infection	32	30
Bacterial infections NEC	6	3
Herpes zoster/varicella	5	4
Lower respiratory tract and lung infections	3	2
Neisseria infections	3	0
Tinea infections	4	3
Viral infections NEC	3	2
MUSCULOSKELETAL AND CONNECTIVE TISSUE DISORDERS		
Joint related signs and symptoms	6	5
NERVOUS SYSTEM DISORDERS		
Memory loss (excluding dementia)	3	1
Parasthesias and Dyesthesias	4	3
RENAL AND URINARY DISORDERS		
Bladder and urethral symptoms	4	3
REPRODUCTIVE SYSTEM AND BREAST DISORDERS		
Erection and ejaculation conditions and disorders	3	2
RESPIRATORY, THORACIC AND MEDIASTINAL DISORDERS		
Upper respiratory tract signs and symptoms	9	5
SKIN AND SUBCUTANEOUS TISSUE DISORDERS		
Acnes	3	2
Alopecias	2	1
Lipodystrophies	4	3
Nail and nail bed conditions (excluding infections and infestations)	6	2

Clinical Studies (14)]. Therefore, maraviroc can be taken with or without food at the recommended dose [*see Dosage and Administration (2)*].

Distribution

Maraviroc is bound (approximately 76%) to human plasma proteins, and shows moderate affinity for albumin and alpha-1 acid glycoprotein. The volume of distribution of maraviroc is approximately 194L.

Metabolism

Studies in humans and in vitro studies using human liver microsomes and expressed enzymes have demonstrated that maraviroc is principally metabolized by the cytochrome P450 system to metabolites that are essentially inactive against HIV-1. In vitro studies indicate that CYP3A is the major enzyme responsible for maraviroc metabolism. In vitro studies also indicate that polymorphic enzymes CYP2C9, CYP2D6 and CYP2C19 do not contribute significantly to the metabolism of maraviroc.

Maraviroc is the major circulating component ($\sim$42% drug-related radioactivity) following a single oral dose of 300 mg[^{14}C]-maraviroc. The most significant circulating metabolite in humans is a secondary amine ($\sim$22% radioactivity) formed by N-dealkylation. This polar metabolite has no significant pharmacological activity. Other metabolites are products of mono-oxidation and are only minor components of plasma drug-related radioactivity.

Excretion

The terminal half-life of maraviroc following oral dosing to steady state in healthy subjects was 14–18 hours. A mass balance/excretion study was conducted using a single 300mg dose of ^{14}C-labeled maraviroc. Approximately 20% of the radiolabel was recovered in the urine and 76% was recovered in the feces over 168 hours. Maraviroc was the major component present in urine (mean of 8% dose) and feces (mean of 25% dose). The remainder was excreted as metabolites.

Hepatic Impairment

Maraviroc is primarily metabolized and eliminated by the liver. A study compared the pharmacokinetics of a single 300 mg dose of SELZENTRY in subjects with mild (Child-Pugh Class A, n=8), and moderate (Child-Pugh Class B, n=8) hepatic impairment to pharmacokinetics in healthy subjects (n=8). The mean Cmax and AUC were 11% and 25% higher, respectively, for subjects with mild hepatic impairment, and 32% and 46% higher, respectively, for subjects with moderate hepatic impairment compared to subjects with normal hepatic function. These changes do not warrant a dose adjustment. Maraviroc concentrations are higher when SELZENTRY 150 mg is administered with a potent CYP3A inhibitor compared to following administration of 300 mg without a CYP3A inhibitor, so patients with moderate hepatic impairment who receive SELZENTRY 150 mg with a potent CYP3A inhibitor should be monitored closely for maraviroc-associated adverse events. The pharmacokinetics of maraviroc have not been studied in subjects with severe hepatic impairment [*see Warnings and Precautions (5.1)*].

Renal Impairment

A study compared the pharmacokinetics of a single 300 mg dose of SELZENTRY in subjects with severe renal impairment (CLcr <30 mL/min, n=6) and end-stage renal disease (ESRD) (n=6) to healthy volunteers (n=6). Geometric mean ratios for maraviroc C_{max} and AUC_{inf} were 2.4-fold and 3.2-fold higher respectively for subjects with severe renal impairment, and 1.7-fold and 2.0-fold higher respectively for subjects with ESRD as compared to subjects with normal renal function in this study. Hemodialysis had a minimal effect on maraviroc clearance and exposure in subjects with ESRD. Exposures observed in subjects with severe renal impairment and ESRD were within the range observed in previous SELZENTRY 300 mg single-dose studies in healthy volunteers with normal renal function. However, maraviroc exposures in the subjects with normal renal function in this study were 50% lower than that observed in previous studies. Based on the results of this study, no dose adjustment is recommended for patients with renal impairment receiving SELZENTRY without a potent CYP3A inhibitor or inducer. However, if patients with severe renal impairment or ESRD experience any symptoms of postural hypotension while taking SELZENTRY 300 mg twice daily, their dose should be reduced to 150 mg twice daily [*see Dosage and Administration (2.2); Warnings and Precautions (5.2)*].

In addition, the study compared the pharmacokinetics of multiple dose SELZENTRY in combination with saquinavir/ritonavir 1000/100 mg twice daily (a potent CYP3A inhibitor combination) for 7 days in subjects with mild renal impairment (CLcr >50 and ≤80 mL/min, n=6) and moderate renal impairment (CLcr ≥30 and ≤50 mL/min, n=6) to healthy volunteers with normal renal function (n=6). Subjects received 150 mg of SELZENTRY at different dose frequencies (healthy volunteers – every 12 hours; mild renal

impairment – every 24 hours; moderate renal impairment – every 48 hours). Compared to healthy volunteers (dosed every 12 hours), geometric mean ratios for maraviroc AUC_{tau}, C_{max} and C_{min} were 50% higher, 20% higher and 43% lower, respectively for subjects with mild renal impairment (dosed every 24 hours). Geometric mean ratios for maraviroc AUC_{tau}, C_{max} and C_{min} were 16% higher, 29% lower and 85% lower, respectively for subjects with moderate renal impairment (dosed every 48 hours) compared to healthy volunteers (dosed every 12 hours). Based on the data from this study, no adjustment in dose is recommended for patients with mild or moderate renal impairment [*see Dosage and Administration (2.2)*].

Effect of Concomitant Drugs on the Pharmacokinetics of Maraviroc

Maraviroc is a substrate of CYP3A and Pgp and hence its pharmacokinetics are likely to be modulated by inhibitors and inducers of these enzymes/transporters. The CYP3A/Pgp inhibitors ketoconazole, lopinavir/ritonavir, ritonavir, darunavir/ritonavir, saquinavir/ritonavir and atazanavir ± ritonavir all increased the C_{max} and AUC of maraviroc [see Table 10]. The CYP3A inducers rifampin, etravirine and efavirenz decreased the C_{max} and AUC of maraviroc [see Table 10].

Tipranavir/ritonavir (net CYP3A inhibitor/Pgp inducer) did not affect the steady state pharmacokinetics of maraviroc (see Table 10). Co-trimoxazole and tenofovir did not affect the pharmacokinetics of maraviroc.

[See table 10 at top of next page]

Effect of Maraviroc on the Pharmacokinetics of Concomitant Drugs

Maraviroc is unlikely to inhibit the metabolism of coadministered drugs metabolized by the following cytochrome P enzymes (CYP1A2, CYP2B6, CYP2C8, CYP2C9, CYP2C19, and CYP3A) because maraviroc did not inhibit activity of those enzymes at clinically relevant concentrations in vitro. Maraviroc does not induce CYP1A2 in vitro.

In vitro results indicate that maraviroc could inhibit P-glycoprotein in the gut and may thus affect bioavailability of certain drugs.

Drug interaction studies were performed with maraviroc and other drugs likely to be coadministered or commonly used as probes for pharmacokinetic interactions [see Table 6]. Maraviroc had no effect on the pharmacokinetics of zidovudine or lamivudine. Maraviroc decreased the C_{min} and AUC of raltegravir by 27% and 37%, respectively, which is not clinically significant. Maraviroc had no clinically relevant effect on the pharmacokinetics of midazolam, the oral contraceptives ethinylestradiol and levonorgestrel, no effect on the urinary 6β-hydroxycortisol/cortisol ratio, suggesting no induction of CYP3A in vivo. Maraviroc had no effect on the debrisoquine metabolic ratio (MR) at 300 mg twice daily or less in vivo and did not cause inhibition of CYP2D6 in

---

Table 6 Maximum Shift in Laboratory Test Values (Without Regard to Baseline) Incidence ≥2% of Grade 3–4 Abnormalities (ACTG Criteria) Study A4001026 (96 Weeks)

Laboratory Parameter Preferred Term	Limit	SELZENTRY 300 Twice daily + zidovudine/lamivudine N =353* %	Efavirenz 600 mg QD + zidovudine/lamivudine N =350* %
Aspartate aminotransferase	>5.0× ULN	4.0	4.0
Alanine aminotransferase	>5.0× ULN	3.9	4.0
Creatine kinase		3.9	4.8
Amylase	>2.0× ULN	4.3	6.0
Absolute neutrophil count	<750/mm^3	5.7	4.9
Hemoglobin	<7.0 g/dL	2.9	2.3

*N = total number of subjects evaluable for laboratory abnormalities. Percentages based on total subjects evaluated for each laboratory parameter. If the same subject in a given treatment group had >1 occurrence of the same abnormality, only the most severe is counted.

Table 7 Treatment-Experienced Subjects with Virologic Success by C_{min} Quartile (Q1–Q4)

	150 mg BID (with CYP3A inhibitors)			300 mg BID (without CYP3A inhibitors)		
	n	Median C_{min}	% subjects with virologic success	n	Median C_{min}	% subjects with virologic success
Placebo	160	-	30.6	35	-	28.6
Q1	78	33	52.6	22	13	50.0
Q2	77	87	63.6	22	29	68.2
Q3	78	166	78.2	22	46	63.6
Q4	78	279	74.4	22	97	68.2

Table 9 Mean Maraviroc Pharmacokinetic Parameters

	Maraviroc dose	N	AUC_{12} (ng.h/Ml)	C_{max} (ng/mL)	C_{min} (ng/mL)
Healthy volunteers (phase 1)	300 mg twice daily	64	2908	888	43.1
Asymptomatic HIV subjects (phase 2a)	300 mg twice daily	8	2550	618	33.6
Treatment-experienced HIV subjects (phase 3)*	300 mg twice daily	94	1513	266	37.2
	150 mg twice daily (+ CYP3A inhibitor)	375	2463	332	101
Treatment-naïve HIV subjects (phase 2b/3)*	300 mg twice daily	344	1865	287	60

* The estimated exposure is lower compared to other studies possibly due to sparse sampling, food effect, compliance and concomitant medications.

vitro until concentrations >100µM. However, there was 234% increase in debrisoquine MR on treatment compared to baseline at 600 mg once daily, suggesting potential inhibition of CYP2D6 at higher dose.

12.4 Microbiology

Mechanism of Action

Maraviroc is a member of a therapeutic class called CCR5 co-receptor antagonists. Maraviroc selectively binds to the human chemokine receptor CCR5 present on the cell membrane, preventing the interaction of HIV-1 gp120 and CCR5 necessary for CCR5-tropic HIV-1 to enter cells. CXCR4-tropic and dual-tropic HIV-1 entry is not inhibited by maraviroc.

Antiviral Activity in Cell Culture

Maraviroc inhibits the replication of CCR5-tropic laboratory strains and primary isolates of HIV-1 in models of acute peripheral blood leukocyte infection. The mean EC_{50} value (50% effective concentration) for maraviroc against HIV-1 group M isolates (subtypes A to J and circulating recombinant form AE) and group O isolates ranged from 0.1 to 4.5 nM (0.05 to 2.3 ng/mL) in cell culture.

When used with other antiretroviral agents in cell culture, the combination of maraviroc was not antagonistic with NNRTIs (delavirdine, efavirenz and nevirapine), NRTIs (abacavir, didanosine, emtricitabine, lamivudine, stavudine, tenofovir, zalcitabine and zidovudine), or protease inhibitors (amprenavir, atazanavir, darunavir, indinavir, lopinavir, nelfinavir, ritonavir, saquinavir and tipranavir). Maraviroc was additive/synergistic with the HIV fusion inhibitor enfuvirtide. Maraviroc was not active against CXCR4-tropic and dual-tropic viruses (EC_{50} value >10 µM). The antiviral activity of maraviroc against HIV-2 has not been evaluated.

Resistance in Cell Culture

HIV-1 variants with reduced susceptibility to maraviroc have been selected in cell culture, following serial passage of two CCR5-tropic viruses (CC1/85 and RU570). The maraviroc-resistant viruses remained CCR5-tropic with no evidence of a change from a CCR5-tropic virus to a CXCR4-using virus. Two amino acid residue substitutions in the V3-loop region of the HIV-1 envelope glycoprotein (gp160), A316T and I323V (HXB2 numbering), were shown to be necessary for the maraviroc-resistant phenotype in the HIV-1 isolate CC1/85. In the RU570 isolate a 3-amino acid residue deletion in the V3 loop, ΔQAI (HXB2 positions 315–317), was associated with maraviroc resistance. The relevance of the specific gp120 mutations observed in maraviroc-resistant isolates selected in cell culture to clinical maraviroc resistance is not known. Maraviroc-resistant viruses were characterized phenotypically by concentration response curves that did not reach 100% inhibition in phenotypic drug assays, rather than increases in EC_{50} values.

Cross-resistance in Cell Culture

Maraviroc had antiviral activity against HIV-1 clinical isolates resistant to NNRTIs, NRTIs, PIs and the fusion inhibitor enfuvirtide in cell culture (EC_{50} values ranged from 0.7 to 8.9 nM (0.36 to 4.57 ng/mL)). Maraviroc-resistant viruses that emerged in cell culture remained susceptible to the enfuvirtide and the protease inhibitor saquinavir.

Clinical Resistance

Virologic failure on maraviroc can result from genotypic and phenotypic resistance to maraviroc, through outgrowth of undetected CXCR4-using virus present before maraviroc treatment (see *Tropism* below), through resistance to background therapy drugs (Table 11), or due to low exposure to maraviroc [see *Clinical Pharmacology (12.2)*].

Antiretroviral treatment-experienced subjects (Studies A4001027 and A4001028)

Week 48 data from treatment-experienced subjects failing maraviroc-containing regimens with CCR5-tropic virus (n=58) have identified 22 viruses that had decreased susceptibility to maraviroc characterized in phenotypic drug assays by concentration response curves that did not reach 100% inhibition. Additionally, CCR5-tropic virus from 2 of these treatment failure subjects had ≥3-fold shifts in EC_{50} values for maraviroc at the time of failure.

Fifteen of these viruses were sequenced in the gp120 encoding region and multiple amino acid substitutions with unique patterns in the heterogeneous V3 loop region were detected. Changes at either amino acid position 308 or 323 (HXB2 numbering) were seen in the V3 loop in 7 of the subjects with decreased maraviroc susceptibility. Substitutions outside the V3 loop of gp120 may also contribute to reduced susceptibility to maraviroc.

Antiretroviral treatment-naïve subjects (Study A4001026)

Treatment-naïve subjects receiving SELZENTRY had more virologic failures and more treatment emergent resistance to the background regimen drugs compared to those receiving efavirenz (Table 11).

[See table 11 at top of next page]

In an as-treated analysis of treatment-naïve subjects at 96 weeks, 32 subjects failed a maraviroc-containing regimen with CCR5-tropic virus and had a tropism result at failure; 7 of these subjects had evidence of maraviroc phenotypic re-

sistance defined as concentration response curves that did not reach 95% inhibition. One additional subject had a ≥3-fold shift in the EC_{50} value for maraviroc at the time of failure. A clonal analysis of the V3 loop amino acid envelope sequences was performed from 6 of the 7 subjects. Changes in V3 loop amino acid sequence differed between each of these different subjects, even for those infected with the same virus clade suggesting that that there are multiple diverse pathways to maraviroc resistance. The subjects who

failed with CCR5-tropic virus and without a detectable maraviroc shift in susceptibility were not evaluated for genotypic resistance.

Of the 32 maraviroc virologic failures failing with CCR5-tropic virus, 20 (63%) also had genotypic and/or phenotypic resistance to background drugs in the regimen (lamivudine, zidovudine).

Tropism

In both treatment-experienced and treatment-naïve subjects, detection of CXCR4-using virus prior to initiation of

Table 10 Effect of Coadministered Agents on the Pharmacokinetics of Maraviroc

Coadministered drug and dose	N	Maraviroc Dose	Ratio (90% CI) of maraviroc pharmacokinetic parameters with/without coadministered drug (no effect = 1.00)		
			C_{min}	AUC_{tau}	Cmax
CYP3A and/or P-gp Inhibitors					
Ketoconazole 400 mg QD	12	100 mg BID	3.75 (3.01, 4.69)	5.00 (3.98, 6.29)	3.38 (2.38, 4.78)
Ritonavir 100 mg BID	8	100 mg BID	4.55 (3.37, 6.13)	2.61 (1.92, 3.56)	1.28 (0.79, 2.09)
Saquinavir (soft gel capsules)/ ritonavir 1000 mg/100 mg BID	11	100 mg BID	11.3 (8.96, 14.1)	9.77 (7.87, 12.14)	4.78 (3.41, 6.71)
Lopinavir/ritonavir 400 mg/100 mg BID	11	300 mg BID	9.24 (7.98, 10.7)	3.95 (3.43, 4.56)	1.97 (1.66, 2.34)
Atazanavir 400 mg QD	12	300 mg BID	4.19 (3.65, 4.80)	3.57 (3.30, 3.87)	2.09 (1.72, 2.55)
Atazanavir/ritonavir 300 mg/100 mg QD	12	300 mg BID	6.67 (5.78, 7.70)	4.88 (4.40, 5.41)	2.67 (2.32, 3.08)
Darunavir/ritonavir 600 mg/100 mg BID	12	150 mg BID	8.00 (6.35, 10.1)	4.05 2.94, 5.59	2.29 (1.46, 3.59)
CYP3A and/or P-gp Inducers					
Efavirenz 600 mg QD	12	100 mg BID	0.55 (0.43, 0.72)	0.552 (0.492, 0.620)	0.486 (0.377, 0.626)
Efavirenz 600 mg QD	12	200 mg BID (+efavirenz): 100 mg BID (alone)	1.09 (0.89, 1.35)	1.15 (0.98, 1.35)	1.16 (0.87, 1.55)
Rifampicin 600 mg QD	12	100 mg BID	0.22 (0.17, 0.28)	0.368 (0.328, 0.413)	0.335 (0.260, 0.431)
Rifampicin 600 mg QD	12	200 mg BID (+rifampicin): 100 mg BID (alone)	0.66 (0.54, 0.82)	1.04 (0.89, 1.22)	0.97 (0.72, 1.29)
Etravirine 200 mg BID	14	300 mg BID	0.609 (0.525, 0.707)	0.468 (0.381, 0.576)	0.400 (0.282, 0.566)
Nevirapine* 200 mg BID (+ lamivudine 150 mg BID, tenofovir 300 mg QD)	8	300 mg SD	-	1.01 (0.65, 1.55)	1.54 (0.94, 2.51)
CYP3A and/or P-gp Inhibitors and Inducers					
Lopinavir/ritonavir + efavirenz 400 mg/100 mg BID + 600 mg QD	11	300 mg BID	6.29 (4.72, 8.39)	2.53 (2.24, 2.87)	1.25 (1.01, 1.55)
Saquinavir (soft gel capsules) /ritonavir + efavirenz 1000 mg/100 mg BID + 600 mg QD	11	100 mg BID	8.42 (6.46, 10.97)	5.00 (4.26, 5.87)	2.26 (1.64, 3.11)
Darunavir/ritonavir + etravirine 600 mg/100 mg BID + 200 mg BID	10	150 mg BID	5.27 (4.51, 6.15)	3.10 (2.57, 3.74)	1.77 (1.20, 2.60)
Tipranavir/ritonavir 500 mg/200 mg BID	12	150 mg BID	1.80 (1.55, 2.09)	1.02 (0.850, 1.23)	0.86 (0.61, 1.21)
Other					
Raltegravir 400 mg BID	17	300 mg BID	0.90 (0.85, 0.96)	0.86 (0.80, 0.92)	0.79 (0.67, 0.94)

*** Compared to historical data**

therapy has been associated with a reduced virologic response to maraviroc.

Antiretroviral treatment-experienced subjects

In the majority of cases, treatment failure on maraviroc was associated with detection of CXCR4-using virus (i.e., CXCR4-or dual/mixed-tropic) which was not detected by the tropism assay prior to treatment. CXCR4-using virus was detected at failure in approximately 55% of subjects who failed treatment on maraviroc by week 48, as compared to 9% of subjects who experienced treatment failure in the placebo arm. To investigate the likely origin of the on-treatment CXCR4-using virus, a detailed clonal analysis was conducted on virus from 20 representative subjects (16 subjects from the maraviroc arms and 4 subjects from the placebo arm) in whom CXCR4-using virus was detected at treatment failure. From analysis of amino acid sequence differences and phylogenetic data, it was determined that CXCR4-using virus in these subjects emerged from a low level of pre-existing CXCR4-using virus not detected by the tropism assay (which is population-based) prior to treatment rather than from a co-receptor switch from CCR5-tropic virus to CXCR4-using virus resulting from mutation in the virus.

Detection of CXCR4-using virus prior to initiation of therapy has been associated with a reduced virological response to maraviroc. Furthermore, subjects failing maraviroc BID at week 48 with CXCR4-using virus had a lower median increase in CD4+ cell counts from baseline (+41 cells/mm^3) than those subjects failing with CCR5-tropic virus (+162 cells/mm^3). The median increase in CD4+ cell count in subjects failing in the placebo arm was +7 cells/mm^3.

Antiretroviral treatment-naïve subjects

In a 96-week study of antiretroviral treatment-naïve subjects, 14% (12/85) who had CCR5-tropic virus at screening with an enhanced sensitivity tropism assay (Trofile®) and failed therapy on maraviroc had CXCR4-using virus at the time of treatment failure. A detailed clonal analysis was conducted in two previously antiretroviral treatment-naïve subjects enrolled in a Phase 2a monotherapy study who had CXCR4-using virus detected after 10 days treatment with maraviroc. Consistent with the detailed clonal analysis conducted in treatment-experienced subjects, the CXCR4-using variants appear to emerge from outgrowth of a pre-existing undetected CXCR4-using virus. Screening with an enhanced sensitivity tropism assay reduced the number of maraviroc virologic failures with CXCR4- or dual/mixed-tropic virus at failure to 12 compared to 24 when screening with the original tropism assay. All but one (11/12; 92%) of the maraviroc failures failing with CXCR4 or dual/mixed-tropic virus also had genotypic and phenotypic resistance to the background drug lamivudine at failure and 33% (4/12) developed zidovudine-associated resistance substitutions. Subjects who had CCR5-tropic virus at baseline and failed maraviroc therapy with CXCR4-using virus had a median increase in CD4+ cell counts from baseline of +113 cells/mm^3 while those subjects failing with CCR5-tropic virus had an increase of +135 cells/mm^3. The median increase in CD4+ cell count in subjects failing in the efavirenz arm was + 95 cells/mm^3.

13 NONCLINICAL TOXICOLOGY

13.1 Carcinogenesis, Mutagenesis, Impairment of Fertility

Carcinogenesis

Long-term oral carcinogenicity studies of maraviroc were carried out in rasH2 transgenic mice (6 months) and in rats for up to 96 weeks (females) and 104 weeks (males). No drug-related increases in tumor incidence were found in mice at 1500 mg/kg/day and in male and female rats at 900 mg/kg/day. The highest exposures in rats were approximately 11 times those observed in humans at the therapeutic dose of 300 mg twice daily for the treatment of HIV-1 infection.

Mutagenesis

Maraviroc was not genotoxic in the reverse mutation bacterial test (Ames test in Salmonella and E. coli), a chromosome aberration test in human lymphocytes and rat bone marrow micronucleus test.

Impairment of Fertility

Maraviroc did not impair mating or fertility of male or female rats and did not affect sperm of treated male rats at approximately 20-fold higher exposures (AUC) than in humans given the recommended 300 mg twice daily dose.

14 CLINICAL STUDIES

The clinical efficacy and safety of SELZENTRY is derived from analyses of data from three ongoing studies in adult subjects infected with CCR5-tropic HIV-1: A4001027 and A4001028, in antiretroviral treatment-experienced adult subjects and A4001026 in treatment-naïve subjects. These studies are supported by a 48-week study in antiretroviral treatment-experienced adult subjects infected with dual/mixed-tropic HIV-1, A4001029.

14.1 Studies in CCR5-tropic, Treatment-Experienced Subjects

Studies A4001027 and A4001028 are ongoing, double-blind, randomized, placebo-controlled, multicenter studies in subjects infected with CCR5-tropic HIV-1. Subjects were required to have an HIV-1 RNA of greater than 5,000 copies/mL despite at least 6 months of prior therapy with at least one agent from three of the four antiretroviral drug classes [≥1 nucleoside reverse transcriptase inhibitors (NRTI), ≥1 non-nucleoside reverse transcriptase inhibitors (NNRTI), ≥2 protease inhibitors (PI), and/or enfuvirtide] or documented resistance to at least one member of each class. All subjects received an optimized background regimen consisting of 3 to 6 antiretroviral agents (excluding low-dose ritonavir) selected on the basis of the subject's prior treatment history and baseline genotypic and phenotypic viral resistance measurements. In addition to the optimized background regimen, subjects were then randomized in a 2:2:1 ratio to maraviroc 300 mg once daily, maraviroc 300 mg twice daily, or placebo. Doses were adjusted based on background therapy as described in *Dosing and Administration*, Table 1.

In the pooled analysis for A4001027 and A4001028, the demographics and baseline characteristics of the treatment groups were comparable (Table 12). Of the 1043 subjects with a CCR5 tropism result at screening, 7.6% had a dual/

Table 11 Development of Resistance to MVC or EFV and Background Drugs in Antiretroviral Treatment-Naïve Trial A4001026 for Patients with CCR5-tropic Virus at Screening using Enhanced Sensitivity Trofile® Assay

	MVC	EFV
Total N in Dataset (As-Treated)	273	241
Total Virologic Failures (As-Treated)	85(31%)	56 (23%)
Evaluable Virologic Failures with Post Baseline Genotypic and Phenotypic Data	73	43
• Lamivudine Resistance	39 (53%)	13 (30%)
• Zidovudine Resistance	2 (3%)	0
• Efavirenz Resistance	--	23 (53%)
• Phenotypic Resistance to MVC*	19 (26 %)	

*Includes subjects failing with CXCR4- or dual/mixed-tropism because these viruses are not intrinsically susceptible to maraviroc.

Table 12 Demographic and Baseline Characteristics of Subjects in Studies A4001027 and A4001028

	SELZENTRY BID N = 426	Placebo N = 209
Age (years) Mean (Range)	46.3 (21–73)	45.7 (29–72)
Sex		
Male	382 (89.7%)	185 (88.5%)
Female	44 (10.3%)	24 (11.5%)
Race		
White	363 (85.2%)	178 (85.2%)
Black	51 (12.0%)	26 (12.4%)
Other	12 (2.8%)	5 (2.4%)
Region		
U.S.	276 (64.8%)	135 (64.6%)
Non-U.S.	150 (35.2%)	74 (35.4%)
Subjects with Previous Enfuvirtide Use	142 (33.3%)	62 (29.7)
Subjects with Enfuvirtide as Part of OBT	182 (42.7%)	91 (43.5%)
Baseline Plasma HIV-1 RNA (log$_{10}$ copies/mL) Mean (Range)	4.85 (2.96–6.88)	4.86 (3.46–7.07)
Subjects with Screening Viral Load ≥100,000 copies/mL	179 (42.0%)	84 (40.2%)
Baseline CD4+ Cell Count (cells/mm^3) Median (Range)	167 (2–820)	171 (1–675)
Subjects with Baseline CD4+ Cell Count ≤200 cells/mm^3)	250 (58.7%)	118 (56.5%)
Subjects with Overall Susceptibility Score (OSS):[a]		
0	57 (13.4%)	35 (16.7%)
1	136 (31.9%)	44 (21.1%)
2	104 (24.4%)	59 (28.2%)
≥3	125 (29.3%)	66 (31.6%)
Subjects with enfuvirtide resistance mutations	90 (21.2%)	45 (21.5%)
Median Number of Resistance-Associated:[b]		
PI mutations	10	10
NNRTI mutations	1	1
NRTI mutations	6	6

a OSS -Sum of active drugs in OBT based on combined information from genotypic and phenotypic testing.
b Resistance mutations based on IAS guidelines[1]

Table 13 Outcomes of Randomized Treatment at Week 48 Studies A4001027 and A4001028

Outcome	SELZENTRY BID N=426	PLACEBO N=209	Mean Difference
Mean change from Baseline to Week 48 in HIV-1 RNA (log$_{10}$ copies/mL)	-1.84	-0.78	-1.05
<400 copies/mL at Week 48	239 (56%)	47 (22%)	34%
<50 copies/mL at Week 48	194 (46%)	35 (17%)	29%
Discontinuations			
Insufficient Clinical Response	97 (23%)	113 (54%)	
Adverse Events	19 (4%)	11 (5%)	
Other	27 (6%)	18 (9%)	
Subjects with treatment-emergent CDC Category C events	22 (5%)	16 (8%)	
Deaths (during study or within 28 days of last dose)	9 (2%)[a]	1 (0.5%)	

[a] One additional subject died while receiving open-label maraviroc therapy subsequent to discontinuing double-blind placebo due to insufficient response

Table 14 Demographic and Baseline Characteristics of Subjects in Study A4001026

	SELZENTRY 300 mg BID + zidovudine/lamivudine (N=360)	Efavirenz 600 mg QD + zidovudine/lamivudine (N=361)
Age (years)		
Mean	36.7	37.4
Range	20–69	18–77
Female n (%)	104 (29)	102 (28)
Race, n.(%)		
White	204 (57)	198 (55)
Black	123 (34)	133 (37)
Asian	6 (2)	5 (1)
Other	27 (8)	25 (7)
Median (Range) CD4 cell count (cells/µL)	241 (5–1422)	254 (8–1053)
Median (Range) HIV-1 RNA (log$_{10}$ copies/mL)	4.9 (3–7)	4.9 (3–7)

Table 15: Study Outcome (Snapshot) at Week 96 Using Enhanced Sensitivity Assay[†]

Outcome at week 96*	SELZENTRY 300 mg BID + zidovudine/lamivudine N = 311 n (%)	Efavirenz 600 mg QD +zidovudine/lamivudine N = 303 n (%)
Virologic Responders: (HIV-1 RNA <400 copies/mL)	199 (64)	195 (64)
Virologic Failure:		
• Non-sustained HIV-1 RNA Suppression	39 (13)	22 (7)
• HIV-1 RNA Never Suppressed	9(3)	1(<1)
Virologic Responders: (HIV-1 RNA <50 copies/mL)	183 (59)	190 (63)
Virologic Failure:		
• Non-sustained HIV-1 RNA Suppression	43 (14)	25 (8)
• HIV-1 RNA Never Suppressed	21 (7)	3 (1)
Discontinuations due to:		
• Adverse Events	19 (6)	47 (16)
• Death	2 (1)	2 (1)
Other[1]	43 (14)	36 (12)

* Week 48 results: Virologic responders (<400): 228/311 (73%) in SELZENTRY, 219/303 (72%) in Efavirenz
Virologic responders (<50): 213/311 (69 %) in SELZENTRY, 207/303 (68%) in Efavirenz
[†] The total number of subjects (Ns) in Table 15 represents the subjects who had a CCR5-tropic virus in the reanalysis of screening samples using the more sensitive tropism assay. This reanalysis reclassified approximately 15% of subjects shown in Table 14 as having Dual/Mixed- or CXCR4-tropic virus. These numbers are different than those presented in table 14 because the numbers in Table 14 reflect the subjects with CCR5-tropic virus according to the original tropism assay.
1 Other reasons for discontinuation include lost to follow-up, withdrawn, protocol violation, and other.

mixed tropism result at the baseline visit 4 to 6 weeks later. This illustrates the background change from CCR5 to dual/mixed tropism result over time in this treatment-experienced population, prior to a change in antiretroviral regimen or administration of a CCR5 co-receptor antagonist.

[See table 12 on previous page]
The week 48 results for the pooled Studies A4001027 and A4001028 are shown in Table 13.
[See table 13 at left]
After 48 weeks of therapy, the proportion of subjects with HIV-1 RNA <400 copies/mL receiving maraviroc compared to placebo was 56% and 22%, respectively. The mean changes in plasma HIV-1 RNA from baseline to week 48 were −1.84 log$_{10}$ copies/mL for subjects receiving maraviroc + OBT compared to −0.78 log$_{10}$ copies/mL for subjects receiving OBT only. The mean increase in CD4+ counts was higher on maraviroc twice daily + OBT (124 cells/mm^3) than on placebo + OBT (60 cells/mm^3).

14.2 Study in Dual/Mixed-tropic, Treatment-Experienced Subjects

Study A4001029 was an exploratory, randomized, double-blind, multicenter trial to determine the safety and efficacy of maraviroc in subjects infected with dual/mixed co-receptor tropic HIV-1. The inclusion/exclusion criteria were similar to those for Studies A4001027 and A4001028 above and the subjects were randomized in a 1:1:1 ratio to SELZENTRY once daily, SELZENTRY twice daily, or placebo. No increased risk of infection or HIV disease progression was observed in the subjects who received SELZENTRY. SELZENTRY use was not associated with a significant decrease in HIV-1 RNA compared to placebo in these subjects and no adverse effect on CD4 count was noted.

14.3 Study in Treatment-Naïve Subjects

Study A4001026 is an ongoing, randomized, double-blind, multicenter study in subjects infected with CCR5-tropic HIV-1 classified by the original Trofile® tropism assay. Subjects were required to have plasma HIV-1 RNA ≥2000 copies/mL and could not have: 1) previously received any antiretroviral therapy for >14 days, 2) an active or recent opportunistic infection or a suspected primary HIV-1 infection, or 3) phenotypic or genotypic resistance to zidovudine, lamivudine, or efavirenz. Subjects were randomized in a 1:1:1 ratio to maraviroc 300 mg once daily, maraviroc 300 mg twice daily, or efavirenz 600 mg once daily, each in combination with zidovudine/lamivudine. The efficacy and safety of SELZENTRY are based on the comparison of SELZENTRY twice daily versus efavirenz. In a pre-planned interim analysis at 16 weeks, the maraviroc 300mg once per day treatment arm failed to meet the pre-specified criteria for demonstrating non-inferiority and was discontinued.
The demographic and baseline characteristics of the maraviroc and efavirenz treatment groups were comparable (Table 14). Subjects were stratified by screening HIV-1 RNA levels and by geographic region. The median CD4 cell counts and mean HIV-1 RNA at baseline were similar for both treatment groups.
[See table 14 above]
The treatment outcomes at 96 weeks for study A4001026 are shown in Table 15. Treatment outcomes are based on reanalysis of the screening samples using a more sensitive tropism assay, Enhanced sensitivity Trofile® HIV tropism assay, which became available after the week 48 analysis, approximately 15% of the subjects identified as CCR5-tropic in the original analysis had Dual/Mixed- or CXCR4-tropic virus. Screening with enhanced sensitivity version of the Trofile® tropism assay reduced the number of maraviroc virologic failures with CXCR4- or Dual/Mixed-tropic virus at failure to 12 compared to 24 when screening with the original Trofile® HIV tropism assay.
[See table 15 at left]
The median increase from baseline in CD4+ cell counts at week 96 was 184 cells/mm^3 for the SELZENTRY arm compared to 155 cells/mm^3 for the efavirenz arm.

15 REFERENCES

[1]IAS-USA Drug Resistance Mutations Figures http://www.iasusa.org/pub/topics/2006/issue3/125.pdf

16 HOW SUPPLIED/STORAGE AND HANDLING

SELZENTRY film-coated tablets are available as follows:
150 and 300 mg tablets are blue, biconvex, oval, film-coated tablets debossed with "Pfizer" on one side and "MVC 150" or "MVC 300" on the other.
Bottle packs 150 mg tablets
• 60 tablets (NDC 0069-0807-60)
Bottle packs 300 mg tablets
• 60 tablets (NDC 0069-0808-60)
SELZENTRY film-coated tablets should be stored at 25°C (77°F); excursions permitted between 15°C and 30°C (59°F–86°F) [see USP Controlled Room Temperature].
Shelf life is 24 months.

17 PATIENT COUNSELING INFORMATION

See Medication Guide.
Patients should be informed that if they develop signs or symptoms of hepatitis or allergic reaction following use of SELZENTRY (rash, skin or eyes look yellow, dark urine,

vomiting, abdominal pain), they should stop SELZENTRY and seek medical evaluation immediately [see *Warnings and Precautions (5.1)*].

Patients should be informed that SELZENTRY is not a cure for HIV infection and patients may still develop illnesses associated with HIV infection, including opportunistic infections. The use of SELZENTRY has not been shown to reduce the risk of transmission of HIV to others through sexual contact, sharing needles or blood contamination.

Patients should be advised that it is important to:
• remain under the care of a physician when using SELZENTRY;
• take SELZENTRY every day as prescribed and in combination with other antiretroviral drugs;
• report to their physician the use of any other prescription or nonprescription medication or herbal products;
• inform their physician if they are pregnant, plan to become pregnant or become pregnant while taking SELZENTRY;
• not change the dose or dosing schedule of SELZENTRY or any antiretroviral medication without consulting their physician.

Patients should be advised that it is important to take all their anti-HIV medicines as prescribed and at the same time(s) each day.

Patients should be advised that when their SELZENTRY supply starts to run low, they should ask their doctor or pharmacist for a refill.

Patients should be advised that if they forget to take a dose, they should take the next dose of SELZENTRY as soon as possible and then take their next scheduled dose at its regular time. If it is less than 6 hours before their next scheduled dose, they should not take the missed dose and should instead wait and take the next dose at the regular time.

Caution should be used when administering SELZENTRY in patients with a history of postural hypotension or on concomitant medication known to lower blood pressure. Patients should be advised that if they experience dizziness while taking SELZENTRY, they should avoid driving or operating machinery.

Distributed by
Pfizer Labs
Division of Pfizer Inc, NY NY 10017
Trofile® is a registered trademark of Monogram Biosciences, Inc.
LAB-0357-5.0

MEDICATION GUIDE

SELZENTRY® (sell-ZEN-tree) Tablets (maraviroc)

Read the Medication Guide that comes with SELZENTRY before you start taking it and each time you get a refill. There may be new information. This information does not take the place of talking with your health care provider about your medical condition or treatment.

What is the most important information I should know about SELZENTRY?

Serious side effects have occurred with SELZENTRY, including liver problems (liver toxicity). An allergic reaction may happen before liver problems occur. Stop taking SELZENTRY and call your health care provider right away if you get any of the following symptoms:
• an itchy rash on your body (allergic reaction)
• yellowing of your skin or whites of your eyes (jaundice)
• dark (tea-colored) urine
• vomiting
• upper right stomach area (abdominal) pain

What is SELZENTRY?

SELZENTRY is an anti-HIV medicine called a CCR5 antagonist. HIV (Human Immunodeficiency Virus) is the virus that causes AIDS (Acquired Immune Deficiency Syndrome). SELZENTRY is used with other anti-HIV medicines in adults with CCR5-tropic HIV-1 infection.

Use of SELZENTRY is not recommended in people with dual/mixed or CXCR4-tropic HIV-1.
• SELZENTRY will not cure HIV infection.
• People taking SELZENTRY may still develop infections, including opportunistic infections or other conditions that happen with HIV infection.
• It is very important that you stay under the care of your health care provider during treatment with SELZENTRY.
• The long-term effects of SELZENTRY are not known at this time.

SELZENTRY has not been studied in children less than 16 years of age.

Does SELZENTRY lower the risk of passing HIV to other people?

No, SELZENTRY does not lower the risk of passing HIV to other people through sexual contact, sharing needles, or being exposed to your blood.
• Continue to practice safer sex.
• Use latex or polyurethane condoms or other barrier methods to lower the chance of sexual contact with any body fluids. This includes semen from a man, vaginal secretions from a woman, or blood.
• Never re-use or share needles.
• Ask your health care provider if you have any questions about safer sex or how to prevent passing HIV to other people.

How does SELZENTRY work?

HIV enters cells in your blood by attaching itself to structures on the surface of the cell called receptors. SELZENTRY blocks a specific receptor called CCR5 that CCR5-tropic HIV-1 uses to enter CD4 or T-cells in your blood. Your health care provider will do a blood test to see if you have been infected with CCR5-tropic HIV-1 before prescribing SELZENTRY for you.
• When used with other anti-HIV medicines, SELZENTRY may:
  • reduce the amount of HIV in your blood. This is called "viral load".
  • increase the number of white blood cells called T (CD4) cells.

SELZENTRY does not work in all people with CCR5-tropic HIV-1 infection.

Who should not take SELZENTRY?

People with severe kidney problems or who are on hemodialysis and are taking certain other medications should not take SELZENTRY. Talk to your healthcare provider before taking this medicine if you have kidney problems.

What should I tell my health care provider before taking SELZENTRY?

Before you take SELZENTRY, tell your health care provider if you:
• have liver problems including a history of hepatitis B or C.
• have heart problems.
• have kidney problems.
• have low blood pressure or take medicines to lower blood pressure.
• have any other medical condition.
• are pregnant or plan to become pregnant. It is not known if SELZENTRY may harm your unborn baby.
  Antiretroviral Pregnancy Registry. There is a pregnancy registry for women who take antiviral medicines during pregnancy. The purpose of the registry is to collect information about the health of you and your baby. Talk to your health care provider about how you can take part in this registry.
• are breastfeeding or plan to breastfeed. It is recommended that HIV-positive women should not breastfeed their babies. This is because of the chance of passing HIV to your baby. You should not breastfeed if you are taking SELZENTRY because the risk to your baby is unknown. Talk with your health care provider about the best way to feed your baby.

Tell your health care provider about all the medicines you take, including prescription and non-prescription medicines, vitamins and herbal supplements. Certain other medicines may affect the levels of SELZENTRY in your blood. Your health care provider may need to change your dose of SELZENTRY when you take it with certain medicines.

The levels of SELZENTRY in your blood may change and your health care provider may need to adjust your dose of SELZENTRY when taking any of the following medications together with SELZENTRY:

-darunavir (Prezista®)	-delavirdine (Rescriptor®)
-lopinavir/ritonavir (Kaletra®, Norvir®)	-ketoconazole (Nizoral®)
-atazanavir (Reyataz®)	-itraconazole (Sporanox®)
-saquinavir (Invirase®)	-clarithromycin (Biaxin®)
-nelfinavir (Viracept®)	-nefazodone (Serzone®)
-indinavir (Crixivan®)	-telithromycin (Ketek®)
-fosamprenavir (Lexiva®)	-efavirenz (Sustiva®, Atripla®)
-etravirine (Intelence®)	-rifampin (Rifadin®, Rifater®)
-carbamezepine (Tegretol®)	-phenobarbital (Luminal®)
-phenytoin (Dilantin®)	
-Ritonavir (Norvir®)	

Do not take products that contain St. John's Wort (hypericum perforatum). St. John's Wort may lower the levels of SELZENTRY in your blood so that it will not work to treat your CCR5-tropic HIV infection.

Know the medicines you take. Keep a list of your medicines. Show the list to your health care provider and pharmacist when you get a new medicine.

How should I take SELZENTRY?

Take SELZENTRY exactly as prescribed by your health care provider. SELZENTRY comes in 150 mg and 300 mg tablets. Your health care provider will prescribe the dose that is right for you.
• Take SELZENTRY 2 times a day.
• Swallow SELZENTRY tablets whole. Do not chew the tablets.
• Take SELZENTRY tablets with or without food.
• Always take SELZENTRY with other anti-HIV drugs as prescribed by your health care provider.

Do not change your dose or stop taking SELZENTRY or your other anti-HIV medicines without first talking with your health care provider.
• If you take too much SELZENTRY, call your health care provider or the poison control center right away.
• If you forget to take SELZENTRY, take the next dose of SELZENTRY as soon as possible and then take your next scheduled dose at its regular time. If it is less than 6 hours before your next dose, do not take the missed dose. Wait and take the next dose at the regular time. Do not take a double dose to make up for a missed dose.
• It is very important to take all your anti-HIV medicines as prescribed. This can help your medicines work better. It also lowers the chance that your medicines will stop working to fight HIV (drug resistance).
• When your SELZENTRY supply starts to run low, ask your health care provider or pharmacist for a refill. This is very important because the amount of virus in your blood may increase and SELZENTRY could stop working if it is stopped for even a short period of time.

What are the possible side effects of SELZENTRY?

There have been serious side effects when SELZENTRY has been given with other anti-HIV drugs including:
• **Liver problems.** See "What is the most important information I should know about SELZENTRY?"
• **Heart problems** including heart attack.
• **Low blood pressure when standing up (postural hypotension).** Low blood pressure when standing up can cause dizziness or fainting. Do not drive a car or operate heavy machinery if you have dizziness while taking SELZENTRY.
• **Changes in your immune system.** A condition called Immune Reconstitution Syndrome can happen when you start taking HIV medicines. Your immune system may get stronger and could begin to fight infections that have been hidden in your body such as pneumonia, herpes virus or tuberculosis. Tell your health care provider if you develop new symptoms after starting your HIV medicines.
• **Possible chance of infection or cancer.** SELZENTRY affects other immune system cells and therefore may possibly increase your chance for getting other infections or cancer.

The most common side effects of SELZENTRY include colds, cough, fever, rash, and dizziness.

Tell your health care provider about any side effect that bothers you or does not go away.

These are not all of the side effects with SELZENTRY. For more information, ask your health care provider or pharmacist.

Call your doctor for medical advice about side effects. You may report side effects to FDA at 1-800-FDA-1088.

How should I store SELZENTRY?
• Store SELZENTRY tablets at room temperature from 59°F to 86°F (15°C to 30°C).
• Safely throw away medicine that is out of date or that you no longer need.

Keep SELZENTRY and all medicines out of the reach of children.

General information about SELZENTRY

Medicines are sometimes prescribed for conditions that are not mentioned in Medication Guides. Do not use SELZENTRY for a condition for which it was not prescribed. Do not give SELZENTRY to other people, even if they have the same symptoms you have. It may harm them. This Medication Guide summarizes the most important information about SELZENTRY. If you would like more information, talk with your health care provider. You can ask your health care provider or pharmacist for more information about SELZENTRY that is written for health professionals. For more information, go to www.selzentry.com.

What are the ingredients in SELZENTRY?

Active ingredient: maraviroc

Inactive ingredients: microcrystalline cellulose, dibasic calcium phosphate (anhydrous), sodium starch glycolate, magnesium stearate

Film-coat: FD&C blue #2 aluminum lake, soya lecithin, polyethylene glycol (macrogol 3350), polyvinyl alcohol, talc and titanium dioxide

Revised May 2010

The brands listed are the trademarks or registered marks of their respective owners and are not trademarks of Pfizer.

Distributed by
Pfizer Labs
Division of Pfizer Inc, NY, NY 10017
LAB-0358-5.0

This Medication Guide has been approved by the US Food and Drug Administration.

TRIZIVIR® ℞

[*trī′ zə-vir*]

(abacavir sulfate, lamivudine,and zidovudine)

Tablets

WARNINGS

TRIZIVIR contains 3 nucleoside analogues (abacavir sulfate, lamivudine, and zidovudine) and is intended only for patients whose regimen would otherwise include these 3 components.

Hypersensitivity Reactions: Serious and sometimes fatal hypersensitivity reactions have been associated with abacavir sulfate, a component of TRIZIVIR. Hypersensitivity to abacavir is a multi-organ clinical syndrome usually characterized by a sign or symptom in 2 or more of the following groups: (1) fever, (2) rash, (3) gastrointestinal (including nausea, vomiting, diarrhea, or abdominal pain), (4) constitutional (including generalized malaise, fatigue, or achiness), and (5) respiratory (including dyspnea, cough, or pharyngitis). Discontinue TRIZIVIR as soon as a hypersensitivity reaction is suspected.

Patients who carry the HLA-B*5701 allele are at high risk for experiencing a hypersensitivity reaction to abacavir. Prior to initiating therapy with abacavir, screening for the HLA-B*5701 allele is recommended; this approach has been found to decrease the risk of hypersensitivity reaction. Screening is also recommended prior to reinitiation of abacavir in patients of unknown HLA-B*5701 status who have previously tolerated abacavir. HLA-B*5701-negative patients may develop a suspected hypersensitivity reaction to abacavir; however, this occurs significantly less frequently than in HLA-B*5701-positive patients.

Regardless of HLA-B*5701 status, permanently discontinue TRIZIVIR if hypersensitivity cannot be ruled out, even when other diagnoses are possible.

Following a hypersensitivity reaction to abacavir, NEVER restart TRIZIVIR or any other abacavir-containing product because more severe symptoms can occur within hours and may include life-threatening hypotension and death.

Reintroduction of TRIZIVIR or any other abacavir-containing product, even in patients who have no identified history or unrecognized symptoms of hypersensitivity to abacavir therapy, can result in serious or fatal hypersensitivity reactions. Such reactions can occur within hours (see WARNINGS and PRECAUTIONS: Information for Patients).

Hematologic Toxicity: Zidovudine has been associated with hematologic toxicity including neutropenia and severe anemia, particularly in patients with advanced Human Immunodeficiency Virus (HIV-1) disease (see WARNINGS). Prolonged use of zidovudine has been associated with symptomatic myopathy.

Lactic Acidosis and Severe Hepatomegaly: Lactic acidosis and severe hepatomegaly with steatosis, including fatal cases, have been reported with the use of nucleoside analogues alone or in combination, including abacavir, lamivudine, zidovudine, and other antiretrovirals (see WARNINGS).

Exacerbations of Hepatitis B: Severe acute exacerbations of hepatitis B have been reported in patients who are co-infected with hepatitis B virus (HBV) and HIV-1 and have discontinued lamivudine, which is one component of TRIZIVIR. Hepatic function should be monitored closely with both clinical and laboratory follow-up for at least several months in patients who discontinue TRIZIVIR and are co-infected with HIV-1 and HBV. If appropriate, initiation of anti-hepatitis B therapy may be warranted (see WARNINGS).

DESCRIPTION

TRIZIVIR: TRIZIVIR Tablets contain the following 3 synthetic nucleoside analogues: abacavir sulfate (ZIAGEN®), lamivudine (also known as EPIVIR® or 3TC), and zidovudine (also known as RETROVIR®, azidothymidine, or ZDV) with inhibitory activity against HIV-1.

TRIZIVIR Tablets are for oral administration. Each film-coated tablet contains the active ingredients 300 mg of abacavir as abacavir sulfate, 150 mg of lamivudine, and 300 mg of zidovudine, and the inactive ingredients magnesium stearate, microcrystalline cellulose, and sodium starch glycolate. The tablets are coated with a film (OPADRY® green 03B11434) that is made of FD&C Blue No. 2, hypromellose, polyethylene glycol, titanium dioxide, and yellow iron oxide.

Abacavir Sulfate: The chemical name of abacavir sulfate is (1*S*,*cis*)-4-[2-amino-6-(cyclopropylamino)-9*H*-purin-9-yl]-2-cyclopentene-1-methanol sulfate (salt) (2:1). Abacavir sulfate is the enantiomer with *1S, 4R* absolute configuration on the cyclopentene ring. It has a molecular formula of $(C_{14}H_{18}N_6O)_2 \bullet H_2SO_4$ and a molecular weight of 670.76 daltons. It has the following structural formula:

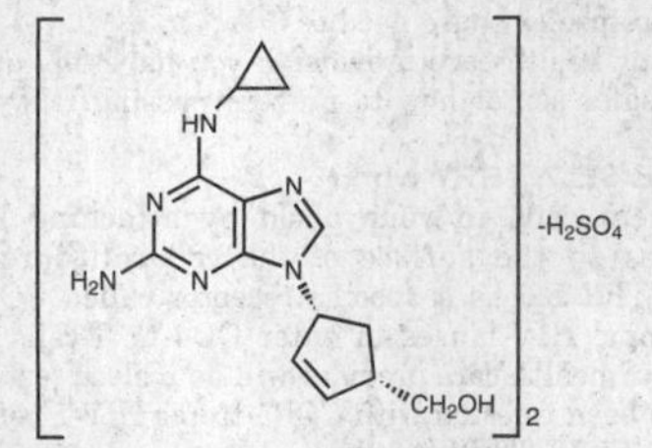

Abacavir sulfate is a white to off-white solid with a solubility of approximately 77 mg/mL in distilled water at 25°C. In vivo, abacavir sulfate dissociates to its free base, abacavir. In this insert, all dosages for ZIAGEN (abacavir sulfate) are expressed in terms of abacavir.

Lamivudine: The chemical name of lamivudine is (2R,cis)-4-amino-1-(2-hydroxymethyl-1,3-oxathiolan-5-yl)-(1H)-pyrimidin-2-one. Lamivudine is the (-)enantiomer of a dideoxy analogue of cytidine. Lamivudine has also been referred to as (-)2′,3′-dideoxy, 3′-thiacytidine. It has a molecular formula of $C_8H_{11}N_3O_3S$ and a molecular weight of 229.3 daltons. It has the following structural formula:

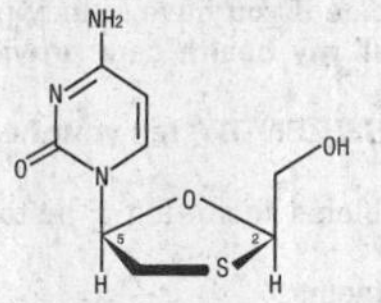

Lamivudine is a white to off-white crystalline solid with a solubility of approximately 70 mg/mL in water at 20°C.

Zidovudine: The chemical name of zidovudine is 3′-azido-3′-deoxythymidine. It has a molecular formula of $C_{10}H_{13}N_5O_4$ and a molecular weight of 267.24 daltons. It has the following structural formula:

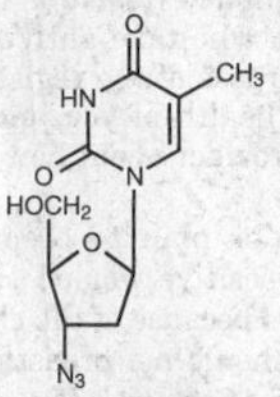

Zidovudine is a white to beige, crystalline solid with a solubility of 20.1 mg/mL in water at 25°C.

MICROBIOLOGY

Mechanism of Action:

Abacavir: Abacavir is a carbocyclic synthetic nucleoside analogue. Abacavir is converted by cellular enzymes to the active metabolite, carbovir triphosphate (CBV-TP), an analogue of deoxyguanosine-5′-triphosphate (dGTP). CBV-TP inhibits the activity of HIV-1 reverse transcriptase (RT) both by competing with the natural substrate dGTP and by its incorporation into viral DNA. The lack of a 3′-OH group in the incorporated nucleotide analogue prevents the formation of the 5′ to 3′ phosphodiester linkage essential for DNA chain elongation, and therefore, the viral DNA growth is terminated. CBV-TP is a weak inhibitor of cellular DNA polymerases α, β, and γ.

Lamivudine: Lamivudine is a synthetic nucleoside analogue. Intracellularly, lamivudine is phosphorylated to its active 5′-triphosphate metabolite, lamivudine triphosphate (3TC-TP). The principal mode of action of 3TC-TP is inhibition of RT via DNA chain termination after incorporation of the nucleotide analogue. 3TC-TP is a weak inhibitor of cellular DNA polymerases α, β, and γ.

Zidovudine: Zidovudine is a synthetic nucleoside analogue. Intracellularly, zidovudine is phosphorylated to its active 5′-triphosphate metabolite, zidovudine triphosphate (ZDV-TP). The principal mode of action of ZDV-TP is inhibition of RT via DNA chain termination after incorporation of the nucleotide analogue. ZDV-TP is a weak inhibitor of the cellular DNA polymerases α and γ and has been reported to be incorporated into the DNA of cells in culture.

Antiviral Activity:

Abacavir: The antiviral activity of abacavir against HIV-1 was evaluated against a T-cell tropic laboratory strain HIV-1_{IIIB} in lymphoblastic cell lines, a monocyte/macrophage tropic laboratory strain HIV-1_{BaL} in primary monocytes/macrophages, and clinical isolates in peripheral blood mononuclear cells. The concentration of drug necessary to effect viral replication by 50 percent (EC_{50}) ranged from 3.7 to 5.8 μM (1 μM = 0.28 mcg/mL) and 0.07 to 1.0 μM against HIV-1_{IIIB} and HIV-1_{BaL}, respectively, and was 0.26 ± 0.18 μM against 8 clinical isolates. The EC_{50} values of abacavir against different HIV-1 clades (A-G) ranged from 0.0015 to 1.05 μM, and against HIV-2 isolates, from 0.024 to 0.49 μM. Abacavir had synergistic activity in cell culture in combination with the nucleoside reverse transcriptase inhibitor (NRTI) zidovudine, the non-nucleoside reverse transcriptase inhibitor (NNRTI) nevirapine, and the protease inhibitor (PI) amprenavir; and additive activity in combination with the NRTIs didanosine, emtricitabine, lamivudine, stavudine, tenofovir, and zalcitabine. Ribavirin (50 μM) had no effect on the anti–HIV-1 activity of abacavir in cell culture.

Lamivudine: The antiviral activity of lamivudine against HIV-1 was assessed in a number of cell lines (including monocytes and fresh human peripheral blood lymphocytes) using standard susceptibility assays. EC_{50} values were in the range of 0.003 to 15 μM (1 μM = 0.23 mcg/mL). HIV-1 from therapy-naive subjects with no amino acid substitutions associated with resistance gave median EC_{50} values of 0.429 μM (range: 0.200 to 2.007 μM) from Virco (n = 92 baseline samples from COLA40263) and 2.35 μM (1.37 to 3.68 μM) from Monogram Biosciences (n = 135 baseline samples from ESS30009). The EC_{50} values of lamivudine against different HIV-1 clades (A-G) ranged from 0.001 to 0.120 μM, and against HIV-2 isolates from 0.003 to 0.120 μM in peripheral blood mononuclear cells. Ribavirin (50 μM) decreased the anti-HIV-1 activity of lamivudine by 3.5 fold in MT-4 cells.

Zidovudine: The antiviral activity of zidovudine against HIV-1 was assessed in a number of cell lines (including monocytes and fresh human peripheral blood lymphocytes). The EC_{50} and EC_{90} values for zidovudine were 0.01 to 0.49 μM (1 μM = 0.27 mcg/mL) and 0.1 to 9 μM, respectively. HIV-1 from therapy-naive subjects with no amino acid substitutions associated with resistance gave median EC_{50} values of 0.011 μM (range: 0.005 to 0.110 μM) from Virco (n = 92 baseline samples from COLA40263) and 0.0017 μM (0.006 to 0.0340 μM) from Monogram Biosciences (n = 135 baseline samples from ESS30009). The EC_{50} values of zidovudine against different HIV-1 clades (A-G) ranged from 0.00018 to 0.02 μM, and against HIV-2 isolates from 0.00049 to 0.004 μM. In cell culture drug combination studies, zidovudine demonstrates synergistic activity with the NRTIs abacavir, didanosine, lamivudine, and zalcitabine; the NNRTIs delavirdine and nevirapine; and the PIs indinavir, nelfinavir, ritonavir, and saquinavir; and additive activity with interferon alfa. Ribavirin has been found to inhibit the phosphorylation of zidovudine in cell culture.

Resistance:

HIV-1 isolates with reduced sensitivity to abacavir, lamivudine, or zidovudine have been selected in cell culture and were also obtained from patients treated with abacavir, lamivudine, and zidovudine, or the combination of lamivudine and zidovudine.

Abacavir: Genotypic analysis of isolates selected in cell culture and recovered from abacavir-treated patients demonstrated that amino acid substitutions K65R, L74V, Y115F, and M184V/I in HIV-1 RT contributed to abacavir resistance. In a study of subjects receiving abacavir once or twice daily in combination with lamivudine and efavirenz once daily, 39% (7/18) of the isolates from patients who experienced virologic failure in the abacavir once-daily arm had a >2.5-fold decrease in abacavir susceptibility with a median-fold decrease of 1.3 (range 0.5 to 11) compared with 29% (5/17) of the failure isolates in the twice-daily arm with a median-fold decrease of 0.92 (range 0.7 to 13).

Lamivudine: Genotypic analysis of isolates selected in cell culture and recovered from lamivudine-treated patients showed that the resistance was due to a specific amino acid substitution in the HIV-1 RT at codon 184 changing the methionine to either isoleucine or valine (M184V/I).

Zidovudine: Genotypic analyses of the isolates selected in cell culture and recovered from zidovudine-treated patients showed mutations in the HIV-1 RT gene resulting in 6 amino acid substitutions (M41L, D67N, K70R, L210W, T215Y or F, and K219Q) that confer zidovudine resistance. In general, higher levels of resistance were associated with greater number of mutations. In some patients harboring zidovudine-resistant virus at baseline, phenotypic sensitivity to zidovudine was restored by 12 weeks of treatment with lamivudine and zidovudine. Combination therapy with lamivudine plus zidovudine delayed the emergence of substitutions conferring resistance to zidovudine.

Cross-Resistance:

Cross-resistance has been observed among NRTIs.

Abacavir: Isolates containing abacavir resistance-associated amino acid substitutions, namely, K65R, L74V, Y115F, and M184V, exhibited cross-resistance to didanosine, emtricitabine, lamivudine, tenofovir, and zalcitabine in cell culture and in patients. The K65R substitution can confer resistance to abacavir, didanosine, emtricitabine, lamivudine, stavudine, tenofovir, and zalcitabine; the L74V substitution can confer resistance to abacavir, didanosine, and zalcitabine; and the M184V substitution can confer resistance to abacavir, didanosine, emtricitabine, lamivudine, and zalcitabine. An increasing number of thymidine analogue mutations (TAMs: M41L, D67N, K70R, L210W, T215Y/F, K219E/R/H/Q/N) is associated with a progressive reduction in abacavir susceptibility.

Lamivudine: Cross-resistance to abacavir, didanosine, tenofovir, and zalcitabine has been observed in some patients harboring lamivudine-resistant HIV-1 isolates. In some patients treated with zidovudine plus didanosine or zalcitabine, isolates resistant to multiple drugs, including lamivudine, have emerged (see under Zidovudine below). Cross-resistance between lamivudine and zidovudine has not been reported.

Zidovudine: In a study of 167 HIV-infected patients, isolates (n = 2) with multi-drug resistance to didanosine, lamivudine, stavudine, zalcitabine, and zidovudine were recovered from patients treated for ≥1 year with zidovudine plus didanosine or zidovudine plus zalcitabine. The pattern of resistance-associated amino acid substitutions with such combination therapies was different (A62V, V75I, F77L, F116Y, Q151M) from the pattern with zidovudine monotherapy, with the Q151M substitution being most commonly associated with multi-drug resistance. The substitution at codon 151 in combination with substitutions at 62, 75, 77, and 116 results in a virus with reduced susceptibility to didanosine, lamivudine, stavudine, zalcitabine, and zidovudine. TAMs are selected by zidovudine and confer cross-resistance to abacavir, didanosine, stavudine, tenofovir, and zalcitabine.

CLINICAL PHARMACOLOGY

Pharmacokinetics in Adults:

TRIZIVIR: In a single-dose, 3-way crossover bioavailability study of 1 TRIZIVIR Tablet versus 1 ZIAGEN Tablet (300 mg), 1 EPIVIR Tablet (150 mg), plus 1 RETROVIR Tablet (300 mg) administered simultaneously in healthy subjects (n = 24), there was no difference in the extent of absorption, as measured by the area under the plasma concentration-time curve (AUC) and maximal peak concentration (C_{max}), of all 3 components. One TRIZIVIR Tablet was bioequivalent to 1 ZIAGEN Tablet (300 mg), 1 EPIVIR Tablet (150 mg), plus 1 RETROVIR Tablet (300 mg) following single-dose administration to fasting healthy subjects (n = 24).

Abacavir: Following oral administration, abacavir is rapidly absorbed and extensively distributed. Binding of abacavir to human plasma proteins is approximately 50%. Binding of abacavir to plasma proteins was independent of concentration. Total blood and plasma drug-related radioactivity concentrations are identical, demonstrating that abacavir readily distributes into erythrocytes. The primary routes of elimination of abacavir are metabolism by alcohol dehydrogenase to form the 5'-carboxylic acid and glucuronyl transferase to form the 5'-glucuronide.

Lamivudine: Following oral administration, lamivudine is rapidly absorbed and extensively distributed. Binding to plasma protein is low. Approximately 70% of an intravenous dose of lamivudine is recovered as unchanged drug in the urine. Metabolism of lamivudine is a minor route of elimination. In humans, the only known metabolite is the transsulfoxide metabolite (approximately 5% of an oral dose after 12 hours).

Zidovudine: Following oral administration, zidovudine is rapidly absorbed and extensively distributed. Binding to plasma protein is low. Zidovudine is eliminated primarily by hepatic metabolism. The major metabolite of zidovudine is 3'-azido-3'-deoxy-5'-O-β-D-glucopyranuronosylthymidine (GZDV). GZDV area under the curve (AUC) is about 3-fold greater than the zidovudine AUC. Urinary recovery of zidovudine and GZDV accounts for 14% and 74% of the dose following oral administration, respectively. A second metabolite, 3'-amino-3'-deoxythymidine (AMT), has been identified in plasma. The AMT AUC was one fifth of the zidovudine AUC.

In humans, abacavir, lamivudine, and zidovudine are not significantly metabolized by cytochrome P450 enzymes.

The pharmacokinetic properties of abacavir, lamivudine, and zidovudine in fasting patients are summarized in Table 1.

[See table 1 above]

Effect of Food on Absorption of TRIZIVIR:

TRIZIVIR may be administered with or without food. Administration with food in a single-dose bioavailability study resulted in lower C_{max}, similar to results observed previously for the reference formulations. The average [90% CI] decrease in abacavir, lamivudine, and zidovudine C_{max} was 32% [24% to 38%], 18% [10% to 25%], and 28% [13% to 40%], respectively, when administered with a high-fat meal, compared with administration under fasted conditions. Administration of TRIZIVIR with food did not alter the extent of abacavir, lamivudine, and zidovudine absorption (AUC), as compared with administration under fasted conditions (n = 24).

Table 1. Pharmacokinetic Parameters* for Abacavir, Lamivudine, and Zidovudine in Adults

Parameter	Abacavir		Lamivudine		Zidovudine	
Oral bioavailability (%)	86 ± 25	n = 6	86 ± 16	n = 12	64 ± 10	n = 5
Apparent volume of distribution (L/kg)	0.86 ± 0.15	n = 6	1.3 ± 0.4	n = 20	1.6 ± 0.6	n = 8
Systemic clearance (L/hr/kg)	0.80 ± 0.24	n = 6	0.33 ± 0.06	n = 20	1.6 ± 0.6	n = 6
Renal clearance (L/hr/kg)	.007 ± .008	n = 6	0.22 ± 0.06	n = 20	0.34 ± 0.05	n = 9
Elimination half-life (hr)[†]	1.45 ± 0.32	n = 20	5 to 7		0.5 to 3	

*Data presented as mean ± standard deviation except where noted.
[†]Approximate range.

Table 2. Effect of Coadministered Drugs on Abacavir, Lamivudine, and Zidovudine AUC*
Note: ROUTINE DOSE MODIFICATION OF ABACAVIR, LAMIVUDINE, AND ZIDOVUDINE IS NOT WARRANTED WITH COADMINISTRATION OF THE FOLLOWING DRUGS.

Drugs That May Alter Lamivudine Blood Concentrations

Coadministered Drug and Dose	Lamivudine Dose	n	Lamivudine Concentrations		Concentration of Coadministered Drug
			AUC	Variability	
Nelfinavir 750 mg q 8 hr × 7 to 10 days	single 150 mg	11	↑10%	95% CI: 1% to 20%	↔
Trimethoprim 160 mg/ Sulfamethoxazole 800 mg daily × 5 days	single 300 mg	14	↑43%	90% CI: 32% to 55%	↔

Drugs That May Alter Zidovudine Blood Concentrations

Coadministered Drug and Dose	Zidovudine Dose	n	Zidovudine Concentrations		Concentration of Coadministered Drug
			AUC	Variability	
Atovaquone 750 mg q 12 hr with food	200 mg q 8 hr	14	↑31%	Range 23% to 78%[†]	↔
Fluconazole 400 mg daily	200 mg q 8 hr	12	↑74%	95% CI: 54% to 98%	Not Reported
Methadone 30 to 90 mg daily	200 mg q 4 hr	9	↑43%	Range 16% to 64%[†]	↔
Nelfinavir 750 mg q 8 hr × 7 to 10 days	single 200 mg	11	↓35%	Range 28% to 41%	↔
Probenecid 500 mg q 6 hr × 2 days	2 mg/kg q 8 hr × 3 days	3	↑106%	Range 100% to 170%[†]	Not Assessed
Ritonavir 300 mg q 6 hr × 4 days	200 mg q 8 hr × 4 days	9	↓25%	95% CI: 15% to 34%	↔
Valproic acid 250 mg or 500 mg q 8 hr × 4 days	100 mg q 8 hr × 4 days	6	↑80%	Range 64% to 130%[†]	Not Assessed

Drugs That May Alter Abacavir Blood Concentrations

Coadministered Drug and Dose	Abacavir Dose	n	Abacavir Concentrations		Concentration of Coadministered Drug
			AUC	Variability	
Ethanol 0.7 g/kg	single 600 mg	24	↑41%	90% CI: 35% to 48%	↔

↑ = Increase; ↓ = Decrease; ↔ = no significant change; AUC = area under the concentration versus time curve; CI = confidence interval.
*See PRECAUTIONS: Drug Interactions for additional information on drug interactions.
[†]Estimated range of percent difference.

Special Populations:

Impaired Renal Function:

TRIZIVIR: Because lamivudine and zidovudine require dose adjustment in the presence of renal insufficiency, TRIZIVIR is not recommended for use in patients with creatinine clearance <50 mL/min (see PRECAUTIONS).

Impaired Hepatic Function:

TRIZIVIR: A reduction in the daily dose of zidovudine may be necessary in patients with mild to moderate impaired hepatic function or liver cirrhosis. Abacavir is contraindicated in patients with moderate to severe hepatic impairment and dose reduction is required in patients with mild hepatic impairment. Because TRIZIVIR is a fixed-dose combination that cannot be adjusted for this patient population, TRIZIVIR is contraindicated for patients with impaired hepatic function.

Pregnancy: See PRECAUTIONS: Pregnancy.

Abacavir and Lamivudine: No data are available on the pharmacokinetics of abacavir or lamivudine during pregnancy.

Zidovudine: Zidovudine pharmacokinetics have been studied in a Phase 1 study of 8 women during the last trimester of pregnancy. As pregnancy progressed, there was no evidence of drug accumulation. The pharmacokinetics of zidovudine were similar to that of nonpregnant adults. Consistent with passive transmission of the drug across the

Table 3. Outcomes of Randomized Treatment Through Week 48 (CNA3005)

Outcome	ZIAGEN plus Lamivudine/Zidovudine (n = 262)	Indinavir plus Lamivudine/Zidovudine (n = 265)
Responder*	49%	50%
Virologic failure†	31%	28%
Discontinued due to adverse reactions	10%	12%
Discontinued due to other reasons‡	11%	10%

* Patients achieved and maintained confirmed HIV-1 RNA <400 copies/mL.
† Includes viral rebound and failure to achieve confirmed <400 copies/mL by Week 48.
‡ Includes consent withdrawn, lost to follow up, protocol violations, those with missing data, clinical progression, and other.

Table 4. Proportions of Responders Through Week 48 By Screening Plasma HIV-1 RNA Levels (CNA3005)

Screening HIV-1 RNA (copies/mL)	ZIAGEN plus Lamivudine/Zidovudine (n = 262)		Indinavir plus Lamivudine/Zidovudine (n = 265)	
	<400 copies/mL	n	<400 copies/mL	n
≥10,000-≤100,000	50%	166	48%	165
>100,000	48%	96	52%	100

placenta, zidovudine concentrations in neonatal plasma at birth were essentially equal to those in maternal plasma at delivery. Although data are limited, methadone maintenance therapy in 5 pregnant women did not appear to alter zidovudine pharmacokinetics. In a nonpregnant adult population, a potential for interaction has been identified (see CLINICAL PHARMACOLOGY: Drug Interactions).

Nursing Mothers: See PRECAUTIONS: Nursing Mothers.

Abacavir: No data are available on the pharmacokinetics of abacavir in nursing mothers.

Lamivudine: Samples of breast milk obtained from 20 mothers receiving lamivudine monotherapy (300 mg twice daily) or combination therapy (150 mg lamivudine twice daily and 300 mg zidovudine twice daily) had measurable concentrations of lamivudine.

Zidovudine: After administration of a single dose of 200 mg zidovudine to 13 HIV-infected women, the mean concentration of zidovudine was similar in human milk and serum.

Pediatric Patients:

TRIZIVIR: TRIZIVIR is not intended for use in pediatric patients. TRIZIVIR should not be administered to adolescents who weigh less than 40 kg because it is a fixed-dose tablet that cannot be dose adjusted for this patient population (see PRECAUTIONS: Pediatric Use).

Geriatric Patients: The pharmacokinetics of abacavir, lamivudine, and zidovudine have not been studied in patients over 65 years of age.

Gender:

Abacavir: A population pharmacokinetic analysis in HIV-1-infected male (n = 304) and female (n = 67) patients showed no gender differences in abacavir AUC normalized for lean body weight.

Lamivudine and Zidovudine: A pharmacokinetic study in healthy male (n = 12) and female (n = 12) subjects showed no gender differences in zidovudine exposure (AUC∞) or lamivudine (AUC∞) normalized for body weight.

Race:

Abacavir: There are no significant differences between blacks and Caucasians in abacavir pharmacokinetics.

Lamivudine: There are no significant racial differences in lamivudine pharmacokinetics.

Zidovudine: The pharmacokinetics of zidovudine with respect to race have not been determined.

Drug Interactions: See PRECAUTIONS: Drug Interactions. The drug interactions described are based on studies conducted with the individual nucleoside analogues. In humans, abacavir, lamivudine, and zidovudine are not significantly metabolized by cytochrome P450 enzymes; therefore, it is unlikely that clinically significant drug interactions will occur with drugs metabolized through these pathways.

Abacavir: Due to the common metabolic pathways of abacavir and zidovudine via glucuronyl transferase, 15 HIV-1-infected patients were enrolled in a crossover study evaluating single doses of abacavir (600 mg), lamivudine (150 mg), and zidovudine (300 mg) alone or in combination. Analysis showed no clinically relevant changes in the pharmacokinetics of abacavir with the addition of lamivudine or zidovudine or the combination of lamivudine and zidovudine. Lamivudine exposure (AUC decreased 15%) and zidovudine exposure (AUC increased 10%) did not show clinically relevant changes with concurrent abacavir.

In a study of 11 HIV-1-infected patients receiving methadone-maintenance therapy (40 mg and 90 mg daily), with 600 mg of ZIAGEN twice daily (twice the currently recommended dose), oral methadone clearance increased 22% (90% CI: 6% to 42%). This alteration will not result in a methadone dose modification in the majority of patients; however, an increased methadone dose may be required in a small number of patients.

Lamivudine and Zidovudine: No clinically significant alterations in lamivudine or zidovudine pharmacokinetics were observed in 12 asymptomatic HIV-1-infected adult patients given a single dose of zidovudine (200 mg) in combination with multiple doses of lamivudine (300 mg q 12 hr).

[See table 2 on previous page]

Ribavirin: In vitro data indicate ribavirin reduces phosphorylation of lamivudine, stavudine, and zidovudine. However, no pharmacokinetic (e.g., plasma concentrations or intracellular triphosphorylated active metabolite concentrations) or pharmacodynamic (e.g., loss of HIV-1/HCV virologic suppression) interaction was observed when ribavirin and lamivudine (n = 18), stavudine (n = 10), or zidovudine (n = 6) were coadministered as part of a multi-drug regimen to HIV-1/HCV co-infected patients (see WARNINGS).

INDICATIONS AND USAGE

TRIZIVIR is indicated in combination with other antiretrovirals or alone for the treatment of HIV-1 infection.

Additional important information on the use of TRIZIVIR for treatment of HIV-1 infection:

- TRIZIVIR is one of multiple products containing abacavir. Before starting TRIZIVIR, review medical history for prior exposure to any abacavir-containing product in order to avoid reintroduction in a patient with a history of hypersensitivity to abacavir.
- Limited data exist on the use of TRIZIVIR alone in patients with higher baseline viral load levels (>100,000 copies/mL, see Description of Clinical Studies).

Description of Clinical Studies:

TRIZIVIR: The following study was conducted with the individual components of TRIZIVIR (see CLINICAL PHARMACOLOGY for information about bioequivalence of TRIZIVIR).

CNA3005 was a multicenter, double-blind, controlled study in which 562 HIV-1-infected, therapy-naive adults were randomized to receive either ZIAGEN (300 mg twice daily) plus COMBIVIR® (lamivudine 150 mg/zidovudine 300 mg twice daily), or indinavir (800 mg 3 times a day) plus COMBIVIR twice daily. The study was stratified at randomization by pre-entry plasma HIV-1 RNA 10,000 to 100,000 copies/mL and plasma HIV-1 RNA >100,000 copies/mL. Study participants were male (87%), Caucasian (73%), black (15%), and Hispanic (9%). At baseline the median age was 36 years, the median pretreatment CD4+ cell count was 360 cells/mm^3, and median plasma HIV-1 RNA was 4.8 $\log_{10}$ copies/mL. Proportions of patients with plasma HIV-1 RNA <400 copies/mL (using Roche AMPLICOR HIV-1 MONITOR® Test) through 48 weeks of treatment are summarized in Table 3.

[See table 3 above]

Treatment response by plasma HIV-1 RNA strata is shown in Table 4.

[See table 4 above]

In subjects with baseline viral load >100,000 copies/mL, percentages of patients with HIV-1 RNA levels <50 copies/mL were 31% in the group receiving abacavir vs. 45% in the group receiving indinavir.

Through Week 48, an overall mean increase in CD4+ cell count of about 150 cells/mm^3 was observed in both treatment arms. Through Week 48, 9 subjects (3.4%) in the group receiving abacavir sulfate (6 CDC classification C events and 3 deaths) and 3 subjects (1.5%) in the group receiving indinavir (2 CDC classification C events and 1 death) experienced clinical disease progression.

CONTRAINDICATIONS

TRIZIVIR Tablets are contraindicated in patients with previously demonstrated hypersensitivity to abacavir or to any other component of the product (see WARNINGS).

NEVER restart TRIZIVIR or any other abacavir-containing product following a hypersensitivity reaction to abacavir, regardless of HLA-B*5701 status (see WARNINGS, PRECAUTIONS, and ADVERSE REACTIONS).

TRIZIVIR Tablets are contraindicated in patients with hepatic impairment (see CLINICAL PHARMACOLOGY).

WARNINGS

Hypersensitivity Reaction: Serious and sometimes fatal hypersensitivity reactions have been associated with TRIZIVIR and other abacavir-containing products. Patients who carry the HLA-B*5701 allele are at high risk for experiencing a hypersensitivity reaction to abacavir. Prior to initiating therapy with abacavir, screening for the HLA-B*5701 allele is recommended; this approach has been found to decrease the risk of a hypersensitivity reaction. Screening is also recommended prior to reinitiation of abacavir in patients of unknown HLA-B*5701 status who have previously tolerated abacavir. For HLA-B*5701-positive patients, treatment with an abacavir-containing regimen is not recommended and should be considered only with close medical supervision and under exceptional circumstances when the potential benefit outweighs the risk.

HLA-B*5701-negative patients may develop a hypersensitivity reaction to abacavir; however, this occurs significantly less frequently than in HLA-B*5701-positive patients. Regardless of HLA-B*5701 status, permanently discontinue TRIZIVIR if hypersensitivity cannot be ruled out, even when other diagnoses are possible.

Important information on signs and symptoms of hypersensitivity, as well as clinical management, is presented below.

Signs and Symptoms of Hypersensitivity: Hypersensitivity to abacavir is a multi-organ clinical syndrome usually characterized by a sign or symptom in 2 or more of the following groups.

Group 1: Fever
Group 2: Rash
Group 3: Gastrointestinal (including nausea, vomiting, diarrhea, or abdominal pain)
Group 4: Constitutional (including generalized malaise, fatigue, or achiness)
Group 5: Respiratory (including dyspnea, cough, or pharyngitis)

Hypersensitivity to abacavir following the presentation of a single sign or symptom has been reported infrequently.

Hypersensitivity to abacavir was reported in approximately 8% of 2,670 patients (n = 206) in 9 clinical trials (range: 2% to 9%) with enrollment from November 1999 to February 2002. Data on time to onset and symptoms of suspected hypersensitivity were collected on a detailed data collection module. The frequencies of symptoms are shown in Figure 1. Symptoms usually appeared within the first 6 weeks of treatment with abacavir, although the reaction may occur at any time during therapy. Median time to onset was 9 days; 89% appeared within the first 6 weeks; 95% of patients reported symptoms from 2 or more of the 5 groups listed above.

A recent study with ZIAGEN used double-blind ascertainment of suspected hypersensitivity reactions. During the blinded portion of the study, suspected hypersensitivity to abacavir was reported by investigators in 9% of 324 patients in the abacavir group and 3% of 325 patients in the zidovudine group.

[See figure 1 at top of next page]

Other less common signs and symptoms of hypersensitivity include lethargy, myolysis, edema, abnormal chest x-ray findings (predominantly infiltrates, which can be localized), and paresthesia. Anaphylaxis, liver failure, renal failure, hypotension, adult respiratory distress syndrome, respiratory failure, and death have occurred in association with hypersensitivity reactions.

Physical findings associated with hypersensitivity to abacavir in some patients include lymphadenopathy, mucous membrane lesions (conjunctivitis and mouth ulcerations), and rash. The rash usually appears maculopapular or urticarial, but may be variable in appearance. There have been reports of erythema multiforme. Hypersensitivity reactions have occurred without rash.

Laboratory abnormalities associated with hypersensitivity to abacavir in some patients include elevated liver function tests, elevated creatine phosphokinase, elevated creatinine, and lymphopenia.

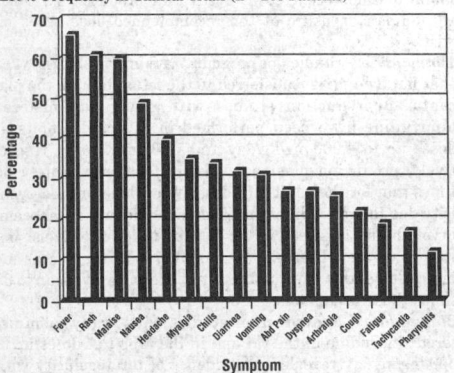

Figure 1. Hypersensitivity-Related Symptoms Reported with ≥10% Frequency in Clinical Trials (n = 206 Patients)

Clinical Management of Hypersensitivity: Discontinue TRIZIVIR as soon as a hypersensitivity reaction is suspected. To minimize the risk of a life-threatening hypersensitivity reaction, permanently discontinue TRIZIVIR if hypersensitivity cannot be ruled out, even when other diagnoses are possible (e.g., acute onset respiratory diseases such as pneumonia, bronchitis, pharyngitis, or influenza; gastroenteritis; or reactions to other medications). Following a hypersensitivity reaction to abacavir, NEVER restart TRIZIVIR or any other abacavir-containing product because more severe symptoms can occur within hours and may include life-threatening hypotension and death.

When therapy with TRIZIVIR has been discontinued for reasons other than symptoms of a hypersensitivity reaction, and if reinitiation of abacavir is under consideration, carefully evaluate the reason for discontinuation to ensure that the patient did not have symptoms of a hypersensitivity reaction. If the patient is of unknown HLA-B*5701 status, screening for the allele is recommended prior to reinitiation of TRIZIVIR.

If hypersensitivity cannot be ruled out, DO NOT reintroduce TRIZIVIR or any other abacavir-containing product. Even in the absence of the HLA-B*5701 allele, it is important to permanently discontinue abacavir and not rechallenge with abacavir if a hypersensitivity reaction cannot be ruled out on clinical grounds, due to the potential for a severe or even fatal reaction.

If symptoms consistent with hypersensitivity are not identified, reintroduction can be undertaken with continued monitoring for symptoms of a hypersensitivity reaction. Make patients aware that a hypersensitivity reaction can occur with reintroduction of abacavir and that abacavir reintroduction needs to be undertaken only if medical care can be readily accessed by the patient or others.

*Risk Factor: HLA-B*5701 Allele:* Studies have shown that carriage of the HLA-B*5701 allele is associated with a significantly increased risk of a hypersensitivity reaction to abacavir.

CNA106030 (PREDICT-1), a randomized, double-blind study, evaluated the clinical utility of prospective HLA-B*5701 screening on the incidence of abacavir hypersensitivity reaction in abacavir-naive HIV-1-infected adults (n = 1,650). In this study, use of pre-therapy screening for the HLA-B*5701 allele and exclusion of subjects with this allele reduced the incidence of clinically suspected abacavir hypersensitivity reactions from 7.8% (66/847) to 3.4% (27/803). Based on this study, it is estimated that 61% of patients with the HLA-B*5701 allele will develop a clinically suspected hypersensitivity reaction during the course of abacavir treatment compared with 4% of patients who do not have the HLA-B*5701 allele.

Screening for carriage of the HLA-B*5701 allele is recommended prior to initiating treatment with abacavir. Screening is also recommended prior to reinitiation of abacavir in patients of unknown HLA-B*5701 status who have previously tolerated abacavir. For HLA-B*5701-positive patients, initiating or reinitiating treatment with an abacavir-containing regimen is not recommended and should be considered only with close medical supervision and under exceptional circumstances where potential benefit outweighs the risk.

Skin patch testing is used as a research tool and should not be used to aid in the clinical diagnosis of abacavir hypersensitivity.

In any patient treated with abacavir, the clinical diagnosis of hypersensitivity reaction must remain the basis of clinical decision-making. Even in the absence of the HLA-B*5701 allele, it is important to permanently discontinue abacavir and not rechallenge with abacavir if a hypersensitivity reaction cannot be ruled out on clinical grounds, due to the potential for a severe or even fatal reaction.

Abacavir Hypersensitivity Reaction Registry: An Abacavir Hypersensitivity Registry has been established to facilitate reporting of hypersensitivity reactions and collection of information on each case. Physicians should register patients by calling 1-800-270-0425.

Lactic Acidosis/Severe Hepatomegaly With Steatosis: Lactic acidosis and severe hepatomegaly with steatosis, including fatal cases, have been reported with the use of nucleoside analogues alone or in combination, including abacavir, lamivudine, zidovudine, and other antiretrovirals. A majority of these cases have been in women. Obesity and prolonged nucleoside exposure may be risk factors. Particular caution should be exercised when administering TRIZIVIR to any patient with known risk factors for liver disease; however, cases have also been reported in patients with no known risk factors. Treatment with TRIZIVIR should be suspended in any patient who develops clinical or laboratory findings suggestive of lactic acidosis or pronounced hepatotoxicity (which may include hepatomegaly and steatosis even in the absence of marked transaminase elevations).

Bone Marrow Suppression: Since TRIZIVIR contains zidovudine, TRIZIVIR should be used with caution in patients who have bone marrow compromise evidenced by granulocyte count <1,000 cells/mm^3 or hemoglobin <9.5 g/dL. Frequent blood counts are strongly recommended in patients with advanced HIV-1 disease who are treated with TRIZIVIR. For HIV-1-infected individuals and patients with asymptomatic or early HIV-1 disease, periodic blood counts are recommended.

Myopathy: Myopathy and myositis, with pathological changes similar to that produced by HIV-1 disease, have been associated with prolonged use of zidovudine, and therefore may occur with therapy with TRIZIVIR.

Posttreatment Exacerbations of Hepatitis: In clinical trials in non-HIV-1-infected patients treated with lamivudine for chronic HBV, clinical and laboratory evidence of exacerbations of hepatitis have occurred after discontinuation of lamivudine. These exacerbations have been detected primarily by serum ALT elevations in addition to re-emergence of HBV DNA. Although most events appear to have been self-limited, fatalities have been reported in some cases. Similar events have been reported from post-marketing experience after changes from lamivudine-containing HIV-1 treatment regimens to non-lamivudine-containing regimens in patients infected with both HIV-1 and HBV. The causal relationship to discontinuation of lamivudine treatment is unknown. Patients should be closely monitored with both clinical and laboratory follow-up for at least several months after stopping treatment. There is insufficient evidence to determine whether re-initiation of lamivudine alters the course of posttreatment exacerbations of hepatitis.

Use With Interferon- and Ribavirin-Based Regimens: In vitro studies have shown ribavirin can reduce the phosphorylation of pyrimidine nucleoside analogues such as lamivudine and zidovudine, components of TRIZIVIR. Although no evidence of a pharmacokinetic or pharmacodynamic interaction (e.g., loss of HIV-1/HCV virologic suppression) was seen when ribavirin was coadministered with lamivudine or zidovudine in HIV-1/HCV co-infected patients (see CLINICAL PHARMACOLOGY: Drug Interactions), **hepatic decompensation (some fatal) has occurred in HIV-1/HCV co-infected patients receiving combination antiretroviral therapy for HIV-1 and interferon alfa with or without ribavirin.** Patients receiving interferon alfa with or without ribavirin and TRIZIVIR should be closely monitored for treatment-associated toxicities, especially hepatic decompensation, neutropenia, and anemia. Discontinuation of TRIZIVIR should be considered as medically appropriate. Dose reduction or discontinuation of interferon alfa, ribavirin, or both should also be considered if worsening clinical toxicities are observed, including hepatic decompensation (e.g., Childs Pugh >6) (see the complete prescribing information for interferon and ribavirin).

Other: TRIZIVIR contains fixed doses of 3 nucleoside analogues: abacavir, lamivudine, and zidovudine and should not be administered concomitantly with abacavir, lamivudine, emtricitabine, or zidovudine. TRIZIVIR should also not be administered concomitantly with the fixed-dose combination drugs: lamivudine/zidovudine (COMBIVIR), abacavir and lamivudine (EPZICOM®), or emtricitabine and tenofovir (TRUVADA®).

Because TRIZIVIR is a fixed-dose tablet, it should not be prescribed for adolescents who weigh less than 40 kg or other patients requiring dosage adjustment.

The complete prescribing information for all agents being considered for use with TRIZIVIR should be consulted before combination therapy with TRIZIVIR is initiated.

PRECAUTIONS

Therapy-Experienced Patients:

Abacavir: In clinical trials, patients with prolonged prior NRTI exposure or who had HIV-1 isolates that contained multiple mutations conferring resistance to NRTIs had limited response to abacavir. The potential for cross-resistance between abacavir and other NRTIs should be considered when choosing new therapeutic regimens in therapy-experienced patients (see MICROBIOLOGY: Cross-Resistance).

Patients With HIV-1 and Hepatitis B Virus Co-infection:

Lamivudine: Safety and efficacy of lamivudine have not been established for treatment of chronic hepatitis B in patients dually infected with HIV-1 and HBV. In non-HIV-1-infected patients treated with lamivudine for chronic hepatitis B, emergence of lamivudine-resistant HBV has been detected and has been associated with diminished treatment response (see EPIVIR-HBV® package insert for additional information). Emergence of hepatitis B virus variants associated with resistance to lamivudine has also been reported in HIV-1-infected patients who have received lamivudine-containing antiretroviral regimens in the presence of concurrent infection with hepatitis B virus.

Patients With Impaired Renal Function:

TRIZIVIR: Since TRIZIVIR is a fixed-dose tablet and the dosage of the individual components cannot be altered, patients with creatinine clearance <50 mL/min should not receive TRIZIVIR.

Patients With Impaired Hepatic Function:

TRIZIVIR: TRIZIVIR is contraindicated in patients with hepatic impairment since it is a fixed-dose tablet and the dosage of the individual components cannot be altered.

Immune Reconstitution Syndrome: Immune reconstitution syndrome has been reported in patients treated with combination antiretroviral therapy, including TRIZIVIR. During the initial phase of combination antiretroviral treatment, patients whose immune system responds may develop an inflammatory response to indolent or residual opportunistic infections (such as *Mycobacterium avium* infection, cytomegalovirus, *Pneumocystis jirovecii* pneumonia [PCP], or tuberculosis), which may necessitate further evaluation and treatment.

Fat Redistribution: Redistribution/accumulation of body fat including central obesity, dorsocervical fat enlargement (buffalo hump), peripheral wasting, facial wasting, breast enlargement, and "cushingoid appearance" have been observed in patients receiving antiretroviral therapy. The mechanism and long-term consequences of these events are currently unknown. A causal relationship has not been established.

Myocardial Infarction: In a published prospective, observational, epidemiological study designed to investigate the rate of myocardial infarction in patients on combination antiretroviral therapy, the use of abacavir within the previous 6 months was correlated with an increased risk of myocardial infarction (MI).[1] In a sponsor-conducted pooled analysis of clinical trials, no excess risk of MI was observed in abacavir-treated subjects as compared with control subjects. In totality, the available data from the observational cohort and from clinical trials are inconclusive.

As a precaution, the underlying risk of coronary heart disease should be considered when prescribing antiretroviral therapies, including abacavir, and action taken to minimize all modifiable risk factors (e.g., hypertension, hyperlipidemia, diabetes mellitus, and smoking).

Information for Patients:

Abacavir: Hypersensitivity Reaction: Inform patients:
- that a Medication Guide and Warning Card summarizing the symptoms of the abacavir hypersensitivity reaction and other product information will be dispensed by the pharmacist with each new prescription and refill of TRIZIVIR, and encourage the patient to read the Medication Guide and Warning Card every time to obtain any new information that may be present about TRIZIVIR. (The complete text of the Medication Guide is reprinted at the end of this document.)
- to carry the Warning Card with them.
- how to identify a hypersensitivity reaction (see WARNINGS and MEDICATION GUIDE).
- that if they develop symptoms consistent with a hypersensitivity reaction they should call their doctor right away to determine if they should stop taking TRIZIVIR.
- that a hypersensitivity reaction can worsen and lead to hospitalization or death if TRIZIVIR is not immediately discontinued.
- to not restart TRIZIVIR or any other abacavir-containing product following a hypersensitivity reaction because more severe symptoms can occur within hours and may include life-threatening hypotension and death.
- that a hypersensitivity reaction is usually reversible if it is detected promptly and TRIZIVIR is stopped right away.
- that if they have interrupted TRIZIVIR for reasons other than symptoms of hypersensitivity (for example, those who have an interruption in drug supply), a serious or fatal hypersensitivity reaction may occur with reintroduction of abacavir.
- to not restart TRIZIVIR or any other abacavir-containing product without medical consultation and that restarting abacavir needs to be undertaken only if medical care can be readily accessed by the patient or others.

- TRIZIVIR should not be coadministered with COMBIVIR, EMTRIVA™, EPIVIR, EPIVIR-HBV, EPZICOM, RETROVIR, TRUVADA, or ZIAGEN.

Lamivudine: Patients co-infected with HIV-1 and HBV should be informed that deterioration of liver disease has occurred in some cases when treatment with lamivudine was discontinued. Patients should be advised to discuss any changes in regimen with their physician.

Zidovudine: Patients should be informed that the important toxicities associated with zidovudine are neutropenia and/or anemia. They should be told of the extreme importance of having their blood counts followed closely while on therapy, especially for patients with advanced HIV-1 disease.

TRIZIVIR: Inform patients that some HIV-1 medicines, including TRIZIVIR can cause a rare, but serious condition called lactic acidosis with liver enlargement (hepatomegaly).

TRIZIVIR is not a cure for HIV-1 infection and patients may continue to experience illnesses associated with HIV-1 infection, including opportunistic infections. Patients should remain under the care of a physician when using TRIZIVIR. Advise patients that the use of TRIZIVIR has not been shown to reduce the risk of transmission of HIV-1 to others through sexual contact or blood contamination.

Inform patients that redistribution or accumulation of body fat may occur in patients receiving antiretroviral therapy and that the cause and long-term health effects of these conditions are not known at this time.

TRIZIVIR Tablets are for oral ingestion only.

Patients should be advised of the importance of taking TRIZIVIR exactly as it is prescribed.

Drug Interactions:

TRIZIVIR: No clinically significant changes to pharmacokinetic parameters were observed for abacavir, lamivudine, or zidovudine when administered together.

Abacavir: Abacavir has no effect on the pharmacokinetic properties of ethanol. Ethanol decreases the elimination of abacavir causing an increase in overall exposure (see CLINICAL PHARMACOLOGY: Drug Interactions).

The addition of methadone has no clinically significant effect on the pharmacokinetic properties of abacavir. In a study of 11 HIV-1-infected patients receiving methadone-maintenance therapy (40 mg and 90 mg daily), with 600 mg of ZIAGEN twice daily (twice the currently recommended dose), oral methadone clearance increased 22% (90% CI: 6% to 42%). This alteration will not result in a methadone dose modification in the majority of patients; however, an increased methadone dose may be required in a small number of patients.

Lamivudine: Trimethoprim (TMP) 160 mg/sulfamethoxazole (SMX) 800 mg once daily has been shown to increase lamivudine exposure (AUC). The effect of higher doses of TMP/SMX on lamivudine pharmacokinetics has not been investigated (see CLINICAL PHARMACOLOGY).

Lamivudine and zalcitabine may inhibit the intracellular phosphorylation of one another. Therefore, use of TRIZIVIR in combination with zalcitabine is not recommended.

Zidovudine: Coadministration of ganciclovir, interferon-alfa, and other bone marrow suppressive or cytotoxic agents may increase the hematologic toxicity of zidovudine. Concomitant use of zidovudine with stavudine should be avoided since an antagonistic relationship has been demonstrated in vitro. In addition, concomitant use of zidovudine with doxorubicin or ribavirin should be avoided because an antagonistic relationship has also been demonstrated in vitro.

See CLINICAL PHARMACOLOGY for additional drug interactions.

Carcinogenesis, Mutagenesis, and Impairment of Fertility:
Carcinogenicity:

Abacavir: Abacavir was administered orally at 3 dosage levels to separate groups of mice and rats in 2-year carcinogenicity studies. Results showed an increase in the incidence of malignant and non-malignant tumors. Malignant tumors occurred in the preputial gland of males and the clitoral gland of females of both species, and in the liver of female rats. In addition, non-malignant tumors also occurred in the liver and thyroid gland of female rats.

Lamivudine: Long-term carcinogenicity studies with lamivudine in mice and rats showed no evidence of carcinogenic potential at exposures up to 10 times (mice) and 58 times (rats) those observed in humans at the recommended therapeutic dose for HIV-1 infection.

Zidovudine: Zidovudine was administered orally at 3 dosage levels to separate groups of mice and rats (60 females and 60 males in each group). Initial single daily doses were 30, 60, and 120 mg/kg/day in mice and 80, 220, and 600 mg/kg/day in rats. The doses in mice were reduced to 20, 30, and 40 mg/kg/day after day 90 because of treatment-related anemia, whereas in rats only the high dose was reduced to 450 mg/kg per day on day 91 and then to 300 mg/kg/day on day 279.

In mice, 7 late-appearing (after 19 months) vaginal neoplasms (5 nonmetastasizing squamous cell carcinomas, 1 squamous cell papilloma, and 1 squamous polyp) occurred in animals given the highest dose. One late-appearing squamous cell papilloma occurred in the vagina of a middle-dose animal. No vaginal tumors were found at the lowest dose. In rats, 2 late-appearing (after 20 months), nonmetastasizing vaginal squamous cell carcinomas occurred in animals given the highest dose. No vaginal tumors occurred at the low or middle dose in rats. No other drug-related tumors were observed in either sex of either species.

At doses that produced tumors in mice and rats, the estimated drug exposure (as measured by AUC) was approximately 3 times (mouse) and 24 times (rat) the estimated human exposure at the recommended therapeutic dose of 100 mg every 4 hours.

Two transplacental carcinogenicity studies were conducted in mice. One study administered zidovudine at doses of 20 mg/kg/day or 40 mg/kg/day from gestation day 10 through parturition and lactation with dosing continuing in offspring for 24 months postnatally. At these doses, exposures were approximately 3 times the estimated human exposure at the recommended doses. After 24 months at the 40-mg/kg/day dose, an increase in incidence of vaginal tumors was noted with no increase in tumors in the liver or lung or any other organ in either gender. These findings are consistent with results of the standard oral carcinogenicity study in mice, as described earlier. A second study administered zidovudine at maximum tolerated doses of 12.5 mg/day or 25 mg/day (~1,000 mg/kg nonpregnant body weight or ~450 mg/kg of term body weight) to pregnant mice from days 12 through 18 of gestation. There was an increase in the number of tumors in the lung, liver, and female reproductive tracts in the offspring of mice receiving the higher dose level of zidovudine.

It is not known how predictive the results of rodent carcinogenicity studies may be for humans.

Mutagenicity:

Abacavir: Abacavir induced chromosomal aberrations both in the presence and absence of metabolic activation in an in vitro cytogenetic study in human lymphocytes. Abacavir was mutagenic in the absence of metabolic activation, although it was not mutagenic in the presence of metabolic activation in an L5178Y/TK$^{+/-}$ mouse lymphoma assay. Abacavir was clastogenic in males and not clastogenic in females in an in vivo mouse bone marrow micronucleus assay. Abacavir was not mutagenic in bacterial mutagenicity assays in the presence and absence of metabolic activation.

Lamivudine: Lamivudine was mutagenic in an L5178Y/TK$^{+/-}$ mouse lymphoma assay and clastogenic in a cytogenetic assay using cultured human lymphocytes. Lamivudine was negative in a microbial mutagenicity assay, in an in vitro cell transformation assay, in a rat micronucleus test, in a rat bone marrow cytogenetic assay, and in an assay for unscheduled DNA synthesis in rat liver.

Zidovudine: Zidovudine was mutagenic in an L5178Y/TK$^{+/-}$ mouse lymphoma assay, positive in an in vitro cell transformation assay, clastogenic in a cytogenetic assay using cultured human lymphocytes, and positive in mouse and rat micronucleus tests after repeated doses. It was negative in a cytogenetic study in rats given a single dose.

Impairment of Fertility:

Abacavir: Abacavir had no adverse effects on the mating performance or fertility of male and female rats at a dose approximately 8 times the human exposure at the recommended dose based on body surface area comparisons.

Lamivudine: In a study of reproductive performance, lamivudine, administered to male and female rats at doses up to 130 times the usual adult dose based on body surface area considerations, revealed no evidence of impaired fertility judged by conception rates and no effect on the survival, growth, and development to weaning of the offspring.

Zidovudine: Zidovudine, administered to male and female rats at doses up to 7 times the usual adult dose based on body surface area considerations, had no effect on fertility judged by conception rates.

Pregnancy: Pregnancy Category C. There are no adequate and well-controlled studies of TRIZIVIR in pregnant women. Reproduction studies with abacavir, lamivudine, and zidovudine have been performed in animals (see Abacavir, Lamivudine, and Zidovudine sections below). TRIZIVIR should be used during pregnancy only if the potential benefits outweigh the risks.

Abacavir: Studies in pregnant rats showed that abacavir is transferred to the fetus through the placenta. Fetal malformations (increased incidences of fetal anasarca and skeletal malformations) and developmental toxicity (depressed fetal body weight and reduced crown-rump length) were observed in rats at a dose which produced 35 times the human exposure, based on AUC. Embryonic and fetal toxicities (increased resorptions, decreased fetal body weights) and toxicities to the offspring (increased incidence of stillbirth and lower body weights) occurred at half of the above-mentioned dose in separate fertility studies conducted in rats. In the

rabbit, no developmental toxicity and no increases in fetal malformations occurred at doses that produced 8.5 times the human exposure at the recommended dose based on AUC.

Lamivudine: Studies in pregnant rats and rabbits showed that lamivudine is transferred to the fetus through the placenta. Reproduction studies with orally administered lamivudine have been performed in rats and rabbits at doses up to 4,000 mg/kg/day and 1,000 mg/kg/day, respectively, producing plasma levels up to approximately 35 times that for the adult HIV dose. No evidence of teratogenicity due to lamivudine was observed. Evidence of early embryolethality was seen in the rabbit at exposure levels similar to those observed in humans, but there was no indication of this effect in the rat at exposure levels up to 35 times those in humans.

Zidovudine: Reproduction studies with orally administered zidovudine in the rat and in the rabbit at doses up to 500 mg/kg/day revealed no evidence of teratogenicity with zidovudine. Zidovudine treatment resulted in embryo/fetal toxicity as evidenced by an increase in the incidence of fetal resorptions in rats given 150 or 450 mg/kg/day and rabbits given 500 mg/kg/day. The doses used in the teratology studies resulted in peak zidovudine plasma concentrations (after one half of the daily dose) in rats 66 to 226 times, and in rabbits 12 to 87 times, mean steady-state peak human plasma concentrations (after one sixth of the daily dose) achieved with the recommended daily dose (100 mg every 4 hours). In an additional teratology study in rats, a dose of 3,000 mg/kg/day (very near the oral median lethal dose in rats of approximately 3,700 mg/kg) caused marked maternal toxicity and an increase in the incidence of fetal malformations. This dose resulted in peak zidovudine plasma concentrations 350 times peak human plasma concentrations. No evidence of teratogenicity was seen in this experiment at doses of 600 mg/kg/day or less. Two rodent carcinogenicity studies were conducted (see Carcinogenesis, Mutagenesis, and Impairment of Fertility).

Antiretroviral Pregnancy Registry: To monitor maternal-fetal outcomes of pregnant women exposed to TRIZIVIR or other antiretroviral agents, an Antiretroviral Pregnancy Registry has been established. Physicians are encouraged to register patients by calling 1-800-258-4263.

Nursing Mothers: The Centers for Disease Control and Prevention recommend that HIV-1-infected mothers not breastfeed their infants to avoid risking postnatal transmission of HIV-1 infection.

Abacavir, Lamivudine, and Zidovudine: Lamivudine and zidovudine are excreted in human breast milk; abacavir and lamivudine are secreted into the milk of lactating rats.

Because of both the potential for HIV-1 transmission and the potential for serious adverse reactions in nursing infants, **mothers should be instructed not to breastfeed if they are receiving TRIZIVIR.**

Pediatric Use: TRIZIVIR is not intended for use in pediatric patients. TRIZIVIR should not be administered to adolescents who weigh less than 40 kg because it is a fixed-dose tablet that cannot be adjusted for this patient population.

Therapy-Experienced Pediatric Patients: A randomized, double-blind study, CNA3006, compared ZIAGEN plus lamivudine and zidovudine versus lamivudine and zidovudine in pediatric patients, most of whom were extensively pretreated with nucleoside analogue antiretroviral agents. Patients in this study had a limited response to abacavir.

Geriatric Use: Clinical studies of abacavir, lamivudine, and zidovudine did not include sufficient numbers of patients aged 65 and over to determine whether they respond differently from younger patients. In general, dose selection for an elderly patient should be cautious, reflecting the greater frequency of decreased hepatic, renal, or cardiac function, and of concomitant disease or other drug therapy. TRIZIVIR is not recommended for patients with impaired renal function (i.e., creatinine clearance <50 mL/min; see PRECAUTIONS: Patients with Impaired Renal Function and DOSAGE AND ADMINISTRATION).

ADVERSE REACTIONS

Hypersensitivity Reaction: Serious and sometimes fatal hypersensitivity reactions have been associated with abacavir sulfate, a component of TRIZIVIR (see WARNINGS and PRECAUTIONS: Information for Patients).

Treatment-emergent clinical adverse reactions (rated by the investigator as moderate or severe) with a ≥5% frequency during therapy with abacavir 300 mg twice daily, lamivudine 150 mg twice daily, and zidovudine 300 mg twice daily compared with indinavir 800 mg 3 times daily, lamivudine 150 mg twice daily, and zidovudine 300 mg twice daily from CNA3005 are listed in Table 5.

Table 5. Treatment-Emergent (All Causality) Adverse Reactions of at Least Moderate Intensity (Grades 2-4, ≥5% Frequency) in Therapy-Naive Adults (CNA3005) Through 48 Weeks of Treatment

Adverse Reaction	ZIAGEN plus Lamivudine/Zidovudine (n = 262)	Indinavir plus Lamivudine/Zidovudine (n = 264)
Nausea	19%	17%
Headache	13%	9%
Malaise and fatigue	12%	12%
Nausea and vomiting	10%	10%
Hypersensitivity reaction	8%	2%
Diarrhea	7%	5%
Fever and/or chills	6%	3%
Depressive disorders	6%	4%
Musculoskeletal pain	5%	7%
Skin rashes	5%	4%
Ear/nose/throat infections	5%	4%
Viral respiratory infections	5%	5%
Anxiety	5%	3%
Renal signs/symptoms	<1%	5%
Pain (non-site-specific)	<1%	5%

Five patients receiving abacavir in study CNA3005 experienced worsening of pre-existing depression compared to none in the indinavir arm. The background rates of pre-existing depression were similar in the 2 treatment arms.
Laboratory Abnormalities: Laboratory abnormalities in study CNA3005 are listed in Table 6.
[See table 6 above]
Other Adverse Events: In addition to adverse reactions in Tables 5 and 6, other adverse events observed in the expanded access program for abacavir were pancreatitis and increased GGT.
Observed During Clinical Practice: The following events have been identified during post-approval use of abacavir, lamivudine, and/or zidovudine. Because they are reported voluntarily from a population of unknown size, estimates of frequency cannot be made. These events have been chosen for inclusion due to a combination of their seriousness, frequency of reporting, or potential causal connection to lamivudine and/or zidovudine.
Abacavir:
Cardiovascular: Myocardial infarction.
Skin: Suspected Stevens-Johnson syndrome (SJS) and toxic epidermal necrolysis (TEN) have been reported in patients receiving abacavir primarily in combination with medications known to be associated with SJS and TEN, respectively. Because of the overlap of clinical signs and symptoms between hypersensitivity to abacavir and SJS and TEN, and the possibility of multiple drug sensitivities in some patients, abacavir should be discontinued and not restarted in such cases.
There have also been reports of erythema multiforme with abacavir use.
Abacavir, Lamivudine, and/or Zidovudine:
Body as a Whole: Redistribution/accumulation of body fat (see PRECAUTIONS: Fat Redistribution).
Cardiovascular: Cardiomyopathy.
Digestive: Stomatitis.
Endocrine and Metabolic: Gynecomastia, hyperglycemia.
Gastrointestinal: Anorexia and/or decreased appetite, abdominal pain, dyspepsia, oral mucosal pigmentation.
General: Vasculitis, weakness.
Hemic and Lymphatic: Aplastic anemia, anemia (including pure red cell aplasia and severe anemias progressing on therapy), lymphadenopathy, splenomegaly, thrombocytopenia.
Hepatic and Pancreatic: Lactic acidosis and hepatic steatosis, elevated bilirubin, elevated transaminases, pancreatitis, posttreatment exacerbation of hepatitis B (see WARNINGS).
Hypersensitivity: Sensitization reactions (including anaphylaxis), urticaria.
Musculoskeletal: Arthralgia, myalgia, muscle weakness, CPK elevation, rhabdomyolysis.
Nervous: Dizziness, paresthesia, peripheral neuropathy, seizures.
Psychiatric: Insomnia and other sleep disorders.
Respiratory: Abnormal breath sounds/wheezing.
Skin: Alopecia, erythema multiforme, Stevens-Johnson syndrome.

OVERDOSAGE

Abacavir: There is no known antidote for abacavir. It is not known whether abacavir can be removed by peritoneal dialysis or hemodialysis.

Table 6. Treatment-Emergent Laboratory Abnormalities (Grades 3-4) in Study CNA3005

	Number of Subjects by Treatment Group	
Grade 3/4 Laboratory Abnormalities	ZIAGEN plus Lamivudine/Zidovudine (n = 262)	Indinavir plus Lamivudine/Zidovudine (n = 264)
Elevated CPK (>4 × ULN)	18 (7%)	18 (7%)
ALT (>5.0 × ULN)	16 (6%)	16 (6%)
Neutropenia (<750/mm^3)	13 (5%)	13 (5%)
Hypertriglyceridemia (>750 mg/dL)	5 (2%)	3 (1%)
Hyperamylasemia (>2.0 × ULN)	5 (2%)	1 (<1%)
Hyperglycemia (>13.9 mmol/L)	2 (<1%)	2 (<1%)
Anemia (Hgb ≤6.9 g/dL)	0 (0%)	3 (1%)

ULN = Upper limit of normal.
n = Number of patients assessed.

Lamivudine: One case of an adult ingesting 6 grams of lamivudine was reported; there were no clinical signs or symptoms noted and hematologic tests remained normal. Because a negligible amount of lamivudine was removed via (4-hour) hemodialysis, continuous ambulatory peritoneal dialysis, and automated peritoneal dialysis, it is not known if continuous hemodialysis would provide clinical benefit in a lamivudine overdose event.
Zidovudine: Acute overdoses of zidovudine have been reported in pediatric patients and adults. These involved exposures up to 50 grams. The only consistent findings were nausea and vomiting. Other reported occurrences included headache, dizziness, drowsiness, lethargy, and confusion. Hematologic changes were transient. All patients recovered. Hemodialysis and peritoneal dialysis appear to have a negligible effect on the removal of zidovudine, while elimination of its primary metabolite, GZDV, is enhanced.

DOSAGE AND ADMINISTRATION

A Medication Guide and Warning Card that provide information about recognition of hypersensitivity reactions should be dispensed with each new prescription and refill. To facilitate reporting of hypersensitivity reactions and collection of information on each case, an Abacavir Hypersensitivity Registry has been established. Physicians should register patients by calling 1-800-270-0425.
The recommended oral dose of TRIZIVIR for adults and adolescents is 1 tablet twice daily. TRIZIVIR is not recommended in adolescents who weigh less than 40 kg because it is a fixed-dose tablet.
Dose Adjustment: Because it is a fixed-dose tablet, TRIZIVIR should not be prescribed for patients requiring dosage adjustment such as those with creatinine clearance <50 mL/min, patients with hepatic impairment, or patients experiencing dose-limiting adverse events.

HOW SUPPLIED

TRIZIVIR is available as tablets. Each tablet contains 300 mg of abacavir as abacavir sulfate, 150 mg of lamivudine, and 300 mg of zidovudine. The tablets are blue-green capsule-shaped, film-coated, and imprinted with GX LL1 on one side with no markings on the reverse side. They are packaged as follows:
Bottles of 60 Tablets (NDC 0173-0691-00).
Store at 25°C (77°F); excursions permitted to 15° to 30°C (59° to 86°F) (see USP Controlled Room Temperature).

ANIMAL TOXICOLOGY

Myocardial degeneration was found in mice and rats following administration of abacavir for 2 years. The systemic exposures were equivalent to 7 to 24 times the expected systemic exposure in humans. The clinical relevance of this finding has not been determined.

REFERENCE

1. Data Collection on Adverse Events of Anti-HIV Drugs (D:A:D) Study Group. *Lancet.* 2008;371 (9622): 1417-1426.

MEDICATION GUIDE

TRIZIVIR® (TRY-zih-veer) Tablets
Generic name: abacavir (uh-BACK-ah-veer) sulfate, lamivudine (la-MIV-yoo-deen), and zidovudine (zahy-doh-vyoo-deen)
Read the Medication Guide that comes with TRIZIVIR before you start taking it and each time you get a refill because there may be new information. This information does not take the place of talking to your doctor about your medical condition or your treatment. Be sure to carry your TRIZIVIR Warning Card with you at all times.
What is the most important information I should know about TRIZIVIR?
• **Serious Allergic Reaction to Abacavir.** TRIZIVIR contains abacavir (also contained in ZIAGEN® and EPZICOM®). Patients taking TRIZIVIR may have a serious allergic re-

action (hypersensitivity reaction) that can cause death. **Your risk of this allergic reaction is much higher if you have a gene variation called HLA-B*5701 than if you do not. Your doctor can determine with a blood test if you have this gene variation. If you get a symptom from 2 or more of the following groups while taking TRIZIVIR, call your doctor right away to determine if you should stop taking this medicine.**

	Symptom(s)
Group 1	Fever
Group 2	Rash
Group 3	Nausea, vomiting, diarrhea, abdominal (stomach area) pain
Group 4	Generally ill feeling, extreme tiredness, or achiness
Group 5	Shortness of breath, cough, sore throat

A list of these symptoms is on the Warning Card your pharmacist gives you. Carry this Warning Card with you. **If you stop TRIZIVIR because of an allergic reaction, NEVER take TRIZIVIR (abacavir sulfate, lamivudine, and zidovudine) or any other abacavir-containing medicine (ZIAGEN, EPZICOM) again.** If you take TRIZIVIR or any other abacavir-containing medicine again after you have had an allergic reaction, **WITHIN HOURS** you may get **life-threatening symptoms** that may include **very low blood pressure** or **death.**
If you stop TRIZIVIR, for any other reason, even for a few days, and you are not allergic to TRIZIVIR, talk with your doctor before taking it again. Taking TRIZIVIR again can cause a serious or life-threatening reaction, even if you never had an allergic reaction to it before. If your doctor tells you that you can take TRIZIVIR again, **start taking it when you are around medical help or people who can call a doctor if you need one.**
• **Blood problems.** RETROVIR®, one of the medicines in TRIZIVIR, can cause serious blood cell problems. These include reduced numbers of white blood cells (neutropenia) and extremely reduced numbers of red blood cells (anemia). These blood cell problems are especially likely to happen in patients with advanced human immunodeficiency virus (HIV) disease or AIDS. Your doctor should be checking your blood cell counts regularly while you are taking TRIZIVIR. This is especially important if you have advanced HIV or AIDS. This is to make sure that any blood cell problems are found quickly.
• **Lactic Acidosis. Some HIV medicines, including TRIZIVIR, can cause a rare but serious condition called lactic acidosis with liver enlargement (hepatomegaly).** Nausea and tiredness that don't get better may be symptoms of lactic acidosis. In some cases this condition can cause death. Women, overweight people, and people who have taken HIV medicines like TRIZIVIR for a long time have a higher chance of getting lactic acidosis and liver enlargement. Lactic acidosis is a medical emergency and must be treated in the hospital.
• **Worsening of hepatitis B virus (HBV) infection.** Patients with HBV infection who take TRIZIVIR and then stop it, may get "flare-ups" of their hepatitis. "Flare-up" is when the disease suddenly returns in a worse way than before. If you have HBV infection, your doctor should closely monitor your liver function for several months after stopping TRIZIVIR. You may need to take anti-HBV medicines.
• **Muscle weakness (myopathy).** RETROVIR, one of the medicines in TRIZIVIR, can cause muscle weakness. This can be a serious problem.

- Use with interferon- and ribavirin-based regimens. Worsening of liver disease (sometimes resulting in death) has occurred in patients infected with both HIV and hepatitis C virus who are taking anti-HIV medicines and are also being treated for hepatitis C with interferon with or without ribavirin. If you are taking TRIZIVIR as well as interferon with or without ribavirin and you experience side effects, be sure to tell your doctor.

TRIZIVIR can have other serious side effects. Be sure to read the section below entitled "What are the possible side effects of TRIZIVIR?"

What is TRIZIVIR?
TRIZIVIR is a prescription medicine used to treat HIV infection. TRIZIVIR includes 3 medicines: ZIAGEN (abacavir), EPIVIR® (lamivudine or 3TC), and RETROVIR® (zidovudine, AZT, or ZDV). See the end of this Medication Guide for a complete list of ingredients in TRIZIVIR. All 3 of these medicines are called nucleoside analogue reverse transcriptase inhibitors (NRTIs). When used together, they help lower the amount of HIV in your blood. This helps to keep your immune system as healthy as possible so it can fight infection.

Different combinations of medicines are used to treat HIV infection. You and your doctor should discuss which combination of medicines is best for you.

- **TRIZIVIR does not cure HIV infection or AIDS.** We do not know if TRIZIVIR will help you live longer or have fewer of the medical problems that people get with HIV or AIDS. It is very important that you see your doctor regularly while you are taking TRIZIVIR.
- **TRIZIVIR does not lower the risk of passing HIV to other people through sexual contact, sharing needles, or being exposed to your blood.** For your health and the health of others, it is important to always practice safe sex by using a latex or polyurethane condom or other barrier method to lower the chance of sexual contact with semen, vaginal secretions, or blood. Never use or share dirty needles.

Who should not take TRIZIVIR?
Do not take TRIZIVIR if you:
- have ever had a serious allergic reaction (a hypersensitivity reaction) to TRIZIVIR or any other medicine (ZIAGEN, EPZICOM) that has abacavir as an ingredient. See the end of this Medication Guide for a complete list of ingredients in TRIZIVIR.
- have a liver that does not function properly
- are an adolescent who weighs less than 90 pounds.

Before starting TRIZIVIR, tell your doctor about all your medical problems, including if you:
- have been tested and know whether or not you have a particular gene variation called HLA-B*5701.
- are pregnant or planning to become pregnant. We do not know if TRIZIVIR will harm your unborn child. You and your doctor will need to decide if TRIZIVIR is right for you. If you use TRIZIVIR while you are pregnant, talk to your doctor about how you can be on the Antiviral Pregnancy Registry for TRIZIVIR.
- are breastfeeding. Some of the ingredients in TRIZIVIR can be passed to your baby in your breast milk. It is not known if they could harm your baby. Also, mothers with HIV should not breastfeed because HIV can be passed to the baby in the breast milk.
- have liver problems including hepatitis B virus infection.
- have kidney problems.
- have low blood cell counts (bone marrow problem). Ask your doctor if you are not sure.
- have heart problems, smoke, or suffer from diseases that increase your risk of heart disease such as high blood pressure, high cholesterol, or diabetes.

Tell your doctor about all the medicines you take, including prescription and nonprescription medicines, vitamins, and herbal supplements. Especially tell your doctor if you take any of the following medicines*:
- methadone
- trimethoprim (TMP/sulfamethoxazole [SMX] [BACTRIM®, SEPTRA®])
- ganciclovir (CYTOVENE®, DHPG)
- interferon-alfa
- doxorubicin (ADRIAMYCIN®)
- ribavirin (COPEGUS®, REBETOL®, VIRAZOLE®)
- any bone marrow suppressive medicines or cytotoxic medicines. Ask your doctor if you are not sure.
- any of the following anti-HIV medicines: COMBIVIR® (lamivudine and zidovudine), EMTRIVA® (emtricitabine), EPIVIR or EPIVIR-HBV® (lamivudine, 3TC), EPZICOM (abacavir sulfate and lamivudine), HIVID® (zalcitabine, ddC), RETROVIR (zidovudine, AZT, or ZDV), TRUVADA® (emtricitabine and tenofovir), ZERIT® (stavudine, d4T), or ZIAGEN (abacavir sulfate).

How should I take TRIZIVIR?
Take TRIZIVIR by mouth exactly as your doctor prescribes it. The usual dosage is 1 tablet twice a day. Do not skip doses.
- You can take TRIZIVIR with or without food.

- If you miss a dose of TRIZIVIR, take the missed dose right away. Then, take the next dose at the usual scheduled time.
- Do not let your TRIZIVIR run out. If you stop your anti-HIV medicines, even for a short time, the amount of virus in your blood may increase and the virus may become harder to treat.
- Starting TRIZIVIR again can cause a serious allergic reaction or life-threatening reaction, even if you have never had an allergic reaction to it before. If you run out of TRIZIVIR even for a few days, you must ask your doctor if you can start TRIZIVIR again. If your doctor tells you that you can take TRIZIVIR again, start taking it when you are around medical help or people who can call a doctor if you need one.
- If you take too much TRIZIVIR, call your doctor or poison control center right away.

What should I avoid while taking TRIZIVIR?
Do not take COMBIVIR (lamivudine and zidovudine), EPIVIR (lamivudine, 3TC), EPZICOM (abacavir sulfate and lamivudine), RETROVIR (zidovudine, AZT, or ZDV), or ZIAGEN (abacavir sulfate) while taking TRIZIVIR. These medicines are already in TRIZIVIR.

Avoid doing things that can spread HIV infection, as TRIZIVIR does not stop you from passing the HIV infection to others.
- Do not share needles or other injection equipment.
- Do not share personal items that can have blood or body fluids on them, like toothbrushes and razor blades.
- Do not have any kind of sex without protection. Always practice safe sex by using a latex or polyurethane condom or other barrier method to lower the chance of sexual contact with semen, vaginal secretions, or blood.
- Do not breastfeed. Some of the medicines in TRIZIVIR can be passed to babies in breast milk and could harm the baby. Also, mothers with HIV should not breastfeed because HIV can be passed to the baby in the breast milk.

What are the possible side effects of TRIZIVIR?
TRIZIVIR can cause the following serious side effects. See "What is the most important information I should know about TRIZIVIR?" at the beginning of this Medication Guide.
- Serious allergic reaction that can cause death.
- Lactic acidosis with liver enlargement (hepatomegaly) that can cause death.
- Worsening of HBV infection. (See "What is the most important information I should know about TRIZIVIR?" at the beginning of this Medication Guide.)
- Blood problems.
- Muscle weakness.
- Changes in immune system. When you start taking HIV medicines, your immune system may get stronger and could begin to fight infections that have been hidden in your body, such as pneumonia, herpes virus, or tuberculosis. If you have new symptoms after starting your HIV medicines, be sure to tell your doctor.
- Changes in body fat. These changes have happened in patients taking antiretroviral medicines like TRIZIVIR. The changes may include an increased amount of fat in the upper back and neck ("buffalo hump"), breast, and around the back, chest, and stomach area. Loss of fat from the legs, arms, and face may also happen. The cause and long-term health effects of these conditions are not known.

Some HIV medicines including TRIZIVIR may increase your risk of heart attack. If you have heart problems, smoke, or suffer from diseases that increase your risk of heart disease such as high blood pressure, high cholesterol, or diabetes, tell your doctor.

The most common adverse events (≥5%) of at least moderate intensity associated with the use of TRIZIVIR include nausea, headache, weakness or tiredness, vomiting, hypersensitivity reaction, diarrhea, fever and/or chills, depression, muscle and joint pain, skin rashes, ear/nose/throat infections, cold symptoms, and nervousness.

This list of side effects is not complete. Call your doctor for medical advice about side effects. You may report side effects to FDA at 1-800-FDA-1088.

How should I store TRIZIVIR?
- Store TRIZIVIR between 59° to 86°F (15° to 30°C).
- Keep TRIZIVIR and all medicines out of the reach of children.

General information for safe and effective use of TRIZIVIR
Medicines are sometimes prescribed for conditions that are not mentioned in Medication Guides. Do not use TRIZIVIR for a condition for which it was not prescribed. Do not give TRIZIVIR to other people, even if they have the same symptoms that you have. It may harm them.

This Medication Guide summarizes the most important information about TRIZIVIR. If you would like more information, talk with your doctor. You can ask your doctor or pharmacist for the information that is written for healthcare professionals or call 1-888-825-5249.

What are the ingredients in TRIZIVIR?
Active ingredients: abacavir sulfate, lamivudine, and zidovudine
Inactive ingredients: Each film-coated TRIZIVIR Tablet contains the inactive ingredients magnesium stearate, microcrystalline cellulose, and sodium starch glycolate. The tablets are coated with a film (OPADRY® green 03B11434) that is made of FD&C Blue No. 2, hypromellose, polyethylene glycol, titanium dioxide, and yellow iron oxide.
This Medication Guide has been approved by the US Food and Drug Administration.
March 2009
TRZ:1MG

COMBIVIR, EPIVIR, EPZICOM, RETROVIR, TRIZIVIR, and ZIAGEN are registered trademarks of GlaxoSmithKline.

*The brands listed are trademarks of their respective owners and are not trademarks of GlaxoSmithKline. The makers of these brands are not affiliated with and do not endorse GlaxoSmithKline or its products.

GlaxoSmithKline
Research Triangle Park, NC 27709
Lamivudine is manufactured under agreement from
Shire Pharmaceuticals Group plc
Basingstoke, UK
©2009, GlaxoSmithKline. All rights reserved.
March 2009
TRZ:1PI

ZIAGEN®
[zī'ə-jin]
(abacavir sulfate)
Tablets and Oral Solution   ℞

HIGHLIGHTS OF PRESCRIBING INFORMATION
These highlights do not include all the information needed to use ZIAGEN safely and effectively. See full prescribing information for ZIAGEN.
ZIAGEN® (abacavir sulfate) Tablets and Oral Solution
Initial U.S. Approval: 1998

> **WARNING: HYPERSENSITIVITY REACTIONS/LACTIC ACIDOSIS AND SEVERE HEPATOMEGALY**
> *See full prescribing information for complete boxed warning.*
> - Serious and sometimes fatal hypersensitivity reactions have been associated with ZIAGEN (abacavir sulfate). (5.1)
> - Hypersensitivity to abacavir is a multi-organ clinical syndrome. (5.1)
> - Patients who carry the HLA-B*5701 allele are at high risk for experiencing a hypersensitivity reaction to abacavir. (5.1)
> - Discontinue ZIAGEN as soon as a hypersensitivity reaction is suspected. Regardless of HLA-B*5701 status, permanently discontinue ZIAGEN if hypersensitivity cannot be ruled out, even when other diagnoses are possible. (5.1)
> - Following a hypersensitivity reaction to abacavir, NEVER restart ZIAGEN or any other abacavir-containing product. (5.1)
> - Lactic acidosis and severe hepatomegaly with steatosis, including fatal cases, have been reported with the use of nucleoside analogues. (5.2)

——RECENT MAJOR CHANGES——

Boxed Warning	July 2008
Dosage and Administration (2.2)	December 2008
Warnings and Precautions (5.1, 5.5)	July 2008

——INDICATIONS AND USAGE——
ZIAGEN, a nucleoside analogue, is indicated in combination with other antiretroviral agents for the treatment of HIV-1 infection. (1)
——DOSAGE AND ADMINISTRATION——
- A medication guide and warning card should be dispensed with each new prescription and refill. (2)
- Adults: 600 mg daily, administered as either 300 mg twice daily or 600 mg once daily. (2.1)
- Pediatric Patients Aged 3 Months and Older: Dose should be calculated on body weight (kg) and should not exceed 300 mg twice daily. (2.2)
- Patients With Hepatic Impairment: Mild hepatic impairment – 200 mg twice daily; moderate/severe hepatic impairment – contraindicated. (2.3)
——DOSAGE FORMS AND STRENGTHS——
Tablets: 300 mg, scored; Oral Solution: 20 mg/mL (3)
——CONTRAINDICATIONS——
- Previously demonstrated hypersensitivity to abacavir. (4, 5.1)
- Moderate or severe hepatic impairment. (4)

WARNINGS AND PRECAUTIONS

- Hypersensitivity: Serious and sometimes fatal hypersensitivity reactions have been associated with ZIAGEN and other abacavir-containing products. Read full prescribing information section 5.1 before prescribing ZIAGEN. (5.1)
- Lactic acidosis and severe hepatomegaly with steatosis have been reported with the use of nucleoside analogues. (5.2)
- Immune reconstitution syndrome (5.3) and redistribution/accumulation of body fat have been reported in patients treated with combination antiretroviral therapy. (5.4)

ADVERSE REACTIONS

- The most commonly reported adverse reactions of at least moderate intensity (incidence ≥10%) in adult HIV-1 clinical studies were nausea, headache, malaise and fatigue, nausea and vomiting, and dreams/sleep disorders. (6.1)
- The most commonly reported adverse reactions of at least moderate intensity (incidence ≥5%) in pediatric HIV-1 clinical studies were fever and/or chills, nausea and vomiting, skin rashes, and ear/nose/throat infections. (6.1)

To report SUSPECTED ADVERSE REACTIONS, contact GlaxoSmithKline at 1-888-825-5249 or FDA at 1-800-FDA-1088 or www.fda.gov/medwatch.

DRUG INTERACTIONS

- Ethanol: Decreases elimination of abacavir. (7)
- Methadone: An increased methadone dose may be required in a small number of patients. (7)

Revised: December 2008
ZGN:2PI

See 17 for PATIENT COUNSELING INFORMATION and Medication Guide

Revised: 06/2009

FULL PRESCRIBING INFORMATION: CONTENTS*

WARNING: RISK OF HYPERSENSITIVITY REACTIONS, LACTIC ACIDOSIS, AND SEVERE HEPATOMEGALY

* Sections or subsections omitted from the full prescribing information are not listed

FULL PRESCRIBING INFORMATION

WARNING: RISK OF HYPERSENSITIVITY REACTIONS, LACTIC ACIDOSIS, AND SEVERE HEPATOMEGALY

Serious and sometimes fatal hypersensitivity reactions have been associated with ZIAGEN (abacavir sulfate). Hypersensitivity to abacavir is a multi-organ clinical syndrome usually characterized by a sign or symptom in 2 or more of the following groups: (1) fever, (2) rash, (3) gastrointestinal (including nausea, vomiting, diarrhea, or abdominal pain), (4) constitutional (including generalized malaise, fatigue, or achiness), and (5) respiratory (including dyspnea, cough, or pharyngitis). Discontinue ZIAGEN as soon as a hypersensitivity reaction is suspected.

Patients who carry the HLA-B*5701 allele are at high risk for experiencing a hypersensitivity reaction to abacavir. Prior to initiating therapy with abacavir, screening for the HLA-B*5701 allele is recommended; this approach has been found to decrease the risk of hypersensitivity reaction. Screening is also recommended prior to reinitiation of abacavir in patients of unknown HLA-B*5701 status who have previously tolerated abacavir. HLA-B*5701-negative patients may develop a suspected hypersensitivity reaction to abacavir; however, this occurs significantly less frequently than in HLA-B*5701-positive patients.

Regardless of HLA-B*5701 status, permanently discontinue ZIAGEN if hypersensitivity cannot be ruled out, even when other diagnoses are possible.

Following a hypersensitivity reaction to abacavir, NEVER restart ZIAGEN or any other abacavir-containing product because more severe symptoms can occur within hours and may include life-threatening hypotension and death.

Reintroduction of ZIAGEN or any other abacavir-containing product, even in patients who have no identified history or unrecognized symptoms of hypersensitivity to abacavir therapy, can result in serious or fatal hypersensitivity reactions. Such reactions can occur within hours [see Warnings and Precautions (5.1)].

Lactic acidosis and severe hepatomegaly with steatosis, including fatal cases, have been reported with the use of nucleoside analogues alone or in combination, including ZIAGEN and other antiretrovirals [see Warnings and Precautions (5.2)].

1 INDICATIONS AND USAGE

ZIAGEN Tablets and Oral Solution, in combination with other antiretroviral agents, are indicated for the treatment of human immunodeficiency virus (HIV-1) infection.

Additional important information on the use of ZIAGEN for treatment of HIV-1 infection:

- ZIAGEN is one of multiple products containing abacavir. Before starting ZIAGEN, review medical history for prior exposure to any abacavir-containing product in order to avoid reintroduction in a patient with a history of hypersensitivity to abacavir.

2 DOSAGE AND ADMINISTRATION

- A Medication Guide and Warning Card that provide information about recognition of hypersensitivity reactions should be dispensed with each new prescription and refill. To facilitate reporting of hypersensitivity reactions and collection of information on each case, an Abacavir Hypersensitivity Registry has been established. Physicians should register patients by calling 1-800-270-0425.
- ZIAGEN may be taken with or without food.

2.1 Adult Patients

The recommended oral dose of ZIAGEN for adults is 600 mg daily, administered as either 300 mg twice daily or 600 mg once daily, in combination with other antiretroviral agents.

2.2 Pediatric Patients

The recommended oral dose of ZIAGEN Oral Solution in HIV-1-infected pediatric patients aged 3 months and older is 8 mg/kg twice daily (up to a maximum of 300 mg twice daily) in combination with other antiretroviral agents.

ZIAGEN is also available as a scored tablet for HIV-1-infected pediatric patients weighing greater than or equal to 14 kg for whom a solid dosage form is appropriate. Before prescribing ZIAGEN Tablets, children should be assessed for the ability to swallow tablets. If a child is unable to reliably swallow ZIAGEN Tablets, the oral solution formulation should be prescribed. The recommended oral dosage of ZIAGEN Tablets for HIV-1-infected pediatric patients is presented in Table 1.

[See table above]

Table 1. Dosing Recommendations for ZIAGEN Tablets in Pediatric Patients

Weight (kg)	Dosage Regimen Using Scored Tablet		Total Daily Dose
	AM Dose	PM Dose	
14 to 21	½ tablet (150 mg)	½ tablet (150 mg)	300 mg
>21 to <30	½ tablet (150 mg)	1 tablet (300 mg)	450 mg
≥30	1 tablet (300 mg)	1 tablet (300 mg)	600 mg

2.3 Patients with Hepatic Impairment

The recommended dose of ZIAGEN in patients with mild hepatic impairment (Child-Pugh score 5 to 6) is 200 mg twice daily. To enable dose reduction, ZIAGEN Oral Solution (10 mL twice daily) should be used for the treatment of these patients. The safety, efficacy, and pharmacokinetic properties of abacavir have not been established in patients with moderate to severe hepatic impairment; therefore, ZIAGEN is contraindicated in these patients.

3 DOSAGE FORMS AND STRENGTHS

ZIAGEN Tablets, containing abacavir sulfate equivalent to 300 mg abacavir, are yellow, biconvex, scored, capsule-shaped, film-coated, and imprinted with "GX 623" on both sides.

ZIAGEN Oral Solution, each mL containing abacavir sulfate equivalent to 20 mg of abacavir, is a clear to opalescent, yellowish, strawberry-banana-flavored liquid.

4 CONTRAINDICATIONS

ZIAGEN is contraindicated in patients with previously demonstrated hypersensitivity to abacavir or any other component of the products. NEVER restart ZIAGEN or any other abacavir-containing product following a hypersensitivity reaction to abacavir, regardless of HLA-B*5701 status [see Warnings and Precautions (5.1), Adverse Reactions (6)]. ZIAGEN is contraindicated in patients with moderate or severe hepatic impairment.

5 WARNINGS AND PRECAUTIONS

5.1 Hypersensitivity Reaction

Serious and sometimes fatal hypersensitivity reactions have been associated with ZIAGEN and other abacavir-containing products. Patients who carry the HLA-B*5701 allele are at high risk for experiencing a hypersensitivity reaction to abacavir. Prior to initiating therapy with abacavir, screening for the HLA-B*5701 allele is recommended; this approach has been found to decrease the risk of a hypersensitivity reaction. Screening is also recommended prior to reinitiation of abacavir in patients of unknown HLA-B*5701 status who have previously tolerated abacavir. For HLA-B*5701-positive patients, treatment with an abacavir-containing regimen is not recommended and should be considered only with close medical supervision and under exceptional circumstances when the potential benefit outweighs the risk.

HLA-B*5701-negative patients may develop a hypersensitivity reaction to abacavir; however, this occurs significantly less frequently than in HLA-B*5701-positive patients. Regardless of HLA-B*5701 status, permanently discontinue ZIAGEN if hypersensitivity cannot be ruled out, even when other diagnoses are possible.

Important information on signs and symptoms of hypersensitivity, as well as clinical management, is presented below.

Signs and Symptoms of Hypersensitivity: Hypersensitivity to abacavir is a multi-organ clinical syndrome usually characterized by a sign or symptom in 2 or more of the following groups.

Group 1: Fever

Group 2: Rash

Group 3: Gastrointestinal (including nausea, vomiting, diarrhea, or abdominal pain)

Group 4: Constitutional (including generalized malaise, fatigue, or achiness)

Group 5: Respiratory (including dyspnea, cough, or pharyngitis)

Hypersensitivity to abacavir following the presentation of a single sign or symptom has been reported infrequently.

Hypersensitivity to abacavir was reported in approximately 8% of 2,670 patients (n = 206) in 9 clinical trials (range: 2% to 9%) with enrollment from November 1999 to February 2002. Data on time to onset and symptoms of suspected hypersensitivity were collected on a detailed data collection module. The frequencies of symptoms are shown in Figure 1. Symptoms usually appeared within the first 6 weeks of treatment with abacavir, although the reaction may occur at any time during therapy. Median time to onset was 9 days; 89% appeared within the first 6 weeks; 95% of patients reported symptoms from 2 or more of the 5 groups listed above.

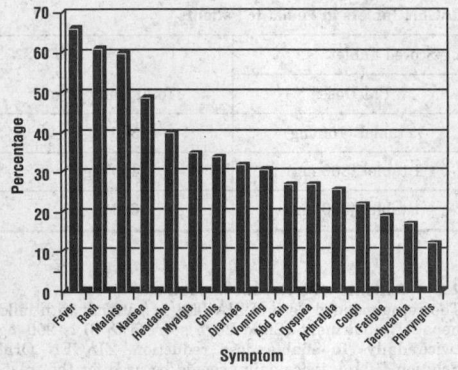

Figure 1. Hypersensitivity-Related Symptoms Reported With ≥10% Frequency in Clinical Trials (n = 206 Patients)

Other less common signs and symptoms of hypersensitivity include lethargy, myolysis, edema, abnormal chest x-ray findings (predominantly infiltrates, which can be localized), and paresthesia. Anaphylaxis, liver failure, renal failure, hypotension, adult respiratory distress syndrome, respiratory failure, and death have occurred in association with hypersensitivity reactions. In one study, 4 patients (11%) receiving ZIAGEN 600 mg once daily experienced hypotension with a hypersensitivity reaction compared with 0 patients receiving ZIAGEN 300 mg twice daily.

Physical findings associated with hypersensitivity to abacavir in some patients include lymphadenopathy, mucous membrane lesions (conjunctivitis and mouth ulcerations), and rash. The rash usually appears maculopapular or urticarial, but may be variable in appearance. There have been reports of erythema multiforme. Hypersensitivity reactions have occurred without rash.

Laboratory abnormalities associated with hypersensitivity to abacavir in some patients include elevated liver function tests, elevated creatine phosphokinase, elevated creatinine, and lymphopenia.

Clinical Management of Hypersensitivity: Discontinue ZIAGEN as soon as a hypersensitivity reaction is suspected. To minimize the risk of a life-threatening hypersensitivity reaction, permanently discontinue ZIAGEN if hypersensitivity cannot be ruled out, even when other diagnoses are possible (e.g., acute onset respiratory diseases such as pneumonia, bronchitis, pharyngitis, or influenza; gastroenteritis; or reactions to other medications).

Following a hypersensitivity reaction to abacavir, NEVER restart ZIAGEN or any other abacavir-containing product because more severe symptoms can occur within hours and may include life-threatening hypotension and death.

When therapy with ZIAGEN has been discontinued for reasons other than symptoms of a hypersensitivity reaction, and if reinitiation of ZIAGEN or any other abacavir-containing product is under consideration, carefully evaluate the reason for discontinuation of ZIAGEN to ensure that the patient did not have symptoms of a hypersensitivity reaction. If the patient is of unknown HLA-B*5701 status, screening for the allele is recommended prior to reinitiation of ZIAGEN.

If hypersensitivity cannot be ruled out, DO NOT reintroduce ZIAGEN or any other abacavir-containing product. Even in the absence of the HLA-B*5701 allele, it is important to permanently discontinue abacavir and not rechallenge with abacavir if a hypersensitivity reaction cannot be ruled out on clinical grounds, due to the potential for a severe or even fatal reaction.

If symptoms consistent with hypersensitivity are not identified, reintroduction can be undertaken with continued monitoring for symptoms of a hypersensitivity reaction. Make patients aware that a hypersensitivity reaction can occur with reintroduction of ZIAGEN or any other abacavir-containing product and that reintroduction of ZIAGEN or any other abacavir-containing product needs to be undertaken only if medical care can be readily accessed by the patient or others.

*Risk Factor: HLA-B*5701 Allele:* Studies have shown that carriage of the HLA-B*5701 allele is associated with a significantly increased risk of a hypersensitivity reaction to abacavir.

CNA106030 (PREDICT-1), a randomized, double-blind study, evaluated the clinical utility of prospective HLA-B*5701 screening on the incidence of abacavir hypersensitivity reaction in abacavir-naive HIV-1-infected adults (n = 1,650). In this study, use of pre-therapy screening for the HLA-B*5701 allele and exclusion of subjects with this allele reduced the incidence of clinically suspected abacavir hypersensitivity reactions from 7.8% (66/847) to 3.4% (27/803). Based on this study, it is estimated that 61% of patients with the HLA-B*5701 allele will develop a clini-

cally suspected hypersensitivity reaction during the course of abacavir treatment compared with 4% of patients who do not have the HLA-B*5701 allele.

Screening for carriage of the HLA-B*5701 allele is recommended prior to initiating treatment with abacavir. Screening is also recommended prior to reinitiation of abacavir in patients of unknown HLA-B*5701 status who have previously tolerated abacavir. For HLA-B*5701-positive patients, initiating or reinitiating treatment with an abacavir-containing regimen is not recommended and should be considered only with close medical supervision and under exceptional circumstances where potential benefit outweighs the risk.

Skin patch testing is used as a research tool and should not be used to aid in the clinical diagnosis of abacavir hypersensitivity.

In any patient treated with abacavir, the clinical diagnosis of hypersensitivity reaction must remain the basis of clinical decision-making. Even in the absence of the HLA-B*5701 allele, it is important to permanently discontinue abacavir and not rechallenge with abacavir if a hypersensitivity reaction cannot be ruled out on clinical grounds, due to the potential for a severe or even fatal reaction.

Abacavir Hypersensitivity Reaction Registry: An Abacavir Hypersensitivity Registry has been established to facilitate reporting of hypersensitivity reactions and collection of information on each case. Physicians should register patients by calling 1-800-270-0425.

5.2 Lactic Acidosis/Severe Hepatomegaly With Steatosis

Lactic acidosis and severe hepatomegaly with steatosis, including fatal cases, have been reported with the use of nucleoside analogues alone or in combination, including abacavir and other antiretrovirals. A majority of these cases have been in women. Obesity and prolonged nucleoside exposure may be risk factors. Particular caution should be exercised when administering ZIAGEN to any patient with known risk factors for liver disease; however, cases have also been reported in patients with no known risk factors. Treatment with ZIAGEN should be suspended in any patient who develops clinical or laboratory findings suggestive of lactic acidosis or pronounced hepatotoxicity (which may include hepatomegaly and steatosis even in the absence of marked transaminase elevations).

5.3 Immune Reconstitution Syndrome

Immune reconstitution syndrome has been reported in patients treated with combination antiretroviral therapy, including ZIAGEN. During the initial phase of combination antiretroviral treatment, patients whose immune systems respond may develop an inflammatory response to indolent or residual opportunistic infections (such as *Mycobacterium avium* infection, cytomegalovirus, *Pneumocystis jirovecii* pneumonia [PCP], or tuberculosis), which may necessitate further evaluation and treatment.

5.4 Fat Redistribution

Redistribution/accumulation of body fat including central obesity, dorsocervical fat enlargement (buffalo hump), peripheral wasting, facial wasting, breast enlargement, and "cushingoid appearance" have been observed in patients receiving antiretroviral therapy. The mechanism and long-term consequences of these events are currently unknown. A causal relationship has not been established.

5.5 Myocardial Infarction

In a published prospective, observational, epidemiological study designed to investigate the rate of myocardial infarction in patients on combination antiretroviral therapy, the use of abacavir within the previous 6 months was correlated with an increased risk of myocardial infarction (MI).[1] In a sponsor-conducted pooled analysis of clinical trials, no excess risk of myocardial infarction was observed in abacavir-treated subjects as compared with control subjects. In totality, the available data from the observational cohort and from clinical trials are inconclusive.

As a precaution, the underlying risk of coronary heart disease should be considered when prescribing antiretroviral therapies, including abacavir, and action taken to minimize all modifiable risk factors (e.g., hypertension, hyperlipidemia, diabetes mellitus, and smoking).

6   ADVERSE REACTIONS

• Serious and sometimes fatal hypersensitivity reactions have been associated with ZIAGEN (abacavir sulfate). In one study, once-daily dosing of ZIAGEN was associated with more severe hypersensitivity reactions *[see Warnings and Precautions (5.1)]*.

6.1 Clinical Trials Experience

Because clinical trials are conducted under widely varying conditions, adverse reaction rates observed in the clinical trials of a drug cannot be directly compared with rates in the clinical trials of another drug and may not reflect the rates observed in practice.

Adults: *Therapy-Naive Adults:* Treatment-emergent clinical adverse reactions (rated by the investigator as moderate or severe) with a greater than or equal to 5% frequency

during therapy with ZIAGEN 300 mg twice daily, lamivudine 150 mg twice daily, and efavirenz 600 mg daily compared with zidovudine 300 mg twice daily, lamivudine 150 mg twice daily, and efavirenz 600 mg daily from CNA30024 are listed in Table 2.

Table 2. Treatment-Emergent (All Causality) Adverse Reactions of at Least Moderate Intensity (Grades 2-4, ≥5% Frequency) in Therapy-Naive Adults (CNA30024*) Through 48 Weeks of Treatment

Adverse Reaction	ZIAGEN plus Lamivudine plus Efavirenz (n = 324)	Zidovudine plus Lamivudine plus Efavirenz (n = 325)
Dreams/sleep disorders	10%	10%[†]
Drug hypersensitivity	9%	<1%[†]
Headaches/migraine	7%	11%
Nausea	7%	11%
Fatigue/malaise	7%	10%
Diarrhea	7%	6%
Rashes	6%	12%
Abdominal pain/gastritis/ gastrointestinal signs and symptoms	6%	8%
Depressive disorders	6%	6%
Dizziness	6%	6%
Musculoskeletal pain	6%	5%
Bronchitis	4%	5%
Vomiting	2%	9%

* This study used double-blind ascertainment of suspected hypersensitivity reactions. During the blinded portion of the study, suspected hypersensitivity to abacavir was reported by investigators in 9% of 324 patients in the abacavir group and 3% of 325 patients in the zidovudine group.

[†] Ten (3%) cases of suspected drug hypersensitivity were reclassified as not being due to abacavir following unblinding.

Treatment-emergent clinical adverse reactions (rated by the investigator as moderate or severe) with a greater than or equal to 5% frequency during therapy with ZIAGEN 300 mg twice daily, lamivudine 150 mg twice daily, and zidovudine 300 mg twice daily compared with indinavir 800 mg 3 times daily, lamivudine 150 mg twice daily, and zidovudine 300 mg twice daily from CNA3005 are listed in Table 3.

Table 3. Treatment-Emergent (All Causality) Adverse Reactions of at Least Moderate Intensity (Grades 2-4, ≥5% Frequency) in Therapy-Naive Adults (CNA3005) Through 48 Weeks of Treatment

Adverse Reaction	ZIAGEN plus Lamivudine/ Zidovudine (n = 262)	Indinavir plus Lamivudine/ Zidovudine (n = 264)
Nausea	19%	17%
Headache	13%	9%
Malaise and fatigue	12%	12%
Nausea and vomiting	10%	10%
Hypersensitivity reaction	8%	2%
Diarrhea	7%	5%
Fever and/or chills	6%	3%
Depressive disorders	6%	4%
Musculoskeletal pain	5%	7%
Skin rashes	5%	4%
Ear/nose/throat infections	5%	4%
Viral respiratory infections	5%	5%
Anxiety	5%	3%
Renal signs/symptom	<1%	5%
Pain (non-site-specific)	<1%	5%

Five patients receiving ZIAGEN in CNA3005 experienced worsening of pre-existing depression compared with none in the indinavir arm. The background rates of pre-existing depression were similar in the 2 treatment arms.

ZIAGEN Once Daily Versus ZIAGEN Twice Daily (CNA30021): Treatment-emergent clinical adverse reactions (rated by the investigator as at least moderate) with a greater than or equal to 5% frequency during therapy with ZIAGEN 600 mg once daily or ZIAGEN 300 mg twice daily both in combination with lamivudine 300 mg once daily and efavirenz 600 mg once daily from CNA30021 were similar. For hypersensitivity reactions, patients receiving ZIAGEN once daily showed a rate of 9% in comparison with a rate of 7% for patients receiving ZIAGEN twice daily. However, patients receiving ZIAGEN 600 mg once daily, experienced a significantly higher incidence of severe drug hypersensitivity reactions and severe diarrhea compared with patients who received ZIAGEN 300 mg twice daily. Five percent (5%) of patients receiving ZIAGEN 600 mg once daily had severe drug hypersensitivity reactions compared with 2% of patients receiving ZIAGEN 300 mg twice daily. Two percent (2%) of patients receiving ZIAGEN 600 mg once daily had severe diarrhea while none of the patients receiving ZIAGEN 300 mg twice daily had this event.

Laboratory Abnormalities: Laboratory abnormalities (Grades 3-4) in therapy-naive adults during therapy with ZIAGEN 300 mg twice daily, lamivudine 150 mg twice daily, and efavirenz 600 mg daily compared with zidovudine 300 mg twice daily, lamivudine 150 mg twice daily, and efavirenz 600 mg daily from CNA30024 are listed in Table 4.

Table 4. Laboratory Abnormalities (Grades 3-4) in Therapy-Naive Adults (CNA30024) Through 48 Weeks of Treatment

Grade 3/4 Laboratory Abnormalities	ZIAGEN plus Lamivudine plus Efavirenz (n = 324)	Zidovudine plus Lamivudine plus Efavirenz (n = 325)
Elevated CPK (>4 × ULN)	8%	8%
Elevated ALT (>5 × ULN)	6%	6%
Elevated AST (>5 × ULN)	6%	5%
Hypertriglyceridemia (>750 mg/dL)	6%	5%
Hyperamylasemia (>2 × ULN)	4%	5%
Neutropenia (ANC <750/mm³)	2%	4%
Anemia (Hgb ≤6.9 gm/dL)	<1%	2%
Thrombocytopenia (Platelets <50,000/mm³)	1%	<1%
Leukopenia (WBC ≤1,500/mm³)	<1%	2%

ULN = Upper limit of normal.

n = Number of patients assessed.

Laboratory abnormalities in CNA3005 are listed in Table 5.

Table 5. Treatment-Emergent Laboratory Abnormalities (Grades 3-4) in CNA3005

Grade 3/4 Laboratory Abnormalities	ZIAGEN plus Lamivudine/ Zidovudine (n = 262)	Indinavir plus Lamivudine/ Zidovudine (n = 264)
Elevated CPK (>4 × ULN)	18 (7%)	18 (7%)
ALT (>5.0 × ULN)	16 (6%)	16 (6%)
Neutropenia (<750/mm³)	13 (5%)	13 (5%)
Hypertriglyceridemia (>750 mg/dL)	5 (2%)	3 (1%)
Hyperamylasemia (>2.0 × ULN)	5 (2%)	1 (<1%)
Hyperglycemia (>13.9 mmol/L)	2 (<1%)	2 (<1%)
Anemia (Hgb ≤6.9 g/dL)	0 (0%)	3 (1%)

ULN = Upper limit of normal.

n = Number of patients assessed.

The frequencies of treatment-emergent laboratory abnormalities were comparable between treatment groups in CNA30021.

Pediatric Patients: *Therapy-Experienced Pediatric Patients:* Treatment-emergent clinical adverse reactions (rated by the investigator as moderate or severe) with a greater than or equal to 5% frequency during therapy with ZIAGEN 8 mg/kg twice daily, lamivudine 4 mg/kg twice daily, and zidovudine 180 mg/m² twice daily compared with lamivudine 4 mg/kg twice daily and zidovudine 180 mg/m² twice daily from CNA3006 are listed in Table 6.

Table 6. Treatment-Emergent (All Causality) Adverse Reactions of at Least Moderate Intensity (Grades 2-4, ≥5% Frequency) in Therapy-Experienced Pediatric Patients (CNA3006) Through 16 Weeks of Treatment

Adverse Reaction	ZIAGEN plus Lamivudine plus Zidovudine (n = 102)	Lamivudine plus Zidovudine (n = 103)
Fever and/or chills	9%	7%
Nausea and vomiting	9%	2%
Skin rashes	7%	1%
Ear/nose/throat infections	5%	1%
Pneumonia	4%	5%
Headache	1%	5%

Laboratory Abnormalities: In Study CNA3006, laboratory abnormalities (anemia, neutropenia, liver function test abnormalities, and CPK elevations) were observed with similar frequencies as in a study of therapy-naive adults (CNA30024). Mild elevations of blood glucose were more frequent in pediatric patients receiving ZIAGEN (CNA3006) as compared with adult patients (CNA30024).

Other Adverse Events: In addition to adverse reactions and laboratory abnormalities reported in Tables 2, 3, 4, 5, and 6, other adverse reactions observed in the expanded access program were pancreatitis and increased GGT.

6.2 Postmarketing Experience

In addition to adverse reactions reported from clinical trials, the following reactions have been identified during postmarketing use of ZIAGEN. Because they are reported voluntarily from a population of unknown size, estimates of frequency cannot be made. These reactions have been chosen for inclusion due to a combination of their seriousness, frequency of reporting, or potential causal connection to ZIAGEN.

Body as a Whole: Redistribution/accumulation of body fat.
Cardiovascular: Myocardial infarction.
Hepatic: Lactic acidosis and hepatic steatosis.
Skin: Suspected Stevens-Johnson syndrome (SJS) and toxic epidermal necrolysis (TEN) have been reported in patients receiving abacavir primarily in combination with medications known to be associated with SJS and TEN, respectively. Because of the overlap of clinical signs and symptoms between hypersensitivity to abacavir and SJS and TEN, and the possibility of multiple drug sensitivities in some patients, abacavir should be discontinued and not restarted in such cases.
There have also been reports of erythema multiforme with abacavir use.

7   DRUG INTERACTIONS

Ethanol: Abacavir has no effect on the pharmacokinetic properties of ethanol. Ethanol decreases the elimination of abacavir causing an increase in overall exposure *[see Clinical Pharmacology (12.3)].*
Methadone: The addition of methadone has no clinically significant effect on the pharmacokinetic properties of abacavir. In a study of 11 HIV-1-infected patients receiving methadone-maintenance therapy with 600 mg of ZIAGEN twice daily (twice the currently recommended dose), oral methadone clearance increased *[see Clinical Pharmacology (12.3)].* This alteration will not result in a methadone dose modification in the majority of patients; however, an increased methadone dose may be required in a small number of patients.

8   USE IN SPECIFIC POPULATIONS

8.1   Pregnancy

Pregnancy Category C. Studies in pregnant rats showed that abacavir is transferred to the fetus through the placenta. Fetal malformations (increased incidences of fetal anasarca and skeletal malformations) and developmental toxicity (depressed fetal body weight and reduced crown-rump length) were observed in rats at a dose which produced 35 times the human exposure, based on AUC. Embryonic and fetal toxicities (increased resorptions, decreased fetal body weights) and toxicities to the offspring (increased incidence of stillbirth and lower body weights) occurred at half of the above-mentioned dose in separate fertility studies conducted in rats. In the rabbit, no developmental toxicity and no increases in fetal malformations occurred at doses that produced 8.5 times the human exposure at the recommended dose based on AUC.
There are no adequate and well-controlled studies in pregnant women. ZIAGEN should be used during pregnancy only if the potential benefits outweigh the risk.
Antiretroviral Pregnancy Registry: To monitor maternal-fetal outcomes of pregnant women exposed to ZIAGEN, an Antiretroviral Pregnancy Registry has been established. Physicians are encouraged to register patients by calling 1-800-258-4263.

8.3   Nursing Mothers

The Centers for Disease Control and Prevention recommend that HIV-1-infected mothers not breastfeed their infants to avoid risking postnatal transmission of HIV-1 infection. Although it is not known if abacavir is excreted in human milk, abacavir is secreted into the milk of lactating rats. Because of both the potential for HIV-1 transmission and the potential for serious adverse reactions in nursing infants, mothers should be instructed not to breastfeed if they are receiving ZIAGEN.

8.4   Pediatric Use

The safety and effectiveness of ZIAGEN have been established in pediatric patients 3 months to 13 years of age. Use of ZIAGEN in these age groups is supported by pharmacokinetic studies and evidence from adequate and well-controlled studies of ZIAGEN in adults and pediatric patients *[see Dosage and Administration (2.2), Clinical Pharmacology (12.3), Clinical Studies (14.2)].*

8.5   Geriatric Use

Clinical studies of ZIAGEN did not include sufficient numbers of patients aged 65 and over to determine whether they respond differently from younger patients. In general, dose selection for an elderly patient should be cautious, reflecting the greater frequency of decreased hepatic, renal, or cardiac function, and of concomitant disease or other drug therapy.

10   OVERDOSAGE

There is no known antidote for ZIAGEN. It is not known whether abacavir can be removed by peritoneal dialysis or hemodialysis.

11   DESCRIPTION

ZIAGEN is the brand name for abacavir sulfate, a synthetic carbocyclic nucleoside analogue with inhibitory activity against HIV-1. The chemical name of abacavir sulfate is (1S,cis)-4-[2-amino-6-(cyclopropylamino)-9H-purin-9-yl]-2-cyclopentene-1-methanol sulfate (salt) (2:1). Abacavir sulfate is the enantiomer with 1S, 4R absolute configuration on the cyclopentene ring. It has a molecular formula of $(C_{14}H_{16}N_6O)_2 \cdot H_2SO_4$ and a molecular weight of 670.76 daltons. It has the following structural formula:

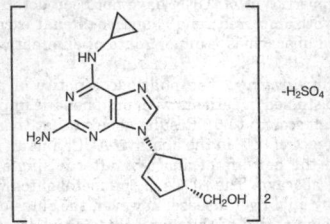

Abacavir sulfate is a white to off-white solid with a solubility of approximately 77 mg/mL in distilled water at 25°C. It has an octanol/water (pH 7.1 to 7.3) partition coefficient (log P) of approximately 1.20 at 25°C.
ZIAGEN Tablets are for oral administration. Each tablet contains abacavir sulfate equivalent to 300 mg of abacavir as active ingredient and the following inactive ingredients: colloidal silicon dioxide, magnesium stearate, microcrystalline cellulose, and sodium starch glycolate. The tablets are coated with a film that is made of hypromellose, polysorbate 80, synthetic yellow iron oxide, titanium dioxide, and triacetin.
ZIAGEN Oral Solution is for oral administration. Each milliliter (1 mL) of ZIAGEN Oral Solution contains abacavir sulfate equivalent to 20 mg of abacavir (i.e., 20 mg/mL) as active ingredient and the following inactive ingredients: artificial strawberry and banana flavors, citric acid (anhydrous), methylparaben and propylparaben (added as preservatives), propylene glycol, saccharin sodium, sodium citrate (dihydrate), sorbitol solution, and water.
In vivo, abacavir sulfate dissociates to its free base, abacavir. All dosages for ZIAGEN are expressed in terms of abacavir.

12   CLINICAL PHARMACOLOGY

12.1   Mechanism of Action

Abacavir is an antiviral agent *[See Clinical Pharmacology (12.4)].*

12.3   Pharmacokinetics

Pharmacokinetics in Adults: The pharmacokinetic properties of abacavir have been studied in asymptomatic, HIV-1-infected adult patients after administration of a single intravenous (IV) dose of 150 mg and after single and multiple oral doses. The pharmacokinetic properties of abacavir were independent of dose over the range of 300 to 1,200 mg/day.
Absorption and Bioavailability: Abacavir was rapidly and extensively absorbed after oral administration. The geometric mean absolute bioavailability of the tablet was 83%. After oral administration of 300 mg twice daily in 20 patients, the steady-state peak serum abacavir concentration (C_{max}) was 3.0 ± 0.89 mcg/mL (mean ± SD) and $AUC_{(0-12 \ hr)}$ was 6.02 ± 1.73 mcg•hr/mL. After oral administration of a

single dose of 600 mg of abacavir in 20 patients, C_{max} was 4.26 ± 1.19 mcg/mL (mean ± SD) and AUC_∞ was 11.95 ± 2.51 mcg•hr/mL.

Distribution: The apparent volume of distribution after IV administration of abacavir was 0.86 ± 0.15 L/kg, suggesting that abacavir distributes into extravascular space. In 3 subjects, the CSF $AUC_{(0\text{-}6\ hr)}$ to plasma abacavir $AUC_{(0\text{-}6\ hr)}$ ratio ranged from 27% to 33%.

Binding of abacavir to human plasma proteins is approximately 50%. Binding of abacavir to plasma proteins was independent of concentration. Total blood and plasma drug-related radioactivity concentrations are identical, demonstrating that abacavir readily distributes into erythrocytes.

Metabolism: In humans, abacavir is not significantly metabolized by cytochrome P450 enzymes. The primary routes of elimination of abacavir are metabolism by alcohol dehydrogenase (to form the 5′-carboxylic acid) and glucuronyl transferase (to form the 5′-glucuronide). The metabolites do not have antiviral activity. In vitro experiments reveal that abacavir does not inhibit human CYP3A4, CYP2D6, or CYP2C9 activity at clinically relevant concentrations.

Elimination: Elimination of abacavir was quantified in a mass balance study following administration of a 600-mg dose of ^{14}C-abacavir: 99% of the radioactivity was recovered, 1.2% was excreted in the urine as abacavir, 30% as the 5′-carboxylic acid metabolite, 36% as the 5′-glucuronide metabolite, and 15% as unidentified minor metabolites in the urine. Fecal elimination accounted for 16% of the dose.

In single-dose studies, the observed elimination half-life ($t_{1/2}$) was 1.54 ± 0.63 hours. After intravenous administration, total clearance was 0.80 ± 0.24 L/hr/kg (mean ± SD).

Effects of Food on Oral Absorption: Bioavailability of abacavir tablets was assessed in the fasting and fed states. There was no significant difference in systemic exposure (AUC_∞) in the fed and fasting states; therefore, ZIAGEN Tablets may be administered with or without food. Systemic exposure to abacavir was comparable after administration of ZIAGEN Oral Solution and ZIAGEN Tablets. Therefore, these products may be used interchangeably.

Special Populations: *Renal Impairment:* The pharmacokinetic properties of ZIAGEN have not been determined in patients with impaired renal function. Renal excretion of unchanged abacavir is a minor route of elimination in humans.

Hepatic Impairment: The pharmacokinetics of abacavir have been studied in patients with mild hepatic impairment (Child-Pugh score 5 to 6). Results showed that there was a mean increase of 89% in the abacavir AUC, and an increase of 58% in the half-life of abacavir after a single dose of 600 mg of abacavir. The AUCs of the metabolites were not modified by mild liver disease; however, the rates of formation and elimination of the metabolites were decreased. A dose of 200 mg (provided by 10 mL of ZIAGEN Oral Solution) administered twice daily is recommended for patients with mild liver disease. The safety, efficacy, and pharmacokinetics of abacavir have not been studied in patients with moderate or severe hepatic impairment, therefore ZIAGEN is contraindicated in these patients.

Pediatric Patients: The pharmacokinetics of abacavir have been studied after either single or repeat doses of ZIAGEN in 68 pediatric patients. Following multiple-dose administration of ZIAGEN 8 mg/kg twice daily, steady-state $AUC_{(0\text{-}12\ hr)}$ and C_{max} were 9.8 ± 4.56 mcg•hr/mL and 3.71 ± 1.36 mcg/mL (mean ± SD), respectively *[see Use in Specific Populations (8.4)]*. In addition, to support dosing of ZIAGEN scored tablet (300 mg) for pediatric patients 14 to greater than 30 kg, analysis of actual and simulated pharmacokinetic data indicated comparable exposures are expected following administration of 300 mg scored tablet and the 8 mg/kg dosing regimen using oral solution.

Geriatric Patients: The pharmacokinetics of ZIAGEN have not been studied in patients over 65 years of age.

Gender: A population pharmacokinetic analysis in HIV-1-infected male (n = 304) and female (n = 67) patients showed no gender differences in abacavir AUC normalized for lean body weight.

Race: There are no significant differences between blacks and Caucasians in abacavir pharmacokinetics.

Drug Interactions: In human liver microsomes, abacavir did not inhibit cytochrome P450 isoforms (2C9, 2D6, 3A4). Based on these data, it is unlikely that clinically significant drug interactions will occur between abacavir and drugs metabolized through these pathways.

Lamivudine and/or Zidovudine: Due to the common metabolic pathways of abacavir and zidovudine via glucuronyl transferase, 15 HIV-1-infected patients were enrolled in a crossover study evaluating single doses of abacavir (600 mg), lamivudine (150 mg), and zidovudine (300 mg) alone or in combination. Analysis showed no clinically relevant changes in the pharmacokinetics of abacavir with the addition of lamivudine or zidovudine or the combination of lamivudine and zidovudine. Lamivudine exposure (AUC decreased 15%) and zidovudine exposure (AUC increased 10%) did not show clinically relevant changes with concurrent abacavir.

Ethanol: Due to their common metabolic pathways via alcohol dehydrogenase, the pharmacokinetic interaction between abacavir and ethanol was studied in 24 HIV-1-infected male patients. Each patient received the following treatments on separate occasions: a single 600-mg dose of abacavir, 0.7 g/kg ethanol (equivalent to 5 alcoholic drinks), and abacavir 600 mg plus 0.7 g/kg ethanol. Coadministration of ethanol and abacavir resulted in a 41% increase in abacavir AUC_∞ and a 26% increase in abacavir $t_{1/2}$. In males, abacavir had no effect on the pharmacokinetic properties of ethanol, so no clinically significant interaction is expected in men. This interaction has not been studied in females.

Methadone: In a study of 11 HIV-1-infected patients receiving methadone-maintenance therapy (40 mg and 90 mg daily), with 600 mg of ZIAGEN twice daily (twice the currently recommended dose), oral methadone clearance increased 22% (90% CI 6% to 42%). This alteration will not result in a methadone dose modification in the majority of patients; however, an increased methadone dose may be required in a small number of patients. The addition of methadone had no clinically significant effect on the pharmacokinetic properties of abacavir.

12.4 Microbiology

Abacavir is a carbocyclic synthetic nucleoside analogue. Abacavir is converted by cellular enzymes to the active metabolite, carbovir triphosphate (CBV-TP), an analogue of deoxyguanosine-5′-triphosphate (dGTP). CBV-TP inhibits the activity of HIV-1 reverse transcriptase (RT) both by competing with the natural substrate dGTP and by its incorporation into viral DNA. The lack of a 3′-OH group in the incorporated nucleotide analogue prevents the formation of the 5′ to 3′ phosphodiester linkage essential for DNA chain elongation, and therefore, the viral DNA growth is terminated. CBV-TP is a weak inhibitor of cellular DNA polymerases α, β, and γ.

Antiviral Activity: The antiviral activity of abacavir against HIV-1 was evaluated against a T-cell tropic laboratory strain HIV-1_{IIIB} in lymphoblastic cell lines, a monocyte/macrophage tropic laboratory strain HIV-1_{BaL} in primary monocytes/macrophages, and clinical isolates in peripheral blood mononuclear cells. The concentration of drug necessary to effect viral replication by 50 percent (EC_{50}) ranged from 3.7 to 5.8 μM (1 μM = 0.28 mcg/mL) and 0.07 to 1.0 μM against HIV-1_{IIIB} and HIV-1_{BaL}, respectively, and was 0.26 ± 0.18 μM against 8 clinical isolates. The EC_{50} values of abacavir against different HIV-1 clades (A-G) ranged from 0.0015 to 1.05 μM, and against HIV-2 isolates, from 0.024 to 0.49 μM. Abacavir had synergistic activity in cell culture in combination with the nucleoside reverse transcriptase inhibitor (NRTI) zidovudine, the non-nucleoside reverse transcriptase inhibitor (NNRTI) nevirapine, and the protease inhibitor (PI) amprenavir; and additive activity in combination with the NRTIs didanosine, emtricitabine, lamivudine, stavudine, tenofovir, and zalcitabine. Ribavirin (50 μM) had no effect on the anti–HIV-1 activity of abacavir in cell culture.

Resistance: HIV-1 isolates with reduced susceptibility to abacavir have been selected in cell culture and were also obtained from patients treated with abacavir. Genotypic analysis of isolates selected in cell culture and recovered from abacavir-treated patients demonstrated that amino acid substitutions K65R, L74V, Y115F, and M184V/I in RT contributed to abacavir resistance. In a study of therapy-naive adults receiving ZIAGEN 600 mg once daily (n = 384) or 300 mg twice daily (n = 386), in a background regimen of lamivudine 300 mg once daily and efavirenz 600 mg once daily (CNA30021), the incidence of virologic failure at 48 weeks was similar between the 2 groups (11% in both arms). Genotypic (n = 38) and phenotypic analyses (n = 35) of virologic failure isolates from this study showed that the RT substitutions that emerged during abacavir once-daily and twice-daily therapy were K65R, L74V, Y115F, and M184V/I. The substitution M184V/I was the most commonly observed substitution in virologic failure isolates from patients receiving abacavir once daily (56%, 10/18) and twice daily (40%, 8/20).

Thirty-nine percent (7/18) of the isolates from patients who experienced virologic failure in the abacavir once-daily arm had a greater than 2.5-fold decrease in abacavir susceptibility with a median-fold decrease of 1.3 (range 0.5 to 11) compared with 29% (5/17) of the failure isolates in the twice-daily arm with a median-fold decrease of 0.92 (range 0.7 to 13).

Cross-Resistance: Cross-resistance has been observed among NRTIs. Isolates containing abacavir resistance-associated substitutions, namely, K65R, L74V, Y115F, and M184V, exhibited cross-resistance to didanosine, emtricitabine, lamivudine, tenofovir, and zalcitabine in cell culture and in patients. The K65R substitution can confer resistance to abacavir, didanosine, emtricitabine, lamivudine, stavudine, tenofovir, and zalcitabine; the L74V substitution can confer resistance to abacavir, didanosine, and zalcitabine; and the M184V substitution can confer resistance to abacavir, didanosine, emtricitabine, lamivudine, and zalcitabine. An increasing number of thymidine analogue mutations (TAMs: M41L, D67N, K70R, L210W, T215Y/F, K219E/R/H/Q/N) is associated with a progressive reduction in abacavir susceptibility.

13 NONCLINICAL TOXICOLOGY

13.1 Carcinogenesis, Mutagenesis, Impairment of Fertility

Abacavir was administered orally at 3 dosage levels to separate groups of mice and rats in 2-year carcinogenicity studies. Results showed an increase in the incidence of malignant and non-malignant tumors. Malignant tumors occurred in the preputial gland of males and the clitoral gland of females of both species, and in the liver of female rats. In addition, non-malignant tumors also occurred in the liver and thyroid gland of female rats. These observations were made at systemic exposures in the range of 6 to 32 times the human exposure at the recommended dose. It is not known how predictive the results of rodent carcinogenicity studies may be for humans.

Abacavir induced chromosomal aberrations both in the presence and absence of metabolic activation in an in vitro cytogenetic study in human lymphocytes. Abacavir was mutagenic in the absence of metabolic activation, although it was not mutagenic in the presence of metabolic activation in an L5178Y mouse lymphoma assay. Abacavir was clastogenic in males and not clastogenic in females in an in vivo mouse bone marrow micronucleus assay.

Abacavir was not mutagenic in bacterial mutagenicity assays in the presence and absence of metabolic activation.

Abacavir had no adverse effects on the mating performance or fertility of male and female rats at a dose approximately 8 times the human exposure at the recommended dose based on body surface area comparisons.

13.2 Animal Toxicology and/or Pharmacology

Myocardial degeneration was found in mice and rats following administration of abacavir for 2 years. The systemic exposures were equivalent to 7 to 24 times the expected systemic exposure in humans. The clinical relevance of this finding has not been determined.

14 CLINICAL STUDIES

14.1 Adults

Therapy-Naive Adults: CNA30024 was a multicenter, double-blind, controlled study in which 649 HIV-1-infected, therapy-naive adults were randomized and received either ZIAGEN (300 mg twice daily), lamivudine (150 mg twice daily), and efavirenz (600 mg once daily) or zidovudine (300 mg twice daily), lamivudine (150 mg twice daily), and efavirenz (600 mg once daily). The duration of double-blind treatment was at least 48 weeks. Study participants were: male (81%), Caucasian (51%), black (21%), and Hispanic (26%). The median age was 35 years, the median pretreatment CD4+ cell count was 264 cells/mm^3, and median plasma HIV-1 RNA was 4.79 $\log_{10}$ copies/mL. The outcomes of randomized treatment are provided in Table 7.

Table 7. Outcomes of Randomized Treatment Through Week 48 (CNA30024)

Outcome	ZIAGEN plus Lamivudine plus Efavirenz (n = 324)	Zidovudine plus Lamivudine plus Efavirenz (n = 325)
Responder*	69% (73%)	69% (71%)
Virologic failures†	6%	4%
Discontinued due to adverse reactions	14%	16%
Discontinued due to other reasons‡	10%	11%

* Patients achieved and maintained confirmed HIV-1 RNA ≤50 copies/mL (<400 copies/mL) through Week 48 (Roche AMPLICOR Ultrasensitive HIV-1 MONITOR® standard test 1.0 PCR).

† Includes viral rebound, insufficient viral response according to the investigator, and failure to achieve confirmed ≤50 copies/mL by Week 48.

‡ Includes consent withdrawn, lost to follow up, protocol violations, those with missing data, clinical progression, and other.

After 48 weeks of therapy, the median CD4+ cell count increases from baseline were 209 cells/mm^3 in the group receiving ZIAGEN and 155 cells/mm^3 in the zidovudine group. Through Week 48, 8 subjects (2%) in the group receiving ZIAGEN (5 CDC classification C events and 3 deaths) and 5 subjects (2%) on the zidovudine arm (3 CDC classification C events and 2 deaths) experienced clinical disease progression.

CNA3005 was a multicenter, double-blind, controlled study in which 562 HIV-1-infected, therapy-naive adults were randomized to receive either ZIAGEN (300 mg twice daily) plus COMBIVIR (lamivudine 150 mg/zidovudine 300 mg twice daily), or indinavir (800 mg 3 times a day) plus COMBIVIR twice daily. The study was stratified at randomization by pre-entry plasma HIV-1 RNA 10,000 to 100,000 copies/mL and plasma HIV-1 RNA greater than 100,000 copies/mL. Study participants were male (87%), Caucasian (73%), black (15%), and Hispanic (9%). At baseline the median age was 36 years, the median baseline CD4+ cell count was 360 cells/mm^3, and median baseline plasma HIV-1 RNA was 4.8 log$_{10}$ copies/mL. Proportions of patients with plasma HIV-1 RNA less than 400 copies/mL (using Roche AMPLICOR HIV-1 MONITOR Test) through 48 weeks of treatment are summarized in Table 8.

Table 8. Outcomes of Randomized Treatment Through Week 48 (CNA3005)

Outcome	ZIAGEN plus Lamivudine/ Zidovudine (n = 262)	Indinavir plus Lamivudine/ Zidovudine (n = 265)
Responder*	49%	50%
Virologic failure†	31%	28%
Discontinued due to adverse reactions	10%	12%
Discontinued due to other reasons‡	11%	10%

* Patients achieved and maintained confirmed HIV-1 RNA <400 copies/mL.

† Includes viral rebound and failure to achieve confirmed <400 copies/mL by Week 48.

‡ Includes consent withdrawn, lost to follow up, protocol violations, those with missing data, clinical progression, and other.

Treatment response by plasma HIV-1 RNA strata is shown in Table 9.

Table 9. Proportions of Responders Through Week 48 By Screening Plasma HIV-1 RNA Levels (CNA3005)

Screening HIV-1 RNA (copies/mL)	ZIAGEN plus Lamivudine/ Zidovudine (n = 262)		Indinavir plus Lamivudine/ Zidovudine (n = 265)	
	<400 copies/mL	n	<400 copies/mL	n
≥10,000-≤100,000	50%	166	48%	165
>100,000	48%	96	52%	100

In subjects with baseline viral load greater than 100,000 copies/mL, percentages of patients with HIV-1 RNA levels less than 50 copies/mL were 31% in the group receiving abacavir vs. 45% in the group receiving indinavir. Through Week 48, an overall mean increase in CD4+ cell count of about 150 cells/mm^3 was observed in both treatment arms. Through Week 48, 9 subjects (3.4%) in the group receiving abacavir sulfate (6 CDC classification C events and 3 deaths) and 3 subjects (1.5%) in the group receiving indinavir (2 CDC classification C events and 1 death) experienced clinical disease progression.

CNA30021 was an international, multicenter, double-blind, controlled study in which 770 HIV-1-infected, therapy-naive adults were randomized and received either abacavir 600 mg once daily or abacavir 300 mg twice daily, both in combination with lamivudine 300 mg once daily and efavirenz 600 mg once daily. The double-blind treatment duration was at least 48 weeks. Study participants had a mean age of 37 years, were: male (81%), Caucasian (54%), black (27%), and American Hispanic (15%). The median baseline CD4+ cell count was 262 cells/mm^3 (range 21 to 918 cells/mm^3) and the median baseline plasma HIV-1 RNA was 4.89 log$_{10}$ copies/mL (range: 2.60 to 6.99 log$_{10}$ copies/mL).

The outcomes of randomized treatment are provided in Table 10.

Table 10. Outcomes of Randomized Treatment Through Week 48 (CNA30021)

Outcome	ZIAGEN 600 mg q.d. plus EPIVIR plus Efavirenz (n = 384)	ZIAGEN 300 mg b.i.d. plus EPIVIR plus Efavirenz (n = 386)
Responder*	64% (71%)	65% (72%)
Virologic failure†	11% (5%)	11% (5%)
Discontinued due to adverse reactions	13%	11%
Discontinued due to other reasons‡	11%	13%

* Patients achieved and maintained confirmed HIV-1 RNA <50 copies/mL (<400 copies/mL) through Week 48 (Roche AMPLICOR Ultrasensitive HIV-1 MONITOR standard test version 1.0).

† Includes viral rebound, failure to achieve confirmed <50 copies/mL (<400 copies/mL) by Week 48, and insufficient viral load response.

‡ Includes consent withdrawn, lost to follow up, protocol violations, clinical progression, and other.

After 48 weeks of therapy, the median CD4+ cell count increases from baseline were 188 cells/mm^3 in the group receiving abacavir 600 mg once daily and 200 cells/mm^3 in the group receiving abacavir 300 mg twice daily. Through Week 48, 6 subjects (2%) in the group receiving ZIAGEN 600 mg once daily (4 CDC classification C events and 2 deaths) and 10 subjects (3%) in the group receiving ZIAGEN 300 mg twice daily (7 CDC classification C events and 3 deaths) experienced clinical disease progression. None of the deaths were attributed to study medications.

14.2 Pediatric Patients

Therapy-Experienced Pediatric Patients: CNA3006 was a randomized, double-blind study comparing ZIAGEN 8 mg/kg twice daily plus lamivudine 4 mg/kg twice daily plus zidovudine 180 mg/m^2 twice daily versus lamivudine 4 mg/kg twice daily plus zidovudine 180 mg/m^2 twice daily. Two hundred and five therapy-experienced pediatric patients were enrolled: female (56%), Caucasian (17%), black (50%), Hispanic (30%), median age of 5.4 years, baseline CD4+ cell percent greater than 15% (median = 27%), and median baseline plasma HIV-1 RNA of 4.6 log$_{10}$ copies/mL. Eighty percent and 55% of patients had prior therapy with zidovudine and lamivudine, respectively, most often in combination. The median duration of prior nucleoside analogue therapy was 2 years. At 16 weeks the proportion of patients responding based on plasma HIV-1 RNA less than or equal to 400 copies/mL was significantly higher in patients receiving ZIAGEN plus lamivudine plus zidovudine compared with patients receiving lamivudine plus zidovudine, 13% versus 2%, respectively. Median plasma HIV-1 RNA changes from baseline were -0.53 log$_{10}$ copies/mL in the group receiving ZIAGEN plus lamivudine plus zidovudine compared with -0.21 log$_{10}$ copies/mL in the group receiving lamivudine plus zidovudine. Median CD4+ cell count increases from baseline were 69 cells/mm^3 in the group receiving ZIAGEN plus lamivudine plus zidovudine and 9 cells/mm^3 in the group receiving lamivudine plus zidovudine.

15 REFERENCES

1. Data Collection on Adverse Events of Anti-HIV Drugs (D:A:D) Study Group. *Lancet.* 2008;371 (9622):1417-1426.

16 HOW SUPPLIED/STORAGE AND HANDLING

ZIAGEN Tablets, containing abacavir sulfate equivalent to 300 mg abacavir are yellow, biconvex, scored, capsule-shaped, film-coated, and imprinted with "GX 623" on both sides. They are packaged as follows:
Bottles of 60 tablets (NDC 0173-0661-01).
Unit dose blister packs of 60 tablets (NDC 0173-0661-00). Each pack contains 6 blister cards of 10 tablets each.
Store at controlled room temperature of 20° to 25°C (68° to 77°F) (see USP).
ZIAGEN Oral Solution is a clear to opalescent, yellowish, strawberry-banana-flavored liquid. Each mL of the solution contains abacavir sulfate equivalent to 20 mg of abacavir. It is packaged in plastic bottles as follows:
Bottles of 240 mL (NDC 0173-0664-00) with child-resistant closure. This product does not require reconstitution.
Store at controlled room temperature of 20° to 25°C (68° to 77°F) (see USP). DO NOT FREEZE. May be refrigerated.

17 PATIENT COUNSELING INFORMATION

See Medication Guide. (17.2)

17.1 Information About Therapy With ZIAGEN

Hypersensitivity Reaction: Inform patients:
• that a Medication Guide and Warning Card summarizing the symptoms of the abacavir hypersensitivity reaction and other product information will be dispensed by the pharmacist with each new prescription and refill of ZIAGEN, and encourage the patient to read the Medication Guide and Warning Card every time to obtain any new information that may be present about ZIAGEN. (The complete text of the Medication Guide is reprinted at the end of this document.)
• to carry the Warning Card with them.
• how to identify a hypersensitivity reaction [see Medication Guide (17.2)].
• that if they develop symptoms consistent with a hypersensitivity reaction they should call their doctor right away to determine if they should stop taking ZIAGEN.
• that a hypersensitivity reaction can worsen and lead to hospitalization or death if ZIAGEN is not immediately discontinued.
• that in one study, more severe hypersensitivity reactions were seen when ZIAGEN was dosed 600 mg once daily.
• to not restart ZIAGEN or any other abacavir-containing product following a hypersensitivity reaction because more severe symptoms can occur within hours and may include life-threatening hypotension and death.
• that a hypersensitivity reaction is usually reversible if it is detected promptly and ZIAGEN is stopped right away.
• that if they have interrupted ZIAGEN for reasons other than symptoms of hypersensitivity (for example, those who have an interruption in drug supply), a serious or fatal hypersensitivity reaction may occur with reintroduction of abacavir.
• to not restart ZIAGEN or any other abacavir-containing product without medical consultation and that restarting abacavir needs to be undertaken only if medical care can be readily accessed by the patient or others.
• ZIAGEN should not be coadministered with EPZICOM® or TRIZIVIR®.
Lactic Acidosis/Hepatomegaly: Inform patients that some HIV medicines, including ZIAGEN, can cause a rare, but serious condition called lactic acidosis with liver enlargement (hepatomegaly).
Redistribution/Accumulation of Body Fat: Inform patients that redistribution or accumulation of body fat may occur in patients receiving antiretroviral therapy and that the cause and long-term health effects of these conditions are not known at this time.
Information About HIV-1 Infection: ZIAGEN is not a cure for HIV-1 infection and patients may continue to experience illnesses associated with HIV-1 infection, including opportunistic infections. Patients should remain under the care of a physician when using ZIAGEN. Advise patients that the use of ZIAGEN has not been shown to reduce the risk of transmission of HIV-1 to others through sexual contact or blood contamination. Patients should be informed to take all HIV medications exactly as prescribed.

17.2 FDA Approved Patient Labeling

MEDICATION GUIDE

ZIAGEN® (ZY-uh-jen) Tablets
ZIAGEN® Oral Solution
Generic name: abacavir (uh-BACK-ah-veer) sulfate tablets and oral solution
Read the Medication Guide that comes with ZIAGEN before you start taking it and each time you get a refill because there may be new information. This information does not take the place of talking to your doctor about your medical condition or your treatment. Be sure to carry your ZIAGEN Warning Card with you at all times.
What is the most important information I should know about ZIAGEN?
• **Serious Allergic Reaction to Abacavir.** ZIAGEN contains abacavir (also contained in EPZICOM and TRIZIVIR®). Patients taking ZIAGEN may have a serious allergic reaction (hypersensitivity reaction) that can cause death. **Your risk of this allergic reaction is much higher if you have a gene variation called HLA-B*5701 than if you do not. Your doctor can determine with a blood test if you have this gene variation. If you get a symptom from 2 or more of the following groups while taking ZIAGEN, call your doctor right away to determine if you should stop taking this medicine.**

	Symptom(s)
Group 1	Fever
Group 2	Rash
Group 3	Nausea, vomiting, diarrhea, abdominal (stomach area) pain
Group 4	Generally ill feeling, extreme tiredness, or achiness
Group 5	Shortness of breath, cough, sore throat

A list of these symptoms is on the Warning Card your pharmacist gives you. Carry this Warning Card with you.
If you stop ZIAGEN because of an allergic reaction, NEVER take ZIAGEN (abacavir sulfate) or any other

abacavir-containing medicine (EPZICOM and TRIZIVIR) again. If you take ZIAGEN or any other abacavir-containing medicine again after you have had an allergic reaction, WITHIN HOURS you may get life-threatening symptoms that may include **very low blood pressure** or **death.**
If you stop ZIAGEN for any other reason, even for a few days and you are not allergic to ZIAGEN, talk with your doctor before taking it again. Taking ZIAGEN again can cause a serious allergic or life-threatening reaction, even if you never had an allergic reaction to it before. If your doctor tells you that you can take ZIAGEN again, **start taking it when you are around medical help or people who can call a doctor if you need one.**

- **Lactic Acidosis.** Some human immunodeficiency virus (HIV) medicines, including ZIAGEN, can cause a rare but serious condition called lactic acidosis with liver enlargement (hepatomegaly). Nausea and tiredness that don't get better may be symptoms of lactic acidosis. In some cases this condition can cause death. Women, overweight people, and people who have taken HIV medicines like ZIAGEN for a long time have a higher chance of getting lactic acidosis and liver enlargement. Lactic acidosis is a medical emergency and must be treated in the hospital.

ZIAGEN can have other serious side effects. Be sure to read the section below entitled "What are the possible side effects of ZIAGEN?"

What is ZIAGEN?

ZIAGEN is a prescription medicine used to treat HIV infection. ZIAGEN is taken by mouth as a tablet or a strawberry-banana-flavored liquid. ZIAGEN is a medicine called a nucleoside analogue reverse transcriptase inhibitor (NRTI). ZIAGEN is always used with other anti-HIV medicines. When used in combination with these other medicines, ZIAGEN helps lower the amount of HIV found in your blood. This helps to keep your immune system as healthy as possible so that it can help fight infection.
Different combinations of medicines are used to treat HIV infection. You and your doctor should discuss which combination of medicines is best for you.

- **ZIAGEN does not cure HIV infection or AIDS.** We do not know if ZIAGEN will help you live longer or have fewer of the medical problems that people get with HIV or AIDS. It is very important that you see your doctor regularly while you are taking ZIAGEN.
- **ZIAGEN does not lower the risk of passing HIV to other people** through sexual contact, sharing needles, or being exposed to your blood. For your health and the health of others, it is important to always practice safe sex by using a latex or polyurethane condom or other barrier method to lower the chance of sexual contact with semen, vaginal secretions, or blood. Never use or share dirty needles.

ZIAGEN has not been studied in children under 3 months of age or in adults over 65 years of age.

Who should not take ZIAGEN?

Do not take ZIAGEN if you:

- have ever had a serious allergic reaction (a hypersensitivity reaction) to ZIAGEN or any other medicine that has abacavir as one of its ingredients (EPZICOM and TRIZIVIR). See the end of this Medication Guide for a complete list of ingredients in ZIAGEN.
- have a liver that does not function properly.

Before starting ZIAGEN, tell your doctor about all of your medical conditions, including if you:

- have been tested and know whether or not you have a particular gene variation called HLA-B*5701.
- are pregnant or planning to become pregnant. We do not know if ZIAGEN will harm your unborn child. You and your doctor will need to decide if ZIAGEN is right for you. If you use ZIAGEN while you are pregnant, talk to your doctor about how you can be on the Antiviral Pregnancy Registry for ZIAGEN.
- are breastfeeding. We do not know if ZIAGEN can be passed to your baby in your breast milk and whether it could harm your baby. Also, mothers with HIV should not breastfeed because HIV can be passed to the baby in the breast milk.
- have liver problems.
- have heart problems, smoke, or suffer from diseases that increase your risk of heart disease such as high blood pressure, high cholesterol, or diabetes.

Tell your doctor about all the medicines you take, including prescription and nonprescription medicines, vitamins, and herbal supplements. Especially tell your doctor if you take:

- methadone
- EPZICOM (abacavir sulfate and lamivudine) and TRIZIVIR (abacavir sulfate, lamivudine, and zidovudine).

How should I take ZIAGEN?

- **Take ZIAGEN by mouth exactly as your doctor prescribes it.** Your doctor will tell you the right dose to take. The usual dose is 1 tablet twice a day or 2 tablets once a day. Do not skip doses.
- Children aged 3 months and older can also take ZIAGEN. The child's healthcare professional will decide the right

dose and formulation based on the child's weight. The dose should not exceed the recommended adult dose.

- **You can take ZIAGEN with or without food.**
- If you miss a dose of ZIAGEN, take the missed dose right away. Then, take the next dose at the usual time.
- Do not let your ZIAGEN run out.
- Starting ZIAGEN again can cause a serious allergic or life-threatening reaction, even if you never had an allergic reaction to it before. If you run out of ZIAGEN even for a few days, you must ask your doctor if you can start ZIAGEN again. If your doctor tells you that you can take ZIAGEN again, start taking it when you are around medical help or people who can call a doctor if you need one.
- If you stop your anti-HIV drugs, even for a short time, the amount of virus in your blood may increase and the virus may become harder to treat.
- If you take too much ZIAGEN, call your doctor or poison control center right away.

What should I avoid while taking ZIAGEN?

- Do not take EPZICOM (abacavir sulfate and lamivudine) or TRIZIVIR (abacavir sulfate, lamivudine, and zidovudine) while taking ZIAGEN. Some of these medicines are already in ZIAGEN.

Avoid doing things that can spread HIV infection, as ZIAGEN does not stop you from passing the HIV infection to others.

- Do not share needles or other injection equipment.
- Do not share personal items that can have blood or body fluids on them, like toothbrushes and razor blades.
- Do not have any kind of sex without protection. Always practice safe sex by using a latex or polyurethane condom or other barrier method to lower the chance of sexual contact with semen, vaginal secretions, or blood.
- Do not breastfeed. We do not know if ZIAGEN can be passed to your baby in your breast milk and whether it could harm your baby. Also, mothers with HIV should not breastfeed because HIV can be passed to the baby in the breast milk.

What are the possible side effects of ZIAGEN?

ZIAGEN can cause the following serious side effects:

- **Serious allergic reaction that can cause death.** (See "What is the most important information I should know about ZIAGEN?" at the beginning of this Medication Guide.)
- **Lactic acidosis with liver enlargement (hepatomegaly) that can cause death.** (See "What is the most important information I should know about ZIAGEN?" at the beginning of this Medication Guide.)
- **Changes in immune system.** When you start taking HIV medicines, your immune system may get stronger and could begin to fight infections that have been hidden in your body, such as pneumonia, herpes virus, or tuberculosis. If you have new symptoms after starting your HIV medicines, be sure to tell your doctor.
- **Changes in body fat.** These changes have happened in patients taking antiretroviral medicines like ZIAGEN. The changes may include an increased amount of fat in the upper back and neck ("buffalo hump"), breast, and around the back, chest, and stomach area. Loss of fat from the legs, arms, and face may also happen. The cause and long-term health effects of these conditions are not known.

Some HIV medicines including ZIAGEN may increase your risk of heart attack. If you have heart problems, smoke, or suffer from diseases that increase your risk of heart disease such as high blood pressure, high cholesterol, or diabetes, tell your doctor.
The most common side effects of ZIAGEN include nausea, vomiting, tiredness, headache, diarrhea, trouble sleeping, fever and chills, and loss of appetite. Most of these side effects did not cause people to stop taking ZIAGEN.
This list of side effects is not complete. Call your doctor for medical advice about side effects. You may report side effects to FDA at 1-800-FDA-1088.

How should I store ZIAGEN?

- Store ZIAGEN at room temperature, between 68° to 77°F (20° to 25°C). Do not freeze ZIAGEN.
- Keep ZIAGEN and all medicines out of the reach of children.

General information for safe and effective use of ZIAGEN

Medicines are sometimes prescribed for conditions that are not mentioned in Medication Guides. Do not use ZIAGEN for a condition for which it was not prescribed. Do not give ZIAGEN to other people, even if they have the same symptoms that you have. It may harm them.
This Medication Guide summarizes the most important information about ZIAGEN. If you would like more information, talk with your doctor. You can ask your doctor or pharmacist for the information that is written for healthcare professionals or call 1-888-825-5249.

What are the ingredients in ZIAGEN?

Tablets: Each tablet contains abacavir sulfate equivalent to 300 mg of abacavir as active ingredient and the following inactive ingredients: colloidal silicon dioxide, magnesium

stearate, microcrystalline cellulose, and sodium starch glycolate. The film-coating is made of hypromellose, polysorbate 80, synthetic yellow iron oxide, titanium dioxide, and triacetin.
Oral Solution: Each milliliter (1 mL) of ZIAGEN Oral Solution contains abacavir sulfate equivalent to 20 mg of abacavir (i.e., 20 mg/mL) as active ingredient and the following inactive ingredients: artificial strawberry and banana flavors, citric acid (anhydrous), methylparaben and propylparaben (added as preservatives), propylene glycol, saccharin sodium, sodium citrate (dihydrate), sorbitol solution, and water.
This Medication Guide has been approved by the US Food and Drug Administration.
GlaxoSmithKline
Research Triangle Park, NC 27709
©2009, GlaxoSmithKline. All rights reserved.
January 2009
ZGN:2MG

Warner Chilcott (US), LLC
100 ENTERPRISE DRIVE
ROCKAWAY, NJ 07866

Direct Inquiries to:
For Product Information:
(800) 521-8813
www.wcrx.com
For Medical Information:
(800) 521-8813
For A Medical Emergency:
(800) 521-8813
After Hours and Weekends:
(877) 740-5015
For All Other Inquiries:
(800) 521-8813
www.wcrx.com

Following is a list of Warner Chilcott products:

DORYX® ℞
(Doxycycline Hyclate Delayed-Release Tablets, USP), 75 mg, 100 mg and 150 mg

ESTRACE® Vaginal Cream ℞
(estradiol vaginal cream, USP, 0.01%)

ESTRACE® Tablets, 0.5 mg, 1 mg, 2 mg ℞
(estradiol tablets, USP)

ESTROSTEP® Fe ℞
(Norethindrone Acetate and Ethinyl Estradiol Tablets, USP and Ferrous Fumarate Tablets)

FEMCON® Fe ℞
(norethindrone and ethinyl estradiol tablets, chewable and ferrous fumarate tablets)

FEMHRT®, 0.5 mg/2.5 mcg, 1 mg/5 mcg ℞
(norethindrone acetate/ethinyl estradiol tablets)

FEMRING®, 0.05 mg/day, 0.10 mg/day ℞
(estradiol acetate vaginal ring)

FEMTRACE®, 0.45 mg, 0.9 mg, 1.8 mg ℞
(estradiol acetate tablets)

LOESTRIN® 24 Fe ℞
(norethindrone acetate and ethinyl estradiol tablets, USP and ferrous fumarate tablets)

OVCON® 35, 0.4/35 ℞
(Norethindrone and Ethinyl Estradiol Tablets, USP)

OVCON® 50, 1.0 mg/0.05 mg ℞
(Norethindrone and Ethinyl Estradiol Tablets, USP)

SARAFEM® (fluoxetine hydrochloride tablets) ℞

ACTONEL® ℞
[ăk'ō-nĕl]
(risedronate sodium)
Tablets

HIGHLIGHTS OF PRESCRIBING INFORMATION

These highlights do not include all the information needed to use ACTONEL safely and effectively. See full prescribing information for ACTONEL.
ACTONEL® (risedronate sodium) tablets
Initial U.S. Approval: 1998

───────RECENT MAJOR CHANGES───────

Contraindications (4)	12/2009
Warnings and Precautions (5.1, 5.3)	12/2009

───────INDICATIONS AND USAGE───────

ACTONEL is a bisphosphonate indicated for:
- Treatment and prevention of postmenopausal osteoporosis (1.1),

- Treatment to increase bone mass in men with osteoporosis (1.2),
- Treatment and prevention of glucocorticoid-induced osteoporosis (1.3),
- Treatment of Paget's disease (1.4).

————————DOSAGE AND ADMINISTRATION————————

Must be taken with plain water (6 to 8 oz) at least 30 minutes before the first food or drink of the day; do not lie down for 30 minutes (2)

Treatment of Osteoporosis in Postmenopausal Women: 5 mg daily, 35 mg once a week, 75 mg taken on two consecutive days each month, or 150 mg once a month (2.1)

Prevention of Osteoporosis in Postmenopausal Women: 5 mg daily, or 35 mg once a week (2.2)

Men with Osteoporosis: 35 mg once a week (2.3)

Treatment and Prevention of Glucocorticoid-Induced Osteoporosis: 5 mg daily (2.4)

Paget's Disease: 30 mg daily for 2 months (2.5)

————————DOSAGE FORMS AND STRENGTHS————————

Tablets: 5, 30, 35, 75, and 150 mg (3)

————————CONTRAINDICATIONS————————

- Abnormalities of the esophagus which delay esophageal emptying such as stricture or achalasia (4, 5.1)
- Inability to stand or sit upright for at least 30 minutes (4, 5.1)
- Hypocalcemia (4, 5.2)
- Known hypersensitivity to any component of this product (4, 6.2)

————————WARNINGS AND PRECAUTIONS————————

- Severe irritation of the upper gastrointestinal (GI) mucosa can occur. Dosing instructions should be followed and caution should be used in patients with active upper GI disease. Discontinue use if new or worsening symptoms occur (5.1).
- Hypocalcemia may worsen and must be corrected prior to use (5.2).
- Osteonecrosis of the jaw has been reported rarely (5.3).
- Severe bone, joint, or muscle pain may occur. Consider discontinuing use if severe symptoms develop (5.4, 6.2).
- Before initiating treatment in patients with glucocorticoid-induced osteoporosis, sex steroid hormonal status of both men and women should be ascertained and appropriate replacement considered (5.6).
- Bisphosphonates may interfere with bone-imaging agents (5.7).

————————ADVERSE REACTIONS————————

Most common adverse reactions reported in >10% of patients treated with ACTONEL and with a higher frequency than placebo are: back pain, arthralgia, abdominal pain, and dyspepsia (6.1).

Hypersensitivity reactions (angioedema, generalized rash, bullous skin reactions), and eye inflammation (iritis, uveitis) have been reported rarely (6.2).

To report SUSPECTED ADVERSE REACTIONS, contact Warner Chilcott at 1-800-836-0658 or FDA at 1-800-FDA-1088 or www.fda.gov/medwatch.

————————DRUG INTERACTIONS————————•

Calcium, antacids, or oral medications containing divalent cations interfere with the absorption of ACTONEL (7.1).

————————USE IN SPECIFIC POPULATIONS————————

ACTONEL is not recommended for use in patients with severe renal impairment (creatinine clearance <30 mL/min) (5.5, 8.6, 12.3).

ACTONEL is not indicated for use in pediatric patients (8.4).

See 17 for PATIENT COUNSELING INFORMATION and FDA-approved patient labeling.

Revised: 03/2010

————————————————————————————————————

FULL PRESCRIBING INFORMATION

1   INDICATIONS AND USAGE

1.1   Postmenopausal Osteoporosis

ACTONEL is indicated for the treatment and prevention of osteoporosis in postmenopausal women. In postmenopausal women with osteoporosis, ACTONEL reduces the incidence of vertebral fractures and a composite endpoint of nonvertebral osteoporosis-related fractures [see Clinical Studies (14.1, 14.2)].

1.2   Osteoporosis in Men

ACTONEL is indicated for treatment to increase bone mass in men with osteoporosis.

1.3   Glucocorticoid-Induced Osteoporosis

ACTONEL is indicated for the treatment and prevention of glucocorticoid-induced osteoporosis in men and women who are either initiating or continuing systemic glucocorticoid treatment (daily dosage of ≥ 7.5 mg prednisone or equivalent) for chronic diseases. Patients treated with glucocorticoids should receive adequate amounts of calcium and vitamin D.

1.4   Paget's Disease

ACTONEL is indicated for treatment of Paget's disease of bone in men and women.

2   DOSAGE AND ADMINISTRATION

ACTONEL should be taken at least 30 minutes before the first food or drink of the day other than water.

To facilitate delivery to the stomach, ACTONEL should be swallowed while the patient is in an upright position and with a full glass of plain water (6 to 8 oz). Patients should not lie down for 30 minutes after taking the medication [see Warnings and Precautions (5.1)].

Patients should receive supplemental calcium and vitamin D if dietary intake is inadequate [see Warnings and Precautions (5.2)]. Calcium supplements and calcium-, aluminum-, and magnesium-containing medications may interfere with the absorption of ACTONEL and should be taken at a different time of the day. ACTONEL is not recommended for use in patients with severe renal impairment (creatinine clearance <30 mL/min). No dosage adjustment is necessary in patients with a creatinine clearance ≥30 mL/min or in the elderly.

2.1   Treatment of Postmenopausal Osteoporosis [see Indications and Usage (1.1)]

The recommended regimen is:
- one 5 mg tablet orally, taken daily
  or
- one 35 mg tablet orally, taken once a week
  or
- one 75 mg tablet orally, taken on two consecutive days for a total of two tablets each month
  or
- one 150 mg tablet orally, taken once a month

2.2   Prevention of Postmenopausal Osteoporosis [see Indications and Usage (1.1)]

The recommended regimen is:
- one 5 mg tablet orally, taken daily
  or
- one 35 mg tablet orally, taken once a week
  or
- alternatively, one 75 mg tablet orally, taken on two consecutive days for a total of two tablets each month may be considered
  or
- alternatively, one 150 mg tablet orally, taken once a month may be considered

2.3   Treatment to Increase Bone Mass in Men with Osteoporosis [see Indications and Usage (1.2)]

The recommended regimen is:
- one 35 mg tablet orally, taken once a week

2.4   Treatment and Prevention of Glucocorticoid-Induced Osteoporosis [see Indications and Usage (1.3)]

The recommended regimen is:
- one 5 mg tablet orally, taken daily

2.5   Treatment of Paget's Disease [see Indications and Usage (1.4)]

The recommended treatment regimen is 30 mg orally once daily for 2 months. Retreatment may be considered (following post-treatment observation of at least 2 months) if relapse occurs, or if treatment fails to normalize serum alkaline phosphatase. For retreatment, the dose and duration of therapy are the same as for initial treatment. No data are available on more than 1 course of retreatment.

3   DOSAGE FORMS AND STRENGTHS

- 5 mg film-coated, oval, yellow tablet with RSN on 1 face and 5 mg on the other.
- 30 mg film-coated, oval, white tablet with RSN on 1 face and 30 mg on the other.
- 35 mg film-coated, oval, orange tablet with RSN on 1 face and 35 mg on the other.
- 75 mg film-coated, oval, pink tablet with RSN on 1 face and 75 mg on the other.
- 150 mg film-coated, oval, blue tablet with RSN on 1 face and 150 mg on the other.

4   CONTRAINDICATIONS

- Abnormalities of the esophagus which delay esophageal emptying such as stricture or achalasia [see Warnings and Precautions (5.1)]
- Inability to stand or sit upright for at least 30 minutes [see Dosage and Administration (2), Warnings and Precautions (5.1)]
- Hypocalcemia [see Warnings and Precautions (5.2)]
- Known hypersensitivity to any component of this product [see Adverse Reactions (6.2)]

5   WARNINGS AND PRECAUTIONS

5.1   Upper Gastrointestinal Adverse Reactions

ACTONEL, like other bisphosphonates administered orally, may cause local irritation of the upper gastrointestinal mucosa. Because of these possible irritant effects and a potential for worsening of the underlying disease, caution should be used when ACTONEL is given to patients with active upper gastrointestinal problems (such as known Barrett's esophagus, dysphagia, other esophageal diseases, gastritis, duodenitis or ulcers) [see Contraindications (4), Adverse Reactions (6.1), Information for Patients (17.1)].

Esophageal adverse experiences, such as esophagitis, esophageal ulcers and esophageal erosions, occasionally with bleeding and rarely followed by esophageal stricture or perforation, have been reported in patients receiving treatment with oral bisphosphonates. In some cases, these have been severe and required hospitalization. Physicians should therefore be alert to any signs or symptoms signaling a possible esophageal reaction and patients should be instructed to discontinue ACTONEL and seek medical attention if they develop dysphagia, odynophagia, retrosternal pain or new or worsening heartburn.

The risk of severe esophageal adverse experiences appears to be greater in patients who lie down after taking oral bisphosphonates and/or who fail to swallow it with the recommended full glass (6-8 oz) of water, and/or who continue to take oral bisphosphonates after developing symptoms suggestive of esophageal irritation. Therefore, it is very important that the full dosing instructions are provided to, and understood by, the patient [see Dosage and Administration

(2)]. In patients who cannot comply with dosing instructions due to mental disability, therapy with ACTONEL should be used under appropriate supervision.

There have been post-marketing reports of gastric and duodenal ulcers with oral bisphosphonate use, some severe and with complications, although no increased risk was observed in controlled clinical trials.

5.2 Mineral Metabolism

Hypocalcemia and other disturbances of bone and mineral metabolism should be effectively treated before starting ACTONEL therapy. Adequate intake of calcium and vitamin D is important in all patients, especially in patients with Paget's disease in whom bone turnover is significantly elevated [*see Contraindications (4), Adverse Reactions (6.1), Information for Patients (17.1)*].

5.3 Jaw Osteonecrosis

Osteonecrosis of the jaw (ONJ), which can occur spontaneously, is generally associated with tooth extraction and/or local infection with delayed healing, and has been reported in patients taking bisphosphonates, including ACTONEL. Known risk factors for osteonecrosis of the jaw include invasive dental procedures (e.g., tooth extraction, dental implants, boney surgery), diagnosis of cancer, concomitant therapies (e.g., chemotherapy, corticosteroids), poor oral hygiene, and co-morbid disorders (e.g., periodontal and/or other pre-existing dental disease, anemia, coagulopathy, infection, ill-fitting dentures).

For patients requiring invasive dental procedures, discontinuation of bisphosphonate treatment may reduce the risk for ONJ. Clinical judgment of the treating physician and/or oral surgeon should guide the management plan of each patient based on individual benefit/risk assessment.

Patients who develop osteonecrosis of the jaw while on bisphosphonate therapy should receive care by an oral surgeon. In these patients, extensive dental surgery to treat ONJ may exacerbate the condition. Discontinuation of bisphosphonate therapy should be considered based on individual benefit/risk assessment. [*see Adverse Reactions (6.2)*]

5.4 Musculoskeletal Pain

In postmarketing experience, there have been reports of severe and occasionally incapacitating bone, joint, and/or muscle pain in patients taking bisphosphonates [*see Adverse Reactions (6.2)*]. The time to onset of symptoms varied from one day to several months after starting the drug. Most patients had relief of symptoms after stopping medication. A subset had recurrence of symptoms when rechallenged with the same drug or another bisphosphonate. Consider discontinuing use if severe symptoms develop.

5.5 Renal Impairment

ACTONEL is not recommended for use in patients with severe renal impairment (creatinine clearance <30 mL/min).

5.6 Glucocorticoid-Induced Osteoporosis

Before initiating ACTONEL treatment for the treatment and prevention of glucocorticoid-induced osteoporosis, the sex steroid hormonal status of both men and women should be ascertained and appropriate replacement considered.

5.7 Laboratory Test Interactions

Bisphosphonates are known to interfere with the use of bone-imaging agents. Specific studies with ACTONEL have not been performed.

6 ADVERSE REACTIONS

6.1 Clinical Studies Experience

Because clinical trials are conducted under widely varying conditions, adverse reaction rates observed in the clinical trials of a drug cannot be directly compared to rates in the clinical trials of another drug and may not reflect the rates observed in practice.

Treatment of Postmenopausal Osteoporosis

Daily Dosing

The safety of ACTONEL 5 mg once daily in the treatment of postmenopausal osteoporosis was assessed in four randomized, double-blind, placebo-controlled multinational trials of 3232 women aged 38 to 85 years with postmenopausal osteoporosis. The duration of the trials was up to three years, with 1619 patients exposed to placebo and 1613 patients exposed to ACTONEL 5 mg. Patients with pre-existing gastrointestinal disease and concomitant use of non-steroidal anti-inflammatory drugs, proton pump inhibitors, and H_2 antagonists were included in these clinical trials. All women received 1000 mg of elemental calcium plus vitamin D supplementation up to 500 IU per day if their 25-hydroxyvitamin D_3 level was below normal at baseline.

The incidence of all-cause mortality was 2.0% in the placebo group and 1.7% in the ACTONEL 5 mg daily group. The incidence of serious adverse events was 24.6% in the placebo group and 27.2% in the ACTONEL 5 mg group. The percentage of patients who withdrew from the study due to adverse events was 15.6% in the placebo group and 14.8% in the ACTONEL 5 mg group. Table 1 lists adverse events from the Phase 3 postmenopausal osteoporosis trials reported in ≥5% of patients. Adverse events are shown without attribution of causality.

Table 1
Adverse Events Occurring at a Frequency ≥5% in Either Treatment Group Combined Phase 3 Postmenopausal Osteoporosis Treatment Trials

Body System	Placebo N = 1619 %	5 mg ACTONEL N = 1613 %
Body as a Whole		
Infection	29.9	31.1
Back Pain	26.1	28.0
Accidental Injury	16.8	16.9
Pain	14.0	14.1
Abdominal Pain	9.9	12.2
Flu Syndrome	11.6	10.5
Headache	10.8	9.9
Asthenia	4.5	5.4
Neck Pain	4.7	5.4
Chest Pain	5.1	5.0
Allergic Reaction	5.9	3.8
Cardiovascular System		
Hypertension	9.8	10.5
Digestive System		
Constipation	12.6	12.9
Diarrhea	10.0	10.8
Dyspepsia	10.6	10.8
Nausea	11.2	10.5
Metabolic & Nutritional Disorders		
Peripheral Edema	8.8	7.7
Musculoskeletal System		
Arthralgia	22.1	23.7
Arthritis	10.1	9.6
Traumatic Bone Fracture	12.3	9.3
Joint Disorder	5.3	7.0
Myalgia	6.2	6.7
Bone Pain	4.8	5.3
Nervous System		
Dizziness	5.7	7.1
Depression	6.1	6.8
Insomnia	4.6	5.0
Respiratory System		
Bronchitis	10.4	10.0
Sinusitis	9.1	8.7
Rhinitis	5.1	6.2
Pharyngitis	5.0	6.0
Increased Cough	6.3	5.9
Skin and Appendages		
Rash	7.1	7.9
Special Senses		
Cataract	5.7	6.5
Urogenital System		
Urinary Tract Infection	10.4	11.1

Gastrointestinal Adverse Events: The incidence of adverse events in the placebo and ACTONEL 5 mg daily groups were: abdominal pain (9.9% vs. 12.2%), diarrhea (10.0% vs. 10.8%), dyspepsia (10.6% vs. 10.8%), and gastritis (2.3% vs. 2.7%). Duodenitis and glossitis have been reported uncommonly in the ACTONEL 5 mg daily group (0.1% to 1%). In patients with active upper gastrointestinal disease at baseline, the incidence of upper gastrointestinal adverse events was similar between the placebo and ACTONEL 5 mg daily groups.

Musculoskeletal Adverse Events: The incidence of adverse events in the placebo and ACTONEL 5 mg daily groups were: back pain (26.1% vs. 28.0%), arthralgia (22.1% vs. 23.7%), myalgia (6.2% vs. 6.7%), and bone pain (4.8% vs. 5.3%).

Laboratory Test Findings: Throughout the Phase 3 studies, transient decreases from baseline in serum calcium (<1%) and serum phosphate (<3%) and compensatory increases in serum PTH levels (<30%) were observed within 6 months in patients in osteoporosis clinical trials treated with ACTONEL 5 mg once daily. There were no significant differences in serum calcium, phosphate, or PTH levels between placebo and ACTONEL 5 mg once daily at 3 years. Serum calcium levels below 8 mg/dL were observed in 18 patients, 9 (0.5%) in each treatment arm (placebo and ACTONEL 5 mg once daily). Serum phosphorus levels below 2 mg/dL were observed in 14 patients, 3 (0.2%) treated with placebo and 11 (0.6%) treated with ACTONEL 5 mg once daily. There have been rare reports (<0.1%) of abnormal liver function tests.

Endoscopic Findings: In the ACTONEL clinical trials, endoscopic evaluation was encouraged in any patient with moderate-to-severe gastrointestinal complaints, while maintaining the blind. Endoscopies were performed on equal numbers of patients between the placebo and treated groups [75 (14.5%) placebo; 75 (11.9%) ACTONEL]. Clinically important findings (perforations, ulcers, or bleeding) among this symptomatic population were similar between groups (51% placebo; 39% ACTONEL).

Once-a-Week Dosing

The safety of ACTONEL 35 mg once-a-week in the treatment of postmenopausal osteoporosis was assessed in a 1-year, double-blind, multicenter study comparing ACTONEL 5 mg daily and ACTONEL 35 mg once-a-week in postmenopausal women aged 50 to 95 years. The duration of the trials was one year, with 480 patients exposed to ACTONEL 5 mg daily and 485 exposed to ACTONEL 35 mg once-a-week. Patients with pre-existing gastrointestinal disease and concomitant use of non-steroidal anti-inflammatory drugs, proton pump inhibitors, and H_2 antagonists were included in these clinical trials. All women received 1000 mg of elemental calcium plus vitamin D supplementation up to 500 IU per day if their 25-hydroxyvitamin D_3 level was below normal at baseline.

The incidence of all-cause mortality was 0.4% in the ACTONEL 5 mg daily group and 1.0% in the ACTONEL 35 mg once-a-week group. The incidence of serious adverse events was 7.1% in the ACTONEL 5 mg daily group and 8.2% in the ACTONEL 35 mg once-a-week group. The percentage of patients who withdrew from the study due to adverse events was 11.9% in the ACTONEL 5 mg daily group and 11.5% in the ACTONEL 35 mg once-a-week group. The overall safety and tolerability profiles of the two dosing regimens were similar.

Gastrointestinal Adverse Events: The incidence of gastrointestinal adverse events was similar between the ACTONEL 5 mg daily group and the ACTONEL 35 mg once-a-week group: dyspepsia (6.9% vs. 7.6%), diarrhea (6.3% vs. 4.9%), and abdominal pain (7.3% vs. 7.6%).

Musculoskeletal Adverse Events: Arthralgia was reported in 11.5% of patients in the ACTONEL 5 mg daily group and 14.2% of patients in the ACTONEL 35 mg once-a-week group. Myalgia was reported by 4.6% of patients in the ACTONEL 5 mg daily group and 6.2% of patients in the ACTONEL 35 mg once-a-week group.

Laboratory Test Findings: The mean percent changes from baseline at 12 months were similar between the ACTONEL 5 mg daily and ACTONEL 35 mg once-a-week groups, respectively, for serum calcium (0.4% vs. 0.7%), phosphate (-3.8% vs. -2.6%) and PTH (6.4% vs. 4.2%).

Monthly Dosing

Two Consecutive Days per Month

The safety of ACTONEL 75 mg administered on two consecutive days per month for the treatment of postmenopausal osteoporosis was assessed in a double-blind, multicenter study in postmenopausal women aged 50 to 86 years. The duration of the trial was two years; 613 patients were exposed to ACTONEL 5 mg daily and 616 were exposed to ACTONEL 75 mg two consecutive days per month. Patients with pre-existing gastrointestinal disease and concomitant use of non-steroidal anti-inflammatory drugs, proton pump inhibitors, and H_2 antagonists were included in this clinical trial. All women received 1000 mg of elemental calcium plus 400 to 800 IU of vitamin D supplementation per day.

The incidence of all-cause mortality was 1.0% for the ACTONEL 5 mg daily group and 0.5% for the ACTONEL 75 mg two consecutive days per month group. The incidence of serious adverse events was 10.8% in the ACTONEL 5 mg daily group and 14.4% in the ACTONEL 75 mg two consecutive days per month group. The percentage of patients who withdrew from treatment due to adverse events was 14.2% in the ACTONEL 5 mg daily group and 13.0% in the ACTONEL 75 mg two consecutive days per month group. The overall safety and tolerability profiles of the two dosing regimens were similar.

Acute Phase Reactions: Symptoms consistent with acute phase reaction have been reported with bisphosphonate use. The overall incidence of acute phase reaction was 3.6% of patients on ACTONEL 5 mg daily and 7.6% of patients on ACTONEL 75 mg two consecutive days per month. These incidence rates are based on reporting of any of 33 acute phase reaction-like symptoms within 5 days of the first dose. Fever or influenza-like illness with onset within the same period were reported by 0.0% of patients on ACTONEL 5 mg daily and 0.6% of patients on ACTONEL 75 mg two consecutive days per month.

Gastrointestinal Adverse Events: The ACTONEL 75 mg two consecutive days per month group resulted in a higher incidence of discontinuation due to vomiting (1.0% vs. 0.2%) and diarrhea (1.0% vs. 0.3%) compared to the ACTONEL 5 mg daily group. Most of these events occurred within a few days of dosing.

Ocular Adverse Events: None of the patients treated with ACTONEL 75 mg two consecutive days per month reported ocular inflammation such as uveitis, scleritis, or iritis; 1 patient treated with ACTONEL 5 mg daily reported uveitis.

Laboratory Test Findings: When ACTONEL 5 mg daily and ACTONEL 75 mg two consecutive days per month were compared in postmenopausal women with osteoporosis, the mean percent changes from baseline at 24 months were 0.2% and 0.8% for serum calcium, -1.9% and -1.3% for phosphate, and -10.4% and -17.2% for PTH, respectively. Compared to the ACTONEL 5 mg daily group, ACTONEL 75 mg two consecutive days per month resulted in a slightly higher incidence of hypocalcemia at the end of the first month of treatment (4.5% vs. 3.0%). Thereafter, the incidence of hypocalcemia with these regimens was similar at approximately 2%.

Once-a-Month
The safety of ACTONEL 150 mg administered once a month for the treatment of postmenopausal osteoporosis was assessed in a double-blind, multicenter study in postmenopausal women aged 50 to 88 years. The duration of the trial was one year, with 642 patients exposed to ACTONEL 5 mg daily and 650 exposed to ACTONEL 150 mg once-a-month. Patients with pre-existing gastrointestinal disease and concomitant use of non-steroidal anti-inflammatory drugs, proton pump inhibitors, and H_2 antagonists were included in this clinical trial. All women received 1000 mg of elemental calcium plus up to 1000 IU of vitamin D supplementation per day.

The incidence of all-cause mortality was 0.5% for the ACTONEL 5 mg daily group and 0.0% for the ACTONEL 150 mg once-a-month group. The incidence of serious adverse events was 4.2% in the ACTONEL 5 mg daily group and 6.2% in the ACTONEL 150 mg once-a-month group. The percentage of patients who withdrew from treatment due to adverse events was 9.5% in the ACTONEL 5 mg daily group and 8.6% in the ACTONEL 150 mg once-a-month group. The overall safety and tolerability profiles of the two dosing regimens were similar.

Acute Phase Reactions: Symptoms consistent with acute phase reaction have been reported with bisphosphonate use. The overall incidence of acute phase reaction was 1.1% in the ACTONEL 5 mg daily group and 5.2% in the ACTONEL 150 mg once-a-month group. These incidence rates are based on reporting of any of 33 acute phase reaction-like symptoms within 3 days of the first dose and for a duration of 7 days or less. Fever or influenza-like illness with onset within the same period were reported by 0.2% of patients on ACTONEL 5 mg daily and 1.4% of patients on ACTONEL 150 mg once-a-month.

Gastrointestinal Adverse Events: A greater percentage of patients experienced diarrhea with ACTONEL 150 mg once-a-month compared to 5 mg daily (8.2% vs. 4.7%, respectively). The ACTONEL 150 mg once-a-month group resulted in a higher incidence of discontinuation due to abdominal pain upper (2.5% vs. 1.4%) and diarrhea (0.8% vs. 0.0%) compared to the ACTONEL 5 mg daily regimen. All of these events occurred within a few days of the first dose. The incidence of vomiting that led to discontinuation was the same in both groups (0.3% vs. 0.3%).

Ocular Adverse Events: None of the patients treated with ACTONEL 150 mg once-a-month reported ocular inflammation such as uveitis, scleritis, or iritis; 2 patients treated with ACTONEL 5 mg daily reported iritis.

Laboratory Test Findings: When ACTONEL 5 mg daily and ACTONEL 150 mg once-a-month were compared in postmenopausal women with osteoporosis, the mean percent changes from baseline at 12 months were 0.1% and 0.3% for serum calcium, -2.3% and -2.3% for phosphate, and 8.3% and 4.8% for PTH, respectively. Compared to the ACTONEL 5 mg daily regimen, ACTONEL 150 mg once-a-month resulted in a slightly higher incidence of hypocalcemia at the end of the first month of treatment (0.2% vs. 2.2%). Thereafter, the incidence of hypocalcemia with these regimens was similar at approximately 2%.

Prevention of Postmenopausal Osteoporosis

Daily Dosing
The safety of ACTONEL 5 mg daily in the prevention of postmenopausal osteoporosis was assessed in two randomized, double-blind, placebo-controlled trials. In one study of postmenopausal women aged 37 to 82 years without osteoporosis, the use of estrogen replacement therapy in both placebo- and ACTONEL-treated patients was included. The duration of the trial was one year, with 259 exposed to placebo and 261 patients exposed to ACTONEL 5 mg. The second study included postmenopausal women aged 44 to 63 years without osteoporosis. The duration of the trial was one year, with 125 exposed to placebo and 129 patients exposed to ACTONEL 5 mg. All women received 1000 mg of elemental calcium per day.

In the trial with estrogen replacement therapy, the incidence of all-cause mortality was 1.5% for the placebo group and 0.4% for the ACTONEL 5 mg group. The incidence of serious adverse events was 8.9% in the placebo group and 5.4% in the ACTONEL 5 mg group. The percentage of patients who withdrew from treatment due to adverse events was 18.9% in the placebo group and 10.3% in the ACTONEL 5 mg group. Constipation was reported by 1.9% of the placebo group and 6.5% of ACTONEL 5 mg group.

In the second trial, the incidence of all-cause mortality was 0.0% for both groups. The incidence of serious adverse events was 17.6% in the placebo group and 9.3% in the ACTONEL 5 mg group. The percentage of patients who withdrew from treatment due to adverse events was 6.4% in the placebo group and 5.4% in the ACTONEL 5 mg group. Nausea was reported by 6.4% of patients in the placebo group and 13.2% of patients in the ACTONEL 5 mg group.

Once-a-Week Dosing
There were no deaths in a 1-year, double-blind, placebo-controlled study of ACTONEL 35 mg once a week for prevention of bone loss in 278 postmenopausal women without osteoporosis. More treated subjects on ACTONEL reported arthralgia (placebo 7.8%; ACTONEL 13.9%), myalgia (placebo 2.1%; ACTONEL 5.1%), and nausea (placebo 4.3%; ACTONEL 7.3%) than subjects on placebo.

Treatment to Increase Bone Mass in Men with Osteoporosis

In a 2-year, double-blind, multicenter study, 284 men with osteoporosis were treated with placebo (N = 93) or ACTONEL 35 mg once-a-week (N = 191). The overall safety and tolerability profile of ACTONEL in men with osteoporosis was similar to the adverse events reported in the ACTONEL postmenopausal osteoporosis clinical trials, with the addition of benign prostatic hyperplasia (placebo 3%; ACTONEL 35 mg 5%), nephrolithiasis (placebo 0%; ACTONEL 35 mg 3%), and arrhythmia (placebo 0%; ACTONEL 35 mg 2%).

Treatment and Prevention of Glucocorticoid-Induced Osteoporosis
The safety of ACTONEL 5 mg daily in the treatment and prevention of glucocorticoid-induced osteoporosis was assessed in two randomized, double-blind, placebo-controlled multinational trials of 344 patients [male (123) and female (221)] aged 18 to 85 years who had recently initiated oral glucocorticoid therapy (≤ 3 months, prevention study) or were on long-term oral glucocorticoid therapy (≥ 6 months, treatment study). The duration of the trials was one year, with 170 patients exposed to placebo and 174 patients exposed to ACTONEL 5 mg daily. Patients in one study received 1000 mg elemental calcium plus 400 IU of vitamin D supplementation per day; patients in the other study received 500 mg calcium supplementation per day.

The incidence of all-cause mortality was 2.9% in the placebo group and 1.1% in the ACTONEL 5 mg daily group. The incidence of serious adverse events was 33.5% in the placebo group and 30.5% in the ACTONEL 5 mg daily group. The percentage of patients who withdrew from the study due to adverse events was 8.8% in the placebo group and 7.5% in the ACTONEL 5 mg daily group. Back pain was reported in 8.8% of patients in the placebo group and 17.8% of patients in the ACTONEL 5 mg daily group. Arthralgia was reported in 14.7% of patients in the placebo group and 24.7% of patients in the ACTONEL 5 mg daily group.

Treatment of Paget's Disease
ACTONEL has been studied in 392 patients with Paget's disease of bone. As in trials of ACTONEL for other indications, the adverse experiences reported in the Paget's disease trials have generally been mild or moderate, have not required discontinuation of treatment, and have not appeared to be related to patient age, gender, or race.

The safety of ACTONEL was assessed in a randomized, double-blind, active-controlled study of 122 patients aged 34 to 85 years. The duration of the trial was 540 days, with 61 patients exposed to ACTONEL and 61 patients exposed to Didronel. The adverse event profile was similar for ACTONEL and Didronel: 6.6% (4/61) of patients treated with ACTONEL 30 mg daily for 2 months discontinued treatment due to adverse events, compared to 8.2% (5/61) of patients treated with Didronel 400 mg daily for 6 months. Table 2 lists adverse events reported in ≥5% of ACTONEL-treated patients in Phase 3 Paget's disease trials. Adverse events shown are considered to be possibly or probably causally related in at least one patient.

Table 2
Adverse Events Reported in ≥5% of ACTONEL-Treated Patients* in Phase 3 Paget's Disease Trials

Body System	30 mg/day × 2 months ACTONEL % (N = 61)	400 mg/day × 6 months DIDRONEL % (N = 61)
Body as a Whole		
Flu Syndrome	9.8	1.6
Chest Pain	6.6	3.3
Gastrointestinal		
Diarrhea	19.7	14.8
Abdominal Pain	11.5	8.2
Nausea	9.8	9.8
Constipation	6.6	8.2
Metabolic and Nutritional Disorders		
Peripheral Edema	8.2	6.6
Musculoskeletal		
Arthralgia	32.8	29.5
Nervous		
Headache	18.0	16.4
Dizziness	6.6	4.9
Skin and Appendages		
Rash	11.5	8.2

*Considered to be possibly or probably causally related in at least one patient.

Gastrointestinal Adverse Events: During the first year of the study (treatment and nontreatment follow-up), the proportion of patients who reported upper gastrointestinal adverse events was similar between the treatment groups; no patients reported severe upper gastrointestinal adverse events. The incidence of diarrhea was 19.7% in the ACTONEL group and 14.8% in the Didronel group; none were serious or resulted in withdrawal.
Ocular Adverse Events: Three patients who received ACTONEL 30 mg daily experienced acute iritis in 1 supportive study. All 3 patients recovered from their events; however, in 1 of these patients, the event recurred during ACTONEL treatment and again during treatment with pamidronate. All patients were effectively treated with topical steroids.

6.2   Postmarketing Experience
Because these adverse reactions are reported voluntarily from a population of uncertain size, it is not always possible to reliably estimate their frequency or establish a causal relationship to drug exposure.

Hypersensitivity Reactions
Hypersensitivity and skin reactions have been reported rarely, including angioedema, generalized rash and bullous skin reactions, some severe.

Gastrointestinal Adverse Events
Events involving upper gastrointestinal irritation, such as esophagitis and esophageal or gastric ulcers, have been reported [see Warnings and Precautions (5.1)].

Musculoskeletal Pain
Bone, joint, or muscle pain, described as severe or incapacitating, have been reported rarely [see Warnings and Precautions (5.4)].

Eye Inflammation
Reactions of eye inflammation including iritis and uveitis have been reported rarely.

Jaw Osteonecrosis
Osteonecrosis of the jaw has been reported rarely [see Warnings and Precautions (5.3)].

7   DRUG INTERACTIONS
No specific drug-drug interaction studies were performed. Risedronate is not metabolized and does not induce or inhibit hepatic microsomal drug-metabolizing enzymes (e.g. Cytochrome P450).

7.1   Calcium Supplements/Antacids
Co-administration of ACTONEL and calcium, antacids, or oral medications containing divalent cations will interfere with the absorption of ACTONEL.

7.2   Hormone Replacement Therapy
One study of about 500 early postmenopausal women has been conducted to date in which treatment with ACTONEL 5 mg daily plus estrogen replacement therapy was compared to estrogen replacement therapy alone. Exposure to study drugs was approximately 12 to 18 months and the primary endpoint was change in BMD. If considered appropriate, ACTONEL may be used concomitantly with hormone replacement therapy.

7.3   Aspirin/Nonsteroidal Anti-Inflammatory Drugs
Of over 5700 patients enrolled in the ACTONEL Phase 3 osteoporosis studies, aspirin use was reported by 31% of patients, 24% of whom were regular users (3 or more days per week). Forty-eight percent of patients reported NSAID use, 21% of whom were regular users. Among regular aspirin or NSAID users, the incidence of upper gastrointestinal adverse experiences in placebo-treated patients (24.8%) was similar to that in ACTONEL-treated patients (24.5%).

7.4   H₂ Blockers and Proton Pump Inhibitors (PPIs)
Of over 5700 patients enrolled in the ACTONEL Phase 3 osteoporosis studies, 21% used H_2 blockers and/or PPIs. Among these patients, the incidence of upper gastrointestinal adverse experiences in the placebo-treated patients was similar to that in ACTONEL-treated patients.

8   USE IN SPECIFIC POPULATIONS
8.1   Pregnancy
Pregnancy Category C: There are no adequate and well-controlled studies of ACTONEL in pregnant women.

ACTONEL should be used during pregnancy only if the potential benefit justifies the potential risk to the mother and fetus.

Bisphosphonates are incorporated into the bone matrix, from which they are gradually released over periods of weeks to years. The amount of bisphosphonate incorporation into adult bone, and hence, the amount available for release back into the systemic circulation, is directly related to the dose and duration of bisphosphonate use. There are no data on fetal risk in humans. However, there is a theoretical risk of fetal harm, predominantly skeletal, if a woman becomes pregnant after completing a course of bisphosphonate therapy. The impact of variables such as time between cessation of bisphosphonate therapy to conception, the particular bisphosphonate used, and the route of administration (intravenous versus oral) on this risk has not been studied.

In animal studies, pregnant rats received risedronate sodium during organogenesis at doses 1 to 26 times the human dose of 30 mg/day. Survival of neonates was decreased in rats treated during gestation with oral doses approximately 5 times the human dose and body weight was decreased in neonates from dams treated with approximately 26 times the human dose. The number of fetuses exhibiting incomplete ossification of sternebrae or skull from dams treated with approximately 2.5 times the human dose was significantly increased compared to controls. Both incomplete ossification and unossified sternebrae were increased in rats treated with oral doses approximately 5 times the human dose. A low incidence of cleft palate was observed in fetuses from female rats treated with oral doses approximately equal to the human dose. The relevance of this finding to human use of ACTONEL is unclear.

No significant fetal ossification effects were seen in rabbits treated with oral doses approximately 7 times the human dose (the highest dose tested). However, 1 of 14 litters were aborted and 1 of 14 litters were delivered prematurely.

Similar to other bisphosphonates, treatment during mating and gestation with doses of risedronate sodium approximately the same as the 30 mg/day human dose resulted in periparturient hypocalcemia and mortality in pregnant rats allowed to deliver.

Dosing multiples provided above are based on the recommended human dose of 30 mg/day and normalized using body surface area (mg/m^2). Actual animal doses were 3.2, 7.1 and 16 mg/kg/day in the rat and 10 mg/kg/day in the rabbit.

8.3 Nursing Mothers

Risedronate was detected in feeding pups exposed to lactating rats for a 24-hour period post-dosing, indicating a small degree of lacteal transfer. It is not known whether ACTONEL is excreted in human milk. Because many drugs are excreted in human milk and because of the potential for serious adverse reactions in nursing infants from ACTONEL, a decision should be made whether to discontinue nursing or to discontinue the drug, taking into account the importance of the drug to the mother.

8.4 Pediatric Use

ACTONEL is not indicated for use in pediatric patients.

The safety and effectiveness of risedronate was assessed in a one-year, randomized, double-blind, placebo controlled study of 143 pediatric patients (94 received risedronate) with osteogenesis imperfecta (OI). The enrolled population was predominantly patients with mild osteogenesis imperfecta (85% Type-I), aged 4 to <16 years, 50% male and 82% Caucasian, with a mean lumbar spine BMD Z-score of -2.08 (2.08 standard deviations below the mean for age-matched controls). Patients received either a 2.5 mg (≤30 kg body weight) or 5 mg (>30 kg body weight) daily oral dose. After one year, an increase in lumbar spine BMD in the risedronate group compared to the placebo group was observed. However, treatment with risedronate did not result in a reduction in the risk of fracture in pediatric patients with osteogenesis imperfecta. In ACTONEL-treated subjects, no mineralization defects were noted in paired bone biopsy specimens obtained at baseline and month 12.

The overall safety profile of risedronate in OI patients treated for up to 12 months was generally similar to that of adults with osteoporosis. However, there was an increased incidence of vomiting compared to placebo. In this study, vomiting was observed in 15% of children treated with risedronate and 6% of patients treated with placebo. Other adverse events reported in ≥10% of patients treated with risedronate and with a higher frequency than placebo were: pain in the extremity (21% with risedronate versus 16% with placebo), headache (20% versus 8%), back pain (17% versus 10%), pain (15% versus 10%), upper abdominal pain (11% versus 8%), and bone pain (10% versus 4%).

8.5 Geriatric Use

Of the patients receiving ACTONEL in postmenopausal osteoporosis studies [*see Clinical Studies (14)*], 47% were between 65 and 75 years of age, and 17% were over 75. The corresponding proportions were 26% and 11% in glucocorticoid-induced osteoporosis trials, and 40% and 26% in Paget's disease trials. No overall differences in efficacy between geriatric and younger patients were observed in these studies. In the male osteoporosis trial, 28% of patients receiving ACTONEL were between 65 and 75 years of age and 9% were over 75. The lumbar spine BMD response for ACTONEL compared to placebo was 5.6% for subjects <65 years and 2.9% for subjects ≥65 years. No overall differences in safety between geriatric and younger patients were observed in the ACTONEL trials, but greater sensitivity of some older individuals cannot be ruled out.

8.6 Renal Impairment

ACTONEL is not recommended for use in patients with severe renal impairment (creatinine clearance <30 mL/min) because of lack of clinical experience. No dosage adjustment is necessary in patients with a creatinine clearance ≥30 mL/min.

8.7 Hepatic Impairment

No studies have been performed to assess risedronate's safety or efficacy in patients with hepatic impairment. Risedronate is not metabolized in human liver preparations. Dosage adjustment is unlikely to be needed in patients with hepatic impairment.

10 OVERDOSAGE

Decreases in serum calcium and phosphorus following substantial overdose may be expected in some patients. Signs and symptoms of hypocalcemia may also occur in some of these patients. Milk or antacids containing calcium should be given to bind ACTONEL and reduce absorption of the drug.

In cases of substantial overdose, gastric lavage may be considered to remove unabsorbed drug. Standard procedures that are effective for treating hypocalcemia, including the administration of calcium intravenously, would be expected to restore physiologic amounts of ionized calcium and to relieve signs and symptoms of hypocalcemia.

Lethality after single oral doses was seen in female rats at 903 mg/kg and male rats at 1703 mg/kg. The minimum lethal dose in mice and rabbits was 4000 mg/kg and 1000 mg/kg, respectively. These values represent 320 to 620 times the 30 mg human dose based on surface area (mg/m^2).

11 DESCRIPTION

ACTONEL (risedronate sodium) tablets is a pyridinyl bisphosphonate that inhibits osteoclast-mediated bone resorption and modulates bone metabolism. Each ACTONEL tablet for oral administration contains the equivalent of 5, 30, 35, 75, or 150 mg of anhydrous risedronate sodium in the form of the hemi-pentahydrate with small amounts of monohydrate. The empirical formula for risedronate sodium hemi-pentahydrate is $C_7H_{10}NO_7P_2Na \cdot 2.5\ H_2O$. The chemical name of risedronate sodium is [1-hydroxy-2-(3-pyridinyl)ethylidene]bis[phosphonic acid] monosodium salt. The chemical structure of risedronate sodium hemi-pentahydrate is the following:

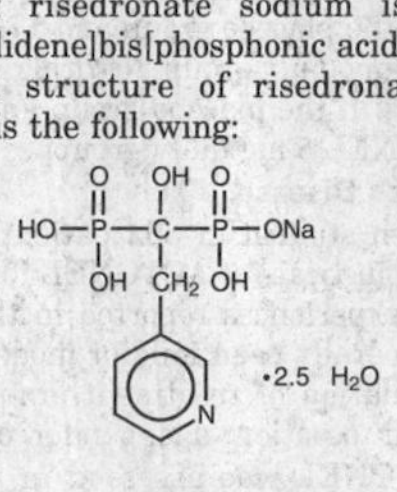

Molecular Weight:
Anhydrous: 305.10
Hemi-pentahydrate: 350.13

Risedronate sodium is a fine, white to off-white, odorless, crystalline powder. It is soluble in water and in aqueous solutions, and essentially insoluble in common organic solvents.

Inactive Ingredients

All dose strengths contain: crospovidone, hydroxypropyl cellulose, hypromellose, magnesium stearate, microcrystalline cellulose, polyethylene glycol, silicon dioxide, titanium dioxide.

Dose strength-specific ingredients include: 5 mg—ferric oxide yellow, lactose monohydrate; 30 mg—lactose monohydrate; 35 mg—ferric oxide red, ferric oxide yellow, lactose monohydrate; 75 mg—ferric oxide red; 150 mg—FD&C blue #2 aluminum lake.

12 CLINICAL PHARMACOLOGY

12.1 Mechanism of Action

ACTONEL has an affinity for hydroxyapatite crystals in bone and acts as an antiresorptive agent. At the cellular level, ACTONEL inhibits osteoclasts. The osteoclasts adhere normally to the bone surface, but show evidence of reduced active resorption (e.g., lack of ruffled border). Histomorphometry in rats, dogs, and minipigs showed that ACTONEL treatment reduces bone turnover (activation frequency, i.e., the rate at which bone remodeling sites are activated) and bone resorption at remodeling sites.

12.2 Pharmacodynamics

ACTONEL treatment decreases the elevated rate of bone turnover that is typically seen in postmenopausal osteoporosis. In clinical trials, administration of ACTONEL to postmenopausal women resulted in decreases in biochemical markers of bone turnover, including urinary deoxypyridinoline/creatinine and urinary collagen cross-linked N-telopeptide (markers of bone resorption) and serum bone-specific alkaline phosphatase (a marker of bone formation). At the 5 mg dose, decreases in deoxypyridinoline/creatinine were evident within 14 days of treatment. Changes in bone formation markers were observed later than changes in resorption markers, as expected, due to the coupled nature of bone resorption and bone formation; decreases in bone-specific alkaline phosphatase of about 20% were evident within 3 months of treatment. Bone turnover markers reached a nadir of about 40% below baseline values by the sixth month of treatment and remained stable with continued treatment for up to 3 years. Bone turnover is decreased as early as 14 days and maximally within about 6 months of treatment, with achievement of a new steady-state that more nearly approximates the rate of bone turnover seen in premenopausal women. In a 1-year study comparing daily versus weekly oral dosing regimens of ACTONEL for the treatment of osteoporosis in postmenopausal women, ACTONEL 5 mg daily and ACTONEL 35 mg once-a-week decreased urinary collagen cross-linked N-telopeptide by 60% and 61%, respectively. In addition, serum bone-specific alkaline phosphatase was also reduced by 42% and 41% in the ACTONEL 5 mg daily and ACTONEL 35 mg once-a-week groups, respectively. When postmenopausal women with osteoporosis were treated for 1 year with ACTONEL 5 mg daily or ACTONEL 75 mg two consecutive days per month, urinary collagen cross-linked N-telopeptide was decreased by 54% and 52%, respectively, and serum bone-specific alkaline phosphatase was reduced by 36% and 35%, respectively. In a 1–year study comparing ACTONEL 5 mg daily versus ACTONEL 150 mg once a month in women with postmenopausal osteoporosis, urinary collagen cross-linked N-telopeptide was decreased by 52% and 49%, respectively, and serum bone-specific alkaline phosphatase was reduced by 31% and 32%, respectively.

Osteoporosis in Men

In a 2-year study of men with osteoporosis, treatment with ACTONEL 35 mg once-a-week resulted in a mean decrease from baseline compared to placebo of 16% (placebo 20%; ACTONEL 35 mg 37%) for the bone resorption marker urinary collagen cross-linked N-telopeptide, 45% (placebo -6%; ACTONEL 35 mg 39%) for the bone resorption marker serum C-telopeptide, and 27% (placebo -2%; ACTONEL 35 mg 25%) for the bone formation marker serum bone-specific alkaline phosphatase.

Glucocorticoid-Induced Osteoporosis

Osteoporosis with glucocorticoid use occurs as a result of inhibited bone formation and increased bone resorption resulting in net bone loss. ACTONEL decreases bone resorption without directly inhibiting bone formation.

In two 1-year clinical trials in the treatment and prevention of glucocorticoid-induced osteoporosis, ACTONEL 5 mg decreased urinary collagen cross-linked N-telopeptide (a marker of bone resorption), and serum bone-specific alkaline phosphatase (a marker of bone formation) by 50% to 55% and 25% to 30%, respectively, within 3 to 6 months after initiation of therapy.

Paget's Disease

Paget's disease of bone is a chronic, focal skeletal disorder characterized by greatly increased and disordered bone remodeling. Excessive osteoclastic bone resorption is followed by osteoblastic new bone formation, leading to the replacement of the normal bone architecture by disorganized, enlarged, and weakened bone structure.

In pagetic patients treated with ACTONEL 30 mg daily for 2 months, bone turnover returned to normal in a majority of patients as evidenced by significant reductions in serum alkaline phosphatase (a marker of bone formation), and in urinary hydroxyproline/creatinine and deoxypyridinoline/creatinine (markers of bone resorption).

12.3 Pharmacokinetics

Absorption

Based on simultaneous modeling of serum and urine data, peak absorption after an oral dose is achieved at ~ 1 hour (Tmax) and occurs throughout the upper gastrointestinal tract. The fraction of the dose absorbed is independent of dose over the range studied (single dose, from 2.5 mg to 30 mg; multiple dose, from 2.5 mg to 5 mg). Steady-state conditions in the serum are observed within 57 days of daily dosing. Mean absolute oral bioavailability of the 30 mg tablet is 0.63% (90% CI: 0.54% to 0.75%) and is comparable to a solution.

Food Effect

The extent of absorption of a 30 mg dose (three 10 mg tablets) when administered 0.5 hours before breakfast is reduced by 55% compared to dosing in the fasting state (no food or drink for 10 hours prior to or 4 hours after dosing). Dosing 1 hour prior to breakfast reduces the extent of absorption by 30% compared to dosing in the fasting state. Dosing either 0.5 hours prior to breakfast or 2 hours after dinner (evening meal) results in a similar extent of absorption. ACTONEL is effective when administered at least 30 minutes before breakfast.

Distribution

The mean steady-state volume of distribution for risedronate is 13.8 L/kg in humans. Human plasma protein binding of drug is about 24%. Preclinical studies in rats and dogs dosed intravenously with single doses of [^{14}C] risedronate indicate that approximately 60% of the dose is distributed to bone. The remainder of the dose is excreted in the urine. After multiple oral dosing in rats, the uptake of risedronate in soft tissues was in the range of 0.001% to 0.01%.

Metabolism

There is no evidence of systemic metabolism of risedronate.

Excretion

In young healthy subjects, approximately half of the absorbed dose of risedronate was excreted in urine within 24 hours, and 85% of an intravenous dose was recovered in the urine over 28 days. Based on simultaneous modeling of serum and urine data, mean renal clearance was 105 mL/min (CV = 34%) and mean total clearance was 122 mL/min (CV = 19%), with the difference primarily reflecting nonrenal clearance or clearance due to adsorption to bone. The renal clearance is not concentration dependent, and there is a linear relationship between renal clearance and creatinine clearance. Unabsorbed drug is eliminated unchanged in feces. In osteopenic postmenopausal women, the terminal exponential half-life was 561 hours, mean renal clearance was 52 mL/min (CV=25%), and mean total clearance was 73 mL/min (CV=15%).

Specific Populations

Pediatric: ACTONEL is not indicated for use in pediatric patients (*see Pediatric Use [8.4]*).

Gender: Bioavailability and pharmacokinetics following oral administration are similar in men and women.

Geriatric: Bioavailability and disposition are similar in elderly (>60 years of age) and younger subjects. No dosage adjustment is necessary.

Race: Pharmacokinetic differences due to race have not been studied.

Renal Impairment: Risedronate is excreted unchanged primarily via the kidney. As compared to persons with normal renal function, the renal clearance of risedronate was decreased by about 70% in patients with creatinine clearance of approximately 30 mL/min. ACTONEL is not recommended for use in patients with severe renal impairment (creatinine clearance <30 mL/min) because of lack of clinical experience. No dosage adjustment is necessary in patients with a creatinine clearance ≥30 mL/min.

Hepatic Impairment: No studies have been performed to assess risedronate's safety or efficacy in patients with hepatic impairment. Risedronate is not metabolized in rat, dog, and human liver preparations. Insignificant amounts (<0.1% of intravenous dose) of drug are excreted in the bile in rats. Therefore, dosage adjustment is unlikely to be needed in patients with hepatic impairment.

Drug Interactions: No specific drug-drug interaction studies were performed. Risedronate is not metabolized and does not induce or inhibit hepatic microsomal drug-metabolizing enzymes (Cytochrome P450) [*see Drug Interactions (7)*].

13   NONCLINICAL TOXICOLOGY

13.1   Carcinogenesis, Mutagenesis, Impairment of Fertility

Carcinogenesis

In a 104-week carcinogenicity study, rats were administered daily oral doses up to approximately 8 times the maximum recommended human daily dose. There were no significant drug-induced tumor findings in male or female rats. The high dose male group was terminated early in the study (Week 93) due to excessive toxicity, and data from this group were not included in the statistical evaluation of the study results. In an 80-week carcinogenicity study, mice were administered daily oral doses approximately 6.5 times the human dose. There were no significant drug-induced tumor findings in male or female mice.

Mutagenesis

Risedronate did not exhibit genetic toxicity in the following assays: *In vitro* bacterial mutagenesis in *Salmonella* and *E. coli* (Ames assay), mammalian cell mutagenesis in CHO/HGPRT assay, unscheduled DNA synthesis in rat hepatocytes and an assessment of chromosomal aberrations *in vivo* in rat bone marrow. Risedronate was positive in a chromosomal aberration assay in CHO cells at highly cytotoxic concentrations (>675 mcg/mL, survival of 6% to 7%). When the assay was repeated at doses exhibiting appropriate cell survival (29%), there was no evidence of chromosomal damage.

Impairment of Fertility

In female rats, ovulation was inhibited at an oral dose approximately 5 times the human dose. Decreased implantation was noted in female rats treated with doses approximately 2.5 times the human dose. In male rats, testicular

and epididymal atrophy and inflammation were noted at approximately 13 times the human dose. Testicular atrophy was also noted in male rats after 13 weeks of treatment at oral doses approximately 5 times the human dose. There was moderate-to-severe spermatid maturation block after 13 weeks in male dogs at an oral dose approximately 8 times the human dose. These findings tended to increase in severity with increased dose and exposure time.

Dosing multiples provided above are based on the recommended human dose of 30 mg/day and normalized using body surface area (mg/m^2). Actual doses were 24 mg/kg/day in rats, 32 mg/kg/day in mice, and 8, 16 and 40 mg/kg/day in dogs.

13.2   Animal Toxicology and/or Pharmacology

Risedronate demonstrated potent anti-osteoclast, antiresorptive activity in ovariectomized rats and minipigs. Bone mass and biomechanical strength were increased dose-dependently at daily oral doses up to 4 and 25 times the human recommended oral dose of 5 mg for rats and minipigs, respectively. Risedronate treatment maintained the positive correlation between BMD and bone strength and did not have a negative effect on bone structure or mineralization. In intact dogs, risedronate induced positive bone balance at the level of the bone remodeling unit at oral doses ranging from 0.5 to 1.5 times the 5 mg/day human daily dose.

In dogs treated with an oral dose approximately 5 times the human daily dose, risedronate caused a delay in fracture healing of the radius. The observed delay in fracture healing is similar to other bisphosphonates. This effect did not occur at a dose approximately 0.5 times the human daily dose.

The Schenk rat assay, based on histologic examination of the epiphyses of growing rats after drug treatment, demonstrated that risedronate did not interfere with bone mineralization even at the highest dose tested, which was approximately 3500 times the lowest antiresorptive dose in this model (1.5 mcg/kg/day) and approximately 800 times the human daily dose of 5 mg. This indicates that ACTONEL administered at the therapeutic dose is unlikely to induce osteomalacia.

Dosing multiples provided above are based on the recommended human dose of 5 mg/day and normalized using body surface area (mg/m^2).

14   CLINICAL STUDIES

14.1   Treatment of Osteoporosis in Postmenopausal Women

The fracture efficacy of ACTONEL 5 mg daily in the treatment of postmenopausal osteoporosis was demonstrated in 2 large, randomized, placebo-controlled, double-blind studies that enrolled a total of almost 4000 postmenopausal women under similar protocols. The Multinational study (VERT MN) (ACTONEL 5 mg, N = 408) was conducted primarily in Europe and Australia; a second study was conducted in North America (VERT NA) (ACTONEL 5 mg, N = 821). Patients were selected on the basis of radiographic evidence of previous vertebral fracture, and therefore, had established disease. The average number of prevalent vertebral fractures per patient at study entry was 4 in VERT

MN, and 2.5 in VERT NA, with a broad range of baseline BMD levels. All patients in these studies received supplemental calcium 1000 mg/day. Patients with low 25-hydroxyvitamin D$_3$ levels (approximately 40 nmol/L or less) also received supplemental vitamin D 500 IU/day.

Effect on Vertebral Fractures

Fractures of previously undeformed vertebrae (new fractures) and worsening of pre-existing vertebral fractures were diagnosed radiographically; some of these fractures were also associated with symptoms (i.e., clinical fractures). Spinal radiographs were scheduled annually and prospectively planned analyses were based on the time to a patient's first diagnosed fracture. The primary endpoint for these studies was the incidence of new and worsening vertebral fractures across the period of 0 to 3 years. ACTONEL 5 mg daily significantly reduced the incidence of new and worsening vertebral fractures and of new vertebral fractures in both VERT NA and VERT MN at all time points (Table 3). The reduction in risk seen in the subgroup of patients who had 2 or more vertebral fractures at study entry was similar to that seen in the overall study population.

[See table 3 above]

Effect on Osteoporosis-Related Nonvertebral Fractures

In VERT MN and VERT NA, a prospectively planned efficacy endpoint was defined consisting of all radiographically confirmed fractures of skeletal sites accepted as associated with osteoporosis. Fractures at these sites were collectively referred to as osteoporosis-related nonvertebral fractures. ACTONEL 5 mg daily significantly reduced the incidence of nonvertebral osteoporosis-related fractures over 3 years in VERT NA (8% vs. 5%; relative risk reduction 39%) and reduced the fracture incidence in VERT MN from 16% to 11%. There was a significant reduction from 11% to 7% when the studies were combined, with a corresponding 36% reduction in relative risk. Figure 1 shows the overall results as well as the results at the individual skeletal sites for the combined studies.

Table 3
The Effect of ACTONEL on the Risk of Vertebral Fractures

VERT NA	Proportion of Patients with Fracture (%)[a]		Absolute Risk Reduction (%)	Relative Risk Reduction (%)
	Placebo N = 678	ACTONEL 5 mg N = 696		
New and Worsening				
0-1 Year	7.2	3.9	3.3	49
0-2 Years	12.8	8.0	4.8	42
0-3 Years	18.5	13.9	4.6	33
New				
0-1 Year	6.4	2.4	4.0	65
0-2 Years	11.7	5.8	5.9	55
0-3 Years	16.3	11.3	5.0	41
VERT MN	Placebo N = 346	ACTONEL 5 mg N = 344	Absolute Risk Reduction (%)	Relative Risk Reduction (%)
New and Worsening				
0-1 Year	15.3	8.2	7.1	50
0-2 Years	28.3	13.9	14.4	56
0-3 Years	34.0	21.8	12.2	46
New				
0-1 Year	13.3	5.6	7.7	61
0-2 Years	24.7	11.6	13.1	59
0-3 Years	29.0	18.1	10.9	49

[a] Calculated by Kaplan-Meier methodology.

Figure 1
Nonvertebral Osteoporosis-Related Fractures
Cumulative Incidence Over 3 Years
Combined VERT MN and VERT NA

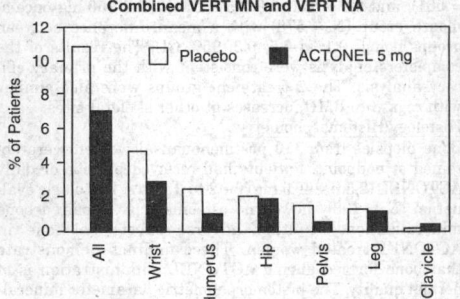

Effect on Bone Mineral Density

The results of 4 randomized, placebo-controlled trials in women with postmenopausal osteoporosis (VERT MN,

Table 4
Mean Percent Increase in BMD from Baseline in Patients Taking ACTONEL 5 mg or Placebo at Endpoint[a]

	VERT MN[b]		VERT NA[b]		BMD MN[c]		BMD NA[c]	
	Placebo N = 323	5 mg N = 323	Placebo N = 599	5 mg N = 606	Placebo N = 161	5 mg N = 148	Placebo N = 191	5 mg N = 193
Lumbar Spine	1.0	6.6	0.8	5.0	0.0	4.0	0.2	4.8
Femoral Neck	-1.4	1.6	-1.0	1.4	-1.1	1.3	0.1	2.4
Femoral Trochanter	-1.9	3.9	-0.5	3.0	-0.6	2.5	1.3	4.0
Midshaft Radius	-1.5*	0.2*	-1.2*	0.1*	ND		ND	

[a] The endpoint value is the value at the study's last time point for all patients who had BMD measured at that time; otherwise the last post-baseline BMD value prior to the study's last time point is used.
[b] The duration of the studies was 3 years.
[c] The duration of the studies was 1.5 to 2 years.
*BMD of the midshaft radius was measured in a subset of centers in VERT MN (placebo, N = 222; 5 mg, N = 214) and VERT NA (placebo, N = 310; 5 mg, N = 306).
ND = analysis not done

VERT NA, BMD MN, BMD NA) demonstrate that ACTONEL 5 mg daily increases BMD at the spine, hip, and wrist compared to the effects seen with placebo. Table 4 displays the significant increases in BMD seen at the lumbar spine, femoral neck, femoral trochanter, and midshaft radius in these trials compared to placebo. Thus, overall ACTONEL reverses the loss of BMD, a central factor in the progression of osteoporosis. In both VERT studies (VERT MN and VERT NA), ACTONEL 5 mg daily produced increases in lumbar spine BMD that were progressive over the 3 years of treatment, and were statistically significant relative to baseline and to placebo at 6 months and at all later time points.
[See table 4 above]
ACTONEL 35 mg once-a-week (N = 485) was shown to be non-inferior to ACTONEL 5 mg daily (N = 480) in a 1-year, double-blind, multicenter study of postmenopausal women with osteoporosis. In the primary efficacy analysis of completers, the mean increases from baseline in lumbar spine BMD at 1 year were 4.0% (3.7, 4.3; 95% confidence interval [CI]) in the 5 mg daily group (N = 391) and 3.9% (3.6, 4.3; 95% CI) in the 35 mg once-a-week group (N = 387) and the mean difference between 5 mg daily and 35 mg once-a-week was 0.1% (-0.4, 0.6; 95% CI). The results of the intent-to-treat analysis with the last observation carried forward were consistent with the primary efficacy analysis of completers. The 2 treatment groups were also similar with regard to BMD increases at other skeletal sites.
In a double-blind, multicenter study of postmenopausal women with osteoporosis, treatment with ACTONEL 75 mg two consecutive days per month (N = 616) was shown to be non-inferior to ACTONEL 5 mg daily (N = 613). In the primary efficacy analysis of completers, the mean increases from baseline in lumbar spine BMD at 1 year were 3.6% (3.3, 3.9; 95% CI) in the 5 mg daily group (N = 527) and 3.4% (3.1, 3.7; 95% CI) in the 75 mg two days per month group (N = 524) with a mean difference between groups being 0.2% (-0.2, 0.6; 95% CI). The results of the intent-to-treat analysis with the last observation carried forward were consistent with the primary efficacy analysis of completers. The 2 treatment groups were also similar with regard to BMD increases at other skeletal sites.
ACTONEL 150 mg once-a-month (N = 650) was shown to be non-inferior to ACTONEL 5 mg daily (N = 642) in a 1-year, double-blind, multicenter study of postmenopausal women with osteoporosis. The primary efficacy analysis was conducted in all randomized patients with baseline and post-baseline lumbar spine BMD values (modified intent-to-treat population) using last observation carried forward. The mean increases from baseline in lumbar spine BMD at 1 year were 3.4% (3.0, 3.8; 95% CI) in the 5 mg daily group (N = 561), and 3.5% (3.1, 3.9; 95% CI) in the 150 mg once-a-month group (N = 578) with a mean difference between groups being -0.1% (-0.5, 0.3; 95% CI). The results of the completers analysis were consistent with the primary efficacy analysis. The 2 treatment groups were also similar with regard to BMD increases at other skeletal sites.
Histology/Histomorphometry
Bone biopsies from 110 postmenopausal women were obtained at endpoint. Patients had received placebo or daily ACTONEL (2.5 mg or 5 mg) for 2 to 3 years. Histologic evaluation (N = 103) showed no osteomalacia, impaired bone mineralization, or other adverse effects on bone in ACTONEL-treated women. These findings demonstrate that bone formed during ACTONEL administration is of normal quality. The histomorphometric parameter mineralizing surface, an index of bone turnover, was assessed based upon baseline and post-treatment biopsy samples from 21 treated with placebo and 23 patients treated with ACTONEL 5 mg. Mineralizing surface decreased moder-

ately in ACTONEL-treated patients (median percent change: placebo, -21%; ACTONEL 5 mg, -74%), consistent with the known effects of treatment on bone turnover.
Effect on Height
In the two 3-year osteoporosis treatment studies, standing height was measured yearly by stadiometer. Both ACTONEL and placebo-treated groups lost height during the studies. Patients who received ACTONEL had a statistically significantly smaller loss of height than those who received placebo. In VERT MN, the median annual height change was -2.4 mm/yr in the placebo group compared to -1.3 mm/yr in the ACTONEL 5 mg daily group. In VERT NA, the median annual height change was -1.1 mm/yr in the placebo group compared to -0.7 mm/yr in the ACTONEL 5 mg daily group.

14.2 Prevention of Osteoporosis in Postmenopausal Women
ACTONEL 5 mg daily prevented bone loss in a majority of postmenopausal women (age range 42 to 63 years) within 3 years of menopause in a 2-year, double-blind, placebo-controlled study in 383 patients (ACTONEL 5 mg, N = 129). All patients in this study received supplemental calcium 1000 mg/day. Increases in BMD were observed as early as 3 months following initiation of ACTONEL treatment. ACTONEL 5 mg daily produced significant mean increases in BMD at the lumbar spine, femoral neck, and trochanter compared to placebo at the end of the study (Figure 2). ACTONEL 5 mg daily was also effective in patients with lower baseline lumbar spine BMD (more than 1 SD below the premenopausal mean) and in those with normal baseline lumbar spine BMD. Bone mineral density at the distal radius decreased in both ACTONEL and placebo-treated women following 1 year of treatment.

Figure 2
Change in BMD from Baseline
2-Year Prevention Study

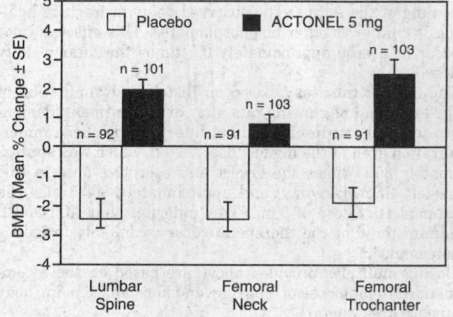

ACTONEL 35 mg once-a-week prevented bone loss in postmenopausal women (age range 44 to 64 years) without osteoporosis in a 1-year, double-blind, placebo-controlled study in 278 patients (ACTONEL 35 mg, N = 136). All patients were supplemented with 1000 mg elemental calcium and 400 IU vitamin D per day. The primary efficacy measure was the percent change in lumbar spine BMD from baseline after 1 year of treatment using LOCF (last observation carried forward). ACTONEL 35 mg once-a-week resulted in a statistically significant mean difference from placebo in lumbar spine BMD of +2.9% (least square mean for placebo -1.05%; risedronate +1.83%). ACTONEL 35 mg once-a-week also showed a statistically significant mean difference from placebo in BMD at the total proximal femur of

+1.5% (placebo -0.53%; risedronate +1.01%), femoral neck of +1.2% (placebo -1.00%; risedronate +0.22%), and trochanter of +1.8% (placebo -0.74%; risedronate +1.07%).
Combined Administration with Hormone Replacement Therapy
The effects of combining ACTONEL 5 mg daily with conjugated estrogen 0.625 mg daily (N = 263) were compared to the effects of conjugated estrogen alone (N = 261) in a 1-year, randomized, double-blind study of women ages 37 to 82 years, who were on average 14 years postmenopausal. The BMD results for this study are presented in Table 5.

Table 5
Percent Change from Baseline in BMD
After 1 Year of Treatment

	Estrogen 0.625 mg N = 261	ACTONEL 5 mg + Estrogen 0.625 mg N = 263
Lumbar Spine	4.6 ± 0.20	5.2 ± 0.23
Femoral Neck	1.8 ± 0.25	2.7 ± 0.25
Femoral Trochanter	3.2 ± 0.28	3.7 ± 0.25
Midshaft Radius	0.4 ± 0.14	0.7 ± 0.17
Distal Radius	1.7 ± 0.24	1.6 ± 0.28

Values shown are mean (±SEM) percent change from baseline.

Histology/Histomorphometry
Bone biopsies from 53 postmenopausal women were obtained at endpoint. Patients had received ACTONEL 5 mg plus estrogen or estrogen alone once daily for 1 year. Histologic evaluation (N = 47) demonstrated that the bone of patients treated with ACTONEL plus estrogen was of normal lamellar structure and normal mineralization. The histomorphometric parameter mineralizing surface, a measure of bone turnover, was assessed based upon baseline and post-treatment biopsy samples from 12 patients treated with ACTONEL plus estrogen and 12 treated with estrogen alone. Mineralizing surface decreased in both treatment groups (median percent change: ACTONEL plus estrogen, -79%; estrogen alone, -50%), consistent with the known effects of these agents on bone turnover.

14.3 Men with Osteoporosis
The effects of ACTONEL 35 mg once-a-week on BMD were examined in a 2-year, double-blind, placebo-controlled, multinational study in 285 men with osteoporosis (ACTONEL, N = 192). The patients had a mean age of 60.6 years (range 36 to 84 years) and 95% were Caucasian. At baseline, mean lumbar spine T-score was -3.2 and mean femoral neck T-score was -2.4. All patients in the study had either, 1) a BMD T-score ≤-2 at the femoral neck and ≤-1 at the lumbar spine, or 2) a BMD T-score ≤-1 at the femoral neck and ≤-2.5 at the lumbar spine. All patients were supplemented with calcium 1000 mg/day and vitamin D 400 to 500 IU/day. ACTONEL 35 mg once-a-week produced significant mean increases in BMD at the lumbar spine, femoral neck, trochanter, and total hip compared to placebo after 2 years of treatment (treatment difference: lumbar spine, 4.5%; femoral neck, 1.1%; trochanter, 2.2%; total proximal femur, 1.5%).

14.4 Glucocorticoid-Induced Osteoporosis
Bone Mineral Density
Two 1-year, double-blind, placebo-controlled trials in patients who were taking ≥7.5 mg/day of prednisone or equivalent demonstrated that ACTONEL 5 mg daily was effective in the prevention and treatment of glucocorticoid-induced osteoporosis in men and women who were either initiating or continuing glucocorticoid therapy. The efficacy of ACTONEL therapy for glucocorticoid-induced osteoporosis beyond one year has not been studied.
The prevention study enrolled 228 patients (ACTONEL 5 mg, N = 76) (18 to 85 years of age), each of whom had initiated glucocorticoid therapy (mean daily dose of prednisone 21 mg) within the previous 3 months (mean duration of use prior to study 1.8 months) for rheumatic, skin, and pulmonary diseases. The mean lumbar spine BMD was normal at baseline (average T-score -0.7). All patients in this study received supplemental calcium 500 mg/day. By the third month of treatment, and continuing through the year-long treatment, the placebo group experienced losses in BMD at the lumbar spine, femoral neck, and trochanter, while BMD was maintained or increased in the ACTONEL 5 mg group. At each skeletal site there were statistically significant differences between the placebo group and the ACTONEL 5 mg group at all timepoints (Months 3, 6, 9, and 12). The treatment differences increased with continued treatment. Although BMD increased at the distal radius in the ACTONEL 5 mg group compared to the placebo group, the difference was not statistically significant. The differences between placebo and ACTONEL 5 mg after 1 year were

3.8% at the lumbar spine, 4.1% at the femoral neck, and 4.6% at the trochanter, as shown in Figure 3. The results at these skeletal sites were similar to the overall results when the subgroups of men and postmenopausal women, but not premenopausal women, were analyzed separately. ACTONEL was effective at the lumbar spine, femoral neck, and trochanter regardless of age (<65 vs. ≥65), gender, prior and concomitant glucocorticoid dose, or baseline BMD. Positive treatment effects were also observed in patients taking glucocorticoids for a broad range of rheumatologic disorders, the most common of which were rheumatoid arthritis, temporal arteritis, and polymyalgia rheumatica.

The treatment study of similar design enrolled 290 patients (ACTONEL 5 mg, N = 100) (19 to 85 years of age) with continuing, long-term (≥6 months) use of glucocorticoids (mean duration of use prior to study 60 months; mean daily dose of prednisone 15 mg) for rheumatic, skin, and pulmonary diseases. The baseline mean lumbar spine BMD was low (1.63 SD below the young healthy population mean), with 28% of the patients more than 2.5 SD below the mean. All patients in this study received supplemental calcium 1000 mg/day and vitamin D 400 IU/day.

After 1 year of treatment, the BMD of the placebo group was within ±1% of baseline levels at the lumbar spine, femoral neck, and trochanter. ACTONEL 5 mg increased BMD at the lumbar spine (2.9%), femoral neck (1.8%), and trochanter (2.4%). The differences between ACTONEL and placebo were 2.7% at the lumbar spine, 1.9% at the femoral neck, and 1.6% at the trochanter as shown in Figure 4. The differences were statistically significant for the lumbar spine and femoral neck, but not at the femoral trochanter. ACTONEL was similarly effective on lumbar spine BMD regardless of age (<65 vs. ≥65), gender, or pre-study glucocorticoid dose. Positive treatment effects were also observed in patients taking glucocorticoids for a broad range of rheumatologic disorders, the most common of which were rheumatoid arthritis, temporal arteritis, and polymyalgia rheumatica.

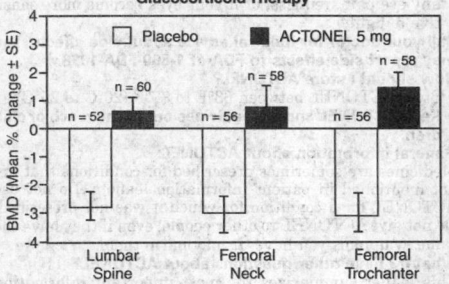

Figure 3
Change in BMD from Baseline
Patients Recently Initiating
Glucocorticoid Therapy

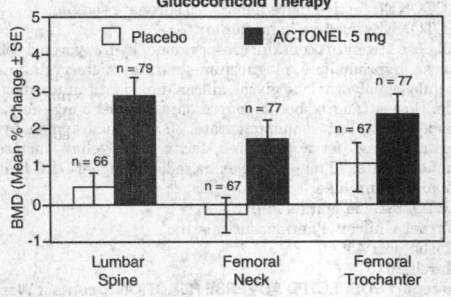

Figure 4
Change in BMD from Baseline
Patients on Long-Term
Glucocorticoid Therapy

Vertebral Fractures
In the prevention study of patients initiating glucocorticoids, the incidence of vertebral fractures at 1 year was reduced from 17% in the placebo group to 6% in the ACTONEL group. In the treatment study of patients continuing glucocorticoids, the incidence of vertebral fractures was reduced from 15% in the placebo group to 5% in the ACTONEL group (Figure 5). The statistically significant reduction in vertebral fracture incidence in the analysis of the combined studies corresponded to an absolute risk reduction of 11% and a relative risk reduction of 70%. All vertebral fractures were diagnosed radiographically; some of

these fractures also were associated with symptoms (i.e., clinical fractures).

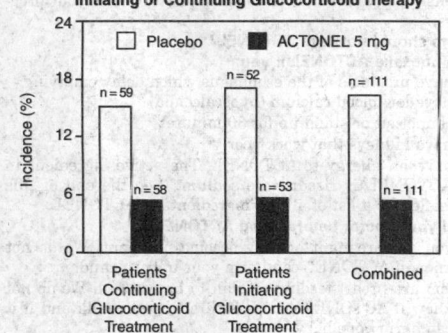

Figure 5
Incidence of Vertebral Fractures in Patients
Initiating or Continuing Glucocorticoid Therapy

Histology/Histomorphometry
Bone biopsies from 40 patients on glucocorticoid therapy were obtained at endpoint. Patients had received placebo or daily ACTONEL (2.5 mg or 5 mg) for 1 year. Histologic evaluation (N = 33) showed that bone formed during treatment with ACTONEL was of normal lamellar structure and normal mineralization, with no bone or marrow abnormalities observed. The histomorphometric parameter mineralizing surface, a measure of bone turnover, was assessed based upon baseline and post-treatment biopsy samples from 10 patients treated with ACTONEL 5 mg. Mineralizing surface decreased 24% (median percent change) in these patients. Only a small number of placebo-treated patients had both baseline and post-treatment biopsy samples, precluding a meaningful quantitative assessment.

14.5   Treatment of Paget's Disease
The efficacy of ACTONEL was demonstrated in 2 clinical studies involving 120 men and 65 women. In a double-blind, active-controlled study of patients with moderate-to-severe Paget's disease (serum alkaline phosphatase levels of at least 2 times the upper limit of normal), patients were treated with ACTONEL 30 mg daily for 2 months or Didronel® (etidronate disodium) 400 mg daily for 6 months. At Day 180, 77% (43/56) of ACTONEL-treated patients achieved normalization of serum alkaline phosphatase levels, compared to 10.5% (6/57) of patients treated with Didronel (p<0.001). At Day 540, 16 months after discontinuation of therapy, 53% (17/32) of ACTONEL-treated patients and 14% (4/29) of Didronel-treated patients with available data remained in biochemical remission.

During the first 180 days of the active-controlled study, 85% (51/60) of ACTONEL-treated patients demonstrated a ≥75% reduction from baseline in serum alkaline phosphatase excess (difference between measured level and midpoint of the normal range) with 2 months of treatment compared to 20% (12/60) in the Didronel-treated group with 6 months of treatment (p<0.001). Changes in serum alkaline phosphatase excess over time (shown in Figure 6) were significant following only 30 days of treatment, with a 36% reduction in serum alkaline phosphatase excess at that time compared to only a 6% reduction seen with Didronel treatment at the same time point (p<0.01).

[See figure 6 at top of next column]

Response to ACTONEL therapy was similar in patients with mild to very severe Paget's disease. Table 6 shows the mean percent reduction from baseline at Day 180 in excess serum alkaline phosphatase in patients with mild, moderate, or severe disease.

[See table 6 above]

Response to ACTONEL therapy was similar between patients who had previously received anti-pagetic therapy and those who had not. In the active-controlled study, 4 patients previously non-responsive to 1 or more courses of antipagetic therapy (calcitonin, Didronel) responded to treat-

Table 6
Mean Percent Reduction from Baseline at Day 180 in
Total Serum Alkaline Phosphatase Excess by Disease Severity

Subgroup: Baseline Disease Severity (AP)	ACTONEL 30 mg			DIDRONEL 400 mg		
	n	Baseline Serum AP (U/L)*	Mean % Reduction	n	Baseline Serum AP (U/L)*	Mean % Reduction
>2, <3× ULN	32	271.6 ± 5.3	-88.1	22	277.9 ± 7.45	-44.6
≥3, <7× ULN	14	475.3 ± 28.8	-87.5	25	480.5 ± 26.44	-35.0
≥7× ULN	8	1336.5 ± 134.19	-81.8	6	1331.5 ± 167.58	-47.2

*Values shown are mean ± SEM; ULN = upper limit of normal.

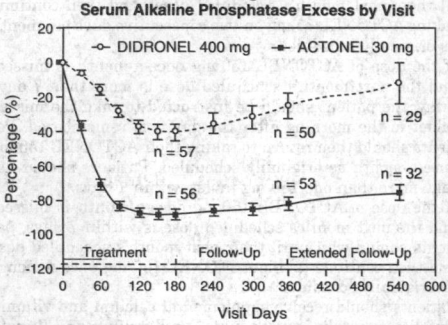

Figure 6
Mean Percent Change from Baseline in
Serum Alkaline Phosphatase Excess by Visit

ment with ACTONEL 30 mg daily (defined by at least a 30% change from baseline). Each of these patients achieved at least 90% reduction from baseline in serum alkaline phosphatase excess, with 3 patients achieving normalization of serum alkaline phosphatase levels.

Histomorphometry of the bone was studied in 14 patients with bone biopsies: 9 patients had biopsies from pagetic bone lesions and 5 patients from non-pagetic bone. Bone biopsy results in non-pagetic bone did not reveal osteomalacia, impairment of bone remodeling, or induction of a significant decline in bone turnover in patients treated with ACTONEL.

16   HOW SUPPLIED/STORAGE AND HANDLING
ACTONEL is available as follows:
5 mg film-coated, oval, yellow tablets with RSN on 1 face and 5 mg on the other.
NDC 0149-0471-01 bottle of 30
NDC 0149-0471-03 bottle of 2000
30 mg film-coated, oval, white tablets with RSN on 1 face and 30 mg on the other.
NDC 0149-0470-01 bottle of 30
35 mg film-coated, oval, orange tablets with RSN on 1 face and 35 mg on the other.
NDC 0149-0472-01 dose pack of 4
NDC 0149-0472-04 dose pack of 12
75 mg film-coated, oval, pink tablets with RSN on 1 face and 75 mg on the other.
NDC 0149-0477-01 dose pack of 2
150 mg film-coated, oval, blue tablets with RSN on 1 face and 150 mg on the other.
NDC 0149-0478-01 dose pack of 1
NDC 0149-0478-03 dose pack of 3
Store at controlled room temperature 20° to 25°C (68° to 77°F) [see USP].

17   PATIENT COUNSELING INFORMATION
[See FDA-Approved Patient Labeling (17.1)]
The patient should be informed to pay particular attention to the dosing instructions as clinical benefits may be compromised by failure to take the drug according to instructions. Specifically, ACTONEL should be taken at least 30 minutes before the first food or drink of the day other than water.

To facilitate delivery to the stomach, and thus reduce the potential for esophageal irritation, patients should take ACTONEL while in an upright position (sitting or standing) with a full glass of plain water (6 to 8 oz). Patients should not lie down for 30 minutes after taking the medication [see Warnings and Precautions (5.1)]. Patients should not chew or suck on the tablet because of a potential for oropharyngeal irritation.

Patients should be instructed that if they develop symptoms of esophageal irritation (such as difficulty or pain upon swallowing, retrosternal pain or severe persistent or worsening heartburn) they should consult their physician before continuing ACTONEL.

Patients should be instructed that if they miss a dose of ACTONEL 35 mg once a week, they should take 1 tablet on the morning after they remember and return to taking

1 tablet once a week, as originally scheduled on their chosen day. Patients should not take 2 tablets on the same day.

If one or both tablets of ACTONEL 75 mg on two consecutive days per month are missed, and the next month's scheduled doses are more than 7 days away, the patient should be instructed as follows:

- If both tablets are missed, take one ACTONEL 75 mg tablet in the morning after the day it is remembered and then the other tablet on the next consecutive morning.
- If only one ACTONEL 75 mg tablet is missed, take the missed tablet in the morning after the day it is remembered.

Patients should then return to taking their ACTONEL 75 mg on two consecutive days per month as originally scheduled. Patients should not take more than two 75 mg tablets within 7 days.

If one or both tablets of ACTONEL 75 mg on two consecutive days per month are missed, and the next month's scheduled doses are within 7 days, patients should wait until their next month's scheduled doses and then continue taking ACTONEL 75 mg on two consecutive days per month as originally scheduled.

If the dose of ACTONEL 150 mg once-a-month is missed, and the next month's scheduled dose is more than 7 days away, the patient should be instructed to take the missed tablet in the morning after the day it is remembered. Patients should then return to taking their ACTONEL 150 mg once-a-month as originally scheduled. Patients should not take more than one 150 mg tablet within 7 days.

If the dose of ACTONEL 150 mg once-a-month is missed, and the next month's scheduled dose is within 7 days, patients should wait until their next month's scheduled dose and then continue taking ACTONEL 150 mg once-a-month as originally scheduled.

Patients should receive supplemental calcium and vitamin D if dietary intake is inadequate [*see Warnings and Precautions (5.2)*]. Calcium supplements or calcium-, aluminum-, and magnesium-containing medications may interfere with the absorption of ACTONEL and should be taken at a different time of the day, as with food.

Weight-bearing exercise should be considered along with the modification of certain behavioral factors, such as excessive cigarette smoking, and/or alcohol consumption, if these factors exist.

Physicians should instruct their patients to read the Patient Information before starting therapy with ACTONEL 5 mg, 35 mg, 75 mg, or 150 mg and to re-read it each time the prescription is renewed.

Patients should be reminded to give all of their health care providers an accurate medication history. Instruct patients to tell all of their health care providers that they are taking ACTONEL. Patients should be instructed that any time they have a medical problem they think may be from ACTONEL, they should talk to their doctor.

Covered under one or more of U.S. Patent Nos. 5,583,122; 5,994,329; 6,015,801; 6,096,342; 6,165,513; 6,410,520; 6,432,932; 6,465,443; and 6,562,974.

Mfg. by: Warner Chilcott Puerto Rico LLC,
Manati, Puerto Rico 00674
or
Norwich Pharmaceuticals, Inc.,
North Norwich, NY 13814
or
Chinoin Pharmaceutical and Chemical Works Private Co. Ltd
Veresegyhaz, Hungary
Mkt. by: Warner Chilcott Pharmaceuticals Inc.,
Mason, OH 45040

17.1 FDA-Approved Patient Labeling

Patient Information
ACTONEL® (AK-toh-nel) Tablets
ACTONEL (risedronate sodium) tablets 5 mg,
ACTONEL (risedronate sodium) tablets 35 mg,
ACTONEL (risedronate sodium) tablets 75 mg, and
ACTONEL (risedronate sodium) tablets 150 mg for Osteoporosis

Read this information carefully before you start to use your medicine. Read the information you get every time you get more medicine. There may be new information. This information does not take the place of talking with your healthcare provider about your medical condition or your treatment. If you have any questions or are not sure about something, ask your healthcare provider or pharmacist.

What is the most important information I should know about ACTONEL?

ACTONEL may cause problems in your stomach and esophagus (the tube that connects the mouth and the stomach), such as trouble swallowing (dysphagia), heartburn (esophagitis), and ulcers. You might feel pain in your bones, joints, or muscles (See "What are the Possible Side Effects of ACTONEL?").

You must follow the instructions exactly for ACTONEL to work and to lower the chance of serious side effects. (See "How should I take ACTONEL?").

What is ACTONEL?

ACTONEL is a prescription medicine used:

- to prevent and treat osteoporosis in postmenopausal women.
- to increase bone mass in men with osteoporosis.
- to prevent and treat osteoporosis in men and women that is caused by treatment with steroid medicines such as prednisone.
- to treat Paget's disease of bone in men and women. The treatment for Paget's disease is very different than for osteoporosis and uses a different dose of ACTONEL. This leaflet does not cover using ACTONEL for Paget's disease. If you have Paget's disease, ask your healthcare provider how to use ACTONEL.

ACTONEL may reverse bone loss by stopping more loss of bone and increasing bone strength in most people who take it, even though they won't be able to see or feel a difference. ACTONEL helps lower the risk of breaking bones (fractures). Your healthcare provider may measure the thickness (density) of your bones or do other tests to check your progress.

Who should not take ACTONEL?

Do not take ACTONEL if you:

- have problems of the esophagus which delay emptying
- have low blood calcium (hypocalcemia)
- cannot sit or stand up for 30 minutes
- have kidneys that work poorly
- have an allergy to ACTONEL. The active ingredient in ACTONEL is risedronate sodium. (See the end of this leaflet for a list of all the ingredients in ACTONEL.)

Tell your doctor before using ACTONEL if:

- you are pregnant or may become pregnant. We do not know if ACTONEL can harm your unborn child.
- you are breast-feeding or plan to breast-feed. We do not know if ACTONEL can pass through your milk and if it can harm your baby.
- you have kidney problems. ACTONEL may not be right for you.

Tell your doctor about all the medicines you take, including prescription and non-prescription medicines, vitamins and herbal supplements. ACTONEL can interact with other medicines. Keep a list of all the medicines you take. Show it to all your healthcare providers, including your dentist and pharmacist, each time you get a new medicine.

How should I take ACTONEL?

The following instructions apply to all patients taking ACTONEL:

- Take ACTONEL exactly as prescribed by your healthcare provider.
- Take ACTONEL first thing in the morning before you eat or drink anything except plain water.
- Take ACTONEL while you are sitting up or standing.
- Take ACTONEL with 6 to 8 ounces (about 1 cup) of plain water. Do **not** take it with any other drink besides plain water.
- Swallow ACTONEL whole. **Do not chew** the tablet or keep it in your mouth to melt or dissolve.
- After taking ACTONEL you must wait at least 30 minutes **BEFORE**:
  - lying down. You may sit, stand, or do normal activities like read the newspaper or take a walk.
  - eating or drinking anything except plain water.
  - taking vitamins, calcium, or antacids. Take vitamins, calcium, and antacids at a different time of the day from when you take ACTONEL.
- Keep taking ACTONEL for as long as your healthcare provider tells you.
- For ACTONEL to treat your osteoporosis or keep you from getting osteoporosis, you have to take it exactly as prescribed.
- If you miss a dose of ACTONEL, call your healthcare provider for instructions.
- If you take more than your prescribed dose of ACTONEL, call your healthcare provider right away.
- Your healthcare provider may tell you to take calcium and vitamin D supplements and to exercise.

What is my ACTONEL schedule?

ACTONEL tablets are made in 4 different dosages (amounts). How often you should take your tablet depends upon the dosage that your doctor has prescribed (recommended) for you.

- 5 mg tablets are yellow. One tablet should be taken every day in the morning.
- 35 mg tablets are orange. One tablet should be taken once a week in the morning.
- 75 mg tablets are pink. One tablet should be taken in the morning two days in a row every month.
- 150 mg tablets are blue. One tablet should be taken once a month in the morning.

If you miss your dose in the morning, do not take it later in the day. You should call your healthcare provider for instructions.

What should I avoid while taking ACTONEL?

- Do not eat or drink anything except water before you take ACTONEL and for at least 30 minutes after you take it. See "How should I take ACTONEL?".
- Do not lie down for at least 30 minutes after you take ACTONEL.
- Foods and some vitamin supplements and medicines can stop your body from absorbing (using) ACTONEL. Therefore, do not take anything other than plain water at or near the time you take ACTONEL.

What are the possible side effects of ACTONEL?

Stop taking ACTONEL and tell your healthcare provider right away if:

- swallowing is difficult or painful
- you have chest pain
- you have very bad heartburn or it doesn't get better

Possible serious side effects may include:

- esophagus or stomach problems, including ulcers, pain, or trouble swallowing. Tell your healthcare provider if you have pain or discomfort in your stomach or esophagus.
- low calcium and other mineral disturbances. If you already have one (or more) of these problems, it should be corrected before taking ACTONEL.
- pain in bones, joints or muscles, sometimes severe. Pain may start as soon as one day or up to several months after starting ACTONEL.
- jaw-bone problems in some people, which may include infection and slower healing after teeth are pulled. Tell your healthcare providers, including your dentist, right away if you have these symptoms.

Common side effects include the following:

- back and joint pain
- upset stomach and abdominal (stomach area) pain
- short-lasting, mild flu-like symptoms, which are reported with the monthly doses and usually get better after the first dose.

Other possible side effects may include:

- **Allergic and severe skin reactions.** Tell your healthcare provider if you develop any symptoms of an allergic reaction including: rash (with or without blisters), hives, or swelling of the face, lips, tongue, or throat. **Get medical help right away if you have trouble breathing or swallowing.**
- **Eye inflammation.** Tell your healthcare provider if you get any eye pain, redness, or if your eyes become more sensitive to light.

Call your doctor for medical advice about side effects. You may report side effects to FDA at 1-800-FDA-1088.

How should I store ACTONEL?

- Store ACTONEL between 68°F to 77°F (20°C to 25°C).
- **Keep ACTONEL and all medicines out of the reach of children.**

General information about ACTONEL:

Medicines are sometimes prescribed for conditions that are not mentioned in patient information leaflets. Do not use ACTONEL for a condition for which it was not prescribed. Do not give ACTONEL to other people, even if they have the same symptoms you have. It may harm them.

What if I have other questions about ACTONEL?

This leaflet summarizes the most important information about ACTONEL for osteoporosis. If you have more questions about ACTONEL, ask your healthcare provider or pharmacist. They can give you information written for healthcare professionals. For more information, call 1-877-**ACTONEL** (toll-free) or visit our web site at www.actonel.com.

What are the ingredients of ACTONEL?

ACTONEL (active ingredient): risedronate sodium.
ACTONEL (inactive ingredients):
All dose strengths contain: crospovidone, hydroxypropyl cellulose, hypromellose, magnesium stearate, microcrystalline cellulose, polyethylene glycol, silicon dioxide, titanium dioxide. Dose-strength specific ingredients include: 5 mg—ferric oxide yellow, lactose monohydrate; 30 mg—lactose monohydrate; 35 mg—ferric oxide red, ferric oxide yellow, lactose monohydrate; 75 mg—ferric oxide red; 150 mg—FD&C blue #2 aluminum lake.

ACTONEL® is marketed by:
Warner Chilcott Pharmaceuticals Inc.,
Mason, OH 45040
March 2010

To report SUSPECTED ADVERSE REACTIONS, contact Warner Chilcott at 1-800-836-0658 or FDA at 1-800-FDA-1088 or www.fda.gov/medwatch.

ASACOL® ℞

[*āce 'ah-kol*]
(mesalamine)
Delayed-Release Tablets

DESCRIPTION

Each **Asacol** delayed-release tablet for oral administration contains 400 mg of mesalamine, an anti-inflammatory drug. The **Asacol** delayed-release tablets are coated with acrylic based resin, Eudragit S (methacrylic acid copolymer B, NF), which dissolves at pH 7 or greater, releasing mesalamine in the terminal ileum and beyond for topical anti-inflammatory action in the colon. Mesalamine has the chemical name 5-amino-2-hydroxybenzoic acid; its structural formula is:

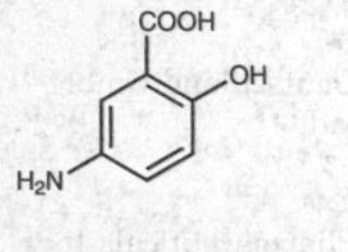

Molecular Weight: 153.1
Molecular Formula: $C_7H_7NO_3$

Inactive Ingredients: Each tablet contains colloidal silicon dioxide, dibutyl phthalate, edible black ink, iron oxide red, iron oxide yellow, lactose monohydrate, magnesium stearate, methacrylic acid copolymer B (Eudragit S), polyethylene glycol, povidone, sodium starch glycolate, and talc.

CLINICAL PHARMACOLOGY

Mesalamine is thought to be the major therapeutically active part of the sulfasalazine molecule in the treatment of ulcerative colitis. Sulfasalazine is converted to equimolar amounts of sulfapyridine and mesalamine by bacterial action in the colon. The usual oral dose of sulfasalazine for active ulcerative colitis is 3 to 4 grams daily in divided doses, which provides 1.2 to 1.6 grams of mesalamine to the colon.

The mechanism of action of mesalamine (and sulfasalazine) is unknown, but appears to be topical rather than systemic. Mucosal production of arachidonic acid (AA) metabolites, both through the cyclooxygenase pathways, i.e., prostanoids, and through the lipoxygenase pathways, i.e., leukotrienes (LTs) and hydroxyeicosatetraenoic acids (HETEs), is increased in patients with chronic inflammatory bowel disease, and it is possible that mesalamine diminishes inflammation by blocking cyclooxygenase and inhibiting prostaglandin (PG) production in the colon.

Pharmacokinetics: **Asacol** tablets are coated with an acrylic-based resin that delays release of mesalamine until it reaches the terminal ileum and beyond. This has been demonstrated in human studies conducted with radiological and serum markers. Approximately 28% of the mesalamine in **Asacol** tablets is absorbed after oral ingestion, leaving the remainder available for topical action and excretion in the feces. Absorption of mesalamine is similar in fasted and fed subjects. The absorbed mesalamine is rapidly acetylated in the gut mucosal wall and by the liver, It is excreted mainly by the kidney as N-acetyl-5-aminosalicylic acid.

Mesalamine from orally administered **Asacol** tablets appears to be more extensively absorbed than the mesalamine released from sulfasalazine. Maximum plasma levels of mesalamine and N-acetyl-5-aminosalicylic acid following multiple **Asacol** doses are about 1.5 to 2 times higher than those following an equivalent dose of mesalamine in the form of sulfasalazine. Combined mesalamine and N-acetyl-5-aminosalicylic acid AUC's and urine drug dose recoveries following multiple doses of **Asacol** tablets are about 1.3 to 1.5 times higher than those following an equivalent dose of mesalamine in the form of sulfasalazine.

The t_{max} for mesalamine and its metabolite, N-acetyl-5-aminosalicylic acid, is usually delayed, reflecting the delayed release, and ranges from 4 to 12 hours. The half-lives of elimination ($t1/2_{elm}$) for mesalamine and N-acetyl-5-aminosalicylic acid are usually about 12 hours, but are variable, ranging from 2 to 15 hours. There is a large intersubject variability in the plasma concentrations of mesalamine and N-acetyl-5-aminosalicylic acid and in their elimination half-lives following administration of **Asacol** tablets.

Clinical Studies:

Mildly to moderately active ulcerative colitis: Two placebo-controlled studies have demonstrated the efficacy of **Asacol** tablets in patients with mildly to moderately active ulcerative colitis. In one randomized, double-blind, multi-center trial of 158 patients, **Asacol** doses of 1.6 g/day and 2.4 g/day were compared to placebo. At the dose of 2.4 g/day, **Asacol** tablets reduced the disease activity, with 21 of 43 (49%) **Asacol** patients showing improvement in sigmoidoscopic appearance of the bowel compared to 12 of 44 (27%) placebo patients ($p = 0.048$). In addition, significantly more patients in the **Asacol** 2.4 g/day group showed improvement in rectal bleeding and stool frequency. The 1.6 g/day dose did not produce consistent evidence of effectiveness.

In a second randomized, double-blind, placebo-controlled clinical trial of 6 weeks duration in 87 ulcerative colitis patients, **Asacol** tablets, at a dose of 4.8 g/day, gave sigmoidoscopic improvement in 28 of 38 (74%) patients compared to 10 of 38 (26%) placebo patients ($p < 0.001$). Also, more patients in the **Asacol** 4.8 g/day group showed improvement in overall symptoms.

Maintenance of remission of ulcerative colitis: A 6-month, randomized, double-blind, placebo-controlled, multi-center study involved 264 patients treated with **Asacol** 0.8 g/day (n = 90), 1.6 g/day (n = 87), or placebo (n = 87). The proportion of patients treated with 0.8 g/day who maintained endoscopic remission was not statistically significant compared to placebo. In the intention to treat (ITT) analysis of all 174 patients treated with **Asacol** 1.6 g/day or placebo, **Asacol** maintained endoscopic remission of ulcerative colitis in 61 of 87 (70.1%) of patients, compared to 42 of 87 (48.3%) of placebo recipients ($p = 0.005$).

A pooled efficacy analysis of 4 maintenance trials compared **Asacol**, at doses of 0.8 g/day to 2.8 g/day, with sulfasalazine, at doses of 2 g/day to 4 g/day (n = 200). Treatment success was 59 of 98 (59%) for **Asacol** and 70 of 102 (69%) for sulfasalazine, a non-significant difference.

Study to assess the effect on male fertility: The effect of **Asacol** (mesalamine) on sulfasalazine-induced impairment of male fertility was examined in an open-label study. Nine patients (age < 40 years) with chronic ulcerative colitis in clinical remission on sulfasalazine 2 g/day to 3 g/day were crossed over to an equivalent **Asacol** dose (0.8 g/day to 1.2 g/day) for 3 months. Improvement in sperm count ($p < 0.02$) and morphology ($p < 0.02$) occurred in all cases. Improvement in sperm motility ($p < 0.001$) occurred in 8 of the 9 patients.

INDICATIONS AND USAGE

Asacol tablets are indicated for the treatment of mildly to moderately active ulcerative colitis and for the maintenance of remission of ulcerative colitis.

CONTRAINDICATIONS

Asacol tablets are contraindicated in patients with hypersensitivity to salicylates or to any of the components of the **Asacol** tablet.

PRECAUTIONS

General: Patients with pyloric stenosis may have prolonged gastric retention of **Asacol** tablets which could delay release of mesalamine in the colon.

Exacerbation of the symptoms of colitis has been reported in 3% of **Asacol**-treated patients in controlled clinical trials. This acute reaction, characterized by cramping, abdominal pain, bloody diarrhea, and occasionally by fever, headache, malaise, pruritus, rash, and conjunctivitis, has been reported after the initiation of **Asacol** tablets as well as other mesalamine products. Symptoms usually abate when **Asacol** tablets are discontinued.

Some patients who have experienced a hypersensitivity reaction to sulfasalazine may have a similar reaction to **Asacol** tablets or to other compounds which contain or are converted to mesalamine.

Renal: Renal impairment, including minimal change nephropathy, acute and chronic interstitial nephritis, and, rarely, renal failure has been reported in patients taking **Asacol** tablets as well as other compounds which contain or are converted to mesalamine. In animal studies (rats, dogs), the kidney is the principal target organ for toxicity. At doses of approximately 750 mg/kg to 1000 mg/kg [15 to 20 times the administered recommended human dose (based on a 50 kg person) on a mg/kg basis and 3 to 4 times on a mg/m^2 basis], mesalamine causes renal papillary necrosis. **Therefore, caution should be exercised when using Asacol (or other compounds which contain or are converted to mesalamine or its metabolites) in patients with known renal dysfunction or history of renal disease. It is recommended that all patients have an evaluation of renal function prior to initiation of Asacol tablets and periodically while on Asacol therapy.**

Use in Hepatic Impairment: There have been reports of hepatic failure in patients with pre existing liver disease who have been administered mesalamine. Caution should be exercised when administering **Asacol** to patients with liver disease.

Information for Patients: Patients should be instructed to swallow the **Asacol** tablets whole, taking care not to break, cut, or chew the tablets, because the coating is an important part of the delayed-release formulation. In 2% to 3% of patients in clinical studies, intact or partially intact tablets have been reported in the stool. If this occurs repeatedly, patients should contact their physician.

Patients with ulcerative colitis should be made aware that ulcerative colitis rarely remits completely, and that the risk of relapse can be substantially reduced by continued administration of **Asacol** at a maintenance dosage.

Drug Interactions: There are no known drug interactions.

Carcinogenesis, Mutagenesis, Impairment of Fertility: Dietary mesalamine was not carcinogenic in rats at doses as high as 480 mg/kg/day, or in mice at 2000 mg/kg/day. These doses are 2.4 and 5.1 times the maximum recommended human maintenance dose of **Asacol** of 1.6 g/day (32 mg/kg/day if 50 kg weight assumed or 1184 mg/m^2), respectively, based on body surface area. Mesalamine was negative in the Ames assay for mutagenesis, negative for induction of sister chromatid exchanges (SCE) and chrornosornal aberrations in Chinese hamster ovary cells *in vitro*, and negative for induction of micronuclei (MN) in mouse bone marrow polychromatic erythrocytes. Mesalamine, at oral doses up to 480 mg/kg/day (about 1.6 times the recommended human treatment dose on a body surface area basis), was found to have no effect on fertility or reproductive performance of male and female rats.

Pregnancy: Pregnancy Category C: There are no adequate and well controlled studies of **Asacol** use in pregnant women. Limited published human data on mesalamine show no increase in the overall rate of congenital malformations. Some data show an increased rate of preterm birth, stillbirth, and low birth weight; however, these adverse pregnancy outcomes are also associated with active inflammatory bowel disease. Animal reproduction studies of mesalamine found no evidence of fetal harm. However, dibutyl phthalate (DBP) is an inactive ingredient in **Asacol's** enteric coating, and in animal studies at doses >190 times the human dose based on body surface area, maternal DBP was associated with external and skeletal malformations and adverse effects on the male reproductive system. **Asacol** should be used during pregnancy only if the potential benefit justifies the potential risk to the fetus.

Mesalamine crosses the placenta. In prospective and retrospective studies of over 600 women exposed to mesalamine during pregnancy, the observed rate of congenital malformations was not increased above the background rate in the general population. Some data show an increased rate of preterm birth, stillbirth, and low birth weight, but it is unclear whether this was due to underlying maternal disease, drug exposure, or both, as active inflammatory bowel disease is also associated with adverse pregnancy outcomes.

Reproduction studies with mesalamine were performed during organogenesis in rats and rabbits at oral doses up to 480 mg/kg/day. There was no evidence of impaired fertility or harm to the fetus. These mesalamine doses were about 1.6 times (rat) and 3.2 times (rabbit) the recommended human dose, based on body surface area.

Dibutyl phthalate (DBP) is an inactive ingredient in **Asacol's** enteric coating. The human daily intake of DBP from the maximum recommended dose of **Asacol** tablets is about 21 mg. Published reports in rats show that male rat offspring exposed in utero to DBP (≥100 mg/kg/day, approximately 39 times the human dose based on body surface area), display reproductive system aberrations compatible with disruption of androgenic dependent development. The clinical significance of this finding in rats is unknown. At higher dosages (≥500 mg/kg/day, approximately 194 times the human dose based on body surface area), additional effects, including cryptorchidism, hypospadias, atrophy or agenesis of sex accessory organs, testicular injury, reduced daily sperm production, permanent retention of nipples, and decreased anogenital distance are noted. Female offspring are unaffected. High doses of DBP, administered to pregnant rats was associated with increased incidences of developmental abnormalities, such as cleft palate (≥630 mg/kg/day, about 244 times the human dose, based on body surface area) and skeletal abnormalities (≥750 mg/kg/day, about 290 times the human dose based on body surface area) in the offspring.

Nursing Mothers: Mesalamine and its N-acetyl metabolite are excreted into human milk. In published lactation studies, maternal mesalamine doses from various oral and rectal formulations and products ranged from 500 mg to 3 g daily. The concentration of mesalamine in milk ranged from non-detectable to 0.11 mg/L. The concentration of the N-acetyl-5-aminosalicylic acid metabolite ranged from 5 to 18.1 mgIL. Based on these concentrations, estimated infant daily doses for an exclusively breastfed infant are 0 - 0.017 mg/kg/day of mesalamine and 0.75-2.72 mg/kg/day of N-acetyl-5-aminosalicylic acid. Caution should be exercised when **Asacol** is administered to a nursing woman.

Dibutyl phthalate (DBP), an inactive ingredient in the enteric coating of **Asacol** tablets, and its primary metabolite mono-butyl phthalate (MBP) are excreted into human milk. In pregnant rats, DBP causes fetal reproductive system aberrations/malformations in male offspring [see PRECAUTIONS, Pregnancy]. The clinical significance of this is has not been determined.

Pediatric Use: Safety and effectiveness of **Asacol** tablets in pediatric patients have not been established.

Geriatric Use: Clinical studies of **Asacol** did not include sufficient numbers of subjects aged 65 and over to determine whether they respond differently from younger subjects. Other reported clinical experience has not identified differences in responses between the elderly and younger patients. In general, the greater frequency of decreased hepatic, renal, or cardiac function, and of concomitant disease or other drug therapy in elderly patients should be considered when prescribing **Asacol**. Reports from uncontrolled clinical studies and post-marketing reporting systems suggest a higher incidence of blood dyscrasias, i.e., agranulocytosis, neutropenia, pancytopenia, in subjects receiving **Asacol** who are 65 years or older. Caution should be taken to closely monitor blood cell counts during drug therapy.

This drug is known to be substantially excreted by the kidney, and the risk of toxic reactions to this drug may be greater in patients with impaired renal function. Because elderly patients are more likely to have decreased renal function, care should be taken when prescribing this drug therapy. As stated in the PRECAUTIONS section, it is recommended that all patients have an evaluation of renal function prior to initiation of **Asacol** tablets and periodically while on **Asacol** therapy.

ADVERSE REACTIONS

Asacol tablets have been evaluated in 3685 inflammatory bowel disease patients (most patients with ulcerative colitis) in controlled and open-label studies. Adverse events seen in clinical trials with **Asacol** tablets have generally been mild and reversible. Adverse events presented in the following sections may occur regardless of length of therapy and similar events have been reported in short- and long-term studies and in the post-marketing setting.

In two short-term (6 weeks) placebo-controlled clinical studies involving 245 patients, 155 of whom were randomized to **Asacol** tablets, five (3.2%) of the **Asacol** patients discontinued **Asacol** therapy because of adverse events as compared to two (2.2%) of the placebo patients. Adverse reactions leading to withdrawal from **Asacol** tablets included (each in one patient): diarrhea and colitis flare; dizziness, nausea, joint pain, and headache; rash, lethargy and constipation; dry mouth, malaise, lower back discomfort, mild disorientation, mild indigestion and cramping; headache, nausea, aching, vomiting, muscle cramps, a stuffy head, plugged ears, and fever.

Adverse events occurring in **Asacol**-treated patients at a frequency of 2% or greater in the two short-term, double-blind, placebo-controlled trials mentioned above are listed in Table 1 below. Overall, the incidence of adverse events seen with **Asacol** tablets was similar to placebo.

Table 1
Frequency (%) of Common Adverse Events Reported
in Ulcerative Colitis Patients Treated with
Asacol Tablets or Placebo in Short-Term (6-Week)
Double-Blind Controlled Studies

Event	Placebo (n = 87)	Asacol tablets (n = 152)
Headache	36	35
Abdominal pain	14	18
Eructation	15	16
Pain	8	14
Nausea	15	13
Pharyngitis	9	11
Dizziness	8	8
Asthenia	15	7
Diarrhea	9	7
Back pain	5	7
Fever	8	6
Rash	3	6
Dyspepsia	1	6
Rhinitis	5	5
Arthralgia	3	5
Hypertonia	3	5
Vomiting	2	5
Constipation	1	5
Flatulence	7	3
Dysmenorrhea	3	3
Chest pain	2	3
Chills	2	3
Flu syndrome	2	3
Peripheral edema	2	3
Myalgia	1	3
Sweating	1	3
Colitis exacerbation	0	3
Pruritus	0	3
Acne	1	2
Increased cough	1	2
Malaise	1	2
Arthritis	0	2
Conjunctivitis	0	2
Insomnia	0	2

Of these adverse events, only rash showed a consistently higher frequency with increasing **Asacol** dose in these studies.

In a 6-month placebo-controlled maintenance trial involving 264 patients, 177 of whom were randomized to **Asacol** tablets, six (3.4%) of the **Asacol** patients discontinued **Asacol** therapy because of adverse events, as compared to four (4.6%) of the placebo patients. Adverse reactions leading to withdrawal from **Asacol** tablets included (each in one patient): anxiety; headache; pruritus; decreased libido; rheumatoid arthritis; and stomatitis and asthenia.

In the 6-month placebo-controlled maintenance trial, the incidence of adverse events seen with **Asacol** tablets was sim-

ilar to that seen with placebo. In addition to events listed in Table 1, the following adverse events occurred in **Asacol**-treated patients at a frequency of 2% or greater in this study: abdominal enlargement, anxiety, bronchitis, ear disorder, ear pain, gastroenteritis, gastrointestinal hemorrhage, infection, joint disorder, migraine, nervousness, paresthesia, rectal disorder, rectal hemorrhage, sinusitis, stool abnormalities, tenesmus, urinary frequency, vasodilation, and vision abnormalities.

In 3342 patients in uncontrolled clinical studies, the following adverse events occurred at a frequency of 5% or greater and appeared to increase in frequency with increasing dose: asthenia, fever, flu syndrome, pain, abdominal pain, back pain, flatulence, gastrointestinal bleeding, arthralgia, and rhinitis.

In addition to the adverse events listed above, the following events have been reported in clinical studies, literature reports, and postmarketing use of products which contain (or have been metabolized to) mesalamine. Because many of these events were reported voluntarily from a population of unknown size, estimates of frequency cannot be made. These events have been chosen for inclusion due to their seriousness or potential causal connection to mesalamine:

Body as a Whole: Neck pain, facial edema, edema, lupus-like syndrome, drug fever (rare).

Cardiovascular: Pericarditis (rare), myocarditis (rare).

Gastrointestinal: Anorexia, pancreatitis, gastritis, increased appetite, cholecystitis, dry mouth, oral ulcers, perforated peptic ulcer (rare), bloody diarrhea. There have been rare reports of hepatotoxicity including, jaundice, cholestatic jaundice, hepatitis, and possible hepatocellular damage including liver necrosis and liver failure. Some of these cases were fatal. Asymptomatic elevations of liver enzymes which usually resolve during continued use or with discontinuation of the drug have also been reported. One case of Kawasaki-like syndrome which included changes in liver enzymes was also reported.

Hematologic: Agranulocytosis (rare), aplastic anemia (rare), thrombocytopenia, eosinophilia, leukopenia, anemia, lymphadenopathy.

Musculoskeletal: Gout.

Nervous: Depression, somnolence, emotional lability, hyperesthesia, vertigo, confusion, tremor, peripheral neuropathy (rare), transverse myelitis (rare), Guillain-Barré syndrome (rare).

Respiratory/Pulmonary: Eosinophilic pneumonia, interstitial pneumonitis, asthma exacerbation, pleuritis.

Skin: Alopecia, psoriasis (rare), pyoderma gangrenosum (rare), dry skin, erythema nodosum, urticaria.

Special Senses: Eye pain, taste perversion, blurred vision, tinnitus.

Urogenital: Renal Failure (rare), interstitial nephritis, minimal change nephropathy (See also Renal subsection in PRECAUTIONS). Dysuria, urinary urgency, hematuria, epididymitis, menorrhagia.

Laboratory Abnormalities: Elevated AST (SGOT) or ALT (SGPT), elevated alkaline phosphatase, elevated GGT, elevated LDH, elevated bilirubin, elevated serum creatinine and BUN.

DRUG ABUSE AND DEPENDENCY

Abuse: None reported.

Dependency: Drug dependence has not been reported with chronic administration of mesalamine.

OVERDOSAGE

Two cases of pediatric overdosage have been reported. A 3-year-old male who ingested 2 grams of **Asacol** tablets was treated with ipecac and activated charcoal: no adverse events occurred. Another 3-year-old male, approximately 16 kg, ingested an unknown amount of a maximum of 24 grams of **Asacol** crushed in solution (i.e., uncoated mesalamine); he was treated with orange juice and activated charcoal, and experienced no adverse events. In dogs, single doses of 6 grams of delayed-release **Asacol** tablets resulted in renal papillary necrosis but were not fatal. This was approximately 12.5 times the recommended human dose (based on a dose of 2.4 g/day in a 50 kg person). Single oral doses of uncoated mesalamine in mice and rats of 5000 mg/kg and 4595 mg/kg, respectively, or of 3000 mg/kg in cynomolgus monkeys, caused significant lethality.

DOSAGE AND ADMINISTRATION

For the treatment of mildly to moderately active ulcerative colitis: The usual dosage in adults is two 400-mg tablets to be taken three times a day for a total daily dose of 2.4 grams for a duration of 6 weeks.

For the maintenance of remission of ulcerative colitis: The recommended dosage in adults is 1.6 grams daily, in divided doses. Treatment duration in the prospective, well-controlled trial was 6 months.

Two **Asacol** 400 mg tablets have not been shown to be bioequivalent to one **Asacol**® HD (mesalamine) delayed-release 800 mg tablet.

HOW SUPPLIED

Asacol tablets are available as red-brown, capsule-shaped tablets containing 400 mg mesalamine and imprinted "Asacol NE" in black.

NDC 0149-0752-15 Bottle of 180

Store at controlled room temperature 20°- 25°C (68°- 77°F) [See USP].

Manufactured by:
Warner Chilcott Deutschland GmbH
D-64331 Weiterstadt
Germany
Marketed by:
Warner Chilcott Pharmaceuticals Inc.
Mason, OH 45040
1-800-836-0658
Under license from Medeva Pharma Suisse AG (registered trademark owner).
U.S. Patent Nos. 5,541,170 and 5,541,171
To report SUSPECTED ADVERSE REACTIONS, contact Warner Chilcott at 1-800-836-0658 or FDA at 1-800-FDA-1088 or www.fda.gov/medwatch.
REVISED May 2010

ASACOL® HD   ℞
(mesalamine)
delayed-release tablet for oral administration

HIGHLIGHTS OF PRESCRIBING INFORMATION
These highlights do not include all the information needed to use Asacol HD safely and effectively. See full prescribing information for Asacol HD.
Asacol® HD (mesalamine) delayed-release tablet for oral administration
Initial U.S. Approval: 1987

———————INDICATIONS AND USAGE———————
- Asacol HD is a locally acting aminosalicylate indicated for the treatment of moderately active ulcerative colitis. Safety and effectiveness of Asacol HD beyond 6 weeks has not been established. (1)

————DOSAGE AND ADMINISTRATION————
- Two 800 mg tablets three times daily for 6 weeks (2)
- Asacol HD should be swallowed whole without cutting, breaking, or chewing (2)
- One Asacol HD 800 mg tablet has not been shown to be bioequivalent to two Asacol® (mesalamine) delayed-release 400 mg tablets (2)

————DOSAGE FORMS AND STRENGTHS————
- 800 mg delayed-release tablet (3)

————————CONTRAINDICATIONS————————
- History of hypersensitivity to salicylates or aminosalicylates or to any component of the Asacol HD tablet (4)

————WARNINGS AND PRECAUTIONS————
- Renal impairment may occur. Monitor renal function at the beginning of treatment and periodically during therapy (5.1)
- Acute exacerbation of colitis symptoms can occur (5.2)
- Patients with pyloric stenosis may have prolonged gastric retention of Asacol HD tablets (5.4)
- Use caution with pre-existing liver disease (5.5)

————————ADVERSE REACTIONS————————
- The most common adverse reactions (observed in >2% of patients) were headache, nausea, nasopharyngitis, abdominal pain, and worsening of ulcerative colitis (6.1)
- **To report SUSPECTED ADVERSE REACTIONS, contact Warner Chilcott at 1-800-836-0658 or FDA at 1-800-FDA-1088 or www.fda.gov/medwatch**

————USE IN SPECIFIC POPULATIONS————
- Use with caution in patients with renal disease (5.1)
- Pregnancy: May cause fetal harm, based on animal data for dibutyl phthalate (inactive ingredient in Asacol HD enteric coating) (8.1)
- Nursing Mothers: Caution should be excercised when administered to a nursing woman (8.3)
- Monitor blood cell counts in geriatric patients (8.5)

See 17 for PATIENT COUNSELING INFORMATION.
Revised: May 2010

FULL PRESCRIBING INFORMATION: CONTENTS*
FULL PRESCRIBING INFORMATION
1   INDICATIONS AND USAGE
2   DOSAGE AND ADMINISTRATION
3   DOSAGE FORMS AND STRENGTHS
4   CONTRAINDICATIONS
5   WARNINGS AND PRECAUTIONS
    5.1   Renal Impairment
    5.2   Exacerbation of Ulcerative Colitis Symptoms
    5.3   Hypersensitivity
    5.4   Pyloric Stenosis
    5.5   Use in Hepatic Impairment
6   ADVERSE REACTIONS
    6.1   Clinical Trials Experience
    6.2   Adverse Reaction Information from Other Sources

*Sections or subsections omitted from the full prescribing information are not listed.

FULL PRESCRIBING INFORMATION

1 INDICATIONS AND USAGE

Asacol HD is indicated for the treatment of moderately active ulcerative colitis. Safety and effectiveness of Asacol HD beyond 6 weeks has not been established.

2 DOSAGE AND ADMINISTRATION

For the treatment of moderately active ulcerative colitis, the recommended dose of Asacol HD in adults is two 800 mg tablets to be taken three times daily with or without food, for a total daily dose of 4.8 g, for a duration of 6 weeks. Asacol HD use beyond 6 weeks has not been evaluated. Asacol HD should be swallowed whole without cutting, breaking, or chewing. One Asacol HD 800 mg tablet has not been shown to be bioequivalent to two Asacol 400 mg tablets *[see Clinical Pharmacology (12.3)]*.

3 DOSAGE FORMS AND STRENGTHS

Asacol HD delayed-release tablets are available as red-brown, capsule-shaped tablets containing 800 mg mesalamine and imprinted with "PG 800" in black.

4 CONTRAINDICATIONS

Asacol HD is contraindicated in patients with hypersensitivity to salicylates or aminosalicylates or to any of the components of Asacol HD tablets.

5 WARNINGS AND PRECAUTIONS

5.1 Renal Impairment

Renal impairment, including minimal change nephropathy, acute and chronic interstitial nephritis, and, rarely, renal failure, has been reported in patients taking products such as Asacol HD that contain or are converted to mesalamine. It is recommended that all patients have an evaluation of renal function prior to initiation of Asacol HD and periodically while on therapy. Exercise caution when using Asacol HD in patients with known renal dysfunction or history of renal disease.

In animal studies (rats, mice, dogs), the kidney was the principal organ for toxicity *[see Nonclinical Toxicology (13.2)]*.

5.2 Exacerbation of Ulcerative Colitis Symptoms

Exacerbation of the symptoms of colitis has been reported in 2.3% of Asacol HD-treated patients in controlled clinical trials. This acute reaction, characterized by cramping, abdominal pain, bloody diarrhea, and occasionally by fever, headache, malaise, pruritus, rash, and conjunctivitis, has been reported after the initiation of Asacol HD tablets as well as other mesalamine products. Symptoms usually abate when Asacol HD tablets are discontinued.

5.3 Hypersensitivity

Some patients who have experienced a hypersensitivity reaction to sulfasalazine may have a similar reaction to Asacol HD tablets or to other compounds that contain or are converted to mesalamine.

5.4 Pyloric Stenosis

Patients with pyloric stenosis may have prolonged gastric retention of Asacol HD tablets, which could delay release of mesalamine in the colon.

5.5 Use in Hepatic Impairment

There have been reports of hepatic failure in patients with pre-existing liver disease who have been administered mesalamine. Caution should be exercised when administering Asacol HD to patients with liver disease.

6 ADVERSE REACTIONS

The most serious adverse reactions seen in Asacol HD clinical trials or with other products that contain or are metabolized to mesalamine were:

- Renal impairment, including renal failure (rare) *[see Warnings and Precautions (5.1)]*
- Acute exacerbation of colitis *[see Warnings and Precautions (5.2)]*
- Hypersensitivity reactions *[see Warnings and Precautions (5.3)]*

6.1 Clinical Trials Experience

Because clinical trials are conducted under widely varying conditions, adverse reaction rates observed in the clinical trials of a drug cannot be directly compared to rates in the clinical trials of another drug and may not reflect the rates observed in practice.

Asacol HD has been evaluated in 896 patients with ulcerative colitis in controlled studies. Three six-week, active-controlled studies were conducted comparing Asacol HD 4.8 g/day with Asacol (mesalamine) 2.4 g/day as control in patients with mildly to moderately active ulcerative colitis. In these studies, 727 patients were dosed with the Asacol HD tablet and 732 patients were dosed with the Asacol 400 mg tablet. (One Asacol HD 800 mg tablet has not been shown to be bioequivalent to two Asacol 400 mg tablets *[see Clinical Pharmacology (12.3)]*.)

The most common reactions reported in the Asacol HD group were headache (4.7%), nausea (2.8%), nasopharyngitis (2.5%), abdominal pain (2.3%), exacerbation of ulcerative colitis (2.3%), diarrhea (1.7%), and dyspepsia (1.7%); Table 1 enumerates adverse drug reactions that occurred in the three studies. The most common reactions in the primary efficacy population of patients with moderately active ulcerative colitis (602 patients dosed with Asacol HD and 618 patients dosed with the Asacol 400 mg tablet) were the same as all treated patients. The majority of adverse reactions with Asacol HD in the double-blind, active-controlled trials were mild or moderate in severity and were reversible.

Discontinuations due to adverse reactions occurred in 3.9% of patients in the Asacol HD group and in 4.2% of patients in the Asacol 400 mg tablet comparator group. The most common cause for discontinuation was gastrointestinal symptoms associated with ulcerative colitis.

Severe adverse reactions occurred in 7.6% of patients in the Asacol HD group and in 7.6% of patients in the Asacol 400 mg tablet comparator group. Most of these reactions were gastrointestinal symptoms related to ulcerative colitis. Serious adverse reactions occurred in 0.8% of patients in the Asacol HD group and in 1.8% of patients in the Asacol 400 mg tablet comparator group. The majority involved the gastrointestinal system.

Table 1. Adverse Reactions Occurring in 1% or More of All Treated Patients (Three studies combined; Intent-to-treat population)

MedDRA Preferred Term	Asacol* 2.4g/day (400 mg Tablet) N=732)	Asacol HD* 4.8g/day (800 mg Tablet) N=727)
Headache	4.9 %	4.7 %
Nausea	2.9 %	2.8 %
Nasopharyngitis	1.4 %	2.5 %
Abdominal pain	2.3 %	2.3 %
Ulcerative Colitis	2.7 %	2.3 %
Diarrhea	1.9 %	1.7 %
Dyspepsia	0.8 %	1.7 %
Vomiting	1.6 %	1.4 %
Flatulence	0.7 %	1.2 %
Influenza	1.2 %	1.0 %
Pyrexia	1.2 %	0.7 %
Cough	1.4 %	0.3 %

N = number of patients within specified treatment group
% = percentage of patients in category and treatment group
* One Asacol HD 800 mg tablet has not been shown to be bioequivalent to two Asacol 400 mg tablets *[see Clinical Pharmacology (12.3)]*.

6.2 Adverse Reaction Information from Other Sources

In addition to the adverse reactions reported above in clinical trials involving the Asacol HD tablet, the adverse events listed below have been reported in controlled clinical trials, open label studies, literature reports, or foreign and domestic marketing experience with Asacol 400 mg tablets or other products that contain or are metabolized to mesalamine. Because these reactions are reported voluntarily from a population of uncertain size, it is not always possible to reliably estimate their frequency or establish a causal relationship to drug exposure.

Body as a Whole: Facial edema, edema, peripheral edema, asthenia, chills, infection, malaise, pain, neck pain, chest pain, back pain, abdominal enlargement, lupus-like syndrome, drug fever (rare).

Cardiovascular: Pericarditis (rare), pericardial effusion, myocarditis (rare), vasodilation, migraine.

Gastrointestinal: Dry mouth, stomatitis, oral ulcers, anorexia, increased appetite, eructation, pancreatitis, cholecystitis, gastritis, gastroenteritis, gastrointestinal bleeding, perforated peptic ulcer (rare), constipation, hemorrhoids, rectal hemorrhage, bloody diarrhea, tenesmus, stool abnormality.

Hepatic: There have been rare reports of hepatotoxicity, including jaundice, cholestatic jaundice, hepatitis, and possible hepatocellular damage including liver necrosis and liver failure. Some of these cases were fatal. Asymptomatic elevations of liver enzymes which usually resolve during continued use or with discontinuation of the drug have also been reported. One case of Kawasaki-like syndrome, that included changes in liver enzymes, was also reported.

Hematologic: Agranulocytosis (rare), aplastic anemia (rare), anemia, thrombocytopenia, leukopenia, eosinophilia, lymphadenopathy.

Musculoskeletal: Gout, rheumatoid arthritis, arthritis, arthralgia, joint disorder, myalgia, hypertonia.

Neurological/Psychiatric: Anxiety, depression, somnolence, insomnia, nervousness, confusion, emotional lability, dizziness, vertigo, tremor, paresthesia, hyperesthesia, peripheral neuropathy (rare), Guillain-Barré syndrome (rare), and transverse myelitis (rare).

Respiratory/Pulmonary: Sinusitis, rhinitis, pharyngitis, asthma exacerbation, pleuritis, bronchitis, eosinophilic pneumonia, interstitial pneumonitis.

Skin: Alopecia, psoriasis (rare), pyoderma gangrenosum (rare), erythema nodosum, acne, dry skin, sweating, pruritus, urticaria, rash.

Special Senses: Ear pain, tinnitus, ear congestion, ear disorder, conjunctivitis, eye pain, blurred vision, vision abnormality, taste perversion.

Renal/Urogenital: Renal failure (rare), interstitial nephritis, minimal change nephropathy *[see Warnings and Precautions (5.1)]*, dysuria, urinary frequency and urgency, hematuria, epididymitis, decreased libido, dysmenorrhea, menorrhagia.

Laboratory Abnormalities: Elevated AST (SGOT) or ALT (SGPT), elevated alkaline phosphatase, elevated GGT, elevated LDH, elevated bilirubin, elevated serum creatinine and BUN.

7 DRUG INTERACTIONS

No formal drug interaction studies have been performed using Asacol HD with other drugs.

8 USE IN SPECIFIC POPULATIONS

8.1 Pregnancy

Pregnancy Category C: There are no adequate well controlled studies of Asacol HD use in pregnant women. Limited published human data on mesalamine show no increase in the overall rate of congenital malformations. Some data show an increased rate of preterm birth, stillbirth, and low birth weight; however, these adverse pregnancy outcomes are also associated with active inflammatory bowel disease. Animal reproduction studies of mesalamine found no evidence of fetal harm. However, dibutyl phthalate (DBP) is an inactive ingredient in Asacol HD's enteric coating, and in animal studies at doses >80 times the human dose based on body surface area, maternal DBP was associated with external and skeletal malformations and adverse effects on the male reproductive system. Asacol HD should be used during pregnancy only if the potential benefit justifies the potential risk to the fetus.

Mesalamine crosses the placenta. In prospective and retrospective studies of over 600 women exposed to mesalamine during pregnancy, the observed rate of congenital malformations was not increased above the background rate in the general population. Some data show an increased rate of preterm birth, stillbirth, and low birth weight, but it is unclear whether this was due to underlying maternal disease, drug exposure, or both, as active inflammatory bowel disease is also associated with adverse pregnancy outcomes.

Reproduction studies with mesalamine were performed during organogenesis in rats and rabbits at oral doses up to 480 mg/kg/day. There was no evidence of impaired fertility or harm to the fetus. These mesalamine doses were about 1.6 times (rat) and 3.2 times (rabbit) the recommended human dose, based on body surface area.

Dibutyl phthalate (DBP) is an inactive ingredient in Asacol HD's enteric coating. The human daily intake of DBP from the maximum recommended dose of Asacol HD tablets is about 48 mg. Published reports in rats show that male rat offspring exposed in utero to DBP (≥100 mg/kg/day, approximately 17 times the human dose based on body surface area), display reproductive system aberrations compatible with disruption of androgenic dependent development. The clinical significance of this finding in rats is unknown. At higher dosages (≥500 mg/kg/day, approximately 84 times the human dose based on body surface area), additional effects, including cryptorchidism, hypospadias, atrophy or agenesis of sex accessory organs, testicular injury, reduced daily sperm production, permanent retention of nipples, and decreased anogenital distance are noted. Female offspring are unaffected. High doses of DBP, administered to pregnant rats was associated with increased incidences of developmental abnormalities, such as cleft palate (≥630 mg/kg/day, about 106 times the human dose, based on body surface area) and skeletal abnormalities (≥750 mg/kg/day, about 127 times the human dose based on body surface area) in the offspring.

8.3 Nursing Mothers

Mesalamine and its N-acetyl metabolite are excreted into human milk. In published lactation studies, maternal mesalamine doses from various oral and rectal formulations and products ranged from 500 mg to 3 g daily. The concentration of mesalamine in milk ranged from non-detectable to 0.11 mg/L. The concentration of the N-acetyl-5-aminosalicylic acid metabolite ranged from 5 to 18.1 rng/L. Based on these concentrations, estimated infant daily doses for an exclusively breastfed infant are 0-0.017 mg/kg/day of mesalamine and 0.75-2.72 mg/kg/day of N-acetyl-5-aminosalicylic acid. Caution should be exercised when Asacol HD is administered to a nursing woman.

Dibutyl phthalate (DBP), an inactive ingredient in the enteric coating of Asacol HD tablets, and its primary metabolite mono-butyl phthalate (MBP) are excreted into human milk. In pregnant rats, DBP causes fetal reproductive system aberrations in male offspring *[see Pregnancy (8.1)]*. The clinical significance of this has not been determined.

8.4 Pediatric Use

Safety and effectiveness of Asacol HD in pediatric patients have not been established.

8.5 Geriatric Use

Clinical studies of Asacol HD did not include sufficient numbers of subjects aged 65 and over to determine whether they respond differently than younger subjects. Other reported clinical experience has not identified differences in response between the elderly and younger patients. In general, the greater frequency of decreased hepatic, renal, or cardiac function, and of concomitant disease or other drug therapy in elderly patients should be considered when prescribing Asacol HD. Reports from uncontrolled clinical studies and postmarketing reporting systems for Asacol (mesalamine) suggested a higher incidence of blood dyscrasias, i.e., agranulocytosis, neutropenia, pancytopenia, in patients who were 65 years or older. Caution should be taken to closely monitor blood cell counts during mesalamine therapy.

Mesalamine is known to be substantially excreted by the kidney, and the risk of toxic reactions to this drug may be greater in patients with impaired renal function. Because elderly patients are more likely to have decreased renal function, care should be taken when prescribing this drug therapy. It is recommended that all patients have an evaluation of renal function prior to initiation of Asacol HD therapy and periodically while on Asacol HD therapy *[see Warnings and Precautions (5.1)]*.

10 OVERDOSAGE

There is no specific antidote for mesalamine overdose and treatment for suspected acute severe toxicity with Asacol HD should be symptomatic and supportive. This may include prevention of further gastrointestinal tract absorption, correction of fluid electrolyte imbalance, and maintaining adequate renal function. Asacol HD is a pH dependent delayed release product and this factor should be considered when treating a suspected overdose.

Single oral doses of 5000 mg/kg mesalamine suspension in mice (approximately 4.2 times the recommended human dose of Asacol HD based on body surface area), 4595 mg/kg in rats (approximately 7.8 times the recommended human dose of Asacol HD based on body surface area) and 3000 mg/kg in cynomolgus monkeys (approximately 10 times the recommended human dose of Asacol HD based on body surface area) were lethal.

11 DESCRIPTION

Each Asacol HD delayed-release tablet for oral administration contains 800 mg of mesalamine, an anti-inflammatory drug. Asacol HD delayed-release tablets have an outer protective coat consisting of a combination of acrylic based resins, Eudragit S (methacrylic acid copolymer B, NF) and Eudragit L (methacrylic acid copolymer A, NF). The inner coat consists of an acrylic based resin, Eudragit S, which dissolves at pH 7 or greater, releasing mesalamine in the terminal ileum and beyond for topical anti-inflammatory action in the colon. Mesalamine (also referred to as 5-aminosalicylic acid or 5-ASA) has the chemical name 5-amino-2-hydroxybenzoic acid; its structural formula is:

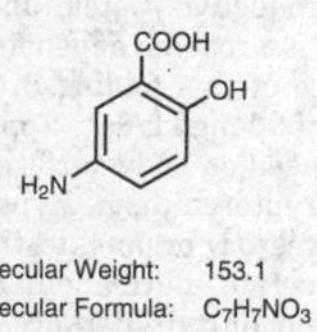

Molecular Weight: 153.1
Molecular Formula: $C_7H_7NO_3$

Inactive Ingredients: Each tablet contains colloidal silicon dioxide, dibutyl phthalate, edible black ink, ferric oxide red, ferric oxide yellow, lactose monohydrate, magnesium stearate, methacrylic acid copolymer B (Eudragit S), methacrylic acid copolymer A (Eudragit L), polyethylene glycol, povidone, sodium starch glycolate, and talc.

12 CLINICAL PHARMACOLOGY

12.1 Mechanism of Action

The mechanism of action of mesalamine is unknown, but appears to be topical rather than systemic. Mucosal production of arachidonic acid (AA) metabolites, both through the cyclooxygenase pathways, i.e., prostanoids, and through the lipoxygenase pathways, i.e., leukotrienes (LTs) and hydroxyeicosatetraenoic acids (HETEs), is increased in patients with chronic inflammatory bowel disease, and it is possible that mesalamine diminishes inflammation by blocking cyclooxygenase and inhibiting prostaglandin (PG) production in the colon.

12.3 Pharmacokinetics

Plasma concentrations of mesalamine (5-aminosalicylic acid; 5-ASA) and its metabolite, N-acetyl-5-aminosalicylic acid (N-Ac-5-ASA) are highly variable following administration of Asacol HD tablets. The time to peak plasma concentration (t_{max}) is prolonged for mesalamine and N-Ac-5-ASA with the median values from various studies ranging from 10 to 16 hours, reflecting the delayed-release characteristics. Based on cumulative urinary recovery of mesalamine and N-Ac-5-ASA from single dose studies in healthy volunteers, approximately 20% of the orally administered mesalamine in Asacol HD tablets is systemically absorbed. The absorbed mesalamine is rapidly acetylated in the gut mucosal wall and by the liver to N-Ac-5-ASA which is excreted mainly by the kidney. The PK parameters following administration of 1600 mg three times daily in healthy subjects are shown in Table 2.

Table 2. Mean (± S.D.) PK parameters in healthy subjects following administration of two 800 mg tablets three times daily for 6 days (n=16)

	Mesalamine	N-Ac-5-ASA
AUC_{tau} (mcg h/mL)	20 ± 14	25 ± 11
C_{max} (mcg/mL)	5.0 ± 4.0	4.6 ± 2.5
$t_{1/2}$ (h)	12.6 ± 10.9*	23.6 ± 11.2#

* n=11, # n=6

A high fat meal does not affect the extent of systemic exposure to mesalamine after single-dose administration of Asacol HD, but mesalamine C_{max} decreases by 47% and t_{max} is delayed by 14 hours under fed conditions.

One Asacol HD 800 mg tablet has not been shown to be bioequivalent to two Asacol 400 mg tablets. In a single dose, cross-over pharmacokinetic study in 20 healthy volunteers, the mean mesalamine C_{max} was 36% lower and the mean mesalamine AUC was 25% lower with administration of one Asacol HD 800 mg tablet relative to two Asacol 400 mg tablets. Because the mechanism of action of mesalamine appears to be topical, the impact of these differences in measures of systemic exposure on clinical efficacy is not known.

13 NONCLINICAL TOXICOLOGY

13.1 Carcinogenesis, Mutagenesis, Impairment of Fertility

Dietary mesalamine was not carcinogenic in rats at doses as high as 480 mg/kg/day, or in mice at 2000 mg/kg/day. These doses are approximately 0.8 and 1.7 times the 4.8 g/day Asacol HD dose (based on body surface area). Mesalamine was not genotoxic in the Ames test, the Chinese hamster ovary cell chromosomal aberration assay, and the mouse micronucleus test. Mesalamine, at oral doses up to 480 mg/kg/day (about 0.8 times the recommended human treatment dose based on body surface area), was found to have no effect on fertility or reproductive performance of male and female rats.

13.2 Animal Toxicology and/or Pharmacology

In animal studies (rats, mice, dogs), the kidney was the principal organ for toxicity. (In the following, comparisons of animal dosing to recommended human dosing are based on body surface area and a 4.8 g/day dose for a 50 kg person.)

Mesalamine causes renal papillary necrosis in rats at single doses of approximately 750 mg/kg to 1000 mg/kg (1.3 to 1.7 times the recommended human dose). Doses of 170 and 360 mg/kg/day (about 0.3 and 0.6 times the recommended human dose) given to rats for six months produced papillary necrosis, papillary edema, tubular degeneration, tubular mineralization, and urothelial hyperplasia.

In mice, oral doses of 4000 mg/kg/day (approximately 3.4 times the recommended human dose) for three months produced tubular nephrosis, multifocal/diffuse tubulo-interstitial inflammation, and multifocal/diffuse papillary necrosis.

In dogs, single doses of 6000 mg (approximately 6.25 times the recommended human dose) of delayed-release mesalamine tablets resulted in renal papillary necrosis but were not fatal. Renal changes have occurred in dogs given chronic administration of mesalamine at doses of 80 mg/kg/day (0.5 times the recommended human dose).

14 CLINICAL STUDIES

14.1 Moderately Active Ulcerative Colitis

The efficacy of Asacol HD at 4.8 g/day was studied in a six-week, randomized, double-blind, active-controlled study in 772 patients with moderately active ulcerative colitis (UC). Moderately active UC was defined as a Physician's Global Assessment (PGA) score of 2; the PGA is a four-point scale (0-3) that encompasses the clinical assessments of rectal bleeding, stool frequency, and sigmoidoscopy findings.

Patients were randomized 1:1 to the Asacol HD 4.8 g/day group (two Asacol HD tablets three times a day) or the Asacol (mesalamine) 2.4 g/day group (two Asacol 400 mg tablets three times a day). (One Asacol HD 800 mg tablet has not been shown to be bioequivalent to two Asacol 400 mg tablets *[see Clinical Pharmacology (12.3)]*.)

Patients characteristically had a history of previous use of oral 5-ASAs (86%), steroids (41%), and rectal therapies (49%), and demonstrated clinical symptoms of three or more stools over normal per day (87%) and obvious blood in the stool most or all of the time (70%). The study population was primarily Caucasian (97%), had a mean age of 43 years (8% aged 65 years or older), and included slightly more males (56%) than females (44%).

The primary endpoint was treatment success defined as improvement from baseline to Week 6 based on the PGA. Treatment success rates were similar in the two groups: 70% in the Asacol HD group and 66% in the Asacol group (difference: 5%; 95% CI: [-1.9%, 11.2%]).

A second controlled study supported the efficacy of Asacol HD at 4.8 g/day. Treatment success was 72% in patients with moderately active UC treated with Asacol HD.

16 HOW SUPPLIED/STORAGE AND HANDLING

Asacol HD tablets are available as red-brown, capsule-shaped tablets containing 800 mg mesalamine and imprinted with "PG 800" in black.

NDC 0149-0783-01 Bottle of 180

Store at controlled room temperature 20° to 25°C (68° to 77°F) [See USP].

17 PATIENT COUNSELING INFORMATION

- Instruct patients to swallow the Asacol HD tablets whole, taking care not to break, cut, or chew the tablets, because the coating is an important part of the delayed-release formulation.
- Inform patients that if they are switching from a previous oral mesalamine therapy to Asacol HD they should discontinue their previous oral mesalamine therapy and follow the dosing instructions for Asacol HD. Inform patients that they should not substitute one Asacol HD tablet with two Asacol 400 mg tablets *[see Dosage Forms and Strengths (3) and Clinical Pharmacology (12.3)]*.
- Inform patients that intact, partially intact, and/or tablet shells have been reported in the stool. Instruct patients to contact their physician if this occurs repeatedly.
- Instruct patients to protect Asacol HD tablets from moisture. Instruct patients to close the container tightly and to leave any desiccant pouches present in the bottle along with the tablets.
- Advise women who are pregnant, breastfeeding, or of childbearing potential that Asacol HD contains dibutyl phthalate, which caused malformations and adverse effects on the male reproductive system in animal studies. Dibutyl phthalate is excreted in human milk.

Manufactured by:
Warner Chilcott Deutschland GmbH
D-64331 Weiterstadt
Germany
Marketed by:
Warner Chilcott Pharmaceuticals Inc.
Mason, OH 45040
1-800-836-0658
Under license from Medeva Pharma Suisse AG (registered trademark owner).
U.S. Patent Nos. 5,541,170; 5,541,171; and 6,893,662 and other patents pending.

DIDRONEL® ℞
[dī′drō-nĕl]
(etidronate disodium)

DESCRIPTION

Didronel tablets contain 400 mg of etidronate disodium, the disodium salt of (1-hydroxyethylidene) diphosphonic acid, for oral administration. This compound, also known as EHDP, regulates bone metabolism. It is a white powder, highly soluble in water, with a molecular weight of 250 and the following structural formula:

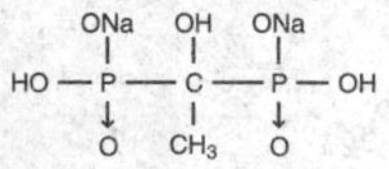

Inactive Ingredients: Each tablet contains magnesium stearate, microcrystalline cellulose, and starch.

CLINICAL PHARMACOLOGY

Didronel acts primarily on bone. It can inhibit the formation, growth, and dissolution of hydroxyapatite crystals and their amorphous precursors by chemisorption to calcium phosphate surfaces. Inhibition of crystal resorption occurs at lower doses than are required to inhibit crystal growth. Both effects increase as the dose increases.

Didronel is not metabolized. The amount of drug absorbed after an oral dose is approximately 3%. In normal subjects, plasma half-life ($t_{1/2}$) of etidronate, based on non-compartmental pharmacokinetics is 1 to 6 hours. Within 24 hours, approximately half the absorbed dose is excreted in urine; the remainder is distributed to bone compartments from which it is slowly eliminated. Animal studies have yielded bone clearance estimates up to 165 days. In humans, the residence time on bone may vary due to such factors as specific metabolic condition and bone type. Unabsorbed drug is excreted intact in the feces. Preclinical studies indicate etidronate disodium does not cross the blood-brain barrier.

Didronel therapy does not adversely affect serum levels of parathyroid hormone or calcium.

Paget's Disease: Paget's disease of bone (osteitis deformans) is an idiopathic, progressive disease characterized by abnormal and accelerated bone metabolism in one or more bones. Signs and symptoms may include bone pain and/or deformity, neurologic disorders, elevated cardiac output and other vascular disorders, and increased serum alkaline phosphatase and/or urinary hydroxyproline levels. Bone fractures are common in patients with Paget's disease.

Didronel slows accelerated bone turnover (resorption and accretion) in pagetic lesions and, to a lesser extent, in normal bone. This has been demonstrated histologically, scintigraphically, biochemically, and through calcium kinetic and balance studies. Reduced bone turnover is often accompanied by symptomatic improvement, including reduced bone pain. Also, the incidence of pagetic fractures may be reduced, and elevated cardiac output and other vascular disorders may be improved by **Didronel** therapy.

Heterotopic Ossification: Heterotopic ossification, also referred to as myositis ossificans (circumscripta, progressiva or traumatica), ectopic calcification, periarticular ossification, or paraosteoarthropathy, is characterized by metaplastic osteogenesis. It usually presents with signs of localized inflammation or pain, elevated skin temperature, and redness. When tissues near joints are involved, functional loss may also be present.

Heterotopic ossification may occur for no known reason as in myositis ossificans progressiva or may follow a wide variety of surgical, occupational, and sports trauma (e.g., hip arthroplasty, spinal cord injury, head injury, burns, and severe thigh bruises). Heterotopic ossification has also been observed in non-traumatic conditions (e.g., infections of the central nervous system, peripheral neuropathy, tetanus, biliary cirrhosis, Peyronie's disease, as well as in association with a variety of benign and malignant neoplasms).

Clinical trials have demonstrated the efficacy of **Didronel** in heterotopic ossification following total hip replacement, or due to spinal cord injury.

—*Heterotopic ossification complicating total hip replacement* typically develops radiographically 3 to 8 weeks postoperatively in the pericapsular area of the affected hip joint. The overall incidence is about 50%; about one-third of these cases are clinically significant.

—*Heterotopic ossification due to spinal cord injury* typically develops radiographically 1 to 4 months after injury. It occurs below the level of injury, usually at major joints. The overall incidence is about 40%; about one-half of these cases are clinically significant.

Didronel chemisorbs to calcium hydroxyapatite crystals and their amorphous precursors, blocking the aggregation, growth, and mineralization of these crystals. This is thought to be the mechanism by which **Didronel** prevents or retards heterotopic ossification. There is no evidence **Didronel** affects mature heterotopic bone.

INDICATIONS AND USAGE

Didronel is indicated for the treatment of symptomatic Paget's disease of bone and in the prevention and treatment of heterotopic ossification following total hip replacement or due to spinal cord injury. **Didronel** is not approved for the treatment of osteoporosis.

Paget's Disease: **Didronel** is indicated for the treatment of symptomatic Paget's disease of bone. **Didronel** therapy usually arrests or significantly impedes the disease process as evidenced by:

—Symptomatic relief, including decreased pain and/or increased mobility (experienced by 3 out of 5 patients).
—Reductions in serum alkaline phosphatase and urinary hydroxyproline levels (30% or more in 4 out of 5 patients).
—Histomorphometry showing reduced numbers of osteoclasts and osteoblasts, and more lamellar bone formation.
—Bone scans showing reduced radionuclide uptake at pagetic lesions.

In addition, reductions in pagetically elevated cardiac output and skin temperature have been observed in some patients.

In many patients, the disease process will be suppressed for a period of at least 1 year following cessation of therapy. The upper limit of this period has not been determined.

The effects of the **Didronel** treatment in patients with asymptomatic Paget's disease have not been studied. However, **Didronel** treatment of such patients may be warranted if extensive involvement threatens irreversible neurologic damage, major joints, or major weight-bearing bones.

Heterotopic Ossification: **Didronel** is indicated in the prevention and treatment of heterotopic ossification following total hip replacement or due to spinal cord injury.

Didronel reduces the incidence of clinically important heterotopic bone by about two-thirds. Among those patients who form heterotopic bone, **Didronel** retards the progression of immature lesions and reduces the severity by at least half. Follow-up data (at least 9 months posttherapy) suggest these benefits persist.

In total hip replacement patients, **Didronel** does not promote loosening of the prosthesis or impede trochanteric reattachment.

In spinal cord injury patients, **Didronel** does not inhibit fracture healing or stabilization of the spine.

CONTRAINDICATIONS

- Abnormalities of the esophagus which delay esophageal emptying such as stricture or achalasia.
- Known hypersensitivity to etidronate disodium or in patients with clinically overt osteomalacia.

WARNINGS

General: Upper Gastrointestinal Adverse Reactions: **Didronel**, like other bisphosphonates administered orally, may cause local irritation of the upper gastrointestinal mucosa. Because of these possible irritant effects and a potential for worsening of the underlying disease, caution should be used when **Didronel** is given to patients with active upper gastrointestinal problems (such as known Barrett's esophagus, dysphagia, other esophageal diseases, gastritis, duodenitis or ulcers).

Esophageal adverse experiences, such as esophagitis, esophageal ulcers and esophageal erosions, occasionally with bleeding and rarely followed by esophageal stricture or perforation, have been reported in patients receiving treatment with oral bisphosphonates. In some cases, these have been severe and required hospitalization. Physicians should therefore be alert to any signs or symptoms signaling a possible esophageal reaction and patients should be instructed to discontinue **Didronel** and seek medical attention if they develop dysphagia, odynophagia, retrosternal pain or new or worsening heartburn.

The risk of severe esophageal adverse experiences appears to be greater in patients who lie down after taking oral bisphosphonates and/or who fail to swallow it with the recommended full glass (6-8 oz) of water, and/or who continue to take oral bisphosphonates after developing symptoms suggestive of esophageal irritation. Therefore, it is very important that the full dosing instructions are provided to, and understood by, the patient [see **DOSAGE AND ADMINISTRATION**]. In patients who cannot comply with dosing instructions due to mental disability, therapy with **Didronel** should be used under appropriate supervision.

There have been post-marketing reports of gastric and duodenal ulcers with oral bisphosphonate use, some severe and with complications, although no increased risk was observed in controlled clinical trials.

Paget's Disease: In Paget's patients the response to therapy may be of slow onset and continue for months after **Didronel** therapy is discontinued. Dosage should not be increased prematurely. A 90-day drug-free interval should be provided between courses of therapy.

Heterotopic Ossification: No specific warnings.

PRECAUTIONS

General: Patients should maintain an adequate nutritional status, particularly an adequate intake of calcium and vitamin D.

Therapy has been withheld from some patients with enterocolitis since diarrhea may be experienced, particularly at higher doses.

Didronel is not metabolized and is excreted intact via the kidney. Hyperphosphatemia may occur at doses of 10 to 20 mg/kg/day, apparently as a result of drug-related increases in tubular reabsorption of phosphate. Serum phosphate levels generally return to normal 2 to 4 weeks post-therapy. There is no experience to specifically guide treatment in patients with impaired renal function. **Didronel** dosage should be reduced when reductions in glomerular filtration rates are present. Patients with renal impairment should be closely monitored. In approximately 10% of patients in clinical trials of **Didronel® I. V. Infusion** (etidronate disodium) for hypercalcemia of malignancy, occasional, mild-to-moderate abnormalities in renal function (increases of > 0.5 mg/dl serum creatinine) were observed during or immediately after treatment.

Didronel suppresses bone turnover, and may retard mineralization of osteoid laid down during the bone accretion process. These effects are dose and time dependent. Osteoid, which may accumulate noticeably at doses of 10 to 20 mg/kg/day, mineralizes normally posttherapy. In patients with fractures, especially of long bones, it may be advisable to delay or interrupt treatment until callus is evident.

Osteonecrosis of the jaw (ONJ): ONJ, which can occur spontaneously, is generally associated with tooth extraction and/or local infection with delayed healing, and has been reported in patients taking bisphosphonates, including **Didronel**. Known risk factors for osteonecrosis of the jaw include invasive dental procedures (e.g., tooth extraction, dental implants, boney surgery), diagnosis of cancer, concomitant therapies (e.g., chemotherapy, corticosteroids), poor oral hygiene, and co-morbid disorders (e.g., periodontal and/or other pre-existing dental disease, anemia, coagulopathy, infection, ill-fitting dentures).

For patients requiring invasive dental procedures, discontinuation of bisphosphonate treatment may reduce the risk for ONJ. Clinical judgment of the treating physician and/or oral surgeon should guide the management plan of each patient based on individual benefit/risk assessment.

Patients who develop osteonecrosis of the jaw while on bisphosphonate therapy should receive care by an oral surgeon. In these patients, extensive dental surgery to treat ONJ may exacerbate the condition. Discontinuation of bisphosphonate therapy should be considered based on individual benefit/risk assessment.

Musculoskeletal Pain:
In postmarketing experience, there have been infrequent reports of severe and occasionally incapacitating bone, joint, and/or muscle pain in patients taking bisphosphonates (see **ADVERSE REACTIONS**). The time to onset of symptoms varied from one day to several months after starting the drug. Most patients had relief of symptoms after stopping medication. A subset had recurrence of symptoms when rechallenged with the same drug or another bisphosphonate.

Paget's Disease: In Paget's patients, treatment regimens exceeding the recommended (see **DOSAGE AND ADMINISTRATION**) daily maximum dose of 20 mg/kg or continuous administration of medication for periods greater than 6 months may be associated with osteomalacia and an increased risk of fracture.

Long bones predominantly affected by lytic lesions, particularly in those patients unresponsive to **Didronel** therapy, may be especially prone to fracture.

Patients with predominantly lytic lesions should be monitored radiographically and biochemically to permit termination of **Didronel** in those patients unresponsive to treatment.

Drug Interactions: There have been isolated reports of patients experiencing increases in their prothrombin times when etidronate was added to warfarin therapy. The majority of these reports concerned variable elevations in prothrombin times without clinically significant sequelae. Although the relevance of these reports and any mechanism of coagulation alterations is unclear, patients on warfarin should have their prothrombin time monitored.

Carcinogenesis: Long-term studies in rats have indicated that **Didronel** is not carcinogenic.

Pregnancy: Teratogenic Effects: Pregnancy Category C. In teratology and developmental toxicity studies conducted in rats and rabbits treated with dosages of up to 100 mg/kg (5 to 20 times the clinical dose), no adverse or teratogenic effects have been observed in the offspring. Etidronate disodium has been shown to cause skeletal abnormalities in rats when given at oral dose levels of 300 mg/kg (15 to 60 times the human dose). Other effects on the offspring (including decreased live births) are at dosages that cause significant toxicity in the parent generation and are 25 to 200 times the human dose. The skeletal effects are thought to be the result of the pharmacological effects of the drug on bone. Bisphosphonates are incorporated into the bone matrix, from which they are gradually released over periods of weeks to years. The amount of bisphosphonate incorporation into adult bone, and hence, the amount available for release back into the systemic circulation, is directly related to the dose and duration of bisphosphonate use. There are no data on fetal risk in humans. However, there is a theoretical risk of fetal harm, predominantly skeletal, if a woman becomes pregnant after completing a course of bisphosphonate therapy. The impact of variables such as time between cessation of bisphosphonate therapy to conception, the particular bisphosphonate used, and the route of administration (intravenous versus oral) on this risk has not been studied.

There are no adequate and well-controlled studies in pregnant women. **Didronel** (etidronate disodium) should be used during pregnancy only if the potential benefit justifies the potential risk to the fetus.

Nursing Mothers: It is not known whether this drug is excreted in human milk. Because many drugs are excreted in human milk, caution should be exercised when **Didronel** is administered to a nursing woman.

Pediatric Use: Safety and effectiveness in pediatric patients have not been established. Pediatric patients have been treated with **Didronel,** at doses recommended for adults, to prevent heterotopic ossifications or soft tissue calcifications. A rachitic syndrome has been reported infrequently at doses of 10 mg/kg/day and more for prolonged periods approaching or exceeding a year. The epiphyseal radiologic changes associated with retarded mineralization of new osteoid and cartilage, and occasional symptoms reported, have been reversible when medication is discontinued.

Geriatric Use: Clinical studies of **Didronel** did not include sufficient numbers of subjects aged 65 and over to determine whether they respond differently from younger subjects. Other reported clinical experience has not identified differences in responses between elderly and younger patients. In general, dose selection for an elderly patient should be cautious, reflecting the greater frequency of decreased hepatic, renal, or cardiac function, and of concomitant disease or other drug therapy. This drug is known to be substantially excreted by the kidney, and the risk of toxic reactions to this drug may be greater in patients with impaired renal function. Because elderly patients are more likely to have decreased renal function, care should be taken when prescribing this drug therapy. As stated in **PRECAUTIONS, Didronel** dosage should be reduced when reductions in glomerular filtration rates are present. In addition, patients with renal impairment should be closely monitored.

ADVERSE REACTIONS

The incidence of gastrointestinal complaints (diarrhea, nausea) is the same for **Didronel** at 5 mg/kg/day as for placebo, about 1 patient in 15. At 10 to 20 mg/kg/day the incidence may increase to 2 or 3 in 10. These complaints are often alleviated by dividing the total daily dose.

Paget's Disease: In Paget's patients, increased or recurrent bone pain at pagetic sites, and/or the onset of pain at previously asymptomatic sites has been reported. At 5 mg/kg/day about 1 patient in 10 (versus 1 in 15 in the placebo group) report these phenomena. At higher doses the incidence rises to about 2 in 10. When therapy continues, pain resolves in some patients but persists in others.

Heterotopic Ossification: No specific adverse reactions.

Worldwide Postmarketing Experience: The worldwide postmarketing experience for etidronate disodium reflects its use in the following approved indications: Paget's disease, heterotopic ossification, and hypercalcemia of malignancy. It also reflects the use of etidronate disodium for osteoporosis where approved in countries outside the US. Other adverse events that have been reported and were thought to be possibly related to etidronate disodium include the following: alopecia; arthropathies, including arthralgia and arthritis; bone fracture; esophagitis; glossitis; hypersensitivity reactions, including angioedema, follicular eruption, macular rash, maculopapular rash, pruritus, Stevens-Johnson syndrome, and urticaria; osteomalacia; neuropsychiatric events, including amnesia, confusion, depression, and hallucination; and paresthesias.

In patients receiving etidronate disodium, there have been rare reports of agranulocytosis, pancytopenia, and a report of leukopenia with recurrence on rechallenge. In addition, there have been rare reports of exacerbation of asthma. Exacerbation of existing peptic ulcer disease including perforation has been reported rarely.

In osteoporosis clinical trials, headache, gastritis, leg cramps, and arthralgia occurred at a significantly greater incidence in patients who received etidronate as compared with those who received placebo.

OVERDOSAGE

Clinical experience with acute **Didronel** overdosage is extremely limited. Decreases in serum calcium following substantial overdosage may be expected in some patients. Signs and symptoms of hypocalcemia also may occur in some of these patients. Some patients may develop vomiting. In one event, an 18-year-old female who ingested an estimated single dose of 4000 to 6000 mg (67 to 100 mg/kg) of **Didronel** was reported to be mildly hypocalcemic (7.52 mg/dl) and experienced paresthesia of the fingers. Hypocalcemia resolved 6 hours after lavage and treatment with intravenous calcium gluconate. A 92-year-old female who accidentally received 1600 mg of etidronate disodium per day for 3.5 days experienced marked diarrhea and required treatment for electrolyte imbalance. Orally administered etidronate disodium may cause hematologic abnormalities in some patients (see **ADVERSE REACTIONS**).

Etidronate disodium suppresses bone turnover and may retard mineralization of osteoid laid down during the bone accretion process. These effects are dose and time dependent. Osteoid which may accumulate noticeably at doses of 10 to 20 mg/kg/day of chronic, continuous dosing mineralizes normally posttherapy.

Prolonged continuous treatment (chronic overdosage) has been reported to cause nephrotic syndrome and fracture.

Gastric lavage may remove unabsorbed drug. Standard procedures for treating hypocalcemia, including the administration of Ca^{++} intravenously, would be expected to restore physiologic amounts of ionized calcium and relieve signs and symptoms of hypocalcemia. Such treatment has been effective.

DOSAGE AND ADMINISTRATION

Didronel should be taken as a single, oral dose. As with other bisphosphonates, it is recommended that **Didronel** should be swallowed with a full glass of water (6 to 8 oz). Patients should not lie down after taking the medication. However, should gastrointestinal discomfort occur, the dose may be divided. To maximize absorption, patients should avoid taking the following items within two hours of dosing:

—Food, especially food high in calcium, such as milk or milk products.

—Vitamins with mineral supplements or antacids which are high in metals such as calcium, iron, magnesium, or aluminum.

Paget's Disease: **Initial Treatment Regimens:** 5 to 10 mg/kg/day, not to exceed 6 months, or 11 to 20 mg/kg/day, not to exceed 3 months.

The recommended initial dose is 5 mg/kg/day for a period not to exceed 6 months. Doses above 10 mg/kg/day should be reserved for when 1) lower doses are ineffective or 2) there is an overriding need to suppress rapid bone turnover (especially when irreversible neurologic damage is possible) or reduce elevated cardiac output. Doses in excess of 20 mg/kg/day are not recommended.

Retreatment Guidelines: Retreatment should be initiated only after 1) a **Didronel**-free period of at least 90 days and 2) there is biochemical, symptomatic or other evidence of active disease process. It is advisable to monitor patients every 3 to 6 months although some patients may go drug free for extended periods. Retreatment regimens are the same as for initial treatment. For most patients the original dose will be adequate for retreatment. If not, consideration should be given to increasing the dose within the recommended guidelines.

Heterotopic Ossification: The following treatment regimens have been shown to be effective:

—Total Hip Replacement Patients: 20 mg/kg/day for 1 month before and 3 months after surgery (4 months total).

—Spinal Cord Injured Patients: 20 mg/kg/day for 2 weeks followed by 10 mg/kg/day for 10 weeks (12 weeks total). **Didronel** therapy should begin as soon as medically feasible following the injury, preferably prior to evidence of heterotopic ossification.

Retreatment has not been studied.

HOW SUPPLIED

Didronel is available as 400-mg, white, scored, capsule-shaped tablets with "N E" on one face and "406" on the other.

NDC 0149-0406-60 bottle of 60

Store at 25°C (77°F); excursions permitted to 15-30°C (59-86°F)

[see USP Controlled Room Temperature]

Mfg. by:
Norwich Pharmaceuticals, Inc.
North Norwich, NY 13814
Mkt. by:
Warner Chilcott Pharmaceuticals Inc., Mason, OH 45040
1-800-836-0658
REVISED MARCH 2010

To report SUSPECTED ADVERSE REACTIONS, contact Warner Chilcott at 1-800-836-0658 or FDA at 1-800-FDA-1088 or www.fda.gov/medwatch.

WellSpring Pharmaceutical Corporation

5911 N. HONORE AVENUE, STE. 211
SARASOTA, FL 34243

Direct Inquiries to:
phone (941) 312-4727
fax (941) 312-4738

DIBENZYLINE ℞

[dī-bĕnz-ĭ-lēn]
phenoxybenzamine hydrochloride
capsule 10mg
adrenergic, *alpha*-receptor-blocking agent

DESCRIPTION

Each Dibenzyline capsule, with red cap and body, is imprinted WPC 001 and 10 mg, and contains 10 mg of Phenoxybenzamine Hydrochloride USP. Inactive ingredients consist of D&C Red No. 33, FD&C Red No. 3, FD&C Yellow No. 6, Gelatin NF, Lactose NF, Sodium Lauryl Sulfate NF and Silicon Dioxide NF.

Dibenzyline is N-(2-Chloroethyl)-N-(1-methyl-2-phenoxyethyl)benzylamine hydrochloride:

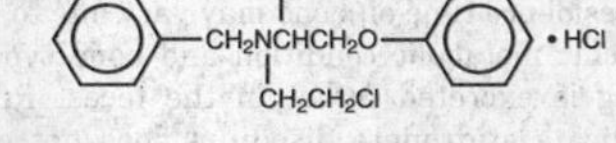

Phenoxybenzamine hydrochloride is a colorless, crystalline powder with a molecular weight of 340.3, which melts between 136°and 141°C. It is soluble in water, alcohol and chloroform; insoluble in ether.

CLINICAL PHARMACOLOGY

Dibenzyline (phenoxybenzamine hydrochloride) is a long-acting, adrenergic, *alpha*-receptor-blocking agent, which can produce and maintain "chemical sympathectomy" by oral administration. It increases blood flow to the skin, mucosa and abdominal viscera, and lowers both supine and erect blood pressures. It has no effect on the parasympathetic system.

Twenty to 30 percent of orally administered phenoxybenzamine appears to be absorbed in the active form.[1]

The half-life of orally administered phenoxybenzamine hydrochloride is not known; however, the half-life of intravenously administered drug is approximately 24 hours. Demonstrable effects with intravenous administration persist for at least 3 to 4 days, and the effects of daily administration are cumulative for nearly a week.[1]

INDICATION AND USAGE

Dibenzyline is indicated in the treatment of pheochromocytoma, to control episodes of hypertension and sweating. If tachycardia is excessive, it may be necessary to use a *beta*-blocking agent concomitantly.

CONTRAINDICATIONS

Conditions where a fall in blood pressure may be undesirable; hypersensitivity to the drug or any of its components.

WARNING

Dibenzyline-induced *alpha*-adrenergic blockade leaves *beta*-adrenergic receptors unopposed. Compounds that stimulate both types of receptors may, therefore, produce an exaggerated hypotensive response and tachycardia.

PRECAUTIONS

General—Administer with caution in patients with marked cerebral or coronary arteriosclerosis or renal damage. Adrenergic blocking effect may aggravate symptoms of respiratory infections.

Drug Interactions[2]

Dibenzyline (phenoxybenzamine hydrochloride) may interact with compounds that stimulate both *alpha*- and *beta*-adrenergic receptors (i.e., epinephrine) to produce an exaggerated hypotensive response and tachycardia. (See WARNING.)

Dibenzyline blocks hyperthermia production by levarterenol, and blocks hypothermia production by reserpine.

Carcinogenesis and Mutagenesis

Case reports of carcinoma in humans after long-term treatment with phenoxybenzamine have been reported. Hence long-term use of phenoxybenzamine is not recommended.[3, 4]

Carefully weigh the benefits and risks before prescribing this drug.

Phenoxybenzamine hydrochloride showed *in vitro* mutagenic activity in the Ames test and mouse lymphoma assay; it did not show mutagenic activity *in vivo* in the micronucleus test in mice. In rats and mice, repeated intraperitoneal administration of phenoxybenzamine hydrochloride (three times per week for up to 52 weeks) resulted in peritoneal sarcomas. Chronic oral dosing in rats (for up to 2 years) produced malignant tumors of the small intestine and non-glandular stomach, as well as ulcerative and/or erosive gastritis of the glandular stomach. Whereas squamous cell carcinomas of the non-glandular stomach were observed at all tested doses of phenoxybenzamine hydrochloride, there was a no-observed-effect-level of 10 mg/kg for tumors (carcinomas and sarcomas) of the small intestine. This dose is, on a body surface area basis, about twice the maximum recommended human dosage of 20 mg b.i.d.

Pregnancy

Teratogenic Effects - Pregnancy Category C

Adequate reproductive studies in animals have not been performed with Dibenzyline (phenoxybenzamine hydrochloride). It is also not known whether Dibenzyline can cause fetal harm when administered to a pregnant woman. Dibenzyline should be given to a pregnant woman only if clearly needed.

Nursing Mothers

It is not known whether this drug is excreted in human milk. Because many drugs are excreted in human milk, and because of the potential for serious adverse reactions from phenoxybenzamine hydrochloride, a decision should be made whether to discontinue nursing or to discontinue the drug, taking into account the importance of the drug to the mother.

Pediatric Use

Safety and effectiveness in pediatric patients have not been established.

ADVERSE REACTIONS

The following adverse reactions have been observed, but there are insufficient data to support an estimate of their frequency.

Autonomic Nervous System*: Postural hypotension, tachycardia, inhibition of ejaculation, nasal congestion, miosis.

*These so-called "side effects" are actually evidence of adrenergic blockade and vary according to the degree of blockade.

Miscellaneous: Gastrointestinal irritation, drowsiness, fatigue.

To report SUSPECTED ADVERSE REACTIONS, contact WellSpring Pharmaceutical Corporation at 1-866-337-4500 or FDA at 1-800-FDA-1088 or www.fda.gov/medwatch.

OVERDOSAGE

SYMPTOMS—These are largely the result of blocking of the sympathetic nervous system and of the circulating epinephrine. They may include postural hypotension, resulting in dizziness or fainting; tachycardia, particularly postural; vomiting; lethargy; shock.

TREATMENT

When symptoms and signs of overdosage exist, discontinue the drug. Treatment of circulatory failure, if present, is a prime consideration. In cases of mild overdosage, recumbent position with legs elevated usually restores cerebral circulation. In the more severe cases, the usual measures to combat shock should be instituted. Usual pressor agents are *not* effective. Epinephrine is contraindicated because it stimulates both *alpha-* and *beta*-receptors; since *alpha*-receptors are blocked, the net effect of epinephrine administration is vasodilation and a further drop in blood pressure (epinephrine reversal).

The patient may have to be kept flat for 24 hours or more in the case of overdose, as the effect of the drug is prolonged. Leg bandages and an abdominal binder may shorten the period of disability.

I.V. Infusion of levarterenol bitartrate** may be used to combat severe hypotensive reactions, because it stimulates *alpha*-receptors primarily. Although Dibenzyline (phenoxybenzamine hydrochloride) is an *alpha*-adrenergic blocking agent, a sufficient dose of levarterenol bitartrate will overcome this effect.

The oral LD_{50} for phenoxybenzamine hydrochloride is approximately 2000 mg/kg in rats and approximately 500 mg/kg in guinea pigs.

DOSAGE AND ADMINISTRATION

The dosage should be adjusted to fit the needs of each patient. Small initial doses should be *slowly* increased until the desired effect is obtained or the side effects from blockade become troublesome. *After each increase, the patient should be observed on that level before instituting another increase.* The dosage should be carried to a point where symptomatic relief and/or objective improvement are obtained, but not so high that the side effects from blockade become troublesome.

Initially, 10 mg of Dibenzyline (phenoxybenzamine hydrochloride) twice a day. Dosage should be increased every other day, usually to 20 to 40 mg 2 or 3 times a day, until an optimal dosage is obtained, as judged by blood pressure control.

Long-term use of phenoxybenzamine is not recommended (see PRECAUTIONS Carciongenesis and Mutagenesis)

STORAGE

Store at 25°C (77°F); excursions permitted to 15°-30°C (59°-86°F) [See USP Controlled Room Temperature].

HOW SUPPLIED

Dibenzyline (phenoxybenzamine hydrochloride) capsules, 10 mg, in bottles of 100 (NDC 65197-001-01).

REFERENCES

- Weiner, N.: Drugs That Inhibit Adrenergic Nerves and Block Adrenergic Receptors, in Goodman, L., and Gilman, A., *The Pharmacological Basis of Therapeutics*, ed. 6, New York, Macmillan Publishing Co., 1980, p. 179; p. 182.
- Martin, E.W.: *Drug Interactions Index 1978/1979*, Philadelphia, J.B. Lippincott Co., 1978, pp. 209-210.
- Nettesheim O, Hoffken G, Gahr M, Breidert M: Haematemesis and dysphagia in a 20-year-old woman with congenital spine malformation and situs inversus partialis [German]. Zeitschrift fur Gastroenterologie. 2003; 41(4): 319-24.
- Vaidyanathan S, Mansour P, Soni BM, Hughes PL, Singh G: Chronic lymphocytic leukaemia, synchronous small cell carcinoma and squamous neoplasia of the urinary bladder in a paraplegic man following long-term phenoxybenzamine therapy. Spinal Cord. 2006;44(3): 188-91.

** Available as Levophed® Bitartrate (brand of norepinephrine bitartrate) from Abbott Laboratories.

DATE OF ISSUANCE MARCH 2009

Manufactured for
WellSpring Pharmaceutical Corporation
Sarasota, FL 34243 USA
By WellSpring Pharmaceutical
Canada Corp.
Oakville, Ontario L6H 1M5 Canada
Rev. 03/09

Shown in Product Identification Guide, page 321

DYRENIUM® ℞

(triamterene USP)

Capsules 50 mg and 100 mg potassium-sparing diuretic

WARNINGS

Abnormal elevation of serum potassium levels (greater than or equal to 5.5 mEq/liter) can occur with all potassium-sparing agents, including Dyrenium. Hyperkalemia is more likely to occur in patients with renal impairment and diabetes (even without evidence of renal impairment), and in the elderly or severely ill. Since uncorrected hyperkalemia may be fatal, serum potassium levels must be monitored at frequent intervals especially in patients receiving Dyrenium, when dosages are changed or with any illness that may influence renal function.

DESCRIPTION

Each capsule for oral use, with opaque red cap and body, contains Triamterene USP, 50 or 100 mg, and is imprinted with the product name, DYRENIUM, strength (50 mg or 100 mg) and WPC 002 (for the 50-mg strength) and WPC 003 (for the 100-mg strength). Inactive ingredients consist of D&C Red No. 33, FD&C Yellow No. 6, Gelatin NF, Lactose NF, Magnesium Stearate NF, Sodium Lauryl Sulfate NF, Titanium Dioxide USP and Silicon Dioxide NF.

Triamterene is 2,4,7-triamino-6-phenyl-pteridine:

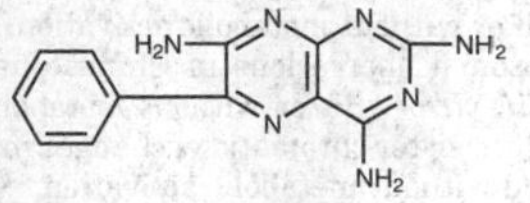

Its molecular weight is 253.27. At 50°C, triamterene is slightly soluble in water. It is soluble in dilute ammonia, dilute aqueous sodium hydroxide and dimethylformamide. It is sparingly soluble in methanol.

CLINICAL PHARMACOLOGY

Triamterene has a unique mode of action; it inhibits the reabsorption of sodium ions in exchange for potassium and hydrogen ions at that segment of the distal tubule under the control of adrenal mineralocorticoids (especially aldosterone). This activity is not directly related to aldosterone secretion or antagonism; it is a result of a direct effect on the renal tubule.

The fraction of filtered sodium reaching this distal tubular exchange site is relatively small, and the amount which is exchanged depends on the level of mineralocorticoid activity. Thus, the degree of natriuresis and diuresis produced by inhibition of the exchange mechanism is necessarily limited. Increasing the amount of available sodium and the level of mineralocorticoid activity by the use of more proximally acting diuretics will increase the degree of diuresis and potassium conservation.

Triamterene occasionally causes increases in serum potassium which can result in hyperkalemia. It does not produce alkalosis, because it does not cause excessive excretion of titratable acid and ammonium.

Triamterene has been shown to cross the placental barrier and appear in the cord blood of animals.

Pharmacokinetics

Onset of action is 2 to 4 hours after ingestion. In normal volunteers the mean peak serum levels were 30 ng/mL at 3 hours. The average percent of drug recovered in the urine (0 to 48 hours) was 21%. Triamterene is primarily metabolized to the sulfate conjugate of hydroxytriamterene. Both the plasma and urine levels of this metabolite greatly exceed triamterene levels. Triamterene is rapidly absorbed, with somewhat less than 50% of the oral dose reaching the urine. Most patients will respond to Dyrenium (triamterene) during the first day of treatment.

Maximum therapeutic effect, however, may not be seen for several days. Duration of diuresis depends on several factors, especially renal function, but it generally tapers off 7 to 9 hours after administration.

INDICATIONS AND USAGE

Dyrenium (triamterene) is indicated in the treatment of edema associated with congestive heart failure, cirrhosis of the liver and the nephrotic syndrome; steroid-induced edema, idiopathic edema and edema due to secondary hyperaldosteronism.

Dyrenium may be used alone or with other diuretics, either for its added diuretic effect or its potassium-sparing potential. It also promotes increased diuresis when patients prove resistant or only partially responsive to thiazides or other diuretics because of secondary hyperaldosteronism.

Usage in Pregnancy. The routine use of diuretics in an otherwise healthy woman is inappropriate and exposes mother and fetus to unnecessary hazard. Diuretics do not prevent development of toxemia of pregnancy, and there is no satisfactory evidence that they are useful in the treatment of developed toxemia.

Edema during pregnancy may arise from pathological causes or from the physiologic and mechanical consequences of pregnancy. Diuretics are indicated in pregnancy (however, see PRECAUTIONS below) when edema is due to pathologic causes, just as they are in the absence of pregnancy. Dependent edema in pregnancy, resulting from restriction of venous return by the expanded uterus, is properly treated through elevation of the lower extremities and use of support hose; use of diuretics to lower intravascular volume in this case is illogical and unnecessary. There is hypervolemia during normal pregnancy which is harmful to neither the fetus nor the mother (in the absence of cardiovascular disease), but which is associated with edema, including generalized edema, in the majority of pregnant women. If this edema produces discomfort, increased recumbency will often provide relief. In rare instances, this edema may cause extreme discomfort which is not relieved by rest. In these cases, a short course of diuretics may provide relief and may be appropriate.

CONTRAINDICATIONS

Anuria. Severe or progressive kidney disease or dysfunction, with the possible exception of nephrosis. Severe hepatic disease. Hypersensitivity to the drug or any of its components.

Dyrenium (triamterene) should not be used in patients with pre-existing elevated serum potassium, as is sometimes seen in patients with impaired renal function or azotemia, or in patients who develop hyperkalemia while on the drug. Patients should not be placed on dietary potassium supplements, potassium salts or potassium-containing salt substitutes in conjunction with Dyrenium.

Dyrenium should not be given to patients receiving other potassium-sparing agents, such as spironolactone, amiloride hydrochloride, or other formulations containing triamterene. Two deaths have been reported in patients receiving concomitant spironolactone and Dyrenium or Dyazide®. Although dosage recommendations were exceeded in one case and in the other serum electrolytes were not properly monitored, these two drugs should not be given concomitantly.

WARNINGS

Abnormal elevation of serum potassium levels (greater than or equal to 5.5 mEq/liter) can occur with all potassium-sparing agents, including Dyrenium. Hyperkalemia is more likely to occur in patients with renal impairment and diabetes (even without evidence of renal impairment), and in the elderly or severely ill. Since uncorrected hyperkalemia may be fatal, serum potassium levels must be monitored at frequent intervals especially in patients receiving Dyrenium, when dosages are changed or with any illness that may influence renal function.

There have been isolated reports of hypersensitivity reactions; therefore, patients should be observed regularly for the possible occurrence of blood dyscrasias, liver damage or other idiosyncratic reactions.

Periodic BUN and serum potassium determinations should be made to check kidney function, especially in patients with suspected or confirmed renal insufficiency. It is particularly important to make serum potassium determinations in elderly or diabetic patients receiving the drug; these patients should be observed carefully for possible serum potassium increases.

If hyperkalemia is present or suspected, an electrocardiogram should be obtained. If the ECG shows no widening of the QRS or arrhythmia in the presence of hyperkalemia, it is usually sufficient to discontinue Dyrenium (triamterene) and any potassium supplementation, and substitute a thiazide alone. Sodium polystyrene sulfonate (Kayexalate®, Sanofi Synthelabo) may be administered to enhance the excretion of excess potassium. **The presence of a widened QRS complex or arrhythmia in association with hyperkalemia requires prompt additional therapy.** For tachyarrhythmia, infuse 44 mEq of sodium bicarbonate or 10 mL of 10% calcium gluconate or calcium chloride over several minutes. For asystole, bradycardia or A-V block transvenous pacing is also recommended.

The effect of calcium and sodium bicarbonate is transient and repeated administration may be required. When indicated by the clinical situation, excess K+ may be removed by dialysis or oral or rectal administration of Kayexalate®. Infusion of glucose and insulin has also been used to treat hyperkalemia.

PRECAUTIONS

General
Dyrenium (triamterene) tends to conserve potassium rather than to promote the excretion as do many diuretics and, occasionally, can cause increases in serum potassium which, in some instances, can result in hyperkalemia. In rare instances, hyperkalemia has been associated with cardiac irregularities.

Electrolyte imbalance often encountered in such diseases as congestive heart failure, renal disease or cirrhosis may be aggravated or caused independently by any effective diuretic agent including Dyrenium. The use of full doses of a diuretic when salt intake is restricted can result in a low-salt syndrome.

Triamterene can cause mild nitrogen retention, which is reversible upon withdrawal of the drug, and is seldom observed with intermittent (every-other-day) therapy.

Triamterene may cause a decreasing alkali reserve, with the possibility of metabolic acidosis.

By the very nature of their illness, cirrhotics with splenomegaly sometimes have marked variations in their blood. Since triamterene is a weak folic acid antagonist, it may contribute to the appearance of megaloblastosis in cases where folic acid stores have been depleted. Therefore, periodic blood studies in these patients are recommended. They should also be observed for exacerbations of underlying liver disease.

Triamterene has elevated uric acid, especially in persons predisposed to gouty arthritis.

Triamterene has been reported in renal stones in association with other calculus components. Dyrenium should be used with caution in patients with histories of renal stones.

Information for Patients
To help avoid stomach upset, it is recommended that the drug be taken after meals.

If a single daily dose is prescribed, it may be preferable to take it in the morning to minimize the effect of increased frequency of urination on nighttime sleep.

If a dose is missed, the patient should not take more than the prescribed dose at the next dosing interval.

Laboratory Tests
Hyperkalemia will rarely occur in patients with adequate urinary output, but it is a possibility if large doses are used for considerable periods of time. If hyperkalemia is observed, Dyrenium (triamterene) should be withdrawn. The normal adult range of serum potassium is 3.5 to 5.0 mEq per liter, with 4.5 mEq often being used for a reference point. Potassium levels persistently above 6 mEq per liter require careful observation and treatment. Normal potassium levels tend to be higher in neonates (7.7 mEq per liter) than in adults. Serum potassium levels do not necessarily indicate true body potassium concentration. A rise in plasma pH may cause a decrease in plasma potassium concentration and an increase in the intracellular potassium concentration. Because Dyrenium conserves potassium, it has been theorized that in patients who have received intensive therapy or are given the drug for prolonged periods, a rebound kaliuresis could occur upon abrupt withdrawal. In such patients, withdrawal of Dyrenium should be gradual.

Drug Interactions
Caution should be used when lithium and diuretics are used concomitantly because diuretic-induced sodium loss may reduce the renal clearance of lithium and increase serum lithium levels with risk of lithium toxicity. Patients receiving such combined therapy should have serum lithium levels monitored closely and the lithium dosage adjusted if necessary.

A possible interaction resulting in acute renal failure has been reported in a few subjects when indomethacin, a nonsteroidal anti-inflammatory agent, was given with triamterene. Caution is advised in administering nonsteroidal anti-inflammatory agents with triamterene.

The effects of the following drugs may be potentiated when given together with triamterene: antihypertensive medication, other diuretics, preanesthetic and anesthetic agents, skeletal muscle relaxants (nondepolarizing).

Potassium-sparing agents should be used with caution in conjunction with angiotensin-converting enzyme (ACE) inhibitors due to an increased risk of hyperkalemia.

The following agents, given together with triamterene, may promote serum potassium accumulation and possibly result in hyperkalemia because of the potassium-sparing nature of triamterene, especially in patients with renal insufficiency: blood from blood bank (may contain up to 30 mEq of potassium per liter of plasma or up to 65 mEq per liter of whole blood when stored for more than 10 days); low-salt milk (may contain up to 60 mEq of potassium per liter); potassium-containing medications (such as parenteral penicillin G potassium); salt substitutes (most contain substantial amounts of potassium).

Dyrenium (triamterene) may raise blood glucose levels; for adult-onset diabetes, dosage adjustments of hypoglycemic agents may be necessary during and/or after therapy; concurrent use with chlorpropamide may increase the risk of severe hyponatremia.

Drug/Laboratory Test Interactions
Triamterene and quinidine have similar fluorescence spectra; thus, triamterene will interfere with the fluorescent measurement of quinidine.

Carcinogenesis, Mutagenesis, Impairment of Fertility
Carcinogenesis: In studies conducted under the auspices of the National Toxicology Program, groups of rats were fed diets containing 0, 150, 300 or 600 ppm of triamterene, and groups of mice were fed diets containing 0, 100, 200 or 400 ppm triamterene. Male and female rats exposed to the highest tested concentration received triamterene at about 25 and 30 mg/kg/day, respectively. Male and female mice exposed to the highest tested concentration received triamterene at about 45 and 60 mg/kg/day, respectively.

There was an increased incidence of hepatocellular neoplasia (primarily adenomas) in male and female mice at the highest dosage level. These doses represent 7.5× and 10× the Maximum Recommended Human Dose (MRHD) of 300 mg/kg/day (or 6 mg/kg/day based on a 50 kg patient) for male and female mice, respectively, when based on body weight and 0.7× and 0.9× the MRHD when based on body-surface area.

Although hepatocellular neoplasia (exclusively adenomas) in the rat study was limited to triamterene-exposed males, incidence was not dose dependent and there was no statistically significant difference from control incidence at any dose level.

Mutagenesis: Triamterene was not mutagenic in bacteria (Salmonella typhimurium strains TA98, TA100, TA1535 or TA1537) with or without metabolic activation. It did not induce chromosomal aberrations in Chinese hamster ovary (CHO) cells *in vitro* with or without metabolic activation, but it did induce sister chromatid exchanges in CHO cells *in vitro* with and without metabolic activation.

Impairment of Fertility: Studies of the effects of triamterene on animal reproductive function have not been conducted.

Pregnancy: Category C
Teratogenic Effects:
Reproduction studies have been performed in rats at doses as high as 20 times the Maximum Recommended Human Dose (MRHD) on the basis of body weight, and 6 times the MRHD on the basis of body-surface area, without evidence of harm to the fetus due to triamterene. Because animal reproduction studies are not always predictive of human response, this drug should be used during pregnancy only if clearly needed.

Nonteratogenic Effects:
Triamterene has been shown to cross the placental barrier and appear in cord blood. The use of triamterene in pregnant women requires that the anticipated benefits be weighed against possible hazards to the fetus. These possible hazards include adverse reactions which have occurred in the adult.

Nursing Mothers:
Triamterene has not been studied in nursing mothers. Triamterene appears in animal milk and is likely present in human milk. If use of the drug product is deemed essential, the patient should stop nursing.

Pediatric Use:
Safety and effectiveness in pediatric patients have not been established.

ADVERSE REACTIONS

Adverse effects are listed in decreasing order of frequency; however, the most serious adverse effects are listed first, regardless of frequency. All adverse effects occur rarely (that is, 1 in 1000, or less).
Hypersensitivity: anaphylaxis, rash, photosensitivity.
Metabolic: hyperkalemia, hypokalemia.
Renal: azotemia, elevated BUN and creatinine, renal stones, acute interstitial nephritis (rare), acute renal failure (one case of irreversible renal failure has been reported).
Gastrointestinal: jaundice and/or liver enzyme abnormalities, nausea and vomiting, diarrhea.
Hematologic: thrombocytopenia, megaloblastic anemia.
Central Nervous System: weakness, fatigue, dizziness, headache, dry mouth.

To report SUSPECTED ADVERSE REACTIONS, contact WellSpring Pharmaceutical Corporation at 1-866-337-4500 or FDA at 1-800-FDA-1088 or www.fda.gov/medwatch.

OVERDOSAGE

In the event of overdosage, it can be theorized that electrolyte imbalance would be the major concern, with particular attention to possible hyperkalemia. Other symptoms that might be seen would be nausea and vomiting, other G.I. disturbances and weakness. It is conceivable that some hypotension could occur. As with an overdose of any drug, immediate evacuation of the stomach should be induced through emesis and gastric lavage. Careful evaluation of the electrolyte pattern and fluid balance should be made. There is no specific antidote.

Reversible acute renal failure following ingestion of 50 tablets of a product containing a combination of 50 mg triamterene and 25 mg hydrochlorothiazide has been reported.

The oral LD50 in mice is 380 mg/kg. The amount of drug in a single dose ordinarily associated with symptoms of overdose or likely to be life-threatening is not known.

Although triamterene is 67% protein bound, there may be some benefit to dialysis in cases of overdosage.

DOSAGE AND ADMINISTRATION

Adult Dosage
Dosage should be titrated to the needs of the individual patient. When used alone, the usual starting dose is 100 mg twice daily after meals. When combined with another diuretic or antihypertensive agent, the total daily dosage of each agent should usually be lowered initially and then adjusted to the patient's needs. The total daily dosage should not exceed 300 mg. Please refer to PRECAUTIONS–General.

When Dyrenium (triamterene) is added to other diuretic therapy or when patients are switched to Dyrenium from other diuretics, all potassium supplementation should be discontinued.

HOW SUPPLIED

Capsules: 50 mg in bottles of 100, and 100 mg in bottles of 100.

STORAGE
Store at 25°C (77°F); excursions permitted to 15°-30°C (59°-86°F) [See USP Controlled Room Temperature]. Dispense in a tight, light resistant container.
50 mg 100s: NDC 65197-002-01
100 mg 100s: NDC 65197-003-01
DATE OF ISSUANCE MARCH 2009
©WellSpring, 2009
Manufactured for
WellSpring Pharmaceutical Corporation
Sarasota, FL 34243 USA
By WellSpring Pharmaceutical Canada Corp.
Oakville, Ontario L6H 1M5 Canada
Rev. 03/09
Shown in Product Identification Guide, page 321

Wyeth Pharmaceuticals
A Division of Pfizer
235 EAST 42ND STREET
NEW YORK, NY 10017-5755

For Medical Information, Contact:
(800) 438-1985
24 hours a day, 7 days a week
Distribution:
1855 Shelby Oaks Drive North
Memphis, TN 38134
(901) 387-5200
Customer Service:
(800) 533-4535

For updates to the product information listed below, please check the Pfizer Web site, http://www.pfizerpro.com, or call (800) 438-1985. For complete product listing, please see the Manufacturers' Index.

BENEFIX®
[bĕn-ē-fĭks]   ℞
[Coagulation Factor IX (Recombinant)]
For Intravenous Use, Lyophilized Powder for Reconstitution

HIGHLIGHTS OF PRESCRIBING INFORMATION
These highlights do not include all the information needed to use BeneFIX safely and effectively. See full prescribing information for BeneFIX.
BeneFIX [Coagulation Factor IX (Recombinant)]
For Intravenous Use, Lyophilized Powder for Reconstitution
Initial U.S. Approval: 1997

─────────INDICATIONS AND USAGE─────────
BeneFIX is an antihemophilic factor (recombinant) indicated for:
• Control and prevention of bleeding episodes in adult and pediatric patients with hemophilia B. (1.1)
• Peri-operative management in adult and pediatric patients with hemophilia B. (1.2)

──────DOSAGE AND ADMINISTRATION──────
For Intravenous Use only
The initial estimated dose may be determined using the following formula: (2)
Required units = body weight (kg) × desired factor IX increase (IU/dL or % of normal) × reciprocal of observed recovery (IU/kg per IU/dL)
Average Recovery: Adult and Pediatric (<15 years) Patients
In clinical studies with adult and pediatric (<15 years) patients, one IU of BeneFIX per kilogram of body weight increased the circulating activity of factor IX as follows:
• Adults: 0.8 ± 0.2 IU/dL [range 0.4 to 1.2 IU/dL]. (2.3)
• Pediatric: 0.7 ± 0.3 IU/dL [range 0.2 to 2.1 IU/dL]. (2.3)
Dosing of BeneFIX may differ from that of plasma-derived factor IX products.
Dosage and duration of treatment with BeneFIX depends on the severity of the factor IX deficiency, the location and extent of bleeding, and the patient's clinical condition, age and recovery of factor IX. (2.1)

──────DOSAGE FORMS AND STRENGTHS──────
BeneFIX lyophilized powder is available as 250, 500, 1000, or 2000 IU in single-use vials. (3)

──────────CONTRAINDICATIONS──────────
BeneFIX is contraindicated in patients who have manifested life-threatening, immediate hypersensitivity reactions, including anaphylaxis, to the product or its components, including hamster protein. (4)

────────WARNINGS AND PRECAUTIONS────────
• Anaphylaxis and severe hypersensitivity reactions are possible. Should symptoms occur, treatment with the product should be discontinued, and emergency treatment should be sought. (5.2)
• BeneFIX has been associated with the development of thromboembolic complications, including patients receiving continuous infusion through a central venous catheter. (5.3)
• Development of activity-neutralizing antibodies has been detected in patients receiving factor IX-containing products. If expected plasma factor IX activity levels are not attained, or if patient presents with allergic reaction, or if bleeding is not controlled with an expected dose, an assay that measures factor IX inhibitor concentration should be performed. (5.5)
• Patients may develop hypersensitivity to hamster (CHO) protein as BeneFIX contains trace amounts. (5.2)

──────────ADVERSE REACTIONS──────────
The most common adverse reactions (incidence >5%) from clinical trials were nausea, injection site reaction, injection site pain, headache, dizziness and rash. (6.1)
To report SUSPECTED ADVERSE REACTIONS, contact Wyeth Pharmaceuticals Inc. at 1-800-934-5556 or FDA at 1-800-FDA-1088 or www.fda.gov/medwatch

──────────DRUG INTERACTIONS──────────
None known. (7)

────────USE IN SPECIFIC POPULATIONS────────
• On average, lower recovery has been observed in pediatric patients (<15 years). A dose adjustment may be needed. (12.3, 14)
See 17 for PATIENT COUNSELING INFORMATION and FDA-approved patient labeling

Revised: 06/2010

FULL PRESCRIBING INFORMATION: CONTENTS*
1   INDICATIONS AND USAGE
   1.1   Control and Prevention of Bleeding Episodes in Hemophilia B
   1.2   Peri-operative Management in Patients with Hemophilia B
2   DOSAGE AND ADMINISTRATION
   2.1   General Considerations for Administration
   2.2   Method of Calculating Initial Estimated Dose
   2.3   Dosing Guide for Control and Prevention of Bleeding Episodes and Peri-operative Management
   2.4   Instructions for Use
   2.5   Preparation and Reconstitution
   2.6   Administration (Intravenous Injection)
3   DOSAGE FORMS AND STRENGTHS
4   CONTRAINDICATIONS
5   WARNINGS AND PRECAUTIONS
   5.1   General
   5.2   Anaphylaxis and Severe Hypersensitivity Reactions
   5.3   Thromboembolic Complications
   5.4   Nephrotic Syndrome
   5.5   Neutralizing Antibodies (Immunogenicity)
   5.6   Monitoring Laboratory Tests
6   ADVERSE REACTIONS
   6.1   Clinical Trials Experience
   6.2   Post-marketing Experience
7   DRUG INTERACTIONS
8   USE IN SPECIFIC POPULATIONS
   8.1   Pregnancy
   8.2   Labor and Delivery
   8.3   Nursing Mothers
   8.4   Pediatric Use
   8.5   Geriatric Use
10   OVERDOSAGE
11   DESCRIPTION
12   CLINICAL PHARMACOLOGY
   12.1   Mechanism of Action
   12.2   Pharmacodynamics
   12.3   Pharmacokinetics
13   NONCLINICAL TOXICOLOGY
   13.1   Carcinogenesis, Mutagenesis, Impairment of Fertility
14   CLINICAL STUDIES
15   REFERENCES
16   HOW SUPPLIED/STORAGE AND HANDLING
   16.1   How Supplied
   16.2   Storage and Handling
17   PATIENT COUNSELING INFORMATION
   17.1   Allergic-type Hypersensitivity Reactions
   17.2   Neutralizing Antibodies (Inhibitors)
   17.3   FDA-Approved Patient Labeling
*Sections or subsections omitted from the full prescribing information are not listed

---

FULL PRESCRIBING INFORMATION

1   INDICATIONS AND USAGE
1.1   Control and Prevention of Bleeding Episodes in Hemophilia B
BeneFIX®, Coagulation Factor IX (Recombinant), is indicated for the control and prevention of bleeding episodes in adult and pediatric patients with hemophilia B (congenital factor IX deficiency or Christmas disease).
1.2   Peri-operative Management in Patients with Hemophilia B
BeneFIX, Coagulation Factor IX (Recombinant), is indicated for peri-operative management in adult and pediatric patients with hemophilia B.
BeneFIX, Coagulation Factor IX (Recombinant), is **NOT** indicated for:
a. treatment of other factor deficiencies (e.g., factors II, VII, VIII, and X),
b. treatment of hemophilia A patients with inhibitors to factor VIII,
c. reversal of coumarin-induced anticoagulation,
d. treatment of bleeding due to low levels of liver-dependent coagulation factors.

2   DOSAGE AND ADMINISTRATION
2.1   General Considerations for Administration
For Intravenous Use after Reconstitution
• **Treatment with BeneFIX, Coagulation Factor IX (Recombinant), should be initiated under the supervision of a physician experienced in the treatment of hemophilia B.**

• Each vial of BeneFIX has the rFIX potency in the International Units (IU) stated on the vial.
• Dosage and duration of treatment for all factor IX products depend on the severity of the factor IX deficiency, the location and extent of bleeding, and the patient's clinical condition, age and recovery of factor IX.
To ensure that the desired factor IX activity level has been achieved, precise monitoring using the factor IX activity assay is advised. Doses should be titrated using the factor IX activity, pharmacokinetic parameters, such as half-life and recovery, as well as taking the clinical situation into consideration in order to adjust the dose as appropriate.
Dosing of BeneFIX may differ from that of plasma-derived factor IX products [see Clinical Pharmacology (12)]. **Subjects at the low end of the observed factor IX recovery may require upward dosage adjustment of BeneFIX to as much as two times (2X) the initial empirically calculated dose in order to achieve the intended rise in circulating factor IX activity.**
The safety and efficacy of BeneFIX administration by continuous infusion have not been established [see Warnings and Precautions (5)].
2.2   Method of Calculating Initial Estimated Dose
The method of calculating the factor IX dose is shown in Table 1.

Table 1

number of factor IX IU required (IU)	=	body weight (kg)	×	desired factor IX increase (% or IU/dL)	×	reciprocal of observed recovery (IU/kg per IU/dL)

Average Recovery Adult Patients in Clinical Trial
In adult PTPs, on average, one International Unit (IU) of BeneFIX per kilogram of body weight increased the circulating activity of factor IX by 0.8 ± 0.2 IU/dL (range 0.4 to 1.2 IU/dL). The method of dose estimation is illustrated in Table 2. If you use 0.8 IU/dL average increase of factor IX per IU/kg body weight administered, then:

Table 2

number of factor IX IU required (IU)	=	body weight (kg)	×	desired factor IX increase (% or IU/dL)	×	1.3 (IU/kg per IU/dL)

Average Recovery Pediatric Patients (<15 years) in Clinical Trial
In pediatric patients, on average, one international unit of BeneFIX per kilogram of body weight increased the circulating activity of factor IX by 0.7 ± 0.3 IU/dL (range 0.2 to 2.1 IU/dL; median of 0.6 IU/dL per IU/kg). The method of dose estimation is illustrated in Table 3. If you use 0.7 IU/dL average increase of factor IX per IU/kg body weight administered, then:

Table 3

number of factor IX IU required (IU)	=	body weight (kg)	×	desired factor IX increase (% or IU/dL)	×	1.4 (IU/kg per IU/dL)

Doses administered should be titrated to the patient's clinical response. Patients may vary in their pharmacokinetic (e.g., half-life, in vivo recovery) and clinical responses to BeneFIX. Although the dose can be estimated by the calculations above, it is highly recommended that, whenever possible, appropriate laboratory tests, including serial factor IX activity assays, be performed.
2.3   Dosing Guide for Control and Prevention of Bleeding Episodes and Peri-operative Management
[See table at top of next page]
2.4   Instructions for Use
BeneFIX is administered by intravenous (IV) infusion after reconstitution of the lyophilized powder with the supplied pre-filled diluent (0.234% sodium chloride solution) syringe. Patients should follow the specific reconstitution and administration procedures provided by their physicians.
For instructions, patients should follow the recommendations in the FDA-Approved Patient Labeling [see Patient Counseling Information (17.3)].
Reconstitution, product administration, and handling of the administration set must be done with caution. Discard all equipment, including any reconstituted BeneFIX product, in an appropriate container. Place needles used for

venopuncture in a sharps container after single use. Percutaneous puncture with a needle contaminated with blood from an infected patient can transmit infectious viruses including HIV (AIDS) and hepatitis. Obtain immediate medical attention if injury occurs.

2.5   Preparation and Reconstitution

The procedures below are provided as general guidelines for the reconstitution and administration of BeneFIX.

Preparation

1. Always wash your hands before performing the following procedures.
2. Aseptic technique (meaning clean and germ-free) should be used during the reconstitution procedure.
3. Use all components in the reconstitution and administration of this product as soon as possible after opening their sterile containers to minimize unnecessary exposure to the atmosphere.

Note: If you use more than one vial of BeneFIX per infusion, each vial should be reconstituted according to the following instructions. The diluent syringe should be removed leaving the vial adapter in place, and a separate large luer lock syringe may be used to draw back the reconstituted contents of each vial. Do not detach the diluent syringes or the large luer lock syringe until you are ready to attach the large luer lock syringe to the next vial adapter.

Reconstitution

1. Allow the vial of lyophilized BeneFIX and the pre-filled diluent syringe to reach room temperature.
2. Remove the plastic flip-top cap from the BeneFIX vial to expose the central portions of the rubber stopper.

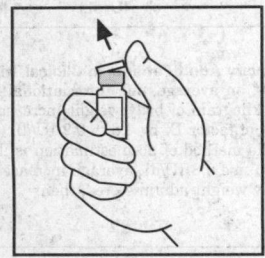

3. Wipe the top of the vial with the alcohol swab provided, or use another antiseptic solution, and allow to dry. After cleaning, do not touch the rubber stopper with your hand or allow it to touch any surface.
4. Peel back the cover from the clear plastic vial adapter package. **Do not remove the adapter from the package.**
5. Place the vial on a flat surface. While holding the adapter in the package, place the vial adapter over the vial and press down firmly on the package until the adapter spike penetrates the vial stopper.

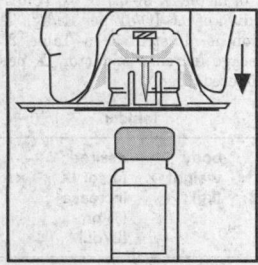

6. Grasp the plunger rod as shown in the diagram. Avoid contact with the shaft of the plunger rod. Attach the threaded end of the plunger rod to the diluent syringe plunger by pushing and turning firmly.

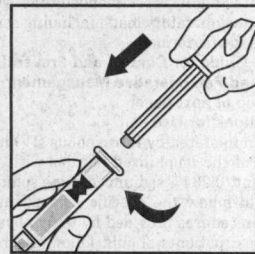

7. Break off the tamper-resistant plastic-tip cap from the diluent syringe by snapping the perforation of the cap. Do not touch the inside of the cap or the syringe tip. The diluent syringe may need to be recapped (if not administering reconstituted BeneFIX immediately), so place

the cap on its top on a clean surface in a spot where it would be least likely to become environmentally contaminated.

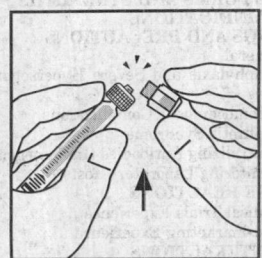

8. Lift the package away from the adapter and discard the package.

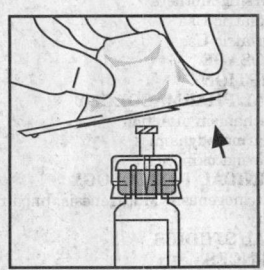

9. Place the vial on a flat surface. Connect the diluent syringe to the vial adapter by inserting the tip into the adapter opening while firmly pushing and turning the syringe clockwise until secured.

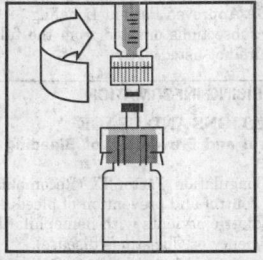

10. Slowly depress the plunger rod to inject all the diluent into the BeneFIX vial.

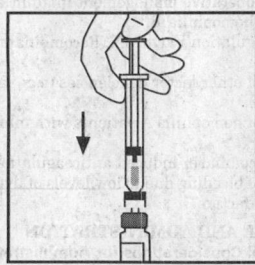

11. Without removing the syringe, **gently** swirl the contents of the vial until the powder is dissolved.
   Note: The final solution should be inspected visually for particulate matter before administration. The solu-

tion should appear clear and colorless. If it is not, the solution should be discarded and a new kit should be used.

12. Invert the vial and slowly draw the solution into the syringe.

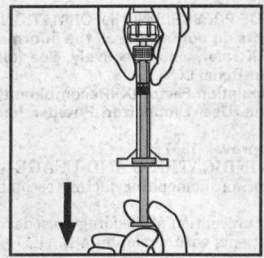

13. Detach the syringe from the vial adapter by gently pulling and turning the syringe counter-clockwise. Discard the vial with the adapter attached.
   Note: If the solution is not to be used immediately, the syringe cap should be carefully replaced. Do not touch the syringe tip or the inside of the cap.

BeneFIX, when reconstituted, contains polysorbate-80, which is known to increase the rate of di-(2-ethylhexyl)phthalate (DEHP) extraction from polyvinyl chloride (PVC). This should be considered during the preparation and administration of BeneFIX, including storage time elapsed in a PVC container following reconstitution. It is important that the recommendations for dosage and administration be followed closely [see Dosage and Administration (2)].

2.6   Administration (Intravenous Injection)

For Intravenous Use only after Reconstitution

BeneFIX is administered by intravenous (IV) infusion after reconstitution with the pre-filled diluent (0.234% sodium chloride solution) syringe.

• BeneFIX should be inspected for particulate matter and discoloration prior to administration, whenever solution and container permit.
• The reconstituted solution may be stored at room temperature prior to administration, but BeneFIX should be administered within 3 hours. BeneFIX should be administered using the tubing provided in this kit, and the pre-filled diluent syringe provided, or a single sterile disposable plastic syringe. In addition, the solution should be withdrawn from the vial using the vial adapter.
• A dose of BeneFIX may be administered over a period of several minutes. The rate of administration, however, should be adapted to the comfort level of each individual patient.

1. Attach the syringe to the luer end of the infusion set tubing provided.
2. Apply a tourniquet and prepare the injections site by wiping the skin well with an alcohol swab provided in the kit.

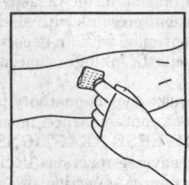

3. Perform venipuncture. Insert the needle on the infusion set tubing into the vein, and remove the tourniquet. The reconstituted BeneFIX product should be injected

Table 4

Type of Hemorrhage	Circulating Factor IX Activity Required [% or (IU/dL)]	Dosing Interval [hours]	Duration of Therapy [days]
Minor			
Uncomplicated hemarthroses, superficial muscle, or soft tissue	20-30	12-24	1-2
Moderate			Treat until bleeding stops and healing begins, about 2 to 7 days
Intramuscle or soft tissue with dissection, mucous membranes, dental extractions, or hematuria	25-50	12-24	
Major			
Pharynx, retropharynx, retroperitoneum, CNS, surgery	50-100	12-24	7-10

Adapted from: Roberts and Eberst[1]

intravenously over several minutes. The rate of administration should be determined by the patient's comfort level.

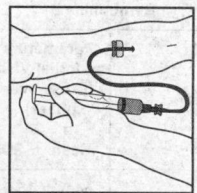

Reconstituted BeneFIX should not be administered in the same tubing or container with other medicinal products. Agglutination of red blood cells in the tubing/syringe has been reported with the administration of BeneFIX. No adverse events have been reported in association with this observation. To minimize the possibility of agglutination, it is important to limit the amount of blood entering the tubing. Blood should not enter the syringe. If red blood cell agglutination is observed in the tubing or syringe, discard all material (tubing, syringe and BeneFIX solution) and resume administration with a new package.

Following completion of BeneFIX treatment, remove the infusion set and discard. Dispose of all unused solution, empty vial(s), and used needles and syringes in an appropriate container for throwing away waste that might hurt others if not handled properly.

The safety and efficacy of administration by continuous infusion have not been established [see Warnings and Precautions (5)].

3 DOSAGE FORMS AND STRENGTHS

BeneFIX is supplied as a white lyophilized powder in the following dosages:
- 250 IU
- 500 IU
- 1000 IU
- 2000 IU

4 CONTRAINDICATIONS

BeneFIX is contraindicated in patients who have manifested life-threatening, immediate hypersensitivity reactions, including anaphylaxis, to the product or its components, including hamster protein.

5 WARNINGS AND PRECAUTIONS

5.1 General
The clinical response to BeneFIX may vary. If bleeding is not controlled with the recommended dose, the plasma level of factor IX should be determined, and a sufficient dose of BeneFIX should be administered to achieve a satisfactory clinical response. If the patient's plasma factor IX level fails to increase as expected or if bleeding is not controlled after the expected dose, the presence of an inhibitor (neutralizing antibodies) should be suspected, and appropriate testing performed [see Warnings and Precautions (5.6)].

5.2 Anaphylaxis and Severe Hypersensitivity Reactions
Allergic type hypersensitivity reactions, including anaphylaxis, have been reported with BeneFIX and have manifested as pruritus, rash, urticaria, hives, facial swelling, dizziness, hypotension, nausea, chest discomfort, cough, dyspnea, wheezing, flushing, discomfort (generalized) and fatigue. Frequently, these events have occurred in close temporal association with the development of factor IX inhibitors. Advise patients to discontinue use of the product and contact their physician and/or seek immediate emergency care.

BeneFIX contains trace amounts of hamster (CHO) proteins. Patients treated with this product may develop hypersensitivity to these non-human mammalian proteins.

5.3 Thromboembolic Complications
The safety and efficacy of BeneFIX administration by continuous infusion have not been established [see Dosage and Administration (2)]. There have been post-marketing reports of thrombotic events in patients receiving continuous-infusion BeneFIX through a central venous catheter, including life-threatening superior vena cava (SVC) syndrome in critically ill neonates [see Adverse Reactions (6)].

5.4 Nephrotic Syndrome
Nephrotic syndrome has been reported following immune tolerance induction with factor IX products in hemophilia B patients with factor IX inhibitors and a history of allergic reactions to factor IX. The safety and efficacy of using BeneFIX for immune tolerance induction have not been established.

5.5 Neutralizing Antibodies (Immunogenicity)
Patients using BeneFIX should be monitored for the development of factor IX inhibitors by appropriate clinical observations and laboratory tests. Inhibitors have been reported following administration of BeneFIX [see Clinical Pharmacology (12)]. If expected plasma factor IX activity levels are not attained, or if bleeding is not controlled with an expected dose, an assay that measures factor IX inhibitor concentration should be performed.

Patients with factor IX inhibitors may be at an increased risk of anaphylaxis upon subsequent challenge with factor IX.[2] Patients experiencing allergic reactions should be evaluated for the presence of an inhibitor. Patients should be observed closely for signs and symptoms of acute hypersensitivity reactions, particularly during the early phases of initial exposure to product. **Because of the potential for allergic reactions with factor IX concentrates, the initial (approximately 10-20) administrations of factor IX should be performed under medical supervision where proper medical care for allergic reactions could be provided.**

5.6 Monitoring Laboratory Tests
- Patients should be monitored for factor IX activity levels by the one-stage clotting assay to confirm that adequate factor IX levels have been achieved and maintained, when clinically indicated [see Dosage and Administration (2)].
- Patients should be monitored for the development of inhibitors if expected factor IX activity plasma levels are not attained, or if bleeding is not controlled with the recommended dose of BeneFIX. Assays used to determine if factor IX inhibitor is present should be titered in Bethesda Units (BUs).

6 ADVERSE REACTIONS

The most serious adverse reactions are systemic hypersensitivity reactions, including bronchospastic reactions and/or hypotension and anaphylaxis and the development of high-titer inhibitors necessitating alternative treatments to factor IX replacement therapy.

The most common adverse reactions observed in clinical trials (frequency > 5% of PTPs or PUPs) were headaches, dizziness, nausea, injections site reaction, injection site pain and skin-related hypersensitivity reactions (e.g., rash, hives).

6.1 Clinical Trials Experience
Because clinical trials are conducted under widely varying conditions, adverse reaction rates observed in the clinical trials of a drug cannot be directly compared to rates in the clinical trials of another drug and may not reflect the rates observed in clinical practice.

During uncontrolled open-label clinical studies with BeneFIX, Coagulation Factor IX (Recombinant), conducted in previously treated patients (PTPs), 113 adverse reactions with known or unknown relation to BeneFIX therapy were reported among 38.5% (25 of 65) of subjects (with some subjects reporting more than one event) who received a total of 7,573 infusions. These adverse reactions are summarized in Table 5.

Table 5: Adverse Reactions Reported for PTPs*

Body System	Adverse Reaction	Number of patients (%)
Blood and lymphatic system disorders	Factor IX inhibition[1]	1 (1.5%)
Eye disorders	Blurred vision	1 (1.5%)
Gastrointestinal disorders	Nausea	4 (6.2%)
	Vomiting	1 (1.5%)
General disorders and administration site conditions	Injection site reaction	5 (7.7%)
	Injection site pain	4 (6.2%)
	Fever	2 (3.1%)
Infections and infestations	Cellulitis at IV site	1 (1.5%)
	Phlebitis at IV site	1 (1.5%)
Nervous system disorders	Headache	7 (10.8%)
	Dizziness	5 (7.7%)
	Taste perversion (altered taste)	3 (4.6%)
	Shaking	1 (1.5%)
	Drowsiness	1 (1.5%)

Renal and urinary disorders	Renal infarct[2]	1 (1.5%)
Respiratory, thoracic and mediastinal disorders	Dry cough	1 (1.5%)
	Hypoxia	1 (1.5%)
	Chest tightness	1 (1.5%)
Skin and subcutaneous disorders	Rash	4 (6.2%)
	Hives	2 (3.1%)
Vascular disorders	Flushing	2 (3.1%)

* Adverse reactions reported within 72 hours of an infusion of BeneFIX.
[1] Low-titer transient inhibitor formation.
[2] The renal infarct developed in a hepatitis C antibody-positive patient 12 days after a dose of BeneFIX for a bleeding episode. The relationship of the infarct to the prior administration of BeneFIX is uncertain.

In the 63 previously untreated patients (PUPs), who received a total of 5,538 infusions, 10 adverse reactions were reported among 9.5% of the patients (6 out of 63) having known or unknown relationship to BeneFIX. These events are summarized in Table 6.

Table 6: Adverse Reactions Reported for PUPs*

Body System	Adverse Reaction	Number of Patients (%)
Blood and lymphatic system disorders	Factor IX inhibition[1]	2 (3.2%)
General disorders and administration site conditions	Injection site reaction	1 (1.6%)
	Chills	1 (1.6%)
Respiratory, thoracic and mediastinal disorders	Dyspnea (respiratory distress)	2 (3.2%)
Skin and subcutaneous disorders	Hives	3 (4.8%)
	Rash	1 (1.6%)

* Adverse reactions reported within 72 hours of an infusion of BeneFIX.
[1] Two subjects developed high-titer inhibitor formation during treatment with BeneFIX.

For adverse reactions thought to be related to the administration of BeneFIX, the rate of infusion should be decreased or the infusion stopped.

Immunogenicity
In clinical studies with 65 PTPs (defined as having more than 50 exposure days), a low-titer inhibitor was observed in one patient. The inhibitor was transient, the patient continued on study and had normal factor IX recovery pharmacokinetics at study completion (approximately 15 months after inhibitor detection).

In clinical studies with pediatric PUPs, inhibitor development was observed in 2 out of 63 patients (3.2%), both were high-titer (> 5 BU) inhibitors detected after 7 and 15 exposure days, respectively. Both patients were withdrawn from the study.

6.2 Post-marketing Experience
The following post-marketing adverse reactions have been reported for BeneFIX: inadequate factor IX recovery, inadequate therapeutic response, inhibitor development [see Clinical Pharmacology (12)], anaphylaxis [see Warnings and Precautions (5.2)], angioedema, dyspnea, hypotension, and thrombosis.

Because these reactions are reported voluntarily from a population of uncertain size, it is not always possible to reliably estimate their frequency or establish a causal relationship to drug exposure.

The safety and efficacy of BeneFIX administration by continuous infusion have not been established [see Warnings and Precautions (5.3)]. There have been post-marketing reports of thrombotic events, including life-threatening SVC syndrome in critically ill neonates, while receiving continuous-infusion BeneFIX through a central venous catheter. Cases of peripheral thrombophlebitis and DVT have also been reported. In some, BeneFIX was administered via **continuous infusion, which is not an approved method of administration** [see Dosage and Administration (2)].

7 DRUG INTERACTIONS

None known.

8 USE IN SPECIFIC POPULATIONS

8.1 Pregnancy

Pregnancy Category C

Animal reproduction and lactation studies have not been conducted with BeneFIX, Coagulation Factor IX (Recombinant). It is not known whether BeneFIX can affect reproductive capacity or cause fetal harm when given to pregnant women. BeneFIX should be administered to pregnant and lactating women only if needed.

8.2 Labor and Delivery

There is no information available on the effect of factor IX replacement therapy on labor and delivery. Use only if needed.

8.3 Nursing Mothers

It is not known whether this drug is excreted into human milk. Because many drugs are excreted into human milk, caution should be exercised if BeneFIX is administered to nursing mothers.

Use only if needed.

8.4 Pediatric Use

Safety, efficacy, and pharmacokinetics of BeneFIX have been evaluated in previously treated (PTP) and previously untreated pediatric patients (PUP) [see Dosage and Administration (2), Clinical Pharmacology (12), Clinical Studies (14) and Adverse Reactions (6)]. On average, lower recovery has been observed in pediatric patients (<15 years). A dose adjustment may be needed [see Dosage and Administration (2) and Clinical Pharmacology (12)].

8.5 Geriatric Use

Clinical studies of BeneFIX did not include sufficient numbers of subjects aged 65 and over to determine whether they respond differently from younger subjects. Dose selection for an elderly patient should be individualized [see Dosage and Administration (2)].

10 OVERDOSAGE

No symptoms of overdose have been reported.

11 DESCRIPTION

BeneFIX, Coagulation Factor IX (Recombinant), is a purified protein produced by recombinant DNA. It has a primary amino acid sequence that is identical to the Ala[148] allelic form of plasma-derived factor IX, and has structural and functional characteristics similar to those of endogenous factor IX. BeneFIX is produced by a genetically engineered Chinese hamster ovary (CHO) cell line that is extensively characterized. No human or animal proteins are added during the purification and formulation processes of BeneFIX.

BeneFIX is not derived from human blood and contains no preservatives, and the manufacture of BeneFIX includes no added animal or human components. The stored cell banks are free of human blood or plasma products. The CHO cell line secretes recombinant factor IX into a defined cell culture medium that does not contain any proteins derived from animal or human sources, and the recombinant factor IX is purified by a chromatography purification process that does not require a monoclonal antibody step. The process also includes a membrane nanofiltration step that has the ability to retain molecules with apparent molecular weights >70,000 Da (such as large proteins and viral particles). BeneFIX is a single component by SDS-polyacrylamide gel electrophoresis evaluation. The potency (in International Units, IU) is determined using an in vitro one-stage clotting assay against the World Health Organization (WHO) International Standard for Factor IX concentrate. One International Unit is the amount of factor IX activity present in 1 mL of pooled, normal human plasma. The specific activity of BeneFIX is greater than or equal to 200 IU per milligram of protein.

BeneFIX is formulated as a sterile, nonpyrogenic, lyophilized powder preparation. BeneFIX is intended for intravenous (IV) injection. It is available in single-use vials containing the labeled amount of factor IX activity, expressed in IU. Each vial contains nominally 250, 500, 1000

or 2000 IU of Coagulation Factor IX (Recombinant). After reconstitution of the lyophilized drug product, the concentrations of excipients are 0.234% sodium chloride, 8 mM L-histidine, 0.8% sucrose, 208 mM glycine, 0.004% polysorbate 80. All dosage strengths yield a clear, colorless solution upon reconstitution.

12 CLINICAL PHARMACOLOGY

12.1 Mechanism of Action

BeneFIX temporarily replaces the missing clotting factor IX that is needed for effective hemostasis.

12.2 Pharmacodynamics

The activated partial thromboplastin time (aPTT) is prolonged in people with hemophilia B. Treatment with factor IX concentrate may normalize the aPTT by temporarily replacing the factor IX. The administration of BeneFIX, Coagulation Factor IX (Recombinant), increases plasma levels of factor IX, and can temporarily correct the coagulation defect in these patients.

12.3 Pharmacokinetics

After single intravenous (IV) doses of 50 IU/kg of previously marketed BeneFIX, Coagulation Factor IX (Recombinant) [reconstituted with Sterile Water for Injection], in 37 previously treated adult patients (>15 years), each given as a 10-minute infusion, the mean increase from pre-infusion level in circulating factor IX activity was 0.8 ± 0.2 IU/dL per IU/kg infused (range 0.4 to 1.4 IU/dL per IU/kg) and the mean biologic half-life was 18.8 ± 5.4 hours (range 11 to 36 hours). In the original randomized, cross-over pharmacokinetic study in previously treated patients (PTPs), the in vivo recovery using previously marketed BeneFIX was statistically significantly less (28% lower, p<0.05) than the recovery using a highly purified plasma-derived factor IX product (pdFIX). A summary of pharmacokinetic data for BeneFIX and pdFIX are presented in Table 7.

Table 7: Pharmacokinetic Parameter Estimates for BeneFIX and pdFIX in Previously Treated Patients with Hemophilia B

Parameter	BeneFIX, n = 11 Mean ± SD	pdFIX, n = 11 Mean ± SD
AUC_∞ (IU•hr/dL)	548 ± 92	928 ± 191
$t_{1/2}$ (hr)	18.1 ± 5.1	17.7 ± 5.3
CL (mL/hr/kg)	8.62 ± 1.7	6.00 ± 1.4
K-value (IU/dL per IU/kg)	0.84 ± 0.30	1.17 ± 0.26
In vivo Recovery (%)	37.8 ± 14.0	52.6 ± 12.4

Abbreviations: AUC_∞ = area under the plasma concentration-time curve from time zero to infinity; K-value = incremental recovery; $t_{1/2}$ = plasma elimination half-life; CL = clearance; SD = standard deviation.

There was no significant difference in biological half-life. Structural differences of the BeneFIX molecule compared with pdFIX were shown to contribute to the lower recovery. In subsequent evaluations for up to 24 months, the pharmacokinetic parameters were similar to the initial results.

In a subsequent randomized, cross-over pharmacokinetic study, BeneFIX reconstituted in 0.234% sodium chloride diluent was shown to be pharmacokinetically equivalent to the previously marketed BeneFIX (reconstituted with Sterile Water for Injection) in 24 previously treated patients (≥12 years) at a dose of 75 IU/kg. In addition, pharmacokinetic parameters were followed up in 23 previously treated patients after repeated administration of BeneFIX for six months and found to be unchanged compared with those obtained at the initial evaluation. A summary of pharmacokinetic data are presented in Table 8:

Table 8: Pharmacokinetic Parameter Estimates for BeneFIX at Baseline (Cross-over phase) and Month 6 (Follow-up phase) in Previously Treated Patients with Hemophilia B

Parameter	Parameters at Initial Visit (Cross-over phase), n = 24 Mean ± SD	Parameters at Month 6 (Follow-up phase) n = 23 Mean ± SD
C_{max} (IU/dL)	54.5 ± 15.0	57.3 ± 13.2
AUC_∞ (IU•hr/dL)	940 ± 237	923 ± 205
$t_{1/2}$ (hr)	22.4 ± 5.3	23.8 ± 6.5
CL (mL/hr/kg)	8.47 ± 2.12	8.54 ± 2.04
K-value (IU/dL per IU/kg)	0.73 ± 0.20	0.76 ± 0.18
In vivo Recovery (%)	34.5 ± 9.3	36.8 ± 8.7

Abbreviations: AUC_∞ = area under the plasma concentration-time curve from time zero to infinity; AUC_t = area under the plasma concentration-time curve from zero to the last measurable concentration; C_{max} = peak concentration; K-value = incremental recovery; $t_{1/2}$ = plasma elimination half-life; CL = clearance; SD = standard deviation.

Pediatric Patients (≤15 years)

Nineteen (19) previously treated pediatric patients (range 4 to ≤15 years) underwent pharmacokinetic evaluations for up to 24 months. Fifty-eight previously untreated patients [PUPs] less than 15 years of age at baseline underwent at least one recovery assessment within 30 minutes post-infusion in the presence or absence of hemorrhage during the study. A total of 202 recovery assessments collected during the 60-month period from these 58 PUPs are combined with 19 recovery assessments from PTPs and were summarized by age group in Table 9. There was one recovery assessment in a neonate, which had a value of 0.46 IU/dL per IU/kg. The overall mean recovery and FIX elimination half-life values were 0.7 ± 0.3 IU/dL per IU/kg and 20.2 ± 4.0 hours, respectively.

[See table 9 below]

Data from 57 PUP subjects who underwent repeat recovery testing for up to 60 months demonstrated that the average incremental FIX recovery was consistent over time, as shown in Figure 1.

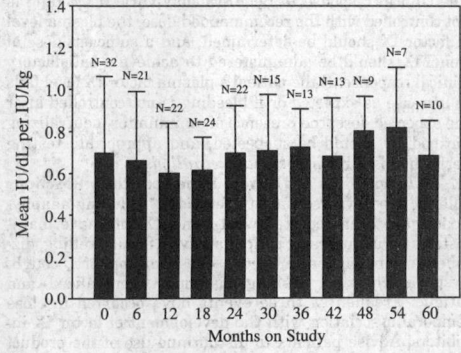

Figure 1. Average Incremental rFIX Recovery over Time

13 NONCLINICAL TOXICOLOGY

13.1 Carcinogenesis, Mutagenesis, Impairment of Fertility

BeneFIX, Coagulation Factor IX (Recombinant), has been shown to be nonmutagenic in the Ames assay and non-clastogenic in a chromosomal aberrations assay. No investigations on carcinogenesis or impairment of fertility have been conducted.

14 CLINICAL STUDIES

Efficacy of BeneFIX has been evaluated in clinical studies in which a total of 128 subjects received BeneFIX either for the treatment of bleeding episodes on an on-demand basis, for the prevention of bleeds (prophylaxis) or for management of hemostasis in the surgical setting (surgical prophylaxis).

Fifty-six PTPs and sixty-three PUPs were treated for bleeding episodes on an on-demand basis or for the prevention of bleeds (see Tables 9 and 10). The PTPs were followed over a median interval of 24 months (mean 23.4 ± 5.3 months) and for a median of 83.5. The PUPs were followed over a median interval of 37 months (mean 38.1 ± 16.4 months) and for a median of 89 exposure days.

Fifty-five PTPs and fifty-four PUPs received BeneFIX for the treatment of bleeding episodes (see Table 10). Bleeding

Table 9: Summary of BeneFIX Pharmacokinetic Parameters in Pediatric Patients

Age Group	n	K-value (IU/dL per IU/kg)	$t_{1/2}$(h)
Infants (≥1 month to <2 years)	33	0.7 ± 0.4 (0.2, 2.1)	ND
Children (≥2 years to <12 years)	61	0.7 ± 0.2 (0.2, 1.5)	19.8 ± 4.0 (14, 27)[a]
Adolescents (≥12 years to ≤15 years)	9	0.8 ± 0.3 (0.4, 1.4)	21.1 ± 4.5 (15, 28)[b]

[a] n = 13
[b] n =6

Data presented are mean ± standard deviation (min, max).

Abbreviations: ND = not determined; K-value = incremental recovery; $t_{1/2}$ = terminal phase elimination half-life.

Note: The columns are not mutually exclusive; individual patients may be listed under more than 1 age category.

episodes that were managed successfully included hemarthrosis and bleeding in soft tissue and muscle. Data concerning the severity of bleeding episodes were not reported. In the PTPs, 88% of total infusions administrated for on-demand treatment were rated as an "excellent" or "good" response.

[See table 10 at right]

A total of 20 PTPs were treated with BeneFIX for secondary prophylaxis (the regular administration of FIX replacement therapy to prevent bleeding in patients who may have already demonstrated clinical evidence of hemophilic arthropathy or joint disease) at some regular interval during the study with a mean of 2.0 infusions per week (see Table 11). Thirty-two PUPs were administered BeneFIX for routine (primary and secondary) prophylaxis (see Table 11). Twenty-four PUPs were administered BeneFIX at least twice weekly, and eight PUPs were administered BeneFIX once weekly. Seven PTPs experienced a total of 26 spontaneous bleeding episodes within 48 hours after an infusion. Six spontaneous bleeds within 48 hours after an infusion were reported in 5 PUPs. Prophylaxis therapy was rated as "excellent" or "effective" in 93% of PTPs receiving prophylaxis one to two times per week.

[See table 11 at right]

Management of hemostasis was evaluated in the surgical setting in both PTPs and PUPs (see Table 12). Thirty-six surgical procedures have been performed in 28 PTPs with 23 major surgical procedures performed (including 6 complicated dental extractions). Thirty surgical procedures have been performed in 23 PUPs. Twenty-eight of these procedures were considered minor. Hemostasis was maintained throughout the surgical period; however, one PTP subject required evacuation of a surgical wound-site hematoma, and another PTP subject who received BeneFIX after a tooth extraction required further surgical intervention due to oozing at the extraction site. There was no clinical evidence of thrombotic complications in any of the subjects.

Among the PTP surgery subjects, the median increase in circulating factor IX activity was 0.7 IU/dL per IU/kg infused (range 0.3–1.2 IU/dL; mean 0.8 ± 0.2 IU/dL per IU/kg). The median elimination half-life for the PTP surgery subjects was 19.4 hours (range 10–37 hours; mean 21.3 ± 8.1 hours).

[See table 12 at right]

Nine of the major surgical procedures were performed in 8 PUPs using a continuous-infusion regimen. Five of the surgical procedures were performed in PUPs using a continuous-infusion regimen over 3 to 5 days. Although circulating factor IX levels targeted to restore and maintain hemostasis were achieved with both pulse replacement and continuous infusion regimens, clinical trial experience with continuous infusion of BeneFIX for surgical prophylaxis in hemophilia B has been too limited to establish the safety and clinical efficacy of administration of the product by continuous infusion.

All subjects participating in the PTP, PUP and surgery studies were monitored for clinical evidence of thrombosis [see Warnings and Precautions (5)]. No thrombotic complications were reported in PUPs or surgery subjects. One PTP subject experienced a renal infarct 12 days after a dose of BeneFIX for a bleeding episode; the relationship of the infarct to the prior administration of BeneFIX is uncertain. Laboratory studies of thrombogenecity (fibrinopeptide A and prothrombin fragment 1 + 2) were obtained in 41 PTPs and 7 surgery subjects prior to infusion and up to 24 hours following infusion. The results of these studies were inconclusive. Out of 29 PTP subjects noted to have elevated fibrinopeptide A levels post-infusion of BeneFIX, 22 also had elevated levels at baseline. Surgery subjects showed no evidence of significant increase in coagulation activation.

15 REFERENCES

1. Roberts HR, Eberst ME. Current management of hemophilia B. Hematol Oncol Clin North Am. 1993;7(6): 1269-1280.
2. Shapiro AD, Ragni MV, Lusher JM, et al. Safety and efficacy of monoclonal antibody purified factor IX concentrate in previously untreated patients with hemophilia B. Thromb Haemost. 1996;75(1):30-35.

16 HOW SUPPLIED/STORAGE AND HANDLING

16.1 How Supplied

BeneFIX, Coagulation Factor IX (Recombinant), is supplied in single-use vials which contain nominally 250, 500, 1000 or 2000 IU per vial (NDC 58394-003-06, 58394-002-06, 58394-001-06, and 58394-008-02, respectively) with sterile pre-filled diluent syringe, vial adapter reconstitution device, sterile infusion set, and two (2) alcohol swabs, one bandage and one gauze pad. Actual factor IX activity in IU is stated on the label of each vial.

16.2 Storage and Handling

Product as packaged for sale: BeneFIX, Coagulation Factor IX (Recombinant), Store under refrigeration at a temperature of 2 to 8°C (36 to 46°F).

Prior to the expiration date, BeneFIX may also be stored at room temperature not to exceed 25°C (77°F) for up to 6 months.

Advise patient to make note of the date the product was placed at room temperature in the space provided on the outer carton.

Do not put the product back into the refrigerator at the end of the 6-month period. Use it immediately or discard.

Do not freeze to prevent damage to the diluent syringe. Do not use BeneFIX after the expiration date on the label.

Product after reconstitution: The product does not contain a preservative and should be used within 3 hours.

17 PATIENT COUNSELING INFORMATION

17.1 Allergic-type Hypersensitivity Reactions

Allergic-type hypersensitivity reactions are possible. Inform patients of the early signs of hypersensitivity reactions [including hives (rash with itching), generalized urticaria, tightness of the chest, wheezing, hypotension] and anaphylaxis. Advise patients to discontinue use of the product and contact their physicians if these symptoms occur.

17.2 Neutralizing Antibodies (Inhibitors)

Advise patients to contact their physician or treatment facility for further treatment and/or assessment if they experience a lack of a clinical response to factor IX replacement therapy, as in some cases this may be a manifestation of an inhibitor.

17.3 FDA-Approved Patient Labeling

BeneFIX®

(BEN-uh-fiks)

[Coagulation Factor IX (Recombinant)]

Please read this Patient Leaflet carefully before using BeneFIX and each time you get a refill. There may be new information. This Patient Leaflet does not take the place of talking with your doctor about your medical condition or your treatment.

What is BeneFIX?

BeneFIX is an injectable medicine that is used to help control and prevent bleeding in people with hemophilia B. Hemophilia B is also called congenital factor IX deficiency or Christmas disease.

BeneFIX is **NOT** used to treat hemophilia A.

What should I tell my doctor before using BeneFIX?

Tell your doctor and pharmacist about all of the medicines you take, including all prescription and non-prescription medicines, such as over-the-counter medicines, supplements, or herbal medicines.

Table 10: Efficacy of BeneFIX for on-demand treatment of PTPs and PUPs

	Median dose: IU/kg (range)	Rate of bleeds resolved with 1 infusion	Response to 1st Infusion Rating[c]		
			Excellent/Good	Moderate	No Response
PTPs N=55[a]	42.8 (6.5-224.6)	81%	90.9%	7.1%	0.7%
PUPs N=54[b]	62.7 (8.2-292)	75%	94.1%	2.9%	1.0%

[a] One subject discontinued the study after one month of treatment due to bleeding episodes that were difficult to control; he did not have a detectable inhibitor.

[b] Three subjects were not successfully treated including one episode in a subject due to delayed time to infusion and insufficient dosing and in 2 subjects due to inhibitor formation.

[c] Response ratings not provided for 1.3% and 2% of 1st infusions for PTPs and PUPs, respectively.

Table 11: Efficacy of Prophylaxis of BeneFIX in PTPs and PUPs

Total exposure (infusions)		Duration of prophylaxis (months) (mean ± SD)	Dose IU/kg (mean ± SD)	Spontaneous bleeds within 48 hrs of infusion	Response rating[a]		
					Excellent	Effective	Inadequate
PTPs 20	2985	18.2 ± 8.4[b]	40.3 ± 15.2[b]	28	56.0%	37.1%	4.3%
PUPs 32	3158	14.4 ± 8.1	73.3 ± 33.1	6	91.3%	6.4%	1.7%

[a] Response ratings provided at approximately 3-month intervals. In total, 116 and 172 assessments reported for PTPs and PUPs, respectively. Response ratings not provided for 2.6% and 0.6% of intervals for PTPs and PUPs, respectively.

[b] N = 19

Table 12: Efficacy of BeneFIX for Surgical Procedures in PTPs and PUPs

Surgery Type	Number of Procedures (Number of Subjects)	Response		
		Excellent/Good	Moderate	No Response
Previously Treated Patients				
Ankle surgery	2 (2)	2 (100%)	-	-
Hip prosthesis implant (right)	1 (1)	1 (100%)	-	-
Knee arthroplasty (2 bilateral, 1 right)	3 (3)	3 (100%)	-	-
Knee arthroscopic synovectomy	2 (2)[a]	1 (50%)	-	-
Liver transplantation (orthotopic)	1 (1)	1 (100%)	-	-
Splenectomy	1 (1)	1 (100%)	-	-
External fixation device removal (wrist)	1 (1)	1 (100%)	-	-
Hernia repair	3 (2)	3 (100%)	-	-
Subacromial decompression (left)	1 (1)	1 (100%)	-	-
Calf debridement, dental extraction[b]	1 (1)	1 (100%)	-	-
Lymph node removal, dental extraction[b]	1 (1)	1 (100%)	-	-
Left heel cord lengthening	1 (1)	1 (100%)	-	-
Dental procedures[c]	12 (11)	11 (92%)	1 (8%)	-
Minor procedures	6 (6)	6 (100%)	-	-
Previously Untreated Patients				
Hernia repair	2 (2)	2 (100%)	-	-
Minor procedures	28 (21)[a]	27 (96%)	-	-

[a] Response assessment not provided for 1 procedure.

[b] Includes pulse and continuous-infusion regimens; CI counted as 1 procedure in this summary.

[c] Includes complicated extractions (6), clearance, and fillings.

Tell your doctor about all of your medical conditions, including if you:
- are pregnant or planning to become pregnant. It is not known if BeneFIX may harm your unborn baby.
- are breastfeeding. It is not known if BeneFIX passes into the milk and if it can harm your baby.

How should I infuse BeneFIX?
The initial administrations of BeneFIX should be administered under proper medical supervision, where proper medical care for severe allergic reactions could be provided.
See the step-by-step instructions for infusing BeneFIX at the end of this leaflet. You should always follow the specific instructions given by your doctor. The steps listed below are general guidelines for using BeneFIX. If you are unsure of the procedures, please call your doctor or pharmacist before using.
Call your doctor right away if bleeding is not controlled after using BeneFIX.
Your doctor will prescribe the dose that you should take. Your doctor may need to test your blood from time to time. BeneFIX should not be administered by continuous infusion.

What if I take too much BeneFIX?
Call your doctor if you take too much BeneFIX.

What are the possible side effects of BeneFIX?
Allergic reactions may occur with BeneFIX. Call your doctor or get emergency treatment right away if you have any of the following symptoms:
wheezing
difficulty breathing
chest tightness
turning blue (look at lips and gums)
fast heartbeat
swelling of the face
faintness
rash
hives
Your body can also make antibodies, called "inhibitors," against BeneFIX, which may stop BeneFIX from working properly.
Some common side effects of BeneFIX are nausea, injection site reaction, injection site pain, headache, dizziness and rash.
BeneFIX may increase the risk of thromboembolism (abnormal blood clots) in your body if you have risk factors for developing blood clots, including an indwelling venous catheter through which BeneFIX is given by continuous infusion. There have been reports of severe blood clotting events, including life-threatening blood clots in critically ill neonates, while receiving continuous-infusion BeneFIX through a central venous catheter. The safety and efficacy of BeneFIX administration by continuous infusion have not been established.
These are not all the possible side effects of BeneFIX.
Tell your doctor about any side effect that bothers you or that does not go away.

How should I store BeneFIX?
DO NOT FREEZE BeneFIX. Store BeneFIX in the refrigerator at 36° to 46°F (2° to 8°C). BeneFIX may also be stored at room temperature (below 77°F) for up to 6 months, until the expiration date.
If you store BeneFIX at room temperature, be careful to write down the date you put BeneFIX at room temperature, so you know when to throw it out.
There is a space provided on the outer carton for you to write the date.
At the end of the 6-month period, the product should not be put back into the refrigerator, but should be used immediately or discarded. Freezing should be avoided to prevent damage to the pre-filled diluent syringe.
Throw away any unused BeneFIX after the expiration date. BeneFIX does not contain a preservative. After reconstituting BeneFIX, you can store it at room temperature for up to 3 hours. If you have not used it in 3 hours, throw it away. Store the diluent syringe at 36° to 77°F (2° to 25°C).
Do not use BeneFIX if the reconstituted solution is not clear and colorless.

What else should I know about BeneFIX?
Medicines are sometimes prescribed for purposes other than those listed here. Do not use BeneFIX for a condition for which it was not prescribed. Do not share BeneFIX with other people, even if they have the same symptoms that you have.
This Patient Leaflet summarizes the most important information about BeneFIX. If you would like more information, talk with your doctor. You can ask your doctor or pharmacist for information about BeneFIX that was written for health-care professionals.

Instructions for Using BeneFIX
BeneFIX is supplied as a powder. Before it can be infused in your vein (intravenous injection), you must reconstitute the powder by mixing it with the liquid diluent supplied. The liquid diluent is 0.234% sodium chloride. BeneFIX should

be reconstituted and infused using the infusion set, diluent, syringe, and adapter provided in this kit, and by following the directions below.

RECONSTITUTION
Always wash your hands before performing the following steps. Try to keep everything clean and germ-free while you are reconstituting BeneFIX. Once you open the vials, you should finish reconstituting BeneFIX as soon as possible. This will help keep the infusion set materials germ-free.
Note: If you use more than one vial of BeneFIX per infusion, reconstitute each vial according to steps 1 through 13.
1. Let the vial of BeneFIX and the pre-filled diluent syringe reach room temperature.
2. Remove the plastic flip-top cap from the BeneFIX vial to show the center part of the rubber stopper.

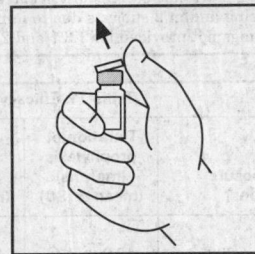

3. Wipe the top of the vial with the alcohol swab provided, or use another antiseptic solution, and allow to dry. After cleaning, do not touch the rubber stopper with your hand or allow it to touch any surface.
4. Peel back the cover from the clear plastic vial adapter package. **Do not remove the adapter from the package.**
5. Place the vial on a flat surface. While holding the adapter in the package, place the vial adapter over the vial. Press down firmly on the package until the adapter snaps into place on top of the vial, with the adapter spike penetrating the vial stopper.

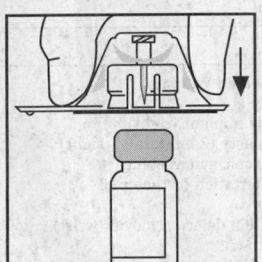

6. Grasp the plunger rod as shown in the picture below. Do not touch the shaft of the plunger rod. Attach the threaded end of the plunger rod to the diluent syringe plunger by pushing and turning firmly.

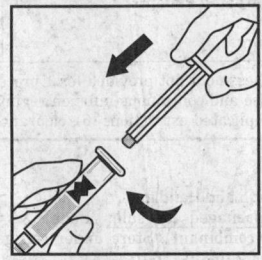

7. Break off the tamper-resistant, plastic-tip cap from the diluent syringe by snapping the perforation of the cap. Do not touch the inside of the cap or the syringe tip. The diluent syringe may need to be recapped (if reconstituted BeneFIX is not used immediately), so place the cap on its tip on a clean surface in a spot where it will stay clean.
[See first figure at top of next column]
8. Lift the package away from the adapter and discard the package.
[See second figure in next column]
9. Place the vial on a flat surface. Connect the diluent syringe to the vial adapter by inserting the tip of the syringe into the adapter opening while firmly pushing and turning the syringe clockwise until the connection is secured.
[See third figure in next column]
10. Slowly push the plunger rod to inject all the diluent into the BeneFIX vial.
[See fourth figure in next column]

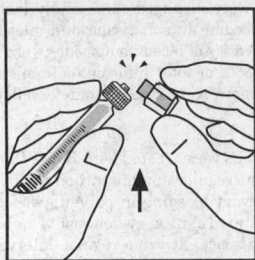

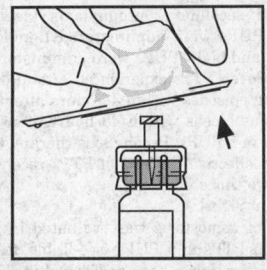

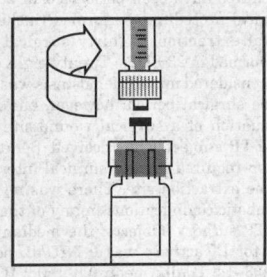

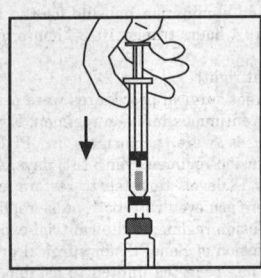

11. With the syringe still connected to the adapter, **gently** swirl the contents of the vial until the powder is dissolved.
   Look at the final solution before infusing it. The solution should be clear to colorless. If it is not, throw away the solution and use a new kit.
12. Make sure the syringe plunger rod is still fully pressed down, then turn over the vial. Slowly pull the solution into the syringe. Turn the syringe upward again and remove any air bubbles by gently tapping the syringe with your finger and slowly pushing air out of the syringe.
   If you reconstituted more than one vial of BeneFIX, remove the diluent syringe from the vial adapter and leave the vial adapter attached to the vial. Quickly attach a separate large luer lock syringe and pull the reconstituted solution as instructed above. Repeat this procedure with each vial in turn. Do not detach the diluent syringes or the large luer lock syringe until you are ready to attach the large luer lock syringe to the next vial adapter.

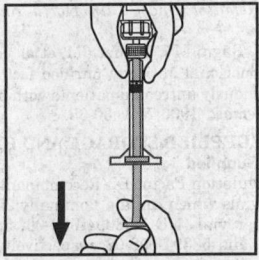

13. Remove the syringe from the vial adapter by gently pulling and turning the syringe counter-clockwise. Throw away the vial with the adapter attached.

If you are not using the solution right away, you should carefully replace the syringe cap. Do not touch the syringe tip or the inside of the cap.

BeneFIX should be infused within 3 hours after reconstitution. The reconstituted solution may be stored at room temperature prior to infusion.

INFUSION (Intravenous Injection)

Continuous infusion is **not** an approved way to administer BeneFIX.

Your doctor or healthcare professional should teach you how to infuse BeneFIX. Once you learn how to self-infuse, you can follow the instructions in this insert.

1. Attach the syringe to the luer end of the provided infusion set tubing.
2. Apply a tourniquet and prepare the injection site by wiping the skin well with an alcohol swab provided in the kit.

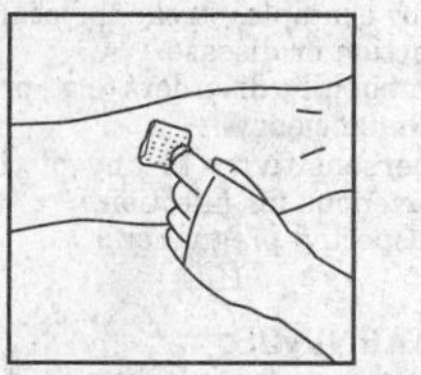

3. Insert the butterfly needle of the infusion set tubing into your vein as instructed by your doctor or healthcare provider. Remove the tourniquet. Infuse the reconstituted BeneFIX product over several minutes. Your comfort level should determine the rate of infusion.

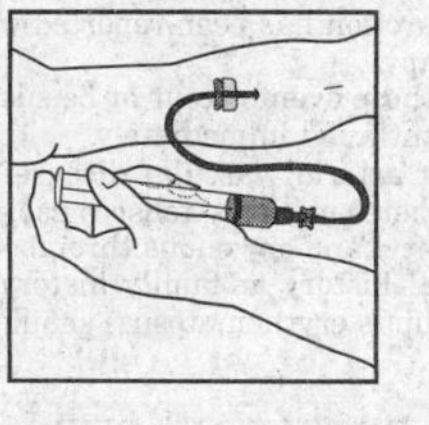

Clumping of red blood cells in the tubing/syringe has been reported with the administration of BeneFIX. No adverse events have been reported in association with this observation. To minimize the possibility of clumping it is important to limit the amount of blood entering the tubing. Blood should not enter the syringe.

Note: If red blood cell clumping is observed in the tubing or syringe, discard all material (tubing, syringe and BeneFIX solution) and continue administration with a new package.

4. After infusing BeneFIX, remove the infusion set and discard. The amount of drug product left in the infusion set will not affect your treatment. Dispose of all unused solution, the empty vial(s), and the used needles and syringes in an appropriate container used for throwing away waste that might hurt others if not handled properly.

It is a good idea to record the lot number from the BeneFIX vial label every time you use BeneFIX. You can use the peel-off label found on the vial to record the lot number.

If you have any questions or concerns about BeneFIX, ask your doctor or healthcare provider.

Wyeth®

Wyeth Pharmaceuticals Inc. W10526C006
Philadelphia, PA 19101 ET01
US Govt. License No. 3 Rev 06/10

PREMARIN® ℞

[*prĕ-mă-rĭn*]

Intravenous

(conjugated estrogens, USP) for injection

Specially prepared for Intravenous & Intramuscular use

NOTE: PATIENT INFORMATION LEAFLET ATTACHED.

Rx only

WARNINGS

ENDOMETRIAL CANCER

Adequate diagnostic measures, including endometrial sampling when indicated, should be undertaken to rule out malignancy in all cases of undiagnosed persistent or recurring abnormal vaginal bleeding. (See **WARNINGS, Malignant neoplasms, Endometrial cancer.**)

CARDIOVASCULAR AND OTHER RISKS

Estrogens with or without progestins should not be used for the prevention of cardiovascular disease or dementia. (See **CLINICAL STUDIES** and **WARNINGS, Cardiovascular disorders** and **Dementia.**)

The estrogen alone substudy of the Women's Health Initiative (WHI) reported increased risks of stroke and deep vein thrombosis (DVT) in postmenopausal women (50 to 79 years of age) during 6.8 years and 7.1 years, respectively, of treatment with daily oral conjugated estrogens (CE 0.625 mg), relative to placebo. (See **CLINICAL STUDIES** and **WARNINGS, Cardiovascular disorders.**)

The estrogen plus progestin substudy of WHI reported increased risks of myocardial infarction, stroke, invasive breast cancer, pulmonary emboli, and DVT in postmenopausal women (50 to 79 years of age) during 5.6 years of treatment with daily CE 0.625 mg combined with medroxyprogesterone acetate (MPA 2.5 mg), relative to placebo. (See **CLINICAL STUDIES** and **WARNINGS, Cardiovascular disorders** and Malignant neoplasms, Breast cancer.)

The Women's Health Initiative Memory Study (WHIMS), a substudy of WHI, reported an increased risk of developing probable dementia in postmenopausal women 65 years of age or older during 5.2 years of treatment with daily CE 0.625 mg alone and during 4 years of treatment with CE 0.625 mg combined with MPA 2.5 mg, relative to placebo. It is unknown whether this finding applies to younger postmenopausal women. (See **CLINICAL STUDIES** and **WARNINGS, Dementia** and **PRECAUTIONS, Geriatric Use.**)

In the absence of comparable data, these risks should be assumed to be similar for other doses of CE and MPA and other combinations and dosage forms of estrogens and progestins. Because of these risks, estrogens with or without progestins should be prescribed at the lowest effective doses and for the shortest duration consistent with treatment goals and risks for the individual woman.

DESCRIPTION

Premarin® Intravenous (conjugated estrogens, USP) for injection contains a mixture of conjugated estrogens obtained exclusively from natural sources, occurring as the sodium salts of water-soluble estrogen sulfates blended to represent the average composition of materials derived from pregnant mares' urine. It is a mixture of sodium estrone sulfate and sodium equilin sulfate. It contains as concomitant components, as sodium sulfate conjugates, 17α-dihydroequilin, 17α-estradiol, and 17β-dihydroequilin.

Each Secule® vial contains 25 mg of conjugated estrogens, USP, in a sterile lyophilized cake which also contains lactose 200 mg, sodium citrate 12.2 mg, and simethicone 0.2 mg. The pH is adjusted with sodium hydroxide or hydrochloric acid. The reconstituted solution is suitable for intravenous or intramuscular injection.

CLINICAL PHARMACOLOGY

Endogenous estrogens are largely responsible for the development and maintenance of the female reproductive system and secondary sexual characteristics. Although circulating estrogens exist in a dynamic equilibrium of metabolic interconversions, estradiol is the principal intracellular human estrogen and is substantially more potent than its metabolites, estrone and estriol, at the receptor level. The primary source of estrogen in normally cycling adult women is the ovarian follicle, which secretes 70 to 500 mcg of estradiol daily, depending on the phase of the menstrual cycle. After menopause, most endogenous estrogen is produced by conversion of androstenedione, secreted by the adrenal cortex, to estrone by peripheral tissues. Thus, estrone and the sulfate-conjugated form, estrone sulfate, are the most abundant circulating estrogen in postmenopausal women.

Estrogens act through binding to nuclear receptors in estrogen-responsive tissues. To date, two estrogen receptors have been identified. These vary in proportion from tissue to tissue.

Circulating estrogens modulate the pituitary secretion of the gonadotropins, luteinizing hormone (LH) and follicle stimulating hormone (FSH) through a negative feedback mechanism. Estrogens act to reduce the elevated levels of these gonadotropins seen in postmenopausal women.

Pharmacokinetics

A. Absorption

Conjugated estrogens are water-soluble and are well-absorbed through the skin, mucous membranes, and gastrointestinal tract after release from the drug formulation.

B. Distribution

The distribution of exogenous estrogens is similar to that of endogenous estrogens. Estrogens are widely distributed in the body and are generally found in higher concentration in the sex hormone target organs. Estrogens circulate in the blood largely bound to sex hormone-binding globulin (SHBG) and albumin.

C. Metabolism

Exogenous estrogens are metabolized in the same manner as endogenous estrogens. Circulating estrogens exist in a dynamic equilibrium of metabolic interconversions. These transformations take place mainly in the liver. Estradiol is converted reversibly to estrone, and both can be converted to estriol, which is the major urinary metabolite. Estrogens also undergo enterohepatic recirculation via sulfate and glucuronide conjugation in the liver, biliary secretion of conjugates into the intestine, and hydrolysis in the intestine followed by reabsorption. In postmenopausal women a significant proportion of the circulating estrogens exists as sulfate conjugates, especially estrone sulfate, which serves as a circulating reservoir for the formation of more active estrogens.

D. Excretion

Estradiol, estrone, and estriol are excreted in the urine, along with glucuronide and sulfate conjugates.

E. Special Populations

No pharmacokinetic studies were conducted in special populations, including patients with renal or hepatic impairment.

F. Drug Interactions

Data from a single-dose drug-drug interaction study involving oral conjugated estrogens and medroxyprogesterone acetate indicate that the pharmacokinetic dispositions of both drugs are not altered when the drugs are coadministered. No other clinical drug-drug interaction studies have been conducted with conjugated estrogens.

In vitro and in vivo studies have shown that estrogens are metabolized partially by cytochrome P450 3A4 (CYP3A4). Therefore, inducers or inhibitors of CYP3A4 may affect estrogen drug metabolism. Inducers of CYP3A4, such as St. John's Wort preparations (Hypericum perforatum), phenobarbital, carbamazepine, and rifampin, may reduce plasma concentrations of estrogens, possibly resulting in a decrease in therapeutic effects and/or changes in the uterine bleeding profile. Inhibitors of CYP3A4, such as erythromycin, clarithromycin, ketoconazole, itraconazole, ritonavir and grapefruit juice, may increase plasma concentrations of estrogens and may result in side effects.

CLINICAL STUDIES

Women's Health Initiative Studies

The Women's Health Initiative (WHI) enrolled approximately 27,000 predominantly healthy postmenopausal women in two substudies to assess the risks and benefits of either the use of daily oral conjugated estrogens (CE 0.625 mg) alone or in combination with medroxyprogesterone acetate (MPA 2.5 mg) compared to placebo in the prevention of certain chronic diseases. The primary endpoint was the incidence of coronary heart disease (CHD) (nonfatal myocardial infarction [MI], silent MI and CHD death), with invasive breast cancer as the primary adverse outcome. A "global index" included the earliest occurrence of CHD, invasive breast cancer, stroke, pulmonary embolism (PE), endometrial cancer (only in CE/MPA substudy), colorectal cancer, hip fracture, or death due to other causes. The study did not evaluate the effects of CE tablets or CE/MPA on menopausal symptoms.

The estrogen alone substudy was stopped early because an increased risk of stroke was observed, and it was deemed that no further information would be obtained regarding the risks and benefits of estrogen alone in predetermined primary endpoints. Results of the estrogen alone substudy, which included 10,739 women (average age of 63 years, range 50 to 79; 75.3 percent White, 15.1 percent Black, 6.1 percent Hispanic, 3.6 percent Other) after an average follow-up of 6.8 years, are presented in Table 1.

[See table 1 at top of next page]

For those outcomes included in the WHI "global index" that reached statistical significance, the absolute excess risk per 10,000 women-years in the group treated with CE alone were 12 more strokes while the absolute risk reduction per 10,000 women-years was 6 fewer hip fractures. The absolute excess risk of events included in the "global index" was a nonsignificant 2 events per 10,000 women-years. There was no difference between the groups in terms of all-cause mortality. (See **BOXED WARNINGS, WARNINGS,** and **PRECAUTIONS.**)

Final centrally adjudicated results for CHD events and centrally adjudicated results for invasive breast cancer incidence from the estrogen alone substudy, after an average follow-up of 7.1 years, reported no overall difference for primary CHD events (nonfatal MI, silent MI and CHD death) and invasive breast cancer incidence in women receiving CE alone compared with placebo (see Table 1).

Centrally adjudicated results for stroke events from the estrogen alone substudy, after an average follow-up of 7.1 years, reported no significant difference in distribution of stroke subtype or severity, including fatal strokes, in women receiving CE alone compared to placebo. Estrogen alone increased the risk of ischemic stroke, and this excess was present in all subgroups of women examined (see Table 1).

The estrogen plus progestin substudy was also stopped early. According to the predefined stopping rule, after an average follow-up of 5.2 years of treatment, the increased risk of breast cancer and cardiovascular events exceeded the specified benefits included in the "global index." The

TABLE 1. RELATIVE AND ABSOLUTE RISK SEEN IN THE ESTROGEN ALONE SUBSTUDY OF WHI

Event	Relative Risk CE vs. Placebo (95% nCI[a])	Placebo n = 5,429	CE n = 5,310
		Absolute Risk per 10,000 Women-Years	
CHD events[b]	0.95 (0.79-1.16)	56	53
Non-fatal MI[b]	*0.91 (0.73-1.14)*	*43*	*41*
CHD death[b]	*1.01 (0.71-1.43)*	*16*	*16*
Stroke[b]	1.37 (1.09-1.73)	33	45
Ischemic[b]	*1.55 (1.19-2.01)*	*25*	*38*
Deep vein thrombosis[b,d]	1.47 (1.06-2.06)	15	23
Pulmonary embolism[b]	1.37 (0.90-2.07)	10	14
Invasive breast cancer[b]	0.80 (0.62-1.04)	34	28
Colorectal cancer[c]	1.08 (0.75-1.55)	16	17
Hip fracture[c]	0.61 (0.41-0.91)	17	11
Vertebral fractures[c,d]	0.62 (0.42-0.93)	17	11
Total fractures[c,d]	0.70 (0.63-0.79)	195	139
Death due to other causes[c,e]	1.08 (0.88-1.32)	50	53
Overall mortality[c,d]	1.04 (0.88-1.22)	78	81
Global Index[c,f]	1.01 (0.91-1.12)	190	192

[a] Nominal confidence intervals unadjusted for multiple looks and multiple comparisons.
[b] Results are based on centrally adjudicated data for an average follow-up of 7.1 years.
[c] Results are based on an average follow-up of 6.8 years.
[d] Not included in Global Index.
[e] All deaths, except from breast or colorectal cancer, definite/probable CHD, PE or cerebrovascular disease.
[f] A subset of the events was combined in a "global index," defined as the earliest occurrence of CHD events, invasive breast cancer, stroke, pulmonary embolism, colorectal cancer, hip fracture, or death due to other causes.

TABLE 2. RELATIVE AND ABSOLUTE RISK SEEN IN THE ESTROGEN PLUS PROGESTIN SUBSTUDY OF WHI AT AN AVERAGE OF 5.6 YEARS[a]

Event	Relative Risk CE/MPA vs. Placebo (95% nCI[b])	Placebo n = 8,102	CE n = 8,506
		Absolute Risk per 10,000 Women-Years	
CHD events	1.24 (1.00-1.54)	33	39
Non-fatal MI	*1.28 (1.00-1.63)*	*25*	*31*
CHD death	*1.10 (0.70-1.75)*	*8*	*8*
All strokes	1.31 (1.02-1.68)	24	31
Ischemic stroke	1.44 (1.09-1.90)	18	26
Deep vein thrombosis	1.95 (1.43-2.67)	13	26
Pulmonary embolism	2.13 (1.45-3.11)	8	18
Invasive breast cancer[c]	1.24 (1.01-1.54)	33	41
Invasive colorectal cancer	0.56 (0.38-0.81)	16	9
Endometrial cancer	0.81 (0.48-1.36)	7	6
Cervical cancer	1.44 (0.47-4.42)	1	2
Hip fracture	0.67 (0.47-0.96)	16	11
Vertebral fractures	0.65 (0.46-0.92)	17	11
Lower arm/wrist fractures	0.71 (0.59-0.85)	62	44
Total fractures	0.76 (0.69-0.83)	199	152

[a] Results are based on centrally adjudicated data. Mortality data was not part of the adjudicated data; however, data at 5.2 years of follow-up showed no difference between the groups in terms of all-cause mortality (RR 0.98, 95 percent nCI 0.82-1.18).
[b] Nominal confidence intervals unadjusted for multiple looks and multiple comparisons.
[c] Includes metastatic and non-metastatic breast cancer, with the exception of in situ breast cancer.

absolute excess risk of events included in the "global index" was 19 per 10,000 women-years (relative risk [RR] 1.15, 95 percent nCI 1.03-1.28).

For those outcomes included in the WHI "global index" that reached statistical significance after 5.6 years of follow-up, the absolute excess risks per 10,000 women years in the group treated with CE/MPA were 6 more CHD events, 7 more strokes, 10 more PEs, and 8 more invasive breast cancers, while the absolute risk reductions per 10,000 women-years were 7 fewer colorectal cancers and 5 fewer hip fractures. (See **BOXED WARNINGS, WARNINGS,** and **PRECAUTIONS.**)

Results of the estrogen plus progestin substudy, which included 16,608 women (average age of 63 years, range 50 to 79; 83.9 percent White, 6.8 percent Black, 5.4 percent Hispanic, 3.9 percent Other) are presented in Table 2. These results reflect centrally adjudicated data after an average follow-up of 5.6 years.

[See table 2 above]

Women's Health Initiative Memory Study

The estrogen alone Women's Health Initiative Memory Study (WHIMS), a substudy of WHI, enrolled 2,947 predominantly healthy postmenopausal women 65 years of age and older (45 percent, age 65 to 69 years; 36 percent, 70 to 74 years; 19 percent, 75 years of age and older) to evaluate the effects of daily CE 0.625 mg on the incidence of probable dementia (primary outcome) compared with placebo.

After an average follow-up of 5.2 years, 28 women in the estrogen alone group (37 per 10,000 women-years) and 19 in the placebo group (25 per 10,000 women-years) were diagnosed with probable dementia. The relative risk of probable dementia in the estrogen alone group was 1.49 (95 percent CI 0.83-2.66) compared to placebo. It is unknown whether these findings apply to younger postmenopausal women. (See **BOXED WARNINGS, WARNINGS, Dementia** and **PRECAUTIONS, Geriatric Use.**)

The estrogen plus progestin WHIMS substudy enrolled 4,532 predominantly healthy postmenopausal women 65 years of age and older (47 percent, age 65 to 69 years; 35 percent, 70 to 74 years; 18 percent, 75 years of age and older) to evaluate the effects of daily CE/MPA 0.625 mg conjugated estrogens/2.5 mg medroxyprogesterone acetate on the incidence of probable dementia (primary outcome) compared with placebo. It is unknown whether these findings apply to younger postmenopausal women. (See **BOXED WARNINGS, WARNINGS, Dementia** and **PRECAUTIONS, Geriatric Use.**)

After an average follow-up of 4 years, 40 women in the estrogen plus progestin group (45 per 10,000 women-years) and 21 in the placebo group (22 per 10,000 women-years) were diagnosed with probable dementia. The relative risk of probable dementia in the hormone therapy group was 2.05 (95 percent CI 1.21-3.48) compared to placebo.

When data from the two populations were pooled as planned in the WHIMS protocol, the reported overall relative risk for probable dementia was 1.76 (95% CI 1.19-2.60). Differences between groups became apparent in the first year of treatment. It is unknown whether these findings apply to younger postmenopausal women. (See **BOXED WARNINGS, WARNINGS, Dementia** and **PRECAUTIONS, Geriatric Use.**)

INDICATIONS AND USAGE

Premarin Intravenous (conjugated estrogens, USP) for injection is indicated in the treatment of abnormal uterine bleeding due to hormonal imbalance in the absence of organic pathology.

Premarin Intravenous is indicated for short-term use only, to provide a rapid and temporary increase in estrogen levels.

CONTRAINDICATIONS

Premarin Intravenous therapy should not be used in individuals with any of the following conditions:
1. Undiagnosed abnormal genital bleeding.
2. Known, suspected, or history of cancer of the breast.
3. Known or suspected estrogen-dependent neoplasia.
4. Active deep vein thrombosis, pulmonary embolism or a history of these conditions.
5. Active or recent (within past year) arterial thromboembolic disease (for example, stroke, myocardial infarction).
6. Liver dysfunction or disease.
7. Known thrombophilic disorders (e.g., protein C, protein S, or antitrhombin deficiency).
8. Known hypersensitivity to any of the ingredients in Premarin Intravenous for injection.
9. Known or suspected pregnancy.

WARNINGS

See **BOXED WARNINGS**.

Premarin Intravenous for injection is indicated for short-term use. However, warnings, precautions and adverse reactions associated with oral Premarin treatment should be taken into account.

1. Cardiovascular disorders

An increased risk of stroke and deep vein thrombosis (DVT) has been reported with estrogen alone therapy.

An increased risk of stroke, DVT, pulmonary embolism, and myocardial infarction has been reported with estrogen plus progestin therapy.

Should any of these events occur or be suspected, estrogens should be discontinued immediately.

Risk factors for arterial vascular disease (for example, hypertension, diabetes mellitus, tobacco use, hypercholesterolemia, and obesity) and/or venous thromboembolism (for example, personal history or family history of VTE, obesity, and systemic lupus erythematosus) should be managed appropriately.

a. Stroke

In the Women's Health Initiative (WHI) estrogen alone substudy, a statistically significant increased risk of stroke was reported in women receiving daily conjugated estrogens (CE 0.625 mg) compared to placebo (44 versus 32 per 10,000 women-years). The increase in risk was demonstrated in year 1 and persisted. (See **CLINICAL STUDIES**.)

In the estrogen plus progestin substudy of WHI, a statistically significant increased risk of stroke was reported in women receiving daily CE 0.625 mg plus medroxyporogesterone acetate (MPA 2.5 mg) compared to placebo (31 versus 24 per 10,000 women-years). The increase in risk was demonstrated after the first year and persisted. (See **CLINICAL STUDIES**.)

b. Coronary heart disease

In the estrogen alone substudy of WHI, no overall effect on coronary heart disease (CHD) events (defined as nonfatal myocardial infarction [MI], silent MI, or CHD death) was reported in women receiving estrogen alone compared to placebo. (See **CLINICAL STUDIES**.)

In the estrogen plus progestin substudy of WHI, no statistically significant increase of CHD events was reported in women receiving CE/MPA compared to placebo (39 versus 33 per 10,000 women-years). An increase in relative risk was demonstrated in year 1, and a trend toward decreasing relative risk was reported in years 2 through 5.

In postmenopausal women with documented heart disease (n = 2,763, average age 66.7 years), in a controlled clinical trial of secondary prevention of cardiovascular disease (Heart and Estrogen/progestin Replacement Study; HERS), treatment with daily CE 0.625 mg/MPA 2.5 mg demonstrated no cardiovascular benefit. During an average follow-up of 4.1 years, treatment with CE/MPA did not reduce the overall rate of CHD events in postmenopausal women with established coronary heart disease. There were more CHD events in the CE/MPA-treated group than in the placebo group in year one, but not during the subsequent years. Two thousand three hundred and twenty-one (2,321) women from the original HERS trial agreed to participate in an open-label extension of HERS, HERS II. Average follow-up in HERS II was an additional 2.7 years, for a total of 6.8 years overall. Rates of CHD events were comparable among women in the CE/MPA group and the placebo group in the HERS, the HERS II, and overall.

c. Venous thromboembolism (VTE)

In the estrogen alone substudy of WHI, the risk of VTE (DVT and pulmonary embolism [PE]), was reported to be increased for women receiving daily CE compared to placebo (30 versus 22 per 10,000 women-years), although only the increased risk of DVT reached statistical significance (23 versus 15 per 10,000 women-years). The increase in VTE risk was demonstrated during the first 2 years. (See **CLINICAL STUDIES**.)

In the estrogen plus progestin substudy of WHI, a statistically significant 2-fold greater rate of VTE was reported in women receiving daily CE/MPA compared to placebo (35 versus 17 per 10,000 women-years). Statistically significant increases in risk for both DVT (26 versus 13 per 10,000 women-years) and PE (18 versus 8 per 10,000 women-years) were also demonstrated. The increase in VTE risk was demonstrated during the first year and persisted. (See **CLINICAL STUDIES**.)

2. Malignant neoplasms

a. Endometrial cancer

An increased risk of endometrial cancer has been reported with the use of unopposed estrogen therapy in women with a uterus. The reported endometrial cancer risk among unopposed estrogen users is about 2 to 12 times greater than in non-users, and appears dependent on duration of treatment and on estrogen dose. Most studies show no significant increased risk associated with use of estrogens for less than 1 year. The greatest risk appears associated with prolonged use, with increased risks of 15- to 24-fold for 5 to 10 years or more and this risk has been shown to persist for at least 8 to 15 years after estrogen therapy is discontinued.

b. Breast cancer

The most important randomized clinical trial providing information about this issue in estrogen alone users is the Women's Health Initiative (WHI) substudy of daily conjugated estrogens (CE 0.625 mg). In the estrogen alone substudy of WHI, after an average of 7.1 years of follow-up, daily CE 0.625 mg was not associated with an increased risk of invasive breast cancer (relative risk [RR] 0.80, 95 percent nominal confidence interval [nCI] 0.62-1.04). (See **CLINICAL STUDIES**.)

The most important randomized clinical trial providing information about this issue in estrogen plus progestin users is the Women's Health Initiative (WHI) substudy of daily CE 0.625 mg plus medroxyprogesterone acetate (MPA 2.5 mg). In the estrogen plus progestin substudy, after a mean follow-up of 5.6 years, the WHI substudy reported an increased risk of breast cancer in women who took daily CE/MPA. In this substudy, prior use of estrogen alone or estrogen plus progestin therapy was reported by 26 percent of the women. The relative risk of invasive breast cancer was 1.24 (95 percent nCI 1.01-1.54), and the absolute risk was 41 versus 33 cases per 10,000 women-years, for estrogen plus progestin compared with placebo, respectively. Among women who reported prior use of hormone therapy, the relative risk of invasive breast cancer was 1.86, and the absolute risk was 46 versus 25 cases per 10,000 women-years, for estrogen plus progestin compared with placebo. Among women who reported no prior use of hormone therapy, the relative risk of invasive breast cancer was 1.09, and the absolute risk was 40 versus 36 cases per 10,000 women-years for estrogen plus progestin compared with placebo. In the same substudy, invasive breast cancers were larger and diagnosed at a more advanced stage in the estrogen plus progestin group compared with the placebo group. Metastatic disease was rare, with no apparent difference between the two groups. Other prognostic factors, such as histologic subtype, grade and hormone receptor status did not differ between the groups. (See **CLINICAL STUDIES**.)

The results from observational studies are generally consistent with those of the WHI clinical trial. Observational studies have also reported an increased risk of breast cancer for estrogen plus progestin therapy, and a smaller increased risk for estrogen alone therapy, after several years of use. The risk increased with duration of use, and appeared to return to baseline over about 5 years after stopping treatment (only the observational studies have substantial data on risk after stopping). Observational studies also suggest that the risk of breast cancer was greater, and became apparent earlier, with estrogen plus progestin therapy as compared to estrogen alone therapy. However, these studies have not found significant variation in the risk of breast cancer among different estrogens or among different estrogen plus progestin combinations, doses, or routes of administration.

The use of estrogen alone and estrogen plus progestin has been reported to result in an increase in abnormal mammograms requiring further evaluation.

All women should receive yearly breast examinations by a healthcare provider and perform monthly breast self-examinations. In addition, mammography examinations should be scheduled based on patient age, risk factors, and prior mammogram results.

3. Dementia

In the estrogen alone Women's Health Initiative Memory Study (WHIMS), a substudy of WHI, a population of 2,947 hysterectomized women 65 to 79 years of age was randomized to daily conjugated estrogens (CE 0.625 mg) or placebo. In the estrogen plus progestin WHIMS substudy, a population of 4,532 postmenopausal women 65 to 79 years of age was randomized to daily CE 0.625 mg plus medroxyprogesterone acetate (MPA 2.5 mg) or placebo.

In the estrogen alone substudy, after an average follow-up of 5.2 years, 28 women in the estrogen alone group and 19 women in the placebo group were diagnosed with probable dementia. The relative risk of probable dementia for CE alone versus placebo was 1.49 (95 percent CI 0.83-2.66). The absolute risk of probable dementia for CE alone versus placebo was 37 versus 25 cases per 10,000 women-years.

In the estrogen plus progestin substudy, after an average follow-up of 4 years, 40 women in the estrogen plus progestin group and 21 women in the placebo group were diagnosed with probable dementia. The relative risk of probable dementia for estrogen plus progestin versus placebo was 2.05 (95 percent CI 1.21-3.48). The absolute risk of probable dementia for CE/MPA versus placebo was 45 versus 22 cases per 10,000 women-years.

When data from the two populations were pooled as planned in the WHIMS protocol, the reported overall relative risk for probable dementia was 1.76 (95 percent CI 1.19-2.60). Since both substudies were conducted in women 65 to 79 years of age, it is unknown whether these findings apply to younger postmenopausal women. (See **BOXED WARNINGS** and **PRECAUTIONS, Geriatric Use**.)

4. Gallbladder disease

A 2- to 4-fold increase in the risk of gallbladder disease requiring surgery in postmenopausal women receiving postmenopausal estrogens has been reported.

5. Hypercalcemia

Estrogen administration may lead to severe hypercalcemia in patients with breast cancer and bone metastases. If hypercalcemia occurs, use of the drug should be stopped and appropriate measures taken to reduce the serum calcium level.

6. Visual abnormalities

Retinal vascular thrombosis has been reported in patients receiving estrogens. Discontinue medication pending examination if there is sudden partial or complete loss of vision, or a sudden onset of proptosis, diplopia, or migraine. If examination reveals papilledema or retinal vascular lesions, estrogens should be permanently discontinued.

7. Angioedema

Exogenous estrogens may induce or exacerbate symptoms of angioedema, particularly in women with hereditary angioedema.

PRECAUTIONS

A. General

Premarin Intravenous for injection is indicated for short-term use. However, warnings, precautions and adverse reactions associated with oral Premarin treatment should be taken into account.

1. Addition of a progestin when a woman has not had a hysterectomy

Studies of the addition of a progestin for 10 or more days of a cycle of estrogen administration or daily with estrogen in a continuous regimen have reported a lowered incidence of endometrial hyperplasia than would be induced by estrogen treatment alone. Endometrial hyperplasia may be a precursor to endometrial cancer.

There are, however, possible risks which may be associated with the use of progestins with estrogens compared to estrogen-alone regimens. These include a possible increased risk of breast cancer, adverse effects on lipoprotein metabolism (lowering HDL, raising LDL) and impairment of glucose tolerance.

2. Elevated blood pressure

In a small number of case reports, substantial increases in blood pressure have been attributed to idiosyncratic reactions to estrogens. In a large, randomized, placebo-controlled clinical trial, a generalized effect of estrogen therapy on blood pressure was not seen. Blood pressure should be monitored at regular intervals with estrogen use.

3. Hypertriglyceridemia

In patients with pre-existing hypertriglyceridemia, estrogen therapy may be associated with elevations of plasma triglycerides leading to pancreatitis and other complications. Consider discontinuation of treatment if pancreatitis or other complications develop.

4. Impaired liver function and past history of cholestatic jaundice

Estrogens may be poorly metabolized in patients with impaired liver function. For patients with a history of cholestatic jaundice associated with past estrogen use or with pregnancy, caution should be exercised, and in the case of recurrence, medication should be discontinued.

5. Hypothyroidism

Estrogen administration leads to increased thyroid-binding globulin (TBG) levels. Patients with normal thyroid function can compensate for the increased TBG by making more thyroid hormone, thus maintaining free T_4 and T_3 serum concentrations in the normal range. Patients dependent on thyroid hormone replacement therapy who are also receiving estrogens may require increased doses of their thyroid replacement therapy. These patients should have their thyroid function monitored in order to maintain their free thyroid hormone levels in an acceptable range.

6. Fluid retention

Estrogens may cause some degree of fluid retention. Patients with conditions that might be influenced by this factor, such as a cardiac or renal dysfunction, warrant careful observation when estrogens are prescribed.

7. Hypocalcemia

Estrogens should be used with caution in individuals with severe hypocalcemia.

8. Ovarian cancer

The estrogen plus progestin substudy of WHI reported a non-statistically significant increased risk of ovarian cancer. After an average follow-up of 5.6 years, the relative risk for ovarian cancer for CE/MPA versus placebo was 1.58 (95 percent nCI 0.77-3.24). The absolute risk for CE/MPA versus placebo was 4.2 versus 2.7 cases per 10,000 women-years. In some epidemiologic studies, the use of estrogen-only products has been associated with an increased risk of ovarian cancer over multiple years of use. However, the duration of exposure associated with increased risk is not consistent across all epidemiologic studies and some report no association.

9. Exacerbation of endometriosis

Endometriosis may be exacerbated with administration of estrogen therapy.

A few cases of malignant transformation of residual endometrial implants have been reported in women treated post-hysterectomy with estrogen alone therapy. For patients known to have residual endometriosis post-hysterectomy, the addition of progestin should be considered.

10. Exacerbation of other conditions

Estrogen therapy may cause an exacerbation of asthma, diabetes mellitus, epilepsy, migraine, porphyria, systemic lupus erythematosus, and hepatic hemangiomas and should be used with caution in women with these conditions.

B. Patient Information

Physicians are advised to discuss the contents of the **PATIENT INFORMATION** leaflet with patients who are being treated with Premarin Intravenous.

C. Laboratory Tests

Estrogen administration should be guided by clinical response at the lowest dose, rather than laboratory monitoring.

D. Drug/Laboratory Test Interactions

1. Accelerated prothrombin time, partial thromboplastin time, and platelet aggregation time; increased platelet count; increased factors II, VII antigen, VIII antigen, VIII coagulant activity, IX, X, XII, VII-X complex, II-VII-X complex, and beta-thromboglobulin; decreased levels of anti-factor Xa and antithrombin III, decreased antithrombin III activity; increased levels of fibrinogen and fibrinogen activity; increased plasminogen antigen and activity.

2. Increased thyroid-binding globulin (TBG) leading to increased circulating total thyroid hormone, as measured by protein-bound iodine (PBI), T_4 levels (by column or by radioimmunoassay) or T_3 levels by radioimmunoassay. T_3 resin uptake is decreased, reflecting the elevated TBG. Free T_4 and free T_3 concentrations are unaltered. Patients on thyroid replacement therapy may require higher doses of thyroid hormone.

3. Other binding proteins may be elevated in serum, i.e., corticosteroid binding globulin (CBG), sex hormone-binding globulin (SHBG), leading to increased total circulating corticosteroids and sex steroids respectively. Free hormone concentrations may be decreased. Other plasma proteins may be increased (angiotensinogen/renin substrate, alpha-1-antitrypsin, ceruloplasmin).

4. Increased plasma HDL and HDL_2 subfraction concentrations, reduced LDL cholesterol concentration, increased triglyceride levels.

5. Impaired glucose tolerance.

E. Carcinogenesis, Mutagenesis, and Impairment of Fertility

(See **BOXED WARNINGS, WARNINGS,** and **PRECAUTIONS**.)

Long-term continuous administration of natural and synthetic estrogens in certain animal species increases the frequency of carcinomas of the breast, uterus, cervix, vagina, testis, and liver.

F. Pregnancy

Premarin Intravenous should not be used during pregnancy. (See **CONTRAINDICATIONS**.)

G. Nursing Mothers

Premarin Intravenous should not be used during lactation. Estrogen administration to nursing mothers has been shown to decrease the quantity and quality of breast milk. Detectable amounts of estrogens have been identified in the milk of mothers receiving the drug.

H. Pediatric Use

Estrogen therapy has been used for the induction of puberty in adolescents with some forms of pubertal delay. Safety and effectiveness in pediatric patients have not otherwise been established.

Large and repeated doses of estrogen over an extended time period have been shown to accelerate epiphyseal closure, which could result in short adult stature if treatment is initiated before the completion of physiologic puberty in normally developing children. If estrogen is administered to patients whose bone growth is not complete, periodic monitoring of bone maturation and effects on epiphyseal centers is recommended during estrogen administration. Estrogen treatment of prepubertal girls also induces premature breast development and vaginal cornification, and may induce vaginal bleeding. In boys, estrogen treatment may modify the normal pubertal process and induce gynecomastia. (See **INDICATIONS AND USAGE** and **DOSAGE AND ADMINISTRATION.**)

I. Geriatric Use

There have not been sufficient numbers of geriatric patients involved in studies utilizing Premarin to determine whether those over 65 years of age differ from younger subjects in their response to Premarin.

In the estrogen alone substudy of the Women's Health Initiative (WHI) study, 46 percent (n=4,943) were 65 years of age and older, while 7.1 percent (n=767) were 75 years of age and older. There was a higher relative risk (daily conjugated estrogens [CE 0.625 mg] versus placebo) of stroke in women less than 75 years of age compared to women 75 years of age and older.

In the estrogen alone Women's Health Initiative Memory Study (WHIMS), a substudy of WHI, a population of 2,947 hysterectomized women, 65 to 79 years of age, was randomized to daily CE 0.625 mg or placebo. After an average follow-up of 5.2 years, the relative risk (CE versus placebo) of probable dementia was 1.49 (95 percent CI 0.83-2.66). The absolute risk of developing probable dementia with estrogen alone was 37 versus 25 cases per 10,000 women-years compared with placebo.

Of the total number of subjects in the estrogen plus progestin substudy of the Women's Health Initiative study, 44 percent (n=7,320) were 65 years of age and older, while 6.6 percent (n=1,095) were 75 years and older. In women 75 years of age and older compared to women less than 74 years of age, there was a higher relative risk of nonfatal stroke and invasive breast cancer in the estrogen plus progestin group versus placebo. In women greater than 75, the increased risk of nonfatal stroke and invasive breast cancer observed in the estrogen plus progestin group compared to placebo was 75 versus 24 per 10,000 women-years and 52 versus 12 per 10,000 women-years, respectively.

In the estrogen plus progestin WHIMS substudy, a population of 4,532 postmenopausal women, 65 to 79 years of age, was randomized to daily CE 0.625 mg/MPA 2.5 mg or placebo. In the estrogen plus progestin group, after an average follow-up of 4 years, the relative risk (CE/MPA versus placebo) of probable dementia was 2.05 (95 percent CI 1.21-3.48). The absolute risk of developing probable dementia with CE/MPA was 45 versus 22 cases per 10,000 women-years compared with placebo.

Seventy-nine percent of the cases of probable dementia occurred in women that were older than 70 for the CE alone group, and 82 percent of the cases of probable dementia occurred in women who were older than 70 in the CE/MPA group. The most common classification of probable dementia in both the treatment groups and placebo groups was Alzheimer's disease.

When data from the two populations were pooled as planned in the WHIMS protocol, the reported overall relative risk for probable dementia was 1.76 (95 percent CI 1.19-2.60). Since both substudies were conducted in women 65 to 79 years of age, it is unknown whether these findings apply to younger postmenopausal women. (See **BOXED WARNINGS** and **WARNINGS, Dementia**.)

ADVERSE REACTIONS

See **BOXED WARNINGS, WARNINGS,** and **PRECAUTIONS.**

Premarin Intravenous for injection is indicated for short-term use. However, the warnings, precautions and adverse reactions associated with oral Premarin treatment should be taken into account.

The following adverse reactions have been reported with estrogen and/or progestin therapy.

1. Genitourinary system.
Abnormal uterine bleeding/spotting.
Dysmenorrhea/pelvic pain.
Increase in size of uterine leiomyomata.
Vaginitis, including vaginal candidiasis.
Change in amount of cervical secretion.
Change in cervical ectropion.
Ovarian cancer.
Endometrial hyperplasia.
Endometrial cancer.

2. Breasts.
Tenderness, enlargement, pain, discharge, galactorrhea.
Fibrocystic breast changes
Breast cancer.

3. Cardiovascular.
Deep and superficial venous thrombosis.
Pulmonary embolism.
Thrombophlebitis.
Myocardial infarction.
Stroke.
Increase in blood pressure.

4. Gastrointestinal.
Nausea, vomiting.
Abdominal cramps, bloating.
Cholestatic jaundice.
Increased incidence of gallbladder disease.
Pancreatitis.
Enlargement of hepatic hemangiomas.
Ischemic colitis.

5. Skin.
Chloasma or melasma that may persist when drug is discontinued.
Erythema multiforme.
Erythema nodosum.
Hemorrhagic eruption.
Loss of scalp hair.
Hirsutism.
Pruritus.
Rash.

6. Eyes.
Retinal vascular thrombosis.
Intolerance to contact lenses.

7. Central Nervous System.
Headache.
Migraine.
Dizziness.
Mental depression.
Exacerbation of chorea.
Nervousness.
Exacerbation of epilepsy.
Dementia.
Possible growth potentiation of benign meningioma.

8. Miscellaneous.
Increase or decrease in weight.
Glucose intolerance.
Aggravation of porphyria.
Edema.
Arthralgia.
Leg cramps.
Changes in libido.
Anaphylactoid/anaphylactic reactions.
Urticaria.
Angioedema.
Hypocalcemia (preexisting condition).
Injection site pain.
Injection site edema.
Phlebitis (injection site).
Exacerbation of asthma.
Increased triglycerides.

OVERDOSAGE

Overdosage of estrogen may cause nausea and vomiting, breast tenderness, abdominal pain, drowsiness/fatigue, and withdrawal bleeding may occur in females. Treatment of overdose consists of discontinuation of Premarin therapy with institution of appropriate symptomatic care.

DOSAGE AND ADMINISTRATION

For treatment of abnormal uterine bleeding due to hormonal imbalance in the absence of organic pathology:

One 25 mg injection, intravenously or intramuscularly. Intravenous use is preferred since more rapid response can be expected from this mode of administration. Repeat in 6 to 12 hours if necessary. The use of Premarin Intravenous for injection does not preclude the advisability of other appropriate measures.

One should adhere to the usual precautionary measures governing intravenous administration. Injection should be made SLOWLY to obviate the occurrence of flushes.

Infusion of Premarin Intravenous for injection with other agents is not generally recommended. In emergencies, however, when an infusion has already been started it may be expedient to make the injection into the tubing just distal to the infusion needle. If so used, compatibility of solutions must be considered.

COMPATIBILITY OF SOLUTIONS: Premarin Intravenous is compatible with normal saline, dextrose, and invert sugar solutions. **It is not compatible with protein hydrolysate, ascorbic acid, or any solution with an acid pH.**

DIRECTIONS FOR STORAGE AND RECONSTITUTION
STORAGE BEFORE RECONSTITUTION: Store package in refrigerator, 2° to 8°C (36° to 46°F).
TO RECONSTITUTE: Reconstitute Premarin® Intravenous with 5 mL of Sterile Water for Injection, USP. Introduce the sterile diluent slowly against the side of SECULE® vial and agitate gently. **Do not shake violently. Use immediately after reconstitution.**

HOW SUPPLIED

NDC 0046-0749-05–Each package provides one SECULE® vial containing 25 mg of conjugated estrogens, USP, for injection (also lactose 200 mg, sodium citrate 12.2 mg, and simethicone 0.2 mg). The pH is adjusted with sodium hydroxide or hydrochloric acid.

Premarin Intravenous (conjugated estrogens, USP) for injection is prepared by cryodesiccation.

SECULE®-Registered trademark to designate a vial containing an injectable preparation in dry form.

PATIENT INFORMATION

Premarin® Intravenous (conjugated estrogens, USP) for injection

Read this PATIENT INFORMATION which describes the benefit and major risks of your treatment, as well as how and when treatment should be used. This information does not take the place of talking to your healthcare provider about your medical condition or your treatment.

What is the most important information I should know about Premarin Intravenous (an estrogen mixture)?
- Estrogens increase the chance of getting cancer of the uterus.
  Report any unusual vaginal bleeding right away while you are taking Premarin. Vaginal bleeding after menopause may be a warning sign of cancer of the uterus (womb). Your healthcare provider should check any unusual vaginal bleeding to find out the cause.
- Do not use estrogens with or without progestins to prevent heart disease, heart attacks, strokes, or dementia.
  Using estrogens with or without progestins may increase your chance of getting heart attacks, strokes, breast cancer, and blood clots. Using estrogens, with or without progestins, may increase your chance of getting dementia, based on a study of women age 65 years or older. You and your healthcare provider should talk regularly about whether you still need treatment with estrogens.

What is Premarin Intravenous?
Premarin Intravenous is a medicine that contains a mixture of estrogen hormones.

Premarin Intravenous is used to:
- Treat certain types of abnormal uterine bleeding due to hormonal imbalance when your doctor has found no other cause of bleeding.

Who should not use Premarin Intravenous?
Premarin Intravenous should not be used if you:
- **Have unusual vaginal bleeding that has not been evaluated by your healthcare provider.**
- **Currently have or have had certain cancers.**
  Estrogens may increase the chance of getting certain types of cancers, including cancer of the breast or uterus. If you have or have had cancer, talk with your healthcare provider about whether you should use Premarin Intravenous.
- **Had a stroke or heart attack in the past year.**
- **Currently have or have had blood clots.**
- **Currently have or have had liver problems.**
- **Have been diagnosed with a bleeding disorder.**
- **Are allergic to Premarin Intravenous or any of its ingredients.**
  See the list of ingredients in Premarin Intravenous at the end of this leaflet.
- **Think you may be pregnant.**

Tell your healthcare provider:
- **If you are breast feeding.** The hormones in Premarin Intravenous can pass into your milk.
- **About all of your medical problems.** Your healthcare provider may need to check you more carefully if you have certain conditions, such as asthma (wheezing), epilepsy (seizures), migraine, endometriosis, lupus, problems with your heart, liver, thyroid, kidneys, or have high calcium levels in your blood.
- **About all the medicines you take,** including prescription and nonprescription medicines, vitamins, and herbal supplements. Some medicines may affect how Premarin Intravenous works.

What are the possible side effects of Premarin Intravenous?
Premarin Intravenous is for short-term use only. However, the risks associated with oral Premarin treatment should be taken into account.

Side effects are grouped by how serious they are and how often they happen when you are treated.

Serious but less common side effects include:
- Breast cancer
- Cancer of the uterus
- Stroke
- Heart attack
- Blood clots
- Dementia

- Gallbladder disease
- Ovarian cancer
- High blood pressure
- Liver problems
- High blood sugar
- Enlargement of benign tumors of the uterus ("fibroids")

Some of the warning signs of these serious side effects include:

- Breast lumps
- Unusual vaginal bleeding
- Dizziness and faintness
- Changes in speech
- Severe headaches
- Chest pain
- Shortness of breath
- Pains in your legs
- Changes in vision
- Vomiting
- Yellowing of the skin, eyes or nail beds

Call your healthcare provider right away if you get any of these warning signs, or any other unusual symptoms that concern you.

Less serious but common side effects include:

- Headache
- Breast pain
- Irregular vaginal bleeding or spotting
- Stomach/abdominal cramps, bloating
- Nausea and vomiting
- Hair loss
- Fluid retention
- Vaginal yeast infection

These are not all the possible side effects of Premarin. For more information, ask your healthcare provider or pharmacist.

What can I do to lower my chances of getting a serious side effect with Premarin Intravenous?

- If you have high blood pressure, high cholesterol (fat in the blood), diabetes, are overweight, or if you use tobacco, you may have higher chances for getting heart disease. Ask your healthcare provider for ways to lower your chances for getting heart disease.

General information about the safe and effective use of Premarin Intravenous

Medicines are sometimes prescribed for conditions that are not mentioned in patient information leaflets. Do not use Premarin Intravenous for conditions for which it was not prescribed. Do not give Premarin Intravenous to other people, even if they have the same symptoms you have. It may harm them. **Keep Premarin Intravenous out of the reach of children.**

This leaflet provides a summary of the most important information about Premarin Intravenous. If you would like more information, talk with your healthcare provider or pharmacist. You can ask for information about Premarin Intravenous that is written for health professionals. You can get more information by calling the toll free number 1-800-934-5556.

What are the ingredients in Premarin IV?

Premarin Intravenous for injection contains a mixture of conjugated estrogens, which are a mixture of sodium estrone sulfate and sodium equilin sulfate and other components including sodium sulfate conjugates: 17α-dihydroequilin, 17α-estradiol, and 17β-dihydroequilin. Premarin Intravenous for injection also contains lactose, sodium citrate, simethicone, and sodium hydroxide or hydrochloric acid in dry form. The reconstituted solution is suitable for intravenous or intramuscular injection.

Each Premarin Intravenous (conjugated estrogens, USP) for injection package provides 25 mg of conjugated estrogens, USP, in dry form for intravenous or intramuscular use.

This product's label may have been updated. For current package insert and further product information, please visit www.wyeth.com or call our medical communications department toll-free at 1-800-934-5556.

Wyeth®
Wyeth Pharmaceuticals Inc.
Philadelphia, PA 19101
W10411C013
ET01
Rev 06/10
TEAR HERE

PATIENT INFORMATION

Premarin®
Intravenous
(conjugated estrogens, USP) for injection
Rx only

Read this PATIENT INFORMATION which describes the benefit and major risks of your treatment, as well as how and when treatment should be used. This information does not take the place of talking to your healthcare provider about your medical condition or your treatment.

What is the most important information I should know about Premarin Intravenous (an estrogen mixture)?

- Estrogens increase the chance of getting cancer of the uterus.
  Report any unusual vaginal bleeding right away while you are taking Premarin. Vaginal bleeding after menopause may be a warning sign of cancer of the uterus (womb). Your healthcare provider should check any unusual vaginal bleeding to find out the cause.
- Do not use estrogens with or without progestins to prevent heart disease, heart attacks, strokes, or dementia.
  Using estrogens, with or without progestins, may increase your chance of getting heart attacks, strokes, breast cancer, and blood clots. Using estrogens, with or without progestins, may increase your chance of getting dementia, based on a study of women age 65 years or older. You and your healthcare provider should talk regularly about whether you still need treatment with estrogens.

What is Premarin Intravenous?
Premarin Intravenous is a medicine that contains a mixture of estrogen hormones.

Premarin Intravenous is used to:

- Treat certain types of abnormal uterine bleeding due to hormonal imbalance when your doctor has found no other cause of bleeding.

Who should not use Premarin Intravenous?
Premarin Intravenous should not be used if you:

- **Have unusual vaginal bleeding that has not been evaluated by your healthcare provider.**
- **Currently have or have had certain cancers.**
  Estrogens may increase the chance of getting certain types of cancers, including cancer of the breast or uterus. If you have or have had cancer, talk with your healthcare provider about whether you should use Premarin Intravenous.
- **Had a stroke or heart attack in the past year.**
- **Currently have or have had blood clots.**
- **Currently have or have had liver problems.**
- **Have been diagnosed with a bleeding disorder.**
- **Are allergic to Premarin Intravenous or any of its ingredients.**
  See the list of ingredients in Premarin Intravenous at the end of this leaflet.
- **Think you may be pregnant.**

Tell your healthcare provider:

- **If you are breast feeding.** The hormones in Premarin Intravenous can pass into your milk.
- **About all of your medical problems.** Your healthcare provider may need to check you more carefully if you have certain conditions, such as asthma (wheezing), epilepsy (seizures), migraine, endometriosis, lupus, problems with your heart, liver, thyroid, kidneys, or have high calcium levels in your blood.
- **About all the medicines you take,** including prescription and nonprescription medicines, vitamins, and herbal supplements. Some medicines may affect how Premarin Intravenous works.

What are the possible side effects of Premarin Intravenous?
Premarin Intravenous is for short-term use only. However, the risks associated with oral Premarin treatment should be taken into account.
Side effects are grouped by how serious they are and how often they happen when you are treated.
Serious but less common side effects include:

- Breast cancer
- Cancer of the uterus
- Stroke
- Heart attack
- Blood clots
- Dementia
- Gallbladder disease
- Ovarian cancer
- High blood pressure
- Liver problems
- High blood sugar
- Enlargement of benign tumors of the uterus ("fibroids")

Some of the warning signs of these serious side effects include:

- Breast lumps
- Unusual vaginal bleeding
- Dizziness and faintness
- Changes in speech
- Severe headaches
- Chest pain
- Shortness of breath
- Pains in your legs
- Changes in vision
- Vomiting
- Yellowing of the skin, eyes or nail beds

Call your healthcare provider right away if you get any of these warning signs, or any other unusual symptoms that concern you.
Less serious but common side effects include:

- Headache
- Breast pain
- Irregular vaginal bleeding or spotting
- Stomach/abdominal cramps, bloating
- Nausea and vomiting
- Hair loss
- Fluid retention
- Vaginal yeast infection

These are not all the possible side effects of Premarin. For more information, ask your healthcare provider or pharmacist.

What can I do to lower my chances of getting a serious side effect with Premarin Intravenous?

- If you have high blood pressure, high cholesterol (fat in the blood), diabetes, are overweight, or if you use tobacco, you may have higher chances for getting heart disease. Ask your healthcare provider for ways to lower your chances for getting heart disease.

General information about the safe and effective use of Premarin Intravenous

Medicines are sometimes prescribed for conditions that are not mentioned in patient information leaflets. Do not use Premarin Intravenous for conditions for which it was not prescribed. Do not give Premarin Intravenous to other people, even if they have the same symptoms you have. It may harm them. **Keep Premarin Intravenous out of the reach of children.**

This leaflet provides a summary of the most important information about Premarin Intravenous. If you would like more information, talk with your healthcare provider or pharmacist. You can ask for information about Premarin Intravenous that is written for health professionals. You can get more information by calling the toll free number 1-800-934-5556.

What are the ingredients in Premarin IV?
Premarin Intravenous for injection contains a mixture of conjugated estrogens, which are a mixture of sodium estrone sulfate and sodium equilin sulfate and other components including sodium sulfate conjugates: 17α-dihydroequilin, 17α-estradiol, and 17β-dihydroequilin. Premarin Intravenous for injection also contains lactose, sodium citrate, simethicone, and sodium hydroxide or hydrochloric acid in dry form. The reconstituted solution is suitable for intravenous or intramuscular injection.

Each Premarin Intravenous (conjugated estrogens, USP) for injection package provides 25 mg of conjugated estrogens, USP, in dry form for intravenous or intramuscular use.

This product's label may have been updated. For current package insert and further product information, please visit www.wyeth.com or call our medical communications department toll-free at 1-800-934-5556.

Wyeth®
Wyeth Pharmaceuticals Inc.
Philadelphia, PA 19101
W10411C013
ET01
Rev 06/10

PREMARIN®   ℞
[prĕ-mă-rĭn]
(conjugated estrogens tablets, USP)
Rx only

WARNINGS
ENDOMETRIAL CANCER
Adequate diagnostic measures, including endometrial sampling when indicated, should be undertaken to rule out malignancy in all cases of undiagnosed persistent or recurring abnormal vaginal bleeding. (See **WARNINGS, Malignant neoplasms, Endometrial cancer.**)
CARDIOVASCULAR AND OTHER RISKS
Estrogens with or without progestins should not be used for the prevention of cardiovascular disease or dementia. (See **CLINICAL STUDIES** and **WARNINGS, Cardiovascular disorders** and **Dementia.**)
The estrogen alone substudy of the Women's Health Initiative (WHI) reported increased risks of stroke and deep vein thrombosis (DVT) in postmenopausal women (50 to 79 years of age) during 6.8 years and 7.1 years, respectively, of treatment with daily oral conjugated estrogens (CE 0.625 mg), relative to placebo. (See **CLINICAL STUDIES** and **WARNINGS, Cardiovascular disorders.**)
The estrogen plus progestin substudy of WHI reported increased risks of myocardial infarction, stroke, invasive breast cancer, pulmonary emboli, and DVT in postmenopausal women (50 to 79 years of age) during 5.6

TABLE 1. PHARMACOKINETIC PARAMETERS FOR PREMARIN®

Pharmacokinetic Profile of Unconjugated Estrogens Following a Dose of 1×0.625 mg

PK Parameter Arithmetic Mean (%CV)	C_{max} (pg/mL)	t_{max} (h)	$t_{1/2}$ (h)	AUC (pg•h/mL)
Estrone	87 (33)	9.6 (33)	50.7 (35)	5557 (59)
Baseline-adjusted estrone	64 (42)	9.6 (33)	20.2 (40)	1723 (52)
Equilin	31 (38)	7.9 (32)	12.9 (112)	602 (54)

Pharmacokinetic Profile of Conjugated Estrogens Following a Dose of 1×0.625 mg

PK Parameter Arithmetic Mean (%CV)	C_{max} (ng/mL)	t_{max} (h)	$t_{1/2}$ (h)	AUC (ng•h/mL)
Total Estrone	2.7 (43)	6.9 (25)	26.7 (33)	75 (52)
Baseline-adjusted total estrone	2.5 (45)	6.9 (25)	14.8 (35)	46 (48)
Total Equilin	1.8 (56)	5.6 (45)	11.4 (31)	27 (56)

Pharmacokinetic Profile of Unconjugated Estrogens Following a Dose of 1×1.25 mg

PK Parameter Arithmetic Mean (%CV)	C_{max} (pg/mL)	t_{max} (h)	$t_{1/2}$ (h)	AUC (pg•h/mL)
Estrone	124 (30)	10.0 (32)	38.1 (37)	6332 (44)
Baseline-adjusted estrone	102 (35)	10.0 (32)	19.7 (48)	3159 (53)
Equilin	59 (43)	8.8 (36)	10.9 (47)	1182 (42)

Pharmacokinetic Profile of Conjugated Estrogens Following a Dose of 1×1.25 mg

PK Parameter Arithmetic Mean (%CV)	C_{max} (ng/mL)	t_{max} (h)	$t_{1/2}$ (h)	AUC (ng•h/mL)
Total Estrone	4.5 (39)	8.2 (58)	26.5 (40)	109 (46)
Baseline-adjusted total estrone	4.3 (41)	8.2 (58)	17.5 (41)	87 (44)
Total equilin	2.9 (42)	6.8 (49)	12.5 (34)	48 (51)

TABLE 2. SUMMARY TABULATION OF THE NUMBER OF HOT FLUSHES PER DAY– MEAN VALUES AND COMPARISONS BETWEEN THE ACTIVE TREATMENT GROUPS AND THE PLACEBO GROUP: PATIENTS WITH AT LEAST 7 MODERATE TO SEVERE FLUSHES PER DAY OR AT LEAST 50 PER WEEK AT BASELINE, LAST OBSERVATION CARRIED FORWARD (LOCF)

Treatment (No. of Patients) Time Period (week)	Baseline Mean ± SD	Observed Mean ± SD	Mean Change ± SD	p-Values vs. Placebo[a]
0.625 mg CE (n = 27)				
4	12.29 ± 3.89	1.95 ± 2.77	-10.34 ± 4.73	<0.001
12	12.29 ± 3.89	0.75 ± 1.82	-11.54 ± 4.62	<0.001
0.45 mg CE (n = 32)				
4	12.25 ± 5.04	5.04 ± 5.31	-7.21 ± 4.75	<0.001
12	12.25 ± 5.04	2.32 ± 3.32	-9.93 ± 4.64	<0.001
0.3 mg CE (n = 30)				
4	13.77 ± 4.78	4.65 ± 3.71	-9.12 ± 4.71	<0.001
12	13.77 ± 4.78	2.52 ± 3.23	-11.25 ± 4.60	<0.001
Placebo (n = 28)				
4	11.69 ± 3.87	7.89 ± 5.28	-3.80 ± 4.71	–
12	11.69 ± 3.87	5.71 ± 5.22	-5.98 ± 4.60	–

a: Based on analysis of covariance with treatment as factor and baseline as covariate.

years of treatment with daily CE 0.625 mg combined with medroxyprogesterone acetate (MPA 2.5 mg), relative to placebo. (See **CLINICAL STUDIES** and **WARNINGS, Cardiovascular disorders** and **Malignant neoplasms, Breast cancer**.)

The Women's Health Initiative Memory Study (WHIMS), a substudy of WHI, reported an increased risk of developing probable dementia in postmenopausal women 65 years of age or older during 5.2 years of treatment with daily CE 0.625 mg alone and during 4 years of treatment with daily CE 0.625 mg combined with MPA 2.5 mg, relative to placebo. It is unknown whether this finding applies to younger postmenopausal women. (See **CLINICAL STUDIES** and **WARNINGS, Dementia** and **PRECAUTIONS, Geriatric Use**.)

In the absence of comparable data, these risks should be assumed to be similar for other doses of CE and MPA and other combinations and dosage forms of estrogens and progestins. Because of these risks, estrogens with or without progestins should be prescribed at the lowest effective doses and for the shortest duration consistent with treatment goals and risks for the individual woman.

DESCRIPTION

PREMARIN® (conjugated estrogens tablets, USP) for oral administration contains a mixture of conjugated estrogens obtained exclusively from natural sources, occurring as the sodium salts of water-soluble estrogen sulfates blended to represent the average composition of material derived from pregnant mares' urine. It is a mixture of sodium estrone sulfate and sodium equilin sulfate. It contains as concomitant components, as sodium sulfate conjugates, 17α-dihydroequilin, 17α-estradiol, and 17β-dihydroequilin.

Tablets for oral administration are available in 0.3 mg, 0.45 mg, 0.625 mg, 0.9 mg, and 1.25 mg strengths of conjugated estrogens.

PREMARIN 0.3 mg, 0.45 mg, 0.625 mg, 0.9 mg, and 1.25 mg tablets also contain the following inactive ingredients: calcium phosphate tribasic, carnauba wax, hydroxypropyl cellulose, hypromellose, lactose monohydrate, magnesium stearate, microcrystalline cellulose, polyethylene glycol, powdered cellulose, sucrose, and titanium dioxide.

— 0.3 mg tablets also contain: D&C Yellow No. 10 and FD&C Blue No. 2.
— 0.45 mg tablets also contain: FD&C Blue No. 2.
— 0.625 mg tablets also contain: FD&C Blue No. 2 and FD&C Red No. 40.
— 0.9 mg tablets also contain: D&C Red No. 30 and D&C Red No. 7.
— 1.25 mg tablets also contain: black iron oxide, D&C Yellow No. 10 and FD&C Yellow No. 6.

PREMARIN tablets comply with USP Dissolution Test criteria as outlined below:

PREMARIN 1.25 mg tablets	USP Dissolution Test 4
PREMARIN 0.3 mg, 0.45 mg and 0.625 mg tablets	USP Dissolution Test 5
PREMARIN 0.9 mg tablets	USP Dissolution Test 6

CLINICAL PHARMACOLOGY

Endogenous estrogens are largely responsible for the development and maintenance of the female reproductive system and secondary sexual characteristics. Although circulating estrogens exist in a dynamic equilibrium of metabolic interconversions, estradiol is the principal intracellular human estrogen and is substantially more potent than its metabolites, estrone and estriol, at the receptor level.

The primary source of estrogen in normally cycling adult women is the ovarian follicle, which secretes 70 to 500 mcg of estradiol daily, depending on the phase of the menstrual cycle. After menopause, most endogenous estrogen is produced by conversion of androstenedione, secreted by the adrenal cortex, to estrone by peripheral tissues. Thus, estrone and the sulfate-conjugated form, estrone sulfate, are the most abundant circulating estrogens in postmenopausal women.

Estrogens act through binding to nuclear receptors in estrogen-responsive tissues. To date, two estrogen receptors have been identified. These vary in proportion from tissue to tissue.

Circulating estrogens modulate the pituitary secretion of the gonadotropins, luteinizing hormone (LH) and follicle stimulating hormone (FSH), through a negative feedback mechanism. Estrogens act to reduce the elevated levels of these gonadotropins seen in postmenopausal women.

Pharmacokinetics

A. Absorption

Conjugated estrogens are water-soluble and are well-absorbed from the gastrointestinal tract after release from the drug formulation. The PREMARIN tablet releases conjugated estrogens slowly over several hours. Table 1 summarizes the mean pharmacokinetic parameters for unconjugated and conjugated estrogens following administration of 1×0.625 mg and 1×1.25 mg tablets to healthy postmenopausal women.

The pharmacokinetics of PREMARIN 0.45 mg and 1.25 mg tablets were assessed following a single dose with a high-fat breakfast and with fasting administration. The C_{max} and AUC of estrogens were altered approximately 3-13%. The changes to C_{max} and AUC are not considered clinically meaningful.

[See table 1 above]

B. Distribution

The distribution of exogenous estrogens is similar to that of endogenous estrogens. Estrogens are widely distributed in the body and are generally found in higher concentration in the sex hormone target organs. Estrogens circulate in the blood largely bound to sex hormone binding globulin (SHBG) and albumin.

C. Metabolism

Exogenous estrogens are metabolized in the same manner as endogenous estrogens. Circulating estrogens exist in a dynamic equilibrium of metabolic interconversions. These transformations take place mainly in the liver. Estradiol is converted reversibly to estrone, and both can be converted to estriol, which is the major urinary metabolite. Estrogens also undergo enterohepatic recirculation via sulfate and glucuronide conjugation in the liver, biliary secretion of conjugates into the intestine, and hydrolysis in the intestine followed by reabsorption. In postmenopausal women a significant proportion of the circulating estrogens exists as sulfate conjugates, especially estrone sulfate, which serves as a circulating reservoir for the formation of more active estrogens.

D. Excretion

Estradiol, estrone, and estriol are excreted in the urine, along with glucuronide and sulfate conjugates.

E. Special Populations

No pharmacokinetic studies were conducted in special populations, including patients with renal or hepatic impairment.

F. Drug Interactions

Data from a single-dose drug-drug interaction study involving conjugated estrogens and medroxyprogesterone acetate indicate that the pharmacokinetic dispositions of both drugs are not altered when the drugs are coadministered. No other clinical drug-drug interaction studies have been conducted with conjugated estrogens.

In vitro and in vivo studies have shown that estrogens are metabolized partially by cytochrome P450 3A4 (CYP3A4). Therefore, inducers or inhibitors of CYP3A4 may affect estrogen drug metabolism. Inducers of CYP3A4, such as St. John's Wort preparations (Hypericum perforatum), phenobarbital, carbamazepine, and rifampin, may reduce plasma concentrations of estrogens, possibly resulting in a decrease in therapeutic effects and/or changes in the uterine bleeding profile. Inhibitors of CYP3A4, such as erythromycin, clarithromycin, ketoconazole, itraconazole, ritonavir and grapefruit juice, may increase plasma concentrations of estrogens and may result in side effects.

CLINICAL STUDIES

Effects on vasomotor symptoms

In the first year of the Health and Osteoporosis, Progestin and Estrogen (HOPE) Study, a total of 2,805 postmenopausal women (average age 53.3 ± 4.9 years) were randomly assigned to one of eight treatment groups, receiving either placebo or conjugated estrogens, with or without medroxyprogesterone acetate. Efficacy for vasomotor symptoms was assessed during the first 12 weeks of treatment in a subset of symptomatic women (n = 241) who had at least

seven moderate to severe hot flushes daily, or at least 50 moderate to severe hot flushes during the week before randomization. PREMARIN (0.3 mg, 0.45 mg, and 0.625 mg tablets) was shown to be statistically better than placebo at weeks 4 and 12 for relief of both the frequency and severity of moderate to severe vasomotor symptoms. Table 2 shows the adjusted mean number of hot flushes in the PREMARIN 0.3 mg, 0.45 mg, and 0.625 mg and placebo treatment groups over the initial 12-week period.
[See table 2 on previous page]

Effects on vulvar and vaginal atrophy
Results of vaginal maturation indexes at cycles 6 and 13 showed that the differences from placebo were statistically significant (p < 0.001) for all treatment groups (conjugated estrogens alone and conjugated estrogens/medroxyprogesterone acetate treatment groups).

Effects on bone mineral density
Health and Osteoporosis, Progestin and Estrogen (HOPE) Study
The HOPE study was a double-blind, randomized, placebo/active-drug-controlled, multicenter study of healthy postmenopausal women with an intact uterus. Subjects (mean age 53.3 ± 4.9 years) were 2.3 ± 0.9 years on average since menopause and took one 600-mg tablet of elemental calcium (Caltrate™) daily. Subjects were not given Vitamin D supplements. They were treated with PREMARIN 0.625 mg, 0.45 mg, 0.3 mg, or placebo. Prevention of bone loss was assessed by measurement of bone mineral density (BMD), primarily at the anteroposterior lumbar spine (L_2 to L_4). Secondarily, BMD measurements of the total body, femoral neck, and trochanter were also analyzed. Serum osteocalcin, urinary calcium, and N-telopeptide were used as bone turnover markers (BTM) at cycles 6, 13, 19, and 26.

Intent-to-treat subjects
All active treatment groups showed significant differences from placebo in each of the four BMD endpoints at cycles 6, 13, 19, and 26. The mean percent increases in the primary efficacy measure (L_2 to L_4 BMD) at the final on-therapy evaluation (cycle 26 for those who completed and the last available evaluation for those who discontinued early) were 2.46 percent with 0.625 mg, 2.26 percent with 0.45 mg, and 1.13 percent with 0.3 mg. The placebo group showed a mean percent decrease from baseline at the final evaluation of 2.45 percent. These results show that the lower dosages of PREMARIN were effective in increasing L_2 to L_4 BMD compared with placebo, and therefore support the efficacy of the lower doses.

The analysis for the other three BMD endpoints yielded mean percent changes from baseline in femoral trochanter that were generally larger than those seen for L_2 to L_4, and changes in femoral neck and total body that were generally smaller than those seen for L_2 to L_4. Significant differences between groups indicated that each of the PREMARIN treatments was more effective than placebo for all three of these additional BMD endpoints. With regard to femoral neck and total body, the active treatment groups all showed mean percent increases in BMD, while placebo treatment was accompanied by mean percent decreases. For femoral trochanter, each of the PREMARIN dose groups showed a mean percent increase that was significantly greater than the small increase seen in the placebo group. The percent changes from baseline to final evaluation are shown in Table 3.
[See table 3 above]

Figure 1 shows the cumulative percentage of subjects with changes from baseline equal to or greater than the value shown on the x-axis.

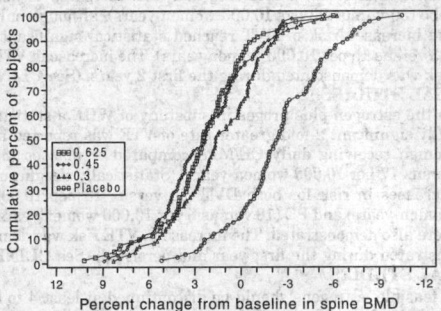

Figure 1. CUMULATIVE PERCENT OF SUBJECTS WITH CHANGES FROM BASELINE IN SPINE BMD OF GIVEN MAGNITUDE OR GREATER IN PREMARIN® AND PLACEBO GROUPS

The mean percent changes from baseline in L_2 to L_4 BMD for women who completed the bone density study are shown with standard error bars by treatment group in Figure 2. Significant differences between each of the PREMARIN dos-

TABLE 3. PERCENT CHANGE IN BONE MINERAL DENSITY: COMPARISON BETWEEN ACTIVE AND PLACEBO GROUPS IN THE INTENT-TO-TREAT POPULATION, LOCF

Region Evaluated Treatment Group[a]	No. of Subjects	Baseline (g/cm^2) Mean ± SD	Change from Baseline (%) Adjusted Mean ± SE	p-Value vs Placebo
L_2 to L_4 BMD				
0.625	83	1.17 ± 0.15	2.46 ± 0.37	<0.001
0.45	91	1.13 ± 0.15	2.26 ± 0.35	<0.001
0.3	87	1.14 ± 0.15	1.13 ± 0.36	<0.001
Placebo	85	1.14 ± 0.14	-2.45 ± 0.36	
Total Body BMD				
0.625	84	1.15 ± 0.08	0.68 ± 0.17	<0.001
0.45	91	1.14 ± 0.08	0.74 ± 0.16	<0.001
0.3	87	1.14 ± 0.07	0.40 ± 0.17	<0.001
Placebo	85	1.13 ± 0.08	-1.50 ± 0.17	
Femoral Neck BMD				
0.625	84	0.91 ± 0.14	1.82 ± 0.45	<0.001
0.45	91	0.89 ± 0.13	1.84 ± 0.44	<0.001
0.3	87	0.86 ± 0.11	0.62 ± 0.45	<0.001
Placebo	85	0.88 ± 0.14	-1.72 ± 0.45	
Femoral Trochanter BMD				
0.625	84	0.78 ± 0.13	3.82 ± 0.58	<0.001
0.45	91	0.76 ± 0.12	3.16 ± 0.56	0.003
0.3	87	0.75 ± 0.10	3.05 ± 0.57	0.005
Placebo	85	0.75 ± 0.12	0.81 ± 0.58	

a: Identified by dosage (mg) of PREMARIN or placebo.

TABLE 4. RELATIVE AND ABSOLUTE RISK SEEN IN THE ESTROGEN ALONE SUBSTUDY OF WHI

Event	Relative Risk CE vs. Placebo (95% nCI[a])	Placebo n = 5,429 Absolute Risk per 10,000 Women-Years	CE n = 5,310 Absolute Risk per 10,000 Women-Years
CHD events[b]	0.95 (0.79-1.16)	56	53
Non-fatal MI[b]	*0.91 (0.73-1.14)*	*43*	*40*
CHD death[b]	*1.01 (0.71-1.43)*	*16*	*16*
Stroke[b]	1.37 (1.09-1.73)	33	45
Ischemic[b]	*1.55 (1.19-2.01)*	*25*	*38*
Deep vein thrombosis[b,d]	1.47 (1.06-2.06)	15	23
Pulmonary embolism[b]	1.37 (0.90-2.07)	10	14
Invasive breast cancer[b]	0.80 (0.62-1.04)	34	28
Colorectal cancer[c]	1.08 (0.75-1.55)	16	17
Hip fracture[c]	0.61 (0.41-0.91)	17	11
Vertebral fractures[c,d]	0.62 (0.42-0.93)	17	11
Total fractures[c,d]	0.70 (0.63-0.79)	195	139
Death due to other causes[c,e]	1.08 (0.88-1.32)	50	53
Overall mortality[c,d]	1.04 (0.88-1.22)	78	81
Global Index[c,f]	1.01 (0.91-1.12)	190	192

[a] Nominal confidence intervals unadjusted for multiple looks and multiple comparisons.
[b] Results are based on centrally adjudicated data for an average follow-up of 7.1 years.
[c] Results are based on average follow-up of 6.8 years.
[d] Not included in Global Index.
[e] All deaths, except from breast or colorectal cancer, definite/probable CHD, PE or cerebrovascular disease.
[f] A subset of the events was combined in a "global index," defined as the earliest occurrence of CHD events, invasive breast cancer, stroke, pulmonary embolism, colorectal cancer, hip fracture, or death due to other causes.

age groups and placebo were found at cycles 6, 13, 19, and 26.

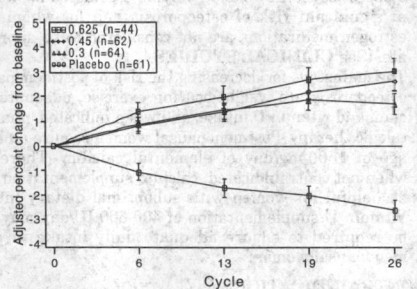

Figure 2. ADJUSTED MEAN (SE) PERCENT CHANGE FROM BASELINE AT EACH CYCLE IN SPINE BMD: SUBJECTS COMPLETING IN PREMARIN® GROUPS AND PLACEBO

The bone turnover markers serum osteocalcin and urinary N-telopeptide significantly decreased (p < 0.001) in all active-treatment groups at cycles 6, 13, 19, and 26 compared with the placebo group. Larger mean decreases from baseline were seen with the active groups than with the placebo group. Significant differences from placebo were seen less frequently in urine calcium.

Women's Health Initiative Studies
The Women's Health Initiative (WHI) enrolled approximately 27,000 predominantly healthy postmenopausal women in two substudies to assess the risks and benefits of either the use of daily oral conjugated estrogens (CE 0.625 mg) alone or in combination with medroxyprogesterone acetate (MPA 2.5 mg) compared to placebo in the prevention of certain chronic diseases. The primary endpoint was the incidence of coronary heart disease [CHD] (nonfatal myocardial infarction [MI], silent MI and CHD death), with invasive breast cancer as the primary adverse outcome. A "global index" included the earliest occurrence of CHD, invasive breast cancer, stroke, pulmonary embolism (PE), endometrial cancer (only in CE/MPA substudy), colorectal cancer, hip fracture, or death due to other causes. The study did not evaluate the effects of CE or CE/MPA on menopausal symptoms.

The estrogen alone substudy was stopped early because an increased risk of stroke was observed, and it was deemed that no further information would be obtained regarding the risks and benefits of estrogen alone in predetermined primary endpoints. Results of the estrogen alone substudy, which included 10,739 women (average age of 63 years, range 50 to 79; 75.3 percent White, 15.1 percent Black, 6.1 percent Hispanic, 3.6 percent Other) after an average follow-up of 6.8 years, are presented in Table 4.
[See table 4 above]

For those outcomes included in the WHI "global index" that reached statistical significance, the absolute excess risk per 10,000 women-years in the group treated with CE alone were 12 more strokes while the absolute risk reduction per 10,000 women-years was 6 fewer hip fractures. The absolute excess risk of events included in the "global index" was a nonsignificant 2 events per 10,000 women-years. There was no difference between the groups in terms of all-cause mortality. (See **BOXED WARNINGS**, **WARNINGS**, and **PRECAUTIONS**.)

Final centrally adjudicated results for CHD events and centrally adjudicated results for invasive breast cancer

TABLE 5. RELATIVE AND ABSOLUTE RISK SEEN IN THE ESTROGEN PLUS PROGESTIN SUBSTUDY OF WHI AT AN AVERAGE OF 5.6 YEARS[a]

Event	Relative Risk CE/MPA vs. Placebo (95% nCI[b])	Placebo n = 8,102	CE/MPA n = 8,506
		Absolute Risk per 10,000 Women-years	
CHD events	1.24 (1.00-1.54)	33	39
Non-fatal MI	*1.28 (1.00-1.63)*	*25*	*31*
CHD death	*1.10 (0.70-1.75)*	*8*	*8*
All strokes	1.31 (1.02-1.68)	24	31
Ischemic Stroke	*1.44 (1.09-1.90)*	*18*	*26*
Deep vein thrombosis	1.95 (1.43-2.67)	13	26
Pulmonary embolism	2.13 (1.45-3.11)	8	18
Invasive breast cancer[c]	1.24 (1.01-1.54)	33	41
Invasive colorectal cancer	0.56 (0.38-0.81)	16	9
Endometrial cancer	0.81 (0.48-1.36)	7	6
Cervical cancer	1.44 (0.47-4.42)	1	2
Hip fracture	0.67 (0.47-0.96)	16	11
Vertebral fractures	0.65 (0.46-0.92)	17	11
Lower arm/wrist fractures	0.71 (0.59-0.85)	62	44
Total fractures	0.76 (0.69-0.83)	199	152

[a] Results are based on centrally adjudicated data. Mortality data was not part of the adjudicated data; however, data at 5.2 years of follow-up showed no difference between the groups in terms of all-cause mortality (RR 0.98, 95 percent nCI 0.82-1.18).

[b] Nominal confidence intervals unadjusted for multiple looks and multiple comparisons.

[c] Includes metastatic and non-metastatic breast cancer, with the exception of in situ breast cancer.

incidence from the estrogen alone substudy, after an average follow-up of 7.1 years, reported no overall difference for primary CHD events (nonfatal MI, silent MI and CHD death) and invasive breast cancer incidence in women receiving CE alone compared with placebo (see Table 4).

Centrally adjudicated results for stroke events from the estrogen alone substudy, after an average follow-up of 7.1 years, reported no significant difference in distribution of stroke subtype or severity, including fatal strokes, in women receiving CE alone compared to placebo. Estrogen alone increased the risk of ischemic stroke, and this excess was present in all subgroups of women examined (see Table 4).

The estrogen plus progestin substudy was also stopped early. According to the predefined stopping rule, after an average follow-up of 5.2 years of treatment, the increased risk of breast cancer and cardiovascular events exceeded the specified benefits included in the "global index." The absolute excess risk of events included in the "global index" was 19 per 10,000 women-years (relative risk [RR] 1.15, 95 percent nCI 1.03-1.28).

For those outcomes included in the WHI "global index" that reached statistical significance after 5.6 years of follow-up, the absolute excess risks per 10,000 women years in the group treated with CE/MPA were 6 more CHD events, 7 more strokes, 10 more PEs, and 8 more invasive breast cancers, while the absolute risk reductions per 10,000 women-years were 7 fewer colorectal cancers and 5 fewer hip fractures. (See **BOXED WARNINGS, WARNINGS,** and **PRECAUTIONS.**)

Results of the estrogen plus progestin substudy, which included 16,608 women (average age of 63 years, range 50 to 79; 83.9 percent White, 6.8 percent Black, 5.4 percent Hispanic, 3.9 percent Other), are presented in Table 5. These results reflect centrally adjudicated data after an average follow-up of 5.6 years.

[See table 5 above]

Women's Health Initiative Memory Study

The estrogen alone Women's Health Initiative Memory Study (WHIMS), a substudy of WHI, enrolled 2,947 predominantly healthy postmenopausal women 65 years of age and older (45 percent, age 65 to 69 years; 36 percent, 70 to 74 years; 19 percent, 75 years of age and older) to evaluate the effects of daily CE 0.625 mg on the incidence of probable dementia (primary outcome) compared with placebo.

After an average follow-up of 5.2 years, 28 women in the estrogen alone group (37 per 10,000 women-years) and 19 in the placebo group (25 per 10,000 women-years) were diagnosed with probable dementia. The relative risk of probable dementia in the estrogen alone group was 1.49 (95 percent CI 0.83–2.66) compared to placebo. It is unknown whether these findings apply to younger postmenopausal women. (See **BOXED WARNINGS, WARNINGS, Dementia** and **PRECAUTIONS, Geriatric Use.**)

The estrogen plus progestin WHIMS substudy enrolled 4,532 predominantly healthy postmenopausal women 65 years of age and older (47 percent, age 65 to 69 years; 35 percent, 70 to 74 years; 18 percent, 75 years of age and older) to evaluate the effects of CE/MPA 0.625 mg conjugated estrogens/2.5 mg medroxyprogesterone acetate daily on the incidence of probable dementia (primary outcome) compared with placebo.

After an average follow-up of 4 years, 40 women in the estrogen plus progestin group (45 per 10,000 women-years) and 21 in the placebo group (22 per 10,000 women-years)

were diagnosed with probable dementia. The relative risk of probable dementia in the hormone therapy group was 2.05 (95 percent CI 1.21–3.48) compared to placebo. It is unknown whether these findings apply to younger postmenopausal women. (See **BOXED WARNINGS, WARNINGS, Dementia** and **PRECAUTIONS, Geriatric Use.**)

When data from the two populations were pooled as planned in the WHIMS protocol, the reported overall relative risk for probable dementia was 1.76 (95 percent CI 1.19-2.60). Differences between groups became apparent in the first year of treatment. It is unknown whether these findings apply to younger postmenopausal women. (See **BOXED WARNINGS, WARNINGS, Dementia** and **PRECAUTIONS, Geriatric Use.**)

INDICATIONS AND USAGE

PREMARIN therapy is indicated in the:

1. Treatment of moderate to severe vasomotor symptoms due to menopause.
2. Treatment of moderate to severe symptoms of vulvar and vaginal atrophy due to menopause. When prescribing solely for the treatment of symptoms of vulvar and vaginal atrophy, topical vaginal products should be considered.
3. Treatment of hypoestrogenism due to hypogonadism, castration or primary ovarian failure.
4. Treatment of breast cancer (for palliation only) in appropriately selected women and men with metastatic disease.
5. Treatment of advanced androgen-dependent carcinoma of the prostate (for palliation only).
6. Prevention of postmenopausal osteoporosis. When prescribing solely for the prevention of postmenopausal osteoporosis, therapy should only be considered for women at significant risk of osteoporosis and for whom non-estrogen medications are not considered to be appropriate. (See **CLINICAL STUDIES.**)

The mainstays for decreasing the risk of postmenopausal osteoporosis are weight-bearing exercise, adequate calcium and vitamin D intake, and when indicated, pharmacologic therapy. Postmenopausal women require an average of 1500 mg/day of elemental calcium. Therefore, when not contraindicated, calcium supplementation may be helpful for women with suboptimal dietary intake. Vitamin D supplementation of 400-800 IU/day may also be required to ensure adequate daily intake in postmenopausal women.

CONTRAINDICATIONS

PREMARIN therapy should not be used in individuals with any of the following conditions:

1. Undiagnosed abnormal genital bleeding.
2. Known, suspected, or history of cancer of the breast except in appropriately selected patients being treated for metastatic disease.
3. Known or suspected estrogen-dependent neoplasia.
4. Active deep vein thrombosis, pulmonary embolism or a history of these conditions.
5. Active or recent (within the past year) arterial thromboembolic disease (for example, stroke, myocardial infarction).
6. Liver dysfunction or disease.
7. Known thrombophilic disorders (e.g., protein C, protein S, or antithrombin deficiency).

8. Known hypersensitivity to any of the ingredients in PREMARIN.
9. Known or suspected pregnancy.

WARNINGS

See **BOXED WARNINGS.**

1. Cardiovascular disorders

An increased risk of stroke and deep vein thrombosis (DVT) has been reported with estrogen alone therapy.

An increased risk of stroke, DVT, pulmonary embolism, and myocardial infarction has been reported with estrogen plus progestin therapy.

Should any of these events occur or be suspected, estrogens with or without progestins should be discontinued immediately.

Risk factors for arterial vascular disease (for example, hypertension, diabetes mellitus, tobacco use, hypercholesterolemia, and obesity) and/or venous thromboembolism (for example, personal history or family history of VTE, obesity, and systemic lupus erythematosus) should be managed appropriately.

a. Stroke

In the Women's Health Initiative (WHI) estrogen alone substudy, a statistically significant increased risk of stroke was reported in women receiving daily conjugated estrogens (CE 0.625 mg) compared to placebo (44 versus 32 per 10,000 women-years). The increase in risk was demonstrated in year one and persisted. (See **CLINICAL STUDIES.**)

In the estrogen plus progestin substudy of WHI, a statistically significant increased risk of stroke was reported in women receiving daily CE 0.625 mg plus medroxyprogesterone acetate (MPA 2.5 mg) compared to placebo (31 versus 24 per 10,000 women-years). The increase in risk was demonstrated after the first year and persisted. (See **CLINICAL STUDIES.**)

b. Coronary heart disease

In the estrogen alone substudy of WHI, no overall effect on coronary heart disease (CHD) events (defined as nonfatal myocardial infarction [MI], silent MI, or CHD death) was reported in women receiving estrogen alone compared to placebo. (See **CLINICAL STUDIES.**)

In the estrogen plus progestin substudy of WHI, no statistically significant increase of CHD events was reported in women receiving CE/MPA compared to placebo (39 versus 33 per 10,000 women years). An increase in relative risk was demonstrated in year 1, and a trend toward decreasing relative risk was reported in years 2 through 5.

In postmenopausal women with documented heart disease (n = 2,763, average age 66.7 years), in a controlled clinical trial of secondary prevention of cardiovascular disease (Heart and Estrogen/progestin Replacement Study; HERS), treatment with daily CE 0.625 mg/MPA 2.5 mg demonstrated no cardiovascular benefit. During an average follow-up of 4.1 years, treatment with CE/MPA did not reduce the overall rate of CHD events in postmenopausal women with established coronary heart disease. There were more CHD events in the CE/MPA-treated group than in the placebo group in year one, but not during the subsequent years. Two thousand three hundred and twenty one (2,321) women from the original HERS trial agreed to participate in an open-label extension of HERS, HERS II. Average follow-up in HERS II was an additional 2.7 years, for a total of 6.8 years overall. Rates of CHD events were comparable among women in the CE/MPA group and the placebo group in the HERS, the HERS II, and overall.

c. Venous thromboembolism (VTE)

In the estrogen alone substudy of WHI, the risk of VTE (DVT and pulmonary embolism [PE]), was reported to be increased for women receiving daily CE compared to placebo (30 versus 22 per 10,000 women-years), although only the increased risk of DVT reached statistical significance (23 versus 15 per 10,000 women years). The increase in VTE risk was demonstrated during the first 2 years. (See **CLINICAL STUDIES.**)

In the estrogen plus progestin substudy of WHI, a statistically significant 2-fold greater rate of VTE was reported in women receiving daily CE/MPA compared to placebo (35 versus 17 per 10,000 women-years). Statistically significant increases in risk for both DVT (26 versus 13 per 10,000 women-years) and PE (18 versus 8 per 10,000 women-years) were also demonstrated. The increase in VTE risk was demonstrated during the first year and persisted. (See **CLINICAL STUDIES.**)

If feasible, estrogens should be discontinued at least 4 to 6 weeks before surgery of the type associated with an increased risk of thromboembolism, or during periods of prolonged immobilization.

2. Malignant neoplasms

a. Endometrial cancer

An increased risk of endometrial cancer has been reported with the use of unopposed estrogen therapy in women with a uterus. The reported endometrial cancer risk among unopposed estrogen users with an intact uterus is about 2 to 12 times greater than in non-users, and appears dependent on duration of treatment and on estrogen dose. Most studies show no significant increased risk associated with the use of estrogens for less than 1 year. The greatest risk appears associated with prolonged use, with increased risks of 15- to 24-fold for 5 to 10 years or more, and this risk has been shown to persist for at least 8 to 15 years after estrogen therapy is discontinued.

Clinical surveillance of all women using estrogen plus progestin therapy is important. Adequate diagnostic measures, including endometrial sampling when indicated, should be undertaken to rule out malignancy in all cases of undiagnosed persistent or recurring abnormal vaginal bleeding. There is no evidence that the use of natural estrogens results in a different endometrial risk profile than synthetic estrogens of equivalent estrogen dose. Adding a progestin to postmenopausal estrogen therapy has been shown to reduce the risk of endometrial hyperplasia, which may be a precursor to endometrial cancer.

b. Breast cancer

The most important randomized clinical trial providing information about this issue in estrogen alone users is the Women's Health Initiative (WHI) substudy of daily conjugated estrogens (CE 0.625 mg). In the estrogen alone substudy of WHI, after an average 7.1 years of follow-up, daily CE 0.625 mg was not associated with an increased risk of invasive breast cancer (relative risk [RR] 0.80, 95 percent nominal confidence interval [nCI] 0.62-1.04). (see CLINICAL STUDIES).

The most important randomized clinical trial providing information about this issue in estrogen plus progestin users is the Women's Health Initiative (WHI) substudy of daily CE 0.625 mg plus medroxyprogesterone acetate (MPA 2.5 mg). In the estrogen plus progestin substudy, after a mean follow-up of 5.6 years, the WHI substudy reported an increased risk of breast cancer in women who took daily CE/MPA. In this substudy, prior use of estrogen alone or estrogen plus progestin therapy was reported by 26 percent of the women. The relative risk of invasive breast cancer was 1.24 (95 percent nCI 1.01-1.54), and the absolute risk was 41 versus 33 cases per 10,000 women-years, for estrogen plus progestin compared with placebo, respectively. Among women who reported prior use of hormone therapy, the relative risk of invasive breast cancer was 1.86, and the absolute risk was 46 versus 25 cases per 10,000 women-years, for CE/MPA compared with placebo. Among women who reported no prior use of hormone therapy, the relative risk of invasive breast cancer was 1.09, and the absolute risk was 40 versus 36 cases per 10,000 women-years for estrogen plus progestin compared with placebo. In the same substudy, invasive breast cancers were larger and diagnosed at a more advanced stage in the CE/MPA group compared with the placebo group. Metastatic disease was rare, with no apparent difference between the two groups. Other prognostic factors, such as histologic subtype, grade and hormone receptor status did not differ between the groups. (See CLINICAL STUDIES.)

The results from observational studies are generally consistent with those of the WHI clinical trial. Observational studies have also reported an increased risk of breast cancer for estrogen plus progestin therapy, and a smaller increased risk for estrogen alone therapy, after several years of use. The risk increased with duration of use, and appeared to return to baseline over about 5 years after stopping treatment (only the observational studies have substantial data on risk after stopping). Observational studies also suggest that the risk of breast cancer was greater, and became apparent earlier, with estrogen plus progestin therapy as compared to estrogen alone therapy. However, these studies have not found significant variation in the risk of breast cancer among different estrogen plus progestin combinations, doses, or routes of administration.

The use of estrogen alone and estrogen plus progestin has been reported to result in an increase in abnormal mammograms requiring further evaluation.

All women should receive yearly breast examinations by a healthcare provider and perform monthly breast self-examinations. In addition, mammography examinations should be scheduled based on patient age, risk factors, and prior mammogram results.

3. Dementia

In the estrogen alone Women's Health Initiative Memory Study (WHIMS), a substudy of WHI, a population of 2,947 hysterectomized women 65 to 79 years of age was randomized to daily conjugated estrogens (CE 0.625 mg) or placebo. In the estrogen plus progestin WHIMS substudy, a population of 4,532 postmenopausal women 65 to 79 years of age was randomized to daily CE 0.625 mg plus medroxyprogesterone acetate (MPA 2.5 mg) or placebo.

In the estrogen alone substudy, after an average follow-up of 5.2 years, 28 women in the estrogen alone group and 19 women in the placebo group were diagnosed with probable dementia. The relative risk of probable dementia for CE alone versus placebo was 1.49 (95 percent CI 0.83-2.66). The absolute risk of probable dementia for CE alone versus pla-

cebo was 37 versus 25 cases per 10,000 women-years. (See CLINICAL STUDIES and PRECAUTIONS, Geriatric Use.)

In the estrogen plus progestin substudy, after an average follow-up of 4 years, 40 women in the CE/MPA group and 21 women in the placebo group were diagnosed with probable dementia. The relative risk of probable dementia for CE/MPA versus placebo was 2.05 (95 percent CI 1.21-3.48). The absolute risk of probable dementia for CE/MPA versus placebo was 45 versus 22 cases per 10,000 women-years. (See CLINICAL STUDIES and PRECAUTIONS, Geriatric Use.)

When data from the two populations were pooled as planned in the WHIMS protocol, the reported overall relative risk for probable dementia was 1.76 (95 percent CI 1.19-2.60). Since both substudies were conducted in women 65 to 79 years of age, it is unknown whether these findings apply to younger postmenopausal women. (See BOXED WARNINGS and PRECAUTIONS, Geriatric Use.)

4. Gallbladder Disease

A 2- to 4-fold increase in the risk of gallbladder disease requiring surgery in postmenopausal women receiving estrogens has been reported.

5. Hypercalcemia

Estrogen administration may lead to severe hypercalcemia in patients with breast cancer and bone metastases. If hypercalcemia occurs, use of the drug should be stopped and appropriate measures taken to reduce the serum calcium level.

6. Visual abnormalities

Retinal vascular thrombosis has been reported in patients receiving estrogens. Discontinue medication pending examination if there is sudden partial or complete loss of vision, or a sudden onset of proptosis, diplopia, or migraine. If examination reveals papilledema or retinal vascular lesions, estrogens should be permanently discontinued.

7. Angioedema

Exogenous estrogens may induce or exacerbate symptoms of angioedema, particularly in women with hereditary angioedema.

PRECAUTIONS

A. General

1. Addition of a progestin when a woman has not had a hysterectomy

Studies of the addition of a progestin for 10 or more days of a cycle of estrogen administration, or daily with estrogen in a continuous regimen, have reported a lowered incidence of endometrial hyperplasia than would be induced by estrogen treatment alone. Endometrial hyperplasia may be a precursor to endometrial cancer.

There are, however, possible risks that may be associated with the use of progestins with estrogens compared to estrogen-alone regimens. These include: a possible increased risk of breast cancer, adverse effects on lipoprotein metabolism (lowering HDL, raising LDL) and impairment of glucose tolerance.

2. Elevated blood pressure

In a small number of case reports, substantial increases in blood pressure have been attributed to idiosyncratic reactions to estrogens. In a large, randomized, placebo-controlled clinical trial, a generalized effect of estrogen therapy on blood pressure was not seen. Blood pressure should be monitored at regular intervals during estrogen use.

3. Hypertriglyceridemia

In patients with pre-existing hypertriglyceridemia, estrogen therapy may be associated with elevations of plasma triglycerides leading to pancreatitis and other complications. Consider discontinuation of treatment if pancreatitis or other complications develop.

In the HOPE study, the mean percent increase from baseline in serum triglycerides after one year of treatment with PREMARIN 0.625 mg, 0.45 mg, and 0.3 mg compared with placebo were 34.3, 30.2, 25.1, and 10.7, respectively. After two years of treatment, the mean percent changes were 47.6, 32.5, 19.0, and 5.5, respectively.

4. Impaired liver function and past history of cholestatic jaundice

Estrogens may be poorly metabolized in patients with impaired liver function. For patients with a history of cholestatic jaundice associated with past estrogen use or with pregnancy, caution should be exercised, and in the case of recurrence, medication should be discontinued.

5. Hypothyroidism

Estrogen administration leads to increased thyroid-binding globulin (TBG) levels. Patients with normal thyroid function can compensate for the increased TBG by making more thyroid hormone, thus maintaining free T_4 and T_3 serum concentrations in the normal range. Patients dependent on thyroid hormone replacement therapy who are also receiving estrogens may require increased doses of their thyroid replacement therapy. These patients should have their thyroid function monitored in order to maintain their free thyroid hormone levels in an acceptable range.

6. Fluid retention

Estrogens may cause some degree of fluid retention. Patients with conditions that might be influenced by this factor, such as cardiac or renal dysfunction, warrant careful observation when estrogens are prescribed.

7. Hypocalcemia

Estrogens should be used with caution in individuals with severe hypocalcemia.

8. Ovarian cancer

The estrogen plus progestin substudy of WHI reported a non-statistically significant increased risk of ovarian cancer. After an average follow-up of 5.6 years, the relative risk for ovarian cancer for CE/MPA versus placebo was 1.58 (95 percent nCI 0.77-3.24). The absolute risk for CE/MPA versus placebo was 4.2 versus 2.7 cases per 10,000 women-years. In some epidemiologic studies, the use of estrogens-progestin and estrogen-only products has been associated with an increased risk of ovarian cancer over multiple years of use. However, the duration of exposure associated with increased risk is not consistent across all epidemiologic studies and some report no association.

9. Exacerbation of endometriosis

Endometriosis may be exacerbated with administration of estrogen therapy.

A few cases of malignant transformation of residual endometrial implants have been reported in women treated post-hysterectomy with estrogen alone therapy. For patients known to have residual endometriosis post-hysterectomy, the addition of progestin should be considered.

10. Exacerbation of other conditions

Estrogen therapy may cause an exacerbation of asthma, diabetes mellitus, epilepsy, migraine, porphyria, systemic lupus erythematosus, and hepatic hemangiomas and should be used with caution in patients with these conditions.

B. Patient Information

Physicians are advised to discuss the contents of the PATIENT INFORMATION leaflet with patients for whom they prescribe PREMARIN.

C. Laboratory Tests

Serum follicle stimulating hormone and estradiol levels have not been shown to be useful in the management of moderate to severe vasomotor symptoms and moderate to severe symptoms of vulvar and vaginal atrophy.

Laboratory parameters may be useful in guiding dosage for the treatment of hypoestrogenism due to hypogonadism, castration and primary ovarian failure.

D. Drug/Laboratory Test Interactions

1. Accelerated prothrombin time, partial thromboplastin time, and platelet aggregation time; increased platelet count; increased factors II, VII antigen, VIII antigen, VIII coagulant activity, IX, X, XII, VII-X complex, II-VII-X complex, and beta-thromboglobulin; decreased levels of anti-factor Xa and antithrombin III, decreased antithrombin III activity; increased levels of fibrinogen and fibrinogen activity; increased plasminogen antigen and activity.

2. Increased thyroid binding globulin (TBG) levels leading to increased circulating total thyroid hormone levels as measured by protein-bound iodine (PBI), T_4 levels (by column or by radioimmunoassay) or T_3 levels by radioimmunoassay. T_3 resin uptake is decreased, reflecting the elevated TBG. Free T_4 and free T_3 concentrations are unaltered. Patients on thyroid replacement therapy may require higher doses of thyroid hormone.

3. Other binding proteins may be elevated in serum, i.e., corticosteroid binding globulin (CBG), sex hormone binding globulin (SHBG), leading to increased total circulating corticosteroids and sex steroids, respectively. Free hormone concentrations may be decreased. Other plasma proteins may be increased (angiotensinogen/renin substrate, alpha-1-antitrypsin, ceruloplasmin).

4. Increased plasma HDL and HDL_2 cholesterol subfraction concentrations, reduced LDL cholesterol concentrations, increased triglyceride levels.

5. Impaired glucose tolerance.

E. Carcinogenesis, Mutagenesis, Impairment of Fertility (See BOXED WARNINGS, WARNINGS, and PRECAUTIONS.)

Long-term continuous administration of natural and synthetic estrogens in certain animal species increases the frequency of carcinomas of the breast, uterus, cervix, vagina, testis, and liver.

F. Pregnancy

PREMARIN should not be used during pregnancy. (See CONTRAINDICATIONS.)

G. Nursing Mothers

PREMARIN should not be used during lactation. Estrogen administration to nursing mothers has been shown to decrease the quantity and quality of the milk. Detectable amounts of estrogens have been identified in the milk of mothers receiving this drug.

H. Pediatric Use

Estrogen therapy has been used for the induction of puberty in adolescents with some forms of pubertal delay. Safety and effectiveness in pediatric patients have not otherwise been established.

Large and repeated doses of estrogen over an extended time period have been shown to accelerate epiphyseal closure, which could result in short stature if treatment is initiated before the completion of physiologic puberty in normally developing children. If estrogen is administered to patients whose bone growth is not complete, periodic monitoring of bone maturation and effects on epiphyseal centers is recommended during estrogen administration.

Estrogen treatment of prepubertal girls also induces premature breast development and vaginal cornification, and may induce vaginal bleeding. In boys, estrogen treatment may modify the normal pubertal process and induce gynecomastia. (See **INDICATIONS AND USAGE** and **DOSAGE AND ADMINISTRATION**.)

I. Geriatric Use

With respect to efficacy in the approved indications, there have not been sufficient numbers of geriatric patients involved in studies utilizing PREMARIN to determine whether those over 65 years of age differ from younger subjects in their response to PREMARIN.

In the estrogen alone substudy of the Women's Health Initiative (WHI) study, 46 percent (n=4,943) were 65 years of age and older, while 7.1 percent (n=767) were 75 years of age and older. There was a higher relative risk (daily conjugated estrogens [CE 0.625 mg] versus placebo) of stroke in women less than 75 years of age compared to women 75 years and older.

In the estrogen alone Women's Health Initiative Memory Study (WHIMS), a substudy of WHI, a population of 2,947 hysterectomized women, 65 to 79 years of age, was randomized to daily CE 0.625 mg or placebo. After an average follow-up of 5.2 years, the relative risk (CE versus placebo) of probable dementia was 1.49 (95 percent CI 0.83-2.66). The absolute risk of developing probable dementia with estrogen alone was 37 versus 25 cases per 10,000 women-years compared with placebo.

Of the total number of subjects in the estrogen plus progestin substudy of the Women's Health Initiative study, 44 percent (n=7,320) were 65 years of age and older, while 6.6 percent (n=1,095) were 75 years and older. In women 75 years of age and older compared to women less than 74 years of age, there was a higher relative risk of nonfatal stroke and invasive breast cancer in the estrogen plus progestin group versus placebo. In women greater than 75, the increased risk of nonfatal stroke and invasive breast cancer observed in the estrogen plus progestin group compared to placebo was 75 versus 24 per 10,000 women-years and 52 versus 12 per 10,000 women years, respectively.

In the estrogen plus progestin substudy of WHIMS, a population of 4,532 postmenopausal women, 65 to 79 years of age, was randomized to daily CE 0.625 mg/MPA 2.5 mg or placebo. In the estrogen plus progestin group, after an average follow-up of 4 years, the relative risk (CE/MPA versus placebo) of probable dementia was 2.05 (95 percent CI 1.21-3.48). The absolute risk of developing probable dementia with CE/MPA was 45 versus 22 cases per 10,000 women-years compared with placebo.

Seventy-nine percent of the cases of probable dementia occurred in women that were older than 70 for the CE alone group, and 82 percent of the cases of probable dementia occurred in women who were older than 70 in the CE/MPA group. The most common classification of probable dementia in both the treatment groups and placebo groups was Alzheimer's disease.

When data from the two populations were pooled as planned in the WHIMS protocol, the reported overall relative risk for probable dementia was 1.76 (95 percent CI 1.19-2.60). Since both substudies were conducted in women 65 to 79 years of age, it is unknown whether these findings apply to younger postmenopausal women. (See **BOXED WARNINGS** and **WARNINGS, Dementia**.)

ADVERSE REACTIONS

See **BOXED WARNINGS**, **WARNINGS**, and **PRECAUTIONS**.

Because clinical trials are conducted under widely varying conditions, adverse reaction rates observed in the clinical trials of a drug cannot be directly compared to rates in the clinical trials of another drug and may not reflect the rates observed in practice.

During the first year of a 2-year clinical trial with 2,333 postmenopausal women between 40 and 65 years of age (88% Caucasian), 1,012 women were treated with conjugated estrogens and 332 were treated with placebo. Table 6 summarizes adverse events that occurred at a rate of ≥ 5%.

[See table 6 below]

The following additional adverse reactions have been reported with estrogen and/or progestin therapy:

1. Genitourinary system
Abnormal uterine bleeding/spotting
Dysmenorrhea/pelvic pain
Increase in size of uterine leiomyomata
Vaginitis, including vaginal candidiasis
Change in amount of cervical secretion
Change in cervical ectropion
Ovarian cancer
Endometrial hyperplasia
Endometrial cancer

2. Breasts
Tenderness, enlargement, pain, discharge, galactorrhea
Fibrocystic breast changes
Breast cancer

3. Cardiovascular
Deep and superficial venous thrombosis
Pulmonary embolism
Thrombophlebitis
Myocardial infarction
Stroke
Increase in blood pressure

4. Gastrointestinal
Nausea, vomiting
Abdominal cramps, bloating
Cholestatic jaundice
Increased incidence of gallbladder disease
Pancreatitis
Enlargement of hepatic hemangiomas
Ischemic colitis

5. Skin
Chloasma or melasma that may persist when drug is discontinued
Erythema multiforme
Erythema nodosum
Hemorrhagic eruption
Loss of scalp hair
Hirsutism
Pruritus, rash

6. Eyes
Retinal vascular thrombosis
Intolerance to contact lenses

7. Central Nervous System
Headache
Migraine
Dizziness
Mental depression
Exacerbation of chorea
Nervousness
Mood disturbances
Irritability
Exacerbation of epilepsy
Dementia
Possible growth potentiation of benign meningioma

8. Miscellaneous
Increase or decrease in weight
Glucose intolerance
Aggravation of porphyria
Edema
Arthralgias
Leg cramps
Changes in libido
Urticaria, angioedema, anaphylactoid/anaphylactic reactions
Hypocalcemia (preexisting condition)
Exacerbation of asthma
Increased triglycerides

OVERDOSAGE

Overdosage of estrogen may cause nausea and vomiting, breast tenderness, abdominal pain, drowsiness/fatigue and withdrawal bleeding may occur in females. Treatment of overdose consists of discontinuation of PREMARIN together with institution of appropriate symptomatic care.

DOSAGE AND ADMINISTRATION

When estrogen is prescribed for a postmenopausal woman with a uterus, progestin should also be initiated to reduce the risk of endometrial cancer. A woman without a uterus does not need progestin. Use of estrogen, alone or in combination with a progestin, should be with the lowest effective dose and for the shortest duration consistent with treatment goals and risks for the individual woman. Patients should be reevaluated periodically as clinically appropriate (for example at 3-month to 6-month intervals) to determine if treatment is still necessary (see **BOXED WARNINGS** and **WARNINGS**). For women with a uterus, adequate diagnostic measures, such as endometrial sampling, when indicated, should be undertaken to rule out malignancy in cases of undiagnosed persistent or recurring abnormal vaginal bleeding.

PREMARIN may be taken without regard to meals.

1. For treatment of moderate to severe vasomotor symptoms and/or moderate to severe symptoms of vulvar and vaginal atrophy due to menopause:
   When prescribing solely for the treatment of moderate to severe symptoms of vulvar and vaginal atrophy, topical vaginal products should be considered.
   Patients should be treated with the lowest effective dose. Generally, women should be started at 0.3 mg PREMARIN daily. Subsequent dosage adjustment may be made based upon the individual patient response. This dose should be periodically reassessed by the healthcare provider.

TABLE 6. NUMBER (%) OF PATIENTS REPORTING ≥5% TREATMENT EMERGENT ADVERSE EVENTS

Body System	—Conjugated Estrogens Treatment Group—			
Adverse event	0.625 mg	0.45 mg	0.3 mg	Placebo
	(n = 348)	(n = 338)	(n = 326)	(n = 332)
Any adverse event	323 (93%)	305 (90%)	292 (90%)	281 (85%)
Body as a Whole				
Abdominal pain	56 (16%)	50 (15%)	54 (17%)	37 (11%)
Accidental injury	21 (6%)	41 (12%)	20 (6%)	29 (9%)
Asthenia	25 (7%)	23 (7%)	25 (8%)	16 (5%)
Back pain	49 (14%)	43 (13%)	43 (13%)	39 (12%)
Flu syndrome	37 (11%)	38 (11%)	33 (10%)	35 (11%)
Headache	90 (26%)	109 (32%)	96 (29%)	93 (28%)
Infection	61 (18%)	75 (22%)	74 (23%)	74 (22%)
Pain	58 (17%)	61 (18%)	66 (20%)	61 (18%)
Digestive System				
Diarrhea	21 (6%)	25 (7%)	19 (6%)	21 (6%)
Dyspepsia	33 (9%)	32 (9%)	36 (11%)	46 (14%)
Flatulence	24 (7%)	23 (7%)	18 (6%)	9 (3%)
Nausea	32 (9%)	21 (6%)	21 (6%)	30 (9%)
Musculoskeletal System				
Arthralgia	47 (14%)	42 (12%)	22 (7%)	39 (12%)
Leg cramps	19 (5%)	23 (7%)	11 (3%)	7 (2%)
Myalgia	18 (5%)	18 (5%)	29 (9%)	25 (8%)
Nervous System				
Depression	25 (7%)	27 (8%)	17 (5%)	22 (7%)
Dizziness	19 (5%)	20 (6%)	12 (4%)	17 (5%)
Insomnia	21 (6%)	25 (7%)	24 (7%)	33 (10%)
Nervousness	12 (3%)	17 (5%)	6 (2%)	7 (2%)
Respiratory System				
Cough increased	13 (4%)	22 (7%)	14 (4%)	14 (4%)
Pharyngitis	35 (10%)	35 (10%)	40 (12%)	38 (11%)
Rhinitis	21 (6%)	30 (9%)	31 (10%)	42 (13%)
Sinusitis	22 (6%)	36 (11%)	24 (7%)	24 (7%)
Upper respiratory infection	42 (12%)	34 (10%)	28 (9%)	35 (11%)
Skin and Appendages				
Pruritus	14 (4%)	17 (5%)	16 (5%)	7 (2%)
Urogenital System				
Breast pain	38 (11%)	41 (12%)	24 (7%)	29 (9%)
Leukorrhea	18 (5%)	22 (7%)	13 (4%)	9 (3%)
Vaginal hemorrhage	47 (14%)	14 (4%)	7 (2%)	0
Vaginal moniliasis	20 (6%)	18 (5%)	17 (5%)	6 (2%)
Vaginitis	24 (7%)	20 (6%)	16 (5%)	4 (1%)

PREMARIN therapy may be given continuously, with no interruption in therapy, or in cyclical regimens (regimens such as 25 days on drug followed by five days off drug), as is medically appropriate on an individualized basis.

2. For prevention of postmenopausal osteoporosis:
When prescribing solely for the prevention of postmenopausal osteoporosis, therapy should be considered only for women at significant risk of osteoporosis and for whom non-estrogen medications are not considered to be appropriate. Patients should be treated with the lowest effective dose. Generally, women should be started at 0.3 mg PREMARIN daily. Subsequent dosage adjustment may be made based upon the individual clinical and bone mineral density responses. This dose should be periodically reassessed by the healthcare provider.
PREMARIN therapy may be given continuously, with no interruption in therapy, or in cyclical regimens (regimens such as 25 days on drug followed by five days off drug), as is medically appropriate on an individualized basis.

3. For treatment of female hypoestrogenism due to hypogonadism, castration, or primary ovarian failure:
Female hypogonadism—0.3 mg or 0.625 mg daily, administered cyclically (e.g., three weeks on and one week off). Doses are adjusted depending on the severity of symptoms and responsiveness of the endometrium.
In clinical studies of delayed puberty due to female hypogonadism, breast development was induced by doses as low as 0.15 mg. The dosage may be gradually titrated upward at 6-to-12 month intervals as needed to achieve appropriate bone age advancement and eventual epiphyseal closure. Clinical studies suggest that doses of 0.15 mg, 0.3 mg, and 0.6 mg are associated with mean ratios of bone age advancement to chronological age progression ($\Delta BA/\Delta CA$) of 1.1, 1.5, and 2.1, respectively. (PREMARIN in the dose strength of 0.15 mg is not available commercially). Available data suggest that chronic dosing with 0.625 mg is sufficient to induce artificial cyclic menses with sequential progestin treatment and to maintain bone mineral density after skeletal maturity is achieved. Female castration or primary ovarian failure—1.25 mg daily, cyclically. Adjust dosage, upward or downward, according to severity of symptoms and response of the patient. For maintenance, adjust dosage to lowest level that will provide effective control.

4. For treatment of breast cancer, for palliation only, in appropriately selected women and men with metastatic disease:
Suggested dosage is 10 mg three times daily, for a period of at least three months.

5. For treatment of advanced androgen-dependent carcinoma of the prostate, for palliation only:
1.25 mg to 2 × 1.25 mg three times daily. The effectiveness of therapy can be judged by phosphatase determinations as well as by symptomatic improvement of the patient.

HOW SUPPLIED

PREMARIN® (conjugated estrogens tablets, USP)
— Each oval green tablet contains 0.3 mg, in bottles of 100 (NDC 0046-1100-81) and 1,000 (NDC 0046-1100-91).
— Each oval blue tablet contains 0.45 mg, in bottles of 100 (NDC 0046-1101-81).
— Each oval maroon tablet contains 0.625 mg, in bottles of 100 (NDC 0046-1102-81) and 1,000 (NDC 0046-1102-91).
— Each oval white tablet contains 0.9 mg, in bottles of 100 (NDC 0046-1103-81).
— Each oval yellow tablet contains 1.25 mg, in bottles of 100 (NDC 0046-1104-81) and 1,000 (NDC 0046-1104-91).
The appearance of these tablets is a trademark of Wyeth Pharmaceuticals.
Store at 20°-25°C (68°-77°F); excursions permitted to 15°-30°C (59°-86°F) [see USP Controlled Room Temperature].
Dispense in a well-closed container, as defined in the USP.

PATIENT INFORMATION

PREMARIN®
(conjugated estrogens tablets, USP)
Read this PATIENT INFORMATION before you start taking PREMARIN and read what you get each time you refill your PREMARIN prescription. There may be new information. This information does not take the place of talking to your healthcare provider about your medical condition or your treatment.

What is the most important information I should know about PREMARIN (an estrogen mixture)?
• Estrogens increase the chance of getting cancer of the uterus.
Report any unusual vaginal bleeding right away while you are taking PREMARIN. Vaginal bleeding after menopause may be a warning sign of cancer of the uterus (womb). Your healthcare provider should check any unusual vaginal bleeding to find out the cause.

• Do not use estrogens with or without progestins to prevent heart disease, heart attacks, strokes, or dementia.
Using estrogens, with or without progestins, may increase your chance of getting heart attacks, strokes, breast cancer, and blood clots. Using estrogens, with or without progestins, may increase your chance of getting dementia, based on a study of women age 65 years or older. You and your healthcare provider should talk regularly about whether you still need treatment with PREMARIN.

What is PREMARIN?
PREMARIN is a medicine that contains a mixture of estrogen hormones.
PREMARIN is used after menopause to:
• **Reduce moderate to severe hot flashes.** Estrogens are hormones made by a woman's ovaries. The ovaries normally stop making estrogens when a woman is between 45 and 55 years old. This drop in body estrogen levels causes the "change of life" or menopause (the end of monthly menstrual periods). Sometimes both ovaries are removed during an operation before natural menopause takes place. The sudden drop in estrogen levels causes "surgical menopause."
When the estrogen levels begin dropping, some women get very uncomfortable symptoms, such as feelings of warmth in the face, neck, and chest, or sudden strong feelings of heat and sweating ("hot flashes" or "hot flushes"). In some women the symptoms are mild, and they will not need to take estrogens. In other women, symptoms can be more severe. You and your healthcare provider should talk regularly about whether you still need treatment with PREMARIN.
• **Treat moderate to severe dryness, itching, and burning, in and around the vagina.** You and your healthcare provider should talk regularly about whether you still need treatment with PREMARIN to control these problems. If you use PREMARIN only to treat your dryness, itching, and burning in and around your vagina, talk with your healthcare provider about whether a topical vaginal product would be better for you.
• **Help reduce your chances of getting osteoporosis (thin weak bones).** Osteoporosis from menopause is a thinning of the bones that makes them weaker and easier to break. If you use PREMARIN only to prevent osteoporosis due to menopause, talk with your healthcare provider about whether a different treatment or medicine without estrogens might be better for you. You and your healthcare provider should talk regularly about whether you should continue with PREMARIN.
Weight-bearing exercise, like walking or running, and taking calcium and vitamin D supplements may also lower your chances for getting postmenopausal osteoporosis. It is important to talk about exercise and supplements with your healthcare provider before starting them.
PREMARIN is also used to:
• **Treat certain conditions in women before menopause if their ovaries do not make enough estrogen naturally.**
• **Ease symptoms of certain cancers that have spread through the body, in men and women.**
Who should not take PREMARIN?
Do not start taking PREMARIN if you:
• **Have unusual vaginal bleeding.**
• **Currently have or have had certain cancers.** Estrogens may increase the chance of getting certain types of cancers, including cancer of the breast or uterus. If you have or have had cancer, talk with your healthcare provider about whether you should take PREMARIN.
• **Had a stroke or heart attack in the past year.**
• **Currently have or have had blood clots.**
• **Currently have or have had liver problems.**
• **Have been diagnosed with a bleeding disorder.**
• **Are allergic to PREMARIN tablets or any of its ingredients.** See the list of ingredients in PREMARIN at the end of this leaflet.
• **Think you may be pregnant.**
Tell your healthcare provider:
• **If you are breast feeding.** The hormones in PREMARIN can pass into your milk.
• **About all of your medical problems.** Your healthcare provider may need to check you more carefully if you have certain conditions, such as asthma (wheezing), epilepsy (seizures), migraine, endometriosis, lupus, problems with your heart, liver, thyroid, kidneys, or have high calcium levels in your blood.
• **About all the medicines you take,** including prescription and nonprescription medicines, vitamins, and herbal supplements. Some medicines may affect how PREMARIN works. PREMARIN may also affect how your other medicines work.
• **If you are going to have surgery or will be on bedrest.** You may need to stop taking estrogens.

How should I take PREMARIN?
• Take one PREMARIN tablet at the same time each day.
• If you miss a dose, take it as soon as possible. If it is almost time for your next dose, skip the missed dose and go back to your normal schedule. Do not take 2 doses at the same time.
• Estrogens should be used at the lowest dose possible for your treatment only as long as needed. You and your healthcare provider should talk regularly (for example, every 3 to 6 months) about the dose you are taking and whether you still need treatment with PREMARIN.
What are the possible side effects of PREMARIN?
Side effects are grouped by how serious they are and how often they happen when you are treated.
Serious but less common side effects include:
• Breast cancer
• Cancer of the uterus
• Stroke
• Heart attack
• Blood clots
• Dementia
• Gallbladder disease
• Ovarian cancer
• High blood pressure
• Liver problems
• High blood sugar
• Enlargement of benign tumors of the uterus ("fibroids")
Some of the warning signs of these serious side effects include:
• Breast lumps
• Unusual vaginal bleeding
• Dizziness and faintness
• Changes in speech
• Severe headaches
• Chest pain
• Shortness of breath
• Pains in your legs
• Changes in vision
• Vomiting
• Yellowing of the skin, eyes or nail beds
Call your healthcare provider right away if you get any of these warning signs, or any other unusual symptoms that concern you.
Less serious but common side effects include:
• Headache
• Breast pain
• Irregular vaginal bleeding or spotting
• Stomach/abdominal cramps, bloating
• Nausea and vomiting
• Hair loss
• Fluid retention
• Vaginal yeast infection
These are not all the possible side effects of PREMARIN. For more information, ask your healthcare provider or pharmacist.
What can I do to lower my chances of getting a serious side effect with PREMARIN?
• Talk with your healthcare provider regularly about whether you should continue taking PREMARIN.
• If you have a uterus, talk to your healthcare provider about whether the addition of a progestin is right for you. The addition of a progestin is generally recommended for women with a uterus to reduce the chance of getting cancer of the uterus.
• See your healthcare provider right away if you get vaginal bleeding while taking PREMARIN.
• Have a breast exam and mammogram (breast X-ray) every year unless your healthcare provider tells you something else. If members of your family have had breast cancer or if you have ever had breast lumps or an abnormal mammogram, you may need to have breast exams more often.
• If you have high blood pressure, high cholesterol (fat in the blood), diabetes, are overweight, or if you use tobacco, you may have higher chances for getting heart disease. Ask your healthcare provider for ways to lower your chances for getting heart disease.
General information about the safe and effective use of PREMARIN
Medicines are sometimes prescribed for conditions that are not mentioned in patient information leaflets. Do not take PREMARIN for conditions for which it was not prescribed. Do not give PREMARIN to other people, even if they have the same symptoms you have. It may harm them.
Keep PREMARIN out of the reach of children.
This leaflet provides a summary of the most important information about PREMARIN. If you would like more information, talk with your healthcare provider or pharmacist. You can ask for information about PREMARIN that is written for health professionals. You can get more information by calling the toll free number 800-934-5556.
What are the ingredients in PREMARIN?
PREMARIN contains a mixture of conjugated estrogens, which are a mixture of sodium estrone sulfate and sodium

equilin sulfate and other components including sodium sulfate conjugates, 17 α-dihydroequilin, 17 α-estradiol, and 17 β-dihydroequilin.

PREMARIN 0.3 mg, 0.45 mg, 0.625 mg, 0.9 mg, and 1.25 mg tablets also contain the following inactive ingredients: calcium phosphate tribasic, carnauba wax, hydroxypropyl cellulose, hypromellose, lactose monohydrate, magnesium stearate, microcrystalline cellulose, polyethylene glycol, powdered cellulose, sucrose and titanium dioxide.

The tablets come in different strengths and each strength tablet is a different color. The color ingredients are:
— 0.3 mg tablet (green color): D&C Yellow No. 10 and FD&C Blue No. 2.
— 0.45 mg tablet (blue color): FD&C Blue No. 2.
— 0.625 mg tablet (maroon color): FD&C Blue No. 2 and FD&C Red No. 40.
— 0.9 mg tablet (white color): D&C Red No. 30 and D&C Red No. 7.
— 1.25 mg tablet (yellow color): black iron oxide, D&C Yellow No. 10, and FD&C Yellow No. 6.

The appearance of these tablets is a trademark of Wyeth Pharmaceuticals.

Store at Controlled Room Temperature 20°–25°C (68°–77°F).

This product's label may have been updated. For current package insert and further product information, please visit www.wyeth.com or call our medical communications department toll-free at 1-800-934-5556.

Wyeth®
Wyeth Pharmaceuticals Inc.
Philadelphia, PA 19101
W10405C027
ET01
Rev 05/10
Shown in Product Identification Guide, page 321

PREMARIN VAGINAL CREAM   ℞
[prĕ-mă-rĭn]
(conjugated estrogens)
Vaginal Cream

HIGHLIGHTS OF PRESCRIBING INFORMATION
These highlights do not include all the information needed to use PREMARIN Vaginal Cream safely and effectively. See full prescribing information for PREMARIN Vaginal Cream. PREMARIN (conjugated estrogens) Vaginal Cream.
Initial U.S. Approval: 1946

> **WARNING: CARDIOVASCULAR DISORDERS, ENDO-METRIAL CANCER, BREAST CANCER and PROBABLE DEMENTIA**
> *See full prescribing information for complete boxed warning.*
> **Estrogen-Alone Therapy**
> - **There is an increased risk of endometrial cancer in a woman with a uterus who uses unopposed estrogens (5.3)**
> - **Estrogen-alone therapy should not be used for the prevention of cardiovascular disease or dementia (5.2, 5.4)**
> - **The Women's Health Initiative (WHI) estrogen-alone substudy reported increased risks of stroke and deep vein thrombosis (DVT) (5.2)**
> - **The WHI Memory Study (WHIMS) estrogen-alone ancillary study of WHI reported an increased risk of probable dementia in postmenopausal women 65 years of age and older (5.4)**
> **Estrogen Plus Progestin Therapy**
> - **Estrogen plus progestin therapy should not be used for the prevention of cardiovascular disease or dementia (5.2, 5.4)**
> - **The WHI estrogen plus progestin substudy reported increased risks of stroke, DVT, pulmonary embolism, and myocardial infarction (5.2)**
> - **The WHI estrogen plus progestin substudy reported increased risks of invasive breast cancer (5.3)**
> - **The WHIMS estrogen plus progestin ancillary study of WHI reported an increased risk of probable dementia in postmenopausal women 65 years of age and older (5.4)**

---RECENT MAJOR CHANGES---
Contraindications (4)   05/2010
Warnings and Precautions
   Angioedema (5.16)   02/2010

---INDICATIONS AND USAGE---
PREMARIN (conjugated estrogens) Vaginal Cream is a mixture of estrogens indicated for:
- Treatment of Atrophic Vaginitis and Kraurosis Vulvae (1.1)

- Treatment of Moderate to Severe Dyspareunia, a Symptom of Vulvar and Vaginal Atrophy, due to Menopause (1.2)

---DOSAGE AND ADMINISTRATION---
- Cyclic administration of 0.5 to 2 g intravaginally [daily for 21 days then off for 7 days] for Treatment of Atrophic Vaginitis and Kraurosis Vulvae (2.2)
- Cyclic administration of 0.5 g intravaginally [daily for 21 days then off for 7 days] for Treatment of Moderate to Severe Dyspareunia, a Symptom of Vulvar and Vaginal Atrophy, due to Menopause (2.3)
- Twice-weekly administration of 0.5 g intravaginally [for example, Monday and Thursday] for Treatment of Moderate to Severe Dyspareunia, a Symptom of Vulvar and Vaginal Atrophy, due to Menopause (2.3)

---DOSAGE FORMS AND STRENGTHS---
- Each gram contains 0.625 mg conjugated estrogens, USP (3)
- *Combination package:* Each contains a net wt. 1.5 oz (42.5 g) tube with one plastic applicator calibrated in 0.5 g increments to a maximum of 2 g (3)

---CONTRAINDICATIONS---
- Undiagnosed abnormal genital bleeding (4)
- Known, suspected, or history of breast cancer (4, 5.3)
- Known or suspected estrogen-dependent neoplasia (4, 5.3)
- Active deep vein thrombosis, pulmonary embolism or a history of these conditions (4, 5.2)
- Active arterial thromboembolic disease (for example, stroke, myocardial infarction) or a history of these conditions (4, 5.2)
- Known liver dysfunction or disease (4, 5.10)
- Known thrombophilic disorders (e.g., protein C, protein S, or antithrombin deficiency) (4)
- Known or suspected pregnancy (4, 8.1)

---WARNINGS AND PRECAUTIONS---
- Estrogens increase the risk of gallbladder disease (5.5)
- Discontinue estrogen if severe hypercalcemia, loss of vision, severe hypertriglyceridemia or cholestatic jaundice occurs (5.6, 5.7, 5.10, 5.11)
- Monitor thyroid function in women on thyroid replacement therapy (5.12, 5.20)

---ADVERSE REACTIONS---
In a prospective, randomized, placebo-controlled, double-blind study, the most common adverse reactions ≥ 5 percent are headache, infection, abdominal pain, back pain, accidental injury, and vaginitis (6.1, 14.1).

To report SUSPECTED ADVERSE REACTIONS, contact Wyeth Pharmaceuticals Inc. at 1-800-934-5556 or FDA at 1-800-FDA-1088 or www.fda.gov/medwatch

---DRUG INTERACTIONS---
Inducers and/or inhibitors of CYP3A4 may affect estrogen drug metabolism (7)

---USE IN SPECIFIC POPULATIONS---
- Nursing Women: Estrogen administration to nursing women has been shown to decrease the quantity and quality of breast milk (8.3)
- Geriatric Use: An increased risk of probable dementia in women over 65 years of age was reported in the Women's Health Initiative Memory ancillary studies of the Women's Health Initiative (5.4, 8.5)

See 17 for PATIENT COUNSELING INFORMATION and FDA-approved patient labeling.

Revised: 05/2010

FULL PRESCRIBING INFORMATION: CONTENTS*
WARNING: CARDIOVASCULAR DISORDERS, ENDOME-TRIAL CANCER, BREAST CANCER AND PROBABLE DEMENTIA

* Sections or subsections omitted from the full prescribing information are not listed

---

FULL PRESCRIBING INFORMATION

> **WARNING: CARDIOVASCULAR DISORDERS, ENDO-METRIAL CANCER, BREAST CANCER AND PROBABLE DEMENTIA**
>
> **Estrogen-Alone Therapy**
> **Endometrial Cancer**
> **There is an increased risk of endometrial cancer in a woman with a uterus who uses unopposed estrogens. Adding a progestin to estrogen therapy has been shown to reduce the risk of endometrial hyperplasia, which may be a precursor to endometrial cancer. Adequate diagnostic measures, including directed or random endometrial sampling when indicated, should be undertaken to rule out malignancy in postmenopausal women with undiagnosed persistent or recurring abnormal genital bleeding [see Warnings and Precautions (5.3)].**
> **Cardiovascular Disorders and Probable Dementia**
> **Estrogen-alone therapy should not be used for the prevention of cardiovascular disease or dementia [see Warnings and Precautions (5.2, 5.4), and Clinical Studies (14.2, 14.3)].**
> **The Women's Health Initiative (WHI) estrogen-alone substudy reported increased risks of stroke and deep vein thrombosis (DVT) in postmenopausal women (50 to 79 years of age) during 7.1 years of treatment with daily oral conjugated estrogens (CE) [0.625 mg], relative to placebo [see Warnings and Precautions (5.2), and Clinical Studies (14.2)].**
> **The WHI Memory Study (WHIMS) estrogen alone ancillary study of WHI reported an increased risk of developing probable dementia in postmenopausal women 65 years of age or older during 5.2 years of treatment with daily CE (0.625 mg) alone, relative to placebo. It is unknown whether this finding applies to younger postmenopausal women [see Warnings and Precautions (5.4), Use in Specific Populations (8.5), and Clinical Studies (14.3)].**
> **In the absence of comparable data, these risks should be assumed to be similar for other doses of CE and other dosage forms of estrogens.**

Estrogens with or without progestins should be prescribed at the lowest effective doses and for the shortest duration consistent with treatment goals and risks for the individual woman.

Estrogen Plus Progestin Therapy

Cardiovascular Disorders and Probable Dementia

Estrogen plus progestin therapy should not be used for the prevention of cardiovascular disease or dementia [see Warnings and Precautions (5.2, 5.4), and Clinical Studies (14.2, 14.3)].

The WHI estrogen plus progestin substudy reported increased risks of DVT, pulmonary embolism, stroke and myocardial infarction in postmenopausal women (50 to 79 years of age) during 5.6 years of treatment with daily oral CE (0.625 mg) combined with medroxyprogesterone acetate (MPA) [2.5 mg], relative to placebo [see Warnings and Precautions (5.2), and Clinical Studies (14.2)].

The WHIMS estrogen plus progestin ancillary study of the WHI, reported an increased risk of developing probable dementia in postmenopausal women 65 years of age or older during 4 years of treatment with daily CE (0.625 mg) combined with MPA (2.5 mg), relative to placebo. It is unknown whether this finding applies to younger postmenopausal women [see Warnings and Precautions (5.4), Use in Specific Populations (8.5), and Clinical Studies (14.3)].

Breast Cancer

The WHI estrogen plus progestin substudy also demonstrated an increased risk of invasive breast cancer [see Warnings and Precautions (5.3), and Clinical Studies (14.2)].

In the absence of comparable data, these risks should be assumed to be similar for other doses of CE and MPA, and other combinations and dosage forms of estrogens and progestins.

Estrogens with or without progestins should be prescribed at the lowest effective doses and for the shortest duration consistent with treatment goals and risks for the individual woman.

1 INDICATIONS AND USAGE

1.1 Treatment of Atrophic Vaginitis and Kraurosis Vulvae

1.2 Treatment of Moderate to Severe Dyspareunia, a Symptom of Vulvar and Vaginal Atrophy, due to Menopause

2 DOSAGE AND ADMINISTRATION

2.1 General Dosing Information

Generally, when estrogen is prescribed for a postmenopausal woman with a uterus, a progestin should also be considered to reduce the risk of endometrial cancer.

A woman without a uterus does not need a progestin. In some cases, however, hysterectomized women with a history of endometriosis may need a progestin [see Warnings and Precautions (5.3, 5.15)].

Use of estrogen-alone, or in combination with a progestin, should be with the lowest effective dose and for the shortest duration consistent with treatment goals and risks for the individual woman. Postmenopausal women should be re-evaluated periodically as clinically appropriate to determine if treatment is still necessary.

2.2 Treatment of Atrophic Vaginitis and Kraurosis Vulvae

PREMARIN Vaginal Cream is administered intravaginally in a cyclic regimen (daily for 21 days and then off for 7 days). Generally, women should be started at the 0.5 g dosage strength. Dosage adjustments (0.5 to 2 g) may be made based on individual response [see Dosage Forms and Strengths (3)].

2.3 Treatment of Moderate to Severe Dyspareunia, a Symptom of Vulvar and Vaginal Atrophy, due to Menopause

PREMARIN Vaginal Cream (0.5 g) is administered intravaginally in a twice-weekly (for example, Monday and Thursday) continuous regimen or in a cyclic regimen of 21 days of therapy followed by 7 days off of therapy [see Dosage Forms and Strengths (3)].

3 DOSAGE FORMS AND STRENGTHS

Each gram contains 0.625 mg conjugated estrogens, USP. *Combination package:* Each contains a net wt. 1.5 oz (42.5 g) tube with one plastic applicator calibrated in 0.5 g increments to a maximum of 2 g.

4 CONTRAINDICATIONS

PREMARIN Vaginal Cream therapy should not be used in women with any of the following conditions:
- Undiagnosed abnormal genital bleeding
- Known, suspected, or history of breast cancer
- Known or suspected estrogen-dependent neoplasia
- Active deep vein thrombosis, pulmonary embolism or a history of these conditions

- Active arterial thromboembolic disease (for example, stroke, and myocardial infarction), or a history of these conditions
- Known liver dysfunction or disease
- Known thrombophilic disorders (e.g., protein C, protein S, or antithrombin deficiency)
- Known or suspected pregnancy

5 WARNINGS AND PRECAUTIONS

5.1 Risks From Systemic Absorption

Systemic absorption occurs with the use of PREMARIN Vaginal Cream. The warnings, precautions, and adverse reactions associated with oral PREMARIN treatment should be taken into account.

5.2 Cardiovascular Disorders

An increased risk of stroke and deep vein thrombosis (DVT) has been reported with estrogen-alone therapy. An increased risk of pulmonary embolism, DVT, stroke and myocardial infarction has been reported with estrogen plus progestin therapy. Should any of these occur or be suspected, estrogens with or without progestins should be discontinued immediately.

Risk factors for arterial vascular disease (for example, hypertension, diabetes mellitus, tobacco use, hypercholesterolemia, and obesity) and/or venous thromboembolism (for example, personal history of venous thromboembolism [VTE], obesity, and systemic lupus erythematosus) should be managed appropriately.

Stroke

In the Women's Health Initiative (WHI) estrogen-alone substudy, a statistically significant increased risk of stroke was reported in women 50 to 79 years of age receiving daily CE (0.625 mg) compared to women in the same age group receiving placebo (45 versus 33 per 10,000 women-years). The increase in risk was demonstrated in year one and persisted [see Clinical Studies (14.2)]. Should a stroke occur or be suspected, estrogens should be discontinued immediately.

Subgroup analyses of women 50 to 59 years of age suggest no increased risk of stroke for those women receiving CE (0.625 mg) versus those receiving placebo (18 versus 21 per 10,000 women-years).[1]

In the WHI estrogen plus progestin substudy, a statistically significant increased risk of stroke was reported in all women receiving daily CE (0.625 mg) plus MPA (2.5 mg) compared to placebo (33 versus 25 per 10,000 women-years) [see Clinical Studies (14.2)]. The increase in risk was demonstrated after the first year and persisted.[1]

Coronary Heart Disease

In the WHI estrogen-alone substudy, no overall effect on coronary heart disease (CHD) events (defined as nonfatal myocardial infarction [MI], silent MI, or CHD death) was reported in women receiving estrogen-alone compared to placebo[2] [see Clinical Studies (14.2)].

Subgroup analyses of women 50 to 59 years of age suggest a statistically non-significant reduction in CHD events (CE 0.625 mg compared to placebo) in women with less than 10 years since menopause (8 versus 16 per 10,000 women-years).[1]

In the WHI estrogen plus progestin substudy, there was a statistically non-significant increased risk of CHD events in women receiving daily CE (0.625 mg) plus MPA (2.5 mg) compared to women receiving placebo (41 versus 34 per 10,000 women-years).[1] An increase in relative risk was demonstrated in year 1, and a trend toward decreasing relative risk was reported in years 2 through 5 [see Clinical Studies (14.2)].

In postmenopausal women with documented heart disease (n = 2,763), average age 66.7 years, in a controlled clinical trial of secondary prevention of cardiovascular disease (Heart and Estrogen/Progestin Replacement Study [HERS]), treatment with daily CE (0.625 mg) plus MPA (2.5 mg) demonstrated no cardiovascular benefit. During an average follow-up of 4.1 years, treatment with CE plus MPA did not reduce the overall rate of CHD events in postmenopausal women with established coronary heart disease. There were more CHD events in the CE plus MPA-treated group than in the placebo group in year 1, but not during subsequent years. Two thousand, three hundred and twenty-one (2,321) women from the original HERS trial agreed to participate in an open label extension of HERS, HERS II. Average follow-up in HERS II was an additional 2.7 years, for a total of 6.8 years overall. Rates of CHD events were comparable among women in the CE (0.625 mg) plus MPA (2.5 mg) group and the placebo group in HERS, HERS II, and overall.

Venous Thromboembolism (VTE)

In the WHI estrogen-alone substudy, the risk of VTE (DVT and pulmonary embolism [PE]) was increased for women receiving daily CE (0.625 mg) compared to placebo (30 versus 22 per 10,000 women-years), although only the increased risk of DVT reached statistical significance (23 versus 15 per 10,000 women-years). The increase in VTE risk was

demonstrated during the first 2 years[3] [see Clinical Studies (14.2)]. Should a VTE occur or be suspected, estrogens should be discontinued immediately.

In the WHI estrogen plus progestin substudy, a statistically significant 2-fold greater rate of VTE was reported in women receiving daily CE (0.625 mg) plus MPA (2.5 mg) compared to women receiving placebo (35 versus 17 per 10,000 women-years). Statistically significant increases in risk for both DVT (26 versus 13 per 10,000 women-years) and PE (18 versus 8 per 10,000 women-years) were also demonstrated. The increase in VTE risk was observed during the first year and persisted[4] [see Clinical Studies (14.2)]. Should a VTE occur or be suspected, estrogens should be discontinued immediately.

If feasible, estrogens should be discontinued at least 4 to 6 weeks before surgery of the type associated with an increased risk of thromboembolism, or during periods of prolonged immobilization.

5.3 Malignant Neoplasms

Endometrial Cancer

An increased risk of endometrial cancer has been reported with the use of unopposed estrogen therapy in a woman with a uterus. The reported endometrial cancer risk among unopposed estrogen users is about 2- to 12-fold greater than in non-users, and appears dependent on duration of treatment and on estrogen dose. Most studies show no significant increased risk associated with use of estrogens for less than 1 year. The greatest risk appears to be associated with prolonged use, with increased risks of 15- to 24-fold for 5 to 10 years or more, and this risk has been shown to persist for at least 8 to 15 years after estrogen therapy is discontinued.

Clinical surveillance of all women using estrogen-alone or estrogen plus progestin therapy is important. Adequate diagnostic measures, including directed or random endometrial sampling when indicated, should be undertaken to rule out malignancy in postmenopausal women with undiagnosed persistent or recurring abnormal genital bleeding.

There is no evidence that the use of natural estrogens results in a different endometrial risk profile than synthetic estrogens of equivalent estrogen dose. Adding a progestin to postmenopausal estrogen therapy has been shown to reduce the risk of endometrial hyperplasia, which may be a precursor to endometrial cancer.

In a 52-week clinical trial using PREMARIN Vaginal Cream alone (0.5 g inserted twice weekly or daily for 21 days, then off for 7 days), there was no evidence of endometrial hyperplasia or endometrial carcinoma.

Breast Cancer

The most important randomized clinical trial providing information about breast cancer in estrogen-alone users is the Women's Health Initiative (WHI) substudy of daily CE (0.625 mg). In the WHI estrogen-alone substudy, after an average follow-up of 7.1 years, daily CE (0.625 mg) was not associated with an increased risk of invasive breast cancer [relative risk (RR) 0.80][5] [see Clinical Studies (14.2)].

The most important randomized clinical trial providing information about breast cancer in estrogen plus progestin users is the WHI substudy of daily CE (0.625 mg) plus MPA (2.5 mg). After a mean follow-up of 5.6 years, the estrogen plus progestin substudy reported an increased risk of breast cancer in women who took daily CE plus MPA. In this substudy, prior use of estrogen-alone or estrogen plus progestin therapy was reported by 26 percent of the women. The relative risk of invasive breast cancer was 1.24, and the absolute risk was 41 versus 33 cases per 10,000 women-years, for estrogen plus progestin compared with placebo.[6] Among women who reported prior use of hormone therapy, the relative risk of invasive breast cancer was 1.86, and the absolute risk was 46 versus 25 cases per 10,000 women-years for estrogen plus progestin compared with placebo. Among women who reported no prior use of hormone therapy, the relative risk of invasive breast cancer was 1.09, and the absolute risk was 40 versus 36 cases per 10,000 women-years for estrogen plus progestin compared with placebo. In the same substudy, invasive breast cancers were larger and diagnosed at a more advanced stage in the CE (0.625 mg) plus MPA (2.5 mg) group compared with the placebo group. Metastatic disease was rare, with no apparent difference between the two groups. Other prognostic factors, such as histologic subtype, grade and hormone receptor status did not differ between the groups [see Clinical Studies (14.2)].

Consistent with the WHI clinical trial, observational studies have also reported an increased risk of breast cancer for estrogen plus progestin therapy, and a smaller increased risk for estrogen-alone therapy, after several years of use. The risk increased with duration of use, and appeared to return to baseline over about 5 years after stopping treatment (only the observational studies have substantial data on risk after stopping). Observational studies also suggest that the risk of breast cancer was greater, and became apparent earlier, with estrogen plus progestin therapy as compared to estrogen-alone therapy. However, these studies have not generally found significant variation in the risk of breast cancer among different estrogen plus progestin combinations, doses, or routes of administration.

Table 1: Number (%) of Patients Reporting Treatment Emergent Adverse Events ≥ 5 Percent Only

Body System[a] Adverse Event	Treatment			
	PVC 21/7 (n=143)	Placebo 21/7 (n=72)	PVC 2×/wk (n=140)	Placebo 2×/wk (n=68)
	Number (%) of Patients with Adverse Event			
Any Adverse Event	95 (66.4)	45 (62.5)	97 (69.3)	46 (67.6)
Body As A Whole				
Abdominal Pain	11 (7.7)	2 (2.8)	9 (6.4)	6 (8.8)
Accidental Injury	4 (2.8)	5 (6.9)	9 (6.4)	3 (4.4)
Asthenia	8 (5.6)	0	2 (1.4)	1 (1.5)
Back Pain	7 (4.9)	3 (4.2)	13 (9.3)	5 (7.4)
Headache	16 (11.2)	9 (12.5)	25 (17.9)	12 (17.6)
Infection	7 (4.9)	5 (6.9)	16 (11.4)	5 (7.4)
Pain	10 (7.0)	3 (4.2)	4 (2.9)	4 (5.9)
Cardiovascular System				
Vasodilatation	5 (3.5)	4 (5.6)	7 (5.0)	1 (1.5)
Digestive System				
Diarrhea	4 (2.8)	2 (2.8)	10 (7.1)	1 (1.5)
Nausea	5 (3.5)	4 (5.6)	3 (2.1)	3 (4.4)
Musculoskeletal System				
Arthralgia	5 (3.5)	5 (6.9)	6 (4.3)	4 (5.9)
Nervous System				
Insomnia	6 (4.2)	3 (4.2)	4 (2.9)	4 (5.9)
Respiratory System				
Cough Increased	0	1 (1.4)	7 (5.0)	3 (4.4)
Pharyngitis	3 (2.1)	2 (2.8)	7 (5.0)	3 (4.4)
Sinusitis	1 (0.7)	3 (4.2)	2 (1.4)	4 (5.9)
Skin And Appendages	12 (8.4)	7 (9.7)	16 (11.4)	3 (4.4)
Urogenital System				
Breast Pain	8 (5.6)	1 (1.4)	4 (2.9)	0
Leukorrhea	3 (2.1)	2 (2.8)	4 (2.9)	6 (8.8)
Vaginitis	8 (5.6)	3 (4.2)	7 (5.0)	3 (4.4)

[a] Body system totals are not necessarily the sum of the individual adverse events, since a patient may report two or more different adverse events in the same body system.

The use of estrogen-alone and estrogen plus progestin therapy has been reported to result in an increase in abnormal mammograms, requiring further evaluation.

All women should receive yearly breast examinations by a healthcare provider and perform monthly breast self-examinations. In addition, mammography examinations should be scheduled based on patient age, risk factors, and prior mammogram results.

Ovarian Cancer

The WHI estrogen plus progestin substudy reported a statistically non-significant increased risk of ovarian cancer. After an average follow-up of 5.6 years, the relative risk for ovarian cancer for CE plus MPA versus placebo, was 1.58 (95 percent nCI 0.77-3.24). The absolute risk for CE plus MPA versus placebo was 4 versus 3 cases per 10,000 women-years.[7] In some epidemiologic studies, the use of estrogen-plus progestin and estrogen-only products has been associated with an increased risk of ovarian cancer over multiple years of use. However, the duration of exposure associated with increased risk is not consistent across all epidemiologic studies, and some report no association.

5.4   Probable Dementia

In the estrogen-alone Women's Health Initiative Memory Study (WHIMS), an ancillary study of WHI, a population of 2,947 hysterectomized women 65 to 79 years of age was randomized to daily CE (0.625 mg) or placebo.

In the WHIMS estrogen-alone ancillary study, after an average follow-up of 5.2 years, 28 women in the estrogen-alone group and 19 women in the placebo group were diagnosed

with probable dementia. The relative risk of probable dementia for CE-alone versus placebo was 1.49 (95 percent nCI 0.83-2.66). The absolute risk of probable dementia for CE-alone versus placebo was 37 versus 25 cases per 10,000 women-years[8] *[see Use in Specific Populations (8.3), and Clinical Studies (14.3)].*

In the WHIMS estrogen plus progestin ancillary study, a population of 4,532 postmenopausal women 65 to 79 years of age was randomized to daily CE (0.625 mg) plus MPA (2.5 mg) or placebo.

After an average follow-up of 4 years, 40 women in the CE plus MPA group and 21 women in the placebo group were diagnosed with probable dementia. The relative risk of probable dementia for CE plus MPA versus placebo was 2.05 (95 percent nCI 1.21-3.48). The absolute risk of probable dementia for CE plus MPA versus placebo was 45 versus 22 cases per 10,000 women-years[8] *[see Use in Specific Populations (8.3), and Clinical Studies (14.3)].*

When data from the two populations were pooled as planned in the WHIMS protocol, the reported overall relative risk for probable dementia was 1.76 (95 percent nCI 1.19-2.60). Since both substudies were conducted in women 65 to 79 years of age, it is unknown whether these findings apply to younger postmenopausal women[8] *[see Use in Specific Populations (8.5), and Clinical Studies (14.3)].*

5.5   Gallbladder Disease

A 2- to 4-fold increase in the risk of gallbladder disease requiring surgery in postmenopausal women receiving estrogens has been reported.

5.6   Hypercalcemia

Estrogen administration may lead to severe hypercalcemia in women with breast cancer and bone metastases. If hypercalcemia occurs, use of the drug should be stopped and appropriate measures taken to reduce the serum calcium level.

5.7   Visual Abnormalities

Retinal vascular thrombosis has been reported in patients receiving estrogens. Discontinue medication pending examination if there is sudden partial or complete loss of vision, or a sudden onset of proptosis, diplopia, or migraine. If examination reveals papilledema or retinal vascular lesions, estrogens should be permanently discontinued.

5.8   Addition of a Progestin When a Woman Has Not Had a Hysterectomy

Studies of the addition of a progestin for 10 or more days of a cycle of estrogen administration or daily with estrogen in a continuous regimen have reported a lowered incidence of endometrial hyperplasia than would be induced by estrogen treatment alone. Endometrial hyperplasia may be a precursor to endometrial cancer.

There are, however, possible risks that may be associated with the use of progestins with estrogens compared to estrogen-alone regimens. These include an increased risk of breast cancer.

5.9   Elevated Blood Pressure

In a small number of case reports, substantial increases in blood pressure have been attributed to idiosyncratic reactions to estrogens. In a large, randomized, placebo-controlled clinical trial, a generalized effect of estrogen therapy on blood pressure was not seen.

5.10   Hypertriglyceridemia

In patients with pre-existing hypertriglyceridemia, estrogen therapy may be associated with elevations of plasma triglycerides leading to pancreatitis. Consider discontinuation of treatment if pancreatitis occurs.

5.11   Hepatic Impairment and/or Past History of Cholestatic Jaundice

Estrogens may be poorly metabolized in women with impaired liver function. For women with a history of cholestatic jaundice associated with past estrogen use or with pregnancy, caution should be exercised, and in the case of recurrence, medication should be discontinued.

5.12   Hypothyroidism

Estrogen administration leads to increased thyroid-binding globulin (TBG) levels. Women with normal thyroid function can compensate for the increased TBG by making more thyroid hormone, thus maintaining free T_4 and T_3 serum concentrations in the normal range. Women dependent on thyroid hormone replacement therapy who are also receiving estrogens may require increased doses of their thyroid replacement therapy. These women should have their thyroid function monitored in order to maintain their free thyroid hormone levels in an acceptable range.

5.13   Fluid Retention

Estrogens may cause some degree of fluid retention. Patients with conditions that might be influenced by this factor, such as cardiac or renal dysfunction, warrant careful observation when estrogens are prescribed.

5.14   Hypocalcemia

Estrogens should be used with caution in individuals with hypoparathyroidism as estrogen-induced hypocalcemia may occur.

5.15   Exacerbation of Endometriosis

A few cases of malignant transformation of residual endometrial implants have been reported in women treated post-hysterectomy with estrogen-alone therapy. For women known to have residual endometriosis post-hysterectomy, the addition of progestin should be considered.

5.16   Angioedema

Exogenous estrogens may induce or exacerbate symptoms of angioedema, particularly in women with hereditary angioedema.

5.17   Exacerbation of Other Conditions

Estrogen therapy may cause an exacerbation of asthma, diabetes mellitus, epilepsy, migraine, porphyria, systemic lupus erythematosus, and hepatic hemangiomas and should be used with caution in women with these conditions.

5.18   Effects on Barrier Contraception

PREMARIN Vaginal Cream exposure has been reported to weaken latex condoms. The potential for PREMARIN Vaginal Cream to weaken and contribute to the failure of condoms, diaphragms, or cervical caps made of latex or rubber should be considered.

5.19   Laboratory Tests

Serum follicle stimulating hormone and estradiol levels have not been shown to be useful in the management of moderate to severe symptoms of vulvar and vaginal atrophy.

5.20   Drug-Laboratory Test Interactions

Accelerated prothrombin time, partial thromboplastin time, and platelet aggregation time; increased platelet count; increased factors II, VII antigen, VIII antigen, VIII coagulant activity, IX, X, XII, VII-X complex, II-VII-X complex, and beta-thromboglobulin; decreased levels of antifactor Xa and antithrombin III, decreased antithrombin III activity; increased levels of fibrinogen and fibrinogen activity; increased plasminogen antigen and activity.

Increased thyroid-binding globulin (TBG) leading to increased circulating total thyroid hormone, as measured by protein-bound iodine (PBI), T_4 levels (by column or by radioimmunoassay) or T_3 levels by radioimmunoassay. T_3 resin uptake is decreased, reflecting the elevated TBG. Free T_4 and free T_3 concentrations are unaltered. Women on thyroid replacement therapy may require higher doses of thyroid hormone.

Other binding proteins may be elevated in serum, for example, corticosteroid binding globulin (CBG), sex hormone-binding globulin (SHBG), leading to increased total circulating corticosteroids and sex steroids, respectively. Free hormone concentrations, such as testosterone and estradiol, may be decreased. Other plasma proteins may be increased (angiotensinogen/renin substrate, alpha-1-antitrypsin, ceruloplasmin).

Increased plasma HDL and HDL_2 cholesterol subfraction concentrations, reduced LDL cholesterol concentrations, increased triglyceride levels.

Impaired glucose tolerance.

6 ADVERSE REACTIONS

The following serious adverse reactions are discussed elsewhere in the labeling:

- Cardiovascular Disorders [see Boxed Warning, Warnings and Precautions (5.2)]
- Endometrial Cancer [see Boxed Warning, Warnings and Precautions (5.3)]

6.1 Clinical Study Experience

Because clinical trials are conducted under widely varying conditions, adverse reaction rates observed in the clinical trial of a drug cannot be directly compared to rates in the clinical trials of another drug and may not reflect the rates observed in practice.

In a 12-week, randomized, double-blind, placebo-controlled trial of PREMARIN Vaginal Cream (PVC), a total of 423 postmenopausal women received at least 1 dose of study medication and were included in all safety analyses: 143 women in the PVC-21/7 treatment group (0.5 g PVC daily for 21 days, then 7 days off), 72 women in the matching placebo treatment group; 140 women in the PVC-2×/wk treatment group (0.5 g PVC twice weekly), 68 women in the matching placebo treatment group. A 40-week, open-label extension followed, in which a total of 394 women received treatment with PVC, including those subjects randomized at baseline to placebo. In this study, the most common adverse reactions ≥ 5 percent are shown below (Table 1) [see Clinical Studies (14.1)].

[See table 1 at top of previous page]

6.2 Postmarketing Experience

The following adverse reactions have been reported with PREMARIN Vaginal Cream. Because these reactions are reported voluntarily from a population of uncertain size, it is not always possible to reliably estimate their frequency or establish a causal relationship to drug exposure.

Genitourinary System

Abnormal uterine bleeding/spotting, dysmenorrhea/pelvic pain, increase in size of uterine leiomyomata, vaginitis (including vaginal candidiasis), change in cervical secretion, cystitis-like syndrome, application site reactions of vulvovaginal discomfort, (including burning, irritation, and genital pruritus), endometrial hyperplasia, endometrial cancer, precocious puberty, leukorrhea.

Breasts

Tenderness, enlargement, pain, discharge, fibrocystic breast changes, breast cancer, gynecomastia in males.

Cardiovascular

Deep venous thrombosis, pulmonary embolism, myocardial infarction, stroke, increase in blood pressure.

Gastrointestinal

Nausea, vomiting, abdominal cramps, bloating, increased incidence of gallbladder disease.

Skin

Chloasma that may persist when drug is discontinued, loss of scalp hair, hirsutism, rash.

Eyes

Retinal vascular thrombosis, intolerance to contact lenses.

Central Nervous System

Headache, migraine, dizziness, mental depression, nervousness, mood disturbances, irritability, dementia.

Miscellaneous

Increase or decrease in weight, glucose intolerance, edema, arthralgias, leg cramps, changes in libido, urticaria, anaphylactic reactions, exacerbation of asthma, increased triglycerides, hypersensitivity.

Additional postmarketing adverse reactions have been reported in patients receiving other forms of hormone therapy.

7 DRUG INTERACTIONS

No formal drug interaction studies have been conducted for PREMARIN Vaginal Cream.

Table 2: Mean ± SD Pharmacokinetic Parameters of PREMARIN Following Daily Administration (7 Days) of PREMARIN Vaginal Cream 0.5 g in 24 Postmenopausal Women

Pharmacokinetic Profiles of Unconjugated Estrogens PREMARIN Vaginal Cream 0.5 g			
PK Parameters Arithmetic Mean ± SD	C_{max} (pg/mL)	T_{max} (hr)	AUC_{ss} (pg·hr/mL)
Estrone	42.0 ± 13.9	7.4 ± 6.2	826 ± 295
Baseline-adjusted estrone	21.9 ± 13.1	7.4 ± 6.2	365 ± 255
Estradiol	12.8 ± 16.6	8.5 ± 6.2	231 ± 285
Baseline-adjusted estradiol	9.14 ± 14.7	8.5 ± 6.2	161 ± 252

Pharmacokinetic Profiles of Conjugated Estrogens PREMARIN Vaginal Cream 0.5 g			
PK Parameters Arithmetic Mean ± SD	C_{max} (ng/mL)	T_{max} (hr)	AUC_{ss} (ng·hr/mL)
Total estrone	0.60 ± 0.32	6.0 ± 4.0	9.75 ± 4.99
Baseline-adjusted total estrone	0.40 ± 0.28	6.0 ± 4.0	5.79 ± 3.7
Total estradiol	0.04 ± 0.04	7.7 ± 5.9	0.70 ± 0.42
Baseline-adjusted total estradiol	0.04 ± 0.04	7.7 ± 6.0	0.49 ± 0.38
Total equilin	0.12 ± 0.15	6.1 ± 4.7	3.09 ± 1.37

7.1 Metabolic Interactions

In vitro and *in vivo* studies have shown that estrogens are metabolized partially by cytochrome P450 3A4 (CYP3A4). Therefore, inducers or inhibitors of CYP3A4 may affect estrogen drug metabolism. Inducers of CYP3A4, such as St. John's Wort (*Hypericum perforatum*) preparations, phenobarbital, carbamazepine, and rifampin, may reduce plasma concentrations of estrogens, possibly resulting in a decrease in therapeutic effects and/or changes in the uterine bleeding profile. Inhibitors of CYP3A4, such as erythromycin, clarithromycin, ketoconazole, itraconazole, ritonavir and grapefruit juice, may increase plasma concentrations of estrogens and may result in side effects.

8 USE IN SPECIFIC POPULATIONS

8.1 Pregnancy

PREMARIN Vaginal Cream should not be used during pregnancy [see Contraindications (4)]. There appears to be little or no increased risk of birth defects in children born to women who have used estrogens and progestins as an oral contraceptive inadvertently during early pregnancy.

8.3 Nursing Mothers

PREMARIN Vaginal Cream should not be used during lactation. Estrogen administration to nursing mothers has been shown to decrease the quantity and quality of the breast milk. Detectable amounts of estrogens have been identified in the breast milk of mothers receiving estrogens. Caution should be exercised when PREMARIN Vaginal Cream is administered to a nursing woman.

8.4 Pediatric Use

PREMARIN Vaginal Cream is not indicated in children. Clinical studies have not been conducted in the pediatric population.

8.5 Geriatric Use

There have not been sufficient numbers of geriatric women involved in clinical studies utilizing PREMARIN Vaginal Cream to determine whether those over 65 years of age differ from younger subjects in their response to PREMARIN Vaginal Cream.

The Women's Health Initiative Study

In the Women's Health Initiative (WHI) estrogen-alone substudy (daily conjugated estrogens 0.625 mg versus placebo), there was a higher relative risk of stroke in women greater than 65 years of age [see Clinical Studies (14.2)].

In the WHI estrogen plus progestin substudy, there was a higher relative risk of nonfatal stroke and invasive breast cancer in women greater than 65 years of age [see Clinical Studies (14.2)].

The Women's Health Initiative Memory Study

In the Women's Health Initiative Memory Study (WHIMS) of postmenopausal women 65 to 79 years of age, there was an increased risk of developing probable dementia in women receiving estrogen-alone or estrogen plus progestin when compared to placebo [see Clinical Studies (14.3)]. Since both ancillary studies were conducted in women 65 to 79 years of age, it is unknown whether these findings apply to younger postmenopausal women[8] [see Clinical Studies (14.3)].

8.6 Renal Impairment

The effect of renal impairment on the pharmacokinetics of PREMARIN Vaginal Cream has not been studied.

8.7 Hepatic Impairment

The effect of hepatic impairment on the pharmacokinetics of PREMARIN Vaginal Cream has not been studied.

10 OVERDOSAGE

Overdosage of estrogen may cause nausea and vomiting, breast tenderness, dizziness, abdominal pain, drowsiness/fatigue, and withdrawal bleeding in women. Treatment of overdose consists of discontinuation of PREMARIN therapy with institution of appropriate symptomatic care.

11 DESCRIPTION

Each gram of PREMARIN (conjugated estrogens) Vaginal Cream contains 0.625 mg conjugated estrogens, USP in a nonliquefying base containing cetyl esters wax, cetyl alcohol, white wax, glyceryl monostearate, propylene glycol monostearate, methyl stearate, benzyl alcohol, sodium lauryl sulfate, glycerin, and mineral oil. PREMARIN Vaginal Cream is applied intravaginally.

PREMARIN Vaginal Cream contains a mixture of conjugated estrogens obtained exclusively from natural sources, occurring as the sodium salts of water-soluble estrogen sulfates blended to represent the average composition of material derived from pregnant mares' urine. It is a mixture of sodium estrone sulfate and sodium equilin sulfate. It contains as concomitant components, sodium sulfate conjugates, 17 α-dihydroequilin, 17 α-estradiol, and 17 β-dihydroequilin.

12 CLINICAL PHARMACOLOGY

12.1 Mechanism of Action

Endogenous estrogens are largely responsible for the development of the female reproductive system and secondary sexual characteristics. Although circulating estrogens exist in a dynamic equilibrium of metabolic interconversions, estradiol is the principal intracellular human estrogen and is substantially more potent than its metabolites, estrone and estriol, at the receptor level.

The primary source of estrogen in normally cycling adult women is the ovarian follicle, which secretes 70 to 500 mcg of estradiol daily, depending on the phase of the menstrual cycle. After menopause, most endogenous estrogen is produced by conversion of androstenedione, which is secreted by the adrenal cortex, to estrone by peripheral tissues. Thus, estrone and the sulfate-conjugated form, estrone sulfate, are the most abundant circulating estrogens in postmenopausal women.

Estrogens act through binding to nuclear receptors in estrogen-responsive tissues. To date, two estrogen receptors have been identified. These vary in proportion from tissue to tissue.

Circulating estrogens modulate the pituitary secretion of the gonadotropins, luteinizing hormone (LH) and follicle stimulating hormone (FSH), through a negative feedback mechanism. Estrogens act to reduce the elevated levels of these gonadotropins seen in postmenopausal women.

12.2 Pharmacodynamics

Currently, there are no pharmacodynamic data known for PREMARIN Vaginal Cream.

12.3 Pharmacokinetics

Absorption

Conjugated estrogens are water soluble and are well-absorbed through the skin, mucous membranes, and the gastrointestinal (GI) tract. The vaginal delivery of estrogens circumvents first-pass metabolism.

Table 3: Mean Change in Most Bothersome Symptom of Dyspareunia Compared to Placebo MITT Population[a]

Dyspareunia*	PVC 0.5 g 2×/wk[b]	Placebo 0.5 g 2×/wk[b]	PVC 0.5 g 21/7[c]	Placebo 0.5 g 21/7[c]
Baseline				
n	52	22	50	18
mean (SD)*	2.43 (0.76)	2.28 (1.04)	2.26 (0.99)	2.32 (0.88)
Week 12				
n	52	21	50	18
mean (SD)*	0.88 (0.96)	1.63 (1.16)	0.77 (1.05)	1.92 (1.03)
Change from Baseline at Week 12				
n	52	21	50	18
LS mean[d] (SD)*	-1.45 (0.16)	-0.69 (0.24)	-1.51 (0.17)	-0.36 (0.26)
P-value vs. Placebo	0.01[e]	—	<0.001[f]	—

[a] Women at baseline had ≤5 percent superficial cells on a vaginal smear, a vaginal pH >5.0, and who identified dyspareunia as the most bothersome symptom.
[b] PVC 2×/wk = apply PVC twice a week
[c] PVC 21/7 = apply PVC for 21 days and then 7 days of no therapy
[d] Least square mean from ANCOVA adjusting for study site and baseline dyspareunia
[e] Comparison of PVC 2×/wk with placebo 2×/wk
[f] Comparison of PVC 21/7 with placebo 21/7
* Symptom Assessment Scale: 0 (none), 1 (mild), 2 (moderate), 3 (severe).

Table 4: Relative and Absolute Risk Seen in the Estrogen-Alone Substudy of WHI[a]

Event	Relative Risk CE vs. Placebo (95% nCI[b])	CE n = 5,310	Placebo n = 5,429
		Absolute Risk per 10,000 Women-Years	
CHD events[c]	0.95 (0.78–1.16)	54	57
Non-fatal MI[c]	*0.91 (0.73–1.14)*	*40*	*43*
CHD death[c]	*1.01 (0.71–1.43)*	*16*	*16*
All Stroke[c]	1.33 (1.05–1.68)	45	33
Ischemic[c]	*1.55 (1.19–2.01)*	*38*	*25*
Deep vein thrombosis[c,d]	1.47 (1.06–2.06)	23	15
Pulmonary embolism[c]	1.37 (0.90–2.07)	14	10
Invasive breast cancer[c]	0.80 (0.62–1.04)	28	34
Colorectal cancer[e]	1.08 (0.75–1.55)	17	16
Hip fracture[c]	0.65 (0.45–0.94)	12	19
Vertebral fractures[c,d]	0.64 (0.44–0.93)	11	18
Lower arm/wrist fractures[c,d]	0.58 (0.47–0.72)	35	59
Total fractures[c,d]	0.71 (0.64–0.80)	144	197
Death due to other causes[e,f]	1.08 (0.88–1.32)	53	50
Overall mortality[c,d]	1.04 (0.88–1.22)	79	75
Global Index[g]	1.02 (0.92–1.13)	206	201

[a] Adapted from numerous WHI publications. WHI publications can be viewed at www.nhlbi.nih.gov/whi.
[b] Nominal confidence intervals unadjusted for multiple looks and multiple comparisons.
[c] Results are based on centrally adjudicated data for an average follow-up of 7.1 years.
[d] Not included in "global index."
[e] Results are based on an average follow-up of 6.8 years.
[f] All deaths, except from breast or colorectal cancer, definite/probable CHD, PE or cerebrovascular disease.
[g] A subset of the events was combined in a "global index" defined as the earliest occurrence of CHD events, invasive breast cancer, stroke, pulmonary embolism, colorectal cancer, hip fracture, or death due to other causes.

A bioavailability study was conducted in 24 postmenopausal women with atrophic vaginitis. The mean (SD) pharmacokinetic parameters for unconjugated estrone, unconjugated estradiol, total estrone, total estradiol and total equilin following 7 once-daily doses of PREMARIN Vaginal Cream 0.5 g is shown in Table 2.
[See table 2 at top of previous page]

Distribution
The distribution of exogenous estrogens is similar to that of endogenous estrogens. Estrogens are widely distributed in the body and are generally found in higher concentration in the sex hormone target organs. Estrogens circulate in the blood largely bound to sex hormone-binding globulin (SHBG) and albumin.

Metabolism
Exogenous estrogens are metabolized in the same manner as endogenous estrogens. Circulating estrogens exist in a dynamic equilibrium of metabolic interconversions. These transformations take place mainly in the liver. Estradiol is converted reversibly to estrone, and both can be converted to estriol, which is a major urinary metabolite. Estrogens also undergo enterohepatic recirculation via sulfate and glucuronide conjugation in the liver, biliary secretion of conjugates into the intestine, and hydrolysis in the intestine followed by reabsorption. In postmenopausal women, a significant portion of the circulating estrogens exists as sulfate conjugates, especially estrone sulfate, which serves as a circulating reservoir for the formation of more active estrogens.

Excretion
Estradiol, estrone, and estriol are excreted in the urine, along with glucuronide and sulfate conjugates.

Specific Populations
No pharmacokinetic studies were conducted in specific populations, including patients with renal or hepatic impairment.

13   NONCLINICAL TOXICOLOGY
13.1   Carcinogenesis, Mutagenesis, Impairment of Fertility
Long-term continuous administration of natural and synthetic estrogens in certain animal species increases the frequency of carcinomas of the breast, uterus, cervix, vagina, testis, and liver.

14   CLINICAL STUDIES
14.1   Effects on Vulvar and Vaginal Atrophy
A 12-week, prospective, randomized, double-blind placebo-controlled study was conducted to compare the safety and efficacy of 2 PREMARIN Vaginal Cream (PVC) regimens 0.5 g (0.3 mg CE) administered twice weekly and 0.5 g (0.3 mg CE) administered sequentially for 21 days on drug followed by 7 days off drug to matching placebo regimens in the treatment of moderate to severe symptoms of vulvar and vaginal atrophy due to menopause. The initial 12-week, double-blind, placebo-controlled phase was followed by an open-label phase to assess endometrial safety through week 52. The study randomized 423 generally healthy postmenopausal women between 44 to 77 years of age (mean 57.8 years), who at baseline had ≤ 5 percent superficial cells on a vaginal smear, a vaginal pH ≥ 5.0, and who identified a most bothersome moderate to severe symptom of vulvar and vaginal atrophy. The majority (92.2 percent) of the women were Caucasian (n = 390); 7.8 percent were Other (n = 33). All subjects were assessed for improvement in the mean change from baseline to Week 12 for the co-primary efficacy variables of: most bothersome symptom of vulvar and vaginal atrophy (defined as the moderate to severe symptom that had been identified by the woman as most bothersome to her at baseline); percentage of vaginal superficial cells and percentage of vaginal parabasal cells; and vaginal pH.
In the 12-week, double-blind phase, a statistically significant mean change between baseline and Week 12 in the symptom of dyspareunia was observed for both of the PREMARIN Vaginal Cream regimens (0.5 g twice weekly and 0.5 g daily for 21 days, then 7 days off) compared to matching placebo, see Table 3. Also demonstrated for each PREMARIN Vaginal Cream regimen compared to placebo was a statistically significant increase in the percentage of superficial cells at Week 12 (28 percent and 26 percent, respectively, compared to 3 percent and 1 percent for matching placebo), a statistically significant decrease in parabasal cells (-61 percent and -58 percent, respectively, compared to -21 percent and -7 percent for matching placebo) and statistically significant mean reduction between baseline and Week 12 in vaginal pH (-1.62 and -1.57, respectively, compared to -0.36 and -0.26 for matching placebo).
Endometrial safety was assessed by endometrial biopsy for all randomly assigned subjects at week 52. For the 155 subjects (83 on the 21/7 regimen, 72 on the twice-weekly regimen) completing the 52-week period with complete follow-up and evaluable endometrial biopsies, there were no reports of endometrial hyperplasia or endometrial carcinoma.
[See table 3 above]

14.2   Women's Health Initiative Studies
The Women's Health Initiative (WHI) enrolled approximately 27,000 predominantly healthy postmenopausal women in two substudies to assess the risks and benefits of daily oral CE (0.625 mg)-alone or in combination with MPA (2.5 mg) compared to placebo in the prevention of certain chronic diseases. The primary endpoint was the incidence of coronary heart disease [(CHD) defined as nonfatal myocardial infarction (MI), silent MI and CHD death], with invasive breast cancer as the primary adverse outcome. A "global index" included the earliest occurrence of CHD, invasive breast cancer, stroke, pulmonary embolism (PE), endometrial cancer (only in the CE plus MPA substudy),

colorectal cancer, hip fracture, or death due to other causes. These substudies did not evaluate the effects of CE or CE plus MPA on menopausal symptoms.

WHI Estrogen-Alone Substudy

The WHI estrogen-alone substudy was stopped early because an increased risk of stroke was observed, and it was deemed that no further information would be obtained regarding the risks and benefits of estrogen alone in predetermined primary endpoints.

Results of the estrogen-alone substudy, which included 10,739 women (average age of 63 years, range 50 to 79; 75.3 percent White, 15.1 percent Black, 6.1 percent Hispanic, 3.6 percent Other) after an average follow-up of 7.1 years, are presented in Table 4.

[See table 4 on previous page]

For those outcomes included in the WHI "global index" that reached statistical significance, the absolute excess risk per 10,000 women-years in the group treated with CE-alone was 12 more strokes while the absolute risk reduction per 10,000 women-years was 7 fewer hip fractures.[9] The absolute excess risk of events included in the "global index" was a non-significant 5 events per 10,000 women-years. There was no difference between the groups in terms of all-cause mortality *[see Boxed Warnings, and Warnings and Precautions (5)].*

No overall difference for primary CHD events (nonfatal MI, silent MI and CHD death) and invasive breast cancer incidence in women receiving CE-alone compared with placebo was reported in final centrally adjudicated results from the estrogen-alone substudy, after an average follow up of 7.1 years.

Centrally adjudicated results for stroke events from the estrogen-alone substudy, after an average follow-up of 7.1 years, reported no significant difference in distribution of stroke subtype or severity, including fatal strokes, in women receiving CE-alone compared to placebo. Estrogen-alone increased the risk for ischemic stroke, and this excess risk was present in all subgroups of women examined, see Table 4.[10]

Timing of the initiation of estrogen therapy relative to the start of menopause may affect the overall risk benefit profile. The WHI estrogen-alone substudy stratified by age showed in women 50-59 years of age, a non-significant trend toward reduced risk for CHD *[HR 0.63 (95 percent CI 0.36-1.09)]* and overall mortality *[HR 0.71 (95 percent CI 0.46-1.11)].*

WHI Estrogen Plus Progestin Substudy

The WHI estrogen plus progestin substudy was stopped early. According to the predefined stopping rule, after an average follow-up of 5.6 years of treatment, the increased risk of breast cancer and cardiovascular events exceeded the specified benefits included in the "global index." The absolute excess risk of events included in the "global index" was 19 per 10,000 women-years.

For those outcomes included in the WHI "global index" that reached statistical significance after 5.6 years of follow-up, the absolute excess risks per 10,000 women-years in the group treated with CE plus MPA were 7 more CHD events, 8 more strokes, 10 more PEs, and 8 more invasive breast cancers, while the absolute risk reductions per 10,000 women-years were 6 fewer colorectal cancers and 5 fewer hip fractures.

Results of the estrogen plus progestin substudy, which included 16,608 women (average 63 years of age, range 50 to 79; 83.9 percent White, 6.8 percent Black, 5.4 percent Hispanic, 3.9 percent Other) are presented in Table 5. These results reflect centrally adjudicated data after an average follow-up of 5.6 years.

[See table 5 above]

Timing of the initiation of estrogen therapy relative to the start of menopause may affect the overall risk benefit profile. The WHI estrogen plus progestin substudy stratified by age showed in women 50-59 years of age, a non-significant trend toward reduced risk for overall mortality *[HR 0.69 (95 percent CI 0.44-1.07)].*

14.3 Women's Health Initiative Memory Study

The estrogen-alone Women's Health Initiative Memory Study (WHIMS), an ancillary study of WHI, enrolled 2,947 predominantly healthy hysterectomized postmenopausal women 65 to 79 years of age and older (45 percent were 65 to 69 years of age; 36 percent were 70 to 74 years of age; 19 percent were 75 years of age and older) to evaluate the effects of daily CE (0.625 mg) on the incidence of probable dementia (primary outcome) compared to placebo.

After an average follow-up of 5.2 years, the relative risk of *probable dementia* for CE-alone versus placebo was 1.49 (95 percent CI 0.83-2.66). The absolute risk of probable dementia for CE-alone versus placebo was 37 versus 25 cases per 10,000 women-years. Probable dementia as defined in this study included Alzheimer's disease (AD), vascular dementia (VaD) and mixed types (having features of both AD and VaD). The most common classification of probable dementia in both the treatment and placebo groups was AD. Since the ancillary study was conducted in women 65 to 79

years of age, it is unknown whether these findings apply to younger postmenopausal women *[see Warnings and Precautions (5.4), and Use in Specific Populations (8.3)].*

The WHIMS estrogen plus progestin substudy enrolled 4,532 predominantly healthy postmenopausal women 65 years of age and older (47 percent were 65 to 69 years of age; 35 percent were 70 to 74 years; 18 percent were 75 years of age and older) to evaluate the effects of daily CE (0.625 mg) plus MPA (2.5 mg) on the incidence of probable dementia (primary outcome) compared to placebo.

After an average follow-up of 4 years, the relative risk of probable dementia for CE (0.625 mg) plus MPA (2.5 mg) versus placebo was 2.05 (95 percent CI 1.21-3.48). The absolute risk of probable dementia for CE (0.625 mg) plus MPA (2.5 mg) versus placebo was 45 versus 22 per 10,000 women-years. Probable dementia as defined in this study included AD, VaD and mixed types (having features of both AD and VaD). The most common classification of probable dementia in both the treatment and placebo groups was AD. Since the ancillary study was conducted in women 65 to 79 years of age, it is unknown whether these findings apply to younger postmenopausal women *[see Warnings and Precautions (5.4), and Use in Specific Populations (8.5)].*

When data from the two populations were pooled as planned in the WHIMS protocol, the reported overall relative risk for probable dementia was 1.76 (95 percent CI 1.19-2.60). Differences between groups became apparent in the first year of treatment. It is unknown whether these findings apply to younger postmenopausal women *[see Warnings and Precautions (5.4), and Use in Specific Populations (8.5)].*

15 REFERENCES

1. Rossouw JE, et al. Postmenopausal Hormone Therapy and Risk of Cardiovascular Disease by Age and Years Since Menopause. *JAMA.* 2007;297:1465-1477.
2. Hsia J, et al. Conjugated Equine Estrogens and Coronary Heart Disease. *Arch Int Med.* 2006;166:357-365.
3. Curb JD, et al. Venous Thrombosis and Conjugated Equine Estrogen in Women Without a Uterus. *Arch Int Med.* 2006;166:772-780.
4. Cushman M, et al. Estrogen Plus Progestin and Risk of Venous Thrombosis. *JAMA.* 2004;292:1573-1580.
5. Stefanick ML, et al. Effects of Conjugated Equine Estrogens on Breast Cancer and Mammography Screening in Postmenopausal Women With Hysterectomy. *JAMA.* 2006;295:1647-1657.
6. Chlebowski RT, et al. Influence of Estrogen Plus Progestin on Breast Cancer and Mammography in Healthy Postmenopausal Women. *JAMA.* 2003;289:3234-3253.
7. Anderson GL, et al. Effects of Estrogen Plus Progestin on Gynecologic Cancers and Associated Diagnostic Procedures. *JAMA.* 2003;290:1739-1748.
8. Shumaker SA, et al. Conjugated Equine Estrogens and Incidence of Probable Dementia and Mild Cognitive Impairment in Postmenopausal Women. *JAMA.* 2004;291:2947-2958.
9. Jackson RD, et al. Effects of Conjugated Equine Estrogen on Risk of Fractures and BMD in Postmenopausal Women With Hysterectomy: Results From the Women's Health Initiative Randomized Trial. *J Bone Miner Res.* 2006;21:817-828.
10. Hendrix SL, et al. Effects of Conjugated Equine Estrogen on Stroke in the Women's Health Initiative. *Circulation.* 2006;113:2425-2434.

16 HOW SUPPLIED/STORAGE AND HANDLING

16.1 How Supplied

PREMARIN (conjugated estrogens) Vaginal Cream—Each gram contains 0.625 mg conjugated estrogens, USP.

Combination package: Each contains a net wt. 1.5 oz (42.5 g) tube with one plastic applicator calibrated in 0.5 g increments to a maximum of 2 g (NDC 0046-0872-93).

16.2 Storage and Handling

Store at 20° to 25°C (68° to 77°F); excursions permitted to 15° to 30°C (59° to 86°F) *[see USP Controlled Room Temperature].*

17 PATIENT COUNSELING INFORMATION

See Section 17.5 for FDA-Approved Patient Labeling.

17.1 Vaginal Bleeding

Inform postmenopausal women of the importance of reporting vaginal bleeding to their healthcare provider as soon as possible *[see Warnings and Precautions (5.3)].*

Table 5: Relative and Absolute Risk Seen in the Estrogen Plus Progestin Substudy of WHI at an Average of 5.6 Years[a,b]

Event	Relative Risk CE/MPA vs. Placebo (95% nCI[c])	CE/MPA n = 8,506	Placebo n = 8,102
		Absolute Risk per 10,000 Women-Years	
CHD events	1.23 (0.99–1.53)	41	34
Non-fatal MI	*1.28 (1.00–1.63)*	*31*	*25*
CHD death	*1.10 (0.70–1.75)*	*8*	*8*
All Strokes	1.31 (1.03–1.68)	33	25
Ischemic stroke	*1.44 (1.09–1.90)*	*26*	*18*
Deep vein thrombosis[d]	1.95 (1.43–2.67)	26	13
Pulmonary embolism	2.13 (1.45–3.11)	18	8
Invasive breast cancer[e]	1.24 (1.01–1.54)	41	33
Colorectal cancer	0.61 (0.42–0.87)	10	16
Endometrial cancer[d]	0.81 (0.48–1.36)	6	7
Cervical cancer[d]	1.44 (0.47–4.42)	2	1
Hip fracture	0.67 (0.47–0.96)	11	16
Vertebral fractures[d]	0.65 (0.46–0.92)	11	17
Lower arm/wrist fractures[d]	0.71 (0.59–0.85)	44	62
Total fractures[d]	0.76 (0.69–0.83)	152	199
Overall Mortality[f]	1.00 (0.83–1.19)	52	52
Global Index[g]	1.13 (1.02–1.25)	184	165

[a] Adapted from numerous WHI publications. WHI publications can be viewed at www.nhlbi.nih.gov/whi.
[b] Results are based on centrally adjudicated data.
[c] Nominal confidence intervals unadjusted for multiple looks and multiple comparisons.
[d] Not included in "global index."
[e] Includes metastatic and non-metastatic breast cancer, with the exception of *in situ* cancer.
[f] All deaths, except from breast or colorectal cancer, definite/probable CHD, PE or cerebrovascular disease.
[g] A subset of the events was combined in a "global index" defined as the earliest occurrence of CHD events, invasive breast cancer, stroke, pulmonary embolism, colorectal cancer, hip fracture, or death due to other causes.

17.2 Possible Serious Adverse Reactions With Estrogens

Inform postmenopausal women of possible serious adverse reactions of estrogen therapy including Cardiovascular Disorders, Malignant Neoplasms, and Probable Dementia *[see Warnings and Precautions (5.2, 5.3, 5.4)]*.

17.3 Possible Less Serious But Common Adverse Reactions With Estrogens

Inform postmenopausal women of possible less serious but common adverse reactions of estrogen therapy such as headache, breast pain and tenderness, nausea and vomiting.

17.4 Instructions for Use of Applicator

1. Remove cap from tube.
2. Screw nozzle end of applicator onto tube.

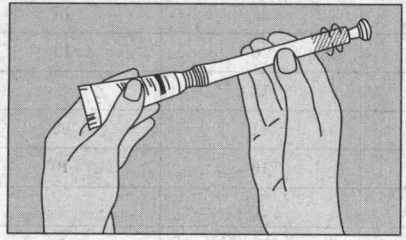

3. *Gently* squeeze tube from the *bottom* to force sufficient cream into the barrel to provide the prescribed dose. Use the marked stopping points on the applicator to measure the correct dose, as prescribed by your healthcare provider.
4. Unscrew applicator from tube.

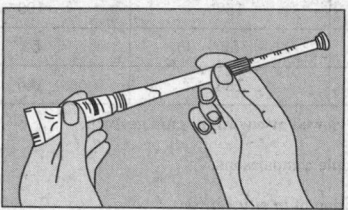

5. Lie on back with knees drawn up. To deliver medication, gently insert applicator deeply into vagina and press plunger downward to its original position.

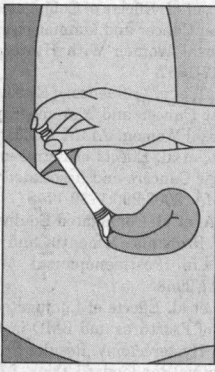

TO CLEANSE: Pull plunger to remove it from barrel. Wash with mild soap and warm water.
DO NOT BOIL OR USE HOT WATER.

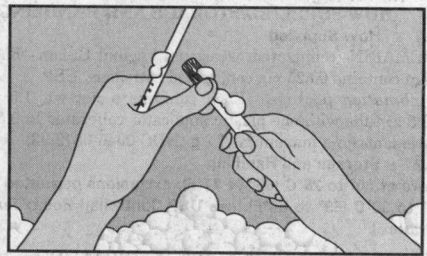

17.5 FDA-Approved Patient Labeling
PREMARIN® (conjugated estrogens) Vaginal Cream
Read this PATIENT INFORMATION before you start using PREMARIN Vaginal Cream and read what you get each time you refill your PREMARIN Vaginal Cream prescrip-

tion. There may be new information. This information does not take the place of talking to your healthcare provider about your menopausal symptoms and their treatment.

What is the most important information I should know about PREMARIN Vaginal Cream (an estrogen mixture)?
- Using estrogen-alone may increase your chance of getting cancer of the uterus (womb)
  Report any unusual vaginal bleeding right away while you are using PREMARIN Vaginal Cream. Vaginal bleeding after menopause may be a warning sign of cancer of the uterus (womb). Your healthcare provider should check any unusual vaginal bleeding to find the cause.
- Do not use estrogen-alone to prevent heart disease, heart attacks, strokes or dementia (decline in brain function)
- Using estrogen-alone may increase your chances of getting strokes or blood clots
- Using estrogen-alone may increase your chance of getting dementia, based on a study of women 65 years or older
- Do not use estrogens with progestins to prevent heart disease, heart attacks, or dementia
- Using estrogens with progestins may increase your chances of getting heart attacks, strokes, breast cancer, or blood clots
- Using estrogens with progestins may increase your chance of getting dementia, based on a study of women age 65 years or older
- You and your healthcare provider should talk regularly about whether you still need treatment with PREMARIN Vaginal Cream

---

What is PREMARIN Vaginal Cream?
PREMARIN Vaginal Cream is a medicine that contains a mixture of estrogen hormones.

What is PREMARIN Vaginal Cream used for?
PREMARIN Vaginal Cream is used after menopause to:
- **Treat menopausal changes in and around the vagina**
  You and your healthcare provider should talk regularly about whether you still need treatment with PREMARIN Vaginal Cream to control these problems.
- **Treat painful intercourse caused by menopausal changes of the vagina**

Who should not use PREMARIN Vaginal Cream?
Do not start using PREMARIN Vaginal Cream if you:
- **Have unusual vaginal bleeding**
- **Currently have or have had certain cancers**
  Estrogens may increase the chance of getting certain types of cancers, including cancer of the breast or uterus. If you have or have had cancer, talk with your healthcare provider about whether you should use PREMARIN Vaginal Cream.
- **Had a stroke or heart attack**
- **Currently have or have had blood clots**
- **Currently have or have had liver problems**
- **Have been diagnosed with a bleeding disorder**
- **Are allergic to PREMARIN Vaginal Cream or any of its ingredients**
  See the list of ingredients in PREMARIN Vaginal Cream at the end of this leaflet.
- **Think you may be pregnant**

Tell your healthcare provider:
- **If you have any unusual vaginal bleeding**
  Vaginal bleeding after menopause may be a warning sign of cancer of the uterus (womb). Your healthcare provider should check any unusual vaginal bleeding to find the cause.
- **About all of your medical problems**
  Your healthcare provider may need to check you more carefully if you have certain conditions, such as asthma (wheezing), epilepsy (seizures), diabetes, migraine, endometriosis, lupus, or problems with your heart, liver, thyroid, kidneys, or have high calcium levels in your blood.
- **About all the medicines you take**
  This includes prescription and nonprescription medicines, vitamins, and herbal supplements. Some medicines may affect how PREMARIN Vaginal Cream works. PREMARIN Vaginal Cream may also affect how your other medicines work.
- **If you are going to have surgery or will be on bedrest**
  You may need to stop using PREMARIN Vaginal Cream.
- **If you are breast feeding**
  The hormones in PREMARIN Vaginal Cream can pass into your milk.

How should I use PREMARIN Vaginal Cream?
PREMARIN Vaginal Cream is a cream that you place in your vagina with the applicator provided with the cream.
- Take the dose recommended by your healthcare provider and talk to him or her about how well that dose is working for you

- Estrogens should be used at the lowest dose possible for your treatment only as long as needed. You and your healthcare provider should talk regularly (for example, every 3 to 6 months) about the dose you are taking and whether you still need treatment with PREMARIN Vaginal Cream
1. Remove cap from tube.
2. Screw nozzle end of applicator onto tube.

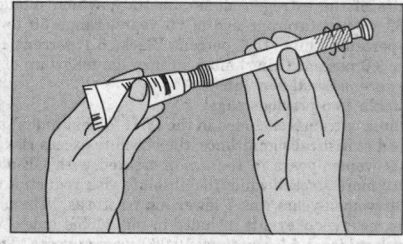

3. *Gently* squeeze tube from the *bottom* to force sufficient cream into the barrel to provide the prescribed dose. Use the marked stopping points on the applicator to measure the correct dose, as prescribed by your healthcare provider.
4. Unscrew applicator from tube.

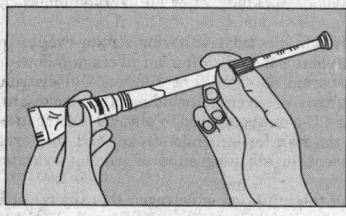

5. Lie on back with knees drawn up. To deliver medication, gently insert applicator deeply into vagina and press plunger downward to its original position.

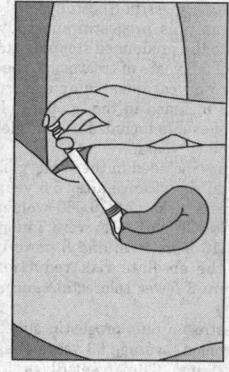

TO CLEANSE: Pull plunger to remove it from barrel. Wash with mild soap and warm water.
DO NOT BOIL OR USE HOT WATER.

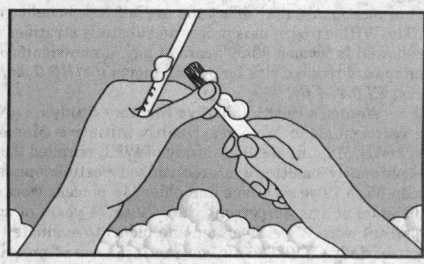

What are the possible side effects of PREMARIN Vaginal Cream?
PREMARIN Vaginal Cream is only used in and around the vagina; however, the risks associated with oral estrogens should be taken into account.
Side effects are grouped by how serious they are and how often they happen when you are treated.
Serious, but less common side effects include:
- Breast cancer
- Cancer of the uterus

- Stroke
- Heart attack
- Blood clots
- Dementia
- Gallbladder disease
- Ovarian cancer
- High blood pressure
- Liver problems
- High blood sugar
- Enlargement of benign tumors of the uterus ("fibroids")

Some of the warning signs of these serious side effects include:
- Breast lumps
- Unusual vaginal bleeding
- Dizziness and faintness
- Changes in speech
- Severe headaches
- Chest pain
- Shortness of breath
- Pains in your legs
- Changes in vision
- Vomiting
- Yellowing of the skin, eyes, or nail beds

Call your healthcare provider right away if you get any of these warning signs, or any other unusual symptoms that concern you.

Less serious, but common, side effects include:
- Headache
- Breast pain
- Irregular vaginal bleeding or spotting
- Stomach/abdominal cramps, bloating
- Nausea and vomiting
- Hair loss
- Fluid retention
- Vaginal yeast infection
- Reactions from inserting PREMARIN Vaginal Cream, such as vaginal burning, irritation, and itching

These are not all the possible side effects of PREMARIN Vaginal Cream. For more information, ask your healthcare provider or pharmacist for advice about side effects. You may report side effects to FDA at 1-800-FDA-1088.

What can I do to lower my chances of getting a serious side effect with PREMARIN Vaginal Cream?
- Talk with your healthcare provider regularly about whether you should continue using PREMARIN Vaginal Cream
- If you have a uterus, talk with your healthcare provider about whether the addition of a progestin is right for you. The addition of a progestin is generally recommended for a woman with a uterus to reduce the chance of getting cancer of the uterus. See your healthcare provider right away if you get vaginal bleeding while using PREMARIN Vaginal Cream
- Have a pelvic exam, breast exam and mammogram (breast X-ray) every year unless your healthcare provider tells you something else. If members of your family have had breast cancer or if you have ever had breast lumps or an abnormal mammogram, you may need to have breast exams more often
- If you have high blood pressure, high cholesterol (fat in the blood), diabetes, are overweight, or if you use tobacco, you may have higher chances for getting heart disease. Ask your healthcare provider for ways to lower your chances for getting heart disease

General information about the safe and effective use of PREMARIN Vaginal Cream
Medicines are sometimes prescribed for conditions that are not mentioned in patient information leaflets. Do not use PREMARIN Vaginal Cream for conditions for which it was not prescribed. Do not give PREMARIN Vaginal Cream to other people, even if they have the same symptoms you have. It may harm them. **Keep PREMARIN Vaginal Cream out of the reach of children.**

Latex or rubber condoms, diaphragms and cervical caps may be weakened and fail when they come into contact with PREMARIN Vaginal Cream.

This leaflet provides a summary of the most important information about PREMARIN Vaginal Cream. If you would like more information, talk with your healthcare provider or pharmacist. You can ask for information about PREMARIN Vaginal Cream that is written for health professionals. You can get more information by calling the toll free number 1-800-934-5556.

What are the ingredients in PREMARIN Vaginal Cream?
PREMARIN Vaginal Cream contains a mixture of conjugated estrogens, which are a mixture of sodium estrone sulfate and sodium equilin sulfate and other components, including sodium sulfate conjugates: 17 α-dihydroequilin, 17 α-estradiol, and 17 β-dihydroequilin. PREMARIN Vaginal Cream also contains cetyl esters wax, cetyl alcohol, white wax, glyceryl monostearate, propylene glycol monostearate, methyl stearate, benzyl alcohol, sodium lauryl sulfate, glycerin, and mineral oil.

PREMARIN (conjugated estrogens) Vaginal Cream—Each gram contains 0.625 mg conjugated estrogens, USP.
Combination package: Each contains a net wt. 1.5 oz (42.5 g) tube with one plastic applicator calibrated in 0.5 g increments to a maximum of 2 g (NDC 0046-0872-93).
Store at 20° to 25°C (68° to 77°F); excursions permitted to 15° to 30°C (59° to 86°F) [see USP Controlled Room Temperature].
Wyeth®
Wyeth Pharmaceuticals Inc.
Philadelphia, PA 19101
<<TEAR HERE
PATIENT INFORMATION
PREMARIN® (conjugated estrogens) Vaginal Cream
Read this PATIENT INFORMATION before you start using PREMARIN Vaginal Cream and read what you get each time you refill your PREMARIN Vaginal Cream prescription. There may be new information. This information does not take the place of talking to your healthcare provider about your menopausal symptoms and their treatment.

What is the most important information I should know about PREMARIN Vaginal Cream (an estrogen mixture)?
- Using estrogen-alone may increase your chance of getting cancer of the uterus (womb)
  Report any unusual vaginal bleeding right away while you are using PREMARIN Vaginal Cream. Vaginal bleeding after menopause may be a warning sign of cancer of the uterus (womb). Your healthcare provider should check any unusual vaginal bleeding to find the cause.
- Do not use estrogen-alone to prevent heart disease, heart attacks, strokes or dementia (decline in brain function)
- Using estrogen-alone may increase your chances of getting strokes or blood clots
- Using estrogen-alone may increase your chance of getting dementia, based on a study of women age 65 years or older
- Do not use estrogens with progestins to prevent heart disease, heart attacks, or dementia
- Using estrogens with progestins may increase your chances of getting heart attacks, strokes, breast cancer, or blood clots
- Using estrogens with progestins may increase your chance of getting dementia, based on a study of women age 65 years or older
- You and your healthcare provider should talk regularly about whether you still need treatment with PREMARIN Vaginal Cream

---

What is PREMARIN Vaginal Cream?
PREMARIN Vaginal Cream is a medicine that contains a mixture of estrogen hormones.
What is PREMARIN Vaginal Cream used for?
PREMARIN Vaginal Cream is used after menopause to:
- **Treat menopausal changes in and around the vagina**
  You and your healthcare provider should talk regularly about whether you still need treatment with PREMARIN Vaginal Cream to control these problems.
- **Treat painful intercourse caused by menopausal changes of the vagina**
Who should not use PREMARIN Vaginal Cream?
Do not start using PREMARIN Vaginal Cream if you:
- **Have unusual vaginal bleeding**
- **Currently have or have had certain cancers**
  Estrogens may increase the chance of getting certain types of cancers, including cancer of the breast or uterus. If you have or have had cancer, talk with your healthcare provider about whether you should use PREMARIN Vaginal Cream.
- **Had a stroke or heart attack**
- **Currently have or have had blood clots**
- **Currently have or have had liver problems**
- **Have been diagnosed with a bleeding disorder**
- **Are allergic to PREMARIN Vaginal Cream or any of its ingredients**
  See the list of ingredients in PREMARIN Vaginal Cream at the end of this leaflet.
- **Think you may be pregnant**
Tell your healthcare provider:
- **If you have any unusual vaginal bleeding**
  Vaginal bleeding after menopause may be a warning sign of cancer of the uterus (womb). Your healthcare provider should check any unusual vaginal bleeding to find the cause.
- **About all of your medical problems**
  Your healthcare provider may need to check you more carefully if you have certain conditions, such as asthma (wheezing), epilepsy (seizures), diabetes, migraine, endometriosis, lupus, or problems with your heart, liver, thyroid, kidneys, or have high calcium levels in your blood.

- **About all the medicines you take**
  This includes prescription and nonprescription medicines, vitamins, and herbal supplements. Some medicines may affect how PREMARIN Vaginal Cream works. PREMARIN Vaginal Cream may also affect how your other medicines work.
- **If you are going to have surgery or will be on bedrest**
  You may need to stop using PREMARIN Vaginal Cream.
- **If you are breast feeding**
  The hormones in PREMARIN Vaginal Cream can pass into your milk.
How should I use PREMARIN Vaginal Cream?
PREMARIN Vaginal Cream is a cream that you place in your vagina with the applicator provided with the cream.
- Take the dose recommended by your healthcare provider and talk to him or her about how well that dose is working for you
- Estrogens should be used at the lowest dose possible for your treatment only as long as needed. You and your healthcare provider should talk regularly (for example, every 3 to 6 months) about the dose you are taking and whether you still need treatment with PREMARIN Vaginal Cream
1. Remove cap from tube.
2. Screw nozzle end of applicator onto tube.

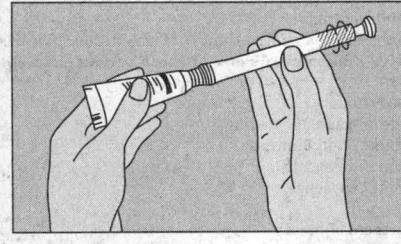

3. *Gently* squeeze tube from the *bottom* to force sufficient cream into the barrel to provide the prescribed dose. Use the marked stopping points on the applicator to measure the correct dose, as prescribed by your healthcare provider.
4. Unscrew applicator from tube.

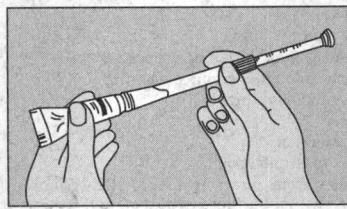

5. Lie on back with knees drawn up. To deliver medication, gently insert applicator deeply into vagina and press plunger downward to its original position.

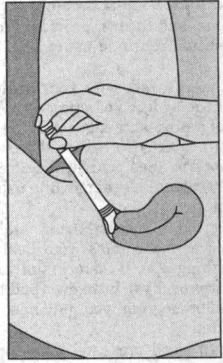

TO CLEANSE: Pull plunger to remove it from barrel. Wash with mild soap and warm water.
DO NOT BOIL OR USE HOT WATER.

[See figure at top of next page]
What are the possible side effects of PREMARIN Vaginal Cream?
PREMARIN Vaginal Cream is only used in and around the vagina; however, the risks associated with oral estrogens should be taken into account.
Side effects are grouped by how serious they are and how often they happen when you are treated.

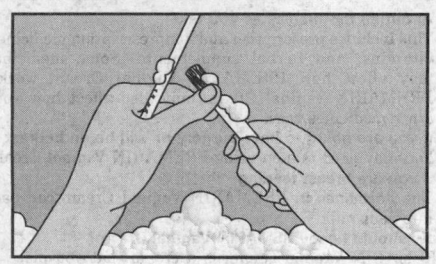

Serious, but less common side effects include:
- Breast cancer
- Cancer of the uterus
- Stroke
- Heart attack
- Blood clots
- Dementia
- Gallbladder disease
- Ovarian cancer
- High blood pressure
- Liver problems
- High blood sugar
- Enlargement of benign tumors of the uterus ("fibroids")

Some of the warning signs of these serious side effects include:
- Breast lumps
- Unusual vaginal bleeding
- Dizziness and faintness
- Changes in speech
- Severe headaches
- Chest pain
- Shortness of breath
- Pains in your legs
- Changes in vision
- Vomiting
- Yellowing of the skin, eyes, or nail beds

Call your healthcare provider right away if you get any of these warning signs, or any other unusual symptoms that concern you.

Less serious, but common, side effects include:
- Headache
- Breast pain
- Irregular vaginal bleeding or spotting
- Stomach/abdominal cramps, bloating
- Nausea and vomiting
- Hair loss
- Fluid retention
- Vaginal yeast infection
- Reactions from inserting PREMARIN Vaginal Cream, such as vaginal burning, irritation, and itching

These are not all the possible side effects of PREMARIN Vaginal Cream. For more information, ask your healthcare provider or pharmacist for advice about side effects. You may report side effects to FDA at 1-800-FDA-1088.

What can I do to lower my chances of getting a serious side effect with PREMARIN Vaginal Cream?
- Talk with your healthcare provider regularly about whether you should continue using PREMARIN Vaginal Cream
- If you have a uterus, talk with your healthcare provider about whether the addition of a progestin is right for you. The addition of a progestin is generally recommended for a woman with a uterus to reduce the chance of getting cancer of the uterus. See your healthcare provider right away if you get vaginal bleeding while using PREMARIN Vaginal Cream
- Have a pelvic exam, breast exam and mammogram (breast X-ray) every year unless your healthcare provider tells you something else. If members of your family have had breast cancer or if you have ever had breast lumps or an abnormal mammogram, you may need to have breast exams more often
- If you have high blood pressure, high cholesterol (fat in the blood), diabetes, are overweight, or if you use tobacco, you may have higher chances for getting heart disease. Ask your healthcare provider for ways to lower your chances for getting heart disease

General information about the safe and effective use of PREMARIN Vaginal Cream

Medicines are sometimes prescribed for conditions that are not mentioned in patient information leaflets. Do not use PREMARIN Vaginal Cream for conditions for which it was not prescribed. Do not give PREMARIN Vaginal Cream to other people, even if they have the same symptoms you have. It may harm them. **Keep PREMARIN Vaginal Cream out of the reach of children.**

Latex or rubber condoms, diaphragms and cervical caps may be weakened and fail when they come into contact with PREMARIN Vaginal Cream.

This leaflet provides a summary of the most important information about PREMARIN Vaginal Cream. If you would like more information, talk with your healthcare provider or pharmacist. You can ask for information about PREMARIN Vaginal Cream that is written for health professionals. You can get more information by calling the toll free number 1-800-934-5556.

What are the ingredients in PREMARIN Vaginal Cream

PREMARIN Vaginal Cream contains a mixture of conjugated estrogens, which are a mixture of sodium estrone sulfate and sodium equilin sulfate and other components, including sodium sulfate conjugates: 17 α-dihydroequilin, 17 α-estradiol, and 17 β-dihydroequilin. PREMARIN Vaginal Cream also contains cetyl esters wax, cetyl alcohol, white wax, glyceryl monostearate, propylene glycol monostearate, methyl stearate, benzyl alcohol, sodium lauryl sulfate, glycerin, and mineral oil.

PREMARIN (conjugated estrogens) Vaginal Cream—Each gram contains 0.625 mg conjugated estrogens, USP.

Combination package: Each contains a net wt. 1.5 oz (42.5 g) tube with one plastic applicator calibrated in 0.5 g increments to a maximum of 2 g (NDC 0046-0872-93).

Store at 20° to 25°C (68° to 77°F); excursions permitted to 15° to 30°C (59° to 86°F) [see USP Controlled Room Temperature].

This product's label may have been updated. For current package insert and further product information, please visit www.wyeth.com or call our medical communications department toll-free at 1-800-934-5556.

Wyeth®
Wyeth Pharmaceuticals Inc.
Philadelphia, PA 19101
W10413C022
ET01
Rev 05/10

PREMPRO® ℞
[prĕm-prō]
(conjugated estrogens/medroxyprogesterone acetate tablets)

PREMPHASE® ℞
[prĕm-făz]
(conjugated estrogens plus medroxyprogesterone acetate tablets)

HIGHLIGHTS OF PRESCRIBING INFORMATION
These highlights do not include all the information needed to use PREMPRO/PREMPHASE safely and effectively. See full prescribing information for PREMPRO/PREMPHASE.
PREMPRO® (conjugated estrogens/medroxyprogesterone acetate tablets)
PREMPHASE® (conjugated estrogens plus medroxyprogesterone acetate tablets)
Initial U.S. Approval: 1995

WARNING: CARDIOVASCULAR DISORDERS, BREAST CANCER, ENDOMETRIAL CANCER and PROBABLE DEMENTIA
See full prescribing information for complete Boxed Warning.
Estrogen Plus Progestin Therapy
- Estrogen plus progestin therapy should not be used for the prevention of cardiovascular disease or dementia (5.1, 5.3)
- The Women's Health Initiative (WHI) estrogen plus progestin substudy reported increased risks of stroke, deep vein thrombosis (DVT), pulmonary embolism, and myocardial infarction (5.1)
- The WHI estrogen plus progestin substudy reported increased risks of invasive breast cancer (5.2)
- The WHI Memory Study (WHIMS) estrogen plus progestin ancillary study of WHI reported an increased risk of probable dementia in postmenopausal women 65 years of age and older (5.3)
Estrogen-Alone Therapy
- There is an increased risk of endometrial cancer in a woman with a uterus who uses unopposed estrogens (5.2)
- Estrogen-alone therapy should not be used for the prevention of cardiovascular disease or dementia (5.1, 5.3)
- The WHI estrogen-alone substudy reported increased risks of stroke and DVT (5.1)
- The WHIMS estrogen-alone ancillary study of WHI reported an increased risk of probable dementia in postmenopausal women 65 years of age and older (5.3)

———RECENT MAJOR CHANGES———
Warnings and Precautions
Angioedema (5.15)   02/2010
———INDICATIONS AND USAGE———
PREMPRO/PREMPHASE is an estrogen/progestin indicated in women with intact uteri for:
- Treatment of Moderate to Severe Vasomotor Symptoms due to Menopause (1.1)
- Treatment of Moderate to Severe Vulvar and Vaginal Atrophy due to Menopause (1.2)
- Prevention of Postmenopausal Osteoporosis (1.3)
———DOSAGE AND ADMINISTRATION———
PREMPRO: one tablet containing conjugated estrogens (CE) plus medroxyprogesterone acetate (MPA) taken orally once daily (2).
PREMPHASE: one maroon tablet containing 0.625 mg CE taken orally on days 1 through 14, and one light-blue tablet containing 0.625 mg CE plus 5.0 mg MPA taken orally on days 15 through 28 (2).
———DOSAGE FORMS AND STRENGTHS———
PREMPRO Tablets (not scored): 0.3 mg CE plus 1.5 mg MPA, 0.45 mg CE plus 1.5 mg MPA, 0.625 mg CE plus 2.5 mg MPA, 0.625 mg CE plus 5 mg MPA.
PREMPHASE Tablets (not scored): 0.625 mg CE, 0.625 mg CE plus 5 mg MPA.
———CONTRAINDICATIONS———
- Undiagnosed abnormal genital bleeding (4)
- Known, suspected, or history of breast cancer (4, 5.2)
- Known or suspected estrogen-dependent neoplasia (4, 5.2)
- Active deep vein thrombosis, pulmonary embolism or a history of these conditions (4, 5.1)
- Active arterial thromboembolic disease (for example, stroke and myocardial infarction) or a history of these conditions (4, 5.1)
- Known liver dysfunction or disease (4, 5.10)
- Known or suspected pregnancy (4, 8.1)
———WARNINGS AND PRECAUTIONS———
- Estrogens increase the risk of gallbladder disease (5.4)
- Discontinue estrogen if severe hypercalcemia, loss of vision, severe hypertriglyceridemia or cholestatic jaundice occurs (5.5, 5.6, 5.9, 5.10)
- Monitor thyroid function in women on thyroid replacement therapy (5.11, 5.18)
———ADVERSE REACTIONS———
In a prospective, randomized, placebo-controlled, double-blind study, the most common adverse reactions ≥ 5 percent are: vaginal hemorrhage, vaginitis, vaginal monoliasis, dysmenorrhea, breast enlargement, breast pain and leg cramps (6.1).
To report SUSPECTED ADVERSE REACTIONS, contact Wyeth Pharmaceuticals Inc. at 1-800-934-5556 or FDA at 1-800-FDA-1088 or www.fda.gov/medwatch
———DRUG INTERACTIONS———
- Inducers and/or inhibitors of CYP3A4 may affect estrogen drug metabolism (7)
- Aminoglutethimide administered concomitantly with MPA may significantly depress the bioavailability of medroxyprogesterone acetate (7)
———USE IN SPECIFIC POPULATIONS———
- Nursing Women: Estrogen administration to nursing women has been shown to decrease the quantity and quality of breast milk (8.3)
- Geriatric Use: An increased risk of probable dementia in women over 65 years of age was reported in the Women's Health Initiative Memory ancillary studies of the Women's Health Initiative (5.3, 8.5)
See 17 for PATIENT COUNSELING INFORMATION and FDA-approved patient labeling

Revised: 02/2010

FULL PRESCRIBING INFORMATION: CONTENTS*
WARNING: CARDIOVASCULAR DISORDERS, BREAST CANCER, ENDOMETRIAL CANCER and PROBABLE DEMENTIA
1   INDICATIONS AND USAGE
    1.1   Treatment of Moderate to Severe Vasomotor Symptoms due to Menopause
    1.2   Treatment of Moderate to Severe Vulvar and Vaginal Atrophy due to Menopause
    1.3   Prevention of Postmenopausal Osteoporosis
2   DOSAGE AND ADMINISTRATION
    2.1   General Dosing Information
    2.2   Treatment of Moderate to Severe Vasomotor Symptoms due to Menopause
    2.3   Treatment of Moderate to Severe Vulvar and Vaginal Atrophy due to Menopause
    2.4   Prevention of Postmenopausal Osteoporosis
3   DOSAGE FORMS AND STRENGTHS
4   CONTRAINDICATIONS
5   WARNINGS AND PRECAUTIONS
    5.1   Cardiovascular Disorders

FULL PRESCRIBING INFORMATION

WARNING: CARDIOVASCULAR DISORDERS, BREAST CANCER, ENDOMETRIAL CANCER and PROBABLE DEMENTIA
Estrogen Plus Progestin Therapy
Cardiovascular Disorders and Probable Dementia
Estrogen plus progestin therapy should not be used for the prevention of cardiovascular disease or dementia *[see Warnings and Precautions (5.1, 5.3), and Clinical Studies (14.6, 14.7)]*.
The Women's Health Initiative (WHI) estrogen plus progestin substudy reported an increased risk of deep vein thrombosis (DVT), pulmonary embolism, stroke and myocardial infarction in postmenopausal women (50 to 79 years of age) during 5.6 years of treatment with daily oral conjugated estrogen (CE) [0.625 mg] combined with medroxyprogesterone acetate (MPA) [2.5 mg], relative to placebo *[see Warnings and Precautions (5.1), and Clinical Studies (14.6)]*.
The WHI Memory Study (WHIMS) estrogen plus progestin ancillary study of the WHI reported an increased risk of developing probable dementia in postmenopausal women 65 years of age or older during 4 years of treatment with daily CE (0.625 mg) combined with MPA (2.5 mg), relative to placebo. It is unknown whether this finding applies to younger postmenopausal women *[see Warnings and Precautions (5.3), Use in Specific Populations (8.5), and Clinical Studies (14.7)]*.

Breast Cancer
The WHI estrogen plus progestin substudy demonstrated an increased risk of invasive breast cancer *[see Warnings and Precautions (5.2), and Clinical Studies (14.6)]*.
In the absence of comparable data, these risks should be assumed to be similar for other doses of CE and MPA and other combinations and dosage forms of estrogens and progestins.
Estrogens with or without progestins should be prescribed at the lowest effective doses and for the shortest duration consistent with treatment goals and risks for the individual woman.
Estrogen-Alone Therapy
Endometrial Cancer
There is an increased risk of endometrial cancer in a woman with a uterus who uses unopposed estrogens. Adding a progestin to estrogen therapy has been shown to reduce the risk of endometrial hyperplasia, which may be a precursor to endometrial cancer. Adequate diagnostic measures, including directed or random endometrial sampling when indicated, should be undertaken to rule out malignancy in postmenopausal women with undiagnosed persistent or recurring abnormal genital bleeding *[see Warnings and Precautions (5.2)]*.
Cardiovascular Disorders and Probable Dementia
Estrogen-alone therapy should not be used for the prevention of cardiovascular disease or dementia *[see Warnings and Precautions (5.1, 5.3), and Clinical Studies (14.6, 14.7)]*.
The WHI estrogen-alone substudy reported increased risks of stroke and deep vein thrombosis (DVT) in postmenopausal women (50 to 79 years of age) during 7.1 years of treatment with daily oral CE (0.625 mg), relative to placebo *[see Warnings and Precautions (5.1), and Clinical Studies (14.6)]*.
The WHIMS estrogen-alone ancillary study of WHI reported an increased risk of developing probable dementia in postmenopausal women 65 years of age or older during 5.2 years of treatment with daily CE (0.625 mg)-alone, relative to placebo. It is unknown whether this finding applies to younger postmenopausal women *[see Warnings and Precautions (5.3), Use in Specific Populations (8.5), and Clinical Studies (14.7)]*.
In the absence of comparable data, these risks should be assumed to be similar for other doses of CE and other dosage forms of estrogens.
Estrogens with or without progestins should be prescribed at the lowest effective doses and for the shortest duration consistent with treatment goals and risks for the individual woman.

1 INDICATIONS AND USAGE

1.1 Treatment of Moderate to Severe Vasomotor Symptoms due to Menopause
1.2 Treatment of Moderate to Severe Vulvar and Vaginal Atrophy due to Menopause
1.3 Prevention of Postmenopausal Osteoporosis

2 DOSAGE AND ADMINISTRATION

2.1 General Dosing Information
Use of estrogen-alone, or in combination with a progestin, should be with the lowest effective dose and for the shortest duration consistent with treatment goals and risks for the individual woman. Postmenopausal women should be re-evaluated periodically as clinically appropriate to determine if treatment is still necessary.
2.2 Treatment of Moderate to Severe Vasomotor Symptoms due to Menopause
PREMPRO therapy consists of a single tablet to be taken orally once daily.
PREMPHASE therapy consists of two separate tablets: one maroon 0.625 mg Premarin (conjugated estrogens) tablet taken daily on days 1 through 14 and one light-blue tablet containing 0.625 mg conjugated estrogens and 5 mg of medroxyprogesterone acetate taken on days 15 through 28.
2.3 Treatment of Moderate to Severe Vulvar and Vaginal Atrophy due to Menopause
PREMPRO therapy consists of a single tablet to be taken orally once daily.
PREMPHASE therapy consists of two separate tablets: one maroon 0.625 mg Premarin [conjugated estrogens (CE)] tablet taken daily on days 1 through 14 and one light-blue tablet containing 0.625 mg CE and 5 mg of medroxyprogesterone acetate (MPA) taken on days 15 through 28. When prescribing solely for the treatment of moderate to severe vulvar and vaginal atrophy, topical vaginal products should be considered.
2.4 Prevention of Postmenopausal Osteoporosis
PREMPRO therapy consists of a single tablet to be taken orally once daily.

PREMPHASE therapy consists of two separate tablets: one maroon 0.625 mg Premarin (conjugated estrogens) tablet taken daily on days 1 through 14 and one light-blue tablet containing 0.625 mg conjugated estrogens and 5 mg of medroxyprogesterone acetate taken on days 15 through 28.

3 DOSAGE FORMS AND STRENGTHS

PREMPRO (conjugated estrogens/medroxyprogesterone acetate tablets)

Tablet Strength	Tablet Shape/Color	Imprint
0.3 mg CE plus 1.5 mg MPA	oval/cream	PREMPRO 0.3/1.5
0.45 mg CE plus 1.5 mg MPA	oval/gold	PREMPRO 0.45/1.5
0.625 mg CE plus 2.5 mg MPA	oval/peach	PREMPRO
0.625 mg CE plus 5 mg MPA	oval/light blue	W 0.625/5

PREMPHASE (conjugated estrogens plus medroxyprogesterone acetate tablets)

Tablet Strength	Tablet Shape/Color	Imprint
0.625 mg CE	oval/maroon (14 tablets)	PREMARIN 0.625
0.625 mg CE plus 5 mg MPA	oval/light-blue (14 tablets)	W 0.625/5

4 CONTRAINDICATIONS

PREMPRO or PREMPHASE therapy should not be used in women with any of the following conditions:
• Undiagnosed abnormal genital bleeding
• Known, suspected, or history of breast cancer
• Known or suspected estrogen-dependent neoplasia
• Active deep vein thrombosis, pulmonary embolism or a history of these conditions
• Active arterial thromboembolic disease (for example, stroke and myocardial infarction), or a history of these conditions
• Known liver dysfunction or disease
• Known or suspected pregnancy

5 WARNINGS AND PRECAUTIONS

5.1 Cardiovascular Disorders
An increased risk of pulmonary embolism, deep vein thrombosis (DVT), stroke and myocardial infarction has been reported with estrogen plus progestin therapy. An increased risk of stroke and DVT has been reported with estrogen-alone therapy. Should any of these occur or be suspected, estrogens with or without progestins should be discontinued immediately.
Risk factors for arterial vascular disease (for example, hypertension, diabetes mellitus, tobacco use, hypercholesterolemia, and obesity) and/or venous thromboembolism (for example, personal history of venous thromboembolism [VTE], obesity, and systemic lupus erythematosus) should be managed appropriately.
Stroke
In the Women's Health Initiative (WHI) estrogen plus progestin substudy, a statistically significant increased risk of stroke was reported in all women receiving daily CE (0.625 mg) plus MPA (2.5 mg) compared to placebo (33 versus 25 per 10,000 women-years) *[see Clinical Studies (14.6)]*. The increase in risk was demonstrated after the first year and persisted.[1] Should a stroke occur or be suspected, estrogen plus progestin therapy should be discontinued immediately.
In the WHI estrogen-alone substudy, a statistically significant increased risk of stroke was reported in women 50 to 79 years of age receiving daily CE (0.625 mg) compared to women in the same age group receiving placebo (45 versus 33 per 10,000 women-years). The increase in risk was demonstrated in year one and persisted *[see Clinical Studies (14.6)]*.
Subgroup analyses of women 50 to 59 years of age suggest no increased risk of stroke for those women receiving CE (0.625 mg) versus those receiving placebo (18 versus 21 per 10,000 women-years).[1]
Coronary Heart Disease
In the WHI estrogen plus progestin substudy, there was a statistically non-significant increased risk of CHD events reported in women receiving daily CE (0.625 mg) plus MPA (2.5 mg) compared to women receiving placebo (41 versus 34 per 10,000 women-years).[1] An increase in relative risk was demonstrated in year 1, and a trend toward decreasing relative risk was reported in years 2 through 5 *[see Clinical Studies (14.6)]*.

In the WHI estrogen-alone substudy, no overall effect on coronary heart disease (CHD) events (defined as nonfatal myocardial infarction [MI], silent MI, or CHD death) was reported in women receiving estrogen-alone compared to placebo[2] *[see Clinical Studies (14.6)].*

Subgroup analyses of women 50 to 59 years of age suggest a statistically non-significant reduction in CHD events (CE 0.625 mg compared to placebo) in women with less than 10 years since menopause (8 versus 16 per 10,000 women-years).[1]

In postmenopausal women with documented heart disease (n = 2,763), average age 66.7 years, in a controlled clinical trial of secondary prevention of cardiovascular disease (Heart and Estrogen/Progestin Replacement Study [HERS]), treatment with daily CE (0.625 mg) plus MPA (2.5 mg) demonstrated no cardiovascular benefit. During an average follow-up of 4.1 years, treatment with CE plus MPA did not reduce the overall rate of CHD events in postmenopausal women with established coronary heart disease. There were more CHD events in the CE plus MPA-treated group than in the placebo group in year 1, but not during subsequent years. Two thousand, three hundred and twenty-one (2,321) women from the original HERS trial agreed to participate in an open label extension of HERS, HERS II. Average follow-up in HERS II was an additional 2.7 years, for a total of 6.8 years overall. Rates of CHD events were comparable among women in the CE (0.625 mg) plus MPA (2.5 mg) group and the placebo group in HERS, HERS II, and overall.

Venous Thromboembolism (VTE)

In the WHI estrogen plus progestin substudy, a statistically significant 2-fold greater rate of VTE (DVT and pulmonary embolism [PE]) was reported in women receiving daily CE (0.625 mg) plus MPA (2.5 mg) compared to women receiving placebo (35 versus 17 per 10,000 women-years). Statistically significant increases in risk for both DVT (26 versus 13 per 10,000 women-years) and PE (18 versus 8 per 10,000 women-years) were also demonstrated. The increase in VTE risk was demonstrated during the first year and persisted[3] *[see Clinical Studies (14.6)].* Should a VTE occur or be suspected, estrogens should be discontinued immediately.

In the WHI estrogen-alone substudy, the risk of VTE (DVT and pulmonary embolism [PE]) was increased for women receiving daily CE (0.625 mg) compared to placebo (30 versus 22 per 10,000 women-years), although only the increased risk of DVT reached statistical significance (23 versus 15 per 10,000 women-years). The increase in VTE risk was demonstrated during the first 2 years[4] *[see Clinical Studies (14.6)].*

If feasible, estrogens should be discontinued at least 4 to 6 weeks before surgery of the type associated with an increased risk of thromboembolism, or during periods of prolonged immobilization.

5.2 Malignant Neoplasms

Endometrial Cancer

Endometrial hyperplasia (a possible precursor of endometrial cancer) has been reported to occur at a rate of approximately 1 percent or less with PREMPRO or PREMPHASE. An increased risk of endometrial cancer has been reported with the use of unopposed estrogen therapy in a woman with a uterus. The reported endometrial cancer risk among unopposed estrogen users is about 2 to 12 times greater than in nonusers, and appears dependent on duration of treatment and on estrogen dose. Most studies show no significant increased risk associated with use of estrogens for less than 1 year. The greatest risk appears to be associated with prolonged use, with increased risks of 15- to 24-fold for 5 to 10 years or more, and this risk has been shown to persist for at least 8 to 15 years after estrogen therapy is discontinued.

Clinical surveillance of all women using estrogen-alone or estrogen plus progestin therapy is important. Adequate diagnostic measures, including directed or random endometrial sampling when indicated, should be undertaken to rule out malignancy in postmenopausal women with undiagnosed persistent or recurring abnormal genital bleeding.

There is no evidence that the use of natural estrogens results in a different endometrial risk profile than synthetic estrogens of equivalent estrogen dose. Adding a progestin to estrogen therapy in postmenopausal women has been shown to reduce the risk of endometrial hyperplasia, which may be a precursor to endometrial cancer.

Breast Cancer

The most important randomized clinical trial providing information about breast cancer in estrogen plus progestin users is the Women's Health Initiative (WHI) substudy of daily CE (0.625 mg) plus MPA (2.5 mg). After a mean follow-up of 5.6 years, the estrogen plus progestin WHI substudy reported an increased risk of breast cancer in women who took daily CE plus MPA. In this substudy, prior use of estrogen-alone or estrogen plus progestin therapy was reported by 26 percent of the women. The relative risk of invasive breast cancer was 1.24, and the absolute risk was 41 versus 33 cases per 10,000 women-years, for estrogen plus progestin compared with placebo.[5] Among women who reported prior use of hormone therapy, the relative risk of invasive breast cancer was 1.86, and the absolute risk was 46 versus 25 cases per 10,000 women-years, for estrogen plus progestin compared with placebo. Among women who reported no prior use of hormone therapy, the relative risk of invasive breast cancer was 1.09, and the absolute risk was 40 versus 36 cases per 10,000 women-years for estrogen plus progestin compared with placebo. In the same substudy, invasive breast cancers were larger and diagnosed at a more advanced stage in the CE (0.625 mg) plus MPA (2.5 mg) group compared with the placebo group. Metastatic disease was rare, with no apparent difference between the two groups. Other prognostic factors, such as histologic subtype, grade and hormone receptor status did not differ between the groups *[see Clinical Studies (14.6)].*

The most important randomized clinical trial providing information about breast cancer in estrogen-alone users is the Women's Health Initiative (WHI) substudy of daily CE (0.625 mg). In the WHI estrogen-alone substudy, after an average follow-up of 7.1 years, daily CE (0.625 mg) was not associated with an increased risk of invasive breast cancer *[relative risk (RR) 0.80]*[6] *[see Clinical Studies (14.6)].*

Consistent with the WHI clinical trials, observational studies have also reported an increased risk of breast cancer for estrogen plus progestin therapy, and a smaller increased risk for estrogen-alone therapy, after several years of use. The risk increased with duration of use, and appeared to return to baseline over about 5 years after stopping treatment (only the observational studies have substantial data on risk after stopping). Observational studies also suggest that the risk of breast cancer was greater, and became apparent earlier, with estrogen plus progestin therapy as compared to estrogen-alone therapy. However, these studies have not found significant variation in the risk of breast cancer among different estrogen plus progestin combinations, doses, or routes of administration.

The use of estrogen-alone and estrogen plus progestin has been reported to result in an increase in abnormal mammograms requiring further evaluation.

All women should receive yearly breast examinations by a healthcare provider and perform monthly breast self-examinations. In addition, mammography examinations should be scheduled based on patient age, risk factors, and prior mammogram results.

Ovarian Cancer

The WHI estrogen plus progestin substudy reported a statistically non-significant increased risk of ovarian cancer. After an average follow-up of 5.6 years, the relative risk for ovarian cancer for CE plus MPA versus placebo was 1.58 (95 percent nCI 0.77-3.24). The absolute risk for CE plus MPA versus placebo was 4 versus 3 cases per 10,000 women-years.[7] In some epidemiologic studies, the use of estrogen-only products, in particular for 5 or more years, has been associated with an increased risk of ovarian cancer. However, the duration of exposure associated with increased risk is not consistent across all epidemiologic studies, and some report no association.

5.3 Probable Dementia

In the estrogen plus progestin Women's Health Initiative Memory Study (WHIMS), an ancillary study of WHI, a population of 4,532 postmenopausal women 65 to 79 years of age was randomized to daily CE (0.625 mg) plus MPA (2.5 mg) or placebo.

In the WHIMS estrogen plus progestin ancillary study, after an average follow-up of 4 years, 40 women in the CE plus MPA group and 21 women in the placebo group were diagnosed with probable dementia. The relative risk of probable dementia for CE plus MPA versus placebo was 2.05 (95 percent nCI 1.21-3.48). The absolute risk of probable dementia for CE plus MPA versus placebo was 45 versus 22 cases per 10,000 women-years[8] *[see Use in Specific Populations (8.5), and Clinical Studies (14.7)].*

In the WHIMS estrogen-alone ancillary study of WHI, a population of 2,947 hysterectomized women 65 to 79 years of age was randomized to daily CE (0.625 mg) or placebo.

In the WHIMS estrogen-alone ancillary study, after an average follow-up of 5.2 years, 28 women in the estrogen-alone group and 19 women in the placebo group were diagnosed with probable dementia. The relative risk of probable dementia for CE-alone versus placebo was 1.49 (95 percent nCI 0.83-2.66). The absolute risk of probable dementia for CE-alone versus placebo was 37 versus 25 cases per 10,000 women-years[8] *[see Use in Specific Populations (8.5), and Clinical Studies (14.7)].*

When data from the two populations in the WHIMS estrogen-alone and estrogen plus progestin ancillary studies were pooled as planned in the WHIMS protocol, the reported overall relative risk for probable dementia was 1.76 (95 percent nCI 1.19-2.60). Since both ancillary studies were conducted in women 65 to 79 years of age, it is unknown whether these findings apply to younger postmenopausal women[8] *[see Use in Specific Populations (8.5), and Clinical Studies (14.7)].*

5.4 Gallbladder Disease

A 2- to 4-fold increase in the risk of gallbladder disease requiring surgery in postmenopausal women receiving estrogens has been reported.

5.5 Hypercalcemia

Estrogen administration may lead to severe hypercalcemia in women with breast cancer and bone metastases. If hypercalcemia occurs, use of the drug should be stopped and appropriate measures taken to reduce the serum calcium level.

5.6 Visual Abnormalities

Retinal vascular thrombosis has been reported in women receiving estrogens. Discontinue medication pending examination if there is sudden partial or complete loss of vision, or a sudden onset of proptosis, diplopia, or migraine. If examination reveals papilledema or retinal vascular lesions, estrogens should be permanently discontinued.

5.7 Addition of a Progestin When a Woman Has Not Had a Hysterectomy

Studies of the addition of a progestin for 10 or more days of a cycle of estrogen administration or daily with estrogen in a continuous regimen have reported a lowered incidence of endometrial hyperplasia than would be induced by estrogen treatment alone. Endometrial hyperplasia may be a precursor to endometrial cancer.

There are, however, possible risks that may be associated with the use of progestins with estrogens compared to estrogen-alone regimens. These include an increased risk of breast cancer.

5.8 Elevated Blood Pressure

In a small number of case reports, substantial increases in blood pressure have been attributed to idiosyncratic reactions to estrogens. In a large, randomized, placebo-controlled clinical trial, a generalized effect of estrogen therapy on blood pressure was not seen.

5.9 Hypertriglyceridemia

In women with pre-existing hypertriglyceridemia, estrogen therapy may be associated with elevations of plasma triglycerides leading to pancreatitis. Consider discontinuation of treatment if pancreatitis occurs.

5.10 Hepatic Impairment and/or Past History of Cholestatic Jaundice

Estrogens may be poorly metabolized in women with impaired liver function. For women with a history of cholestatic jaundice associated with past estrogen use or with pregnancy, caution should be exercised, and in the case of recurrence, medication should be discontinued.

5.11 Hypothyroidism

Estrogen administration leads to increased thyroid-binding globulin (TBG) levels. Women with normal thyroid function can compensate for the increased TBG by making more thyroid hormone, thus maintaining free T_4 and T_3 serum concentrations in the normal range. Women dependent on thyroid hormone replacement therapy who are also receiving estrogens may require increased doses of their thyroid replacement therapy. These women should have their thyroid function monitored in order to maintain their free thyroid hormone levels in an acceptable range.

5.12 Fluid Retention

Estrogens plus progestins may cause some degree of fluid retention. Women with conditions that might be influenced by this factor, such as cardiac or renal dysfunction, warrant careful observation when estrogens are prescribed.

5.13 Hypocalcemia

Estrogen therapy should be used with caution in women with hypoparathyroidism as estrogen-induced hypocalcemia may occur.

5.14 Exacerbation of Endometriosis

A few cases of malignant transformation of residual endometrial implants have been reported in women treated posthysterectomy with estrogen-alone therapy. For women known to have residual endometriosis post-hysterectomy, the addition of progestin should be considered.

5.15 Angioedema

Exogenous estrogens may induce or exacerbate symptoms of angioedema, particularly in women with hereditary angioedema.

5.16 Exacerbation of Other Conditions

Estrogen therapy may cause an exacerbation of asthma, diabetes mellitus, epilepsy, migraine, porphyria, systemic lupus erythematosus, and hepatic hemangiomas and should be used with caution in women with these conditions.

5.17 Laboratory Tests

Serum follicle stimulating hormone and estradiol levels have not been shown to be useful in the management of moderate to severe vasomotor symptoms and moderate to severe symptoms of vulvar and vaginal atrophy.

5.18 Drug-Laboratory Test Interactions

Accelerated prothrombin time, partial thromboplastin time, and platelet aggregation time; increased platelet count; increased factors II, VII antigen, VIII antigen, VIII coagulant activity, IX, X, XII, VII-X complex, II-VII-X complex, and beta-thromboglobulin; decreased levels of antifactor Xa and antithrombin III, decreased antithrombin III activity; increased levels of fibrinogen and fibrinogen activity; increased plasminogen antigen and activity.

Increased thyroid-binding globulin (TBG) leading to increased circulating total thyroid hormone, as measured by protein-bound iodine (PBI), T_4 levels (by column or by radioimmunoassay), or T_3 levels by radioimmunoassay. T_3 resin uptake is decreased, reflecting the elevated TBG. Free T_4 and free T_3 concentrations are unaltered. Women on thyroid replacement therapy may require higher doses of thyroid hormone.

Other binding proteins may be elevated in serum, for example, corticosteroid binding globulin (CBG), sex hormone binding globulin (SHBG), leading to increased total circulating corticosteroids and sex steroids, respectively. Free hormone concentrations, such as testosterone and estradiol, may be decreased. Other plasma proteins may be increased (angiotensinogen/renin substrate, alpha-1-antitrypsin, ceruloplasmin).

Increased plasma HDL and HDL_2 cholesterol subfraction concentrations, reduced LDL cholesterol concentrations, increased triglyceride levels.

Impaired glucose tolerance.

6 ADVERSE REACTIONS

The following serious adverse reactions are discussed elsewhere in the labeling:
- Cardiovascular Disorders [see Boxed Warning, Warnings and Precautions (5.1)]
- Breast Cancer [see Boxed Warning, Warnings and Precautions, Malignant Neoplasms (5.2)]

6.1 Clinical Study Experience

Because clinical trials are conducted under widely varying conditions, adverse reaction rates observed in the clinical trial of a drug cannot be directly compared to rates in the clinical trials of another drug and may not reflect the rates observed in practice.

In a 1-year clinical trial that included 678 postmenopausal women treated with PREMPRO and 351 postmenopausal women treated with PREMPHASE, the following adverse events occurred at a rate ≥ 5 percent, see Table 1.

TABLE 1: ALL TREATMENT EMERGENT STUDY EVENTS REGARDLESS OF DRUG RELATIONSHIP REPORTED AT A FREQUENCY ≥ 5%

Body System Adverse event	PREMPRO 0.625 mg/ 2.5 mg continuous (n = 340)	PREMPRO 0.625 mg/ 5 mg continuous (n = 338)	PREMPHASE 0.625 mg/ 5 mg sequential (n = 351)
Body As A Whole			
abdominal pain	16%	21%	23%
accidental injury	5%	4%	5%
asthenia	6%	8%	10%
back pain	14%	13%	16%
flu syndrome	10%	13%	12%
headache	36%	28%	37%
infection	16%	16%	18%
pain	11%	13%	12%
pelvic pain	4%	5%	5%
Digestive System			
diarrhea	6%	6%	5%
dyspepsia	6%	6%	5%
flatulence	8%	9%	8%
nausea	11%	9%	11%
Metabolic and Nutritional			
peripheral edema	4%	4%	3%
Musculoskeletal System			
arthralgia	9%	7%	9%
leg cramps	3%	4%	5%
Nervous System			
depression	6%	11%	11%
dizziness	5%	3%	4%
hypertonia	4%	3%	3%
Respiratory System			
pharyngitis	11%	11%	13%
rhinitis	8%	6%	8%
sinusitis	8%	7%	7%
Skin and Appendages			
pruritus	10%	8%	5%
rash	4%	6%	4%
Urogenital System			
breast pain	33%	38%	32%
cervix disorder	4%	4%	5%
dysmenorrhea	8%	5%	13%
leukorrhea	6%	5%	9%
vaginal hemorrhage	2%	1%	3%
vaginitis	7%	7%	5%

TABLE 2: PERCENT OF PATIENTS WITH TREATMENT EMERGENT STUDY EVENTS REGARDLESS OF DRUG RELATIONSHIP REPORTED AT A FREQUENCY ≥ 5% DURING STUDY YEAR 1

Body System Adverse event	Prempro 0.625 mg/2.5 mg continuous (n = 331)	Prempro 0.45 mg/1.5 mg continuous (n = 331)	Prempro 0.3 mg/1.5 mg continuous (n = 327)	Placebo daily (n = 332)
Any adverse event	92%	89%	90%	85%
Body As A Whole				
abdominal pain	17%	16%	13%	11%
accidental injury	10%	9%	9%	9%
asthenia	8%	8%	6%	5%
back pain	12%	13%	12%	12%
flu syndrome	8%	11%	10%	11%
headache	28%	29%	33%	28%
infection	21%	19%	18%	22%
pain	14%	15%	20%	18%
Digestive System				
diarrhea	7%	7%	6%	6%
dyspepsia	8%	8%	8%	14%
flatulence	7%	8%	5%	3%
nausea	7%	10%	8%	9%
Musculoskeletal System				
arthralgia	9%	13%	10%	12%
leg cramps	7%	5%	4%	2%
myalgia	5%	5%	4%	8%
Nervous System				
anxiety	4%	5%	2%	4%
depression	11%	5%	8%	7%
dizziness	3%	5%	5%	5%
insomnia	6%	7%	6%	10%
nervousness	3%	2%	2%	2%
Respiratory System				
cough increased	8%	5%	6%	4%
pharyngitis	11%	8%	9%	11%
rhinitis	8%	9%	10%	13%
sinusitis	8%	8%	10%	7%
upper respiratory infection	10%	9%	11%	11%
Skin and Appendages				
pruritus	4%	5%	5%	2%
Urogenital System				
breast enlargement	5%	3%	2%	<1%
breast pain	26%	21%	13%	9%
dysmenorrhea	5%	6%	3%	<1%
leukorrhea	4%	5%	3%	3%
vaginal hemorrhage	6%	4%	2%	0%
vaginal moniliasis	8%	7%	4%	2%
vaginitis	5%	6%	4%	1%

During the first year of a 2-year clinical trial with postmenopausal women between 40 and 65 years of age (88% Caucasian), 989 postmenopausal women received continuous regimens of PREMPRO, and 332 received placebo tablets. Table 2 summarizes adverse events that occurred at a rate ≥ 5 percent in at least 1 treatment group.

[See table 2 above]

6.2 Postmarketing Experience

The following adverse reactions have been reported with PREMPRO or PREMPHASE. Because these reactions are reported voluntarily from a population of uncertain size, it is not always possible to reliably estimate the frequency or establish a causal relationship to drug exposure.

Genitourinary System
Abnormal uterine bleeding, dysmenorrhea/pelvic pain, increase in size of uterine leiomyomata, vaginitis, vaginal candidiasis, amenorrhea, changes in cervical secretion, ovarian cancer, endometrial hyperplasia, endometrial cancer.

Breasts
Tenderness, enlargement, pain, nipple discharge, galactorrhea, fibrocystic breast changes, breast cancer.

Cardiovascular
Deep and superficial venous thrombosis, pulmonary embolism, superficial thrombophlebitis, myocardial infarction, stroke, increase in blood pressure.

Gastrointestinal
Nausea, vomiting, abdominal pain, bloating, cholestatic jaundice, increased incidence of gallbladder disease, pancreatitis, changes in appetite, ischemic colitis.

Skin
Chloasma or melasma that may persist when drug is discontinued, erythema multiforme, erythema nodosum, loss of scalp hair, hirsutism, pruritus, urticaria, rash, acne.

Eyes
Retinal vascular thrombosis, intolerance of contact lenses.

Central Nervous System (CNS)
Headache, migraine, dizziness, mental depression, exacerbation of chorea, mood disturbances, anxiety, irritability, exacerbation of epilepsy, dementia, growth potentiation of benign meningioma.

Miscellaneous
Increase or decrease in weight, arthralgia, glucose intolerance, edema, changes in libido, angioedema, anaphylactoid/anaphylactic reactions, exacerbation of asthma, increased triglycerides, hypersensitivity.

Additional postmarketing adverse reactions have been reported in patients receiving other forms of hormone therapy.

7 DRUG INTERACTIONS

Data from a single-dose drug-drug interaction study involving conjugated estrogens and medroxyprogesterone acetate indicate that the pharmacokinetic disposition of both drugs is not altered when the drugs are coadministered. No other clinical drug-drug interaction studies have been conducted with CE plus MPA.

7.1 Metabolic Interactions

In vitro and *in vivo* studies have shown that estrogens are metabolized partially by cytochrome P450 3A4 (CYP3A4). Therefore, inducers or inhibitors of CYP3A4 may affect estrogen drug metabolism. Inducers of CYP3A4, such as St. John's Wort (*Hypericum perforatum*) preparations, phenobarbital, carbamazepine, and rifampin, may reduce plasma concentrations of estrogens, possibly resulting in a decrease in therapeutic effects and/or changes in the uterine bleeding profile. Inhibitors of CYP3A4, such as erythromycin, clarithromycin, ketoconazole, itraconazole, ritonavir and grapefruit juice, may increase plasma concentrations of estrogens and may result in side effects.

Aminoglutethimide administered concomitantly with MPA may significantly depress the bioavailability of MPA.

8 USE IN SPECIFIC POPULATIONS

8.1 Pregnancy

PREMPRO and PREMPHASE should not be used during pregnancy [see Contraindications (4)]. There appears to be little or no increased risk of birth defects in children born to women who have used estrogens and progestins as an oral contraceptive inadvertently during early pregnancy.

8.3 Nursing Mothers

PREMPRO and PREMPHASE should not be used during lactation. Estrogen administration to nursing mothers has been shown to decrease the quantity and quality of the breast milk. Detectable amounts of estrogen and progestin

TABLE 3: PHARMACOKINETIC PARAMETERS FOR UNCONJUGATED AND CONJUGATED ESTROGENS (CE) AND MEDROXYPROGESTERONE ACETATE (MPA)

DRUG	2 × 0.625 mg CE/2.5 mg MPA Combination Tablets (n = 54)				2 × 0.625 mg CE/5 mg MPA Combination Tablets (n = 51)			
PK Parameter Arithmetic Mean (%CV)	C_{max} (pg/mL)	t_{max} (h)	$t_{1/2}$ (h)	AUC (pg•h/mL)	C_{max} (pg/mL)	t_{max} (h)	$t_{1/2}$ (h)	AUC (pg•h/mL)
Unconjugated Estrogens								
Estrone	175	7.6	31.6	5358	124	10	62.2	6303
	(23)	(24)	(23)	(34)	(43)	(35)	(137)	(40)
BA* -Estrone	159	7.6	16.9	3313	104	10	26.0	3136
	(26)	(24)	(34)	(40)	(49)	(35)	(100)	(51)
Equilin	71	5.8	9.9	951	54	8.9	15.5	1179
	(31)	(34)	(35)	(43)	(43)	(34)	(53)	(56)
PK Parameter Arithmetic Mean (%CV)	C_{max} (ng/mL)	t_{max} (h)	$t_{1/2}$ (h)	AUC (ng•h/mL)	C_{max} (ng/mL)	t_{max} (h)	$t_{1/2}$ (h)	AUC (ng•h/mL)
Conjugated Estrogens								
Total Estrone	6.6	6.1	20.7	116	6.3	9.1	23.6	151
	(38)	(28)	(34)	(59)	(48)	(29)	(36)	(42)
BA* -Total Estrone	6.4	6.1	15.4	100	6.2	9.1	20.6	139
	(39)	(28)	(34)	(57)	(48)	(29)	(35)	(40)
Total Equilin	5.1	4.6	11.4	50	4.2	7.0	17.2	72
	(45)	(35)	(25)	(70)	(52)	(36)	(131)	(50)
PK Parameter Arithmetic Mean (%CV)	C_{max} (ng/mL)	t_{max} (h)	$t_{1/2}$ (h)	AUC (ng•h/mL)	C_{max} (ng/mL)	t_{max} (h)	$t_{1/2}$ (h)	AUC (ng•h/mL)
Medroxyprogesterone Acetate								
MPA	1.5	2.8	37.6	37	4.8	2.4	46.3	102
	(40)	(54)	(30)	(30)	(31)	(50)	(39)	(28)

BA* = Baseline adjusted
C_{max} = peak plasma concentration
t_{max} = time peak concentration occurs
$t_{1/2}$ = apparent terminal-phase disposition half-life (0.693/λ_z)
AUC = total area under the concentration-time curve

have been identified in the breast milk of mothers receiving these drugs. Caution should be exercised when PREMPRO or PREMPHASE is administered to a nursing woman.

8.4   Pediatric Use
PREMPRO and PREMPHASE are not indicated in children. Clinical studies have not been conducted in the pediatric population.

8.5   Geriatric Use
There have not been sufficient numbers of geriatric women involved in clinical studies utilizing PREMPRO or PREMPHASE to determine whether those over 65 years of age differ from younger subjects in their response to PREMPRO or PREMPHASE.

The Women's Health Initiative Study
In the Women's Health Initiative (WHI) estrogen plus progestin substudy (daily conjugated estrogens 0.625 mg plus medroxyprogesterone acetate 2.5 mg), there was a higher relative risk of nonfatal stroke and invasive breast cancer in women greater than 65 years of age [see Clinical Studies (14.6)].
In the WHI estrogen-alone substudy (daily CE [0.625 mg] versus placebo), there was a higher relative risk of stroke in women greater than 65 years of age [see Clinical Studies (14.6)].

The Women's Health Initiative Memory Study
In the Women's Health Initiative Memory Study (WHIMS) of postmenopausal women 65 to 79 years of age, there was an increased risk of developing probable dementia in women receiving estrogen plus progestin or estrogen-alone when compared to placebo. It is unknown whether this finding applies to younger postmenopausal women [see Clinical Studies (14.7)].
Since both ancillary studies were conducted in women 65 to 79 years of age, it is unknown whether these findings apply to younger postmenopausal women[8] [see Clinical Studies (14.7)].

8.6   Renal Impairment
The effects of renal impairment on PREMPRO or PREMPHASE pharmacokinetics have not been studied.

8.7   Hepatic Impairment
The effects of hepatic impairment on PREMPRO or PREMPHASE pharmacokinetics have not been studied.

10   OVERDOSAGE
Overdosage of estrogen or estrogen plus progestin may cause nausea and vomiting, breast tenderness, abdominal pain, drowsiness/fatigue, and withdrawal bleeding may occur in women. Treatment of overdose consists of discontinuation of PREMPRO or PREMPHASE therapy with institution of appropriate symptomatic care.

11   DESCRIPTION
Premarin (conjugated estrogens tablets, USP) for oral administration contains a mixture obtained exclusively from natural sources, occurring as the sodium salts of water-soluble estrogen sulfates blended to represent the average composition of material derived from pregnant mares' urine. It is a mixture of sodium estrone sulfate and sodium equilin sulfate. It contains as concomitant components, as sodium sulfate conjugates, 17 α-dihydroequilin, 17 α-estradiol and 17 β-dihydroequilin.
Medroxyprogesterone acetate is a derivative of progesterone. It is a white to off-white, odorless, crystalline powder, stable in air, melting between 200°C and 210°C. It is freely soluble in chloroform, soluble in acetone and in dioxane, sparingly soluble in alcohol and in methanol, slightly soluble in ether, and insoluble in water. The chemical name for MPA is pregn-4-ene-3, 20-dione, 17-(acetyloxy)-6-methyl-, (6α)-. Its molecular formula is $C_{24}H_{34}O_4$, with a molecular weight of 386.53. Its structural formula is:

PREMPRO 0.3 mg/1.5 mg and 0.45 mg/1.5 mg tablets contain the following inactive ingredients: calcium phosphate tribasic, microcrystalline cellulose, hypromellose, hydroxypropyl cellulose, sucrose, Eudragit NE 30D, lactose monohydrate, magnesium stearate, polyethylene glycol, povidone, titanium dioxide, yellow iron oxide, and black iron oxide.
PREMPRO 0.625 mg/2.5 mg tablets contain the following inactive ingredients: calcium phosphate tribasic, calcium sulfate, carnauba wax, cellulose, glyceryl monooleate, lactose, magnesium stearate, methylcellulose, pharmaceutical glaze, polyethylene glycol, sucrose, povidone, titanium dioxide, red ferric oxide, and black iron oxide.
PREMPRO 0.625 mg/5 mg tablets contain the following inactive ingredients: calcium phosphate tribasic, calcium sulfate, carnauba wax, cellulose, glyceryl monooleate, lactose, magnesium stearate, methylcellulose, pharmaceutical glaze, polyethylene glycol, sucrose, povidone, titanium dioxide, FD&C Blue No. 2, and black iron oxide.

PREMPHASE
Each maroon Premarin tablets for oral administration contain 0.625 mg of conjugated estrogens and the following inactive ingredients: calcium phosphate tribasic, hydroxypropyl cellulose, microcrystalline cellulose, powdered cellulose, hypromellose, lactose monohydrate, magnesium stearate, polyethylene glycol, sucrose, titanium dioxide, FD&C Blue No. 2, and FD&C Red No. 40. These tablets comply with USP Dissolution Test 5.
Each light-blue tablet for oral administration contains 0.625 mg of conjugated estrogens, 5 mg of medroxyprogesterone acetate, and the following inactive ingredients: calcium phosphate tribasic, calcium sulfate, carnauba wax, cellulose, glyceryl monooleate, lactose, magnesium stearate, methylcellulose, pharmaceutical glaze, polyethylene glycol, sucrose, povidone, titanium dioxide, FD&C Blue No. 2, and black iron oxide.

PREMPRO

Tablet Strength	Tablet Color Contains
0.3 mg/1.5 mg	Yellow ferric oxide and black iron oxide
0.45 mg/1.5 mg	Yellow ferric oxide and black iron oxide
0.625 mg/2.5 mg	Red ferric oxide and black iron oxide
0.625 mg/5 mg	FD&C Blue No. 2 and black iron oxide

PREMPHASE

Tablet Strength	Tablet Color Contains
0.625 mg	FD&C Blue No. 2 and FD&C Red No. 40
0.625 mg/5 mg	FD&C Blue No. 2 and black iron oxide

12   CLINICAL PHARMACOLOGY
12.1   Mechanism of Action
Endogenous estrogens are largely responsible for the development and maintenance of the female reproductive system and secondary sexual characteristics. Although circulating estrogens exist in a dynamic equilibrium of metabolic interconversions, estradiol is the principal intracellular human estrogen and is substantially more potent than its metabolites, estrone and estriol, at the receptor level.
The primary source of estrogen in normally cycling adult women is the ovarian follicle, which secretes 70 to 500 mcg of estradiol daily, depending on the phase of the menstrual cycle. After menopause, most endogenous estrogen is produced by conversion of androstenedione, which is secreted by the adrenal cortex, to estrone in the peripheral tissues. Thus, estrone and the sulfate-conjugated form, estrone sulfate, are the most abundant circulating estrogens in postmenopausal women.
Estrogens act through binding to nuclear receptors in estrogen-responsive tissues. To date, two estrogen receptors have been identified. These vary in proportion from tissue to tissue.
Circulating estrogens modulate the pituitary secretion of the gonadotropins, luteinizing hormone (LH) and follicle stimulating hormone (FSH), through a negative feedback mechanism. Estrogens act to reduce the elevated levels of these gonadotropins seen in postmenopausal women.
Parenterally administered medroxyprogesterone acetate (MPA) inhibits gonadotropin production, which in turn prevents follicular maturation and ovulation; although available data indicate that this does not occur when the usually recommended oral dosage is given as single daily doses. MPA may achieve its beneficial effect on the endometrium in part by decreasing nuclear estrogen receptors and suppression of epithelial DNA synthesis in endometrial tissue. Androgenic and anabolic effects of MPA have been noted, but the drug is apparently devoid of significant estrogenic activity.

12.2   Pharmacodynamics
Currently, there are no pharmacodynamic data known for PREMPRO or PREMPHASE tablets.

12.3   Pharmacokinetics
Absorption
PREMPRO and PREMPHASE contain a formulation of medroxyprogesterone acetate (MPA) that is immediately released and conjugated estrogens that are slowly released over several hours.
Conjugated estrogens are water-soluble and are well-absorbed from the gastrointestinal tract after release from the drug formulation. MPA is well absorbed from the gastrointestinal tract. Table 3 and Table 4 summarize the mean pharmacokinetic parameters for select unconjugated and conjugated estrogens and medroxyprogesterone acetate following administration of PREMPRO to healthy, postmenopausal women.
[See table 3 above]

TABLE 4. PHARMACOKINETIC PARAMETERS FOR UNCONJUGATED AND CONJUGATED ESTROGENS (CE) AND MEDROXYPROGESTERONE ACETATE (MPA)

DRUG	4×0.45 mg CE/1.5 mg MPA Combination (n = 65)			
PK Parameter Arithmetic Mean (%CV)	C_{max} (pg/mL)	t_{max} (h)	$t_{1/2}$ (h)	AUC (pg•h/mL)
Unconjugated Estrogens				
Estrone	149 (35)	8.9 (35)	37.5 (35)	6641 (39)
BA* -Estrone	130 (40)	8.9 (35)	21.2 (35)	3799 (47)
Equilin	83 (38)	8.3 (48)	15.9 (44)	1889 (40)
PK Parameter Arithmetic Mean (%CV)	C_{max} (ng/mL)	t_{max} (h)	$t_{1/2}$ (h)	AUC (ng•h/mL)
Conjugated Estrogens				
Total Estrone	5.4 (49)	7.9 (48)	22.4 (53)	119 (48)
BA* -Total Estrone	5.2 (48)	7.9 (48)	15.1 (29)	100 (47)
Total Equilin	4.3 (42)	6.5 (45)	11.6 (31)	74 (48)
PK Parameter Arithmetic Mean (%CV)	C_{max} (ng/mL)	t_{max} (h)	$t_{1/2}$ (h)	AUC (ng•h/mL)
Medroxyprogesterone Acetate				
MPA	0.7 (66)	2.0 (52)	26.2 (35)	5.0 (61)

BA* = Baseline adjusted
C_{max} = peak plasma concentration
t_{max} = time peak concentration occurs
$t_{1/2}$ = apparent terminal-phase disposition half-life $(0.693/\lambda_z)$
AUC = total area under the concentration-time curve

TABLE 5: SUMMARY TABULATION OF THE NUMBER OF HOT FLUSHES PER DAY – MEAN VALUES AND COMPARISONS BETWEEN THE ACTIVE TREATMENT GROUPS AND THE PLACEBO GROUP – PATIENTS WITH AT LEAST 7 MODERATE TO SEVERE FLUSHES PER DAY OR AT LEAST 50 PER WEEK AT BASELINE, LAST OBSERVATION CARRIED FORWARD (LOCF)

Treatment[a] (No. of Patients) Time Period (week)	No. of Hot Flushes/Day			
	Baseline Mean ± SD	Observed Mean ± SD	Mean Change ± SD	p-Values vs. Placebo[b]
0.625 mg/2.5 mg (n = 34)				
4	11.98 ± 3.54	3.19 ± 3.74	-8.78 ± 4.72	<0.001
12	11.98 ± 3.54	1.16 ± 2.22	-10.82 ± 4.61	<0.001
0.45 mg/1.5 mg (n = 29)				
4	12.61 ± 4.29	3.64 ± 3.61	-8.98 ± 4.74	<0.001
12	12.61 ± 4.29	1.69 ± 3.36	-10.92 ± 4.63	<0.001
0.3 mg/1.5 mg (n = 33)				
4	11.30 ± 3.13	3.70 ± 3.29	-7.60 ± 4.71	<0.001
12	11.30 ± 3.13	1.31 ± 2.82	-10.00 ± 4.60	<0.001
Placebo (n = 28)				
4	11.69 ± 3.87	7.89 ± 5.28	-3.80 ± 4.71	-
12	11.69 ± 3.87	5.71 ± 5.22	-5.98 ± 4.60	-

[a] Identified by dosage (mg) of Premarin/MPA or placebo.
[b] There were no statistically significant differences between the 0.625 mg/2.5 mg, 0.45 mg/1.5 mg, and 0.3 mg/1.5 mg groups at any time period.

TABLE 6: INCIDENCE OF ENDOMETRIAL HYPERPLASIA AFTER ONE YEAR OF TREATMENT

	Groups			
	PREMPRO 0.625 mg/2.5 mg	PREMPRO 0.625 mg/5 mg	PREMPHASE 0.625 mg/5 mg	Premarin 0.625 mg
Total number of patients	340	338	351	347
Number of patients with evaluable biopsies	279	274	277	283
No. (%) of patients with biopsies:				
• All focal and non-focal hyperplasia	2 (<1)*	0 (0)*	3 (1)*	57 (20)
• Excluding focal cystic hyperplasia	2 (<1)*	0 (0)*	1 (<1)*	25 (8)

*Significant (p < 0.001) in comparison with Premarin (0.625 mg) alone.

Food-Effect: Single dose studies in healthy, postmenopausal women were conducted to investigate any potential drug interaction when PREMPRO or PREMPHASE is administered with a high-fat breakfast. Administration with food decreased the C_{max} of total estrone by 18 to 34 percent and increased total equilin C_{max} by 38 percent compared to the fasting state, with no other effect on the rate or extent of absorption of other conjugated or unconjugated estrogens. Administration with food approximately doubles MPA C_{max} and increases MPA AUC by approximately 20 to 30 percent.
Dose Proportionality: The C_{max} and AUC values for MPA observed in two separate pharmacokinetic studies conducted with 2 PREMPRO 0.625 mg/2.5 mg or 2 PREMPRO or PREMPHASE 0.625 mg/5 mg tablets exhibited nonlinear dose proportionality; doubling the MPA dose from 2×2.5 to 2×5 mg increased the mean C_{max} and AUC by 3.2- and 2.8-fold, respectively.

The dose proportionality of estrogens and medroxyprogesterone acetate was assessed by combining pharmacokinetic data across another two studies totaling 61 healthy, postmenopausal women. Single conjugated estrogens doses of 2×0.3 mg, 2×0.45 mg, or 2×0.625 mg were administered either alone or in combination with medroxyprogesterone acetate doses of 2×1.5 mg or 2×2.5 mg. Most of the estrogen components demonstrated dose proportionality; however, several estrogen components did not. Medroxyprogesterone acetate pharmacokinetic parameters increased in a dose-proportional manner.

Distribution
The distribution of exogenous estrogens is similar to that of endogenous estrogens. Estrogens are widely distributed in the body and are generally found in higher concentrations in the sex hormone target organs. Estrogens circulate in the blood largely bound to sex hormone-binding globulin (SHBG) and albumin. MPA is approximately 90 percent bound to plasma proteins, but does not bind to SHBG.

Metabolism
Exogenous estrogens are metabolized in the same manner as endogenous estrogens. Circulating estrogens exist in a dynamic equilibrium of metabolic interconversions. These transformations take place mainly in the liver. Estradiol is converted reversibly to estrone, and both can be converted to estriol, which is a major urinary metabolite. Estrogens also undergo enterohepatic recirculation via sulfate and glucuronide conjugation in the liver, biliary secretion of conjugates into the intestine, and hydrolysis in the intestine followed by reabsorption. In postmenopausal women, a significant portion of the circulating estrogens exists as sulfate conjugates, especially estrone sulfate, which serves as a circulating reservoir for the formation of more active estrogens. Metabolism and elimination of MPA occur primarily in the liver via hydroxylation, with subsequent conjugation and elimination in the urine.

Excretion
Estradiol, estrone, and estriol are excreted in the urine, along with glucuronide and sulfate conjugates. Most metabolites of MPA are excreted as glucuronide conjugates, with only minor amounts excreted as sulfates.

Specific Populations
No pharmacokinetic studies were conducted in specific populations, including patients with renal or hepatic impairment.

13 NONCLINICAL TOXICOLOGY

13.1 Carcinogenesis, Mutagenesis, Impairment of Fertility
Long-term continuous administration of natural and synthetic estrogens in certain animal species increases the frequency of carcinomas of the breasts, uterus, cervix, vagina, testis, and liver.

14 CLINICAL STUDIES

14.1 Effects on Vasomotor Symptoms
In the first year of the Health and Osteoporosis, Progestin and Estrogen (HOPE) Study, a total of 2,805 postmenopausal women (average age 53.3 ± 4.9 years) were randomly assigned to one of eight treatment groups of either placebo or conjugated estrogens, with or without medroxyprogesterone acetate. Efficacy for vasomotor symptoms was assessed during the first 12 weeks of treatment in a subset of symptomatic women (n = 241) who had at least seven moderate to severe hot flushes daily, or at least 50 moderate to severe hot flushes during the week before randomization. With PREMPRO 0.625 mg/2.5 mg, 0.45 mg/1.5 mg, and 0.3 mg/1.5 mg, the relief of both the frequency and severity of moderate-to-severe vasomotor symptoms was shown to be statistically improved compared to placebo at weeks 4 and 12. Table 5 shows the adjusted mean number of hot flushes in the PREMPRO 0.625 mg/2.5 mg, 0.45 mg/1.5 mg, 0.3 mg/1.5 mg, and placebo groups during the initial 12-week period.
[See table 5 above]

14.2 Effects on Vulvar and Vaginal Atrophy
Results of vaginal maturation indexes at cycles 6 and 13 showed that the differences from placebo were statistically significant (p < 0.001) for all treatment groups.

14.3 Effects on the Endometrium
In a 1-year clinical trial of 1,376 women (average age 54 ± 4.6 years) randomized to PREMPRO 0.625 mg/2.5 mg (n = 340), PREMPRO 0.625 mg/5 mg (n = 338), PREMPHASE 0.625 mg/5 mg (n = 351), or Premarin 0.625 mg alone (n = 347), results of evaluable biopsies at 12 months (n = 279, 274, 277, and 283, respectively) showed a reduced risk of endometrial hyperplasia in the two PREMPRO treatment groups (less than 1 percent) and in the PREMPHASE treatment group (less than 1 percent; 1 percent when focal hyperplasia was included) compared to the Premarin group (8 percent; 20 percent when focal hyperplasia was included), see Table 6.
[See table 6 above]

In the first year of the Health and Osteoporosis, Progestin and Estrogen (HOPE) Study, 2,001 women (average age 53.3 ± 4.9 years), of whom 88 percent were Caucasian, were treated with either Premarin 0.625 mg alone (n = 348), Premarin 0.45 mg alone (n = 338), Premarin 0.3 mg alone (n = 326) or PREMPRO 0.625 mg/2.5 mg (n = 331), PREMPRO 0.45 mg/1.5 mg (n = 331) or PREMPRO 0.3 mg/1.5 mg (n = 327). Results of evaluable endometrial biopsies at 12 months showed a reduced risk of endometrial hyperplasia or cancer in the PREMPRO treatment groups compared with the corresponding Premarin alone treatment groups, except for the PREMPRO 0.3 mg/1.5 mg and Premarin 0.3 mg alone groups, in each of which there was only 1 case, see Table 7.

No endometrial hyperplasia or cancer was noted in those patients treated with the continuous combined regimens who continued for a second year in the osteoporosis and metabolic substudy of the HOPE study, see Table 8.
[See table 7 at top of next page]
[See table 8 on next page]

14.4 Effects on Uterine Bleeding or Spotting

The effects of PREMPRO on uterine bleeding or spotting, as recorded on daily diary cards, were evaluated in 2 clinical trials. Results are shown in Figures 1 and 2.

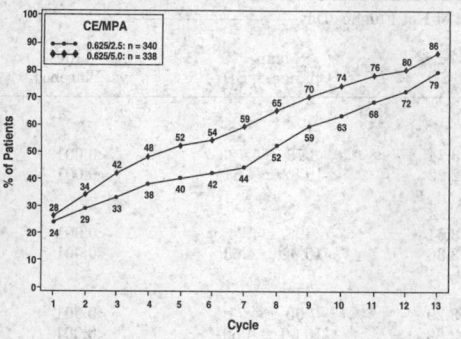

FIGURE 1. PATIENTS WITH CUMULATIVE AMENORRHEA OVER TIME PERCENTAGES OF WOMEN WITH NO BLEEDING OR SPOTTING AT A GIVEN CYCLE THROUGH CYCLE 13 INTENT-TO-TREAT POPULATION, LOCF

Note: The percentage of patients who were amenorrheic in a given cycle and through cycle 13 is shown. If data were missing, the bleeding value from the last reported day was carried forward (LOCF).

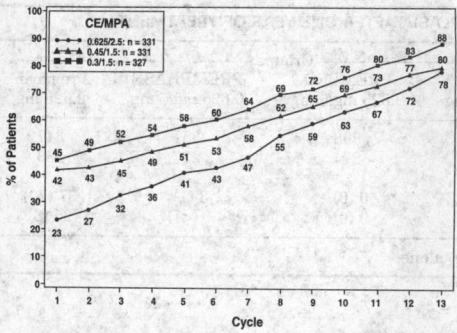

FIGURE 2. PATIENTS WITH CUMULATIVE AMENORRHEA OVER TIME PERCENTAGES OF WOMEN WITH NO BLEEDING OR SPOTTING AT A GIVEN CYCLE THROUGH CYCLE 13 INTENT-TO-TREAT POPULATION, LOCF

Note: The percentage of patients who were amenorrheic in a given cycle and through cycle 13 is shown. If data were missing, the bleeding value from the last reported day was carried forward (LOCF).

14.5 Effects on Bone Mineral Density

Health and Osteoporosis, Progestin and Estrogen (HOPE) Study

The HOPE study was a double-blind, randomized, placebo/active-drug-controlled, multicenter study of healthy post-menopausal women with an intact uterus. Subjects (mean age 53.3 ± 4.9 years) were 2.3 ± 0.9 years on average since menopause and took one 600 mg tablet of elemental calcium (Caltrate™) daily. Subjects were not given Vitamin D supplements. They were treated with PREMPRO 0.625 mg/2.5 mg, 0.45 mg/1.5 mg or 0.3 mg/1.5 mg, comparable doses of Premarin alone, or placebo. Prevention of bone loss was assessed by measurement of bone mineral density (BMD), primarily at the anteroposterior lumbar spine (L_2 to L_4). Secondarily, BMD measurements of the total body, femoral neck, and trochanter were also analyzed. Serum osteocalcin, urinary calcium, and N-telopeptide were used as bone turn-over markers (BTM) at cycles 6, 13, 19, and 26.

Intent-to-treat subjects

All active treatment groups showed significant differences from placebo in each of the four BMD endpoints. These significant differences were seen at cycles 6, 13, 19, and 26. The percent changes from baseline to final evaluation are shown in Table 9.

[See table 9 at right]

Figure 3 shows the cumulative percentage of subjects with percent changes from baseline in spine BMD equal to or greater than the percent change shown on the x-axis.

[See figure 3 at top of next page]

The mean percent changes from baseline in L2 to L4 BMD for women who completed the bone density study are shown with standard error bars by treatment group in Figure 4. Significant differences between each of the PREMPRO dos-

age groups and placebo were found at cycles 6, 13, 19, and 26.

[See figure 4 on next page]

The bone turnover markers, serum osteocalcin and urinary N-telopeptide, significantly decreased ($p < 0.001$) in all active-treatment groups at cycles 6, 13, 19, and 26 compared with the placebo group. Larger mean decreases from baseline were seen with the active groups than with the placebo group. Significant differences from placebo were seen less frequently in urine calcium; only with PREMPRO

0.625 mg/2.5 mg and 0.45 mg/1.5 mg were there significantly larger mean decreases than with placebo at 3 or more of the 4 time points.

14.6 Women's Health Initiative Studies

The Women's Health Initiative (WHI) enrolled approximately 27,000 predominantly healthy post-menopausal women in two substudies to assess the risks and benefits of daily oral CE (0.625 mg)-alone or in combination with MPA (2.5 mg) compared to placebo in the prevention of certain chronic diseases. The primary endpoint was the incidence of

TABLE 7: INCIDENCE OF ENDOMETRIAL HYPERPLASIA/CANCER[a] AFTER ONE YEAR OF TREATMENT[b]

Patient	Prempro 0.625 mg/ 2.5 mg	Premarin 0.625 mg	Prempro 0.45 mg/ 1.5 mg	Premarin 0.45 mg	Prempro 0.3 mg/ 1.5 mg	Premarin 0.3 mg
Total number of patients	331	348	331	338	327	326
Number of patients with evaluable biopsies	278	249	272	279	271	269
No. (%) of patients with biopsies:						
• Hyperplasia/cancer[a] (consensus[c])	0 (0)[d]	20 (8)	1 (<1)[a,d]	9 (3)	1 (<1)[e]	1 (<1)[a]

[a] All cases of hyperplasia/cancer were endometrial hyperplasia except for 1 patient in the Premarin 0.3 mg group diagnosed with endometrial cancer based on endometrial biopsy and 1 patient in the Premarin/MPA 0.45 mg/1.5 mg group diagnosed with endometrial cancer based on endometrial biopsy.
[b] Two (2) primary pathologists evaluated each endometrial biopsy. Where there was lack of agreement on the presence or absence of hyperplasia/cancer between the two, a third pathologist adjudicated (consensus).
[c] For an endometrial biopsy to be counted as consensus endometrial hyperplasia or cancer, at least 2 pathologists had to agree on the diagnosis.
[d] Significant ($p < 0.05$) in comparison with corresponding dose of Premarin alone.
[e] Non-significant in comparison with corresponding dose of Premarin alone.

TABLE 8: OSTEOPOROSIS AND METABOLIC SUBSTUDY, INCIDENCE OF ENDOMETRIAL HYPERPLASIA/CANCER[a] AFTER TWO YEARS OF TREATMENT[b]

Patient	Prempro 0.625 mg/ 2.5 mg	Premarin 0.625 mg	Prempro 0.45 mg/ 1.5 mg	Premarin 0.45 mg	Prempro 0.3 mg/ 1.5 mg	Premarin 0.3 mg
Total number of patients	75	65	75	74	79	73
Number of patients with evaluable biopsies	62	55	69	67	75	63
No. (%) of patients with biopsies:						
• Hyperplasia/cancer[a] (consensus[c])	0 (0)[d]	15 (27)	0 (0)[d]	10 (15)	0 (0)[d]	2 (3)

[a] All cases of hyperplasia/cancer were endometrial hyperplasia in patients who continued for a second year in the osteoporosis and metabolic substudy of the HOPE study.
[b] Two (2) primary pathologists evaluated each endometrial biopsy. Where there was lack of agreement on the presence or absence of hyperplasia/cancer between the two, a third pathologist adjudicated (consensus).
[c] For an endometrial biopsy to be counted as consensus endometrial hyperplasia or cancer, at least 2 pathologists had to agree on the diagnosis.
[d] Significant ($p < 0.05$) in comparison with corresponding dose of Premarin alone.

TABLE 9: PERCENT CHANGE IN BONE MINERAL DENSITY: COMPARISON BETWEEN ACTIVE AND PLACEBO GROUPS IN THE INTENT-TO-TREAT POPULATION, LOCF

Region Evaluated Treatment Group[a]	No. of Subjects	Baseline (g/cm²) Mean ± SD	Change from Baseline (%) Adjusted Mean ± SE	p-Value vs. Placebo
L_2 to L_4 BMD				
0.625/2.5	81	1.14 ± 0.16	3.28 ± 0.37	<0.001
0.45/1.5	89	1.16 ± 0.14	2.18 ± 0.35	<0.001
0.3/1.5	90	1.14 ± 0.15	1.71 ± 0.35	<0.001
Placebo	85	1.14 ± 0.14	-2.45 ± 0.36	
Total body BMD				
0.625/2.5	81	1.14 ± 0.08	0.87 ± 0.17	<0.001
0.45/1.5	89	1.14 ± 0.07	0.59 ± 0.17	<0.001
0.3/1.5	91	1.13 ± 0.08	0.60 ± 0.16	<0.001
Placebo	85	1.13 ± 0.08	-1.50 ± 0.17	
Femoral neck BMD				
0.625/2.5	81	0.89 ± 0.14	1.62 ± 0.46	<0.001
0.45/1.5	89	0.89 ± 0.12	1.48 ± 0.44	<0.001
0.3/1.5	91	0.86 ± 0.11	1.31 ± 0.43	<0.001
Placebo	85	0.88 ± 0.14	-1.72 ± 0.45	
Femoral trochanter BMD				
0.625/2.5	81	0.77 ± 0.14	3.35 ± 0.59	0.002
0.45/1.5	89	0.76 ± 0.12	2.84 ± 0.57	0.011
0.3/1.5	91	0.76 ± 0.12	3.93 ± 0.56	<0.001
Placebo	85	0.75 ± 0.12	0.81 ± 0.58	

[a] Identified by dosage (mg/mg) of Premarin/MPA or placebo.

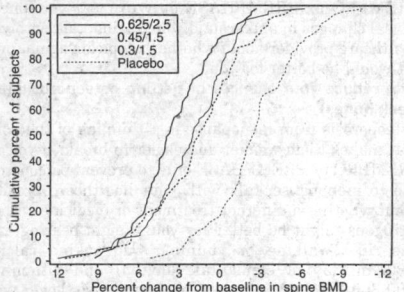

FIGURE 3. CUMULATIVE PERCENT OF SUBJECTS WITH CHANGES FROM BASELINE IN SPINE BMD OF GIVEN MAGNITUDE OR GREATER IN PREMARIN/MPA AND PLACEBO GROUPS

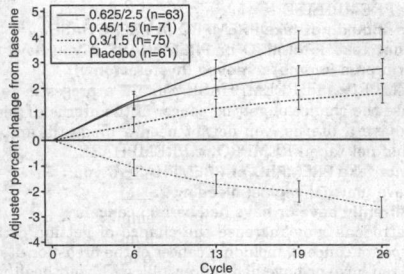

FIGURE 4. ADJUSTED MEAN (SE) PERCENT CHANGE FROM BASELINE AT EACH CYCLE IN SPINE BMD: SUBJECTS COMPLETING IN PREMARIN/MPA GROUPS AND PLACEBO

coronary heart disease [(CHD) defined as non-fatal myocardial infarction (MI), silent MI and CHD death], with invasive breast cancer as the primary adverse outcome. A "global index" included the earliest occurrence of CHD, invasive breast cancer, stroke, pulmonary embolism (PE), endometrial cancer (only in the CE plus MPA substudy), colorectal cancer, hip fracture, or death due to other causes. These substudies did not evaluate the effects of CE plus MPA or CE on menopausal symptoms.

WHI Estrogen Plus Progestin Substudy
The WHI estrogen plus progestin substudy was stopped early. According to the predefined stopping rule, after an average follow-up of 5.6 years of treatment, the increased risk of breast cancer and cardiovascular events exceeded the specified benefits included in the "global index." The absolute excess risk of events included in the "global index" was 19 per 10,000 women-years.
For those outcomes included in the WHI "global index" that reached statistical significance after 5.6 years of follow-up, the absolute excess risks per 10,000 women-years in the group treated with CE plus MPA were 7 more CHD events, 8 more strokes, 10 more PEs, and 8 more invasive breast cancers, while the absolute risk reductions per 10,000 women-years were 6 fewer colorectal cancers and 5 fewer hip fractures.
Results of the estrogen plus progestin substudy, which included 16,608 women (average 63 years of age, range 50 to 79; 83.9 percent White, 6.8 percent Black, 5.4 percent Hispanic, 3.9 percent Other) are presented in Table 10. These results reflect centrally adjudicated data after an average follow-up of 5.6 years.
[See table 10 above]
Timing of the initiation of estrogen therapy relative to the start of menopause may affect the overall risk benefit profile. The WHI estrogen plus progestin substudy stratified by age showed in women 50-59 years of age, a non-significant trend toward reduced risk for overall mortality [HR 0.69 (95 percent CI 0.44-1.07)].

WHI Estrogen-Alone Substudy
The WHI estrogen-alone substudy was stopped early because an increased risk of stroke was observed, and it was deemed that no further information would be obtained regarding the risks and benefits of estrogen alone in predetermined primary endpoints.
Results of the estrogen-alone substudy, which included 10,739 women (average age of 63 years, range 50 to 79; 75.3 percent White, 15.1 percent Black, 6.1 percent Hispanic, 3.6 percent Other) after an average follow-up of 7.1 years, are presented in Table 11.
[See table 11 at right]
For those outcomes included in the WHI "global index" that reached statistical significance, the absolute excess risk per 10,000 women-years in the group treated with CE-alone was 12 more strokes while the absolute risk reduction per 10,000 women-years was 7 fewer hip fractures.[9] The absolute excess risk of events included in the "global index" was a non-significant 5 events per 10,000 women-years. There

TABLE 10: Relative and Absolute Risk Seen In The Estrogen Plus Progestin Substudy of WHI at an Average of 5.6 Years[a,b]

Event	Relative Risk CE/MPA vs. Placebo (95% nCI[b])	CE/MPA n = 8,506	Placebo n = 8,102
		Absolute Risk per 10,000 Women-Years	
CHD events	1.23 (0.99–1.53)	41	34
Non-fatal MI[c]	*1.28 (1.00–1.63)*	*31*	*25*
CHD death	*1.10 (0.70–1.75)*	*8*	*8*
All Strokes	1.31 (1.03–1.68)	33	25
Ischemic stroke	*1.44 (1.09–1.90)*	*26*	*18*
Deep vein thrombosis[d]	1.95 (1.43–2.67)	26	13
Pulmonary embolism	2.13 (1.45–3.11)	18	8
Invasive breast cancer[e]	1.24 (1.01–1.54)	41	33
Colorectal cancer	0.61 (0.42–0.87)	10	16
Endometrial cancer[d]	0.81 (0.48–1.36)	6	7
Cervical cancer[d]	1.44 (0.47–4.42)	2	1
Hip fracture[c]	0.67 (0.47–0.96)	11	16
Vertebral fractures[d]	0.65 (0.46–0.92)	11	17
Lower arm/wrist fractures[d]	0.71 (0.59–0.85)	44	62
Total fractures[d]	0.76 (0.69–0.83)	152	199
Overall Mortality[f]	1.00 (0.83–1.19)	52	52
Global Index[g]	1.13 (1.02–1.25)	184	165

[a] Adapted from numerous WHI publications. WHI publications can be viewed at www.nhlbi.nih.gov/whi.
[b] Results are based on centrally adjudicated data.
[c] Nominal confidence intervals unadjusted for multiple looks and multiple comparisons.
[d] Not included in "global index."
[e] Includes metastatic and non-metastatic breast cancer, with the exception of *in situ* breast cancer.
[f] All deaths, except from breast or colorectal cancer, definite/probable CHD, PE or cerebrovascular disease.
[g] A subset of the events was combined in a "global index" defined as the earliest occurrence of CHD events, invasive breast cancer, stroke, pulmonary embolism, colorectal cancer, hip fracture, or death due to other causes.

Table 11: Relative and Absolute Risk Seen in the Estrogen-Alone Substudy of WHI[a]

Event	Relative Risk CE vs. Placebo (95% nCI[b])	CE n = 5,310	Placebo n = 5,429
		Absolute Risk per 10,000 Women-Years	
CHD events[c]	0.95 (0.78–1.16)	54	57
Non-fatal MI[c]	*0.91 (0.73–1.14)*	*40*	*43*
CHD death[c]	*1.01 (0.71–1.43)*	*16*	*16*
All Stroke[c]	1.33 (1.05–1.68)	45	33
Ischemic[c]	*1.55 (1.19–2.01)*	*38*	*25*
Deep vein thrombosis[c,d]	1.47 (1.06–2.06)	23	15
Pulmonary embolism[c]	1.37 (0.90–2.07)	14	10
Invasive breast cancer[c]	0.80 (0.62–1.04)	28	34
Colorectal cancer[e]	1.08 (0.75–1.55)	17	16
Hip fracture[c]	0.65 (0.45–0.94)	12	19
Vertebral fractures[c,d]	0.64 (0.44–0.93)	11	18
Lower arm/wrist fractures[c,d]	0.58 (0.47–0.72)	35	59
Total fractures[c,d]	0.71 (0.64–0.80)	144	197
Death due to other causes[e,f]	1.08 (0.88–1.32)	53	50
Overall mortality[c,d]	1.04 (0.88–1.22)	79	75
Global Index[g]	1.02 (0.92–1.13)	206	201

[a] Adapted from numerous WHI publications. WHI publications can be viewed at www.nhlbi.nih.gov/whi.
[b] Nominal confidence intervals unadjusted for multiple looks and multiple comparisons.
[c] Results are based on centrally adjudicated data for an average follow-up of 7.1 years.
[d] Not included in "global index."
[e] Results are based on an average follow-up of 6.8 years.
[f] All deaths, except from breast or colorectal cancer, definite/probable CHD, PE or cerebrovascular disease.
[g] A subset of the events was combined in a "global index" defined as the earliest occurrence of CHD events, invasive breast cancer, stroke, pulmonary embolism, colorectal cancer, hip fracture, or death due to other causes.

was no difference between the groups in terms of all-cause mortality [see Boxed Warnings, and Warnings and Precautions (5)].
No overall difference for primary CHD events (nonfatal MI, silent MI and CHD death) and invasive breast cancer incidence in women receiving CE-alone compared with placebo was reported in final centrally adjudicated results from the estrogen-alone substudy, after an average follow-up of 7.1 years.
Centrally adjudicated results for stroke events from the estrogen-alone substudy, after an average follow-up of 7.1 years, reported no significant difference in distribution of stroke subtype or severity, including fatal strokes, in women receiving CE-alone compared to placebo. Estrogen-alone increased the risk for ischemic stroke, and this excess risk was present in all subgroups of women examined, see Table 10.[10]
Timing of the initiation of estrogen therapy relative to the start of menopause may affect the overall risk benefit profile. The WHI estrogen-alone substudy stratified by age showed in women 50-59 years of age, a non-significant trend

toward reduced risk for CHD [HR 0.63 (95 percent CI 0.36-1.09)] and overall mortality [HR 0.71 (95 percent CI 0.46-1.11)].

14.7   Women's Health Initiative Memory Study
The estrogen plus progestin Women's Health Initiative Memory Study (WHIMS), an ancillary study of WHI, enrolled 4,532 predominantly healthy postmenopausal women 65 years of age and older (47 percent were 65 to 69 years of age; 35 percent were 70 to 74 years of age; and 18 percent were 75 years of age and older) to evaluate the effects of daily CE (0.625 mg) plus MPA (2.5 mg) on the incidence of probable dementia (primary outcome) compared to placebo. After an average follow-up of 4 years, the relative risk of probable dementia for CE (0.625 mg) plus MPA (2.5 mg) versus placebo was 2.05 (95 percent CI 1.21-3.48). The absolute risk of probable dementia for CE (0.625 mg) plus MPA (2.5 mg) versus placebo was 45 versus 22 cases per 10,000 women-years. Probable dementia as defined in this study included Alzheimer's disease (AD), vascular dementia (VaD) and mixed types (having features of both AD and VaD). The most common classification of probable dementia in the

treatment group and the placebo group was AD. Since the ancillary study was conducted in women 65 to 79 years of age, it is unknown whether these findings apply to younger postmenopausal women [see Warnings and Precautions (5.3), and Use in Specific Populations (8.5)].

The WHIMS estrogen-alone ancillary study of WHI, enrolled 2,947 predominantly healthy hysterectomized postmenopausal women 65 to 79 years of age and older (45 percent were 65 to 69 years of age; 36 percent were 70 to 74 years of age; 19 percent were 75 years of age and older) to evaluate the effects of daily CE (0.625 mg) on the incidence of probable dementia (primary outcome) compared to placebo.

After an average follow-up of 5.2 years, the relative risk of probable dementia for CE-alone versus placebo was 1.49 (95 percent CI 0.83-2.66). The absolute risk of probable dementia for CE-alone versus placebo was 37 versus 25 cases per 10,000 women-years. Probable dementia as defined in this study included Alzheimer's disease (AD), vascular dementia (VaD) and mixed types (having features of both AD and VaD). The most common classification of probable dementia in both the treatment and placebo groups was AD. Since the ancillary study was conducted in women 65 to 79 years of age, it is unknown whether these findings apply to younger postmenopausal women [see Warnings and Precautions (5.3), and Use in Specific Populations (8.5)].

When data from the two populations were pooled as planned in the WHIMS protocol, the reported overall relative risk for probable dementia was 1.76 (95 percent CI 1.19-2.60). Differences between groups became apparent in the first year of treatment. It is unknown whether these findings apply to younger postmenopausal women [see Warnings and Precautions (5.3), and Use in Special Populations (8.5)].

15   REFERENCES

1. Rossouw JE, et al. Postmenopausal Hormone Therapy and Risk of Cardiovascular Disease by Age and Years Since Menopause. JAMA. 2007;297:1465-1477.
2. Hsia J, et al. Conjugated Equine Estrogens and Coronary Heart Disease. Arch Int Med. 2006;166:357-365.
3. Cushman M, et al. Estrogen Plus Progestin and Risk of Venous Thrombosis. JAMA. 2004;292:1573-1580.
4. Curb JD, et al. Venous Thrombosis and Conjugated Equine Estrogen in Women Without a Uterus. Arch Int Med. 2006;166:772-780.
5. Chlebowski RT, et al. Influence of Estrogen Plus Progestin on Breast Cancer and Mammography in Healthy Postmenopausal Women. JAMA. 2003;289:3234-3253.
6. Stefanick ML, et al. Effects of Conjugated Equine Estrogens on Breast Cancer and Mammography Screening in Postmenopausal Women With Hysterectomy. JAMA. 2006;295:1647-1657.
7. Anderson GL, et al. Effects of Estrogen Plus Progestin on Gynecologic Cancers and Associated Diagnostic Procedures. JAMA. 2003;290:1739-1748.
8. Shumaker SA, et al. Conjugated Equine Estrogens and Incidence of Probable Dementia and Mild Cognitive Impairment in Postmenopausal Women. JAMA. 2004;291:2947-2958.
9. Jackson RD, et al. Effects of Conjugated Equine Estrogen on Risk of Fractures and BMD in Postmenopausal Women With Hysterectomy: Results From the Women's Health Initiative Randomized Trial. J Bone Miner Res. 2006;21:817-828.
10. Hendrix SL, et al. Effects of Conjugated Equine Estrogen on Stroke in the Women's Health Initiative. Circulation. 2006;113:2425-2434.

16   HOW SUPPLIED/STORAGE AND HANDLING
16.1   How Supplied
PREMPRO therapy consists of a single tablet to be taken once daily.
PREMPRO 0.3 mg/1.5 mg
NDC 0046-1105-11, carton includes 1 blister card containing 28 oval, cream tablets.
PREMPRO 0.45 mg/1.5 mg
NDC 0046-1106-11, carton includes 1 blister card containing 28 oval, gold tablets.
PREMPRO 0.625 mg/2.5 mg
NDC 0046-0875-06, carton includes 3 EZ DIAL® dispensers each containing 28 oval, peach tablets.
NDC 0046-0875-11, carton includes 1 blister card containing 28 oval, peach tablets.
PREMPRO 0.625 mg/5 mg
NDC 0046-0975-06, carton includes 3 EZ DIAL dispensers each containing 28 oval, light-blue tablets.
NDC 0046-0975-11, carton includes 1 blister card containing 28 oval, light-blue tablets.
PREMPHASE therapy consists of two separate tablets; one maroon Premarin tablet taken daily on days 1 through 14 and one light-blue tablet taken on days 15 through 28.
NDC 0046-2579-11, carton includes 1 blister card containing 28 tablets (14 oval, maroon Premarin tablets and 14 oval, light-blue tablets).

The appearance of PREMPRO tablets is a trademark of Wyeth Pharmaceuticals.
The appearance of PREMARIN tablets is a trademark of Wyeth Pharmaceuticals.
The appearance of the conjugated estrogens/medroxyprogesterone acetate combination tablets is a trademark.
16.2   Storage and Handling
Store at 20°-25°C (68°-77°F); excursions permitted to 15°-30°C (59°-86°F) [see USP Controlled Room Temperature].

17   PATIENT COUNSELING INFORMATION
See Section 17.4 for FDA-Approved Patient Labeling.
17.1   Abnormal Vaginal Bleeding
Inform postmenopausal women of the importance of reporting abnormal vaginal bleeding to their healthcare provider as soon as possible [see Warnings and Precautions (5.2)].
17.2   Possible Serious Adverse Reactions With Estrogen Plus Progestin Therapy
Inform postmenopausal women of possible serious adverse reactions of estrogen plus progestin therapy including Cardiovascular Disorders, Malignant Neoplasms, and Probable Dementia [see Warnings and Precautions (5.1, 5.2, 5.3)].
17.3   Possible Less Serious But Common Adverse Reactions With Estrogen Plus Progestin Therapy
Inform postmenopausal women of possible less serious but common adverse reactions of estrogen plus progestin therapy such as headache, breast pain and tenderness, nausea and vomiting.
17.4   FDA-Approved Patient Labeling
PREMPRO®
(Conjugated Estrogens/Medroxyprogesterone Acetate Tablets)
PREMPHASE®
(Conjugated Estrogens plus Medroxyprogesterone Acetate Tablets)
Read this PATIENT INFORMATION before you start taking PREMPRO or PREMPHASE and read what you get each time you refill your PREMPRO or PREMPHASE prescription. There may be new information. This information does not take the place of talking to your health-care provider about your medical condition or your treatment.

What is the most important information I should know about PREMPRO and PREMPHASE (combinations of estrogens and a progestin)?

- Do not use estrogens with progestins to prevent heart disease, heart attacks, strokes, or dementia (decline of brain function)
- Using estrogens with progestins may increase your chances of getting heart attacks, strokes, breast cancer, or blood clots
- Using estrogens with progestins may increase your chance of getting dementia, based on a study of women age 65 years or older
- Do not use estrogen-alone to prevent heart disease, heart attacks, or dementia
- Using estrogen-alone may increase your chance of getting cancer of the uterus (womb)
- Using estrogen-alone may increase your chances of getting strokes or blood clots
- Using estrogen-alone may increase your chance of getting dementia, based on a study of women age 65 years or older
- You and your healthcare provider should talk regularly about whether you still need treatment with PREMPRO or PREMPHASE

What is PREMPRO or PREMPHASE?
PREMPRO or PREMPHASE are medicines that contain two kinds of hormones, estrogens and a progestin.
PREMPRO or PREMPHASE is used after menopause to:
- **Reduce moderate to severe hot flashes**
Estrogens are hormones made by a woman's ovaries. The ovaries normally stop making estrogens when a woman is between 45 and 55 years old. This drop in body estrogen levels causes the "change of life" or menopause (the end of monthly menstrual periods). Sometimes, both ovaries are removed during an operation before natural menopause takes place. The sudden drop in estrogen levels causes "surgical menopause."
When the estrogen levels begin dropping, some women get very uncomfortable symptoms, such as feelings of warmth in the face, neck, and chest, or sudden strong feelings of heat and sweating ("hot flashes" or "hot flushes"). In some women the symptoms are mild, and they will not need to take estrogens. In other women, symptoms can be more severe.
- **Treat menopausal changes in and around the vagina**
You and your healthcare provider should talk regularly about whether you still need treatment with PREMPRO or PREMPHASE to control these problems. If you use

PREMPRO or PREMPHASE only to treat your menopausal changes in and around your vagina, talk with your healthcare provider about whether a topical vaginal product would be better for you.
- **Help reduce your chances of getting osteoporosis (thin weak bones)**
Osteoporosis from menopause is a thinning of the bones that makes them weaker and easier to break. If you use PREMPRO or PREMPHASE only to prevent osteoporosis due to menopause, talk with your healthcare provider about whether a different treatment or medicine without estrogens might be better for you. Weight-bearing exercise, like walking or running, and taking calcium (1500 mg/day of elemental calcium) and vitamin D (400-800 IU/day) supplements may also lower your chances of getting postmenopausal osteoporosis. It is important to talk about exercise and supplements with your healthcare provider before starting them.
You and your healthcare provider should talk regularly about whether you still need treatment with PREMPRO or PREMPHASE.
Who should not take PREMPRO or PREMPHASE?
Do not take PREMPRO or PREMPHASE if you have had your uterus (womb) removed (hysterectomy).
PREMPRO and PREMPHASE contain a progestin to decrease the chance of getting cancer of the uterus. If you do not have a uterus, you do not need a progestin and you should not take PREMPRO or PREMPHASE.
Do not take PREMPRO or PREMPHASE if you:
- **Have unusual vaginal bleeding**
- **Currently have or have had certain cancers**
Estrogens may increase the chance of getting certain types of cancers, including cancer of the breast or uterus. If you have or have had cancer, talk with your healthcare provider about whether you should use PREMPRO or PREMPHASE.
- **Had a stroke or heart attack**
- **Currently have or have had blood clots**
- **Currently have or have had liver problems**
- **Are allergic to PREMPRO or PREMPHASE or any of their ingredients**
See the end of this leaflet for a list of ingredients in PREMPRO and PREMPHASE.
- **Think you may be pregnant**
Tell your healthcare provider
- **If you have any unusual vaginal bleeding**
Vaginal bleeding after menopause may be a warning sign of cancer of the uterus (womb). Your healthcare provider should check any unusual vaginal bleeding to find out the cause.
- **About all of your medical problems**
Your healthcare provider may need to check you more carefully if you have certain conditions, such as asthma (wheezing), epilepsy (seizures), diabetes, migraine, endometriosis, lupus, problems with your heart, liver, thyroid, kidneys, or have high calcium levels in your blood.
- **About all the medicines you take**
This includes prescription and nonprescription medicines, vitamins, and herbal supplements. Some medicines may affect how PREMPRO or PREMPHASE works. PREMPRO or PREMPHASE may also affect how your other medicines work.
- **If you are going to have surgery or will be on bedrest**
You may need to stop taking estrogens and progestins.
- **If you are breastfeeding**
The hormones in PREMPRO and PREMPHASE can pass into your milk.
How should I take PREMPRO or PREMPHASE?
- Take one PREMPRO or PREMPHASE tablet at the same time each day
- If you miss a dose, take it as soon as possible
If it is almost time for your next dose, skip the missed dose and go back to your normal schedule. Do not take 2 doses at the same time.
- Estrogens should be used at the lowest dose possible for your treatment only as long as needed
You and your healthcare provider should talk regularly (for example, every 3 to 6 months) about the dose you are taking and whether you still need treatment with PREMPRO or PREMPHASE.
What are the possible side effects of PREMPRO or PREMPHASE?
Side effects are grouped by how serious they are and how often they happen when you are treated.
Serious, but less common side effects:
- Breast cancer
- Cancer of the uterus
- Stroke
- Heart attack
- Blood clots
- Dementia
- Gallbladder disease
- Ovarian cancer
- High blood pressure

- Liver problems
- High blood sugar
- Enlargement of benign tumors of the uterus ("fibroids")
- Mental depression

Some of the warning signs of these serious side effects include:

- Breast lumps
- Unusual vaginal bleeding
- Dizziness and faintness
- Changes in speech
- Severe headaches
- Chest pain
- Shortness of breath
- Pains in your legs
- Changes in vision
- Vomiting
- Yellowing of the skin, eyes or nail beds

Call your healthcare provider right away if you get any of these warning signs, or any other unusual symptoms that concern you.

Less serious, but common side effects include:

- Headache
- Breast pain
- Irregular vaginal bleeding or spotting
- Stomach/abdominal cramps/bloating
- Nausea and vomiting
- Hair loss
- Fluid retention
- Vaginal yeast infection

These are not all the possible side effects of PREMPRO or PREMPHASE. For more information, ask your healthcare provider or pharmacist for advice about side effects. You may report side effects to FDA at 1-800-FDA-1088.

What can I do to lower my chances of getting a serious side effect with PREMPRO or PREMPHASE?

- Talk with your healthcare provider regularly about whether you should continue taking PREMPRO or PREMPHASE
- See your healthcare provider right away if you get vaginal bleeding while taking PREMPRO or PREMPHASE
- Have a pelvic exam, breast exam and mammogram (breast X-ray) every year unless your healthcare provider tells you something else
  If members of your family have had breast cancer or if you have ever had breast lumps or an abnormal mammogram, you may need to have breast exams more often.
- If you have high blood pressure, high cholesterol (fat in the blood), diabetes, are overweight, or if you use tobacco, you may have higher chances for getting heart disease
  Ask your healthcare provider for ways to lower your chances of getting heart disease.

General Information about the safe and effective use of PREMPRO and PREMPHASE

Medicines are sometimes prescribed for conditions that are not mentioned in patient information leaflets. Do not take PREMPRO or PREMPHASE for conditions for which it was not prescribed. Do not give PREMPRO or PREMPHASE to other people, even if they have the same symptoms you have. It may harm them.

Keep PREMPRO and PREMPHASE out of the reach of children.

This leaflet provides a summary of the most important information about PREMPRO and PREMPHASE. If you would like more information, talk with your healthcare provider or pharmacist. You can ask for information about PREMPRO and PREMPHASE that is written for health professionals by calling the toll free number 800-934-5556.

What are the ingredients in PREMPRO and PREMPHASE?

PREMPRO contains the same conjugated estrogens found in Premarin, which are a mixture of sodium estrone sulfate and sodium equilin sulfate and other components, including sodium sulfate conjugates, 17α-dihydroequilin, 17α-estradiol and 17β-dihydroequilin. PREMPRO also contains either 1.5, 2.5, or 5 mg of medroxyprogesterone acetate. PREMPRO 0.3 mg/1.5 mg and 0.45 mg/1.5 mg tablets also contain calcium phosphate tribasic, microcrystalline cellulose, lactose monohydrate, hypromellose, magnesium stearate, polyethylene glycol, sucrose, hydroxypropyl cellulose, Eudragit NE 30D, povidone, titanium dioxide, yellow iron oxide, and black iron oxide.

PREMPRO 0.625 mg/2.5 mg and 0.625 mg/5 mg tablets also contain calcium phosphate tribasic, calcium sulfate, carnauba wax, cellulose, glyceryl monooleate, lactose, magnesium stearate, methylcellulose, pharmaceutical glaze, polyethylene glycol, sucrose, povidone, titanium dioxide, black iron oxide, and FD&C Blue No. 2 or red ferric oxide.

PREMPHASE is two separate tablets. One tablet (maroon color) is 0.625 mg of Premarin, which is a mixture of sodium estrone sulfate and sodium equilin sulfate and other components, including sodium sulfate conjugates, 17 α-dihydroequilin, 17 α-estradiol and 17 β-dihydroequilin. The maroon tablet also contains calcium phosphate tribasic, hydroxypropyl cellulose, microcrystalline cellulose, powdered cellulose, hypromellose, lactose monohydrate, magne-

sium stearate, polyethylene glycol, sucrose, titanium dioxide, FD&C Blue No. 2, FD&C Red No. 40. The second tablet (light-blue color) contains 0.625 mg of the same ingredients as the maroon color tablet plus 5 mg of medroxyprogesterone acetate. The light-blue tablet also contains calcium phosphate tribasic, calcium sulfate, carnauba wax, cellulose, glyceryl monooleate, lactose, magnesium stearate, methylcellulose, pharmaceutical glaze, polyethylene glycol, sucrose, povidone, titanium dioxide, FD&C Blue No. 2, and black iron oxide.

PREMPRO therapy consists of a single tablet to be taken once daily.

PREMPRO 0.3 mg/1.5 mg

Blister Card—Each carton includes 1 blister card containing 28 oval, cream tablets. Each tablet contains 0.3 mg of the conjugated estrogens found in Premarin tablets and 1.5 mg of medroxyprogesterone acetate for oral administration.

PREMPRO 0.45 mg/1.5 mg

Blister Card—Each carton includes 1 blister card containing 28 oval, gold tablets. Each tablet contains 0.45 mg of the conjugated estrogens found in Premarin tablets and 1.5 mg of medroxyprogesterone acetate for oral administration.

PREMPRO 0.625 mg/2.5 mg

EZ DIAL dispenser—Each carton includes 3 EZ DIAL® dispensers containing 28 tablets. One EZ DIAL dispenser contains 28 oval, peach tablets. Each tablet contains 0.625 mg of the conjugated estrogens found in Premarin tablets and 2.5 mg of medroxyprogesterone acetate for oral administration.

Blister Card—Each carton includes 1 blister card containing 28 oval, peach tablets. Each tablet contains 0.625 mg of the conjugated estrogens found in Premarin tablets and 2.5 mg of medroxyprogesterone acetate for oral administration.

PREMPRO 0.625 mg/5 mg

EZ DIAL dispenser—Each carton includes 3 EZ DIAL dispensers containing 28 tablets. One EZ DIAL dispenser contains 28 oval, light-blue tablets. Each tablet contains 0.625 mg of the conjugated estrogens found in Premarin tablets and 5 mg of medroxyprogesterone acetate for oral administration.

Blister Card - Each carton includes 1 blister card containing 28 oval, light-blue tablets. Each tablet contains 0.625 mg of the conjugated estrogens found in Premarin tablets and 5 mg of medroxyprogesterone acetate for oral administration.

PREMPHASE therapy consists of two separate tablets; one maroon Premarin tablet taken daily on days 1 through 14 and one light-blue tablet taken on days 15 through 28.

Each carton includes 1 blister pack containing 28 tablets. One blister pack contains 14 oval, maroon Premarin tablets containing 0.625 mg of conjugated estrogens and 14 oval, light-blue tablets that contain 0.625 mg of the conjugated estrogens found in Premarin tablets and 5 mg of medroxyprogesterone acetate for oral administration.

The appearance of PREMPRO tablets is a trademark of Wyeth Pharmaceuticals.

The appearance of PREMARIN tablets is a trademark of Wyeth Pharmaceuticals. The appearance of the conjugated estrogens/medroxyprogesterone acetate combination tablets is a trademark.

Store at 20°-25°C (68°-77°F); excursions permitted to 15°-30°C (59°-86°F) [see USP Controlled Room Temperature].

United States Patent Number 5,547,948 (PREMPRO).

This product's label may have been updated. For current package insert and further product information, please visit www.wyeth.com or call our medical communications department toll-free at 1-800-934-5556.

Wyeth®

Wyeth Pharmaceuticals Inc.
Philadelphia, PA 19101
W10537C006
ET01
Rev 02/10

Shown in Product Identification Guide, page 321

PREVNAR® 13   ℞
[prĕv' năr]
Pneumococcal 13-valent Conjugate Vaccine
[Diphtheria CRM$_{197}$ Protein]]
Suspension for intramuscular injection

HIGHLIGHTS OF PRESCRIBING INFORMATION
These highlights do not include all the information needed to use PREVNAR 13 safely and effectively. See full prescribing information for PREVNAR 13.
PREVNAR 13 (Pneumococcal 13-valent Conjugate Vaccine [Diphtheria CRM$_{197}$ Protein])
Suspension for intramuscular injection
Initial U.S. Approval: 2010

————INDICATIONS AND USAGE————
Prevnar 13 is a vaccine approved for use in children 6 weeks through 5 years of age (prior to the 6th birthday).
Prevnar 13 is indicated for active immunization for the prevention of invasive disease caused by *Streptococcus pneumoniae* serotypes 1, 3, 4, 5, 6A, 6B, 7F, 9V, 14, 18C, 19A, 19F and 23F.
Prevnar 13 is also indicated for the prevention of otitis media caused by *Streptococcus pneumoniae* serotypes 4, 6B, 9V, 14, 18C, 19F, and 23F. No otitis media efficacy data are available for serotypes 1, 3, 5, 6A, 7F, and 19A. (1)
————DOSAGE AND ADMINISTRATION————
The four-dose immunization series consists of a 0.5 mL intramuscular injection administered at 2, 4, 6, and 12-15 months of age. (2.3)
————DOSAGE FORMS AND STRENGTHS————
0.5 mL suspension for intramuscular injection, supplied in a single-dose pre-filled syringe. (3)
————CONTRAINDICATIONS————
Severe allergic reaction (e.g., anaphylaxis) to any component of Prevnar 13, Prevnar (Pneumococcal 7-valent Conjugate Vaccine [Diphtheria CRM$_{197}$ Protein]) or any diphtheria toxoid-containing vaccine. (4)
————WARNINGS AND PRECAUTIONS————
Apnea following intramuscular vaccination has been observed in some infants born prematurely. Decisions about when to administer an intramuscular vaccine, including Prevnar 13, to infants born prematurely should be based on consideration of the individual infant's medical status, and the potential benefits and possible risks of vaccination. (5.4)
————ADVERSE REACTIONS————
The most commonly reported solicited adverse reactions (≥20 %) in U.S. clinical trials with Prevnar 13 were redness, swelling and tenderness at the injection site, fever, decreased appetite, irritability, increased sleep, and decreased sleep. (6.1)
To report SUSPECTED ADVERSE REACTIONS, contact Wyeth Pharmaceuticals Inc. at 1-800-934-5556 or VAERS at 1-800-822-7967 or http://vaers.hhs.gov.
————DRUG INTERACTIONS————
- Do not mix with any other vaccine in the same syringe. (7.1)
- Immunosuppressive therapies may reduce immune response to Prevnar 13. (7.2)
————USE IN SPECIFIC POPULATIONS————
Safety and effectiveness of Prevnar 13 in children below the age of 6 weeks or on or after the 6th birthday have not been established. Prevnar 13 is not approved for use in children in these age groups. (8.4)
See 17 for PATIENT COUNSELING INFORMATION
Revised: 04/2010

FULL PRESCRIBING INFORMATION: CONTENTS*

17 PATIENT COUNSELING INFORMATION
17.1 Potential Benefits and Risks
17.2 Adverse Reactions

* Sections or subsections omitted from the full prescribing information are not listed

FULL PRESCRIBING INFORMATION

1 INDICATIONS AND USAGE

Prevnar 13™ is a vaccine approved for use in children 6 weeks through 5 years of age (prior to the 6th birthday).

Prevnar 13 is indicated for active immunization for the prevention of invasive disease caused by *Streptococcus pneumoniae* serotypes 1, 3, 4, 5, 6A, 6B, 7F, 9V, 14, 18C, 19A, 19F and 23F.

Prevnar 13 is also indicated for the prevention of otitis media caused by *Streptococcus pneumoniae* serotypes 4, 6B, 9V, 14, 18C, 19F, and 23F. No otitis media efficacy data are available for serotypes 1, 3, 5, 6A, 7F, and 19A.

2 DOSAGE AND ADMINISTRATION

For intramuscular injection only.

2.1 Preparation for Administration

Since this product is a suspension containing an adjuvant, shake vigorously immediately prior to use to obtain a homogenous, white suspension in the vaccine container. Do not use the vaccine, if it cannot be resuspended. Parenteral drug products should be inspected visually for particulate matter and discoloration prior to administration *[see Description (11)]*. This product should not be used if particulate matter or discoloration is found.

Do not mix Prevnar 13 with other vaccines/products in the same syringe.

2.2 Administration Information

Do not inject intravenously, intradermally, or subcutaneously.

Each 0.5 mL dose is to be injected intramuscularly. The preferred sites for injection are the anterolateral aspect of the thigh in infants or the deltoid muscle of the upper arm in toddlers and young children. The vaccine should not be injected in the gluteal area or areas where there may be a major nerve trunk and/or blood vessel.

2.3 Vaccine Schedule for Infants and Toddlers

Prevnar 13 is to be administered as a four-dose series at 2, 4, 6, and 12-15 months of age.

Table 1: Vaccination Schedule for Infants and Toddlers

Dose	Dose 1*†	Dose 2†	Dose 3†	Dose 4‡
Age at Dose	2 months	4 months	6 months	12-15 months

* Dose 1 may be given as early as 6 weeks of age.
† The recommended dosing interval is 4 to 8 weeks.
‡ The fourth dose should be administered at approximately 12-15 months of age, and at least 2 months after the third dose.

2.4 Vaccine Schedule for Unvaccinated Children ≥7 Months of Age

For children who are beyond the age of the routine infant schedule and have not received Prevnar or Prevnar 13, the following catch-up schedule applies:

Table 2: Vaccine Schedule for Unvaccinated Children ≥7 Months of Age

Age at First Dose	Total Number of 0.5 mL Doses
7-11 months of age	3*
12-23 months of age	2†
24 months through 5 years of age (prior to the 6th birthday)	1

* The first 2 doses at least 4 weeks apart; third dose after the one-year birthday, separated from the second dose by at least 2 months.
† Two doses at least 2 months apart.

The immune responses induced by this catch-up schedule may result in lower antibody concentrations for some serotypes, compared to antibody concentrations following 4 doses of Prevnar 13 (given at 2, 4, 6, and 12 to 15 months). In children 24 months through 5 years of age, the catch-up schedule may result in lower antibody concentrations for some serotypes, compared to antibody concentrations following 3 doses of Prevnar 13 (given at 2, 4, and 6 months). The clinical relevance of these lower antibody responses is not known.

2.5 Prevnar 13 Vaccine Schedule for Children Previously Vaccinated With Prevnar (*Streptococcus pneumoniae* serotypes 4, 6B, 9V, 14, 18C, 19F, and 23F)

Children who have received one or more doses of Prevnar may complete the 4-dose immunization series with Prevnar 13. Children 15 months through 5 years of age who have received 4 doses of Prevnar may receive one dose of Prevnar 13 to elicit immune responses to the six additional serotypes. This catch-up dose of Prevnar 13 should be administered with an interval of at least 8 weeks after the fourth dose of Prevnar. The immune responses induced by this Prevnar 13 transition schedule may result in lower antibody concentrations for the 6 additional serotypes (types 1, 3, 5, 6A, 7F, and 19A), compared to antibody concentrations following 4 doses of Prevnar 13 (given at 2, 4, 6, and 12 to 15 months). The clinical relevance of these lower antibody responses is not known.

3 DOSAGE FORMS AND STRENGTHS

Prevnar 13 is a suspension for intramuscular injection available in 0.5 mL single-dose pre-filled syringes.

4 CONTRAINDICATIONS

Severe allergic reaction (e.g., anaphylaxis) to any component of Prevnar 13, Prevnar or any diphtheria toxoid-containing vaccine.

5 WARNINGS AND PRECAUTIONS

5.1 Management of Allergic Reactions or Other Adverse Reactions

Before administration of any dose, all precautions should be taken to prevent allergic or any other adverse reactions. This includes a review of the patient's immunization history for possible sensitivity to the vaccine or similar vaccines and for previous vaccination-related adverse reactions in order to determine the existence of any contraindication to immunization with Prevnar 13 and to allow an assessment of risks and benefits. Epinephrine and other appropriate agents used for the control of immediate allergic reactions must be immediately available should an acute anaphylactic reaction occur following the administration of the vaccine.

5.2 Limitations of Vaccine Effectiveness

Prevnar 13 may not protect all individuals receiving the vaccine. Prevnar 13 will not protect against *Streptococcus pneumoniae* serotypes that are not in the vaccine or serotypes unrelated to those in the vaccine. It will also not protect against other microorganisms. This vaccine does not treat active infection.

Protection against otitis media is expected to be substantially lower than protection against invasive disease. In addition, because otitis media is caused by many organisms other than the 7 serotypes of *Streptococcus pneumoniae* included in the indication, protection against all causes of otitis media is expected to be lower than for pneumococcal otitis media caused by these 7 vaccine serotypes *[see Clinical Studies (14.2)]*.

The duration of protection from immunization is not known.

5.3 Altered Immunocompetence

Data on the safety and effectiveness of Prevnar 13 when administered to children in specific groups at higher risk for invasive pneumococcal disease (e.g., children with congenital or acquired splenic dysfunction, HIV infection, malignancy, nephrotic syndrome) are not available.

Children in these groups may have reduced antibody response to active immunization due to impaired immune responsiveness. Vaccination in high-risk groups should be considered on an individual basis *[see Drug Interactions (7.2)]*.

The use of pneumococcal conjugate vaccine does not replace the use of 23-valent pneumococcal polysaccharide vaccine (PPV23) in children ≥24 months of age with sickle cell disease, asplenia, HIV infection, chronic illness or who are otherwise immunocompromised.

5.4 Premature Infants

Apnea following intramuscular vaccination has been observed in some infants born prematurely. Decisions about when to administer an intramuscular vaccine, including Prevnar 13, to infants born prematurely should be based on consideration of the individual infant's medical status, and the potential benefits and possible risks of vaccination.

6 ADVERSE REACTIONS

Because clinical trials are conducted under widely varying conditions, adverse-reaction rates observed in the clinical trials of a vaccine cannot be directly compared to rates in the clinical trials of another vaccine and may not reflect the rates observed in practice. As with any vaccine, there is the possibility that broad use of Prevnar 13 could reveal adverse reactions not observed in clinical trials.

6.1 Clinical Trials Experience With Prevnar 13

The safety of Prevnar 13 was evaluated in 13 clinical trials in which 4,729 infants and toddlers received at least one dose of Prevnar 13 and 2,760 infants and toddlers received at least one dose of Prevnar active control. Safety data for

Table 3: Percentage of U.S. Infant and Toddler Subjects Reporting Solicited Local Reactions at the Prevnar 13 or Prevnar Injection Sites Within 7 Days After Each Vaccination at 2, 4, 6, and 12-15 Months of Age[a]

Graded Local Reaction[c]	Dose 1 Prevnar 13 (N[b]=1375-1612)	Dose 1 Prevnar (N[b]=516-606)	Dose 2 Prevnar 13 (N[b]=1069-1331)	Dose 2 Prevnar (N[b]=405-510)	Dose 3 Prevnar 13 (N[b]=998-1206)	Dose 3 Prevnar (N[b]=348-446)	Dose 4 Prevnar 13 (N[b]=874-1060)	Dose 4 Prevnar (N[b]=283-379)
Redness[c]								
Any	24.3	26.0	33.3	29.7	37.1	36.6	42.3	45.5
Mild	23.1	25.2	31.9	28.7	35.3	35.3	39.5	42.7
Moderate	2.2	1.5	2.7	2.2	4.6	5.1	9.6	13.4*
Severe	0	0	0	0	0	0	0	0
Swelling[c]								
Any	20.1	20.7	25.2	22.5	26.8	28.4	31.6	36.0*
Mild	17.2	18.7	23.8	20.5	25.2	27.5	29.4	33.8
Moderate	4.9	3.9	3.7	4.9	3.8	5.8	8.3	11.2*
Severe	0	0	0.1	0	0	0	0	0
Tenderness								
Any	62.5	64.5	64.7	62.9	59.2	60.8	57.8	62.5
Interferes with limb movement	10.4	9.6	9.0	10.5	8.4	9.0	6.9	5.7

* Statistically significant difference p < 0.05
[a] Data are from three primary U.S. safety studies (the U.S. phase II infant study, the pivotal U.S. non-inferiority study, and the U.S. consistency study). All infants received concomitant routine infant immunizations. Concomitant vaccines and pneumococcal conjugate vaccines were administered in different limbs.
[b] Number of subjects reporting Yes for at least 1 day or No for all days.
[c] Diameters were measured in caliper units of whole numbers from 1 to 14 or 14+. One caliper unit = 0.5 cm. Measurements were rounded up to the nearest whole number. Intensity of induration and erythema were then characterized as Mild (0.5-2.0 cm), Moderate (2.5-7.0 cm), or Severe (>7.0 cm).

the first three doses are available for all 13 infant studies; dose 4 data are available for 10 studies; and data for the 6-month follow-up are available for 7 studies. The vaccination schedule and concomitant vaccinations used in these infant trials were consistent with country-specific recommendations and local clinical practice. There were no substantive differences in demographic characteristics between the vaccine groups. By race, 84.0% of subjects were White, 6.0% were Black or African-American, 5.8% were Asian and 3.8% were of 'Other' race (most of these being biracial). Overall, 52.3% of subjects were male infants.

Three studies in the U.S. evaluated the safety of Prevnar 13 when administered concomitantly with routine U.S. pediatric vaccinations at 2, 4, 6, and 12-15 months of age. Solicited local and systemic adverse events were recorded daily by parents/guardians using an electronic diary for 7 consecutive days following each vaccination. For unsolicited adverse events, study subjects were monitored from administration of the first dose until one month after the infant series, and for one month after the administration of the toddler dose. Information regarding unsolicited and serious adverse events, newly diagnosed chronic medical conditions, and hospitalizations since the last visit were collected during the clinic visit for the fourth-study dose and during a scripted telephone interview 6 months after the fourth-study dose. Serious adverse events were also collected throughout the study period. Overall, the safety data show a similar proportion of Prevnar 13 and Prevnar subjects reporting serious adverse events. Among U.S. study subjects, a similar proportion of Prevnar 13 and Prevnar recipients reported solicited local and systemic adverse reactions as well as unsolicited adverse events.

Serious Adverse Events in All Infant and Toddler Clinical Studies
Serious adverse events were collected throughout the study period for all 13 clinical trials. This reporting period is longer than the 30-day post-vaccination period used in some vaccine trials. The longer reporting may have resulted in serious adverse events being reported in a higher percentage of subjects than for other vaccines. Serious adverse events reported following vaccination in infants and toddlers occurred in 8.2% among Prevnar 13 recipients and 7.2% among Prevnar recipients. Serious adverse events observed during different study periods for Prevnar 13 and Prevnar respectively were: 1) 3.7% and 3.5% from dose 1 to the bleed after the infant series; 2) 3.6% and 2.7% from the bleed after the infant series to the toddler dose; 3) 0.9% and 0.8% from the toddler dose to the bleed after the toddler dose and 4) 2.5% and 2.8% during the 6 month follow up period after the last dose.

The most commonly reported serious adverse events were in the 'Infections and infestations' system organ class including bronchiolitis (0.9%, 1.1%), gastroenteritis, (0.9%, 0.9%), and pneumonia (0.9%, 0.5%) for Prevnar 13 and Prevnar respectively.

There were 3 (0.063%) deaths among Prevnar 13 recipients, and 1 (0.036%) death in Prevnar recipients, all as a result of sudden infant death syndrome (SIDS). These SIDS rates are consistent with published age specific background rates of SIDS from the year 2000.

There was 1 hypotonic-hyporesponsive episode adverse reaction reported (0.015%).

Solicited Adverse Reactions in the Three U.S. Infant and Toddler Studies
A total of 1,907 subjects received at least 1 dose of Prevnar 13 and 701 subjects received at least one dose of Prevnar in the three U.S. studies. Most subjects were White (77.3%), 14.2% were Black or African-American, and 1.7% were Asian; 79.1% of subjects were non-Hispanic and non-Latino and 14.6% were Hispanic or Latino. Overall, 53.6% of subjects were male infants.

The incidence and severity of solicited adverse reactions that occurred within 7 days following each dose of Prevnar 13 or Prevnar administered to U.S. infants and toddlers are shown in Tables 3 and 4.

[See table 3 at top of previous page]
[See table 4 above]

Unsolicited Adverse Reactions in the Three U.S. Infant and Toddler Safety Studies
The following were determined to be adverse drug reactions based on experience with Prevnar 13 in clinical trials:
Reactions occurring in greater than 1% of infants and toddlers: diarrhea, vomiting, and rash.
Reactions occurring in less than 1% of infants and toddlers: crying, hypersensitivity reaction (including face edema, dyspnea, and bronchospasm), seizures (including febrile seizures), and urticaria or urticaria-like rash.

Safety Assessments in the Catch-Up Studies
In a catch-up study conducted in Poland, 354 children (7 months through 5 years of age) receiving at least one dose of Prevnar 13 were also monitored for safety. All subjects in this study were White and non-Hispanic. Overall, 49.6% of subjects were male infants. The incidence and severity of solicited adverse reactions that occurred within 4 days fol-

lowing each dose of Prevnar 13 administered to pneumococcal-vaccine naïve children 7 months through 5 years of age are shown in Tables 5 and 6.
[See table 5 above]
[See table 6 at top of next page]
A U.S. study evaluated the use of Prevnar 13 in children previously immunized with Prevnar. In this open label trial,

284 healthy children 15 through 59 months of age previously vaccinated with at least 3 doses of Prevnar, received 1 or 2 doses of Prevnar 13. Children 15 months through 23 months of age (group 1) received 2 doses, and children 24 months through 59 months of age (group 2) received one dose. Most subjects were White (75.0%), 15.8% were Black or African-American, and 1.6% were Asian; 86.6% of

Table 4: Percentage of U.S. Infant and Toddler Subjects Reporting Solicited Systemic Adverse Reactions Within 7 Days After Each Vaccination at 2, 4, 6, and 12-15 Months of Age[a,b]

Graded Systemic Events	Dose 1		Dose 2		Dose 3		Dose 4	
	Prevnar 13 (N[a]=1360-1707)	Prevnar (N[a]=497-640)	Prevnar 13 (N[a]=1084-1469)	Prevnar (N[a]=409-555)	Prevnar 13 (N[a]=997-1361)	Prevnar (N[a]=354-521)	Prevnar 13 (N[a]=850-1227)	Prevnar (N[a]=278-436)
Fever[c]								
Any	24.3	22.1	36.5	32.8	30.3	31.6	31.9	30.6
Mild	23.6	21.7	34.9	31.6	29.1	30.2	30.3	30.0
Moderate	1.1	0.6	3.4	2.8	4.2	3.3	4.4	4.6
Severe	0.1	0.2	0.1	0.3	0.1	0.7	1.0	0
Decreased appetite	48.3	43.6	47.8	43.6	47.6	47.6	51.0	49.4
Irritability	85.6	83.6	84.8	80.4	79.8	80.8	80.4	77.8
Increased sleep	71.5	71.5	66.6	63.4	57.7	55.2	48.7	55.1
Decreased sleep	42.5	40.6	45.6	43.7	46.5	47.7	45.3	40.3

[a] Number of subjects reporting Yes for at least 1 day or No for all days.
[b] Data are from three primary U.S. safety studies (the U.S. phase II infant study, the pivotal U.S. non-inferiority study, and the U.S. consistency study). All infants received concomitant routine infant immunizations. Concomitant vaccines and pneumococcal conjugate vaccines were administered in different limbs.
[d] Fever gradings: Mild (≥38°C but ≤39°C), Moderate (>39°C but ≤40°C), and Severe (> 40°C). No other systemic event other than fever was graded. Parents reported the use of antipyretic medication to treat or prevent symptoms in 62 to 75% of subjects after any of the 4 doses. There were no statistical differences between the Prevnar 13 and Prevnar groups.

Table 5: Percentage of Subjects 7 Months Through 5 Years of Age Reporting Solicited Local Reactions Within 4 Days After Each Catch-Up Prevnar 13 Vaccination[a]

Graded Local Reaction	7 through 11 months			12 through 23 months		24 months through 5 years
	Dose 1 N[b]=86 %	Dose 2 N[b]=86-87 %	Dose 3 N[b]=78-82 %	Dose 1 N[b]=108-110 %	Dose 2 N[b]=98-106 %	Dose 1 N[b]=147-149 %
Redness[c]						
Any	48.8	46.0	37.8	70.0	54.7	50.0
Mild	41.9	40.2	31.3	55.5	44.7	37.4
Moderate	16.3	9.3	12.5	38.2	25.5	25.7
Severe	0.0	0.0	0.0	0.0	0.0	0.0
Swelling[c]						
Any	36.0	32.2	25.0	44.5	41.0	36.9
Mild	32.6	28.7	20.5	36.7	36.2	28.2
Moderate	11.6	14.0	11.3	24.8	12.1	20.3
Severe	0.0	0.0	0.0	0.0	0.0	0.0
Tenderness						
Any	15.1	15.1	15.2	33.3	43.7	42.3
Interferes with limb movement	1.2	3.5	6.4	0.0	4.1	4.1

[a] Study conducted in Poland.
[b] Number of subjects reporting Yes for at least 1 day or No for all days.
[c] Diameters were measured in caliper units of whole numbers from 1 to 14 or 14+. One caliper unit = 0.5 cm. Measurements were rounded up to the nearest whole number. Intensity of redness and swelling were then characterized as Mild (0.5-2.0 cm), Moderate (2.5-7.0 cm), or Severe (>7.0 cm).

Table 6: Percentage of Subjects 7 Months Through 5 Years of Age Reporting Solicited Systemic Adverse Reactions Within 4 Days After Each Catch-Up Prevnar 13 Vaccination[a]

	7 through 11 months			12 through 23 months		24 months through 5 years
Systemic Reaction	Dose 1 N[b]=86-87 %	Dose 2 N[b]=86-87 %	Dose 3 N[b]=78-81 %	Dose 1 N[b]=108 %	Dose 2 N[b]=98-100 %	Dose 1 N[b]=147-148 %
Fever[c]						
Mild	3.4	8.1	5.1	3.7	5.1	0.7
Moderate	1.2	2.3	1.3	0.9	0.0	0.7
Severe	0.0	0.0	0.0	0.0	0.0	0.0
Decreased appetite	19.5	17.2	17.5	22.2	25.5	16.3
Irritability	24.1	34.5	24.7	30.6	34.0	14.3
Increased sleep	9.2	9.3	2.6	13.0	10.1	11.6
Decreased sleep	24.1	18.4	15.0	19.4	20.4	6.8

[a] Study conducted in Poland.
[b] Number of subjects reporting Yes for at least 1 day or No for all days.
[c] Fever gradings: Mild (≥38°C but ≤39°C), Moderate (>39°C but ≤40°C), and Severe (> 40°C). No other systemic event other than fever was graded.

Table 7: Percentage of Subjects 15 Months Through 59 Months of Age, Previously Vaccinated with 3 or 4 Prior Infant Doses of Prevnar, Reporting Solicited Local Reactions Within 7 Days After One Supplemental Prevnar 13 Vaccination

	15 months through 23 months[a]		24 months through 59 months[b]
Graded Local Reaction	1 dose Prevnar 13 3 prior Prevnar doses N[c]=28-32 %	1 dose Prevnar 13 4 prior Prevnar doses N[c]=62-76 %	1 dose Prevnar 13 3 or 4 prior Prevnar doses N[c]=138-155 %
Redness[d]			
Any	46.9	36.6	34.9
Mild	31.0	31.4	31.5
Moderate	22.6	7.9	9.9
Severe	0.0	0.0	0.0
Swelling[d]			
Any	35.5	21.2	22.2
Mild	26.7	18.8	20.3
Moderate	13.8	7.7	5.7
Severe	0.0	0.0	0.0
Tenderness			
Any	53.1	50.0	61.9
Interferes with limb movement	10.3	6.3	10.6

[a] Dose 2 data not shown.
[b] The data for this age group are only represented as a single result as 95% of children received 4 doses of Prevnar prior to enrollment.
[c] Number of subjects reporting Yes for at least 1 day or No for all days.
[d] Diameters were measured in caliper units of whole numbers from 1 to 14 or 14+. One caliper unit = 0.5 cm. Measurements were rounded up to the nearest whole number. Intensity of redness and swelling were then characterized as Mild (0.5-2.0 cm), Moderate (2.5-7.0 cm), or Severe (>7.0 cm).

subjects were non-Hispanic and non-Latino and 13.4% were Hispanic or Latino. Overall, 54.0% of subjects were male infants.

The incidence and severity of solicited adverse reactions that occurred within 7 days following one dose of Prevnar 13 administered to children 15 months through 59 months of age are shown in Tables 7 and 8.
[See table 7 above]
[See table 8 at top of next page]

6.2   Clinical Trials Experience With Prevnar®
The safety experience with Prevnar is relevant to Prevnar 13 because the two vaccines share common components.
Generally, the adverse reactions reported in clinical trials with Prevnar 13 were also reported in clinical trials with Prevnar.

Overall, the safety of Prevnar was evaluated in a total of five clinical studies in the U.S. in which 18,168 infants and children received a total of 58,699 doses of vaccine at 2, 4, 6, and 12-15 months of age.
Adverse events reported in clinical trials with Prevnar include:
Bronchiolitis, UTI, acute gastroenteritis, asthma, aspiration, breath holding, influenza, inguinal hernia repair, viral syndrome, URI, croup, thrush, wheezing, choking, conjunctivitis, pharyngitis, colic, colitis, congestive heart failure, roseola, sepsis.

6.3   Post-marketing Experience With Prevnar
The following adverse reactions have been reported through passive surveillance since market introduction of Prevnar and therefore, are considered adverse reactions for Prevnar

13 as well. Because these events are reported voluntarily from a population of uncertain size, it is not always possible to reliably estimate its frequency or establish a causal relationship to the vaccine.
Administrative site conditions: Injection-site dermatitis, injection-site pruritus, injection-site urticaria
Blood and lymphatic system disorders: Lymphadenopathy localized to the region of the injection site
Immune system disorders: Anaphylactic/anaphylactoid reaction including shock
Skin and subcutaneous tissue disorders: Angioneurotic edema, erythema multiforme
Respiratory: Apnea
The safety of Prevnar given concomitantly with other vaccines as part of routine care was assessed in a three-year observational study performed at Northern California Kaiser Permanente in which 65,927 children received three doses of Prevnar in the first year of life. Primary safety outcomes analyses included an evaluation of pre-defined adverse events occurring in temporal relationship to immunization. Rates of adverse events occurring within various time periods post-vaccination (e.g., 0-2, 0-7, 0-14, and 0-30 days) were compared to the rates of those events occurring within a control time window (i.e., 31-60 days). Secondary safety outcomes analyses included comparisons to a historical control population of infants (1995-1996, N=40,223) prior to the introduction of Prevnar. In addition, the study included extended follow-up of subjects originally enrolled in the NCKP efficacy trial (N=37,866).
The primary safety outcomes analyses did not demonstrate a consistently elevated risk of healthcare utilization for croup, gastroenteritis, allergic reactions, seizures, wheezing diagnoses, or breath-holding across doses, healthcare settings, or multiple time windows. As in prelicensure trials, fever was associated with Prevnar administration. In analyses of secondary safety outcomes, the adjusted relative risk of hospitalization for reactive airways disease was 1.23 (95% CI: 1.11, 1.35). Potential confounders, such as differences in concomitantly administered vaccines, yearly variation in respiratory infections, or secular trends in reactive airways disease incidence, could not be controlled. Extended follow-up of subjects originally enrolled in the NCKP efficacy trial revealed no increased risk of reactive airways disease among Prevnar recipients. In general, the study results support the previously described safety profile of Prevnar.

7   DRUG INTERACTIONS
7.1   Concomitant Immunizations
In clinical trials, Prevnar 13 was administered concomitantly with the following U.S. licensed vaccines: Pediarix [Diphtheria and Tetanus Toxoids and Acellular Pertussis Adsorbed, Hepatitis B (Recombinant) and Inactivated Poliovirus Vaccine Combined] (DTaP-HBV-IPV) and ActHIB [Haemophilus b Conjugate Vaccine (Tetanus Toxoid Conjugate)] (PRP-T) for the first three doses and with PedvaxHIB [Haemophilus b Conjugate Vaccine (Meningococcal Protein Conjugate)] (PRP-OMP), M-M-R II [Measles, Mumps, Rubella Virus Vaccine Live] (MMR) and Varivax [Varicella Virus Vaccine Live], or ProQuad [Measles, Mumps, Rubella and Varicella Virus Vaccine Live] (MMRV) and VAQTA [Hepatitis A vaccine, Inactivated] (HepA) for dose 4 [see Clinical Studies (14.2)].
When Prevnar 13 is administered at the same time as another injectable vaccine(s), the vaccines should always be administered with different syringes and given at different injection sites.
Do not mix Prevnar 13 with other vaccines/products in the same syringe.
7.2   Immunosuppressive Therapies
Children with impaired immune responsiveness due to the use of immunosuppressive therapy (including irradiation, corticosteroids, antimetabolites, alkylating agents, and cytotoxic agents) may not respond optimally to active immunization.

8   USE IN SPECIFIC POPULATIONS
8.1   Pregnancy
Pregnancy Category C
Animal reproduction studies have not been conducted with Prevnar 13. It is also not known whether Prevnar 13 can cause fetal harm when administered to a pregnant woman or whether it can affect reproductive capacity.
8.4   Pediatric Use
Safety and effectiveness of Prevnar 13 in children below the age of 6 weeks or on or after the 6th birthday have not been established. Prevnar 13 is not approved for use in children in these age groups [see Dosage and Administration (2)].
Immune responses elicited by Prevnar 13 among infants born prematurely have not been specifically studied.
8.5   Geriatric Use
The safety and effectiveness of Prevnar 13 in geriatric populations have not been established.

Prevnar 13 is not to be used as a substitute for 23-valent pneumococcal polysaccharide vaccine (PPV23) in geriatric populations.

10 OVERDOSAGE

Overdose with Prevnar 13 is unlikely due to its presentation as a pre-filled syringe. However, there have been reports of overdose with Prevnar 13 defined as subsequent doses administered closer than recommended to the previous dose. In general, adverse events reported with overdose are consistent with those which have been reported with doses given in the recommended schedules of Prevnar 13.

11 DESCRIPTION

Prevnar 13, Pneumococcal 13-valent Conjugate Vaccine (Diphtheria CRM$_{197}$ Protein) is a sterile suspension of saccharides of the capsular antigens of *Streptococcus pneumoniae* serotypes 1, 3, 4, 5, 6A, 6B, 7F, 9V, 14, 18C, 19A, 19F, and 23F, individually linked to non-toxic diphtheria CRM$_{197}$ protein. Each serotype is grown in soy peptone broth. The individual polysaccharides are purified through centrifugation, precipitation, ultrafiltration, and column chromatography. The polysaccharides are chemically activated to make saccharides, which are directly conjugated by reductive amination to the protein carrier CRM$_{197}$, to form the glycoconjugate. CRM$_{197}$ is a nontoxic variant of diphtheria toxin isolated from cultures of *Corynebacterium diphtheriae* strain C7 (β197) grown in a casamino acids and yeast extract-based medium. CRM$_{197}$ is purified through ultrafiltration, ammonium sulfate precipitation, and ion-exchange chromatography. The individual glycoconjugates are purified by ultrafiltration and column chromatography and analyzed for saccharide to protein ratios, molecular size, free saccharide, and free protein.

The individual glycoconjugates are compounded to formulate Prevnar 13. Potency of the formulated vaccine is determined by quantification of each of the saccharide antigens and by the saccharide to protein ratios in the individual glycoconjugates. Each 0.5 mL dose of the vaccine is formulated to contain approximately 2.2 µg of each of *Streptococcus pneumoniae* serotypes 1, 3, 4, 5, 6A, 7F, 9V, 14, 18C, 19A, 19F, 23F saccharides, 4.4 µg of 6B saccharides, 34 µg CRM$_{197}$ carrier protein, 100 µg polysorbate 80, 295 µg succinate buffer and 125 µg aluminum as aluminum phosphate adjuvant.

The tip cap and rubber plunger of the pre-filled syringe do not contain latex.

12 CLINICAL PHARMACOLOGY

A serum anti-capsular polysaccharide antibody concentration of 0.35 µg/mL measured one month after the third dose as a single antibody reference concentration was used to estimate the effectiveness of Prevnar 13 against IPD. The assay used for this determination is a standardized ELISA involving pre-absorption of the test sera with pneumococcal C-polysaccharide and serotype 22F polysaccharide to reduce non-specific background reactivity. The single antibody reference value was based on pooled efficacy estimates from three placebo-controlled IPD efficacy trials with either Prevnar or the investigational 9-valent CRM$_{197}$ conjugate pneumococcal polysaccharide vaccine. This reference concentration is only applicable on a population basis and cannot be used to predict protection against IPD on an individual basis. Functional antibodies elicited by the vaccine (as measured by opsonophagocytic assay [OPA]) were also evaluated.

12.1 Mechanism of Action

B-cells produce antibodies in response to antigenic stimulation via T-dependent and T-independent mechanisms. Prevnar 13, comprised of polysaccharides conjugated to a carrier protein, elicits a T-cell dependent immune response. Protein carrier-specific T-cells provide the signals needed for maturation of the B-cell response and generation of B-cell memory. This type of response induces immune memory and elicits booster responses on re-exposure in infants and young children to pneumococcal polysaccharides.

13 NONCLINICAL TOXICOLOGY

13.1 Carcinogenesis, Mutagenesis, Impairment of Fertility

Prevnar 13 has not been evaluated for any carcinogenic or mutagenic potential, or impairment of fertility.

14 CLINICAL STUDIES

14.1 Prevnar Efficacy Data

Invasive Pneumococcal Disease (IPD)

Prevnar was licensed in the U.S. in 2000, following a randomized, double-blind clinical trial in a multiethnic population at Northern California Kaiser Permanente (NCKP) from October 1995 through August 20, 1998, in which 37,816 infants were randomized to receive either Prevnar or a control vaccine (an investigational meningococcal group C conjugate vaccine [MnCC]) at 2, 4, 6, and 12-15 months of age. In this study, the efficacy of Prevnar against invasive disease due to *S. pneumoniae* in cases accrued during this period was 100% in both the per-protocol and intent-to-treat

Table 8: Percentage of U.S. Subjects 15 Months Through 59 Months of Age, Previously Vaccinated with 3 or 4 Prior Infant Prevnar Doses, Reporting Solicited Systemic Adverse Reactions Within 7 Days After One Supplemental Prevnar 13 Vaccination

Systemic Reaction	15 months through 23 months[a]		24 months through 59 months[b]
	1 dose Prevnar 13 3 prior Prevnar doses N^c=28-33 %	1 dose Prevnar 13 4 prior Prevnar doses N^c=62-75 %	1 dose Prevnar 13 3 or 4 prior Prevnar doses N^c=138-151 %
Fever[d]			
Mild	10.7	18.8	5.1
Moderate	7.1	3.2	0.7
Severe	0.0	0.0	0.7
Decreased appetite	56.7	36.2	24.8
Irritability	66.7	57.3	39.7
Increased sleep	30.0	33.8	15.9
Decreased sleep	22.6	22.7	14.0

[a] Dose 2 data not shown.
[b] The data for this age group are only represented as a single result as 95 % of children received 4 doses of Prevnar prior to enrollment.
[c] Number of subjects reporting Yes for at least 1 day or No for all days.
[d] Fever gradings: Mild (≥38°C but ≤39°C), Moderate (>39°C but ≤40°C), and Severe (> 40°C). No other systemic event other than fever was graded.

Table 9: Percentage of Subjects With Anti-capsular Antibody Concentration ≥0.35 µg/mL One Month After Dose 3, U.S. Pivotal Non-inferiority Study*[†]

Serotype	Prevnar 13 N=249-252 (95% CI)	Prevnar N=250-252 (95% CI)	Difference in % responders (95% CI)
Prevnar Serotypes			
4	94.4 (90.9, 96.9)	98.0 (95.4, 99.4)	-3.6 (-7.3, -0.1)
6B	87.3 (82.5, 91.1)	92.8 (88.9, 95.7)	-5.5 (-10.9, -0.1)
9V	90.5 (86.2, 93.8)	98.4 (96.0, 99.6)	-7.9 (-12.4, -4.0)
14	97.6 (94.9, 99.1)	97.2 (94.4, 98.9)	0.4 (-2.7, 3.5)
18C	96.8 (93.8, 98.6)	98.4 (96.0, 99.6)	-1.6 (-4.7, 1.2)
19F	98.0 (95.4, 99.4)	97.6 (99.4, 99.1)	0.4 (-2.4, 3.4)
23F	90.5 (86.2, 93.8)	94.0 (90.4, 96.6)	-3.6 (-8.5, 1.2)
Additional Serotypes[††]			
1	95.6 (92.3, 97.8)	††	2.8 (-1.3, 7.2)
3	63.5 (57.1, 69.4)	††	-29.3 (-36.2, -22.4)
5	89.7 (85.2, 93.1)	††	-3.1 (-8.3, 1.9)
6A	96.0 (92.8, 98.1)	††	3.2 (-0.8, 7.6)
7F	98.4 (96.0, 99.6)	††	5.6 (1.9, 9.7)
19A	98.4 (96.0, 99.6)	††	5.6 (1.9, 9.7)

* Non-inferiority was met when the lower bound of the 95% CI for the difference between groups (Prevnar 13 minus Prevnar) was greater than -10%.
† Antibody measured by a standardized ELISA involving pre-absorption of the test sera with pneumococcal C-polysaccharide and serotype 22F polysaccharide to reduce non-specific background reactivity.
†† Comparison for the 6 additional serotypes was to the lowest responder of the 7 common serotypes in Prevnar recipients, which for this analysis was serotype 6B (92.8%; 95% CI: 88.9, 95.7).

analyses (95% CI: 75.4%-100% and 81.7%-100%, respectively). Data accumulated through an extended follow-up period to April 20, 1999, resulted in similar efficacy estimates of 97.4% in the per-protocol analysis and 93.9% in the intent-to-treat analysis (95% CI: 82.7%-99.9% and 79.6%-98.5%, respectively).

Acute Otitis Media (AOM)

The efficacy of Prevnar against otitis media was assessed in two clinical trials: a trial in Finnish infants at the National Public Health Institute and the pivotal-efficacy trial in U.S. infants at Northern California Kaiser Permanente (NCKP). The Finnish Otitis Media (FinOM) trial was a randomized, double-blind trial in which 1,662 infants were equally randomized to receive either Prevnar or a control vaccine

Recombivax HB (Hepatitis B vaccine (Recombinant) [Hep B]) at 2, 4, 6, and 12-15 months of age. In this study, conducted between December 1995 and March 1999, parents of study participants were asked to bring their children to the study clinics if the child had respiratory infections or symptoms suggesting acute otitis media (AOM). If AOM was diagnosed, tympanocentesis was performed, and the middle-ear fluid was cultured. If *S. pneumoniae* was isolated, serotyping was performed; the primary endpoint was efficacy against AOM episodes caused by vaccine serotypes in the per-protocol population. In the NCKP trial, the efficacy of Prevnar against otitis media was assessed from the beginning of the trial in October 1995 through April 1998. The otitis media analysis included 34,146 infants randomized to

Table 10: Pneumococcal OPA Geometric Mean Titers One Month After the Third Dose-Evaluable Immunogenicity Population, U.S. Pivotal Non-inferiority Study*

Serotype	Prevnar 13 N=91-94 (95% CI)	Prevnar N=89-94 (95% CI)
Prevnar Serotypes		
4	359 (276, 468)	536 (421, 681)
6B	1055 (817, 1361)	1514 (1207, 1899)
9V	4035 (2933, 5553)	3259 (2288, 4641)
14	1240 (935, 1646)	1481 (1133, 1934)
18C	276 (210, 361)	376 (292, 484)
19F	54 (40, 74)	45 (34, 60)
23F	791 (605, 1034)	924 (709, 1204)
Additional Serotypes		
1	52 (39, 69)	4 (4, 5)
3	121 (92, 158)	7 (5, 9)
5	91 (67, 123)	4 (4, 4)
6A	980 (783, 1226)	100 (66, 152)
7F	9494 (7339, 12281)	128 (80, 206)
19A	152 (105, 220)	7 (5, 9)

* The OPA (opsonophagocytic activity) assay measures the ability of immune sera, in conjunction with complement, to mediate the uptake and killing of *S. pneumoniae* by phagocytic cells.

Table 11: Pneumococcal IgG GMCs (µg/mL) One Month After Dose 4, U.S. Pivotal Non-inferiority Study*†

Serotype	Prevnar 13 N=232-236 (95% CI)	Prevnar N=222-223 (95% CI)	GMC Ratio (95% CI)
Prevnar Serotypes			
4	3.73 (3.28, 4.24)	5.49 (4.91, 6.13)	0.68 (0.57, 0.80)
6B	11.53 (9.99, 13.30)	15.63 (13.80, 17.69)	0.74 (0.61, 0.89)
9V	2.62 (2.34, 2.94)	3.63 (3.25, 4.05)	0.72 (0.62, 0.85)
14	9.11 (7.95, 10.45)	12.72 (11.22, 14.41)	0.72 (0.60, 0.86)
18C	3.20 (2.82, 3.64)	4.70 (4.18, 5.28)	0.68 (0.57, 0.81)
19F	6.60 (5.85, 7.44)	5.60 (4.87, 6.43)	1.18 (0.98, 1.41)
23F	5.07 (4.41, 5.83)	7.84 (6.91, 8.90)	0.65 (0.54, 0.78)
Additional Serotypes††			
1	5.06 (4.43, 5.80)	††	1.40 (1.17, 1.66)
3	0.94 (0.83, 1.05)	††	0.26 (0.22, 0.30)
5	3.72 (3.31, 4.18)	††	1.03 (0.87, 1.20)
6A	8.20 (7.30, 9.20)	††	2.26 (1.93, 2.65)
7F	5.67 (5.01, 6.42)	††	1.56 (1.32, 1.85)
19A	8.55 (7.64, 9.56)	††	2.36 (2.01, 2.76)

* Non-inferiority was declared if the lower limit of the 2-sided 95% CI for Geometric Mean Ratio (Prevnar 13:Prevnar) was greater than 0.5.
† Antibody measured by a standardized ELISA involving pre-absorption of the test sera with pneumococcal C-polysaccharide and serotype 22F polysaccharide to reduce non-specific background reactivity.
†† Comparison for the 6 additional serotypes was to the lowest responder of the 7 common serotypes in Prevnar recipients, which for this analysis was serotype 9V (3.63; 95% CI 3.25, 4.05).

receive either Prevnar (N=17,070), or the control vaccine (N=17,076), at 2, 4, 6, and 12-15 months of age. In this trial, no routine tympanocentesis was performed, and no standard definition of otitis media was used by study physicians. The primary otitis media endpoint was efficacy against all otitis media episodes in the per-protocol population.

The vaccine efficacy against AOM episodes due to vaccine serotypes assessed in the Finnish trial, was 57% (95% CI: 44%-67%) in the per-protocol population and 54% (95% CI: 41%-64%) in the intent-to-treat population. The vaccine ef-

ficacy against AOM episodes due to vaccine-related serotypes (6A, 9N, 18B, 19A, 23A), also assessed in the Finnish trial, was 51% (95% CI: 27, 67) in the per-protocol population and 44% (95% CI: 20, 62) in the intent-to-treat population. There was a nonsignificant increase in AOM episodes caused by serotypes unrelated to the vaccine in the per-protocol population, compared to children who received the control vaccine, suggesting that children who received Prevnar appeared to be at increased risk of otitis media due to pneumococcal serotypes not represented in the vaccine.

However, vaccination with Prevnar reduced pneumococcal otitis media episodes overall. In the NCKP trial, in which the endpoint was all otitis media episodes regardless of etiology, vaccine efficacy was 7% (95% CI: 4%-10%) and 6% (95% CI: 4%-9%), respectively, in the per-protocol and intent-to-treat analyses. Several other otitis media endpoints were also assessed in the two trials.

Recurrent AOM, defined as 3 episodes in 6 months or 4 episodes in 12 months, was reduced by 9% in both the per-protocol and intent-to-treat populations (95% CI: 3%-15% in per-protocol and 95% CI: 4%-14% in intent-to-treat) in the NCKP trial; a similar trend was observed in the Finnish trial. The NCKP trial also demonstrated a 20% reduction (95% CI: 2, 35) in the placement of tympanostomy tubes in the per-protocol population and a 21% reduction (95% CI: 4, 34) in the intent-to-treat population. Data from the NCKP trial accumulated through an extended follow-up period to April 20, 1999, in which a total of 37,866 children were included (18,925 in Prevnar group and 18,941 in MnCC control group), resulted in similar otitis media efficacy estimates for all endpoints.

14.2   Evaluation of Prevnar 13 Effectiveness
Prevnar 13 effectiveness against invasive pneumococcal disease was inferred from comparative studies to a U.S. licensed 7-valent pneumococcal conjugate vaccine, Prevnar, in which Prevnar 13 elicited immune responses as measured by antipolysaccharide binding and functional OPA antibodies. These studies were designed to evaluate immunologic non-inferiority of Prevnar 13 to Prevnar.

Clinical trials have been conducted in the U.S. using a 2, 4, 6, and 12 to 15 month schedule.

The pivotal U.S. non-inferiority study was a randomized, double-blind, active-controlled trial in which 2 month-old infants were randomly assigned to receive either Prevnar 13 or Prevnar in a 1:1 ratio. The 2 vaccine groups were well balanced with respect to race, ethnicity, and age and weight at enrollment. Most subjects were White (69.1%), 19.6% were Black or African-American, and 2.4% were Asian; 82.1% of subjects were non-Hispanic and non-Latino and 17.3% were Hispanic or Latino. Overall, 54.0% of subjects were male infants.

In the pivotal U.S. non-inferiority study, immune responses were compared in subjects receiving either Prevnar 13 or Prevnar using a set of non-inferiority criteria. Co-primary endpoints included the percentage of subjects with serum pneumococcal anti-capsular polysaccharide IgG ≥0.35 µg/mL measured one month after the third dose and serum pneumococcal anti-capsular polysaccharide IgG geometric mean concentrations (GMCs) one month after the fourth dose. The assay used for this determination was a standardized ELISA involving pre-absorption of the test sera with pneumococcal C-polysaccharide and serotype 22F polysaccharide to reduce non-specific background reactivity. Responses to the 7 common serotypes in Prevnar 13 and Prevnar recipients were compared directly. Responses to the 6 additional serotypes in Prevnar 13 recipients were each compared to the lowest response observed among the Prevnar serotypes in Prevnar recipients.

Pneumococcal Immune Responses Following Three Doses
In the pivotal U.S. non-inferiority study, the non-inferiority criterion for the proportion of subjects with pneumococcal anti-capsular polysaccharide IgG antibody concentrations ≥0.35 µg/mL one month after the third dose was met for 10 of the 13 serotypes. The exceptions were serotypes 6B, 9V, and 3. Although the response to serotypes 6B and 9V did not meet the pre-specified non-inferiority criterion, the differences were marginal. The clinical relevance of these differences, if any, is unknown.

The percentage of infants achieving pneumococcal anticapsular polysaccharide IgG antibody concentrations ≥0.35 µg/mL one month after the third dose is shown below (Table 9).
[See table 9 on previous page]
Functional OPA antibody responses were elicited for all 13 serotypes, as shown in Table 10.
[See table 10 above]

Pneumococcal Immune Responses Following Four Doses
In the pivotal U.S. non-inferiority study, post-dose 4 antibody concentrations were higher for all 13 serotypes than those achieved after the third dose. The non-inferiority criterion for pneumococcal anti-capsular polysaccharide GMCs after 4 doses was met for 12 of the 13 pneumococcal serotypes. The non-inferiority criterion was not met for the response to serotype 3 (Table 11).
[See table 11 at left]
Following the 4th dose, the functional OPA response for each serotype was quantitatively greater than the response following the 3rd dose (see Table 12).
[See table 12 at top of next page]

Table 12: Pneumococcal OPA Geometric Mean Titers One Month After the Fourth Dose-Evaluable Toddler Immunogenicity Population, U.S. Pivotal Non-inferiority Study*

Serotype	Prevnar 13 N=88-92 (95% CI)		Prevnar N=92-96 (95% CI)	
Prevnar Serotypes				
4	1180	(847, 1643)	1492	(1114, 1999)
6B	3100	(2337, 4111)	4066	(3243, 5098)
9V	11856	(8810, 15955)	18032	(14125, 23021)
14	2002	(1453, 2760)	2366	(1871, 2992)
18C	993	(754, 1308)	1722	(1327, 2236)
19F	200	(144, 276)	167	(121, 230)
23F	2723	(1961, 3782)	4982	(3886, 6387)
Additional Serotypes				
1	164	(114, 237)	5	(4, 6)
3	380	(300, 482)	12	(9, 16)
5	300	(229, 393)	5	(4, 6)
6A	2242	(1707, 2945)	539	(375, 774)
7F	11629	(9054, 14938)	268	(165, 436)
19A	1024	(774, 1355)	29	(19, 44)

* The OPA (opsonophagocytic activity) assay measures the ability of immune sera, in conjunction with complement, to mediate the uptake and killing of *S. pneumoniae* by phagocytic cells.

Table 13: Pneumococcal Anti-capsular Polysaccharide IgG Antibody Geometric Mean Concentrations (µg/mL) One Month After the Final Prevnar 13 Catch-Up Dose in Pneumococcal Vaccine Naïve Children 7 Months through 5 Years of Age by Age Group, Poland Catch-Up Study

Serotype	3 doses Prevnar 13 7 through 11 months N=83-84 (95% CI)		2 doses Prevnar 13 12 through 23 months N=104-110 (95% CI)		1 dose Prevnar 13 24 months through 5 years N=135-152 (95% CI)	
1	2.88	(2.44, 3.39)	2.74	(2.37, 3.16)	1.78	(1.52, 2.08)
3	1.94	(1.68, 2.24)	1.86	(1.60, 2.15)	1.42	(1.23, 1.64)
4	3.63	(3.11, 4.23)	4.28	(3.78, 4.86)	3.37	(2.95, 3.85)
5	2.85	(2.34, 3.46)	2.16	(1.89, 2.47)	2.33	(2.05, 2.64)
6A	3.72	(3.12, 4.45)	2.62	(2.25, 3.06)	2.96	(2.52, 3.47)
6B	4.77	(3.90, 5.84)	3.38	(2.81, 4.06)	3.41	(2.80, 4.16)
7F	5.30	(4.54, 6.18)	5.99	(5.40, 6.65)	4.92	(4.26, 5.68)
9V	2.56	(2.21, 2.96)	3.08	(2.69, 3.53)	2.67	(2.32, 3.07)
14	8.04	(6.95, 9.30)	6.45	(5.48, 7.59)	2.24	(1.71, 2.93)
18C	2.77	(2.39, 3.23)	3.71	(3.29, 7.19)	2.56	(2.17, 3.03)
19A	4.77	(4.28, 5.33)	4.94	(4.31, 5.65)	6.03	(5.22, 6.97)
19F	2.88	(2.35, 3.54)	3.07	(2.68, 3.51)	2.53	(2.14, 2.99)
23F	2.16	(1.82, 2.55)	1.98	(1.64, 2.39)	1.55	(1.31, 1.85)

Simultaneous Administration With Other Vaccines
The concomitant administration of routine U.S. infant vaccines *[see Drug Interactions (7.1)]* with Prevnar 13 was evaluated in two studies: the U.S. pivotal non-inferiority study *[see Clinical Studies (14.2), Pneumococcal Immune Responses Following Three Doses]* and the U.S. lot consistency study. In the lot consistency study, subjects were randomly assigned to receive one of 3 lots of Prevnar 13 or Prevnar in a 2:2:2:1 ratio. The total number of infants vaccinated was *663* (U.S. non-inferiority study) and 1699 (U.S. lot consistency study). Immune *responses to concomitant vaccine* antigens were compared in infants receiving Prevnar and Prevnar 13. Responses to diphtheria toxoid, tetanus toxoid, pertussis, polio types 1, 2, and 3, hepatitis B, PRP-T, PRP-OMP, measles, and varicella antigens in Prevnar 13 recipients were similar to those in Prevnar recipients. Based on limited data, responses to mumps and rubella antigens in Prevnar 13 recipients were similar to those in Prevnar recipients.

Previously Unvaccinated Older Infants and Children
In an open-label descriptive study of Prevnar 13 in Poland, children 7 through 11 months of age, 12 through 23 months of age and 24 months through 5 years of age (prior to the 6th birthday) who were naïve to pneumococcal conjugate vaccine, were given 3, 2 or 1 dose of Prevnar 13 respectively, according to the age-appropriate schedules in Table 1. Serum IgG concentrations were measured one month after the final dose in each age group and the data are shown in Table 13.
[See table 13 above]

Children Previously Vaccinated with Prevnar
In an open-label descriptive study in the U.S., children previously vaccinated with 3 or 4 doses of Prevnar, received 2 doses of Prevnar 13 (children 15 through 23 months of age) or 1 dose of Prevnar 13 (children 24 months through 59 months of age). The data following one dose of Prevnar 13 in children 24 months through 59 months of age are shown in Table 14.

Table 14: Pneumococcal Anti-capsular Polysaccharide IgG Antibody Geometric Mean Concentrations (µg/mL) One Month After One Prevnar 13 Catch-Up Dose in Children 24 through 59 Months of Age With 3 or 4 Prior Doses of Prevnar, U.S. Catch-Up Study

Serotype	1 dose Prevnar 13 24 months through 59 months N=173-175 (95% CI)	
1	2.43	(2.15, 2.75)
3	1.38	(1.17, 1.61)
5	2.13	(1.89, 2.41)
6A	12.96	(11.04, 15.21)
7F	4.22	(3.74, 4.77)
19A	14.18	(12.37, 16.25)

16   HOW SUPPLIED/STORAGE AND HANDLING
Pre-filled Syringe, 1 Dose (10 per package) – NDC 0005-1971-02.
Store refrigerated at +2°C to +8°C (36°F to 46°F).
The tip cap and rubber plunger of the pre-filled syringe do not contain latex.
Do not freeze. Discard if the vaccine has been frozen.

17   PATIENT COUNSELING INFORMATION
17.1   Potential Benefits and Risks
Prior to administration of this vaccine, the healthcare professional should inform the parent, guardian, or other responsible adult of the potential benefits and risks to the patient *[see Warnings and Precautions (5) and Adverse Reactions (6)]*, and the importance of completing the immunization series unless contraindicated.
17.2   Adverse Reactions
Instruct parents, guardians, or other responsible adults to report any suspected adverse reactions to their healthcare professional.

Wyeth®
Wyeth Pharmaceuticals Inc.
Philadelphia, PA 19101
U.S. Govt. License No. 3
W10543C003
ET01
Rev 04/10
CPT Code 90670
United States Patent Number: 5,614,382.

PRISTIQ®   R
[*pris-TEEK*]
(desvenlafaxine)
Extended-Release Tablets, Oral

HIGHLIGHTS OF PRESCRIBING INFORMATION
These highlights do not include all the information needed to use PRISTIQ safely and effectively. See full prescribing information for PRISTIQ.
PRISTIQ® (desvenlafaxine) Extended-Release Tablets, oral
Initial U.S. Approval: 2008

WARNING: SUICIDALITY AND ANTIDEPRESSANT DRUGS
See full prescribing information for complete boxed warning.
Increased risk of suicidal thinking and behavior in children, adolescents and young adults taking antidepressants for major depressive disorder (MDD) and other psychiatric disorders. PRISTIQ is not approved for use in pediatric patients (5.1).

—————RECENT MAJOR CHANGES—————
Dosage and Administration, Switching Patients From Other Antidepressants to PRISTIQ (2.5)   11/2009

—————INDICATIONS AND USAGE—————
PRISTIQ, a selective serotonin and norepinephrine reuptake inhibitor (SNRI), is indicated for the treatment of major depressive disorder [MDD] (1).

————DOSAGE AND ADMINISTRATION————
• Recommended dose: 50 mg once daily with or without food (2.1).
• There was no evidence that doses greater than 50 mg/day confer any additional benefit (2.1).
• When discontinuing treatment, gradual dose reduction is recommended whenever possible (2.1 and 5.9).
• Tablets should be taken whole; do not divide, crush, chew, or dissolve (2.1).
• Renal Impairment: The recommended dose in patients with moderate renal impairment is 50 mg/day. The recommended dose in patients with severe renal impairment

and end-stage renal disease (ESRD) is 50 mg every other day. The dose should not be escalated in patients with moderate or severe renal impairment or ESRD (2.2).
- Hepatic Impairment: Dose escalation above 100 mg/day is not recommended (2.2).

DOSAGE FORMS AND STRENGTHS
- PRISTIQ tablets are available as 50 and 100 mg tablets (3).
- Each tablet contains 76 mg or 152 mg of desvenlafaxine succinate equivalent to 50 mg or 100 mg of desvenlafaxine (3).

CONTRAINDICATIONS
- Hypersensitivity to desvenlafaxine succinate, venlafaxine hydrochloride or any excipients in the PRISTIQ formulation (4.1).
- Do not use with an MAOI or within 14 days of stopping an MAOI. Allow 7 days after stopping PRISTIQ before starting an MAOI (4.2).

WARNINGS AND PRECAUTIONS
- **Clinical Worsening/Suicide Risk:** Monitor for clinical worsening and suicide risk (5.1).
- **Serotonin Syndrome or Neuroleptic Malignant Syndrome (NMS)-like Reactions:** Serotonin syndrome or NMS-like reactions have been reported with SSRIs and SNRIs. Discontinue PRISTIQ and initiate supportive treatment (5.2).
- **Elevated Blood Pressure:** Has occurred with PRISTIQ. Hypertension should be controlled before initiating treatment. Monitor blood pressure regularly during treatment (5.3).
- **Abnormal Bleeding:** PRISTIQ may increase the risk of bleeding events. Patients should be cautioned about the risk of bleeding associated with the concomitant use of PRISTIQ and NSAIDs, aspirin, or other drugs that affect coagulation (5.4).
- **Narrow-angle Glaucoma:** Mydriasis has occurred with PRISTIQ. Patients with raised intraocular pressure or those at risk of angle-closure glaucoma should be monitored (5.5).
- **Activation of Mania/Hypomania:** Has occurred. Use cautiously in patients with Bipolar Disorder. Caution patients about the risk of activation of mania/hypomania (5.6).
- **Cardiovascular/Cerebrovascular Disease:** Use cautiously in patients with cardiovascular or cerebrovascular disease (5.7).
- **Cholesterol and Triglyceride Elevation:** Have occurred. Use cautiously in patients with lipid metabolism disorders. Consider monitoring serum cholesterol and triglyceride (5.8).
- **Discontinuation Symptoms:** Have occurred. Taper the dose when possible and monitor for discontinuation symptoms (5.9).
- **Renal Impairment:** Reduces the clearance of PRISTIQ. Dosage adjustment is necessary in severe and ESRD. In moderate renal impairment, the dose should not exceed 50 mg/day (5.10).
- **Seizure:** Can occur. Use cautiously in patients with seizure disorder (5.11).
- **Hyponatremia:** Can occur in association with SIADH (5.12).
- **Drugs Containing Desvenlafaxine or Venlafaxine:** Should not be used concomitantly with PRISTIQ (5.13).
- **Interstitial Lung Disease and Eosinophilic Pneumonia:** Can occur (5.14).

ADVERSE REACTIONS
Adverse reactions in patients in short-term fixed-dose studies (incidence ≥ 5% and twice the rate of placebo in the 50 or 100 mg dose groups) were: nausea, dizziness, insomnia, hyperhidrosis, constipation, somnolence, decreased appetite, anxiety, and specific male sexual function disorders (6.1).
To report SUSPECTED ADVERSE REACTIONS, contact Wyeth Pharmaceuticals Inc. at 1-800-934-5556 or FDA at 1-800-FDA-1088 or www.fda.gov/medwatch

USE IN SPECIFIC POPULATIONS
- Dosage adjustment is recommended in patients with severe renal impairment and end-stage renal disease. The dose should not be escalated in moderate to severe impairment or in ESRD (2.2, 8.6 and 12.6).
- There is an increased incidence of orthostatic hypotension in PRISTIQ treated patients ≥ 65 years (6.1 and 8.5).
- For elderly patients, the possibility of reduced renal clearance of desvenlafaxine should be considered when determining dose (2.2).
- Only administer PRISTIQ to pregnant or breastfeeding women if the expected benefits outweigh the possible risks (8.1 and 8.3).

See 17 for PATIENT COUNSELING INFORMATION and the FDA-approved Medication Guide.

Revised: 05/2010

FULL PRESCRIBING INFORMATION

> **WARNING: SUICIDALITY AND ANTIDEPRESSANT DRUGS**
>
> Antidepressants increased the risk compared to placebo of suicidal thinking and behavior (suicidality) in children, adolescents, and young adults in short-term studies of Major Depressive Disorder (MDD) and other psychiatric disorders. Anyone considering the use of PRISTIQ® or any other antidepressant in a child, adolescent, or young adult must balance this risk with the clinical need. Short-term studies did not show an increase in the risk of suicidality with antidepressants compared to placebo in adults beyond age 24; there was a reduction in risk with antidepressants compared to placebo in adults aged 65 and older. Depression and certain other psychiatric disorders are themselves associated with increases in the risk of suicide. Patients of all ages who are started on antidepressant therapy should be monitored appropriately and observed closely for clinical worsening, suicidality, or unusual changes in behavior. Families and caregivers should be advised of the need for close observation and communication with the prescriber. PRISTIQ is not approved for use in pediatric patients [see Warnings and Precautions (5.1), Use in Specific Populations (8.4), and Patient Counseling Information (17.1)].

1 INDICATIONS AND USAGE

PRISTIQ, a selective serotonin and norepinephrine reuptake inhibitor (SNRI), is indicated for the treatment of major depressive disorder (MDD) [see Clinical Studies (14) and Dosage and Administration (2.1)]. The efficacy of PRISTIQ has been established in four 8-week, placebo-controlled studies of outpatients who met DSM-IV criteria for major depressive disorder.

A major depressive episode (DSM-IV) implies a prominent and relatively persistent (nearly every day for at least 2 weeks) depressed or dysphoric mood that usually interferes with daily functioning, and includes at least 5 of the following 9 symptoms: depressed mood, loss of interest in usual activities, significant change in weight and/or appetite, insomnia or hypersomnia, psychomotor agitation or retardation, increased fatigue, feelings of guilt or worthlessness, slowed thinking or impaired concentration, or a suicide attempt or suicidal ideation.

2 DOSAGE AND ADMINISTRATION

2.1 Initial Treatment of Major Depressive Disorder
The recommended dose for PRISTIQ is 50 mg once daily, with or without food.

In clinical studies, doses of 50-400 mg/day were shown to be effective, although no additional benefit was demonstrated at doses greater than 50 mg/day and adverse events and discontinuations were more frequent at higher doses.

When discontinuing therapy, gradual dose reduction is recommended whenever possible to minimize discontinuation symptoms [see Dosage and Administration (2.4) and Warnings and Precautions (5.9)].

PRISTIQ should be taken at approximately the same time each day. Tablets must be swallowed whole with fluid and not divided, crushed, chewed, or dissolved.

2.2 Special Populations
Pregnant women during the third trimester

Neonates exposed to SNRIs or SSRIs late in the third trimester have developed complications requiring prolonged hospitalization, respiratory support, and tube feeding [see Use in Specific Populations (8.1)]. When treating pregnant women with PRISTIQ during the third trimester, the physician should carefully consider the potential risks and benefits of treatment. The physician may consider tapering PRISTIQ in the third trimester.

Patients with renal impairment

No dosage adjustment is necessary in patients with mild renal impairment (24-hr CrCl = 50-80 mL/min).

The recommended dose in patients with moderate renal impairment (24-hr CrCl = 30-50 mL/min) is 50 mg per day. The recommended dose in patients with severe renal impairment (24-hr CrCl < 30 mL/min) or end-stage renal disease (ESRD) is 50 mg every other day. Supplemental doses should not be given to patients after dialysis. The doses should not be escalated in patients with moderate or severe renal impairment, or ESRD [see Warnings and Precautions (5.10), Use in Specific Populations (8.6) and Clinical Pharmacology (12.6)].

Patients with hepatic impairment

The recommended dose in patients with hepatic impairment is 50 mg/day. Dose escalation above 100 mg/day is not recommended [see Clinical Pharmacology (12.6)].

Elderly patients

No dosage adjustment is required solely on the basis of age; however, the possibility of reduced renal clearance of PRISTIQ should be considered when determining the dose [see Use in Specific Populations (8.5) and Clinical Pharmacology (12.6)].

2.3   Maintenance/Continuation/Extended Treatment

It is generally agreed that acute episodes of major depressive disorder require several months or longer of sustained pharmacologic therapy. However, the longer-term efficacy of PRISTIQ at a dose of 50 mg/day that was effective in short-term, controlled studies has not been studied. Patients should be periodically reassessed to determine the need for continued treatment.

2.4   Discontinuing PRISTIQ

Symptoms associated with discontinuation of PRISTIQ, other SNRIs and SSRIs have been reported [see Warnings and Precautions (5.9)]. Patients should be monitored for these symptoms when discontinuing treatment. A gradual reduction in the dose rather than abrupt cessation is recommended whenever possible. If intolerable symptoms occur following a decrease in the dose or upon discontinuation of treatment, then resuming the previously prescribed dose may be considered. Subsequently, the physician may continue decreasing the dose, but at a more gradual rate.

2.5   Switching Patients From Other Antidepressants to PRISTIQ

Discontinuation symptoms have been reported when switching patients from other antidepressants, including venlafaxine, to PRISTIQ. Tapering of the initial antidepressant may be necessary to minimize discontinuation symptoms [see Contraindications (4.2)].

2.6   Switching Patients To or From a Monoamine Oxidase Inhibitor (MAOI)

At least 14 days must elapse between discontinuation of an MAOI and initiation of therapy with PRISTIQ. In addition, at least 7 days must be allowed after stopping PRISTIQ before starting an MAOI [see Contraindications (4.2)].

3   DOSAGE FORMS AND STRENGTHS

PRISTIQ® (desvenlafaxine) Extended-Release Tablets are available as 50 and 100 mg tablets.

50 mg, light pink, square pyramid tablet debossed with "W" over "50" on the flat side

100 mg, reddish-orange, square pyramid tablet debossed with "W" over "100" on the flat side

4   CONTRAINDICATIONS

4.1   Hypersensitivity

Hypersensitivity to desvenlafaxine succinate, venlafaxine hydrochloride or to any excipients in the PRISTIQ formulation.

4.2   Monoamine Oxidase Inhibitors

PRISTIQ must not be used concomitantly in patients taking monoamine oxidase inhibitors (MAOIs) or in patients who have taken MAOIs within the preceding 14 days due to the risk of serious, sometimes fatal, drug interactions with SNRI or SSRI treatment or with other serotonergic drugs. These interactions have been associated with symptoms that include tremor, myoclonus, diaphoresis, nausea, vomiting, flushing, dizziness, hyperthermia with features resembling neuroleptic malignant syndrome, seizures, rigidity, autonomic instability with possible rapid fluctuations of vital signs, and mental status changes that include extreme agitation progressing to delirium and coma. Based on the half-life of desvenlafaxine, at least 7 days should be allowed after stopping PRISTIQ before starting an MAOI [see Dosage and Administration (2.6)].

5   WARNINGS AND PRECAUTIONS

5.1   Clinical Worsening and Suicide Risk

Patients with major depressive disorder (MDD), both adult and pediatric, may experience worsening of their depression and/or the emergence of suicidal ideation and behavior (suicidality) or unusual changes in behavior, whether or not they are taking antidepressant medications, and this risk may persist until significant remission occurs. Suicide is a known risk of depression and certain other psychiatric disorders, and these disorders themselves are the strongest predictors of suicide. There has been a long-standing concern, however, that antidepressants may have a role in inducing worsening of depression and the emergence of suicidality in certain patients during the early phases of treatment. Pooled analyses of short-term placebo-controlled studies of antidepressant drugs (SSRIs and others) showed that these drugs increase the risk of suicidal thinking and behavior (suicidality) in children, adolescents, and young adults (ages 18-24) with major depressive disorder (MDD) and other psychiatric disorders. Short-term studies did not

show an increase in the risk of suicidality with antidepressants compared to placebo in adults beyond age 24; there was a reduction with antidepressants compared to placebo in adults aged 65 and older.

The pooled analyses of placebo-controlled studies in children and adolescents with MDD, obsessive compulsive disorder (OCD), or other psychiatric disorders included a total of 24 short-term studies of 9 antidepressant drugs in over 4,400 patients. The pooled analyses of placebo-controlled studies in adults with MDD or other psychiatric disorders included a total of 295 short-term studies (median duration of 2 months) of 11 antidepressant drugs in over 77,000 patients. There was considerable variation in risk of suicidality among drugs, but a tendency toward an increase in the younger patients for almost all drugs studied. There were differences in absolute risk of suicidality across the different indications, with the highest incidence in MDD. The risk differences (drug vs. placebo), however, were relatively stable within age strata and across indications. These risk differences (drug-placebo difference in the number of cases of suicidality per 1000 patients treated) are provided in Table 1.

Table 1

Age Range	Drug-Placebo Difference in Number of Cases of Suicidality per 1000 Patients Treated
	Increases Compared to Placebo
<18	14 additional cases
18-24	5 additional cases
	Decreases Compared to Placebo
25-64	1 fewer case
≥65	6 fewer cases

No suicides occurred in any of the pediatric studies. There were suicides in the adult studies, but the number was not sufficient to reach any conclusion about drug effect on suicide.

It is unknown whether the suicidality risk extends to longer-term use, i.e., beyond several months. However, there is substantial evidence from placebo-controlled maintenance studies in adults with depression that the use of antidepressants can delay the recurrence of depression.

All patients being treated with antidepressants for any indication should be monitored appropriately and observed closely for clinical worsening, suicidality, and unusual changes in behavior, especially during the initial few months of a course of drug therapy, or at times of dose changes, either increases or decreases.

The following symptoms, anxiety, agitation, panic attacks, insomnia, irritability, hostility, aggressiveness, impulsivity, akathisia (psychomotor restlessness), hypomania, and mania, have been reported in adult and pediatric patients being treated with antidepressants for major depressive disorder as well as for other indications, both psychiatric and nonpsychiatric. Although a causal link between the emergence of such symptoms and either the worsening of depression and/or the emergence of suicidal impulses has not been established, there is concern that such symptoms may represent precursors to emerging suicidality.

Consideration should be given to changing the therapeutic regimen, including possibly discontinuing the medication, in patients whose depression is persistently worse, or who are experiencing emergent suicidality or symptoms that might be precursors to worsening depression or suicidality, especially if these symptoms are severe, abrupt in onset, or were not part of the patient's presenting symptoms.

If the decision has been made to discontinue treatment, medication should be tapered, as rapidly as is feasible, but with recognition that abrupt discontinuation can be associated with certain symptoms [see Warnings and Precautions (5.9) and Dosage and Administration (2.3) for a description of the risks of discontinuation of PRISTIQ].

Families and caregivers of patients being treated with antidepressants for major depressive disorder or other indications, both psychiatric and nonpsychiatric, should be alerted about the need to monitor patients for the emergence of agitation, irritability, unusual changes in behavior, and the other symptoms described above, as well as the emergence of suicidality, and to report such symptoms immediately to healthcare providers. Such monitoring should include daily observation by families and caregivers. Prescriptions for PRISTIQ should be written for the smallest quantity of tablets consistent with good patient management, in order to reduce the risk of overdose.

Screening patients for bipolar disorder

A major depressive episode may be the initial presentation of bipolar disorder. It is generally believed (though not established in controlled studies) that treating such an episode with an antidepressant alone may increase the likelihood of precipitation of a mixed/manic episode in patients at risk for bipolar disorder. Whether any of the symptoms described above represent such a conversion is unknown. However, prior to initiating treatment with an antidepressant, patients with depressive symptoms should be adequately screened to determine if they are at risk for bipolar disorder; such screening should include a detailed psychiatric history, including a family history of suicide, bipolar disorder, and depression. It should be noted that PRISTIQ is not approved for use in treating bipolar depression.

5.2   Serotonin Syndrome or Neuroleptic Malignant Syndrome (NMS)-like Reactions

The development of a potentially life-threatening serotonin syndrome or Neuroleptic Malignant Syndrome (NMS)-like reactions have been reported with SNRIs and SSRIs alone, including PRISTIQ treatment, but particularly with concomitant use of serotonergic drugs (including triptans) with drugs which impair metabolism of serotonin (including MAOIs), or with antipsychotics or other dopamine antagonists. Serotonin syndrome symptoms may include mental status changes (e.g., agitation, hallucinations, coma), autonomic instability (e.g., tachycardia, labile blood pressure, hyperthermia), neuromuscular aberrations (e.g., hyperreflexia, incoordination) and/or gastrointestinal symptoms (e.g., nausea, vomiting, diarrhea). Serotonin syndrome, in its most severe form can resemble neuroleptic malignant syndrome, which includes hyperthermia, muscle rigidity, autonomic instability with possible rapid fluctuation of vital signs, and mental status changes. Patients should be monitored for the emergence of serotonin syndrome or NMS-like signs and symptoms.

The concomitant use of PRISTIQ with MAOIs intended to treat depression is contraindicated [see Contraindications (4.2)].

If concomitant treatment of PRISTIQ with a 5-hydroxytryptamine receptor agonist (triptan) is clinically warranted, careful observation of the patient is advised, particularly during treatment initiation and dose increases. The concomitant use of PRISTIQ with serotonin precursors (such as tryptophan) is not recommended.

Treatment with PRISTIQ and any concomitant serotonergic or antidopaminergic agents, including antipsychotics, should be discontinued immediately if the above events occur and supportive symptomatic treatment should be initiated.

5.3   Elevated Blood Pressure

Patients receiving PRISTIQ should have regular monitoring of blood pressure since increases in blood pressure were observed in clinical studies. Pre-existing hypertension should be controlled before initiating treatment with PRISTIQ. Caution should be exercised in treating patients with pre-existing hypertension or other underlying conditions that might be compromised by increases in blood pressure. Cases of elevated blood pressure requiring immediate treatment have been reported with PRISTIQ.

Sustained hypertension

Sustained blood pressure increases could have adverse consequences. For patients who experience a sustained increase in blood pressure while receiving PRISTIQ, either dose reduction or discontinuation should be considered [see Adverse Reactions (6.1)]. Treatment with PRISTIQ at all doses from 50 mg/day to 400 mg/day in controlled studies was associated with sustained hypertension, defined as treatment-emergent supine diastolic blood pressure (SDBP) ≥ 90 mm Hg and ≥ 10 mm Hg above baseline for 3 consecutive on-therapy visits (see Table 2). Analyses of patients in PRISTIQ controlled studies who met criteria for sustained hypertension revealed a consistent increase in the proportion of patients who developed sustained hypertension. This was seen at all doses with a suggestion of a higher rate at 400 mg/day.

Table 2: Proportion of Patients with Sustained Elevation of Supine Diastolic Blood Pressure

Treatment Group	Proportion of Patients with Sustained Hypertension
Placebo	0.5%
PRISTIQ 50 mg/day	1.3%
PRISTIQ 100 mg/day	0.7%
PRISTIQ 200 mg/day	1.1%
PRISTIQ 400 mg/day	2.3%

Table 3: Common Adverse Reactions: Percentage of Patients (≥ 2% in any Fixed-Dose Group) in MDD 8-Week Placebo-Controlled Studies[a]

System Organ Class Preferred Term	Percentage of Patients Reporting Reaction				
	Placebo	PRISTIQ			
		50 mg	100 mg	200 mg	400 mg
Cardiac disorders					
Palpitations	2	1	3	2	3
Tachycardia	1	1	<1	1	2
Blood pressure increased	1	1	1	2	2
Gastrointestinal disorders					
Nausea	10	22	26	36	41
Dry mouth	9	11	17	21	25
Diarrhea	9	11	9	7	5
Constipation	4	9	9	10	14
Vomiting	3	3	4	6	9
General disorders and administration site conditions					
Fatigue	4	7	7	10	11
Chills	1	1	<1	3	4
Feeling jittery	1	1	2	3	3
Asthenia	1	1	2	1	1
Metabolism and nutrition disorders					
Decreased appetite	2	5	8	10	10
Weight decreased	1	2	1	1	2
Nervous system disorders					
Dizziness	5	13	10	15	16
Somnolence	4	4	9	12	12
Headache	23	20	22	29	25
Tremor	2	2	3	9	9
Paraesthesia	1	2	2	1	3
Disturbance in attention	<1	<1	1	2	1
Psychiatric disorders					
Insomnia	6	9	12	14	15
Anxiety	2	3	5	4	4
Nervousness	1	<1	1	2	2
Irritability	1	2	2	2	2
Abnormal dreams	1	2	3	2	4

(Table continued on next page)

5.4 Abnormal Bleeding

SSRIs and SNRIs, including PRISTIQ, may increase the risk of bleeding events. Concomitant use of aspirin, nonsteroidal anti-inflammatory drugs, warfarin, and other anticoagulants may add to this risk. Case reports and epidemiological studies (case-control and cohort design) have demonstrated an association between use of drugs that interfere with serotonin reuptake and the occurrence of gastrointestinal bleeding. Bleeding events related to SSRIs and SNRIs have ranged from ecchymosis, hematoma, epistaxis, and petechiae to life-threatening hemorrhages. Patients should be cautioned about the risk of bleeding associated with the concomitant use of PRISTIQ and NSAIDs, aspirin, or other drugs that affect coagulation or bleeding.

5.5 Narrow-angle Glaucoma

Mydriasis has been reported in association with PRISTIQ; therefore, patients with raised intraocular pressure or those at risk of acute narrow-angle glaucoma (angle-closure glaucoma) should be monitored.

5.6 Activation of Mania/Hypomania

During all MDD and VMS (vasomotor symptoms) phase 2 and phase 3 studies, mania was reported for approximately 0.1% of patients treated with PRISTIQ. Activation of mania/hypomania has also been reported in a small proportion of patients with major affective disorder who were treated with other marketed antidepressants. As with all antidepressants, PRISTIQ should be used cautiously in patients with a history or family history of mania or hypomania.

5.7 Cardiovascular/Cerebrovascular Disease

Caution is advised in administering PRISTIQ to patients with cardiovascular, cerebrovascular, or lipid metabolism disorders [see Adverse Reactions (6.1)]. Increases in blood pressure and small increases in heart rate were observed in clinical studies with PRISTIQ. PRISTIQ has not been evaluated systematically in patients with a recent history of myocardial infarction, unstable heart disease, uncontrolled hypertension, or cerebrovascular disease. Patients with

these diagnoses, except for cerebrovascular disease, were excluded from clinical studies.

5.8 Serum Cholesterol and Triglyceride Elevation

Dose-related elevations in fasting serum total cholesterol, LDL (low density lipoprotein) cholesterol, and triglycerides were observed in the controlled studies. Measurement of serum lipids should be considered during treatment with PRISTIQ [see Adverse Reactions (6.1)].

5.9 Discontinuation of Treatment with PRISTIQ

Discontinuation symptoms have been systematically and prospectively evaluated in patients treated with PRISTIQ during clinical studies in Major Depressive Disorder. Abrupt discontinuation or dose reduction has been associated with the appearance of new symptoms that include dizziness, nausea, headache, irritability, insomnia, diarrhea, anxiety, fatigue, abnormal dreams, and hyperhidrosis. In general, discontinuation events occurred more frequently with longer duration of therapy.

During marketing of SNRIs (Serotonin and Norepinephrine Reuptake Inhibitors), and SSRIs (Selective Serotonin Reuptake Inhibitors), there have been spontaneous reports of adverse events occurring upon discontinuation of these drugs, particularly when abrupt, including the following: dysphoric mood, irritability, agitation, dizziness, sensory disturbances (e.g., paresthesia, such as electric shock sensations), anxiety, confusion, headache, lethargy, emotional lability, insomnia, hypomania, tinnitus, and seizures. While these events are generally self-limiting, there have been reports of serious discontinuation symptoms.

Patients should be monitored for these symptoms when discontinuing treatment with PRISTIQ. A gradual reduction in the dose rather than abrupt cessation is recommended whenever possible. If intolerable symptoms occur following a decrease in the dose or upon discontinuation of treatment, then resuming the previously prescribed dose may be considered. Subsequently, the physician may continue decreasing the dose, but at a more gradual rate [see Dosage and Administration (2.4) and Adverse Reactions (6.1)].

5.10 Renal Impairment

In patients with moderate or severe renal impairment or end-stage renal disease (ESRD) the clearance of PRISTIQ was decreased, thus prolonging the elimination half-life of the drug. As a result, there were potentially clinically significant increases in exposures to PRISTIQ [see Clinical Pharmacology (12.6)]. Dosage adjustment (50 mg every other day) is necessary in patients with severe renal impairment or ESRD. The doses should not be escalated in patients with moderate or severe renal impairment or ESRD [see Dosage and Administration (2.2)].

5.11 Seizure

Cases of seizure have been reported in pre-marketing clinical studies with PRISTIQ. PRISTIQ has not been systematically evaluated in patients with a seizure disorder. Patients with a history of seizures were excluded from pre-marketing clinical studies. PRISTIQ should be prescribed with caution in patients with a seizure disorder.

5.12 Hyponatremia

Hyponatremia may occur as a result of treatment with SSRIs and SNRIs, including PRISTIQ. In many cases, this hyponatremia appears to be the result of the syndrome of inappropriate antidiuretic hormone secretion (SIADH). Cases with serum sodium lower than 110 mmol/L have been reported. Elderly patients may be at greater risk of developing hyponatremia with SSRIs and SNRIs. Also, patients taking diuretics or who are otherwise volume depleted can be at greater risk [see Use in Specific Populations (8.5) and Clinical Pharmacology (12.6)]. Discontinuation of PRISTIQ should be considered in patients with symptomatic hyponatremia and appropriate medical intervention should be instituted.

Signs and symptoms of hyponatremia include headache, difficulty concentrating, memory impairment, confusion, weakness, and unsteadiness, which can lead to falls. Signs and symptoms associated with more severe and/or acute cases have included hallucination, syncope, seizure, coma, respiratory arrest, and death.

5.13 Co-administration of Drugs Containing Desvenlafaxine and Venlafaxine

Desvenlafaxine is the major active metabolite of venlafaxine. Products containing desvenlafaxine and products containing venlafaxine should not be used concomitantly with PRISTIQ.

5.14 Interstitial Lung Disease and Eosinophilic Pneumonia

Interstitial lung disease and eosinophilic pneumonia associated with venlafaxine (the parent drug of PRISTIQ) therapy have been rarely reported. The possibility of these adverse events should be considered in patients treated with PRISTIQ who present with progressive dyspnea, cough, or chest discomfort. Such patients should undergo a prompt medical evaluation, and discontinuation of PRISTIQ should be considered.

6 ADVERSE REACTIONS

The following adverse reactions are discussed in greater detail in other sections of the label;

Table 3 (cont.): Common Adverse Reactions: Percentage of Patients (≥ 2% in any Fixed-Dose Group) in MDD 8-Week Placebo-Controlled Studies[a]

System Organ Class Preferred Term	Percentage of Patients Reporting Reaction				
	Placebo	PRISTIQ			
		50 mg	100 mg	200 mg	400 mg
Renal and urinary disorders					
Urinary hesitation	0	<1	1	2	2
Respiratory, thoracic and mediastinal disorders					
Yawning	<1	1	1	4	3
Skin and subcutaneous tissue disorders					
Hyperhidrosis	4	10	11	18	21
Rash	<1	1	1	2	<1
Special Senses					
Vision blurred	1	3	4	4	4
Mydriasis	<1	2	2	6	6
Tinnitus	1	2	1	1	2
Dysgeusia	1	1	1	1	2
Vascular disorders					
Hot flush	<1	1	1	2	2

a: Percentage based on the number of patients (placebo, n = 636; PRISTIQ 50 mg, n = 317; PRISTIQ 100 mg, n = 424; PRISTIQ 200 mg, n = 307; PRISTIQ 400 mg, n = 317).

Table 4: Sexual Function Disorders: Adverse Reactions (≥ 2% in Men[a] or Women[b] in any PRISTIQ Group) During the On-Therapy Period

System Organ Class Preferred Term	Placebo	PRISTIQ			
		50 mg	100 mg	200 mg	400 mg
Men only					
Anorgasmia	0	0	3	5	8
Libido decreased	1	4	5	6	3
Orgasm abnormal	0	0	1	2	3
Ejaculation delayed	<1	1	5	7	6
Erectile dysfunction	1	3	6	8	11
Ejaculation disorder	0	0	1	2	5
Ejaculation failure	0	1	0	2	2
Sexual dysfunction	0	1	0	0	2
Women only					
Anorgasmia	0	1	1	0	3

a: Percentage based on the number of men (placebo, n = 239; PRISTIQ 50 mg, n = 108; PRISTIQ 100 mg, n = 157; PRISTIQ 200 mg, n = 131; PRISTIQ 400 mg, n = 154).
b: Percentage based on the number of women (placebo, n = 397; PRISTIQ 50 mg, n = 209; PRISTIQ 100 mg, n = 267; PRISTIQ 200 mg, n = 176; PRISTIQ 400 mg, n = 163).

• Hypersensitivity [see Contraindications (4.1)]
• Effects on blood pressure [see Warnings and Precautions (5.3)]
• Abnormal bleeding [see Warnings and Precautions (5.4)]
• Mydriasis [see Warnings and Precautions (5.5)]
• Hypomania and mania [see Warnings and Precautions (5.6)]
• Serum cholesterol and triglyceride elevation [see Warnings and Precautions (5.8)]
• Seizure [see Warnings and Precautions (5.11)]

6.1 Clinical Studies Experience
The most commonly observed adverse reactions in PRISTIQ treated MDD patients in short-term fixed-dose studies (incidence ≥ 5% and at least twice the rate of placebo in the 50 or 100 mg dose groups) were: nausea, dizziness, insomnia, hyperhidrosis, constipation, somnolence, decreased appetite, anxiety, and specific male sexual function disorders.

Adverse reactions reported as reasons for discontinuation of treatment
Combined across 8-week placebo-controlled pre-marketing studies for major depressive disorder, 12% of the 1,834 patients who received PRISTIQ (50-400 mg) discontinued treatment due to an adverse event, compared with 3% of the 1,116 placebo-treated patients in those studies. At the recommended dose of 50 mg, the discontinuation rate due to an adverse event for PRISTIQ (4.1%) was similar to the rate for placebo (3.8%). For the 100 mg dose of PRISTIQ the discontinuation rate due to an adverse event was 8.7%.

The most common adverse reactions leading to discontinuation in at least 2% of the PRISTIQ treated patients in the short-term studies, up to 8 weeks, were: nausea (4%); dizziness, headache and vomiting (2% each); in the long-term study, up to 9 months, the most common was vomiting (2%).

Patient exposure
PRISTIQ was evaluated for safety in 3,292 patients diagnosed with major depressive disorder who participated in multiple-dose pre-marketing studies, representing 1,289 patient-years of exposure. Among these 3,292 PRISTIQ treated patients, 1,834 patients were exposed to PRISTIQ in 8-week, placebo-controlled studies at doses ranging from 50 to 400 mg/day. Out of the 1,834 patients, 687 PRISTIQ treated patients continued into a 10-month open-label study. Of the total 3,292 patients exposed to at least one dose of PRISTIQ, 1,070 were exposed to PRISTIQ for 6 months, representing 842 patient-years of exposure, and 274 were exposed for one year, representing 241 patient-years of exposure.

Because clinical studies are conducted under widely varying conditions, adverse reaction rates observed in the clinical studies of a drug cannot be directly compared to rates in the clinical studies of another drug and may not reflect the rates observed in practice.

Common adverse reactions in placebo-controlled MDD studies
Table 3 shows the incidence of common adverse reactions that occurred in ≥ 2% of PRISTIQ treated MDD patients at any dose in the 8-week, placebo-controlled, fixed dose, pre-marketing clinical studies. In general, the adverse reactions were most frequent in the first week of treatment.
[See table 3 on previous page and at left]

Sexual function adverse reactions
Table 4 shows the incidence of sexual function adverse reactions that occurred in ≥ 2% of PRISTIQ treated MDD patients in any fixed-dose group (8-week, placebo-controlled, fixed and flexible-dose, pre-marketing clinical studies).
[See table 4 at left]

Other adverse reactions observed in pre-marketing clinical studies
Other infrequent adverse reactions, not described elsewhere in section 6.1, occurring at an incidence of < 2% in MDD patients treated with PRISTIQ were:
Immune system disorders—Hypersensitivity.
Investigations—Weight increased, liver function test abnormal, blood prolactin increased.
Nervous system disorders—Convulsion, syncope, extrapyramidal disorder.
Musculoskeletal and connective tissue disorders—Musculoskeletal stiffness.
Psychiatric disorders—Depersonalization, hypomania.
Respiratory, thoracic and mediastinal disorders—Epistaxis.
Vascular disorders—Orthostatic hypotension.
In clinical studies, there were uncommon reports of ischemic cardiac adverse events, including myocardial ischemia, myocardial infarction, and coronary occlusion requiring revascularization; these patients had multiple underlying cardiac risk factors. More patients experienced these events during PRISTIQ treatment as compared to placebo [see Warnings and Precautions (5.7)].

Discontinuation events
Adverse events reported in association with abrupt discontinuation, dose reduction or tapering of treatment in MDD clinical studies at a rate of ≥ 5% include: dizziness, nausea, headache, irritability, insomnia, diarrhea, anxiety, abnormal dreams, fatigue, and hyperhidrosis. In general, discontinuation events occurred more frequently with longer duration of therapy [see Dosage and Administration (2.4) and Warnings and Precautions (5.9)].

Laboratory, ECG and vital sign changes observed in MDD clinical studies
The following changes were observed in placebo-controlled, short-term, pre-marketing MDD studies with PRISTIQ.
Lipids
Elevations in fasting serum total cholesterol, LDL (low density lipoproteins) cholesterol, and triglycerides occurred in the controlled studies. Some of these abnormalities were considered potentially clinically significant [see Warnings and Precautions (5.8)].
The percentage of patients who exceeded a predetermined threshold value is shown in Table 5.
[See table 5 at top of next page]
Proteinuria
Proteinuria, greater than or equal to trace, was observed in the fixed-dose controlled studies (see Table 6). This proteinuria was not associated with increases in BUN or creatinine and was generally transient.

Table 6: Incidence (%) of Patients with Proteinuria in the Fixed-dose Clinical Studies

	Placebo	PRISTIQ			
		50 mg	100 mg	200 mg	400 mg
Proteinuria	4	6	8	5	7

ECG changes
Electrocardiograms were obtained from 1,492 PRISTIQ treated patients with major depressive disorder and 984 placebo-treated patients in clinical studies lasting up to 8 weeks. No clinically relevant differences were observed

Table 5: Incidence (%) of Patients With Lipid Abnormalities of Potential Clinical Significance*

	Placebo	PRISTIQ			
		50 mg	100 mg	200 mg	400 mg
Total Cholesterol *(Increase of ≥ 50 mg/dl and an absolute value of ≥ 261 mg/dl)	2	3	4	4	10
LDL Cholesterol *(Increase ≥ 50 mg/dl and an absolute value of ≥ 190 mg/dl)	0	1	0	1	2
Triglycerides, fasting *(Fasting: ≥ 327 mg/dl)	3	2	1	4	6

Table 7: Mean Changes in Vital Signs at Final on Therapy for All Short-term, Fixed-dose Controlled Studies

	Placebo	PRISTIQ			
		50 mg	100 mg	200 mg	400 mg
Blood pressure					
Supine systolic bp (mm Hg)	-1.4	1.2	2.0	2.5	2.1
Supine diastolic bp (mm Hg)	-0.6	0.7	0.8	1.8	2.3
Pulse rate					
Supine pulse (bpm)	-0.3	1.3	1.3	0.9	4.1
Weight (kg)	0.0	-0.4	-0.6	-0.9	-1.1

between PRISTIQ treated and placebo-treated patients for QT, QTc, PR, and QRS intervals. In a thorough QTc study with prospectively determined criteria, desvenlafaxine did not cause QT prolongation. No difference was observed between placebo and desvenlafaxine treatments for the QRS interval.

Vital sign changes
Table 7 summarizes the changes that were observed in placebo-controlled, short-term, pre-marketing studies with PRISTIQ in patients with MDD (doses 50 to 400 mg).
[See table 7 above]
At the final on-therapy assessment in the 6-month, double-blind, placebo-controlled phase of a long-term study in patients who had responded to PRISTIQ during the initial 12-week, open-label phase, there was no statistical difference in mean weight change between PRISTIQ and placebo-treated patients.

Orthostatic hypotension
In the short-term, placebo-controlled clinical studies with doses of 50-400 mg, systolic orthostatic hypotension (decrease ≥ 30 mm Hg from supine to standing position) occurred more frequently in patients ≥ 65 years of age receiving PRISTIQ (8.0%, 7/87) versus placebo (2.5%, 1/40), compared to patients < 65 years of age receiving PRISTIQ (0.9%, 18/1,937) versus placebo (0.7%, 8/1,218).

6.2 Adverse Reactions Identified During Post-Approval Use
The following adverse reaction has been identified during post-approval use of PRISTIQ. Because post-approval reactions are reported voluntarily from a population of uncertain size, it is not always possible to reliably estimate their frequency or establish a causal relationship to drug exposure:
Skin and subcutaneous tissue disorders—Angioedema.

6.3 Adverse Reactions Reported With Other SNRIs
Although the following are not considered adverse reactions for PRISTIQ, they are adverse reactions for other SNRIs and may also occur with PRISTIQ: gastrointestinal bleeding, hallucinations, photosensitivity reactions and severe cutaneous reactions (such as Stevens-Johnson Syndrome, toxic epidermal necrolysis, and/or erythema multiforme).

7 DRUG INTERACTIONS
7.1 Central Nervous System (CNS)-Active Agents
The risk of using PRISTIQ in combination with other CNS-active drugs has not been systematically evaluated. Consequently, caution is advised when PRISTIQ is taken in combination with other CNS-active drugs [see *Warnings and Precautions (5.13)*].

7.2 Monoamine Oxidase Inhibitors (MAOI)
Adverse reactions, some of which were serious, have been reported in patients who have recently been discontinued from a monoamine oxidase inhibitor (MAOI) and started on antidepressants with pharmacological properties similar to PRISTIQ (SNRIs or SSRIs), or who have recently had SNRI or SSRI therapy discontinued prior to initiation of an MAOI [see *Contraindications (4.2)*].

7.3 Serotonergic Drugs
Based on the mechanism of action of PRISTIQ and the potential for serotonin syndrome, caution is advised when PRISTIQ is co-administered with other drugs that may affect the serotonergic neurotransmitter systems [see *Warnings and Precautions (5.2)*].

7.4 Drugs that Interfere with Hemostasis (e.g., NSAIDs, Aspirin, and Warfarin)
Serotonin release by platelets plays an important role in hemostasis. Epidemiological studies of case-control and cohort design that have demonstrated an association between use of psychotropic drugs that interfere with serotonin reuptake and the occurrence of upper gastrointestinal bleeding. These studies have also shown that concurrent use of an NSAID or aspirin may potentiate this risk of bleeding. Altered anticoagulant effects, including increased bleeding, have been reported when SSRIs and SNRIs are co-administered with warfarin. Patients receiving warfarin therapy should be carefully monitored when PRISTIQ is initiated or discontinued.

7.5 Ethanol
A clinical study has shown that desvenlafaxine does not increase the impairment of mental and motor skills caused by ethanol. However, as with all CNS-active drugs, patients should be advised to avoid alcohol consumption while taking PRISTIQ.

7.6 Potential for Other Drugs to Affect Desvenlafaxine
Inhibitors of CYP3A4 (ketoconazole)
CYP3A4 is a minor pathway for the metabolism of PRISTIQ. In a clinical study, ketoconazole (200 mg BID) increased the area under the concentration vs. time curve (AUC) of PRISTIQ (400 mg single dose) by about 43% and C_{max} by about 8%. Concomitant use of PRISTIQ with potent inhibitors of CYP3A4 may result in higher concentrations of PRISTIQ.
Inhibitors of other CYP enzymes
Based on *in vitro* data, drugs that inhibit CYP isozymes 1A1, 1A2, 2A6, 2D6, 2C8, 2C9, 2C19, and 2E1 are not expected to have significant impact on the pharmacokinetic profile of PRISTIQ.

7.7 Potential for Desvenlafaxine to Affect Other Drugs
Drugs metabolized by CYP2D6 (desipramine)
In vitro studies showed minimal inhibitory effect of desvenlafaxine on CYP2D6.
Clinical studies have shown that desvenlafaxine does not have a clinically relevant effect on CYP2D6 metabolism at the dose of 100 mg daily. When desvenlafaxine succinate was administered at a dose of 100 mg daily in conjunction with a single 50 mg dose of desipramine, a CYP2D6 substrate, the C_{max} and AUC of desipramine increased approximately 25% and 17%, respectively. When 400 mg (8 times the recommended 50 mg dose) was administered, the C_{max} and AUC of desipramine increased approximately 50% and 90%, respectively. Concomitant use of desvenlafaxine with a drug metabolized by CYP2D6 can result in higher concentrations of that drug.

Drugs metabolized by CYP3A4 (midazolam)
In vitro, desvenlafaxine does not inhibit or induce the CYP3A4 isozyme.
In a clinical study, PRISTIQ 400 mg daily (8 times the recommended 50 mg dose) was co-administered with a single 4 mg dose of midazolam (a CYP3A4 substrate). The AUC and C_{max} of midazolam decreased by approximately 31% and 16%, respectively. Concomitant use of PRISTIQ with a drug metabolized by CYP3A4 can result in lower exposures to that drug.
Drugs metabolized by CYP1A2, 2A6, 2C8, 2C9 and 2C19
In vitro, desvenlafaxine does not inhibit CYP1A2, 2A6, 2C8, 2C9, and 2C19 isozymes and would not be expected to affect the pharmacokinetics of drugs that are metabolized by these CYP isozymes.

7.8 P-glycoprotein Transporter
In vitro, desvenlafaxine is not a substrate or an inhibitor for the P-glycoprotein transporter.
The pharmacokinetics of PRISTIQ are unlikely to be affected by drugs that inhibit the P-glycoprotein transporter, and desvenlafaxine is not likely to affect the pharmacokinetics of drugs that are substrates of the P-glycoprotein transporter.

7.9 Electroconvulsive Therapy
There are no clinical data establishing the risks and/or benefits of electroconvulsive therapy combined with PRISTIQ treatment.

8 USE IN SPECIFIC POPULATIONS
8.1 Pregnancy
Patients should be advised to notify their physician if they become pregnant or intend to become pregnant during therapy.
Teratogenic effects – Pregnancy Category C
When desvenlafaxine succinate was administered orally to pregnant rats and rabbits during the period of organogenesis, there was no evidence of teratogenicity in rats at any doses tested, up to 10 times a human dose of 100 mg/day (on a mg/m² basis) in rats, and up to 15 times a human dose of 100 mg/day (on a mg/m² basis) in rabbits. However, fetal weights were decreased in rats, with a no-effect dose 10 times a human dose of 100 mg/day (on a mg/m² basis).
When desvenlafaxine succinate was administered orally to pregnant rats throughout gestation and lactation, there was a decrease in pup weights and an increase in pup deaths during the first four days of lactation. The cause of these deaths is not known. The no-effect dose for rat pup mortality was 10 times a human dose of 100 mg/day (on a mg/m² basis). Post-weaning growth and reproductive performance of the progeny were not affected by maternal treatment with desvenlafaxine at a dose 29 times a human dose of 100 mg/day (on a mg/m² basis).
There are no adequate and well-controlled studies of PRISTIQ in pregnant women. Therefore, PRISTIQ should be used during pregnancy only if the potential benefits justify the potential risks.
Non-teratogenic effects
Neonates exposed to SNRIs (Serotonin and Norepinephrine Reuptake Inhibitors), or SSRIs (Selective Serotonin Reuptake Inhibitors), late in the third trimester have developed complications requiring prolonged hospitalization, respiratory support, and tube feeding. Such complications can arise immediately upon delivery. Reported clinical findings have included respiratory distress, cyanosis, apnea, seizures, temperature instability, feeding difficulty, vomiting, hypoglycemia, hypotonia, hypertonia, hyperreflexia, tremor, jitteriness, irritability, and constant crying. These features are consistent with either a direct toxic effect of SSRIs and SNRIs or, possibly, a drug discontinuation syndrome. It should be noted that, in some cases, the clinical picture is consistent with serotonin syndrome [see *Warnings and Precautions (5.2)*]. When treating a pregnant woman with PRISTIQ during the third trimester, the physician should carefully consider the potential risks and benefits of treatment [see *Dosage and Administration (2.2)*].

8.2 Labor and Delivery
The effect of PRISTIQ on labor and delivery in humans is unknown. PRISTIQ should be used during labor and delivery only if the potential benefits justify the potential risks.

8.3 Nursing Mothers
Desvenlafaxine (O-desmethylvenlafaxine) is excreted in human milk. Because of the potential for serious adverse reactions in nursing infants from PRISTIQ, a decision should be made whether or not to discontinue nursing or to discontinue the drug, taking into account the importance of the drug to the mother. Only administer PRISTIQ to breast-feeding women if the expected benefits outweigh any possible risk.

8.4 Pediatric Use
Safety and effectiveness in the pediatric population have not been established [see *Box Warning and Warnings and*

Precautions (5.1)]. Anyone considering the use of PRISTIQ in a child or adolescent must balance the potential risks with the clinical need.

8.5 Geriatric Use

Of the 3,292 patients in clinical studies with PRISTIQ, 5% were 65 years of age or older. No overall differences in safety or efficacy were observed between these patients and younger patients; however, in the short-term, placebo-controlled studies, there was a higher incidence of systolic orthostatic hypotension in patients ≥ 65 years of age compared to patients < 65 years of age treated with PRISTIQ [*see Adverse Reactions (6)*]. For elderly patients, possible reduced renal clearance of desvenlafaxine should be considered when determining dose [*see Dosage and Administration (2.2) and Clinical Pharmacology (12.6)*]. If PRISTIQ is poorly tolerated, every other day dosing can be considered. SSRIs and SNRIs, including PRISTIQ, have been associated with cases of clinically significant hyponatremia in elderly patients, who may be at greater risk for this adverse event [*see Warnings and Precautions (5.12)*].

Greater sensitivity of some older individuals cannot be ruled out.

8.6 Renal Impairment

In subjects with renal impairment the clearance of PRISTIQ was decreased. In subjects with severe renal impairment (24-hr CrCl < 30 mL/min) and end-stage renal disease, elimination half-lives were significantly prolonged, increasing exposures to PRISTIQ; therefore, dosage adjustment is recommended in these patients [*see Dosage and Administration (2.2) and Clinical Pharmacology (12.6)*].

8.7 Hepatic Impairment

The mean $t_{1/2}$ changed from approximately 10 hours in healthy subjects and subjects with mild hepatic impairment to 13 and 14 hours in moderate and severe hepatic impairment, respectively. The recommended dose in patients with hepatic impairment is 50 mg/day. Dose escalation above 100 mg/day is not recommended [*see Clinical Pharmacology (12.6)*].

9 DRUG ABUSE AND DEPENDENCE

9.1 Controlled Substance

Desvenlafaxine is not a controlled substance.

9.2 Abuse and Dependence

Although PRISTIQ has not been systematically studied in preclinical or clinical studies for its potential for abuse, no indication of drug-seeking behavior was seen in the clinical studies. However, it is not possible to predict on the basis of pre-marketing experience, the extent to which a CNS-active drug will be misused, diverted, and/or abused once marketed. Consequently, physicians should carefully evaluate patients for a history of drug abuse and follow such patients closely, observing them for signs of misuse or abuse of PRISTIQ (e.g., development of tolerance, incrementation of dose, drug-seeking behavior).

10 OVERDOSAGE

10.1 Human Experience with Overdosage

There is limited clinical experience with desvenlafaxine succinate overdosage in humans. In pre-marketing clinical studies, no cases of fatal acute overdose of desvenlafaxine were reported.

Among the patients included in the MDD pre-marketing studies of PRISTIQ, there were four adults who ingested desvenlafaxine succinate (4000 mg [desvenlafaxine alone], 900, 1800 and 5200 mg [in combination with other drugs]); all patients recovered. In addition, one patient's 11-month-old child accidentally ingested 600 mg of desvenlafaxine succinate, was treated, and recovered. The adverse reactions reported within 5 days of an overdose > 600 mg that were possibly related to PRISTIQ included: headache, vomiting, agitation, dizziness, nausea, constipation, diarrhea, dry mouth, paresthesia, and tachycardia.

Desvenlafaxine (PRISTIQ) is the major active metabolite of venlafaxine. Overdose experience reported with venlafaxine (the parent drug of PRISTIQ) is presented below; the identical information can be found in the *Overdosage* section of the venlafaxine package insert.

In postmarketing experience, overdose with venlafaxine (the parent drug of PRISTIQ) has occurred predominantly in combination with alcohol and/or other drugs. The most commonly reported events in overdosage include tachycardia, changes in level of consciousness (ranging from somnolence to coma), mydriasis, seizures, and vomiting. Electrocardiogram changes (e.g., prolongation of QT interval, bundle branch block, QRS prolongation), sinus and ventricular tachycardia, bradycardia, hypotension, rhabdomyolysis, vertigo, *liver necrosis, serotonin* syndrome, and death have been reported.

Published retrospective studies report that venlafaxine overdosage may be associated with an increased risk of fatal outcomes compared to that observed with SSRI antidepressant products, but lower than that for tricyclic antidepressants. Epidemiological studies have shown that venlafaxine-treated patients have a higher pre-existing burden of suicide risk factors than SSRI-treated patients. The extent to which the finding of an increased risk of fatal outcomes can be attributed to the toxicity of venlafaxine in overdosage, as opposed to some characteristic(s) of venlafaxine-treated patients, is not clear.

Prescriptions for PRISTIQ should be written for the smallest quantity of tablets consistent with good patient management, in order to reduce the risk of overdose.

10.2 Management of Overdosage

Treatment should consist of those general measures employed in the management of overdosage with any SSRI/SNRI.

Ensure an adequate airway, oxygenation, and ventilation. Monitor cardiac rhythm and vital signs. General supportive and symptomatic measures are also recommended. Gastric lavage with a large-bore orogastric tube with appropriate airway protection, if needed, may be indicated if performed soon after ingestion or in symptomatic patients. Activated charcoal should be administered.

Induction of emesis is not recommended. Because of the moderate volume of distribution of this drug, forced diuresis, dialysis, hemoperfusion, and exchange transfusion are unlikely to be of benefit. No specific antidotes for desvenlafaxine are known.

In managing an overdose, consider the possibility of multiple drug involvement. The physician should consider contacting a poison control center for additional information on the treatment of any overdose. Telephone numbers for certified poison control centers are listed in the Physicians Desk Reference® (PDR).

11 DESCRIPTION

PRISTIQ is an extended-release tablet for oral administration that contains desvenlafaxine succinate, a structurally novel SNRI for the treatment of MDD. Desvenlafaxine (O-desmethylvenlafaxine) is the major active metabolite of the antidepressant venlafaxine, a medication used to treat major depressive, generalized anxiety, social anxiety and panic disorders.

Desvenlafaxine is designated *RS*-4-[2-dimethylamino-1-(1-hydroxycyclohexyl)ethyl]phenol and has the empirical formula of $C_{16}H_{25}NO_2$ (free base) and $C_{16}H_{25}NO_2 \bullet C_4H_6O_4 \bullet H_2O$ (succinate monohydrate). Desvenlafaxine succinate monohydrate has a molecular weight of 399.48. The structural formula is shown below.

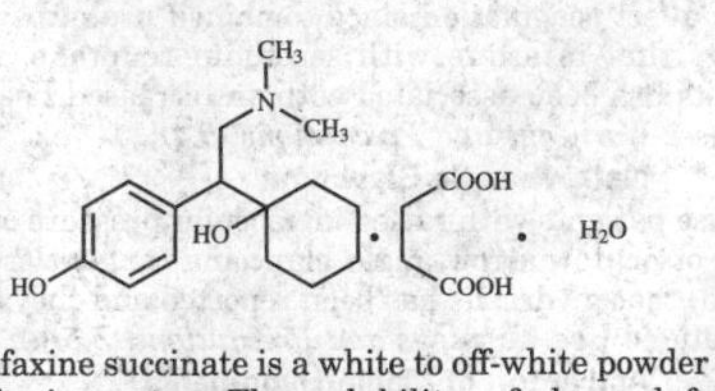

Desvenlafaxine succinate is a white to off-white powder that is soluble in water. The solubility of desvenlafaxine succinate is pH dependent. Its octanol:aqueous system (at pH 7.0) partition coefficient is 0.21.

PRISTIQ is formulated as an extended-release tablet for once-a-day oral administration.

Each tablet contains 76 or 152 mg of desvenlafaxine succinate equivalent to 50 or 100 mg of desvenlafaxine, respectively.

Inactive ingredients for the 50 mg tablet consist of hypromellose, microcrystalline cellulose, talc, magnesium stearate and film coating, which consists of polyvinyl alcohol, polyethylene glycol, talc, titanium dioxide, and iron oxides.

Inactive ingredients for the 100 mg tablet consist of hypromellose, microcrystalline cellulose, talc, magnesium stearate and film coating, which consists of polyvinyl alcohol, polyethylene glycol, talc, titanium dioxide, iron oxide and FD&C yellow #6.

12 CLINICAL PHARMACOLOGY

12.1 Mechanism of Action

Non-clinical studies have shown that desvenlafaxine succinate is a potent and selective serotonin and norepinephrine reuptake inhibitor (SNRI). The clinical efficacy of desvenlafaxine succinate is thought to be related to the potentiation of these neurotransmitters in the central nervous system.

12.2 Pharmacodynamics

Desvenlafaxine lacked significant affinity for numerous receptors, including muscarinic-cholinergic, H_1-histaminergic, or α_1-adrenergic receptors *in vitro*. PRISTIQ also lacked monoamine oxidase (MAO) inhibitory activity.

12.3 Pharmacokinetics

The single-dose pharmacokinetics of desvenlafaxine are linear and dose-proportional in a dose range of 100 to 600 mg/day. The mean terminal half-life, $t_{1/2}$, is approximately 11 hours. With once-daily dosing, steady-state plasma concentrations are achieved within approximately 4-5 days. At steady-state, multiple-dose accumulation of desvenlafaxine is linear and predictable from the single-dose pharmacokinetic profile.

12.4 Absorption and Distribution

The absolute oral bioavailability of PRISTIQ after oral administration is about 80%. Mean time to peak plasma concentrations (T_{max}) is about 7.5 hours after oral administration.

A food-effect study involving administration of PRISTIQ to healthy subjects under fasting and fed conditions (high-fat meal) indicated that the C_{max} was increased about 16% in the fed state, while the AUCs were similar. This difference is not clinically significant; therefore, PRISTIQ can be taken without regard to meals [*see Dosage and Administration (2.1)*].

The plasma protein binding of desvenlafaxine is low (30%) and is independent of drug concentration. The desvenlafaxine volume of distribution at steady-state following intravenous administration is 3.4 L/kg, indicating distribution into nonvascular compartments.

12.5 Metabolism and Elimination

Desvenlafaxine is primarily metabolized by conjugation (mediated by UGT isoforms) and, to a minor extent, through oxidative metabolism. CYP3A4 is the cytochrome P450 isozyme mediating the oxidative metabolism (N-demethylation) of desvenlafaxine. The CYP2D6 metabolic pathway is not involved, and after administration of 100 mg, the pharmacokinetics of desvenlafaxine was similar in subjects with CYP2D6 poor and extensive metabolizer phenotype. Approximately 45% of desvenlafaxine is excreted unchanged in urine at 72 hours after oral administration. Approximately 19% of the administered dose is excreted as the glucuronide metabolite and < 5% as the oxidative metabolite (N,O-didesmethylvenlafaxine) in urine.

12.6 Special Populations

Age

In a study of healthy subjects administered doses of up to 300 mg, there was an approximate 32% increase in C_{max} and a 55% increase in AUC in subjects older than 75 years of age (n = 17), compared with subjects 18 to 45 years of age (n = 16). Subjects 65 to 75 years of age (n = 15) had no change in C_{max}, but an approximately 32% increase in AUC, compared to subjects 18 to 45 years of age [*see Dosage and Administration (2.2)*].

Gender

In a study of healthy subjects administered doses of up to 300 mg, women had an approximately 25% higher C_{max} and an approximately 10% higher AUC than age-matched men. No adjustment of dosage on the basis of gender is needed.

Race

Pharmacokinetic analysis showed that race (White, n = 466; Black, n = 97; Hispanic, n = 39; Other, n = 33) had no apparent effect on the pharmacokinetics of PRISTIQ. No adjustment of dosage on the basis of race is needed.

Hepatic insufficiency

The disposition of desvenlafaxine succinate after administration of 100 mg was studied in subjects with mild (Child-Pugh A, n = 8), moderate (Child-Pugh B, n = 8), and severe (Child-Pugh C, n = 8) hepatic impairment and to healthy subjects (n = 12).

Average AUC was increased by approximately 31% and 35% in patients with moderate and severe hepatic impairment, respectively, as compared to healthy subjects. Average AUC values were similar in subjects with mild hepatic impairment and healthy subjects (< 5% difference).

Systemic clearance (CL/F) was decreased by approximately 20% and 36% in patients with moderate and severe hepatic impairment, respectively, as compared to healthy subjects. CL/F values were comparable in mild hepatic impairment and healthy subjects (< 5% difference).

The mean $t_{1/2}$ changed from approximately 10 hours in healthy subjects and subjects with mild hepatic impairment to 13 and 14 hours in moderate and severe hepatic impairment, respectively. The recommended dose in patients with hepatic impairment is 50 mg/day. Dose escalation above 100 mg/day is not recommended [*see Use in Specific Populations (8.7)*].

Renal insufficiency

The disposition of desvenlafaxine after administration of 100 mg was studied in subjects with mild (n = 9), moderate (n = 8), severe (n = 7) and end-stage renal disease [ESRD] (n = 9) requiring dialysis and in healthy, age-matched control subjects (n = 8). Elimination was significantly correlated with creatinine clearance. Increases in AUCs of about 42% in mild renal impairment (24-hr CrCl = 50-80 mL/min), about 56% in moderate renal impairment (24-hr CrCl = 30-50 mL/min), about 108% in severe renal impairment (24-hr CrCl ≤ 30 mL/min), and about 116% in ESRD subjects were observed, compared with healthy, age-matched control subjects.

The mean terminal half-life ($t_{1/2}$) was prolonged from 11.1 hours in the control subjects to approximately 13.5, 15.5, 17.6, and 22.8 hours in mild, moderate, severe renal impairment and ESRD subjects, respectively. Less than 5% of the drug in the body was cleared during a standard 4-hour hemodialysis procedure.

The recommended dose in patients with moderate renal impairment is 50 mg per day. Dosage adjustment (50 mg every other day) is recommended in patients with severe renal impairment or ESRD. Doses should not be escalated in patients with moderate or severe renal impairment, or ESRD [*see Dosage and Administration (2.2) and Use in Specific Populations (8.6)*].

13 NONCLINICAL TOXICOLOGY

13.1 Carcinogenesis, Mutagenesis, Impairment of Fertility

Carcinogenesis

Desvenlafaxine succinate administered by oral gavage to mice and rats for 2 years did not increase the incidence of tumors in either study.

Mice received desvenlafaxine succinate at dosages up to 500/300 mg/kg/day (dosage lowered after 45 weeks of dosing). The 300 mg/kg/day dose is 15 times a human dose of 100 mg/day on a mg/m^2 basis.

Rats received desvenlafaxine succinate at dosages up to 300 mg/kg/day (males) or 500 mg/kg/day (females). The highest dose is 29 (males) or 48 (females) times a human dose of 100 mg/day on a mg/m^2 basis.

Mutagenesis

Desvenlafaxine was not mutagenic in the *in vitro* bacterial mutation assay (Ames test) and was not clastogenic in an *in vitro* chromosome aberration assay in cultured CHO cells, an *in vivo* mouse micronucleus assay, or an *in vivo* chromosome aberration assay in rats. Additionally, desvenlafaxine was not genotoxic in the *in vitro* CHO mammalian cell forward mutation assay and was negative in the *in vitro* BALB/c-3T3 mouse embryo cell transformation assay.

Impairment of fertility

Reduced fertility was observed in a study in which both male and female rats received desvenlafaxine succinate. This effect was noted at oral doses approximately 10 times a human dose of 100 mg/day on a mg/m^2 basis. There was no effect on fertility at oral doses approximately 3 times a human dose of 100 mg/day on a mg/m^2 basis.

14 CLINICAL STUDIES

The efficacy of PRISTIQ as a treatment for depression was established in four 8-week, randomized, double-blind, placebo-controlled, fixed-dose studies (at doses of 50 mg/day to 400 mg/day) in adult outpatients who met the Diagnostic and Statistical Manual of Mental Disorders (DSM-IV) criteria for major depressive disorder. In the first study, patients received 100 mg (n = 114), 200 mg (n = 116), or 400 mg (n = 113) of PRISTIQ once daily, or placebo (n = 118). In a second study, patients received either 200 mg (n = 121) or 400 mg (n = 124) of PRISTIQ once daily, or placebo (n = 124). In two additional studies, patients received 50 mg (n = 150 and n = 164) or 100 mg (n = 147 and n = 158) of PRISTIQ once daily, or placebo (n = 150 and n = 161).

PRISTIQ showed superiority over placebo as measured by improvement in the 17-item Hamilton Rating Scale for Depression (HAM-D$_{17}$) total score in four studies and overall improvement, as measured by the Clinical Global Impressions Scale - Improvement (CGI-I), in three of the four studies. In studies directly comparing 50 mg/day and 100 mg/day there was no suggestion of a greater effect with the higher dose and adverse events and discontinuations were more frequent at higher doses [*see Dosage and Administration (2.1)*].

Analyses of the relationships between treatment outcome and age and treatment outcome and gender did not suggest any differential responsiveness on the basis of these patient characteristics. There was insufficient information to determine the effect of race on outcome in these studies.

16 HOW SUPPLIED/STORAGE AND HANDLING

PRISTIQ® (desvenlafaxine) Extended-Release Tablets are available as follows:

50 mg, light pink, square pyramid tablet debossed with "W" (over) "50" on the flat side

NDC 0008-1211-14, bottle of 14 tablets in unit-of-use package

NDC 0008-1211-30, bottle of 30 tablets in unit-of-use package

NDC 0008-1211-01, bottle of 90 tablets in unit-of-use package

NDC 0008-1211-50, 10 blisters of 10 (HUD)

100 mg, reddish-orange, square pyramid tablet debossed with "W" (over) "100" on the flat side

NDC 0008-1222-14, bottle of 14 tablets in unit-of-use package

NDC 0008-1222-30, bottle of 30 tablets in unit-of-use package

NDC 0008-1222-01, bottle of 90 tablets in unit-of-use package

NDC 0008-1222-50, 10 blisters of 10 (HUD)

Store at 20° to 25°C (68° to 77°F); excursions permitted to 15° to 30°C (59° to 86°F) [see USP Controlled Room Temperature].

Each tablet contains 76 or 152 mg of desvenlafaxine succinate equivalent to 50 or 100 mg of desvenlafaxine, respectively.

The unit-of-use package is intended to be dispensed as a unit.

The appearance of these tablets is a trademark of Wyeth Pharmaceuticals.

U.S. Patent No. 6,673,838; 7,291,347.

17 PATIENT COUNSELING INFORMATION

Advise patients, their families, and their caregivers about the benefits and risks associated with treatment with PRISTIQ and counsel them in its appropriate use.

Advise patients, their families, and their caregivers to read the Medication Guide and assist them in understanding its contents. The complete text of the Medication Guide is reprinted at the end of this document.

17.1 Suicide Risk

Advise patients, their families and caregivers to look for the emergence of suicidality, especially early during treatment and when the dose is adjusted up or down [*see Box Warning and Warnings and Precautions (5.1)*].

17.2 Concomitant Medication

Advise patients taking PRISTIQ not to use concomitantly other products containing desvenlafaxine or venlafaxine. Healthcare professionals should instruct patients not to take PRISTIQ with an MAOI or within 14 days of stopping an MAOI and to allow 7 days after stopping PRISTIQ before starting an MAOI [*see Contraindications (4.2)*].

17.3 Serotonin Syndrome or Neuroleptic Malignant Syndrome (NMS)-like Reactions

Caution patients about the risk of serotonin syndrome or Neuroleptic Malignant Syndrome (NMS)-like reactions, particularly with the concomitant use of PRISTIQ and triptans, tramadol, tryptophan supplements, other serotonergic agents, or antipsychotic drugs [*see Warnings and Precautions (5.2) and Drug Interactions (7.3)*].

17.4 Elevated Blood Pressure

Advise patients that they should have regular monitoring of blood pressure when taking PRISTIQ [*see Warnings and Precautions (5.3)*].

17.5 Abnormal Bleeding

Patients should be cautioned about the concomitant use of PRISTIQ and NSAIDs, aspirin, warfarin, or other drugs that affect coagulation since combined use of psychotropic drugs that interfere with serotonin reuptake and these agents has been associated with an increased risk of bleeding [*see Warnings and Precautions (5.4)*].

17.6 Narrow-angle Glaucoma

Advise patients with raised intraocular pressure or those at risk of acute narrow-angle glaucoma (angle-closure glaucoma) that mydriasis has been reported and they should be monitored [*see Warnings and Precautions (5.5)*].

17.7 Activation of Mania/Hypomania

Advise patients, their families and caregivers to observe for signs of activation of mania/hypomania [*see Warnings and Precautions (5.6)*].

17.8 Cardiovascular/Cerebrovascular Disease

Caution is advised in administering PRISTIQ to patients with cardiovascular, cerebrovascular, or lipid metabolism disorders [*see Adverse Reactions (6.1) and Warnings and Precautions (5.7)*].

17.9 Serum Cholesterol and Triglyceride Elevation

Advise patients that elevations in total cholesterol, LDL and triglycerides may occur and that measurement of serum lipids may be considered [*see Warnings and Precautions (5.8)*].

17.10 Discontinuation

Advise patients not to stop taking PRISTIQ without talking first with their healthcare professional. Patients should be aware that discontinuation effects may occur when stopping PRISTIQ [*see Warnings and Precautions (5.9) and Adverse Reactions (6.1)*].

17.11 Switching Patients From Other Antidepressants to PRISTIQ

Discontinuation symptoms have been reported when switching patients from other antidepressants, including venlafaxine, to PRISTIQ. Tapering of the initial antidepressant may be necessary to minimize discontinuation symptoms.

17.12 Interference with Cognitive and Motor Performance

Caution patients about operating hazardous machinery, including automobiles, until they are reasonably certain that PRISTIQ therapy does not adversely affect their ability to engage in such activities.

17.13 Alcohol

Advise patients to avoid alcohol while taking PRISTIQ [*see Drug Interactions (7.5)*].

17.14 Allergic Reactions

Advise patients to notify their physician if they develop allergic phenomena such as rash, hives, swelling, or difficulty breathing.

17.15 Pregnancy

Advise patients to notify their physician if they become pregnant or intend to become pregnant during therapy [*see Use in Specific Populations (8.1)*].

17.16 Nursing

Advise patients to notify their physician if they are breastfeeding an infant [*see Use in Specific Populations (8.3)*].

17.17 Residual Inert Matrix Tablet

Patients receiving PRISTIQ may notice an inert matrix tablet passing in the stool or via colostomy. Patients should be informed that the active medication has already been absorbed by the time the patient sees the inert matrix tablet.

MEDICATION GUIDE

PRISTIQ® (pris-**TEEK**) Extended-Release Tablets (desvenlafaxine)

Antidepressant Medicines, Depression and Other Serious Mental Illnesses, and Suicidal Thoughts or Actions

Read the Medication Guide that comes with your or your family member's antidepressant medicine. This Medication Guide is only about the risk of suicidal thoughts and actions with antidepressant medicines.

Talk to your, or your family member's, healthcare provider about:

- all risks and benefits of treatment with antidepressant medicines
- all treatment choices for depression or other serious mental illness

What is the most important information I should know about antidepressant medicines, depression and other serious mental illnesses, and suicidal thoughts or actions?

1. **Antidepressant medicines may increase suicidal thoughts or actions in some children, teenagers, and young adults within the first few months of treatment.**
2. **Depression and other serious mental illnesses are the most important causes of suicidal thoughts and actions. Some people may have a particularly high risk of having suicidal thoughts or actions.** These include people who have (or have a family history of) bipolar illness (also called manic-depressive illness) or suicidal thoughts or actions.
3. **How can I watch for and try to prevent suicidal thoughts and actions in myself or a family member?**

- Pay close attention to any changes, especially sudden changes, in mood, behaviors, thoughts, or feelings. This is very important when an antidepressant medicine is started or when the dose is changed.
- Call the healthcare provider right away to report new or sudden changes in mood, behavior, thoughts, or feelings.
- Keep all follow-up visits with the healthcare provider as scheduled. Call the healthcare provider between visits as needed, especially if you have concerns about symptoms.

Call a healthcare provider right away if you or your family member has any of the following symptoms, especially if they are new, worse, or worry you:

- thoughts about suicide or dying
- attempts to commit suicide
- new or worse depression
- new or worse anxiety
- feeling very agitated or restless
- panic attacks
- trouble sleeping (insomnia)
- new or worse irritability
- acting aggressive, being angry, or violent
- acting on dangerous impulses
- an extreme increase in activity and talking (mania)
- other unusual changes in behavior or mood

What else do I need to know about antidepressant medicines?

- Never stop an antidepressant medicine without first talking to a healthcare provider. Stopping an antidepressant medicine suddenly can cause other symptoms.
- **Antidepressants are medicines used to treat depression and other illnesses.** It is important to discuss all the risks of treating depression and also the risks of not treating it. Patients and their families or other caregivers should discuss all treatment choices with the healthcare provider, not just the use of antidepressants.
- **Antidepressant medicines have other side effects.** Talk to the healthcare provider about the side effects of the medicine prescribed for you or your family member.
- **Antidepressant medicines can interact with other medicines.** Know all of the medicines that you or your family member takes. Keep a list of all medicines to show the healthcare provider. Do not start new medicines without first checking with your healthcare provider.
- **Not all antidepressant medicines prescribed for children are FDA approved for use in children.** Talk to your child's healthcare provider for more information.

This Medication Guide has been approved by the U.S. Food and Drug Administration for all antidepressants.

Important Information about PRISTIQ® Extended-Release Tablets

Read the patient information that comes with PRISTIQ before you take PRISTIQ and each time you refill your prescription. There may be new information. If you have questions, ask your healthcare provider. This information does not take the place of talking with your healthcare provider about your medical condition or treatment.

What is PRISTIQ?
- PRISTIQ is a prescription medicine used to treat depression. PRISTIQ belongs to a class of medicines known as SNRIs (or serotonin-norepinephrine reuptake inhibitors).
- PRISTIQ has not been studied or approved for use in children and adolescents.

Who should not take PRISTIQ?
Do not take PRISTIQ if you:
- are allergic to desvenlafaxine, venlafaxine or any of the ingredients in PRISTIQ. See the end of this Medication Guide for a complete list of ingredients in PRISTIQ.
- currently take or have taken within the last 14 days, any medicine known as an MAOI. Taking an MAOI with certain other medicines, including PRISTIQ, can cause serious or even life-threatening side effects. Also, you must wait at least 7 days after you stop taking PRISTIQ before you take any MAOI.

What should I tell my healthcare provider before taking PRISTIQ?
Tell your healthcare provider about all your medical conditions, including if you:
- have high blood pressure
- have heart problems
- have high cholesterol or high triglycerides
- have a history of a stroke
- have glaucoma
- have kidney problems
- have liver problems
- have or had bleeding problems
- have or had seizures or convulsions
- have mania or bipolar disorder
- have low sodium levels in your blood
- are pregnant or plan to become pregnant. It is not known if PRISTIQ will harm your unborn baby.
- are breastfeeding. PRISTIQ can pass into your breast milk and may harm your baby. Talk with your healthcare provider about the best way to feed your baby if you take PRISTIQ.

Serotonin syndrome or neuroleptic malignant syndrome (NMS)-like reactions
Rare, but potentially life-threatening, conditions called serotonin syndrome or Neuroleptic Malignant Syndrome (NMS)-like reactions can happen when medicines such as PRISTIQ are taken with certain other medicines. Serotonin syndrome or NMS-like reactions can cause serious changes in how your brain, muscles and digestive system work.

Especially tell your healthcare provider if you take the following:
- medicines to treat migraine headaches known as triptans
- medicines used to treat mood disorders, including tricyclics, lithium, selective serotonin reuptake inhibitors (SSRIs), or serotonin norepinephrine reuptake inhibitors (SNRIs)
- silbutramine
- tramadol
- St. John's Wort
- MAOIs (including linezolid, an antibiotic)
- tryptophan supplements

Ask your healthcare provider if you are not sure if you are taking any of these medicines.

Before you take PRISTIQ with any of these medicines, talk to your healthcare provider about serotonin syndrome. See "What are the possible side effects of PRISTIQ?"

PRISTIQ contains the medicine desvenlafaxine. Do not take PRISTIQ with other medicines containing venlafaxine or desvenlafaxine.

How should I take PRISTIQ?
- Take PRISTIQ exactly as your healthcare provider has told you.
- Take PRISTIQ at about the same time each day.
- PRISTIQ may be taken either with or without food.
- Swallow PRISTIQ tablets whole, with fluid. Do not crush, cut, chew, or dissolve PRISTIQ tablets because the tablets are time-released.
- When you take PRISTIQ, you may see something in your stool that looks like a tablet. This is the empty shell from the tablet after the medicine has been absorbed by your body.
- It is common for antidepressant medicines such as PRISTIQ to take several weeks before you start to feel better. Do not stop taking PRISTIQ if you do not feel results right away.

- Do not stop taking or change the dose of PRISTIQ without talking with your healthcare provider, even if you feel better.
- Talk with your healthcare provider about how long you should use PRISTIQ. Take PRISTIQ for as long as your healthcare provider tells you to.
- If you miss a dose of PRISTIQ, take it as soon as you remember. If it is almost time for your next dose, skip the missed dose. Do not try to "make up" for the missed dose by taking two doses at the same time.
- Do not take more PRISTIQ than prescribed by your healthcare provider. If you take more PRISTIQ than the amount prescribed, contact your healthcare provider right away.
- In case of an overdose of PRISTIQ, call your healthcare provider or poison control center, or go to the emergency room right away.

Switching from other antidepressants
Side effects from discontinuing antidepressant medication have occurred when patients switched from other antidepressants, including venlafaxine, to PRISTIQ. Your doctor may gradually reduce the dose of your initial antidepressant medication to help to reduce these side effects.

What should I avoid while taking PRISTIQ?
- Do not drive a car or operate machinery until you know how PRISTIQ affects you.
- Avoid drinking alcohol while taking PRISTIQ.

What are the possible side effects of PRISTIQ?
PRISTIQ can cause serious side effects, including:
- See the beginning of this Medication Guide – Antidepressant Medicines, Depression and other Serious Mental Illnesses, and Suicidal Thoughts or Actions.
- Serotonin syndrome or neuroleptic malignant syndrome (NMS)-like reactions. See "What should I tell my healthcare provider before taking PRISTIQ?"
  Get medical help right away if you think that you have these syndromes. Signs and symptoms of these syndromes may include one or more of the following:

- restlessness
- hallucinations (seeing and hearing things that are not real)
- loss of coordination
- fast heart beat
- increased body temperature
- muscle stiffness
- increase in blood pressure
- diarrhea
- coma
- nausea
- vomiting
- confusion

PRISTIQ may also cause other serious side effects, including:
- **New or worsened high blood pressure (hypertension).** Your healthcare provider should monitor your blood pressure before and while you are taking PRISTIQ. If you have high blood pressure, it should be controlled before you start taking PRISTIQ.
- **Abnormal bleeding or bruising.** PRISTIQ and other SNRIs/SSRIs may cause you to have an increased chance of bleeding. Taking aspirin, NSAIDs (non-steroidal anti-inflammatory drugs), or blood thinners may add to this risk. Tell your healthcare provider right away about any unusual bleeding or bruising.
- **Glaucoma (increased eye pressure)**
- **Increased cholesterol and triglyceride levels in your blood**
- **Symptoms when stopping PRISTIQ (discontinuation symptoms).** Side effects may occur when stopping PRISTIQ (discontinuation symptoms), especially when therapy is stopped suddenly. Your healthcare provider may want to decrease your dose slowly to help avoid side effects. Some of these side effects may include:

- dizziness
- nausea
- headache
- irritability
- sleeping problems (insomnia)
- anxiety
- abnormal dreams
- tiredness
- sweating
- diarrhea

- **Seizures (convulsions)**
- **Low sodium levels in your blood.** Symptoms of this may include: headache, difficulty concentrating, memory changes, confusion, weakness and unsteadiness on your feet. In severe or more sudden cases, symptoms can include: hallucinations (seeing or hearing things that are not real), fainting, seizures and coma. If not treated, severe low sodium levels could be fatal.

Contact your healthcare provider if you think you have any of these side effects.

Common side effects with PRISTIQ include:

- nausea
- headache
- dry mouth
- sweating
- dizziness
- insomnia
- constipation
- loss of appetite
- sleepiness
- tiredness
- diarrhea
- vomiting
- anxiety
- tremor
- dilated pupils
- decreased sex drive
- delayed orgasm and ejaculation

These are not all the possible side effects of PRISTIQ. Tell your healthcare provider about any side effect that bothers you or does not go away. Call your doctor for medical advice about side effects. You may report side effects to FDA at 1-800-FDA-1088. For more information on these and other side effects associated with PRISTIQ, talk to your healthcare provider, visit our web site at www.pristiq.com or call our toll-free number at 1-888-PRISTIQ (774-7847).

How should I store PRISTIQ?
- Store PRISTIQ at 68° to 77°F (20° to 25°C).
- Do not use PRISTIQ after the expiration date (EXP), which is on the container. The expiration date refers to the last day of that month.
- Keep PRISTIQ and all medicines out of the reach of children.

General Information about the safe and effective use of PRISTIQ
Medicines are sometimes used for conditions that are not mentioned in Medication Guides. Do not use PRISTIQ for a condition for which it was not prescribed. Do not give PRISTIQ to other people, even if they have the same symptoms that you have. It may harm them.

This Medication Guide summarizes the most important information about PRISTIQ. If you would like more information, talk with your healthcare provider. You can ask your pharmacist or healthcare provider for information about PRISTIQ that is written for healthcare professionals. For more information, go to www.pristiq.com or call 1-888-PRISTIQ (774-7847).

What are the ingredients in PRISTIQ?
Active ingredient: desvenlafaxine
Inactive ingredients: For the 50 mg tablet, hypromellose, microcrystalline cellulose, talc, magnesium stearate and film coating, which consists of polyvinyl alcohol, polyethylene glycol, talc, titanium dioxide, and iron oxides.
For the 100 mg tablet, hypromellose, microcrystalline cellulose, talc, magnesium stearate, a film coating which consists of polyvinyl alcohol, polyethylene glycol, talc, titanium dioxide, iron oxide and FD&C yellow #6.
This Medication Guide has been approved by the U.S. Food and Drug Administration.
Issued July 2009.

Contact Information
Please visit our web site at www.pristiq.com, or call our toll-free number 1-888-PRISTIQ (774-7847) to receive more information.

This product's label may have been updated. For current package insert and further product information, please visit www.wyeth.com or call our medical communications department toll-free at 1-800-934-5556.

Wyeth®
Wyeth Pharmaceuticals Inc.
Philadelphia, PA 19101

W10529C014
ET01
Rev 05/10

MEDICATION GUIDE
PRISTIQ® (pris-**TEEK**) Extended-Release Tablets (desvenlafaxine)
Antidepressant Medicines, Depression and Other Serious Mental Illnesses, and Suicidal Thoughts or Actions
Read the Medication Guide that comes with your or your family member's antidepressant medicine. This Medication Guide is only about the risk of suicidal thoughts and actions with antidepressant medicines.
Talk to your, or your family member's, healthcare provider about:
- all risks and benefits of treatment with antidepressant medicines
- all treatment choices for depression or other serious mental illness

What is the most important information I should know about antidepressant medicines, depression and other serious mental illnesses, and suicidal thoughts or actions?
1. Antidepressant medicines may increase suicidal thoughts or actions in some children, teenagers, and young adults within the first few months of treatment.
2. Depression and other serious mental illnesses are the most important causes of suicidal thoughts and actions. Some people may have a particularly high risk of having

suicidal thoughts or actions. These include people who have (or have a family history of) bipolar illness (also called manic-depressive illness) or suicidal thoughts or actions.

3. **How can I watch for and try to prevent suicidal thoughts and actions in myself or a family member?**
- Pay close attention to any changes, especially sudden changes, in mood, behaviors, thoughts, or feelings. This is very important when an antidepressant medicine is started or when the dose is changed.
- Call the healthcare provider right away to report new or sudden changes in mood, behavior, thoughts, or feelings.
- Keep all follow-up visits with the healthcare provider as scheduled. Call the healthcare provider between visits as needed, especially if you have concerns about symptoms.

Call a healthcare provider right away if you or your family member has any of the following symptoms, especially if they are new, worse, or worry you:

- thoughts about suicide or dying
- attempts to commit suicide
- new or worse depression
- new or worse anxiety
- feeling very agitated or restless
- panic attacks
- trouble sleeping (insomnia)
- new or worse irritability
- acting aggressive, being angry, or violent
- acting on dangerous impulses
- an extreme increase in activity and talking (mania)
- other unusual changes in behavior or mood

What else do I need to know about antidepressant medicines?
- Never stop an antidepressant medicine without first talking to a healthcare provider. Stopping an antidepressant medicine suddenly can cause other symptoms.
- **Antidepressants are medicines used to treat depression and other illnesses.** It is important to discuss all the risks of treating depression and also the risks of not treating it. Patients and their families or other caregivers should discuss all treatment choices with the healthcare provider, not just the use of antidepressants.
- **Antidepressant medicines have other side effects.** Talk to the healthcare provider about the side effects of the medicine prescribed for you or your family member.
- **Antidepressant medicines can interact with other medicines.** Know all of the medicines that you or your family member takes. Keep a list of all medicines to show the healthcare provider. Do not start new medicines without first checking with your healthcare provider.
- **Not all antidepressant medicines prescribed for children are FDA approved for use in children.** Talk to your child's healthcare provider for more information.

This Medication Guide has been approved by the U.S. Food and Drug Administration for all antidepressants.

Important Information about PRISTIQ® Extended-Release Tablets

Read the patient information that comes with PRISTIQ before you take PRISTIQ and each time you refill your prescription. There may be new information. If you have questions, ask your healthcare provider. This information does not take the place of talking with your healthcare provider about your medical condition or treatment.

What is PRISTIQ?
- PRISTIQ is a prescription medicine used to treat depression. PRISTIQ belongs to a class of medicines known as SNRIs (or serotonin-norepinephrine reuptake inhibitors).
- PRISTIQ has not been studied or approved for use in children and adolescents.

Who should not take PRISTIQ?
Do not take PRISTIQ if you:
- are allergic to desvenlafaxine, venlafaxine or any of the ingredients in PRISTIQ. See the end of this Medication Guide for a complete list of ingredients in PRISTIQ.
- currently take or have taken within the last 14 days, any medicine known as an MAOI. Taking an MAOI with certain other medicines, including PRISTIQ, can cause serious or even life-threatening side effects. Also, you must wait at least 7 days after you stop taking PRISTIQ before you take any MAOI.

What should I tell my healthcare provider before taking PRISTIQ?
Tell your healthcare provider about all your medical conditions, including if you:
- have high blood pressure
- have heart problems
- have high cholesterol or high triglycerides
- have a history of a stroke
- have glaucoma

- have kidney problems
- have liver problems
- have or had bleeding problems
- have or had seizures or convulsions
- have mania or bipolar disorder
- have low sodium levels in your blood
- are pregnant or plan to become pregnant. It is not known if PRISTIQ will harm your unborn baby.
- are breastfeeding. PRISTIQ can pass into your breast milk and may harm your baby. Talk with your healthcare provider about the best way to feed your baby if you take PRISTIQ.

Serotonin syndrome or neuroleptic malignant syndrome (NMS)-like reactions
Rare, but potentially life-threatening, conditions called serotonin syndrome or Neuroleptic Malignant Syndrome (NMS)-like reactions can happen when medicines such as PRISTIQ are taken with certain other medicines. Serotonin syndrome or NMS-like reactions can cause serious changes in how your brain, muscles and digestive system work.
Especially tell your healthcare provider if you take the following:
- medicines to treat migraine headaches known as triptans
- medicines used to treat mood disorders, including tricyclics, lithium, selective serotonin reuptake inhibitors (SSRIs), or serotonin norepinephrine reuptake inhibitors (SNRIs)
- silbutramine
- tramadol
- St. John's Wort
- MAOIs (including linezolid, an antibiotic)
- tryptophan supplements

Ask your healthcare provider if you are not sure if you are taking any of these medicines.
Before you take PRISTIQ with any of these medicines, talk to your healthcare provider about serotonin syndrome. See "What are the possible side effects of PRISTIQ?"
PRISTIQ contains the medicine desvenlafaxine. Do not take PRISTIQ with other medicines containing venlafaxine or desvenlafaxine.

How should I take PRISTIQ?
- Take PRISTIQ exactly as your healthcare provider has told you.
- Take PRISTIQ at about the same time each day.
- PRISTIQ may be taken either with or without food.
- Swallow PRISTIQ tablets whole, with fluid. Do not crush, cut, chew, or dissolve PRISTIQ tablets because the tablets are time-released.
- When you take PRISTIQ, you may see something in your stool that looks like a tablet. This is the empty shell from the tablet after the medicine has been absorbed by your body.
- It is common for antidepressant medicines such as PRISTIQ to take several weeks before you start to feel better. Do not stop taking PRISTIQ if you do not feel results right away.
- Do not stop taking or change the dose of PRISTIQ without talking with your healthcare provider, even if you feel better.
- Talk with your healthcare provider about how long you should use PRISTIQ. Take PRISTIQ for as long as your healthcare provider tells you to.
- If you miss a dose of PRISTIQ, take it as soon as you remember. If it is almost time for your next dose, skip the missed dose. Do not try to "make up" for the missed dose by taking two doses at the same time.
- Do not take more PRISTIQ than prescribed by your healthcare provider. If you take more PRISTIQ than the amount prescribed, contact your healthcare provider right away.
- In case of an overdose of PRISTIQ, call your healthcare provider or poison control center, or go to the emergency room right away.

Switching from other antidepressants
Side effects from discontinuing antidepressant medication have occurred when patients switched from other antidepressants, including venlafaxine, to PRISTIQ. Your doctor may gradually reduce the dose of your initial antidepressant medication to help to reduce these side effects.

What should I avoid while taking PRISTIQ?
- Do not drive a car or operate machinery until you know how PRISTIQ affects you.
- Avoid drinking alcohol while taking PRISTIQ.

What are the possible side effects of PRISTIQ?
PRISTIQ can cause serious side effects, including:
- See the beginning of this Medication Guide – Antidepressant Medicines, Depression and other Serious Mental Illnesses, and Suicidal Thoughts or Actions.
- Serotonin syndrome or neuroleptic malignant syndrome (NMS)-like reactions. See "What should I tell my healthcare provider before taking PRISTIQ?"
Get medical help right away if you think that you have these syndromes. Signs and symptoms of these syndromes may include one or more of the following:

- restlessness
- hallucinations (seeing and hearing things that are not real)
- loss of coordination
- fast heart beat
- increased body temperature
- muscle stiffness
- increase in blood pressure
- diarrhea
- coma
- nausea
- vomiting
- confusion

PRISTIQ may also cause other serious side effects, including:
- **New or worsened high blood pressure (hypertension).** Your healthcare provider should monitor your blood pressure before and while you are taking PRISTIQ. If you have high blood pressure, it should be controlled before you start taking PRISTIQ.
- **Abnormal bleeding or bruising.** PRISTIQ and other SNRIs/SSRIs may cause you to have an increased chance of bleeding. Taking aspirin, NSAIDs (non-steroidal anti-inflammatory drugs), or blood thinners may add to this risk. Tell your healthcare provider right away about any unusual bleeding or bruising.
- **Glaucoma (increased eye pressure)**
- **Increased cholesterol and triglyceride levels in your blood**
- **Symptoms when stopping PRISTIQ (discontinuation symptoms).** Side effects may occur when stopping PRISTIQ (discontinuation symptoms), especially when therapy is stopped suddenly. Your healthcare provider may want to decrease your dose slowly to help avoid side effects. Some of these side effects may include:

- dizziness
- nausea
- headache
- irritability
- sleeping problems (insomnia)
- anxiety
- abnormal dreams
- tiredness
- sweating
- diarrhea

- Seizures (convulsions)
- Low sodium levels in your blood. Symptoms of this may include: headache, difficulty concentrating, memory changes, confusion, weakness and unsteadiness on your feet. In severe or more sudden cases, symptoms can include: hallucinations (seeing or hearing things that are not real), fainting, seizures and coma. If not treated, severe low sodium levels could be fatal.

Contact your healthcare provider if you think you have any of these side effects.
Common side effects with PRISTIQ include:

- nausea
- headache
- dry mouth
- sweating
- dizziness
- insomnia
- constipation
- loss of appetite
- sleepiness
- tiredness
- diarrhea
- vomiting
- anxiety
- tremor
- dilated pupils
- decreased sex drive
- delayed orgasm and ejaculation

These are not all the possible side effects of PRISTIQ. Tell your healthcare provider about any side effect that bothers you or does not go away. Call your doctor for medical advice about side effects. You may report side effects to FDA at 1-800-FDA-1088. For more information on these and other side effects associated with PRISTIQ, talk to your healthcare provider, visit our web site at www.pristiq.com or call our toll-free number at 1-888-PRISTIQ (774-7847).

How should I store PRISTIQ?
- Store PRISTIQ at 68° to 77°F (20° to 25°C).
- Do not use PRISTIQ after the expiration date (EXP), which is on the container. The expiration date refers to the last day of that month.
- Keep PRISTIQ and all medicines out of the reach of children.

General Information about the safe and effective use of PRISTIQ

Medicines are sometimes used for conditions that are not mentioned in Medication Guides. Do not use PRISTIQ for a condition for which it was not prescribed. Do not give PRISTIQ to other people, even if they have the same symptoms that you have. It may harm them.

This Medication Guide summarizes the most important information about PRISTIQ. If you would like more information, talk with your healthcare provider. You can ask your pharmacist or healthcare provider for information about PRISTIQ that is written for healthcare professionals. For more information, go to www.pristiq.com or call 1-888-PRISTIQ (774-7847).

What are the ingredients in PRISTIQ?
Active ingredient: desvenlafaxine
Inactive ingredients: For the 50 mg tablet, hypromellose, microcrystalline cellulose, talc, magnesium stearate and film coating, which consists of polyvinyl alcohol, polyethylene glycol, talc, titanium dioxide, and iron oxides.
For the 100 mg tablet, hypromellose, microcrystalline cellulose, talc, magnesium stearate, a film coating which consists of polyvinyl alcohol, polyethylene glycol, talc, titanium dioxide, iron oxide and FD&C yellow #6.
This Medication Guide has been approved by the U.S. Food and Drug Administration.

Issued July 2009.

Contact Information
Please visit our web site at www.pristiq.com, or call our toll-free number 1-888-PRISTIQ (774-7847) to receive more information.

This product's label may have been updated. For current package insert and further product information, please visit www.wyeth.com or call our medical communications department toll-free at 1-800-934-5556.

Wyeth®
Wyeth Pharmaceuticals Inc.
Philadelphia, PA 19101

W10530P007
Rev 02/10

Shown in Product Identification Guide, page 321

TORISEL KIT ℞

[*tōr-ĭ-sĕl*]
(temsirolimus)
injection, for intravenous infusion only

HIGHLIGHTS OF PRESCRIBING INFORMATION
These highlights do not include all the information needed to use TORISEL® safely and effectively. See full prescribing information for TORISEL.

TORISEL Kit (temsirolimus) injection, for intravenous infusion only
Initial U.S. Approval: 2007

──────RECENT MAJOR CHANGES──────
Dosage and Administration, Dose Modification Guidelines (2.4)	07/2010
Contraindications (4)	07/2010
Warnings and Precautions, Hepatic Impairment (5.2)	07/2010

──────INDICATIONS AND USAGE──────
TORISEL® is a kinase inhibitor indicated for the treatment of advanced renal cell carcinoma. (1)

──────DOSAGE AND ADMINISTRATION──────
- The recommended dose of TORISEL is 25 mg infused over a 30-60 minute period once a week. Treat until disease progression or unacceptable toxicity. (2.1)
- Antihistamine pre-treatment is recommended. (2.2)
- Dose reduction is required in patients with mild hepatic impairment. (2.4)
- TORISEL (temsirolimus) injection vial contents must first be diluted with the enclosed diluent before diluting the resultant solution with 250 mL of 0.9% sodium chloride injection. (2.5)

──────DOSAGE FORMS AND STRENGTHS──────
TORISEL injection, 25 mg/mL supplied with DILUENT for TORISEL®. (3)

──────CONTRAINDICATIONS──────
TORISEL is contraindicated in patients with bilirubin >1.5 × ULN. (4)

──────WARNINGS AND PRECAUTIONS──────
- To treat hypersensitivity reactions stop TORISEL and treat with an antihistamine. TORISEL may be restarted at physician discretion at a slower rate. (5.1)

- Hepatic Impairment: Use caution when treating patients with mild hepatic impairment and reduce dose. (2.4, 5.2)
- Hyperglycemia and hyperlipemia are likely and may require treatment. Monitor glucose and lipid profiles. (5.3, 5.6)
- Infections may result from immunosuppression. (5.4)
- Monitor for symptoms or radiographic changes of interstitial lung disease (ILD). If ILD is suspected, discontinue TORISEL, and consider use of corticosteroids and/or antibiotics. (5.5)
- Bowel perforation may occur. Evaluate fever, abdominal pain, bloody stools, and/or acute abdomen promptly. (5.7)
- Renal failure, sometimes fatal, has occurred. Monitor renal function at baseline and while on TORISEL. (5.8)
- Due to abnormal wound healing, use TORISEL with caution in the perioperative period. (5.9)
- Live vaccinations and close contact with those who received live vaccines should be avoided. (5.13)
- Women of childbearing potential should be advised of the potential hazard to the fetus and to avoid becoming pregnant. (5.14)

──────ADVERSE REACTIONS──────
The most common adverse reactions (incidence ≥30%) are rash, asthenia, mucositis, nausea, edema, and anorexia. The most common laboratory abnormalities (incidence ≥30%) are anemia, hyperglycemia, hyperlipemia, hypertriglyceridemia, elevated alkaline phosphatase, elevated serum creatinine, lymphopenia, hypophosphatemia, thrombocytopenia, elevated AST, and leukopenia. (6)

To report SUSPECTED ADVERSE REACTIONS, contact Wyeth Pharmaceuticals Inc. at 1-800-934-5556 or FDA at 1-800-FDA-1088 or www.fda.gov/medwatch

──────DRUG INTERACTIONS──────
Strong inducers of CYP3A4/5 and inhibitors of CYP3A4 may affect concentrations of the primary metabolite of TORISEL. If alternatives cannot be used, dose modifications of TORISEL are recommended. (7.1, 7.2)

See 17 for PATIENT COUNSELING INFORMATION
Revised: 09/2010

FULL PRESCRIBING INFORMATION: CONTENTS*

17 PATIENT COUNSELING INFORMATION
*Sections or subsections omitted from the full prescribing information are not listed

FULL PRESCRIBING INFORMATION

1 INDICATIONS AND USAGE
TORISEL is indicated for the treatment of advanced renal cell carcinoma.

2 DOSAGE AND ADMINISTRATION
2.1 Advanced Renal Cell Carcinoma
The recommended dose of TORISEL for advanced renal cell carcinoma is 25 mg infused over a 30-60 minute period once a week.
Treatment should continue until disease progression or unacceptable toxicity occurs.
2.2 Premedication
Patients should receive prophylactic intravenous diphenhydramine 25 to 50 mg (or similar antihistamine) approximately 30 minutes before the start of each dose of TORISEL [*see Hypersensitivity Reactions (5.1)*].
2.3 Dosage Interruption/Adjustment
TORISEL should be held for absolute neutrophil count (ANC) < 1,000/mm³, platelet count < 75,000/mm³, or NCI CTCAE grade 3 or greater adverse reactions. Once toxicities have resolved to grade 2 or less, TORISEL may be restarted with the dose reduced by 5 mg/week to a dose no lower than 15 mg/week.
2.4 Dose Modification Guidelines
Hepatic Impairment: Use caution when treating patients with hepatic impairment. If TORISEL must be given in patients with mild hepatic impairment (bilirubin > 1–1.5 × ULN or AST > ULN but bilirubin ≤ ULN), reduce the dose of TORISEL to 15 mg/week. TORISEL is contraindicated in patients with bilirubin > 1.5 × ULN [*see Contraindications (4), Warnings and Precautions (5.2) and Use in Specific Populations (8.7)*].
Concomitant Strong CYP3A4 Inhibitors: The concomitant use of strong CYP3A4 inhibitors should be avoided (e.g. ketoconazole, itraconazole, clarithromycin, atazanavir, indinavir, nefazodone, nelfinavir, ritonavir, saquinavir, telithromycin, and voriconazole). Grapefruit juice may also increase plasma concentrations of sirolimus (a major metabolite of temsirolimus) and should be avoided. If patients must be co-administered a strong CYP3A4 inhibitor, based on pharmacokinetic studies, a TORISEL dose reduction to 12.5 mg/week should be considered. This dose of TORISEL is predicted to adjust the AUC to the range observed without inhibitors. However, there are no clinical data with this dose adjustment in patients receiving strong CYP3A4 inhibitors. If the strong inhibitor is discontinued, a washout period of approximately 1 week should be allowed before the TORISEL dose is adjusted back to the dose used prior to initiation of the strong CYP3A4 inhibitor [*see Drug Interactions (7.2)*].
Concomitant Strong CYP3A4 Inducers: The use of concomitant strong CYP3A4 inducers should be avoided (e.g. dexamethasone, phenytoin, carbamazepine, rifampin, rifabutin, rifampacin, phenobarbital). If patients must be co-administered a strong CYP3A4 inducer, based on pharmacokinetic studies, a TORISEL dose increase from 25 mg/week up to 50 mg/week should be considered. This dose of TORISEL is predicted to adjust the AUC to the range observed without inducers. However, there are no clinical data with this dose adjustment in patients receiving strong CYP3A4 inducers. If the strong inducer is discontinued the temsirolimus dose should be returned to the dose used prior to initiation of the strong CYP3A4 inducer [*see Drug Interactions (7.1)*].
2.5 Instructions for Preparation and Administration
TORISEL must be stored under refrigeration at 2°-8°C (36°-46°F) and protected from light. During handling and preparation of admixtures, TORISEL should be protected from excessive room light and sunlight.
Parenteral drug products should be inspected visually for particulate matter and discoloration prior to administration, whenever solution and container permit.
In order to minimize the patient exposure to the plasticizer DEHP (di-2-ethylhexyl phthalate), which may be leached from PVC infusion bags or sets, the final TORISEL dilution for infusion should be stored in bottles (glass, polypropylene) or plastic bags (polypropylene, polyolefin) and administered through polyethylene-lined administration sets.
Dilution:
In preparing the TORISEL administration solution, follow this two-step dilution process in an aseptic manner.
Step 1:
Inject 1.8 mL of DILUENT for TORISEL® into the vial of TORISEL (temsirolimus) injection (25 mg/mL). The TORISEL (temsirolimus) vial contains an overfill of 0.2 mL (30 mg/1.2 mL). Due to the intentional overfill in the TORISEL injection vial, the drug concentration of the resulting solution will be 10 mg/mL. A total volume of 3 mL will be obtained including the overfill. Mix well by inversion of the vial. Allow sufficient time for air bubbles to subside. This 10 mg/mL drug solution/diluent mixture must be further diluted as described in Step 2 below.

The solution is clear to slightly turbid, colorless to yellow, and free from visual particulates. The 10 mg/mL drug solution/diluent mixture is stable for up to 24 hours at controlled room temperature.

Step 2:
Withdraw the required amount of temsirolimus from the 10 mg/mL drug solution/diluent mixture prepared in Step 1. Inject rapidly into a 250 mL container (glass, polyolefin, or polyethylene) of 0.9% sodium chloride injection. Mix the admixture by inversion of the bag or bottle. Avoid excessive shaking as this may cause foaming.

Administration:
• The sodium chloride injection container should be composed of non-DEHP containing materials, such as glass, polyolefin or polyethylene, and the administration set should consist of non-DEHP tubing to avoid extraction of di-(2-ethylhexyl) phthalate (DEHP). TORISEL contains polysorbate 80, which is known to increase the rate of di-(2-ethylhexyl) phthalate (DEHP) extraction from PVC.
• An in-line polyethersulfone filter with a pore size of not greater than 5 microns is recommended for administration.
• The final diluted solution of TORISEL is intravenously infused over a 30-60 minute period once a week. The use of an infusion pump is the preferred method of administration to ensure accurate delivery of the drug.
• Administration of the final diluted infusion solution should be completed within six hours from the time that the drug solution/diluent mixture is added to the sodium chloride injection.

Compatibilities and Incompatibilities
Undiluted TORISEL injection should not be added directly to aqueous infusion solutions. Direct addition of TORISEL injection to aqueous solutions will result in precipitation of drug. Always combine TORISEL injection with DILUENT for TORISEL® before adding to infusion solutions. It is recommended that TORISEL be administered in 0.9% sodium chloride injection after combining with diluent. The stability of TORISEL in other infusion solutions has not been evaluated. Addition of other drugs or nutritional agents to admixtures of TORISEL in sodium chloride injection has not been evaluated and should be avoided. Temsirolimus is degraded by both acids and bases, and thus combinations of temsirolimus with agents capable of modifying solution pH should be avoided.

3 DOSAGE FORMS AND STRENGTHS
TORISEL (temsirolimus) is supplied as a kit consisting of the following:
TORISEL (temsirolimus) injection (25 mg/mL). The TORISEL vial includes an overfill of 0.2 mL.
DILUENT for TORISEL®. The DILUENT vial includes a deliverable volume of 1.8 mL.

4 CONTRAINDICATIONS
TORISEL is contraindicated in patients with bilirubin >1.5 × ULN [see Warnings and Precautions (5.2)].

5 WARNINGS AND PRECAUTIONS
5.1 Hypersensitivity Reactions
Hypersensitivity reactions manifested by symptoms including, but not limited to, anaphylaxis, dyspnea, flushing, and chest pain have been observed with TORISEL.
TORISEL should be used with caution in persons with known hypersensitivity to temsirolimus or its metabolites (including sirolimus), polysorbate 80, or to any other component (including the excipients) of TORISEL.
An H_1 antihistamine should be administered to patients before the start of the intravenous temsirolimus infusion. TORISEL should be used with caution in patients with known hypersensitivity to an antihistamine, or patients who cannot receive an antihistamine for other medical reasons.
If a patient develops a hypersensitivity reaction during the TORISEL infusion, the infusion should be stopped and the patient should be observed for at least 30 to 60 minutes (depending on the severity of the reaction). At the discretion of the physician, treatment may be resumed with the administration of an H_1-receptor antagonist (such as diphenhydramine), if not previously administered [see Dosage and Administration (2.2)], and/or an H_2-receptor antagonist (such as intravenous famotidine 20 mg or intravenous ranitidine 50 mg) approximately 30 minutes before restarting the TORISEL infusion. The infusion may then be resumed at a slower rate (up to 60 minutes).

5.2 Hepatic Impairment
The safety and pharmacokinetics of TORISEL were evaluated in a dose escalation phase 1 study in 110 patients with normal or varying degrees of hepatic impairment. Patients with baseline bilirubin >1.5 × ULN experienced greater toxicity than patients with baseline bilirubin ≤1.5 × ULN when treated with TORISEL. The overall frequency of ≥ grade 3 adverse reactions and deaths, including deaths due to progressive disease, were greater in patients with

Table 1 – Adverse Reactions Reported in at Least 10% of Patients Who Received 25 mg IV TORISEL or IFN-α in the Randomized Trial

Adverse Reaction	TORISEL 25 mg n=208		IFN-α n=200	
	All Grades* n (%)	Grades 3&4* n (%)	All Grades* n (%)	Grades 3&4* n (%)
Any	208 (100)	139 (67)	199 (100)	155 (78)
General disorders				
Asthenia	106 (51)	23 (11)	127 (64)	52 (26)
Edema[a]	73 (35)	7 (3)	21 (11)	1 (1)
Pain	59 (28)	10 (5)	31 (16)	4 (2)
Pyrexia	50 (24)	1 (1)	99 (50)	7 (4)
Weight Loss	39 (19)	3 (1)	50 (25)	4 (2)
Headache	31 (15)	1 (1)	30 (15)	0 (0)
Chest Pain	34 (16)	2 (1)	18 (9)	2 (1)
Chills	17 (8)	1 (1)	59 (30)	3 (2)
Gastrointestinal disorders				
Mucositis[b]	86 (41)	6 (3)	19 (10)	0 (0)
Anorexia	66 (32)	6 (3)	87 (44)	8 (4)
Nausea	77 (37)	5 (2)	82 (41)	9 (5)
Diarrhea	56 (27)	3 (1)	40 (20)	4 (2)
Abdominal Pain	44 (21)	9 (4)	34 (17)	3 (2)
Constipation	42 (20)	0 (0)	36 (18)	1 (1)
Vomiting	40 (19)	4 (2)	57 (29)	5 (3)
Infections				
Infections[e]	42 (20)	6 (3)	19 (10)	4 (2)
Urinary tract infection[d]	31 (15)	3 (1)	24 (12)	3 (2)
Pharyngitis	25 (12)	0 (0)	3 (2)	0 (0)
Rhinitis	20 (10)	0 (0)	4 (2)	
Musculoskeletal and connective tissue disorders				
Back Pain	41 (20)	6 (3)	28 (14)	7 (4)
Arthralgia	37 (18)	2 (1)	29 (15)	2 (1)
Myalgia	16 (8)	1 (1)	29 (15)	2 (1)
Respiratory, thoracic and mediastinal disorders				
Dyspnea	58 (28)	18 (9)	48 (24)	11 (6)
Cough	53 (26)	2 (1)	29 (15)	0 (0)
Epistaxis	25 (12)	0 (0)	7 (4)	0 (0)
Skin and subcutaneous tissue disorders				
Rash[e]	97 (47)	10 (5)	14 (7)	0 (0)
Pruritus	40 (19)	1 (1)	16 (8)	0 (0)
Nail Disorder	28 (14)	0 (0)	1 (1)	0 (0)
Dry Skin	22 (11)	1 (1)	14 (7)	0 (0)
Acne	21 (10)	0 (0)	2 (1)	
Nervous system disorders				
Dysgeusia[f]	41 (20)	0 (0)	17 (9)	0 (0)
Insomnia	24 (12)	1 (1)	30 (15)	0 (0)
Depression	9 (4)	0 (0)	27 (14)	4 (2)

* Common Toxicity Criteria for Adverse Events (CTCAE), Version 3.0.
[a] Includes edema, facial edema, and peripheral edema
[b] Includes aphthous stomatitis, glossitis, mouth ulceration, mucositis, and stomatitis
[e] Includes infections not otherwise specified (NOS) and the following infections that occurred infrequently as distinct entities: abscess, bronchitis, cellulitis, herpes simplex, and herpes zoster
[d] Includes cystitis, dysuria, hematuria, urinary frequency, and urinary tract infection
[e] Includes eczema, exfoliative dermatitis, maculopapular rash, pruritic rash, pustular rash, rash (NOS), and vesiculobullous rash
[f] Includes taste loss and taste perversion

baseline bilirubin >1.5 × ULN. TORISEL is contraindicated in patients with bilirubin >1.5 × ULN due to increased risk of death [see Contraindications (4)].
Use caution when treating patients with mild hepatic impairment. Concentrations of temsirolimus and its metabolite sirolimus were increased in patients with elevated AST or bilirubin levels. If TORISEL must be given in patients with mild hepatic impairment (bilirubin >1–1.5 × ULN or AST >ULN but bilirubin ≤ ULN), reduce the dose of TORISEL to 15 mg/week [see Dosage and Administration (2.4)].

5.3 Hyperglycemia/Glucose Intolerance
The use of TORISEL is likely to result in increases in serum glucose. In the phase 3 trial, 89% of patients receiving TORISEL had at least one elevated serum glucose while on treatment, and 26% of patients reported hyperglycemia as an adverse event. This may result in the need for an increase in the dose of, or initiation of, insulin and/or oral hypoglycemic agent therapy. Serum glucose should be tested before and during treatment with TORISEL. Patients should be advised to report excessive thirst or any increase in the volume or frequency of urination.

5.4 Infections
The use of TORISEL may result in immunosuppression. Patients should be carefully observed for the occurrence of infections, including opportunistic infections [see Adverse Reactions (6.1)].

5.5 Interstitial Lung Disease
Cases of interstitial lung disease, some resulting in death, occurred in patients who received TORISEL. Some patients were asymptomatic with infiltrates detected on computed tomography scan or chest radiograph. Others presented with symptoms such as dyspnea, cough, hypoxia, and fever. Some patients required discontinuation of TORISEL and/or treatment with corticosteroids and/or antibiotics, while some patients continued treatment without additional intervention. Patients should be advised to report promptly any new or worsening respiratory symptoms.

5.6 Hyperlipemia
The use of TORISEL is likely to result in increases in serum triglycerides and cholesterol. In the phase 3 trial, 87% of patients receiving TORISEL had at least one elevated serum cholesterol value and 83% had at least one elevated serum triglyceride value. This may require initiation, or

increase in the dose, of lipid-lowering agents. Serum cholesterol and triglycerides should be tested before and during treatment with TORISEL.

5.7 Bowel Perforation
Cases of fatal bowel perforation occurred in patients who received TORISEL. These patients presented with fever, abdominal pain, metabolic acidosis, bloody stools, diarrhea, and/or acute abdomen. Patients should be advised to report promptly any new or worsening abdominal pain or blood in their stools.

5.8 Renal Failure
Cases of rapidly progressive and sometimes fatal acute renal failure not clearly related to disease progression occurred in patients who received TORISEL. Some of these cases were not responsive to dialysis.

5.9 Wound Healing Complications
Use of TORISEL has been associated with abnormal wound healing. Therefore, caution should be exercised with the use of TORISEL in the perioperative period.

5.10 Intracerebral Hemorrhage
Patients with central nervous system tumors (primary CNS tumor or metastases) and/or receiving anticoagulation therapy may be at an increased risk of developing intracerebral bleeding (including fatal outcomes) while receiving TORISEL.

5.11 Co-administration with Inducers or Inhibitors of CYP3A Metabolism
Agents Inducing CYP3A Metabolism:
Strong inducers of CYP3A4/5 such as dexamethasone, carbamazepine, phenytoin, phenobarbital, rifampin, rifabutin, and rifampacin may decrease exposure of the active metabolite, sirolimus. If alternative treatment cannot be administered, a dose adjustment should be considered. St. John's Wort may decrease TORISEL plasma concentrations unpredictably. Patients receiving TORISEL should not take St. John's Wort concomitantly [see Dosage and Administration (2.4) and Drug Interactions (7.1)].
Agents Inhibiting CYP3A Metabolism:
Strong CYP3A4 inhibitors such as atazanavir, clarithromycin, indinavir, itraconazole, ketoconazole, nefazodone, nelfinavir, ritonavir, saquinavir, and telithromycin may increase blood concentrations of the active metabolite sirolimus. If alternative treatments cannot be administered, a dose adjustment should be considered [see Dosage and Administration (2.4) and Drug Interactions (7.2)].

5.12 Concomitant use of TORISEL with sunitinib
The combination of TORISEL and sunitinib resulted in dose-limiting toxicity. Dose-limiting toxicities (Grade 3/4 erythematous maculopapular rash, and gout/cellulitis requiring hospitalization) were observed in two out of three patients treated in the first cohort of a phase 1 study at doses of TORISEL 15 mg IV per week and sunitinib 25 mg oral per day (Days 1-28 followed by a 2-week rest).

5.13 Vaccinations
The use of live vaccines and close contact with those who have received live vaccines should be avoided during treatment with TORISEL. Examples of live vaccines are: intranasal influenza, measles, mumps, rubella, oral polio, BCG, yellow fever, varicella, and TY21a typhoid vaccines.

5.14 Pregnancy
Pregnancy Category D
Temsirolimus administered daily as an oral formulation caused embryo-fetal and intrauterine toxicities in rats and rabbits at human sub-therapeutic exposures. Embryo-fetal adverse effects in rats consisted of reduced fetal weight and reduced ossifications, and in rabbits included reduced fetal weight, omphalocele, bifurcated sternabrae, notched ribs, and incomplete ossifications.
In rats, the intrauterine and embryo-fetal adverse effects were observed at the oral dose of 2.7 mg/m²/day (approximately 0.04-fold the AUC in cancer patients at the human recommended dose). In rabbits, the intrauterine and embryo-fetal adverse effects were observed at the oral dose of ≥7.2 mg/m²/day (approximately 0.12-fold the AUC in cancer patients at the recommended human dose).
Women of childbearing potential should be advised to avoid becoming pregnant throughout treatment and for 3 months after TORISEL therapy has stopped. Temsirolimus can cause fetal harm when administered to a pregnant woman. If this drug is used during pregnancy, or if the patient becomes pregnant while taking this drug, the patient should be apprised of the potential hazard to the fetus.
Men should be counseled regarding the effects of TORISEL on the fetus and sperm prior to starting treatment [see Nonclinical Toxicology (13.1)]. Men with partners of childbearing potential should use reliable contraception throughout treatment and are recommended to continue this for 3 months after the last dose of TORISEL.

5.15 Monitoring Laboratory Tests
In the randomized, phase 3 trial, complete blood counts (CBCs) were checked weekly, and chemistry panels were checked every two weeks. Laboratory monitoring for patients receiving TORISEL may need to be performed more or less frequently at the physician's discretion.

Table 2 – Incidence of Selected Laboratory Abnormalities in Patients Who Received 25 mg IV TORISEL or IFN-α in the Randomized Trial

Laboratory Abnormality	TORISEL 25 mg n=208		IFN-α n=200	
	All Grades* n (%)	Grades 3&4* n (%)	All Grades* n (%)	Grades 3&4* n (%)
Any	208 (100)	162 (78)	195 (98)	144 (72)
Hematology				
Hemoglobin Decreased	195 (94)	41 (20)	180 (90)	43 (22)
Lymphocytes Decreased**	110 (53)	33 (16)	106 (53)	48 (24)
Neutrophils Decreased**	39 (19)	10 (5)	58 (29)	19 (10)
Platelets Decreased	84 (40)	3 (1)	51 (26)	0 (0)
Leukocytes Decreased	67 (32)	1 (1)	93 (47)	11 (6)
Chemistry				
Alkaline Phosphatase Increased	141 (68)	7 (3)	111 (56)	13 (7)
AST Increased	79 (38)	5 (2)	103 (52)	14 (7)
Creatinine Increased	119 (57)	7 (3)	97 (49)	2 (1)
Glucose Increased	186 (89)	33 (16)	128 (64)	6 (3)
Phosphorus Decreased	102 (49)	38 (18)	61 (31)	17 (9)
Total Bilirubin Increased	16 (8)	2 (1)	25 (13)	4 (2)
Total Cholesterol Increased	181 (87)	5 (2)	95 (48)	2 (1)
Triglycerides Increased	173 (83)	92 (44)	144 (72)	69 (35)
Potassium Decreased	43 (21)	11 (5)	15 (8)	0 (0)

*NCI CTC version 3.0
**Grade 1 toxicity may be under-reported for lymphocytes and neutrophils

Table 3 – Adverse Reactions in Patients With Advanced Malignancies Plus Normal or Impaired Hepatic Function

Hepatic Function*	TORISEL Dose Range	Adverse Reactions Grade ≥ 3** n (%)	Death*** n (%)
Normal (n=25)	25–175	20 (8.0)	2 (8.0)
Mild (n=39)	10–25	32 (82.1)	5 (12.8)
Moderate (n=20)	10–25	19 (95.0)	8 (40.0)
Severe (n=24)	7.5–15	23 (95.8)	13 (54.2)
Liver Transplant (n=2)	10	1 (50.0)	0 (0)

* Hepatic Function Groups: normal = bilirubin and AST ≤ULN; mild = bilirubin >1–1.5 × ULN or AST >ULN but bilirubin ≤ULN; moderate = bilirubin >1.5-3 × ULN; severe = bilirubin >3 × ULN; liver transplant = any bilirubin and AST.
** Common Terminology Criteria for Adverse Events, version 3.0, including all causality.
*** Includes deaths due to progressive disease and adverse reactions.

6 ADVERSE REACTIONS
The following serious adverse reactions have been associated with TORISEL in clinical trials and are discussed in greater detail in other sections of the label [see Warnings and Precautions (5)].
Hypersensitivity Reactions [see Warnings and Precautions (5.1)]
Hyperglycemia/Glucose Intolerance [see Warnings and Precautions (5.3)]
Interstitial Lung Disease [see Warnings and Precautions (5.5)]
Hyperlipemia [see Warnings and Precautions (5.6)]
Bowel Perforation [see Warnings and Precautions (5.7)]
Renal Failure [see Warnings and Precautions (5.8)]
The most common (≥ 30%) adverse reactions observed with TORISEL are rash, asthenia, mucositis, nausea, edema, and anorexia. The most common (≥ 30%) laboratory abnormalities observed with TORISEL are anemia, hyperglycemia, hyperlipemia, hypertriglyceridemia, lymphopenia, elevated alkaline phosphatase, elevated serum creatinine, hypophosphatemia, thrombocytopenia, elevated AST, and leukopenia.

6.1 Clinical Trials Experience
Because clinical trials are conducted under widely varying conditions, the adverse reaction rates observed cannot be directly compared to rates in other trials and may not reflect the rates observed in clinical practice.
In the Phase 3 randomized, open-label study of interferon alfa (IFN-α) alone, TORISEL alone, and TORISEL and IFN-α, a total of 616 patients were treated. Two hundred patients received IFN-α weekly, 208 received TORISEL 25 mg weekly, and 208 patients received a combination of TORISEL and IFN-α weekly [see Clinical Studies (14)].
Treatment with the combination of TORISEL 15 mg and IFN-α was associated with an increased incidence of multiple adverse reactions and did not result in a significant increase in overall survival when compared with IFN-α alone.

Table 1 shows the percentage of patients experiencing treatment emergent adverse reactions. Reactions reported in at least 10% of patients who received TORISEL 25 mg alone or IFN-α alone are listed. Table 2 shows the percentage of patients experiencing selected laboratory abnormalities. Data for the same adverse reactions and laboratory abnormalities in the IFN-α alone arm are shown for comparison.
[See table 1 at top of previous page]
The following selected adverse reactions were reported less frequently (<10%).
Gastrointestinal Disorders-Fatal bowel perforation occurred in 1 patient (1%).
Eye Disorders-Conjunctivitis (including lacrimation disorder) occurred in 15 patients (7%).
Immune System-Allergic/Hypersensitivity reactions occurred in 18 patients (9%).
Angioneurotic edema-type reactions have been observed in some patients who received TORISEL and ACE inhibitors concomitantly.
Infections-Pneumonia occurred in 17 patients (8%); upper respiratory tract infection occurred in 14 patients (7%).
General Disorders and Administration Site Conditions-Impaired wound healing occurred in 3 patients (1%).
Respiratory, Thoracic and Mediastinal Disorders-Interstitial lung disease occurred in 5 patients (2%), including rare fatalities.
Vascular-Hypertension occurred in 14 patients (7%); venous thromboembolism (including deep vein thrombosis and pulmonary embolus) occurred in 5 patients (2%); thrombophlebitis occurred in 2 patients (1%).
[See table 2 above]

6.2 Post-marketing and Other Clinical Experience
The following adverse reactions have been identified during postapproval use of TORISEL. Because these reactions are reported voluntarily from a population of uncertain size, it is not possible to readily estimate their frequency or establish a causal relationship to drug exposure.

There have been reports of rhabdomyolysis in patients who received TORISEL.

7 DRUG INTERACTIONS

7.1 Agents Inducing CYP3A Metabolism

Co-administration of TORISEL with rifampin, a potent CYP3A4/5 inducer, had no significant effect on temsirolimus C_{max} (maximum concentration) and AUC (area under the concentration versus the time curve) after intravenous administration, but decreased sirolimus C_{max} by 65% and AUC by 56% compared to TORISEL treatment alone. If alternative treatment cannot be administered, a dose adjustment should be considered [*see Dosage and Administration (2.4)*].

7.2 Agents Inhibiting CYP3A Metabolism

Co-administration of TORISEL with ketoconazole, a potent CYP3A4 inhibitor, had no significant effect on temsirolimus C_{max} or AUC; however, sirolimus AUC increased 3.1-fold, and C_{max} increased 2.2-fold compared to TORISEL alone. If alternative treatment cannot be administered, a dose adjustment should be considered [*see Dosage and Administration (2.4)*].

7.3 Interactions with Drugs Metabolized by CYP2D6

The concentration of desipramine, a CYP2D6 substrate, was unaffected when 25 mg of TORISEL was co-administered. No clinically significant effect is anticipated when temsirolimus is co-administered with agents that are metabolized by CYP2D6 or CYP3A4.

8 USE IN SPECIFIC POPULATIONS

8.1 Pregnancy

Pregnancy Category D [*see Warnings and Precautions (5.14)*].

8.3 Nursing Mothers

It is not known whether TORISEL is excreted into human milk, and due to the potential for tumorigenicity shown for sirolimus (active metabolite of TORISEL) in animal studies, a decision should be made whether to discontinue nursing or discontinue TORISEL, taking into account the importance of the drug to the mother.

8.4 Pediatric Use

The safety and effectiveness of TORISEL in pediatric patients have not been established.

8.5 Geriatric Use

Clinical studies of TORISEL did not include sufficient numbers of subjects aged 65 and older to determine whether they respond differently from younger subjects.

8.6 Renal Impairment

No clinical studies were conducted with TORISEL in patients with decreased renal function. Less than 5% of total radioactivity was excreted in the urine following a 25 mg intravenous dose of [^{14}C]-labeled temsirolimus in healthy subjects. Renal impairment is not expected to markedly influence drug exposure, and no dosage adjustment of TORISEL is recommended in patients with renal impairment.

TORISEL has not been studied in patients undergoing hemodialysis.

8.7 Hepatic Impairment

TORISEL was evaluated in a dose escalation phase 1 study in 110 patients with normal or varying degrees of hepatic impairment as defined by AST and bilirubin levels and patients with liver transplant (Table 3).

Patients with moderate and severe hepatic impairment had increased rates of adverse reactions and deaths, including deaths due to progressive disease, during the study (Table 3).

[See table 3 on previous page]

TORISEL is contraindicated in patients with bilirubin >1.5 × ULN [*see Contraindications (4), and Warnings and Precautions (5.2)*]. Use caution when treating patients with mild hepatic impairment. If TORISEL must be given in patients with mild hepatic impairment (bilirubin >1–1.5 × ULN **or** AST ≥ULN but bilirubin ≤ULN), reduce the dose of TORISEL to 15 mg/week [*see Dosage and Administration (2.4)*]. Because there is a need for dosage adjustment based upon hepatic function, assessment of AST and bilirubin levels is recommended before initiation of TORISEL and periodically thereafter.

10 OVERDOSAGE

There is no specific treatment for TORISEL intravenous overdose. TORISEL has been administered to patients with cancer in phase 1 and 2 trials with repeated intravenous doses as high as 220 mg/m^2. The risk of several serious adverse events, including thrombosis, bowel perforation, interstitial lung disease (ILD), seizure, and psychosis, is increased with doses of TORISEL greater than 25 mg.

11 DESCRIPTION

Temsirolimus, an inhibitor of mTOR, is an antineoplastic agent.

Temsirolimus is a white to off-white powder with a molecular formula of $C_{56}H_{87}NO_{16}$ and a molecular weight of 1030.30. It is non-hygroscopic. Temsirolimus is practically insoluble in water and soluble in alcohol. It has no ionizable functional groups, and its solubility is independent of pH.

The chemical name of temsirolimus is (3*S*,6*R*,7*E*,9*R*,10*R*,12*R*,14*S*,15*E*,17*E*,19*E*,21*S*,23*S*,26*R*,27*R*,34a*S*)-9,10,12,13,14,21,22,23,24,25,26,27,32,33,34,34a-Hexadecahydro-9,27-dihydroxy-3-[(1*R*)-2-[(1*S*,3*R*,4*R*)-4-hydroxy-3-methoxycyclohexyl]-1-methylethyl]-10,21-dimethoxy-6,8,12,14,20,26-hexamethyl-23,27-epoxy-3*H*-pyrido[2,1-*c*][1,4]oxaazacyclohentriacontine-1,5,11,28,29(4*H*,6*H*,31*H*)-pentone 4′-[2,2-bis(hydroxymethyl)propionate]; or Rapamycin, 42-[3-hydroxy-2-(hydroxymethyl)-2-methylpropanoate].

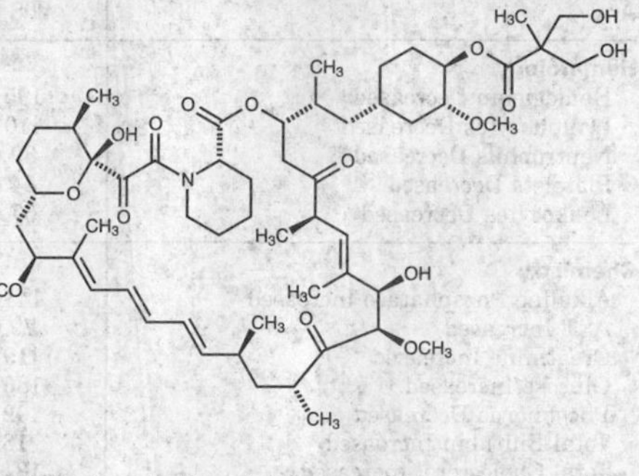

TORISEL (temsirolimus) injection, 25 mg/mL, is a clear, colorless to light yellow, non-aqueous, ethanolic, sterile solution. TORISEL (temsirolimus) injection requires two dilutions prior to intravenous infusion. TORISEL (temsirolimus) injection should be diluted only with the supplied DILUENT for TORISEL®.

DILUENT for TORISEL® is a sterile, non-aqueous solution that is supplied with TORISEL injection, as a kit.

TORISEL (temsirolimus) injection, 25 mg/mL:

Active ingredient: temsirolimus (25 mg/mL)

Inactive ingredients: dehydrated alcohol (39.5% w/v), *dl*-alpha-tocopherol (0.075% w/v), propylene glycol (50.3% w/v), and anhydrous citric acid (0.0025% w/v).

DILUENT for TORISEL®

Inactive ingredients: polysorbate 80 (40.0% w/v), polyethylene glycol 400 (42.8% w/v) and dehydrated alcohol (19.9% w/v).

After the TORISEL (temsirolimus) injection vial has been diluted with DILUENT for TORISEL®, in accordance with the instructions in section 2.5, the solution contains 35.2% alcohol.

TORISEL (temsirolimus) injection and DILUENT for TORISEL® are filled in clear glass vials with butyl rubber stoppers.

12 CLINICAL PHARMACOLOGY

12.1 Mechanism of Action

Temsirolimus is an inhibitor of mTOR (mammalian target of rapamycin). Temsirolimus binds to an intracellular protein (FKBP-12), and the protein-drug complex inhibits the activity of mTOR that controls cell division. Inhibition of mTOR activity resulted in a G1 growth arrest in treated tumor cells. When mTOR was inhibited, its ability to phosphorylate p70S6k and S6 ribosomal protein, which are downstream of mTOR in the PI3 kinase/AKT pathway was blocked. In *in vitro* studies using renal cell carcinoma cell lines, temsirolimus inhibited the activity of mTOR and resulted in reduced levels of the hypoxia-inducible factors HIF-1 and HIF-2 alpha, and the vascular endothelial growth factor.

12.2 Pharmacodynamics

Effects on Electrocardiogram There were no clinically relevant QT changes observed at the recommended dose for TORISEL. In a randomized, crossover study, 58 healthy subjects received TORISEL 25 mg, placebo, and a single oral dose of moxifloxacin 400 mg. A supratherapeutic TORISEL dose was not studied in this randomized QT trial. The largest difference between the upper bound 2-sided 90% CI for the mean difference between TORISEL and placebo-corrected QT interval was less than 10 ms. In a different trial in 69 patients with a hematologic malignancy, TORISEL doses up to 175 mg were studied. No patient with a normal QTcF at baseline had an increase in QTcF>60 ms. Additionally, there were no patients with a QTcF interval greater than 500 ms.

12.3 Pharmacokinetics

Absorption

Following administration of a single 25 mg dose of TORISEL in patients with cancer, mean temsirolimus C_{max} in whole blood was 585 ng/mL (coefficient of variation, CV =14%), and mean AUC in blood was 1627 ng•h/mL (CV=26%). Typically C_{max} occurred at the end of infusion. Over the dose range of 1 mg to 25 mg, temsirolimus exposure increased in a less than dose proportional manner while sirolimus exposure increased proportionally with dose. Following a single 25 mg intravenous dose in patients with cancer, sirolimus AUC was 2.7-fold that of temsirolimus AUC, due principally to the longer half-life of sirolimus.

Distribution

Following a single 25 mg intravenous dose, mean steady-state volume of distribution of temsirolimus in whole blood of patients with cancer was 172 liters. Both temsirolimus and sirolimus are extensively partitioned into formed blood elements.

Metabolism

Cytochrome P450 3A4 is the major isozyme responsible for the formation of five temsirolimus metabolites. Sirolimus, an active metabolite of temsirolimus, is the principal metabolite in humans following intravenous treatment. The remainder of the metabolites account for less than 10% of radioactivity in the plasma. In human liver microsomes temsirolimus was an inhibitor of CYP2D6 and 3A4. However, there was no effect observed in vivo when temsirolimus was administered with desipramine (a CYP2D6 substrate), and no effect is anticipated with substrates of CYP3A4 metabolism.

Elimination

Elimination is primarily via the feces. After a single IV dose of [^{14}C]-temsirolimus approximately 82% of total radioactivity was eliminated within 14 days, with 4.6% and 78% of the administered radioactivity recovered in the urine and feces, respectively. Following a single 25 mg dose of TORISEL in patients with cancer, temsirolimus mean (CV) systemic clearance was 16.2 (22%) L/h. Temsirolimus exhibits a biexponential decline in whole blood concentrations and the mean half-lives of temsirolimus and sirolimus were 17.3 hr and 54.6 hr, respectively.

Effects of Age and Gender

In population pharmacokinetic-based data analyses, no relationship was apparent between drug exposure and patient age or gender.

13 NONCLINICAL TOXICOLOGY

13.1 Carcinogenesis, Mutagenesis, Impairment of Fertility

Carcinogenicity studies have not been conducted with temsirolimus. However, sirolimus, the major metabolite of temsirolimus in humans, was carcinogenic in mice and rats. The following effects were reported in mice and/or rats in the carcinogenicity studies conducted with sirolimus: lymphoma, hepatocellular adenoma and carcinoma, and testicular adenoma.

Temsirolimus was not genotoxic in a battery of *in vitro* (bacterial reverse mutation in *Salmonella typhimurium* and *Escherichia coli*, forward mutation in mouse lymphoma cells, and chromosome aberrations in Chinese hamster ovary cells) and *in vivo* (mouse micronucleus) assays.

In male rats, the following fertility effects were observed: decreased number of pregnancies, decreased sperm concentration and motility, decreased reproductive organ weights, and testicular tubular degeneration. These effects were observed at oral temsirolimus doses ≥ 3 mg/m^2/day (approximately 0.2-fold the human recommended intravenous dose). Fertility was absent at 30 mg/m^2/day.

In female rats, an increased incidence of pre- and post-implantation losses occurred at oral doses ≥ 4.2 mg/m^2/day (approximately 0.3-fold the human recommended intravenous dose), resulting in decreased numbers of live fetuses.

14 CLINICAL STUDIES

A phase 3, multi-center, three-arm, randomized, open-label study was conducted in previously untreated patients with advanced renal cell carcinoma (clear cell and non-clear cell histologies). The objectives were to compare Overall Survival (OS), Progression-Free Survival (PFS), Objective Response Rate (ORR), and safety in patients receiving IFN-α to those receiving TORISEL or TORISEL plus IFN-α. Patients in this study had 3 or more of 6 pre-selected prognostic risk factors (less than one year from time of initial RCC diagnosis to randomization, Karnofsky performance status of 60 or 70, hemoglobin less than the lower limit of normal, corrected calcium of greater than 10 mg/dL, lactate dehydrogenase > 1.5 times the upper limit of normal, more than one metastatic organ site). Patients were stratified for prior nephrectomy status within three geographic regions and were randomly assigned (1:1:1) to receive IFN-α alone (n=207), TORISEL alone (25 mg weekly; n=209), or the combination arm (n=210).

The ITT population for this interim analysis included 626 patients. Demographics were comparable between the three treatment arms with regard to age, gender, and race. The mean age of all groups was 59 years (range 23-86). Sixty-nine percent were male and 31% were female. The racial distribution for all groups was 91% White, 4% Black, 2% Asian, and 3% other. Sixty-seven percent of patients had a history of prior nephrectomy.

The median duration of treatment in the TORISEL arm was 17 weeks (range 1-126 weeks). The median duration of treatment on the IFN arm was 8 weeks (range 1-124 weeks).

There was a statistically significant improvement in OS (time from randomization to death) in the TORISEL 25 mg

Table 4 – Summary of Efficacy Results of TORISEL vs. IFN-α

Parameter	TORISEL n = 209	IFN-α n = 207	P-value[a]	Hazard Ratio (95% CI)[b]
Median Overall Survival Months (95% CI)	10.9 (8.6, 12.7)	7.3 (6.1, 8.8)	0.0078*	0.73 (0.58, 0.92)
Median Progression-Free Survival Months (95% CI)	5.5 (3.9, 7.0)	3.1 (2.2, 3.8)	0.0001**	0.66 (0.53, 0.81)
Overall Response Rate % (95% CI)	8.6 (4.8, 12.4)	4.8 (1.9, 7.8)	0.1232**[c]	NA

CI = confidence interval; NA = not applicable
* A comparison is considered statistically significant if the p-value is <0.0159 (O'Brien-Fleming boundary at 446 deaths).
** Not adjusted for multiple comparisons.
a. Based on log-rank test stratified by prior nephrectomy and region.
b. Based on Cox proportional hazard model stratified by prior nephrectomy and region.
c. Based on Cochran-Mantel-Haenszel test stratified by prior nephrectomy and region.

arm compared to IFN-α. The combination of TORISEL 15 mg and IFN-α did not result in a significant increase in overall survival when compared with IFN-α alone. Figure 1 is a Kaplan-Meier plot of OS in this study. The evaluations of PFS (time from randomization to disease progression or death) and ORR, were based on blinded independent radiologic assessment of tumor response. Efficacy results are summarized in Table 4.
[See table 4 above]

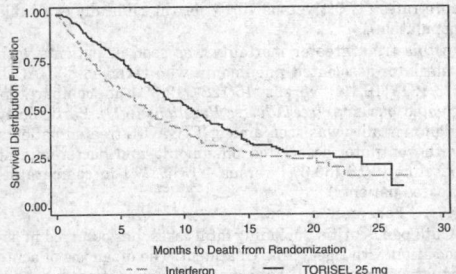

Figure 1: Kaplan-Meier Curves for Overall Survival – TORISEL vs. IFN

15   REFERENCES

1. NIOSH Alert: Preventing occupational exposures to antineoplastic and other hazardous drugs in healthcare settings. 2004. U.S. Department of Health and Human Services, Public Health Service, Centers for Disease Control and Prevention, National Institute for Occupational Safety and Health, DHHS (NIOSH) Publication No. 2004-165.
2. OSHA Technical Manual, TED 1-0.15A, Section VI: Chapter 2. Controlling Occupational Exposure to Hazardous Drugs. OSHA, 1999. http://www.osha.gov/dts/osta/otm/otm_vi/otm_vi_2.html
3. American Society of Health-System Pharmacists. (2006) ASHP Guidelines on Handling Hazardous Drugs. Am J Health-syst Pharm. 2006;63:1172-1193.
4. Polovich, M., White, J. M., & Kelleher, L.O. (eds.) 2005. Chemotherapy and biotherapy guidelines and recommendations for practice (2nd. ed.) Pittsburgh, PA: Oncology Nursing Society.

16   HOW SUPPLIED/STORAGE AND HANDLING

NDC 0008-1179-01 TORISEL® (temsirolimus) injection, 25 mg/mL.

Each kit is supplied in a single carton containing one single-use vial of 25 mg/mL of temsirolimus and one DILUENT vial which includes a deliverable volume of 1.8 mL, and must be stored at 2°-8°C (36°-46°F).

Protect from light.

17   PATIENT COUNSELING INFORMATION

• Allergic (Hypersensitivity) Reactions
Patients should be informed of the possibility of serious allergic reactions, including anaphylaxis, despite premedication with antihistamines, and to immediately report any facial swelling or difficulty breathing [see Warnings and Precautions (5.1)].

• Increased Blood Glucose Levels
Patients are likely to experience increased blood glucose levels while taking TORISEL. This may result in the need for initiation of, or increase in the dose of, insulin and/or hypoglycemic agents. Patients should be directed to report any excessive thirst or frequency of urination to their physician [see Warnings and Precautions (5.3)].

• Infections
Patients should be informed that they may be more susceptible to infections while being treated with TORISEL [see Warnings and Precautions (5.4)].

• Interstitial Lung Disease
Patients should be warned of the possibility of developing interstitial lung disease, a chronic inflammation of the lungs, which may rarely result in death [see Warnings and Precautions (5.5)]. Patients should be directed to report promptly any new or worsening respiratory symptoms to their physician.

• Increased Blood Triglycerides and/or Cholesterol
Patients are likely to experience elevated triglycerides and/or cholesterol during TORISEL treatment. This may require initiation of, or increase in the dose of, lipid-lowering agents [see Warnings and Precautions (5.6)].

• Bowel Perforation
Patients should be warned of the possibility of bowel perforation. Patients should be directed to report promptly any new or worsening abdominal pain or blood in their stools [see Warnings and Precautions (5.7)].

• Renal Failure
Patients should be informed of the risk of renal failure [see Warnings and Precautions (5.8)].

• Wound Healing Complications
Patients should be advised of the possibility of abnormal wound healing if they have surgery within a few weeks of initiating therapy or during therapy [see Warnings and Precautions (5.9)].

• Intracerebral Bleeding
Patients with CNS tumors and/or receiving anticoagulants should be informed of the increased risk of developing intracerebral bleeding (including fatal outcomes) while on TORISEL [see Warnings and Precautions (5.10)].

• Medications that can interfere with TORISEL
Some medicines can interfere with the breakdown or metabolism of TORISEL. In particular, patients should be directed to inform their physician if they are taking any of the following: Protease inhibitors, anti-epileptic medicines including carbamazepine, phenytoin, and barbiturates, St. John's Wort, rifampicin, rifabutin, nefazodone or selective serotonin re-uptake inhibitors used to treat depression, antibiotics or antifungal medicines used to treat infections [see Warnings and Precautions (5.11)].

• Vaccinations
Patients should be advised that vaccinations may be less effective while being treated with TORISEL. In addition, the use of live vaccines, and close contact with those who have received live vaccines, while on TORISEL should be avoided [see Warnings and Precautions (5.13)].

• Pregnancy
TORISEL can cause fetal harm. Women of childbearing potential should be advised to avoid becoming pregnant throughout treatment and for 3 months after TORISEL therapy has stopped. Men with partners of childbearing potential should use reliable contraception throughout treatment and are recommended to continue this for 3 months after the last dose of TORISEL [see Warnings and Precautions (5.14)].

Wyeth®
Wyeth Pharmaceuticals Inc.
Philadelphia, PA 19101
Manufactured for: Wyeth Pharmaceuticals Inc. Philadelphia, PA 19101
TORISEL® (temsirolimus) injection is manufactured by: Pierre Fabre Medicament Production, Aquitaine Pharm International, Avenue du Bearn, F64320 Idron, France
DILUENT for TORISEL® is manufactured by: Ben Venue Laboratories, Inc., Bedford, Ohio 44146-0568

W10524C011
ET01
Rev 09/10

————RECENT MAJOR CHANGES————

Warnings and Precautions	
All-Cause Mortality (5.1)	7/2010
Mortality Imbalance and Lower Cure Rates in Ventilator-Associated Pneumonia (5.4)	7/2010
Pancreatitis (5.5)	7/2010

————INDICATIONS AND USAGE————
TYGACIL is a tetracycline class antibacterial indicated in patients 18 years of age and older for:
• Complicated skin and skin structure infections (1.1)
• Complicated intra-abdominal infections (1.2)
• Community-acquired bacterial pneumonia (1.3)

————DOSAGE AND ADMINISTRATION————
• Initial dose of 100 mg, followed by 50 mg every 12 hours administered intravenously over approximately 30 to 60 minutes. (2.1)
• Severe hepatic impairment (Child Pugh C): Initial dose of 100 mg followed by 25 mg every 12 hours. (2.2)

————DOSAGE FORMS AND STRENGTHS————
50 mg lyophilized powder for reconstitution in a single-dose 5 mL vial. (3)

————CONTRAINDICATIONS————
Known hypersensitivity to tigecycline. (4)

————WARNINGS AND PRECAUTIONS————
• An increase in all-cause mortality has been observed across Phase 3 and 4 clinical trials in TYGACIL-treated patients versus comparator. The cause of this increase has not been established. This increase in all-cause mortality should be considered when selecting among treatment options. (5.1)
• Anaphylaxis/anaphylactoid reactions have been reported with TYGACIL, and may be life-threatening. Exercise caution in patients with known hypersensitivity to tetracyclines. (5.2)
• Hepatic dysfunction and liver failure have been reported with TYGACIL. (5.3)
• Lower cure rates and higher mortality were seen when patients with ventilator-associated pneumonia were treated with TYGACIL. (5.4)
• Pancreatitis, including fatalities, has been reported with TYGACIL. If pancreatitis is suspected, then consider stopping TYGACIL. (5.5)
• TYGACIL may cause fetal harm when administered to a pregnant woman. (5.6)
• The use of TYGACIL during tooth development may cause permanent discoloration of the teeth. (5.7)
• Clostridium difficile associated diarrhea: evaluate if diarrhea occurs. (5.8)

————ADVERSE REACTIONS————
The most common adverse reactions (incidence >5%) are nausea, vomiting, diarrhea, abdominal pain, headache, and increased SGPT. (6.1)
To report SUSPECTED ADVERSE REACTIONS, contact Wyeth Pharmaceuticals Inc. at 1-800-934-5556 or FDA at 1-800-FDA-1088 or www.fda.gov/medwatch

————DRUG INTERACTIONS————
• Suitable anticoagulation test should be monitored if TYGACIL is administered to patients receiving warfarin. (7.1)

————USE IN SPECIFIC POPULATIONS————
• Pediatrics: Use in patients under 18 years of age is not recommended. (8.4)

See 17 for PATIENT COUNSELING INFORMATION
                                      Revised: 07/2010

FULL PRESCRIBING INFORMATION: CONTENTS*

* Sections or subsections omitted from the full prescribing information are not listed

FULL PRESCRIBING INFORMATION

1 INDICATIONS AND USAGE

TYGACIL is a tetracycline-class antibacterial indicated for the treatment of infections caused by susceptible isolates of the designated microorganisms in the conditions listed below for patients 18 years of age and older:

1.1 Complicated Skin and Skin Structure Infections

Complicated skin and skin structure infections caused by *Escherichia coli, Enterococcus faecalis* (vancomycin-susceptible isolates), *Staphylococcus aureus* (methicillin-susceptible and -resistant isolates), *Streptococcus agalactiae, Streptococcus anginosus* grp. (includes *S. anginosus, S. intermedius,* and *S. constellatus*), *Streptococcus pyogenes, Enterobacter cloacae, Klebsiella pneumoniae,* and *Bacteroides fragilis*.

1.2 Complicated Intra-abdominal Infections

Complicated intra-abdominal infections caused by *Citrobacter freundii, Enterobacter cloacae, Escherichia coli, Klebsiella oxytoca, Klebsiella pneumoniae, Enterococcus faecalis* (vancomycin-susceptible isolates), *Staphylococcus aureus* (methicillin-susceptible and -resistant isolates), *Streptococcus anginosus* grp. (includes *S. anginosus, S. intermedius,* and *S. constellatus*), *Bacteroides fragilis, Bacteroides thetaiotaomicron, Bacteroides uniformis, Bacteroides vulgatus, Clostridium perfringens,* and *Peptostreptococcus micros.*

1.3 Community-Acquired Bacterial Pneumonia

Community-acquired bacterial pneumonia caused by *Streptococcus pneumoniae* (penicillin-susceptible isolates), including cases with concurrent bacteremia, *Haemophilus influenzae* (beta-lactamase negative isolates), and *Legionella pneumophila*.

1.4 Usage

To reduce the development of drug-resistant bacteria and maintain the effectiveness of TYGACIL and other antibacterial drugs, TYGACIL should be used only to treat or prevent infections that are proven or strongly suspected to be caused by susceptible bacteria. When culture and susceptibility information are available, they should be considered in selecting or modifying antibacterial therapy. In the absence of such data, local epidemiology and susceptibility patterns may contribute to the empiric selection of therapy. Appropriate specimens for bacteriological examination should be obtained in order to isolate and identify the causative organisms and to determine their susceptibility to tigecycline. TYGACIL may be initiated as empiric monotherapy before results of these tests are known.

2 DOSAGE AND ADMINISTRATION

2.1 General Dosage and Administration

The recommended dosage regimen for TYGACIL is an initial dose of 100 mg, followed by 50 mg every 12 hours. Intravenous infusions of TYGACIL should be administered over approximately 30 to 60 minutes every 12 hours.

The recommended duration of treatment with TYGACIL for complicated skin and skin structure infections or for complicated intra-abdominal infections is 5 to 14 days. The recommended duration of treatment with TYGACIL for community-acquired bacterial pneumonia is 7 to 14 days. The duration of therapy should be guided by the severity and site of the infection and the patient's clinical and bacteriological progress.

2.2 Patients With Hepatic Impairment

No dosage adjustment is warranted in patients with mild to moderate hepatic impairment (Child Pugh A and Child Pugh B). In patients with severe hepatic impairment (Child Pugh C), the initial dose of TYGACIL should be 100 mg followed by a reduced maintenance dose of 25 mg every 12 hours. Patients with severe hepatic impairment (Child Pugh C) should be treated with caution and monitored for treatment response *[see Clinical Pharmacology (12.3) and Use in Specific Populations (8.6)]*.

2.3 Preparation and Handling

Each vial of TYGACIL should be reconstituted with 5.3 mL of 0.9% Sodium Chloride Injection, USP, 5% Dextrose Injection, USP, or Lactated Ringer's Injection, USP to achieve a concentration of 10 mg/mL of tigecycline. (Note: Each vial contains a 6% overage. Thus, 5 mL of reconstituted solution is equivalent to 50 mg of the drug.) The vial should be gently swirled until the drug dissolves. Withdraw 5 mL of the reconstituted solution from the vial and add to a 100 mL intravenous bag for infusion (for a 100 mg dose, reconstitute two vials; for a 50 mg dose, reconstitute one vial). The maximum concentration in the intravenous bag should be 1 mg/mL. The reconstituted solution should be yellow to orange in color; if not, the solution should be discarded. Parenteral drug products should be inspected visually for particulate matter and discoloration (e.g., green or black) prior to administration. Once reconstituted, TYGACIL may be stored at room temperature for up to 24 hours (up to 6 hours in the vial and the remaining time in the intravenous bag). Alternatively, TYGACIL mixed with 0.9% Sodium Chloride Injection, USP or 5% Dextrose Injection, USP may be stored refrigerated at 2° to 8°C (36° to 46°F) for up to 48 hours following immediate transfer of the reconstituted solution into the intravenous bag.

TYGACIL may be administered intravenously through a dedicated line or through a Y-site. If the same intravenous line is used for sequential infusion of several drugs, the line should be flushed before and after infusion of TYGACIL with 0.9% Sodium Chloride Injection, USP, 5% Dextrose Injection, USP or Lactated Ringer's Injection, USP. Injection should be made with an infusion solution compatible with tigecycline and with any other drug(s) administered via this common line.

Compatibilities

Compatible intravenous solutions include 0.9% Sodium Chloride Injection, USP, 5% Dextrose Injection, USP, and Lactated Ringer's Injection, USP. When administered through a Y-site, TYGACIL is compatible with the following drugs or diluents when used with either 0.9% Sodium Chloride Injection, USP or 5% Dextrose Injection, USP: amikacin, dobutamine, dopamine HCl, gentamicin, haloperidol, Lactated Ringer's, lidocaine HCl, metoclopramide, morphine, norepinephrine, piperacillin/tazobactam (EDTA formulation), potassium chloride, propofol, ranitidine HCl, theophylline, and tobramycin.

Incompatibilities

The following drugs should not be administered simultaneously through the same Y-site as TYGACIL: amphotericin B, amphotericin B lipid complex, diazepam, esomeprazole and omeprazole.

3 DOSAGE FORMS AND STRENGTHS

Each single-dose 5 mL glass vial and 10 mL glass vial contain 50 mg of tigecycline as an orange lyophilized powder for reconstitution.

4 CONTRAINDICATIONS

TYGACIL is contraindicated for use in patients who have known hypersensitivity to tigecycline.

5 WARNINGS AND PRECAUTIONS

5.1 All-Cause Mortality

An increase in all-cause mortality has been observed across Phase 3 and 4 clinical trials in TYGACIL-treated patients versus comparator-treated patients. In all 13 Phase 3 and 4 trials that included a comparator, death occurred in 4.0% (150/3788) of patients receiving TYGACIL and 3.0% (110/3646) of patients receiving comparator drugs. In a pooled analysis of these trials, based on a random effects model by trial weight, an adjusted risk difference of all-cause mortality was 0.6% (95% CI 0.1, 1.2) between TYGACIL and comparator-treated patients. The cause of this increase has not been established. This increase in all-cause mortality should be considered when selecting among treatment options *[see Warnings and Precautions (5.4) and Adverse Reactions (6.1)]*.

5.2 Anaphylaxis/Anaphylactoid Reactions

Anaphylaxis/anaphylactoid reactions have been reported with nearly all antibacterial agents, including TYGACIL, and may be life-threatening. TYGACIL is structurally similar to tetracycline-class antibiotics and should be administered with caution in patients with known hypersensitivity to tetracycline-class antibiotics.

5.3 Hepatic Effects

Increases in total bilirubin concentration, prothrombin time and transaminases have been seen in patients treated with tigecycline. Isolated cases of significant hepatic dysfunction and hepatic failure have been reported in patients being treated with tigecycline. Some of these patients were receiving multiple concomitant medications. Patients who develop abnormal liver function tests during tigecycline therapy should be monitored for evidence of worsening hepatic function and evaluated for risk/benefit of continuing tigecycline therapy. Adverse events may occur after the drug has been discontinued.

5.4 Mortality Imbalance and Lower Cure Rates in Ventilator-Associated Pneumonia

A trial of patients with hospital acquired pneumonia failed to demonstrate the efficacy of TYGACIL. In this trial, patients were randomized to receive TYGACIL (100 mg initially, then 50 mg every 12 hours) or a comparator. In addition, patients were allowed to receive specified adjunctive therapies. The sub-group of patients with ventilator-associated pneumonia who received TYGACIL had lower cure rates (47.9% versus 70.1% for the clinically evaluable population).

In this trial, greater mortality was seen in patients with ventilator-associated pneumonia who received TYGACIL (25/131 [19.1%] versus 15/122 [12.3%] in comparator-treated patients) *[see Adverse Reactions (6.1)]*. Particularly high mortality was seen among TYGACIL-treated patients with ventilator-associated pneumonia and bacteremia at baseline (9/18 [50.0%] versus 1/13 [7.7%] in comparator-treated patients).

5.5 Pancreatitis

Acute pancreatitis, including fatal cases, has occurred in association with tigecycline treatment. The diagnosis of acute pancreatitis should be considered in patients taking tigecycline who develop clinical symptoms, signs, or laboratory abnormalities suggestive of acute pancreatitis. Cases have been reported in patients without known risk factors for pancreatitis. Patients usually improve after tigecycline discontinuation. Consideration should be given to the cessation of the treatment with tigecycline in cases suspected of having developed pancreatitis *[see Adverse Reactions (6.2)]*.

5.6 Use During Pregnancy

TYGACIL may cause fetal harm when administered to a pregnant woman. If the patient becomes pregnant while taking tigecycline, the patient should be apprised of the potential hazard to the fetus. Results of animal studies indicate that tigecycline crosses the placenta and is found in fetal tissues. Decreased fetal weights in rats and rabbits (with associated delays in ossification) and fetal loss in rabbits have been observed with tigecycline *[see Use in Specific Populations (8.1)]*.

5.7 Tooth Development

The use of TYGACIL during tooth development (last half of pregnancy, infancy, and childhood to the age of 8 years) may cause permanent discoloration of the teeth (yellow-gray-brown). Results of studies in rats with TYGACIL have shown bone discoloration. TYGACIL should not be used during tooth development unless other drugs are not likely to be effective or are contraindicated.

5.8 *Clostridium difficile* Associated Diarrhea

Clostridium difficile associated diarrhea (CDAD) has been reported with use of nearly all antibacterial agents, including TYGACIL, and may range in severity from mild diarrhea to fatal colitis. Treatment with antibacterial agents alters the normal flora of the colon leading to overgrowth of *C. difficile*.

C. difficile produces toxins A and B which contribute to the development of CDAD. Hypertoxin producing strains of *C. difficile* cause increased morbidity and mortality, as these infections can be refractory to antimicrobial therapy and may require colectomy. CDAD must be considered in all patients who present with diarrhea following antibiotic use. Careful medical history is necessary since CDAD has been reported to occur over two months after the administration of antibacterial agents.

If CDAD is suspected or confirmed, ongoing antibiotic use not directed against *C. difficile* may need to be discontinued. Appropriate fluid and electrolyte management, protein supplementation, antibiotic treatment of *C. difficile*, and surgical evaluation should be instituted as clinically indicated.

5.9 Patients With Intestinal Perforation
Caution should be exercised when considering TYGACIL monotherapy in patients with complicated intra-abdominal infections (cIAI) secondary to clinically apparent intestinal perforation. In cIAI studies (n=1642), 6 patients treated with TYGACIL and 2 patients treated with imipenem/cilastatin presented with intestinal perforations and developed sepsis/septic shock. The 6 patients treated with TYGACIL had higher APACHE II scores (median = 13) versus the 2 patients treated with imipenem/cilastatin (APACHE II scores = 4 and 6). Due to differences in baseline APACHE II scores between treatment groups and small overall numbers, the relationship of this outcome to treatment cannot be established.

5.10 Tetracycline-Class Effects
TYGACIL is structurally similar to tetracycline-class antibiotics and may have similar adverse effects. Such effects may include: photosensitivity, pseudotumor cerebri, and anti-anabolic action (which has led to increased BUN, azotemia, acidosis, and hyperphosphatemia). As with tetracyclines, pancreatitis has been reported with the use of TYGACIL [see Warnings and Precautions (5.5)].

5.11 Superinfection
As with other antibacterial drugs, use of TYGACIL may result in overgrowth of non-susceptible organisms, including fungi. Patients should be carefully monitored during therapy. If superinfection occurs, appropriate measures should be taken.

5.12 Development of Drug-Resistant Bacteria
Prescribing TYGACIL in the absence of a proven or strongly suspected bacterial infection is unlikely to provide benefit to the patient and increases the risk of the development of drug-resistant bacteria.

6 ADVERSE REACTIONS
6.1 Clinical Trials Experience
Because clinical trials are conducted under widely varying conditions, adverse reaction rates observed in the clinical trials of a drug cannot be directly compared to rates in the clinical trials of another drug and may not reflect the rates observed in practice.

In clinical trials, 2514 patients were treated with TYGACIL. TYGACIL was discontinued due to adverse reactions in 7% of patients compared to 6% for all comparators. Table 1 shows the incidence of treatment-emergent adverse reactions through test of cure reported in ≥2% of patients in these trials.

Table 1. Incidence (%) of Adverse Reactions Through Test of Cure Reported in ≥2% of Patients Treated in Clinical Studies

Body System Adverse Reactions	TYGACIL (N=2514)	Comparators[a] (N=2307)
Body as a Whole		
Abdominal pain	6	4
Abscess	3	3
Asthenia	3	2
Headache	6	7
Infection	8	5
Cardiovascular System		
Phlebitis	3	4
Digestive System		
Diarrhea	12	11
Dyspepsia	2	2
Nausea	26	13
Vomiting	18	9
Hemic and Lymphatic System		
Anemia	4	5
Metabolic and Nutritional		
Alkaline Phosphatase Increased	4	3
Amylase Increased	3	2
Bilirubinemia	2	1
BUN Increased	3	1
Healing Abnormal	4	3
Hypoproteinemia	5	3
SGOT Increased[b]	4	5
SGPT Increased[b]	5	5
Nervous System		
Dizziness	3	3
Skin and Appendages		
Rash	3	4

[a] Vancomycin/Aztreonam, Imipenem/Cilastatin, Levofloxacin, Linezolid.
[b] LFT abnormalities in TYGACIL-treated patients were reported more frequently in the post therapy period than those in comparator-treated patients, which occurred more often on therapy.

In all 13 Phase 3 and 4 trials that included a comparator, death occurred in 4.0% (150/3788) of patients receiving TYGACIL and 3.0% (110/3646) of patients receiving com-

Table 2. Patients with Outcome of Death by Infection Type

Infection Type	TYGACIL n/N	%	Comparator n/N	%	Risk Difference* % (95% CI)
cSSSI	12/834	1.4	6/813	0.7	0.7 (-0.3, 1.7)
cIAI	42/1382	3.0	31/1393	2.2	0.8 (-0.4, 2.0)
CAP	12/424	2.8	11/422	2.6	0.2 (-2.0, 2.4)
HAP	66/467	14.1	57/467	12.2	1.9 (-2.4, 6.3)
Non-VAP[a]	41/336	12.2	42/345	12.2	0.0 (-4.9, 4.9)
VAP[a]	25/131	19.1	15/122	12.3	6.8 (-2.1, 15.7)
RP	11/128	8.6	2/43	4.7	3.9 (-4.0, 11.9)
DFI	7/553	1.3	3/508	0.6	0.7 (-0.5, 1.8)
Overall Adjusted	150/3788	4.0	110/3646	3.0	0.6 (0.1, 1.2)**

CAP = Community-acquired pneumonia; cIAI = Complicated intra-abdominal infections; cSSSI = Complicated skin and skin structure infections; HAP = Hospital-acquired pneumonia; VAP = Ventilator-associated pneumonia; RP = Resistant pathogens; DFI = Diabetic foot infections.
* The difference between the percentage of patients who died in TYGACIL and comparator treatment groups. The 95% CI for each infection type was calculated using the normal approximation method without continuity correction.
** Overall adjusted (random effects model by trial weight) risk difference estimate and 95% CI.
[a] These are subgroups of the HAP population.
Note: The studies include 300, 305, 900 (cSSSI), 301, 306, 315, 316, 400 (cIAI), 308 and 313 (CAP), and 311 (HAP), 307 [Resistant gram-positive pathogen study in patients with MRSA or Vancomycin-Resistant Enterococcus (VRE)], and 319 (DFI with and without osteomyelitis).

parator drugs. In a pooled analysis of these trials, based on a random effects model by trial weight, an adjusted risk difference of all-cause mortality was 0.6% (95% CI 0.1, 1.2) between TYGACIL and comparator-treated patients (see Table 2). The cause of the imbalance has not been established. Generally, deaths were the result of worsening infection, complications of infection or underlying co-morbidities.
[See table 2 above]
In comparative clinical studies, infection-related serious adverse events were more frequently reported for subjects treated with TYGACIL (7%) versus comparators (6%). Serious adverse events of sepsis/septic shock were more frequently reported for subjects treated with TYGACIL (2%) versus comparators (1%). Due to baseline differences between treatment groups in this subset of patients, the relationship of this outcome to treatment cannot be established [see Warnings and Precautions (5.9)].
The most common treatment-emergent adverse reactions were nausea and vomiting which generally occurred during the first 1–2 days of therapy. The majority of cases of nausea and vomiting associated with TYGACIL and comparators were either mild or moderate in severity. In patients treated with TYGACIL, nausea incidence was 26% (17% mild, 8% moderate, 1% severe) and vomiting incidence was 18% (11% mild, 6% moderate, 1% severe).
In patients treated for complicated skin and skin structure infections (cSSSI), nausea incidence was 35% for TYGACIL and 9% for vancomycin/aztreonam; vomiting incidence was 20% for TYGACIL and 4% for vancomycin/aztreonam. In patients treated for complicated intra-abdominal infections (cIAI), nausea incidence was 25% for TYGACIL and 21% for imipenem/cilastatin; vomiting incidence was 20% for TYGACIL and 15% for imipenem/cilastatin. In patients treated for community-acquired bacterial pneumonia (CABP), nausea incidence was 24% for TYGACIL and 8% for levofloxacin; vomiting incidence was 16% for TYGACIL and 6% for levofloxacin.
Discontinuation from tigecycline was most frequently associated with nausea (1%) and vomiting (1%). For comparators, discontinuation was most frequently associated with nausea (<1%).
The following adverse reactions were reported infrequently (<2%) in patients receiving TYGACIL in clinical studies:
Body as a Whole: injection site inflammation, injection site pain, injection site reaction, septic shock, allergic reaction, chills, injection site edema, injection site phlebitis
Cardiovascular System: thrombophlebitis
Digestive System: anorexia, jaundice, abnormal stools
Metabolic/Nutritional System: increased creatinine, hypocalcemia, hypoglycemia, hyponatremia
Special Senses: taste perversion
Hemic and Lymphatic System: partial thromboplastin time (aPTT), prolonged prothrombin time (PT), eosinophilia, increased international normalized ratio (INR), thrombocytopenia
Skin and Appendages: pruritus
Urogenital System: vaginal moniliasis, vaginitis, leukorrhea

6.2 Post-Marketing Experience
The following adverse reactions have been identified during postapproval use of TYGACIL. Because these reactions are reported voluntarily from a population of uncertain size, it is not always possible to reliably estimate their frequency or establish causal relationship to drug exposure.
• anaphylaxis/anaphylactoid reactions
• acute pancreatitis
• hepatic cholestasis, and jaundice

7 DRUG INTERACTIONS
7.1 Warfarin
Prothrombin time or other suitable anticoagulation test should be monitored if tigecycline is administered with warfarin [see Clinical Pharmacology (12.3)].
7.2 Oral Contraceptives
Concurrent use of antibacterial drugs with oral contraceptives may render oral contraceptives less effective.

8 USE IN SPECIFIC POPULATIONS
8.1 Pregnancy
Teratogenic Effects—Pregnancy Category D [see Warnings and Precautions (5.6)]
Tigecycline was not teratogenic in the rat or rabbit. In preclinical safety studies, ^{14}C-labeled tigecycline crossed the placenta and was found in fetal tissues, including fetal bony structures. The administration of tigecycline was associated with slight reductions in fetal weights and an increased incidence of minor skeletal anomalies (delays in bone ossification) at exposures of 5 times and 1 times the human daily dose based on AUC in rats and rabbits, respectively (28 mcg•hr/mL and 6 mcg•hr/mL at 12 and 4 mg/kg/day). An increased incidence of fetal loss was observed at maternotoxic doses in the rabbits with exposure equivalent to human dose.
There are no adequate and well-controlled studies of tigecycline in pregnant women. TYGACIL should be used during pregnancy only if the potential benefit justifies the potential risk to the fetus.

8.3 Nursing Mothers
Results from animal studies using ^{14}C-labeled tigecycline indicate that tigecycline is excreted readily via the milk of lactating rats. Consistent with the limited oral bioavailability of tigecycline, there is little or no systemic exposure to tigecycline in nursing pups as a result of exposure via maternal milk.
It is not known whether this drug is excreted in human milk. Because many drugs are excreted in human milk, caution should be exercised when TYGACIL is administered to a nursing woman [see Warnings and Precautions (5.7)].

8.4 Pediatric Use
Safety and effectiveness in pediatric patients below the age of 18 years have not been established. Because of effects on tooth development, use in patients under 8 years of age is not recommended [see Warnings and Precautions (5.7)].

8.5 Geriatric Use
Of the total number of subjects who received TYGACIL in Phase 3 clinical studies (n=2514), 664 were 65 and over, while 288 were 75 and over. No unexpected overall differences in safety or effectiveness were observed between these subjects and younger subjects, but greater sensitivity to adverse events of some older individuals cannot be ruled out. No significant difference in tigecycline exposure was observed between healthy elderly subjects and younger subjects following a single 100 mg dose of tigecycline [see Clinical Pharmacology (12.3)].

8.6 Hepatic Impairment
No dosage adjustment is warranted in patients with mild to moderate hepatic impairment (Child Pugh A and Child Pugh B). In patients with severe hepatic impairment (Child Pugh C), the initial dose of tigecycline should be 100 mg followed by a reduced maintenance dose of 25 mg every 12

hours. Patients with severe hepatic impairment (Child Pugh C) should be treated with caution and monitored for treatment response *[see Clinical Pharmacology (12.3) and Dosage and Administration (2.2)]*.

10 OVERDOSAGE

No specific information is available on the treatment of overdosage with tigecycline. Intravenous administration of TYGACIL at a single dose of 300 mg over 60 minutes in healthy volunteers resulted in an increased incidence of nausea and vomiting. In single-dose intravenous toxicity studies conducted with tigecycline in mice, the estimated median lethal dose (LD_{50}) was 124 mg/kg in males and 98 mg/kg in females. In rats, the estimated LD_{50} was 106 mg/kg for both sexes. Tigecycline is not removed in significant quantities by hemodialysis.

11 DESCRIPTION

TYGACIL (tigecycline) is a tetracycline derivative (a glycylcycline) for intravenous infusion. The chemical name of tigecycline is (4*S*,4a*S*,5a*R*,12a*S*)-9-[2-(*tert*-butylamino)acetamido]-4,7-bis(dimethylamino)-1,4,4a,5,5a,6,11,12a-octahydro-3,10,12,12a-tetrahydroxy-1,11-dioxo-2-naphthacenecarboxamide. The empirical formula is $C_{29}H_{39}N_5O_8$ and the molecular weight is 585.65.

The following represents the chemical structure of tigecycline:

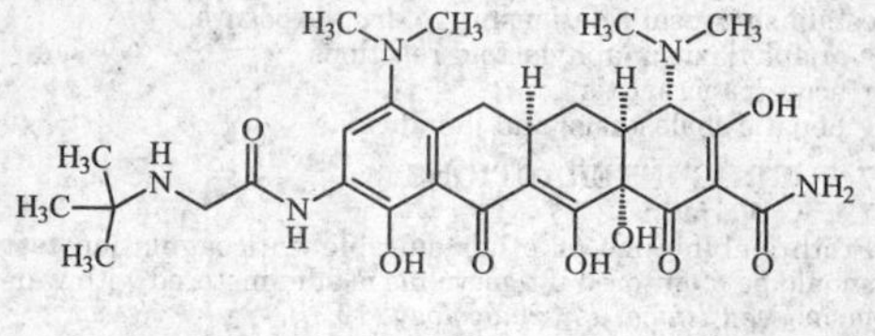

TYGACIL is an orange lyophilized powder or cake. Each TYGACIL vial contains 50 mg tigecycline lyophilized powder for reconstitution for intravenous infusion and 100 mg of lactose monohydrate. The pH is adjusted with hydrochloric acid, and if necessary sodium hydroxide. The product does not contain preservatives.

12 CLINICAL PHARMACOLOGY

12.1 Mechanism of Action

Tigecycline is an antibacterial drug *[see Clinical Pharmacology (12.4)]*.

12.3 Pharmacokinetics

The mean pharmacokinetic parameters of tigecycline after single and multiple intravenous doses based on pooled data from clinical pharmacology studies are summarized in Table 3. Intravenous infusions of tigecycline were administered over approximately 30 to 60 minutes.

Table 3. Mean (CV%) Pharmacokinetic Parameters of Tigecycline

	Single Dose 100 mg (N=224)	Multiple Dose[a] 50 mg every 12h (N=103)
C_{max} (mcg/mL)[b]	1.45 (22%)	0.87 (27%)
C_{max} (mcg/mL)[c]	0.90 (30%)	0.63 (15%)
AUC (mcg•h/mL)	5.19 (36%)	—
AUC_{0-24h} (mcg•h/mL)	—	4.70 (36%)
C_{min} (mcg/mL)	—	0.13 (59%)
$t_{1/2}$ (h)	27.1 (53%)	42.4 (83%)
CL (L/h)	21.8 (40%)	23.8 (33%)
CL_r (mL/min)	38.0 (82%)	51.0 (58%)
V_{ss} (L)	568 (43%)	639 (48%)

[a] 100 mg initially, followed by 50 mg every 12 hours
[b] 30-minute infusion
[c] 60-minute infusion

Distribution

The *in vitro* plasma protein binding of tigecycline ranges from approximately 71% to 89% at concentrations observed in clinical studies (0.1 to 1.0 mcg/mL). The steady-state volume of distribution of tigecycline averaged 500 to 700 L (7 to 9 L/kg), indicating tigecycline is extensively distributed beyond the plasma volume and into the tissues.

Following the administration of tigecycline 100 mg followed by 50 mg every 12 hours to 33 healthy volunteers, the tigecycline AUC_{0-12h} (134 mcg•h/mL) in alveolar cells was approximately 78-fold higher than the AUC_{0-12h} in the serum, and the AUC_{0-12h} (2.28 mcg•h/mL) in epithelial lining fluid was approximately 32% higher than the AUC_{0-12h} in serum. The AUC_{0-12h} (1.61 mcg•h/mL) of tigecycline in skin blister fluid was approximately 26% lower than the AUC_{0-12h} in the serum of 10 healthy subjects.

In a single-dose study, tigecycline 100 mg was administered to subjects prior to undergoing elective surgery or medical procedure for tissue extraction. Concentrations at 4 hours after tigecycline administration were higher in gallbladder (38-fold, n=6), lung (3.7-fold, n=5), and colon (2.3-fold, n=6), and lower in synovial fluid (0.58-fold, n=5), and bone (0.35-fold, n=6) relative to serum. The concentration of tigecycline in these tissues after multiple doses has not been studied.

Metabolism

Tigecycline is not extensively metabolized. *In vitro* studies with tigecycline using human liver microsomes, liver slices, and hepatocytes led to the formation of only trace amounts of metabolites. In healthy male volunteers receiving ^{14}C-tigecycline, tigecycline was the primary ^{14}C-labeled material recovered in urine and feces, but a glucuronide, an N-acetyl metabolite, and a tigecycline epimer (each at no more than 10% of the administered dose) were also present.

Elimination

The recovery of total radioactivity in feces and urine following administration of ^{14}C-tigecycline indicates that 59% of the dose is eliminated by biliary/fecal excretion, and 33% is excreted in urine. Approximately 22% of the total dose is excreted as unchanged tigecycline in urine. Overall, the primary route of elimination for tigecycline is biliary excretion of unchanged tigecycline and its metabolites. Glucuronidation and renal excretion of unchanged tigecycline are secondary routes.

Specific Populations

Patients with Hepatic Impairment

In a study comparing 10 patients with mild hepatic impairment (Child Pugh A), 10 patients with moderate hepatic impairment (Child Pugh B), and 5 patients with severe hepatic impairment (Child Pugh C) to 23 age and weight matched healthy control subjects, the single-dose pharmacokinetic disposition of tigecycline was not altered in patients with mild hepatic impairment. However, systemic clearance of tigecycline was reduced by 25% and the half-life of tigecycline was prolonged by 23% in patients with moderate hepatic impairment (Child Pugh B). Systemic clearance of tigecycline was reduced by 55%, and the half-life of tigecycline was prolonged by 43% in patients with severe hepatic impairment (Child Pugh C). Dosage adjustment is necessary in patients with severe hepatic impairment (Child Pugh C) *[see Use in Specific Populations (8.6) and Dosage and Administration (2.2)]*.

Patients with Renal Impairment

A single dose study compared 6 subjects with severe renal impairment (creatinine clearance <30 mL/min), 4 end stage renal disease (ESRD) patients receiving tigecycline 2 hours before hemodialysis, 4 ESRD patients receiving tigecycline 1 hour after hemodialysis, and 6 healthy control subjects. The pharmacokinetic profile of tigecycline was not significantly altered in any of the renally impaired patient groups, nor was tigecycline removed by hemodialysis. No dosage adjustment of TYGACIL is necessary in patients with renal impairment or in patients undergoing hemodialysis.

Geriatric Patients

No significant differences in pharmacokinetics were observed between healthy elderly subjects (n=15, age 65-75; n=13, age >75) and younger subjects (n=18) receiving a single 100-mg dose of TYGACIL. Therefore, no dosage adjustment is necessary based on age *[see Use in Specific Populations (8.5)]*.

Gender

In a pooled analysis of 38 women and 298 men participating in clinical pharmacology studies, there was no significant difference in the mean (±SD) tigecycline clearance between women (20.7±6.5 L/h) and men (22.8±8.7 L/h). Therefore, no dosage adjustment is necessary based on gender.

Race

In a pooled analysis of 73 Asian subjects, 53 Black subjects, 15 Hispanic subjects, 190 White subjects, and 3 subjects classified as "other" participating in clinical pharmacology studies, there was no significant difference in the mean (±SD) tigecycline clearance among the Asian subjects (28.8±8.8 L/h), Black subjects (23.0±7.8 L/h), Hispanic subjects (24.3±6.5 L/h), White subjects (22.1±8.9 L/h), and "other" subjects (25.0±4.8 L/h). Therefore, no dosage adjustment is necessary based on race.

Drug Interactions

TYGACIL (100 mg followed by 50 mg every 12 hours) and digoxin (0.5 mg followed by 0.25 mg, orally, every 24 hours) were coadministered to healthy subjects in a drug interaction study. Tigecycline slightly decreased the C_{max} of digoxin by 13%, but did not affect the AUC or clearance of digoxin. This small change in C_{max} did not affect the steady-state pharmacodynamic effects of digoxin as measured by changes in ECG intervals. In addition, digoxin did not affect the pharmacokinetic profile of tigecycline. Therefore, no dosage adjustment of either drug is necessary when TYGACIL is administered with digoxin.

Concomitant administration of TYGACIL (100 mg followed by 50 mg every 12 hours) and warfarin (25 mg single-dose) to healthy subjects resulted in a decrease in clearance of R-warfarin and S-warfarin by 40% and 23%, an increase in C_{max} by 38% and 43% and an increase in AUC by 68% and 29%, respectively. Tigecycline did not significantly alter the effects of warfarin on INR. In addition, warfarin did not affect the pharmacokinetic profile of tigecycline. However, prothrombin time or other suitable anticoagulation test should be monitored if tigecycline is administered with warfarin.

In vitro studies in human liver microsomes indicate that tigecycline does not inhibit metabolism mediated by any of the following 6 cytochrome P450 (CYP) isoforms: 1A2, 2C8, 2C9, 2C19, 2D6, and 3A4. Therefore, TYGACIL is not expected to alter the metabolism of drugs metabolized by these enzymes. In addition, because tigecycline is not extensively metabolized, clearance of tigecycline is not expected to be affected by drugs that inhibit or induce the activity of these CYP450 isoforms.

12.4 Microbiology

Mechanism of Action

Tigecycline, a glycylcycline, inhibits protein translation in bacteria by binding to the 30S ribosomal subunit and blocking entry of amino-acyl tRNA molecules into the A site of the ribosome. This prevents incorporation of amino acid residues into elongating peptide chains. Tigecycline carries a glycylamido moiety attached to the 9-position of minocycline. The substitution pattern is not present in any naturally occurring or semisynthetic tetracycline and imparts certain microbiologic properties to tigecycline. In general, tigecycline is considered bacteriostatic; however, TYGACIL has demonstrated bactericidal activity against isolates of *S. pneumoniae* and *L. pneumophila*.

Mechanism(s) of Resistance

To date there has been no cross-resistance observed between tigecycline and other antibacterials. Tigecycline is not affected by the two major tetracycline-resistance mechanisms, ribosomal protection and efflux. Additionally, tigecycline is not affected by resistance mechanisms such as beta-lactamases (including extended spectrum beta-lactamases), target-site modifications, macrolide efflux pumps or enzyme target changes (e.g. gyrase/topoisomerases). Tigecycline resistance in some bacteria (e.g. *Acinetobacter calcoaceticus-Acinetobacter baumannii* complex) is associated with multi-drug resistant (MDR) efflux pumps.

Interaction with Other Antimicrobials

In vitro studies have not demonstrated antagonism between tigecycline and other commonly used antibacterials.

Tigecycline has been shown to be active against most of the following bacteria, both *in vitro* and in clinical infections *[see Indications and Usage (1)]*.

Facultative Gram-positive bacteria
Enterococcus faecalis (vancomycin-susceptible isolates)
Staphylococcus aureus (methicillin-susceptible and -resistant isolates)
Streptococcus agalactiae
Streptococcus anginosus grp. (includes *S. anginosus, S. intermedius,* and *S. constellatus*)
Streptococcus pneumoniae (penicillin-susceptible isolates)
Streptococcus pyogenes

Facultative Gram-negative bacteria
Citrobacter freundii
Enterobacter cloacae
Escherichia coli
Haemophilus influenzae (beta-lactamase negative isolates)
Klebsiella oxytoca
Klebsiella pneumoniae
Legionella pneumophila

Anaerobic bacteria
Bacteroides fragilis
Bacteroides thetaiotaomicron
Bacteroides uniformis
Bacteroides vulgatus
Clostridium perfringens
Peptostreptococcus micros

At least 90% of the following bacteria exhibit *in vitro* minimum inhibitory concentrations (MICs) that are at concentrations that are achievable using the prescribed dosing regimens. However, the clinical significance of this is unknown because the safety and effectiveness of tigecycline in treating clinical infections due to these bacteria have not been established in adequate and well-controlled clinical trials.

Facultative Gram-positive bacteria
Enterococcus avium
Enterococcus casseliflavus
Enterococcus faecalis (vancomycin-resistant isolates)
Enterococcus faecium (vancomycin-susceptible and -resistant isolates)
Enterococcus gallinarum
Listeria monocytogenes
Staphylococcus epidermidis (methicillin-susceptible and -resistant isolates)

Staphylococcus haemolyticus
Facultative Gram-negative bacteria
*Acinetobacter baumannii**
Aeromonas hydrophila
Citrobacter koseri
Enterobacter aerogenes
Haemophilus influenzae (ampicillin-resistant)
Haemophilus parainfluenzae
Pasteurella multocida
Serratia marcescens
Stenotrophomonas maltophilia
Anaerobic bacteria
Bacteroides distasonis
Bacteroides ovatus
Peptostreptococcus spp.
Porphyromonas spp.
Prevotella spp.
Other bacteria
Mycobacterium abscessus
Mycobacterium fortuitum

*There have been reports of the development of tigecycline resistance in *Acinetobacter* infections seen during the course of standard treatment. Such resistance appears to be attributable to an MDR efflux pump mechanism. While monitoring for relapse of infection is important for all infected patients, more frequent monitoring in this case is suggested. If relapse is suspected, blood and other specimens should be obtained and cultured for the presence of bacteria. All bacterial isolates should be identified and tested for susceptibility to tigecycline and other appropriate antimicrobials.

Susceptibility Test Methods
When available, the clinical microbiology laboratory should provide cumulative results of the *in vitro* susceptibility test results for antimicrobial drugs used in local hospitals and practice areas to the physician as periodic reports that describe the susceptibility profile of nosocomial and community-acquired pathogens. These reports should aid the physician in selecting the most effective antimicrobial.

Dilution Techniques
Quantitative methods are used to determine antimicrobial minimum inhibitory concentrations (MICs). These MICs provide estimates of the susceptibility of bacteria to antimicrobial compounds. The MICs should be determined using a standardized procedure based on dilution methods (broth, agar, or microdilution)[1,3,4] or equivalent using standardized inoculum and concentrations of tigecycline. For broth dilution tests for aerobic organisms, MICs must be determined in testing medium that is fresh (<12h old). The MIC values should be interpreted according to the criteria provided in Table 4.

Diffusion Techniques
Quantitative methods that require measurement of zone diameters also provide reproducible estimates of the susceptibility of bacteria to antimicrobial compounds. The standardized procedure[2,4] requires the use of standardized inoculum concentrations. This procedure uses paper disks impregnated with 15 mcg tigecycline to test the susceptibility of bacteria to tigecycline. Interpretation involves correlation of the diameter obtained in the disk test with the MIC for tigecycline. Reports from the laboratory providing results of the standard single-disk susceptibility test with a 15 mcg tigecycline disk should be interpreted according to the criteria in Table 4.

Anaerobic Techniques
Anaerobic susceptibility testing with tigecycline should be done by the agar dilution method[3] since quality control parameters for broth-dilution are not established.
[See table 4 above]

A report of "Susceptible" indicates that the pathogen is likely to be inhibited if the antimicrobial compound reaches the concentrations usually achievable. A report of "Intermediate" indicates that the result should be considered equivocal, and, if the microorganism is not fully susceptible to alternative, clinically feasible drugs, the test should be repeated. This category implies possible clinical applicability in body sites where the drug is physiologically concentrated or in situations where high dosage of drug can be used. This category also provides a buffer zone that prevents small uncontrolled technical factors from causing major discrepancies in interpretation. A report of "Resistant" indicates that the pathogen is not likely to be inhibited if the antimicrobial compound reaches the concentrations usually achievable; other therapy should be selected.

Quality Control
As with other susceptibility techniques, the use of laboratory control microorganisms is required to control the technical aspects of the laboratory standardized procedures.[1,2,3,4] Standard tigecycline powder should provide the MIC values provided in Table 5. For the diffusion technique using the 15 mcg tigecycline disk the criteria provided in Table 5 should be achieved.
[See table 5 at right]

13 NONCLINICAL TOXICOLOGY

13.1 Carcinogenesis, Mutagenesis, Impairment of Fertility
Lifetime studies in animals have not been performed to evaluate the carcinogenic potential of tigecycline. No mutagenic or clastogenic potential was found in a battery of tests, including *in vitro* chromosome aberration assay in Chinese

Table 4. Susceptibility Test Result Interpretive Criteria for Tigecycline

Pathogen	Minimum Inhibitory Concentrations (mcg/mL) S	I	R	Disk Diffusion (zone diameters in mm) S	I	R
Staphylococcus aureus (including methicillin-resistant isolates)	≤0.5[a]	-	-	≥19	-	-
Streptococcus spp. other than *S. pneumoniae*	≤0.25[a]	-	-	≥19	-	-
Streptococcus pneumoniae	≤0.06[a]	-	-	≥19	-	-
Enterococcus faecalis (vancomycin-susceptible isolates)	≤0.25[a]	-	-	≥19	-	-
Enterobacteriaceae[b]	≤2	4	≥8	≥19	15-18	≤14
Haemophilus influenzae	≤0.25[a]	-	-	≥19	-	-
Anaerobes[c]	≤4	8	≥16	n/a	n/a	n/a

[a] The current absence of resistant isolates precludes defining any results other than "Susceptible." Isolates yielding MIC results suggestive of "Nonsusceptible" category should be submitted to reference laboratory for further testing.
[b] Tigecycline has decreased *in vitro* activity against *Morganella* spp, *Proteus* spp. and *Providencia* spp.
[c] Agar dilution

Table 5. Acceptable Quality Control Ranges for Susceptibility Testing

QC organism	Minimum Inhibitory Concentrations (mcg/mL)	Disk Diffusion (zone diameters in mm)
Staphylococcus aureus ATCC 25923	Not Applicable	20-25
Staphylococcus aureus ATCC 29213	0.03-0.25	Not Applicable
Escherichia coli ATCC 25922	0.03-0.25	20-27
Enterococcus faecalis ATCC 29212	0.03-0.12	Not Applicable
Streptococcus pneumoniae ATCC 49619	0.016-0.12	23-29
Haemophilus influenzae ATCC 49247	0.06-0.5	23-31
Bacteroides fragilis[a] ATCC 25285	0.12-1	Not Applicable
Bacteroides thetaiotaomicron[a] ATCC 29741	0.5-2	Not Applicable
Eubacterium lentum[a] ATCC 43055	0.06-0.5	Not Applicable
Clostridium difficile[a] ATCC 70057	0.12-1	Not Applicable

ATCC = American Type Culture Collection
[a] Agar dilution

Table 7. Clinical Cure Rates By Infecting Pathogen in Microbiologically Evaluable Patients with Complicated Skin and Skin Structure Infections[a]

Pathogen	TYGACIL n/N (%)	Vancomycin/Aztreonam n/N (%)
Escherichia coli	29/36 (80.6)	26/30 (86.7)
Enterobacter cloacae	10/12 (83.3)	15/15 (100)
Enterococcus faecalis (vancomycin-susceptible only)	15/21 (71.4)	19/24 (79.2)
Klebsiella pneumoniae	12/14 (85.7)	15/16 (93.8)
Methicillin-susceptible *Staphylococcus aureus* (MSSA)	124/137 (90.5)	113/120 (94.2)
Methicillin-resistant *Staphylococcus aureus* (MRSA)	79/95 (83.2)	46/57 (80.7)
Streptococcus agalactiae	8/8 (100)	11/14 (78.6)
Streptococcus anginosus grp.[b]	17/21 (81.0)	9/10 (90.0)
Streptococcus pyogenes	31/32 (96.9)	24/27 (88.9)
Bacteroides fragilis	7/9 (77.8)	4/5 (80.0)

[a] Two cSSSI pivotal studies and two Resistant Pathogen studies
[b] Includes *Streptococcus anginosus*, *Streptococcus intermedius*, and *Streptococcus constellatus*

hamster ovary (CHO) cells, *in vitro* forward mutation assay in CHO cells (HGRPT locus), *in vitro* forward mutation assays in mouse lymphoma cells, and *in vivo* mouse micronucleus assay. Tigecycline did not affect mating or fertility in rats at exposures up to 5 times the human daily dose based on AUC (28mcg•hr/mL at 12 mg/kg/day). In female rats, there were no compound-related effects on ovaries or estrous cycles at exposures up to 5 times the human daily dose based on AUC.

13.2 Animal Toxicology and/or Pharmacology
In two week studies, decreased erythrocytes, reticulocytes, leukocytes, and platelets, in association with bone marrow hypocellularity, have been seen with tigecycline at exposures of 8 times and 10 times the human daily dose based on AUC in rats and dogs, (AUC of approximately 50 and 60 mcg•hr/mL at doses of 30 and 12 mg/kg/day) respectively. These alterations were shown to be reversible after two weeks of dosing.

14 CLINICAL STUDIES

14.1 Complicated Skin and Skin Structure Infections
TYGACIL was evaluated in adults for the treatment of complicated skin and skin structure infections (cSSSI) in two randomized, double-blind, active-controlled, multinational, multicenter studies (Studies 300 and 305). These studies compared TYGACIL (100 mg intravenous initial dose followed by 50 mg every 12 hours) with vancomycin (1 g intravenous every 12 hours)/aztreonam (2 g intravenous every 12 hours) for 5 to 14 days. Patients with complicated deep soft tissue infections including wound infections and cellulitis (≥10 cm, requiring surgery/drainage or with complicated underlying disease), major abscesses, infected ulcers, and burns were enrolled in the studies. The primary efficacy endpoint was the clinical response at the test of cure (TOC) visit in the co-primary populations of the clinically evaluable (CE) and clinical modified intent-to-treat (c-mITT) patients. See Table 6. Clinical cure rates at TOC by pathogen in the microbiologically evaluable patients are presented in Table 7.

Table 6. Clinical Cure Rates from Two Studies in Complicated Skin and Skin Structure Infections after 5 to 14 Days of Therapy

	TYGACIL[a] n/N (%)	Vancomycin/Aztreonam[b] n/N (%)
Study 300		
CE	165/199 (82.9)	163/198 (82.3)
c-mITT	209/277 (75.5)	200/260 (76.9)
Study 305		
CE	200/223 (89.7)	201/213 (94.4)
c-mITT	220/261 (84.3)	225/259 (86.9)

[a] 100 mg initially, followed by 50 mg every 12 hours
[b] Vancomycin (1 g every 12 hours)/Aztreonam (2 g every 12 hours)

[See table 7 above]

Table 9. Clinical Cure Rates By Infecting Pathogen in Microbiologically Evaluable Patients with Complicated Intra-abdominal Infections[a]

Pathogen	TYGACIL n/N (%)	Imipenem/Cilastatin n/N (%)
Citrobacter freundii	12/16 (75.0)	3/4 (75.0)
Enterobacter cloacae	15/17 (88.2)	16/17 (94.1)
Escherichia coli	284/336 (84.5)	297/342 (86.8)
Klebsiella oxytoca	19/20 (95.0)	17/19 (89.5)
Klebsiella pneumoniae	42/47 (89.4)	46/53 (86.8)
Enterococcus faecalis	29/38 (76.3)	35/47 (74.5)
Methicillin-susceptible Staphylococcus aureus (MSSA)	26/28 (92.9)	22/24 (91.7)
Methicillin-resistant Staphylococcus aureus (MRSA)	16/18 (88.9)	1/3 (33.3)
Streptococcus anginosus grp.[b]	101/119 (84.9)	60/79 (75.9)
Bacteroides fragilis	68/88 (77.3)	59/73 (80.8)
Bacteroides thetaiotaomicron	36/41 (87.8)	31/36 (86.1)
Bacteroides uniformis	12/17 (70.6)	14/16 (87.5)
Bacteroides vulgatus	14/16 (87.5)	4/6 (66.7)
Clostridium perfringens	18/19 (94.7)	20/22 (90.9)
Peptostreptococcus micros	13/17 (76.5)	8/11 (72.7)

[a] Two cIAI pivotal studies and two Resistant Pathogen studies
[b] Includes Streptococcus anginosus, Streptococcus intermedius, and Streptococcus constellatus

Table 10. Clinical Cure Rates from Two Studies in Community-Acquired Bacterial Pneumonia after 7 to 14 Days of Total Therapy

	TYGACIL[a] n/N (%)	Levofloxacin[b] n/N (%)	95% CI[c]
Study 308[d]			
CE	125/138 (90.6)	136/156 (87.2)	(-4.4, 11.2)
c-mITT	149/191 (78)	158/203 (77.8)	(-8.5, 8.9)
Study 313			
CE	128/144 (88.9)	116/136 (85.3)	(-5.0, 12.2)
c-mITT	170/203 (83.7)	163/200 (81.5)	(-5.6, 10.1)

[a] 100 mg initially, followed by 50 mg every 12 hours
[b] Levofloxacin (500 mg intravenous every 12 or 24 hours)
[c] 95% confidence interval for the treatment difference
[d] After at least 3 days of intravenous therapy, a switch to oral levofloxacin (500 mg daily) was permitted for both treatment arms in Study 308.

Table 11. Clinical Cure Rates By Infecting Pathogen in Microbiologically Evaluable Patients with Community-Acquired Bacterial Pneumonia[a]

Pathogen	TYGACIL n/N (%)	Levofloxacin n/N (%)
Haemophilus influenzae	14/17 (82.4)	13/16 (81.3)
Legionella pneumophila	10/10 (100.0)	6/6 (100.0)
Streptococcus pneumoniae (penicillin-susceptible only)[b]	44/46 (95.7)	39/44 (88.6)

[a] Two CABP studies
[b] Includes cases of concurrent bacteremia [cure rates of 20/22 (90.9%) versus 13/18 (72.2%) for TYGACIL and levofloxacin respectively]

Table 12. Post-hoc Analysis of Clinical Cure Rates in Patients with Community-Acquired Bacterial Pneumonia Based on Risk of Mortality[a]

	TYGACIL n/N (%)	Levofloxacin n/N (%)	95% CI[b]
Study 308[c]			
CE			
Higher risk			
Yes	93/103 (90.3)	84/102 (82.4)	(-2.3, 18.2)
No	32/35 (91.4)	52/54 (96.3)	(-20.8, 7.1)
c-mITT			
Higher risk			
Yes	111/142 (78.2)	100/134 (74.6)	(-6.9, 14)
No	38/49 (77.6)	58/69 (84.1)	(-22.8, 8.7)
Study 313			
CE			
Higher risk			
Yes	95/107 (88.8)	68/85 (80)	(-2.2, 20.3)
No	33/37 (89.2)	48/51 (94.1)	(-21.1, 8.6)
c-mITT			
Higher risk			
Yes	112/134 (83.6)	93/120 (77.5)	(-4.2, 16.4)
No	58/69 (84.1)	70/80 (87.5)	(-16.2, 8.8)

[a] Patients at higher risk of death include patients with any one of the following: ≥50 year of age; PSI score ≥3; or bacteremia due to Streptococcus pneumoniae
[b] 95% confidence interval for the treatment difference
[c] After at least 3 days of intravenous therapy, a switch to oral levofloxacin (500 mg daily) was permitted for both treatment arms in Study 308.

14.2 Complicated Intra-abdominal Infections

TYGACIL was evaluated in adults for the treatment of complicated intra-abdominal infections (cIAI) in two randomized, double-blind, active-controlled, multinational, multicenter studies (Studies 301 and 306). These studies compared TYGACIL (100 mg intravenous initial dose followed by 50 mg every 12 hours) with imipenem/cilastatin (500 mg intravenous every 6 hours) for 5 to 14 days. Patients with complicated diagnoses including appendicitis, cholecystitis, diverticulitis, gastric/duodenal perforation, intra-abdominal abscess, perforation of intestine, and peritonitis were enrolled in the studies. The primary efficacy endpoint was the clinical response at the TOC visit for the co-primary populations of the microbiologically evaluable (ME) and the microbiologic modified intent-to-treat (m-mITT) patients. See Table 8. Clinical cure rates at TOC by pathogen in the microbiologically evaluable patients are presented in Table 9.

Table 8. Clinical Cure Rates from Two Studies in Complicated Intra-abdominal Infections after 5 to 14 Days of Therapy

	TYGACIL[a] n/N (%)	Imipenem/Cilastatin[b] n/N (%)
Study 301		
ME	199/247 (80.6)	210/255 (82.4)
m-mITT	227/309 (73.5)	244/312 (78.2)
Study 306		
ME	242/265 (91.3)	232/258 (89.9)
m-mITT	279/322 (86.6)	270/319 (84.6)

[a] 100 mg initially, followed by 50 mg every 12 hours
[b] Imipenem/Cilastatin (500 mg every 6 hours)

[See table 9 above]

14.3 Community-Acquired Bacterial Pneumonia

TYGACIL was evaluated in adults for the treatment of community-acquired bacterial pneumonia (CABP) in two randomized, double-blind, active-controlled, multinational, multicenter studies (Studies 308 and 313). These studies compared TYGACIL (100 mg intravenous initial dose followed by 50 mg every 12 hours) with levofloxacin (500 mg intravenous every 12 or 24 hours). In one study (Study 308), after at least 3 days of intravenous therapy, a switch to oral levofloxacin (500 mg daily) was permitted for both treatment arms. Total therapy was 7 to 14 days. Patients with community-acquired bacterial pneumonia who required hospitalization and intravenous therapy were enrolled in the studies. The primary efficacy endpoint was the clinical response at the test of cure (TOC) visit in the co-primary populations of the clinically evaluable (CE) and clinical modified intent-to-treat (c-mITT) patients. See Table 10. Clinical cure rates at TOC by pathogen in the microbiologically evaluable patients are presented in Table 11.

[See table 10 at left]
[See table 11 at left]

To further evaluate the treatment effect of tigecycline, a post-hoc analysis was conducted in CABP patients with a higher risk of mortality, for whom the treatment effect of antibiotics is supported by historical evidence. The higher-risk group included CABP patients from the two studies with any of the following factors:
- Age ≥50 years
- PSI score ≥3
- Streptococcus pneumoniae bacteremia

The results of this analysis are shown in Table 12. Age ≥50 was the most common risk factor in the higher-risk group.
[See table 12 at left]

15 REFERENCES

1. Clinical and Laboratory Standards Institute (CLSI). Methods for Dilution Antimicrobial Susceptibility Tests for Bacteria that Grow Aerobically – 8th ed. Approved Standard, CLSI document M07-A8, CLSI, 940 West Valley Road, Suite 1400, Wayne, PA 19087-1898. January 2009.
2. Clinical and Laboratory Standards Institute (CLSI). Performance Standards for Antimicrobial Disk Diffusion Susceptibility Tests – 10th ed. Approved Standard, CLSI document M02-A10, CLSI, 940 West Valley Road, Suite 1400, Wayne, PA 19087-1898. January 2009.
3. Clinical and Laboratory Standards Institute (CLSI). Methods for Antimicrobial Susceptibility Testing of Anaerobic Bacteria – 7th ed. Approved Standard, CLSI document M11-A7, CLSI, 940 West Valley Road, Suite 1400, Wayne, PA 19087-1898. January 2007.
4. Clinical and Laboratory Standards Institute (CLSI). Performance Standards for Antimicrobial Susceptibility Testing – 19th Informational Supplement. Approved Standard, CLSI document M100-S19, CLSI, 940 West Valley Road, Suite 1400, Wayne, PA 19087-1898. January 2009.

16 HOW SUPPLIED/STORAGE AND HANDLING

TYGACIL (tigecycline) for injection is supplied in a single-dose 5 mL glass vial or 10 mL glass vial, each containing 50 mg tigecycline lyophilized powder for reconstitution.
Supplied:

5 mL—10 vials/box. NDC 0008-4990-02

10 mL—10 vials/box. NDC 0008-4990-20

Prior to reconstitution, TYGACIL should be stored at 20° to 25°C (68° to 77°F); excursions permitted to 15° to 30°C (59° to 86°F). [See USP Controlled Room Temperature.] Once reconstituted, TYGACIL may be stored at room temperature for up to 24 hours (up to 6 hours in the vial and the remaining time in the intravenous bag. Alternatively, TYGACIL mixed with 0.9% Sodium Chloride Injection, USP or 5% Dextrose Injection, USP may be stored refrigerated at 2° to 8°C (36° to 46°F) for up to 48 hours following immediate transfer of the reconstituted solution into the intravenous bag. Reconstituted solution must be transferred and further diluted for intravenous infusion.

U.S. Patent Numbers: RE40086; RE40183; 5,284,963; 5,530,117; 5,675,030; and 7,365,087.

17 PATIENT COUNSELING INFORMATION

- Patients should be counseled that antibacterial drugs including TYGACIL should only be used to treat bacterial infections. They do not treat viral infections (e.g., the common cold). When TYGACIL is prescribed to treat a bacterial infection, patients should be told that although it is common to feel better early in the course of therapy, the medication should be taken exactly as directed. Skipping doses or not completing the full course of therapy may (1) decrease the effectiveness of the immediate treatment and (2) increase the likelihood that bacteria will develop resistance and will not be treatable by TYGACIL or other antibacterial drugs in the future.
- Diarrhea is a common problem caused by antibiotics which usually ends when the antibiotic is discontinued. Sometimes after starting treatment with antibiotics, patients can develop watery and bloody stools (with or without stomach cramps and fever) even as late as two or more months after having taken the last dose of the antibiotic. If this occurs, patients should contact their physician as soon as possible.

This product's label may have been updated. For current package insert and further product information, please visit www.wyeth.com or call our medical communications department toll-free at 1-800-934-5556.

Wyeth®
Manufactured for:
Wyeth Pharmaceuticals Inc.
Philadelphia, PA 19101
By:
Wyeth Pharmaceuticals Inc.
Philadelphia, PA 19101
Or
Patheon Italia S.p.A.
20052 Monza, Italy

W10521C016
ET01
Rev 07/10

XYNTHA™   ℞
[ZIN-tha]
[Antihemophilic Factor (Recombinant),
Plasma/Albumin-Free]
For Intravenous Use, Freeze-Dried Powder

HIGHLIGHTS OF PRESCRIBING INFORMATION

These highlights do not include all the information needed to use XYNTHA™ safely and effectively. See full prescribing information for XYNTHA™.

XYNTHA™ [Antihemophilic Factor (Recombinant), Plasma/Albumin-Free] For Intravenous Use, Freeze-Dried Powder
Initial U.S. Approval: 2008

─────── INDICATIONS AND USAGE ───────

XYNTHA is an antihemophilic factor indicated for:

- Control and prevention of bleeding episodes in patients with hemophilia A (1.1)
- Surgical prophylaxis in patients with hemophilia A (1.2)

─────── DOSAGE AND ADMINISTRATION ───────

The required dosage is determined using the following formula: (2)

Required units = body weight (kg) × desired factor VIII rise (IU/dL or % of normal) × 0.5 (IU/kg per IU/dL)

Frequency of intravenous injection of the reconstituted product is determined by the type of bleeding episode and the recommendation of the treating physician. (2.1, 2.2)

─────── DOSAGE FORMS AND STRENGTHS ───────

XYNTHA powder is available as 250, 500, 1000, or 2000 IU in single-use vials. (3)

─────── CONTRAINDICATIONS ───────

None.

─────── WARNINGS AND PRECAUTIONS ───────

- Anaphylaxis and severe hypersensitivity reactions are possible. Should such reactions occur, treatment with the product should be discontinued, and appropriate treatment should be administered. (5.1)
- Development of activity-neutralizing antibodies has been detected in patients receiving factor VIII-containing products. If expected plasma factor VIII activity levels are not attained, or if bleeding is not controlled with an appropriate dose, an assay that measures factor VIII inhibitor concentration should be performed. (5.2, 5.4)
- Patients may develop hypersensitivity to hamster protein, which is present in trace amounts in the product. (5.3)

─────── ADVERSE REACTIONS ───────

The most common adverse reaction in Study 1 (24% of subjects) is headache and in Study 2 is pyrexia (41% of subjects). (6.1)

Two out of 89 subjects (who completed ≥ 50 exposure days) developed an inhibitor during the course of the study. The observation of 2 inhibitors in 89 subjects who completed ≥ 50 exposure days was consistent with a 95% probability that the inhibitor formation rate with XYNTHA is less than 4.17% using a Bayesian analysis. (6.1)

To report SUSPECTED ADVERSE REACTIONS, contact Wyeth Pharmaceuticals, Inc. at 1-800-934-5556 or FDA at 1-800-FDA-1088 or www.fda.gov/medwatch

─────── DRUG INTERACTIONS ───────

None.

─────── USE IN SPECIFIC POPULATIONS ───────

Limited pharmacokinetic data (N=7) on the use of XYNTHA in pediatric subjects are available. (8.4)

See 17 for PATIENT COUNSELING INFORMATION and FDA-approved patient labeling

Revised: 04/2008

FULL PRESCRIBING INFORMATION: CONTENTS*

FULL PRESCRIBING INFORMATION

1 INDICATIONS AND USAGE

1.1 Control of Bleeding Episodes in Hemophilia A

XYNTHA Antihemophilic Factor (Recombinant), Plasma/Albumin-Free is indicated for the control and prevention of bleeding episodes in patients with hemophilia A (congenital factor VIII deficiency or classic hemophilia).

XYNTHA does not contain von Willebrand factor, and therefore is not indicated in von Willebrand's disease.

1.2 Surgical Prophylaxis in Patients with Hemophilia A

XYNTHA Antihemophilic Factor (Recombinant), Plasma/Albumin-Free is indicated for surgical prophylaxis in patients with hemophilia A.

2 DOSAGE AND ADMINISTRATION

Treatment with XYNTHA Antihemophilic Factor (Recombinant), Plasma/Albumin-Free should be initiated under the supervision of a physician experienced in the treatment of hemophilia A.

Dosage and duration of treatment depend on the severity of the factor VIII deficiency, the location and extent of bleeding, and the patient's clinical condition. Doses administered should be titrated to the patient's clinical response. In the presence of an inhibitor, higher doses may be required.[1]

One International Unit (IU) of factor VIII activity corresponds approximately to the quantity of factor VIII in one milliliter of normal human plasma. The calculation of the required dosage of factor VIII is based upon the empirical finding that, on average, 1 IU of factor VIII per kg body weight raises the plasma factor VIII activity by approximately 2 IU/dL.[2] The required dosage is determined using the following formula:

Required units = body weight (kg) × desired factor VIII rise (IU/dL or % of normal) × 0.5 (IU/kg per IU/dL)

The labeled potency of XYNTHA is based on the European Pharmacopoeia chromogenic substrate assay, in which the Wyeth manufacturing standard has been calibrated using a one-stage clotting assay. This method of potency assignment is intended to harmonize XYNTHA with clinical monitoring using a one-stage clotting assay [see Clinical Pharmacology (12.3)].

2.1 Control of Bleeding Episodes

In the case of the following bleeding events, consideration should be given to maintaining the factor VIII activity at or above the plasma levels (in % of normal or in IU/dL) outlined below for the indicated period.

The following chart can be used to guide dosing in bleeding episodes:

Type of Bleeding Episode	Factor VIII Level Required (IU/dL or % of normal)	Frequency of Doses/Duration of Therapy
Minor Early hemarthrosis, minor muscle or oral bleeds.	20–40	Repeat every 12-24 hours as necessary until resolved. At least 1 day, depending upon the severity of the bleeding episode.
Moderate Bleeding into muscles. Mild head trauma. Bleeding into the oral cavity.	30–60	Repeat infusion every 12-24 hours for 3-4 days or until adequate local hemostasis is achieved.
Major Gastrointestinal bleeding. Intracranial, intra-abdominal or intrathoracic bleeding. Fractures.	60–100	Repeat infusion every 8-24 hours until bleeding is resolved.

2.2 Surgical Prophylaxis in Patients with Hemophilia A

In the case of the following bleeding events, consideration should be given to maintaining the factor VIII activity at or above the plasma levels (in % of normal or in IU/dL) outlined below for the indicated period. Monitoring of replacement therapy by means of plasma factor VIII activity is recommended, particularly for surgical intervention.

The following chart can be used to guide dosing in surgery:

Type of Bleeding Episode	Factor VIII Level Required (IU/dL or % of normal)	Frequency of Doses/Duration of Therapy
Minor		
Minor operations, including tooth extraction.	30–60	Repeat infusion every 12-24 hours for 3-4 days or until adequate local hemostasis is achieved. For tooth extraction, a single infusion plus oral antifibrinolytic therapy within 1 hour may be sufficient.
Major		
Major operations.	60–100	Repeat infusion every 8-24 hours until threat is resolved, or in the case of surgery, until adequate local hemostasis and wound healing are achieved.

2.3 Instructions for Use

XYNTHA is administered by intravenous (IV) infusion after reconstitution of the freeze-dried powder with the supplied pre-filled diluent (0.9% Sodium Chloride solution) syringe. Patients should follow the specific reconstitution and administration procedures provided by their physicians. For instructions, patients should follow the recommendations in the *FDA-Approved Patient Labeling (17.6)*. The procedures below are provided as general guidelines for the reconstitution and administration of XYNTHA.

2.4 Preparation and Reconstitution

Preparation

1. Always wash your hands before performing the following procedures.
2. Aseptic technique (meaning clean and germ-free) should be used during the reconstitution procedure.
3. All components used in the reconstitution and administration of this product should be used as soon as possible after opening their sterile containers to minimize unnecessary exposure to the atmosphere.

Note: If you use more than one vial of XYNTHA per infusion, each vial should be reconstituted according to the following instructions. The diluent syringe should be removed, leaving the vial adapter in place, and a separate large luer lock syringe may be used to draw back the reconstituted contents of each vial. Do not detach the diluent syringes or the large luer lock syringe until you are ready to attach the large luer lock syringe to the next vial adapter.

Reconstitution

1. Allow the vials of freeze-dried XYNTHA and the pre-filled diluent syringe to reach room temperature.
2. Remove the plastic flip-top cap from the XYNTHA vial to expose the central portions of the rubber stopper.

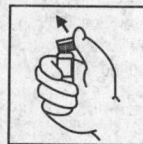

3. Wipe the top of the vial with the alcohol swab provided, or use another antiseptic solution, and allow to dry. After cleaning, do not touch the rubber stopper with your hand or allow it to touch any surface.
4. Peel back the cover from the clear plastic vial adapter package. **Do not remove the adapter from the package.**
5. Place the vial on a flat surface. While holding the adapter package, place the vial adapter over the vial and press down firmly on the package until the adapter spike penetrates the vial stopper.

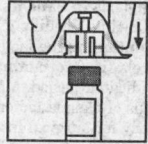

6. Grasp the plunger rod as shown in the diagram. Avoid contact with the shaft of the plunger rod. Attach the threaded end of the plunger rod to the diluent syringe plunger by pushing and turning firmly.

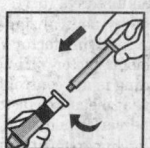

7. Break off the tamper-resistant plastic tip cap from the diluent syringe by snapping the perforation of the cap. Do not touch the inside of the cap or the syringe tip. The diluent syringe may need to be recapped (if not administering reconstituted XYNTHA immediately), so place the cap on its top on a clean surface in a spot where it would be least likely to become environmentally contaminated.

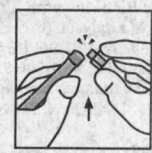

8. Lift the package away from the adapter and discard the package.

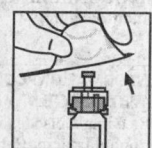

9. Place the vial on a flat surface. Connect the diluent syringe to the vial adapter by inserting the tip into the adapter opening while firmly pushing and turning the syringe clockwise until secured.

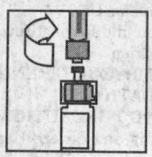

10. Slowly depress the plunger rod to inject all the diluent into the XYNTHA vial.

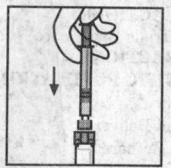

11. Without removing the syringe, **gently** swirl the contents of the vial until the powder is dissolved.
    Note: The final solution should be inspected visually for particulate matter before administration. The solution should be clear to slightly opalescent and colorless. If it is not, the solution should be discarded and a new kit should be used.
12. Invert the vial and slowly draw the solution into the syringe.

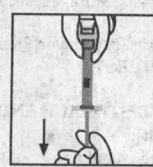

13. Detach the syringe from the vial adapter by gently pulling and turning the syringe counter-clockwise. Discard the vial with the adapter attached.
    Note: If the solution is not to be used immediately, the syringe cap should be carefully replaced. Do not touch the syringe tip or the inside of the cap.

The reconstituted solution may be stored at room temperature prior to administration, but should be administered within 3 hours.

XYNTHA, when reconstituted, contains polysorbate 80, which is known to increase the rate of di-(2-ethylhexyl)phthalate (DEHP) extraction from polyvinyl chloride (PVC). This should be considered during the preparation and administration of XYNTHA, including storage time elapsed in a PVC container following reconstitution. It is important that the recommendations in *Dosage and Administration (2)* be followed closely.

2.5 Administration

XYNTHA is administered by intravenous (IV) infusion after reconstitution with the supplied pre-filled diluent (0.9% Sodium Chloride solution, 4 mL) syringe. Parenteral drug products should be inspected for particulate matter and discoloration prior to administration, whenever solution and container permit.

XYNTHA should be administered using the tubing provided in this kit and the pre-filled diluent syringe provided, or a single sterile disposable plastic syringe. In addition, the solution should be withdrawn from the vial using the vial adapter.

1. Attach the syringe to the luer end of the infusion set tubing provided.
2. Apply a tourniquet and prepare the injections site by wiping the skin well with an alcohol swab provided in the kit.

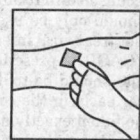

3. Perform venipuncture. Insert the needle on the infusion set tubing into the vein, and remove the tourniquet. The reconstituted XYNTHA product should be injected intravenously over several minutes. The rate of administration should be determined by the patient's comfort level.

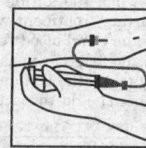

Reconstituted XYNTHA should not be administered in the same tubing or container with other medicinal products.[3]

Following completion of XYNTHA treatment, remove the infusion set and discard. Dispose of all unused solution, the empty vial(s), and the used needles and syringes in an appropriate container for throwing away waste that might hurt others if not handled properly.

3 DOSAGE FORMS AND STRENGTHS

XYNTHA is supplied as a white to off-white powder in the following dosages:
- 250 IU
- 500 IU
- 1000 IU
- 2000 IU

4 CONTRAINDICATIONS

None.

5 WARNINGS AND PRECAUTIONS

5.1 Anaphylaxis and Severe Hypersensitivity Reactions

Allergic type hypersensitivity reactions are possible. Patients should be informed of the early signs or symptoms of hypersensitivity reactions [including hives (rash with itching), generalized urticaria, tightness of the chest, wheezing, and hypotension] and anaphylaxis. Patients should be advised to discontinue use of the product and contact their physicians if these symptoms occur.

5.2 Neutralizing Antibodies

The occurrence of neutralizing antibodies (inhibitors) is well known in the treatment of patients with hemophilia A. Inhibitors have been detected in patients receiving factor VIII-containing products. Inhibitors are common in previously untreated patients[4, 5, 6] and have been observed in previously treated patients on factor VIII products.[7, 8, 9, 10, 11, 12] Patients using coagulation factor VIII products, including XYNTHA, should be monitored for the development of factor VIII inhibitors. If expected factor VIII activity plasma levels are not attained, or if bleeding is not controlled with an appropriate dose, an assay should be performed to determine if a factor VIII inhibitor is present. If detected, inhibitors should be titered in Bethesda Units (BU).

5.3 Formation of Antibodies to Hamster Protein

XYNTHA contains trace amounts of hamster proteins. Patients treated with this product could develop hypersensitivity to these non-human mammalian proteins.

5.4 Monitoring: Laboratory Tests

When clinically indicated, patients should have plasma factor VIII activity levels monitored by the one-stage clotting assay to confirm that adequate factor VIII levels have been achieved and are maintained [see *Dosage and Administration (2)*].

It is recommended that individual factor VIII values for recovery and, if clinically indicated, other pharmacokinetic characteristics be used to guide dosing and administration.

6   ADVERSE REACTIONS
6.1   Clinical Trials Experience
Because clinical trials are conducted under widely varying conditions, adverse reaction rates observed in the clinical trials of a drug cannot be directly compared to rates in the clinical trials of another drug and may not reflect the rates observed in clinical practice.

In Study 1, a pivotal phase 3 study in which previously treated patients (PTPs) with hemophilia A received XYNTHA for routine prophylaxis and on-demand treatment, 94 subjects received at least one dose of XYNTHA, resulting in a total of 6,775 infusions [see *Clinical Studies (14)*].

Study 2 is an on-going open-label, single-arm study of at least 25 evaluable PTPs with severe or moderately severe hemophilia A (factor VIII activity in plasma [FVIII:C] ≤ 2%) who require elective major surgery and are planned to receive XYNTHA replacement therapy for at least 6 days post-surgery. Twenty-two subjects received at least one dose of XYNTHA, resulting in 766 infusions [see *Clinical Studies (14)*].

In Study 1 (safety and efficacy study), the most frequently reported treatment-emergent adverse reaction was headache (24% of subjects). Other adverse reactions reported in ≥ 5% of subjects were: nausea (6%), diarrhea (5%), asthenia (5%) and pyrexia (5%). No subject developed anti-CHO or anti-TN8.2 antibodies.

In Study 2 (surgery study), the most frequently reported treatment-emergent adverse reaction was pyrexia (41% of subjects). Other adverse reactions reported in ≥ 5% of subjects were: headache (9%), nausea (9%), diarrhea (5%), vomiting (5%) and asthenia (5%). The adverse reactions reported in either study were considered mild or moderate in severity.

Immunogenicity is discussed below.

Immunogenicity

In Study 1, the incidence of FVIII inhibitors to XYNTHA was the primary safety endpoint. Two subjects with inhibitors were observed in 89 subjects (2.2%) who completed ≥ 50 exposure days. These results were consistent with the pre-specified endpoint that no more than 2 inhibitors may be observed in at least 81 subjects.

In a Bayesian statistical analysis, results from this study were used to update PTP results from a prior supporting study using XYNTHA manufactured at the initial facility, where one *de novo* and two recurrent inhibitors were observed in 110 subjects, and the experience with predecessor product (1 inhibitor in 113 subjects). This Bayesian analysis indicates that the population (true) inhibitor rate for XYNTHA, the estimate of the 95% upper limit of the true inhibitor rate, was 4.17% (see Table 1).

[See table 1 above]

7   DRUG INTERACTIONS
None known.

8   USE IN SPECIFIC POPULATIONS
8.1   Pregnancy
Pregnancy Category C

Animal reproduction studies have not been conducted with XYNTHA Antihemophilic Factor (Recombinant), Plasma/Albumin-Free. It is also not known whether XYNTHA can cause fetal harm when administered to a pregnant woman or can affect reproduction capacity. XYNTHA should be given to a pregnant woman only if clinically indicated.

8.2   Labor and Delivery
There is no information available on the effect of factor VIII replacement therapy on labor and delivery.

8.3   Nursing Mothers
It is not known whether this drug is excreted into human milk. Because many drugs are excreted into human milk, caution should be exercised if XYNTHA is administered to nursing mothers.

8.4   Pediatric Use
A study of XYNTHA in previously treated patients less than 6 years of age is currently ongoing.

Pharmacokinetics of XYNTHA was studied in 7 previously treated patients 12-16 years of age. Pharmacokinetic parameters in these patients were similar to those obtained for adults after a dose of 50 IU/kg. For these 7 patients, the mean (± SD) C_{max} and AUC_∞ were 1.09 ± 0.21 IU/mL and 11.5 ± 5.2 IU·h/mL, respectively. The mean clearance and plasma half-life values were 5.23 ± 2.36 mL/h/kg and 8.03 ± 2.44 hours (range 3.52–10.6 hours), respectively. The mean K-value and *in vivo* recoveries were 2.18 ± 0.41 IU/dL per IU/kg and 112 ± 23%, respectively.

8.5   Geriatric Use
Clinical studies of XYNTHA did not include subjects aged 65 and over. In general, dose selection for an elderly patient should be individualized.

Table 1: Bayesian Posterior Distribution of Inhibitor Rate

FVIII Inhibitor Nijmegen Result (BU/mL)	Number of Inhibitors	Number of Subjects Analyzed	Observed Inhibitor Rate (%)	Alpha[a]	Beta[b]	Posterior Probability[c]	95% Upper Limit of Inhibitor Rate (%)[d]
				---Posterior Beta Distribution Characteristics---			
≥0.6	2	89	2.25	4.5	197	0.9613	4.17

[a] Prior alpha of 2.5 plus the number of observed inhibitors.
[b] Prior beta of 110 plus the number of subjects analyzed minus the number of observed inhibitors.
[c] Posterior probability is the probability that the true inhibitor rate is less than the upper acceptable limit of 4.4%. A posterior probability greater than 0.95 is deemed acceptable.
[d] The 95% upper limit of the true inhibitor rate (the maximum rate calculated with at least 95% probability) based on the posterior distribution. An inhibitor rate less than 4.4% is deemed acceptable.

10   OVERDOSAGE
No symptoms of overdose have been reported.

11   DESCRIPTION
Antihemophilic Factor (Recombinant), Plasma/Albumin-Free, the active ingredient in XYNTHA, is a recombinant coagulation factor VIII produced by recombinant DNA technology for use in therapy of factor VIII deficiency. The Antihemophilic Factor (Recombinant), Plasma/Albumin-Free in XYNTHA is a purified glycoprotein, with an approximate molecular mass of 170 kDa consisting of 1,438 amino acids, which does not contain the B-domain.[13] The amino acid sequence of Antihemophilic Factor (Recombinant), Plasma/Albumin-Free in XYNTHA is comparable to the 90 + 80 kDa form of human factor VIII.

The Antihemophilic Factor (Recombinant), Plasma/Albumin-Free in XYNTHA is secreted by a genetically engineered Chinese hamster ovary (CHO) cell line. The cell line is grown in a chemically defined cell culture medium that contains recombinant insulin, but does not contain any materials derived from human or animal sources. The Antihemophilic Factor (Recombinant), Plasma/Albumin-Free in XYNTHA is purified by a process that uses a series of chromatography steps, one of which is based on affinity chromatography using a patented synthetic peptide affinity ligand.[14] The process also includes a solvent-detergent viral inactivation step and a virus-retaining nanofiltration step. The potency expressed in International Units (IU) is determined using the chromogenic assay of the European Pharmacopoeia. The Wyeth manufacturing reference standard for potency has been calibrated against the World Health Organization (WHO) International Standard for factor VIII activity using the one-stage clotting assay. The specific activity of XYNTHA is 5,500 to 9,900 IU per milligram of protein.

XYNTHA is formulated as a sterile, nonpyrogenic, preservative-free, freeze-dried powder preparation for intravenous (IV) injection. Each single-use vial contains nominally 250, 500, 1000 or 2000 IU of XYNTHA. Upon reconstitution, the product is a clear to slightly opalescent, colorless solution that contains sodium chloride, sucrose, L-histidine, calcium chloride and polysorbate 80.

12   CLINICAL PHARMACOLOGY
12.1   Mechanism of Action
Factor VIII is the specific clotting factor deficient in patients with hemophilia A (classical hemophilia).[15] Activated factor VIII acts as a cofactor for activated factor IX, accelerating the conversion of factor X to activated factor X.[15] Activated factor X converts prothrombin into thrombin.[15] Thrombin then converts fibrinogen into fibrin, and a clot is formed.[15] Factor VIII activity is greatly reduced in patients with hemophilia A, and, therefore, replacement therapy is necessary. The administration of XYNTHA increases plasma levels of factor VIII activity and can temporarily correct the coagulation defect in these patients.

12.2   Pharmacodynamics
The administration of XYNTHA increases plasma levels of factor VIII activity and can temporarily correct the coagulation defect in hemophilia A patients.

12.3   Pharmacokinetics
In a pivotal crossover clinical study, 30 evaluable previously treated patients [PTP] (≥ 12 years) received a single infusion of 50 IU/kg of XYNTHA followed by a full-length recombinant FVIII (FLrFVIII, Advate®) or a single infusion of FLrFVIII followed by XYNTHA in a randomized crossover design. The one-stage clotting assay method was used to determine the concentrations of these two products in blood. XYNTHA was shown to be pharmacokinetically equivalent to FLrFVIII as the 90% confidence intervals for XYNTHA-to-FLrFVIII ratios of the mean values of C_{max} and AUC_∞ were within pre-established limits of 80% to 125%. The pharmacokinetic parameters of XYNTHA in the above group of patients are summarized in Table 2.

In addition, 25 PTPs received a single infusion of 50 IU/kg of XYNTHA for a 6-month follow-up PK study. The pharmacokinetic parameters were comparable between baseline and month 6, indicating no time-dependent changes in the pharmacokinetic properties of XYNTHA; the 90% confidence intervals for XYNTHA 6 month-to-baseline ratios of the mean values of C_{max} and AUC_∞ were within pre-established limits of 80% to 125%.

Table 2: Pharmacokinetic Parameter Estimates for XYNTHA at Baseline (Cross-over phase) and Month 6 (Follow-up phase) in Previously Treated Patients with Hemophilia A

Parameter	Parameters at Initial Visit (Crossover phase, n = 30) Mean ± SD	Parameters at Month 6 (Follow-up phase, n = 25) Mean ± SD
C_{max} (IU/mL)	1.08 ± 0.22	1.24 ± 0.42
AUC_∞ (IU•hr/mL)	13.5 ± 5.6	15.0 ± 7.5
$t_{1/2}$ (hr)	11.2 ± 5.0	11.8 ± 6.2*
CL (mL/hr/kg)	4.51 ± 2.23	4.04 ± 1.87
K-value (IU/dL per IU/kg)	2.15 ± 0.44	2.47 ± 0.84
In vivo Recovery (%)	103 ± 21	116 ± 40

Abbreviations: AUC_∞ = area under the plasma concentration-time curve from zero to infinity; C_{max} = peak concentration; K-value = incremental recovery; $t_{1/2}$ = plasma elimination half-life; CL = clearance; n = number of subjects; SD = standard deviation.
* One subject was excluded from the calculation due to lack of a well-defined terminal phase.

13   NONCLINICAL TOXICOLOGY
13.1   Carcinogenesis, Mutagenesis, Impairment of Fertility
No studies have been conducted with XYNTHA to assess its mutagenic or carcinogenic potential. XYNTHA has been shown to be comparable to the predecessor product with respect to its biochemical and physicochemical properties, as well as its non-clinical *in vivo* pharmacology and toxicology. By inference, predecessor product and XYNTHA would be expected to have equivalent mutagenic and carcinogenic potential. The predecessor product has been shown to be non-genotoxic in the mouse micronucleus assay. No studies have been conducted in animals to assess impairment of fertility or fetal development.

13.2   Animal Toxicology and/or Pharmacology
Preclinical studies evaluating XYNTHA in hemophilia A dogs without inhibitors demonstrated safe and effective restoration of hemostasis. XYNTHA demonstrated a toxicological profile that was similar to the toxicological profile observed with the predecessor product. Toxicity associated with XYNTHA was primarily associated with anti-FVIII neutralizing antibody generation first detectable at 15 days of repeat dosing in high (approximately 735 IU/kg/day) level-dosed, non-human primates.

14   CLINICAL STUDIES
The efficacy of XYNTHA was evaluated in Study 1, in which subjects received XYNTHA on a prophylaxis treatment regimen, with on-demand treatment administered as clinically indicated. Ninety-four (94) subjects were enrolled and treated with at least one dose, and all are included in the intent-to-treat (ITT) population. Eighty-nine (89) subjects accrued ≥ 50 exposure days. From the 94 subjects enrolled, thirty (30) evaluable subjects participated in the PK study and received at least 1 PK dose. Twenty-five (25) evaluable subjects with FVIII:C ≤ 1% completed both the first (PK1) and the second (PK2) assessments [see *Clinical*

Pharmacology (12.3)]. Median age for the 94 treated subjects was 24 years (mean 27.7 and range 12-60 years). All subjects had ≥ 150 previous exposure days with baseline FVIII activity level of ≤ 2%.

In the open-label safety and efficacy period, all 94 subjects received XYNTHA for routine prophylaxis at the dose of 30 ± 5 IU/kg 3 times a week with provisions for dose escalation based on pre-specified criteria. Seven (7) dose escalations were prescribed for 6 subjects during the course of the study. Forty-three (43) of ninety-four (94), i.e. 45.7%, subjects reported no bleeding while on routine prophylaxis. The median annualized bleeding rate (ABR) for all bleeding episodes was 1.9 (mean 3.9, range 0 to 42.1).

Fifty-three (53) of 94 subjects received XYNTHA for on-demand treatment for a total of 187 bleeding episodes (Table 3). Seven of these bleeding episodes occurred in subjects prior to switching to a prophylaxis treatment regimen. One hundred ten of one hundred eighty (110/180) bleeds (61.1%) occurred ≤ 48 hours after the last dose and 38.9% (70 of 180 bleeds) occurred > 48 hours after the last dose. The majority of bleeds reported to occur ≤ 48 hours after the last prophylaxis dose were traumatic (64 of 110 bleeds; 58.2%). Forty-two (42) of 70 bleeds (60%) reported to occur > 48 hours after the last prophylaxis dose were spontaneous. The on-demand treatment dosing regimen was determined by the investigator. The median dose for on-demand treatment was 30.6 IU/kg (range, 6.4 to 74.4 IU/kg).

[See table 3 above]

The majority of bleeding episodes (173/187; 92.5%) resolved with 1 or 2 infusions. Subjects rated the outcomes of infusions on a pre-specified four (4) point hemostatic efficacy scale. One hundred thirty-two (132) of 187 bleeding episodes (70.6%) treated with XYNTHA were rated excellent or good in their response to initial treatment, 45 (24.1%) were rated moderate. Five [5] (2.7%) were rated no response, and 5 (2.7%) were not rated.

[See table 4 at right]

In an ongoing, open-label study of XYNTHA in surgical prophylaxis, 21 of at least 25 evaluable PTPs with severe or moderately severe (FVIII:C ≤ 2%) hemophilia A undergoing major surgical procedures received XYNTHA. One (1) subject received XYNTHA for a pre-surgery pharmacokinetic assessment only and had not undergone surgery.

The results of an interim analysis on 21 of the 25 planned evaluable subjects who had undergone major surgical procedures (13 total knee replacements, 1 hip replacement, 3 synovectomies, 1 left ulnar nerve transposition release, 1 ventral hernia repair/scar revision, 1 knee arthroscopy, 1 revision and debridement of the knee after a total knee replacement) are presented in Table 5. For the 21 surgical subjects, investigator's ratings of efficacy at the end of surgery and at the end of the initial postoperative period were excellent or good for all assessments. All reported blood loss during the intra-operative and postoperative periods was rated normal with the exception of one subject who experienced iatrogenic bleeding.

Table 5: Summary of Hemostatic Efficacy

Time of Hemostatic Efficacy Assessment	Excellent	Good	Number of subjects
End of surgery	14 (67%)	7 (33%)	21
End of initial postoperative period[a]	16 (84%)	3 (16%)	19

[a] Conclusion of initial postoperative period is date of discharge or postoperative Day 6, whichever occurs later.

15   REFERENCES

1. Nilsson IM, Berntorp EE and Freiburghaus C. Treatment of patients with factor VIII and IX inhibitors. *Thromb Haemost.* 1993;70(1):56-59.
2. Hoyer LW. Hemophilia A. *N Engl J Med.* 1994;330: 38-47.
3. Juhlin F. Stability and Compatibility of Reconstituted Recombinant Factor VIII SQ, 250 IU/ml, in a System for Continuous Infusion. Pharmacia Document 9610224, 1996.
4. Ehrenforth S, Kreuz W, Scharrer I, et al. Incidence of development of factor VIII and factor IX inhibitors in hemophiliacs. *Lancet.* 1992;339:594-598.
5. Lusher J, Arkin S, Abildgaard CF, Schwartz RS, the Kogenate PUP Study Group. Recombinant factor VIII for the treatment of previously untreated patients with hemophilia A. *N Engl J Med.* 1993;328:453-459.
6. Bray GL, Gomperts ED, Courter S, et al. A multicenter study of recombinant factor VIII (Recombinate): safety, efficacy, and inhibitor risk in previously untreated patients with hemophilia A. *Blood.* 1994;83(9):2428-2435.
7. Kessler C, Sachse K. Factor VIII:C inhibitor associated with monoclonal-antibody purified FVIII concentrate. *Lancet.* 1990;335:1403.
8. Schwartz RS, Abildgaard CF, Aledort LM, et al. Human recombinant DNA-derived antihemophilic factor (factor VIII) in the treatment of hemophilia A. *N Engl J Med.* 1990;323:1800-1805.
9. White GC II, Courter S, Bray GL, et al. A multicenter study of recombinant Factor VIII (Recombinate™) in previously treated patients with hemophilia A. *Thromb Haemost.* 1997;77(4):660-667.
10. Gruppo R, Chen H, Schroth P, et al. Safety and immunogenicity of recombinant factor VIII (Recombinate™) in previously untreated patients: A 7.3 year update. *Haemophilia.* 1998;4:228 (Abstract No. 291, XXIII Congress of the WFH, The Hague).
11. Scharrer I, Bray GL, Neutzling O. Incidence of inhibitors in haemophilia A patients - a review of recent studies of recombinant and plasma-derived factor VIII concentrates. *Haemophilia.* 1999;5:145-154.
12. Abshire TC, Brackmann HH, Scharrer I, et al. Sucrose formulated recombinant human antihemophilic Factor VIII is safe and efficacious for treatment of hemophilia A in home therapy: Results of a multicenter, international, clinical investigation. *Thromb Haemost.* 2000;83(6): 811-816.
13. Sandberg H, Almstedt A, Brandt J, Castro VM, Gray E, Holmquist L, et al. Structural and Functional Characterization of B-Domain Deleted Recombinant Factor VIII. *Sem Hematol.* 2001;38 (Suppl. 4):4-12.
14. Kelley BD, Tannatt M, Magnusson R, Hagelberg S. Development and Validation of an Affinity Chromatography Step Using a Peptide Ligand for cGMP Production of Factor VIII. *Biotechnol Bioeng.* 2004;87(3):400-412.
15. Mann KG and Ziedens KB. Overview of Hemostasis. In: Lee CA, Berntorp EE and Hoots WK, eds. *Textbook of Hemophilia.* USA, Blackwell Publishing; 2005:1-4.

16   HOW SUPPLIED/STORAGE AND HANDLING

16.1   How Supplied

XYNTHA™ Antihemophilic Factor (Recombinant), Plasma/Albumin-Free is supplied in kits that include single-use (Freeze-Dried) vials that contain nominally 250, 500, 1000, or 2000 IU per vial:

250 IU Kit: NDC 58394-012-01
500 IU Kit: NDC 58394-013-01
1000 IU Kit: NDC 58394-014-01
2000 IU Kit: NDC 58394-015-01

Actual factor VIII activity in IU is stated on the label of each XYNTHA Antihemophilic Factor (Recombinant), Plasma/Albumin-Free vial.

In addition, each XYNTHA Antihemophilic Factor (Recombinant), Plasma/Albumin-Free kit contains: one pre-filled diluent syringe containing 4 mL 0.9% Sodium Chloride with plunger rod for assembly, one vial adapter, one sterile infusion set, two alcohol swabs, one bandage, one gauze, and one package insert.

16.2   Storage and Handling

Product as packaged for sale: XYNTHA Antihemophilic Factor (Recombinant), Plasma/Albumin-Free should be stored under refrigeration at a temperature of 2° to 8°C (36° to 46°F). XYNTHA may also be stored at room temperature not to exceed 25°C (77°F) for up to 3 months, until the expiration date. The patient should write in the space provided on the outer carton, the date the product was placed at room temperature. At the end of the 3-month period, the product should not be put back into the refrigerator, but should be used immediately or discarded. The diluent syringe may be stored at 2° to 25°C (36° to 77°F). Freezing should be avoided to prevent damage to the pre-filled diluent syringe. During storage, avoid prolonged exposure of XYNTHA vial to light. Do not use XYNTHA after the expiration date on the label.

Product after reconstitution: The reconstituted solution may be stored at room temperature prior to administration. The product does not contain a preservative and should be used within 3 hours.

United States Patent Numbers: 4,868,112; 5,733,873; 5,919,766; 6,005,082; 6,492,105; 5,831,026; 5,378,612.

17   PATIENT COUNSELING INFORMATION

17.1   Allergic-type Hypersensitivity Reactions

Allergic-type hypersensitivity reactions are possible. Patients should be informed of the early signs of hypersensitivity reactions [including hives (rash with itching), generalized urticaria, tightness of the chest, wheezing, hypotension] and anaphylaxis. Patients should be advised to discontinue use of the product and contact their physicians if these symptoms occur.

17.2   Neutralizing Antibodies (Inhibitors)

Patients should be advised to contact their physician or treatment facility for further treatment and/or assessment, if they experience a lack of a clinical response to factor VIII replacement therapy, as this may be a manifestation of an inhibitor.

17.3   Pregnancy

Female patients should be advised to notify their physician if they become pregnant or intend to become pregnant during therapy.

17.4   Nursing

Patients should be advised to notify their physician if they are breastfeeding.

17.5   Usage While Traveling

Based on their current regimen, individuals with hemophilia using XYNTHA should be advised to bring an adequate supply of XYNTHA for anticipated treatment when traveling. Patients should be advised to consult with their healthcare professional prior to travel.

17.6   FDA-Approved Patient Labeling

XYNTHA ™ (ZIN-tha)

[ANTIHEMOPHILIC FACTOR (RECOMBINANT), PLASMA/ALBUMIN-FREE]

Please read this Patient Information carefully before using XYNTHA and each time you get a refill. There may be new information. This leaflet does not take the place of talking with your doctor about your medical problems or your treatment.

What is XYNTHA?

XYNTHA is an injectable medicine that is used to help control and prevent bleeding in people with hemophilia A. Hemophilia A is also called classic hemophilia.

Table 3: Time Interval Between Last Prophylaxis Dose of XYNTHA and Start of Bleed

≤ 24 hrs		> 24 ≤ 48 hrs		> 48 ≤ 72 hrs		> 72 hrs		Unknown[a]		Total Bleeding Episodes
Spon	Traum	Spon	Traum	Spon	Traum	Spon	Traum	Spon	Traum	
13	20	33	44	24	12	18	16	3	4	187

[a] Bleeds with unknown start time or bleeds in which previous prophylaxis dose was before the start of the safety and efficacy period of the study. Abbreviations: Spon = spontaneous new bleed; Traum = new bleed due to trauma; hrs = hours.

Table 4: Summary of Response to Infusions to Treat New Bleeding Episode by Number of Infusions Needed for Resolution

Response to 1st Infusion	--------------------Number of Infusions (%)--------------------					Total Number of Bleeds
	1	2	3	4	> 4	
Excellent	42 (95.5)	2 (4.5)	0 (0.0)	0 (0.0)	0 (0.0)	44
Good	69 (78.4)	16 (18.2)	3 (3.4)	0 (0.0)	0 (0.0)	88
Moderate	24 (53.3)	16 (35.6)	2 (4.4)	0 (0.0)	3 (6.7)	45
No Response	0 (0.0)	0 (0.0)	2 (40.0)	2 (40.0)	1 (20.0)	5
Not Assessed	4 (80.0)	0 (0.0)	0 (0.0)	1 (20.0)	0 (0.0)	5[a]
Total	139 (74.3)	34 (18.2)	7 (3.7)	3 (1.6)	4 (2.1)	187

[a] Includes 1 infusion with commercial FVIII that occurred before routine prophylaxis began.

XYNTHA is not used to treat von Willebrand's disease.

What should I tell my doctor before using XYNTHA?

Tell your doctor about all of your medical conditions, including if you:

• are pregnant or planning to become pregnant. It is not known if XYNTHA may harm your unborn baby.

• are breastfeeding. It is not known if XYNTHA passes into your milk and if it can harm your baby.

Tell your doctor and pharmacist about all of the medicines you take, including all prescription and non-prescription medicines, such as over-the-counter medicines, supplements, or herbal remedies.

How should I infuse XYNTHA?

See the step-by-step instructions for infusing XYNTHA at the end of this leaflet. You should always follow the specific instructions given by your doctor. The steps listed below are general guidelines for using XYNTHA. If you are unsure of the procedures, please call your doctor or pharmacist before using.

Call your doctor right away if bleeding is not controlled after using XYNTHA.

Your doctor will prescribe the dose that you should take.

Your doctor may need to take blood tests from time to time.

Talk to your doctor before traveling. You should plan to bring enough XYNTHA for your treatment during this time.

What if I take too much XYNTHA?

Call your doctor if you take too much XYNTHA.

What are the possible side effects of XYNTHA?

Allergic reactions may occur with XYNTHA. Call your doctor or get emergency treatment right away if you have any of the following symptoms:

wheezing

difficulty breathing

chest tightness

turning blue (look at lips and gums)

fast heartbeat

swelling of the face

faintness

rash

hives

Your body can also make antibodies, called "inhibitors," against XYNTHA, which may stop XYNTHA from working properly.

Some common side effects of XYNTHA are headache, fever, nausea, vomiting, diarrhea, or weakness.

These are not all the possible side effects of XYNTHA.

Tell your doctor about any side effect that bothers you or that does not go away.

How should I store XYNTHA?

Do not freeze XYNTHA.

Store XYNTHA in the refrigerator at 36° to 46°F (2° to 8°C). XYNTHA can last at room temperature (below 77°F) for up to 3 months. If you store XYNTHA at room temperature, be careful to write down the date you put XYNTHA at room temperature, so you will know when to throw it out. There is a space on the carton for you to write the date.

Throw away any unused XYNTHA after the expiration date.

After reconstituting XYNTHA, you can store it at room temperature for up to 3 hours. If you have not used it in 3 hours, throw it away.

Store the diluent syringe at 36° to 77°F (2° to 25°C).

Do not use reconstituted XYNTHA if it is not clear to slightly opalescent and colorless.

What else should I know about XYNTHA?

Medicines are sometimes prescribed for purposes other than those listed here. Do not use XYNTHA for a condition for which it is not prescribed. Do not share XYNTHA with other people, even if they have the same symptoms that you have. This leaflet summarizes the most important information about XYNTHA. If you would like more information, talk to your doctor. You can ask your doctor or pharmacist for information about XYNTHA that was written for healthcare professionals.

Instructions for Using XYNTHA

XYNTHA is supplied as a powder. Before it can be infused in your vein (intravenous injection), you must reconstitute the powder by mixing it with the liquid diluent supplied. The liquid diluent is 0.9% Sodium Chloride. XYNTHA should be reconstituted and infused using the infusion set, diluent, syringe, and adapter provided in this kit, and by following the directions below.

RECONSTITUTION

Always wash your hands before doing the following steps. Try to keep everything clean and germ-free while you are reconstituting XYNTHA. Once you open the vials, you should finish reconstituting XYNTHA as soon as possible. This will help to keep them germ-free.

Note: If you use more than one vial of XYNTHA for each infusion, reconstitute each vial according to steps 1 through 11.

1. Let the vial of XYNTHA and the pre-filled diluent syringe reach room temperature.

2. Remove the plastic flip-top cap from the XYNTHA vial to show the center part of the rubber stopper.

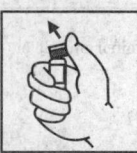

3. Wipe the top of the vial with the alcohol swab provided, or use another antiseptic solution, and allow to dry. After cleaning, do not touch the rubber stopper with your hand or allow it to touch any surface.

4. Peel back the cover from the clear plastic vial adapter package. **Do not remove the adapter from the package.**

5. Place the vial on a flat surface. While holding the adapter in the package, place the vial adapter over the vial. Press down firmly on the package until the adapter snaps into place on top of the vial, with the adapter spike going into the vial stopper.

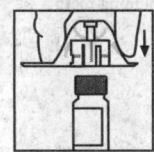

6. Grasp the plunger rod as shown in the picture below. Do not touch the shaft of the plunger rod. Attach the threaded end of the plunger rod to the diluent syringe plunger by pushing and turning firmly.

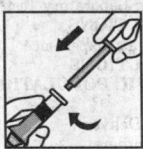

7. Break off the tamper-resistant, plastic-tip cap from the diluent syringe by snapping the perforation of the cap. Do not touch the inside of the cap or the syringe tip. The diluent syringe may need to be recapped (if reconstituted XYNTHA is not used immediately), so place the cap on its top on a clean surface in a spot where it will stay clean.

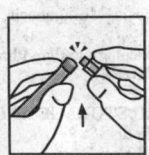

8. Lift the package cover away from the adapter and discard the package.

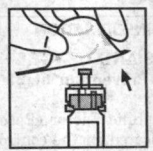

9. Place the vial on a flat surface. Connect the diluent syringe to the vial adapter by inserting the tip of the syringe into the adapter opening while firmly pushing and turning the syringe clockwise until the connection is secured.

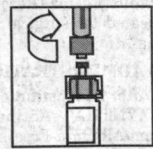

10. Slowly push the plunger rod to inject all the diluent into the XYNTHA vial.

[See figure at top of next column]

11. With the syringe still connected to the adapter, **gently** swirl the contents of the vial until the powder is dissolved.

Look at the final solution before infusing it. The solution should be clear to slightly opalescent and colorless. If it is not, throw away the solution and use a new kit.

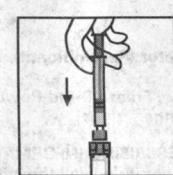

12. Make sure the syringe plunger rod is still fully pressed down, then turn over the vial. Slowly pull the solution into the syringe. Turn the syringe upward again and remove any air bubbles by gently tapping the syringe with your finger and slowly pushing air out of the syringe.

If you reconstituted more than one vial of XYNTHA, remove the diluent syringe from the vial adapter and leave the vial adapter attached to the vial. Quickly attach a separate large luer lock syringe and pull the reconstituted solution as instructed above. Repeat this procedure with each vial in turn. Do not detach the diluent syringes or the large luer lock syringe until you are ready to attach the large luer lock syringe to the next vial adapter.

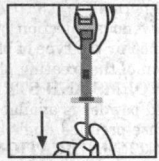

13. Remove the syringe from the vial adapter by gently pulling and turning the syringe counterclockwise. Throw away the vial with the adapter attached.

If you are not using the solution right away, you should carefully replace the syringe cap. Do not touch the syringe tip or the inside of the cap.

XYNTHA should be infused within 3 hours after reconstitution. The reconstituted solution may be stored at room temperature prior to infusion.

INFUSION (Intravenous Injection)

Your doctor or healthcare professional should teach you how to infuse XYNTHA. Once you learn how to self-infuse, you can follow the instructions in this insert.

1. Attach the syringe to the luer end of the provided infusion set tubing.

2. Apply a tourniquet and prepare the injection site by wiping the skin well with an alcohol swab provided in the kit.

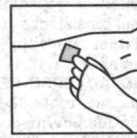

3. Insert the butterfly needle of the infusion set tubing into your vein as instructed by your doctor or healthcare professional. Remove the tourniquet. Infuse the reconstituted XYNTHA product over several minutes. Your comfort level should determine the rate of infusion.

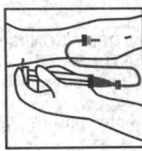

4. After infusing XYNTHA, remove the infusion set and discard. The amount of drug product left in the infusion set will not affect your treatment. Dispose of all unused solution, the empty vial(s), and the used needles and syringes in an appropriate container used for throwing away waste that might hurt others if not handled properly.

It is a good idea to record the lot number from the XYNTHA vial label every time you use XYNTHA. You can use the peel-off label found on the vial to record the lot number.

This Patient Package Insert has been approved by the U.S. Food and Drug Administration.

Wyeth®

Wyeth Pharmaceuticals Inc.

Philadelphia, PA 19101

W10528C004

ET01

Rev 04/08

Type of Bleeding Episode	Factor VIII Level Required (IU/dL or % of normal)	Frequency of Doses/Duration of Therapy
Minor		
Early hemarthrosis, minor muscle or oral bleeds.	20–40	Repeat every 12-24 hours as necessary until resolved. At least 1 day, depending upon the severity of the bleeding episode.
Moderate		
Bleeding into muscles. Mild head trauma. Bleeding into the oral cavity.	30–60	Repeat infusion every 12-24 hours for 3-4 days or until adequate local hemostasis is achieved.
Major		
Gastrointestinal bleeding. Intracranial, intra-abdominal or intrathoracic bleeding. Fractures.	60–100	Repeat infusion every 8-24 hours until bleeding is resolved.

Type of Surgery	Factor VIII Level Required (IU/dL or % of normal)	Frequency of Doses/Duration of Therapy
Minor		
Minor operations, including tooth extraction.	30–60	Repeat infusion every 12-24 hours for 3-4 days or until adequate local hemostasis is achieved. For tooth extraction, a single infusion plus oral antifibrinolytic therapy within 1 hour may be sufficient.
Major		
Major operations.	60–100	Repeat infusion every 8-24 hours until threat is resolved, or in the case of surgery, until adequate local hemostasis and wound healing are achieved.

XYNTHA ℞

[*ZIN-tha*]

[Antihemophilic Factor (Recombinant), Plasma/Albumin-Free]
For Intravenous Use, Freeze-Dried Powder in Prefilled Dual-Chamber Syringe

HIGHLIGHTS OF PRESCRIBING INFORMATION

These highlights do not include all the information needed to use XYNTHA safely and effectively. See full prescribing information for XYNTHA.

XYNTHA [Antihemophilic Factor (Recombinant), Plasma/Albumin-Free] For Intravenous Use, Freeze-Dried Powder in Prefilled Dual-Chamber Syringe
Initial U.S. Approval: 2008

INDICATIONS AND USAGE

XYNTHA is an Antihemophilic (Recombinant) Factor indicated for:
- Control and prevention of bleeding episodes in patients with hemophilia A (1.1)
- Surgical prophylaxis in patients with hemophilia A (1.2)

DOSAGE AND ADMINISTRATION

For intravenous use after reconstitution only (2)
- The required dosage is determined using the following formula:
  Required units = body weight (kg) × desired factor VIII rise (IU/dL or % of normal) × 0.5 (IU/kg per IU/dL)
- Frequency of intravenous injection of the reconstituted product is determined by the type of bleeding episode and the recommendation of the treating physician. (2.1, 2.2)

DOSAGE FORMS AND STRENGTHS

XYNTHA freeze-dried powder is available as:
3000 IU in a single-use prefilled dual-chamber syringe. (3)

CONTRAINDICATIONS

None.

WARNINGS AND PRECAUTIONS

- Anaphylaxis and severe hypersensitivity reactions are possible. Should such reactions occur, treatment with the product should be discontinued, and appropriate treatment should be administered. (5.1)
- Development of activity-neutralizing antibodies has been detected in patients receiving factor VIII-containing products. If expected plasma factor VIII activity levels are not attained, or if bleeding is not controlled with an appropriate dose, an assay that measures factor VIII inhibitor concentration should be performed. (5.2, 5.4)
- Patients may develop hypersensitivity to hamster protein, which is present in trace amounts in the product. (5.3)

ADVERSE REACTIONS

The most common adverse reaction in Study 1 is headache (24% of subjects) and in Study 2 is pyrexia (41% of subjects). (6.1)

Two out of 89 subjects (who completed ≥ 50 exposure days) developed an inhibitor during the course of the study. The observation of 2 inhibitors in 89 subjects who completed ≥ 50 exposure days was consistent with a 95% probability that the inhibitor formation rate with XYNTHA is less than 4.17% using a Bayesian analysis. (6.1)

To report SUSPECTED ADVERSE REACTIONS, contact Wyeth Pharmaceuticals, Inc. at 1-800-934-5556 or FDA at 1-800-FDA-1088 or www.fda.gov/medwatch

DRUG INTERACTIONS

None.

USE IN SPECIFIC POPULATIONS

Pregnancy: No human or animal data. Use only if clearly needed. (8.1)

See 17 for PATIENT COUNSELING INFORMATION and FDA-approved patient labeling

Revised: 08/2010

FULL PRESCRIBING INFORMATION: CONTENTS*

* Sections or subsections omitted from the full prescribing information are not listed

FULL PRESCRIBING INFORMATION

1 INDICATIONS AND USAGE

1.1 Control and Prevention of Bleeding Episodes in Hemophilia A

XYNTHA Antihemophilic Factor (Recombinant), Plasma/Albumin-Free is indicated for the control and prevention of bleeding episodes in patients with hemophilia A (congenital factor VIII deficiency or classic hemophilia).

XYNTHA does not contain von Willebrand factor, and therefore is not indicated in patients with von Willebrand's disease.

1.2 Surgical Prophylaxis in Patients with Hemophilia A

XYNTHA Antihemophilic Factor (Recombinant), Plasma/Albumin-Free is indicated for surgical prophylaxis in patients with hemophilia A.

2 DOSAGE AND ADMINISTRATION

For Intravenous Use After Reconstitution

Treatment with XYNTHA Antihemophilic Factor (Recombinant), Plasma/Albumin-Free should be initiated under the supervision of a physician experienced in the treatment of hemophilia A.

Dosage and duration of treatment depend on the severity of the factor VIII deficiency, the location and extent of bleeding, and the patient's clinical condition. Doses administered should be titrated to the patient's clinical response. In the presence of an inhibitor, higher doses may be required.[1]

One International Unit (IU) of factor VIII activity corresponds approximately to the quantity of factor VIII in one milliliter of normal human plasma. The calculation of the required dosage of factor VIII is based upon the empirical finding that, on average, 1 IU of factor VIII per kg body weight raises the plasma factor VIII activity by approximately 2 IU/dL.[2] The required dosage is determined using the following formula:

Required units = body weight (kg) × desired factor VIII rise (IU/dL or % of normal) × 0.5 (IU/kg per IU/dL)

The labeled potency of XYNTHA is based on the European Pharmacopoeia chromogenic substrate assay, in which the Wyeth manufacturing standard has been calibrated using a one-stage clotting assay. This method of potency assignment is intended to harmonize XYNTHA with clinical monitoring using a one-stage clotting assay [*see Clinical Pharmacology (12.3)*].

2.1 Control and Prevention of Bleeding Episodes

In the case of the following bleeding events, consideration should be given to maintaining the factor VIII activity at or above the plasma levels (in % of normal or in IU/dL) outlined below for the indicated period.

The following chart can be used to guide dosing in bleeding episodes:

[See first table above]

2.2 Surgical Prophylaxis in Patients with Hemophilia A

In the case of the following bleeding events, consideration should be given to maintaining the factor VIII activity at or above the plasma levels (in % of normal or in IU/dL) outlined below for the indicated period. Monitoring of replacement therapy by means of plasma factor VIII activity is recommended, particularly for surgical intervention.

The following chart can be used to guide dosing in surgery:

[See second table above]

2.3 Instructions for Use

XYNTHA is administered by intravenous (IV) infusion after reconstitution of the freeze-dried powder with the diluent (0.9% Sodium Chloride). Both the XYNTHA powder and the diluent are supplied within the prefilled dual-chamber syringe.

Patients should follow the specific reconstitution and administration procedures provided by their physicians. For instructions, patients should follow the recommendations in the *FDA-Approved Patient Labeling (17)*. The procedures below are provided as general guidelines for the reconstitution and administration of XYNTHA.

Additional instructions are provided after *Administration 2.5* that detail the use of a XYNTHA Prefilled Dual-Chamber Syringe and a XYNTHA vial or multiple XYNTHA Prefilled Dual-Chamber Syringes [*see Use of a XYNTHA Vial Kit and a XYNTHA Prefilled Dual-Chamber Syringe Kit (2.6)*, and *Multiple XYNTHA Prefilled Dual-Chamber Syringe Reconstitution to a 10 cc or Larger Luer Lock Syringe (2.7)*].

Note: If the patient uses more than one vial and/or prefilled dual-chamber syringe of XYNTHA per infusion, each vial and/or syringe should be reconstituted according to the instructions for that respective product kit. A separate 10 cc or larger luer lock syringe (not included in this kit) may be used to draw back the reconstituted contents of each vial or syringe.

2.4   Preparation and Reconstitution

Preparation

1. Always wash your hands before performing the following procedures.
2. Use aseptic technique (clean and germ-free) during the reconstitution procedure.
3. Use all components for the reconstitution and administration of this product as soon as possible after opening their sterile containers to minimize unnecessary exposure to the atmosphere.

Reconstitution

1. Allow the prefilled dual-chamber syringe of freeze-dried XYNTHA to reach room temperature.
2. Remove the contents of the XYNTHA Prefilled Dual-Chamber Syringe Kit and place on a clean surface, making sure you have all the supplies you will need.
3. Grasp the plunger rod as shown in the following diagram. Avoid contact with the shaft of the plunger rod. Screw the plunger rod firmly into the opening in the finger rest of the XYNTHA Prefilled Dual-Chamber Syringe by pushing and turning firmly until resistance is felt (approximately 2 turns).

Note: Throughout the reconstitution process, it is important to keep the XYNTHA Prefilled Dual-Chamber Syringe upright to prevent possible leakage.

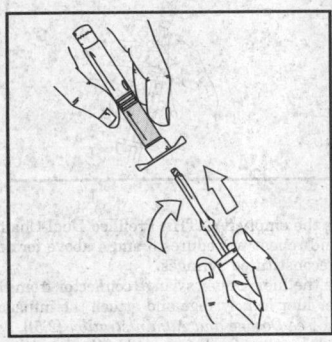

4. Holding the XYNTHA Prefilled Dual-Chamber Syringe upright, remove the white tamper-evident seal by bending the seal right to left (or a gentle rocking motion) to break the perforation of the cap and expose the grey rubber tip cap of the XYNTHA Prefilled Dual-Chamber Syringe.

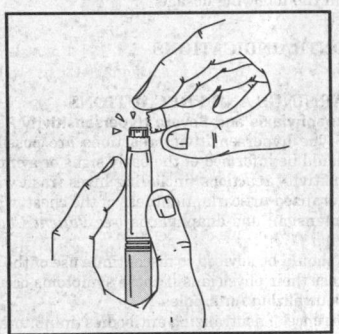

5. Remove the protective blue vented sterile cap from its package.
   While holding the XYNTHA Prefilled Dual-Chamber Syringe upright, remove the grey rubber tip cap and replace it with the protective blue vented cap (prevents pressure build-up). Avoid touching the open end of both the syringe and the protective blue vented cap.

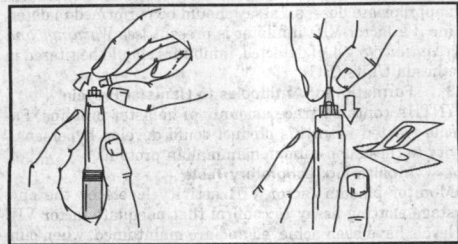

6. **Gently and slowly** advance the plunger rod by pushing until the two stoppers inside the XYNTHA Prefilled Dual-Chamber Syringe meet, and all of the diluent is transferred to the chamber containing the XYNTHA powder.

Note: To prevent the escape of fluid from the tip of the syringe, the plunger rod should not be pushed with excessive force.

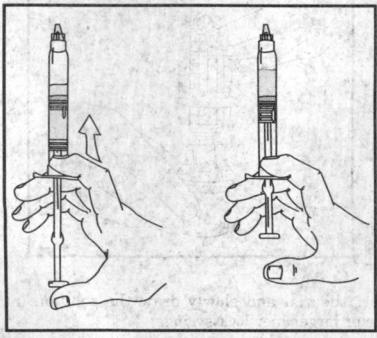

7. With the XYNTHA Prefilled Dual-Chamber Syringe remaining upright, swirl **gently** several times until the powder is dissolved.

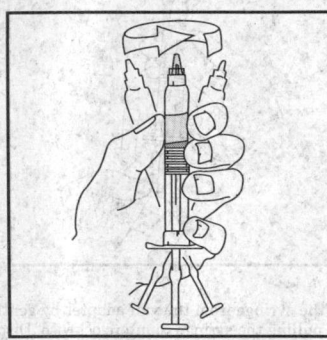

Note: The final solution should be inspected visually for particulate matter before administration. The solution should be clear to slightly opalescent and colorless. If it is not, the solution should be discarded and a new kit should be used.

8. Holding the XYNTHA Prefilled Dual-Chamber Syringe in an upright position, slowly advance the plunger rod until most, but not all, of the air is removed from the drug product chamber.

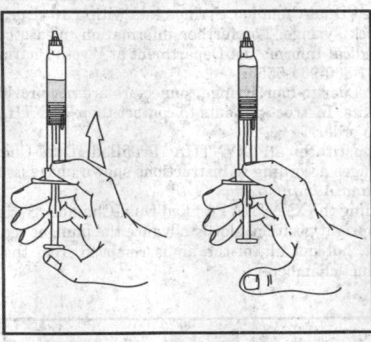

The reconstituted solution may be stored at room temperature prior to administration, but should be administered within 3 hours after reconstitution or removal of the grey rubber tip cap.

If the solution is not used immediately, the syringe should be stored upright and the protective blue vent cap should remain on the XYNTHA Prefilled Dual-Chamber Syringe until ready to infuse.

XYNTHA, when reconstituted, contains polysorbate 80, which is known to increase the rate of di-(2-ethylhexyl)phthalate (DEHP) extraction from polyvinyl chloride (PVC). This should be considered during the preparation and administration of XYNTHA, including storage time elapsed in a PVC container following reconstitution. It is important that the recommendations in *Dosage and Administration (2)* be followed closely.

Note: The tubing of the infusion set included with this kit does not contain DEHP.

2.5   Administration

XYNTHA is administered by intravenous (IV) infusion after reconstitution of the freeze-dried powder with the diluent (0.9% Sodium Chloride). Both the XYNTHA powder and the diluent are supplied within the prefilled dual-chamber syringe. Parenteral drug products should be inspected visually for particulate matter and discoloration prior to administration, whenever solution and container permit.

XYNTHA, as provided in the prefilled dual-chamber syringe, should routinely be administered using the infusion set included in the kit.

1. After removing the protective blue vented cap, firmly attach the intravenous infusion set provided in the kit onto the XYNTHA Prefilled Dual-Chamber Syringe.

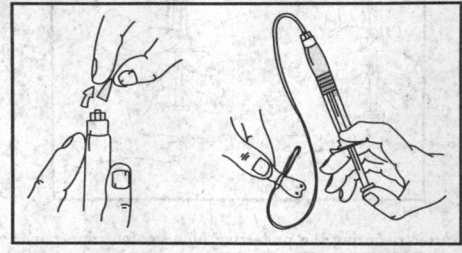

2. Apply a tourniquet and prepare the injection site by wiping the skin well with an alcohol swab provided in the kit.
3. Remove the protective needle cover and perform venipuncture. Insert the needle on the infusion set tubing into the vein, and remove the tourniquet. The reconstituted XYNTHA product should be injected intravenously over several minutes. The rate of administration should be determined by the patient's comfort level. As with any intravenous administration, always verify proper needle placement.

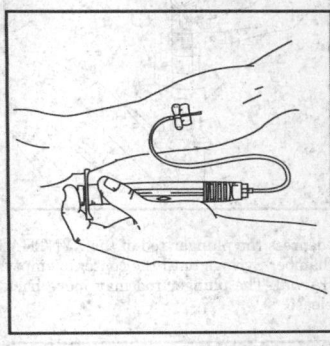

Reconstituted XYNTHA should not be administered in the same tubing or container with other medicinal products.[3]

4. After infusing XYNTHA, remove the infusion set and discard. The amount of drug product left in the infusion set will not affect treatment.

Note: Dispose of all unused solution, the empty XYNTHA Prefilled Dual-Chamber Syringe, and other used medical supplies in an appropriate container for medical waste that might hurt others if not handled properly.

2.6   Use of a XYNTHA Vial Kit and a XYNTHA Prefilled Dual-Chamber Syringe Kit

These instructions are for the use of only one XYNTHA vial kit and one XYNTHA Prefilled Dual-Chamber Syringe Kit. For further information, please contact the Medical Information Department at Wyeth Pharmaceuticals, 1-800-934-5556.

1. Reconstitute the XYNTHA vial using the instructions included with the kit. Detach the empty diluent syringe from the vial adapter by gently turning and pulling the syringe counterclockwise, leaving the contents in the vial and the vial adapter in place.

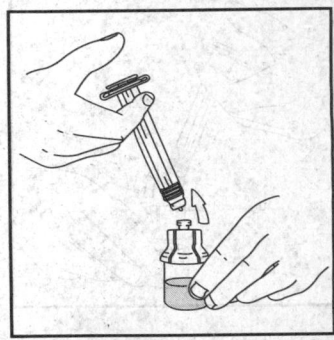

2. Reconstitute the XYNTHA Prefilled Dual-Chamber Syringe using the instructions included with the kit,

remembering to remove most, but not all, of the air from the drug product chamber.

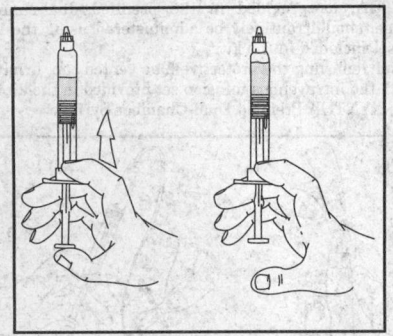

3. After removing the protective blue vented cap, connect the XYNTHA Prefilled Dual-Chamber Syringe to the vial adapter by inserting the tip into the adapter opening while firmly pushing and turning the syringe clockwise until secured.

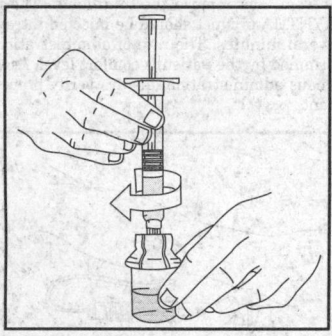

4. Slowly depress the plunger rod of the XYNTHA Prefilled Dual-Chamber Syringe until the contents empty into the XYNTHA vial. The plunger rod may move back slightly after release.

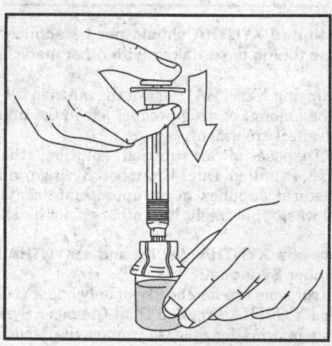

5. Detach and discard the empty XYNTHA Prefilled Dual-Chamber Syringe from the vial adapter.
   Note: If the syringe turns without detaching from the vial adapter, grasp the white collar and turn.

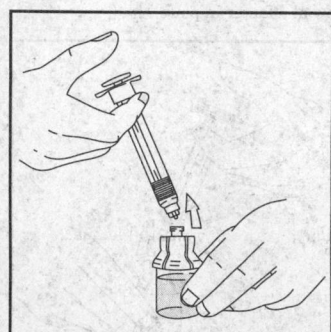

6. Connect a sterile 10 cc or larger luer lock syringe to the vial adapter. You may want to inject some air into the vial to make withdrawing the vial contents easier.

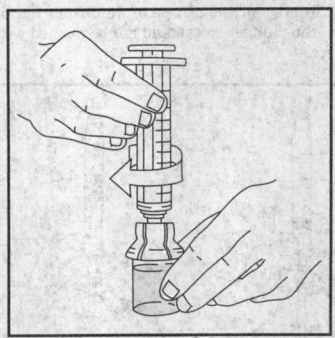

7. Invert the vial and slowly draw the solution into the 10 cc or larger luer lock syringe.

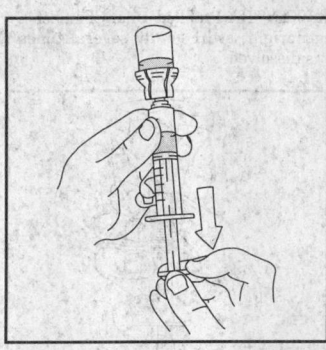

8. Detach the syringe from the vial adapter by gently turning and pulling the syringe counterclockwise. Discard the vial with the adapter attached.
9. Attach the infusion set to the 10 cc or larger luer lock syringe as directed [*see Dosage and Administration (2.5)*].
   Note: Dispose of all unused solution, the empty XYNTHA Prefilled Dual-Chamber Syringe, and other used medical supplies in an appropriate container for medical waste that might hurt others if not handled properly.

2.7   Multiple XYNTHA Prefilled Dual-Chamber Syringe Reconstitution to a 10 cc or Larger Luer Lock Syringe
The instructions below are for the use of multiple XYNTHA Prefilled Dual-Chamber Syringe kits with a 10 cc or larger luer lock syringe. For further information, please contact the Medical Information Department at Wyeth Pharmaceuticals, 1-800-934-5556.
Note: Luer-to-luer syringe connectors are not provided in these kits. Instruct patients to contact their XYNTHA supplier to order.
1. Reconstitute all XYNTHA Prefilled Dual-Chamber Syringes according to instructions shown above [*see Dosage and Administration (2.4)*].
   Holding the XYNTHA Prefilled Dual-Chamber Syringe in an upright position, slowly advance the plunger rod until most, but not all, of the air is removed from the drug product chamber.

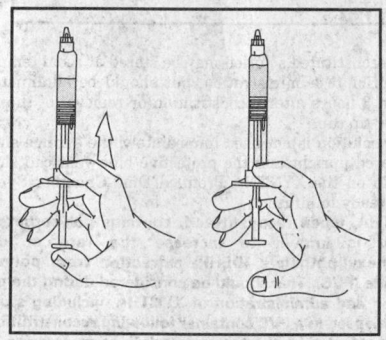

2. Remove the luer-to-luer syringe connector from its package.
3. After removing the protective blue vented cap, connect a sterile 10 cc or larger luer lock syringe to one opening (port) in the syringe connector and the XYNTHA Prefilled Dual-Chamber Syringe to the remaining open port on the opposite end.

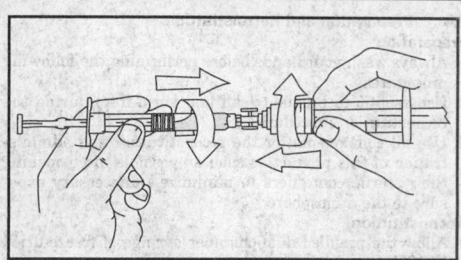

4. With the XYNTHA Prefilled Dual-Chamber Syringe on top, slowly depress the plunger rod until the contents empty into the 10 cc or larger luer lock syringe.

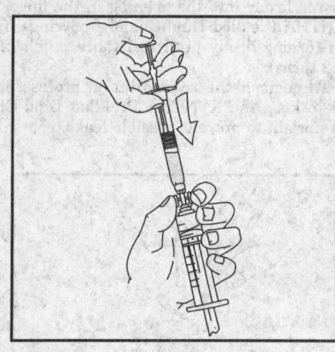

5. Remove the empty XYNTHA Prefilled Dual-Chamber Syringe and repeat procedures 3 and 4 above for any additional reconstituted syringes.
6. Remove the luer-to-luer syringe connector from the 10 cc or larger luer lock syringe and attach the infusion set as directed [*see Dosage and Administration (2.5)*].
   Note: Dispose of all unused solution, the empty XYNTHA Prefilled Dual-Chamber Syringe(s), and other used medical supplies in an appropriate container for medical waste that might hurt others if not handled properly.

3   DOSAGE FORMS AND STRENGTHS
XYNTHA is supplied as a white to off-white freeze-dried powder in the following dosage:
● 3000 IU

4   CONTRAINDICATIONS
None.

5   WARNINGS AND PRECAUTIONS
5.1   Anaphylaxis and Severe Hypersensitivity Reactions
Allergic type hypersensitivity reactions are possible. Patients should be informed of the early signs or symptoms of hypersensitivity reactions [including hives (rash with itching), generalized urticaria, tightness of the chest, wheezing, and hypotension] and anaphylaxis [*see Patient Counseling Information (17)*].
Patients should be advised to discontinue use of the product and contact their physicians if these symptoms occur.
5.2   Neutralizing Antibodies
The occurrence of neutralizing antibodies (inhibitors) is well known in the treatment of patients with hemophilia A. Inhibitors have been detected in patients receiving factor VIII-containing products. Inhibitors are common in previously untreated patients [4,5,6] and have been observed in previously treated patients on factor VIII products.[7,8,9,10,11,12] Patients using coagulation factor VIII products, including XYNTHA, should be monitored for the development of factor VIII inhibitors. If expected factor VIII activity plasma levels are not attained, or if bleeding is not controlled with an appropriate dose, an assay should be performed to determine if a factor VIII inhibitor is present [*see Warnings and Precautions (5.4)*]. If detected, inhibitors should be titered in Bethesda Units (BU).
5.3   Formation of Antibodies to Hamster Protein
XYNTHA contains trace amounts of hamster proteins. Patients treated with this product could develop hypersensitivity to these non-human mammalian proteins.
5.4   Monitoring: Laboratory Tests
● Monitor plasma factor VIII activity levels by the one-stage clotting assay to confirm that adequate factor VIII levels have been achieved and are maintained, when clinically indicated [*see Dosage and Administration (2)*].
● It is recommended that individual factor VIII values for recovery and, if clinically indicated, other pharmacokinetic characteristics be used to guide dosing and administration.

- Monitor for development of factor VIII inhibitors. Perform assay to determine if factor VIII inhibitor is present when expected factor VIII activity plasma levels are not attained, or when bleeding is not controlled with the expected dose of XYNTHA. Use Bethesda Units (BU) to titer inhibitors.

6 ADVERSE REACTIONS

The most common adverse reaction in study 1 is headache (24% of subjects) and in study 2 is pyrexia (41% of subjects).

6.1 Clinical Trials Experience

Because clinical trials are conducted under widely varying conditions, adverse reaction rates observed in the clinical trials of a drug cannot be directly compared to rates in the clinical trials of another drug and may not reflect the rates observed in clinical practice.

Study 1 is a pivotal phase 3 (safety and efficacy) study in which previously treated patients (PTPs) with hemophilia A received XYNTHA for routine prophylaxis and on-demand treatment, 94 subjects received at least one dose of XYNTHA, resulting in a total of 6,775 infusions [*see Clinical Studies (14)*]. In Study 1, the most frequently reported treatment-emergent adverse reaction was headache (24% of subjects). Other adverse reactions reported in ≥ 5% of subjects were: nausea (6%), diarrhea (5%), asthenia (5%) and pyrexia (5%). No subject developed anti-CHO or anti-TN8.2 antibodies.

Study 2 (surgery) is an on-going, open-label, single-arm study of at least 25 evaluable PTPs with severe or moderately severe hemophilia A (factor VIII activity in plasma [FVIII:C] ≤ 2%) who required elective major surgery and were planned to receive XYNTHA replacement therapy for at least 6 days post-surgery. Twenty-two subjects received at least one dose of XYNTHA, resulting in 766 infusions [*see Clinical Studies (14)*].

In Study 2, the most frequently reported treatment-emergent adverse reaction was pyrexia (41% of subjects). Other adverse reactions reported in ≥ 5% of subjects were: headache (9%), nausea (9%), diarrhea (5%), vomiting (5%) and asthenia (5%). The adverse reactions reported in either study were considered mild or moderate in severity.

Immunogenicity

In Study 1, the incidence of FVIII inhibitors to XYNTHA was the primary safety endpoint. Two subjects with inhibitors were observed in 89 subjects (2.2%) who completed ≥ 50 exposure days. These results were consistent with the pre-specified endpoint that no more than 2 inhibitors may be observed in at least 81 subjects.

In a Bayesian statistical analysis, results from this study were used to update PTP results from a prior supporting study using XYNTHA manufactured at the initial facility, where one *de novo* and two recurrent inhibitors were observed in 110 subjects, and the experience with predecessor product (1 inhibitor in 113 subjects). This Bayesian analysis indicates that the population (true) inhibitor rate for XYNTHA, the estimate of the 95% upper limit of the true inhibitor rate, was 4.17% (see Table 1).

[See table above]

Table 1: Bayesian Posterior Distribution of Inhibitor Rate

FVIII Inhibitor Nijmegen Result (BU/mL)	Number of Inhibitors	Number of Subjects Analyzed	Observed Inhibitor Rate (%)	---Posterior Beta Distribution Characteristics--- Alpha[a]	Beta[b]	Posterior Probability[c]	95% Upper Limit of Inhibitor Rate (%)[d]
≥0.6	2	89	2.25	4.5	197	0.9613	4.17

[a] Prior alpha of 2.5 plus the number of observed inhibitors.
[b] Prior beta of 110 plus the number of subjects analyzed minus the number of observed inhibitors.
[c] Posterior probability is the probability that the true inhibitor rate is less than the upper acceptable limit of 4.4%. A posterior probability greater than 0.95 is deemed acceptable.
[d] The 95% upper limit of the true inhibitor rate (the maximum rate calculated with at least 95% probability) based on the posterior distribution. An inhibitor rate less than 4.4% is deemed acceptable.

Table 2: Pharmacokinetic Parameter Estimates for XYNTHA at Baseline (Cross-over phase) and Month 6 (Follow-up phase) in Previously Treated Patients with Hemophilia A

Parameter	Parameters at Initial Visit (Crossover phase, n = 30) Mean ± SD	Parameters at Month 6 (Follow-up phase, n = 25) Mean ± SD
C_{max} (IU/mL)	1.08 ± 0.22	1.24 ± 0.42
AUC_{∞} (IU•hr/mL)	13.5 ± 5.6	15.0 ± 7.5
$t_{1/2}$ (hr)	11.2 ± 5.0	11.8 ± 6.2*
CL (mL/hr/kg)	4.51 ± 2.23	4.04 ± 1.87
K-value (IU/dL per IU/kg)	2.15 ± 0.44	2.47 ± 0.84
In vivo Recovery (%)	103 ± 21	116 ± 40

Abbreviations: AUC_{∞} = area under the plasma concentration-time curve from zero to infinity; Cmax = peak concentration; K-value = incremental recovery; $t_{1/2}$ = plasma elimination half-life; CL = clearance; n = number of subjects; SD = standard deviation.
*One subject was excluded from the calculation due to lack of a well-defined terminal phase.

7 DRUG INTERACTIONS

None known.

8 USE IN SPECIFIC POPULATIONS

8.1 Pregnancy

Pregnancy Category C

Animal reproduction studies have not been conducted with XYNTHA Antihemophilic Factor (Recombinant), Plasma/Albumin-Free. It is also not known whether XYNTHA can cause fetal harm when administered to a pregnant woman or can affect reproduction capacity. XYNTHA should be given to a pregnant woman only if clinically indicated.

8.2 Labor and Delivery

There is no information available on the effect of factor VIII replacement therapy on labor and delivery. XYNTHA should be used only if clinically indicated.

8.3 Nursing Mothers

It is not known whether this drug is excreted into human milk. Because many drugs are excreted into human milk, caution should be exercised if XYNTHA is administered to nursing mothers. XYNTHA should be given to nursing mothers only if clinically indicated.

8.4 Pediatric Use

A study of XYNTHA in previously treated patients less than 6 years of age is currently ongoing.

Pharmacokinetics of XYNTHA was studied in 7 previously treated patients *12-16* years of age. Pharmacokinetic parameters in these patients were *similar to those* obtained for adults after a dose of 50 IU/kg. For these 7 patients, the mean (± SD) C_{max} and AUC_{∞} were 1.09 ± 0.21 IU/mL and 11.5 ± 5.2 IU•h/mL, respectively. The mean clearance and plasma half-life values were 5.23 ± 2.36 mL/h/kg and 8.03 ± 2.44 hours (range 3.52–10.6 hours), respectively. The mean K-value and *in vivo* recoveries were 2.18 ± 0.41 IU/dL per IU/kg and 112 ± 23%, respectively.

8.5 Geriatric Use

Clinical studies of XYNTHA did not include subjects aged 65 and over. In general, dose selection for an elderly patient should be individualized.

11 DESCRIPTION

Antihemophilic Factor (Recombinant), Plasma/Albumin-Free, the active ingredient in XYNTHA, is a recombinant coagulation factor VIII produced by recombinant DNA technology for use in therapy of factor VIII deficiency. The Antihemophilic Factor (Recombinant), Plasma/Albumin-Free in XYNTHA is a purified glycoprotein, with an approximate molecular mass of 170 kDa consisting of 1,438 amino acids, which does not contain the B-domain.[13] The amino acid sequence of Antihemophilic Factor (Recombinant), Plasma/Albumin-Free in XYNTHA is comparable to the 90 + 80 kDa form of human factor VIII.

The Antihemophilic Factor (Recombinant), Plasma/Albumin-Free in XYNTHA is secreted by a genetically engineered Chinese hamster ovary (CHO) cell line. The cell line is grown in a chemically defined cell culture medium that contains recombinant insulin, but does not contain any materials derived from human or animal sources. The Antihemophilic Factor (Recombinant), Plasma/Albumin-Free in XYNTHA is purified by a process that uses a series of chromatography steps, one of which is based on affinity chromatography using a patented synthetic peptide affinity ligand.[14] The process also includes a solvent-detergent viral inactivation step and a virus-retaining nanofiltration step. The potency expressed in International Units (IU) is determined using the chromogenic assay of the European Pharmacopoeia. The Wyeth manufacturing reference standard for potency has been calibrated against the World Health Organization (WHO) International Standard for factor VIII activity using the one-stage clotting assay. The specific activity of XYNTHA is 5,500 to 9,900 IU per milligram of protein.

XYNTHA is formulated as a sterile, nonpyrogenic, preservative-free, freeze-dried powder preparation for intravenous (IV) injection. Each single-use prefilled dual-chamber syringe contains nominally 3000 IU of XYNTHA. Upon reconstitution, the product is a clear to slightly opalescent, colorless solution that contains sodium chloride, sucrose, L-histidine, calcium chloride and polysorbate 80.

12 CLINICAL PHARMACOLOGY

12.1 Mechanism of Action

Factor VIII is the specific clotting factor deficient in patients with hemophilia A (classical hemophilia).[15] Activated factor VIII acts as a cofactor for activated factor IX, accelerating the conversion of factor X to activated factor X.[15] Activated factor X converts prothrombin into thrombin.[15] Thrombin then converts fibrinogen into fibrin, and a clot is formed.[15] Factor VIII activity is greatly reduced in patients with hemophilia A, and, therefore, replacement therapy is necessary. The administration of XYNTHA increases plasma levels of factor VIII activity and can temporarily correct the coagulation defect in these patients.

12.2 Pharmacodynamics

The administration of XYNTHA increases plasma levels of factor VIII activity and can temporarily correct the coagulation defect in hemophilia A patients.

12.3 Pharmacokinetics

In a pivotal crossover clinical study, 30 evaluable previously treated patients [PTP] (≥ 12 years) received a single infusion of 50 IU/kg of XYNTHA followed by a full-length recombinant FVIII (FLrFVIII, Advate®) or a single infusion of FLrFVIII followed by XYNTHA in a randomized crossover design. The one-stage clotting assay method was used to determine the concentrations of these two products in blood. XYNTHA was shown to be pharmacokinetically equivalent to FLrFVIII as the 90% confidence intervals for XYNTHA-to-FLrFVIII ratios of the mean values of C_{max} and AUC_{∞} were within pre-established limits of 80% to 125%. The pharmacokinetic parameters of XYNTHA in the above group of patients are summarized in Table 2.

In addition, 25 PTPs received a single infusion of 50 IU/kg of XYNTHA for a 6-month follow-up PK study. The pharmacokinetic parameters were comparable between baseline and month 6, indicating no time-dependent changes in the pharmacokinetic properties of XYNTHA; the 90% confidence intervals for XYNTHA 6 month-to-baseline ratios of the mean values of C_{max} and AUC_{∞} were within pre-established limits of 80% to 125%.

[See table 2 above]

13 NONCLINICAL TOXICOLOGY

13.1 Carcinogenesis, Mutagenesis, Impairment of Fertility

No studies have been conducted with XYNTHA to assess its mutagenic or carcinogenic potential. XYNTHA has been shown to be comparable to the predecessor product with respect to its biochemical and physicochemical properties, as well as its non-clinical *in vivo* pharmacology and toxicology. By inference, predecessor product and XYNTHA would be expected to have equivalent mutagenic and carcinogenic potential. The predecessor product has been shown to be nongenotoxic in the mouse micronucleus assay. No studies have been conducted in animals to assess impairment of fertility or fetal development.

13.2 Animal Toxicology and/or Pharmacology

Preclinical studies evaluating XYNTHA in hemophilia A dogs without inhibitors demonstrated safe and effective restoration of hemostasis. XYNTHA demonstrated a toxicological profile that was similar to the toxicological profile observed with the predecessor product. Toxicity associated with XYNTHA was primarily associated with anti-FVIII neutralizing antibody generation first detectable at 15 days of repeat dosing in high (approximately 735 IU/kg/day) level-dosed, non-human primates.

Table 3: Time Interval Between Last Prophylaxis Dose of XYNTHA and Start of Bleed

≤ 24 hrs		> 24 ≤ 48 hrs		> 48 ≤ 72 hrs		> 72 hrs		Unknown[a]		Total Bleeding Episodes
Spon	Traum	Spon	Traum	Spon	Traum	Spon	Traum	Spon	Traum	
13	20	33	44	24	12	18	16	3	4	187

[a] Bleeds with unknown start time or bleeds in which previous prophylaxis dose was before the start of the safety and efficacy period of the study. Abbreviations: Spon = spontaneous new bleed; Traum = new bleed due to trauma; hrs = hours.

Table 4: Summary of Response to Infusions to Treat New Bleeding Episode by Number of Infusions Needed for Resolution

Response to 1st Infusion	Number of Infusions (%)					Total Number of Bleeds
	1	2	3	4	> 4	
Excellent	42 (95.5)	2 (4.5)	0 (0.0)	0 (0.0)	0 (0.0)	44
Good	69 (78.4)	16 (18.2)	3 (3.4)	0 (0.0)	0 (0.0)	88
Moderate	24 (53.3)	16 (35.6)	2 (4.4)	0 (0.0)	3 (6.7)	45
No Response	0 (0.0)	0 (0.0)	2 (40.0)	2 (40.0)	1 (20.0)	5
Not Assessed	4 (80.0)	0 (0.0)	0 (0.0)	1 (20.0)	0 (0.0)	5[a]
Total	139 (74.3)	34 (18.2)	7 (3.7)	3 (1.6)	4 (2.1)	187

[a] Includes 1 infusion with commercial FVIII that occurred before routine prophylaxis began.

14   CLINICAL STUDIES

The efficacy of XYNTHA was evaluated in Study 1, in which subjects received XYNTHA on a prophylaxis treatment regimen, with on-demand treatment administered as clinically indicated. Ninety-four (94) subjects were enrolled and treated with at least one dose, and all are included in the intent-to-treat (ITT) population. Eighty-nine (89) subjects accrued ≥ 50 exposure days. From the 94 subjects enrolled, thirty (30) evaluable subjects participated in the PK study and received at least 1 PK dose. Twenty-five (25) evaluable subjects with FVIII:C ≤ 1% completed both the first (PK1) and the second (PK2) assessments [see Clinical Pharmacology (12.3)]. Median age for the 94 treated subjects was 24 years (mean 27.7 and range 12-60 years). All subjects had ≥ 150 previous exposure days with baseline FVIII activity level of ≤ 2%.

In the open-label safety and efficacy period, all 94 subjects received XYNTHA for routine prophylaxis at the dose of 30 ± 5 IU/kg 3 times a week with provisions for dose escalation based on pre-specified criteria. Seven (7) dose escalations were prescribed for 6 subjects during the course of the study. Forty-three (43) of ninety-four (94), i.e. 45.7%, subjects reported no bleeding while on routine prophylaxis. The median annualized bleeding rate (ABR) for all bleeding episodes was 1.9 (mean 3.9, range 0 to 42.1).

Fifty-three (53) of 94 subjects received XYNTHA for on-demand treatment for a total of 187 bleeding episodes (Table 3). Seven of these bleeding episodes occurred in subjects prior to switching to a prophylaxis treatment regimen. One hundred ten of one hundred eighty (110/180) bleeds (61.1%) occurred ≤ 48 hours after the last dose and 38.9% (70 of 180 bleeds) occurred > 48 hours after the last dose. The majority of bleeds reported to occur ≤ 48 hours after the last prophylaxis dose were traumatic (64 of 110 bleeds; 58.2%). Forty-two (42) of 70 bleeds (60%) reported to occur > 48 hours after the last prophylaxis dose were spontaneous. The on-demand treatment dosing regimen was determined by the investigator. The median dose for on-demand treatment was 30.6 IU/kg (range, 6.4 to 74.4 IU/kg).

[See table 3 above]

The majority of bleeding episodes (173/187; 92.5%) resolved with 1 or 2 infusions. Subjects rated the outcomes of infusions on a pre-specified four (4) point hemostatic efficacy scale. One hundred thirty-two (132) of 187 bleeding episodes (70.6%) treated with XYNTHA were rated excellent or good in their response to initial treatment, 45 (24.1%) were rated moderate. Five [5] (2.7%) were rated no response, and 5 (2.7%) were not rated.

[See table 4 above]

In an on-going, open-label study of XYNTHA in surgical prophylaxis, 21 of at least 25 evaluable PTPs with severe or moderately severe (FVIII:C ≤ 2%) hemophilia A undergoing major surgical procedures received XYNTHA. One (1) subject received XYNTHA for a pre-surgery pharmacokinetic assessment only and had not undergone surgery.

The results of an interim analysis on 21 of the 25 planned evaluable subjects who had undergone major surgical procedures (13 total knee replacements, 1 hip replacement, 3 synovectomies, 1 left ulnar nerve transposition release, 1 ventral hernia repair/scar revision, 1 knee arthroscopy, 1 revision and debridement of the knee after a total knee replacement) are presented in Table 5. For the 21 surgical subjects, investigator's ratings of efficacy at the end of surgery and at the end of the initial postoperative period were excellent or good for all assessments. All reported blood loss during the intra-operative and postoperative periods was rated normal with the exception of one subject who experienced iatrogenic bleeding.

Table 5: Summary of Hemostatic Efficacy

Time of Hemostatic Efficacy Assessment	Excellent	Good	Number of subjects
End of surgery	14 (67%)	7 (33%)	21
End of initial postoperative period[a]	16 (84%)	3 (16%)	19

[a] Conclusion of initial postoperative period is date of discharge or postoperative Day 6, whichever occurs later.

15   REFERENCES

1. Nilsson IM, Berntorp EE and Freiburghaus C. Treatment of patients with factor VIII and IX inhibitors. Thromb Haemost. 1993;70(1):56-59.
2. Hoyer LW. Hemophilia A. N Engl J Med. 1994;330:38-47.
3. Juhlin F. Stability and Compatibility of Reconstituted Recombinant Factor VIII SQ, 250 IU/ml, in a System for Continuous Infusion. Pharmacia Document 9610224, 1996.
4. Ehrenforth S, Kreuz W, Scharrer I, et al. Incidence of development of factor VIII and factor IX inhibitors in hemophiliacs. Lancet. 1992;339:594-598.
5. Lusher J, Arkin S, Abildgaard CF, Schwartz RS, the Kogenate PUP Study Group. Recombinant factor VIII for the treatment of previously untreated patients with hemophilia A. N Engl J Med. 1993;328:453-459.
6. Bray GL, Gomperts ED, Courter S, et al. A multicenter study of recombinant factor VIII (Recombinate): safety, efficacy, and inhibitor risk in previously untreated patients with hemophilia A. Blood. 1994;83(9):2428-2435.
7. Kessler C, Sachse K. Factor VIII:C inhibitor associated with monoclonal-antibody purified FVIII concentrate. Lancet. 1990;335:1403.
8. Schwartz RS, Abildgaard CF, Aledort LM, et al. Human recombinant DNA-derived antihemophilic factor (factor VIII) in the treatment of hemophilia A. N Engl J Med. 1990;323:1800-1805.
9. White GC II, Courter S, Bray GL, et al. A multicenter study of recombinant factor VIII (Recombinate™) in previously treated patients with hemophilia A. Thromb Haemost. 1997;77(4):660-667.
10. Gruppo R, Chen H, Schroth P, et al. Safety and immunogenicity of recombinant factor VIII (Recombinate™) in previously untreated patients: A 7.3 year update. Haemophilia. 1998;4:228 (Abstract No. 291, XXIII Congress of the WFH, The Hague).
11. Scharrer I, Bray GL, Neutzling O. Incidence of inhibitors in haemophilia A patients - a review of recent studies of recombinant and plasma-derived factor VIII concentrates. Haemophilia. 1999;5:145-154.
12. Abshire TC, Brackmann HH, Scharrer I, et al. Sucrose formulated recombinant human antihemophilic Factor VIII is safe and efficacious for treatment of hemophilia A in home therapy: Results of a multicenter, international, clinical investigation. Thromb Haemost. 2000;83(6):811-816.
13. Sandberg H, Almstedt A, Brandt J, Castro VM, Gray E, Holmquist L, et al. Structural and Functional Characterization of B-Domain Deleted Recombinant Factor VIII. Sem Hematol. 2001;38 (Suppl. 4):4-12.
14. Kelley BD, Tannatt M, Magnusson R, Hagelberg S. Development and Validation of an Affinity Chromatography Step Using a Peptide Ligand for cGMP Production of Factor VIII. Biotechnol Bioeng. 2004;87(3):400-412.
15. Mann KG and Ziedens KB. Overview of Hemostasis. In: Lee CA, Berntorp EE and Hoots WK, eds. Textbook of Hemophilia. USA, Blackwell Publishing; 2005:1-4.

16   HOW SUPPLIED/STORAGE AND HANDLING

16.1   How Supplied

XYNTHA® Antihemophilic Factor (Recombinant), Plasma/Albumin-Free is supplied in a kit that includes the XYNTHA freeze-dried powder that contain nominally 3000 IU and 4 mL 0.9% Sodium Chloride solution for reconstitution in a prefilled dual-chamber syringe:

3000 IU Kit: NDC 58394-016-03

In addition, each XYNTHA Antihemophilic Factor (Recombinant), Plasma/Albumin-Free Kit contains: one plunger rod for assembly, one sterile infusion set, two alcohol swabs, one bandage, one gauze pad, one vented sterile cap, and one package insert.

XYNTHA® Antihemophilic Factor (Recombinant), Plasma/Albumin-Free is also supplied in kits that include single-use vials that contain nominally 250, 500, 1000, or 2000 IU of freeze-dried powder per vial:

250 IU Kit: NDC 58394-012-01
500 IU Kit: NDC 58394-013-01
1000 IU Kit: NDC 58394-014-01
2000 IU Kit: NDC 58394-015-01

Actual factor VIII activity in IU is stated on the label of each XYNTHA Antihemophilic Factor (Recombinant), Plasma/Albumin-Free prefilled dual-chamber syringe or vial.

16.2   Storage and Handling

Product as Packaged for Sale:

• Store XYNTHA under refrigeration at a temperature of 2° to 8°C (36° to 46°F) for up to 36 months from the date of manufacture until the expiration date stated on the label. XYNTHA may also be stored at room temperature not to exceed 25°C (77°F) for up to 3 months.

• The starting date at room temperature storage should be clearly recorded in the space provided on the outer carton. At the end of the 3-month period, the product must not be put back into the refrigerator, but must be used immediately or discarded.

• Do not use XYNTHA after the expiration date stated on the label or after 3 months when stored at room temperature, whichever is earlier.

• Do not freeze, to prevent damage to the XYNTHA Prefilled Dual-Chamber Syringe.

• During storage, avoid prolonged exposure of XYNTHA to light.

Product After Reconstitution:

• Administer XYNTHA within 3 hours after reconstitution or after removal of the grey rubber tip cap from the XYNTHA Prefilled Dual-Chamber Syringe. The reconstituted solution may be stored at room temperature prior to administration.

17   PATIENT COUNSELING INFORMATION

See Patient Product Information and Instructions for Using XYNTHA.

Advise patients to report any adverse reactions or problems following XYNTHA administration to their physician or healthcare provider.

• Advise patients that allergic-type hypersensitivity reactions are possible and inform them of the early signs of hypersensitivity reactions [including hives (rash with itching), generalized urticaria, tightness of the chest, wheezing, hypotension] and anaphylaxis. Advise patients to discontinue use of the product and contact their physicians if these symptoms occur.

• Advise patients to contact their physician or treatment facility for further treatment and/or assessment, if they experience a lack of a clinical response to factor VIII replacement therapy, as this may be a manifestation of an inhibitor.

• Advise female patients to notify their physician if they become pregnant or intend to become pregnant during therapy.

• Advise nursing mothers to notify their physician if they are breastfeeding.

• Advise patients that local irritation may occur when infusing XYNTHA after the reconstitution in the prefilled dual-chamber syringe.

- Advise patients to consult with their healthcare professional prior to travel and to bring an adequate supply of XYNTHA, based on their current regimen, for anticipated treatment when traveling.

FDA-APPROVED PATIENT LABELING

Patient Product Information (PPI)

XYNTHA (ZIN-tha)

[ANTIHEMOPHILIC FACTOR (RECOMBINANT), PLASMA/ ALBUMIN-FREE]

Please read this Patient Information carefully before using XYNTHA and each time you get a refill. There may be new information. This leaflet does not take the place of talking with your doctor about your medical problems or your treatment.

What is XYNTHA?

XYNTHA is an injectable medicine that is used to help control and prevent bleeding in people with hemophilia A. Hemophilia A is also called classic hemophilia.

XYNTHA is not used to treat von Willebrand's disease.

What should I tell my doctor before using XYNTHA?

Tell your doctor about all of your medical conditions, including if you:

- are pregnant or planning to become pregnant. It is not known if XYNTHA may harm your unborn baby.
- are breastfeeding. It is not known if XYNTHA passes into your milk and if it can harm your baby.

Tell your doctor and pharmacist about all of the medicines you take, including all prescription and non-prescription medicines, such as over-the-counter medicines, supplements, or herbal remedies.

How should I infuse XYNTHA?

See the step-by-step instructions for infusing XYNTHA at the end of this leaflet. You should always follow the specific instructions given by your doctor. The steps listed below are general guidelines for using XYNTHA. If you are unsure of the procedures, please call your doctor or pharmacist before using.

Call your doctor right away if bleeding is not controlled after using XYNTHA.

Your doctor will prescribe the dose that you should take.

Your doctor may need to take blood tests from time to time. Talk to your doctor before traveling. You should plan to bring enough XYNTHA for your treatment during this time.

What if I take too much XYNTHA?

Call your doctor if you take too much XYNTHA.

What are the possible side effects of XYNTHA?

Allergic reactions may occur with XYNTHA. Call your doctor or get emergency treatment right away if you have any of the following symptoms:

- **wheezing**
- **difficulty breathing**
- **chest tightness**
- **turning blue (look at lips and gums)**
- **fast heartbeat**
- **swelling of the face**
- **faintness**
- **rash**
- **hives**

Your body can also make antibodies, called "inhibitors," against XYNTHA, which may stop XYNTHA from working properly. Consult with your healthcare provider to make sure you are carefully monitored with blood tests for the development of inhibitors to factor VIII.

Some common side effects of XYNTHA are headache, fever, nausea, vomiting, diarrhea, or weakness. These are not all the possible side effects of XYNTHA.

Tell your doctor about any side effect that bothers you or that does not go away.

How should I store XYNTHA?

Do not freeze XYNTHA and protect from light.

Store the XYNTHA Prefilled Dual-Chamber Syringe in the refrigerator at 36° to 46°F (2° to 8°C). XYNTHA can last at room temperature (below 77°F) for up to 3 months. If you store XYNTHA at room temperature, be careful to write down the date you put XYNTHA at room temperature, so you will know when to throw it away. There is a space on the carton for you to write the date.

Throw away any unused XYNTHA after the expiration date.

Infuse XYNTHA within 3 hours after reconstitution or after removal of the grey rubber tip cap from the prefilled dual-chamber syringe. You may store the reconstituted solution at room temperature prior to infusion. If you have not used it in 3 hours, throw it away.

Do not use reconstituted XYNTHA if it is not clear to slightly opalescent and colorless.

Disposal of all XYNTHA materials, whether reconstituted or not, must be done using an appropriate medical waste container. Contact your healthcare professional if you need additional instructions.

What else should I know about XYNTHA?

Medicines are sometimes prescribed for purposes other than those listed here. Do not use XYNTHA for a condition for which it is not prescribed. Do not share XYNTHA with other people, even if they have the same symptoms that you have.

This leaflet summarizes the most important information about XYNTHA. If you would like more information, talk to your doctor. You can ask your doctor or pharmacist for information about XYNTHA that was written for healthcare professionals.

Instructions for Using XYNTHA

XYNTHA is supplied as a freeze-dried powder. Before it can be infused in your vein (intravenous injection), you must reconstitute the powder by mixing it with the 0.9% Sodium Chloride solution. Both the XYNTHA powder and the 0.9% Sodium Chloride solution are supplied in one prefilled dual-chamber syringe. XYNTHA should be reconstituted and infused using the infusion set provided in this kit. Please follow the directions below for the proper use of this product. Additional instructions for using XYNTHA are provided after **INFUSION (Intravenous Injection)** that detail the use of a XYNTHA Prefilled Dual-Chamber Syringe and a XYNTHA vial or multiple XYNTHA Prefilled Dual-Chamber Syringes.

PREPARATION AND RECONSTITUTION

Preparation

1. Always wash your hands before performing the following procedures.
2. Use aseptic technique (clean and germ-free) during the reconstitution procedure.
3. Use all components for the reconstitution and administration of this product as soon as possible after opening their sterile containers to minimize unnecessary exposure to the atmosphere.

Reconstitution

1. Allow the prefilled dual-chamber syringe of freeze-dried XYNTHA to reach room temperature.
2. Remove the contents of the XYNTHA Prefilled Dual-Chamber Syringe Kit and place on a clean surface, making sure you have all the supplies you will need.
3. Grasp the plunger rod as shown in the following diagram. Avoid contact with the shaft of the plunger rod. Screw the plunger rod firmly into the opening in the finger rest of the XYNTHA Prefilled Dual-Chamber Syringe by pushing and turning firmly until resistance is felt (approximately 2 turns).
   Note: Throughout the reconstitution process, it is important to keep the XYNTHA Prefilled Dual-Chamber Syringe upright to prevent possible leakage.

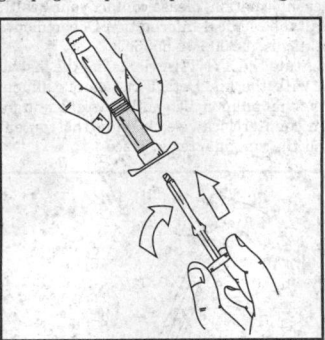

4. Holding the XYNTHA Prefilled Dual-Chamber Syringe upright, remove the white tamper-evident seal by bending the seal right to left (or a gentle rocking motion) to break the perforation of the cap and expose the grey rubber tip cap of the XYNTHA Prefilled Dual-Chamber Syringe.

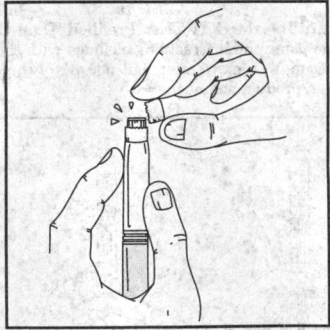

5. Remove the protective blue vented sterile cap from its package.
   While holding the XYNTHA Prefilled Dual-Chamber Syringe upright, remove the grey rubber tip cap and replace it with the protective blue vented cap (prevents pressure build-up). Avoid touching the open end of both the syringe and the protective blue vented cap.

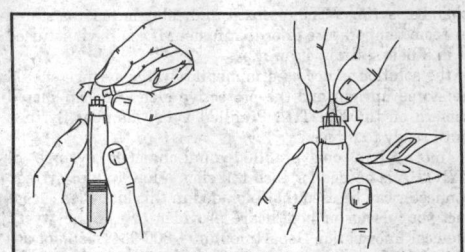

6. **Gently and slowly** advance the plunger rod by pushing until the two stoppers inside the XYNTHA Prefilled Dual-Chamber Syringe meet, and all of the diluent is transferred to the chamber containing the XYNTHA powder.
   Note: To prevent the escape of fluid from the tip of the syringe, the plunger rod should not be pushed with excessive force.

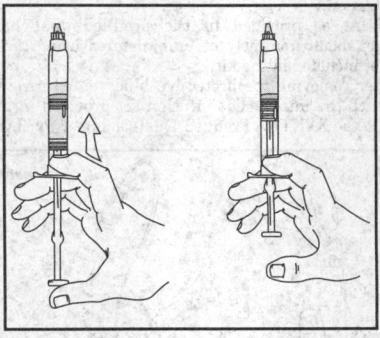

7. With the XYNTHA Prefilled Dual-Chamber Syringe remaining upright, swirl **gently** several times until the powder is dissolved.

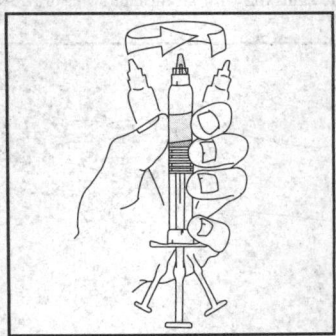

Note: Look carefully at the solution in the XYNTHA Prefilled Dual-Chamber Syringe. The solution should be clear to slightly opalescent and colorless. If it is not, the solution should be discarded and a new kit should be used.

8. Holding the XYNTHA Prefilled Dual-Chamber Syringe in an upright position, slowly advance the plunger rod until most, but not all, of the air is removed from the drug product chamber.

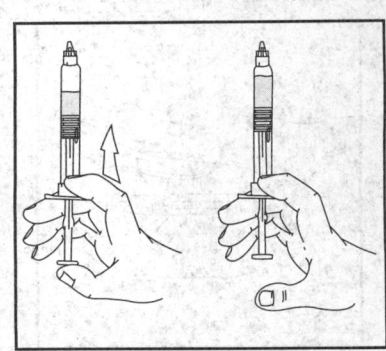

XYNTHA should be infused within 3 hours after reconstitution or removal of the grey tip cap from the prefilled dual-chamber syringe. The reconstituted solution may be stored at room temperature prior to infusion. If you have not used it in 3 hours, throw it away.

If the solution is not used immediately, the syringe should be stored upright and the protective blue vent cap should remain on the XYNTHA Prefilled Dual-Chamber Syringe until ready to infuse.

If more than one prefilled dual-chamber syringe of XYNTHA is needed for each infusion, a luer-to-luer syringe connector can be used (not included in this kit). Please contact your doctor or healthcare provider, or call the Wyeth Medical Information Department at 1-800-934-5556, for additional information.

INFUSION (Intravenous Injection)

Your doctor or healthcare professional should teach you how to infuse XYNTHA. Once you learn how to self-infuse, you can follow the instructions in this insert.

XYNTHA is administered by intravenous (IV) infusion after reconstitution of the freeze-dried powder with the diluent (0.9% Sodium Chloride). Both the XYNTHA powder and the diluent are supplied within the prefilled dual-chamber syringe. Once reconstituted, XYNTHA should be inspected visually for particulate matter and discoloration prior to administration.

XYNTHA, as provided in the prefilled dual-chamber syringe, should routinely be administered using the infusion set included in the kit.

1. After removing the protective blue vented cap, firmly attach the intravenous infusion set provided in the kit onto the XYNTHA Prefilled Dual-Chamber Syringe.

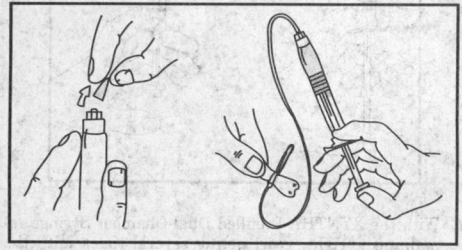

2. Apply a tourniquet and prepare the injection site by wiping the skin well with an alcohol swab provided in the kit.

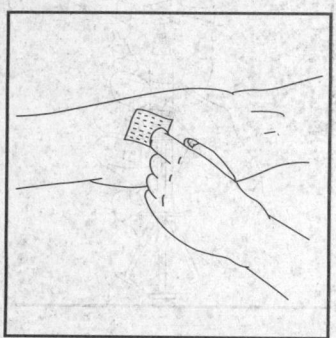

3. Remove the protective needle cover and insert the butterfly needle of the infusion set tubing into your vein as instructed by your doctor or healthcare professional. Remove the tourniquet. Infuse the reconstituted XYNTHA product over several minutes. Your comfort level should determine the rate of infusion.

   As with any intravenous administration, always verify proper needle placement.

   Discuss this procedure with your health care provider.

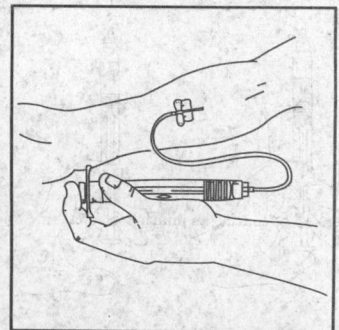

Reconstituted XYNTHA should not be administered in the same tubing or container with other medicinal products.

4. After infusing XYNTHA, remove the infusion set and discard. The amount of drug product left in the infusion set will not affect your treatment.

   Note: Dispose of all unused solution, the empty XYNTHA Prefilled Dual-Chamber Syringe, and other used medical supplies in an appropriate container used for throwing away medical waste that might hurt others if not handled properly.

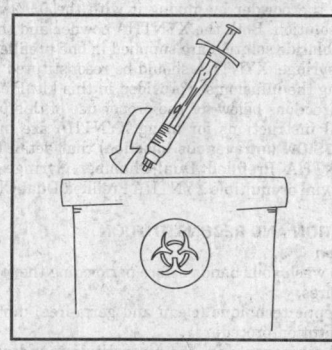

It is a good idea to record the lot number from the XYNTHA Prefilled Dual-Chamber Syringe label every time you use XYNTHA. You can use the peel-off label found on the XYNTHA Prefilled Dual-Chamber Syringe to record the lot number.

ADDITIONAL INSTRUCTIONS FOR USING XYNTHA

XYNTHA is also supplied in kits that include single-use vials with freeze-dried powder and prefilled diluent syringes. If you use more than one vial and/or prefilled dual-chamber syringe of XYNTHA per infusion, each vial and/or syringe should be reconstituted according to the specific directions for that respective product kit. A separate, 10 cc or larger luer lock syringe (not included in this kit) may be used to draw back the reconstituted contents of each vial or syringe.

Use of a XYNTHA Vial Kit and a XYNTHA Prefilled Dual-Chamber Syringe Kit

These instructions are for the use of only one XYNTHA vial kit and one XYNTHA Prefilled Dual-Chamber Syringe Kit. For further information, please contact your healthcare provider or call the Medical Information Department at Wyeth Pharmaceuticals, 1-800-934-5556.

1. Reconstitute the XYNTHA vial using the instructions included with the kit. Detach the empty diluent syringe from the vial adapter by gently turning and pulling the syringe counterclockwise, leaving the contents in the vial and the vial adapter in place.

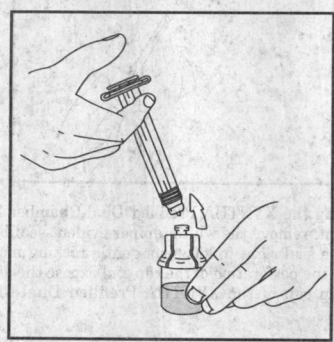

2. Reconstitute the XYNTHA Prefilled Dual-Chamber Syringe using the instructions included with the kit, remembering to remove most, but not all, of the air from the drug product chamber.

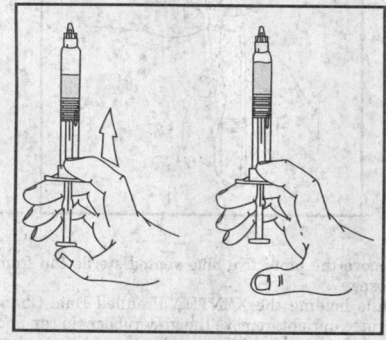

3. After removing the protective blue vented cap, connect the XYNTHA Prefilled Dual-Chamber Syringe to the

vial adapter by inserting the tip into the adapter opening while firmly pushing and turning the syringe clockwise until secured.

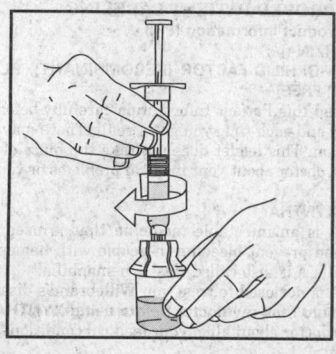

4. Slowly depress the plunger rod of the XYNTHA Prefilled Dual-Chamber Syringe until the contents empty into the XYNTHA vial. The plunger rod may move back slightly after release.

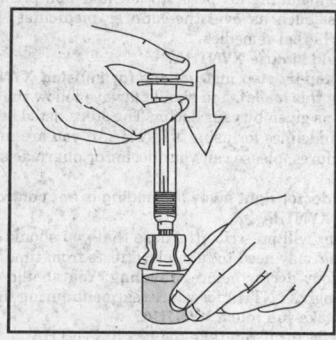

5. Detach and discard the empty XYNTHA Prefilled Dual-Chamber Syringe from the vial adapter.
   Note: If the syringe turns without detaching from the vial adapter, grasp the white collar and turn.

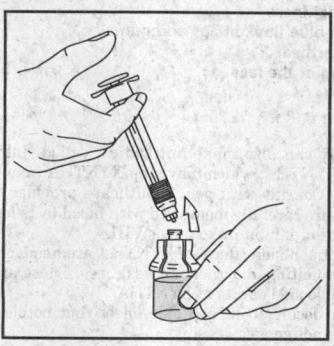

6. Connect a sterile 10 cc or larger luer lock syringe to the vial adapter. You may want to inject some air into the vial to make withdrawing the vial contents easier.

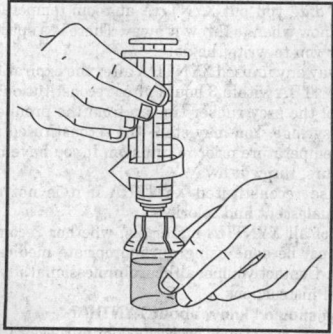

7. Invert the vial and slowly draw the solution into the 10 cc or larger luer lock syringe.

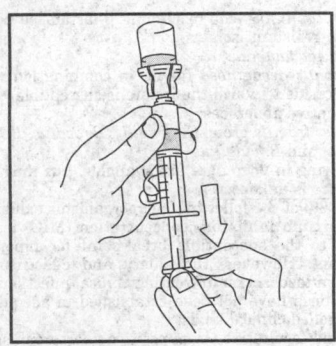

8. Detach the syringe from the vial adapter by gently turning and pulling the syringe counterclockwise. Discard the vial with the adapter attached.
9. Attach the infusion set to the 10 cc or larger luer lock syringe as directed [see Dosage and Administration (2.5)].
   Note: Dispose of all unused solution, the empty XYNTHA Prefilled Dual-Chamber Syringe, and other used medical supplies in an appropriate container for throwing away medical waste that might hurt others if not handled properly.

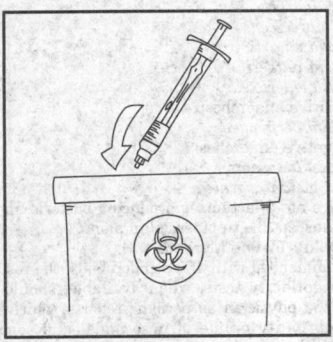

Multiple XYNTHA Prefilled Dual-Chamber Syringe Reconstitution to a 10 cc or Larger Luer Lock Syringe
The instructions below are for the use of multiple XYNTHA Prefilled Dual-Chamber Syringe kits with a 10 cc or larger luer lock syringe. For further information, please contact your healthcare provider or call the Medical Information Department at Wyeth Pharmaceuticals, 1-800-934-5556.
Note: Luer-to-luer syringe connectors are not provided in the kits. Contact your XYNTHA supplier to order.
1. Reconstitute all XYNTHA Prefilled Dual-Chamber Syringes according to instructions described in **PREPARATION AND RECONSTITUTION** section. Holding the XYNTHA Prefilled Dual-Chamber Syringe in an upright position, slowly advance the plunger rod until most, but not all, of the air is removed from the drug product chamber.

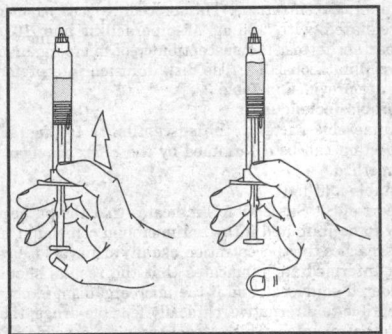

2. Remove the luer-to-luer syringe connector from its package.
3. After removing the protective blue vented cap, connect a sterile 10 cc or larger luer lock syringe to one opening (port) in the syringe connector and the XYNTHA Prefilled Dual-Chamber Syringe to the remaining open port on the opposite end.

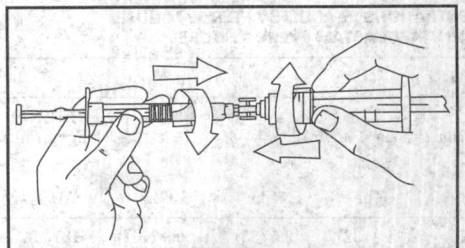

4. With the XYNTHA Prefilled Dual-Chamber Syringe on top, slowly depress the plunger rod until the contents empty into the 10 cc or larger luer lock syringe.

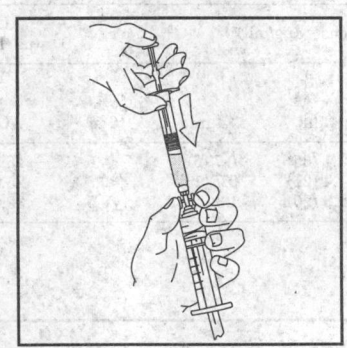

5. Remove the empty XYNTHA Prefilled Dual-Chamber Syringe and repeat procedures 3 and 4 above for any additional reconstituted syringes.
6. Remove the luer-to-luer syringe connector from the 10 cc or larger luer lock syringe and attach the infusion set as directed [see **INFUSION** section].
   Note: Dispose of all unused solution, the empty XYNTHA Prefilled Dual-Chamber Syringes, and other used medical supplies in an appropriate container for throwing away medical waste that might hurt others if not handled properly.

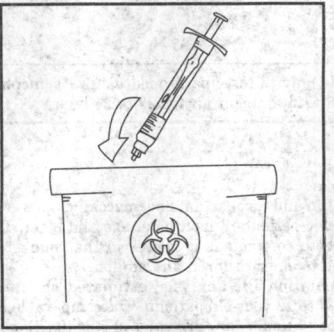

This Patient Package Insert has been approved by the U.S. Food and Drug Administration.

This product's label may have been updated. For current package insert and further product information, please visit www.wyeth.com or call our medical communications department toll-free at 1-800-934-5556.

Wyeth®
Wyeth Pharmaceuticals Inc.
Philadelphia, PA 19101
W10547C002
ET01
Rev 08/10

ZOSYN®   ℞
[zō'sĭn]
(Piperacillin and Tazobactam for Injection, USP)
Rx only

To reduce the development of drug-resistant bacteria and maintain the effectiveness of Zosyn (piperacillin and tazobactam) injection and other antibacterial drugs, Zosyn (piperacillin and tazobactam) should be used only to treat or prevent infections that are proven or strongly suspected to be caused by bacteria.

DESCRIPTION
Zosyn (piperacillin and tazobactam for injection, USP) is an injectable antibacterial combination product consisting of the semisynthetic antibiotic piperacillin sodium and the β-lactamase inhibitor tazobactam sodium for intravenous administration.

Piperacillin sodium is derived from D(-)-α-aminobenzyl-penicillin. The chemical name of piperacillin sodium is sodium (2S,5R,6R)-6-[(R)-2-(4-ethyl-2,3-dioxo-1-piperazine-carboxamido)-2-phenylacetamido]-3,3-dimethyl-7-oxo-4-thia-1-azabicyclo[3.2.0]heptane-2-carboxylate. The chemical formula is $C_{23}H_{26}N_5NaO_7S$ and the molecular weight is 539.5. The chemical structure of piperacillin sodium is:

Tazobactam sodium, a derivative of the penicillin nucleus, is a penicillanic acid sulfone. Its chemical name is sodium (2S,3S,5R)-3-methyl-7-oxo-3-(1H-1,2,3-triazol-1-ylmethyl)-4-thia-1-azabicyclo[3.2.0]heptane-2-carboxylate-4,4-dioxide. The chemical formula is $C_{10}H_{11}N_4NaO_5S$ and the molecular weight is 322.3. The chemical structure of tazobactam sodium is:

Zosyn, piperacillin/tazobactam parenteral combination, is a white to off-white sterile, cryodesiccated powder consisting of piperacillin and tazobactam as their sodium salts packaged in glass vials. The formulation also contains edetate disodium dihydrate (EDTA) and sodium citrate.
Each Zosyn 2.25 g single dose vial contains an amount of drug sufficient for withdrawal of piperacillin sodium equivalent to 2 grams of piperacillin and tazobactam sodium equivalent to 0.25 g of tazobactam. The product also contains 0.5 mg of EDTA per vial.
Each Zosyn 3.375 g single dose vial contains an amount of drug sufficient for withdrawal of piperacillin sodium equivalent to 3 grams of piperacillin and tazobactam sodium equivalent to 0.375 g of tazobactam. The product also contains 0.75 mg of EDTA per vial.
Each Zosyn 4.5 g single dose vial contains an amount of drug sufficient for withdrawal of piperacillin sodium equivalent to 4 grams of piperacillin and tazobactam sodium equivalent to 0.5 g of tazobactam. The product also contains 1 mg of EDTA per vial.
Zosyn (piperacillin and tazobactam for injection, USP) contains a total of 2.79 mEq (64 mg) of sodium (Na⁺) per gram of piperacillin in the combination product.

CLINICAL PHARMACOLOGY
Adults
Peak plasma concentrations of piperacillin and tazobactam are attained immediately after completion of an intravenous infusion of Zosyn. Piperacillin plasma concentrations, following a 30-minute infusion of Zosyn, were similar to those attained when equivalent doses of piperacillin were administered alone, with mean peak plasma concentrations of approximately 134, 242 and 298 µg/mL for the 2.25 g, 3.375 g and 4.5 g Zosyn (piperacillin/tazobactam) doses, respectively. The corresponding mean peak plasma concentrations of tazobactam were 15, 24 and 34 µg/mL, respectively. Following a 30-minute I.V. infusion of 3.375 g Zosyn every 6 hours, steady-state plasma concentrations of piperacillin and tazobactam were similar to those attained after the first dose. In like manner, steady-state plasma concentrations were not different from those attained after the first dose when 2.25 g or 4.5 g doses of Zosyn were administered via 30-minute infusions every 6 hours. Steady-state plasma concentrations after 30-minute infusions every 6 hours are provided in **Table 1**.
Following single or multiple Zosyn doses to healthy subjects, the plasma half-life of piperacillin and of tazobactam ranged from 0.7 to 1.2 hours and was unaffected by dose or duration of infusion.
Piperacillin is metabolized to a minor microbiologically active desethyl metabolite. Tazobactam is metabolized to a single metabolite that lacks pharmacological and antibacterial activities. Both piperacillin and tazobactam are eliminated via the kidney by glomerular filtration and tubular secretion. Piperacillin is excreted rapidly as unchanged drug with 68% of the administered dose excreted in the urine. Tazobactam and its metabolite are eliminated primarily by renal excretion with 80% of the administered dose excreted as unchanged drug and the remainder as the single metabolite. Piperacillin, tazobactam and desethyl piperacillin are also secreted into the bile.

TABLE 1 STEADY STATE MEAN PLASMA CONCENTRATIONS IN ADULTS AFTER 30-MINUTE INTRAVENOUS INFUSION OF PIPERACILLIN/TAZOBACTAM EVERY 6 HOURS

PIPERACILLIN

Piperacillin/ Tazobactam Dose[a]	No. of Evaluable Subjects	Plasma Concentrations** (µg/mL)						AUC** (µg•hr/mL)
		30 min	1 hr	2 hr	3 hr	4 hr	6 hr	AUC_{0-6}
2.25 g	8	134 (14)	57 (14)	17.1 (23)	5.2 (32)	2.5 (35)	0.9 (14)[b]	131 (14)
3.375 g	6	242 (12)	106 (8)	34.6 (20)	11.5 (19)	5.1 (22)	1.0 (10)	242 (10)
4.5 g	8	298 (14)	141 (19)	46.6 (28)	16.4 (29)	6.9 (29)	1.4 (30)	322 (16)

TAZOBACTAM

Piperacillin/ Tazobactam Dose[a]	No. of Evaluable Subjects	Plasma Concentrations** (µg/mL)						AUC** (µg•hr/mL)
		30 min	1 hr	2 hr	3 hr	4 hr	6 hr	AUC_{0-6}
2.25 g	8	14.8 (14)	7.2 (22)	2.6 (30)	1.1 (35)	0.7 (6)[c]	<0.5	16.0 (21)
3.375 g	6	24.2 (14)	10.7 (7)	4.0 (18)	1.4 (21)	0.7 (16)[b]	<0.5	25.0 (8)
4.5 g	8	33.8 (15)	17.3 (16)	6.8 (24)	2.8 (25)	1.3 (30)	<0.5	39.8 (15)

**Numbers in parentheses are coefficients of variation (CV%).
a: Piperacillin and tazobactam were given in combination.
b: N = 4
c: N = 3

TABLE 2 SUSCEPTIBILITY INTERPRETIVE CRITERIA FOR PIPERACILLIN/TAZOBACTAM

Pathogen	Susceptibility Test Result Interpretive Criteria					
	Minimal Inhibitory Concentration (MIC in µg/mL)			Disk Diffusion (Zone Diameter in mm)		
	S	I	R	S	I	R
Enterobacteriaceae and Acinetobacter baumanii	≤ 16	32-64	≥ 128	≥ 21	18-20	≤ 17
Haemophilus influenzae[a]	≤ 1	-	≥ 2	-	-	-
Pseudomonas aeruginosa	≤ 64	-	≥ 128	≥ 18	-	≤ 17
Staphylococcus aureus	≤ 8	-	≥ 16	≥ 20	-	≤ 19
Bacteroides fragilis group	≤ 32	64	≥ 128	-	-	-

a: These interpretive criteria for *Haemophilus influenzae* are applicable only to tests performed using Haemophilus Test Medium inoculated with a direct colony suspension and incubated at 35°C in ambient air for 20 to 24 hours.

Both piperacillin and tazobactam are approximately 30% bound to plasma proteins. The protein binding of either piperacillin or tazobactam is unaffected by the presence of the other compound. Protein binding of the tazobactam metabolite is negligible.

Piperacillin and tazobactam are widely distributed into tissues and body fluids including intestinal mucosa, gallbladder, lung, female reproductive tissues (uterus, ovary, and fallopian tube), interstitial fluid, and bile. Mean tissue concentrations are generally 50% to 100% of those in plasma. Distribution of piperacillin and tazobactam into cerebrospinal fluid is low in subjects with non-inflamed meninges, as with other penicillins.

After the administration of single doses of piperacillin/tazobactam to subjects with renal impairment, the half-life of piperacillin and of tazobactam increases with decreasing creatinine clearance. At creatinine clearance below 20 mL/min, the increase in half-life is twofold for piperacillin and fourfold for tazobactam compared to subjects with normal renal function. Dosage adjustments for Zosyn are recommended when creatinine clearance is below 40 mL/min in patients receiving the usual recommended daily dose of Zosyn (piperacillin and tazobactam for injection, USP). (See **DOSAGE AND ADMINISTRATION** section for specific recommendations for the treatment of patients with renal insufficiency.)

Hemodialysis removes 30% to 40% of a piperacillin/tazobactam dose with an additional 5% of the tazobactam dose removed as the tazobactam metabolite. Peritoneal dialysis removes approximately 6% and 21% of the piperacillin and tazobactam doses, respectively, with up to 16% of the tazobactam dose removed as the tazobactam metabolite. For dosage recommendations for patients undergoing hemodialysis, see **DOSAGE AND ADMINISTRATION** section.

The half-life of piperacillin and of tazobactam increases by approximately 25% and 18%, respectively, in patients with hepatic cirrhosis compared to healthy subjects. However, this difference does not warrant dosage adjustment of Zosyn due to hepatic cirrhosis.

[See table 1 above]

Pediatrics
Piperacillin and tazobactam pharmacokinetics were studied in pediatric patients 2 months of age and older. The clearance of both compounds is slower in the younger patients compared to older children and adults.

In a population PK analysis, estimated clearance for 9 month-old to 12 year-old patients was comparable to adults, with a population mean (SE) value of 5.64 (0.34) mL/min/kg. The piperacillin clearance estimate is 80% of this value for pediatric patients 2-9 months old. In patients younger than 2 months of age, clearance of piperacillin is slower compared to older children; however, it is not adequately characterized for dosing recommendations. The population mean (SE) for piperacillin distribution volume is 0.243 (0.011) L/kg and is independent of age.

Microbiology
Piperacillin sodium exerts bactericidal activity by inhibiting septum formation and cell wall synthesis of susceptible bacteria. In vitro, piperacillin is active against a variety of gram-positive and gram-negative aerobic and anaerobic bacteria. Tazobactam sodium has little clinically relevant in vitro activity against bacteria due to its reduced affinity to penicillin-binding proteins. It is, however, a β-lactamase inhibitor of the Richmond-Sykes class III (Bush class 2b & 2b') penicillinases and cephalosporinases. It varies in its ability to inhibit class II and IV (2a & 4) penicillinases. Tazobactam does not induce chromosomally-mediated β-lactamases at tazobactam concentrations achieved with the recommended dosage regimen.

Piperacillin/tazobactam has been shown to be active against most strains of the following microorganisms both in vitro and in clinical infections as described in the **INDICATIONS AND USAGE** section.

Aerobic and facultative Gram-positive microorganisms:
Staphylococcus aureus (excluding methicillin and oxacillin-resistant isolates)
Aerobic and facultative Gram-negative microorganisms:
Acinetobacter baumanii
Escherichia coli

Haemophilus influenzae (excluding β-lactamase negative, ampicillin-resistant isolates)
Klebsiella pneumoniae
Pseudomonas aeruginosa (given in combination with an aminoglycoside to which the isolate is susceptible)
Gram-negative anaerobes:
Bacteroides fragilis group (*B. fragilis, B. ovatus, B. thetaiotaomicron,* and *B. vulgatus*)
The following in vitro data are available, **but their clinical significance is unknown.**
At least 90% of the following microorganisms exhibit an in vitro minimum inhibitory concentration (MIC) less than or equal to the susceptible breakpoint for piperacillin/tazobactam. However, the safety and effectiveness of piperacillin/tazobactam in treating clinical infections due to these bacteria have not been established in adequate and well-controlled clinical trials.
Aerobic and facultative Gram-positive microorganisms:
Enterococcus faecalis (ampicillin or penicillin-susceptible isolates only)
Staphylococcus epidermidis (excluding methicillin and oxacillin-resistant isolates)
Streptococcus agalactiae[†]
Streptococcus pneumoniae[†] (penicillin-susceptible isolates only)
Streptococcus pyogenes[†]
Viridans group streptococci[†]
Aerobic and facultative Gram-negative microorganisms:
Citrobacter koseri
Moraxella catarrhalis
Morganella morganii
Neisseria gonorrhoeae
Proteus mirabilis
Proteus vulgaris
Serratia marcescens
Providencia stuartii
Providencia rettgeri
Salmonella enterica
Gram-positive anaerobes:
Clostridium perfringens
Gram-negative anaerobes:
Bacteroides distasonis
Prevotella melaninogenica
[†] These are not β-lactamase producing bacteria and, therefore, are susceptible to piperacillin alone.

Susceptibility Testing Methods
As is recommended with all antimicrobials, the results of in vitro susceptibility tests, when available, should be provided to the physician as periodic reports, which describe the susceptibility profile of nosocomial and community-acquired pathogens. These reports should aid the physician in selecting the most effective antimicrobial.
Dilution Techniques:
Quantitative methods are used to determine antimicrobial minimum inhibitory concentrations (MICs). These MICs provide estimates of the susceptibility of bacteria to antimicrobial compounds. The MICs should be determined using a standardized procedure. Standardized procedures are based on a dilution method (broth or agar) or equivalent with standardized inoculum concentrations and standardized concentrations of piperacillin and tazobactam powders.[1,2] MIC values should be determined using serial dilutions of piperacillin combined with a fixed concentration of 4 µg/mL tazobactam. The MIC values obtained should be interpreted according to criteria provided in **Table 2.**
Diffusion Technique:
Quantitative methods that require measurement of zone diameters also provide reproducible estimates of the susceptibility of bacteria to antimicrobial compounds. One such standardized procedure[1,3] requires the use of standardized inoculum concentrations. This procedure uses paper disks impregnated with 100 µg of piperacillin and 10 µg of tazobactam to test the susceptibility of microorganisms to piperacillin/tazobactam. The disk diffusion interpreted criteria are provided in **Table 2.**
Anaerobic Techniques
For anaerobic bacteria, the susceptibility to piperacillin/tazobactam can be determined by the reference agar dilution method.[4]
[See table 2 at left]
A report of S ("Susceptible") indicates that the pathogen is likely to be inhibited if the antimicrobial compound in the blood reaches the concentration usually achievable. A report of I ("Intermediate") indicates that the results should be considered equivocal, and if the microorganism is not fully susceptible to alternative, clinically feasible drugs, the test should be repeated. This category implies possible clinical applicability in body sites where the drug is physiologically concentrated or in situations where high dosage of drug can be used. This category also provides a buffer zone, which prevents small, uncontrolled technical factors from causing major discrepancies in interpretation. A report of R ("Resistant") indicates that the pathogen is not likely to be inhibited if the antimicrobial compound in the blood reaches the concentration usually achievable; other therapy should be considered.

Quality Control
Standardized susceptibility test procedures require the use of quality control microorganisms to control the technical aspects of the test procedures.[1,2,3,4] Standard piperacillin/tazobactam powder should provide the following ranges of values noted in **Table 3**. Quality control microorganisms are specific strains of microorganisms with intrinsic biological properties relating to resistance mechanisms and their genetic expression within the microorganism; the specific strains used for microbiological quality control are not clinically significant.
[See table 3 at right]

TABLE 3 ACCEPTABLE QUALITY CONTROL RANGES FOR PIPERACILLIN/TAZOBACTAM TO BE USED IN VALIDATION OF SUSCEPTIBILITY TEST RESULTS

	Acceptable Quality Control Ranges	
QC Strain	Minimum Inhibitory Concentration Range (MIC in µg/mL)	Disk Diffusion Zone Diameter Ranges in mm
Escherichia coli ATCC 25922	1-4	24-30
Escherichia coli ATCC 35218	0.5-2	24-30
Pseudomonas aeruginosa ATCC 27853	1-8	25-33
Haemophilus influenzae[a] ATCC 49247	0.06-0.5	-
Staphylococcus aureus ATCC 29213	0.25-2	-
Staphylococcus aureus ATCC 25923	-	27-36
Bacteroides fragilis ATCC 25285	0.12-0.5	-
Bacteroides thetaiotaomicron ATCC 29741	4-16	-

a: This quality control range for *Haemophilus influenzae* is applicable only to tests performed using Haemophilus Test Medium inoculated with a direct colony suspension and incubated at 35°C in ambient air for 20 to 24 hours.

INDICATIONS AND USAGE

Zosyn (piperacillin and tazobactam for injection, USP) is indicated for the treatment of patients with moderate to severe infections caused by piperacillin-resistant, piperacillin/tazobactam-susceptible, β-lactamase producing strains of the designated microorganisms in the specified conditions listed below:

Appendicitis (complicated by rupture or abscess) and peritonitis caused by piperacillin-resistant, β-lactamase producing strains of *Escherichia coli* or the following members of the *Bacteroides fragilis* group: *B. fragilis, B. ovatus, B. thetaiotaomicron*, or *B. vulgatus*. The individual members of this group were studied in less than 10 cases.

Uncomplicated and complicated skin and skin structure infections, including cellulitis, cutaneous abscesses and ischemic/diabetic foot infections caused by piperacillin-resistant, β-lactamase producing strains of *Staphylococcus aureus*.

Postpartum endometritis or pelvic inflammatory disease caused by piperacillin-resistant, β-lactamase producing strains of *Escherichia coli*.

Community-acquired pneumonia (moderate severity only) caused by piperacillin-resistant, β-lactamase producing strains of *Haemophilus influenzae*.

Nosocomial pneumonia (moderate to severe) caused by piperacillin-resistant, β-lactamase producing strains of *Staphylococcus aureus* and by piperacillin/tazobactam-susceptible *Acinetobacter baumanii, Haemophilus influenzae, Klebsiella pneumoniae*, and *Pseudomonas aeruginosa* (Nosocomial pneumonia caused by *P. aeruginosa* should be treated in combination with an aminoglycoside). (See **DOSAGE AND ADMINISTRATION**.)

Zosyn (piperacillin and tazobactam for injection, USP) is indicated only for the specified conditions listed above. Infections caused by piperacillin-susceptible organisms, for which piperacillin has been shown to be effective, are also amenable to Zosyn treatment due to its piperacillin content. The tazobactam component of this combination product does not decrease the activity of the piperacillin component against piperacillin-susceptible organisms. Therefore, the treatment of mixed infections caused by piperacillin-susceptible organisms and piperacillin-resistant, β-lactamase producing organisms susceptible to Zosyn should not require the addition of another antibiotic. (See **DOSAGE AND ADMINISTRATION**.)

Zosyn is useful as presumptive therapy in the indicated conditions prior to the identification of causative organisms because of its broad spectrum of bactericidal activity against gram-positive and gram-negative aerobic and anaerobic organisms.

Appropriate cultures should usually be performed before initiating antimicrobial treatment in order to isolate and identify the organisms causing infection and to determine their susceptibility to Zosyn. Antimicrobial therapy should be adjusted, if appropriate, once the results of culture(s) and antimicrobial susceptibility testing are known.

To reduce the development of drug-resistant bacteria and maintain the effectiveness of Zosyn (piperacillin and tazobactam) injection and other antibacterial drugs, Zosyn (piperacillin and tazobactam) should be used only to treat or prevent infections that are proven or strongly suspected to be caused by susceptible bacteria. When culture and susceptibility information are available, they should be considered in selecting or modifying antibacterial therapy. In the absence of such data, local epidemiology and susceptibility patterns may contribute to the empiric selection of therapy.

CONTRAINDICATIONS

Zosyn is contraindicated in patients with a history of allergic reactions to any of the penicillins, cephalosporins, or β-lactamase inhibitors.

WARNINGS

SERIOUS AND OCCASIONALLY FATAL HYPERSENSITIVITY (ANAPHYLACTIC/ANAPHYLACTOID) REACTIONS (INCLUDING SHOCK) HAVE BEEN REPORTED IN PATIENTS RECEIVING THERAPY WITH PENICILLINS INCLUDING ZOSYN. THESE REACTIONS ARE MORE LIKELY TO OCCUR IN INDIVIDUALS WITH A HISTORY OF PENICILLIN HYPERSENSITIVITY OR A HISTORY OF SENSITIVITY TO MULTIPLE ALLERGENS. THERE HAVE BEEN REPORTS OF INDIVIDUALS WITH A HISTORY OF PENICILLIN HYPERSENSITIVITY WHO HAVE EXPERIENCED SEVERE REACTIONS WHEN TREATED WITH CEPHALOSPORINS. BEFORE INITIATING THERAPY WITH ZOSYN, CAREFUL INQUIRY SHOULD BE MADE CONCERNING PREVIOUS HYPERSENSITIVITY REACTIONS TO PENICILLINS, CEPHALOSPORINS, OR OTHER ALLERGENS. IF AN ALLERGIC REACTION OCCURS, ZOSYN SHOULD BE DISCONTINUED AND APPROPRIATE THERAPY INSTITUTED. **SERIOUS ANAPHYLACTIC/ANAPHYLACTOID REACTIONS (INCLUDING SHOCK) REQUIRE IMMEDIATE EMERGENCY TREATMENT WITH EPINEPHRINE. OXYGEN, INTRAVENOUS STEROIDS, AND AIRWAY MANAGEMENT, INCLUDING INTUBATION, SHOULD ALSO BE ADMINISTERED AS INDICATED.**

Clostridium difficile associated diarrhea (CDAD) has been reported with use of nearly all antibacterial agents, including Zosyn, and may range in severity from mild diarrhea to fatal colitis. Treatment with antibacterial agents alters the normal flora of the colon leading to overgrowth of *C. difficile*.

C. difficile produces toxins A and B which contribute to the development of CDAD. Hypertoxin producing strains of *C. difficile* cause increased morbidity and mortality, as these infections can be refractory to antimicrobial therapy and may require colectomy. CDAD must be considered in all patients who present with diarrhea following antibiotic use. Careful medical history is necessary since CDAD has been reported to occur over two months after the administration of antibacterial agents.

If CDAD is suspected or confirmed, ongoing antibiotic use not directed against *C. difficile* may need to be discontinued. Appropriate fluid and electrolyte management, protein supplementation, antibiotic treatment of *C. difficile*, and surgical evaluation should be instituted as clinically indicated.

PRECAUTIONS

General

Bleeding manifestations have occurred in some patients receiving β-lactam antibiotics, including piperacillin. These reactions have sometimes been associated with abnormalities of coagulation tests such as clotting time, platelet aggregation and prothrombin time, and are more likely to occur in patients with renal failure. If bleeding manifestations occur, Zosyn (piperacillin and tazobactam for injection, USP) should be discontinued and appropriate therapy instituted.

The possibility of the emergence of resistant organisms that might cause superinfections should be kept in mind. If this occurs, appropriate measures should be taken.

As with other penicillins, patients may experience neuromuscular excitability or convulsions if higher than recommended doses are given intravenously (particularly in the presence of renal failure).

Zosyn contains a total of 2.79 mEq (64 mg) of Na^+ per gram of piperacillin in the combination product. This should be considered when treating patients requiring restricted salt intake. Periodic electrolyte determinations should be performed in patients with low potassium reserves, and the possibility of hypokalemia should be kept in mind with patients who have potentially low potassium reserves and who are receiving cytotoxic therapy or diuretics.

As with other semisynthetic penicillins, piperacillin therapy has been associated with an increased incidence of fever and rash in cystic fibrosis patients.

In patients with creatinine clearance ≤ 40 mL/min and dialysis patients (hemodialysis and CAPD), the intravenous dose should be adjusted to the degree of renal function impairment. (See **DOSAGE AND ADMINISTRATION**.)

Prescribing Zosyn (piperacillin and tazobactam) in the absence of a proven or strongly suspected bacterial infection or a prophylactic indication is unlikely to provide benefit to the patient and increases the risk of development of drug-resistant bacteria.

Information for Patients

Patients should be counseled that antibacterial drugs including Zosyn should only be used to treat bacterial infections. They do not treat viral infections (e.g., the common cold). When Zosyn is prescribed to treat a bacterial infection, patients should be told that although it is common to feel better early in the course of therapy, the medication should be taken exactly as directed. Skipping doses or not completing the full course of therapy may (1) decrease the effectiveness of the immediate treatment and (2) increase the likelihood that bacteria will develop resistance and will not be treatable by Zosyn or other antibacterial drugs in the future.

Diarrhea is a common problem caused by antibiotics which usually ends when the antibiotic is discontinued. Sometimes after starting treatment with antibiotics, patients can develop watery and bloody stools (with or without stomach cramps and fever) even as late as two or more months after having taken the last dose of the antibiotic. If this occurs, patients should contact their physician as soon as possible.

Laboratory Tests

Periodic assessment of hematopoietic function should be performed, especially with prolonged therapy, ie, ≥ 21 days. (See **ADVERSE REACTIONS, Adverse Laboratory Events**.)

Drug Interactions

Aminoglycosides

The mixing of beta-lactam antibiotics with aminoglycosides *in vitro* can result in substantial inactivation of the aminoglycoside. However, amikacin and gentamicin have been shown to be compatible *in vitro* with reformulated Zosyn containing EDTA supplied in vials or bulk pharmacy containers in certain diluents at specific concentrations for a simultaneous Y-site infusion. (See **DOSAGE AND ADMINISTRATION**.) Reformulated Zosyn containing EDTA is not compatible with tobramycin for simultaneous coadministration via Y-site infusion.

The inactivation of aminoglycosides in the presence of penicillin-class drugs has been recognized. It has been postulated that penicillin-aminoglycoside complexes form; these complexes are microbiologically inactive and of unknown toxicity. Sequential administration of Zosyn with tobramycin to patients with normal renal function and mild to moderate renal impairment has been shown to modestly decrease serum concentrations of tobramycin but does not significantly affect tobramycin pharmacokinetics. When aminoglycosides are administered in combination with piperacillin to patients with end-stage renal disease requiring hemodialysis, the concentrations of the aminoglycosides (especially tobramycin) may be significantly altered and should be monitored. Since aminoglycosides are not equally susceptible to inactivation by piperacillin, consideration should be given to the choice of the aminoglycoside when administered in combination with piperacillin to these patients.

Probenecid

Probenecid administered concomitantly with Zosyn prolongs the half-life of piperacillin by 21% and that of tazobactam by 71%.

Vancomycin

No pharmacokinetic interactions have been noted between Zosyn and vancomycin.

Heparin

Coagulation parameters should be tested more frequently and monitored regularly during simultaneous administration of high doses of heparin, oral anticoagulants, or other drugs that may affect the blood coagulation system or the thrombocyte function.

Vecuronium

Piperacillin when used concomitantly with vecuronium has been implicated in the prolongation of the neuromuscular blockade of vecuronium. Zosyn (piperacillin/tazobactam) could produce the same phenomenon if given along with vecuronium. Due to their similar mechanism of action, it is expected that the neuromuscular blockade produced by any of the non-depolarizing muscle relaxants could be prolonged in the presence of piperacillin. (See package insert for vecuronium bromide.)

Methotrexate

Limited data suggests that co-administration of methotrexate and piperacillin may reduce the clearance of methotrexate due to competition for renal secretion. The impact of tazobactam on the elimination of methotrexate has not been evaluated. If concurrent therapy is necessary, serum concentrations of methotrexate as well as the signs and symptoms of methotrexate toxicity should be frequently monitored.

Drug/Laboratory Test Interactions

As with other penicillins, the administration of Zosyn® (piperacillin and tazobactam for injection, USP) may result in a false-positive reaction for glucose in the urine using a copper-reduction method (CLINITEST®). It is recommended that glucose tests based on enzymatic glucose oxidase reactions (such as DIASTIX® or TES-TAPE®) be used.

There have been reports of positive test results using the Bio-Rad Laboratories Platelia *Aspergillus* EIA test in patients receiving piperacillin/tazobactam injection who were subsequently found to be free of *Aspergillus* infection. Cross-reactions with non-*Aspergillus* polysaccharides and polyfuranoses with the Bio-Rad Laboratories Platelia *Aspergillus* EIA test have been reported.

Therefore, positive test results in patients receiving piperacillin/tazobactam should be interpreted cautiously and confirmed by other diagnostic methods.

Carcinogenesis, Mutagenesis, Impairment of Fertility

Long-term carcinogenicity studies in animals have not been conducted with piperacillin/tazobactam, piperacillin, or tazobactam.

Piperacillin/Tazobactam

Piperacillin/tazobactam was negative in microbial mutagenicity assays at concentrations up to 14.84/1.86 µg/plate. Piperacillin/tazobactam was negative in the unscheduled DNA synthesis (UDS) test at concentrations up to 5689/711 µg/mL. Piperacillin/tazobactam was negative in a mammalian point mutation (Chinese hamster ovary cell HPRT) assay at concentrations up to 8000/1000 µg/mL. Piperacillin/tazobactam was negative in a mammalian cell (BALB/c-3T3) transformation assay at concentrations up to 8/1 µg/mL. In vivo, piperacillin/tazobactam did not induce chromosomal aberrations in rats dosed I.V. with 1500/187.5 mg/kg; this dose is similar to the maximum recommended human daily dose on a body-surface-area basis (mg/m^2).

Piperacillin

Piperacillin was negative in microbial mutagenicity assays at concentrations up to 50 µg/plate. There was no DNA damage in bacteria (Rec assay) exposed to piperacillin at concentrations up to 200 µg/disk. Piperacillin was negative in the UDS test at concentrations up to 10,000 µg/mL. In a mammalian point mutation (mouse lymphoma cells) assay, piperacillin was positive at concentrations ≥2500 µg/mL. Piperacillin was negative in a cell (BALB/c-3T3) transformation assay at concentrations up to 3000 µg/mL. In vivo, piperacillin did not induce chromosomal aberrations in mice at I.V. doses up to 2000 mg/kg/day or rats at I.V. doses up to 1500 mg/kg/day. These doses are half (mice) or similar (rats) to the maximum recommended human daily dose based on body-surface area (mg/m^2). In another in vivo test, there was no dominant lethal effect when piperacillin was administered to rats at I.V. doses up to 2000 mg/kg/day, which is similar to the maximum recommended human daily dose based on body-surface area (mg/m^2). When mice were administered piperacillin at I.V. doses up to 2000 mg/kg/day, which is half the maximum recommended human daily dose based on body-surface area (mg/m^2), urine from these animals was not mutagenic when tested in a microbial mutagenicity assay. Bacteria injected into the peritoneal

cavity of mice administered piperacillin at I.V. doses up to 2000 mg/kg/day did not show increased mutation frequencies.

Tazobactam

Tazobactam was negative in microbial mutagenicity assays at concentrations up to 333 µg/plate. Tazobactam was negative in the UDS test at concentrations up to 2000 µg/mL. Tazobactam was negative in a mammalian point mutation (Chinese hamster ovary cell HPRT) assay at concentrations up to 5000 µg/mL. In another mammalian point mutation (mouse lymphoma cells) assay, tazobactam was positive at concentrations ≥3000 µg/mL. Tazobactam was negative in a cell (BALB/c-3T3) transformation assay at concentrations up to 900 µg/mL. In an in vitro cytogenetics (Chinese hamster lung cells) assay, tazobactam was negative at concentrations up to 3000 µg/mL. In vivo, tazobactam did not induce chromosomal aberrations in rats at I.V. doses up to 5000 mg/kg, which is 23 times the maximum recommended human daily dose based on body-surface area (mg/m^2).

Pregnancy

Teratogenic effects—Pregnancy Category B

Piperacillin/tazobactam

Reproduction studies have been performed in rats and have revealed no evidence of impaired fertility due to piperacillin/tazobactam administered up to a dose which is similar to the maximum recommended human daily dose based on body-surface area (mg/m^2).

Teratology studies have been performed in mice and rats and have revealed no evidence of harm to the fetus due to piperacillin/tazobactam administered up to a dose which is 1 to 2 times and 2 to 3 times the human dose of piperacillin and tazobactam, respectively, based on body-surface area (mg/m^2).

Piperacillin and tazobactam cross the placenta in humans.

Piperacillin

Reproduction and teratology studies have been performed in mice and rats and have revealed no evidence of impaired fertility or harm to the fetus due to piperacillin administered up to a dose which is half (mice) or similar (rats) to the maximum recommended human daily dose based on body-surface area (mg/m^2).

Tazobactam

Reproduction studies have been performed in rats and have revealed no evidence of impaired fertility due to tazobactam administered at doses up to 3 times the maximum recommended human daily dose based on body-surface area (mg/m^2).

Teratology studies have been performed in mice and rats and have revealed no evidence of harm to the fetus due to tazobactam administered at doses up to 6 and 14 times, respectively, the human dose based on body-surface area (mg/m^2). In rats, tazobactam crosses the placenta. Concentrations in the fetus are less than or equal to 10% of those found in maternal plasma.

There are, however, no adequate and well-controlled studies with the piperacillin/tazobactam combination or with piperacillin or tazobactam alone in pregnant women. Because animal reproduction studies are not always predictive of the human response, this drug should be used during pregnancy only if clearly needed.

Nursing Mothers

Piperacillin is excreted in low concentrations in human milk; tazobactam concentrations in human milk have not been studied. Caution should be exercised when Zosyn (piperacillin and tazobactam for injection, USP) is administered to a nursing woman.

Pediatric Use

Use of Zosyn in pediatric patients 2 months of age or older with appendicitis and/or peritonitis is supported by evidence from well-controlled studies and pharmacokinetic studies in adults and in pediatric patients. This includes a prospective, randomized, comparative, open-label clinical trial with 542 pediatric patients 2-12 years of age with complicated intra-abdominal infections, in which 273 pediatric patients received piperacillin/tazobactam. Safety and efficacy in pediatric patients less than 2 months of age have not been established (see **CLINICAL PHARMACOLOGY** and **DOSAGE AND ADMINISTRATION**).

There are no dosage recommendations for Zosyn in pediatric patients with impaired renal function.

Geriatric Use

Patients over 65 years are **not** at an increased risk of developing adverse effects solely because of age. However, dosage should be adjusted in the presence of renal insufficiency. (See **DOSAGE AND ADMINISTRATION**.)

In general, dose selection for an elderly patient should be cautious, usually starting at the low end of the dosing range, reflecting the greater frequency of decreased hepatic, renal, or cardiac function, and of concomitant disease or other drug therapy.

Zosyn contains 64 mg (2.79 mEq) of sodium per gram of piperacillin in the combination product. At the usual recommended doses, patients would receive between 768 and 1024 mg/day (33.5 and 44.6 mEq) of sodium. The geriatric

population may respond with a blunted natriuresis to salt loading. This may be clinically important with regard to such diseases as congestive heart failure.

This drug is known to be substantially excreted by the kidney, and the risk of toxic reactions to this drug may be greater in patients with impaired renal function. Because elderly patients are more likely to have decreased renal function, care should be taken in dose selection, and it may be useful to monitor renal function.

ADVERSE REACTIONS

Adverse Events From Clinical Trials

During the initial clinical investigations, 2621 patients worldwide were treated with Zosyn (piperacillin and tazobactam for injection, USP) in phase 3 trials. In the key North American clinical trials (n=830 patients), 90% of the adverse events reported were mild to moderate in severity and transient in nature. However, in 3.2% of the patients treated worldwide, Zosyn was discontinued because of adverse events primarily involving the skin (1.3%), including rash and pruritus; the gastrointestinal system (0.9%), including diarrhea, nausea, and vomiting; and allergic reactions (0.5%).

Adverse local reactions that were reported, irrespective of relationship to therapy with Zosyn, were phlebitis (1.3%), injection site reaction (0.5%), pain (0.2%), inflammation (0.2%), thrombophlebitis (0.2%), and edema (0.1%).

Based on patients from the North American trials (n=1063), the events with the highest incidence in patients, irrespective of relationship to Zosyn therapy, were diarrhea (11.3%); headache (7.7%); constipation (7.7%); nausea (6.9%); insomnia (6.6%); rash (4.2%), including maculopapular, bullous, urticarial, and eczematoid; vomiting (3.3%); dyspepsia (3.3%); pruritus (3.1%); stool changes (2.4%); fever (2.4%); agitation (2.1%); pain (1.7%); moniliasis (1.6%); hypertension (1.6%); dizziness (1.4%); abdominal pain (1.3%); chest pain (1.3%); edema (1.2%); anxiety (1.2%); rhinitis (1.2%); and dyspnea (1.1%).

Additional adverse systemic clinical events reported in 1.0% or less of the patients in the initial North American trials are listed below within each body system.

Autonomic nervous system—hypotension, ileus, syncope
Body as a whole—rigors, back pain, malaise
Cardiovascular—tachycardia, including supraventricular and ventricular; bradycardia; arrhythmia, including atrial fibrillation, ventricular fibrillation, cardiac arrest, cardiac failure, circulatory failure, myocardial infarction
Central nervous system—tremor, convulsions, vertigo
Gastrointestinal—melena, flatulence, hemorrhage, gastritis, hiccough, ulcerative stomatitis

Pseudomembranous colitis was reported in one patient during the clinical trials. The onset of pseudomembranous colitis symptoms may occur during or after antibacterial treatment. (See **WARNINGS**.)

Hearing and Vestibular System—tinnitus
Hypersensitivity—anaphylaxis
Metabolic and Nutritional—symptomatic hypoglycemia, thirst
Musculoskeletal—myalgia, arthralgia
Platelets, Bleeding, Clotting—mesenteric embolism, purpura, epistaxis, pulmonary embolism (See **PRECAUTIONS, General**).
Psychiatric—confusion, hallucination, depression
Reproductive, Female—leukorrhea, vaginitis
Respiratory—pharyngitis, pulmonary edema, bronchospasm, coughing
Skin and Appendages—genital pruritus, diaphoresis
Special senses—taste perversion
Urinary—retention, dysuria, oliguria, hematuria, incontinence
Vision—photophobia
Vascular (extracardiac)—flushing

Nosocomial Pneumonia Trials

In a completed study of nosocomial lower respiratory tract infections, 222 patients were treated with Zosyn in a dosing regimen of 4.5 g every 6 hours in combination with an aminoglycoside and 215 patients were treated with imipenem/cilastatin (500 mg/500 mg q6h) in combination with an aminoglycoside. In this trial, treatment-emergent adverse events were reported by 402 patients, 204 (91.9%) in the piperacillin/tazobactam group and 198 (92.1%) in the imipenem/cilastatin group. Twenty-five (11.0%) patients in the piperacillin/tazobactam group and 14 (6.5%) in the imipenem/cilastatin group (p > 0.05) discontinued treatment due to an adverse event.

In this study of Zosyn in combination with an aminoglycoside, adverse events that occurred in more than 1% patients and were considered by the investigator to be drug-related were: diarrhea (17.6%), fever (2.7%), vomiting (2.7%), urinary tract infection (2.7%), rash (2.3%), abdominal pain (1.8%), generalized edema (1.8%), moniliasis (1.8%), nausea (1.8%), oral moniliasis (1.8%), BUN increased (1.8%), creatinine increased (1.8%), peripheral edema (1.8%), abdomen enlarged (1.4%), headache (1.4%), constipation (1.4%), liver function tests abnormal (1.4%), thrombocythemia (1.4%), excoriations (1.4%), and sweating (1.4%).

Drug-related adverse events reported in 1% or less of patients in the nosocomial pneumonia study of Zosyn with an aminoglycoside were: acidosis, acute kidney failure, agitation, alkaline phosphatase increased, anemia, asthenia, atrial fibrillation, chest pain, CNS depression, colitis, confusion, convulsion, cough increased, thrombocytopenia, dehydration, depression, diplopia, drug level decreased, dry mouth, dyspepsia, dysphagia, dyspnea, dysuria, eosinophilia, fungal dermatitis, gastritis, glossitis, grand mal convulsion, hematuria, hyperglycemia, hypernatremia, hypertension, hypertonia, hyperventilation, hypochromic anemia, hypoglycemia, hypokalemia, hyponatremia, hypophosphatemia, hypoxia, ileus, injection site edema, injection site pain, injection site reaction, kidney function abnormal, leukocytosis, leukopenia, local reaction to procedure, melena, pain, prothrombin decreased, pruritus, respiratory disorder, SGOT increased, SGPT increased, sinus bradycardia, somnolence, stomatitis, stupor, tremor, tachycardia, ventricular extrasystoles, and ventricular tachycardia.

In a previous nosocomial pneumonia study conducted with a dosing regimen of 3.375 g given every 4 hours with an aminoglycoside, the following adverse events, irrespective of drug relationship, were observed: diarrhea (20%); constipation (8.4%); agitation (7.1%); nausea (5.8%); headache (4.5%); insomnia (4.5%); oral thrush (3.9%); erythematous rash (3.9%); anxiety (3.2%); fever (3.2%); pain (3.2%); pruritus (3.2%); hiccough (2.6%); vomiting (2.6%); dyspepsia (1.9%); edema (1.9%); fluid overload (1.9%); stool changes (1.9%); anorexia (1.3%); cardiac arrest (1.3%); confusion (1.3%); diaphoresis (1.3%); duodenal ulcer (1.3%); flatulence (1.3%); hypertension (1.3%); hypotension (1.3%); inflammation at injection site (1.3%); pleural effusion (1.3%); pneumothorax (1.3%); rash, not otherwise specified (1.3%); supraventricular tachycardia (1.3%); thrombophlebitis (1.3%); and urinary incontinence (1.3%).

Adverse events irrespective of drug relationship observed in 1% or less of patients in the above study with Zosyn and an aminoglycoside included: aggressive reaction (combative), angina, asthenia, atelectasis, balanoposthitis, cerebrovascular accident, chest pain, conjunctivitis, deafness, dyspnea, earache, ecchymosis, fecal incontinence, gastric ulcer, gout, hemoptysis, hypoxia, pancreatitis, perineal irritation/pain, urinary tract infection with trichomonas, vitamin B_{12} deficiency anemia, xerosis, and yeast in urine.

Pediatrics

Studies of Zosyn in pediatric patients suggest a similar safety profile to that seen in adults. In a prospective, randomized, comparative, open-label clinical trial of pediatric patients with severe intra-abdominal infections (including appendicitis and/or peritonitis), 273 patients were treated with Zosyn (112.5 mg/kg every 8 hours) and 269 patients were treated with cefotaxime (50 mg/kg) plus metronidazole (7.5 mg/kg) every 8 hours. In this trial, treatment-emergent adverse events were reported by 146 patients, 73 (26.7%) in the Zosyn group and 73 (27.1%) in the cefotaxime/metronidazole group. Six patients (2.2%) in the Zosyn group and 5 patients (1.9%) in the cefotaxime/metronidazole group discontinued due to an adverse event.

In this study, adverse events that were reported in more than 1% of patients, irrespective of relationship to therapy with Zosyn were: diarrhea (7.0%), fever (4.8%), vomiting (3.7%), local reaction (3.3%), abscess (2.2%), sepsis (2.2%), abdominal pain (1.8%), infection (1.8%), bloody diarrhea (1.1%), pharyngitis (1.5%), constipation (1.1%) and SGOT increase (1.1%).

Adverse events reported in 1% or less of pediatric patients receiving Zosyn are consistent with adverse events reported in adults.

Additional controlled studies in pediatric patients showed a similar safety profile as that described above.

Post-Marketing Experience

Additional adverse events reported from worldwide marketing experience with Zosyn, occurring under circumstances where causal relationship to Zosyn is uncertain:

Gastrointestinal—hepatitis, cholestatic jaundice

Hematologic—hemolytic anemia, anemia, thrombocytosis, agranulocytosis, pancytopenia

Immune—hypersensitivity reactions, anaphylactic/anaphylactoid reactions (including shock)

Infections—candidal superinfections

Renal—interstitial nephritis, renal failure

Skin and Appendages—erythema multiforme, Stevens-Johnson syndrome, toxic epidermal necrolysis

Post-marketing experience with Zosyn in pediatric patients suggests a similar safety profile to that seen in adults.

Adverse Laboratory Events (Seen During Clinical Trials)

Of the studies reported, including that of nosocomial lower respiratory tract infections in which a higher dose of Zosyn (piperacillin and tazobactam for injection, USP) was used in combination with an aminoglycoside, changes in laboratory parameters, without regard to drug relationship, include:

TABLE 4

Aminoglycoside	Zosyn Dose (grams)	Zosyn Diluent Volume (mL)	Aminoglycoside Concentration Range* (mg/mL)	Acceptable Diluents
Amikacin	2.25, 3.375, 4.5	50, 100, 150	1.75-7.5	0.9% Sodium Chloride or 5% Dextrose
Gentamicin	2.25, 3.375, 4.5	100, 150	0.7-3.32	0.9% Sodium Chloride

* The concentration ranges in Table 4 are based on administration of the aminoglycoside in divided doses (10-15 mg/kg/day in two daily doses for amikacin and 3-5 mg/kg/day in three daily doses for gentamicin). Administration of amikacin or gentamicin in a single daily dose or in doses exceeding those stated above via Y-site with Zosyn containing EDTA has not been evaluated. See package insert for each aminoglycoside for complete Dosage and Administration instructions.

Recommended Dosing of Zosyn in Patients with Normal Renal Function and Renal Insufficiency (As total grams piperacillin/tazobactam)

Renal Function (Creatinine Clearance, mL/min)	All Indications (except nosocomial pneumonia)	Nosocomial Pneumonia
>40 mL/min	3.375 q 6 h	4.5 q 6 h
20-40 mL/min*	2.25 q 6 h	3.375 q 6 h
<20 mL/min*	2.25 q 8 h	2.25 q 6 h
Hemodialysis**	2.25 q 12 h	2.25 q 8 h
CAPD	2.25 q 12 h	2.25 q 8 h

*Creatinine clearance for patients not receiving hemodialysis
** 0.75 g should be administered following each hemodialysis session on hemodialysis days

Hematologic—decreases in hemoglobin and hematocrit, thrombocytopenia, increases in platelet count, eosinophilia, leukopenia, neutropenia. The leukopenia/neutropenia associated with Zosyn administration appears to be reversible and most frequently associated with prolonged administration, ie, ≥21 days of therapy. These patients were withdrawn from therapy; some had accompanying systemic symptoms (eg, fever, rigors, chills).

Coagulation—positive direct Coombs' test, prolonged prothrombin time, prolonged partial thromboplastin time

Hepatic—transient elevations of AST (SGOT), ALT (SGPT), alkaline phosphatase, bilirubin

Renal—increases in serum creatinine, blood urea nitrogen

Urinalysis—proteinuria, hematuria, pyuria

Additional laboratory events include abnormalities in electrolytes (ie, increases and decreases in sodium, potassium, and calcium), hyperglycemia, decreases in total protein or albumin, blood glucose decreased, gamma-glutamyltransferase increased, hypokalemia, and bleeding time prolonged.

The following adverse reaction has also been reported for PIPRACIL® (piperacillin for injection):

Skeletal—prolonged muscle relaxation (See **PRECAUTIONS, Drug Interactions**.)

Piperacillin therapy has been associated with an increased incidence of fever and rash in cystic fibrosis patients.

OVERDOSAGE

There have been postmarketing reports of overdose with piperacillin/tazobactam. The majority of those events experienced, including nausea, vomiting, and diarrhea, have also been reported with the usual recommended dosages. Patients may experience neuromuscular excitability or convulsions if higher than recommended doses are given intravenously (particularly in the presence of renal failure).

Treatment should be supportive and symptomatic according the patient's clinical presentation. Excessive serum concentrations of either piperacillin or tazobactam may be reduced by hemodialysis. Following a single 3.375 g dose of piperacillin/tazobactam, the percentage of the piperacillin and tazobactam dose removed by hemodialysis was approximately 31% and 39%, respectively. (See **CLINICAL PHARMACOLOGY**.)

DOSAGE AND ADMINISTRATION

Zosyn should be administered by intravenous infusion over 30 minutes.

The usual total daily dose of Zosyn for adults is 3.375 g every six hours totaling 13.5 g (12.0 g piperacillin/1.5 g tazobactam).

Nosocomial Pneumonia

Initial presumptive treatment of patients with nosocomial pneumonia should start with Zosyn at a dosage of 4.5 g every six hours plus an aminoglycoside, totaling 18.0 g (16.0 g piperacillin/2.0 g tazobactam). Treatment with the aminoglycoside should be continued in patients from whom *Pseudomonas aeruginosa* is isolated. If *Pseudomonas aeruginosa* is not isolated, the aminoglycoside may be discontinued at the discretion of the treating physician.

Due to the *in vitro* inactivation of the aminoglycoside by beta-lactam antibiotics, Zosyn and the aminoglycoside are recommended for separate administration. Zosyn and the aminoglycoside should be reconstituted, diluted, and administered separately when concomitant therapy with aminoglycosides is indicated. (See **PRECAUTIONS, Drug Interactions.**)

In circumstances where co-administration via Y-site is necessary, reformulated Zosyn containing EDTA supplied in vials or bulk pharmacy containers is compatible for simultaneous coadministration via Y-site infusion only with the following aminoglycosides under the following conditions:

The following compatibility information does not apply to the Zosyn (piperacillin/tazobactam) formulation not containing EDTA. This information does not apply to Zosyn in Galaxy® containers. Refer to the package insert for Zosyn Galaxy containers for instructions.

[See table 4 above]

Zosyn is not compatible with tobramycin for simultaneous coadministration via Y-site infusion. Compatibility of Zosyn with other aminoglycosides has not been established. Only the concentration and diluents for amikacin or gentamicin with the dosages of Zosyn listed above have been established as compatible for coadministration via Y-site infusion. Simultaneous coadministration via Y-site infusion in any manner other than listed above may result in inactivation of the aminoglycoside by Zosyn.

Renal Insufficiency

In patients with renal insufficiency (Creatinine Clearance ≤ 40 mL/min), the intravenous dose of Zosyn (piperacillin and tazobactam for injection, USP) should be adjusted to the degree of actual renal function impairment. In patients with nosocomial pneumonia receiving concomitant aminoglycoside therapy, the aminoglycoside dosage should be adjusted according to the recommendations of the manufacturer. The recommended daily doses of Zosyn for patients with renal insufficiency are as follows:

[See second table above]

For patients on hemodialysis, the maximum dose is 2.25 g every twelve hours for all indications other than nosocomial pneumonia and 2.25 g every eight hours for nosocomial pneumonia. Since hemodialysis removes 30% to 40% of the administered dose, an additional dose of 0.75 g Zosyn should be administered following each dialysis period on hemodialysis days. No additional dosage of Zosyn is necessary for CAPD patients.

Duration of Therapy

The usual duration of Zosyn treatment is from seven to ten days. However, the recommended duration of Zosyn treatment of nosocomial pneumonia is 7 to 14 days. In all conditions, the duration of therapy should be guided by the severity of the infection and the patient's clinical and bacteriological progress.

Pediatric Patients

For children with appendicitis and/or peritonitis 9 months of age or older, weighing up to 40 kg, and with normal renal function, the recommended Zosyn dosage is 100 mg piperacillin/12.5 mg tazobactam per kilogram of body weight, every 8 hours. For pediatric patients between 2 months and 9 months of age, the recommended Zosyn dosage based on pharmacokinetic modeling, is 80 mg piperacillin/10 mg tazobactam per kilogram of body weight, every 8 hours (see **PRECAUTIONS, General, Pediatric Use** and **CLINICAL PHARMACOLOGY**). Pediatric patients weighing over 40 kg and with normal renal function should receive the adult dose. There are no dosage recommendations for Zosyn in pediatric patients with impaired renal function.

Directions for Reconstitution and Dilution for Use

Intravenous Administration

For conventional vials, reconstitute Zosyn per gram of piperacillin with 5 mL of a compatible reconstitution diluent from the list provided below.

2.25 g, 3.375 g, and 4.5 g Zosyn should be reconstituted with 10 mL, 15 mL, and 20 mL, respectively. Swirl until dissolved.

Pharmacy vials should be used immediately after reconstitution. Discard any unused portion after 24 hours if stored at room temperature (20°C to 25°C [68°F to 77°F]), or after 48 hours if stored at refrigerated temperature (2°C to 8°C [36°F to 46°F]).

Compatible Reconstitution Diluents
0.9% Sodium Chloride for Injection
Sterile Water for Injection‡
Dextrose 5%
Bacteriostatic Saline/Parabens
Bacteriostatic Water/Parabens
Bacteriostatic Saline/Benzyl Alcohol
Bacteriostatic Water/Benzyl Alcohol
Reconstituted Zosyn solution should be further diluted (recommended volume per dose of 50 mL to 150 mL) in a compatible intravenous solution listed below. Administer by infusion over a period of at least 30 minutes. During the infusion it is desirable to discontinue the primary infusion solution.

Compatible Intravenous Solutions
0.9% Sodium Chloride for Injection
Sterile Water for Injection‡
Dextrose 5%
Dextran 6% in Saline
Lactated Ringer's Solution (Compatible **only** with reformulated Zosyn containing EDTA)
‡Maximum recommended volume per dose of Sterile Water for Injection is 50 mL.

Zosyn should not be mixed with other drugs in a syringe or infusion bottle since compatibility has not been established.

Zosyn is not chemically stable in solutions that contain only sodium bicarbonate and solutions that significantly alter the pH.

Zosyn should not be added to blood products or albumin hydrolysates.

Zosyn can be used in ambulatory intravenous infusion pumps.

Stability of Zosyn Following Reconstitution

Zosyn is stable in glass and plastic containers (plastic syringes, I.V. bags and tubing) when used with compatible diluents.

Pharmacy vials should be used immediately after reconstitution. Discard any unused portion after 24 hours if stored at room temperature (20°C to 25°C [68°F to 77°F]), or after 48 hours if stored at refrigerated temperature (2°C to 8°C [36°F to 46°F]). Vials should not be frozen after reconstitution.

Stability studies in the I.V. bags have demonstrated chemical stability (potency, pH of reconstituted solution and clarity of solution) for up to 24 hours at room temperature and up to one week at refrigerated temperature. Zosyn contains no preservatives. Appropriate consideration of aseptic technique should be used.

Stability of Zosyn in an ambulatory intravenous infusion pump has been demonstrated for a period of 12 hours at room temperature. Each dose was reconstituted and diluted to a volume of 37.5 mL or 25 mL. One-day supplies of dosing solution were aseptically transferred into the medication reservoir (I.V. bags or cartridge). The reservoir was fitted to a preprogrammed ambulatory intravenous infusion pump per the manufacturer's instructions. Stability of Zosyn is not affected when administered using an ambulatory intravenous infusion pump.

Parenteral drug products should be inspected visually for particulate matter and discoloration prior to administration, whenever solution and container permit.

HOW SUPPLIED

Zosyn® (piperacillin and tazobactam for injection, USP) is supplied in the following sizes:

Each Zosyn 2.25 g vial provides piperacillin sodium equivalent to 2 grams of piperacillin and tazobactam sodium

equivalent to 0.25 g of tazobactam. Each vial contains 5.58 mEq (128 mg) of sodium. Supplied 10 per box—NDC 0206-8852-16

Each Zosyn 3.375 g vial provides piperacillin sodium equivalent to 3 grams of piperacillin and tazobactam sodium equivalent to 0.375 g of tazobactam. Each vial contains 8.38 mEq (192 mg) of sodium. Supplied 10 per box—NDC 0206-8854-16

Each Zosyn 4.5 g vial provides piperacillin sodium equivalent to 4 grams of piperacillin and tazobactam sodium equivalent to 0.5 g of tazobactam. Each vial contains 11.17 mEq (256 mg) of sodium. Supplied 10 per box—NDC 0206-8855-16

Zosyn vials should be stored at controlled room temperature (20°C to 25°C [68°F to 77°F]) prior to reconstitution.

Also Available

Zosyn® (piperacillin and tazobactam injection) in Galaxy® Container (PL 2040 Plastic) is supplied as a frozen, iso-osmotic, sterile, nonpyrogenic solution in single dose plastic containers as follows:

2.25 g (piperacillin sodium equivalent to 2 g piperacillin/tazobactam sodium equivalent to 0.25 g tazobactam) in 50 mL. Each container has 5.58 mEq (128 mg) of sodium. Supplied 24/box—NDC 0206-8860-02

3.375 g (piperacillin sodium equivalent to 3 g piperacillin/tazobactam sodium equivalent to 0.375 g tazobactam) in 50 mL. Each container has 8.38 mEq (192 mg) of sodium. Supplied 24/box—NDC 0206-8861-02

4.5 g (piperacillin sodium equivalent to 4 g piperacillin/tazobactam sodium equivalent to 0.5 g tazobactam) in 100 mL. Each container has 11.17 mEq (256 mg) of sodium. Supplied 12/box—NDC 0206-8862-02

Also Available

Zosyn (piperacillin and tazobactam for injection, USP) is supplied as a powder in the pharmacy bulk vial as follows: 40.5 g pharmacy bulk vial containing piperacillin sodium equivalent to 36 grams of piperacillin and tazobactam sodium equivalent to 4.5 grams of tazobactam. Each pharmacy bulk vial contains 100.4 mEq (2,304 mg) of sodium. NDC 0206-8859-10.

REFERENCES

1. National Committee for Clinical Laboratory Standards, Performance Standards for Antimicrobial Susceptibility Testing; 13th Informational Supplement. NCCLS document M100-S13. NCCLS, Wayne, PA, 2003.
2. National Committee for Clinical Laboratory Standards, Methods for Dilution Antimicrobial Susceptibility Test for Bacteria that Grow Aerobically; Approved Standard—5th Edition. NCCLS document M7-A5. NCCLS, Wayne, PA, 2000.
3. National Committee for Clinical Laboratory Standards, Performance Standards for Antimicrobial Disk Susceptibility Test; Approved Standard—8th Edition. NCCLS document M2-A8. NCCLS, Wayne, PA, 2003.
4. National Committee for Clinical Laboratory Standards, Methods for Antimicrobial Susceptibility Testing of Anaerobic Bacteria; Approved Standard—5th ed. NCCLS document M11-A5. NCCLS, Wayne, PA, 2001.

CLINITEST® and DIASTIX® are registered trademarks of Ames Division, Miles Laboratories, Inc.

TES-TAPE® is a registered trademark of Eli Lilly and Company.

Galaxy® is a registered trademark of Baxter International, Inc.

United States Patent Numbers: 6,900,184 and 6,207,661

This product's label may have been updated. For current package insert and further product information, please visit www.wyeth.com or call our medical communications department toll-free at 1-800-934-5556.

Wyeth®
Wyeth Pharmaceuticals Inc.
Philadelphia, PA 19101
W10414C011
ET01
Rev 09/09

Angelini Labopharm LLC

**202 CARNEGIE CENTER, SUITE 107
PRINCETON, NJ 08540**

Telephone: 1-877-345-6177

OLEPTRO™   ℞

[Oh-LEP-troe]
**(trazodone hydrochloride)
extended-release tablets**

HIGHLIGHTS OF PRESCRIBING INFORMATION

These highlights do not include all the information needed to use Oleptro safely and effectively. See full prescribing information for Oleptro.

**OLEPTRO (trazodone hydrochloride) extended-release tablets
Initial U.S. Approval: 1981**

> **WARNING: SUICIDALITY AND ANTIDEPRESSANT DRUGS**
> *See full prescribing information for complete boxed warning.*
> Increased risk of suicidal thinking and behavior in children, adolescents and young adults taking antidepressants for major depressive disorder (MDD) and other psychiatric disorders. Oleptro is not approved for use in pediatric patients (5.1).

INDICATIONS AND USAGE

Oleptro is indicated for the treatment of major depressive disorder (1).
• Efficacy was established in one 8-week trial of Oleptro as well as in trials of trazodone immediate release formulation in patients with major depressive disorder (14).

DOSAGE AND ADMINISTRATION

• Starting dose: 150 mg once daily. May be increased by 75 mg per day every three days. Maximum dose: 375 mg per day (2).
• Dosing at the same time every day in the late evening, preferably at bedtime, on an empty stomach (2).
• Tablets should be swallowed whole or broken in half along the score line, and should not be chewed or crushed (2).
• When discontinued, gradual dose reduction is recommended (2).

DOSAGE FORMS AND STRENGTHS

Bisectable tablets of 150 mg or 300 mg (3).

CONTRAINDICATIONS

None (4).

WARNINGS AND PRECAUTIONS

• Clinical Worsening/Suicide Risk: Monitor for clinical worsening and suicidal thinking and behavior (5.1).
• Serotonin Syndrome or Neuroleptic Malignant Syndrome-like Reactions: Have been reported with antidepressants. Discontinue Oleptro and initiate supportive treatment (5.2).
• Activation of Mania/Hypomania: Screen for bipolar disorder and monitor for mania/hypomania (5.3).
• QT Prolongation: Increases the QT interval. Avoid use with drugs that also increase the QT interval and in patients with risk factors for prolonged QT interval (5.4).
• Use in Patients with Heart Disease: Use with caution in patients with cardiac disease (5.5).
• Orthostatic Hypotension and Syncope: Have occurred. Warn patients of risk and symptoms of hypotension (5.6).
• Abnormal Bleeding: May increase the risk of bleeding. Use with NSAIDs, aspirin, or other drugs that affect coagulation may compound this risk (5.7).
• Interaction with MAOIs: Do not use concomitantly or within 14 days of monoamine oxidase inhibitors (5.8).
• Priapism: Has occurred. Warn male patients of this risk and how/when to seek medical attention (5.9).
• Hyponatremia: Can occur in association with SIADH (5.10).
• Potential for Cognitive and Motor Impairment: Has potential to impair judgment, thinking, and motor skills. Advise patients to use caution when operating machinery (5.11).
• Discontinuation Symptoms: May occur with abrupt discontinuation and include anxiety and sleep disturbance. Upon discontinuation, taper Oleptro and monitor for symptoms (5.12).

ADVERSE REACTIONS

Most common adverse reactions (incidence ≥5% and twice that of placebo) are: somnolence/sedation, dizziness, constipation, vision blurred (6).

To report SUSPECTED ADVERSE REACTIONS, contact Labopharm at 1-877-345-6177 or FDA at 1-800-FDA-1088 or www.fda.gov/medwatch.

DRUG INTERACTIONS

• Monoamine Oxidase Inhibitors: Should not be used concomitantly with Oleptro (5.8, 7).
• CNS Depressants: Trazodone may enhance effects of alcohol, barbiturates, or other CNS depressants (7).
• CYP3A4 Inhibitors: May necessitate lower dose of Oleptro (7).
• CYP3A4 Inducers (e.g., carbamazepine): May necessitate higher dose of Oleptro (7).
• Digoxin or Phenytoin: Monitor for increased serum levels (7).
• Warfarin: Monitor for increased or decreased prothrombin time (7).
• Serotonergic Medications: Serotonin syndrome has been reported (5.2, 7).
• NSAIDs, Aspirin or other Anticoagulants: Potential for increased risk of bleeding (5.7, 7).

USE IN SPECIFIC POPULATIONS

- Pregnancy: Based on animal data, may cause fetal harm (8.1).
- Nursing Mothers: Use with caution (8.3).
- Pediatric Patients: Oleptro is not approved in pediatric patients (8.4).
- Renal or Hepatic Impairment: Use with caution (8.6, 8.7).

See 17 for PATIENT COUNSELING INFORMATION as well as Medication Guide.

Revised: 06/2010

FULL PRESCRIBING INFORMATION: CONTENTS*

FULL PRESCRIBING INFORMATION

WARNING: SUICIDALITY AND ANTIDEPRESSANT DRUGS

Antidepressants increased the risk compared to placebo of suicidal thinking and behavior (suicidality) in children, adolescents, and young adults in short-term studies of major depressive disorder (MDD) and other psychiatric disorders. Anyone considering the use of Oleptro or any other antidepressant in a child, adolescent, or young adult must balance this risk with the clinical need. Short-term studies did not show an increase in the risk of suicidality with antidepressants compared to placebo in adults beyond age 24; there was a reduction in risk with antidepressants compared to placebo in adults aged 65 and older. Depression and certain other psychiatric disorders are themselves associated with increases in the risk of suicide. Patients of all ages who are started on antidepressant therapy should be monitored appropriately and observed closely for clinical worsening, suicidality, or unusual changes in behavior. Families and caregivers should be advised of the need for close observation and communication with the prescriber. Oleptro is not approved for use in pediatric patients [see *Warnings and Precautions (5.1) and Patient Counseling Information (17.1)*].

1 INDICATIONS AND USAGE

Oleptro™ is indicated for the treatment of major depressive disorder (MDD) in adults. The efficacy of Oleptro has been established in a trial of outpatients with MDD as well as in trials with the immediate release formulation of trazodone [see *Clinical Studies (14)*].

2 DOSAGE AND ADMINISTRATION

Dose Selection

The recommended starting dose of Oleptro is 150 mg once daily in adults. The dose may be increased by 75 mg/day every three days (i.e., start 225 mg on Day 4 of therapy). The maximum daily dose should not exceed 375 mg.

- Oleptro tablets should be taken orally at the same time every day, in the late evening preferably at bedtime, on an empty stomach.
- Once an adequate response has been achieved, dosage may be gradually reduced, with subsequent adjustment depending on therapeutic response.
- Patients should be monitored for withdrawal symptoms when discontinuing treatment with trazodone hydrochloride. The dose should be gradually reduced whenever possible [see *Warnings and Precautions (5.12)*].

Maintenance Treatment

The efficacy of Oleptro for the maintenance treatment of MDD has not been evaluated. While there is no body of evidence available to answer the question of how long a patient treated with Oleptro should continue the drug, it is generally recommended that treatment be continued for several months after an initial response. Patients should be maintained on the lowest effective dose and be periodically reassessed to determine the continued need for maintenance treatment.

Important Administration Instructions

Oleptro tablets are scored to provide flexibility in dosing. Oleptro can be swallowed whole or administered as a half tablet by breaking the tablet along the score line. Breaking the tablet in half does not affect the controlled-release properties of the tablet.

In order to maintain its controlled-release properties, Oleptro should not be chewed or crushed.

3 DOSAGE FORMS AND STRENGTHS

Oleptro tablets are available in the following strengths:

- Oleptro bisectable tablets containing 150 mg of trazodone hydrochloride (yellowish-beige, capsule-shaped tablet, coated and scored on both sides with DDS 080 printed on one side)
- Oleptro bisectable tablets containing 300 mg of trazodone hydrochloride (beige-orange, capsule-shaped tablet, coated and scored on both sides with DDS 081 printed on one side)

4 CONTRAINDICATIONS

None.

5 WARNINGS AND PRECAUTIONS

5.1 Clinical Worsening and Suicide Risk

Patients with major depressive disorder (MDD), both adult and pediatric, may experience worsening of their depression and/or the emergence of suicidal ideation and behavior (suicidality) or unusual changes in behavior, whether or not they are taking antidepressant medications, and this risk may persist until significant remission occurs. Suicide is a known risk of depression and certain other psychiatric disorders and these disorders themselves are the strongest predictors of suicide. There has been a long standing concern, however, that antidepressants may have a role in inducing worsening of depression and the emergence of suicidality in certain patients during the early phases of treatment. Pooled analyses of short-term placebo-controlled trials of antidepressant drugs (SSRIs and others) showed that these drugs increase the risk of suicidal thinking and behavior (suicidality) in children, adolescents, and young adults (ages 18–24) with MDD and other psychiatric disorders. Short-term studies did not show an increase in the risk of suicidality with antidepressants compared to placebo in adults beyond age 24; there was a reduction with antidepressants compared to placebo in adults aged 65 and older. The pooled analyses of placebo-controlled trials in children and adolescents with MDD, obsessive compulsive disorder (OCD), or other psychiatric disorders included a total of 24 short-term trials of 9 antidepressant drugs in over 4,400 patients. The pooled analyses of placebo-controlled trials in adults with MDD or other psychiatric disorders included a total of 295 short-term trials (median duration of 2 months) of 11 antidepressant drugs in over 77,000 patients. There was considerable variation in risk of suicidality among drugs, but a tendency toward an increase in the younger patients for almost all drugs studied. There were differences in absolute risk of suicidality across the different indications, with the highest incidence in MDD. The risk differences (drug vs. placebo), however, were relatively stable within age strata and across indications. These risk differences (drug-placebo difference in the number of cases of suicidality per 1,000 patients treated) are provided in Table 1.

Table 1

Age Range	Drug-Placebo Difference in Number of Cases of Suicidality per 1,000 Patients Treated
	Increases Compared to Placebo
< 18	14 additional cases
18–24	5 additional cases
	Decreases Compared to Placebo
25–64	1 fewer case
≥ 65	6 fewer cases

No suicides occurred in any of the pediatric trials. There were suicides in the adult trials, but the number was not sufficient to reach any conclusion about drug effect on suicide.

It is unknown whether the suicidality risk extends to longer-term use, i.e., beyond several months. However, there is substantial evidence from placebo-controlled maintenance trials in adults with depression that the use of antidepressants can delay the recurrence of depression.

All patients being treated with antidepressants for any indication should be monitored appropriately and observed closely for clinical worsening, suicidality, and unusual changes in behavior, especially during the initial few months of a course of drug therapy, or at times of dose changes, either increases or decreases.

The following symptoms, anxiety, agitation, panic attacks, insomnia, irritability, hostility, aggressiveness, impulsivity, akathisia (psychomotor restlessness), hypomania, and mania, have been reported in adult and pediatric patients being treated with antidepressants for major depressive disorder as well as for other indications, both psychiatric and nonpsychiatric. Although a causal link between the emergence of such symptoms and either the worsening of depression and/or the emergence of suicidal impulses has not been established, there is concern that such symptoms may represent precursors to emerging suicidality.

Consideration should be given to changing the therapeutic regimen, including possibly discontinuing the medication, in patients whose depression is persistently worse, or who are experiencing emergent suicidality or symptoms that might be precursors to worsening depression or suicidality, especially if these symptoms are severe, abrupt in onset, or were not part of the patient's presenting symptoms.

Families and caregivers of patients being treated with antidepressants for major depressive disorder or other indications, both psychiatric and nonpsychiatric, should be alerted about the need to monitor patients for the emergence of agitation, irritability, unusual changes in behavior, and the other symptoms described above, as well as the emergence of suicidality, and to report such symptoms immediately to health care providers. Such monitoring should include daily observation by families and caregivers. Prescriptions for Oleptro should be written for the smallest quantity of tablets consistent with good patient management, in order to reduce the risk of overdose.

5.2 Serotonin Syndrome or Neuroleptic Malignant Syndrome (NMS)-like Reactions

The development of a potentially life-threatening serotonin syndrome or neuroleptic malignant syndrome (NMS)-like reactions have been reported with antidepressants alone and may occur with trazodone treatment, but particularly with concomitant use of other serotoninergic drugs (including SSRIs, SNRIs and triptans) and with drugs that impair metabolism of serotonin (including monoamine oxidase inhibitors [MAOIs]), or with antipsychotics or other dopamine antagonists. Serotonin syndrome symptoms may include mental status changes (e.g., agitation, hallucinations, and coma), autonomic instability (e.g., tachycardia, labile blood pressure, and hyperthermia), neuromuscular aberrations (e.g., hyperreflexia, incoordination) and/or gastrointestinal symptoms (e.g., nausea, vomiting, and diarrhea). Serotonin syndrome, in its most severe form, can resemble neuroleptic malignant syndrome, which includes hyperthermia, muscle rigidity, autonomic instability with possible rapid fluctuation of vital signs, and mental status changes.

Treatment with Oleptro and any concomitant serotonergic or antidopaminergic agents, including antipsychotics, should be discontinued immediately if the above reactions occur and supportive symptomatic treatment should be initiated.

Oleptro should not be used within 14 days of an MAOI [see *Warnings and Precautions (5.8) and Drug Interactions (7)*].

If concomitant treatment with Oleptro and an SSRI, SNRI or a 5-hydroxytryptamine receptor agonist (triptan) is clinically warranted, careful observation of the patient is advised, particularly during treatment initiation and dose increases.

The concomitant use of Oleptro with serotonin precursors (such as tryptophan) is not recommended.

5.3 Screening Patients for Bipolar Disorder and Monitoring for Mania/Hypomania

A major depressive episode may be the initial presentation of bipolar disorder. It is generally believed (though not established in controlled trials) that treating such an episode with an antidepressant alone may increase the likelihood of precipitation of a mixed/manic episode in patients at risk for bipolar disorder. Whether any of the symptoms described for clinical worsening and suicide risk represent such a conversion is unknown. However, prior to initiating treatment with an antidepressant, patients with depressive symptoms should be adequately screened to determine if they are at risk for bipolar disorder; such screening should include a detailed psychiatric history, including a family history of suicide, bipolar disorder, and depression. It should be noted that Oleptro is not approved for use in treating bipolar depression.

5.4 QT Prolongation and Risk of Sudden Death

Trazodone is known to prolong the QT/QTc interval. Some drugs that prolong the QT/QTc interval can cause Torsades de Pointes with sudden, unexplained death. The relationship of QT prolongation is clearest for larger increases (20 msec and greater), but it is possible that smaller QT/QTc prolongations may also increase risk, especially in susceptible individuals, such as those with hypokalemia, hypomagnesemia, or a genetic predisposition to prolonged QT/QTc.

Although Torsades de Pointes has not been observed with the use of Oleptro at recommended doses in premarketing trials, experience is too limited to rule out an increased risk. However, there have been postmarketing reports of Torsades de Pointes with the immediate-release form of trazodone (in the presence of multiple confounding factors), even at doses of 100 mg per day or less.

5.5 Use in Patients with Heart Disease

Trazodone hydrochloride is not recommended for use during the initial recovery phase of myocardial infarction.

Caution should be used when administering Oleptro to patients with cardiac disease and such patients should be closely monitored, since antidepressant drugs (including trazodone hydrochloride) may cause cardiac arrhythmias. QT prolongation has been reported with trazodone therapy *[see Warnings and Precautions (5.4)]*. Clinical studies in patients with pre-existing cardiac disease indicate that trazodone hydrochloride may be arrhythmogenic in some patients in that population. Arrhythmias identified include isolated PVCs, ventricular couplets, tachycardia with syncope, and Torsades de Pointes. Postmarketing events have been reported at doses of 100 mg or less with the immediate-release form of trazodone.

Concomitant administration of drugs that prolong the QT interval or that are inhibitors of CYP3A4 may increase the risk of cardiac arrhythmia.

5.6 Orthostatic Hypotension and Syncope

Hypotension, including orthostatic hypotension and syncope has been reported in patients receiving trazodone hydrochloride. Concomitant use with an antihypertensive may require a reduction in the dose of the antihypertensive drug.

5.7 Abnormal Bleeding

Postmarketing data have shown an association between use of drugs that interfere with serotonin reuptake and the occurrence of gastrointestinal (GI) bleeding. While no association between trazodone and bleeding events, in particular GI bleeding, was shown, patients should be cautioned about potential risk of bleeding associated with the concomitant use of trazodone and NSAIDs, aspirin, or other drugs that affect coagulation or bleeding. Other bleeding events related to SSRIs and SNRIs have ranged from ecchymosis, hematoma, epistaxis, and petechiae to life-threatening hemorrhages.

5.8 Interaction with MAOIs

In patients receiving serotonergic drugs in combination with a monoamine oxidase inhibitor (MAOI), there have been reports of serious, sometimes fatal reactions including hyperthermia, rigidity, myoclonus, autonomic instability with rapid fluctuation in vital signs, and mental status changes that include extreme agitation progressing to delirium and coma. These reactions have also been reported in patients who have recently discontinued antidepressant treatment and have been started on an MAOI. Some cases presented with features resembling neuroleptic malignant syndrome. Furthermore, limited animal data on the effects of combined use of serotonergic antidepressants and MAOIs suggest that these drugs may act synergistically to elevate blood pressure and evoke behavioral excitation. Therefore, it is recommended that Oleptro should not be used in combination with an MAOI or within 14 days of discontinuing treatment with an MAOI. Similarly, at least 14 days should be allowed after stopping Oleptro before starting an MAOI.

5.9 Priapism

Rare cases of priapism (painful erections greater than 6 hours in duration) were reported in men receiving trazodone. Priapism, if not treated promptly, can result in irreversible damage to the erectile tissue. Men who have an erection lasting greater than 6 hours, whether painful or not, should immediately discontinue the drug and seek emergency medical attention *[see Adverse Reactions (6.2) and Overdosage (10)]*.

Trazodone should be used with caution in men who have conditions that might predispose them to priapism (e.g., sickle cell anemia, multiple myeloma, or leukemia), or in men with anatomical deformation of the penis (e.g., angulation, cavernosal fibrosis, or Peyronie's disease).

5.10 Hyponatremia

Hyponatremia may occur as a result of treatment with antidepressants. In many cases, this hyponatremia appears to be the result of the syndrome of inappropriate antidiuretic hormone secretion (SIADH). Cases with serum sodium lower than 110 mmol/L have been reported. Elderly patients may be at greater risk of developing hyponatremia with antidepressants. Also, patients taking diuretics or who are otherwise volume-depleted can be at greater risk. Discontinuation of Oleptro should be considered in patients with symptomatic hyponatremia and appropriate medical intervention should be instituted.

Signs and symptoms of hyponatremia include headache, difficulty concentrating, memory impairment, confusion, weakness, and unsteadiness, which can lead to falls. Signs and symptoms associated with more severe and/or acute cases have included hallucination, syncope, seizure, coma, respiratory arrest, and death.

5.11 Potential for Cognitive and Motor Impairment

Oleptro may cause somnolence or sedation and may impair the mental and/or physical ability required for the performance of potentially hazardous tasks. Patients should be cautioned about operating hazardous machinery, including automobiles, until they are reasonably certain that the drug treatment does not affect them adversely.

5.12 Discontinuation Symptoms

Withdrawal symptoms including anxiety, agitation and sleep disturbances, have been reported with trazodone. Clinical experience suggests that the dose should be gradually reduced before complete discontinuation of the treatment.

6 ADVERSE REACTIONS

The following serious adverse reactions are described elsewhere in the labeling:

- Clinical Worsening and Suicide Risk *[see Boxed Warning and Warnings and Precautions (5.1)]*
- Serotonin Syndrome or NMS-like Reactions *[see Warnings and Precautions (5.2)]*
- QT Prolongation and Risk of Sudden Death *[see Warnings and Precautions (5.4)]*
- Orthostatic Hypotension *[see Warnings and Precautions (5.6)]*
- Abnormal bleeding events *[see Warnings and Precautions (5.7)]*
- Priapism *[see Warnings and Precautions (5.9)]*
- Hyponatremia *[see Warnings and Precautions (5.10)]*
- Cognitive and Motor Impairment *[see Warnings and Precautions (5.11)]*
- Discontinuation symptoms *[see Warnings and Precautions (5.12)]*

The most common adverse reactions (reported in ≥5% and at twice the rate of placebo) are: somnolence/sedation, dizziness, constipation, vision blurred.

Table 2 presents the summary of adverse events (AEs) leading to discontinuation of Oleptro treatment with an incidence of at least 1% and at least twice that for placebo.

Table 2: AEs with discontinuation as action taken (≥1% incidence and incidence 2× placebo)

	Oleptro N = 202
Somnolence/Sedation	8 (4.0%)
Dizziness	7 (3.5%)
Confusional state	2 (1.0%)
Coordination abnormal	2 (1.0%)
Headache	2 (1.0%)
Nausea	2 (1.0%)
Balance disorder/Gait disturbance	2 (1.0%)

6.1 Clinical Studies Experience

The data described below reflects exposure in a clinical trial of 406 patients, including 204 exposed to placebo and 202 exposed to Oleptro. Patients were between 18-80 years of age and 69.3% and 67.5% of patients had at least one previous episode of depression in the last 24 months in the placebo and active-treated group, respectively. In individual patients, doses were flexible and ranged from 150 to 375 mg per day. The mean daily dose during the 6-week treatment period was 310 mg. The tablets were administered orally and were given once a day for a total duration of 8 weeks, including the titration period.

Because clinical trials are conducted under widely varying conditions, adverse reaction rates observed in the clinical trials of a drug cannot be directly compared to rates in the clinical trials of another drug and may not reflect the rates observed in practice.

Table 3 presents the summary of all treatment emergent AEs that occurred at an incidence of ≥ 5% in the Oleptro group, whether considered by the clinical investigator to be related to the study drug or not.

Table 3: Most Common Treatment Emergent Adverse Events (≥ 5% of Patients on Active Treatment)

Preferred Term	Placebo N = 204	Oleptro N = 202
Somnolence/Sedation	39 (19%)	93 (46%)
Headache	55 (27%)	67 (33%)
Dry mouth	26 (13%)	51 (25%)
Dizziness	25 (12%)	50 (25%)
Nausea	26 (13%)	42 (21%)
Fatigue	17 (8%)	30 (15%)
Diarrhea	23 (11%)	19 (9%)
Constipation	4 (2%)	16 (8%)
Back pain	7 (3%)	11 (5%)
Vision blurred	0 (0%)	11 (5%)

Sexual Dysfunction

Adverse events related to sexual dysfunction (regardless of causality) were reported by 4.9% and 1.5% of patients treated with Oleptro and placebo, respectively. In the Oleptro group, ejaculation disorders occurred in 1.5% of patients, decreased libido occurred in 1.5% of patients, and erectile dysfunction and abnormal orgasm < 1% of patients.

Vital Signs and Weight

There were no notable changes in vital signs (blood pressure, respiratory rate, pulse) or weight in either treatment group.

Following is a list of treatment-emergent adverse reactions with an incidence of ≥ 1% to < 5% (i.e., less common) in patients treated with Oleptro. This listing is not intended to include reactions (i) already listed in previous tables or elsewhere in the labeling (ii) for which the association with treatment is remote, (iii) which were so general as to be uninformative, and (iv) which were not considered to have significant clinical implications. Reactions are classified by body-system using the following definitions: frequent adverse reactions are those occurring in at least 1/100 patients; infrequent adverse reactions are those occurring in less than 1/100 patients.

Ear and Labyrinth Disorders—*Infrequent:* hypoacusis, tinnitus, vertigo

Eye Disorders—*Frequent:* visual disturbance; *Infrequent:* dry eye, eye pain, photophobia

Gastrointestinal Disorders—*Frequent:* abdominal pain, vomiting; *Infrequent:* reflux esophagitis

General Disorders and Administration Site Conditions—*Frequent:* edema; *Infrequent:* gait disturbance

Immune System Disorders—*Infrequent:* hypersensitivity

Musculoskeletal and Connective Tissue Disorders—*Frequent:* musculoskeletal complaints, myalgia; *Infrequent:* muscle twitching

Nervous System Disorders—*Frequent:* coordination abnormal, dysgeusia, memory impairment, migraine, paraesthesia, tremor; *Infrequent:* amnesia, aphasia, hypoesthesia, speech disorder

Psychiatric Disorders—*Frequent:* agitation, confusional state, disorientation

Renal and Urinary Disorders—*Frequent:* micturition urgency; *Infrequent:* bladder pain, urinary incontinence

Respiratory, Thoracic and Mediastinal Disorders—*Frequent:* dyspnea

Skin and Subcutaneous Tissue Disorders—*Frequent:* night sweats; *Infrequent:* acne, hyperhidrosis, photosensitivity reaction

Vascular Disorders—*Infrequent:* flushing

6.2 Postmarketing Experience

Spontaneous reports regarding trazodone hydrochloride received from postmarketing experience include the following: abnormal dreams, agitation, alopecia, anxiety, aphasia, apnea, ataxia, breast enlargement or engorgement, cardiospasm, cerebrovascular accident, chills, cholestasis, clitorism, congestive heart failure, diplopia, edema, extrapyramidal symptoms, grand mal seizures, hallucinations, hemolytic anemia, hirsutism, hyperbilirubinemia, increased amylase, increased salivation, insomnia, leukocytosis, leukonychia, jaundice, lactation, liver enzyme alterations, methemoglobinemia, nausea/vomiting (most frequently), paresthesia, paranoid reaction, priapism *[see Warnings and Precautions (5.9) and Patient Counseling Information (17.1)]*, pruritus, psoriasis, psychosis, rash, stupor, inappropriate ADH syndrome, tardive dyskinesia, unexplained death, urinary incontinence, urinary retention, urticaria, vasodilation, vertigo, and weakness.

Cardiovascular system effects which have been reported include the following: conduction block, orthostatic hypotension and syncope, palpitations, bradycardia, atrial fibrillation, myocardial infarction, cardiac arrest, arrhythmia, ventricular ectopic activity, including ventricular tachycardia and QT prolongation. In postmarketing surveillance, prolonged QT interval, Torsades de Pointes, and ventricular tachycardia have been reported with the immediate-release form of trazodone at doses of 100 mg per day or less *[see Warnings and Precautions (5.4)]*.

7 DRUG INTERACTIONS

MAOIs

MAOIs should not be used within 14 days of Oleptro *[see Warnings and Precautions (5.8)]*.

Central Nervous System (CNS) Depressants

Trazodone may enhance the response to alcohol, barbiturates, and other CNS depressants.

Cytochrome P450 3A4 Inhibitors

In vitro drug metabolism studies suggest that there is a potential for drug interactions when trazodone is given with cytochrome P450 3A4 (CYP3A4) inhibitors. The effect of short-term administration of ritonavir (200 mg twice daily, 4 doses) on the pharmacokinetics of a single dose of trazodone (50 mg) has been studied in 10 healthy subjects. The C_{max} of trazodone increased by 34%, the AUC increased 2.4-fold, the half-life increased by 2.2-fold, and the clearance decreased by 52%. Adverse effects including nausea, hypotension, and syncope were observed when ritonavir and trazodone were co-administered. It is likely that ketoconazole, indinavir, and other CYP3A4 inhibitors such as itraconazole may lead to substantial increases in trazodone plasma concentrations with the potential for adverse effects. If trazodone is used with a potent CYP3A4 inhibitor, the risk of cardiac arrhythmia may be increased *[see Warnings and Precautions (5.4)]* and a lower dose of trazodone should be considered.

Cytochrome P450 Inducers (e.g., carbamazepine)

Carbamazepine induces CYP3A4. Following co-administration of carbamazepine 400 mg per day with trazodone 100 mg to 300 mg daily, carbamazepine reduced plasma concentrations of trazodone and m-chlorophenylpiperazine (an active metabolite) by 76% and 60% respectively, compared to pre-carbamazepine values. Patients should be closely monitored to see if there is a need for an increased dose of trazodone when taking both drugs.

Digoxin and Phenytoin

Increased serum digoxin or phenytoin levels have been reported in patients receiving trazodone concurrently with either of these drugs. Monitor serum levels and adjust dosages as needed.

Serotonergic Drugs

Based on the mechanism of action of Oleptro and the potential for serotonin syndrome, caution is advised when Oleptro is co-administered with other drugs that may affect the neurotransmitter systems *[see Warnings and Precautions (5.2)]*.

NSAIDs, Aspirin, or Other Drugs Affecting Coagulation or Bleeding

Due to a possible association between serotonin modulating drugs and gastrointestinal bleeding, patients should be monitored for and cautioned about the potential risk of bleeding associated with the concomitant use of trazodone and NSAIDs, aspirin, or other drugs that affect coagulation or bleeding *[see Warnings and Precautions (5.7)]*.

Warfarin

There have been reports of altered (either increased or decreased) prothrombin times in taking both warfarin and trazodone.

8 USE IN SPECIFIC POPULATIONS

8.1 Pregnancy

Pregnancy Category C

Trazodone hydrochloride has been shown to cause increased fetal resorption and other adverse effects on the fetus in two studies using the rat when given at dose levels approximately 30-50 times the proposed maximum human dose. There was also an increase in congenital anomalies in one of three rabbit studies at approximately 15–50 times the maximum human dose. There are no adequate and well-controlled studies in pregnant women. Oleptro should be used during pregnancy only if the potential benefit justifies the potential risk to the fetus.

8.3 Nursing Mothers

Trazodone and/or its metabolites have been found in the milk of lactating rats, suggesting that the drug may be secreted in human milk. Caution should be exercised when Oleptro is administered to a nursing woman.

8.4 Pediatric Use

Safety and effectiveness in the pediatric population have not been established *[see Boxed Warning and Warnings and Precautions (5.1)]*. Oleptro should not be used in children or adolescents.

8.5 Geriatric Use

Of 202 patients treated with Oleptro in the clinical trial, there were 9 patients older than 65. No overall differences in safety or effectiveness were observed between these subjects and younger subjects, and other reported clinical literature and experience with trazodone have not identified differences in responses between elderly and younger patients. However, as experience in the elderly with Oleptro is limited, it should be used with caution in geriatric patients.

Antidepressants have been associated with cases of clinically significant hyponatremia in elderly patients who may be at greater risk for this adverse reaction *[see Warnings and Precautions (5.10)]*.

8.6 Renal Impairment

Oleptro has not been studied in patients with renal impairment. Trazodone should be used with caution in this population.

8.7 Hepatic Impairment

Oleptro has not been studied in patients with hepatic impairment. Trazodone should be used with caution in this population.

9 DRUG ABUSE AND DEPENDENCE

9.1 Controlled Substance

Oleptro is not a controlled substance.

9.2 Abuse

Although trazodone hydrochloride has not been systematically studied in preclinical or clinical studies for its potential for abuse, no indication of drug-seeking behavior was seen in the clinical studies with Oleptro. However, it is difficult to predict the extent to which a CNS-active drug will be misused, diverted, and abused. Consequently, physicians should carefully evaluate patients for a history of drug abuse and follow such patients closely, observing them for signs of misuse or abuse of trazodone hydrochloride (e.g., development of tolerance, incrementation of dose, drug-seeking behavior).

10 OVERDOSAGE

10.1 Human Experience

It is expected that the health risks associated with overdose of Oleptro are most likely similar to those for trazodone immediate-release formulations.

Death from overdose has occurred in patients ingesting trazodone and other CNS depressant drugs concurrently (alcohol; alcohol and chloral hydrate and diazepam; amobarbital; chlordiazepoxide; or meprobamate).

The most severe reactions reported to have occurred with overdose of trazodone alone have been priapism, respiratory arrest, seizures, and ECG changes, including QT prolongation. The reactions reported most frequently have been drowsiness and vomiting. Overdosage may cause an increase in incidence or severity of any of the reported adverse reactions.

10.2 Management of Overdose

There is no specific antidote for Oleptro overdose.

Treatment should consist of those general measures employed in the management of overdosage with any drug effective in the treatment of major depressive disorder.

Ensure an adequate airway, oxygenation and ventilation. Monitor cardiac rhythm and vital signs.

General supportive and symptomatic measures are also recommended. Induction of emesis is not recommended. Gastric lavage with a large bore orogastric tube with appropriate airway protection, if needed, may be indicated if performed soon after ingestion, or in symptomatic patients. Activated charcoal should be administered. Forced diuresis may be useful in facilitating elimination of the drug.

In managing overdosage, consider the possibility of multiple drug involvement. The physician should consider contacting a poison control center for additional information on the treatment of any overdose.

11 DESCRIPTION

Oleptro (trazodone hydrochloride) is a triazolopyridine. It is a white, odorless crystalline powder which is freely soluble in water.

Chemical Name: 2-[3-[4-(*m*-Chlorophenyl)-1-piperazinyl] propyl]-*s*-triazolo[4,3-*a*]pyridin-3(2*H*)-one monohydrochloride

Structural Formula:

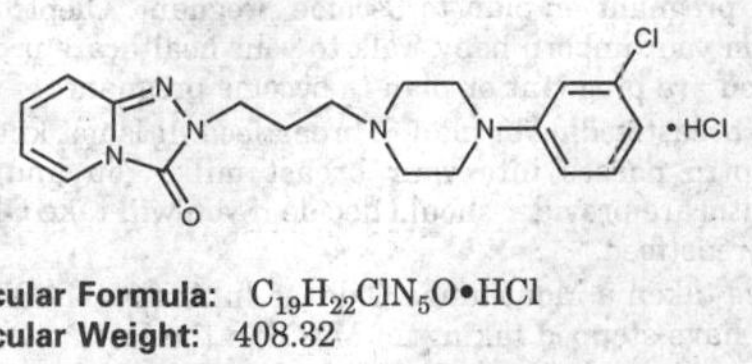

Molecular Formula: $C_{19}H_{22}ClN_5O{\bullet}HCl$

Molecular Weight: 408.32

Oleptro tablets containing 150 mg or 300 mg of trazodone hydrochloride are designed to release their drug content over a 24-hour period and are intended for once-a-day dosing.

Inactive Ingredients:

Hydroxypropyl distarch phosphate (Contramid®)
Hypromellose
Sodium stearyl fumarate
Colloidal silicon dioxide
Iron Oxide Yellow
Iron Oxide Red
Talc
Polyethylene Glycol 3350
Titanium Dioxide
Polyvinyl Alcohol
Black ink (food grade)

12 CLINICAL PHARMACOLOGY

12.1 Mechanism of Action

The mechanism of trazodone's antidepressant action is not fully understood, but is thought to be related to its potentiation of serotonergic activity in the CNS.

12.2 Pharmacodynamics

Preclinical studies have shown that trazodone selectively inhibits neuronal reuptake of serotonin and acts as an antagonist at 5-HT-2A/2C serotonin receptors.

Trazodone is not a monoamine oxidase inhibitor and, unlike amphetamine-type drugs, does not stimulate the central nervous system.

Trazodone antagonizes alpha 1-adrenergic receptors, a property which may be associated with postural hypotension.

12.3 Pharmacokinetics

Steady state AUC of Trazodone is equivalent after administration of Trazodone 100 mg immediate release (IR) three (3) times a day (mean $\pm$ SD AUC_{ss} = 33058 $\pm$ 8006 ng*h/mL) and Oleptro 300 mg once daily (mean $\pm$ SD AUC_{ss} = 29131 $\pm$ 9931 ng*h/mL) for one week. Steady State C_{max} and C_{min} of trazodone were not equivalent after administration of trazodone 100 mg IR 3 times a day (mean $\pm$ SD $C_{max,ss}$ = 3118 $\pm$ 758 ng/mL, $C_{min,ss}$ = 843 $\pm$ 274 ng/mL) and Oleptro 300 mg once daily (mean $\pm$ SD $C_{max,ss}$ = 1812 $\pm$ 621 ng/mL, $C_{min,ss}$ = 674 $\pm$ 355 ng/mL) for one week.

Absorption

Trazodone is well absorbed after oral administration, without selective localization in any tissue. Following single-dose administration of Oleptro 300 mg tablets under fasting conditions, a mean peak trazodone plasma concentration (C_{max}) of 1188 $\pm$ 362 ng/mL was reported at a median T_{max} of 9 hours post-dose. When Oleptro 300 mg tablets are taken shortly after ingestion of a high-fat meal, C_{max} increases by about 86% compared to taking it under fasting conditions. However, $AUC_{0-\infty}$ and T_{max} are not significantly affected by food.

Oleptro tablets are dose proportional following single-dose administration of doses ranging from 75 mg to 375 mg as intact or bisected tablets.

Metabolism

In vitro studies in human liver microsomes show that trazodone is metabolized, via oxidative cleavage, to an active metabolite, m-chlorophenylpiperazine (mCPP) by CYP3A4. Other metabolic pathways that may be involved in the metabolism of trazodone have not been well characterized. Trazodone is extensively metabolized; less than 1% of an oral dose is excreted unchanged in the urine.

Elimination

Elimination is predominantly renal, with 70 to 75% of an oral dose being recovered in the urine within the first 72 hours of ingestion. Following single-dose administration of Oleptro 300 mg tablets, a mean apparent terminal half-life of 10 hours was reported.

Protein Binding

Trazodone is 89 to 95% protein bound *in vitro* at concentrations attained with therapeutic doses in humans.

13 NONCLINICAL TOXICOLOGY

13.1 Carcinogenesis, Mutagenesis, Impairment of Fertility

No drug- or dose-related occurrence of carcinogenesis was evident in rats receiving trazodone in daily oral doses up to 300 mg/kg for 18 months.

14 CLINICAL STUDIES

The efficacy and safety of Oleptro were established from trials of the immediate release formulation as well as a randomized, double-blind, two-arm study comparing the efficacy and safety of Oleptro and placebo in the treatment of unipolar major depressive disorder.

The Oleptro trial was a multi-center, parallel-design study of outpatients meeting DSM-IV criteria for major depressive disorder (MDD). This study consisted of a Baseline Phase (screening and washout) and a double-blind Randomized Phase (randomization to Oleptro (n=206) or placebo (n=206)). The total study duration, including washout of prohibited medications, was approximately 11 weeks; the total duration of the randomized treatment phase was 8 weeks (titration: 2 weeks and treatment: 6 weeks). Rescue medication for MDD was not allowed during the study. Patients were between 18 and 80 years of age. Of this population, 25 patients were 65 years old or older. The mean age of the population was 44 years; 64% were female. The primary efficacy endpoint in this study was change from baseline in HAMD-17 total score.

A statistically significant difference in the HAMD-17 score was demonstrated at 8 weeks between the Oleptro group and the placebo group.

16 HOW SUPPLIED/STORAGE AND HANDLING

Oleptro 150 mg is a yellowish-beige, capsule-shaped extended-release tablet, coated and scored on both sides with DDS 080 printed on one side. It is supplied as follows:
Bottles of 30 tablets NDC 43595-080-03
Oleptro 300 mg is a beige-orange, capsule-shaped extended-release tablet, coated and scored on both sides with DDS 081 printed on one side. It is supplied as follows:
Bottles of 30 tablets NDC 43595-081-03
Store at room temperature (15–30°C) in tight, light-resistant containers.

17 PATIENT COUNSELING INFORMATION
See Medication Guide (17.2).

17.1 Information for Patients
Prescribers or other health professionals should inform patients, their families, and their caregivers about the benefits and risks associated with treatment with Oleptro and should counsel them in its appropriate use.
Patients should be warned that:
- There is a potential for increased risk of suicidal thoughts especially in children, teenagers and young adults.
- The following symptoms should be reported to the physician: anxiety, agitation, panic attacks, insomnia, irritability, hostility, aggressiveness, impulsivity, akathisia, hypomania and mania.
- They should inform their physician if they have a history of bipolar disorder, cardiac disease or myocardial infarction.
- Serotonin syndrome could occur and symptoms may include changes in mental status (e.g., agitation, hallucinations, and coma), autonomic instability (e.g., tachycardia, labile blood pressure, and hyperthermia), neuromuscular aberrations (e.g., hyperreflexia, incoordination) and/or gastrointestinal symptoms (e.g., nausea, vomiting, and diarrhea).
- Trazodone hydrochloride has been associated with the occurrence of priapism.
- There is a potential for hypotension, including orthostatic hypotension and syncope.
- There is a potential risk of bleeding (including life-threatening hemorrhages) and bleeding related events (including ecchymosis, hematoma, epistaxis, and petechiae) with the concomitant use of trazodone hydrochloride and NSAIDs, aspirin, or other drugs that affect coagulation or bleeding.
- Withdrawal symptoms including anxiety, agitation and sleep disturbances, have been reported with trazodone. Clinical experience suggests that the dose should be gradually reduced.
Patients should be counseled that:
- Oleptro may cause somnolence or sedation and may impair the mental and/or physical ability required for the performance of potentially hazardous tasks. Patients should be cautioned about operating hazardous machinery, including automobiles until they are reasonably certain that the drug treatment does not affect them.
- Trazodone may enhance the response to alcohol, barbiturates, and other CNS depressants.
- Women who intend to become pregnant or who are breastfeeding should discuss with a physician whether they should continue to use Oleptro, since use in pregnant and nursing women is not recommended.
<u>Important Administration Instructions:</u>
- Oleptro should be swallowed whole or broken in half along the score line.
- In order to maintain its controlled-release properties, it should not be chewed or crushed.
- Oleptro should be taken at the same time every day, in the late evening preferably at bedtime, on an empty stomach.
Labopharm Europe Limited
Unit 5, The Seapoint Building
44/45 Clontarf Road, Dublin 3, IRELAND.
© 2010, Labopharm Europe Limited. All rights reserved.
U.S. Patent 6,607,748
Oleptro™ is a trademark of Labopharm Inc.
Contramid® is a registered trademark of Labopharm Inc.
[June 2010]
17.2 MEDICATION GUIDE
Oleptro™ (Oh-LEP-troe)
(trazodone hydrochloride) extended-release tablets
Read the Medication Guide that comes with Oleptro before you start taking it and each time you get a refill. There may

be new information. This information does not take the place of talking to your healthcare provider about your medical condition or treatment. Talk to your healthcare provider or pharmacist if there is something you do not understand or you want to learn about Oleptro.
What is the most important information I should know about Oleptro?
Antidepressant medicines, depression or other serious mental illnesses, and suicidal thoughts or actions:
Talk to your healthcare provider about:
- All risks and benefits of treatment with antidepressant medicines
- All treatment choices for depression or other serious mental illnesses
1. **Antidepressant medicines may increase suicidal thoughts or actions in some children, teenagers, and young adults within the first few months of treatment.**
2. **Depression and other serious mental illnesses are the most important causes of suicidal thoughts and actions. Some people may have a higher risk of having suicidal thoughts or actions.** These include people who have or have a family history of bipolar illness (also called manic-depressive illness) or suicidal thoughts or actions.
3. **How can I watch for and try to prevent suicidal thoughts and actions?**
- Pay close attention to any changes, especially sudden changes in mood, behaviors, thoughts, or feelings. This is very important when an antidepressant medicine is started or when the dose is changed.
- Call your healthcare provider right away to report new or sudden changes in mood, behavior, thoughts or feelings.
- Keep all follow-up visits with your healthcare provider as scheduled. Call your healthcare provider between visits as needed, especially if you are worried about symptoms.
Call a healthcare provider right away if you have any of the following symptoms, especially if they are new, worse, or worry you:
- Thoughts about suicide or dying
- Attempts to commit suicide
- New or worse depression
- New or worse anxiety
- Feeling very agitated or restless
- Panic attacks
- Trouble sleeping (insomnia)
- New or worse irritability
- Acting aggressive, being angry or violent
- Acting on dangerous impulses
- An extreme increase in activity and talking (mania)
- Other unusual changes in behavior or mood
What else do I need to know about antidepressant medicines?
- **Never stop an antidepressant medicine without first talking to a healthcare provider.** Stopping an antidepressant medicine suddenly can cause other symptoms.
- **Antidepressants are medicines used to treat depression and other illnesses.** It is important to discuss all the risks of treating depression and also the risks of not treating it. You should discuss all treatment choices with your healthcare provider, not just the use of antidepressants.
- **Antidepressant medicines have other side effects.** Talk to your healthcare provider about the side effects of your medicines.
- **Antidepressant medicines can interact with other medicines.** Know all of the medicines that you take. Keep a list of all medicines to show your healthcare provider. Do not start new medicines without first checking with your healthcare provider.
4. **Oleptro is not approved for use in children.** Talk to your healthcare provider for more information.
What is Oleptro?
Oleptro is a prescription medicine taken 1 time a day to treat major depressive disorder in adults.
What should I tell my healthcare provider before taking Oleptro?
Before you take Oleptro, tell your healthcare provider if you:
- Have heart problems, including QT prolongation or a family history of it
- Have ever had a heart attack
- Have bipolar disorder
- Have liver or kidney problems
- Have other serious medical conditions
- Are pregnant or plan to become pregnant. Oleptro may harm your unborn baby. Talk to your healthcare provider if you are pregnant or plan to become pregnant.
- Are breastfeeding or plan to breastfeed. It is not known if Oleptro passes into your breast milk. You and your healthcare provider should decide if you will take Oleptro or breastfeed.
- Have taken a Monoamine Oxidase Inhibitor (MAOI) or if you have stopped taking an MAOI in the last 2 weeks.

Tell your healthcare provider about all the medicines you take, including prescription and non-prescription medicines, vitamins, and herbal supplements.
Using Oleptro with certain other medicines can affect each other causing serious side effects.
Know the medicines you take. Keep a list of them and show it to your healthcare provider and pharmacist when you get a new medicine.
How should I take Oleptro?
- Take Oleptro exactly as your healthcare provider tells you.
- Oleptro should be taken 1 time a day.
- Oleptro should be taken at the same time each day in the late evening, if possible at bedtime, on an empty stomach.
- Do not stop taking Oleptro without talking to your healthcare provider.
- Oleptro should be swallowed whole or broken in half along the score line. Do not chew or crush Oleptro. Tell your healthcare provider if you cannot swallow Oleptro either whole or as a half tablet.
What should I avoid while taking Oleptro?
- Do not drive, operate heavy machinery, or do other dangerous activities until you know how Oleptro affects you. Oleptro can slow your thinking and motor skills.
- Do not drink alcohol or take other medicines that make you sleepy or dizzy while taking Oleptro until you talk with your healthcare provider. Oleptro may make your sleepiness or dizziness worse if you take it with alcohol or other medicines that cause sleepiness or dizziness.
What are the possible side effects of Oleptro?
Oleptro can cause serious side effects or death. See "What is the most important information I should know about Oleptro?"
Serious side effects include:
- Serotonin syndrome. Symptoms of serotonin syndrome include: agitation, hallucinations, problems with coordination, fast heartbeat, tight muscles, trouble walking, nausea, vomiting, diarrhea.
- Feeling high or in a very good mood, then becoming irritable, or having too much energy, feeling like you have to keep talking or do not sleep (Mania).
- Irregular or fast heartbeat or faint (QT prolongation).
- Low blood pressure. You feel dizzy or faint when you change positions (go from sitting to standing).
- Unusual bruising or bleeding.
- Erection lasting for more than 6 hours (Priapism).
- Low sodium in your blood (Hyponatremia). Symptoms of hyponatremia include: headache, feeling weak, feeling confused, trouble concentrating, memory problems and feeling unsteady when you walk.
Get medical help right away, if you have any of the symptoms listed above.
The most common side effects of Oleptro include:
- Sleepiness
- Dizziness
- Constipation
- Blurry vision
Tell your healthcare provider if you have any side effect that bothers you or that does not go away.
These are not all the possible side effects of Oleptro. For more information, ask your healthcare provider or pharmacist.
Call your doctor for medical advice about side effects. You may report side effects to FDA at 1-800-FDA-1088.
How should I store Oleptro?
- Store Oleptro between 59°F to 86°F (15°C to 30°C)
- Keep in tight container
- Keep out of the light
Keep Oleptro and all medicines out of the reach of children.
General information about Oleptro.
Medicines are sometimes prescribed for purposes other than those listed in a Medication Guide. Do not use Oleptro for a condition for which it was not prescribed. Do not give Oleptro to other people, even if they have the same symptoms that you have. It may harm them.
This Medication Guide summarizes the most important information about Oleptro. If you would like more information, talk with your healthcare provider. You can ask your pharmacist or healthcare provider for information about Oleptro that is written for health professionals.
For more information, go to www.oleptro.com or call 1-877-345-6177.
What are the ingredients in Oleptro?
Active ingredient: trazodone hydrochloride
Inactive ingredients: hydroxypropyl distarch phosphate (Contramid®), hypromellose, sodium stearyl fumarate, colloidal silicon dioxide, iron oxide yellow, iron oxide red, talc, polyethylene glycol 3350, titanium dioxide, polyvinyl alcohol, black ink (food grade).
This Medication Guide has been approved by the U.S. Food and Drug Administration.
Labopharm Europe Limited
Unit 5, The Seapoint Building
44/45 Clontarf Road, Dublin 3, IRELAND

AstraZeneca LP
WILMINGTON, DE 19850-5437

For Product Full Prescribing Information, Business Information, Medical Information, Adverse Drug Experiences, and Customer Service:
Information Center
1-800-236-9933
For Product Ordering:
Trade Customer Service
1-800-842-9920
For Product Full Prescribing Information:
Internet: www.astrazeneca-us.com

ATACAND®   ℞
[ăt'-ă-kănd]
(candesartan cilexetil)
TABLETS

HIGHLIGHTS OF PRESCRIBING INFORMATION
These highlights do not include all the information needed to use ATACAND safely and effectively. See full prescribing information for ATACAND.
ATACAND® (candesartan cilexetil) TABLETS
INITIAL U.S. APPROVAL: 1998

WARNING: USE IN PREGNANCY: *See Full Prescribing Information for complete boxed warning.*
When used in pregnancy during the second and third trimesters, drugs that act directly on the renin-angiotensin system can cause injury and even death to the developing fetus. When pregnancy is detected, ATACAND should be discontinued as soon as possible. See WARNINGS AND PRECAUTIONS, Fetal/Neonatal Morbidity and Mortality (5.1).

——————RECENT MAJOR CHANGES——————
Dosage and Administration: pediatric hypertension 1 to < 17 years of age (2.2). 10/2009
——————INDICATIONS AND USAGE——————
ATACAND is an angiotensin II receptor blocker (ARB) indicated for:
• Treatment of hypertension in adults and children 1 to < 17 years of age (1.1).
• Treatment of heart failure (NYHA class II-IV); ATACAND reduces cardiovascular death and heart failure hospitalization (1.2).
——————DOSAGE AND ADMINISTRATION——————
[See table above]
——————DOSAGE FORMS AND STRENGTHS——————
Tablets 4 mg, 8 mg, 16 mg, 32 mg (3).
——————CONTRAINDICATIONS——————
Known hypersensitivity to product components (4).
——————WARNINGS AND PRECAUTIONS——————
• Avoid fetal (in utero) and neonatal exposure (5.1).
• Children < 1 year of age must not receive ATACAND for hypertension (5.2).
• Observe for signs and symptoms of hypotension (5.3).
• Use with caution in patients with impaired hepatic (5.4) or renal (5.5) function.
• Hyperkalemia may occur in heart failure patients treated with ATACAND (5.6).
——————ADVERSE REACTIONS——————
• Most common adverse reactions which caused adult patients to discontinue therapy for:
• Hypertension were headache (0.6%) and dizziness (0.3%) (6.1).
• Heart Failure were hypotension (4.1%) (5.3), abnormal renal function (6.3%) (5.5), and hyperkalemia (2.4%) (5.6).
• Most common adverse reactions (incidence ≥ 2% and greater than placebo) are back pain, dizziness, upper respiratory tract infection, pharyngitis and rhinitis (6.1).
To report SUSPECTED ADVERSE REACTIONS contact AstraZeneca LP at 1–800–236–9933 or FDA at 1-800-FDA-1088 or www.fda.gov/medwatch.
——————DRUG INTERACTIONS——————
• Lithium: Reversible increases in serum lithium concentrations and toxicity (7).
——————USE IN SPECIFIC POPULATIONS——————
• *Nursing Mothers:* Either nursing or drug should be discontinued (8.3).

	Starting Dose	Dose Range	Target Maintenance Dose
Adult Hypertension (2.1)	16 mg tablet once daily	8-32 mg tablet total daily dose	–
Pediatric Hypertension (1 to < 6 years) (2.2)	0.20 mg/kg oral suspension once daily	0.05-0.4 mg/kg oral suspension once daily or consider divided dose	-
Pediatric Hypertension (6 to < 17 years) (2.2)	< 50 kg 4–8 mg tablet once daily > 50 kg 8–16 mg tablet once daily	< 50 kg 4–16 mg tablet once daily or consider divided dose > 50 kg 4–32 mg tablet once daily or consider divided dose	–
Adult Heart Failure (2.3)	4 mg tablet once daily		32 mg tablet once daily*

* The target dose is 32 mg once daily, which is achieved by doubling the dose at approximately 2-week intervals, as tolerated by patient

• *Pediatrics:* Children < 1 year of age must not receive ATACAND for hypertension (5.2). Inhibitors of the renin-angiotensin system can cause renal abnormalities in neonatal animals (12.3).
• *Geriatrics:* No overall difference in efficacy or safety vs. younger adult patients, but greater sensitivity of some older individuals cannot be ruled out (8.5).
See 17 for PATIENT COUNSELING INFORMATION
Revised: 10/2009

FULL PRESCRIBING INFORMATION: CONTENTS*
WARNING: USE IN PREGNANCY:
RECENT MAJOR CHANGES
1 INDICATIONS AND USAGE
   1.1 Hypertension
   1.2 Heart Failure
2 DOSAGE AND ADMINISTRATION
   2.1 Adult Hypertension
   2.2 Pediatric Hypertension 1 to < 17 Years of age
   2.3 Adult Heart Failure
3 DOSAGE FORMS AND STRENGTHS
4 CONTRAINDICATIONS
5 WARNINGS AND PRECAUTIONS
   5.1 Fetal/Neonatal Morbidity and Mortality
   5.2 Morbidity in Infants
   5.3 Hypotension
   5.4 Impaired Hepatic Function
   5.5 Renal Function Deterioration
   5.6 Hyperkalemia
6 ADVERSE REACTIONS
   6.1 Clinical Studies Experience
   6.2 Postmarketing Experience
   6.3 Laboratory Test Findings
7 DRUG INTERACTIONS
8 USE IN SPECIFIC POPULATIONS
   8.1 Pregnancy
   8.2 Labor and Delivery
   8.3 Nursing Mothers
   8.4 Pediatric Use
   8.5 Geriatric Use
10 OVERDOSAGE
11 DESCRIPTION
12 CLINICAL PHARMACOLOGY
   12.1 Mechanism of Action
   12.2 Pharmacodynamics
   12.3 Pharmacokinetics
13 NONCLINICAL TOXICOLOGY
   13.1 Carcinogenesis, Mutagenesis, Impairment of Fertility
14 CLINICAL STUDIES
   14.1 Hypertension
   14.2 Heart Failure
16 HOW SUPPLIED/STORAGE AND HANDLING
17 PATIENT COUNSELING INFORMATION
* Sections or subsections omitted from the full prescribing information are not listed

---

FULL PRESCRIBING INFORMATION

WARNING: USE IN PREGNANCY:
When used in pregnancy during the second and third trimesters, drugs that act directly on the renin-angiotensin system can cause injury and even death to the developing fetus. When pregnancy is detected, ATACAND should be discontinued as soon as possible *[see WARNINGS AND PRECAUTIONS, Fetal/Neonatal Morbidity and Mortality (5.1)].*

---

1 INDICATIONS AND USAGE
1.1 Hypertension
ATACAND is indicated for the treatment of hypertension in adults and children 1 to < 17 years of age. It may be used alone or in combination with other antihypertensive agents.

1.2 Heart Failure
ATACAND is indicated for the treatment of heart failure (NYHA class II-IV) in adults with left ventricular systolic dysfunction (ejection fraction ≤ 40%) to reduce cardiovascular death and to reduce heart failure hospitalizations *[see CLINICAL STUDIES (14.2)].* ATACAND also has an added effect on these outcomes when used with an ACE inhibitor.

2 DOSAGE AND ADMINISTRATION
2.1 Adult Hypertension
Dosage must be individualized. Blood pressure response is dose related over the range of 2 to 32 mg. The usual recommended starting dose of ATACAND is 16 mg once daily when it is used as monotherapy in patients who are not volume depleted. ATACAND can be administered once or twice daily with total daily doses ranging from 8 mg to 32 mg. Larger doses do not appear to have a greater effect, and there is relatively little experience with such doses. Most of the antihypertensive effect is present within 2 weeks, and maximal blood pressure reduction is generally obtained within 4 to 6 weeks of treatment with ATACAND.
No initial dosage adjustment is necessary for elderly patients, for patients with mildly impaired renal function, or for patients with mildly impaired hepatic function *[see CLINICAL PHARMACOLOGY (12.3)].* In patients with moderate hepatic impairment, consideration should be given to initiation of ATACAND at a lower dose *[see CLINICAL PHARMACOLOGY (12.3)].* For patients with possible depletion of intravascular volume (eg, patients treated with diuretics, particularly those with impaired renal function), ATACAND should be initiated under close medical supervision and consideration should be given to administration of a lower dose *[see WARNINGS AND PRECAUTIONS (5.3)].* ATACAND may be administered with or without food.
If blood pressure is not controlled by ATACAND alone, a diuretic may be added. ATACAND may be administered with other antihypertensive agents.
2.2 Pediatric Hypertension 1 to < 17 Years of age
ATACAND may be administered once daily or divided into two equal doses. Adjust the dosage according to blood pressure response. For patients with possible depletion of intravascular volume (e.g., patients treated with diuretics, particularly those with impaired renal function), initiate ATACAND under close medical supervision and consider administration of a lower dose *[see WARNINGS AND PRECAUTIONS (5.3)].*
Children 1 to < 6 years of age:
The dose range is 0.05 to 0.4 mg/kg per day. The recommended starting dose is 0.20 mg/kg (oral suspension).
Children 6 to < 17 years of age:
For those less than 50 kg, the dose range is 2 to 16 mg per day. The recommended starting dose is 4 to 8 mg.
For those greater than 50 kg, the dose range is 4 to 32 mg per day. The recommended starting dose is 8 to 16 mg.
Doses above 0.4 mg/kg (1 to < 6 year olds) or 32 mg (6 to < 17 year olds) have not been studied in pediatric patients *[see CLINICAL STUDIES (14.1)].*
An antihypertensive effect is usually present within 2 weeks, with full effect generally obtained within 4 weeks of treatment with ATACAND.
Children < 1 year of age must not receive ATACAND for hypertension.
All pediatric patients with a glomerular filtration rate less than 30 mL/min/1.73m² should not receive ATACAND since ATACAND has not been studied in this population *[see WARNINGS AND PRECAUTIONS (5.2)].*
For children who cannot swallow tablets, an oral suspension may be substituted *[see Preparation of Oral Suspension].*
Preparation of Oral Suspension:
ATACAND oral suspension can be prepared in concentrations within the range of 0.1 to 2.0 mg/mL. Typically, a concentration of 1 mg/mL will be suitable for the prescribed dose. Any strength of ATACAND tablets can be used in the preparation of the suspension.

Follow the steps below for preparation of the suspension. The number of tablets and volume of vehicle specified below will yield 160 mL of a 1 mg/mL suspension.
• Prepare the vehicle by adding equal volumes of *Ora-Plus® (80 mL) and *Ora-Sweet SF® (80 mL) or, alternatively, use *,†Ora-Blend SF® (160 mL).
• Add a small amount of vehicle to the required number of ATACAND tablets (five 32 mg tablets) and grind into a smooth paste using a mortar and pestle.
• Add the paste to a preparation vessel of suitable size.
• Rinse the mortar and pestle clean using the vehicle and add this to the vessel. Repeat, if necessary.
• Prepare the final volume by adding the remaining vehicle.
• Mix thoroughly.
• Dispense into suitably sized amber PET bottles.
• Label with an expiry date of 100 days and include the following instructions:
Store at room temperature (below 30°C/86°F). Use within 30 days after first opening. Do not use after the expiry date stated on the bottle.
Do not freeze.
Shake well before each use.
*Ora-Plus®, Ora-Sweet SF®, and Ora-Blend SF® are registered trademarks of Paddock Laboratories, Inc.
†Supplied as a 50/50% pre-mix of Ora-Plus® and Ora-Sweet SF®.

2.3 Adult Heart Failure

The recommended initial dose for treating heart failure is 4 mg once daily. The target dose is 32 mg once daily, which is achieved by doubling the dose at approximately 2-week intervals, as tolerated by the patient.

3 DOSAGE FORMS AND STRENGTHS

4 mg are white to off-white, circular/biconvex-shaped, non-film-coated scored tablets, coded ACF on one side and 004 on the other.

8 mg are light pink, circular/biconvex-shaped, non-film-coated scored tablets, coded ACG on one side and 008 on the other.

16 mg are pink, circular/biconvex-shaped, non-film-coated scored tablets, coded ACH on one side and 016 on the other.

32 mg are pink, circular/biconvex-shaped, non-film-coated scored tablets, coded ACL on one side and 032 on the other.

4 CONTRAINDICATIONS

ATACAND is contraindicated in patients who are hypersensitive to any component of this product.

5 WARNINGS AND PRECAUTIONS

5.1 Fetal/Neonatal Morbidity and Mortality

Drugs that act directly on the renin-angiotensin system can cause fetal and neonatal morbidity and death when administered to pregnant women. Several dozen cases have been reported in the world literature in patients who were taking angiotensin-converting enzyme inhibitors. Post-marketing experience has identified reports of fetal and neonatal toxicity in babies born to women treated with ATACAND during pregnancy. When pregnancy is detected, ATACAND should be discontinued as soon as possible.

The use of drugs that act directly on the renin-angiotensin system during the second and third trimesters of pregnancy has been associated with fetal and neonatal injury, including hypotension, neonatal skull hypoplasia, anuria, reversible or irreversible renal failure, and death. Oligohydramnios has also been reported, presumably resulting from decreased fetal renal function; oligohydramnios in this setting has been associated with fetal limb contractures, craniofacial deformation, and hypoplastic lung development. Prematurity, intrauterine growth retardation, and patent ductus arteriosus have also been reported, although it is not clear whether these occurrences were due to exposure to the drug.

These adverse effects do not appear to have resulted from intrauterine drug exposure that has been limited to the first trimester. Mothers whose embryos and fetuses are exposed to an angiotensin II receptor antagonist only during the first trimester should be so informed. Nonetheless, when patients become pregnant, physicians should have the patient discontinue the use of ATACAND as soon as possible. Rarely (probably less often than once in every thousand pregnancies), no alternative to a drug acting on the renin-angiotensin system will be found. In these rare cases, the mothers should be apprised of the potential hazards to their fetuses, and serial ultrasound examinations should be performed to assess the intra-amniotic environment.

If oligohydramnios is observed, ATACAND should be discontinued unless it is considered life saving for the mother. Contraction stress testing (CST), a nonstress test (NST), or biophysical profiling (BPP) may be appropriate, depending upon the week of pregnancy. Patients and physicians should be aware, however, that oligohydramnios may not appear until after the fetus has sustained irreversible injury.

Infants with histories of *in utero* exposure to an angiotensin II receptor antagonist should be closely observed for hypotension, oliguria, and hyperkalemia. If oliguria occurs, attention should be directed toward support of blood pressure and renal perfusion. Exchange transfusion or dialysis may be required as means of reversing hypotension and/or substituting for disordered renal function.

Oral doses ≥10 mg of candesartan cilexetil/kg/day administered to pregnant rats during late gestation and continued through lactation were associated with reduced survival and an increased incidence of hydronephrosis in the offspring. The 10-mg/kg/day dose in rats is approximately 2.8 times the maximum recommended daily human dose (MRHD) of 32 mg on a mg/m^2 basis (comparison assumes human body weight of 50 kg). Candesartan cilexetil given to pregnant rabbits at an oral dose of 3 mg/kg/day (approximately 1.7 times the MRHD on a mg/m^2 basis) caused maternal toxicity (decreased body weight and death) but, in surviving dams, had no adverse effects on fetal survival, fetal weight, or external, visceral, or skeletal development. No maternal toxicity or adverse effects on fetal development were observed when oral doses up to 1000 mg of candesartan cilexetil/kg/day (approximately 138 times the MRHD on a mg/m^2 basis) were administered to pregnant mice.

5.2 Morbidity in Infants

Children < 1 year of age must not receive ATACAND for hypertension. The consequences of administering drugs that act directly on the renin-angiotensin system (RAS) can have effects on the development of immature kidneys.

5.3 Hypotension

In adult or children patients with an activated renin-angiotensin system, such as volume- and/or salt-depleted patients (eg, those being treated with diuretics), symptomatic hypotension may occur. These conditions should be corrected prior to administration of ATACAND, or the treatment should start under close medical supervision [see DOSAGE AND ADMINISTRATION (2.1)].

If hypotension occurs, the patients should be placed in the supine position and, if necessary, given an intravenous infusion of normal saline. A transient hypotensive response is not a contraindication to further treatment which usually can be continued without difficulty once the blood pressure has stabilized.

Caution should be observed when initiating therapy in patients with heart failure. Patients with heart failure given ATACAND commonly have some reduction in blood pressure. In patients with symptomatic hypotension this may require temporarily reducing the dose of ATACAND, or diuretic, or both, and volume repletion. In the CHARM program, hypotension was reported in 18.8% of patients on ATACAND versus 9.8% of patients on placebo. The incidence of hypotension leading to drug discontinuation in ATACAND-treated patients was 4.1% compared with 2.0% in placebo-treated patients.

Monitoring of blood pressure is recommended during dose escalation and periodically thereafter.

Major Surgery/Anesthesia

Hypotension may occur during major surgery and anesthesia in patients treated with angiotensin II receptor antagonists, including ATACAND, due to blockade of the renin-angiotensin system. Very rarely, hypotension may be severe such that it may warrant the use of intravenous fluids and/or vasopressors.

5.4 Impaired Hepatic Function

Based on pharmacokinetic data which demonstrate significant increases in candesartan AUC and C_{max} in patients with moderate hepatic impairment, a lower initiating dose should be considered for patients with moderate hepatic impairment [see CLINICAL PHARMACOLOGY (12.3)].

5.5 Renal Function Deterioration

As a consequence of inhibiting the renin-angiotensin-aldosterone system, changes in renal function may be anticipated in some individuals treated with ATACAND. In patients whose renal function may depend upon the activity of the renin-angiotensin-aldosterone system (eg, patients with severe heart failure), treatment with angiotensin-converting enzyme inhibitors and angiotensin receptor antagonists has been associated with oliguria and/or progressive azotemia and (rarely) with acute renal failure and/or death. Similar results may be anticipated in patients treated with ATACAND [see CLINICAL PHARMACOLOGY (12.3)].

In studies of ACE inhibitors in patients with unilateral or bilateral renal artery stenosis, increases in serum creatinine or blood urea nitrogen (BUN) have been reported. There has been no long-term use of ATACAND in patients with unilateral or bilateral renal artery stenosis, but similar results may be expected.

In heart failure patients treated with ATACAND, increases in serum creatinine may occur. Dosage reduction or discontinuation of the diuretic or ATACAND, and volume repletion may be required. In the CHARM program, the incidence of abnormal renal function (e.g., creatinine increase) was 12.5% in patients treated with ATACAND versus 6.3% in patients treated with placebo. The incidence of abnormal renal function (eg, creatinine increase) leading to drug discontinuation in ATACAND-treated patients was 6.3% compared with 2.9% in placebo-treated patients. Evaluation of patients with heart failure should always include assessment of renal function and volume status. Monitoring of serum creatinine is recommended during dose escalation and periodically thereafter.

Pediatrics—ATACAND has not been studied in children with estimated glomerular filtration rate < 30 mL/min/1.73m^2.

5.6 Hyperkalemia

In heart failure patients treated with ATACAND, hyperkalemia may occur, especially when taken concomitantly with ACE inhibitors and potassium-sparing diuretics such as spironolactone. In the CHARM program, the incidence of hyperkalemia was 6.3% in patients treated with ATACAND versus 2.1% in patients treated with placebo. The incidence of hyperkalemia leading to drug discontinuation in ATACAND-treated patients was 2.4% compared with 0.6% in placebo-treated patients. During treatment with ATACAND in patients with heart failure, monitoring of serum potassium is recommended during dose escalation and periodically thereafter.

6 ADVERSE REACTIONS

6.1 Clinical Studies Experience

Because clinical studies are conducted under widely varying conditions, adverse reaction rates observed in the clinical studies of a drug cannot be directly compared to rates in the clinical studies of another drug and may not reflect the rates observed in practice.

Adult Hypertension

ATACAND has been evaluated for safety in more than 3600 patients/subjects, including more than 3200 patients treated for hypertension. About 600 of these patients were studied for at least 6 months and about 200 for at least 1 year. In general, treatment with ATACAND was well tolerated. The overall incidence of adverse events reported with ATACAND was similar to placebo.

The rate of withdrawals due to adverse events in all trials in patients (7510 total) was 3.3% (ie, 108 of 3260) of patients treated with ATACAND as monotherapy and 3.5% (ie, 39 of 1106) of patients treated with placebo. In placebo-controlled trials, discontinuation of therapy due to clinical adverse events occurred in 2.4% (ie, 57 of 2350) of patients treated with ATACAND and 3.4% (ie, 35 of 1027) of patients treated with placebo.

The most common reasons for discontinuation of therapy with ATACAND were headache (0.6%) and dizziness (0.3%).

The adverse events that occurred in placebo-controlled clinical trials in at least 1% of patients treated with ATACAND and at a higher incidence in candesartan cilexetil (n = 2350) than placebo (n = 1027) patients included back pain (3% vs. 2%), dizziness (4% vs. 3%), upper respiratory tract infection (6% vs. 4%), pharyngitis (2% vs. 1%), and rhinitis (2% vs. 1%).

The following adverse events occurred in placebo-controlled clinical trials at a more than 1% rate but at about the same or greater incidence in patients receiving placebo compared to ATACAND: fatigue, peripheral edema, chest pain, headache, bronchitis, coughing, sinusitis, nausea, abdominal pain, diarrhea, vomiting, arthralgia, albuminuria.

Other potentially important adverse events that have been reported, whether or not attributed to treatment, with an incidence of 0.5% or greater from the 3260 patients worldwide treated in clinical trials with ATACAND are listed below. It cannot be determined whether these events were causally related to ATACAND. **Body as a Whole:** asthenia, fever; **Central and Peripheral Nervous System:** paresthesia, vertigo; **Gastrointestinal System Disorder:** dyspepsia, gastroenteritis; **Heart Rate and Rhythm Disorders:** tachycardia, palpitation; **Metabolic and Nutritional Disorders:** creatine phosphokinase increased, hyperglycemia, hypertriglyceridemia, hyperuricemia; **Musculoskeletal System Disorders:** myalgia; **Platelet/Bleeding-Clotting Disorders:** epistaxis; **Psychiatric Disorders:** anxiety, depression, somnolence; **Respiratory System Disorders:** dyspnea; **Skin and Appendages Disorders:** rash, sweating increased; **Urinary System Disorders:** hematuria.

Other reported events seen less frequently included angina pectoris, myocardial infarction, and angioedema.

Adverse events occurred at about the same rates in men and women, older and younger patients, and black and non-black patients.

Pediatric Hypertension

Among children in clinical studies, 1 in 93 children age 1 to < 6 and 3 in 240 age 6 to < 17 experienced worsening renal disease. The association between candesartan and exacerbation of the underlying condition could not be excluded.

Heart Failure

The adverse event profile of ATACAND in adult heart failure patients was consistent with the pharmacology of the drug and the health status of the patients. In the CHARM program, comparing ATACAND in total daily doses up to

32 mg once daily (n=3803) with placebo (n=3796), 21.0% of patients discontinued ATACAND for adverse events vs. 16.1% of placebo patients.

6.2 Postmarketing Experience

The following adverse reactions were identified during post-approval use of ATACAND. Because these reactions are reported voluntarily from a population of uncertain size, it is not always possible to reliably estimate their frequency or establish a causal relationship to drug exposure.

The following have been very rarely reported in post-marketing experience:

Digestive: Abnormal hepatic function and hepatitis.

Hematologic: Neutropenia, leukopenia, and agranulocytosis.

Metabolic and Nutritional Disorders: hyperkalemia, hyponatremia.

Renal: renal impairment, renal failure.

Skin and Appendages Disorders: Pruritus and urticaria.

Rare reports of rhabdomyolysis have been reported in patients receiving angiotensin II receptor blockers.

6.3 Laboratory Test Findings

Hypertension

In controlled clinical trials, clinically important changes in standard laboratory parameters were rarely associated with the administration of ATACAND.

Creatinine, Blood Urea Nitrogen

Minor increases in blood urea nitrogen (BUN) and serum creatinine were observed infrequently.

Hyperuricemia

Hyperuricemia was rarely found (19 or 0.6% of 3260 patients treated with ATACAND and 5 or 0.5% of 1106 patients treated with placebo).

Hemoglobin and Hematocrit

Small decreases in hemoglobin and hematocrit (mean decreases of approximately 0.2 grams/dL and 0.5 volume percent, respectively) were observed in patients treated with ATACAND alone but were rarely of clinical importance. Anemia, leukopenia, and thrombocytopenia were associated with withdrawal of one patient each from clinical trials.

Potassium

A small increase (mean increase of 0.1 mEq/L) was observed in patients treated with ATACAND alone but was rarely of clinical importance. One patient from a congestive heart failure trial was withdrawn for hyperkalemia (serum potassium = 7.5 mEq/L). This patient was also receiving spironolactone *[see WARNINGS AND PRECAUTIONS (5.6)]*.

Liver Function Tests

Elevations of liver enzymes and/or serum bilirubin were observed infrequently. Five patients assigned to ATACAND in clinical trials were withdrawn because of abnormal liver chemistries. All had elevated transaminases. Two had mildly elevated total bilirubin, but one of these patients was diagnosed with Hepatitis A.

Heart Failure

In the CHARM program, small increases in serum creatinine (mean increase 0.2 mg/dL in candesartan-treated patients and 0.1 mg/dL in placebo-treated patients) and serum potassium (mean increase 0.15 mEq/L in ATACAND-treated patients and 0.02 mEq/L in placebo-treated patients), and small decreases in hemoglobin (mean decrease 0.5 gm/dL in ATACAND-treated patients and 0.3 gm/dL in placebo-treated patients) and hematocrit (mean decrease 1.6% in ATACAND-treated patients and 0.9% in placebo-treated patients) were observed.

7 DRUG INTERACTIONS

No significant drug interactions have been reported in studies of candesartan cilexetil given with other drugs such as glyburide, nifedipine, digoxin, warfarin, hydrochlorothiazide, and oral contraceptives in healthy volunteers, or given with enalapril to patients with heart failure (NYHA class II and III). Because candesartan is not significantly metabolized by the cytochrome P450 system and at therapeutic concentrations has no effects on P450 enzymes, interactions with drugs that inhibit or are metabolized by those enzymes would not be expected.

Lithium

Reversible increases in serum lithium concentrations and toxicity have been reported during concomitant administration of lithium with ACE inhibitors, and with some angiotensin II receptor antagonists. An increase in serum lithium concentration has been reported during concomitant administration of lithium with ATACAND, so careful monitoring of serum lithium levels is recommended during concomitant use.

8 USE IN SPECIFIC POPULATIONS

8.1 Pregnancy

Pregnancy Categories C (first trimester) *and D* (second and third trimesters) *[see WARNINGS AND PRECAUTIONS (5.1)]*.

8.2 Labor and Delivery

The effect of ATACAND on labor and delivery in humans is unknown *[see WARNINGS AND PRECAUTIONS (5.1)]*.

8.3 Nursing Mothers

It is not known whether candesartan is excreted in human milk, but candesartan has been shown to be present in rat milk. Because of the potential for adverse effects on the nursing infant, a decision should be made whether to discontinue nursing or discontinue ATACAND, taking into account the importance of the drug to the mother.

8.4 Pediatric Use

The antihypertensive effects of ATACAND were evaluated in hypertensive children 1 to < 17 years of age in randomized, double-blind clinical studies *[see CLINICAL STUDIES (14.1)]*. The pharmacokinetics of ATACAND have been evaluated in pediatric patients 1 to < 17 years of age *[see Pharmacokinetics (12.3)]*.

Children < 1 year of age must not receive ATACAND for hypertension *[see WARNINGS AND PRECAUTIONS (5.2)]*.

8.5 Geriatric Use

Hypertension

Of the total number of subjects in clinical studies of ATACAND, 21% (683/3260) were 65 and over, while 3% (87/3260) were 75 and over. No overall differences in safety or effectiveness were observed between these subjects and younger adult subjects, and other reported clinical experience has not identified differences in responses between the elderly and younger patients, but greater sensitivity of some older individuals cannot be ruled out. In a placebo-controlled trial of about 200 elderly hypertensive patients (ages 65 to 87 years), administration of candesartan cilexetil was well tolerated and lowered blood pressure by about 12/6 mm Hg more than placebo.

Heart Failure

Of the 7599 patients with heart failure in the CHARM program, 4343 (57%) were age 65 years or older and 1736 (23%) were 75 years or older. In patients ≥ 75 years of age, the incidence of drug discontinuations due to adverse events was higher for those treated with ATACAND or placebo compared with patients <75 years of age. In these patients, the most common adverse events leading to drug discontinuation at an incidence of at least 3%, and more frequent with ATACAND than placebo, were abnormal renal function (7.9% vs. 4.0%), hypotension (5.2% vs. 3.2%) and hyperkalemia (4.2% vs. 0.9%). In addition to monitoring of serum creatinine, potassium, and blood pressure during dose escalation and periodically thereafter, greater sensitivity of some older individuals with heart failure must be considered.

10 OVERDOSAGE

No lethality was observed in acute toxicity studies in mice, rats, and dogs given single oral doses of up to 2000 mg/kg of candesartan cilexetil. In mice given single oral doses of the primary metabolite, candesartan, the minimum lethal dose was greater than 1000 mg/kg but less than 2000 mg/kg.

The most likely manifestation of overdosage with ATACAND would be hypotension, dizziness, and tachycardia; bradycardia could occur from parasympathetic (vagal) stimulation. If symptomatic hypotension should occur, supportive treatment should be instituted.

Candesartan cannot be removed by hemodialysis.

Treatment: To obtain up-to-date information about the treatment of overdose, consult your Regional Poison Control Center. Telephone numbers of certified poison control centers are listed in the *Physicians' Desk Reference (PDR)*. In managing overdose, consider the possibilities of multiple-drug overdoses, drug-drug interactions, and altered pharmacokinetics in your patient.

11 DESCRIPTION

ATACAND (candesartan cilexetil), a prodrug, is hydrolyzed to candesartan during absorption from the gastrointestinal tract. Candesartan is a selective AT_1 subtype angiotensin II receptor antagonist.

Candesartan cilexetil, a nonpeptide, is chemically described as (±)-1-Hydroxyethyl 2-ethoxy-1-[*p*-(*o*-1*H*-tetrazol-5-ylphenyl)benzyl]-7-benzimidazolecarboxylate, cyclohexyl carbonate (ester).

Its empirical formula is $C_{33}H_{34}N_6O_6$, and its structural formula is:

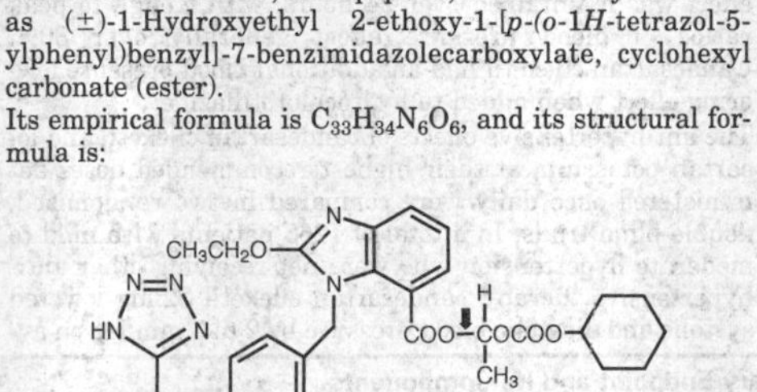

site of ester hydrolysis.

Candesartan cilexetil is a white to off-white powder with a molecular weight of 610.67. It is practically insoluble in water and sparingly soluble in methanol. Candesartan cilexetil is a racemic mixture containing one chiral center at the cyclohexyloxycarbonyloxy ethyl ester group. Following oral administration, candesartan cilexetil undergoes hydrolysis at the ester link to form the active drug, candesartan, which is achiral.

ATACAND is available for oral use as tablets containing either 4 mg, 8 mg, 16 mg, or 32 mg of candesartan cilexetil and the following inactive ingredients: hydroxypropyl cellulose, polyethylene glycol, lactose, corn starch, carboxymethylcellulose calcium, and magnesium stearate. Ferric oxide (reddish brown) is added to the 8-mg, 16-mg, and 32-mg tablets as a colorant.

12 CLINICAL PHARMACOLOGY

12.1 Mechanism of Action

Angiotensin II is formed from angiotensin I in a reaction catalyzed by angiotensin-converting enzyme (ACE, kininase II). Angiotensin II is the principal pressor agent of the renin-angiotensin system, with effects that include vasoconstriction, stimulation of synthesis and release of aldosterone, cardiac stimulation, and renal reabsorption of sodium. Candesartan blocks the vasoconstrictor and aldosterone-secreting effects of angiotensin II by selectively blocking the binding of angiotensin II to the AT_1 receptor in many tissues, such as vascular smooth muscle and the adrenal gland. Its action is, therefore, independent of the pathways for angiotensin II synthesis.

There is also an AT_2 receptor found in many tissues, but AT_2 is not known to be associated with cardiovascular homeostasis. Candesartan has much greater affinity (>10,000-fold) for the AT_1 receptor than for the AT_2 receptor.

Blockade of the renin-angiotensin system with ACE inhibitors, which inhibit the biosynthesis of angiotensin II from angiotensin I, is widely used in the treatment of hypertension. ACE inhibitors also inhibit the degradation of bradykinin, a reaction also catalyzed by ACE. Because candesartan does not inhibit ACE (kininase II), it does not affect the response to bradykinin. Whether this difference has clinical relevance is not yet known. Candesartan does not bind to or block other hormone receptors or ion channels known to be important in cardiovascular regulation.

Blockade of the angiotensin II receptor inhibits the negative regulatory feedback of angiotensin II on renin secretion, but the resulting increased plasma renin activity and angiotensin II circulating levels do not overcome the effect of candesartan on blood pressure.

12.2 Pharmacodynamics

Candesartan inhibits the pressor effects of angiotensin II infusion in a dose-dependent manner. After 1 week of once daily dosing with 8 mg of candesartan cilexetil, the pressor effect was inhibited by approximately 90% at peak with approximately 50% inhibition persisting for 24 hours.

Plasma concentrations of angiotensin I and angiotensin II, and plasma renin activity (PRA), increased in a dose-dependent manner after single and repeated administration of candesartan cilexetil to healthy subjects, hypertensive, and heart failure patients. ACE activity was not altered in healthy subjects after repeated candesartan cilexetil administration. The once-daily administration of up to 16 mg of candesartan cilexetil to healthy subjects did not influence plasma aldosterone concentrations, but a decrease in the plasma concentration of aldosterone was observed when 32 mg of candesartan cilexetil was administered to hypertensive patients. In spite of the effect of candesartan cilexetil on aldosterone secretion, very little effect on serum potassium was observed.

Hypertension

Adults

In multiple-dose studies with hypertensive patients, there were no clinically significant changes in metabolic function, including serum levels of total cholesterol, triglycerides, glucose, or uric acid. In a 12-week study of 161 patients with non-insulin-dependent (type 2) diabetes mellitus and hypertension, there was no change in the level of HbA_{1c}.

Heart Failure

In heart failure patients, candesartan ≥ 8 mg resulted in decreases in systemic vascular resistance and pulmonary capillary wedge pressure.

12.3 Pharmacokinetics

Distribution

The volume of distribution of candesartan is 0.13 L/kg. Candesartan is highly bound to plasma proteins (>99%) and does not penetrate red blood cells. The protein binding is constant at candesartan plasma concentrations well above the range achieved with recommended doses. In rats, it has been demonstrated that candesartan crosses the blood-brain barrier poorly, if at all. It has also been demonstrated in rats that candesartan passes across the placental barrier and is distributed in the fetus.

Metabolism and Excretion

Total plasma clearance of candesartan is 0.37 mL/min/kg, with a renal clearance of 0.19 mL/min/kg. When candesartan is administered orally, about 26% of the dose is excreted unchanged in urine. Following an oral dose of ^{14}C-labeled candesartan cilexetil, approximately 33% of radioactivity is recovered in urine and approximately 67%

in feces. Following an intravenous dose of ^{14}C-labeled candesartan, approximately 59% of radioactivity is recovered in urine and approximately 36% in feces. Biliary excretion contributes to the elimination of candesartan.

Adults

Candesartan cilexetil is rapidly and completely bioactivated by ester hydrolysis during absorption from the gastrointestinal tract to candesartan, a selective AT_1 subtype angiotensin II receptor antagonist. Candesartan is mainly excreted unchanged in urine and feces (via bile). It undergoes minor hepatic metabolism by O-deethylation to an inactive metabolite. The elimination half-life of candesartan is approximately 9 hours. After single and repeated administration, the pharmacokinetics of candesartan are linear for oral doses up to 32 mg of candesartan cilexetil. Candesartan and its inactive metabolite do not accumulate in serum upon repeated once-daily dosing.

Following administration of candesartan cilexetil, the absolute bioavailability of candesartan was estimated to be 15%. After tablet ingestion, the peak serum concentration (C_{max}) is reached after 3 to 4 hours. Food with a high fat content does not affect the bioavailability of candesartan after candesartan cilexetil administration.

Pediatrics

In children 1 to 17 years of age, plasma levels are greater than 10–fold higher at peak (approximately 4 hours) than 24 hours after a single dose.

Children 1 to < 6 years of age, given 0.2 mg/kg had exposure similar to adults given 8 mg.

Children > 6 years of age had exposure similar to adults given the same dose.

The pharmacokinetics (C_{max} and AUC) were not modified by age, sex or body weight.

Candesartan cilexetil pharmacokinetics have not been investigated in pediatric patients less than 1 year of age.

From the dose-ranging studies of candesartan cilexetil, there was a dose related increase in plasma candesartan concentrations.

The renin-angiotensin system (RAS) plays a critical role in kidney development. RAS blockade has been shown to lead to abnormal kidney development in very young mice. Children < 1 year of age must not receive ATACAND. Administering drugs that act directly on the renin-angiotensin system (RAS) can alter normal renal development.

Geriatric and Sex

The pharmacokinetics of candesartan have been studied in the elderly (≥ 65 years) and in both sexes. The plasma concentration of candesartan was higher in the elderly (C_{max} was approximately 50% higher, and AUC was approximately 80% higher) compared to younger subjects administered the same dose. The pharmacokinetics of candesartan were linear in the elderly, and candesartan and its inactive metabolite did not accumulate in the serum of these subjects upon repeated, once-daily administration. No initial dosage adjustment is necessary *[see DOSAGE AND ADMINISTRATION (2)]*. There is no difference in the pharmacokinetics of candesartan between male and female subjects.

Renal Insufficiency

In hypertensive patients with renal insufficiency, serum concentrations of candesartan were elevated. After repeated dosing, the AUC and C_{max} were approximately doubled in patients with severe renal impairment (creatinine clearance <30 mL/min/1.73m^2) compared to patients with normal kidney function. The pharmacokinetics of candesartan in hypertensive patients undergoing hemodialysis are similar to those in hypertensive patients with severe renal impairment. Candesartan cannot be removed by hemodialysis. No initial dosage adjustment is necessary in patients with renal insufficiency *[see DOSAGE AND ADMINISTRATION (2.1)]*.

In heart failure patients with renal impairment, AUC_{0-72h} was 36% and 65% higher in mild and moderate renal impairment, respectively. C_{max} was 15% and 55% higher in mild and moderate renal impairment, respectively.

Pediatrics:

ATACAND pharmacokinetics have not been determined in children with renal insufficiency.

Hepatic Insufficiency

The pharmacokinetics of candesartan were compared in patients with mild and moderate hepatic impairment to matched healthy volunteers following a single oral dose of 16 mg candesartan cilexetil. The increase in AUC for candesartan was 30% in patients with mild hepatic impairment (Child-Pugh A) and 145% in patients with moderate hepatic impairment (Child-Pugh B). The increase in C_{max} for candesartan was 56% in patients with mild hepatic impairment and 73% in patients with moderate hepatic impairment. The pharmacokinetics after candesartan cilexetil administration have not been investigated in patients with severe hepatic impairment. No initial dosage adjustment is necessary in patients with mild hepatic impairment. In hypertensive patients with moderate hepatic impairment, consideration should be given to initiation of ATACAND at a lower dose *[see DOSAGE AND ADMINISTRATION (2.1)]*.

Heart Failure

The pharmacokinetics of candesartan were linear in patients with heart failure (NYHA class II and III) after candesartan cilexetil doses of 4, 8, and 16 mg. After repeated dosing, the AUC was approximately doubled in these patients compared with healthy, younger patients. The pharmacokinetics in heart failure patients is similar to that in healthy elderly volunteers [see DOSAGE AND ADMINISTRATION (2.3)].

13 NONCLINICAL TOXICOLOGY

13.1 Carcinogenesis, Mutagenesis, Impairment of Fertility

There was no evidence of carcinogenicity when candesartan cilexetil was orally administered to mice and rats for up to 104 weeks at doses up to 100 and 1000 mg/kg/day, respectively. Rats received the drug by gavage, whereas mice received the drug by dietary administration. These (maximally-tolerated) doses of candesartan cilexetil provided systemic exposures to candesartan (AUCs) that were, in mice, approximately 7 times and, in rats, more than 70 times the exposure in man at the maximum recommended daily human dose (32 mg).

Candesartan and its O-deethyl metabolite tested positive for genotoxicity in the *in vitro* Chinese hamster lung (CHL) chromosomal aberration assay. Neither compound tested positive in the Ames microbial mutagenesis assay or the *in vitro* mouse lymphoma cell assay. Candesartan (but not its O-deethyl metabolite) was also evaluated *in vivo* in the mouse micronucleus test and *in vitro* in the Chinese hamster ovary (CHO) gene mutation assay, in both cases with negative results. Candesartan cilexetil was evaluated in the Ames test, the *in vitro* mouse lymphoma cell and rat hepatocyte unscheduled DNA synthesis assays and the *in vivo* mouse micronucleus test, in each case with negative results. Candesartan cilexetil was not evaluated in the CHL chromosomal aberration or CHO gene mutation assay.

Fertility and reproductive performance were not affected in studies with male and female rats given oral doses of up to 300 mg/kg/day (83 times the maximum daily human dose of 32 mg on a body surface area basis).

14 CLINICAL STUDIES

14.1 Hypertension

Adult

The antihypertensive effects of ATACAND were examined in 14 placebo-controlled trials of 4- to 12-weeks duration, primarily at daily doses of 2 to 32 mg per day in patients with baseline diastolic blood pressures of 95 to 114 mm Hg. Most of the trials were of candesartan cilexetil as a single agent, but it was also studied as add-on to hydrochlorothiazide and amlodipine. These studies included a total of 2350 patients randomized to one of several doses of candesartan cilexetil and 1027 to placebo. Except for a study in diabetics, all studies showed significant effects, generally dose related, of 2 to 32 mg on trough (24 hour) systolic and diastolic pressures compared to placebo, with doses of 8 to 32 mg giving effects of about 8-12/4-8 mm Hg. There were no exaggerated first-dose effects in these patients. Most of the antihypertensive effect was seen within 2 weeks of initial dosing and the full effect in 4 weeks. With once-daily dosing, blood pressure effect was maintained over 24 hours, with trough to peak ratios of blood pressure effect generally over 80%. Candesartan cilexetil had an additional blood pressure lowering effect when added to hydrochlorothiazide.

The antihypertensive effects of candesartan cilexetil and losartan potassium at their highest recommended doses administered once daily were compared in two randomized, double-blind trials. In a total of 1268 patients with mild to moderate hypertension who were not receiving other antihypertensive therapy, candesartan cilexetil 32 mg lowered systolic and diastolic blood pressure by 2 to 3 mm Hg on average more than losartan potassium 100 mg, when measured at the time of either peak or trough effect. The antihypertensive effects of twice daily dosing of either candesartan cilexetil or losartan potassium were not studied.

The antihypertensive effect was similar in men and women and in patients older and younger than 65. Candesartan was effective in reducing blood pressure regardless of race, although the effect was somewhat less in blacks (usually a low-renin population). This has been generally true for angiotensin II antagonists and ACE inhibitors.

In long-term studies of up to 1 year, the antihypertensive effectiveness of candesartan cilexetil was maintained, and there was no rebound after abrupt withdrawal.

There were no changes in the heart rate of patients treated with candesartan cilexetil in controlled trials.

Pediatric

The antihypertensive effects of ATACAND were evaluated in hypertensive children 1 to < 6 years old and 6 to < 17 years of age in two randomized, double-blind multicenter, 4-week dose ranging studies. There were 93 patients 1 to < 6 years of age, 74% of whom had renal disease, that were randomized to receive an oral dose of candesartan cilexetil suspension 0.05, 0.20 or 0.40 mg/kg once daily. The primary method of analysis was slope of the change in systolic blood pressure (SBP) as a function of dose. Since there was no placebo group, the change from baseline likely overestimates the true magnitude of blood pressure effect. Nevertheless, SBP and diastolic blood pressure (DBP) decreased 6.0/5.2 to 12.0/11.1 mmHg from baseline across the three doses of candesartan.

In children 6 to < 17 years, 240 patients were randomized to receive either placebo or low, medium, or high doses of ATACAND in a ratio of 1: 2: 2: 2. For children who weighed < 50 kg the doses of ATACAND were 2, 8, or 16 mg once daily. For those > 50 kg the ATACAND doses were 4, 16 or 32 mg once daily. Those enrolled were 47% Black and 29% were female; mean age +/- SD was 12.9 +/- 2.6 years.

The placebo subtracted effect at trough for sitting systolic blood pressure/sitting diastolic blood pressure for the different doses were from 4.9/3.0 to 7.5/7.2 mmHg.

In children 6 to < 17 years there was a trend for a lesser blood pressure effect for Blacks compared to other patients. There were too few individuals in the age group of 1-6 years old to determine whether Blacks respond differently than other patients to ATACAND.

14.2 Heart Failure

Candesartan was studied in two heart failure outcome studies: 1. The Candesartan in Heart failure: Assessment of Reduction in Mortality and morbidity trial in patients intolerant of ACE inhibitors (CHARM–Alternative), 2. CHARM–Added in patients already receiving ACE inhibitors. Both studies were international double-blind, placebo-controlled trials in patients with NYHA class II - IV heart failure and LVEF ≤40%. In both trials, patients were randomized to placebo or ATACAND (initially 4-8 mg once daily, titrated as tolerated to 32 mg once daily) and followed for up to 4 years. Patients with serum creatinine > 3 mg/dL, serum potassium > 5.5 mEq/L, symptomatic hypotension or known bilateral renal artery stenosis were excluded. The primary end point in both trials was time to either cardiovascular death or hospitalization for heart failure.

CHARM–Alternative included 2028 subjects not receiving an ACE inhibitor due to intolerance. The mean age was 67 years and 32% were female, 48% were NYHA II, 49% were NYHA III, 4% were NYHA IV, and the mean ejection fraction was 30%. Sixty-two percent had a history of myocardial infarction, 50% had a history of hypertension, and 27% had diabetes. Concomitant drugs at baseline were diuretics (85%), digoxin (46%), beta-blockers (55%), and spironolactone (24%). The mean daily dose of ATACAND was approximately 23 mg and 59% of subjects on treatment received 32 mg once daily.

After a median follow-up of 34 months, there was a 23% reduction in the risk of cardiovascular death or heart failure hospitalization on ATACAND (p<0.001), with both components contributing to the overall effect (Table 1).

[See table 1 at bottom left]

In CHARM–Added, 2548 subjects receiving an ACE inhibitor were randomized to ATACAND or placebo. The specific ACE inhibitor and dose were at the discretion of the investigators, who were encouraged to titrate patients to doses known to be effective in clinical outcome trials, subject to patient tolerability. Forced titration to maximum tolerated doses of ACE inhibitor was not required.

The mean age was 64 years and 21% were female, 24% were NYHA II, 73% were NYHA III, 3% were NYHA IV, and the mean ejection fraction was 28%. Fifty-six percent had a history of myocardial infarction, 48% had a history of hypertension, and 30% had diabetes. Concomitant drugs at baseline in addition to ACE inhibitors were diuretics (90%), digoxin (58%), beta-blockers (55%), and spironolactone

Table 1. CHARM — Alternative: Primary Endpoint and its Components

Endpoint (time to first event)	ATACAND (n=1013)	Placebo (n=1015)	Hazard Ratio (95% CI)	p-value (logrank)
CV death or heart failure hospitalization	334	406	0.77 (0.67–0.89)	<0.001
CV death	219	252	0.85 (0.71–1.02)	0.072
Heart failure hospitalization	207	286	0.68 (0.57–0.81)	<0.001

Table 2. CHARM — Added: Primary Endpoint and its Components

Endpoint (time to first event)	ATACAND (n=1276)	Placebo (n=1272)	Hazard Ratio (95% CI)	p-value (logrank)
CV death or heart failure hospitalization	483	538	0.85 (0.75–0.96)	0.011
CV death	302	347	0.84 (0.72–0.98)	0.029
Heart failure hospitalization	309	356	0.83 (0.71–0.96)	0.014

(17%). The mean daily dose of ATACAND was approximately 24 mg and 61% of subjects on treatment received 32 mg once daily.

After a median follow-up of 41 months, there was a 15% reduction in the risk of cardiovascular death or heart failure hospitalization on ATACAND (p=0.011), with both components contributing to the overall effect (Table 2). There was no evident relationship between dose of ACE inhibitor and the benefit of ATACAND.

[See table 2 above]

In these two studies, the benefit of ATACAND in reducing the risk of CV death or heart failure hospitalization (18% p<0.001) was evident in major subgroups (see Figure), and in patients on other combinations of cardiovascular and heart failure treatments, including ACE inhibitors and beta-blockers.

Figure. CV Death or Heart Failure Hospitalization in Subgroups – LV Systolic Dysfunction Trials

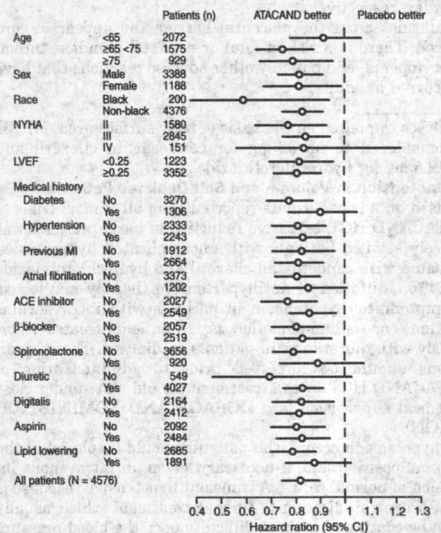

16   HOW SUPPLIED/STORAGE AND HANDLING

No. 3782—Tablets ATACAND, 4 mg, are white to off-white, circular/biconvex-shaped, non-film-coated scored tablets, coded ACF on one side and 004 on the other. They are supplied as follows:
NDC 0186-0004-31 unit of use bottles of 30.
No. 3780—Tablets ATACAND, 8 mg, are light pink, circular/biconvex-shaped, non-film-coated scored tablets, coded ACG on one side and 008 on the other. They are supplied as follows:
NDC 0186-0008-31 unit of use bottles of 30.
No. 3781—Tablets ATACAND, 16 mg, are pink, circular/biconvex-shaped, non-film-coated scored tablets, coded ACH on one side and 016 on the other. They are supplied as follows:
NDC 0186-0016-31 unit of use bottles of 30
NDC 0186-0016-54 unit of use bottles of 90
NDC 0186-0016-28 unit dose packages of 100.
No. 3791—Tablets ATACAND, 32 mg, are pink, circular/biconvex-shaped, non-film-coated scored tablets, coded ACL on one side and 032 on the other. They are supplied as follows:
NDC 0186-0032-31 unit of use bottles of 30
NDC 0186-0032-54 unit of use bottles of 90
NDC 0186-0032-28 unit dose packages of 100.
Storage
Store at 25°C (77°F); excursions permitted to 15-30°C (59-86°F) [see USP Controlled Room Temperature]. Keep container tightly closed.

17   PATIENT COUNSELING INFORMATION

Pregnancy—Female patients of childbearing age should be told about the consequences of second- and third-trimester exposure to drugs that act on the renin-angiotensin system, and they should also be told that these consequences do not appear to have resulted from intrauterine drug exposure that has been limited to the first trimester. These patients should be asked to report pregnancies to their physicians as soon as possible.

Post-menarche adolescents should be questioned on a regular basis as to changes in menstrual pattern and the possibility of pregnancy.

Manufactured under the license
from Takeda Pharmaceutical Company, Ltd.
by: AstraZeneca AB, S-151 85 Södertälje, Sweden
for: AstraZeneca LP, Wilmington, DE 19850
Made in Sweden
Rev. 10/09
ATACAND is a trademark of the AstraZeneca group of companies.
©AstraZeneca 2009
Shown in Product Identification Guide, page 321

ATACAND HCT®   ℞
[ăt ă-kănd]
(candesartan cilexetil-hydrochlorothiazide)
Tablets

USE IN PREGNANCY
When used in pregnancy during the second and third trimesters, drugs that act directly on the renin-angiotensin system can cause injury and even death to the developing fetus. When pregnancy is detected, ATACAND HCT should be discontinued as soon as possible. See **WARNINGS, Fetal/Neonatal Morbidity and Mortality.**

DESCRIPTION

ATACAND HCT (candesartan cilexetil-hydrochlorothiazide) combines an angiotensin II receptor (type AT_1) antagonist and a diuretic, hydrochlorothiazide.

Candesartan cilexetil, a nonpeptide, is chemically described as (±)-1-Hydroxyethyl 2-ethoxy-1-[p-(o-1H-tetrazol-5-ylphenyl)benzyl]-7-benzimidazolecarboxylate, cyclohexyl carbonate (ester).

Its empirical formula is $C_{33}H_{34}N_6O_6$, and its structural formula is

↓ site of ester hydrolysis.

Candesartan cilexetil is a white to off-white powder with a molecular weight of 610.67. It is practically insoluble in water and sparingly soluble in methanol. Candesartan cilexetil is a racemic mixture containing one chiral center at the cyclohexyloxycarbonyloxy ethyl ester group. Following oral administration, candesartan cilexetil undergoes hydrolysis at the ester link to form the active drug, candesartan, which is achiral.

Hydrochlorothiazide is 6-chloro-3,4-dihydro-2H-1,2,4-benzothiadiazine-7-sulfonamide 1,1-dioxide. Its empirical formula is $C_7H_8ClN_3O_4S_2$ and its structural formula is

Hydrochlorothiazide is a white, or practically white, crystalline powder with a molecular weight of 297.72, which is slightly soluble in water, but freely soluble in sodium hydroxide solution.

ATACAND HCT is available for oral administration in three tablet strengths of candesartan cilexetil and hydrochlorothiazide.

ATACAND HCT 16-12.5 contains 16 mg of candesartan cilexetil and 12.5 mg of hydrochlorothiazide. ATACAND HCT 32-12.5 contains 32 mg of candesartan cilexetil and 12.5 mg of hydrochlorothiazide. ATACAND HCT 32-25 contains 32 mg of candesartan cilexetil and 25 mg of hydrochlorothiazide. The inactive ingredients of the tablets are carboxymethylcellulose calcium, hydroxypropyl cellulose, lactose monohydrate, magnesium stearate, corn starch, polyethylene glycol 8000, and ferric oxide (yellow). Ferric oxide (reddish brown) is also added to the 16-12.5 mg and 32-25 mg tablets as colorant.

CLINICAL PHARMACOLOGY
Mechanism of Action

Angiotensin II is formed from angiotensin I in a reaction catalyzed by angiotensin-converting enzyme (ACE, kininase II). Angiotensin II is the principal pressor agent of the renin-angiotensin system, with effects that include vasoconstriction, stimulation of synthesis and release of aldosterone, cardiac stimulation, and renal reabsorption of sodium. Candesartan blocks the vasoconstrictor and aldosterone-secreting effects of angiotensin II by selectively blocking the binding of angiotensin II to the AT_1 receptor in many tissues, such as vascular smooth muscle and the adrenal gland. Its action is, therefore, independent of the pathways for angiotensin II synthesis.

There is also an AT_2 receptor found in many tissues, but AT_2 is not known to be associated with cardiovascular homeostasis. Candesartan has much greater affinity (>10,000-fold) for the AT_1 receptor than for the AT_2 receptor.

Blockade of the renin-angiotensin system with ACE inhibitors, which inhibit the biosynthesis of angiotensin II from angiotensin I, is widely used in the treatment of hypertension. ACE inhibitors also inhibit the degradation of bradykinin, a reaction also catalyzed by ACE. Because candesartan does not inhibit ACE (kininase II), it does not affect the response to bradykinin. Whether this difference has clinical relevance is not yet known. Candesartan does not bind to or block other hormone receptors or ion channels known to be important in cardiovascular regulation.

Blockade of the angiotensin II receptor inhibits the negative regulatory feedback of angiotensin II on renin secretion, but the resulting increased plasma renin activity and angiotensin II circulating levels do not overcome the effect of candesartan on blood pressure.

Hydrochlorothiazide is a thiazide diuretic. Thiazides affect the renal tubular mechanisms of electrolyte reabsorption, directly increasing excretion of sodium and chloride in approximately equivalent amounts. Indirectly, the diuretic action of hydrochlorothiazide reduces plasma volume, with consequent increases in plasma renin activity, increases in aldosterone secretion, increases in urinary potassium loss, and decreases in serum potassium. The renin-aldosterone link is mediated by angiotensin II, so coadministration of an angiotensin II receptor antagonist tends to reverse the potassium loss associated with these diuretics.

The mechanism of the antihypertensive effect of thiazides is unknown.

Pharmacokinetics
General
Candesartan Cilexetil

Candesartan cilexetil is rapidly and completely bioactivated by ester hydrolysis during absorption from the gastrointestinal tract to candesartan, a selective AT_1 subtype angiotensin II receptor antagonist. Candesartan is mainly excreted unchanged in urine and feces (via bile). It undergoes minor hepatic metabolism by O-deethylation to an inactive metabolite. The elimination half-life of candesartan is approximately 9 hours. After single and repeated administration, the pharmacokinetics of candesartan are linear for oral doses up to 32 mg of candesartan cilexetil. Candesartan and its inactive metabolite do not accumulate in serum upon repeated once-daily dosing.

Following administration of candesartan cilexetil, the absolute bioavailability of candesartan was estimated to be 15%. After tablet ingestion, the peak serum concentration (C_{max}) is reached after 3 to 4 hours. Food with a high fat content does not affect the bioavailability of candesartan after candesartan cilexetil administration.

Hydrochlorothiazide
When plasma levels have been followed for at least 24 hours, the plasma half-life has been observed to vary between 5.6 and 14.8 hours.

Metabolism and Excretion
Candesartan Cilexetil

Total plasma clearance of candesartan is 0.37 mL/min/kg, with a renal clearance of 0.19 mL/min/kg. When candesartan is administered orally, about 26% of the dose is excreted unchanged in urine. Following an oral dose of ^{14}C-labeled candesartan cilexetil, approximately 33% of radioactivity is recovered in urine and approximately 67% in feces. Following an intravenous dose of ^{14}C-labeled candesartan, approximately 59% of radioactivity is recovered in urine and approximately 36% in feces. Biliary excretion contributes to the elimination of candesartan.

Hydrochlorothiazide
Hydrochlorothiazide is not metabolized but is eliminated rapidly by the kidney. At least 61% of the oral dose is eliminated unchanged within 24 hours.

Distribution

Candesartan Cilexetil

The volume of distribution of candesartan is 0.13 L/kg. Candesartan is highly bound to plasma proteins (>99%) and does not penetrate red blood cells. The protein binding is constant at candesartan plasma concentrations well above the range achieved with recommended doses. In rats, it has been demonstrated that candesartan crosses the blood-brain barrier poorly, if at all. It has also been demonstrated in rats that candesartan passes across the placental barrier and is distributed in the fetus.

Hydrochlorothiazide

Hydrochlorothiazide crosses the placental but not the blood-brain barrier and is excreted in breast milk.

Special Populations

Pediatric

The pharmacokinetics of candesartan cilexetil have not been investigated in patients <18 years of age.

Geriatric

The pharmacokinetics of candesartan have been studied in the elderly ($\geq$ 65 years). The plasma concentration of candesartan was higher in the elderly (C_{max} was approximately 50% higher, and AUC was approximately 80% higher) compared to younger subjects administered the same dose. The pharmacokinetics of candesartan were linear in the elderly, and candesartan and its inactive metabolite did not accumulate in the serum of these subjects upon repeated, once-daily administration. No initial dosage adjustment is necessary. (See **DOSAGE AND ADMINISTRATION**.)

Gender

There is no difference in the pharmacokinetics of candesartan between male and female subjects.

Renal Insufficiency

In hypertensive patients with renal insufficiency, serum concentrations of candesartan were elevated. After repeated dosing, the AUC and C_{max} were approximately doubled in patients with severe renal impairment (creatinine clearance <30 mL/min/1.73m²) compared to patients with normal kidney function. The pharmacokinetics of candesartan in hypertensive patients undergoing hemodialysis are similar to those in hypertensive patients with severe renal impairment. Candesartan cannot be removed by hemodialysis. No initial dosage adjustment is necessary in patients with renal insufficiency.

Thiazide diuretics are eliminated by the kidney, with a terminal half-life of 5-15 hours. In a study of patients with impaired renal function (mean creatinine clearance of 19 mL/min), the half-life of hydrochlorothiazide elimination was lengthened to 21 hours. (See **DOSAGE AND ADMINISTRATION**.)

Hepatic Insufficiency

The pharmacokinetics of candesartan were compared in patients with mild (Child-Pugh A) or moderate (Child-Pugh B) hepatic impairment to matched healthy volunteers following a single dose of 16 mg candesartan cilexetil. The AUC for candesartan in patients with mild and moderate hepatic impairment was increased 30% and 145% respectively. The C_{max} for candesartan was increased 56% and 73% respectively. The pharmacokinetics of candesartan in severe hepatic impairment have not been studied. No dose adjustment is recommended for patients with mild hepatic impairment. In patients with moderate hepatic impairment, consideration should be given to initiation of ATACAND at a lower dose, such as 8 mg. If a lower starting dose is selected for candesartan cilexetil, ATACAND HCT is not recommended for initial titration because the appropriate initial starting dose of candesartan cilexetil cannot be given. (See **DOSAGE AND ADMINISTRATION**).

Thiazide diuretics should be used with caution in patients with hepatic impairment. (See **DOSAGE AND ADMINISTRATION**.)

Pharmacodynamics

Candesartan Cilexetil

Candesartan inhibits the pressor effects of angiotensin II infusion in a dose-dependent manner. After 1 week of once-daily dosing with 8 mg of candesartan cilexetil, the pressor effect was inhibited by approximately 90% at peak with approximately 50% inhibition persisting for 24 hours.

Plasma concentrations of angiotensin I and angiotensin II, and plasma renin activity (PRA), increased in a dose-dependent manner after single and repeated administration of candesartan cilexetil to healthy subjects and hypertensive patients. ACE activity was not altered in healthy subjects after repeated candesartan cilexetil administration. The once-daily administration of up to 16 mg of candesartan cilexetil to healthy subjects did not influence plasma aldosterone concentrations, but a decrease in the plasma concentration of aldosterone was observed when 32 mg of candesartan cilexetil was administered to hypertensive patients. In spite of the effect of candesartan cilexetil on aldosterone secretion, very little effect on serum potassium was observed.

In multiple-dose studies with hypertensive patients, there were no clinically significant changes in metabolic function including serum levels of total cholesterol, triglycerides, glucose, or uric acid. In a 12-week study of 161 patients with non-insulin-dependent (type 2) diabetes mellitus and hypertension, there was no change in the level of HbA_{1c}.

Hydrochlorothiazide

After oral administration of hydrochlorothiazide, diuresis begins within 2 hours, peaks in about 4 hours and lasts about 6 to 12 hours.

Clinical Trials

Candesartan Cilexetil-Hydrochlorothiazide

Of 12 controlled clinical trials involving 4588 patients, 5 were double-blind, placebo controlled and evaluated the antihypertensive effects of single entities vs the combination. These 5 trials, of 8 to 12 weeks duration, randomized 3037 hypertensive patients. Doses ranged from 2 to 32 mg candesartan cilexetil and from 6.25 to 25 mg hydrochlorothiazide administered once daily in various combinations.

The combination of candesartan cilexetil-hydrochlorothiazide resulted in placebo-adjusted decreases in sitting systolic and diastolic blood pressures of 14-18/8-11 mm Hg at doses of 16-12.5 mg and 32-12.5 mg. The combination of candesartan cilexetil and hydrochlorothiazide 32-25 mg resulted in placebo-adjusted decreases in sitting systolic and diastolic blood pressures of 16-19/9-11 mm Hg. The placebo corrected trough to peak ratio was evaluated in a study of candesartan cilexetil-hydrochlorothiazide 32-12.5 mg and was 88%.

Most of the antihypertensive effect of the combination of candesartan cilexetil and hydrochlorothiazide was seen in 1 to 2 weeks with the full effect observed within 4 weeks. In long-term studies of up to 1 year, the blood pressure lowering effect of the combination was maintained. The antihypertensive effect was similar regardless of age or gender, and overall response to the combination was similar in black and non-black patients. No appreciable changes in heart rate were observed with combination therapy in controlled trials.

INDICATIONS AND USAGE

ATACAND HCT is indicated for the treatment of hypertension. This fixed dose combination is not indicated for initial therapy (see **DOSAGE AND ADMINISTRATION**).

CONTRAINDICATIONS

ATACAND HCT is contraindicated in patients who are hypersensitive to any component of this product.

Because of the hydrochlorothiazide component, this product is contraindicated in patients with anuria or hypersensitivity to other sulfonamide-derived drugs.

WARNINGS

Fetal/Neonatal Morbidity and Mortality

Drugs that act directly on the renin-angiotensin system can cause fetal and neonatal morbidity and death when administered to pregnant women. Several dozen cases have been reported in the world literature in patients who were taking angiotensin-converting enzyme inhibitors. Post-marketing experience has identified reports of fetal and neonatal toxicity in babies born to women treated with candesartan cilexetil during pregnancy. Because candesartan cilexetil is a component of ATACAND HCT, when pregnancy is detected, ATACAND HCT should be discontinued as soon as possible.

The use of drugs that act directly on the renin-angiotensin system during the second and third trimesters of pregnancy has been associated with fetal and neonatal injury, including hypotension, neonatal skull hypoplasia, anuria, reversible or irreversible renal failure, and death. Oligohydramnios has also been reported, presumably resulting from decreased fetal renal function; oligohydramnios in this setting has been associated with fetal limb contractures, craniofacial deformation, and hypoplastic lung development. Prematurity, intrauterine growth retardation, and patent ductus arteriosus have also been reported, although it is not clear whether these occurrences were due to exposure to the drug.

These adverse effects do not appear to have resulted from intrauterine drug exposure that has been limited to the first trimester. Mothers whose embryos and fetuses are exposed to an angiotensin II receptor antagonist only during the first trimester should be so informed. Nonetheless, when patients become pregnant, physicians should have the patient discontinue the use of ATACAND HCT as soon as possible.

Rarely (probably less often than once in every thousand pregnancies), no alternative to a drug acting on the renin-angiotensin system will be found. In these rare cases, the mothers should be apprised of the potential hazards to their fetuses, and serial ultrasound examinations should be performed to assess the intra-amniotic environment.

If oligohydramnios is observed, ATACAND HCT should be discontinued unless it is considered life saving for the mother. Contraction stress testing (CST), a nonstress test (NST), or biophysical profiling (BPP) may be appropriate, depending upon the week of pregnancy. Patients and physicians should be aware, however, that oligohydramnios may not appear until after the fetus has sustained irreversible injury.

Infants with histories of *in utero* exposure to an angiotensin II receptor antagonist should be closely observed for hypotension, oliguria, and hyperkalemia. If oliguria occurs, attention should be directed toward support of blood pressure and renal perfusion. Exchange transfusion or dialysis may be required as means of reversing hypotension and/or substituting for disordered renal function.

Candesartan Cilexetil-Hydrochlorothiazide

There was no evidence of teratogenicity or other adverse effects on embryo-fetal development when pregnant mice, rats or rabbits were treated orally with candesartan cilexetil alone or in combination with hydrochlorothiazide. For mice, the maximum dose of candesartan cilexetil was 1000 mg/kg/day (about 150 times the maximum recommended daily human dose [MRHD][1]). For rats, the maximum dose of candesartan cilexetil was 100 mg/kg/day (about 31 times the MRHD[1]). For rabbits, the maximum dose of candesartan cilexetil was 1 mg/kg/day (a maternally toxic dose that is about half the MRHD[1]). In each of these studies, hydrochlorothiazide was tested at the same dose level (10 mg/kg/day, about 4, 8, and 15 times the MRHD[1] in mouse, rats, and rabbit, respectively). There was no evidence of harm to the rat or mouse fetus or embryo in studies in which hydrochlorothiazide was administered alone to the pregnant rat or mouse at doses of up to 1000 and 3000 mg/kg/day, respectively.

Thiazides cross the placental barrier and appear in cord blood. There is a risk of fetal or neonatal jaundice, thrombocytopenia, and possibly other adverse reactions that have occurred in adults.

---

[1] Doses compared on the basis of body surface area. MRHD considered to be 32 mg for candesartan cilexetil and 12.5 mg for hydrochlorothiazide.

Hypotension in Volume- and Salt-Depleted Patients

Based on adverse events reported from all clinical trials of ATACAND HCT, excessive reduction of blood pressure was rarely seen in patients with uncomplicated hypertension treated with candesartan cilexetil and hydrochlorothiazide (0.4%). Initiation of antihypertensive therapy may cause symptomatic hypotension in patients with intravascular volume- or sodium-depletion, eg, in patients treated vigorously with diuretics or in patients on dialysis. These conditions should be corrected prior to administration of ATACAND HCT, or the treatment should start under close medical supervision (see **DOSAGE AND ADMINISTRATION**).

If hypotension occurs, the patients should be placed in the supine position and, if necessary, given an intravenous infusion of normal saline. A transient hypotensive response is not a contraindication to further treatment which usually can be continued without difficulty once the blood pressure has stabilized.

Hydrochlorothiazide

Impaired Hepatic Function

Thiazide diuretics should be used with caution in patients with impaired hepatic function or progressive liver disease, since minor alterations of fluid and electrolyte balance may precipitate hepatic coma.

Hypersensitivity Reaction

Hypersensitivity reactions to hydrochlorothiazide may occur in patients with or without a history of allergy or bronchial asthma, but are more likely in patients with such a history.

Systemic Lupus Erythematosus

Thiazide diuretics have been reported to cause exacerbation or activation of systemic lupus erythematosus.

Lithium Interaction

Lithium generally should not be given with thiazides (see **PRECAUTIONS, Drug Interactions, Hydrochlorothiazide, Lithium**).

PRECAUTIONS

General

Candesartan Cilexetil-Hydrochlorothiazide

In clinical trials of various doses of candesartan cilexetil and hydrochlorothiazide, the incidence of hypertensive patients who developed hypokalemia (serum potassium <3.5 mEq/L) was 2.5% versus 2.1% for placebo; the incidence of hyperkalemia (serum potassium >5.7 mEq/L) was 0.4% versus 1.0% for placebo. No patient receiving ATACAND HCT 16-12.5 mg or 32-12.5 mg was discontinued due to increases or decreases in serum potassium. Overall, the combination of candesartan cilexetil and hydrochlorothiazide had no clinically significant effect on serum potassium.

Candesartan

Major Surgery/Anesthesia - Hypotension may occur during major surgery and anesthesia in patients treated with angiotensin II receptor antagonists, including candesartan, due to blockade of the renin-angiotensin system. Very rarely, hypotension may be severe such that it may warrant the use of intravenous fluids and/or vasopressors.

Hydrochlorothiazide
Periodic determination of serum electrolytes to detect possible electrolyte imbalance should be performed at appropriate intervals.

All patients receiving thiazide therapy should be observed for clinical signs of fluid or electrolyte imbalance: namely, hyponatremia, hypochloremic alkalosis, and hypokalemia. Serum and urine electrolyte determinations are particularly important when the patient is vomiting excessively or receiving parenteral fluids. Warning signs or symptoms of fluid and electrolyte imbalance, irrespective of cause, include dryness of mouth, thirst, weakness, lethargy, drowsiness, restlessness, confusion, seizures, muscle pains or cramps, muscular fatigue, hypotension, oliguria, tachycardia, and gastrointestinal disturbances such as nausea and vomiting.

Hypokalemia may develop, especially with brisk diuresis, when severe cirrhosis is present, or after prolonged therapy. Interference with adequate oral electrolyte intake will also contribute to hypokalemia. Hypokalemia may cause cardiac arrhythmia and may also sensitize or exaggerate the response of the heart to the toxic effects of digitalis (eg, increased ventricular irritability).

Although any chloride deficit is generally mild and usually does not require specific treatment, except under extraordinary circumstances (as in liver disease or renal disease), chloride replacement may be required in the treatment of metabolic alkalosis.

Dilutional hyponatremia may occur in edematous patients in hot weather; appropriate therapy is water restriction, rather than administration of salt, except in rare instances when the hyponatremia is life-threatening. In actual salt depletion, appropriate replacement is the therapy of choice. Hyperuricemia may occur or acute gout may be precipitated in certain patients receiving thiazide therapy.

In diabetic patients dosage adjustments of insulin or oral hypoglycemic agents may be required. Hyperglycemia may occur with thiazide diuretics. Thus latent diabetes mellitus may become manifest during thiazide therapy.

The antihypertensive effects of the drug may be enhanced in the post-sympathectomy patient.

If progressive renal impairment becomes evident consider withholding or discontinuing diuretic therapy.

Thiazides have been shown to increase the urinary excretion of magnesium; this may result in hypomagnesemia.

Thiazides may decrease urinary calcium excretion. Thiazides may cause intermittent and slight elevation of serum calcium in the absence of known disorders of calcium metabolism. Marked hypercalcemia may be evidence of hidden hyperparathyroidism. Thiazides should be discontinued before carrying out tests for parathyroid function.

Increases in cholesterol and triglyceride levels may be associated with thiazide diuretic therapy.

Impaired Renal Function
Candesartan Cilexetil
As a consequence of inhibiting the renin-angiotensin-aldosterone system, changes in renal function may be anticipated in susceptible individuals treated with candesartan cilexetil. In patients whose renal function may depend upon the activity of the renin-angiotensin-aldosterone system (eg, patients with severe congestive heart failure), treatment with angiotensin-converting enzyme inhibitors and angiotensin receptor antagonists has been associated with oliguria and/or progressive azotemia and (rarely) with acute renal failure and/or death. Similar results may be anticipated in patients treated with candesartan cilexetil. (See **CLINICAL PHARMACOLOGY, Special Populations.**)

In studies of ACE inhibitors in patients with unilateral or bilateral renal artery stenosis, increases in serum creatinine or blood urea nitrogen (BUN) have been reported. There has been no long-term use of candesartan cilexetil in patients with unilateral or bilateral renal artery stenosis, but similar results may be expected.

Hydrochlorothiazide
Thiazides should be used with caution in severe renal disease. In patients with renal disease, thiazides may precipitate azotemia. Cumulative effects of the drug may develop in patients with impaired renal function.

Impaired Hepatic Function
Candesartan Cilexetil
Based on pharmacokinetic data significant increases in candesartan AUC and C_{max} in patients with moderate hepatic impairment have been demonstrated. (See **CLINICAL PHARMACOLOGY, Special Populations.**)

Information for Patients
Pregnancy
Female patients of childbearing age should be told about the consequences of second- and third-trimester exposure to drugs that act on the renin-angiotensin system, and they should also be told that these consequences do not appear to

have resulted from intrauterine drug exposure that has been limited to the first trimester. These patients should be asked to report pregnancies to their physicians as soon as possible.

Symptomatic Hypotension
A patient receiving ATACAND HCT should be cautioned that lightheadedness can occur, especially during the first days of therapy, and that it should be reported to the prescribing physician. The patients should be told that if syncope occurs, ATACAND HCT should be discontinued until the physician has been consulted.

All patients should be cautioned that inadequate fluid intake, excessive perspiration, diarrhea, or vomiting can lead to an excessive fall in blood pressure, with the same consequences of lightheadedness and possible syncope.

Potassium Supplements
A patient receiving ATACAND HCT should be told not to use potassium supplements or salt substitutes containing potassium without consulting the prescribing physician.

Drug Interactions
Candesartan Cilexetil
No significant drug interactions have been reported in studies of candesartan cilexetil given with other drugs such as glyburide, nifedipine, digoxin, warfarin, hydrochlorothiazide, and oral contraceptives in healthy volunteers. Because candesartan is not significantly metabolized by the cytochrome P450 system and at therapeutic concentrations has no effects on P450 enzymes, interactions with drugs that inhibit or are metabolized by those enzymes would not be expected.

Lithium - Reversible increases in serum lithium concentrations and toxicity have been reported during concomitant administration of lithium with ACE inhibitors, and with some angiotensin II receptor antagonists. An increase in serum lithium concentration has been reported during concomitant administration of lithium with candesartan cilexetil, so careful monitoring of serum lithium levels is recommended during concomitant use.

Hydrochlorothiazide
When administered concurrently the following drugs may interact with thiazide diuretics:

Alcohol, barbiturates, or narcotics - Potentiation of orthostatic hypotension may occur.

Antidiabetic drugs (oral agents and insulin) - Dosage adjustment of the antidiabetic drug may be required.

Other antihypertensive drugs - Additive effect or potentiation.

Cholestyramine and colestipol resins - Absorption of hydrochlorothiazide is impaired in the presence of anionic exchange resins. Single doses of either cholestyramine or colestipol resins bind the hydrochlorothiazide and reduce its absorption from the gastrointestinal tract by up to 85 and 43 percent, respectively.

Corticosteroids, ACTH—Intensified electrolyte depletion, particularly hypokalemia.

Pressor amines (eg, norepinephrine)—Possible decreased response to pressor amines but not sufficient to preclude their use.

Skeletal muscle relaxants, nondepolarizing (eg, tubocurarine)—Possible increased responsiveness to the muscle relaxant.

Lithium - Generally should not be given with diuretics. Diuretic agents reduce the renal clearance of lithium and add a high risk of lithium toxicity. Refer to the package insert for lithium preparations before use of such preparations with ATACAND HCT.

Non-steroidal Anti-inflammatory Drugs - In some patients, the administration of a non-steroidal anti-inflammatory agent can reduce the diuretic, natriuretic, and antihypertensive effects of loop, potassium-sparing and thiazide diuretics. Therefore, when ATACAND HCT and non-steroidal anti-inflammatory agents are used concomitantly, the patient should be observed closely to determine if the desired effect of the diuretic is obtained.

Carcinogenesis, Mutagenesis, Impairment of Fertility
No carcinogenicity studies have been conducted with the combination of candesartan cilexetil and hydrochlorothiazide. There was no evidence of carcinogenicity when candesartan cilexetil was orally administered to mice and rats for up to 104 weeks at doses up to 100 and 1000 mg/kg/day, respectively. Rats received the drug by gavage whereas mice received the drug by dietary administration. These (maximally-tolerated) doses of candesartan cilexetil provided systemic exposures to candesartan (AUCs) that were, in mice, approximately 7 times and, in rats, more than 70 times the exposure in man at the maximum recommended daily human dose (32 mg). Two-year feeding studies in mice and rats conducted under the auspices of the National Toxicology Program (NTP) uncovered no evidence of a carcinogenic potential of hydrochlorothiazide in female mice (at doses of up to approximately 600 mg/kg/day) or in male and female rats (at

doses of up to approximately 100 mg/kg/day). The NTP, however, found equivocal evidence for hepatocarcinogenicity in male mice.

Candesartan cilexetil or candesartan (the active metabolite), in combination with hydrochlorothiazide, tested positive *in vitro* in the Chinese hamster lung (CHL) chromosomal aberration assay and mouse lymphoma mutagenicity assay. The candesartan cilexetil/hydrochlorothiazide combination tested negative for mutagenicity in bacteria (Ames test), for unscheduled DNA synthesis in rat liver, for chromosomal aberrations in rat bone marrow and for micronuclei in mouse bone marrow.

Both candesartan and its O-deethyl metabolite tested positive for genotoxicity in the *in vitro* CHL chromosomal aberration assay. Neither compound tested positive in the Ames microbial mutagenesis assay or in the *in vitro* mouse lymphoma cell assay. Candesartan (but not its O-deethyl metabolite) was also evaluated *in vivo* in the mouse micronucleus test and *in vitro* in the Chinese hamster ovary (CHO) gene mutation assay, in both cases with negative results. Candesartan cilexetil was evaluated in the Ames test, the *in vitro* mouse lymphoma cell assay, the *in vivo* rat hepatocyte unscheduled DNA synthesis assay and the *in vivo* mouse micronucleus test, in each case with negative results. Candesartan cilexetil was not evaluated in the CHL chromosomal aberration or CHO gene mutation assays.

When hydrochlorothiazide was tested alone, positive results were obtained *in vitro* in the CHO sister chromatid exchange (clastogenicity) and mouse lymphoma cell (mutagenicity) assays and in the *Aspergillus nidulans* nondisjunciton assay. Hydrochlorothiazide was not genotoxic *in vitro* in the Ames test for point mutations and the CHO test for chromosomal aberrations, or *in vivo* in assays using mouse germinal cell chromosomes, Chinese hamster bone marrow chromosomes, and the Drosophila sex-linked recessive lethal trait gene.

No fertility studies have been conducted with the combination of candesartan cilexetil and hydrochlorothiazide. Fertility and reproductive performance were not affected in studies with male and female rats given oral doses of up to 300 mg candesartan cilexetil/kg/day (83 times the maximum daily human dose of 32 mg on a body surface area basis). Hydrochlorothiazide had no adverse effects on the fertility of mice and rats of either sex in studies wherein these species were exposed, via their diet, to doses of up to 100 and 4 mg/kg, respectively, prior to conception and throughout gestation.

Pregnancy
Pregnancy Categories C (first trimester) *and D* (second and third trimesters). See **WARNINGS, Fetal/Neonatal Morbidity and Mortality.**

Nursing Mothers
It is not known whether candesartan is excreted in human milk, but candesartan has been shown to be present in rat milk. Thiazides appear in human milk. Because of the potential for adverse effects on the nursing infant, a decision should be made whether to discontinue nursing or discontinue the drug, taking into account the importance of the drug to the mother.

Pediatric Use
Safety and effectiveness in pediatric patients have not been established.

Geriatric Use
Of the total number of subjects in all clinical studies of ATACAND HCT (2831), 611 (22%) were 65 and over, while 94 (3%) were 75 and over. No overall differences in safety or effectiveness were observed between these subjects and younger subjects. Other reported clinical experience has not identified differences in responses between the elderly and younger patients, but greater sensitivity of some older individuals cannot be ruled out.

Hydrochlorothiazide is known to be substantially excreted by the kidney, and the risk of toxic reactions to this drug may be greater in patients with impaired renal function.

ADVERSE REACTIONS
Candesartan Cilexetil-Hydrochlorothiazide
ATACAND HCT has been evaluated for safety in more than 2800 patients treated for hypertension. More than 750 of these patients were studied for at least six months and more than 500 patients were treated for at least one year. Adverse experiences have generally been mild and transient in nature and have only infrequently required discontinuation of therapy. The overall incidence of adverse events reported with ATACAND HCT was comparable to placebo. The overall frequency of adverse experiences was not related to dose, age, gender, or race.

In placebo-controlled trials that included 1089 patients treated with various combinations of candesartan cilexetil (doses of 2-32 mg) and hydrochlorothiazide (doses of 6.25-25 mg) and 592 patients treated with placebo, adverse events, whether or not attributed to treatment, occurring in greater than 2% of patients treated with ATACAND HCT and that were more frequent for ATACAND HCT than placebo were: ***Respiratory System Disorder:*** upper respiratory tract infection (3.6% vs 3.0%); ***Body as a Whole:*** back pain (3.3% vs 2.4%); influenza-like symptoms (2.5% vs 1.9%); ***Central/Peripheral Nervous System:*** dizziness (2.9% vs 1.2%).

The frequency of headache was greater than 2% (2.9%) in patients treated with ATACAND HCT but was less frequent than the rate in patients treated with placebo (5.2%).

Other adverse events that have been reported, whether or not attributed to treatment, with an incidence of 0.5% or greater from the more than 2800 patients worldwide treated with ATACAND HCT included: ***Body as a Whole:*** inflicted injury, fatigue, pain, chest pain, peripheral edema, asthenia; ***Central and Peripheral Nervous System:*** vertigo, paresthesia, hypesthesia; ***Respiratory System Disorders:*** bronchitis, sinusitis, pharyngitis, coughing, rhinitis, dyspnea; ***Musculoskeletal System Disorders:*** arthralgia, myalgia, arthrosis, arthritis, leg cramps, sciatica; ***Gastrointestinal System Disorders:*** nausea, abdominal pain, diarrhea, dyspepsia, gastritis, gastroenteritis, vomiting; ***Metabolic and Nutritional Disorders:*** hyperuricemia, hyperglycemia, hypokalemia, increased BUN, creatine phosphokinase increased; ***Urinary System Disorders:*** urinary tract infection, hematuria, cystitis; ***Liver/Biliary System Disorders:*** hepatic function abnormal, increased transaminase levels; ***Heart Rate and Rhythm Disorders:*** tachycardia, palpitation, extrasystoles, bradycardia; ***Psychiatric Disorders:*** depression, insomnia, anxiety; ***Cardiovascular Disorders:*** ECG abnormal; ***Skin and Appendages Disorders:*** eczema, sweating increased, pruritus, dermatitis, rash; ***Platelet/Bleeding-Clotting Disorders:*** epistaxis; ***Resistance Mechanism Disorders:*** infection, viral infection; ***Vision Disorders:*** conjunctivitis; ***Hearing and Vestibular Disorders:*** tinnitus.

Reported events seen less frequently than 0.5% included angina pectoris, myocardial infarction and angioedema.

Candesartan Cilexetil

Other adverse experiences that have been reported with candesartan cilexetil, without regard to causality, were: ***Body as a Whole:*** fever; ***Metabolic and Nutritional Disorders:*** hypertriglyceridemia; ***Psychiatric Disorders:*** somnolence; ***Urinary System Disorders:*** albuminuria.

Post-Marketing Experience

The following have been very rarely reported in post-marketing experience with candesartan cilexetil:

Digestive: Abnormal hepatic function and hepatitis.

Hematologic: Neutropenia, leukopenia, and agranulocytosis.

Metabolic and Nutritional Disorders: hyperkalemia, hyponatremia.

Renal: renal impairment, renal failure.

Skin and Appendages Disorders: Pruritus and urticaria.

Rare reports of rhabdomyolysis have been reported in patients receiving angiotensin II receptor blockers.

Hydrochlorothiazide

Other adverse experiences that have been reported with hydrochlorothiazide, without regard to causality, are listed below:

Body As A Whole: weakness; ***Cardiovascular:*** hypotension including orthostatic hypotension (may be aggravated by alcohol, barbiturates, narcotics or antihypertensive drugs); ***Digestive:*** pancreatitis, jaundice (intrahepatic cholestatic jaundice), sialadenitis, cramping, constipation, gastric irritation, anorexia; ***Hematologic:*** aplastic anemia, agranulocytosis, leukopenia, hemolytic anemia, thrombocytopenia; ***Hypersensitivity:*** anaphylactic reactions, necrotizing angiitis (vasculitis and cutaneous vasculitis), respiratory distress including pneumonitis and pulmonary edema, photosensitivity, urticaria, purpura; ***Metabolic:*** electrolyte imbalance, glycosuria; ***Musculoskeletal:*** muscle spasm; ***Nervous System/Psychiatric:*** restlessness; ***Renal:*** renal failure, renal dysfunction, interstitial nephritis; ***Skin:*** erythema multiforme including Stevens-Johnson syndrome, exfoliative dermatitis including toxic epidermal necrolysis, alopecia; ***Special Senses:*** transient blurred vision, xanthopsia; ***Urogenital:*** impotence.

Laboratory Test Findings

In controlled clinical trials, clinically important changes in standard laboratory parameters were rarely associated with the administration of ATACAND HCT.

Creatinine, Blood Urea Nitrogen—Minor increases in blood urea nitrogen (BUN) and serum creatinine were observed infrequently. One patient was discontinued from ATACAND HCT due to increased BUN. No patient was discontinued due to an increase in serum creatinine.

Hemoglobin and Hematocrit—Small decreases in hemoglobin and hematocrit (mean decreases of approximately 0.2 g/dL and 0.4 volume percent, respectively) were observed in patients treated with ATACAND HCT, but were rarely of clinical importance.

Potassium—A small decrease (mean decrease of 0.1 mEq/L) was observed in patients treated with ATACAND HCT. In placebo-controlled trials, hypokalemia was reported in 0.4% of patients treated with ATACAND HCT as compared to 1.0% of patients treated with hydrochlorothiazide or 0.2% of patients treated with placebo.

Liver Function Tests—Occasional elevations of liver enzymes and/or serum bilirubin have occurred.

OVERDOSAGE

Candesartan Cilexetil – Hydrochlorothiazide

No lethality was observed in acute toxicity studies in mice, rats and dogs given single oral doses of up to 2000 mg/kg of candesartan cilexetil or in rats given single oral doses of up to 2000 mg/kg of candesartan cilexetil in combination with 1000 mg/kg of hydrochlorothiazide. In mice given single oral doses of the primary metabolite, candesartan, the minimum lethal dose was greater than 1000 mg/kg but less than 2000 mg/kg.

Limited data are available in regard to overdosage with candesartan cilexetil in humans. The most likely manifestations of overdosage with candesartan cilexetil would be hypotension, dizziness, and tachycardia; bradycardia could occur from parasympathetic (vagal) stimulation. If symptomatic hypotension should occur, supportive treatment should be initiated. For hydrochlorothiazide, the most common signs and symptoms observed are those caused by electrolyte depletion (hypokalemia, hypochloremia, hyponatremia) and dehydration resulting from excessive diuresis. If digitalis has also been administered, hypokalemia may accentuate cardiac arrhythmias.

Candesartan cannot be removed by hemodialysis. The degree to which hydrochlorothiazide is removed by hemodialysis has not been established.

Treatment

To obtain up-to-date information about the treatment of overdose, consult your Regional Poison Control Center. Telephone numbers of certified poison control centers are listed in the *Physicians' Desk Reference (PDR)*. In managing overdose, consider the possibilities of multiple-drug overdoses, drug-drug interactions, and altered pharmacokinetics in your patient.

DOSAGE AND ADMINISTRATION

The usual recommended starting dose of candesartan cilexetil is 16 mg once daily when it is used as monotherapy in patients who are not volume depleted. ATACAND can be administered once or twice daily with total daily doses ranging from 8 mg to 32 mg. Patients requiring further reduction in blood pressure should be titrated to 32 mg. Doses larger than 32 mg do not appear to have a greater blood pressure lowering effect.

Hydrochlorothiazide is effective in doses of 12.5 to 50 mg once daily.

To minimize dose-independent side effects, it is usually appropriate to begin combination therapy only after a patient has failed to achieve the desired effect with monotherapy.

The side effects (See **WARNINGS**) of candesartan cilexetil are generally rare and apparently independent of dose; those of hydrochlorothiazide are a mixture of dose-dependent phenomena (primarily hypokalemia) and dose-independent phenomena (eg, pancreatitis), the former much more common than the latter.

Therapy with any combination of candesartan cilexetil and hydrochlorothiazide will be associated with both sets of dose-independent side effects.

Replacement Therapy: The combination may be substituted for the titrated components.

Dose Titration by Clinical Effect: A patient whose blood pressure is not controlled on 25 mg of hydrochlorothiazide once daily can expect an incremental effect from ATACAND HCT 16-12.5 mg. A patient whose blood pressure is controlled on 25 mg of hydrochlorothiazide but is experiencing decreases in serum potassium can expect the same or incremental blood pressure effects from ATACAND HCT 16-12.5 mg and serum potassium may improve.

A patient whose blood pressure is not controlled on 32 mg of ATACAND can expect incremental blood pressure effects from ATACAND HCT 32-12.5 mg and then 32-25 mg. The maximal antihypertensive effect of any dose of ATACAND HCT can be expected within 4 weeks of initiating that dose.

Patients with Renal Impairment: The usual regimens of therapy with ATACAND HCT may be followed as long as the patient's creatinine clearance is > 30 mL/min. In patients with more severe renal impairment, loop diuretics are preferred to thiazides, so ATACAND HCT is not recommended.

Patients with Hepatic Impairment: The usual regimens of therapy with ATACAND HCT may be followed in patients with mild hepatic impairment. In patients with moderate hepatic impairment, consideration should be given to initiation of ATACAND at a lower dose, such as 8 mg. If a lower starting dose is selected for candesartan cilexetil, ATACAND HCT is not recommended for initial titration because the appropriate initial starting dose of candesartan cilexetil cannot be given. (See **CLINICAL PHARMACOLOGY, Special Populations, Hepatic Insufficiency**).

Thiazide diuretics should be used with caution in patients with hepatic impairment; therefore, care should be exercised with dosing of ATACAND HCT.

ATACAND HCT may be administered with other antihypertensive agents.

ATACAND HCT may be administered with or without food.

HOW SUPPLIED

No. 3825—Tablets ATACAND HCT 16-12.5, are peach, oval, biconvex, non-film-coated tablets, scored on both sides and coded with ACS on one side. They are supplied as follows:

NDC 0186-0162-28 unit dose packages of 100.

NDC 0186-0162-54 unit of use bottles of 90.

No. 3826—Tablets ATACAND HCT 32-12.5, are yellow, oval, biconvex, non-film-coated tablets, scored on both sides and coded with ACJ on one side. They are supplied as follows:

NDC 0186-0322-28 unit dose packages of 100.

NDC 0186-0322-54 unit of use bottles of 90.

No. 3899—Tablets ATACAND HCT 32-25, are pink, oval, biconvex, non-film-coated tablets, scored on both sides and coded with ACD on one side. They are supplied as follows:

NDC 0186–0324–54 unit of use bottles of 90.

Storage:

Store at 25°C (77°F); excursions permitted to 15-30°C (59-86°F) [see USP Controlled Room Temperature]. Keep container tightly closed.

ATACAND HCT is a trademark of the AstraZeneca group of companies

©AstraZeneca 2008

Manufactured under the license from Takeda Pharmaceutical Company, Ltd.

by: AstraZeneca AB, S-151 85 Södertälje, Sweden

for: AstraZeneca LP, Wilmington, DE 19850

Made in Sweden

Shown in Product Identification Guide, page 321

Bristol-Myers Squibb Company

P.O. BOX 4500
PRINCETON, NJ 08543-4500

For Medical Information Contact:
Generally:
Bristol-Myers Squibb Medical Information Department
P.O. Box 4500
Princeton, NJ 08543-4500
(800) 321-1335 between 8:00 AM-8:00 PM EST
To report SUSPECTED ADVERSE REACTIONS, Contact Bristol-Myers Squibb Company at
(800) 721-5072
Sales and Ordering:
Orders may be placed by:
Calling your purchase orders in toll-free between
8:30 AM-5:00 PM EST:
(800) 631-5244
Mailing your purchase orders to:
Bristol-Myers Squibb U.S. Pharmaceuticals
Attn: Customer Service
P.O. Box 4500
Princeton, NJ 08543-4500
Faxing your purchase orders in:
(800) 277-0988

Product information on these pages reflects product labeling on September 1, 2010. Current information on products of Bristol-Myers Squibb may be obtained at www.bms.com or www.pdr.net

ABILIFY® ℞
[a-BIL-ĭ-fī]
(aripiprazole)
Tablets
ABILIFY DISCMELT®
(aripiprazole)
Orally Disintegrating Tablets
ABILIFY®
(aripiprazole)
Oral Solution
ABILIFY®
(aripiprazole)
Injection FOR INTRAMUSCULAR USE ONLY

HIGHLIGHTS OF PRESCRIBING INFORMATION

These highlights do not include all the information needed to use ABILIFY safely and effectively. See full prescribing information for ABILIFY.

ABILIFY® (aripiprazole) Tablets
ABILIFY DISCMELT® (aripiprazole) Orally Disintegrating Tablets
ABILIFY® (aripiprazole) Oral Solution
ABILIFY® (aripiprazole) Injection FOR INTRAMUSCULAR USE ONLY
Initial U.S. Approval: 2002

WARNINGS: INCREASED MORTALITY IN ELDERLY PATIENTS WITH DEMENTIA-RELATED PSYCHOSIS and SUICIDALITY AND ANTIDEPRESSANT DRUGS

See full prescribing information for complete boxed warning.
- **Elderly patients with dementia-related psychosis treated with antipsychotic drugs are at an increased risk of death. ABILIFY is not approved for the treatment of patients with dementia-related psychosis. (5.1)**
- **Children, adolescents, and young adults taking antidepressants for major depressive disorder (MDD) and other psychiatric disorders are at increased risk of suicidal thinking and behavior. (5.2)**

---RECENT MAJOR CHANGES---

Indications and Usage, Pediatric (6 to 17 years), Irritability Associated with Autistic Disorder (1.4)   11/2009
Dosage and Administration, Pediatric (6 to 17 years), Irritability Associated with Autistic Disorder (2.4)   11/2009
Warnings and Precautions, Leukopenia, Neutropenia, and Agranulocytosis (5.7)   07/2009

---INDICATIONS AND USAGE---

ABILIFY (aripiprazole) is an atypical antipsychotic indicated
as oral formulations for the:
Treatment of schizophrenia (1.1)
- Adults: Efficacy was established in four 4-6 week trials and one maintenance trial in patients with schizophrenia (14.1)
- Adolescents (ages 13-17): Efficacy was established in one 6-week trial in patients with schizophrenia (14.1)
Acute treatment of manic or mixed episodes associated with bipolar I disorder as monotherapy and as an adjunct to lithium or valproate (1.2)
- Adults: Efficacy was established in four 3-week monotherapy trials and one 6-week adjunctive trial in patients with manic or mixed episodes (14.2)
- Pediatric Patients (ages 10-17): Efficacy was established in one 4-week monotherapy trial in patients with manic or mixed episodes (14.2)
Maintenance treatment of bipolar I disorder (1.2)
- Adults: Efficacy was established in one maintenance trial (14.2)
Adjunctive treatment of major depressive disorder (MDD) (1.3)
- Adults: Efficacy was established in two 6-week trials in patients with MDD who had an inadequate response to antidepressant therapy during the current episode (14.3)
Treatment of irritability associated with autistic disorder (1.4)
- Pediatric Patients (ages 6-17 years): Efficacy was established in two 8-week trials in patients with autistic disorder (14.4)
as an injection for the:
Acute treatment of agitation associated with schizophrenia or bipolar I disorder (1.5)
- Adults: Efficacy was established in three 24-hour trials in agitated patients with schizophrenia or manic/mixed episodes of bipolar I disorder (14.5)

---DOSAGE AND ADMINISTRATION---

[See table above]
- Oral formulations: Administer once daily without regard to meals (2)
- IM injection: Wait at least 2 hours between doses. Maximum daily dose 30 mg (2.5)

---DOSAGE FORMS AND STRENGTHS---

- Tablets: 2 mg, 5 mg, 10 mg, 15 mg, 20 mg, and 30 mg (3)
- Orally Disintegrating Tablets: 10 mg and 15 mg (3)
- Oral Solution: 1 mg/mL (3)
- Injection: 9.75 mg/1.3 mL single-dose vial (3)

---CONTRAINDICATIONS---

Known hypersensitivity to ABILIFY (aripiprazole) (4)

---WARNINGS AND PRECAUTIONS---

- *Elderly Patients with Dementia-Related Psychosis:* Increased incidence of cerebrovascular adverse events (eg, stroke, transient ischemic attack, including fatalities) (5.1)
- *Suicidality and Antidepressants:* Increased risk of suicidality in children, adolescents, and young adults with major depressive disorder (5.2)
- *Neuroleptic Malignant Syndrome:* Manage with immediate discontinuation and close monitoring (5.3)
- *Tardive Dyskinesia:* Discontinue if clinically appropriate (5.4)
- *Hyperglycemia and Diabetes Mellitus:* Monitor glucose regularly in patients with and at risk for diabetes (5.5)
- *Orthostatic Hypotension:* Use with caution in patients with known cardiovascular or cerebrovascular disease (5.6)
- *Leukopenia, Neutropenia, and Agranulocytosis:* have been reported with antipsychotics including ABILIFY. Patients with a history of a clinically significant low white blood cell count (WBC) or a drug-induced leukopenia/neutropenia should have their complete blood count (CBC) monitored frequently during the first few months

	Initial Dose	Recommended Dose	Maximum Dose
Schizophrenia – adults (2.1)	10-15 mg/day	10-15 mg/day	30 mg/day
Schizophrenia – adolescents (2.1)	2 mg/day	10 mg/day	30 mg/day
Bipolar mania – adults: monotherapy or as an adjunct to lithium or valproate (2.2)	15 mg/day	15 mg/day	30 mg/day
Bipolar mania – pediatric patients: monotherapy or as an adjunct to lithium or valproate (2.2)	2 mg/day	10 mg/day	30 mg/day
As an adjunct to antidepressants for the treatment of major depressive disorder – adults (2.3)	2-5 mg/day	5-10 mg/day	15 mg/day
Irritability associated with autistic disorder – pediatric patients (2.4)	2 mg/day	5-10 mg/day	15 mg/day
Agitation associated with schizophrenia or bipolar mania – adults (2.5)	9.75 mg/1.3 mL injected IM		30 mg/day injected IM

of therapy and discontinuation of ABILIFY (aripiprazole) should be considered at the first sign of a clinically significant decline in WBC in the absence of other causative factors (5.7)
- *Seizures/Convulsions:* Use cautiously in patients with a history of seizures or with conditions that lower the seizure threshold (5.8)
- *Potential for Cognitive and Motor Impairment:* Use caution when operating machinery (5.9)
- *Suicide:* The possibility of a suicide attempt is inherent in schizophrenia and bipolar disorder. Closely supervise high-risk patients (5.11)

---ADVERSE REACTIONS---

Commonly observed adverse reactions (incidence ≥5% and at least twice that for placebo) were (6.2):
- Adult patients with schizophrenia: akathisia
- Pediatric patients (13 to 17 years) with schizophrenia: extrapyramidal disorder, somnolence, and tremor
- Adult patients (monotherapy) with bipolar mania: akathisia, sedation, restlessness, tremor, and extrapyramidal disorder
- Adult patients (adjunctive therapy with lithium or valproate) with bipolar mania: akathisia, insomnia, and extrapyramidal disorder
- Pediatric patients (10 to 17 years) with bipolar mania: somnolence, extrapyramidal disorder, fatigue, nausea, akathisia, blurred vision, salivary hypersecretion, and dizziness
- Adult patients with major depressive disorder (adjunctive treatment to antidepressant therapy): akathisia, restlessness, insomnia, constipation, fatigue, and blurred vision
- Pediatric patients (6 to 17 years) with autistic disorder: sedation, fatigue, vomiting, somnolence, tremor, pyrexia, drooling, decreased appetite, salivary hypersecretion, extrapyramidal disorder, and lethargy
- Adult patients with agitation associated with schizophrenia or bipolar mania: nausea

To report SUSPECTED ADVERSE REACTIONS, contact Bristol-Myers Squibb at 1-800-721-5072 or FDA at 1-800-FDA-1088 or www.fda.gov/medwatch

---DRUG INTERACTIONS---

- *Strong CYP3A4 (eg, ketoconazole) or CYP2D6 (eg, fluoxetine) inhibitors will increase* ABILIFY drug concentrations; reduce ABILIFY dose by one-half when used concomitantly (2.6, 7.1), except when used as adjunctive treatment with antidepressants (2.6)
- *CYP3A4 inducers (eg, carbamazepine) will decrease* ABILIFY drug concentrations; double ABILIFY dose when used concomitantly (2.6, 7.1)

See 17 for PATIENT COUNSELING INFORMATION and Medication Guide

Revised: 11/2009

FULL PRESCRIBING INFORMATION: CONTENTS*
WARNINGS: INCREASED MORTALITY IN ELDERLY PATIENTS WITH DEMENTIA-RELATED PSYCHOSIS AND SUICIDALITY AND ANTIDEPRESSANT DRUGS

16 HOW SUPPLIED/STORAGE AND HANDLING
16.1 How Supplied
16.2 Storage
17 PATIENT COUNSELING INFORMATION
17.1 Information for Patients
* Sections or subsections omitted from the full prescribing information are not listed

FULL PRESCRIBING INFORMATION

WARNINGS: INCREASED MORTALITY IN ELDERLY PATIENTS WITH DEMENTIA-RELATED PSYCHOSIS and SUICIDALITY AND ANTIDEPRESSANT DRUGS
Elderly patients with dementia-related psychosis treated with antipsychotic drugs are at an increased risk of death. Analyses of seventeen placebo-controlled trials (modal duration of 10 weeks), largely in patients taking atypical antipsychotic drugs, revealed a risk of death in drug-treated patients of between 1.6 to 1.7 times the risk of death in placebo-treated patients. Over the course of a typical 10-week controlled trial, the rate of death in drug-treated patients was about 4.5%, compared to a rate of about 2.6% in the placebo group. Although the causes of death were varied, most of the deaths appeared to be either cardiovascular (eg, heart failure, sudden death) or infectious (eg, pneumonia) in nature. Observational studies suggest that, similar to atypical antipsychotic drugs, treatment with conventional antipsychotic drugs may increase mortality. The extent to which the findings of increased mortality in observational studies may be attributed to the antipsychotic drug as opposed to some characteristic(s) of the patients is not clear. ABILIFY (aripiprazole) is not approved for the treatment of patients with dementia-related psychosis [see WARNINGS AND PRECAUTIONS (5.1)].

Antidepressants increased the risk compared to placebo of suicidal thinking and behavior (suicidality) in children, adolescents, and young adults in short-term studies of major depressive disorder (MDD) and other psychiatric disorders. Anyone considering the use of adjunctive ABILIFY or any other antidepressant in a child, adolescent, or young adult must balance this risk with the clinical need. Short-term studies did not show an increase in the risk of suicidality with antidepressants compared to placebo in adults beyond age 24; there was a reduction in risk with antidepressants compared to placebo in adults aged 65 and older. Depression and certain other psychiatric disorders are themselves associated with increases in the risk of suicide. Patients of all ages who are started on antidepressant therapy should be monitored appropriately and observed closely for clinical worsening, suicidality, or unusual changes in behavior. Families and caregivers should be advised of the need for close observation and communication with the prescriber. ABILIFY is not approved for use in pediatric patients with depression [see WARNINGS AND PRECAUTIONS (5.2)].

1 INDICATIONS AND USAGE

1.1 Schizophrenia
ABILIFY (aripiprazole) is indicated for the treatment of schizophrenia. The efficacy of ABILIFY was established in four 4-6 week trials in adults and one 6-week trial in adolescents (13 to 17 years). Maintenance efficacy was demonstrated in one trial in adults and can be extrapolated to adolescents [see CLINICAL STUDIES (14.1)].

1.2 Bipolar I Disorder
Monotherapy
ABILIFY is indicated for the acute and maintenance treatment of manic and mixed episodes associated with bipolar I disorder. Efficacy was established in four 3-week monotherapy trials in adults and one 4-week monotherapy trial in pediatric patients (10 to 17 years). Maintenance efficacy was demonstrated in a monotherapy trial in adults and can be extrapolated to pediatric patients (10 to 17 years) [see CLINICAL STUDIES (14.2)].

Adjunctive Therapy
ABILIFY is indicated as an adjunctive therapy to either lithium or valproate for the acute treatment of manic and mixed episodes associated with bipolar I disorder. Efficacy was established in one 6-week adjunctive trial in adults and can be extrapolated to pediatric patients (10 to 17 years) [see CLINICAL STUDIES (14.2)].

1.3 Adjunctive Treatment of Major Depressive Disorder
ABILIFY is indicated for use as an adjunctive therapy to antidepressants for the treatment of major depressive disorder (MDD). Efficacy was established in two 6-week trials in adults with MDD who had an inadequate response to antidepressant therapy during the current episode [see CLINICAL STUDIES (14.3)].

1.4 Irritability Associated with Autistic Disorder
ABILIFY is indicated for the treatment of irritability associated with autistic disorder. Efficacy was established in two 8-week trials in pediatric patients (aged 6 to 17 years) with irritability associated with autistic disorder (including symptoms of aggression towards others, deliberate self-injuriousness, temper tantrums, and quickly changing moods) [see CLINICAL STUDIES (14.4)].

1.5 Agitation Associated with Schizophrenia or Bipolar Mania
ABILIFY (aripiprazole) Injection is indicated for the acute treatment of agitation associated with schizophrenia or bipolar disorder, manic or mixed. "Psychomotor agitation" is defined in DSM-IV as "excessive motor activity associated with a feeling of inner tension". Patients experiencing agitation often manifest behaviors that interfere with their diagnosis and care (eg, threatening behaviors, escalating or urgently distressing behavior, or self-exhausting behavior), leading clinicians to the use of intramuscular antipsychotic medications to achieve immediate control of the agitation. Efficacy was established in three short-term (24-hour) trials in adults [see CLINICAL STUDIES (14.5)].

1.6 Special Considerations in Treating Pediatric Schizophrenia, Bipolar I Disorder, and Irritability Associated with Autistic Disorder
Psychiatric disorders in children and adolescents are often serious mental disorders with variable symptom profiles that are not always congruent with adult diagnostic criteria. It is recommended that psychotropic medication therapy for pediatric patients only be initiated after a thorough diagnostic evaluation has been conducted and careful consideration given to the risks associated with medication treatment. Medication treatment for pediatric patients with schizophrenia, bipolar I disorder, and irritability associated with autistic disorder is indicated as part of a total treatment program that often includes psychological, educational, and social interventions.

2 DOSAGE AND ADMINISTRATION
2.1 Schizophrenia
Adults
Dose Selection: The recommended starting and target dose for ABILIFY is 10 mg/day or 15 mg/day administered on a once-a-day schedule without regard to meals. ABILIFY has been systematically evaluated and shown to be effective in a dose range of 10 mg/day to 30 mg/day, when administered as the tablet formulation; however, doses higher than 10 mg/day or 15 mg/day were not more effective than 10 mg/day or 15 mg/day. Dosage increases should generally not be made before 2 weeks, the time needed to achieve steady-state [see CLINICAL STUDIES (14.1)].
Maintenance Treatment: Maintenance of efficacy in schizophrenia was demonstrated in a trial involving patients with schizophrenia who had been symptomatically stable on other antipsychotic medications for periods of 3 months or longer. These patients were discontinued from those medications and randomized to either ABILIFY 15 mg/day or placebo, and observed for relapse [see CLINICAL STUDIES (14.1)]. Patients should be periodically reassessed to determine the continued need for maintenance treatment.

Adolescents
Dose Selection: The recommended target dose of ABILIFY is 10 mg/day. Aripiprazole was studied in adolescent patients 13 to 17 years of age with schizophrenia at daily doses of 10 mg and 30 mg. The starting daily dose of the tablet formulation in these patients was 2 mg, which was titrated to 5 mg after 2 days and to the target dose of 10 mg after 2 additional days. Subsequent dose increases should be administered in 5 mg increments. The 30 mg/day dose was not shown to be more efficacious than the 10 mg/day dose. ABILIFY can be administered without regard to meals [see CLINICAL STUDIES (14.1)].
Maintenance Treatment: The efficacy of ABILIFY for the maintenance treatment of schizophrenia in the adolescent population has not been evaluated. While there is no body of evidence available to answer the question of how long the adolescent patient treated with ABILIFY should be maintained on the drug, maintenance efficacy can be extrapolated from adult data along with comparisons of aripiprazole pharmacokinetic parameters in adult and pediatric patients. Thus, it is generally recommended that responding patients be continued beyond the acute response, but at the lowest dose needed to maintain remission. Patients should be periodically reassessed to determine the need for maintenance treatment.

Switching from Other Antipsychotics
There are no systematically collected data to specifically address switching patients with schizophrenia from other antipsychotics to ABILIFY or concerning concomitant administration with other antipsychotics. While immediate discontinuation of the previous antipsychotic treatment may be acceptable for some patients with schizophrenia, more gradual discontinuation may be most appropriate for others. In all cases, the period of overlapping antipsychotic administration should be minimized.

2.2 Bipolar I Disorder
Adults
Dose Selection: The recommended starting and target dose is 15 mg given once daily as monotherapy or as adjunctive therapy with lithium or valproate. ABILIFY (aripiprazole) may be given without regard to meals. The dose may be increased to 30 mg/day based on clinical response. The safety of doses above 30 mg/day has not been evaluated in clinical trials [see CLINICAL STUDIES (14.2)].
Maintenance Treatment: Maintenance of efficacy in bipolar I disorder was demonstrated in a trial involving patients who had been symptomatically stable on ABILIFY Tablets (15 mg/day or 30 mg/day, as monotherapy) for at least 6 consecutive weeks. These patients were discontinued from those medications and randomized to either ABILIFY, at the same dose they were stabilized on, or placebo, and observed for relapse [see CLINICAL STUDIES (14.2)].
Patients should be periodically reassessed to determine the continued need for maintenance treatment.

Pediatric Patients
Dose Selection: The efficacy of ABILIFY has been established in the treatment of pediatric patients 10 to 17 years of age with bipolar I disorder at doses of 10 mg/day or 30 mg/day. The recommended target dose of ABILIFY is 10 mg/day, as monotherapy or as adjunctive therapy with lithium or valproate. The starting daily dose of the tablet formulation in these patients was 2 mg/day, which was titrated to 5 mg/day after 2 days and to the target dose of 10 mg/day after 2 additional days. Subsequent dose increases should be administered in 5 mg/day increments. ABILIFY can be administered without regard to meals. [See CLINICAL STUDIES (14.2).]
Maintenance Treatment: The efficacy of ABILIFY for the maintenance treatment of bipolar I disorder in the pediatric population has not been evaluated. While there is no body of evidence available to answer the question of how long the pediatric patient treated with ABILIFY should be maintained, maintenance efficacy can be extrapolated from adult data along with comparisons of aripiprazole pharmacokinetic parameters in adult and pediatric patients. Thus, responding patients may be considered for continued treatment beyond the acute response at the lowest dose required to maintain remission. Patients should be periodically reassessed to determine the continued need for maintenance treatment.

2.3 Adjunctive Treatment of Major Depressive Disorder
Adults
Dose Selection: The recommended starting dose for ABILIFY as adjunctive treatment for patients already taking an antidepressant is 2 mg/day to 5 mg/day. The efficacy of ABILIFY as an adjunctive therapy for major depressive disorder was established within a dose range of 2 mg/day to 15 mg/day. Dose adjustments of up to 5 mg/day should occur gradually, at intervals of no less than 1 week [see CLINICAL STUDIES (14.3)].
Maintenance Treatment: The efficacy of ABILIFY for the adjunctive maintenance treatment of major depressive disorder has not been evaluated. While there is no body of evidence available to answer the question of how long the patient treated with ABILIFY should be maintained, patients should be periodically reassessed to determine the continued need for maintenance treatment.

2.4 Irritability Associated with Autistic Disorder
Pediatric Patients
Dose Selection: The efficacy of aripiprazole has been established in the treatment of pediatric patients 6 to 17 years of age with irritability associated with autistic disorder at doses of 5 mg/day to 15 mg/day. The dosage of ABILIFY should be individualized according to tolerability and response.
Dosing should be initiated at 2 mg/day. The dose should be increased to 5 mg/day, with subsequent increases to 10 mg/day or 15 mg/day if needed. Dose adjustments of up to 5 mg/day should occur gradually, at intervals of no less than 1 week [see CLINICAL STUDIES (14.4)].
Maintenance Treatment: The efficacy of ABILIFY for the maintenance treatment of irritability associated with autistic disorder has not been evaluated. While there is no body of evidence available to answer the question of how long the patient treated with ABILIFY should be maintained, patients should be periodically reassessed to determine the continued need for maintenance treatment.

2.5 Agitation Associated with Schizophrenia or Bipolar Mania (Intramuscular Injection)
Adults
Dose Selection: The recommended dose in these patients is 9.75 mg. The effectiveness of aripiprazole injection in controlling agitation in schizophrenia and bipolar mania was demonstrated over a dose range of 5.25 mg to 15 mg. No additional benefit was demonstrated for 15 mg compared to 9.75 mg. A lower dose of 5.25 mg may be considered when clinical factors warrant. If agitation warranting a second dose persists following the initial dose, cumulative doses up to a total of 30 mg/day may be given. However, the efficacy of repeated doses of aripiprazole injection in agitated patients has not been systematically evaluated in controlled

clinical trials. The safety of total daily doses greater than 30 mg or injections given more frequently than every 2 hours have not been adequately evaluated in clinical trials [see CLINICAL STUDIES (14.5)].

If ongoing aripiprazole therapy is clinically indicated, oral aripiprazole in a range of 10 mg/day to 30 mg/day should replace aripiprazole injection as soon as possible [see DOSAGE AND ADMINISTRATION (2.1 and 2.2)].

Administration of ABILIFY Injection

To administer ABILIFY (aripiprazole) Injection, draw up the required volume of solution into the syringe as shown in Table 1. Discard any unused portion.

Table 1: ABILIFY Injection Dosing Recommendations

Single-Dose	Required Volume of Solution
5.25 mg	0.7 mL
9.75 mg	1.3 mL
15 mg	2 mL

ABILIFY Injection is intended for intramuscular use only. Do not administer intravenously or subcutaneously. Inject slowly, deep into the muscle mass.

Parenteral drug products should be inspected visually for particulate matter and discoloration prior to administration, whenever solution and container permit.

2.6   Dosage Adjustment

Dosage adjustments in adults are not routinely indicated on the basis of age, gender, race, or renal or hepatic impairment status [see USE IN SPECIFIC POPULATIONS (8.4-8.10)].

Dosage adjustment for patients taking aripiprazole concomitantly with strong CYP3A4 inhibitors: When concomitant administration of aripiprazole with strong CYP3A4 inhibitors such as ketoconazole or clarithromycin is indicated, the aripiprazole dose should be reduced to one-half the usual dose. When the CYP3A4 inhibitor is withdrawn from the combination therapy, the aripiprazole dose should then be increased [see DRUG INTERACTIONS (7.1)].

Dosage adjustment for patients taking aripiprazole concomitantly with potential CYP2D6 inhibitors: When concomitant administration of potential CYP2D6 inhibitors such as quinidine, fluoxetine, or paroxetine with aripiprazole occurs, aripiprazole dose should be reduced at least to one-half of its normal dose. When the CYP2D6 inhibitor is withdrawn from the combination therapy, the aripiprazole dose should then be increased [see DRUG INTERACTIONS (7.1)]. When adjunctive ABILIFY is administered to patients with major depressive disorder, ABILIFY should be administered without dosage adjustment as specified in DOSAGE AND ADMINISTRATION (2.3).

Dosage adjustment for patients taking potential CYP3A4 inducers: When a potential CYP3A4 inducer such as carbamazepine is added to aripiprazole therapy, the aripiprazole dose should be doubled. Additional dose increases should be based on clinical evaluation. When the CYP3A4 inducer is withdrawn from the combination therapy, the aripiprazole dose should be reduced to 10 mg to 15 mg [see DRUG INTERACTIONS (7.1)].

2.7   Dosing of Oral Solution

The oral solution can be substituted for tablets on a mg-per-mg basis up to the 25 mg dose level. Patients receiving 30 mg tablets should receive 25 mg of the solution [see CLINICAL PHARMACOLOGY (12.3)].

2.8   Dosing of Orally Disintegrating Tablets

The dosing for ABILIFY Orally Disintegrating Tablets is the same as for the oral tablets [see DOSAGE AND ADMINISTRATION (2.1, 2.2, 2.3, and 2.4)].

3   DOSAGE FORMS AND STRENGTHS

ABILIFY® (aripiprazole) Tablets are available as described in Table 2.

[See table above]

ABILIFY DISCMELT® (aripiprazole) Orally Disintegrating Tablets are available as described in Table 3.

Table 3: ABILIFY DISCMELT Orally Disintegrating Tablet Presentations

Tablet Strength	Tablet Color/Shape	Tablet Markings
10 mg	pink (with scattered specks) round	"A" and "640" "10"
15 mg	yellow (with scattered specks) round	"A" and "641" "15"

Table 2: ABILIFY Tablet Presentations

Tablet Strength	Tablet Color/Shape	Tablet Markings
2 mg	green modified rectangle	"A-006" and "2"
5 mg	blue modified rectangle	"A-007" and "5"
10 mg	pink modified rectangle	"A-008" and "10"
15 mg	yellow round	"A-009" and "15"
20 mg	white round	"A-010" and "20"
30 mg	pink round	"A-011" and "30"

ABILIFY® (aripiprazole) Oral Solution (1 mg/mL) is a clear, colorless to light yellow solution, supplied in child-resistant bottles along with a calibrated oral dosing cup.

ABILIFY® (aripiprazole) Injection for Intramuscular Use is a clear, colorless solution available as a ready-to-use, 9.75 mg/1.3 mL (7.5 mg/mL) solution in clear, Type 1 glass vials.

4   CONTRAINDICATIONS

Known hypersensitivity reaction to ABILIFY. Reactions have ranged from pruritus/urticaria to anaphylaxis [see ADVERSE REACTIONS (6.3)].

5   WARNINGS AND PRECAUTIONS

5.1   Use in Elderly Patients with Dementia-Related Psychosis

Increased Mortality

Elderly patients with dementia-related psychosis treated with antipsychotic drugs are at an increased risk of death. ABILIFY (aripiprazole) is not approved for the treatment of patients with dementia-related psychosis [see BOXED WARNING].

Cerebrovascular Adverse Events, Including Stroke

In placebo-controlled clinical studies (two flexible dose and one fixed dose study) of dementia-related psychosis, there was an increased incidence of cerebrovascular adverse events (eg, stroke, transient ischemic attack), including fatalities, in aripiprazole-treated patients (mean age: 84 years; range: 78-88 years). In the fixed-dose study, there was a statistically significant dose response relationship for cerebrovascular adverse events in patients treated with aripiprazole. Aripiprazole is not approved for the treatment of patients with dementia-related psychosis [see also BOXED WARNING].

Safety Experience in Elderly Patients with Psychosis Associated with Alzheimer's Disease

In three, 10-week, placebo-controlled studies of aripiprazole in elderly patients with psychosis associated with Alzheimer's disease (n=938; mean age: 82.4 years; range: 56-99 years), the treatment-emergent adverse events that were reported at an incidence of ≥3% and aripiprazole incidence at least twice that for placebo were lethargy [placebo 2%, aripiprazole 5%], somnolence (including sedation) [placebo 3%, aripiprazole 8%], and incontinence (primarily, urinary incontinence) [placebo 1%, aripiprazole 5%], excessive salivation [placebo 0%, aripiprazole 4%], and lightheadedness [placebo 1%, aripiprazole 4%].

The safety and efficacy of ABILIFY in the treatment of patients with psychosis associated with dementia have not been established. If the prescriber elects to treat such patients with ABILIFY, vigilance should be exercised, particularly for the emergence of difficulty swallowing or excessive somnolence, which could predispose to accidental injury or aspiration [see also BOXED WARNING].

5.2   Clinical Worsening of Depression and Suicide Risk

Patients with major depressive disorder (MDD), both adult and pediatric, may experience worsening of their depression and/or the emergence of suicidal ideation and behavior (suicidality) or unusual changes in behavior, whether or not they are taking antidepressant medications, and this risk may persist until significant remission occurs. Suicide is a known risk of depression and certain other psychiatric disorders, and these disorders themselves are the strongest predictors of suicide. There has been a long-standing concern, however, that antidepressants may have a role in inducing worsening of depression and the emergence of suicidality in certain patients during the early phases of treatment. Pooled analyses of short-term placebo-controlled trials of antidepressant drugs (SSRIs and others) showed that these drugs increase the risk of suicidal thinking and behavior (suicidality) in children, adolescents, and young adults (ages 18-24) with MDD and other psychiatric disorders. Short-term studies did not show an increase in the risk of suicidality with antidepressants compared to placebo in adults beyond age 24; there was a reduction with antidepressants compared to placebo in adults aged 65 and older.

The pooled analyses of placebo-controlled trials in children and adolescents with MDD, Obsessive Compulsive Disorder (OCD), or other psychiatric disorders included a total of 24 short-term trials of 9 antidepressant drugs in over 4400 patients. The pooled analyses of placebo-controlled trials in adults with MDD or other psychiatric disorders included a total of 295 short-term trials (median duration of 2 months) of 11 antidepressant drugs in over 77,000 patients. There was considerable variation in risk of suicidality among drugs, but a tendency toward an increase in the younger patients for almost all drugs studied. There were differences in absolute risk of suicidality across the different indications, with the highest incidence in MDD. The risk differences (drug vs. placebo), however, were relatively stable within age strata and across indications. These risk differences (drug-placebo difference in the number of cases of suicidality per 1000 patients treated) are provided in Table 4.

Table 4:

Age Range	Drug-Placebo Difference in Number of Cases of Suicidality per 1000 Patients Treated
	Increases Compared to Placebo
<18	14 additional cases
18-24	5 additional cases
	Decreases Compared to Placebo
25-64	1 fewer case
≥65	6 fewer cases

No suicides occurred in any of the pediatric trials. There were suicides in the adult trials, but the number was not sufficient to reach any conclusion about drug effect on suicide.

It is unknown whether the suicidality risk extends to longer-term use, ie, beyond several months. However, there is substantial evidence from placebo-controlled maintenance trials in adults with depression that the use of antidepressants can delay the recurrence of depression.

All patients being treated with antidepressants for any indication should be monitored appropriately and observed closely for clinical worsening, suicidality, and unusual changes in behavior, especially during the initial few months of a course of drug therapy, or at times of dose changes, either increases or decreases.

The following symptoms, anxiety, agitation, panic attacks, insomnia, irritability, hostility, aggressiveness, impulsivity, akathisia (psychomotor restlessness), hypomania, and mania, have been reported in adult and pediatric patients being treated with antidepressants for MDD as well as for other indications, both psychiatric and nonpsychiatric. Although a causal link between the emergence of such symptoms and either the worsening of depression and/or the emergence of suicidal impulses has not been established, there is concern that such symptoms may represent precursors to emerging suicidality.

Consideration should be given to changing the therapeutic regimen, including possibly discontinuing the medication, in patients whose depression is persistently worse, or who are experiencing emergent suicidality or symptoms that might be precursors to worsening depression or suicidality, especially if these symptoms are severe, abrupt in onset, or were not part of the patient's presenting symptoms.

Families and caregivers of patients being treated with antidepressants for major depressive disorder or other indications, both psychiatric and nonpsychiatric, should be alerted about the need to monitor patients for the emergence of agitation, irritability, unusual changes in behavior, and the other symptoms described above, as well as the emergence of suicidality, and to report such symptoms immediately to healthcare providers. Such monitoring should include daily observation by families and caregivers.

Prescriptions for ABILIFY (aripiprazole) should be written for the smallest quantity of tablets consistent with good patient management, in order to reduce the risk of overdose.

Screening Patients for Bipolar Disorder: A major depressive episode may be the initial presentation of bipolar disorder. It is generally believed (though not established in controlled trials) that treating such an episode with an antidepressant alone may increase the likelihood of precipitation of a mixed/manic episode in patients at risk for bipolar disorder. Whether any of the symptoms described above represent such a conversion is unknown. However, prior to initiating treatment with an antidepressant, patients with depressive symptoms should be adequately screened to determine if they are at risk for bipolar disorder; such screening should include a detailed psychiatric history, including a family history of suicide, bipolar disorder, and depression.

It should be noted that ABILIFY is not approved for use in treating depression in the pediatric population.

5.3   Neuroleptic Malignant Syndrome (NMS)
A potentially fatal symptom complex sometimes referred to as Neuroleptic Malignant Syndrome (NMS) may occur with administration of antipsychotic drugs, including aripiprazole. Rare cases of NMS occurred during aripiprazole treatment in the worldwide clinical database. Clinical manifestations of NMS are hyperpyrexia, muscle rigidity, altered mental status, and evidence of autonomic instability (irregular pulse or blood pressure, tachycardia, diaphoresis, and cardiac dysrhythmia). Additional signs may include elevated creatine phosphokinase, myoglobinuria (rhabdomyolysis), and acute renal failure.

The diagnostic evaluation of patients with this syndrome is complicated. In arriving at a diagnosis, it is important to exclude cases where the clinical presentation includes both serious medical illness (eg, pneumonia, systemic infection) and untreated or inadequately treated extrapyramidal signs and symptoms (EPS). Other important considerations in the differential diagnosis include central anticholinergic toxicity, heat stroke, drug fever, and primary central nervous system pathology.

The management of NMS should include: 1) immediate discontinuation of antipsychotic drugs and other drugs not essential to concurrent therapy; 2) intensive symptomatic treatment and medical monitoring; and 3) treatment of any concomitant serious medical problems for which specific treatments are available. There is no general agreement about specific pharmacological treatment regimens for uncomplicated NMS.

If a patient requires antipsychotic drug treatment after recovery from NMS, the potential reintroduction of drug therapy should be carefully considered. The patient should be carefully monitored, since recurrences of NMS have been reported.

5.4   Tardive Dyskinesia
A syndrome of potentially irreversible, involuntary, dyskinetic movements may develop in patients treated with antipsychotic drugs. Although the prevalence of the syndrome appears to be highest among the elderly, especially elderly women, it is impossible to rely upon prevalence estimates to predict, at the inception of antipsychotic treatment, which patients are likely to develop the syndrome. Whether antipsychotic drug products differ in their potential to cause tardive dyskinesia is unknown.

The risk of developing tardive dyskinesia and the likelihood that it will become irreversible are believed to increase as the duration of treatment and the total cumulative dose of antipsychotic drugs administered to the patient increase. However, the syndrome can develop, although much less commonly, after relatively brief treatment periods at low doses.

There is no known treatment for established cases of tardive dyskinesia, although the syndrome may remit, partially or completely, if antipsychotic treatment is withdrawn. Antipsychotic treatment, itself, however, may suppress (or partially suppress) the signs and symptoms of the syndrome and, thereby, may possibly mask the underlying process. The effect that symptomatic suppression has upon the long-term course of the syndrome is unknown.

Given these considerations, ABILIFY should be prescribed in a manner that is most likely to minimize the occurrence of tardive dyskinesia. Chronic antipsychotic treatment should generally be reserved for patients who suffer from a chronic illness that (1) is known to respond to antipsychotic drugs and (2) for whom alternative, equally effective, but potentially less harmful treatments are not available or appropriate. In patients who do require chronic treatment, the smallest dose and the shortest duration of treatment producing a satisfactory clinical response should be sought. The need for continued treatment should be reassessed periodically.

If signs and symptoms of tardive dyskinesia appear in a patient on ABILIFY (aripiprazole), drug discontinuation should be considered. However, some patients may require treatment with ABILIFY despite the presence of the syndrome.

5.5   Hyperglycemia and Diabetes Mellitus
Hyperglycemia, in some cases extreme and associated with ketoacidosis or hyperosmolar coma or death, has been reported in patients treated with atypical antipsychotics. There have been few reports of hyperglycemia in patients treated with ABILIFY [see ADVERSE REACTIONS (6.2, 6.3)]. Although fewer patients have been treated with ABILIFY, it is not known if this more limited experience is the sole reason for the paucity of such reports. Assessment of the relationship between atypical antipsychotic use and glucose abnormalities is complicated by the possibility of an increased background risk of diabetes mellitus in patients with schizophrenia and the increasing incidence of diabetes mellitus in the general population. Given these confounders, the relationship between atypical antipsychotic use and hyperglycemia-related adverse events is not completely understood. However, epidemiological studies which did not include ABILIFY suggest an increased risk of treatment-emergent hyperglycemia-related adverse events in patients treated with the atypical antipsychotics included in these studies. Because ABILIFY was not marketed at the time these studies were performed, it is not known if ABILIFY is associated with this increased risk. Precise risk estimates for hyperglycemia-related adverse events in patients treated with atypical antipsychotics are not available.

Patients with an established diagnosis of diabetes mellitus who are started on atypical antipsychotics should be monitored regularly for worsening of glucose control. Patients with risk factors for diabetes mellitus (eg, obesity, family history of diabetes) who are starting treatment with atypical antipsychotics should undergo fasting blood glucose testing at the beginning of treatment and periodically during treatment. Any patient treated with atypical antipsychotics should be monitored for symptoms of hyperglycemia including polydipsia, polyuria, polyphagia, and weakness. Patients who develop symptoms of hyperglycemia during treatment with atypical antipsychotics should undergo fasting blood glucose testing. In some cases, hyperglycemia has resolved when the atypical antipsychotic was discontinued; however, some patients required continuation of antidiabetic treatment despite discontinuation of the suspect drug.

5.6   Orthostatic Hypotension
Aripiprazole may cause orthostatic hypotension, perhaps due to its α_1-adrenergic receptor antagonism. The incidence of orthostatic hypotension-associated events from short-term, placebo-controlled trials of adult patients on oral ABILIFY (n=2467) included (aripiprazole incidence, placebo incidence) orthostatic hypotension (1%, 0.3%), postural dizziness (0.5%, 0.3%), and syncope (0.5%, 0.4%); of pediatric patients 6 to 17 years of age (n=611) on oral ABILIFY included orthostatic hypotension (0.5%, 0%), postural dizziness (0.3%, 0%), and syncope (0.2%, 0%); and of patients on ABILIFY Injection (n=501) included orthostatic hypotension (0.6%, 0%), postural dizziness (0.2%, 0.5%), and syncope (0.4%, 0%).

The incidence of a significant orthostatic change in blood pressure (defined as a decrease in systolic blood pressure $\geq$20 mmHg accompanied by an increase in heart rate $\geq$25 when comparing standing to supine values) for aripiprazole was not meaningfully different from placebo (aripiprazole incidence, placebo incidence): in adult oral aripiprazole-treated patients (4%, 2%), in pediatric oral aripiprazole-treated patients aged 6 to 17 years (0.2%, 1%), or in aripiprazole injection-treated patients (3%, 2%).

Aripiprazole should be used with caution in patients with known cardiovascular disease (history of myocardial infarction or ischemic heart disease, heart failure or conduction abnormalities), cerebrovascular disease, or conditions which would predispose patients to hypotension (dehydration, hypovolemia, and treatment with antihypertensive medications).

If parenteral benzodiazepine therapy is deemed necessary in addition to aripiprazole injection treatment, patients should be monitored for excessive sedation and for orthostatic hypotension [see DRUG INTERACTIONS (7.3)].

5.7   Leukopenia, Neutropenia, and Agranulocytosis
Class Effect: In clinical trial and/or postmarketing experience, events of leukopenia/neutropenia have been reported temporally related to antipsychotic agents, including ABILIFY. Agranulocytosis has also been reported.

Possible risk factors for leukopenia/neutropenia include pre-existing low white blood cell count (WBC) and history of drug-induced leukopenia/neutropenia. Patients with a history of a clinically significant low WBC or drug-induced leukopenia/neutropenia should have their complete blood count (CBC) monitored frequently during the first few months of therapy and discontinuation of ABILIFY should be considered at the first sign of a clinically significant decline in WBC in the absence of other causative factors.

Patients with clinically significant neutropenia should be carefully monitored for fever or other symptoms or signs of infection and treated promptly if such symptoms or signs occur. Patients with severe neutropenia (absolute neutrophil count <1000/mm^3) should discontinue ABILIFY (aripiprazole) and have their WBC followed until recovery.

5.8   Seizures/Convulsions
In short-term, placebo-controlled trials, seizures/convulsions occurred in 0.1% (3/2467) of adult patients treated with oral aripiprazole, in 0.2% (1/611) of pediatric patients (6 to 17 years), and in 0.2% (1/501) of adult aripiprazole injection-treated patients.

As with other antipsychotic drugs, aripiprazole should be used cautiously in patients with a history of seizures or with conditions that lower the seizure threshold, eg, Alzheimer's dementia. Conditions that lower the seizure threshold may be more prevalent in a population of 65 years or older.

5.9   Potential for Cognitive and Motor Impairment
ABILIFY, like other antipsychotics, may have the potential to impair judgment, thinking, or motor skills. For example, in short-term, placebo-controlled trials, somnolence (including sedation) was reported as follows (aripiprazole incidence, placebo incidence): in adult patients (n=2467) treated with oral ABILIFY (11%, 6%), in pediatric patients ages 6 to 17 (n=611) (24%, 6%), and in adult patients (n=501) on ABILIFY Injection (9%, 6%). Somnolence (including sedation) led to discontinuation in 0.3% (8/2467) of adult patients and 3% (15/611) of pediatric patients (6 to 17 years) on oral ABILIFY in short-term, placebo-controlled trials, but did not lead to discontinuation of any adult patients on ABILIFY Injection.

Despite the relatively modest increased incidence of these events compared to placebo, patients should be cautioned about operating hazardous machinery, including automobiles, until they are reasonably certain that therapy with ABILIFY does not affect them adversely.

5.10   Body Temperature Regulation
Disruption of the body's ability to reduce core body temperature has been attributed to antipsychotic agents. Appropriate care is advised when prescribing aripiprazole for patients who will be experiencing conditions which may contribute to an elevation in core body temperature, (eg, exercising strenuously, exposure to extreme heat, receiving concomitant medication with anticholinergic activity, or being subject to dehydration) [see ADVERSE REACTIONS (6.3)].

5.11   Suicide
The possibility of a suicide attempt is inherent in psychotic illnesses, bipolar disorder, and major depressive disorder, and close supervision of high-risk patients should accompany drug therapy. Prescriptions for ABILIFY should be written for the smallest quantity consistent with good patient management in order to reduce the risk of overdose [see ADVERSE REACTIONS (6.2, 6.3)].

In two 6-week placebo-controlled studies of aripiprazole as adjunctive treatment of major depressive disorder, the incidences of suicidal ideation and suicide attempts were 0% (0/371) for aripiprazole and 0.5% (2/366) for placebo.

5.12   Dysphagia
Esophageal dysmotility and aspiration have been associated with antipsychotic drug use, including ABILIFY. Aspiration pneumonia is a common cause of morbidity and mortality in elderly patients, in particular those with advanced Alzheimer's dementia. Aripiprazole and other antipsychotic drugs should be used cautiously in patients at risk for aspiration pneumonia [see WARNINGS AND PRECAUTIONS (5.1) and ADVERSE REACTIONS (6.3)].

5.13   Use in Patients with Concomitant Illness
Clinical experience with ABILIFY in patients with certain concomitant systemic illnesses is limited [see USE IN SPECIFIC POPULATIONS (8.6, 8.7)].

ABILIFY has not been evaluated or used to any appreciable extent in patients with a recent history of myocardial infarction or unstable heart disease. Patients with these diagnoses were excluded from premarketing clinical studies [see WARNINGS AND PRECAUTIONS (5.1, 5.6)].

6   ADVERSE REACTIONS
6.1   Overall Adverse Reactions Profile
The following are discussed in more detail in other sections of the labeling:

• Use in Elderly Patients with Dementia-Related Psychosis [see BOXED WARNING and WARNINGS AND PRECAUTIONS (5.1)]
• Clinical Worsening of Depression and Suicide Risk [see BOXED WARNING and WARNINGS AND PRECAUTIONS (5.2)]
• Neuroleptic Malignant Syndrome (NMS) [see WARNINGS AND PRECAUTIONS (5.3)]
• Tardive Dyskinesia [see WARNINGS AND PRECAUTIONS (5.4)]
• Hyperglycemia and Diabetes Mellitus [see WARNINGS AND PRECAUTIONS (5.5)]

- Orthostatic Hypotension [see WARNINGS AND PRECAUTIONS (5.6)]
- Leukopenia, Neutropenia, and Agranulocytosis [see WARNINGS AND PRECAUTIONS (5.7)]
- Seizures/Convulsions [see WARNINGS AND PRECAUTIONS (5.8)]
- Potential for Cognitive and Motor Impairment [see WARNINGS AND PRECAUTIONS (5.9)]
- Body Temperature Regulation [see WARNINGS AND PRECAUTIONS (5.10)]
- Suicide [see WARNINGS AND PRECAUTIONS (5.11)]
- Dysphagia [see WARNINGS AND PRECAUTIONS (5.12)]
- Use in Patients with Concomitant Illness [see WARNINGS AND PRECAUTIONS (5.13)]

The most common adverse reactions in adult patients in clinical trials (≥10%) were nausea, vomiting, constipation, headache, dizziness, akathisia, anxiety, insomnia, and restlessness.

The most common adverse reactions in the pediatric clinical trials (≥10%) were somnolence, headache, vomiting, extrapyramidal disorder, fatigue, increased appetite, insomnia, nausea, nasopharyngitis, and weight increased.

Aripiprazole has been evaluated for safety in 13,543 adult patients who participated in multiple-dose, clinical trials in schizophrenia, bipolar disorder, major depressive disorder, Dementia of the Alzheimer's type, Parkinson's disease, and alcoholism, and who had approximately 7619 patient-years of exposure to oral aripiprazole and 749 patients with exposure to aripiprazole injection. A total of 3390 patients were treated with oral aripiprazole for at least 180 days and 1933 patients treated with oral aripiprazole had at least 1 year of exposure.

Aripiprazole has been evaluated for safety in 920 patients (6 to 17 years) who participated in multiple-dose, clinical trials in schizophrenia, bipolar mania, or autistic disorder and who had approximately 517 patient-years of exposure to oral aripiprazole. A total of 465 pediatric patients were treated with oral aripiprazole for at least 180 days and 117 pediatric patients treated with oral aripiprazole had at least 1 year of exposure.

The conditions and duration of treatment with aripiprazole (monotherapy and adjunctive therapy with antidepressants or mood stabilizers) included (in overlapping categories) double-blind, comparative and noncomparative open-label studies, inpatient and outpatient studies, fixed- and flexible-dose studies, and short- and longer-term exposure. Adverse events during exposure were obtained by collecting volunteered adverse events, as well as results of physical examinations, vital signs, weights, laboratory analyses, and ECG. Adverse experiences were recorded by clinical investigators using terminology of their own choosing. In the tables and tabulations that follow, MedDRA dictionary terminology has been used to classify reported adverse events into a smaller number of standardized event categories, in order to provide a meaningful estimate of the proportion of individuals experiencing adverse events.

The stated frequencies of adverse reactions represent the proportion of individuals who experienced at least once, a treatment-emergent adverse event of the type listed. An event was considered treatment emergent if it occurred for the first time or worsened while receiving therapy following baseline evaluation. There was no attempt to use investigator causality assessments; ie, all events meeting the defined criteria, regardless of investigator causality are included. Throughout this section, adverse reactions are reported. These are adverse events that were considered to be reasonably associated with the use of ABILIFY (aripiprazole) (adverse drug reactions) based on the comprehensive assessment of the available adverse event information. A causal association for ABILIFY often cannot be reliably established in individual cases.

The figures in the tables and tabulations cannot be used to predict the incidence of side effects in the course of usual medical practice where patient characteristics and other factors differ from those that prevailed in the clinical trials. Similarly, the cited frequencies cannot be compared with figures obtained from other clinical investigations involving different treatment, uses, and investigators. The cited figures, however, do provide the prescriber with some basis for estimating the relative contribution of drug and nondrug factors to the adverse reaction incidence in the population studied.

6.2 Clinical Studies Experience
Adult Patients with Schizophrenia
The following findings are based on a pool of five placebo-controlled trials (four 4-week and one 6-week) in which oral aripiprazole was administered in doses ranging from 2 mg/day to 30 mg/day.
Adverse Reactions Associated with Discontinuation of Treatment
Overall, there was little difference in the incidence of discontinuation due to adverse reactions between aripiprazole-treated (7%) and placebo-treated (9%) patients. The types of

adverse reactions that led to discontinuation were similar for the aripiprazole-treated and placebo-treated patients.
Commonly Observed Adverse Reactions
The only commonly observed adverse reaction associated with the use of aripiprazole in patients with schizophrenia (incidence of 5% or greater and aripiprazole incidence at least twice that for placebo) was akathisia (aripiprazole 8%; placebo 4%).
Adult Patients with Bipolar Mania
Monotherapy
The following findings are based on a pool of 3-week, placebo-controlled, bipolar mania trials in which oral aripiprazole was administered at doses of 15 mg/day or 30 mg/day.
Adverse Reactions Associated with Discontinuation of Treatment
Overall, in patients with bipolar mania, there was little difference in the incidence of discontinuation due to adverse reactions between aripiprazole-treated (11%) and placebo-treated (10%) patients. The types of adverse reactions that led to discontinuation were similar between the aripiprazole-treated and placebo-treated patients.
Commonly Observed Adverse Reactions
Commonly observed adverse reactions associated with the use of aripiprazole in patients with bipolar mania (incidence of 5% or greater and aripiprazole incidence at least twice that for placebo) are shown in Table 5.

Table 5: Commonly Observed Adverse Reactions in Short-Term, Placebo-Controlled Trials of Adult Patients with Bipolar Mania Treated with Oral ABILIFY Monotherapy

| Preferred Term | Percentage of Patients Reporting Reaction | |
	Aripiprazole (n=917)	Placebo (n=753)
Akathisia	13	4
Sedation	8	3
Restlessness	6	3
Tremor	6	3
Extrapyramidal Disorder	5	2

Less Common Adverse Reactions in Adults
Table 6 enumerates the pooled incidence, rounded to the nearest percent, of adverse reactions that occurred during acute therapy (up to 6 weeks in schizophrenia and up to 3 weeks in bipolar mania), including only those reactions that occurred in 2% or more of patients treated with aripiprazole (doses ≥2 mg/day) and for which the incidence in patients treated with aripiprazole was greater than the incidence in patients treated with placebo in the combined dataset.

Table 6: Adverse Reactions in Short-Term, Placebo-Controlled Trials in Adult Patients Treated with Oral ABILIFY

| System Organ Class Preferred Term | Percentage of Patients Reporting Reaction[a] | |
	Aripiprazole (n=1843)	Placebo (n=1166)
Eye Disorders		
Blurred Vision	3	1
Gastrointestinal Disorders		
Nausea	15	11
Constipation	11	7
Vomiting	11	6
Dyspepsia	9	7
Dry Mouth	5	4
Toothache	4	3
Abdominal Discomfort	3	2
Stomach Discomfort	3	2
General Disorders and Administration Site Conditions		
Fatigue	6	4
Pain	3	2
Musculoskeletal and Connective Tissue Disorders		
Musculoskeletal Stiffness	4	3
Pain in Extremity	4	2
Myalgia	2	1
Muscle Spasms	2	1
Nervous System Disorders		
Headache	27	23
Dizziness	10	7
Akathisia	10	4
Sedation	7	4
Extrapyramidal Disorder	5	3
Tremor	5	3
Somnolence	5	3
Psychiatric Disorders		
Agitation	19	17

Insomnia	18	13
Anxiety	17	13
Restlessness	5	3
Respiratory, Thoracic, and Mediastinal Disorders		
Pharyngolaryngeal Pain	3	2
Cough	3	2

[a] Adverse reactions reported by at least 2% of patients treated with oral aripiprazole, except adverse reactions which had an incidence equal to or less than placebo.

An examination of population subgroups did not reveal any clear evidence of differential adverse reaction incidence on the basis of age, gender, or race.
Adult Patients with Adjunctive Therapy with Bipolar Mania
The following findings are based on a placebo-controlled trial of adult patients with bipolar disorder in which aripiprazole was administered at doses of 15 mg/day or 30 mg/day as adjunctive therapy with lithium or valproate.
Adverse Reactions Associated with Discontinuation of Treatment
In a study of patients who were already tolerating either lithium or valproate as monotherapy, discontinuation rates due to adverse reactions were 12% for patients treated with adjunctive aripiprazole compared to 6% for patients treated with adjunctive placebo. The most common adverse drug reactions associated with discontinuation in the adjunctive aripiprazole-treated compared to placebo-treated patients were akathisia (5% and 1%, respectively) and tremor (2% and 1%, respectively).
Commonly Observed Adverse Reactions
The commonly observed adverse reactions associated with adjunctive aripiprazole and lithium or valproate in patients with bipolar mania (incidence of 5% or greater and incidence at least twice that for adjunctive placebo) were: akathisia, insomnia, and extrapyramidal disorder.
Less Common Adverse Reactions in Adult Patients with Adjunctive Therapy in Bipolar Mania
Table 7 enumerates the incidence, rounded to the nearest percent, of adverse reactions that occurred during acute treatment (up to 6 weeks), including only those reactions that occurred in 2% or more of patients treated with adjunctive aripiprazole (doses of 15 mg/day or 30 mg/day) and lithium or valproate and for which the incidence in patients treated with this combination was greater than the incidence in patients treated with placebo plus lithium or valproate.

Table 7: Adverse Reactions in a Short-Term, Placebo-Controlled Trial of Adjunctive Therapy in Patients with Bipolar Disorder

| System Organ Class Preferred Term | Percentage of Patients Reporting Reaction[a] | |
	Aripiprazole + Li or Val* (n=253)	Placebo + Li or Val* (n=130)
Gastrointestinal Disorders		
Nausea	8	5
Vomiting	4	0
Salivary Hypersecretion	4	2
Dry Mouth	2	1
Infections and Infestations		
Nasopharyngitis	3	2
Investigations		
Weight Increased	2	1
Nervous System Disorders		
Akathisia	19	5
Tremor	9	6
Extrapyramidal Disorder	5	1
Dizziness	4	1
Sedation	4	2
Psychiatric Disorders		
Insomnia	8	4
Anxiety	4	1
Restlessness	2	1

[a] Adverse reactions reported by at least 2% of patients treated with oral aripiprazole, except adverse reactions which had an incidence equal to or less than placebo.
*Lithium or Valproate

Pediatric Patients (13 to 17 years) with Schizophrenia
The following findings are based on one 6-week placebo-controlled trial in which oral aripiprazole was administered in doses ranging from 2 mg/day to 30 mg/day.
Adverse Reactions Associated with Discontinuation of Treatment
The incidence of discontinuation due to adverse reactions between aripiprazole-treated and placebo-treated pediatric patients (13 to 17 years) was 5% and 2%, respectively.

Commonly Observed Adverse Reactions
Commonly observed adverse reactions associated with the use of aripiprazole in adolescent patients with schizophrenia (incidence of 5% or greater and aripiprazole incidence at least twice that for placebo) were extrapyramidal disorder, somnolence, and tremor.

Pediatric Patients (10 to 17 years) with Bipolar Mania
The following findings are based on one 4-week placebo-controlled trial in which oral aripiprazole was administered in doses of 10 mg/day or 30 mg/day.
Adverse Reactions Associated with Discontinuation of Treatment
The incidence of discontinuation due to adverse reactions between aripiprazole-treated and placebo-treated pediatric patients (10 to 17 years) was 7% and 2%, respectively.
Commonly Observed Adverse Reactions
Commonly observed adverse reactions associated with the use of aripiprazole in pediatric patients with bipolar mania (incidence of 5% or greater and aripiprazole incidence at least twice that for placebo) are shown in Table 8.

Table 8: Commonly Observed Adverse Reactions in Short-Term, Placebo-Controlled Trials of Pediatric Patients (10 to 17 years) with Bipolar Mania Treated with Oral ABILIFY

| Preferred Term | Percentage of Patients Reporting Reaction | |
	Aripiprazole (n=197)	Placebo (n=97)
Somnolence	23	3
Extrapyramidal Disorder	20	3
Fatigue	11	4
Nausea	11	4
Akathisia	10	2
Blurred Vision	8	0
Salivary Hypersecretion	6	0
Dizziness	5	1

Pediatric Patients (6 to 17 years) with Autistic Disorder
The following findings are based on two 8-week, placebo-controlled trials in which oral aripiprazole was administered in doses of 2 mg/day to 15 mg/day.
Adverse Reactions Associated with Discontinuation of Treatment
The incidence of discontinuation due to adverse reactions between aripiprazole-treated and placebo-treated pediatric patients (6 to 17 years) was 10% and 8%, respectively.
Commonly Observed Adverse Reactions
Commonly observed adverse reactions associated with the use of aripiprazole in pediatric patients with autistic disorder (incidence of 5% or greater and aripiprazole incidence at least twice that for placebo) are shown in Table 9.

Table 9: Commonly Observed Adverse Reactions in Short-Term, Placebo-Controlled Trials of Pediatric Patients (6 to 17 years) with Autistic Disorder Treated with Oral ABILIFY

| Preferred Term | Percentage of Patients Reporting Reaction | |
	Aripiprazole (n=212)	Placebo (n=101)
Sedation	21	4
Fatigue	17	2
Vomiting	14	7
Somnolence	10	4
Tremor	10	0
Pyrexia	9	1
Drooling	9	0
Decreased Appetite	7	2
Salivary Hypersecretion	6	1
Extrapyramidal Disorder	6	0
Lethargy	5	0

Less Common Adverse Reactions in Pediatric Patients (6 to 17 years) with Schizophrenia, Bipolar Mania, or Autistic Disorder
Table 10 enumerates the pooled incidence, rounded to the nearest percent, of adverse reactions that occurred during acute therapy (up to 6 weeks in schizophrenia, up to 4 weeks in bipolar mania, and up to 8 weeks in autistic disorder), including only those reactions that occurred in 1% or more of pediatric patients treated with aripiprazole (doses ≥2 mg/day) and for which the incidence in patients treated with aripiprazole was greater than the incidence in patients treated with placebo.

Table 10: Adverse Reactions in Short-Term, Placebo-Controlled Trials of Pediatric Patients (6 to 17 years) Treated with Oral ABILIFY

| System Organ Class Preferred Term | Percentage of Patients Reporting Reaction[a] | |
	Aripiprazole (n=611)	Placebo (n=298)
Eye Disorders		
Blurred Vision	3	0
Gastrointestinal Disorders		
Vomiting	9	7
Nausea	8	4
Diarrhea	5	3
Salivary Hypersecretion	4	1
Abdominal Pain Upper	3	2
Constipation	3	2
Dry Mouth	1	0
General Disorders and Administration Site Conditions		
Fatigue	10	2
Pyrexia	5	1
Irritability	1	0
Thirst	1	0
Infections and Infestations		
Nasopharyngitis	6	3
Investigations		
Weight Increased	2	1
Metabolism and Nutrition Disorders		
Increased Appetite	7	3
Decreased Appetite	4	2
Musculoskeletal and Connective Tissue Disorders		
Arthralgia	1	0
Musculoskeletal Stiffness	1	0
Nervous System Disorders		
Somnolence	16	4
Extrapyramidal Disorder	14	2
Headache	13	12
Sedation	8	1
Akathisia	6	1
Tremor	6	1
Drooling	4	0
Dizziness	3	1
Lethargy	2	0
Dystonia	1	0
Dyskinesia	1	0
Hypersomnia	1	0
Reproductive System and Breast Disorders		
Dysmenorrhoea*	2	1
Respiratory, Thoracic, and Mediastinal Disorders		
Rhinorrhoea	2	1
Skin and Subcutaneous Tissue Disorders		
Rash	2	1

[a] Adverse reactions reported by at least 1% of pediatric patients treated with oral aripiprazole, except adverse reactions which had an incidence equal to or less than placebo.
* Adjusted for gender.

Adult Patients Receiving ABILIFY (aripiprazole) as Adjunctive Treatment of Major Depressive Disorder
The following findings are based on a pool of two placebo-controlled trials of patients with major depressive disorder in which aripiprazole was administered at doses of 2 mg to 20 mg as adjunctive treatment to continued antidepressant therapy.
Adverse Reactions Associated with Discontinuation of Treatment
The incidence of discontinuation due to adverse reactions was 6% for adjunctive aripiprazole-treated patients and 2% for adjunctive placebo-treated patients.
Commonly Observed Adverse Reactions
The commonly observed adverse reactions associated with the use of adjunctive aripiprazole in patients with major depressive disorder (incidence of 5% or greater and aripiprazole incidence at least twice that for placebo) were: akathisia, restlessness, insomnia, constipation, fatigue, and blurred vision.
Less Common Adverse Reactions in Adult Patients with Major Depressive Disorder
Table 11 enumerates the pooled incidence, rounded to the nearest percent, of adverse reactions that occurred during acute therapy (up to 6 weeks), including only those adverse reactions that occurred in 2% or more of patients treated with adjunctive aripiprazole (doses ≥2 mg/day) and for which the incidence in patients treated with adjunctive aripiprazole was greater than the incidence in patients treated with adjunctive placebo in the combined dataset.

Table 11: Adverse Reactions in Short-Term, Placebo-Controlled Adjunctive Trials in Patients with Major Depressive Disorder

| System Organ Class Preferred Term | Percentage of Patients Reporting Reaction[a] | |
	Aripiprazole+ADT* (n=371)	Placebo+ADT* (n=366)
Eye Disorders		
Blurred Vision	6	1
Gastrointestinal Disorders		
Constipation	5	2
General Disorders and Administration Site Conditions		
Fatigue	8	4
Feeling Jittery	3	1
Infections and Infestations		
Upper Respiratory Tract Infection	6	4
Investigations		
Weight Increased	3	2
Metabolism and Nutrition Disorders		
Increased Appetite	3	2
Musculoskeletal and Connective Tissue Disorders		
Arthralgia	4	3
Myalgia	3	1
Nervous System Disorders		
Akathisia	25	4
Somnolence	6	4
Tremor	5	4
Sedation	4	2
Dizziness	4	2
Disturbance in Attention	3	1
Extrapyramidal Disorder	2	0
Psychiatric Disorders		
Restlessness	12	2
Insomnia	8	2

[a] Adverse reactions reported by at least 2% of patients treated with adjunctive aripiprazole, except adverse reactions which had an incidence equal to or less than placebo.
* Antidepressant Therapy

Patients with Agitation Associated with Schizophrenia or Bipolar Mania (Intramuscular Injection)
The following findings are based on a pool of three placebo-controlled trials of patients with agitation associated with schizophrenia or bipolar mania in which aripiprazole injection was administered at doses of 5.25 mg to 15 mg.
Adverse Reactions Associated with Discontinuation of Treatment
Overall, in patients with agitation associated with schizophrenia or bipolar mania, there was little difference in the incidence of discontinuation due to adverse reactions between aripiprazole-treated (0.8%) and placebo-treated (0.5%) patients.
Commonly Observed Adverse Reactions
There was one commonly observed adverse reaction (nausea) associated with the use of aripiprazole injection in patients with agitation associated with schizophrenia and bipolar mania (incidence of 5% or greater and aripiprazole incidence at least twice that for placebo).
Less Common Adverse Reactions in Patients with Agitation Associated with Schizophrenia or Bipolar Mania
Table 12 enumerates the pooled incidence, rounded to the nearest percent, of adverse reactions that occurred during acute therapy (24-hour), including only those adverse reactions that occurred in 2% or more of patients treated with aripiprazole injection (doses ≥5.25 mg/day) and for which the incidence in patients treated with aripiprazole injection was greater than the incidence in patients treated with placebo in the combined dataset.

Table 12: Adverse Reactions in Short-Term, Placebo-Controlled Trials in Patients Treated with ABILIFY Injection

| System Organ Class Preferred Term | Percentage of Patients Reporting Reaction[a] | |
	Aripiprazole (n=501)	Placebo (n=220)
Cardiac Disorders		
Tachycardia	2	<1
Gastrointestinal Disorders		
Nausea	9	3
Vomiting	3	1
General Disorders and Administration Site Conditions		
Fatigue	2	1
Nervous System Disorders		
Headache	12	7

Dizziness	8	5
Somnolence	7	4
Sedation	3	2
Akathisia	2	0

[a] Adverse reactions reported by at least 2% of patients treated with aripiprazole injection, except adverse reactions which had an incidence equal to or less than placebo.

Dose-Related Adverse Reactions

Schizophrenia

Dose response relationships for the incidence of treatment-emergent adverse events were evaluated from four trials in adult patients with schizophrenia comparing various fixed doses (2 mg/day, 5 mg/day, 10 mg/day, 15 mg/day, 20 mg/day, and 30 mg/day) of oral aripiprazole to placebo. This analysis, stratified by study, indicated that the only adverse reaction to have a possible dose response relationship, and then most prominent only with 30 mg, was somnolence [including sedation]; (incidences were placebo, 7.1%; 10 mg, 8.5%; 15 mg, 8.7%; 20 mg, 7.5%; 30 mg, 12.6%).

In the study of pediatric patients (13 to 17 years of age) with schizophrenia, three common adverse reactions appeared to have a possible dose response relationship: extrapyramidal disorder (incidences were placebo, 5.0%; 10 mg, 13.0%; 30 mg, 21.6%); somnolence (incidences were placebo, 6.0%; 10 mg, 11.0%; 30 mg, 21.6%); and tremor (incidences were placebo, 2.0%; 10 mg, 2.0%; 30 mg, 11.8%).

Bipolar Mania

In the study of pediatric patients (10 to 17 years of age) with bipolar mania, four common adverse reactions had a possible dose response relationship at 4 weeks; extrapyramidal disorder (incidences were placebo, 3.1%; 10 mg, 12.2%; 30 mg, 27.3%); somnolence (incidences were placebo, 3.1%; 10 mg, 19.4%; 30 mg, 26.3%); akathisia (incidences were placebo, 2.1%; 10 mg, 8.2%; 30 mg, 11.1%); and salivary hypersecretion (incidences were placebo, 0%; 10 mg, 3.1%; 30 mg, 8.1%).

Autistic Disorder

In a study of pediatric patients (6 to 17 years of age) with autistic disorder, one common adverse reaction had a possible dose response relationship: fatigue (incidences were placebo, 0%; 5 mg, 3.8%; 10 mg, 22.0%; 15 mg, 18.5%).

Extrapyramidal Symptoms

Schizophrenia

In short-term, placebo-controlled trials in schizophrenia in adults, the incidence of reported EPS-related events, excluding events related to akathisia, for aripiprazole-treated patients was 13% vs. 12% for placebo; and the incidence of akathisia-related events for aripiprazole-treated patients was 8% vs. 4% for placebo. In the short-term, placebo-controlled trial of schizophrenia in pediatric (13 to 17 years) patients, the incidence of reported EPS-related events, excluding events related to akathisia, for aripiprazole-treated patients was 25% vs. 7% for placebo; and the incidence of akathisia-related events for aripiprazole-treated patients was 9% vs. 6% for placebo.

Objectively collected data from those trials was collected on the Simpson Angus Rating Scale (for EPS), the Barnes Akathisia Scale (for akathisia), and the Assessments of Involuntary Movement Scales (for dyskinesias). In the adult schizophrenia trials, the objectively collected data did not show a difference between aripiprazole and placebo, with the exception of the Barnes Akathisia Scale (aripiprazole, 0.08; placebo, -0.05). In the pediatric (13 to 17 years) schizophrenia trial, the objectively collected data did not show a difference between aripiprazole and placebo, with the exception of the Simpson Angus Rating Scale (aripiprazole, 0.24; placebo, -0.29).

Similarly, in a long-term (26-week), placebo-controlled trial of schizophrenia in adults, objectively collected data on the Simpson Angus Rating Scale (for EPS), the Barnes Akathisia Scale (for akathisia), and the Assessments of Involuntary Movement Scales (for dyskinesias) did not show a difference between aripiprazole and placebo.

Bipolar Mania

In the short-term, placebo-controlled trials in bipolar mania in adults, the incidence of reported EPS-related events, excluding events related to akathisia, for monotherapy aripiprazole-treated patients was 16% vs. 8% for placebo and the incidence of akathisia-related events for monotherapy aripiprazole-treated patients was 13% vs. 4% for placebo. In the 6-week, placebo-controlled trial in bipolar mania for adjunctive therapy with lithium or valproate, the incidence of reported EPS-related events, excluding events related to akathisia for adjunctive aripiprazole-treated patients was 15% vs. 8% for adjunctive placebo and the incidence of akathisia-related events for adjunctive aripiprazole-treated patients was 19% vs. 5% for adjunctive placebo. In the short-term, placebo-controlled trial in bipolar mania in pediatric (10 to 17 years) patients, the incidence of reported EPS-related events, excluding events related to akathisia, for aripiprazole-treated patients was 26% vs. 5% for placebo and the incidence of akathisia-related events for aripiprazole-treated patients was 10% vs. 2% for placebo.

In the adult bipolar mania trials with monotherapy aripiprazole, the Simpson Angus Rating Scale and the Barnes Akathisia Scale showed a significant difference between aripiprazole and placebo (aripiprazole, 0.50; placebo, -0.01 and aripiprazole, 0.21; placebo, -0.05). Changes in the Assessments of Involuntary Movement Scales were similar for the aripiprazole and placebo groups. In the bipolar mania trials with aripiprazole as adjunctive therapy with either lithium or valproate, the Simpson Angus Rating Scale and the Barnes Akathisia Scale showed a significant difference between adjunctive aripiprazole and adjunctive placebo (aripiprazole, 0.73; placebo, 0.07 and aripiprazole, 0.30; placebo, 0.11). Changes in the Assessments of Involuntary Movement Scales were similar for adjunctive aripiprazole and adjunctive placebo. In the pediatric (10 to 17 years) short-term bipolar mania trial, the Simpson Angus Rating Scale showed a significant difference between aripiprazole and placebo (aripiprazole, 0.90; placebo, -0.05). Changes in the Barnes Akathisia Scale and the Assessments of Involuntary Movement Scales were similar for the aripiprazole and placebo groups.

Major Depressive Disorder

In the short-term, placebo-controlled trials in major depressive disorder, the incidence of reported EPS-related events, excluding events related to akathisia, for adjunctive aripiprazole-treated patients was 8% vs. 5% for adjunctive placebo-treated patients; and the incidence of akathisia-related events for adjunctive aripiprazole-treated patients was 25% vs. 4% for adjunctive placebo-treated patients.

In the major depressive disorder trials, the Simpson Angus Rating Scale and the Barnes Akathisia Scale showed a significant difference between adjunctive aripiprazole and adjunctive placebo (aripiprazole, 0.31; placebo, 0.03 and aripiprazole, 0.22; placebo, 0.02). Changes in the Assessments of Involuntary Movement Scales were similar for the adjunctive aripiprazole and adjunctive placebo groups.

Autistic Disorder

In the short-term, placebo-controlled trials in autistic disorder in pediatric patients (6 to 17 years), the incidence of reported EPS-related events, excluding events related to akathisia, for aripiprazole-treated patients was 18% vs. 2% for placebo and the incidence of akathisia-related events for aripiprazole-treated patients was 3% vs. 9% for placebo.

In the pediatric (6 to 17 years) short-term autistic disorder trials, the Simpson Angus Rating Scale showed a significant difference between aripiprazole and placebo (aripiprazole, 0.1; placebo, -0.4). Changes in the Barnes Akathisia Scale and the Assessments of Involuntary Movement Scales were similar for the aripiprazole and placebo groups.

Agitation Associated with Schizophrenia or Bipolar Mania

In the placebo-controlled trials in patients with agitation associated with schizophrenia or bipolar mania, the incidence of reported EPS-related events excluding events related to akathisia for aripiprazole-treated patients was 2% vs. 2% for placebo and the incidence of akathisia-related events for aripiprazole-treated patients was 2% vs. 0% for placebo. Objectively collected data on the Simpson Angus Rating Scale (for EPS) and the Barnes Akathisia Scale (for akathisia) for all treatment groups did not show a difference between aripiprazole and placebo.

Dystonia

Class Effect: Symptoms of dystonia, prolonged abnormal contractions of muscle groups, may occur in susceptible individuals during the first few days of treatment. Dystonic symptoms include: spasm of the neck muscles, sometimes progressing to tightness of the throat, swallowing difficulty, difficulty breathing, and/or protrusion of the tongue. While these symptoms can occur at low doses, they occur more frequently and with greater severity with high potency and at higher doses of first generation antipsychotic drugs. An elevated risk of acute dystonia is observed in males and younger age groups.

Laboratory Test Abnormalities

A between group comparison for 3-week to 6-week, placebo-controlled trials in adults or 4-week to 8-week, placebo-controlled trials in pediatric patients (6 to 17 years) revealed no medically important differences between the aripiprazole and placebo groups in the proportions of patients experiencing potentially clinically significant changes in routine serum chemistry, hematology, or urinalysis parameters. Similarly, there were no aripiprazole/placebo differences in the incidence of discontinuations for changes in serum chemistry, hematology, or urinalysis in adult or pediatric patients.

In the 6-week trials of aripiprazole as adjunctive therapy for major depressive disorder, there were no clinically important differences between the adjunctive aripiprazole-treated and adjunctive placebo-treated patients in the median change from baseline in prolactin, fasting glucose, HDL, LDL, or total cholesterol measurements. The median % change from baseline in triglycerides was 5% for adjunctive aripiprazole-treated patients vs. 0% for adjunctive placebo-treated patients.

In a long-term (26-week), placebo-controlled trial there were no medically important differences between the aripiprazole and placebo patients in the mean change from baseline in prolactin, fasting glucose, triglyceride, HDL, LDL, or total cholesterol measurements.

Weight Gain

In 4-week to 6-week trials in adults with schizophrenia, there was a slight difference in mean weight gain between aripiprazole and placebo patients (+0.7 kg vs. -0.05 kg, respectively) and also a difference in the proportion of patients meeting a weight gain criterion of ≥7% of body weight [aripiprazole (8%) compared to placebo (3%)]. In a 6-week trial in pediatric patients (13 to 17 years) with schizophrenia, there was a slight difference in mean weight gain between aripiprazole and placebo patients (+0.13 kg vs. -0.83 kg, respectively) and also a difference in the proportion of patients meeting a weight gain criterion of ≥7% of body weight [aripiprazole (5%) compared to placebo (1%)].

In 3-week trials in adults with mania with monotherapy aripiprazole, the mean weight gain for aripiprazole and placebo patients was 0.1 kg vs. 0.0 kg, respectively. The proportion of patients meeting a weight gain criterion of ≥7% of body weight was aripiprazole (2%) compared to placebo (3%). In the 6-week trial in mania with aripiprazole as adjunctive therapy with either lithium or valproate, the mean weight gain for aripiprazole and placebo patients was 0.6 kg vs. 0.2 kg, respectively. The proportion of patients meeting a weight gain criterion of ≥7% of body weight with adjunctive aripiprazole was 3% compared to adjunctive placebo 4%.

In the trials adding aripiprazole to antidepressants, patients first received 8 weeks of antidepressant treatment followed by 6 weeks of adjunctive aripiprazole or placebo in addition to their ongoing antidepressant treatment. The mean weight gain with adjunctive aripiprazole was 1.7 kg vs. 0.4 kg with adjunctive placebo. The proportion of patients meeting a weight gain criterion of ≥7% of body weight was 5% with adjunctive aripiprazole compared to 1% with adjunctive placebo.

In the two short term, placebo-controlled trials in patients (6 to 17 years) with autistic disorder, the mean increase in body weight in the aripiprazole group was 1.6 kg vs. 0.4 kg in the placebo group. The proportion of patients meeting a weight gain criterion of ≥7% of body weight was 26% in aripiprazole group compared to 7% in placebo group.

Table 13 provides the weight change results from a long-term (26-week), placebo-controlled study of aripiprazole in adults with schizophrenia, both mean change from baseline and proportions of patients meeting a weight gain criterion of ≥7% of body weight relative to baseline, categorized by BMI at baseline. Although there was no mean weight increase, the aripiprazole group tended to show more patients with a ≥7% weight gain.

[See table 13 above]

Table 13: Weight Change Results Categorized by BMI at Baseline: Placebo-Controlled Study in Schizophrenia, Safety Sample

	BMI <23		BMI 23-27		BMI >27	
	Placebo (n=54)	Aripiprazole (n=59)	Placebo (n=48)	Aripiprazole (n=39)	Placebo (n=49)	Aripiprazole (n=53)
Mean change from baseline (kg)	-0.5	-0.5	-0.6	-1.3	-1.5	-2.1
% with ≥7% increase BW	3.7%	6.8%	4.2%	5.1%	4.1%	5.7%

Table 14 provides the weight change results from a long-term (52-week) study of aripiprazole in adults with schizophrenia, both mean change from baseline and proportions of patients meeting a weight gain criterion of ≥7% of body weight relative to baseline, categorized by BMI at baseline:

Table 14: Weight Change Results Categorized by BMI at Baseline: Active-Controlled Study in Schizophrenia, Safety Sample

	BMI <23 (n=314)	BMI 23-27 (n=265)	BMI >27 (n=260)
Mean change from baseline (kg)	2.6	1.4	-1.2
% with ≥7% increase BW	30%	19%	8%

ECG Changes

Between group comparisons for a pooled analysis of placebo-controlled trials in patients with schizophrenia, bipolar mania, or major depressive disorder revealed no significant differences between oral aripiprazole and placebo in the proportion of patients experiencing potentially important changes in ECG parameters. Aripiprazole was associated with a median increase in heart rate of 2 beats per minute compared to no increase among placebo patients.

In the pooled, placebo-controlled trials in patients with agitation associated with schizophrenia or bipolar mania, there were no significant differences between aripiprazole injection and placebo in the proportion of patients experiencing potentially important changes in ECG parameters, as measured by standard 12-lead ECGs.

Additional Findings Observed in Clinical Trials

Adverse Reactions in Long-Term, Double-Blind, Placebo-Controlled Trials

The adverse reactions reported in a 26-week, double-blind trial comparing oral ABILIFY and placebo in patients with schizophrenia were generally consistent with those reported in the short-term, placebo-controlled trials, except for a higher incidence of tremor [8% (12/153) for ABILIFY vs. 2% (3/153) for placebo]. In this study, the majority of the cases of tremor were of mild intensity (8/12 mild and 4/12 moderate), occurred early in therapy (9/12 ≤49 days), and were of limited duration (7/12 ≤10 days). Tremor infrequently led to discontinuation (<1%) of ABILIFY. In addition, in a long-term (52-week), active-controlled study, the incidence of tremor was 5% (40/859) for ABILIFY. A similar profile was observed in a long-term study in bipolar disorder.

Other Adverse Reactions Observed During the Premarketing Evaluation of Aripiprazole

Following is a list of MedDRA terms that reflect adverse reactions as defined in *ADVERSE REACTIONS (6.1)* reported by patients treated with oral aripiprazole at multiple doses ≥2 mg/day during any phase of a trial within the database of 13,543 adult patients. All events assessed as possible adverse drug reactions have been included with the exception of more commonly occurring events. In addition, medically/clinically meaningful adverse reactions, particularly those that are likely to be useful to the prescriber or that have pharmacologic plausibility, have been included. Events already listed in other parts of *ADVERSE REACTIONS (6)*, or those considered in *WARNINGS AND PRECAUTIONS (5)* or *OVERDOSAGE (10)* have been excluded. Although the reactions reported occurred during treatment with aripiprazole, they were not necessarily caused by it.

Events are further categorized by MedDRA system organ class and listed in order of decreasing frequency according to the following definitions: those occurring in at least 1/100 patients (only those not already listed in the tabulated results from placebo-controlled trials appear in this listing); those occurring in 1/100 to 1/1000 patients; and those occurring in fewer than 1/1000 patients.

Adults - Oral Administration

Blood and Lymphatic System Disorders:

≥1/1000 patients and <1/100 patients - leukopenia, neutropenia, thrombocytopenia

Cardiac Disorders:

≥1/1000 patients and <1/100 patients - bradycardia, palpitations, cardiopulmonary failure, myocardial infarction, cardio-respiratory arrest, atrioventricular block, extrasystoles, sinus tachycardia, atrial fibrillation, angina pectoris, myocardial ischemia; *<1/1000 patients* - atrial flutter, supraventricular tachycardia, ventricular tachycardia

Eye Disorders:

≥1/1000 patients and <1/100 patients - photophobia, diplopia, eyelid edema, photopsia

Gastrointestinal Disorders:

≥1/1000 patients and <1/100 patients - gastroesophageal reflux disease, swollen tongue, esophagitis; *<1/1000 patients* - pancreatitis

General Disorders and Administration Site Conditions:

≥1/100 patients - asthenia, peripheral edema, chest pain; *≥1/1000 patients and <1/100 patients* - face edema, angioedema; *<1/1000 patients* - hypothermia

Hepatobiliary Disorders:

<1/1000 patients - hepatitis, jaundice

Immune System Disorders:

≥1/1000 patients and <1/100 patients - hypersensitivity

Injury, Poisoning, and Procedural Complications:

≥1/100 patients - fall; *≥1/1000 patients and <1/100 patients* - self mutilation; *<1/1000 patients* - heat stroke

Investigations:

≥1/100 patients - weight decreased, creatine phosphokinase increased; *≥1/1000 patients and <1/100 patients* - hepatic enzyme increased, blood glucose increased, blood prolactin increased, blood urea increased, electrocardiogram QT prolonged, blood creatinine increased, blood bilirubin increased; *<1/1000 patients* - blood lactate dehydrogenase increased, glycosylated hemoglobin increased, gamma-glutamyl transferase increased

Metabolism and Nutrition Disorders:

≥1/1000 patients and <1/100 patients - hyperlipidemia, anorexia, diabetes mellitus (including blood insulin increased, carbohydrate tolerance decreased, diabetes mellitus non-insulin-dependent, glucose tolerance impaired, glycosuria, glucose urine, glucose urine present), hyperglycemia, hypokalemia, hyponatremia, hypoglycemia, polydipsia; *<1/1000 patients* - diabetic ketoacidosis

Musculoskeletal and Connective Tissue Disorders:

≥1/1000 patients and <1/100 patients - muscle rigidity, muscular weakness, muscle tightness, mobility decreased; *<1/1000 patients* - rhabdomyolysis

Nervous System Disorders:

≥1/100 patients - coordination abnormal; *≥1/1000 patients and <1/100 patients* - speech disorder, parkinsonism, memory impairment, cogwheel rigidity, cerebrovascular accident, hypokinesia, tardive dyskinesia, hypotonia, myoclonus, hypertonia, akinesia, bradykinesia; *<1/1000 patients* - Grand Mal convulsion, choreoathetosis

Psychiatric Disorders:

≥1/100 patients - suicidal ideation; *≥1/1000 patients and <1/100 patients* - aggression, loss of libido, suicide attempt, hostility, libido increased, anger, anorgasmia, delirium, intentional self injury, completed suicide, tic, homicidal ideation; *<1/1000 patients* - catatonia, sleep walking

Renal and Urinary Disorders:

≥1/1000 patients and <1/100 patients - urinary retention, polyuria, nocturia

Reproductive System and Breast Disorders:

≥1/1000 patients and <1/100 patients - menstruation irregular, erectile dysfunction, amenorrhea, breast pain; *<1/1000 patients* - gynaecomastia, priapism

Respiratory, Thoracic, and Mediastinal Disorders:

≥1/100 patients - nasal congestion, dyspnea, pneumonia aspiration

Skin and Subcutaneous Tissue Disorders:

≥1/100 patients - rash (including erythematous, exfoliative, generalized, macular, maculopapular, papular rash; acneiform, allergic, contact, exfoliative, seborrheic dermatitis, neurodermatitis, and drug eruption), hyperhydrosis; *≥1/1000 patients and <1/100 patients* - pruritus, photosensitivity reaction, alopecia, urticaria

Vascular Disorders:

≥1/100 patients - hypertension; *≥1/1000 patients and <1/100 patients* - hypotension

Pediatric Patients - Oral Administration

Most adverse events observed in the pooled database of 920 pediatric patients aged 6 to 17 years were also observed in the adult population. Additional adverse reactions observed in the pediatric population are listed below.

Gastrointestinal Disorders:

≥1/1000 patients and <1/100 patients - tongue dry, tongue spasm

Investigations:

≥1/100 patients - blood insulin increased

Nervous System Disorders:

≥1/1000 patients and <1/100 patients - sleep talking

Skin and Subcutaneous Tissue Disorders:

≥1/1000 patients and <1/100 patients - hirsutism

Adults - Intramuscular Injection

Most adverse reactions observed in the pooled database of 749 adult patients treated with aripiprazole injection, were also observed in the adult population treated with oral aripiprazole. Additional adverse reactions observed in the aripiprazole injection population are listed below.

General Disorders and Administration Site Conditions:

≥1/100 patients - injection site reaction; *≥1/1000 patients and <1/100 patients* - venipuncture site bruise

6.3 Postmarketing Experience

The following adverse reactions have been identified during postapproval use of ABILIFY (aripiprazole). Because these reactions are reported voluntarily from a population of uncertain size, it is not always possible to establish a causal relationship to drug exposure: rare occurrences of allergic reaction (anaphylactic reaction, angioedema, laryngospasm, pruritus/urticaria, or oropharyngeal spasm), and blood glucose fluctuation.

7 DRUG INTERACTIONS

Given the primary CNS effects of aripiprazole, caution should be used when ABILIFY (aripiprazole) is taken in combination with other centrally-acting drugs or alcohol.

Due to its alpha adrenergic antagonism, aripiprazole has the potential to enhance the effect of certain antihypertensive agents.

7.1 Potential for Other Drugs to Affect ABILIFY

Aripiprazole is not a substrate of CYP1A1, CYP1A2, CYP2A6, CYP2B6, CYP2C8, CYP2C9, CYP2C19, or CYP2E1 enzymes. Aripiprazole also does not undergo direct glucuronidation. This suggests that an interaction of aripiprazole with inhibitors or inducers of these enzymes, or other factors, like smoking, is unlikely.

Both CYP3A4 and CYP2D6 are responsible for aripiprazole metabolism. Agents that induce CYP3A4 (eg, carbamazepine) could cause an increase in aripiprazole clearance and lower blood levels. Inhibitors of CYP3A4 (eg, ketoconazole) or CYP2D6 (eg, quinidine, fluoxetine, or paroxetine) can inhibit aripiprazole elimination and cause increased blood levels.

Ketoconazole and Other CYP3A4 Inhibitors

Coadministration of ketoconazole (200 mg/day for 14 days) with a 15 mg single dose of aripiprazole increased the AUC of aripiprazole and its active metabolite by 63% and 77%, respectively. The effect of a higher ketoconazole dose (400 mg/day) has not been studied. When ketoconazole is given concomitantly with aripiprazole, the aripiprazole dose should be reduced to one-half of its normal dose. Other strong inhibitors of CYP3A4 (itraconazole) would be expected to have similar effects and need similar dose reductions; moderate inhibitors (erythromycin, grapefruit juice) have not been studied. When the CYP3A4 inhibitor is withdrawn from the combination therapy, the aripiprazole dose should be increased.

Quinidine and Other CYP2D6 Inhibitors

Coadministration of a 10 mg single dose of aripiprazole with quinidine (166 mg/day for 13 days), a potent inhibitor of CYP2D6, increased the AUC of aripiprazole by 112% but decreased the AUC of its active metabolite, dehydro-aripiprazole, by 35%. Aripiprazole dose should be reduced to one-half of its normal dose when quinidine is given concomitantly with aripiprazole. Other significant inhibitors of CYP2D6, such as fluoxetine or paroxetine, would be expected to have similar effects and should lead to similar dose reductions. When the CYP2D6 inhibitor is withdrawn from the combination therapy, the aripiprazole dose should be increased. When adjunctive ABILIFY is administered to patients with major depressive disorder, ABILIFY should be administered without dosage adjustment as specified in *DOSAGE AND ADMINISTRATION (2.3)*.

Carbamazepine and Other CYP3A4 Inducers

Coadministration of carbamazepine (200 mg twice daily), a potent CYP3A4 inducer, with aripiprazole (30 mg/day) resulted in an approximate 70% decrease in C_{max} and AUC values of both aripiprazole and its active metabolite, dehydro-aripiprazole. When carbamazepine is added to aripiprazole therapy, aripiprazole dose should be doubled. Additional dose increases should be based on clinical evaluation. When carbamazepine is withdrawn from the combination therapy, the aripiprazole dose should be reduced.

7.2 Potential for ABILIFY to Affect Other Drugs

Aripiprazole is unlikely to cause clinically important pharmacokinetic interactions with drugs metabolized by cytochrome P450 enzymes. In *in vivo* studies, 10 mg/day to 30 mg/day doses of aripiprazole had no significant effect on metabolism by CYP2D6 (dextromethorphan), CYP2C9 (warfarin), CYP2C19 (omeprazole, warfarin), and CYP3A4 (dextromethorphan) substrates. Additionally, aripiprazole and dehydro-aripiprazole did not show potential for altering CYP1A2-mediated metabolism *in vitro*.

No effect of aripiprazole was seen on the pharmacokinetics of lithium or valproate.

Alcohol

There was no significant difference between aripiprazole coadministered with ethanol and placebo coadministered with ethanol on performance of gross motor skills or stimulus response in healthy subjects. As with most psychoactive medications, patients should be advised to avoid alcohol while taking ABILIFY.

7.3 Drugs Having No Clinically Important Interactions with ABILIFY

Famotidine

Coadministration of aripiprazole (given in a single dose of 15 mg) with a 40 mg single dose of the H_2 antagonist famotidine, a potent gastric acid blocker, decreased the solubility of aripiprazole and, hence, its rate of absorption, reducing by 37% and 21% the C_{max} of aripiprazole and dehydro-aripiprazole, respectively, and by 13% and 15%, respectively, the extent of absorption (AUC). No dosage adjustment of aripiprazole is required when administered concomitantly with famotidine.

IMPORTANT NOTICE: Updated drug information is sent bi-monthly via the PDR® Update Insert. For *monthly* email updates, register at PDR.net.

Valproate

When valproate (500 mg/day-1500 mg/day) and aripiprazole (30 mg/day) were coadministered, at steady-state the C_{max} and AUC of aripiprazole were decreased by 25%. No dosage adjustment of aripiprazole is required when administered concomitantly with valproate.

When aripiprazole (30 mg/day) and valproate (1000 mg/day) were coadministered, at steady-state there were no clinically significant changes in the C_{max} or AUC of valproate. No dosage adjustment of valproate is required when administered concomitantly with aripiprazole.

Lithium

A pharmacokinetic interaction of aripiprazole with lithium is unlikely because lithium is not bound to plasma proteins, is not metabolized, and is almost entirely excreted unchanged in urine. Coadministration of therapeutic doses of lithium (1200 mg/day-1800 mg/day) for 21 days with aripiprazole (30 mg/day) did not result in clinically significant changes in the pharmacokinetics of aripiprazole or its active metabolite, dehydro-aripiprazole (C_{max} and AUC increased by less than 20%). No dosage adjustment of aripiprazole is required when administered concomitantly with lithium.

Coadministration of aripiprazole (30 mg/day) with lithium (900 mg/day) did not result in clinically significant changes in the pharmacokinetics of lithium. No dosage adjustment of lithium is required when administered concomitantly with aripiprazole.

Lamotrigine

Coadministration of 10 mg/day to 30 mg/day oral doses of aripiprazole for 14 days to patients with bipolar I disorder had no effect on the steady-state pharmacokinetics of 100 mg/day to 400 mg/day lamotrigine, a UDP-glucuronosyltransferase 1A4 substrate. No dosage adjustment of lamotrigine is required when aripiprazole is added to lamotrigine.

Dextromethorphan

Aripiprazole at doses of 10 mg/day to 30 mg/day for 14 days had no effect on dextromethorphan's O-dealkylation to its major metabolite, dextrorphan, a pathway dependent on CYP2D6 activity. Aripiprazole also had no effect on dextromethorphan's N-demethylation to its metabolite 3-methoxymorphinan, a pathway dependent on CYP3A4 activity. No dosage adjustment of dextromethorphan is required when administered concomitantly with aripiprazole.

Warfarin

Aripiprazole 10 mg/day for 14 days had no effect on the pharmacokinetics of R-warfarin and S-warfarin or on the pharmacodynamic end point of International Normalized Ratio, indicating the lack of a clinically relevant effect of aripiprazole on CYP2C9 and CYP2C19 metabolism or the binding of highly protein-bound warfarin. No dosage adjustment of warfarin is required when administered concomitantly with aripiprazole.

Omeprazole

Aripiprazole 10 mg/day for 15 days had no effect on the pharmacokinetics of a single 20 mg dose of omeprazole, a CYP2C19 substrate, in healthy subjects. No dosage adjustment of omeprazole is required when administered concomitantly with aripiprazole.

Lorazepam

Coadministration of lorazepam injection (2 mg) and aripiprazole injection (15 mg) to healthy subjects (n=40: 35 males and 5 females; ages 19-45 years old) did not result in clinically important changes in the pharmacokinetics of either drug. No dosage adjustment of aripiprazole is required when administered concomitantly with lorazepam. However, the intensity of sedation was greater with the combination as compared to that observed with aripiprazole alone and the orthostatic hypotension observed was greater with the combination as compared to that observed with lorazepam alone [see WARNINGS AND PRECAUTIONS (5.6)].

Escitalopram

Coadministration of 10 mg/day oral doses of aripiprazole for 14 days to healthy subjects had no effect on the steady-state pharmacokinetics of 10 mg/day escitalopram, a substrate of CYP2C19 and CYP3A4. No dosage adjustment of escitalopram is required when aripiprazole is added to escitalopram.

Venlafaxine

Coadministration of 10 mg/day to 20 mg/day oral doses of aripiprazole for 14 days to healthy subjects had no effect on the steady-state pharmacokinetics of venlafaxine and O-desmethylvenlafaxine following 75 mg/day venlafaxine XR, a CYP2D6 substrate. No dosage adjustment of venlafaxine is required when aripiprazole is added to venlafaxine.

Fluoxetine, Paroxetine, and Sertraline

A population pharmacokinetic analysis in patients with major depressive disorder showed no substantial change in plasma concentrations of fluoxetine (20 mg/day or 40 mg/day), paroxetine CR (37.5 mg/day or 50 mg/day), or sertraline (100 mg/day or 150 mg/day) dosed to steady-state. The steady-state plasma concentrations of fluoxetine and norfluoxetine increased by about 18% and 36%, respectively, and concentrations of paroxetine decreased by about 27%. The steady-state plasma concentrations of sertraline and desmethylsertraline were not substantially changed when these antidepressant therapies were coadministered with aripiprazole. Aripiprazole dosing was 2 mg/day to 15 mg/day (when given with fluoxetine or paroxetine) or 2 mg/day to 20 mg/day (when given with sertraline).

8 USE IN SPECIFIC POPULATIONS

In general, no dosage adjustment for ABILIFY (aripiprazole) is required on the basis of a patient's age, gender, race, smoking status, hepatic function, or renal function [see DOSAGE AND ADMINISTRATION (2.5)].

8.1 Pregnancy

Pregnancy Category C: In animal studies, aripiprazole demonstrated developmental toxicity, including possible teratogenic effects in rats and rabbits.

Pregnant rats were treated with oral doses of 3 mg/kg/day, 10 mg/kg/day, and 30 mg/kg/day (1 times, 3 times, and 10 times the maximum recommended human dose [MRHD] on a mg/m^2 basis) of aripiprazole during the period of organogenesis. Gestation was slightly prolonged at 30 mg/kg. Treatment caused a slight delay in fetal development, as evidenced by decreased fetal weight (30 mg/kg), undescended testes (30 mg/kg), and delayed skeletal ossification (10 mg/kg and 30 mg/kg). There were no adverse effects on embryofetal or pup survival. Delivered offspring had decreased body weights (10 mg/kg and 30 mg/kg), and increased incidences of hepatodiaphragmatic nodules and diaphragmatic hernia at 30 mg/kg (the other dose groups were not examined for these findings). A low incidence of diaphragmatic hernia was also seen in the fetuses exposed to 30 mg/kg. Postnatally, delayed vaginal opening was seen at 10 mg/kg and 30 mg/kg and impaired reproductive performance (decreased fertility rate, corpora lutea, implants, live fetuses, and increased post-implantation loss, likely mediated through effects on female offspring) was seen at 30 mg/kg. Some maternal toxicity was seen at 30 mg/kg; however, there was no evidence to suggest that these developmental effects were secondary to maternal toxicity.

In pregnant rats receiving aripiprazole injection intravenously (3 mg/kg/day, 9 mg/kg/day, and 27 mg/kg/day) during the period of organogenesis, decreased fetal weight and delayed skeletal ossification were seen at the highest dose, which also caused some maternal toxicity.

Pregnant rabbits were treated with oral doses of 10 mg/kg/day, 30 mg/kg/day, and 100 mg/kg/day (2 times, 3 times, and 11 times human exposure at MRHD based on AUC and 6 times, 19 times, and 65 times the MRHD based on mg/m^2) of aripiprazole during the period of organogenesis. Decreased maternal food consumption and increased abortions were seen at 100 mg/kg. Treatment caused increased fetal mortality (100 mg/kg), decreased fetal weight (30 mg/kg and 100 mg/kg), increased incidence of a skeletal abnormality (fused sternebrae at 30 mg/kg and 100 mg/kg), and minor skeletal variations (100 mg/kg).

In pregnant rabbits receiving aripiprazole injection intravenously (3 mg/kg/day, 10 mg/kg/day, and 30 mg/kg/day) during the period of organogenesis, the highest dose, which caused pronounced maternal toxicity, resulted in decreased fetal weight, increased fetal abnormalities (primarily skeletal), and decreased fetal skeletal ossification. The fetal no-effect dose was 10 mg/kg, which produced 5 times the human exposure at the MRHD based on AUC and is 6 times the MRHD based on mg/m^2.

In a study in which rats were treated with oral doses of 3 mg/kg/day, 10 mg/kg/day, and 30 mg/kg/day (1 times, 3 times, and 10 times the MRHD on a mg/m^2 basis) of aripiprazole perinatally and postnatally (from day 17 of gestation through day 21 postpartum), slight maternal toxicity and slightly prolonged gestation were seen at 30 mg/kg. An increase in stillbirths and decreases in pup weight (persisting into adulthood) and survival were seen at this dose.

In rats receiving aripiprazole injection intravenously (3 mg/kg/day, 8 mg/kg/day, and 20 mg/kg/day) from day 6 of gestation through day 20 postpartum, an increase in stillbirths was seen at 8 mg/kg and 20 mg/kg, and decreases in early postnatal pup weights and survival were seen at 20 mg/kg. These doses produced some maternal toxicity. There were no effects on postnatal behavioral and reproductive development.

There are no adequate and well-controlled studies in pregnant women. It is not known whether aripiprazole can cause fetal harm when administered to a pregnant woman or can affect reproductive capacity. Aripiprazole should be used during pregnancy only if the potential benefit outweighs the potential risk to the fetus.

8.2 Labor and Delivery

The effect of aripiprazole on labor and delivery in humans is unknown.

8.3 Nursing Mothers

Aripiprazole was excreted in milk of rats during lactation. It is not known whether aripiprazole or its metabolites are excreted in human milk. It is recommended that women receiving aripiprazole should not breast-feed.

8.4 Pediatric Use

Safety and effectiveness in pediatric patients with major depressive disorder or agitation associated with schizophrenia or bipolar mania have not been established.

Safety and effectiveness in pediatric patients with schizophrenia were established in a 6-week, placebo-controlled clinical trial in 202 pediatric patients aged 13 to 17 years [see INDICATIONS AND USAGE (1.1), DOSAGE AND ADMINISTRATION (2.1), ADVERSE REACTIONS (6.2), and CLINICAL STUDIES (14.1)]. Although maintenance efficacy in pediatric patients has not been systematically evaluated, maintenance efficacy can be extrapolated from adult data along with comparisons of aripiprazole pharmacokinetic parameters in adult and pediatric patients.

Safety and effectiveness in pediatric patients with bipolar mania were established in a 4-week, placebo-controlled clinical trial in 197 pediatric patients aged 10 to 17 years [see INDICATIONS AND USAGE (1.2), DOSAGE AND ADMINISTRATION (2.2), ADVERSE REACTIONS (6.2), and CLINICAL STUDIES (14.2)]. Although maintenance efficacy in pediatric patients has not been systematically evaluated, maintenance efficacy can be extrapolated from adult data along with comparisons of aripiprazole pharmacokinetic parameters in adult and pediatric patients.

The efficacy of adjunctive ABILIFY (aripiprazole) with concomitant lithium or valproate in the treatment of manic or mixed episodes in pediatric patients has not been systematically evaluated. However, such efficacy and lack of pharmacokinetic interaction between aripiprazole and lithium or valproate can be extrapolated from adult data, along with comparisons of aripiprazole pharmacokinetic parameters in adult and pediatric patients.

Safety and effectiveness in pediatric patients demonstrating irritability associated with autistic disorder were established in two 8-week, placebo-controlled clinical trials in 212 pediatric patients aged 6 to 17 years [see INDICATIONS AND USAGE (1.4), DOSAGE AND ADMINISTRATION (2.4), ADVERSE REACTIONS (6.2), and CLINICAL STUDIES (14.4)]. Maintenance efficacy in pediatric patients has not been systematically evaluated.

The pharmacokinetics of aripiprazole and dehydro-aripiprazole in pediatric patients 10 to 17 years of age were similar to those in adults after correcting for the differences in body weights.

8.5 Geriatric Use

In formal single-dose pharmacokinetic studies (with aripiprazole given in a single dose of 15 mg), aripiprazole clearance was 20% lower in elderly (≥65 years) subjects compared to younger adult subjects (18 to 64 years). There was no detectable age effect, however, in the population pharmacokinetic analysis in schizophrenia patients. Also, the pharmacokinetics of aripiprazole after multiple doses in elderly patients appeared similar to that observed in young, healthy subjects. No dosage adjustment is recommended for elderly patients [see also BOXED WARNING and WARNINGS AND PRECAUTIONS (5.1)].

Of the 13,543 patients treated with oral aripiprazole in clinical trials, 1073 (8%) were ≥65 years old and 799 (6%) were ≥75 years old. The majority (81%) of the 1073 patients were diagnosed with Dementia of the Alzheimer's type.

Placebo-controlled studies of oral aripiprazole in schizophrenia, bipolar mania, or major depressive disorder did not include sufficient numbers of subjects aged 65 and over to determine whether they respond differently from younger subjects.

Of the 749 patients treated with aripiprazole injection in clinical trials, 99 (13%) were ≥65 years old and 78 (10%) were ≥75 years old. Placebo-controlled studies of aripiprazole injection in patients with agitation associated with schizophrenia or bipolar mania did not include sufficient numbers of subjects aged 65 and over to determine whether they respond differently from younger subjects.

Studies of elderly patients with psychosis associated with Alzheimer's disease have suggested that there may be a different tolerability profile in this population compared to younger patients with schizophrenia [see also BOXED WARNING and WARNINGS AND PRECAUTIONS (5.1)]. The safety and efficacy of ABILIFY in the treatment of patients with psychosis associated with Alzheimer's disease has not been established. If the prescriber elects to treat such patients with ABILIFY, vigilance should be exercised.

8.6 Renal Impairment

In patients with severe renal impairment (creatinine clearance <30 mL/min), C_{max} of aripiprazole (given in a single dose of 15 mg) and dehydro-aripiprazole increased by 36% and 53%, respectively, but AUC was 15% lower for aripiprazole and 7% higher for dehydro-aripiprazole. Renal excretion of both unchanged aripiprazole and dehydro-aripiprazole is less than 1% of the dose. No dosage adjustment is required in subjects with renal impairment.

8.7 Hepatic Impairment

In a single-dose study (15 mg of aripiprazole) in subjects with varying degrees of liver cirrhosis (Child-Pugh Classes A, B, and C), the AUC of aripiprazole, compared to healthy subjects, increased 31% in mild HI, increased 8% in moderate HI, and decreased 20% in severe HI. None of these differences would require dose adjustment.

8.8 Gender

C_{max} and AUC of aripiprazole and its active metabolite, dehydro-aripiprazole, are 30% to 40% higher in women than in men, and correspondingly, the apparent oral clearance of aripiprazole is lower in women. These differences, however, are largely explained by differences in body weight (25%) between men and women. No dosage adjustment is recommended based on gender.

8.9 Race

Although no specific pharmacokinetic study was conducted to investigate the effects of race on the disposition of aripiprazole, population pharmacokinetic evaluation revealed no evidence of clinically significant race-related differences in the pharmacokinetics of aripiprazole. No dosage adjustment is recommended based on race.

8.10 Smoking

Based on studies utilizing human liver enzymes *in vitro*, aripiprazole is not a substrate for CYP1A2 and also does not undergo direct glucuronidation. Smoking should, therefore, not have an effect on the pharmacokinetics of aripiprazole. Consistent with these *in vitro* results, population pharmacokinetic evaluation did not reveal any significant pharmacokinetic differences between smokers and nonsmokers. No dosage adjustment is recommended based on smoking status.

9 DRUG ABUSE AND DEPENDENCE

9.1 Controlled Substance

ABILIFY (aripiprazole) is not a controlled substance.

9.2 Abuse and Dependence

Aripiprazole has not been systematically studied in humans for its potential for abuse, tolerance, or physical dependence. In physical dependence studies in monkeys, withdrawal symptoms were observed upon abrupt cessation of dosing. While the clinical trials did not reveal any tendency for any drug-seeking behavior, these observations were not systematic and it is not possible to predict on the basis of this limited experience the extent to which a CNS-active drug will be misused, diverted, and/or abused once marketed. Consequently, patients should be evaluated carefully for a history of drug abuse, and such patients should be observed closely for signs of ABILIFY misuse or abuse (eg, development of tolerance, increases in dose, drug-seeking behavior).

10 OVERDOSAGE

MedDRA terminology has been used to classify the adverse reactions.

10.1 Human Experience

A total of 76 cases of deliberate or accidental overdosage with oral aripiprazole have been reported worldwide. These include overdoses with oral aripiprazole alone and in combination with other substances. No fatality was reported from these cases. Of the 44 cases with known outcome, 33 cases recovered without sequelae and one case recovered with sequelae (mydriasis and feeling abnormal). The largest known case of acute ingestion with a known outcome involved 1080 mg of oral aripiprazole (36 times the maximum recommended daily dose) in a patient who fully recovered. Included in the 76 cases are 10 cases of deliberate or accidental overdosage in children (age 12 and younger) involving oral aripiprazole ingestions up to 195 mg with no fatalities.

Common adverse reactions (reported in at least 5% of all overdose cases) reported with oral aripiprazole overdosage (alone or in combination with other substances) include vomiting, somnolence, and tremor. Other clinically important signs and symptoms observed in one or more patients with aripiprazole overdoses (alone or with other substances) include acidosis, aggression, aspartate aminotransferase increased, atrial fibrillation, bradycardia, coma, confusional state, convulsion, blood creatine phosphokinase increased, depressed level of consciousness, hypertension, hypokalemia, hypotension, lethargy, loss of consciousness, QRS complex prolonged, QT prolonged, pneumonia aspiration, respiratory arrest, status epilepticus, and tachycardia.

10.2 Management of Overdosage

No specific information is available on the treatment of overdose with aripiprazole. An electrocardiogram should be obtained in case of overdosage and if QT interval prolongation is present, cardiac monitoring should be instituted. Otherwise, management of overdose should concentrate on supportive therapy, maintaining an adequate airway, oxygenation and ventilation, and management of symptoms. Close medical supervision and monitoring should continue until the patient recovers.

Charcoal: In the event of an overdose of ABILIFY, an early charcoal administration may be useful in partially preventing the absorption of aripiprazole. Administration of 50 g of activated charcoal, one hour after a single 15 mg oral dose of aripiprazole, decreased the mean AUC and C_{max} of aripiprazole by 50%.

Hemodialysis: Although there is no information on the effect of hemodialysis in treating an overdose with aripiprazole, hemodialysis is unlikely to be useful in overdose management since aripiprazole is highly bound to plasma proteins.

11 DESCRIPTION

Aripiprazole is a psychotropic drug that is available as ABILIFY® (aripiprazole) Tablets, ABILIFY DISCMELT® (aripiprazole) Orally Disintegrating Tablets, ABILIFY® (aripiprazole) Oral Solution, and ABILIFY® (aripiprazole) Injection, a solution for intramuscular injection. Aripiprazole is 7-[4-[4-(2,3-dichlorophenyl)-1-piperazinyl] butoxy]-3,4-dihydrocarbostyril. The empirical formula is $C_{23}H_{27}Cl_2N_3O_2$ and its molecular weight is 448.38. The chemical structure is:

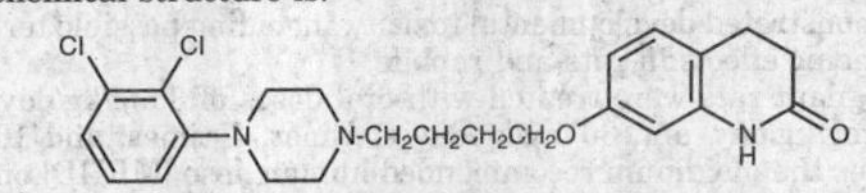

ABILIFY Tablets are available in 2 mg, 5 mg, 10 mg, 15 mg, 20 mg, and 30 mg strengths. Inactive ingredients include cornstarch, hydroxypropyl cellulose, lactose monohydrate, magnesium stearate, and microcrystalline cellulose. Colorants include ferric oxide (yellow or red) and FD&C Blue No. 2 Aluminum Lake.

ABILIFY DISCMELT Orally Disintegrating Tablets are available in 10 mg and 15 mg strengths. Inactive ingredients include acesulfame potassium, aspartame, calcium silicate, croscarmellose sodium, crospovidone, crème de vanilla (natural and artificial flavors), magnesium stearate, microcrystalline cellulose, silicon dioxide, tartaric acid, and xylitol. Colorants include ferric oxide (yellow or red) and FD&C Blue No. 2 Aluminum Lake.

ABILIFY Oral Solution is a clear, colorless to light yellow solution available in a concentration of 1 mg/mL. The inactive ingredients for this solution include disodium edetate, fructose, glycerin, dl-lactic acid, methylparaben, propylene glycol, propylparaben, sodium hydroxide, sucrose, and purified water. The oral solution is flavored with natural orange cream and other natural flavors.

ABILIFY Injection is available in single-dose vials as a ready-to-use, 9.75 mg/1.3 mL (7.5 mg/mL) clear, colorless, sterile, aqueous solution for intramuscular use only. Inactive ingredients for this solution include 150 mg/mL of sulfobutylether β-cyclodextrin (SBECD), tartaric acid, sodium hydroxide, and water for injection.

12 CLINICAL PHARMACOLOGY

12.1 Mechanism of Action

The mechanism of action of aripiprazole, as with other drugs having efficacy in schizophrenia, bipolar disorder, major depressive disorder, irritability associated with autistic disorder, and agitation associated with schizophrenia or bipolar disorder, is unknown. However, it has been proposed that the efficacy of aripiprazole is mediated through a combination of partial agonist activity at D_2 and 5-HT_{1A} receptors and antagonist activity at 5-HT_{2A} receptors. Actions at receptors other than D_2, 5-HT_{1A}, and 5-HT_{2A} may explain some of the other clinical effects of aripiprazole (eg, the orthostatic hypotension observed with aripiprazole may be explained by its antagonist activity at adrenergic alpha$_1$ receptors).

12.2 Pharmacodynamics

Aripiprazole exhibits high affinity for dopamine D_2 and D_3, serotonin 5-HT_{1A} and 5-HT_{2A} receptors (K_i values of 0.34 nM, 0.8 nM, 1.7 nM, and 3.4 nM, respectively), moderate affinity for dopamine D_4, serotonin 5-HT_{2C} and 5-HT_7, alpha$_1$-adrenergic and histamine H_1 receptors (K_i values of 44 nM, 15 nM, 39 nM, 57 nM, and 61 nM, respectively), and moderate affinity for the serotonin reuptake site (K_i=98 nM). Aripiprazole has no appreciable affinity for cholinergic muscarinic receptors (IC_{50}>1000 nM). Aripiprazole functions as a partial agonist at the dopamine D_2 and the serotonin 5-HT_{1A} receptors, and as an antagonist at serotonin 5-HT_{2A} receptor.

12.3 Pharmacokinetics

ABILIFY activity is presumably primarily due to the parent drug, aripiprazole, and to a lesser extent, to its major metabolite, dehydro-aripiprazole, which has been shown to have affinities for D_2 receptors similar to the parent drug and represents 40% of the parent drug exposure in plasma. The mean elimination half-lives are about 75 hours and 94 hours for aripiprazole and dehydro-aripiprazole, respectively. Steady-state concentrations are attained within 14 days of dosing for both active moieties. Aripiprazole accumulation is predictable from single-dose pharmacokinetics. At steady-state, the pharmacokinetics of aripiprazole are dose-proportional. Elimination of aripiprazole is mainly through hepatic metabolism involving two P450 isozymes, CYP2D6 and CYP3A4.

Pharmacokinetic studies showed that ABILIFY DISCMELT Orally Disintegrating Tablets are bioequivalent to ABILIFY Tablets.

ORAL ADMINISTRATION

Absorption

Tablet: Aripiprazole is well absorbed after administration of the tablet, with peak plasma concentrations occurring within 3 hours to 5 hours; the absolute oral bioavailability of the tablet formulation is 87%. ABILIFY (aripiprazole) can be administered with or without food. Administration of a 15 mg ABILIFY Tablet with a standard high-fat meal did not significantly affect the C_{max} or AUC of aripiprazole or its active metabolite, dehydro-aripiprazole, but delayed T_{max} by 3 hours for aripiprazole and 12 hours for dehydro-aripiprazole.

Oral Solution: Aripiprazole is well absorbed when administered orally as the solution. At equivalent doses, the plasma concentrations of aripiprazole from the solution were higher than that from the tablet formulation. In a relative bioavailability study comparing the pharmacokinetics of 30 mg aripiprazole as the oral solution to 30 mg aripiprazole tablets in healthy subjects, the solution to tablet ratios of geometric mean C_{max} and AUC values were 122% and 114%, respectively *[see DOSAGE AND ADMINISTRATION (2.6)]*. The single-dose pharmacokinetics of aripiprazole were linear and dose-proportional between the doses of 5 mg to 30 mg.

Distribution

The steady-state volume of distribution of aripiprazole following intravenous administration is high (404 L or 4.9 L/kg), indicating extensive extravascular distribution. At therapeutic concentrations, aripiprazole and its major metabolite are greater than 99% bound to serum proteins, primarily to albumin. In healthy human volunteers administered 0.5 mg/day to 30 mg/day aripiprazole for 14 days, there was dose-dependent D_2 receptor occupancy indicating brain penetration of aripiprazole in humans.

Metabolism and Elimination

Aripiprazole is metabolized primarily by three biotransformation pathways: dehydrogenation, hydroxylation, and N-dealkylation. Based on *in vitro* studies, CYP3A4 and CYP2D6 enzymes are responsible for dehydrogenation and hydroxylation of aripiprazole, and N-dealkylation is catalyzed by CYP3A4. Aripiprazole is the predominant drug moiety in the systemic circulation. At steady-state, dehydro-aripiprazole, the active metabolite, represents about 40% of aripiprazole AUC in plasma.

Approximately 8% of Caucasians lack the capacity to metabolize CYP2D6 substrates and are classified as poor metabolizers (PM), whereas the rest are extensive metabolizers (EM). PMs have about an 80% increase in aripiprazole exposure and about a 30% decrease in exposure to the active metabolite compared to EMs, resulting in about a 60% higher exposure to the total active moieties from a given dose of aripiprazole compared to EMs. Coadministration of ABILIFY with known inhibitors of CYP2D6, such as quinidine or fluoxetine in EMs, approximately doubles aripiprazole plasma exposure, and dose adjustment is needed *[see DRUG INTERACTIONS (7.1)]*. The mean elimination half-lives are about 75 hours and 146 hours for aripiprazole in EMs and PMs, respectively. Aripiprazole does not inhibit or induce the CYP2D6 pathway.

Following a single oral dose of [^{14}C]-labeled aripiprazole, approximately 25% and 55% of the administered radioactivity was recovered in the urine and feces, respectively. Less than 1% of unchanged aripiprazole was excreted in the urine and approximately 18% of the oral dose was recovered unchanged in the feces.

INTRAMUSCULAR ADMINISTRATION

In two pharmacokinetic studies of aripiprazole injection administered intramuscularly to healthy subjects, the median times to the peak plasma concentrations were at 1 hour and 3 hours. A 5 mg intramuscular injection of aripiprazole had an absolute bioavailability of 100%. The geometric mean maximum concentration achieved after an intramuscular dose was on average 19% higher than the C_{max} of the oral tablet. While the systemic exposure over 24 hours was generally similar between aripiprazole injection given intramuscularly and after oral tablet administration, the aripiprazole AUC in the first 2 hours after an intramuscular injection was 90% greater than the AUC after the same dose as a tablet. In stable patients with schizophrenia or schizoaffective disorder, the pharmacokinetics of aripiprazole after intramuscular administration were linear over a dose range of 1 mg to 45 mg. Although the metabolism of aripiprazole injection was not systematically evaluated, the intramuscular route of administration would not be expected to alter the metabolic pathways.

13 NONCLINICAL TOXICOLOGY

13.1 Carcinogenesis, Mutagenesis, Impairment of Fertility

Carcinogenesis

Lifetime carcinogenicity studies were conducted in ICR mice and in Sprague-Dawley (SD) and F344 rats. Aripiprazole was administered for 2 years in the diet at doses of 1 mg/kg/day, 3 mg/kg/day, 10 mg/kg/day, and

30 mg/kg/day to ICR mice and 1 mg/kg/day, 3 mg/kg/day, and 10 mg/kg/day to F344 rats (0.2 times to 5 times and 0.3 times to 3 times the maximum recommended human dose [MRHD] based on mg/m^2, respectively). In addition, SD rats were dosed orally for 2 years at 10 mg/kg/day, 20 mg/kg/day, 40 mg/kg/day, and 60 mg/kg/day (3 times to 19 times the MRHD based on mg/m^2). Aripiprazole did not induce tumors in male mice or rats. In female mice, the incidences of pituitary gland adenomas and mammary gland adenocarcinomas and adenoacanthomas were increased at dietary doses of 3 mg/kg/day to 30 mg/kg/day (0.1 times to 0.9 times human exposure at MRHD based on AUC and 0.5 times to 5 times the MRHD based on mg/m^2). In female rats, the incidence of mammary gland fibroadenomas was increased at a dietary dose of 10 mg/kg/day (0.1 times human exposure at MRHD based on AUC and 3 times the MRHD based on mg/m^2); and the incidences of adrenocortical carcinomas and combined adrenocortical adenomas/carcinomas were increased at an oral dose of 60 mg/kg/day (14 times human exposure at MRHD based on AUC and 19 times the MRHD based on mg/m^2).

Proliferative changes in the pituitary and mammary gland of rodents have been observed following chronic administration of other antipsychotic agents and are considered prolactin-mediated. Serum prolactin was not measured in the aripiprazole carcinogenicity studies. However, increases in serum prolactin levels were observed in female mice in a 13-week dietary study at the doses associated with mammary gland and pituitary tumors. Serum prolactin was not increased in female rats in 4-week and 13-week dietary studies at the dose associated with mammary gland tumors. The relevance for human risk of the findings of prolactin-mediated endocrine tumors in rodents is unknown.

Mutagenesis

The mutagenic potential of aripiprazole was tested in the *in vitro* bacterial reverse-mutation assay, the *in vitro* bacterial DNA repair assay, the *in vitro* forward gene mutation assay in mouse lymphoma cells, the *in vitro* chromosomal aberration assay in Chinese hamster lung (CHL) cells, the *in vivo* micronucleus assay in mice, and the unscheduled DNA synthesis assay in rats. Aripiprazole and a metabolite (2,3-DCPP) were clastogenic in the *in vitro* chromosomal aberration assay in CHL cells with and without metabolic activation. The metabolite, 2,3-DCPP, produced increases in numerical aberrations in the *in vitro* assay in CHL cells in the absence of metabolic activation. A positive response was obtained in the *in vivo* micronucleus assay in mice; however, the response was due to a mechanism not considered relevant to humans.

Impairment of Fertility

Female rats were treated with oral doses of 2 mg/kg/day, 6 mg/kg/day, and 20 mg/kg/day (0.6 times, 2 times, and 6 times the maximum recommended human dose [MRHD] on a mg/m^2 basis) of aripiprazole from 2 weeks prior to mating through day 7 of gestation. Estrus cycle irregularities and increased corpora lutea were seen at all doses, but no impairment of fertility was seen. Increased pre-implantation loss was seen at 6 mg/kg and 20 mg/kg and decreased fetal weight was seen at 20 mg/kg.

Male rats were treated with oral doses of 20 mg/kg/day, 40 mg/kg/day, and 60 mg/kg/day (6 times, 13 times, and 19 times the MRHD on a mg/m^2 basis) of aripiprazole from 9 weeks prior to mating through mating. Disturbances in spermatogenesis were seen at 60 mg/kg and prostate atrophy was seen at 40 mg/kg and 60 mg/kg, but no impairment of fertility was seen.

13.2 Animal Toxicology and/or Pharmacology

Aripiprazole produced retinal degeneration in albino rats in a 26-week chronic toxicity study at a dose of 60 mg/kg and in a 2-year carcinogenicity study at doses of 40 mg/kg and 60 mg/kg. The 40 mg/kg and 60 mg/kg doses are 13 times and 19 times the maximum recommended human dose (MRHD) based on mg/m^2 and 7 times to 14 times human exposure at MRHD based on AUC. Evaluation of the retinas of albino mice and of monkeys did not reveal evidence of retinal degeneration. Additional studies to further evaluate the mechanism have not been performed. The relevance of this finding to human risk is unknown.

14 CLINICAL STUDIES

14.1 Schizophrenia

Adults

The efficacy of ABILIFY (aripiprazole) in the treatment of schizophrenia was evaluated in five short-term (4-week and 6-week), placebo-controlled trials of acutely relapsed inpatients who predominantly met DSM-III/IV criteria for schizophrenia. Four of the five trials were able to distinguish aripiprazole from placebo, but one study, the smallest, did not. Three of these studies also included an active control group consisting of either risperidone (one trial) or haloperidol (two trials), but they were not designed to allow for a comparison of ABILIFY and the active comparators.

In the four positive trials for ABILIFY, four primary measures were used for assessing psychiatric signs and symp-

toms. The Positive and Negative Syndrome Scale (PANSS) is a multi-item inventory of general psychopathology used to evaluate the effects of drug treatment in schizophrenia. The PANSS positive subscale is a subset of items in the PANSS that rates seven positive symptoms of schizophrenia (delusions, conceptual disorganization, hallucinatory behavior, excitement, grandiosity, suspiciousness/persecution, and hostility). The PANSS negative subscale is a subset of items in the PANSS that rates seven negative symptoms of schizophrenia (blunted affect, emotional withdrawal, poor rapport, passive apathetic withdrawal, difficulty in abstract thinking, lack of spontaneity/flow of conversation, stereotyped thinking). The Clinical Global Impression (CGI) assessment reflects the impression of a skilled observer, fully familiar with the manifestations of schizophrenia, about the overall clinical state of the patient.

In a 4-week trial (n=414) comparing two fixed doses of ABILIFY (aripiprazole) (15 mg/day or 30 mg/day) to placebo, both doses of ABILIFY were superior to placebo in the PANSS total score, PANSS positive subscale, and CGI-severity score. In addition, the 15 mg dose was superior to placebo in the PANSS negative subscale.

In a 4-week trial (n=404) comparing two fixed doses of ABILIFY (20 mg/day or 30 mg/day) to placebo, both doses of ABILIFY were superior to placebo in the PANSS total score, PANSS positive subscale, PANSS negative subscale, and CGI-severity score.

In a 6-week trial (n=420) comparing three fixed doses of ABILIFY (10 mg/day, 15 mg/day, or 20 mg/day) to placebo, all three doses of ABILIFY were superior to placebo in the PANSS total score, PANSS positive subscale, and the PANSS negative subscale.

In a 6-week trial (n=367) comparing three fixed doses of ABILIFY (2 mg/day, 5 mg/day, or 10 mg/day) to placebo, the 10 mg dose of ABILIFY was superior to placebo in the PANSS total score, the primary outcome measure of the study. The 2 mg and 5 mg doses did not demonstrate superiority to placebo on the primary outcome measure.

In a fifth study, a 4-week trial (n=103) comparing ABILIFY in a range of 5 mg/day to 30 mg/day to placebo, ABILIFY was only significantly different compared to placebo in a responder analysis based on the CGI-severity score, a primary outcome for that trial.

Thus, the efficacy of 10 mg, 15 mg, 20 mg, and 30 mg daily doses was established in two studies for each dose. Among these doses, there was no evidence that the higher dose groups offered any advantage over the lowest dose group of these studies.

An examination of population subgroups did not reveal any clear evidence of differential responsiveness on the basis of age, gender, or race.

A longer-term trial enrolled 310 inpatients or outpatients meeting DSM-IV criteria for schizophrenia who were, by history, symptomatically stable on other antipsychotic medications for periods of 3 months or longer. These patients were discontinued from their antipsychotic medications and randomized to ABILIFY 15 mg/day or placebo for up to 26 weeks of observation for relapse. Relapse during the double-blind phase was defined as CGI-Improvement score of ≥5 (minimally worse), scores ≥5 (moderately severe) on the hostility or uncooperativeness items of the PANSS, or ≥20% increase in the PANSS total score. Patients receiving ABILIFY 15 mg/day experienced a significantly longer time to relapse over the subsequent 26 weeks compared to those receiving placebo.

Pediatric Patients

The efficacy of ABILIFY (aripiprazole) in the treatment of schizophrenia in pediatric patients (13 to 17 years of age) was evaluated in one 6-week, placebo-controlled trial of outpatients who met DSM-IV criteria for schizophrenia and had a PANSS score ≥70 at baseline. In this trial (n=302) comparing two fixed doses of ABILIFY (10 mg/day or 30 mg/day) to placebo, ABILIFY was titrated starting from 2 mg/day to the target dose in 5 days in the 10 mg/day treatment arm and in 11 days in the 30 mg/day treatment arm. Both doses of ABILIFY were superior to placebo in the PANSS total score, the primary outcome measure of the study. The 30 mg/day dosage was not shown to be more efficacious than the 10 mg/day dose. Although maintenance efficacy in pediatric patients has not been systematically evaluated, maintenance efficacy can be extrapolated from adult data along with comparisons of aripiprazole pharmacokinetic parameters in adult and pediatric patients.

14.2 Bipolar Disorder

Monotherapy

Adults

The efficacy of ABILIFY in the acute treatment of manic episodes was established in four 3-week, placebo-controlled trials in hospitalized patients who met the DSM-IV criteria for bipolar I disorder with manic or mixed episodes. These studies included patients with or without psychotic features and two of the studies also included patients with or without a rapid-cycling course.

The primary instrument used for assessing manic symptoms was the Young Mania Rating Scale (Y-MRS), an 11-item clinician-rated scale traditionally used to assess the degree of manic symptomatology (irritability, disruptive/aggressive behavior, sleep, elevated mood, speech, increased activity, sexual interest, language/thought disorder, thought content, appearance, and insight) in a range from 0 (no manic features) to 60 (maximum score). A key secondary instrument included the Clinical Global Impression - Bipolar (CGI-BP) Scale.

In the four positive, 3-week, placebo-controlled trials (n=268; n=248; n=480; n=485) which evaluated ABILIFY in a range of 15 mg to 30 mg, once daily (with a starting dose of 15 mg/day in two studies and 30 mg/day in two studies), ABILIFY (aripiprazole) was superior to placebo in the reduction of Y-MRS total score and CGI-BP Severity of Illness score (mania). In the two studies with a starting dose of 15 mg/day, 48% and 44% of patients were on 15 mg/day at endpoint. In the two studies with a starting dose of 30 mg/day, 86% and 85% of patients were on 30 mg/day at endpoint.

A trial was conducted in patients meeting DSM-IV criteria for bipolar I disorder with a recent manic or mixed episode who had been stabilized on open-label ABILIFY and who had maintained a clinical response for at least 6 weeks. The first phase of this trial was an open-label stabilization period in which inpatients and outpatients were clinically stabilized and then maintained on open-label ABILIFY (15 mg/day or 30 mg/day, with a starting dose of 30 mg/day) for at least 6 consecutive weeks. One hundred sixty-one outpatients were then randomized in a double-blind fashion, to either the same dose of ABILIFY they were on at the end of the stabilization and maintenance period or placebo and were then monitored for manic or depressive relapse. During the randomization phase, ABILIFY was superior to placebo on time to the number of combined affective relapses (manic plus depressive), the primary outcome measure for this study. The majority of these relapses were due to manic rather than depressive symptoms. There is insufficient data to know whether ABILIFY is effective in delaying the time to occurrence of depression in patients with bipolar I disorder.

An examination of population subgroups did not reveal any clear evidence of differential responsiveness on the basis of age and gender; however, there were insufficient numbers of patients in each of the ethnic groups to adequately assess inter-group differences.

Pediatric Patients

The efficacy of ABILIFY in the treatment of bipolar I disorder in pediatric patients (10 to 17 years of age) was evaluated in one four-week placebo-controlled trial (n=296) of outpatients who met DSM-IV criteria for bipolar I disorder manic or mixed episodes with or without psychotic features and had a Y-MRS score ≥20 at baseline. This double-blind, placebo-controlled trial compared two fixed doses of ABILIFY (10 mg/day or 30 mg/day) to placebo. The ABILIFY dose was started at 2 mg/day, which was titrated to 5 mg/day after 2 days, and to the target dose in 5 days in the 10 mg/day treatment arm and in 13 days in the 30 mg/day treatment arm. Both doses of ABILIFY were superior to placebo in change from baseline to week 4 on the Y-MRS total score. Although maintenance efficacy in pediatric patients has not been systematically evaluated, maintenance efficacy can be extrapolated from adult data along with comparisons of aripiprazole pharmacokinetic parameters in adult and pediatric patients.

Adjunctive Therapy

The efficacy of adjunctive ABILIFY with concomitant lithium or valproate in the treatment of manic or mixed episodes was established in a 6-week, placebo-controlled study (n=384) with a 2-week lead-in mood stabilizer monotherapy phase in adult patients who met DSM-IV criteria for bipolar I disorder. This study included patients with manic or mixed episodes and with or without psychotic features. Patients were initiated on open-label lithium (0.6 mEq/L to 1.0 mEq/L) or valproate (50 µg/mL to 125 µg/mL) at therapeutic serum levels, and remained on stable doses for 2 weeks. At the end of 2 weeks, patients demonstrating inadequate response (Y-MRS total score ≥16 and ≤25% improvement on the Y-MRS total score) to lithium or valproate were randomized to receive either aripiprazole (15 mg/day or an increase to 30 mg/day as early as day 7) or placebo as adjunctive therapy with open-label lithium or valproate. In the 6-week placebo-controlled phase, adjunctive ABILIFY starting at 15 mg/day with concomitant lithium or valproate (in a therapeutic range of 0.6 mEq/L to 1.0 mEq/L or 50 µg/mL to 125 µg/mL, respectively) was superior to lithium or valproate with adjunctive placebo in the reduction of the Y-MRS total score and CGI-BP Severity of Illness score (mania). Seventy-one percent of the patients coadministered valproate and 62% of the patients coadministered lithium were on 15 mg/day at 6-week endpoint.

Although the efficacy of adjunctive ABILIFY with concomitant lithium or valproate in the treatment of manic or mixed episodes in pediatric patients has not been systemat-

Table 15: ABILIFY Tablet Presentations

Tablet Strength	Tablet Color/Shape	Tablet Markings	Pack Size	NDC Code
2 mg	green modified rectangle	"A-006" and "2"	Bottle of 30	59148-006-13
5 mg	blue modified rectangle	"A-007" and "5"	Bottle of 30	59148-007-13
			Blister of 100	59148-007-35
10 mg	pink modified rectangle	"A-008" and "10"	Bottle of 30	59148-008-13
			Blister of 100	59148-008-35
15 mg	yellow round	"A-009" and "15"	Bottle of 30	59148-009-13
			Blister of 100	59148-009-35
20 mg	white round	"A-010" and "20"	Bottle of 30	59148-010-13
			Blister of 100	59148-010-35
30 mg	pink round	"A-011" and "30"	Bottle of 30	59148-011-13
			Blister of 100	59148-011-35

Table 16: ABILIFY DISCMELT Orally Disintegrating Tablet Presentations

Tablet Strength	Tablet Color	Tablet Markings	Pack Size	NDC Code
10 mg	pink (with scattered specks)	"A" and "640" "10"	Blister of 30	59148-640-23
15 mg	yellow (with scattered specks)	"A" and "641" "15"	Blister of 30	59148-641-23

ically evaluated, such efficacy can be extrapolated from adult data along with comparisons of aripiprazole pharmacokinetic parameters in adult and pediatric patients.

14.3 Adjunctive Treatment of Major Depressive Disorder
Adults

The efficacy of ABILIFY (aripiprazole) in the adjunctive treatment of major depressive disorder (MDD) was demonstrated in two short-term (6-week), placebo-controlled trials of adult patients meeting DSM-IV criteria for MDD who had had an inadequate response to prior antidepressant therapy (1 to 3 courses) in the current episode and who had also demonstrated an inadequate response to 8 weeks of prospective antidepressant therapy (paroxetine controlled-release, venlafaxine extended-release, fluoxetine, escitalopram, or sertraline). Inadequate response for prospective treatment was defined as less than 50% improvement on the 17-item version of the Hamilton Depression Rating Scale (HAMD17), minimal HAMD17 score of 14, and a Clinical Global Impressions Improvement rating of no better than minimal improvement. Inadequate response to prior treatment was defined as less than 50% improvement as perceived by the patient after a minimum of 6 weeks of antidepressant therapy at or above the minimal effective dose.

The primary instrument used for assessing depressive symptoms was the Montgomery-Asberg Depression Rating Scale (MADRS), a 10-item clinician-rated scale used to assess the degree of depressive symptomatology (apparent sadness, reported sadness, inner tension, reduced sleep, reduced appetite, concentration difficulties, lassitude, inability to feel, pessimistic thoughts, and suicidal thoughts). The key secondary instrument was the Sheehan Disability Scale (SDS), a 3-item self-rated instrument used to assess the impact of depression on three domains of functioning (work/school, social life, and family life) with each item scored from 0 (not at all) to 10 (extreme).

In the two trials (n=381, n=362), ABILIFY was superior to placebo in reducing mean MADRS total scores. In one study, ABILIFY was also superior to placebo in reducing the mean SDS score.

In both trials, patients received ABILIFY adjunctive to antidepressants at a dose of 5 mg/day. Based on tolerability and efficacy, doses could be adjusted by 5 mg increments, one week apart. Allowable doses were: 2 mg/day, 5 mg/day, 10 mg/day, 15 mg/day, and for patients who were not on potent CYP2D6 inhibitors fluoxetine and paroxetine, 20 mg/day. The mean final dose at the end point for the two trials was 10.7 mg/day and 11.4 mg/day.

An examination of population subgroups did not reveal evidence of differential response based on age, choice of prospective antidepressant, or race. With regard to gender, a smaller mean reduction on the MADRS total score was seen in males than in females.

14.4 Irritability Associated with Autistic Disorder
Pediatric Patients

The efficacy of ABILIFY (aripiprazole) in the treatment of irritability associated with autistic disorder was established in two 8-week, placebo-controlled trials in pediatric patients (6 to 17 years of age) who met the DSM-IV criteria for autistic disorder and demonstrated behaviors such as tantrums, aggression, self-injurious behavior, or a combination of these problems. Over 75% of these subjects were under 13 years of age.

Efficacy was evaluated using two assessment scales: the Aberrant Behavior Checklist (ABC) and the Clinical Global Impression-Improvement (CGI-I) scale. The primary outcome measure in both trials was the change from baseline to endpoint in the Irritability subscale of the ABC (ABC-I). The ABC-I subscale measured the emotional and behavioral symptoms of irritability in autistic disorder, including aggression towards others, deliberate self-injuriousness, temper tantrums, and quickly changing moods.

The results of these trials are as follows:

In one of the 8-week, placebo-controlled trials, children and adolescents with autistic disorder (n=98), aged 6 to 17 years, received daily doses of placebo or ABILIFY 2 mg/day to 15 mg/day. ABILIFY, starting at 2 mg/day with increases allowed up to 15 mg/day based on clinical response, significantly improved scores on the ABC-I subscale and on the CGI-I scale compared with placebo. The mean daily dose of ABILIFY at the end of 8-week treatment was 8.6 mg/day.

In the other 8-week, placebo-controlled trial in children and adolescents with autistic disorder (n=218), aged 6 to 17 years, three fixed doses of ABILIFY (5 mg/day, 10 mg/day, or 15 mg/day) were compared to placebo. ABILIFY dosing started at 2 mg/day and was increased to 5 mg/day after one week. After a second week, it was increased to 10 mg/day for patients in the 10 mg and 15 mg dose arms, and after a third week, it was increased to 15 mg/day in the 15 mg/day treatment arm. All three doses of ABILIFY significantly improved scores on the ABC-I subscale compared with placebo.

14.5 Agitation Associated with Schizophrenia or Bipolar Mania

The efficacy of intramuscular aripiprazole for injection for the treatment of agitation was established in three short-term (24-hour), placebo-controlled trials in agitated inpatients from two diagnostic groups: schizophrenia and bipolar I disorder (manic or mixed episodes, with or without psychotic features). Each of the trials included a single active comparator treatment arm of either haloperidol injection (schizophrenia studies) or lorazepam injection (bipolar mania study). Patients could receive up to three injections during the 24-hour treatment periods; however, patients could not receive the second injection until after the initial

2-hour period when the primary efficacy measure was assessed. Patients enrolled in the trials needed to be: (1) judged by the clinical investigators as clinically agitated and clinically appropriate candidates for treatment with intramuscular medication, and (2) exhibiting a level of agitation that met or exceeded a threshold score of $\geq$15 on the five items comprising the Positive and Negative Syndrome Scale (PANSS) Excited Component (ie, poor impulse control, tension, hostility, uncooperativeness, and excitement items) with at least two individual item scores $\geq$4 using a 1-7 scoring system (1 = absent, 4 = moderate, 7 = extreme). In the studies, the mean baseline PANSS Excited Component score was 19, with scores ranging from 15 to 34 (out of a maximum score of 35), thus suggesting predominantly moderate levels of agitation with some patients experiencing mild or severe levels of agitation. The primary efficacy measure used for assessing agitation signs and symptoms in these trials was the change from baseline in the PANSS Excited Component at 2 hours post-injection. A key secondary measure was the Clinical Global Impression of Improvement (CGI-I) Scale. The results of the trials follow:

In a placebo-controlled trial in agitated inpatients predominantly meeting DSM-IV criteria for schizophrenia (n=350), four fixed aripiprazole injection doses of 1 mg, 5.25 mg, 9.75 mg, and 15 mg were evaluated. At 2 hours post-injection, the 5.25 mg, 9.75 mg, and 15 mg doses were statistically superior to placebo in the PANSS Excited Component and on the CGI-I Scale.

In a second placebo-controlled trial in agitated inpatients predominantly meeting DSM-IV criteria for schizophrenia (n=445), one fixed aripiprazole injection dose of 9.75 mg was evaluated. At 2 hours post-injection, aripiprazole for injection was statistically superior to placebo in the PANSS Excited Component and on the CGI-I Scale.

In a placebo-controlled trial in agitated inpatients meeting DSM-IV criteria for bipolar I disorder (manic or mixed) (n=291), two fixed aripiprazole injection doses of 9.75 mg and 15 mg were evaluated. At 2 hours post-injection, both doses were statistically superior to placebo in the PANSS Excited Component.

Examination of population subsets (age, race, and gender) did not reveal any differential responsiveness on the basis of these subgroupings.

16 HOW SUPPLIED/STORAGE AND HANDLING
16.1 How Supplied

ABILIFY® (aripiprazole) Tablets have markings on one side and are available in the strengths and packages listed in Table 15.
[See table 15 above]

ABILIFY DISCMELT® (aripiprazole) Orally Disintegrating Tablets are round tablets with markings on either side. ABILIFY DISCMELT is available in the strengths and packages listed in Table 16.
[See table 16 at left]

ABILIFY® (aripiprazole) Oral Solution (1 mg/mL) is supplied in child-resistant bottles along with a calibrated oral dosing cup. ABILIFY Oral Solution is available as follows:
150 mL bottle   NDC 59148-013-15
ABILIFY® (aripiprazole) Injection for intramuscular use is available as a ready-to-use, 9.75 mg/1.3 mL (7.5 mg/mL) solution in clear, Type 1 glass vials as follows:
9.75 mg/1.3 mL single-dose vial   NDC 59148-016-65

16.2 Storage
Tablets

Store at 25° C (77° F); excursions permitted between 15° C to 30° C (59° F to 86° F) [see USP Controlled Room Temperature].

Oral Solution

Store at 25° C (77° F); excursions permitted between 15° C to 30° C (59° F to 86° F) [see USP Controlled Room Temperature]. Opened bottles of ABILIFY Oral Solution can be used for up to 6 months after opening, but not beyond the expiration date on the bottle. The bottle and its contents should be discarded after the expiration date.

Injection

Store at 25° C (77° F); excursions permitted between 15° C to 30° C (59° F to 86° F) [see USP Controlled Room Temperature]. Protect from light by storing in the original container. Retain in carton until time of use.

17 PATIENT COUNSELING INFORMATION

See Medication Guide

17.1 Information for Patients

Physicians are advised to discuss the following issues with patients for whom they prescribe ABILIFY:

Increased Mortality in Elderly Patients with Dementia-Related Psychosis

Patients and caregivers should be advised that elderly patients with dementia-related psychoses treated with antipsychotic drugs are at increased risk of death. ABILIFY is not approved for elderly patients with dementia-related psychosis [see WARNINGS AND PRECAUTIONS (5.1)].

Clinical Worsening of Depression and Suicide Risk

Patients, their families, and their caregivers should be encouraged to be alert to the emergence of anxiety, agitation, panic attacks, insomnia, irritability, hostility, aggressiveness, impulsivity, akathisia (psychomotor restlessness), hypomania, mania, other unusual changes in behavior, worsening of depression, and suicidal ideation, especially early during antidepressant treatment and when the dose is adjusted up or down. Families and caregivers of patients should be advised to look for the emergence of such symptoms on a day-to-day basis, since changes may be abrupt. Such symptoms should be reported to the patient's prescriber or health professional, especially if they are severe, abrupt in onset, or were not part of the patient's presenting symptoms. Symptoms such as these may be associated with an increased risk for suicidal thinking and behavior and indicate a need for very close monitoring and possibly changes in the medication *[see WARNINGS AND PRECAUTIONS (5.2)]*.

Prescribers or other health professionals should inform patients, their families, and their caregivers about the benefits and risks associated with treatment with ABILIFY (aripiprazole) and should counsel them in its appropriate use. A patient Medication Guide about "Antidepressant Medicines, Depression and other Serious Mental Illness, and Suicidal Thoughts or Actions" is available for ABILIFY. The prescriber or health professional should instruct patients, their families, and their caregivers to read the Medication Guide and should assist them in understanding its contents. Patients should be given the opportunity to discuss the contents of the Medication Guide and to obtain answers to any questions they may have. It should be noted that ABILIFY is not approved as a single agent for treatment of depression and has not been evaluated in pediatric major depressive disorder.

Use of Orally Disintegrating Tablet

Do not open the blister until ready to administer. For single tablet removal, open the package and peel back the foil on the blister to expose the tablet. Do not push the tablet through the foil because this could damage the tablet. Immediately upon opening the blister, using dry hands, remove the tablet and place the entire ABILIFY DISCMELT Orally Disintegrating Tablet on the tongue. Tablet disintegration occurs rapidly in saliva. It is recommended that ABILIFY DISCMELT be taken without liquid. However, if needed, it can be taken with liquid. Do not attempt to split the tablet.

Interference with Cognitive and Motor Performance

Because aripiprazole may have the potential to impair judgment, thinking, or motor skills, patients should be cautioned about operating hazardous machinery, including automobiles, until they are reasonably certain that aripiprazole therapy does not affect them adversely *[see WARNINGS AND PRECAUTIONS (5.9)]*.

Pregnancy

Patients should be advised to notify their physician if they become pregnant or intend to become pregnant during therapy with ABILIFY *[see USE IN SPECIFIC POPULATIONS (8.1)]*.

Nursing

Patients should be advised not to breast-feed an infant if they are taking ABILIFY *[see USE IN SPECIFIC POPULATIONS (8.3)]*.

Concomitant Medication

Patients should be advised to inform their physicians if they are taking, or plan to take, any prescription or over-the-counter drugs, since there is a potential for interactions *[see DRUG INTERACTIONS (7)]*.

Alcohol

Patients should be advised to avoid alcohol while taking ABILIFY *[see DRUG INTERACTIONS (7.2)]*.

Heat Exposure and Dehydration

Patients should be advised regarding appropriate care in avoiding overheating and dehydration *[see WARNINGS AND PRECAUTIONS (5.10)]*.

Sugar Content

Patients should be advised that each mL of ABILIFY Oral Solution contains 400 mg of sucrose and 200 mg of fructose.

Phenylketonurics

Phenylalanine is a component of aspartame. Each ABILIFY DISCMELT Orally Disintegrating Tablet contains the following amounts: 10 mg - 1.12 mg phenylalanine and 15 mg - 1.68 mg phenylalanine.

Tablets manufactured by Bristol-Myers Squibb Company, Princeton, NJ 08543 USA

Orally Disintegrating Tablets, Oral Solution, and Injection manufactured by Bristol-Myers Squibb Company, Princeton, NJ 08543 USA

Distributed and marketed by Otsuka America Pharmaceutical, Inc, Rockville, MD 20850 USA

Marketed by Bristol-Myers Squibb Company, Princeton, NJ 08543 USA

US Patent Nos: 5,006,528; 6,977,257; and 7,115,587

ABILIFY (aripiprazole) is a trademark of Otsuka Pharmaceutical Company.

1239550A7 0309L-2745A

D6-B0001-11-09   Rev November 2009

© 2009, Otsuka Pharmaceutical Co, Ltd, Tokyo, 101-8535 Japan

MEDICATION GUIDE

ABILIFY® (a-BIL-i-fi)

Generic name: aripiprazole

Antidepressant Medicines, Depression and other Serious Mental Illnesses, and Suicidal Thoughts or Actions

Read the Medication Guide that comes with your or your family member's antidepressant medicine. This Medication Guide is only about the risk of suicidal thoughts and actions with antidepressant medicines. **Talk to your, or your family member's, healthcare provider about:**

• all risks and benefits of treatment with antidepressant medicines

• all treatment choices for depression or other serious mental illness

What is the most important information I should know about antidepressant medicines, depression and other serious mental illnesses, and suicidal thoughts or actions?

1. Antidepressant medicines may increase suicidal thoughts or actions in some children, teenagers, and young adults within the first few months of treatment.

2. Depression and other serious mental illnesses are the most important causes of suicidal thoughts and actions. Some people may have a particularly high risk of having suicidal thoughts or actions. These include people who have (or have a family history of) bipolar illness (also called manic-depressive illness) or suicidal thoughts or actions.

3. How can I watch for and try to prevent suicidal thoughts and actions in myself or a family member?

• Pay close attention to any changes, especially sudden changes, in mood, behaviors, thoughts, or feelings. This is very important when an antidepressant medicine is started or when the dose is changed.

• Call the healthcare provider right away to report new or sudden changes in mood, behavior, thoughts, or feelings.

• Keep all follow-up visits with the healthcare provider as scheduled. Call the healthcare provider between visits as needed, especially if you have concerns about symptoms.

Call a healthcare provider right away if you or your family member has any of the following symptoms, especially if they are new, worse, or worry you:

• thoughts about suicide or dying

• attempts to commit suicide

• new or worse depression

• new or worse anxiety

• feeling very agitated or restless

• panic attacks

• trouble sleeping (insomnia)

• new or worse irritability

• acting aggressive, being angry, or violent

• acting on dangerous impulses

• an extreme increase in activity and talking (mania)

• other unusual changes in behavior or mood

What else do I need to know about antidepressant medicines?

• **Never stop an antidepressant medicine without first talking to a healthcare provider.** Stopping an antidepressant medicine suddenly can cause other symptoms.

• **Antidepressants are medicines used to treat depression and other illnesses.** It is important to discuss all the risks of treating depression and also the risks of not treating it. Patients and their families or other caregivers should discuss all treatment choices with the healthcare provider, not just the use of antidepressants.

• **Antidepressant medicines have other side effects.** Talk to the healthcare provider about the side effects of the medicine prescribed for you or your family member.

• **Antidepressant medicines can interact with other medicines.** Know all of the medicines that you or your family member takes. Keep a list of all medicines to show the healthcare provider. Do not start new medicines without first checking with your healthcare provider.

• **Not all antidepressant medicines prescribed for children are FDA approved for use in children.** Talk to your child's healthcare provider for more information.

This Medication Guide has been approved by the U.S. Food and Drug Administration for all antidepressants.

It should be noted that ABILIFY is approved to be added to an antidepressant when the response from the antidepressant alone is not adequate. ABILIFY is not approved for pediatric patients with depression.

Call your doctor for medical advice about side effects. You may report side effects to FDA at 1-800-FDA-1088.

ABILIFY is a trademark of Otsuka Pharmaceutical Company.

1239550A7 0309L-2745C

D6-B0001-11-09   Rev November 2009

© 2009, Otsuka Pharmaceutical Co, Ltd, Tokyo, 101-8535 Japan

Shown in Product Identification Guide, page 321

ATRIPLA®   ℞

[uh TRIP luh]

(efavirenz/emtricitabine/tenofovir disoproxil fumarate) tablets

HIGHLIGHTS OF PRESCRIBING INFORMATION

These highlights do not include all the information needed to use ATRIPLA safely and effectively. See full prescribing information for ATRIPLA.

ATRIPLA® **(efavirenz/emtricitabine/tenofovir disoproxil fumarate) tablets**

Initial U.S. Approval: 2006

WARNINGS: LACTIC ACIDOSIS/SEVERE HEPATO-MEGALY WITH STEATOSIS and POST TREATMENT EXACERBATION OF HEPATITIS B

See full prescribing information for complete boxed warning.

• **Lactic acidosis and severe hepatomegaly with steatosis, including fatal cases, have been reported with the use of nucleoside analogs, including tenofovir disoproxil fumarate, a component of ATRIPLA. (5.1)**

• **ATRIPLA is not approved for the treatment of chronic hepatitis B virus (HBV) infection. Severe acute exacerbations of hepatitis B have been reported in patients coinfected with HBV and HIV-1 who have discontinued EMTRIVA or VIREAD, two of the components of ATRIPLA. Hepatic function should be monitored closely in these patients. If appropriate, initiation of anti-hepatitis B therapy may be warranted. (5.2)**

——————RECENT MAJOR CHANGES——————

Boxed Warning	1/2010
Warnings and Precautions	
Patients Coinfected with HIV-1 and HBV (5.2)	1/2010
New Onset or Worsening Renal Impairment (5.7)	1/2010
Reproductive Risk Potential (5.8)	5/2010
Decrease in Bone Mineral Density (5.11)	1/2010
Hepatotoxicity (5.10)	5/2010

——————INDICATIONS AND USAGE——————

ATRIPLA, a combination of 2 nucleoside analog HIV-1 reverse transcriptase inhibitors and 1 non-nucleoside HIV-1 reverse transcriptase inhibitor, is indicated for use alone as a complete regimen or in combination with other antiretroviral agents for the treatment of HIV-1 infection in adults. (1)

——————DOSAGE AND ADMINISTRATION——————

• Recommended dose: One tablet once daily taken orally on an empty stomach, preferably at bedtime. (2)

• Dose in renal impairment: Should not be administered in patients with creatinine clearance <50 mL/min. (2)

——————DOSAGE FORMS AND STRENGTHS——————

Tablet containing 600 mg of efavirenz, 200 mg of emtricitabine and 300 mg of tenofovir disoproxil fumarate. (3)

——————CONTRAINDICATIONS——————

• Previously demonstrated hypersensitivity (e.g., Stevens-Johnson syndrome, erythema multiforme, or toxic skin eruptions) to efavirenz, a component of ATRIPLA. (4.1)

• For some drugs, competition for CYP3A by efavirenz could result in inhibition of their metabolism and create the potential for serious and/or life-threatening adverse reactions (e.g., cardiac arrhythmias, prolonged sedation, or respiratory depression). (4.2)

——————WARNINGS AND PRECAUTIONS——————

• Serious psychiatric symptoms: Immediate medical evaluation is recommended. (5.5, 6.1)

• Nervous system symptoms (NSS): NSS are frequent, usually begin 1–2 days after initiating therapy and resolve in 2–4 weeks. Dosing at bedtime may improve tolerability. NSS are not predictive of onset of psychiatric symptoms. (2, 5.6)

• New onset or worsening renal impairment: Can include acute renal failure and Fanconi syndrome. Assess creatinine clearance (CrCl) before initiating treatment with ATRIPLA. Monitor CrCl and serum phosphorus in patients at risk. Avoid administering ATRIPLA with concurrent or recent use of nephrotoxic drugs. (5.7)

• Pregnancy: Fetal harm can occur when administered to a pregnant woman during the first trimester. Women should be apprised of the potential harm to the fetus. (5.8)

• Rash: Discontinue if severe rash develops. (5.9, 6.1)

• Hepatotoxicity: Monitor liver function tests before and during treatment in patients with underlying hepatic disease, including hepatitis B or C coinfection, marked transaminase elevations, or who are taking medications associated with liver toxicity. Among reported cases of hepatic failure, a few occurred in patients with no pre-existing hepatic disease. (5.10, 6.3, 8.6)

- Decreases in bone mineral density (BMD): Consider monitoring BMD in patients with a history of pathological fracture or who are at risk for osteopenia. (5.11)
- Convulsions: Use caution in patients with a history of seizures. (5.12)
- Immune reconstitution syndrome: May necessitate further evaluation and treatment. (5.13)
- Redistribution/accumulation of body fat: Observed in patients receiving antiretroviral therapy. (5.14)
- Coadministration with other products: Do not use with drugs containing efavirenz, emtricitabine or tenofovir disoproxil fumarate including SUSTIVA, TRUVADA, EMTRIVA, VIREAD; or with drugs containing lamivudine. Do not administer in combination with HEPSERA. (5.4)

---ADVERSE REACTIONS---

Most common adverse reactions (incidence ≥10%) observed in an active-controlled clinical study of efavirenz, emtricitabine, and tenofovir DF are diarrhea, nausea, fatigue, headache, dizziness, depression, insomnia, abnormal dreams, and rash. (6)

To report SUSPECTED ADVERSE REACTIONS, contact Gilead Sciences, Inc. at 1-800-GILEAD-5 or FDA at 1-800-FDA-1088 or www.fda.gov/medwatch

---DRUG INTERACTIONS---

- Efavirenz: Coadministration of efavirenz can alter the concentrations of other drugs and other drugs may alter the concentrations of efavirenz. The potential for drug-drug interactions must be considered before and during therapy. (4.2, 7.1, 12.3)
- Didanosine: Tenofovir disoproxil fumarate increases didanosine concentrations. Use with caution and monitor for evidence of didanosine toxicity (e.g., pancreatitis, neuropathy) when coadministered. Consider dose reductions or discontinuations of didanosine if warranted. (7.2)
- Atazanavir: Coadministration of ATRIPLA and atazanavir or atazanavir/ritonavir is not recommended. (7.3)
- Lopinavir/ritonavir: Coadministration increases tenofovir concentrations. Monitor for evidence of tenofovir toxicity. (7.3)

---USE IN SPECIFIC POPULATIONS---

- Pregnancy: Women should avoid pregnancy while receiving ATRIPLA (efavirenz/emtricitabine/tenofovir disoproxil fumarate) and for 12 weeks after discontinuation. (5.8)
- Nursing mothers: Women infected with HIV should be instructed not to breast-feed. (8.3)
- Hepatic impairment: Use caution in patients with hepatic impairment. (5.10, 8.6)
- Pediatrics: Safety and efficacy not established in patients less than 18 years of age. (2, 8.4)

See 17 for PATIENT COUNSELING INFORMATION and FDA-approved patient labeling

Revised: 05/2010

FULL PRESCRIBING INFORMATION: CONTENTS*
WARNINGS: LACTIC ACIDOSIS/SEVERE HEPATOMEGALY WITH STEATOSIS AND POST TREATMENT EXACERBATION OF HEPATITIS B
1   INDICATIONS AND USAGE
2   DOSAGE AND ADMINISTRATION
3   DOSAGE FORMS AND STRENGTHS
4   CONTRAINDICATIONS
    4.1   Hypersensitivity
    4.2   Contraindicated Drugs
5   WARNINGS AND PRECAUTIONS
    5.1   Lactic Acidosis/Severe Hepatomegaly with Steatosis
    5.2   Patients Coinfected with HIV-1 and HBV
    5.3   Drug Interactions
    5.4   Coadministration with Related Products
    5.5   Psychiatric Symptoms
    5.6   Nervous System Symptoms
    5.7   New Onset or Worsening Renal Impairment
    5.8   Reproductive Risk Potential
    5.9   Rash
    5.10 Hepatotoxicity
    5.11 Decreases in Bone Mineral Density
    5.12 Convulsions
    5.13 Immune Reconstitution Syndrome
    5.14 Fat Redistribution
6   ADVERSE REACTIONS
    6.1   Adverse Reactions from Clinical Trials Experience
    6.2   Laboratory Abnormalities
    6.3   Postmarketing Experience
7   DRUG INTERACTIONS
    7.1   Efavirenz
    7.2   Emtricitabine and Tenofovir Disoproxil Fumarate
    7.3   Efavirenz, Emtricitabine and Tenofovir Disoproxil Fumarate
    7.4   Efavirenz Assay Interference
8   USE IN SPECIFIC POPULATIONS
    8.1   Pregnancy
    8.3   Nursing Mothers
    8.4   Pediatric Use
    8.5   Geriatric Use
    8.6   Hepatic Impairment
    8.7   Renal Impairment
10 OVERDOSAGE
11 DESCRIPTION
12 CLINICAL PHARMACOLOGY
    12.1 Mechanism of Action
    12.3 Pharmacokinetics
    12.4 Microbiology
13 NONCLINICAL TOXICOLOGY
    13.1 Carcinogenesis, Mutagenesis, Impairment of Fertility

13.2 Animal Toxicology and/or Pharmacology
14 CLINICAL STUDIES
16 HOW SUPPLIED/STORAGE AND HANDLING
17 PATIENT COUNSELING INFORMATION AND FDA-APPROVED PATIENT LABELING
    17.1 Drug Interactions
    17.2 Information for Patients
    17.3 Lactic Acidosis/Severe Hepatomegaly with Steatosis
    17.4 Patients Coinfected with HIV-1 and HBV
    17.5 New Onset or Worsening Renal Impairment
    17.6 Decreases in Bone Mineral Density
    17.7 Dosing Instructions
    17.8 Nervous System Symptoms
    17.9 Psychiatric Symptoms
    17.10 Rash
    17.11 Reproductive Risk Potential
* Sections or subsections omitted from the full prescribing information are not listed

---

FULL PRESCRIBING INFORMATION

> **WARNINGS: LACTIC ACIDOSIS/SEVERE HEPATO-MEGALY WITH STEATOSIS AND POST TREATMENT EXACERBATION OF HEPATITIS B**
> Lactic acidosis and severe hepatomegaly with steatosis, including fatal cases, have been reported with the use of nucleoside analogs, including tenofovir disoproxil fumarate, a component of ATRIPLA, in combination with other antiretrovirals *[See Warnings and Precautions (5.1)]*.
> ATRIPLA (efavirenz/emtricitabine/tenofovir disoproxil fumarate) is not approved for the treatment of chronic hepatitis B virus (HBV) infection and the safety and efficacy of ATRIPLA have not been established in patients coinfected with HBV and HIV-1. Severe acute exacerbations of hepatitis B have been reported in patients who have discontinued EMTRIVA or VIREAD, which are components of ATRIPLA. Hepatic function should be monitored closely with both clinical and laboratory follow-up for at least several months in patients who are coinfected with HIV-1 and HBV and discontinue ATRIPLA. If appropriate, initiation of anti-hepatitis B therapy may be warranted *[See Warnings and Precautions (5.2)]*.

1   INDICATIONS AND USAGE

ATRIPLA® is indicated for use alone as a complete regimen or in combination with other antiretroviral agents for the treatment of HIV-1 infection in adults.

2   DOSAGE AND ADMINISTRATION

Adults: The dose of ATRIPLA is one tablet once daily taken orally on an empty stomach. Dosing at bedtime may improve the tolerability of nervous system symptoms.
Pediatrics: ATRIPLA is not recommended for use in patients <18 years of age.
Renal Impairment: Because ATRIPLA is a fixed-dose combination, it should not be prescribed for patients requiring dosage adjustment such as those with moderate or severe renal impairment (creatinine clearance <50 mL/min).

3   DOSAGE FORMS AND STRENGTHS

ATRIPLA is available as tablets. Each tablet contains 600 mg of efavirenz, 200 mg of emtricitabine and 300 mg of tenofovir disoproxil fumarate (tenofovir DF, which is equivalent to 245 mg of tenofovir disoproxil). The tablets are pink, capsule-shaped, film-coated, debossed with "123" on one side and plain-faced on the other side.

4   CONTRAINDICATIONS

4.1   Hypersensitivity

ATRIPLA is contraindicated in patients with previously demonstrated clinically significant hypersensitivity (e.g., Stevens-Johnson syndrome, erythema multiforme, or toxic skin eruptions) to efavirenz, a component of ATRIPLA.

4.2   Contraindicated Drugs

For some drugs, competition for CYP3A by efavirenz could result in inhibition of their metabolism and create the potential for serious and/or life-threatening adverse reactions (e.g., cardiac arrhythmias, prolonged sedation, or respiratory depression). Drugs that are contraindicated with ATRIPLA are listed in Table 1.
[See table 1 at left]

5   WARNINGS AND PRECAUTIONS

5.1   Lactic Acidosis/Severe Hepatomegaly with Steatosis

Lactic acidosis and severe hepatomegaly with steatosis, including fatal cases, have been reported with the use of nucleoside analogs including tenofovir DF, a component of ATRIPLA, in combination with other antiretrovirals.

Table 1: Drugs That Are Contraindicated or Not Recommended for Use With ATRIPLA

Drug Class: Drug Name	Clinical Comment
Antifungal: voriconazole	Efavirenz significantly decreases voriconazole plasma concentrations, and coadministration may decrease the therapeutic effectiveness of voriconazole. Also, voriconazole significantly increases efavirenz plasma concentrations, which may increase the risk of efavirenz-associated side effects. Because ATRIPLA is a fixed-dose combination product, the dose of efavirenz cannot be altered. *[See Clinical Pharmacology (12.3) Tables 5 and 6]*
Ergot derivatives (dihydroergotamine, ergonovine, ergotamine, methylergonovine)	Potential for serious and/or life-threatening reactions such as acute ergot toxicity characterized by peripheral vasospasm and ischemia of the extremities and other tissues.
Benzodiazepines: midazolam, triazolam	Potential for serious and/or life-threatening reactions such as prolonged or increased sedation or respiratory depression.
Calcium channel blocker: bepridil	Potential for serious and/or life-threatening reactions such as cardiac arrhythmias.
GI motility agent: cisapride	Potential for serious and/or life-threatening reactions such as cardiac arrhythmias.
Neuroleptic: pimozide	Potential for serious and/or life-threatening reactions such as cardiac arrhythmias.
St. John's wort (*Hypericum perforatum*)	May lead to loss of virologic response and possible resistance to efavirenz or to the class of non-nucleoside reverse transcriptase inhibitors (NNRTIs).

A majority of these cases have been in women. Obesity and prolonged nucleoside exposure may be risk factors. Particular caution should be exercised when administering nucleoside analogs to any patient with known risk factors for liver disease; however, cases have also been reported in patients with no known risk factors. Treatment with ATRIPLA (efavirenz/emtricitabine/tenofovir disoproxil fumarate) should be suspended in any patient who develops clinical or laboratory findings suggestive of lactic acidosis or pronounced hepatotoxicity (which may include hepatomegaly and steatosis even in the absence of marked transaminase elevations).

5.2 Patients Coinfected with HIV-1 and HBV

It is recommended that all patients with HIV-1 be tested for the presence of chronic HBV before initiating antiretroviral therapy. ATRIPLA is not approved for the treatment of chronic HBV infection, and the safety and efficacy of ATRIPLA have not been established in patients coinfected with HBV and HIV-1. Severe acute exacerbations of hepatitis B have been reported in patients who are coinfected with HBV and HIV-1 and have discontinued emtricitabine or tenofovir DF, two of the components of ATRIPLA. In some patients infected with HBV and treated with emtricitabine, the exacerbations of hepatitis B were associated with liver decompensation and liver failure. Patients who are coinfected with HIV-1 and HBV should be closely monitored with both clinical and laboratory follow up for at least several months after stopping treatment with ATRIPLA. If appropriate, initiation of anti-hepatitis B therapy may be warranted.

ATRIPLA should not be administered with HEPSERA® (adefovir dipivoxil) *[See Drug Interactions (7.2)]*.

5.3 Drug Interactions

Efavirenz plasma concentrations may be altered by substrates, inhibitors, or inducers of CYP3A. Likewise, efavirenz may alter plasma concentrations of drugs metabolized by CYP3A *[See Contraindications (4.2), Drug Interactions (7.1)]*.

5.4 Coadministration with Related Products

Related drugs not for coadministration with ATRIPLA include EMTRIVA (emtricitabine), VIREAD (tenofovir DF), TRUVADA (emtricitabine/tenofovir DF), and SUSTIVA (efavirenz), which contain the same active components as ATRIPLA. Due to similarities between emtricitabine and lamivudine, ATRIPLA should not be coadministered with drugs containing lamivudine, including Combivir (lamivudine/zidovudine), Epivir, or Epivir-HBV (lamivudine), Epzicom (abacavir sulfate/lamivudine), or Trizivir (abacavir sulfate/lamivudine/zidovudine).

5.5 Psychiatric Symptoms

Serious psychiatric adverse experiences have been reported in patients treated with efavirenz. In controlled trials of 1008 subjects treated with regimens containing efavirenz for a mean of 2.1 years and 635 subjects treated with control regimens for a mean of 1.5 years, the frequency (regardless of causality) of specific serious psychiatric events among subjects who received efavirenz or control regimens, respectively, were: severe depression (2.4%, 0.9%), suicidal ideation (0.7%, 0.3%), nonfatal suicide attempts (0.5%, 0%), aggressive behavior (0.4%, 0.5%), paranoid reactions (0.4%, 0.3%), and manic reactions (0.2%, 0.3%). When psychiatric symptoms similar to those noted above were combined and evaluated as a group in a multifactorial analysis of data from Study AI266006 (006), treatment with efavirenz was associated with an increase in the occurrence of these selected psychiatric symptoms. Other factors associated with an increase in the occurrence of these psychiatric symptoms were history of injection drug use, psychiatric history, and receipt of psychiatric medication at study entry; similar associations were observed in both the efavirenz and control treatment groups. In Study 006, onset of new serious psychiatric symptoms occurred throughout the study for both efavirenz-treated and control-treated subjects. One percent of efavirenz-treated subjects discontinued or interrupted treatment because of one or more of these selected psychiatric symptoms. There have also been occasional postmarketing reports of death by suicide, delusions, and psychosis-like behavior, although a causal relationship to the use of efavirenz cannot be determined from these reports. Patients with serious psychiatric adverse experiences should seek immediate medical evaluation to assess the possibility that the symptoms may be related to the use of efavirenz, and if so, to determine whether the risks of continued therapy outweigh the benefits *[See Adverse Reactions (6)]*.

5.6 Nervous System Symptoms

Fifty-three percent (531/1008) of subjects receiving efavirenz in controlled trials reported central nervous system symptoms (any grade, regardless of causality) compared to 25% (156/635) of subjects receiving control regimens. These symptoms included dizziness (28.1% of the 1008 subjects), insomnia (16.3%), impaired concentration (8.3%), somnolence (7.0%), abnormal dreams (6.2%), and hallucinations (1.2%). Other reported symptoms were euphoria, confusion, agitation, amnesia, stupor, abnormal thinking, and depersonalization. The majority of these symptoms were mild-moderate (50.7%); symptoms were severe in 2.0% of subjects. Overall, 2.1% of subjects discontinued therapy as a result. These symptoms usually begin during the first or second day of therapy and generally resolve after the first 2–4 weeks of therapy. After 4 weeks of therapy, the prevalence of nervous system symptoms of at least moderate severity ranged from 5% to 9% in subjects treated with regimens containing efavirenz and from 3% to 5% in subjects treated with a control regimen. Patients should be informed that these common symptoms were likely to improve with continued therapy and were not predictive of subsequent onset of the less frequent psychiatric symptoms *[See Warnings and Precautions (5.5)]*. Dosing at bedtime may improve the tolerability of these nervous system symptoms *[See Dosage and Administration (2)]*.

Analysis of long-term data from Study 006, (median follow-up 180 weeks, 102 weeks, and 76 weeks for subjects treated with efavirenz + zidovudine + lamivudine, efavirenz + indinavir, and indinavir + zidovudine + lamivudine, respectively) showed that, beyond 24 weeks of therapy, the incidences of new-onset nervous system symptoms among efavirenz-treated subjects were generally similar to those in the indinavir-containing control arm.

Patients receiving ATRIPLA (efavirenz/emtricitabine/tenofovir disoproxil fumarate) should be alerted to the potential for additive central nervous system effects when ATRIPLA is used concomitantly with alcohol or psychoactive drugs.

Patients who experience central nervous system symptoms such as dizziness, impaired concentration, and/or drowsiness should avoid potentially hazardous tasks such as driving or operating machinery.

5.7 New Onset or Worsening Renal Impairment

Emtricitabine and tenofovir are principally eliminated by the kidney; however, efavirenz is not. Since ATRIPLA is a combination product and the dose of the individual components cannot be altered, patients with creatinine clearance <50 mL/min should not receive ATRIPLA.

Renal impairment, including cases of acute renal failure and Fanconi syndrome (renal tubular injury with severe hypophosphatemia), has been reported with the use of tenofovir DF *[See Adverse Reactions (6.3)]*.

It is recommended that creatinine clearance be calculated in all patients prior to initiating therapy and as clinically appropriate during therapy with ATRIPLA. Routine monitoring of calculated creatinine clearance and serum phosphorus should be performed in patients at risk for renal impairment, including patients who have previously experienced renal events while receiving HEPSERA.

ATRIPLA should be avoided with concurrent or recent use of a nephrotoxic agent.

5.8 Reproductive Risk Potential

Pregnancy Category D: Efavirenz may cause fetal harm when administered during the first trimester to a pregnant woman. Pregnancy should be avoided in women receiving ATRIPLA. Barrier contraception must always be used in combination with other methods of contraception (e.g., oral or other hormonal contraceptives). Because of the long half-life of efavirenz, use of adequate contraceptive measures for 12 weeks after discontinuation of ATRIPLA is recommended. Women of childbearing potential should undergo pregnancy testing before initiation of ATRIPLA. If this drug is used during the first trimester of pregnancy, or if the patient becomes pregnant while taking this drug, the patient should be apprised of the potential harm to the fetus.

There are no adequate and well-controlled studies of ATRIPLA in pregnant women. ATRIPLA should be used during pregnancy only if the potential benefit justifies the potential risk to the fetus, such as in pregnant women without other therapeutic options.

Antiretroviral Pregnancy Registry: To monitor fetal outcomes of pregnant women, an Antiretroviral Pregnancy Registry has been established. Physicians are encouraged to register patients who become pregnant by calling (800) 258-4263.

Efavirenz: As of July 2009, the Antiretroviral Pregnancy Registry has received prospective reports of 661 pregnancies exposed to efavirenz-containing regimens, nearly all of which were first-trimester exposures (606 pregnancies). Birth defects occurred in 14 of 501 live births (first-trimester exposure) and 2 of 55 live births (second/third-trimester exposure). One of these prospectively reported defects with first-trimester exposure was a neural tube defect. A single case of anophthalmia with first-trimester exposure to efavirenz has also been prospectively reported; however, this case included severe oblique facial clefts and amniotic banding, a known association with anophthalmia. There have been six retrospective reports of findings consistent with neural tube defects, including meningomyelocele. All mothers were exposed to efavirenz-containing regimens in the first trimester. Although a causal relationship of these events to the use of efavirenz has not been established, similar defects have been observed in preclinical studies of efavirenz.

Malformations have been observed in 3 of 20 fetuses/infants from efavirenz-treated cynomolgus monkeys (versus 0 of 20 concomitant controls) in a developmental toxicity study. The pregnant monkeys were dosed throughout pregnancy (postcoital days 20–150) with efavirenz 60 mg/kg daily, a dose which resulted in plasma drug concentrations similar to those in humans given 600 mg/day of efavirenz. Anencephaly and unilateral anophthalmia were observed in one fetus, microophthalmia was observed in another fetus, and cleft palate was observed in a third fetus. Efavirenz crosses the placenta in cynomolgus monkeys and produces fetal blood concentrations similar to maternal blood concentrations. Efavirenz has been shown to cross the placenta in rats and rabbits and produces fetal blood concentrations of efavirenz similar to maternal concentrations. An increase in fetal resorptions was observed in rats at efavirenz doses that produced peak plasma concentrations and AUC values in female rats equivalent to or lower than those achieved in humans given 600 mg once daily of efavirenz. Efavirenz produced no reproductive toxicities when given to pregnant rabbits at doses that produced peak plasma concentrations similar to and AUC values approximately half of those achieved in humans given 600 mg once daily of efavirenz.

5.9 Rash

In controlled clinical trials, 26% (266/1008) of subjects treated with 600 mg efavirenz experienced new-onset skin rash compared with 17% (111/635) of subjects treated in control groups. Rash associated with blistering, moist desquamation, or ulceration occurred in 0.9% (9/1008) of subjects treated with efavirenz. The incidence of Grade 4 rash (e.g., erythema multiforme, Stevens-Johnson syndrome) in subjects treated with efavirenz in all studies and expanded access was 0.1%. Rashes are usually mild-to-moderate maculopapular skin eruptions that occur within the first 2 weeks of initiating therapy with efavirenz (median time to onset of rash in adults was 11 days) and, in most subjects continuing therapy with efavirenz, rash resolves within 1 month (median duration, 16 days). The discontinuation rate for rash in clinical trials was 1.7% (17/1008). ATRIPLA can be reinitiated in patients interrupting therapy because of rash. ATRIPLA (efavirenz/emtricitabine/tenofovir disoproxil fumarate) should be discontinued in patients developing severe rash associated with blistering, desquamation, mucosal involvement, or fever. Appropriate antihistamines and/or corticosteroids may improve the tolerability and hasten the resolution of rash.

Experience with efavirenz in subjects who discontinued other antiretroviral agents of the NNRTI class is limited. Nineteen subjects who discontinued nevirapine because of rash have been treated with efavirenz. Nine of these subjects developed mild-to-moderate rash while receiving therapy with efavirenz, and two of these subjects discontinued because of rash.

5.10 Hepatotoxicity

Monitoring of liver enzymes before and during treatment is recommended for patients with underlying hepatic disease, including hepatitis B or C infection; patients with marked transaminase elevations; and patients treated with other medications associated with liver toxicity *[See also Warnings and Precautions (5.2)]*. A few of the postmarketing reports of hepatic failure occurred in patients with no preexisting hepatic disease or other identifiable risk factors *[See Adverse Reactions (6.3)]*. Liver enzyme monitoring should also be considered for patients without pre-existing hepatic dysfunction or other risk factors. In patients with persistent elevations of serum transaminases to greater than five times the upper limit of the normal range, the benefit of continued therapy with ATRIPLA needs to be weighed against the unknown risks of significant liver toxicity *[See Adverse Reactions (6.2)]*.

5.11 Decreases in Bone Mineral Density

Bone mineral density (BMD) monitoring should be considered for HIV-1 infected subjects who have a history of pathologic bone fracture or are at risk for osteopenia. Although the effect of supplementation with calcium and vitamin D was not studied, such supplementation may be beneficial for all patients. If bone abnormalities are suspected then appropriate consultation should be obtained.

In a 144-week study of treatment-naive subjects receiving tenofovir DF, decreases in BMD were seen at the lumbar spine and hip in both arms of the study. At Week 144, there was a significantly greater mean percentage decrease from baseline in BMD at the lumbar spine in subjects receiving tenofovir DF + lamivudine + efavirenz compared with subjects receiving stavudine + lamivudine + efavirenz. Changes in BMD at the hip were similar between the two treatment groups. In both groups, the majority of the reduction in BMD occurred in the first 24–48 weeks of the study and this reduction was sustained through 144 weeks. Twenty-eight percent of tenofovir DF-treated subjects vs. 21% of the comparator subjects lost at least 5% of BMD at the spine or 7%

of BMD at the hip. Clinically relevant fractures (excluding fingers and toes) were reported in 4 subjects in the tenofovir DF group and 6 subjects in the comparator group. Tenofovir DF was associated with significant increases in biochemical markers of bone metabolism (serum bone-specific alkaline phosphatase, serum osteocalcin, serum C-telopeptide, and urinary N-telopeptide), suggesting increased bone turnover. Serum parathyroid hormone levels and 1,25 Vitamin D levels were also higher in subjects receiving tenofovir DF. The effects of tenofovir DF-associated changes in BMD and biochemical markers on long-term bone health and future fracture risk are unknown. For additional information, consult the tenofovir DF prescribing information.

Cases of osteomalacia (associated with proximal renal tubulopathy and which may contribute to fractures) have been reported in association with the use of tenofovir DF [See Adverse Reactions (6.3)].

5.12 Convulsions

Convulsions have been observed in patients receiving efavirenz, generally in the presence of known medical history of seizures. Caution must be taken in any patient with a history of seizures.

Patients who are receiving concomitant anticonvulsant medications primarily metabolized by the liver, such as phenytoin and phenobarbital, may require periodic monitoring of plasma levels [See Drug Interactions (7.3)].

5.13 Immune Reconstitution Syndrome

Immune reconstitution syndrome has been reported in patients treated with combination antiretroviral therapy, including the components of ATRIPLA (efavirenz/emtricitabine/tenofovir disoproxil fumarate). During the initial phase of combination antiretroviral treatment, patients whose immune system responds may develop an inflammatory response to indolent or residual opportunistic infections [such as Mycobacterium avium infection, cytomegalovirus, Pneumocystis jirovecii pneumonia (PCP), or tuberculosis], which may necessitate further evaluation and treatment.

5.14 Fat Redistribution

Redistribution/accumulation of body fat including central obesity, dorsocervical fat enlargement (buffalo hump), peripheral wasting, facial wasting, breast enlargement, and "cushingoid appearance" have been observed in patients receiving antiretroviral therapy. The mechanism and long-term consequences of these events are currently unknown. A causal relationship has not been established.

6 ADVERSE REACTIONS

Efavirenz, Emtricitabine and Tenofovir Disoproxil Fumarate: The following adverse reactions are discussed in other sections of the labeling:

- Lactic Acidosis/Severe Hepatomegaly with Steatosis [See Boxed Warning, Warnings and Precautions (5.1)].
- Severe Acute Exacerbations of Hepatitis B [See Boxed Warning, Warnings and Precautions (5.2)].
- Psychiatric Symptoms [See Warnings and Precautions (5.5)].
- Nervous System Symptoms [See Warnings and Precautions (5.6)].
- New Onset or Worsening Renal Impairment [See Warnings and Precautions (5.7)].
- Rash [See Warnings and Precautions (5.9)].
- Hepatotoxicity [See Warnings and Precautions (5.10)].
- Decreases in Bone Mineral Density [See Warnings and Precautions (5.11)].
- Immune Reconstitution Syndrome [See Warnings and Precautions (5.13)].
- Drug Interactions [See Contraindications (4.2), Warnings and Precautions (5.3) and Drug Interactions (7)].

For additional safety information about SUSTIVA (efavirenz), EMTRIVA (emtricitabine), or VIREAD (tenofovir DF) in combination with other antiretroviral agents, consult the prescribing information for these products.

6.1 Adverse Reactions from Clinical Trials Experience

Because clinical trials are conducted under widely varying conditions, adverse reaction rates observed in the clinical trials of a drug cannot be directly compared to rates in the clinical trials of another drug and may not reflect the rates observed in practice.

Study 934

Study 934 was an open-label active-controlled study in which 511 antiretroviral-naive subjects received either emtricitabine + tenofovir DF administered in combination with efavirenz (N=257) or zidovudine/lamivudine administered in combination with efavirenz (N=254).

The most common adverse reactions (incidence ≥ 10%, any severity) occurring in Study 934 include diarrhea, nausea, fatigue, headache, dizziness, depression, insomnia, abnormal dreams, and rash. Adverse reactions observed in Study 934 were generally consistent with those seen in previous studies of the individual components (Table 2).

Table 2: Selected Treatment-Emergent Adverse Reactions* (Grades 2–4) Reported in ≥5% in Either Treatment Group in Study 934 (0–144 Weeks)

	FTC + TDF + EFV[†]	AZT/3TC + EFV
	N=257	N=254
Gastrointestinal Disorder		
Diarrhea	9%	5%
Nausea	9%	7%
Vomiting	2%	5%
General Disorders and Administration Site Condition		
Fatigue	9%	8%
Infections and Infestations		
Sinusitis	8%	4%
Upper respiratory tract infections	8%	5%
Nasopharyngitis	5%	3%
Nervous System Disorders		
Headache	6%	5%
Dizziness	8%	7%
Psychiatric Disorders		
Anxiety	5%	4%
Depression	9%	7%
Insomnia	5%	7%
Skin and Subcutaneous Tissue Disorders		
Rash Event[‡]	7%	9%

* Frequencies of adverse reactions are based on all treatment-emergent adverse events, regardless of relationship to study drug.
† From Weeks 96 to 144 of the study, subjects received emtricitabine/tenofovir DF administered in combination with efavirenz in place of emtricitabine + tenofovir DF with efavirenz.
‡ Rash event includes rash, exfoliative rash, rash generalized, rash macular, rash maculo-papular, rash pruritic, and rash vesicular.

Study 073

In Study 073, subjects with stable, virologic suppression on antiretroviral therapy and no history of virologic failure were randomized to receive ATRIPLA (efavirenz/emtricitabine/tenofovir disoproxil fumarate) or to stay on their baseline regimen. The adverse reactions observed in Study 073 were generally consistent with those seen in Study 934 and those seen with the individual components of ATRIPLA when each was administered in combination with other antiretroviral agents.

Efavirenz, Emtricitabine, or Tenofovir Disoproxil Fumarate In addition to the adverse reactions in Study 934 and Study 073 the following adverse reactions were observed in clinical trials of efavirenz, emtricitabine, or tenofovir DF in combination with other antiretroviral agents.

Efavirenz: The most significant adverse reactions observed in subjects treated with efavirenz are nervous system symptoms [See Warnings and Precautions (5.6)], psychiatric symptoms [See Warnings and Precautions (5.5)], and rash [See Warnings and Precautions (5.9)].

Selected adverse reactions of moderate-severe intensity observed in ≥2% of efavirenz-treated subjects in two controlled clinical trials included pain, impaired concentration, abnormal dreams, somnolence, anorexia, dyspepsia, abdominal pain, nervousness, and pruritus.

Pancreatitis has also been reported, although a causal relationship with efavirenz has not been established. Asymptomatic increases in serum amylase levels were observed in a significantly higher number of subjects treated with efavirenz 600 mg than in control subjects.

Emtricitabine and Tenofovir Disoproxil Fumarate: Adverse reactions that occurred in at least 5% of treatment-experienced or treatment-naive subjects receiving emtricitabine or tenofovir DF with other antiretroviral agents in clinical trials include arthralgia, increased cough, dyspepsia, fever, myalgia, pain, abdominal pain, back pain, paresthesia, peripheral neuropathy (including peripheral neuritis and neuropathy), pneumonia, rhinitis and rash event (including rash, pruritus, maculopapular rash, urticaria, vesiculobullous rash, pustular rash and allergic reaction).

Skin discoloration has been reported with higher frequency among emtricitabine-treated subjects; it was manifested by hyperpigmentation on the palms and/or soles and was generally mild and asymptomatic. The mechanism and clinical significance are unknown.

6.2 Laboratory Abnormalities

Efavirenz, Emtricitabine and Tenofovir Disoproxil Fumarate: Laboratory abnormalities observed in Study 934 were generally consistent with those seen in previous studies (Table 3).

Table 3: Significant Laboratory Abnormalities Reported in ≥1% of Subjects in Either Treatment Group in Study 934 (0–144 Weeks)

	FTC + TDF + EFV*	AZT/3TC + EFV
	(N=257)	(N=254)
Any ≥ Grade 3 Laboratory Abnormality	30%	26%
Fasting Cholesterol (>240 mg/dL)	22%	24%
Creatine Kinase (M: >990 U/L) (F: >845 U/L)	9%	7%
Serum Amylase (>175 U/L)	8%	4%
Alkaline Phosphatase (>550 U/L)	1%	0%
AST (M: >180 U/L) (F: >170 U/L)	3%	3%
ALT (M: >215 U/L) (F: >170 U/L)	2%	3%
Hemoglobin (<8.0 mg/dL)	0%	4%
Hyperglycemia (>250 mg/dL)	2%	1%
Hematuria (>75 RBC/HPF)	3%	2%
Glycosuria (≥3+)	<1%	1%
Neutrophils (<750/mm^3)	3%	5%
Fasting Triglycerides (>750 mg/dL)	4%	2%

* From Weeks 96 to 144 of the study, subjects received emtricitabine/tenofovir DF administered in combination with efavirenz in place of emtricitabine + tenofovir DF with efavirenz.

Laboratory abnormalities observed in Study 073 were generally consistent with those in Study 934.

In addition to the laboratory abnormalities described for Study 934 (Table 3), Grade 3/4 elevations of bilirubin (>2.5 × ULN), pancreatic amylase (>2.0 × ULN), serum glucose (<40 or >250 mg/dL), and serum lipase (>2.0 × ULN) occurred in up to 3% of subjects treated with emtricitabine or tenofovir DF with other antiretroviral agents in clinical trials.

Hepatic Events: In Study 934, 19 subjects treated with efavirenz, emtricitabine, and tenofovir DF and 20 subjects treated with efavirenz and fixed-dose zidovudine/lamivudine were hepatitis B surface antigen or hepatitis C antibody positive. Among these coinfected subjects, one subject (1/19) in the efavirenz, emtricitabine and tenofovir DF arm had elevations in transaminases to greater than five times ULN through 144 weeks. In the fixed-dose zidovudine/lamivudine arm, two subjects (2/20) had elevations in transaminases to greater than five times ULN through 144 weeks. No HBV and/or HCV coinfected subject discontinued from the study due to hepatobiliary disorders [See Warnings and Precautions (5.10)].

6.3 Postmarketing Experience

The following adverse reactions have been identified during postapproval use of efavirenz, emtricitabine, or tenofovir DF. Because postmarketing reactions are reported voluntarily from a population of uncertain size, it is not always possible to reliably estimate their frequency or establish a causal relationship to drug exposure.

Efavirenz:

Cardiac Disorders
Palpitations

Ear and Labyrinth Disorders
Tinnitus

Endocrine Disorders
Gynecomastia

Eye Disorders
Abnormal vision

Gastrointestinal Disorders
Constipation, malabsorption
General Disorders and Administration Site Conditions
Asthenia
Hepatobiliary Disorders
Hepatic enzyme increase, hepatic failure, hepatitis. A few of the postmarketing reports of hepatic failure, including cases in patients with no pre-existing hepatic disease or other identifiable risk factors, were characterized by a fulminant course, progressing in some cases to transplantation or death.
Immune System Disorders
Allergic reactions
Metabolism and Nutrition Disorders
Redistribution/accumulation of body fat [See Warnings and Precautions (5.14)], hypercholesterolemia, hypertriglyceridemia
Musculoskeletal and Connective Tissue Disorders
Arthralgia, myalgia, myopathy
Nervous System Disorders
Abnormal coordination, ataxia, cerebellar coordination and balance disturbances, convulsions, hypoesthesia, paresthesia, neuropathy, tremor
Psychiatric Disorders
Aggressive reactions, agitation, delusions, emotional lability, mania, neurosis, paranoia, psychosis, suicide
Respiratory, Thoracic and Mediastinal Disorders
Dyspnea
Skin and Subcutaneous Tissue Disorders
Flushing, erythema multiforme, photoallergic dermatitis, Stevens-Johnson syndrome
Emtricitabine: No postmarketing adverse reactions have been identified for inclusion in this section.
Tenofovir Disoproxil Fumarate:
Immune System Disorders
Allergic reaction, including angioedema
Metabolism and Nutrition Disorders
Lactic acidosis, hypokalemia, hypophosphatemia
Respiratory, Thoracic, and Mediastinal Disorders
Dyspnea
Gastrointestinal Disorders
Pancreatitis, increased amylase, abdominal pain
Hepatobiliary Disorders
Hepatic steatosis, hepatitis, increased liver enzymes (most commonly AST, ALT, gamma GT)
Skin and Subcutaneous Tissue Disorders
Rash
Musculoskeletal and Connective Tissue Disorders
Rhabdomyolysis, osteomalacia (manifested as bone pain and which may contribute to fractures), muscular weakness, myopathy
Renal and Urinary Disorders
Acute renal failure, renal failure, acute tubular necrosis, Fanconi syndrome, proximal renal tubulopathy, interstitial nephritis (including acute cases), nephrogenic diabetes insipidus, renal insufficiency, increased creatinine, proteinuria, polyuria
General Disorders and Administration Site Conditions
Asthenia
The following adverse reactions, listed under the body system headings above, may occur as a consequence of proximal renal tubulopathy: rhabdomyolysis, osteomalacia, hypokalemia, muscular weakness, myopathy, hypophosphatemia.

7   DRUG INTERACTIONS
This section describes clinically relevant drug interactions with ATRIPLA (efavirenz/emtricitabine/tenofovir disoproxil fumarate). Drug interaction studies are described elsewhere in the labeling [See Clinical Pharmacology (12.3)].

7.1   Efavirenz
Efavirenz has been shown in vivo to induce CYP3A. Other compounds that are substrates of CYP3A may have decreased plasma concentrations when coadministered with efavirenz. In vitro studies have demonstrated that efavirenz inhibits CYP2C9, 2C19, and 3A4 isozymes in the range of observed efavirenz plasma concentrations. Coadministration of efavirenz with drugs primarily metabolized by these isozymes may result in altered plasma concentrations of the coadministered drug. Therefore, appropriate dose adjustments may be necessary for these drugs.
Drugs that induce CYP3A activity (e.g., phenobarbital, rifampin, rifabutin) would be expected to increase the clearance of efavirenz resulting in lowered plasma concentrations.

7.2   Emtricitabine and Tenofovir Disoproxil Fumarate
Since emtricitabine and tenofovir are primarily eliminated by the kidneys, coadministration of ATRIPLA with drugs that reduce renal function or compete for active tubular secretion may increase serum concentrations of emtricitabine, tenofovir, and/or other renally eliminated drugs. Some examples include, but are not limited to, acyclovir, adefovir dipivoxil, cidofovir, ganciclovir, valacyclovir, and valganciclovir.

Table 4: Established and Other Potentially Significant* Drug Interactions: Alteration in Dose or Regimen May Be Recommended Based on Drug Interaction Studies or Predicted Interaction

Concomitant Drug Class: Drug Name	Effect	Clinical Comment
Antiretroviral agents		
Protease inhibitor: atazanavir	↓ atazanavir concentration ↑ tenofovir concentration	Coadministration of atazanavir with ATRIPLA is not recommended. Coadministration of atazanavir with either efavirenz or tenofovir DF decreases plasma concentrations of atazanavir. The combined effect of efavirenz plus tenofovir DF on atazanavir plasma concentrations is not known. Also, atazanavir has been shown to increase tenofovir concentrations. There are insufficient data to support dosing recommendations for atazanavir or atazanavir/ritonavir in combination with ATRIPLA.
Protease inhibitor: fosamprenavir calcium	↓ amprenavir concentration	Fosamprenavir (unboosted): Appropriate doses of fosamprenavir and ATRIPLA with respect to safety and efficacy have not been established. Fosamprenavir/ritonavir: An additional 100 mg/day (300 mg total) of ritonavir is recommended when ATRIPLA is administered with fosamprenavir/ritonavir once daily. No change in the ritonavir dose is required when ATRIPLA is administered with fosamprenavir plus ritonavir twice daily.
Protease inhibitor: indinavir	↓ indinavir concentration	The optimal dose of indinavir, when given in combination with efavirenz, is not known. Increasing the indinavir dose to 1000 mg every 8 hours does not compensate for the increased indinavir metabolism due to efavirenz.
Protease inhibitor: lopinavir/ritonavir	↓ lopinavir concentration ↑ tenofovir concentration	A dose increase of lopinavir/ritonavir to 600/150 mg (3 tablets) twice daily may be considered when used in combination with efavirenz in treatment-experienced patients where decreased susceptibility to lopinavir is clinically suspected (by treatment history or laboratory evidence). **Patients should be monitored for tenofovir-associated adverse reactions. ATRIPLA should be discontinued in patients who develop tenofovir-associated adverse reactions.**
Protease inhibitor: ritonavir	↑ ritonavir concentration ↑ efavirenz concentration	When ritonavir 500 mg every 12 hours was coadministered with efavirenz 600 mg once daily, the combination was associated with a higher frequency of adverse clinical experiences (e.g., dizziness, nausea, paresthesia) and laboratory abnormalities (elevated liver enzymes). Monitoring of liver enzymes is recommended when ATRIPLA is used in combination with ritonavir.
Protease inhibitor: saquinavir	↓ saquinavir concentration	Should not be used as sole protease inhibitor in combination with ATRIPLA.
CCR5 co-receptor antagonist: Maraviroc	↓ maraviroc concentration	Efavirenz decreases plasma concentrations of maraviroc. Refer to the full prescribing information for maraviroc for guidance on coadministration with ATRIPLA.
NRTI: didanosine	↑ didanosine concentration	Higher didanosine concentrations could potentiate didanosine-associated adverse reactions, including pancreatitis and neuropathy. **In adults weighing >60 kg, the didanosine dose should be reduced to 250 mg if coadministered with ATRIPLA. Data are not available to recommend a dose adjustment of didanosine for patients weighing <60 kg. Coadministration of ATRIPLA and didanosine should be undertaken with caution and patients receiving this combination should be monitored closely for didanosine-associated adverse reactions. For additional information, please consult the Videx/Videx EC (didanosine) prescribing information.**

(Table continued on next page)

Coadministration of tenofovir DF and didanosine should be undertaken with caution and patients receiving this combination should be monitored closely for didanosine-associated adverse reactions. Didanosine should be discontinued in patients who develop didanosine-associated adverse reactions [for didanosine dosing adjustment recommendations, see Table 4]. Suppression of CD4+ cell counts has been observed in patients receiving tenofovir DF with didanosine 400 mg daily.
Lopinavir/ritonavir has been shown to increase tenofovir concentrations. The mechanism of this interaction is unknown. Patients receiving lopinavir/ritonavir with

ATRIPLA (efavirenz/emtricitabine/tenofovir disoproxil fumarate) should be monitored for tenofovir-associated adverse reactions. ATRIPLA should be discontinued in patients who develop tenofovir-associated adverse reactions [See Table 4].
Coadministration of atazanavir with ATRIPLA is not recommended since coadministration of atazanavir with either efavirenz or tenofovir DF has been shown to decrease plasma concentrations of atazanavir. Also, atazanavir has been shown to increase tenofovir concentrations. There are insufficient data to support dosing recommendations for atazanavir or atazanavir/ritonavir in combination with ATRIPLA [See Table 4].

Table 4 *(cont.)*: Established and Other Potentially Significant* Drug Interactions: Alteration in Dose or Regimen May Be Recommended Based on Drug Interaction Studies or Predicted Interaction

Concomitant Drug Class: Drug Name	Effect	Clinical Comment
Other agents		
Anticoagulant: warfarin	↑ or ↓ warfarin concentration	Plasma concentrations and effects potentially increased or decreased by efavirenz.
Anticonvulsants: carbamazepine phenytoin phenobarbital	↓ carbamazepine concentration ↓ efavirenz concentration ↓ anticonvulsant concentration ↓ efavirenz concentration	There are insufficient data to make a dose recommendation for ATRIPLA. Alternative anticonvulsant treatment should be used. Potential for reduction in anticonvulsant and/or efavirenz plasma levels; periodic monitoring of anticonvulsant plasma levels should be conducted.
Antidepressant: sertraline	↓ sertraline concentration	Increases in sertraline dose should be guided by clinical response.
Antifungals: itraconazole	↓ itraconazole concentration ↓ hydroxy-itraconazole concentration	Since no dose recommendation for itraconazole can be made, alternative antifungal treatment should be considered.
ketoconazole	↓ ketoconazole concentration	Drug interaction studies with ATRIPLA and ketoconazole have not been conducted. Efavirenz has the potential to decrease plasma concentrations of ketoconazole.
posaconazole	↓ posaconazole concentration	Avoid concomitant use unless the benefit outweighs the risks.
Anti-infective: clarithromycin	↓ clarithromycin concentration ↑ 14-OH metabolite concentration	Clinical significance unknown. In uninfected volunteers, 46% developed rash while receiving efavirenz and clarithromycin. No dose adjustment of ATRIPLA is recommended when given with clarithromycin. Alternatives to clarithromycin, such as azithromycin, should be considered. Other macrolide antibiotics, such as erythromycin, have not been studied in combination with ATRIPLA.
Antimycobacterial: rifabutin	↓ rifabutin concentration	Increase daily dose of rifabutin by 50%. Consider doubling the rifabutin dose in regimens where rifabutin is given 2 or 3 times a week.
Antimycobacterial: rifampin	↓ efavirenz concentration	Clinical significance of reduced efavirenz concentration is unknown. Dosing recommendations for concomitant use of ATRIPLA and rifampin have not been established.
Calcium channel blockers: diltiazem	↓ diltiazem concentration ↓ desacetyl diltiazem concentration ↓ N-monodesmethyl diltiazem concentration	Diltiazem dose adjustments should be guided by clinical response (refer to the full prescribing information for diltiazem). No dose adjustment of ATRIPLA is necessary when administered with diltiazem.
Others (eg, felodipine, nicardipine, nifedipine, verapamil)	↓ calcium channel blocker	No data are available on the potential interactions of efavirenz with other calcium channel blockers that are substrates of CYP3A. The potential exists for reduction in plasma concentrations of the calcium channel blocker. Dose adjustments should be guided by clinical response (refer to the full prescribing information for the calcium channel blocker).
HMG-CoA reductase inhibitors: atorvastatin pravastatin simvastatin	↓ atorvastatin concentration ↓ pravastatin concentration ↓ simvastatin concentration	Plasma concentrations of atorvastatin, pravastatin, and simvastatin decreased with efavirenz. Consult the full prescribing information for the HMG-CoA reductase inhibitor for guidance on individualizing the dose.

(Table continued on next page)

7.3 Efavirenz, Emtricitabine and Tenofovir Disoproxil Fumarate

Other important drug interaction information for ATRIPLA (efavirenz/emtricitabine/tenofovir disoproxil fumarate) is summarized in Table 1 and Table 4. The drug interactions described are based on studies conducted with efavirenz, emtricitabine or tenofovir DF as individual agents or are potential drug interactions; no drug interaction studies have been conducted using ATRIPLA [for pharmacokinetics data see *Clinical Pharmacology (12.3)*, Tables 5–9]. The tables include potentially significant interactions, but are not all inclusive.

[See table 4 above and on 3477]

7.4 Efavirenz Assay Interference

Cannabinoid Test Interaction: Efavirenz does not bind to cannabinoid receptors. False-positive urine cannabinoid test results have been observed in non-HIV-infected volunteers receiving efavirenz when the Microgenics Cedia DAU Multi-Level THC assay was used for screening. Negative results were obtained when more specific confirmatory testing was performed with gas chromatography/mass spectrometry. For more information, please consult the SUSTIVA prescribing information.

8 USE IN SPECIFIC POPULATIONS

8.1 Pregnancy

Pregnancy Category D [See Warnings and Precautions (5.8)]

8.3 Nursing Mothers

The Centers for Disease Control and Prevention recommend that HIV-1-infected mothers not breast-feed their infants to avoid risking postnatal transmission of HIV-1. Studies in rats have demonstrated that both efavirenz and tenofovir are secreted in milk. It is not known whether efavirenz, emtricitabine, or tenofovir is excreted in human milk. Because of both the potential for HIV-1 transmission and the potential for serious adverse reactions in nursing infants, **mothers should be instructed not to breast-feed if they are receiving ATRIPLA.**

8.4 Pediatric Use

ATRIPLA (efavirenz/emtricitabine/tenofovir disoproxil fumarate) is not recommended for patients less than 18 years of age because it is a fixed-dose combination tablet containing a component, tenofovir DF, for which safety and efficacy have not been established in this age group.

8.5 Geriatric Use

Clinical studies of efavirenz, emtricitabine, or tenofovir DF did not include sufficient numbers of subjects aged 65 and over to determine whether they respond differently from younger subjects. In general, dose selection for the elderly patients should be cautious, keeping in mind the greater frequency of decreased hepatic, renal, or cardiac function, and of concomitant disease or other drug therapy.

8.6 Hepatic Impairment

The pharmacokinetics of efavirenz have not been adequately studied in subjects with hepatic impairment. Because of the extensive cytochrome P450-mediated metabolism of efavirenz and limited clinical experience in patients with hepatic impairment, caution should be exercised in administering ATRIPLA to these patients [See Warnings and Precautions (5.10)].

8.7 Renal Impairment

Because ATRIPLA (efavirenz/emtricitabine/tenofovir disoproxil fumarate) is a fixed-dose combination, it should not be prescribed for patients requiring dosage adjustment such as those with moderate or severe renal impairment (creatinine clearance <50 mL/min) [See Warnings and Precautions (5.7)].

10 OVERDOSAGE

If overdose occurs, the patient should be monitored for evidence of toxicity, including monitoring of vital signs and observation of the patient's clinical status; standard supportive treatment should then be applied as necessary. Administration of activated charcoal may be used to aid removal of unabsorbed efavirenz. Hemodialysis can remove both emtricitabine and tenofovir DF (refer to detailed information below), but is unlikely to significantly remove efavirenz from the blood.

Efavirenz: Some patients accidentally taking 600 mg twice daily have reported increased nervous system symptoms. One patient experienced involuntary muscle contractions.

Emtricitabine: Limited clinical experience is available at doses higher than the therapeutic dose of emtricitabine. In one clinical pharmacology study single doses of emtricitabine 1200 mg were administered to 11 subjects. No severe adverse reactions were reported.

Hemodialysis treatment removes approximately 30% of the emtricitabine dose over a 3-hour dialysis period starting within 1.5 hours of emtricitabine dosing (blood flow rate of 400 mL/min and a dialysate flow rate of 600 mL/min). It is not known whether emtricitabine can be removed by peritoneal dialysis.

Tenofovir Disoproxil Fumarate: Limited clinical experience at doses higher than the therapeutic dose of tenofovir DF 300 mg is available. In one study, 600 mg tenofovir DF was administered to 8 subjects orally for 28 days, and no severe adverse reactions were reported. The effects of higher doses are not known.

Tenofovir is efficiently removed by hemodialysis with an extraction coefficient of approximately 54%. Following a single 300 mg dose of tenofovir DF, a 4-hour hemodialysis session removed approximately 10% of the administered tenofovir dose.

11 DESCRIPTION

ATRIPLA is a fixed-dose combination tablet containing efavirenz, emtricitabine, and tenofovir disoproxil fumarate (tenofovir DF). SUSTIVA is the brand name for efavirenz, a non-nucleoside reverse transcriptase inhibitor. EMTRIVA is the brand name for emtricitabine, a synthetic nucleoside analog of cytidine. VIREAD is the brand name for tenofovir DF, which is converted *in vivo* to tenofovir, an acyclic nucleoside phosphonate (nucleotide) analog of adenosine 5′-monophosphate. VIREAD and EMTRIVA are the components of TRUVADA.

ATRIPLA tablets are for oral administration. Each tablet contains 600 mg of efavirenz, 200 mg of emtricitabine, and 300 mg of tenofovir DF (which is equivalent to 245 mg of tenofovir disoproxil) as active ingredients. The tablets include the following inactive ingredients: croscarmellose sodium, hydroxypropyl cellulose, magnesium stearate, microcrystalline cellulose, and sodium lauryl sulfate. The tablets are film-coated with a coating material containing black iron oxide, polyethylene glycol, polyvinyl alcohol, red iron oxide, talc, and titanium dioxide.

Efavirenz: Efavirenz is chemically described as (S)-6-chloro-4-(cyclopropylethynyl)-1,4-dihydro-4-(trifluoromethyl)-2H-3,1-benzoxazin-2-one. Its molecular formula is $C_{14}H_9ClF_3NO_2$ and its structural formula is:

Efavirenz is a white to slightly pink crystalline powder with a molecular mass of 315.68. It is practically insoluble in water (<10 μg/mL).

Emtricitabine: The chemical name of emtricitabine is 5-fluoro-1-(2R,5S)-[2-(hydroxymethyl)-1,3-oxathiolan-5-

yl]cytosine. Emtricitabine is the (-) enantiomer of a thio analog of cytidine, which differs from other cytidine analogs in that it has a fluorine in the 5-position.

It has a molecular formula of $C_8H_{10}FN_3O_3S$ and a molecular weight of 247.24. It has the following structural formula:

Emtricitabine is a white to off-white crystalline powder with a solubility of approximately 112 mg/mL in water at 25 °C.

Tenofovir Disoproxil Fumarate: Tenofovir DF is a fumaric acid salt of the *bis*-isopropoxycarbonyloxymethyl ester derivative of tenofovir. The chemical name of tenofovir disoproxil fumarate is 9-[(R)-2-[[bis[[(isopropoxycarbonyl)oxy]-methoxy]phosphinyl]methoxy]propyl]adenine fumarate (1:1). It has a molecular formula of $C_{19}H_{30}N_5O_{10}P$ • $C_4H_4O_4$ and a molecular weight of 635.52. It has the following structural formula:

Tenofovir DF is a white to off-white crystalline powder with a solubility of 13.4 mg/mL in water at 25 °C.

12 CLINICAL PHARMACOLOGY

For additional information on Mechanism of Action, Antiviral Activity, Resistance and Cross Resistance, please consult the SUSTIVA, EMTRIVA and VIREAD prescribing information.

12.1 Mechanism of Action

ATRIPLA (efavirenz/emtricitabine/tenofovir disoproxil fumarate) is a fixed-dose combination of antiviral drugs efavirenz, emtricitabine and tenofovir disoproxil fumarate. *[See Clinical Pharmacology (12.4)].*

12.3 Pharmacokinetics

ATRIPLA: One ATRIPLA tablet is bioequivalent to one SUSTIVA tablet (600 mg) plus one EMTRIVA capsule (200 mg) plus one VIREAD tablet (300 mg) following single-dose administration to fasting healthy subjects (N=45).

Efavirenz: In HIV-1 infected subjects time-to-peak plasma concentrations were approximately 3–5 hours and steady-state plasma concentrations were reached in 6–10 days. In 35 HIV-1 infected subjects receiving efavirenz 600 mg once daily, steady-state C_{max} was 12.9 ± 3.7 µM (mean ± SD), C_{min} was 5.6 ± 3.2 µM, and AUC was 184 ± 73 µM•hr. Efavirenz is highly bound (approximately 99.5–99.75%) to human plasma proteins, predominantly albumin. Following administration of ^{14}C-labeled efavirenz, 14–34% of the dose was recovered in the urine (mostly as metabolites) and 16–61% was recovered in feces (mostly as parent drug). *In vitro* studies suggest CYP3A and CYP2B6 are the major isozymes responsible for efavirenz metabolism. Efavirenz has been shown to induce CYP enzymes, resulting in induction of its own metabolism. Efavirenz has a terminal half-life of 52–76 hours after single doses and 40–55 hours after multiple doses.

Emtricitabine: Following oral administration, emtricitabine is rapidly absorbed with peak plasma concentrations occurring at 1–2 hours post-dose. Following multiple dose oral administration of emtricitabine to 20 HIV-1-infected subjects, the steady-state plasma emtricitabine C_{max} was 1.8 ± 0.7 µg/mL (mean ± SD) and the AUC over a 24-hour dosing interval was 10.0 ± 3.1 µg•hr/mL. The mean steady state plasma trough concentration at 24 hours post-dose was 0.09 µg/mL. The mean absolute bioavailability of emtricitabine was 93%. *In vitro* binding of emtricitabine to human plasma proteins is <4% and is independent of concentration over the range of 0.02–200 µg/mL. Following administration of radiolabelled emtricitabine, approximately 86% is recovered in the urine and 13% is recovered as metabolites. The metabolites of emtricitabine include 3′-sulfoxide diastereomers and their glucuronic acid conjugate. Emtricitabine is eliminated by a combination of glomerular filtration and active tubular secretion with a renal clearance in adults with normal renal function of 213 ± 89 mL/min (mean ± SD). Following a single oral dose, the plasma emtricitabine half-life is approximately 10 hours.

Tenofovir Disoproxil Fumarate: Following oral administration of a single 300 mg dose of tenofovir DF to HIV-1 infected subjects in the fasted state, maximum serum concentrations (C_{max}) were achieved in 1.0 ± 0.4 hrs (mean ± SD) and C_{max} and AUC values were 296 ± 90 ng/mL and 2287 ± 685 ng•hr/mL, respectively. The oral bioavailability of tenofovir from tenofovir DF in fasted subjects is approximately 25%. *In vitro* binding of tenofovir to human plasma proteins is <0.7% and is independent of concentration over the range of 0.01–25 µg/mL. Approximately 70–80% of the intravenous dose of tenofovir is recovered as unchanged drug in the urine. Tenofovir is eliminated by a combination of glomerular filtration and active tubular secretion with a renal clearance in adults with normal renal function of 243 ± 33 mL/min (mean ± SD). Following a single oral dose, the terminal elimination half-life of tenofovir is approximately 17 hours.

Effects of Food on Oral Absorption

ATRIPLA (efavirenz/emtricitabine/tenofovir disoproxil fumarate) has not been evaluated in the presence of food. Administration of efavirenz tablets with a high fat meal increased the mean AUC and C_{max} of efavirenz by 28% and 79%, respectively, compared to administration in the fasted state. Compared to fasted administration, dosing of tenofovir DF and emtricitabine in combination with either a high fat meal or a light meal increased the mean AUC and C_{max} of tenofovir by 35% and 15%, respectively, without affecting emtricitabine exposures *[See Dosage and Administration (2) and Patient Counseling Information (17.3)].*

Special Populations

Race

Efavirenz: The pharmacokinetics of efavirenz in HIV-1 infected subjects appear to be similar among the racial groups studied.

Emtricitabine: No pharmacokinetic differences due to race have been identified following the administration of emtricitabine.

Tenofovir Disoproxil Fumarate: There were insufficient numbers from racial and ethnic groups other than Caucasian to adequately determine potential pharmacokinetic differences among these populations following the administration of tenofovir DF.

Gender

Efavirenz, Emtricitabine, and Tenofovir Disoproxil Fumarate: Efavirenz, emtricitabine, and tenofovir pharmacokinetics are similar in male and female subjects.

Pediatric and Geriatric Patients

Pharmacokinetic studies of tenofovir DF have not been performed in pediatric subjects (<18 years). Efavirenz has not been studied in pediatric subjects below 3 years of age or who weigh less than 13 kg. Emtricitabine has been studied in pediatric subjects from 3 months to 17 years of age. ATRIPLA is not recommended for pediatric administration.

Pharmacokinetics of efavirenz, emtricitabine and tenofovir have not been fully evaluated in the elderly (>65 years) *[See Use in Specific Populations (8)].*

Patients with Impaired Renal Function

Efavirenz: The pharmacokinetics of efavirenz have not been studied in subjects with renal insufficiency; however, less than 1% of efavirenz is excreted unchanged in the urine, so the impact of renal impairment on efavirenz elimination should be minimal.

Emtricitabine and Tenofovir Disoproxil Fumarate: The pharmacokinetics of emtricitabine and tenofovir DF are altered in subjects with renal impairment. In subjects with creatinine clearance <50 mL/min, C_{max} and $AUC_{0-\infty}$ of emtricitabine and tenofovir were increased *[See Warnings and Precautions (5.7)].*

Patients with Hepatic Impairment

Efavirenz: The pharmacokinetics of efavirenz have not been adequately studied in subjects with hepatic impairment *[See Warnings and Precautions (5.10) and Use in Specific Populations (8.6)].*

Emtricitabine: The pharmacokinetics of emtricitabine have not been studied in subjects with hepatic impairment; however, emtricitabine is not significantly metabolized by liver enzymes, so the impact of liver impairment should be limited.

Tenofovir Disoproxil Fumarate: The pharmacokinetics of tenofovir following a 300 mg dose of tenofovir DF have been studied in non-HIV-infected subjects with moderate to severe hepatic impairment. There were no substantial alterations in tenofovir pharmacokinetics in subjects with hepatic impairment compared with unimpaired subjects.

Assessment of Drug Interactions

The drug interaction studies described were conducted with efavirenz, emtricitabine, or tenofovir DF as individual agents; no drug interaction studies have been conducted using ATRIPLA (efavirenz/emtricitabine/tenofovir disoproxil fumarate).

Efavirenz: The steady-state pharmacokinetics of efavirenz and tenofovir were unaffected when efavirenz and tenofovir DF were administered together versus each agent dosed alone. Specific drug interaction studies have not been performed with efavirenz and NRTIs other than tenofovir, lamivudine, and zidovudine. Clinically significant interactions would not be expected based on NRTIs elimination pathways.

Efavirenz has been shown *in vivo* to cause hepatic enzyme induction, thus increasing the biotransformation of some drugs metabolized by CYP3A. *In vitro* studies have shown

---

Table 4 *(cont.)*: Established and Other Potentially Significant* Drug Interactions: Alteration in Dose or Regimen May Be Recommended Based on Drug Interaction Studies or Predicted Interaction

Concomitant Drug Class: Drug Name	Effect	Clinical Comment
Other agents (continued)		
Hormonal contraceptives: Oral: Ethinyl estradiol/Norgestimate	↓ active metabolites of norgestimate	A reliable method of barrier contraception must be used in addition to hormonal contraceptives. Efavirenz had no effect on ethinyl estradiol concentrations, but progestin levels (norelgestromin and levonorgestrel) were markedly decreased. No effect of ethinyl estradiol/norgestimate on efavirenz plasma concentrations was observed.
Implant: Etonogestrel	↓ etonogestrel	A reliable method of barrier contraception must be used in addition to hormonal contraceptives. The interaction between etonogestrel and efavirenz has not been studied. Decreased exposure of etonogestrel may be expected. There have been postmarketing reports of contraceptive failure with etonogestrel in efavirenz-exposed patients.
Immunosuppressants: Cyclosporine, tacrolimus, sirolimus, and others metabolized by CYP3A	↓ immuno-suppressant	Decreased exposure of the immunosuppressant may be expected due to CYP3A induction by efavirenz. These immunosuppressants are not anticipated to affect exposure of efavirenz. Dose adjustments of the immunosuppressant may be required. Close monitoring of immunosuppressant concentrations for at least 2 weeks (until stable concentrations are reached) is recommended when starting or stopping treatment with ATRIPLA.
Narcotic analgesic: methadone	↓ methadone concentration	Coadministration of efavirenz in HIV-1 infected individuals with a history of injection drug use resulted in decreased plasma levels of methadone and signs of opiate withdrawal. Methadone dose was increased by a mean of 22% to alleviate withdrawal symptoms. Patients should be monitored for signs of withdrawal and their methadone dose increased as required to alleviate withdrawal symptoms.

*This table is not all inclusive.

Table 5: Drug Interactions: Changes in Pharmacokinetic Parameters for Efavirenz in the Presence of the Coadministered Drug

Coadministered Drug	Dose of Coadministered Drug (mg)	Efavirenz Dose (mg)	N	Mean % Change of Efavirenz Pharmacokinetic Parameters* (90% CI)		
				C_{max}	AUC	C_{min}
Indinavir	800 mg q8h × 14 days	200 mg qd × 14 days	11	↔	↔	↔
Lopinavir/ritonavir	400/100 mg q12h × 9 days	600 mg qd × 9 days	11, 12[†]	↔	↓ 16 (↓ 38 to ↑ 15)	↓ 16 (↓ 42 to ↑ 20)
Nelfinavir	750 mg q8h × 7 days	600 mg qd × 7 days	10	↓ 12 (↓ 32 to ↑ 13)[‡]	↓ 12 (↓ 35 to ↑ 18)[‡]	↓ 21 (↓ 53 to ↑ 33)
Ritonavir	500 mg q12h × 8 days	600 mg qd × 10 days	9	↑ 14 (↑ 4 to ↑ 26)	↑ 21 (↑ 10 to ↑ 34)	↑ 25 (↑ 7 to ↑ 46)[‡]
Saquinavir SGC[§]	1200 mg q8h × 10 days	600 mg qd × 10 days	13	↓ 13 (↓ 5 to ↓ 20)	↓ 12 (↓ 4 to ↓ 19)	↓ 14 (↓ 2 to ↓ 24)[‡]
Clarithromycin	500 mg q12h × 7 days	400 mg qd × 7 days	12	↑ 11 (↑ 3 to ↑ 19)	↔	↔
Itraconazole	200 mg q12h × 14 days	600 mg qd × 28 days	16	↔	↔	↔
Rifabutin	300 mg qd × 14 days	600 mg qd × 14 days	11	↔	↔	↓ 12 (↓ 24 to ↑ 1)
Rifampin	600 mg × 7 days	600 mg qd × 7 days	12	↓ 20 (↓ 11 to ↓ 28)	↓ 26 (↓ 15 to ↓ 36)	↓ 32 (↓ 15 to ↓ 46)
Atorvastatin	10 mg qd × 4 days	600 mg qd × 15 days	14	↔	↔	↔
Pravastatin	40 mg qd × 4 days	600 mg qd × 15 days	11	↔	↔	↔
Simvastatin	40 mg qd × 4 days	600 mg qd × 15 days	14	↓ 12 (↓ 28 to ↑ 8)	↔	↓ 12 (↓ 25 to ↑ 3)
Carbamazepine	200 mg qd × 3 days, 200 mg bid × 3 days, then 400 mg qd × 15 days	600 mg qd × 35 days	14	↓ 21 (↓ 15 to ↓ 26)	↓ 36 (↓ 32 to ↓ 40)	↓ 47 (↓ 41 to ↓ 53)
Diltiazem	240 mg × 14 days	600 mg qd × 28 days	12	↑ 16 (↑ 6 to ↑ 26)	↑ 11 (↑ 5 to ↑ 18)	↑ 13 (↑ 1 to ↑ 26)
Sertraline	50 mg qd × 14 days	600 mg qd × 14 days	13	↑ 11 (↑ 6 to ↑ 16)	↔	↔
Voriconazole	400 mg po q12h × 1 day then 200 mg po q12h × 8 days	400 mg qd × 9 days	NA	↑ 38[¶]	↑ 44[¶]	NA
Voriconazole	300 mg po q12h days 2–7	300 mg qd × 7 days	NA	↓ 14[#] (↓ 7 to ↓ 21)	↔[#]	NA
Voriconazole	400 mg po q12h days 2–7	300 mg qd × 7 days	NA	↔[#]	↑ 17[#] (↑ 6 to ↑ 29)	NA

NA = not available
* Increase = ↑; Decrease = ↓; No Effect = ↔
† Parallel-group design; N for efavirenz + lopinavir/ritonavir, N for efavirenz alone.
‡ 95% CI
§ Soft Gelatin Capsule.
¶ 90% CI not available
# Relative to steady-state administration of efavirenz (600 mg once daily for 9 days).

that efavirenz inhibited CYP isozymes 2C9, 2C19, and 3A4 with K_i values (8.5–17 μM) in the range of observed efavirenz plasma concentrations. In *in vitro* studies, efavirenz did not inhibit CYP2E1 and inhibited CYP2D6 and CYP1A2 (K_i values 82–160 μM) only at concentrations well above those achieved clinically. Coadministration of efavirenz with drugs primarily metabolized by 2C9, 2C19, and 3A4 isozymes may result in altered plasma concentrations of the coadministered drug. Drugs which induce CYP3A activity would be expected to increase the clearance of efavirenz resulting in lowered plasma concentrations. Drug interaction studies were performed with efavirenz and other drugs likely to be coadministered or drugs commonly used as probes for pharmacokinetic interaction. There was no clinically significant interaction observed between efavirenz and zidovudine, lamivudine, azithromycin, fluconazole, lorazepam, cetirizine, or paroxetine. Single

doses of famotidine or an aluminum and magnesium antacid with simethicone had no effects on efavirenz exposures. The effects of coadministration of efavirenz on C_{max}, AUC, and C_{min} are summarized in Table 5 (effect of other drugs on efavirenz) and Table 6 (effect of efavirenz on other drugs). For information regarding clinical recommendations see *Drug Interactions (7)*.
[See table 5 above]
[See table 6 on pages 3479 and 3480]
Emtricitabine and Tenofovir Disoproxil Fumarate: The steady-state pharmacokinetics of emtricitabine and tenofovir were unaffected when emtricitabine and tenofovir DF were administered together versus each agent dosed alone.
In vitro and clinical pharmacokinetic drug-drug interaction studies have shown that the potential for CYP mediated interactions involving emtricitabine and tenofovir with other medicinal products is low.

Emtricitabine and tenofovir are primarily excreted by the kidneys by a combination of glomerular filtration and active tubular secretion. No drug-drug interactions due to competition for renal excretion have been observed; however, coadministration of emtricitabine and tenofovir DF with drugs that are eliminated by active tubular secretion may increase concentrations of emtricitabine, tenofovir, and/or the coadministered drug.
Drugs that decrease renal function may increase concentrations of emtricitabine and/or tenofovir.
No clinically significant drug interactions have been observed between emtricitabine and famciclovir, indinavir, stavudine, tenofovir DF or zidovudine. Similarly, no clinically significant drug interactions have been observed between tenofovir DF and abacavir, efavirenz, emtricitabine, entecavir, indinavir, lamivudine, lopinavir/ritonavir, methadone, nelfinavir, oral contraceptives, ribavirin, saquinavir/ritonavir or tacrolimus in studies conducted in healthy volunteers.
Following multiple dosing to HIV-negative subjects receiving either chronic methadone maintenance therapy, oral contraceptives, or single doses of ribavirin, steady-state tenofovir pharmacokinetics were similar to those observed in previous studies, indicating a lack of clinically significant drug interactions between these agents and tenofovir DF. The effects of coadministered drugs on the C_{max}, AUC, and C_{min} of tenofovir are shown in Table 7. The effects of coadministration of tenofovir DF on C_{max}, AUC, and C_{min} of coadministered drugs are shown in Table 8 and Table 9.
[See table 7 at top of page 3481]
[See table 8 on page 3481]
Coadministration of tenofovir DF with didanosine results in changes in the pharmacokinetics of didanosine that may be of clinical significance. Table 9 summarizes the effects of tenofovir DF on the pharmacokinetics of didanosine. Concomitant dosing of tenofovir DF with didanosine buffered tablets or enteric-coated capsules significantly increases the C_{max} and AUC of didanosine. When didanosine 250 mg enteric-coated capsules were administered with tenofovir DF, systemic exposures of didanosine were similar to those seen with the 400 mg enteric-coated capsules alone under fasted conditions. The mechanism of this interaction is unknown [for didanosine dosing adjustment recommendations see *Drug Interactions (7.3)*, Table 4].
[See table 9 at top of page 3482]

12.4 Microbiology
Mechanism of Action
Efavirenz: Efavirenz is a non-nucleoside reverse transcriptase (RT) inhibitor of HIV-1. Efavirenz activity is mediated predominantly by noncompetitive inhibition of HIV-1 reverse transcriptase (RT). HIV-2 RT and human cellular DNA polymerases α, β, γ, and δ are not inhibited by efavirenz.
Emtricitabine: Emtricitabine, a synthetic nucleoside analog of cytidine, is phosphorylated by cellular enzymes to form emtricitabine 5'-triphosphate. Emtricitabine 5'-triphosphate inhibits the activity of the HIV-1 RT by competing with the natural substrate deoxycytidine 5'-triphosphate and by being incorporated into nascent viral DNA which results in chain termination. Emtricitabine 5'-triphosphate is a weak inhibitor of mammalian DNA polymerase α, β, ε, and mitochondrial DNA polymerase γ.
Tenofovir Disoproxil Fumarate: Tenofovir DF is an acyclic nucleoside phosphonate diester analog of adenosine monophosphate. Tenofovir DF requires initial diester hydrolysis for conversion to tenofovir and subsequent phosphorylations by cellular enzymes to form tenofovir diphosphate. Tenofovir diphosphate inhibits the activity of HIV-1 RT by competing with the natural substrate deoxyadenosine 5'-triphosphate and, after incorporation into DNA, by DNA chain termination. Tenofovir diphosphate is a weak inhibitor of mammalian DNA polymerases α, β, and mitochondrial DNA polymerase γ.
Antiviral Activity
Efavirenz, Emtricitabine, and Tenofovir Disoproxil Fumarate: In combination studies evaluating the antiviral activity in cell culture of emtricitabine and efavirenz together, efavirenz and tenofovir together, and emtricitabine and tenofovir together, additive to synergistic antiviral effects were observed.
Efavirenz: The concentration of efavirenz inhibiting replication of wild-type laboratory adapted strains and clinical isolates in cell culture by 90–95% (EC_{90-95}) ranged from 1.7–25 nM in lymphoblastoid cell lines, peripheral blood mononuclear cells, and macrophage/monocyte cultures. Efavirenz demonstrated additive antiviral activity against HIV-1 in cell culture when combined with non-nucleoside reverse transcriptase inhibitors (NNRTIs) (delavirdine and nevirapine), nucleoside reverse transcriptase inhibitors (NRTIs) (abacavir, didanosine, lamivudine, stavudine, zalcitabine, and zidovudine), protease inhibitors (PIs) (amprenavir, indinavir, lopinavir, nelfinavir, ritonavir, and saquinavir), and the fusion inhibitor enfuvirtide. Efavirenz

Table 6: Drug Interactions: Changes in Pharmacokinetic Parameters for Coadministered Drug in the Presence of Efavirenz

Coadministered Drug	Dose of Coadministered Drug (mg)	Efavirenz Dose (mg)	N	Mean % Change of Coadministered Drug Pharmacokinetic Parameters* (90% CI)		
				C_{max}	AUC	C_{min}
Atazanavir	400 mg qd with a light meal d 1–20	600 mg qd with a light meal d 7–20	27	↓ 59 (↓ 49 to ↓ 67)	↓ 74 (↓ 68 to ↓ 78)	↓ 93 (↓ 90 to ↓ 95)
	400 mg qd d 1–6, then 300 mg qd d 7–20 with ritonavir 100 mg qd and a light meal	600 mg qd 2 h after atazanavir and ritonavir d 7–20	13	↑ 14[†] (↓ 17 to ↑ 58)	↑ 39[†] (↑ 2 to ↑ 88)	↑ 48[†] (↑ 24 to ↑ 76)
	300 mg qd/ritonavir 100 mg qd d 1–10 (pm), then 400 mg qd/ritonavir 100 mg qd d 11–24 (pm) (simultaneous with efavirenz)	600 mg qd with a light snack d 11–24 (pm)	14	↑ 17 (↑ 8 to ↑ 27)	↔	↓ 42 (↓ 31 to ↓ 51)
Indinavir	1000 mg q8h × 10 days	600 mg qd × 10 days	20			
	After morning dose			↔[‡]	↓ 33[‡] (↓ 26 to ↓ 39)	↓ 39[‡] (↓ 24 to ↓ 51)
	After afternoon dose			↔[‡]	↓ 37[‡] (↓ 26 to ↓ 46)	↓ 52[‡] (↓ 47 to ↓ 57)
	After evening dose			↓ 29[‡] (↓ 11 to ↓ 43)	↓ 46[‡] (↓ 37 to ↓ 54)	↓ 57[‡] (↓ 50 to ↓ 63)
Lopinavir/ritonavir	400/100 mg q12h × 9 days	600 mg qd × 9 days	11, 7[§]	↔[¶]	↓ 19[¶] (↓ 36 to ↑ 3)	↓ 39[¶] (↓ 3 to ↓ 62)
Nelfinavir	750 mg q8h × 7 days	600 mg qd × 7 days	10	↑ 21 (↑ 10 to ↑ 33)	↑ 20 (↑ 8 to ↑ 34)	↔
Metabolite AG-1402				↓ 40 (↓ 30 to ↓ 48)	↓ 37 (↓ 25 to ↓ 48)	↓ 43 (↓ 21 to ↓ 59)
Ritonavir	500 mg q12h × 8 days	600 mg qd × 10 days	11			
	After AM dose			↑ 24 (↑ 12 to ↑ 38)	↑ 18 (↑ 6 to ↑ 33)	↑ 42 (↑ 9 to ↑ 86)[#]
	After PM dose			↔	↔	↑ 24 (↑ 3 to ↑ 50)[#]
Saquinavir SGC[P]	1200 mg q8h × 10 days	600 mg qd × 10 days	12	↓ 50 (↓ 28 to ↓ 66)	↓ 62 (↓ 45 to ↓ 74)	↓ 56 (↓ 16 to ↓ 77)[#]
Maraviroc	100 mg bid	600 mg qd	12	↓ 51 (↓ 37 to ↓ 62)	↓ 45 (↓ 38 to ↓ 51)	↓ 45 (↓ 28 to ↓ 57)
Clarithromycin	500 mg q12h × 7 days	400 mg qd × 7 days	11	↓ 26 (↓ 15 to ↓ 35)	↓ 39 (↓ 30 to ↓ 46)	↓ 53 (↓ 42 to ↓ 63)
14-OH metabolite				↑ 49 (↑ 32 to ↑ 69)	↑ 34 (↑ 18 to ↑ 53)	↑ 26 (↑ 9 to ↑ 45)
Itraconazole	200 mg q12h × 28 days	600 mg qd × 14 days	18	↓ 37 (↓ 20 to ↓ 51)	↓ 39 (↓ 21 to ↓ 53)	↓ 44 (↓ 27 to ↓ 58)
Hydroxy-itraconazole				↓ 35 (↓ 12 to ↓ 52)	↓ 37 (↓ 14 to ↓ 55)	↓ 43 (↓ 18 to ↓ 60)
Posaconazole	400 mg (oral suspension) bid × 10 and 20 days	400 mg qd × 10 and 20 days	11	↓ 45 (↓ 34 to ↓ 53)	↓ 50 (↓ 40 to ↓ 57)	NA
Rifabutin	300 mg qd × 14 days	600 mg qd × 14 days	9	↓ 32 (↓ 15 to ↓ 46)	↓ 38 (↓ 28 to ↓ 47)	↓ 45 (↓ 31 to ↓ 56)
Atorvastatin	10 mg qd × 4 days	600 mg qd × 15 days	14	↓ 14 (↓ 1 to ↓ 26)	↓ 43 (↓ 34 to ↓ 50)	↓ 69 (↓ 49 to ↓ 81)
Total active (including metabolites)				↓ 15 (↓ 2 to ↓ 26)	↓ 32 (↓ 21 to ↓ 41)	↓ 48 (↓ 23 to ↓ 64)
Pravastatin	40 mg qd × 4 days	600 mg qd × 15 days	13	↓ 32 (↓ 59 to ↑ 12)	↓ 44 (↓ 26 to ↓ 57)	↓ 19 (↓ 0 to ↓ 35)

(Table continued on next page)

demonstrated additive to antagonistic antiviral activity in cell culture with atazanavir. Efavirenz demonstrated antiviral activity against clade B and most non-clade B isolates (subtypes A, AE, AG, C, D, F, G, J, and N), but had reduced antiviral activity against group O viruses. Efavirenz is not active against HIV-2.

Emtricitabine: The antiviral activity in cell culture of emtricitabine against laboratory and clinical isolates of HIV-1 was assessed in lymphoblastoid cell lines, the MAGI-CCR5 cell line, and peripheral blood mononuclear cells. The 50% effective concentration (EC$_{50}$) values for emtricitabine were in the range of 0.0013–0.64 μM (0.0003–0.158 μg/mL). In drug combination studies of emtricitabine with NRTIs (abacavir, lamivudine, stavudine, zalcitabine, and zidovudine), NNRTIs (delavirdine, efavirenz, and nevirapine), and PIs (amprenavir, nelfinavir, ritonavir, and saquinavir), additive to synergistic effects were observed. Emtricitabine displayed antiviral activity in cell culture against HIV-1 clades A, B, C, D, E, F, and G (EC$_{50}$ values ranged from 0.007–0.075 μM) and showed strain specific activity against HIV-2 (EC$_{50}$ values ranged from 0.007–1.5 μM).

Tenofovir Disoproxil Fumarate: The antiviral activity in cell culture of tenofovir against laboratory and clinical isolates of HIV-1 was assessed in lymphoblastoid cell lines, primary monocyte/macrophage cells and peripheral blood lymphocytes. The EC$_{50}$ values for tenofovir were in the range of

Table 6 *(cont.)*: Drug Interactions: Changes in Pharmacokinetic Parameters for Coadministered Drug in the Presence of Efavirenz

Coadministered Drug	Dose of Coadministered Drug (mg)	Efavirenz Dose (mg)	N	Mean % Change of Coadministered Drug Pharmacokinetic Parameters* (90% CI)		
				C_{max}	AUC	C_{min}
Simvastatin	40 mg qd × 4 days	600 mg qd × 15 days	14	↓ 72 (↓ 63 to ↓ 79)	↓ 68 (↓ 62 to ↓ 73)	↓ 45 (↓ 20 to ↓ 62)
Total active (including metabolites)				↓ 68 (↓ 55 to ↓ 78)	↓ 60 (↓ 52 to ↓ 68)	NA[ß]
Carbamazepine	200 mg qd × 3 days, 200 mg bid × 3 days, then 400 mg qd × 29 days	600 mg qd × 14 days	12	↓ 20 (↓ 15 to ↓ 24)	↓ 27 (↓ 20 to ↓ 33)	↓ 35 (↓ 24 to ↓ 44)
Epoxide metabolite				↔	↔	↓ 13 (↓ 30 to ↑ 7)
Diltiazem	240 mg × 21 days	600 mg qd × 14 days	13	↓ 60 (↓ 50 to ↓ 68)	↓ 69 (↓ 55 to ↓ 79)	↓ 63 (↓ 44 to ↓ 75)
Desacetyl diltiazem				↓ 64 (↓ 57 to ↓ 69)	↓ 75 (↓ 59 to ↓ 84)	↓ 62 (↓ 44 to ↓ 75)
N-monodesmethyl diltiazem				↓ 28 (↓ 7 to ↓ 44)	↓ 37 (↓ 17 to ↓ 52)	↓ 37 (↓ 17 to ↓ 52)
Ethinyl estradiol/ Norgestimate	0.035 mg/0.25 mg × 14 days	600 mg qd × 14 days				
Ethinyl estradiol			21	↔	↔	↔
Norelgestromin			21	↓ 46 (↓ 39 to ↓ 52)	↓ 64 (↓ 62 to ↓ 67)	↓ 82 (↓ 79 to ↓ 85)
Levonorgestrel			6	↓ 80 (↓ 77 to ↓ 83)	↓ 83 (↓ 79 to ↓ 87)	↓ 86 (↓ 80 to ↓ 90)
Methadone	Stable maintenance 35–100 mg daily	600 mg qd × 14–21 days	11	↓ 45 (↓ 25 to ↓ 59)	↓ 52 (↓ 33 to ↓ 66)	NA
Sertraline	50 mg qd × 14 days	600 mg qd × 14 days	13	↓ 29 (↓ 15 to ↓ 40)	↓ 39 (↓ 27 to ↓ 50)	↓ 46 (↓ 31 to ↓ 58)
Voriconazole	400 mg po q12h × 1 day then 200 mg po q12h × 8 days	400 mg qd × 9 days	NA	↓ 61[à]	↓ 77[à]	NA
	300 mg po q12h days 2–7	300 mg qd × 7 days	NA	↓ 36[è] (↓ 21 to ↓ 49)	↓ 55[è] (↓ 45 to ↓ 62)	NA
	400 mg po q12h days 2–7	300 mg qd × 7 days	NA	↑ 23[è] (↓ 1 to ↑ 53)	↓ 7[è] (↓ 23 to ↑ 13)	NA

NA = not available

* Increase = ↑; Decrease = ↓; No Effect = ↔
† Compared with atazanavir 400 mg qd alone.
‡ Comparator dose of indinavir was 800 mg q8h × 10 days.
§ Parallel-group design; N for efavirenz + lopinavir/ritonavir, N for lopinavir/ritonavir alone.
¶ Values are for lopinavir. The pharmacokinetics of ritonavir 100 mg q12h are unaffected by concurrent efavirenz.
# 95% CI
Þ Soft Gelatin Capsule
ß Not available because of insufficient data.
à 90% CI not available
è Relative to steady-state administration of voriconazole (400 mg for 1 day, then 200 mg po q12h for 2 days).

0.04–8.5 µM. In drug combination studies of tenofovir with NRTIs (abacavir, didanosine, lamivudine, stavudine, zalcitabine, and zidovudine), NNRTIs (delavirdine, efavirenz, and nevirapine), and PIs (amprenavir, indinavir, nelfinavir, ritonavir, and saquinavir), additive to synergistic effects were observed. Tenofovir displayed antiviral activity in cell culture against HIV-1 clades A, B, C, D, E, F, G and O (EC_{50} values ranged from 0.5–2.2 µM) and showed strain specific activity against HIV-2 (EC_{50} values ranged from 1.6 µM to 5.5 µM).

Resistance

Efavirenz, Emtricitabine, and Tenofovir Disoproxil Fumarate: HIV-1 isolates with reduced susceptibility to the combination of emtricitabine and tenofovir have been selected in cell culture and in clinical studies. Genotypic analysis of these isolates identified the M184V/I and/or K65R amino acid substitutions in the viral RT.

In a clinical study of treatment-naive subjects *[Study 934, see Clinical Studies (14)]* resistance analysis was performed on HIV-1 isolates from all confirmed virologic failure subjects with >400 copies/mL of HIV-1 RNA at Week 144 or early discontinuations. Genotypic resistance to efavirenz, predominantly the K103N substitution, was the most common form of resistance that developed. Resistance to efavirenz occurred in 13/19 analyzed subjects in the emtricitabine + tenofovir DF group and in 21/29 analyzed subjects in the zidovudine/lamivudine fixed-dose combina-

tion group. The M184V amino acid substitution, associated with resistance to emtricitabine and lamivudine, was observed in 2/19 analyzed subject isolates in the emtricitabine + tenofovir DF group and in 10/29 analyzed subject isolates in the zidovudine/lamivudine group. Through 144 weeks of Study 934, no subjects developed a detectable K65R substitution in their HIV-1 as analyzed through standard genotypic analysis.

In a clinical study of treatment-naive subjects, isolates from 8/47 (17%) analyzed subjects receiving tenofovir DF developed the K65R substitution through 144 weeks of therapy; 7 of these occurred in the first 48 weeks of treatment and one at Week 96. In treatment experienced subjects, 14/304 (5%) of tenofovir DF treated subjects with virologic failure through Week 96 showed >1.4 fold (median 2.7) reduced susceptibility to tenofovir. Genotypic analysis of the resistant isolates showed a substitution in the HIV-1 RT gene resulting in the K65R amino acid substitution.

Efavirenz: Clinical isolates with reduced susceptibility in cell culture to efavirenz have been obtained. The most frequently observed amino acid substitution in clinical studies with efavirenz is K103N (54%). One or more RT substitutions at amino acid positions 98, 100, 101, 103, 106, 108, 188, 190, 225, 227, and 230 were observed in subjects failing treatment with efavirenz in combination with other antiretrovirals. Other resistance substitutions observed to emerge commonly included L100I (7%), K101E/Q/R (14%), V108I (11%), G190S/T/A (7%), P225H (18%), and M230I/L (11%).

HIV-1 isolates with reduced susceptibility to efavirenz (>380-fold increase in EC_{90} value) emerged rapidly under selection in cell culture. Genotypic characterization of these viruses identified single amino acid substitutions L100I or V179D, double substitutions L100I/V108I, and triple substitutions L100I/V179D/Y181C in RT.

Emtricitabine: Emtricitabine-resistant isolates of HIV-1 have been selected in cell culture and in clinical studies. Genotypic analysis of these isolates showed that the reduced susceptibility to emtricitabine was associated with a substitution in the HIV-1 RT gene at codon 184 which resulted in an amino acid substitution of methionine by valine or isoleucine (M184V/I).

Tenofovir Disoproxil Fumarate: HIV-1 isolates with reduced susceptibility to tenofovir have been selected in cell culture. These viruses expressed a K65R substitution in RT and showed a 2–4 fold reduction in susceptibility to tenofovir.

Cross Resistance

Efavirenz, Emtricitabine, and Tenofovir Disoproxil Fumarate: Cross-resistance has been recognized among NNRTIs. Cross resistance has also been recognized among certain NRTIs. The M184V/I and/or K65R substitutions selected in cell culture by the combination of emtricitabine and tenofovir are also observed in some HIV-1 isolates from subjects failing treatment with tenofovir in combination with either lamivudine or emtricitabine, and either abacavir or didanosine. Therefore, cross-resistance among these drugs may occur in patients whose virus harbors either or both of these amino acid substitutions.

Efavirenz: Clinical isolates previously characterized as efavirenz-resistant were also phenotypically resistant in cell culture to delavirdine and nevirapine compared to baseline. Delavirdine- and/or nevirapine-resistant clinical viral isolates with NNRTI resistance-associated substitutions (A98G, L100I, K101E/P, K103N/S, V106A, Y181X, Y188X, G190X, P225H, F227L, or M230L) showed reduced susceptibility to efavirenz in cell culture. Greater than 90% of NRTI-resistant isolates tested in cell culture retained susceptibility to efavirenz.

Emtricitabine: Emtricitabine-resistant isolates (M184V/I) were cross-resistant to lamivudine and zalcitabine but retained susceptibility in cell culture to didanosine, stavudine, tenofovir, zidovudine, and NNRTIs (delavirdine, efavirenz, and nevirapine). HIV-1 isolates containing the K65R substitution, selected *in vivo* by abacavir, didanosine, tenofovir, and zalcitabine, demonstrated reduced susceptibility to inhibition by emtricitabine. Viruses harboring substitutions conferring reduced susceptibility to stavudine and zidovudine (M41L, D67N, K70R, L210W, T215Y/F, and K219Q/E) or didanosine (L74V) remained sensitive to emtricitabine.

Tenofovir Disoproxil Fumarate: The K65R substitution selected by tenofovir is also selected in some HIV-1 infected patients treated with abacavir, didanosine, or zalcitabine. HIV-1 isolates with the K65R substitution also showed reduced susceptibility to emtricitabine and lamivudine. Therefore, cross-resistance among these drugs may occur in patients whose virus harbors the K65R substitution. HIV-1 isolates from patients (N=20) whose HIV-1 expressed a mean of 3 zidovudine-associated RT amino acid substitutions (M41L, D67N, K70R, L210W, T215Y/F, or K219Q/E/N) showed a 3.1-fold decrease in the susceptibility to tenofovir. Subjects whose virus expressed an L74V substitution without zidovudine resistance associated substitutions (N=8) had reduced response to VIREAD. Limited data are available for patients whose virus expressed a Y115F substitution (N=3), Q151M substitution (N=2), or T69 insertion (N=4), all of whom had a reduced response.

13 NONCLINICAL TOXICOLOGY
13.1 Carcinogenesis, Mutagenesis, Impairment of Fertility

Efavirenz: Long-term carcinogenicity studies in mice and rats were carried out with efavirenz. Mice were dosed with 0, 25, 75, 150, or 300 mg/kg/day for 2 years. Incidences of hepatocellular adenomas and carcinomas and pulmonary alveolar/bronchiolar adenomas were increased above background in females. No increases in tumor incidence above background were seen in males. In studies in which rats were administered efavirenz at doses of 0, 25, 50, or 100 mg/kg/day for 2 years, no increases in tumor incidence above background were observed. The systemic exposure (based on AUCs) in mice was approximately 1.7-fold that in humans receiving the 600-mg/day dose. The exposure in rats was lower than that in humans. The mechanism of the carcinogenic potential is unknown. In genetic toxicology assays, efavirenz showed no evidence of mutagenic or clastogenic activity in a battery of *in vitro* and *in vivo* studies. These included bacterial mutation assays in *S. typhimurium* and *E. coli*, mammalian mutation assays in Chinese hamster ovary cells, chromosome aberration assays in human peripheral blood lymphocytes or Chinese hamster ovary cells, and an *in vivo* mouse bone marrow micronucleus assay. Given the lack of genotoxic activity of efavirenz, the relevance to humans of neoplasms in efavirenz-treated mice is not known.

Efavirenz did not impair mating or fertility of male or female rats, and did not affect sperm of treated male rats. The reproductive performance of offspring born to female rats given efavirenz was not affected. As a result of the rapid clearance of efavirenz in rats, systemic drug exposures achieved in these studies were equivalent to or below those achieved in humans given therapeutic doses of efavirenz.

Emtricitabine: In long-term carcinogenicity studies of emtricitabine, no drug-related increases in tumor incidence were found in mice at doses up to 750 mg/kg/day (26 times the human systemic exposure at the therapeutic dose of 200 mg/day) or in rats at doses up to 600 mg/day (31 times the human systemic exposure at the therapeutic dose).

Emtricitabine was not genotoxic in the reverse mutation bacterial test (Ames test), mouse lymphoma or mouse micronucleus assays.

Emtricitabine did not affect fertility in male rats at approximately 140-fold or in male and female mice at approximately 60-fold higher exposures (AUC) than in humans given the recommended 200 mg daily dose. Fertility was normal in the offspring of mice exposed daily from before birth (*in utero*) through sexual maturity at daily exposures (AUC) of approximately 60-fold higher than human exposures at the recommended 200 mg daily dose.

Table 7: Drug Interactions: Changes in Pharmacokinetic Parameters for Tenofovir in the Presence of the Coadministered Drug*,†

Coadministered Drug	Dose of Coadministered Drug (mg)	N	Mean % Change of Tenofovir Pharmacokinetic Parameters‡ (90% CI)		
			C_max	AUC	C_min
Atazanavir§	400 once daily × 14 days	33	↑ 14 (↑ 8 to ↑ 20)	↑ 24 (↑ 21 to ↑ 28)	↑ 22 (↑ 15 to ↑ 30)
Didanosine (enteric-coated)	400 once	25	↔	↔	↔
Didanosine (buffered)	250 or 400 once daily × 7 days	14	↔	↔	↔
Lopinavir/ritonavir	400/100 twice daily × 14 days	24		↑ 32 (↑ 25 to ↑ 38)	↑ 51 (↑ 37 to ↑ 66)

* All interaction studies conducted in healthy volunteers.
† Subjects received tenofovir DF 300 mg once daily.
‡ Increase = ↑; Decrease = ↓; No Effect = ↔
§ Reyataz Prescribing Information

Table 8: Drug Interactions: Changes in Pharmacokinetic Parameters for Coadministered Drug in the Presence of Tenofovir Disoproxil Fumarate*,†

Coadministered Drug	Dose of Coadministered Drug (mg)	N	Mean % Change of Coadministered Drug Pharmacokinetic Parameters‡ (90% CI)		
			C_max	AUC	C_min
Atazanavir§	400 once daily × 14 days	34	↓ 21 (↓ 27 to ↓ 14)	↓ 25 (↓ 30 to ↓ 19)	↓ 40 (↓ 48 to ↓ 32)
	Atazanavir/ritonavir 300/100 once daily × 42 days	10	↓ 28 (↓ 50 to ↑ 5)	↓ 25¶ (↓ 42 to ↓ 3)	↓ 23¶ (↓ 46 to ↑ 10)
Lopinavir	Lopinavir/ritonavir 400/100 twice daily × 14 days	24	↔	↔	↔
Ritonavir	Lopinavir/ritonavir 400/100 twice daily × 14 days	24	↔	↔	↔

* All interaction studies conducted in healthy volunteers.
† Subjects received tenofovir DF 300 mg once daily.
‡ Increase = ↑; Decrease = ↓; No Effect = ↔
§ Reyataz Prescribing Information
¶ In HIV-infected patients, addition of tenofovir DF to atazanavir 300 mg plus ritonavir 100 mg, resulted in AUC and C_min values of atazanavir that were 2.3- and 4-fold higher than the respective values observed for atazanavir 400 mg when given alone.

Tenofovir Disoproxil Fumarate: Long-term oral carcinogenicity studies of tenofovir DF in mice and rats were carried out at exposures up to approximately 16 times (mice) and 5 times (rats) those observed in humans at the therapeutic dose for HIV-1 infection. At the high dose in female mice, liver adenomas were increased at exposures 16 times that in humans. In rats, the study was negative for carcinogenic findings at exposures up to 5 times that observed in humans at the therapeutic dose.

Tenofovir DF was mutagenic in the *in vitro* mouse lymphoma assay and negative in an *in vitro* bacterial mutagenicity test (Ames test). In an *in vivo* mouse micronucleus assay, tenofovir DF was negative when administered to male mice.

There were no effects on fertility, mating performance or early embryonic development when tenofovir DF was administered to male rats at a dose equivalent to 10 times the human dose based on body surface area comparisons for 28 days prior to mating and to female rats for 15 days prior to mating through day seven of gestation. There was, however, an alteration of the estrous cycle in female rats.

13.2 Animal Toxicology and/or Pharmacology

Efavirenz: Nonsustained convulsions were observed in 6 of 20 monkeys receiving efavirenz at doses yielding plasma AUC values 4- to 13-fold greater than those in humans given the recommended dose.

Tenofovir Disoproxil Fumarate: Tenofovir and tenofovir DF administered in toxicology studies to rats, dogs and monkeys at exposures (based on AUCs) greater than or equal to 6-fold those observed in humans caused bone toxicity. In monkeys the bone toxicity was diagnosed as osteomalacia. Osteomalacia observed in monkeys appeared to be reversible upon dose reduction or discontinuation of tenofovir. In rats and dogs, the bone toxicity manifested as reduced bone mineral density. The mechanism(s) underlying bone toxicity is unknown.

Evidence of renal toxicity was noted in 4 animal species administered tenofovir and tenofovir DF. Increases in serum creatinine, BUN, glycosuria, proteinuria, phosphaturia and/or calciuria and decreases in serum phosphate were observed to varying degrees in these animals. These toxicities were noted at exposures (based on AUCs) 2–20 times higher than those observed in humans. The relationship of the renal abnormalities, particularly the phosphaturia, to the bone toxicity is not known.

14 CLINICAL STUDIES

Clinical Study 934 supports the use of ATRIPLA (efavirenz/emtricitabine/tenofovir disoproxil fumarate) tablets in antiretroviral treatment-naive HIV-1-infected patients. Additional data in support of the use of ATRIPLA in treatment-naive patients can be found in the prescribing information for VIREAD.

Clinical Study 073 provides clinical experience in subjects with stable, virologic suppression and no history of virologic failure who switched from their current regimen to ATRIPLA.

In antiretroviral treatment-experienced patients, the use of ATRIPLA tablets may be considered for patients with HIV-1 strains that are expected to be susceptible to the components of ATRIPLA as assessed by treatment history or by genotypic or phenotypic testing [See Clinical Pharmacology (12.4)].

Study 934: Data through 144 weeks are reported for Study 934, a randomized, open-label, active-controlled multicenter study comparing emtricitabine + tenofovir DF administered in combination with efavirenz versus zidovudine/lamivudine fixed-dose combination administered in combination with efavirenz in 511 antiretroviral-naive subjects.

Table 9: Drug Interactions: Changes in Pharmacokinetic Parameters for Didanosine in the Presence of Tenofovir Disoproxil Fumarate*,†

Didanosine Dose (mg)/Method of Administration‡	Tenofovir DF Method of Administration†,‡	N	Mean % Change (90% CI) vs. Didanosine 400 mg Alone, Fasted§	
			C_{max}	AUC
Buffered tablets				
400 once daily¶ × 7 days	Fasted 1 hour after didanosine	14	↑ 28 (↑ 11 to ↑ 48)	↑ 44 (↑ 31 to ↑ 59)
Enteric coated capsules				
400 once, fasted	With food, 2 hr after didanosine	26	↑ 48 (↑ 25 to ↑ 76)	↑ 48 (↑ 31 to ↑ 67)
400 once, with food	Simultaneously with didanosine	26	↑ 64 (↑ 41 to ↑ 89)	↑ 60 (↑ 44 to ↑ 79)
250 once, fasted	With food, 2 hr after didanosine	28	↓ 10 (↓ 22 to ↑ 3)	↔
250 once, fasted	Simultaneously with didanosine	28	↔	↑ 14 (0 to ↑ 31)
250 once, with food	Simultaneously with didanosine	28	↓ 29 (↓ 39 to ↓ 18)	↓ 11 (↓ 23 to ↑ 2)

* All interaction studies conducted in healthy volunteers.
† Subjects received tenofovir DF 300 mg once daily.
‡ Administration with food was with a light meal (~373 kcal, 20% fat).
§ Increase = ↑; Decrease = ↓; No Effect = ↔
¶ Includes 4 subjects weighing <60 kg receiving ddI 250 mg.

Table 10: Outcomes of Randomized Treatment at Weeks 48 and 144 (Study 934)

Outcomes	At Week 48		At Week 144	
	FTC + TDF +EFV (N=244)	AZT/3TC +EFV (N=243)	FTC + TDF +EFV (N=227)*	AZT/3TC +EFV (N=229)*
Responder†	84%	73%	71%	58%
Virologic failure‡	2%	4%	3%	6%
Rebound	1%	3%	2%	5%
Never suppressed	0%	0%	0%	0%
Change in antiretroviral regimen	1%	1%	1%	1%
Death	<1%	1%	1%	1%
Discontinued due to adverse event	4%	9%	5%	12%
Discontinued for other reasons§	10%	14%	20%	22%

* Subjects who were responders at Week 48 or Week 96 (HIV-1 RNA <400 copies/mL) but did not consent to continue study after Week 48 or Week 96 were excluded from analysis.
† Subjects achieved and maintained confirmed HIV-1 RNA <400 copies/mL through Weeks 48 and 144.
‡ Includes confirmed viral rebound and failure to achieve confirmed HIV-1 RNA <400 copies/mL through Weeks 48 and 144.
§ Includes lost to follow-up, patient withdrawal, noncompliance, protocol violation and other reasons.

From weeks 96 to 144 of the study, subjects received emtricitabine/tenofovir DF fixed-dose combination with efavirenz in place of emtricitabine + tenofovir DF with efavirenz. Subjects had a mean age of 38 years (range 18–80), 86% were male, 59% were Caucasian and 23% were Black. The mean baseline CD4+ cell count was 245 cells/mm³ (range 2–1191) and median baseline plasma HIV-1 RNA was 5.01 $\log_{10}$ copies/mL (range 3.56–6.54). Subjects were stratified by baseline CD4+ cell count (< or ≥ 200 cells/mm³) and 41% had CD4+ cell counts <200 cells/mm³. Fifty-one percent (51%) of subjects had baseline viral loads >100,000 copies/mL. Treatment outcomes through 48 and 144 weeks for those subjects who did not have efavirenz resistance at baseline (n=487) are presented in Table 10.
[See table 10 above]
Through Week 48, 84% and 73% of subjects in the emtricitabine + tenofovir DF group and the zidovudine/lamivudine group, respectively, achieved and maintained HIV-1 RNA <400 copies/mL (71% and 58% through Week 144). The difference in the proportion of subjects who achieved and maintained HIV-1 RNA <400 copies/mL through 48 weeks largely results from the higher number of discontinuations due to adverse events and other reasons in the zidovudine/lamivudine group in this open-label study. In addition, 80% and 70% of subjects in the emtricitabine + tenofovir DF group and the zidovudine/lamivudine group, respectively, achieved and maintained HIV-1 RNA <50 copies/mL through Week 48 (64% and 56% through Week 144). The mean increase from baseline in CD4+ cell count was 190 cells/mm³ in the emtricitabine + tenofovir DF group and 158 cells/mm³ in the zidovudine/lamivudine group at Week 48 (312 and 271 cells/mm³ at Week 144).
Through 48 weeks, 7 subjects in the emtricitabine + tenofovir DF group and 5 subjects in the zidovudine/lamivudine group experienced a new CDC Class C event (10 and 6 subjects through 144 weeks).
Study 073: Study 073 was a 48-week open-label, randomized clinical trial in subjects with stable, virologic suppression on combination antiretroviral therapy consisting of at least two nucleoside reverse transcriptase inhibitors (NR-TIs) administered in combination with a protease inhibitor (with or without ritonavir) or a non-nucleoside reverse transcriptase inhibitor (NNRTI).
To be enrolled, subjects were to have HIV-1 RNA <200 copies/mL for at least 12 weeks on their current regimen prior to study entry with no known HIV-1 substitutions conferring resistance to the components of ATRIPLA (efavirenz/emtricitabine/tenofovir disoproxil fumarate) and no history of virologic failure.

The study compared the efficacy of switching to ATRIPLA (efavirenz/emtricitabine/tenofovir disoproxil fumarate) or staying on the baseline antiretroviral regimen (SBR). Subjects were randomized in a 2:1 ratio to switch to ATRIPLA (N=203) or stay on SBR (N=97). Subjects had a mean age of 43 years (range 22 to 73 years), 88% were male, 68% were white, 29% were black or African-American, and 3% were of other races. At baseline, median CD4+ cell count was 516 cells/mm³ and 96% had HIV-1 RNA <50 copies/mL. The median time since onset of antiretroviral therapy was 3 years and 88% of subjects were receiving their first antiretroviral regimen at study enrollment.
At Week 48, 89% and 87% of subjects who switched to ATRIPLA (efavirenz/emtricitabine/tenofovir disoproxil fumarate) maintained HIV RNA <200 copies/mL and <50 copies/mL, respectively, compared to 88% and 85% who remained on SBR; this difference was not statistically significant. No changes in CD4+ cell counts from baseline to Week 48 were observed in either treatment arm.

16 HOW SUPPLIED/STORAGE AND HANDLING
ATRIPLA tablets are pink, capsule-shaped, film-coated, debossed with "123" on one side and plain-faced on the other side. Each bottle contains 30 tablets (NDC 15584-0101-1) and silica gel desiccant, and is closed with a child-resistant closure.
Store at 25 °C (77 °F); excursions permitted to 15–30 °C (59–86 °F) *[See USP Controlled Room Temperature]*.
• Keep container tightly closed.
• Dispense only in original container.
• Do not use if seal over bottle opening is broken or missing.

17 PATIENT COUNSELING INFORMATION AND FDA-APPROVED PATIENT LABELING
17.1 Drug Interactions
A statement to patients and healthcare providers is included on the product's bottle labels: *ALERT: Find out about medicines that should NOT be taken with ATRIPLA.* ATRIPLA may interact with some drugs; therefore, patients should be advised to report to their doctor the use of any other prescription, nonprescription medication, or herbal products, particularly St. John's wort.
17.2 Information for Patients
Patients should be advised that:
• ATRIPLA is not a cure for HIV-1 infection and that they may continue to experience illnesses associated with HIV-1 infection, including opportunistic infections. Patients should remain under the care of a physician when using ATRIPLA.
• The use of ATRIPLA has not been shown to reduce the risk of transmission of HIV-1 to others through sexual contact or blood contamination. Patients should be advised to continue to practice safer sex and to use latex or polyurethane condoms to lower the chance of sexual contact with any body fluids such as semen, vaginal secretions or blood. Patients should be advised never to re-use or share needles.
• The long term effects of ATRIPLA are unknown.
• Redistribution or accumulation of body fat may occur in patients receiving antiretroviral therapy and that the cause and long-term health effects of these conditions are not known.
• ATRIPLA should not be coadministered with SUSTIVA, EMTRIVA, VIREAD, or TRUVADA, or drugs containing lamivudine, including Combivir, Epivir, Epivir-HBV, Epzicom, or Trizivir.
• ATRIPLA should not be administered with HEPSERA *[See Warnings and Precautions (5.2)]*.
17.3 Lactic Acidosis/Severe Hepatomegaly with Steatosis
Patients should be informed that lactic acidosis and severe hepatomegaly with steatosis, including fatal cases, have been reported. Treatment will be suspended in any patients who develop clinical symptoms suggestive of lactic acidosis or pronounced hepatotoxicity (including nausea, vomiting, unusual or unexpected stomach discomfort, and weakness) *[See Warnings and Precautions (5.1)]*.
17.4 Patients Coinfected with HIV-1 and HBV
Patients with HIV-1 should be tested for hepatitis B virus (HBV) before initiating antiretroviral therapy.
Patients should be advised that severe acute exacerbations of hepatitis B have been reported in patients who are coinfected with HBV and HIV-1 and have discontinued EMTRIVA (emtricitabine) or VIREAD (tenofovir DF), which are components of ATRIPLA.
17.5 New Onset or Worsening Renal Impairment
Renal impairment, including cases of acute renal failure and Fanconi syndrome, has been reported. ATRIPLA should be avoided with concurrent or recent use of a nephrotoxic agent *[See Warnings and Precautions (5.7)]*.
17.6 Decreases in Bone Mineral Density
Patients should be informed that decreases in bone mineral density have been observed with the use of tenofovir DF. Bone mineral density monitoring may be performed in patients who have a history of pathologic bone fracture or are at risk for osteopenia *[See Warnings and Precautions (5.11)]*.

17.7 Dosing Instructions

Patients should be advised to take ATRIPLA (efavirenz/emtricitabine/tenofovir disoproxil fumarate) orally on an empty stomach and that it is important to take ATRIPLA on a regular dosing schedule to avoid missing doses.

17.8 Nervous System Symptoms

Patients should be informed that central nervous system symptoms (NSS) including dizziness, insomnia, impaired concentration, drowsiness, and abnormal dreams are commonly reported during the first weeks of therapy with efavirenz. Dosing at bedtime may improve the tolerability of these symptoms, which are likely to improve with continued therapy. Patients should be alerted to the potential for additive effects when ATRIPLA is used concomitantly with alcohol or psychoactive drugs. Patients should be instructed that if they experience NSS they should avoid potentially hazardous tasks such as driving or operating machinery [See Warnings and Precautions (5.6), and Dosage and Administration (2)].

17.9 Psychiatric Symptoms

Patients should be informed that serious psychiatric symptoms including severe depression, suicide attempts, aggressive behavior, delusions, paranoia, and psychosis-like symptoms have been reported in patients receiving efavirenz. If they experience severe psychiatric adverse experiences they should seek immediate medical evaluation. Patients should be advised to inform their physician of any history of mental illness or substance abuse [See Warnings and Precautions (5.5)].

17.10 Rash

Patients should be informed that a common side effect is rash. Rashes usually go away without any change in treatment. However, since rash may be serious, patients should be advised to contact their physician promptly if rash occurs.

17.11 Reproductive Risk Potential

Women receiving ATRIPLA should be instructed to avoid pregnancy [See Warnings and Precautions (5.8)]. A reliable form of barrier contraception must always be used in combination with other methods of contraception, including oral or other hormonal contraception. Because of the long half-life of efavirenz, use of adequate contraceptive measures for 12 weeks after discontinuation of ATRIPLA is recommended. Women should be advised to notify their physician if they become pregnant or plan to become pregnant while taking ATRIPLA. If this drug is used during the first trimester of pregnancy, or if the patient becomes pregnant while taking this drug, she should be apprised of the potential harm to the fetus.

FDA-APPROVED PATIENT LABELING

Patient Information

ATRIPLA® (uh TRIP luh) Tablets

ALERT: Find out about medicines that should NOT be taken with ATRIPLA.

Please also read the section "MEDICINES YOU SHOULD NOT TAKE WITH ATRIPLA."

Generic name: efavirenz, emtricitabine and tenofovir disoproxil fumarate

(eh FAH vih renz, em tri SIT uh bean and te NOE' fo veer dye soe PROX il FYOU mar ate)

Read the Patient Information that comes with ATRIPLA before you start taking it and each time you get a refill since there may be new information. This information does not take the place of talking to your healthcare provider about your medical condition or treatment. You should stay under a healthcare provider's care when taking ATRIPLA. **Do not change or stop your medicine without first talking with your healthcare provider.** Talk to your healthcare provider or pharmacist if you have any questions about ATRIPLA.

What is the most important information I should know about ATRIPLA?

- Some people who have taken medicine like ATRIPLA (which contains nucleoside analogs) have developed a serious condition called lactic acidosis (build up of an acid in the blood). Lactic acidosis can be a medical emergency and may need to be treated in the hospital. **Call your healthcare provider right away if you get the following signs or symptoms of lactic acidosis:**
  - You feel very weak or tired.
  - You have unusual (not normal) muscle pain.
  - You have trouble breathing.
  - You have stomach pain with nausea and vomiting.
  - You feel cold, especially in your arms and legs.
  - You feel dizzy or lightheaded.
  - You have a fast or irregular heartbeat.
- Some people who have taken medicines like ATRIPLA have developed serious liver problems called hepatotoxicity, with liver enlargement (hepatomegaly) and fat in the liver (steatosis). **Call your healthcare provider right away if you get the following signs or symptoms of liver problems:**
  - Your skin or the white part of your eyes turns yellow (jaundice).
  - Your urine turns dark.
  - Your bowel movements (stools) turn light in color.

- You don't feel like eating food for several days or longer.
- You feel sick to your stomach (nausea).
- You have lower stomach area (abdominal) pain.
- **You may be more likely to get lactic acidosis or liver problems** if you are female, very overweight (obese), or have been taking nucleoside analog-containing medicines, like ATRIPLA (efavirenz/emtricitabine/tenofovir disoproxil fumarate), for a long time.
- **If you also have hepatitis B virus (HBV) infection and you stop taking ATRIPLA, you may get a "flare-up" of your hepatitis. A "flare-up" is when the disease suddenly returns in a worse way than before.** Patients with HBV who stop taking ATRIPLA need close medical follow-up for several months, including medical exams and blood tests to check for hepatitis that could be getting worse. ATRIPLA is not approved for the treatment of HBV, so you must discuss your HBV therapy with your healthcare provider.

What is ATRIPLA?

ATRIPLA contains 3 medicines, SUSTIVA® (efavirenz), EMTRIVA® (emtricitabine) and VIREAD® (tenofovir disoproxil fumarate also called tenofovir DF) combined in one pill. EMTRIVA and VIREAD are HIV-1 (human immunodeficiency virus) nucleoside analog reverse transcriptase inhibitors (NRTIs) and SUSTIVA is an HIV-1 non-nucleoside analog reverse transcriptase inhibitor (NNRTI). VIREAD and EMTRIVA are the components of TRUVADA®. ATRIPLA can be used alone as a complete regimen, or in combination with other anti-HIV-1 medicines to treat people with HIV-1 infection. ATRIPLA is for adults age 18 and over. ATRIPLA has not been studied in children under age 18 or adults over age 65.

HIV infection destroys CD4+ T cells, which are important to the immune system. The immune system helps fight infection. After a large number of T cells are destroyed, acquired immune deficiency syndrome (AIDS) develops.

ATRIPLA helps block HIV-1 reverse transcriptase, a viral chemical in your body (enzyme) that is needed for HIV-1 to multiply. ATRIPLA lowers the amount of HIV-1 in the blood (viral load). ATRIPLA may also help to increase the number of T cells (CD4+ cells), allowing your immune system to improve. Lowering the amount of HIV-1 in the blood lowers the chance of death or infections that happen when your immune system is weak (opportunistic infections).

Does ATRIPLA cure HIV-1 or AIDS?

ATRIPLA does not cure HIV-1 infection or AIDS. The long-term effects of ATRIPLA are not known at this time. People taking ATRIPLA may still get opportunistic infections or other conditions that happen with HIV-1 infection. Opportunistic infections are infections that develop because the immune system is weak. Some of these conditions are pneumonia, herpes virus infections, and *Mycobacterium avium complex* (MAC) infection. **It is very important that you see your healthcare provider regularly while taking ATRIPLA.**

Does ATRIPLA reduce the risk of passing HIV-1 to others?

ATRIPLA has not been shown to lower your chance of passing HIV-1 to other people through sexual contact, sharing needles, or being exposed to your blood.

- **Do not share needles or other injection equipment.**
- **Do not share personal items that can have blood or body fluids on them, like toothbrushes or razor blades.**
- **Do not have any kind of sex without protection.** Always practice safer sex by using a latex or polyurethane condom or other barrier to reduce the chance of sexual contact with semen, vaginal secretions, or blood.

Who should not take ATRIPLA?

Together with your healthcare provider, you need to decide whether ATRIPLA is right for you.

Do not take ATRIPLA if you are allergic to ATRIPLA or any of its ingredients. The active ingredients of ATRIPLA are efavirenz, emtricitabine, and tenofovir DF. See the end of this leaflet for a complete list of ingredients.

What should I tell my healthcare provider before taking ATRIPLA?

Tell your healthcare provider if you:

- **Are pregnant or planning to become pregnant** (see "What should I avoid while taking ATRIPLA?").
- **Are breastfeeding** (see "What should I avoid while taking ATRIPLA?").
- **Have kidney problems or are undergoing kidney dialysis treatment.**
- **Have bone problems.**
- **Have liver problems, including hepatitis B virus infection.** Your healthcare provider may want to do tests to check your liver while you take ATRIPLA.
- **Have ever had mental illness or are using drugs or alcohol.**
- **Have ever had seizures or are taking medicine for seizures.**

What important information should I know about taking other medicines with ATRIPLA?

ATRIPLA may change the effect of other medicines, including the ones for HIV-1, and may cause serious side effects. Your healthcare provider may change your other medicines or change their doses. Other medicines, including herbal

products, may affect ATRIPLA (efavirenz/emtricitabine/tenofovir disoproxil fumarate). For this reason, **it is very important to** let all your healthcare providers and pharmacists know what medications, herbal supplements, or vitamins you are taking.

MEDICINES YOU SHOULD NOT TAKE WITH ATRIPLA

- The following medicines may cause serious and life-threatening side effects when taken with ATRIPLA. You should not take any of these medicines while taking ATRIPLA: Vascor (bepridil), Propulsid (cisapride), Versed (midazolam), Orap (pimozide), Halcion (triazolam), ergot medications (for example, Wigraine and Cafergot).
- ATRIPLA also should not be used with Combivir (lamivudine/zidovudine), EMTRIVA, Epivir, Epivir-HBV (lamivudine), Epzicom (abacavir sulfate/lamivudine), Trizivir (abacavir sulfate/lamivudine/zidovudine), SUSTIVA, TRUVADA, or VIREAD.
- Vfend (voriconazole) should not be taken with ATRIPLA since it may lose its effect or may increase the chance of having side effects from ATRIPLA.
- **Do not take St. John's wort (*Hypericum perforatum*), or products containing St. John's wort with ATRIPLA.** St. John's wort is an herbal product sold as a dietary supplement. Talk with your healthcare provider if you are taking or are planning to take St. John's wort. Taking St. John's wort may decrease ATRIPLA levels and lead to increased viral load and possible resistance to ATRIPLA or cross-resistance to other anti-HIV-1 drugs.
- ATRIPLA should not be used with HEPSERA® (adefovir dipivoxil).

It is also important to tell your healthcare provider if you are taking any of the following:

- Fortovase, Invirase (saquinavir), Biaxin (clarithromycin), Noxafil (posaconazole), or Sporanox (itraconazole); **these medicines may need to be replaced with another medicine when taken with ATRIPLA.**
- Calcium channel blockers such as Cardizem or Tiazac (diltiazem), Covera HS or Isoptin (verapamil) and others; Crixivan (indinavir), Selzentry (maraviroc); the immunosuppressant medicines cyclosporine (Gengraf, Neoral, Sandimmune, and others), Prograf (tacrolimus), or Rapamune (sirolimus); Methadone; Mycobutin (rifabutin); Rifampin; cholesterol-lowering medicines such as Lipitor (atorvastatin), Pravachol (pravastatin sodium), and Zocor (simvastatin); or Zoloft (sertraline); **these medicines may need to have their dose changed when taken with ATRIPLA.**
- Videx, Videx EC (didanosine); tenofovir DF (a component of ATRIPLA) may increase the amount of didanosine in your blood, which could result in more side effects. **You may need to be monitored more carefully** if you are taking ATRIPLA and didanosine together. Also, the dose of didanosine may need to be changed.
- Reyataz (atazanavir sulfate) or Kaletra (lopinavir/ritonavir); these medicines may increase the amount of tenofovir DF (a component of ATRIPLA) in your blood, which could result in more side effects. Reyataz is not recommended with ATRIPLA. **You may need to be monitored more carefully** if you are taking ATRIPLA and Kaletra together. Also, the dose of Kaletra may need to be changed.
- Medicine for seizures [for example, Dilantin (phenytoin), Tegretol (carbamazepine), or phenobarbital]; your healthcare provider may want to switch you to another medicine or check drug levels in your blood from time to time.

These are not all the medicines that may cause problems if you take ATRIPLA. Be sure to tell your healthcare provider about all medicines that you take.

Keep a complete list of all the prescription and nonprescription medicines as well as any herbal remedies that you are taking, how much you take, and how often you take them. Make a new list when medicines or herbal remedies are added or stopped, or if the dose changes. Give copies of this list to all of your healthcare providers and pharmacists **every** time you visit your healthcare provider or fill a prescription. This will give your healthcare provider a complete picture of the medicines you use. Then he or she can decide the best approach for your situation.

How should I take ATRIPLA?

- Take the exact amount of ATRIPLA your healthcare provider prescribes. Never change the dose on your own. Do not stop this medicine unless your healthcare provider tells you to stop.
- You should take ATRIPLA on an empty stomach.
- Swallow ATRIPLA with water.
- Taking ATRIPLA at bedtime may make some side effects less bothersome.
- Do not miss a dose of ATRIPLA. If you forget to take ATRIPLA, take the missed dose right away, unless it is almost time for your next dose. Do not double the next dose. Carry on with your regular dosing schedule. If you need help in planning the best times to take your medicine, ask your healthcare provider or pharmacist.
- If you believe you took more than the prescribed amount of ATRIPLA, contact your local poison control center or emergency room right away.
- Tell your healthcare provider if you start any new medicine or change how you take old ones. Your doses may need adjustment.

- When your ATRIPLA (efavirenz/emtricitabine/tenofovir disoproxil fumarate) supply starts to run low, get more from your healthcare provider or pharmacy. This is very important because the amount of virus in your blood may increase if the medicine is stopped for even a short time. The virus may develop resistance to ATRIPLA and become harder to treat.
- Your healthcare provider may want to do blood tests to check for certain side effects while you take ATRIPLA.

What should I avoid while taking ATRIPLA?

- **Women should not become pregnant while taking ATRIPLA and for 12 weeks after stopping it.** Serious birth defects have been seen in the babies of animals and women treated with efavirenz (a component of ATRIPLA) during pregnancy. It is not known whether efavirenz caused these defects. **Tell your healthcare provider right away if you are pregnant.** Also talk with your healthcare provider if you want to become pregnant.
- Women should not rely only on hormone-based birth control, such as pills, injections, or implants, because ATRIPLA may make these contraceptives ineffective. Women must use a reliable form of barrier contraception, such as a condom or diaphragm, even if they also use other methods of birth control. Efavirenz, a component of ATRIPLA, may remain in your blood for a time after therapy is stopped. Therefore, you should continue to use contraceptive measures for 12 weeks after you stop taking ATRIPLA.
- **Do not breast-feed if you are taking ATRIPLA.** The Centers for Disease Control and Prevention recommend that mothers with HIV not breast-feed because they can pass the HIV through their milk to the baby. Also, ATRIPLA may pass through breast milk and cause serious harm to the baby. Talk with your healthcare provider if you are breast-feeding. You should stop breast-feeding or may need to use a different medicine.
- Taking ATRIPLA with alcohol or other medicines causing similar side effects as ATRIPLA, such as drowsiness, may increase those side effects.
- Do not take any other medicines, including prescription and nonprescription medicines and herbal products, without checking with your healthcare provider.
- **Avoid doing things that can spread HIV-1 infection** since ATRIPLA does not stop you from passing the HIV-1 infection to others.

What are the possible side effects of ATRIPLA?

ATRIPLA may cause the following serious side effects:

- **Lactic acidosis** (buildup of an acid in the blood). Lactic acidosis can be a medical emergency and may need to be treated in the hospital. **Call your healthcare provider right away if you get signs of lactic acidosis.** (See "What is the most important information I should know about ATRIPLA?")
- **Serious liver problems (hepatotoxicity)**, with liver enlargement (hepatomegaly) and fat in the liver (steatosis). Call your healthcare provider right away if you get any signs of liver problems. (See "What is the most important information I should know about ATRIPLA?")
- **"Flare-ups" of hepatitis B virus (HBV) infection**, in which the disease suddenly returns in a worse way than before, can occur if you have HBV and you stop taking ATRIPLA. Your healthcare provider will monitor your condition for several months after stopping ATRIPLA if you have both HIV-1 and HBV infection and may recommend treatment for your HBV. ATRIPLA is not approved for the treatment of hepatitis B virus infection. If you have advanced liver disease and stop treatment with ATRIPLA, the "flare-up" of hepatitis B may cause your liver function to decline.
- **Serious psychiatric problems.** A small number of patients may experience severe depression, strange thoughts, or angry behavior while taking ATRIPLA. Some patients have thoughts of suicide and a few have actually committed suicide. These problems may occur more often in patients who have had mental illness. Contact your healthcare provider right away if you think you are having these psychiatric symptoms, so your healthcare provider can decide if you should continue to take ATRIPLA.
- **Kidney problems** (including decline or failure of kidney function). If you have had kidney problems in the past or take other medicines that can cause kidney problems, your healthcare provider should do regular blood tests to check your kidneys. Symptoms that may be related to kidney problems include a high volume of urine, thirst, muscle pain, and muscle weakness.
- **Other serious liver problems.** Some patients have experienced serious liver problems including liver failure resulting in transplantation or death. Most of these serious side effects occurred in patients with a chronic liver disease such as hepatitis infection, but there have also been a few reports in patients without any existing liver disease.
- **Changes in bone mineral density (thinning bones).** Laboratory tests show changes in the bones of patients treated with tenofovir DF, a component of ATRIPLA. Some HIV patients treated with tenofovir DF developed thinning of the bones (osteopenia) which could lead to fractures. If you have had bone problems in the past, your healthcare provider may need to do tests to check your bone mineral density or may prescribe medicines to help your bone mineral density. Additionally, bone pain and softening of the bone (which may contribute to fractures) may occur as a consequence of kidney problems.

Common side effects:

Patients may have dizziness, headache, trouble sleeping, drowsiness, trouble concentrating, and/or unusual dreams during treatment with ATRIPLA (efavirenz/emtricitabine/tenofovir disoproxil fumarate). These side effects may be reduced if you take ATRIPLA at bedtime on an empty stomach. They also tend to go away after you have taken the medicine for a few weeks. If you have these common side effects, such as dizziness, it does not mean that you will also have serious psychiatric problems, such as severe depression, strange thoughts, or angry behavior. Tell your healthcare provider right away if any of these side effects continue or if they bother you. It is possible that these symptoms may be more severe if ATRIPLA is used with alcohol or mood altering (street) drugs.

If you are dizzy, have trouble concentrating, or are drowsy, avoid activities that may be dangerous, such as driving or operating machinery.

Rash may be common. Rashes usually go away without any change in treatment. In a small number of patients, rash may be serious. If you develop a rash, call your healthcare provider right away.

Other common side effects include tiredness, upset stomach, vomiting, gas, and diarrhea.

Other possible side effects with ATRIPLA:

- Changes in body fat. Changes in body fat develop in some patients taking anti-HIV-1 medicine. These changes may include an increased amount of fat in the upper back and neck ("buffalo hump"), in the breasts, and around the trunk. Loss of fat from the legs, arms, and face may also happen. The cause and long-term health effects of these fat changes are not known.
- Skin discoloration (small spots or freckles) may also happen with ATRIPLA.
- In some patients with advanced HIV infection (AIDS), signs and symptoms of inflammation from previous infections may occur soon after anti-HIV treatment is started. It is believed that these symptoms are due to an improvement in the body's immune response, enabling the body to fight infections that may have been present with no obvious symptoms. If you notice any symptoms of infection, please inform your doctor immediately.
- Additional side effects are inflammation of the pancreas, allergic reaction (including swelling of the face, lips, tongue, or throat), shortness of breath, pain, stomach pain, weakness and indigestion.

Tell your healthcare provider or pharmacist if you notice any side effects while taking ATRIPLA.

Contact your healthcare provider before stopping ATRIPLA because of side effects or for any other reason.

This is not a complete list of side effects possible with ATRIPLA. Ask your healthcare provider or pharmacist for a more complete list of side effects of ATRIPLA and all the medicines you will take.

How do I store ATRIPLA?

- **Keep ATRIPLA and all other medicines out of reach of children.**
- Store ATRIPLA at room temperature 77 °F (25 °C).
- Keep ATRIPLA in its original container and keep the container tightly closed.
- Do not keep medicine that is out of date or that you no longer need. If you throw any medicines away make sure that children will not find them.

General information about ATRIPLA:

Medicines are sometimes prescribed for conditions that are not mentioned in patient information leaflets. Do not use ATRIPLA for a condition for which it was not prescribed. Do not give ATRIPLA to other people, even if they have the same symptoms you have. It may harm them.

This leaflet summarizes the most important information about ATRIPLA. If you would like more information, talk with your healthcare provider. You can ask your healthcare provider or pharmacist for information about ATRIPLA that is written for health professionals.

Do not use ATRIPLA if the seal over bottle opening is broken or missing.

What are the ingredients of ATRIPLA?

Active Ingredients: efavirenz, emtricitabine, and tenofovir disoproxil fumarate

Inactive Ingredients: croscarmellose sodium, hydroxypropyl cellulose, microcrystalline cellulose, magnesium stearate, sodium lauryl sulfate. The film coating contains black iron oxide, polyethylene glycol, polyvinyl alcohol, red iron oxide, talc, and titanium dioxide.

℞ Only

May 2010

ATRIPLA is a trademark of Bristol-Myers Squibb & Gilead Sciences, LLC. EMTRIVA, TRUVADA, HEPSERA and VIREAD are trademarks of Gilead Sciences, Inc. SUSTIVA is a trademark of Bristol-Myers Squibb Pharma Company. Reyataz and Videx are trademarks of Bristol-Myers Squibb Company. Pravachol is a trademark of ER Squibb & Sons, LLC. Other brands listed are the trademarks of their respective owners.

SF-B0001-05-10   21-927-GS-007
ST5650   May 2010

Shown in Product Identification Guide, page 321

BARACLUDE® ℞

[BEAR ah klude]
(entecavir)
Tablets

BARACLUDE®

(entecavir)
Oral Solution

HIGHLIGHTS OF PRESCRIBING INFORMATION

These highlights do not include all the information needed to use BARACLUDE safely and effectively. See full prescribing information for BARACLUDE.

BARACLUDE® (entecavir) Tablets
BARACLUDE® (entecavir) Oral Solution
Initial U.S. Approval: 2005

WARNINGS: SEVERE ACUTE EXACERBATIONS OF HEPATITIS B, PATIENTS CO-INFECTED WITH HIV AND HBV, and LACTIC ACIDOSIS AND HEPATOMEGALY

See full prescribing information for complete boxed warning.

- **Severe acute exacerbations of hepatitis B have been reported in patients who have discontinued anti-hepatitis B therapy, including entecavir. Hepatic function should be monitored closely for at least several months after discontinuation. Initiation of anti-hepatitis B therapy may be warranted. (5.1)**
- **BARACLUDE is not recommended for patients co-infected with human immunodeficiency virus (HIV) and hepatitis B virus (HBV) who are not also receiving highly active antiretroviral therapy (HAART), because of the potential for the development of resistance to HIV nucleoside reverse transcriptase inhibitors. (5.2)**
- **Lactic acidosis and severe hepatomegaly with steatosis, including fatal cases, have been reported with the use of nucleoside analogues. (5.3)**

INDICATIONS AND USAGE

BARACLUDE (entecavir) is a nucleoside analogue indicated for the treatment of chronic hepatitis B virus infection in adults with evidence of active viral replication and either evidence of persistent elevations in serum aminotransferases (ALT or AST) or histologically active disease. (1)

DOSAGE AND ADMINISTRATION

- Nucleoside-treatment-naïve (≥16 years old): 0.5 mg once daily. (2.1)
- Lamivudine-refractory or known lamivudine or telbivudine resistance mutations (≥16 years old): 1 mg once daily. (2.1)
- Renal impairment: Dosage adjustment is recommended if creatinine clearance is less than 50 mL/min. (2.2)
- BARACLUDE (entecavir) should be administered on an empty stomach. (2)

DOSAGE FORMS AND STRENGTHS

- Tablets: 0.5 mg and 1 mg (3, 16)
- Oral solution: 0.05 mg/mL (3, 16)

CONTRAINDICATIONS

- None. (4)

WARNINGS AND PRECAUTIONS

- Severe acute exacerbations of hepatitis B virus infection after discontinuation: Monitor hepatic function closely for at least several months. (5.1, 6.1)
- Co-infection with HIV: BARACLUDE is not recommended unless the patient is also receiving HAART. (5.2)
- Lactic acidosis and severe hepatomegaly with steatosis: If suspected, treatment should be suspended. (5.3)

ADVERSE REACTIONS

- Most common adverse reactions (≥3%, all severity grades) are headache, fatigue, dizziness, and nausea. (6.1)

To report SUSPECTED ADVERSE REACTIONS, contact Bristol-Myers Squibb at 1-800-721-5072 or FDA at 1-800-FDA-1088 or www.fda.gov/medwatch

USE IN SPECIFIC POPULATIONS

- Pregnancy: Pregnancy registry available. Enroll patients by calling 1-800-258-4263. (8.1)
- Nursing mothers: Discontinue nursing or BARACLUDE taking into consideration the importance of BARACLUDE to the mother. (8.3)

See 17 for PATIENT COUNSELING INFORMATION and FDA-approved patient labeling

Revised: 07/2009

FULL PRESCRIBING INFORMATION: CONTENTS*
WARNINGS: SEVERE ACUTE EXACERBATIONS OF HEPATITIS B, PATIENTS CO-INFECTED WITH HIV AND HBV, and LACTIC ACIDOSIS AND HEPATOMEGALY

FULL PRESCRIBING INFORMATION

WARNINGS: SEVERE ACUTE EXACERBATIONS OF HEPATITIS B, PATIENTS CO-INFECTED WITH HIV AND HBV, and LACTIC ACIDOSIS AND HEPATOMEGALY
Severe acute exacerbations of hepatitis B have been reported in patients who have discontinued anti-hepatitis B therapy, including entecavir. Hepatic function should be monitored closely with both clinical and laboratory follow-up for at least several months in patients who discontinue anti-hepatitis B therapy. If appropriate, initiation of anti-hepatitis B therapy may be warranted [see *Warnings and Precautions (5.1)*].
Limited clinical experience suggests there is a potential for the development of resistance to HIV (human immunodeficiency virus) nucleoside reverse transcriptase inhibitors if BARACLUDE (entecavir) is used to treat chronic hepatitis B virus (HBV) infection in patients with HIV infection that is not being treated. Therapy with BARACLUDE is not recommended for HIV/HBV co-infected patients who are not also receiving highly active antiretroviral therapy (HAART) [see *Warnings and Precautions (5.2)*].
Lactic acidosis and severe hepatomegaly with steatosis, including fatal cases, have been reported with the use of nucleoside analogues alone or in combination with antiretrovirals [see *Warnings and Precautions (5.3)*].

1 INDICATIONS AND USAGE
BARACLUDE® (entecavir) is indicated for the treatment of chronic hepatitis B virus infection in adults with evidence of active viral replication and either evidence of persistent elevations in serum aminotransferases (ALT or AST) or histologically active disease.
The following points should be considered when initiating therapy with BARACLUDE:
• This indication is based on histologic, virologic, biochemical, and serologic responses in nucleoside-treatment-naïve and lamivudine-resistant adult subjects with HBeAg-positive or HBeAg-negative chronic HBV infection with compensated liver disease [see *Clinical Studies (14)*].
• Limited data are available in adult subjects with HIV/HBV co-infection who have received prior lamivudine therapy [see *Warnings and Precautions (5.2)* and *Clinical Studies (14)*].
• BARACLUDE has not been evaluated in patients with decompensated liver disease.

2 DOSAGE AND ADMINISTRATION
BARACLUDE should be administered on an empty stomach (at least 2 hours after a meal and 2 hours before the next meal).

2.1 Recommended Dosage
The recommended dose of BARACLUDE for chronic hepatitis B virus infection in nucleoside-treatment-naïve adults and adolescents 16 years of age and older is 0.5 mg once daily.
The recommended dose of BARACLUDE in adults and adolescents (at least 16 years of age) with a history of hepatitis B viremia while receiving lamivudine or known lamivudine or telbivudine resistance mutations rtM204I/V with or without rtL180M, rtL80I/V, or rtV173L is 1 mg once daily. BARACLUDE (entecavir) Oral Solution contains 0.05 mg of entecavir per milliliter. Therefore, 10 mL of the oral solution provides a 0.5-mg dose and 20 mL provides a 1-mg dose of entecavir.

2.2 Renal Impairment
In subjects with renal impairment, the apparent oral clearance of entecavir decreased as creatinine clearance decreased [see *Clinical Pharmacology (12.3)*]. Dosage adjustment is recommended for patients with creatinine clearance less than 50 mL/min, including patients on hemodialysis or continuous ambulatory peritoneal dialysis (CAPD), as shown in Table 1. The once-daily dosing regimens are preferred.

Table 1: Recommended Dosage of BARACLUDE in Patients with Renal Impairment

Creatinine Clearance (mL/min)	Usual Dose (0.5 mg)	Lamivudine-Refractory (1 mg)
≥50	0.5 mg once daily	1 mg once daily
30 to <50	0.25 mg once daily[a] **OR** 0.5 mg every 48 hours	0.5 mg once daily **OR** 1 mg every 48 hours
10 to <30	0.15 mg once daily[a] **OR** 0.5 mg every 72 hours	0.3 mg once daily[a] **OR** 1 mg every 72 hours
<10 Hemodialysis[b] or CAPD	0.05 mg once daily[a] **OR** 0.5 mg every 7 days	0.1 mg once daily[a] **OR** 1 mg every 7 days

[a] For doses less than 0.5 mg, BARACLUDE Oral Solution is recommended.
[b] If administered on a hemodialysis day, administer BARACLUDE after the hemodialysis session.

2.3 Hepatic Impairment
No dosage adjustment is necessary for patients with hepatic impairment.

2.4 Duration of Therapy
The optimal duration of treatment with BARACLUDE (entecavir) for patients with chronic hepatitis B virus infection and the relationship between treatment and long-term outcomes such as cirrhosis and hepatocellular carcinoma are unknown.

3 DOSAGE FORMS AND STRENGTHS
• BARACLUDE 0.5-mg film-coated tablets are white to off-white, triangular-shaped and debossed with "BMS" on one side and "1611" on the other side.
• BARACLUDE 1-mg film-coated tablets are pink, triangular-shaped and debossed with "BMS" on one side and "1612" on the other side.
• BARACLUDE oral solution, 0.05-mg/mL, is a ready-to-use, orange-flavored, clear, colorless to pale yellow aqueous solution.

4 CONTRAINDICATIONS
None.

5 WARNINGS AND PRECAUTIONS
5.1 Severe Acute Exacerbations of Hepatitis B
Severe acute exacerbations of hepatitis B have been reported in patients who have discontinued anti-hepatitis B therapy, including entecavir [see *Adverse Reactions (6.1)*]. Hepatic function should be monitored closely with both clinical and laboratory follow-up for at least several months in patients who discontinue anti-hepatitis B therapy. If appropriate, initiation of anti-hepatitis B therapy may be warranted.

5.2 Patients Co-infected with HIV and HBV
BARACLUDE (entecavir) has not been evaluated in HIV/HBV co-infected patients who were not simultaneously receiving effective HIV treatment. Limited clinical experience suggests there is a potential for the development of resistance to HIV nucleoside reverse transcriptase inhibitors if BARACLUDE is used to treat chronic hepatitis B virus infection in patients with HIV infection that is not being treated [see *Clinical Pharmacology (12.4)*]. Therefore, therapy with BARACLUDE is not recommended for HIV/HBV co-infected patients who are not also receiving HAART. Before initiating BARACLUDE therapy, HIV antibody testing should be offered to all patients. BARACLUDE has not been studied as a treatment for HIV infection and is not recommended for this use.

5.3 Lactic Acidosis and Severe Hepatomegaly with Steatosis
Lactic acidosis and severe hepatomegaly with steatosis, including fatal cases, have been reported with the use of nucleoside analogues alone or in combination with antiretrovirals.
A majority of these cases have been in women. Obesity and prolonged nucleoside exposure may be risk factors. Particular caution should be exercised when administering nucleoside analogues to any patient with known risk factors for liver disease; however, cases have also been reported in patients with no known risk factors. Treatment with BARACLUDE should be suspended in any patient who develops clinical or laboratory findings suggestive of lactic acidosis or pronounced hepatotoxicity (which may include hepatomegaly and steatosis even in the absence of marked transaminase elevations).

6 ADVERSE REACTIONS
The following adverse reactions are discussed in other sections of the labeling:
• Exacerbations of hepatitis after discontinuation of treatment [see *Boxed Warning, Warnings and Precautions (5.1)*].
• Lactic acidosis and severe hepatomegaly with steatosis [see *Boxed Warning, Warnings and Precautions (5.3)*].

6.1 Clinical Trial Experience
Because clinical trials are conducted under widely varying conditions, adverse reaction rates observed in the clinical trials of a drug cannot be directly compared to rates in the clinical trials of another drug and may not reflect the rates observed in practice.
Assessment of adverse reactions is based on four studies (AI463014, AI463022, AI463026, and AI463027) in which 1720 subjects with chronic hepatitis B virus infection received double-blind treatment with BARACLUDE 0.5 mg/day (n=679), BARACLUDE 1 mg/day (n=183), or lamivudine (n=858) for up to 2 years. Median duration of therapy was 69 weeks for BARACLUDE-treated subjects and 63 weeks for lamivudine-treated subjects in Studies AI463022 and AI463027 and 73 weeks for BARACLUDE-treated subjects and 51 weeks for lamivudine-treated subjects in Studies AI463026 and AI463014. The safety profiles of BARACLUDE and lamivudine were comparable in these studies. The safety profile of BARACLUDE 1 mg (n=51) in HIV/HBV co-infected subjects enrolled in Study AI463038 was similar to that of placebo (n=17) through 24 weeks of blinded treatment and similar to that seen in non-HIV infected subjects [see *Warnings and Precautions (5.2)*].
The most common adverse reactions of any severity (≥3%) with at least a possible relation to study drug for BARACLUDE-treated subjects were headache, fatigue, dizziness, and nausea. The most common adverse reactions among lamivudine-treated subjects were headache, fatigue, and dizziness. One percent of BARACLUDE-treated subjects in these four studies compared with 4% of lamivudine-treated subjects discontinued for adverse events or abnormal laboratory test results.
Clinical adverse reactions of moderate-severe intensity and considered at least possibly related to treatment occurring during therapy in four clinical studies in which BARACLUDE was compared with lamivudine are presented in Table 2.
[See table 2 at top of next page]
Laboratory Abnormalities
Frequencies of selected treatment-emergent laboratory abnormalities reported during therapy in four clinical trials of BARACLUDE compared with lamivudine are listed in Table 3.
[See table 3 on next page]
Among BARACLUDE-treated subjects in these studies, on-treatment ALT elevations greater than 10 times the upper limit of normal (ULN) and greater than 2 times baseline generally resolved with continued treatment. A majority of these exacerbations were associated with a ≥2 $\log_{10}$/mL

reduction in viral load that preceded or coincided with the ALT elevation. Periodic monitoring of hepatic function is recommended during treatment.

Exacerbations of Hepatitis after Discontinuation of Treatment [see also *Warnings and Precautions (5.1)*]

An exacerbation of hepatitis or ALT flare was defined as ALT greater than 10 times ULN and greater than 2 times the subject's reference level (minimum of the baseline or last measurement at end of dosing). For all subjects who discontinued treatment (regardless of reason), Table 4 presents the proportions of subjects in each study who experienced post-treatment ALT flares. In these studies, a subset of subjects was allowed to discontinue treatment at or after 52 weeks if they achieved a protocol-defined response to therapy. If BARACLUDE (entecavir) is discontinued without regard to treatment response, the rate of post-treatment flares could be higher.

Table 4: Exacerbations of Hepatitis During Off-Treatment Follow-up, Subjects in Studies AI463022, AI463027, and AI463026

	Subjects with ALT Elevations >10 × ULN and >2 × Reference[a]	
	BARACLUDE	Lamivudine
Nucleoside-naïve		
HBeAg-positive	4/174 (2%)	13/147 (9%)
HBeAg-negative	24/302 (8%)	30/270 (11%)
Lamivudine-refractory	6/52 (12%)	0/16

[a] Reference is the minimum of the baseline or last measurement at end of dosing. Median time to off-treatment exacerbation was 23 weeks for BARACLUDE-treated subjects and 10 weeks for lamivudine-treated subjects.

6.2 Postmarketing Experience

The following adverse reactions have been reported during postmarketing use of BARACLUDE. Because these reactions were reported voluntarily from a population of unknown size, it is not possible to reliably estimate their frequency or establish a causal relationship to BARACLUDE exposure.

Immune system disorders: Anaphylactoid reaction.
Skin and subcutaneous tissue disorders: Alopecia, rash.

7 DRUG INTERACTIONS

Since entecavir is primarily eliminated by the kidneys [see *Clinical Pharmacology (12.3)*], coadministration of BARACLUDE with drugs that reduce renal function or compete for active tubular secretion may increase serum concentrations of either entecavir or the coadministered drug. Coadministration of entecavir with lamivudine, adefovir dipivoxil, or tenofovir disoproxil fumarate did not result in significant drug interactions. The effects of coadministration of BARACLUDE with other drugs that are renally eliminated or are known to affect renal function have not been evaluated, and patients should be monitored closely for adverse events when BARACLUDE is coadministered with such drugs.

8 USE IN SPECIFIC POPULATIONS

8.1 Pregnancy

Pregnancy Category C.

There are no adequate and well-controlled studies of BARACLUDE in pregnant women. When pregnant rats and rabbits received entecavir at 28 and 212 times the human exposure at the highest human dose, there were no signs of embryofetal toxicity. Because animal reproduction studies are not always predictive of human response, BARACLUDE should be used during pregnancy only if clearly needed and after careful consideration of the risks and benefits.

Pregnancy Registry: To monitor fetal outcomes of pregnant women exposed to entecavir, a pregnancy registry has been established. Healthcare providers are encouraged to register patients by calling 1-800-258-4263.

Developmental toxicity studies were performed in rats and rabbits. There were no signs of embryofetal or maternal toxicity when pregnant animals received oral entecavir at approximately 28 (rat) and 212 (rabbit) times the human exposure achieved at the highest recommended human dose of 1 mg/day. In rats, maternal toxicity, embryofetal toxicity (resorptions), lower fetal body weights, tail and vertebral malformations, reduced ossification (vertebrae, sternebrae, and phalanges), and extra lumbar vertebrae and ribs were observed at exposures 3100 times those in humans. In rabbits, embryofetal toxicity (resorptions), reduced ossification (hyoid), and an increased incidence of 13th rib were observed at exposures 883 times those in humans. In a peripostnatal study, no adverse effects on offspring occurred when rats received oral entecavir at exposures greater than 94 times those in humans.

Table 2: Clinical Adverse Reactions[a] of Moderate-Severe Intensity (Grades 2-4) Reported in Four Entecavir Clinical Trials Through 2 Years

Body System/ Adverse Reaction	Nucleoside-Naïve[b]		Lamivudine-Refractory[c]	
	BARACLUDE 0.5 mg n=679	Lamivudine 100 mg n=668	BARACLUDE 1 mg n=183	Lamivudine 100 mg n=190
Any Grade 2-4 adverse reaction[a]	15%	18%	22%	23%
Gastrointestinal				
Diarrhea	<1%	0	1%	0
Dyspepsia	<1%	<1%	1%	0
Nausea	<1%	<1%	<1%	2%
Vomiting	<1%	<1%	<1%	0
General				
Fatigue	1%	1%	3%	3%
Nervous System				
Headache	2%	2%	4%	1%
Dizziness	<1%	<1%	0	1%
Somnolence	<1%	<1%	0	0
Psychiatric				
Insomnia	<1%	<1%	0	<1%

[a] Includes events of possible, probable, certain, or unknown relationship to treatment regimen.
[b] Studies AI463022 and AI463027.
[c] Includes Study AI463026 and the BARACLUDE 1-mg and lamivudine treatment arms of Study AI463014, a Phase 2 multinational, randomized, double-blind study of three doses of BARACLUDE (0.1, 0.5, and 1 mg) once daily versus continued lamivudine 100 mg once daily for up to 52 weeks in subjects who experienced recurrent viremia on lamivudine therapy.

Table 3: Selected Treatment-Emergent[a] Laboratory Abnormalities Reported in Four Entecavir Clinical Trials Through 2 Years

Test	Nucleoside-Naïve[b]		Lamivudine-Refractory[c]	
	BARACLUDE 0.5 mg n=679	Lamivudine 100 mg n=668	BARACLUDE 1 mg n=183	Lamivudine 100 mg n=190
Any Grade 3-4 laboratory abnormality[d]	35%	36%	37%	45%
ALT >10 × ULN and >2 × baseline	2%	4%	2%	11%
ALT >5.0 × ULN	11%	16%	12%	24%
Albumin <2.5 g/dL	<1%	<1%	0	2%
Total bilirubin >2.5 × ULN	2%	2%	3%	2%
Lipase ≥2.1 × ULN	7%	6%	7%	7%
Creatinine >3.0 × ULN	0	0	0	0
Confirmed creatinine increase ≥0.5 mg/dL	1%	1%	2%	1%
Hyperglycemia, fasting >250 mg/dL	2%	1%	3%	1%
Glycosuria[e]	4%	3%	4%	6%
Hematuria[f]	9%	10%	9%	6%
Platelets <50,000/mm³	<1%	<1%	<1%	<1%

[a] On-treatment value worsened from baseline to Grade 3 or Grade 4 for all parameters except albumin (any on-treatment value <2.5 g/dL), confirmed creatinine increase ≥0.5 mg/dL, and ALT >10 × ULN and >2 × baseline.
[b] Studies AI463022 and AI463027.
[c] Includes Study AI463026 and the BARACLUDE 1-mg and lamivudine treatment arms of Study AI463014, a Phase 2 multinational, randomized, double-blind study of three doses of BARACLUDE (0.1, 0.5, and 1 mg) once daily versus continued lamivudine 100 mg once daily for up to 52 weeks in subjects who experienced recurrent viremia on lamivudine therapy.
[d] Includes hematology, routine chemistries, renal and liver function tests, pancreatic enzymes, and urinalysis.
[e] Grade 3 = 3+, large, ≥ 500 mg/dL; Grade 4 = 4+, marked, severe.
[f] Grade 3 = 3+, large; Grade 4 = ≥ 4+, marked, severe, many.
ULN = upper limit of normal

8.2 Labor and Delivery

There are no studies in pregnant women and no data on the effect of BARACLUDE (entecavir) on transmission of HBV from mother to infant. Therefore, appropriate interventions should be used to prevent neonatal acquisition of HBV.

8.3 Nursing Mothers

It is not known whether BARACLUDE is excreted into human milk; however, entecavir is excreted into the milk of rats. Because many drugs are excreted into human milk and because of the potential for serious adverse reactions in nursing infants from BARACLUDE, a decision should be made to discontinue nursing or to discontinue BARACLUDE taking into consideration the importance of continued hepatitis B therapy to the mother and the known benefits of breastfeeding.

8.4 Pediatric Use

Safety and effectiveness of entecavir in pediatric patients below the age of 16 years have not been established.

8.5 Geriatric Use

Clinical studies of BARACLUDE did not include sufficient numbers of subjects aged 65 years and over to determine whether they respond differently from younger subjects. Entecavir is substantially excreted by the kidney, and the risk of toxic reactions to this drug may be greater in patients with impaired renal function. Because elderly patients are more likely to have decreased renal function,

care should be taken in dose selection, and it may be useful to monitor renal function [see *Dosage and Administration (2.2)*].

8.6 Use in Racial/Ethnic Groups

Clinical studies of BARACLUDE (entecavir) did not include sufficient numbers of subjects from some racial/ethnic minorities (black/African American, Hispanic) to determine whether they respond differently to treatment with the drug. There are no significant racial differences in entecavir pharmacokinetics.

8.7 Renal Impairment

Dosage adjustment of BARACLUDE is recommended for patients with creatinine clearance less than 50 mL/min, including patients on hemodialysis or CAPD [see *Dosage and Administration (2.2)* and *Clinical Pharmacology (12.3)*].

Liver transplant recipients: The safety and efficacy of BARACLUDE in liver transplant recipients are unknown. If BARACLUDE treatment is determined to be necessary for a liver transplant recipient who has received or is receiving an immunosuppressant that may affect renal function, such as cyclosporine or tacrolimus, renal function must be carefully monitored both before and during treatment with BARACLUDE [see *Dosage and Administration (2.2)* and *Clinical Pharmacology (12.3)*].

10 OVERDOSAGE

There is limited experience of entecavir overdosage reported in patients. Healthy subjects who received single entecavir

doses up to 40 mg or multiple doses up to 20 mg/day for up to 14 days had no increase in or unexpected adverse events. If overdose occurs, the patient must be monitored for evidence of toxicity, and standard supportive treatment applied as necessary.
Following a single 1-mg dose of entecavir, a 4-hour hemodialysis session removed approximately 13% of the entecavir dose.

11 DESCRIPTION

BARACLUDE® (entecavir) is the tradename for entecavir, a guanosine nucleoside analogue with selective activity against HBV. The chemical name for entecavir is 2-amino-1,9-dihydro-9-[(*1S,3R,4S*)-4-hydroxy-3-(hydroxymethyl)-2-methylenecyclopentyl]-6*H*-purin-6-one, monohydrate. Its molecular formula is $C_{12}H_{15}N_5O_3 \cdot H_2O$, which corresponds to a molecular weight of 295.3. Entecavir has the following structural formula:

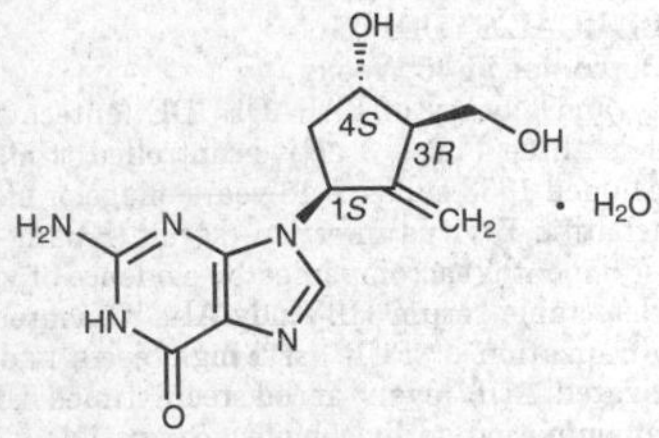

Entecavir is a white to off-white powder. It is slightly soluble in water (2.4 mg/mL), and the pH of the saturated solution in water is 7.9 at 25° ± 0.5° C.
BARACLUDE film-coated tablets are available for oral administration in strengths of 0.5 mg and 1 mg of entecavir. BARACLUDE 0.5-mg and 1-mg film-coated tablets contain the following inactive ingredients: lactose monohydrate, microcrystalline cellulose, crospovidone, povidone, and magnesium stearate. The tablet coating contains titanium dioxide, hypromellose, polyethylene glycol 400, polysorbate 80 (0.5-mg tablet only), and iron oxide red (1-mg tablet only). BARACLUDE Oral Solution is available for oral administration as a ready-to-use solution containing 0.05 mg of entecavir per milliliter. BARACLUDE Oral Solution contains the following inactive ingredients: maltitol, sodium citrate, citric acid, methylparaben, propylparaben, and orange flavor.

12 CLINICAL PHARMACOLOGY

12.1 Mechanism of Action

Entecavir is an antiviral drug [see *Clinical Pharmacology (12.4)*].

12.3 Pharmacokinetics

The single- and multiple-dose pharmacokinetics of entecavir were evaluated in healthy subjects and subjects with chronic hepatitis B virus infection.

Absorption

Following oral administration in healthy subjects, entecavir peak plasma concentrations occurred between 0.5 and 1.5 hours. Following multiple daily doses ranging from 0.1 to 1.0 mg, C_{max} and area under the concentration-time curve (AUC) at steady state increased in proportion to dose. Steady state was achieved after 6 to 10 days of once-daily administration with approximately 2-fold accumulation. For a 0.5-mg oral dose, C_{max} at steady state was 4.2 ng/mL and trough plasma concentration (C_{trough}) was 0.3 ng/mL. For a 1-mg oral dose, C_{max} was 8.2 ng/mL and C_{trough} was 0.5 ng/mL.
In healthy subjects, the bioavailability of the tablet was 100% relative to the oral solution. The oral solution and tablet may be used interchangeably.
Effects of food on oral absorption: Oral administration of 0.5 mg of entecavir with a standard high-fat meal (945 kcal, 54.6 g fat) or a light meal (379 kcal, 8.2 g fat) resulted in a delay in absorption (1.0-1.5 hours fed vs. 0.75 hours fasted), a decrease in C_{max} of 44%-46%, and a decrease in AUC of 18%-20% [see *Dosage and Administration (2)*].

Distribution

Based on the pharmacokinetic profile of entecavir after oral dosing, the estimated apparent volume of distribution is in excess of total body water, suggesting that entecavir is extensively distributed into tissues.
Binding of entecavir to human serum proteins *in vitro* was approximately 13%.

Metabolism and Elimination

Following administration of ^{14}C-entecavir in humans and rats, no oxidative or acetylated metabolites were observed. Minor amounts of phase II metabolites (glucuronide and sulfate conjugates) were observed. Entecavir is not a substrate, inhibitor, or inducer of the cytochrome P450 (CYP450) enzyme system [see *Drug Interactions*, below].
After reaching peak concentration, entecavir plasma concentrations decreased in a bi-exponential manner with a terminal elimination half-life of approximately 128-149 hours. The observed drug accumulation index is approximately 2-fold with once-daily dosing, suggesting an effective accumulation half-life of approximately 24 hours.
Entecavir is predominantly eliminated by the kidney with urinary recovery of unchanged drug at steady state ranging from 62% to 73% of the administered dose. Renal clearance is independent of dose and ranges from 360 to 471 mL/min suggesting that entecavir undergoes both glomerular filtration and net tubular secretion [see *Drug Interactions (7)*].

Special Populations

Gender: There are no significant gender differences in entecavir pharmacokinetics.
Race: There are no significant racial differences in entecavir pharmacokinetics.
Elderly: The effect of age on the pharmacokinetics of entecavir was evaluated following administration of a single 1-mg oral dose in healthy young and elderly volunteers. Entecavir AUC was 29.3% greater in elderly subjects compared to young subjects. The disparity in exposure between elderly and young subjects was most likely attributable to differences in renal function. Dosage adjustment of BARACLUDE (entecavir) should be based on the renal function of the patient, rather than age [see *Dosage and Administration (2.2)*].
Pediatrics: Pharmacokinetic studies have not been conducted in children.
Renal impairment: The pharmacokinetics of entecavir following a single 1-mg dose were studied in subjects (without chronic hepatitis B virus infection) with selected degrees of renal impairment, including subjects whose renal impairment was managed by hemodialysis or continuous ambulatory peritoneal dialysis (CAPD). Results are shown in Table 5 [see *Dosage and Administration (2.2)*].
[See table 5 above]

Table 5: Pharmacokinetic Parameters in Subjects with Selected Degrees of Renal Function

	Renal Function Group					
	Baseline Creatinine Clearance (mL/min)					
	Unimpaired >80 n=6	Mild >50-≤80 n=6	Moderate 30-50 n=6	Severe <30 n=6	Severe Managed with Hemodialysis[a] n=6	Severe Managed with CAPD n=4
C_{max} (ng/mL)	8.1	10.4	10.5	15.3	15.4	16.6
(CV%)	(30.7)	(37.2)	(22.7)	(33.8)	(56.4)	(29.7)
$AUC_{(0-T)}$ (ng•h/mL)	27.9	51.5	69.5	145.7	233.9	221.8
(CV)	(25.6)	(22.8)	(22.7)	(31.5)	(28.4)	(11.6)
CLR (mL/min)	383.2	197.9	135.6	40.3	NA	NA
(SD)	(101.8)	(78.1)	(31.6)	(10.1)		
CLT/F (mL/min)	588.1	309.2	226.3	100.6	50.6	35.7
(SD)	(153.7)	(62.6)	(60.1)	(29.1)	(16.5)	(19.6)

[a] Dosed immediately following hemodialysis.
CLR = renal clearance; CLT/F = apparent oral clearance.

Following a single 1-mg dose of entecavir administered 2 hours before the hemodialysis session, hemodialysis removed approximately 13% of the entecavir dose over 4 hours. CAPD removed approximately 0.3% of the dose over 7 days [see *Dosage and Administration (2.2)*].
Hepatic impairment: The pharmacokinetics of entecavir following a single 1-mg dose were studied in subjects (without chronic hepatitis B virus infection) with moderate or severe hepatic impairment (Child-Pugh Class B or C). The pharmacokinetics of entecavir were similar between hepatically impaired and healthy control subjects; therefore, no dosage adjustment of BARACLUDE is recommended for patients with hepatic impairment.
Post-liver transplant: The safety and efficacy of BARACLUDE in liver transplant recipients are unknown. However, in a small pilot study of entecavir use in HBV-infected liver transplant recipients on a stable dose of cyclosporine A (n=5) or tacrolimus (n=4), entecavir exposure was approximately 2-fold the exposure in healthy subjects with normal renal function. Altered renal function contributed to the increase in entecavir exposure in these subjects. The potential for pharmacokinetic interactions between entecavir and cyclosporine A or tacrolimus was not formally evaluated [see *Use in Specific Populations (8.7)*].

Drug Interactions

The metabolism of entecavir was evaluated in *in vitro* and *in vivo* studies. Entecavir is not a substrate, inhibitor, or inducer of the cytochrome P450 (CYP450) enzyme system. At concentrations up to approximately 10,000-fold higher than those obtained in humans, entecavir inhibited none of the major human CYP450 enzymes 1A2, 2C9, 2C19, 2D6, 3A4, 2B6, and 2E1. At concentrations up to approximately 340-fold higher than those observed in humans, entecavir did not induce the human CYP450 enzymes 1A2, 2C9, 2C19, 3A4, 3A5, and 2B6. The pharmacokinetics of entecavir are unlikely to be affected by coadministration with agents that are either metabolized by, inhibit, or induce the CYP450 system. Likewise, the pharmacokinetics of known CYP substrates are unlikely to be affected by coadministration of entecavir.
The steady-state pharmacokinetics of entecavir and coadministered drug were not altered in interaction studies of entecavir with lamivudine, adefovir dipivoxil, and tenofovir disoproxil fumarate [see *Drug Interactions (7)*].

12.4 Microbiology

Mechanism of Action

Entecavir, a guanosine nucleoside analogue with activity against HBV polymerase, is efficiently phosphorylated to the active triphosphate form, which has an intracellular half-life of 15 hours. By competing with the natural substrate deoxyguanosine triphosphate, entecavir triphosphate functionally inhibits all three activities of the HBV polymerase (reverse transcriptase, rt): (1) base priming, (2) reverse transcription of the negative strand from the pregenomic messenger RNA, and (3) synthesis of the positive strand of HBV DNA. Entecavir triphosphate is a weak inhibitor of cellular DNA polymerases α, β, and δ and mitochondrial DNA polymerase γ with K_i values ranging from 18 to >160 μM.

Antiviral Activity

Entecavir inhibited HBV DNA synthesis (50% reduction, EC_{50}) at a concentration of 0.004 μM in human HepG2 cells transfected with wild-type HBV. The median EC_{50} value for entecavir against lamivudine-resistant HBV (rtL180M, rtM204V) was 0.026 μM (range 0.010-0.059 μM).
The coadministration of HIV nucleoside/nucleotide reverse transcriptase inhibitors (NRTIs) with BARACLUDE (entecavir) is unlikely to reduce the antiviral efficacy of BARACLUDE against HBV or of any of these agents against HIV. In HBV combination assays in cell culture, abacavir, didanosine, lamivudine, stavudine, tenofovir, or zidovudine were not antagonistic to the anti-HBV activity of entecavir over a wide range of concentrations. In HIV antiviral assays, entecavir was not antagonistic to the cell culture anti-HIV activity of these six NRTIs or emtricitabine at concentrations greater than 100 times the C_{max} of entecavir using the 1-mg dose.

Antiviral Activity against HIV

A comprehensive analysis of the inhibitory activity of entecavir against a panel of laboratory and clinical HIV type 1 (HIV-1) isolates using a variety of cells and assay conditions yielded EC_{50} values ranging from 0.026 to >10 μM; the lower EC_{50} values were observed when decreased levels of virus were used in the assay. In cell culture, entecavir selected for an M184I substitution in HIV reverse transcriptase at micromolar concentrations, confirming inhibitory pressure at high entecavir concentrations. HIV variants containing the M184V substitution showed loss of susceptibility to entecavir.

Resistance

In Cell Culture

In cell-based assays, 8- to 30-fold reductions in entecavir phenotypic susceptibility were observed for lamivudine-resistant strains. Further reductions (>70-fold) in entecavir phenotypic susceptibility required the presence of amino acid substitutions rtM204I/V with or without rtL180M along with additional substitutions at residues rtT184, rtS202, or rtM250, or a combination of these substitutions with or without an rtI169 substitution in the HBV polymerase.

Clinical Studies

Nucleoside-naïve subjects: Genotypic evaluations were performed on evaluable samples (>300 copies/mL serum HBV DNA) from 562 subjects who were treated with BARACLUDE for up to 96 weeks in nucleoside-naïve studies (AI463022, AI463027, and rollover study AI463901). By Week 96, evidence of emerging amino acid substitution

Table 6: Histologic Improvement and Change in Ishak Fibrosis Score at Week 48, Nucleoside-Naïve Subjects in Studies AI463022 and AI463027

	Study AI463022 (HBeAg-Positive)		Study AI463027 (HBeAg-Negative)	
	BARACLUDE 0.5 mg n=314[a]	Lamivudine 100 mg n=314[a]	BARACLUDE 0.5 mg n=296[a]	Lamivudine 100 mg n=287[a]
Histologic Improvement (Knodell Scores)				
Improvement[b]	72%*	62%	70%*	61%
No improvement	21%	24%	19%	26%
Ishak Fibrosis Score				
Improvement[c]	39%	35%	36%	38%
No change	46%	40%	41%	34%
Worsening[c]	8%	10%	12%	15%
Missing Week 48 biopsy	7%	14%	10%	13%

[a] Subjects with evaluable baseline histology (baseline Knodell Necroinflammatory Score ≥2).
[b] ≥2-point decrease in Knodell Necroinflammatory Score from baseline with no worsening of the Knodell Fibrosis Score.
[c] For Ishak Fibrosis Score, improvement = ≥1-point decrease from baseline and worsening = ≥1-point increase from baseline.
* p<0.05

rtS202G with rtM204V and rtL180M substitutions was detected in the HBV of 2 subjects (2/562 = <1%), and 1 of them experienced virologic rebound (≥1 $\log_{10}$ increase above nadir). In addition, emerging amino acid substitutions at rtM204I/V and rtL180M, rtL80I, or rtV173L, which conferred decreased phenotypic susceptibility to entecavir in the absence of rtT184, rtS202, or rtM250 changes, were detected in the HBV of 3 subjects (3/562 = <1%) who experienced virologic rebound. For subjects who continued treatment beyond 48 weeks, 75% (202/269) had HBV DNA <300 copies/mL at end of dosing (up to 96 weeks).

HBeAg-positive (n=243) and -negative (n=39) treatment-naïve subjects who failed to achieve the study-defined complete response by 96 weeks were offered continued entecavir treatment in a rollover study. Complete response for HBeAg-positive was <0.7 MEq/mL (approximately 7 × 10^5 copies/mL) serum HBV DNA and HBeAg loss and, for HBeAg-negative was <0.7 MEq/mL HBV DNA and ALT normalization. Subjects received 1 mg entecavir once daily for up to an additional 144 weeks. Of these 282 subjects, 141 HBeAg-positive and 8 HBeAg-negative subjects entered the long-term follow-up rollover study and were evaluated for entecavir resistance. Of the 149 subjects entering the rollover study, 88% (131/149), 92% (137/149), and 92% (137/149) attained serum HBV DNA <300 copies/mL by Weeks 144, 192, and 240 (including end of dosing), respectively. No novel entecavir resistance-associated substitutions were identified in a comparison of the genotypes of evaluable isolates with their respective baseline isolates. The cumulative probability of developing rtT184, rtS202, or rtM250 entecavir resistance-associated substitutions (in the presence of rtM204V and rtL180M substitutions) at Weeks 48, 96, 144, 192, and 240 was 0.2%, 0.5%, 1.2%, 1.2%, and 1.2%, respectively.

Lamivudine-refractory subjects: Genotypic evaluations were performed on evaluable samples from 190 subjects treated with BARACLUDE (entecavir) for up to 96 weeks in studies of lamivudine-refractory HBV (AI463026, AI463014, AI463015, and rollover study AI463901). By Week 96, resistance-associated amino acid substitutions at rtS202, rtT184, or rtM250, with or without rtI169 changes, in the presence of amino acid substitutions rtM204I/V with or without rtL180M, rtL80V, or rtV173L/M emerged in the HBV from 22 subjects (22/190 = 12%), 16 of whom experienced virologic rebound (≥1 $\log_{10}$ increase above nadir) and 4 of whom were never suppressed <300 copies/mL. The HBV from 4 of these subjects had entecavir resistance substitutions at baseline and acquired further changes on entecavir treatment. In addition to the 22 subjects, 3 subjects experienced virologic rebound with the emergence of rtM204I/V and rtL180M, rtL80V, or rtV173L/M. For isolates from subjects who experienced virologic rebound with the emergence of resistance substitutions (n=19), the median fold-change in entecavir EC_{50} values from reference was 19-fold at baseline and 106-fold at the time of virologic rebound. For subjects who continued treatment beyond 48 weeks, 40% (31/77) had HBV DNA <300 copies/mL at end of dosing (up to 96 weeks).

Lamivudine-refractory subjects (n=157) who failed to achieve the study-defined complete response by Week 96 were offered continued entecavir treatment. Subjects received 1 mg entecavir once daily for up to an additional 144 weeks. Of these subjects, 80 subjects entered the long-term follow-up study and were evaluated for entecavir resistance. By Weeks 144, 192, and 240 (including end of dosing), 34% (27/80), 35% (28/80), and 36% (29/80), respectively, attained HBV DNA <300 copies/mL. The cumulative probability of developing rtT184, rtS202, or rtM250 entecavir resistance-associated substitutions (in the presence of rtM204I/V with or without rtL180M substitutions) at Weeks 48, 96, 144, 192, and 240 was 6.2%, 15%, 36.3%, 46.6%, and 51.5%, respectively. The HBV of 6 subjects developed rtA181C/G/S/T amino acid substitutions while receiving entecavir, and of these, 4 developed entecavir resistance-associated substitutions at rtT184, rtS202, or rtM250 and 1 had an rtT184S substitution at baseline. Of 7 subjects whose HBV had an rtA181 substitution at baseline, 2 also had substitutions at rtT184, rtS202, or rtM250 at baseline and another 2 developed them while on treatment with entecavir.

Cross-resistance

Cross-resistance has been observed among HBV nucleoside analogues. In cell-based assays, entecavir had 8- to 30-fold less inhibition of HBV DNA synthesis for HBV containing lamivudine and telbivudine resistance substitutions rtM204I/V with or without rtL180M than for wild-type HBV. Substitutions rtM204I/V with or without rtL180M, rtL80I/V, or rtV173L, which are associated with lamivudine and telbivudine resistance, also confer decreased phenotypic susceptibility to entecavir. The efficacy of entecavir against HBV harboring adefovir resistance-associated substitutions has not been established in clinical trials. HBV isolates from lamivudine-refractory subjects failing entecavir therapy were susceptible in cell culture to adefovir but remained resistant to lamivudine. Recombinant HBV genomes encoding adefovir resistance-associated substitutions at either rtN236T or rtA181V had 0.3- and 1.1- fold shifts in susceptibility to entecavir in cell culture, respectively.

13 NONCLINICAL TOXICOLOGY

13.1 Carcinogenesis, Mutagenesis, Impairment of Fertility

Long-term oral carcinogenicity studies of entecavir in mice and rats were carried out at exposures up to approximately 42 times (mice) and 35 times (rats) those observed in humans at the highest recommended dose of 1 mg/day. In mouse and rat studies, entecavir was positive for carcinogenic findings.

In mice, lung adenomas were increased in males and females at exposures 3 and 40 times those in humans. Lung carcinomas in both male and female mice were increased at exposures 40 times those in humans. Combined lung adenomas and carcinomas were increased in male mice at exposures 3 times and in female mice at exposures 40 times those in humans. Tumor development was preceded by pneumocyte proliferation in the lung, which was not observed in rats, dogs, or monkeys administered entecavir, supporting the conclusion that lung tumors in mice may be a species-specific event. Hepatocellular carcinomas were increased in males and combined liver adenomas and carcinomas were also increased at exposures 42 times those in humans. Vascular tumors in female mice (hemangiomas of ovaries and uterus and hemangiosarcomas of spleen) were increased at exposures 40 times those in humans. In rats, hepatocellular adenomas were increased in females at exposures 24 times those in humans; combined adenomas and carcinomas were also increased in females at exposures 24 times those in humans. Brain gliomas were induced in both males and females at exposures 35 and 24 times those in humans. Skin fibromas were induced in females at exposures 4 times those in humans.

It is not known how predictive the results of rodent carcinogenicity studies may be for humans.

Entecavir was clastogenic to human lymphocyte cultures. Entecavir was not mutagenic in the Ames bacterial reverse mutation assay using *S. typhimurium* and *E. coli* strains in the presence or absence of metabolic activation, a mammalian-cell gene mutation assay, and a transformation assay with Syrian hamster embryo cells. Entecavir was also negative in an oral micronucleus study and an oral DNA repair study in rats. In reproductive toxicology studies, in which animals were administered entecavir at up to 30 mg/kg for up to 4 weeks, no evidence of impaired fertility was seen in male or female rats at systemic exposures greater than 90 times those achieved in humans at the highest recommended dose of 1 mg/day. In rodent and dog toxicology studies, seminiferous tubular degeneration was observed at exposures 35 times or greater than those achieved in humans. No testicular changes were evident in monkeys.

14 CLINICAL STUDIES

14.1 Outcomes at 48 Weeks

The safety and efficacy of BARACLUDE (entecavir) were evaluated in three Phase 3 active-controlled trials. These studies included 1633 subjects 16 years of age or older with chronic hepatitis B virus infection (serum HBsAg-positive for at least 6 months) accompanied by evidence of viral replication (detectable serum HBV DNA, as measured by the bDNA hybridization or PCR assay). Subjects had persistently elevated ALT levels at least 1.3 times ULN and chronic inflammation on liver biopsy compatible with a diagnosis of chronic viral hepatitis. The safety and efficacy of BARACLUDE were also evaluated in a study of 68 subjects co-infected with HBV and HIV.

Nucleoside-naïve subjects with compensated liver disease

HBeAg-positive: Study AI463022 was a multinational, randomized, double-blind study of BARACLUDE 0.5 mg once daily versus lamivudine 100 mg once daily for a minimum of 52 weeks in 709 (of 715 randomized) nucleoside-naïve subjects with chronic hepatitis B virus infection and detectable HBeAg. The mean age of subjects was 35 years, 75% were male, 57% were Asian, 40% were Caucasian, and 13% had previously received interferon-α. At baseline, subjects had a mean Knodell Necroinflammatory Score of 7.8, mean serum HBV DNA as measured by Roche COBAS Amplicor® PCR assay was 9.66 $\log_{10}$ copies/mL, and mean serum ALT level was 143 U/L. Paired, adequate liver biopsy samples were available for 89% of subjects.

HBeAg-negative (anti-HBe-positive/HBV DNA-positive): Study AI463027 was a multinational, randomized, double-blind study of BARACLUDE 0.5 mg once daily versus lamivudine 100 mg once daily for a minimum of 52 weeks in 638 (of 648 randomized) nucleoside-naïve subjects with HBeAg-negative (HBeAb-positive) chronic hepatitis B virus infection. The mean age of subjects was 44 years, 76% were male, 39% were Asian, 58% were Caucasian, and 13% had previously received interferon-α. At baseline, subjects had a mean Knodell Necroinflammatory Score of 7.8, mean serum HBV DNA as measured by Roche COBAS Amplicor PCR assay was 7.58 $\log_{10}$ copies/mL, and mean serum ALT level was 142 U/L. Paired, adequate liver biopsy samples were available for 88% of subjects.

In Studies AI463022 and AI463027, BARACLUDE was superior to lamivudine on the primary efficacy endpoint of Histologic Improvement, defined as a 2-point or greater reduction in Knodell Necroinflammatory Score with no worsening in Knodell Fibrosis Score at Week 48, and on the secondary efficacy measures of reduction in viral load and ALT normalization. Histologic Improvement and change in Ishak Fibrosis Score are shown in Table 6. Selected virologic, biochemical, and serologic outcome measures are shown in Table 7.

[See table 6 above]
[See table 7 at top of next page]

Histologic Improvement was independent of baseline levels of HBV DNA or ALT.

Lamivudine-refractory subjects

Study AI463026 was a multinational, randomized, double-blind study of BARACLUDE in 286 (of 293 randomized) subjects with lamivudine-refractory chronic hepatitis B virus infection. Subjects receiving lamivudine at study entry either switched to BARACLUDE 1 mg once daily (with neither a washout nor an overlap period) or continued on lamivudine 100 mg for a minimum of 52 weeks. The mean age of subjects was 39 years, 76% were male, 37% were Asian, 62% were Caucasian, and 52% had previously received interferon-α. The mean duration of prior lamivudine therapy was 2.7 years, and 85% had lamivudine resistance mutations at baseline by an investigational line probe assay. At baseline, subjects had a mean Knodell Necroinflammatory Score of 6.5, mean serum HBV DNA as measured by Roche COBAS Amplicor PCR assay was 9.36 $\log_{10}$ copies/mL, and mean serum ALT level was 128 U/L. Paired, adequate liver biopsy samples were available for 87% of subjects.

BARACLUDE (entecavir) was superior to lamivudine on a primary endpoint of Histologic Improvement (using the Knodell Score at Week 48). These results and change in Ishak Fibrosis Score are shown in Table 8. Table 9 shows selected virologic, biochemical, and serologic endpoints.

Table 8: Histologic Improvement and Change in Ishak Fibrosis Score at Week 48, Lamivudine-Refractory Subjects in Study AI463026

	BARACLUDE 1 mg n=124[a]	Lamivudine 100 mg n=116[a]
Histologic Improvement (Knodell Scores)		
Improvement[b]	55%*	28%
No improvement	34%	57%
Ishak Fibrosis Score		
Improvement[c]	34%*	16%
No change	44%	42%
Worsening[c]	11%	26%
Missing Week 48 biopsy	11%	16%

[a] Subjects with evaluable baseline histology (baseline Knodell Necroinflammatory Score ≥2).
[b] ≥2-point decrease in Knodell Necroinflammatory Score from baseline with no worsening of the Knodell Fibrosis Score.
[c] For Ishak Fibrosis Score, improvement = ≥1-point decrease from baseline and worsening = ≥1-point increase from baseline.
*p<0.01

Table 9: Selected Virologic, Biochemical, and Serologic Endpoints at Week 48, Lamivudine-Refractory Subjects in Study AI463026

	BARACLUDE 1 mg n=141	Lamivudine 100 mg n=145
HBV DNA[a]		
Proportion undetectable (<300 copies/mL)	19%*	1%
Mean change from baseline ($\log_{10}$ copies/mL)	-5.11*	-0.48
ALT normalization (≤1 × ULN)	61%*	15%
HBeAg seroconversion	8%	3%

[a] Roche COBAS Amplicor PCR assay (LLOQ = 300 copies/mL).
*p<0.0001

Histologic Improvement was independent of baseline levels of HBV DNA or ALT.

14.2 Outcomes beyond 48 Weeks

The optimal duration of therapy with BARACLUDE is unknown. According to protocol-mandated criteria in the Phase 3 clinical trials, subjects discontinued BARACLUDE or lamivudine treatment after 52 weeks according to a definition of response based on HBV virologic suppression (<0.7 MEq/mL by bDNA assay) and loss of HBeAg (in HBeAg-positive subjects) or ALT <1.25 × ULN (in HBeAg-negative subjects) at Week 48. Subjects who achieved virologic suppression but did not have serologic response (HBeAg-positive) or did not achieve ALT <1.25 × ULN (HBeAg-negative) continued blinded dosing through 96 weeks or until the response criteria were met. These protocol-specified subject management guidelines are not intended as guidance for clinical practice.

Nucleoside-naïve subjects: Among nucleoside-naïve, HBeAg-positive subjects (Study AI463022), 243 (69%) BARACLUDE-treated subjects and 164 (46%) lamivudine-treated subjects continued blinded treatment for up to 96 weeks. Of those continuing blinded treatment in Year 2, 180 (74%) BARACLUDE subjects and 60 (37%) lamivudine subjects achieved HBV DNA <300 copies/mL by PCR at the end of dosing (up to 96 weeks). 193 (79%) BARACLUDE subjects achieved ALT ≤1 × ULN compared to 112 (68%) lamivudine subjects, and HBeAg seroconversion occurred in 26 (11%) BARACLUDE subjects and 20 (12%) lamivudine subjects.

Among nucleoside-naïve, HBeAg-positive subjects, 74 (21%) BARACLUDE subjects and 67 (19%) lamivudine subjects met the definition of response at Week 48, discontinued study drugs, and were followed off treatment for 24 weeks.

Among BARACLUDE responders, 26 (35%) subjects had HBV DNA <300 copies/mL, 55 (74%) subjects had ALT ≤1 ×

ULN, and 56 (76%) subjects sustained HBeAg seroconversion at the end of follow-up. Among lamivudine responders, 20 (30%) subjects had HBV DNA <300 copies/mL, 41 (61%) subjects had ALT ≤1 × ULN, and 47 (70%) subjects sustained HBeAg seroconversion at the end of follow-up.

Among nucleoside-naïve, HBeAg-negative subjects (Study AI463027), 26 (8%) BARACLUDE-treated subjects and 28 (9%) lamivudine-treated subjects continued blinded treatment for up to 96 weeks. In this small cohort continuing treatment in Year 2, 22 BARACLUDE (entecavir) and 16 lamivudine subjects had HBV DNA <300 copies/mL by PCR, and 7 and 6 subjects, respectively, had ALT ≤1 × ULN at the end of dosing (up to 96 weeks).

Among nucleoside-naïve, HBeAg-negative subjects, 275 (85%) BARACLUDE subjects and 245 (78%) lamivudine subjects met the definition of response at Week 48, discontinued study drugs, and were followed off treatment for 24 weeks. In this cohort, very few subjects in each treatment arm had HBV DNA <300 copies/mL by PCR at the end of follow-up. At the end of follow-up, 126 (46%) BARACLUDE subjects and 84 (34%) lamivudine subjects had ALT ≤1 × ULN.

Lamivudine-refractory subjects: Among lamivudine-refractory subjects (Study AI463026), 77 (55%) BARACLUDE-treated subjects and 3 (2%) lamivudine subjects continued blinded treatment for up to 96 weeks. In this cohort of BARACLUDE subjects, 31 (40%) subjects achieved HBV DNA <300 copies/mL, 62 (81%) subjects had ALT ≤1 × ULN, and 8 (10%) subjects demonstrated HBeAg seroconversion at the end of dosing.

14.3 Special Populations

Patients Co-infected with HIV and HBV

Study AI463038 was a randomized, double-blind, placebo-controlled study of BARACLUDE versus placebo in 68 subjects co-infected with HIV and HBV who experienced recurrence of HBV viremia while receiving a lamivudine-containing highly active antiretroviral (HAART) regimen. Subjects continued their lamivudine-containing HAART regimen (lamivudine dose 300 mg/day) and were assigned to add either BARACLUDE 1 mg once daily (51 subjects) or placebo (17 subjects) for 24 weeks followed by an open-label phase for an additional 24 weeks where all subjects received BARACLUDE. At baseline, subjects had a mean serum HBV DNA level by PCR of 9.13 $\log_{10}$ copies/mL. Ninety-nine percent of subjects were HBeAg-positive at baseline, with a mean baseline ALT level of 71.5 U/L. Median HIV RNA level remained stable at approximately 2 $\log_{10}$ copies/mL through 24 weeks of blinded therapy. Virologic and biochemical endpoints at Week 24 are shown in Table 10. There are no data in patients with HIV/HBV co-infection who have not received prior lamivudine therapy. BARACLUDE has not been evaluated in HIV/HBV co-infected patients who were

not simultaneously receiving effective HIV treatment [see *Warnings and Precautions (5.2)*].

Table 10: Virologic and Biochemical Endpoints at Week 24, Study AI463038

	BARACLUDE 1 mg[a] n=51	Placebo[a] n=17
HBV DNA[b]		
Proportion undetectable (<300 copies/mL)	6%	0
Mean change from baseline ($\log_{10}$ copies/mL)	-3.65*	+0.11
ALT normalization (≤1 × ULN)	34%[c]	8%[c]

[a] All subjects also received a lamivudine-containing HAART regimen.
[b] Roche COBAS Amplicor PCR assay (LLOQ = 300 copies/mL).
[c] Percentage of subjects with abnormal ALT (>1 × ULN) at baseline who achieved ALT normalization (n=35 for BARACLUDE and n=12 for placebo).
*p<0.0001

For subjects originally assigned to BARACLUDE, at the end of the open-label phase (Week 48), 8% of subjects had HBV DNA <300 copies/mL by PCR, the mean change from baseline HBV DNA by PCR was -4.20 $\log_{10}$ copies/mL, and 37% of subjects with abnormal ALT at baseline had ALT normalization (≤1 × ULN).

16 HOW SUPPLIED/STORAGE AND HANDLING

BARACLUDE® (entecavir) Tablets and Oral Solution are available in the following strengths and configurations in plastic bottles with child-resistant closures:
[See second table above]

BARACLUDE Oral Solution is a ready-to-use product; dilution or mixing with water or any other solvent or liquid product is not recommended. Each bottle of the oral solution is accompanied by a dosing spoon that is calibrated in 1-mL increments up to 10 mL [see *Patient Counseling Information (17.1)*].

Storage

BARACLUDE Tablets should be stored in a tightly closed container at 25° C (77° F); excursions permitted between 15-30° C (59-86° F) [see USP Controlled Room Temperature].

BARACLUDE Oral Solution should be stored in the outer carton at 25° C (77° F); excursions permitted between 15-30° C (59-86° F) [see USP Controlled Room Temperature]. Protect from light. After opening, the oral solution can be used up to the expiration date on the bottle. The bottle and its contents should be discarded after the expiration date.

Table 7: Selected Virologic, Biochemical, and Serologic Endpoints at Week 48, Nucleoside-Naïve Subjects in Studies AI463022 and AI463027

	Study AI463022 (HBeAg-Positive)		Study AI463027 (HBeAg-Negative)	
	BARACLUDE 0.5 mg n=354	Lamivudine 100 mg n=355	BARACLUDE 0.5 mg n=325	Lamivudine 100 mg n=313
HBV DNA[a]				
Proportion undetectable (<300 copies/mL)	67%*	36%	90%*	72%
Mean change from baseline ($\log_{10}$ copies/mL)	-6.86*	-5.39	-5.04*	-4.53
ALT normalization (≤1 × ULN)	68%*	60%	78%*	71%
HBeAg seroconversion	21%	18%	NA	NA

[a] Roche COBAS Amplicor PCR assay (LLOQ = 300 copies/mL).
*p<0.05

Product Strength and Dosage Form	Description	Quantity	NDC Number
0.5-mg film-coated tablet	White to off-white, triangular-shaped tablet, debossed with "BMS" on one side and "1611" on the other side.	30 tablets 90 tablets	0003-1611-12 0003-1611-13
1.0-mg film-coated tablet	Pink, triangular-shaped tablet, debossed with "BMS" on one side and "1612" on the other side.	30 tablets	0003-1612-12
0.05-mg/mL oral solution	Ready-to-use, orange-flavored, clear, colorless to pale yellow aqueous solution in a 260-mL bottle.	210 mL	0003-1614-12

17 PATIENT COUNSELING INFORMATION

See *FDA-Approved Patient Labeling (17.4)*.

17.1 Information about Treatment

Physicians should inform their patients of the following important points when initiating BARACLUDE (entecavir) treatment:

- Patients should remain under the care of a physician while taking BARACLUDE. They should discuss any new symptoms or concurrent medications with their physician.
- Patients should be advised that treatment with BARACLUDE has not been shown to reduce the risk of transmission of HBV to others through sexual contact or blood contamination.
- Patients should be advised to take BARACLUDE on an empty stomach (at least 2 hours after a meal and 2 hours before the next meal).
- Patients using the oral solution should be instructed to hold the dosing spoon in a vertical position and fill it gradually to the mark corresponding to the prescribed dose. Rinsing of the dosing spoon with water is recommended after each daily dose.

17.2 Post-treatment Exacerbation of Hepatitis

Patients should be informed that deterioration of liver disease may occur in some cases if treatment is discontinued, and that they should discuss any change in regimen with their physician.

17.3 HIV/HBV Co-infection

Patients should be offered HIV antibody testing before starting BARACLUDE therapy. They should be informed that if they have HIV infection and are not receiving effective HIV treatment, BARACLUDE may increase the chance of HIV resistance to HIV medication.

Bristol-Myers Squibb Company
Princeton, NJ 08543 USA
1195459A8
F0-B0001-07-09 Rev July 2009

17.4 FDA-approved Patient Labeling

BARACLUDE® (BEAR ah klude)
(generic name = **entecavir**)
Tablets and Oral Solution

Read the Patient Information that comes with BARACLUDE before you start taking it and each time you get a refill. There may be new information. This information does not take the place of talking with your healthcare provider about your medical condition or treatment.

What is the most important information I should know about BARACLUDE?

1. **Your hepatitis B virus infection may get worse or become very serious if you stop BARACLUDE.**
   - Take BARACLUDE exactly as prescribed.
   - Do not run out of BARACLUDE.
   - Do not stop BARACLUDE without talking to your healthcare provider.

   Your healthcare provider will need to monitor your health and do regular blood tests to check your liver if you stop BARACLUDE. Tell your healthcare provider right away about any new or unusual symptoms that you notice after you stop taking BARACLUDE.
2. **If you have or get HIV (human immunodeficiency virus) infection be sure to discuss your treatment with your doctor.** If you are taking BARACLUDE to treat chronic hepatitis B and are not taking medicines for your HIV at the same time, some HIV treatments that you take in the future may be less likely to work. You are advised to get an HIV test before you start taking BARACLUDE and anytime after that when there is a chance you were exposed to HIV. BARACLUDE will not help your HIV infection.
3. **Some people who have taken medicines like BARACLUDE (a nucleoside analogue) have developed a serious condition called lactic acidosis** (buildup of an acid in the blood). Lactic acidosis is a serious medical emergency that can lead to death. Lactic acidosis must be treated in the hospital. **Call your healthcare provider right away if you get any of the following signs of lactic acidosis.**
   - You feel very weak or tired.
   - You have unusual (not normal) muscle pain.
   - You have trouble breathing.
   - You have stomach pain with nausea and vomiting.
   - You feel cold, especially in your arms and legs.
   - You feel dizzy or light-headed.
   - You have a fast or irregular heartbeat.
4. **Some people who have taken medicines like BARACLUDE have developed serious liver problems called hepatotoxicity,** with liver enlargement (hepatomegaly) and fat in the liver (steatosis). **Call your healthcare provider right away if you get any of the following signs of liver problems.**
   - Your skin or the white part of your eyes turns yellow (jaundice).
   - Your urine turns dark.
   - Your bowel movements (stools) turn light in color.
   - You don't feel like eating food for several days or longer.
   - You feel sick to your stomach (nausea).
   - You have lower stomach pain.

What is BARACLUDE (entecavir)?

BARACLUDE is a prescription medicine used for chronic infection with hepatitis B virus (HBV) in adults who also have active liver damage.

- BARACLUDE will not cure HBV.
- BARACLUDE may lower the amount of HBV in the body.
- BARACLUDE may lower the ability of HBV to multiply and infect new liver cells.
- BARACLUDE may improve the condition of your liver.
- It is not known whether BARACLUDE will reduce your chances of getting liver cancer or liver damage (cirrhosis), which may be caused by chronic HBV infection.

It is important to stay under your healthcare provider's care while taking BARACLUDE. Some people, especially those who have already been treated with certain other medicines for HBV infection, may develop resistance to BARACLUDE. These people may have less benefit from treatment with BARACLUDE and may have worsening of hepatitis after resistant virus appears. Your healthcare provider will test the level of the hepatitis B virus in your blood regularly.

Does BARACLUDE lower the risk of passing HBV to others?

BARACLUDE does not stop you from spreading HBV to others by sex, sharing needles, or being exposed to your blood. Talk with your healthcare provider about safe sexual practices that protect your partner. Never share needles. Do not share personal items that can have blood or body fluids on them, like toothbrushes or razor blades. A shot (vaccine) is available to protect people at risk from becoming infected with HBV.

Who should not take BARACLUDE?

Do not take BARACLUDE if you are allergic to any of its ingredients. The active ingredient in BARACLUDE is entecavir. See the end of this leaflet for a complete list of ingredients in BARACLUDE. Tell your healthcare provider if you think you have had an allergic reaction to any of these ingredients.

BARACLUDE has not been studied in children and is not recommended for anyone less than 16 years old.

What should I tell my healthcare provider before I take BARACLUDE?

Tell your healthcare provider about all of your medical conditions, including if you:

- **have kidney problems.** Your BARACLUDE dose or dose schedule may need to be adjusted.
- **are pregnant or planning to become pregnant.** It is not known if BARACLUDE is safe to use during pregnancy. It is not known whether BARACLUDE helps prevent a pregnant mother from passing HBV to her baby. You and your healthcare provider will need to decide if BARACLUDE is right for you. If you use BARACLUDE while you are pregnant, talk to your healthcare provider about the BARACLUDE Pregnancy Registry.
- **are breast-feeding.** It is not known if BARACLUDE can pass into your breast milk or if it can harm your baby. Do not breast-feed if you are taking BARACLUDE.

Tell your healthcare provider about all the medicines you take including prescription and nonprescription medicines, vitamins, and herbal supplements. BARACLUDE may interact with other medicines that leave the body through the kidneys.

Know the medicines you take. Keep a list of your medicines with you to show your healthcare provider and pharmacist.

How should I take BARACLUDE?

- Take BARACLUDE exactly as prescribed. Your healthcare provider will tell you how much BARACLUDE to take. Your dose will depend on whether you have been treated for HBV infection before and what medicine you took. The usual dose of BARACLUDE Tablets is either 0.5 mg (one white tablet) or 1 mg (one pink tablet) once daily by mouth. The usual dose of BARACLUDE Oral Solution is either 10 mL or 20 mL once daily by mouth. Your dose may be lower or you may take BARACLUDE less often than once a day if you have kidney problems.
- **Take BARACLUDE once a day on an empty stomach** to help it work better. Empty stomach means at least 2 hours after a meal and at least 2 hours before the next meal. To help you remember to take your BARACLUDE, try to take it at the same time each day.
- If you are taking BARACLUDE Oral Solution, carefully measure your dose with the spoon provided, as follows:
  1. Hold the spoon in a vertical (upright) position and fill it gradually to the mark corresponding to the prescribed dose. Holding the spoon with the volume marks facing you, check that it has been filled to the proper mark.
  2. Swallow the medicine directly from the measuring spoon.
  3. After each use, rinse the spoon with water and allow it to air dry.

  If you lose the spoon, call your pharmacist or healthcare provider for instructions.
- **Do not change your dose or stop taking BARACLUDE (entecavir) without talking to your healthcare provider. Your hepatitis B symptoms may get worse or become very serious if you stop taking BARACLUDE.** After you stop taking BARACLUDE, it is important to stay under your healthcare provider's care. Your healthcare provider will need to do regular blood tests to check your liver.
- **If you forget to take BARACLUDE,** take it as soon as you remember and then take your next dose at its regular time. If it is almost time for your next dose, skip the missed dose. Do not take two doses at the same time. Call your healthcare provider or pharmacist if you are not sure what to do.
- When your supply of BARACLUDE starts to run low, get more from your healthcare provider or pharmacy. **Do not run out of BARACLUDE (entecavir).**
- **If you take more than the prescribed dose of BARACLUDE,** call your healthcare provider right away.

What are the possible side effects of BARACLUDE?

BARACLUDE may cause the following serious side effects (see "What is the most important information I should know about BARACLUDE?"):

- **a worse or very serious hepatitis if you stop taking it.**
- **lactic acidosis and liver problems.**

The most common side effects of BARACLUDE are headache, tiredness, dizziness, and nausea. Less common side effects include diarrhea, indigestion, vomiting, sleepiness, and trouble sleeping. There have also been occasional reports of rash and hair loss. In some patients, the results of blood tests that measure how the liver or pancreas is working may worsen.

These are not all the side effects of BARACLUDE. The list of side effects is **not** complete at this time because BARACLUDE is still under study. Report any new or continuing symptom to your healthcare provider. If you have questions about side effects, ask your healthcare provider. Your healthcare provider may be able to help you manage these side effects.

How should I store BARACLUDE?

- Store BARACLUDE Tablets or Oral Solution at room temperature, 59° to 86° F (15° to 30° C). They do not require refrigeration. Do not store BARACLUDE Tablets in a damp place such as a bathroom medicine cabinet or near the kitchen sink.
- Keep the container tightly closed. BARACLUDE Oral Solution should be stored in the original carton and protected from light.
- **Keep BARACLUDE and all medicines out of the reach of children and pets at all times.** Do not keep medicine that is out of date or that you no longer need. Dispose of unused medicines through community take-back disposal programs when available or place BARACLUDE in an unrecognizable closed container in the household trash.

General information about BARACLUDE: Medicines are sometimes prescribed for conditions other than those described in patient information leaflets. Do not use BARACLUDE for a condition for which it was not prescribed. Do not give BARACLUDE to other people, even if they have the same symptoms you have. It may harm them.

The leaflet summarizes the most important information about BARACLUDE. If you would like more information, talk with your healthcare provider. You can ask your healthcare provider or pharmacist for information about BARACLUDE that is written for healthcare professionals. You can also call 1-800-321-1335 or visit the BARACLUDE website at *www.Baraclude.com*.

What are the ingredients in BARACLUDE?

Active Ingredient: entecavir

Inactive Ingredients in BARACLUDE Tablets: lactose monohydrate, microcrystalline cellulose, crospovidone, povidone, magnesium stearate, titanium dioxide, hypromellose, polyethylene glycol 400, polysorbate 80 (0.5-mg tablet only), and iron oxide red (1-mg tablet only).

Inactive Ingredients in BARACLUDE Oral Solution: maltitol, sodium citrate, citric acid, methylparaben, propylparaben, and orange flavor.

Bristol-Myers Squibb Company
Princeton, NJ 08543 USA

This Patient Information Leaflet has been approved by the U.S. Food and Drug Administration.

1195459A8
F0-B0001-07-09 Rev July 2009

Shown in Product Identification Guide, page 321

ERBITUX® ℞

[ER-be-tux]
(cetuximab)
Solution for Intravenous Infusion

HIGHLIGHTS OF PRESCRIBING INFORMATION

These highlights do not include all the information needed to use ERBITUX safely and effectively. See full prescribing information for ERBITUX.

ERBITUX® (cetuximab)
Solution for intravenous infusion
Initial U.S. Approval: 2004

WARNING: SERIOUS INFUSION REACTIONS and CARDIOPULMONARY ARREST
See full prescribing information for complete boxed warning.

- Serious infusion reactions, some fatal, occurred in approximately 3% of patients. (5.1)
- Cardiopulmonary arrest and/or sudden death occurred in 2% of patients receiving Erbitux in combination with radiation therapy. (5.2, 5.6)

——————RECENT MAJOR CHANGES——————
Indications and Usage
Colorectal Cancer (1.2)   07/2009

——————INDICATIONS AND USAGE——————
Erbitux® is an epidermal growth factor receptor (EGFR) antagonist indicated for treatment of:
Head and Neck Cancer
- Locally or regionally advanced squamous cell carcinoma of the head and neck in combination with radiation therapy. (1.1, 14.1)
- Recurrent or metastatic squamous cell carcinoma of the head and neck progressing after platinum-based therapy. (1.1, 14.1)
Colorectal Cancer
- As a single agent, EGFR-expressing metastatic colorectal cancer after failure of both irinotecan- and oxaliplatin-based regimens or in patients who are intolerant to irinotecan-based regimens. (1.2, 14.2)
- In combination with irinotecan, EGFR-expressing metastatic colorectal carcinoma in patients who are refractory to irinotecan-based chemotherapy. Approval is based on objective response rate; no data are available demonstrating an improvement in increased survival. (1.2, 14.2)
- Retrospective subset analyses of metastatic or advanced colorectal cancer trials have not shown a treatment benefit for Erbitux in patients whose tumors had *KRAS* mutations in codon 12 or 13. Use of Erbitux is not recommended for the treatment of colorectal cancer with these mutations. (1.2, 12.1, 14.2)

——————DOSAGE AND ADMINISTRATION——————
- Premedicate with an H_1 antagonist. (2.3)
- Administer 400 mg/m^2 initial dose as a 120-minute intravenous infusion followed by 250 mg/m^2 weekly infused over 60 minutes. (2.1, 2.2)
- Initiate Erbitux (cetuximab) one week prior to initiation of radiation therapy. (2.1)
- Reduce the infusion rate by 50% for NCI CTC Grade 1 or 2 infusion reactions and non-serious NCI CTC Grades 3–4 infusion reactions. (2.4)
- Permanently discontinue for serious infusion reactions. (2.4)
- Withhold infusion for severe, persistent acneform rash. Reduce dose for recurrent, severe rash. (2.4)

——————DOSAGE FORMS AND STRENGTHS——————
- 100 mg/50 mL, single-use vial (3)
- 200 mg/100 mL, single-use vial (3)

——————CONTRAINDICATIONS——————
None (4)

——————WARNINGS AND PRECAUTIONS——————
- **Infusion Reactions:** Immediately stop and permanently discontinue Erbitux for serious infusion reactions. Monitor patients following infusion. (5.1)
- **Cardiopulmonary Arrest:** Closely monitor serum electrolytes during and after Erbitux. (5.2, 5.6)
- **Pulmonary Toxicity:** Interrupt therapy for acute onset or worsening of pulmonary symptoms. (5.3)
- **Dermatologic Toxicity:** Limit sun exposure. Monitor for inflammatory or infectious sequelae. (2.4, 5.4)

——————ADVERSE REACTIONS——————
The most common adverse reactions (incidence ≥25%) are: cutaneous adverse reactions (including rash, pruritus, and nail changes), headache, diarrhea, and infection. (6)
To report SUSPECTED ADVERSE REACTIONS, contact Bristol-Myers Squibb at 1-800-721-5072 or FDA at 1-800-FDA-1088 or www.fda.gov/medwatch

——————USE IN SPECIFIC POPULATIONS——————
- **Pregnancy:** Administer Erbitux to a pregnant woman only if the potential benefit justifies the potential risk to the fetus. (8.1)
- **Nursing Mothers:** Discontinue nursing during and for 60 days following treatment with Erbitux. (8.3)

See 17 for PATIENT COUNSELING INFORMATION
                                          Revised: 03/2010

FULL PRESCRIBING INFORMATION: CONTENTS*
HIGHLIGHTS OF PRESCRIBING INFORMATION
FULL PRESCRIBING INFORMATION
WARNING: SERIOUS INFUSION REACTIONS AND CARDIOPULMONARY ARREST

FULL PRESCRIBING INFORMATION

WARNING: SERIOUS INFUSION REACTIONS and CARDIOPULMONARY ARREST
Infusion Reactions: Serious infusion reactions occurred with the administration of Erbitux in approximately 3% of patients in clinical trials, with fatal outcome reported in less than 1 in 1000. [See *Warnings and Precautions (5.1)* and *Adverse Reactions (6).*] Immediately interrupt and permanently discontinue Erbitux infusion for serious infusion reactions. [See *Warnings and Precautions (5.1)* and *Dosage and Administration (2.4).*]
Cardiopulmonary Arrest: Cardiopulmonary arrest and/or sudden death occurred in 2% of 208 patients with squamous cell carcinoma of the head and neck treated with radiation therapy and Erbitux. Closely monitor serum electrolytes, including serum magnesium, potassium, and calcium, during and after Erbitux. [See *Warnings and Precautions (5.2, 5.6).*]

---

1 INDICATIONS AND USAGE
1.1 Squamous Cell Carcinoma of the Head and Neck (SCCHN)
Erbitux® (cetuximab) is indicated in combination with radiation therapy for the initial treatment of locally or regionally advanced squamous cell carcinoma of the head and neck. [See *Clinical Studies (14.1).*]
Erbitux, as a single agent, is indicated for the treatment of patients with recurrent or metastatic squamous cell carcinoma of the head and neck for whom prior platinum-based therapy has failed. [See *Clinical Studies (14.1).*]
1.2 Colorectal Cancer
Erbitux, as a single agent, is indicated for the treatment of epidermal growth factor receptor (EGFR)-expressing metastatic colorectal cancer after failure of both irinotecan- and oxaliplatin-based regimens. Erbitux, as a single agent, is also indicated for the treatment of EGFR-expressing metastatic colorectal cancer in patients who are intolerant to irinotecan-based regimens. [See *Clinical Studies (14.2)* and *Warnings and Precautions (5.7).*]
Erbitux, in combination with irinotecan, is indicated for the treatment of EGFR-expressing metastatic colorectal carcinoma in patients who are refractory to irinotecan-based chemotherapy. The effectiveness of Erbitux (cetuximab) in combination with irinotecan is based on objective response rates. Currently, no data are available that demonstrate an improvement in disease-related symptoms or increased survival with Erbitux in combination with irinotecan for the treatment of EGFR-expressing, metastatic colorectal carcinoma. [See *Clinical Studies (14.2)* and *Warnings and Precautions (5.7).*]
Retrospective subset analyses of metastatic or advanced colorectal cancer trials have not shown a treatment benefit for Erbitux in patients whose tumors had *KRAS* mutations in codon 12 or 13. Use of Erbitux is not recommended for the treatment of colorectal cancer with these mutations [see *Clinical Studies (14.2)* and *Clinical Pharmacology (12.1)*].

2 DOSAGE AND ADMINISTRATION
2.1 Squamous Cell Carcinoma of the Head and Neck
Erbitux in combination with radiation therapy:
- The recommended initial dose is 400 mg/m^2 administered one week prior to initiation of a course of radiation therapy as a 120-minute intravenous infusion (maximum infusion rate 10 mg/min).
- The recommended subsequent weekly dose (all other infusions) is 250 mg/m^2 infused over 60 minutes (maximum infusion rate 10 mg/min) for the duration of radiation therapy (6–7 weeks). Complete Erbitux administration 1 hour prior to radiation therapy.
Erbitux monotherapy:
- The recommended initial dose is 400 mg/m^2 administered as a 120-minute intravenous infusion (maximum infusion rate 10 mg/min).
- The recommended subsequent weekly dose (all other infusions) is 250 mg/m^2 infused over 60 minutes (maximum infusion rate 10 mg/min) until disease progression or unacceptable toxicity.

2.2 Colorectal Cancer
- The recommended initial dose, either as monotherapy or in combination with irinotecan, is 400 mg/m^2 administered as a 120-minute intravenous infusion (maximum infusion rate 10 mg/min).
- The recommended subsequent weekly dose, either as monotherapy or in combination with irinotecan, is 250 mg/m^2 infused over 60 minutes (maximum infusion rate 10 mg/min) until disease progression or unacceptable toxicity.

2.3 Recommended Premedication
Premedicate with an H_1 antagonist (eg, 50 mg of diphenhydramine) intravenously 30–60 minutes prior to the first dose; premedication should be administered for subsequent Erbitux doses based upon clinical judgment and presence/severity of prior infusion reactions.

2.4 Dose Modifications
Infusion Reactions
Reduce the infusion rate by 50% for NCI CTC Grade 1 or 2 and non-serious NCI CTC Grades 3–4 infusion reactions. Immediately and permanently discontinue Erbitux for serious infusion reactions requiring medical intervention and/or hospitalization. [See *Warnings and Precautions (5.1).*]
Dermatologic Toxicity
Recommended dose modifications for severe (NCI CTC Grade 3 or 4) acneform rash are specified in Table 1. [See *Warnings and Precautions (5.4).*]
[See table 1 at top of next page]
2.5 Preparation for Administration
Do not administer Erbitux as an intravenous push or bolus. Administer via infusion pump or syringe pump. Do not exceed an infusion rate of 10 mg/min.
Administer through a low protein binding 0.22-micrometer in-line filter.
Parenteral drug products should be inspected visually for particulate matter and discoloration prior to administration, whenever solution and container permit.
The solution should be clear and colorless and may contain a small amount of easily visible, white, amorphous, cetuximab particulates. **Do not shake or dilute.**

3 DOSAGE FORMS AND STRENGTHS
100 mg/50 mL, single-use vial
200 mg/100 mL, single-use vial

4 CONTRAINDICATIONS
None.

5 WARNINGS AND PRECAUTIONS
5.1 Infusion Reactions
Serious infusion reactions, requiring medical intervention and immediate, permanent discontinuation of Erbitux, included rapid onset of airway obstruction (bronchospasm, stridor, hoarseness), hypotension, shock, loss of consciousness, myocardial infarction, and/or cardiac arrest. Severe (NCI CTC Grades 3 and 4) infusion reactions occurred in 2–5% of 1373 patients in clinical trials, with fatal outcome in 1 patient.

Table 1: Erbitux Dose Modification Guidelines for Rash

Severe Acneform Rash	Erbitux	Outcome	Erbitux Dose Modification
1st occurrence	Delay infusion 1 to 2 weeks	Improvement No Improvement	Continue at 250 mg/m² Discontinue Erbitux
2nd occurrence	Delay infusion 1 to 2 weeks	Improvement No Improvement	Reduce dose to 200 mg/m² Discontinue Erbitux
3rd occurrence	Delay infusion 1 to 2 weeks	Improvement No Improvement	Reduce dose to 150 mg/m² Discontinue Erbitux
4th occurrence	Discontinue Erbitux		

Table 2: Incidence of Selected Adverse Events (≥10%) in Patients with Locoregionally Advanced SCCHN

Body System Preferred Term	Erbitux plus Radiation (n=208)		Radiation Therapy Alone (n=212)	
	Grades 1–4	Grades 3 and 4	Grades 1–4	Grades 3 and 4
	% of Patients			
Body as a Whole				
Asthenia	56	4	49	5
Fever[1]	29	1	13	1
Headache	19	<1	8	<1
Infusion Reaction[2]	15	3	2	0
Infection	13	1	9	1
Chills[1]	16	0	5	0
Digestive				
Nausea	49	2	37	2
Emesis	29	2	23	4
Diarrhea	19	2	13	1
Dyspepsia	14	0	9	1
Metabolic/Nutritional				
Weight Loss	84	11	72	7
Dehydration	25	6	19	8
Alanine Transaminase, high[3]	43	2	21	1
Aspartate Transaminase, high[3]	38	1	24	1
Alkaline Phosphatase, high[3]	33	<1	24	0
Respiratory				
Pharyngitis	26	3	19	4
Skin/Appendages				
Acneform Rash[4]	87	17	10	1
Radiation Dermatitis	86	23	90	18
Application Site Reaction	18	0	12	1
Pruritus	16	0	4	0

[1] Includes cases also reported as infusion reaction.
[2] Infusion reaction is defined as any event described at any time during the clinical study as "allergic reaction" or "anaphylactoid reaction", or any event occurring on the first day of dosing described as "allergic reaction", "anaphylactoid reaction", "fever", "chills", "chills and fever", or "dyspnea".
[3] Based on laboratory measurements, not on reported adverse events, the number of subjects with tested samples varied from 205–206 for Erbitux plus Radiation arm; 209–210 for Radiation alone.
[4] Acneform rash is defined as any event described as "acne", "rash", "maculopapular rash", "pustular rash", "dry skin", or "exfoliative dermatitis".

Approximately 90% of severe infusion reactions occurred with the first infusion despite premedication with antihistamines.

Monitor patients for 1 hour following Erbitux (cetuximab) infusions in a setting with resuscitation equipment and other agents necessary to treat anaphylaxis (eg, epinephrine, corticosteroids, intravenous antihistamines, bronchodilators, and oxygen). Monitor longer to confirm resolution of the event in patients requiring treatment for infusion reactions.

Immediately and permanently discontinue Erbitux in patients with serious infusion reactions. [See *Boxed Warning* and *Dosage and Administration (2.4)*.]

5.2 Cardiopulmonary Arrest

Cardiopulmonary arrest and/or sudden death occurred in 4 (2%) of 208 patients treated with radiation therapy and Erbitux as compared to none of 212 patients treated with radiation therapy alone in a randomized, controlled trial in patients with SCCHN. Three patients with prior history of coronary artery disease died at home, with myocardial infarction as the presumed cause of death. One of these patients had arrhythmia and one had congestive heart failure. Death occurred 27, 32, and 43 days after the last dose of Erbitux. One patient with no prior history of coronary artery disease died one day after the last dose of Erbitux. Carefully consider use of Erbitux in combination with radiation therapy in head and neck cancer patients with a history of coronary artery disease, congestive heart failure, or arrhythmia in light of these risks. Closely monitor serum electrolytes, including serum magnesium, potassium, and calcium, during and after Erbitux. [See *Boxed Warning* and *Warnings and Precautions (5.6)*.]

5.3 Pulmonary Toxicity

Interstitial lung disease (ILD), including 1 fatality, occurred in 4 of 1570 (<0.5%) patients receiving Erbitux (cetuximab) in clinical trials. Interrupt Erbitux for acute onset or worsening of pulmonary symptoms. Permanently discontinue Erbitux for confirmed ILD.

5.4 Dermatologic Toxicity

Dermatologic toxicities, including acneform rash, skin drying and fissuring, paronychial inflammation, infectious sequelae (for example *S. aureus* sepsis, abscess formation, cellulitis, blepharitis, conjunctivitis, keratitis, cheilitis), and hypertrichosis occurred in patients receiving Erbitux therapy. Acneform rash occurred in 76–88% of 1373 patients receiving Erbitux in clinical trials. Severe acneform rash occurred in 1–17% of patients.

Acneform rash usually developed within the first two weeks of therapy and resolved in a majority of the patients after cessation of treatment, although in nearly half, the event continued beyond 28 days. Monitor patients receiving Erbitux for dermatologic toxicities and infectious sequelae. Instruct patients to limit sun exposure during Erbitux therapy. [See *Dose Modifications (2.4)*.]

5.5 Use of Erbitux in Combination With Radiation and Cisplatin

The safety of Erbitux in combination with radiation therapy and cisplatin has not been established. Death and serious cardiotoxicity were observed in a single-arm trial with Erbitux, radiation therapy, and cisplatin (100 mg/m²) in patients with locally advanced SCCHN. Two of 21 patients died, one as a result of pneumonia and one of an unknown cause. Four patients discontinued treatment due to adverse

events. Two of these discontinuations were due to cardiac events.

5.6 Hypomagnesemia and Electrolyte Abnormalities

In patients evaluated during clinical trials, hypomagnesemia occurred in 55% of patients (199/365) receiving Erbitux (cetuximab) and was severe (NCI CTC Grades 3 and 4) in 6–17%. The onset of hypomagnesemia and accompanying electrolyte abnormalities occurred days to months after initiation of Erbitux. Periodically monitor patients for hypomagnesemia, hypocalcemia, and hypokalemia, during and for at least 8 weeks following the completion of Erbitux. Replete electrolytes as necessary.

5.7 Epidermal Growth Factor Receptor (EGFR) Expression and Response

Because expression of EGFR has been detected in nearly all SCCHN tumor specimens, patients enrolled in the head and neck cancer clinical studies were not required to have immunohistochemical evidence of EGFR tumor expression prior to study entry.

Patients enrolled in the colorectal cancer clinical studies were required to have immunohistochemical evidence of EGFR tumor expression. Primary tumor or tumor from a metastatic site was tested with the DakoCytomation EGFR pharmDx™ test kit. Specimens were scored based on the percentage of cells expressing EGFR and intensity (barely/faint, weak-to-moderate, and strong). Response rate did not correlate with either the percentage of positive cells or the intensity of EGFR expression.

6 ADVERSE REACTIONS

The following adverse reactions are discussed in greater detail in other sections of the label:

- Infusion reactions [See *Boxed Warning* and *Warnings and Precautions (5.1)*.]
- Cardiopulmonary arrest [See *Boxed Warning* and *Warnings and Precautions (5.2)*.]
- Pulmonary toxicity [See *Warnings and Precautions (5.3)*.]
- Dermatologic toxicity [See *Warnings and Precautions (5.4)*.]
- Hypomagnesemia and Electrolyte Abnormalities [See *Warnings and Precautions (5.6)*.]

The most common adverse reactions with Erbitux (incidence ≥25%) are cutaneous adverse reactions (including rash, pruritus, and nail changes), headache, diarrhea, and infection.

The most serious adverse reactions with Erbitux are infusion reactions, cardiopulmonary arrest, dermatologic toxicity and radiation dermatitis, sepsis, renal failure, interstitial lung disease, and pulmonary embolus.

Across all studies, Erbitux was discontinued in 3–10% of patients because of adverse reactions.

6.1 Clinical Trials Experience

Because clinical trials are conducted under widely varying conditions, adverse reaction rates observed in the clinical trials of a drug cannot be directly compared to rates in the clinical trials of another drug and may not reflect the rates observed in practice.

The data below reflect exposure to Erbitux in 1373 patients with colorectal cancer or SCCHN in randomized Phase 3 (Studies 1 and 3) or Phase 2 (Studies 2 and 4) trials treated at the recommended dose and schedule for a median of 7 to 14 weeks. [See *Clinical Studies (14)*.]

Infusion reactions: Infusion reactions, which included pyrexia, chills, rigors, dyspnea, bronchospasm, angioedema, urticaria, hypertension, and hypotension occurred in 15–21% of patients across studies. Grades 3 and 4 infusion reactions occurred in 2–5% of patients; infusion reactions were fatal in 1 patient.

Infections: The incidence of infection was variable across studies, ranging from 13–35%. Sepsis occurred in 1–4% of patients.

Renal: Renal failure occurred in 1% of patients with colorectal cancer.

Squamous Cell Carcinoma of the Head and Neck

Table 2 contains selected adverse events in 420 patients receiving radiation therapy either alone or with Erbitux for locally or regionally advanced SCCHN in Study 1. Erbitux was administered at the recommended dose and schedule (400 mg/m² initial dose, followed by 250 mg/m² weekly). Patients received a median of 8 infusions (range 1–11).

[See table 2 at left]

The incidence and severity of mucositis, stomatitis, and xerostomia were similar in both arms of the study.

Late Radiation Toxicity

The overall incidence of late radiation toxicities (any grade) was higher in Erbitux in combination with radiation therapy compared with radiation therapy alone. The following sites were affected: salivary glands (65% versus 56%), larynx (52% versus 36%), subcutaneous tissue (49% versus 45%), mucous membrane (48% versus 39%), esophagus (44% versus 35%), skin (42% versus 33%). The incidence of Grade 3 or 4 late radiation toxicities was similar between the radiation therapy alone and the Erbitux plus radiation treatment groups.

Colorectal Cancer

Table 3 contains selected adverse events in 562 patients receiving best supportive care (BSC) alone or with Erbitux (cetuximab) monotherapy for metastatic colorectal cancer in Study 3. Erbitux was administered at the recommended dose and schedule (400 mg/m² initial dose, followed by 250 mg/m² weekly).

[See table 3 at right]

The most frequently reported adverse events in 354 patients treated with Erbitux plus irinotecan in clinical trials were acneform rash (88%), asthenia/malaise (73%), diarrhea (72%), and nausea (55%). The most common Grades 3–4 adverse events included diarrhea (22%), leukopenia (17%), asthenia/malaise (16%), and acneform rash (14%).

6.2 Immunogenicity

As with all therapeutic proteins, there is potential for immunogenicity. Immunogenic responses to cetuximab were assessed using either a double antigen radiometric assay or an ELISA assay. Due to limitations in assay performance and sampling timing, the incidence of antibody development in patients receiving Erbitux has not been adequately determined. Non-neutralizing anti-cetuximab antibodies were detected in 5% (49 of 1001) of evaluable patients without apparent effect on the safety or antitumor activity of Erbitux.

The incidence of antibody formation is highly dependent on the sensitivity and specificity of the assay. Additionally, the observed incidence of antibody (including neutralizing antibody) positivity in an assay may be influenced by several factors including assay methodology, sample handling, timing of sample collection, concomitant medications, and underlying disease. For these reasons, comparison of the incidence of antibodies to Erbitux with the incidence of antibodies to other products may be misleading.

6.3 Postmarketing Experience

The following adverse reaction has been identified during post-approval use of Erbitux. Because this reaction was reported from a population of uncertain size, it was not always possible to reliably estimate its frequency or establish a causal relationship to drug exposure.

• Aseptic meningitis

7 DRUG INTERACTIONS

A drug interaction study was performed in which Erbitux was administered in combination with irinotecan. There was no evidence of any pharmacokinetic interactions between Erbitux and irinotecan.

8 USE IN SPECIFIC POPULATIONS

8.1 Pregnancy

Pregnancy Category C

There are no adequate and well-controlled studies of Erbitux in pregnant women. Based on animal models, EGFR has been implicated in the control of prenatal development and may be essential for normal organogenesis, proliferation, and differentiation in the developing embryo. Human IgG is known to cross the placental barrier; therefore, Erbitux may be transmitted from the mother to the developing fetus, and has the potential to cause fetal harm when administered to pregnant women. Erbitux should be used during pregnancy only if the potential benefit justifies the potential risk to the fetus.

Pregnant cynomolgus monkeys were treated weekly with 0.4 to 4 times the recommended human dose of cetuximab (based on body surface area) during the period of organogenesis (gestation day [GD] 20–48). Cetuximab was detected in the amniotic fluid and in the serum of embryos from treated dams at GD 49. No fetal malformations or other teratogenic effects occurred in offspring. However, significant increases in embryolethality and abortions occurred at doses of approximately 1.6 to 4 times the recommended human dose of cetuximab (based on total body surface area).

8.3 Nursing Mothers

It is not known whether Erbitux is secreted in human milk. IgG antibodies, such as Erbitux, can be excreted in human milk. Because many drugs are excreted in human milk and because of the potential for serious adverse reactions in nursing infants from Erbitux, a decision should be made whether to discontinue nursing or to discontinue the drug, taking into account the importance of the drug to the mother. If nursing is interrupted, based on the mean half-life of cetuximab [see *Clinical Pharmacology (12.3)*], nursing should not be resumed earlier than 60 days following the last dose of Erbitux.

8.4 Pediatric Use

The safety and effectiveness of Erbitux in pediatric patients have not been established. The pharmacokinetics of cetuximab have not been studied in pediatric populations.

8.5 Geriatric Use

Of the 1062 patients who received Erbitux with irinotecan or Erbitux monotherapy in five studies of advanced colorectal cancer, 363 patients were 65 years of age or older. No overall differences in safety or efficacy were observed between these patients and younger patients.

Table 3: Incidence of Selected Adverse Events Occurring in ≥10% of Patients with Advanced Colorectal Carcinoma[1] Treated with Erbitux Monotherapy

Body System Preferred Term	Erbitux plus BSC (n=288)		BSC alone (n=274)	
	Any Grades[2]	Grades 3 and 4	Any Grades	Grades 3 and 4
	% of Patients			
Dermatology				
Rash/Desquamation	89	12	16	<1
Dry Skin	49	0	11	0
Pruritus	40	2	8	0
Other-Dermatology	27	1	6	1
Nail Changes	21	0	4	0
Body as a Whole				
Fatigue	89	33	76	26
Fever	30	1	18	<1
Infusion Reactions[3]	20	5		
Rigors, Chills	13	<1	4	0
Pain				
Abdominal Pain	59	14	52	16
Pain-Other	51	16	34	7
Headache	33	4	11	0
Bone Pain	15	3	7	2
Pulmonary				
Dyspnea	48	16	43	12
Cough	29	2	19	1
Gastrointestinal				
Constipation	46	4	38	5
Diarrhea	39	2	20	2
Vomiting	37	6	29	6
Stomatitis	25	1	10	<1
Other-Gastrointestinal	23	10	18	8
Mouth Dryness	11	0	4	0
Infection				
Infection without neutropenia	35	13	17	6
Neurology				
Insomnia	30	1	15	1
Confusion	15	6	9	2
Anxiety	14	2	8	1
Depression	13	1	6	<1

[1] Adverse reactions occurring more frequently in Erbitux-treated patients compared with controls.
[2] Adverse events were graded using the NCI CTC, V 2.0.
[3] Infusion reaction is defined as any event (chills, rigors, dyspnea, tachycardia, bronchospasm, chest tightness, swelling, urticaria, hypotension, flushing, rash, hypertension, nausea, angioedema, pain, pruritus, sweating, tremors, shaking, cough, visual disturbances, or other) recorded by the investigator as infusion-related.
BSC = best supportive care

Clinical studies of Erbitux (cetuximab) conducted in patients with head and neck cancer did not include sufficient number of subjects aged 65 and over to determine whether they respond differently from younger subjects. Of the 208 patients with head and neck cancer who received Erbitux with radiation therapy, 45 patients were 65 years of age or older.

10 OVERDOSAGE

The maximum single dose of Erbitux administered is 1000 mg/m² in one patient. No adverse events were reported for this patient.

11 DESCRIPTION

Erbitux (cetuximab) is a recombinant, human/mouse chimeric monoclonal antibody that binds specifically to the extracellular domain of the human epidermal growth factor receptor (EGFR). Cetuximab is composed of the Fv regions of a murine anti-EGFR antibody with human IgG1 heavy and kappa light chain constant regions and has an approximate molecular weight of 152 kDa. Cetuximab is produced in mammalian (murine myeloma) cell culture.

Erbitux is a sterile, clear, colorless liquid of pH 7.0 to 7.4, which may contain a small amount of easily visible, white, amorphous cetuximab particulates. Erbitux is supplied at a concentration of 2 mg/mL in either 100 mg (50 mL) or 200 mg (100 mL), single-use vials. Cetuximab is formulated in a preservative-free solution containing 8.48 mg/mL sodium chloride, 1.88 mg/mL sodium phosphate dibasic heptahydrate, 0.41 mg/mL sodium phosphate monobasic monohydrate, and Water for Injection, USP.

12 CLINICAL PHARMACOLOGY

12.1 Mechanism of Action

The epidermal growth factor receptor (EGFR, HER1, c-ErbB-1) is a transmembrane glycoprotein that is a member of a subfamily of type I receptor tyrosine kinases including EGFR, HER2, HER3, and HER4. The EGFR is constitutively expressed in many normal epithelial tissues, including the skin and hair follicle. Expression of EGFR is also detected in many human cancers including those of the head and neck, colon, and rectum.

Cetuximab binds specifically to the EGFR on both normal and tumor cells, and competitively inhibits the binding of epidermal growth factor (EGF) and other ligands, such as transforming growth factor–alpha. *In vitro* assays and *in vivo* animal studies have shown that binding of cetuximab to the EGFR blocks phosphorylation and activation of receptor-associated kinases, resulting in inhibition of cell growth, induction of apoptosis, and decreased matrix metalloproteinase and vascular endothelial growth factor production. Signal transduction through the EGFR results in activation of wild-type KRAS protein. However, in cells with activating *KRAS* somatic mutations, the mutant KRAS protein is continuously active and appears independent of EGFR regulation.

In vitro, cetuximab can mediate antibody-dependent cellular cytotoxicity (ADCC) against certain human tumor types. *In vitro* assays and *in vivo* animal studies have shown that cetuximab inhibits the growth and survival of tumor cells that express the EGFR. No anti-tumor effects of cetuximab were observed in human tumor xenografts lacking EGFR expression. The addition of cetuximab to radiation therapy or irinotecan in human tumor xenograft models in mice resulted in an increase in anti-tumor effects compared to radiation therapy or chemotherapy alone.

12.3 Pharmacokinetics

Erbitux administered as monotherapy or in combination with concomitant chemotherapy or radiation therapy exhibits nonlinear pharmacokinetics. The area under the concentration time curve (AUC) increased in a greater than dose proportional manner while clearance of cetuximab decreased from 0.08 to 0.02 L/h/m² as the dose increased from 20 to 200 mg/m², and at doses >200 mg/m², it appeared to plateau. The volume of the distribution for cetuximab appeared to be independent of dose and approximated the vascular space of 2–3 L/m².

Following the recommended dose regimen (400 mg/m² initial dose; 250 mg/m² weekly dose), concentrations of cetuximab reached steady-state levels by the third weekly infusion with mean peak and trough concentrations across studies ranging from 168 to 235 and 41 to 85 μg/mL, respectively. The mean half-life of cetuximab was approximately 112 hours (range 63–230 hours). The pharmacokinetics of cetuximab were similar in patients with SCCHN and those with colorectal cancer.

Table 4: Study 1: Clinical Efficacy in Locoregionally Advanced SCCHN

	Erbitux + Radiation (n=211)	Radiation Alone (n=213)	Hazard Ratio (95% CI[a])	Stratified Log-rank p-value
Locoregional control				
Median duration (months)	24.4	14.9	0.68 (0.52–0.89)	0.005
Overall survival				
Median duration (months)	49.0	29.3	0.74 (0.57–0.97)	0.03

[a] CI = confidence interval

Table 5: Retrospective Analyses of Treatment Effect in the Subset of Patients with mCRC Containing _KRAS_ Mutations Enrolled in Randomized Clinical Trials

Population (n: ITT[1])	Treatment	Number of Patients with KRAS Results (% ITT)	Number of Patients with _KRAS_ mutant (mAb[2]/control)	Effect of mAb on Endpoints: _KRAS_ Mutant[3]
1st line treatment mCRC (1198)	FOLFIRI ± Erbitux	540 (45%)	105/87	**PFS[2]: no difference** OS[2]: no difference ORR[2]: decreased
1st line treatment mCRC (337)	FOLFOX-4 ± Erbitux	233 (69%)	52/47	ORR: decreased PFS: decreased OS: no difference
1st line treatment mCRC (1053)	oxaliplatin or irinotecan-based chemotherapy, bevacizumab ± panitumumab	oxaliplatin 664 (81%)	135/125	**PFS: decreased** OS: no difference ORR: increased
		irinotecan 201 (87%)	47/39	**ORR: decreased** PFS: decreased OS: decreased
1st line treatment mCRC (736)	bevacizumab, capecitabine, oxaliplatin ± Erbitux	528 (72%)	98/108	**PFS: decreased** OS: decreased ORR: decreased
2nd line treatment mCRC (1298)	irinotecan ± Erbitux	300 (23%)	49/59	**OS: decreased** PFS: no difference ORR: increased
Study 3 3rd line treatment mCRC (572)	BSC ± Erbitux	394 (69%)	81/83	**OS: no difference** PFS: no difference ORR: increased
3rd line treatment mCRC (463)	BSC ± panitumumab	427 (92%)	84/100	**PFS: no difference** OS: no difference ORR: no difference

[1] ITT: intent-to-treat.
[2] mAb: EGFR monoclonal antibody; PFS: progression-free survival; ORR: overall response rate; OS: overall survival.
[3] Results from the primary efficacy endpoint are in bold. A given endpoint is designated as "decreased" if there was a numerically smaller result and as "increased" if there was a numerically higher result in the mAb group than in the control group.

Based on a population pharmacokinetic analysis, female patients with colorectal cancer had a 25% lower intrinsic clearance of cetuximab than male patients. Qualitatively similar, but smaller gender differences in cetuximab clearance were observed in patients with SCCHN. The gender differences in clearance do not necessitate any alteration of dosing because of a similar safety profile.

13 NONCLINICAL TOXICOLOGY
13.1 Carcinogenesis, Mutagenesis, Impairment of Fertility
Long-term animal studies have not been performed to test cetuximab for carcinogenic potential, and no mutagenic or clastogenic potential of cetuximab was observed in the _Salmonella-Escherichia coli_ (Ames) assay or in the _in vivo_ rat micronucleus test. Menstrual cyclicity was impaired in female cynomolgus monkeys receiving weekly doses of 0.4 to 4 times the human dose (based on total body surface area). Cetuximab-treated animals exhibited increased incidences of irregular or absent cycles, as compared to control animals. These effects were initially noted beginning week 25 of cetuximab treatment and continued through the 6-week recovery period. In this same study, there were no effects of cetuximab treatment on measured male fertility parameters (ie, serum testosterone levels and analysis of sperm counts, viability, and motility) as compared to control male monkeys. It is not known if cetuximab can impair fertility in humans.
13.2 Animal Pharmacology and/or Toxicology
In cynomolgus monkeys, cetuximab, when administered at doses of approximately 0.4 to 4 times the weekly human exposure (based on total body surface area), resulted in dermatologic findings, including inflammation at the injection site and desquamation of the external integument. At the highest dose level, the epithelial mucosa of the nasal passage, esophagus, and tongue were similarly affected, and degenerative changes in the renal tubular epithelium occurred. Deaths due to sepsis were observed in 50% (5/10) of the animals at the highest dose level beginning after approximately 13 weeks of treatment.

14 CLINICAL STUDIES
14.1 Squamous Cell Carcinoma of the Head and Neck (SCCHN)
Study 1 was a randomized, multicenter, controlled trial of 424 patients with locally or regionally advanced SCCHN. Patients with Stage III/IV SCCHN of the oropharynx, hypopharynx, or larynx with no prior therapy were randomized (1:1) to receive either Erbitux (cetuximab) plus radiation therapy or radiation therapy alone. Stratification factors were Karnofsky Performance Status (60–80 versus 90–100), nodal stage (N0 versus N+), tumor stage (T1–3 versus T4 using American Joint Committee on Cancer 1998 staging criteria), and radiation therapy fractionation (concomitant boost versus once-daily versus twice-daily). Radiation therapy was administered for 6–7 weeks as once daily, twice daily, or concomitant boost. Erbitux was administered as a 400 mg/m² initial dose beginning one week prior to initiation of radiation therapy, followed by 250 mg/m² weekly administered 1 hour prior to radiation therapy for the duration of radiation therapy (6–7 weeks).
Of the 424 randomized patients, the median age was 57 years, 80% were male, 83% were Caucasian, and 90% had baseline Karnofsky Performance Status ≥80. There were 258 patients enrolled in US sites (61%). Sixty percent of patients had oropharyngeal, 25% laryngeal, and 15% hy-

popharyngeal primary tumors; 28% had AJCC T4 tumor stage. Fifty-six percent of the patients received radiation therapy with concomitant boost, 26% received once-daily regimen, and 18% twice-daily regimen.
The main outcome measure of this trial was duration of locoregional control. Overall survival was also assessed. Results are presented in Table 4.
[See table 4 at left]
Study 2 was a single-arm, multicenter clinical trial in 103 patients with recurrent or metastatic SCCHN. All patients had documented disease progression within 30 days of a platinum-based chemotherapy regimen. Patients received a 20-mg test dose of Erbitux (cetuximab) on Day 1, followed by a 400-mg/m² initial dose, and 250 mg/m² weekly until disease progression or unacceptable toxicity.
The median age was 57 years, 82% were male, 100% Caucasian, and 62% had a Karnofsky Performance Status of ≥80.
The objective response rate was 13% (95% confidence interval 7%–21%). Median duration of response was 5.8 months (range 1.2–5.8 months).
14.2 Colorectal Cancer
Erbitux Clinical Trials in EGFR-Expressing, Recurrent, Metastatic Colorectal Cancer
Study 3 was a multicenter, open-label, randomized, clinical trial conducted in 572 patients with EGFR-expressing, previously treated, recurrent, metastatic colorectal cancer (mCRC). Patients were randomized (1:1) to receive either Erbitux plus best supportive care (BSC) or BSC alone. Erbitux was administered as a 400-mg/m² initial dose, followed by 250 mg/m² weekly until disease progression or unacceptable toxicity.
Of the 572 randomized patients, the median age was 63 years, 64% were male, 89% were Caucasian, and 77% had baseline ECOG Performance Status of 0–1. All patients were to have received and progressed on prior therapy including an irinotecan-containing regimen and an oxaliplatin-containing regimen.
The main outcome measure of the study was overall survival. The results are presented in Figure 1.

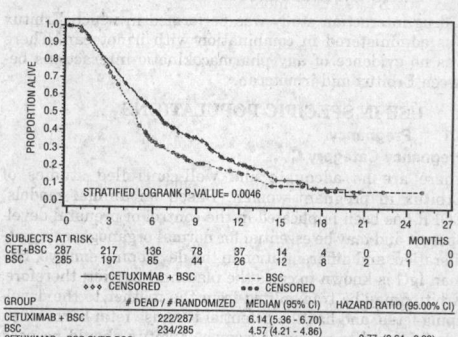

Figure 1: Kaplan Meier Curve for Overall Survival in Patients with Metastatic Colorectal Cancer

	# DEAD / # RANDOMIZED	MEDIAN (95% CI)	HAZARD RATIO (95.00% CI)
CETUXIMAB + BSC	222/287	6.14 (5.36 - 6.70)	
BSC	234/285	4.57 (4.21 - 4.86)	
CETUXIMAB + BSC OVER BSC			0.77 (0.64 - 0.92)

Study 4 was a multicenter, clinical trial conducted in 329 patients with EGFR-expressing recurrent mCRC. Patients were randomized (2:1) to receive either Erbitux plus irinotecan (218 patients) or Erbitux monotherapy (111 patients). Erbitux was administered as a 400-mg/m² initial dose, followed by 250 mg/m² weekly until disease progression or unacceptable toxicity. In the Erbitux plus irinotecan arm, irinotecan was added to Erbitux using the same dose and schedule for irinotecan as the patient had previously failed. Acceptable irinotecan schedules were 350 mg/m² every 3 weeks, 180 mg/m² every 2 weeks, or 125 mg/m² weekly times four doses every 6 weeks. Of the 329 patients, the median age was 59 years, 63% were male, 98% were Caucasian, and 88% had baseline Karnofsky Performance Status ≥80. Approximately two-thirds had previously failed oxaliplatin treatment.
The efficacy of Erbitux plus irinotecan or Erbitux monotherapy, based on durable objective responses, was evaluated in all randomized patients and in two pre-specified subpopulations: irinotecan refractory patients, and irinotecan and oxaliplatin failures. In patients receiving Erbitux plus irinotecan, the objective response rate was 23% (95% confidence interval 18%–29%), median duration of response was 5.7 months, and median time to progression was 4.1 months. In patients receiving Erbitux monotherapy, the objective response rate was 11% (95% confidence interval 6%–18%), median duration of response was 4.2 months, and median time to progression was 1.5 months. Similar response rates were observed in the pre-defined subsets in both the combination arm and monotherapy arm of the study.
Lack of Efficacy of Anti-EGFR Monoclonal Antibodies in Patients With mCRC Containing _KRAS_ Mutations
Retrospective analyses as presented in Table 5 across seven randomized clinical trials suggest that anti-EGFR

monoclonal antibodies are not effective for the treatment of patients with mCRC containing *KRAS* mutations. In these trials, patients received standard of care (ie, BSC or chemotherapy) and were randomized to receive either an anti-EGFR antibody (cetuximab or panitumumab) or no additional therapy. In all studies, investigational tests were used to detect *KRAS* mutations in codon 12 or 13. The percentage of study populations for which *KRAS* status was assessed ranged from 23% to 92%. [See *Clinical Pharmacology (12.1)*.]

[See table 5 on previous page]

16   HOW SUPPLIED/STORAGE AND HANDLING

Erbitux® (cetuximab) is supplied at a concentration of 2 mg/mL as a 100 mg/50 mL, single-use vial or as a 200 mg/100 mL, single-use vial as a sterile, preservative-free, injectable liquid.

NDC 66733-948-23   100 mg/50 mL, single-use vial, individually packaged in a carton

NDC 66733-958-23   200 mg/100 mL, single-use vial, individually packaged in a carton

Store vials under refrigeration at 2° C to 8° C (36° F to 46° F). **Do not freeze.** Increased particulate formation may occur at temperatures at or below 0° C. This product contains no preservatives. Preparations of Erbitux in infusion containers are chemically and physically stable for up to 12 hours at 2° C to 8° C (36° F to 46° F) and up to 8 hours at controlled room temperature (20° C to 25° C; 68° F to 77° F). Discard any remaining solution in the infusion container after 8 hours at controlled room temperature or after 12 hours at 2° C to 8° C. Discard any unused portion of the vial.

17   PATIENT COUNSELING INFORMATION

Advise patients:

• To report signs and symptoms of infusion reactions such as fever, chills, or breathing problems.

• Of the potential risks of using Erbitux during pregnancy or nursing and of the need to use adequate contraception in both males and females during and for 6 months following the last dose of Erbitux therapy.

• That nursing is not recommended during, and for 2 months following the last dose of Erbitux therapy.

• To limit sun exposure (use sunscreen, wear hats) while receiving and for 2 months following the last dose of Erbitux.

Erbitux® is a registered trademark of ImClone Systems Incorporated.

Manufactured by ImClone Systems Incorporated, Branchburg, NJ 08876

Distributed and Marketed by Bristol-Myers Squibb Company, Princeton, NJ 08543

Copyright ©2010 ImClone Systems Incorporated and Bristol-Myers Squibb Company.

All rights reserved.

1236886A6   ER-B0001-03-10   Rev March 2010

Shown in Product Identification Guide, page 321

ONGLYZA   ℞
[*on-GLY-zah*]
(saxagliptin)
tablets

HIGHLIGHTS OF PRESCRIBING INFORMATION

These highlights do not include all the information needed to use ONGLYZA safely and effectively. See full prescribing information for ONGLYZA.

ONGLYZA (saxagliptin) tablets
Initial U.S. Approval: 2009

————————INDICATIONS AND USAGE————————

ONGLYZA is a dipeptidyl peptidase-4 inhibitor indicated as an adjunct to diet and exercise to improve glycemic control in adults with type 2 diabetes mellitus. (1.1)

Important limitations of use:

• Should not be used for the treatment of type 1 diabetes mellitus or diabetic ketoacidosis. (1.2)

• Has not been studied in combination with insulin. (1.2)

————————DOSAGE AND ADMINISTRATION————————

• The recommended dose is 2.5 mg or 5 mg once daily taken regardless of meals. (2.1)

• 2.5 mg daily is recommended for patients with moderate or severe renal impairment, or end-stage renal disease (CrCl ≤50 mL/min). Assess renal function prior to initiation of ONGLYZA and periodically thereafter. (2.2)

• 2.5 mg daily is recommended for patients also taking strong cytochrome P450 3A4/5 (CYP3A4/5) inhibitors (e.g., ketoconazole). (2.3, 7.2)

————————DOSAGE FORMS AND STRENGTHS————————

• Tablets: 5 mg and 2.5 mg (3)

————————CONTRAINDICATIONS————————

• None. (4)

————————WARNINGS AND PRECAUTIONS————————

• When used with an insulin secretagogue (e.g., sulfonylurea), a lower dose of the insulin secretagogue may be required to reduce the risk of hypoglycemia. (5.1)

• There have been no clinical studies establishing conclusive evidence of macrovascular risk reduction with ONGLYZA (saxagliptin) or any other antidiabetic drug. (5.2)

————————ADVERSE REACTIONS————————

• Adverse reactions reported in ≥5% of patients treated with ONGLYZA and more commonly than in patients treated with placebo are: upper respiratory tract infection, urinary tract infection, and headache. (6.1)

• Peripheral edema was reported more commonly in patients treated with the combination of ONGLYZA and a thiazolidinedione (TZD) than in patients treated with the combination of placebo and TZD. (6.1)

• Hypoglycemia was reported more commonly in patients treated with the combination of ONGLYZA and sulfonylurea than in patients treated with the combination of placebo and sulfonylurea. (6.1)

• Hypersensitivity-related events (e.g., urticaria, facial edema) were reported more commonly in patients treated with ONGLYZA than in patients treated with placebo. (6.1)

To report SUSPECTED ADVERSE REACTIONS, contact Bristol-Myers Squibb at 1-800-721-5072 or FDA at 1-800-FDA-1088 or *www.fda.gov/medwatch*

————————DRUG INTERACTIONS————————

• Coadministration with strong CYP3A4/5 inhibitors (e.g., ketoconazole) significantly increases saxagliptin concentrations. Recommend limiting ONGLYZA dose to 2.5 mg once daily. (2.3, 7.2)

————————USE IN SPECIFIC POPULATIONS————————

• There are no adequate and well-controlled studies in pregnant women. (8.1)

• Safety and effectiveness of ONGLYZA in pediatric patients below the age of 18 have not been established. (8.4)

See 17 for PATIENT COUNSELING INFORMATION and FDA-approved patient labeling

Revised: 07/2009

FULL PRESCRIBING INFORMATION: CONTENTS*

FULL PRESCRIBING INFORMATION

1   INDICATIONS AND USAGE

1.1   Monotherapy and Combination Therapy

ONGLYZA (saxagliptin) is indicated as an adjunct to diet and exercise to improve glycemic control in adults with type 2 diabetes mellitus. [See *Clinical Studies (14)*.]

1.2   Important Limitations of Use

ONGLYZA should not be used for the treatment of type 1 diabetes mellitus or diabetic ketoacidosis, as it would not be effective in these settings.

ONGLYZA (saxagliptin) has not been studied in combination with insulin.

2   DOSAGE AND ADMINISTRATION

2.1   Recommended Dosing

The recommended dose of ONGLYZA is 2.5 mg or 5 mg once daily taken regardless of meals.

2.2   Patients with Renal Impairment

No dosage adjustment for ONGLYZA is recommended for patients with mild renal impairment (creatinine clearance [CrCl] >50 mL/min).

The dose of ONGLYZA is 2.5 mg once daily for patients with moderate or severe renal impairment, or with end-stage renal disease (ESRD) requiring hemodialysis (creatinine clearance [CrCl] ≤50 mL/min). ONGLYZA should be administered following hemodialysis. ONGLYZA has not been studied in patients undergoing peritoneal dialysis.

Because the dose of ONGLYZA should be limited to 2.5 mg based upon renal function, assessment of renal function is recommended prior to initiation of ONGLYZA and periodically thereafter. Renal function can be estimated from serum creatinine using the Cockcroft-Gault formula or Modification of Diet in Renal Disease formula. [See *Clinical Pharmacology (12.3)*.]

2.3   Strong CYP3A4/5 Inhibitors

The dose of ONGLYZA is 2.5 mg once daily when coadministered with strong cytochrome P450 3A4/5 (CYP3A4/5) inhibitors (e.g., ketoconazole, atazanavir, clarithromycin, indinavir, itraconazole, nefazodone, nelfinavir, ritonavir, saquinavir, and telithromycin). [See *Drug Interactions (7.2)* and *Clinical Pharmacology (12.3)*.]

3   DOSAGE FORMS AND STRENGTHS

• ONGLYZA (saxagliptin) 5 mg tablets are pink, biconvex, round, film-coated tablets with "5" printed on one side and "4215" printed on the reverse side, in blue ink.

• ONGLYZA (saxagliptin) 2.5 mg tablets are pale yellow to light yellow, biconvex, round, film-coated tablets with "2.5" printed on one side and "4214" printed on the reverse side, in blue ink.

4   CONTRAINDICATIONS

None.

5   WARNINGS AND PRECAUTIONS

5.1   Use with Medications Known to Cause Hypoglycemia

Insulin secretagogues, such as sulfonylureas, cause hypoglycemia. Therefore, a lower dose of the insulin secretagogue may be required to reduce the risk of hypoglycemia when used in combination with ONGLYZA. [See *Adverse Reactions (6.1)*.]

5.2   Macrovascular Outcomes

There have been no clinical studies establishing conclusive evidence of macrovascular risk reduction with ONGLYZA or any other antidiabetic drug.

6   ADVERSE REACTIONS

6.1   Clinical Trials Experience

Because clinical trials are conducted under widely varying conditions, adverse reaction rates observed in the clinical trials of a drug cannot be directly compared to rates in the clinical trials of another drug and may not reflect the rates observed in practice.

Monotherapy and Add-On Combination Therapy

In two placebo-controlled monotherapy trials of 24-weeks duration, patients were treated with ONGLYZA 2.5 mg daily, ONGLYZA 5 mg daily, and placebo. Three 24-week, placebo-controlled, add-on combination therapy trials were also conducted: one with metformin, one with a thiazolidinedione (pioglitazone or rosiglitazone), and one with glyburide. In these three trials, patients were randomized to add-on therapy with ONGLYZA 2.5 mg daily, ONGLYZA 5 mg daily, or placebo. A saxagliptin 10 mg treatment arm was included in one of the monotherapy trials and in the add-on combination trial with metformin.

In a prespecified pooled analysis of the 24-week data (regardless of glycemic rescue) from the two monotherapy trials, the add-on to metformin trial, the add-on to thiazolidinedione (TZD) trial, and the add-on to glyburide trial, the overall incidence of adverse events in patients treated with ONGLYZA 2.5 mg and ONGLYZA 5 mg was similar to placebo (72.0% and 72.2% versus 70.6%, respectively). Discontinuation of therapy due to adverse events occurred in 2.2%, 3.3%, and 1.8% of patients receiving ONGLYZA 2.5 mg, ONGLYZA 5 mg, and placebo, respectively. The most common adverse events (reported in at least 2 patients treated with ONGLYZA 2.5 mg or at least 2 patients treated with ONGLYZA 5 mg) associated with premature discontinuation of therapy included lymphopenia (0.1% and 0.5% versus 0%, respectively), rash (0.2% and 0.3% versus 0.3%), blood creatinine increased (0.3% and 0% versus 0%), and blood creatine phosphokinase increased (0.1% and 0.2% versus 0%). The adverse reactions in this pooled analysis reported (regardless of investigator assessment of causality) in ≥5% of patients treated with ONGLYZA 5 mg, and more commonly than in patients treated with placebo are shown in Table 1.

Table 1: Adverse Reactions (Regardless of Investigator Assessment of Causality) in Placebo-Controlled Trials* Reported in ≥5% of Patients Treated with ONGLYZA 5 mg and More Commonly than in Patients Treated with Placebo

	Number (%) of Patients	
	ONGLYZA 5 mg N=882	Placebo N=799
Upper respiratory tract infection	68 (7.7)	61 (7.6)
Urinary tract infection	60 (6.8)	49 (6.1)
Headache	57 (6.5)	47 (5.9)

*The 5 placebo-controlled trials include two monotherapy trials and one add-on combination therapy trial with each of the following: metformin, thiazolidinedione, or glyburide. Table shows 24-week data regardless of glycemic rescue.

In patients treated with ONGLYZA (saxagliptin) 2.5 mg, headache (6.5%) was the only adverse reaction reported at a rate ≥5% and more commonly than in patients treated with placebo.

In this pooled analysis, adverse reactions that were reported in ≥2% of patients treated with ONGLYZA 2.5 mg or ONGLYZA 5 mg and ≥1% more frequently compared to placebo included: sinusitis (2.9% and 2.6% versus 1.6%, respectively), abdominal pain (2.4% and 1.7% versus 0.5%), gastroenteritis (1.9% and 2.3% versus 0.9%), and vomiting (2.2% and 2.3% versus 1.3%).

In the add-on to TZD trial, the incidence of peripheral edema was higher for ONGLYZA 5 mg versus placebo (8.1% and 4.3%, respectively). The incidence of peripheral edema for ONGLYZA 2.5 mg was 3.1%. None of the reported adverse reactions of peripheral edema resulted in study drug discontinuation. Rates of peripheral edema for ONGLYZA 2.5 mg and ONGLYZA 5 mg versus placebo were 3.6% and 2% versus 3% given as monotherapy, 2.1% and 2.1% versus 2.2% given as add-on therapy to metformin, and 2.4% and 1.2% versus 2.2% given as add-on therapy to glyburide.

The incidence rate of fractures was 1.0 and 0.6 per 100 patient-years, respectively, for ONGLYZA (pooled analysis of 2.5 mg, 5 mg, and 10 mg) and placebo. The incidence rate of fracture events in patients who received ONGLYZA did not increase over time. Causality has not been established and nonclinical studies have not demonstrated adverse effects of saxagliptin on bone.

An event of thrombocytopenia, consistent with a diagnosis of idiopathic thrombocytopenic purpura, was observed in the clinical program. The relationship of this event to ONGLYZA is not known.

Adverse Reactions Associated with ONGLYZA Coadministered with Metformin in Treatment-Naive Patients with Type 2 Diabetes

Table 2 shows the adverse reactions reported (regardless of investigator assessment of causality) in ≥5% of patients participating in an additional 24-week, active-controlled trial of coadministered ONGLYZA and metformin in treatment-naive patients.

Table 2: Initial Therapy with Combination of ONGLYZA and Metformin in Treatment-Naive Patients: Adverse Reactions Reported (Regardless of Investigator Assessment of Causality) in ≥5% of Patients Treated with Combination Therapy of ONGLYZA 5 mg Plus Metformin (and More Commonly than in Patients Treated with Metformin Alone)

	Number (%) of Patients	
	ONGLYZA 5 mg + Metformin* N=320	Metformin* N=328
Headache	24 (7.5)	17 (5.2)
Nasopharyngitis	22 (6.9)	13 (4.0)

*Metformin was initiated at a starting dose of 500 mg daily and titrated up to a maximum of 2000 mg daily.

Hypoglycemia

Adverse reactions of hypoglycemia were based on all reports of hypoglycemia; a concurrent glucose measurement was not required. In the add-on to glyburide study, the overall incidence of reported hypoglycemia was higher for ONGLYZA 2.5 mg and ONGLYZA 5 mg (13.3% and 14.6%) versus placebo (10.1%). The incidence of confirmed hypoglycemia in this study, defined as symptoms of hypoglycemia accompanied by a fingerstick glucose value of ≤50 mg/dL, was 2.4% and 0.8% for ONGLYZA (saxagliptin) 2.5 mg and ONGLYZA 5 mg and 0.7% for placebo. The incidence of reported hypoglycemia for ONGLYZA 2.5 mg and ONGLYZA 5 mg versus placebo given as monotherapy was 4.0% and 5.6% versus 4.1%, respectively, 7.8% and 5.8% versus 5% given as add-on therapy to metformin, and 4.1% and 2.7% versus 3.8% given as add-on therapy to TZD. The incidence of reported hypoglycemia was 3.4% in treatment-naive patients given ONGLYZA 5 mg plus metformin and 4.0% in patients given metformin alone.

Hypersensitivity Reactions

Hypersensitivity-related events, such as urticaria and facial edema in the 5-study pooled analysis up to Week 24 were reported in 1.5%, 1.5%, and 0.4% of patients who received ONGLYZA 2.5 mg, ONGLYZA 5 mg, and placebo, respectively. None of these events in patients who received ONGLYZA required hospitalization or were reported as life-threatening by the investigators. One saxagliptin-treated patient in this pooled analysis discontinued due to generalized urticaria and facial edema.

Vital Signs

No clinically meaningful changes in vital signs have been observed in patients treated with ONGLYZA.

Laboratory Tests

Absolute Lymphocyte Counts

There was a dose-related mean decrease in absolute lymphocyte count observed with ONGLYZA. From a baseline mean absolute lymphocyte count of approximately 2200 cells/microL, mean decreases of approximately 100 and 120 cells/microL with ONGLYZA 5 mg and 10 mg, respectively, relative to placebo were observed at 24 weeks in a pooled analysis of five placebo-controlled clinical studies. Similar effects were observed when ONGLYZA 5 mg was given in initial combination with metformin compared to metformin alone. There was no difference observed for ONGLYZA 2.5 mg relative to placebo. The proportion of patients who were reported to have a lymphocyte count ≤750 cells/microL was 0.5%, 1.5%, 1.4%, and 0.4% in the saxagliptin 2.5 mg, 5 mg, 10 mg, and placebo groups, respectively. In most patients, recurrence was not observed with repeated exposure to ONGLYZA although some patients had recurrent decreases upon rechallenge that led to discontinuation of ONGLYZA. The decreases in lymphocyte count were not associated with clinically relevant adverse reactions.

The clinical significance of this decrease in lymphocyte count relative to placebo is not known. When clinically indicated, such as in settings of unusual or prolonged infection, lymphocyte count should be measured. The effect of ONGLYZA on lymphocyte counts in patients with lymphocyte abnormalities (e.g., human immunodeficiency virus) is unknown.

Platelets

ONGLYZA did not demonstrate a clinically meaningful or consistent effect on platelet count in the six, double-blind, controlled clinical safety and efficacy trials.

7 DRUG INTERACTIONS

7.1 Inducers of CYP3A4/5 Enzymes

Rifampin significantly decreased saxagliptin exposure with no change in the area under the time-concentration curve (AUC) of its active metabolite, 5-hydroxy saxagliptin. The plasma dipeptidyl peptidase-4 (DPP4) activity inhibition over a 24-hour dose interval was not affected by rifampin. Therefore, dosage adjustment of ONGLYZA is not recommended. [See *Clinical Pharmacology (12.3)*.]

7.2 Inhibitors of CYP3A4/5 Enzymes

Moderate Inhibitors of CYP3A4/5

Diltiazem increased the exposure of saxagliptin. Similar increases in plasma concentrations of saxagliptin are anticipated in the presence of other moderate CYP3A4/5 inhibitors (e.g., amprenavir, aprepitant, erythromycin, fluconazole, fosamprenavir, grapefruit juice, and verapamil); however, dosage adjustment of ONGLYZA is not recommended. [See *Clinical Pharmacology (12.3)*.]

Strong Inhibitors of CYP3A4/5

Ketoconazole significantly increased saxagliptin exposure. Similar significant increases in plasma concentrations of saxagliptin are anticipated with other strong CYP3A4/5 inhibitors (e.g., atazanavir, clarithromycin, indinavir, itraconazole, nefazodone, nelfinavir, ritonavir, saquinavir, and telithromycin). The dose of ONGLYZA should be limited to 2.5 mg when coadministered with a strong CYP3A4/5 inhibitor. [See *Dosage and Administration (2.3)* and *Clinical Pharmacology (12.3)*.]

8 USE IN SPECIFIC POPULATIONS

8.1 Pregnancy

Pregnancy Category B

There are no adequate and well-controlled studies in pregnant women. Because animal reproduction studies are not always predictive of human response, ONGLYZA, like other antidiabetic medications, should be used during pregnancy only if clearly needed.

Saxagliptin was not teratogenic at any dose tested when administered to pregnant rats and rabbits during periods of organogenesis. Incomplete ossification of the pelvis, a form of developmental delay, occurred in rats at a dose of 240 mg/kg, or approximately 1503 and 66 times human exposure to saxagliptin and the active metabolite, respectively, at the maximum recommended human dose (MRHD) of 5 mg. Maternal toxicity and reduced fetal body weights were observed at 7986 and 328 times the human exposure at the MRHD for saxagliptin and the active metabolite, respectively. Minor skeletal variations in rabbits occurred at a maternally toxic dose of 200 mg/kg, or approximately 1432 and 992 times the MRHD. When administered to rats in combination with metformin, saxagliptin was not teratogenic nor embryolethal at exposures 21 times the saxagliptin MRHD. Combination administration of metformin with a higher dose of saxagliptin (109 times the saxagliptin MRHD) was associated with craniorachischisis (a rare neural tube defect characterized by incomplete closure of the skull and spinal column) in two fetuses from a single dam. Metformin exposures in each combination were 4 times the human exposure of 2000 mg daily.

Saxagliptin administered to female rats from gestation day 6 to lactation day 20 resulted in decreased body weights in male and female offspring only at maternally toxic doses (exposures ≥1629 and 53 times saxagliptin and its active metabolite at the MRHD). No functional or behavioral toxicity was observed in offspring of rats administered saxagliptin at any dose.

Saxagliptin crosses the placenta into the fetus following dosing in pregnant rats.

8.3 Nursing Mothers

Saxagliptin is secreted in the milk of lactating rats at approximately a 1:1 ratio with plasma drug concentrations. It is not known whether saxagliptin is secreted in human milk. Because many drugs are secreted in human milk, caution should be exercised when ONGLYZA (saxagliptin) is administered to a nursing woman.

8.4 Pediatric Use

Safety and effectiveness of ONGLYZA in pediatric patients have not been established.

8.5 Geriatric Use

In the six, double-blind, controlled clinical safety and efficacy trials of ONGLYZA, 634 (15.3%) of the 4148 randomized patients were 65 years and over, and 59 (1.4%) patients were 75 years and over. No overall differences in safety or effectiveness were observed between patients ≥65 years old and the younger patients. While this clinical experience has not identified differences in responses between the elderly and younger patients, greater sensitivity of some older individuals cannot be ruled out.

Saxagliptin and its active metabolite are eliminated in part by the kidney. Because elderly patients are more likely to have decreased renal function, care should be taken in dose selection in the elderly based on renal function. [See *Dosage and Administration (2.2)* and *Clinical Pharmacology (12.3)*.]

10 OVERDOSAGE

In a controlled clinical trial, once-daily, orally-administered ONGLYZA in healthy subjects at doses up to 400 mg daily for 2 weeks (80 times the MRHD) had no dose-related clinical adverse reactions and no clinically meaningful effect on QTc interval or heart rate.

In the event of an overdose, appropriate supportive treatment should be initiated as dictated by the patient's clinical status. Saxagliptin and its active metabolite are removed by hemodialysis (23% of dose over 4 hours).

11 DESCRIPTION

Saxagliptin is an orally-active inhibitor of the DPP4 enzyme.

Saxagliptin monohydrate is described chemically as (1*S*,3*S*,5*S*)-2-[(2*S*)-2-Amino-2-(3-hydroxytricyclo[3.3.1.1^{3,7}]dec-1-yl)acetyl]-2-azabicyclo[3.1.0]hexane-3-carbonitrile, monohydrate or (1*S*,3*S*,5*S*)-2-[(2*S*)-2-Amino-2-(3-hydroxyadamantan-1-yl)acetyl]-2-azabicyclo[3.1.0]hexane-3-carbonitrile hydrate. The empirical formula is $C_{18}H_{25}N_3O_2 \cdot H_2O$ and the molecular weight is 333.43. The structural formula is:

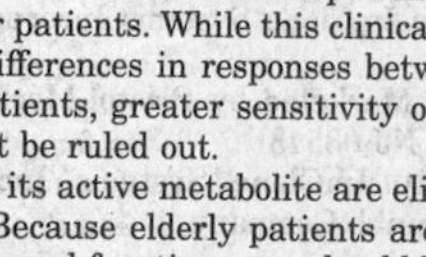

Saxagliptin monohydrate is a white to light yellow or light brown, non-hygroscopic, crystalline powder. It is sparingly soluble in water at 24°C ± 3°C, slightly soluble in ethyl acetate, and soluble in methanol, ethanol, isopropyl alcohol, acetonitrile, acetone, and polyethylene glycol 400 (PEG 400).

Each film-coated tablet of ONGLYZA for oral use contains either 2.79 mg saxagliptin hydrochloride (anhydrous) equivalent to 2.5 mg saxagliptin or 5.58 mg saxagliptin hydrochloride (anhydrous) equivalent to 5 mg saxagliptin and the following inactive ingredients: lactose monohydrate, microcrystalline cellulose, croscarmellose sodium, and magnesium stearate. In addition, the film coating contains the following inactive ingredients: polyvinyl alcohol, polyethylene glycol, titanium dioxide, talc, and iron oxides

12 CLINICAL PHARMACOLOGY

12.1 Mechanism of Action

Increased concentrations of the incretin hormones such as glucagon-like peptide-1 (GLP-1) and glucose-dependent insulinotropic polypeptide (GIP) are released into the bloodstream from the small intestine in response to meals. These hormones cause insulin release from the pancreatic beta cells in a glucose-dependent manner but are inactivated by the dipeptidyl peptidase-4 (DPP4) enzyme within minutes. GLP-1 also lowers glucagon secretion from pancreatic alpha cells, reducing hepatic glucose production. In patients with type 2 diabetes, concentrations of GLP-1 are reduced but the insulin response to GLP-1 is preserved. Saxagliptin is a competitive DPP4 inhibitor that slows the inactivation of the incretin hormones, thereby increasing their bloodstream concentrations and reducing fasting and postprandial glucose concentrations in a glucose-dependent manner in patients with type 2 diabetes mellitus.

12.2 Pharmacodynamics

In patients with type 2 diabetes mellitus, administration of ONGLYZA (saxagliptin) inhibits DPP4 enzyme activity for a 24-hour period. After an oral glucose load or a meal, this DPP4 inhibition resulted in a 2- to 3-fold increase in circulating levels of active GLP-1 and GIP, decreased glucagon concentrations, and increased glucose-dependent insulin secretion from pancreatic beta cells. The rise in insulin and decrease in glucagon were associated with lower fasting glucose concentrations and reduced glucose excursion following an oral glucose load or a meal.

Cardiac Electrophysiology

In a randomized, double-blind, placebo-controlled, 4-way crossover, active comparator study using moxifloxacin in 40 healthy subjects, ONGLYZA was not associated with clinically meaningful prolongation of the QTc interval or heart rate at daily doses up to 40 mg (8 times the MRHD).

12.3 Pharmacokinetics

The pharmacokinetics of saxagliptin and its active metabolite, 5-hydroxy saxagliptin were similar in healthy subjects and in patients with type 2 diabetes mellitus. The C_{max} and AUC values of saxagliptin and its active metabolite increased proportionally in the 2.5 to 400 mg dose range. Following a 5 mg single oral dose of saxagliptin to healthy subjects, the mean plasma AUC values for saxagliptin and its active metabolite were 78 ng•h/mL and 214 ng•h/mL, respectively. The corresponding plasma C_{max} values were 24 ng/mL and 47 ng/mL, respectively. The average variability (%CV) for AUC and C_{max} for both saxagliptin and its active metabolite was less than 25%.

No appreciable accumulation of either saxagliptin or its active metabolite was observed with repeated once-daily dosing at any dose level. No dose- and time-dependence were observed in the clearance of saxagliptin and its active metabolite over 14 days of once-daily dosing with saxagliptin at doses ranging from 2.5 to 400 mg.

Absorption

The median time to maximum concentration (T_{max}) following the 5 mg once daily dose was 2 hours for saxagliptin and 4 hours for its active metabolite. Administration with a high-fat meal resulted in an increase in T_{max} of saxagliptin by approximately 20 minutes as compared to fasted conditions. There was a 27% increase in the AUC of saxagliptin when given with a meal as compared to fasted conditions. ONGLYZA may be administered with or without food.

Distribution

The *in vitro* protein binding of saxagliptin and its active metabolite in human serum is negligible. Therefore, changes in blood protein levels in various disease states (e.g., renal or hepatic impairment) are not expected to alter the disposition of saxagliptin.

Metabolism

The metabolism of saxagliptin is primarily mediated by cytochrome P450 3A4/5 (CYP3A4/5). The major metabolite of saxagliptin is also a DPP4 inhibitor, which is one-half as potent as saxagliptin. Therefore, strong CYP3A4/5 inhibitors and inducers will alter the pharmacokinetics of saxagliptin and its active metabolite. [See *Drug Interactions (7)*.]

Excretion

Saxagliptin is eliminated by both renal and hepatic pathways. Following a single 50 mg dose of ^{14}C-saxagliptin, 24%, 36%, and 75% of the dose was excreted in the urine as saxagliptin, its active metabolite, and total radioactivity, respectively. The average renal clearance of saxagliptin (~230 mL/min) was greater than the average estimated glomerular filtration rate (~120 mL/min), suggesting some active renal excretion. A total of 22% of the administered radioactivity was recovered in feces representing the fraction of the saxagliptin dose excreted in bile and/or unabsorbed drug from the gastrointestinal tract. Following a single oral dose of ONGLYZA (saxagliptin) 5 mg to healthy subjects, the mean plasma terminal half-life ($t_{1/2}$) for saxagliptin and its active metabolite was 2.5 and 3.1 hours, respectively.

Specific Populations

Renal Impairment

A single-dose, open-label study was conducted to evaluate the pharmacokinetics of saxagliptin (10 mg dose) in subjects with varying degrees of chronic renal impairment (N=8 per group) compared to subjects with normal renal function. The study included patients with renal impairment classified on the basis of creatinine clearance as mild (>50 to ≤80 mL/min), moderate (30 to ≤50 mL/min), and severe (<30 mL/min), as well as patients with end-stage renal disease on hemodialysis. Creatinine clearance was estimated from serum creatinine based on the Cockcroft-Gault formula:

$$CrCl = \frac{[140 - \text{age (years)}] \times \text{weight (kg)} \; \{\times 0.85 \text{ for female patients}\}}{[72 \times \text{serum creatinine (mg/dL)}]}$$

The degree of renal impairment did not affect the C_{max} of saxagliptin or its active metabolite. In subjects with mild renal impairment, the AUC values of saxagliptin and its active metabolite were 20% and 70% higher, respectively, than AUC values in subjects with normal renal function. Because increases of this magnitude are not considered to be clinically relevant, dosage adjustment in patients with mild renal impairment is not recommended. In subjects with moderate or severe renal impairment, the AUC values of saxagliptin and its active metabolite were up to 2.1- and 4.5-fold higher, respectively, than AUC values in subjects with normal renal function. To achieve plasma exposures of saxagliptin and its active metabolite similar to those in patients with normal renal function, the recommended dose is 2.5 mg once daily in patients with moderate and severe renal impairment, as well as in patients with end-stage renal disease requiring hemodialysis. Saxagliptin is removed by hemodialysis.

Hepatic Impairment

In subjects with hepatic impairment (Child-Pugh classes A, B, and C), mean C_{max} and AUC of saxagliptin were up to 8% and 77% higher, respectively, compared to healthy matched controls following administration of a single 10 mg dose of saxagliptin. The corresponding C_{max} and AUC of the active metabolite were up to 59% and 33% lower, respectively, compared to healthy matched controls. These differences are not considered to be clinically meaningful. No dosage adjustment is recommended for patients with hepatic impairment.

Body Mass Index

No dosage adjustment is recommended based on body mass index (BMI) which was not identified as a significant covariate on the apparent clearance of saxagliptin or its active metabolite in the population pharmacokinetic analysis.

Gender

No dosage adjustment is recommended based on gender. There were no differences observed in saxagliptin pharmacokinetics between males and females. Compared to males, females had approximately 25% higher exposure values for the active metabolite than males, but this difference is unlikely to be of clinical relevance. Gender was not identified as a significant covariate on the apparent clearance of saxagliptin and its active metabolite in the population pharmacokinetic analysis.

Geriatric

No dosage adjustment is recommended based on age alone. Elderly subjects (65-80 years) had 23% and 59% higher geometric mean C_{max} and geometric mean AUC values, respectively, for saxagliptin than young subjects (18-40 years). Differences in active metabolite pharmacokinetics between elderly and young subjects generally reflected the differences observed in saxagliptin pharmacokinetics. The difference between the pharmacokinetics of saxagliptin and the active metabolite in young and elderly subjects is likely due to multiple factors including declining renal function and metabolic capacity with increasing age. Age was not identified as a significant covariate on the apparent clearance of saxagliptin and its active metabolite in the population pharmacokinetic analysis.

Pediatric

Studies characterizing the pharmacokinetics of saxagliptin in pediatric patients have not been performed.

Race and Ethnicity

No dosage adjustment is recommended based on race. The population pharmacokinetic analysis compared the pharmacokinetics of saxagliptin and its active metabolite in 309 Caucasian subjects with 105 non-Caucasian subjects (consisting of six racial groups). No significant difference in the pharmacokinetics of saxagliptin and its active metabolite were detected between these two populations.

Drug-Drug Interactions

In Vitro Assessment of Drug Interactions

The metabolism of saxagliptin is primarily mediated by CYP3A4/5.

In *in vitro* studies, saxagliptin and its active metabolite did not inhibit CYP1A2, 2A6, 2B6, 2C9, 2C19, 2D6, 2E1, or 3A4, or induce CYP1A2, 2B6, 2C9, or 3A4. Therefore, saxagliptin is not expected to alter the metabolic clearance of coadministered drugs that are metabolized by these enzymes. Saxagliptin is a P-glycoprotein (P-gp) substrate but is not a significant inhibitor or inducer of P-gp.

The *in vitro* protein binding of saxagliptin and its active metabolite in human serum is negligible. Thus, protein binding would not have a meaningful influence on the pharmacokinetics of saxagliptin or other drugs.

In Vivo Assessment of Drug Interactions

Effects of Saxagliptin on Other Drugs

In studies conducted in healthy subjects, as described below, saxagliptin did not meaningfully alter the pharmacokinetics of metformin, glyburide, pioglitazone, digoxin, simvastatin, diltiazem, or ketoconazole.

Metformin: Coadministration of a single dose of saxagliptin (100 mg) and metformin (1000 mg), an hOCT-2 substrate, did not alter the pharmacokinetics of metformin in healthy subjects. Therefore, ONGLYZA (saxagliptin) is not an inhibitor of hOCT-2-mediated transport.

Glyburide: Coadministration of a single dose of saxagliptin (10 mg) and glyburide (5 mg), a CYP2C9 substrate, increased the plasma C_{max} of glyburide by 16%; however, the AUC of glyburide was unchanged. Therefore, ONGLYZA does not meaningfully inhibit CYP2C9-mediated metabolism.

Pioglitazone: Coadministration of multiple once-daily doses of saxagliptin (10 mg) and pioglitazone (45 mg), a CYP2C8 substrate, increased the plasma C_{max} of pioglitazone by 14%; however, the AUC of pioglitazone was unchanged.

Digoxin: Coadministration of multiple once-daily doses of saxagliptin (10 mg) and digoxin (0.25 mg), a P-gp substrate, did not alter the pharmacokinetics of digoxin. Therefore, ONGLYZA is not an inhibitor or inducer of P-gp-mediated transport.

Simvastatin: Coadministration of multiple once-daily doses of saxagliptin (10 mg) and simvastatin (40 mg), a CYP3A4/5 substrate, did not alter the pharmacokinetics of simvastatin. Therefore, ONGLYZA is not an inhibitor or inducer of CYP3A4/5-mediated metabolism.

Diltiazem: Coadministration of multiple once-daily doses of saxagliptin (10 mg) and diltiazem (360 mg long-acting formulation at steady state), a moderate inhibitor of CYP3A4/5, increased the plasma C_{max} of diltiazem by 16%; however, the AUC of diltiazem was unchanged.

Ketoconazole: Coadministration of a single dose of saxagliptin (100 mg) and multiple doses of ketoconazole (200 mg every 12 hours at steady state), a strong inhibitor of CYP3A4/5 and P-gp, decreased the plasma C_{max} and AUC of ketoconazole by 16% and 13%, respectively.

Effects of Other Drugs on Saxagliptin

Metformin: Coadministration of a single dose of saxagliptin (100 mg) and metformin (1000 mg), an hOCT-2 substrate, decreased the C_{max} of saxagliptin by 21%; however, the AUC was unchanged.

Glyburide: Coadministration of a single dose of saxagliptin (10 mg) and glyburide (5 mg), a CYP2C9 substrate, increased the C_{max} of saxagliptin by 8%; however, the AUC of saxagliptin was unchanged.

Pioglitazone: Coadministration of multiple once-daily doses of saxagliptin (10 mg) and pioglitazone (45 mg), a CYP2C8 (major) and CYP3A4 (minor) substrate, did not alter the pharmacokinetics of saxagliptin.

Digoxin: Coadministration of multiple once-daily doses of saxagliptin (10 mg) and digoxin (0.25 mg), a P-gp substrate, did not alter the pharmacokinetics of saxagliptin.

Simvastatin: Coadministration of multiple once-daily doses of saxagliptin (10 mg) and simvastatin (40 mg), a CYP3A4/5 substrate, increased the C_{max} of saxagliptin by 21%; however, the AUC of saxagliptin was unchanged.

Diltiazem: Coadministration of a single dose of saxagliptin (10 mg) and diltiazem (360 mg long-acting formulation at steady state), a moderate inhibitor of CYP3A4/5, increased the C_{max} of saxagliptin by 63% and the AUC by 2.1-fold. This was associated with a corresponding decrease in the C_{max} and AUC of the active metabolite by 44% and 36%, respectively.

Ketoconazole: Coadministration of a single dose of saxagliptin (100 mg) and ketoconazole (200 mg every 12 hours at steady state), a strong inhibitor of CYP3A4/5 and P-gp, increased the C_{max} for saxagliptin by 62% and the AUC by 2.5-fold. This was associated with a corresponding decrease in the C_{max} and AUC of the active metabolite by 95% and 91%, respectively.

In another study, coadministration of a single dose of saxagliptin (20 mg) and ketoconazole (200 mg every 12 hours at steady state), increased the C_{max} and AUC of

Table 3: Glycemic Parameters at Week 24 in a Placebo-Controlled Study of ONGLYZA Monotherapy in Patients with Type 2 Diabetes*

Efficacy Parameter	ONGLYZA 2.5 mg N=102	ONGLYZA 5 mg N=106	Placebo N=95
Hemoglobin A1C (%)	N=100	N=103	N=92
Baseline (mean)	7.9	8.0	7.9
Change from baseline (adjusted mean[†])	−0.4	−0.5	+0.2
Difference from placebo (adjusted mean[†])	−0.6[‡]	−0.6[‡]	
95% Confidence Interval	(−0.9, −0.3)	(−0.9, −0.4)	
Percent of patients achieving A1C <7%	35% (35/100)	38%[§] (39/103)	24% (22/92)
Fasting Plasma Glucose (mg/dL)	N=101	N=105	N=92
Baseline (mean)	178	171	172
Change from baseline (adjusted mean[†])	−15	−9	+6
Difference from placebo (adjusted mean[†])	−21[§]	−15[§]	
95% Confidence Interval	(−31, −10)	(−25, −4)	
2-hour Postprandial Glucose (mg/dL)	N=78	N=84	N=71
Baseline (mean)	279	278	283
Change from baseline (adjusted mean[†])	−45	−43	−6
Difference from placebo (adjusted mean[†])	−39[¶]	−37[§]	
95% Confidence Interval	(−61, −16)	(−59, −15)	

* Intent-to-treat population using last observation on study or last observation prior to metformin rescue therapy for patients needing rescue.
† Least squares mean adjusted for baseline value.
‡ p-value <0.0001 compared to placebo
§ p-value <0.05 compared to placebo
¶ Significance was not tested for the 2-hour PPG for the 2.5 mg dose of ONGLYZA.

saxagliptin by 2.4-fold and 3.7-fold, respectively. This was associated with a corresponding decrease in the C_{max} and AUC of the active metabolite by 96% and 90%, respectively.
Rifampin: Coadministration of a single dose of saxagliptin (5 mg) and rifampin (600 mg QD at steady state) decreased the C_{max} and AUC of saxagliptin by 53% and 76%, respectively, with a corresponding increase in C_{max} (39%) but no significant change in the plasma AUC of the active metabolite.
Omeprazole: Coadministration of multiple once-daily doses of saxagliptin (10 mg) and omeprazole (40 mg), a CYP2C19 (major) and CYP3A4 substrate, an inhibitor of CYP2C19, and an inducer of MRP-3, did not alter the pharmacokinetics of saxagliptin.
Aluminum hydroxide + magnesium hydroxide + simethicone: Coadministration of a single dose of saxagliptin (10 mg) and a liquid containing aluminum hydroxide (2400 mg), magnesium hydroxide (2400 mg), and simethicone (240 mg) decreased the C_{max} of saxagliptin by 26%; however, the AUC of saxagliptin was unchanged.
Famotidine: Administration of a single dose of saxagliptin (10 mg) 3 hours after a single dose of famotidine (40 mg), an inhibitor of hOCT-1, hOCT-2, and hOCT-3, increased the C_{max} of saxagliptin by 14%; however, the AUC of saxagliptin was unchanged.

13 NONCLINICAL TOXICOLOGY

13.1 Carcinogenesis, Mutagenesis, Impairment of Fertility

Saxagliptin did not induce tumors in either mice (50, 250, and 600 mg/kg) or rats (25, 75, 150, and 300 mg/kg) at the highest doses evaluated. The highest doses evaluated in mice were equivalent to approximately 870 (males) and 1165 (females) times the human exposure at the MRHD of 5 mg/day. In rats, exposures were approximately 355 (males) and 2217 (females) times the MRHD.
Saxagliptin was not mutagenic or clastogenic with or without metabolic activation in an *in vitro* Ames bacterial assay, an *in vitro* cytogenetics assay in primary human lymphocytes, an *in vivo* oral micronucleus assay in rats, an *in vivo* oral DNA repair study in rats, and an oral *in vivo/in vitro* cytogenetics study in rat peripheral blood lymphocytes. The active metabolite was not mutagenic in an *in vitro* Ames bacterial assay.
In a rat fertility study, males were treated with oral gavage doses for 2 weeks prior to mating, during mating, and up to scheduled termination (approximately 4 weeks total) and females were treated with oral gavage doses for 2 weeks prior to mating through gestation day 7. No adverse effects on fertility were observed at exposures of approximately 603 (males) and 776 (females) times the MRHD. Higher doses that elicited maternal toxicity also increased fetal resorptions (approximately 2069 and 6138 times the MRHD). Additional effects on estrous cycling, fertility, ovulation, and implantation were observed at approximately 6138 times the MRHD.

13.2 Animal Toxicology

Saxagliptin produced adverse skin changes in the extremities of cynomolgus monkeys (scabs and/or ulceration of tail, digits, scrotum, and/or nose). Skin lesions were reversible at ≥20 times the MRHD but in some cases were irreversible

and necrotizing at higher exposures. Adverse skin changes were not observed at exposures similar to (1 to 3 times) the MRHD of 5 mg. Clinical correlates to skin lesions in monkeys have not been observed in human clinical trials of saxagliptin.

14 CLINICAL STUDIES

ONGLYZA has been studied as monotherapy and in combination with metformin, glyburide, and thiazolidinedione (pioglitazone and rosiglitazone) therapy. ONGLYZA (saxagliptin) has not been studied in combination with insulin.
A total of 4148 patients with type 2 diabetes mellitus were randomized in six, double-blind, controlled clinical trials conducted to evaluate the safety and glycemic efficacy of ONGLYZA. A total of 3021 patients in these trials were treated with ONGLYZA. In these trials, the mean age was 54 years, and 71% of patients were Caucasian, 16% were Asian, 4% were black, and 9% were of other racial groups. An additional 423 patients, including 315 who received ONGLYZA, participated in a placebo-controlled, dose-ranging study of 6 to 12 weeks in duration.
In these six, double-blind trials, ONGLYZA was evaluated at doses of 2.5 mg and 5 mg once daily. Three of these trials also evaluated a saxagliptin dose of 10 mg daily. The 10 mg daily dose of saxagliptin did not provide greater efficacy than the 5 mg daily dose. Treatment with ONGLYZA at all doses produced clinically relevant and statistically significant improvements in hemoglobin A1c (A1C), fasting plasma glucose (FPG), and 2-hour postprandial glucose (PPG) following a standard oral glucose tolerance test (OGTT), compared to control. Reductions in A1C were seen across subgroups including gender, age, race, and baseline BMI.
ONGLYZA was not associated with significant changes from baseline in body weight or fasting serum lipids compared to placebo.

14.1 Monotherapy

A total of 766 patients with type 2 diabetes inadequately controlled on diet and exercise (A1C ≥7% to ≤10%) participated in two 24-week, double-blind, placebo-controlled trials evaluating the efficacy and safety of ONGLYZA monotherapy.
In the first trial, following a 2-week single-blind diet, exercise, and placebo lead-in period, 401 patients were randomized to 2.5 mg, 5 mg, or 10 mg of ONGLYZA or placebo. Patients who failed to meet specific glycemic goals during the study were treated with metformin rescue therapy, added on to placebo or ONGLYZA. Efficacy was evaluated at the last measurement prior to rescue therapy for patients needing rescue. Dose titration of ONGLYZA was not permitted.
Treatment with ONGLYZA 2.5 mg and 5 mg daily provided significant improvements in A1C, FPG, and PPG compared to placebo (Table 3). The percentage of patients who discontinued for lack of glycemic control or who were rescued for meeting prespecified glycemic criteria was 16% in the ONGLYZA 2.5 mg treatment group, 20% in the ONGLYZA 5 mg treatment group, and 26% in the placebo group.
[See table 3 above]
A second 24-week monotherapy trial was conducted to assess a range of dosing regimens for ONGLYZA. Treatment-

naive patients with inadequately controlled diabetes (A1C ≥7% to ≤10%) underwent a 2-week, single-blind diet, exercise, and placebo lead-in period. A total of 365 patients were randomized to 2.5 mg every morning, 5 mg every morning, 2.5 mg with possible titration to 5 mg every morning, or 5 mg every evening of ONGLYZA (saxagliptin), or placebo. Patients who failed to meet specific glycemic goals during the study were treated with metformin rescue therapy added on to placebo or ONGLYZA; the number of patients randomized per treatment group ranged from 71 to 74.
Treatment with either ONGLYZA 5 mg every morning or 5 mg every evening provided significant improvements in A1C versus placebo (mean placebo-corrected reductions of −0.4% and −0.3%, respectively). Treatment with ONGLYZA 2.5 mg every morning also provided significant improvement in A1C versus placebo (mean placebo-corrected reduction of −0.4%).

14.2 Combination Therapy

Add-On Combination Therapy with Metformin

A total of 743 patients with type 2 diabetes participated in this 24-week, randomized, double-blind, placebo-controlled trial to evaluate the efficacy and safety of ONGLYZA in combination with metformin in patients with inadequate glycemic control (A1C ≥7% and ≤10%) on metformin alone. To qualify for enrollment, patients were required to be on a stable dose of metformin (1500-2550 mg daily) for at least 8 weeks.
Patients who met eligibility criteria were enrolled in a single-blind, 2-week, dietary and exercise placebo lead-in period during which patients received metformin at their pre-study dose, up to 2500 mg daily, for the duration of the study. Following the lead-in period, eligible patients were randomized to 2.5 mg, 5 mg, or 10 mg of ONGLYZA or placebo in addition to their current dose of open-label metformin. Patients who failed to meet specific glycemic goals during the study were treated with pioglitazone rescue therapy, added on to existing study medications. Dose titrations of ONGLYZA and metformin were not permitted. ONGLYZA 2.5 mg and 5 mg add-on to metformin provided significant improvements in A1C, FPG, and PPG compared with placebo add-on to metformin (Table 4). Mean changes from baseline for A1C over time and at endpoint are shown in Figure 1. The proportion of patients who discontinued for lack of glycemic control or who were rescued for meeting prespecified glycemic criteria was 15% in the ONGLYZA 2.5 mg add-on to metformin group, 13% in the ONGLYZA 5 mg add-on to metformin group, and 27% in the placebo add-on to metformin group.
[See table 4 at top of next page]

Figure 1: Mean Change from Baseline in A1C in a Placebo-Controlled Trial of ONGLYZA as Add-On Combination Therapy with Metformin*

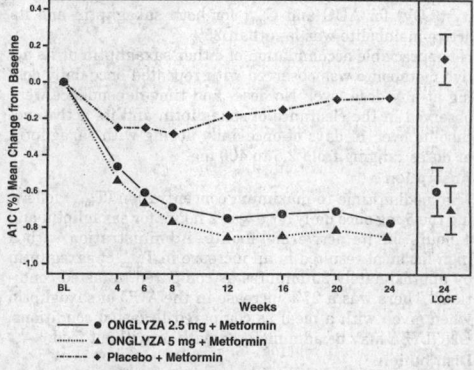

* Includes patients with a baseline and week 24 value.
Week 24 (LOCF) includes intent-to-treat population using last observation on study prior to pioglitazone rescue therapy for patients needing rescue. Mean change from baseline is adjusted for baseline value.

Add-On Combination Therapy with a Thiazolidinedione

A total of 565 patients with type 2 diabetes participated in this 24-week, randomized, double-blind, placebo-controlled trial to evaluate the efficacy and safety of ONGLYZA in combination with a thiazolidinedione (TZD) in patients with inadequate glycemic control (A1C ≥7% to ≤10.5%) on TZD alone. To qualify for enrollment, patients were required to be on a stable dose of pioglitazone (30-45 mg once daily) or rosiglitazone (4 mg once daily or 8 mg either once daily or in two divided doses of 4 mg) for at least 12 weeks.
Patients who met eligibility criteria were enrolled in a single-blind, 2-week, dietary and exercise placebo lead-in period during which patients received TZD at their pre-study dose for the duration of the study. Following the lead-in period, eligible patients were randomized to 2.5 mg or 5 mg of ONGLYZA or placebo in addition to their current dose of TZD. Patients who failed to meet specific glycemic

goals during the study were treated with metformin rescue, added on to existing study medications. Dose titration of ONGLYZA (saxagliptin) or TZD was not permitted during the study. A change in TZD regimen from rosiglitazone to pioglitazone at specified, equivalent therapeutic doses was permitted at the investigator's discretion if believed to be medically appropriate.

ONGLYZA 2.5 mg and 5 mg add-on to TZD provided significant improvements in A1C, FPG, and PPG compared with placebo add-on to TZD (Table 5). The proportion of patients who discontinued for lack of glycemic control or who were rescued for meeting prespecified glycemic criteria was 10% in the ONGLYZA 2.5 mg add-on to TZD group, 6% for the ONGLYZA 5 mg add-on to TZD group, and 10% in the placebo add-on to TZD group.

[See table 5 at right]

Add-On Combination Therapy with Glyburide

A total of 768 patients with type 2 diabetes participated in this 24-week, randomized, double-blind, placebo-controlled trial to evaluate the efficacy and safety of ONGLYZA in combination with a sulfonylurea (SU) in patients with inadequate glycemic control at enrollment (A1C ≥7.5% to ≤10%) on a submaximal dose of SU alone. To qualify for enrollment, patients were required to be on a submaximal dose of SU for 2 months or greater. In this study, ONGLYZA in combination with a fixed, intermediate dose of SU was compared to titration to a higher dose of SU.

Patients who met eligibility criteria were enrolled in a single-blind, 4-week, dietary and exercise lead-in period, and placed on glyburide 7.5 mg once daily. Following the lead-in period, eligible patients with A1C ≥7% to ≤10% were randomized to either 2.5 mg or 5 mg of ONGLYZA add-on to 7.5 mg glyburide or to placebo plus a 10 mg total daily dose of glyburide. Patients who received placebo were eligible to have glyburide up-titrated to a total daily dose of 15 mg. Up-titration of glyburide was not permitted in patients who received ONGLYZA 2.5 mg or 5 mg. Glyburide could be down-titrated in any treatment group once during the 24-week study period due to hypoglycemia as deemed necessary by the investigator. Approximately 92% of patients in the placebo plus glyburide group were up-titrated to a final total daily dose of 15 mg during the first 4 weeks of the study period. Patients who failed to meet specific glycemic goals during the study were treated with metformin rescue, added on to existing study medication. Dose titration of ONGLYZA was not permitted during the study.

In combination with glyburide, ONGLYZA 2.5 mg and 5 mg provided significant improvements in A1C, FPG, and PPG compared with the placebo plus up-titrated glyburide group (Table 6). The proportion of patients who discontinued for lack of glycemic control or who were rescued for meeting prespecified glycemic criteria was 18% in the ONGLYZA 2.5 mg add-on to glyburide group, 17% in the ONGLYZA 5 mg add-on to glyburide group, and 30% in the placebo plus up-titrated glyburide group.

[See table 6 at top of next page]

Coadministration with Metformin in Treatment-Naive Patients

A total of 1306 treatment-naive patients with type 2 diabetes mellitus participated in this 24-week, randomized, double-blind, placebo-controlled trial to evaluate the efficacy and safety of ONGLYZA coadministered with metformin in patients with inadequate glycemic control (A1C ≥8% to ≤12%) on diet and exercise alone. Patients were required to be treatment-naive to be enrolled in this study.

Patients who met eligibility criteria were enrolled in a single-blind, 1-week, dietary and exercise placebo lead-in period. Patients were randomized to one of four treatment arms: ONGLYZA 5 mg + metformin 500 mg, saxagliptin 10 mg + metformin 500 mg, saxagliptin 10 mg + placebo, or metformin 500 mg + placebo. ONGLYZA was dosed once daily. In the 3 treatment groups using metformin, the metformin dose was up-titrated weekly in 500 mg per day increments, as tolerated, to a maximum of 2000 mg per day based on FPG. Patients who failed to meet specific glycemic goals during the studies were treated with pioglitazone rescue as add-on therapy.

Coadministration of ONGLYZA 5 mg plus metformin provided significant improvements in A1C, FPG, and PPG compared with placebo plus metformin (Table 7).

[See table 7 on next page]

16   HOW SUPPLIED/STORAGE AND HANDLING

How Supplied

ONGLYZA™ (saxagliptin) tablets have markings on both sides and are available in the strengths and packages listed in Table 8.

[See table 8 on next page]

Storage and Handling

Store at 20°-25°C (68°-77°F); excursions permitted to 15°-30°C (59°-86°F) [see USP Controlled Room Temperature].

Table 4: Glycemic Parameters at Week 24 in a Placebo-Controlled Study of ONGLYZA as Add-On Combination Therapy with Metformin*

Efficacy Parameter	ONGLYZA 2.5 mg + Metformin N=192	ONGLYZA 5 mg + Metformin N=191	Placebo + Metformin N=179
Hemoglobin A1C (%)	N=186	N=186	N=175
Baseline (mean)	8.1	8.1	8.1
Change from baseline (adjusted mean†)	−0.6	−0.7	+0.1
Difference from placebo (adjusted mean†)	−0.7‡	−0.8‡	
95% Confidence Interval	(−0.9, −0.5)	(−1.0, −0.6)	
Percent of patients achieving A1C <7%	37%§ (69/186)	44%§ (81/186)	17% (29/175)
Fasting Plasma Glucose (mg/dL)	N=188	N=187	N=176
Baseline (mean)	174	179	175
Change from baseline (adjusted mean†)	−14	−22	+1
Difference from placebo (adjusted mean†)	−16§	−23§	
95% Confidence Interval	(−23, −9)	(−30, −16)	
2-hour Postprandial Glucose (mg/dL)	N=155	N=155	N=135
Baseline (mean)	294	296	295
Change from baseline (adjusted mean†)	−62	−58	−18
Difference from placebo (adjusted mean†)	−44§	−40§	
95% Confidence Interval	(−60, −27)	(−56, −24)	

* Intent-to-treat population using last observation on study or last observation prior to pioglitazone rescue therapy for patients needing rescue.
† Least squares mean adjusted for baseline value.
‡ p-value <0.0001 compared to placebo + metformin
§ p-value <0.05 compared to placebo + metformin

Table 5: Glycemic Parameters at Week 24 in a Placebo-Controlled Study of ONGLYZA as Add-On Combination Therapy with a Thiazolidinedione*

Efficacy Parameter	ONGLYZA 2.5 mg + TZD N=195	ONGLYZA 5 mg + TZD N=186	Placebo + TZD N=184
Hemoglobin A1C (%)	N=192	N=183	N=180
Baseline (mean)	8.3	8.4	8.2
Change from baseline (adjusted mean†)	−0.7	−0.9	−0.3
Difference from placebo (adjusted mean†)	−0.4§	−0.6‡	
95% Confidence Interval	(−0.6, −0.2)	(−0.8, −0.4)	
Percent of patients achieving A1C <7%	42%§ (81/192)	42%§ (77/184)	26% (46/180)
Fasting Plasma Glucose (mg/dL)	N=193	N=185	N=181
Baseline (mean)	163	160	162
Change from baseline (adjusted mean†)	−14	−17	−3
Difference from placebo (adjusted mean†)	−12§	−15§	
95% Confidence Interval	(−20, −3)	(−23, −6)	
2-hour Postprandial Glucose (mg/dL)	N=156	N=134	N=127
Baseline (mean)	296	303	291
Change from baseline (adjusted mean†)	−55	−65	−15
Difference from placebo (adjusted mean†)	−40§	−50§	
95% Confidence Interval	(−56, −24)	(−66, −34)	

* Intent-to-treat population using last observation on study or last observation prior to metformin rescue therapy for patients needing rescue.
† Least squares mean adjusted for baseline value.
‡ p-value <0.0001 compared to placebo p-value + TZD
§ p-value <0.05 compared to placebo + TZD

---

17   PATIENT COUNSELING INFORMATION

See FDA-approved patient labeling.

17.1   Instructions

Patients should be informed of the potential risks and benefits of ONGLYZA (saxagliptin) and of alternative modes of therapy. Patients should also be informed about the importance of adherence to dietary instructions, regular physical activity, periodic blood glucose monitoring and A1C testing, recognition and management of hypoglycemia and hyperglycemia, and assessment of diabetes complications. During periods of stress such as fever, trauma, infection, or surgery, medication requirements may change and patients should be advised to seek medical advice promptly.

Physicians should instruct their patients to read the Patient Package Insert before starting ONGLYZA therapy and to re-read it each time the prescription is renewed. Patients should be instructed to inform their doctor or pharmacist if they develop any unusual symptom or if any existing symptom persists or worsens.

17.2   Laboratory Tests

Patients should be informed that response to all diabetic therapies should be monitored by periodic measurements of blood glucose and A1C, with a goal of decreasing these levels toward the normal range. A1C is especially useful for evaluating long-term glycemic control. Patients should be informed of the potential need to adjust their dose based on changes in renal function tests over time.

Manufactured by:
Bristol-Myers Squibb Company
Princeton, NJ 08543 USA
Marketed by:
Bristol-Myers Squibb Company
Princeton, NJ 08543
and
AstraZeneca Pharmaceuticals LP
Wilmington, DE 19850
1256316 1256317 SA-B0001-07-09   Iss July 2009

PATIENT INFORMATION
ONGLYZA (on-GLY-zah)
(saxagliptin)
tablets

Read the Patient Information that comes with ONGLYZA (saxagliptin) before you start taking it and each time you get a refill. There may be new information. This patient leaflet does not take the place of talking with your healthcare provider about your medical condition or treatment.

What is ONGLYZA?

ONGLYZA is a prescription medicine used with diet and exercise to control high blood sugar (hyperglycemia) in adults with type 2 diabetes.

ONGLYZA (saxagliptin) lowers blood sugar by helping the body increase the level of insulin after meals.

ONGLYZA is unlikely to cause your blood sugar to be lowered to a dangerous level (hypoglycemia) because it does not work well when your blood sugar is low.

ONGLYZA has not been studied in children younger than 18 years old.

What should I tell my healthcare provider before taking ONGLYZA?

Before you take ONGLYZA, tell your healthcare provider about all of your medical conditions, including if you:

- have type 1 diabetes. ONGLYZA should not be used to treat people with type 1 diabetes.
- have a history or risk for diabetic ketoacidosis (high levels of certain acids, known as ketones, in the blood or urine). ONGLYZA should not be used for the treatment of diabetic ketoacidosis.
- have kidney problems.
- are taking insulin. ONGLYZA has not been studied with insulin.
- are pregnant or plan to become pregnant. It is not known if ONGLYZA will harm your unborn baby. If you are pregnant, talk with your healthcare provider about the best way to control your blood sugar while you are pregnant.
- are breast-feeding or plan to breast-feed. ONGLYZA may be passed in your milk to your baby. Talk with your healthcare provider about the best way to feed your baby while you take ONGLYZA.

Tell your healthcare provider about all the medicines you take, including prescription and nonprescription medicines, vitamins, and herbal supplements. Know the medicines you take. Keep a list of your medicines and show it to your healthcare provider and pharmacist when you get a new medicine.

ONGLYZA may affect the way other medicines work, and other medicines may affect how ONGLYZA works. Contact your healthcare provider if you will be starting or stopping certain other types of medications, such as antibiotics, or medicines that treat fungus or HIV/AIDS, because your dose of ONGLYZA might need to be changed.

How should I take ONGLYZA?

- Take ONGLYZA by mouth one time each day exactly as directed by your healthcare provider. Do not change your dose without talking to your healthcare provider.
- ONGLYZA can be taken with or without food.
- During periods of stress on the body, such as:
  - fever
  - trauma
  - infection
  - surgery

  Contact your healthcare provider right away as your medication needs may change.
- Your healthcare provider should test your blood to measure how well your kidneys work. You may need a lower dose of ONGLYZA if your kidneys are not working well.
- Your healthcare provider may prescribe ONGLYZA along with other medicines that lower blood sugar.
- Follow your healthcare provider's instructions for treating blood sugar that is too low (hypoglycemia). Talk to your healthcare provider if low blood sugar is a problem for you.
- If you miss a dose of ONGLYZA, take it as soon as you remember. If it is almost time for your next dose, skip the missed dose. Just take the next dose at your regular time. Do not take two doses at the same time unless your healthcare provider tells you to do so. Talk to your healthcare provider if you have questions about a missed dose.
- If you take too much ONGLYZA, call your healthcare provider or Poison Control Center at 1-800-222-1222, or go to the nearest hospital emergency room right away.

What are the possible side effects of ONGLYZA?

Common side effects of ONGLYZA include:

- upper respiratory tract infection
- urinary tract infection
- headache

Low blood sugar (hypoglycemia) may become worse in people who already take another medication to treat diabetes, such as sulfonylureas. Tell your healthcare provider if you take other diabetes medicines. If you have symptoms of low blood sugar, you should check your blood sugar and treat if low, then call your healthcare provider. Symptoms of low blood sugar include:

- shaking
- sweating
- rapid heartbeat
- change in vision
- hunger
- headache
- change in mood

Swelling or fluid retention in your hands, feet, or ankles (peripheral edema) may become worse in people who also take a thiazolidinedione to treat diabetes. If you do not know whether you are already on this type of medication, ask your healthcare provider.

Table 6: Glycemic Parameters at Week 24 in a Placebo-Controlled Study of ONGLYZA as Add-On Combination Therapy with Glyburide*

Efficacy Parameter	ONGLYZA 2.5 mg + Glyburide 7.5 mg N=248	ONGLYZA 5 mg + Glyburide 7.5 mg N=253	Placebo + Up-Titrated Glyburide N=267
Hemoglobin A1C (%)	N=246	N=250	N=264
Baseline (mean)	8.4	8.5	8.4
Change from baseline (adjusted mean[†])	−0.5	−0.6	[‡]+0.1
Difference from up-titrated glyburide (adjusted mean[†])	−0.6[‡]	−0.7[‡]	
95% Confidence Interval	(−0.8, −0.5)	(−0.9, −0.6)	
Percent of patients achieving A1C <7%	22%[§] (55/246)	23%[§] (57/250)	9% (24/264)
Fasting Plasma Glucose (mg/dL)	N=247	N=252	N=265
Baseline (mean)	170	175	174
Change from baseline (adjusted mean[†])	−7	−10	+1
Difference from up-titrated glyburide (adjusted mean[†])	−8[§]	−10[§]	
95% Confidence Interval	(−14, −1)	(−17, −4)	
2-hour Postprandial Glucose (mg/dL)	N=195	N=202	N=206
Baseline (mean)	309	315	323
Change from baseline (adjusted mean[†])	−31	−34	+8
Difference from up-titrated glyburide (adjusted mean[†])	−38[§]	−42[§]	
95% Confidence Interval	(−50, −27)	(−53, −31)	

* Intent-to-treat population using last observation on study or last observation prior to metformin rescue therapy for patients needing rescue.
† Least squares mean adjusted for baseline value.
‡ p-value <0.0001 compared to placebo + up-titrated glyburide
§ p-value <0.05 compared to placebo + up-titrated glyburide

Table 7: Glycemic Parameters at Week 24 in a Placebo-Controlled Trial of ONGLYZA Coadministration with Metformin in Treatment-Naive Patients*

Efficacy Parameter	ONGLYZA 5 mg + Metformin N=320	Placebo + Metformin N=328
Hemoglobin A1C (%)	N=306	N=313
Baseline (mean)	9.4	9.4
Change from baseline (adjusted mean[†])	−2.5	−2.0
Difference from placebo + metformin (adjusted mean[†])	−0.5[‡]	
95% Confidence Interval	(−0.7, −0.4)	
Percent of patients achieving A1C <7%	60%[§] (185/307)	41% (129/314)
Fasting Plasma Glucose (mg/dL)	N=315	N=320
Baseline (mean)	199	199
Change from baseline (adjusted mean[†])	−60	−47
Difference from placebo + metformin (adjusted mean[†])	−13[§]	
95% Confidence Interval	(−19, −6)	
2-hour Postprandial Glucose (mg/dL)	N=146	N=141
Baseline (mean)	340	355
Change from baseline (adjusted mean[†])	−138	−97
Difference from placebo + metformin (adjusted mean[†])	−41[§]	
95% Confidence Interval	(−57, −25)	

* Intent-to-treat population using last observation on study or last observation prior to pioglitazone rescue therapy for patients needing rescue.
† Least squares mean adjusted for baseline value.
‡ p-value <0.0001 compared to placebo + metformin
§ p-value <0.05 compared to placebo + metformin

Table 8: ONGLYZA Tablet Presentations

Tablet Strength	Film-Coated Tablet Color/Shape	Tablet Markings	Package Size	NDC Code
5 mg	pink biconvex, round	"5" on one side and "4215" on the reverse, in blue ink	Bottles of 30 Bottles of 90 Bottles of 500 Blister of 100	0003-4215-11 0003-4215-21 0003-4215-31 0003-4215-41
2.5 mg	pale yellow to light yellow biconvex, round	"2.5" on one side and "4214" on the reverse, in blue ink	Bottles of 30 Bottles of 90	0003-4214-11 0003-4214-21

Allergic (hypersensitivity) reactions, such as rash, hives, and swelling of the face, lips, and throat. If you have these symptoms, stop taking ONGLYZA (saxagliptin) and call your healthcare provider right away.

These are not all of the possible side effects of ONGLYZA (saxagliptin). Tell your healthcare provider if you have any side effects that bother you or that do not go away. For more information, ask your healthcare provider.

IMPORTANT NOTICE: Updated drug information is sent bi-monthly via the PDR® Update Insert. For *monthly* email updates, register at PDR.net.

Call your healthcare provider for medical advice about side effects. You may report side effects to the FDA at 1-800-FDA-1088.

How should I store ONGLYZA (saxagliptin)?
Store ONGLYZA between 68° to 77°F (20° to 25°C).

Keep ONGLYZA and all medicines out of the reach of children.

General information about the use of ONGLYZA
Medicines are sometimes prescribed for conditions that are not mentioned in patient leaflets. Do not use ONGLYZA for a condition for which it was not prescribed. Do not give ONGLYZA to other people, even if they have the same symptoms you have. It may harm them.

This patient leaflet summarizes the most important information about ONGLYZA. If you would like to know more information about ONGLYZA, talk with your healthcare provider. You can ask your healthcare provider for additional information about ONGLYZA that is written for healthcare professionals. For more information, go to www.ONGLYZA.com or call 1-800-ONGLYZA.

What are the ingredients of ONGLYZA?
Active ingredient: saxagliptin
Inactive ingredients: lactose monohydrate, microcrystalline cellulose, croscarmellose sodium, and magnesium stearate. In addition, the film coating contains the following inactive ingredients: polyvinyl alcohol, polyethylene glycol, titanium dioxide, talc, and iron oxides.

What is type 2 diabetes?
Type 2 diabetes is a condition in which your body does not make enough insulin, and the insulin that your body produces does not work as well as it should. Your body can also make too much sugar. When this happens, sugar (glucose) builds up in the blood. This can lead to serious medical problems.
The main goal of treating diabetes is to lower your blood sugar to a normal level.
High blood sugar can be lowered by diet and exercise, and by certain medicines when necessary.
ONGLYZA (saxagliptin) tablets
Manufactured by:
Bristol-Myers Squibb Company
Princeton, NJ 08543 USA
Marketed by:
Bristol-Myers Squibb Company
Princeton, NJ 08543
and
AstraZeneca Pharmaceuticals LP
Wilmington, DE 19850
1256316   1256317   SA-B0001-07-09   Iss July 2009
Shown in Product Identification Guide, page 321

ORENCIA®   ℞
[oh-REN-see-ah]
(abatacept)
Lyophilized Powder for Intravenous Infusion

HIGHLIGHTS OF PRESCRIBING INFORMATION
These highlights do not include all the information needed to use ORENCIA safely and effectively. See full prescribing information for ORENCIA.
ORENCIA (abatacept)
Lyophilized Powder for Intravenous Infusion
Initial U.S. Approval: 2005

————————INDICATIONS AND USAGE————————
ORENCIA is a selective T cell costimulation modulator indicated for:
Adult Rheumatoid Arthritis (RA) (1.1)
• moderately to severely active RA in adults. ORENCIA may be used as monotherapy or concomitantly with DMARDs other than TNF antagonists (1.1).
Juvenile Idiopathic Arthritis (1.2)
• moderately to severely active polyarticular juvenile idiopathic arthritis in pediatric patients 6 years of age and older. ORENCIA may be used as monotherapy or concomitantly with MTX (1.2).
Important Limitations of Use (1.3)
• should not be given concomitantly with TNF antagonists (1.3, 5.1).

————————DOSAGE AND ADMINISTRATION————————
Adult RA (2.1)

Body Weight of Patient	Dose	Number of Vials
<60 kg	500 mg	2
60 to 100 kg	750 mg	3
>100 kg	1000 mg	4

Juvenile Idiopathic Arthritis (2.2)
• Pediatric patients weighing less than 75 kg receive 10 mg/kg based on the patient's body weight. Pediatric pa-

---

tients weighing 75 kg or more should be administered ORENCIA (abatacept) following the adult dosing regimen, not to exceed a maximum dose of 1000 mg (2.2).
General Dosing Information (2)
• Administer as a 30-minute intravenous infusion (2)
• Following initial dose, give at 2 and 4 weeks, then every 4 weeks (2)
• Prepare ORENCIA using only the silicone-free disposable syringe (2.3)

————————DOSAGE FORMS AND STRENGTHS————————
• 250 mg single-use vial (3)

————————CONTRAINDICATIONS————————
• None (4)

————————WARNINGS AND PRECAUTIONS————————
• Concomitant use with a TNF antagonist can increase the risk of infections and serious infections (5.1)
• Hypersensitivity, anaphylaxis, and anaphylactoid reactions (5.2)
• Patients with a history of recurrent infections or underlying conditions predisposing to infections may experience more infections (5.3, 8.5)
• Discontinue if a serious infection develops (5.3)
• Screen for latent TB infection prior to initiating therapy. Patients testing positive should be treated prior to initiating ORENCIA (5.3)
• Live vaccines should not be given concurrently or within 3 months of discontinuation (5.4)
• Patients with juvenile idiopathic arthritis should be brought up to date with all immunizations prior to ORENCIA therapy (5.4)
• Based on its mechanism of action, ORENCIA may blunt the effectiveness of some immunizations (5.4)
• COPD patients may develop more frequent respiratory adverse events (5.5)

————————ADVERSE REACTIONS————————
Most common adverse events (≥10%) are headache, upper respiratory tract infection, nasopharyngitis, and nausea (6.1).

To report SUSPECTED ADVERSE REACTIONS, contact Bristol-Myers Squibb at 1-800-721-5072 or FDA at 1-800-FDA-1088 or www.fda.gov/medwatch

————————USE IN SPECIFIC POPULATIONS————————
• Pregnancy: Registry available. Based on animal data, may cause fetal harm (8.1).

See 17 for PATIENT COUNSELING INFORMATION and FDA-approved patient labeling
                                                            Revised: 08/2009

FULL PRESCRIBING INFORMATION

1 INDICATIONS AND USAGE
1.1 Adult Rheumatoid Arthritis (RA)
ORENCIA® (abatacept) is indicated for reducing signs and symptoms, inducing major clinical response, inhibiting the progression of structural damage, and improving physical function in adult patients with moderately to severely active rheumatoid arthritis. ORENCIA may be used as monotherapy or concomitantly with disease-modifying antirheumatic drugs (DMARDs) other than tumor necrosis factor (TNF) antagonists.
1.2 Juvenile Idiopathic Arthritis
ORENCIA is indicated for reducing signs and symptoms in pediatric patients 6 years of age and older with moderately to severely active polyarticular juvenile idiopathic arthritis. ORENCIA may be used as monotherapy or concomitantly with methotrexate (MTX).
1.3 Important Limitations of Use
ORENCIA should not be administered concomitantly with TNF antagonists. ORENCIA is not recommended for use concomitantly with other biologic rheumatoid arthritis (RA) therapy, such as anakinra.

2 DOSAGE AND ADMINISTRATION
2.1 Adult Rheumatoid Arthritis
For adult patients with RA, ORENCIA should be administered as a 30-minute intravenous infusion utilizing the weight range-based dosing specified in Table 1. Following the initial administration, ORENCIA should be given at 2 and 4 weeks after the first infusion and every 4 weeks thereafter. ORENCIA may be used as monotherapy or concomitantly with DMARDs other than TNF antagonists.
For pediatric juvenile idiopathic arthritis, a dose calculated based on each patient's body weight is used [see *Dosage and Administration (2.2)*].

Table 1:   Dose of ORENCIA in Adult RA

Body Weight of Patient	Dose	Number of Vials[a]
<60 kg	500 mg	2
60 to 100 kg	750 mg	3
>100 kg	1000 mg	4

[a] Each vial provides 250 mg of abatacept for administration.

2.2 Juvenile Idiopathic Arthritis
The recommended dose of ORENCIA for patients 6 to 17 years of age with juvenile idiopathic arthritis who weigh less than 75 kg is 10 mg/kg calculated based on the patient's body weight at each administration. Pediatric patients weighing 75 kg or more should be administered ORENCIA following the adult dosing regimen, not to exceed a maximum dose of 1000 mg. ORENCIA should be administered as a 30-minute intravenous infusion. Following the initial administration, ORENCIA should be given at 2 and 4 weeks after the first infusion and every 4 weeks thereafter. Any unused portions in the vials must be immediately discarded.
2.3 Preparation and Administration Instructions
Use aseptic technique.
ORENCIA is provided as a lyophilized powder in preservative-free, single-use vials. Each ORENCIA vial provides 250 mg of abatacept for administration. The ORENCIA powder in each vial must be reconstituted with 10 mL of Sterile Water for Injection, USP, using **ONLY the SILICONE-FREE DISPOSABLE SYRINGE PROVIDED WITH EACH VIAL** and an 18- to 21-gauge needle. After reconstitution, the concentration of abatacept in the vial will be 25 mg/mL. If the ORENCIA powder is accidentally reconstituted using a siliconized syringe, the solution may develop a few translucent particles. Discard any solutions prepared using siliconized syringes.
If the **SILICONE-FREE DISPOSABLE SYRINGE** is dropped or becomes contaminated, use a new **SILICONE-FREE**

DISPOSABLE SYRINGE from inventory. For information on obtaining additional **SILICONE-FREE DISPOSABLE SYRINGES**, contact Bristol-Myers Squibb 1-800-ORENCIA.

During reconstitution, to minimize foam formation in solutions of ORENCIA (abatacept), the vial should be rotated with gentle swirling until the contents are completely dissolved. Avoid prolonged or vigorous agitation. DO NOT SHAKE. Upon complete dissolution of the lyophilized powder, the vial should be vented with a needle to dissipate any foam that may be present. The solution should be clear and colorless to pale yellow. Do not use if opaque particles, discoloration, or other foreign particles are present.

1) To reconstitute the ORENCIA powder, remove the flip-top from the vial and wipe the top with an alcohol swab. Insert the syringe needle into the vial through the center of the rubber stopper and direct the stream of Sterile Water for Injection, USP, to the glass wall of the vial. Do not use the vial if the vacuum is not present. Rotate the vial with gentle swirling until the contents are completely dissolved.
2) Upon complete dissolution of the lyophilized powder, the vial should be vented with a needle to dissipate any foam that may be present. After reconstitution, each milliliter will contain 25 mg (250 mg/10 mL).
3) The reconstituted ORENCIA solution must be further diluted to 100 mL as follows. From a 100 mL infusion bag or bottle, withdraw a volume of 0.9% Sodium Chloride Injection, USP, equal to the volume of the reconstituted ORENCIA solution required for the patient's dose. Slowly add the reconstituted ORENCIA solution into the infusion bag or bottle using the same SILICONE-FREE DISPOSABLE SYRINGE PROVIDED WITH EACH VIAL. Gently mix. DO NOT SHAKE THE BAG OR BOTTLE. The final concentration of abatacept in the bag or bottle will depend upon the amount of drug added, but will be no more than 10 mg/mL. Any unused portions in the vials must be immediately discarded.
4) Prior to administration, the ORENCIA solution should be inspected visually for particulate matter and discoloration. Discard the solution if any particulate matter or discoloration is observed.
5) The entire, fully diluted ORENCIA solution should be administered over a period of 30 minutes and must be administered with an infusion set and a **STERILE, NON-PYROGENIC, LOW-PROTEIN-BINDING FILTER** (pore size of 0.2 μm to 1.2 μm).
6) The infusion of the fully diluted ORENCIA solution must be completed within 24 hours of reconstitution of the ORENCIA vials. The fully diluted ORENCIA solution may be stored at room temperature or refrigerated at 2°C to 8°C (36°F to 46°F) before use.
7) ORENCIA should not be infused concomitantly in the same intravenous line with other agents. No physical or biochemical compatibility studies have been conducted to evaluate the coadministration of ORENCIA with other agents.

3 DOSAGE FORMS AND STRENGTHS

250 mg single-use vial

4 CONTRAINDICATIONS

None.

5 WARNINGS AND PRECAUTIONS

5.1 Concomitant Use with TNF Antagonists

In controlled clinical trials in patients with adult RA, patients receiving concomitant ORENCIA and TNF antagonist therapy experienced more infections (63%) and serious infections (4.4%) compared to patients treated with only TNF antagonists (43% and 0.8%, respectively) [see *Adverse Reactions (6.1)*]. These trials failed to demonstrate an important enhancement of efficacy with concomitant administration of ORENCIA with TNF antagonist; therefore, concurrent therapy with ORENCIA and a TNF antagonist is not recommended. While transitioning from TNF antagonist therapy to ORENCIA therapy, patients should be monitored for signs of infection.

5.2 Hypersensitivity

Of 2688 patients with adult RA treated with ORENCIA in clinical trials, there were two cases of anaphylaxis or anaphylactoid reactions. Other events potentially associated with drug hypersensitivity, such as hypotension, urticaria, and dyspnea, each occurred in less than 0.9% of ORENCIA-treated patients. Of the 190 patients with juvenile idiopathic arthritis treated with ORENCIA in clinical trials, there was one case of a hypersensitivity reaction (0.5%). Appropriate medical support measures for the treatment of hypersensitivity reactions should be available for immediate use in the event of a reaction [see *Adverse Reactions (6.1, 6.2)*].

5.3 Infections

Physicians should exercise caution when considering the use of ORENCIA (abatacept) in patients with a history of recurrent infections, underlying conditions which may predispose them to infections, or chronic, latent, or localized infections. Patients who develop a new infection while undergoing treatment with ORENCIA should be monitored closely. Administration of ORENCIA should be discontinued if a patient develops a serious infection [see *Adverse Reactions (6.1)*]. A higher rate of serious infections has been observed in adult RA patients treated with concurrent TNF antagonists and ORENCIA [see *Warnings and Precautions (5.1)*].

Prior to initiating immunomodulatory therapies, including ORENCIA, patients should be screened for latent tuberculosis infection with a tuberculin skin test. ORENCIA has not been studied in patients with a positive tuberculosis screen, and the safety of ORENCIA in individuals with latent tuberculosis infection is unknown. Patients testing positive in tuberculosis screening should be treated by standard medical practice prior to therapy with ORENCIA.

Antirheumatic therapies have been associated with hepatitis B reactivation. Therefore, screening for viral hepatitis should be performed in accordance with published guidelines before starting therapy with ORENCIA. In clinical studies with ORENCIA, patients who screened positive for hepatitis were excluded from study.

5.4 Immunizations

Live vaccines should not be given concurrently with ORENCIA or within 3 months of its discontinuation. No data are available on the secondary transmission of infection from persons receiving live vaccines to patients receiving ORENCIA. The efficacy of vaccination in patients receiving ORENCIA is not known. Based on its mechanism of action, ORENCIA may blunt the effectiveness of some immunizations.

It is recommended that patients with juvenile idiopathic arthritis be brought up to date with all immunizations in agreement with current immunization guidelines prior to initiating ORENCIA therapy.

5.5 Use in Patients with Chronic Obstructive Pulmonary Disease (COPD)

Adult COPD patients treated with ORENCIA developed adverse events more frequently than those treated with placebo, including COPD exacerbations, cough, rhonchi, and dyspnea. Use of ORENCIA in patients with RA and COPD should be undertaken with caution and such patients should be monitored for worsening of their respiratory status [see *Adverse Reactions (6.1)*].

5.6 Immunosuppression

The possibility exists for drugs inhibiting T cell activation, including ORENCIA, to affect host defenses against infections and malignancies since T cells mediate cellular immune responses. The impact of treatment with ORENCIA on the development and course of malignancies is not fully understood [see *Adverse Reactions (6.1)*]. In clinical trials in patients with adult RA, a higher rate of infections was seen in ORENCIA-treated patients compared to placebo [see *Adverse Reactions (6.1)*].

6 ADVERSE REACTIONS

6.1 Clinical Studies Experience in Adult RA

Because clinical trials are conducted under widely varying and controlled conditions, adverse reaction rates observed in clinical trials of a drug cannot be directly compared to rates in the clinical trials of another drug and may not predict the rates observed in a broader patient population in clinical practice.

The data described herein reflect exposure to ORENCIA in patients with active RA in placebo-controlled studies (1955 patients with ORENCIA, 989 with placebo). The studies had either a double-blind, placebo-controlled period of 6 months (258 patients with ORENCIA, 133 with placebo) or 1 year (1697 patients with ORENCIA, 856 with placebo). A subset of these patients received concomitant biologic DMARD therapy, such as a TNF blocking agent (204 patients with ORENCIA, 134 with placebo).

The majority of patients in RA clinical studies received one or more of the following concomitant medications with ORENCIA: MTX, nonsteroidal anti-inflammatory drugs (NSAIDs), corticosteroids, TNF blocking agents, azathioprine, chloroquine, gold, hydroxychloroquine, leflunomide, sulfasalazine, and anakinra.

The most serious adverse reactions were serious infections and malignancies.

The most commonly reported adverse events (occurring in ≥10% of patients treated with ORENCIA) were headache, upper respiratory tract infection, nasopharyngitis, and nausea.

The adverse events most frequently resulting in clinical intervention (interruption or discontinuation of ORENCIA) were due to infection. The most frequently reported infections resulting in dose interruption were upper respiratory tract infection (1.0%), bronchitis (0.7%), and herpes zoster (0.7%). The most frequent infections resulting in discontinuation were pneumonia (0.2%), localized infection (0.2%), and bronchitis (0.1%).

Infections

In the placebo-controlled trials, infections were reported in 54% of ORENCIA-treated patients and 48% of placebo-treated patients. The most commonly reported infections (reported in 5-13% of patients) were upper respiratory tract infection, nasopharyngitis, sinusitis, urinary tract infection, influenza, and bronchitis. Other infections reported in fewer than 5% of patients at a higher frequency (>0.5%) with ORENCIA (abatacept) compared to placebo, were rhinitis, herpes simplex, and pneumonia [see *Warnings and Precautions (5.3)*].

Serious infections were reported in 3.0% of patients treated with ORENCIA and 1.9% of patients treated with placebo. The most common (0.2-0.5%) serious infections reported with ORENCIA were pneumonia, cellulitis, urinary tract infection, bronchitis, diverticulitis, and acute pyelonephritis [see *Warnings and Precautions (5.3)*].

Malignancies

In the placebo-controlled portions of the clinical trials (1955 patients treated with ORENCIA for a median of 12 months), the overall frequencies of malignancies were similar in the ORENCIA- and placebo-treated patients (1.3% and 1.1%, respectively). However, more cases of lung cancer were observed in ORENCIA-treated patients (4, 0.2%) than placebo-treated patients (0). In the cumulative ORENCIA clinical trials (placebo-controlled and uncontrolled, open-label) a total of 8 cases of lung cancer (0.21 cases per 100 patient-years) and 4 lymphomas (0.10 cases per 100 patient-years) were observed in 2688 patients (3827 patient-years). The rate observed for lymphoma is approximately 3.5-fold higher than expected in an age- and gender-matched general population based on the Surveillance, Epidemiology, and End Results Database.[1] Patients with RA, particularly those with highly active disease, are at a higher risk for the development of lymphoma. Other malignancies included skin, breast, bile duct, bladder, cervical, endometrial, lymphoma, melanoma, myelodysplastic syndrome, ovarian, prostate, renal, thyroid, and uterine cancers [see *Warnings and Precautions (5.6)*]. The potential role of ORENCIA in the development of malignancies in humans is unknown.

Infusion-Related Reactions and Hypersensitivity Reactions

Acute infusion-related events (adverse reactions occurring within 1 hour of the start of the infusion) in Studies III, IV, and V [see *Clinical Studies (14.1)*] were more common in the ORENCIA-treated patients than the placebo patients (9% for ORENCIA, 6% for placebo). The most frequently reported events (1-2%) were dizziness, headache, and hypertension.

Acute infusion-related events that were reported in >0.1% and ≤1% of patients treated with ORENCIA included cardiopulmonary symptoms, such as hypotension, increased blood pressure, and dyspnea; other symptoms included nausea, flushing, urticaria, cough, hypersensitivity, pruritus, rash, and wheezing. Most of these reactions were mild to moderate. Fewer than 1% of ORENCIA-treated patients discontinued due to an acute infusion-related event. In controlled trials, 6 ORENCIA-treated patients compared to 2 placebo-treated patients discontinued study treatment due to acute infusion-related events.

Of 2688 patients treated with ORENCIA in clinical trials, there were two cases of anaphylaxis or anaphylactoid reactions. Other events potentially associated with drug hypersensitivity, such as hypotension, urticaria, and dyspnea, each occurred in less than 0.9% of ORENCIA-treated patients and generally occurred within 24 hours of ORENCIA infusion. Appropriate medical support measures for the treatment of hypersensitivity reactions should be available for immediate use in the event of a reaction [see *Warnings and Precautions (5.2)*].

Adverse Reactions in Patients with COPD

In Study V [see *Clinical Studies (14.1)*], there were 37 patients with chronic obstructive pulmonary disease (COPD) who were treated with ORENCIA and 17 COPD patients who were treated with placebo. The COPD patients treated with ORENCIA developed adverse events more frequently than those treated with placebo (97% vs 88%, respectively). Respiratory disorders occurred more frequently in ORENCIA-treated patients compared to placebo-treated patients (43% vs 24%, respectively) including COPD exacerbation, cough, rhonchi, and dyspnea. A greater percentage of ORENCIA-treated patients developed a serious adverse event compared to placebo-treated patients (27% vs 6%), including COPD exacerbation (3 of 37 patients [8%]) and pneumonia (1 of 37 patients [3%]) [see *Warnings and Precautions (5.5)*].

Other Adverse Reactions

Adverse events occurring in 3% or more of patients and at least 1% more frequently in ORENCIA-treated patients during placebo-controlled RA studies are summarized in Table 2.

Table 2: Adverse Events Occurring in 3% or More of Patients and at Least 1% More Frequently in ORENCIA-Treated Patients During Placebo-Controlled RA Studies

Adverse Event (Preferred Term)	ORENCIA (n=1955)[a] Percentage	Placebo (n=989)[b] Percentage
Headache	18	13
Nasopharyngitis	12	9
Dizziness	9	7
Cough	8	7
Back pain	7	6
Hypertension	7	4
Dyspepsia	6	4
Urinary tract infection	6	5
Rash	4	3
Pain in extremity	3	2

[a] Includes 204 patients on concomitant biologic DMARDs (adalimumab, anakinra, etanercept, or infliximab).

[b] Includes 134 patients on concomitant biologic DMARDs (adalimumab, anakinra, etanercept, or infliximab).

Immunogenicity

Antibodies directed against the entire abatacept molecule or to the CTLA-4 portion of abatacept were assessed by ELISA assays in RA patients for up to 2 years following repeated treatment with ORENCIA (abatacept). Thirty-four of 1993 (1.7%) patients developed binding antibodies to the entire abatacept molecule or to the CTLA-4 portion of abatacept. Because trough levels of abatacept can interfere with assay results, a subset analysis was performed. In this analysis it was observed that 9 of 154 (5.8%) patients that had discontinued treatment with ORENCIA for over 56 days developed antibodies.

Samples with confirmed binding activity to CTLA-4 were assessed for the presence of neutralizing antibodies in a cell-based luciferase reporter assay. Six of 9 (67%) evaluable patients were shown to possess neutralizing antibodies.

No correlation of antibody development to clinical response or adverse events was observed.

The data reflect the percentage of patients whose test results were positive for antibodies to abatacept in specific assays. The observed incidence of antibody (including neutralizing antibody) positivity in an assay is highly dependent on several factors, including assay sensitivity and specificity, assay methodology, sample handling, timing of sample collection, concomitant medication, and underlying disease. For these reasons, comparison of the incidence of antibodies to abatacept with the incidence of antibodies to other products may be misleading.

Clinical Experience in MTX-Naive Patients

Study VI was an active-controlled clinical trial in MTX-naive patients [see *Clinical Studies (14.1)*]. The safety experience in these patients was consistent with Studies I-V.

6.2 Clinical Studies Experience in Juvenile Idiopathic Arthritis

In general, the adverse events in pediatric patients were similar in frequency and type to those seen in adult patients [see *Warnings and Precautions (5), Adverse Reactions (6)*]. ORENCIA has been studied in 190 pediatric patients, 6 to 17 years of age, with polyarticular juvenile idiopathic arthritis. Overall frequency of adverse events in the 4-month, lead-in, open-label period of the study was 70%; infections occurred at a frequency of 36% [see *Clinical Studies (14.2)*]. The most common infections were upper respiratory tract infection and nasopharyngitis. The infections resolved without sequelae, and the types of infections were consistent with those commonly seen in outpatient pediatric populations. Other events that occurred at a prevalence of at least 5% were headache, nausea, diarrhea, cough, pyrexia, and abdominal pain.

A total of 6 serious adverse events (acute lymphocytic leukemia, ovarian cyst, varicella infection, disease flare [2], and joint wear) were reported during the initial 4 months of treatment with ORENCIA.

Of the 190 patients with juvenile idiopathic arthritis treated with ORENCIA in clinical trials, there was one case of a hypersensitivity reaction (0.5%). During Periods A, B, and C, acute infusion-related reactions occurred at a frequency of 4%, 2%, and 3%, respectively, and were consistent with the types of events reported in adults.

Upon continued treatment in the open-label extension period, the types of adverse events were similar in frequency and type to those seen in adult patients, except for a single patient diagnosed with multiple sclerosis while on open-label treatment.

Immunogenicity

Antibodies directed against the entire abatacept molecule or to the CTLA-4 portion of abatacept were assessed by ELISA assays in patients with juvenile idiopathic arthritis following repeated treatment with ORENCIA (abatacept) throughout the open-label period. For patients who were withdrawn from therapy for up to 6 months during the double-blind period, the rate of antibody formation to the CTLA-4 portion of the molecule was 41% (22/54), while for those who remained on therapy the rate was 13% (7/54). The presence of antibodies was generally transient and titers were low. The presence of antibodies was not associated with adverse events, changes in efficacy, or an effect on serum concentrations of abatacept. For patients who were withdrawn from ORENCIA during the double-blind period for up to 6 months, no serious acute infusion-related events were observed upon re-initiation of ORENCIA therapy.

6.3 Postmarketing Experience

Adverse reactions have been reported during the postapproval use of ORENCIA. Because these reactions are reported voluntarily from a population of uncertain size, it is not always possible to reliably estimate their frequency or establish a causal relationship to ORENCIA. Based on the postmarketing experience with ORENCIA in adult RA patients, the adverse event profile of ORENCIA does not differ from that listed/discussed above in Section 6.1 in adults.

7 DRUG INTERACTIONS

7.1 TNF Antagonists

Concurrent administration of a TNF antagonist with ORENCIA has been associated with an increased risk of serious infections and no significant additional efficacy over use of the TNF antagonists alone. Concurrent therapy with ORENCIA and TNF antagonists is not recommended [see *Warnings and Precautions (5.1)*].

7.2 Other Biologic RA Therapy

There is insufficient experience to assess the safety and efficacy of ORENCIA administered concurrently with other biologic RA therapy, such as anakinra, and therefore such use is not recommended.

7.3 Blood Glucose Testing

Parenteral drug products containing maltose can interfere with the readings of blood glucose monitors that use test strips with glucose dehydrogenase pyrroloquinolinequinone (GDH-PQQ). The GDH-PQQ based glucose monitoring systems may react with the maltose present in ORENCIA, resulting in falsely elevated blood glucose readings on the day of infusion. When receiving ORENCIA, patients that require blood glucose monitoring should be advised to consider methods that do not react with maltose, such as those based on glucose dehydrogenase nicotine adenine dinucleotide (GDH-NAD), glucose oxidase, or glucose hexokinase test methods.

8 USE IN SPECIFIC POPULATIONS

8.1 Pregnancy

Pregnancy Category C

There are no adequate and well-controlled studies of ORENCIA use in pregnant women. Abatacept has been shown to cross the placenta in animals, and in animal reproduction studies alterations in immune function occurred. ORENCIA should be used during pregnancy only if the potential benefit to the mother justifies the potential risk to the fetus.

Abatacept was not teratogenic when administered to pregnant mice at doses up to 300 mg/kg and in pregnant rats and rabbits at doses up to 200 mg/kg daily representing approximately 29 times the exposure associated with the maximum recommended human dose (MRHD) of 10 mg/kg based on AUC (area under the time-concentration curve).

Abatacept administered to female rats every three days during early gestation and throughout the lactation period, produced no adverse effects in offspring at doses up to 45 mg/kg, representing 3 times the exposure associated with the MRHD of 10 mg/kg based on AUC. However, at 200 mg/kg, 11 times the MRHD exposure, alterations in immune function were observed consisting of a 9-fold increase in T-cell dependent antibody response in female pups and thyroid inflammation in one female pup. It is not known whether these findings indicate a risk for development of autoimmune diseases in humans exposed *in utero* to abatacept. However, exposure to abatacept in the juvenile rat, which may be more representative of the fetal immune system state in the human, resulted in immune system abnormalities including inflammation of the thyroid and pancreas [see *Nonclinical Toxicology (13.2)*].

Pregnancy Registry: To monitor maternal-fetal outcomes of pregnant women exposed to ORENCIA, a pregnancy registry has been established. Healthcare professionals are encouraged to register patients and pregnant women are encouraged to enroll themselves by calling 1-877-311-8972.

8.3 Nursing Mothers

It is not known whether ORENCIA is excreted into human milk or absorbed systemically after ingestion by a nursing infant. However, abatacept was excreted in rat milk. Because many drugs are excreted in human milk, and because of the potential for serious adverse reactions in nursing infants from ORENCIA (abatacept), a decision should be made whether to discontinue nursing or to discontinue the drug, taking into account the importance of the drug to the mother.

8.4 Pediatric Use

ORENCIA is indicated for reducing signs and symptoms in pediatric patients with moderately to severely active polyarticular juvenile idiopathic arthritis ages 6 years and older. ORENCIA may be used as monotherapy or concomitantly with MTX.

Studies in juvenile rats exposed to ORENCIA prior to immune system maturity have shown immune system abnormalities including an increase in the incidence of infections leading to death as well as inflammation of the thyroid and pancreas [see *Nonclinical Toxicology (13.2)*]. Studies in adult mice and monkeys have not demonstrated similar findings. As the immune system of the rat is undeveloped in the first few weeks after birth, the relevance of these results to humans greater than 6 years of age (where the immune system is largely developed) is unknown.

The safety and effectiveness of ORENCIA in pediatric patients below 6 years of age have not been established. Therefore, ORENCIA is not recommended for use in patients below the age of 6 years.

Safety and efficacy of ORENCIA in pediatric patients for uses other than juvenile idiopathic arthritis have not been established.

8.5 Geriatric Use

A total of 323 patients 65 years of age and older, including 53 patients 75 years and older, received ORENCIA in clinical studies. No overall differences in safety or effectiveness were observed between these patients and younger patients, but these numbers are too low to rule out differences. The frequency of serious infection and malignancy among ORENCIA-treated patients over age 65 was higher than for those under age 65. Because there is a higher incidence of infections and malignancies in the elderly population in general, caution should be used when treating the elderly.

10 OVERDOSAGE

ORENCIA is administered as an intravenous infusion under medically controlled conditions. Doses up to 50 mg/kg have been administered without apparent toxic effect. In case of overdosage, it is recommended that the patient be monitored for any signs or symptoms of adverse reactions and appropriate symptomatic treatment instituted.

11 DESCRIPTION

ORENCIA (abatacept) is a soluble fusion protein that consists of the extracellular domain of human cytotoxic T-lymphocyte-associated antigen 4 (CTLA-4) linked to the modified Fc (hinge, CH2, and CH3 domains) portion of human immunoglobulin G1 (IgG1). Abatacept is produced by recombinant DNA technology in a mammalian cell expression system. The apparent molecular weight of abatacept is 92 kilodaltons.

ORENCIA is supplied as a sterile, white, preservative-free, lyophilized powder for parenteral administration. Following reconstitution with 10 mL of Sterile Water for Injection, USP, the solution of ORENCIA is clear, colorless to pale yellow, with a pH range of 7.2 to 7.8. Each single-use vial of ORENCIA provides 250 mg abatacept, 500 mg maltose, 17.2 mg monobasic sodium phosphate, and 14.6 mg sodium chloride for administration.

12 CLINICAL PHARMACOLOGY

12.1 Mechanism of Action

Abatacept, a selective costimulation modulator, inhibits T cell (T lymphocyte) activation by binding to CD80 and CD86, thereby blocking interaction with CD28. This interaction provides a costimulatory signal necessary for full activation of T lymphocytes. Activated T lymphocytes are implicated in the pathogenesis of RA and are found in the synovium of patients with RA.

In vitro, abatacept decreases T cell proliferation and inhibits the production of the cytokines TNF alpha (TNFα), interferon-γ, and interleukin-2. In a rat collagen-induced arthritis model, abatacept suppresses inflammation, decreases anti-collagen antibody production, and reduces antigen specific production of interferon-γ. The relationship of these biological response markers to the mechanisms by which ORENCIA exerts its effects in RA is unknown.

12.2 Pharmacodynamics

In clinical trials with ORENCIA at doses approximating 10 mg/kg, decreases were observed in serum levels of soluble interleukin-2 receptor (sIL-2R), interleukin-6 (IL-6), rheumatoid factor (RF), C-reactive protein (CRP), matrix metalloproteinase-3 (MMP3), and TNFα. The relationship of these biological response markers to the mechanisms by which ORENCIA exerts its effects in RA is unknown.

12.3 Pharmacokinetics

Healthy Adults and Adult RA

The pharmacokinetics of abatacept were studied in healthy adult subjects after a single 10 mg/kg intravenous infusion and in RA patients after multiple 10 mg/kg intravenous infusions (see Table 3).

Table 3: Pharmacokinetic Parameters (Mean, Range) in Healthy Subjects and RA Patients After 10 mg/kg Intravenous Infusion(s)

PK Parameter	Healthy Subjects (After 10 mg/kg Single Dose) n=13	RA Patients (After 10 mg/kg Multiple Doses[a]) n=14
Peak Concentration (C_{max}) [mcg/mL]	292 (175-427)	295 (171-398)
Terminal half-life ($t_{1/2}$) [days]	16.7 (12-23)	13.1 (8-25)
Systemic clearance (CL) [mL/h/kg]	0.23 (0.16-0.30)	0.22 (0.13-0.47)
Volume of distribution (Vss) [L/kg]	0.09 (0.06-0.13)	0.07 (0.02-0.13)

[a] Multiple intravenous infusions were administered at days 1, 15, 30, and monthly thereafter.

The pharmacokinetics of abatacept in RA patients and healthy subjects appeared to be comparable. In RA patients, after multiple intravenous infusions, the pharmacokinetics of abatacept showed proportional increases of C_{max} and AUC over the dose range of 2 mg/kg to 10 mg/kg. At 10 mg/kg, serum concentration appeared to reach a steady-state by day 60 with a mean (range) trough concentration of 24 (1 to 66) mcg/mL. No systemic accumulation of abatacept occurred upon continued repeated treatment with 10 mg/kg at monthly intervals in RA patients.

Population pharmacokinetic analyses in RA patients revealed that there was a trend toward higher clearance of abatacept with increasing body weight. Age and gender (when corrected for body weight) did not affect clearance. Concomitant MTX, NSAIDs, corticosteroids, and TNF blocking agents did not influence abatacept clearance.

No formal studies were conducted to examine the effects of either renal or hepatic impairment on the pharmacokinetics of abatacept.

Juvenile Idiopathic Arthritis

In patients 6 to 17 years of age, the mean (range) steady-state serum peak and trough concentrations of abatacept were 217 (57 to 700) and 11.9 (0.15 to 44.6) mcg/mL. Population pharmacokinetic analyses of the serum concentration data showed that clearance of abatacept increased with baseline body weight. The estimated mean (range) clearance of abatacept in the juvenile idiopathic arthritis patients was 0.4 (0.20 to 1.12) mL/h/kg. After accounting for the effect of body weight, the clearance of abatacept was not related to age and gender. Concomitant methotrexate, corticosteroids, and NSAIDs were also shown not to influence abatacept clearance.

13 NONCLINICAL TOXICOLOGY
13.1 Carcinogenesis, Mutagenesis, Impairment of Fertility

In a mouse carcinogenicity study, weekly subcutaneous injections of 20, 65, or 200 mg/kg of abatacept administered for up to 84 weeks in males and 88 weeks in females were associated with increases in the incidence of malignant lymphomas (all doses) and mammary gland tumors (intermediate- and high-dose in females). The mice from this study were infected with murine leukemia virus and mouse mammary tumor virus. These viruses are associated with an increased incidence of lymphomas and mammary gland tumors, respectively, in immunosuppressed mice. The doses used in these studies produced exposures 0.8, 2.0, and 3.0 times higher, respectively, than the exposure associated with the maximum recommended human dose (MRHD) of 10 mg/kg based on AUC (area under the time-concentration curve). The relevance of these findings to the clinical use of ORENCIA (abatacept) is unknown.

In a one-year toxicity study in cynomolgus monkeys, abatacept was administered intravenously once weekly at doses up to 50 mg/kg (producing 9 times the MRHD exposure based on AUC). Abatacept was not associated with any significant drug-related toxicity. Reversible pharmacological effects consisted of minimal transient decreases in serum IgG and minimal to severe lymphoid depletion of germinal centers in the spleen and/or lymph nodes. No evidence of lymphomas or preneoplastic morphologic changes was observed, despite the presence of a virus (lymphocryptovirus) known to cause these lesions in immunosuppressed monkeys within the time frame of this study. The relevance of these findings to the clinical use of ORENCIA is unknown. No mutagenic potential of abatacept was observed in the *in vitro* bacterial reverse mutation (Ames) or Chinese hamster ovary/hypoxanthine guanine phosphoribosyl-transferase (CHO/HGPRT) forward point mutation assays with or without metabolic activation, and no chromosomal aberrations were observed in human lymphocytes treated with abatacept with or without metabolic activation.

Abatacept had no adverse effects on male or female fertility in rats at doses up to 200 mg/kg every three days (11 times the MRHD exposure based on AUC).

13.2 Animal Toxicology and/or Pharmacology

A juvenile animal study was conducted in rats dosed with abatacept from 4 to 94 days of age in which an increase in the incidence of infections leading to death occurred at all doses compared with controls. Altered T-cell subsets including increased T-helper cells and reduced T-regulatory cells were observed. In addition, inhibition of T-cell-dependent antibody responses (TDAR) was observed. Upon following these animals into adulthood, lymphocytic inflammation of the thyroid and pancreatic islets was observed.

In studies of adult mice and monkeys, inhibition of TDAR was apparent. However, infection and mortality, altered T-helper cells, and inflammation of thyroid and pancreas were not observed.

14 CLINICAL STUDIES
14.1 Adult Rheumatoid Arthritis

The efficacy and safety of ORENCIA (abatacept) were assessed in six randomized, double-blind, controlled studies (five placebo-controlled and one active-controlled) in patients ≥18 years of age with active RA diagnosed according to American College of Rheumatology (ACR) criteria. Studies I, II, III, IV, and VI required patients to have at least 12 tender and 10 swollen joints at randomization. Study V did not require any specific number of tender or swollen joints. ORENCIA or placebo treatment was given intravenously at weeks 0, 2, and 4 and then every 4 weeks thereafter.

Study I evaluated ORENCIA as monotherapy in 122 patients with active RA who had failed at least one non-biologic DMARD or etanercept. In Study II and Study III, the efficacy and safety of ORENCIA were assessed in patients with an inadequate response to MTX and who were continued on their stable dose of MTX. In Study IV, the efficacy and safety of ORENCIA were assessed in patients with an inadequate response to a TNF blocking agent, with the TNF blocking agent discontinued prior to randomization; other DMARDs were permitted. Study V primarily assessed safety in patients with active RA requiring additional intervention in spite of current therapy with DMARDs; all DMARDs used at enrollment were continued. Patients in Study V were not excluded for comorbid medical conditions. In Study VI, the efficacy and safety of ORENCIA were assessed in MTX-naive patients with RA of less than 2 years disease duration. In Study VI, patients previously naive to MTX were randomized to receive ORENCIA plus MTX or MTX plus placebo.

Study I patients were randomized to receive one of three doses of ORENCIA (0.5, 2, or 10 mg/kg) or placebo ending at week 8. Study II patients were randomized to receive ORENCIA 2 or 10 mg/kg or placebo for 12 months. Study III, IV, V, and VI patients were randomized to receive a dose of ORENCIA based on weight range or placebo for 12 months (Studies III, V, and VI) or 6 months (Study IV). The dose of ORENCIA was 500 mg for patients weighing less than 60 kg, 750 mg for patients weighing 60 to 100 kg, and 1000 mg for patients weighing greater than 100 kg.

Clinical Response

The percent of ORENCIA-treated patients achieving ACR 20, 50, and 70 response and major clinical response in Studies I, III, IV, and VI are shown in Table 4. ORENCIA-treated patients had higher ACR 20, 50, and 70 response rates at 6 months compared to placebo-treated patients. Month 6 ACR response rates in Study II for the 10 mg/kg group were similar to the ORENCIA group in Study III.

In Studies III and IV, improvement in the ACR 20 response rate versus placebo was observed within 15 days in some patients and within 29 days versus MTX in Study VI. In Studies II, III, and VI, ACR response rates were maintained to 12 months in ORENCIA-treated patients. ACR responses were maintained up to three years in the open-label extension of Study II.

In Study VI, a greater proportion of patients treated with ORENCIA plus MTX achieved a low level of disease activity as measured by a DAS28-CRP less than 2.6 at 12 months compared to those treated with MTX plus placebo (Table 4). Of patients treated with ORENCIA plus MTX who achieved DAS28-CRP less than 2.6, 54% had no active joints, 17% had one active joint, 7% had two active joints, and 22% had three or more active joints, where an active joint was a joint that was rated as tender or swollen or both.

[See table 4 at left]

The results of the components of the ACR response criteria for Studies III and IV are shown in Table 5. In ORENCIA-treated patients, greater improvement was seen in all ACR response criteria components through 6 and 12 months than in placebo-treated patients.

[See table 5 at top of next page]

The percent of patients achieving the ACR 50 response for Study III by visit is shown in Figure 1. The time course for the ORENCIA group in Study VI was similar to that in Study III.

[See figure 1 at top of next page]

ORENCIA-treated patients experienced greater improvement than placebo-treated patients in morning stiffness.

Radiographic Response

In Study III and Study VI, structural joint damage was assessed radiographically and expressed as change from baseline in the Genant-modified Total Sharp Score (TSS) and its components, the Erosion Score (ES) and Joint Space Narrowing (JSN) score. ORENCIA/MTX slowed the progression of structural damage compared to placebo/MTX after 12 months of treatment as shown in Table 6.

[See table 6 on next page]

In the open-label extension of Study III, 75% of patients initially randomized to ORENCIA/MTX and 65% of patients initially randomized to placebo/MTX were evaluated radio-

Table 4: Clinical Responses in Controlled Trials

	Percent of Patients							
	Inadequate Response to DMARDs		Inadequate Response to MTX		Inadequate Response to TNF Blocking Agent		MTX-Naive	
	Study I		Study III		Study IV		Study VI	
Response Rate	ORN[a] n=32	PBO n=32	ORN[b] +MTX n=424	PBO +MTX n=214	ORN[b] +DMARDs n=256	PBO +DMARDs n=133	ORN[b] +MTX n=256	PBO +MTX n=253
ACR 20								
Month 3	53%	31%	62%***	37%	46%***	18%	64%*	53%
Month 6	NA	NA	68%***	40%	50%***	20%	75%**	62%
Month 12	NA	NA	73%***	40%	NA	NA	76%***	62%
ACR 50								
Month 3	16%	6%	32%***	8%	18%**	6%	40%***	23%
Month 6	NA	NA	40%***	17%	20%***	4%	53%***	38%
Month 12	NA	NA	48%***	18%	NA	NA	57%***	42%
ACR 70								
Month 3	6%	0	13%***	3%	6%*	1%	19%**	10%
Month 6	NA	NA	20%***	7%	10%***	2%	32%**	20%
Month 12	NA	NA	29%***	6%	NA	NA	43%***	27%
Major Clinical Response[c]	NA	NA	14%***	2%	NA	NA	27%***	12%
DAS28-CRP <2.6[d]								
Month 12	NA	NA	NA	NA	NA	NA	41%***	23%

* p<0.05, ORENCIA (ORN) vs placebo (PBO) or MTX.
** p<0.01, ORENCIA vs placebo or MTX.
*** p<0.001, ORENCIA vs placebo or MTX.
[a] 10 mg/kg.
[b] Dosing based on weight range [see *Dosage and Administration (2.1)*].
[c] Major clinical response is defined as achieving an ACR 70 response for a continuous 6-month period.
[d] Refer to text for additional description of remaining joint activity.

Figure 1: Percent of Patients Achieving ACR 50 Response by Visit* (Study III)

Time Course of ACR 50 Response
Inadequate Response to MTX (Study III)

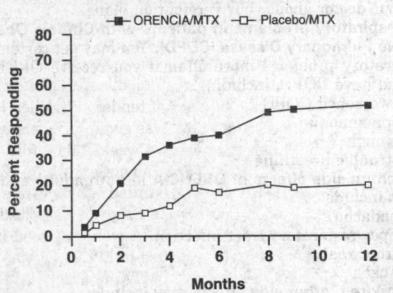

* The same patients may not have responded at each time point.

graphically at Year 2. As shown in Table 6, progression of structural damage in ORENCIA/MTX-treated patients was further reduced in the second year of treatment.
Following 2 years of treatment with ORENCIA/MTX, 51% of patients had no progression of structural damage as defined by a change in the TSS of zero or less compared with baseline. Fifty-six percent (56%) of ORENCIA/MTX-treated patients had no progression during the first year compared to 45% of placebo/MTX-treated patients. In their second year of treatment with ORENCIA/MTX, more patients had no progression than in the first year (65% vs 56%).

Physical Function Response and Health-Related Outcomes
Improvement in physical function was measured by the Health Assessment Questionnaire Disability Index (HAQ-DI). In the HAQ-DI, ORENCIA (abatacept) emonstrated greater improvement from baseline versus placebo in Studies II-V and versus MTX in Study VI. The results from Studies II and III are shown in Table 7. Similar results were observed in Study V compared to placebo and in Study VI compared to MTX. During the open-label period of Study II, the improvement in physical function has been maintained for up to 3 years.
[See table 7 at right]
Health-related quality of life was assessed by the SF-36 questionnaire at 6 months in Studies II, III, and IV and at 12 months in Studies II and III. In these studies, improvement was observed in the ORENCIA group as compared with the placebo group in all 8 domains of the SF-36 as well as the Physical Component Summary (PCS) and the Mental Component Summary (MCS).

14.2   Juvenile Idiopathic Arthritis
The safety and efficacy of ORENCIA were assessed in a three-part study including an open-label extension in children with polyarticular juvenile idiopathic arthritis (JIA). Patients 6 to 17 years of age (n=190) with moderately to severely active polyarticular JIA who had an inadequate response to one or more DMARDs, such as MTX or TNF antagonists, were treated. Patients had a disease duration of approximately 4 years with moderately to severely active disease at study entry, as determined by baseline counts of active joints (mean, 16) and joints with loss of motion (mean, 16); patients had elevated C-reactive protein (CRP) levels (mean, 3.2 mg/dL) and ESR (mean, 32 mm/h). The patients enrolled had subtypes of JIA that at disease onset included Oligoarticular (16%), Polyarticular (64%; 20% were rheumatoid factor positive), and Systemic (20%). At study entry, 74% of patients were receiving MTX (mean dose, 13.2 mg/m^2 per week) and remained on a stable dose of MTX (those not receiving MTX did not initiate MTX treatment during the study).
In Period A (open-label, lead-in), patients received 10 mg/kg (maximum 1000 mg per dose) intravenously on days 1, 15, 29, and monthly thereafter. Response was assessed utilizing the ACR Pediatric 30 definition of improvement, defined as ≥30% improvement in at least 3 of the 6 JIA core set variables and ≥30% worsening in not more than 1 of the 6 JIA core set variables. Patients demonstrating an ACR Pedi 30 response at the end of Period A were randomized into the double-blind phase (Period B) and received either ORENCIA or placebo for 6 months or until disease flare. Disease flare was defined as a ≥30% worsening in at least 3 of the 6 JIA core set variables with ≥30% improvement in not more than 1 of the 6 JIA core set variables; ≥2 cm of worsening of the Physician or Parent Global Assessment was necessary if used as 1 of the 3 JIA core set variables used to define flare, and worsening in ≥2 joints was necessary if the number of active joints or joints with limitation of motion was used as 1 of the 3 JIA core set variables used to define flare.
At the conclusion of Period A, pediatric ACR 30/50/70 responses were 65%, 50%, and 28%, respectively. Pediatric ACR 30 responses were similar in all subtypes of JIA studied.
During the double-blind randomized withdrawal phase (Period B), ORENCIA-treated patients experienced signifi-

cantly fewer disease flares compared to placebo-treated patients (20% vs 53%); 95% CI of the difference (15%, 52%). The risk of disease flare among patients continuing on ORENCIA (abatacept) was less than one third than that for patients withdrawn from ORENCIA treatment (hazard ratio=0.31, 95% CI [0.16, 0.59]). Among patients who received ORENCIA throughout the study (Period A, Period B, and the open-label extension Period C), the proportion of pediatric ACR 30/50/70 responders has remained consistent for 1 year.

15   REFERENCES

1. Ries LAG, Eisner MP, Kosary CL, et al. SEER Cancer Statistics Review, 1975-2001, National Cancer Institute. Bethesda, MD, http://seer.cancer.gov/csr/1975_2001/. Accessed 2004.

16   HOW SUPPLIED/STORAGE AND HANDLING
ORENCIA® (abatacept) lyophilized powder for intravenous infusion is supplied as an individually packaged, single-use vial with a silicone-free disposable syringe. The product is available in the following strength: NDC 0003-2187-10, providing 250 mg of abatacept in a 15-mL vial.
Storage
Store in a refrigerator, 2°C to 8°C (36°F to 46°F). Do not use beyond the expiration date. Protect the vials from light by storing in the original package until time of use.

Table 5:   Components of ACR Response at 6 Months

	Inadequate Response to MTX				Inadequate Response to TNF Blocking Agent			
	Study III				Study IV			
	ORENCIA +MTX n=424		Placebo +MTX n=214		ORENCIA +DMARDs n=256		Placebo +DMARDs n=133	
Component (median)	Baseline	Month 6	Baseline	Month 6	Baseline	Month 6	Baseline	Month 6
Number of tender joints (0-68)	28	7***	31	14	30	13***	31	24
Number of swollen joints (0-66)	19	5***	20	11	21	10***	20	14
Pain[a]	67	27***	70	50	73	43**	74	64
Patient global assessment[a]	66	29***	64	48	71	44***	73	63
Disability index[b]	1.75	1.13***	1.75	1.38	1.88	1.38***	2.00	1.75
Physician global assessment[a]	69	21***	68	40	71	32***	69	54
CRP (mg/dL)	2.2	0.9***	2.1	1.8	3.4	1.3***	2.8	2.3

** p<0.01, ORENCIA vs placebo, based on mean percent change from baseline.
*** p<0.001, ORENCIA vs placebo, based on mean percent change from baseline.
[a] Visual analog scale: 0 = best, 100 = worst.
[b] Health Assessment Questionnaire: 0 = best, 3 = worst; 20 questions; 8 categories: dressing and grooming, arising, eating, walking, hygiene, reach, grip, and activities.

Table 6:   Mean Radiographic Changes in Study III[a] and Study VI[b]

Parameter	ORENCIA/MTX	Placebo/MTX	Differences	P-value[d]
Study III				
First Year				
TSS	1.07	2.43	1.36	<0.01
ES	0.61	1.47	0.86	<0.01
JSN score	0.46	0.97	0.51	<0.01
Second Year				
TSS	0.48	0.74[c]	–	–
ES	0.23	0.22[c]	–	–
JSN score	0.25	0.51[c]	–	–
Study VI				
First Year				
TSS	0.6	1.1	0.5	0.04

[a] Patients with an inadequate response to MTX.
[b] MTX-naive patients.
[c] Patients received 1 year of placebo/MTX followed by 1 year of ORENCIA/MTX.
[d] Based on a nonparametric ANCOVA model.

Table 7:   Mean Improvement from Baseline in Health Assessment Questionnaire Disability Index (HAQ-DI)

| | Inadequate Response to Methotrexate | | | |
| | Study II | | Study III | |
HAQ Disability Index	ORENCIA[a] +MTX (n=115)	Placebo +MTX (n=119)	ORENCIA[b] +MTX (n=422)	Placebo +MTX (n=212)
Baseline (Mean)	0.98[c]	0.97[c]	1.69[d]	1.69[d]
Mean Improvement Year 1	0.40[c,***]	0.15[c]	0.66[d,***]	0.37[d]

*** p<0.001, ORENCIA vs placebo.
[a] 10 mg/kg.
[b] Dosing based on weight range [see Dosage and Administration (2.1)].
[c] Modified Health Assessment Questionnaire: 0 = best, 3 = worst; 8 questions; 8 categories: dressing and grooming, arising, eating, walking, hygiene, reach, grip, and activities.
[d] Health Assessment Questionnaire: 0 = best, 3 = worst; 20 questions; 8 categories: dressing and grooming, arising, eating, walking, hygiene, reach, grip, and activities.

17   PATIENT COUNSELING INFORMATION

See FDA-Approved Patient Labeling (17.7).

17.1   Concomitant Use With Biologic Medications for RA

Patients should be informed that they should not receive ORENCIA (abatacept) treatment concomitantly with a TNF antagonist, such as adalimumab, etanercept, and infliximab because such combination therapy may increase their risk for infections [see *Indications and Usage (1.3), Warnings and Precautions (5.1),* and *Drug Interactions (7.1)*], and that they should not receive ORENCIA concomitantly with other biologic RA therapy, such as anakinra because there is not enough information to assess the safety and efficacy of such combination therapy [see *Indications and Usage (1.3),* and *Drug Interactions (7.2)*].

17.2   Hypersensitivity

Patients should be instructed to immediately tell their healthcare professional if they experience symptoms of an allergic reaction during or for the first day after the administration of ORENCIA [see *Warnings and Precautions (5.2)*].

17.3   Infections

Patients should be asked if they have a history of recurrent infections, have underlying conditions which may predispose them to infections, or have chronic, latent, or localized infections. Patients should be asked if they have had tuberculosis (TB), a positive skin test for TB, or recently have been in close contact with someone who has had TB. Patients should be instructed that they may be tested for TB before they receive ORENCIA. Patients should be informed to tell their healthcare professional if they develop an infection during therapy with ORENCIA [see *Warnings and Precautions (5.3)*].

17.4   Immunizations

Patients should be informed that live vaccines should not be given concurrently with ORENCIA or within 3 months of its discontinuation. Caregivers of patients with juvenile idiopathic arthritis should be informed that the patient should be brought up to date with all immunizations in agreement with current immunization guidelines prior to initiating ORENCIA therapy and to discuss with their healthcare provider how best to handle future immunizations once ORENCIA therapy has been initiated [see *Warnings and Precautions (5.4)*].

17.5   Pregnancy and Nursing Mothers

Patients should be informed that ORENCIA has not been studied in pregnant women or nursing mothers so the effects of ORENCIA on pregnant women or nursing infants are not known. Patients should be instructed to tell their healthcare professional if they are pregnant, become pregnant, or are thinking about becoming pregnant [see *Use in Specific Populations (8.1)*]. Patients should be instructed to tell their healthcare professional if they plan to breast-feed their infant [see *Use in Specific Populations (8.3)*].

17.6   Blood Glucose Testing

Patients should be asked if they have diabetes. Maltose contained in ORENCIA can give falsely elevated blood glucose readings with certain blood glucose monitors on the day of ORENCIA infusion. If a patient is using such a monitor, the patient should be advised to discuss with their healthcare professional methods that do not react with maltose [see *Drug Interactions (7.3)*].

Bristol-Myers Squibb Company
Princeton, NJ 08543 U.S.A.

B5-B0001-08-09   1251507A1   Rev August 2009

17.7   FDA-Approved Patient Labeling

PATIENT INFORMATION
ORENCIA® (oh-REN-see-ah)
(abatacept)

Read this Patient Information before you start receiving ORENCIA and each time before you are scheduled to receive ORENCIA. The information may have changed. This leaflet does not take the place of talking with your doctor about your medical condition or your treatment.

What is ORENCIA?

ORENCIA is a prescription medicine that reduces signs and symptoms in:

- adults with moderate to severe rheumatoid arthritis (RA), including those who have not been helped enough by other medicines for RA. ORENCIA may prevent further damage to your bones and joints and may help your ability to perform daily activities.
- children and adolescents 6 years of age and older with moderate to severe polyarticular juvenile idiopathic arthritis (JIA).

In RA and JIA, ORENCIA can reduce pain and joint inflammation, but it can also make your immune system less able to fight infection. ORENCIA can make you more likely to get infections or make any infection you have worse. It is important to tell your doctor if you think you have any infections.

ORENCIA has not been studied in children under 6 years of age.

What should I tell my doctor before treatment with ORENCIA (abatacept)?

Before you receive ORENCIA you should tell your doctor about all your medical conditions, including if you:

- have any kind of infection even if it is small (such as an open cut or sore), or an infection that is in your whole body (such as the flu). If you have an infection when taking ORENCIA, you may have a higher chance for getting serious side effects.
- have an infection that will not go away or a history of infections that keep coming back.
- have had tuberculosis (TB), a positive skin test for TB, or you recently have been in close contact with someone who has had TB. If you get any of the symptoms of TB (a dry cough that doesn't go away, weight loss, fever, night sweats) call your doctor right away. Before you start ORENCIA, your doctor may examine you for TB or perform a skin test.
- have or have had viral hepatitis. Before you use ORENCIA, your doctor may examine you for hepatitis.
- have a history of chronic obstructive pulmonary (lung) disease (COPD).
- are scheduled to have surgery.
- are allergic to any of the ingredients in ORENCIA. See the end of this leaflet for a list of the ingredients in ORENCIA.
- recently received a vaccination or are scheduled for any vaccination. If you are receiving ORENCIA, you should not take live vaccines.
- have diabetes and use a blood glucose monitor to check your blood sugar (blood glucose) levels. ORENCIA contains maltose, a type of sugar that can give false high blood sugar readings with certain types of blood glucose monitors, on the day of ORENCIA infusion. Your doctor may tell you to use a different way to monitor your blood sugar levels.
- are pregnant or planning to become pregnant. It is not known if ORENCIA can harm your unborn baby. Bristol-Myers Squibb Company has a registry for pregnant women exposed to ORENCIA. The purpose of this registry is to check the health of the pregnant mother and her child. Patients are encouraged to call the registry themselves or ask their doctors to contact the registry for them by calling 1-877-311-8972.
- are breast-feeding. ORENCIA can pass into breast milk. Women who are breast-feeding should talk to their doctor about whether or not to use ORENCIA.

Tell your doctor about all the medicines you take, including prescription and non-prescription medicines, vitamins, and herbal supplements. Do not start taking any new medicine without talking with your doctor.

Especially tell your doctor if you take other biologic medicines to treat RA or JIA that may affect your immune system, such as:

- Enbrel® (etanercept)
- Humira® (adalimumab)
- Remicade® (infliximab)
- Kineret® (anakinra)
- Rituxan® (rituximab)

You may have a higher chance of getting a serious infection if you take ORENCIA with other biologic medicines for your RA or JIA.

Know the medicines you take. Keep a list of your medicines and show it to your doctor and pharmacist when you get a new prescription.

How will I receive ORENCIA?

- You will be given ORENCIA by a healthcare provider through a needle placed in a vein (IV or intravenous infusion) in your arm. It takes about 30 minutes to give you the full dose of medicine.
- You will receive ORENCIA 2 weeks and 4 weeks after the first dose. You will then receive ORENCIA every 4 weeks.
- If you miss your appointment to receive ORENCIA, ask your doctor when to schedule your next dose.

What are the possible side effects of ORENCIA?

ORENCIA can cause serious side effects including:

- **Serious infections.** Patients receiving ORENCIA have a higher chance of getting infections including pneumonia, and other infections caused by viruses, bacteria, or fungi. Call your doctor right away if you feel sick or get any of the following symptoms of infection, which may be early signs of a serious infection:
  - a fever
  - feel very tired
  - have a cough
  - have flu-like symptoms
  - warm, red, or painful skin
- **Allergic reactions.** Allergic reactions can happen on the day of treatment or the day after receiving ORENCIA. Tell your doctor or get emergency medical help right away if you have hives, swollen face, eyelids, lips, tongue, throat, or trouble breathing.
- **Cancer (malignancies).** Certain kinds of cancer have been reported in patients receiving ORENCIA. It is not known

if ORENCIA (abatacept) increases your chance of getting certain kinds of cancer.

- **Vaccinations.** You should not receive ORENCIA with certain types of vaccines (live vaccines). ORENCIA may also cause some vaccinations to be less effective. Talk with your doctor about your vaccination plans.
- **Respiratory problems in patients with Chronic Obstructive Pulmonary Disease (COPD).** You may get certain respiratory problems more often if you receive ORENCIA and have COPD, including:
  - worsened COPD
  - pneumonia
  - cough
  - trouble breathing

Common side effects of ORENCIA in both adults and children include:

- headache
- upper respiratory tract infection
- sore throat
- nausea

In children, other side effects may include:

- diarrhea
- cough
- fever
- abdominal pain

Tell your doctor if you have any side effect that bothers you or that does not go away. These are not all the possible side effects of ORENCIA. For more information, ask your doctor or pharmacist.

Call your doctor for medical advice about side effects. You may report side effects to FDA at 1-800-FDA-1088.

General information about ORENCIA

Medicines are sometimes prescribed for conditions that are not mentioned in patient information leaflets. Do not use ORENCIA for a condition for which it was not prescribed. This patient information leaflet summarizes the most important information that you need to know about ORENCIA. If you would like more information, talk to your doctor.

You can ask your pharmacist or doctor for information about ORENCIA that is written for health professionals. For more information, go to www.ORENCIA.com or the company internet site at www.BMS.com or call 1-800-ORENCIA toll-free.

What are the ingredients in ORENCIA?

Active ingredient: abatacept

Inactive ingredients: maltose, monobasic sodium phosphate, sodium chloride for administration

Enbrel®, Humira®, Remicade®, Kineret®, and Rituxan® are trademarks of their respective companies.

Bristol-Myers Squibb Company
Princeton, NJ 08543 U.S.A.

B5-B0001-08-09   1251507A1   Rev August 2009
Shown in Product Identification Guide, page 321

PLAVIX   ℞

[*PLA-vix*]
(clopidogrel bisulfate)
tablets

HIGHLIGHTS OF PRESCRIBING INFORMATION
These highlights do not include all the information needed to use PLAVIX safely and effectively. See full prescribing information for PLAVIX.
PLAVIX (clopidogrel bisulfate) tablets
Initial U.S. Approval: 1997

WARNING: DIMINISHED EFFECTIVENESS IN POOR METABOLIZERS

See full prescribing information for complete boxed warning.

- **Effectiveness of Plavix depends on activation to an active metabolite by the cytochrome P450 (CYP) system, principally CYP2C19. (5.1)**
- **Poor metabolizers treated with Plavix at recommended doses exhibit higher cardiovascular event rates following acute coronary syndrome (ACS) or percutaneous coronary intervention (PCI) than patients with normal CYP2C19 function. (12.5)**
- **Tests are available to identify a patient's CYP2C19 genotype and can be used as an aid in determining therapeutic strategy. (12.5)**
- **Consider alternative treatment or treatment strategies in patients identified as CYP2C19 poor metabolizers. (2.3, 5.1)**

————RECENT MAJOR CHANGES————

Boxed Warning   03/2010
Dosage and Administration (2.3, 2.4)   08/2010
Warnings and Precautions (5.1, 5.2, 5.3) 08/2010

————INDICATIONS AND USAGE————

Plavix is a P2Y$_{12}$ platelet inhibitor indicated for:
- Acute coronary syndrome
  - For patients with non-ST-segment elevation ACS [unstable angina (UA)/ non-ST-elevation myocardial infarction (NSTEMI)] including patients who are to be

managed medically and those who are to be managed with coronary revascularization, Plavix has been shown to decrease the rate of a combined endpoint of cardiovascular death, myocardial infarction (MI), or stroke as well as the rate of a combined endpoint of cardiovascular death, MI, stroke, or refractory ischemia. (1.1)

- For patients with ST-elevation myocardial infarction (STEMI), Plavix has been shown to reduce the rate of death from any cause and the rate of a combined endpoint of death, re-infarction, or stroke. The benefit for patients who undergo primary PCI is unknown. (1.1)

• Recent myocardial infarction (MI), recent stroke, or established peripheral arterial disease. Plavix has been shown to reduce the combined endpoint of new ischemic stroke (fatal or not), new MI (fatal or not), and other vascular death. (1.2)

──────────**DOSAGE AND ADMINISTRATION**──────────
• Acute coronary syndrome (2.1)
- Non-ST-segment elevation ACS (UA/NSTEMI): 300 mg loading dose followed by 75 mg once daily, in combination with aspirin (75-325 mg once daily)
- STEMI: 75 mg once daily, in combination with aspirin (75-325 mg once daily), with or without a loading dose and with or without thrombolytics
• Recent MI, recent stroke, or established peripheral arterial disease: 75 mg once daily (2.2)

──────────**DOSAGE FORMS AND STRENGTHS**──────────
Tablets: 75 mg, 300 mg (3)

──────────**CONTRAINDICATIONS**──────────
• Active pathological bleeding, such as peptic ulcer or intracranial hemorrhage (4.1)
• Hypersensitivity to clopidogrel or any component of the product (4.2)

──────────**WARNINGS AND PRECAUTIONS**──────────
• Reduced effectiveness in impaired CYP2C19 function: Avoid concomitant use with drugs that are strong or moderate CYP2C19 inhibitors (e.g., omeprazole). (5.1)
• Bleeding: Plavix (clopidogrel bisulfate) increases risk of bleeding. Discontinue 5 days prior to elective surgery. (5.2)
• Discontinuation of Plavix: Premature discontinuation increases risk of cardiovascular events. (5.3)
• Recent transient ischemic attack or stroke: Combination use of Plavix and aspirin in these patients was not shown to be more effective than Plavix alone, but was shown to increase major bleeding. (5.4)
• Thrombotic thrombocytopenic purpura (TTP): TTP has been reported with Plavix, including fatal cases. (5.5)

──────────**ADVERSE REACTIONS**──────────
Bleeding, including life-threatening and fatal bleeding, is the most commonly reported adverse reaction. (6.1)

To report SUSPECTED ADVERSE REACTIONS, contact Bristol-Myers Squibb/ Sanofi Pharmaceuticals Partnership at 1-800-633-1610 or FDA at 1-800-FDA-1088 or www.fda.gov/medwatch.

──────────**DRUG INTERACTIONS**──────────
• Nonsteroidal anti-inflammatory drugs (NSAIDs): Combination use increases risk of gastrointestinal bleeding. (7.2)
• Warfarin: Combination use increases risk of bleeding. (7.3)

──────────**USE IN SPECIFIC POPULATIONS**──────────
Nursing mothers: Discontinue drug or nursing, taking into consideration importance of drug to mother. (8.3)
See 17 for PATIENT COUNSELING INFORMATION.
Revised: August 2010

FULL PRESCRIBING INFORMATION: CONTENTS*

FULL PRESCRIBING INFORMATION

┌───┐
WARNING: DIMINISHED EFFECTIVENESS IN POOR METABOLIZERS

The effectiveness of Plavix (clopidogrel bisulfate) is dependent on its activation to an active metabolite by the cytochrome P450 (CYP) system, principally CYP2C19 *[see Warnings and Precautions (5.1)]*. Plavix at recommended doses forms less of that metabolite and has a smaller effect on platelet function in patients who are CYP2C19 poor metabolizers. Poor metabolizers with acute coronary syndrome or undergoing percutaneous coronary intervention treated with Plavix at recommended doses exhibit higher cardiovascular event rates than do patients with normal CYP2C19 function. Tests are available to identify a patient's CYP2C19 genotype; these tests can be used as an aid in determining therapeutic strategy *[see Clinical Pharmacology (12.5)]*. Consider alternative treatment or treatment strategies in patients identified as CYP2C19 poor metabolizers *[see Dosage and Administration (2.3)]*.
└───┘

1 INDICATIONS AND USAGE

1.1 Acute Coronary Syndrome (ACS)

• For patients with non-ST-segment elevation ACS [unstable angina (UA)/non-ST-elevation myocardial infarction (NSTEMI)], including patients who are to be managed medically and those who are to be managed with coronary revascularization, Plavix has been shown to decrease the rate of a combined endpoint of cardiovascular death, myocardial infarction (MI), or stroke as well as the rate of a combined endpoint of cardiovascular death, MI, stroke, or refractory ischemia.

• For patients with ST-elevation myocardial infarction (STEMI), Plavix has been shown to reduce the rate of death from any cause and the rate of a combined endpoint of death, re-infarction, or stroke. The benefit for patients who undergo primary percutaneous coronary intervention is unknown.

The optimal duration of Plavix therapy in ACS is unknown.

1.2 Recent MI, Recent Stroke, or Established Peripheral Arterial Disease

For patients with a history of recent myocardial infarction (MI), recent stroke, or established peripheral arterial disease, Plavix has been shown to reduce the rate of a combined endpoint of new ischemic stroke (fatal or not), new MI (fatal or not), and other vascular death.

2 DOSAGE AND ADMINISTRATION

2.1 Acute Coronary Syndrome

Plavix can be administered with or without food *[see Clinical Pharmacology (12.3)]*

• For patients with non-ST-elevation ACS (UA/NSTEMI), initiate Plavix with a single 300 mg oral loading dose and then continue at 75 mg once daily. Initiate aspirin (75-325 mg once daily) and continue in combination with Plavix *[see Clinical Studies (14.1)]*.

• For patients with STEMI, the recommended dose of Plavix is 75 mg once daily orally, administered in combination with aspirin (75-325 mg once daily), with or without thrombolytics. Plavix (clopidogrel bisulfate) may be initiated with or without a loading dose *[see Clinical Studies (14.1)]*.

2.2 Recent MI, Recent Stroke, or Established Peripheral Arterial Disease

The recommended daily dose of Plavix is 75 mg once daily orally, with or without food *[see Clinical Pharmacology (12.3)]*.

2.3 CYP2C19 Poor Metabolizers

CYP2C19 poor metabolizer status is associated with diminished antiplatelet response to clopidogrel. Although a higher dose regimen in poor metabolizers increases antiplatelet response *[see Clinical Pharmacology (12.5)]*, an appropriate dose regimen for this patient population has not been established.

2.4 Use with Proton Pump Inhibitors (PPI)

Omeprazole, a moderate CYP2C19 inhibitor, reduces the pharmacological activity of Plavix. Avoid using omeprazole concomitantly or 12 hours apart with Plavix. Consider using another acid-reducing agent with less CYP2C19 inhibitory activity. A higher dose regimen of clopidogrel concomitantly administered with omeprazole increases antiplatelet response; an appropriate dose regimen has not been established *[see Warnings and Precautions (5.1), Drug Interactions (7.1) and Clinical Pharmacology (12.5)]*.

3 DOSAGE FORMS AND STRENGTHS

• 75 mg tablets: Pink, round, biconvex, film-coated tablets debossed with "75" on one side and "1171" on the other
• 300 mg tablets: Pink, oblong, film-coated tablets debossed with "300" on one side and "1332" on the other

4 CONTRAINDICATIONS

4.1 Active Bleeding

Plavix is contraindicated in patients with active pathological bleeding such as peptic ulcer or intracranial hemorrhage.

4.2 Hypersensitivity

Plavix is contraindicated in patients with hypersensitivity (e.g., anaphylaxis) to clopidogrel or any component of the product *[see Adverse Reactions (6.2)]*.

5 WARNINGS AND PRECAUTIONS

5.1 Diminished Antiplatelet Activity Due to Impaired CYP2C19 Function

Clopidogrel is a prodrug. Inhibition of platelet aggregation by clopidogrel is due to an active metabolite. The metabolism of clopidogrel to its active metabolite can be impaired by genetic variations in CYP2C19 *[see Boxed Warning]* and by concomitant medications that interfere with CYP2C19. Avoid concomitant use of Plavix and strong or moderate CYP2C19 inhibitors.

Omeprazole, a moderate CYP2C19 inhibitor, has been shown to reduce the pharmacological activity of Plavix if given concomitantly or if given 12 hours apart. Consider using another acid-reducing agent with less CYP2C19 inhibitory activity. Pantoprazole, a weak CYP2C19 inhibitor, had less effect on the pharmacological activity of Plavix than omeprazole *[see Drug Interactions (7.1) and Dosage and Administration (2.4)]*.

5.2 General Risk of Bleeding

Thienopyridines, including Plavix, increase the risk of bleeding. If a patient is to undergo surgery and an antiplatelet effect is not desired, discontinue Plavix five days prior to surgery. In patients who stopped therapy more than five days prior to CABG the rates of major bleeding were similar (event rate 4.4% Plavix + aspirin; 5.3% placebo + aspirin). In patients who remained on therapy within five days of CABG, the major bleeding rate was 9.6% for Plavix + aspirin, and 6.3% for placebo + aspirin.

Thienopyridines inhibit platelet aggregation for the lifetime of the platelet (7-10 days), so withholding a dose will not be useful in managing a bleeding event or the risk of bleeding associated with an invasive procedure. Because the half-life of clopidogrel's active metabolite is short, it may be possible to restore hemostasis by administering exogenous platelets; however, platelet transfusions within 4 hours of the loading dose or 2 hours of the maintenance dose may be less effective.

5.3 Discontinuation of Plavix

Avoid lapses in therapy, and if Plavix must be temporarily discontinued, restart as soon as possible. Premature discontinuation of Plavix may increase the risk of cardiovascular events.

5.4 Patients with Recent Transient Ischemic Attack (TIA) or Stroke

In patients with recent TIA or stroke who are at high risk for recurrent ischemic events, the combination of aspirin and Plavix (clopidogrel bisulfate) has not been shown to be more effective than Plavix alone, but the combination has been shown to increase major bleeding.

5.5   Thrombotic Thrombocytopenic Purpura (TTP)
TTP, sometimes fatal, has been reported following use of Plavix, sometimes after a short exposure (<2 weeks). TTP is a serious condition that requires urgent treatment including plasmapheresis (plasma exchange). It is characterized by thrombocytopenia, microangiopathic hemolytic anemia (schistocytes [fragmented RBCs] seen on peripheral smear), neurological findings, renal dysfunction, and fever *[see Adverse Reactions (6.2)]*.

6   ADVERSE REACTIONS
The following serious adverse reactions are discussed below and elsewhere in the labeling:
• Bleeding *[see Warnings and Precautions (5.2)]*
• Thrombotic thrombocytopenic purpura *[see Warnings and Precautions (5.5)]*

6.1   Clinical Studies Experience
Because clinical trials are conducted under widely varying conditions and durations of follow up, adverse reaction rates observed in the clinical trials of a drug cannot be directly compared to rates in the clinical trials of another drug and may not reflect the rates observed in practice.

Plavix has been evaluated for safety in more than 54,000 patients, including over 21,000 patients treated for 1 year or more. The clinically important adverse reactions observed in trials comparing Plavix plus aspirin to placebo plus aspirin and trials comparing Plavix alone to aspirin alone are discussed below.

Bleeding
CURE
In CURE, Plavix use with aspirin was associated with an increase in major bleeding (primarily gastrointestinal and at puncture sites) compared to placebo with aspirin (see Table 1). The incidence of intracranial hemorrhage (0.1%) and fatal bleeding (0.2%) were the same in both groups. Other bleeding events that were reported more frequently in the clopidogrel group were epistaxis, hematuria, and bruise. The overall incidence of bleeding is described in Table 1. [See table 1 above]

Ninety-two percent (92%) of the patients in the CURE study received heparin or low molecular weight heparin (LMWH), and the rate of bleeding in these patients was similar to the overall results.

COMMIT
In COMMIT, similar rates of major bleeding were observed in the Plavix and placebo groups, both of which also received aspirin (see Table 2).

Table 2:   Incidence of Bleeding Events in COMMIT (% patients)

Type of bleeding	Plavix (+ aspirin) (n=22961)	Placebo (+ aspirin) (n=22891)	p-value
Major* noncerebral or cerebral bleeding**	0.6	0.5	0.59
Major noncerebral	0.4	0.3	0.48
Fatal	0.2	0.2	0.90
Hemorrhagic stroke	0.2	0.2	0.91
Fatal	0.2	0.2	0.81
Other noncerebral bleeding (non-major)	3.6	3.1	0.005
Any noncerebral bleeding	3.9	3.4	0.004

* Major bleeds were cerebral bleeds or non-cerebral bleeds thought to have caused death or that required transfusion.
**The relative rate of major noncerebral or cerebral bleeding was independent of age. Event rates for Plavix + aspirin by age were: <60 years = 0.3%, ≥60 to <70 years = 0.7%, ≥70 years = 0.8%. Event rates for placebo + aspirin by age were: <60 years = 0.4%, ≥60 to <70 years = 0.6%, ≥70 years = 0.7%.

CAPRIE (Plavix vs. Aspirin)
In CAPRIE, gastrointestinal hemorrhage occurred at a rate of 2.0% in those taking Plavix vs. 2.7% in those taking aspirin; bleeding requiring hospitalization occurred in 0.7% and 1.1%, respectively. The incidence of intracranial hemorrhage was 0.4% for Plavix compared to 0.5% for aspirin. Other bleeding events that were reported more frequently in the Plavix group were epistaxis and hematoma.

Other Adverse Events
In CURE and CHARISMA, which compared Plavix plus aspirin to aspirin alone, there was no difference in the rate of adverse events (other than bleeding) between Plavix and placebo.

Table 1:   CURE Incidence of Bleeding Complications (% patients)

Event	Plavix (+ aspirin)* (n=6259)	Placebo (+ aspirin)* (n=6303)	p-value
Major bleeding[†]	3.7[‡]	2.7[§]	0.001
Life-threatening bleeding	2.2	1.8	0.13
Fatal	0.2	0.2	
5 g/dL hemoglobin drop	0.9	0.9	
Requiring surgical intervention	0.7	0.7	
Hemorrhagic strokes	0.1	0.1	
Requiring inotropes	0.5	0.5	
Requiring transfusion (≥4 units)	1.2	1.0	
Other major bleeding	1.6	1.0	0.005
Significantly disabling	0.4	0.3	
Intraocular bleeding with significant loss of vision	0.05	0.03	
Requiring 2-3 units of blood	1.3	0.9	
Minor bleeding[¶]	5.1	2.4	<0.001

* Other standard therapies were used as appropriate.
† Life-threatening and other major bleeding.
‡ Major bleeding event rate for Plavix + aspirin was dose-dependent on aspirin: <100 mg = 2.6%; 100-200 mg = 3.5%; >200 mg = 4.9%.
   Major bleeding event rates for Plavix + aspirin by age were: <65 years = 2.5%, ≥65 to <75 years = 4.1%, ≥75 years = 5.9%.
§ Major bleeding event rate for placebo + aspirin was dose-dependent on aspirin: <100 mg = 2.0%; 100-200 mg = 2.3%; >200 mg = 4.0%.
   Major bleeding event rates for placebo + aspirin by age were: <65 years = 2.1%, ≥65 to <75 years = 3.1%, ≥75 years = 3.6%.
¶ Led to interruption of study medication.

Table 3:   Comparison of Clopidogrel Active Metabolite Exposure and Platelet Inhibition with and without Proton Pump Inhibitors, Omeprazole and Pantoprazole

Plavix plus	% Change from Plavix (300 mg/75 mg) alone					
	C_{max} (ng/mL)		AUC		Platelet Inhibition[†] (%)	
	Day 1	Day 5	Day 1	Day 5**	Day 1	Day 5
Omeprazole* 80 mg	↓46%	↓42%	↓45%	↓40%	↓39%	↓21%
Pantoprazole 80 mg	↓24%	↓28%	↓20%	↓14%	↓15%	↓11%

† Inhibition of platelet aggregation with 5 mcM ADP.
* Similar results seen when Plavix and omeprazole were administered 12 hours apart.
**AUC at Day 5 is AUC_{0-24}.

In CAPRIE, which compared Plavix (clopidogrel bisulfate) to aspirin, pruritus was more frequently reported in those taking Plavix. No other difference in the rate of adverse events (other than bleeding) was reported.

6.2   Postmarketing Experience
The following adverse reactions have been identified during post-approval use of Plavix. Because these reactions are reported voluntarily from a population of an unknown size, it is not always possible to reliably estimate their frequency or establish a causal relationship to drug exposure.

• *Blood and lymphatic system disorders:* Agranulocytosis, aplastic anemia/ pancytopenia, thrombotic thrombocytopenic purpura (TTP)
• *Gastrointestinal disorders:* Gastrointestinal and retroperitoneal hemorrhage with fatal outcome, colitis (including ulcerative or lymphocytic colitis), pancreatitis, stomatitis
• *General disorders and administration site condition:* Fever, hemorrhage of operative wound
• *Hepato-biliary disorders:* Acute liver failure, hepatitis (non-infectious), abnormal liver function test
• *Immune system disorders:* Hypersensitivity reactions, anaphylactoid reactions, serum sickness
• *Musculoskeletal, connective tissue and bone disorders:* Musculoskeletal bleeding, myalgia, arthralgia, arthritis
• *Nervous system disorders:* Taste disorders, fatal intracranial bleeding
• *Eye disorders:* Eye (conjunctival, ocular, retinal) bleeding
• *Psychiatric disorders:* Confusion, hallucinations
• *Respiratory, thoracic and mediastinal disorders:* Bronchospasm, interstitial pneumonitis, respiratory tract bleeding
• *Renal and urinary disorders:* Glomerulopathy, increased creatinine levels
• *Skin and subcutaneous tissue disorders:* Maculopapular or erythematous rash, urticaria, bullous dermatitis, eczema, toxic epidermal necrolysis, Stevens-Johnson syndrome, angioedema, erythema multiforme, skin bleeding, lichen planus
• *Vascular disorders:* Vasculitis, hypotension

7   DRUG INTERACTIONS
7.1   CYP2C19 Inhibitors
Clopidogrel is metabolized to its active metabolite in part by CYP2C19. Concomitant use of drugs that inhibit the activity of this enzyme results in reduced plasma concentrations of the active metabolite of clopidogrel and a reduction in platelet inhibition *[see Warnings and Precautions (5.1) and Dosage and Administration (2.4)]*.

Proton Pump Inhibitors (PPI)
A study was conducted with Plavix (clopidogrel bisulfate) (300 mg loading dose followed by 75 mg/day) administered with a high dose (80 mg/day) of omeprazole. As shown in Table 3 below, with concomitant dosing of omeprazole, exposure (C_{max} and AUC) to the clopidogrel active metabolite and platelet inhibition were substantially reduced. Similar reductions in exposure to the clopidogrel active metabolite and platelet inhibition were observed when Plavix and omeprazole were administered 12 hours apart (data not shown). There are no adequate studies of a lower dose of omeprazole or a higher dose of Plavix in comparison with the approved dose of Plavix.

A study was conducted using Plavix (300 mg loading dose followed by 75 mg/day) and a high dose (80 mg/day) of pantoprazole, a PPI with less CYP2C19 inhibitory activity than omeprazole. The plasma concentrations of the clopidogrel active metabolite and the degree of platelet inhibition were less than observed with Plavix alone but were greater than observed when omeprazole 80 mg was coadministered with 300 mg loading dose followed by 75 mg/day of Plavix (Table 3).
[See table 3 above]

7.2   Nonsteroidal Anti-Inflammatory Drugs (NSAIDs)
Coadministration of Plavix and NSAIDs increases the risk of gastrointestinal bleeding.

7.3   Warfarin (CYP2C9 Substrates)
Although the administration of clopidogrel 75 mg per day did not modify the pharmacokinetics of S-warfarin (a CYP2C9 substrate) or INR in patients receiving long-term warfarin therapy, coadministration of Plavix with warfarin increases the risk of bleeding because of independent effects on hemostasis.

However, at high concentrations *in vitro*, clopidogrel inhibits CYP2C9.

8   USE IN SPECIFIC POPULATIONS
8.1   Pregnancy
Pregnancy Category B
Reproduction studies performed in rats and rabbits at doses up to 500 and 300 mg/kg/day, respectively (65 and 78 times the recommended daily human dose, respectively, on a mg/m^2 basis), revealed no evidence of impaired fertility or fetotoxicity due to clopidogrel. There are, however, no adequate and well-controlled studies in pregnant women. Because animal reproduction studies are not always predictive of a human response, Plavix should be used during pregnancy only if clearly needed.

8.3   Nursing Mothers
Studies in rats have shown that clopidogrel and/or its metabolites are excreted in the milk. It is not known whether this drug is excreted in human milk. Because many drugs are excreted in human milk and because of the potential for serious adverse reactions in nursing infants from clopidogrel, a decision should be made whether to discontinue nursing or to discontinue the drug, taking into account the importance of the drug to the mother.

8.4   Pediatric Use
Safety and effectiveness in the pediatric population have not been established.

8.5   Geriatric Use
Of the total number of subjects in the CAPRIE and CURE controlled clinical studies, approximately 50% of patients treated with Plavix (clopidogrel bisulfate) were 65 years of age and older, and 15% were 75 years and older. In COMMIT, approximately 58% of the patients treated with Plavix were 60 years and older, 26% of whom were 70 years and older.
The observed risk of thrombotic events with clopidogrel plus aspirin versus placebo plus aspirin by age category is provided in Figures 2 and 5 for the CURE and COMMIT trials, respectively [*see Clinical Studies (14.1)*]. The observed risk of bleeding events with clopidogrel plus aspirin versus placebo plus aspirin by age category is provided in Tables 1 and 2 for the CURE and COMMIT trials, respectively [*see Adverse Reactions (6.1)*]. No dosage adjustment is necessary in elderly patients.

8.6   Renal Impairment
Experience is limited in patients with severe and moderate renal impairment [*see Clinical Pharmacology (12.2)*].

8.7   Hepatic Impairment
No dosage adjustment is necessary in patients with hepatic impairment [*see Clinical Pharmacology (12.2)*].

10   OVERDOSAGE
Platelet inhibition by Plavix is irreversible and will last for the life of the platelet. Overdose following clopidogrel administration may result in bleeding complications. A single oral dose of clopidogrel at 1500 or 2000 mg/kg was lethal to mice and to rats and at 3000 mg/kg to baboons. Symptoms of acute toxicity were vomiting, prostration, difficult breathing, and gastrointestinal hemorrhage in animals.
Based on biological plausibility, platelet transfusion may restore clotting ability.

11   DESCRIPTION
Plavix (clopidogrel bisulfate) is a thienopyridine class inhibitor of P2Y$_{12}$ ADP platelet receptors. Chemically it is methyl (+)-(*S*)-α-(2-chlorophenyl)-6,7-dihydrothieno[3,2-c] pyridine-5(4*H*)-acetate sulfate (1:1). The empirical formula of clopidogrel bisulfate is $C_{16}H_{16}ClNO_2S \bullet H_2SO_4$ and its molecular weight is 419.9.
The structural formula is as follows:

Clopidogrel bisulfate is a white to off-white powder. It is practically insoluble in water at neutral pH but freely soluble at pH 1. It also dissolves freely in methanol, dissolves sparingly in methylene chloride, and is practically insoluble in ethyl ether. It has a specific optical rotation of about +56°.
Plavix for oral administration is provided as either pink, round, biconvex, debossed, film-coated tablets containing 97.875 mg of clopidogrel bisulfate which is the molar equivalent of 75 mg of clopidogrel base or pink, oblong, debossed film-coated tablets containing 391.5 mg of clopidogrel bisulfate which is the molar equivalent of 300 mg of clopidogrel base.
Each tablet contains hydrogenated castor oil, hydroxypropylcellulose, mannitol, microcrystalline cellulose and polyethylene glycol 6000 as inactive ingredients. The pink film coating contains ferric oxide, hypromellose 2910, lactose monohydrate, titanium dioxide and triacetin. The tablets are polished with Carnauba wax.

Table 4:   Active Metabolite Pharmacokinetics and Antiplatelet Responses by CYP2C19 Metabolizer Status

	Dose	Ultrarapid (n=10)	Extensive (n=10)	Intermediate (n=10)	Poor (n=10)
C$_{max}$ (ng/mL)	300 mg (24 h)	24 (10)	32 (21)	23 (11)	11 (4)
	600 mg (24 h)	36 (13)	44 (27)	39 (23)	17 (6)
	75 mg (Day 5)	12 (6)	13 (7)	12 (5)	4 (1)
	150 mg (Day 5)	16 (9)	19 (5)	18 (7)	7 (2)
IPA (%)*	300 mg (24 h)	40 (21)	39 (28)	37 (21)	24 (26)
	600 mg (24 h)	51 (28)	49 (23)	56 (22)	32 (25)
	75 mg (Day 5)	56 (18)	58 (19)	60 (18)	37 (23)
	150 mg (Day 5)	68 (18)	73 (9)	74 (14)	61 (14)
VASP-PRI (%)[†]	300 mg (24 h)	73 (12)	68 (16)	78 (12)	91 (12)
	600 mg (24 h)	51 (20)	48 (20)	56 (26)	85 (14)
	75 mg (Day 5)	40 (9)	39 (14)	50 (16)	83 (13)
	150 mg (Day 5)	20 (10)	24 (10)	29 (11)	61 (18)

Values are mean (SD).
* Inhibition of platelet aggregation with 5mcM ADP; larger value indicates greater platelet inhibition.
[†] Vasodilator-stimulated phosphoprotein – platelet reactivity index; smaller value indicates greater platelet inhibition.

Table 5:   Outcome Events in the CURE Primary Analysis

Outcome	Plavix (+ aspirin)* (n=6259)	Placebo (+ aspirin)* (n=6303)	Relative Risk Reduction (%) (95% CI)
Primary outcome (Cardiovascular death, MI, stroke)	582 (9.3%)	719 (11.4%)	20% (10.3, 27.9) p<0.001
All Individual Outcome Events:[†]			
CV death	318 (5.1%)	345 (5.5%)	7% (-7.7, 20.6)
MI	324 (5.2%)	419 (6.6%)	23% (11.0, 33.4)
Stroke	75 (1.2%)	87 (1.4%)	14% (-17.7, 36.6)

* Other standard therapies were used as appropriate.
[†] The individual components do not represent a breakdown of the primary and co-primary outcomes, but rather the total number of subjects experiencing an event during the course of the study.

12   CLINICAL PHARMACOLOGY
12.1   Mechanism of Action
Clopidogrel is an inhibitor of platelet activation and aggregation through the irreversible binding of its active metabolite to the P2Y$_{12}$ class of ADP receptors on platelets.
12.2   Pharmacodynamics
Clopidogrel must be metabolized by CYP450 enzymes to produce the active metabolite that inhibits platelet aggregation. The active metabolite of clopidogrel selectively inhibits the binding of adenosine diphosphate (ADP) to its platelet P2Y$_{12}$ receptor and the subsequent ADP-mediated activation of the glycoprotein GPIIb/IIIa complex, thereby inhibiting platelet aggregation. This action is irreversible. Consequently, platelets exposed to clopidogrel's active metabolite are affected for the remainder of their lifespan (about 7 to 10 days). Platelet aggregation induced by agonists other than ADP is also inhibited by blocking the amplification of platelet activation by released ADP.
Dose-dependent inhibition of platelet aggregation can be seen 2 hours after single oral doses of Plavix (clopidogrel bisulfate). Repeated doses of 75 mg Plavix per day inhibit ADP-induced platelet aggregation on the first day, and inhibition reaches steady state between Day 3 and Day 7. At steady state, the average inhibition level observed with a dose of 75 mg Plavix per day was between 40% and 60%. Platelet aggregation and bleeding time gradually return to baseline values after treatment is discontinued, generally in about 5 days.
Geriatric Patients
Elderly (≥75 years) and young healthy subjects had similar effects on platelet aggregation.
Renally-Impaired Patients
After repeated doses of 75 mg Plavix per day, patients with severe renal impairment (creatinine clearance from 5 to 15 mL/min) and moderate renal impairment (creatinine clearance from 30 to 60 mL/min) showed low (25%) inhibition of ADP-induced platelet aggregation.
Hepatically-Impaired Patients
After repeated doses of 75 mg Plavix per day for 10 days in patients with severe hepatic impairment, inhibition of ADP-induced platelet aggregation was similar to that observed in healthy subjects.
Gender
In a small study comparing men and women, less inhibition of ADP-induced platelet aggregation was observed in women.
12.3   Pharmacokinetics
Clopidogrel is a prodrug and is metabolized to a pharmacologically active metabolite and inactive metabolites.

Absorption
After single and repeated oral doses of 75 mg per day, clopidogrel is rapidly absorbed. Absorption is at least 50%, based on urinary excretion of clopidogrel metabolites.
Effect of Food
Plavix can be administered with or without food. In a study in healthy male subjects when Plavix (clopidogrel bisulfate) 75 mg per day was given with a standard breakfast, mean inhibition of ADP-induced platelet aggregation was reduced by less than 9%. The active metabolite AUC$_{0-24}$ was unchanged in the presence of food, while there was a 57% decrease in active metabolite C$_{max}$. Similar results were observed when a Plavix 300 mg loading dose was administered with a high-fat breakfast.
Metabolism
Clopidogrel is extensively metabolized by two main metabolic pathways: one mediated by esterases and leading to hydrolysis into an inactive carboxylic acid derivative (85% of circulating metabolites) and one mediated by multiple cytochrome P450 enzymes. Cytochromes first oxidize clopidogrel to a 2-oxo-clopidogrel intermediate metabolite. Subsequent metabolism of the 2-oxo-clopidogrel intermediate metabolite results in formation of the active metabolite, a thiol derivative of clopidogrel. This metabolic pathway is mediated by CYP2C19, CYP3A, CYP2B6 and CYP1A2. The active thiol metabolite binds rapidly and irreversibly to platelet receptors, thus inhibiting platelet aggregation for the lifespan of the platelet.
The C$_{max}$ of the active metabolite is twice as high following a single 300 mg clopidogrel loading dose as it is after four days of 75 mg maintenance dose. C$_{max}$ occurs approximately 30 to 60 minutes after dosing. In the 75 to 300 mg dose range, the pharmacokinetics of the active metabolite deviates from dose proportionality: increasing the dose by a factor of four results in 2.0- and 2.7-fold increases in C$_{max}$ and AUC, respectively.
Elimination
Following an oral dose of ^{14}C-labeled clopidogrel in humans, approximately 50% of total radioactivity was excreted in urine and approximately 46% in feces over the 5 days post-dosing. After a single, oral dose of 75 mg, clopidogrel has a half-life of approximately 6 hours. The half-life of the active metabolite is about 30 minutes.
12.5   Pharmacogenomics
CYP2C19 is involved in the formation of both the active metabolite and the 2-oxo-clopidogrel intermediate metabolite. Clopidogrel active metabolite pharmacokinetics and antiplatelet effects, as measured by *ex vivo* platelet aggregation

assays, differ according to CYP2C19 genotype. Genetic variants of other CYP450 enzymes may also affect the formation of clopidogrel's active metabolite.

The CYP2C19*1 allele corresponds to fully functional metabolism while the CYP2C19*2 and *3 alleles are nonfunctional. CYP2C19*2 and *3 account for the majority of reduced function alleles in white (85%) and Asian (99%) poor metabolizers. Other alleles associated with absent or reduced metabolism are less frequent, and include, but are not limited to, CYP2C19*4, *5, *6, *7, and *8. A patient with poor metabolizer status will possess two loss-of-function alleles as defined above. Published frequencies for poor CYP2C19 metabolizer genotypes are approximately 2% for whites, 4% for blacks and 14% for Chinese. Tests are available to determine a patient's CYP2C19 genotype.

A crossover study in 40 healthy subjects, 10 each in the four CYP2C19 metabolizer groups, evaluated pharmacokinetic and antiplatelet responses using 300 mg followed by 75 mg per day and 600 mg followed by 150 mg per day, each for a total of 5 days. Decreased active metabolite exposure and diminished inhibition of platelet aggregation were observed in the poor metabolizers as compared to the other groups. When poor metabolizers received the 600 mg/150 mg regimen, active metabolite exposure and antiplatelet response were greater than with the 300 mg/75 mg regimen (see Table 4). An appropriate dose regimen for this patient population has not been established in clinical outcome trials.
[See table 4 at top of previous page]

Some published studies suggest that intermediate metabolizers have decreased active metabolite exposure and diminished antiplatelet effects.

The relationship between CYP2C19 genotype and Plavix (clopidogrel bisulfate) treatment outcome was evaluated in retrospective analyses of Plavix-treated subjects in CHARISMA (n=2428) and TRITON-TIMI 38 (n=1477), and in several published cohort studies. In TRITON-TIMI 38 and the majority of the cohort studies, the combined group of patients with either intermediate or poor metabolizer status had a higher rate of cardiovascular events (death, myocardial infarction, and stroke) or stent thrombosis compared to extensive metabolizers. In CHARISMA and one cohort study, the increased event rate was observed only in poor metabolizers.

13 NONCLINICAL TOXICOLOGY

13.1 Carcinogenesis, Mutagenesis, Impairment of Fertility

There was no evidence of tumorigenicity when clopidogrel was administered for 78 weeks to mice and 104 weeks to rats at dosages up to 77 mg/kg per day, which afforded plasma exposures >25 times that in humans at the recommended daily dose of 75 mg.

Clopidogrel was not genotoxic in four *in vitro* tests (Ames test, DNA-repair test in rat hepatocytes, gene mutation assay in Chinese hamster fibroblasts, and metaphase chromosome analysis of human lymphocytes) and in one *in vivo* test (micronucleus test by oral route in mice).

Clopidogrel was found to have no effect on fertility of male and female rats at oral doses up to 400 mg/kg per day (52 times the recommended human dose on a mg/m^2 basis).

14 CLINICAL STUDIES

The clinical evidence of the efficacy of Plavix is derived from three double-blind trials involving 77,599 patients. The CAPRIE study (Clopidogrel vs. Aspirin in Patients at Risk of Ischemic Events) was a comparison of Plavix to aspirin. The CURE (Clopidogrel in Unstable Angina to Prevent Recurrent Ischemic Events) and the COMMIT/CCS-2 (Clopidogrel and Metoprolol in Myocardial Infarction Trial/Second Chinese Cardiac Study) studies were comparisons of Plavix to placebo, given in combination with aspirin and other standard therapy. The CHARISMA (Clopidogrel for High Atherothrombotic Risk Ischemic Stabilization, Management, and Avoidance) study (n=15,603) also compared Plavix to placebo, given in combination with aspirin and other standard therapy.

14.1 Acute Coronary Syndrome

CURE

The CURE study included 12,562 patients with ACS without ST-elevation (UA or NSTEMI) and presenting within 24 hours of onset of the most recent episode of chest pain or symptoms consistent with ischemia. Patients were required to have either ECG changes compatible with new ischemia (without ST-elevation) or elevated cardiac enzymes or troponin I or T to at least twice the upper limit of normal. The patient population was largely Caucasian (82%) and included 38% women, and 52% patients ≥65 years of age. Patients were randomized to receive Plavix (300-mg loading dose followed by 75 mg once daily) or placebo, and were treated for up to one year. Patients also received aspirin (75-325 mg once daily) and other standard therapies such as heparin. The use of GPIIb/IIIa inhibitors was not permitted for three days prior to randomization.

The number of patients experiencing the primary outcome (CV death, MI, or stroke) was 582 (9.3%) in the Plavix-

treated group and 719 (11.4%) in the placebo-treated group, a 20% relative risk reduction (95% CI of 10%-28%; p<0.001) for the Plavix-treated group (see Table 5).
[See table 5 on previous page]

Most of the benefit of Plavix occurred in the first two months, but the difference from placebo was maintained throughout the course of the trial (up to 12 months) (see Figure 1).

Figure 1: Cardiovascular Death, Myocardial Infarction, and Stroke in the CURE Study

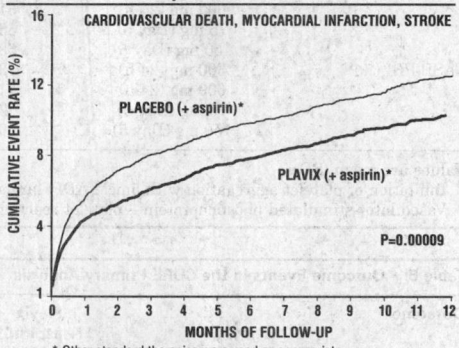

* Other standard therapies were used as appropriate.

In CURE, the use of Plavix (clopidogrel bisulfate) was associated with a lower incidence of CV death, MI or stroke in patient populations with different characteristics, as shown in Figure 2. The benefits associated with Plavix were independent of the use of other acute and long-term cardiovascular therapies, including heparin/LMWH, intravenous glycoprotein IIb/IIIa (GPIIb/IIIa) inhibitors, lipid-lowering drugs, beta-blockers, and ACE-inhibitors. The efficacy of Plavix was observed independently of the dose of aspirin (75-325 mg once daily). The use of oral anticoagulants, non-study anti-platelet drugs, and chronic NSAIDs was not allowed in CURE.

Figure 2: Hazard Ratio for Patient Baseline Characteristics and On-Study Concomitant Medications/Interventions for the CURE Study

Baseline Characteristics		N	Percent Events PLAVIX (+aspirin)*	Percent Events Placebo (+aspirin)*	PLAVIX Better	Placebo Better
Overall		12562	9.3	11.4		
Diagnosis	Non-Q-W	3295	12.7	15.5		
	UnstAng	8298	7.3	8.7		
	Other	968	15.1	19.7		
Age	<65	5996	5.2	7.6		
	65-74	4136	10.2	12.4		
	≥75	2430	17.8	19.2		
Gender	Male	7726	9.1	11.9		
	Female	4836	9.5	10.7		
Race	Caucas	10308	9.1	11.0		
	Non-Cauc	2250	10.1	13.2		
Elev Card Enzy	No	9381	8.8	10.9		
	Yes	3176	10.7	13.0		
ST Depr >1.0mm	No	7273	7.5	8.9		
	Yes	5288	11.8	14.8		
Diabetes	No	9721	7.9	9.9		
	Yes	2840	14.2	16.7		
Previous MI	No	8517	7.8	9.5		
	Yes	4044	12.5	15.4		
Previous Stroke	No	12055	8.9	11.0		
	Yes	506	17.9	22.4		
Concomitant Medication / Therapy						
Heparin/LMWH	No	951	4.9	7.7		
	Yes	11611	9.5	11.7		
Aspirin	<100mg	1927	8.5	9.7		
	100-200mg	7428	9.2	10.9		
	>200mg	3201	9.9	13.7		
GPIIb/IIIa Antag	No	11739	8.9	10.8		
	Yes	823	15.7	19.2		
Beta-Blocker	No	2032	9.9	12.0		
	Yes	10530	9.2	11.3		
ACEI	No	4813	6.3	8.1		
	Yes	7749	11.2	13.5		
Lipid-Lowering	No	4461	10.9	13.1		
	Yes	8101	8.4	10.5		
PTCA/CABG	No	7977	8.1	10.0		
	Yes	4585	11.4	13.8		

*Other standard therapies were used as appropriate.

Hazard Ratio (95% CI) 0.4 0.6 0.8 1.0 1.2

The use of Plavix in CURE was associated with a decrease in the use of thrombolytic therapy (71 patients [1.1%] in the Plavix group, 126 patients [2.0%] in the placebo group; relative risk reduction of 43%), and GPIIb/IIIa inhibitors (369 patients [5.9%] in the Plavix group, 454 patients [7.2%] in the placebo group, relative risk reduction of 18%). The use of Plavix in CURE did not affect the number of patients treated with CABG or PCI (with or without stenting), (2253 patients [36.0%] in the Plavix group, 2324 patients [36.9%] in the placebo group; relative risk reduction of 4.0%).

COMMIT

In patients with STEMI, the safety and efficacy of Plavix were evaluated in the randomized, placebo-controlled, double-blind study, COMMIT. COMMIT included 45,852

patients presenting within 24 hours of the onset of the symptoms of myocardial infarction with supporting ECG abnormalities (*i.e.*, ST-elevation, ST-depression or left bundle-branch block). Patients were randomized to receive Plavix (clopidogrel bisulfate) (75 mg once daily) or placebo, in combination with aspirin (162 mg per day), for 28 days or until hospital discharge, whichever came first.

The primary endpoints were death from any cause and the first occurrence of re-infarction, stroke or death.

The patient population included 28% women, 58% age ≥60 years (26% age ≥70 years), 55% patients who received thrombolytics, 68% who received ACE-inhibitors, and only 3% who underwent PCI.

As shown in Table 6 and Figures 3 and 4 below, Plavix significantly reduced the relative risk of death from any cause by 7% (p=0.029), and the relative risk of the combination of re-infarction, stroke or death by 9% (p=0.002).
[See table 6 at top of next page]

Figure 3: Cumulative Event Rates for Death in the COMMIT Study*

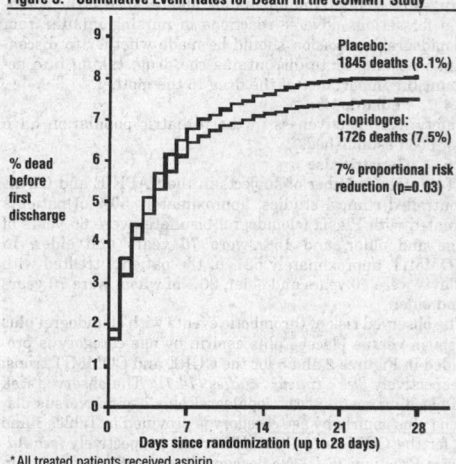

* All treated patients received aspirin.

Figure 4: Cumulative Event Rates for the Combined Endpoint Re-Infarction, Stroke or Death in the COMMIT Study*

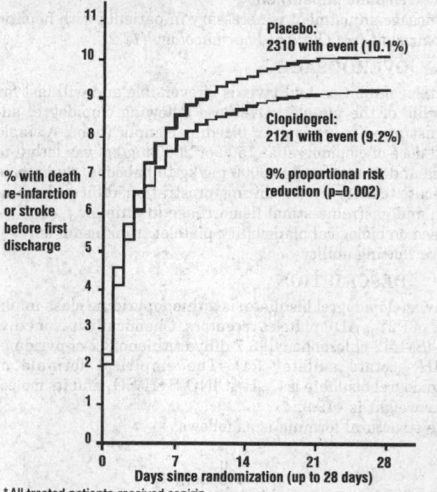

* All treated patients received aspirin.

The effect of Plavix did not differ significantly in various pre-specified subgroups as shown in Figure 5. The effect was also similar in non-prespecified subgroups including those based on infarct location, Killip class or prior MI history (see Figure 6). Such subgroup analyses should be interpreted cautiously.
[See figure 5 at top of next page]
[See figure 6 on next page]

14.2 Recent Myocardial Infarction, Recent Stroke, or Established Peripheral Arterial Disease

CAPRIE

The CAPRIE trial was a 19,185-patient, 304-center, international, randomized, double-blind, parallel-group study comparing Plavix (75 mg daily) to aspirin (325 mg daily). The patients randomized had: 1) recent histories of myocardial infarction (within 35 days); 2) recent histories of ischemic stroke (within 6 months) with at least a week of residual neurological signs; or 3) established peripheral arterial disease. Patients received randomized treatment for an average of 1.6 years (maximum of 3 years).

The trial's primary outcome was the time to first occurrence of new ischemic stroke (fatal or not), new myocardial

Figure 5: Effects of Adding Plavix to Aspirin on the Combined Primary Endpoint across Baseline and Concomitant Medication Subgroups for the COMMIT Study

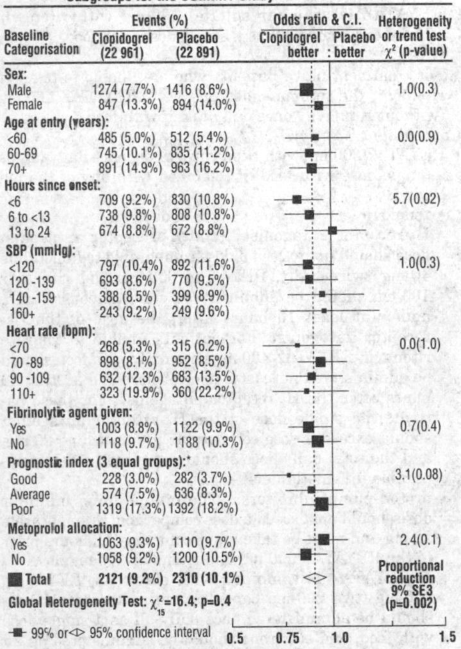

* Three similar-sized prognostic index groups were based on absolute risk of primary composite outcome for each patient calculated from baseline prognostic variables (excluding allocated treatments) with a Cox regression model.

Figure 6: Effects of Adding Plavix to Aspirin in the Non-Prespecified Subgroups in the COMMIT Study

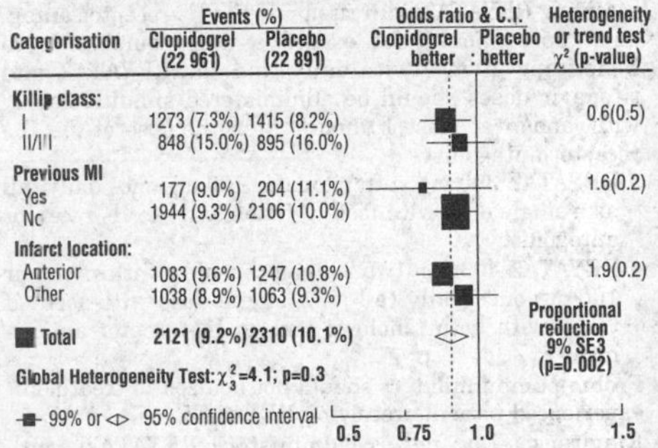

infarction (fatal or not), or other vascular death. Deaths not easily attributable to nonvascular causes were all classified as vascular.

Table 7: Outcome Events in the CAPRIE Primary Analysis

Patients	Plavix n=9599	aspirin n=9586
Ischemic stroke (fatal or not)	438 (4.6%)	461 (4.8%)
MI (fatal or not)	275 (2.9%)	333 (3.5%)
Other vascular death	226 (2.4%)	226 (2.4%)
Total	939 (9.8%)	1020 (10.6%)

As shown in the table, Plavix (clopidogrel bisulfate) was associated with a lower incidence of outcome events, primarily MI. The overall relative risk reduction (9.8% vs. 10.6%) was 8.7%, p=0.045. Similar results were obtained when all-cause mortality and all-cause strokes were counted instead of vascular mortality and ischemic strokes (risk reduction 6.9%). In patients who survived an on-study stroke or myocardial infarction, the incidence of subsequent events was lower in the Plavix group.

The curves showing the overall event rate are shown in Figure 7. The event curves separated early and continued to diverge over the 3-year follow-up period.

[See figure 7 at top of next column]

The statistical significance favoring Plavix over aspirin was marginal (p=0.045). However, because aspirin is itself effective in reducing cardiovascular events in patients with recent myocardial infarction or stroke, the effect of Plavix is substantial.

Table 6: Outcome Events in the COMMIT Analysis

Event	Plavix (+ aspirin) (N=22961)	Placebo (+ aspirin) (N=22891)	Odds ratio (95% CI)	p-value
Composite endpoint: Death, MI, or Stroke*	2121 (9.2%)	2310 (10.1%)	0.91 (0.86, 0.97)	0.002
Death	1726 (7.5%)	1845 (8.1%)	0.93 (0.87, 0.99)	0.029
Non-fatal MI**	270 (1.2%)	330 (1.4%)	0.81 (0.69, 0.95)	0.011
Non-fatal Stroke**	127 (0.6%)	142 (0.6%)	0.89 (0.70, 1.13)	0.33

* The difference between the composite endpoint and the sum of death+non-fatal MI+non-fatal stroke indicates that 9 patients (2 clopidogrel and 7 placebo) suffered both a non-fatal stroke and a non-fatal MI.
**Non-fatal MI and non-fatal stroke exclude patients who died (of any cause).

Figure 7: Fatal or Non-Fatal Vascular Events in the CAPRIE Study

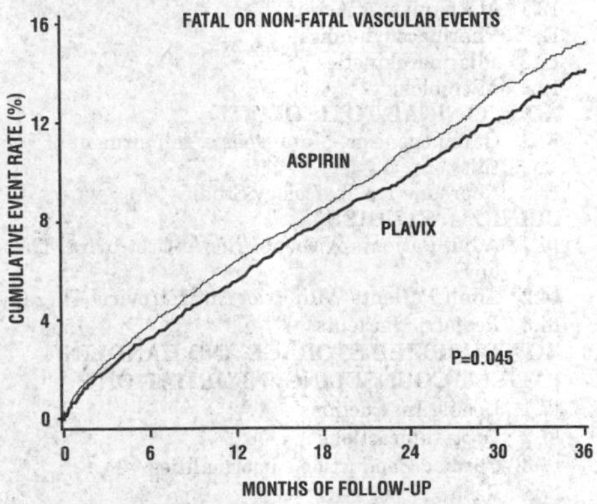

The CAPRIE trial included a population that was randomized on the basis of 3 entry criteria. The efficacy of Plavix (clopidogrel bisulfate) relative to aspirin was heterogeneous across these randomized subgroups (p=0.043). It is not clear whether this difference is real or a chance occurrence. Although the CAPRIE trial was not designed to evaluate the relative benefit of Plavix over aspirin in the individual patient subgroups, the benefit appeared to be strongest in patients who were enrolled because of peripheral vascular disease (especially those who also had a history of myocardial infarction) and weaker in stroke patients. In patients who were enrolled in the trial on the sole basis of a recent myocardial infarction, Plavix was not numerically superior to aspirin.

14.3 Lack of Established Benefit of Plavix plus Aspirin in Patients with Multiple Risk Factors or Established Vascular Disease

CHARISMA

The CHARISMA trial was a 15,603 subject, randomized, double-blind, parallel group study comparing Plavix (75 mg daily) to placebo for prevention of ischemic events in patients with vascular disease or multiple risk factors for atherosclerosis. All subjects were treated with aspirin 75-162 mg daily. The mean duration of treatment was 23 months. The study failed to demonstrate a reduction in the occurrence of the primary endpoint, a composite of CV death, MI, or stroke. A total of 534 (6.9%) patients in the Plavix group versus 573 (7.4%) patients in the placebo group experienced a primary outcome event (p=0.22). Bleeding of all severities was more common in the subjects randomized to Plavix.

16 HOW SUPPLIED/STORAGE AND HANDLING

Plavix (clopidogrel bisulfate) 75 mg tablets are available as pink, round, biconvex, film-coated tablets debossed with "75" on one side and "1171" on the other. Tablets are provided as follows:

NDC 63653-1171-6	Bottles of 30
NDC 63653-1171-1	Bottles of 90
NDC 63653-1171-5	Bottles of 500
NDC 63653-1171-3	Blisters of 100

Plavix (clopidogrel bisulfate) 300 mg tablets are available as pink, oblong, film-coated tablets debossed with "300" on one side and "1332" on the other. Tablets are provided as follows:

NDC 63653-1332-2	Unit-dose packages of 30
NDC 63653-1332-3	Unit-dose packages of 100

Store at 25° C (77° F); excursions permitted to 15°–30° C (59°–86° F) [see USP Controlled Room Temperature].

17 PATIENT COUNSELING INFORMATION
17.1 Benefits and Risks
• Summarize the effectiveness features and potential side effects of Plavix.

• Tell patients to take Plavix (clopidogrel bisulfate) exactly as prescribed.
• Remind patients not to discontinue Plavix (clopidogrel bisulfate) without first discussing it with the physician who prescribed Plavix.

17.2 Bleeding
Inform patients that they:
• will bruise and bleed more easily.
• will take longer than usual to stop bleeding.
• should report any unanticipated, prolonged, or excessive bleeding, or blood in their stool or urine.

17.3 Other Signs and Symptoms Requiring Medical Attention
• Inform patients that TTP is a rare but serious condition that has been reported with Plavix and other drugs in this class of drugs.
• Instruct patients to get prompt medical attention if they experience any of the following symptoms that cannot otherwise be explained: fever, weakness, extreme skin paleness, purple skin patches, yellowing of the skin or eyes, or neurological changes.

17.4 Invasive Procedures
Instruct patients to:
• inform physicians and dentists that they are taking Plavix before any invasive procedure is scheduled.
• tell the doctor performing the invasive procedure to talk to the prescribing health care professional before stopping Plavix.

17.5 Concomitant Medications
Ask patients to list all prescription medications, over-the-counter medications, or dietary supplements they are taking or plan to take, including prescription or over-the-counter omeprazole, so the physician knows about other treatments that may affect how Plavix works (e.g., warfarin and NSAIDs) [see Warnings and Precautions (5)].

Distributed by:
Bristol-Myers Squibb/Sanofi Pharmaceuticals Partnership
Bridgewater, NJ 08807
Plavix® is a registered trademark.

B1-B0001-08-10   August 2010
Shown in Product Identification Guide, page 322

REYATAZ®   ℞
[*RAY-ah-taz*]
(atazanavir sulfate)
Capsules

HIGHLIGHTS OF PRESCRIBING INFORMATION
These highlights do not include all the information needed to use REYATAZ safely and effectively. See full prescribing information for REYATAZ.
REYATAZ® (atazanavir sulfate) Capsules
Initial U.S. Approval: 2003

————RECENT MAJOR CHANGES————

Indications and Usage (1)	11/2009
Contraindications (4)	04/2010

————INDICATIONS AND USAGE————
REYATAZ is a protease inhibitor indicated for use in combination with other antiretroviral agents for the treatment of HIV-1 infection. (1)

————DOSAGE AND ADMINISTRATION————
• *Treatment-naive patients:* REYATAZ 300 mg with ritonavir 100 mg once daily with food or REYATAZ 400 mg once daily with food. When coadministered with tenofovir, the recommended dose is REYATAZ 300 mg with ritonavir 100 mg. (2.1)
• *Treatment-experienced patients:* REYATAZ 300 mg with ritonavir 100 mg once daily with food. (2.1)
• *Pediatric patients (6 to less than 18 years of age):* Dosage is based on body weight not to exceed the adult dose. (2.2)
• *Concomitant therapy:* Dosing modifications may be required. (2.1, 7)
• *Renal impairment:* Dosing modifications may be required. (2.3)

- *Hepatic impairment:* Dosing modifications may be required. (2.4)

DOSAGE FORMS AND STRENGTHS

- Capsules: 100 mg, 150 mg, 200 mg, 300 mg. (3, 16)

CONTRAINDICATIONS

- REYATAZ (atazanavir sulfate) is contraindicated in patients with previously demonstrated hypersensitivity (eg, Stevens-Johnson syndrome, erythema multiforme, or toxic skin eruptions) to any of the components of this product. (4)
- Coadministration with alfuzosin, triazolam, orally administered midazolam, ergot derivatives, rifampin, irinotecan, lovastatin, simvastatin, indinavir, cisapride, pimozide, St. John's wort, and sildenafil when dosed as REVATIO®. (4)

WARNINGS AND PRECAUTIONS

- *Cardiac conduction abnormalities:* PR interval prolongation may occur in some patients. Use with caution in patients with preexisting conduction system disease or when administered with other drugs that may prolong the PR interval. (5.2, 6.4, 7.3, 12.2, 17.3)
- *Rash:* Discontinue if severe rash develops. (5.3, 6.4, 17.4)
- *Hyperbilirubinemia:* Most patients experience asymptomatic increases in indirect bilirubin, which is reversible upon discontinuation. Do not dose reduce. If a concomitant transaminase increase occurs, evaluate for alternative etiologies. (5.4, 6.2)
- *Hepatotoxicity:* Patients with hepatitis B or C are at risk of increased transaminases or hepatic decompensation. Monitor liver function tests prior to therapy and during treatment. (2.4, 5.5, 6.3, 6.4, 8.8)
- *Nephrolithiasis* has been reported. Consider temporary interruption or discontinuation. (5.6, 6.4)
- Patients receiving REYATAZ (atazanavir sulfate) may develop new onset or exacerbations of diabetes mellitus/hyperglycemia (5.7, 6.4), immune reconstitution syndrome (5.8), and redistribution/accumulation of body fat. (5.9)
- *Hemophilia:* Spontaneous bleeding may occur and additional factor VIII may be required. (5.10)

ADVERSE REACTIONS

Most common adverse reactions (≥2%) are nausea, jaundice/scleral icterus, rash, headache, abdominal pain, vomiting, insomnia, peripheral neurologic symptoms, dizziness, myalgia, diarrhea, depression, and fever. (6.1, 6.2)

To report SUSPECTED ADVERSE REACTIONS, contact Bristol-Myers Squibb at 1-800-721-5072 or FDA at 1-800-FDA-1088 or www.fda.gov/medwatch

DRUG INTERACTIONS

Coadministration of REYATAZ can alter the concentration of other drugs and other drugs may alter the concentration of atazanavir. The potential drug-drug interactions must be considered prior to and during therapy. (4, 5.1, 7, 12.3)

USE IN SPECIFIC POPULATIONS

- *Pregnancy:* Use only if the potential benefit justifies the potential risk to the fetus. Physicians are encouraged to register patients in the Antiretroviral Pregnancy Registry by calling 1-800-258-4263. (8.1)
- *Nursing mothers* should be instructed not to breast-feed due to the potential for postnatal HIV transmission. (8.3)
- *Hepatitis B or C co-infection:* Monitor liver enzymes. (5.5, 6.3)
- *Renal impairment:* Do not use in treatment-experienced patients with end stage renal disease managed with hemodialysis. (2.3, 8.7)
- *Hepatic impairment:* Do not use REYATAZ in patients with severe hepatic impairment. REYATAZ/ritonavir is not recommended. (2.4, 8.8)

See 17 for PATIENT COUNSELING INFORMATION and FDA-approved patient labeling

Revised: 04/2010

FULL PRESCRIBING INFORMATION: CONTENTS*

FULL PRESCRIBING INFORMATION

1 INDICATIONS AND USAGE

REYATAZ® (atazanavir sulfate) is indicated in combination with other antiretroviral agents for the treatment of HIV-1 infection. This indication is based on analyses of plasma HIV-1 RNA levels and CD4+ cell counts from controlled studies of 96 weeks duration in antiretroviral-naive and 48 weeks duration in antiretroviral-treatment-experienced adult and pediatric patients at least 6 years of age.

The following points should be considered when initiating therapy with REYATAZ:

- In Study AI424-045 REYATAZ/ritonavir and lopinavir/ritonavir were similar for the primary efficacy outcome measure of time-averaged difference in change from baseline in HIV RNA level. This study was not large enough to reach a definitive conclusion that REYATAZ/ritonavir and lopinavir/ritonavir are equivalent on the secondary efficacy outcome measure of proportions below the HIV RNA lower limit of detection [see *Clinical Studies (14.2)*].
- The number of baseline primary protease inhibitor mutations affects the virologic response to REYATAZ/ritonavir [see *Clinical Pharmacology (12.4)*].

2 DOSAGE AND ADMINISTRATION

General Dosing Recommendations:

- REYATAZ Capsules must be taken with food.
- The recommended oral dosage of REYATAZ depends on the treatment history of the patient and the use of other coadministered drugs. When coadministered with H₂-receptor antagonists or proton-pump inhibitors, dose separation may be required [see *Dosage and Administration (2.1)*].
- When coadministered with didanosine buffered or enteric-coated formulations, REYATAZ should be given (with food) 2 hours before or 1 hour after didanosine.
- REYATAZ without ritonavir is not recommended for treatment-experienced patients with prior virologic failure [see *Clinical Studies (14)*].
- Efficacy and safety of REYATAZ with ritonavir in doses greater than 100 mg once daily have not been established. The use of higher ritonavir doses might alter the safety profile of atazanavir (cardiac effects, hyperbilirubinemia) and, therefore, is not recommended. Prescribers should consult the complete prescribing information for NORVIR® (ritonavir) when using this agent.

2.1 Recommended Adult Dosage

Dose Recommendations for Therapy-Naive Patients

- For treatment-naive patients, the recommended dosage is REYATAZ (atazanavir sulfate) 300 mg with ritonavir 100 mg once daily (all as a single dose with food).

OR

- For treatment-naive patients who are unable to tolerate ritonavir, the recommended dosage is REYATAZ 400 mg (without ritonavir) once daily taken with food.

Concomitant Therapy:

- REYATAZ 300 mg with ritonavir 100 mg once daily (all as a single dose with food) if combined with any of the following:
  - tenofovir
  - H₂-receptor antagonist: The H₂-receptor antagonist dose should not exceed a dose comparable to famotidine 40 mg twice daily. REYATAZ 300 mg and ritonavir 100 mg should be administered simultaneously with, and/or at least 10 hours after, the dose of the H₂-receptor antagonist. For patients unable to tolerate ritonavir, REYATAZ 400 mg once daily with food should be administered at least 2 hours before and at least 10 hours after the H₂-receptor antagonist. For these patients, no single dose of the H₂-receptor antagonist should exceed a dose comparable to famotidine 20 mg, and the total daily dose should not exceed a dose comparable to famotidine 40 mg.
  - proton-pump inhibitors: The proton-pump inhibitor dose should not exceed a dose comparable to omeprazole 20 mg and must be taken approximately 12 hours prior to the REYATAZ 300 mg and ritonavir 100 mg dose.
- If REYATAZ is combined with efavirenz, REYATAZ 400 mg (two 200-mg capsules) with ritonavir 100 mg should be administered once daily all as a single dose with food, and efavirenz should be administered on an empty stomach, preferably at bedtime.

Dose Recommendations for Therapy-Experienced Patients

REYATAZ 300 mg with ritonavir 100 mg once daily (all as a single dose with food).

Concomitant Therapy:

- Whenever an H₂-receptor antagonist is given to a patient receiving REYATAZ with ritonavir, the H₂-receptor antagonist dose should not exceed a dose comparable to famotidine 20 mg twice daily, and the REYATAZ and ritonavir doses should be administered simultaneously with, and/or at least 10 hours after, the dose of the H₂-receptor antagonist.
  - REYATAZ 300 mg with ritonavir 100 mg once daily (all as a single dose with food) if taken with an H₂-receptor antagonist.
  - REYATAZ 400 mg (two 200-mg capsules) with ritonavir 100 mg once daily (all as a single dose with food) if taken with both tenofovir and an H₂-receptor antagonist.
- Proton-pump inhibitors should not be used in treatment-experienced patients receiving REYATAZ.
- Efavirenz: Do not coadminister REYATAZ with efavirenz in treatment-experienced patients due to decreased atazanavir exposure.

[For these drugs and other antiretroviral agents for which dosing modification may be appropriate, see *Drug Interactions (7)*.]

2.2 Recommended Pediatric Dosage

The recommended dosage of REYATAZ for pediatric patients (6 to less than 18 years of age) is based on body weight and should not exceed the recommended adult dosage. REYATAZ Capsules must be taken with food. The data are insufficient to recommend dosing of REYATAZ for any of the following: (1) patients less than 6 years of age, (2) without ritonavir in patients less than 13 years of age, and (3) treatment-experienced pediatric patients with body weight less than 25 kg.

Therapy-Naive Pediatric Patients

The recommended dosage of REYATAZ with ritonavir in treatment-naive patients at least 6 years of age is shown in Table 1.

For treatment-naive patients at least 13 years of age and at least 39 kg, who are unable to tolerate ritonavir, the recommended dose is REYATAZ 400 mg (without ritonavir) once daily with food.

[See table 1 at top of next page]

Therapy-Experienced Pediatric Patients

The recommended dosage of REYATAZ with ritonavir in treatment-experienced patients at least 6 years of age is shown in Table 2.

[See table 2 on next page]

2.3 Renal Impairment

For patients with renal impairment, including those with severe renal impairment who are not managed with hemodialysis, no dose adjustment is required for REYATAZ. Treatment-naive patients with end stage renal disease managed with hemodialysis should receive REYATAZ 300 mg with ritonavir 100 mg. REYATAZ should not be administered to HIV-treatment-experienced patients with end stage renal disease managed with hemodialysis. [See *Use in Specific Populations (8.7)*.]

2.4   Hepatic Impairment

REYATAZ (atazanavir sulfate) should be used with caution in patients with mild-to-moderate hepatic impairment. For patients with moderate hepatic impairment (Child-Pugh Class B) who have not experienced prior virologic failure, a dose reduction to 300 mg once daily should be considered. REYATAZ should not be used in patients with severe hepatic impairment (Child-Pugh Class C). REYATAZ/ritonavir has not been studied in subjects with hepatic impairment and is not recommended. [See *Warnings and Precautions (5.5)* and *Use in Specific Populations (8.8)*.]

3   DOSAGE FORMS AND STRENGTHS

- 100 mg capsule with blue cap and white body, printed with white ink "BMS 100 mg" on the cap and with blue ink "3623" on the body.
- 150 mg capsule with blue cap and powder blue body, printed with white ink "BMS 150 mg" on the cap and with blue ink "3624" on the body.
- 200 mg capsule with blue cap and blue body, printed with white ink "BMS 200 mg" on the cap and with white ink "3631" on the body.
- 300 mg capsule with red cap and blue body, printed with white ink "BMS 300 mg" on the cap and with white ink "3622" on the body.

4   CONTRAINDICATIONS

REYATAZ (atazanavir sulfate) is contraindicated:

- in patients with previously demonstrated clinically significant hypersensitivity (eg, Stevens-Johnson syndrome, erythema multiforme, or toxic skin eruptions) to any of the components of this product.
- when coadministered with drugs that are highly dependent on CYP3A or UGT1A1 for clearance, and for which elevated plasma concentrations are associated with serious and/or life-threatening events. These and other contraindicated drugs are listed in Table 3.

[See table 3 at right]

5   WARNINGS AND PRECAUTIONS

5.1   Drug Interactions

See Table 3 for a listing of drugs that are contraindicated for use with REYATAZ due to potentially life-threatening adverse events, significant drug interactions, or loss of virologic activity. [See *Contraindications (4)*.] Please refer to Table 13 for established and other potentially significant drug interactions [see *Drug Interactions (7.3)*].

5.2   Cardiac Conduction Abnormalities

Atazanavir has been shown to prolong the PR interval of the electrocardiogram in some patients. In healthy volunteers and in patients, abnormalities in atrioventricular (AV) conduction were asymptomatic and generally limited to first-degree AV block. There have been rare reports of second-degree AV block and other conduction abnormalities [see *Adverse Reactions (6.4)* and *Overdosage (10)*]. In clinical trials that included electrocardiograms, asymptomatic first-degree AV block was observed in 5.9% of atazanavir-treated patients (n=920), 5.2% of lopinavir/ritonavir-treated patients (n=252), 10.4% of nelfinavir-treated patients (n=48), and 3.0% of efavirenz-treated patients (n=329). In Study AI424-045, asymptomatic first-degree AV block was observed in 5% (6/118) of atazanavir/ritonavir-treated patients and 5% (6/116) of lopinavir/ritonavir-treated patients who had on-study electrocardiogram measurements. Because of limited clinical experience in patients with preexisting conduction system disease (eg, marked first-degree AV block or second- or third-degree AV block), atazanavir should be used with caution in these patients. [See *Clinical Pharmacology (12.2)*.]

Atazanavir in combination with diltiazem increased diltiazem plasma concentration by 2-fold with an additive effect on the PR interval. When used in combination with atazanavir, a dose reduction of diltiazem by one half should be considered and ECG monitoring is recommended. In a pharmacokinetic study between atazanavir 400 mg once daily and atenolol 50 mg once daily, no clinically significant additive effect of atazanavir and atenolol on the PR interval was observed. Dose adjustment of atenolol is not required when used in combination with atazanavir. [See *Drug Interactions (7)* and *Clinical Pharmacology (12.2)*.] Pharmacokinetic studies between atazanavir and other drugs that prolong the PR interval including beta blockers [other than atenolol, see *Drug Interactions (7)*], verapamil, and digoxin have not been performed. An additive effect of atazanavir and these drugs cannot be excluded; therefore, caution should be exercised when atazanavir is given concurrently with these drugs, especially those that are metabolized by CYP3A (eg, verapamil).

5.3   Rash

In controlled clinical trials, rash (all grades, regardless of causality) occurred in approximately 20% of patients treated with REYATAZ. The median time to onset of rash in clinical studies was 7.3 weeks and the median duration of rash was 1.4 weeks. Rashes were generally mild-to-moderate maculopapular skin eruptions. Treatment-emergent adverse reactions of moderate or severe rash (occurring at a rate of ≥2%) are presented for the individual clinical studies [see *Adverse Reactions (6.1)*]. Dosing with REYATAZ (atazanavir sulfate) was often continued without interruption in patients who developed rash. The discontinuation rate for rash in clinical trials was <1%. REYATAZ should be discontinued if severe rash develops. Cases of Stevens-Johnson syndrome, erythema multiforme, and toxic skin eruptions have been reported in patients receiving REYATAZ. [See *Contraindications (4)*.]

5.4   Hyperbilirubinemia

Most patients taking REYATAZ (atazanavir sulfate) experience asymptomatic elevations in indirect (unconjugated) bilirubin related to inhibition of UDP-glucuronosyl

---

Table 1:   Dosage for Treatment-Naive Pediatric Patients (6 to less than 18 years of age) for REYATAZ Capsules with ritonavir

Body Weight		REYATAZ dose[a,b] (mg)	ritonavir dose[b] (mg)
(kg)	(lbs)		
15 to less than 25	33 to less than 55	150	80[c]
25 to less than 32	55 to less than 70	200	100[c]
32 to less than 39	70 to less than 86	250	100[d]
at least 39	at least 86	300	100[d]

[a] The recommended dosage of REYATAZ can be achieved using a combination of commercially available capsule strengths.
[b] The dosage of REYATAZ and ritonavir was calculated as follows:
- 15 kg to less than 20 kg: REYATAZ 8.5 mg/kg with ritonavir 4 mg/kg once daily with food.
- at least 20 kg: REYATAZ 7 mg/kg with ritonavir 4 mg/kg once daily with food not to exceed REYATAZ 300 mg and ritonavir 100 mg.

[c] Ritonavir liquid.
[d] Ritonavir capsule or liquid.

Table 2:   Dosage for Treatment-Experienced Pediatric Patients (6 to less than 18 years of age) for REYATAZ Capsules with ritonavir

Body Weight		REYATAZ dose[a,b] (mg)	ritonavir dose[b] (mg)
(kg)	(lbs)		
25 to less than 32	55 to less than 70	200	100[c]
32 to less than 39	70 to less than 86	250	100[c]
at least 39	at least 86	300	100[c]

[a] The recommended dosage of REYATAZ can be achieved using a combination of commercially available capsule strengths.
[b] The dosage was calculated as REYATAZ 7 mg/kg with ritonavir 4 mg/kg once daily with food not to exceed REYATAZ 300 mg and ritonavir 100 mg.
[c] Ritonavir capsule or liquid.

Table 3:   Drugs That Are Contraindicated with REYATAZ (atazanavir) (Information in the table applies to REYATAZ with or without ritonavir, unless otherwise indicated)

Drug Class	Drugs within class that are contraindicated with REYATAZ	Clinical Comment
Alpha 1-Adrenoreceptor Antagonist	Alfuzosin	Potential for increased alfuzosin concentrations, which can result in hypotension.
Antimycobacterials	Rifampin	Rifampin substantially decreases plasma concentrations of atazanavir, which may result in loss of therapeutic effect and development of resistance.
Antineoplastics	Irinotecan	Atazanavir inhibits UGT1A1 and may interfere with the metabolism of irinotecan, resulting in increased irinotecan toxicities.
Benzodiazepines	Triazolam, orally administered midazolam[a]	Triazolam and orally administered midazolam are extensively metabolized by CYP3A4. Coadministration of triazolam or orally administered midazolam with REYATAZ may cause large increases in the concentration of these benzodiazepines. Potential for serious and/or life-threatening events such as prolonged or increased sedation or respiratory depression.
Ergot Derivatives	Dihydroergotamine, ergotamine, ergonovine, methylergonovine	Potential for serious and/or life-threatening events such as acute ergot toxicity characterized by peripheral vasospasm and ischemia of the extremities and other tissues.
GI Motility Agent	Cisapride	Potential for serious and/or life-threatening reactions such as cardiac arrhythmias.
Herbal Products	St. John's wort (*Hypericum perforatum*)	Patients taking REYATAZ should not use products containing St. John's wort because coadministration may be expected to reduce plasma concentrations of atazanavir. This may result in loss of therapeutic effect and development of resistance.
HMG-CoA Reductase Inhibitors	Lovastatin, simvastatin	Potential for serious reactions such as myopathy including rhabdomyolysis.
Neuroleptic	Pimozide	Potential for serious and/or life-threatening reactions such as cardiac arrhythmias.
PDE5 Inhibitor	Sildenafil[b] when dosed as REVATIO® for the treatment of pulmonary arterial hypertension	A safe and effective dose in combination with REYATAZ has not been established for sildenafil (REVATIO®) when used for the treatment of pulmonary hypertension. There is increased potential for sildenafil-associated adverse events (which include visual disturbances, hypotension, priapism, and syncope).
Protease Inhibitors	Indinavir	Both REYATAZ and indinavir are associated with indirect (unconjugated) hyperbilirubinemia.

[a] See *Drug Interactions, Table 13 (7)* for parenterally administered midazolam.
[b] See *Drug Interactions, Table 13 (7)* for sildenafil when dosed as VIAGRA® for erectile dysfunction.

transferase (UGT). This hyperbilirubinemia is reversible upon discontinuation of REYATAZ (atazanavir sulfate). Hepatic transaminase elevations that occur with hyperbilirubinemia should be evaluated for alternative etiologies. No long-term safety data are available for patients experiencing persistent elevations in total bilirubin >5 times ULN. Alternative antiretroviral therapy to REYATAZ may be considered if jaundice or scleral icterus associated with bilirubin elevations presents cosmetic concerns for patients. Dose reduction of atazanavir is not recommended since long-term efficacy of reduced doses has not been established. [See *Adverse Reactions (6.1, 6.2)*.]

5.5 Hepatotoxicity

Caution should be exercised when administering REYATAZ to patients with hepatic impairment because atazanavir concentrations may be increased. [See *Dosage and Administration (2.4)*.] Patients with underlying hepatitis B or C viral infections or marked elevations in transaminases before treatment may be at increased risk for developing further transaminase elevations or hepatic decompensation. In these patients, appropriate laboratory testing should be conducted prior to initiating therapy with REYATAZ and these patients should be monitored during treatment. [See *Adverse Reactions (6.3)* and *Use in Specific Populations (8.8)*.]

5.6 Nephrolithiasis

Cases of nephrolithiasis were reported during postmarketing surveillance in HIV-infected patients receiving REYATAZ therapy. Because these events were reported voluntarily during clinical practice, estimates of frequency cannot be made. If signs or symptoms of nephrolithiasis occur, temporary interruption or discontinuation of therapy may be considered. [See *Adverse Reactions (6.4)*.]

5.7 Diabetes Mellitus/Hyperglycemia

New-onset diabetes mellitus, exacerbation of preexisting diabetes mellitus, and hyperglycemia have been reported during postmarketing surveillance in HIV-infected patients receiving protease inhibitor therapy. Some patients required either initiation or dose adjustments of insulin or oral hypoglycemic agents for treatment of these events. In some cases, diabetic ketoacidosis has occurred. In those patients who discontinued protease inhibitor therapy, hyperglycemia persisted in some cases. Because these events have been reported voluntarily during clinical practice, estimates of frequency cannot be made and a causal relationship between protease inhibitor therapy and these events has not been established. [See *Adverse Reactions (6.4)*.]

5.8 Immune Reconstitution Syndrome

Immune reconstitution syndrome has been reported in patients treated with combination antiretroviral therapy, including REYATAZ. During the initial phase of combination antiretroviral treatment, patients whose immune system responds may develop an inflammatory response to indolent or residual opportunistic infections (such as *Mycobacterium avium* infection, cytomegalovirus, *Pneumocystis jiroveci* pneumonia, or tuberculosis), which may necessitate further evaluation and treatment.

5.9 Fat Redistribution

Redistribution/accumulation of body fat including central obesity, dorsocervical fat enlargement (buffalo hump), peripheral wasting, facial wasting, breast enlargement, and "cushingoid appearance" have been observed in patients receiving antiretroviral therapy. The mechanism and long-term consequences of these events are currently unknown. A causal relationship has not been established.

5.10 Hemophilia

There have been reports of increased bleeding, including spontaneous skin hematomas and hemarthrosis, in patients with hemophilia type A and B treated with protease inhibitors. In some patients additional factor VIII was given. In more than half of the reported cases, treatment with protease inhibitors was continued or reintroduced. A causal relationship between protease inhibitor therapy and these events has not been established.

5.11 Resistance/Cross-Resistance

Various degrees of cross-resistance among protease inhibitors have been observed. Resistance to atazanavir may not preclude the subsequent use of other protease inhibitors. [See *Clinical Pharmacology (12.4)*.]

6   ADVERSE REACTIONS

The following adverse reactions are discussed in greater detail in other sections of the labeling:

- cardiac conduction abnormalities [see *Warnings and Precautions (5.2)*]
- rash [see *Warnings and Precautions (5.3)*]
- hyperbilirubinemia [see *Warnings and Precautions (5.4)*]
- nephrolithiasis [see *Warnings and Precautions (5.6)*]

Because clinical trials are conducted under widely varying conditions, adverse reaction rates observed in the clinical trials of a drug cannot be directly compared to rates in the clinical trials of another drug and may not reflect the rates observed in practice.

6.1   Clinical Trial Experience in Adults

Treatment-Emergent Adverse Reactions in Treatment-Naive Patients

The safety profile of REYATAZ (atazanavir sulfate) in treatment-naive adults is based on 1625 HIV-1 infected patients in clinical trials. 536 patients received REYATAZ 300 mg with ritonavir 100 mg and 1089 patients received REYATAZ 400 mg or higher (without ritonavir).

The most common adverse reactions are nausea, jaundice/scleral icterus, and rash.

Selected clinical adverse reactions of moderate or severe intensity reported in ≥2% of treatment-naive patients receiving combination therapy including REYATAZ 300 mg with ritonavir 100 mg and REYATAZ 400 mg (without ritonavir) are presented in Tables 4 and 5, respectively.

Table 4:   Selected Treatment-Emergent Adverse Reactions[a] of Moderate or Severe Intensity Reported in ≥2% of Adult Treatment-Naive Patients,[b] Study AI424-138

	96 weeks[c] REYATAZ 300 mg with ritonavir 100 mg (once daily) and tenofovir with emtricitabine[d] (n=441)	96 weeks[c] lopinavir 400 mg with ritonavir 100 mg (twice daily) and tenofovir with emtricitabine[d] (n=437)
Digestive System		
Nausea	4%	8%
Jaundice/ scleral icterus	5%	*
Diarrhea	2%	12%
Skin and Appendages		
Rash	3%	2%

* None reported in this treatment arm.
[a] Includes events of possible, probable, certain, or unknown relationship to treatment regimen.
[b] Based on the regimen containing REYATAZ.
[c] Median time on therapy.
[d] As a fixed-dose combination: 300 mg tenofovir, 200 mg emtricitabine once daily.

[See table 5 at bottom left]

Treatment-Emergent Adverse Reactions in Treatment-Experienced Patients

The safety profile of REYATAZ (atazanavir sulfate) in treatment-experienced adults is based on 119 HIV-1 infected patients in clinical trials.

The most common adverse reactions are jaundice/scleral icterus and myalgia.

Selected clinical adverse reactions of moderate or severe intensity reported in ≥2% of treatment-experienced patients receiving REYATAZ/ritonavir are presented in Table 6.

Table 6:   Selected Treatment-Emergent Adverse Reactions[a] of Moderate or Severe Intensity Reported in ≥2% of Adult Treatment-Experienced Patients,[b] Study AI424-045

	48 weeks[c] REYATAZ/ritonavir 300/100 mg once daily + tenofovir + NRTI (n=119)	48 weeks[c] lopinavir/ritonavir 400/100 mg twice daily[d] + tenofovir + NRTI (n=118)
Body as a Whole		
Fever	2%	*
Digestive System		
Jaundice/ scleral icterus	9%	*
Diarrhea	3%	11%
Nausea	3%	2%
Nervous System		
Depression	2%	<1%
Musculoskeletal System		
Myalgia	4%	*

* None reported in this treatment arm.
[a] Includes events of possible, probable, certain, or unknown relationship to treatment regimen.
[b] Based on the regimen containing REYATAZ.
[c] Median time on therapy.
[d] As a fixed-dose combination.

Laboratory Abnormalities in Treatment-Naive Patients

The percentages of adult treatment-naive patients treated with combination therapy including REYATAZ (atazanavir sulfate) 300 mg with ritonavir 100 mg and REYATAZ 400 mg (without ritonavir) with Grade 3–4 laboratory abnormalities are presented in Tables 7 and 8, respectively.

[See table 7 at top of next page]
[See table 8 on next page]

Laboratory Abnormalities in Treatment-Experienced Patients

The percentages of adult treatment-experienced patients treated with combination therapy including REYATAZ/ritonavir with Grade 3–4 laboratory abnormalities are presented in Table 9.

[See table 9 on next page]

Lipids, Change from Baseline in Treatment-Naive Patients

For Study AI424-138 and Study AI424-034, changes from baseline in LDL-cholesterol, HDL-cholesterol, total cholesterol, and triglycerides are shown in Tables 10 and 11, respectively.

Table 5:   Selected Treatment-Emergent Adverse Reactions[a] of Moderate or Severe Intensity Reported in ≥2% of Adult Treatment-Naive Patients,[b] Studies AI424-034, AI424-007, and AI424-008

	Study AI424-034 64 weeks[c] REYATAZ 400 mg once daily + lamivudine + zidovudine[e] (n=404)	Study AI424-034 64 weeks[c] efavirenz 600 mg once daily + lamivudine + zidovudine[e] (n=401)	Studies AI424-007, -008 120 weeks[c,d] REYATAZ 400 mg once daily + stavudine + lamivudine or didanosine (n=279)	Studies AI424-007, -008 73 weeks[c,d] nelfinavir 750 mg TID or 1250 mg BID + stavudine + lamivudine or didanosine (n=191)
Body as a Whole				
Headache	6%	6%	1%	2%
Digestive System				
Nausea	14%	12%	6%	4%
Jaundice/scleral icterus	7%	*	7%	*
Vomiting	4%	7%	3%	3%
Abdominal pain	4%	4%	4%	2%
Diarrhea	1%	2%	3%	16%
Nervous System				
Insomnia	3%	3%	<1%	*
Dizziness	2%	7%	<1%	*
Peripheral neurologic symptoms	<1%	1%	4%	3%
Skin and Appendages				
Rash	7%	10%	5%	1%

* None reported in this treatment arm.
[a] Includes events of possible, probable, certain, or unknown relationship to treatment regimen.
[b] Based on regimens containing REYATAZ.
[c] Median time on therapy.
[d] Includes long-term follow-up.
[e] As a fixed-dose combination: 150 mg lamivudine, 300 mg zidovudine twice daily.

IMPORTANT NOTICE: Updated drug information is sent bi-monthly via the PDR® Update Insert. For *monthly* email updates, register at PDR.net.

[See table 10 at top of next page]
[See table 11 on next page]

Lipids, Change from Baseline in Treatment-Experienced Patients

For Study AI424-045, changes from baseline in LDL-cholesterol, HDL-cholesterol, total cholesterol, and triglycerides are shown in Table 12. The observed magnitude of dyslipidemia was less with REYATAZ/ritonavir than with lopinavir/ritonavir. However, the clinical impact of such findings has not been demonstrated.

[See table 12 on next page]

6.2   Clinical Trial Experience in Pediatric Patients

The safety and tolerability of REYATAZ (atazanavir sulfate) Capsules with and without ritonavir have been established in pediatric patients at least 6 years of age from the open-label, multicenter clinical trial PACTG 1020A. Use of REYATAZ in pediatric patients less than 6 years of age is under investigation.

The safety profile of REYATAZ in pediatric patients (6 to less than 18 years of age) was comparable to that observed in clinical studies of REYATAZ in adults. The most common Grade 2–4 adverse events (≥5%, regardless of causality) reported in pediatric patients were cough (21%), fever (19%), rash (14%), jaundice/scleral icterus (13%), diarrhea (8%), vomiting (8%), headache (7%), and rhinorrhea (6%). Asymptomatic second-degree atrioventricular block was reported in 2% of patients. The most common Grade 3–4 laboratory abnormality was elevation of total bilirubin (≥3.2 mg/dL) which occurred in 49% of pediatric patients. All other Grade 3–4 laboratory abnormalities occurred with a frequency of less than 3%.

6.3   Patients Co-infected With Hepatitis B and/or Hepatitis C Virus

Liver function tests should be monitored in patients with a history of hepatitis B or C.

In study AI424-138, 60 patients treated with REYATAZ/ritonavir 300 mg/100 mg once daily, and 51 patients treated with lopinavir/ritonavir 400 mg/100 mg twice daily, each with fixed dose tenofovir-emtricitabine, were seropositive for hepatitis B and/or C at study entry. ALT levels >5 times ULN developed in 10% (6/60) of the REYATAZ/ritonavir-treated patients and 8% (4/50) of the lopinavir/ritonavir-treated patients. AST levels >5 times ULN developed in 10% (6/60) of the REYATAZ/ritonavir-treated patients and none (0/50) of the lopinavir/ritonavir-treated patients.

In study AI424-045, 20 patients treated with REYATAZ/ritonavir 300 mg/100 mg once daily, and 18 patients treated with lopinavir/ritonavir 400 mg/100 mg twice daily, were seropositive for hepatitis B and/or C at study entry. ALT levels >5 times ULN developed in 25% (5/20) of the REYATAZ/ritonavir-treated patients and 6% (1/18) of the lopinavir/ritonavir-treated patients. AST levels >5 times ULN developed in 10% (2/20) of the REYATAZ/ritonavir-treated patients and 6% (1/18) of the lopinavir/ritonavir-treated patients.

In studies AI424-008 and AI424-034, 74 patients treated with 400 mg of REYATAZ (atazanavir sulfate) once daily, 58 who received efavirenz, and 12 who received nelfinavir were seropositive for hepatitis B and/or C at study entry. ALT levels >5 times the upper limit of normal (ULN) developed in 15% of the REYATAZ-treated patients, 14% of the efavirenz-treated patients, and 17% of the nelfinavir-treated patients. AST levels >5 times ULN developed in 9% of the REYATAZ-treated patients, 5% of the efavirenz-treated patients, and 17% of the nelfinavir-treated patients. Within atazanavir and control regimens, no difference in frequency of bilirubin elevations was noted between seropositive and seronegative patients. [See *Warnings and Precautions (5.5).*]

6.4   Postmarketing Experience

The following events have been identified during postmarketing use of REYATAZ. Because these reactions are reported voluntarily from a population of unknown size, it is not always possible to reliably estimate their frequency or establish a causal relationship to drug exposure.

Body as a Whole: edema

Cardiovascular System: second-degree AV block, third-degree AV block, left bundle branch block, QTc prolongation [see *Warnings and Precautions (5.2)*]

Gastrointestinal System: pancreatitis

Hepatic System: hepatic function abnormalities

Hepatobiliary Disorders: cholelithiasis, cholecystitis, cholestasis

Metabolic System and Nutrition Disorders: diabetes mellitus, hyperglycemia [see *Warnings and Precautions (5.7)*]

Musculoskeletal System: arthralgia

Renal System: nephrolithiasis [see *Warnings and Precautions (5.6)*]

Skin and Appendages: alopecia, maculopapular rash [see *Contraindications (4)* and *Warnings and Precautions (5.3)*], pruritus

Table 7:   Grade 3–4 Laboratory Abnormalities Reported in ≥2% of Adult Treatment-Naive Patients,[a] Study AI424-138

Variable	Limit[c]	96 weeks[b] REYATAZ 300 mg with ritonavir 100 mg (once daily) and tenofovir with emtricitabine[d] (n=441)	96 weeks[b] lopinavir 400 mg with ritonavir 100 mg (twice daily) and tenofovir with emtricitabine[d] (n=437)
Chemistry	High		
SGOT/AST	≥5.1 × ULN	3%	1%
SGPT/ALT	≥5.1 × ULN	3%	2%
Total Bilirubin	≥2.6 × ULN	44%	<1%
Lipase	≥2.1 × ULN	2%	2%
Creatine Kinase	≥5.1 × ULN	8%	7%
Total Cholesterol	≥240 mg/dL	11%	25%
Hematology	Low		
Neutrophils	<750 cells/mm^3	5%	2%

[a] Based on the regimen containing REYATAZ.
[b] Median time on therapy.
[c] ULN = upper limit of normal.
[d] As a fixed-dose combination: 300 mg tenofovir, 200 mg emtricitabine once daily.

Table 8:   Grade 3–4 Laboratory Abnormalities Reported in ≥2% of Adult Treatment-Naive Patients,[a] Studies AI424-034, AI424-007, and AI424-008

Variable	Limit[d]	Study AI424-034 64 weeks[b] REYATAZ 400 mg once daily + lamivudine + zidovudine[e] (n=404)	Study AI424-034 64 weeks[b] efavirenz 600 mg once daily + lamivudine + zidovudine[e] (n=401)	Studies AI424-007, -008 120 weeks[b,c] REYATAZ 400 mg once daily + stavudine + lamivudine or + stavudine + didanosine (n=279)	Studies AI424-007, -008 73 weeks[b,c] nelfinavir 750 mg TID or 1250 mg BID + stavudine + lamivudine or + stavudine + didanosine (n=191)
Chemistry	High				
SGOT/AST	≥5.1 × ULN	2%	2%	7%	5%
SGPT/ALT	≥5.1 × ULN	4%	3%	9%	7%
Total Bilirubin	≥2.6 × ULN	35%	<1%	47%	3%
Amylase	≥2.1 × ULN	*	*	14%	10%
Lipase	≥2.1 × ULN	<1%	1%	4%	5%
Creatine Kinase	≥5.1 × ULN	6%	6%	11%	9%
Total Cholesterol	≥240 mg/dL	6%	24%	19%	48%
Triglycerides	≥751 mg/dL	<1%	3%	4%	2%
Hematology	Low				
Hemoglobin	<8.0 g/dL	5%	3%	<1%	4%
Neutrophils	<750 cells/mm^3	7%	9%	3%	7%

* None reported in this treatment arm.
[a] Based on regimen(s) containing REYATAZ.
[b] Median time on therapy.
[c] Includes long-term follow-up.
[d] ULN = upper limit of normal.
[e] As a fixed-dose combination: 150 mg lamivudine, 300 mg zidovudine twice daily.

Table 9:   Grade 3–4 Laboratory Abnormalities Reported in ≥2% of Adult Treatment-Experienced Patients, Study AI424-045[a]

Variable	Limit[c]	48 weeks[b] REYATAZ/ritonavir 300/100 mg once daily + tenofovir + NRTI (n=119)	48 weeks[b] lopinavir/ritonavir 400/100 mg twice daily[d] + tenofovir + NRTI (n=118)
Chemistry	High		
SGOT/AST	≥5.1 × ULN	3%	3%
SGPT/ALT	≥5.1 × ULN	4%	3%
Total Bilirubin	≥2.6 × ULN	49%	<1%
Lipase	≥2.1 × ULN	5%	6%
Creatine Kinase	≥5.1 × ULN	8%	8%
Total Cholesterol	≥240 mg/dL	25%	26%
Triglycerides	≥751 mg/dL	8%	12%
Glucose	≥251 mg/dL	5%	<1%
Hematology	Low		
Platelets	<50,000 cells/mm^3	2%	3%
Neutrophils	<750 cells/mm^3	7%	8%

[a] Based on regimen(s) containing REYATAZ.
[b] Median time on therapy.
[c] ULN = upper limit of normal.
[d] As a fixed-dose combination.

7   DRUG INTERACTIONS

See also *Contraindications (4)* and *Clinical Pharmacology (12.3).*

7.1   Potential for REYATAZ to Affect Other Drugs

Atazanavir is an inhibitor of CYP3A and UGT1A1. Coadministration of REYATAZ (atazanavir sulfate) and drugs primarily metabolized by CYP3A or UGT1A1 may result in increased plasma concentrations of the other drug that could increase or prolong its therapeutic and adverse effects.

Table 10: Lipid Values, Mean Change from Baseline, Study AI424-138

| | REYATAZ/ritonavir[a,b] | | | | | | lopinavir/ritonavir[b,c] | | | | | |
| | Baseline mg/dL (n=428[e]) | Week 48 | | Week 96 | | Baseline mg/dL (n=424[e]) | Week 48 | | Week 96 | |
		mg/dL (n=372[e])	Change[d] (n=372[e])	mg/dL (n=342[e])	Change[d] (n=342[e])		mg/dL (n=335[e])	Change[d] (n=335[e])	mg/dL (n=291[e])	Change[d] (n=291[e])
LDL-Cholesterol[f]	92	105	+14%	105	+14%	93	111	+19%	110	+17%
HDL-Cholesterol[f]	37	46	+29%	44	+21%	36	48	+37%	46	+29%
Total Cholesterol[f]	149	169	+13%	169	+13%	150	187	+25%	186	+25%
Triglycerides[f]	126	145	+15%	140	+13%	129	194	+52%	184	+50%

[a] REYATAZ 300 mg with ritonavir 100 mg once daily with the fixed-dose combination: 300 mg tenofovir, 200 mg emtricitabine once daily.
[b] Values obtained after initiation of serum lipid-reducing agents were not included in these analyses. At baseline, serum lipid-reducing agents were used in 1% in the lopinavir/ritonavir treatment arm and 1% in the REYATAZ/ritonavir arm. Through Week 48, serum lipid-reducing agents were used in 8% in the lopinavir/ritonavir treatment arm and 2% in the REYATAZ/ritonavir arm. Through Week 96, serum lipid-reducing agents were used in 10% in the lopinavir/ritonavir treatment arm and 3% in the REYATAZ/ritonavir arm.
[c] Lopinavir 400 mg with ritonavir 100 mg twice daily with the fixed-dose combination 300 mg tenofovir, 200 mg emtricitabine once daily.
[d] The change from baseline is the mean of within-patient changes from baseline for patients with both baseline and Week 48 or Week 96 values and is not a simple difference of the baseline and Week 48 or Week 96 mean values, respectively.
[e] Number of patients with LDL-cholesterol measured.
[f] Fasting.

Table 11: Lipid Values, Mean Change from Baseline, Study AI424-034

| | REYATAZ[a,b] | | | efavirenz[b,c] | | |
	Baseline mg/dL (n=383[e])	Week 48 mg/dL (n=283[e])	Week 48 Change[d] (n=272[e])	Baseline mg/dL (n=378[e])	Week 48 mg/dL (n=264[e])	Week 48 Change[d] (n=253[e])
LDL-Cholesterol[f]	98	98	+1%	98	114	+18%
HDL-Cholesterol[f]	39	43	+13%	38	46	+24%
Total Cholesterol	164	168	+2%	162	195	+21%
Triglycerides[f]	138	124	-9%	129	168	+23%

[a] REYATAZ 400 mg once daily with the fixed-dose combination: 150 mg lamivudine, 300 mg zidovudine twice daily.
[b] Values obtained after initiation of serum lipid-reducing agents were not included in these analyses. At baseline, serum lipid-reducing agents were used in 0% in the efavirenz treatment arm and <1% in the REYATAZ arm. Through Week 48 serum lipid-reducing agents were used in 3% in the efavirenz treatment arm and 1% in the REYATAZ arm.
[c] Efavirenz 600 mg once daily with the fixed-dose combination: 150 mg lamivudine, 300 mg zidovudine twice daily.
[d] The change from baseline is the mean of within-patient changes from baseline for patients with both baseline and Week 48 values and is not a simple difference of the baseline and Week 48 mean values.
[e] Number of patients with LDL-cholesterol measured.
[f] Fasting.

Table 12: Lipid Values, Mean Change from Baseline, Study AI424-045

| | REYATAZ/ritonavir[a,b] | | | lopinavir/ritonavir[b,c] | | |
	Baseline mg/dL (n=111[e])	Week 48 mg/dL (n=75[e])	Week 48 Change[d] (n=74[e])	Baseline mg/dL (n=108[e])	Week 48 mg/dL (n=76[e])	Week 48 Change[d] (n=73[e])
LDL-Cholesterol[f]	108	98	-10%	104	103	+1%
HDL-Cholesterol	40	39	-7%	39	41	+2%
Total Cholesterol	188	170	-8%	181	187	+6%
Triglycerides[f]	215	161	-4%	196	224	+30%

[a] REYATAZ 300 mg once daily + ritonavir + tenofovir + 1 NRTI.
[b] Values obtained after initiation of serum lipid-reducing agents were not included in these analyses. At baseline, serum lipid-reducing agents were used in 4% in the lopinavir/ritonavir treatment arm and 4% in the REYATAZ/ritonavir arm. Through Week 48, serum lipid-reducing agents were used in 19% in the lopinavir/ritonavir treatment arm and 8% in the REYATAZ/ritonavir arm.
[c] Lopinavir/ritonavir (400/100 mg) BID + tenofovir + 1 NRTI.
[d] The change from baseline is the mean of within-patient changes from baseline for patients with both baseline and Week 48 values and is not a simple difference of the baseline and Week 48 mean values.
[e] Number of patients with LDL-cholesterol measured.
[f] Fasting.

Atazanavir is a weak inhibitor of CYP2C8. Caution should be used when REYATAZ (atazanavir sulfate) without ritonavir is coadministered with drugs highly dependent on CYP2C8 with narrow therapeutic indices (eg, paclitaxel, repaglinide). When REYATAZ with ritonavir is coadministered with substrates of CYP2C8, clinically significant interactions are not expected. [See *Clinical Pharmacology, Table 14 (12.3).*]

The magnitude of CYP3A-mediated drug interactions on coadministered drug may change when REYATAZ is coadministered with ritonavir. See the complete prescribing information for NORVIR® (ritonavir) for information on drug interactions with ritonavir.

7.2   Potential for Other Drugs to Affect Atazanavir
Atazanavir is a CYP3A4 substrate; therefore, drugs that induce CYP3A4 may decrease atazanavir plasma concentrations and reduce REYATAZ's therapeutic effect.

Atazanavir solubility decreases as pH increases. Reduced plasma concentrations of atazanavir are expected if proton-pump inhibitors, antacids, buffered medications, or H₂-receptor antagonists are administered with atazanavir.

7.3   Established and Other Potentially Significant Drug Interactions
Table 13 provides dosing recommendations as a result of drug interactions with REYATAZ (atazanavir sulfate). These recommendations are based on either drug interaction studies or predicted interactions due to the expected magnitude of interaction and potential for serious events or loss of efficacy.
[See table 13 on pages 3517 through 3521]

7.4   Drugs with No Observed or Predicted Interactions with REYATAZ
Clinically significant interactions are not expected between atazanavir and substrates of CYP2C19, CYP2C9, CYP2D6, CYP2B6, CYP2A6, CYP1A2, or CYP2E1. Clinically significant interactions are not expected between atazanavir when administered with ritonavir and substrates of CYP2C8. See the complete prescribing information for NORVIR® for information on other potential drug interactions with ritonavir.

Based on known metabolic profiles, clinically significant drug interactions are not expected between REYATAZ (atazanavir sulfate) and fluvastatin, pravastatin, dapsone, trimethoprim/sulfamethoxazole, azithromycin, or erythromycin. REYATAZ does not interact with substrates of CYP2D6 (eg, nortriptyline, desipramine, metoprolol). Additionally, no clinically significant drug interactions were observed when REYATAZ was coadministered with methadone, fluconazole, acetaminophen, or atenolol. [See *Clinical Pharmacology, Tables 16* and *17 (12.3).*]

8   USE IN SPECIFIC POPULATIONS

8.1   Pregnancy
Pregnancy Category B
There are no adequate and well controlled studies of atazanavir use during pregnancy. Cases of lactic acidosis syndrome and symptomatic hyperlactatemia have occurred in pregnant women using REYATAZ in combination with nucleoside analogues. In animal reproduction and pre- and post-natal development studies, there was no evidence of adverse fetal effects or teratogenicity. Because animal reproduction studies are not always predictive of human response, REYATAZ should be used during pregnancy only if clearly needed.

Cases of lactic acidosis syndrome, sometimes fatal, and symptomatic hyperlactatemia have been reported in patients (including pregnant women) receiving REYATAZ in combination with nucleoside analogues. Nucleoside analogues are associated with an increased risk of lactic acidosis syndrome. In addition, hyperbilirubinemia occurred frequently during treatment with REYATAZ. It is not known whether REYATAZ administered during pregnancy will exacerbate physiological hyperbilirubinemia or increase the risk of kernicterus in neonates and young infants. In the prepartum period, additional monitoring and alternative therapy should be considered.

In animal reproduction studies, there was no evidence of teratogenicity in offspring born to animals exposed to atazanavir levels one (in rabbits) to two times (in rats) those observed at the human clinical dose (400 mg once daily). In pre- and post-natal development studies in rats, there were no adverse effects on offspring following maternal exposure to atazanavir levels equivalent to those in humans taking 400 mg once daily. Weight loss and weight gain suppression occurred in pups with maternal atazanavir exposures two times the human exposure at 400 mg once daily; however, maternal toxicity also occurred at this exposure level.

Antiretroviral Pregnancy Registry: To monitor maternal-fetal outcomes of pregnant women exposed to REYATAZ, an Antiretroviral Pregnancy Registry has been established. Physicians are encouraged to register patients by calling 1-800-258-4263.

8.3   Nursing Mothers
The Centers for Disease Control and Prevention recommend that HIV-infected mothers not breast-feed their infants to avoid risking postnatal transmission of HIV. It is not known whether atazanavir is present in human milk. Because of both the potential for HIV transmission and the potential for serious adverse reactions in nursing infants, **mothers should be instructed not to breast-feed if they are taking REYATAZ.**

8.4   Pediatric Use
REYATAZ should not be administered to pediatric patients below the age of 3 months due to the risk of kernicterus.

The safety, activity, and pharmacokinetic profiles of REYATAZ in pediatric patients ages 3 months to less than 6 years have not been established.

The safety, pharmacokinetic profile, and virologic response of REYATAZ were evaluated in pediatric patients in an open-label, multicenter clinical trial PACTG 1020A [see *Clinical Pharmacology (12.3)* and *Clinical Studies (14.3)*]. The safety profile in pediatric patients was comparable to that observed in adults [see *Adverse Reactions (6.2)*]. Please see *Dosage and Administration (2.2)* for dosing recommendations for pediatric patients 6 years of age and older.

8.5   Geriatric Use
Clinical studies of REYATAZ did not include sufficient numbers of patients aged 65 and over to determine whether they respond differently from younger patients. Based on a comparison of mean single-dose pharmacokinetic values for C_{max} and AUC, a dose adjustment based upon age is not recommended. In general, appropriate caution should be exercised in the administration and monitoring of REYATAZ in elderly patients reflecting the greater frequency of decreased hepatic, renal, or cardiac function, and of concomitant disease or other drug therapy.

8.6   Age/Gender
A study of the pharmacokinetics of atazanavir was performed in young (n=29; 18–40 years) and elderly (n=30; ≥65

Table 13: Established and Other Potentially Significant Drug Interactions: Alteration in Dose or Regimen May Be Recommended Based on Drug Interaction Studies[a] or Predicted Interactions (Information in the table applies to REYATAZ with or without ritonavir, unless otherwise indicated)

Concomitant Drug Class: Specific Drugs	Effect on Concentration of Atazanavir or Concomitant Drug	Clinical Comment
HIV Antiviral Agents		
Nucleoside Reverse Transcriptase Inhibitors (NRTIs): didanosine buffered formulations enteric-coated (EC) capsules	↓ atazanavir ↓ didanosine	Coadministration of REYATAZ with didanosine buffered tablets resulted in a marked decrease in atazanavir exposure. It is recommended that REYATAZ be given (with food) 2 h before or 1 h after didanosine buffered formulations. Simultaneous administration of didanosine EC and REYATAZ with food results in a decrease in didanosine exposure. Thus, REYATAZ and didanosine EC should be administered at different times.
Nucleotide Reverse Transcriptase Inhibitors: tenofovir disoproxil fumarate	↓ atazanavir ↑ tenofovir	Tenofovir may decrease the AUC and C_{min} of atazanavir. When coadministered with tenofovir, it is recommended that REYATAZ 300 mg be given with ritonavir 100 mg and tenofovir 300 mg (all as a single daily dose with food). **REYATAZ without ritonavir should not be coadministered with tenofovir.** REYATAZ increases tenofovir concentrations. The mechanism of this interaction is unknown. Higher tenofovir concentrations could potentiate tenofovir-associated adverse events, including renal disorders. Patients receiving REYATAZ and tenofovir should be monitored for tenofovir-associated adverse events.
Non-nucleoside Reverse Transcriptase Inhibitors (NNRTIs): efavirenz	↓ atazanavir	Efavirenz decreases atazanavir exposure. *In treatment-naive patients:* If REYATAZ is combined with efavirenz, REYATAZ 400 mg (two 200-mg capsules) with ritonavir 100 mg should be administered once daily all as a single dose with food, and efavirenz 600 mg should be administered once daily on an empty stomach, preferably at bedtime. *In treatment-experienced patients:* Do not coadminister REYATAZ with efavirenz in treatment-experienced patients due to decreased atazanavir exposure.
Non-nucleoside Reverse Transcriptase Inhibitors: nevirapine	↓ atazanavir ↑ nevirapine	Do not coadminister REYATAZ with nevirapine because: • Nevirapine substantially decreases atazanavir exposure. • Potential risk for nevirapine associated toxicity due to increased nevirapine exposures.
Protease Inhibitors: saquinavir (soft gelatin capsules)	↑ saquinavir	Appropriate dosing recommendations for this combination, with or without ritonavir, with respect to efficacy and safety have not been established. In a clinical study, saquinavir 1200 mg coadministered with REYATAZ 400 mg and tenofovir 300 mg (all given once daily) plus nucleoside analogue reverse transcriptase inhibitors did not provide adequate efficacy [see *Clinical Studies (14.2)*].
Protease Inhibitors: ritonavir	↑ atazanavir	If REYATAZ is coadministered with ritonavir, it is recommended that REYATAZ 300 mg once daily be given with ritonavir 100 mg once daily with food. See the complete prescribing information for NORVIR® (ritonavir) for information on drug interactions with ritonavir.
Protease Inhibitors: others	↑ other protease inhibitor	*REYATAZ/ritonavir:* Although not studied, the coadministration of REYATAZ/ritonavir and other protease inhibitors would be expected to increase exposure to the other protease inhibitor. Such coadministration is not recommended.
Other Agents		
Antacids and buffered medications	↓ atazanavir	Reduced plasma concentrations of atazanavir are expected if antacids, including buffered medications, are administered with REYATAZ. REYATAZ should be administered 2 hours before or 1 hour after these medications.
Antiarrhythmics: amiodarone, bepridil, lidocaine (systemic), quinidine	↑ amiodarone, bepridil, lidocaine (systemic), quinidine	Coadministration with REYATAZ has the potential to produce serious and/or life-threatening adverse events and has not been studied. Caution is warranted and therapeutic concentration monitoring of these drugs is recommended if they are used concomitantly with REYATAZ (atazanavir sulfate).
Anticoagulants: warfarin	↑ warfarin	Coadministration with REYATAZ has the potential to produce serious and/or life-threatening bleeding and has not been studied. It is recommended that INR (International Normalized Ratio) be monitored.

(Table continued on next page)

years) healthy subjects. There were no clinically important pharmacokinetic differences observed due to age or gender.

8.7 Impaired Renal Function

In healthy subjects, the renal elimination of unchanged atazanavir was approximately 7% of the administered dose. REYATAZ (atazanavir sulfate) has been studied in adult subjects with severe renal impairment (n=20), including those on hemodialysis, at multiple doses of 400 mg once daily. The mean atazanavir C_{max} was 9% lower, AUC was 19% higher, and C_{min} was 96% higher in subjects with severe renal impairment not undergoing hemodialysis (n=10), than in age, weight, and gender matched subjects with nor-

mal renal function. Atazanavir was not appreciably cleared during hemodialysis. In a 4-hour dialysis session, 2.1% of the administered dose was removed. When atazanavir was administered either prior to, or following hemodialysis (n=10), the geometric means for C_{max}, AUC, and C_{min} were approximately 25 to 43% lower compared to subjects with normal renal function. The mechanism of this decrease is unknown. REYATAZ (atazanavir sulfate) should not be administered to HIV-treatment experienced patients with end stage renal disease managed with hemodialysis. [See *Dosage and Administration (2.3)*.]

8.8 Impaired Hepatic Function

Atazanavir is metabolized and eliminated primarily by the liver. REYATAZ (atazanavir sulfate) has been studied in adult subjects with moderate to severe hepatic impairment (14 Child-Pugh B and 2 Child-Pugh C subjects) after a single 400-mg dose. The mean $AUC_{(0-\infty)}$ was 42% greater in subjects with impaired hepatic function than in healthy volunteers. The mean half-life of atazanavir in hepatically impaired subjects was 12.1 hours compared to 6.4 hours in healthy volunteers. Increased concentrations of atazanavir are expected in patients with moderately or severely impaired hepatic function. The pharmacokinetics of REYATAZ in combination with ritonavir have not been studied in subjects with hepatic impairment. REYATAZ should not be administered to patients with severe hepatic impairment. REYATAZ/ritonavir is not recommended for use in patients with hepatic impairment. [See *Dosage and Administration (2.4)* and *Warnings and Precautions (5.5)*.]

10 OVERDOSAGE

Human experience of acute overdose with REYATAZ is limited. Single doses up to 1200 mg have been taken by healthy volunteers without symptomatic untoward effects. A single self-administered overdose of 29.2 g of REYATAZ in an HIV-infected patient (73 times the 400-mg recommended dose) was associated with asymptomatic bifascicular block and PR interval prolongation. These events resolved spontaneously. At high doses that lead to high drug exposures, jaundice due to indirect (unconjugated) hyperbilirubinemia (without associated liver function test changes) or PR interval prolongation may be observed. [See *Warnings and Precautions (5.2, 5.4)* and *Clinical Pharmacology (12.2)*.]

Treatment of overdosage with REYATAZ should consist of general supportive measures, including monitoring of vital signs and ECG, and observations of the patient's clinical status. If indicated, elimination of unabsorbed atazanavir should be achieved by emesis or gastric lavage. Administration of activated charcoal may also be used to aid removal of unabsorbed drug. There is no specific antidote for overdose with REYATAZ. Since atazanavir is extensively metabolized by the liver and is highly protein bound, dialysis is unlikely to be beneficial in significant removal of this medicine.

11 DESCRIPTION

REYATAZ® (atazanavir sulfate) is an azapeptide inhibitor of HIV-1 protease.

The chemical name for atazanavir sulfate is (3S,8S,9S,12S)-3,12-Bis(1,1-dimethylethyl)-8-hydroxy-4,11-dioxo-9-(phenylmethyl)-6-[[4-(2-pyridinyl)phenyl] methyl]-2,5,6,10,13-pentaazatetradecanedioic acid dimethyl ester, sulfate (1:1). Its molecular formula is $C_{38}H_{52}N_6O_7 \cdot H_2SO_4$, which corresponds to a molecular weight of 802.9 (sulfuric acid salt). The free base molecular weight is 704.9. Atazanavir sulfate has the following structural formula:

Atazanavir sulfate is a white to pale yellow crystalline powder. It is slightly soluble in water (4–5 mg/mL, free base equivalent) with the pH of a saturated solution in water being about 1.9 at $24 \pm 3°$ C.

REYATAZ Capsules are available for oral administration in strengths containing the equivalent of 100 mg, 150 mg, 200 mg, or 300 mg of atazanavir as atazanavir sulfate and the following inactive ingredients: crospovidone, lactose monohydrate, and magnesium stearate. The capsule shells contain the following inactive ingredients: gelatin, FD&C Blue #2, titanium dioxide, black iron oxide, red iron oxide, and yellow iron oxide. The capsules are printed with ink containing shellac, titanium dioxide, FD&C Blue #2, isopropyl alcohol, ammonium hydroxide, propylene glycol, n-butyl alcohol, simethicone, and dehydrated alcohol.

12   CLINICAL PHARMACOLOGY

12.1   Mechanism of Action

Atazanavir is an antiviral drug [see *Clinical Pharmacology* (12.4)].

12.2   Pharmacodynamics

Effects on Electrocardiogram

Concentration- and dose-dependent prolongation of the PR interval in the electrocardiogram has been observed in healthy volunteers receiving atazanavir. In a placebo-controlled study (AI424-076), the mean (±SD) maximum change in PR interval from the predose value was 24 (±15) msec following oral dosing with 400 mg of atazanavir (n=65) compared to 13 (±11) msec following dosing with placebo (n=67). The PR interval prolongations in this study were asymptomatic. There is limited information on the potential for a pharmacodynamic interaction in humans between atazanavir and other drugs that prolong the PR interval of the electrocardiogram. [See *Warnings and Precautions (5.2)*.]

Electrocardiographic effects of atazanavir were determined in a clinical pharmacology study of 72 healthy subjects. Oral doses of 400 mg and 800 mg were compared with placebo; there was no concentration-dependent effect of atazanavir on the QTc interval (using Fridericia's correction). In 1793 HIV-infected patients receiving antiretroviral regimens, QTc prolongation was comparable in the atazanavir and comparator regimens. No atazanavir-treated healthy subject or HIV-infected patient in clinical trials had a QTc interval >500 msec. [See *Warnings and Precautions (5.2)*.]

In a pharmacokinetic study between atazanavir 400 mg once daily and diltiazem 180 mg once daily, a CYP3A substrate, there was a 2-fold increase in the diltiazem plasma concentration and an additive effect on the PR interval. In a pharmacokinetic study between atazanavir 400 mg once daily and atenolol 50 mg once daily, there was no substantial additive effect of atazanavir and atenolol on the PR interval. [See *Warnings and Precautions (5.2)*.]

12.3   Pharmacokinetics

The pharmacokinetics of atazanavir were evaluated in healthy adult volunteers and in HIV-infected patients after administration of REYATAZ (atazanavir sulfate) 400 mg once daily and after administration of REYATAZ 300 mg with ritonavir 100 mg once daily (see Table 14).

[See table 14 at top of page 3522.]

Figure 1 displays the mean plasma concentrations of atazanavir at steady state after REYATAZ 400 mg once daily (as two 200-mg capsules) with a light meal and after REYATAZ 300 mg (as two 150-mg capsules) with ritonavir 100 mg once daily with a light meal in HIV-infected adult patients.

Figure 1:   Mean (SD) Steady-State Plasma Concentrations of Atazanavir 400 mg (n=13) and 300 mg with Ritonavir (n=10) for HIV-Infected Adult Patients

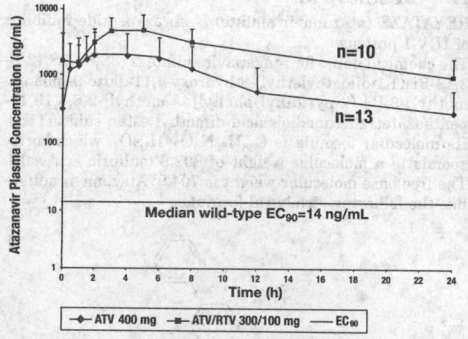

Absorption

Atazanavir is rapidly absorbed with a T_{max} of approximately 2.5 hours. Atazanavir demonstrates nonlinear pharmacokinetics with greater than dose-proportional increases in AUC and C_{max} values over the dose range of 200–800 mg once daily. Steady-state is achieved between Days 4 and 8, with an accumulation of approximately 2.3-fold.

Food Effect

Administration of REYATAZ with food enhances bioavailability and reduces pharmacokinetic variability. Administration of a single 400-mg dose of REYATAZ with a light meal (357 kcal, 8.2 g fat, 10.6 g protein) resulted in a 70% increase in AUC and 57% increase in C_{max} relative to the fasting state. Administration of a single 400-mg dose of REYATAZ with a high-fat meal (721 kcal, 37.3 g fat, 29.4 g protein) resulted in a mean increase in AUC of 35% with no change in C_{max} relative to the fasting state. Administration of REYATAZ (atazanavir sulfate) with either a light meal or high-fat meal decreased the coefficient of variation of AUC and C_{max} by approximately one half compared to the fasting state.

Coadministration of a single 300-mg dose of REYATAZ (atazanavir sulfate) and a 100-mg dose of ritonavir with a light meal (336 kcal, 5.1 g fat, 9.3 g protein) resulted in a 33% increase in the AUC and a 40% increase in both the C_{max} and the 24-hour concentration of atazanavir relative to the fasting state.

Coadministration with a high-fat meal (951 kcal, 54.7 g fat, 35.9 g protein) did not affect the AUC of atazanavir relative to fasting conditions and the C_{max} was within 11% of fasting values. The 24-hour concentration following a high-fat meal was increased by approximately 33% due to delayed absorption; the median T_{max} increased from 2.0 to 5.0 hours. Co-administration of REYATAZ (atazanavir sulfate) with ritonavir with either a light or a high-fat meal decreased the coefficient of variation of AUC and C_{max} by approximately 25% compared to the fasting state.

Distribution

Atazanavir is 86% bound to human serum proteins and protein binding is independent of concentration. Atazanavir binds to both alpha-1-acid glycoprotein (AAG) and albumin to a similar extent (89% and 86%, respectively). In a multiple-dose study in HIV-infected patients dosed with REYATAZ 400 mg once daily with a light meal for 12 weeks,

Table 13 *(cont.)*: Established and Other Potentially Significant Drug Interactions: Alteration in Dose or Regimen May Be Recommended Based on Drug Interaction Studies[a] or Predicted Interactions (Information in the table applies to REYATAZ with or without ritonavir, unless otherwise indicated)

Concomitant Drug Class: Specific Drugs	Effect on Concentration of Atazanavir or Concomitant Drug	Clinical Comment
Antidepressants: tricyclic antidepressants	↑ tricyclic antidepressants	Coadministration with REYATAZ has the potential to produce serious and/or life-threatening adverse events and has not been studied. Concentration monitoring of these drugs is recommended if they are used concomitantly with REYATAZ.
trazodone	↑ trazodone	Concomitant use of trazodone and REYATAZ with or without ritonavir may increase plasma concentrations of trazodone. Adverse events of nausea, dizziness, hypotension, and syncope have been observed following coadministration of trazodone and ritonavir. If trazodone is used with a CYP3A4 inhibitor such as REYATAZ, the combination should be used with caution and a lower dose of trazodone should be considered.
Antifungals: ketoconazole, itraconazole	**REYATAZ/ritonavir:** ↑ ketoconazole ↑ itraconazole	Coadministration of ketoconazole has only been studied with REYATAZ without ritonavir (negligible increase in atazanavir AUC and C_{max}). Due to the effect of ritonavir on ketoconazole, high doses of ketoconazole and itraconazole (>200 mg/day) should be used cautiously with REYATAZ/ritonavir.
Antifungals: voriconazole	Effect is unknown	Coadministration of voriconazole with REYATAZ, with or without ritonavir, has not been studied. Administration of voriconazole with ritonavir 100 mg every 12 hours decreased voriconazole steady-state AUC by an average of 39%. Voriconazole should not be administered to patients receiving REYATAZ/ritonavir, unless an assessment of the benefit/risk to the patient justifies the use of voriconazole. Coadministration of voriconazole with REYATAZ (without ritonavir) may increase atazanavir concentrations; however, no data are available.
Antigout: colchicine	↑ colchicine	REYATAZ should not be coadministered with colchicine to patients with renal or hepatic impairment. ***Recommended dosage of colchicine when administered with REYATAZ:*** **Treatment of gout flares:** 0.6 mg (1 tablet) for 1 dose, followed by 0.3 mg (half tablet) 1 hour later. Not to be repeated before 3 days. **Prophylaxis of gout flares:** If the original regimen was 0.6 mg *twice* a day, the regimen should be adjusted to 0.3 mg *once a day*. If the original regimen was 0.6 mg *once* a day, the regimen should be adjusted to 0.3 mg *once every other day*. **Treatment of familial Mediterranean fever (FMF):** Maximum daily dose of 0.6 mg (may be given as 0.3 mg twice a day).
Antimycobacterials: rifabutin	↑ rifabutin	A rifabutin dose reduction of up to 75% (eg, 150 mg every other day or 3 times per week) is recommended. Increased monitoring for rifabutin-associated adverse reactions including neutropenia is warranted.
Benzodiazepines: parenterally administered midazolam[b]	↑ midazolam	Concomitant use of parenteral midazolam with REYATAZ may increase plasma concentrations of midazolam. Coadministration should be done in a setting which ensures close clinical monitoring and appropriate medical management in case of respiratory depression and/or prolonged sedation. Dosage reduction for midazolam should be considered, especially if more than a single dose of midazolam is administered. Coadministration of oral midazolam with REYATAZ is CONTRAINDICATED.
Calcium channel blockers: diltiazem	↑ diltiazem and desacetyl-diltiazem	Caution is warranted. A dose reduction of diltiazem by 50% should be considered. ECG monitoring is recommended. Coadministration of REYATAZ/ritonavir with diltiazem has not been studied.
eg, felodipine, nifedipine, nicardipine, and verapamil	↑ calcium channel blocker	Caution is warranted. Dose titration of the calcium channel blocker should be considered. ECG monitoring is recommended.

(Table continued on next page)

Table 13 (cont.): Established and Other Potentially Significant Drug Interactions: Alteration in Dose or Regimen May Be Recommended Based on Drug Interaction Studies[a] or Predicted Interactions (Information in the table applies to REYATAZ with or without ritonavir, unless otherwise indicated)

Concomitant Drug Class: Specific Drugs	Effect on Concentration of Atazanavir or Concomitant Drug	Clinical Comment
Endothelin receptor antagonists: bosentan	↓ atazanavir ↑ bosentan	Plasma concentrations of atazanavir may be decreased when bosentan is administered with REYATAZ without ritonavir. Coadministration of bosentan and REYATAZ without ritonavir is not recommended. **Coadministration of bosentan in patients on REYATAZ/ritonavir:** For patients who have been receiving REYATAZ/ritonavir for at least 10 days, start bosentan at 62.5 mg once daily or every other day based on individual tolerability. **Coadministration of REYATAZ/ritonavir in patients on bosentan:** Discontinue bosentan at least 36 hours before starting REYATAZ/ritonavir. At least 10 days after starting REYATAZ/ritonavir, resume bosentan at 62.5 mg once daily or every other day based on individual tolerability.
HMG-CoA reductase inhibitors: atorvastatin, rosuvastatin	↑ atorvastatin ↑ rosuvastatin	Use the lowest possible dose of atorvastatin or rosuvastatin with careful monitoring, or consider other HMG-CoA reductase inhibitors such as pravastatin or fluvastatin in combination with REYATAZ (with or without ritonavir). The risk of myopathy, including rhabdomyolysis, may be increased when HIV protease inhibitors, including REYATAZ, are used in combination with these drugs.
H₂-Receptor antagonists	↓ atazanavir	Plasma concentrations of atazanavir were substantially decreased when REYATAZ 400 mg once daily was administered simultaneously with famotidine 40 mg twice daily, which may result in loss of therapeutic effect and development of resistance. **In treatment-naive patients:** REYATAZ 300 mg with ritonavir 100 mg once daily with food should be administered simultaneously with, and/or at least 10 hours after, a dose of the H₂-receptor antagonist. An H₂-receptor antagonist dose comparable to famotidine 20 mg once daily up to a dose comparable to famotidine 40 mg twice daily can be used with REYATAZ 300 mg with ritonavir 100 mg in treatment-naive patients. OR For patients unable to tolerate ritonavir, REYATAZ 400 mg once daily with food should be administered at least 2 hours before and at least 10 hours after a dose of the H₂-receptor antagonist. No single dose of the H₂-receptor antagonist should exceed a dose comparable to famotidine 20 mg, and the total daily dose should not exceed a dose comparable to famotidine 40 mg. **In treatment-experienced patients:** Whenever an H₂-receptor antagonist is given to a patient receiving REYATAZ with ritonavir, the H₂-receptor antagonist dose should not exceed a dose comparable to famotidine 20 mg twice daily, and the REYATAZ and ritonavir doses should be administered simultaneously with, and/or at least 10 hours after, the dose of the H₂-receptor antagonist. • REYATAZ 300 mg with ritonavir 100 mg once daily (all as a single dose with food) if taken with an H₂-receptor antagonist. • REYATAZ 400 mg with ritonavir 100 mg once daily (all as a single dose with food) if taken with both tenofovir and an H₂-receptor antagonist.
Hormonal contraceptives: ethinyl estradiol and norgestimate or norethindrone	↓ ethinyl estradiol ↑ norgestimate[c] ↑ ethinyl estradiol ↑ norethindrone[d]	Use with caution if coadministration of REYATAZ or REYATAZ/ritonavir with oral contraceptives is considered. If an oral contraceptive is administered with REYATAZ plus ritonavir, it is recommended that the oral contraceptive contain at least 35 mcg of ethinyl estradiol. If REYATAZ is administered without ritonavir, the oral contraceptive should contain no more than 30 mcg of ethinyl estradiol. Potential safety risks include substantial increases in progesterone exposure. The long-term effects of increases in concentration of the progestational agent are unknown and could increase the risk of insulin resistance, dyslipidemia, and acne. Coadministration of REYATAZ or REYATAZ/ritonavir with other hormonal contraceptives (eg, contraceptive patch, contraceptive vaginal ring, or injectable contraceptives) or oral contraceptives containing progestagens other than norethindrone or norgestimate, or less than 25 mcg of ethinyl estradiol, has not been studied; therefore, alternative methods of contraception are recommended.

(Table continued on next page)

atazanavir was detected in the cerebrospinal fluid and semen. The cerebrospinal fluid/plasma ratio for atazanavir (n=4) ranged between 0.0021 and 0.0226 and seminal fluid/plasma ratio (n=5) ranged between 0.11 and 4.42.

Metabolism

Atazanavir is extensively metabolized in humans. The major biotransformation pathways of atazanavir in humans consisted of monooxygenation and dioxygenation. Other minor biotransformation pathways for atazanavir or its metabolites consisted of glucuronidation, N-dealkylation, hydrolysis, and oxygenation with dehydrogenation. Two minor metabolites of atazanavir in plasma have been characterized. Neither metabolite demonstrated *in vitro* antiviral activity. *In vitro* studies using human liver microsomes suggested that atazanavir is metabolized by CYP3A.

Elimination

Following a single 400-mg dose of ^{14}C-atazanavir, 79% and 13% of the total radioactivity was recovered in the feces and urine, respectively. Unchanged drug accounted for approximately 20% and 7% of the administered dose in the feces and urine, respectively. The mean elimination half-life of atazanavir in healthy volunteers (n=214) and HIV-infected adult patients (n=13) was approximately 7 hours at steady state following a dose of 400 mg daily with a light meal.

Special Populations

Pediatrics

The pharmacokinetic data from pediatric patients receiving REYATAZ (atazanavir sulfate) Capsules with ritonavir based on body surface area are presented in Table 15.

Table 15: Steady-State Pharmacokinetics of Atazanavir with ritonavir in HIV-Infected Pediatric Patients (6 to less than 18 years of age) in the Fed State

	205 mg/m² atazanavir with 100 mg/m² ritonavir once daily Age Range (years)	
	at least 6 to 13 (n=17)	at least 13 to 18 (n=10)
Dose mg		
Median	200	400
[min-max]	[150–400]	[250–500]
C_{max} ng/mL		
Geometric mean (CV%)	4451 (33)	3711 (46)
AUC ng•h/mL		
Geometric mean (CV%)	42503 (36)	44970 (34)
C_{min} ng/mL		
Geometric mean (CV%)	535 (62)	1090 (60)

Drug Interaction Data

Atazanavir is a metabolism-dependent CYP3A inhibitor, with a K_{inact} value of 0.05 to 0.06 min^{-1} and K_i value of 0.84 to 1.0 µM. Atazanavir is also a direct inhibitor for UGT1A1 (K_i=1.9 µM) and CYP2C8 (K_i=2.1 µM).

Atazanavir has been shown *in vivo* not to induce its own metabolism, nor to increase the biotransformation of some drugs metabolized by CYP3A. In a multiple-dose study, REYATAZ decreased the urinary ratio of endogenous 6β-OH cortisol to cortisol versus baseline, indicating that CYP3A production was not induced.

Drug interaction studies were performed with REYATAZ and other drugs likely to be coadministered and some drugs commonly used as probes for pharmacokinetic interactions. The effects of coadministration of REYATAZ on the AUC, C_{max}, and C_{min} are summarized in Tables 16 and 17. For information regarding clinical recommendations, see *Drug Interactions (7)*.

[See table 16 on pages 3523 and 3524]
[See table 17 on pages 3525 and 3526]

12.4 Microbiology

Mechanism of Action

Atazanavir (ATV) is an azapeptide HIV-1 protease inhibitor (PI). The compound selectively inhibits the virus-specific processing of viral Gag and Gag-Pol polyproteins in HIV-1 infected cells, thus preventing formation of mature virions.

Antiviral Activity in Cell Culture

Atazanavir exhibits anti-HIV-1 activity with a mean 50% effective concentration (EC_{50}) in the absence of human serum of 2 to 5 nM against a variety of laboratory and clinical HIV-1 isolates grown in peripheral blood mononuclear cells, macrophages, CEM-SS cells, and MT-2 cells. ATV has activity against HIV-1 Group M subtype viruses A, B, C, D, AE, AG, F, G, and J isolates in cell culture. ATV has variable activity against HIV-2 isolates (1.9 to 32 nM), with EC_{50} values above the EC_{50} values of failure isolates. Two-drug combination antiviral activity studies with ATV showed no antagonism in cell culture with NNRTIs (delavirdine, efavirenz, and nevirapine), PIs (amprenavir, indinavir, lopinavir, nelfinavir, ritonavir, and saquinavir), NRTIs (abacavir, didanosine, emtricitabine, lamivudine, stavudine, tenofovir, zalcitabine, and zidovudine), the HIV-1 fusion inhibitor enfuvirtide, and two compounds used in the treatment of viral hepatitis, adefovir and ribavirin, without enhanced cytotoxicity.

Resistance

In Cell Culture: HIV-1 isolates with a decreased susceptibility to ATV have been selected in cell culture and obtained from patients treated with ATV or atazanavir/ritonavir (ATV/RTV). HIV-1 isolates with 93- to 183-fold reduced susceptibility to ATV from three different viral strains were selected in cell culture by 5 months. The substitutions in these HIV-1 viruses that contributed to ATV resistance include I50L, N88S, I84V, A71V, and M46I. Changes were also observed at the protease cleavage sites following drug selection. Recombinant viruses containing the I50L substitution without other major PI substitutions were growth impaired and displayed increased susceptibility in cell culture to other PIs (amprenavir, indinavir, lopinavir, nelfinavir, ritonavir, and saquinavir). The I50L and I50V substitutions yielded selective resistance to ATV and amprenavir, respectively, and did not appear to be cross-resistant.

Clinical Studies of Treatment-Naive Patients: Comparison of Ritonavir-Boosted REYATAZ vs. Unboosted REYATAZ: Study AI424-089 compared REYATAZ (atazanavir sulfate) 300 mg once daily with ritonavir 100 mg vs. REYATAZ 400 mg once daily when administered with lamivudine and extended-release stavudine in HIV-infected treatment-naive patients. A summary of the number of virologic failures and virologic failure isolates with ATV resistance in each arm is shown in Table 18.

Table 18: Summary of Virologic Failures[a] at Week 96 in Study AI424-089: Comparison of Ritonavir Boosted REYATAZ vs. Unboosted REYATAZ: Randomized Patients

	REYATAZ 300 mg + ritonavir 100 mg (n=95)	REYATAZ 400 mg (n=105)
Virologic Failure (≥50 copies/mL) at Week 96	15 (16%)	34 (32%)
Virologic Failure with Genotypes and Phenotypes Data	5	17
Virologic Failure Isolates with ATV-resistance at Week 96	0/5 (0%)[b]	4/17 (24%)[b]
Virologic Failure Isolates with I50L Emergence at Week 96[c]	0/5 (0%)[b]	2/17 (12%)[b]
Virologic Failure Isolates with Lamivudine Resistance at Week 96	2/5 (40%)[b]	11/17 (65%)[b]

[a] Virologic failure includes patients who were never suppressed through Week 96 and on study at Week 96, had virologic rebound or discontinued due to insufficient viral load response.

[b] Percentage of Virologic Failure Isolates with genotypic and phenotypic data.

[c] Mixture of I50I/L emerged in 2 other ATV 400 mg-treated patients. Neither isolate was phenotypically resistant to ATV.

Clinical Studies of Treatment-Naive Patients Receiving REYATAZ 300 mg With Ritonavir 100 mg: In Phase III study AI424-138, an as-treated genotypic and phenotypic analysis was conducted on samples from patients who experienced virologic failure (HIV-1 RNA ≥400 copies/mL) or discontinued before achieving suppression on ATV/RTV (n=39; 9%) and LPV/RTV (n=39; 9%) through 96 weeks of treatment. In the ATV/RTV arm, one of the virologic failure isolates had a 56-fold decrease in ATV susceptibility emerge on therapy with the development of PI resistance-associated substitutions L10F, V32I, K43T, M46I, A71I, G73S, I85I/V, and L90M. The NRTI resistance-associated substitution M184V also emerged on treatment in this isolate conferring emtricitabine resistance. Two ATV/RTV-virologic failure isolates had baseline phenotypic ATV resistance and IAS-defined major PI resistance-associated substitutions at baseline. The I50L substitution emerged on study in one of these failure isolates and was associated with a 17-fold decrease in ATV susceptibility from baseline and the other failure isolate with baseline ATV resistance and PI substitutions (M46M/I and I84I/V) had additional IAS-defined major PI substitutions (V32I, M46I, and I84V) emerge on ATV treatment associated with a 3-fold decrease in ATV susceptibility from baseline. Five of the treatment failure isolates in the ATV/RTV arm developed phenotypic emtricitabine resistance with the emergence of either the M184I (n=1) or the M184V (n=4) substitution on therapy and none developed phenotypic tenofovir disoproxil resistance. In the LPV/RTV arm, one of the virologic failure pa-

tient isolates had a 69-fold decrease in LPV susceptibility emerge on therapy with the development of PI substitutions L10V, V11I, I54V, G73S, and V82A in addition to baseline PI substitutions L10L/I, V32I, I54I/V, A71I, G73G/S, V82V/A, L89V, and L90M. Six LPV/RTV virologic failure isolates developed the M184V substitution and phenotypic emtricitabine resistance and two developed phenotypic tenofovir disoproxil resistance.

Clinical Studies of Treatment-Naive Patients Receiving REYATAZ (atazanavir sulfate) 400 mg Without Ritonavir: ATV-resistant clinical isolates from treatment-naive patients who experienced virologic failure on REYATAZ 400 mg treatment without ritonavir often developed an I50L substitution (after an average of 50 weeks of ATV therapy), often in combination with an A71V substitution, but also developed one or more other PI substitutions (eg, V32I, L33F, G73S, V82A, I85V, or N88S) with or without the I50L substitution. In treatment-naive patients, viral isolates that developed the I50L substitution, without other major PI substitutions, showed phenotypic resistance to ATV but retained in cell culture susceptibility to other PIs (amprenavir, indinavir, lopinavir, nelfinavir, ritonavir, and saquinavir); however, there are no clinical data available to demonstrate the effect of the I50L substitution on the efficacy of subsequently administered PIs.

Clinical Studies of Treatment-Experienced Patients: In studies of treatment-experienced patients treated with ATV or ATV/RTV, most ATV-resistant isolates from patients who experienced virologic failure developed substitutions that were associated with resistance to multiple PIs and displayed decreased susceptibility to multiple PIs. The most

common protease substitutions to develop in the viral isolates of patients who failed treatment with ATV 300 mg once daily and RTV 100 mg once daily (together with tenofovir and an NRTI) included V32I, L33F/V/I, E35D/G, M46I/L, I50L, F53L/V, I54V, A71V/T/I, G73S/T/C, V82A/T/L, I85V, and L89V/Q/M/T. Other substitutions that developed on ATV/RTV treatment including E34K/A/Q, G48V, I84V, N88S/D/T, and L90M occurred in less than 10% of patient isolates. Generally, if multiple PI resistance substitutions were present in the HIV-1 virus of the patient at baseline, ATV resistance developed through substitutions associated with resistance to other PIs and could include the development of the I50L substitution. The I50L substitution has been detected in treatment-experienced patients experiencing virologic failure after long-term treatment. Protease cleavage site changes also emerged on ATV treatment but their presence did not correlate with the level of ATV resistance.

Cross-Resistance

Cross-resistance among PIs has been observed. Baseline phenotypic and genotypic analyses of clinical isolates from ATV clinical trials of PI-experienced patients showed that isolates cross-resistant to multiple PIs were cross-resistant to ATV. Greater than 90% of the isolates with substitutions that included I84V or G48V were resistant to ATV. Greater than 60% of isolates containing L90M, G73S/T/C, A71V/T, I54V, M46I/L, or a change at V82 were resistant to ATV, and 38% of isolates containing a D30N substitution in addition to other changes were resistant to ATV. Isolates resistant to ATV were also cross-resistant to other PIs with >90% of the isolates[a] resistant to indinavir, lopinavir, nelfinavir,

Table 13 (cont.): Established and Other Potentially Significant Drug Interactions: Alteration in Dose or Regimen May Be Recommended Based on Drug Interaction Studies[a] or Predicted Interactions (Information in the table applies to REYATAZ with or without ritonavir, unless otherwise indicated)

Concomitant Drug Class: Specific Drugs	Effect on Concentration of Atazanavir or Concomitant Drug	Clinical Comment
Immunosuppressants: cyclosporin, sirolimus, tacrolimus	↑ immunosuppressants	Therapeutic concentration monitoring is recommended for immunosuppressant agents when coadministered with REYATAZ (atazanavir sulfate).
Inhaled beta agonist: salmeterol	↑ salmeterol	Coadministration of salmeterol with REYATAZ is not recommended. Concomitant use of salmeterol and REYATAZ may result in increased risk of cardiovascular adverse events associated with salmeterol, including QT prolongation, palpitations, and sinus tachycardia.
Inhaled/nasal steroid: fluticasone	**REYATAZ** ↑ fluticasone	Concomitant use of fluticasone propionate and REYATAZ (without ritonavir) may increase plasma concentrations of fluticasone propionate. Use with caution. Consider alternatives to fluticasone propionate, particularly for long-term use.
	REYATAZ/ritonavir ↑ fluticasone	Concomitant use of fluticasone propionate and REYATAZ/ritonavir may increase plasma concentrations of fluticasone propionate, resulting in significantly reduced serum cortisol concentrations. Systemic corticosteroid effects, including Cushing's syndrome and adrenal suppression, have been reported during postmarketing use in patients receiving ritonavir and inhaled or intranasally administered fluticasone propionate. Coadministration of fluticasone propionate and REYATAZ/ritonavir is not recommended unless the potential benefit to the patient outweighs the risk of systemic corticosteroid side effects [see *Warnings and Precautions (5.1)*].
Macrolide antibiotics: clarithromycin	↑ clarithromycin ↓ 14-OH clarithromycin ↑ atazanavir	Increased concentrations of clarithromycin may cause QTc prolongations; therefore, a dose reduction of clarithromycin by 50% should be considered when it is coadministered with REYATAZ. In addition, concentrations of the active metabolite 14-OH clarithromycin are significantly reduced; consider alternative therapy for indications other than infections due to *Mycobacterium avium* complex. Coadministration of REYATAZ/ritonavir with clarithromycin has not been studied.
Opioids: Buprenorphine	↑ buprenorphine ↑ norbuprenorphine	Coadministration of buprenorphine and REYATAZ with or without ritonavir increases the plasma concentration of buprenorphine and norbuprenorphine. Coadministration of REYATAZ plus ritonavir with buprenorphine warrants clinical monitoring for sedation and cognitive effects. A dose reduction of buprenorphine may be considered. Coadministration of buprenorphine and REYATAZ with ritonavir is not expected to decrease atazanavir plasma concentrations. Coadministration of buprenorphine and REYATAZ without ritonavir may decrease atazanavir plasma concentrations. REYATAZ without ritonavir should not be coadministered with buprenorphine.

(Table continued on next page)

ritonavir, and saquinavir, and 80% resistant to amprenavir. In treatment-experienced patients, PI-resistant viral isolates that developed the I50L substitution in addition to other PI resistance-associated substitution were also cross-resistant to other PIs.

Baseline Genotype/Phenotype and Virologic Outcome Analyses

Genotypic and/or phenotypic analysis of baseline virus may aid in determining ATV susceptibility before initiation of ATV/RTV therapy. An association between virologic response at 48 weeks and the number and type of primary PI resistance-associated substitutions detected in baseline HIV-1 isolates from antiretroviral-experienced patients receiving ATV/RTV once daily or lopinavir (LPV)/RTV twice daily in Study AI424-045 is shown in Table 19.

Overall, both the number and type of baseline PI substitutions affected response rates in treatment-experienced patients. In the ATV/RTV group, patients had lower response rates when 3 or more baseline PI substitutions, including a substitution at position 36, 71, 77, 82, or 90, were present compared to patients with 1–2 PI substitutions, including one of these substitutions.

Table 19: HIV RNA Response by Number and Type of Baseline PI Substitution, Antiretroviral-Experienced Patients in Study AI424-045, As-Treated Analysis

	Virologic Response = HIV RNA <400 copies/mL[b]	
Number and Type of Baseline PI Substitutions[a]	ATV/RTV (n=110)	LPV/RTV (n=113)
3 or more primary PI substitutions including:[c]		
D30N	75% (6/8)	50% (3/6)
M36I/V	19% (3/16)	33% (6/18)
M46I/L/T	24% (4/17)	23% (5/22)
I54V/L/T/M/A	31% (5/16)	31% (5/16)
A71V/T/I/G	34% (10/29)	39% (12/31)
G73S/A/C/T	14% (1/7)	38% (3/8)
V77I	47% (7/15)	44% (7/16)
V82A/F/T/S/I	29% (6/21)	27% (7/26)
I84V/A	11% (1/9)	33% (2/6)
N88D	63% (5/8)	67% (4/6)
L90M	10% (2/21)	44% (11/25)
Number of baseline primary PI substitutions[a]		
All patients, as-treated	58% (64/110)	59% (67/113)
0–2 PI substitutions	75% (50/67)	75% (50/67)
3–4 PI substitutions	41% (14/34)	43% (12/28)
5 or more PI substitutions	0% (0/9)	28% (5/18)

[a] Primary substitutions include any change at D30, V32, M36, M46, I47, G48, I50, I54, A71, G73, V77, V82, I84, N88, and L90.
[b] Results should be interpreted with caution because the subgroups were small.
[c] There were insufficient data (n<3) for PI substitutions V32I, I47V, G48V, I50V, and F53L.

The response rates of antiretroviral-experienced patients in Study AI424-045 were analyzed by baseline phenotype (shift in susceptibility in cell culture relative to reference, Table 20). The analyses are based on a select patient population with 62% of patients receiving an NNRTI-based regimen before study entry compared to 35% receiving a PI-based regimen. Additional data are needed to determine clinically relevant break points for REYATAZ (atazanavir sulfate).

Table 20: Baseline Phenotype by Outcome, Antiretroviral-Experienced Patients in Study AI424-045, As-Treated Analysis

	Virologic Response = HIV RNA <400 copies/mL[b]	
Baseline Phenotype[a]	ATV/RTV (n=111)	LPV/RTV (n=111)
0–2	71% (55/78)	70% (56/80)
>2–5	53% (8/15)	44% (4/9)
>5–10	13% (1/8)	33% (3/9)
>10	10% (1/10)	23% (3/13)

[a] Fold change susceptibility in cell culture relative to the wild-type reference.
[b] Results should be interpreted with caution because the subgroups were small.

13 NONCLINICAL TOXICOLOGY

13.1 Carcinogenesis, Mutagenesis, Impairment of Fertility

Two-year carcinogenicity studies in mice and rats were conducted with atazanavir. At the high dose in female mice, the incidence of benign hepatocellular adenomas was increased at systemic exposures 7.2-fold higher than those in humans at the recommended 400-mg clinical dose. There were no increases in the incidence of tumors in male mice at any dose in the study. In rats, no significant positive trends in the incidence of neoplasms occurred at systemic exposures up to 5.7-fold higher than those in humans at the recommended 400-mg clinical dose. The clinical relevance of the carcinogenic findings in female mice is unknown.

Atazanavir tested positive in an *in vitro* clastogenicity test using primary human lymphocytes, in the absence and presence of metabolic activation. Atazanavir tested negative in the *in vitro* Ames reverse-mutation assay, *in vivo* micronucleus and DNA repair tests in rats, and *in vivo* DNA damage test in rat duodenum (comet assay).

13.2 Reproductive Toxicology Studies

At the systemic drug exposure levels (AUC) equal to (in male rats) or two times (in female rats) those at the human clinical dose (400 mg once daily), atazanavir did not produce significant effects on mating, fertility, or early embryonic development.

Table 13 (cont.): Established and Other Potentially Significant Drug Interactions: Alteration in Dose or Regimen May Be Recommended Based on Drug Interaction Studies[a] or Predicted Interactions (Information in the table applies to REYATAZ with or without ritonavir, unless otherwise indicated)

Concomitant Drug Class: Specific Drugs	Effect on Concentration of Atazanavir or Concomitant Drug	Clinical Comment
PDE5 inhibitors: sildenafil, tadalafil, vardenafil	↑ sildenafil ↑ tadalafil ↑ vardenafil	Coadministration with REYATAZ has not been studied but may result in an increase in PDE5 inhibitor-associated adverse events, including hypotension, syncope, visual disturbances, and priapism. **Use of PDE5 inhibitors for pulmonary arterial hypertension (PAH):** Use of REVATIO® (sildenafil) for the treatment of pulmonary hypertension (PAH) is contraindicated with REYATAZ [see *Contraindications (4)*]. The following dose adjustments are recommended for the use of ADCIRCA® (tadalafil) with REYATAZ: Coadministration of ADCIRCA® in patients on REYATAZ (with or without ritonavir): • For patients receiving REYATAZ (with or without ritonavir) for at least one week, start ADCIRCA® at 20 mg once daily. Increase to 40 mg once daily based on individual tolerability. Coadministration of REYATAZ (with or without ritonavir) in patients on ADCIRCA®: • Avoid the use of ADCIRCA® when starting REYATAZ (with or without ritonavir). Stop ADCIRCA® at least 24 hours before starting REYATAZ (with or without ritonavir). At least one week after starting REYATAZ (with or without ritonavir), resume ADCIRCA® at 20 mg once daily. Increase to 40 mg once daily based on individual tolerability. **Use of PDE5 inhibitors for erectile dysfunction:** Use VIAGRA® (sildenafil) with caution at reduced doses of 25 mg every 48 hours with increased monitoring for adverse events. Use CIALIS® (tadalafil) with caution at reduced doses of 10 mg every 72 hours with increased monitoring for adverse events. **REYATAZ/ritonavir:** Use LEVITRA® (vardenafil) with caution at reduced doses of no more than 2.5 mg every 72 hours with increased monitoring for adverse events. **REYATAZ:** Use LEVITRA® (vardenafil) with caution at reduced doses of no more than 2.5 mg every 24 hours with increased monitoring for adverse events.
Proton-pump inhibitors: omeprazole	↓ atazanavir	Plasma concentrations of atazanavir were substantially decreased when REYATAZ 400 mg or REYATAZ 300 mg/ritonavir 100 mg once daily was administered with omeprazole 40 mg once daily, which may result in loss of therapeutic effect and development of resistance. **In treatment-naive patients:** The proton-pump inhibitor dose should not exceed a dose comparable to omeprazole 20 mg and must be taken approximately 12 hours prior to the REYATAZ 300 mg with ritonavir 100 mg dose. **In treatment-experienced patients:** Proton-pump inhibitors should not be used in treatment-experienced patients receiving REYATAZ.

[a] For magnitude of interactions see *Clinical Pharmacology, Tables 16 and 17 (12.3)*.
[b] See *Contraindications (4), Table 3* for orally administered midazolam.
[c] In combination with atazanavir 300 mg and ritonavir 100 mg once daily.
[d] In combination with atazanavir 400 mg once daily.

14 CLINICAL STUDIES

14.1 Adult Patients Without Prior Antiretroviral Therapy

Study AI424-138: *a 96-week study comparing the antiviral efficacy and safety of atazanavir/ritonavir with lopinavir/ritonavir, each in combination with fixed-dose tenofovir-emtricitabine in HIV-1 infected treatment naive subjects.* Study AI424-138 is a 96-week open-label, randomized, multicenter study, comparing REYATAZ (atazanavir sulfate) (300 mg once daily) with ritonavir (100 mg once daily) to lopinavir with ritonavir (400/100 mg twice daily), each in combination with fixed-dose tenofovir with emtricitabine (300/200 mg once daily), in 878 antiretroviral treatment-naive treated patients. Patients had a mean age of 36 years (range: 19–72), 49% were Caucasian, 18% Black, 9% Asian, 23% Hispanic/Mestizo/mixed race, and 68% were male. The median baseline plasma CD4+ cell count was 204 cells/mm[3] (range: 2 to 810 cells/mm[3]) and the mean baseline plasma HIV-1 RNA level was 4.94 log10 copies/mL (range: 2.60 to 5.88 log10 copies/mL). Treatment response and outcomes through Week 96 are presented in Table 21.

Table 14: Steady-State Pharmacokinetics of Atazanavir in Healthy Subjects or HIV-Infected Patients in the Fed State

Parameter	400 mg once daily		300 mg with ritonavir 100 mg once daily	
	Healthy Subjects (n=14)	HIV-Infected Patients (n=13)	Healthy Subjects (n=28)	HIV-Infected Patients (n=10)
C_{max} (ng/mL)				
Geometric mean (CV%)	5199 (26)	2298 (71)	6129 (31)	4422 (58)
Mean (SD)	5358 (1371)	3152 (2231)	6450 (2031)	5233 (3033)
T_{max} (h)				
Median	2.5	2.0	2.7	3.0
AUC (ng•h/mL)				
Geometric mean (CV%)	28132 (28)	14874 (91)	57039 (37)	46073 (66)
Mean (SD)	29303 (8263)	22262 (20159)	61435 (22911)	53761 (35294)
T-half (h)				
Mean (SD)	7.9 (2.9)	6.5 (2.6)	18.1 (6.2)[a]	8.6 (2.3)
C_{min} (ng/mL)				
Geometric mean (CV%)	159 (88)	120 (109)	1227 (53)	636 (97)
Mean (SD)	218 (191)	273 (298)[b]	1441 (757)	862 (838)

[a] n=26.
[b] n=12.

Table 21: Outcomes of Treatment Through Week 96 (Study AI424-138)

Outcome	REYATAZ 300 mg + ritonavir 100 mg (once daily) with tenofovir/emtricitabine (once daily)[a] (n=441) 96 Weeks	lopinavir 400 mg + ritonavir 100 mg (twice daily) with tenofovir/emtricitabine (once daily)[a] (n=437) 96 Weeks
Responder[b,c,d]	75%	68%
Virologic failure[e]	17%	19%
Rebound	8%	10%
Never suppressed through Week 96	9%	9%
Death	1%	1%
Discontinued due to adverse event	3%	5%
Discontinued for other reasons[f]	4%	7%

[a] As a fixed-dose combination: 300 mg tenofovir, 200 mg emtricitabine once daily.
[b] Patients achieved HIV RNA <50 copies/mL at Week 96. Roche Amplicor®, v1.5 ultra-sensitive assay.
[c] Pre-specified ITT analysis at Week 48 using as-randomized cohort: ATV/RTV 78% and LPV/RTV 76% [difference estimate: 1.7% (95% confidence interval: -3.8%, 7.1%)].
[d] Pre-specified ITT analysis at Week 96 using as-randomized cohort: ATV/RTV 74% and LPV/RTV 68% [difference estimate: 6.1% (95% confidence interval: 0.3%, 12.0%)].
[e] Includes viral rebound and failure to achieve confirmed HIV RNA <50 copies/mL through Week 96.
[f] Includes lost to follow-up, patient's withdrawal, noncompliance, protocol violation, and other reasons.

Through 96 weeks of therapy, the proportion of responders among patients with high viral loads (ie, baseline HIV RNA ≥100,000 copies/mL) was comparable for the REYATAZ/ritonavir (165 of 223 patients, 74%) and lopinavir/ritonavir (148 of 222 patients, 67%) arms. At 96 weeks, the median increase from baseline in CD4+ cell count was 261 cells/mm³ for the REYATAZ/ritonavir arm and 273 cells/mm³ for the lopinavir/ritonavir arm.
Study AI424-034: REYATAZ once daily compared to efavirenz once daily, each in combination with fixed-dose lamivudine + zidovudine twice daily. Study AI424-034 was a randomized, double-blind, multicenter trial comparing REYATAZ (atazanavir sulfate) (400 mg once daily) to efavirenz (600 mg once daily), each in combination with a fixed-dose combination of lamivudine (3TC) (150 mg) and zidovudine (ZDV) (300 mg) given twice daily, in 810 antiretroviral treatment-naive patients. Patients had a mean age of 34 years (range: 18 to 73), 36% were Hispanic, 33% were Caucasian, and 65% were male. The mean baseline CD4+ cell count was 321 cells/mm³ (range: 64 to 1424 cells/mm³) and the mean baseline plasma HIV-1 RNA level was 4.8 $\log_{10}$ copies/mL (range: 2.2 to 5.9 $\log_{10}$ copies/mL). Treatment response and outcomes through Week 48 are presented in Table 22.

Table 22: Outcomes of Randomized Treatment Through Week 48 (Study AI424-034)

Outcome	REYATAZ 400 mg once daily + lamivudine + zidovudine[d] (n=405)	efavirenz 600 mg once daily + lamivudine + zidovudine[d] (n=405)
Responder[a]	67% (32%)	62% (37%)
Virologic failure[b]	20%	21%
Rebound	17%	16%
Never suppressed through Week 48	3%	5%
Death	–	<1%
Discontinued due to adverse event	5%	7%
Discontinued for other reasons[c]	8%	10%

[a] Patients achieved and maintained confirmed HIV RNA <400 copies/mL (<50 copies/mL) through Week 48. Roche Amplicor® HIV-1 Monitor™ Assay, test version 1.0 or 1.5 as geographically appropriate.
[b] Includes viral rebound and failure to achieve confirmed HIV RNA <400 copies/mL through Week 48.
[c] Includes lost to follow-up, patient's withdrawal, noncompliance, protocol violation, and other reasons.
[d] As a fixed-dose combination: 150 mg lamivudine, 300 mg zidovudine twice daily.

Through 48 weeks of therapy, the proportion of responders among patients with high viral loads (ie, baseline HIV RNA ≥100,000 copies/mL) was comparable for the REYATAZ (atazanavir sulfate) and efavirenz arms. The mean increase from baseline in CD4+ cell count was 176 cells/mm³ for the REYATAZ arm and 160 cells/mm³ for the efavirenz arm.
Study AI424-008: REYATAZ 400 mg once daily compared to REYATAZ 600 mg once daily, and compared to nelfinavir 1250 mg twice daily, each in combination with stavudine and lamivudine twice daily. Study AI424-008 was a 48-week, randomized, multicenter trial, blinded to dose of REYATAZ, comparing REYATAZ at two dose levels (400 mg and 600 mg once daily) to nelfinavir (1250 mg twice daily), each in combination with stavudine (40 mg) and lamivudine (150 mg) given twice daily, in 467 antiretroviral treatment-naive patients. Patients had a mean age of 35 years (range: 18 to 69), 55% were Caucasian, and 63% were male. The mean baseline CD4+ cell count was 295 cells/mm³ (range: 4 to 1003 cells/mm³) and the mean baseline plasma HIV-1 RNA level was 4.7 $\log_{10}$ copies/mL (range: 1.8 to 5.9 $\log_{10}$ copies/mL). Treatment response and outcomes through Week 48 are presented in Table 23.

Table 23: Outcomes of Randomized Treatment Through Week 48 (Study AI424-008)

Outcome	REYATAZ 400 mg once daily + lamivudine + stavudine (n=181)	nelfinavir 1250 mg twice daily + lamivudine + stavudine (n=91)
Responder[a]	67% (33%)	59% (38%)
Virologic failure[b]	24%	27%

Rebound	14%	14%
Never suppressed through Week 48	10%	13%
Death	<1%	–
Discontinued due to adverse event	1%	3%
Discontinued for other reasons[c]	7%	10%

[a] Patients achieved and maintained confirmed HIV RNA <400 copies/mL (<50 copies/mL) through Week 48. Roche Amplicor® HIV-1 Monitor™ Assay, test version 1.0 or 1.5 as geographically appropriate.
[b] Includes viral rebound and failure to achieve confirmed HIV RNA <400 copies/mL through Week 48.
[c] Includes lost to follow-up, patient's withdrawal, noncompliance, protocol violation, and other reasons.

Through 48 weeks of therapy, the mean increase from baseline in CD4+ cell count was 234 cells/mm³ for the REYATAZ (atazanavir sulfate) 400-mg arm and 211 cells/mm³ for the nelfinavir arm.

14.2 Adult Patients With Prior Antiretroviral Therapy
Study AI424-045: REYATAZ once daily + ritonavir once daily compared to REYATAZ once daily + saquinavir (soft gelatin capsules) once daily, and compared to lopinavir + ritonavir twice daily, each in combination with tenofovir + one NRTI. Study AI424-045 is an ongoing, randomized, multicenter trial comparing REYATAZ (300 mg once daily) with ritonavir (100 mg once daily) to REYATAZ (400 mg once daily) with saquinavir soft gelatin capsules (1200 mg once daily), and to lopinavir + ritonavir (400/100 mg twice daily), each in combination with tenofovir and one NRTI, in 347 (of 358 randomized) patients who experienced virologic failure on HAART regimens containing PIs, NRTIs, and NNRTIs. The mean time of prior exposure to antiretrovirals was 139 weeks for PIs, 283 weeks for NRTIs, and 85 weeks for NNRTIs. The mean age was 41 years (range: 24 to 74); 60% were Caucasian, and 78% were male. The mean baseline CD4+ cell count was 338 cells/mm³ (range: 14 to 1543 cells/mm³) and the mean baseline plasma HIV-1 RNA level was 4.4 $\log_{10}$ copies/mL (range: 2.6 to 5.88 $\log_{10}$ copies/mL).
Treatment outcomes through Week 48 for the REYATAZ/ritonavir and lopinavir/ritonavir treatment arms are presented in Table 24. REYATAZ/ritonavir and lopinavir/ritonavir were similar for the primary efficacy outcome measure of time-averaged difference in change from baseline in HIV RNA level. Study AI424-045 was not large enough to reach a definitive conclusion that REYATAZ/ritonavir and lopinavir/ritonavir are equivalent on the secondary efficacy outcome measure of proportions below the HIV RNA lower limit of detection. [See *Clinical Pharmacology*, Tables 19 and 20 (12.4).]
[See table 24 at top of page 3527]
No patients in the REYATAZ/ritonavir treatment arm and three patients in the lopinavir/ritonavir treatment arm experienced a new-onset CDC Category C event during the study.
In Study AI424-045, the mean change from baseline in plasma HIV-1 RNA for REYATAZ 400 mg with saquinavir (n=115) was -1.55 $\log_{10}$ copies/mL, and the time-averaged difference in change in HIV-1 RNA levels versus lopinavir/ritonavir was 0.33. The corresponding mean increase in CD4+ cell count was 72 cells/mm³. Through 48 weeks of treatment, the proportion of patients in this treatment arm with plasma HIV-1 RNA <400 (<50) copies/mL was 38% (26%). In this study, coadministration of REYATAZ and saquinavir did not provide adequate efficacy [see *Drug Interactions (7)*].
Study AI424-045 also compared changes from baseline in lipid values. [See *Adverse Reactions (6.1)*.]
Study AI424-043: Study AI424-043 was a randomized, open-label, multicenter trial comparing REYATAZ (400 mg once daily) to lopinavir/ritonavir (400/100 mg twice daily), each in combination with two NRTIs, in 300 patients who experienced virologic failure to only one prior PI-containing regimen. Through 48 weeks, the proportion of patients with plasma HIV-1 RNA <400 (<50) copies/mL was 49% (35%) for patients randomized to REYATAZ (n=144) and 69% (53%) for patients randomized to lopinavir/ritonavir (n=146). The mean change from baseline was -1.59 $\log_{10}$ copies/mL in the REYATAZ treatment arm and -2.02 $\log_{10}$ copies/mL in the lopinavir/ritonavir arm. Based on the results of this study, REYATAZ without ritonavir is inferior to lopinavir/ritonavir in PI-experienced patients with prior virologic failure and is not recommended for such patients.

14.3 Pediatric Patients
Assessment of the pharmacokinetics, safety, tolerability, and efficacy of REYATAZ is based on data from the open-label, multicenter clinical trial PACTG 1020A conducted in patients from 3 months to 21 years of age. In this study, 182 patients (83 antiretroviral-naive and 99 antiretroviral-experienced) received once daily REYATAZ, with or without ritonavir, in combination with two NRTIs.
Ninety-nine patients (6 to less than 18 years of age) treated with the REYATAZ capsule formulation, with or without

ritonavir, were evaluated. In this cohort, the overall proportions of antiretroviral-naive and -experienced patients with HIV RNA <400 copies/mL at week 24 were 68% (28/41) and 33% (19/58), respectively. The overall proportions of antiretroviral-naive and -experienced patients with HIV RNA <50 copies/mL at week 24 were 59% (24/41) and 24% (14/58), respectively. The median increase from baseline in absolute CD4 count at 20 weeks of therapy was 171 cells/mm³ in antiretroviral-naive patients and 116 cells/mm³ in antiretroviral-experienced patients.

16   HOW SUPPLIED/STORAGE AND HANDLING

REYATAZ® (atazanavir sulfate) Capsules are available in the following strengths and configurations of plastic bottles with child-resistant closures.
[See second table on page 3527]
REYATAZ (atazanavir sulfate) Capsules should be stored at 25° C (77° F); excursions permitted to 15–30° C (59–86° F) [see USP Controlled Room Temperature].

17   PATIENT COUNSELING INFORMATION

A statement to patients and healthcare providers is included on the product's bottle label: **ALERT: Find out about medicines that should NOT be taken with REYATAZ.** FDA-Approved Patient Labeling is available for REYATAZ. Patients should be informed that REYATAZ is not a cure for HIV infection and that they may continue to develop opportunistic infections and other complications associated with HIV disease. Patients should be told that there are currently no data demonstrating that therapy with REYATAZ can reduce the risk of transmitting HIV to others through sexual contact.

17.1   Dosing Instructions

Patients should be told that sustained decreases in plasma HIV RNA have been associated with a reduced risk of progression to AIDS and death. Patients should remain under the care of a physician while using REYATAZ. Patients should be advised to take REYATAZ with food every day and take other concomitant antiretroviral therapy as prescribed. REYATAZ must always be used in combination with other antiretroviral drugs. Patients should not alter the dose or discontinue therapy without consulting with their doctor. If a dose of REYATAZ is missed, patients should take the dose as soon as possible and then return to their normal schedule. However, if a dose is skipped the patient should not double the next dose.

17.2   Drug Interactions

REYATAZ may interact with some drugs; therefore, patients should be advised to report to their doctor the use of any other prescription, nonprescription medication, or herbal products, particularly St. John's wort.
Patients receiving a PDE5 inhibitor and atazanavir should be advised that they may be at an increased risk of PDE5 inhibitor-associated adverse events including hypotension, syncope, visual disturbances, and priapism, and should promptly report any symptoms to their doctor.
Patients should be informed that REVATIO® (used to treat pulmonary arterial hypertension) is contraindicated with REYATAZ and that dose adjustments are necessary when REYATAZ is used with CIALIS®, LEVITRA® or VIAGRA® (used to treat erectile dysfunction), or ADCIRCA® (used to treat pulmonary arterial hypertension).

17.3   Cardiac Conduction Abnormalities

Patients should be informed that atazanavir may produce changes in the electrocardiogram (eg, PR prolongation). Patients should consult their physician if they are experiencing symptoms such as dizziness or lightheadedness.

17.4   Rash

Patients should be informed that mild rashes without other symptoms have been reported with REYATAZ use. These rashes go away within two weeks with no change in treatment. However, there have been a few reports of severe skin reactions (eg, Stevens-Johnson syndrome, erythema multiforme, and toxic skin eruptions) with REYATAZ use. Patients developing signs or symptoms of severe skin reactions or hypersensitivity reactions (including, but not limited to, severe rash or rash accompanied by one or more of the following: fever, general malaise, muscle or joint aches, blisters, oral lesions, conjunctivitis, facial edema, hepatitis, eosinophilia, granulocytopenia, lymphadenopathy, and renal dysfunction) must discontinue REYATAZ and seek medical evaluation immediately.

17.5   Hyperbilirubinemia

Patients should be informed that asymptomatic elevations in indirect bilirubin have occurred in patients receiving REYATAZ. This may be accompanied by yellowing of the skin or whites of the eyes and alternative antiretroviral therapy may be considered if the patient has cosmetic concerns.

17.6   Fat Redistribution

Patients should be informed that redistribution or accumulation of body fat may occur in patients receiving antiretroviral therapy including protease inhibitors and that the cause and long-term health effects of these conditions are not known at this time. It is unknown whether long-term use of REYATAZ (atazanavir sulfate) will result in a lower incidence of lipodystrophy than with other protease inhibitors.

FDA-Approved Patient Labeling
Patient Information
REYATAZ® (RAY-ah-taz)
(generic name = **atazanavir sulfate**)
Capsules

ALERT: Find out about medicines that should NOT be taken with REYATAZ (atazanavir sulfate). Read the section "What important information should I know about taking REYATAZ with other medicines?"
Read the Patient Information that comes with REYATAZ before you start using it and each time you get a refill. There may be new information. This leaflet provides a summary about REYATAZ and does not include everything

Table 16: Drug Interactions: Pharmacokinetic Parameters for Atazanavir in the Presence of Coadministered Drugs[a]

Coadministered Drug	Coadministered Drug Dose/Schedule	REYATAZ Dose/Schedule	Ratio (90% Confidence Interval) of Atazanavir Pharmacokinetic Parameters with/without Coadministered Drug; No Effect = 1.00		
			C_{max}	AUC	C_{min}
atenolol	50 mg QD, d 7–11 (n=19) and d 19–23	400 mg QD, d 1–11 (n=19)	1.00 (0.89, 1.12)	0.93 (0.85, 1.01)	0.74 (0.65, 0.86)
clarithromycin	500 mg BID, d 7–10 (n=29) and d 18–21	400 mg QD, d 1–10 (n=29)	1.06 (0.93, 1.20)	1.28 (1.16, 1.43)	1.91 (1.66, 2.21)
didanosine (ddI) (buffered tablets) plus stavudine (d4T)[b]	ddI: 200 mg × 1 dose, d4T: 40 mg × 1 dose (n=31)	400 mg × 1 dose simultaneously with ddI and d4T (n=31)	0.11 (0.06, 0.18)	0.13 (0.08, 0.21)	0.16 (0.10, 0.27)
	ddI: 200 mg × 1 dose, d4T: 40 mg × 1 dose (n=32)	400 mg × 1 dose 1 h after ddI + d4T (n=32)	1.12 (0.67, 1.18)	1.03 (0.64, 1.67)	1.03 (0.61, 1.73)
ddI (enteric-coated [EC] capsules)[c]	400 mg d 8 (fed) (n=34)	400 mg QD, d 2–8 (n=34)	1.03 (0.93, 1.14)	0.99 (0.91, 1.08)	0.98 (0.89, 1.08)
	400 mg d 19 (fed) (n=31)	300 mg/ritonavir 100 mg QD, d 9–19 (n=31)	1.04 (1.01, 1.07)	1.00 (0.96, 1.03)	0.87 (0.82, 0.92)
diltiazem	180 mg QD, d 7–11 (n=30) and d 19–23	400 mg QD, d 1–11 (n=30)	1.04 (0.96, 1.11)	1.00 (0.95, 1.05)	0.98 (0.90, 1.07)
efavirenz	600 mg QD, d 7–20 (n=27)	400 mg QD, d 1–20 (n=27)	0.41 (0.33, 0.51)	0.26 (0.22, 0.32)	0.07 (0.05, 0.10)
	600 mg QD, d 7–20 (n=13)	400 mg QD, d 1–6 (n=23) then 300 mg/ritonavir 100 mg QD, 2 h before efavirenz, d 7–20 (n=13)	1.14 (0.83, 1.58)	1.39 (1.02, 1.88)	1.48 (1.24, 1.76)
	600 mg QD, d 11–24 (pm) (n=14)	300 mg QD/ritonavir 100 mg QD, d 1–10 (pm) (n=22), then 400 mg QD/ritonavir 100 mg QD, d 11–24 (pm), (simultaneous with efavirenz) (n=14)	1.17 (1.08, 1.27)	1.00 (0.91, 1.10)	0.58 (0.49, 0.69)
famotidine	40 mg BID, d 7–12 (n=15)	400 mg QD, d 1–6 (n=45), d 7–12 (simultaneous administration) (n=15)	0.53 (0.34, 0.82)	0.59 (0.40, 0.87)	0.58 (0.37, 0.89)
	40 mg BID, d 7–12 (n=14)	400 mg QD (pm), 1–6 (n=14), d 7–12 (10 h after, 2 h before famotidine) (n=14)	1.08 (0.82, 1.41)	0.95 (0.74, 1.21)	0.79 (0.60, 1.04)
	40 mg BID, d 11–20 (n=14)[d]	300 mg QD/ritonavir 100 mg QD, d 1–10 (n=46), d 11–20[d] (simultaneous administration) (n=14)	0.86 (0.79, 0.94)	0.82 (0.75, 0.89)	0.72 (0.64, 0.81)
	20 mg BID, d 11–17 (n=18)	300 mg QD/ritonavir 100 mg QD/tenofovir 300 mg QD, d 1–10 (am) (n=39), d 11–17 (am) (simultaneous administration with am famotidine) (n=18)[e,f]	0.91 (0.84, 0.99)	0.90 (0.82, 0.98)	0.81 (0.69, 0.94)
	40 mg QD (pm), d 18–24 (n=20)	300 mg QD/ritonavir 100 mg QD/tenofovir 300 mg QD, d 1–10 (am) (n=39), d 18–24 (am) (12 h after pm famotidine) (n=20)[f]	0.89 (0.81, 0.97)	0.88 (0.80, 0.96)	0.77 (0.63, 0.93)
	40 mg BID, d 18–24 (n=18)	300 mg QD/ritonavir 100 mg QD/tenofovir 300 mg QD, d 1–10 (am) (n=39), d 18–24 (am) (10 h after pm famotidine and 2 h before am famotidine) (n=18)[f]	0.74 (0.66, 0.84)	0.79 (0.70, 0.88)	0.72 (0.63, 0.83)
	40 mg BID, d 11–20 (n=15)	300 mg QD/ritonavir 100 mg QD, d 1–10 (am) (n=46), then 400 mg QD/ritonavir 100 mg QD, d 11–20 (am) (n=15)	1.02 (0.87, 1.18)	1.03 (0.86, 1.22)	0.86 (0.68, 1.08)
fluconazole	200 mg QD, d 11–20 (n=29)	300 mg QD/ritonavir 100 mg QD, d 1–10 (n=19), d 11–20 (n=29)	1.03 (0.95, 1.11)	1.04 (0.95, 1.13)	0.98 (0.85, 1.13)

(Table continued on next page)

Table 16 (cont.): Drug Interactions: Pharmacokinetic Parameters for Atazanavir in the Presence of Coadministered Drugs[a]

Coadministered Drug	Coadministered Drug Dose/Schedule	REYATAZ Dose/Schedule	Ratio (90% Confidence Interval) of Atazanavir Pharmacokinetic Parameters with/without Coadministered Drug; No Effect = 1.00		
			C_{max}	AUC	C_{min}
ketoconazole	200 mg QD, d 7–13 (n=14)	400 mg QD, d 1–13 (n=14)	0.99 (0.77, 1.28)	1.10 (0.89, 1.37)	1.03 (0.53, 2.01)
nevirapine[g,h]	200 mg BID, d 1–23 (n=23)	300 mg QD/ ritonavir 100 mg QD, d 4–13, then 400 mg QD/ ritonavir 100 mg QD, d 14–23 (n=23)[i]	0.72 (0.60, 0.86) 1.02 (0.85, 1.24)	0.58 (0.48, 0.71) 0.81 (0.65, 1.02)	0.28 (0.20, 0.40) 0.41 (0.27, 0.60)
omeprazole	40 mg QD, d 7–12 (n=16)[j] 40 mg QD, d 11–20 (n=15)[j] 20 mg QD, d 17–23 (am) (n=13) 20 mg QD, d 17–23 (am) (n=14)	400 mg QD, d 1–6 (n=48), d 7–12 (n=16) 300 mg QD/ ritonavir 100 mg QD, d 1–20 (n=15) 300 mg QD/ ritonavir 100 mg QD, d 7–16 (pm) (n=27), d 17–23 (pm) (n=13)[k,l] 300 mg QD/ ritonavir 100 mg QD, d 7–16 (am) (n=27), then 400 mg QD/ritonavir 100 mg QD, d 17–23 (am) (n=14)[m,n]	0.04 (0.04, 0.05) 0.28 (0.24, 0.32) 0.61 (0.46, 0.81) 0.69 (0.58, 0.83)	0.06 (0.05, 0.07) 0.24 (0.21, 0.27) 0.58 (0.44, 0.75) 0.70 (0.57, 0.86)	0.05 (0.03, 0.07) 0.22 (0.19, 0.26) 0.54 (0.41, 0.71) 0.69 (0.54, 0.88)
rifabutin	150 mg QD, d 15–28 (n=7)	400 mg QD, d 1–28 (n=7)	1.34 (1.14, 1.59)	1.15 (0.98, 1.34)	1.13 (0.68, 1.87)
rifampin	600 mg QD, d 17–26 (n=16)	300 mg QD/ ritonavir 100 mg QD, d 7–16 (n=48), d 17–26 (n=16)	0.47 (0.41, 0.53)	0.28 (0.25, 0.32)	0.02 (0.02, 0.03)
ritonavir[o]	100 mg QD, d 11–20 (n=28)	300 mg QD, d 1–20 (n=28)	1.86 (1.69, 2.05)	3.38 (3.13, 3.63)	11.89 (10.23, 13.82)
tenofovir[p]	300 mg QD, d 9–16 (n=34) 300 mg QD, d 15–42 (n=10)	400 mg QD, d 2–16 (n=34) 300 mg/ ritonavir 100 mg QD, d 1–42 (n=10)	0.79 (0.73, 0.86) 0.72[q] (0.50, 1.05)	0.75 (0.70, 0.81) 0.75[q] (0.58, 0.97)	0.60 (0.52, 0.68) 0.77[q] (0.54, 1.10)

[a] Data provided are under fed conditions unless otherwise noted.
[b] All drugs were given under fasted conditions.
[c] 400 mg ddI EC and REYATAZ were administered together with food on Days 8 and 19.
[d] REYATAZ 300 mg plus ritonavir 100 mg once daily coadministered with famotidine 40 mg twice daily resulted in atazanavir geometric mean C_{max} that was similar and AUC and C_{min} values that were 1.79- and 4.46-fold higher relative to REYATAZ 400 mg once daily alone.
[e] Similar results were noted when famotidine 20 mg BID was administered 2 hours after and 10 hours before atazanavir 300 mg and ritonavir 100 mg plus tenofovir 300 mg.
[f] Atazanavir/ritonavir/tenofovir was administered after a light meal.
[g] Study was conducted in HIV-infected individuals.
[h] Compared with atazanavir 400 mg historical data without nevirapine (n=13), the ratio of geometric means (90% confidence intervals) for C_{max}, AUC, and C_{min} were 1.42 (0.98, 2.05), 1.64 (1.11, 2.42), and 1.25 (0.66, 2.36), respectively, for atazanavir/ritonavir 300/100 mg; and 2.02 (1.42, 2.87), 2.28 (1.54, 3.38), and 1.80 (0.94, 3.45), respectively, for atazanavir/ritonavir 400/100 mg.
[i] Parallel group design; n=23 for atazanavir/ritonavir plus nevirapine, n=22 for atazanavir 300 mg/ritonavir 100 mg without nevirapine. Subjects were treated with nevirapine prior to study entry.
[j] Omeprazole 40 mg was administered on an empty stomach 2 hours before REYATAZ.
[k] Omeprazole 20 mg was administered 30 minutes prior to a light meal in the morning and REYATAZ 300 mg plus ritonavir 100 mg in the evening after a light meal, separated by 12 hours from omeprazole.
[l] REYATAZ 300 mg plus ritonavir 100 mg once daily separated by 12 hours from omeprazole 20 mg daily resulted in increases in atazanavir geometric mean AUC (10%) and C_{min} (2.4-fold), with a decrease in C_{max} (29%) relative to REYATAZ 400 mg once daily in the absence of omeprazole (study days 1–6).
[m] Omeprazole 20 mg was given 30 minutes prior to a light meal in the morning and REYATAZ 400 mg plus ritonavir 100 mg once daily after a light meal, 1 hour after omeprazole. Effects on atazanavir concentrations were similar when REYATAZ 400 mg plus ritonavir 100 mg was separated from omeprazole 20 mg by 12 hours.
[n] REYATAZ 400 mg plus ritonavir 100 mg once daily administered with omeprazole 20 mg once daily resulted in increases in atazanavir geometric mean AUC (32%) and C_{min} (3.3-fold), with a decrease in C_{max} (26%) relative to REYATAZ 400 mg once daily in the absence of omeprazole (study days 1–6).
[o] Compared with atazanavir 400 mg QD historical data, administration of atazanavir/ritonavir 300/100 mg QD increased the atazanavir geometric mean values of C_{max}, AUC, and C_{min} by 18%, 103%, and 671%, respectively.
[p] Note that similar results were observed in studies where administration of tenofovir and REYATAZ was separated by 12 hours.
[q] Ratio of atazanavir plus ritonavir plus tenofovir to atazanavir plus ritonavir. Atazanavir 300 mg plus ritonavir 100 mg results in higher atazanavir exposure than atazanavir 400 mg (see footnote [o]). The geometric mean values of atazanavir pharmacokinetic parameters when coadministered with ritonavir and tenofovir were: C_{max} = 3190 ng/mL, AUC = 34459 ng•h/mL, and C_{min} = 491 ng/mL. Study was conducted in HIV-infected individuals.

there is to know about your medicine. This information does not take the place of talking with your healthcare provider about your medical condition or treatment.

What is REYATAZ (atazanavir sulfate)?
REYATAZ is a prescription medicine used with other anti-HIV medicines to treat people who are infected with the human immunodeficiency virus (HIV). HIV is the virus that causes acquired immune deficiency syndrome (AIDS). REYATAZ (atazanavir sulfate) is a type of anti-HIV medicine called a protease inhibitor. HIV infection destroys CD4+ (T) cells, which are important to the immune system. The immune system helps fight infection. After a large number of (T) cells are destroyed, AIDS develops. REYATAZ helps to block HIV protease, an enzyme that is needed for the HIV virus to multiply. REYATAZ (atazanavir sulfate) may lower the amount of HIV in your blood, help your body keep its supply of CD4+ (T) cells, and reduce the risk of death and illness associated with HIV.

Does REYATAZ cure HIV or AIDS?
REYATAZ does not cure HIV infection or AIDS. At present there is no cure for HIV infection. People taking REYATAZ may still get opportunistic infections or other conditions that happen with HIV infection. Opportunistic infections are infections that develop because the immune system is weak. Some of these conditions are pneumonia, herpes virus infections, and *Mycobacterium avium* complex (MAC) infections. **It is very important that you see your healthcare provider regularly while taking REYATAZ.**
REYATAZ does not lower your chance of passing HIV to other people through sexual contact, sharing needles, or being exposed to your blood. For your health and the health of others, it is important to always practice safer sex by using a latex or polyurethane condom or other barrier to lower the chance of sexual contact with semen, vaginal secretions, or blood. Never use or share dirty needles.

Who should not take REYATAZ?
Do not take REYATAZ if you:
- **are taking certain medicines.** (See "What important information should I know about taking REYATAZ with other medicines?") Serious life-threatening side effects or death may happen. Before you take REYATAZ, tell your healthcare provider about all medicines you are taking or planning to take. These include other prescription and nonprescription medicines, vitamins, and herbal supplements.
- **are allergic to REYATAZ or to any of its ingredients.** The active ingredient is atazanavir sulfate. See the end of this leaflet for a complete list of ingredients in REYATAZ. Tell your healthcare provider if you think you have had an allergic reaction to any of these ingredients.

What should I tell my healthcare provider before I take REYATAZ?
Tell your healthcare provider:
- **If you are pregnant or planning to become pregnant.** It is not known if REYATAZ can harm your unborn baby. Pregnant women have experienced serious side effects when taking REYATAZ with other HIV medicines called nucleoside analogues. You and your healthcare provider will need to decide if REYATAZ is right for you. If you use REYATAZ while you are pregnant, talk to your healthcare provider about the Antiretroviral Pregnancy Registry.
- **If you are breast-feeding.** You should not breast-feed if you are HIV-positive because of the chance of passing HIV to your baby. Also, it is not known if REYATAZ can pass into your breast milk and if it can harm your baby. If you are a woman who has or will have a baby, talk with your healthcare provider about the best way to feed your baby.
- **If you have liver problems or are infected with the hepatitis B or C virus.** See "What are the possible side effects of REYATAZ?"
- **If you have end stage kidney disease** managed with hemodialysis.
- **If you have diabetes.** See "What are the possible side effects of REYATAZ?"
- **If you have hemophilia.** See "What are the possible side effects of REYATAZ?"
- **About all the medicines you take** including prescription and nonprescription medicines, vitamins, and herbal supplements. Keep a list of your medicines with you to show your healthcare provider. For more information, see "What important information should I know about taking REYATAZ with other medicines?" and "Who should not take REYATAZ?" Some medicines can cause serious side effects if taken with REYATAZ.

How should I take REYATAZ?
- **Take REYATAZ once every day exactly as instructed by your healthcare provider.** Your healthcare provider will prescribe the amount of REYATAZ that is right for you.
  - For adults who have never taken anti-HIV medicines before, the dose is 300 mg once daily with 100 mg of NORVIR® once daily taken with food. For adults who are unable to tolerate ritonavir, 400 mg (two 200-mg capsules) once daily (without NORVIR®) taken with food is recommended.
  - For adults who have taken anti-HIV medicines in the past, the usual dose is 300 mg plus 100 mg of NORVIR® (ritonavir) once daily taken with food.
- Your dose will depend on your liver function and on the other anti-HIV medicines that you are taking. REYATAZ is always used with other anti-HIV medicines. If you are taking REYATAZ with SUSTIVA® (efavirenz) or with VIREAD® (tenofovir disoproxil fumarate), you should also be taking NORVIR® (ritonavir).
- **Always take REYATAZ with food** (a meal or snack) to help it work better. Swallow the capsules whole. **Do not open the capsules.** Take REYATAZ at the same time each day.

- If you are taking antacids or didanosine (VIDEX® or VIDEX® EC), take REYATAZ (atazanavir sulfate) 2 hours before or 1 hour after these medicines.
- If you are taking medicines for indigestion, heartburn, or ulcers such as AXID® (nizatidine), PEPCID AC® (famotidine), TAGAMET® (cimetidine), ZANTAC® (ranitidine), AcipHex® (rabeprazole), NEXIUM® (esomeprazole), PREVACID® (lansoprazole), PRILOSEC® (omeprazole), or PROTONIX® (pantoprazole), talk to your healthcare provider.
- Do not change your dose or stop taking REYATAZ without first talking with your healthcare provider. It is important to stay under a healthcare provider's care while taking REYATAZ.
- When your supply of REYATAZ starts to run low, get more from your healthcare provider or pharmacy. It is important not to run out of REYATAZ. The amount of HIV in your blood may increase if the medicine is stopped for even a short time.
- If you miss a dose of REYATAZ, take it as soon as possible and then take your next scheduled dose at its regular time. If, however, it is within 6 hours of your next dose, do not take the missed dose. Wait and take the next dose at the regular time. Do not double the next dose. It is important that you do not miss any doses of REYATAZ or your other anti-HIV medicines.
- If you take more than the prescribed dose of REYATAZ, call your healthcare provider or poison control center right away.

Can children take REYATAZ?
Dosing recommendations are available for children 6 years of age and older for REYATAZ Capsules. Dosing recommendations are not available for children from 3 months to less than 6 years of age. REYATAZ should not be used in babies under the age of 3 months.

What are the possible side effects of REYATAZ?
The following list of side effects is **not** complete. Report any new or continuing symptoms to your healthcare provider. If you have questions about side effects, ask your healthcare provider. Your healthcare provider may be able to help you manage these side effects.

The following side effects have been reported with REYATAZ:
- **mild rash** (redness and itching) without other symptoms sometimes occurs in patients taking REYATAZ, most often in the first few weeks after the medicine is started. Rashes usually go away within 2 weeks with no change in treatment. Tell your healthcare provider if rash occurs.
- **severe rash:** In a small number of patients, a rash can develop that is associated with other symptoms which could be serious and potentially cause death.

If you develop a rash with any of the following symptoms stop using REYATAZ and call your healthcare provider right away:
- shortness of breath
- general ill feeling or "flu-like" symptoms
- fever
- muscle or joint aches
- conjunctivitis (red or inflamed eyes, like "pink eye")
- blisters
- mouth sores
- swelling of your face
- **yellowing of the skin or eyes.** These effects may be due to increases in bilirubin levels in the blood (bilirubin is made by the liver). Call your healthcare provider if your skin or the white part of your eyes turn yellow. Although these effects may not be damaging to your liver, skin, or eyes, it is important to tell your healthcare provider promptly if they occur.
- **a change in the way your heart beats (heart rhythm change).** Call your healthcare provider right away if you get dizzy or lightheaded. These could be symptoms of a heart problem.
- **diabetes and high blood sugar (hyperglycemia)** sometimes happen in patients taking protease inhibitor medicines like REYATAZ. Some patients had diabetes before taking protease inhibitors while others did not. Some patients may need changes in their diabetes medicine.
- **if you have liver disease** including hepatitis B or C, your liver disease may get worse when you take anti-HIV medicines like REYATAZ.
- **kidney stones** have been reported in patients taking REYATAZ. If you develop signs or symptoms of kidney stones (pain in your side, blood in your urine, pain when you urinate) tell your healthcare provider promptly.
- **some patients with hemophilia** have increased bleeding problems with protease inhibitors like REYATAZ.
- **changes in body fat.** These changes may include an increased amount of fat in the upper back and neck ("buffalo hump"), breast, and around the trunk. Loss of fat from the legs, arms, and face may also happen. The cause and long-term health effects of these conditions are not known at this time.

Other common side effects of REYATAZ (atazanavir sulfate) taken with other anti-HIV medicines include nausea; headache; stomach pain; vomiting; diarrhea; depression; fever; dizziness; trouble sleeping; numbness, tingling, or burning of hands or feet; and muscle pain.

Gallbladder disorders (which may include gallstones and gallbladder inflammation) have been reported in patients taking REYATAZ (atazanavir sulfate).

Table 17: Drug Interactions: Pharmacokinetic Parameters for Coadministered Drugs in the Presence of REYATAZ[a]

Coadministered Drug	Coadministered Drug Dose/Schedule	REYATAZ Dose/Schedule	Ratio (90% Confidence Interval) of Coadministered Drug Pharmacokinetic Parameters with/without REYATAZ; No Effect = 1.00		
			C_{max}	AUC	C_{min}
acetaminophen	1 gm BID, d 1–20 (n=10)	300 mg QD/ ritonavir 100 mg QD, d 11–20 (n=10)	0.87 (0.77, 0.99)	0.97 (0.91, 1.03)	1.26 (1.08, 1.46)
atenolol	50 mg QD, d 7–11 (n=19) and d 19–23	400 mg QD, d 1–11 (n=19)	1.34 (1.26, 1.42)	1.25 (1.16, 1.34)	1.02 (0.88, 1.19)
clarithromycin	500 mg BID, d 7–10 (n=21) and d 18–21	400 mg QD, d 1–10 (n=21)	1.50 (1.32, 1.71) OH-clarithromycin: 0.28 (0.24, 0.33)	1.94 (1.75, 2.16) OH-clarithromycin: 0.30 (0.26, 0.34)	2.60 (2.35, 2.88) OH-clarithromycin: 0.38 (0.34, 0.42)
didanosine (ddI) (buffered tablets) plus stavudine (d4T)[b]	ddI: 200 mg × 1 dose, d4T: 40 mg × 1 dose (n=31)	400 mg × 1 dose simultaneous with ddI and d4T (n=31)	ddI: 0.92 (0.84, 1.02) d4T: 1.08 (0.96, 1.22)	ddI: 0.98 (0.92, 1.05) d4T: 1.00 (0.97, 1.03)	NA d4T: 1.04 (0.94, 1.16)
ddI (enteric-coated [EC] capsules)[c]	400 mg d 1 (fasted), d 8 (fed) (n=34)	400 mg QD, d 2–8 (n=34)	0.64 (0.55, 0.74)	0.66 (0.60, 0.74)	1.13 (0.91, 1.41)
	400 mg d 1 (fasted), d 19 (fed) (n=31)	300 mg QD/ ritonavir 100 mg QD, d 9–19 (n=31)	0.62 (0.52, 0.74)	0.66 (0.59, 0.73)	1.25 (0.92, 1.69)
diltiazem	180 mg QD, d 7–11 (n=28) and d 19–23	400 mg QD, d 1–11 (n=28)	1.98 (1.78, 2.19) desacetyl-diltiazem: 2.72 (2.44, 3.03)	2.25 (2.09, 2.16) desacetyl-diltiazem: 2.65 (2.45, 2.87)	2.42 (2.14, 2.73) desacetyl-diltiazem: 2.21 (2.02, 2.42)
ethinyl estradiol & norethindrone[d]	Ortho-Novum® 7/7/7 QD, d 1–29 (n=19)	400 mg QD, d 16–29 (n=19)	ethinyl estradiol: 1.15 (0.99, 1.32) norethindrone: 1.67 (1.42, 1.96)	ethinyl estradiol: 1.48 (1.31, 1.68) norethindrone: 2.10 (1.68, 2.62)	ethinyl estradiol: 1.91 (1.57, 2.33) norethindrone: 3.62 (2.57, 5.09)
ethinyl estradiol & norgestimate[e]	Ortho Tri-Cyclen® QD, d 1–28 (n=18), then Ortho Tri-Cyclen® LO QD, d 29–42[f] (n=14)	300 mg QD/ritonavir 100 mg QD, d 29–42 (n=14)	ethinyl estradiol: 0.84 (0.74, 0.95) 17-deacetyl norgestimate:[g] 1.68 (1.51, 1.88)	ethinyl estradiol: 0.81 (0.75, 0.87) 17-deacetyl norgestimate:[g] 1.85 (1.67, 2.05)	ethinyl estradiol: 0.63 (0.55, 0.71) 17-deacetyl norgestimate:[g] 2.02 (1.77, 2.31)
fluconazole	200 mg QD, d 1–10 (n=11) and 200 mg QD, d 11–20 (n=29)	300 mg QD/ ritonavir 100 mg QD, d 11–20 (n=29)	1.05 (0.99, 1.10)	1.08 (1.02, 1.15)	1.07 (1.00, 1.15)
methadone	Stable maintenance dose, d 1–15 (n=16)	400 mg QD, d 2–15 (n=16)	(R)-methadone[h] 0.91 (0.84, 1.0) total: 0.85 (0.78, 0.93)	(R)-methadone[h] 1.03 (0.95, 1.10) total: 0.94 (0.87, 1.02)	(R)-methadone[h] 1.11 (1.02, 1.20) total: 1.02 (0.93, 1.12)
nevirapine[i,j]	200 mg BID, d 1–23 (n=23)	300 mg QD/ ritonavir 100 mg QD, d 4–13, then	1.17 (1.09, 1.25)	1.25 (1.17, 1.34)	1.32 (1.22, 1.43)
		400 mg QD/ ritonavir 100 mg QD, d 14–23 (n=23)	1.21 (1.11, 1.32)	1.26 (1.17, 1.36)	1.35 (1.25, 1.47)
omeprazole[k]	40 mg single dose, d 7 and d 20 (n=16)	400 mg QD, d 1–12 (n=16)	1.24 (1.04, 1.47)	1.45 (1.20, 1.76)	NA

(Table continued on next page)

Table 17 *(cont.)*: Drug Interactions: Pharmacokinetic Parameters for Coadministered Drugs in the Presence of REYATAZ[a]

Coadministered Drug	Coadministered Drug Dose/Schedule	REYATAZ Dose/ Schedule	Ratio (90% Confidence Interval) of Coadministered Drug Pharmacokinetic Parameters with/without REYATAZ; No Effect = 1.00		
			C_{max}	AUC	C_{min}
rifabutin	300 mg QD, d 1–10 then 150 mg QD, d 11–20 (n=3) 150 mg twice weekly, d 1–15 (n=7)	600 mg QD,[l] d 11–20 (n=3) 300 mg QD/ ritonavir 100 mg QD, d 1–17 (n=7)	1.18 (0.94, 1.48) 25-O-desacetyl-rifabutin: 8.20 (5.90, 11.40) 2.49[m] (2.03, 3.06) 25-O-desacetyl-rifabutin: 7.77 (6.13, 9.83)	2.10 (1.57, 2.79) 25-O-desacetyl-rifabutin: 22.01 (15.97, 30.34) 1.48[m] (1.19, 1.84) 25-O-desacetyl-rifabutin: 10.90 (8.14, 14.61)	3.43 (1.98, 5.96) 25-O-desacetyl-rifabutin: 75.6 (30.1, 190.0) 1.40[m] (1.05, 1.87) 25-O-desacetyl-rifabutin: 11.45 (8.15, 16.10)
rosiglitazone[n]	4 mg single dose, d 1, 7, 17 (n=14)	400 mg QD, d 2–7, then 300 mg QD/ ritonavir 100 mg QD, d 8–17 (n=14)	1.08 (1.03, 1.13) 0.97 (0.91, 1.04)	1.35 (1.26, 1.44) 0.83 (0.77, 0.89)	NA NA
saquinavir[o] (soft gelatin capsules)	1200 mg QD, d 1–13 (n=7)	400 mg QD, d 7–13 (n=7)	4.39 (3.24, 5.95)	5.49 (4.04, 7.47)	6.86 (5.29, 8.91)
tenofovir[p]	300 mg QD, d 9–16 (n=33) and d 24–30 (n=33) 300 mg QD, d 1–7 (pm) (n=14) d 25–34 (pm) (n=12)	400 mg QD, d 2–16 (n=33) 300 mg QD/ ritonavir 100 mg QD, d 25–34 (am) (n=12)[q]	1.14 (1.08, 1.20) 1.34 (1.20, 1.51)	1.24 (1.21, 1.28) 1.37 (1.30, 1.45)	1.22 (1.15, 1.30) 1.29 (1.21, 1.36)
lamivudine + zidovudine	150 mg lamivudine + 300 mg zidovudine BID, d 1–12 (n=19)	400 mg QD, d 7–12 (n=19)	lamivudine: 1.04 (0.92, 1.16) zidovudine: 1.05 (0.88, 1.24) zidovudine glucuronide: 0.95 (0.88, 1.02)	lamivudine: 1.03 (0.98, 1.08) zidovudine: 1.05 (0.96, 1.14) zidovudine glucuronide: 1.00 (0.97, 1.03)	lamivudine: 1.12 (1.04, 1.21) zidovudine: 0.69 (0.57, 0.84) zidovudine glucuronide: 0.82 (0.62, 1.08)

[a] Data provided are under fed conditions unless otherwise noted.
[b] All drugs were given under fasted conditions.
[c] 400 mg ddI EC and REYATAZ were administered together with food on Days 8 and 19.
[d] Upon further dose normalization of ethinyl estradiol 25 mcg with atazanavir relative to ethinyl estradiol 35 mcg without atazanavir, the ratio of geometric means (90% confidence intervals) for C_{max}, AUC, and C_{min} were 0.82 (0.73, 0.92), 1.06 (0.95, 1.17), and 1.35 (1.11, 1.63), respectively.
[e] Upon further dose normalization of ethinyl estradiol 35 mcg with atazanavir/ritonavir relative to ethinyl estradiol 25 mcg without atazanavir/ritonavir, the ratio of geometric means (90% confidence intervals) for C_{max}, AUC, and C_{min} were 1.17 (1.03, 1.34), 1.13 (1.05, 1.22), and 0.88 (0.77, 1.00), respectively.
[f] All subjects were on a 28 day lead-in period; one full cycle of Ortho Tri-Cyclen®. Ortho Tri-Cyclen® contains 35 mcg of ethinyl estradiol. Ortho Tri-Cyclen® LO contains 25 mcg of ethinyl estradiol. Results were dose normalized to an ethinyl estradiol dose of 35 mcg.
[g] 17-deacetyl norgestimate is the active component of norgestimate.
[h] (R)-methadone is the active isomer of methadone.
[i] Study was conducted in HIV-infected individuals.
[j] Subjects were treated with nevirapine prior to study entry.
[k] Omeprazole was used as a metabolic probe for CYP2C19. Omeprazole was given 2 hours after REYATAZ on Day 7; and was given alone 2 hours after a light meal on Day 20.
[l] Not the recommended therapeutic dose of atazanavir.
[m] When compared to rifabutin 150 mg QD alone d1-10 (n=14). Total of Rifabutin + 25-O-desacetyl-rifabutin: AUC 2.19 (1.78, 2.69).
[n] Rosiglitazone used as a probe substrate for CYP2C8.
[o] The combination of atazanavir and saquinavir 1200 mg QD produced daily saquinavir exposures similar to the values produced by the standard therapeutic dosing of saquinavir at 1200 mg TID. However, the C_{max} is about 79% higher than that for the standard dosing of saquinavir (soft gelatin capsules) alone at 1200 mg TID.
[p] Note that similar results were observed in a study where administration of tenofovir and REYATAZ was separated by 12 hours.
[q] Administration of tenofovir and REYATAZ was temporally separated by 12 hours.
NA = not available.

What important information should I know about taking REYATAZ (atazanavir sulfate) with other medicines?
Do not take REYATAZ if you take the following medicines (not all brands may be listed; tell your healthcare provider about all the medicines you take). REYATAZ may cause serious, life-threatening side effects or death when used with these medicines.
- Ergot medicines: dihydroergotamine, ergonovine, ergotamine, and methylergonovine such as CAFERGOT®, MIGRANAL®, D.H.E. 45®, ergotrate maleate, METHERGINE®, and others (used for migraine headaches).
- ORAP® (pimozide, used for Tourette's disorder).

- PROPULSID® (cisapride, used for certain stomach problems).
- Triazolam, also known as HALCION® (used for insomnia).
- Midazolam, also known as VERSED® (used for sedation), when taken by mouth.
Do not take the following medicines with REYATAZ (atazanavir sulfate) because of possible serious side effects:
- CAMPTOSAR® (irinotecan, used for cancer).
- CRIXIVAN® (indinavir, used for HIV infection). Both REYATAZ and CRIXIVAN sometimes cause increased levels of bilirubin in the blood.

- Cholesterol-lowering medicines MEVACOR® (lovastatin) or ZOCOR® (simvastatin).
- UROXATRAL® (alfuzosin, used to treat benign enlargement of the prostate).
- REVATIO® (sildenafil, used to treat pulmonary arterial hypertension).
Do not take the following medicines with REYATAZ (atazanavir sulfate) because they may lower the amount of REYATAZ in your blood. This may lead to an increased HIV viral load. Resistance to REYATAZ or cross-resistance to other HIV medicines may develop:
- Rifampin (also known as RIMACTANE®, RIFADIN®, RIFATER®, or RIFAMATE®, used for tuberculosis).
- St. John's wort (*Hypericum perforatum*), an herbal product sold as a dietary supplement, or products containing St. John's wort.
- VIRAMUNE® (nevirapine, used for HIV infection).
The following medicines are not recommended with REYATAZ:
- SEREVENT DISKUS® (salmeterol) and ADVAIR® (salmeterol with fluticasone), used to treat asthma, emphysema/chronic obstructive pulmonary disease also known as COPD.
Do not take the following medicine if you are taking REYATAZ and NORVIR® together:
- VFEND® (voriconazole).
The following medicines may require your healthcare provider to monitor your therapy more closely (for some medicines a change in the dose or dose schedule may be needed):
- CIALIS® (tadalafil), LEVITRA® (vardenafil), or VIAGRA® (sildenafil), used to treat erectile dysfunction. REYATAZ may increase the chances of serious side effects that can happen with CIALIS, LEVITRA, or VIAGRA. Do not use CIALIS, LEVITRA, or VIAGRA while you are taking REYATAZ unless your healthcare provider tells you it is okay.
- ADCIRCA® (tadalafil) or TRACLEER® (bosentan), used to treat pulmonary arterial hypertension.
- LIPITOR® (atorvastatin) or CRESTOR® (rosuvastatin). There is an increased chance of serious side effects if you take REYATAZ with this cholesterol-lowering medicine.
- Medicines for abnormal heart rhythm: CORDARONE® (amiodarone), lidocaine, quinidine (also known as CARDIOQUIN®, QUINIDEX®, and others).
- MYCOBUTIN® (rifabutin, an antibiotic used to treat tuberculosis).
- BUPRENEX®, SUBUTEX®, SUBOXONE®, (buprenorphine or buprenorphine/naloxone, used to treat pain and addiction to narcotic painkillers).
- VASCOR® (bepridil, used for chest pain).
- COUMADIN® (warfarin).
- Tricyclic antidepressants such as ELAVIL® (amitriptyline), NORPRAMIN® (desipramine), SINEQUAN® (doxepin), SURMONTIL® (trimipramine), TOFRANIL® (imipramine), or VIVACTIL® (protriptyline).
- Medicines to prevent organ transplant rejection: SANDIMMUNE® or NEORAL® (cyclosporin), RAPAMUNE® (sirolimus), or PROGRAF® (tacrolimus).
- The antidepressant trazodone (DESYREL® and others).
- Fluticasone propionate (FLONASE®, FLOVENT®), given by nose or inhaled to treat allergic symptoms or asthma. Your doctor may choose not to keep you on fluticasone, especially if you are also taking NORVIR®.
- Colchicine (COLCRYS®), used to prevent or treat gout or treat familial Mediterranean fever.
The following medicines may require a change in the dose or dose schedule of either REYATAZ or the other medicine:
- INVIRASE® (saquinavir).
- NORVIR® (ritonavir).
- SUSTIVA® (efavirenz).
- Antacids or buffered medicines.
- VIDEX® (didanosine).
- VIREAD® (tenofovir disoproxil fumarate).
- MYCOBUTIN® (rifabutin).
- Calcium channel blockers such as CARDIZEM® or TIAZAC® (diltiazem), COVERA-HS® or ISOPTIN SR® (verapamil) and others.
- BIAXIN® (clarithromycin).
- Medicines for indigestion, heartburn, or ulcers such as AXID® (nizatidine), PEPCID AC® (famotidine), TAGAMET® (cimetidine), or ZANTAC® (ranitidine).
Talk to your healthcare provider about choosing an effective method of contraception. REYATAZ may affect the safety and effectiveness of hormonal contraceptives such as birth control pills or the contraceptive patch. Hormonal contraceptives do not prevent the spread of HIV to others.
Remember:
1. **Know all the medicines you take.**
2. **Tell your healthcare provider about all the medicines you take.**
3. **Do not start a new medicine without talking to your healthcare provider.**
How should I store REYATAZ?
- Store REYATAZ Capsules at room temperature, 59° to 86° F (15° to 30° C). Do **not** store this medicine in a damp place such as a bathroom medicine cabinet or near the kitchen sink.

IMPORTANT NOTICE: Updated drug information is sent bi-monthly via the PDR® Update Insert. For *monthly* email updates, register at PDR.net.

Table 24: Outcomes of Treatment Through Week 48 in Study AI424-045 (Patients with Prior Antiretroviral Experience)

Outcome	REYATAZ 300 mg + ritonavir 100 mg once daily + tenofovir + 1 NRTI (n=119)	lopinavir/ritonavir (400/100 mg) twice daily + tenofovir + 1 NRTI (n=118)	Difference[a] (REYATAZ-lopinavir/ ritonavir) (CI)
HIV RNA Change from Baseline ($\log_{10}$ copies/mL)[b]	-1.58	-1.70	+0.12[c] (-0.17, 0.41)
CD4+ Change from Baseline (cells/mm³)[d]	116	123	-7 (-67, 52)
Percent of Patients Responding[e]			
HIV RNA <400 copies/mL[b]	55%	57%	-2.2% (-14.8%, 10.5%)
HIV RNA <50 copies/mL[b]	38%	45%	-7.1% (-19.6%, 5.4%)

[a] Time-averaged difference through Week 48 for HIV RNA; Week 48 difference in HIV RNA percentages and CD4+ mean changes, REYATAZ/ritonavir vs lopinavir/ritonavir; CI = 97.5% confidence interval for change in HIV RNA; 95% confidence interval otherwise.
[b] Roche Amplicor® HIV-1 Monitor™ Assay, test version 1.5.
[c] Protocol-defined primary efficacy outcome measure.
[d] Based on patients with baseline and Week 48 CD4+ cell count measurements (REYATAZ/ritonavir, n=85; lopinavir/ritonavir, n=93).
[e] Patients achieved and maintained confirmed HIV-1 RNA <400 copies/mL (<50 copies/mL) through Week 48.

Product Strength*	Capsule Shell Color (cap/body)	Markings on Capsule (ink color)		Capsules per Bottle	NDC Number
		cap	body		
100 mg	blue/white	BMS 100 mg (white)	3623 (blue)	60	0003-3623-12
150 mg	blue/powder blue	BMS 150 mg (white)	3624 (blue)	60	0003-3624-12
200 mg	blue/blue	BMS 200 mg (white)	3631 (white)	60	0003-3631-12
300 mg	red/blue	BMS 300 mg (white)	3622 (white)	30	0003-3622-12

*atazanavir equivalent as atazanavir sulfate.

- Keep your medicine in a tightly closed container.
- Keep all medicines out of the reach of children and pets at all times. Do not keep medicine that is out of date or that you no longer need. Dispose of unused medicines through community take-back disposal programs when available or place REYATAZ (atazanavir sulfate) in an unrecognizable, closed container in the household trash.

General information about REYATAZ
This medicine was prescribed for your particular condition. Do not use REYATAZ for another condition. Do not give REYATAZ to other people, even if they have the same symptoms you have. It may harm them. **Keep REYATAZ and all medicines out of the reach of children and pets.**
This summary does not include everything there is to know about REYATAZ. Medicines are sometimes prescribed for conditions that are not mentioned in patient information leaflets. Remember no written summary can replace careful discussion with your healthcare provider. If you would like more information, talk with your healthcare provider or you can call 1-800-321-1335.

What are the ingredients in REYATAZ?
Active Ingredient: atazanavir sulfate
Inactive Ingredients: Crospovidone, lactose monohydrate (milk sugar), magnesium stearate, gelatin, FD&C Blue #2, and titanium dioxide.

VIDEX® and REYATAZ® are registered trademarks of Bristol-Myers Squibb Company. COUMADIN® and SUSTIVA® are registered trademarks of Bristol-Myers Squibb Pharma Company. DESYREL® is a registered trademark of Mead Johnson and Company. Other brands listed are the trademarks of their respective owners and are not trademarks of Bristol-Myers Squibb Company.
Bristol-Myers Squibb Company
Princeton, NJ 08543 USA
1246226A7   F1-B0001-04-10   Rev April 2010

Shown in Product Identification Guide, page 322

SPRYCEL®
[sprī-cell]
(dasatinib)
Tablet for Oral Use

HIGHLIGHTS OF PRESCRIBING INFORMATION
These highlights do not include all the information needed to use SPRYCEL safely and effectively. See full prescribing information for SPRYCEL.

SPRYCEL® (dasatinib) Tablet for Oral Use
Initial U.S. Approval: 2006

————RECENT MAJOR CHANGES————
Indications and Usage (1)   05/2009
Dosage and Administration (2)   05/2009
Warnings and Precautions, Fluid Retention (5.3)   05/2009

————INDICATIONS AND USAGE————
SPRYCEL is a kinase inhibitor indicated for
- treatment of adults with chronic, accelerated, or myeloid or lymphoid blast phase chronic myeloid leukemia (CML) with resistance or intolerance to prior therapy including imatinib. (1, 14)
- treatment of adults with Philadelphia chromosome-positive acute lymphoblastic leukemia (Ph+ ALL) with resistance or intolerance to prior therapy. (1, 14)

————DOSAGE AND ADMINISTRATION————
- Chronic phase CML: 100 mg once daily. (2)
- Accelerated phase CML, myeloid or lymphoid blast phase CML, or Ph+ ALL: 140 mg once daily. (2)

Administered orally, with or without a meal. Tablets should not be crushed or cut. (2)

————DOSAGE FORMS AND STRENGTHS————
Tablets: 20 mg, 50 mg, 70 mg, and 100 mg. (3, 16)

————CONTRAINDICATIONS————
None. (4)

————WARNINGS AND PRECAUTIONS————
- *Myelosuppression:* Severe thrombocytopenia, neutropenia, and anemia may occur and require dose interruption or reduction. Monitor complete blood counts regularly. (2.3, 5.1, 6.1)
- *Bleeding Related Events (mostly associated with severe thrombocytopenia):* CNS hemorrhages, including fatalities, have occurred. Severe gastrointestinal hemorrhage may require treatment interruptions and transfusions. Use SPRYCEL (dasatinib) with caution in patients requiring medications that inhibit platelet function or anticoagulants. (5.2, 6.1)
- *Fluid Retention:* SPRYCEL is associated with fluid retention, sometimes severe, including ascites, edema, and pleural and pericardial effusions. Manage with appropriate supportive care measures. (5.3, 6.1)
- *QT Prolongation:* Use SPRYCEL with caution in patients who have or may develop prolongation of the QT interval. (5.4)

- Fetal harm may occur when administered to a pregnant woman. Women should be advised of the potential hazard to the fetus and to avoid becoming pregnant. (5.5, 8.1)

————ADVERSE REACTIONS————
Most common adverse reactions (≥20%) included myelosuppression, fluid retention events, diarrhea, headache, dyspnea, skin rash, fatigue, nausea, and hemorrhage. (6.1)
To report SUSPECTED ADVERSE REACTIONS, contact Bristol-Myers Squibb at 1-800-721-5072 or FDA at 1-800-FDA-1088 or www.fda.gov/medwatch

————DRUG INTERACTIONS————
- *CYP3A4 Inhibitors:* May increase dasatinib drug levels and should be avoided. If coadministration cannot be avoided, monitor closely and consider reducing SPRYCEL dose. (2.1, 7.1)
- *CYP3A4 Inducers:* May decrease dasatinib drug levels. If coadministration cannot be avoided, consider increasing SPRYCEL dose. (2.1, 7.2)
- *Antacids:* May decrease dasatinib drug levels. Avoid simultaneous administration. If needed, administer the antacid at least 2 hours prior to or 2 hours after the dose of SPRYCEL. (7.2)
- *H_2 Antagonists/Proton Pump Inhibitors:* May decrease dasatinib drug levels. Consider antacids in place of H_2 antagonists or proton pump inhibitors. (7.2)

————USE IN SPECIFIC POPULATIONS————
- *Hepatic Impairment:* Use SPRYCEL with caution in patients with hepatic impairment. (8.6)

See 17 for PATIENT COUNSELING INFORMATION and FDA-approved patient labeling

Revised: 06/2009

FULL PRESCRIBING INFORMATION: CONTENTS*
1   INDICATIONS AND USAGE
2   DOSAGE AND ADMINISTRATION
  2.1   Dose Modification
  2.2   Dose Escalation
  2.3   Dose Adjustment for Adverse Reactions
3   DOSAGE FORMS AND STRENGTHS
4   CONTRAINDICATIONS
5   WARNINGS AND PRECAUTIONS
  5.1   Myelosuppression
  5.2   Bleeding Related Events
  5.3   Fluid Retention
  5.4   QT Prolongation
  5.5   Use in Pregnancy
6   ADVERSE REACTIONS
  6.1   Chronic Myeloid Leukemia (CML)
  6.2   Philadelphia Chromosome-Positive Acute Lymphoblastic Leukemia (Ph+ ALL)
  6.3   Additional Data From Clinical Trials
7   DRUG INTERACTIONS
  7.1   Drugs That May Increase Dasatinib Plasma Concentrations
  7.2   Drugs That May Decrease Dasatinib Plasma Concentrations
  7.3   Drugs That May Have Their Plasma Concentration Altered By Dasatinib
8   USE IN SPECIFIC POPULATIONS
  8.1   Pregnancy
  8.3   Nursing Mothers
  8.4   Pediatric Use
  8.5   Geriatric Use
  8.6   Hepatic Impairment
  8.7   Renal Impairment
10   OVERDOSAGE
11   DESCRIPTION
12   CLINICAL PHARMACOLOGY
  12.1   Mechanism of Action
  12.3   Pharmacokinetics
13   NONCLINICAL TOXICOLOGY
  13.1   Carcinogenesis, Mutagenesis, Impairment of Fertility
14   CLINICAL STUDIES
  14.1   Chronic Phase CML
  14.2   Advanced Phase CML and Ph+ ALL
15   REFERENCES
16   HOW SUPPLIED/STORAGE AND HANDLING
  16.1   How Supplied
  16.2   Storage
  16.3   Handling and Disposal
17   PATIENT COUNSELING INFORMATION
  17.1   Bleeding
  17.2   Myelosuppression
  17.3   Fluid Retention
  17.4   Pregnancy
  17.5   Gastrointestinal Complaints
  17.6   Pain
  17.7   Fatigue
  17.8   Rash
  17.9   Lactose
  17.10   FDA-Approved Patient Labeling
* Sections or subsections omitted from the full prescribing information are not listed

Table 1: Dose Adjustments for Neutropenia and Thrombocytopenia

Chronic Phase CML (starting dose 100 mg once daily)	ANC* <0.5 × 10^9/L or Platelets <50 × 10^9/L	1. Stop SPRYCEL until ANC ≥1.0 × 10^9/L and platelets ≥50 × 10^9/L. 2. Resume treatment with SPRYCEL at the original starting dose if recovery occurs in ≤7 days. 3. If platelets <25 × 10^9/L or recurrence of ANC <0.5 × 10^9/L for >7 days, repeat Step 1 and resume SPRYCEL at a reduced dose of 80 mg once daily (second episode) or discontinue (third episode).
Accelerated Phase CML, Blast Phase CML and Ph+ ALL (starting dose 140 mg once daily)	ANC* <0.5 × 10^9/L or Platelets <10 × 10^9/L	1. Check if cytopenia is related to leukemia (marrow aspirate or biopsy). 2. If cytopenia is unrelated to leukemia, stop SPRYCEL until ANC ≥1.0 × 10^9/L and platelets ≥20 × 10^9/L and resume at the original starting dose. 3. If recurrence of cytopenia, repeat Step 1 and resume SPRYCEL at a reduced dose of 100 mg once daily (second episode) or 80 mg once daily (third episode). 4. If cytopenia is related to leukemia, consider dose escalation to 180 mg once daily.

*ANC: absolute neutrophil count

FULL PRESCRIBING INFORMATION

1 INDICATIONS AND USAGE

SPRYCEL® (dasatinib) is indicated for the treatment of adults with chronic, accelerated, or myeloid or lymphoid blast phase chronic myeloid leukemia (CML) with resistance or intolerance to prior therapy including imatinib.

SPRYCEL is also indicated for the treatment of adults with Philadelphia chromosome-positive acute lymphoblastic leukemia (Ph+ ALL) with resistance or intolerance to prior therapy.

2 DOSAGE AND ADMINISTRATION

The recommended starting dosage of SPRYCEL for chronic phase CML is 100 mg administered orally once daily. The recommended starting dosage of SPRYCEL for accelerated phase CML, myeloid or lymphoid blast phase CML, or Ph+ ALL is 140 mg administered orally once daily. Tablets should not be crushed or cut; they should be swallowed whole. SPRYCEL can be taken with or without a meal, either in the morning or in the evening.

In clinical studies, treatment with SPRYCEL was continued until disease progression or until no longer tolerated by the patient. The effect of stopping treatment after the achievement of a complete cytogenetic response (CCyR) has not been investigated.

2.1 Dose Modification

Concomitant Strong CYP3A4 inducers: The use of concomitant strong CYP3A4 inducers may decrease dasatinib plasma concentrations and should be avoided (eg, dexamethasone, phenytoin, carbamazepine, rifampin, rifabutin, phenobarbital). St. John's Wort may decrease dasatinib plasma concentrations unpredictably and should be avoided. If patients must be coadministered a strong CYP3A4 inducer, based on pharmacokinetic studies, a SPRYCEL dose increase should be considered. If the dose of SPRYCEL is increased, the patient should be monitored carefully for toxicity [see *Drug Interactions (7.2)*].

Concomitant Strong CYP3A4 inhibitors: CYP3A4 inhibitors (eg, ketoconazole, itraconazole, clarithromycin, atazanavir, indinavir, nefazodone, nelfinavir, ritonavir, saquinavir, telithromycin, and voriconazole) may increase dasatinib plasma concentrations. Grapefruit juice may also increase plasma concentrations of dasatinib and should be avoided.

Selection of an alternate concomitant medication with no or minimal enzyme inhibition potential, if possible, is recommended. If SPRYCEL must be administered with a strong CYP3A4 inhibitor, a dose decrease should be considered. Based on pharmacokinetic studies, a dose decrease to 20 mg daily should be considered for patients taking SPRYCEL 100 mg daily. For patients taking SPRYCEL 140 mg daily, a dose decrease to 40 mg daily should be considered.These reduced doses of SPRYCEL are predicted to adjust the area under the curve (AUC) to the range observed without CYP3A4 inhibitors. However, there are no clinical data with these dose adjustments in patients receiving strong CYP3A4 inhibitors. If SPRYCEL is not tolerated after dose reduction, either the strong CYP3A4 inhibitor must be discontinued, or SPRYCEL should be stopped until treatment with the inhibitor has ceased. When the strong inhibitor is discontinued, a washout period of approximately 1 week should be allowed before the SPRYCEL dose is increased. [See *Drug Interactions (7.1)*.]

2.2 Dose Escalation

In clinical studies of adult CML and Ph+ ALL patients, dose escalation to 140 mg once daily (chronic phase CML) or 180 mg once daily (advanced phase CML and Ph+ ALL) was allowed in patients who did not achieve a hematologic or cytogenetic response at the recommended starting dosage.

2.3 Dose Adjustment for Adverse Reactions

Myelosuppression

In clinical studies, myelosuppression was managed by dose interruption, dose reduction, or discontinuation of study therapy. Hematopoietic growth factor has been used in patients with resistant myelosuppression. Guidelines for dose modifications are summarized in Table 1.

[See table 1 above]

Non-hematological adverse reactions

If a severe non-hematological adverse reaction develops with SPRYCEL (dasatinib) use, treatment must be withheld until the event has resolved or improved.Thereafter, treatment can be resumed as appropriate at a reduced dose depending on the initial severity of the event.

3 DOSAGE FORMS AND STRENGTHS

SPRYCEL (dasatinib) Tablets are available as 20-mg, 50-mg, 70-mg, and 100-mg white to off-white, biconvex, film-coated tablets. [See *How Supplied (16.1)*.]

4 CONTRAINDICATIONS

None.

5 WARNINGS AND PRECAUTIONS

5.1 Myelosuppression

Treatment with SPRYCEL is associated with severe (NCI CTC Grade 3 or 4) thrombocytopenia, neutropenia, and anemia. Their occurrence is more frequent in patients with advanced phase CML or Ph+ ALL than in chronic phase CML. Complete blood counts should be performed weekly for the first 2 months and then monthly thereafter, or as clinically indicated. Myelosuppression was generally reversible and usually managed by withholding SPRYCEL temporarily or dose reduction [see *Dosage and Administration (2.3)* and *Adverse Reactions (6.1)*]. In a dose-optimization study in patients with chronic phase CML, Grade 3 or 4 myelosuppression was reported less frequently in patients treated with 100 mg once daily than in patients treated with other dosing regimens.

5.2 Bleeding Related Events

In addition to causing thrombocytopenia in human subjects, dasatinib caused platelet dysfunction *in vitro*. In all clinical studies, severe central nervous system (CNS) hemorrhages, including fatalities, occurred in 1% of patients receiving SPRYCEL. Severe gastrointestinal hemorrhage occurred in 4% of patients and generally required treatment interruptions and transfusions. Other cases of severe hemorrhage occurred in 2% of patients. Most bleeding events were associated with severe thrombocytopenia.

Patients were excluded from participation in initial SPRYCEL clinical studies if they took medications that inhibit platelet function or anticoagulants. In subsequent trials, the use of anticoagulants, aspirin, and non-steroidal anti-inflammatory drugs (NSAIDs) was allowed concurrently with SPRYCEL if the platelet count was >50,000–75,000. Caution should be exercised if patients are required to take medications that inhibit platelet function or anticoagulants.

5.3 Fluid Retention

SPRYCEL is associated with fluid retention. In all clinical studies, severe fluid retention was reported in 10% of patients, including pleural and pericardial effusion reported in 7% and 1% of patients, respectively. Severe ascites and generalized edema were each reported in <1% of patients. Severe pulmonary edema was reported in 1% of patients. Patients who develop symptoms suggestive of pleural effusion such as dyspnea or dry cough should be evaluated by chest X-ray. Severe pleural effusion may require thoracentesis and oxygen therapy. Fluid retention events were typically managed by supportive care measures that include diuretics or short courses of steroids. In dose-optimization studies, fluid retention events were reported less frequently with once daily dosing than with other dosing regimens.

5.4 QT Prolongation

In vitro data suggest that dasatinib has the potential to prolong cardiac ventricular repolarization (QT interval). In 865 patients with leukemia from five single-arm studies, the mean changes in QTcF from baseline were 4–6 msec; the upper 95% confidence intervals (CIs) for all mean changes from baseline were <7 msec. Of the 2182 patients treated with SPRYCEL (dasatinib) in clinical studies, 14 (<1%) patients had QTc prolongation reported as an adverse reaction. Twenty-one patients (1%) experienced a QTcF >500 msec.

SPRYCEL should be administered with caution to patients who have or may develop prolongation of QTc. These include patients with hypokalemia or hypomagnesemia, patients with congenital long QT syndrome, patients taking anti-arrhythmic medicines or other medicinal products that lead to QT prolongation, and cumulative high-dose anthracycline therapy. Hypokalemia or hypomagnesemia should be corrected prior to SPRYCEL administration.

5.5 Use in Pregnancy

Pregnancy Category D

SPRYCEL may cause fetal harm when administered to a pregnant woman. In nonclinical studies, at plasma concentrations below those observed in humans receiving therapeutic doses of dasatinib, embryo-fetal toxicities, including skeletal malformations, were observed in rats and rabbits. There are no adequate and well-controlled studies of SPRYCEL in pregnant women. Women of childbearing potential should be advised to avoid becoming pregnant while receiving treatment with SPRYCEL [see *Use in Specific Populations (8.1)*].

6 ADVERSE REACTIONS

The following adverse reactions are discussed in greater detail in other sections of the labeling:

- Myelosuppression [see *Dosage and Administration (2.3)* and *Warnings and Precautions (5.1)*].
- Bleeding related events [see *Warnings and Precautions (5.2)*].
- Fluid retention [see *Warnings and Precautions (5.3)*].
- QT prolongation [see *Warnings and Precautions (5.4)*].

Because clinical trials are conducted under widely varying conditions, adverse reaction rates observed in the clinical trials of a drug cannot be directly compared to rates in the clinical trials of another drug and may not reflect the rates observed in practice.

The data described below reflect exposure to SPRYCEL in 2182 patients with CML or Ph+ ALL in clinical studies with a minimum of 2 years follow-up (starting dosage 100 mg once daily, 140 mg once daily, 50 mg twice daily, or 70 mg twice daily). The median duration of therapy was 15 months (range 0.03–36 months).

The majority of SPRYCEL-treated patients experienced adverse reactions at some time. Drug was discontinued for adverse reactions in 15% of patients in chronic phase CML, 16% in accelerated phase CML, 15% in myeloid blast phase CML, 8% in lymphoid blast phase CML, and 8% in Ph+ ALL. In a dose-optimization study in patients with chronic phase CML, the rate of discontinuation for adverse reaction was lower in patients treated with 100 mg once daily than in patients treated with other dosing regimens (10% and 16%, respectively).

The most frequently reported adverse reactions (reported in ≥20% of patients) included myelosuppression, fluid retention events, diarrhea, headache, dyspnea, skin rash, fatigue, nausea, and hemorrhage.

The most frequently reported serious adverse reactions included pleural effusion (11%), gastrointestinal bleeding (4%), febrile neutropenia (4%), dyspnea (3%), pneumonia (3%), pyrexia (3%), diarrhea (3%), infection (2%), congestive heart failure/cardiac dysfunction (2%), pericardial effusion (1%), and CNS hemorrhage (1%).

6.1 Chronic Myeloid Leukemia (CML)

The median duration of treatment for patients with chronic phase CML who received 100 mg once daily was 24 months (range 1–33 months). The median duration of treatment for patients with advanced phase CML who received 140 mg once daily was 15 months (range 0.03–36 months) for accelerated phase CML, 3 months (range 0.03–29 months) for myeloid blast phase CML, and 3 months (range 0.1–10 months) for lymphoid blast CML.

Adverse reactions (excluding laboratory abnormalities) that were reported in at least 10% of the patients with CML who received the recommended starting doses of SPRYCEL are shown by disease phase in Table 2.

[See table 2 at top of next page]

Laboratory Abnormalities

Myelosuppression was commonly reported in all patient populations.The frequency of Grade 3 or 4 neutropenia, thrombocytopenia, and anemia was higher in patients with advanced phase CML than in chronic phase CML (Table 3).

Myelosuppression was reported in patients with normal baseline laboratory values as well as in patients with pre-existing laboratory abnormalities.

In patients who experienced severe myelosuppression, recovery generally occurred following dose interruption or reduction; permanent discontinuation of treatment occurred in 5% of patients [see *Warnings and Precautions (5.1)*].

Grade 3 or 4 elevations of transaminase or bilirubin and Grade 3 or 4 hypocalcemia, hypokalemia, and hypophosphatemia were reported in patients with all phases of CML but were reported with an increased frequency in patients with myeloid or lymphoid blast phase CML. Elevations in transaminase or bilirubin were usually managed with dose reduction or interruption. Patients developing Grade 3 or 4 hypocalcemia during the course of SPRYCEL (dasatinib) therapy often had recovery with oral calcium supplementation.

Laboratory abnormalities reported in patients with CML who received the recommended starting doses of SPRYCEL are shown by disease phase in Table 3.

[See table 3 at right]

6.2 Philadelphia Chromosome-Positive Acute Lymphoblastic Leukemia (Ph+ ALL)

A total of 135 patients with Ph+ ALL were treated with SPRYCEL in clinical studies. The median duration of treatment was 3 months (range 0.03–31 months). The safety profile of patients with Ph+ ALL was similar to those with lymphoid blast phase CML. The most frequently reported adverse reactions included fluid retention events such as pleural effusion (24%) and superficial edema (19%), and gastrointestinal disorders such as diarrhea (31%), nausea (24%), and vomiting (16%). Hemorrhage (19%), pyrexia (17%), rash (16%), and dyspnea (16%) were also frequently reported. The most frequently reported serious adverse reactions included pleural effusion (11%), gastrointestinal bleeding (7%), febrile neutropenia (6%), infection (5%), pyrexia (4%), pneumonia (3%), diarrhea (3%), nausea (2%), vomiting (2%), and colitis (2%).

6.3 Additional Data From Clinical Trials

The following adverse reactions were reported in patients in the SPRYCEL clinical studies at a frequency of ≥10%, 1%–<10%, 0.1%–<1%, or <0.1%. These events are included on the basis of clinical relevance.

Gastrointestinal Disorders: 1%–<10% – mucosal inflammation (including mucositis/stomatitis), dyspepsia, abdominal distension, constipation, gastritis, colitis (including neutropenic colitis), oral soft tissue disorder; 0.1%–<1% – ascites, dysphagia, anal fissure, upper gastrointestinal ulcer, esophagitis, pancreatitis.

General Disorders and Administration Site Conditions: 1%–<10% – asthenia, pain, chest pain, chills; 0.1%–<1% – malaise, temperature intolerance.

Skin and Subcutaneous Tissue Disorders: 1%–<10% – pruritus, alopecia, acne, dry skin, hyperhidrosis, urticaria, dermatitis (including eczema); 0.1%–<1% – pigmentation disorder, skin ulcer, bullous conditions, photosensitivity, nail disorder, acute febrile neutrophilic dermatosis, panniculitis, palmar-plantar erythrodysesthesia syndrome.

Respiratory, Thoracic, and Mediastinal Disorders: ≥10% – cough; 1%–<10% – lung infiltration, pneumonitis, pulmonary hypertension; 0.1%–<1% – asthma, bronchospasm; <0.1% – acute respiratory distress syndrome.

Nervous System Disorders: 1%–<10% – neuropathy (including peripheral neuropathy), dizziness, dysgeusia, somnolence; 0.1%–<1% – amnesia, tremor, syncope; <0.1% – convulsion, cerebrovascular accident, transient ischemic attack.

Blood and Lymphatic System Disorders: 1%–<10% – pancytopenia; <0.1% – aplasia pure red cell.

Musculoskeletal and Connective Tissue Disorders: 1%–<10% – muscular inflammation, muscular weakness, musculoskeletal stiffness; 0.1%–<1% – rhabdomyolysis; <0.1% – tendonitis.

Investigations: 1%–<10% – weight increased, weight decreased; 0.1%–<1% – blood creatine phosphokinase increased.

Infections and Infestations: 1%–<10% – pneumonia (including bacterial, viral, and fungal), upper respiratory tract infection/inflammation, herpes virus infection, enterocolitis infection, sepsis (including fatal outcomes).

Metabolism and Nutrition Disorders: 1%–<10% – anorexia, appetite disturbances, hyperuricemia; <0.1% – hypoalbuminemia.

Cardiac Disorders: 1%–<10% – arrhythmia (including tachycardia), palpitations; 0.1%–<1% – angina pectoris, cardiomegaly, pericarditis, ventricular arrhythmia (including ventricular tachycardia), myocardial infarction; <0.1% – cor pulmonale, myocarditis, acute coronary syndrome.

Eye Disorders: 1%–<10% – visual disorder (including visual disturbance, vision blurred, and visual acuity reduced), dry eye; 0.1%–<1% – conjunctivitis.

Vascular Disorders: 1%–<10% – flushing, hypertension; 0.1%–<1% – hypotension, thrombophlebitis; <0.1% – livedo reticularis.

Table 2: Adverse Reactions Reported in ≥10% of Patients in SPRYCEL Clinical Studies of CML

Preferred Term	100 mg Once Daily Chronic (n=165)		140 mg Once Daily Accelerated (n=157)		Myeloid Blast (n=74)		Lymphoid Blast (n=33)	
	All Grades	Grade 3/4	All Grades	Grade 3/4	All Grades	Grade 3/4	All Grades	Grade 3/4
	Percent (%) of Patients							
Fluid Retention	34	4	35	8	34	7	21	6
Superficial localized edema	18	0	18	1	14	0	3	0
Pleural effusion	18	2	21	7	20	7	21	6
Generalized edema	3	0	1	0	3	0	0	0
Pericardial effusion	2	1	3	1	0	0	0	0
Congestive heart failure/cardiac dysfunction[a]	0	0	0	0	4	0	0	0
Pulmonary edema	0	0	1	0	4	3	0	0
Headache	33	1	27	1	18	1	15	3
Diarrhea	27	2	31	3	20	5	18	0
Fatigue	24	2	19	2	20	1	9	3
Dyspnea	20	2	20	3	15	3	3	3
Musculoskeletal pain	19	2	11	0	8	1	0	0
Nausea	18	1	19	1	23	1	21	3
Skin rash[b]	17	2	15	0	16	1	21	0
Myalgia	13	0	7	1	7	1	3	0
Arthralgia	12	1	10	0	5	1	0	0
Infection (including bacterial, viral, fungal, and non-specified)	12	1	10	6	14	7	9	0
Abdominal pain	12	1	6	0	8	3	3	0
Hemorrhage	11	1	26	8	19	9	24	9
Gastrointestinal bleeding	2	1	8	6	9	7	9	3
CNS bleeding	0	0	1	1	0	0	3	3
Vomiting	7	1	11	1	12	0	15	0
Pyrexia	5	1	11	2	18	3	6	0
Febrile neutropenia	1	1	4	4	12	12	12	12

[a] Includes ventricular dysfunction, cardiac failure, cardiac failure congestive, cardiomyopathy, congestive cardiomyopathy, diastolic dysfunction, ejection fraction decreased, and ventricular failure.
[b] Includes drug eruption, erythema, erythema multiforme, erythrosis, exfoliative rash, generalized erythema, genital rash, heat rash, milia, rash, rash erythematous, rash follicular, rash generalized, rash macular, rash maculopapular, rash papular, rash pruritic, rash pustular, skin exfoliation, skin irritation, urticaria vesiculosa, and rash vesicular.

Table 3: CTC Grade 3/4 Laboratory Abnormalities in Clinical Studies of CML

	Chronic Phase CML	Advanced Phase CML		
		140 mg Once Daily		
	100 mg Once Daily (n=165)	Accelerated Phase (n=157)	Myeloid Blast Phase (n=74)	Lymphoid Blast Phase (n=33)
	Percent (%) of Patients			
Hematology Parameters				
Neutropenia	36	58	77	79
Thrombocytopenia	23	63	78	85
Anemia	13	47	74	52
Biochemistry Parameters				
Hypophosphatemia	10	13	12	18
Hypokalemia	2	7	11	15
Hypocalcemia	<1	4	9	12
Elevated SGPT (ALT)	0	2	5	3
Elevated SGOT (AST)	<1	0	4	3
Elevated Bilirubin	<1	1	3	6
Elevated Creatinine	0	2	8	0

CTC grades: neutropenia (Grade 3 ≥0.5–<1.0 × 10^9/L, Grade 4 <0.5 × 10^9/L); thrombocytopenia (Grade 3 ≥25–<50 × 10^9/L, Grade 4 <25 × 10^9/L); anemia (hemoglobin Grade 3 ≥65–<80 g/L, Grade 4 <65 g/L); elevated creatinine (Grade 3 >3–6 × upper limit of normal range [ULN], Grade 4 >6 × ULN); elevated bilirubin (Grade 3 >3–10 × ULN, Grade 4 >10 × ULN); elevated SGOT or SGPT (Grade 3 >5–20 × ULN, Grade 4 >20 × ULN); hypocalcemia (Grade 3 <7.0–6.0 mg/dL, Grade 4 <6.0 mg/dL); hypophosphatemia (Grade 3 <2.0–1.0 mg/dL, Grade 4 <1.0 mg/dL); hypokalemia (Grade 3 <3.0–2.5 mmol/L, Grade 4 <2.5 mmol/L).

Psychiatric Disorders: 1%–<10% – insomnia, depression; 0.1%–<1% – anxiety, affect lability, confusional state, libido decreased.

Reproductive System and Breast Disorders: 0.1%–<1% – gynecomastia, menstruation irregular.

Injury, Poisoning, and Procedural Complications: 1%–<10% – contusion.

Ear and Labyrinth Disorders: 1%–<10% – tinnitus; 0.1%–<1% – vertigo.

Hepatobiliary Disorders: 0.1%–<1% – cholestasis, cholecystitis, hepatitis.

Renal and Urinary Disorders: 0.1%–<1% – urinary frequency, renal failure, proteinuria.

Neoplasms Benign, Malignant, and Unspecified: 0.1%–<1% – tumor lysis syndrome.

Immune System Disorders: 0.1%–<1% – hypersensitivity (including erythema nodosum).

7 DRUG INTERACTIONS

7.1 Drugs That May Increase Dasatinib Plasma Concentrations

CYP3A4 Inhibitors: Dasatinib is a CYP3A4 substrate. In a study of 18 patients with solid tumors, 20-mg SPRYCEL once daily coadministered with 200 mg of ketoconazole twice daily increased the dasatinib C_{max} and AUC by four- and five-fold, respectively. Concomitant use of SPRYCEL (dasatinib) and drugs that inhibit CYP3A4 may increase exposure to dasatinib and should be avoided. In patients receiving treatment with SPRYCEL, close monitoring for toxicity and a SPRYCEL dose reduction should be considered if systemic administration of a potent CYP3A4 inhibitor cannot be avoided [see *Dosage and Administration (2.1)*].

7.2 Drugs That May Decrease Dasatinib Plasma Concentrations

CYP3A4 Inducers: When a single morning dose of SPRYCEL was administered following 8 days of continuous evening administration of 600 mg of rifampin, a potent CYP3A4 inducer, the mean C_{max} and AUC of dasatinib were decreased by 81% and 82%, respectively. Alternative agents with less enzyme induction potential should be considered. If SPRYCEL must be administered with a CYP3A4 inducer, a dose increase in SPRYCEL should be considered [see *Dosage and Administration (2.1)*].

Antacids: Nonclinical data demonstrate that the solubility of dasatinib is pH dependent. In a study of 24 healthy subjects, administration of 30 mL of aluminum hydroxide/magnesium hydroxide 2 hours prior to a single 50-mg dose of SPRYCEL was associated with no relevant change in dasatinib AUC; however, the dasatinib C_{max} increased 26%. When 30 mL of aluminum hydroxide/magnesium hydroxide was administered to the same subjects concomitantly with a 50-mg dose of SPRYCEL, a 55% reduction in dasatinib AUC and a 58% reduction in C_{max} were observed. Simultaneous administration of SPRYCEL with antacids should be avoided. If antacid therapy is needed, the antacid dose should be administered at least 2 hours prior to or 2 hours after the dose of SPRYCEL.

H_2 Antagonists/Proton Pump Inhibitors: Long-term suppression of gastric acid secretion by H_2 antagonists or proton pump inhibitors (eg, famotidine and omeprazole) is likely to reduce dasatinib exposure. In a study of 24 healthy subjects, administration of a single 50-mg dose of SPRYCEL 10 hours following famotidine reduced the AUC and C_{max} of dasatinib by 61% and 63%, respectively. The concomitant use of H_2 antagonists or proton pump inhibitors with SPRYCEL is not recommended. The use of antacids should be considered in place of H_2 antagonists or proton pump inhibitors in patients receiving SPRYCEL therapy.

7.3 Drugs That May Have Their Plasma Concentration Altered By Dasatinib

CYP3A4 Substrates: Single-dose data from a study of 54 healthy subjects indicate that the mean C_{max} and AUC of simvastatin, a CYP3A4 substrate, were increased by 37% and 20%, respectively, when simvastatin was administered in combination with a single 100-mg dose of SPRYCEL. Therefore, CYP3A4 substrates known to have a narrow therapeutic index such as alfentanil, astemizole, terfenadine, cisapride, cyclosporine, fentanyl, pimozide, quinidine, sirolimus, tacrolimus, or ergot alkaloids (ergotamine, dihydroergotamine) should be administered with caution in patients receiving SPRYCEL.

8 USE IN SPECIFIC POPULATIONS

8.1 Pregnancy

Pregnancy Category D

SPRYCEL may cause fetal harm when administered to a pregnant woman. There are no adequate and well-controlled studies of SPRYCEL in pregnant women. Women of childbearing potential should be advised of the potential hazard to the fetus and to avoid becoming pregnant. If SPRYCEL is used during pregnancy, or if the patient becomes pregnant while taking SPRYCEL, the patient should be apprised of the potential hazard to the fetus.

In nonclinical studies, at plasma concentrations below those observed in humans receiving therapeutic doses of dasatinib, embryo-fetal toxicities were observed in rats and rabbits. Fetal death was observed in rats. In both rats and rabbits, the lowest doses of dasatinib tested (rat: 2.5 mg/kg/day [15 mg/m^2/day] and rabbit: 0.5 mg/kg/day [6 mg/m^2/day]) resulted in embryo-fetal toxicities. These doses produced maternal AUCs of 105 ng•hr/mL (0.3-fold the human AUC in females at a dose of 70 mg twice daily) and 44 ng•hr/mL (0.1-fold the human AUC) in rats and rabbits, respectively. Embryo-fetal toxicities included skeletal malformations at multiple sites (scapula, humerus, femur, radius, ribs, clavicle), reduced ossification (sternum; thoracic, lumbar, and sacral vertebrae; forepaw phalanges; pelvis; and hyoid body), edema, and microhepatia.

8.3 Nursing Mothers

It is unknown whether SPRYCEL is excreted in human milk. Because many drugs are excreted in human milk and because of the potential for serious adverse reactions in nursing infants from SPRYCEL, a decision should be made whether to discontinue nursing or to discontinue the drug, taking into account the importance of the drug to the mother.

8.4 Pediatric Use

The safety and efficacy of SPRYCEL (dasatinib) in patients less than 18 years of age have not been established.

8.5 Geriatric Use

Of the 2182 patients in clinical studies of SPRYCEL, 547 (25%) were 65 years of age and over and 105 (5%) were 75 years of age and over. No differences in efficacy were observed between older and younger patients. While the safety profile of SPRYCEL in the geriatric population was similar to that in the younger population, patients aged 65 years and older are more likely to experience fluid retention events and dyspnea.

8.6 Hepatic Impairment

The effect of hepatic impairment on the pharmacokinetics of dasatinib was evaluated in healthy volunteers with normal liver function and patients with moderate (Child-Pugh class B) and severe (Child-Pugh class C) hepatic impairment. Compared to the healthy volunteers with normal hepatic function, the dose normalized pharmacokinetic parameters were decreased in the patients with hepatic impairment.

No dosage adjustment is necessary in patients with hepatic impairment [see *Clinical Pharmacology (12.3)*]. Caution is recommended when administering SPRYCEL to patients with hepatic impairment.

8.7 Renal Impairment

There are currently no clinical studies with SPRYCEL in patients with impaired renal function. Less than 4% of dasatinib and its metabolites are excreted via the kidney.

10 OVERDOSAGE

Experience with overdose of SPRYCEL in clinical studies is limited to isolated cases. Overdosage of 280 mg per day for 1 week was reported in two patients and both developed severe myelosuppression and bleeding. Since SPRYCEL is associated with severe myelosuppression [see *Warnings and Precautions (5.1)* and *Adverse Reactions (6.1)*], patients who ingested more than the recommended dosage should be closely monitored for myelosuppression and appropriate supportive treatment given.

Acute overdose in animals was associated with cardiotoxicity. Evidence of cardiotoxicity included ventricular necrosis and valvular/ventricular/atrial hemorrhage at single doses ≥100 mg/kg (600 mg/m^2) in rodents. There was a tendency for increased systolic and diastolic blood pressure in monkeys at single doses ≥10 mg/kg (120 mg/m^2).

11 DESCRIPTION

SPRYCEL (dasatinib) is a kinase inhibitor. The chemical name for dasatinib is N-(2-chloro-6-methylphenyl)-2-[[6-[4-(2-hydroxyethyl)-1-piperazinyl]-2-methyl-4-pyrimidinyl]amino]-5-thiazolecarboxamide, monohydrate. The molecular formula is $C_{22}H_{26}ClN_7O_2S \bullet H_2O$, which corresponds to a formula weight of 506.02 (monohydrate). The anhydrous free base has a molecular weight of 488.01. Dasatinib has the following chemical structure:

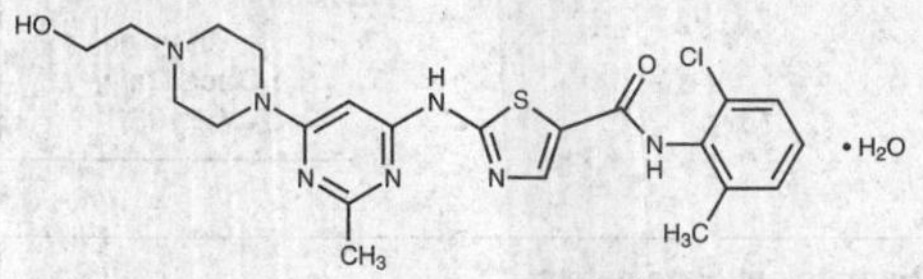

Dasatinib is a white to off-white powder. The drug substance is insoluble in water and slightly soluble in ethanol and methanol. SPRYCEL tablets are white to off-white, biconvex, film-coated tablets containing dasatinib, with the following inactive ingredients: lactose monohydrate, microcrystalline cellulose, croscarmellose sodium, hydroxypropyl cellulose, and magnesium stearate. The tablet coating consists of hypromellose, titanium dioxide, and polyethylene glycol.

12 CLINICAL PHARMACOLOGY

12.1 Mechanism of Action

Dasatinib, at nanomolar concentrations, inhibits the following kinases: BCR-ABL, SRC family (SRC, LCK, YES, FYN), c-KIT, EPHA2, and PDGFRβ. Based on modeling studies, dasatinib is predicted to bind to multiple conformations of the ABL kinase.

In vitro, dasatinib was active in leukemic cell lines representing variants of imatinib mesylate sensitive and resistant disease. Dasatinib inhibited the growth of chronic myeloid leukemia (CML) and acute lymphoblastic leukemia (ALL) cell lines overexpressing BCR-ABL. Under the conditions of the assays, dasatinib was able to overcome imatinib resistance resulting from BCR-ABL kinase domain mutations, activation of alternate signaling pathways involving the SRC family kinases (LYN, HCK), and multi-drug resistance gene overexpression.

12.3 Pharmacokinetics

Absorption

Maximum plasma concentrations (C_{max}) of dasatinib are observed between 0.5 and 6 hours (T_{max}) following oral administration. Dasatinib exhibits dose proportional increases in AUC and linear elimination characteristics over the dose range of 15 mg to 240 mg/day. The overall mean terminal half-life of dasatinib is 3–5 hours.

Data from a study of 54 healthy subjects administered a single, 100-mg dose of dasatinib 30 minutes following consumption of a high-fat meal resulted in a 14% increase in the mean AUC of dasatinib. The observed food effects were not clinically relevant.

Distribution

In patients, dasatinib has an apparent volume of distribution of 2505 L, suggesting that the drug is extensively distributed in the extravascular space. Binding of dasatinib and its active metabolite to human plasma proteins *in vitro* was approximately 96% and 93%, respectively, with no concentration dependence over the range of 100–500 ng/mL.

Metabolism

Dasatinib is extensively metabolized in humans, primarily by the cytochrome P450 enzyme 3A4. CYP3A4 was the primary enzyme responsible for the formation of the active metabolite. Flavin-containing monooxygenase 3 (FMO-3) and uridine diphosphate-glucuronosyltransferase (UGT) enzymes are also involved in the formation of dasatinib metabolites.

The exposure of the active metabolite, which is equipotent to dasatinib, represents approximately 5% of the dasatinib AUC. This indicates that the active metabolite of dasatinib is unlikely to play a major role in the observed pharmacology of the drug. Dasatinib also had several other inactive oxidative metabolites.

Dasatinib is a weak time-dependent inhibitor of CYP3A4. At clinically relevant concentrations, dasatinib does not inhibit CYP1A2, 2A6, 2B6, 2C8, 2C9, 2C19, 2D6, or 2E1. Dasatinib is not an inducer of human CYP enzymes.

Elimination

Elimination is primarily via the feces. Following a single oral dose of [^{14}C]-labeled dasatinib, approximately 4% and 85% of the administered radioactivity was recovered in the urine and feces, respectively, within 10 days. Unchanged dasatinib accounted for 0.1% and 19% of the administered dose in urine and feces, respectively, with the remainder of the dose being metabolites.

Effects of Age and Gender

Pharmacokinetic analyses of demographic data indicate that there are no clinically relevant effects of age and gender on the pharmacokinetics of dasatinib.

Hepatic Impairment

Dasatinib doses of 50 mg and 20 mg were evaluated in eight patients with moderate (Child-Pugh class B) and seven patients with severe (Child-Pugh class C) hepatic impairment, respectively. Matched controls with normal hepatic function (n=15) were also evaluated and received a dasatinib dose of 70 mg. Compared to subjects with normal liver function, patients with moderate hepatic impairment had decreases in dose normalized C_{max} and AUC by 47% and 8%, respectively. Patients with severe hepatic impairment had dose normalized C_{max} decreased by 43% and AUC decreased by 28% compared to the normal controls.

These differences in C_{max} and AUC are not clinically relevant. Dose adjustment is not necessary in patients with hepatic impairment.

13 NONCLINICAL TOXICOLOGY

13.1 Carcinogenesis, Mutagenesis, Impairment of Fertility

Carcinogenicity studies were not performed with dasatinib. Dasatinib was clastogenic when tested *in vitro* in Chinese hamster ovary cells, with and without metabolic activation. Dasatinib was not mutagenic when tested in an *in vitro* bacterial cell assay (Ames test) and was not genotoxic in an *in vivo* rat micronucleus study.

The effects of dasatinib on male and female fertility have not been studied. However, results of repeat-dose toxicity studies in multiple species indicate the potential for dasatinib to impair reproductive function and fertility. Effects evident in male animals included reduced size and secretion of seminal vesicles, and immature prostate, seminal vesicle, and testis. The administration of dasatinib resulted in uterine inflammation and mineralization in monkeys, and cystic ovaries and ovarian hypertrophy in rodents.

14 CLINICAL STUDIES

The efficacy and safety of SPRYCEL (dasatinib) were investigated in adult patients with CML or Ph+ ALL whose disease was resistant to or who were intolerant to imatinib: 1158 patients had chronic phase CML, 858 patients had accelerated phase, myeloid blast phase, or lymphoid blast phase CML, and 130 patients had Ph+ ALL. In a clinical study in chronic phase CML, resistance to imatinib was defined as failure to achieve a complete hematologic response (CHR; after 3 months), major cytogenetic response (MCyR; after 6 months), or complete cytogenetic response (CCyR; after 12 months); or loss of a previous molecular response (with concurrent ≥10% increase in Ph+ metaphases), cytogenetic response, or hematologic response. Imatinib intolerance was defined as inability to tolerate 400 mg or more of imatinib per day or discontinuation of imatinib because of toxicity.

Results described below are based on a minimum of 2 years follow-up after the start of SPRYCEL therapy in patients with a median time from initial diagnosis of approximately

5 years. Across all studies, 48% of patients were women, 81% were white, 15% were black or Asian, 25% were 65 years of age or older, and 5% were 75 years of age or older. Most patients had long disease histories with extensive prior treatment, including imatinib, cytotoxic chemotherapy, interferon, and stem cell transplant. Overall, 80% of patients had imatinib-resistant disease and 20% of patients were intolerant to imatinib. The maximum imatinib dose had been 400–600 mg/day in about 60% of the patients and >600 mg/day in 40% of the patients.

The primary efficacy endpoint in chronic phase CML was MCyR, defined as elimination (CCyR) or substantial diminution (by at least 65%, partial cytogenetic response) of Ph+ hematopoietic cells. The primary efficacy endpoint in accelerated phase, myeloid blast phase, lymphoid blast phase CML, and Ph+ ALL was major hematologic response (MaHR), defined as either a CHR or no evidence of leukemia (NEL).

14.1 Chronic Phase CML

Dose-Optimization Study: A randomized, open-label study was conducted in patients with chronic phase CML to evaluate the efficacy and safety of SPRYCEL (dasatinib) administered once daily compared with SPRYCEL administered twice daily. Patients with significant cardiac diseases, including myocardial infarction within 6 months, congestive heart failure within 3 months, significant arrhythmias, or QTc prolongation were excluded from the study. The primary efficacy endpoint was MCyR in patients with imatinib-resistant CML. A total of 670 patients, of whom 497 had imatinib-resistant disease, were randomized to the SPRYCEL 100 mg once daily, 140 mg once daily, 50 mg twice daily, or 70 mg twice daily group. Median duration of treatment was 22 months.

Efficacy was achieved across all SPRYCEL treatment groups with the once daily schedule demonstrating comparable efficacy (non-inferiority) to the twice daily schedule on the primary efficacy endpoint (difference in MCyR 1.9%; 95% CI [-6.8%–10.6%]).

Efficacy results are presented in Table 4 for patients with chronic phase CML who received the recommended starting dose of 100 mg once daily. Additional efficacy results in this patient population are described after the table. Results for all patients with chronic phase CML, regardless of dosage (a starting dosage of 100 mg once daily, 140 mg once daily, 50 mg twice daily, or 70 mg twice daily), were consistent with those for patients treated with 100 mg once daily.

Table 4: Efficacy of SPRYCEL in Chronic Phase CML

	100 mg Once Daily (n=167)
CHR[a] % (95% CI)	92% (86–95)
MCyR[b] % (95% CI)	63% (56–71)
CCyR % (95% CI)	50% (42–58)

[a] CHR (response confirmed after 4 weeks): WBC ≤ institutional ULN, platelets <450,000/mm^3, no blasts or promyelocytes in peripheral blood, <5% myelocytes plus metamyelocytes in peripheral blood, basophils in peripheral blood <20%, and no extramedullary involvement.
[b] MCyR combines both complete (0% Ph+ metaphases) and partial (>0%–35%) responses.

In the SPRYCEL 100 mg once daily group, median time to MCyR was 2.9 months (95% CI: [2.8–3.0]). Based on the Kaplan-Meier estimates, 93% (95% CI: [88%–98%]) of patients who had achieved an MCyR maintained that response for 18 months. The estimated rate of progression-free survival and overall survival in all patients treated with 100 mg once daily was 80% (95% CI: [73%–87%]) and 91% (95% CI: [86%–96%]), respectively, at 2 years.

14.2 Advanced Phase CML and Ph+ ALL

Dose-Optimization Study: One randomized open-label study was conducted in patients with advanced phase CML (accelerated phase CML, myeloid blast phase CML, or lymphoid blast phase CML) to evaluate the efficacy and safety of SPRYCEL administered once daily compared with SPRYCEL administered twice daily. The primary efficacy endpoint was MaHR. A total of 611 patients were randomized to either the SPRYCEL 140 mg once daily or 70 mg twice daily group. Median duration of treatment was approximately 6 months for both treatment groups. The once daily schedule demonstrated comparable efficacy (non-inferiority) to the twice daily schedule on the primary efficacy endpoint.

The efficacy and safety of SPRYCEL were also investigated in patients with Ph+ ALL in one randomized study (starting dosage 140 mg once daily or 70 mg twice daily) and one single-arm study (starting dosage 70 mg twice daily). The primary efficacy endpoint was MaHR. A total of 130 patients were enrolled in these studies. The median duration of therapy was 3 months.

Response rates are presented in Table 5.
[See table 5 above]

Table 5: Efficacy of SPRYCEL in Advanced Phase CML and Ph+ ALL

	140 mg Once Daily			
	Accelerated (n=158)	Myeloid Blast (n=75)	Lymphoid Blast (n=33)	Ph+ ALL (n=40)
MaHR[a]	66%	28%	42%	38%
(95% CI)	(59–74)	(18–40)	(26–61)	(23–54)
CHR[a]	47%	17%	21%	33%
(95% CI)	(40–56)	(10–28)	(9–39)	(19–49)
NEL[a]	19%	11%	21%	5%
(95% CI)	(13–26)	(5–20)	(9–39)	(1–17)
MCyR[b]	39%	28%	52%	70%
(95% CI)	(31–47)	(18–40)	(34–69)	(54–83)
CCyR	32%	17%	39%	50%
(95% CI)	(25–40)	(10–28)	(23–58)	(34–66)

[a] Hematologic response criteria (all responses confirmed after 4 weeks): Major hematologic response: (MaHR) = complete hematologic response (CHR) + no evidence of leukemia (NEL).
CHR: WBC ≤ institutional ULN, ANC ≥1000/mm^3, platelets ≥100,000/mm^3, no blasts or promyelocytes in peripheral blood, bone marrow blasts ≤5%, <5% myelocytes plus metamyelocytes in peripheral blood, basophils in peripheral blood <20%, and no extramedullary involvement.
NEL: same criteria as for CHR but ANC ≥500/mm^3 and <1000/mm^3, or platelets ≥20,000/mm^3 and ≤100,000/mm^3.
[b] MCyR combines both complete (0% Ph+ metaphases) and partial (>0%–35%) responses.
CI = confidence interval ULN = upper limit of normal range.

Table 6: SPRYCEL Trade Presentations

NDC Number	Strength	Description	Tablets per Bottle
0003-0527-11	20 mg	white to off-white, biconvex, round, film-coated tablet with "BMS" debossed on one side and "527" on the other side	60
0003-0528-11	50 mg	white to off-white, biconvex, oval, film-coated tablet with "BMS" debossed on one side and "528" on the other side	60
0003-0524-11	70 mg	white to off-white, biconvex, round, film-coated tablet with "BMS" debossed on one side and "524" on the other side	60
0003-0852-22	100 mg	white to off-white, biconvex, oval, film-coated tablet with "BMS 100" debossed on one side and "852" on the other side	30

In the SPRYCEL (dasatinib) 140 mg once daily group, the median time to MaHR was 1.9 months for patients with accelerated phase CML, 1.9 months for patients with myeloid blast phase CML, and 1.8 months for patients with lymphoid blast phase CML.

In patients with myeloid blast phase CML, the median duration of MaHR was 8 months and 9 months for the 140 mg once daily group and the 70 mg twice daily group, respectively. In patients with lymphoid blast phase CML, the median duration of MaHR was 5 months and 8 months for the 140 mg once daily group and the 70 mg twice daily group, respectively. In patients with Ph+ ALL who were treated with SPRYCEL 140 mg once daily, the median duration of MaHR was 4.6 months. The medians of progression-free survival for patients with Ph+ ALL treated with SPRYCEL 140 mg once daily and 70 mg twice daily were 4.0 months and 3.5 months, respectively.

15 REFERENCES

1. NIOSH Alert: Preventing occupational exposures to antineoplastic and other hazardous drugs in healthcare settings. 2004. U.S. Department of Health and Human Services, Public Health Service, Centers for Disease Control and Prevention, National Institute for Occupational Safety and Health, DHHS (NIOSH) Publication No. 2004–165.
2. OSHA Technical Manual, TED 1-0.15A, Section VI: Chapter 2. Controlling Occupational Exposure to Hazardous Drugs. OSHA, 1999, http://www.osha.gov/dts/osta/otm/otm_vi/otm_vi_2.html.
3. American Society of Health-System Pharmacists. ASHP guidelines on handling hazardous drugs. *Am J Health-Syst Pharm.* (2006) 63:1172–1193.
4. Polovich M, White JM, Kelleher LO (eds). 2005. Chemotherapy and biotherapy guidelines and recommendations for practice (2nd ed). Pittsburgh, PA: Oncology Nursing Society.

16 HOW SUPPLIED/STORAGE AND HANDLING

16.1 How Supplied

SPRYCEL® (dasatinib) tablets are available as described in Table 6.
[See table 6 above]

16.2 Storage

SPRYCEL® tablets should be stored at 25° C (77° F); excursions permitted between 15°–30° C (59°–86° F) [see USP Controlled Room Temperature].

16.3 Handling and Disposal

Procedures for proper handling and disposal of anticancer drugs should be considered. Several guidelines on this subject have been published [see *References (15)*].

SPRYCEL (dasatinib) tablets consist of a core tablet (containing the active drug substance), surrounded by a film coating to prevent exposure of pharmacy and clinical personnel to the active drug substance. However, if tablets are inadvertently crushed or broken, pharmacy and clinical personnel should wear disposable chemotherapy gloves. Personnel who are pregnant should avoid exposure to crushed or broken tablets.

17 PATIENT COUNSELING INFORMATION

See *FDA-Approved Patient Labeling (17.10)*.

17.1 Bleeding

Patients should be informed of the possibility of serious bleeding and to report immediately any signs or symptoms suggestive of hemorrhage (unusual bleeding or easy bruising).

17.2 Myelosuppression

Patients should be informed of the possibility of developing low blood cell counts; they should be instructed to report immediately should fever develop, particularly in association with any suggestion of infection.

17.3 Fluid Retention

Patients should be informed of the possibility of developing fluid retention (swelling, weight gain, or shortness of breath) and to seek medical attention if those symptoms arise.

17.4 Pregnancy

Patients should be informed that dasatinib may cause fetal harm when administered to a pregnant woman. Women should be advised of the potential hazard to the fetus and to avoid becoming pregnant. If SPRYCEL is used during pregnancy, or if the patient becomes pregnant while taking SPRYCEL, the patient should be apprised of the potential hazard to the fetus [see *Warnings and Precautions (5.5)*].

17.5 Gastrointestinal Complaints

Patients should be informed that they may experience nausea, vomiting, or diarrhea with SPRYCEL. If these symptoms are significant, they should seek medical attention.

17.6 Pain

Patients should be informed that they may experience headache or musculoskeletal pain with SPRYCEL. If these symptoms are significant, they should seek medical attention.

17.7 Fatigue

Patients should be informed that they may experience fatigue with SPRYCEL (dasatinib). If this symptom is significant, they should seek medical attention.

17.8 Rash

Patients should be informed that they may experience skin rash with SPRYCEL. If this symptom is significant, they should seek medical attention.

17.9 Lactose

Patients should be informed that SPRYCEL contains 135 mg of lactose monohydrate in a 100-mg daily dose and 189 mg of lactose monohydrate in a 140-mg daily dose.

Manufactured by:
Bristol-Myers Squibb Company
Princeton, NJ 08543 USA

1237674A6   DS-B0001-06-09   Rev June 2009

17.10   FDA-Approved Patient Labeling

PATIENT INFORMATION
SPRYCEL® (dasatinib) Tablets
What is SPRYCEL?
SPRYCEL® (dasatinib) is a prescription medicine used to treat adults who have:

- chronic myeloid leukemia (CML) who are no longer benefitting from, or cannot tolerate, prior treatment including GLEEVEC® (imatinib mesylate).
- Philadelphia chromosome positive acute lymphoblastic leukemia (Ph+ ALL) who are no longer benefitting from, or cannot tolerate, prior treatment.

How does SPRYCEL work?
The active ingredient of SPRYCEL is dasatinib. Dasatinib reduces the activity of one or more proteins responsible for the uncontrolled growth of the leukemia cells of patients with CML or Ph+ ALL. This reduction allows the bone marrow to resume production of normal red cells, white cells, and platelets.

Who should not take SPRYCEL?
- SPRYCEL is currently not recommended for patients who have not previously had a trial of GLEEVEC® (imatinib mesylate).
- Women who are pregnant or planning to become pregnant should not take SPRYCEL (see below).

What should I tell my healthcare provider before I take SPRYCEL?
Tell your healthcare provider about all of your medical conditions, including if you:

- are pregnant or planning to become pregnant. SPRYCEL may harm an unborn baby. Women should avoid becoming pregnant while undergoing treatment with SPRYCEL. Tell your healthcare provider *immediately* if you become pregnant or plan to become pregnant while taking SPRYCEL.
- are breast-feeding. It is not known if SPRYCEL can pass into your breast milk or if it can harm your baby. Do not breast feed if you are taking SPRYCEL.
- are a sexually active male. Men who take SPRYCEL are advised to use a condom to avoid pregnancy in their partner.
- have a liver or heart problem.
- are lactose intolerant.

Tell your healthcare provider about all the medicines you take, including prescription and non-prescription medicines, vitamins, antacids, and herbal supplements.
SPRYCEL is eliminated from your body through the liver. The use of certain other medicines may alter the levels of SPRYCEL in your bloodstream. Likewise, levels of other medicines in your bloodstream can be affected by SPRYCEL. Such changes can increase the side effects, or reduce the activity of the medicines you are taking, including SPRYCEL.

- Medicines that increase the amount of SPRYCEL in your bloodstream are NIZORAL® (ketoconazole), SPORANOX® (itraconazole), NORVIR® (ritonavir), REYATAZ® (atazanavir sulfate), CRIXIVAN® (indinavir), VIRACEPT® (nelfinavir), INVIRASE® (saquinavir), KETEK® (telithromycin), E-MYCIN® (erythromycin), and BIAXIN® (clarithromycin).
- Medicines that decrease the amount of SPRYCEL in your bloodstream are DECADRON® (dexamethasone), DILANTIN® (phenytoin), TEGRETOL® (carbamazepine), RIMACTANE® (rifampin), and LUMINAL® (phenobarbital).
- Medicines whose blood levels might be altered by SPRYCEL are SANDIMMUNE® (cyclosporine), ALFENTA® (alfentanil), FENTANYL® (fentanyl), ORAP® (pimozide), RAPAMUNE® (sirolimus), PROGRAF® (tacrolimus), and ERGOMAR® (ergotamine).

SPRYCEL is best absorbed from your stomach into your bloodstream in the presence of stomach acid. You should avoid taking medicines that reduce stomach acid such as TAGAMET® (cimetidine), PEPCID® (famotidine), ZANTAC® (ranitidine), PRILOSEC® (omeprazole), PROTONIX® (pantoprazole sodium), NEXIUM® (esomeprazole), ACIPHEX® (rabeprazole), or PREVACID®

(lansoprazole) while taking SPRYCEL (dasatinib). Medicines that neutralize stomach acid, such as MAALOX® (aluminum hydroxide/magnesium hydroxide), TUMS® (calcium carbonate), or ROLAIDS® (calcium carbonate and magnesia) may be taken up to 2 hours before or 2 hours after SPRYCEL.

Since SPRYCEL therapy may cause bleeding, tell your healthcare provider if you are using blood thinners, such as COUMADIN® (warfarin sodium) or aspirin.

Know the medicines you take. Keep a list of your medicines and show it to your healthcare provider and pharmacist when you get a new medicine.

How do I take SPRYCEL?
Take SPRYCEL exactly as prescribed by your healthcare provider.

- If you have chronic phase CML, the usual dose is 100 mg (one 100-mg tablet or two 50-mg tablets) once daily, either in the morning or in the evening.
- If you have accelerated or blast crisis CML or Ph+ ALL, the usual dose is 140 mg (two 70-mg tablets) once daily, either in the morning or in the evening.
- Take SPRYCEL with or without a meal. Try to take SPRYCEL at the same time each day.
- Swallow SPRYCEL tablets whole with water. Do not break, cut, or crush the tablets.
- Do not drink grapefruit juice while taking SPRYCEL.
- **Depending on your response to treatment and any side effects that you may experience, your healthcare provider may adjust your dose of SPRYCEL upward or downward, or may temporarily discontinue SPRYCEL.**
- **You should not change your dose or stop taking SPRYCEL without first talking with your healthcare provider.**
- **If you miss a dose of SPRYCEL,** take your next scheduled dose at its regular time. Do not take two doses at the same time. Call your healthcare provider or pharmacist if you are not sure what to do.
- **If you have accidentally taken more than the prescribed dose of SPRYCEL,** call your healthcare provider right away.

What are the possible side effects of SPRYCEL?
The following information describes the most important side effects of SPRYCEL. It is not a comprehensive list of all side effects recorded in clinical trials with SPRYCEL. You should report any unusual symptoms to your healthcare provider.

- **Low Blood Counts:** SPRYCEL may cause low red blood cell counts (anemia), low white blood cell counts (neutropenia), and low platelet counts (thrombocytopenia). Your healthcare provider will check your blood counts regularly during treatment with SPRYCEL and may adjust your dose of SPRYCEL or withhold the drug temporarily in the event your blood counts drop too low. **Notify your healthcare provider immediately if you develop a fever while taking SPRYCEL.**
- **Bleeding:** SPRYCEL may cause bleeding. The most serious bleeding events observed in clinical studies included bleeding into the brain leading to death in 1% of patients, and bleeding from the gastrointestinal tract. Less severe events included bleeding from the nose, the gums, bruising of the skin, and excessive menstrual bleeding. **Tell your healthcare provider immediately if you have any bleeding or bruising while taking SPRYCEL.**
- **Fluid Retention:** SPRYCEL may cause fluid to accumulate in your legs and around your eyes. In more severe cases, fluid may accumulate in the lining of your lungs, the sac around your heart, or your abdominal cavity. **Notify your healthcare provider immediately if you experience swelling, weight gain, or increasing shortness of breath while taking SPRYCEL.**

Other common side effects of SPRYCEL therapy include diarrhea, headache, shortness of breath, skin rash, fatigue, and nausea. Tell your healthcare provider if you have any side effects.

How will I know if SPRYCEL is working?
How well you respond to SPRYCEL therapy may depend on several factors, including the phase of your disease and prior treatments. General treatment goals for patients treated with SPRYCEL include a reduction in the number of leukemia cells and improvement of the blood cell counts. While you are on SPRYCEL, your healthcare provider will monitor these responses through routine blood tests.

How should I store SPRYCEL?
- Store SPRYCEL (dasatinib) Tablets at room temperature, 59° to 86° F (15° to 30° C).
- **Keep SPRYCEL and all medicines out of the reach of children and pets.**

General information about SPRYCEL: Medicines are sometimes prescribed for purposes other than those listed in the patient information leaflet. Do not use SPRYCEL for a condition for which it is not prescribed. Do not give SPRYCEL to other people even if they have the same symptoms you have. It may harm them.

This patient information leaflet summarizes the most important information about SPRYCEL. If you would like

more information, talk with your healthcare provider. You can ask your healthcare provider or pharmacist for information about SPRYCEL (dasatinib) that is written for healthcare professionals. You can visit *www.sprycel.com* or call 1-800-332-2056.

What are the ingredients in SPRYCEL?
Active Ingredient: dasatinib
Inactive Ingredients: lactose monohydrate, microcrystalline cellulose, croscarmellose sodium, hydroxypropyl cellulose, and magnesium stearate. The tablet coating consists of hypromellose, titanium dioxide, and polyethylene glycol.

REYATAZ® is a registered trademark of Bristol-Myers Squibb Company. COUMADIN® is a registered trademark of Bristol-Myers Squibb Pharma Company. Other brands listed are the trademarks of their respective owners and are not trademarks of Bristol-Myers Squibb Company.
Manufactured by:
Bristol-Myers Squibb Company
Princeton, NJ 08543 USA
1237674A6   DS-B0001-06-09   Rev June 2009
Shown in Product Identification Guide, page 322

SUSTIVA®   ℞
[*sus-TEE-vah*]
(efavirenz)
capsules and tablets

HIGHLIGHTS OF PRESCRIBING INFORMATION
These highlights do not include all the information needed to use SUSTIVA safely and effectively. See full prescribing information for SUSTIVA.
SUSTIVA® (efavirenz) capsules and tablets
Initial U.S. Approval: 1998
————————**RECENT MAJOR CHANGES**————————

Warnings and Precautions, Reproductive Risk Potential (5.6)	3/2010
Warnings and Precautions, Hepatotoxicity (5.8)	3/2010

————————**INDICATIONS AND USAGE**————————
SUSTIVA is a non-nucleoside reverse transcriptase inhibitor indicated in combination with other antiretroviral agents for the treatment of human immunodeficiency virus type 1 infection. (1)
————————**DOSAGE AND ADMINISTRATION**————————
- SUSTIVA should be taken orally once daily on an empty stomach, preferably at bedtime. (2)
- Recommended adult dose: 600 mg. (2.1)
- With voriconazole, increase voriconazole maintenance dose to 400 mg every 12 hours and decrease SUSTIVA dose to 300 mg once daily using the capsule formulation. (2.1)

[See table at top of next page]
————————**DOSAGE FORMS AND STRENGTHS**————————
- Capsules: 200 mg and 50 mg. (3)
- Tablets: 600 mg. (3)
————————**CONTRAINDICATIONS**————————
- SUSTIVA is contraindicated in patients with previously demonstrated hypersensitivity (eg, Stevens-Johnson syndrome, erythema multiforme, or toxic skin eruptions) to any of the components of this product. (4.1)
- For some drugs, competition for CYP3A by efavirenz could result in inhibition of their metabolism and create the potential for serious and/or life-threatening adverse reactions (eg, cardiac arrhythmias, prolonged sedation, or respiratory depression). (4.2)
————————**WARNINGS AND PRECAUTIONS**————————
- *Do not use as a single agent* or add on as a sole agent to a failing regimen. Consider potential for cross resistance when choosing other agents. (5.2)
- Not recommended with ATRIPLA, which contains efavirenz, emtricitabine, and tenofovir disoproxil fumarate. (5.3)
- *Serious psychiatric symptoms:* Immediate medical evaluation is recommended for serious psychiatric symptoms such as severe depression or suicidal ideation. (5.4, 17.5)
- *Nervous system symptoms* (NSS): NSS are frequent, usually begin 1-2 days after initiating therapy and resolve in 2-4 weeks. Dosing at bedtime may improve tolerability. NSS are not predictive of onset of psychiatric symptoms. (5.5, 6.1, 17.4)
- *Pregnancy:* Fetal harm can occur when administered to a pregnant woman during the first trimester. Women should be apprised of the potential harm to the fetus. (5.6, 17.7)
- *Hepatotoxicity:* Monitor liver function tests before and during treatment in patients with underlying hepatic disease, including hepatitis B or C coinfection, marked transaminase elevations, or who are taking medications associated with liver toxicity. Among reported cases of hepatic failure, a few occurred in patients with no pre-existing hepatic disease. (5.8, 6.1, 8.6)

- *Rash:* Rash usually begins within 1-2 weeks after initiating therapy and resolves within 4 weeks. Discontinue if severe rash develops. (5.7, 6.1, 17.6)
- *Convulsions:* Use caution in patients with a history of seizures. (5.9)
- *Lipids:* Total cholesterol and triglyceride elevations. Monitor before therapy and periodically thereafter. (5.10)
- *Immune reconstitution syndrome:* May necessitate further evaluation and treatment. (5.11)
- *Redistribution/accumulation of body fat:* Observed in patients receiving antiretroviral therapy. (5.12, 17.8)

---------------------ADVERSE REACTIONS---------------------

Most common adverse reactions (>5%, moderate-severe) are rash, dizziness, nausea, headache, fatigue, insomnia, and vomiting. (6)

To report SUSPECTED ADVERSE REACTIONS, contact Bristol-Myers Squibb at 1-800-721-5072 or FDA at 1-800-FDA-1088 or www.fda.gov/medwatch

---------------------DRUG INTERACTIONS---------------------

Coadministration of efavirenz can alter the concentrations of other drugs and other drugs may alter the concentrations of efavirenz. The potential for drug-drug interactions must be considered before and during therapy. (4.2, 7.1, 12.3)

---------------------USE IN SPECIFIC POPULATIONS---------------------

- *Pregnancy:* Women should avoid pregnancy during SUSTIVA (efavirenz) therapy and for 12 weeks after discontinuation. (5.6)
- *Nursing mothers:* Women infected with HIV should be instructed not to breast-feed. (8.3)
- *Hepatic impairment:* Use caution in patients with hepatic impairment. (5.8, 8.6)
- *Pediatric patients:* The incidence of rash was higher than in adults. (5.7, 6.1, 6.2, 8.4)

See 17 for PATIENT COUNSELING INFORMATION and FDA-approved patient labeling

Revised: 03/2010

FULL PRESCRIBING INFORMATION: CONTENTS*

Pediatric Patients at Least 3 Years and at Least 10 kg (2.2)

kg	lbs	dose	kg	lbs	dose
10–<15	22–<33	200 mg	25–<32.5	55–<71.5	350 mg
15–<20	33–<44	250 mg	32.5–<40	71.5–<88	400 mg
20–<25	44–<55	300 mg	at least 40	at least 88	600 mg

FULL PRESCRIBING INFORMATION

1 INDICATIONS AND USAGE

SUSTIVA® (efavirenz) in combination with other antiretroviral agents is indicated for the treatment of human immunodeficiency virus type 1 (HIV-1) infection. This indication is based on two clinical trials of at least one year duration that demonstrated prolonged suppression of HIV RNA [see *Clinical Studies (14)*].

2 DOSAGE AND ADMINISTRATION

2.1 Adults

The recommended dosage of SUSTIVA (efavirenz) is 600 mg orally, once daily, in combination with a protease inhibitor and/or nucleoside analogue reverse transcriptase inhibitors (NRTIs). It is recommended that SUSTIVA be taken on an empty stomach, preferably at bedtime. The increased efavirenz concentrations observed following administration of SUSTIVA with food may lead to an increase in frequency of adverse reactions [see *Clinical Pharmacology (12.3)*]. Dosing at bedtime may improve the tolerability of nervous system symptoms [see *Warnings and Precautions (5.5), Adverse Reactions (6.1)*, and *Patient Counseling Information (17.4)*].

Concomitant Antiretroviral Therapy

SUSTIVA must be given in combination with other antiretroviral medications [see *Indications and Usage (1), Warnings and Precautions (5.2), Drug Interactions (7.1)*, and *Clinical Pharmacology (12.3)*].

Dosage Adjustment

If SUSTIVA is coadministered with voriconazole, the voriconazole maintenance dose should be increased to 400 mg every 12 hours and the SUSTIVA dose should be decreased to 300 mg once daily using the capsule formulation (one 200-mg and two 50-mg capsules or six 50-mg capsules). SUSTIVA tablets should not be broken. See *Drug Interactions (7.1, Table 7)* and *Clinical Pharmacology (12.3, Tables 8 and 9)*.

2.2 Pediatric Patients

It is recommended that SUSTIVA be taken on an empty stomach, preferably at bedtime. Table 1 describes the recommended dose of SUSTIVA for pediatric patients 3 years of age or older and weighing between 10 and 40 kg [see *Use in Specific Populations (8.4)*]. The recommended dosage of SUSTIVA for pediatric patients weighing greater than 40 kg is 600 mg once daily.

Table 1: Pediatric Dose to be Administered Once Daily

Body Weight		SUSTIVA Dose (mg)
kg	lbs	
10 to less than 15	22 to less than 33	200
15 to less than 20	33 to less than 44	250
20 to less than 25	44 to less than 55	300
25 to less than 32.5	55 to less than 71.5	350
32.5 to less than 40	71.5 to less than 88	400
at least 40	at least 88	600

3 DOSAGE FORMS AND STRENGTHS

- *Capsules*
200-mg capsules are gold color, reverse printed with "SUSTIVA" on the body and imprinted "200 mg" on the cap.
50-mg capsules are gold color and white, printed with "SUSTIVA" on the gold color cap and reverse printed "50 mg" on the white body.
- *Tablets*
600-mg tablets are yellow, capsular-shaped, film-coated tablets, with "SUSTIVA" printed on both sides.

4 CONTRAINDICATIONS

4.1 Hypersensitivity

SUSTIVA is contraindicated in patients with previously demonstrated clinically significant hypersensitivity (eg, Stevens-Johnson syndrome, erythema multiforme, or toxic skin eruptions) to any of the components of this product.

4.2 Contraindicated Drugs

For some drugs, competition for CYP3A by efavirenz could result in inhibition of their metabolism and create the potential for serious and/or life-threatening adverse reactions (eg, cardiac arrhythmias, prolonged sedation, or respiratory depression). Drugs that are contraindicated with SUSTIVA are listed in Table 2.

Table 2: Drugs That Are Contraindicated or Not Recommended for Use With SUSTIVA

Drug Class: Drug Name	Clinical Comment
Antimigraine: ergot derivatives (dihydroergotamine, ergonovine, ergotamine, methylergonovine)	Potential for serious and/or life-threatening reactions such as acute ergot toxicity characterized by peripheral vasospasm and ischemia of the extremities and other tissues.
Benzodiazepines: midazolam, triazolam	Potential for serious and/or life-threatening reactions such as prolonged or increased sedation or respiratory depression.
Calcium channel blocker: bepridil	Potential for serious and/or life-threatening reactions such as cardiac arrhythmias.
GI motility agent: cisapride	Potential for serious and/or life-threatening reactions such as cardiac arrhythmias.
Neuroleptic: pimozide	Potential for serious and/or life-threatening reactions such as cardiac arrhythmias.
St. John's wort (*Hypericum perforatum*)	May lead to loss of virologic response and possible resistance to efavirenz or to the class of non-nucleoside reverse transcriptase inhibitors (NNRTI).

5 WARNINGS AND PRECAUTIONS

5.1 Drug Interactions

Efavirenz plasma concentrations may be altered by substrates, inhibitors, or inducers of CYP3A. Likewise, efavirenz may alter plasma concentrations of drugs metabolized by CYP3A [see *Contraindications (4.2)* and *Drug Interactions (7.1)*].

5.2 Resistance

SUSTIVA (efavirenz) must not be used as a single agent to treat HIV-1 infection or added on as a sole agent to a failing regimen. Resistant virus emerges rapidly when efavirenz is administered as monotherapy. The choice of new antiretroviral agents to be used in combination with efavirenz should take into consideration the potential for viral cross-resistance.

5.3 Coadministration with Related Products

Coadministration of SUSTIVA with ATRIPLA (efavirenz 600 mg/emtricitabine 200 mg/tenofovir disoproxil fumarate 300 mg) is not recommended, since efavirenz is one of its active ingredients.

5.4 Psychiatric Symptoms

Serious psychiatric adverse experiences have been reported in patients treated with SUSTIVA. In controlled trials of 1008 patients treated with regimens containing SUSTIVA for a mean of 2.1 years and 635 patients treated with control regimens for a mean of 1.5 years, the frequency (regardless of causality) of specific serious psychiatric events among patients who received SUSTIVA or control regimens, respectively, were severe depression (2.4%, 0.9%), suicidal ideation (0.7%, 0.3%), nonfatal suicide attempts (0.5%, 0), aggressive behavior (0.4%, 0.5%), paranoid reactions (0.4%, 0.3%), and manic reactions (0.2%, 0.3%). When psychiatric symptoms similar to those noted above were combined and evaluated as a group in a multifactorial analysis of data from Study 006, treatment with efavirenz was associated with an increase in the occurrence of these selected psychiatric symptoms. Other factors associated with an increase in the occurrence of these psychiatric symptoms were history of injection drug use, psychiatric history, and receipt of psychiatric medication at study entry; similar associations were observed in both the SUSTIVA and control treatment groups. In Study 006, onset of new serious psychiatric symptoms occurred throughout the study for both SUSTIVA-treated and control-treated patients. One percent of SUSTIVA-treated patients discontinued or interrupted treatment because of one or more of these selected psychiatric symptoms. There have also been occasional post-marketing reports of death by suicide, delusions, and psychosis-like behavior, although a causal relationship to the use of SUSTIVA (efavirenz) cannot be determined from these reports. Patients with serious psychiatric adverse experiences should seek immediate medical evaluation to assess the possibility that the symptoms may be related to the use of SUSTIVA, and if so, to determine whether the risks of continued therapy outweigh the benefits. See *Adverse Reactions (6.1)*.

5.5 Nervous System Symptoms

Fifty-three percent (531/1008) of patients receiving SUSTIVA in controlled trials reported central nervous system symptoms (any grade, regardless of causality) compared to 25% (156/635) of patients receiving control regimens [see *Adverse Reactions (6.1, Table 4)*]. These symptoms included, but were not limited to, dizziness (28.1% of the 1008 patients), insomnia (16.3%), impaired concentration (8.3%), somnolence (7.0%), abnormal dreams (6.2%), and hallucinations (1.2%). These symptoms were severe in 2.0% of patients, and 2.1% of patients discontinued therapy as a result. These symptoms usually begin during the first or second day of therapy and generally resolve after the first 2-4 weeks of therapy. After 4 weeks of therapy, the prevalence of nervous system symptoms of at least moderate severity ranged from 5% to 9% in patients treated with regimens containing SUSTIVA and from 3% to 5% in patients treated with a control regimen. Patients should be informed that these common symptoms were likely to improve with continued therapy and were not predictive of subsequent onset of the less frequent psychiatric symptoms [see *Warnings and Precautions (5.4)*]. Dosing at bedtime may improve the tolerability of these nervous system symptoms [see *Dosage and Administration (2)*].

Analysis of long-term data from Study 006 (median follow-up 180 weeks, 102 weeks, and 76 weeks for patients treated with SUSTIVA + zidovudine + lamivudine, SUSTIVA + indinavir, and indinavir + zidovudine + lamivudine, respectively) showed that, beyond 24 weeks of therapy, the incidences of new-onset nervous system symptoms among SUSTIVA-treated patients were generally similar to those in the indinavir-containing control arm.

Patients receiving SUSTIVA should be alerted to the potential for additive central nervous system effects when SUSTIVA is used concomitantly with alcohol or psychoactive drugs.

Patients who experience central nervous system symptoms such as dizziness, impaired concentration, and/or drowsiness should avoid potentially hazardous tasks such as driving or operating machinery.

5.6 Reproductive Risk Potential

Pregnancy Category D. Efavirenz may cause fetal harm when administered during the first trimester to a pregnant woman. Pregnancy should be avoided in women receiving SUSTIVA. Barrier contraception must always be used in combination with other methods of contraception (eg, oral or other hormonal contraceptives). Because of the long half-life of efavirenz, use of adequate contraceptive measures for 12 weeks after discontinuation of SUSTIVA is recommended. Women of childbearing potential should undergo pregnancy testing before initiation of SUSTIVA. If this drug is used during the first trimester of pregnancy, or if the patient becomes pregnant while taking this drug, the patient should be apprised of the potential harm to the fetus.

There are no adequate and well-controlled studies in pregnant women. SUSTIVA should be used during pregnancy only if the potential benefit justifies the potential risk to the fetus, such as in pregnant women without other therapeutic options.

Antiretroviral Pregnancy Registry: To monitor fetal outcomes of pregnant women exposed to SUSTIVA, an Antiretroviral Pregnancy Registry has been established. Physicians are encouraged to register patients by calling 1-800-258-4263.

As of July 2009, the Antiretroviral Pregnancy Registry has received prospective reports of 661 pregnancies exposed to efavirenz-containing regimens, nearly all of which were first-trimester exposures (606 pregnancies). Birth defects occurred in 14 of 501 live births (first-trimester exposure) and 2 of 55 live births (second/third-trimester exposure). One of these prospectively reported defects with first-trimester exposure was a neural tube defect. A single case of anophthalmia with first-trimester exposure to efavirenz has also been prospectively reported; however, this case included severe oblique facial clefts and amniotic banding, a known association with anophthalmia. There have been six retrospective reports of findings consistent with neural tube defects, including meningomyelocele. All mothers were exposed to efavirenz-containing regimens in the first trimester. Although a causal relationship of these events to the use of SUSTIVA has not been established, similar defects have been observed in preclinical studies of efavirenz.

Malformations have been observed in 3 of 20 fetuses/infants from efavirenz-treated cynomolgus monkeys (versus 0 of 20 concomitant controls) in a developmental toxicity study. The pregnant monkeys were dosed throughout pregnancy (postcoital days 20-150) with efavirenz 60 mg/kg daily, a dose which resulted in plasma drug concentrations similar to those in humans given 600 mg/day of SUSTIVA (efavirenz). Anencephaly and unilateral anophthalmia were observed in one fetus, microophthalmia was observed in another fetus, and cleft palate was observed in a third fetus. Efavirenz crosses the placenta in cynomolgus monkeys and produces fetal blood concentrations similar to maternal blood concentrations. Efavirenz has been shown to cross the placenta in rats and rabbits and produces fetal blood concentrations of efavirenz similar to maternal concentrations. An increase in fetal resorptions was observed in rats at efavirenz doses that produced peak plasma concentrations and AUC values in female rats equivalent to or lower than those achieved in humans given 600 mg once daily of SUSTIVA. Efavirenz produced no reproductive toxicities when given to pregnant rabbits at doses that produced peak plasma concentrations similar to and AUC values approximately half of those achieved in humans given 600 mg once daily of SUSTIVA.

5.7 Rash

In controlled clinical trials, 26% (266/1008) of patients treated with 600 mg SUSTIVA experienced new-onset skin rash compared with 17% (111/635) of patients treated in control groups [see *Adverse Reactions (6.1, Table 5)*]. Rash associated with blistering, moist desquamation, or ulceration occurred in 0.9% (9/1008) of patients treated with SUSTIVA. The incidence of Grade 4 rash (eg, erythema multiforme, Stevens-Johnson syndrome) in patients treated with SUSTIVA in all studies and expanded access was 0.1%. Rashes are usually mild-to-moderate maculopapular skin eruptions that occur within the first 2 weeks of initiating therapy with efavirenz (median time to onset of rash in adults was 11 days) and, in most patients continuing therapy with efavirenz, rash resolves within 1 month (median duration, 16 days). The discontinuation rate for rash in clinical trials was 1.7% (17/1008). SUSTIVA can be reinitiated in patients interrupting therapy because of rash. SUSTIVA should be discontinued in patients developing severe rash associated with blistering, desquamation, mucosal involvement, or fever. Appropriate antihistamines and/or corticosteroids may improve the tolerability and hasten the resolution of rash.

Rash was reported in 26 of 57 pediatric patients (46%) treated with SUSTIVA (efavirenz) capsules [see *Adverse Reactions (6.1, 6.2)*]. One pediatric patient experienced Grade 3 rash (confluent rash with fever), and two patients had Grade 4 rash (erythema multiforme). The median time to onset of rash in pediatric patients was 8 days. Prophylaxis with appropriate antihistamines before initiating therapy with SUSTIVA in pediatric patients should be considered.

5.8 Hepatotoxicity

Monitoring of liver enzymes before and during treatment is recommended for patients with underlying hepatic disease, including hepatitis B or C infection; patients with marked transaminase elevations; and patients treated with other medications associated with liver toxicity [see *Adverse Reactions (6.1)* and *Use in Specific Populations (8.6)*]. A few of the postmarketing reports of hepatic failure occurred in patients with no pre-existing hepatic disease or other identifiable risk factors [see *Adverse Reactions (6.3)*]. Liver enzyme monitoring should also be considered for patients without pre-existing hepatic dysfunction or other risk factors. In patients with persistent elevations of serum transaminases to greater than five times the upper limit of the normal range, the benefit of continued therapy with SUSTIVA needs to be weighed against the unknown risks of significant liver toxicity.

5.9 Convulsions

Convulsions have been observed in patients receiving efavirenz, generally in the presence of known medical history of seizures [see *Nonclinical Toxicology (13.2)*]. Caution must be taken in any patient with a history of seizures. Patients who are receiving concomitant anticonvulsant medications primarily metabolized by the liver, such as phenytoin and phenobarbital, may require periodic monitoring of plasma levels [see *Drug Interactions (7.1)*].

5.10 Lipid Elevations

Treatment with SUSTIVA has resulted in increases in the concentration of total cholesterol and triglycerides [see *Adverse Reactions (6.1)*]. Cholesterol and triglyceride testing should be performed before initiating SUSTIVA therapy and at periodic intervals during therapy.

5.11 Immune Reconstitution Syndrome

Immune reconstitution syndrome has been reported in patients treated with combination antiretroviral therapy, including SUSTIVA. During the initial phase of combination

Table 3: Selected Treatment-Emergent[a] Adverse Reactions of Moderate or Severe Intensity Reported in ≥2% of SUSTIVA-Treated Patients in Studies 006 and ACTG 364

Adverse Reactions	Study 006 LAM-, NNRTI-, and Protease Inhibitor-Naive Patients			Study ACTG 364 NRTI-experienced, NNRTI- and Protease Inhibitor-Naive Patients		
	SUSTIVA[b] + ZDV/LAM (n=412) 180 weeks[c]	SUSTIVA[b] + Indinavir (n=415) 102 weeks[c]	Indinavir + ZDV/LAM (n=401) 76 weeks[c]	SUSTIVA[b] + Nelfinavir + NRTIs (n=64) 71.1 weeks[c]	SUSTIVA[b] + NRTIs (n=65) 70.9 weeks[c]	Nelfinavir + NRTIs (n=66) 62.7 weeks[c]
Body as a Whole						
Fatigue	8%	5%	9%	0	2%	3%
Pain	1%	2%	8%	13%	6%	17%
Central and Peripheral Nervous System						
Dizziness	9%	9%	2%	2%	6%	6%
Headache	8%	5%	3%	5%	2%	3%
Insomnia	7%	7%	2%	0	0	2%
Concentration impaired	5%	3%	<1%	0	0	0
Abnormal dreams	3%	1%	0	—	—	—
Somnolence	2%	2%	<1%	0	0	0
Anorexia	1%	<1%	<1%	0	2%	2%
Gastrointestinal						
Nausea	10%	6%	24%	3%	2%	2%
Vomiting	6%	3%	14%	—	—	—
Diarrhea	3%	5%	6%	14%	3%	9%
Dyspepsia	4%	4%	6%	0	0	2%
Abdominal pain	2%	2%	5%	3%	3%	3%
Psychiatric						
Anxiety	2%	4%	<1%	—	—	—
Depression	5%	4%	<1%	3%	0	5%
Nervousness	2%	2%	0	2%	0	2%
Skin & Appendages						
Rash[d]	11%	16%	5%	9%	5%	9%
Pruritus	<1%	1%	1%	9%	5%	9%

[a] Includes adverse events at least possibly related to study drug or of unknown relationship for Study 006. Includes all adverse events regardless of relationship to study drug for Study ACTG 364.
[b] SUSTIVA provided as 600 mg once daily.
[c] Median duration of treatment.
[d] Includes erythema multiforme, rash, rash erythematous, rash follicular, rash maculopapular, rash petechial, rash pustular, and urticaria for Study 006 and macules, papules, rash, erythema, redness, inflammation, allergic rash, urticaria, welts, hives, itchy, and pruritus for ACTG 364.
— = Not Specified.
ZDV = zidovudine, LAM = lamivudine.

antiretroviral treatment, patients whose immune system responds may develop an inflammatory response to indolent or residual opportunistic infections [such as *Mycobacterium avium* infection, cytomegalovirus, *Pneumocystis jiroveci* pneumonia (PCP), or tuberculosis], which may necessitate further evaluation and treatment.

5.12 Fat Redistribution

Redistribution/accumulation of body fat including central obesity, dorsocervical fat enlargement (buffalo hump), peripheral wasting, facial wasting, breast enlargement, and "cushingoid appearance" have been observed in patients receiving antiretroviral therapy. The mechanism and long-term consequences of these events are currently unknown. A causal relationship has not been established.

6 ADVERSE REACTIONS

The most significant adverse reactions observed in patients treated with SUSTIVA (efavirenz) are:

- psychiatric symptoms [see *Warnings and Precautions (5.4)*],
- nervous system symptoms [see *Warnings and Precautions (5.5)*],
- rash [see *Warnings and Precautions (5.7)*].

The most common (>5% in either efavirenz treatment group) adverse reactions of at least moderate severity among patients in Study 006 treated with SUSTIVA in combination with zidovudine/lamivudine or indinavir were rash, dizziness, nausea, headache, fatigue, insomnia, and vomiting.

6.1 Clinical Trials Experience in Adults

Because clinical studies are conducted under widely varying conditions, the adverse reaction rates reported cannot be directly compared to rates in other clinical studies and may not reflect the rates observed in clinical practice.

Selected clinical adverse reactions of moderate or severe intensity observed in ≥2% of SUSTIVA-treated patients in two controlled clinical trials are presented in Table 3.

[See table 3 at top of previous page]

Pancreatitis has been reported, although a causal relationship with efavirenz has not been established. Asymptomatic increases in serum amylase levels were observed in a significantly higher number of patients treated with efavirenz 600 mg than in control patients (see *Laboratory Abnormalities*).

Nervous System Symptoms

For 1008 patients treated with regimens containing SUSTIVA and 635 patients treated with a control regimen in controlled trials, Table 4 lists the frequency of symptoms of different degrees of severity and gives the discontinuation rates for one or more of the following nervous system symptoms: dizziness, insomnia, impaired concentration, somnolence, abnormal dreaming, euphoria, confusion, agitation, amnesia, hallucinations, stupor, abnormal thinking, and depersonalization [see *Warnings and Precautions (5.5)*]. The frequencies of specific central and peripheral nervous system symptoms are provided in Table 3.

Table 4: Percent of Patients with One or More Selected Nervous System Symptoms[a,b]

Percent of Patients with:	SUSTIVA 600 mg Once Daily (n=1008) %	Control Groups (n=635) %
Symptoms of any severity	52.7	24.6
Mild symptoms[c]	33.3	15.6
Moderate symptoms[d]	17.4	7.7
Severe symptoms[e]	2.0	1.3
Treatment discontinuation as a result of symptoms	2.1	1.1

[a] Includes events reported regardless of causality.
[b] Data from Study 006 and three Phase 2/3 studies.
[c] "Mild" = Symptoms which do not interfere with patient's daily activities.
[d] "Moderate" = Symptoms which may interfere with daily activities.
[e] "Severe" = Events which interrupt patient's usual daily activities.

Psychiatric Symptoms

Serious psychiatric adverse experiences have been reported in patients treated with SUSTIVA. In controlled trials, psychiatric symptoms observed at a frequency of >2% among patients treated with SUSTIVA or control regimens, respectively, were depression (19%, 16%), anxiety (13%, 9%), and nervousness (7%, 2%).

Rash

For 1008 adults and 57 pediatric patients treated with regimens containing SUSTIVA and 635 patients treated with a control regimen in controlled trials, the frequency of rash by

Table 5: Percent of Patients with Treatment-Emergent Rash[a,b]

Percent of Patients with:	Description of Rash Grade[c]	SUSTIVA 600 mg Once Daily Adults (n=1008) %	SUSTIVA Pediatric Patients (n=57) %	Control Groups Adults (n=635) %
Rash of any grade	—	26.3	45.6	17.5
Grade 1 rash	Erythema, pruritus	10.7	8.8	9.8
Grade 2 rash	Diffuse maculopapular rash, dry desquamation	14.7	31.6	7.4
Grade 3 rash	Vesiculation, moist desquamation, ulceration	0.8	1.8	0.3
Grade 4 rash	Erythema multiforme, Stevens-Johnson syndrome, toxic epidermal necrolysis, necrosis requiring surgery, exfoliative dermatitis	0.1	3.5	0.0
Treatment discontinuation as a result of rash	—	1.7	8.8	0.3

[a] Includes events reported regardless of causality.
[b] Data from Study 006 and three Phase 2/3 studies.
[c] NCI Grading System.

Table 6: Selected Grade 3-4 Laboratory Abnormalities Reported in ≥2% of SUSTIVA-Treated Patients in Studies 006 and ACTG 364

Variable	Limit	Study 006 LAM-, NNRTI-, and Protease Inhibitor-Naive Patients			Study ACTG 364 NRTI-experienced, NNRTI- and Protease Inhibitor-Naive Patients		
		SUSTIVA[a] + ZDV/LAM (n=412) 180 weeks[b]	SUSTIVA[a] + Indinavir (n=415) 102 weeks[b]	Indinavir + ZDV/LAM (n=401) 76 weeks[b]	SUSTIVA[a] + Nelfinavir + NRTIs (n=64) 71.1 weeks[b]	SUSTIVA[a] + NRTIs (n=65) 70.9 weeks[b]	Nelfinavir + NRTIs (n=66) 62.7 weeks[b]
Chemistry							
ALT	>5 × ULN	5%	8%	5%	2%	6%	3%
AST	>5 × ULN	5%	6%	5%	6%	8%	8%
GGT[c]	>5 × ULN	8%	7%	3%	5%	0	5%
Amylase	>2 × ULN	4%	4%	1%	0	6%	2%
Glucose	>250 mg/dL	3%	3%	3%	5%	2%	3%
Triglycerides[d]	≥751 mg/dL	9%	6%	6%	11%	8%	17%
Hematology							
Neutrophils	<750/mm³	10%	3%	5%	2%	3%	2%

[a] SUSTIVA provided as 600 mg once daily.
[b] Median duration of treatment.
[c] Isolated elevations of GGT in patients receiving SUSTIVA may reflect enzyme induction not associated with liver toxicity.
[d] Nonfasting.
ZDV = zidovudine, LAM = lamivudine, ULN = Upper limit of normal, ALT = alanine aminotransferase, AST = aspartate aminotransferase, GGT = gamma-glutamyltransferase.

NCI grade and the discontinuation rates as a result of rash in clinical studies are provided in Table 5 [see *Warnings and Precautions (5.7)*].

[See table 5 above]

As seen in Table 5, rash is more common in pediatric patients and more often of higher grade (ie, more severe) [see *Warnings and Precautions (5.7)*].

Experience with SUSTIVA (efavirenz) in patients who discontinued other antiretroviral agents of the NNRTI class is limited. Nineteen patients who discontinued nevirapine because of rash have been treated with SUSTIVA. Nine of these patients developed mild-to-moderate rash while receiving therapy with SUSTIVA, and two of these patients discontinued because of rash.

Laboratory Abnormalities

Selected Grade 3-4 laboratory abnormalities reported in ≥2% of SUSTIVA-treated patients in two clinical trials are presented in Table 6.

[See table 6 above]

Patients Coinfected with Hepatitis B or C

Liver function tests should be monitored in patients with a history of hepatitis B and/or C. In the long-term data set from Study 006, 137 patients treated with SUSTIVA-containing regimens (median duration of therapy, 68 weeks) and 84 treated with a control regimen (median duration, 56 weeks) were seropositive at screening for hepatitis B (surface antigen positive) and/or C (hepatitis C antibody positive). Among these coinfected patients, elevations in AST to greater than five times ULN developed in 13% of patients in the SUSTIVA arms and 7% of those in the control arm, and elevations in ALT to greater than five times ULN developed in 20% of patients in the SUSTIVA arms and 7% of patients in the control arm. Among coinfected patients, 3% of those treated with SUSTIVA-containing regimens and 2% in the

control arm discontinued from the study because of liver or biliary system disorders [see *Warnings and Precautions (5.8)*].

Lipids

Increases from baseline in total cholesterol of 10-20% have been observed in some uninfected volunteers receiving SUSTIVA (efavirenz). In patients treated with SUSTIVA + zidovudine + lamivudine, increases from baseline in nonfasting total cholesterol and HDL of approximately 20% and 25%, respectively, were observed. In patients treated with SUSTIVA + indinavir, increases from baseline in nonfasting cholesterol and HDL of approximately 40% and 35%, respectively, were observed. Nonfasting total cholesterol levels ≥240 mg/dL and ≥300 mg/dL were reported in 34% and 9%, respectively, of patients treated with SUSTIVA + zidovudine + lamivudine; 54% and 20%, respectively, of patients treated with SUSTIVA + indinavir; and 28% and 4%, respectively, of patients treated with indinavir + zidovudine + lamivudine. The effects of SUSTIVA on triglycerides and LDL in this study were not well characterized since samples were taken from nonfasting patients. The clinical significance of these findings is unknown [see *Warnings and Precautions (5.10)*].

6.2 Clinical Trial Experience in Pediatric Patients

Clinical adverse experiences observed in ≥10% of 57 pediatric patients aged 3 to 16 years who received SUSTIVA capsules, nelfinavir, and one or more NRTIs in Study ACTG 382 [see *Use In Specific Populations (8.4)*] were rash (46%), diarrhea/loose stools (39%), fever (21%), cough (16%), dizziness/lightheaded/fainting (16%), ache/pain/discomfort (14%), nausea/vomiting (12%), and headache (11%). The incidence of nervous system symptoms was 18% (10/57). One patient experienced Grade 3 rash, two patients had Grade 4 rash, and five patients (9%) discontinued because of rash [see *Warnings and Precautions (5.7)* and *Adverse Reactions (6.1, Table 5)*].

Table 7: Established[a] and Other Potentially Significant[b] Drug Interactions: Alteration in Dose or Regimen May Be Recommended Based on Drug Interaction Studies or Predicted Interaction

Concomitant Drug Class: Drug Name	Effect	Clinical Comment
Antiretroviral agents		
Protease inhibitor: Fosamprenavir calcium	↓ amprenavir	Fosamprenavir (unboosted): Appropriate doses of the combinations with respect to safety and efficacy have not been established. Fosamprenavir/ritonavir: An additional 100 mg/day (300 mg total) of ritonavir is recommended when SUSTIVA is administered with fosamprenavir/ritonavir once daily. No change in the ritonavir dose is required when SUSTIVA is administered with fosamprenavir plus ritonavir twice daily.
Protease inhibitor: Atazanavir	↓ atazanavir[a]	*Treatment-naive patients:* When coadministered with SUSTIVA, the recommended dose of atazanavir is 400 mg with ritonavir 100 mg (together once daily with food) and SUSTIVA 600 mg (once daily on an empty stomach, preferably at bedtime). *Treatment-experienced patients:* Coadministration of SUSTIVA and atazanavir is not recommended.
Protease inhibitor: Indinavir	↓ indinavir[a]	The optimal dose of indinavir, when given in combination with SUSTIVA, is not known. Increasing the indinavir dose to 1000 mg every 8 hours does not compensate for the increased indinavir metabolism due to SUSTIVA. When indinavir at an increased dose (1000 mg every 8 hours) was given with SUSTIVA (600 mg once daily), the indinavir AUC and C_{min} were decreased on average by 33-46% and 39-57%, respectively, compared to when indinavir (800 mg every 8 hours) was given alone.
Protease inhibitor: Lopinavir/ritonavir	↓ lopinavir[a]	Lopinavir/ritonavir tablets should not be administered once-daily in combination with SUSTIVA. In antiretroviral-naive patients, lopinavir/ritonavir tablets can be used twice daily in combination with SUSTIVA with no dose adjustment. A dose increase of lopinavir/ritonavir tablets to 600/150 mg (3 tablets) twice daily may be considered when used in combination with SUSTIVA in treatment-experienced patients where decreased susceptibility to lopinavir is clinically suspected (by treatment history or laboratory evidence). A dose increase of lopinavir/ritonavir oral solution to 533/133 mg (6.5 mL) twice daily taken with food is recommended when used in combination with SUSTIVA.
Protease inhibitor: Ritonavir	↑ ritonavir[a] ↑ efavirenz[a]	When ritonavir 500 mg q12h was coadministered with SUSTIVA 600 mg once daily, the combination was associated with a higher frequency of adverse clinical experiences (eg, dizziness, nausea, paresthesia) and laboratory abnormalities (elevated liver enzymes). Monitoring of liver enzymes is recommended when SUSTIVA is used in combination with ritonavir.
Protease inhibitor: Saquinavir	↓ saquinavir[a]	Should not be used as sole protease inhibitor in combination with SUSTIVA.
CCR5 co-receptor antagonist: Maraviroc	↓ maraviroc[a]	Refer to the full prescribing information for maraviroc for guidance on coadministration with efavirenz.
Other agents		
Anticoagulant: Warfarin	↑ or ↓ warfarin	Plasma concentrations and effects potentially increased or decreased by SUSTIVA.
Anticonvulsants: Carbamazepine	↓ carbamazepine[a] ↓ efavirenz[a]	There are insufficient data to make a dose recommendation for efavirenz. Alternative anticonvulsant treatment should be used.
Phenytoin Phenobarbital	↓ anticonvulsant ↓ efavirenz	Potential for reduction in anticonvulsant and/or efavirenz plasma levels; periodic monitoring of anticonvulsant plasma levels should be conducted.
Antidepressant: Sertraline	↓ sertraline[a]	Increases in sertraline dosage should be guided by clinical response.

(Table continued on next page)

6.3 Postmarketing Experience

The following adverse reactions have been identified during postapproval use of SUSTIVA (efavirenz). Because these reactions are reported voluntarily from a population of unknown size, it is not always possible to reliably estimate their frequency or establish a causal relationship to drug exposure.

Body as a Whole: allergic reactions, asthenia, redistribution/accumulation of body fat [see *Warnings and Precautions (5.12)*]

Central and Peripheral Nervous System: abnormal coordination, ataxia, cerebellar coordination and balance disturbances, convulsions, hypoesthesia, paresthesia, neuropathy, tremor

Endocrine: gynecomastia

Gastrointestinal: constipation, malabsorption

Cardiovascular: flushing, palpitations

Liver and Biliary System: hepatic enzyme increase, hepatic failure, hepatitis. A few of the postmarketing reports of hepatic failure, including cases in patients with no preexisting hepatic disease or other identifiable risk factors, were characterized by a fulminant course, progressing in some cases to transplantation or death.

Metabolic and Nutritional: hypercholesterolemia, hypertriglyceridemia

Musculoskeletal: arthralgia, myalgia, myopathy

Psychiatric: aggressive reactions, agitation, delusions, emotional lability, mania, neurosis, paranoia, psychosis, suicide

Respiratory: dyspnea

Skin and Appendages: erythema multiforme, photoallergic dermatitis, Stevens-Johnson syndrome

Special Senses: abnormal vision, tinnitus

7 DRUG INTERACTIONS

7.1 Drug-Drug Interactions

Efavirenz has been shown *in vivo* to induce CYP3A. Other compounds that are substrates of CYP3A may have decreased plasma concentrations when coadministered with SUSTIVA (efavirenz). *In vitro* studies have demonstrated that efavirenz inhibits CYP2C9, 2C19, and 3A4 isozymes in the range of observed efavirenz plasma concentrations. Coadministration of efavirenz with drugs primarily metabolized by these isozymes may result in altered plasma concentrations of the coadministered drug. Therefore, appropriate dose adjustments may be necessary for these drugs.

Drugs that induce CYP3A activity (eg, phenobarbital, rifampin, rifabutin) would be expected to increase the clearance of efavirenz resulting in lowered plasma concentrations. Drug interactions with SUSTIVA are summarized in Tables 2 and 7 [for pharmacokinetics data see *Clinical Pharmacology (12.3, Tables 8 and 9)*]. The tables include potentially significant interactions, but are not all inclusive. [See table 7 at left and on next page]

Other Drugs

Based on the results of drug interaction studies [see *Clinical Pharmacology (12.3, Tables 8 and 9)*], no dosage adjustment is recommended when SUSTIVA (efavirenz) is given with the following: aluminum/magnesium hydroxide antacids, azithromycin, cetirizine, famotidine, fluconazole, lamivudine, lorazepam, nelfinavir, paroxetine, tenofovir disoproxil fumarate, and zidovudine.

Specific drug interaction studies have not been performed with SUSTIVA and NRTIs other than lamivudine and zidovudine. Clinically significant interactions would not be expected since the NRTIs are metabolized via a different route than efavirenz and would be unlikely to compete for the same metabolic enzymes and elimination pathways.

7.2 Cannabinoid Test Interaction

Efavirenz does not bind to cannabinoid receptors. False-positive urine cannabinoid test results have been observed in non-HIV-infected volunteers receiving SUSTIVA when the Microgenics CEDIA DAU Multi-Level THC assay was used for screening. Negative results were obtained when more specific confirmatory testing was performed with gas chromatography/mass spectrometry.

Of the three assays analyzed (Microgenics CEDIA DAU Multi-Level THC assay, Cannabinoid Enzyme Immunoassay [Diagnostic Reagents, Inc], and AxSYM Cannabinoid Assay), only the Microgenics CEDIA DAU Multi-Level THC assay showed false-positive results. The other two assays provided true-negative results. The effects of SUSTIVA on cannabinoid screening tests other than these three are unknown. The manufacturers of cannabinoid assays should be contacted for additional information regarding the use of their assays with patients receiving efavirenz.

8 USE IN SPECIFIC POPULATIONS

8.1 Pregnancy

Pregnancy Category D: See *Warnings and Precautions (5.6)*.

8.3 Nursing Mothers

The Centers for Disease Control and Prevention recommend that HIV-infected mothers not breast-feed their infants to avoid risking postnatal transmission of HIV. Although it is not known if efavirenz is secreted in human milk, efavirenz is secreted into the milk of lactating rats. Because of the potential for HIV transmission and the potential for serious adverse effects in nursing infants, mothers should be instructed not to breast-feed if they are receiving SUSTIVA.

8.4 Pediatric Use

ACTG 382 is an ongoing, open-label study in 57 NRTI-experienced pediatric patients to characterize the safety, pharmacokinetics, and antiviral activity of SUSTIVA in combination with nelfinavir (20-30 mg/kg three times daily) and NRTIs. Mean age was 8 years (range 3-16). SUSTIVA has not been studied in pediatric patients below 3 years of age or who weigh less than 13 kg. At 48 weeks, the type and frequency of adverse experiences was generally similar to that of adult patients with the exception of a higher incidence of rash, which was reported in 46% (26/57) of pediatric patients compared to 26% of adults, and a higher frequency of Grade 3 or 4 rash reported in 5% (3/57) of pediatric patients compared to 0.9% of adults [see *Warnings and Precautions (5.7)* and *Adverse Reactions (6.1, Table 5; 6.2)*].

The starting dose of SUSTIVA was 600 mg once daily adjusted to body size, based on weight, targeting AUC levels in the range of 190-380 μM•h [see *Dosage and Administration (2.2)*]. The pharmacokinetics of efavirenz in pediatric patients were similar to the pharmacokinetics in adults who received 600-mg daily doses of SUSTIVA. In 48 pediatric patients receiving the equivalent of a 600-mg dose of SUSTIVA, steady-state C_{max} was 14.2 ± 5.8 μM (mean ± SD), steady-state C_{min} was 5.6 ± 4.1 μM, and AUC was 218 ± 104 μM•h.

8.5 Geriatric Use

Clinical studies of SUSTIVA did not include sufficient numbers of subjects aged 65 years and over to determine whether they respond differently from younger subjects. In general, dose selection for an elderly patient should be

Table 7 (cont.): Established[a] and Other Potentially Significant[b] Drug Interactions: Alteration in Dose or Regimen May Be Recommended Based on Drug Interaction Studies or Predicted Interaction

Concomitant Drug Class: Drug Name	Effect	Clinical Comment
Antifungals: Voriconazole	↓ voriconazole[a] ↑ efavirenz[a]	SUSTIVA and voriconazole must not be coadministered at standard doses. Efavirenz significantly decreases voriconazole plasma concentrations, and coadministration may decrease the therapeutic effectiveness of voriconazole. Also, voriconazole significantly increases efavirenz plasma concentrations, which may increase the risk of SUSTIVA-associated side effects. When voriconazole is coadministered with SUSTIVA, voriconazole maintenance dose should be increased to 400 mg every 12 hours and SUSTIVA dose should be decreased to 300 mg once daily using the capsule formulation. SUSTIVA tablets should not be broken. [See *Dosage and Administration (2.1)* and *Clinical Pharmacology (12.3, Tables 8* and *9).*]
Itraconazole	↓ itraconazole[a] ↓ hydroxyitraconazole[a]	Since no dose recommendation for itraconazole can be made, alternative antifungal treatment should be considered.
Ketoconazole	↓ ketoconazole	Drug interaction studies with SUSTIVA and ketoconazole have not been conducted. SUSTIVA has the potential to decrease plasma concentrations of ketoconazole.
Posaconazole	↓ posaconazole[a]	Avoid concomitant use unless the benefit outweighs the risks.
Anti-infective: Clarithromycin	↓ clarithromycin[a] ↑ 14-OH metabolite[a]	Plasma concentrations decreased by SUSTIVA; clinical significance unknown. In uninfected volunteers, 46% developed rash while receiving SUSTIVA and clarithromycin. No dose adjustment of SUSTIVA is recommended when given with clarithromycin. Alternatives to clarithromycin, such as azithromycin, should be considered (see *Other Drugs*, following table). Other macrolide antibiotics, such as erythromycin, have not been studied in combination with SUSTIVA.
Antimycobacterial: Rifabutin	↓ rifabutin[a]	Increase daily dose of rifabutin by 50%. Consider doubling the rifabutin dose in regimens where rifabutin is given 2 or 3 times a week.
Rifampin	↓ efavirenz[a]	Clinical significance of reduced efavirenz concentrations is unknown. Dosing recommendations for concomitant use of SUSTIVA and rifampin have not been established.
Calcium channel blockers: Diltiazem	↓ diltiazem[a] ↓ desacetyl diltiazem[a] ↓ N-monodesmethyl diltiazem[a]	Diltiazem dose adjustments should be guided by clinical response (refer to the full prescribing information for diltiazem). No dose adjustment of efavirenz is necessary when administered with diltiazem.
Others (eg, felodipine, nicardipine, nifedipine, verapamil)	↓ calcium channel blocker	No data are available on the potential interactions of efavirenz with other calcium channel blockers that are substrates of CYP3A. The potential exists for reduction in plasma concentrations of the calcium channel blocker. Dose adjustments should be guided by clinical response (refer to the full prescribing information for the calcium channel blocker).
HMG-CoA reductase inhibitors: Atorvastatin Pravastatin Simvastatin	↓ atorvastatin[a] ↓ pravastatin[a] ↓ simvastatin[a]	Plasma concentrations of atorvastatin, pravastatin, and simvastatin decreased. Consult the full prescribing information for the HMG-CoA reductase inhibitor for guidance on individualizing the dose.
Hormonal contraceptives: Oral Ethinyl estradiol/ Norgestimate	↓ active metabolites of norgestimate[a]	A reliable method of barrier contraception must be used in addition to hormonal contraceptives. Efavirenz had no effect on ethinyl estradiol concentrations, but progestin levels (norelgestromin and levonorgestrel) were markedly decreased. No effect of ethinyl estradiol/norgestimate on efavirenz plasma concentrations was observed.
Implant Etonogestrel	↓ etonogestrel	A reliable method of barrier contraception must be used in addition to hormonal contraceptives. The interaction between etonogestrel and efavirenz has not been studied. Decreased exposure of etonogestrel may be expected. There have been postmarketing reports of contraceptive failure with etonogestrel in efavirenz-exposed patients.
Immunosuppressants: Cyclosporine, tacrolimus, sirolimus, and others metabolized by CYP3A	↓ immunosuppressant	Decreased exposure of the immunosuppressant may be expected due to CYP3A induction. These immunosuppressants are not anticipated to affect exposure of efavirenz. Dose adjustments of the immunosuppressant may be required. Close monitoring of immunosuppressant concentrations for at least 2 weeks (until stable concentrations are reached) is recommended when starting or stopping treatment with efavirenz.
Narcotic analgesic: Methadone	↓ methadone[a]	Coadministration in HIV-infected individuals with a history of injection drug use resulted in decreased plasma levels of methadone and signs of opiate withdrawal. Methadone dose was increased by a mean of 22% to alleviate withdrawal symptoms. Patients should be monitored for signs of withdrawal and their methadone dose increased as required to alleviate withdrawal symptoms.

[a] See *Clinical Pharmacology (12.3, Tables 8* and *9)* for magnitude of established interactions.
[b] This table is not all-inclusive.

cautious, reflecting the greater frequency of decreased hepatic, renal, or cardiac function and of concomitant disease or other therapy.

8.6 Hepatic Impairment
The pharmacokinetics of efavirenz have not been adequately studied in patients with hepatic impairment. Because of the extensive cytochrome P450-mediated metabolism of efavirenz and limited clinical experience in patients with hepatic impairment, caution should be exercised in administering SUSTIVA (efavirenz) to these patients [see *Warnings and Precautions (5.8)*].

10 OVERDOSAGE
Some patients accidentally taking 600 mg twice daily have reported increased nervous system symptoms. One patient experienced involuntary muscle contractions.
Treatment of overdose with SUSTIVA should consist of general supportive measures, including monitoring of vital signs and observation of the patient's clinical status. Administration of activated charcoal may be used to aid removal of unabsorbed drug. There is no specific antidote for overdose with SUSTIVA. Since efavirenz is highly protein bound, dialysis is unlikely to significantly remove the drug from blood.

11 DESCRIPTION
SUSTIVA® (efavirenz) is an HIV-1 specific, non-nucleoside, reverse transcriptase inhibitor (NNRTI). Efavirenz is chemically described as (S)-6-chloro-4-(cyclopropylethynyl)-1,4-dihydro-4-(trifluoromethyl)-2H-3,1-benzoxazin-2-one. Its empirical formula is $C_{14}H_9ClF_3NO_2$ and its structural formula is:

Efavirenz is a white to slightly pink crystalline powder with a molecular mass of 315.68. It is practically insoluble in water (<10 microgram/mL).
Capsules: SUSTIVA is available as capsules for oral administration containing either 50 mg or 200 mg of efavirenz and the following inactive ingredients: lactose monohydrate, magnesium stearate, sodium lauryl sulfate, and sodium starch glycolate. The capsule shell contains the following inactive ingredients and dyes: gelatin, sodium lauryl sulfate, titanium dioxide, and/or yellow iron oxide. The capsule shells may also contain silicon dioxide. The capsules are printed with ink containing carmine 40 blue, FD&C Blue No. 2, and titanium dioxide.
Tablets: SUSTIVA is available as film-coated tablets for oral administration containing 600 mg of efavirenz and the following inactive ingredients: croscarmellose sodium, hydroxypropyl cellulose, lactose monohydrate, magnesium stearate, microcrystalline cellulose, and sodium lauryl sulfate. The film coating contains Opadry Yellow and Opadry Clear. The tablets are polished with carnauba wax and printed with purple ink, Opacode WB.

12 CLINICAL PHARMACOLOGY
12.1 Mechanism of Action
Efavirenz is an antiviral drug [see *Clinical Pharmacology (12.4)*].
12.3 Pharmacokinetics
Absorption
Peak efavirenz plasma concentrations of 1.6-9.1 µM were attained by 5 hours following single oral doses of 100 mg to 1600 mg administered to uninfected volunteers. Dose-related increases in C_{max} and AUC were seen for doses up to 1600 mg; the increases were less than proportional suggesting diminished absorption at higher doses.
In HIV-1-infected patients at steady state, mean C_{max}, mean C_{min}, and mean AUC were dose proportional following 200-mg, 400-mg, and 600-mg daily doses. Time-to-peak plasma concentrations were approximately 3-5 hours and steady-state plasma concentrations were reached in 6-10 days. In 35 patients receiving SUSTIVA 600 mg once daily, steady-state C_{max} was 12.9 ± 3.7 µM (mean ± SD), steady-state C_{min} was 5.6 ± 3.2 µM, and AUC was 184 ± 73 µM•h.
Effect of Food on Oral Absorption:
Capsules: Administration of a single 600-mg dose of efavirenz capsules with a high-fat/high-caloric meal (894 kcal, 54 g fat, 54% calories from fat) or a reduced-fat/normal-caloric meal (440 kcal, 2 g fat, 4% calories from fat) was associated with a mean increase of 22% and 17% in efavirenz $AUC_∞$ and a mean increase of 39% and 51% in efavirenz C_{max}, respectively, relative to the exposures achieved when given under fasted conditions. See *Dosage and Administration (2)* and *Patient Counseling Information (17.3)*.
Tablets: Administration of a single 600-mg efavirenz tablet with a high-fat/high-caloric meal (approximately 1000 kcal, 500-600 kcal from fat) was associated with a 28% increase in mean $AUC_∞$ of efavirenz and a 79% increase in

Table 8: Effect of Efavirenz on Coadministered Drug Plasma C_{max}, AUC, and C_{min}

Coadministered Drug	Dose	Efavirenz Dose	Number of Subjects	C_{max} (90% CI)	AUC (90% CI)	C_{min} (90% CI)
Atazanavir	400 mg qd with a light meal d 1-20	600 mg qd with a light meal d 7-20	27	↓ 59% (49-67%)	↓ 74% (68-78%)	↓ 93% (90-95%)
	400 mg qd d 1-6, then 300 mg qd d 7-20 with ritonavir 100 mg qd and a light meal	600 mg qd 2 h after atazanavir and ritonavir d 7-20	13	↑ 14%[a] (↓ 17-↑ 58%)	↑ 39%[a] (2-88%)	↑ 48%[a] (24-76%)
	300 mg qd/ritonavir 100 mg qd d 1-10 (pm), then 400 mg qd/ritonavir 100 mg qd d 11-24 (pm) (simultaneous with efavirenz)	600 mg qd with a light snack d 11-24 (pm)	14	↑ 17% (8-27%)	↔	↓ 42% (31-51%)
Indinavir	1000 mg q8h × 10 days	600 mg qd × 10 days	20			
	After morning dose			↔[b]	↓ 33%[b] (26-39%)	↓ 39%[b] (24-51%)
	After afternoon dose			↔[b]	↓ 37%[b] (26-46%)	↓ 52%[b] (47-57%)
	After evening dose			↓ 29%[b] (11-43%)	↓ 46%[b] (37-54%)	↓ 57%[b] (50-63%)
Lopinavir/ ritonavir	400/100 mg capsule q12h × 9 days	600 mg qd × 9 days	11,7[c]	↔[d]	↓ 19%[d] (↓ 36-↑ 3%)	↓ 39%[d] (3-62%)
	600/150 mg tablet q12h × 10 days with efavirenz compared to 400/100 mg q12h alone	600 mg qd × 9 days	23	↑ 36%[d] (28-44%)	↑ 36%[d] (28-44%)	↑ 32%[d] (21-44%)
Nelfinavir	750 mg q8h × 7 days	600 mg qd × 7 days	10	↑ 21% (10-33%)	↑ 20% (8-34%)	↔
Metabolite AG-1402				↓ 40% (30-48%)	↓ 37% (25-48%)	↓ 43% (21-59%)
Ritonavir	500 mg q12h × 8 days	600 mg qd × 10 days	11			
	After AM dose			↑ 24% (12-38%)	↑ 18% (6-33%)	↑ 42% (9-86%)[e]
	After PM dose			↔	↔	↑ 24% (3-50%)[e]
Saquinavir SGC[f]	1200 mg q8h × 10 days	600 mg qd × 10 days	12	↓ 50% (28-66%)	↓ 62% (45-74%)	↓ 56% (16-77%)[e]
Lamivudine	150 mg q12h × 14 days	600 mg qd × 14 days	9	↔	↔	↑ 265% (37-873%)
Tenofovir[g]	300 mg qd	600 mg qd × 14 days	29	↔	↔	↔
Zidovudine	300 mg q12h × 14 days	600 mg qd × 14 days	9	↔	↔	↑ 225% (43-640%)
Maraviroc	100 mg bid	600 mg qd	12	↓ 51% (37-62%)	↓ 45% (38-51%)	↓ 45% (28-57%)
Azithromycin	600 mg single dose	400 mg qd × 7 days	14	↑ 22% (4-42%)	↔	NA
Clarithromycin	500 mg q12h × 7 days	400 mg qd × 7 days	11	↓ 26% (15-35%)	↓ 39% (30-46%)	↓ 53% (42-63%)
14-OH metabolite				↑ 49% (32-69%)	↑ 34% (18-53%)	↑ 26% (9-45%)
Fluconazole	200 mg × 7 days	400 mg qd × 7 days	10	↔	↔	↔
Itraconazole	200 mg q12h × 28 days	600 mg qd × 14 days	18	↓ 37% (20-51%)	↓ 39% (21-53%)	↓ 44% (27-58%)
Hydroxy-itraconazole				↓ 35% (12-52%)	↓ 37% (14-55%)	↓ 43% (18-60%)

(Table continued on next page)

mean C_{max} of efavirenz relative to the exposures achieved under fasted conditions. See *Dosage and Administration (2)* and *Patient Counseling Information (17.3)*.

Distribution

Efavirenz is highly bound (approximately 99.5-99.75%) to human plasma proteins, predominantly albumin. In HIV-1 infected patients (n=9) who received SUSTIVA 200 to 600 mg once daily for at least one month, cerebrospinal fluid concentrations ranged from 0.26 to 1.19% (mean 0.69%) of the corresponding plasma concentration. This proportion is approximately 3-fold higher than the non-protein-bound (free) fraction of efavirenz in plasma.

Metabolism

Studies in humans and *in vitro* studies using human liver microsomes have demonstrated that efavirenz is principally metabolized by the cytochrome P450 system to hydroxyl-ated metabolites with subsequent glucuronidation of these hydroxylated metabolites. These metabolites are essentially inactive against HIV-1. The *in vitro* studies suggest that CYP3A and CYP2B6 are the major isozymes responsible for efavirenz metabolism.

Efavirenz has been shown to induce CYP enzymes, resulting in the induction of its own metabolism. Multiple doses of 200-400 mg per day for 10 days resulted in a lower than predicted extent of accumulation (22-42% lower) and a shorter terminal half-life of 40-55 hours (single dose half-life 52-76 hours).

Elimination

Efavirenz has a terminal half-life of 52-76 hours after single doses and 40-55 hours after multiple doses. A one-month mass balance/excretion study was conducted using 400 mg per day with a ^{14}C-labeled dose administered on Day 8. Approximately 14-34% of the radiolabel was recovered in the urine and 16-61% was recovered in the feces. Nearly all of the urinary excretion of the radiolabeled drug was in the form of metabolites. Efavirenz accounted for the majority of the total radioactivity measured in feces.

Special Populations

Gender and race: The pharmacokinetics of efavirenz in patients appear to be similar between men and women and among the racial groups studied.

Renal impairment: The pharmacokinetics of efavirenz have not been studied in patients with renal insufficiency; however, less than 1% of efavirenz is excreted unchanged in the urine, so the impact of renal impairment on efavirenz elimination should be minimal.

Drug Interaction Studies

Efavirenz has been shown *in vivo* to cause hepatic enzyme induction, thus increasing the biotransformation of some drugs metabolized by CYP3A. *In vitro* studies have shown that efavirenz inhibited CYP isozymes 2C9, 2C19, and 3A4 with K_i values (8.5-17 μM) in the range of observed efavirenz plasma concentrations. In *in vitro* studies, efavirenz did not inhibit CYP2E1 and inhibited CYP2D6 and CYP1A2 (K_i values 82-160 μM) only at concentrations well above those achieved clinically. The inhibitory effect on CYP3A is expected to be similar between 200-mg, 400-mg, and 600-mg doses of efavirenz. Coadministration of efavirenz with drugs primarily metabolized by 2C9, 2C19, and 3A isozymes may result in altered plasma concentrations of the coadministered drug. Drugs which induce CYP3A activity would be expected to increase the clearance of efavirenz resulting in lowered plasma concentrations.

Drug interaction studies were performed with efavirenz and other drugs likely to be coadministered or drugs commonly used as probes for pharmacokinetic interaction. The effects of coadministration of efavirenz on the C_{max}, AUC, and C_{min} are summarized in Table 8 (effect of efavirenz on other drugs) and Table 9 (effect of other drugs on efavirenz). For information regarding clinical recommendations see *Contraindications (4.2)* and *Drug Interactions (7.1)*.

[See table 8 at left and on next page]
[See table 9 on pages 3540 and 3541]

12.4 Microbiology

Mechanism of Action

Efavirenz (EFV) is an NNRTI of HIV-1. EFV activity is mediated predominantly by noncompetitive inhibition of HIV-1 reverse transcriptase (RT). HIV-2 RT and human cellular DNA polymerases α, β, γ, and δ are not inhibited by EFV.

Antiviral Activity in Cell Culture

The concentration of EFV inhibiting replication of wild-type laboratory adapted strains and clinical isolates in cell culture by 90-95% (EC_{90-95}) ranged from 1.7 to 25 nM in lymphoblastoid cell lines, peripheral blood mononuclear cells (PBMCs), and macrophage/monocyte cultures. EFV demonstrated antiviral activity against clade B and most non-clade B isolates (subtypes A, AE, AG, C, D, F, G, J, N), but had reduced antiviral activity against group O viruses. EFV demonstrated additive antiviral activity without cytotoxicity against HIV-1 in cell culture when combined with the NNRTIs delavirdine (DLV) and nevirapine (NVP), NRTIs (abacavir, didanosine, emtricitabine, lamivudine [LAM], stavudine, tenofovir, zalcitabine, zidovudine [ZDV]), PIs (amprenavir, indinavir [IDV], lopinavir, nelfinavir, ritonavir, saquinavir), and the fusion inhibitor enfuvirtide. EFV demonstrated additive to antagonistic antiviral activity in cell culture with atazanavir. EFV was not antagonistic with adefovir, used for the treatment of hepatitis B virus infection, or ribavirin, used in combination with interferon for the treatment of hepatitis C virus infection.

Resistance

In cell culture

In cell culture, HIV-1 isolates with reduced susceptibility to EFV (>380-fold increase in EC_{90} value) emerged rapidly in the presence of drug. Genotypic characterization of these viruses identified single amino acid substitutions L100I or V179D, double substitutions L100I/V108I, and triple substitutions L100I/V179D/Y181C in RT.

Clinical studies

Clinical isolates with reduced susceptibility in cell culture to EFV have been obtained. One or more RT substitutions at amino acid positions 98, 100, 101, 103, 106, 108, 188, 190, 225, and 227 were observed in patients failing treatment with EFV in combination with IDV, or with ZDV plus LAM. The mutation K103N was the most frequently observed. Long-term resistance surveillance (average 52 weeks, range 4-106 weeks) analyzed 28 matching baseline and virologic failure isolates. Sixty-one percent (17/28) of these failure isolates had decreased EFV susceptibility in cell culture with a median 88-fold change in EFV susceptibility (EC_{50} value) from reference. The most frequent NNRTI substitution to develop in these patient isolates was K103N (54%). Other NNRTI substitutions that developed included L100I (7%), K101E/Q/R (14%), V108I (11%), G190S/T/A (7%), P225H (18%), and M230I/L (11%).

Cross-Resistance

Cross-resistance among NNRTIs has been observed. Clinical isolates previously characterized as EFV-resistant were also phenotypically resistant in cell culture to DLV and NVP compared to baseline. DLV- and/or NVP-resistant clinical viral isolates with NNRTI resistance-associated substitutions (A98G, L100I, K101E/P, K103N/S, V106A, Y181X, Y188X, G190X, P225H, F227L, or M230L) showed reduced susceptibility to EFV in cell culture. Greater than 90% of NRTI-resistant clinical isolates tested in cell culture retained susceptibility to EFV.

13   NONCLINICAL TOXICOLOGY

13.1   Carcinogenesis, Mutagenesis, Impairment of Fertility

Long-term carcinogenicity studies in mice and rats were carried out with efavirenz. Mice were dosed with 0, 25, 150, or 300 mg/kg/day for 2 years. Incidences of hepatocellular adenomas and carcinomas and pulmonary alveolar/bronchiolar adenomas were increased above background in females. No increases in tumor incidence above background were seen in males. In studies in which rats were administered efavirenz at doses of 0, 25, 50, or 100 mg/kg/day for 2 years, no increases in tumor incidence above background were observed. The systemic exposure (based on AUCs) in mice was approximately 1.7-fold that in humans receiving the 600-mg/day dose. The exposure in rats was lower than that in humans. The mechanism of the carcinogenic potential is unknown. However, in genetic toxicology assays, efavirenz showed no evidence of mutagenic or clastogenic activity in a battery of in vitro and in vivo studies. These included bacterial mutation assays in S. typhimurium and E. coli, mammalian mutation assays in Chinese hamster ovary cells, chromosome aberration assays in human peripheral blood lymphocytes or Chinese hamster ovary cells, and an in vivo mouse bone marrow micronucleus assay. Given the lack of genotoxic activity of efavirenz, the relevance to humans of neoplasms in efavirenz-treated mice is not known.

Efavirenz did not impair mating or fertility of male or female rats, and did not affect sperm of treated male rats. The reproductive performance of offspring born to female rats given efavirenz was not affected. As a result of the rapid clearance of efavirenz in rats, systemic drug exposures achieved in these studies were equivalent to or below those achieved in humans given therapeutic doses of efavirenz.

13.2   Animal Toxicology

Nonsustained convulsions were observed in 6 of 20 monkeys receiving efavirenz at doses yielding plasma AUC values 4- to 13-fold greater than those in humans given the recommended dose [see Warnings and Precautions (5.9)].

14   CLINICAL STUDIES

Study 006, a randomized, open-label trial, compared SUSTIVA (600 mg once daily) + zidovudine (ZDV, 300 mg q12h) + lamivudine (LAM, 150 mg q12h) or SUSTIVA (600 mg once daily) + indinavir (IDV, 1000 mg q8h) with indinavir (800 mg q8h) + zidovudine (300 mg q12h) + lamivudine (150 mg q12h). Twelve hundred sixty-six patients (mean age 36.5 years [range 18-81], 60% Caucasian, 83% male) were enrolled. All patients were efavirenz-, lamivudine-, NNRTI-, and PI-naive at study entry. The median baseline CD4+ cell count was 320 cells/mm³ and the median baseline HIV-1 RNA level was 4.8 $\log_{10}$ copies/mL. Treatment outcomes with standard assay (assay limit 400 copies/mL) through 48 and 168 weeks are shown in Table 10. Plasma HIV RNA levels were quantified with standard (assay limit 400 copies/mL) and ultrasensitive (assay limit 50 copies/mL) versions of the AMPLICOR HIV-1 MONITOR assay. During the study, version 1.5 of the assay was introduced in Europe to enhance detection of non-clade B virus.

[See table 10 on page 3541]

Table 8 (cont.): Effect of Efavirenz on Coadministered Drug Plasma C_{max}, AUC, and C_{min}

Coadministered Drug	Dose	Efavirenz Dose	Number of Subjects	Coadministered Drug (mean % change) C_{max} (90% CI)	AUC (90% CI)	C_{min} (90% CI)
Posaconazole	400 mg (oral suspension) bid × 10 and 20 days	400 mg qd × 10 and 20 days	11	↓ 45% (34-53%)	↓ 50% (40-57%)	NA
Rifabutin	300 mg qd × 14 days	600 mg qd × 14 days	9	↓ 32% (15-46%)	↓ 38% (28-47%)	↓ 45% (31-56%)
Voriconazole	400 mg po q12h × 1 day, then 200 mg po q12h × 8 days	400 mg qd × 9 days	NA	↓ 61%[h]	↓ 77%[h]	NA
	300 mg po q12h days 2-7	300 mg qd × 7 days	NA	↓ 36%[i] (21-49%)	↓ 55%[i] (45-62%)	NA
	400 mg po q12h days 2-7	300 mg qd × 7 days	NA	↑ 23%[i] (↓ 1-↑ 53%)	↓ 7%[i] (↓ 23-↑ 13%)	NA
Atorvastatin	10 mg qd × 4 days	600 mg qd × 15 days	14	↓ 14% (1-26%)	↓ 43% (34-50%)	↓ 69% (49-81%)
Total active (including metabolites)				↓ 15% (2-26%)	↓ 32% (21-41%)	↓ 48% (23-64%)
Pravastatin	40 mg qd × 4 days	600 mg qd × 15 days	13	↓ 32% (↓ 59-↑ 12%)	↓ 44% (26-57%)	↓ 19% (0-35%)
Simvastatin	40 mg qd × 4 days	600 mg qd × 15 days	14	↓ 72% (63-79%)	↓ 68% (62-73%)	↓ 45% (20-62%)
Total active (including metabolites)				↓ 68% (55-78%)	↓ 60% (52-68%)	NA[j]
Carbamazepine	200 mg qd × 3 days, 200 mg bid × 3 days, then 400 mg qd × 29 days	600 mg qd × 14 days	12	↓ 20% (15-24%)	↓ 27% (20-33%)	↓ 35% (24-44%)
Epoxide metabolite				↔	↔	↓ 13% (↓ 30-↑ 7%)
Cetirizine	10 mg single dose	600 mg qd × 10 days	11	↓ 24% (18-30%)	↔	NA
Diltiazem	240 mg × 21 days	600 mg qd × 14 days	13	↓ 60% (50-68%)	↓ 69% (55-79%)	↓ 63% (44-75%)
Desacetyl diltiazem				↓ 64% (57-69%)	↓ 75% (59-84%)	↓ 62% (44-75%)
N-monodesmethyl diltiazem				↓ 28% (7-44%)	↓ 37% (17-52%)	↓ 37% (17-52%)
Ethinyl estradiol/ Norgestimate	0.035 mg/0.25 mg × 14 days	600 mg qd × 14 days				
Ethinyl estradiol			21	↔	↔	↔
Norelgestromin			21	↓ 46% (39-52%)	↓ 64% (62-67%)	↓ 82% (79-85%)
Levonorgestrel			6	↓ 80% (77-83%)	↓ 83% (79-87%)	↓ 86% (80-90%)
Lorazepam	2 mg single dose	600 mg qd × 10 days	12	↑ 16% (2-32%)	↔	NA
Methadone	Stable maintenance 35-100 mg daily	600 mg qd × 14-21 days	11	↓ 45% (25-59%)	↓ 52% (33-66%)	NA
Paroxetine	20 mg qd × 14 days	600 mg qd × 14 days	16	↔	↔	↔
Sertraline	50 mg qd × 14 days	600 mg qd × 14 days	13	↓ 29% (15-40%)	↓ 39% (27-50%)	↓ 46% (31-58%)

↑ Indicates increase
↓ Indicates decrease
↔ Indicates no change or a mean increase or decrease of <10%.
[a] Compared with atazanavir 400 mg qd alone.
[b] Comparator dose of indinavir was 800 mg q8h × 10 days.
[c] Parallel-group design; n for efavirenz + lopinavir/ritonavir, n for lopinavir/ritonavir alone.
[d] Values are for lopinavir; the pharmacokinetics of ritonavir in this study were unaffected by concurrent efavirenz.
[e] 95% CI.
[f] Soft Gelatin Capsule.
[g] Tenofovir disoproxil fumarate.
[h] 90% CI not available.
[i] Relative to steady-state administration of voriconazole (400 mg for 1 day, then 200 mg po q12h for 2 days).
[j] Not available because of insufficient data.
NA = not available.

For patients treated with SUSTIVA + zidovudine + lamivudine, SUSTIVA + indinavir, or indinavir + zidovudine + lamivudine, the percentage of responders with HIV-1 RNA <50 copies/mL was 65%, 50%, and 45%, respectively,

Table 9: Effect of Coadministered Drug on Efavirenz Plasma C_{max}, AUC, and C_{min}

Coadministered Drug	Dose	Efavirenz Dose	Number of Subjects	Efavirenz (mean % change) C_{max} (90% CI)	AUC (90% CI)	C_{min} (90% CI)
Indinavir	800 mg q8h × 14 days	200 mg qd × 14 days	11	↔	↔	↔
Lopinavir/ ritonavir	400/100 mg q12h × 9 days	600 mg qd × 9 days	11,12[a]	↔	↓ 16% (↓ 38-↑ 15%)	↓ 16% (↓ 42-↑ 20%)
Nelfinavir	750 mg q8h × 7 days	600 mg qd × 7 days	10	↓ 12% (↓ 32-↑ 13%)[b]	↓ 12% (↓ 35-↑ 18%)[b]	↓ 21% (↓ 53-↑ 33%)
Ritonavir	500 mg q12h × 8 days	600 mg qd × 10 days	9	↑ 14% (4-26%)	↑ 21% (10-34%)	↑ 25% (7-46%)[b]
Saquinavir SGC[c]	1200 mg q8h × 10 days	600 mg qd × 10 days	13	↓ 13% (5-20%)	↓ 12% (4-19%)	↓ 14% (2-24%)[b]
Tenofovir[d]	300 mg qd	600 mg qd × 14 days	30	↔	↔	↔
Azithromycin	600 mg single dose	400 mg qd × 7 days	14	↔	↔	↔
Clarithromycin	500 mg q12h × 7 days	400 mg qd × 7 days	12	↑ 11% (3-19%)	↔	↔
Fluconazole	200 mg × 7 days	400 mg qd × 7 days	10	↔	↑ 16% (6-26%)	↑ 22% (5-41%)
Itraconazole	200 mg q12h × 14 days	600 mg qd × 28 days	16	↔	↔	↔
Rifabutin	300 mg qd × 14 days	600 mg qd × 14 days	11	↔	↔	↓ 12% (↓ 24-↑ 1%)
Rifampin	600 mg × 7 days	600 mg qd × 7 days	12	↓ 20% (11-28%)	↓ 26% (15-36%)	↓ 32% (15-46%)
Voriconazole	400 mg po q12h × 1 day, then 200 mg po q12h × 8 days	400 mg qd × 9 days	NA	↑ 38%[e]	↑ 44%[e]	NA
	300 mg po q12h days 2-7	300 mg qd × 7 days	NA	↓ 14%[f] (7-21%)	↔[f]	NA
	400 mg po q12h days 2-7	300 mg qd × 7 days	NA	↔[f]	↑ 17%[f] (6-29%)	NA
Atorvastatin	10 mg qd × 4 days	600 mg qd × 15 days	14	↔	↔	↔
Pravastatin	40 mg qd × 4 days	600 mg qd × 15 days	11	↔	↔	↔
Simvastatin	40 mg qd × 4 days	600 mg qd × 15 days	14	↓ 12% (↓ 28-↑ 8%)	↔	↓ 12% (↓ 25-↑ 3%)

(Table continued on next page)

through 48 weeks, and 43%, 31%, and 23%, respectively, through 168 weeks. A Kaplan-Meier analysis of time to loss of virologic response (HIV RNA <400 copies/mL) suggests that both the trends of virologic response and differences in response continue through 4 years.

ACTG 364 is a randomized, double-blind, placebo-controlled, 48-week study in NRTI-experienced patients who had completed two prior ACTG studies. One-hundred ninety-six patients (mean age 41 years [range 18-76], 74% Caucasian, 88% male) received NRTIs in combination with SUSTIVA (efavirenz) (600 mg once daily), or nelfinavir (NFV, 750 mg three times daily), or SUSTIVA (600 mg once daily) + nelfinavir in a randomized, double-blinded manner. The mean baseline CD4+ cell count was 389 cells/mm[3] and mean baseline HIV-1 RNA level was 8130 copies/mL. Upon entry into the study, all patients were assigned a new open-label NRTI regimen, which was dependent on their previous NRTI treatment experience. There was no significant difference in the mean CD4+ cell count among treatment groups; the overall mean increase was approximately 100 cells at 48 weeks among patients who continued on study regimens. Treatment outcomes are shown in Table 11. Plasma HIV RNA levels were quantified with the AMPLICOR HIV-1 MONITOR assay using a lower limit of quantification of 500 copies/mL.

[See table 11 on next page]

A Kaplan-Meier analysis of time to treatment failure through 72 weeks demonstrates a longer duration of virologic suppression (HIV RNA <500 copies/mL) in the SUSTIVA-containing treatment arms.

16 HOW SUPPLIED/STORAGE AND HANDLING
16.1 Capsules
SUSTIVA® (efavirenz) capsules are available as follows:
Capsules 200 mg are gold color, reverse printed with "SUSTIVA" on the body and imprinted "200 mg" on the cap.
    Bottles of 90   NDC 0056-0474-92
Capsules 50 mg are gold color and white, printed with "SUSTIVA" on the gold color cap and reverse printed "50 mg" on the white body.
    Bottles of 30   NDC 0056-0470-30
16.2 Tablets
SUSTIVA® (efavirenz) tablets are available as follows:
Tablets 600 mg are yellow, capsular-shaped, film-coated tablets, with "SUSTIVA" printed on both sides.
    Bottles of 30   NDC 0056-0510-30
16.3 Storage
SUSTIVA capsules and SUSTIVA tablets should be stored at 25° C (77° F); excursions permitted to 15°–30° C (59°–86° F) [see USP Controlled Room Temperature].

17 PATIENT COUNSELING INFORMATION
See *FDA-Approved Patient Labeling.*
17.1 Drug Interactions
A statement to patients and healthcare providers is included on the product's bottle labels: *ALERT: Find out about medicines that should NOT be taken with SUSTIVA.*
SUSTIVA may interact with some drugs; therefore, patients should be advised to report to their doctor the use of any other prescription, nonprescription medication, or herbal products, particularly St. John's wort.

17.2 General Information for Patients
Patients should be informed that SUSTIVA is not a cure for HIV-1 infection and that they may continue to experience illnesses associated with HIV-1 infection, including opportunistic infections. Patients should remain under the care of a physician while taking SUSTIVA (efavirenz). Patients should be told that the use of SUSTIVA has not been shown to reduce the risk of transmitting HIV-1 to others through sexual contact or blood contamination.
17.3 Dosing Instructions
Patients should be advised to take SUSTIVA every day as prescribed. SUSTIVA must always be used in combination with other antiretroviral drugs. Patients should be advised to take SUSTIVA on an empty stomach, preferably at bedtime. Taking SUSTIVA with food increases efavirenz concentrations and may increase the frequency of adverse reactions. Dosing at bedtime may improve the tolerability of nervous system symptoms [see *Dosage and Administration (2)* and *Adverse Reactions (6.1)*].
17.4 Nervous System Symptoms
Patients should be informed that central nervous system symptoms (NSS) including dizziness, insomnia, impaired concentration, drowsiness, and abnormal dreams are commonly reported during the first weeks of therapy with SUSTIVA [see *Warnings and Precautions (5.5)*]. Dosing at bedtime may improve the tolerability of these symptoms, which are likely to improve with continued therapy. Patients should be alerted to the potential for additive effects when SUSTIVA is used concomitantly with alcohol or psychoactive drugs. Patients should be instructed that if they experience NSS they should avoid potentially hazardous tasks such as driving or operating machinery.
17.5 Psychiatric Symptoms
Patients should be informed that serious psychiatric symptoms including severe depression, suicide attempts, aggressive behavior, delusions, paranoia, and psychosis-like symptoms have been reported in patients receiving SUSTIVA [see *Warnings and Precautions (5.4)*]. If they experience severe psychiatric adverse experiences they should seek immediate medical evaluation. Patients should be advised to inform their physician of any history of mental illness or substance abuse.
17.6 Rash
Patients should be informed that a common side effect is rash [see *Warnings and Precautions (5.7)*]. Rashes usually go away without any change in treatment. However, since rash may be serious, patients should be advised to contact their physician promptly if rash occurs.
17.7 Reproductive Risk Potential
Women receiving SUSTIVA should be instructed to avoid pregnancy [see *Warnings and Precautions (5.6)*]. A reliable form of barrier contraception must always be used in combination with other methods of contraception, including oral or other hormonal contraception. Because of the long half-life of efavirenz, use of adequate contraceptive measures for 12 weeks after discontinuation of SUSTIVA is recommended. Women should be advised to notify their physician if they become pregnant or plan to become pregnant while taking SUSTIVA. If this drug is used during the first trimester of pregnancy, or if the patient becomes pregnant while taking this drug, she should be apprised of the potential harm to the fetus.
17.8 Fat Redistribution
Patients should be informed that redistribution or accumulation of body fat may occur in patients receiving antiretroviral therapy and that the cause and long-term health effects of these conditions are not known [see *Warnings and Precautions (5.12)*].

FDA-Approved Patient Labeling
Patient Information
SUSTIVA® (sus-TEE-vah)
[efavirenz (eh-FAH-vih-rehnz)]
capsules and tablets
ALERT: Find out about medicines that should NOT be taken with SUSTIVA.
Please also read the section "MEDICINES YOU SHOULD NOT TAKE WITH SUSTIVA."
Read this information before you start taking SUSTIVA. Read it again each time you refill your prescription, in case there is any new information. This leaflet provides a summary about SUSTIVA and does not include everything there is to know about your medicine. This information is not meant to take the place of talking with your doctor.
What is SUSTIVA?
SUSTIVA is a medicine used in combination with other medicines to help treat infection with Human Immunodeficiency Virus type 1 (HIV-1), the virus that causes AIDS (acquired immune deficiency syndrome). SUSTIVA is a type of anti-HIV drug called a "non-nucleoside reverse transcriptase inhibitor" (NNRTI). NNRTIs are not used in the treatment of Human Immunodeficiency Virus type 2 (HIV-2) infection.

SUSTIVA (efavirenz) works by lowering the amount of HIV-1 in the blood (viral load). SUSTIVA must be taken with other anti-HIV medicines. When taken with other anti-HIV medicines, SUSTIVA has been shown to reduce viral load and increase the number of CD4+ cells, a type of immune cell in blood. SUSTIVA may not have these effects in every patient.

SUSTIVA does not cure HIV or AIDS. People taking SUSTIVA may still develop other infections and complications. Therefore, it is very important that you stay under the care of your doctor.

SUSTIVA has not been shown to reduce the risk of passing HIV to others. Therefore, continue to practice safe sex, and do not use or share dirty needles.

What are the possible side effects of SUSTIVA?

Serious psychiatric problems. A small number of patients experience severe depression, strange thoughts, or angry behavior while taking SUSTIVA. Some patients have thoughts of suicide and a few have actually committed suicide. These problems tend to occur more often in patients who have had mental illness. Contact your doctor right away if you think you are having these psychiatric symptoms, so your doctor can decide if you should continue to take SUSTIVA (efavirenz).

Common side effects. Many patients have dizziness, trouble sleeping, drowsiness, trouble concentrating, and/or unusual dreams during treatment with SUSTIVA. These side effects may be reduced if you take SUSTIVA at bedtime on an empty stomach. They also tend to go away after you have taken the medicine for a few weeks. If you have these common side effects, such as dizziness, it does not mean that you will also have serious psychiatric problems, such as severe depression, strange thoughts, or angry behavior. Tell your doctor right away if any of these side effects continue or if they bother you. It is possible that these symptoms may be more severe if SUSTIVA is used with alcohol or mood altering (street) drugs.

If you are dizzy, have trouble concentrating, or are drowsy, avoid activities that may be dangerous, such as driving or operating machinery.

Rash is common. Rashes usually go away without any change in treatment. In a small number of patients, rash may be serious. If you develop a rash, call your doctor right away. **Rash may be a serious problem in some children.** Tell your child's doctor right away if you notice rash or any other side effects while your child is taking SUSTIVA.

Other common side effects include tiredness, upset stomach, vomiting, and diarrhea. Some patients taking SUSTIVA have experienced increased levels of lipids (cholesterol and triglycerides) in the blood.

Changes in body fat. Changes in body fat develop in some patients taking anti-HIV medicine. These changes may include an increased amount of fat in the upper back and neck ("buffalo hump"), in the breasts, and around the trunk. Loss of fat from the legs, arms, and face may also happen. The cause and long-term health effects of these fat changes are not known.

Liver problems. Some patients taking SUSTIVA have experienced serious liver problems including liver failure resulting in transplantation or death. Most of these serious side effects occurred in patients with a chronic liver disease such as hepatitis infection, but there have also been a few reports in patients without any existing liver disease.

Tell your doctor or healthcare provider if you notice any side effects while taking SUSTIVA.

Contact your doctor before stopping SUSTIVA because of side effects or for any other reason.

This is not a complete list of side effects possible with SUSTIVA. Ask your doctor or pharmacist for a more complete list of side effects of SUSTIVA and all the medicines you will take.

How should I take SUSTIVA?

General Information

- You should take SUSTIVA on an empty stomach, preferably at bedtime.
- Swallow SUSTIVA with water.
- Taking SUSTIVA with food increases the amount of medicine in your body, which may increase the frequency of side effects.
- Taking SUSTIVA at bedtime may make some side effects less bothersome.
- SUSTIVA must be taken in combination with other anti-HIV medicines. If you take only SUSTIVA, the medicine may stop working.
- Do not miss a dose of SUSTIVA. If you forget to take SUSTIVA, take the missed dose right away, unless it is almost time for your next dose. Do not double the next dose. Carry on with your regular dosing schedule. If you need help in planning the best times to take your medicine, ask your doctor or pharmacist.
- Take the exact amount of SUSTIVA your doctor prescribes. Never change the dose on your own. Do not stop this medicine unless your doctor tells you to stop.

Table 9 (cont.): Effect of Coadministered Drug on Efavirenz Plasma C_{max}, AUC, and C_{min}

Coadministered Drug	Dose	Efavirenz Dose	Number of Subjects	Efavirenz (mean % change) C_{max} (90% CI)	AUC (90% CI)	C_{min} (90% CI)
Aluminum hydroxide 400 mg, magnesium hydroxide 400 mg, plus simethicone 40 mg	30 mL single dose	400 mg single dose	17	↔	↔	NA
Carbamazepine	200 mg qd × 3 days, 200 mg bid × 3 days, then 400 mg qd × 15 days	600 mg qd × 35 days	14	↓ 21% (15-26%)	↓ 36% (32-40%)	↓ 47% (41-53%)
Cetirizine	10 mg single dose	600 mg qd × 10 days	11	↔	↔	↔
Diltiazem	240 mg × 14 days	600 mg qd × 28 days	12	↑ 16% (6-26%)	↑ 11% (5-18%)	↑ 13% (1-26%)
Famotidine	40 mg single dose	400 mg single dose	17	↔	↔	NA
Paroxetine	20 mg qd × 14 days	600 mg qd × 14 days	12	↔	↔	↔
Sertraline	50 mg qd × 14 days	600 mg qd × 14 days	13	↑ 11% (6-16%)	↔	↔

↑ Indicates increase
↓ Indicates decrease
↔ Indicates no change or a mean increase or decrease of <10%.
[a] Parallel-group design; n for efavirenz + lopinavir/ritonavir, n for efavirenz alone.
[b] 95% CI.
[c] Soft Gelatin Capsule.
[d] Tenofovir disoproxil fumarate.
[e] 90% CI not available.
[f] Relative to steady-state administration of efavirenz (600 mg once daily for 9 days).
NA = not available.

Table 10: Outcomes of Randomized Treatment Through 48 and 168 Weeks, Study 006

Outcome	SUSTIVA + ZDV + LAM (n=422) Week 48	Week 168	SUSTIVA + IDV (n=429) Week 48	Week 168	IDV + ZDV + LAM (n=415) Week 48	Week 168
Responder[a]	69%	48%	57%	40%	50%	29%
Virologic failure[b]	6%	12%	15%	20%	13%	19%
Discontinued for adverse events	7%	8%	6%	8%	16%	20%
Discontinued for other reasons[c]	17%	31%	22%	32%	21%	32%
CD4+ cell count (cells/mm³)						
Observed subjects (n)	(279)	(205)	(256)	(158)	(228)	(129)
Mean change from baseline	190	329	191	319	180	329

[a] Patients achieved and maintained confirmed HIV-1 RNA <400 copies/mL through Week 48 or Week 168.
[b] Includes patients who rebounded, patients who were on study at Week 48 and failed to achieve confirmed HIV-1 RNA <400 copies/mL at time of discontinuation, and patients who discontinued due to lack of efficacy.
[c] Includes consent withdrawn, lost to follow-up, noncompliance, never treated, missing data, protocol violation, death, and other reasons. Patients with HIV-1 RNA levels <400 copies/mL who chose not to continue in the voluntary extension phases of the study were censored at date of last dose of study medication.

Table 11: Outcomes of Randomized Treatment Through 48 Weeks, Study ACTG 364*

Outcome	SUSTIVA + NFV + NRTIs (n=65)	SUSTIVA + NRTIs (n=65)	NFV + NRTIs (n=66)
HIV-1 RNA <500 copies/mL[a]	71%	63%	41%
HIV-1 RNA ≥500 copies/mL[b]	17%	34%	54%
CDC Category C Event	2%	0%	0%
Discontinuations for adverse events[c]	3%	3%	5%
Discontinuations for other reasons[d]	8%	0%	0%

*For some patients, Week 56 data were used to confirm the status at Week 48.
[a] Subjects achieved virologic response (two consecutive viral loads <500 copies/mL) and maintained it through Week 48.
[b] Includes viral rebound and failure to achieve confirmed HIV-1 RNA <500 copies/mL by Week 48.
[c] See *Adverse Reactions (6.1)* for a safety profile of these regimens.
[d] Includes loss to follow-up, consent withdrawn, noncompliance.

- If you believe you took more than the prescribed amount of SUSTIVA (efavirenz), contact your local Poison Control Center or emergency room right away.
- Tell your doctor if you start any new medicine or change how you take old ones. Your doses may need adjustment.
- When your SUSTIVA supply starts to run low, get more from your doctor or pharmacy. This is very important because the amount of virus in your blood may increase if the medicine is stopped for even a short time. The virus may develop resistance to SUSTIVA and become harder to treat.
- Your doctor may want to do blood tests to check for certain side effects while you take SUSTIVA (efavirenz).

Capsules
- The dose of SUSTIVA capsules for adults is 600 mg (three 200-mg capsules, taken together) once a day by mouth. The dose of SUSTIVA for children may be lower (see **Can children take SUSTIVA?**).

Tablets
- The dose of SUSTIVA tablets for adults is 600 mg (one tablet) once a day by mouth.

Can children take SUSTIVA?
Yes, children who are able to swallow capsules can take SUSTIVA. Rash may be a serious problem in some children. Tell your child's doctor right away if you notice rash or any other side effects while your child is taking SUSTIVA. The dose of SUSTIVA for children may be lower than the dose for adults. Capsules containing lower doses of SUSTIVA are available. Your child's doctor will determine the right dose based on your child's weight.

Who should not take SUSTIVA?
Do not take SUSTIVA if you are allergic to the active ingredient, efavirenz, or to any of the inactive ingredients. Your doctor and pharmacist have a list of the inactive ingredients.

What should I avoid while taking SUSTIVA?
- **Women should not become pregnant while taking SUSTIVA and for 12 weeks after stopping it.** Serious birth defects have been seen in the offspring of animals and women treated with SUSTIVA during pregnancy. It is not known whether SUSTIVA caused these defects. **Tell your doctor right away if you are pregnant.** Also talk with your doctor if you want to become pregnant.
- Women should not rely only on hormone-based birth control, such as pills, injections, or implants, because SUSTIVA may make these contraceptives ineffective. Women must use a reliable form of barrier contraception, such as a condom or diaphragm, even if they also use other methods of birth control. SUSTIVA may remain in your blood for a time after therapy is stopped. Therefore, you should continue to use contraceptive measures for 12 weeks after you stop taking SUSTIVA.
- **Do not breast-feed if you are taking SUSTIVA.** The Centers for Disease Control and Prevention recommend that mothers with HIV not breast-feed because they can pass the HIV through their milk to the baby. Also, SUSTIVA may pass through breast milk and cause serious harm to the baby. Talk with your doctor if you are breast-feeding. You may need to stop breast-feeding or use a different medicine.
- Taking SUSTIVA with alcohol or other medicines causing similar side effects as SUSTIVA, such as drowsiness, may increase those side effects.

- Do not take any other medicines without checking with your doctor. These medicines include prescription and nonprescription medicines and herbal products, especially St. John's wort (*Hypericum perforatum*).

Before using SUSTIVA (efavirenz), tell your doctor if you
- **have problems with your liver or have hepatitis.** Your doctor may want to do tests to check your liver while you take SUSTIVA.
- **have ever had mental illness or are using drugs or alcohol.**
- **have ever had seizures or are taking medicine for seizures** [for example, Dilantin (phenytoin), Tegretol (carbamazepine), or phenobarbital]. Your doctor may want to switch you to another medicine or check drug levels in your blood from time to time.

What important information should I know about taking other medicines with SUSTIVA?
SUSTIVA may change the effect of other medicines, including ones for HIV, and cause serious side effects. Your doctor may change your other medicines or change their doses. Other medicines, including herbal products, may affect SUSTIVA. For this reason, it is very important to:
- let all your doctors and pharmacists know that you take SUSTIVA.
- tell your doctors and pharmacists about all medicines you take. This includes those you buy over-the-counter and herbal or natural remedies.

Bring all your prescription and nonprescription medicines as well as any herbal remedies that you are taking when you see a doctor, or make a list of their names, how much you take, and how often you take them. This will give your doctor a complete picture of the medicines you use. Then he or she can decide the best approach for your situation.

Taking SUSTIVA with St. John's wort (*Hypericum perforatum*), an herbal product sold as a dietary supplement, or products containing St. John's wort is not recommended. Talk with your doctor if you are taking or are planning to take St. John's wort. Taking St. John's wort may decrease SUSTIVA levels and lead to increased viral load and possible resistance to SUSTIVA or cross-resistance to other anti-HIV drugs.

MEDICINES YOU SHOULD NOT TAKE WITH SUSTIVA
The following medicines may cause serious and life-threatening side effects when taken with SUSTIVA. You should not take any of these medicines while taking SUSTIVA:
- Vascor (bepridil)
- Propulsid (cisapride)
- Versed (midazolam)
- Orap (pimozide)
- Halcion (triazolam)
- Ergot medications (for example, Wigraine and Cafergot)

The following medicine should not be taken with SUSTIVA since it contains efavirenz, the active ingredient in SUSTIVA:
- ATRIPLA (efavirenz, emtricitabine, tenofovir disoproxil fumarate)

The following medicines may need to be replaced with another medicine when taken with SUSTIVA:
- Fortovase, Invirase (saquinavir)
- Biaxin (clarithromycin)
- Carbatrol, Tegretol (carbamazepine)
- Noxafil (posaconazole)

- Sporanox (itraconazole)
- REYATAZ (atazanavir sulfate), if this is not the first time you are receiving treatment for your HIV infection

The following medicines may require a change in the dose of either SUSTIVA (efavirenz) or the other medicine:
- Calcium channel blockers such as Cardizem or Tiazac (diltiazem), Covera HS or Isoptin SR (verapamil), and others.
- The cholesterol-lowering medicines Lipitor (atorvastatin), PRAVACHOL (pravastatin sodium), and Zocor (simvastatin).
- Crixivan (indinavir)
- Kaletra (lopinavir/ritonavir)
- Methadone
- Mycobutin (rifabutin)
- REYATAZ (atazanavir sulfate). If you are taking SUSTIVA and REYATAZ, you should also be taking Norvir (ritonavir).
- Rifadin (rifampin) or the rifampin-containing medicines Rifamate and Rifater.
- Selzentry (maraviroc)
- Vfend (voriconazole) and SUSTIVA must not be taken together at standard doses. Some doses of voriconazole can be taken at the same time as a lower dose of SUSTIVA, but you must check with your doctor first.
- Zoloft (sertraline)
- The immunosuppressant medicines cyclosporine (Gengraf, Neoral, Sandimmune, and others), Prograf (tacrolimus), or Rapamune (sirolimus).

These are not all the medicines that may cause problems if you take SUSTIVA. Be sure to tell your doctor about all medicines that you take.

General advice about SUSTIVA:
Medicines are sometimes prescribed for conditions that are not mentioned in patient information leaflets. Do not use SUSTIVA for a condition for which it was not prescribed. Do not give SUSTIVA to other people, even if they have the same symptoms you have. It may harm them.
Keep SUSTIVA at room temperature (77° F) in the bottle given to you by your pharmacist. The temperature can range from 59° to 86° F.
Keep SUSTIVA out of the reach of children.
This leaflet summarizes the most important information about SUSTIVA. If you would like more information, talk with your doctor. You can ask your pharmacist or doctor for the full prescribing information about SUSTIVA, or you can visit the SUSTIVA website at http://www.sustiva.com or call 1-800-321-1335.

SECTION 6

DIETARY SUPPLEMENTS

This section presents information on natural remedies and nutritional supplements marketed under the Dietary Supplement Health and Education Act (DSHEA) of 1994. The information on each product described has been provided by the manufacturer and contains the latest information available when *PDR®* went to press. Listings are arranged alphabetically by manufacturer; late submissions appear alphabetically by manufacturer at the end of this section.

The function of the Publisher is solely the compilation, organization, and distribution of this information on natural remedies and nutritional supplements. The Publisher does not assume, and expressly disclaims, any obligation to obtain and include any information on natural remedies and nutritional supplements other than that provided to it by the manufacturers. It should be understood that by making this material available, the Publisher is not advocating the use of any product described herein, nor is the Publisher responsible for misuse of a product due to typographical error. Additional information on any natural remedy and/or nutritional supplement product may be obtained from the manufacturer.

Products found in this section include herbal preparations, vitamins, minerals, and other substances intended to supplement the diet. The descriptions of these products are designed to provide the information necessary for informed use. Dietary supplements marketed under the DSHEA do not receive formal evaluation or approval from the FDA. The following disclaimer applies to all product information listed in this section, as mandated by the federal government: *These statements have not been evaluated by the Food and Drug Administration. This product is not intended to diagnose, treat, cure, or prevent any disease.*

4Life Research USA, LLC

9850 SOUTH 300 WEST
SANDY, UT 84070

Direct Inquiries to:
(801) 562-3600
Fax: (801) 562-3611
productsupport@4life.com
www.4life.com

4LIFE TRANSFER FACTOR®
TRI-FACTOR® FORMULA

PRODUCT DESCRIPTION

4Life Transfer Factor Tri-Factor Formula combines proprietary transfer factors and NanoFactor® molecules extracted from bovine colostrum and chicken egg yolk sources. These molecules contain antigen information which educates, enhances, and helps maintain immune system balance.

TECHNICAL DESCRIPTION

Transfer factors are molecules that communicate antigenic immunological information intercellularly and from a donor to a recipient. They support immune function through cell mediated immunity. Transfers factors, which carry antigen specific information to which all tested immune cells respond, are produced by mononuclear cells and serve to support and improve immune function through cell mediated pathways. Mammalian transfer factors, including those of humans are small molecules between 3,500 and 10,000 daltons.[1, 2] Transfer factors are polypeptides that consist of 40 to 44 amino acids [3] and have a conserved region and a variable region. From a molecular biological standpoint, these two properties are analogous to antibodies, however transfer factors' functions of cell mediated immunity (CMI) and non-specific immunological activity differ almost completely from the functions of antibodies. The molecules that have a molecular weight of less than 3,500 daltons modulate immune response but they do not transfer delayed-type hypersensitivity (DTH).[1]

4Life's transfer factors are sourced from the ultra-filtration of colostrum and from egg yolks.[4, 5] The molecules obtained from the spray dried ultra-filtrate of bovine colostrum are of two classes; the transfer factors present in the ultra-filtrate of ≤10,000 daltons and the nanofraction molecules that are present in the nano-filtrate of ≤ 3,500 daltons.

Transfer factors were first discovered in 1949 by H. Sherwood Lawrence when he demonstrated that CMI could be transferred from one individual to another by way of low molecular weight extracts of white blood cells. Transfer factors could transfer DTH of a specific form from a skin test positive individual to a skin test negative individual who subsequent to the transfer would skin test positive for that antigen.[6] In a subsequent study in 1955 he demonstrated that DTH could be passed serially, first from a skin test positive individual to a test negative individual, who became test positive, then 6 months later from the second individual to another test negative individual who became test positive.[7] At the time antibodies were the focus of immune research and little was known of the importance of DTH and of the involvement of T-cells in immune response. Transfer factors promote wellness via cell mediated immunity. These compounds are components of colostrum, an infant's first meal. They bridge the generational gap by passing cell mediated immunity from mother to infant.

BIOLOGICAL AND PHYSIOLOGICAL ACTION

Transfer factors' preparations contain more than 200 different moieties of polypeptide molecules with a molecular weight of <10,000 daltons; each moiety potentially having a great number of epitotic variations. These antigen specific factors are synthesized in monocytes and stored in the cytoplasm or on the cell membrane. A significant body of evidence indicates that the primary biological function of transfer factors is to recruit and specifically sensitize previously uncommitted lymphocytes. These sensitized T-lymphocytes initiate the events of cell-mediated immunity, thereby, promoting immunity not only at the site of antigen challenge but also throughout the body.[8] The effect of transfer factors on antigen mediated immunity, via B-cells, is not completely understood; however, clinical studies have reported an increase in particular antibodies, such as IgA and IgG, during transfer factor administration. Clinical studies have demonstrated that transfer factors' unique ability to express DTH and promote cell-mediated immunity can be transferred from a sensitized donor to a non-immune recipient.[1, 9] This antigen specific effect is well documented and is likely produced through activation

of the CD3-antigen site of T-cells, increased macrophage activation, and interleukin production—which can also enhance natural killer cell function.[1, 10]

Although the exact mechanism of action is unknown, research has shown that transfer factors will bind to antigens. However, the antigen specificity that is "transferred" to recipients is mediated by T-lymphocytes.[3] Current structure function models propose that transfer factors have a variable region and a conserved amino acid region, which determines the antigenic specificity for an estimated 8^{18} epitopes [1] and serves as a binding target for immune cell receptors, respectively.[2, 11] These highly conserved regions presumably allow transfer factors to be administered across a species barrier without any loss of potency. In fact, research has demonstrated that bovine transfer factors are structurally analogous to human-derived transfer factors with equivalent physiological activity. This is further supported by several studies, which used transfer factors extracted from bovine lymph nodes and colostrum to confer cell-mediated immunity to specific antigens in animals and human recipients.[12, 13]

Although most clinical trials with transfer factors have used parental administration; oral administration has also demonstrated successful transfer of DTH and cell mediated immunity in recipients.[14] Dose response studies, which compare various routes of administration, have been performed in both human and animals. Results of these experiments refute any arguments that the acidic or enzymatic environment of the gastrointestinal tract effects oral administration of transfer factors.[14]

CLINICAL AND EXPERIMENTAL STUDIES
Natural Killer Cell Activity

Peripheral blood mononuclear cells were isolated and pooled from several healthy donors. Sixty thousand cells were added to each well of a 96-well microtiter plate. Various immune modulating ingredients, including 4Life Transfer Factor® Tri-Factor® Formula, were added to select wells on the plate and a 48 hour incubation started. At the end of the incubation period 30 thousand K562 cells were added to each well. MTT assay techniques were used to determine the cytotoxic index. The various 4Life Transfer Factor products resulted in cytotoxic indices of 80-98%. By comparison, mononuclear cells incubated with IL-2 for the same 48 hour period produced a cytotoxic index of 88%.

CD4 T Helper Cell Research

Multiple studies were performed using the FDA-approved diagnostic CD4 T Helper cell assay kit and/or a T Cell Memory (CD8) assay kit under development by the same company. Similar to the NK cell research described above these *in vitro* studies were performed on 96-well microtiter plates measuring ATP production via a luciferase-based luminescence reaction.

The CD4 assay utilizes PHA-stimulated cells isolated from whole blood via the use of Dynabeads™. An 18 hour incubation of these isolated, stimulated CD4 cells with the 4Life Transfer Factor products has resulted in a modulation of immune cell activity as exhibited by a decrease in ATP production without a negative impact on cell viability. It is hypothesized that this reduction in ATP production is a result of a redirection in immune cell focus, essentially diminishing the distraction induced by the addition of PHA to the microtiter wells.

Salivary Secretory IgA–Preliminary Investigation

Twenty-four subjects naive to transfer factor supplementation were enrolled in a small-scale, preliminary study. Twenty-one were included in the final analysis. Salivary samples were collected from each subject weekly at roughly the same time of day and day of the week. Saliva was collected over a 5 minute period via passive drool while subjects chewed on a piece of Parafilm™. The samples were put on ice and then frozen at -70°C until assay. The commercial Salimetrics™ salivary IgA assay kit was used for analysis. Subjects were given 4Life Transfer Factor Tri-Factor formula at 2 capsules per day for two weeks and then transitioned to 4Life Transfer Factor® RioVida® Tri-Factor® formula at 60ml per day for an additional 2 weeks. At the end of the 4 week supplementation period the group showed an average 73% increase in salivary secretory IgA (SIgA) production over their baseline value. Furthermore, none of the 21 subjects showed a SIgA production rate less than their baseline value at the end of the study.

Wellness Research

A study conducted with 30 college students found that either 15 or 30 days of transfer factor administered according to label dose helped them maintain their health. Those that took the product for 30 days showed a prolonged health maintenance than those who took it for only 15 days.[15]

Longevity Studies

Two studies on the effects of 4Life Transfer Factor products on longevity were conducted. An initial, preliminary study was done on mice. This was followed up with a more intricate study on a small group of older men.

Groups of 20 mice each were compared in terms of organ weights, serum immune parameters, strength (dynamometer and hanging time), and isoproterenol-induced salivary hyperplasia. One group was injected with 4mg/kg of a product containing transfer factors. The treatment group showed improvements in all the aforementioned parameters. Isoproterenol-induced salivary gland hyperplasia declines with age. This diminished response is thought to be a consequence of decreased lymphoid cellular regulation of somatic tissue growth. The increased hyperplasia seen in the treatment animals approximated that seen in younger, untreated mice. There were no significant changes noted in height, weight, or rectal temperature between the two groups.[16]

Based on the results of this study an additional study was undertaken in 11 older men aged 55-73. Subjects were given 3 capsules per day of a product containing transfer factors 5 days a week for 6 weeks. At the end of the six week study period a determination of biological age using the Kiev method [17, 18] showed a reduction of approximately four years. There were significant improvements in several parameters of cardiovascular function, hearing, balance, vital lung capacity, ability to hold their breath, and some subjective measures.[16]

Safety

In a study of acute toxicity rats were assessed for fourteen days following a single gavage of 4Life Transfer Factor. Five female SD rats were each gavaged with a dose of 2,000mg/kg. No treatment-related mortalities occurred and there were no clinical signs of toxicity. No significant difference in body weights occurred. No gross lesions were found at necropsy in any of the animals. Thus, acute toxicity is considered to be greater than 2,000mg/kg.

Since the discovery of transfer factors in 1949 there have been no reports of allergic reactions [1] or of any side effects resulting from long-term use of 10 years or more.

The use of transfer factors is contraindicated in persons receiving immunosuppressive therapy, though actual interactions have not been documented.

HOW SUPPLIED

4Life Transfer Factor® can be found in the following products:

4Life Transfer Factor® Tri-Factor® Formula
4Life Transfer Factor Plus® Tri-Factor® Formula
4Life Transfer Factor® RioVida® Tri-Factor® Formula
4Life Transfer Factor® RioVida® Burst™ Tri-Factor® Formula
4Life Transfer Factor® Chewable Tri-Factor® Formula
4Life Transfer Factor® Classic
4Life Transfer Factor® Immune Spray
4Life Transfer Factor® KBU™
4Life Transfer Factor® Kids
4Life Transfer Factor® Belle Vie®
4Life Transfer Factor® Cardio
4Life Transfer Factor® GluCoach®
4Life Transfer Factor® MalePro®
4Life Transfer Factor® ReCall®

REFERENCES

1. Fudenberg, H. and G. Pizza, Progress in Drug Research, 1994. **42**: p. 309-400.
2. Lawrence, H.S. and W. Borkowsky, Biotherapy, 1996. **9**(1-3): p. 1-5.
3. Kirkpatrick, C.H., Mol Med, 2000. **6**(4): p. 332-41.
4. Hennen, W. and D. Lisonbee, U.P. Office, Editor. 2002, 4Life Research, LC: USA.
5. Wilson, G. and G. Paddock, U.P. Office, Editor. 1989, Amtron, Inc.: USA.
6. Lawrence, H.S., Proc Soc Exp Biol Med, 1949. **71**(4): p. 516-22.
7. Lawrence, H.S., J Clin Invest, 1955. **34**(2): p. 219-30.
8. Levin, A.S., L.E. Spitler, and H.H. Fudenberg, Annu Rev Med, 1973. **24**: p. 175-208.
9. Fudenberg, H. and H. Fudenberg, Ann Rev Pharmacol Toxicol, 1989. **29**: p. 475-516.
10. See, D., S. Mason, and R. Roshan, Immunol Invest, 2002. **31**(2): p. 137-53.
11. Dwyer, J.M., Biotherapy, 1996. **9**(1-3): p. 7-11.
12. Wilson, G.B., R.T. Newell, and N.M. Burdash, Cell Immunol, 1979. **47**(1): p. 1-18.
13. Radosevich, J.K., G.H. Scott, and G.B. Olson, Am J Vet Res, 1985. **46**(4): p. 875-8.
14. Kirkpatrick, C.H., Biotherapy, 1996. **9**(1-3): p. 13-6.
15. Klimov, V. and E. Oganova, in *Euromedica-Hannover 2004.* 2004: Hannover, Germany. p. 15-16.
16. Chizhov, A., et al., in *Euromedica. Hanover.* 2007: Hanover, Germany.
17. Agadzhanian, N., et al., ATMA, 1996.
18. Chebotarev, D., Annals of Gerontology and Geriatrics, 1984.

These statements have not been evaluated by the Food and Drug Administration. This product is not intended to diagnose, treat, cure of prevent any disease.

Alto Pharmaceuticals, Inc.

P.O. BOX 271150
TAMPA, FL 33688-1150
3172 LAKE ELLEN DRIVE
TAMPA, FL 33618

Direct Inquiries to:
John J. Cullaro
Customer Service
ALTOPHARM@AOL.COM
Tel (800) 330-2891
Fax (813) 968-0527

ZINC-220® CAPSULES
[zĭnk]
(zinc sulfate 220 mg.)

COMPOSITION

Each opaque blue and pink capsule contains zinc sulfate 220 mg. delivering 78.5 mg. of elemental zinc. Zinc-220 Capsules do not contain dextrose or glucose. Inactive Ingredients dicalcium phosphate, cellulose, magnesium stearate, magnesium trisilicate and gelatin (capsule shell).

ACTION AND USES

Zinc-220 Capsules are indicated as a dietary supplement. Normal growth and tissue repair are directly dependent upon an adequate supply of zinc in the diet. Zinc functions as an integral part of a number of enzymes important to protein and carbohydrate metabolism. Zinc-220 Capsules are recommended for deficiencies or the prevention of deficiencies of zinc.

WARNINGS

Zinc-220 if administered in stat dosages of 2 grams (9 capsules) will cause an emetic effect. This product should not be used by pregnant or lactating women.

PRECAUTION

It is recommended that Zinc-220 Capsules be taken with meals or milk to avoid gastric distress.

DOSAGE

One capsule daily with milk or meals. One capsule daily provides approximately 523% times the recommended adult requirement for zinc.

HOW SUPPLIED

Product	NDC	SIZE
Zinc-220® Capsules	0731-0401-06	Unit Dose Boxes ... 100 (5×10×2)

Each Zinc-220® capsule is identified by the "ALTO" logo on one side and the number "401" on the other side of the capsule.

ALTO® Pharmaceuticals, Inc.

Shown in Product Identification Guide, page 305

Beach Pharmaceuticals

Division of Beach Products, Inc.
5220 SOUTH MANHATTAN AVENUE
TAMPA, FL 33611

Direct Inquiries to:
Richard Stephen Jenkins
(813) 839-6565
FAX (813) 837-2511

BEELITH Tablets
MAGNESIUM SUPPLEMENT
with PYRIDOXINE HCl
Each tablet supplies 362 mg (30 mEq) of magnesium and 25 mg of pyridoxine hydrochloride.

DESCRIPTION

Each tablet contains magnesium oxide 600 mg and pyridoxine hydrochloride (Vitamin B₆) 25 mg equivalent to Vitamin B₆ 20 mg. Each tablet yields 362 mg of magnesium and supplies 90% of the Adult U.S. Recommended Daily Allowance (RDA) for magnesium and 1000% of the Adult RDA for Vitamin B₆.

INACTIVE INGREDIENTS

FD&C Yellow No. 6, hydroxypropyl methylcellulose, magnesium stearate, microcrystalline cellulose, polyethylene glycol, sodium starch glycolate, titanium dioxide. May also contain D&C Yellow No. 10, FD&C Yellow No. 5 (Tartrazine), hydroxypropyl cellulose, polydextrose, stearic acid and/or triacetin.

INDICATIONS

As a dietary supplement for patients with magnesium and/or Vitamin B₆ deficiencies resulting from malnutrition, alcoholism, magnesium depleting drugs, chemotherapy, and inadequate nutritional intake or absorption. Also, increases urinary magnesium levels.

DOSAGE

One tablet daily or as directed by a physician.

DRUG INTERACTION PRECAUTION

Do not take this product if you are presently taking a prescription drug without consulting your physician or other health professional.

WARNINGS

Do not take this product if you are presently taking a prescription drug without consulting your physician or other health professional. Ask a physician before use if you have kidney disease or if you are on a magnesium-restricted diet. Excessive dosage may cause laxation. If pregnant or breast-feeding, ask a health professional before use. Keep out of the reach of children.

HOW SUPPLIED

Golden yellow, film-coated tablet with the letters **BP** and the number **132** imprinted on each tablet. Packaged in bottles of 100 (Item No. 0486-1132-01) tablets.

Shown in Product Identification Guide, page 307

J.R. Carlson Laboratories, Inc.

15 COLLEGE DRIVE
ARLINGTON HEIGHTS, IL 60004-1985

Direct Inquiries to:
Customer Service
(888) 234-5656
FAX: (847) 255-1605
www.carlsonlabs.com
For Medical Information Contact:
In Emergencies:
Customer Service
(888) 234-5656
FAX: (847) 255-1605

DDROPS
Dietary Supplement

DESCRIPTION

Pure, natural liquid vitamin D3 simply drops onto your food or tongue. Carlson Ddrops is highly concentrated: receive 400 IU, 1000 IU, 2000 IU or 4000 IU in only 1 drop. Vitamin D supports healthy immune system function, supports a healthy mood and promotes muscle strength.*
Ingredient: Vitamin D3
Other Ingredient: Fractionated Coconut Oil

DIRECTIONS

Take 1 drop (0.027 ml) once or twice daily or as directed by your health care professional. May be put on food or mixed in other liquids such as water or juice.

WARNINGS

KEEP OUT OF REACH OF CHILDREN. BOTTLE SHOULD BE STORED UPRIGHT BETWEEN 60°F AND 85°F.

HOW SUPPLIED

Supplied in 10 ml bottles 400 IU, 1000 IU, 2000 IU and 4000 IU
*These statements have not been evaluated by the FDA. These products are not intended to diagnose, treat, cure or present diseases.

Shown in Product Identification Guide, page 307

MED OMEGA™ FISH OIL 2800
[mĕd ōmĕga]
ORANGE FLAVOR
100 ML. (3.3 FL.OZ.)

DESCRIPTION

Supplement Facts		
Serving Size 1 Teaspoonful (5 ml)		Servings Per Container 20
Each Teaspoonful Contains		% D.V.
Calories (energy)	40	
Calories from Fat	40	
Total Fat	4 g	6%★
Saturated Fat	1 g	5%★
Polyunsaturated Fat	2 g	†
Monounsaturated Fat	1 g	†
Cholesterol	15 mg	5%
Vitamin E (d-Alpha Tocopherol)	10 IU	33%
Omega-3 Fatty Acids	2.8 g [2800 mg]	†
EPA (Eicosapentaenoic Acid)	1.2 g [1200 mg]	†
DHA (Docosahexaenoic Acid)	1.2 g [1200 mg]	†
Other Omega-3 Fatty acids	.4 g [400 mg]	†

★ Percent Daily Value is based on a 2000 calorie diet
† Daily Value (D.V.) not established

Other Ingredients: Natural orange flavor, natural tocopherols.
Promotes Heart, Brain & Joint Health*
From Norway:
The finest fish oil from deep, cold ocean-water fish. Concentrated to supply 2800 mg (2.8 grams) of total omega 3's per teaspoonful. Bottled in Norway to ensure maximum freshness. Refreshing natural orange taste.
PURITY GUARANTEED
This product is regularly tested (using AOAC international protocols) for freshness, potency and purity by an independent, FDA-registered laboratory and has been determined to be fresh, fully-potent and free of detrimental levels of mercury, cadmium, lead, PCB's and 28 other contaminants.

DIRECTIONS

Take one teaspoonful daily AT MEALTIME. Try it on popcorn & salads.
REFRIGERATE: To retain freshness after initially opening the bottle, keep refrigerated and preferably use within 60 days.

> *** This Statement has not been evaluated by the FDA. This product is not intended to diagnose, treat, cure or prevent any disease.**

Manufactured & bottled in Norway for
J.R. Carlson Laboratories, Inc.
Arlington Hts., IL 60004-1985
888-234-5656 • 847-255-1600 • www.carlsonlabs.com

CARLSON NORWEGIAN COD LIVER OIL
8.4 FL OZ (250 ml)
Dietary Supplement

DESCRIPTION

Carlson Cod Liver Oil comes from the livers of fresh cod fish found in the arctic ocean waters of Norway. The oil is separated from the liver tissues without the use of chemicals. To ensure the freshness of the oil, the air inside the bottle is replaced with nitrogen and natural-source vitamin E is added.

Supplement Facts
Serving Size
1 Teaspoonful (5 ml)

	Amount Per Teaspoonful	% DV
Calories	45	
Calories from Fat	45	
Total Fat	5 g	8%★
Saturated Fat	1 g	5%★
Cholesterol	20 mg	7%
Vitamin A	850 IU	17%
Vitamin D	400 IU	100%
Vitamin E (as d-alpha tocopheryl acetate, d-alpha tocopherol & mixed tocopherols)	10 IU	33%
Omega-3 Fatty Acids	1,100 mg	†
DHA (Docosahexaenoic Acid)	500 mg	†
EPA (Eicosapentaenoic Acid)	400 mg	†
ALA (Alpha Linolenic Acid)	40 mg	†
100% Norwegian Cod Liver Oil	4.6 g	†

★ Percent Daily Values are based on a 2000 calorie diet.
† Daily Value (DV) not established.

Other ingredients: Natural lemon flavor. Omega-3's reported as glyceride units.
Suggested Use: Take one teaspoonful daily AT MEALTIME. After initially opening the bottle, keep refrigerated and preferably use within 100 days.

PURITY GUARANTEED
This product is regularly tested (using AOAC international protocols) for freshness, potency and purity by an independent, FDA-registered laboratory and has been determined to be fresh, fully-potent and free of detrimental levels of mercury, cadmium, lead, PCB's and 28 other contaminants. Manufactured and bottled in Norway for J.R. Carlson Laboratories, Inc.

Arlington Hts., IL 60004-1985 • 847-255-1600 • 888-234-5656

SUPER OMEGA-3 GEMS™ FISH OIL CONCENTRATE
Dietary Supplement

DESCRIPTION
Medical Scientists Internationally are encouraging people to eat more fish. Fish body oil is the **MAJOR SOURCE** of the polyunsaturated Omega-3's **EPA** and **DHA**.
For those individuals who do not eat an oily fish diet, Carlson offers Omega-3's in easy-to-swallow soft gelatin capsules. Carlson **SUPER OMEGA-3 GEMS™** soft gels contain 1000 mg (1 gram) of a special concentrate of fish body oils from deep, cold water fish which are especially rich in the important Omega-3's EPA and DHA.
To Promote Cardiovascular, Joint, Brain & Vision Health**

Supplement Facts	Serving Size 1 Soft Gel	
	Amount Per Soft Gel	% DV
Calories	9	
Calories from Fat	9	
Total Fat	1 g	2%★
Vitamin E Natural (d-Alpha Tocopherol)	10 IU	33%
Omega-3 Fatty Acids (from fish oil)	600 mg	†
EPA (Eicosapentaenoic Acid)	300 mg	†
DHA (Docosahexaenoic Acid)	200 mg	†
Other Omega-3's	100 mg	†

★ Percent Daily Values are based on a 2,000 calorie diet.
† Daily Value (DV) not established.

Other Ingredients: Soft Gel Shell: Beef gelatin, glycerin, water.
Suggested Use: Take one to six soft gels daily, AT MEALTIME.

PURITY GUARANTEED
This product is regularly tested (using AOAC international protocols) for freshness, potency and purity by an independent, FDA-registered laboratory and has been determined to be fresh, fully-potent and free of detrimental levels of mercury, cadmium, lead, PCB's and 28 other contaminants. Preservative-free. Cholesterol-free. Gluten-free.
Distributed by Carlson Division of J.R. Carlson Laboratories, Inc., Arlington Heights, IL 60004-1985
888-234-5656 • www.carlsonlabs.com

> ** This Statement has not been evaluated by the FDA. This product is not intended to diagnose, treat, cure or prevent any disease.

CPH International Corp.
P.O. Box 11439
Oakland, CA 94611
U.S.A.

E-MAIL: CPHINTL@SBCGLOBAL.NET
FAX: (510) 352-6009

ALOPEX®/ROMIXON®/BETACARIN®/ SITOPRESIL®

DESCRIPTION
Androgenetic alopecia is the most common type of hair loss in men and women. The dermal papilla of the hair follicle over-expresses 5-alpha-reductase activity may results in alopecia. Natural beta-sitosterol and L-carnitine may be recommended for keeping a normal and healthy hair growth by up-regulation of proliferation and down-regulation of appotosis in follicular keratinocytes.*

INGREDIENTS
Beta-SIT® beta-sitosterol, Natu-Carin® L-carnitine, Alpha-Lipoic acid. Urtica Dioica Extract, Horsetail Extract, Kelp, Biotin, Zinc, Selenium, Magnesium Stearate, Stearic Acid, Cellulose, Silicon Dioxide, Food Colors.

RECOMMENDED USE
Take one tablet twice daily with water for adults.

WARNINGS
Consult a physician prior to use if pregnant or lactating, or taking a prescription medication.

HOW SUPPLIED
Bottle of 30.
*These statements have not been evaluated by the Food and Drug Administration. These products are not intended to diagnose, treat, cure or prevent any disease.

CATASOD®-OCUXTRA/OPTIGOLD®/ MACUTEIN MEGA-30MG PLUS MCT

DESCRIPTION
Lutein and Zeaxanthin are natural macular pigments found in human lenses and retinas. The MCT contained in Mega-30mg may enhance the absorption of lutein and zeaxanthin in intestinal lumen.*

INGREDIENTS
Lutein/Zeaxanthin, Vitamins & Minerals, MCT (Mega-30mg tablets), Cellulose, Stearic Acid, Silicon Dioxide, Magnesium Stearate, Potato Starch, HPMC, Food Colors.

RECOMMENDED USE
Take one 5mg tablet twice daily or one Mega-30mg per day with water for adults.

WARNINGS
Consult a physician prior to use if pregnant or lactating, or taking a prescription medication.

HOW SUPPLIED
Bottle of 30.
*These statements have not been evaluated by the Food and Drug Administration. These products are not intended to diagnose, treat, cure or prevent any disease.

SANITIN®/CERICAR®/CARMENTIN®/ DEMENCERIN®

DESCRIPTION
Acetyl-L-Carnitine may be related to healthy cognitive function through delaying the mitochondrial decay of aging. Omegalon® DHA is contaminant free (heavy metals, PCBs) and free of fishy smell.*

INGREDIENTS
Alcarin® Acetyl-L-Carnitine, Alpha-GPC Soy Extract, NATU-SOY-PS® Phosphatidyl Serine, Omegalon® DHA, Yeast RNA, L-Glutamic Acid, L-Tyrosine, L-Aspartic Acid, Vitamin B1, B6 & B12, Biotin, Soybean Oil, Gelatin, Glycerin, Water, Food Colors.

RECOMMENDED USE
Take one capsule twice daily with water for adults.

WARNINGS
Consult a physician prior to use if pregnant or lactating, or taking a prescription medication.

HOW SUPPLIED
Bottle of 30.
*These statements have not been evaluated by the Food and Drug Administration. These products are not intended to diagnose, treat, cure or prevent any disease.

SANOLIP®/TIOWAX®/WAXANER®/ NERVOX-NEUTROPIN®/NEUROFIT-MEGA®

DESCRIPTION
Natural hexacosanol may be related to the secretion of neurotrophic factors including NGF, IGF and BDNF on nerve regeneration. Alpha-lipoic acid is a natural antioxidant for maintaining healthy nervous functions.*

INGREDIENTS
Waxanol® hexacosanol, Alpha-lipoic acid, Nucleotides, Vitamin B1, B3 & B12, Olive Oil, Lecithin, Beeswax, Gelatin, Glycerin, Water, and Food Colors.

RECOMMENDED USE
Take one capsule twice daily with water for adults.

WARNINGS
Consult a physician prior to use if pregnant or lactating, or taking a prescription medication.

HOW SUPPLIED
Bottle of 30.
*These statements have not been evaluated by the Food and Drug Administration. not intended to diagnose, treat, cure or prevent any disease.

SERICAN®/UROPLAX®/PROSERIL®/ SITOMIX®

DESCRIPTION
Lower urinary tract symptoms (LUTS) attributable to benign prostatic hyperplasia (BPH) are the most common medical problems in aged men. Natural beta-sitosterol and some phytochemicals are recommended as daily supplements for the health of human prostate and urinary tracts.*

INGREDIENTS
Beta-SIT® beta-sitosterol, Quercetin, Stinging Nettle ext., Goldenrod ext., Juniper berry Ext., Pumpkin seed oil, Buchu ext, Soybean Oil, Beeswax, Gelatin, Glycerin, Water, Food Colors.

RECOMMENDED USE
Take one capsule twice daily with water for men.

WARNINGS
Consult a physician prior to use if taking a prescription medication.

HOW SUPPLIED
Bottle of 30.
*These statements have not been evaluated by the Food and Drug Administration. These products are not intended to diagnose, treat, cure or prevent any disease.

TOFIPAN®/TOFIPAN-Z®/FIBRINASE-PMS®/ ANDROMON®

DESCRIPTION

Natural dehydroepiandrosterone and vitex agnus-castus herbal extract may be recommended for menopausal women. TOFIPAN-Z is developed for aged men to support a healthy endocrinal system.*

INGREDIENTS

Natural dehydroepiandrosterone, vitex agnus-castus, herbs, Silicon Dioxide, Cellulose, Magnesium Stearate, Gelatin, Food Colors.

RECOMMENDED USE

Take one capsule twice daily with water for adults.

WARNINGS

Consult a physician prior to use if pregnant or lactating, or taking a prescription medication.

HOW SUPPLIED

Bottle of 30.
*These statements have not been evaluated by the Food and Drug Administration. These products are not intended to diagnose, treat, cure or prevent any disease.

XANTASIL®/NEOASTER®/VASCULAX®/ CHOROXAN®

DESCRIPTION

Age-related macular degeneration complicated by choroidal neovascularization (CNV) is the leading cause to severe vision loss and blindness. Astaxanthin is a natural red pigment produced by algae, which may be related to a wide variety of protective activities for choroidal and retinal tissues.*

INGREDIENTS

Astaxanthin, Quercetin, Omegalon® DHA, Lutein/ Zeaxanthin, Vit. A, C, E, B-Complex, Zinc, Manganese, Copper, Selenium, MCT, Soybean Oil, Beeswax, Gelatin, Glycerin, Water, Food Colors.

RECOMMENDED USE

Take one capsule twice daily with water for adults.

WARNINGS

Consult a physician prior to use if pregnant or lactating, or taking a prescription medication.

HOW SUPPLIED

Bottle of 30.
*These statements have not been evaluated by the Food and Drug Administration. These products are not intended to diagnose, treat, cure or prevent any disease.

Immunotec Inc.

300 JOSEPH CARRIER
VAUDREUIL-DORION, QC
CANADA J7V 5V5

For Direct Inquiries Contact:
450-424-9992 Ext 4453

IMMUNOCAL®
Nutraceutical
Glutathione precursor (Bonded cysteine™ supplement)
Powder Sachets

DESCRIPTION and CLINICAL PHARMACOLOGY

IMMUNOCAL® is a U.S. patented natural food protein isolate in the FDA category of GRAS (generally recognized as safe) which assists the body in maintaining optimal concentrations of glutathione (GSH) by supplying the precursors required for intracellular glutathione synthesis. It is clinically proven to raise glutathione values.

Glutathione is a tripeptide made intracellularly from its constituent amino acids L-glutamate, L-cysteine and glycine. The sulfhydryl (thiol) group (SH) of cysteine is responsible for the biological activity of glutathione. Provision of this amino acid is the rate-limiting factor in glutathione synthesis by the cells since bioavailable cysteine is relatively rare in foodstuffs

Immunocal® is a bovine whey protein isolate specially prepared so as to provide a rich source of bioavailable cysteine. Immunocal® can thus be viewed as a cysteine delivery system.

The disulphide bond in cystine is pepsin and trypsin resistant but may be split by heat, low pH or mechanical stress releasing free cysteine. When subject to heat or shearing forces (inherent in most extraction processes), the fragile disulfide bonds within the peptides are broken and the bioavailablility of cysteine is greatly diminished.

Glutathione is a tightly regulated intracellular constituent and is limited in its production by negative feedback inhibition of its own synthesis through the enzyme gamma-glutamylcysteine synthetase, thus greatly minimizing any possibility of overdosage.

Glutathione has multiple functions:

1. It is the major endogenous antioxidant produced by the cells, participating directly in the neutralization of free radicals and reactive oxygen compounds, as well as maintaining exogenous antioxidants such as vitamins C and E in their reduced (active) forms.
2. Through direct conjugation, it detoxifies many xenobiotics (foreign compounds) and carcinogens, both organic and inorganic.
3. It is essential for the immune system to exert its full potential, e.g. (1) modulating antigen presentation to lymphocytes, thereby influencing cytokine production and type of response (cellular or humoral) that develops, (2) enhancing proliferation of lymphocytes thereby increasing magnitude of response, (3) enhancing killing activity of cytotoxic T cells and NK cells, and (4) regulating apoptosis, thereby maintaining control of the immune response.
4. It plays a fundamental role in numerous metabolic and biochemical reactions such as DNA synthesis and repair, protein synthesis, prostaglandin synthesis, amino acid transport and enzyme activation. Thus, most systems in the body can be affected by the state of the glutathione system, especially the immune system, the nervous system, the gastrointestinal system and the lungs.

INDICATIONS AND USAGE

IMMUNOCAL® is a natural food supplement and as such is limited from stating medical claims per se. Statements have not been evaluated by the FDA. As such, this product is thus not intended to diagnose, cure, prevent or treat any disease. Glutathione augmentation is a strategy developed to address states of glutathione deficiency, high oxidative stress, immune deficiency, and xenobiotic overload in which glutathione plays a part in the detoxification of the xenobiotic in question. Glutathione deficiency states include, but are not limited to: HIV/AIDS, infectious hepatitis, certain types of cancers, cataracts, Alzheimer's Disease, Parkinsons, chronic obstructive pulmonary disease, asthma, radiation, poisoning by acetominophen and related agents, malnutritive states, arduous physical stress, aging, and has been associated with sub-optimal immune response. Many clinical pathologies are associated with oxidative stress and are elaborated upon in numerous medical references.

Low glutathione is also strongly implicated in wasting and negative nitrogen balance, notably as seen in cancer, AIDS, sepsis, trauma, burns and even athletic overtraining. Cysteine supplementation can oppose this process and in AIDS, for example, result in improved survival rates.

CONTRAINDICATIONS

IMMUNOCAL® is contraindicated in individuals who develop or have known hypersensitivity to specific milk proteins.

PRECAUTIONS

Each sachet of IMMUNOCAL® contains nine grams of protein. Patients on a protein-restricted diet need to take this into account when calculating their daily protein load. Although a bovine milk derivative, IMMUNOCAL® contains less than 1% lactose and therefore is generally well tolerated by lactose-intolerant individuals.

WARNINGS

Patients undergoing immunosuppressive therapy should discuss the use of this product with their health professional. Individuals with the autosomal-recessive metabolic disorder cystinuria, are at higher risk of developing cysteine nephrolithiasis (1–2% of renal calculi).

ADVERSE REACTIONS

Gastrointestinal bloating and cramps if not sufficiently rehydrated. Transient urticarial-like rash in rare individuals undergoing severe detoxification reaction. Rash abates when product intake stopped or reduced.

OVERDOSAGE

Overdosing on IMMUNOCAL® has not been reported.

DOSAGE AND ADMINISTRATION

For mild to moderate health challenges, 20 grams per day is recommended. Clinical trials in patients with AIDS, COPD, cancer and chronic fatigue syndrome have used 30–40 grams per day without ill effect. IMMUNOCAL® is best administered on an empty stomach or with a light meal. Concomitant intake of another high protein load may adversely affect absorption.

RECONSTITUTION

IMMUNOCAL® is a dehydrated powdered protein isolate. It must be appropriately rehydrated before use. Ideally consumed after mixing. If it is premixed for later consumption, it should be refrigerated and consumed shortly after mixing. DO NOT heat or use a hot liquid to rehydrate the product. DO NOT use a high-speed blender for reconstitution. These methods will decrease the activity of the product.

Proper mixing is imperative. Consult instructions included in packaging.

HOW SUPPLIED

10 grams of bovine milk protein isolate powder per sachet. 30 sachets per box.

STORAGE

Store in a cool dry environment. Refrigeration is not necessary.

Patent no.'s: 5,230,902 - 5,290,571 - 5,456,924 - 5,451,412 - 5,888,552

REFERENCES

1. Baruchel S, Viau G, Olivier R. et al. Nutraceutical modulation of glutathione with a humanized native milk serum protein isolate, Immunocal®: application in AIDS and cancer. In: Oxidative Stress in Cancer, AIDS and Neurodegenerative Diseases. Ed.; Montagnier L, Olivier R, Pasquier C. Marcel Dekker Inc. New York, 447–461, 1998
2. Bounous G, Kongshavn P. Influence of protein type in nutritionally adequate diets on the development of immunity. In Absorption and Utilization of Amino Acids Vol.II. Ed. M. Friedman. CRC Press, Inc., Fla. 2:219–32, 1989
3. Bounous G, Gold P. The biological activity of undenatured whey proteins: role of glutathione. Clin Invest Med 14:296–309, 1991
4. Bounous G, Baruchel S, Falutz J. Gold P. Whey proteins as a food supplement in HIV-seropositive individuals. Clin Invest Med. 16:3; 204–209, 1992
5. Bounous G. Whey protein concentrate (WPC) and glutathione modulation in cancer treatment. Anticancer Res. 20:4785–4792, 2000
6. Bounous G. Immunoenhancing properties of undenatured milk serum protein isolate in HIV patients. Int. Dairy Fed: Whey: 293–305, 1998
7. Bray T, Taylor C. Enhancement of tissue glutathione for antioxidant and immune functions in malnutrition. Biochem. Pharmacol. 47:2113–2123, 1994.
8. Droge W, Holm E. Role of cysteine and glutathione in HIV infection and other diseases associated with muscle wasting and immunological dysfunction. FASEB J: 11(13):1077–1089, 1997
9. Herzenberg LA, De Rosa SC, Dubs JG et al. Glutathione deficiency is associated with impaired survival in HIV disease. Proc Natl Acad Sci 94:1967–72, 1997
10. Kennedy R, Konok G, Bounous G et al.. The use of a whey protein concentrate in the treatment of patients with metastatic carcinoma: A phase 1-II clinical study. Anticancer Res. 15:2643–50, 1995
11. Lands LC, Grey VL, Smountas AA. Effect of supplementation with a cysteine donor on muscular performance. J. Appl. Physiol. 87:1381–1385, 1999
12. Locigno R, Castronovo V. Reduced glutathione System: Role in cancer development, prevention and treatment. International Journal of Oncology 19:221–236, 2001
13. Lomaestro B, Malone M. Glutathione in health and disease: pharmacotherapeutic issues. Ann Pharmacother 29: 1263–73, 1995
14. Lothian B, Grey V, Kimoff RJ, Lands. Treatment of obstructive airway disease with a cysteine donor protein supplement: a case report. Chest 117:914–916, 2000
15. Meister A. Glutathione. Ann Rev Biochem 52:711–60, 1983
16. Peterson JD, Herzenberg LA, Vasquez KK, Waltenbaugh C. Glutathione levels in antigen-presenting cells modulate Th1 versus Th2 response patterns. Proc. Natl. Acad. Sci. 95:3071–3076, 1998
17. Tozer RG, Tai P, Falconer W, Ducruet T, Karabadjian A, Bounous G, Molson J, Dröge W. Cysteine-rich protein reverses weight loss in lung cancer patients receiving chemotherapy or radiotherapy. Antioxidants & redox signalling. 10: 395–402, 2008.
18. Watanabe A, Higachi K, Yasumura S. et al. Nutritional modulation of glutathione level and cellular immunity in chronic hepatitis B and C. Hepatology. 24:597A, 1996
19. Witschi A, Reddy S, Stofer B, Lauterberg B. The systemic availability of oral glutathione. Eur. J. Clin. Pharmacol. 43:667–669, 1992.

Manufactured by Immunotec Inc.
Tel: 450-424-9992 Ext. 4453
www.immunocal.com

Kyowa Wellness Co., Ltd.
S-S-I CO., Ltd.
Ishikura Bldg. 3F3
5-2 Oodenma-Cho, Nihonbashi,
Chuo-Ku, Tokyo 103-001, Japan

Direct Inquiries to:
Consumer Relations
Tel: +81-3-3660-1235
Fax: +81-3-3660-1236
URL: http://www.s-s-i.jp

SEN-SEI-RO LIQUID GOLD™
Kyowa's Agaricus blazei Murill Mushroom Extract
100ml liquid
Dietary Supplement

SEN-SEI-RO LIQUID ROYAL™
Kyowa's Agaricus blazei Murill Mushroom Extract
50ml liquid (2 × concentrate of Liquid Gold, v/v)
Dietary Supplement

DESCRIPTION

Sen-Sei-Ro Liquid Gold™, a dietary supplement containing exclusively all natural, standardized extract of the Kyowa's cultured *Agaricus blazei* Murill mushroom is primarily used to reduce symptoms of fatigue, promote vitality and overall well-being, and support immune functions.† Normal immune function necessary for maintenance of vitality, energy, good health, and quality of life can decline with age. Major biomarkers for decreased immune function are diminished natural killer cell (NK) activity and reduced number of lymphocytes and macrophage cells. These cells, primarily attack diseased cells and thereby, maintain body homeostasis, promote health and quality of life. For the past half-century in Brazil and other countries, *Agaricus blazei* Murill mushroom has been used to restore vitality, and energy, and to serve as a potent tonic conducive to general health and aging concerns.†

CLINICAL TRIALS

Preclinical genetic toxicity studies in Ames' test, chromosome aberration, and micronuclei tests were negative. In addition, subchronic toxicity studies in F344 male and female rats and SPF-bred beagle dogs showed no toxicities based on a comprehensive microscopic pathology of all organs in both species. All GLP toxicity studies were in compliance to US, FDA guidelines.

The effectiveness of ABMK22 in Sen-Sei-Ro Gold™ and Sen-Sei-Ro Royal™ for health benefits were tested in several controlled pre- and clinical trials in animals and in humans.† Recent studies in Japan led researchers to report that in humans, ABMK22 in Sen-Sei-Ro Gold™ and Sen-Sei-Ro Royal™ enhanced NK cell activity, promoted maturation and activation of dendritic cells indicated by increased cell kill, elevated expression of CD80 and CD83 expressions (Biotherapy 15(4): 503–507, 2001), increased the number of macrophage (Anticancer Research 17(1A): 274–284, 1997; Japanese Association of Cancer Research, no. 2268, 1999) and tumor necrosis factor TNF-α (Japanese Association of Cancer Research, no. 1406, 1999; Japanese J. Veterinary Clin. Medicine 17(2):31–42, 1998).† Recently, the molecular basis of its potential mechanism(s) of action and the current safety status of the product was published (Jap. J. Complimentary Altern. Med. 6(2):75–87, 2009). Further clinical studies with Sen-Sei-Ro Gold™ and Sen-Sei-Ro Royal™ among 100 cancer patients undergoing chemotherapy in Korea have shown that NK cell activity were significantly enhanced, while NK cell activity in the placebo group was markedly diminished (Int. J. Gynecol. Cancer 14: 589–594, 2004).† This finding is further supported by a retrospective study of 782 cancer patients, who, after consumption of Sen-Sei-Ro products, demonstrated consumer's perception of relief of symptoms and functional well being (Cronbach's alpha: Relief of symptoms, $\alpha = .74$; Functional well being, $\alpha = .91$) (BMC Complimentary and Alternative Medicine, 7:32, 2008). Earlier and recent pre- and clinical studies in Japan and Korea led researchers to report that Kyowa's *Agaricus blazei* Murill mushroom extract can be part of an effective treatment for supporting the immune systems of cancer patients by stimulating the host defense system (Biotherapy 15(4): 503–507, 2001; Carbohydrate Res. 186(2): 267–273, 1989; Japanese J. Pharmacology 662: 265–271, 1994; Agricultural and Biological Chemistry 54: 2889–2905, 1990).†

INGREDIENTS

Each 100ml heat-treated high pressure pack of all natural Kyowa's *Agaricus blazei* Murill water extract is scientifically standardized to contain 300mg% carbohydrate, 700mg% protein, 0mg% fat, 1.4mg% sodium, 0% food quality cellulose, and 4 Kcal energy.

Molecular weights of polysaccharopeptides range between 600~8,000. Water: 99.2g%, includes a variety of amino acids and vitamins (arginine 12mg%, lysine 6mg%, histidine 2mg%, phenylalanine 4mg%, tyrosine 4mg%, leucine 5mg%, isoleucine 3mg%, methionine 1mg%, valine 5mg%, alanine 13mg%, glycine 7mg%, proline 13mg%, glutamic acid 53mg%, serine 6mg%, threonine 5mg%, and asparagine 10mg%).

RECOMMENDED USE

As a dietary supplement, take 1~3 packs per day. Pour the liquid content into a cup or drink directly from the pack. Do not heat the pack either in a microwave oven or heating range or leave the pack open since the product does not contain any preservatives. If warming is necessary, place the pack in warm to mildly hot water for desired length of time. Once the pack is open, drink immediately.

ADVERSE REACTIONS

No subjects have reported any side effects since the dietary supplement was placed for consumers in Japan, and Korea for the past 18, and 10 years, respectively. The use of these dietary supplements (Sen-Sei-Ro Gold™, Royal™, and ABMK22) is generally safe based on FDA's INDA required tripartite genotoxicities, and 28-day subacute toxicity involving a comprehensive microscopic pathology of rats and dogs. In addition, two-year chronic toxicity studies of the products were carried out by Toxicology Research Center, which is both GLP (Good Laboratory Practice) and AAALAC (American Association of Accreditation of Laboratory Animal Certification) certified. Toxicity evaluation of general, CNS, reproductive and developmental, cardiovascular, immunology, and the two-year bioassay for carcinogenicity was negative. Recent clinical studies with 100 cancer patients undergoing chemotherapy in Korea have shown no known side effects or contraindications (Int. J. Gynecol. Cancer 14: 589–594, 2004).†

WARNINGS

Sen-Sei-Ro Liquid Gold™ and Sen-Sei-Ro Liquid Royal™ have not been evaluated in children or pregnant and breast feeding mothers. Both should consult a physician prior to use. Also consult a physician prior to use if taking a prescription medication. **Keep this product out of the reach of children. Do not use if you are pregnant, can become pregnant or are breast feeding.** Quality of the dietary supplement is guaranteed for 2 years from the manufactured date, but for more information, please write or call 81-72-257-8568 or 81-3-3512-5032.

HOW SUPPLIED

Sen-Sei-Ro Liquid Gold™ 100ml and Sen-Sei-Ro Liquid Royal™ 50ml in water extract are high pressure heat sealed. A box contains 30, 100ml packs, and can be purchased directly from company representatives, health food stores, and independent pharmacies. Store at room temperature and avoid any direct heat or sun light.

† These statements have not been evaluated by the Food and Drug Administration. These products are not intended to diagnose, treat, cure or prevent any disease.

Shown in Product Identification Guide, page 310

SEN-SEI-RO POWDER GOLD™
KYOWA'S Agaricus blazei Murill Mushroom
1800mg standard granulated powder
Dietary Supplement

DESCRIPTION

Sen-Sei-Ro Powder Gold™ slim pack, a dietary supplement containing an exclusively all natural and prepared from Kyowa's *Agaricus blazei* Murill mushroom is primarily used to reduce symptoms of fatigue, promote vitality and overall well-being, and support immune functions.† Normal immune function necessary for maintenance of vitality, energy, good health, and quality of life can decline with age. Major biomarkers for decreased immune function are diminished natural killer cell (NK) activity and reduced number of lymphocytes and macrophage cells. These cells, primarily attack diseased cells and thereby, maintain body homeostasis, promote health and quality of life. For the past half-century in Brazil and other countries, *Agaricus blazei* Murill mushroom has been used to restore vitality, and energy, and to serve as a potent tonic conducive to general health and aging concerns.†

CLINICAL TRIALS

Preclinical 2-year chronic cancer bioassay in compliance to FDA GLP Guideline demonstrated no increase in carcinogenicity in all Sen-Sei-Ro treated groups as compared to controls. Furthermore, survival of Sen-Sei-Ro consumed groups were increased by 20–34% over that of controls at the end of life-time feeding studies (2-years) and incidence of cataract in males at the end of 2-year study showed only 20–30% of controls thus demonstrating the highly significant impact of Sen-Sei-Ro on survival rate and prevention of cataracts (*SAS version* 9; p<0.006).†

The effectiveness of Sen-Sei-Ro Powder Gold™ for health benefits was tested in several controlled pre- and clinical trials in animals and in humans.† Recent studies in Japan, and Korea led researchers to report that in humans, Sen-Sei-Ro Powder Gold™ enhanced NK cell activity, increased the number of macrophage cells (Anticancer Research 17 (1A): 274–284, 1997; Japanese Association of Cancer Research, no. 2268, 1999) and tumor necrosis factor TNF-α (Japanese Association of Cancer Research, no. 1406, 1999).† Antitumor effects of Sen-Sei-Ro against various murine and dog tumors were thought to be mediated by stimulation of NK cell activity, increased number of macrophage cells, and increased activity of tumor necrosis factor TNF-α (Japanese J. Veterinary Clin. Medicine 17(2):31–42, 1998).† Recent clinical studies in Japan, and Korea, led researchers to report that *Agaricus blazei* Murill mushroom extract can be part of an effective treatment for supporting the immune systems of cancer patients by stimulating the host defense system (Biotherapy 15(4): 503–507, 2001; Carbohydrate Res. 186(2): 267–273, 1989; Japanese J. Pharmacology 662: 265–271, 1994; Agricultural and Biological Chemistry 54: 2889–2905, 1990).†

INGREDIENTS

Each 1800mg granulated powder in a slim pack contains 488 mg protein, 820 mg carbohydrate, 47 mg fat, 0.19 mg Sodium, 284 mg food grade cellulose, 5.7 kcal energy.

Water: 68mg, includes 0.1 mg Fe, 0.24 mg Ca, 37 mg K, 0.01mg thiamine, 0.04mg ergosterol, 0.59mg niacin.

RECOMMENDED USE

As a dietary supplement, take 1~3 packs per day. Pour the contents into a cup containing warm water or other desirable beverage, mix, and drink. Do not heat the pack either in a microwave oven or heating range or leave the pack open since the product does not contain any preservatives. Once the pack is open, consume immediately.

ADVERSE REACTIONS

No subjects have reported any side effects since the dietary supplement was placed for consumers in Japan and Korea for the past 18, and 10 years, respectively. The use of this dietary supplement is generally safe based on two-year chronic toxicity studies of the product by Toxicology Research Center, which is both GLP (Good Laboratory Practice) and AAALAC (American Association of Accreditation of Laboratory Animal Certification) certified. Toxicity evaluation of general, CNS, reproductive and developmental, cardiovascular, immunology, and the two-year bioassay for carcinogenicity were negative.†

WARNINGS

Sen-Sei-Ro Powder Gold™ has not been evaluated in children or in pregnant and breast feeding mothers. Both should consult a physician prior to use. Also consult a physician prior to use if taking prescription medications. **Keep this product out of the reach of children. Do not use if you are pregnant, can become pregnant or are breast feeding.** Quality of the dietary supplement is guaranteed for 2 years from the manufactured date, but for more information, please write or call 81-72-257-8568 or 81-3-3512-5032.

HOW SUPPLIED

Sen-Sei-Ro Powder Gold™ is high pressure heat sealed. A box contains 30 slim packs each with 1800mg per pack, and can be purchased directly from company representatives, health food stores, and independent pharmacies.

Store at room temperature and avoid any direct heat or sunlight.

†These statements have not been evaluated by the Food and Drug Administration. These products are not intended to diagnose, treat, cure or prevent any disease.

Shown in Product Identification Guide, page 310

Legacy for Life, LLC
P.O. BOX 14510
OKLAHOMA CITY, OK 73113

Direct Inquiries to:
1-800-557.8477
info@legacyforlife.net

www.LegacyforLife.net

www.HyperimmuneEgg.org

i26®
(polyvalent hyperimmune egg)
Dietary Supplement
Hyperimmune Egg (HIE) Powder

DESCRIPTION

i26 (polyvalent "hyperimmune" egg) is whole egg protein(HIE).1 Along with the generation of specific antibodies, increased levels of bioactive molecules are produced.2,3 In vitro, in vivo, and human trials, suggest that the naturally-occurring immune components in hyperimmune egg are utilized by the body to help it achieve immune homeostasis. The biological factors in i26 help the body maintain immune homeostasis by partnering to help it modulate immunological responses, especially those of an autoimmune or inflammatory nature.

BACKGROUND

Upon oral administration of hyperimmune egg, a wide range of immune components, both of a specific and non-specific nature, are passively transferred to the recipient. Although the intact immunoglobulins are confined to the lumen, other smaller, bioactive immune components may work systemically. This may occur: a) indirectly by activating cells in the GALT which then migrate with the appropriate message, or b) by directly crossing the GI barrier and circulating throughout the body to help it appropriately modulate immunological reactions.

STUDIES

Joint Comfort and Flexibility

An open-label clinical trial conducted at The Hospital for Special Surgery in New York, NYC, demonstrated that the daily consumption of 4.5g of HIE resulted in statistically significant changes in the daily aches and discomfort associated with daily life.4 Combining hyperimmune egg with certain forms of glucosamine-HCl results in a synergistic joint support effect.5

Circulatory and Cardiovascular Health

Hyperimmune egg has been demonstrated to help the body control several key indices of cardiovascular health both in vivo, and in a double-blind, placebo-controlled human trial.6,7

Gastrointestinal Health

Administration of hyperimmune egg significantly helps the body support healthy digestive function 8 and intestinal transit.9 It also appears to help maintain overall health of the gastrointestinal lining.10, 11

Maintaining Healthy Weight in Populations At Risk

Hyperimmune egg helps maintain or increase lean muscle mass in individuals experiencing involuntary weight changes.12-14

Quality of Life

Subjects with poor quality of life, that consumed 6.0g of hyperimmune egg showed marked changes in energy, weight, appetite, sleep quality, gastrointestinal and pulmonary areas as well as blood counts.12-14

Enhanced Athletic Performance, Stamina, Recovery

In a randomized, double-blind, placebo-controlled university trial, subjects utilizing 13.5g daily of hyperimmune egg experienced greater athletic performance as measured by endurance, recovery and strength. Hyperimmune egg appeared to help the body lower intrinsic heart rates, and stimulate muscle growth and repair resulting in better performance. Subjects reported higher levels of both anaerobic and aerobic performance, with less effort when using hyperimmune egg.15,16 Professional athletes report similar findings.

INDICATIONS AND USAGE

i26 is defined under the Dietary Supplements Health and Education Act (DSHEA) as a dietary supplement and as such is not intended to diagnose, prevent, treat, or cure disease. An independent panel of experts has conferred self-affirmed GRAS ("generally recognized as safe") status to hyperimmune egg. The FDA has issued a Food Master File Number for this ingredient.

Statements as to function have not been evaluated by the Food and Drug Administration but the following structure function claims for i26 have been submitted to the Agency:

Balances and supports the immune system

Helps the body maintain:

digestive tract health

flexible and healthy joints

healthy levels of cholesterol

cardiovascular function and healthy circulatory systems

Helps increase energy levels

Helps enhance a sense of well-being

Note: Hyperimmune egg may be used concomitantly with prescription medications.

CONTRAINDICATION

Hyperimmune egg is contraindicated in individuals with a history of extreme hypersensitivity or life-threatening allergy to orally administered egg.

PRECAUTIONS

Although reactions are rare, it is prudent for individuals with "sensitive" digestive systems to introduce hyperimmune egg gradually. Start with 0.5g (1/8 of a scoop) of i26/day for 3-4 days successively and double the amount every few days until desired serving is achieved. Diabetics may wish to monitor their blood glucose levels more frequently while introducing hyperimmune egg into their diets, since some individuals appear to reach glucose homeostasis rapidly as they start to approach immune homeostasis.

ADVERSE REACTIONS

Adverse reactions rarely occur. In two randomized double-blind, placebo-controlled trials (one with the US Military, the other at a University) the hyperimmune egg was well-tolerated. There was 82% compliance in a US Military study and 100% compliance in the University study.

ADMINISTRATION

Recommended servings are 4.5g-9g/daily for maintenance, more as desired. Some of the larger bioactive immune components in hyperimmune egg are heat-labile, but other than high temperature foods or beverages, HIE can be added to almost all other foods or beverages (e.g., puddings, yogurts, salads, juices, ice cream, etc.).

The equivalent of one serving (4.5g) of hyperimmune egg is found in: one scoop of i26, 9 capsules, 3 Chewables, 1 scoop of i26 COMPLETE Support, or 2 scoops of i26 FIT.

HOW SUPPLIED

- i26 - pure hyperimmune egg powder (31 servings)
- i26 Capsules – pure hyperimmune egg in capsules (15 servings)
- i26 Chewables- hyperimmune egg in flavored tablets (vanilla, banana) (15 servings)
- i26 COMPLETE Support – hyperimmune egg with vitamins and minerals (chocolate, strawberry, vanilla) (31 servings) [to be reconstituted with liquid]
- i26 FIT – hyperimmune egg with protein, fiber, vitamins and minerals (15 servings)
[to be reconstituted with liquid, preferably skim milk]

Stability and Storage

Store in a dry cool location with the lid tightly shut.

REFERENCES

1 Hens are stimulated multiple times with more than 26 whole inactivated bacteria of human interest including Salmonella, Staphylococcus, Streptococcus, Escherichia coli, Klebsiella pneumoniae, Pseudomonas, Proteus, Propionibacterium acnes, and Hemophilus influenzae.

2 US Patent # 6,420,337 Highly purified cytokine activating factor and methods of use

3 US Patent # 7,083,809 Purified cytokine inhibitory factor

4 Greenblatt HC Adalsteinsson O & L Kagen, Administration to Arthritis Patients of a Dietary Supplement Containing Immune Egg: An Open-Label Pilot Study, 1998 J Med Food 1:171

5 US Patent # 6,706,267 Glucosamine and egg for reducing inflammation

6 Wilborn WH Effect of Immune Egg Protein on Serum Cholesterol in Rabbits on Atherogenic Diets 1997 unpublished

7 Karge WH et al. Pilot Study on the effect of Hyperimmune Egg Protein on Elevated Cholesterol Levels and Cardiovascular Risk Factors 1999 J Med Food 2:51

8 Morningstar MW Hyperimmune Egg Powder For The Treatment Of Irritable Bowel Syndrome: A Case Series 2004 J Chiropr Med 3:12-4

9 Jacoby, HI Moore G and G Wnorowski Inhibition of Diarrhea by Immune Egg: A Castor Oil Mouse Model J Nutr Funct 2001 Med Foods 3:47

10 US Patent # 6,803,035 Anti-diarrheal and method for using the same

11 US Patent # 5,772,999 Method of Preventing, Countering or Reducing NSAID-Induced Gastrointestinal Damage by Administering Milk or Egg Products from Hyperimmunized Animals

12 Ambekar R Chungi V Hyperimmune Egg: Its Ability to Maintain Weight and Lean Muscle Mass in Individuals with Cachexia 1998 unpublished

13 Okullo J An Assessment of Effectiveness and Acceptability of immune26 in the Management of the Sick in Uganda 2002 unpublished

14 Kizito FB Improvements in Quality of Life for HIV/AIDS Patients Using Hyperimmune Egg (Immune 26™) — The TASO Study 3rd Inter AIDS Soc Conf HIV Pathogenesis and Treatment 2005 Abstract No. MoPe11.2C43

15 Scheett TM, et al. Hyperimmune Egg Protein Decreases Submaximal Heart Rate and Increases Peak Power 2007 Med Sci Sports Med Exerc 39:S365

16 Scheett TM, et al. Increased Muscular Strength and Enhanced Muscle Repair with Hyperimmune Egg Protein Supplementation 2007 J Strength Cond Res 21:e41

Shown in Product Identification Guide, page 310

Mericon Industries, Inc.

8819 N. PIONEER ROAD
PEORIA, IL 61615

Direct Inquiries to:
William R. Connelly
(309) 693-2150
FAX: (309) 693-2158

FLORICAL®
[*flor ĭ cal*]
(fluoride and calcium supplement)

ACTIVE INGREDIENTS

Florical contains 3.75mg fluoride (as sodium fluoride) and 145mg calcium (as calcium carbonate)

DESCRIPTION

Otosclerosis is an inherited disease of the small bones of the middle ear. Florical supports the stimulation of bone mineral density and supports the repair of small cracks (microfractures) in the small bones in the otic capsule. The leakage of enzymes that occurs at this time is also neutralized by Florical halting the progression of hearing loss in a large percentage of patients.[1]

SIDE EFFECTS

Gastrointestinal upset, joint pain. Most side effects can be alleviated by staying below 15mg elemental fluoride (4 capsules of Florical).

PRECAUTIONS

Florical should not be used in patients with a known allergy or hypersensitivity to any of its ingredients.

INDICATIONS

Florical may be used in otosclerosis.

DOSAGE

1–4 capsules daily as recommended by your physician. Use only one capsule daily during pregnancy.

These statements have not been evaluated by the FDA. This product is not intended to diagnose, treat, cure, or prevent any disease.

HOW SUPPLIED

Florical® is supplied as tablets or capsules in bottles of 100 or 500

NDC 00394-0102-02 (Capsules 100's)
NDC 00394-0102-05 (Capsules 500's)
NDC 00394-0100-02 (Tablets 100's)
NDC 00394-0100-05 (Tablets 500's)

[1]Causse, JR et al, Sodium Fluoride Therapy, The American Journal of Otology (14) Sep 1993, p. 482.

Shown in Product Identification Guide, page 310

MERIBIN®
(biotin 5mg)

DESCRIPTION

Biotinidase deficiency is an autosomal inherited disorder that is the cause of most cases of late-onset multiple carboxylase deficiency. Affected children usually exhibit seizures, hypotonia, developmental delay, ataxia, hyperventilation and/or coma between one week and two years of age. Visual and hearing abnormalities as well as alopecia, skin rash, conjunctivitis and recurrent infections often occur later.[1]

All symptomatic children have responded to pharmacologic doses of Meribin (biotin 5mg) with resolution of symptoms, with the exception of visual and hearing impairments and severe developmental delay.

ADVERSE REACTIONS

Urticaria and gastrointestinal upset have been reported.

PRECAUTIONS

Meribin should not be used in patients with known allergy or hypersensitivity to any of its ingredients.

INDICATIONS

Meribin is recommended as the product of choice for biotinidase deficiency.

DOSAGE

1 capsule daily. Capsule may be emptied into babies' bottles. Contents of capsule will pass through nipple of baby bottle.

HOW SUPPLIED

MERIBIN (biotin 5mg) is supplied in bottles of 120 capsules (120-day supply)

These statements have not been evaluated by the Food and Drug Administration. This product is not intended to diagnose, treat, cure, or prevent any disease.

[1]Bousounis, D.P., Canfield, P.R., Wolf, B. Reversal of Brain Atrophy with Biotin Treatment in Biotinidase Deficiency. Neuropediatrics 24 (1993) 214-217.

Pharmanex, LLC
75 WEST CENTER STREET
PROVO, UT 84601

For Information and Product Support:
Phone: 1-800-487-1000
Website: www.pharmanex.com

CORDYMAX® Cs-4®
[kŏr-dē-măks CS-4]
Dietary Supplement

DESCRIPTION
CordyMax® Cs-4® (Patent Pending) is a dietary supplement used to reduce symptoms of fatigue, and to promote vitality and overall well-being.* It is an exclusive fermentation product derived from the renowned *Cordyceps sinensis* mushroom.

INGREDIENTS
Each capsule contains 525 mg *Cordyceps sinensis* (Berk.) Sacc. mycelia (*Paecilomyces hepiali* Chen, Cs-4), standardized 0.14% adenosine and 5% mannitol.

RECOMMENDED USE
Take 2 capsules bid or tid with water and food.

WARNINGS
Keep out of reach of children. Consult a physician prior to use if pregnant or breastfeeding, or using anticoagulants, MAO inhibitors, or any other prescription medication. Discontinue use of this product 2 weeks prior to and after surgery.

HOW SUPPLIED
20–30 day supply, 120 count bottle.

LIFEPAK® ANTI-AGING FORMULA
[līf-păk]
Dietary Supplement

DESCRIPTION
LifePak® is a comprehensive nutritional wellness program, delivering the optimum types and amounts of vitamins, minerals, trace elements, antioxidants, and phytonutrients for general health and well-being. LifePak addresses all common nutrient deficiencies, provides key anti-aging nutrients that promote cellular protection, and supports cardiovascular health, bone metabolism, nutrient metabolism, and normal immune function.*

INGREDIENTS
LifePak provides an optimal blend of vitamins, minerals, trace elements, antioxidants, and phytonutrients. Contact Pharmanex for a detailed ingredient list.

RECOMMENDED USE
Take 1 packet bid with water and food.

WARNINGS
Keep this product out of reach of children. Consult a physician prior to use if pregnant or lactating, or taking a prescription medication. Discontinue use of this product 2 weeks prior to and after surgery.

HOW SUPPLIED
60 individual packets, 30 day supply. Additional LifePak® products include: LifePak® nano, Prime, Women, Prenatal, Teen, and Jungamals.

MARINEOMEGA™
[mă-rēn-ō-mě-gă]
Dietary Supplement

DESCRIPTION
MarineOmega™ is a dietary supplement of ultra-pure omega-3 (n-3) fatty acids formulated to promote normal immune function, cardiovascular health, joint mobility, brain function, and skin health*.

INGREDIENTS
Each softgel capsule contains 1,100 mg of Marine Lipid Concentrate (150 mg of EPA, 100 mg of DHA, and 50 mg of other Omega 3 Fatty Acids), 50 mg of krill oil, and 5 IU of Vitamin E (as Natural Mixed Tocopherols).

RECOMMENDED USE
Take 2 softgel capsules bid with water and food.

WARNINGS
Keep this product out of reach of children. Consult a physician if pregnant or lactating, taking anticoagulants, or any other prescription medication. Discontinue use of this product 2 weeks prior to and after surgery.

HOW SUPPLIED
30 day supply, 120 count bottle.

REISHIMAX GLp®
[rīsh-ĭ-măks GL-p]
Dietary Supplement

DESCRIPTION
ReishiMax® GLp is a proprietary, standardized extract of Reishi (*Ganoderma lucidum*) mushroom. ReishiMax supports healthy immune system function by stimulating cell-mediated immunity.*

INGREDIENTS
Each capsule contains 495 mg of standardized Reishi mushroom extract and 5 mg of Reishi cracked spores, standardized to 6% triterpenes and 13.5% polysaccharides.

WARNINGS
Keep out of reach of children. If you are pregnant or nursing, or taking a prescription medication, including immunosuppressive therapies, consult a physician before using this product. Discontinue use of this product 2 weeks prior to and after surgery.

RECOMMENDED USE
Take 1-2 capsules bid with water and food.

HOW SUPPLIED
15-30 day supply, 60 count bottle.

TeGREEN 97®
[tē-grēn 97]
Dietary Supplement

DESCRIPTION
Tegreen® is a standardized, decaffeinated polyphenol extract of fresh green tea leaves, with proven free radical scavenging and antioxidant properties.*

INGREDIENTS
Each 250 mg capsule contains a 20:1 extract of green tea leaves (*Camellia sinensis*) standardized to a minimum 97% pure polyphenols including 162 mg catechins, of which 95 mg is EGCg.

RECOMMENDED USE
Take 1–2 capsules bid with water and food. Maximum recommended dose of 4 capsules daily (1,000 mg). Do not exceed 1,200 mg green tea extract in combination with other green tea-containing supplements.

WARNINGS
Keep out of reach of children. Consult a physician prior to use if pregnant or lactating, taking anticoagulants, or other prescription medications. Discontinue use of this product 2 weeks prior to and after surgery.

HOW SUPPLIED
30-day supply, 30 and 120 count bottles.

---

*These statements have not been evaluated by the Food and Drug Administration. This product is not intended to diagnose, treat, cure or prevent any disease.

Tahitian Noni International, Inc.
333 WEST RIVER PARK DRIVE
PROVO, UT 84604 USA

Direct Inquiries to:
Phone: (801) 234-1000
Website: http://www.tahitiannoni.com

TAHITIAN NONI® ORIGINAL BIOACTIVE

DESCRIPTION
Tahitian Noni® Original Bioactive, an excellent source of bioactive iridoids, made from the fruits of *Morinda citrifolia* L, plant commonly known as noni. It has been demonstrated in various human clinical trials to be safe; increases antioxidant status in heavy smokers; protects DNA from aromatic DNA adducts in heavy smokers; lowers cholesterol, triglyceride, and homocysteine levels while increasing HDL cholesterol in smokers with elevated levels of cholesterol and triglycerides; improved joint health in people with neck pain; increases energy, antioxidant activity and endurance of highly trained athletes; modulates the immune system; lowers blood pressure in hypertensive subjects and does not contain illegal drugs or cause false positive results in performance enhancing drug tests.

Supplement Facts
Serving Size: 1 fluid ounce (30 ml)
Servings Per Container 33

Amount Per Serving	%Daily Value*
Calories 13	
Total Carbohydrate 3g	1%
Surgars 2g	†

*Percent Daily Values are based on a 2,000 calorie diet.
† Daily Value not established.

Ingredients: Reconstituted *Morinda citrifolia* fruit juice from pure juice puree from French Polynesia, natural grape juice concentrate, natural blueberry juice concentrate, and natural flavors. Not made from dried or powdered *Morinda citrifolia*.

HOW SUPPLIED
1 FL. OZ./30 mL daily.
Preferably before meals
Shake well before using and refrigerate after opening
Do not use if seal around cap is broken
Packaged by Tahitian Noni International, Inc.
Provo, UT 84604. USA.

REFERENCES
Tahitian Noni® Original Bioactive is Safe for Consumption. West et al. (2009). *Pacific Health Dialog*, 15 (2), 21-32.
Drinking up to 750 ml Tahitian Noni® Original Bioactive per day found to be safe, reduce the number of illness related events in a human clinical safety study involving 96 subjects.
Tahitian Noni® Original Bioactive Increases Antioxidant Status in Heavy Smokers.
Wang et al. (2009). *Chemistry Central Journal*, 3 (13), 1-5.
A double blind, placebo-controlled, one month trial with 285 people showed that as little as 1 fl. oz. per day lowered free radicals significantly while the placebo had no significant effect
Tahitian Noni® Original Bioactive Lowers Cholesterol and Triglyceride Levels in Current Smokers.
Palu et al., The 47th Annual Meeting of Society for Economic Botany. Chiang Mai, Thailand June 5-9, 2006. Wang et al. (2006). *Circulation* 113: E327.
Bioassays showed Tahitian Noni® Original Bioactive (TNJ) inhibited HMG-CoA Reductase, an enzyme involved in human cholesterol biosynthesis, by 50, 81 and 83%, respectively. A double blind, placebo-controlled clinical trial with 285 current smokers showed that drinking 4 ounces of TNJ daily for 4 weeks caused decreases in average cholesterol (from 235.2/dL to 190.2 mg/dL) and triglycerides and (from 242.5 mg/dL to 193.5 mg/dL).
Tahitian Noni® Original Bioactive Modulates Cholesterol Levels in Nonsmokers.
Palu et al. (2009). AGFD 146. *237th National Meeting of the American Chemical Society*, Salt Lake City, Utah, March 22-26, 2009.
A one month pilot study with 10 adult nonsmokers drinking Tahitian Noni® Original Bioactive showed that drinking 4 ounces modulate the already healthy cholesterol levels to remain within the healthy normal range, but had a mild cholesterol lowering & HDL raising effect in those who were within the high end range of normal, thus indicating an adaptogenic effect.
Tahitian Noni® Original Bioactive Modulates the Immune System and Increases Antioxidant Status.
Ma et al. (2008). Chinese Medical Research & Clinical, 6 (6), 8-10.
In a clinical trial with 12 people, drinking 330 mL Tahitian Noni® Original Bioactive per day for two months was found to increase adaptive immune system activity by 32% and innate immunity system activity by 30%, while it reduced oxidative stress by 19%.
Tahitian Noni® Original Bioactive Lowers High Blood Pressure.
Palu et al. (2008). ACS Symposium Series. Vol. 993: Functional Food and Health (pp. 446-453). American Chemical Society.
Tahitian Noni® Original Bioactive (TNJ) inhibited ACE enzymes and blocked AT_1 and AT_2 receptors concentration-dependently. An open label clinical trial of 10 hypertensive subjects showed consuming 4 ounces of TNJ per day for 1 month lowered average blood pressure from 144/83 (pretest) to 132/76 (post-test) without modification to their lifestyles.

IMPORTANT NOTICE: Updated drug information is sent bi-monthly via the PDR® Update Insert. For *monthly* email updates, register at PDR.net.

Tahitian Noni® Original Bioactive Increases Antioxidant Status and Improves Endurance in Highly Trained Athletes.
Palu et al. 2008. Journal of Medicinal Plant Research, 2 (7), 154-158.
In a placebo-controlled clinical trial involving 40 highly trained athletes, Tahitian Noni® Original Bioactive (TNJ) was shown to increase endurance by 21%, while it increased antioxidant status of the blood by 25%.
Tahitian Noni® Original Bioactive Health Effects on Cervical Spondylosis.
Akinbo et al. (2006). Nigerian Journal of Health and Biomedical Sciences, 5, 6-11.
A one month clinical trial with 90 cervical spondylosis patients found that drinking 30 mL of Tahitian Noni® Original Bioactive (TNJ) per day improved range of movement and pain in addition to further increased benefits from a combination of TNJ and standard therapy.
Tahitian Noni® Original Bioactive Does Not Contain Athletic Banned Substances.
Palu et al. (2008). Journal of Medicinal Plants Research 2(7): 154-158.
A pilot study with 6 people drinking Tahitian Noni® Original Bioactive revealed the absence of all performance-enhancing drugs and substances banned by the World Anti Doping Association.
Tahitian Noni® Original Bioactive Has DNA Protection Effects.
Wang et al. (2007). AACR Annual Meeting April 14-18. Los Angeles, CA
Drinking 1 or 4 ounces of Tahitian Noni® Original Bioactive (TNJ) was shown to reduced the amount of MDA caused DNA damage by 53% in a double-blind, placebo-controlled, one month clinical trial involving 203 current heavy smokers.
Tahitian Noni® Original Bioactive has a positive effect on postmenopausal women.
Langford et al. (2004). The Journal of Alternative and Complementary Medicine, 10, 737-742.
A three month, placebo controlled, pilot study, with 8 postmenopausal women showed that drinking 4 ounces of Tahitian Noni® Original Bioactive improved mood, energy, attenuated hearing loss, and showed evidence of potential anti-osteoporosis effect.
Tahitian Noni® Original Bioactive Is Safe for Human Consumption.
The EFSA Journal 2006, 376: 1-12.
The European Food Safety Authority reports, "it is unlikely that consumption of noni juice, at the observed levels of intake, induces adverse human liver effects."
Tahitian Noni® Original Bioactive Not a Significant Source of Potassium.
A case report stated that the potassium content of noni juice was 56.3 mEq/L, or 65 mg/ounce, and may be a "surreptitious" source of potassium for patients with renal disease. **(Mueller et al. Am J. Kidney Dis. 2000 35: 330–2).** Mueller **(USA Today, March 28, 2000)** clarified his research, stating he did not analyze TNJ (Tahitian Noni® Original Bioactive), but rather a different brand of noni juice and that the amount of potassium was only "as much as you'd get in 2 inches of banana."
Tahitian Noni® Original Bioactive Not a Significant Source of Potassium.
West et al. (2006). International Journal of Food Sciences and Nutrition, 57(7/8), 556-558..
Potassium content of Tahitian Noni® Original Bioactive is 30-50 mg per 1 ounce serving. This is a minor source when compared with bananas, yogurt, and other significant dietary sources of potassium.
Tahitian Noni® Original Bioactive Does Not Contain Vitamin K.
Palu 'AK et al., Am J Hematol 2005 79: 79-82.
Vitamin K has not been detected in Tahitian Noni® Original Bioactive and in noni fruits from Tahiti.
***Source: USDA Nutrient Database for Standard Reference.**
Noni Fruits from Tahiti Contains Iridoids
Deng et al. (2010). Phytochemical Analysis. DOI: 10.1002/pca.1246
Chemical research has revealed that iridoids are the major bioactive phytochemicals in noni fruit from Tahiti. The presence of iridoids and their wide range of biological activities explain the health benefits of Tahitian Noni® Original Bioactive.

Shown in Product Identification Guide, page 319

TAHITIAN NONI® NONI LEAF SERUM

DESCRIPTION
In an exclusive process known only to Tahitian Noni International, we've extracted the juice of the long-treasured noni leaf and made it into a soothing balm. Especially for skin that's been exposed to the elements, this serum will condition and revitalize irritated, wind-chaffed, or sunburned skin with lasting relief.

Ingredients: TAHITIAN NONI® Exclusive Noni Leaf Formula [Purified Water, *Morinda citrifolia* (Noni) Leaf Juice, *Morinda citrifolia* (Noni) Leaf Extract, *Vanilla tahitensis* (Tahitian Vanilla) Fruit Extract], Pentylene Glycol, Propylene Glycol, SD Alcohol 40-B, PEG-400 Laurate and Laureth-4, Sodium Dehydroacetate, Disodium EDTA, Phenoxyethanol, Fragrance, Acrylates/C10-30 Alkyl Acrylate Crosspolymer, Potassium Hydroxide.
Suggested Use: Smooth over irritated skin as needed.
Storage: Keep tightly closed in a dry place; do not expose to excessive heat.

HOW SUPPLIED
1, 3 and 6 packs of cream, 1 oz/30 ml Packaged for Tahitian Noni International, a subsidiary of Morinda, Inc. Provo, UT 84604. USA.

REFERENCES
Tahitian Noni® Leaf Extract Topical Usage Promotes Wound Healing.
Palu et al, (2010). Phytotherapy Research. DOI: 10.1002/ptr.3150.
A noni leaf ethanolic extract demonstrated significant wound healing effects in the mouse cutaneous assay by doubling the wound closure rate with 5.4 CT_{50}.
Tahitian Noni® Leaf Extract Offers Skin Protection.
West et al. (2009). Journal of Natural Medicines, 63 (3), 351-354.
A clinical trial involving 25 people showed that noni leaf extracts protected the skin against ultraviolet (UV) induced redness and swelling by approximately 350%.
Noni Leaf Extracts Taken Internally Promotes Wound Healing.
Nayak BS et al. (2007). *eCAM*, 1-6.
The ethanolic extract from the noni leaf significantly enhanced wound contraction, decreased epithilialization time, and increased hydorxyproline, suggesting that noni leaf extract has wound healing properties.
Noni Leaf Preparation Has Tonic and Antiseptic Effect.
Mannetje L. *Morinda citrifolia* L. in: Plant-Resources of South-East Asia (Edit.: E. Westphal, P. and C. M. Jansen). Pudoc Wageningen 1989, p. 185-187.
A noni leaf preparation is used as a tonic and antiseptic. Leaves are placed directly on wounds and the leaf juice produces painkilling effects.
Noni Leaf Antibacterial Effects
Saludes JP et al. (2002). Phytother Res, 16, 683-685
Ethanol and hexane fractions from *Morinda citrifolia* leaf showed antitubercular activity by killing 89% of the bacteria *in vitro*, comparable to 97% kill by the anti-TB drug Rifampicin at the same concentration.
Noni Leaf Antioxidant Effects
West et al. (2009). International Journal of Food Science and Technology, 44, 2142-2146.
The aqueous infusion prepared from noni leaves from Tahiti exhibited greater radical scavenging (antioxidant) activity than green tea infusion. **Zin et al. (2006). Food Chem, 94, 169-178.** Methanol fractions from defatted noni leaf juice showed strong antioxidant activities comparable to that of alpha-tocopherol

Shown in Product Identification Guide, page 319

Unicity International
THE MAKE LIFE BETTER COMPANY
1201 NORTH 800 EAST
OREM, UT 84097

Direct Inquiries to:
(801) 226-2600
www.unicity.net
science@unicity.net

Products of Unicity International are distributed through independent distributors.

BIO-C™
[*bīō sē*]

DESCRIPTION
Bio-C™ is a vitamin C nutritional supplement.
Bio-C™ is a yellow, water-soluble, crystalline powder pressed into a tablet. Each Bio-C™ tablet consists of a proprietary blend of ascorbyl palmitate, calcium ascorbate, ascorbic acid, magnesium ascorbate and 75 mg of citrus bioflavonoids. In addition to the active ingredients, each 800 mg tablet contains dextrose, microcrystalline cellulose, silicon dioxide, magnesium stearate, and stearic acid.

BENEFITS AND RESEARCH
Vitamin C (ascorbic acid) is a water-soluble vitamin that is used in the body to form cartilage, collagen, muscles and blood vessels. Vitamin C is a potent antioxidant that can protect small molecules such as proteins, carbohydrates, nucleic acids and lipids from damage caused by free radicals that are generated through the course of normal metabolism or through exposure to external toxins and pollutants (e.g. ultraviolet radiation from the sun or smoking). Vitamin C can also regenerate other antioxidants like vitamin E. Additionally, vitamin C is required for the synthesis of carnitine, a molecule involved in the transport of fats across the mitochondrial membrane, as well as the synthesis of norepinephrine, a neurotransmitter.*

USAGE
Take one tablet morning and night with a meal.

SAFETY AND WARNINGS
Bio-C™ is well tolerated. Some gastrointestinal discomfort may be experienced as with any dietary supplement.

HOW SUPPLIED
Available in tablets.

REFERENCES

Carr, AC and Frei B. (1999), American Journal of Clinical Nutrition 96: 1086-1107.
Jacob, RA and Sotoudeh G. (2002), Nutrition in Clinical Care 5: 66-74.
Deruelle F, Baron B. (2008), Journal of Alternative and Complementary Medicine 14:1291-1298.
Levine M, Rumsey SC, Daruwala R, Park JB, Wang Y. (1999), The Journal of the American Medical Association 281: 1415-1423.

* THESE STATEMENTS HAVE NOT BEEN EVALUATED BY THE FOOD AND DRUG ADMINISTRATION. THIS PRODUCT IS NOT INTENDED TO DIAGNOSE, TREAT, CURE, OR PREVENT ANY DISEASE.

BIOS LIFE® CARDIO
[*bī-ōs līf kärd-ē-ō*]
Advanced Fiber and Nutrient Drink

DESCRIPTION
Bios Life® Cardio is a fiber based, vitamin rich nutritional supplement. Bios Life® Cardio contains a blend of soluble and insoluble fibers, phytosterols, policosanol, an extract of *Chrysanthemum morifolium*, vitamins, and minerals that when combined with a healthy diet and exercise may lower total serum cholesterol, lower triglyceride levels and reduce the risk of heart disease.
Bios Life® Cardio is light orange in color. It is a hygroscopic crystalline powder that is generally soluble in water. Each serving of Bios Life® Cardio contains 3 g of fiber, 1 g of phytosterols, 6 mg of policosanol, and 12.5 mg of an extract of *Chrysamthemum morifolium*. In addition to these active ingredients, each serving of Bios Life® Cardio contains maltodextrin, citric acid, orange juice powder, sucralose and orange flavor.

BENEFITS AND RESEARCH
It's estimated that Americans consume 10-12 g of total fiber per day, less than half the amount of the recommended daily intake. Epidemiological and clinical studies have correlated low daily fiber intake with higher incidences of hyperinsulinemia, hypercholesterolemia, and elevated risks of cardiovascular disease.
Bios Life® Cardio is a nutritional supplement designed to increased daily fiber intake. Each serving of Bios Life® Cardio contains three grams of dietary fiber. When taken three times a day this achieves nearly half of the recommended daily value of fiber. Fiber supplementation has been shown to decrease preprandial and postprandial glucose levels and lower LDL cholesterol and apolipoprotein B levels.
In addition to fiber supplementation, Bios Life® Cardio contains a patented blend of phytosterols, policosanol, *Chrysanthemum morifolium*, vitamins and minerals. This blend of ingredients optimizes cholesterol levels through a combination of four mechanisms. First, the soluble fiber matrix prevents cholesterol reabsorption in the gastrointestinal tract through bile-acid sequestration. Second, the phytosterols reduce dietary absorption of cholesterol. Third, policosanol inhibits hepatic synthesis of cholesterol mediated through HMG-CoA reductase. Fourth, *Chrysanthemum morifolium* provides phytonutrients that enhance conversion of cholesterol to 7-α-hydryoxycholesterol. The four mechanisms provide a synergistic approach to optimizing cholesterol levels. Research has shown that this product may serve as a first line treatment option for mild hypercholesterolemia, as well as adjunct therapy for lipid lowering pharmaceutical intervention.

SUGGESTED USAGE
Dissolve the contents of one packet or one scoop into 8 to 10 fl. oz. of liquid (water or juice) and stir vigorously. Drink immediately. Use 15-20 minutes prior to meals up to three times daily.

SAFETY AND WARNINGS

Bios Life® Cardio is well tolerated. There may be mild gastrointestinal discomfort, such as increased flatulence or loose stools, during the first month of initial use due to the increased uptake of dietary fiber. This GI disturbance usually disappears within the first thirty days. If the GI discomfort persists, reduce the number of servings of Bios Life® Cardio. If the GI discomfort further persists, stop taking the product and consult your physician. Taking this product without adequate liquid can result in complications. If you are a diabetic, consult a physician for proper use of this product, as the chromium may reduce the need for medication.

HOW SUPPLIED

Bios Life® Cardio is packaged in single-serving foil packets or in bulk canisters.

REFERENCES

Sprecher, DL and Pearce GL (2002), Metabolism 51: 1166–70.
Verdegem, PJE; Freed, S and Joffe D (2005), American Diabetes Assocation 65th Scientific Sessions, San Diego, CA.
Duenas, V; Duenas, J; Burke, E and Verdegem, PJE (2006), 7th International Conference on Arteriosclerosis, Thrombosis, and Vascular Biology, American Heart Association, Denver, CO.
Verdegem, PJE (2007), Current Topics in Nutraceutical Research 5: 1-6
US Patent 6,933,291.

* THESE STATEMENTS HAVE NOT BEEN EVALUATED BY THE FOOD AND DRUG ADMINISTRATION. THIS PRODUCT IS NOT INTENDED TO DIAGNOSE, TREAT, CURE, OR PREVENT ANY DISEASE.

Shown in Product Identification Guide, page 320

BIOS LIFE® SLIM™

[bī-ōs līf slim]

Advanced Fiber and Nutrient Drink

DESCRIPTION

Bios Life® Slim™ is a fiber-based, vitamin-rich nutritional supplement. Bios Life® Slim™ contains a blend of soluble and insoluble fibers, Unicity® 7× technology, phytosterols, policosanol, an extract of *Chrysanthemum morifolium*, vitamins, and minerals that when combined with a healthy diet and exercise may lower total serum cholesterol, reduce the risk of heart disease and help achieve and maintain a healthy body weight.

Bios Life® Slim™ is light orange in color. It is a hygroscopic crystalline powder that is generally soluble in water. Each serving of Bios Life® Slim™ contains 4 g of fiber, 1 g of phytosterols, 750 mg of Unicity 7×, 6 mg of policosanol and 12.5 mg of an extract of *Chrysanthemum morifolium*. In addition to these active ingredients each serving of Bios Life® Slim™ contains maltodextrin, citric acid, orange juice powder, sucralose and orange flavor.

BENEFITS AND RESEARCH

It's estimated that Americans consume 10-12 g of total fiber per day, less than half the amount of the recommended daily intake. Epidemiological and clinical studies have correlated low daily fiber intake with higher incidences of obesity, hyperinsulinemia, hypercholesterolemia, and elevated risks of cardiovascular disease.

Bios Life® Slim™ is a nutritional supplement designed to increase fiber intake. Each serving of Bios Life® Slim™ contains four grams of fiber. When taken three times a day this achieves half of the recommended daily value of fiber. Fiber supplementation has been shown to decrease preprandial and postprandial glucose levels; lower LDL cholesterol and apolipoprotein B levels; increase satiety and facilitate weight loss.

In addition to fiber supplementation, Bios Life® Slim™ contains a patented blend of phytosterols, policosanol, *Chrysanthemum morifolium*, vitamins and minerals. Bios Life® Slim™ facilitates weight loss through five distinct mechanisms. First, the soluble fiber matrix promotes an increase in satiety. Second, Bios Life® Slim™ improves cholesterol levels. Reduction in LDL content removes a potent inhibitor of lipolysis. Third, Bios Life® Slim™ improves blood glucose levels. Maintaining appropriate serum glucose levels reduces hyperinsulinemia and promotes insulin sensitivity. Reducing insulin levels permits fatty acid oxidation to occur. Fourth, Bios Life® Slim™ restores appropriate leptin signaling. Lastly, Bios Life® Slim™, reduces triglyceride levels allowing for leptin to cross the blood-brain barrier and effect its mechanism of action. Research has shown that this product may serve as a first line treatment option for mild hypercholesterolemia, as well as adjunct therapy for lipid lowering pharmaceutical intervention.

SUGGESTED USAGE

Dissolve the contents of one packet or one scoop into 8 to 10 fl. oz. of liquid (water or juice) and stir vigorously. Drink immediately. Use 15-20 minutes before meals up to three times daily.

SAFETY AND WARNINGS

Bios Life® Slim™ is well tolerated. There may be mild gastrointestinal discomfort, such as increased flatulence or loose stools, during the first month of initial use due to the increased uptake of dietary fiber. This GI disturbance usually disappears within the first thirty days. If the GI discomfort persists, reduce the number of servings of Bios Life® Slim™. If the GI discomfort further persists, stop taking the product and consult your physician. Taking this product without adequate liquid can result in complications. If you are a diabetic, consult a physician for proper use of this product, as the chromium may reduce the need for medication.

HOW SUPPLIED

Bios Life® Slim™ is packaged in single-serving foil packets or in bulk canisters.

REFERENCES

Sprecher, DL and Pearce GL (2002), Metabolism 51: 1166-70.
Verdegem, PJE; Freed, S and Joffe D (2005), American Diabetes Assocation 65th Scientific Sessions, San Diego, CA.
Slavin, JL, (2005) Nutrition 21: 411-418.
Delzenne NM, Cani PD, (2005) Current Opinion Clincal Nutrition & Metabolic Care 8: 636-640
Duenas, V; Duenas, J; Burke, E and Verdegem, PJE (2006), 7th International Conference on Arteriosclerosis, Thrombosis, and Vascular Biology, American Heart Association, Denver, CO.
Verdegem, PJE (2007), Current Topics in Nutraceutical Research 5: 1-6
US Patent 6,933,291.

* THESE STATEMENTS HAVE NOT BEEN EVALUATED BY THE FOOD AND DRUG ADMINISTRATION. THIS PRODUCT IS NOT INTENDED TO DIAGNOSE, TREAT, CURE, OR PREVENT ANY DISEASE.

Shown in Product Identification Guide, page 320

BONEMATE® PLUS

[bōn-māt plŭs]

Advanced Bone Health Formula

DESCRIPTION

BoneMate® Plus is specially formulated to help maintain optimal bone health.* It contains three forms of calcium and vitamin D to maximize absorption and aid in the support of healthy bones, teeth, nerves, heart, and muscle tissue.

BoneMate® Plus is a light gray in color and is soluble in water. Each serving of BoneMate® Plus contains the following active ingredients 600mg of calcium, 300mg of magnesium, 30 mg of vitamin C, 2000 IU of vitamin D, 0.5mg of boron, 5 mg of zinc, 1mg of manganese, 1mg of copper, and 20mg of vitamin K. In addition, it also contains the inactive ingredients microcrystalline cellulose, croscarmellose sodium, and magnesium stearate.

BENEFITS AND RESEARCH

Calcium is the most common mineral in the body. Almost 99% of the calcium in our body is found in the bones and teeth. Bone is a dynamic tissue that is constantly being remodeled throughout our lives. A chronically low calcium intake in growing individuals may prevent the attainment of optimal peak bone mass. Once peak bone mass has been achieved, inadequate calcium intake may contribute to accelerated bone loss and eventually to osteoporosis.

Vitamin D, a secosteroid that is produced by the body upon exposure to the sun, is required for optimal calcium absorption. To ensure that calcium absorption is not limited by inadequate vitamin D levels, BoneMate® Plus contains 2000 IU of vitamin D per serving. In addition to facilitating calcium absorption, Vitamin D has been shown to target over 2000 different genes in the body. Vitamin D deficiency has been associated with increased risks for heart disease, stroke, diabetes, depression, osteoarthritis, chronic pain, and osteoporosis.

USAGE

Take two tablets twice daily with a meal.

SAFETY AND WARNINGS

BoneMate® Plus is well tolerated. Some gastrointestinal discomfort may be experienced as with any dietary supplement. The Food and Nutrition Board of the Institute of Medicine has set the tolerable upper level (UL) of intake for calcium in adults at 2,500 milligrams (mg) of calcium/day.

HOW SUPPLIED

Available as tablets or as a powder.

REFERENCES

Weaver CM, Heaney RP. Calcium. In: Shils M, Olson JA, Shike M, Ross AC, eds. Modern Nutrition in Health and Disease. 9th ed. Baltimore: Williams & Wilkins; 1999: 141-155.
Heaney RP. Calcium, dairy products and osteoporosis. J Am Coll Nutr. 2000;19(2 Suppl):83S-99S.
Food and Nutrition Board, Institute of Medicine. Calcium. Dietary Reference Intakes: Calcium, Phosphorus, Magnesium, Vitamin D, and Fluoride. Washington, D.C.: National Academy Press; 1997:71-145.
Reid IR. Therapy of osteoporosis: calcium, vitamin D, and exercise. Am J Med Sci 1996;312:278-86. Food and Nutrition Board, Institute of Medicine. Calcium. Dietary Reference Intakes: Calcium, Phosphorus, Magnesium, Vitamin D, and Fluoride. Washington, D.C.: National Academy Press; 1997:71-145.

* THESE STATEMENTS HAVE NOT BEEN EVALUATED BY THE FOOD AND DRUG ADMINISTRATION. THIS PRODUCT IS NOT INTENDED TO DIAGNOSE, TREAT, CURE, OR PREVENT ANY DISEASE.

CARDIO-BASICS™

Caring for your heart*

DESCRIPTION

Cardio-Basics™ is a nutritional supplement that combines multivitamins, minerals and antioxidants to support the cardiovascular system.

Cardio-Basics™ is a light orange, water-soluble powder pressed into tablets. Each tablet of Cardio-Basics™ contains the following vitamins, minerals, amino acids and antioxidants: beta-carotene (vitamin A), thiamine (vitamin B1), riboflavin (vitamin B2), niacin (vitamin B3), calcium d-pantothenate (vitamin B5), pyridoxine hydrochloride (vitamin B6), folate (vitamin B9), cyanocobalamin (vitamin B12), ascorbic acid and ascorbyl palmitate (vitamin C), cholecalciferol (vitamin D), d-alpha-tocopherol (vitamin E), biotin, calcium, chromium, copper, magnesium, manganese, molybdenum, phosphorus, potassium, selenium, sodium, zinc, L-arginine, L-carnitine, L-cysteine, L-lysine, L-proline, inositol, coenzyme Q10, and maritime pine extract. In addition to those active ingredients each tablet also contains microcrystalline cellulose, sucrose, fatty acid esters, silicon dioxide, magnesium stearate, and maltodextrin.

BENEFITS AND RESEARCH

According to the Center for Disease Control and Prevention, one American will die every minute as a result of heart disease. Narrowing of the arterial walls can lead to blocked blood flow to the brain. A healthy lifestyle including being physically active, not smoking, and making good food choices can lead to a reduction of heart disease. Cardio-Basics™ provides the vitamins, minerals and antioxidants needed for a healthy heart. In clinical studies, participants using Cardio-Basics™ and Bio-C™ saw a significant reduction in arterial wall thickness, removal of calcification deposits and a reduced risk for cardiovascular disease when compared to the placebo group. Cardio-Basics™ provides the body with the necessary vitamins and minerals needed to support a healthy vascular system.*

SUGGESTED USE

Take two tablets daily with food.

SAFETY AND WARNINGS

Cardio-Basics™ is well tolerated. Some gastrointestinal discomfort may be experienced as with any dietary supplement.

HOW SUPPLIED

Available in tablets

REFERENCES

Niedzwiekcki, A, Rath, M. (1996) Journal of Applied Nutrition, 48: 67-78.
Jeejeebhoy, F, Keith, M, Freeman, M, Barr, A, McCall, M, Kurian, R, Mazer, D, Errett, L, (2002), American Heart Journal 143: 1092-1100.
Verdgem, PJE, Lonky, S, Curley, S. (2005) 7th Conference on Arteriosclerosis, Thrombosis and Vascular Biology.
Lloyd-Jones D, Adams R, Carnethon M, DeSimone G, Ferguson TB, Flegal K, Ford E, Furie K, Go A, Greenlund K, Haase N, Hailpern S, Ho M, Howard V, Kissela B, Kittner S, Lackland D, Lisabeth L, Marelli A, McDermott M, Meigs J, Mozaffarian D, Nichol G, O'Donnell C, Roger V, Rosamond W, Sacco R, Sorlie P, Stafford R, Steinberger J, Hong Y; (2009) Circulation, 119: 480-486.

* THESE STATEMENTS HAVE NOT BEEN EVALUATED BY THE FOOD AND DRUG ADMINISTRATION. THIS PRODUCT IS NOT INTENDED TO DIAGNOSE, TREAT, CURE, OR PREVENT ANY DISEASE.

CARDIO-ESSENTIALS

Caring for your heart*

DESCRIPTION

Cardio-Essentials is a nutritional supplement for the heart. Cardio-Essentials contains Coenzyme Q-10, L-carnitine, L-taurine and Hawthorn berry.

Cardio-Essentials is a light tan, water-soluble powder. Each capsule of Cardio-Essentials contains 100 mg of Coenzyme Q-10 and 3.5 g of a blend of L-carnitine, L-taurine, and Hawthorn berry. In addition to those active ingredients, each capsule also contains silicon dioxide, stearic acid and calcium silicate.

BENEFITS AND RESEARCH
One of the leading causes of congestive heart failure (CHF), left ventricular dysfunction, affects approximately 1.5% of the population in the United States. CHF patients with left ventricular dysfunction have reduced levels of Coenzyme Q-10, L-carnitine and L-taurine and have an enlarged left ventricle. In a clinical study, the combination of L-carnitine, L-taurine, and Coenzyme Q10 was shown to benefit congestive heart failure patients by reducing left ventricular size. These ingredients are known to be important in providing adequate energy for heart muscle. Cardio-Essentials provides adequate amounts of these ingredients, i.e. 100 mg of CoQ10 and Hawthorn extract is traditionally used in supporting the heart function.

SUGGESTED USE
Take three capsules twice a day with food.

SAFETY AND WARNINGS
Cardio-Essentials is well tolerated. Some gastrointestinal discomfort may be experienced as with any dietary supplement.

HOW SUPPLIED
Available in capsules

REFERENCES
Jeejeebhoy, F et al (2002), American Heart Journal 143 1092–1100.
* THESE STATEMENTS HAVE NOT BEEN EVALUATED BY THE FOOD AND DRUG ADMINISTRATION. THIS PRODUCT IS NOT INTENDED TO DIAGNOSE, TREAT, CURE, OR PREVENT ANY DISEASE.

CM PLEX™ AND CM PLEX™ CREAM
[CM plĕks]
Proprietary fatty acid blend to help alleviate symptoms of osteoarthritis*

DESCRIPTION
CM Plex and CM Plex Cream are a softgel and topical cream, respectively, that contain a proprietary blend of cetylated fatty acids, soy and fish oil.
CM Plex is an opaque powder that is insoluble in water. One softgel capsule of CM Plex contains 350 mg of cetylated fatty acids, 160 mg of soy oil and 25 mg of salmon oil. In addition to these active ingredients, each softgel capsule contains glycerin and St. John's Bread.
CM Plex Cream is an off-white powder that is insoluble in water. One gram of CM Plex Cream contains 7.7 mg of cetylated fatty acids and olive oil. In addition to these active ingredients CM Plex Cream also contains glyceryl stearate, glycerin, lecithin, tocopheryl acetate, benzyl alcohol, phenoxyethanol, carbomer, PEG-100 stearate, sodium hydroxide, methylparaben, propylparaben, butylparaben, ethylparaben, isobutylparaben and citrus aurantium bergamia (Bergamot) fruit oil.

BENEFITS AND RESEARCH
Cetyl myristoleate and related fatty acids have been proven to improve joint health through their anti-inflammatory effects. A clinical study indicated that subjects exhibited improvements in knee flexion compared to placebo. A second study indicated the cream is effective for improving knee range of motion, ability to climb stairs, rise from a chair and walk, balance, strength, and endurance.*

SUGGESTED USE
Softgels: Take one to two softgels three times daily with meals.
Cream: Apply generously onto clean skin and gently massage until the cream disappears. Repeat 3 to 4 times daily as necessary. For maximum results combine both products.

SAFETY AND WARNINGS
CM Plex Softgels and Cream are well tolerated. Some gastrointestinal discomfort may be experienced with CM Plex Softgels as with any dietary supplement.

HOW SUPPLIED
CM Plex is available in soft gels and as a topical cream.

REFERENCES
Hesslink, R et al (2002), Journal of Rheumatology 29, 1708–1712.
Kraemer, WJ et al (2004), Journal of Rheumatology 31, 767–774.
* THESE STATEMENTS HAVE NOT BEEN EVALUATED BY THE FOOD AND DRUG ADMINISTRATION. THIS PRODUCT IS NOT INTENDED TO DIAGNOSE, TREAT, CURE, OR PREVENT ANY DISEASE.
Shown in Product Identification Guide, page 321

IMMUNIZEN®
[ĭm mōō nĭ zĕn]

DESCRIPTION
Immunizen® is a nutritional supplement for boosting the immune system.
Immunizen® is a modestly water soluble, white crystalline powder. Immunizen® consists of a proprietary ingredient blend of colostrum, arabinogalactan, 1,3, 1,6 yeast beta-glucans and lactoferrin. In addition to the active ingredients, each 835 mg capsule of Immunizen® contains natural gelatin, stearic acid and silicon dioxide.

BENEFITS AND RESEARCH
Immunizen® combines the positive immune modulating effects of colostrum, arabinogalactans, yeast beta-glucans and lactoferrin to boost your body's natural defenses to foreign antigens. Colostrum is composed of immunoglobulins that bolster the body's immune system by providing immunity against various pathogens.
Beta-glucans are generally derived from the cell walls of the yeast species *Saccharomyces cerevisiae*. Beta-glucans are potent immuno-modulating agents that prime both the innate and adaptive immune systems.

USAGE
Take six capsules with water one to two hours before a meal for 10 days as needed.

SAFETY AND WARNINGS
Immunizen® is well tolerated. Some gastrointestinal discomfort may be experienced as with any dietary supplement.

HOW SUPPLIED
Available in capsules.

REFERENCES
Lilius EM, Marnila P. (2001), Current Opinion in Infectious Diseases 14:295-300.
Hammarström L, Weiner CK. (2008), Advances in Experimental Medicine and Biology 606: 321-343.
Chan GC, Chan WK, Sze DM. (2009), The Journal of Hematology and Oncology, 2: 25-
* THESE STATEMENTS HAVE NOT BEEN EVALUATED BY THE FOOD AND DRUG ADMINISTRATION. THIS PRODUCT IS NOT INTENDED TO DIAGNOSE, TREAT, CURE, OR PREVENT ANY DISEASE.

OMEGALIFE-3™
[ōmĕgā-līf 3]
Omega-3 Fatty Acid Supplementation

DESCRIPTION
OmegaLife-3™ is a blend of omega-3 fatty acids designed to help maintain healthy cardiovascular and cerebral function as well as aiding in the prevention of age-related macular degeneration.
OmegaLife-3™ is an amber-colored, semi-viscous, fat-soluble liquid. Each serving of OmegaLife-3™ contains the following active ingredients 800 mg eicosapentaenoic acid (EPA), 400 mg docosahexaenoic acid (DHA), and vitamin E. In addition, it also contains the inactive ingredients gelatin, glycerin, purified water, and orange oil. OmegaLife-3™ has been molecularly distilled to ensure exceptionally pure oil and includes orange oil to prevent a fishy after taste.

BENEFITS AND RESEARCH
Clinical research suggests that fish oil can help support proper brain and visual function. In 2002 the FDA approved supplementation of DHA in infant formula. DHA is potentially important in fetal and infant neural development, in that DHA and arachidonic acid have been shown to be incorporated into brain and retinal cell membranes—particularly during the third trimester and early infant life.
DHA is the predominant structural fatty acid in the central nervous system and in the retina of the eyes.
EPA supports the synthesis of important compounds in the body. EPA is the precursor of thromboxane and leukotriene, compounds involved in supporting healthy circulation. They also promote healthy blood vessels.*
Evidence is accumulating that increasing intakes of EPA and DHA can decrease the risk of cardiovascular disease by preventing arrhythmias, decreasing the risk of thrombosis, decreasing triglyceride levels, slowing the growth of atherosclerotic plaque, and decreasing inflammation.*
The U.S. Food and Drug Administration (FDA) has stated that, "Supportive but not conclusive research shows that consumption of EPA and DHA omega-3 fatty acids may reduce the risk of coronary heart disease."

USAGE
Take two softgels per day with a meal.

SAFETY AND WARNINGS
OmegaLife-3™ is well tolerated. Some gastrointestinal discomfort may be experienced as with any dietary supplement. Common side effects include a "fishy" taste upon eructation.

HOW SUPPLIED
Available in softgels.

REFERENCES
Barter P, Ginsberg HN. Effectiveness of combined statin plus omega-3 fatty acid therapy for mixed dyslipidemia. Am J Cardiol. 2008 Oct 15:102(8):1040-5.
Lee JH, Harris WS, et al. Omega-3 fatty acids for cardioprotection. Mayo Clin Proc. 2008 Mar;83(3):324-32.
SanGiovanni JP, Chew EY, Sperduto RD, et al. The relationship of dietary omega-3 long-chain polyunsaturated fatty acid intake with incident age-related macular degeneration: AREDS report no. 23. Arch Ophthalmol. 2008 Sep;126(9): 1274-9.
SanGiovanni JP, Parra-Cabrera S, Colditz GA, Berkey CS, Dwyer JT. Meta-analysis of dietary essential fatty acids and long-chain polyunsaturated fatty acids as they relate to visual resolution acuity in healthy preterm infants. Pediatrics 2000;105:1292-8.
Kris-Etherton PM, Harris WS, Appel LJ. Omega-3 fatty acids and cardiovascular disease: new recommendations from the American Heart Association. Arterioscler Thromb Vasc Biol. 2003;23(2):151-152.
* THESE STATEMENTS HAVE NOT BEEN EVALUATED BY THE FOOD AND DRUG ADMINISTRATION. THIS PRODUCT IS NOT INTENDED TO DIAGNOSE, TREAT, CURE, OR PREVENT ANY DISEASE.

BIOS LIFE® VISION ESSENTIALS™
[bī-ōs līf vizh-uhn ē-sen-shuhls]

Clinically proven to support healthy eyes and vision.*

DESCRIPTION
Bios Life® Vision Essentials™ is a nutritional supplement for maintaining healthy eyes. Bios Life® Vision Essentials™contains vitamin C, vitamin E, zinc, natural beta carotene, lutein, zeaxanthin, and anthocyanidins from wild bilberry, wild blueberry, strawberry, cranberry, elderberry and raspberries.
Bios Life® Vision Essentials™ is a purple crystalline powder that is water soluble. In addition to the active ingredients vitamin C, vitamin E, zinc, natural beta carotene, lutein, zeaxanthin, and anthocyanidins from wild bilberry, wild blueberry, strawberry, cranberry, elderberry and raspberries, each 425 mg capsule contains silicon dioxide, microcrystalline cellulose and is packaged in vegetarian capsules.

BENEFITS AND RESEARCH
Antioxidants from the carotenoid chemical family, such as beta carotene, lutein and zeaxanthin, play an important role in eye health. Clinical studies have demonstrated that lutein and zeaxanthin are concentrated to the retina and lens of the eye. Low concentrations of these compounds in the retina are associated with age-related macular degeneration (AMD). Supplementation with high levels of lutein can restore the lutein concentration in the retina. Further supplementation of vitamins C and E and A (in the form of beta-carotene) along with zinc, and copper delayed the onset of AMD. Additional support for the eyes comes from a proprietary berry blend included in Bios Life® Vision Essentials™. This proprietary berry blend contains anthocyanidins, anti-oxidant compounds that support the vasculature within the eye, reducing the risk for diabetic retinopathies.

USAGE
Take two capsules per day with a meal.

SAFETY AND WARNINGS
Bios Life® Vision Essentials™ is well tolerated. Some gastrointestinal discomfort may be experienced as with any dietary supplement.

HOW SUPPLIED
Available in vegetarian capsules.

REFERENCES
Krishnadev N, Meleth AD, Chew EY (2010) "Nutritional supplements for age-related macular degeneration." Current Opinion in Opthamology 21:184-189.
Ma L, Lin XM, Zou ZY, Xu XR, Li Y, Xu R. (2009) "A 12-week lutein supplementation improves visual function in Chinese people with long-term computer display light exposure." British Journal of Nutrition 102: 186-190.
Yagi, A, Fujimoto, K, Michihiro, K, Goh, B, Tsi, D, Nagai, H, (2009) "The effect of lutein supplementation on visual fatigue: A psychophysiological analysis". Applied Ergonomics 40:1047-1054.

Age Related Eye Disease Study Group, (2001) "A randomized, placebo-controlled, clinical trial of high-dose supplementation with vitamins C and E, beta carotene, and zinc for age-related macular degeneration and vision loss: AREDS report no. 8". Archives of Ophthalmology. 10: 1417-36.

* THESE STATEMENTS HAVE NOT BEEN EVALUATED BY THE FOOD AND DRUG ADMINISTRATION. THIS PRODUCT IS NOT INTENDED TO DIAGNOSE, TREAT CURE, OR PREVENT ANY DISEASE.

Upsher-Smith Laboratories, Inc.
6701 EVENSTAD DRIVE
MINNEAPOLIS, MN 55369

For Medical Information Contact:
Write: Medical Information Department
or call: (800) 654-2299
(during business hours-8:00 am to 5:00 pm CST)

SLO-NIACIN® TABLETS
[*slow-nI-a-sin*]
(polygel® controlled-release niacin)
Dietary Supplement
250 mg, 500 mg, 750 mg

DESCRIPTION
Slo-Niacin® Tablets are manufactured utilizing a unique, patented polygel® controlled-release delivery system. This exclusive technology assures the gradual and measured release of niacin (nicotinic acid) and is designed to reduce the incidence of flushing and itching commonly associated with niacin use. Slo-Niacin® Tablets are available in 250 mg, 500 mg, and 750 mg strengths.

SUGGESTED USE
Slo-Niacin® is a member of the vitamin B-complex group (nicotinic acid, vitamin B_3) and is suggested as a dietary supplement. This product has the advantage of a slower release of niacin than conventional dosage forms. This may permit its use by those who do not tolerate immediate-release tablets.

DIRECTIONS
250 mg: Adults—one Slo-Niacin® Tablet morning or evening, or as directed by a physician.
500 mg: Adults—one Slo-Niacin® Tablet morning or evening, or as directed by a physician.
750 mg: Adults—one Slo-Niacin® Tablet morning or evening, or as directed by a physician.
Before using more than 500 mg daily, consult a physician.
Note: Slo-Niacin® Tablets may be broken on the score line, but should not be crushed or chewed.
Store at controlled room temperature, 15-30° C (59-86° F).
INFO & TIPS ON FLUSHING
What is flushing?
Flushing is a common side effect of niacin therapy, including Slo-Niacin®. Flushing is associated with temporary itching and tingling, feelings of warmth and headache, particularly when beginning or increasing the dose. These effects seldom require discontinuation of niacin.
Tips to avoid flushing
• Talk to your healthcare professional about taking 1 aspirin or ibuprofen 30 minutes **before** taking Slo-Niacin® Tablets
• Take Slo-Niacin® Tablets with a low-fat snack and cold water
• Take Slo-Niacin® Tablets **before** going to bed
• **Do not** take Slo-Niacin® Tablets with spicy foods, alcohol, coffee, tea, or other hot drinks

CAUTION
Niacin may cause temporary flushing, itching and tingling, feelings of warmth and headache, particularly when beginning, increasing amount or changing brand of niacin. These effects seldom require discontinuing niacin use. Skin rash, upset stomach, and low blood pressure when standing are less common symptoms; if they persist, contact a physician.

WARNINGS
Slo-Niacin® Tablets should not be used by persons with a known sensitivity or allergy to niacin. Persons with heart disease, particularly those who have recurrent chest pain (angina) or who recently suffered a heart attack, should take niacin only under the supervision of a physician. Persons taking high blood pressure or cholesterol-lowering drugs should contact a physician before taking niacin because of possible interactions. Case reports of myopathy (unexplained muscle related complaints, including discomfort, weakness, or tenderness) have been documented with

the use of HMG-CoA Reductase Inhibitors in combination with lipid-altering doses of niacin therapy (≥1 gram of niacin per day). Do not take niacin unless recommended by and taken under the supervision of a physician if you have any of the following conditions: gallbladder disease, gout, arterial bleeding, glaucoma, diabetes, impaired liver function, peptic ulcer, pregnancy or lactating women. Increased uric acid and glucose levels and abnormal liver function tests have been reported in persons taking daily doses of 500 mg or more of niacin.
Discontinue use and consult a physician immediately if any of the following symptoms occur: persistent flu-like symptoms (nausea, vomiting, a general "not well" feeling); loss of appetite; a decrease in urine output associated with dark-colored urine; muscle discomfort such as tender, swollen muscles or muscle weakness; irregular heartbeat; or cloudy or blurry vision.
Keep out of reach of children.

INGREDIENTS
250 mg niacin (nicotinic acid), supplying 1,250% of the Daily Value (DV) for niacin.
500 mg niacin (nicotinic acid), supplying 2,500% of the Daily Value (DV) for niacin.
750 mg niacin (nicotinic acid), supplying 3,750% of the Daily Value (DV) for niacin.
Each tablet also contains: hypromellose, hydrogenated vegetable oil, silicon dioxide, magnesium stearate, glyceryl behenate, Red 40.
UPSHER-SMITH LABORATORIES, INC.
6701 Evenstad Drive
Maple Grove, MN 55369
©2002 Upsher-Smith Laboratories, Inc.
All Rights Reserved.
US Patents 5,126,145 and 5,268,181.
www.slo-niacin.com
1-800-654-2299
100792-02
Revised 0810

USANA Health Sciences, Inc.
3838 WEST PARKWAY BOULEVARD
SALT LAKE CITY, UT 84120-6336

Direct Inquiries to:
Ph: (801) 954 7860
Fax: (801) 954 7658

ACTIVE CALCIUM™

COMPOSITION
Each Active Calcium contains the following minerals:

Vitamin D3 (as Cholecalciferol)	100 IU
Vitamin K (as Phylloquinone)	15 mcg
Calcium (as Calcium Citrate and Carbonate)	200 mg
Magnesium (as Magnesium Citrate, Amino Acid Chelate and Oxide)	100 mg
Boron (as Boron Citrate)	0.33 mg
Silicon (as Silicon Amino Acid Complex)	2.25 mg

ADVANTAGES
Each tablet contains a balanced blend of calcium, magnesium, vitamin D, vitamin K, boron and silicon; six nutrients required for bone development, bone remodeling and skeletal health. This non-prescription product meets USP guidelines for potency (as applicable), uniformity and disintegration, and is manufactured according to pharmaceutical cGMP standards.

RECOMMENDED USE
Take 4 tablets by mouth daily, preferably with meals.

SUPPLIED
Capsule-shaped tablet, mottled greenish-white color, with clear film coating, and with USANA imprint. In bottle of 112 tablets.

CHELATED MINERAL
[*key'-lā-tĕd*]
mineral

COMPOSITION
Each Chelated Mineral contains the following minerals:

Calcium (As Calcium Citrate and Carbonate)	67.5 mg
Iodine (As Potassium Iodide)	75 mcg
Magnesium (As Magnesium Citrate and Amino Acid Chelate)	75 mg
Zinc (As zinc citrate)	5 mg
Selenium (As L-selenomethionine and Amino Acid Complex)	50 mcg
Copper (As Copper Gluconate)	0.5 mg
Manganese (As Manganese Gluconate)	1.25 mg
Chromium (As Chromium Polynicotinate and Picolinate**)	75 mcg
Molybdenum (As Molybdenum Citrate)	1.25 mcg
Boron (As boron citrate)	0.75 mg
Silicon (As Silicon Amino Acid Complex)	1 mg
Vanadium (As Vanadium Citrate)	10 mcg
Ultra trace Minerals	0.75 mg

**Licensed under U.S. Patent 4,315,927.

ADVANTAGES
Each tablet contains a complete and balanced blend of essential minerals in bioavailable forms. The Chelated Mineral is designed to be taken with USANA's Mega Antioxidant to provide a full complement of essential nutrients required for health. This non-prescription product meets USP guidelines for potency (as applicable), uniformity and disintegration, and is manufactured according to pharmaceutical cGMP standards.

RECOMMENDED USE
Take two (2) tablets twice daily, preferably with food.

SUPPLIED
Oblong shaped tablets, off-white color, with clear film coating with USANA imprint. In bottle of 112 tablets

---

COQUINONE® 30
[*cō'-kwi-nōn*]

COMPOSITION
Each CoQuinone 30 capsule contains the following:

Coenzyme Q10	30 mg
Alpha Lipoic Acid	12.5 mg

ADVANTAGES
CoQuinone 30 contains a hydrosoluble form of Coenzyme Q_{10} (CoQ_{10}) that is 2.5 times more bioavailable than material supplied in dry tablet/capsule formulas. The higher blood levels of CoQ_{10} supplied enhance mitochondrial production of ATP. CoQ_{10} is a rate-limiting factor in the electron transport chain involved in mitochondrial production of ATP. It is also involved in neutralizing free radicals generated during ATP production. As such, CoQ_{10} helps the body maintain healthy skeletal and cardiac muscle. Alpha lipoic acid is included in the formula as a lipid-soluble antioxidant to recycle CoQ_{10} from the prooxidant form to the antioxidant form. This non-prescription product meets USP guidelines for potency (where applicable), uniformity and disintegration, and is manufactured according to cGMP standards.

RECOMMENDED USE
Take 1 or 2 capsules by mouth daily.

SUPPLIED
Oval shaped, soft gelatin capsule, annatto-colored, opaque, imprinted with USANA in white edible ink. Capsules contain an orange colored liquid. In bottle of 56 soft-gel capsules.

MEGA ANTIOXIDANT
[*mě-gă aenti-ŏx'-si-dĕnt*]

COMPOSITION
Each Mega Antioxidant contains the following vitamins and Minerals:

Vitamin A (as beta carotene)	3,750 IU
Vitamin C (as Calcium, Potassium, Magnesium, & Zinc Ascorbates)	325 mg
Vitamin D3 (as Cholecalciferol)	450 IU
Vitamin E (as D-alpha Tocopheryl Succinate)	100 IU
Vitamin K (as Phylloquinone)	15 mcg
Thiamin (as Thiamine HCL)	6.75 mg
Riboflavin	6.75 mg
Niacin and Niacinamide	10 mg
Vitamin B6 (as Pyridoxine HCL)	8 mg
Folate (as Folic Acid)	250 mcg
Vitamin B12 (as Cyanocobalamin)	50 mcg
Biotin	75 mcg
Pantothenic Acid (as D-Calcium Pantothenate)	22.5 mg
Olivol ® (Olive Extract)	7.5 mg
Mixed Natural Tocopherols (D-gamma, D-delta, D-beta Tocopherol)	8.5 mg

Bioflavonoid complex (Rutin, Quercetin, Hesperidin, Green Tea Extract-Decaffeinate, Pomegranate Extract, Cinnamon Extract, Bilberry Extract)	49.5 mg
Inositol	37.5 mg
Choline Bitartrate	25 mg
N-Acetyl L-Cysteine	25 mg
Bromelain	12.5 mg
Alpha-Lipoic Acid	5 mg
Coenzyme Q10	3 mg
Turmeric Extract	3.75 mg
Lutein	150 mcg
Lycopene	250 mcg
Broccoli Concentrate	3.75 mg

ADVANTAGES

A comprehensive and balanced formula containing the essential vitamins and antioxidants at levels substantially higher than RDA amounts. In addition to the traditionally recognized essential nutrients, the formula contains a unique blend of dietary antioxidants including carotenoids, a bioflavonoid complex, a glutathione complex, and USANA's patented Olivol™ to provide full-spectrum antioxidant protection. This formula is designed to be taken with USANA's Chelated Mineral to provide a full compliment of essential nutrients required for health. This non-prescription product meets USP guidelines for potency (as applicable), uniformity and disintegration, and is manufactured according to pharmaceutical cGMP standards.

RECOMMENDED USE

Take two (2) tablets twice daily, preferably with food.

SUPPLIED

Oblong shaped tablets, mottled orange-brown color, with clear film coating with USANA imprint. In bottle of 112 tablets.

PROCOSA II

COMPOSITION

Each Procosa II tablet contains the following:
Vitamin C (As Calcium Ascorbate)	75 mg
Manganese (As Manganese Gluconate)	1.25 mg
Glucosamine Sulfate 2KCl (From Shrimp & Crab Shells)	500 mg
Turmeric Extract (*Curcuma longa L.*, Root)	125 mg
Silicon (As Silicon Amino Acid Complex)	0.75 mg

ADVANTAGES

A comprehensive joint health formula which combines a widely researched, clinically studied dose of Glucosamine Sulfate with Vitamin C, Manganese, and Silicon; three additional nutrients, necessary for the maintenance of healthy cartilage.

Procosa II also contains Turmeric Extract, a potent antioxidant that supports the body's inflammatory response processes. This non-prescription product meets USP guidelines for potency (as applicable), uniformity and disintegration and is manufactured according to pharmaceutical GMP standards.

RECOMMENDED USE

Take two tablets twice daily, preferably with meals

SUPPLIED

Oblong, orange-colored tablet, scored on one side. In bottle of 120 tablets.

PROFLAVANOL® C 100
[prō-flă' vi-nol]

COMPOSITION

Each Proflavanol C 100 tablet contains the following:
| Vitamin C (As Calcium, Potassium, Magnesium, Zinc Ascorbates) | 300 mg |
| Grape Seed Extract (*Vitis Vinifera L.*, Seeds) | 100 mg |

ADVANTAGES

A potent antioxidant formula combining the proanthocyanidins (bioflavonoids) from standardized grape seed extract with vitamin C in the form of ascorbate salts and ascorbyl palmitate. Proflavanol C 100 is designed to be taken as a stand-alone antioxidant, or preferably in combination with USANA's Mega Antioxidant and Chelated Mineral to provide additional antioxidant protection. This non-prescription product meets USP guidelines for potency (where applicable), uniformity and disintegration, and is manufactured according to pharmaceutical cGMP standards.

RECOMMENDED USE

Take 1–3 tablets by mouth daily.

SUPPLIED

Oblong, bilayer tablet, with clear film coating, with USANA imprint. In bottles of 56 tablets.

Westlake Laboratories, Inc.
24700 CENTER RIDGE ROAD
CLEVELAND, OH 44145

Direct Inquiries to:
Customer Service
(888) WSTLAKE (978–5253)
Fax (440) 835–2177
Internet: www.westlake-labs.com

AUTHIA® CREAM
TTFD & Methyl B₁₂ Supplement

DESCRIPTION

Thiamine (Vitamin B$_1$) disulfide and methyl Vitamin B$_{12}$ is a pink liposomal cream for topical application designed for transdermal delivery (TD) of the two vitamins. It has a mild odor due to its sulfur content.

CLINICAL OBSERVATIONS

TD application is a more efficient way of administering these vitamins and they are solely responsible for any therapeutic benefit from the cream. Use of TTFD has been shown to result in clinical improvement in 8 of 10 autistic children in a pilot study.

CONTRAINDICATIONS

None known other than a rare sensitivity to excipients in the cream. (Paraben Free)

ADVERSE REACTIONS

Occasional localized rash may result at the site of application. An abnormal metabolism of the patient may create a skunk-like odor. This gradually disappears as clinical improvement occurs and can often be modified by taking 10 mg of Biotin daily.

DOSAGE

¼ tsp. (approximately 1 ml) of AUTHIA® CREAM topically will provide a pharmacological dose of 1000 mcg methyl cobalamin and 50 mg TTFD. Usual dose is once to twice daily.

HOW SUPPLIED

AUTHIA® CREAM is supplied in a 2 oz. plastic tube that does not require refrigeration.
Also available in enteric coated tablets.
Covered by U.S. Patent Number 6,585,996
Shown in Product Identification Guide, page 321

BEVITAMEL®
[bĕ-vĭt 'ə-mĕl]
Melatonin-B-Vitamin Supplement

DESCRIPTION

Each tablet contains:

	Amount	% U.S. RDA*
Melatonin	3 mg	***
Methylcobalamin (Vitamin B12)	1000 µg	16667
Folic Acid	400 µg	100

* U.S. Recommended Daily Amount (RDA) established by the U.S. Food and Drug Administration (FDA).
*** The U.S.RDA has not been established by the U.S. FDA.

INDICATIONS

Bevitamel can be used to enhance the natural sleep process. Vitamin B12 and Folic Acid can be used to assist the metabolism of blood homocysteine.

CONTRAINDICATIONS

Product NOT intended for the treatment of Pernicious anemia

WARNINGS

Keep out of reach of children and store in a cool dry place. Tamper-resistant package, do not use if outer seal is missing or broken.

PRECAUTIONS

The dose size and timing may need to be adjusted by the physician to provide maximum effect for individual patients.
Individuals taking other medications, or with autoimmune, seizure or endocrine disorders and pregnant or lactating women, should consult a physician prior to use.

ADVERSE REACTIONS

None known.

DOSAGE AND ADMINISTRATION

One tablet sub-lingual approximately 30 minutes before bedtime as directed by a physician. Fractional tablets may be taken when indicated.

OVERDOSAGE

None known.

HOW SUPPLIED

BEVITAMEL is supplied as a pink bisected sub-lingual tablet (60 per bottle).
Shown in Product Identification Guide, page 321

ALCOHOL-FREE PRODUCTS

The following is a selection of alcohol-free products grouped by therapeutic category. This list is not comprehensive. Generic and alternate brands may exist. Always check product labeling for definitive information on specific ingredients.

Analgesics

Advil Children's Suspension	Wyeth Consumer
APAP Elixir	Bio-Pharm
Motrin Children's Suspension	McNeil Consumer
Motrin Infants' Suspension	McNeil Consumer
Silapap Infant's Drops	Silarx
Tylenol Children's Suspension	McNeil Consumer
Tylenol Extra Strength Solution	McNeil Consumer
Tylenol Infant's Suspension	McNeil Consumer

Antiasthmatic Agent

Dy-G Liquid	Cypress

Anticonvulsant

Zarontin Syrup	Pfizer

Antiviral Agent

Epivir Oral Solution	GlaxoSmithKline

Cough/Cold/Allergy Preparations

Accuhist PDX Drops Solution	Tiber
Alacol Solution	Ballay
Alacol DM Syrup	Ballay
Allanhist PDX Syrup	Allan
Andehist DM NR Syrup	Cypress
Andehist NR Syrup	Cypress
Aridex Solution	Gentex
Aridex-D Solution	Gentex
Baltussin Solution	Ballay
Banophen Elixir	Major
Benadryl Allergy Solution	Pfizer Consumer
Bromaline Syrup	Rugby
Bromaline DM Elixir	Rugby
Bromhist PDX Solution	Cypress
Bromhist Pediatric Solution	Cypress
Bromhist-DM Pediatric Syrup	Cypress
Bromhist-DM Solution	Cypress
Bromhist-NR Solution	Cypress
Bromhist-PDX Syrup	Cypress
Bromphenex DM Solution	Breckenridge
Bromphenex HD Solution	Breckenridge
Bromplex DM Solution	Prasco
Bromplex HD Solution	Prasco
Bromtuss DM Solution	Breckenridge
Broncotron Liquid	Seyer Pharmatec
Broncotron-D Suspension	Seyer Pharmatec
B-Tuss Liquid	Blansett

Carbaphen 12 Ped Suspension	Gil
Carbaphen 12 Suspension	Gil
Carbatuss Liquid	GM
Carbatuss-12 Suspension	GM
Carbatuss-CL Solution	GM
Carbetaplex Solution	Breckenridge
Carbetaplex TS Suspension	Breckenridge
Carbofed DM Syrup	Quality Care
Cardec DM Solution	Qualitest
Children's Dimetapp Cold & Allergy Solution	Wyeth Consumer
Children's Dimetapp Long Acting Cough Plus Cold Solution	Wyeth Consumer
Children's Dimetapp Nighttime Flu Syrup	Wyeth Consumer
Children's Dimetapp DM Cold & Cough Solution	Wyeth Consumer
Children's Mucinex Cold Solution	Reckitt Benkiser
Children's Mucinex Cough Syrup	Reckitt Benkiser
Children's Mucinex Multi-Symptom Cold & Alcohol Free	Reckitt Benkiser
Children's Mucinex Syrup	Adams
Chlordex GP Syrup	Cypress
Chlor-Mes D Solution	Cypress
Codal-DM Syrup	Cypress
Complete Allergy Elixir	Cardinal Health
Corfen DM Solution	Cypress
Coughtuss Solution	Breckenridge
Crantex HC Syrup	Breckenridge
Crantex Syrup	Breckenridge
Creomulsion Cough Syrup	Summit Industries
Creomulsion for Children Syrup	Summit Industries
Dacex-DM Solution	Cypress
Dallergy Solution	Laser
De-Chlor DM Solution	Cypress
De-Chlor DR Solution	Cypress
Dehistine Syrup	Cypress
Despec Liquid	International Ethical
Dex PC Syrup	Boca Pharmacal
Diabetic Tussin Cough Lozenges	Health Care Products
Diabetic Tussin Night Time Formula Solution	Health Care Products
Diabetic Tussin Solution	Health Care Products
Diabetic Tussin DM Solution	Health Care Products
Diabetic Tussin DM Maximum Strength Liquid	Health Care Products
Diabetic Tussin EX Liquid	Health Care Products
Dimetapp Decongestant Pediatric Drops	Wyeth Consumer

Cough/Cold/Allergy Preparations (Continued)

Donatussin Solution	Laser
Donatussin DC Syrup	Laser
Donatussin DM Solution	Laser
Donatussin DM Suspension	Laser
Donatussin DM Syrup	Laser
Double-Tussin DM Solution	Reese
Dynatuss EX Syrup	Breckenridge
Dynatuss HC Solution	Breckenridge
Father John's Medicine Plus Drops	Oakhurst
Ganidin NR Liquid	Cypress
Gani-Tuss NR Liquid	Cypress
Gani-Tuss-DM NR Liquid	Cypress
Genebronco-D Liquid	PGD
Genecof-HC Liquid	PGD
Genecof-XP Liquid	PGD
Genecof-XP Syrup	PGD
Genedel Syrup	PGD
Genedotuss-DM Liquid	PGD
Genepatuss Liquid	PGD
Genetuss-2 Liquid	PGD
Genexpect-DM Liquid	PGD
Genexpect-PE Liquid	PGD
Genexpect-SF Liquid	PGD
Giltuss Liquid	Gil
Giltuss Pediatric Liquid	Gil
Giltuss Ped-C Solution	Gil
H-C Tussive Syrup	Bryant Ranch
Histinex HC Syrup	Ethex
Histinex PV Syrup	Ethex
Hydramine Elixir	Quality Care
Hydro-Tussin HC Syrup	Ethex
Hydro-Tussin HD Liquid	Ethex
Hydro-Tussin XP Syrup	Ethex
Lodrane D Suspension	ECR
Lohist D Syrup	Larken
Lohist DM Syrup	Larken
Marcof Expectorant Syrup	Marnel
M-Clear Solution	McNeil, R.A.
Mintuss G Syrup	Breckenridge
Mintuss MR Syrup	Breckenridge
Mintuss MS Syrup	Breckenridge
Mintuss NX Solution	Breckenridge
Motrin Cold Children's Suspension	McNeil Consumer
Myhist-DM Solution	Larken
Myhist-PD Solution	Larken
Nalex DH Liquid	Blansett Pharmacal
Nalex-A Liquid	Blansett Pharmacal
Nasop Suspension	Hawthorn
Neotuss S/F Liquid	A.G. Marin

Neotuss-D Liquid	A.G. Marin
Norel DM Liquid	U.S. Pharmaceutical
Organidin NR Liquid	Meda
PediaCare Cough + Cold Children's Liquid	Johnson & Johnson Consumer
PediaCare Decongestant & Cough Liquid	Johnson & Johnson Consumer
PediaCare Long-Acting Cough Solution	Johnson & Johnson Consumer
PediaCare Multi-Symptom Cold Liquid	Johnson & Johnson Consumer
PediaCare Nightrest Liquid	Johnson & Johnson Consumer
Pediahist DM Syrup	Boca Pharmacal
Pedia-Relief Liquid	Major
Phena-HC Solution	GM
Phena-S Liquid	GM
Phena-S 12 Suspension	GM
Poly Hist DM Solution	Poly
Poly Hist HC Solution	Poly
Poly Hist PD Solution	Poly
Poly-Tussin Solution	Poly
Poly-Tussin AC	Poly
Poly-Tussin DHC	Poly
Poly-Tussin DM Syrup	Poly
Poly-Tussin HD Syrup	Poly
Poly-Tussin XP Solution	Poly
Pro-Clear AC Solution	Pro-Pharma
Prolex DM Liquid	Blansett Pharmacal
Pro-Red AC Solution	Pro-Pharma
Q-Tussin Liquid	Qualitest
Q-Tussin DM Liquid	Qualitest
Rescon-DM Liquid	Capellon
Rescon-GG Liquid	Capellon
Rindal HD Liquid	Breckenridge
Rindal HD Plus Solution	Breckenridge
Robitussin Chest Congestion Syrup	Wyeth Consumer
Robitussin Cough & Allergy Solution	Wyeth Consumer
Robitussin Cough & Cold CF Syrup	Wyeth Consumer
Robitussin Cough, Cold & Flu Nighttime Solution	Wyeth Consumer
Robitussin Cough & Congestion Liquid	Wyeth Consumer
Robitussin Cough DM Syrup	Wyeth Consumer
Robitussin Head & Chest Congestion PE Syrup	Wyeth Consumer
Robitussin Pediatric Cough & Cold CF Solution	Wyeth Consumer
Robitussin Pediatric Cough & Cold Long-Acting Solution	Wyeth Consumer
Robitussin Pediatric Night Relief Liquid	Wyeth Consumer
Ru-Tuss DM Solution	Carwin

Scot-Tussin Diabetes CF Liquid	Scot-Tussin
Scot-Tussin DM Solution	Scot-Tussin
Scot-Tussin Expectorant Solution	Scot-Tussin
Scot-Tussin Original Solution	Scot-Tussin
Scot-Tussin Senior Solution	Scot-Tussin
Siladryl Allergy Solution	Silarx
Sildec-PE Solution	Silarx
Sildec PE-DM Solution	Silarx
Siltussin DAS Liquid	Silarx
Siltussin DM DAS Cough Formula Syrup	Silarx
Siltussin SA Syrup	Silarx
Sudafed Children's Cold & Cough Solution	Johnson & Johnson
Sudafed Children's Solution	Johnson & Johnson
Sudatuss DM Syrup	PGD
Sudatuss-2 Liquid	PGD
Sudatuss-SF Liquid	PGD
Triant-HC Solution	Hawthorn
TriTuss Solution	Everett
Tusdec-DM Solution	Cypress
Tusnel Pediatric Solution	Llorens
Tusnel Solution	Llorens
Tussafed-EX Syrup	Everett
Tussafed-EX Pediatric Drops	Everett
Tussafed-HC Syrup	Everett
Tussafed-HCG Solution	Everett
Tussall Solution	Everett
Tussi-Pres Liquid	Kramer-Novis
Tussi-Pres Pediatric Solution	Kramer-Novis
Tylenol Cold Children's Suspension	McNeil Consumer
Tylenol Cold Infants' Drops	McNeil Consumer
Tylenol Cold Plus Cough Children's Suspension	McNeil Consumer
Tylenol Cold Plus Cough Infants' Suspension	McNeil Consumer
Tylenol Flu Children's Suspension	McNeil Consumer
Tylenol Flu Night Time Max Strength Liquid	McNeil Consumer
Tylenol Sinus Children's Suspension	McNeil Consumer
Vazol Solution	Wraser Pharm
Vicks 44E Pediatric Liquid	Procter & Gamble
Vicks 44M Pediatric Liquid	Procter & Gamble
Vicks Dayquil Multi-Symptom Liquid	Procter & Gamble
Vicks Nyquil Children's Liquid	Procter & Gamble
V-Tann Suspension	Breckenridge
Z-Tuss DM Syrup	Magna

Ear/Nose/Throat Products

4-Way Saline Moisturizing Mist Spray	Bristol-Myers
Ayr Baby Saline Spray	Ascher
Bucalcide Spray	Seyer Pharmatec
Bucalsep Solution	Gil
Bucalsep Spray	Gil
Cheracol Sore Throat Spray	Lee
Fresh N Free Solution	Geritrex
Gly-Oxide Solution	GlaxoSmithKline
Listermint Solution	Johnson & Johnson Consumer
Nasal Moist Gel	Blairex
Orajel Baby Day & Night Gel	Del
Orajel Baby Nighttime Teething Pain Medicine Gel	Del
OraMagic Plus Powder	MPM Medical
OraMagicRx Powder	MPM Medical
Tanac Liquid	Del
Throto-Ceptic Spray	S.S.S.
Triaminic Sore Throat Spray	Novartis Consumer
Vicks Sinex Spray	P&G Company
Vicks Sinex 12 Hour Spray	P&G Company
Zilactin Baby Extra Strength Gel	Zila

Gastrointestinal Agents

Axid Solution	Braintree
Colidrops Pediatric Drops	A.G. Marin
Colace Solution	Purdue
Gas Relief Solution	Perrigo
Imogen Liquid	PGD
Kaopectate Advanced Formula Suspension	Pharmacia Consumer
Liqui-Doss Liquid	Ferndale
Mylicon Infants' Drops	Johnson & Johnson/ Merck

Topical Products

Aloe Vesta 2-N-1 Antifungal Ointment	Convatec
Dermatone Lips N Face Protector Ointment	Dermatone
Dermatone Moisturizing Sunblock Cream	Dermatone
Dermatone Skin Protector Cream	Dermatone
Fresh & Pure Douche Solution	Unico
Handclens Solution	Woodward
Neutrogena Acne Wash Liquid	Neutrogena
Neutrogena Antiseptic Solution	Neutrogena
Neutrogena Clear Pore Gel	Neutrogena
Neutrogena T/Derm Liquid	Neutrogena
Neutrogena Toner Solution	Neutrogena
Podiclens Spray	Woodward
Sea Breeze Foaming Face Wash Gel	Clairol
Sportz Bloc Cream	Med-Derm
Tiger Balm Arthritis Rub Lotion	Prince of Peace

Alcohol-Free Products *(Continued)*

Vitamins/Minerals/Supplements

Adaptosode For Stress Liquid	HVS
Adaptosode R+R For Acute Stress Liquid	HVS
Apetigen Elixir	Kramer-Novis
Biosode Liquid	HVS
Detoxosode Products Liquid	HVS
Genesupp-500 Liquid	PGD
Genetect Plus Liquid	PGD
Multi-Delyn Liquid	Silarx
Multi-Delyn w/Iron Liquid	Silarx
Nutrivit Solution	Llorens
Poly-Vi-Sol Drops	Mead Johnson
Poly-Vi-Sol w/Iron Drops	Mead Johnson
Protect Plus Liquid	Gil
Strovite Forte Syrup	Everett
Supervite Liquid	Seyer Pharmatec
Suplevit Liquid	Gil
Tri-Vi-Sol w/Iron Drops	Mead Johnson
Vitafol Syrup	Everett

Miscellaneous

Cytra-2 Solution	Cypress
Cytra-K Solution	Cypress
Fluorinse Solution	Oral B
Namenda Solution	Forest
Primsol Solution	FSC

SUGAR-FREE PRODUCTS

The following is a selection of products by therapeutic category that contain no sugar. When recommending these products to diabetic patients, keep in mind that many may contain sorbitol, alcohol, or other sources of carbohydrates. This list is not all-inclusive and generics and alternate brands may be available. Check product labeling for a current listing of inactive ingredients.

Analgesics

Addaprin Tablets	Dover
Aminofen Tablets	Dover
Back Pain-Off Tablets ‡	Medique
I-Prin Tablets ‡	Medique
Medi-Seltzer Effervescent Tablets	Medique
Methadose Sugar Free Oral Concentrate	Mallinckrodt
Ms.-Aid Tablets ‡	Medique
Children's Silapap Liquid	Silarx

Antacids/Antiflatulants

Alcalak Chewable Tablets*† ‡ §	Medique
Diotame Chewable Tablets*† ‡ §	Medique
Pepto-Bismol Caplets † ‡	Procter & Gamble
Tums Extra Sugar Free Tablets* §	GlaxoSmithKline Consumer

Anti-asthmatic/Respiratory Agent

Jay-Phyl Syrup	JayMac

Antidiarrheal

Imogen Liquid	Pharm Generic

Blood Modifier/Iron Preparation

I.L.X. B-12 Elixir	Kenwood

Corticosteroid

Pediapred Solution* §	UCB

Cough/Cold/Allergy Preparations

Alacol DM Syrup	Ballay
Alacol Solution	Ballay
Aridex Solution	Gentex
Baltussin Solution	Ballay
Bromhist-DM Solution	Cypress
Bromhist Pediatric Solution	Cypress
Bromphenex DM Solution*† §	Breckenridge
Bromplex DM Solution*† §	Prasco
Broncotron Liquid	Seyer Pharmatec
Broncotron-D Suspension	Seyer Pharmatec
B-Tuss Liquid	Blansett
Carbaphen 12 Ped Suspension	Gil
Carbaphen 12 Suspension	Gil
Carbatuss-12 Suspension	GM
Carbatuss-CL Solution	GM
Carbetaplex Liquid* §	Breckenridge
Carbofed DM Liquid	Quality Care
Carbofed DM Syrup	Quality Care
Cardec DM Syrup	Qualitest
Cetafen Cough & Cold Tablets ‡	Hart Health and Safety
Cetafen Cold Tablets ‡	Hart Health and Safety
Cheratussin DAC Liquid	Qualitest
Chlordex GP Syrup	Cypress
Codal-DM Syrup	Cypress
Coldcough PD Syrup* §	Breckenridge
Coldcough Syrup* §	Breckenridge
Coldonyl Tablets	Dover
Corfen DM Solution	Cypress
Crantex Syrup	Breckenridge
Dallergy Drops*† §	Laser
De-Chlor DM Solution	Cypress
De-Chlor DR Solution	Cypress
Despec Liquid	International Ethical
Despec-SF Liquid	International Ethical
Diabetic Tussin	Health Care Products
Diabetic Tussin DM Liquid §	Health Care Products
Diabetic Tussin Solution§	Health Care Products
Diphen Capsules ‡	Medique
Donatussin Solution*† §	Laser
Double Tussin DM Liquid	Reese
Dytan-CS Tablets	Hawthorn
Emagrin Forte Tablets	Otis Clapp & Son
Emagrin Tablets	Otis Clapp & Son
Endacof-PD Solution † §	Larken Laboratories
Ganidin NR Liquid	Cypress
Gani-Tuss NR Liquid	Cypress
Gani-Tuss-DM NR Liquid	Cypress
Genebronco-D Liquid	Pharm Generic
Genecof-HC Liquid	Pharm Generic
Genecof-XP Liquid	Pharm Generic
Genedel Syrup	Pharm Generic

* Contains sorbitol.

† May contain other sugar alcohols (eg, glycerol, isomalt, maltitol, mannitol, xylitol).

‡ May contain other sources of carbohydrates (eg, cellulose, lactose, maltodextrin, polydextrose, starch).

§ May contain natural or artificial flavors.

Sugar-Free Products (Continued)

Cough/Cold/Allergy Preparations (Continued)

Genedotuss-DM Liquid	Pharm Generic
Genelan Liquid	Pharm Generic
Genetuss-2 Liquid	Pharm Generic
Genexpect DM Liquid	Pharm Generic
Genexpect SF Liquid	Pharm Generic
Gilphex TR Tablets	Gil
Giltuss Liquid§	Gil
Giltuss Ped-C Solution§	Gil
Giltuss Pediatric Liquid§	Gil
Giltuss TR Tablets	Gil
Guiadex DM Liquid*† §	Breckenridge
Halotussin AC Liquid	Axiom
Halotussin DAC Solution	Axiom
Lodrane D Suspension	ECR
Lohist-PD Solution*† §	Larken
Marcof Expectorant Syrup	Marnel
Metanx Tablets‡	Pamlab
Nalex DH Liquid	Blansett
Nalex A Liquid	Blansett
Neo DM Drops*† §	Laser
Neo DM Syrup*† §	Laser
Neotuss-D Liquid † §	A.G. Marin
Neotuss S/F Liquid † §	A.G. Marin
Niferex Elixir* ‡ §	Ther-Rx
Organidin NR Tablets ‡	Meda
Phena-HC Solution	GM
Phenabid Tablets	Gil
Phenabid DM Tablets	Gil
Phena-S 12 Suspension	GM
Phena-S Liquid	GM
Poly Hist DM	Poly
Poly Hist PD Solution	Poly
Prolex DM Liquid	Blansett
Rescon-DM Liquid* §	Capellon
Ru-Tuss DM Syrup*† §	Carwin
Scot-Tussin Diabetes CF Liquid	Scot-Tussin
Scot-Tussin Diabetes CF	Scot-Tussin
Scot-Tussin Expectorant Solution	Scot-Tussin
Scot-Tussin Senior Solution	Scot-Tussin
Siladryl Allergy Solution* §	Silarx
Sildec PE-DM Syrup*† §	Silarx
Sildec-PE Syrup*† §	Silarx
Siltussin DAS Liquid*† §	Silarx
Siltussin DM DAS Cough Formula Syrup*† §	Silarx
Siltussin SA Liquid*† §	Silarx
Children's Sudafed PE Cough & Cold Liquid*† §	Pfizer
Children's Sudafed Nasal Decongestant Liquid*† §	Pfizer
Sudatuss-SF Liquid	Pharm Generic
Supress DX Pediatric Drops † §	Kramer-Novis
Suttar-SF Syrup	Gil
Tusdec-DM Solution*† §	Cypress
Tusnel Solution	Llorens
Tussall Solution* §	Everett
Tussi-Pres Liquid † §	Kramer-Novis
Vazol Solution	Wraser
Z-Tuss DM Syrup † §	Magna

Fluoride Preparations

Fluor-A-Day Tablets*† §	Arbor
Fluor-A-Day Liquid	Arbor
Sensodyne with Fluoride Cool Gel*† ‡ §	GlaxoSmithKline Consumer
Sensodyne Tartar Control with Whitening † ‡ §	GlaxoSmithKline Consumer
Sensodyne w/Fluoride Toothpaste Original Flavor*† ‡ §	GlaxoSmithKline Consumer

Laxatives

Benefiber Powder	Novartis
Citrucel Powder ‡ §	GlaxoSmithKline Consumer
Colace Liquid 1% Solution	Purdue Products
Fiber Choice Tablets* ‡ §	GlaxoSmithKline Consumer
Fibro-XL Capsules	Key
Konsyl Easy Mix Formula Powder ‡	Konsyl
Konsyl Orange Powder ‡ §	Konsyl
Konsyl Powder ‡	Konsyl
Metamucil Smooth Texture Powder ‡	Procter & Gamble
Reguloid Powder Regular Flavor ‡	Rugby
Reguloid Powder Orange Flavor ‡ §	Rugby

Mouth/Throat Preparations

Cepacol Dual Relief Sore Throat Spray † §	Combe
Cepacol Sore Throat + Coating Relief Lozenge † §	Combe
Cepacol Sore Throat Lozenges † §	Combe

* Contains sorbitol.

† May contain other sugar alcohols (eg, glycerol, isomalt, maltitol, mannitol, xylitol).

‡ May contain other sources of carbohydrates (eg, cellulose, lactose, maltodextrin, polydextrose, starch).

§ May contain natural or artificial flavors.

Cheracol Sore Throat Spray †	Lee
Chloraseptic Spray*† §	Prestige
Diabetic Tussin Cough Drops † §	Health Care Products
Fisherman's Friend Sugar Free Mint Lozenges*	Physicians Total Care
Fresh N Free Liquid	Geritrex
Listerine Pocketpaks Film ‡ §	Johnson & Johnson
Luden's Sugar Free & Wild Cherry Throat Drops † §	McNeil Consumer
Medikoff Sugar Free Drops †	Medique
N'ice Lozenges* §	Heritage/Insight
Oragesic Solution* §	Parnell
Oragel Dry Mouth Moisturizing Gel*† ‡ §	Del
Orajel Dry Mouth Moisturizing Spray † ‡ §	Del
Sepasoothe Lozenges* ‡ §	Medique
Triaminic Sore Throat Spray*† §	Novartis

Vitamins/Minerals/Supplements

Action Tabs Made for Men ‡	Action Labs
Adaptosode For Stress Liquid	HVS
Adaptosode R+R For Acute Stress Liquid	HVS
Alamag Tablets*† ‡ §	Medique
Alcalak Tablets*† ‡	Medique
Apetigen Elixir*†	Kramer-Novis
Apptrim Capsules	Physician Therapeutics
Apptrim-D Capsules	Physician Therapeutics
Bevitamel Tablets	Westlake
Biosode Liquid	HVS
Biotect Plus Caplet	Gil
Bugs Bunny Complete	Bayer
C&M Caps-375 Capsules	Key
Cal-Cee Tablets	Key
Calcet Plus Tablets	Mission Pharmacal
Calcimin-300 Tablets	Key
Cal-Mint Chewable Tablets*† ‡	Freeda Vitamins
Cerefolin NAC Tablets	Pamlab
Chromacaps ‡	Key
Delta D3 Tablets ‡	Freeda Vitamins
Detoxosode Liquids	HVS
DHEA Capsules	ADH Health Products
Diatx ZN Tablets ‡	Centrix
Diucaps Capsules	Legere
DL-Phen-500 Capsules	Key
Enterex Diabetic Liquid ‡	Victus
Evening Primrose Oil Capsules †	National Vitamin
Ex-L Tablets Tablets ‡	Key
Extress Tablets	Key
Eyetamins Tablets ‡	Rexall Consumer
Fem-Cal Citrate Tablets ‡	Freeda Vitamins
Fem-Cal Tablets ‡	Freeda Vitamins

Fem-Cal Plus Tablets	Freeda Vitamins
Ferrocite Plus Tablets ‡	Breckenridge
Folacin-800 Tablets ‡	Key
Folbee Plus Tablets ‡	Breckenridge
Folbee Tablets ‡	Breckenridge
Folplex 2.2 Tablets ‡	Breckenridge
Foltx Tablets ‡	Pamlab
Gabadone Capsules	Physician Therapeutics
Gram-O-Leci Tablets*† ‡	Freeda Vitamins
Herbal Slim Complex Capsules	ADH Health Products
Hypertensa Capsules ‡	Physician Therapeutics
Lynae Calcium/Vitamin C Chewable Tablets	Boscogen
Lynae Chondroitin/ Glucosamine Capsules	Boscogen
Lynae Ginse-Cool Chewable Tablets	Boscogen
Mag-Ox 400 Tablets	Blaine
Mag-SR Tablets ‡	Cypress
Mag-SR Plus Calcium Tablets ‡	Cypress
Magimin Tablets ‡	Key
Magnacaps Capsules ‡	Key
Mangimin Tablets ‡	Key
Medi-Lyte Tablets ‡	Medique
Metanx Tablets ‡	Pamlab
Multi-Delyn with Iron Liquid †	Silarx
New Life Hair Tablets ‡	Rexall Consumer
Niferex Elixir* ‡ §	Ther-Rx
Nutrisure OTC Tablets	Westlake
Nutrivit Solution*† §	Llorens
Ob Complete Tablets	Vertical
O-Cal Fa Tablets ‡	Pharmics
Os-Cal 500 + D Tablets ‡	GlaxoSmithKline Consumer
Powervites Tablets ‡	Green Turtle Bay Vitamin
Prostaplex Herbal Complex Capsules	ADH Health Products
Protect Plus Liquid	Gil
Protect Plus Liquid NR Softgels	Gil
Pulmona Capsules	Physician Therapeutics
Quintabs-M Tablets ‡	Freeda Vitamins
Replace Capsules ‡	Key
Replace w/o Iron Capsules ‡	Key
Ribo-100 T.D. Capsules	Key
Samolinic Softgels †	Key
Sea Omega 30 Softgels †	Rugby
Sea Omega 50 Softgels †	Rugby
Sentra AM Capsules	Physician Therapeutics
Sentra PM Capsules	Physician Therapeutics
Soy Care for Menopause Capsules	Inverness Medical

Sugar-Free Products (Continued)

Vitamins/Minerals/Supplements (Continued)

Span C Tablets ‡	Freeda Vitamins
Strovite Forte Syrup	Everett
Sunnie Tablets	Green Turtle Bay Vitamin
Sunvite Tablets † ‡	Rexall Naturalist
Super Dec B100 Tablets ‡	Freeda Vitamins
Super Quints B-50 Tablets ‡	Freeda Vitamins
Supervite Liquid	Seyer Pharmatec
Suplevit Liquid	Gil
Theramine Capsules	Physician Therapeutics
Triamin Tablets	Key
Triamino Tablets* ‡	Freeda Vitamins
Ultramino Powder	Freeda Vitamins
Uro-Mag Capsules ‡	Blaine
Vitafol Tablets † ‡	Everett
Vitamin C/Rose Hips Tablets	ADH Health Products
Xtramins Tablets	Key
Yohimbe Power Max 1500 for Women Tablets ‡	Action Labs
Ze Plus Softgel	Everett

Miscellaneous

Acidoll Capsules	Key
Alka-Gest Tablets	Key
Cafergot Tablets ‡	Sandoz
Cytra-2 Solution* §	Cypress
Cytra-K Solution* §	Cypress
Cytra-K Crystals	Cypress
Melatin Tablets ‡	Mason Vitamins
Namenda Solution*† §	Forest
Prosed/DS Tablets ‡	Ferring
Questran Light Powder ‡ §	Par

---

* Contains sorbitol.

† May contain other sugar alcohols (eg, glycerol, isomalt, maltitol, mannitol, xylitol).

‡ May contain other sources of carbohydrates (eg, cellulose, lactose, maltodextrin, polydextrose, starch).

§ May contain natural or artificial flavors.